Pediatrics
16th Edition

This sixteenth edition of PEDIATRICS represents the continuation of Holt's DISEASES OF INFANCY AND CHILDHOOD, originally written in 1896 by the late L. Emmett Holt, Professor of Diseases of Children at Columbia University from 1901 to 1923. Associated with him in several revisions was John Howland, Professor of Pediatrics at Johns Hopkins University from 1912 to 1926. From 1927 until 1962 L. Emmett Holt, Jr. and Rustin McIntosh were responsible for its revision. In 1962 they shared this responsibility with Henry L. Barnett, who edited the fourteenth and fifteenth editions in 1968 and 1972.

Pediatrics

16th Edition

EDITOR

Abraham M. Rudolph, M.D.
Professor of Pediatrics, Physiology, and Obstetrics and
Gynecology and Reproductive Sciences, Neider Profes-
sor of Pediatric Cardiology, and Senior Staff Member,
Cardiovascular Research Institute, University of Cali-
fornia, San Francisco.

CO-EDITORS

Henry L. Barnett, M.D.
Professor, Department of Pediatrics, Albert Einstein College of
Medicine of Yeshiva University, Bronx, New York

Arnold H. Einhorn, M.D.
Professor of Pediatrics, Albert Einstein College of Medicine of
Yeshiva University, Director of Pediatrics Services and Director of
the Pediatric Intensive Care Unit, Bronx Municipal Hospital
Center, Bronx, New York

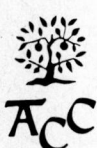

APPLETON-CENTURY-CROFTS/New York

Library of Congress Cataloging in Publication Data

Main entry under title:
Pediatrics.

   In the 15th ed., Barnett's name appeared first
on the t. p.
  Bibliography: p.
  Includes index.
  1. Pediatrics. I. Rudolph, Abraham M.
II. Barnett, Henry L. III. Einhorn, Arnold H.
[DNLM: 1. Pediatrics. WS200 P373]
RJ45.B35 1977   618.9 2   76-56741
ISBN 0-8385-7794-6

PRINTED IN THE UNITED STATES OF AMERICA

Cover design: The Old Typosopher

Associate Editors

Contributors

Mark Abramowicz, M.D.
Assistant Professor of Pediatrics, Albert Einstein College of Medicine of Yeshiva University, Bronx, New York

Chester A. Alper, M.D.
Professor of Pediatrics, The Children's Hospital Medical Center, Harvard Medical School; Scientific Director, Center for Blood Research; Senior Associate in Hematology and Oncology, Children's Hospital Medical Center, Boston, Massachusetts

Claudine Amiel-Tison, M.D.
Centre de Recherches Biologiques Neonatales, Institut National de la Santé et de la Hôpital Recherches Medicales, Association Claude Bernard, Hôpital Port Royal, Université René Descartes, Paris, France

Arthur J. Ammann, M.D.
Director, Pediatric Immunology and Pediatric Clinical Research Center; Associate Professor of Pediatrics, University of California, San Francisco, California

Raymond A. Amoury, M.D.
Katharine Berry Richardson Professor of Pediatric Surgery, The University of Missouri Kansas City School of Medicine; Surgeon-in-Chief, The Children's Mercy Hospital; Consultant in Surgery, Kansas City General Hospital and Medical Center and St. Luke's Hospital of Kansas City, Kansas City, Missouri

Robert L. Anderton, M.D.
601 Fifth Avenue, Yuma, Arizona

Warren A. Andiman, M.D.
Instructor in Pediatrics, Epidemiology, and Public Health, Yale University School of Medicine, New Haven, Connecticut

Leonard Apt, M.D.
Professor of Ophthalmology, Chief of Pediatric Ophthalmology, Jules Stein Eye Institute, University of California at Los Angeles School of Medicine, Los Angeles, California

Irwin M. Arias, M.D.
Vice-Chairman, Department of Medicine; Professor of Medicine; Chief, Division of Gastroenterology-Liver Disease; Director, Liver Research Center, Albert Einstein College of Medicine of Yeshiva University, Bronx, New York

Roberta A. Ballard, M.D.
Adjunct Assistant Professor of Pediatrics, University of California, San Francisco; Chief, Department of Pediatrics, Mount Zion Hospital and Medical Center, San Francisco, California

Myles M. Behrens, M.D., D.Med.Sc.
Chief, Neuro-Ophthalmology Unit; Assistant Professor of Clinical Ophthalmology, Columbia-Presbyterian Medical Center, New York, New York

William R. Bergren, Ph.D.
Professor of Biochemistry, University of Southern California School of Medicine; Division of Medical Genetics, Children's Hospital of Los Angeles, Los Angeles, California

Kenneth I. Berns, M.D., Ph.D.
Professor and Chairman, Department of Immunology and Medical Microbiology, University of Florida, College of Medicine, Gainesville, Florida

Jay Bernstein, M.D.
Director, Department of Anatomic Pathology, William Beaumont Hospital, Royal Oak, Michigan; Visiting Professor of Pathology, Albert Einstein College of Medicine of Yeshiva University, Bronx, New York

Richard Bland, M.D.
Assistant Professor of Pediatrics; Research Staff Member, Cardiovascular Research Institute, University of California, San Francisco, California

Robert M. Blizzard, M.D.
Professor and Chairman, Department of Pediatrics, University of Virginia Medical Center, Charlottesville, Virginia

Alfred M. Bongiovanni, M.D.
Professor of Pediatrics, University of Pennsylvania; Director of Endocrinology, Children's Hospital of Philadelphia, Philadelphia, Pennsylvania; Professor of Pediatrics, University of Ife, Nigeria

William L. Bradford, M.D.
Professor Emeritus of Pediatrics, The University of Rochester School of Medicine and Dentistry, Rochester, New York

June P. Brady, M.B., B.Chir.
Associate Clinical Professor of Pediatrics; Associate Staff Member, Cardiovascular Research Institute, University of California, San Francisco; Director of the Nurseries, Children's Hospital of San Francisco, San Francisco, California

Roscoe O. Brady, M.D.
Chief, Developmental and Metabolic Neurology Branch, National Institute of Neurological and Communicative Disorders and Stroke, National Institutes of Health, Bethesda, Maryland

James B. Brayton, M.D.
Associate Professor of Pediatrics and Laboratory Animal Medicine, The Johns Hopkins University School of Medicine; Pediatrician, The Johns Hopkins Hospital, Baltimore, Maryland

John G. Brooks, M.D.
Assistant Professor of Pediatrics, University of Colorado Medical Center, Denver, Colorado

A. Joseph Brough, M.D.
Associate Adjunct Professor (FT), Affiliated Program in Pathology, Wayne State University School of Medicine; Pathologist in Chief, Department of Laboratory Medicine, Children's Hospital of Michigan, Detroit, Michigan.

Philip A. Brunnell, M.D.
Professor and Chairman, Department of Pediatrics, The University of Texas Health Science Center at San Antonio; Director of Pediatrics, Texas County Hospital District, San Antonio, Texas

Joseph W. Burnett, M.D.
Professor of Medicine in Dermatology, University of Maryland School of Medicine, Baltimore, Maryland

Peter W. Carmel, M.D.
Assistant Professor of Clinical Neurological Surgery, College of Physicians and Surgeons, Columbia University, New York, New York

Charles C. J. Carpenter, M.D.
Professor and Chairman, Department of Medicine, Case Western Reserve University, Cleveland, Ohio

Sidney Carter, M.D.
Professor of Neurology and Pediatrics; Chief, Division of Pediatric Neurology, Columbia University College of Physicians and Surgeons, Presbyterian Hospital, New York, New York

David H. Carver, M.D.
Physician-in-Chief, The Hospital for Sick Children; Chairman and Professor, Department of Pediatrics, The University of Toronto, Toronto, Ontario, Canada

Ranjit K. Chandra, M.D.
Professor of Pediatric Research, Memorial University of Newfoundland; Pediatrician, Janeway Child Health Centre, St. John's Newfoundland, Canada

Dora Chao, M.D.
Clinical Assistant Professor, Baylor College of Medicine, Houston, Texas

J. Julian Chisolm, Jr., M.D.
Associate Professor of Pediatrics, The Johns Hopkins University School of Medicine; Senior Staff Pediatrician, Baltimore City Hospital, Baltimore, Maryland

Abe M. Chutorian, M.D.
Professor of Clinical Neurology and of Pediatrics, Columbia University College of Physicians and Surgeons; Attending Neurologist, Columbia-Presbyterian Medical Center; Consultant in Neurology, Blythedale Children's Hospital, Harlem Hospital Medical Center, New York, New York

Herbert J. Cohen, M.D.
Professor of Pediatrics, Associate Professor of Rehabilitation Medicine, Albert Einstein College of Medicine of Yeshiva University; Director, Rose F. Kennedy Center University Affiliated Facility; Director, Bronx Developmental Services and Center, Bronx, New York

Michael I. Cohen, M.D.
Director, Division of Adolescent Medicine, Department of Pediatrics, Montefiore Hospital and Medical Center; Professor of Pediatrics, Albert Einstein College of Medicine of Yeshiva University, Bronx, New York

James D. Connor, M.D.
Professor of Pediatrics, University of California San Diego School of Medicine, La Jolla, California

Louis Z. Cooper, M.D.
Director, Pediatric Service, The Roosevelt Hospital; Professor of Pediatrics, College of Physicians and Surgeons of Columbia University, New York, New York

David Baird Coursin, M.D.
Director of Research, St. Joseph Hospital, Lancaster, Pennsylvania

Robert K. Creasy, M.D.
Associate Professor of Obstetrics and Gynecology; Associate Staff Member, Cardiovascular Research Institute, University of California, San Francisco, California

Robert G. Crounse, M.D.
Professor of Dermatology; Associate Dean and Chairman, Department of Medical Allied Health Professions, University of North Carolina School of Medicine, Chapel Hill, North Carolina

Edward C. Curnen, Jr., M.D.
Carpentier Professor of Pediatrics, Emeritus, Columbia University College of Physicians and Surgeons; Consultant in Pediatrics, Columbia-Presbyterian Medical Center and St. Luke's Hospital Center; Attending Pediatrician, Harlem Hospital Center, New York, New York

Peter R. Dallman, M.D.
Associate Professor of Pediatrics; Chief, Division of Hematology and Oncology, University of California, San Francisco, California

B. Shannon Danes, M.D.
Associate Professor, Cornell University Medical College; Associate Attending Physician, The New York Hospital, New York, New York

Fredric Daum, M.D.
Division of Adolescent Medicine, Department of Pediatrics, Montefiore Hospital and Medical Center; Assistant Professor of Pediatrics, Albert Einstein College of Medicine, Bronx, New York

Murray Davidson, M.D.
Professor of Pediatrics and Assistant Dean, Albert Einstein College of Medicine; Director of Pediatrics, Bronx-Lebanon Hospital Center, Bronx, New York

William De Myer, M.D.
Professor of Child Neurology, Indiana University School of Medicine, Indianapolis, Indiana

George N. Donnell, M.D.
Winzer Professor and Chairman, Department of Pediatrics, University of Southern California School of Medicine; Physician-in-Chief, Department of Pediatrics, Children's Hospital of Los Angeles; Member, Division of Medical Genetics at Children's Hospital of Los Angeles, Los Angeles, California

John C. Dower, M.D.
Professor of Pediatrics and Director of Pediatric Clinics, University of California, San Francisco, California

John M. Driscoll, M.D.
Associate Professor of Clinical Pediatrics, College of Physicians and Surgeons, Columbia University, New York, New York

Herbert L. Du Pont, M.D.
Professor and Director, Program in Infectious Diseases and Clinical Microbiology, The University of Texas Health Science Center at Houston, The Medical School, Houston, Texas

Vu Van Dzi, M.D.
Instructor in Pediatrics, University of Saigon Faculty of Medicine, Saigon, Republic of Vietnam

Chester M. Edelmann, Jr., M.D.
Professor and Chairman, Department of Pediatrics, Albert Einstein College of Medicine; Director of Pediatric Service, Bronx Municipal Hospital Center, Bronx, New York

Heinz F. Eichenwald, M.D.
William Buchanan Professor and Chairman, Department of Pediatrics, The University of Texas Health Science Center at Dallas, Dallas, Texas

Arnold H. Einhorn, M.D.
Professor of Pediatrics, Albert Einstein College of Medicine of Yeshiva University; Chief, Pediatric Clinical Services and Director of Pediatric Intensive Care Unit, Bronx Municipal Hospital Center, Bronx, New York

Fred J. Epstein, M.D.
Associate Professor of Neurosurgery, New York University School of Medicine, New York, New York

Laurence Finberg, M.D.
Professor and Chairman, Department of Pediatrics, Albert Einstein College of Medicine of Yeshiva University (Montefiore Hospital and Medical Center), Bronx, New York

Delbert A. Fisher, M.D.
Professor of Pediatrics and Medicine, University of California at Los Angeles, Harbor General Hospital Campus, Torrance, California

Alfred L. Florman, M.D.
Professor of Pediatrics, New York University School of Medicine, New York, New York

John M. Freeman, M.D.
Associate Professor of Pediatrics and Neurology, Johns Hopkins School of Medicine; Director, Birth Defects Treatment Center, John F. Kennedy Institute for Habilitation of the Mentally and Physically Handicapped Child; Director, Pediatric Seizure Clinic; Director, Pediatric Neurology, Baltimore, Maryland

Oscar L. Frick, M.D., Ph.D.
Professor of Pediatrics; Director, Allergy-Immunology Research Laboratory, University of California, San Francisco, California

William L. Gaffney, M.D.
Clinical Associate, Jules Stein Eye Institute, University of California, School of Medicine, Los Angeles, California

Pierce Gardner, M.D.
Associate Professor of Medicine and Pediatrics, The University of Chicago; Director, Clinical Training Program in Infectious Diseases, University of Chicago Hospitals and Michael Reese Medical Center, Chicago, Illinois

Lawrence M. Gartner, M.D.
Professor of Pediatrics, Director, Division of Neonatology and Rose F. Kennedy Clinical Research Unit, Albert Einstein College of Medicine of Yeshiva University, Bronx, New York

Anne Hendrick Gaston, M.D.
Director of Nursery Services, Kaiser Foundation Hospital, Oakland; Associate Clinical Professor of Pediatrics, University of California, San Francisco, California

Sydney S. Gellis, M.D.
Professor and Chairman, Department of Pediatrics, Tufts University School of Medicine; Pediatrician-in-Chief, New England Medical Center Hospital-Boston Floating Hospital for Infants and Children, Boston, Massachusetts

Salome Gluecksohn-Waelsch, Ph.D.
Professor and Chairman, Department of Genetics, Albert Einstein College of Medicine of Yeshiva University, Bronx, New York

Arnold Gold, M.D.
Professor of Clinical Neurology; Professor of Clinical Pediatrics, College of Physicians and Surgeons of Columbia University, New York, New York

Eli Gold, M.D.
Professor and Chairman, Department of Pediatrics, University of California, Davis, California

Sidney Goldfischer, M.D.
Professor of Pathology, Albert Einstein College of Medicine; Attending Pathologist, Bronx Municipal Hospital Center, Bronx, New York

George G. Graham, M.D.
Professor of International Health (Human Nutrition), The School of Hygiene and Public Health, The Johns Hopkins University; Associate Professor of Pediatrics, The Johns Hopkins School of Medicine, Baltimore, Maryland; Director of Research, British-American Hospital, Lima, Peru

Dan M. Granoff, M.D.
Assistant Chief of Pediatrics (Infectious Diseases), Valley Medical Center of Fresno, Fresno, California

Melvin Greer, M.D.
Professor and Chairman, Department of Neurology, University of Florida College of Medicine, Gainesville, Florida

Robert H. Gregg, M.D.
Clinical Associate Professor of Pediatrics, Wayne State University School of Medicine; President of Children's Hospital of Michigan, Detroit, Michigan

George A. Gregory, M.D.
Associate Professor of Anesthesiology and Pediatrics, University of California, San Francisco, California

Melvin M. Grumbach, M.D.
Professor and Chairman, Department of Pediatrics; Director of Pediatric Services, University of California, San Francisco, California

Crystie C. Halsted, M.D.
Assistant Professor of Pediatrics, University of California, Davis, California

James F. Hammill, M.D.
Professor of Clinical Neurology, Columbia University College of Physicians and Surgeons; Attending Neurologist, Neurological Institute, Presbyterian Hospital, New York, New York

James B. Hanshaw, M.D.
Professor and Chairman, Department of Pediatrics, University of Massachusetts Medical School, Worcester, Massachusetts

Gordon P. Harper, Jr., M.D.
Assistant in Psychiatry; Assistant in Medicine, Children's Hospital Medical Center; Clinical Instructor in Psychiatry, Harvard Medical School, Boston, Massachusetts

Susan R. Harris, M.D.
Instructor in Medicine, Albert Einstein College of Medicine of Yeshiva University; Assistant Attending Physician, Bronx Municipal Hospital Center, Bronx, New York

Harold E. Harrison, M.D.
Professor of Pediatrics, The Johns Hopkins University School of Medicine; Pediatrician-in-Chief, Baltimore City Hospitals, Baltimore, Maryland

Eileen G. Hasselmeyer, Ph.D., R.N.
Program Director, Pregnancy and Infancy Branch, National Institute of Child Health and Human Development, Bethesda, Maryland

William E. Hathway, M.D.
Professor of Pediatrics, University of Colorado School of Medicine, Denver, Colorado

Richard M. Heller, M.D.
Director of Pediatric Radiology, Vanderbilt University Hospital, Nashville, Tennessee

Walter L. Henley, M.D.
Professor of Pediatrics, Mount Sinai School of Medicine of the City University of New York, New York, New York

Michael A. Heymann, M.D.
Associate Professor of Pediatrics and Obstetrics and Gynecology; Senior Staff Member, Cardiovascular Research Institute, University of California, San Francisco, California

Horace L. Hodes, M.D.
Herbert H. Lehman Professor and Chairman, Department of Pediatrics, Mount Sinai School of Medicine of the City University of New York, New York, New York

Julien I. E. Hoffman, M.D.
Professor of Pediatrics; Senior Staff Member, Cardiovascular Research Institute, University of California, San Francisco, California

Dorothy M. Horstmann, M.D.
Professor of Epidemiology and Pediatrics, Yale University School of Medicine, New Haven, Connecticut

Walter T. Hughes, M.D.
Chief, Infectious Diseases Service, St. Jude Children's Research Hospital; Professor of Pediatrics and Microbiology, University of Tennessee Center for Health Sciences, Memphis, Tennessee

Jane V. Hunt, M.D.
Associate Research Psychologist, Institute of Human Development, University of California, Berkeley; Research Associate, Department of Pediatrics, University of California, San Francisco, California

Norman B. Javitt, M.D., Ph.D.
Professor of Medicine; Head, Division of Gastroenterology, New York Hospital-Cornell Medical Center, New York, New York

Stephen R. Kandall, M.D.
Assistant Professor of Pediatrics, Mount Sinai School of Medicine; Chief, Division of Neonatology, Beth Israel Medical Center, New York, New York

Bary H. Kaplan, M.D., Ph.D.
Associate Professor of Medicine; Assistant Professor of Biochemistry, Albert Einstein College of Medicine of Yeshiva University, Bronx, New York

Selna L. Kaplan, M.D.
Professor of Pediatrics, University of California, San Francisco, California

Michael Katz, M.D.
Professor of Tropical Medicine and of Pediatrics; Head, Division of Tropical Medicine, School of Public Health; Director, Division of Infectious Diseases, Department of Pediatrics, Columbia University College of Physicians and Surgeons; Acting Chairman, Department of Pediatrics and Acting Director, Pediatric Service Presbyterian Hospital (Babies Hospital), New York, New York

Samuel L. Katz, M.D.
Wilburt C. Davison Professor and Chairman, Department of Pediatrics, Duke University Medical Center, Durham, North Carolina

Robert P. Kelch, M.D.
Associate Professor of Pediatrics, University of Michigan, Ann Arbor, Michigan

C. Henry Kempe, M.D.
Professor of Pediatrics and Microbiology; Director of National Center for the Prevention and Treatment of Child Abuse, University of Colorado Medical Center, Denver, Colorado

Joseph A. Kitterman, M.D.
Associate Professor of Pediatrics, University of California, San Francisco, California

Martin B. Kleiman, M.D.
Assistant Professor of Pediatrics; Director, Section of Pediatric Infectious Diseases, Department of Pediatrics, Indiana University School of Medicine, Indianapolis, Indiana

M. Richard Koenigsberger, M.D.
Associate Professor of Clinical Neurology; Associate Professor of Clinical Pediatrics, College of Physicians and Surgeons, Columbia University, New York, New York

Arthur F. Kohrman, M.D.
Professor and Associate Chairman, Department of Human Development, Michigan State University College of Human Medicine, East Lansing, Michigan

Norman Kretchmer, M.D.
Director, National Institute of Child Health and Human Development, National Institutes of Health, Public Health Service, Department of Health, Education and Welfare, Bethesda, Maryland

Saul Krugman, M.D.
Professor of Pediatrics, New York University Medical Center, New York, New York

Karen Kuehl, M.D.
Research Assistant Professor, Biochemistry; Instructor in Pediatrics, University of Virginia School of Medicine, Charlottesville, Virginia

Howard E. Kulin, M.D.
Associate Professor of Pediatrics and Chief, Division of Pediatric Endocrinology, The Milton S. Hershey Medical Center of the Pennsylvania State University, Hershey, Pennsylvania

Peter O. Kwiterovich, Jr., M.D.
Director, Lipid Research Clinic; Assistant Professor of Pediatrics and Medicine, Johns Hopkins University School of Medicine, Baltimore, Maryland

Daniel L. Levin, M.D.
Assistant Professor of Pediatrics, The University of Texas Health Science Center at Dallas, Southwestern Medical School, Dallas, Texas

Selwyn B. Levitt, M.B., B.Ch., F.A.C.S.
Associate Professor of Urology and Pediatrics; Director of the Division of Pediatric Urology and Pediatric Renal Transplantation, Albert Einstein College of Medicine of Yeshiva University and Montefiore Hospital and Medical Center, Bronx, New York

Herman W. Lipow, M.D.
Associate Clinical Professor of Pediatrics; Research Staff Member, Cardiovascular Research Institute, University of California, San Francisco, California

Iris F. Litt, M.D.
Associate Professor of Pediatrics, Albert Einstein College of Medicine of Yeshiva University; Assistant Director, Division of Adolescent Medicine, Department of Pediatrics, Montefiore Hospital and Medical Center, Bronx, New York

Niels L. Low, M.D.
Professor of Clinical Neurology and Clinical Pediatrics, Columbia University College of Physicians and Surgeons; Attending Physician, Presbyterian Hospital; Clinical Director, Blythedale Children's Hospital, New York, New York

Bertram Lubin, M.D.
Director, Division of Hematology-Oncology, Children's Hospital Medical Center of Northern California, Oakland; Assistant Clinical Professor of Pediatrics, University of California, San Francisco, California

Andrew M. Margileth, M.D.
Professor and Associate Chairman, Department of Child Health and Development, George Washington University School of Medicine, Washington, D.C.

Angus M. McBryde, M.D.
Emeritus Professor of Pediatrics, Duke University School of Medicine; Emeritus Director of Nurseries, Duke Medical Center, Durham, North Carolina

George H. McCracken, Jr., M.D.
Professor of Pediatrics, The University of Texas Health Science Center at Dallas, Dallas, Texas

Joseph McGuire, M.D.
Professor of Dermatology, Yale University School of Medicine, New Haven, Connecticut

Donald S. McLaren, M.D.
Professor of Clinical Nutrition, American University of Beirut School of Medicine, Beirut, Lebanon

William C. Mentzer, Jr., M.D.
Associate Professor of Pediatrics, University of California, San Francisco; Chief, Pediatric Hematology, San Francisco General Hospital, San Francisco, California

Claude J. Migeon, M.D.
Professor of Pediatrics, Johns Hopkins University Hospital, Baltimore, Maryland

I. George Miller, Jr., M.D.
Associate Professor of Pediatrics and Epidemiology, Yale University School of Medicine, New Haven, Connecticut

J. Gordon Millichap, M.D.
Professor of Neurology and Pediatrics, Northwestern University Medical School; Pediatric Neurologist, Children's Memorial Hospital and Passavant Memorial Hospital, Chicago, Illinois

Bernard L. Mirkin, Ph.D., M.D.
Professor of Pediatrics and Pharmacology; Director, Division of Clinical Pharmacology, University of Minnesota, Minneapolis, Minnesota

Ralph E. Moloshok, M.D.
Clinical Professor of Pediatrics, Mount Sinai School of Medicine of the City of New York; Attending Pediatrician, Mount Sinai Hospital, New York, New York

Rachel Morecki, M.D.
Assistant Professor of Pathology, Albert Einstein College of Medicine of Yeshiva University, Bronx, New York

James W. Mosley, M.D.
Professor of Medicine and Director, Hepatic Epidemiology Laboratory, Liver Service, University of Southern California, School of Medicine, Los Angeles, California

E. Richard Moxon, M.B., B.Chir., M.R.C.P.
Assistant Professor of Pediatrics, The Johns Hopkins University School of Medicine, Baltimore, Maryland

Patrick Murphy, M.D.
Associate Professor of Medicine and Microbiology, The Johns Hopkins University School of Medicine, Baltimore, Maryland

Andre J. Nahmias, M.D.
Professor of Pediatrics; Chief, Infectious Diseases and Immunology, Emory University School of Medicine, Atlanta, Georgia

Martin A. Nash, M.D.
Assistant Professor of Pediatrics, College of Physicians and Surgeons of Columbia University; Director of Pediatric Nephrology, Babies Hospital, New York, New York

Erwin Neter, M.D.
Professor of Microbiology, The State University of New York at Buffalo School of Medicine; Director of Bacteriology, Children's Hospital, Buffalo, New York

Harold M. Nitowsky, M.D.
Professor of Pediatrics and Genetics, Albert Einstein College of Medicine, Bronx Municipal Hospital Center, Bronx, New York

William L. Nyhan, M.D.
Professor and Chairman, Department of Pediatrics, University of California, San Diego School of Medicine, La Jolla, California

Allan C. Oglesby, M.D., M.P.H.
Assistant Medical Director, Golden Gate Regional Center; Lecturer in Maternal and Child Health, School of Public Health, University of California, Berkeley, California

Anthony S. Pagliara, M.D.
Associate Professor of Pediatrics and Medicine, Washington University School of Medicine, St. Louis, Missouri

Julian T. Parer, M.D., Ph.D.
Assistant Professor of Obstetrics and Gynecology, University of California, San Francisco, California

Milton H. Paul, M.D.
Professor of Pediatrics, Northwestern University Medical School; Director, Division of Cardiology, Willis J. Potts Children's Heart Center, Children's Memorial Hospital, Chicago, Illinois

Elsa Proehl Paulsen, M.A., M.D.
Associate Professor of Pediatrics, Assistant Professor of Biochemistry, University of Virginia School of Medicine, Charlottesville, Virginia; Visiting Associate Professor of Pediatrics, Albert Einstein College of Medicine, Bronx, New York

David C. Peakman, A.I.M.L.T.
Senior Instructor, Department of Biophysics and Genetics, University of Colorado Medical Center and National Jewish Hospital and Research Center, Denver, Colorado

Roger W. Pearson, M.D.
Associate Professor of Dermatology, Rush-Presbyterian-St. Luke's Medical Center, Chicago, Illinois

Roderic H. Phibbs, M.D.
Associate Professor of Pediatrics; Director of the Newborn Nursery; Associate Staff Member, Cardiovascular Research Institute, University of California, San Francisco, California

Larry K. Pickering, M.D.
Assistant Professor of Pediatrics, Program in Infectious Diseases and Clinical Microbiology, The University of Texas Health Science Center at Houston, Medical School, Houston, Texas

Edward L. Pratt, M.D.
Professor and Director, Department of Pediatrics, University of Cincinnati College of Medicine, Cincinnati, Ohio

Helen M. Ranney, M.D.
Professor and Chairman, Department of Medicine, University of California School of Medicine at San Diego, La Jolla, California

Joseph Ransohoff, M.D.
Professor and Chairman, Department of Neurosurgery, New York University School of Medicine; Director of Neurosurgery, University Hospital-New York University Medical Center; Director of Neurological Surgery, Bellevue Hospital Center, New York, New York

Isabelle Rapin, M.D.
Professor of Neurology and Pediatrics (Neurology), Hospital of Albert Einstein College of Medicine, Montefiore Hospital and Medical Center, Bronx, New York

Mark M. Ravitch, M.D.
Professor of Surgery, University of Pittsburgh; Surgeon-in-Chief, Montefiore Hospital of Pittsburgh, Pennsylvania

Edward O. Reiter, M.D.
Assistant Professor of Pediatrics, University of South Florida College of Medicine, All Children's Hospital, St. Petersburg, Florida

Joseph H. Richman, M.D.
Area Medical Director (Silver Spring Area), Montgomery County Health Department of Medicine; Clinical Instructor of Pediatrics, Georgetown University, Washington, D.C.

John B. Robbins, M.D.
Director, Division of Bacterial Projects, Bureau of Biologics, Bethesda, Maryland

Arthur Robinson, M.D.
Professor of Biophysics and Genetics, Professor of Pediatrics, University of Colorado Medical Center; Director of Professional Services, National Jewish Hospital, Denver, Colorado

Juan Rodriguez-Soriano, M.D.
Head, Department of Pediatrics, Hospital Infantil de la Seguridad Social, Bilbao, Spain

Solomon S. Rosenstein, D.D.S.
Professor Emeritus of Dentistry, Columbia University; Consultant in Dental Service, Presbyterian Hospital, Columbia-Presbyterian Medical Center, New York, New York

Griff T. Ross, M.D., Ph.D.
Deputy Director, The Clinical Center, National Institutes of Health, Bethesda, Maryland

Robert J. Ruben, M.D.
Professor and Chairman, Department of Otorhinolaryngology, Albert Einstein College of Medicine of Yeshiva University, Bronx, New York

Abraham M. Rudolph, M.D.
Professor of Pediatrics, Physiology, Obstetrics and Gynecology; Neider Professor of Pediatric Cardiology; Senior Staff Member, Cardiovascular Research Institute, University of California, San Francisco, California

Rhona S. Rudolph, M.B., B.Ch., M.P.H.
Medical Director, Golden Gate Regional Center; Assistant Clinical Professor of Pediatrics, University of California

Thomas V. Santulli, M.D.
Professor of Surgery, Columbia University College of Physicians and Surgeons; Attending Surgeon Columbia-Presbyterian Medical Center; Chief, Pediatric Surgical Service, Babies Hospital, New York, New York

Selma G. Sapir, M.A.
Senior Faculty, Graduate Programs in Learning Disability; Director, Reading/Language Learning Center, Bank Street College of Education, New York, New York

S. Kenneth Schonberg, M.D.
Medical Director, Methadone Maintenance Treatment Program, Montefiore Hospital and Medical Center; Assistant Professor of Pediatrics, Albert Einstein College of Medicine of Yeshiva University, Bronx, New York

John H. Seashore, M.D.
Assistant Professor of Surgery and Pediatrics, Yale University School of Medicine; Attending Surgeon, Yale-New Haven Medical Center, New Haven, Connecticut

William E. Segar, M.D.
Professor and Chairman, Department of Pediatrics, The University of Wisconsin Medical School, Madison, Wisconsin

Dexter S. Y. Seto, M.D.
Associate Professor of Pediatrics, Assistant Professor of Microbiology, The Johns Hopkins University School of Medicine, Baltimore, Maryland

Kenneth Shapiro, M.D.
Senior Resident, Department of Neurological Surgery, Albert Einstein College of Medicine of Yeshiva University, Bronx, New York

Henry R. Shinefield, M.D.
Chief, Department of Pediatrics, Kaiser-Permanente Medical Center; Clinical Professor of Pediatrics, University of California, San Francisco, California

Kenneth Shulman, M.D.
Professor and Chairman, Department of Neurological Surgery, Albert Einstein College of Medicine of Yeshiva University, Bronx, New York

James B. Sidbury, Jr., M.D.
Scientific Director, National Institute of Child Health and Human Development, Bethesda, Maryland

Mervin Silverberg, M.D.
Director, Department of Pediatrics; Chief, Division of Pediatric Gastroenterology, North Shore University Hospital; Professor of Pediatrics, Cornell University Medical College, Manhasset, New York

Frederic N. Silverman, M.D.
Professor of Radiology, Stanford University Medical Center, Stanford, California

Norman H. Silverman, M.D.
Assistant Professor-in-Residence, Department of Pediatrics; Director, Pediatric Non-Invasive Laboratory, University of California, San Francisco, California

Joseph V. Simone, M.D.
Member and Chief, Hematology-Oncology, St. Jude Children's Research Hospital; Associate Professor of Pediatrics, University of Tennessee Center for the Health Sciences, Memphis, Tennessee

David H. Smith, M.D.
Chief, Division of Infectious Diseases, The Children's Hospital Medical Center, Boston, Massachusetts

J. Graham Smith, Jr., M.D.
Professor of Dermatology and Medicine; Chairman, Department of Dermatology, Medical College of Georgia, Augusta, Georgia

Adrian Spitzer, M.D.
Professor of Pediatrics, Director of Pediatric Nephrology, Rose F. Kennedy Center, Albert Einstein College of Medicine of Yeshiva University, Bronx, New York

Paul Stanger, M.D.
Associate Professor of Pediatrics and Pathology, University of California, San Francisco, California

Alex J. Steigman, M.D. and Sc.D. (hon)
Professor of Pediatrics, Mount Sinai School of Medicine, City University of New York, New York, New York

John M. Stein, M.D.
Associate Professor of Surgery, Albert Einstein College of Medicine of Yeshiva University; Chief, Burn Service, Bronx Municipal Hospital Center, Bronx, New York

Philip Sunshine, M.D.
Professor of Pediatrics, Director of Nurseries, Stanford Medical Center, Stanford, California

Lawrence T. Taft, M.D.
Professor and Chairman, Department of Pediatrics, College of Medicine and Dentistry of New Jersey, Rutgers Medical School, Piscataway, New Jersey

William H. Tooley, M.D.
Professor of Pediatrics; Senior Staff Member, Cardiovascular Research Institute, University of California, San Francisco

Judson J. Van Wyk, M.D.
Kenan Professor of Pediatrics; Chief, Division of Pediatric Endocrinology, The University of North Carolina School of Medicine, Chapel Hill, North Carolina

Mary L. Voorhess, M.D.
Professor of Pediatrics, State University of New York at Buffalo; Co-director, Endocrinology Division, Children's Hospital of Buffalo, Buffalo, New York

Diane Wara, M.D.
Assistant Professor of Pediatrics, University of California, San Francisco, California

William B. Weil, Jr., M.D.
Professor and Chairman, Department of Human Development, Michigan State University College of Human Medicine, East Lansing, Michigan

Stuart Weiss, M.D.
Assistant Professor of Clinical Neurology, Washington University School of Medicine, St. Louis, Missouri

Clark D. West, M.D.
Professor of Pediatrics, University of Cincinnati College of Medicine; Associate Director, Children's Hospital Research Foundation, Cincinnati, Ohio

Bernice M. Wilson
Board of Education, Hommocks School, Mamaroneck, New York

Murray Wittner, M.D., Ph.D.
Professor of Pathology and Parasitology, Albert Einstein College of Medicine of Yeshiva University; Director of the Tropical Disease Clinic and Laboratory, Lincoln Hospital; Chief, Tropical Disease Clinic and Laboratory, Bronx Municipal Hospital Center, Bronx, New York

Emanuel Wolinsky, M.D.
Professor of Medicine, Case Western Reserve University; Director of Microbiology, Cleveland Metropolitan General Hospital, Cleveland, Ohio

Richard J. Wurtman, M.D.
Professor of Endocrinology and Metabolism, Laboratory of Neuroendocrine Regulation, Department of Nutrition and Food Sciences, Massachusetts Institute of Technology, Cambridge, Massachusetts

Preface

Since the publication of the fifteenth edition of *Pediatrics* in 1972, there has been an increasing tendency toward specialization in handling the health problems of infants and children. The American Board of Pediatrics has recognized this trend and has approved subspecialty boards in cardiology, allergy, neonatology, nephrology, and hematology-oncology, and is considering others. Books on specific organ systems and special aspects of childhood disorders have also proliferated.

It is not possible, within the confines of a single volume, to provide a comprehensive and detailed review of the total body of knowledge concerning child health. However, there is a great need to delineate current approaches and recent developments for the physician concerned with general aspects of normal child growth and development as well as diseases of infancy and childhood. In this sixteenth edition, we have attempted to present a body of current thought and practice in pediatrics to provide the student and practicing pediatrician with an overview of clinical diagnosis and management. Since many disorders of childhood are related to alterations of normal development, we have attempted, as far as possible, to present normal biologic processes and behavior as a basis for understanding their disturbances in infants and children.

Many people have assisted in the preparation of this sixteenth edition. I particularly appreciate the advice of Dr. Henry Barnett, the editor of the previous two editions, and now a co-editor, and the invaluable assistance of Dr. Arnold Einhorn, also a co-editor. As with the fourteenth and fifteenth editions, the associate editors selected contributors for the sections that they organized, and I gratefully acknowledge the efforts of all these individuals. Because of space limitations, it was necessary in many instances to pare the manuscripts submitted. I have regretfully had to assume this responsibility and apologize to those who spent many hours in preparing the material.

I gratefully acknowledge the invaluable efforts of my wife, Dr. Rhona Rudolph, both as an associate editor, and as an unofficial co-editor. During the preparation of this edition, Susan Axelrod, my editorial assistant, provided inestimable help, and I am also most appreciative of the assistance of Anne Schmid and Muriel Byram. I am also indebted to David Stires and John Cernusca, as well as many other members of the staff of Appleton-Century-Crofts, who have provided valuable advice and guidance.

Abraham M. Rudolph, M.D.
San Francisco
August 1976

Contents

CHAPTER 13   MYCOTIC AND PARASITIC DISEASES

CHAPTER 14   ANOMALIES OF METABOLISM

CHAPTER 24   BLOOD AND BLOOD-FORMING TISSUES   1109

CHAPTER 25   THE RETICULOENDOTHELIOSES   1223

CHAPTER 26   THE KIDNEYS AND URINARY TRACT   1235

CHAPTER 27   CIRCULATORY SYSTEM   1351

CHAPTER 28   THE LUNG   1503

CHAPTER 29 ENDOCRINE SYSTEM   1599

CHAPTER 30 NERVOUS SYSTEM   1733

Color Plates

CHAPTER 17: The Skin

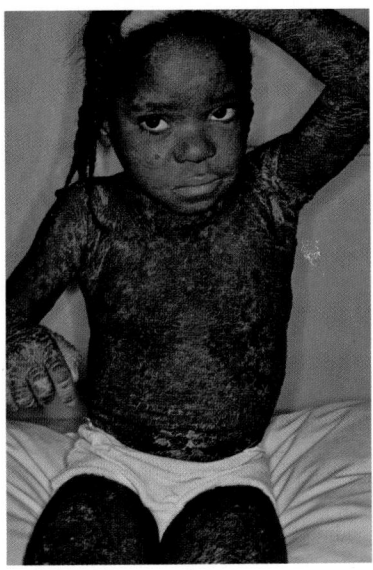

FIG. 3. Epidermolytic hyperkeratosis. A dominantly inherited congenital icthyosis characterized by quill-like scales, characteristic odor, and flexural involvement.

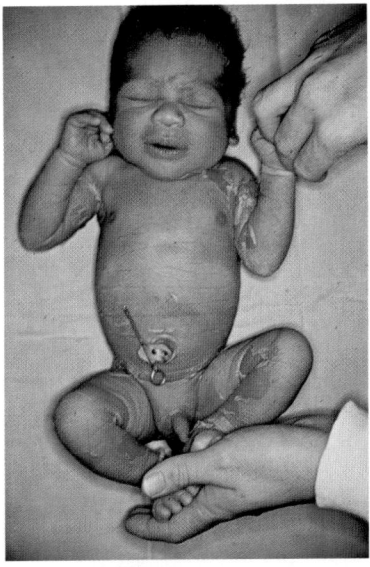

FIG. 4. Epidermolytic hyperkeratosis. This newborn Black child has large erosions where the epidermis has been wiped off. These infants go on to have bullous CIE (epidermolytic hyperkeratosis) and at birth are sometimes mistaken for collodion babies.

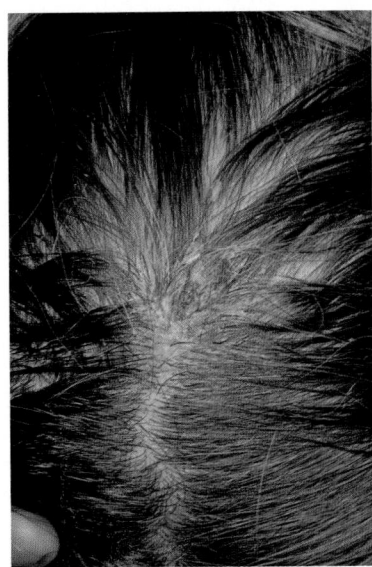

FIG. 10. Nevus sebaceous (Jadassohn) typical yellowish, nodular nevus on scalp at birth in this young adult. Risk of eventual appearance of basal cell epithelioma in this nevus necessitates its removal.

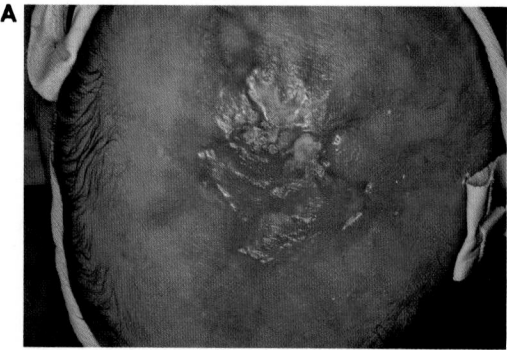

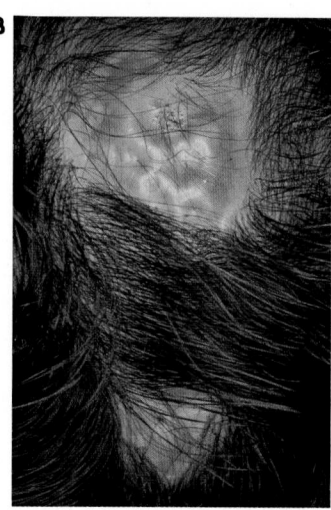

FIG. 11. A. Aplasia cutis congenita in a 2-month-old boy with evidence of earlier erosion of the scalp. B. Aplasia cutis congenita. Multiple lesions with obvious scarring and hair loss. The scarred areas are thought to represent erosions that may have occurred before birth.

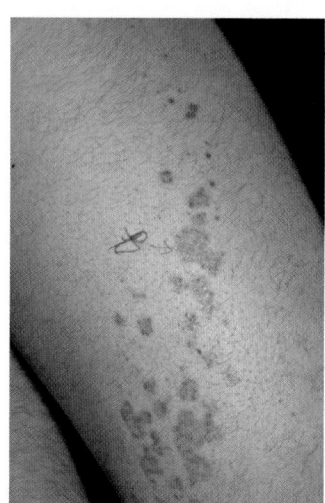

FIG. 12. Porokeratosis of Mibelli. Asymptomatic nevoid malformation, sometimes occurs in a linear pattern.

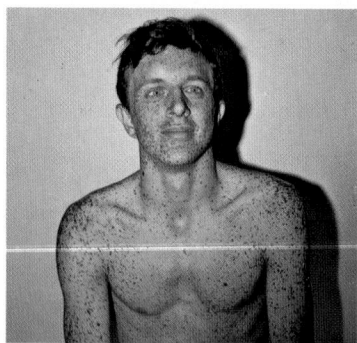

FIG. 45. Multiple lentigines syndrome. This 19-year-old boy has the major findings of the "leopard" syndrome, including congenital deafness and multiple lentigines.

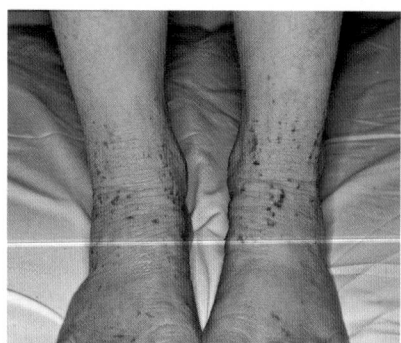

FIG. 48. Flexural eczema in a 9-year-old girl. Lichenification and excoriations are common findings.

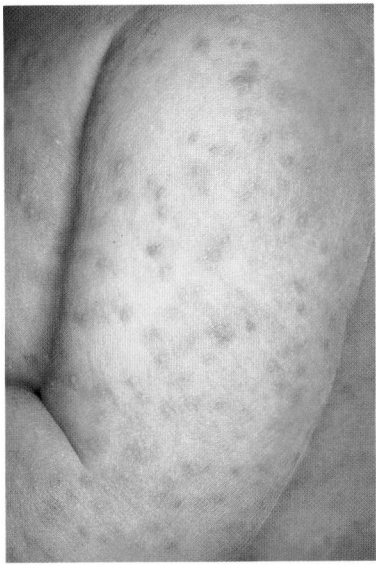

FIG. 56. Erythema neonatorum. Involvement is sometimes extensive, as is shown in this infant. Usually there are also scattered lesions on the face.

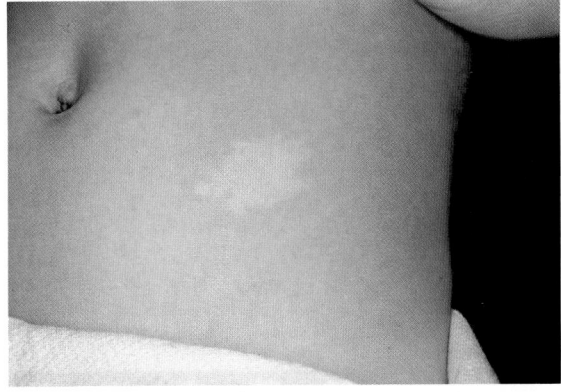

FIG. 57. Adenoma sebaceum. The hypopigmented macules are sometimes a clue to the diagnosis of this disease before the facial papules appear.

CHAPTER 30: The Nervous System

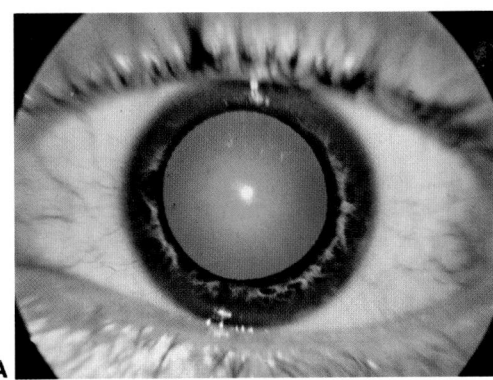

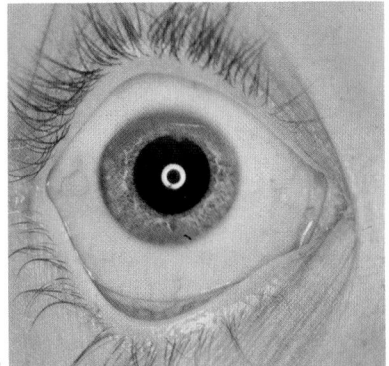

FIG. 44. Kayser-Fleischer ring. A. Complete ring in eye with relatively dark iris. B. Crescents at superior and inferior poles of limbus in an eye with a light iris. (Courtesy of Dr. B. L. Beckerman and I. H. Scheinberg.)

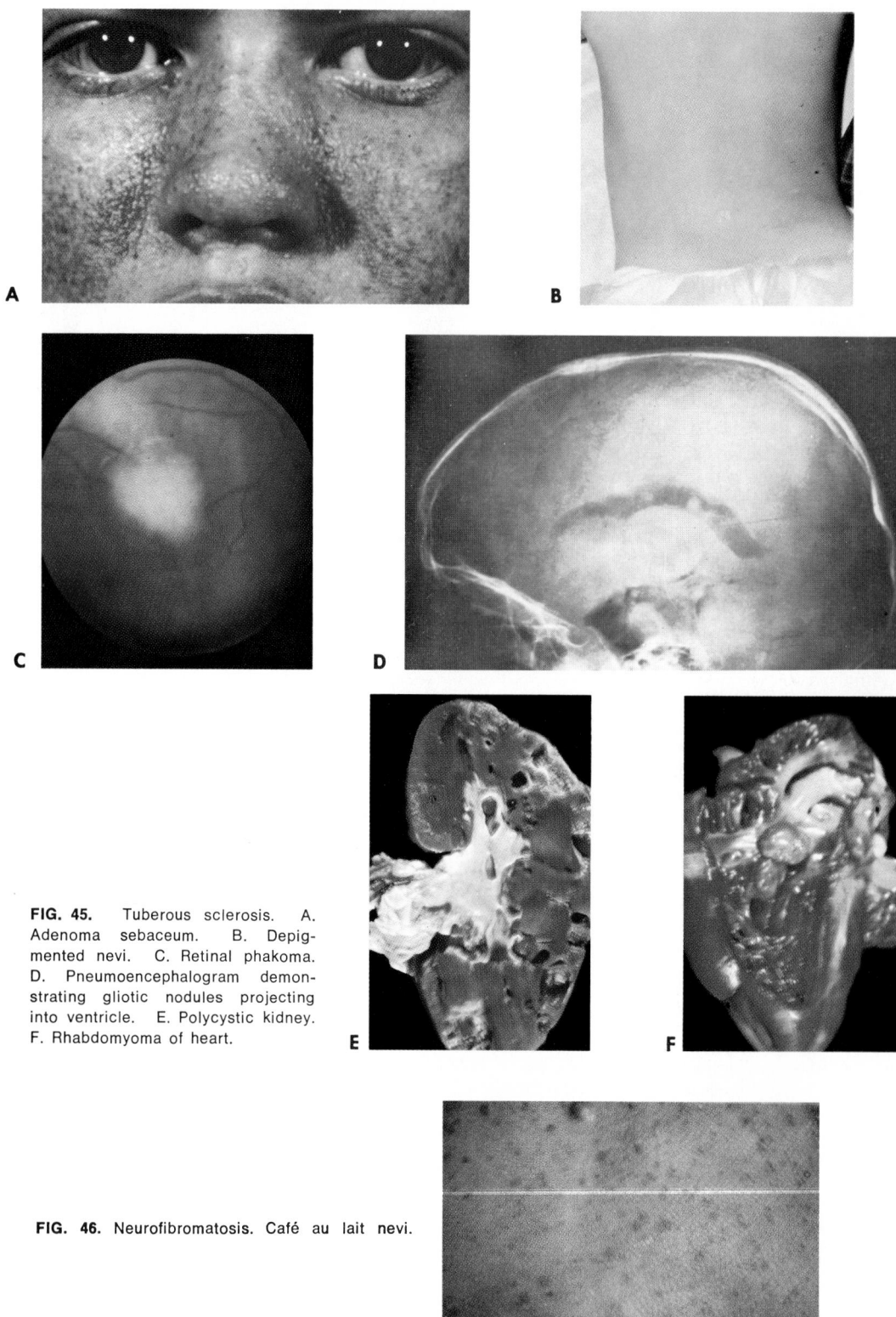

FIG. 45. Tuberous sclerosis. A. Adenoma sebaceum. B. Depigmented nevi. C. Retinal phakoma. D. Pneumoencephalogram demonstrating gliotic nodules projecting into ventricle. E. Polycystic kidney. F. Rhabdomyoma of heart.

FIG. 46. Neurofibromatosis. Café au lait nevi.

The Health Care System

RHONA S. RUDOLPH AND ALLAN C. OGLESBY, *Associate Editors*

HISTORICAL PERSPECTIVE

RHONA S. RUDOLPH AND
ALLAN C. OGLESBY

There has been little humanitarian concern for children generally in Western civilization. In ancient Sparta the city-state claimed the child and decided who would be allowed to survive. Those selected to survive were reared with great care by the city-state and were given special training to increase their usefulness to Sparta. Those who were defective were left to die on a hillside. In Athens the city-state still controlled the life of the child, but the Athenians showed less inclination to kill unwanted children, and it was this society that began to develop a few institutions to benefit children who were not reared by their own families.

In Roman society at the time of the Republic the father, rather than the state, was the power responsible for the child. Those children who were rejected by their fathers became the property of the state and were mutilated to become beggars or to be used as slaves. During the days of the Roman Empire there was more concern for children. Emperor Augustus declared a state subsidy for anyone raising a child in a foster home, and in the fourth century Emperor Constantine provided state funds for needy families with children so that the children could remain in the home.

By the sixth century the Church had begun to show some interest in children, but from the beginning of the Middle Ages little change occurred. In the fifteenth century the first foundling homes began to develop in Europe. In 1538 in England Henry VIII instituted the recording of christenings, births, and deaths which was the beginning in Western civilization of vital statistics. In the seventeenth century we find the founding of the society of St. Vincent de Paul, which declared among its interests the care of children. It was not until the nineteenth century that many activities began to develop that showed an increased concern for the welfare and future of children. The French Revolution emphasized the rights of individuals, and this was reflected in an increasing concern for the care of children.

In the United States the first infant mortality studies were done in Philadelphia in 1871 by the Social Science Association. Two years later the American Medical Association organized a section on obstetrics and diseases of women and children. This was the first time that the medical profession had singled out and emphasized the care of mothers and children. In 1876 the Society for the Prevention of Cruelty to Children was formed, and that same year New York enacted child welfare laws that required the state to intervene when a child was not properly cared for by its family. Public health legislation specifically for children was first enacted in the New York State legislature in 1879; it required New York City to appropriate $10,000 annually to hire doctors and nurses to work with families in an effort to save infants from dying of "summer diarrhea." That same year the American Medical Association formed a section on the diseases of children, which was the first official recognition of pediatrics as a specialty in medicine. In 1888 the American Pediatric Society, one of the first medical specialty organizations in the United States, was formed, its object being "the study of diseases in children."

The first hospital in the United States concerned with the care and treatment of diseases of children was opened in Philadelphia in 1855. Five years later, in 1860, Dr. Abraham Jacobi established the first department of pediatrics; he is rightfully called the father of American pediatrics. Milk stations were started to combat infant diarrhea and improve the nutritional status of infants and children in New York City in 1893. These were the forerunners of the Child Health Conference that continues today. Boston began inspecting school children for communicable diseases in 1894, and this program was considered to be the beginning of school health care in the United States.

In 1902 the federal Bureau of the Census was authorized to issue statistics on births and deaths in the United States; this was the beginning of an effort to collect national vital statistics. In 1908 the New York City Health Department formed the Bureau of Child Hygiene, which was the first separate unit in a health department for the care of mothers and children. One year later the American Association for the Study and Prevention of Infant Mortality was formed. It was not until 1930 that the American Academy of Pediatrics was founded; since then the academy has grown to more than 17,000 members and has assumed a leadership role in establishing standards of child health care.

In 1910 the Flexner report revolutionized medical education in the United States by recommending that it should be the responsibility of the universities, thus significantly changing the scope and quality of the training of American physicians. Also in 1910 President Theodore Roosevelt began the White House Conferences on Children which have been held every decade since that time. The first White House conference was concerned with the care of dependent children, and subsequent ones have also been concerned with national issues such as child welfare standards (1920), child health and protection (1930), and emotional growth and development (1950). In 1970 there were two conferences, one concerned with children and the other with youth through 24 years of age, heralding a new concept of youth as distinguished from majority status. While all these White House conferences dealt with important issues that evoked considerable interest and produced specific recommendations, little direct action has resulted, and many of the goals remain to be achieved.

Also in 1910 recommendations were being heard for a federal agency concerned with children in the United States, and in 1912 the Organic Act created the Children's Bureau, charged by Congress to "investigate and report upon all matters pertaining to the welfare of children and child life among all classes of our people, to investigate the questions of infant mortality, the birth rate, orphanages, juvenile courts, desertion, dangerous occupations, accidents and diseases of children, and employment legislation affecting children in the several states and territories." In 1921 the Maternity and Infant Act was passed by Congress, the first federal grant-in-aid program for health services to mothers and children. This act, also known as the Shepherd-Towner Act, authorized $1.2 million annually to the states to improve health services for mothers during childbearing, as well as for infants. This legislation expired in 1929, which was the year in which the Great Depression began in America. Nevertheless, the Shepherd-Towner Act was considered the blueprint for Title V of the Social Security Act, which was passed in 1935. It was developed as a result of the activities of the National Committee on the Cost of Medical Care, which began its work in 1933 and was concerned with the effects of the Depression on health and other services.

The 6-year interval between the expiration of the Shepherd-Towner Act and the passage of the Social Security Act emphasizes a distressing and recurrent trend toward cutbacks in governmental support of children's services in times of economic stress. Such retrogressive fiscal policies also highlight the contrast between the United States and other countries in both Western Europe and Asia that have tended to view their children and youth as a prime national resource whose needs have high priority when allocating scarce resources.

Children's Bureau, the official government agency concerned with children and women of childbearing age, was designated to administer the financial aid that was authorized to the states in Title V of the Social Security Act. Title V included basic provisions for maternal and child health services to be vested in official health agencies in the states and territories, as well as crippled children's services to be conducted by the official health agencies in 34 states, the state welfare agencies in 9 states, the state departments of education in 4 states, the state university medical schools in 4 states, and special commissions in 4 states. This administrative authority continued until October, 1969, when the Children's Bureau was moved to the Office of Child Development, while its functions were scattered through the Department of Health, Education, and Welfare (HEW). Its authority was transferred to the Maternal and Child Health Service, which in turn was cut back severely in 1973, when its staff was slashed from 130 to 6 members.

With the entry of the United States into World War II in 1941 and the rapid mobilization of manpower, there was increasing concern with the need for services related to childbearing for a transient population of wives of servicemen. In 1943 Congress enacted the Federal Emergency Maternal and Infant Care Program, which provided federal funds for states to purchase medical and hospital care for servicemen's wives and children. This was the largest public medical care program in the United States and was administered through state health departments. This program authorized full payment by the federal government and did not require matching funds from the states. This emergency program was terminated in 1949 when the emergency period for World War II ended; by then it had effectively cared for 1.25 million mothers and 230,000 infants. There was no special planning for continuity of care for this group or for provision of similar civilian services after the emergency ended.

In 1946 federal legislation provided for the National Institute of Mental Health and later other institutes in such fields as heart disease, neurologic disease and blindness, cancer, arthritis and metabolic diseases, dental health, allergy, and infectious diseases. The National Institutes support research, demonstration projects, and training of personnel. In 1961 the National Institute of Child Health and Human Development was established, and it now includes provision of funds for research in child development.

In 1946 the Federal Hospital Survey and Construction Act, also called the Hill-Burton Act, was passed by Congress and provided federal funds for states to study hospital facilities, construct new hospitals, and expand existing hospitals. This made hospital care available for many women who had not previously had the advantage of hospital deliveries, and promoted a significant upgrading of the quality of hospital care. In 1954 the Hill-Burton legislation was extended to provide for persons with chronic illness. Diagnostic services, chronic disease hospitals, rehabilitation centers, and nursing homes were included in the benefits of this legislation.

The Vocational Rehabilitation Act, which was passed in 1954, provided funds for expansion of services, research, and demonstration programs and training of personnel in the field of rehabilitation. In that year the Children's Bureau for the first time provided special grants to develop diagnostic clinics for the mentally retarded in three locations, Washington, Hawaii, and California. In 1957 Congress increased the appropriation for maternal and child health funds and earmarked $1 million for special projects serving mentally retarded children.

In 1963 landmark amendments to Title V of the Social Security Act were passed. These were known as the Mental Retardation Planning Amendments and were "to assist states and communities in preventing and combating mental retardation through expansion and improvement of Maternal and Child Health and Crippled Children's programs through provision of prenatal, maternity, and infant care for individuals with conditions associated with childbearing which may lead to mental retardation, and through planning for comprehensive action to combat mental retardation." Special projects called Maternity and Infant Care (MIC) projects were begun to "help reduce the incidence of mental retardation caused by complications associated with childbearing." In 1965 further amendments to Title V of the Social Security Act provided for special projects for comprehensive health services for school-age and pre-school age children, popularly known as Children and Youth (C and Y) projects (Table 1).

The Office of Economic Opportunity was opened in 1965; it included two significant programs for children. The Head Start program was directed to preschool children of poverty-level families and was based on the premise that early stimulation would prevent environmentally determined developmental lags. The other major program was the Job Corps, which directed its efforts to the poor adolescent, providing opportunities beyond the school experience that would prepare the individual for adult life. Objective evaluation of the effectiveness of these types of intervention has not yet been done, but there is general consensus that these programs have been less successful than their architects had anticipated.

Other milestones of 1965 were Title XVIII (Medicare) and Title XIX (Medicaid) of the Social Security Act, which provided funds for health care for the elderly and for those with low incomes. According to Wallace, the largest current public medical care progrm for children in the United States is Medicaid. In 1966 the Demonstration Cities and Metropolitan Development Act, known as the model cities program, was authorized by Congress; this program had a significant health component that affected many children in poverty areas in urban settings.

The Developmental Disabilities Services and Facilities Construction Act was passed by Congress in 1970. This provided funds to the states for developing and implementing comprehensive and continuing state plans for this group. Included were provisions for services for the developmentally disabled, construction of facilities for services and research, development and demonstration of new or improved techniques of services, construction of university-affiliated facilities for interdisciplinary training of professional personnel, and demonstration and training grants.

In January, 1975, the most recent changes in delivery of social services for children and families and for the aged, blind, and disabled were enacted and signed into law under Title XX of the Social Security Act. This new legislation reduces the federal role in determining the nature and scope of services provided by states receiving federal funds. Congress has authorized $2.5 billion annually to be allotted to the states on the basis of population (the federal ceiling since 1972) and to include protective services to children and adults and family planning services.

While this brief overview suggests an increasing concern for and continuing commitment to health services for children in the United States, it is clear because of the piecemeal way in which services have been developed and have been provided that we still have no comprehensive plan for the health of children, including preventive and health maintenance services. Medical care, not only for the disadvantaged, but also for most children in this country, continues to be crisis-oriented and fragmented, with little concern for the total child and his needs for normal development. The proportion of the national expenditure for personal health care actually spent on children aged 0 to 18 years was 16 percent of $72 billion in 1972, although this group comprised 32 percent of the population at that time.

Although high hopes were generated as a result of some of the legislation previously described and other activities, especially during the 1960s, the demonstrable achievements have not borne out the promise of earlier years. Regrettably, some goals that appeared to be relatively easily accomplished are perhaps further from realization in the 1970s than they were in the 1960s. This is exemplified in the general failure to in-

TABLE 1. Comparison of Per Capita Expenditures for Health Care of Children and Youth in Selected Programs (1967 to 1973)

Program	Expenditure[a]	Year
Job Corps[b]	$344.00	1967–1968
Medicaid[c]	$301.87	1971
Children and youth projects[d]	$128.00	1972–1973
Head Start[e]		1972–1973
Screening & immunization	$27.00–$44.00	
Treatment	$73.00–$98.00	
Total	$100.00–$142.00	
United States, all sources (average)	$146.86	Fiscal 1972

[a] *Annual per capita expenditure for health care of children and/or youth.*
[b] *Data from Bicknell et al.*
[c] *Data from Wallace and Goldstein.*
[d] *Data from Weckwerth.*
[e] *Data from Randolph.*

corporate innovations in methods of health care delivery to children that were tested in demonstration projects during the last decade but have not been widely utilized in either the private or public sector (M and I projects; C and Y projects, neighborhood health centers, etc). Also, we have failed to apply new knowledge and new techniques as fully as we might to prevention of certain widespread conditions. Thus, although scientific advances in the development of effective vaccines against most of the common childhood infectious diseases have occurred since midcentury, we have not eliminated these diseases as significant causes of childhood morbidity in the United States. In fact, despite the hope that measles, rubella, poliomyelitis, and mumps would disappear, they continue to occur sporadically, and as local epidemics. Also, diphtheria, pertussis, and tetanus, against which immunizations were developed much earlier, are still occurring in the United States and have a high degree of prevalence in many developing countries.

INTERNATIONAL CHILD HEALTH

During World War II child health services, like many other services, were in disarray in many parts of the world, particularly in those countries actively engaged in conflict on their own soil. In England, where millions of children were separated from their families and evacuated to the country, and in Western Europe, where large numbers of refugees moved to and fro across the countryside, there could be little semblance of a normal health delivery system. In the same manner the U.S.S.R., which suffered enormous losses and experienced famine in areas of combat, especially in the siege of Leningrad, was not able to concentrate on preventive or health maintenance services. However, concern for child health was alive and was actively demonstrated shortly after the founding of the United Nations by the development of the World Health Organization, UNESCO, and other organizations working collaboratively. The World Health Organization was established with headquarters in Geneva in 1946, with regional offices located in various parts of the world. The major objectives were stated as being to assist in the development of appropriate child health services, in eradication of certain diseases, and in various disease control programs. Among the laudable goals of this organization have been real emphasis on family planning, reduction of infant and maternal mortality, and eradication of malaria and smallpox.

The World Health Organization makes use of large numbers of experts from various countries whose particular experience or skills may be of value in addressing a particular problem. Numerous individuals and teams from the United States have served at various times in efforts such as population control studies in India, Pakistan, and Indonesia, eradication of trachoma in Egypt, and malaria control in developing countries in tropical and subtropical areas. Political considerations have been reflected in a recent reduction in the number of United States consultants utilized by the World Health Organization. It should also be noted that the World Health Organization has not been directly involved in any programs within the continental United States or in the other developed countries. It also has not had an impact in the People's Republic of China, which was not a member of the United Nations until recently.

The World Health Organization has also supported training of health professionals from developing countries, who are expected to return to their own countries to apply their newly acquired skills in dealing with its special health needs and problems within a cultural context with which they are familiar. A major contribution by the World Health Organization has been the convening of expert committees that have prepared technical publications applicable to health planning efforts and delivery of health services throughout the world.

MANPOWER

At least in part, lack of adequate health services for children has been related to lack of manpower in many areas, notably disadvantaged rural areas, urban slums, or agricultural localities with a high proportion of migrant workers. At the same time there has been a significant concentration of extremely well trained medical personnel in large urban centers and affluent suburban areas. Studies of distribution of physicians, including pediatricians, in the United States reveal that while the overall physician-to-population ratio is consistently increasing, regional variations are great. Thus in 1971 Boston had 239 physicians per 100,000 population, while there were some rural areas with only 40 physicians per 100,000, as well as 133 counties with no active physician. There has been an actual decrease in the proportion of primary care physicians over the past decade from 43 percent to 35 percent of those practicing. There have been various estimates of the extent of the national shortage of physicians, some as high as 50,000; the shortage has been reduced in part by increasing the number of graduating medical students from 7,574 in 1966 to 11,862 in 1974, according to the Association of American Medical Colleges. At the same time there has been a great influx of foreign medical graduates, who at present represent 20 percent of all physicians in the United States and who represented 46 percent of newly licensed physicians in 1972. Their presence has contributed significantly to maintaining or increasing the overall physician–patient ratios. However, these physicians also tend to remain in areas with high concentrations of medical manpower.

Concern regarding maldistribution of physicians has led to various congressional and other efforts to initiate remedies, including creation of the National Health Service Corps, which assigns physicians for 1- to 2-year periods of subsidized activity in underserved areas. According to Stimmel, although this provides short-term coverage, it will not provide long-term continuity of care. He also doubts that such exposure will attract physicians to stay in remote areas for longer than the required time. Until recent years there was little concern for recruiting and training professionals and other health workers from minority groups, and many children have been deprived of effective health services because of language or cultural barriers that make community health services inaccessible to them.

Although new roles for health professionals have been developed and new types of health workers have emerged, they unfortunately continue to experience difficulty in many parts of the country in fitting into the health care system. Their training and performance are not standardized in such a way that they can become licensed and function effectively, taking full responsibility for their own participation in providing health care. Career mobility is also limited by lack of uniform standards and by a considerable degree of rivalry between the various new health professionals and those with similar skills who have differing backgrounds. Many other countries around the world have been able to effectively develop and utilize health workers who require less training and skill than we in the United States deem essential for effective health care. The felcher and the midwife in Russia, the barefoot doctor in China, the dia (traditional midwife) in India, and others have contributed significantly to national health care systems. There is a slow and halting growth of reliance on health personnel such as midwives, pediatric nurse practitioners, and others in some parts of the United States, but widespread acceptance is far from a reality. Although over the years a substantial literature has documented patient acceptance and professional competence, the degree of independence of practice of these health personnel depends to a great extent on the laws of individual states. Current political problems center around questions of who should certify the competency of new health professionals and who should supervise or oversee their work.

VITAL STATISTICS: UNITED STATES

RHONA S. RUDOLPH AND
ALLAN C. OGLESBY

Population growth has been a significant concern for the past two decades. The studies of Ehrlich and others (eg, *Population Bomb*) have drawn a great deal of public attention to the so-called population explosion and the potential difficulties inherent therein. Population growth obviously depends on an excess of births over deaths; there has been a trend in recent years for high birth rates, which were previously offset by high death rates, to continue even as mortality has decreased. In 1940 there were 45 million young people under the age of 20 years in the United States. By 1970 there were 80 million young people, of whom 64 million were under the age of 18 years. The birth rate increased steadily until 1971, when it began to decline below its peak of 1957. This has been attributed to a decline in the proportion of women marrying at ages below 24 years, accompanied by an increase in divorce and separation and some impact from liberalized abortion laws. However, the provisional birth rate for 1974 is slightly higher than the final rate for 1973, which reflects a possible reversal of the decline of recent years. This may be attributable to the increasing proportion of women between the ages of 15 and 44 years, the generally accepted child bearing years. According to the Bureau of the Census, the number of women in this age range will increase about 12 percent by 1980; so unless the fertility rate (the number of births per 1,000 women age 15 to 44 years) continues to decline sufficiently to offset these increased numbers, a gradually increasing birth rate is a distinct possibility.

Infant Mortality

It should be noted that definitions of infant mortality are relatively clear, but when one attempts to look at aspects of perinatal mortality, fetal deaths, stillbirths, etc, there is continuing confusion. While the concept of perinatal mortality has developed over the years, definitions have varied from organization to organization and from state to state. In the United States it is generally accepted that the neonatal death rate refers to infants dying during the firt 27 days after birth, and the postnatal death rate refers to those infants dying between the ages of 28 days and 1 year. The rate is based on the number of deaths per 1,000 live births in a given year. Live birth, as defined by the World Health Organization in 1950, is "the complete expulsion or extraction from its mother of a product of conception, irrespective of the duration of pregnancy, which after such separation, breathes or shows any evidence of life such as beating of the heart, pulsation of the umbilical cord or definite movement of voluntary muscles, whether or not the umbilical cord has been cut or the placenta is attached; each product of such a birth is considered live born." In 1950 the World Health Organization defined fetal death as "death prior to the complete expulsion or extraction from its mother of a product of conception, irrespective of the duration of pregnancy; the death is indicated by the fact that after such separation, the fetus does not breathe, show any other evidence of life such as beating of the heart, pulsation of the umbilical cord, or definite movement of voluntary muscles." Many individuals believe that these definitions do not adequately meet today's needs and that revisions are overdue.

The vital statistics for the United States for 1972 and 1973 reveal that there were 15.6 live births per 1,000 population in 1972 and 14.9 per 1,000 in 1973, as opposed to 18.4 in 1970 and 17.8 in 1967. The death rate was 9.5 per 1,000 in 1970 and 9.4 per 1,000 in 1967, 1972, and 1973, thereby diminishing the natural percentage increase in the child population over the 6-year period 1967–1973. However, in one state (California) there was a sharp rise in the birth rate (23 percent) in 1974, and the provisional figures for 1974 suggest that this increase will be reflected in national statitstics, thus suggesting an end to the declining birth rate. Thus the provisional data for 1974 set the birth rate at 15.0 per 1,000 population and the death rate at 9.1 per 1,000.

The infant mortality rate is generally accepted as an indicator of the level of health care services, although it is obviously also strongly influenced by other socioeconomic factors. Infant mortality in the United States in 1935 was 55.7 per 1,000 live births, in 1950 it was

TABLE 2. Infant Mortality Rates per 1,000 Live Births by Age and Race for the United States, 1950, 1960, and 1970–1974[a]

	Total			White			All Other		
Year	Under 1 Year	Under 28 Days	28 Days through 11 Months	Under 1 Year	Under 28 Days	28 Days through 11 Months	Under 1 Year	Under 28 Days	28 Days through 11 Months
1950	29.2	20.5	8.7	26.8	19.4	7.4	44.5	27.5	16.9
1960	26.0	18.7	7.3	22.9	17.2	5.7	43.2	26.9	16.4
1970	20.0	15.1	4.9	17.8	13.8	4.0	30.9	21.4	9.5
1971	19.1	14.2	4.9	17.1	13.0	4.0	28.5	19.6	8.9
1972	18.5	13.6	4.8	16.4	12.4	4.0	27.7	19.2	8.5
1973	17.7	13.0	4.8	15.8	11.8	3.9	26.2	17.9	8.3
1974[b]	16.5	12.1	4.4	14.7	11.1	3.6	24.6	16.6	8.0

[a] Adapted from Wegman M: Annual summary of vital statistics—1974, Pediatrics 56:960, 1975.
[b] Data for 1974 based on a 10% sample of deaths; for all other years, based on final data.

29.2, and in 1965 it was 24.7. By 1973 this figure was down to 17.7, and the provisional infant mortality rate for 1974 is 16.5. There is a significant difference between the infant mortality for white infants and those of other races, so that in 1935 the figure for white children was 51.9 per 1,000 live births and for nonwhites 83.2. By 1950 this figure had dropped to 26.8 for white children and 44.5 for all others; by 1965 the white mortality had dropped to 21.5, while mortality for all others was still as high as 40.3 (Table 2).

The 1974 provisional mortality statistics indicate that for white children under 1 year of age the mortality is 14.7, whereas for others it is 24.6. These figures indicate close to a 2 to 1 mortality for children of other ethnic groups and minorities compared to white children under the age of 1 year; they obviously reflect significant social and economic factors. The overall infant mortality rate of 16.5 for 1974 represents a decline of 7 percent from 1973. It is pointed out by Goldstein that the overall infant mortality rate for the 35 years 1935 to 1970 declined from 55.7 to 19.8, a drop of 64 percent. Approximately three-fourths of this decrease occurred in the first 15 years from 1935 to 1950.

International comparisons are difficult to make. It would be somewhat unrealistic to attempt to compare United States data with those available from other countries that do not keep the kinds of detailed statistics maintained by the Center for Health Statistics and various federal, state, and local agencies. Reporting procedures vary and definitions are not consistent. The United Nations does require a degree of completeness in reporting, and until recently it listed only seven Western Hemisphere countries including the United States and Canada. It is difficult indeed to separate out the influence of medical factors such as prenatal and infant care, delivery of child health services, and child health supervision from environmental, social, and economic factors such as nutrition, housing, and poverty. Nevertheless, the infant mortality rates for 25 countries with populations over 2.5 million reveal that whereas it ranked thirteenth in infant mortality in 1968, United Nations data for 1972 and 1973 rank the United States as sixteenth (Table 3). Although there has been a con-

tinuing general downward trend that has been shared by the United States, our rate is still far from a figure commensurate with our wealth and power. According to Wegman, "what is really remarkable is the continuing decline in countries which already have rates that no pediatrician would have believed possible 25 years

TABLE 3. Infant Mortality Rates for Lowest 24 Countries With Population Over 2,500,000

Area	1973	1974
Sweden	9.6	9.2[a]
Finland	10.0	
Japan	11.3	
Netherlands	11.5	11.0[a]
Denmark	11.5	
Norway	11.8[a]	
Switzerland	13.2[a]	
France	15.5[a]	
Canada	15.6	
German Democratic Republic	16.0	
New Zealand	16.2[a]	
Australia	16.5[a]	
Hong Kong	16.8[a]	17.7[a]
England and Wales	16.9	15.5[a]
Belgium	17.0[a]	
United States	17.7	16.5[a]
Ireland	18.0	
Czechoslovakia	21.2	
German Federal Republic	22.7	
Israel	22.8	
Austria	23.8	23.4[a]
Greece	24.1	24.0[a]
Italy	25.7	
Poland	25.8	23.5[a]

[a] Provisional data.

ago." He also points out that the 15 countries with rates in 1973 that were better than that of the United States had a combined population of 320 million. It is of interest that the provisional infant mortality figures for the United States for 1974 continue to show a proportionately greater decline in deaths in the first 28 days of life (neonatal death rate) than at later ages. This more rapid drop in the neonatal rate than in the postneonatal rate cannot be accounted for by any single medical or non medical factor. It may be speculated that this drop reflects the influence of the increased number of neonatal intensive care units and the regionalization of intensive care services for high-risk newborns. The major causes of death in this age period continue to be related to prematurity and its associated problems, with immaturity, respiratory disorders, congenital malformations, and birth injuries still the leading factors, especially in the first week of life (Table 4). In a Swedish

TABLE 4. Infant Mortality Rates by Age and Selected Causes for the United States, 1964, 1969, and 1974[a]

Age and Cause of Death	1964[b]	1969[c] (est.)	1974 (est.)
Age			
Total under 1 year (Infant)	24.8	20.7	16.5
Under 28 days (Neonatal)	17.9	15.4	12.1
28 days to 11 months (Postnatal)	6.9	5.4	4.4
Cause of death			
Congenital anomalies	3.6	3.2	2.9
Asphyxia of newborn, unspecified	3.7	2.7	1.5
Immaturity, unqualified	3.5	2.7	1.5
Influenza and pneumonia	3.1	2.1	0.9
Birth injuries	0.7	0.7	0.6
Certain gastrointestinal diseases	0.6	0.3	0.3
Other diseases of early infancy	5.8	5.8	5.3
All other causes	3.7	3.4	3.7

[a] *Source: Monthly Vital Statistics Reports.*
[b] *International Classification of Diseases, Seventh Revision.*
[c] *International Classification of Diseases, Eighth Revision, adapted 1965.*

study by Carlgren there was evidence of congenital heart disease in 8 of 1,000 live births, with a mortality of 40 percent by age 15 years. Of these deaths, 87 percent occurred within the first year, which illustrates the importance of early diagnosis and intervention when serious problems are present from birth.

Children Age 1 Through 4 Years

The mortality rate in this age group declined from 150.2 per 100,000 population in 1949 to 84.5 in 1970. As in the infant mortality rates, the figures are higher for groups other than whites, but the decline in mortality among all groups in this period is the same (45 percent). Since 1949 the leading cause of death in this age group has been accidents. The 1968–1970 statistics revealed a mortality due to accidents of 31.5 per 100,000, of a total mortality rate of 85.3. More than one-third of these deaths were due to motor vehicle accidents, and although the overall death rate due to accidents has shown a slight drop through the years, there has been no comparable drop in fatalities due to motor vehicle accidents.

Congenital anomalies are the second leading cause of death in this age group, accounting for a rate of 9.7 per 100,000 in 1968–1970. The third largest group is deaths attributed to influenza and pneumonia (7.6), and the fourth leading cause of death is malignant disease, with leukemia accounting for almost half of these. It is noteworthy that while the reported incidence of malignant diseases in children has increased, the death rate has declined somewhat with the development of new and sophisticated treatment methods. Cardiovascular diseases accounted for a death rate of 2.6 in 1968–1970.

A startling increase in the overall death rate from homicide in the United States from 5.4 per 100,000 in 1950 to 10.5 per 100,000 in 1973 is reflected also in an increase in homicides of children from 0.6 in 1949–1951 to 1.6 in 1968–1970. For 1973, 503 homicides were reported in children under the age of 4 years, accounting for 2.5 percent of homicides in that year. This reflects an apparent increase in child abuse in the United States along with the increase in violent attacks on persons in general.

Children Age 5 Through 14 Years

While the decline in mortality rate in this group was not as large as in the younger age groups (from 66.1 per 100,000 population in 1949 to 41.3 in 1970), it was slightly greater among nonwhites than it was among white children (41 and 37 percent, respectively). Accidents are the leading cause of death in children 5 to 14 years of age, accounting for almost half the deaths (20.1 of 42.0 in 1968–1970). Half of the accidental deaths are related to motor vehicles, and the death rate due to motor vehicle accidents has continually increased for this age group over the past 25 years.

The second leading cause of death in this age group is malignant diseases, with a rate of 6.1 per 100,000 in 1968–1970, with very little evidence of a decline over the years. Leukemia also is the most frequent malignancy in this group, with brain tumors the second most frequent. Congenital anomalies account for the third largest number of deaths, 2.4 in 1968–1970, with no real downward trend since 1949–1951. Cardiovascular diseases, on the other hand, showed a marked decline from 4.6 in 1949–1951 to 1.8 in 1968–1970, largely due to a decline in rheumatic diseases. Deaths due to infections have also declined markedly in the past 25 years.

As previously noted, homicides have increased substantially, and this has included increased deaths of children. However, the death rate from homicide in children 5 to 14 years of age was half that in children under 5 years of age during 1968–1970. There were 481 homicides of children ages 5 to 14 years reported in 1973, almost equal to the number under age 5 years suggesting a dramatic upsurge in mortality due to homicide in the brief period from 1970 to 1973. The percentage of deaths due to homicide of children under 15 years of age was 4.5 percent of all homicides in 1973.

Suicide is a factor in the deaths of an unknown number of young children. There are no valid statistics for the group under 15 years of age, but sociologists infer that suicide is an increasingly serious problem in the very young, as in other age groups. According to Peck and Seiden, the suicide rate for children ages 15 to 24 years has gone from fewer than 5 per 100,000 in the 1940s and 1950s to nearly 10 per 100,000 in 1972, a 100-fold increase. Their studies and those of others reveal a pattern of striving for success on the part of parents coupled with an inability of the children to live up to parental expectations. These children have tended to be unhappy, frustrated, and on poor terms with their families. Nearly half of adolescent suicides in one recent study were involved in some form of drug or alcohol abuse shortly before their deaths, and more than one-half had received psychotherapy or counseling.

Homicide accounted for 5,182 deaths of children ages 15 to 24 years, or more than 25 percent of all deaths due to homicide in 1973. Perhaps even more startling is the fact that 1.7 percent (299) of those arrested for homicide were under age 15 years, while 7,524 (43.3 percent) of those arrested were 15 to 24 years of age. Also of concern to pediatricians is the most recent Federal Bureau of Investigation data regarding crime in general, which revealed that 30 percent of crimes in 1974 were committed by teenagers (16 percent of the population).

When these figures are considered in conjunction with the fact that accidents are still the major cause of death for those 15 to 24 years of age, we are forced to recognize that three of the four leading causes of death at the stage of life where individuals are at or are approaching their physical and intellectual peak are due to violence in one form or another. These figures do not take into account deaths in times of armed conflict. They are an alarming reflection on our alleged progress as a civilization.

In general, reduction in deaths of children and youth in the United States has been due to reduction of deaths from infectious diseases, coupled with improved medical care for mothers and children, new medical and social programs, and higher overall standards of living. However, as exemplified by our poor relative standing, the United States still has a long way to go in overcoming those socioeconomic and other factors standing in the way of achieving at least parity with other developed countries.

Although there are impressive differences in United States mortality statistics by ethnic groups, it has been suggested that such differences are due more to socioeconomic factors than to other factors. Unfortunately, statistics are not readily available identifying mortality and other rates or trends according to socioeconomic rather than ethnic indicators. However, it is known that while the overall mortality rate for black children is considerably higher than for whites, there is close correlation between the mortality figures for black and white children of the same social class and family income level. Such a correlation serves to reinforce the view that health is more than the absence of disease. If the child health care system in the United States is to achieve the objectives of promoting health and preventing illness, in addition to treating disease once it has

occurred, it must at least be ready to acknowledge the palpable differences in access to health care and other aspects of health maintenance between the haves and have-nots in our society. Also, it would be desirable to develop some more refined indicators of a nation's health than its relative mortality statistics.

It is at this juncture that one recognizes certain stumbling blocks to the planning and provision of appropriate health services. In the first place, there is in fact little agreement as to the definition of health and little evidence that the majority of health care providers concerned with children have a common agenda for promoting and protecting health. In spite of innumerable lofty pronouncements that good health is concerned with mental as well as physical health and well-being, an examination of the existing fragmented, piecemeal modes of delivery of services suggests a serious lack of attention to the noble objectives of professional planners. When the health care system is examined in terms of how it operates, it is readily apparent that prevention of disease and promotion of good health have a lesser priority than illness-centered care in most countries of the world and certainly in the United States.

References

Distribution of Physicians in the United States. Chicago, American Medical Association, 1972.

Goldstein H: In Wallace, Gold, Lis (eds): Maternal and Child Health Practice. Springfield, Ill, Charles C Thomas p 84

National Center for Health Statistics: Monthly Vital Statistics Report, Vol. 23, No 13. June 27, 1974

Peck L, Seiden R: Youth suicide. Exchange 3: 1975

Physician Manpower and Distribution: The Primary Care Physician. Washington, DC, Association of American Medical Colleges, 1974, p 4

Sklar J, Berkov B: The American birth rate: evidence of a coming rise. Science 189:693,

Stimmel B: The Congress and health manpower. N Engl J Med 293:68, 1975

Wallace HM, Goldstein H: Child health care in the United States: expenditures and extent of coverage with selected comprehensive services. Pediatrics 55:176, 1975

SOCIAL CHANGES AFFECTING CHILD HEALTH

JOHN DOWER

The fact previously noted that the child population receives a disproportionately low share of the health dollar is not difficult to comprehend when the rapidity of the changes in attitudes toward children is considered.

One of the societal variables that has both a direct and indirect impact on the health of children is socioeconomic status. An unconscionable percentage of children live in economically deprived circumstances. This results in such palpable outcomes as increased neonatal mortality and lead poisoning, to more subtle but equally pervasive problems such as school failure and higher crime rates. Blacks, people of Hispanic origin, and American Indians are all overrepresented among the poor. In addition to economic squalor, the imponderable burden of racial discrimination is present. The poor, both in rural and urban areas, have less access to quality health care because of the maldistribution of health manpower and such other barriers as economic, ethnic, language, and transportation.

The organizational and structural characteristics of a society have a direct impact on the health of children; thus, high-risk infants born in areas where Regional Neonatal Intensive Care Centers exist have a much greater chance of high-quality survival than those born in areas without sophisticated transport and backup facilities. The lack of communitywide organization of health and social services results in massive inequities in both the cost and quality of care.

THE FAMILY STRUCTURE—NUCLEAR, SINGLE, AND EXTENDED FAMILIES

The family is the traditional unit of social organization. There are many definite types of family groups. A polygamous family consists of two or more nuclear families, affiliated by plural marriages, ie, having one married parent in common. The extended family consists of two or more of the nuclear families, affiliated through an extension of the parent-child relationship rather than the husband-wife relationship, ie, by joining the nuclear family of a married adult to that of his parents. The patrilocal extended family, often called the patriarchal family, furnishes an excellent example. It includes, typically, an older man, his wife or wives, his unmarried children, his married sons, and the wives and children of the latter. Three generations, including the nuclear families of father and sons, live under a single roof or in a cluster of adjacent dwellings. Most families deriving their livelihood from farming pursued this pattern until about one generation ago. A new format of family organization is emerging rapidly; this is the single-parent group and is usually composed of the biologic mother and her children. At times, two or more such units combine to form yet another type of family group. The problems of social isolation and multiple caretakers characterize this arrangement, and it is clear that more effective support systems than those in existence are needed for this group. During the sixties, there was the rapid development also of various types of communal living arrangements, both urban and rural, with differing philosophies and organizations, but almost all including children whose rearing was based on the group orientation and structure. It is not known how many children are presently part of such living arrangements.

One of the most profound influences on the structure and function of the family unit has been the continuing trend toward urbanization of society. The physical mobility this imposes contributes to instability. The average American family moves once every five years and while it is true that the majority of these moves are for short distances, there have been dislocations of major

portions of our rural populations to urban slums. A sample of the challenges to family stability resulting from this phenomenon are high unemployment rates, welfare systems that discourage keeping an unemployed father in the household, and the effect of working mothers on the supervision and support of their children.

The increasing numbers of women who work outside the home, coupled with little noticeable increase in planned resources for appropriate child care, presents a problem of some magnitude. Of the 91 million people in the work force, 38 percent are women, an increase from 29 percent in 1950. Of the 64 million children under 18 years, 41 percent have working mothers; of the 6 million under age 6 years, 31 percent. In the past 10 years, 60 percent of the increase in the labor force has been female, and these women are not only those who are single, separated, and widowed. Currently, 53 percent of women in intact families are employed and, while some of these women may work in pursuit of a sense of personal fulfillment, most do so out of economic necessity. The average working mother continues to carry 70 to 80 percent of child care and household duties in addition to her job. Where is the time for the warm, intimate, and continuous relationship with the mother that experts in personality development regard as essential? In other societies, such as the Israeli Kibbutz and China's child care centers, parent surrogates seem to be used successfully.

Another force unbalancing the stability of the nuclear family is divorce. In 1974, both the number and the rate of divorces and annulments continued to increase; more than one million divorces were granted, more than double the number 10 years ago. In 1974, more than one million children were affected by divorce. These figures, when viewed in the context of a decline in the number of and rate of marriages, suggest that alternative life styles are not transient social experiments. The implications in terms of the effects on child rearing can only be speculative, although it is evident that family structure and dynamics do have some direct consequences on health.

For many children affected by the breakup of the family unit because of divorce, death, or desertion, considerable social disorganization results. For some of these children, foster care is a temporary solution. In any given year 350,000 children live in 150,000 foster homes. They are a population at high risk; a high percentage have physical, emotional, and mental handicaps. The mobility from home to home for some of these children precludes good health care, and a pattern of community neglect often replaces parental neglect.

The problem of identifying children in high-risk situations is not simple. Many profitable hours have been spent decrying the lack of availability and accessibility of comprehensive health services for children of the poor, while it was evident that the families in highest need often did not utilize available services. A recent study of health care utilization patterns revealed that the urban poor represent a wide range of family characteristics, problems, and resource utilization patterns.

An attempt at systematic and objective knowledge about these characteristics resulted in the development of a guide for further explorations in differentiating truly high-risk children and their families from families sharing the same disadvantaged neighborhood but apparently in less urgent need of comprehensive health care. The high-need group not only had greater unmet health needs, but also more difficulty in participating in the system, and a higher drop-out rate (Table 5).

THE CHILD AND THE ENVIRONMENT

The societal and family issues noted above have profound effects on how the individual child grows and develops. It is crucial to recognize that these factors impinge on and critically shape the biologic determinants of the individual, but it is also important to reaffirm the dynamic interplay between genetic and environmental factors. This is graphically demonstrated by the striking increase in height and weight of Japanese children in the era following World War II, as compared with their growth prior to that time. A society with a fairly constant genetic pool was growing at a substantially increased rate, presumably due to improved nutritional status. In individual cases the weight of evidence is not as persuasive as in population studies, and often other conceptual prejudices cloud the issue.

The child brings to a family setting a set of biologic and personality characteristics capable of profoundly modifying the ecology of that unit. Chess and her colleagues resurrected previous observations by Aldrich and expanded them into a rational framework when they detailed the behavioral individuality of very young children. Brazelton has designed a Neonatal Assessment Scale to assess a wide variety of behaviors as well as neurologic status of infants. This rediscovery of the newborn as a person and a personality has implications for the management of problems arising in the first few months of life.

The intrauterine environment must be viewed as part of the ecology of the developing fetus. The nutritional status of the mother; her underlying metabolic diseases; her habits, such as smoking, drinking, and drug-taking; and her exposure to environmental hazards may all affect the fetus adversely. Maternal infections, such as syphilis, rubella, cytomegalic inclusion virus, and toxoplasmosis, may cause a wide range of defects and disease in the fetus and infant. During delivery, commonplace inhabitants such as Group B streptococci, or transient pathogens such as herpes simplex virus, may cause life-threatening disease in the neonate. Infants of mothers with diabetes mellitus have high mortality, both in utero and after birth. Their abnormal environment results in a spectrum of morphologic and biochemical changes that pose a direct threat to survival in postnatal life. Large numbers of infants are born addicted to heroin or methadone. The infants, exposed to the drugs continually in utero, manifest withdrawal symptoms after birth. They have an increased mortality, and long-range prognosis for intellectual and behavioral functioning of these infants is not yet clearly elucidated. Infants born to alcoholic mothers have morphologic changes designated as the fetal acohol syndrome and many manifest developmental delay and mental retardation.

Pollution and contamination of the environment have been responsible for poisoning of fetuses and infants. An outbreak of methylmercury poisoning of fetuses in Japanese women was attributed to the consumption of contaminated fish; this resulted from release of methylmercury as a waste product from industrial plants. The mothers showed no toxic signs during pregnancy, yet their offspring were severely affected, with gross impairment of motor and mental development.

The hazards to the health of the child and adolescent, which are largely products of his culture, race, socioeconomic status, and habitat, have been alluded to above. For an expanded view, the reader is referred to a series of monographs by Robert Coles.

HEALTH CARE RESOURCES: ORGANIZATIONAL PATTERNS

In spite of the very high level of concern by a number of professional societies, government agencies, and citizen groups over the issue of the health of children, there is no national policy, no clearly articulated goal, no organizational structure, no control apparatus, and no universal funding mechanism to allow an organized health system to develop. This does not mean that there

TABLE 5. Predictive Matrix for Identification of High Need/Low Utilizers and Low Need/High Utilizers

	Indicator	High Need/Low Utilizers	Low Need/High Utilizers
1.	Number of children	Many (3 or more)	Few (1 or 2)
2.	Family size	Large (over 5)	Small (5 or less)
3.	Father's whereabouts	Separated from family	Lives with family
4.	Household composition	Nuclear	Extended
5.	Children's ages	Includes teenagers	Mostly preteen
6.	Mother's age	Thirties or older	Twenties or younger
7.	Public welfare status	On welfare	Not on welfare
8.	Mother's employment	Not employed	Employed
9.	Residential mobility	Frequent moves	Infrequent moves
10.	Children's grade level	Several below norm	Few or none below norm
11.	School attendance	Many nonmedical absences	Few or no nonmedical absences

From Leopold EA: Pediatrics 53:344, 1974

is a universal failure to deliver services. It does mean that there are often costly duplications, unacceptable omissions, and generally uncontrolled quality in the delivery of health services to children. Nevertheless, a variety of professionals are busily plying their craft toward the advancement of the health of children.

There are numerous arrangements under which children receive care in this country. For the most part they share one feature in common—the care is patient-initiated. The major exception to this is care of the infant during the first year of life, when health supervision visits form the bulk of the encounters.

PRIVATE PRACTICE. Although most critics of the current system view the rubric private practice as the *bête noire* of our system, the fact of the matter is that most encounters children have with physicians occur in a private practice setting. Physicians in private practice tend to aggregate in communities where parents and caretakers possess sufficient means to meet the obligations of the care pattern. This immediately defines the population base as being loaded with intact, middle-class families possessing sufficient financial resources to honor their part of the contract. In return, the physician agrees to supply continuous first-line care and to be available and accessible for the majority of the needs of his patients for health supervision and care during sickness.

HOSPITAL PRACTICE. Children receiving care in hospital settings do so for a variety of reasons. Many families use hospitals as the source of primary care for themselves and their children. The care sought is often crisis-oriented and there is little perception of the value of preventive care. Those using hospitals in municipal areas for primary care frequently have no alternative, as many live in slums or disintegrating neighborhoods where there are few or no physicians. Many low-income families work in marginal employment, without released time for physician visits, so that in order to bring the child to the doctor or hospital the breadwinner must face the cost of lost pay as well as the cost of care. To a large extent this is the cause of the high utilization of hospital emergency rooms, which remain open 24 hours daily, for primary care of the children of the poor, who often have their total health care paid by federal and state funds.

In large teaching and community hospitals there are subpopulations of children who use the specialty clinic for secondary care administered by physicians, providing full- of part-time hospital-based services. These are often children with chronic illnesses, such as cystic fibrosis, or congenital cardiac disease, who attend the clinics for long-range specialized supervision of their chronic condition, but have physicians close to their homes who manage their day-to-day problems.

The *neighborhood health center* movement was launched about 10 years ago, with objectives that were ambitious and broad. Centers were established in areas underserved by health professionals. The programs were designed to provide for comprehensive health care for low-income families residing within defined geographic areas, usually inner-city slums or underserved rural

areas. Mental health services and dental services were designed into most of the programs. Initially, it was envisioned that the communities should control the operations of these centers through the formation of governing boards elected by the residents of the community being served.

Upward of 150 of these centers were funded by federal contracts. In general, they succeeded in the goal of eventually supplying comprehensive health care to low-income families at reasonable costs. The failures were generally on the side of overly ambitious expectations for what community organization could achieve. The long-range contribution of this model is the demonstration that organization of health services can work toward the provision of high-quality care; that populations can be defined; and the relationships of that population and its health professionals can be negotiated in terms of the services needed. The organizational contributions were the demonstration of the applicability of multispecialty group practice to low-income families; the demonstration that a variety of health professionals could be better organized to serve their patients; and that consumer governing boards could interact with professionals.

Substantial numbers of children have been cared for in *Children and Youth Projects* funded to deliver comprehensive care services to low-income children. The projects were usually associated with medical schools, health departments, or hospitals. Again, the use of health care teams, utilizing physicians, nurses, social workers, and psychologists, demonstrated the effectiveness of this approach when a multitude of factors were impinging on the health of the children in the target population.

The *Maternal-Infant Care* (MIC) projects were built around the identification of high-risk pregnant women. Comprehensive services were provided for the mothers during pregnancy and for the mothers and their infants during the first year of life.

One of the problems facing all of these categorical programs was the control and continuity of funding support from governmental agencies; the fragile status of this support was a constant source of anxiety, making it difficult to attract and keep qualified health providers. At the present time, these programs are quite restricted in scope and funding.

Many specialized services for children are supported to a significant degree by *voluntary agencies.* Services for children with hearing and visual handicaps; speech, language, and perceptual problems; mental retardation; and a variety of crippling conditions, diseases, or problems of physical and mental health are supported by the efforts of private agencies. Frequently, such organizations have provided the incentive to the development of programs that have resulted in several desirable ends.

As previously noted, Crippled Children's Programs authorized through federal legislation provide federal and state funds for provision of services to children with a variety of disabilities. These diagnostic and treatment services are administered at the local level in a number of models and with considerable variability, not only in range and scope of services offered, but also in the fiscal constraints on eligibility for assistance in defraying the costs of care for eligible conditions.

PROFESSIONAL ROLES IN THE PROVISION OF CARE TO CHILDREN

THE PHYSICIAN.   What is the role of the physician who cares for children? For the hospital-based teacher and researcher, the task is better defined than that of the practitioner who sees most of his patients in an ambulatory setting. The hospital specialist deals with a population of patients, usually defined by the organ system primarily affected by disease. A substantial portion of the patients in his population are those who would not be alive had they been born 20 to 30 years ago. The task is clear for those engaged in secondary and tertiary care patterns. It is to uncover new knowledge and develop more effective treatment and management strategies. Today many disciplines are involved, each with specialized skills, which contribute to the welfare of the patient and are necessary to effective management. Team dynamics and the decision-making process vary considerably, depending on the personalities involved, but team composition is pragmatically interdisciplinary. Where such resources are available, as in a medical school setting, such team-work is commonplace.

What of the primary care pediatrician, the physician of first contact who maintains continuous availability to his patient population, a population for the most part well but with a substantial percentage of chronic illness and a predictable reservoir of psychosocial dissonance? What resources does he or she command? What organizational patterns can be utilized? With whom and where can he interact? How does he or she find out what skills and knowledge other professionals possess? How does he or she arrive at the point where the total needs of the patients are considered? The answers to these questions will help in determining what the pediatrician of the immediate future should be. The changing nature of the health problems of American youth also affect this decision. Should the pediatrician of the future be a hospital-based consultant specializing in an organ system, or should there be multiple models to pursue? In a large sense society will answer that question but, unless the primary pediatrician of today recongizes the limits of his or her personal skills and knowledge and develops both training programs and organizational models for utilizing the contributions of other professionals, he or she will not serve the broad needs of the patients.

THE EDUCATIONAL REALM—TEACHERS, PSYCHOLOGISTS, SCHOOL HEALTH NURSES.   The current training models for pediatricians largely ignore the fact that, from age 4 or 5 through 18 years, most children spend the major portion of their waking hours in school. There is little reason to doubt that life within the schools has a profound effect on how children act, think, and behave. One of the major tasks of later childhood and adolescence is the acquisition of cognitive skills that are, to a certain extent, school related. How this occurs should be of vital interest to any professional concerned with the health of children.

Teachers are important to the mental health of developing children in a large number of ways; they have the potential of being role models. In addition, they are observers; they become quite competent in recognizing aberrations from the norm in behavior and development. Frequently they are familiar with elements of the family and social history unknown to the physician, and they act as screeners for visual, auditory, and behavioral problems. As a rule, they are cooperative with health personnel and have valuable insights into family dynamics.

Individual schools and almost all school districts have educational and, occasionally, clinical psychologists on their staff. Children who are failing in school usually have contact with psychologists, and frequently an extensive test history is available. The physician should attempt to gather all of the test material about a child who is not performing adequately before he examines the child. In this way, costly duplication of testing may be avoided. *School health programs* are usually under the jurisdiction of local school districts and have, to a large extent, been out of the mainstream of personal health services. They have, in the past, maintained poor liaison with the rest of the system, but there are encouraging signs that changes are in the offing and, in a few areas, creative programs are being launched. It should be expected that, in the next decade, schools will be the locus of imaginative health education and service programs. At one time the school nurse's offices were populated by superannuated bureaucrats whose diagnostic and therapeutic repertoire was limited to aspirin and one-half hour of rest. This was a reflection of the priorities health and school authorities placed on the function. Health education was largely the domain of physical education teachers. Currently, there is widespread ferment and a willingness to attempt different solutions to the problem. The school health nurses have much more rigid criteria for certification, and in some states they are primarily nurse-teachers. The teaching function is broad and includes nutrition, dental hygiene, and human sexuality.

OTHER HEALTH PROFESSIONALS—SOCIAL WORKERS, PHARMACISTS, AND OTHER THERAPISTS.   The contributions of social workers to clinical settings, where large numbers of families in crisis are seen, is of great importance. The clinical setting may be in a large, inner-city, neighborhood health center; a rural health center; or a university clinic where aggregates of children with chronic illness are seen. The physically handicapped and mentally retarded particularly benefit from their services. In these latter areas, physicians often unconsciously harbor guilt feelings over their inability to cure or make better these unfortunate children, and withdraw to an area behind a wall of professionalism. Social workers in these settings function as advocates, primary care psychiatrists, supporters of the families, and problem solvers; they contribute to a broader view of the patient in his world than most physicians possess.

Especially in the teaching hospital, disciplines such as recreation therapy, occupational therapy, and physical therapy have earned an important place in the treatment teams.

NURSE PRACTITIONERS. Recently, steps have been taken to produce a new type of health practitioner, the pediatric Nurse Practitioner. They have been trained in academic health centers and community hospitals in cognitive and practical skills in pediatric history, physical examination, and diagnosis and treatment of minor illness. They are being increasingly accepted in public health clinics, neighborhood health centers, and private practice offices.

The emergence of *clinical pharmacology* as a recognized specialty has supplied the physician with a useful ally. The knowledge of drug action and interaction; the availability of the capability to measure drug levels for important therapeutic agents; the presence of an in-house expert on dosage, duration of action, packaging data, drug profiles, and histories makes the modern pharmacist an indispensable part of the health team. Again, this alliance is generally viable only in a clinic or teaching hospital setting.

References

SOCIAL CHANGES AFFECTING CHILD HEALTH.

Aldrich CA, Aldrich M: Babies are Human Beings. New York, Macmillan, 1938

Bell NW, Vogel EF (eds): A Modern Introduction to the Family. Toronto, Macmillan, 1960

Brazelton TB: Neonatal Behavioral Assessment Scale, Clinics in Developmental Medicine No. 50. London, Spastics International Medical Publications, 1973

Coles R: Children of Crisis. New York, Dell, 1967

Coles R: Children of Crisis: Migrants, Mountaineers, and Sharecroppers. Boston, Little, Brown, 1972

Coles R: Children of Crisis: South Goes North. Boston, Little, Brown 1973

Dingle JH, Badger GF, Jordan WS: Illness in the Home. Cleveland, Press of Western Reserve University, 1964

Eisenberg L: Caring for children and working: dilemmas of contemporary womanhood. Pediatrics 56:24, 1975

LeRiche WH, Milner J: Epidemiology as Medical Ecology. Baltimore, Williams & Wilkins, 1971

Mead M: Determinants of health beleifs and behavoir, III. Cultural determinants. Am J Public Health 51:1552, 1961

THE ROLE OF THE PHYSICIAN IN THE ASSESSMENT OF CHILDREN

Bergman A, Wedgwood RJ: Time-motion study of pediatrics practitioners. Pediatrics 38:254, 1966

Feinstein AR: Clinical judgment. Baltimore, Williams & Wilkins, 1967

Ford LC: Nurse practitioners. Pediatrics 54:533, 1974

Hoekelman R: What constitutes well-baby care? Pediatrics 55:313, 1975

Leopold EA: Whom do we reach? Astudy of health care utilization. Pediatrics 53:341, 1974

McAtee PA, Silver HK: Nurse practitioners for children - past and future. Pediatrics 54:578, 1974

Ott JE: New health professionals in pediatrics. Adv Pediatr 20:39, 1973

Tumulty PA: What is a clinician and what does he do? N Engl J Med 283:20, 1970

ETHICAL ASPECTS OF MANAGEMENT OF INFANTS WITH SEVERE HANDICAPS

JOHN M. FREEMAN

Modern medicine has developed much of the technology to preserve life, but medicine and society are only now beginning to philosophize about the circumstances in which life might not, or should not, be preserved. The development of this philosophy has highlighted ethical dilemmas facing physicians.

A cause for rise of ethical problems is the conflict generated between guiding principles. Two traditional aims of medicine have been the prevention of suffering and the preservation of life. It is the conflict between these two which has raised ethical dilemmas in the management of birth defects. If one is guided solely by the aim of preservation of life at all costs, there is no dilemma; the only decision demanded is which technology to employ. If one is guided solely by the utilitarian principle of prevention of suffering, there is no dilemma; the only decision becomes which suffering to prevent. It is when prevention of suffering may mean loss of life—or preservation of life may require increase in suffering—that ethical dilemmas arise.

The author would hold with the utilitarian principle and be guided primarily by consideration of the relief of suffering. Yet when the principle of the sanctity of life conflicts with relief of suffering, life must be given considerable weight.

If the physician is to concentrate on relief of suffering, he must decide how much suffering is acceptable, and to whom. Who has the right to decide if another's life is acceptable, or if he or she has too much suffering?

Voiced in other terms, it is said that the physician need not employ extraordinary means to preserve life. But this guideline creates the same ethical dilemmas, since the term extraordinary becomes defined by circumstances. The use of a respirator in an elderly person in the terminal stages of cancer may be extraordinary, but its use in a young person with severe pneumonia may be ordinary. The ethical dilemma becomes linked with how a physician defines his patient's situation. In a child with a birth defect, ordinary and extraordinary are also defined by the situation, and the situation is defined by the physician.

Thus ethics must focus less on what is done, or not done and more critically on how and by whom the decision is made to do or not to do. Ethics must focus on what stage of a person's life or suffering is acceptable, and which situations require extraordinary rather than ordinary treatment.

THE DECISION MAKING PROCESS

Most physicians agree that life need not be preserved "at all costs," and that for some patients treatment should consist of caring and relief of suffering rather than vigorous medical intervention. But the decision must be made on the basis of knowledge of the cause and the disease, and that knowledge must be based on correct facts coupled with due attention to the legal implications involved.

The debate over whether all children with meningomyelocele should be treated is an example of current decision-making conflicts. The debate pivots on the questions of which children should be treated and how that decision should be made.

John Lorber has proposed criteria for "selecting" children with spina bifida who should not receive surgical or medical intervention. He states that the child who meets his adverse criteria and thus should not be treated would have had a 60 percent chance of dying despite maximal therapy. If that child had survived, he would have had a 50 percent chance of being retarded, would be paraplegic, incontinent, and would often have a severe degree of kyphosis or scoliosis, deteriorating renal tracts, and fecal incontinence.

On the other hand, others have achieved different results. With similar cases Freeman and others have found an 80 percent chance of survival, and have reported that 80 percent of the survivors have a normal IQ; with kyphosis or scoliosis prevented, or treated; with incontinence managed by ileal loop or catheter; and rectal incontinence managed by regimen. Two-thirds of those children will be up in braces, and ambulatory.

If we are to "select" for surgury—and for life—on the basis of what the future will hold for the child, what set of facts are employed in this selection process? Would the outcome, as delineated by Dr. Lorber, be acceptable or unacceptable, (as he suggests)? If the outcome were to be as found in this country, would that *life* be acceptable—or would the child in question be better off dead?

We should also ask: "acceptable to whom?" Are physicians able to project themselves into the child's situation? Would that life be acceptable to the child? Would it be acceptable to the family? Many children and families adapt and adjust to handicaps which we would not elect for ourselves, and do so, very well. Is the question really one of "Must the life of this individual be acceptable to us?"

Similar reasoning may be applied in the case of the child born with other congenital defects, such as Downs' Syndrome and duodenal atresia. If that child is unwanted by his parents, and his future is to be both retarded from birth and institutionalized in the "classic" institutions for the retarded, would he be better off not treated? If, on the other hand, he could be placed in a loving foster home, or, better yet, be accepted and wanted by his family, and able to relate to life and people, extraordinary means should be employed to preserve his life? And by whom is this decision to be made? The physician? The family? Or both together? And what of society? Should it form a committee or make a policy with respect to same?

Who Makes the Decision

While we may be reaching the day when a competent person may be able to decide to accept or reject therapy, pediatricians are usually dealing with legal incompetents. The infant certainly cannot make these decisions which so profoundly affect his future existence and the quality of his life. Who is to make the decision for him?

The ideal person would know and understand all the facts, would be able to project into the child's future and understand the consequences of the condition for the child and the family, and the effects of the family and society on the child. He would have no prejudices or bias about the disease, and could make a decision which would be in the best interests of the child, the family, and society.

The family traditionally has been assumed to act in the child's best interest, and since it will be required to assume the social and financial burdens of the child, it has been given the major say in the decision. But can family members know and comprehend the consequences of a decision to treat a child with meningomyelocele? Can they comprehend what life will be like with a child who for years will be dependent, and who, despite maximal medical therapy, will always be 'less' than his peers? It is most important that much time be spent with the parents by the physician in attendence, the social worker, and, if possible, by other parents experienced in similar problems to educate them fully to the future. It is also important to realize that parents of a newborn infant with a major malformation or a life-threatening disease may temporarily be in an emotional state in which they are incapable of making a choice, which they in fact might make after they had the time to organize their thoughts and emotions. During this interim period the pediatrician will have to be the advocate for the child.

The physician must try to state the facts about procedures and outcome, and future problems for the child and the family with and without treatment or surgery. He should note that other physicians may have different interpretations of the same facts. He must also inform the family of his bias, for few of us can present the facts in a truly unbiased fashion. In discussing therapy and treatment, the physician must take into account the family's social situation and the community's ability to provide the supporting facilities: social, financial, schooling, and further medical care.

After such a discussion, it is said the family should make the decision. That may be acceptable in the case of a severely defective child, but what about the less affected one? If that child's family decides to have the child operated on, the child receives treatment. If, on the other hand, with equal knowledge, or lack thereof, the family decides not to have the child treated, what then? Some say that we as pediatricians should serve as the child's advocate—but what should we advocate? While we as physicians have greater knowledge of the given condition and its future, do we have greater comprehension of its consequences for the child or for the family? Would a committee or society as a whole have greater knowledge, or comprehension and thus be able to play a role in the decision-making process.

The ethics of decision making may be summarized

briefly: The ethical decision is that *which is best for the child and for the family*. The decision may include the alternative of providing only care and not medical intervention. It must weigh the alternatives between relief of suffering and the preservation of life. It must be based on knowledge of the disease in question and its outcome; of the suffering to be incurred by the child and his family; and what mechanisms may be available to relieve that suffering for both. The decision must recognize the consequences of nonintervention, and, in the case of the child with meningomyelocele, it must include the realization that the untreated child may survive for months or even years. With full comprehension of this information, and its presentation to the family in as unbiased a way as possible, the family and the physician must reason together to achieve the best solution for that individual child.

Bibliography

1. Anonymous: Ethics of selective treatment of spina bifida. Lancet 1: 85-88, 1975
2. Fletcher J: Abortion, euthanasia, and care of defective newborns. New Eng. J. Med. 292: 75-78, 1975
3. Rachels J: Active and passive euthanasia. New Eng. J. Med. 292, 78-80, 1975
4. Freeman JM: Is there a right to die—quickly—? J. Pediat. 80: 904-905, 1972
5. Lorber J: Spina bifida cystica. Archives. Dis. Childhood 47: 854-873, 1972
6. Freeman JM: To treat or not to treat: ethical dilemmas in the management of myelomeningocele. Clin. Neurosurg 20: 134-146, 1973
7. Shurtleff DB et al: Myelodysplasia: decision for death and disability. New Eng. J. Med. 291:1005-1011, 1974
8. Ames MD, Schut L: Results of treatment of 171 consecutive myelomeningoceles—1963-1968. Pediat 50: 466-470, 1972
9. Freeman JM (ed): Practical Management of Meningomyelocele. Univ. Park. Press, Baltimore, Md., 1974

CHAPTER 2

Assessment and Care of The Child

JOHN C. DOWER

THE PEDIATRIC INTERVIEW

Many physicians are convinced that the history of a complaint yields clues to successful diagnosis and management in up to 90 percent of encounters with adult patients. In a general pediatric practice, however, there are substantial differences in the encounter, which bear examination and analysis. The features in common with the history-taking encounter in adults is that the process is essentially one of gathering evidence; the process precedes the physical examination, and data are recorded according to a prescribed format. The important differences are that the history (except in the case of an adolescent patient) is related by an intermediary, the parent; that the identified patient, the child, is not always the real patient; and that the identified problem is often not the real problem. Another essential difference is that the traditional history-taking process and the traditional physical examination are blurred in the pediatric interview. Observation of the child and mother, or family, begins while they are in the waiting room, in passage to the examining room, and during the conduct of the interview. The relationship between the mother and child, their reaction to stress or separation, the developmental status of the child, the appearance of the child, the relationship between the parents, the state of dress and hygiene, the ethnic origin and social class, the appropriateness of discipline and expectations, the warmth of support, and a host of other observations are made prior to the first introduction. In subsequent paragraphs this will be treated more fully.

Communicating with Parents

While the explicit objective of the interview is to elicit information, there are important secondary functions which may have far-reaching implications. The initial encounter with the child and his family sets the tone for the ensuing doctor-patient relationship. The taking of the history should be viewed as the beginning of the management process. Although the focus of concern should be the child-patient, the interview should be family centered. Relationships with the parent(s) are essential. The wisest of pediatricians depends on them to carry out the most rudimentary instructions. Barriers to communication hamper compliance with physician advice.

Communication skills are necessary for this type of endeavor. A set of intellectual biases is a prerequisite to the acquisition of these skills. The prime prerequisite is the recognition of the importance of psychosocial factors in the communications between physicians and parents. Different people require different approaches and styles of interviewing. Since what transpires depends on the success of the communication, something special is demanded of the physician as well as the parent. Both must use words and concepts that are heard and clearly understood by the other. Nonverbal messages must be anticipated and received.

There are obvious barriers and obstacles to communication. There are very human limits to human memory. For physicians who work in clinic settings, the problem of poor communication because of language barriers is readily understood. Some measure of the personal nature of the communication process is gained by sensing how inadequate it is when a third party is interposed. Perhaps it is not so readily grasped that the language physicians use to communicate with each other is totally foreign to parents. The use of medical jargon invariably inhibits good communication and it is good for the soul to have the occasional parent remind a senior physician of this by saying. "Now would you explain that in English?"

A real barrier to good and effective communication occurs when the parent brings a sick child to be evaluated. Parents are invariably anxious and often guilty about whether their actions caused the illness. Remarks such as, "Everytime I let him out without a hat he gets an ear infection," or "If I had dressed her warmer this might not have happened," are typical examples of parental guilt. The physician can often feed this negative feeling by statements such as, "Why didn't you bring him sooner," or "You got her here in the nick of time." Because of experiences such as these parents often shade the truth in their desire to please the physician.

In her comprehensive studies of the communications process between physicians and parents, Korsch makes the crucial point that the first priority is to establish the scope and quality of the anticipated relationship with the patient and family. The nature of the encounter governs this to a certain degree. Is the visit for an acute illness, a consultative evaluation for a major problem, or a well-child supervision visit? The setting and the scheduling of the time allocated for the visit is governed by the anticipated problem. An encounter with an intact family presenting a healthy three month old infant requires a smaller time commitment and a different psychologic set than a conference for an acting-out adolescent from a recently divorced family.

Regardless of the setting for the visit, some amenities should be followed. Korsch's studies of young resident pediatricians in the process of interacting with families revealed that many physicians never introduced themselves. The physician's opening remark frequently put the family on the defense and curtailed straightforward communication. Most families respond positively to a physician who is warm, friendly, and concerned about their child and their fears and anxieties.

Giving families an opportunity to explore their concerns is essential to good communication. This can often be accomplished early in the interview, but in certain circumstances, such as when a mother is extremely anxious, it can be postponed to later in the encounter. At that time she has had an opportunity to see the physician demonstrate his concern, warmth, and skill during the examination of the child and will be more at ease and less guarded about her inner fears. At any rate, the physician's opening gambit frequently sets the style for the remainder of the interview. A non-threatening statement delivered in a warm friendly manner often breaks the ice. One example is, "Good morning Mrs. Jones, I'm Dr. Smith. I'll be examining Peter today. I wonder if you could tell me something about him and why you brought him today?" After she tells the story, the physician can move directly to explore her concerns by asking, "What worried you most about him?" followed by, "Why did that worry you?" The most seasoned physicians continue to be amazed by the responses that follow on the heels of these questions, eg, a simple upper respiratory infection is feared to be tuberculosis because that is the manner in which Grandma started out her disease.

After a patient exploration of her concerns, the physician can then move on to her expectations of the visit. A simple, "What had you hoped we could do for him today?" frequently allows the mother to reveal her real agenda. At this juncture, it is often helpful to ask if she has further questions before proceeding. This strategy of allowing the mother to move swiftly to her concerns is frequently productive and allows the mother to cooperate with the more structured part of the interview, relieved of the anxiety that the doctor will not give her a chance to express her concerns.

During the interview, time should be spent in exploring the emotional and social consequences of the illness and the reaction of the family to the illness. It would be important to know that the mother had quit her job because of the child's illness and that the family was experiencing great financial hardship as a consequence. The hostility that the family is displaying toward the physician and the overprotective attitude on the part of the mother might be better understood in the light of this information. Critical events in the family, such as the death or serious illness of a grandparent, are frequently occasions when a family decompensates and seeks medical advice for a problem they had previously regarded as trivial. This information can be elicited during the review of family structure and living arrangements.

The physician is most effective when a supportive and nonjudgmental attitude is maintained. Exclamations of dismay or disbelief are counterproductive and turn parents off immediately. Expressions such as, "You did what?" or "You took her to a chiropractor?" can reduce a trusting, communicating mother to a pillar of salt capable only of monosyllabic responses for the rest of the interview. A gentle, supportive statement such as, "Massage is frequently helpful for sore muscles. You were wise to do that," can often ease the guilt of a distraught mother who has lost confidence in her ability to parent.

The quality of empathy is a rare natural endowment, and most physicians must work hard to achieve it. Empathy is the ability to place yourself in the other person's position and to experience their reactions as they would. It is not to be confused with its judgmental bedfellows, pity and sympathy. Physicians find such empathetic expressions as, "You can't have had much sleep last night," or, "That must have been frightening to you," extremely supportive when applied at appropriate times. Expressions such as these assure mothers of the human qualities of the physician and transform them to a more willing partner in the ensuing therapeutic adventure.

There is occasional danger in overidentifying with patients and their families. This is particularly true when psychologic and emotional issues of a profound nature are involved. The effective physician always strives to maintain objectivity in dealing with issues of this kind. It is possible to communicate a kind, nonjudgmental, interested attitude without taking sides in family quarrels. Particular care must be taken when parents are angry or displeased with a previous physician or health professional. The responsible course is to ask the family for permission to communicate with the person and to personally telephone for the results of previous studies. There are invariably two sides to the story, and the cooperation of the previous caretaker frequently uncovers valuable data not elicited in the initial history.

In an ideal world, physicians would be kind and omniscient, and patients and families would be intelligent, cooperative, and compliant. In the real world, it is not infrequent for the physician to not like the family on the initial encounter. The physician must be aware of his own set of prejudices and vulnerabilities, and guard against projecting them on families who present as hostile, critical, and demanding. Experience reveals that these qualities are often reactions to fears and anxieties. The physician who can absorb the heat without reflecting it back in the form of covert or overt response is frequently rewarded by observing the relationship take a more constructive turn as the fears and anxieties are slowly dissipated. The true measure of the skill of a physician is to turn the hostile encounter into a relationship of mutual trust and understanding.

A common error is to regard the history-taking process as complete with the termination of the initial interview. In actuality, it is a continuous, dynamic process wherein data are accumulated beginning with the first interview and continuing throughout the physician-patient relationship. History-taking includes what is specifically communicated and what is learned by observation in office or home visits. Indeed, the tragedy of the demise of the house call is that it deprives the physician of seeing how individual families actually function.

Often pediatricians care for children without having the opportunity of meeting their fathers or assessing what sort of relationship the father and mother really have.

Senn and Solnit have defined the objectives of the pediatrician in serving patients as: to enhance normal development, to prevent mental and physical disorders, and to restore the physical and emotional health of the patient. They have adopted a utilitarian synthesis of traditional and problem-oriented approaches in phrasing the tasks of evaluation and management in the following manner:

Correct identification of the patient and the problem (to take a history).
Thorough collection of the evidence (to continue the history and perform examinations).
Accurate assessment of the data (to differentiate, diagnose, and predict).
Solution of the problem (to plan and participate in care and management).

In the preceding paragraphs we have examined the most effective manner in which to communicate with mothers. All evidence points to the observation that mothers relate best to warm, friendly physicians who generate empathy by specifically dealing with their concerns and expectations.

Communicating with Children

The age of the child-patient determines the amount and the level of verbal communication. For the infant and young child, the mother is usually the dominant informant. However, it must not be overlooked that important nonverbal communication takes place between the pediatrician and the child beyond early infancy during the interview. To the 6-month-old on his mother's knee, the pediatrician might be a source of fun and entertainment with his rattle, fuzzy toy, and bell, while to the 10-month-old he might be a strange threat with a new face and deep voice. The toddler and preschool child warily eyes the interloper and makes value judgments based on how he perceives his parents' reaction to the stranger and on his own experience with adults. Even at this age, valuable information can be gained by direct conversation with the child. It is well worth the investment in time to engage in simple play, utilizing the toys in the developmental kit, the physicians instruments. (The stethoscope becomes a telephone, the percussion hammer a hammer, and the otoscope is transformed from an instrument of torture to a magic light.) In addition to supplying the opportunity to observe the child at play, handling the instruments defuses the situation for the imminent examination.

Older school children should be given the chance to tell the physician why they have come to him. They are usually ignorant of what will transpire and invariably anxious and apprehensive. Parents frequently bring children to the doctor under false pretenses. It is the physician's duty to be forthright and honest with the child and to emphasize that his role is to help. The child's age, maturity, cooperation, and level of intelligence are all factors in how the doctor proceeds. In some instances his approach can be direct, in others quite indirect. Patience, flexibility, and sensitivity are all necessary ingredients for successful communication.

The adolescent patient requires special consideration. Whether the patient comes to the physician alone or with a parent, he or she (and the parent) should be informed that the patient will have an opportunity to speak with the physician alone and that absolute confidentiality will be honored. In discussion of problems with the adolescent it is particularly important to maintain a nonjudgmental and supportive attitude. A common error is to push too vigorously for an early and immediate solution to the adolescent's problem. It is not uncommon to have the young patient reveal more than he wished to on the initial interview and then be panicked by his revelations. The wise physician can sense this and hold up the outflow of material at a judicious juncture of the interview. A followup appointment can be made for the same week to reassess the problem and reexplore the wisdom of pursuing loaded material full tilt. Usually the adolescent will adopt a holding pattern for days, weeks, or months, but if trust is established, they usually return for another look at their problem.

Age-specific Variables in the History and Physical Examination

Human development can be viewed as a sequence of discrete stages, each with its own unique attributes, catalyzed into manifest form by a delicate interaction of biologic maturation and experience. We choose to define stages in this continuum and to describe special sets of defining characteristics to each category, with full recognition that they are arbitrary and not always rooted in firm biologic bases. Nevertheless, they prove to be a useful way to observe phenomena. In this section the contacts the pediatrician has with the family will be viewed within the context of the ascending stages of development. The specific tasks of the child, the mother, and the family at these stages will be reviewed; the acceptable behavioral characteristics will be noted; and evidence of minimal and extreme psychopathology will be catalogued (Table 1). In addition, the major issues of health supervision and developmental assessment will be considered for each major stage (Table 2).

THE PRENATAL VISIT

Pregnancy is the first period in the life of the mother and child when a pediatrician may be helpful. It is the usual practice of many pediatricians to meet the parents expecting a baby once or twice before a delivery. The prospective parents get to know the pediatrician and have an opportunity to ask questions about the developing fetus, the physiology of the newborn, the advantages of breastfeeding, and the care of the infant. It gives the pediatrician the opportunity to assess the parents as people and to gain some insight into their personalities, anxieties, expectations, and fears.

TABLE 1. Behavior Characteristics and Psychopathology in Parent–Child Relationships

Tasks in Process	Acceptable Behavior Characteristics	Minimal Psychopathology	Extreme Psychopathology
Newborn and Young Infant (Birth to 6 Months)			
Infant			
To adjust physiologically to extrauterine life To develop appropriate psychologic response To assimilate experientially, with increasing capacity to postpone and accept substitutes	Copes with mechanics of life (eating, sleeping, etc) Body needs urgent Reflexes dominate Establishes symbiotic relationship to mother Sucking behavior predominant Cries when distressed Responds to mouth, skin, sense modalities Functions egocentrically Is completely dependent Low patience tolerance Needs expressed instinctively Develops trust in adult	Feeding and digestive problems Sleep disturbances Excessive sucking activity Excessive motor discharge Excessive crying Excessive irritability Difficult to comfort	Lethargy (depression) Marasmus Cannot be comforted Unresponsive Infantile autism Developmental arrest
Mother			
To sustain baby and self physically and pleasurably To give and get emotional gratification from nurturing To foster and integrate baby's development	Provides feeding and fondling Gets to know baby Has tolerance for baby Promotes sense of trust Learns baby's cues Interacts emotionally with baby Encourages baby's development Has reasonable expectations of baby Develops good working relationship with baby	Indifference to baby Ambivalence toward baby and its needs Self-doubt and anxiety Intolerance of baby's characteristics Overresponds or underresponds to baby Premature or inappropriate expectations Dissatisfaction with role of motherhood	Alienation from baby Severe depression Excessive guilt Complete inability to function in maternal role Overwhelming and incapacitating anxiety Denies or tries to control baby's needs Severe clashes with baby Vents dissatisfactions on baby
Older Infant (6 to 18 Months)			
Infant			
To develop more reliance and self control To differentiate self from mother To make developmental progress	More stable physiologically Increased voluntary motor activity and exploration Higher level of patience tolerance Instinctual needs in better control Strong selective tie to mother Stranger differentiation Increased play, verbalizing, and sensorimotor behavior Discernible social responses Outbursts of negativism and anger Sensory modalities important Emergence of idiosyncratic patterns Demonstrates memory and anticipation Begins to imitate	Excessive crying, anger, and irritability Low frustration tolerance Excessive negativism Finicky eater, sleep disturbances Digestive and elimination problems Distinctive motility patterns (rocking, etc) Delayed development	Frequent tantrums Apathy, immobility, withdrawal Extreme, obsessive finger-sucking, rocking, head-banging No interest in objects, play, or environment Anorexia Psychogenic megacolon Inexpressive of feelings No social discrimination No tie to mother; wary of all adults Infantile autism Failure to thrive Arrested development
Mother			
To provide a healthy physical and emotional climate To foster weaning, training, habits To understand, appreciate, and accept baby	Satisfaction from serving baby Responds appropriately to baby's signs of distress Aware of baby's inborn reaction pattern Has more confidence in own ability	Disappointed in and unaccepting of baby Misses baby's cues Infancy unappealing Impersonal management Attempts to coerce to desired behavior	Neglect or abuse of baby Rejection of the maternal role Severe hostility reactions No attempt to understand or gratify baby Deliberately thwarts baby

TABLE 1. Behavior Characteristics and Psychopathology in Parent–Child Relationships (cont.)

Tasks in Process	Acceptable Behavior Characteristics	Minimal Psychopathology	Extreme Psychopathology
	Gives positive psychologic reassurances (fondling, talking) Shows pleasure in baby Keeps pace with baby's advances Accepts baby's idiosyncrasies	Overanxious or overprotective Mildly depressed or apathetic	Complete withdrawal and separation from baby

Toddler and Preschool Age (Under 5 Years)
Child

Tasks in Process	Acceptable Behavior Characteristics	Minimal Psychopathology	Extreme Psychopathology
To reach physiologic plateaus (motor action, toilet training) To differentiate self and secure sense of autonomy To tolerate separations from mother To develop conceptual frames and ethical values To master instinctual psychologic impulses (oedipal, sexual, guilt) To assimilate and handle socialization and acculturation (aggression relationships, feelings) To learn sex distinctions	Gratification from exercise of neuromotor skills Investigative, imitative, imaginative play Actions somewhat modified by thought Memory good; original thinking Exercises autonomy with body (sphincter control; eating) Dependence on mother and separation fears Behavior identification with parents, siblings, peers Learns speech for communication Awareness of own motives, beginnings of concience Intense feelings of shame, guilt, joy, desire to please Standards of good and bad Sex curiosity and differentiation Dependence, independence, ambivalence Questions birth and death	Poor motor coordination Persistent speech problems Timidity toward people and experiences Fears and night terrors Problems with eating, sleeping, elimination, toileting, weaning Irritability, crying, temper tantrums Partial return to infantile manners Inability to leave mother without panic Fear of strangers Breath-holding spells Lack of interest in other children	Extreme lethargy, passivity, or hypermotility Little or no speech; noncommunicative No response or relationship to people; symbiotic clinging to mother Somatic ills; vomiting, constipation, diarrhea, tics Autism; childhood psychosis Excessive enuresis, fecal soiling, fears Completely infantile behavior Play inhibited or nonconceptualized; absence or excess of autoerotic behavior Obsessive-compulsive behavior, ritual mannerisms Impulsive destructive behavior

Mother

Tasks in Process	Acceptable Behavior Characteristics	Minimal Psychopathology	Extreme Psychopathology
To promote training, habits To aid family and group socialization of child To encourage speech and other learning To reinforce child's sense of autonomy and identity To set a model for ethical conduct To delineate male and female roles	Moderate and flexible in training Shows pleasure and praise for childs advances Encourages and participates with child's ability to play Sets reasonable standards and controls Paces herself to child's capacity Consistent in own behavior, conduct, and ethics Provides emotional reassurance to child Promotes peer play and guided group activity Reinforces child's cognition of male and female roles	Premature, coercive, or censoring training Exacting standards above child's ability to conform Transmits anxiety and tension Unaccepting of child's efforts, intolerant toward failure Overreacts, overprotective, overanxious Despondent, apathetic	Severely coercive, punitive Totally critical and rejecting Overidentification with or overly submissive to child Severe repression of child's need for gratification Deprivation of all stimulations, freedoms, and pleasures Extreme anger and displeasure with child Child assault and abuse Severe depression and withdrawal

School Age and Preadolescence (5 to 12 Years)
Child

Tasks in Process	Acceptable Behavior Characteristics	Minimal Psychopathology	Extreme Psychopathology
To master greater physical prowess To further establish self-identity and sex role To work toward greater independence from parents	General good health, greater body competence, acute sensory perception Pride and self-confidence; less dependence on parents Better impulse control	Anxiety and oversensitivity to new experiences (school, relationships, separation) Lack of attentiveness, learning difficulties, disinterest in learning	Extreme withdrawal, apathy, depression, grief, self-destructive tendencies Complete failure to learn. Speech difficulty, especially stuttering

TABLE 1. Behavior Characteristics and Psychopathology in Parent-Child Relationships (cont.)

Tasks in Process	Acceptable Behavior Characteristics	Minimal Psychopathology	Extreme Psychopathology
To become aware of world at large To develop peer and other relationships To acquire learning, new skills, and a sense of industry	Ambivalence re dependency, separation, and new experiences Accepts own sex role; psychosexual expression in play and fantasy Equates parents with peers and other adults Aware of natural world (life, death, birth, science); subjective but realistic world Competitive but well organized in play; enjoys peer interaction Regard for collective obedience to social laws, rules, and fair play Explores environment; school and neighborhood basic to social learning experience Cognition advancing; intuitive thinking advancing to concrete operational level; responds to teaching Speech becomes reasoning and expressive tool; thinking still egocentric	Acting-out: lying, stealing, temper outbursts; inappropriate social behavior Regressive behavior (wetting soiling, crying, fears) Appearance of compulsive mannerisms (ties, rituals) Somatic illness: eating and sleeping problems, aches, pains, digestive upsets Fear of illness and body injury Difficulties and rivalry with peers, siblings, adults; constant fighting Destructive tendencies strong; temper tantrums Inability or unwillingness to do things for self Moodiness and withdrawal; few friends or personal relationships	Extreme and uncontrollable antisocial behavior (aggression, destruction, chronic lying, stealing, intentional cruelty to animals) Severe obsessive-compulsive behavior (phobias, fantasies, rituals) Inability to distinguish reality from fantasy Excessive sexual exhibitionism, eroticism, sexual assaults on others Extreme somatic illness: failure to thrive, anorexia, obesity, hypocondriasis, abnormal menses Complete absence or deterioration of personal and peer relationships

Parents

Tasks in Process	Acceptable Behavior Characteristics	Minimal Psychopathology	Extreme Psychopathology
To help child's emancipation from parents To reinforce self-identification and independence To provide positive pattern of social and sex role behavior To acclimatize child to world at large To facilitate learning, reasoning, communication and experiencing To promote wholesome moral and ethical values	Ambivalent toward child's separation but encourage independence Mixed feelings about parent-surrogates, but help child to accept them Encourage child to participate outside of home Set appropriate model of social and ethical behavior and standards Take pleasure in child's developing skills and abilities Understand and cope with child's behavior Find other gratifications in life (activity, employment) Supportive toward child as required	Disinclination to separate from child; or prematurely hastening separation Signs of despondency, apathy, hostility Foster fears, dependence, apprehension Disinterested in or rejecting of child Overly critical and censuring; undermine child's confidence Inconsistent in discipline or control; erratic in behavior Offer a restrictive, overly moralistic model	Extreme depression and withdrawal; rejection of child Intense hostility; aggression toward child Uncontrollable fears, anxieties, guilts Complete inability to function in family role Severe moralistic prohibition of child's independent strivings

Puberty and Early Adolescence (12 to 15 Years)
Child

Tasks in Process	Acceptable Behavior Characteristics	Minimal Psychopathology	Extreme Psychopathology
To come to terms with body changes To cope with sexual development and psychosexual drives To establish and confirm sense of identity To learn further re sex role To synthesize personality To struggle for independence and emancipation from family	Heightened physical power, strength, and coordination Occasional psychosomatic and somatopsythic disturbances Maturing sex characteristics and proclivities Review and resolution of oedipal conflicts Inconsistent, unpredictable, and paradoxical behavior	Apprehensions, fears, guilt, and anxiety re sex, health, education Defiant, negative, impulsive, or depressed behavior Frequent somatic or hypochondriacal complaints, or denial of ordinary illnesses Learning irregular or deficient Sexual preoccupation Poor or absent personal relationships with adults or peers	Complete withdrawal into self, extreme depression Acts of delinquency, asceticism, ritualism, overconformity Neuroses, especially phobias; persistent anxiety, compulsions, inhibitions, or constrictive behavior Persistent hypochondriases Sex aberrations Somatic illness: anorexia, colitis, menstrual disorders

TABLE 1. Behavior Characteristics and Psychopathology in Parent-Child Relationships (cont.)

Tasks in Process	Acceptable Behavior Characteristics	Minimal Psychopathology	Extreme Psychopathology
To incorporate learning to the gestalt of living	Exploration and experimentation with self and world Eagerness for peer approval and relationships Strong moral and ethical perceptions Cognitive development accelerated; deductive and inductive reasoning; operational thought Competitive in play; erratic work-play patterns Better use of language and other symbolic material Critical of self and others; self-evaluative Highly ambivalent toward parents Anxiety over loss of parental nurturing Hostility to parents Verbal aggression	Immaturity or precocious behavior; unchanging personality and temperament Unwillingness to assume responsibility of greater autonomy Inability to substitute or postpone gratifications	Complete inability to socialize or work (learning, etc) Psychoses
Parents			
To help child complete emancipation To provide support and understanding To limit child's behavior and set standards To offer favorable and appropriate environment for healthy development To recall own adolescent difficulties; to accept and respect the adolescent's differences or similarities to parents or others To relate to adolescents and adolescence with a constructive sense of humor	Allow and encourage reasonable independence Set fair rules; be consistent Compassionate and understanding; firm but not punitive or derogatory Feel pleasure and pride, occasional guilt and disappointment Have other interests besides child Marital life fulfilled apart from child Occasional expression of intolerance, resentment, envy, or anxiety about adolescent's development	Sense of failure Disappointment greater than joy Indifference to child and family Apathy and depression Persistent intolerance of child Limited interests and self-expression Loss of perspective about childs capacities Occasional direct or vicarious reversion to adolescent impulses Uncertainty about standards regarding sexual behavior and deviant social or personal activity	Severe depression and withdrawal Complete rejection of child and/or family Inability to function in family role Rivalrous, competitive, destructive, and abusive to child Abetting child's acting-out of unacceptable sexual or aggressive impulses for vacarious reasons Perpetuation of incapacitating infantilism in the preadolescent Panic reactions to acceptable standards of sexual behavior, social activity, and assertiveness Compulsive, obsessive, or psychotic behavior

TABLE 2. Suggested Schedule for Preventive Child Health Care[*]

Age	History[†]	Measurements[‡]	Physical Exam	Developmental Landmarks[†§]	Discussion and Guidance[§]	Procedures[‡]	Attending
1 mo	Initial Eating Sleeping Elimination Crying At every visit mother should be asked for questions	Height Weight Head circumference Temperature Evaluation of hearing	Complete[#]	Eyes follow to midline Baby regards face *While prone, lifts head off table*[¶]	Vitamins Sneezing Hiccoughs Straining with bowel movements Irregular respiration Startle reflex Ease and force of urination Night bottle Colic "Spoiling" Accidents	PKU Urinalysis	M.D. and assistant

TABLE 2. Suggested Schedule for Preventive Child Health Care* (cont.)

Age	History†	Measurements‡	Physical Exam	Developmental Landmarks†§	Discussion and Guidance§	Procedures‡	Attending
2 mo	Health Sensori-motor development Eating Sleeping Elimination Happiness	Height Weight Head circumference Temperature	Complete or observation"	*Vocalizes* *Smiles responsively*	Solid foods Immunizations Thumb-sucking	DPT TOPV Urine screening	M.D. and/or assistant
3 mo	Health Eating Sleeping Elimination Crying Other behavior	Height Weight Head circumference Temperature	Complete or observation"	Holds head and chest up to make 90° angle with table Laughs	Feeding Accidents Sleeping without rocking, holding, etc Coping with frustrations		M.D. and/or assistant
4 mo	Health Eating Sleeping Elimination Other behavior Sensorimotor development Current living situation Parent–child interaction	Height Weight Head circumference Temperature	Complete#	Holds head erect and steady when held in sitting position *Squeals* Grasps rattle Eyes follow object for 180°	Feeding Schedule to fit in with family Attitude of father Respiratory infections	DPT TOPV	M.D. and assistant
5 mo	Health Eating Sleeping Elimination Sensorimotor development	Height Weight Temperature	Complete or observation"	*Smiles spontaneously* *Rolls from back to stomach or vice versa* Reaches for object on table	Feeding Vitamins (if not previously mentioned)		MD. and/or assistant
6 mo	Health Eating Sleeping Elimination Other behavior Sensorimotor development	Height Weight Head circumference Temperature Evaluation of hearing	Complete or observation"	No head lag if baby is pulled to sitting position by hands	Feeding Accidents Night crying Fear of strangers Separation anxiety Description of normal micturition	DPT TOPV	M.D. and/or assistant
8 mo to 9 mo	Health Eating Sleeping Elimination Sensorimotor development Behavior	Height Weight Temperature	Complete or screening#	Sits alone for 5 sec after support is released Bears weight momentarily if held with feet on table Looks after fallen object Transfers block from one hand to the other *Feeds self cracker*	Use of cup Eating with fingers Fear of strangers Accidents Need for affection Normal unpleasant behavior Discipline		M.D. and/or assistant

TABLE 2. Suggested Schedule for Preventive Child Health Care* (cont.)

Age	History†	Measurements‡	Physical Exam	Developmental Landmarks†§	Discussion and Guidance§	Procedures‡	Attending
10 mo if last exam at 8 mo	Health Eating Sleeping Elimination Behavior Sensori-motor development Speech development Current living situation Parent–child interaction	Height Weight Temperature	Complete or observa-tion"	*Pulls self to standing po-sition* *Stands holding on to solid object (not human)* Pincer grasp—picks up small object using any part of thumb and fingers in opposition *Says Da-Da or Ma-Ma* Resists toy being pulled away from him *Plays peek-a-boo* Makes attempt to get toy just out of reach *Initial anxiety toward strangers*	Toilet training—when to start Normal drop in appetite Independence vs depen-dency Discipline Instructions for use of syrup of ipecac	Hgb or Hct	M.D. and/or assistant
12 mo	As for 10 mo	Height Weight Head circumference Temperature	Complete #	*Cruises—walks around hold-ing on to furniture* *Stands alone 2–3 sec if outside support is removed* *Bangs together two blocks held one in each hand* *Imitates vocal-ization heard within preced-ing minute* *Plays pat-a-cake*	Negativism Likelihood of respiratory infections "Getting into things" Weaning from bottle Proper dose of vitamins Control of drugs and poisons	Tuberculin test (intra-dermal pre-ferred) Measles Rubella and mumps may be given at this or subsequent visit Urinalysis	M.D. and assistant
15 mo	As for 10 mo	Height Weight Temperature	Complete or observa-tion"	*Walks well* Stoops to recover toys on floor Uses Da-Da and Ma-Ma specifically for correct parent Rolls or tosses ball back to examiner *Indicates wants by pulling, pointing, or appropriate verbalization (not crying)* *Drinks from cup without spil-ling much*	Temper tantrums Obedience		M.D. and/or assistant

TABLE 2. Suggested Schedule for Preventive Child Health Care[*] (cont.)

Age	History[†]	Measurements[‡]	Physical Exam	Developmental Landmarks[†§]	Discussion and Guidance[§]	Procedures[‡]	Attending
18 mo	As for 10 mo	Height Weight Temperature	Complete[#]	Puts one block on another without its falling off *Mimics household chores like dusting or sweeping*	Reaction toward and of siblings Toilet training Speech development	DTP TOPV	M.D. and assistant
21 mo	As for 10 mo Peer reaction	Height Weight Temperature	Complete or observation"	Walks backward and upstairs Feeds self with spoon *Removes article of clothing other than hat* *Says 3 specific words besides Da-Da and Ma-Ma*	Manners "Poor appetite"		M.D. and/or assistant
2 yr	Health Eating Sleeping Elimination Toilet training Sensorimotor development Speech Current living situation Peer and social adjustment	Height Weight Temperature Hearing	Complete[#]	Kicks a ball in front of him with foot without support *Scribbles spontaneously—purposeful marking of more than one stroke on paper* Balances 4 blocks on top of one another *Points correctly to one body part* Dumps small objects out of bottle after demonstration *Does simple tasks in house*	Need for peer companionship Immaturity—inability to share or take turns Care of teeth From this point on, guidance may be indicated by the mother's answers to a questionnaire about behavior and emotional problems	Hgb and/or Hct Urinalysis	M.D. and assistant
2½ yr	As for 2 yr	Height Weight Temperature	Complete[#]	*Throws overhand after demonstration* Names correctly one picture in book, eg, cat or apple Combines 2 words meaningfully	Guidance from questionnaire answers Dental referral Perversity and decisiveness		M.D. and/or assistant
3 yr	As for 2 yr	As for 2 yr Blood pressure	Complete[#]	Jumps in place *Pedals tricycle* Dumps small article out of bottle without demonstration	Guidance from questionnaire answers Sex education	As for 2 yr	M.D. and assistant

TABLE 2. Suggested Schedule for Preventive Child Health Care* (cont.)

Age	History†	Measurements‡	Physical Exam	Developmental Landmarks†§	Discussion and Guidance§	Procedures‡	Attending
				Uses plurals *Washes and dries hands*	Nursery schools— qualifications of a good one Obedience and discipline		
4 yr	As for 2 yr	As for 2 yr Vision ("E" chart) Blood pressure	Complete# Fundus exam	Builds bridge of 3 blocks after demonstration Copies circle and cross *Identifies longer of two lines* Knows first and last names Understands what to do when "tired" *Plays with other children so they interact—tag* *Dresses with supervision*	Guidance from questionnaire answers Kindergarten Use of money Dental care	As for 2 yr	M.D. and assistant
5 yr	As for 2 yr (omit toilet training) Kindergarten	As for 2 yr Vision ("E" chart) Color blindness Audiometer Blood pressure	Complete#	Hops 2 or more times Catches ball thrown 3 ft Dresses without supervision *Can tolerate separation from mother for a few minutes without anxiety*	Guidance from questionnaire answers Readiness for school Span of attention—how to increase it	As for 2 yr TOPV DTP	M.D. and assistant
6 yr	As for 2 yr Peer and adjustment	As for 5 yr (omit color blindness)	Complete#	Bicycle riding Copy a square Draw a man with 6 parts Define 6 simple words, eg, ball, lake, house Name materials of which things are made, eg, spoon, door	Guidance from questionnaire answers School readiness or performance Allowance	As for 2 yr	M.D. and assistant

From 6 years on, annual examinations follow approximately the same pattern. Developmental landmarks are judged by school performance, assumption of responsibilities, and physical maturation. Guidance is more complicated and is summarized below. Immunization includes maintenance of immunity to diphtheria and tetanus. If community situations preclude examination by a physician yearly, it should be accomplished at least every 2 years.

Items to be considered for guidance and discussion after 6 years are:

Posture and prediction of future height, where of concern.
Safety.
Responsibility for household tasks—giving choice and changing often.
Responsibility for money—how to teach.
Independence versus close supervision in out-of-school activities.
Obedience.
Discipline.
Need for praise.
Summer activities—age for going to camp; hometown programs.

Swimming—learn to do it capably.
Responsibility for homework without prodding.
Responsibility for getting to school on time.
Hours of sleep.
TV versus activities requiring child participation.
Sex education—elementary knowledge. Dating and supervision.
Increasing independence during youth.
Competitive athletics—when? Desirability during youth.
Planning for future careers.

*Adapted from Standards of Child Health Care, 2nd ed. American Academy of Pediatrics.
† May be accomplished in part by assistant if physician desires. Much of this may be accomplished in part by appropriate pamphlets or leaflets where deemed desirable.

‡ *Usually accomplished by assistant.*
§ *Age given for landmarks indicates approximate age at which 90% of children have accomplished test. Adapted from Denver Developmental Screening Test. Text should be consulted for details of tests where they are unfamiliar to examiner.*
¶ *Italicized items indicate report of parent may be accepted as proof of accomplishment. May be obtained by an assistant.*
" *Observation of child, completely undressed, by assistant trained to observe respiration, skin, musculature, motor activities, and so forth.*
Obvious deviations from normal must be checked by physician.

This anticipatory guidance is most useful after the seventh month of pregnancy. This is a unique period for a woman—she starts thinking of the fetus as a person, has fantasies about the baby and anxieties about her own performance as a mother. She may have fears about the outcome of the pregnancy, the worst being that the infant will be stillborn or malformed.

During the visit with the pediatrician, the parents-to-be should be encouraged to air their anxieties. The pediatrician should determine whether the pregnancy was planned, what the feelings of the parents were when the pregnancy was first known to them, and how the pregnancy has progressed. Discussion of breastfeeding is useful at this time. For mothers who wish to breast feed, encouragement should be offered. For those not wishing to pursue this mode of nutrition reassurance of the adequacy of artificial feeding should be provided and implanting the seeds of guilt should be avoided.

Mild anxiety is common during pregnancy. The cost of the labor, delivery, and obstetric fees; the fears of being an inadequate mother; the realization that the first baby will alter profoundly the husband-wife relationship, all contribute to this anxiety. Mild depression is not uncommon 3 to 4 days after birth, and the day that mother and infant go home is particularly trying. These feelings are usually transient, and most women adjust well to life at home, particularly if they have some temporary help.

The sensitive pediatrician should be alert to the possiblity of a severe postpartum depression. Some hints in the past history of the mother may exist. A history of a previous depression; a particularly troublesome or complicated pregnancy; a dissolving or unhappy marriage; unexpectedly difficult delivery; or the delivery of the infant on the anniversary of a particularly unhappy period in the life of the mother are all clues to impending problems. A pediatrician who takes the time to sit down with the mother during the first few days after birth, particularly when she has her baby with her, will be rewarded with some valuable insights. Klaus and his colleagues have made important observations on the importance of the first days of life in the relationship between mothers and their infants. This vital period of imprinting is essential to both mother and child. The pediatrician should do all in his power to encourage prolonged contacts of the mother and her infant during this period. Skilled nurses on the postpartum service are valuable observers on how the relationship is progressing and should be consulted.

THE NEWBORN AND YOUNG INFANT

Many pediatricians find that the initial examination of the newborn infant can profitably be done in the presence of the mother and father. The details of the examination often escape the parents, but the pronouncement at the end of the examination that all is well is received with unbounded joy. The details of the newborn examination are covered elsewhere (p. 141). As the pediatrician conducts the examination he may cover specific features that frequently are of concern to parents. The skin is the area first examined closely by the mother and she is invariably upset by the flat red discolorations frequently noted over the eyelids, the bridge of the nose, the nape of the neck, and just below the nose. Parents can be reassured that these *nevi flammeus* will disappear in a matter of months. In black infants a darkly pigmented nevus is frequently present over the sacral and buttocks area and occasionally on the distal extremity as an isolated spot. The so-called *mongolian spot* also fades and disappears during the first year of life. So called flea-bite dermatitis or *erythema toxicum* may appear in the second day of life. It is of brief duration and requires reassurance only.

The appearance of the head and face is often a cause of concern. The soft *caput succedeum,* which represents the presenting part, is fortunately a temporary cause of concern that disappears by absorption in a matter of days. The *cephalhematoma* of the scalp undergoes a process of remodeling over weeks or months, and in the process of recalcification presents an uneven, irregular bony edge. The process of bone remodeling usually results in an acceptable cosmetic result. The anterior fontanelle or *soft spot* is given a wide berth by many mothers. Explanation that it is safe to wash the overlying skin with vigor is all that is required. The scalp may have single or multiple small lacerations resulting from sampling of fetal blood or the attachment of fetal monitoring devices. These heal rapidly without complication. Not infrequently the face and nose is assymetrical because of fetal positioning or face presentation. This is a cause of great parental alarm, but reassurance that all will be well in a matter of days to weeks is well founded. The same may be said for forceps marks along the lateral face and the unilateral facial nerve paresis accompanying them. Infants of prolonged gestational age may show yellow staining of the nails and dry, cracked, peeling skin. This is also a short-lived problem.

The eyes are an area of concern for parents. Not infrequently a chemical conjunctivitis from the silver nitrate prophylaxis is noted. The duration of this problem is usually less than a week and requires only cleaning with a moist cotton ball. Because of the prevalence of gonorrhea and the severe consequences of untreated gonococcal ophthalmitis mothers should be warned that prolonged or purulent conjunctivitis is a reason for the infant to be rechecked prior to the first appointment. Most of these infections prove to be due to *Chlamydia* organisms which, like the gonococcus, are acquired in the vaginal canal. The prognosis for this infection is good. A unilateral or bilateral conjunctival hemorrhage is invariably noted by the mother and requires only reassurance. The most frequent question concerning the eyes is, "When can he see?" The answer is that he can "see" immediately after birth, but that the acquisition of adult vision is a gradual process. The next most frequent question has to do with the color of the infant's eyes. Darkly pigmented irides usually remain that way, and lightly pigmented irides may become darker with time. It is best not to predict what will happen. The occasional "crossing" of eyes in the first few weeks of life is not uncommon and does not presage future problems. An essential part of the newborn examination is to check the red reflex to assure that there are no retinal lesions. It is helpful to practice the ophthalmoscopic examination on normal awake newborns. Do not be surprised to find occasional retinal hemorrhages—these are rapidly absorbed.

Although parents frequently do not admit it, they are concerned with the appearance of the genitalia. In female infants the vulvae are frequently edematous, the clitoris is prominent, and there is a milky vaginal discharge. Assurance that this is a normal finding and pointing out that there is occasionally mild vaginal withdrawal bleeding usually suffices. Needless to say, abnormal clitoromegaly bears investigation for adrenogenital syndrome or androgen stimulation from exogenous sources.

The scrotum of male infants is frequently edematous and may contain small hydroceles that usually resorb rapidly. The occasional breech delivery will have an edematous, hyperemic scrotum that also subsides within days. The uncircumcised prepuce is usually adherent to the glans penis and requires no special care. The circumcised penis requires no special care other than cleanliness. Vaseline gauze during the first several days postcircumcision prevents adherence to the diaper.

The umbilical cord is distasteful to most mothers. The bloated, gelatinous cord undergoes rapid drying and involution, spontaneously falling off in the second week of life. Rarely, the cord is a portal of entry for systemic infection and the cord and stump should be cleaned with alcohol-soaked cotton balls until the area is clean and dry. Mothers can be instructed to seek advice if the cord becomes excessively smelly or periumbilical redness develops. In black infants an umbilical hernia is not uncommon after the cord separates. The majority of these resolve spontaneously by 2 years of age and repeated reassurance is all that is required.

The burden of the rest of the examination must be borne by the physician. This is detailed on p. 141. The findings, which should never be missed on the initial examination, are dermal sinuses (preauricular, cervical, sacral, or midline back), choanal atresia, cleft palate, tracheoesophageal fistula with esophageal atresia, natal teeth, detrocardia, mirror image position of the abdominal contents, hydronephrosis, hypospadius, anal atresia, ambiguous genitalia, club feet, micro- or macrocephaly, Down's syndrome, glaucoma, cataract, retinoblastoma, syndactyly or rudimentary digits, paralysis of an extremity, and, of course, respiratory distress or congestive heart failure. Some of these conditions are of no consequence, but are best recognized by the physician rather than the mother; others are life-threatening and require definitive diagnosis and therapy.

Adaptation of the Mother-Infant Dyad

Now that the parents are reassured of the intactness of their infant, the mother and infant move into an important phase of imprinting or bonding. The provision of rooming-in facilities in the hospital greatly facilitates this process. The mother examines the infant in great detail and in a short time learns his patterns of reacting to hunger, pain, and pleasure. The infant, in turn, learns to respond to his mother.

Since the process of nurturing depends a good deal on the successful establishment of feeding, it is important that the mother be instructed in the feeding process. Mothers who breastfeed are often encouraged and instructed by an interested nursing staff. Problems associated with breastfeeding are anxiety that the milk is not coming in; breast discomfort during the early phase of sucking; difficulty in getting contact between the infant and the breast; the irregularity of the sleep pattern during the first weeks of life; and the mother's anxiety that he is not getting enough to eat. Assuring the mother that all will be well; instructing her in good technique; reassuring her that flexibility in scheduling works best; and pointing out that infants have very individual reaction patterns is often helpful.

The variety of other caretaking procedures provided by the mother during the first weeks of life serves to strengthen the attachment bond. Bathing, diapering, fondling, and talking to the infant provide additional opportunities for learning. The areas which give great anxiety to parents because of their lack of understanding are feeding, sleep patterns, and crying.

Although the feeding pattern of the newborn infant may be erratic, the tendency is to move toward a pattern. Some infants may consume large volumes infrequently, others may feed frequently and consume smaller volumes. In the ideal situation, the breast feeding mother has a fine sense of (what and when her infant needs milk) and when he is content to suck. The hand and mouth activity of the young infant confuses young mothers. They interpret this reflex activity as hunger. (Nutritional requirements are discussed in p. 202).

The amount of time infants sleep is variable. The average total hours of sleep for the first 3 months of life is from 15 to 18 hours daily, with a range from 13 to 20 hours. The periods young infants sleep varies from 2 to 4 hours and usually within a 24-hour period there will be a prolonged sleep of 5 to 6 hours. Unfortunately, this does not always match the diurnal pattern of adults, and the long waking periods often occur during the time the adults wish to sleep. This is a temporary pattern, however, and by 2 or 3 months most infants are sleeping 10 to 12 hours at night, in addition to several long naps during the day. It must be emphasized that there is extreme variability in pattern and predicting what individual infants will do is hazardous. During early infancy mothers who do not have other children should be advised to rest during the day when the infant may tend to have long naps.

The amount of crying young infants do often astonishes new parents. The myth that mothers rapidly determine whether an infant is wet, cold, or hungry by the nature of his cry needs reexamination. The fact is that many infants cry when none of the above conditions maintain, that most of them are easily consoled by fondling and can be put down again in a short period of time. The amount of crying decreases with age.

A syndrome called colic may appear in the first several months of life. Crying is a hallmark of this problem. It tends to be intense, inconsolable, and interminable. The legs are often flexed as the infant acts as though it were experiencing periodic attacks of abdominal pain. Eructation and passing flatus is common. The attacks rarely last past the fourth month. Infants with colic seem to be stimulated by minor sensory input. They are frequently irritable and seem not to derive satisfaction from fondling. The etiology of colic is unknown. There is little question that psychologic stress is present in any household once the syndrome becomes manifest. Management should focus on the entire family setting with efforts to get adequate rest and separation for the mother and periods of unstimulated calm for the infant. Support of the family is essential during the height of the problem. Fortunately, it terminates almost invariably by the fourth month of life.

Signs of Problems

Reference to Table 1 indicates some of the signs of impending or established problems in both the infant and the mother. The implication stands that the infant and the mother have great importance for each other during this critical period. The term *maternal deprivation* has centered on the failure of mothers in the early bonding and attachment behavior. Rutter has pointed out some of the fallacies of regarding the bonding process as essentially monotropic, with the bond of child-mother being of a different kind than bonds formed with others. It is not uncommon to observe rejecting mothers, with young infants who are progressing well in growth and development. Further search usually reveals a grandmother, or uncles and aunts who share a mother-surrogate role.

Intellectual development in the human is clearly related to the quality and amount of experience with different forms of perceptual stimulation in early life. Early language stimulation in terms of amount, type, and clarity of conversation is influential in the development of verbal skills.

Individual differences in children are important in the consideration of children's responses to deprivation. The variability in vulnerability to separation in different children has long been appreciated and apparently is related to the quality of the mother-child relationship prior to the separation. It is clear that "bad" care of infants and children during early life can have "bad" effects, both short-term and long-term.

Preventive Care

The first 6 months after birth represent the period when the infant and mother have the most concentrated experience with the pediatrician (see Table 2). There is a substantial literature on what occurs between the pediatrician and the child and family during this period of time, but surprisingly little data on how these encounters affect the actual health outcomes for these infants. Hoekelman has pointed out that for the variables capable of being measured, there seems to be little difference between who delivers the service, nurse practitioners or pediatricians. In terms of cost, the quantifiable services can be delivered in significantly fewer visits than recommended by the American Academy of Pediatrics. Parent satisfaction and knowledge of child-rearing information was not significantly different between groups receiving 3 visits in the first year and those receiving 6 visits (substantially below the 9 visits recommended by the American Academy of Pediatrics). The most productive strategy might be to focus on families who are clearly in need and yet fail to utilize available health services. Another group of infants who would benefit from increased surveillance are infants suspect or clearly failing in their developmental screens. Haka-Ikse has described such infants where maternal mental illness seems to be the critical factor. Pediatricians are probably aware of this problem, but are often ineffective because of a lack of skills in crisis intervention and counseling of young adults.

The majority of visits in the first 6 months are for health supervision, but frequent unscheduled visits to the office or clinic for trivial complaints should alert one that these are signals of impending problems. If, upon entering the examining room, the mother is sitting immobile and the infant lies swaddled on the examining table 6 feet away, the evidence mounts. After a rapid but careful assessment of the infant, the pediatrician might show his understanding by first reassuring mother about the infant and then saying, "Mothers are often surprised at how much trouble new babies can be." Her response may be an outpouring of resentment that can gently be explored, or a tearful confession that she has never felt so inadequate in her life. In spite of the changing position of women in modern society, our culture still expects women to be effective mothers simply by virtue of their biology and the fact of having undergone the physiologic process of childbirth. If the pediatrician lets her know that we expect it to be a little tough at times, it may allow the mother to discuss what is on her mind without feeling stigmatized or subjected to critical judgment.

An exploration of the family setting can often begin by asking the mother whether she has any help in the care of the baby. This may open the door to clues about an unsatisfactory marital relationship, an overbearing mother-in-law, or an overwhelming isolation. The problem of isolation and depression is particularly prevalent in the very young unmarried mother. Social workers and public health nurses are often supportive in this type of situation. It should be remembered that the consequences of this setting are not only predictive of poor maternal-child attachment, but present the very real potential for child abuse or neglect.

During the first 6 months, the infant receives his first three DPT and TOPV immunizations (Table 7, p 56). Much can be learned about the quality of the maternal-child relationship by observing how the mother reacts to the prospect of a painful intramuscular injection for her infant. A few words of warning to the mothers and an explanation that you would like them to pick up and comfort the infant is often helpful. Mothers should be cautioned that infants may be uncomfortable or even febrile in the 24 hours following immunization. Appropriate doses of acetaminophen can be recommended.

The infant undergoes a rapid increase in both calorie intake and range of foods ingested during the first 6 months. Fads in infant nutrition persist, and many mothers have strong ideas about what constitutes ideal nutrition. Fortunately, the human infant has great tolerance to nutritional irrationality and can thrive on a wide range of styles. Infants in low-income families are at risk for less than optimal nutrition and should be closely monitored.

One of the unheralded but efficacious results of the women's movement has been the trend toward increased breastfeeding, particularly among middle class and counterculture women. Whatever the claims about the merits of artificial formula, there is no question that successful breastfeeding is a uniquely rewarding experience for mothers and infants. Many questions are raised about breastfeeding. Who should breastfeed? Everyone who is emotionally and physically capable. For how long? As long as possible. When to start solid foods? From 4 to 5 months of age. Should vitamins be used? It is probably safer to use vitamin A, D, and C supplements, starting at age 10 days, but this depends on the supply of these vitamins in the diet and in natural sunlight. Do birth control pills cut off the milk supply? No. They may decrease the concentration of fat, protein, and calcium slightly, but this does not significantly affect the infant. Do the hormones from birth control pills pass in the breast milk? Yes, in minute amounts. Will they cause future harm to my baby? I don't know, but I don't believe so. Can I get pregnant while breastfeeding? Yes! Can I prevent allergies in my baby by breastfeeding? The evidence is not clear-cut, but it is a rational idea. Can I go back to work and continue breastfeeding? Yes. If I am taking medication, should I continue to breastfeed? If you are taking anticoagulants, antimicrobials, such as tetracyclines or sulfonamides, thiouracil, radioactive substances, aspirin in therapeutic doses, or antineoplastics agents, do not breastfeed.

How about safety in the first 6 months. The statistics on the number of deaths and injuries in the first 4 years of life in automobile accidents is discouraging. Remind mothers that more infants are killed *inside* of cars than outside. Early commitment to wearing approved restraining devices for children should be encouraged at each visit. Falls from beds and changing tables, burns

from pulled over cups of hot beverages, and drownings from unattended baths are all avoidable with proper parental guidance.

The physical examination in the first 6 months is challenging and enlightening. As is always true in the pediatric examination, keen observation is an absolute requisite. During the first 3 months the infant tolerates separation from the mother reasonably well and can best be examined on the table with the mother within sight, touch, and sound. During the first few months of age, the seasoned clinician can determine rapidly whether the infant can see (by focusing on the face and following) and hear (by turning toward a sound). Actually both of these modalities can reliably be checked by asking the mother about how the infant functions in these areas. The infant's attention can usually be gained by placing the examiner's face about 18 inches from the infant's and engaging in quiet rhythmic tongue clicking. The very young infant greets this maneuver with awe and arrested attention while the 4- to 5-month-old infant often grins broadly and gurgles. If all goes well, what transpires next is one of the almost universal human acts of communication—the adult conducting verbal or linguistic contact with the infant. The voice is soft, high pitched, rhythmic, and punctuated by clucking and lip smacking, while the examiner's face is distorted with raised eyebrows, puckered lips, smiles, and slow head movements. This harlequin behavior is completely accepted by all adults present, whereas in another setting the same behavior would make one a candidate for a locked ward. The infant enjoys it tremendously and while he cooperatively gurgles, the pediatrician deftly palpates the liver edge 1 or 2 cm below the right costal margin; occasionally feels a spleen tip; painlessly slips down into both pelvic gutters where large kidneys are certain to be felt and normal sized kidneys often are located.

The infant survives this 1-to 2-minute maneuver with equanimity and is still gurgling as the pediatrician auscultates the heart. It is not uncommon to hear heart murmurs at this age. The vast majority of them are of no physiologic consequence and shortly disappear (see p1362).The lungs can be adequately auscultated at this juncture and then the femoral arterial pulsations checked. Following this, the hips are flexed and abducted singly with an attempt to obtain a hip click by anterior and posterior movement in and out of the acetabulum. The asymmetry of the folds of the legs is not a good sign of hip dysplasia, but the presence of hip clicks in early infancy arouses suspicion of early hip dysplasia. The remainder of the lower extremity is checked for full foot mobility and questions often arise as to whether the forefoot adduction is a remnant of fetal position or is true metatarsus adductus. If the forefoot can be brought to neutral position without force, watchful waiting is usually safe.

Evaluation of neurologic status is accomplished by a combination of observation, active testing of developmental status, and testing of reflexes and muscle tone (p 153). The young infant is in a state of predominantly flexor tone and the arms and legs are in a position of moderate flexion with the hands tightly clenched. Asymmetry of position or the tone of extremities is suggestive of central neurologic dysfunction. The primitive reflexes, such as the startle response (Moro reflex) and steppage gait when held upright in a weight-bearing position, can be rapidly checked. Pulling the infant to a sitting position from the supine position gives some estimate of the strength of the neck flexors. Signs which at later ages frequently are associated with pathologic states are commonly found in normal newborns and persist for the first few months of life. The Babinski response, transient ankle clonus, myoclonic jerks (particularly in premature infants), the Chvostek response are examples of physical signs in the first few months of life which are usually not associated with central nervous system abnormality.

The genitalia are evaluated by inspection and palpation. In the female, the edema of the vulvae and the prominence of the clitoris recede quite rapidly. Creamy vaginal discharge is not uncommon for the first week or two and rarely a transient bloody discharge or so-called *withdrawal bleeding* is noted during the first several days. The detection of a mass in the vulvae or in the canal should immediately arouse the suspicion of the presence of a gonad. If bilateral, hermaphroditism is a possibility; if unilateral, a normal ovary in an inguinal hernia sac is not uncommon. The vagina should be inspected. Small, glistening tags of vaginal mucosa protruding from the perineal border of the vagina are occasionally noted. These usually extrude and are harmless. They are not to be confused with the rare but serious finding of a grape-cluster appearance of sarcoma botyroides presenting in the vagina.

In the male infant, it is not uncommon for hydrocoeles to persist for weeks or months. Hydrocoeles transilluminate with a pen light. It is understandable that hydrocoeles are frequently mistaken for inguinal hernias. The differentiation on clinical grounds can be made by history (a hernia will be present only part of the time and disappear for the remainder) and the physical examination. On inspection the hernia has the appearance of a pear in the scrotum, with the smaller end located at the external ring, while the hydrocoele will appear as an orange with no proximal connection to the intraabdominal contents. The differentiation is important, since an inguinal hernia presenting before the age of 6 months should be promptly repaired because of the relatively high incidence of incarceration below this age. A hydrocoele can be safely observed.

Even at an early age some male infants may have mobile tests that retreat rapidly into the inguinal canal with stimuli, such as cold or tactile reflexes. The issue of whether a testis is cryptorchid is important because of the surveillance necessary to observe whether it will descend naturally in the first months or years of life, or whether surgery will be necessary. The appearance of the scrotum can often be helpful. When testes have been descended, the scrotum is full and rugated. When the testes have not been in the scrotum, it tends to be small with poorly formed rugae. A helpful maneuver is to block the external canals at the external ring with two fingers of one hand and palpate each side of the scrotum for the presence of the testes. Most often they can be palpated. If one or both testes are not felt, the inguinal canals can be palpated gently, and frequently the errant testes is found. Occasionally, the normal testes will not be palpated discretely, but the happy infant will cry out in pain as the examiner compresses it. More careful examination is usually rewarded by delineating a normal gonad.

The examination of the head, ears, and oral cavity are best left to the last part of the procedure in most children below the age of 3 to 4 years. Even the measurement of head circumference (the largest diameter with the tape fixed at the occiput and, anteriorly, the most prominent portion of the forehead) is annoying to the infant. The head circumference should be measured frequently and charged on a head growth grid during the first year. Infants demonstrating either microcephaly or megalencephaly should be investigated fully. The graph is particularly helpful in detecting slowly evolving hydrocephalus. Head size continues to grow at a rapid pace in the first postnatal year to accommodate the continually growing brain. The anterior and posterior fontanelles gradually close from 9 to 11 months.

The mother can give valuable information concerning her infant's visual apparatus. She can be asked about whether she thinks the infant sees, follows, reacts to bright light, or crosses its eyes. Perhaps the most frequent complaint about the eyes is the mother's fear that the infant is crosseyed. This is most frequently related to the prominent epicanthal folds noted in young infants.The Cover Test (p.1968) is important in the assessment of the infant's ability to focus with both eyes. The detecting of early amblyopia is of prime importance.

A persistent dacrocystitis is occasionally seen as a result of nasolacrimal duct stenosis. This can safely be observed for several months, with the expectation of resolution. Referral to an ophthalmologist is recommended if this persists beyond 6 months of age.

The red reflex should be elicited routinely during the examinations of the first year. Abnormalities of the red reflex or suspicious differences between the reflexes elicited from each eye is reason for a thorough ophthalmoscopic examination or referral, it this cannot be accomplished. Retinoblastoma is a rare tumor, but is often first noted in this simple maneuver.

Routine examination of the oral cavity and nasal passages should be performed. The normal neonate is an obligate nose breather, and any young infant who chronically breathes through the mouth should be suspected of choanal atresia. The tympanic membrane examination in the young infant is best delayed until the very end. The infant almost invariably requires restraint. The ear canal can be straightened for adequate visualization by pulling downward as the earlobe is grasped. This is the opposite direction from that pursued in the examination of older infants, young children, and adolescents. It is essential that the pediatrician learn to distinguish normal landmarks of the tympanic membrane in the first 6 months after birth (p 960). Bluestone offers convincing evidence for the routine use of bulb attachments to the otoscope head to achieve estimates of tympanic membrane mobility.

The oral cavity during the early months of life is usually edentulous, but rarely infants will be born with teeth—most often one or both lower central incisors. These are frequently abnormal and loose and should be extracted. If they appear normal, a dental consultation often assists in making a decision about whether to preserve the teeth.

Pale yellow or whitish cysts measuring 1 to 2 mm, located along the median raphe of the hard palate (Epstein's pearls), are common and usually disappear within the first few months. Larger cystic lesions appearing on the alveolar ridges are less common but alarming to mothers. They can be safely observed. It is important to differentiate these from an early erupting molar with necrotic material appearing at its margins; this may be the initial lesion of histocytosis X and a dental x-ray will reveal the typical lesion of a *floating* tooth.

By far the most common oral lesion is candidiasis (thrush), which characteristically presents as adherent, white, circinate, or plaquelike lesions of the buccal mucosa and tongue. Primary herpetic gingivostomatitis is less common at this age but may be confused with thrush. This disease usually involves the gingiva and lips, is more florid, and is accompanied by systemic signs, such as fever, irritability, and refusal to feed. Thrush is most often asymptomatic.

The faucial tonsils are small during the first 6 months. The usual response to upper respiratory infection manifests itself by intense redness, occasional emanthem, and rarely, exudation. The anterior cervical lymph nodes are rarely enlarged. A persistent midline mass, of pea size or smaller, should arouse the suspicion of a thyroglossal duct cyst; a linear, firm longitudinal mass below the mandible and lateral to the sternocleidomastoid muscles is a candidate for a branchial cleft cyst; a large, soft, rubbery, transilluminating mass extending below the mandible into the anterior cervical triangle should raise the spectre of a cystic hygroma.

During this age, mothers should be taught to hold their infants in their laps with arms, legs, and head restrained for a reliable ear and pharynx examination. For examination of the right ear, the mother sits facing the physician with the infant seated on her lap sideways, facing to her left. Both of the infant's legs can be effectively restrained by tightly clasping them between her knees; both hands and arms by wrapping her right arm around the child and firmly grasping both hands; and the head steadied by her left hand clasping the head firmly against her right upper chest and shoulder. Most mothers can learn this maneuver rapidly with a brief, patient explanation and demonstration. Some cannot because they are unable or unwilling to apply the necessary force to restrain the child. If the physician suspects this, it is best to examine the infant's ears on the examining table under proper restraint. This assures good control, a rapid and effective examination, and the termination of a procedure upsetting to the infant, the mother, and the physician.

No procedure is as threatening to a good relationship between the physician and the child and his mother as the removal of wax from the external canal in order to visualize the tympanic membrane. In the absence of symptoms the risk/benefit seems heavily weighted against aggressive maneuvers. There are those who are advocates of *spooning* out soft wax with a curette, and there are those who are *flushers,* utilizing a variety of syringe devices. The chief disadvantage of spooning is the creation of small tears in the lining epithelium of the external canal, which bleed briefly but briskly, obscuring the field and creating anxiety and resentment in the mother and fear in the infant. Flushing often alters the appearance of the tympanic membrane so that the suspicion of pathology may be aroused when the tympanic membrane is actually normal. In the presence of unexplained fever or symptoms suggestive of middle-ear infection, both tympanic membranes must be adequately visualized and tested for mobility, regardless of the above-noted risks.

THE OLDER INFANT (SIX TO EIGHTEEN MONTHS)

In many ways, this age-span bridges some of the most satisfying and frustrating experiences of parenting. The early tribulations of self-doubt about her own abilities have long disappeared; mother is more confident that she knows her baby better and anticipates his needs; she enjoys her interactions far more because of his increasing repertoire of social responses; and she is moving into a more satisfying relationship with her husband. The father plays an increasing role with the infant and is often delighted with the rapid acquisition of motor skills. The infant goes through a kaleidoscope of experience, which allows him to start the process of differentiating himself from his mother. During this period the infant learns to talk, walk, speak, explore, communicate, and, generally, to expand his horizons. Table 1 outlines the salient developmental landmarks and the signs of minimal and major psychopathology in mother and child during this period. Table 2 offers suggestions for the content of the encounter at various ages during this period; developmental landmarks to be observed; the anticipatory guidance to be offered; the immunization and screening procedures for each age; and suggestions for the appropriate health care professional to supervise the encounter. This portion of the schedule and the frequency of visits is subject to a good deal of variation, depending on the nature of the population, the organization of the health services, the availability of manpower (in some settings pediatric nurse practitioner or physicians assistant could be substituted for the physician), and the habits of the practitioners.

Common problems brought to the pediatrician when the infant is about 8 to 10 months have to do with the infant's increasing differentiation of strangers and the development of an even stronger selective tie to the mother. The pediatrician experiences this phenomena during examinations at this age. An infant who delighted in his antics 2 short months ago regards him with suspicion, and on his approach, buries his head in his mother's shoulder. The experienced physician can utilize a swivel chair on wheels to good advantage. The interview can start with the child on mother's lap and the physician a comfortable distance away. While talking directly to the mother he may place items from the developmental kit in full view, or display his stethoscope or otoscope in a manner that excites curiosity. An occasional eye contact with the child may be made but prolonged eye contact or closing the distance rapidly is usually greeted by retreat. A slow, imperceptible approach is tolerated, increased eye contact accepted, an occasional brief remark addressed to the infant is warily filed, a light and brief touch on the lower extremity regarded suspiciously, a small moving toy presented and proffered, the stethoscope head placed on the foot briefly is accepted, and the remainder of the examination conducted as a *pas de deux,* with the pediatrician responding to the infant's cues, moving rapidly, opportunely, now auscultating, now palpating, now deftly abducting the hips, always observing, chatting and clucking; consoling and cajoling, gathering and filing information.

By now it is obvious that the physical examination in young children and infants is unstructured, opportunistic, performed with good humor and a sense of fun. The pediatrician must have the grace to retreat when the day is lost because the infant is cranky, hungry, tired, in a bad humor, or sick. Common sense is indispensable. Attempts at developmental assessment with an uncooperative infant are fraught with the danger of misinterpretation.

Just as the knowledge of the developmental stage of the infant allows the pediatrician the opportunity to conduct an effective, efficient examination, the problems experienced by parents at specific times allows for anticipatory guidance. Around 1 year of age, many mothers become frustrated with the feeding habits of children. A constructive solution is to advise mothers to allow children to feed themselves finger foods, giving them small allocations that can be replenished when finished. The content of the diet can be monitored and altered.

Somewhere in the second year, mothers are invariably concerned over the decrease in food consumption. "Doctor, he won't eat!" is the paradigm of this complaint. The rational explanation that the relative food requirements for growth are less at this stage rarely satisfies mothers, but the graphic demonstration that the child is still at the 75th percentile for height and weight often does placate her.

Sleep problems continue to plague the parents. The 8-month-old who suddenly starts awakening and engages in demanding behavior; the 16-month-old who can climb out of the crib and does so repeatedly, are typical examples. Removing the night bottle from the crib, and firm, consistent, nonrewarding conduct by the parents should be encouraged. The dynamic underlying these changes in behavior is frequently obscure and transient, but patient interest in arriving at a mutually acceptable attempt at solution solidifies the trust between the parents and the physician.

At all patient visits during this period the issue of accidents and poisonings should be raised. In spite of encouraging progress against the traditional leading poisoner of children, aspirin, it does no harm to remind parents that accidents kill far more children between the ages of 1 and 15 than any of the disease categories. The so-called childproof containers for aspirin, some potentially toxic over-the-counter remedies, and prescription drugs have reduced toxic episodes from these agents. Unfortunately, petroleum distillate products are still readily available in furniture polishes and other products. Before the child is permitted to be ambulant, the home should be childproofed. All cleansers, polishes, medications, should be placed in high inaccessible areas and preferably locked. Gates should guard open staircases, and windows should be securely fastened. Falls are surprisingly common and are not infrequently the cause of severe morbidity and occasionally death.

Mothers need to be reminded that the home is still the site of greatest danger. In addition to poisoning and falls, the dread possibility of fires and drownings needs to be explored. Particularly, in older housing in rural areas where space heaters are still commonly used, fire is a constant problem. Flame-retardant fabrics for children's clothes are slowly becoming more available, but this is secondary prevention at best.

Just as home fires tend to be more prevalent in winter, drownings cluster in the early summer. Children unsupervised at pools and beaches are at high risk. Just as in the younger age groups, mothers need to be encouraged to insist that their infants use approved automobile-seat restraints. Most mothers know it, but it is reasonable to remind them that little boys are at higher risk than girls for accidents around the home.

Developmental Assessment

The task of assessing the development of infants and young children requires a substantial fund of information on ranges of normality, the time of appearance of specific accomplishments, an appreciation of the variables at work in the test situation, a respect for the practical problems existing with all of the developmental tests, and that most elusive quality, experience.

The person utilizing any of the available developmental tests should be very clear about the objectives of the testing and the limitations of the method. If the instrument is used for screening purposes, the examiner must recognize that definitive diagnosis is the responsibility of a higher level of skill. Various tests in common use are presented on p 1768. Some practitioners find the Denver Developmental Screening Test (see p 1768) most valuable during the first 2 to 3 years. Beyond this age, the scales designed by Leavitt and his colleagues prove useful (see Table 3).

During this phase of development it is extremely important to ascertain whether or not the sensory functions of the child are intact. The mother's opinion of

TABLE 3A. Development Assessment Scales

Motor Behavior

Activity

Output—amount of activity. Is the infant very active, moderately active, inactive, etc?
Tempo of movements—fast, slow, etc.
Type of movements:
Coordination of movements.
Abnormal motility patterns such as whirling, flicking, athetoid or choreiform movements, convulsive movements, etc.

Mastery of Motor Skills

Gross motor development—postural control, position, change, locomotion.
Fine motor development—grasping and manipulation of toys, finger skills, etc.

Use of Motor System

To approach people and inanimate objects (by position change or by reaching out).
To flee from, avoid, actively ward off, or get rid of a person, an inanimate object, or a painful stimulus.
To express feelings—*eg,* interest, pleasure, love, anticipation, curiosity, anger, anxiety, fear, aggression, excitement, etc.
In self-stimulating activities—thumb-sucking, hand play, genital play, rocking, hand–foot and foot–mouth play, head–rolling or -banging, biting, etc.

Reactions to People

To the Parent(s)

When and how does the baby turn to the mother? What is the nature of the interchange between mother and baby?
For comfort when in real distress? To share in the pleasure?
Are there frequent visual, social, or body contacts?

To the Examiner

Are there signs of discrimination of the stranger, anxiety, tentativeness in the approach? What can be said about how the baby accepts or initiates a contact? Is there an attempt to engage the examiner in play? Is there behavior that could be called provocative, teasing, or flirtatious? What can be seen in the facial expression, use of vocalization, motor activity, response to play, and use of toys that seems to be directly related to the presence of the examiner?

Language and Communication

Vocalizations and Verbalizations

What sounds are heard? When? How are they used? Are there specific words? Is verbalization inhibited? Is there a change during the course of the test session? Do the sounds seem to be used in a purposive way to communicate something to another person? Are they used to express some feeling? Can the feelings be identified?

Nonverbal Communication

What forms of nonverbal communication are visible? How much gestural language is seen? How effective is this communication? What does the infant understand of the nonverbal communication of the adult?

Comprehension of Language

Does the infant indicate understanding of specific words or tones of voice of the adult? Does he associate word sounds with specific people, actions, objects, or pictorial representations?

Reactions to and Use of Toys (Test Materials)

Amount of interest. Expression of preferences. How are the toys used? What is the reaction to the removal of a toy? The hidden toy? The presentation of two toys simultaneously?
In addition to the adaptive use of toys in play, does one see them being used in the service of contact with the adult? What feelings are visible around the use of toys (pleasure, excitement, discharge of energy, aggression, anger, etc)?
Does the baby see and hear? What is the evidence?
Changes of behavior during test session. Disorganization of behavior with fatigue, frustration, or discomfort? Changes in mood, activity, or responsiveness during test?

Impressions of Parents

Interest and involvement in test. Interaction with baby. Evidences of discomfort or pleasure. Ways of comforting infant.

TABLE 3B. Developmental Charts for Ages 3 to 15 Years*

Ages 3–4 Yr

Activities to be observed:
Climbs stairs with alternating feet.
Begins to button and unbutton.
"What do you like to do that's fun?" (Answers using plurals, personal pronoun, and verbs.)
Responds to command to place toy *in, on,* or *under* table.
Draws a circle when asked to draw a man (girl, boy).
Knows his sex. ("Are you a boy or a girl?")
Gives full name.
Copies a circle already drawn. ("Can you make one like this?")

Activities related by parent:
Feeds self at mealtime.
Takes off shoes and jacket.

Ages 4–5 Yr

Activities to be observed:
Runs and turns without losing balance.
May stand on one leg for at least 10 sec.
Buttons clothes and laces shoes. (Does not tie.)
Counts to 4 by rote.
"Give me 2 sticks." (Able to do so from pile of 4 tongue depressors.)
Draws a man. (Head, 2 appendages, and possibly 2 eyes; no torso yet.)
"You know the days of the week; what day comes after Tuesday?"
Gives appropriate answers to: "What must you do if you are sleepy? Hungry? Cold?"
Copies ÷ in imitation.

Activities related by parent:
Self care at toilet. (May need help with wiping.)
Plays outside for at least 30 minutes.
Dresses self except for tying.

TABLE 3B. Development Charts for Ages 3 to 15 Years* (cont.)

Ages 5–6 Yr

Activities to be observed:
Can catch ball.
Skips smoothly.
Copies a ÷ already drawn.
Tells his age.
Concept of 10 (eg, counts 10 tongue depressors).
   May recite to higher number by rote.
Knows his right and left hands.
Draws recognizable man with at least 8 details.
Can describe favorite television program in some
   detail.

Activities related by parent:
Does simple chores at home (taking out garbage,
   drying silverware, etc).
Goes to school unattended or meets school bus.
Good motor ability but little awareness of
   dangers.

Ages 6–7 Yr

Activities to be observed:
Copies a △
Defines words by use. ("What is an orange?" "To eat.")
Knows if morning or afternoon.
Draws a man with 12 details.
Reads several one-syllable printed words (my,
   dog, see, boy).
Uses pencil for printing name.

Ages 7–8 Yr

Activities to be observed:
Counts by 2's and 5's.
Ties shoes.
Copies a ◇ .
Know what day of the week it is (not date or
   year).
Reads paragraph #1 Durrell:
Reading
Muff is a little yellow kitten. She drinks milk. She sleeps
   on a chair. She does not like to get wet.

Corresponding arithmetic

$$
\begin{array}{cccc}
7 & 6 & 6 & 8 \\
+4 & +7 & -4 & -3 \\
\hline
\end{array}
$$

No evidence of sound substitution in speech (eg,
   fr for *thr*).
Adds and subtracts one-digit numbers.
Draws a man with 16 details.

Ages 8–9 Yr

Activities to be observed:
Defines words better than by use. ("What is an
   orange?" "A fruit.")
Can give an appropriate answer to the following:
"What is the thing for you to do if . . .
—you've broken something that belongs
   to someone else?"
—a playmate hits you without meaning
   to do so?"
Reads paragraph #2 Durrell:

Reading

A little black dog ran away from home. He played with
   two big dogs. They ran away from him. It began to rain. He
   went under a tree. He wanted to go home, but he did not know
   the way. He saw a boy he knew. The boy took him home.

Corresponding arithmetic

$$
\begin{array}{cccc}
 & 45 & & \\
67 & 16 & 14 & 84 \\
+4 & +27 & -8 & -36 \\
\hline
\end{array}
$$

Is learning borrowing and carrying processes in
   addition and subtraction.

Ages 9–10 Yr

Activities to be observed:
Knows the month, day, and year.
Names the months in order (fifteen sec, one
   error).
Makes a sentence with these 3 words in it (1
   of 2; can use words orally in proper context):
   1. work . . . . money . . . . men
   2. boy . . . . river . . . . ball
Reads paragraph #3 Durrell:
Reading
Six boys put up a tent by the side of river. They took
   things to eat with them. When the sun went down, they went
   into the tent to sleep. In the night, a cow came and began to eat
   grass around the tent. The boys were afraid. They thought it
   was a bear.

Corresponding arithmetic

$$
\begin{array}{ccc}
5204 & 23 & 837 \\
-530 & \times 3 & \times 7 \\
\hline
\end{array}
$$

Should comprehend and answer question: "What
   was the cow doing?"
Learning simple multiplication.

Ages 10–12 Yr

Activities to be observed:
Should read and comprehend paragraph #5
   Durrell:
Reading
In 1807, Robert Fulton took the first long trip in a steam-
   boat. He went one hundred and fifty miles up the Hudson
   River. The boat went five miles an hour. This was faster than a
   steamboat had ever gone before. Crowds gathered on both
   banks of the river to see this new kind of boat. They were afraid
   that its noise and splashing would drive away all the fish.

Corresponding arithmetic

$$
\begin{array}{ccc}
420 & & \\
\times 29 & 9)72 & 31)62 \\
\hline
\end{array}
$$

Answer: "What river was the trip made on?"
Ask to write the sentence: "The fishermen did
   not like the boat."
Should do multiplication and simple division.

TABLE 3B. Development Charts for Ages 3 to 15 Years* (cont.)

Ages 12–15 Yr

Activities to be observed:
Reads paragraph #7 Durrell:
Reading

Golf originated in Holland as a game played on ice. The
   game in its present form first appeared in Scotland. It became
   unusually popular and kings found it so enjoyable that it was
   known as "the royal game." James IV, however, thought that
   people neglected their work to indulge in this fascinating sport
   so that it was forbidden in 1457. James relented when he found
   how attractive the game was, and it immediately regained its
   former popularity. Golf spread gradually to other countries,
   being introduced in America in 1890. It has grown in favor until
   there is hardly a town that does not boast of a private or public
   course.

Corresponding arithmetic

$$536)4762 \qquad \begin{array}{r} 1/3 \\ +1/3 \\ \hline \end{array} \qquad \begin{array}{r} 7\ 1/6 \\ -3/4 \\ \hline \end{array}$$

Reduce fractions to lowest forms.

Ask to write sentence: "Golf originated in Hol-
   land as a game played on ice."
Answers questions:
   "Why was golf forbidden by James IV?"
   "Why did he change his mind?"
Does long division; adds and subtracts fractions.

*Adapted from Leavitt SR, Gofman H, Harvin D: Pediatrics 31:499, 1963.

whether the child sees or hears appropriately should always be sought and seriously considered. Screening tests are described in a subsequent section (see p. 57); but it should be noted that major causes of disability, such as amblyopia secondary to muscle imbalance or refractive error and hearing loss secondary to serous otitis media are largely preventable. The fact that screening tests exist should not relieve the pediatrician of the burden of historical probing, keen observation, and skillful physicial examination. A comprehensive schedule for investigating the development of speech, language, and hearing is found in Table 4.

TABLE 4. Speech, Language, and Hearing Communication Chart (Newborn to 18 Months)*

Normal Development Expectancies: Responses to Acoustic Stimuli, Learning of Language, and Speech Output

Age	Activities Responses	Parental Observation	Office Procedures	Interpretations and Meaning
Newborn	Startle reflex to sound, more often to sudden sounds of moderate-to-loud intensity. Arousal responses. Investigators have demonstrated that relatively loud sound will arouse the newborn infant from accustomed sleep state.	Not pertinent	Not pertinent	Not ideal time to test auditory responses. Lack of expected responses bears little relationship to later communication problems. Conditions that apparently lead to auditory or other communicative problems may not become operative until several days after birth. In neurologic terms, clinical motor responses in the early months are relatively simple (gross). At this stage, more complex "apparatus" neurologic pathways (ultimately used for communicative purposes) may or may not be intact.
8 mo	1. Turns head and upper torso toward interesting sounds (at level of quiet conversational voice) 2. Vocalizes with variety of sounds and inflections. Done spontaneously when alone. Gives vocal responses when somebody talks to him, eg, smiles, giggles, coos. 3. Usually responds to familiar sounds (his name, telephone bell, vacuum cleaner, barking dog) and quiets to mother's voice.	1. Have you seen this? 2. What have you heard him say? What noises does he make? 3. What does he do if he hears father's footsteps, the vacuum cleaner, the telephone?	Test at ear level. Baby should seek and find sound source. It is important to test from both sides out of baby's vision range. When baby does respond, reinforcement must be used to hold baby's attention. This is done by immediately repeating stimulus at a louder level while expressing	Response should be prompt. Delayed responses suggest possible hearing involvement. Persistent turning to one side or searching for sound but not identifying appropriate direction of its source suggests hearing problem. Failure to turn quickly in presence of other evidence of hearing suggests developmental lag and need for careful follow-up. Item 3 responses indicate baby's developing ability to "understand" everyday sounds around him (listening and discrimination).

TABLE 4. Speech, Language, and Hearing Communication Chart (Newborn to 18 Months)* (cont.)

Normal Development Expectancies: Responses to Acoustic Stimuli, Learning of Language, and Speech Output

Age	Activities Responses	Parental Observation	Office Procedures	Interpretations and Meaning
	4. Usually awakens when mother talks to him.	4. Does he respond to "no-no"? Does he jiggle to music? 5. Has babbling decreased?	approval of baby.	
12 mo	1. Responds to a number of different sounds, often with different reactions, and seems to recognize them as different, eg, jabbers in response to human voice, may cry when there is thunder, quiet when he hears mother nearby (vacuum cleaner), and frowns when scolded.	1. Direct query and observation. What kinds of sounds and noises does he make when you talk to him? What does he do when he hears a loud noise?		1. Average behavior is similar to 8-mo period (item 3), but responses should indicate more differentiation among speech sounds.
	2. Demonstrates understanding of some words by appropriate behavior, eg, points or looks at familiar objects on request.	2. Try to test with appropriate objects by saying the word quietly without general conversation or instruction.		2. This behavior indicates early differentiation of speech sounds as symbolic meanings.
	3. Uses sounds. "Talks" to toys. This is an enjoyable experience for baby.	3. Direct query and observation. Does he "talk" to himself or make sounds as he plays with his toys?		3. One can look for changes in baby's "talking" as his attention and patterns of play change.
	4. Tries to imitate some simple words.	4. If possible, have mother demonstrate this; he is more used to her manner of speaking.		4. This is evidence of developmental maturation. Many children use a few words at this age. However, babies may not imitate words at 12 mo. Absence of verbal utterance indicates a need to inquire about verbal stimulation at home, parental attitudes, and expectancies, eg, "Do you have time to sit and talk with him and let him jabber back?" "Does his father?"
18 mo	1. Expect some progressive increase in child's vocabulary (more definite words) from what was observable at 12 mo.	1. Query and demonstration. How many understandable words does he use? More or fewer than he used a few months ago?		1. Note any apparent loss of words that were previously used. With a child who has severely impaired hearing, one can expect cessation or regression of previously noted babbling.†
	2. Begins to identify parts of body, eg, may point to nose on request.	2. Demonstration, if possible. The baby should be able to show you his nose or eyes.		2. This is clear evidence of verbal symbolic understanding.
	3. Begins to pay attention to, and identify, various sounds from considerable distance.	3. Note detail of parental anecdotes. It is important that auditory responses are identified without the use of visual cues. What does he do when refrigerator door opens in another room? When ice cream man's bell rings? When there is a fire siren? When you open a box of candy that he cannot see? Does he seem to react to music? With rhythm? Does he like to look at books with you, and turn the page?		3. Whereas at 8–12 mo, baby's auditory attention is limited to close environment, by 18 mo he is responding to wider environment of sound, eg, from another room or from outside the house. If hearing loss has been acquired, he probably will not do this and may show symptoms of regression in speech attempts previously made.

Adapted from Standards of Child Health Care, 2nd ed. American Academy of Pediatrics.
†*This usually happens before 18 mo if the child is, in fact, deaf.*

THE TODDLER AND PRESCHOOL AGE (UNDER 5 YEARS)

During the early months of this period, mothers interpret much of the child's behavior as negative. *The terrible twos* has become part of the maternal lexicon. The child perceives the concept of choice and to many maternally initiated projects he responds with a firm "no!" Skilled mothers recognize this as a sign of a developing sense of autonomy and identity and do not waste time with confrontations. This creates conflicts for the child also. He wishes increasing independence, and can tolerate increasing separation from mother in structured situations. The fragility of this autonomy is best illustrated by the reaction of the toddler lost in a store. Inconsolable grief at the loss and separation is the immediate reaction.

There is increasing socialization with other children, which moves from parallel to participatory play. The level of direct parental supervision decreases and the opportunity for an actual occurrence of accidents increases. As noted in the previous section, falls, fire, drowning, and being struck by automobiles are typical hazards. Specific warnings and discussion of these issues should be part of the health supervision visit.

Toilet training is a task feared by some mothers. They recognize it as a developmental landmark over which they exercise partial control. They wish their child to perform at the right age. As with most other physiologic functions, there is considerable variation in the time when children achieve sphincter control. In general, bowel control precedes bladder control. While there are striking individual differences in tolerance to early training, it is probably best to delay attempts at bowel training to about 18 to 24 months of age. By age 2½ years about 90 percent of girls and 75 percent of boys take responsibility for going to the toilet for defecation. By age 2 years, about two-thirds of all infants will be trained; by 3 years; 90 percent; and by 4 years; 95 percent. There is a great variability in frequency of defecation, some toddlers have three bowel movements a day

and others one every other day, or even less frequently. The habit of giving laxatives to young children routinely is to be condemned. Feeding bran products, once daily, is usually sufficient to regulate bowel frequency. Forced and punitive bowel traning is to be avoided. A mother who is overly concerned about bowel function should be encouraged to adopt a hands-off policy.

Control over urination is acquired much later than bowel control. Daytime control precedes nighttime control by at least several months. About one-half of children have daytime control at age 2 years; 85 percent at age 3 years; 90 percent at 4 years; 95 percent at 5 years. Nighttime control is achieved by two-thirds of the children by age 3 years; 75 percent by 4 years; and 80 percent by 5 years. The proportion with control rises slowly until by age 8½ years 90 percent of children are dry throughout the night.

Sleep disturbances continue into this age range. The increased mobility of the toddler allows him to appear blinking and innocent long after his expected time of sleep. There are multiple variations on this theme, just as there are rituals before placing the child in bed. They are best handled by good-natured firmness and prompt parental accompaniment back to bed. Nighttime crying also demands firmness, parental consistency, and agreement about "waiting it out." Disagreement among parents is frequently the reason for perpetuation of this problem.

Sibling rivalry is often manifest when the toddler finds that his preserve is invaded by an intruder in the form of a new brother and sister. Mothers are disturbed by regressive behavior, such as fecal soiling, wetting, fingersucking, demands to be fed at same time as baby. Most parents are sympathetic to the plight of the older child and with some imaginative and constructive maneuvers bring him into the care process and arrange for special times when he gets undivided attention.

Particular attention to the child's dentition is needed during this period. Training in good hygiene, the avoidance of sucrose-containing foods, and the establishment of regular dental care by age 3 years all contribute

TABLE 5. Suggested Schedule for Preventive Child Dental Health Care*

Age	Developmental Landmarks	Discussion and Guidance	Procedures
Fetal period		Parent education to dental needs Effect of drugs on developing dentition during pregnancy Diet and proper maternal dental care	Brochures and pamphlets from American Dental Association Fluoridated drinking water
Newborn	Edentulous gumpads Infantile swallowing pattern	Parent education to dental needs Effect of drugs on developing dentition during pregnancy Diet and proper maternal health care Congenital anomalies Birth trauma	Thorough oral examination by physician

TABLE 5. Suggested Schedule for Preventive Child Dental Health Care (cont.)

Age	Developmental Landmarks	Discussion and Guidance	Procedures
Birth to 6 mo	Neonatal teeth Lower primary incisor eruption Epstein pearls	Parent education to dental needs Effect of drugs on developing dentition Diet and proper dental care Congenital anomalies Dental arch and oral facial development	Drinking fluoridated water
6 to 30 mo	Eruption sequence and time of eruption Completion of primary dentition Transitional period from infantile to mature swallow Tongue, lip, finger habits Learning and sleeping habits	Effect of drugs on developing dentition Diet and proper dental health care Dental arch and oral facial development Trauma Oral habit patterns Caries	Oral hygiene supervision Oral habit control
30 mo to 6 yr	Complete primary dentition Appearance of spaces between incisors Deep overbite normal Loss of primary incisors	Period of use of complete primary dentition and developmental preparation for permanent teeth Routine periodic visits to dentist Oral manifestations of drug therapy Trauma more likely Temporomandibular joint disturbances Dietary regimen	First visit to dentist Supervision of occlusion and dentofacial development (arch and jaw relationships and space control) Control of abnormal pressure habits Caries control Oral hygiene instruction
6 to 12 yr	Mixed dentition period Eruption of eight permanent incisors and four permanent molars by 8.5 yr Reduction of overbite Loss of primary canines and molars Eruption of premolars by 10.5 to 12 yr Eruption of second molars (12-yr molars)	Periodic dental visits (at least once a year) Caries, soft tissue disturbances Malocclusion Oral manifestations of drug therapy Trauma more likely Temporomandibular joint disturbances (bruxism, clenching, rheumatoid arthritis, and so forth) Dietary regimen Oral effects of puberty	Supervision of dental development (arch and jaw relationships and space control) Optimum time for orthodontic consultation and guidance; possible interceptive procedures Oral hygiene instruction Caries control Soft tissue care

Adapted from Standards of Child Health Care, 2nd ed. American Academy of Pediatrics.

to good dental health. Table 5 presents a suggested schedule for preventive child dental health care.

The majority of nonscheduled visits to the pediatrician during this phase is for acute diseases of the upper and lower respiratory tract. Most of these are due to viral agents and do not require antibiotics. One of the most common bacterial infections is acute suppurative otitis media, most often due to pneumococcus or H. influenzae. Upper and lower respiratory tract allergy is common, and the child who has almost constant rhinorrhea, night cough, nasal itchiness, should be suspect. Gastroenteritis, skin infections, and minor trauma are not infrequent complaints, and among girls pain on micturition, which is not associated with urinary tract infection, is not unusual.

SCHOOL AGE AND PREADOLESCENCE (5 TO 12 YEARS)

During this period of development, the child continues to strive toward greater independence from the family. His peer group becomes increasingly meaningful and more relationships are formed outside of the home. The site at which some of his major life tasks are performed is the school and he becomes increasingly aware of a larger world beyond himself and his family.

He actively works through his own identity and continues to work through his own sex role. While there are some tentative overt explorations with the opposite sex, it is stereotypical for the social group, and peers of the same sex continue to be most important.

The physical vitality and general good health noted at the earlier phase continues. Children let out of school seem to have a universal reaction akin to a first-order chemical reaction. Action, noise, barely controlled zeal are characteristic of this age. It is this barely controlled energy that frequently brings them into conflict with authority—at home with the family, at school with the teachers.

Some mothers and children have extreme difficulty achieving mature separation, and this may manifest itself in school phobia or school refusal (see p. 42). This manifests itself as extreme anxiety on the part of the child at the prospect of separating from the parent, usually the mother. When this problem surfaces, it is almost invariably accompanied by unresolved conflicts within the family, and attempts at dealing with this complaint superficially are doomed to failure.

During the few years prior to puberty, the child is gradually acquiring several new and profound intellectual capacities. He gains an ease in dealing with hypothetical premises that may violate reality. The 12-year-old will accept and think about the following problem: "All three-legged snakes are purple; I am hiding a three-legged snake; guess its color?" The 7-year-old is confused by the fact that the initial premises violate his notion of what is real, and he will not cooperate. The younger child does not appreciate the discontinuity between the self-contained information in a hypothetical problem and the egocentric information he carries with him for more practical challenges. To appreciate that problems can be self-contained entities solved by special rules is a masterful accomplishment not usually achieved until early adolescence. The illustration is useful to emphasize one of Piaget's observations—that the structure of the child's concepts is not only less complex than the adult's, it is also different. The child's thought is not just a simplified version of the adult's. The acceptance of this fact is a great advantage to the pediatrician as he deals with the child throughout this period.

The relationship of the child and the pediatrician changes radically during this period. In the past mother had been the sole historian, the physician was omnipotent. Now the child must be brought more into the information-gathering task. His attitude toward the physician starts to change. He is recognized as part of the adult world, which he views with increasing distrust. Now the physician must intellectually earn what he could cheaply barter for at earlier ages.

The nature of the problem brought to the pediatrician also changes dramatically. The dominance of problems of the respiratory tract is challenged by problems best characterized as psychophysiologic and frankly behavioral. The problem of recurrent abdominal pain is prototypical. The child is about 10 or 11 years and has had recurrent attacks of periumbilical pain for a period of 1 or 2 years. He has had several hospitalizations, numerous radiologic examinations of the gastrointestinal and genitourinary tracts, which have not demonstrated pathology. The pain has prevented school attendance; on occasion he has had headaches or pains in the limbs associated with these attacks. A complete and detailed history and physical examination fail to reveal a significant clue to organic disease, but there are factors pointing toward severe family dysfunction. Further observation reveals dysfunctional communication, unresolved conflicts, and scapegoating within the family unit. Minuchin has skillfully described families who breed psychosomatic problems and suggests methods of intervention. The fact is that abdominal pain, headache, and limb pain can all be due to serious organic disease, but when seen in the context of a dysfunctional family setting, psychophysiologic reactions are the most likely diagnosis.

Certain groups of organic diseases tend to be manifest during this age span. The careful clinician finds that a well-kept growth curve provides excellent clues as to the onset of disease processes. The child with chronic systemic illness tends to follow a pattern of weight loss or stationary weight and less than expected incremental linear growth.

The onset of puberty varies greatly. During this stage of development, the majority of girls will show physical manifestations of the early stages of puberty (see p 1712). The linear growth spurt in girls accompanies the early stages of puberty, in contrast to boys where the linear growth spurt accompanies the early to middle stages of puberty. This explains why most of the girls at this age tower over their male age peers. A frequent concern of mother is a lump in the breast in 10- or 11-year-old girls. It is common for breast development to proceed in a unilateral fashion and the first sign of puberty may be a unilateral breast bud. The pediatrician can reassure the parent that this is the onset of normal puberty, but the task is not complete. The degree of preparation of the child for the ensuing developmental cascade should be determined. While most schools assume the burden of education about sexual development, this is not always so, and the event gives the physician the opportunity to talk to the mother about her attitudes and feelings. A question addressed to the mother like, "Do you recall when your menstrual periods first started?" can be informative about how the mother perceived this event, what her feelings about it were, and how comfortable and supportive she will be with her own daughter.

Problems with school performance tend to emerge at this time. The task of the pediatrician is to help to frame the problem in terms of whether the unacceptable performance is because of inappropriate substrate, that is, that the child does not have the intellectual competence to perform the task, or that the problem is one of poor motivation or emotional blocking. This is not a simple task. So much of the school experience is tied to peer acceptance and approval that aberrations in performance are bound to have repercussions in the emotional realm. Educators and psychologists expect that the pediatrician can tell them whether organic factors are participating in the unsatisfactory performance of the child. Other than the neurocutaneous syndromes associated with mental retardation, such as tuberous sclerosis, neurofibromatosis, Sturge-Weber syndrome, or juvenile hypothyroidism, labels can rarely be found. The status of vision and hearing must be checked accurately, and in the younger child the history should rule out problems of attention such as petit mal. The rare child will show extreme psychopathology manifest by depression, apathy, and withdrawal. Even at this age suicide is a real possibility. The etiology of school failure differs with socioeconomic status and subculture. In the lower socioeconomic groups it is not unusual for children to turn off. The great promise that achievement, conformity, and hard work will pay off in later life with job, status, and independence does not seem to apply to life as they know it. Identifying and helping to "turn on" this type of child is at least as rewarding as the detection of an abdominal mass in an infant, and a good deal harder to achieve.

THE ADOLESCENT

The American Academy of Pediatrics has declared that pediatricians are responsible for the health care needs of children from birth to 21 years of age. Many pediatricians are poorly trained and uncomfortable in the care of adolescent patients. Their practice consists largely of younger children and they are comfortable with the techniques of communicating with the toddler and early school age child. Who is to care for the 44 million young people in the United States between the ages of 12 and 21 years? A problem-oriented approach might be to ask what are the problems of people in this age range.

There are problems related to specific health needs, which require specific health intervention. These represent such problems as unwanted pregnancy; venereal disease; drug and alcohol abuse; accidents, principally motor vehicles; delinquency; school failure; suicide; runaways; and precursors of chronic disease, such as obesity, hypertension, and heart disease.

It is clear that as long as physicians who encounter this age group regard the "school exam" or the "sports exam" as a legal chore, there will be little progress toward addressing these major problems. It is also obvious that many of these problems are societal in nature and not purely medical.

Operational Problems in the Care of Adolescents

Another group of unmet needs deals with how the organization of health care affects adolescents. The majority of the serious problems adolescents would like help with are of a highly confidential nature. Most parents still feel that physicians have a prime responsibility to them and not to the adolescent patient. Young people are acutely aware of this, and the majority of them do not feel that confidentiality is honored by the physician. While some states have laws that protect the confidential nature of communication between physicians and adolescent patients when it involves the treatment of venereal disease or pregnancy, the legal mantle does not shelter the physician and his patient in many other areas, such as contraception.

The right of the adolescent to determine what can or cannot be done to him without his consent is another issue that has serious implications for the relationship of the physician and his adolescent patient. What are the rights of the unmarried teenage woman who is pregnant? Can her mother or her physician force her to undergo a therapeutic abortion? What are the rights of the mentally retarded teenager in regard to hysterectomy or tubal ligation? There are no legal or ethical positions on these questions that achieve universal acceptance. In the absence of resolution of these and other important issues, the pediatrician, the parent, and the adolescent often are cast into antagonist roles inappropriate to a therapeutic relationship.

Interviewing for Specific Problems

The biologic landmark of adolescence is puberty. The acquisition of the ability to reproduce is central to this process. The central social and cultural thrust of this period is to achieve emancipation and independence. This involves separation from parents and preparation for a vocation. The prime psychologic process is to establish and confirm a sense of identity and to synthesize personality with the subculture of that particular time. It bears repetition that the sequence and tempo of these changes vary dramatically among individuals and result in a great degree of individual variation in the time of achievement of these tasks.

How can the pediatrician be a more effective advocate for the adolescent? There are some obvious changes he can make in the organization of his own practice. Setting aside one afternoon or evening for seeing adolescent patients in his office represents a first step. The adolescent can be intensely uncomfortable in a waiting room peopled by infants and preschool children. The reception staff requires special training to emphasize their approach to these patients and the importance of confidentiality.

The supporting staff required will depend to some extent on the socioeconomic group being served and by the interests of the physician. In all groups, it can be anticipated that psychosocial problems will represent a significant proportion of the patient volume. Where problems of school failure form a substantial portion of the volume, the physician requires professionals skilled in other disciplines to assist in the evaluation of the child and family. Some physicians in private practice utilize part-time skills of a social worker and/or an educational psychologist. It requires good management skills to identify the appropriate volume of patients who can be evaluated within a given time span and to predict the amount of ancillary input necessary to provide parents and children with guidance and placement. In many cases, the input of the physician will be minimal. Occasionally, these skills can be obtained from other interested agencies, such as schools or service agencies. The advantage of a central facility is that interprofessional communication is enhanced and the responsibility for outlining a program is clearly in the hands of one person or group.

The conduct of the interview is of crucial importance. In addition to the traditional function of gathering and weighing information, the physician can use the interview for establishing certain ground rules with both the parent and the adolescent. Perhaps the most important message to be delivered is that the pediatrician is the adolescent's physician and that confidentiality will be observed.

An opportunity for both the parent and the adolescent to relate the problem as they see it should be afforded. Some physicians prefer to see the parents separately and then the adolescent. Another method is to see them both concurrently and get some appreciation of the dynamic and style of the family transactions. Depending on the age and maturation of the adolescent, and the cultural background of the family, it may not be wise to separate parent and child during the first visit. In older, sexually mature adolescents, separate interviews and examination are usually helpful. The separate interview implicitly states that separation and independence are facts of life, and explicitly defines the responsibility of the physician to the adolescent.

The history should include specific items not usually included in routine pediatric histories. In female patients, it should be determined, if possible, whether the mother received diethylstilbesterol during the pregnancy because of the probable increased risk of vaginal adenosis in women so treated as fetuses. Many physicians find it of value to have the adolescent fill out a separate history form with specific questions about how they regard the state of their health; some questions about how they perceive themselves in terms of body image ("How do you feel about your weight?"); questions about peer relationships, school performance and work load; career goals; and habits. Specific opportunity should be afforded to give them a choice about talking to the doctor, nurse, or social worker about smoking, venereal disease, future plans, birth control, drugs and alcohol, diet, medication, and exercise.

The physical examination should include visual and hearing screening in addition to a general examination. In sexually active females, a pelvic examination including a Papanicolaou smear, culture for gonococcus, and preparations for examination for trichomonas and yeast made. A nurse attendant is essential in preparing the patient for the examination and to provide support during the examination. While many young women have had previous pelvic examinations, it is best to explain what the procedure entails prior to and during the examination. In some clinic settings where women physicians, nurse midwives, or pediatric nurse practitioners are available, young women patients should be given an opportunity to select a woman caretaker.

Special situations arise with the adolescent patient, which are not commonly encountered with the younger child and require special management The uncommunicative adolescent who slouches in his chair, maintains no eye contact, and answers inquiries in low toned monosyllables is a vexing challenge for the physician. Calm reflection about how the adolescent got to the office in the first place is a helpful first step. One of the prime reasons behind this behavior is anger because of the referral. Most often, the adolescent has had no part in the decision that brings him to the physician. He is there because an anxious or irate parent dragged him there or because school or the court ordered him to appear. He views the physician as part of the system he is failing in, and he bristles with hostility. Letting the patient know that the physician realizes how rough life can be can often be communicated by a supporting comment such as: "You seem pretty angry. I'll bet there are places you'd rather be than here." Frequently this will allow an outpouring of resentment that will give the physician some insight into the patient's feelings and allow him to explore the nature of the real problem.

Occasionally, this strategy does not work and the physician is faced with a virtually mute patient. At times this may be due to poor verbal or communicative skills on the part of the patient, but more often it is a reflection that the patient has "turned off." Pursuit of a long protracted history in the face of this type of reaction is counterproductive and it is surprising how often focusing on a concrete issue for a short time can turn the situation around. It is sometimes helpful to strike a contract with the patient for a certain time period or visit sequence where very specific and concrete issues are to be addressed and resolved.

The mute patient who is angry should be differentiated from the depressed adolescent. The incidence of suicide is relatively high and on the increase in this age group. Early identification and treatment of the depressed patient is the best method of prevention. Depression can be masked under the normal mood swings of adolescence. It is not uncommon for days of intense physical activity and exuberance to be followed by days of long daytime naps and sloth-like dragging about the house. The mood swings tend to be brief, but when a protracted change involving a change of dress to slovenly, a marked decrease and disinterest in school performance, a shutting off of peer contact, and a withdrawal from family and social activities is detected, depression must be considered. Sometimes it comes cloaked in the garb of somatic complaints, acting out, hypochondriasis, or drug taking. Obese adolescents are frequently isolated, fail to achieve normal psychosocial tasks, and become depressed.

Sometimes broaching the subject of suicide directly by asking a question such as, "Many young people when they are down or unhappy think about dying or harming themselves. Have you ever worried about this?" allows the patient to admit the depth of his depression. The management of the patient at risk for suicide requires a commitment to ready availability. In most instances psychiatric consultation is indicated.

At the opposite end of the communication scale from the mute patient is the adolescent who moves rapidly into the area of deep feelings on the first or second interview. This can represent tricky ground for the physician. Frequently, the adolescent on reflection feels that all of his innermost secrets have been divulged, he is frightened by the depth of his own feelings and poor control he has over them, and is ashamed to renew the contact with the physician. The physician can avoid this problem during the interview by controlling the outpouring of material. This can be achieved by insisting on focusing on one issue and when the volume or the nature of the outflow seems to be excessive, to close off the interview and make an appointment for later that week.

The issue of frequency of appointments for the adolescent with psychosocial problems is important. Seeing a patient twice weekly during the initial phases of problem resolution can be very supporting. The interviews do not need to be excessive in length and should be structured so that excessive rambling is not tolerated. After some element of trust has been established the physician can allow the patient some input in the decision about frequency of visits. It is not uncommon for the patient to disappear for a protracted period only to return full of news and exuberance to pick up the relationship. The key qualities for the physician to have are tolerance and patience.

In communication with professional colleagues about their patients, physicians must be circumspect about revealing confidential material. If the physician wishes to communicate with previous physicians, the school, the juvenile court, or other agencies who have dealt with the adolescent in the past, he should ask the patient for his permission and explain the reason for the communication.

COMPLAINT-SPECIFIC VARIABLES

In the previous section, the age of the child was the chief variable. The emphasis was on the developmental tasks characteristic of each specific age for children and their parents; the behavior characteristics which result in the pursuit of task attainment; and the psychopathology characteristic of each age. On this framework, the problems encountered by the pediatric physician in the history and physical examination were considered and tentative solutions suggested. In this section, the encounters of the pediatrician and the child are considered in the context of the complaint or problem which brings the two together. While the last section dealt primarily with routine health supervision and develop-

mental issues, this section deals with how the pediatrician functions in settings where parents or adolescents appear with specific problems. The visit may be occasioned by fear and anxiety on the part of the parent; the desire of an adolescent for advice on birth control; a referral from a school, court, or social agency prompted by failure, truancy, or crime; a harried call from an obstetrician who has a mother with a labor progressing poorly. Each of these encounters requires a different approach, the exercise of different sets of skills, and widely disparate expectations on the part of the parent or adolescent as to what the result of the visit will bring. A few illustrations follow.

The Complicated Labor

The pediatrician should be involved in the labor and delivery of several types of stressed fetuses. (see p 140). There is an increasing tendency for neonatologists to care for these infants in perinatal regional centers. Pediatricians still must be responsible for infants in areas not served by these centers. The pediatrician who refers a stressed infant to a neonatal intensive care unit can continue to play a vital supportive role for the family. While mothers and families are encouraged to visit the units as frequently as possible, there are often barriers to communication beyond the distance barrier, which increase parental anxiety. The primary pediatrician can act as the interpreter and advocate of the family. He knows their strengths, weaknesses, and needs and can provide the support which is so important at that time. By an empathetic and timely presence, he can allow the mother to verbalize her fantasies and be relieved of the terrible isolation she feels at that time. This task is no mere "hand holding"—it is a skill of the most delicate sort, and compassion for which families are eternally grateful.

The Visit for Acute Illness

In the section on the pediatric interview it was duly noted that the concerns and expectations of the parent or child for a particular visit should be routinely explored. This is particularly true of the unscheduled visit where the child is brought in for an acute illness. Mothers frequently have terrible fantasies about what a given illness may represent—a swollen cervical lymph node is leukemia; a headache is meningitis, etc. Concerns and fears can be explored directly and the subsequent physical examination can help assuage irrational concerns.

Even though the duration of this type of visit is brief, the essential features of exploring concerns, ascertaining expectations, giving a diagnosis in simple, nonjargon terms, and outlining a prognosis and treatment plan must be included.

The Well-Child Visit

The problems arising during the first 2 years of life have been outlined in the section on age-specific variables and in Table 2. The specific areas, which should be dealt with in every encounter, are family dynamics particularly looking at maternal support structures; maternal child interaction; current diet; developmental status of the child; height and weight on every visit and head circumference three to four times throughout the first year (these measurements should be plotted on a growth grid); the physical status of the child including clinical evaluation of vision and hearing as determined by physical examination; an updating of the immunization status; anticipatory guidance appropriate for age; and plans for the next visit. Nurse practitioners and physician's assistants can perform the majority of these evaluations, with the pediatrician examining the child at prescribed visits or being used as a consultant by his colleagues when needed.

The Comprehensive Care Visit

Every solo practitioner, group practice, neighborhood health center, or clinic should have a set of baseline data on patients for whom he or it assumes ongoing responsibility. Each group should make the decision on what the minimal data set should be for its particular organizational pattern.

The health assessment should include a history which specifically covers the prenatal, perinatal, and postnatal events; a nutritional history; an immunization history; growth and development assessment including current social and intellectual functioning; a past history including system review, illnesses, accidents, hospitalizations, and operations; a family history; a physical examination including height, weight, head circumference, pulse, respirations, and blood pressure; a hearing and visual screening test; a current developmental screening test; laboratory data which should reflect the risk factors of age, sex, race. An assessment should be made of the problems of the patient including social problems and a plan for resolving or addressing the identified problems articulated.

At the initial visit the physician should advise the parent and child or adolescent of the projected scope of the investigation in terms of time and cost. Procedures that require blood-letting or injections should be carefully examined prior to the actual performance. More complex procedures should be explained in detail as to the necessity of the procedure, and what is hoped to be accomplished; the physician must inform the parent of the risks and the hazards involved.

Referrals and Consultations

The referral communication should be clear about what the referring physician expects to happen as a result of the encounter. A referral usually implies that the patient is referred for a specific problem which the consulting physician will manage for the duration of that problem. The referring physician may continue to administer primary care on an ongoing basis and/or to monitor the underlying problem which stimulated the referral on a day-to-day basis. The decision is usually a mutual one based on the complexity of the problem, the distance separating the patient and the specialist, the styles of the physicians, and the desires of the patient.

Consultations should be sought under the following circumstances:

When the primary care physician is not certain of the diagnosis and/or treatment and he needs more expert opinion.

When the primary care physician has arrived at a diagnosis, but the treatment must come from a specialist in another discipline. An example of this is an infant with pyloric stenosis who requires surgery.

In severe, life-threatening illness such as leukemia. Parents feel more secure when a physician who is an expert in the field has corroborated the diagnosis of a chronic or fatal illness.

When the physician anticipates the wishes of the family for a consultant. This occurs most often when the diagnosis remains in doubt. This allows the physician to select the most competent consultant in the field, rather than having the family surreptitiously consult less competent professionals in their anxiety to do everything possible for their child.

Occasionally complex and obscure disease is found in a child. The symptoms and clinical course do not fit into a neat organ system and the primary care physician must seek out several consultations. This situation requires strength, tact, and wisdom on his part. He is responsible for coordinating the various recommendations, synthesizing the information gained, and making treatment and management decisions. He must take the responsibility for communicating the opinions of the specialists to the family in terms they understand. Deviations from recommendations should be explained to both the parents and the specialists. In the setting of the teaching hospital it is particularly commonplace for parents to fall between the cracks and get little or distorted information. Parents are baffled by the array of students, housestaff, fellows, and attending physicians from various specialty services and disciplines. The most constructive position for the primary physician to assume is that of the physician-manager, where he assumes the responsibility for coordinating, integrating, and implementing the barrage of information and suggestions which swirl about the patient. Every physician is not equipped by training, temperament, or commitment to assume this role, but it is essential that he defines his role clearly for the family and his professional colleagues.

The Chronic Disease Visit

Current best estimates are that there are 3.1 million children, or 1 child in 8 in the age group 6 to 11 years who have one or more significant cardiovascular, neurologic, musculoskeletal, or other physical abnormality. In the age group 12 to 17 years there are an estimated 4.9 million, or 1 out of 5 with such abnormalities. The average pediatric practice will have 7 to 8 percent of its total encounters with children who have chronic conditions.

The type of chronic conditions seen by the pediatrician is headed by allergic diseases; of these, asthma is the most serious. Other chronic conditions of modest frequency are visual and hearing problems, cardiovascular, renal, and neurologic and musculoskeletal problems; and less frequently metabolic problems, such as diabetes mellitus.

The initial interview with the family of a child with a newly diagnosed severe chronic illness is a challenge worthy of the most gifted and sensitive physician. The interview should be conducted with both parents present in intact families, and with the parent and a supporting family member in divorced or separated couples. The setting of the interview is important. It should not be held in an open ward or a corridor, but in a private place where there are no interruptions or diversions. On some occasions, the pediatrician will be in the role of a consultant and will not know the family well. This is an opportunity to take advantage of one of the family's expectations—that is, that they are dealing with an expert who has some answers—and get to know something about how that family functions. The short time this takes allows the family to gain composure and represents a wise investment of time.

The physician then can proceed with an explanation of his findings. Many children with diseases in this category have been seen by multiple physicians during the evolution of the disease, and frequently a diagnosis has not been established. One of the first priorities is to advise the family that a diagnosis has been established. At this time, it is sometimes helpful to attach a qualifier such as, "It is *not* cancer or leukemia." This often is greeted by a great show of relief and at that juncture some of the fears of the parents can be explored.

A full explanation of the anatomic and physiologic consequences of the disease should follow. For some disease processes it is helpful to illustrate this with drawings (if the physician has the slightest talent) or by the use of prepared illustrations from texts. An outline of the treatment plan with an honest assessment of the risks and hazards of further procedures should follow. Parents can usually summon up sufficient courage and stamina to face a hospitalization of some length complicated by painful procedures, but the ultimate prognosis of the child is what really interests them. In dealing with this issue the physician should be candid and honest, but in most cases the positive aspects can be stressed. The most sensitive and circumspect physician can expect a show of grief by one or more of the parents. This can be viewed as therapeutic, and the manner in which other family members behave during this interlude gives the physician insight into how the family deals with stress. Even at this early phase, the physician should recall that families of children with severe chronic illness are at special risk for divorce and separation.

During the course of the acute phases of a newly diagnosed chronic illness, it is not unusual for parents to ask the same set of questions over and over. Inexperienced physicians are often exasperated that after a long and detailed explanation the parents have not absorbed even the most basic information. Parents unconsciously block out long sequences of the physician's monologue because of grief at the announced diagnosis and because their psychic tolerance for more bad news has been exceeded. It does no harm to reinforce the points they missed or suppressed, and it is essential to repeat it in a calm, unhurried manner.

After the critical storm of the first days or weeks following diagnosis is weathered, the far more demanding phase of navigating the uncharted sea of family dynamics is entered. The child must return to his family setting and reenter the process of interaction in an altered state. The nature of his disability conditions his own and his family's response. If he has a visible disfiguring condition such as facial scars following an accident, he will be perceived in a different manner than if he has a disability without visible signs, such as asthma or diabetes mellitus. It is important for the physician to know how the child and his parents "accept" the condition. Parents who "overaccept" the disability tend to coddle, overprotect, and perpetuate overdependence of the child. Those who "underaccept" or "nonaccept" may treat the child with ambivalence and rejection. Either extreme leads to erosion of the child's self-image. The late Bronson Crowthers emphasized how family attitudes affected the functional outcome for children with disability. One family consisted of an extended Italian-American family where the father was a railroad worker. One of their daughters had severe spastic quadriplegia with mild mental retardation. She functioned well in her setting, performing domestic chores and receiving warmth and support from her siblings. The other family was a branch of one of the distinguished New England puritan class. The father had achieved fame as an Ivy League football player and currently was a successful stockbroker. His only son had mild hemiplegia and normal intelligence. Each evening father would drag his reluctant son out on the extensive lawn and they would religiously practice kicking and passing the football. The boy subsequently became seriously depressed.

It is the physician's duty to learn what the child's reaction to his illness is, how the family perceives the child with the illness, and how the child reacts in turn with his family members. This takes time, but it is necessary because it has a direct effect on compliance with treatment plans and functional outcome. Adequate time must be set aside for conferences with the parent and child. The symptoms of the child cause reverberations throughout the family structure. The physical symptoms of the child may allow the family to skirt around intrafamilial conflict under the guise of great concern for the child. The ill child is used as a conflict-avoidance tool.

As the physician becomes more familiar with his patient and family he is in a better position to assess their pattern of adaptation. Several characteristic behavioral patterns are noted in children and adolescents who adapt poorly to their chronic disorder. One group is the fearful, inactive children, who are frequently markedly dependent on their mothers. They usually lack outside friends and interests, and mother cares for their most rudimentary needs. They present a picture of passive-dependent personality development. Children with chronic continuous symptomatology from inflammatory bowel disease frequently present this picture. Another group consists of the overly daring, vigorous young children who engage in prohibited or risk-taking behavior. They employ denial of fear or unpleasant consequences for their acts. Children with hemophilia often adopt this reaction pattern, and it is not uncommon for the adolescent with diabetes mellitus or asthma to ignore their medication schedules. A third pattern of personality maladjustment is the shy withdrawn child who becomes increasingly hostile as an adolescent. These patterns should be looked for, and when identified, the physician should attempt intervention if he has skills in family therapy, or enlist the help of a family therapist. All too often the adolescent with diabetes mellitus who has multiple admissions for ketoacidosis is characterized as having "brittle" diabetes. A look beyond his insulin requirements will frequently reveal a seething, bitter person who denies his difference from others by forgetting to administer his insulin.

There are multiple patterns employed by pediatricians for caring for children with chronic illness. The same pediatrician may employ several different patterns within his practice, depending on the disease and the relationship with the consultant.

The pattern most worthy of well-trained pediatricians is for the pediatrician to assume the responsibility for the total care of the patient. In order to achieve this the pediatrician must satisfy certain criteria, some of which are organizational, but the most important aspects are personal. In the latter category is commitment to the concept of total care. The organizational requirements are that sufficient time be routinely set aside for conferences with the patients and parents; that other professionals be available to the pediatrician in the practice setting—nurse practitioners and social worker constitute one model; and that the pediatrician and the organ specialists he uses for referral understand the system and communicate freely.

The Child in Hospital

The decision to hospitalize a child should be made only after alternative modes of diagnosis and treatment have been considered. There are situations where the indication is clear—the suspected acute abdomen, a poisoning requiring treatment and observation, severe trauma, acute obstructive airway problems, the neonate or young infant suspected of sepsis, the child with meningitis, and many other illnesses. There are other situations where the indications are not clear-cut, such as with infants who are failing to grow at the expected rate, a child with a chronic illness who is not responding in the expected manner to a therapeutic plan. The physician should have clear-cut objectives to be achieved by the hospitalization and they should be explained to the family.

The psychologic impact of hospitalization must be anticipated and steps taken to modify adverse factors. The young child between the ages of 6 months and 4 years appears most vulnerable to the hospital experience. The separation from parents, the unfamiliarity with the hospital setting and procedures, the nursing and support staff who are strangers, the child's fantasies about the meaning of his illness, and his perceptions of parental fear and anxiety make the experience an indelible memory. Regressive behavior is not uncommon following hospitalization. A recurrence of bedwetting or fecal soiling, thumb sucking, night terrors, and fear of parental separation are some of the more obvious sequelae of hospitalization. These can be ameliorated by liberal visiting hours and overnight facilities for parents, special training for the nursing staff in the needs of hospitalized children, a child life program to integrate the recreational and educational activities of the child while in hospital, and when possible a preparation for the hospital experience. The latter may consist of a visit to the hospital prior to admission or a review of printed and illustrated literature designated in the form of a child's book that relates many of the experiences the child will have.

THE MEDICAL RECORD. Every hospitalized child should have a complete history and physical examination recorded. A suggested format follows, but it should be emphasized that the problem-oriented medical record is an equally valid method for presenting patient management data. Debates as to the superiority of one method over the other are based on opinion and preference and not on solid data.

THE HISTORY. The initial history should be as complete as possible (Table 6). However, it is desirable

---

TABLE 6. Suggested Outline for History and Physical Examination of Sick Patient

History

Chief complaint:

Source of history: Mother, father, doctor's note, with estimate of reliability.

Present illness: Chronologically, where possible, with dates. Initial symptom and date of onset; subsequent symptoms; pertinent negative data.

Past history

Birth

Date, where born, birth weight, respirations—spontaneous, or after resuscitation, presentation of fetus.

Parity of mother; term or premature; diet and lab studies during pregnancy; complications of pregnancy (bleeding, toxemic infections, etc); length, type, and complications of delivery; anesthesia during labor.

Table 6 (cont.)

Neonatal period

Cyanosis; pallor; convulsions; jaundice; hemorrhage; birth marks or deformities; respiratory or feeding difficulties.

Nutrition

Breast or bottle-fed—type of formula. Vitamins—type, when started, and when stopped. Orange juice. Age solids started—any food intolerances. Appetite—weight at 1 mo, 6 mo, 1 yr, and present.

Development

Smiled; head up; rolled over; reached for objects; sat without support; stood, with and without support; walked; first tooth; first words. Toilet training—when began and when successfully completed.
Age started school—scholastic and social achievement; present grade in school.

Habits and personality

Hours of sleep, dreams, nightmares; exercise; thumb-sucking; nail-biting; tantrums; breath-holding; tics; enuresis; encopresis; masturbation; pica; social adjustment— hostile, aggressive, submissive, friendly, etc.

Immunization (indicate source of information: health department record, mother, school record). Date, type of reaction, and boosters. Smallpox, diphtheria, pertussis, tetanus, polio (Salk/oral), measles, mumps, rubella; BCG.

Tuberculin tests: tine or PPD.

Previous illnesses (age, severity, complications, and sequelae): Contagion—measles, mumps, varicella, rubella, pertussis, etc. Other medical illnesses—hospitalized? If so, when, where, and for how long, therapy received, final diagnosis. Surgical conditions—date and place of operation. Accidents, fractures, etc.

Allergy: Eczema, asthma, hay fever, hives, food or drug sensitivities to penicillin, sulfas, etc.

System review (list only positives)
Head, eyes, ears, nose, and throat: Headache, head trauma. Eyes—vision, glasses, squint, inflammatory disease. Ears—hearing, otitis, discharge. Nose—discharge, epistaxis. Mouth—gingivitis, condition of teeth, date of last dental visit. Throat—tonsillitis, recurrent pharyngitis.

Respiratory: Chronic cough, frequent URIs, previous pneumonia, exposure to tuberculosis, previous chest x-ray.

Cardiac: History of murmurs, dyspnea, orthopnea, cyanosis, acute rheumatic fever.

Gastrointestinal: Appetite and digestion, bowel habits, character and frequency of stools, jaundice, vomiting, hematemesis, passage of worms.

Genitourinary: Circumcised; dysuria; hematuria; polydipsia; nocturia, frequency. Onset of menarche in females.

Neuromuscular: Tremors, convulsions, weakness or paralysis, polio.

Joints: Arthritis or arthralgia; loss of mobility.

Hematologic disorders: Hemorrhages, anemia, bleeding tendency.

Recent onset of infection

Family history

Parents and grandparents: age, occupation, state of physical and emotional health; if parents are not living, age at death, cause, and nature of symptoms.

Siblings: age, state of health, and where living (if not living, age of death, cause, and nature of symptoms).

Familial illnesses or anomalies: tuberculosis, syphilis, diabetes, cancer, epilepsy, rheumatic fever, allergy, hereditary blood dyscrasias, mental retardation, dystrophies, congenital anomalies, heredo-degenerative diseases.

Family pedigree: if existence of a genetic anomaly is suspected.
  Persons included: Begin pedigree with the patient (identified by arrow—proband or propositus); then include, as a minimum, the following living or dead relatives in this order: siblings (record in order of birth, with eldest on left); parents (father, and male ancestors in general, on left); father's siblings; all descendants of father's siblings; father's parents; mother's siblings; all descendants of mother's siblings; mother's parents; all descendants of case and his siblings.
  Information required: As each relative, living or dead, is added to pedigree, inquire whether or not relative has had: same affliction as propositus, any other chronic disorder or defect.

Table 6 (cont.)

Pedigree symbols

□ Male	○ Female	◇ Sex unknown
⑧ 8 persons, sex unknown	◇ Pregnancy	(□) Adopted
■ Examined, affected with trait	⊡ Examined, negative for trait	□ Reported normal for trait
□s Single	□—○ Marriage	□⚌○ Consanguineous marriage
□-¦-○ Illegitimacy	□⊥○ No offspring	○⌒○ Identical twins
○FR○ Fraternal twins	⊞ Reliability reported to have trait	⊡ Questionably reported to have trait

Small Symbols

□ ○ ◇ Lived less than one day	⊞ ⊕ ⬦ Stillbirth	⊡ ⊙ ◇ Miscarriage

Social history: Living circumstances: place and nature of dwelling; sleeping arrangements; number of persons living in home in addition to parents and children; relation of such persons to family members. *Economic circumstances:* members of family who work; working hours if unusual; general level of economic independence, support from community agencies if any. *Neighborhood circumstances:* available recreational and educational outlets in neighborhood.

Physical Examination

Temperature   Pulse   Respirations
Blood pressure   Surface area (m²)
Weight (kg) (%)   Height (cm) (%)
     percentiles for
     height and weight

(If less than 3%, indicate also age for which height and weight are in 50% group.)
(See percentile charts in Appendix.)
Head circumference   Chest circumference   (Percentiles)
     (%)   (%)

General appearance: age, sex, state of nutrition, attitude, position, sensorium, type of cry or voice, acutely or chronically ill, distress, gait; personality, intelligence, cooperation, interest in environment; gross developmental status for age.

Head: contour, bossing, texture of hair, scalp, fontanels—with dimensions in centimeters, if open, and comment on tension sutures; percussion and auscultation—parotid glands.

Eyes: pupils, sclerae, conjunctivae, extraocular movements, nystagmus, ptosis, squint, photophobia, vision, ophthalmoscopic exam.

Ears: hearing, discharge, canals; examination of drums—color, bulging, light reflex, perforation; mastoid tenderness.

Nose: patency of nares, flaring of alae nasi, discharge, obstruction, mucous membranes, and turbinates—swollen, red, pale, boggy; septum; sinus tenderness (frontal and maxillary).

Mouth and throat: lips: color, dryness, fissures, sores, herpes. *Tongue:* color, moisture, coating, fissures, ulcers, frenulum protrusion. *Breath. Teeth:* number, arrangement, caries. *Gums:* color, hypertrophy, bleeding, ulcers. *Buccal mucosa:* color, exudate, postnasal discharge, lymphoid tissue, palpation of adenoids in infants. *Epiglottis. Tonsils:* size, signs of inflammation, exudate, membrane. *Pillars.*

Neck: flexibility, swelling, thyroid enlargement, trachea in midline.

Lymph glands: size in centimeters, consistency, tenderness, mobility, fluctuation, discrete or matted, GGE.

Spine: curvature, tenderness along spinous process, mobility, CVA tenderness.

Thorax: contour, respiration, rate, regularity, abdominal or thoracic adequacy, and symmetry of expansion.

Lungs: percussion, palpation, fremitus, auscultation.

Cardiovascular: Heart: inspection, precordial bulge, apical heave. Palpation: PMI—diffuse or circumscribed, thrills, shocks. Percussion: heart borders. Auscultation: rhythm, character, and quality of sounds. M1 vs M2 vs A2. Murmurs: time, duration, location, intensity, transmission, alteration with change of position, with patient's exercise. Pulse: radial and femoral—rate and rhythm, volume.

Table 6 (cont.)

Abdomen: Inspection: contour, umbilicus, hernia, distension, veins, visible peristalsis. Percussion: fluid wave, shifting dullness, tympanites, bladder, liver, spleen. Also a good method for localizing point of tenderness. Palpation: tone, tenderness, direct or indirect rebound. Diastasis recti, masses, liver, spleen, kidneys, auscultation of bowel sounds.

Genitalia: Male: prepuce or circumcision, meatus; testes—descent, hydrocele. Female: external examination only—vulva, clitoris, discharge.

Rectal (can be deferred unless this examination is relevant to the child's illness on suspected condition): Fissures, hemorrhoids, prolapse, sphincter tone—masses, tenderness, stool in ampula.

Skin: texture, color, tissue turgor, temperature, moisture, icterus, cyanosis, eruption, scars, ecchymosis, petechiae, spiders, desquamation, hemangiomata, mongolian spots, nevi.

Extremities: tone, color, warmth; clubbing, cyanosis, mobility of joints, hip abduction in infants, with knees flexed. Feet: deformities, decreased ankle movements.

Neurologic

Mental state: intelligence.
Motor: gait, stance, Romberg, muscle power, paresis, paralysis, spasticity, rigidity, flaccidity, clonus, carpopedal spasm, tics, tremors, athetosis, etc.

Tone: on palpation, ballottement, and stretching; flaccidity, hypotonia, hypertonus, spasticity, rigidity, cogwheel phenomenon.

Cranial nerves

I. Smell

II. Sight, visual fields, optic disks—sensory arc of pupillary constriction.

III. Elevation of upper lids. EOM—superior, inferior, medical recti, inferior oblique, motor arc of pupillary constriction (dilation if via cervical sympathetics).

IV. EOM—superior oblique.

V. Motor—muscles of mastication—jaw jerk; jaw deviates to side of lesion; sensory—sensation to face, forehead, lips, tongue buccal mucosa, eyes; sensory arc of corneal reflex.

VI. External rectus.

VII. Peripheral lesion—paralysis of all mimetic muscles, widened palpebral fissure with inability to close eye, often associated with increased tearing; loss of taste on anterior 2/3 of tongue; loss of motor arc or corneal reflex; supranuclear lesion—weakness of lower 1/2 of face; no loss of taste; involuntary expressions of emotion are intact and symmetrical.

VIII. Auditory—hearing—vesticular nystagmus, vertigo.

IX. Taste on posterior 1/3 of tongue—elevation of palate, sensory arc of gag reflex.

X. Swallowing, elevation of epiglottis, movements of vocal cords. Cranial—deviation of uvula away from side of lesion. Spinal—innervates sternomastoid and trapezius; atrophy, drooping, and inability to shrug shoulders; poor head turning against resistance (away from side of weakness).

XI. Tongue movements; tongue atrophy; tongue moves toward side of lesion.

Reflexes: 2+ is normal. Deep tendon biceps, triceps, radial, knee, ankle, Chvostek sign. *Superficial*—abdominal, cremasteric. *Abnormal*—Hoffmann, Babinski, Kerning, Brudzinski, "tache cerebrale." *In infants*—grasp, suck, Moro, root tonic neck.

Sensory system: superficial and deep sensations; pinprick, touch, sense of position, vibratory sense.

Cerebellar signs: incoordination, ataxia, intention tremor, passpointing, dysdiadochokinesia, rebound phenomenon, slurred speech, nystagmus, or extreme lateral gaze.

Special senses: hearing—response to loud sounds, normal voice, whispers; vision—moving lights or objects, charts in older children.

Formulation should include

A brief summary of pertinent history and physical findings.
A discussion of the differential diagnosis, and of the problem as presented by the patient.
The diagnosis or diagnoses.
Plan for diagnostic work-up in order of importance.

Plan

All diagnostic studies planned, diet, therapeutic regimen.

to review the history repeatedly. During the course of a specific illness, certain parts of the history may assume increased importance and require more detailed inquiry. Also, it should be realized that the initial history of an acutely ill child is usually taken at a time when the mother or other informant is under considerable stress, and reviewing the data at a later occasion may yield important additional information. Certain aspects of the history, particularly those concerning psychologic factors, depend upon a relationship between the physician and the family, which takes time to develop. It is apparent that continuity of care, which provides an ongoing relationship, also contributes to better interpretation of the history.

FAMILY HISTORY. It is important to obtain information about the age, physical condition, and state of health of each parent and member of the family. A listing of the mother's pregnancies in chronologic order may provide important information regarding miscarriages and abortions. If any brothers or sisters have died, the date and cause of death should be recorded. Acute illness of recent date in a member of the household may be the source of infection. Of equal importance is the history of chronic infection, particularly tuberculosis, in any household contact. When a heritable condition is suspected, information should be gathered regarding its distribution in the family and among forebears; this applies to a wide spectrum of diseases, including allergy, rheumatic disease, diabetes, renal disease, congenital malformations, inborn errors of metabolism, anomalies of growth and development, degenerative diseases of the nervous system, and mental disorders. Particular attention should be directed to exploring the possibility of consanguineous marriage. A knowledge of the environment may indicate exposure to specific infections, or toxins.

PAST HISTORY. The type of inquiry will depend in large part on the age of the patient. The outline which follows is designed chiefly as a guide in management of problems of the infant.

Pregnancy. The mother should be questioned regarding the duration of pregnancy, her attitude toward it, her health during that period, and any factors which might have had a harmful effect on the child, such as infections, hemorrhage, drugs, or x-ray radiation. The mother's blood group and Rh factor status, if known, should be recorded.

Birth and Neonatal Period. One should inquire about the character of labor, and sedation used, whether delivery was spontaneous or instrumental, prolonged or precipitate—and about the condition and vigor of the infant at birth—whether there was difficulty of resuscitation, early cyanosis, jaundice, eruptions, hemorrhage, or convulsions. Knowledge about the mother's response to the infant after delivery and on returning home may help in understanding subsequent problems in the mother-child relationships.

Feeding. The early feeding history should be explored regarding duration of breastfeeding, reasons for weaning, formulas used for artificial feeding and reasons for changes, and use of vitamin supplements. The child's approximate daily food intake should be ascer-tained, together with information regarding dietary habits. One should ascertain the attitude of the parents toward the child's eating, noting whether the child is forced, entreated, threatened, or rewarded.

Growth and Development. If a height and weight record is not available, one must depend on general statements as to how the child thrived at different periods. A history of dentition serves as an index of maturation. So also does the age when the anterior fontanel closed. Other developmental landmarks should be recorded: the age at which the child first smiled, held his head erect, recognized people or objects, sat alone, stood with support and alone, crawled, walked, used words and sentences. The behavior development of a normal child during the first years is a subject with which the physician should be familiar if he would detect early those differences, often slight at this age, in children whose development is retarded.

PAST ILLNESSES.

Infectious Diseases: The following should be considered: attacks of infectious diseases with details as to duration, severity, and complications.

Respiratory System: Occurrence of respiratory infections along with their severity, manifestations, durations, and complications, such as otitis media, bronchitis, pneumonia.

Cardiovascular System: Occurrence of cyanosis, dyspnea, excessive sweating during infancy, fatigability, syncope, joint pains, and epistaxis.

Gastrointestinal System: History of early feeding difficulties, diarrhea, constipation, abnormalities of the stools (size, odor, color, presence of blood, mucus, or pus), and vomiting; associated with infections or emotional upsets; relation to certain foods; and occasional or habitual.

Genitourinary System: Infections of the urinary tract, hematuria, dysuria, frequency, urgency, dribbling, enuresis, edema, and oliguria; repeated bouts of unexplained fever.

Nervous System: Convulsions; if they have occurred, details regarding circumstances of their occurrence.

Operations and Injuries: Dates, nature, and complications of all operations and serious injuries.

Immunizations: The dates of all immunizations and tests for immunity.

PSYCHOLOGIC INVESTIGATION. Information about a child's general adjustment and about his reaction to a specific illness should be an integral part of the history. The occurrence of such symptoms as restlessness, irritability, tantrums, night terrors, and tics should be noted, as well as indications of how a child gets along with his peers at play and at school and with his siblings and parents. Some indication of the attitude of the parents toward the child can also be obtained from appropriate questions in the history.

PRESENT ILLNESS. As definite a statement as possible should be obtained as to when the child was last quite well, whether the onset of the illness was abrupt or gradual, and with what particular symptoms it began. The mother should then be allowed to give her own account of the illness without interruption. Attention should be paid to the chronology of the appearance of symptoms and each should be traced up to the time of the visit. Medications used should be noted.

THE EXAMINATION. The success of the examination (Table 6) will depend on the approach of the examiner. This is discussed in detail in the previous section. In examining infants, it is helpful to use a pacifier.

GENERAL INSPECTION. In acute disease, much of importance can be learned from simple observation. The following features may serve as examples.

The state of physical development in relation to the child's age should be noted: Is he robust or frail? His posture of choice should be observed—whether he lies on the side, back, or face, the state of flexion of the extremities, and whether the head is drawn back. The type and amount of spontaneous activity may disclose a tendency to spare or protect some part of the body and will reveal whether the child is restless and excitable, or drowsy and apathetic. One may note the color of the skin, whether it is pale or cyanotic or jaundiced, and the presence of rashes or focal lesions, their character and distribution. It is important to observe facial expression, whether it is alert or dull, peaceful or anxious, and whether the features are contracted from time to time as if in pain. Respiratory difficulty may be limited to inspiration, or to expiration, or may involve both phases of respiration. Inspiratory retraction—suprasternal, supracavicular, infrasternal, or intercostal—should be noted. One hemithorax may show an inspiratory lag, or the breathing may be predominantly costal or abdominal in type, suggesting paralysis of one or another group of respiratory muscles. Nasal obstruction is usually accompanied by snorting or mouth breathing.

It is important, though not always easy, to determine whether a child cries from fear or from pain. The cry of pain may be distinctive; it may be accompanied by some attempt at localization, as when a child puts his hand to an inflamed part; but in infancy the pain of acute inflammation is often indicated only by general restlessness and irritability.

MEASUREMENTS. *Body Measurements are of greatest value in chronic diseases.* They also serve as a point of reference for subsequent progress. The important measurements are the head and chest circumferences, the weight, and the body length or height.

In taking the circumference of the head the largest measurement (over the occipital and frontal eminences) is preferable. The measurement of the chest is usually taken over the nipples. The body length of an infant is best taken on a measuring table or with a portable board as the child lies upon his back on the table or a firm bed. For older children a measuring rod or a fixed measuring board is convenient. The measurements should be compared with normal averages.

Pulse, Respiration, and Temperature. The rate, regularity, and quality of the pulse should be noted. In young children, pulse rate is less important than its force and quality. A slow, irregular pulse is always significant; a slight irregularity of the pulse during sleep has no special significance. Furthermore, the pulse rate varies normally with respiration in many children. The pulse rate is greatly increased by slight disturbances; the approach of a stranger or the examination by the physician may cause it to rise 20 or 30 beats. In acute disease, a pulse rate of 150 to 180/minute is often seen when other symptoms are not particularly severe.

The rate, depth, and rhythm of respiration should be noted. The last often cannot be determined except by watching the child attentively for several minutes. In premature and very young infants a rather marked irregularity may be seen. In the very young, it is not to be taken as indicating a cerebral lesion, since newborn infants frequently have irregular respiration. The respiratory rate is proportionately greater in infants than in adults. In pneumonia and acute bronchiolitis it not infrequently rises to 70–80/minute.

In general, the temperature of infants and very young children should be taken in the rectum. In many hospital nurseries for newborn infants, especially in premature units, axillary temperatures are taken as a routine. Under normal conditions the rectal temperature varies between 36.4 and 37.6 C.

Except in young infants, who may have little or no fever even with severe infections, the increase in body temperature from infections or from any other cause tends to be greater in infants and children than it does in adults. Moreover, high fever may be present in cases that are not serious. A continuous or recurring high temperature has greater significance.

Subnormal temperatures are commonly seen in premature infants, in whom the temperature may fall below 35 C. This phenomenon is also seen after defervescence of fevers of various kinds and in wasting diseases.

Blood Pressure. The measurement of blood pressure in infants and children is discussed in chap. 24.

MENTAL DEVELOPMENT. The first examination of every new patient, unless he is acutely or seriously ill, should include an evaluation of his intelligence. In the case of newborn infants, one has little to go on except facial expression. From the second month onward, however, an increasing variety of devices are at hand for determining the stage of mental development at which the patient has arrived for comparison with his chronologic age. These are discussed above (p. 52). The clinician, who is not primarily concerned with the formal calculation of an intelligence quotient, should nevertheless have at his command a sufficiently detailed understanding of the accomplishments a normal infant or child of a given age may be expected to perform, so that he may judge whether his patient is unusually bright, average, or retarded, and may thus be in a better position to evaluate the complaints, responses, and general behavior of his patient.

LOCAL EXAMINATION. Skin. The skin should first be inspected for eruptions, and it is important that the entire skin be examined so that distribution as well as the character of individual lesions may be appreciated. Marked wrinkling or loss of elasticity of the skin is one of the best indications of loss in weight. The rapidity with which a fold of skin and subcutaneous tissue pinched up in the thumb and finger resumes its normal contour when released is a convenient measure of dehydration. Edema may be localized or general, increasing or receding. Any large veins should be noted.

Superficial Lymph Nodes.   All lymph node areas should be examined, not only the cervical, axillary, and inguinal, but also the occipital, posterior cervical, pre- and retroauricular, submental, supraclavicular, and epitrochlear. Many healthy children will have moderate enlargement of the cervical, axillary, or inguinal nodes usually due to minor infections in the regions they drain. However, the cause of marked enlargement of any of these groups, or any enlargement of the epitrochlear nodes, should be thoroughly investigated.

Head.   One should note whether cranial sutures are ossified or unnaturally open or separated; also whether the fontanel is closed or, if open, whether it is depressed or bulging. Craniotabes should be tested for during the first year.

Eyes.   The condition of the conjunctivae and lids should be noted, as well as the presence of ptosis, strabismus, or other paralysis, but particularly the condition of the pupils, whether contracted or dilated, and the nature of their response to light. One should look also for the presence of corneal ulcers or opacities. The sclerae should be examined for jaundice. Examination of the eyegrounds and appraisal of visual acuity should not be neglected simply because the patient is young.

Ears.   Otoscopic examination of the ears must often be preceded by removal of cerumen see p. 963 .This can usually be accomplished by the use of a curette, care being taken to avoid trauma to the canal wall with resultant hemorrhage which may obscure the membrane. Small bits of wax may often be easily removed by means of a cotton applicator dipped in mineral oil. When the canal is filled with impacted cerumen, it is sometimes necessary to syringe the canal with warm water. The normal and abnormal tympanic membrane is described on p. 963 .

Examination of the eardrums should be a part of every routine physical examination; the drums should be carefully followed in all diseases involving the mouth, rhinopharynx, and the lower respiratory tract; in all communicable diseases; and in head trauma. In any acute febrile condition, and particularly when otorrhea already exists, one should look for tenderness or swelling over the mastoid bone.

Screening tests for gross abnormalities of hearing are an important part of the physical examination of infants and children.

Nose.   The appearance of the nasal mucosa should be noted and the character of any nasal discharge determined. In young infants, an abundant discharge tinged with blood should suggest syphilis; in older children, diphtheria. A chronic discharge should suggest paranasal sinusitis; chronic rhinorrhea after head injury, a fracture of the ethmoidal cribiform plate; and a purulent discharge from one side, a foreign body.

Mouth.   The appearance of the mucous membrane of the mouth and gums, as well as the teeth, often may be ascertained by watching the child while he is crying. It should be noted whether the tongue is dry or moist, clear or coated, whether thrush or any other form of stomatitis is present, and whether the gums are congested, swollen, or hemorrhagic. The number, position, and character of the teeth are important. The color of the mucous membrane may be significant. Cyanosis or pallor should be noted. On the mucous membrane of the hard palate may often be found the first local evidence of scarlet fever, in the form of a minute punctate eruption; the cheeks opposite the molar teeth may show the presence of Koplik spots, the earliest reliable sign of measles. The pharynx should be examined for inflammation, exudate, and membrane. The size and appearance of the tonsils should be noted, though size alone is not a reliable index of infection. A thorough though brief inspection of the entire pharynx may be made when the child gags as the tongue depressor is applied to the posterior part of the tongue. In children with laryngeal stridor it is possible in many instances to effect a brief inspection of the posterior structures of the mouth and pharynx during the inspiratory phase of crying, which may even bring an inflamed, edematous epiglottis into view.

Neck.   One should consider the position in which the head is held and the amount of rigidity of the cervical muscles. Considerable information may be derived in diseases of the nervous system by noting the ease with which the head is raised by the patient when the trunk is lifted from the supine to a sitting position.

Chest.   In young children particular importance should be attached to the shape and symmetry of the chest. Rickets and pulmonary or cardiac disease may produce striking alterations in the configuration of the thorax. One should also notice the recession of the soft parts—intercostal spaces, the suprasternal notch, or the epigastrium; the amount of this is usually the best means of judging the severity of dyspnea (see also Chap 15).

Heart.   In patients less than 2 years of age soft murmurs heard over the precordium are frequently functional. Marked sinus arrhythmia is a common finding in children (see also Chap 28).

Abdomen.   In very young patients shifting dullness is not infrequently demonstrable when ascites is absent. With free peritoneal fluid in significant amount, a fluid wave can be due to enlargement of an underlying organ, to weakness of overlying parietes, or to some pathologic structure, such as a tumor or cyst. The vigor of peristaltic activity in the intestinal tract can be judged to some extent by listening for approximately one minute while the stethoscope bell is applied to the abdominal wall in the region of the umbilicus. In infants whose gain in weight has been delayed for any reason, the pattern of intestinal coils often can be seen through the thin abdominal wall, with the slow writhing characteristic of normal peristaltic activity. Deep waves in the epigastrium, moving always from left to right, are gastric in orgin and usually denote pyloric or duodenal obstruction. Abdominal tenderness when present should be carefully evaluated and its distribution localized as soon as possible. The size and position of the liver and spleen are best determined by palpation. The lower border of the right lobe of the liver can usually be made out distinctly in patients less than 2 years of age. If the spleen can be felt easily below the ribs, it is, as a rule, enlarged. Umbilical hernia is common in the first year.

Spine. The spine should be carefully examined to detect variations from the normal, which are recognized by decreases or increases of the normal curves, and by the appearance of abnormal curvatures and protrusions. If found, it should be determined whether these are permanent, or reducible by change of posture.

Extremities. The color of the extremities and the character of the peripheral circulation should be noted, as well as any evidences of edema or hemorrhage in the form of punctuate or larger extravasations. Clubbing of the fingers and toes and any abnormality in the nails or desquamation of palms should be noted. In examining the extremities one should note especially the presence of tenderness, flaccidity, or rigidity of muscles, whether the limbs are wasted or plump, and the degree of muscular power, abnormal swelling on the shaft or near the ends of the bones, as well as the contours of the joints and their range of motion. In the patient of suitable age, provided he is not too ill, the gait and the posture assumed on sitting and standing should be observed.

Palpation of the femoral artery pulsation in the inguinal region should be a part of the physical examination of every patient seen for the first time; the most common cause of absent or weak femoral pulsation is coarctation of the aorta.

Reflexes. The tendon reflexes may be difficult to elicit in an infant at any one examination, and at another they may appear exaggerated. The plantar cutaneous reflex of Babinski in extension is normally present during the first year but takes on increasing pathologic significance thereafter. The abdominal reflexes can be regularly obtained after the age of 6 months and the cremasterics somewhat later; in children superficial reflexes may be active.

Genital Organs. Male children should be examined to determine the presence of hypospadias, phimosis, or undescended testicles. Hydrocele is a frequent condition and may be mistaken for hernia. In the female, it is important to recognize the existence of hymenal imperforation, labial fusion, vaginal atresia, or clitoral enlargement. Every vaginal discharge is significant, and, if purulent, should be examined bacteriologically. In both girls and boys the presence of sexual hair or abnormal pigmentation should be noted.

The obligation of the physician is to make all entries to the medical record legible. The medical record is a legal document used by others for the care of the patient. The enactment of federal legislation creating professional standards review organizations (PSRO) for the purpose of monitoring the quality of care has defined the accountability of physicians for this function; the review of medical records will be one of the forms of quality assurance. The record should include a statement of the problem, detailed history and physical examination, a formulation of diagnosis, a plan of approach, and frequent pertinent progress notes updating the information base, changes in the condition of the patient, success or failure in movement toward the therapeutic plan, the psychologic status of the patient and family. At discharge, a summary statement of the patient's experience during the hospital stay should include a diagnosis, specific treatment, operations or procedures, and a plan for the continuation of the program as an ambulatory patient.

On the day prior to discharge it is helpful to sit down with the parents to review what has transpired. This is the time to allay anxieties, review the management plan, and most important, to allow parents to ask questions. By assuring the parents of his availability, the physician cements his commitment and allows the parents to return home to face the convalescence with some confidence.

The physician's relationship to the child during the hospitalization will be somewhat dependent on the age of the child. Certain principles apply to most situations. The physician should appear optimistic and confident on all occasions. Particularly during hospitalization, the child perceives the physician as omnipotent and capable of controlling all of the forces of pain and discomfort. The child's feeling of helplessness must be recognized and dealt with. Depression and tears not infrequently greet the physician's visit and on occasion he must conduct painful or degrading examinations. Some of this stress can be avoided or minimized by letting the child know that the physician is aware that he or she has feelings and gently exploring them with the child. Trust is gained by cheerfulness, gentleness, honesty, and scrupulous attention to the child's privacy. In teaching settings the discussions about the patient's progress should be done out of sight and hearing of the patient and other patients. It is not uncommon for children to overhear discussion of other patients and think that the discussion refers to them. The choice of language is also important. Words such as "death" and expressions such as "going downhill" are to be avoided at all costs within ear range of children and parents. They serve to feed the fantasies of both and do irreparable harm.

IMMUNIZATION

The success of active immunization programs has resulted in a large number of pediatricians who have never seen a patient with diphtheria, tetanus, or polio, and only rarely will diagnose a child with measles or pertussis. There is little question that the active immunization of infants and children provides an effective tool for the prevention of disease and the promotion of health. A number of vaccines are currently available and can be used in a variety of ways. Several factors should be considered in the design of a schedule for active immunization. These include:

1. The current risk from the disease for which active immunization is available.
2. The efficacy and safety of the vaccines.
3. The most efficient manner in which to utilize these agents.

The Committee on Infectious Disease of the American Academy of Pediatrics (AAP) has proposed a schedule for active immunization of infants and children (Tables 7 and 8). It should be emphasized that these are recommendations, not rules. The Advisory Committee on Immunization Practices of the U.S. Public Health recommends a procedure and schedule that differ in minor ways from those proposed by the AAP Committee. Because of rapid developments in this area, such as the vaccine being developed against *Hemophilus influenzae*, Type B, changes in this schedule are not infrequent.

AGE TO START ACTIVE IMMUNIZATION. Normal infants may commence routine immunization at 2 months of age. The first vaccines administered are DPT (diphtheria and tetanus toxoids combined with pertussis vaccine) and TOPV (trivalent oral polio vaccine). Maternal antibodies against measles, which are acquired transplacentally, can interfere with the effectiveness of measles vaccine administered prior to 12 months of age. For this reason, measles vaccine is usually given at one year of age. In population groups where measles commonly occur during the first year of life, measles vaccine may be given at 6 months of age. It is recommended that a repeat dose be given at the age of 1 year.

IMMUNIZING AGENTS AND DOSAGE. Combined preparations that contain diphtheria and tetanus toxoids, adsorbed, and pertussis vaccine (DPT) are recommended for primary immunization of infants and young children. Because of their enhanced immunogenicity, these depot antigens are preferred over the combined fluid toxoids and pertussis vaccine. The widely held belief that untoward reactions to pertussis increase with age is not supported by evidence. However, there is firm evidence that untoward reactions to diphtheria toxoid do increase with age. The adult type of combined tetanus-diphtheria toxoids (Td) contain a much smaller dose of diphtheria toxoid and is the recommended product for children over 6 years and for adults.

Live oral poliovirus vaccine is recommended because it is easy to administer, has broad immunologic effects (humoral and local secretory antibodies), and its protective effects are persistent and prolonged.

ADMINISTRATION. Mothers and adolescents should be advised of the objectives of immunization, the contents of the intended "shot" or oral preparation, and the short-range side effects, such as fever or local redness. The consent of the mother or adolescent should be obtained before proceeding. A surprising number of young mothers are dedicated to pursuing a natural life style. A few moments invested in an explanation is usually attended by consent. There is not universal agreement over how much to tell parents about the rare, but severe side effects of some of the vaccines. While the doctrine of informed consent is firmly implanted in medical ethics, there is disagreement about full disclosure. Most pediatricians do not recite a lexicon of severe side effects to mothers already distraught about the prospect of a "shot."

The depot antigens should be injected deep into the muscle. The large muscle mass of the lateral thigh is the preferred site, but the deltoid is suitable in older children. Some physicians continue to administer these in the buttock in spite of the known risk of damage to the sciatic nerve. A different site should be used for each injection during the course of primary immunization.

PRECAUTIONS AND CONTRAINDICATIONS TO ROUTINE ACTIVE IMMUNIZATION. Generally during the acute phase of a febrile illness, routine immunization should be deferred. Infections not associated with fever, such as the common cold or uncomplicated upper respiratory infection are not contraindications. The occurrence of severe reactions to DPT, such as fever over 39C, convulsions, or prolonged somnolence should be the occasion for caution in the subsequent administration of these agents. For infants with uncomplicated febrile reactions to DPT, completion of the basic series with fractional doses starting with 0.05 ml has been recommended. It is common practice to reduce the dose by one-half to one-quarter the recommended dose in such children.

Severe encephalopathy rarely has been reported associated with pertussis vaccine. The frequency of this complication associated with immunization is less than that associated with the disease. For this reason, most authorities continue to recommend the routine use of DPT. If a convulsion does occur, no further pertussis immunization should be attempted and DT (without pertussis) should be used.

PERTUSSIS. Pertussis immunization should not be repeated if major complications such as thrombocytopenia or central nervous system disorder follow a DPT injection.

MEASLES, MUMPS, RUBELLA. (Specific contraindications to the use of measles, mumps, and rubella live attenuated vaccines, are pregnancy;) leukemia, lymphoma, or other generalized malignancy associated with immunosuppression; diseases in which cell-mediated immunity is impaired; immunosuppressive therapy (corticosteroids, irradiation, alkylating agents, antimetabolites); severe febrile illness; or recent administration of immune serum globulin, plasma, or blood. Measles, mumps, rubella, and polio vaccine are produced in cell culture systems and may contain trace amounts of cell culture materials. Adverse or hypersensitivity effects have not been reported from the administration of these vaccines. However, when a vaccine such as rubella has been prepared from a variety of cell systems (duck embryo, rabbit kidney) and a child is known to be sensitive to the proteins of one of the species, a product from one of the alternate cell sources should be selected.

INTERRUPTION OF SCHEDULE. Interruption of the recommended schedule with a delay between doses does not interfere with the final immunity achieved. It is not recommended to start the series over regardless of the time elapsed since the previous immunization.

IMMUNIZATION RECORDS. The medical record should contain information as to the agent used, manufacturer, lot number, dose, and site of administration. Reactions and their nature should be recorded,

TABLE 7. Recommended Schedule for Active Immunization of Normal Infants and Children*

2 mo	DTP[†]	TOPV[‡]
4 mo	DTP	TOPV
6 mo	DTP	TOPV
1 yr	Measles[§]	Tuberculin test"
	Rubella[§]	Mumps[§]
1½ yr	DTP	TOPV
4–6 yr	DTP	TOPV
14–16 yr	Td[#] and thereafter every 10 yr	

Adapted from Report of the Committee on Infectious Diseases, 1974. American Academy of Pediatrics.

[†]*DTP—diphtheria and tetanus toxoids combined with pertussis vaccine.*

[‡]*TOPV—trivalent oral poliovirus vaccine. This recommendation is suitable for breast-fed as well as bottle-fed infants.*

[§]*May be given at 1 yr as measles-rubella or measles-mumps-rubella combined vaccines.*

"*Frequency of repeated tuberculin tests depends on risk of exposure of the child and on the prevalence of tuberculosis in the population group. The initial test should be at the time of, or preceding, the measles immunization.*

[#]*Td—combined tetanus and diphtheria toxoids (adult type) for those more than 6 yr of age, in contrast to diphtheria and tetanus (DT), which contains a larger amount of diphtheria antigen. Tetanus toxoid at time of injury: For clean, minor wounds, no booster dose is needed by a fully immunized child unless more than 10 yr have elapsed since the last dose. For contaminated wounds, a booster dose should be given if more than 5 yr have elapsed since the last dose.*

Storage of vaccines: *Because biologics are of varying stability, the manufacturers' recommendations for optimal storage conditions (e.g., temperature, light) should be carefully followed. Failure to observe these precautions may significantly reduce the potency and effectiveness of the vaccines.*

and severe reactions should be reported to the local health department. The medical record should be organized in such a manner that the cumulative immunization record can be displayed in one place, preferably the front of the record. Parents should be encouraged to keep a record of their children's immunizations. There is both costly duplication and incomplete immunization because of faulty memories and lost records.

COMBINED LIVE VIRUS VACCINES AND SIMULTANEOUS ADMINISTRATION OF LIVE VIRUS VACCINES. The concurrent administration of combined live virus vaccines, such as measles-mumps-rubella (MMR) and trivalent oral poliovirus (TOPV, third or fourth feeding), does not interfere with antibody response. Other effective live virus combinations are measles-rubella (MR); rubella-mumps; and measles-smallpox (for jet inoculation in mass inoculation programs).

PRIMARY IMMUNIZATION OF CHILDREN NOT IMMUNIZED IN INFANCY. It is discouraging to frequently discover children who have not been immunized during infancy. The schedule suggested in Table 8 is suggested for these children.

IMMUNIZATION PROCEDURES ON EXPOSURE. It is not uncommon to be faced with a decision about what to do for a susceptible child or adult exposed to an infectious disease for which there is an effective immunizing agent. Clinical judgment is essential in estimating the risk of contracting the disease. The following are guidelines for some of the common diseases, if the risk is judged to be genuine.

MEASLES. Administer live measles vaccine and 0.04 ml/kg Immune Serum Globulin (ISG) at separate sites. An alternative is to give a preventive dose (0.25 ml/kg) of ISG intramuscularly as soon as possible after exposure, followed in 8 to 10 weeks by administration of live vaccine. Children with immune suppression by disease or therapy should receive 20 to 30 ml of ISG intramuscularly immediately.

MUMPS. No prophylaxis is indicated for prepubertal children. Among exposed adults with no history of mumps, about 50 percent will have had inapparent infection and will be immune. Attempts may be made to protect exposed postpubertal males from mumps and the complication of orchitis by the prompt administration of live attentuated mumps virus vaccine. Mumps Hyperimmune Serum Globulin (Human) has *not* demonstrated effectiveness in preventing parotitis or orchitis. Current skin test antigens are not reliable, and their use is not recommended.

RUBELLA. There is no evidence that live virus vaccine given after exposure will prevent illness. In spite of this there is no contraindication to vaccinating recently exposed prepubertal children over 1 year of age. The occasion rises when pregnant women seek counsel because of exposure to children with febrile illness associated with a rash. More often than not, another physician has diagnosed rubella. What to do? Do not give rubella virus vaccine! Serologic tests utilizing a reliable hemagglutination-inhibition (HI) method are commonly available and should be done to determine susceptibility. If the titer indicates a previous infection

TABLE 8. Primary Immunization for Children Not Immunized in Infancy*

1 Through 5 Yr of Age[†]

First visit	DTP, TOPV, tuberculin test
1 mo later	Measles, rubella, mumps
2 mo later	DTP, TOPV
4 mo later	DTP, TOPV
6 to 12 mo later or preschool	DTP, TOPV
Age 14–16 yr	Td—continue every 10 yr

6 Yr of Age and Over[†]

First visit	Td, TOPV, tuberculin test
1 mo later	Measles, rubella, mumps
2 mo later	Td, TOPV
6 to 12 mo later	Td, TOPV
Age 14–16 yr	Td—continue every 10 yr

Adapted from Report of the Committee on Infectious Diseases, 1974. American Academy of Pediatrics.

[†]*Physicians may choose to alter the sequence of these schedules if specific infections are prevalent at the time. For example, measles vaccine might be given on the first visit if an epidemic is under way in the community.*

and immunity, all is well. If antibody is not present the ethics of the patient with regard to therapeutic abortion must be considered. For those women who would not consider interrupting the pregnancy, Immune Serum Globulin (ISG), 20 ml intramuscularly, may be considered despite the conflicting evidence concerning its efficacy in preventing viremia and subsequent fetal infection. A second blood specimen should be obtained 4 weeks later and paired serum specimens (the original and current) run for HI antibody. Antibody detectable in the second specimen indicates rubella infection.

If the initial blood sample is obtained later than 1 week after exposure, the presence of HI antibody may be indicative of past or current infection and further testing is necessary. A second specimen should be obtained in 2 weeks, and the paired serum specimens should be tested for complement fixation (CF) and HI antibody as well as IgM specific antibody. A rising titer of antibody and/or the presence of IgM specific rubella antibody are indicative of current rubella infection. The risks to the fetus should be fully discussed again, and the pregnant woman advised of her options.

PERTUSSIS. Exposed contacts under the age of 4 years, previously immunized against pertussis, should receive a booster dose of vaccine. Since immunity conferred by immunization is not absolute, erythromycin may be added. Contacts not previously immunized should receive chemoprophylaxis using erythromycin for 10 days after the contact is broken or, if the contact cannot be broken, for the duration of the cough in the infected contact. In spite of the fact that its efficacy has not been clearly established, Pertussis Immune Serum Globulin (Human) is still used by some clinicians for unvaccinated exposed infants in a dose of 1.5 ml intramuscularly, repeated once in 5 to 7 days.

References

IMMUNIZATION

Report of the Committee on Infectious Diseases, 17th ed. American Academy of Pediatrics, 1974

Phillips CF: Children out of step with immunization. Pediatrics 55:877, 1975

SCREENING

Traditionally, pediatricians have had a major interest in the prevention of disease; early recognition of disease accompanied by prompt intervention is far more effective than late intervention after symptoms are present. Thus early diagnosis and treatment of congential cretinism is accompanied by better outcomes than when therapy is started after the clinical syndrome has become fully manifest. Interest in prevention has stimulated the development of screening procedures for asymptomatic disease. The demonstration that infants with phenylketonuria (PKU) could be detected in the first weeks of life and that mental retardation could be significantly reduced by the institution of a low phenylalanine diet gave considerable impetus to the establishment of screening procedures.

A broader view of health demands that any consideration of the child must include elements of the entire social milieu in which children develop. This includes, in addition to the physical and emotional environment, the social and educational system of the culture or subculture of any given child. The definition proposed by Lessler encompasses this view:

Screening is the acquiring of preliminary information about characteristics which may be significant to the health, education, or well-being of the individual and which are relevant to his life tasks. The means of data collection must be appropriate and reasonable with regard to the economics of time, money, and resources for dealing with large numbers of persons.

Screening tests sort out apparently well persons who probably do not have a disease from those who probably do have the disease; they are not intended to be diagnostic. Persons with positive or suspicious findings must be referred for definitive diagnosis and necessary treatment.

Mass screening is the large-scale screening of entire population groups. *Selective or prescriptive screening* is the screening of individuals who have a higher probability of harboring the disease in question (for example, screening only blacks for sickle cell disease). *Multiple screening* is the application on one occasion of two or more screening tests to identify two or more diseases. *Multiphasic screening* is the application on one occasion of multiple screening tests to detect a variety of health problems. Multiphasic screening usually refers to a battery of ten or more screening tests. *Surveillance* is the periodic screening of an individual or a group of people to monitor health. *Sensitivity* is the degree of accuracy of a screening test in correctly identifying diseased subjects. *Specificity* is the degree of accuracy of a screening test in correctly identifying nondiseased subjects.

SELECTION OF DISEASE FOR SCREENING. As with any procedure performed on patients, the application of a screening procedure should be justified by meeting certain criteria:

The disease or condition should be serious or potentially so. The issue of cost/effectiveness is of prime importance in screening procedures, and if the disease has little effect on morbidity or mortality, the cost of screening, identification, and follow-up are certain to be excessive. The costs of screening, identification, and follow-up of a child with PKU are relatively small compared to the costs of institutionalizing a profoundly retarded child for many years. The human costs are much more difficult to assess than economic costs, which can be predicted with some accuracy.

Available diagnostic tests or procedures should be capable of differentiating the diseased from borderline or nondiseased individuals. Unfortunately, few diseases fall into such neat categories, and from a practical point of view, individuals who fall into the gray zones between disease and nondisease require periodic follow-up.

The outcome of the disease or condition should be improved if detected and treated in the asymptomatic stage.

The disease should be treatable or controllable. An individual finds little solace in the diagnosis of a disease, during the asymptomatic stage, if the natural history of the disease can-

TABLE 9. Summary of Tentative Screening Recommendations*

	NB	2 mo	4 mo	6 mo	9 mo	12 mo	18 mo	2 yr	4 yr	6 yr	9 yr	12 yr	15 yr
Screening Tests													
PKU and galactosemia†	+	←	←										
Anemia	+	←	←	←	←	+	←	←	←	←		+	←
Sickle cell diseases‡§	+	←	←	←	←								
Hemoglobin S and C traits§"												+	+
Bacteriuria (girls only)									+	+	+	+	+
Hearing					#				+**	+**	+	+	
Vision									+	+	+	+	+
Physical growth	+	+	←	+	←	+	←	+	+	+	+	+	+
Psychomotor development						+	←	←	+				
Lead absorption (high-risk only)						+††	+††	+††	+				
Tuberculosis (high-risk only)						+			+			+	
Interview Questions													
Illness or medication in pregnancy	+	←	←										
Family history of genetic disease	+	←	←	←	←	←	←	←	←				
Abnormalities of delivery	+	←	←										
Social and economic factors affecting health and health care	+	←	←	←	←	+	←	+	←				
Mother's perception of child as "easy–difficult" or "good–bad"	+	+	+	+	+	+	+	+	+	+	+	+	
Psychomotor development		+	+	+	+	+	+	+	+				
Language development			+	+	+	+	+	+	+				
Evidence of sight and hearing		+	+	+	+	+	+						
Relationships with peers and sibs						+	+	+	+	+	+	+	+
Exposure to lead					+	+	+	+	+				
Exposure to tuberculosis	+	←	←	+	+	+	+	+	+	+	+	+	+
Feeding or eating patterns		+	+	+	+	+	+	+				+	+
Bowel movement patterns		+	+	+	+	+	+	+					
Allergic symptoms			+	+	+	+	+	+	+	+	+	+	+
Seizurelike symptoms			+	+	+	+	+	+	+	+	+	+	+
Lower urinary tract symptoms		+	+	+	+	+	+	+	+	+	+	+	+
School progress										+	+	+	+
Dental care									+	+	+	+	+
Sexual behavior												+	+
Drug, alcohol, tobacco use												+	+
Child's perception of self											+	+	+
Immunization status		+	+	+	+	+	+	+	+	+	+	+	+
Physical Examination Items													
Cardiorespiratory signs	+	←											
Gastrointestinal obstruction	+												
Visible congenital anomalies	+	←	←										
Hip dislocation	+	←	←	+	←	←							
Vision and hearing behavior	+	+	+	+	+	+	+	+	+				
Neuromotor development	+	+	+	+	+	+	+	+	+	+			
Mother–child interaction		+	+	+	+	+	+	+	+	+	+		
Strabismus			+	+	+	+	+	+	+				
Serous otitis				+	+	+	+	+	+				
Scoliosis											+	+	+
Breast development											+	+	+
Genital development	+	←	←	←	←	+	←	←			+	+	+
Acne, eczema and other skin disease	+	+	+	+	+	+	+	+	+	+	+	+	+

+ *Do at this age.*

← *Do at this age if not done at previous scheduled age.*

*Adapted from North AF Jr: Pediatrics 54:631, 1974.

† *Other inborn errors may be added with the development of adequate testing and follow up services.*

‡ *Screening should only take place when excellent comprehensive care can be given to all positives.*

§ *Only persons with African, Mediterranean, and certain Latin-American ancestry need be tested.*

" *Testing should take place only with informed consent and when skilled counseling can be ensured.*

Testing with calibrated noisemakers may be added at 9 or 12 mo if skills and resources permit.

** *Hearing should be tested yearly from ages 4 to 8.*

†† *Lead testing should be performed two to three times yearly for children living in high-risk environments.*

not be altered. For this reason, there has been criticism of the sickle cell disease detection programs. On the other hand, inherited metabolic disease carriers, such as for Tay-Sachs disease, can be identified, the pregnancy of high-risk couples (both parent carriers) can be monitored, affected fetuses identified in utero by amniocentesis, and the opportunity for elective abortion offered.

The condition should be relatively prevalent. Prevalence is the frequency with which a disease or condition is found in a given population at a given point in time. The importance of prevalence is that it is inversely related to the cost of case finding. The greater the prevalence, the less is the cost of discovering one case.

Facilities should be available to diagnose and treat individuals who have positive findings on the screening test.

The cost of screening, diagnosis, and treatment during the asymptomatic phase should be outweighed by savings in human suffering and the economic costs incurred, if the problem is not discovered until the symptomatic stage.

The diseases recommended for screening are growing rapidly. Currently they include:

Amblyopia
Anemia
Bacteriuria
Congenital heart disease
Congenital hypothyroidism
Dental problems
Developmental delay
Diabetes mellitus
Galactosemia
Growth retardation
Hearing impairment
Lead poisoning
Learning disorders
Malnutrition
Mental retardation
Obesity
Phenylketonuria
Rubella immunity
Speech and language problems
Tuberculosis
Venereal disease
Visual impairment

Selection of Screening Tests.

The following criteria can be used to judge the usefulness of a particular screening test.

ACCEPTABILITY. The screening test must be acceptable to the person who will perform the screening, to the children to be screened and their parents, and to the practitioners, who will be called upon to diagnose and treat children with positive screening tests. This simply means that all elements of the system should concur on the appropriateness of the test.

RELIABILITY. Reliability is the consistency with which a test or observation measures what it was designed to indicate.

VALIDITY. Validity is the consistency with which positive and negative findings agree with the actual presence or absence of the disease or problem.

Tests that have a high incidence of false-positive results have the disadvantage that a large number of addi-

tional or special diagnostic tests must be done at extra expense and inconvenience. False-negative tests will obviously defeat the purpose of the test, as the condition will not be suspected.

Current State of the Art

A review of current information on screening tests commonly performed in physicians' offices, ambulatory care facilities, schools, and public health clinics reveals the disappointing gap between the theoretical and the real world. A tentative recommendation for screening for a wide variety of problems is presented in Table 9.

EPSDT (Early and Periodic Screening, Diagnosis, and Treatment)

Title XIX (Medicaid), an amendment to the Social Security Act, was passed by Congress in 1965. One of its main objectives was to increase the availability of medical care to low-income groups by paying their medical expenses. The states were mandated to provide Early and Periodic Screening, Diagnosis, and Treatment Programs for all children under 21 years by 1973. If the screening tests indicate the need for further evaluation, the patient must be referred for diagnosis by a physician or clinical facility. The state governments are responsible for administering the EPSDT programs. For a variety of reasons, the programs have been slow getting off the mark, and roughly 10 percent of the 10 million eligible children have been screened. One outcome which is almost certain to come in time, and which is critically needed, is to define the cost and efficiency of large-scale screening programs.

References

Screening

Allen CM, Shinefield H: Automated multiphasic screening. Pediatrics 54:621, 1974

Dixon MS, Jr: EPSDT (early and periodic screening, diagnosis and treatment programs). Pediatrics 54:84, 1974

Edwards PQ: Tuberculin testing of children. Pediatrics 54:628, 1974

Foltz AM, Silver GA: EPSDT. Pediatrics 54:2, 1974

Frankenburg WK: Pediatric screening. Advances in Pediatrics, Vol 20. Chicago, Yearbook Medical Publishers, 1973, 149

Kunin CM: Current status of screening children with urinary tract infection. Pediatrics 54:619, 1974

Lessler K: Screening, screening programs and the pediatrician. Pediatrics 54:608, 1974

Moriarty RW: Screening to prevent lead poisoning. Pediatrics 54:626, 1974

North AF, Jr: Screening in child health care: where are we now and where are we going? Pediatrics 54:631, 1974

Scriver CR: PKU and beyond: when do costs exceed benefits? Pediatrics 54:616, 1974

Sewell EM, O'Hare D, Kendig EL, Jr: The tuberculin test. Pediatrics 54:650, 1974

Starfield B, Holtzman NA: A comparison of effectiveness of screening for phenylketonuria in the United States, United Kingdom and Ireland. N Engl J Med 293:118, 1975

Thorpe H, Werner EE: Developmental screening of pre-school children: a critical review. Pediatrics 53:362, 1974

CHAPTER 3

Normal and Abnormal Psychosocial Development

GORDON HARPER AND JULIUS B. RICHMOND

CHILD DEVELOPMENT

In approaching the subject of child development the pediatrician is faced with a problem not encountered in the study of single organs or organ systems: he must choose a *conceptual framework* within which to organize his observations and set forth his expectations. This need exists for several reasons: in considering the development of the whole child, the areas available for study are so numerous that one must decide where one is going to focus. Even when only one aspect of child development is considered, different cultural values and social expectations make it impossible to have the kind of consensus about what behavior is normal (or even what behavior is important) that we find in discussions of subjects such as physical growth or immunity. There is a similar cultural heterogeneity among students of child development concerning which aspects of child development merit attention and which instruments of assessment are appropriate for following them. Such instruments include the more or less objective tests of discrete behaviors, more abstract formulations of a particular aspect of personality development that are based more on inference than on observation, and the pediatrician's overall assessment of how the whole child is progressing in growth and development, based on his observations of many children.

The various views of children and of how they should be raised are reflected in social discussions, in popular literature, in official publications like the infant care pamphlets of the United States Children's Bureau, and in more formally organized bodies of scientific knowledge. Richmond and Caldwell have reviewed the predominant scientific theories about child development that have influenced the thinking and child-rearing practices of American parents in this century. The *school of social learning*, which was associated with the sociology of social role and with the psychology of learned behavior, focused on the presumed plasticity of the child and the ways in which he was molded by the actions of those around him. Watson, the founder of this school, in words reminiscent of Loyola, said that he could take an infant and produce in him any behaviors desired, simply through reinforcement. Partly in reaction to this concept, the *maturational school* of Gesell devoted many years of work to describing the regular schedule of behaviors emerging from within the child himself. Gesell's work emphasized the autonomy of this development, which was driven from within, and at times seemed to de-emphasize individual differences in favor of the expectation that all children would follow certain timetables of development. The third major school, the *psychoanalytic*, concerned itself with a new aspect of development: unconscious mental processes. It introduced new methods of study that consisted of detailed, often long-term, observations of individual children coupled with the observer's interpretation of what was seen. The psychoanalytic school was concerned with ego psychology, the development of ways of organizing inner emotional life and experiences, and interpersonal theory (the development of relationships with others).

The cognitive development of the child was studied initially by Piaget. Modern behavior theory and therapy have brought other kinds of systematic inquiry to bear on child development and have offered new concepts that have aided physicians, students of child development, and parents in placing their own observations and expectations in a coherent framework.

For the pediatrician the conceptual framework of psychosocial development offered by Erik Erikson is probably the most useful. Erikson draws on various conceptual and empirical schools and also pays close attention to informal folk beliefs and cultural influences. He is concerned with the sequential unfolding of the capacities of the growing child as described by the maturationists. Drawing on the work of cultural anthropologists and his own observations in the field, Erikson stresses the influence of family and culture on the child. He is also concerned with the social meaning of each aspect of child development, the behaviors various cultures and families use to shape and maintain maturation, and the relationships between the individual, the parents, and the larger society. As a psychoanalyst he is explicitly concerned with the conscious and unconscious meaning of the development of drives in early childhood and with the forms that sexual and aggressive energies take as the child's capacities and the circle of significant others expand from infancy to school age. Erikson stresses the role of development in shaping a child's view of himself and its expression in his changing relationships with other people. At the center of his theory of psychosocial development he places a developing series of conscious and unconscious feelings, which he calls inner senses. The word sense is used not as in discussions of perceptual senses but as a pervasive feeling about oneself and one's world, as in the phrases "a sense of basic trust" or "a sense of autonomy."

There are several advantages to using this conceptual framework in pediatrics. It is eminently developmental, setting forth major issues in child growth in sequential terms. It is inclusive; all of the advances in locomotion, prehension, cognition, and social interaction described by other developmentalists are integrated into this view of child development. In fact, Erikson puts the child's intergration of all these parts of himself at the center of the unfolding story of development. In clear, accessible language Erikson presents many of the issues posed in more recondite terms by other students of child development. Also, it is an interactional model that at each stage considers the mutual influences of parents and child on one another and also the interactions between child, family, and society. Finally, Erikson focuses on the growing child's developing sense of who he is (his psychosocial identity), which is the major interest of parents, children, and pediatricians: Who is the child in his own eyes? Who is he in the eyes of his family and others? How does he make a coherent whole of the diverse elements in his constitution, his life experience, and the possibilities open to him in the world? Such concerns are the core of developmental pediatrics and of the psychosocial theory of Erikson.

BIOLOGY OF DEVELOPMENT

Because of his concern with the physical health of the child, the pediatrician will bring to his work an awareness of the biologic factors in development and the need to consider them in assessing all aspects of a child's progress. It is important to consider not only these universal aspects shared by all children but also particular events in a given child's life.

Consideration of biologic factors in development is complicated by the fact that they operate on many levels ranging from anatomic to behavior and psychologic levels; they also interact to varying degrees with factors in the environment, and our knowledge of such interactions is variable and incomplete. For example, we know that the genetic potential for phenylketonuria will express itself in some degree of mental deficiency in most cases in which a child with a deficiency of phenylalanine hydroxylase is exposed to unrestricted amounts of phenylalanine. However, we know little about the extent to which biologic potential is involved in such development as of musical talent or athletic prowess, and still less about the mechanisms through which such skills develop. The work of Thomas and associates has elucidated many constitutional differences in temperament among children; however, we still cannot say with precision to what degree constitutional components contribute to such entities as behavior disorder, learning disability, hyperactivity, antisocial activity, and childhood psychosis. The process of sexual differentiation illustrates the complexity of the biology of development: there are variations (ranging from anatomic and physiologic to behavioral) in the organ or system affected, there is an effect of environment on what is differentiated (invariably present but variably acting), and there are varying degrees of incompleteness in our knowledge of mechanisms. One must maintain proper regard for this incompleteness of our present knowledge in any situation where it might appear that only one set of factors is solely responsible. A wise policy in making a judgment in such instances is to make a wide-ranging search among all possible factors (genetic, physiologic, environmental) and an appropriate acknowledgment that any seemingly final statements are really only provisional, the best that can be formulated with present knowledge.

REGULATION OF DEVELOPMENT

The central questions of child development involve determination of the factors that regulate its rate and scope. Theresa Benedek illustrated both the complexity of the answer and the areas where an answer must be sought when she wrote that "growth, neurophysiological maturation, and psycho-social development are intrinsically interwoven processes." In this discussion we can only indicate some of the ways these several factors interact. The importance of interaction is emhasized when we compare fetal and extrauterine development. Old wives' tales notwithstanding, we know of no factors other than the genetic map, the physiologic environment of the mother's body, and accidents of development such as infection or trauma that can influence the growth of the fetus. But once he is born the child begins a continuing and ever increasing process of participating in his growth that changes the framework within which growth (or failure to grow) must be considered. There is also the fact that to provide her child with what he needs to grow requires much more of the mother postnatally than before birth. Interactions between the growing child and those caring for him, and the degree of matching between them, henceforth become the critical elements in development.

Growth itself brings the development of each organ along to the point where it calls out to be used, in terms of both size and refinement of function; for example, increasing muscle mass and skeletal growth lead to walking and later to riding a bicycle or running races. Frisch's work on the onset of menarche suggests that it is the increase in body bulk, particularly the attainment of a critical ratio of body fat to height, that triggers the hypothalamic-pituitary events of puberty. The child participates in all of this, obviously, in his increasing regulation of what he eats. Negative participation in one's own nutrition is seen in such clinical problems as feeding difficulties in young children (in whom negativism or depression can lead to malnutrition), pica in toddlers, and anorexia nervosa in adolescents, all of which are also related to failed mutuality with the mother.

The dependence of growth on environmental factors other than the availability of food, particularly the personal atmosphere around the child, is still hypothetical. However, clinical experience has shown that children with nonorganic failure to thrive fail to secrete growth hormone and to grow in one environment but resume growth and secretion of growth hormone in another. This observation strongly suggests that the physiologic mechanisms for growth, which have been traced back from pituitary to hypothalamus, probably reach higher still to the cortex, and thence to the child's environment.

The impetus given to growth and development by *neurophysiologic maturation* is well known. Attention to developmental milestones is a cornerstone of child health supervision. Less well recognized are the neurologically determined shifts in cognitive function or in ability to think in new ways that occur continuously, but with dramatic spurts at certain points, eg, between the ages of 5 and 7 years. These changes form the neurobiologic basis for the universal cultural provision for the child to enter some kind of organized education at this stage. Much pediatric diagnostic and counseling effort is concerned with children who are out of step with their peers and with society's expectations during this phase of development. Some of their failure to learn and to adjust to routines in school will be due to developmental lag or deviation in regard to their progression through this 5-to-7 shift. Another neurologic-cognitive set of changes occurs around puberty; it involves improved coordination at tasks involving repeated rhythmic behavior, an alteration in body image, and the beginning of the kind of abstract thinking that Piaget called *formal operations.*

Here again the child's participation is crucial: in order to develop each new potential ability as he acquires it, and thereafter to integrate it, the child must be oriented (from contact with family and peers) to see this new activity as something suited both to his actual abilities and to the expectations others have of his future. He must have enough conflict-free energy available to attempt the untried, and he must be comfortable with his own initiative, his pleasure in taking on something new. Clinical experience is full of examples of children who either are temporarily regressed or are frightened, exhausted, or babied at home and who consequently hold back, whereas if their progress depended on neurophysiologic maturation alone, they would move forward.

Here the contribution of *psychosocial development* to overall development is most clear. The child must be ready, in all the ways listed above, to appropriate or to make his own the developmental skills coming his way. Every parent and pediatrician has experienced situations where children were not ready for a development (eg, for toilet training, even though spinal cord, bladder, and bowel functions indicated that they were). On the positive side, the quality of initiative and pleasure in taking something on in a healthy child for whom life is going well is one of the strongest drives in all development. This drive to do, and to enjoy doing, variously called a sense of mastery or competence or prowess, is easier to recognize in action than to account for in terms of either neurophysiology or psychosocial development. There are analogies in animal studies where repetition and mastery of newly learned tasks can be observed, although some have believed this drive to be specifically human. According to Bronowski, "the most powerful force in the ascent of man is his pleasure in his own skill."

Thus Erikson indicates that at each stage of development, because of growth or maturation or both, a child has *available* new ingredients of his personality that he must *integrate,* making something of them in a way that preserves a feeling of continuity with his previous sense of himself. He borrows from embryology the epigenetic notion that each development must occur at the right time and in the right sequence. The ingredients include elements of physical growth, new large and fine motor skills, sphincter control, and an increasingly elaborate set of cognitive skills (ways of perceiving and using information about the world). In addition to these more or less directly observable capacities, Erikson employs the psychoanalytic concept of *drives* as activating successive stages of development. These drives may be viewed as activating bodily zones that seem to have a sequence of sensory and symbolic importance, modes of using these zones (incorporation, retention, etc), and social modalities or ways of interacting with others (getting, holding on, letting go). At each stage there is an opportunity for a new kind of self-regulation and shared regulation, or mutuality, between the child and those most important to him. Failure to achieve such self-regulation and mutuality leads to a characteristic disturbance at each stage and a corresponding sense of estrangement, including basic mistrust, pervasive shame and doubt, and often crippling guilt. The crucial factor in the outcome for the child is the ratio between the polarities involved, such as basic trust versus mistrust or autonomy versus shame and doubt. Each stage, then, involves a crisis, not in the excited journalistic sense of the word but in the sense of a time when the child hesitates in his growth, more or less beset with fumbling and fear, and the outcome seems in doubt. Then, as Erikson puts it, a resolution occurs in that the child suddenly appears to grow together, both in his person and in his body. He appears more himself, more loving, more relaxed and brighter in his judgment, more activated and activating. In keeping with the epigenetic model, the gains of each stage are seen as the critical building blocks for the developmental tasks of the next.

STAGES OF DEVELOPMENT

INFANCY: BASIC TRUST VERSUS BASIC MISTRUST. The prodigious physical growth of the infant during the first year is accompanied by parallel growth in other areas. Gradual adjustments to life outside the physical and psychologic shelter of the womb are seen in autonomic function, including skin temperature regulation, pulse and respiratory regulation, and even complex behavior cycles like waking and sleeping. Motor skills progress through well-defined stages. The arms and hands, used initially only as part of the generalized startle (Moro) response, are successively brought under specific control. Similar sequences, which Gesell described so well, occur with regard to head and trunk control and use of the legs: kicking and crawling, then passive weight bearing in standing position, and finally standing and walking follow one another in regular order (see also Table 2 , p. 23). As for perceptual skills, the newborn can track visually for fleeting moments, but it is weeks before his eyes work conjugally; it is months before he can recognize specific patterns and later still before he can coordinate what he sees with what he can do with his hands. Piaget has described the ways in which thinking can be traced to its origins in these early sensorimotor activities. Linguistic milestones can be described in the same way.

From a developmental point of view, however, the most crucial aspect of the baby's growth during this time may be said to be the way he is gradually woven into the social fabric—into society, to be sure, but more immediately into a family and most specifically of all into a mutual relationship with the mother or other primary care-giver. In this discussion the term mother will refer to the primary care-giver, whether or not that person is the biologic mother. The mother who strives to meet the infant's needs finds these needs exercising a new kind of influence over the familiar pattern of her day, for the infant is initially more responsive to drives from within than to outside events, and these drives are beyond the mother's control. In contrast, the 1-year-old responds selectively to those around him; he can indicate preferences and tolerate frustration. He has entered into a series of human cycles and has developed sleeping and feeding patterns and times of activity and times of rest. Erikson sees the accomplishment of this degree of *mutality* as the social expression of basic trust, the first of the key inner senses. He traces the line of development of social trust through the young baby's ease of feeding, depth of sleep, and relaxation of bowels; stresses that these visceral expressions of well-being are psychosocial milestones that reflect the infant's "experience of a mutual regulation of his increasingly receptive capacities with the maternal techniques of provision." Three related aspects of basic trust and mutuality can be identified: the infant learns to trust his own ability to regulate his inner needs and not be overwhelmed by them, to trust that others will provide what he needs within reasonable limits, and to trust that those whom he needs will not be driven away by his neediness.

This view of infancy is useful both for what it says about the first year of life and for the insight it gives into this kind of developmental model. The mother provides consistent care for the infant; she becomes "an inner certainty as well as an outer predictability." His relaxation and gradually increasing responsiveness activate her responses to him. His ability to endure longer periods when she is out of sight and her ability to respond to his needs with increasing sophistication and sensitivity reflect parallel development and demonstrate the relationship between a new kind of mutuality and the inner sense of basic trust. The positive feeling about oneself and about what is possible in relationships with others, which is implicit in basic trust, gives life its flavor of optimism and makes possible future development.

Two broader psychosocial aspects of this stage bear emphasis. First, what a child experiences at each stage depends on the social matrix into which he is born. The mother will be able to meet her infant's needs to the extent that her own needs, social, emotional, and material, are met in the world around her. The role of the pediatrician in bringing out and supporting the mother's best functioning is strongly supportive, as he can encourage her and develop her ability to make a good match, which is so much a matter of meeting the baby's basic biologic needs. Second, the attitudes toward the infant of those around him are crucial for his developing sense of who he is. Is he to be valued for himself, or is his role to be delineated by a parental need to relive his or her own past?

Generations of clinicians have concluded (and epidemiologists have begun to support the clinical impressions) that children whose life circumstances in infancy inhibit development of an inner sense of basic trust are at risk for a series of emotional and behavior disorders in later life. These range from recurrent depressive mood or illness to antisocial behavior and disordered relationships in adulthood that are marked either by fear of getting involved emotionally with anyone or by an apparent inability to have anything but frustrating relationships with those from whom one would seek love. The cornerstone on which all preventive psychosocial pediatrics is based can be conceived in this sense to be the alertness of the pediatrician to the amount of developing mutuality or mutual frustration between mother and infant.

TODDLER STAGE: AUTONOMY VERSUS SHAME AND DOUBT.   In the second and third years a number of developments occur that make possible, and that center attention on, the child's development of autonomy or self-regulation. Motor development gives him the capacity to stand, to walk, to get about, and to decide for himself where he wishes to go. Increased manual dexterity coupled with curiosity about everything around him gives him the frequently exasperating capacity to get into everything. The rapid growth of language, once words succeed early cooing and babbling around the first year (see also Table 4 , p. 37), gives him the means to inquire and to reply, using words to indicate what his wishes, feelings, and intentions are. At the same time, maturation of the cortical-spinal tracts mediating voluntary control over bladder and bowel function allows for voluntary control in a previously locally autonomous area. Age 2 years is the average age for acquisition of toilet traning, an area of child training that can become the focus for the larger struggle between parents and child over who controls what and whom. The alternating modalities of holding on and letting go figure prominently here.

For the child the crucial developmental issue is one of control, of discrimination, of regulation of words and actions, of newly felt mastery. There is considerable power felt by the 2-year-old when he can make demands, say "no," and control his sphincters at will. The meaning of this stage in terms of psychosocial identity hinges on the relationship between inner feeling, intent, and the growing capacity for self-control. It is as if the child were asking: Is it within my capacity to control my own body, speech, and feelings, or must I be continually on guard, overcontrolling my shameful self, doubting what I would do, lest others find out that I am no good? Erikson calls this stage the crisis of autonomy versus shame and doubt.The child needs a gentle kind of support from his parents, a reassuring model of shared control that takes account of his abilities but won't let him endanger himself or others if he oversteps his limitations while he learns. The parent must be able to trust the child to learn gradually to control his own social interactions, his emotions, and his body without parental overcontrol or abdication. The pediatrician's task, accordingly, is to help the parents recognize the growth toward a goal, the positive moving forward through the 2-year-old's stubbornness and his seemingly endless negativism. He must help them keep in mind that the healthy personality is not built around absolute self-control nor total indulgence of all whims and desires, as well as that parent and child must relate through appropriate sharing and shared control while they both work toward their common goals of full self-regulation and autonomy in the grown-up child.

PRESCHOOL STAGE: INITIATIVE VERSUS GUILT. For the child between 3 and 6 years of age, growth and maturation open up new areas of experience in several ways. In terms of muscular development, walking, running, jumping, and climbing have become effortless activities. The child can throw a ball and engage in rather elaborate play with peers. Language expands rapidly to the point where the child has all the rules and sufficient vocabulary to speak his language well. Changes emerge in the mode of thinking, and children begin to think imaginatively; play is no longer bound to what has happened around the child. A whole world of fantasy becomes available to the child and can be shared (through language) with other children and adults. For some children imaginary playmates may embody the first use of creative fantasy. Questions about death similarly reflect the child's expanding imaginative capacity and his developing awareness of his physical vulnerability.

Initiative begins to develop at this time and is the characteristic strength relevant to exploring all new areas of life. This inner sense is seen in the pleasure children and adults take in actively approaching people and undertaking new activities and new areas of endeavor. The child, now well in control of his body, can use it to explore and expand his world. The parallel danger is a paralyzing sense of guilt, attaching either to the exuberant actions or the desired goals. Feelings coming from inside, fueled by the newly available fantasy life and by an awareness of a new capacity to win or lose, to harm or be harmed physically, make the newly active child subject to new anxiety and guilt.

The discovery of new genital sensitivity and of fantasies, in which the pleasurable initiative involves parents, leads to the association of much of this guilt and anxiety with sexual wishes and fears. A frightening side of the child's inner life arises here, as fondness for one parent involves rivalry with the other. Partly as a resolution of such wishes and fears in these years, a large part of a child's sexual identification is grounded here. The model of the parents is crucial for this process. Parents frightened by their own or their child's sexuality may overreact in ways that make a child anxious. The pediatrician may be asked questions about punishment or overprotection or about children's sex play, which may reflect the parents' own anxieties. Other parents may be concerned that their children at this age appear frightened or inhibited or show symptoms of anxiety such as phobias or sleep disturbance that seem to have come out of nowhere. Careful assessment of the child and discussion with the parents is indicated, especially with regard to the ways that they are working together and presenting to their children a model of adult mutuality. The parents' awareness of these issues will provide the child the best chance to appropriately integrate his own capacity for initiative, identify with the adults who can use their own initiative caringly and responsibly, and keep on growing.

SCHOOL AGE: INDUSTRY VERSUS INFERIORITY. During the school years major developmental changes occur in the psychosocial area. The child makes a major separation from home and enters a world of school or other preparation for adult work in which he encounters certain arbitrary or standardized demands and opportunities. Through learning to cope with this world of school, and so with the larger world outside, he continues a process begun at home of learning to reconcile his own inner needs with the realities of the world outside. The impersonal rules of children's games, like the rules of language and mathematics, are a part of this learning. The peer group, attracting and pulling the child from his orientation primarily to his family, demands competence in terms of physical prowess and achievement. It will also expose the child to standards not based on achievement, such as assignment to one group or another on the basis of race, religion, or social class. And in school the child will be exposed to more or less standardized learning materials, to a curriculum judged by society to be worthy of learning and possibly relevant to adult life.

The crisis of this age is industry versus inferiority. For each child each of the above areas offers a challenge where he can develop a sense of his own competence vis-à-vis his peers and the physical world and an ability to anticipate his adult role. Each area also offers potential frustration: enhancement of a sense of inferiority, of not having the right forebears, origins, bodily equipment, social skills, or mental ability to make good in every sense that society offers.

The pediatrician's attentiveness in these years to the physical bases of the child's competence (his vision and hearing and his neurologic intactness, especially where minor dysfunction is a possibility) and to the ways that his parents and school support his competence and sense of industry can be highly supportive and beneficial to the child.

ADOLESCENCE: IDENTITY VERSUS IDENTITY CONFUSION. The years of adolescence confront the child with two sets of demands. From inside come the pressures of puberty, manifested as a rapid increase and then a tapering off of linear growth, as well as changes in body proportions, and the pressures of sexual maturation, with the appearance of body, facial, and pubic hair, maturation of the genitalia, and onset of menses in girls. Physical changes are accompanied by internal emotional pressures, including the need to do for oneself and be on one's own while feeling a strong contradictory need to be cared for. Meanwhile, there are external social pressures to conform to peer group norms and to prepare for taking part in the adult world, as an adult.

Related developmental changes within the adolescent involve an increasing emotional separation from parents, coupled with what Erikson called formation of identity. The latter includes consolidation of one's sexual identity (reworking earlier identifications and linking them to newly emerging sexual drives, as well as accepting a changed perception of oneself as a mature sexual being and potential parent), definition of an occupational role that reconciles one's own competence with possibilities actually available in the world, and self-definition within a pluralistic society and all its religious, social, and ideologic possibilities. Such changes clearly involve young people well beyond the years in which pediatricians care for them.

The conflicts involved here are easily pointed out. In an emotionally tumultuous time adolescents experience confusing feelings involving a need for closeness to parents, as well as pressing reasons to keep their distance and even to repudiate parents and parental values. Adolescents are aware of physical and emotional dependence on parents; yet they need to appear, and inwardly to feel, independent. They feel the need to be close to present and future sexual partners; yet they fear a loss of identity in closeness.

The risk at this stage lies in the occurrence of severe identity crises or even acute breakdowns or psychotic episodes in adolescents who cannot resolve previous doubts about their identities. Physiologic and family demands, sexual confusion, and other stresses may also lead to protracted moratoria that may be more or less productive, as when youths suspend cloture on life choices for themselves and explore various alternative possibilities. Such experiences may be considered as experiments and as opportunities for learning, or they may be regarded primarily as running away. In the last two decades the usefulness of this kind of moratorium has been widely recognized; families, educational institutions, and the culture at large have accepted interruptions in various career ladders that would previously have been seen as symptoms of potential failure and would have been discouraged and disapproved.

YOUNG ADULTHOOD: INTIMACY VERSUS ISOLATION. While the stages in the life cycle beyond adolescence lie outside the usual pediatric practice, some attention to them is merited both to complete the view of the life cycle as conceptualized by Erikson and because pediatricians are importantly involved with the parents of their patients, who as young adults must negotiate these life stages.

In beginning relationships with others in the years after adolescence, the young adult must risk that consolidation of identity recently achieved. In the closeness of affectionate intimacy and professional and social competition, one puts one's identity on the line, based on the assumption that it is now secure enough to withstand such risks. There are two dangers here: that intimate, competitive, and combative relationships will not be differentiated but will occur with the same person, and that, one way or another, isolation will take the place of the intimacy that should have developed. In addition to the obvious kind of isolation (people who avoid any contacts that would lead to intimacy), a kind of isolation à deux can exist in relationships that become frozen at this point, with the partners unable to undertake generativity. In addition, young couples or single parents raising children in the kind of isolation frequently imposed by twentieth-century life styles, be it in suburbia or inner city, must attempt to provide the important developmental framework previously described for their infant while consolidating their own precarious hold on adulthood.

MIDDLE ADULTHOOD: GENERATIVITY VERSUS STAGNATION. For the bringing up of children (indeed, for the whole transmission of culture and civilization) this stage is clearly central. It involves the growth of a sense of caring for those in the coming generation and involvement in a generation outside one's own, not necessarily as parents. Erikson coined the term generativity, with apologies for its awkwardness, in an effort to suggest both a concern with generations and the generative act and attitude. Generativity is clearly anticipated in every stage of life, from the infant's need for and gradual interest in and concern for his mother through the preschooler's crucial identification with the same-sex parent to the adolescent's reworking of previous identifications and integrating what had accrued in previous stages with new mature genital capacity and drives.

Pediatricians are strategically located to watch and to help with the growing pains of parents as they bring their children, the products of their intimacy and objects of their generativity, for pediatric attention. Beginning during pregnancy and continuing through the puerperium and the months of early infancy, the pediatrician is usually the professional person most closely in contact with the young mother and, increasingly, the young father. Sensitivity to the previous life experiences and personal strengths and weaknesses they have brought to parenthood, as well as sensitivity to the normal developmental upheavals and conflicts at their time, will enable the pediatrician to provide optimum help to the parents and hence to the child.

LATE ADULTHOOD: INTEGRITY VERSUS DESPAIR. The developmental crisis of the end of life involves a review: there may be a new acceptance of one's whole life as a life that has made sense, a life that gives one a feeling of integrity with one's past, one's aging, and one's relationship to life in one's own life cycle and in general, thus permitting acceptance of the reality of death. Or there may be what Erikson describes as the development of a malignant fear of death, a despair with life, a feeling that time is too short for any attempt to start another life and try out alternate roads to integrity. Erikson relates this last stage of life to the first via the definition of trust (assured reliance on another's integrity) and, relating adult integrity to infantile trust, concludes that "healthy children will not fear life if their elders have integrity enough not to fear death."

PSYCHOSOCIAL ASSESSMENT: PSYCHOLOGIC GROWTH AND DEVELOPMENT

The subjects of assessment and psychopathology will be presented together to emphasize their interconnection. No assessment of psychopathology can be made in a child without consideration of his overall development, and no assessment of development (in particular psychologic development) can be made without an awareness of the pathologic potential of each age and stage. The pediatric task of assessing a child's psychologic growth and development can be described in three parts: *developmental assessment, assessment of mutuality,* and *attempt at empathy* with the child. In the care of the healthy child this approach will increase the pediatrician's ability to give anticipatory guidance to parents, to understand current concerns, and to decide whether what he is observing falls within or outside the range of normal. When an emotional or behavior problem is presented, this approach will help the pediatrician to understand both the problem presented and what can be done to help. The role of understanding what is going on, rather than simply choosing a diagnostic label, is worth emphasizing at the outset for two reasons that have to do with the way children grow. In the first place, the nature of childhood and of growth and development is such that symptoms change over time, so that understanding a situation, rather than finding a diagnostic category into which the child can be fitted, is more true to nature. Second, the negative consequences of labeling, which are worth considering at any age, are especially relevant at an age when the child's concept of himself and his identity in his family's eyes are still in process of formation and when the paramount need of both child and family is a sympathetic understanding of what the meaning of the current situation is to him and his parents.

DEVELOPMENTAL ASSESSMENT

Developmental assessment consists of a review of the three aspects of development mentioned earlier—*growth, neurophysiologic maturation,* and *psychosocial development.* Growth is discussed in detail in Chap 4 . For the purposes of developmental assessment, it is important to determine the growth of the child as compared with his peers, possible illness in the past that may have affected growth, present illness, stage of growth, and what growth potential remains. It is also crucial to assess what meaning all these issues have for the child and the parents.

Neurophysiologic maturation is discussed in Chap 6 . Here we underline its importance for development at several ages. Prematurity affects neurologic maturity, not only in the months after birth but also later, in that children born prematurely are more likely to have gross neurologic syndromes (retardation and cerebral palsy) as well as difficulties in learning and coordination. Degrees of neurophysiologic maturity, even in term infants, may have much to do with variability in establishment of sleep cycles, ability of the child to tolerate increasing intervals between feedings, and ability to organize the flood of perceptual stimuli ranging from touch to noise with which newborns must contend. Constitutional or temperamental differences, on the other hand, are probably not as much a matter of maturity. Neurologic maturity underlies the milestones of development in the first 5 years. Advances in neurologic maturation occur throughout childhood, but especially around the age of entry into school and in the years before and during early adolescence. It must be emphasized that an assessment of the maturity and integrity of the child's whole body, especially his neurologic functioning, must underlie every developmental and psychologic assessment. Surveys of children referred to child guidance centers as emotionally disturbed and studies of children labeled delinquents because of socially deviant behavior indicate a prevalence of neurologic immaturity or impared development many times higher than in the general population.

Psychosocial development is the third aspect of development; it refers, as we have seen above, to what the child makes of his unique combination of growth, neurologic maturation, psychologic endowent, and interactions with those around him. In the following sections we will discuss the assessment of development, including psychosocial development, by ages.

PRENATAL PERIOD. The pediatrician begins assessing the child's potential for development well before he is born. For some children the history will raise the issues of chromosomal disorder, inherited metobolic disease, or acquired intrauterine disease such as rubella. Prenatal diagnosis of many conditions has become possible as a result of development of amniocentesis and techniques for identifying numerous hereditary disorders. New techniques for pregnancy termination, new legal and institutional arrangements, and a climate of opinion increasingly open to therapeutic termination of pregnancy permits prenatal intervention where indicated.

Aside from such particular conditions, however, the prenatal developmental assessment of the unborn child will include certain factors universal to all children. The pediatrician is uniquely suited to explore these and to use what he learns. The relationship he develops with the parents as part of a prenatal pediatric interview offers an opportunity to explore the setting into which the child will be born. The maturity, attitudes to the new child, and life circumstances of the parents can be assessed. The infant born to immature parents or to a single mother or the unwanted child are all at added risk during pregnancy, infancy, and childhood. A review of the early experiences of both parents and their relationships with their own families, as well as an assessment of the present relationship between the parents, will enable the pediatrician to identify those for whom parenthood, as a developmental stage in its own right, will be predictably difficult. Especially relevant is the relationship of the expectant mother with her own mother. In taking this history the pediatrician builds an alliance with the prospective parents as a person interested in them as people in their own right, with feelings that he takes seriously, and also as the parents of his patients.

A pregnancy begun against the wishes of either parent, severe vomiting well past the first trimester or other symptoms possibly indicative of maternal psychologic distress, or the mother's failure to use prenatal medical care should all raise the pediatrician's index of concern.

NEWBORN PERIOD. The physiologic demands of birth and of the period of adaptation to the extrauterine environment are discussed in Chaps 5 and 6. The infant's responses, his maintenance to vital functions, his ability to organize his changing states of alertness and to adjust to the flood of extrauterine stimuli reflect his developmental maturity, the degree of intrauterine nourishment or privation he experienced, the amount of intrapartum stress, and the lingering effects of any maternal medication. After a few days have passed and feeding has been established, his responses bespeak the temperament or activity level with which he is born.

Developmental assessment in the newborn period involves indentifying parents and infants at risk. It begins with appreciation, and sensitive exposition of the parents, of all of the aspects described above. Infants may be at developmental risk in several ways and for many reasons. The effects of gross developmental handicaps and major congenital anomalies or serious chronic illnesses need no elaboration here.

All severely handicapped children run a second developmental risk arising out of their family's inability to integrate the experience of having a handicapped or chronically ill child and to adjust interactions to the child's needs and capacities. Reactions taking the form of either unrealistic expectations of what the child can do or overprotective infantilization and undersocialization of the child are extremely common and probably account for as many funcitional handicaps as the original physical lesions themselves. Yet these problems can be very responsive to intervention by an aware and sensitive pediatrician.

A third type of risk arises from gestational or perinatal insults that compromise an infant's prospects in ways that may not be apparent at birth but that may show up later in developmental delays or deviation or in subtle signs (often first noted by mothers) that all is not well in the quality of the child's interacting. In these cases a careful differential diagnosis includes assessment of temperamental factors, possible current physiologic

distress in the child, and environmental tension in the parents. This requires assessment of several factors, including the infant's competence as an infant, the mother's comfort in managing him, and the state of the interaction between them. The risk here is that only the mother will perceive that there is something different about her child and that it is not simply a very active, demanding quality but a more diffuse difficulty in organizing experience or coordinating responses to it. Reassurance by the physican, without appreciation of the reality she faces, will result in her feeling alienated both from the rapport she looked for in her child and from the community of adults, including the physician. Such maternal alienation then becomes a developmental handicap in its own right.

The frequency with which this kind of difficulty in integrating experience and interactions with the environment may actually follow some innocuous perinatal stress or subclinical infection is unknown. Two lines of evidence argue for the need for attention to such a possibility. One is the frequency of a history of difficult birth or other CNS insult that is seen when retrospective developmental histories of early teenagers with severe emotional and behavior disturbances are reviewed. In many of these cases a second noteworthy indication is the mother's conviction that from an early age something was different about her child. Such evidence is obviously subject to all of the caveats that apply to data collected retrospectively. The other line of evidence deals with differences in school performance, language development, and psychologic test scores in children with histories of severe infantile illness but in whom no gross sequelae were evident and whose neurologic examinations were normal. If the pediatrician acknowledges that such diffuse neurologic handicaps may follow what we have thought to be innocent insults early in development, he can be responsive to the mother's perception that something is awry and help her find ways to manage her different kind of child, thereby making an important prophylactic contribution to mental health.

The social circumstances of the family into which he is born are a fourth major risk for any child. Is there enough money? How realistically have the parents planned? Will the mother's health support the physical and emotional strain of child-raising? Are the new parents part of an extended community that welcomes the child and supports the parents, or are they cut off, isolated, and alone? Are there religious or other beliefs that interfere with proper feeding of the baby? Religious differences between the parents may be exacerbated by the demands imposed in fitting a member of a new generation into the secular and religious order of things. To the extent that family sources of child-rearing standards and lore are not available or satisfactory to them, do the young parents have books and other sources of information to turn to for guidance in raising their child? In recent years the effectiveness of identifying infants at risk on the basis of their parents' social and psychologic situations has been demonstrated in primary care pediatric centers in urban areas. Specially adapted high-intensity services have been effective in preventing illness and developmental attrition.

A fifth kind of risk is that one of a number of factors may interfere with the process of attachment, or bonding, especially between mother and child. Evolution has prepared the newborn and his parents to be exquisitely ready to make attachments to each other. The capacity of imprinting that has been dramatically evident in some avian species exists in humans as well and is increasingly being studied. We know that the early days and even hours of extrauterine life are in many ways a critical time for the establishment of such attachment, that the degree of attachment is reliably observable and persistent, that it probably affects child development in the long run and certainly does so in the early months, and that the process is susceptible to interferences of many kinds that may arise either from the state of the mother or the newborn or from the circumstances around their early contacts.

Among those infants who may be at special risk of defective bonding are all those set off as different by virtue of premature birth, congenital anomaly, or chronic illness that is evident in the neonatal period, as well as all those whom the parents perceive as different either because of the circumstances of delivery or because of some incidental feature of their newborn appearance or behavior. The recognition that such differences exist in the parents' eyes may require unusual perceptiveness and sensitivity on the pediatrician's part. Thus a young mother unaware that the lanugo hair of the newborn is a normal characteristic may fantasize that her child is a throwback to a state not fully human and may become somewhat distant from her child. Or a child born after several fetal losses or stillbirths may be perceived as exceedingly frail, vulnerable, and in need of special care. Such a child may be so overprotected and restricted as to grow up in a way that distorts all aspects of development.

Such factors set the child off from the average and from what the parents had expected. Prematurity and other neonatal conditons requiring hospitalization and separation from the parents at a critical time of bonding, plus the anxiety attendant upon life-threatening illness, even through such illness may not appear life-threatening to professionals, plus the emotional blow of not having produced the anticipated perfect baby—all these factors complicate the early parent–child relationship. Even a minor intervention such as phototherapy for hyperbilirubinemia, with the unexpectedly striking appearance presented by protective eye coverings, can be upsetting to parents and may be recalled years later as the first sign of impending difficulty. Unless dealt with prophylactically by the pediatrician, such experiences can make it impossible for susceptible parents to integrate the new child emotionally, with his own unique features, even when he is a wanted child.

The term *susceptible parents* is useful, as it points to factors in the parents, especially in the mother, that suggest a risk of defective bonding. Among these factors are abnormal ambivalence about this child because of the circumstances of his conception or gestation, a disturbed marital relationship around the time of his birth, his arrival as a psychologic replacement for a previously deceased child, or his identification in the mother's emotions with an ambivalently regarded relative. Major maternal illness, maternal depression, or recent severe losses in the mother's own life all jeopardize the chances for bonding. Appreciation of any of these factors in the mother's situation should raise the pediatrician's index of concern and stimulate him to seek ways to help the new parents at a crucial time.

INFANCY. Developmental assessment in infancy begins with attention to the characteristics of the individual newborn. Thomas, Chess, and Birch, and more recently Brazelton, have demonstrated and stated in clinically relevant terms what mothers and pediatricians have always recognized: namely, that babies differ in disposition or temperament in ways that will influence interactions with care-givers and hence the course of all future development. The continuum runs from the quiet baby who is difficult to stimulate and difficult to arouse, who gives little but may be highly observant of what goes on around him, to the very active easily stimulated baby who may drive the family to distraction because he is so difficult to calm. The mixed or matched relationships between such widely different infants and parents who may themselves be better disposed to manage one or the other kind provide the setting in which mutually satisfying patterns and routines of feeding, sleeping, and other activities must be established.

Most developmental assessment in infancy and early childhood deals with the gradual sequential attainment of a series of behaviors in the areas of adaptive, gross motor, fine motor, language, and social-personal skills that Gesell first spelled out with precision. The timetables of development Gesell presents should not be taken to apply rigidly to all infants. As indicated earlier, individual variation among infants is where developmental assessment begins. But the general direction of development, along each of the five lines identified, holds for each child, and major delays or failures to attain predicted milestones are the first indications of serious pathology, especially when the failures include several of the areas of behavior. The problem may be intrinsic to the child or the result of lack of stimulation or inconsistency of care, or it may be due to some other experience detrimental to development.

Organized tests can assist the clinician in certain aspects of developmental assessment. The Denver Developmental Screening Test is widely used by pediatricians and public health nurses. It is of value as an indicator that something is amiss, as it lists in chronologic sequence the ages at which children, on the average, perform selected tasks in each of four areas (Gross Motor, Fine Motor, Language, and Social Development) and allows charting of the child's current level in easily assimilated form. With this or similar tools and a few simple toys the pediatrician can in about 15 minutes determine a given child's development vis-à-vis his peers and children older and younger. Much of the same material is presented in more comprehensive form in a revision of Gesell's developmental diagnosis by Passamanick and Knobloch. The Bayley Infant Scale is an extension of this kind of instrument. None has definite predictive value, but all assist in determining where the child is functioning at a given time.

Other standardized assessment instruments will become increasingly available. The cognitive developmental observations of Piaget have led Casati and Lezine and Uzgiris and Hunt to develop instruments to measure a child's acquisition of the early forms of sensorimotor intelligence. These tests and others similar to them are already in use by pediatricians and psychologists with special interests in early child development. The proper application of tests by pediatricians and psychologists depends on clinicians' familiarity with the theory and principles involved, not just with the tests themselves. While such instruments assess many aspects of development, the crucial issue in psychosocial development, as indicated earlier, is the emergence of the quality of basic trust. This quality is assessed clinically, not by testing.

On the basis of a relationship with his primary caregiver in which his needs are consistently met and in which he also experiences frustration when appropriate, the infant shows a relaxed, comfortable quality that is reflected in his sleeping, eating, and bowel function. The frequent questions about all aspects of development that mothers ask during routine clinical visits provide the opportunity to ask how the mother and child are getting along together. This leads to questions involving how much the mother is able to trust herself in her caretaking of her child and whether she is able to give him a feeling of personal confidence and gradually confidence in others as well.

TODDLER STAGE. The toddler has the task of integrating all the new behavior changes we have described earlier with a sense of autonomy, which makes for a continuing sense of himself and for mutually satisfying interactions with those around him. The family has the task of responding to his developing capacity to assert himself with some mixture of flexibility and firmness, with judicious permission to do for himself and with faith that his new skills can and will be integrated and made into something coherent. The task of developmental assessment at this stage involves looking at the child's growth not only in terms of specific behaviors but also in terms of the kind of person he is becoming, in particular his ability to make choices for himself and the way in which he fits in with the needs and expectations of those around him. An observation that mother and child are in a power struggle and are losing the ability to enjoy each other suggests problems, even before the issue of toilet training and sphincter control emerges. This area, more than any other, can be the focus for the battle over who is going to control whom and over the degree to which the child will be perceived by his family as being capable of learning to manage his own affairs or as needing to be constantly watched and regulated by others.

Thus developmental assessment at this age pays special attention to the emergence of the ability to say "I want this," or "I don't want that," in ways that are not simply stubborn and negativistic but to which the family can respond positively. The child at this age who never says "I want," who has no choices, who complies passively or asserts himself only in ways that end up in his being prohibited from doing what he wants, cannot be said to be developing positively.

PRESCHOOL STAGE. Around the age of school entry a critical rush of development occurs that for most children results in readiness for the behavior demands and intellectual opportunities of school. White has called this the 5-to-7 shift and has pointed out its neurologic, cognitive, and behavior components. Neurophysiologic maturation provides much of the impetus for this shift, and pediatric assessment of such maturation can play a large part in identifying children with delayed or deviant development for whom school entry at the regular age might offer more frustration and defeat than learning and satifying adaptation. For many of these children special transitional classes would be beneficial, and the pediatrician who is aware of possibly delayed readiness can perform a real service by astute counseling and referral if needed.

In examining the child between 3 and 6 years of age the pediatrician will be attentive to the many new skills he is acquiring: skipping, jumping, riding a tricycle, learning the full use of language, and learning to separate from home and to get along with peers in play situations, nursery school, and kindergarten. The child's ability to relate to, play with, and get along with other children his own age requires careful attention here, as a reflection of his autonomy, of his developing sense of himself, and of the ability of child and parents together to manage the separation involved in the child's movement from the orbit of the family toward the outside.

The quality of initiative can be assessed both historically and by observation in the office. Initiative involves the behaviors of approaching, attacking, undertaking, and grasping any variety of toys, people, and ideas, and also the pleasure a child of this age can take in such activity. Holding back, overconstriction, or lack of pleasure in play and conversation are important diagnostic indicators. Other symptoms at this age include nightmares, preoccupation with themes of mutilation in talk or play, destructiveness, and some kinds of aggressiveness. These reflect anxiety and a new awareness of the body's capacities and vulnerabilities. They can be assessed by history and by direct observation.

Anticipatory guidance can be offered to parents concerning the manifestations of sexual development at this age: discovery of one's genitals and of the sensations there can be anticipated and discussed in relation to the parents' experiences and expectations, and an effort can be made to put self-manipulation into the perspective of normal development. The syndrome of the impossible child who simply cannot be managed by the parents and is impulsive, disobedient, possibly destructive, and a source of agitated concern may appear at this or an earlier or later age. It may be considered one of the forms of severe failed mutuality; it will be discussed later in that context.

SCHOOL AGE. Entrance into school presents another crisis of separation and tells much about the ability of the child and his family to negotiate development in general. Once in school his prior experiences with other children and his idea of himself as one of a group will be reflected in the way he relates to peers and teachers. School performance will reflect another area of development: readiness for sustaining attention, for taking in information by visual and auditory channels, for processing and remembering what is seen and heard, and for learning the specifics of reading and calculation. His teachers and others will evaluate his progress on the basis of the ease and facility with which these skills are acquired. It is important to emphasize that neurologic maturation must coincide with educational expectations if status and self-esteem are to be dependent on performance on standardized tasks that require a certain degree of neurologic organization. Frustration and failure in school have social meanings for the child (What kind of child is he among his peers?) and meanings as to personal intactness and competence (What kind of child is he intrinsically?). The pediatrician who is able to identify a possible perceptual or cognitive handicap in a child early in his educational career, before all of the secondary effects become manifest, and who can help the family and school make the necessary adjustments and arrange appropriate educational placement where indicated, will be doing the child a major service.

An increasingly important part of developmental assessment will be specific tests for neurologic maturity and coordination. Some test items, like tandem walking or diadochokinesia, have long been part of standard neurologic assessment. Tests such as the Lincoln-Ozeretsky test of motor maturity assess systematically many items of coordination, balance, ability at tasks involving rapid repeated actions (sequencing tasks), and eye–hand coordination. Disturbances in these functions are often referred to as minor neurologic signs or soft signs. Yet if they interfere with the child's cognitive ability in school, his ability to play effectively with peers, or his enjoyment of the use of his body in any kind of activity, the problem can be major indeed. Moreover, because the child is not obviously handicapped, the nature of his problem often escapes detection for years, so that without sympathetic clarification of his difficulty he is left to feel that he is at fault, and he does not benefit from whatever practical educational aids might be indicated.

The overall developmental task for the child of primary school age is that of integrating all of the new motor, cognitive, and social potentials of this stage into a personality structure that can channel the initiative of earlier stages into new activities and that can take pleasure in being among, and in measuring oneself against, peers. The pathologic potential here is an overwhelming sense of inferiority, which calls for diagnostic zeal in seeking the basis in his earlier experiences or in his family or in the apparatus he brings to his tasks currently, and which may be handicapping him.

The function of education as preparation for adult work indicates that yet another important factor in the child's developing sense of himself is the kind of message about him and his future that the school conveys to the child. Schools may fill a child with despair or develop in him the dull rigidity that can cover despair; they can offer demonstrations that society's rewards are given to others on the basis of race, religion, or cultural or economic background rather than on the basis of intrinsic worth; or they can indicate that a bright economic future is not available to him. Because forces beyond personal endowment and home environment impinge so heavily on the child at this stage, developmental assessment during the school years must include some knowledge of the nature and quality of the school experience to which he is exposed daily. Especially where the child has school problems, whether these are in the area of learning or behavior, the physician will find it helpful to become personally familiar with both the school and teacher.

ADOLESCENCE. Assessment in adolescence can be considered along several developmental lines. First, with regard to puberty: where is the adolescent with respect to physical maturation, and what is the reaction to it? Again the developmental task is to stay on top of things, to manage to integrate the present physical and physiologic upheavals with the person one was previously. Second, with regard to emotional attachment: developmental progression normally takes the adolescent through intensified relationships with the parent of the same sex on to intense relationships with peers of the same sex (the setting in which individual or group sex play normally occurs) and then to relationships with peers of the opposite sex. Simple questioning and discussion will soon make clear whether an adolescent is moving through this sequence smoothly, tumultuously, or not at all. The adolescent may be either withdrawing from all relationships or developing an intense mutual dependence and hostility with the same-sex parent (especially girls with their mothers). Some will attempt to resolve old issues of caring and protection by leapfrogging from closeness to parents to premature forced intimacy with a peer or older person, giving the appearance of maturity without its substance. Failure to integrate adolescence in general may be seen in lasting hypochondriacal states, in the retention of a childish personal style, in compulsive self-starvation (anorexia nervosa has been called weight phobia or growing-up phobia), or in an inability to manage personal hygiene, especially menses.

Mood and involvement in activities may be useful phenomena to observe as part of this assessment. Swings of mood and initial episodes of noticeable depression may be features of adolescence related to new kinds of self-awareness, bodily changes, and the estrangement from earlier relationships that come with growing up. Withdrawal from peer activities may be conspicuous. The key dimension is the duration of the depression or withdrawal. A period of 1 or 2 months with little interest in relationships or in school may be of little moment in the perspective of all of adolescence. However, a period of withdrawal or depression lasting for a longer period would be a real concern. In general, the physician doing developmental assessment at this age must take a longer view than that of his patient and often that of the parents. He must put the rebelliousness or the need to separate from parental control in perspective, and yet at the same time recognize the malignant possibilities of the more severe forms of withdrawal.

Pediatricians and their patients have long been aware that the physician must like to work with adolescents before he can succeed with them. Not everyone would enjoy the particular demands that adolescents place on their doctors (as on their parents and teachers). Since the quality of the personal relationship has such developmental importance to the adolescent and since his intolerance of simulation is so keen, doctors tend to make a definite choice of this kind of work or else avoid it entirely. Enjoyment of it is not simply a matter of the doctor's own personality; clinical experience under supervision is a major and necessary ingredient in the competence and confidence of the physician caring for adolescents.

For many children with chronic illness early adolescence is marked by deterioration in self-care, as in diabetics who refuse to take their medications. Severe, openly expressed discouragement about life, or covert despair, may be expressed in the form of delinquency, decline in schoolwork, or withdrawal from relationships. Issues are at work here having to do with the meaning, for the adolescent himself, of coming of age as an adult with chronic illness. An illness like diabetes will often be questioned, rejected, and then accepted again on the adolescent's own terms, even when a good adjustment existed before adolescence. Because of the adolescent's cognitive ability to deal with abstractions and to compare his life situation with others that are different from his own, the chronically ill or handicapped adolescent may develop an unusually strong preoccupation with concepts like justice and fate that are always evident in this developmental phase. For the parent, especially for the mother, many of the early issues involved in having a child with a handicap (which can be thought of as part of postpartum mourning) may be reawakened, even though the parent may not fully realize it. The pediatrician, when confronting unexplained problems in an adolescent with chronic illness or handicap, may be able to help himself, his patient, and the family understand what is happening if he explores these issues with them.

Since identity development is the central psychosocial task at this age, the identities available for a given adolescent in his inner life, his family, his community and school, and in the world of adult work are worth attention. Many of the behavior problems of this age can be seen either as desperate attempts to amount to something where few options or only unacceptable options exist in one's family or community or as signs that one has given up the struggle in despair. These problems may or may not be labeled as psychopathologic; they include running away, delinquency, and drug experimentation and abuse. The diagnostic and therapeutic task of the pediatrician is to see the turmoil in perspective and help the youth to resist (and the family to let up on) pressures for early identity foreclosure. He must help the adolescent take advantage of whatever psychosocial moratoria his community offers and his interests and aptitudes suit him for, so that further growth can take place with somewhat less pressure. The decade of the 1960s demonstrated how strong the pressures can be and how tumultuous and often personally distressing the responses of youth can be when the larger society seems to offer few ways for them to express themselves acceptably. The social and political turmoil of that decade touched almost every adolescent struggling to develop his own identity, with far-reaching consequences to many.

MUTUALITY ASSESSMENT

Mutuality refers to the mutual activation of two people by each other. Each gives, as a part of his own development, what the other needs to receive in order to move ahead in his development. To cite an example from early in the life cycle: as the new mother feels her milk come in, learns ways to hold and to nurse that feel comfortable to her and to her infant, and so gains confidence in her own ability as a mother, which is her relevant developmental task, her baby receives the two things he needs for growth—nourishment and a feeling of comfort and security, the beginning of basic trust. He, in turn, by growing, by responding socially, and by fitting into cycles of sleep and waking and quiet and active times of day, gives something to her—objective and concrete confirmation that she is succeeding as a mother. In essence, each assists the other with whatever developmental tasks are at hand

Mutuality assessment can be complicated unless one can emotionally distance oneself. In identifying the developmental tasks at hand, where many data are available about each person's immediate concerns, a conceptual framework is required. Understanding the subtle ways that parents and children can frustrate each other often requires a perceptive history and careful observation. Thus a mother may verbally express concern because her child resists going to kindergarten, while a skilled diagnostician can perceive the subtle and probably unconscious cues by which she conveys the message that home is the only safe place. Or an adolescent who is the youngest child may develop symptoms such as intractable headaches that the empathetic pediatrician may trace to the beginning separation needs of the child whose mother is holding on to him emotionally and is vicariously participating in his turmoil. Therapeutic intervention involves identifying and dealing with the blocks that impede development and helping all parties to restore the mutuality whose loss they are feeling, so that development may resume its normal progression. Understanding the tasks required of both parent and child at each stage of psychosocial development may make such assessment of mutuality easier.

SEVERE FAILED MUTUALITY.   Three especially difficult clinical conditions can be described as examples of failure of mutual regulation between parent and child. They are the impossible child, nonorganic failure to thrive, and child abuse.

IMPOSSIBLE CHILD.   The term impossible child refers to children who are often described with precisely this term by their parents, whom the parents regard as unmanageable in the home because of symptoms such as severe temper tantrums and intensely demanding, impulsive, and aggressive behavior. Parental use of the term may exceed the diagnostic use we make of it here; not everything described as impossible is really impossible. While many of these symptoms (like tantrums) may be developmentally normal at certain ages, the critical diagnostic finding here is the failure of mutuality, the desperate feeling in both parent and child (even though parents are usually the only ones able to express it directly) that life together is becoming impossible. Frequently the history will reveal that such children were the products of difficult pregnancies, that they had feeding and sleeping problems in infancy and often cried inconsolably, and that they progressed to other behavior problems such as tantrums, head banging, and other demanding behavior. Such children may persist in finicky eating habits and disturbed sleep patterns even though major developmental milestones are on schedule. They are frequently healthy and bright, but are unable to relate to their parents in any mutually satisfactory way. Observation will reveal inconsistent, unpredictable parental responses to the child that suggest failed mutuality from an early age. Skilled psychotherapy may be effective in improving the child's behavior and the ability of child and family to get along with each other. In other children with this syndrome neurologic problems of greater or lesser severity may coexist with and contribute to the behavior and interaction disorder. In such cases detailed neurologic assessment and appropriate medication, if indicated, will be a part of treatment.

The psychologic factors involved include the childhood experiences of the parents that have poorly prepared them for parenthood, intense self-doubt and ambivalence toward the child on the mother's part, marital schism depriving the mother of support from the father, and intense uncertainty in the child about the constancy of anything in his world, from parents to himself. The key issue is assessment of how supportive or destructive the family is to the child's own efforts at self-control. For all such parents and children a deliberate restructuring of their environment is a major part of treatment.

The syndrome of pathologic interaction will manifest itself during many pediatric contacts ranging from routine clinical visits to examinations in emergency wards and the specialty services to which such children are brought for assessment. The prognosis is not optimistic in terms of the child's own psychologic development, in terms of the distorted development of the rest of the family, and in potential for violence against or by such a child. Russell and Harper have described a group of such children among severely disturbed delinquent youth, and they may also become chronically seriously impaired adults.

Possibilities for prevention lie in early detection of such serious disturbance in mutuality and relief of identifiable factors in parent and child. Treatment of the syndrome may involve temporary separation of parent and child. Psychotherapeutic help for parent and child must aim at helping each to respond more consistently and supportively to the other. Most important is that the pediatrician recognize and respond to the situation as a serious one with which he and the parents should be concerned. This is not a situation the pediatrician should attempt to deal with unaided; psychiatric consultation and referral will in general be useful.

FAILURE TO THRIVE.   Nonorganic failure to thrive, or psychosocial dwarfism (p. 217) has often been thought of as an illness of deprivation; deprivational dwarfism has at times been used as an equivalent term. Clinical experience suggests that this condition may better be considered a disorder of failed mutuality, especially when it occurs in children over 2 years of age who participate to a major degree in their own feeding. In the older child fear of self-regulation and frustration in developing his own autonomy may underlie the feeding problem and may be related to parental responses that confirm the child's feeling that inner controls are impossible to achieve. Assessment includes reviewing the amount of trust and autonomy the child has developed and defining the areas in which mutuality has failed.

The operation of such mechanisms in infants who fail to thrive is more problematic but is suggested by several factors. In many families only one child of several fails to thrive. In addition, such infants are often dramatically unresponsive on admission to hospitals; they are often difficult to care for, and they constitute a therapeutic challenge to medical and nursing staff.

CHILD ABUSE.   Child abuse is discussed elsewhere at length (p. 827), but in the context of failed mutuality two aspects are relevant. The first has to do with nomenclature and the attitudes it reflects. As a reflection of the overwhelmed and desperate situation in which parents who have become unable to protect their children find themselves, the phrase intentional injury of children is as naive psychologically as it is misleading operationally. The clinical issue is not to make the diagnosis of inflicted injury in a spirit often more prosecutorial than therapeutic, but to attend to the needs for immediate protection and long-term planning for both the injured child or the child at risk and the parents who have been unable to protect him. Fortunately the term battered child is also passing out of clinical use; in addition to the unhelpful emotionality it evokes, it also focuses on the act rather than on the failure to protect. A view focused primarily on the injuries that have occurred distracts clinicians from the context of the family setting and the stresses that may impinge on children at risk of injury who may be in as great a need of protective and other clinical services as those already injured.

The second relevant aspect here has to do with psychologic development in children injured in the home or at risk of such injury or with a past history of such injury. Such children suffer damage to their emotional development that may be less conspicuous but more longlasting than physical trauma and that may contribute after the age of 3 or 4 years to further injury. The most frequent distortions involve damage to the capacity to sustain loving relationships (specifically, a distrust of and flight from personal closeness), a tendency to deal with loss or threatened loss by provocation (often surprisingly infuriating even to usually well-disposed and well-controlled adults), a lowered threshold for impulsive action (including aggression) in interpersonal relations, and in common with children who have known emotional deprivation with or without abuse, a tendency to use sexual contacts to seek care and nurturance. These traits can lead to lifelong patterns of relationships in which one or the other party is forever hurting or being hurt, leaving or being left, or to aggressive disorders and sexual experiences with adults that can be viewed as further abuse but that can also be seen as attempts to regain earlier forms of caring.

INTERVENTION.　The three types of disorder we have discussed have a common potential for serious immediate physical damage to children as well as long-term physical and psychologic harm to them and continuing psychologic distress to their parents. The pediatrician may intervene through immediate assessment of physical risk to the child, through hospitalization where the breakdown of home functioning is so severe that the child cannot be considered safe there, and through physical evaluation and treatment of the child as indicated. Special attention is warranted in all these conditions to possible factors in the child that may have contributed to the failure of mutual regulation. The apparent victim is not served by being seen only as a victim. In one child a metabolic error that made her smell "dirty" even when she was clean contributed to exasperation in her mother, who had particular personal and family reasons to want her baby to be wholesome in every sense.

In addition, psychologic assessment of the child is needed, with particular reference to the foundations of mutuality: basic trust, autonomy, quality of relationships, ways of seeking affection, and ways of dealing with loss. Medical and psychosocial assessment of the parents may reveal stresses such as painful medical conditions, work-related or landlord problems, absence of spouse, or need for day care; intervention may tip the balance for the parents' ability to cope. A team approach including social worker, patient advocate, and psychiatric consultant may be useful. The pediatrician's approach to the parents must remain sympathetic and helpful, avoiding the temptation to view the parents as the source of all the pain and suffering in the case.

Mandatory reporting to the state or other protective agencies is required in most states in situations where physicians or other professionals see children injured or at risk in the home. As a rule such reporting is not an accusation, nor will it lead to charges being pressed against the parents. It does not involve asking for state custody, and it can be and must be shared with parents in a frank and nonjudgmental way (the physician can present himself as an ally in helping the parents to protect the child). To many a clinician's surprise, the act of reporting often strengthens rather than destroys the parents' alliance with the doctor, and it includes legal immunity to the reporting physician against charges of slander or defamation. In some cases placement in foster care or in a residential institution on a long-term or short-term basis may be needed. These decisions need not and generally should not be made on first contact with such a case, but only after evaluation of the total situation and in particular after assessment of the parents' ability to respond to offered assistance.

EMPATHIZING WITH THE CHILD

It is necessary to integrate the developmental and mutuality assessments, as well as knowledge of normal child development, if one is to understand what the child is experiencing in the process of growing up. At times the knowledge that the physician is aware of and empathetic with his situation may result in dramatic improvement, especially where family and child have found no way of understanding troubling symptoms other than to attribute them to the child himself. In some cases a diagnosis of a specific problem can lift a great burden from child and parents alike. For example, if the parent complains that the child "just wants to stare and ignore me," and a diagnosis of petit mal epilepsy is made, or if the child "just won't listen" and is found to have unsuspected hearing loss, the child is no longer seen to be the problem but is seen to be in need of special treatment and care. Other situations may be less amenable to simple solutions. Yet on the basis of his understanding of what it means to have that particular condition, the pediatrician can empathize with the child and convey his understanding to the family. Thus the hyperactive child with an attention disorder who has been seen as never wanting to get down to work may be seen anew as a child trying to cope with impaired ability to screen out competing stimuli.

In other cases where a diagnosis in terms of physiologic factors is not as readily available, or where an existing diagnosis does not seem to account for the child's behavior, the task of empathizing is more difficult, especially when the forces with which the child must contend are emotional. When the pathogenic forces are not as concretely demonstrated as in conditions with an obvious physical basis, it is not as easy to convey the sense of their constraining power. In addition, the feelings involved themselves constitute an obstacle to seeing the problem objectively. The most stressful aspects of the lives of parents and children are likely tied up with symptoms that activate the parents' own fears of loss or aggression or their sexual anxieties. Such emotions will be stirred up by and will help stimulate school phobia, aggressiveness, or adolescent promiscuity in the child. The emotional intensity associated with the clinical problem will accentuate the overall difficulty in recognizing and dealing with the true nature of the presenting complaint.

The basic tasks, however, remain the same: to identify the problems the child is trying to overcome and to avoid the common pitfall of viewing the child himself as the problem when an explanation is lacking. The foremost developmental task at each age is to integrate physical and emotional changes associated with growth and development with past experience, with role and position in the family, and with the prevailing ethos and opportunities of the larger society so as to develop and maintain a coherent and continuing sense of personal identity. *In assessing any troubled child it is a useful initial assumption that the only way he can manage to achieve any integration and sustain a sense of continuous personal identity is through the symptoms he is manifesting.*

In addition to the panicky feeling (often masked by despair and apathy) of not being able to get together all the elements of personal identity, there are specific feeling states that are common to children and adults but distressing in different ways. Feelings of weakness or helplessness or lack of control of one's own body and emotions or important aspects of one's life contribute to feeling endangered or threatened and inferior or inadequate vis-à-vis parents, siblings, and peers. A child's own idea of what he should be, or his view that he is not ready for the next stage or is unwilling to face up to what lies ahead, may arouse particularly strong feelings of being pushed by events, especially at the onset of adolescence. To make these feelings less obvious both to others and to themselves, children try to cope with such feelings in certain recurring ways. The physician may note the bravado and the aggressiveness of the scared child, the attempt to do everything by himself of the child fearing dependency, the desire to be up and about of the child faced with confinement, bed rest, or any other regressive situation, the overconstriction and inhibition of the child afraid things will get out of hand, and the forced adult pose of the child despairing that he will ever really be on his own.

It is important to understand the parental relationship with the child from the point of view of parental development if one is to assist in dealing with such problems. If parents are unable to empathize with the child, or if they are unable or unwilling to try to understand what the child is doing and feeling, while admitting that reasons for his behavior might exist, they are denying him any possibility of emotional support from them. They may cast everything the child does in unsympathetic terms and express negative feelings that clearly indicate that their expectations are low. The parents' view of their child will be determined by their own emotional maturity, their feelings about this particular child, or their ability in general to take another's perspective. However, it may also be influenced by their knowledge of child development and by discussion with a sympathetic and understanding third party, such as the pediatrician, who should be aware that most parents are genuinely interested and concerned and often feel as helpless as their child in dealing with complex and baffling behavior manifestations. It is important that the physician avoid taking sides, as this reduces his ability to help either the child or the parents.

SEXUAL BEHAVIOR

The attitudes of society have probably changed more markedly in the area of overt sexual behavior than in any other area during the past decade. This has been reflected not only in the liberalization of laws relating to sexual activities of adults, but also in increasingly open acknowledgment of the sexual needs and behavior of adolescents. Minors now are able, in many states, to seek prophylactic and therapeutic intervention for sex-related problems without parental consent, and sex information and education are increasingly available to large groups of children and adolescents. Nevertheless, misinformation, ignorance, and folklore still permeate the attitudes of an excessive number of individuals seen in the pediatrician's office, either as adolescent patients, as very young parents of infants and young children, or as concerned older parents not yet fully attuned to the recent sexual revolution. Unfortunately, at times the physician is also not in tune with current mores and manners, and in such cases he can be less than helpful to a young person in need of support. It is important for the pediatrician to recognize that if he cannot be comfortable in dealing with the sexual behavior, problems, and needs of his adolescent patients, or if he believes that he must report their confidences to their parents, he should be aware of alternative resources for them and refer them elsewhere.

As we all now recognize, sexual awareness does not develop de novo in adolescence or preadolescence. It is present from infancy, differing in expression and relative importance at different stages of development. The attitude toward sex of those with whom he is in daily contact is of vital importance to the healthy sexual development of the growing child. We now recognize that children are concerned with sex and sex differences from an early age. By the age of 2.5 years children become aware of anatomic differences, and by the age of 3 years they are beginning to ask questions, often at times or in places that are apt to be embarrassing to some parents or care-givers. In such situations there is a risk that the adult response will suggest to the child that the question or the questioner is bad or wrong. By the age of 4 years most children will be eager for answers to many questions regarding sex differences, the origin of babies, etc. Sex information should be given simply and truthfully, in language the child can understand, and preferably by the parents in a natural response to a child's questions. If his first questions are met with evasion or disapproval, the child may stop asking and may obtain inaccurate information elsewhere or rely on fantasies based on vague or distorted notions. On the other hand, a simple straightforward answer usually satisfies the child, who will return with additional questions as they arise.

It is during the toddler and preschool stages of development that parental attitudes can do considerable harm, such as when parents overemphasize certain behavior, reprimand the child unnecessarily, or laugh at his valid questions. An overenthusiastic attempt to teach modesty may suggest that nudity is wrong. At the same time, many thoughtful persons are becoming concerned about overemphasis on nudity and openness in some homes, which may in some cases lead to preoccupation with sexual differences at an early age. This is especially likely when a small boy becomes concerned with his comparatively small penis and begins to compare himself unfavorably with the ideal of the adult male. Curiosity about sex differences may lead to exploration of each other's genitals and to sex play between small children. It is important to advise parents to avoid expressing shock or disgust when their young children engage in such activities; parental overreactions may be prevented by preparation of the parents in casual discussions during routine clinical visits.

Masturbation as a mode of sexual expression is practiced at all ages and by both sexes. It is rare before the age of 6 months and is not commonly an open activity once the child has learned to be discreet about public behavior. As with other aspects of sexuality, attitudes to masturbation have changed significantly in recent years, with most parents, teachers, and physicians accepting it as normal behavior that should not arouse undue concern unless it becomes excessive and preoccupies the child to the exclusion of other activities. In general, masturbation is no longer as common a complaint of parents to the pediatrician as it was even 10 or 15 years ago. Nevertheless, parents whose religious, moral, or ethnic backgrounds cause differences from the prevailing mores may continue to view masturbation as immoral, sinful, or likely to cause effects as diverse as failure to grow, epilepsy, or insanity. It is essential that the pediatrician be alert to these views and that he make a real effort to treat the parental attitudes before lasting harm is done. Parents must be made to understand that, in general, masturbation does no harm, that it is a fairly universal activity engaged in at one time or another by all children, and that their child is not a pervert.

In situations where masturbation becomes a major preoccupation it does reflect underlying tensions and anxieties. The potential harm lies in the manner in which the masturbation and the underlying stresses are dealt with and possible withdrawal from peer group activities and contacts in order to satisfy the self-stimulatory need. The anxiety and insecurity of the child, exaggerated and perpetuated by parental responses, are likely to create a situation that can be alleviated only through referral for psychotherapy, unless the pediatrician can prevail on the family to pay less attention to the act, avoid threats and punishment, and assist the child in seeking more appropriate sources of satisfaction. Adequate diversion, including physical and social activities that keep the child occupied during the day, may be needed, especially where children spend long unoccupied periods at home. It has been noted that in institutions for the mentally retarded or severely mentally disordered, where excessive masturbation was once the rule rather than the exception, it is now rarely a significant problem provided that structured activity programs are part of the daily routine. This tends to confirm the view that if one type of experience is the major source of pleasure and relief to an individual, it may well become the major outlet for his feelings until other constructive activities are substituted.

Early *adolescent sexuality* may be expressed by increased masturbation or by infatuations with same-sex or opposite-sex adults, as well as in the usual romantic attachments to peers. There is increasing acceptance of the view that sexual experimentation, including some homosexual exploration, is normal in this phase of development and that it should not necessarily arouse excessive parental concern. The need for wise and sympathetic guidance and adequate sex education courses appropriate to the developmental needs of the child or adolescent must not be underestimated at this crucial stage. The pediatrician should be alert to the needs of an adolescent who may be baffled by the turmoil he is experiencing and who may need someone with whom he can discuss his fears that he is somehow different or abnormal, with some assurance that his confidences will be respected. Parental guidance at this stage is of great importance also. Many concerned parents are unable to distance themselves sufficiently and may become so concerned about the sexuality of their children that they deny them privacy, trust, and room to grow, which are so essential to a truly adult sexual adjustment.

EMOTIONAL ADJUSTMENT OF THE HANDICAPPED CHILD AND HIS FAMILY

Although it has frequently been stated by pediatricians, social workers, and psychiatrists that the parents of the child with chronic illness or handicap must learn to accept the illness, a developmental point of view conceptualizes the parents' reaction to having such a child as part of a process that requires understanding and support. The birth of a handicapped child or the development of a handicap or chronic illness in a previously healthy child involves an emotional loss and produces a response akin to mourning. Parental response to chronic handicap, serious illness, or death of a child should be viewed as an adaptive process in which the individual experiences many apparently contradictory feelings, such as sadness, denial, anger, guilt, resignation, and bargaining. These can exist concurrently or sequentially and can culminate in some degree of adjustment or acceptance and renewed coping and involvement with life. The clinician's role in such a situation is to be aware of what the mourning person is going through, to bear with him, to try to help him put his experience in perspective, and at all times to be accepting and supportive of his efforts at coping.

In discussing both handicap and chronic illness with parents it is useful to remember that at some time each set of parents must deal with their sadness, denial, anger and accusation, self-reproach, and guilt. While one can sense, probe, tentatively explore, and facilitate the expression of some feelings, one cannot accelerate the process or force people to deal with more than they are able to at the time. Dissembling of any kind, particularly about prognosis, puts an intolerable burden on physician and parent alike. Candor does not require spelling out every painful detail at once, but it does require giving a generally accurate overall view of things. Many parents will press the physician who attempts to be candid for total prediction and explanation of all aspects of the situation, and it may be extremely difficult for them to accept or understand uncertainty in diagnosis or prognosis. A nonguilty presentation of this uncertainty will aid many parents, as will rational encouragement without undue pessimism or baseless optimism. Thus the physician must endeavor to convey reasonable hopefulness while being as candid as possible (p. 45).

The process of assimilating information of such magnitude takes time and requires several interviews. The physician frequently hears later of tremendously distorted interpretations of his findings and recommendations. This result can stem from a facile expectation that information of high emotional charge can be assimilated at one exposure. Informing the parents that assimilation takes time and arranging to see them again will result in better communication and in prevention of the kinds of secondary disability that can occur when parents have not adequately integrated what has happened. Use of psychiatric or other consultation   - ferral for therapy, if indicated, is an appropriate acknowledgment of the seriousness and difficulty of the process involved and the amount of professional time it can require. The secondary emotional complications of handicap or chronic illness, which occur when this process of assimilation is derailed or left incomplete, will account for as much functional disability as the original problem. Such complications take several forms, including frank emotional rejection of the child. This is easy to recognize, although it manifests itself in various ways, including neglect of medical care, failure to thrive, and childhood depression.

Emotional denial of the illness is also easily recognized, since it manifests itself as failure to use medical care or endless confusion about treatment procedures. Recurrent medical crises occur, as with diabetes, or the child is subjected to unrealistic pressures to behave or perform as if there were no handicap or chronic illness. This may produce a profound sense of frustration, failure, inferiority, and inadequacy in the child, who always feels himself unable to live according to expectations.

Especially for the parent unable to deal with his legitimate disappointment in having a handicapped or chronically ill child, or the parent who already has poorly managed anxieties about physical health, much of his own unconscious hostility to the child will be expressed as overprotection or infantilization, with projection of anger on external factors such as dangers from germs, peers, the neighbors, and school; the child will be overprotected and overrestricted and in the end prevented from developing to his full extent. Many such children are needlessly kept from school, the objects of the constant care of unrealistically devoted parents. Guilt, more or less overt, that has not been integrated but on which a parent has got stuck may play a large part

here. In less blatant cases this syndrome may be more difficult to recognize. The outcome, seen especially in children with retardation, cerebral palsy, or cardiac disease, can be a child more disabled by his experience of growing up than by the original condition. Potentially fatal dangers may be avoided, but the child runs the risk of becoming overly passive, inhibited, and frightened or functionally defective and scapegoated socially. Inwardly he remains terrified of aggression, both his own, which he has never been able to experience, and a more diffuse sense of projected and pervading hostility in the home.

In the process of a family's adapting to a child's handicap, the time of initial recognition of the problem is the most conspicuous time of crisis, but other milestones may be predictably difficult. Crises occur at the usual ages: when school is begun; at pubescence, with increased physical growth, sexual development, and adolescent personality development; at entry into adult life and integration into the community. At any of these times, for reasons particular to each family, the painful experience of the first crisis may be repeated, or new problems may become evident (p. 1774).

PSYCHOLOGIC DISORDERS

Scope of Diagnosis

More than half of the children seen in urban pediatric practice have behavior or personality problems, although only a relatively small number of them are brought to the physician's office with the primary complaint of a psychologic disturbance. It is rare that a single diagnosis adequately reflects a child's situation, and a specific diagnosis is seldom useful without a thorough understanding of the multiple factors contributing to the presenting problem. In general, diagnostic labels in pediatrics have reflected either descriptions of specific syndromes or specific knowledge of pathophysiology, etiology, or effective treatment. In contrast, objective descriptions of the characteristics of behavior disorders and knowledge of their pathophysiology, specific etiology, and therapeutic specificity are lacking in child psychiatry. Some of this deficit is attributable to limitations in our knowledge and will perhaps be overcome as we acquire greater understanding of the biologic bases of neurologic development and the underlying mechanisms for the child's organization of experience.

Continuing definition of previously nonspecific retardation syndromes in terms of metabolic errors, elucidation of the specific biochemical bases of some of the childhood psychoses, and definition of the long-term neuropsychiatric sequelae of early childhood infections, along with identification of late-onset (second-decade) CNS complications of congenital infections such as rubella, raise the possibility of similar mechanisms underlying other disintegrative syndromes. Further elaboration of the contribution of constitutional factors or temperament to development and more precise delineation of learning disabilities and coordination problems in school-age children, including those possibly at risk on the basis of birth history, will enable us to refine our diagnostic skills and develop more effective approaches to treatment. At the same time, we may better understand the extent to which the biology of depressive illness and schizophrenia is manifested in children.

While all of these areas offer opportunities for study, it is likely that they will continue to account for only a small part of the developmental problems that pediatricians are asked to evaluate. The pediatrician who looks only for specific biologic entities among the children he sees will be frustrated, both in primary care and in referral and consultative practice. Assessment, as we have indicated, can best be made in a systematic but holistic way, looking at each component of a child's life (his growth, maturation, personality, family, and community) and endeavoring to understand how they all mesh as he proceeds with his task of integrating them in the normal course of development. This understanding is not intended to mean understanding of the child's emotional development only, as such development cannot be understood without consideration of the entire context in which the child is growing up and the personal and social needs not only of himself but of his family. It is important also to understand the meaning of the child and his symptoms to the family and to know something of their current situation and of how things seem from their point of view.

The pediatrician's understanding of the needs of both child and parents, sympathetically communicated to them, is the cornerstone of successful intervention. Simply conveying to the family a sense of sympathetic awareness of the fact that everyone feels frustrated and exhausted can be a powerful source of support to all of them. Furthermore, when the pediatrician recognizes that the child has problems and approaches him accordingly (rather than viewing the child himself as the problem) he can often provide dramatic relief to all concerned. Within a relationship built on understanding the pediatrician can offer acceptance and hope to the family and child. For many children this leads to a marked change in the atmosphere around them and may result in symptomatic improvement, even where, prior to such understanding, no therapeutic effect resulted from intensive efforts.

Of course the pediatrician can offer not only understanding and a plausible explanation of what has gone on, but specific advice. Parents usually have some capacity to take an objective viewpoint once they understand what has happened and some disposition to make an effort on the child's behalf even when it is inconvenient to them. They usually also have a reservoir of sympathy for the child, even when this is not immediately apparent. In such cases management advice can often be quite effective, and further exploration of feelings around the problem may not be needed to effect change. In other situations the pediatrician must recognize that there are deep-seated needs and problems for which no simple solutions exist and for which the intervention of a skilled psychotherapist is required.

COMMON BEHAVIORAL DISTURBANCES

Appetite Disturbances

Refusal of Food. Of all behavior problems brought to the attention of the pediatrician, those related to *anorexia* or refusal of food are the most common, the most easily prevented, the most readily precipitated, and the most amenable to cure by environmental manipulation. It is a commonplace that as many as 10 to 20 percent of children between 2 and 5 years of age will at some point be brought to the physician with the complaint that they do not eat, despite all sorts of parental efforts to encourage them. It is, in fact, the parental concern and the methods employed by the parents to cajole the resistant child to eat that serve to perpetuate what might have begun as a transient anorexia due to a minor illness or fatigue, perhaps coupled with the normal negativism of a 2- to 3-year-old.

The basic causes of feeding problems related to refusal or faddishness are found in the development of the ego, with associated negativism that may be coupled to a greater or lesser degree with failed mutuality. Some infants will quite suddenly refuse the breast or bottle between 6 and 9 months of age or refuse to eat if not permitted to try to hold the spoon or bottle themselves, which is clearly related to increasing self-determination in the child. By 6 months of age an infant may have firm likes and dislikes and may flatly refuse a new food he does not like or one whose texture or even appearance is not appealing to him. He may also become bored with a certain food if it is offered too frequently. Any attempt to force the rejected or disliked food at this time can lead to permanent refusal of this food or to the beginning of a typical anorexia of the type so commonly seen.

Another important factor in the early development of food refusal is maternal preoccupation with the amount consumed, without regard for such facts as variation in individual appetites, that a child may be ill, uncomfortable, or unhappy, and that dawdling is normal between 9 months and 2 to 3 years of age, whether or not it is convenient for the mother. Simple attempts to persuade the dawdling child to eat can be the beginning of a long saga in which a perfectly normal stage in eating behavior becomes exaggerated and ultimately becomes a fixed anorectic pattern.

The most important single factor in the genesis of appetite problems is attempting to force food. Parents fail to recognize that children cannot be forced to take food and that in a battle over food the child always wins. However, the costs in emotional tension and faulty developmental progression are enormous for both child and parent. Parents use a variety of methods to cajole, entreat, bribe, or threaten their child into eating. These have a range: pleading; offering desserts, candy, or even money; distracting with music, games, and various antics; threats and physical punishment. At the same time many parents will allow the child who does not eat at mealtimes to eat whenever and whatever he wants between meals, so that he has constant snacks and then refuses everything at the regular family meal.

Prevention of this maladaptive pattern begins with an understanding of normal developmental processes, plus the realization that most children have appetites sufficient for their needs, are entitled to an off day when they may not wish to eat, and may have firm likes and dislikes. The child should be allowed to attempt self-feeding, however messily, as soon as he seems ready and should never be forced or persuaded to eat. The pediatrician should be alert to an incipient problem if the mother shows any signs of overconcern in this area and should respond with early intervention in the form of appropriate advice, as well as exploration of a possible basis of failed mutuality for the emerging symptoms.

Treatment must be based on careful and sympathetic discussion with the parents, who must not be made to feel that the physician is critical of their management of the child, and yet must understand that the child will not grow out of it as long as the current management persists. They must also be helped to understand that there is no physical basis for the problem, that no medicines or food supplements are needed, and that the child is not mischievous, disturbed, or ill. All attempts at forcing the child to eat must be stopped, as well as all tricks, inducements, or bribes. The child should be expected to sit with the family at mealtimes, and no food should be given between meals. The child should have his food placed before him without fanfare. He should be free to eat or not to eat and should not be praised when he does eat nor blamed for not eating. When the family meal is complete, his plate should be removed along with the rest and without comment, whether the food was eaten or not. No food should be allowed between meals until a normal eating pattern is reestablished. If the child did not eat at a meal, he should be left without food until the next meal. It is extremely unusual for a second meal to be refused if this procedure is followed. At most, two meals will be refused. It is important to reassure the parents that no healthy child will starve because he is not forced to eat and that as long as no one makes a great fuss he will soon capitulate and begin to eat normally. Thereafter, as long as foods are available and attractive, and as long as there is no undue insistence on any particular food, with respect being shown for his legitimate preferences, the problem should be resolved.

Pica. Many children between the second and fourth years eat everything they can pick up from the floor: dirt, sand, plaster, wood, or coal. They may pick the fuzz from blankets or chew the paint from toys or furniture. The cause is obscure; iron deficiency, with or without anemia, mental deficiency, disturbed mother–child relationship, and boredom are often cited. In severe cases, where potentially harmful materials continue to be ingested, the failure of the child to develop appropriate self-protective eating habits should draw attention to the atmosphere and relationships in the home. Al-though the habit is usually innocuous, it may lead to serious consequences, such as lead poisoning due to eating of old paint (p. 801). Treatment is generally directed toward the underlying cause, if one is evident. In most normally intelligent children it does not persist beyond the fourth year, and when it does it should be viewed as indicative of severe underlying personality disorder. The prevention of the toxic effects of lead is well described elsewhere.

Psychogenic vomiting. Psychogenic vomiting may occur at any age, even in young infants, and may be a symptom of mild emotional maladjustment or one manifestation of a serious neurotic disorder. It may be precipitated by a variety of factors and situations ranging from excessive crying for any reason during the first 3 years through food forcing and excitement to use as an attention-getting device. In the very young infant, air swallowing resulting from prolonged crying appears to be a major factor. When vomiting occurs only with acute excitement or following sudden separation from a parent or on school mornings, it may be viewed as an expression of underlying emotional tensions, and it usually disappears when the precipitating factor is dealt with. Of particular interest is *rumination* (p. 987).

Regardless of the presence of emotional or environmental problems that may seem to account for the symptom, persistence of vomiting in an older child requires a thorough evaluation to rule out physical causes (p. 983). Children with expanding intracranial lesions may at first be thought to have psychogenic vomiting, because the symptom appears only in the morning. The discovery of physical disease does not necessarily imply a causal relationship with a child's vomiting. As a rule, only extreme food hypersensitiveness causes vomiting; the foods that later may cause marked urticaria or angioneurotic edema are usually eaten with pleasure and are retained, and vomiting is unlikely to be due to sensitivity to a particular food.

In school-age children and adolescents, psychogenic vomiting may be an aspect of school phobia, but more often it represents serious unconscious emotional conflicts in child or family; if it is persistent or recurrent it suggests a need for psychotherapy. Referral in such cases may often be delayed because of particularly strong family resistance or because of the desire of the physician to rule out a physiologic cause of the vomiting.

Bladder and Bowel Disorders

At some stage in early development most children will develop minor problems of sphincter control that may include delay in acquiring bowel or bladder control, loss of previously acquired control, deliberate withholding of urine or stools, constipation, frequency of micturition, or temporary refusal to utilize specific toilet facilities. These problems are generally transient and are relatively easily managed.

Enuresis. In general, bladder control during both day and night occurs by 3 to 3.5 years of age, although it should not be expected to be complete prior to 4 years.

Primary enuresis refers to bed-wetting that continues without intermission after the end of the third year. It may be due to delayed maturation of the complex mechanism of bladder control, or it may occur as a manifestation of general emotional immaturity, often associated with other evidence such as prolonged use of baby talk and persistence of immature behaviors. There is frequently a family history of enuresis in parents and siblings. Psychogenic factors also play a part, as coercive measures and parental anxiety will superimpose a psychologic problem on the delay in maturation. Some parents who may themselves have been enuretic may make little effort to adequately train their child, preferring to ascribe the condition to "weak kidneys" or "weak bladder."

Secondary enuresis, which occurs after a dry period had been established, may follow an obvious cause for regression, such as the birth of a sibling or an illness or hospitalization, or a less obvious factor in home or emotional life causing increased anxiety and tension in the child. It may also occur when physiologic causes of frequency are present, such as diabetes mellitus or cystitis. Both primary and secondary enuresis occur during a particular phase of sleep (p. 81). The symptom may be very poorly handled by concerned parents. Corporal punishment, shaming, and scolding serve only to focus his attention on his symptom and to increase the feeling of shame and of being different from other children that leads him into an unhappy seclusive existence. Self-confidence may be severely threatened after the difficulty has persisted for a while.

The child and his environment should be studied before treatment is begun. A careful inquiry into toilet training, especially the time begun and the methods used, is important. Physical examination and simple tests to rule out conditions that are readily apparent are mandatory. However, unless highly specific indications for further investigation exist, procedures involving instrumentation should be avoided. A urinalysis should indicate the presence of infection, and other symptoms generally point to diseases such as diabetes mellitus (p. 694). Emotional complications are unfortunately common, often secondary to extensive medical investigations and procedures so conducted as to increase the child's concerns and heighten his anxiety without providing him any means for dealing with frightening manipulations around a very sensitive and important portion of his anatomy.

Encopresis. Encopresis is the persistence of fecal soiling beyond the age of 2 to 2.5 years in the absence of any organic lesion of the rectum or anus. It is common in children who are severely retarded or seriously emotionally disturbed, in whom it may be associated with enuresis. A similar association is seen in neglected children and in those raised in institutions, where emotional deprivation may be a factor. In general, toilet training may have failed because of inappropriate methods or because of emotional maladjustment on the part of the child. Many children who develop this symptom have been forced to sit for prolonged periods on the toilet, with threats, punishments, and rewards used to force passage of what the parents consider an adequate stool. In some cases parents have been ignorant of the normal pattern for breast-fed children and have resorted to enemas, medication, or other means to obtain more frequent bowel movements.

With the development of the ego, refusal to let go of the bowel movement can begin a pattern of negative behavior that ultimately leads to a serious problem. Similarly, a baby may withhold the stools deliberately after passage of a particularly hard one that caused pain or after painful passage due to the presence of an anal fissure. More often he withholds because he can gain attention and cause considerable parental fuss and anxiety.

Regardless of how the pattern began, by the time most children get to treatment, usually at age 5 years or after, there is marked colonic distension with fecal impaction and overflow incontinence. This syndrome makes purely psychologic treatment irrelevant, and the severe emotional overlay to such a condition makes purely physiologic intervention generally frustrating. Treatment must be based on pediatric-psychiatric collaboration, with simultaneous assessment of the readiness of the bowel and readiness of the child to function with autonomy.

Constipation. The causes and the management of constipation are discussed elsewhere (p. 81); however, it may be pointed out here that psychic factors may be at the root of the difficulty. Unwillingness of the mismanaged child to cooperate with the parents may take this form, and fear of the toilet is at times an underlying factor. The precipitating cause is usually undue concern on the part of the parents over the necessity of a daily bowel movement, a state of mind fostered by laxative manufacturers, by tradition, and sometimes by the physician.

SLEEP DISTURBANCES

Psychologic Disturbances

Most children, sooner or later in the first 4 years of life, develop problems related to sleep. These may include crying, refusal to go to bed, to lie down, or to fall asleep, complicated sleep rituals, and awakening during the night. Such sleep problems are conveniently viewed either as part of normal or natural developmental processes, such as variations in sleep requirements or changes with maturation, or as being related to interaction of environmental and developmental factors, such as sleep refusal or crying during the night.

Many problems related to sleep appear to have their roots in mistaken notions regarding the amount of sleep required by a normal child; there may be attempts at imposition of unrealistic sleep patterns on a healthy infant or toddler whose requirements are less than the parents' expectation. Thus, although most newborn babies sleep most of the day, the 3-month-old infant may be wakeful for considerable periods, and by 1 year only two or three sleep periods are needed by most children.

Some 6-month-old infants sleep little by day, and many children refuse to nap by 18 months to 2 years of age, while others may continue to do so until 3 or 4 years of age. It is normal for children to lie awake talking or playing in bed in the evening and to awaken at 5 or 6 A.M. At the age of 2 to 3 years sleep requirements vary from 8 to 17 hours, averaging 9 to 12 hours nightly.

Waking. Newborn babies awaken for feeding once or twice nightly up to 10 to 16 weeks of age. Settling, or sleeping through the night, reflects CNS maturity; children who have experienced a perinatal insult may be restless, wakeful, or irritable. Where there is maternal anxiety that is reflected in inconsistent handling or where the child does not receive sufficient environmental stimulation, settling may also be delayed. Once it has occurred, night wakenings recur in 50 percent of infants in the second half of the first year; recurrences are usually transient, occurring after changes in the sleeping environment or family environment. Parental anxiety and anger about sleep can compound existing difficulties—a form of failed mutuality.

Resistance to Sleep. Resistance to going to sleep occurs during the second year as part of cognitive and emotional development as the child begins to appreciate the difference between the reassuring daytime world of familiar people and things and the nighttime world of sleep and poorly organized fantasies. Inability to distinguish between temporary absence and total loss leads the child to use transitional objects, such as teddy bears or blankets, to hold on to a part of the daytime world even as he leaves it. Dreams in this period are full of day residues of frightening events and monsters, and they unsettle the child who is as yet unable to distinguish between dreams and reality. Nighttime rituals are developed spontaneously by many parents and children at this age as an aid to organizing what seems unmanageable. Most children discard these rituals shortly after the third birthday.

Refusal to go to bed for one parent and not the other may be due to greater dependence on one or the other and may be dealt with by encouraging both parents to participate in the process and then having them alternate the role. The frightened child who is unable to admit his fears may be helped by sitting quietly with him for a short while, allowing the radio to play softly for a period, or leaving a night light in the hall or in the room. In general, if the parents can be helped to be firm, yet kind, and to leave the child in bed in his room, even though he may be standing up and yelling, the problem will usually settle itself. Unfortunately, because families live at close quarters, or because fathers who work odd hours must sleep, or because neighbors complain, it is not always possible to allow children or infants to cry themselves out, and the problem may be compounded.

Restlessness and Disturbed Sleep. When a child who normally sleeps through the night is restless or cries out, the cause should be investigated, unless it subsides rapidly. Certainly, persistent crying or screaming by such a child requires immediate attention. A change of diaper, reassurance, or brief rocking may suffice, or the child may turn out to be ill and in pain. It is another matter when the child cries or is restless and wakeful night after night. Such a habit must be broken. The child must not be taken into the parental bed, played with, fed snacks, or spanked. He wants company, but he needs to learn that this is not an appropriate time for it.

Talking During Sleep. Talking during sleep is an isolated event in the sleep patterns of most children and adults and seems to reflect anxiety-provoking daytime occurrences. It should not be a cause for alarm unless it recurs frequently, in which case it requires careful assessment of the child's overall situation.

Disorders of Sleep and Arousal

The development of polygraphic recording during sleep has permitted the classification of sleep disturbances according to their association with electrical disorders. All disorders of sleep and arousal occur as maturational lags or deviations in a developmental process whereby poorly organized infantile sleep gradually gets organized into clearly differentiated REM sleep (rapid-eye-movement or dream sleep) and NREM sleep (non-rapid-eye-movement sleep), which occurs at varying depths.

Nocturnal enuresis occurs during an enuretic episode, which is a lightening of depth of sleep prior to the first REM sleep of the night and is characterized by increased skeletal and autonomic activity. The effectiveness of imipramine (which increases lighter NREM sleep and decreases REM sleep) in the treatment of enuresis is understandable in these terms.

Somnambulism and somniloquy occur at least once in 15 percent and recurrently in 1 to 6 percent of the child population; they gradually decrease in frequency as the CNS matures. Episodes begin with the child abruptly sitting up in bed, eyes open, glassy, and unseeing; the child may or may not get out of bed and walk about; he may or may not speak. Episodes last from 15 to 30 sec when sitting in bed and from 5 to 30 minutes when walking occurs. The episode occurs, as do enuretic episodes, as the depth of sleep lightens before the first REM sleep. They are not, then, as folklore would have it, walking dreams. A characteristic electroencephalographic pattern occurs that is held to be reflective of CNS immaturity. No particular psychologic or personality traits are consistently seen in somnambulistic children. For severe intractable somnambulism, diazepam (Valium) is used.

Pavor nocturnus (night terror) differs from nightmares or anxiety dreams in that the child sits bolt upright from sleep, screams, and appears to be staring at an imaginary object; he sweats, is in obvious distress, and breathes heavily. Relaxation and sleep occur only after 10 minutes or longer, and there is no recall in the morning. The episode occurs during intense and sudden arousal from deep sleep and, like somnambulism, responds to diazepam.

Narcolepsy (p.1862), or recurrent daytime episodes of irresistible drowsiness and sleep, is defined as a disorder of sleep, in contrast to the above disturbances, which are disorders of arousal. Electrically, it represents an invasion of REM sleep into daytime wakefulness. The narcoleptic tetrad, which occurs in full form only 10 percent of the time, consists of narcolepsy, cataplexy (sudden loss of muscle tone and falling to the ground while still conscious), sleep paralysis (sudden awareness while falling asleep of the inability to move or cry out), and hypnagogic hallucinations (vivid images occurring at sleep onset). Narcolepsy begins for unknown reasons, generally in adolescence or early adulthood. Among various pharmacologic treatments, amphetamines are the most widely used.

DISTURBANCES OF BODY MOVEMENT

Almost all healthy young children manifest a state of constant activity, the extent of which depends largely on their character and personality. While a degree of activity that may be viewed as normal by one set of parents or by a specific teacher may be annoying or upsetting to others who see it as fidgetiness, restlessness, or even hyperactivity, it is generally not of concern until it becomes so marked as to disrupt learning and other activities. Some children are almost continually in motion—moving, banging, tapping, pulling at their clothing, playing with their fingers or hair, exploring everything around them, and generally displaying a high degree of motor restlessness. This activity will normally be curtailed if the child is deeply involved in a task, and he is usually able to maintain concentration and attention when he wishes, which distinguishes the behavior from that described as the syndrome of hyperkinesis (p. 1764).

Rocking. It is not uncommon for infants to begin rocking in their cribs toward the end of the first year of life. This is frequently attributed to masturbation, but it may occur without evident masturbatory activity. It may be so intense as to rock the crib from one side of the room to the other and may be associated with head-banging. Children with emotional disorders or children experiencing severe deprivation may begin to rock in their cribs, either on hands and knees or in the upright seated position. In general, rocking stops spontaneously after a few months. It may be less annoying if the crib is placed on a carpet to reduce vibrations, and it may stop if the child is moved to a bed.

Head-banging. Head-banging occurs particularly in infants 7 to 12 months of age and is manifested at bedtime, when the child may bang his head rhythmically against the mattress, the side of the crib, the wall, or any other convenient place. It occurs in perfectly normal children as well as in those with mental retardation. The banging may be kept up for 2 or 3 hours at a time, but the child rarely hurts himself even though there may be a localized thickening of the skin and underlying tissues. Like other habits, head-banging is frequently emulated by other youngsters. It may also become a daytime activity in some children, who may retreat to the bathroom to bang their heads on the tile or other hard area. It usually runs a benign course and usually stops spontaneously between the ages of 2 and 3 years. It is rarely seen during waking hours after the fourth year, although it may persist in sleep or in semisleeping states until a much later period. While the cause is obscure, it seems to provide some stimulation to the child. To the extent that head-banging may involve withdrawal from normal relationships when it occurs during waking hours, this symptom is of concern, especially if it is frequent and persists beyond 4 years of age.

Tics. Although the term habit spasm is frequently used as synonymous with tic, it should be discarded; tics are not spasms, but frequently repeated, involuntary movements of parts of the body. They are uncommon in the preschool child, and the incidence peaks in the early prepuberty period. Tics usually involve the face, although almost any part of the body may be involved. Blinking, grimacing, clearing the throat, sniffling, rotating the head, or shrugging the shoulders are among the movements most frequently seen, although a wide variety of other movements, some of them quite complex, may be present in the same child. Tics are usually found associated with other symptoms of emotional tension and insecurity, most frequently in restless, overactive, and easily fatigued youngsters. They occur in children of all degrees of intelligence.

Tics are to be differentiated from chorea, a distinction that is not always easy. Choreic movements have a larger range of excursion and are repeated irregularly, while tics are repeated in the same fashion and seem to have a more purposeful nature. Both types of movement disappear in sleep and are made worse by emotional tension and fatigue. The tic differs from manipulations of the body (such as thumb-sucking or nose-picking) in that it is more rapid, it is involuntary, and it cannot be interrupted. The general motor restlessness seen in anxious, jittery children is different in that the twitching is not consistently localized and does not follow a definite pattern.

The tic may originate as a voluntary, purposeful act, such as a defensive movement against some constant irritation: a tight collar may evoke a twisting of the neck, or an uncomfortable sleeve a shrugging of the shoulders. Blinking may begin with a conjunctivitis and persist after the disappearance of the exciting cause. Imitation of others may also play a role. In a setting of environmental and emotional stress the movement may become detached from the precipitating cause and may persist even though it is no longer useful.

Treatment must be directed at the underlying emotional difficulties rather than at the tic itself. The more the child is made aware of the tic through parental admonition, massage, exercises before a mirror, or electrotherapy, the more the condition is apt to be aggravated. It is important that those in the child's environment stop calling attention to the symptom. Not only will scolding and punishment not stop the tics, they may aggravate matters. The child is usually old enough to discuss his personality problems and to participate in plans for his better adjustment at home, in his recreational life, and if necessary at school. Treatment should be begun as early as possible, as tics are notoriously resistant to treatment when they have persisted over a long period of time, although they may quickly disappear if the conflict can be resolved soon after they have begun. Unfortunately, one tic is apt to be replaced by another or to return at a later date during a period of stress.

BODY MANIPULATIONS

Finger-sucking is important because of the concern it occasions in parents. Sucking of the thumb or other fingers occurs during the first year of life in practically every child, especially when hungry. In the normal hand-to-mouth reaction during the middle and latter months of the first year, sucking the fingers occurs as a result of the sucking reflex. In the well-fed happy infant this should cause no alarm. Restraints are contraindicated, since they often provoke a power contest. Parents have been subjected to many scares regarding the damaging effects of thumb-sucking on the formation of the jaw and alignment of the teeth. Lewis concluded that if the sucking disappears by the time of eruption of the permanent teeth there is no danger of permanent deformity and that deformities already produced will disappear spontaneously. The old wives' tale relating finger-sucking to masturbation, which has been of much concern to parents, has no basis in fact.

Between the second and fifth years finger-sucking is most frequently seen in connection with fatigue, boredom, illness, punishment, and frustrating situations, as the child returns to a more infantile mode of satisfaction. Prohibition and restraint are contraindicated; they tend to fix the habit. Treatment should be directed toward sources of emotional dissatisfaction and toward keeping the child reasonably well occupied. The parent should be reassured of its harmlessness. After the age of 5 or 6 years, thumb-sucking should be viewed a little less casually, as it may lead to distortion of the oral structures and malocclusion, with resultant problems that may be permanent. The symptom is usually a manifestation of a general emotional immaturity and is frequently found associated with other infantile behavior. These children deserve careful study and adequate treatment, including modification of the environment where it is indicated.

Hair-plucking (trichotillomania) may occur in association with finger-sucking and is apt to be evident when the child is angry or frustrated. It tends to disappear after the cause is removed, provided the act is ignored.

Nail-biting (onychophagy) is not common in the first 3 years of life, and although it is frequently encountered in practice it is not often a primary complaint. It usually begins in the early school years and may be a lifelong habit; it appears to affect as many as 50 percent of all schoolchildren. Although nail-biting is said to be a manifestation of anxiety or insecurity, its wide prevalence raises some doubt in this regard. It is true that children (and adults) may begin to bite their nails when they are tense or nervous or in deep thought, but its persistence as a habit in even highly successful well-adjusted individuals must cause some reconsideration of these views. Nail-biting does no harm, but parental and societal attitudes to it certainly may. Treatment should be directed to relieving any clear-cut causes of anxiety. Punishment and restraining devices will do nothing but harm. Nagging and constantly calling the child's attention to his nail-biting will serve only to increase tension. Ridicule and teasing do not work. Treatment of evident emotional maladjustment is slow to affect nail-biting, although other symptoms may disappear quite promptly.

COMPULSIONS

Compulsions in mild form are quite common in children. They consist of such well-known activities as stepping over cracks in the sidewalk and ritualistic games. These are usually of minor importance, especially when seen in well-adjusted children; as a rule they are found in children of school age, the pattern being common to a group of playmates. Handwashing compulsions and obsessive fear of germs are also not uncommon in childhood. Compulsion in a more severe form may occur in an emotionally malfunctioning child, and some children develop numerous complex rituals, such as a particular order in which bedtime activities must be performed. There may be an inability to proceed to another activity until dressed, undressed, or toileted in a particular order or an inability to sleep until doors, windows, lights, and bedclothes have received the required ritualized attention.

Such rituals usually disappear with time, but in some cases they tend to be accentuated or to appear for the first time at adolescence. These tend to be more severe and more complex in character; they are apt to be a factor in school and social maladjustment, as they inhibit completion of assignments and interfere with other activities. These compulsive young people are frequently shy, punctilious, perfectionistic individuals who may recognize the ritualistic and maladaptive quality of their behavior but may be at a loss to modify it voluntarily. These severe forms of compulsion may presage serious emotional disorders. They are not outgrown, and they can lead to crippling of the personality if not recognized and treated through psychiatric referral.

SPEECH AND LANGUAGE DISORDERS

Functional speech disorders must be differentiated from those of organic origin. The latter are benefited by direct attack on the speech defect itself through educative methods or correction of the organic disability if possible. Local conditions affecting the peripheral speech mechanisms, such as defects of the tongue, lips, nose, palate, uvula, teeth, and larynx, may produce characteristic speech defects, as in cleft palate. Tongue-tie is not a cause of speech defect, despite the popular misconception, which fortunately is now waning. Hearing loss, even of mild degree, is a factor in speech disorder, as the child incorrectly reproduces the imperfectly heard word. Therefore in all cases of speech defect the hearing should be carefully investigated. Disorders of the central and peripheral nervous systems and certain endocrine disorders may also produce defects. There are some speech defects that have no organic basis but cannot be classified with those of emotional origin; this group occurs in children who imitate the poor speech they hear at home. The most common functional speech defects are delayed speech, mutism, faulty articulation, and stuttering. All forms are more common in boys than girls.

Delayed development of speech implies lateness in beginning to say single words with meaning and subsequently in putting two and three words together. It may be due to mental retardation, to maturational delay (as in children with slow motor development), or to inadequate exposure to language in the home, or it may reflect an intrinsic developmental language problem. Delayed speech development, peculiarities of speech development, or loss or deterioration of speech may also occur in young children with psychoses. It is important to stress that the understanding of words is of much greater importance than the ability to say them; lateness in speaking distinctly or even in speaking at all should be assessed in the context of the child's ability to understand what is said to him, to point to common objects, and to carry out commands. Many highly intelligent children are late in learning to talk, but the reasons are unclear. There is often a family history of similar delays in these cases. Deafness is of major importance and must always be considered in the presence of any disorders of language acquisition, which should lead to hearing evaluation without delay. If language has not appeared by age 4 years, or if there is any major abnormality of language, a speech pathologist should be consulted.

Mutism usually occurs as a result of congenital or early acquired deafness, but it may exist as a functional disorder. Grossly retarded intellectual development may be a cause. Mutism may also occur as a symptom in hysteria and in certain negativistic children; here it is apt to be transitory. Rarely, young children may not talk for some time after a particularly traumatic anesthesia and tonsillectomy. Temporary aphasia sometimes follows typhoid fever or severe chorea; the condition is usually transient, clearing as the chorea improves, but occasionally it lasts for months.

Faulty articulation may be due to organic causes, to poor training, to poor examples of speech, or to retarded mental development. Frequently it is due to emotional immaturity. Lisping and baby talk are the more common types; they are often associated with other infantile traits.

Stuttering is a frequent form of speech disorder; there are estimated to be about a quarter of a million stuttering children in the United States. The symptoms are well known and will not be described in detail. It has been said that the condition develops as a consequence of the diagnosis, when someone becomes concerned and begins to instruct the child to speak more slowly or more distinctly. Despite much debate and many dogmatic assertions, the interactions of neurologic and emotional problems in the condition remain obscure. The symptom is inconstant; it is apt to worsen in some situations and to be absent in others. A child may stutter at home and not in school, or only in the presence of certain individuals. It is intensified by emotional stress. However, the severe stutterer may be able to sing or recite from memory or count with no difficulty whatsoever. Stuttering is especially apt to begin at emotionally critical periods of the child's life, as at the beginning of school and at puberty.

The misnamed physiologic stuttering in young children between 3 and 4 years of age is a normal feature of the acquisition of speech; it is very common and usually disappears if met calmly and not handled destructively. The pediatrician should explain its benign nature to parents concerned about this pattern and attempt to allay anxiety; parents should stop instructing the child to speak distinctly and ignore his diction.

Established stuttering in older children merits evaluation and treatment by a qualified speech pathologist. The pediatrician can encourage nonpunitive, supportive attitudes in the family by presenting the condition to them as an aspect of that child's makeup that must be accepted as a part of him and that must not be the object of effort, attention, and struggle.

RELATIONSHIPS WITH OTHERS

Problems in relationships with others are a normal part of the development of all children and are a function of their own personalities, parental attitudes (which are in turn, the crystallization of their life experiences), and the larger environment in which the child is growing and maturing. The child's position in the family and the way in which his basic needs are met in the early stages of development will directly affect his responses to the birth of a sibling, to the first day of school, or to the aggression of others. Many later behavior problems are the unfortunate results of poor management of responses that are part and parcel of normal development.

Negativism is a characteristic feature of the normal child from 18 months to 3 years of age. As discussed earlier, in this stage the child is testing his capacity for self-control and self-regulation. He has not yet learned to distinguish between alternatives and cannot clearly differentiate between yes and no, give and take, push and pull. He responds in confused and often contradictory ways, often unable to do what he wants to and refusing to do what he can do. Frequently he seems to delight in doing the opposite of what he is asked; he refuses to hurry, dawdles over dressing or eating, and refuses to lie down, get up, go outdoors, come in, or perform any activity requested by his mother. This may be part of his developing sense of autonomy, his need to assert his own power, or it may be simply a desire to continue doing what he wants to do, without regard to the wishes of others. It is difficult to draw the line between normal and abnormal negativism. Negativism is exaggerated by hunger, fatigue, insecurity, and jealousy, as well as by excessive demands for instant responses or by parental overcontrol or demands for excessively mature behavior.

The pediatrician can assist the family to understand that this behavior is a normal aspect of development and that the child needs freedom to test his developing sense of self in this manner. Needless struggles are frequently prevented by encouraging the parents to avoid setting up situations that precipitate a negative response. Thus asking a 2-year-old if he wishes to go to bed, to bathe, or to toilet is foolhardy unless the parent is genuinely offering him a choice. If it is time to engage in the activity, the parent should simply inform the child of this in a matter-of-fact manner, offering no alternatives. Many parents fail to realize that a child in the midst of an activity may be rightfully resistant to discontinuing it and may react negatively if abruptly interrupted. They should be advised to warn a child to prepare to end his game and should allow a period for doing so prior to announcing another activity. Such simple measures show a child that his interests and concerns merit consideration, and they significantly reduce the confrontations so common in the toddler phase of negativism and avoid development of resultant maladaptive behaviors.

Anger and *resentment* are normal emotions experienced and expressed in different ways at various stages. *Breath-holding spells* are a dramatic expression of anger, closely related to temper tantrums. They are common between 1 and 3 years of age and are rare after 4 years; they are precipitated by thwarting, punishment, or other conflict with the parent. In an attack the child may cry loudly, then hold the breath in expiration for 5 to 20 seconds. He may become mildly to severely cyanotic and may lose consciousness and fall. There is usually prompt recovery, and only rarely are attacks so prolonged as to result in a convulsion secondary to anoxemia. These attacks may cause considerable consternation and excitement, and the child may learn to use them to get his own way. They are best treated by ignoring them, once it is certain that they are typical breath-holding responses and not epilepsy. This differentiation can usually be made by taking a careful history, which for breath-holding usually reveals a precipitating factor followed by crying, breath-holding in expiration, rapid onset of cyanosis, and limpness and convulsion. An epileptic convulsion in a child is rarely preceded by an ordinary cry, the clonic phase is not preceded by limpness, and cyanosis follows rather than precedes the convulsion.

Temper tantrums as an expression of anger usually begin in the toddler or early preschool stage and are coincidental with negativism and the normal aggressiveness of this important transitional phase in development. They may persist until adolescence or even into adult life as an emotional response to frustration. The precipitating factor may be the child's failure to get his own way, attempts to get him to do something he does not want to do, depriving him of some object or action he wants, or jealousy. The child often finds a pattern for his tantrums in some older members of the family. The attacks are usually found in children of overprotective and oversolicitous parents, who encourage them by giving in. The child begins to use the outbursts more or less deliberately to gain his own ends. Children who display tantrums are usually not happy, despite their domination of the home. They seem to resent the submission of their parents and desire someone who can impose reasonable limits on their impulses. They usually display other evidences of emotional instability and immaturity, with the history of maladjustment going back to earlier difficulties in feeding, toilet training, and acquiring skills. Tantrums are apt to be associated with fears and with other evidences of anxiety and tension.

Treatment should aim at providing good physical health and sufficient rest; ill or tired children are notoriously irritable. An environment that provides sufficient freedom from admonitions and prohibitions is important. It is often difficult to provide this in a small apartment where the child cannot find sufficient space to play. Nursery school placement may afford suitable outlets and aid the child in his general social development. If any patent jealousies are present they should be dealt with. The tantrum itself must be handled constructively. Avoidance of situations that are sure to produce the reaction will materially aid in bringing about its cessation. The parent should make full use of the child's easy distractability when a tantrum seems inevitable. Reasoning is futile; signs of alarm or a similar tantrum on the part of the parent serve only to intensify the reaction. Punishment rarely brings about cessation and frequently adds to the anxiety already present in the child. The tantrums should be met with calm firmness; indifference enjoys more success than any method that allows the child to be the center of attention. Proper sympathetic handling at the age of resistance is apt to prevent the persistence of tantrum behavior.

Fear reactions may develop in young infants exposed to sudden loud noises, loss of support, and strange surroundings; fears are not abnormal. Older children develop, through example and education, a realization of danger that results in a way of reacting that avoids harm or injury. The child who has learned the perils of traffic and the inherent dangers of fire is not a fearful child; this is constructive use of fear to avoid real risks.

In children past the age of infancy there may develop fears of darkness, ghosts, thunderstorms, fires, policemen, doctors, and many other things. Mild fears that do not affect the child's daily life are not at all uncommon and may arise out of imitation of adult patterns (as with thunderstorms) and misinterpretation of phenomena that are not understood, such as creaking boards in the house or dim shadows in the dark. If the parent tends to act as if these dangers are real, the child comes to feel that his fears are justified; however, fears that concern the child a great deal and that preoccupy him so much that they interfere with his daily life are rarely on this basis alone. Almost invariably the child displays other symptoms as evidence of emotional disorder. While a great many of the milder fear reactions may occur in relatively well adjusted children and may arise out of anxieties during the critical periods in emotional and social growth and development, severe chronic fear reactions call for careful psychiatric help. It is best not to try to break the child of his fears by forcing him into situations about which he is fearful. His fears should be recognized but not unduly emphasized. If amelioration of what seem to be the more specific etiologic factors in the background is not feasible, much can be done to improve the child's general emotional security. A friendly noncritical ear can do much to build up self-confidence in the child.

Anxiety attacks reflect a state of fearfulness that may appear in waves lasting from a few seconds to an hour or so. These attacks are not rare in children. They usually occur in the evening. Most frequently they are found in preadolescent girls. During the attack the child is filled with dread; she may cling to her parents and seek reassurance. There is tachycardia and palpitation, difficulty in breathing, sweating, and flushing. She may complain of paresthesias, urinary frequency, and an urge to defecate. There is sometimes an aimless burst of motor overactivity. When questioned as to her fears she usually states that something terrible is about to happen and that she may die or faint. There may be only a few attacks, or they may be very frequent. Between attacks the child may be relatively normal or may show constant anxiety. In the latter case she may withdraw from all social contacts, refuse to be left alone, and lose all interest in play and school. Worry about the attacks may accentuate the condition.

Anxiety attacks are apt to occur in a home atmosphere of worry and insecurity. The precipitating factor (an operation, death, or sudden shock) acts as a trigger and is not to be regarded as the cause. Treatment depends on what specific factors are involved in the individual case. The anxiety attack itself is a symptom; the state may be relatively benign, or it may be symptomatic of a more serious type of personality disorder. Because of the frequent somatic complaints during the attack, parents and physicians are apt to interpret it in terms of an organic disorder. It is important to reassure the child and the parents that physical health is good after a careful study. The condition may be confused with paroxysmal tachycardia, in which anxiety is frequent at the beginning of an attack. Chronic hypochondriacal reactions in children may result from mishandling of anxiety attacks.

An *anxiety state* may exist without any individual attacks of anxiety being manifest. The child may be generally apprehensive and may constantly change the fear that is expressed, shifting from fires to kidnapers to physical disease or to preoccupation with the possible illness or death of a parent. The child realizes the unjustifiable nature of his fears but can do little about them.

Jealousy is a normal reaction that is experienced at some point by most normal children. Sometimes the manifestations are not overt, and parents may think that their child has never experienced this normal emotion, which need not be a problem unless it is mismanaged. Jealousy is the result of fear that one is losing something of value—love or a feeling of importance or of being wanted. It is greatly exaggerated by any cause of insecurity, such as overprotection, parental irritability, or domestic friction. The resentment of an older child

whose mother has little time or energy to devote to him after she brings home a new sibling may be due to his interpretation of her fatigue and irritability as withdrawal of love and interest. With the first pangs of jealousy will come increased demandingness, and possibly the onset of a cycle of maternal–child interactions that can only serve to increase the jealous feelings. Behavior regression is not uncommon at such a time, and it is important to prepare parents for it. The best way to avoid such problems is to prevent them by preparing the child for the arrival of a sibling, allowing him to participate in the care of the infant, punctiliously meeting his needs for attention, and recognizing that he needs reassurance that he is loved and wanted. A child should not be moved out of his crib to accommodate the new baby nor be sent off to nursery school at the time of the baby's arrival. These changes should be made well in advance or should be deferred, so that the older child does not infer that he is being ousted in favor of the newcomer.

In the older child jealousy may arise if the parents reprimand him for protecting his toys when the baby snatches them or for some act that is condoned in the younger child because he does not understand that it is wrong. It is difficult for children to understand such differences in treatment, and if they are accompanied by unfavorable comparisons, considerable disturbance may result. Not only do comparisons with siblings cause ill-feeling and enmity, they also lead to feelings of insecurity, inferiority, and rebellion. It is important that parents avoid favoritism and particularly that they avoid making invidious comparisons. There are particular difficulties with twins, who require very careful management if troublesome jealousy is to be avoided. In general, prevention and management of jealousy, while of great importance, can be accomplished in the course of the physician's contacts with the family. When it is allowed to become a serious problem, it can have a permanently damaging effect on the child's character and personality.

ANTISOCIAL BEHAVIOR

The more common forms of antisocial behavior are disobedience, lying, stealing, cruelty to other children and animals, running away from home, destructiveness, truancy, and markedly aggressive behavior toward others. As with other manifestations of childhood personality disorders, the child must be treated rather than the symptom. The physician must be on his guard lest he be pushed into assuming a judicial or disciplinary role; his function is to interpret behavior both from the point of view of organic disease and in its psychologic setting. Through his influence in the home management of a child he may be able to prevent many of these difficulties. The young child, being self-centered, demands and attempts to extract satisfaction of his wishes regardless of others. As he grows older he learns to appreciate property rights, the differences between right and wrong, and truth and untruth, and the rights and feelings of others. What we can expect of him depends on his training and the examples set for him. We cannot condemn the child for stealing coal when the whole family makes forays on the coalyard to get their fuel.

Among the more persistent patterns of antisocial behavior are those in which the disturbance takes the form of rebellion against what may seem to the child and to others an unjust or intolerable situation. After a more or less prolonged period of stress, antisocial behavior may occur as a protest or reaction. The family may be imposing on the child by piling up chores, relegating to him the care of younger children, or providing too many planned after-school activities, music lessons, religious instruction, and the like. The underlying factor may sometimes be found in the school situation— a harsh and unsympathetic teacher or the presence of an unrecognized visual or hearing defect, mental retardation, or specific educational disability that may interfere with his progress and schoolwork. Once the intolerable situation has been uncovered and steps have been taken to correct it, the undesirable behavior usually clears up. A situation less easily solved is that of the emotionally deprived child of neglectful or hostile parents. Here aggressive rebellious behavior may result from anxiety due to the child's feeling of lack of love. Antisocial behavior should be handled in the light of the total setting. Before attempting to handle these problems one should have thorough unbiased information about the personalities, the backgrounds, and the difficulties of the children and their families.

In most of the well-defined chronic aggressive antisocial behavior patterns the pediatrician will find the services of the trained child psychiatrist of great help. He will be of greatest assistance in recognizing the organic and nonorganic factors, in referring the child to the appropriate authority, and in sparing him from undue harshness on the part of those who feel that he is being deliberately bad.

SCHOOL PROBLEMS

School problems associated with learning difficulties and mental retardation have been discussed elsewhere. *Resistance to going to school,* formerly called school phobia, describes the refusal of a child to go to school; it is distinguished from truancy by the fact that the child elects to stay at home. It is generally regarded as a separation problem—as much the parent's as the child's. There are two peak age periods of incidence: around the beginning of school (ages 6 to 8 years) and in early and mid-adolescence. These periods differ greatly with regard to prognosis and severity of underlying psychologic problems. Younger children are likely to return to school without great difficulty and are usually not seriously disturbed; the older group includes many children with severe personality disorders and prepsychotic states. Pediatric concerns are the difficulty of making a diagnosis, since a host of somatic complaints may mask the psychologic problem; and the urgency, especially in the younger group, of an early return to school, since delay is said to contribute to chronicity. In all cases developmental

assessment is indicated; in refractory cases psychiatric referral will be necessary.

Truancy differs from school phobia in that the truant not only absents himself from school without leave but also absents himself from home. Truancy is most frequent in the adolescent age group and is a serious problem in some schools, where large numbers of students may absent themselves from classes, individually or in groups. Habitual truancy, as a symptom of social and educational maladaptation, is a complex problem that requires a thorough review of the entire situation. It may occur when a student is unable to compete with his peers because of inappropriate class placement, severe learning disability, or emotional problems or when the school experience is irrelevant to his social and economic situation. The physician can be helpful as a concerned and informed participant in a broad effort to intervene, but he can do little working alone.

SERIOUS PSYCHIATRIC DISORDERS

DEPRESSION. Depression has long been an underemphasized problem in the general population as well as in children and adolescents. However, in recent years professionals in several fields have become increasingly aware of the importance of underlying depression in many of the behavior symptoms with which they must deal in settings such as schools, shelters for runaways, hospitals, and juvenile correctional facilities, as well as pediatricians' offices. Depression may occur during health or disease and may be of varying degree and duration. Sometimes it is manifested in characteristic ways: by depressed facies that the onlooker perceives as looking sad, unhappy, or depressed; in symptoms such as fatigue, anorexia, insomnia, or loss of libido; by withdrawal from usually pleasurable activities with peers or family, apathy, passivity, or developmental regression; by feelings expressed as being blue or down, by a sense of hopelessness or discouragement with the self, a tendency to self-reproach, or preoccupation with bleak or discouraging events. At other times it may not be evident even to close family members, who may not notice or understand the behavior and feelings of the affected individual.

Depression may be a normal response to loss, illness, or disappointment that lasts for a brief or prolonged period and is characterized by decreased energy, dysphoric mood, and emotional preoccupation with the loss. Such reactive depression does not seriously interfere with day-to-day functioning. Depressive illness, on the other hand, occurs when the symptoms are more pronounced, and it may lead to such complications as psychosis or suicide. A severe and protracted depressive state interferes with life to an extent that can have markedly deleterious effects on the education, social adjustment, and future prospects of a child or adolescent. The term depressive character or depressive personality refers to a chronic, generally subconscious, low sense of self-esteem. This state may predispose the child to a depressive illness in which he may embody, as a part of his most basic sense of himself, the feelings of emptiness and neediness that characterize the depressive state.

The term *masked depression* in children has been used to refer to disorders that are often characterized by antisocial or aggressive behavior and that do not outwardly suggest low self-esteem, but that can be seen retrospectively as a behavior reflection of despair when onset of symptoms is related to a loss. In such cases the relationship of the depressive feelings and the symptomatic behavior may become evident during treatment, or it may become evident if the behavior manifestations disappear when overt depression appears or is unmasked.

Depression that initially occurs as a part of the normal grief process following loss may persist or take severe form. This is especially likely following losses that cannot be acknowledged or successfully grieved. Such loss may be concrete (such as the death of a parent) or symbolic (such as the loss of a more satisfying state of health or period of life) and may be evident and readily discussed or consciously concealed or unconsciously repressed. Clinical experience suggests that the personal meaning of a given loss, the individual's relationship to what has been lost, and his ability to bear losses in general are as important, if not more important, as the objective circumstances of the loss itself in determining how an individual reacts. Many clinicians believe that early life experiences, especially the quality and the continuity of the mother–child relationship, play a critical role in this determination, although there is considerable evidence indicating a strong genetic contribution, at least in depressive illness in adults. One group has found that children who are clinically diagnosed as depressed have a greater incidence of close relatives with depressive illness than do controls.

Anaclitic depression refers to a state of profound apathy, anorexia, and social withdrawal in an infant or toddler who loses his primary caretaker at an age when specific attachments have been made to that person but not to others. Failure to thrive and death can be the outcome in cases in which such a relationship is not reestablished with a new object of attachment. However, the significance of depressive states in the pediatric care of children extend beyond this dramatic syndrome. The behavior manifestations in children may be chronic moodiness or apathy or a persistent lack of zest in moving forward in development. This may take the form of excessive dependency, immature behavior, constant seeking of approval, or being scapegoated. Since most of these symptoms can also be transient reflections of developmental stress in a child who will again move ahead, the diagnostic perspective must be a long one.

Although in many cases clear-cut clinical depression follows some change in the child's world that he experiences as a loss, other symptoms may be more prominent. Thus anorexia may be the only symptom of such reactions, or the only symptom reported to the pediatrician. Additional symptoms may not be appreciated or reported, either because the anorexia is the most conspicuous and troubling to the parents or because a common physical symptom of illness may be a prerequisite to approaching a physician for parents who would be reluctant to seek help for an emotional problem.

In older children and adolescents depression accounts for much missed school, many visits to physicians, and much hospitalization, but it is often undiagnosed. This is because it is difficult for adults to think of children as depressed and because physical symptoms, especially abdominal pain, anorexia, and weight loss, may predominate among the child's and the parents' complaints. Only sensitive inquiry as to the child's emotional life (eg, mood, involvement with peers and in school, and pleasure taken in favorite activities) will clarify the picture. Once the presence of depression is appreciated, a review with parents and child of possibly significant recent losses that might have precipitated the depressive episode is indicated for understanding the illness and for guiding treatment. Frequently, of course, the significant loss or losses will not immediately be apparent to child or parent, and referral for appropriate treatment will be needed.

Certain objective criteria for diagnosis of depressive illness have been suggested; they require that a child must have both dysphoric mood and self-deprecatory ideation and at least two of eight vegetative and behavior symptoms (aggressive behavior, change in attitude toward school or performance in school, decreased socialization, loss of energy, sleep disturbance, somatic complaints, change in appetite or weight) that have been present for more than a month. These symptoms must also represent a change from the child's usual state in order to justify the diagnosis.

It is important that the pediatrician maintain a high degree of sensitivity to the possibility of a depressive syndrome when a child or adolescent exhibits a sudden unexplained change in behavior, attitude, mood, or school performance. He should endeavor to identify precipitating events, especially losses that were difficult to acknowledge or mourn, around the time of onset of symptoms and explore as tactfully as possible aspects of current family functioning, which may indicate whether the child is in some way the carrier of unacknowledged family conflict. The pediatrician should attempt to discuss the issues with child and family if he feels comfortable in this role, or he should seek appropriate consultation or referral if he does not. In any severe or long-lasting depressive illness the pediatrician would be well advised to direct the child and family to an appropriate psychotherapeutic resource without delay.

CONVERSION REACTIONS. In conversion, emotional conflicts are usually expressed (converted) through physical symptoms that may simulate organic illness. Symptoms may be found singly or in almost any conceivable combination; they may be long-lasting or may manifest themselves briefly with abrupt onset and cessation. Symptoms may be largely somatic, or psychic symptoms may predominate. They include many types of disorders of sensation: visual disturbances, including amblyopia, diplopia, and scotomas; deafness, which may be complete or limited only to certain hours or to contacts with certain individuals; disturbances of cutaneous sensation, anesthesia, hyperesthesias or hypoesthesias having no relation to peripheral or segmental nerve distribution; motor disturbances, such as paralyses, limps, or inability to walk, although the legs can be used for other purposes quite normally; choreiform manifestations, atactic features, and speech disturbances, including aphonia, mutism, and stuttering. The visceral symptoms may include vomiting, diarrhea, constipation, and cough and may involve one or more organ systems. Other manifestations include amnesia and convulsive, hysterical, delirious, and stuporous states.

The outstanding characteristic of the conversion reaction is the massiveness of the symptom. The paralyzed limb cannot move at all; the child with hysterical anorexia refuses all food to the point of collapse. The differentiation from organic disease is not always easy, and the difficulty may be increased because of the tendency of conversion reactions to occur as a complication of some organic or constitutional disease. Careful and repeated examination is indicated. Conversion anesthesia is characterized by its distribution, which corresponds to the child's idea rather than to any anatomic nerve distribution. Paralyses are apt to correspond exactly to the anesthetic area. Pharyngeal anesthesia with loss of the gag reflex is a common finding. Generally symptoms occur in such combinations that the diagnosis is clear. The attitude of the child toward his symptoms is also helpful, as he is not apt to be disturbed by the symptoms and at times actually seems to enjoy them. Characteristically the child is unaware of any emotional conflict within himself. He seems contented and more or less happy, and it is difficult to elicit any evidence of anxiety or tension. Thus the symptoms seem to have banished his conflicts from his conscious thinking.

Treatment that does not go beyond consideration of the isolated symptom cannot be considered satisfactory. Hysterical symptoms have a tendency to disappear when no longer needed, or as a result of some sudden shock or suprise. They also have a tendency to recur in the same or other forms unless the underlying difficulties are dealt with. The symptom may disappear if ignored or if suggestion is used. This is often important, especially when the symptom is profoundly affecting the child's daily life or threatening his physical health. However, every attempt should be made to direct the therapeutic approach toward the total child and those with whom he lives.

ANOREXIA NERVOSA. Anorexia nervosa, first described in adults by Gull a century ago, has been increasing in frequency during the past two decades. Although anorexia nervosa formerly occurred primarily in late adolescence and early womanhood, it is now also seen in girls between 9 and 14 years of age. It is rarely seen in males, in whom it is usually a manifestation of a psychotic process. Anorexia nervosa is a serious disorder that rarely may result in death. It is characterized by weight loss of at least 25 to 30 percent of body weight without evident organic basis and is accompanied by distortion either of body image or of appetite. The anorectic believes that she is fat and that her appetite is so overwhelming that if she once starts eating she will not be able to stop. The evidence of her weight loss and of the mirror does not convince her that she is not obese.

The weight loss is associated with increase of body hair, especially on the back and extremities, decreased body temperature to as low as 96 F, decreased pulse rate, lowered blood pressure, lowered leukocyte count, amenorrhea or delayed menses, and a marked degree of hyperactivity with excessive energy output. There is no loss of breast tissue or axillary or pubic hair. The level of blood urea nitrogen tends to be elevated when starvation is severe. Edema sometimes appears when the patients begin to eat after prolonged starvation. Radiographs of the chest may show microcardia. Most writers agree that the disorder is psychologic in origin, with the clinial psychiatric diagnoses ranging from neurosis to psychosis. The approach to treatment also varies with the diagnostic perspective of the therapist, and it may be supportive or quite punitive in some settings.

Characteristically anorexia nervosa begins with a self-imposed diet that gradually leads to extreme restriction of food intake, marked weight loss, a fear of eating, and a concomitant preoccupation with food and diet. There is much bargaining with family and others and much complaining about food, weight, and eating. There is marked distrust and suspicion of others that leads to secrecy about eating, bathroom activities, and exercise. If those in her environment behave inconsistently, this only serves to confirm her belief that people cannot be trusted. Although the initial diet is explained as an effort to reduce, the incipient anorectic's concern about overweight may not be realistic and in most cases is not borne out by photographs or weight records. Despite an emaciated appearance, the patient will deny that she is thin and will stoutly maintain that her abdomen protrudes and that her pipestem extremities are too heavy.

The family setting in which this syndrome develops is usually characterized by emotional unavailability of the mother, to which the child has previously responded by a high degree of conforming behavior. She has usually had a warm, close relationship with her father, and at pubescence this has become increasingly difficult for her to handle emotionally. In some cases the father has seemed to be consciously trying to make up for the maternal unavailability, while in others there has been evidence of a considerable degree of personal psychopathology in the father.

Because of the severe nutritional problem and the tendency of some of these patients to develop circulatory collapse, it is important that initial treatment be in a hospital setting. Circulatory collapse may be heralded by a resting systolic blood pressure reading below 50 mm Hg, which does not rise later in the day. Obviously, in addition to the risk of circulatory collpase and the need to increase food intake, a separation from the environment in which the symptoms developed seems appropriate, at least until the patient can gain some trust in herself and others and until therapeutic intervention with the family can effect changes in the family balance.

Management should be based on understanding,

kindly firmness, consistent demands, low pressure for eating, and great patience. Skilled psychotherapy is essential. There is disagreement over whether recovery should be measured in terms of weight gain alone or in terms of psychologic change in the patient or the family. These patients may be quite manipulative and may engage the staff in obsessive surveillance of covert vomiting or frenetic exercising, which are perceived as dangerous activities. It may be helpful to offer a high-calorie formula as a medication, thereby ensuring some caloric intake and decreasing the concern of ward personnel. Forcing oral feedings should be avoided under all circumstances. If the situation becomes desperate, feedings can be given through an indwelling naso-gastric tube, which, in the rare instances they have to be used, are usually left in place. Intermittent tube feeding should not be used.

It is important that the patient not be given a target weight for discharge, but the patient and her family should be told that many different factors will enter into the decision for discharge. Furthermore, plans for continuing ambulatory treatment must be discussed long before discharge from the hospital. The average length of stay on a psychosomatic unit is 3 months, and this must be followed by continued psychotherapy for the patient and family. With proper management, mortality can be significantly reduced from the previously reported 10 to 15 percent, but the risk to life cannot be ignored when planning a treatment program for a girl with anorexia nervosa. These patients are not only difficult and annoying but also anxiety-provoking. However, the results of successful treatment are highly visible, and the rewards are great, especially for the psychiatrist, who rarely has such concrete evidence of therapeutic success.

PSYCHOSES. The childhood psychoses are rare, and the clinical pictures differ from those seen in adulthood. *Infantile autism* refers to children with profoundly aberrant development from early childhood, particularly with regard to personal relatedness and language development. Symptoms may be apparent early in infancy or after a period of apparently good development lasting from a few months to 2 years. The onset is often after an apparently mild illness, frequently coincident with an environmental change. These children turn away from people and relate more to themselves or to inanimate objects like phonographs, television sets, or toilet bowls; they have an intense intolerance for change. They generally have severely distorted language development, not speaking until quite late or speaking in broken, fragmented sentences; sometimes they never master the use of personal pronouns, especially those referring to themselves. About half these children will never achieve social self-sufficiency. Many of them, who earlier were apparently normal neurologically, go on to develop frank seizure disorder or other signs of major neurologic disease. *Schizophrenic psychosis* in childhood begins later than infantile autism; it resembles adult schizophrenia in that affected children have more nearly normal language development, but exhibit seriously disturbed thought processes and poor rela-

tionships with people. The *disintegrative psychoses*, of which Heller's disease is considered the prototype, occur in children who have had normal development before an insidious psychologic deterioration sets in. Behavior, emotions, and relationships are disturbed, and language may be lost.

In none of these conditions is the etiology known. A congenital or acquired disorder in auditory language processing may underlie infantile autism. The relevance of environmental contributions, including maternal coldness and interruption of relationships, remains moot. A triaxial classification system has been proposed by Rutter and associates, with intellectual level, psychiatric diagnosis, and any associated or etiologic factors listed separately. This approach will facilitate description and classification. Psychiatric evaluation is indicated if it is suspected that a child has any serious emotional disorder. Pediatricians must be careful to avoid the tendency to label any child with aberrant behavior development as retarded without a careful review of symptomatology and overall development. In general, the behavior of a retarded child is akin to that of a younger or less mature normal child, while children with psychoses present behavior manifestations that are quite unusual and unpredictable.

BEHAVIORAL PHARMACOTOXICITY

As the pediatric pharmacopoeia expands, both in efficacy and in potential adverse effects, the pediatrician must include possible pharmacologic toxicity in his assessment of the child with behavior and emotional disorders associated with drug treatment of an existing medical problem. Since a child's behavior is frequently influenced by his illness, by other environmental factors, and by medication, it is difficult to assess the role of drugs in such disorders. A readiness to consider possible drug effects will serve the patient's interests, even if no such effects have previously been reported for the drug being used (p. 92).

Effective drug concentrations may be influenced by many factors besides the amount prescribed, including changes in drug metabolism or target organ sensitivity, onset of puberty, acute illness, and surgery or anesthesia. In addition, changes in the effectivenss of one drug may be due to interactions with another. Attempts at self-regulation of dosage or other changes of compliance may be significant factors in drug levels. Idiosyncratic reactions are particularly difficult to recognize and are especially likely in patients with previously altered central nervous system anatomy or function.

The behavioral side effects of the stimulant medications such as amphetamines and methylphenidate and of the sympathomimetic amines are well known, as are the paradoxic effects of stimulants on some hyperkinetic children. The paradoxic stimulant effect of sedative drugs, especially phenobarbital, has also long been recognized in children below the age of puberty. It occurs variably and is difficult if not impossible to predict in advance of giving the drug. Fortunately the effect does not last once the drug is withdrawn.

Evidence for behavioral toxicity of steroids in children is not well documented. However, these drugs are widely used in children, and there is abundant documentation of such side effects in adults, which suggests that one should seriously consider drug effects when behavior changes occur in children on steroids. In some children with asthma or colitis, increased aggressivity, violent fantasy life, and sadistic forms of play with animals or peers have occurred when they were on steroids and have remitted on withdrawal. Depression and frank psychoses occur in adults as side effects of prolonged administration of steroids; similar symptoms in children receiving these drugs should raise the question of possible drug effect. Drug reactions may occur not only as dose-related reactions but also idiosyncratically (non-dose-related) and during withdrawal of medication. Avoiding selection, wherever possible, of treatment modalities in which systemic absorption of drugs is known to have such effects may avoid issues of behavioral toxicity in many cases.

Anticonvulsive medications are particularly likely to produce serious behavioral side effects. Phenacemide (Phenurone) may exacerbate preexisting behavior disorders and precipitate pronounced depression and aggressiveness. Cerebellar ataxia and nystagmus are familiar signs of diphenylhydantoin (Dilantin) toxicity. In addition, pseudodementia may occur and may or may not be accompanied by the classic cerebellar signs. A syndrome of minor motor status epilepticus, with frequent petit mal, akinetic, and minor motor seizures, may also occur and may suggest a need for additional anticonvulsants when, in fact, withdrawal or change of present medication may be required.

In the presence of suspected behavioral side effects of drugs, the pediatrician will need to weigh the seriousness of the behavior manifestation, the seriousness of the condition for which the drug was prescribed, and the availability of alternate methods of treatment. It is evident that the essential prerequisite for effective management of the syndrome of behavioral pharmacotoxicity is recognition that it may be present.

TREATMENT MODALITIES

BEHAVIOR THERAPY. Various techniques of behavior modification or behavior therapy have been utilized in recent years. These draw on the tradition of directive counseling of parents about their children's behavior disorders, with a variety of specific approaches being used. Behavior therapy techniques include systematic charting of specific behaviors and attempts to analyze precisely those behaviors of child and parents that constitute or sustain the problem, to spell out the consequences of specific behaviors, and to help vacillating parents to respond more consistently to their child. These therapies also utilize techniques such as time-out periods, when a child will sit for a certain time in a familiar place and no other interactions may take place. These techniques, while in many ways still in the exploratory phase, may prove useful to pediatricians who are interested and who are able to invest the time and study necessary to master a specific approach. For others, referral to mental health workers, especially psychologists specializing in this area, will be appropriate.

Behavior therapy has recently been used in a variety of somatic conditions, including seizure disorders. Although these applications are still experimental and are not to be used casually by those who can use them only part-time, they may in the future yield benefits that can be more widely applied. Behavior therapy in an educational setting plays an important part in the education or therapy of children with severe behavior problems associated with autism or severe retardation. Some nonverbal children who have learned to communicate symbolically in this way have later begun to speak.

ENVIRONMENTAL MANIPULATION. For many children developmental assessment will reveal needs that must be met outside the home. Problems in rapport at school or special learning problems will involve pediatricians in consultation with teachers. For a boy with little opportunity to identify with adult men, whose own father may be deceased or out of the home, the pediatrician may wish to recommend that the boy spend time with an uncle or with the Big Brother program. Children with special needs may benefit from programs of therapeutic recreation. The physician who shares with specialists in other disciplines his view of the child's special needs and strengths can be of tremendous help to the child.

Pediatricians can have a role in development of community programs for children with special educational needs. Innovative programs such as drop-in centers for teenagers with no place to go or day care programs for preschoolers or various other services need input from skilled professionals who recognize that provision of adequate and accessible services can prevent a great deal of environmentally related malfunction.

PSYCHOPHARMACOLOGY. Aside from the use of stimulant medication in the minimal cerebral dysfunction and hyperactivity syndromes (p. 1764), the role of medication in behavior disorders in children is small. The *minor tranquilizers* of the benzodiazepine class, such as Valium and Librium, which are widely used and overused in adult medicine, have not found a place in pediatric practice. Major tranquilizers (antipsychotic) with sedative qualities, like chlorpromazine (Thorazine), are used only in severely impulsive children for behavior control rather than for thought disorder, which contrasts with their use in adult psychiatry. How much of their apparent efficacy in such situations is due to placebo effect in the child, tranquilization in those caring for the child, or relief of anxiety in the child has not been ascertained. These drugs also have a place in the management of crises in psychotic children, where their use is more specifically directed at the thought disorder. Because of their unknown effects on growth, and because of serious, often irreversible, neurologic side effects following their long-term use in adults, they should be used for children only in exceptional circumstances. Chlorpromazine, the first of these drugs to appear and the one most thoroughly evaluated in children and adults, is probably as effective as any.

TABLE 1. Suggested Doses of Psychotropic Drugs

Drug	Age	Minimum Daily Dose	Maximum Daily Dose
Imipramine	3-6	not recommended	
(Tofranil)	6-12	30 mg	100 mg
Diphenhydramine	3-6	25 mg	150 mg
(Benadryl)	6-12	50 mg	300 mg
Benztropine mesylate	3-6	1 mg	2 mg
(Cogentin)	6-12	1 mg	2 mg
Chlorpromazine*	3-6	0.5 mg/kg	3.0 mg/kg
(Thorazine)	6-12	25 mg	600 mg
Thioridazine*	3-6	0.5 mg/kg	3.0 mg/kg
(Mellaril)	6-12	25 mg	600 mg
Perphenazine*	3-6	0.05 mg/kg	0.1 mg/kg
(Trilafon)	6-12	2.0 mg	16.0 mg
Fluphenazine*	3-6	0.01 mg/kg	0.05 mg/kg
(Permitil, Prolixin)	6-12	1.0 mg	8.0 mg
Haloperidol*	3-6	0.01 mg/kg	0.03 mg/kg
(Haldol)	6-12	0.75 mg	10 mg

* See text for cautions regarding use of anti-psychotic medication in children.

However, some psychopharmacologists advocate the use of more recently developed major tranquilizers that are more potent. Suggested doses for some of these agents are listed in Table 1.

Divided doses are probably not necessary pharmacologically, as tissue levels accumulate after a few days and are relatively stable; however, divided doses may produce a desired placebo and sedative effect. Parkinsonian and dystonic reactions are less common with the less potent drugs, such as chlorpromazine. They are easily managed with diphenhydramine (Benadryl) or benztropine mesylate (Cogentin) in daily divided doses. Some authors have suggested that antiparkinsonian medications should be given from the outset of therapy and that they are especially indicated in children to prevent the potential resistance of the family to therapy after a frightening reaction. However, an equally strong case can be made for communicative rather than pharmacologic preparation. Even when reactions occur, the indication for the antiparkinsonian agent is generally transient, as the child adjusts to the antipsychotic drug. The overriding principle should be to limit the use of antipsychotic medication, both in dosage and in duration of therapy, to the minimum necessary and to reevaluate a child's need for medication by a periodic trial without drugs. Little is known of the long-term effects of antipsychotic drugs on growing children.

The *tricyclic antidepressants* such as amitriptyline (Elavil) and imipramine (Tofranil) have been little used for depression in children and have not been adequately evaluated in adolescents. Imipramine has been used effectively in the treatment of enuresis; whether its site of action is the brainstem (where it would modify depth of sleep) or the bladder (where it would have a peripheral anticholinergic effect) is unclear. If there is a role for these drugs in the management of childhood depressive phenomena, it is most likely in children with a positive history for depressive illness and with symptoms marking a change from the child's usual state and lasting more than a few weeks. The depression should include both psychologic symptoms (apathy, self-deprecation, hopelessness) and somatic symptoms (altered sleep and appetite). At present the pharmacotherapy of depression in children remains investigational.

With psychoactive drugs, even more than with other medication, the setting in which the drug is given can be as important as the drug itself in determining therapeutic outcome. The relationships among physician, patient, and parent, the expectations of each, and the communications around the drug are also important. Relevant principles include identification of specific target symptoms for which the drug is being given (as opposed to the inevitable wish that the drug will transform the child globally) and anticipation of possible side effects, particularly with the major tranquilizers. Dystonias, which can be acute and frightening to child and family, can be anticipated and treated, and they need not be a reason to stop treatment.

Full communication among all parties (including physician and child) about the purpose of the medication may contrast with the usual practice of leaving it entirely to the parent or nurse who administers medication to talk with the child about it. Some effort should be made to anticipate and elicit the child's feelings about the drug. Common fantasies include fear that a drug, especially one to "calm you down," will immoblize and weaken and fear that a drug "to make you feel better" will operate by "taking away feelings" that a child cannot imagine as separate from himself. Such fantasies stem from the child's poorly developed view of himself, his emotions, and his symptoms, from lay notions espoused by parents in which mental health is seen as the absence of troubling symptoms and feeling, and from a view of treatment as a process of forcing the patient into line, eradicating aspects of the child that he may for good reason be quite unable to imagine forsaking. In the face of such parent–child communication, direct discussion between physician and child is all the more essential. The frequent confusion in both parents and older children and adolescents between the uses and abuses of prescribed medication and of street drugs can also be explored and discussed.

PSYCHIATRIC REFERRAL. Referral to mental health professionals will depend on the nature of the perceived problem, the availability of community mental health services, the pediatrician's knowledge of and relationship with these, his inclination and ability to spend the extra time required for in-depth assessment of problems, and the family's and the child's receptivity to the idea of referral. The last is less determinative, except with adolescents. The health professionals to whom referrals are made can include child psychiatrists and psychologists, other psychiatrists and psychologists without special training in the disorders of childhood, and social workers.

There are no precise diagnostic indications for referral. In general, the following have been useful teaching guides: (1) when a patient is obviously manifesting symptoms of behavior indicative of a major psychiatric disturbance that may be either active or passive; (2) when there are major physiologic disturbances that are presumed to have a psychologic basis (psychosomatic disorders); (3) when it is likely that management will require extended interviews over a considerable period of time and a major reorientation of feelings and attitudes; (4) when the nature of the doctor–patient relationship seems disturbed and this relationship appears to be deteriorating instead of improving; (5) when the physician is uncomfortable in the relationship, cannot identify the reason, and desires clarification as to whether it is desirable for him to continue in the relationship. Referral of a child by a pediatrician to a psychiatric consultant requires a particular balance of frankness and reassurance. The pediatrician must resist the temptation to make it easier for the parent by suggesting that the problem is really quite small or will be easy to take care of. If the problem were small or did not require special help, the pediatrician would not be making the referral.

Uncertainty about referral is often occasioned by the apparent overlap in services provided by the different members of the mental health team, where relationships in training and function among clinicians of different backgrounds are different from those that exist among pediatricians and the ancillary professionals. With the traditional child guidance team the child psychiatrist did clinical evaluations of children and treated them in psychotherapy, the child psychologist provided psychologic testing, and the social worker evaluated and treated (in casework) the parents, usually the mother. However, increasingly these services are not always divided according to those strict professional lines. In his referral practices, therefore, the pediatri-cian must have knowledge of the services offered rather than of the discipline and must be acquainted with the training and competence of clinicians in his area rather than with their professional discipline per se.

Evaluation includes clinical assessment (medical history and physical examination) and especially psychologic assessment of the child and his parents or his entire family. Formal psychologic testing is a part of most evaluations and includes both tests of intellectual competence and projective testing, which attempts to assess unconscious attitudes and feelings by presenting ambiguous pictorial or verbal stimuli and drawing inferences from the child's responses. Formulation of the problem may focus on the child, on the parents, on their interactions, or on the entire family. The pediatrician should be aware that parents who seek corrective help for the child may become anxious and may require support when professionals suggest that aspects of their own lives are part of the problem.

Thus treatment may be offered to any combination of family members. Pharmacotherapy has a small place, and behavior therapies are used increasingly by child mental health professionals. However, psychotherapies that consist of talking to a professional, or with a younger child playing with a professional, continue to be used most widely. The therapist attempts to develop a relationship and to use it therapeutically to increase the child's, the parents', or the family's understanding of the unrecognized distortions in development of relationships causing their problems and to help them learn new ways of managing their difficulties. The duration of treatment may vary from a few weeks to several years, according to the nature of the problem.

Some therapy will be based on the theory that children and adults recreate in current relationships the developmental impasses that led to distortions in their development and functioning. The therapist endeavors to recognize and, by commenting on it, use this repetition of the stressful past. Family therapies are increasingly used; they focus on current relationships and attempt to promote understanding and induce change, with less emphasis being placed on relating behaviors to their origins. Such therapy must be provided by those with specialized training in its application.

HOSPITALIZATION. Hospitalization has traditionally been used only for severely disturbed, often psychotic, youngsters. In situations that are troubling enough to lead to hospitalization, the period of hospital stay is usually longer than intended because of problems of placement or disposition. These, in turn, are due to the inadequacy of any treatment facilities to fill the gap between the child's home and the facilities offering total custodial care in institutions. There is a need for halfway houses that are therapeutically oriented. From the first contact with each child in need of hospitalization, the immediate need is to consider appropriate placement; the long-term requirement is for expansion of our network of facilities so as to provide a continuum of living settings that will be capable of meeting the children's needs as they progress in treatment.

The development of psychosomatic units for children and adolescents includes several hopeful features. These units can be located in general hospitals and can end the medical isolation of psychiatric settings. They can combine the best aspects of psychiatric and pediatric care, they can address themselves to the needs of children with problems hard to categorize as either psychologic or physical and also to the needs of those with psychologic problems that complicate chronic physical illness, and they can legitimize inpatient services, as needed, for a wider group of children than either straight pediatric wards or straight psychiatric hospitals. The special therapeutic advantages of such units are many: separation of the child from a home situation where little change is possible, or hospitalization of mother and child together, as indicated; a chance for the child to learn new ways of relating, in a milieu with other children; a chance for the parents to engage in psychologic work of their own, with the pressure of the sick child at home temporarily lifted; a chance to coordinate medical and psychologic treatments in ways not possible otherwise.

References

Akiskal HS, McKinney WT Jr: Depressive disorders: toward a unified hypothesis. Science 182:20, 1973

Anders TF, Weinstein P: Sleep and its disorders. Pediatrics 50:312, 1972

Anthony EJ, Koupernik C (eds): The Child in His Family: Children at Psychiatric Risk. New York, Wiley, 1974

Benedict R: Patterns of Culture. Boston, Houghton Mifflin, 1934

Birch HF, Gussow JD: Disadvantaged Children: Health, Nutrition, and School Failure. New York, Grune & Stratton, 1970

Blitzer JR, Rollins N, Blackwell A: Children who starve themselves: anorexia nervosa. Psychosom Med 23:369, 1961

Bronfenbrenner U: A Report on Longitudinal Evaluation of Preschool Programs, Vol II, Is Early Intervention Effective? Washington, DC, USDHEW Publication No (OHD) 75-25

Bronowski J: The Ascent of Man. Boston, Little, Brown, 1973

Broverman DM, Klaiber EL, Kobayashi Y, Vogel W: Roles of activation and inhibition in sex differences in cognitive abilities. Psychol Rev 75:23, 1968

Casati I, Lezine I: Administration Manual: The Stages of Sensory-Motor Intelligence in the Child from Birth to Two Years. Paris, Center of Applied Psychology, 1968

Coolidge JC, Silver ML, Tessman E, Waldfogel S: School phobia in adolescence—a manifestation of servere character disturbance. Am J Orthopsychiatry 30:599, 1960

Cytryn L, McKnew DH Jr: Proposed classification of childhood depression. Am J Psychiatry 129:149, 1972

Eisenberg L: The course of childhood schizophrenia. Arch Neurol Psychiatry 78:69, 1957

Erikson E: Childhood and Society, 2nd ed. New York, Norton, 1963

Fraiberg S: The Magic Years. New York, Scribner's, 1959

Freud A: Normality and Pathology in Childhood: Assessments of Development. New York, International Universities Press, 1965

Garrard SD, Richmond JB: Psychological aspects of management of chronic disease in children. In Lief H (ed): Psychological Basis of Medical Practice. New York, Harper & Row, 1963

Graziano AM (ed): Behavior Therapy with Children, Vol 2. Chicago, Aldine, 1975

Griffiths R: The Abilities of Young Children. London, Child Development Research Centre, 1970

Guthrie RD, Wyatt RJ: Biochemistry and schizophrenia. III. A review of childhood psychosis. Schiz Bull 12:18, 1975

Hollingshead AB, Redlich FC: Social Class and Mental Illness. New York, Wiley, 1958

Illingsworth RS: The Normal Child. London, Churchill & Livingstone, 1973

Kanner L: Early infantile autism. J Pediatr 25:211, 1944

Kessler JW: Psychopathology of Childhood. Englewood Cliffs, NJ, Prentice-Hall, 1966

Knobloch H, Pasamanick B: Gesell and Amatruda's Developmental Diagnosis, 3rd ed. New York, Harper & Row, 1974

Langford WS: Anxiety attacks in children. Am J Orthopsychiatry 7:210, 1937

Malmquist CP: Depression in childhood and adolescence. N Engl J Med 284:887, 955, 1971

Maxmen JS, Siberfarb PM, Ferrell RB: Anorexia nervosa: practical initial management in a general hospital. JAMA 229:801, 1974

Minuchin S: Families and Family Therapy. Cambridge, Harvard Univ Press, 1974

Piaget J: The Origins of Intelligence in Children. New York, International Universities Press, 1952

Powell GF, Brasel JA, Blizzard RM: Emotional deprivation and growth retardation simulating idiopathic hypopituitarism. I. Clinical evaluation of the syndrome. N Engl J Med 276:1271, 1967

Redl F: When We Deal with Children. New York, Free Press, 1966

———Wineman D: The Aggressive Child (combined edition of Children Who Hate and Controls from Within). New York, Free Press, 1957

Richmond JB: Disadvantaged children: what have they compelled us to learn? Yale J Biol Med 43:127, 1970

———The State of the Child: Is the Glass Half-empty or Half-full? Am J Orthopsychiatry 44:484, 1974

———Caldwell BM: The impact of theories of child development. Children 9:73, 1962

Robins L: Deviant Children Grown Up. Baltimore, Williams & Wilkins, 1966

Russell DH: Juvenile delinquency. Psychiatr Annals 5:1, 1975

Rutter M: Childhood schizophrenia reconsidered. J Autism Child Schizo 2:315, 1972

———Maternal Deprivation Reassessed. Baltimore, Penguin, 1972

———Graham P, Yule W: A Neuropsychiatric Study in Childhood. London, Heineman, 1970

———Levocici S, Eisenberg L, et al: A tri-axial classification of mental disorders in childhood. J Child Psychol Psychiatry 10:41, 1969

Schmitt BD: School phobia, the great imitator: a pediatrician's viewpoint. Pediatrics 48:433, 1971

Skinner BF: The Behavior of Organisms. New York, Appleton-Century-Crofts, 1938

Solnit AS, Stark MH: Mourning and the birth of a defective child. Psychoanal Study Child 16:000, 1961

Stunkard AJ: From explanation to action in psychosomatic medicine: the case of obesity. Psychosom Med 37:195, 1975

Thomas A, Chess S, Birch HG: Temperament and Behavior Disorders in Children. New York, New York Univ Press, 1968

Uzgiris IC, Hunt JMV: Assessment in Infancy. Urbana, Univ Illinois Press, 1975

Vallarta JM, Bell DB, Reichert A: Progressive encephalopathy due to chronic hydantoin intoxication. Am J Dis Child 128:27, 1974

Waldfogen S, Coolidge JC, Hahn PB: The development, meaning, and management of school phobia. Am J Orthopsychiatry 27:754, 1957

Watson JB: Behaviorism. London, Routledge & Kegan, 1925

Weinberg WA, Rutman J, Sullivan L, Penick EC, Dietz SG: Depression in children referred to an educational diagnostic center: diagnosis and treatment, preliminary report. J Pediatr 83:1065, 1973

CHAPTER 4

Normal and Abnormal Growth

SELNA L. KAPLAN, *Associate Editor*

Growth may be defined as a continuum involving changes in body size and form, complexity of physiologic function, and biologic maturation.* The growth process, in the simplest and in the most complex species, follows a sigmoid curve, with an accelerative phase, decelerative phase, and steady accumulative phase. In the human, three sigmoid growth periods can be described. First, during fetal life there is rapid increase in growth rate until midgestation, with a deceleration as time of birth approaches. Postnatally, incremental growth accelerates briefly, with a decreased but steady state of growth during childhood. The final accelerative phase is seen during puberty, with subsequent deceleration and cessation of linear growth.

Concomitantly, growth of each organ system proceeds at a unique rate and timing (Fig. 1). These processes involve not only hypertrophy and hyperplasia but also functional changes, including development of enzymes and cellular receptors, regulatory control mechanisms, and secretory capacity. Growth of muscle, heart, liver, and kidney follows the general pattern observed for statural changes during human development. In contrast, the brain grows rapidly during the first 2 years, at which time adult size but not maturity is attained. Lymphoid tissue achieves peak growth in the peripubertal period, with a steady decline thereafter. As expected, reproductive organs show the most rapid increases in size and function with onset of puberty. Spatial differences in growth rate exist in that cephalocaudal and distoproximal directions are favored; head growth occurs before neck growth, arm before leg, and hand before upper arm. These sequences are more apparent during fetal development. Postnatally, growth of the head slows, whereas limb growth increases proportionately. There are also individual differences in human growth with respect to absolute size, shape, and physiognomy.

What is normal growth? In essence, for an individual there is no true normal, but rather an average, with an allowable range of variability (3rd to 97th percentile or ± 2 SD from mean values) within the comparison group. The comparison group must be similar to the individual in regard to age, sex, genetic attributes, and socioeconomic or nutritional status. The relative contributions of these factors will be discussed later. Thus an abnormal growth pattern is defined as one in which the

absolute measurement or the rate of growth falls outside these designated limits.

Numerous studies have indicated that growth involves increases in cell size and/or cell number. Total cell number is 1.3×10^9 at 60 days of fetal life, 2×10^{12} at birth, and 6×10^{13} in a 70-kg adult. Thus the

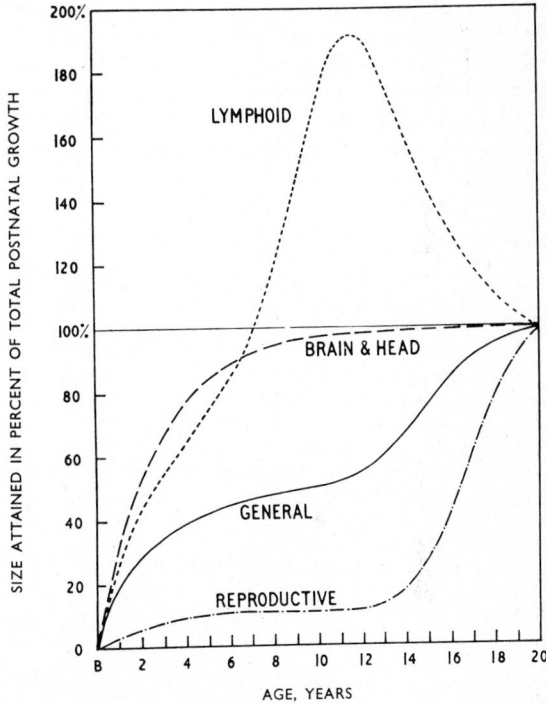

FIG. 1. Postnatal growth curves of four major organ systems are shown. All values are calculated in terms of the size attained at 20 years. General type includes body as a whole, respiratory and digestive organs, kidney, spleen, musculature, and skeleton. (From Tanner: Growth at Adolescence, 1962. Courtesy of Blackwell Scientific Publications.)

major increase in cell number occurs during fetal development, and an increase in cell size is responsible for most of bodily growth during childhood. The elegant studies of Cheek on muscle cell number are supportive in that they show cell number to be 0.22×10^{12} at 2 months postnatally, increasing to only 3.0×10^{12} postpubertally; there is a fivefold increase before puberty and a 10- to 14-fold increase at full development. Muscle cell size is believed to stabilize by 10.5 years, with maximum cell size being attained in males by 20 to 25

---

*Other authors differentiate the terms growth (increase in size or body mass) and development (progression of changes that lead from an undifferentiated state to a highly organized and specialized functional capacity). Such a distinction has value in some contexts; however, the present discussion is better served by using the terms interchangeably or by using the term growth for both processes.

years and at an earlier age in females. Adverse growth factors have differential effects on muscle cell size and number. Decreased cell number is seen with growth hormone deficiency, congenital heart disease, and intrauterine growth retardation. A significant decrease in cell size occurs with congenital hypothyroidism and with protein deprivation. In most pathologic conditions specific treatment reverses the abnormality in cell size and cell number.

GENERAL MEASUREMENTS OF GROWTH

SELNA L. KAPLAN

Growth Charts.   Growth charts have been developed for visualization of the progressive changes in height and weight with age. These charts consider the range of growth, as expressed either in percentiles or as stand-

ard deviations of the mean for average height or weight for age. The percentile curves are derived from a gaussian distribution (bell-shaped curve) of the data. The median or midpoint is the 50th percentile, and the accepted range of average height or weight falls between the 3rd and 97th percentiles (Fig. 2). The standard deviation (SD) charts are based on distribution of data above or below a mean value. The average range falls between +2.0 and −2.0 SD. The median, or 50th percentile, indicates that 50 percent of the measurements of a normal group of children are above and 50 percent are below that point. The range between the 3rd and 97th percentiles, or −2 SD to +2 SD, includes 94 percent of all normal children. Measurements at the 16th percentile are equivalent to −1 SD, at the 3rd percentile to −2 SD, and at the 1st percentile to −3 SD; measurements at the 84th percentile are +1 SD, at the 97th percentile +2 SD, and at the 99th percentile +3 SD (Fig. 3). If the data base used for the growth charts

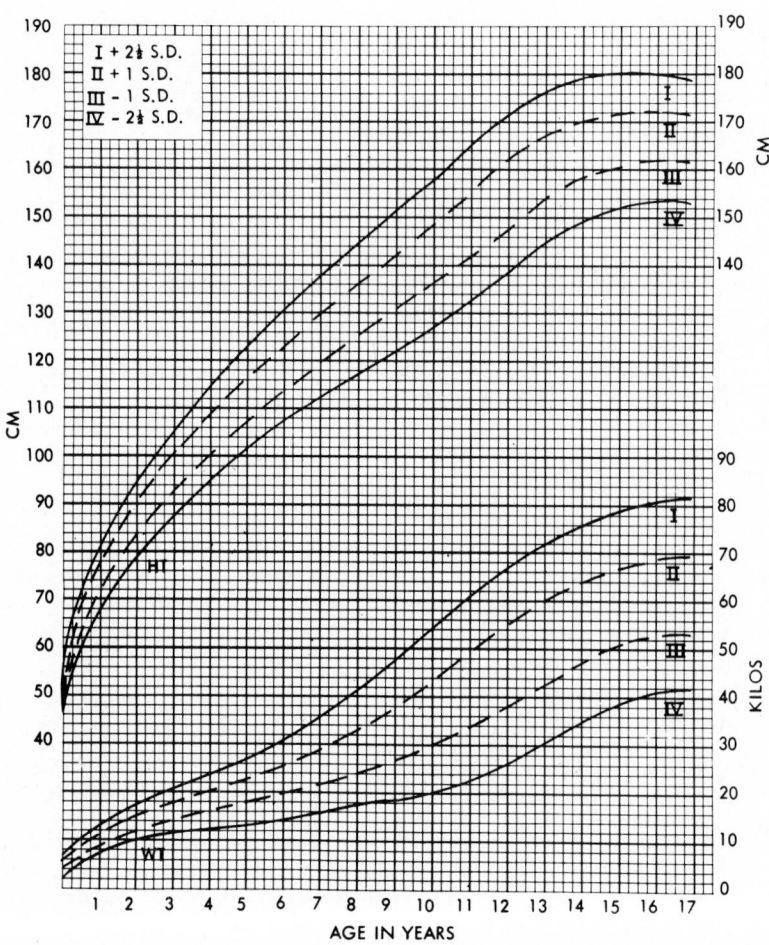

FIG. 2.   Distance growth curves for height of males from birth to 17 years of age are shown. Measurements are plotted as ±2.5 SD from mean of height for age in centimeters. (From Tanner and Whitehouse: Arch Dis Child 51:170, 1976.)

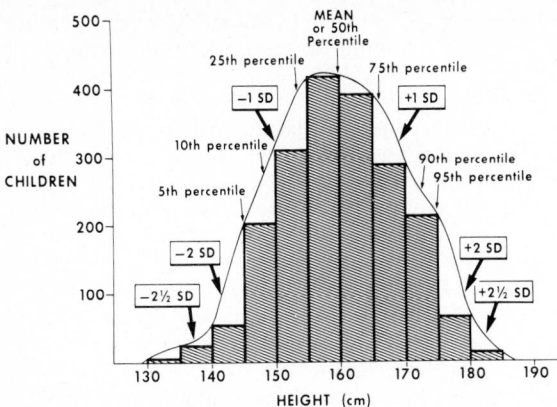

FIG. 3. Graphic representation of the distribution (in percentiles and standard deviations) of the height of 13-year-old males. (Data from HEW survey, HEW Series 11, Number 124, 1973.)

follows a gaussian distribution, percentile or SD charts are comparable. Measurements plotted on either of the growth charts show a similar pattern.

For assessing significant retardation in height, SD curves provide an advantage over percentile curves. Available tables for mean and SD for height for age can be used for quantitative comparison of the degree of retardation in height. Children with significant growth retardation are generally more than −3.5 SD from the mean height for age. Between −2.5 and −3.5 SD from the mean height for age would include those whose retardation in growth is of borderline significance. By the percentile charts, all of these children would be included in the group at or below the 1st percentile. Percentile charts tend to emphasize differences unequally, and major changes at the outer range of curves especially are obscured. The ease of visualization of significant changes should influence the choice of chart. However, systematic recording of height and weight is more important than the type of growth chart used. The validity of the growth data used as the basis for these charts has been criticized with respect to number of children included and appropriateness of the grouping in terms of ethnic and socioeconomic background. Growth charts derived in the United States and England for well-nurtured children of similar socioeconomic backgrounds show no major discrepancies, particularly in height at various ages. The data base for most growth measurements is derived from cross-sectional studies in which each child is measured once. In longitudinal studies the same child is measured yearly. Percentile charts developed by Tanner and Whitehouse and based on longitudinal growth data from English children provide an advantage, particularly for the individual differences in timing of the adolescent growth spurt.

In an extensive cross-sectional study conducted by the United States Public Health Service covering 7,000 normal children, minimal differences in height were observed between children residing in the six geographic areas of the United States. The heights of black and

Caucasian children in the United States have been equivalent in all but one study. Growth charts for children of other ethnic groups are not available at present; the heights of these children should be appropriate for the mean parental height.

Incremental Height Charts. Linear growth can be assessed in terms of increment in height per unit time, ie, centimeters or inches increase per minimum time interval of 6 months to 1 year. These charts emphasize significant deviations from average for age (Fig. 4); they illustrate more vividly the change in growth rate at different age periods, such as the rapid growth rate of the neonate, which decelerates during the first year of life, and the steady growth rate during most of childhood, with the secondary growth spurt at adolescence. These aspects are discussed further in the section on phases of growth.

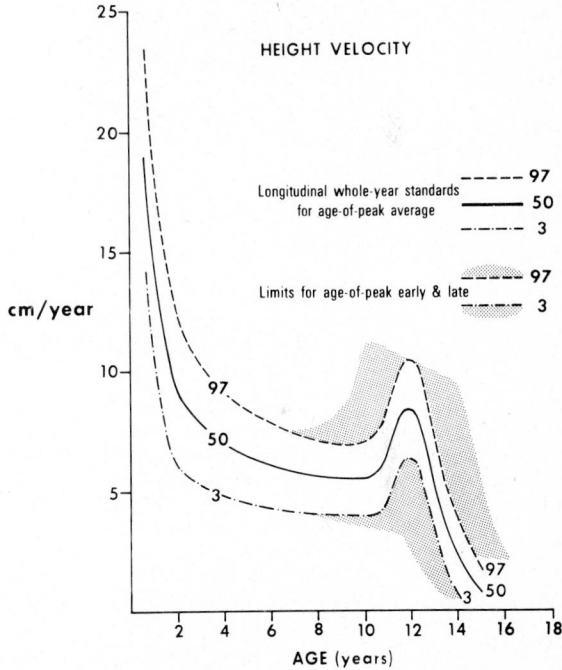

FIG. 4. Incremental growth charts: heights (cm/year) of males from birth to 19 years of age are plotted in percentiles. (From Tanner and Whitehouse: Arch Dis Child 51:170, 1976.)

Daily Variation. Diurnal variations in measurements of height occur, with decreased height in late afternoon. Small differences (2 mm) are noted in measurements taken between morning and early afternoon, but decreases up to 4.6 mm occur between 10 A.M. and 7 P.M. Serial measurements of height should be taken at a similar time of day, but these small differences in height do not significantly affect routine determinations; also, this effect can be overcome in part by ensuring that the child stretches as tall as possible with shoulders relaxed and head erect.

Seasonal Variation. In the Northern Hemisphere maximum growth rate occurs in spring and summer (between March and July); in the Southern Hemisphere it occurs during a similar seasonal period. As a consequence, there may be no increment in growth over a 3-month period in normal children (particularly during the months of September to February). However, a growth rate of less than 4 cm/year or an absolute increase of less than 2.0 cm between March and July is generally abnormal (Fig. 5). In blind or partially sighted children no seasonal changes are apparent, although the yearly growth rate is similar to that of sighted children.

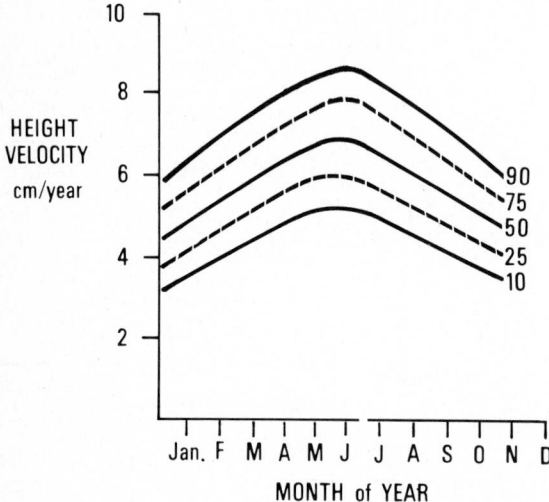

FIG. 5. The slowest and the most rapid periods of growth of prepubertal males are indicated. The measurements (cm/year) were determined during a 6-month interval terminating in the month for which the data are plotted. (Adapted from Marshall: Arch Dis Child 46:414, 1971.)

Genetic Factors. Genetic factors influence growth and final height to a significant degree. There are recognizable differences in height in certain ethnic populations. Genetic differences in adult height exist, as may be judged by the short stature of the Oriental population in the United States and the taller stature of Dutch boys as compared with boys from other European countries. However, the extent to which these differences may be attributable to poor nutrition or other environmental influences is difficult to judge. The height of a child over 3 years of age correlates significantly with median parental height. A parent–child sex-associated (mother–daughter, father–son) correlation in height has been suggested but not established. Correlation in height is best with twins, but it is similar with siblings. Skeletal age is similar in twins and in sex-matched siblings. Children born to parents of average height are said to achieve taller final heights than children born to families in which one parent is tall and the other is short.

Mean parental height (average of both parents'

heights at any age between 25 and 45 years) provides the best correlation for the appropriateness of the height of the child with respect to the familial trend. The mean parental charts developed by Tanner and associates provide a visual method to determine the relationship of the height of the child to parental height. Any child whose height is less than 2.5 SD from mean parental height represents a significant deviation from the normal. Examples of the use of this method of comparison are shown in Figure 6.

Sex. At birth the average length and weight of males are greater than those of females. By 1 year of age there are no sex differences in height and weight. After infancy skeletal age is more advanced in females than in males. The length of the forearm and the growth of the forearm relative to the upper arm are greater in males than in females from 2 years of age to adolescence. The length of the second metacarpal, compared to other hand bones, is greater in females than in males, so that the index finger is often longer than the fourth finger in females.

The most significant sex differences in bodily configuration, exclusive of the development of secondary sex characteristics, occur at puberty. The increase in hip width is more pronounced in females, and the shoulder width and chest breadth in males. In general, leg length relative to trunk length is greater in adolescent males than in adolescent females. Further details are provided in later sections of this chapter.

Secular Trends. Physical growth has increased from the late nineteenth to the middle twentieth century. The maximum height potential was 5 to 10 cm higher for adults in the 1930s than in the 1880s, as demonstrated in studies from the United States, England, the Scandinavian countries, Japan, and Russia. In the last few decades the height increments have decreased. In Sweden, between 1939 and 1971 only a 2.5-cm difference was demonstrated, and lesser increments have been reported in the United States during that time. The mean height of adult males in the United States now is 177.4 $\pm$ 7.0 cm SD, and for adult females 162.8 $\pm$ 6.8 cm SD. Improvements in nutrition, health care, and socioeconomic conditions may be the major factors contributing to these changes in height. The increased mobility of populations with improvement in transportation has led to movement from rural to urban communities. In addition, assortive mating as a consequence of increased migration to other sections of the country and the world may have influenced this secular trend in height. The introduction of new ethnic strains has been suggested as an additional factor. Comparable changes in average weight have been reported.

Children of Multiple-Birth Pregnancies. The discrepancy in birth weight of twins and the normal range for singletons and between the twins themselves has a strong influence on ultimate growth. It was noted in one study that by 8.5 years of age the twin with the lower birth weight was at least 2 inches shorter and 5 pounds lighter than the twin who was heavier at birth. In a recent study describing growth in a large series of twins, retardation in height and weight compared with the

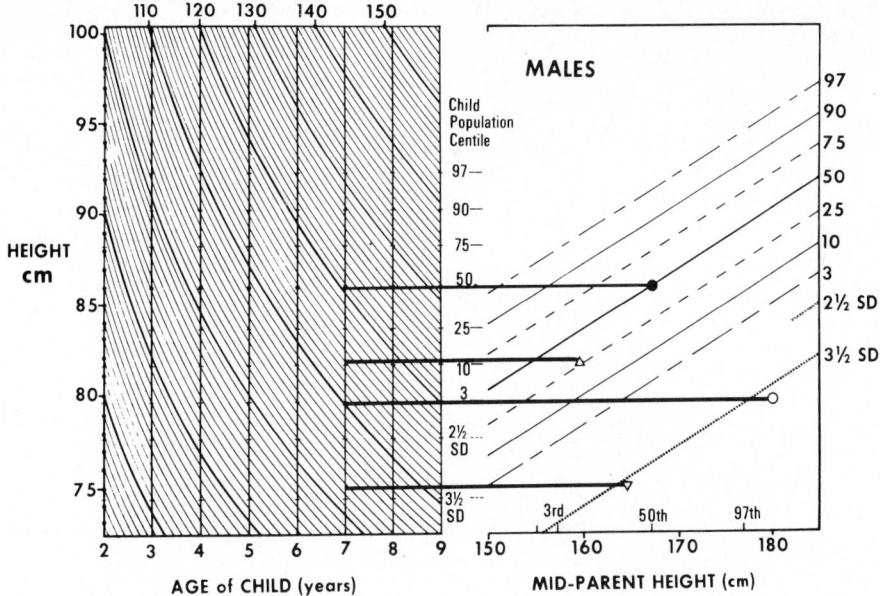

FIG. 6.   Appropriateness of the height of the child to that of the parents (mean mid-parental height) is indicated on the Tanner-Whitehouse chart (Arch Dis Child 45:755, 1970). The point of intersection of the height of the child with the median parental height is shown for 4 children (7-year-old males).

average were present only to 4 years of age. Greater increments in length and weight during the first year of life were noted in the twins as compared with singletons. The sex difference in growth noted in singletons is maintained in male–female twins.

MEASUREMENT OF HEIGHT
Selna L. Kaplan

Infants.   The measuring device should utilize a stationary headboard with a sliding vertical footpiece on the horizontal board to which a metal tape measure is attached. This requires two people, one to hold the head against the board and the second to move the mobile rod against the soles of feet, while the knees are pressed firmly so that they are straight. More than one measurement will improve accuracy. Measurement of the length of an infant on a mattress with a paper or cloth tape is rarely accurate.

Children over 2 Years.   Two types of measuring devices are recommended for meaningful data. One utilizes a metal tape measure on a vertical board attached to the wall, with a grooved horizontal board lowered onto the top of the head to determine height. The second device utilizes a sliding horizontal board, which moves on a rack and pinion with a counterweight attached to give a direct digital readout. This is subject to less variation because of decreased observer error. The measuring rod attached to a weight scale is generally not accurate. The child stands with heels firm against the backboard and flat on the floor, eyes looking straight ahead, and shoulders against the board. The child should be asked to take a deep breath and stretch as tall as possible, but keep the shoulders relaxed. Upward pressure can be applied on the mastoid processes to insure this position is attained. For younger children, a second person may be required to be certain heels are flat and knees are straight.

Prediction.   The estimation of ultimate height is of interest to both parents and children and is often useful to physicians concerned with disorders of growth in children. It has also been invaluable for those with specific career goals in which height restrictions exist, ie, dancer, airline hostess, policeman, or fireman. Several methods have been proposed, all of which have limitations in that the prediction is generally within ± 4 cm of the final actual height. (1) The Bayley-Pinneau method utilizes bone age as an index of the percentage of final height attained. Tables are provided for children with average, retarded, and accelerated growth. The greater the discrepancy between bone age and chronologic age, the more inaccurate the prediction. It cannot be used in any child with a bone age less than 7 years. (2) The Tanner method requires use of a formula and table of coefficients for height in centimeters and chronologic and bone age. (3) The Walker method utilizes a formula and table of constants for height and rate of growth. (4) The Weech formula is based on a correlation of the height at 3 years (H_3) and median parental height (A) with final adult height: $0.545 H_3 + 0.544 A + 14.84$ inches (male); $0.545 H_3 + 0.544 A + 10.09$ inches (female). (5) The Roche method utilizes a formula and table of contents. The height prediction for a 12-year-old male with a bone age of 12 years and height of 152 cm (60 inches) who was 94 cm (37 inches) at 3 years of age and whose median parental height is 167.6 cm (66 inches) is 182.6 cm (71.9 inches) by method 1, 180.6 cm (71.1 inches) by method 2, 179.9 cm (70.8 inches) by method 3, and 180.1 cm (70.9 inches) by method 4.

BODY COMPOSITION
SELNA L. KAPLAN

Cell Size and Number. Implicit in the definition of growth is an increase in cell size and cell number. These aspects of cellular growth are considered in detail by Cheek and associates using the muscle cell as the model. A direct relationship exists between cell number and DNA content of tissue mass, based on the constancy of the DNA/nuclear ratio. Cell size can be determined by DNA/protein ratio, since the ratio, cell protein/cell water content, is constant. Based on these methods, Widdowson has shown a twofold increase in cell size from midgestation to term (Fig. 7), and Cheek has dem-

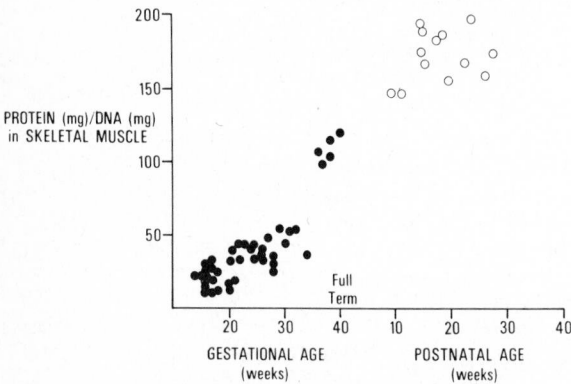

FIG. 7. Ratio of protein/DNA in skeletal muscle before and after birth. (From Davis & Dobbing (eds): Scientific Foundations of Paediatrics, 1974. Courtesy of W.B. Saunders -9 Co.)

onstrated an additional twofold to threefold increase in muscle cell size during childhood. In females maximum cell size and cell number are attained at approximately 10.5 years of age, whereas in males muscle cell size increases steadily until early adulthood. In contrast, the linear increase in cell number in the male parallels that in the female until 10.5 years; a secondary sharp increase in cell number is initiated and sustained in the male throughout adolescence (Fig. 8). Thus in the adolescent male the muscle cell number is greater than that in the female by a ratio of 3:2. This difference may underlie the sex difference in muscle strength that has been reported, particularly at puberty.

Decreased protein intake with adequate caloric intake leads to decreased cell size without affecting cell number. Deficient caloric and protein intake is associated with a decrease in cell number; cell size may increase or remain constant. Hypoxia has a greater effect on cell number than on cell size. Cell number and size also are

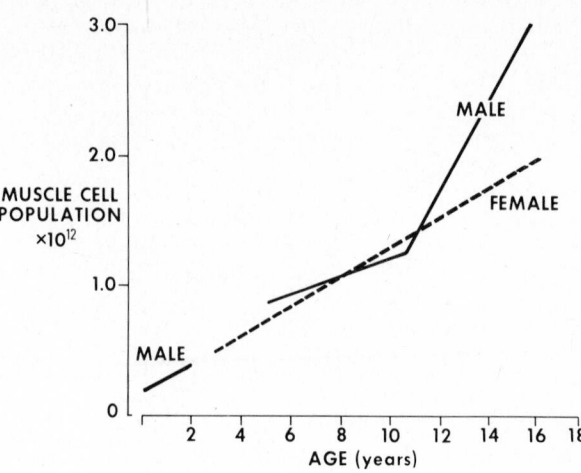

FIG. 8. Muscle cell population (× 10¹²) is plotted against age in years. Note the sex difference and the quadratic relationship or intersection of the two lines at 10.5 years of age. From Cheek: Human Growth, 1968. Courtesy of Lea & Febiger.)

influenced by the hormonal milieu. Growth hormone affects cell number primarily, with a lesser effect on cell size. Thyroxine influences cell size, but its effect varies with the age of the child. Insulin, by stimulation of RNA and cell protein content, increases cell size. Androgens apparently stimulate both cell size and cell number. Present evidence suggests that estrogens may decrease cell multiplication.

In normal growth the action of individual hormones is integrated. The changes described in cell number and cell size have been observed primarily in children with hormonal deficiencies. Furthermore, it is not known if these changes are representative of cell populations in other tissues or organs in the human body.

Lean Body Mass. Lean body mass (LBM) has been shown to be a better index of body mass than total mass, with the variable content of adipose tissue. LBM can be

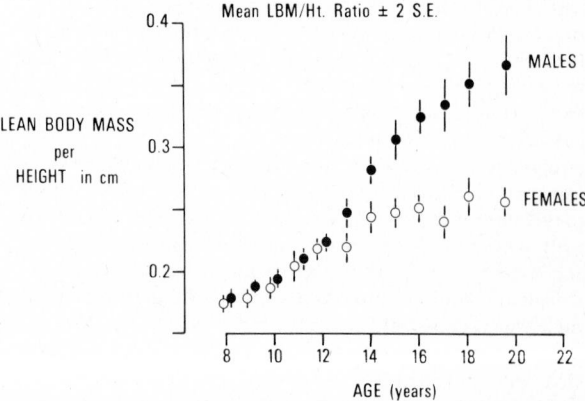

FIG. 9. Mean ratio (+2 SD) of lean body mass (LBM) to height is plotted as a function of age for males and females. (From Forbes: Pediatr Res 6:32, 1972.)

determined by underwater weighing, by measurement of total body water, or by total body distribution of the stable isotope ^{40}K. Using the latter method, Forbes has shown that the ratio of LBM to height increases linearly and is similar in males and females from the age of 7.5 to 12.5 years (Fig. 9). In males the incremental rise is greater during the adolescent period, with a peak ratio being attained by 19 to 20 years of age. In females the maximum ratio is attained at 16 years of age and is two-thirds that of the male, reflecting the increased muscle mass of adolescent males compared with adolescent females. There is also a direct relationship of height to muscle mass.

Adipose Tissue.   Adipose cell number reaches its peak at 1 year of age; thereafter the major increase is by increase in cell size. There is only a fivefold increase in cell number from infancy to adolescence (Fig. 10). A

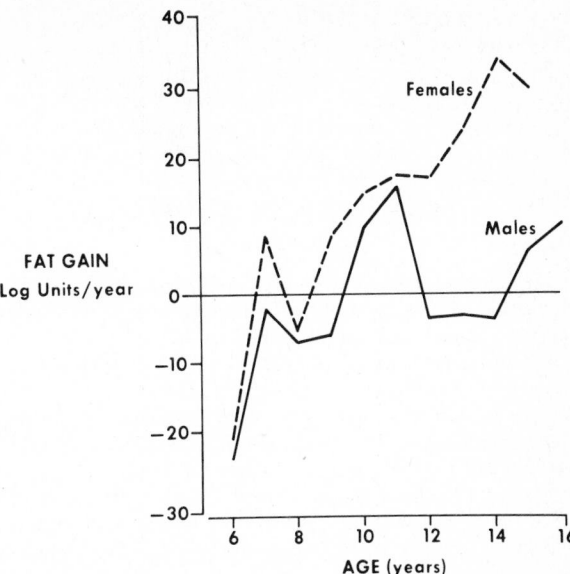

FIG. 11.   Mean increment in thickness of skin fold measured at four sites with calipers in female and male children. (From Tanner: Growth at Adolescence. 1955. Courtesy of Charles C. Thomas.)

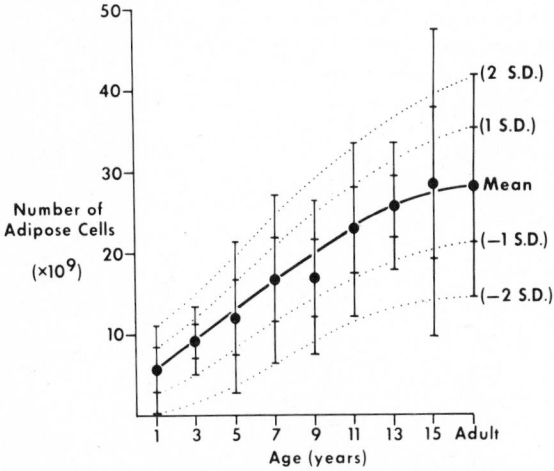

FIG. 10.   Progression in total adipose cell number ($\times$ 10^9) from infancy to adulthood. (From Brook: Lancet 2:624, 1972.)

twofold increase in adipose cell size occurs from midgestation to term, with a lesser increase by 3 to 6 months postnatally. From 4 to 12 years of age cell size remains unchanged. At any age, sex differences are reflected only in adipose cell size, not cell number. In the infant there is proportionately more fat than muscle, with a decrease in thickness of the subcutaneous layer between 1 and 7 years of age. At birth, fat constitutes 16 percent of total body weight; this increases to 22 percent by 2 months of age and is sustained at this level until 1 year of age. A gradual decrease in body fat content to 12.5 to 15.3 percent at 5 years of age has been observed. Up to 6 years of age the percentage of body fat is higher in females than in males. During the preadolescent period from 6 to 10 years of age a slight increase in body fat content has been reported in males but not females. Subsequently the percentage of body fat decreases in males and increases in females (Fig. 11). The fat content of adolescent females averages 24.6 percent, which is twice that of adolescent males. Skin-

fold thickness, determined by Harpenden calipers at four sites, can provide a good index of body fat content when compared with available standards for age.

Brook has demonstrated an increased adipose cell number in children who are obese by the first year of life. Obesity with onset later in childhood is associated primarily with increase in adipose cell size. Advanced bone maturation and linear growth occur only in the early obese group. Growth hormone deficiency and intrauterine growth retardation are associated with a significant decrease in adipose cell number.

Body Weight and Somatotype.   The appropriateness of weight for age can be evaluated by the use of available weight–growth charts. The incremental weight changes related to different age groups are discussed in subsequent sections. The appropriateness of body weight may also be considered in terms of the individual body form, or somatotype, as described by Sheldon. Somatotypes denote differences in the distribution and amount of muscle mass and fat. The endomorph is generally round, with the broader dimensions anterior to posterior. The mesomorph is more muscular and broader in the lateral than in the anterior/posterior diameter. The ectomorph is generally thin and narrow, with limited subcutaneous fat. These differences in bodily form are said not to be established until young adulthood; however, they can be determined in most children.

Chemical Growth.   Changes in the chemical constitution of the body have been discussed in detail elsewhere (p. 261). The nitrogen content reaches its peak at approximately 2 years of age; potassium remains at a steady level. At birth, about 75 percent of body weight is water; by 2 years of age this decreases to about 60 percent and remains stable thereafter. Changes in alkaline phosphatase parallel the height velocity, with higher plasma levels in children than in adults. There is an additional rise during puberty, with a peak that is coincident with a period of maximum height velocity. Inorganic phosphorus is generally higher in children than in adults and increases slightly during puberty.

OSSEOUS DEVELOPMENT

Selna L. Kaplan

Skeletal Maturation. Skeletal maturational age is estimated by bone age determined radiographically; it can provide an assessment of physiologic development distinct from chronologic age. Formation of endochondral bone proceeds by transformation of the primary ossification center of the cartilaginous shaft early in gestation to a calcified cortical form later (Fig. 12). The clavicle and mandible are the first to ossify (at 50 days of gestation), and the long bones ossify by 60 days of gestation. The os calcis and talus are the first epiphyseal centers to appear and are usually present by 23 to 26 weeks of gestation. With progression of gestation the distal femoral, proximal tibial, cuboid, and proximal humeral epiphyses develop in the indicated order, and all six epiphyseal centers are generally present at birth. These

secondary ossification centers develop, mature, and fuse according to a timed sequence from birth to sexual maturity. The attainment of the end stage of skeletal maturation is by fusion of the epiphysis and diaphysis, at which time calcification is complete. The age of appearance of each epiphysis, its increase in size and degree of molding, and its attainment of mature size and fusion with its diaphysis constitute the basis for determination of skeletal age. Several factors influence this determination: Sex: In females, skeletal age is more advanced for chronologic age and less variable than in males. Genetic: Time of appearance of some epiphyses may be familial. Ethnic: European standards are 1 year less advanced than those in the United States; blacks of average height in the United States have a more mature skeletal age than Caucasians. Maturation: Round bones (carpal and tarsal) are subject to asymmetric maturation and more variability in onset of ossification than long bones.

Assessment. There are a number of methods available for assessment of skeletal age; each attempts to compensate for the inherent variabilities. The first three methods require a single radiograph of the hands and wrists; they are used from ages 1 to 13 years. In the newborn a radiograph of the foot and knee is essential,

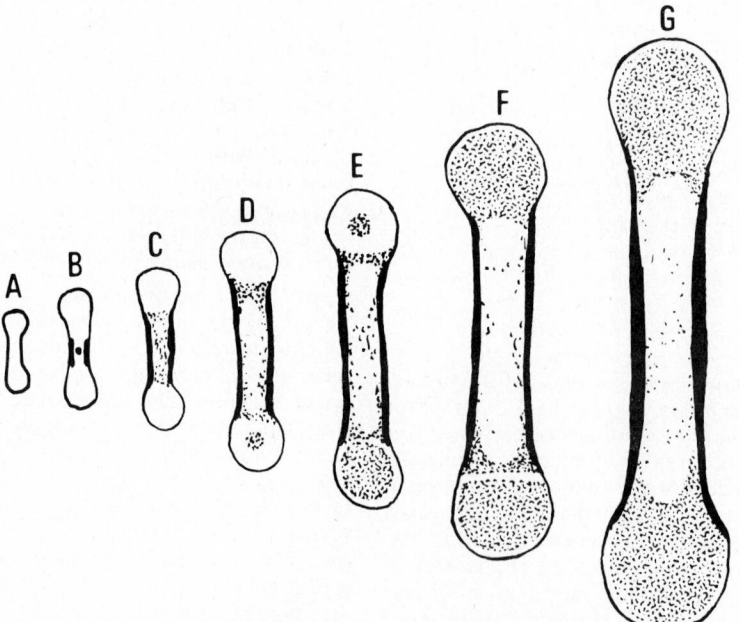

FIG. 12. Growth of long bone: (a) Cartilage model. (b) Primary centre appears in the shaft, and a collar of compact periosteal bone surrounds it. (c) The shaft is ossified, but the ends remain cartilaginous. (d) The marrow cavity appears in the shaft and progressively enlarges. A secondary center eventually appears at one end of the bone. The walls of the shaft are made of compact bone. (e) Another secondary center has appeared. The first has now formed an epiphysis of cancellous bone covered by cartilage and separated from the bony end of the shaft by a cartilaginous epiphyseal plate. (f) The second epiphyseal plate has been overwhelmed by the ossification proceeding into it from the shaft and has been converted into bone. Growth at this plate has ceased, and the epiphysis is said to be closed. (g) The cartilaginous epiphyseal plate at the growing end of the bone continues to grow in thickness for some time, but eventually it, too, is replaced by bone, and growth in length comes to a halt. Throughout the whole process of growth in length, growth in thickness of the shaft has proceeded steadily by apposition from the periosteum.

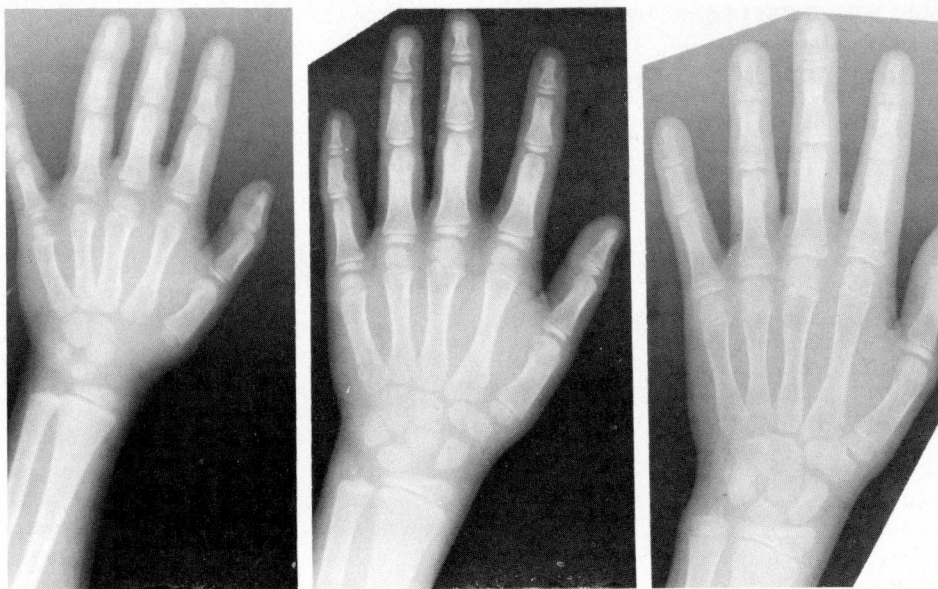

FIG. 13. Radiographs of left hands of 3 male children with skeletal ages of 4.5, 7, and 12.5 years (left to right), according to standards of Greulich and Pyle.

at 3 to 12 months the shoulder is best, and at 12 to 14 years radiographs of the elbow and hip are also useful.

Atlas standards, such as those of Greulich and Pyle, compare the number, shape, and size of the epiphyses of the left hand and wrist with published radiographic standards appropriate for the age and sex of the child. The range of variability is not constant at different ages; standard deviation is 2 to 4 months at 1 to 2 years of age, 6 months at 3 to 4 years of age, and 12 months after 8 years of age. This is the method most frequently used (Fig. 13).

Maturity scoring, as described by Tanner and associates, entails the assignment of one of some nine morphologic stages of development for each epiphysis in the hand and wrist, according to available charts. The maturity score is weighted such that carpal bones constitute 50 percent, radius and ulna 20 percent, and the remainder of the phalanges 30 percent of the final assigned number. A more recent modification of the maturity points method does not include carpal epiphyses in the weighted maturity score. This method provides a quantitative assessment of skeletal age, but it is also more time-consuming. It is more useful for long-term growth studies than for routine evaluation (Fig. 14).

Time of apperance of epiphyses for determining skeletal age is based solely on whether certain epiphyses are present or absent. The limitations with this method are the large differences in time of appearance of some epiphyses, particularly carpal bones. The late appearance of an epiphysis that matures rapidly could result in inconsistencies in estimation of bone age.

Hemiskeleton epiphyseal score for determining skeletal age is similar to the time-of-appearance method, but it utilizes radiographs of the hemiskeleton.

Correlation. A direct correlation between increments in skeletal maturation and percentage of ultimate height achieved per unit time has been demonstrated by Bayley and associates and is the basis for their height prediction tables. There is a sex-specific difference in patterns of skeletal maturity, with earlier achievement of final height in females than in males (Fig. 15).

Children destined to have constitutional delayed adolescence will be shorter than average and will have an equivalent degree of skeletal retardation; the converse is equally true. Obesity in children results in slight advancement in skeletal maturation and height. Hormonal abnormalities usually affect skeletal maturation adversely. Hypothyroidism leads to a more profound retardation in bone age than in height, whereas growth hormone deficiency generally affects bone age and height equally. Excess glucocorticoids induce delayed skeletal developement as well as impaired growth. Sexual precocity, with increased secretion of sex steroids, is associated with an advancement of bone age. Dysharmonic maturation of bone development is seen in patients with congenital malformations, and asymmetric development is seen in those with spastic hemiplegia, rheumatoid arthritis, and hemihypertrophy.

Skeletal development also can reflect other factors that affect growth, such as nutritional deficiencies and severe illnesses. Hewitt and associates have shown that delayed maturation of the carpal bones is a more sensitive index of environmental influences than delays at other epiphyseal centers. Postgrowth arrest lines along the diaphysis of the long bones can also be seen follow-

RADIUS

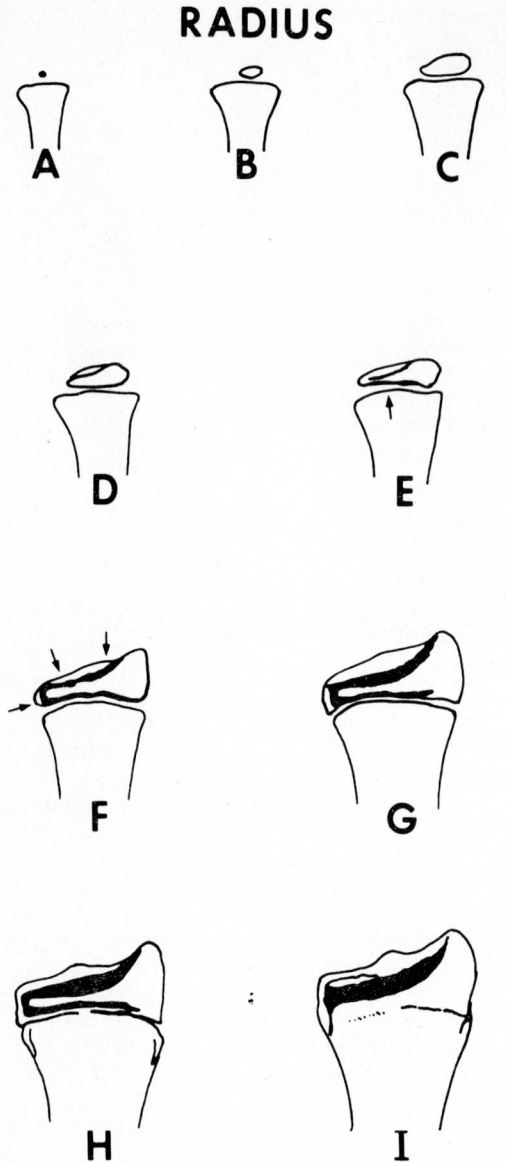

FIG. 14. Maturity scoring system for the epiphysis of the radius is shown. (From Tanner et al: Assessment of Skeletal Maturity and Prediction of Adult Height: TW2 Method, 1975. Courtesy of Academic Press.)

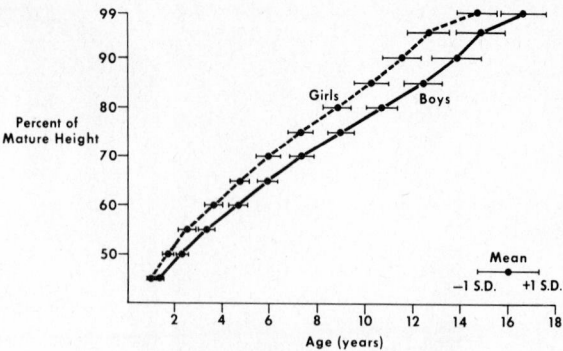

FIG. 15. Percentage of mature height (mean ± 1 SD) attained in males and females from infancy to adolescence. (Adapted from Nicolson and Hanley: Child Dev 24:3, 1953.)

ing severe illnesses or malnutrition. These have been attributed to sustained osteoblastic activity accompanying decreased calcification and bone formation. Subsequent improved clinical status leads to increased osteoblastic activity and thickening of the primary horizontal bony stratum, which becomes visible radiographically as fine horizontal lines proximal to the epiphyseal plate (Fig. 16); these appear before chondrogenesis is reinstituted. Park refers to these as postgrowth arrest lines, since they become visible during the recovery period; similar changes can be observed in teeth. Heavy-metal poisoning produces thickened lines at the epiphyseal ends of long bones, but the pathophysiologic mechanisms differ.

Fetal Skeletal Age. Estimation of fetal age based on epiphyseal centers present at birth or in utero is not generally reliable in view of the wide variability in time of appearance of the epiphyseal centers of the os calcis, talus, distal femur, proximal tibia, cuboid, and proximal humerus during gestation. However, all these epiphyseal centers are present in the full-term neonate. Pryse-Davies and associates have indicated that the appropriateness of ossification, normal, retarded, or advanced, can be assessed on this basis, but not precise fetal age.

Dental Age. Dental age, as judged by gingival eruption of teeth (Fig. 17) (p. 106), is closely correlated with skeletal age. Demirjian and associates have recently shown that the timing of tooth formation, rather than eruption, provides a more reliable index of dental maturity; the former is not affected by mechanical factors such as crowding, impaction, or extraction of teeth. Furthermore, eruption times are restricted to less than 30 months and after 6 years of age. The main disadvantage of the tooth formation method is the requirement for radiographs of the teeth. Filipsson has described a modification of dental age determination based on an individual curve of erupted permanent teeth; dental age is determined by comparison with a mean curve of tooth eruption for age.

PHASES OF GROWTH
Selna L. Kaplan

FETAL GROWTH

The transformation of a fertilized ovum into an embryo and thence to fetus involves increases in cell size, in cell number, and in complexity of function that comprise growth and development. The total body length increases sixfold in the first 4 months of fetal life, and twofold from 6 months to birth. Thus approximately 30 percent of the final height of an individual is attained by birth. Body weight shows similar changes, with a 15-

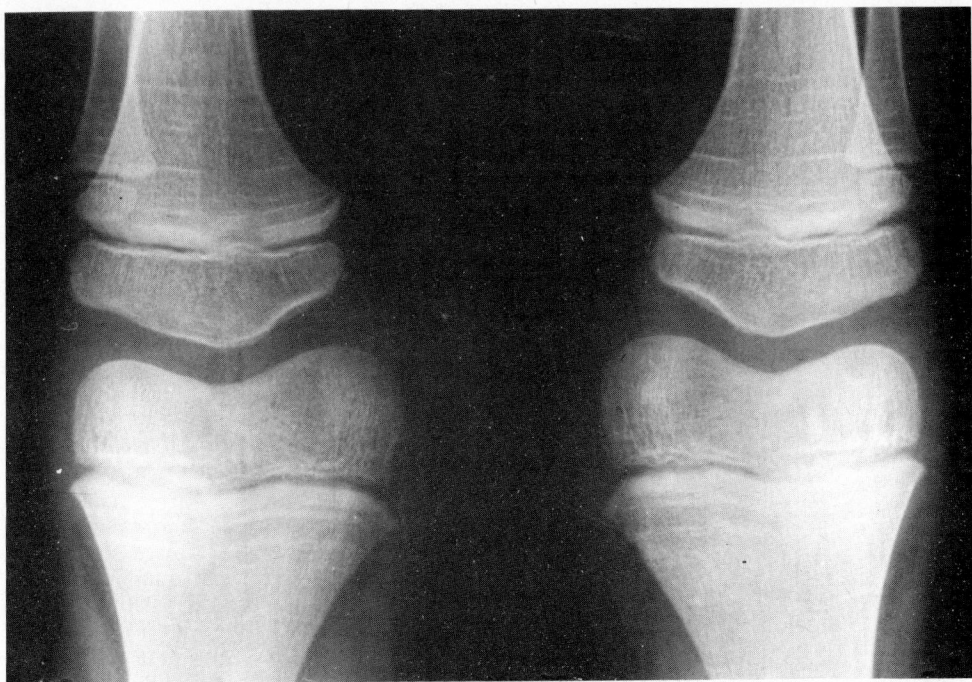

FIG. 16. Radiograph of knees with postgrowth arrest lines visible in diaphyses of femur, tibia, and fibula. (Courtesy of Dr. Charles Gooding.)

fold increase by the fourth month and an additional threefold increase from 6 to 9 months of gestation. A slight deceleration in weight gain occurs during the last weeks of gestation. About 5 percent of final body weight is achieved by the time of birth. Weights of organs such as the brain, liver, heart, lungs, and kidneys in general increase in parallel to the body weight during fetal life, ie, a 12-fold increase by the fourth month and a further threefold increase by term. The ratio organ/brain weight is constant for fetal body weights of 1,000 to 3,500 g. Some organs, such as the pituitary gland, show a greater increase in weight during the last trimester.

Alterations in body composition have been discussed in detail by Widdowson. During the first 2 months of gestation the cartilaginous components represent 80 percent of the solid constituents of the body. There is minimal fat in the fetus until late in the gestational period: 0.1 percent body weight at 15 weeks, 1 percent at 26 weeks, 5 percent at 33 weeks, and 16 percent at term. The percentage of body fat at birth is similar to that of children 5 to 8 years of age. There are corresponding changes in total body water, which comprises 90 percent of body weight at 15 weeks, 81 percent at 33 weeks, and 69 percent at term, a figure slightly lower than the one usually reported. The nitrogen content in the body increases from 1 percent at 15 weeks to 1.8 percent at term.

Ossification is initiated at 8 to 10 weeks of gestation. Concomitant increases in calcium and phosphorus occur with the onset of ossification. The calcium/phosphorus ratio is 1.0 early in gestation and increases to 1.8 at birth. At term, 98 percent of total calcium, 80 percent of phosphorus, and 60 percent of magnesium are found in the body skeleton.

About 30 percent of craniofacial skeletal development is complete by birth, with characteristic human proportions apparent by 12 weeks of gestation. Facial growth is initiated late in gestation, and it is in a rapid growth phase when cranial growth is virtually completed. There is both an increased length of the facial skeleton and a change with respect to the skull.

Hormonal Influences on Growth. *Thyroxine* is synthesized and secreted in the human fetus by 12 weeks of gestation, and its level rises significantly from 18 weeks until term, along with an observed rise in plasma thyroid-stimulating hormone. Fetal linear growth is not affected by thyroxine deficiency, since athyreotic infants are of normal length at birth. However, skeletal maturation is significantly retarded in such infants. Birth weight is normal or above normal, probably as a consequence of accumulated myxedematous fluid. Further details are presented on page 1669.

Growth hormone is secreted early in human gestation (8 weeks), with peak increments during midgestation and elevated levels still present in the serum at term. Present evidence suggests that fetal or maternal growth hormone is not essential for growth of the fetus. Apituitary fetuses, anencephalic fetuses, and children with hypothalamic hypopituitarism with growth hormone deficiency have normal length and weight at birth, as do infants born to mothers with isolated growth hormone deficiency.

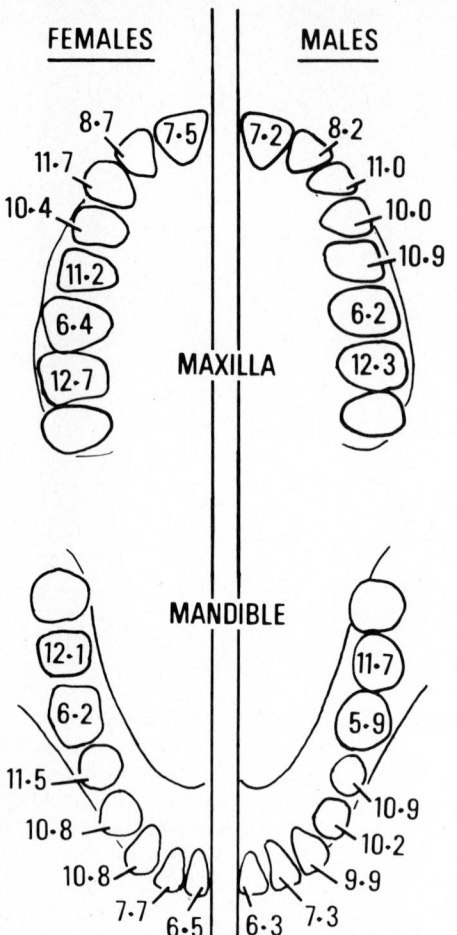

FIG. 17. Mean age of eruption of permanent teeth in males and females. The first teeth to appear are the first molars in the upper and lower jaws. (From Sinclair: Human Growth After Birth, 1973. Courtesy of Oxford University Press.)

Insulin secretion has been demonstrated by 80 days of gestation in the human fetus, concomitant with its localization in the pancreatic islets. A progressive rise in insulin content of pancreatic tissue from 25 weeks to term has been observed. The concentration of insulin in pancreatic tissue is higher in the fetus than in the adult. Insulin may have stimulatory effect on fetal growth, as evidenced by decreased birth length and weight of infants with neonatal diabetes and by the excessive growth seen in infants born to diabetic mothers. Decreased fetal growth has been induced experimentally in fetuses treated during gestation with streptozotocin, a cytotoxic agent of pancreatic beta cells.

Somatomedins (sulfation factors) are peptides considered to be intracellular mediators of growth hormone action, which may affect fetal growth. Children with somatomedin deficiency (Laron dwarfism), who characteristically have elevated serum growth hormone levels,

have significantly decreased birth lengths. The secretory pattern of these peptides during gestation has not been studied. The possible effects of other growth factors on fetal length are unknown at present.

Human chorionic somatomammotropin (HCS) is a polypeptide hormone secreted by the placenta that shares many of the immunochemical, structural, and biologic properties described for human growth hormone. During gestation the increments of HCS in maternal plasma parallel placental growth. Although there is limited transplacental passage, HCS may contribute indirectly to fetal growth. Present evidence suggests that the effect of HCS on maternal metabolism and placental physiology may regulate the availability and transport of nutrients to the fetus during gestation.

GROWTH DURING INFANCY

Physical Proportions. At birth the head is large for the body size, the face is small and round with a small mandible, the chest is rounded, and the abdomen is protuberant. The limbs are short, and the ratio of upper segment to lower segment (crown to pubis/pubis to heel) is high (1.7:1) (Fig. 18).

Linear Growth. The most dramatic growth spurt occurs during the first 2 years after birth. The length of the normal full-term male infant is 50.4 ± 2.0 cm, and the female, 49.7 ± 1.9 cm; there is an increment of 25 to 30 cm during the first year of life and an additional 12 cm by 2 years of age. In general, boys are slightly taller (0.5 cm) and weigh more (0.5 kg) than girls during the first 2 years.

Weight at Birth and During Infancy. Intrauterine environment has major effects on birth weight. Mean birth weight for Caucasian infants is 3.4 kg. The birth weight of Orientals, Mexicans, and black Americans ranges from 2.9 to 3.2 kg. Infants born to tall mothers are reported to be 8 percent heavier than those of short mothers; there is a 16 percent increase in mean birth weight of infants of mothers who are both tall and obese. Babies of multiparous mothers are generally larger than those born to primiparous women, and singleton infants are heavier than infants of multiple births. Drillien has noted that in twins, one-third have normal birth weights of 2.0 to 2.5 kg; the remainder are less than 2 kg. Birth weights in pregnancies with multiple births of 3 to 6 infants are generally 1 to 2 kg. The relationship of low birth weight to survival rate is discussed elsewhere (p. 154).

Maternal nutrition, intrauterine infection, cigarette smoking, alcoholism or drug addiction in the mother, and living at high altitude all lead to decreased birth weight. Low birth weight is seen in association with chromosomal anomalies in the infant, including mongolism and other autosomal trisomies and gonadal dysgenesis. Newborns with growth hormone deficiency are generally of normal birth weight. Birth weights over 4,500 g are unusual. Birth weights of infants of diabetic and prediabetic mothers are generally higher than average; this may be the consequence of increased insulin secretion, as suggested by the observed islet hyper-

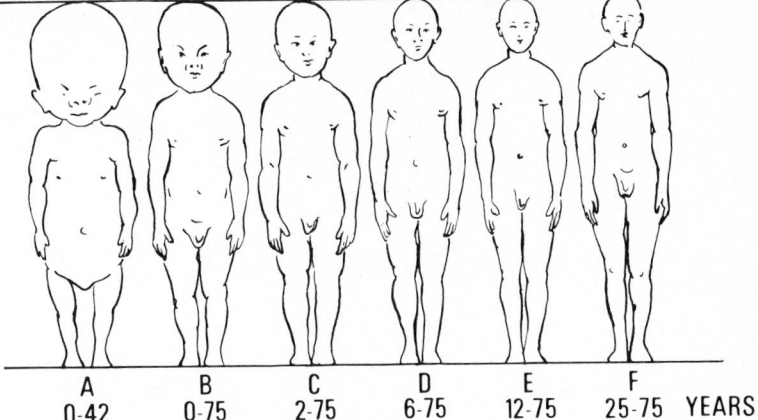

FIG. 18. Relative proportions of head size and body length and ratio of trunk to limbs are shown from the fifth month of fetal life to adulthood. (From Tanner: Human Growth, Vol III, 1960. Courtesy of Pergamon Press.)

plasia in such infants. Further aspects of prenatal factors that affect birth weights of infants are discussed elsewhere.

A 5 to 10 percent loss of weight normally occurs during the first few days after birth, but birth weight is generally regained by the 10th day. This weight loss results from a normal decrease in body water content. During the first 6 months weight increases 0.5 to 1.0 kg/month, and it doubles by the end of that period. By 2 years of age the rate of weight gain has decreased to about 0.2 kg/month. Black children tend to gain weight more rapidly than Caucasian children during the first year, with comparable weight gains thereafter. The consistent gain of weight during infancy provides a useful guide to nutritional status and health of the infant; it is not as sensitive a guide in the older child.

Brain Growth and Development of Neurophysiologic Function. The human brain attains its peak growth phase at birth and during the postnatal period. At birth the brain is only one-sixth its final weight. Dobbing has discussed the differential growth rates of the cellular components and of various areas of the brain. The sequence of brain development is initiated by a rapid increase in neuronal cell number during the 10th to 18th weeks of gestation, at which time the adult cell number is virtually attained. Further development of the neuronal elements is primarily by an increase in dendritic growth and arborization and synaptic connectivity. Spongioblast or glial multiplication constitutes the major growth phase of the brain components during late gestation and at birth. During the latter half of the brain growth period, from birth to 2 years, active myelination occurs. Myelination proceeds rapidly until 4 years of age, and at a more gradual pace until adulthood.

Differential rates of growth of parts of the brain have been described. Most notable is that of the cerebellum, which has a more rapid growth than the forebrain in the postnatal period. At 15 months of age the cerebellum is of adult size, whereas the remainder of the brain is only 65 percent its final adult weight. According to Dobbing, the vulnerability of the brain components to adverse conditions is dependent on the timing of these events. Irradiation, viral infections such as rubella, au-

tosomal anomalies, other congenital anomalies associated with fetal growth retardation, maternal medications, and inborn errors of metabolism, all of which induce major effects during the first trimester, would be expected primarily to decrease neuronal cell development. Maternal malnutrition during the last trimester and neonatal malnutrition such as kwashiorkor affect glial cell number and size predominantly. Hypothyroidism during the fetal and neonatal period affects primarily glial cell development and myelination. Maturation of neurophysiologic function has been documented during the active phase of brain growth. EEG activity first appears at the fifth month of gestation, but sleep–wakefulness stages are not distinguishable until the eighth month. Synchronous hemispheric activity with EEG changes in response to sleep are first evident at 2 months postnatally. Coordinative motor activity is not present until after birth.

These changes can be correlated with development of the regulatory mechanisms for secretion of pituitary hormones in the fetus, neonate, and child. The general pattern is one of elevated serum levels of most of the pituitary hormones in the human fetus during midgestation and late gestation. The development of inhibitory neural circuits results in more controlled secretory patterns by the late neonatal period, comparable to those in the older child and adult. Similarly, sleep-induced growth hormone release and diurnal variation of cortisol are not apparent until 2 months postnatally. Further details of the ontogeny of pituitary hormone secretion are described in a recent review by Grumbach and Kaplan. Circadian rhythmicity also is established during the neonatal period, as discussed by Mills.

Cranial Growth. The growth of the skull parallels in part the rapid brain growth during this age period. At birth the mean head circumference is 35.3 ± 1.2 cm. There is a 5-cm increment during the first 3 months after birth and an additional 6-cm increment during the latter part of the first year of life (Fig. 19). At birth the circumference of the head is greater than that of the chest, and it approaches unity by 1 year. During infancy the growth of the head reflects to some extent normalcy of brain development. Microcephaly generally suggests

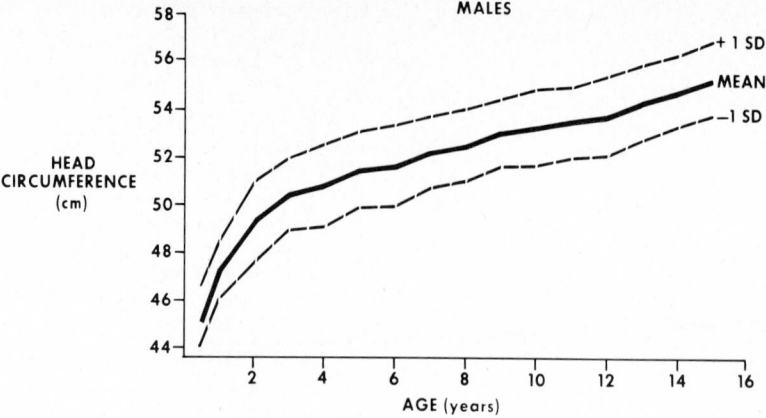

FIG. 19.   Mean ±1 SD for head circumference for age for males. (Adapted from Pryor: J Pediatr 68:615, 1966.

impaired development of the brain, whereas a rapid increase in head size may indicate hydrocephalus or less commonly subdural hematoma, neoplasia, megalocephaly, or other diseases of the cranium. Abnormalities in the shape of the head often result from premature synostosis of sutures, but they may be due to genetic variations such as brachycephaly and dolichocephaly. Asymmetric deformities can result from compression during labor or as a genetic variation. Cranial molding occurs in infants who tend to maintain the head in the same position for long periods of time; this can be altered by changing the position of the child and is of no serious import.

The principal sutures of the skull are generally fused by 5 to 6 months. The lateral fontanelle is usually closed by the sixth week, and the posterior fontanelle is no longer palpable by 4 months of age. The size of the anterior fontanelle may increase during the first few months of life, but it decreases after 6 months. Between 9 and 16 months of age it is no longer palpable, but a small opening may be demonstrated radiographically.

Craniofacial Growth.   The cranial vault increases rapidly, but the face and base of the skull develop at a slower rate. The mandible is small at birth and the two halves fuse during the first year, with additional forward growth (Fig. 20).

Limb Growth.   At birth the bones of the pelvis and the lower limbs are less advanced with respect to their subsequent size than those of the upper limbs and shoulder girdle. This results in more rapid growth of the former in the first year of life. In the neonate the pelvic cavity is small and funnel-shaped, as a result of the more upright position of the ilia and sacrum. By 1 year of age the ilia become thicker and stronger, the curvature of the sacrum increases, and the acetabula are deeper.

Chest.   Transverse and anterior/posterior diameters of the chest are of equal circumference at birth. The transverse diameter increases more rapidly, and at 1 year of age the ratio of transverse diameter to anterior/-posterior diameter is about 1.25:1.

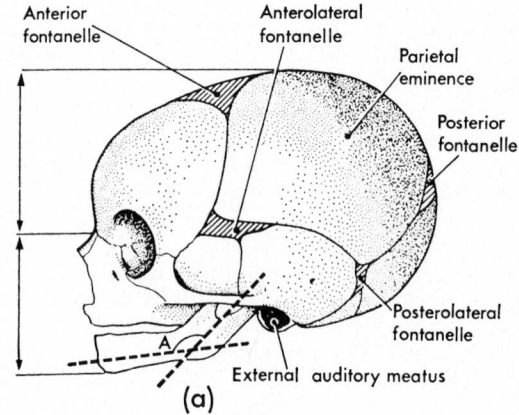

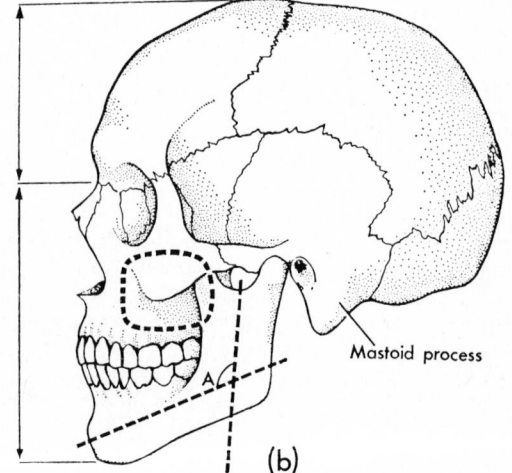

FIG. 20.   Changes in the skull and face from birth to adulthood are shown. Vertical diameter increases, and obliquity of mandibular angle decreases. (From Sinclair: Human Growth After Birth, 2nd ed. 1973. Courtesy of Oxford University Press.)

Abdomen. During the first year of life the circumference of the abdomen is equivalent to that of the chest; by 2 years of life the chest has enlarged more rapidly and the circumference is greater than that of the abdomen.

GROWTH DURING CHILDHOOD

Height and Weight. During childhood there is a general deceleration in the rapid incremental height and weight gains noted during infancy. During the second year height increases by about 12 cm, and weight by about 2.5 kg. Appetite usually decreases during the second year. The increase in physical activity and decreased appetite result in transformation from a pudgy infantile appearance to a more lean and muscular child with a decrease in subcutaneous tissue. With the onset of upright posture there is evidence of protuberant abdomen and mild lordosis. By the third to fifth years the height increment is less, with a rate of 6 to 8 cm/year, and there is a weight gain of about 2 kg/year. During this period the abdomen becomes less prominent. From 6 to 10 years in girls and 6 to 12 years in boys the height increment is generally 6 cm/year, and the weight gain is 3 to 3.5 kg/year. With the greater increase in limb length than in trunk length there is an appropriate change in body proportions. The upper segment is longer than the lower segment by a factor of 1.35 at 3 years of age, 1.14 at 6 years, and 1.0 at 10 years (Fig. 21).

Skull. The head circumference increases less rapidly during the second year of life (2 cm/year), in accordance with the decreased growth of the brain. There is

a limited increase in head circumference up to 12 years of age, generally 2 to 3 cm (Fig. 19). Although the increase in head size is restricted during this age period, there is a significant change in the facial configuration. The length of the skull increases, in association with a forward movement of the position of the mandible. The upper jaw develops rapidly during this period to accommodate dental development. Concurrently, sinus development is noted. Frontal sinuses are apparent radiographically by 2 to 6 years of age, whereas the sphenoid sinuses are not fully developed until late childhood. The maxillary and ethmoid sinuses generally are not radiographically distinguishable until 6 to 10 years of age.

ADOLESCENCE

Growth Pattern. At adolescence bodily transformation involves not only secondary sexual development but also changes in height, body mass and habitus, organ size, and craniofacial proportions. The details of the hormonal and secondary sexual changes are discussed in Chapter 29. The pattern of growth during this period differs in males and females with respect to the relationship of peak height velocity to pubertal staging and to total period of growth. In both sexes a slight deceleration in growth rate occurs in the immediate preadolescent period; it is more pronounced in those who have late onset of puberty (Fig. 22).

In females (Fig. 23) the mean age of onset of puberty is 10.5 years (range 9 to 12 years), as evidenced by breast budding and/or appearance of pubic hair; however, there is no direct relationship of onset of puberty to skeletal age. At the skeletal age of 10 years the female has attained 84 percent of her ultimate height, with the additional 23 to 28 cm to be achieved during the course of pubertal development. Postmenarchal growth is rarely more than 5 to 7.5 cm, so that 95 percent of

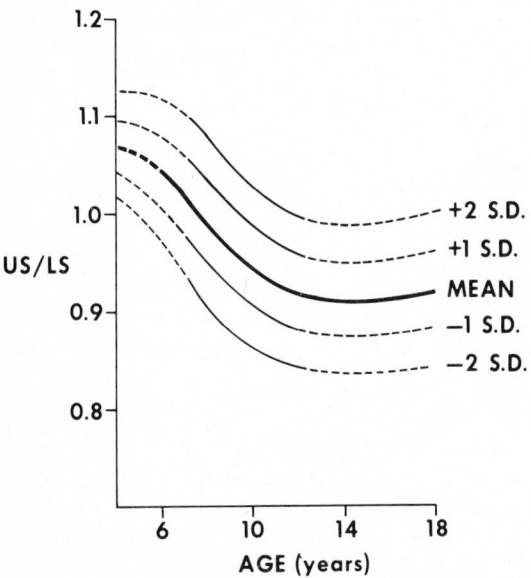

FIG. 21. Body proportions (upper/lower segment) plotted against age in years (combined males and females) for Caucasian and black children. (From McKusick: Heritable Disorders of Connective Tissue 4th ed. 1972. Courtesy of C.V. Mosby.)

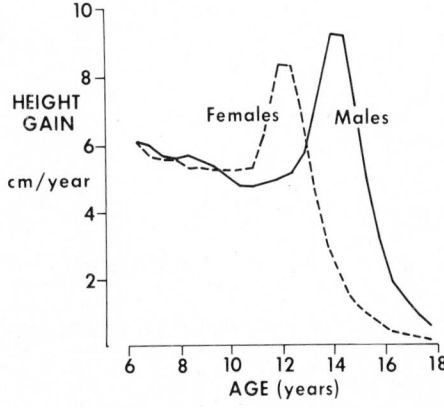

FIG. 22. Maximum height gain (cm/year) is plotted for females and males from peripubertal to pubertal period. Note the slight deceleration in height velocity in males prior to onset of pubertal spurt. (From Tanner: Growth at Adolescence, 1962. Courtesy of Blackwell Scientific Publications.)

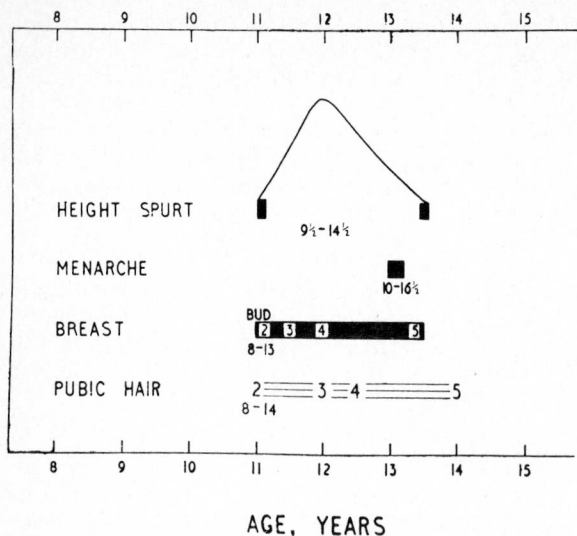

FIG. 23. Diagram of sequence of events at adolescence in females. The range of age of each event is indicated. (From Tanner: Growth at Adolescence, 1962. Courtesy of Blackwell Scientific Publications.)

mature height is generally attained at a skeletal age of 13 years (Fig. 23). Peak height velocity (PHV) in females occurs at a mean age of 12.3 years, with a mean height of 142.5 ± 6.7 cm. PHV is noted approximately 1 year after breast development and 1.4 years before menarche. The magnitude of PHV (mean 8.3 ± 1.2 cm) shows no correlation with chronologic or skeletal age, height, weight, or age at onset of puberty. The age at onset of menarche is inversely related to the magnitude of PHV: the earlier the onset of menarche, the greater the PHV and the growth subsequent to PHV. In other words, girls who mature early will be taller sooner and will attain final height at a younger age. Although PHV is less in those who mature late, their final height is greater due to the longer preadolescent growth period.

In males, pubertal development is normally initiated later than in females (mean age 12 years, range 11 to 16 years), and secondary sexual development occurs at a less mature stage of skeletal development. In males, 84 percent of mature height is attained at a skeletal age of 12 years, and 95 percent of mature height at a skeletal age of 15 years (Fig. 24). In general, physical signs of puberty are well advanced before PHV in males is apparent (mean age 13.9 years). The total growth accumulated during the 4- to 5-year pubertal phase is usually 28 cm. The maximum height achieved during this period is related to skeletal age at onset of puberty, as well as to genetic factors. Awareness of this sex difference in the pattern of incremental growth during adolescence can allay anxiety for parents and adolescents, as well as for the physician.

Concurrently with the appearance of secondary sexual characteristics, other physical bodily changes occur. Body weight increases, with peak weight velocity noted at 30.6 kg in females and 36 kg in males; maximum weight increment occurs earlier in females than in males. A relationship exists between the attainment of a critical weight of 46 kg and the time of onset of menses. Alterations in body composition during adolescence have been discussed earlier in this chapter. During puberty the heart size increases, and many of the abdominal organs hypertrophy. Skeletal changes other than those related to linear height are apparent at this time. In females the width of the hips increases, presumably due to significant growth of the pubic bone and the inferior portion of the ilium and also to the pattern of fat deposition. Acromial (shoulder width) increases are more pronounced in males than in females, and leg length is generally greater in males. The increments in lean body mass and secretion of testosterone during the late adolescent phase in the male may account for the marked increase in muscular strength. Sex differences

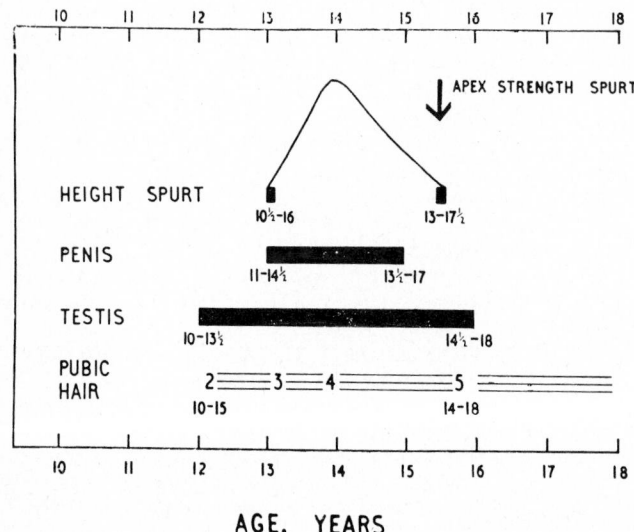

FIG. 24. Diagram of sequence of events at adolescence in males. The range of age of each event is indicated. (From Tanner: Growth at Adolescence, 1962. Courtesy of Blackwell Scientific Publications.)

in strength, as judged by grip and arm pull, have been demonstrated only after 13 years of age. Alteration in craniofacial proportions have been discussed (p. 108). Growth of the mandibular ramus is only 75 percent complete at the onset of puberty. The facial transformation entails not only mandibular growth with a more prominent chin, but also sharpening of the features, with an increased anterior/posterior diameter of the nose. The well-recognized voice changes that occur during puberty in the male are the consequences of growth of the larynx and cricoid cartilages and laryngeal muscles.

ABNORMALITIES THAT INFLUENCE GROWTH

Edward O. Reiter and Selna L. Kaplan

Short Stature

Short stature can be the consequence of genetic variation, intrauterine disease, or a myriad of malformations or chronic diseases. A decleration in the rate of growth to less than 4 cm/year is often of serious import.

GENETIC SHORT STATURE. Genetic or constitutional short stature encompasses those children in whom retardation in height deviates from the mean for age but is appropriate for mean parental height. The range of deviation in height is generally between -1 SD and -3 SD (Fig. 2), but the yearly growth rate is appropriate for age. Retardation in skeletal age of 1 to 2 years is not uncommon. A delay in the onset of adolescent development occurs frequently in this group. As a consequence, by comparison with peers the short stature is magnified in the adolescent with constitutional short stature.

MALNUTRITION. In worldwide perspective, deficient protein caloric intake is the most common cause of growth retardation in childhood and eventual short stature in adults. It has been said that 60 percent of all preschool children in the world have some degree of malnutrition. Poor nutritional status affects not only growth but also physical activity, mental alertness, and resistance to infections. Malnutrition may be a significant factor in the growth failure that is seen in many chronic diseases, as will be discussed later (p. 113). The long-term effects of malnutrition on intellectual development are still in dispute. Decreased brain growth occurs in malnourished infants less than 6 months of age, as has been shown by Winick and Rossi, but Dobbing has suggested that the decreased brain growth observed in infancy affects glial, not neuronal, elements. Recent data by Hansen and associates indicate no evidence of permanent intellectual or bodily impairment in malnourished children treated between 10 months and 4 years of age. Chronic malnutrition of a milder form is said to induce a limited retardation in height and skeletal age, with a reduction in adolescent growth spurt and final adult height.

Trace Metal Deficiency. The importance of trace metal deficiency has only recently been made apparent. Zinc-deficient subjects characteristically have anorexia, growth retardation, and failure of sexual development, which are prominent features of many of the chronic disease entities discussed in this section. Low levels of zinc have been found in patients with illnesses such as chronic infection, varied malabsorption syndromes, cystic fibrosis, cirrhosis, uremic syndrome, and sickle cell disease.

Iron Deficiency. The infant with iron deficiency often has been thought to be chubby and pale and to have normal linear growth and excessive weight growth. Recent studies suggest that considerable weight growth retardation, rather than obesity, is present in severe iron deficiency in childhood, with a hemoglobin level less than 9 g/100 ml, low serum iron, and diminished saturation of transferrin. From 30 to 50 percent of affected children have been noted to be below the 10th percentile in weight; linear growth retardation has also been observed. A spurt of growth in height and weight has been observed after initiation of iron therapy. The pathogenesis of poor weight gain in iron deficiency is unknown. The associated malabsorption syndrome (which occurs secondarily to the iron deficiency), the poor general nutrition, and the anorexia of severe anemia may be contributing factors. Recent observations of elevated levels of urinary norepinephrine suggest one possible mechanism for the diminished appetite, as well as the learning and behavior abnormalities frequently seen in iron-deficient children.

Stimulant Drugs. Stimulant drugs, mainly dextroamphetamine and methylphenidate, are being used with increasing frequency in the treatment of children with hyperkinetic behavior disorders. Limited suppression of height and weight increments has been demonstrated with chronic administration of these medications, especially dextroamphetamine, but also with methylphenidate in high dosages of more than 20 mg/day. Average deficits of 0.5 to 1.3 kg in weight and 1.0 to 1.5 cm in height yearly have occurred over 3-year treatment periods. There seems to be a diminished effect on weight gain with prolonged therapy, but the decrement in height is said to persist. Discontinuation of stimulant drugs during the summer months is associated with about a twofold increment in height and weight velocity. The acceleration of growth during the summer, while diminishing the degree of growth retardation, does not result in a compensatory growth phase to the normal range. The etiology of this growth failure may be related to central appetite suppression. Extensive endocrinologic evaluations have not been performed, although preliminary studies have not demonstrated a depression of growth hormone or insulin secretion.

INTRAUTERINE GROWTH RETARDATION. Intrauterine growth retardation refers to children whose birth weights are low for their gestational ages. The causative factors have been discussed elsewhere — (p.170). These children have a distinctive appearance: they are slender with craniofacial disproportion and sharp, fine facial features. A significant deviation in height from the normal is seen (-3.5 to -5 SD), but the yearly growth rate is usually appropriate. Their final heights are in the range of 137.2 to 152.4 cm.

HORMONAL ABNORMALITIES. In appraisal of a child with short stature, a hormonal deficit is frequently considered, but this is less commonly a causative factor than chronic illness. Deficient secretion of growth hormone or thyroid hormone during childhood (or sex steroids at adolescence) can lead to a decreased rate of growth and short stature. Excess endogenous secretion of glucocorticoids, as in Cushing's syndrome, or exogenous administration, can also induce growth retardation.

Growth Hormone Deficiency. Children with idiopathic growth hormone deficiency have variable degrees of short stature ranging from −3 SD to −10 SD. They are pudgy and immature in appearance; they have normal intelligence, and in general their health status is good. Fifty percent of these children manifest growth retardation within the first year; in the remainder a decreased growth rate may not be apparent until 4 to 10 years. Most of these children continue to grow, although at a reduced rate (2 to 4 cm/year). Diagnosis requires measurement of plasma growth hormone levels after specific stimulation tests, such as insulin-induced hypoglycemia, arginine infusion, or administration of oral L-dopa. Growth hormone stimulation tests are indicated in any child whose height retardation is more than −3.5 SD from mean height for age, whose yearly growth rate is 3 cm or less, or whose height is inappropriate for mean parental height according to the charts of Marshall and Tanner.

Thyroid Hormone Deficiency. In infants with congenital hypothyroidism, physiologic changes precede the development of growth retardation. In children with hypothyroidism due to a dysgenetic or undescended thyroid or with an inborn error of thyroxine metabolism, growth retardation may be pronounced, although other physical signs of hypothyroidism may be less overt. Abnormalities in sexual maturation and/or a decreased growth spurt may be a late manifestation of hypothyroidism due to Hashimoto's thyroiditis in the preadolescent or adolescent female.

Diabetes. Short stature is not an uncommon feature in children with diabetes. There is no general agreement as to whether this is a consequence of poorly controlled insulin therapy or dietary inadequacy or is an inherent characteristic of this disease. Insulin deficiency, as in the neonate with congenital diabetes, does lead to a severe retardation in length and weight.

Glucocorticoid Excess. Growth retardation is often the first manifestation of adrenal hypersecretion of glucocorticoids, as in Cushing's syndrome. Obesity, hypertension, and cushingoid facies appear subsequently. Administration of high doses of glucocorticoids, particulary the synthetic analogues, can induce slowing or even cessation of growth. Compensatory acceleration in growth may be delayed following withdrawal of steroid therapy (Fig. 25). Growth retardation also can be induced by absorption, via the skin, of high concentrations of steroid-containing ointments or of small amounts applied over a prolonged period of time in

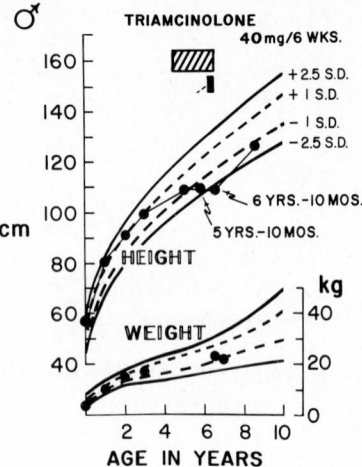

FIG. 25. Prolonged effect of intramuscular triamcinolone on retardation of linear growth. No growth was observed for 10 months after cortisone therapy was discontinued.

children with eczema or psoriasis. Further details of these abnormalities in hormonal secretion are presented in Chapter (29).

CHRONIC DISEASES. Growth failure is often a major clinical manifestation of chronic illness. In some instances the primary disease process is not suspected or diagnosed until the child is evaluated for poor height or weight gain. Renal disease (both glomerular and tubular), gastrointestinal malfunction ranging from abnormalities of swallowing to inflammatory large-bowel disease, congenital heart disease, hematologic disorders, asthma, and cystic fibrosis may all inhibit growth. In addition to the growth processes affected, maturational phenomena such as appearance of secondary sexual characteristics, menarche, and appropriate skeletal development are delayed in the presence of chronic disease. The rate of growth (height and weight velocity) is remarkably constant during childhood; thus a departure should be considered serious and evaluated fully. The poor weight and height gains of the sick child have been attributed to a variety of causes: poor food intake with consequent diminished availability of nutrients (including calories, minerals, vitamins and trace metals), anorexia, vomiting, or malabsorption; poor food utilization due to abnormal vascular perfusion, chronic acidosis, or hypoxia; hypermetabolism due to chronic infection, vascular shunting, or increased cell number per unit tissue mass; psychologic factors including disturbed parent–child interactions; and possible end organ resistance to deficient production of such anabolic hormones as growth hormone, insulin, and somatomedin.

Renal Disease. Many systemic abnormalities arise from a wide spectrum of renal diseases. The uremic syndrome, metabolic acidosis, chronic malnutrition, chronic infection, and interference with bone growth and mineralization all contribute to the growth failure associated with kidney malfunction. The *uremic syndrome* appears in chronic glomerular disease or in end stages of pyelonephritis and other tubular disease and is characterized by anorexia, gastrointestinal malfunction, varied neuropathies, and other systemic features. In these patients growth failure is always present, with undernutrition and caloric insufficiency playing an important role. In view of the anabolic state of the young child, there may be a disparity between his high caloric requirements and his ability to tolerate the accompanying protein and mineral load. This disparity is even more marked in the patient with markedly decreased glomerular function or in the anephric child treated with hemodialysis. Careful supervision of caloric intake is necessary in such patients. Appetite itself, even during efficient dialysis, is not an adequate determinant of caloric requirement. Growth in height is abnormally low at caloric intakes less than 67 percent of the recommended daily allowance (RDA) and ceases at 40 percent of RDA. With protein-free high-calorie supplementation an improved incremental growth pattern can be achieved. Patients with the uremic syndrome may have abnormalities of carbohydrate metabolism, with evidence of peripheral insulin resistance and abnormalities of growth hormone regulation; the relationship of these abnormalities to poor growth or to chronic malnutrition is not yet understood.

Renal Tubular Disease. Children with predominantly tubular disease also may have significant growth failure. In renal tubular acidosis (RTA) of the proximal type, severe growth retardation may be the primary presenting sign. Many of these patients will attain a growth rate in the low normal range with high-dosage bicarbonate therapy (10 to 15 mEq/kg/day). RTA may be a temporary defect, and the children may not require permanent treatment. In contrast, patients with distal tubular acidosis have symptoms such as polydipsia and polyuria, in addition to growth failure, and they respond to lower amounts of bicarbonate (p. 1308).

The secondary effects of renal tubular disease on bone growth, with development of rickets, have been well documented. The patients with RTA reported by Nash and associates did not have radiologic evidence of rickets, although distal RTA has been reported with rickets. In another series of patients with renal tubular and interstitial disease, radiologic and chemical evidence for rickets was described in the presence of growth retardation, in contrast to its absence in the patients with normal growth. Roger and others have suggested that increased vitamin D supplements, as well as increased caloric intake, may be essential to ensure normal growth in such children. The possibility of decreased tubular conversion of 25-hydroxycholecalciferol to the active vitamin D metabolite 1,25-dihydroxycholecalciferol may explain these findings (p. 238). Poor growth can occur in children with chronic urinary tract infections, with or without significant pyelonephritis. The relative roles of subtle abnormalities of renal tubular function, caloric deficiency, and nonspecific effects of chronic infections are not clear.

Diabetes Insipidus. Diabetes insipidus, either of CNS or renal origin, particularly in infancy or early childhood, can lead to poor growth and poor weight gain. The increased requirement for fluids decreases appetite and physical activity. Hyperosmolality may also result in growth retardation.

Cardiac Disease. Significant *congenital cardiac anomalies* commonly lead to decreased height and weight. In most large series reported weight is often more retarded than height. The retardation of growth seems to be more profound in early childhood than in adolescence. Skeletal growth and maturation are also delayed. Growth retardation in early infancy is most marked in shunt-induced congestive heart failure, such as in large nonrestrictive ventricular septal defect, patent ductus arteriosus, transposition of the great vessels, or other left-to-right shunt lesions. Cyanotic cardiac lesions do not have as marked an effect on growth unless the cyanosis is severe and persistent. Prenatal influences that are manifest by other (even minor) anomalies and intrauterine growth retardation may contribute to growth failure. The more severe and prolonged the cardiac failure, the greater the effect on growth.

Acquired cardiac lesions such as myocarditis and cardiomyopathies may produce growth retardation if severe and chronic cardiac failure occurs. The pathogenesis of growth failure with childhood cardiac diseases is not known. Decreased availability of nutrients, because of either poor intake or malabsorption, seems primary, although hypoxia or vascular shunts may be contributory factors. These infants have decreased feeding capacity due to tachypnea and abdominal organomegaly, with consequent limitation of caloric intake; they also have anorexia due to respiratory infection or secondary to malnutrition. Krieger has suggested that the poor nutritional state, as judged by the greater weight retardation than height retardation, is accentuated by hypermetabolism. Thus, even with an apparently reasonable intake for age and weight, these children may become deficient calorically. An excellent growth response has been observed after short-term caloric supplementation.

Cheek and associates have summarized the metabolic abnormalities in infants with congenital cardiac defects. The characteristic findings are diminished muscle cell number, increased cell size, decreased body fat, decreased total body potassium, and decreased turnover of albumin; a mild protein-losing enteropathy is also present. Oxygen consumption is normal when calculated in terms of lean body mass; a positive nitrogen balance, despite poor weight gain, suggests increased pulmonary loss of nitrogen. On the basis of their data, nutritional deficits may not totally explain the growth failure. Hait has indicated that infants with chronic cardiac failure may have abnormalities in carbohydrate metabolism and insulin turnover. Following cardiac surgery an increased rate of growth is frequently seen, although a catch-up growth pattern has not been observed.

Pulmonary Disease. In children with asthma the combination of chronic pulmonary dysfunction and glucocorticoid therapy, with its inherent growth-suppressive effects, can lead to decreased height and weight accretion and proportionate retardation in skeletal maturation and height. Moderate retardation was evident in one group of untreated asthmatic children, 73 percent of whom were below the 50th percentile in height and weight. In general, the degree of growth failure seems to be related to the severity of the asthma. Glucocorticoid administration accentuates this poor growth. There is a clinical suggestion of a larger growth-suppressive effect of synthetic corticosteroids, such as prednisone or dexamethasone, than of equivalent therapeutic doses of cortisone. Alternate-day steroid therapy will ameliorate the growth retardation and may be associated with an accelerated catch-up phase. Patients with chronic pulmonary infections associated with immunologic deficiency syndromes, structural, parenchymal, or great vessel anomalies, or cystic fibrosis have significant growth retardation. This diminution of growth with prolonged infectious processes of multiple types is well known, but is only partially explained by factors such as poor intake, hypermetabolism, and medication.

Cystic Fibrosis. Chronic pulmonary infection with bronchiectasis, pancreatic insufficiency, and exocrine and endocrine inadequacy, as well as nutrient malabsorption and malnutrition, all contribute to decreased growth and late sexual maturation in patients with cystic fibrosis. The falloff in height and weight, as well as the retardation in skeletal maturation, progress throughout childhood and are most marked in the preadolescent period when the growth and developmental spurt are delayed. The eventual adult height is usually in the normal range. The degree of growth retardation seems to be related to the severity and the variability of the pulmonary disease rather than to the pancreatic achylia. The degree of steatorrhea does not correlate well with the growth and development, but in adolescence the

nutritional state seems to improve, with greater lipid tolerance.

Endocrine abnormalities, such as islet cell failure of both alpha and beta cells with decrease of both glucagon and insulin production, do not seem to influence growth patterns. Delayed sexual maturation, with a prepubertal pattern of pituitary gonadotropin secretion evoked by gonadotropin-releasing hormone infusions, has been observed in adolescence. The critical weight hypothesis of Frisch may in part explain the delayed hypothalamic-pituitary maturation in these chronically underweight adolescents.

Gastrointestinal Disorders. Upper gastrointestinal tract disorders usually manifest themselves in early infancy; sucking and swallowing difficulties can cause failure to thrive in the first weeks of life. Dysphagia can result from gross structural abnormalities of the mouth, throat, esophagus, and great vessels, neuromuscular incoordination due to cerebral palsy, cricopharyngeal incoordination, varied myopathies, or acute infectious conditions. Malnutrition and failure to thrive may also occur from lower esophageal abnormalities, such as chalasia, achalasia, or hiatus hernia and esophageal stricture, as well as from pyloric stenosis and other obstructive lesions.

Lower intestinal disorders that commonly lead to growth failure during childhood include inflammatory bowel disease, gluten-induced enteropathy, chronic intractable diarrhea of infancy, and cystic fibrosis. These are characterized by variable degrees of malabsorption of nutrients, vitamins, and trace metals, endogenous protein and amino acid loss, and a chronic relapsing clinical course. Other systemic complications such as arthritis, osteoporosis, iridocyclitis, and dermatoses may occur.

Approximately 20 percent of children with inflamma-

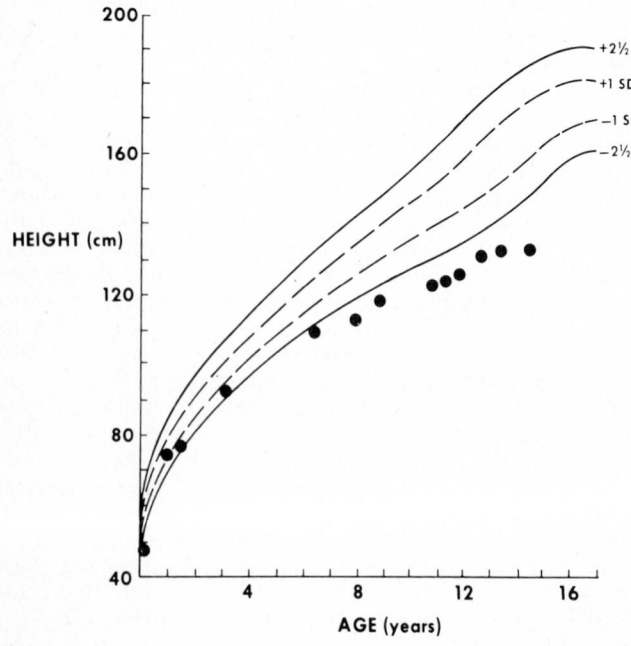

FIG. 26. Growth pattern of a male in whom the diagnosis of regional enteritis was made at 14 years of age.

tory bowel disease, such as ulcerative colitis or Crohn's disease of the small and/or large intestine, have severe growth retardation. Crohn's disease (granulomatous bowel disease) is the more frequent cause of decreased growth in these patients in one-third of whom growth failure may precede by several years the onset of symptoms referable to the gastrointestinal tract (Fig. 26). Corticosteroid therapy induces additional growth failure in some patients. There is often an increased growth rate after operative intervention.

Gluten-induced enteropathy (celiac disease, sprue) very commonly presents with growth failure; in children under 4 years of age weight may be more compromised than height, with about 65 percent of patients showing a weight deficit but only 30 percent having a decrement in height (Fig. 27). In older children growth failure is as common as poor weight gain and delayed sexual maturation. Adherence to a gluten-free diet greatly accelerates growth, with attainment of appropriate height, weight, and skeletal age after a 3-year dietary period. Children with strict gluten restrictions usually maintain a normal height, but poor dietary compliance is associated with continuing severe growth failure.

Chronic liver disease may also lead to growth failure. Cirrhosis, chronic active hepatitis, glycogen storage disease, and Wilson's disease may present with abnormalities of height and weight. Osteoporosis and poor growth have been striking findings in glycogen storage disease, hepatoma, and cirrhosis. Abnormalities in liver metabolism may contribute to the inadequate bone mineralization. It is tempting to speculate that growth retardation in children with severe liver disease may be the consequence of decreased synthesis of somatomedin, an intracellular mediator of growth hormone action.

Hematologic Disorders.　Hemoglobinopathies (such as sickle cell anemia), disorders of hemoglobin synthesis (such as the thalassemia syndromes), and red blood cell enzymatic deficiencies (as in pyruvate kinase deficiency) may be associated with growth retardation. In children

with sickle cell disease, both mean height and weight are below the 25th percentile, sexual maturity is delayed, and there is a concomitant delay of skeletal development. Males with sickle cell trait also are smaller than normal, but females are not. Menarche is late, and subsequent fertility is decreased. Zinc deficiency has been demonstrated in some patients with sickle cell disease. In thalassemia major, poor growth and development may be apparent by 4 years of age (Fig. 28). The presence of other systemic complications, including splenomegaly, hepatomegaly, and facial bone abnormalities, is associated with a more severe degree of retardation in height. Pubertal maturation is strikingly delayed, and ultimate reproductive capability may never be achieved. Iron deposition in the hypothalamus, pituitary, and gonads may be responsible for the observed dysfunction of the reproductive endocrine system, but growth hormone secretion appears to be normal. Hypertransfusion regimens seem to have a beneficial effect on growth.

Bone Diseases.　Defective development of bony cartilage or collagen could result in decreased linear growth. Children with chondrodystrophic bone disease, including achondroplasia and hypochondroplasia, are short and have disproportionate trunk/limb ratios for age. Gross deformities of the spine and limbs lead to decreased growth potential; final height is usually within the range of 107 to 137 cm. Chronic rickets, as seen in vitamin-D-resistant individuals, is associated with short stature. Winters and associates reported the presence of short stature with hypophosphatemia without radiographic evidence of rickets. The deformities of the lower extremities induced by rickets are responsible for the short stature in these children.

Chromosomal and Genetic Disorders.　Intrauterine growth retardation is an inherent characteristic of infants with autosomal abnormalities, gonadal dysgenesis, and other developmental anomalies. The growth pattern during childhood is more variable. The most severe retardation in growth is seen in children with

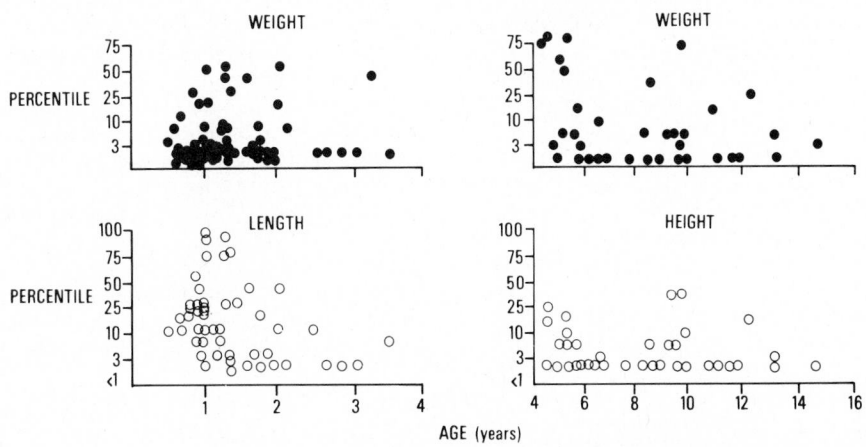

FIG. 27.　Height and weight of children with celiac disease at time of diagnosis: left—less than 4 years of age; right—more than 4 years of age. (From Young and Pringle: Arch Dis Child 46:421, 1971.)

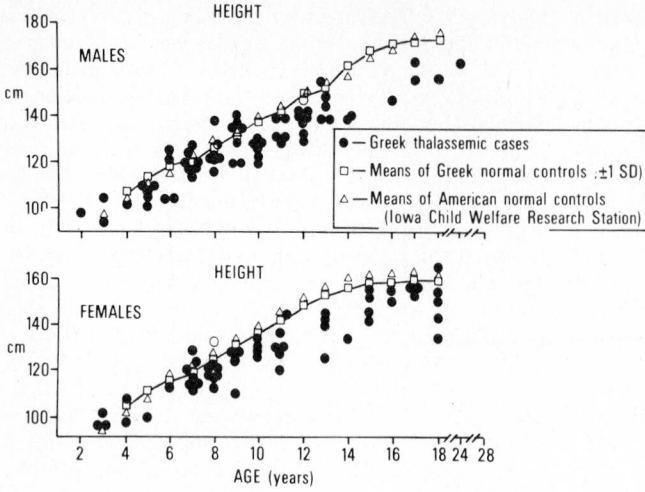

FIG. 28. Height of 138 males and females with thalassemia is compared with that of normal controls. (From Logothetis et al: Pediatrics 50:92, 1972.)

Down's syndrome (trisomy 21). Their deviations in height are apparent at an early age and are in the range −2 to −4 SD from mean height for age. Retention of infantile proportions (trunk/limb ratio) is common. The mean final height is 154 ± 6.7 cm for males and 143 ± 5.9 cm for females. Microcephaly is usual, and facial development remains immature. The skeletal age is generally appropriate for chronologic age. The presence of heart disease or hypothyroidism leads to a more pronounced retardation in height; skeletal age is often more retarded than height in children with Down's syndrome and hypothyroidism.

In one study of handicapped children it was found that children with multiple congenital anomalies do not show a significant decrease in growth rate until 5 years of age. Their height retardation is in the range −1 to −4 SD from mean height for age. A blunted growth spurt is seen at adolescence. Skeletal retardation is usually equivalent to height age. The degree of mental deficiency does not influence the severity of the height or skeletal retardation. Microcephaly associated with narrow facial configuration is common in this group. Van Gelderen observed that children with perinatal cerebral damage and cerebral palsy have severe linear and skeletal retardation, whereas those with postnatal brain damage are usually of normal height; this conflicts with the data of Pryor and Thelander, which show that children with cerebral palsy are within the normal range for height during childhood but have a decreased growth increment during adolescence.

Short stature is a characteristic feature of other distinct syndromes not included in the classification of Pryor and Thelander. Seckel's dwarfism encompasses a group of children with intrauterine growth retardation, microcephaly, sharp facial features with underdeveloped chin, and severe mental deficiency. These children never attain a final height greater than 110 cm. Children with the Prader-Willi syndrome have small hands and feet (acromicria), mild microcephaly, and hypotonia. Growth retardation is moderate (−2 to −4 SD) during childhood, with final height around 150 cm. Delayed or impaired sexual maturation, a blunted

growth spurt at adolescence, and development of massive obesity are common features. Girls with gonadal dysgenesis invariably have moderate growth retardation. They are generally small at birth, but the major deviation in growth from the normal range occurs after 6 to 8 years of age. Final height is in the range of 120 to 140 cm. Deletion of the long arms of the X chromosome is associated with hypogonadism but with normal growth, suggesting that the short arm of the X chromosome may carry the determinant gene for stature in these patients. Short stature is a common feature in patients with a phenotypic form of gonadal dysgenesis referred to as pseudo-Turner's or Noonan's syndrome. Retardation in growth is not characteristic of other forms of male or female pseudohermaphroditism (p. 1695).

Catch-up Growth.   Whatever the etiology of the poor growth seen in sick children, the phenomenon of post illness catch-up growth has been well documented. Following initiation of alkali therapy in renal tubular acidosis or a gluten-free diet in celiac disease, or after discontinuation of glucocorticoid therapy, growth velocity may accelerate far beyond the normal rate, until a child's size more closely approximates its genetically determined magnitude. To a lesser degree skeletal maturation will manifest a similar catch-up. Forbes has mathematically conceptualized the process of catch-up growth, indicating that the integrated velocity excess during the recovery period must match the previous velocity deficit to ensure complete correction of the distorted growth pattern. The rate of catch-up growth is said to vary with the energy value of the food. The mechanism of this rapid accretion of height and weight, along with the appearance of secondary sexual characteristics when age-appropriate, remains obscure.

TALL STATURE
EDWARD O. REITER AND SELNA L. KAPLAN

There are many causes of excessive growth in height during childhood and adolescence. Such clinical entities as Marfan's syndrome, homocystinuria, total lipodystrophy, thyrotoxicosis, sexual precocity, virilization syndromes due to adrenal neoplasms or to adrenogenital syndrome, neurofibromatosis, chromosomal abnormalities such as Klinefelter's syndrome, 48,XXYY syndrome, and 47,XYY syndrome, and hypogonadotropic hypogonadism with eunuchoidal habitus may give rise to increased absolute height or to accelerated height velocity. These causes of overgrowth are discussed elsewhere. Several other syndromes characterized by tall stature are considered in this section. These are constitutional tall stature, gigantism and acromegaly, and cerebral gigantism.

CONSTITUTIONAL TALL STATURE. When the adult height prediction for a girl exceeds 180 cm, based on an assessment of skeletal maturation and the Bayley-Pinneau tables, it is often considered that she will be excessively tall. Concern about final adult height in boys is rarely about overgrowth, but rather about short stature and delayed adolescent maturation. In general, tall children have tall parents, their body proportions are normal, their height has been greater than the 97th percentile since early childhood, and height velocity is within the normal range. Children with constitutional tall stature have normal hypothalamic-pituitary function; specifically, they have appropriate LRF-induced (Luteinizing releasing factor) pituitary gonadotropin release and nonexaggerated pituitary growth hormone secretion in response to various pharmacologic and physiologic stimuli.

Treatment of the excessively tall girl is a therapeutic dilemma for the pediatrician and the endocrinologist. Considerable data suggest that high-dose estrogen therapy will significantly restrict final height to less than the Bayley-Pinneau prediction. The vagaries of height prediction and the ever-present potential of long-term side effects of hormonal therapy should dictate careful consideration of each patient's clinical state, self-image, and desire for treatment. As for height restriction as a cosmetic alteration, the final decision should be made by the parents and the child, not by the physician. A conjugated estrogen preparation (eg, Premarin) is given cyclically; 10 mg/day for 21 days, then no treatment for 8 to 10 days. A progestational agent (5 mg) may be added for the last 5 days of the treatment period. Therapy should be initiated when skeletal age is between 10 and 12 years. Hormonal treatment should be continued until growth ceases, usually when the bone age is between 15 and 16 years. Post menarcheal girls do not usually require exogenous estrogen therapy, as maximum growth after menarche is not more than 5 to 10 cm. The average diminution of final adult height as a result of high-dose estrogen administration appears to be about 4 cm (range 0 to 9 cm).

GIGANTISM AND ACROMEGALY. Excessive growth in height beginning in childhood, or more commonly in early adolescence, and resulting in a final height between 213 and 275 cm characterizes the syndrome of gigantism. Many of the manifestations of acromegaly (including increased body weight gain, acral enlargement and soft tissue growth, excessive diaphoresis, galactorrhea, osteoarthritis, sellar enlargement, headache, and diminished visual acuity and bitemporal homonymous hemianopsia) are present in gigantism, as in acromegaly with onset in late adolescence and in adulthood. Giants, if untreated, have continued growth into the fourth decade, as epiphyses do not fuse and the extremities become extremely long.

Hyperplasia or adenomata of the eosinophilic somatotropes of the pituitary, with excessive production of growth hormone, lead to the changes of gigantism. Adenohypophyseal tumors may develop spontaneously or may respond to abnormal hypothalamic synthesis and release of the as yet unidentified growth hormone releasing factor. Evaluation of growth hormone secretion in acromegalics supports the notion of an abnormality of hypothalamic regulation of the pituitary somatotropes. Treatment of gigantism and acromegaly has involved direct surgical resection, sellar x-irradiation, proton-beam irradiation, cryohypophysectomy, yttrium or gold implants, and transnasal microsurgery. Variable results have been reported, but at present microsurgery is the most promising therapeutic modality. Rapid surgical intervention, after appropriate glucocorticoid administration, is indicated for visual loss, extrasellar growth, increased intracranial pressure, or hemorrhage into the tumor.

CEREBRAL GIGANTISM. Children with accelerated growth in height and weight, macrocrania, acromegalic appearance of the hands and feet, and a nonprogressive cerebral disorder with mental retardation have been grouped into the clinical entity of cerebral gigantism. Birth length and growth during the first years of life are excessive, with a subsequent deceleration of growth rate to follow a channel above, but parallel to, the 97th percentile. Sexual maturation may occur at an earlier than normal chronologic age compatible with the degree of skeletal maturation, which may be similar to or greater than the rate of height increase. Growth hormone secretion and bioactivity are normal in these patients. The physiology of other growth-promoting substances, such as insulin, somatomedin, and sex steroid, has not been systematically evaluated in these children.

References

GENERAL MEASUREMENTS OF GROWTH

Height and weight of children in the United States, 1970, National Center for Health Statistics Series II, Number 104. Washington DC, USDHEW

Height and weight of youths 12–17 years, United States, 1973, National Center for Health Statistics Series II, Number 124, Washington DC, USDHEW

Hunt EE Jr: The developmental genetics of man. In Falkner F (ed): Human Growth. Philadelphia, WB Saunders, 1966, p 76

Marshall WA: Evaluation of growth rate in height over periods less than one year. Arch Dis Child 46:414, 1971

Nicholson AB, Hanley C: Indices of physiological maturity: derivation and interrelationships. Child Dev 24:3, 1953

Pryor HB: Charts of normal body measurements and revised width-weight charts in graphic form. J Pediatr 68:615, 1966

Sinclair D: In Human Growth After Birth, 2nd ed. London, Oxford Univ Press, 1973

Tanner JM: Genetics of human growth. In Tanner JM (ed): Human Growth, Vol 3. New York, Symposium Publications, 1960, p 43

————Whitehouse RH, Takaishi M: Standards from birth to maturity for height, weight, height velocity, and weight velocity, British children 1965. Arch Dis Child 41:454, 1966

————Goldstein H, Whitehouse RH: Standards for children's height at ages 2 to 9 years, allowing for height of parents. Arch Dis Child 45:755, 1970

————Whitehouse RH: Clinical longitudinal standards for height, weight, height velocity, weight velocity, and the stages of puberty. Arch Dis Child 51:170, 1976

Verghese KP, Scott RB, Tiexera G, Ferguson AD: Studies in growth and development. XII. Physical growth in North American Negro children. Pediatrics 44:243, 1969

Whitehouse RH, Tanner JM, Healy MJR: Diurnal variation in stature and sitting height in 12–14 year old boys. Ann Hum Biol 1:103, 1974

Wilson RS: Growth standards for twins from birth to four years. Ann Hum Biol 1:175, 1974

Wingerd J, Schoen EJ, Solomon IL: Growth standards in the first two years of life based on measurements of white and black children in a prepaid health care program. Pediatrics 47:818, 1971

————Solomon IL, Schoen EJ: Parent-specific height standards for pre-adolescent children of three racial groups, with method for rapid determination. Pediatrics 52:555, 1973

————Schoen EJ: Factors influencing length at birth and height at 5 years. Pediatrics 53:737, 1974

Wolanski N: The stature of offspring and the assortative mating of parents. Hum Biol 46:613, 1974

MEASUREMENT OF HEIGHT

Bayer LM, Bayley N: In Growth Diagnosis. Chicago, Univ Chicago Press, 1959

Bayley N, Pinneau SR: Tables for predicting adult height from skeletal age: revised for use with the Greulich-Pyle standards. J Pediatr 40:423, 1952

Roche AF, Wainer H, Thissen D: The RWT method for the prediction of adult stature. Pediatrics 56:1026, 1975

Tanner JM, Whitehouse RH, Marshall WA, Carter, BS: Prediction of adult height from height, bone age and occurrence of menarche, at ages 4–16 with allowance for midparent height. Arch Dis Child 50:14, 1975

————Whitehouse RH, Marshall WA, Healy, MJR, Goldstein H: In Assessment of Skeletal Maturity and Prediction of Adult Height: TW2 Method. New York, Academic, 1975

Walker RN: Standards for somatotyping children. I. Prediction of young adult height from children's growth data. Ann Hum Biol 1:149, 1974

BODY COMPOSITION

Boulton TJC, Dunlop M, Court JM: Adipocyte growth in the first 2 years of life. Aust Paediatr J 10:301, 1974

Brook CGD: Evidence for a sensitive period in adipose-cell replication in man. Lancet 2:624, 1972

Cheek DR, Mellits D, Elliott D: Body water, height, and weight during growth in normal children. Am J Dis Child 112:312, 1966

————Cellular growth hormones, nutrition and time. Pediatrics 41:30, 1968

Forbes GB: Relation of lean body mass to height in children and adolescents. Pediatr Res 6:32, 1972

Frisancho AR, Garn SM, Ascoli W: Childhood retardation resulting in reduction of adult body size due to lesser adolescent skeletal delay. Am J Phys Anthropol 33:325, 1970

Hansen JDL, Freesemann C, Moodie AD, Evans DE: What does nutritional growth retardation imply. Pediatrics 47:299, 1971

Owen GM, Brozek J: Influence of age, sex, and nutrition on body composition during childhood and adolescence. In Faulkner F (ed): Human Growth. Philadelphia, WB Saunders, 1966, p 222

Parizkova J, Roth Z: The assessment of depot fat in children from skinfold thickness measurements by Holtain (Tanner/Whitehouse) caliper. Hum Biol 44:613, 1972

Sandstead HH, Carter JP, House FR, McConnell F, Horton KB, Vander-Zwaag R: Nutritional deficiencies in disadvantaged preschool children. Am J Dis Child 121:455, 1971

Widdowson EM: Changes in body proportions and composition during growth. In Davis SA, Dobbing J (eds): Scientific Foundations of Paediatrics. Philadelphia, WB Saunders, 1974, p 153

Winick M, Rosso P: The effect of severe early malnutrition on cellular growth of the human brain. Pediatr Res 3:181, 1969

SKELETAL MATURATION

Acheson RM, Vicinus JH, Fowler GB: Studies in the reliability of assessing skeletal maturity from x-rays. Part III. Greulich-Pyle atlas and Tanner-Whitehouse method contrasted. Hum Biol 38:204, 1966

———— Maturation of the skeleton. In Falkner F (ed): Human Growth. Philadelphia, WB Saunders, 1966, p 465

Demirjian A, Goldstein H, Tanner JM: A new system of dental age assessment. Hum Biol 45:211, 1973

Filipsson R: A new method for assessment of dental maturity using the individual curve of number of erupted permanent teeth. Ann Hum Biol 2:13, 1975

Greulich WW, Pyle SI: In Radiographic Atlas of Skeletal Development of the Hand and Wrist, 2nd ed. Stanford, Stanford Univ Press, 1959

O'Rahilly R, Gardner E: The initial appearance of ossification in staged human embryos. Am J Anat 134:291, 1972

Pozanski AK, Garn SM, Kuhns LR, Sandusky ST: Dysharmonic maturation of the hand in the congenital malformation syndromes. Am J Phys Anthropol 35:417, 1971

Pryse-Davies J, Smitham JH, Napier KA: Factors influencing development of secondary ossification centers in the fetus and newborn. Arch Dis Child 49:425, 1974

Pyle I, Sontag LW: Variability in onset of ossification in epiphyses and short bones of the extremities. Am J Roentgenol Radium Ther Nucl Med 49:795, 1943

Roche AF: Sex-associated differences in skeletal maturity. Acta Anat 71:321, 1968

Tanner JM, Whitehouse RH, Healy MJR: In A New System for Estimating Skeletal Maturity from the Hand and Wrist with Standards Derived from a Study of 2600 Healthy British Children, Parts I and II. Paris, Centre International de l'Enfance, 1962

Wingerd J, Peritz E, Sproul A: Race and stature differences in the skeletal maturation of the hand and wrist. Ann Hum Biol 1:201, 1974

ADOLESCENCE

Frisch RE, Revelle R: Height and weight at menarche and a hypothesis of critical body weights and adolescent events. Science 169:397, 1970

Johnston FE, Roche AF, Schell LM, Wettenhall HNB: Critical weight at menarche. Critique of a hypothesis. Am J Dis Child 129:19, 1975

Marshall WA: Interrelationships of skeletal maturation, sexual development and somatic growth in man. Ann Hum Biol 1:29, 1974

Onat T, Ertem B: Adolescent female height velocity: relationships to body measurements, sexual and skeletal maturity. Hum Biol 46:199, 1974

Tanner JM: In Growth at Adolescence, 2nd ed. Oxford, Blackwell Scientific, Springfield, Ill, Charles C Thomas, 1962

SHORT STATURE

Cheek DB, Cooke RE: Growth and growth retardation. Ann Rev Med 15:357, 1964

Forbes GB: A note on the mathematics of "catch-up" growth. Pediatr Res 8:929, 1974

Gotlin RW, Mace JW: Diagnosis and management of short stature in childhood and adolescence. Curr Probl Pediatr 11:4,5 1972

Hambridge KM, Hambridge C, Jacobs M, Baum JD: Low levels of zinc in hair, anorexia, poor growth, and hypogeusia in children. Pediatr Res 6:868, 1972

Lacey KA, Parkin JM: The normal short child. Arch Dis Child 49:417, 1974

Prader A, Tanner JM, von Harnack GA: Catch-up growth following illness or starvation. J Pediatr 62:646, 1963

Prasad AD, Oberleas D: Zinc: human nutrition and metabolic effects. Ann Intern Med 73:631, 1970

Pryor HB, Thelander HE: Growth deviations in handicapped children. Clin Pediatr 6:501, 1967

Thelander HE, Pryor HB: Abnormal patterns of growth and development in mongolism. Clin Pediatr 5:493, 1966

IRON DEFICIENCY

Judisch JM, Naiman JL, Oski FA: The fallacy of the fat iron-deficient child. Pediatrics 37:987, 1966

Naiman JL, Oski FA, Diamond LK, Vawter GF, Schwachman H: The gastrointestinal effects of iron-deficiency anemia. Pediatrics 33:83, 1964

Voorhees ML, Stuart MJ, Stockman JA, Oski FA: Iron deficiency anemia and increased urinary norepinephrine excretion. J Pediatr 86:542, 1975

STIMULANT DRUGS

Safer D, Allen R, Barr E: Depression of growth in hyperactive children on stimulant drugs. N Engl J Med 287:27, 1972

———— Allen RP: Factors influencing the suppressive effects of two stimulant drugs on the growth of hyperactive children. Pediatrics 51:660, 1973

———— Allen RP, Barr E: Growth rebound after termination of stimulant drugs. J Pediatr 86:113, 1975

RENAL DISEASE

Lewy JE, New MI: Growth in children with renal failure. Am J Med 58:65, 1975

Lowrie EG, Soeldner JS, Hampers CL, Merrill JP: Glucose metabolism and insulin secretion in uremic, prediabetic, and normal subjects. J Lab Clin Med 76:603, 1970

Nash MA, Torrado AD, Griefer I, Spitzer A, Edelmann CM: Renal tubular acidosis in infants and children. J Pediatr 80:738, 1972

Samaan NA, Freeman RM: Growth hormone levels in severe renal disease. Metabolism 19:102, 1970

Simmons JM, Wilson CJ, Potter DE, Holliday MA: Relation of calorie deficiency to growth failure in children on hemodialysis and the growth response to calorie supplementation. N Engl J Med 285:653, 1971

Stickler GB, Bergen BJ: A review: short stature in renal disease. Pediatr Res 7:978, 1973

CARDIAC DISEASE

Bayer L, Robinson SJ: Growth history of children with congenital heart defects. Am J Dis Child 117:564, 1969

Feldt RH, Stickler GB, Weidman WH: Growth of children with congenital heart disease. Am J Dis Child 117:573, 1969

Fomon SJ, Ziegler EE: Nutritional management of infants with congenital heart disease. Am Heart J 83:581, 1972

Iber FL, Cheek DB, Wolf KP: Nitrogen metabolism in children with congenital cardiac defects and severe growth retardation. Am J Clin Nutr 20:1166, 1967

Krieger I: Growth failure and congenital heart disease. Am J Dis Child 120:497, 1970

Umansky R, Hauck AJ: Factors in the growth of children with patent ductus arteriosus. Pediatrics 30:540, 1962

White RI, Jordan CE, Fischer KC, et al: Delayed skeletal growth and maturation in adolescent congenital heart disease. Invest Radiol 6:326, 1971

PULMONARY DISEASE

Cohen MB, Abram LE: Growth pattern of allergic children. J Allergy 19:165, 1948

Falliers CI, Tan LS, Szentivanyi J, Jorgeson JR, Bukantz SC: Childhood asthma and steroid therapy as influences on growth. Am J Dis Child 105:127, 1963

Snyder RD, Collipp PJ, Greene JS: Growth and ultimate height of children with asthma. Clin Pediatr 6:389, 1967

CYSTIC FIBROSIS

Lapey A, Kattwinkel J, di'Sant Agnese PA, Laster L: Steatorrhea and azotorrhea and their relation to growth and nutrition in adolescents and young adults with cystic fibrosis. J Pediatr 84:328, 1974

Schwachman H, Kulczycki LL, Khaw KT: Studies in cystic fibrosis: 65 patients over 17 years of age. Pediatrics 36:689, 1965

Sproul A, Huang N: Growth patterns in children with cystic fibrosis. J Pediatr 65:664, 1964

Stahl M, Girard J, Rutishauser M, Nars PW, Zuppinger K: Endocrine function of the pancreas in cystic fibrosis: evidence for an impaired glucagon and insulin response following arginine infusion. J Pediatr 84:821, 1974

GASTROINTESTINAL DISORDERS

Ament ME: Malabsorption syndromes in infancy and childhood. Part I. J Pediatr 81:685, 1972

———— Malabsorption syndromes in infancy and childhood. Part II. J Pediatr 81:867, 1972

Barr DGD, Shmerling DH, Prader A: Catch-up growth in malnutrition, studied in celiac disease after institution of gluten-free diet. Pediatr Res 6:521, 1972

Berger M, Gribetz D, Korelitz BI: Growth retardation in children with ulcerative colitis: the effect of medical and surgical therapy. Pediatrics 55:459, 1975

Fine RN, Frasier SD, Donnell GN: Growth in glycogen-storage disease type I. Am J Dis Child 117:169, 1969

Gotlin RW, Bubois RS: Nyctohemeral growth hormone levels in children with growth retardation and inflammatory bowel disease. Gut 14:-191, 1973

McCaffrey TD, Nasr K, Lawrence AM, Kirsner JB: Severe growth retardation in children with inflammatory bowel disease. Pediatrics 45:386, 1970

Sobel EH, Silverman FM, Lee CM Jr: Chronic regional enteritis and growth retardation. Am J Dis Child 103:569, 1962

Young WF, Pringle EM: 110 children with coeliac disease, 1950–1969. Arch Dis Child 46:421, 1971

HEMATOLOGIC DISORDERS

Johnston FE, Hertzog KP, Molina RM: Longitudinal growth in thalassemia major: relationship to hemoglobin level. Am J Dis Child 112:396, 1966

Katz SH, Lubin B, Armstrong D: Growth of adolescents with sickle cell trait. Lancet 1:814, 1974

Kuo B, Zaino E, Roginsky MS: Endocrine function in thalassemia major. J Clin Endocrinol Metab 28:805, 1968

Logothetis J, Loewenson RB, Augoustaki O, Economidou J, Constantoulakis M: Body growth in Cooley's anemia (homozygous beta-thalassemia) with a correlative study as to other aspects of the illness in 138 cases. Pediatrics 50:92, 1972

Whitten CF: Growth status of children with sickle cell anemia. Am J Dis Child 102:355, 1961

TALL STATURE

Gardner LI: The child with "excessive" height prediction. Am J Dis Child 129:17, 1975

Schoen EJ, Solomon IL, Warner O, Wingert J: Estrogen treatment of tall girls. Am J Dis Child 125:71, 1973

Wettenhall HNB, Cahill C, Roche AF: Tall girls: a survey of 15 years of management and treatment. J Pediatr 86:602, 1975

Whitelow JJ, Foster TN, Graham WH: Comparative study of the effects of estradiol valerate on the prepubertal and pubertal female. Am J Obstet Gynecol 97:1041, 1967

GIGANTISM AND ACROMEGALY

Costin G, Fefferman RA, Kogut MD: Hypothalamic gigantism. J Pediatr 83:419, 1973

Haigler ED, Hershman JM, Meador CK: Pituitary gigantism, a case report and review. Arch Intern Med 132:588, 1973

Yen SSC, Siler TM, De Vane GW: Effect of somatostatin in patients with acromegaly. N Engl J Med 290:935, 1974

CEREBRAL GIGANTISM

Ott JE, Robinson A: Cerebral gigantism. Am J Dis Child 117:357, 1969

Sotos JF, Dodge PR, Muirhead D, Crawford JD, Talbot NB: Cerebral gigantism in childhood. A syndrome of excessively rapid growth with acromegalic features and a non-progressive neurologic disorder. N Engl J Med 271:109, 1964

Stephenson JN, Mellinger RC, Manson G: Cerebral gigantism. Pediatrics 41:130, 1968

CHAPTER 5

Prenatal Care and Diagnosis

Robert K. Creasy and Julian T. Parer

Perinatal medicine actually begins with the health status of the mother prior to conception and then proceeds through intrauterine development to postnatal adaptation. Traditionally the role of the obstetrician has ended with delivery of the infant, after which the role of the pediatrician has begun. However, over the past two decades these artificial divisions have broken down to some degree. There has arisen an understanding of the importance of the interrelationships between maternal and fetal well-being and neonatal, childhood, and even adult performance. Although the obstetrician may be primarily responsible to the mother and child during the antenatal period, we now recognize that care should be provided by a team including the internist, the anesthesiologist, the pediatrician, and basic scientists. Through a sharing of knowledge of the various specialties and basic sciences, significant progress has been made in perinatal medicine, placing management and therapy during the perinatal period on a firmer foundation. This foundation will undoubtedly be expanded further in the future, with a resultant decrease in perinatal morbidity and mortality and, hopefully, an improved performance of the adult individual. The following sections on maternal and fetal surveillance techniques will inform the student of pediatrics about problems faced in the antenatal and intrapartum period and how these problems are assessed and managed.

FIRST OBSTETRIC VISIT

PREGNANCY RISK. Optimally, each woman should be assessed prior to conception for factors that might adversely affect the successful outcome of her pregnancy, either for herself or her fetus. Unfortunately at the present time this rarely occurs, unless the patient has had an infertility problem, a previous poor obstetric history, or a potentially life-threatening disease. Therefore the initial visit after conception usually provides the physician with the first opportunity to evaluate the woman fully and possibly to place her in a high-risk category. Some 10 to 20 percent of all pregnancies may be identified at the first visit as being in a group in which the fetus has an increased risk of death before, during, or after birth or increased risk of neurologic impairment later in life. These patients will account for approximately 50 percent of poor perinatal outcome, but as pregnancy advances others will move from the low-risk to the high-risk category. Maternal and fetal reasons for placing a patient in the high-risk category are listed in Table 1. The increased perinatal mortality risks are 2 to 3 times normal for some categories such as

preeclampsia and up to 20 times normal in conditions such as polyhydramnios. Patients in the high-risk category should be seen at frequent intervals, preferably in a center where the various specialties needed for perinatal care are well represented and the maternal and fetal surveillance techniques described later in this chapter are available on a routine basis.

PREMATURE LABOR RISK. Many of the pregnancy risks listed in Table 1 relate to abnormal fetal development due to infections, chromosomal aberration, or im-

TABLE 1. Reasons for Placing a Pregnancy at Risk

Maternal	Fetal
Cardiac disease	Habitual abortion
Chronic hypertension	Polyhydramnios
Renal disease	Prolonged gestation
Preeclampsia	Macrosomia
Diabetes mellitus	Abruptio placenta
Hematologic disorder	Placenta previa
Hx of premature labor	Erythroblastosis fetalis
Hx of I.U.G.R.	Abnormal estriol, HPL
Viral or bacterial infection	Multiple gestation
Gastrointestinal disorder	I.U.G.R.
Malignant disease	Premature rupture of membranes
Primigravida > 35 years	Abnormal presentation
Age < 18 years	Amnionitis
2nd or 3rd trimester bleeding	Abnormal fetal heart rate
Thyroid disorders	Meconium in amniotic fluid
Collagen disease	History of stillbirth
Incompetent cervix Hx	
Hx of Uterine surgery	
Grandmultiparity	
Drug abuse	
Malnourishment	
Pulmonary disorder	

paired growth. It is also important to identify early in pregnancy those individuals at risk of entering labor prematurely. As mentioned below, certain β-adrenergic compounds that are now available are useful in preventing undesirable uterine contractions. These compounds are of value only if premature labor is detected early, before the cervix is significantly effaced or dilated. At present many patients in premature labor are detected too late for these agents to inhibit delivery for a prolonged period. It is thus necessary to detect those at risk and educate them to recognize the subtle signs of premature labor so that it can be detected early. Scoring systems to identify patients at risk of premature labor have been developed. One such system suggested by Papiernick is shown in Table 2. A patient scoring over 6 is at significant risk of developing premature labor and must be handled appropriately.

GESTATIONAL AGE. It is important to record the menstrual history during the first visit, because it frequently becomes vital in interpretation and timing of various testing procedures later in gestation. The expected date of confinement is 280 days from the first day of the last menstruation, but this is true only if the menses are regular, with a periodicity of 28 days. The luteal phase of the menstrual cycle is approximately 14 days; so if the menstrual cycle is 35 days, ovulation has occurred 3 weeks rather than 2 weeks after the first day of the last menses, and the confinement date will be 1 week later. In past years the use of the last menstrual period to calculate the duration of the gestation was frequently questioned, but this was prior to the recognition of the entity of intrauterine fetal growth retardation. We now know that between 30 and 60 percent of all infants born weighing less than 2,500 g (the previously established criterion of prematurity) are actually not premature but are born near term after having sustained intrauterine growth retardation.

Indeed, the menstrual history is reliable in at least 85 percent of pregnancies, and the earlier a patient is seen, the more accurately she will recall the proper date. Immunologic pregnancy tests now used are usually positive within 6 weeks after the last menstrual period; this may be useful in establishing certain limits to gestational age. Undoubtedly the exact dating of the gestation is one of the most important and frequent problems posed for the obstetrician, and it is very important in considering the proper time for indicated premature delivery of the high-risk patient.

PHYSICAL EXAMINATION. Particular attention should be directed to maternal weight prior to conception, for if the prepregnant nutritional status is poor, perinatal outcome is not optimal. A thorough complete physical examination and description of the general body habitus should be performed routinely. The blood pressure should be measured; it will be the basis for follow-up examinations as the pregnancy progresses.

TABLE 2. Coefficient of Risk of Premature Labor

Score	Socioeconomic	Past History	Daily Habits	Current Pregnancy
1	2 children at home Low socioeconomic status	D&C × 1 Less than 1 year last birth	Work outside home	Unusual fatigue
2	Less than 20 years More than 40 years Not married	D&C × 2	Apartment, 3 floors More than 10 cigarettes per day	Less than 12 pounds by 32 weeks Albuminuria Hypertension
3	Very low socioeconomic status Less than 5 feet Less than 100 pounds	D&C × 3	Heavy work Long commute Long tiring trip	Breech at 32 weeks Weight loss of 5 pounds Head engaged < 36 weeks Lower uterine segment formation < 36 weeks
4	Less than 18 years	Pyelonephritis		Vaginal bleeding after 12 weeks Effacement < 36 weeks Dilatation < 36 weeks Uterine irritability
5		Uterine anomaly 2nd trimester abortion Premature delivery		Twins Placenta previa Hydramnios Adominal surgery

The uterine size should be appropriate for the gestational age by history; excessive size must alert one to the possibility of twins. Small uterine size should lead to the consideration of fetal growth retardation or inaccurate dating of the gestation. Clinical pelvimetry is performed to determine pelvic capacity.

LABORATORY TESTS. Routine laboratory tests performed at the initial visit should include the following: hemoglobin or hematocrit; blood type and antibody screen (even if the patient is rhesus-positive, because 4 percent of patients will have antibodies that may make cross-matching of blood difficult); serologic testing for venereal disease; rubella screen (primarily as an index of risk, as well as for vaccination immediately postpartum when a repeat gestation is unlikely to occur for 3 months); urinalysis (if bacteria are present, pyelonephritis and/or premature labor may ensue); Papanicolaou smear of the cervix to rule out cervical neoplastic disease.

EDUCATION. The mean weight gain in pregnancy is 10 to 12 kg, and the patient should be so instructed. Excessive weight gain does not predispose to the development of preeclampsia, as was once thought, but it may place additional strain on the cardiovascular system of the mother. A weight gain of 10 to 12 kg accounts for the weight of the fetus, the placenta, and the amniotic fluid, the increased weight of the breasts and uterus, an increase in circulatory blood volume, and physiologic water retention of about 1 to 2 kg. If the patient is excessively obese, a weight reduction program is not indicated; weight gain in obese patients is generally lower than average. Since the developing fetus receives about 12 percent of the mother's iron stores and the menstruating female is frequently deficient in iron, 30 mg of elemental iron should be taken daily. Iron administration may be delayed until the fourth month, after the nausea that is frequently seen in the first trimester has abated.

The patient should be permitted and even encouraged to maintain normal physical activity and exercise. Coital activity may be continued until labor begins unless there are specific problems such as abnormal vaginal bleeding or premature rupture of the membranes.

Arrangements should be made at the first obstetric visit for the woman to attend education sessions during which she may learn and understand more about her pregnancy. She should attend a pregnancy awareness class early in the first or second trimester, a breast preparation class if she plans to breast-feed the baby, and a preparation for childbirth class to learn how labor normally occurs and how she may be able to assist in the process. These classes are useful to all women, not only to those patients desiring to undergo labor and delivery without analgesia or anesthesia. The more that the pregnant woman understands about what is happening to her own body and to the fetus, the less fear and anxiety will result.

ANTENATAL MATERNAL SURVEILLANCE

Frequency of Examination

There are four main goals of prenatal care: establishment of rapport between physician and patient, education of the patient, early detection of any abnormality that may adversely affect the outcome of the gestation, and assessment of fetal and maternal well-being and appropriate timing of delivery. The frequency of antenatal examination is determined by the presence of risk factors. In the seemingly normal pregnancy the woman should be seen every 3 to 4 weeks during the first and second trimesters, every 2 weeks in the beginning of the third trimester, and every week during the last month of pregnancy. If any abnormalities are detected during the course of the gestation, the frequency of the visits should be increased.

Routine Examination

At each visit the physician should note historical events that have occured since the last visit: the absence or presence of weight gain, the level of blood pressure, the growth of the uterus as measured from the pubic symphysis, the presence of fetal life as determined by fetal activity and/or auscultation of the fetal heart, and the presence or absence of glucose and protein in the urine (first voided morning sample).

Nutrition and Weight Gain

Preferably the pregnant woman should gain 1 to 3 kg in the first trimester and about 0.35 kg each week thereafter. The woman who is malnourished before conception and the pregnant teenager will have to meet their own increased dietary needs as well as those of the developing fetus, and special nutritional counseling is indicated in these cases. Edema is frequently a source of unusual increase in weight; although it does not cause preeclampsia, it may be a sign of preeclampsia. The treatment of choice for women with excessive edema is rest in bed in the left lateral recumbent position for 1 to 2 days. Maternal cardiac output and renal blood flow are improved in this position and perhaps aid in producing the diuresis that results. Diuretic medication and salt restriction are rarely necessary. Prolonged diuretic therapy can be hazardous because it may result in decreased plasma volume and severe electrolyte imbalance. These conditions have been associated with hemorrhagic pancreatitis and maternal death. Also, prolonged diuretic therapy may be associated with hemorrhagic disease of the fetus and newborn and may cause electrolyte imbalances, particularly hyponatremia, in the newborn. If diuretics are necessary they should be used only for short periods. Since much of the mother's weight gain is due to fluid expansion, both within her own tissues and in the developing fetus, sodium retention is necessary for this fluid expansion to remain physiologic. Dietary restrictions should not reduce sodium intake below 2 g/day.

Maternal Blood Pressure

The arterial blood pressure decreases from its normal value (about 120/80 mm Hg) in the first trimester; it is 5 to 10 mm Hg lower in midgestation. In normal pregnancy it rises again in the third trimester to prepregnant values. The patient with a slight elevation of blood pressure during the first trimester whose pressure remains in the range of 120/80 mm Hg in midgestation will frequently develop increased arterial blood pressure in the third trimester; this usually denotes the presence of underlying hypertensive disease. Any known hypertensive patient deserves close scrutiny, since one-third of them will develop preeclampsia (as defined by a blood pressure of 140/90 or higher or a rise of 15 mm Hg in mean pressure, plus proteinuria of over 300 mg/day). Excessive sudden weight gain and edema, which are frequently seen with preeclampsia, are not necessary for the diagnosis.

The renal status of anyone with hypertension should be evaluated early in pregnancy. The usual tests performed are serum creatinine and creatinine clearance and total protein on a 24-hour urine specimen. The normal serum creatinine level during pregnancy is 0.5 to 0.8 mg/100 ml, and a serum creatinine of 1.0 or greater suggests renal disease. The blood urea nitrogen is also lowered in the normal gestation. The creatinine clearance is normally elevated to levels of about 150 ml/min.

If preeclampsia is diagnosed in a previously normal patient or in a patient with underlying hypertensive disease, the woman should be hospitalized and a daily record should be made of 24-hour proteinuria, creatinine clearance, maternal blood pressure, weight gain, and symptomatology. Termination of pregnancy is indicated when there is an uncontrollable elevation of arterial blood pressure, a sudden increase in the daily amount of proteinuria (eg, an increase from 1.5 to 4 g per 24 hours), or a sudden drop of creatinine clearance below 50 ml/min. Patients with underlying renal disease, such as nephrotic syndrome, may also develop superimposed preeclampsia in the presence of preexisting proteinuria; unfortunately the above criteria are of limited value in this particular situation.

Uterine Growth

Serial growth of the uterine fundus should be judged by the same examiner at each prenatal visit. Inappropriate growth for gestational age may indicate intrauterine growth retardation, which necessitates further assessment. Uterine size that is excessive for the gestation suggests a multiple gestation, hydramnios, or possibly error in dating the pregnancy.

Urine Examination

Glycosuria on a random urine sample correlates very poorly with diabetes mellitus since the renal threshold for glucose is decreased during pregnancy. However, repeated glucosuria, or a history of diabetes mellitus in the family, or a history of a previous infant with a birth weight over 9 pounds, is reason for a glucose tolerance test. Since absorption of nutrients in the gastrointestinal tract is frequently delayed during pregnancy and may be unpredictable, an intravenous rather than an oral glucose tolerance test is preferred. The presence of proteinuria in a random sample is an indication for investigation of the urinary tract for undiagnosed infection or renal disease, or the onset of preeclampsia.

Infection

Although viral and bacterial infections may affect the outcome of pregnancy adversely, the exact effect of many infections on gestation is unknown. Rubella infection before 16 weeks of gestation may result in congenital malformations; after that time it may cause fetal growth retardation. Any evidence of a rubella infection must be communicated to the pediatric staff, since live virus may be excreted by the infant for months after birth.

Maternal bacterial infections, such as pneumonia, pyelonephritis, or appendicitis, should be treated appropriately; but there should also be strict attention to any signs of premature labor, which is frequently associated with systemic bacterial infections. Intrauterine bacterial infection of the fetus may occur with intact membranes, but it is rare. If the membranes rupture prematurely and the fetus is mature, delivery should be accomplished within 24 to 48 hours, since maternal and fetal infection rates rise precipitously after that time. If the fetus is immature a conservative course may be followed. In this instance the mother's temperature should be taken every 4 hours, and white blood cell count should be followed. Even a slight rise of temperature should be suspect; a white cell count of over 16,000/mm^3 is usually indicative of chorioamnionitis. Amniotic fluid may be obtained by transabdominal amniocentesis; the presence of polymorphonuclear leukocytes is suggestive but not proof of chorioamnionitis. Prophylactic antibiotic therapy prior to the onset of labor in mothers with premature rupture of membranes has not proved to be useful.

In the last month of gestation a careful examination of the vaginal tract for evidence of herpes simplex vaginalis is indicated, particularly if there are any symptoms. Cultures from suspect lesions should be taken and a Papanicolaou smear performed. The smear may provide evidence of a herpes vaginalis infection prior to the return of the culture report. If active disease or an open lesion is present, delivery should be performed by cesarean section, because infection of the baby during vaginal delivery may cause severe illness leading to serious neurologic disease or death. It is vital that the pediatrician be notified of this disease process prior to delivery.

Third Trimester Bleeding

Vaginal bleeding in the third trimester may be caused by many conditions, such as cervicitis, cervical polyps, and carcinoma of the cervix, but the most important problems confronting the obstetrician are abruptio placentae and placenta previa. Both ultrasound and radioisotopic techniques may be used to determine the location of the placenta. Ultrasound has the advantage that the fetus is not exposed to gamma radiation and also that it may be used to examine the implantation site for evidence of premature separation of the placenta. If ultrasound with B mode is unavailable, the placenta may be localized by the radioactive isotope technique. Albumin labeled with [99] technetium is usually employed, as this radionuclide has a particularly short half-life and albumin does not cross the placental barrier. With abruptio placentae spontaneous labor frequently ensues; otherwise the degree of abruption will dictate the timing and mode of delivery. With placenta previa a conservative course is followed unless the fetus is known to be mature.

Premature Labor

If a patient has a history suggesting an incompetent cervix, examination of the cervix should be performed weekly from about 14 weeks of gestation. Any cervical dilatation before 30 weeks of gestation warrants the placement of a suture around the cervix. The patient who is at risk of premature labor also requires frequent examination. The high association of premaure labor with urinary tract infection calls for routine urine cultures in these patients. The woman should be taught to detect uterine contractions by palpation and to monitor her uterus carefully if she experiences vague lower abdominal discomfort or low back pain or has other symptoms suggesting uterine contractions.

The newer β-adrenergic compounds have been useful in arresting premature labor; they are effective in doses that do not cause serious maternal cardiovascular side effects. They have limited value for long-term delay of delivery if the cervix is dilated more than 3 cm or is more than 80 percent effaced when therapy is first instituted. If premature labor is detected before advanced cervical changes have occurred, β-adrenergic therapy may prolong gestation for several weeks. Three β-adrenergic agents currently undergoing investigation and chemical trial in many countries are ritodrine hydrochloride, isoxsuprine, and orciprenaline. Excessive doses of these drugs may cause maternal tachycardia or hypotension; they should be administered under careful surveillance. High rates of infusion of these drugs into a maternal vein will cause fetal tachycardia.

Intravenous infusion of ethanol has also been used to inhibit premature labor, with partial success. The disorientation and emesis frequently seen with intravenous ethanol treatment make this mode of therapy less desirable and less acceptable to the patient.

ANTENATAL FETAL SURVEILLANCE

Prenatal Genetic Diagnosis

Amniocentesis for genetic diagnosis is usually performed only after appropriate genetic counseling, at approximately 15 weeks of gestation. For some conditions, amniotic fluid cells are cultured over a period of 3 to 4 weeks for subsequent biochemical and/or cytogenetic examination. The success rate in culturing such cells is about 95 percent in most laboratories. The risk of causing termination of the pregnancy by amniocentesis is approximately 0.5 percent.

The incidence of trisomy 21 is about 1.5 percent between 35 and 39 years of age and about 2.5 percent between 40 and 45 years. Other chromosomal abnormalities occur less frequently. More than 50 inborn errors in metabolism can be diagnosed prenatally, and recognition of them in pedigree or in a previous pregnancy is an indication for genetic counseling. Sex-linked disease may be suggested by examination of the amniotic fluid cells for the presence of nuclear sex chromatin to determine sex. However, it is preferable to perform karyotyping for a more accurate determination of fetal sex. It is now also possible to determine the presence of neural tube defects antenatally by measurement of the amount of αfetoprotein in the amniotic fluid. A history of anencephaly or meningomyelocele indicates a potential recurrence rate of approximately 5 percent in a succeeding pregnancy; thus this condition warrants counseling. Recent reports indicate that the diagnosis of hemoglobinopathies can be made in utero by obtaining small amounts of fetal blood at 18 to 22 weeks of gestation. Patients in these categories should receive genetic counseling before 15 weeks of gestation and should make a decision whether to proceed with amniocentesis.

Erythroblastosis Fetalis

The introduction of transabdominal amniocentesis in the management of pregnancies in which Rh antigen immunization has occurred has resulted in an improvement of perinatal mortality in this disease. If the Rh-negative patient has an antibody titer against Rh antigen higher than 1:8, an amniocentesis with spectrophotometric analysis of the fluid is indicated. In the first sensitized pregnancy, a rise in Rh antibody titer correlates with the degree of fetal hemolysis, but in over 85 percent of sensitized pregnancies the Rh titer does not change significantly. Spectrophotometric analysis of amniotic fluid is a more accurate means of assessing the severity of fetal disease. Several techniques are used, but all depend on the fact that indirect bilirubin absorbs light that has a wavelength of 450 mμ. The optical density difference Δ OD at 450 mμ is calculated as depicted in Figure 1. The ΔOD is then used to calculate the severity of the hemolytic process using Liley's original suggestion or a modification thereof. If the ΔOD lies in the lower zone (Fig. 2), either the fetus is not affected by the Rh sensitization of the mother or the degree of fetal hemolysis is minimal, and premature delivery is not indicated. If the ΔOD is in the middle zone, amniocentesis must be repeated at intervals of 1 to 3 weeks, depending on the past obstetric history and the ΔOD reading. If the ΔOD is high, intrauterine fetal transfusion is indicated if the pregnancy is less than 33 weeks of gestation. If the gestation is beyond 34 weeks, the 10 percent risk of fetal death associated with intrauterine fetal transfusion is greater than the risk of premature delivery in a unit with neonatal intensive care facilities, and premature delivery is thus indicated. Delivery by cesarean section is often suggested because these fetuses tolerate the stress of labor poorly.

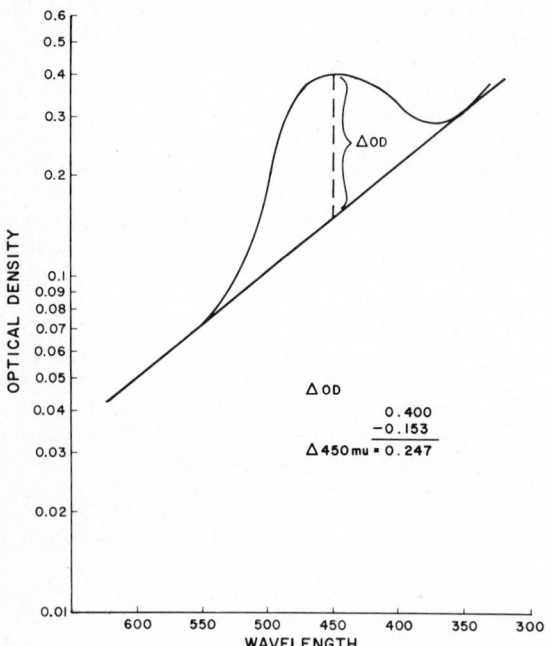

FIG. 1.   Filtered amniotic fluid is examined spectrophotometrically from 650 to 325 mμ, and the curves are plotted on semilogarithmic paper. The optical density difference at 450 mμ is calculated from the observed reading and the density at 450 mμ of a tangential line connecting 525 and 365 mμ (this straight line is obtained in the absence of unconjugated bilirubin, as is the case near term in the nonsensitized patient). The optical density difference in this patient was 0.247.

Although intrauterine fetal transfusion by the transabdominal technique may be attempted as early as 22 to 23 weeks of gestation, the chances of a successful outcome are very low if fetal transfusion is necessary this early. Repeat fetal transfusions are done at intervals of 10 days to 3 weeks up to 33 weeks of gestation.

An amniogram should be performed prior to fetal transfusion to outline the postion of the fetus. Meglumine diatrizoate (Renografin-60), a water-soluble dye, is injected into the amniotic cavity, and often ethyl 10-p-iodophenyl undecylate (Pantopaque), a lipid-soluble agent, is also injected to coat the fetal skin (Fig. 3). Radiologic examination 24 hours later reveals contrast material in the fetal intestines (if swallowing has occurred) and the placental implantation site and the presence or absence of hydrops fetalis. Lack of swallowing indicates fetal death, severe hydrops, or possibly a tracheoesophageal fistula. The contrast material in the fetal intestines is used to direct the placement of the needle when fetal transfusion is performed on the following day.

Fetal Growth and Maturity

Intrauterine fetal growth retardation results in a six- to eightfold increase in perinatal mortality. Many maternal conditions, such as hypertensive renal disease or preeclampsia, are frequently associated with fetal growth retardation, but in many cases there are no indications that fetal growth is likely to be suspect. Therefore it is important to document appropriate fetal growth in all gestations, not only those at risk. Serial increase of fundal size is the most important clinical sign of fetal growth. The size of the uterus parallels gestational age to 24 weeks of gestation, and growth retardation is rarely detected prior to this time. Although estimations of fetal weight are quite good in the average fetal weight range near term, often large differences between estimated and actual fetal weight are noted at the upper and lower ends of the spectrum. If

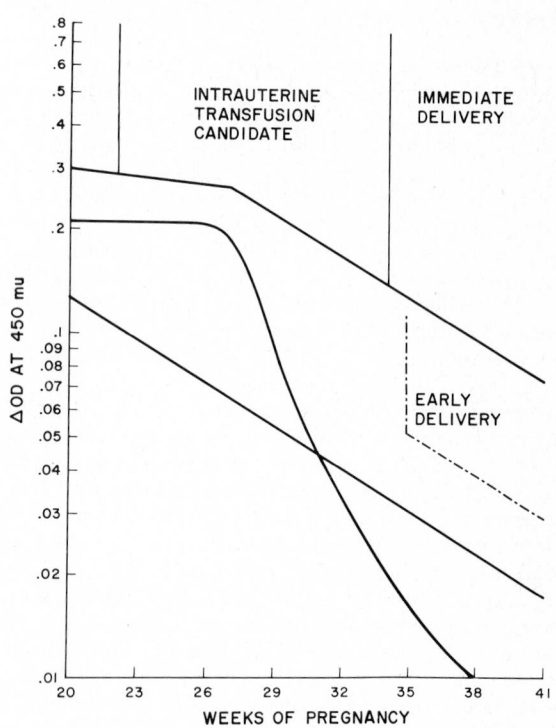

FIG. 2.   The ΔOD at 450 mμ is plotted. The curved line indicates the ΔOD that is obtained in non-rhesus-sensitized patients at various gestational ages (see text for explanation of how this graph is used in management). The ΔOD of 0.247 obtained in Figure 1 at 31 weeks of gestation led to transfusion of the fetus.

there is a lack of progressive uterine growth in a high-risk pregnancy, other techniques are used as described below.

Ultrasound

During the past decade ultrasound has been used with increasing frequency for diagnosis in obstetrics.

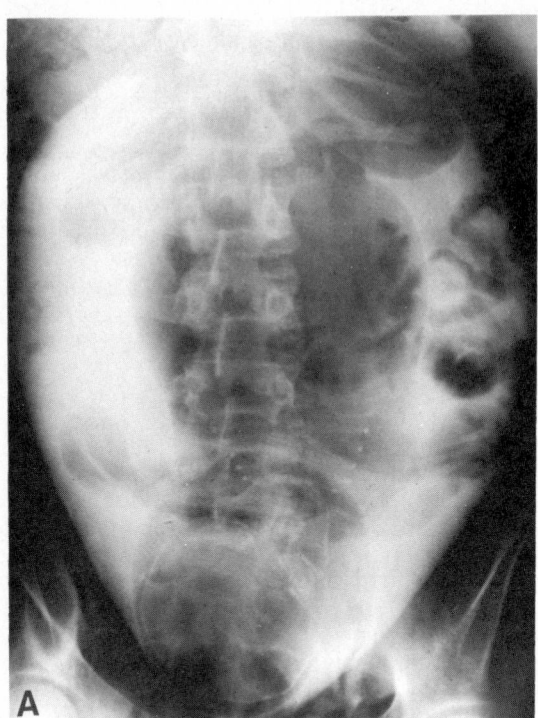

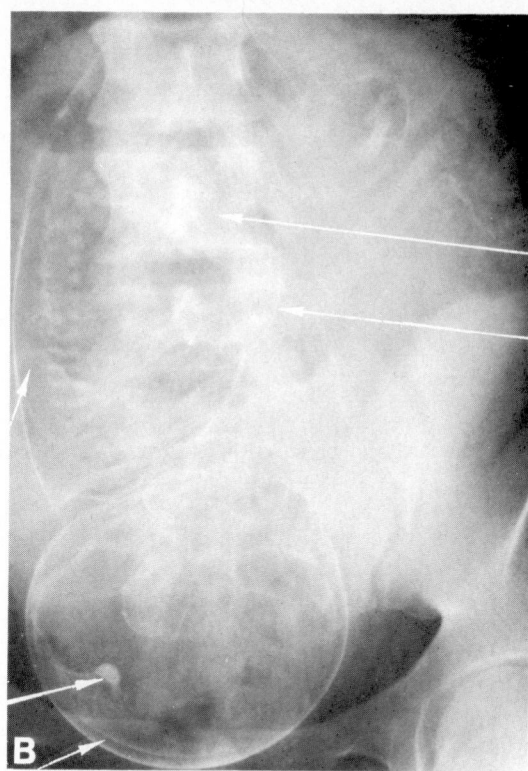

FIG. 3. Part (a) shows an amniogram taken after injecting a water-soluble opaque dye into the amniotic cavity. The fetus is hydropic, as indicated by the swollen abdomen, scalp edema, and buddha position. In (b) the amniogram has been taken after injection of a water-soluble and lipid-soluble dye. The arrows (starting at 9 o'clock and reading counterclockwise) depict excessive edema of the back, a globule of the lipid-soluble dye not yet dispersed and overlying the fetal head, scalp edema, the protuberant abdomen below the thorax, and dye in the fetal intestines. The intestines do not fill the fetal abdomen, thus indicating fetal ascites.

Short pulses of low-intensity high-frequency sound are transmitted from a transducer placed on the abdomen overlying the uterus. Reflections of the sound waves occur at tissue interfaces and echo back to the transmitting transducer where they are displayed as an image on a storage oscilloscope.

A particular mode of display called the B scan is employed to visualize the uterine contents on a cross-sectional basis. After identification of fetal parts, especially the fetal head, an electronic caliper can be applied to the A mode presentation for accurate measurement of the biparietal diameter or other structures of interest (Fig. 4). The crown–rump length of the fetus may be determined early in the gestation and correlated with gestational age with excellent accuracy (Fig. 5). Later the duration of gestation can be estimated by measurement of the biparietal diameter. As biologic variation becomes more pronounced in the last trimester, it is advisable to determine the biparietal diameter at 18 to 24 weeks if accurate dating is desired, such as in a pregnancy that may be terminated prematurely because the mother has diabetes mellitus.

Growth of the fetus may also be followed by serial determinations of the biparietal diameter every 2 to 4 weeks. Normal ranges for weekly increments in biparietal diameters have been reported (Fig. 6). The fetus with a biparietal diameter that is small for gestational age but is showing normal incremental growth would lead one to suspect error in the calculated gestational age. A biparietal diameter that is not increasing normally signifies intrauterine growth retardation of a severe degree, since head growth is among the last parameters to be affected by fetal malnutrition. Recently it has been suggested that determination of abdominal circumference and ratio of head to abdominal circumference may be useful in assessing fetal nutritional and intrauterine fetal growth retardation. Prediction of fetal weight using the ultrasonic techniques has some variability, but it appears to be accurate to within 200 g in the small fetuses, in which clinical estimates are often quite poor.

Following identification of the fetal thorax with the B scan, the transducer may be held stationary, and by switching to the M mode (M = motion), pulsatile structures such as the fetal heart or vessels may be displayed. This is an excellent method to confirm that the fetus is alive.

More recently, gray scale echography has been intro-

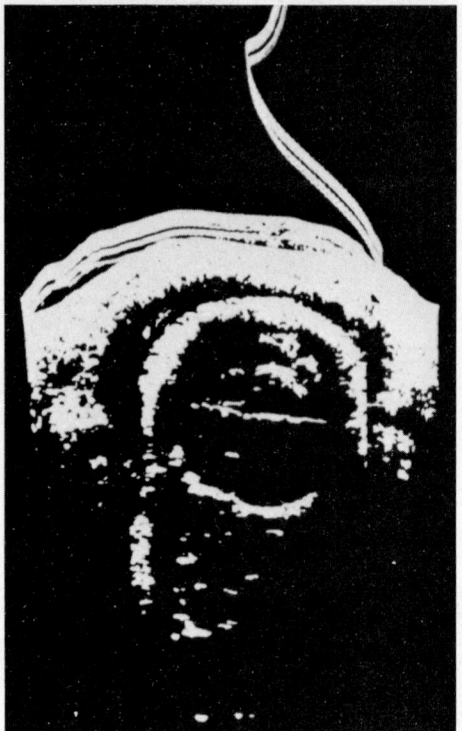

FIG. 4. Sonogram taken at 28 weeks menstrual age showing a transverse section of the fetal head. The continuous midline echo midway between the parietal bones indicates that this is the correct transverse section of the fetal head for determination of the biparietal diameter with the use of the A scan.

duced. The storage tube oscilloscope displays only a constant level of brightness of a signal and fails to give information regarding the magnitude of the echo. However, the echoes may be displayed on photographic film, thus utilizing at least 10 different shades of gray. This permits soft tissue differentiation and evaluation of various fetal organs or anomalies (Figs. 7 and 8).

Diagnostic ultrasound is used mainly to determine fetal age and size, placental localization and size, and abnormalities such as hydatid mole, fetal anomalies, and intrauterine fetal death. Future refinements of this technique should greatly increase its importance in prenatal diagnosis.

Roentgenography

Since the rapid development of ultrasound, it has largely replaced roentgenography as a means to determine gestational age and maturity, but radiologic examination may be used when ultrasound is not available. Amniography is used for fetal transfusions, for the detection of soft tissue anomalies or to rule out uniovular twins (which have a high perinatal mortality rate), or for documentation of tracheoesphageal fistulas. The distal femoral epiphyses may be seen by 32 weeks of gestation and are present at term in most fetuses. Thus absence of these centers suggests immaturity, but their presence does not assure maturity. The proximal tibial epiphysis is seldom seen before 36 weeks of gestation and is present at term in only 50 to 70 percent of fetuses. Fetal crown–rump length is too variable to be useful.

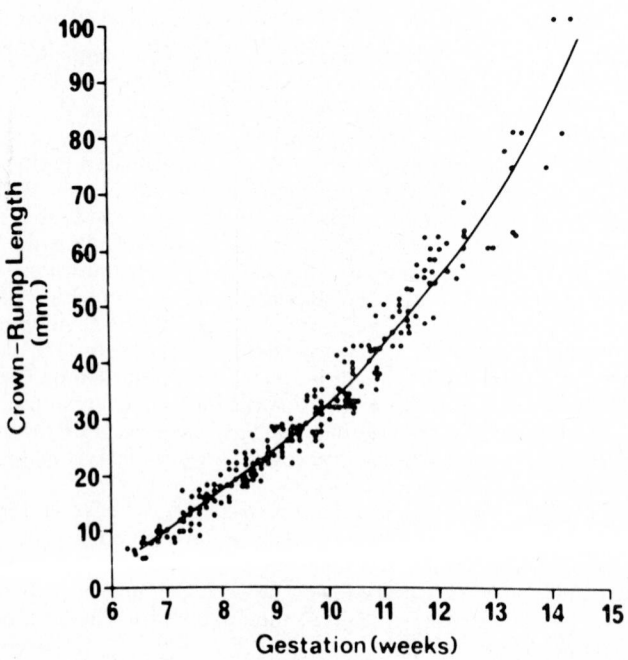

FIG. 5. Relationship between crown–rump length and menstrual age as determined by ultrasound between the sixth and fourteenth weeks of normal pregnancy. (From Robinson: Br Med J 4:28, 1973.)

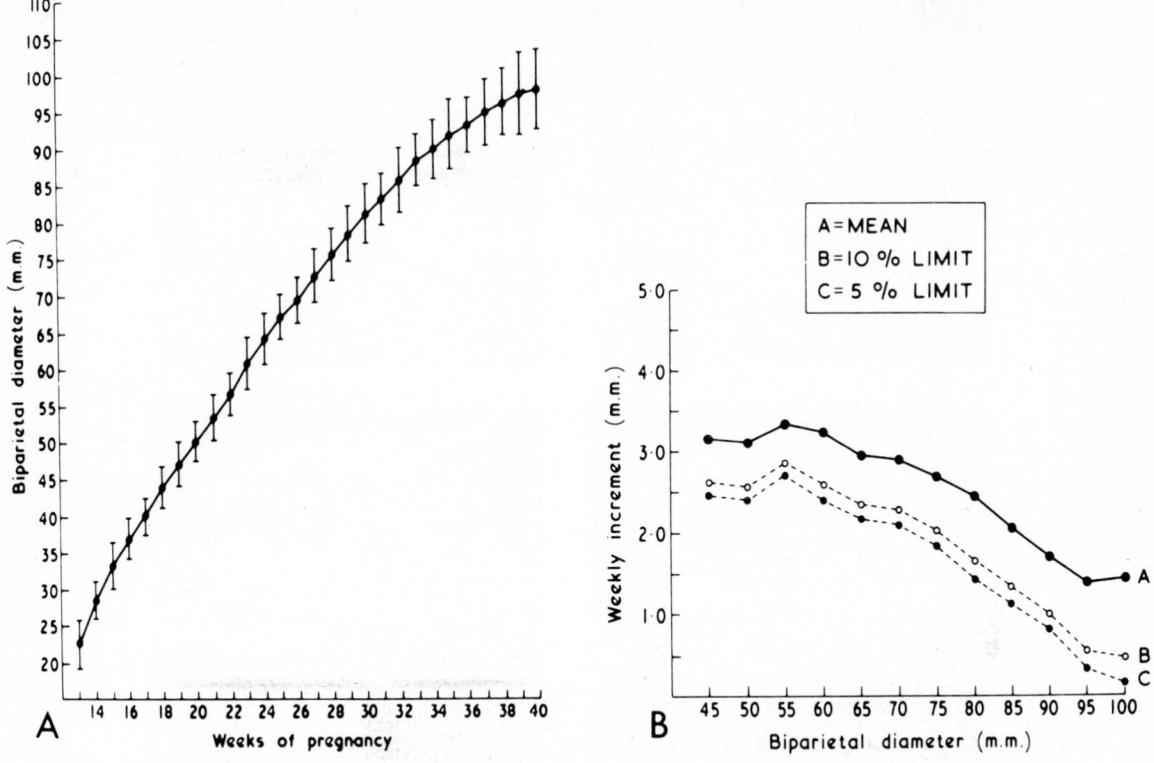

FIG. 6. A: Relationship of mean biparietal diameters (plus or minus 2 SD) from 13 to 40 weeks of menstrual age. B: Mean weekly increments in fetal biparietal diameter with 10 percent and 5 percent limits according to size of the biparietal diameter. This may be used to assess fetal growth rate. (From Campbell: Clin Perinat 1:507, 1974.)

Amniotic Fluid Analysis

Transabdominal amniocentesis is a relatively safe procedure, but it is not free of complications. It should be performed only when indicated, and then cautiously, as lacerations of placental or umbilical vessels may cause fetal hemorrhage and death. It appears that the suprapubic approach is the desired method, rather than the upper abdominal approach, if the presenting part can be definitely elevated above the suprapubic site. If the upper abdominal approach is chosen, placental localization with ultrasound is indicated.

Spectrophotometric analysis of amniotic fluid at 450 mμ, used mainly in patients with Rh-sensitized pregnancies, may also help in estimating duration of gestation. An optical density difference less than 0.01 usually denotes that gestation is beyond 36 weeks, but in 15 percent of pregnancies beyond 36 weeks the OD difference is greater than 0.01. The late decrease in OD difference may reflect increasing ability of the fetal liver to conjugate bilirubin, and thus maturation of the liver. As gestation advances the concentration of creatinine in the amniotic fluid rises. In mothers with normal renal function, a level of 2 mg/dl or more suggests that fetal weight is greater than 2500 g. However, these high levels are noted before 36 weeks in 10 percent of pregnancies. The high creatinine levels have not been explained, but they could reflect increasing fetal muscle mass or renal maturation.

Application of Nile blue sulfate stain to a drop of amniotic fluid may reveal groups of cells that stain orange, which suggests that they contain lipid material. When 10 to 20 percent of the exfoliated cells stain orange, the gestation is usually beyond 38 weeks. The cells may also be examined for morphology; if more than 10 percent of the cells are large and anucleated, the gestation is probably beyond 38 weeks. The origin of these cells is not certain, but they are thought to be derived from fetal skin. With these analyses some insight into fetal weight, fetal renal and hepatic function, and possibly skin maturation can be gained.

Since idiopathic respiratory distress is the leading cause of perinatal mortality, estimation of fetal lung maturation is most important. Phospholipid determinations in amniotic fluid have been useful in this regard. The concentration of lecithin, an important component of surfactant, in the amniotic fluid is thought to reflect the presence of surfactant within the alveoli of the fetal lung and thus to indicate the potential stability of alveolar structure after birth. Two tests are used widely. When the ratio of lecithin to sphingomyelin is greater than 2:1 respiratory distress syndrome is rare after

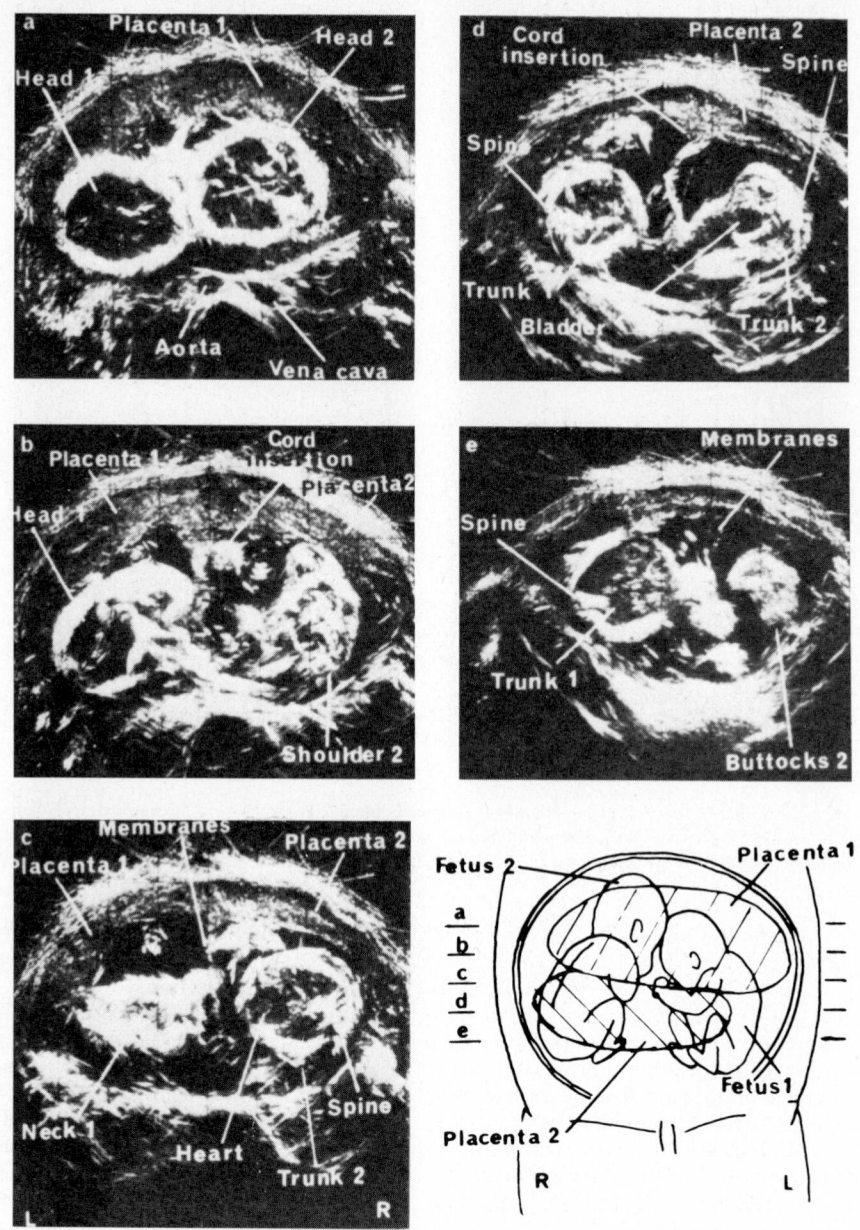

FIG. 7.   Sonogram using gray scale technique of a twin pregnancy at 23 weeks of gestation. Five sonograms are shown, taken at 3-cm intervals, as shown in insert. (From Kossoff et al: Australas Radiol 18:62, 1974.)

birth, but if the ratio is less than 1.5:1 the syndrome is very common. The foam test or shake test is based on the ability of pulmonary surfactant to maintain stable bubble formation. When a positive test is noted in a 1:2 dilution, respiratory distress syndrome is rare; if the test is negative in a 1:1 dilution, there is a 75 percent or greater risk of the disease if the fetus is delivered.

Maternal Blood and Urine Assays

Levels of several enzymes in maternal blood, such as heat-stable akaline phosphatase, diamine oxidase, and oxytocinase, increase throughout gestation, but normal variation is so great that they are not useful for determining fetal age and maturity. Poor fetal growth may be suspected if maternal venous blood or maternal urine estriol levels do not follow the normal rise noted with advancing gestation.

Estriol Determinations

Estriol constitutes the major fraction of the marked estrogen rise that occurs in pregnancy and is a useful index of fetal and placental function. Estriol precursors

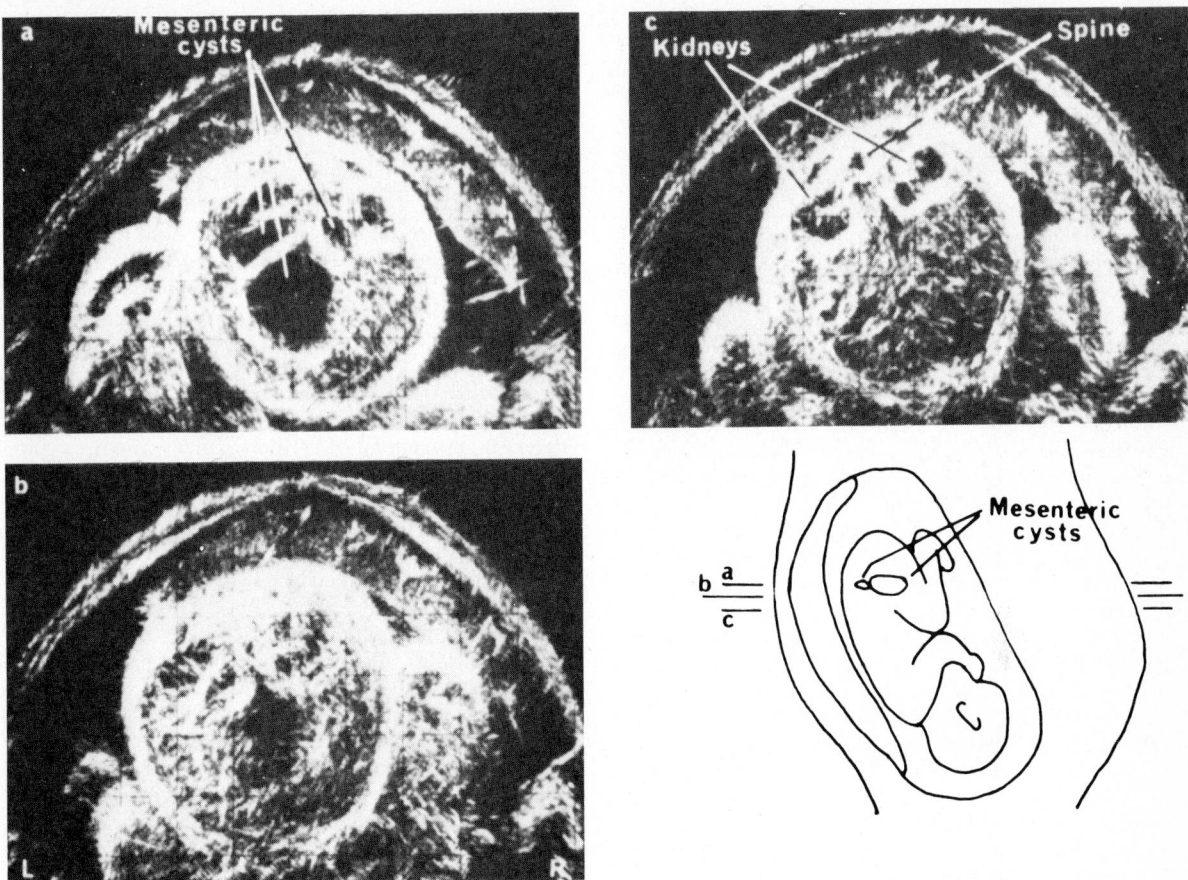

FIG. 8.   Sonogram using gray scale technique demonstrating the presence of abnormal cysts in the fetal abdomen. The three sonograms are spaced 1 cm apart. (From Kossoff et al: Australas Radiol 18:62, 1974.)

are produced mainly by the fetal adrenal gland; they are converted to estriol by the placenta and then excreted by the maternal kidneys. Both these latter processes are very efficient, and excretion is unaffected except in extreme degrees of maternal liver and kidney damage. There is a diurnal variation in excretion; so the hormone is usually measured in a 24-hour urine specimen. Completeness of collection can be assessed in patients with normal renal function from the quantity of creatinine in the urine. The analytical techniques and the percentage of the hormone recovered vary; therefore each laboratory should develop its own normal values for estriol excretion. In the normal pregnancy, daily variation of 20 percent may occur; thus at least three values are required in any pregnancy to establish a trend. If estriol values are normal, and especially if they are rising, a good fetal outcome may be predicted. Values below 2 standard deviations of the mean or values that are falling are more difficult to interpret. They must be regarded as ominous, indicating a compromised fetus, a compromised placenta, or a growth-retarded fetus unless other factors are excluded. However, a number of other conditions may be associated with low estriol determinations. These include anencephaly (due to small or absent fetal adrenals),

fetal adrenal hypoplasia, placental sulfatase deficiency, and maternal ingestion of certain drugs. These drugs fall into three classes: corticosteroids, which can suppress fetal adrenal function; some antibiotics (eg, ampicillin and neomycin, which inhibit maternal processing of estriol); and drugs that affect the analysis, such as mandelamine.

In several high-risk conditions, such as maternal hypertension, preeclampsia, renal disease, intrauterine growth retardation, and postmaturity, estriol levels can be measured twice each week, as levels decline slowly. However, in diabetes mellitus estriol levels may fall within 24 to 48 hours, and sudden fetal death may result; thus daily determinations are needed in this disease.

Low estriol values correlate well with fetal size; this is noticeable in the fetus with intrauterine growth retardation, as determined clinically by failure of fundal height to increase over several weeks. In this instance the low estriol determinations are a source of worry, but they cannot be used to predict impending fetal death. However, such fetuses are more susceptible to asphyxial death in utero than in pregnancies in which higher estriols are present.

Estriol determinations are not usually done before 27

weeks of gestation—the time that fetal survival is likely. In diabetes mellitus sudden unexpected stillbirths are relatively rare before 34 weeks of gestation; so daily determinations are not generally done before then, unless indicated by other complications.

Human Placental Lactogen

Human placental loctogen (HPL) is synthesized and stored in the syncytiotrophoblast during pregnancy. It is a peptide hormone with a biologic half-life of about 30 minutes, and its concentration in maternal serum correlates with placental and fetal weight. Its concentration is related to integrity of placental function, and low values have been found in conditions that affect placental function, such as hypertension, postmaturity, intrauterine growth retardation, and diabetes with vascular disease. In patients with diabetes without vascular disease and in Rh-immunized gestations, HPL values are abnormally high; in both these conditions the placenta may be larger than normal.

There is a large scatter of HPL levels in normal patients, but a fetal danger zone has been categorized; this includes HPL levels below 4 $\mu g/ml$ between 30 and 43 weeks of gestation. In the presence of maternal hypertension there is a striking relationship between stillbirths and low HPL levels; however, in mothers without hypertension stillbirths are poorly predicted by HPL values. A prospective study has shown that the routine use of HPL measurements for screening and management of high-risk pregnancy patients can result in a fivefold decrease in the stillbrith rate.

Amniotic Fluid Meconium

The presence of meconium in the amniotic fluid was at one time considered a sign of fetal distress. It was thought that fetal hypoxia caused gastrointestinal peristalsis and relaxation of the anal sphincter. However, several large studies showed that in the presence of meconium the incidence of neonatal mortality was low, but perinatal mortality was still double that observed in the absence of meconium staining. The presence of meconium in high-risk pregnancies (Tables 1 and 2) was shown to be a more ominous sign; meconium was present in amniotic fluid in up to 20 percent of cases before the onset of labor. Also, about 20 percent of the fetuses had acidemia when the meconium was first detected, and the perinatal mortality rate was as high as 15 percent.

In the antepartum period meconium can be detected by amniocentesis, as described above, or amnioscopy. Amnioscopy involves placing a small cone-shaped trocar with obturator through the vagina and through the cervical os to view the membranes. The presence of a greenish color seen against flecks of vernix or fetal scalp or hair, or the presence of a small amount of amniotic fluid, is considered to represent potential fetal jeopardy. Amnioscopy carries with it a slightly increased incidence of premature rupture of membranes close to term, as well as increased risk of postpartum endometritis. It has been used either in high-risk pregancies near term or in post-term pregnancies to detect the presence

of meconium on a weekly or biweekly basis, and some clinicians have advocated delivery of the fetus at risk on the basis of the presence of meconium. Such a policy is appropriate when the fetus is mature, but other methods must be used to evaluate the immature fetus before induction of labor.

Fetal Heart Rate Changes

Certain patterns of fetal heart rate and R–R interval have been noted to be associated with the subsequent outcome of the fetus. These data were initially gathered in the intrapartum period (see below), but the development of techniques for recording fetal heart rate before labor and rupture of membranes now allows this technique to be used in the antepartum period.

The fetal heart rate can be determined antenatally by detecting movement of cardiovascular structures using ultrasound, by detecting heart sounds using a microphone on the maternal abdomen, or by detecting the fetal electrocardiogram complex peaks from electrodes placed on the maternal abdomen. A rate is calculated for each interval between beats as though the fetal heart maintained that rate for 1 minute, and the data are displayed against time on a strip-chart recorder. A device called a tokodynamometer placed on the maternal abdomen will also detect the frequency and duration (but not intensity) of uterine contractions, and these are also displayed on the same strip recorder.

The information can be used in two ways. First in the so-called stress test or oxytocin challenge test, maternal uterine contractions are induced with a maternal infusion of oxytocin, and the fetal heart rate response to the contractions is noted. The presence of late decelerations (as described later) is considered a positive test, and the fetus is therefore considered at risk for intrauterine asphyxia. The test is considered negative when three uterine contractions of at least 60 seconds duration occur in a 10-minute period and no late decelerations are elicted. A fetus having a negative test is, with rare exceptions, free of risk of intrauterine demise for a further week, except in the most rapidly changing pathologic conditions.

The predictive value of positive tests is high, and before the significance of the positive test was recognized, 10 percent of fetuses that had positive tests were stillborn. However, the test is not absolutely reliable, and false positive results are common, occurring in about 25 percent of tests. In these fetuses, if membranes are ruptured after the test and internal electrodes are placed on the fetal head and the patient is allowed to labor, no evidence of fetal distress throughout the subsequent labor and delivery will be noted. Therefore a negative stress test is highly predictive of fetal well-being, but a positive stress test needs further evaluation, such as an attempt at vaginal delivery if the fetus is mature or confirmation with estriols if the fetus has not attained pulmonary maturity.

A second technique is termed nonstressed heart rate monitoring. Beat-to-beat heart rate and variability and responses of heart rate to fetal movement and spontaneous uterine contractions are monitored. This evaluation is particularly valuable in patients in whom induction of the uterine contractions is absolutely contraindicated, as with placenta previa or previous classical cesarean section, or relatively contraindicated, as in patients with an incompetent cervix, ruptured membranes, or twins.

The use of ultrasound or of phonocardiography to detect fetal heart rate often introduces difficulties because the signal is not as discrete as the R wave of the fetal electrocardiogram. This may result in apparent exaggeration of the variability of fetal heart rate. However, a flat baseline cannot be caused by electronic artifact. The determination of fetal heart rate with electrocardiographic leads on the mother's abdomen usually provides more accurate reproduction of the normal beat-to-beat variability, but it is technically more difficult and cannot be recorded in every patient. Using this test, fetuses may be categorized as reactive or nonreactive. The reactive fetus has a variable baseline heart rate in the normal range and fetal movement causes an acceleration of heart rate. There are also no late decelerations detected with spontaneous uterine contractions. The nonreactive fetus has a flat or silent baseline, which shows no accelerations with fetal movement; in fact, generally no fetal movement is detected, and there may be late decelerations with spontaneous contractions. The fetus with such a nonreactive pattern needs evaluation with other testing, eg, oxytocin challenge test, determination of the presence of amniotic meconium, and estriol estimation.

INTRAPARTUM FETAL SURVEILLANCE

About one-third of all stillbirths occur in the intrapartum period, ie, the fetus dies after the mother has been admitted to the hospital with fetal heart tones present. A number of these babies are so premature that dramatic efforts at salvage have not been made in the face of fetal distress. However, a substantial percentage of deaths occur in term pregnancies, which based on conventional techniques are apparently normal. The purpose of intrapartum fetal surveillance techniques is to reduce this fetal mortality to a minimum and also to reduce morbidity occurring during labor and delivery.

Intrapartum morbidity is primarily due to birth trauma during the actual mechanical process of delivery and to asphyxial damage. In some studies it has been suggested that as many as 5 percent of babies born suffer severe sequelae of neurologic damage due to intrapartum hypoxia.

Traumatic injury to the newborn is largely a result of uncontrollable occurrences in the expulsion stage of labor or a result of injudicious use of certain obstetric techniques. Fetal injury occurring during expulsion usually manifests as central nervous system damage or bleeding due to sudden compression and decompression or as excessive pressure on delicate structures. Usually these problems can be avoided by controlled delivery and adequate anesthesia. Some deliveries are associated with damage to muscle or other soft tissues, peripheral nerves, spinal cord, and skeleton. Much of this can be reduced by the recognition that vaginally delivered abnormal presentations carry a much higher fetal morbidity than simple vertex presentations. There

is now general agreement that heroic attempts to accomplish a difficult delivery with forceps should be rejected, and cesarean section should be performed more freely.

The obstetric management of specific problems will not be discussed, but emphasis is placed upon the recognition and prevention or treatment of those conditions that result in fetal asphyxia during the intrapartum period.

Asphyxia in utero is due to the inadequate transport of oxygen and carbon dioxide across the placenta; it results in hypoxemia, hypercapnia, and metabolic acidosis due to fetal anaerobic glycolysis. The physiologic response of the human fetus to asphyxia is poorly understood, but from data obtained in experimental animals the initial response of the fetus to moderate asphyxia appears to be increased arterial blood pressure and decreased cardiac output and heart rate. The response is probably mediated through the carotid and aortic chemoreceptors and baroreceptors. Blood flow is preferentially maintained to the heart, brain, adrenal glands, and placenta. During more severe asphyxia, cardiac output will decrease further and may be insufficient to protect vital fetal functions.

Compensatory mechanisms during impaired placental exchange that protect the fetus are an increased gradient of oxygen due to a falling umbilical artery oxygen tension, an improved matching of blood flow rates on each side of the placenta, anaerobic glycolysis, and redistribution of fetal organ blood flows.

Three techniques are currently used for evaluating fetal condition during labor: presence of meconium in amniotic fluid, change in fetal heart rate, and fetal acid–base and respiratory gas status.

Amniotic Fluid Meconium

Meconium-stained amiotic fluid has been discussed previously in relation to antenatal fetal monitoring. It is found in about 10 percent of patients in labor. Even in the otherwise apparently normal gestation the presence of meconium carries with it an increased perinatal mortality rate. Its presence in the normal or the high-risk gestation is an indication for more intensive intrapartum or fetal surveillance.

It has not been possible to quantitate the viscosity of meconium, but clinical observations indicate that thick, heavy, viscid meconium is more commonly associated with poor neonatal outcome. This may represent a more severe insult in utero, with more likelihood of intrapartum gasping resulting in aspiration. It is also difficult to remove thick, tenacious meconium from the pharynx and trachea after birth, and there is thus greater danger of aspiration with the onset of air breathing. Immediately after suctioning the nose and pharynx, the vocal cords should be visualized and residual meconium aspirated from the trachea. This has been shown to result in a marked decrease in aspiration pneumonitis in these babies.

Fetal Heart Rate

The availability of continuous beat-to-beat fetal heart rate monitoring has revolutionized our thinking con-

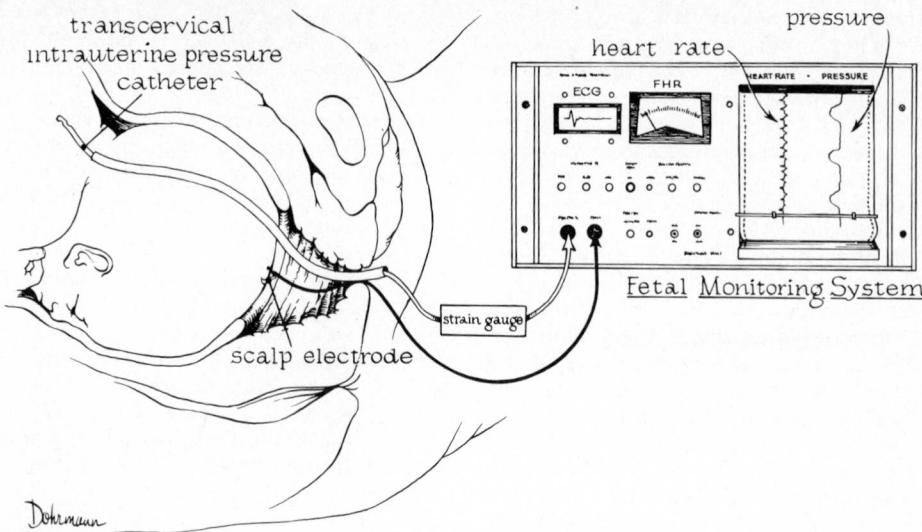

FIG. 9. Schematic representation of components for monitoring fetal heart rate and uterine contractions during labor.

cerning fetal heart rate changes during labor. In the past it was considered that rapid changes in heart rate, particularly a slow fetal heart rate detected by auscultation, was indicative of fetal distress, and a number of operative deliveries were carried out for this indication. Continuous monitoring of fetal heart rate has led us to recognize that rapid changes in fetal heart rate or decreased fetal heart rates are not always associated with fetal hypoxemia. However, we also appreciate that fetal heart rates in the normal range can be associated with severe fetal distress, under certain circumstances.

During labor the fetal electrocardiogram can be recorded by means of a metal clip or spiral applied to the fetal scalp. Since very useful information is gained by relating fetal heart rate changes to uterine contractions, uterine pressure may be measured with an open-ended catheter passed transcervically into the amniotic cavity. Uterine pressure and fetal heart rate are recorded simultaneously. The advantage of the uterine cavity catheter over external monitoring of contractions is that it provides actual levels of pressure achieved during labor and thus accurately indicates the strength of contractions. The technique of internal fetal monitoring is illustrated in Figure 9.

The important characteristics of heart rate for assessment of fetal evaluation are summarized in Table 3. The

TABLE 3. Description of Fetal Heart Tracing

1. Baseline features, between uterine contractions:
   a. Rate
   b. Variability
2. Periodic changes, associated with uterine contractions:
   a. Early decelerations
   b. Late decelerations
   c. Variable decelerations
   d. Accelerations

average normal baseline rate in the fetus is 110 to 160 beats/minute. Both tachycardia and bradycardia may be associated with asphyxiated and depressed infants, but they may be due to other conditions. For example, tachycardia can be caused by fever, prematurity, or the administration of parasympatholytic drugs. Bradycardia may be caused by congenital fetal heart block. However, in the absence of heart block a sudden prolonged bradycardia is always considered to reflect fetal asphyxia.

Baseline variability, or irregularity of the beat-to-beat period, is normal in the fetus. It gives the fetal heart rate tracing a jagged, sawtooth appearance (Fig. 10). Loss of this variability results in a flattening of the baseline and often is associated with fetal asphyxia (Fig. 11). Other conditions associated with loss of beat-to-beat variability are fetal tachycardia, adminstration of centrally depressing drugs, and administration of parasympatholytics. It is also seen in some premature infants and in some anencephalic fetuses.

The second important feature of the fetal heart rate tracing is a periodic change; this is a change occurring in association with a uterine contraction. The four different types of responses are noted in Table 3.

Early decelerations (type 1 dips) (deceleration is a technical term indicating a transient, periodic change as opposed to a baseline change, which is denoted as bradycardia) occur regularly with uterine contractions, and their onset occurs simultaneously with the onset of uterine contraction. This early deceleration has the same waveform as the uterine contraction, but is the mirror image of it. The transient deceleration ceases when the uterine contraction has been completed. These early decelerations may be abolished by atropine and are not associated with fetal asphyxia. Late decelerations (type 2 dips) are somewhat similar to early decelerations in that they occur regularly, they also reflect

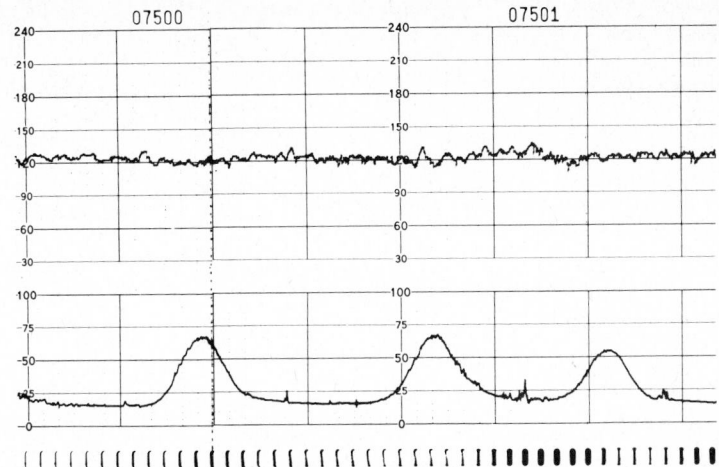

FIG. 10. A normal fetal heart rate and uterine contraction tracing. The upper panel shows fetal heart rate in beats per minute with a normal rate of approximately 120 beats/minute and normal baseline variability. Uterine contractions are depicted in the bottom panel, showing intraamniotic pressure in millimeters of mercury. The paper speed is 3 cm/minute, and each of the dark vertical lines represents 1-minute intervals.

the waveform of the uterine contraction, and they are generally smooth in appearance. However, their time of onset is delayed beyond the beginning of the onset of the uterine contraction, and the nadir of the deceleration lags behind the peak of the contraction (Fig. 12). Late decelerations can be modified but not abolished by atropine. Also, sometimes they may be abolished by administration of oxygen to the mother. They are considered to represent direct effects of fetal asphyxia on the myocardium. Variable decelerations are, as their name implies, variable in shape, time of onset, duration, profundity, and appearance. Frequently they can be

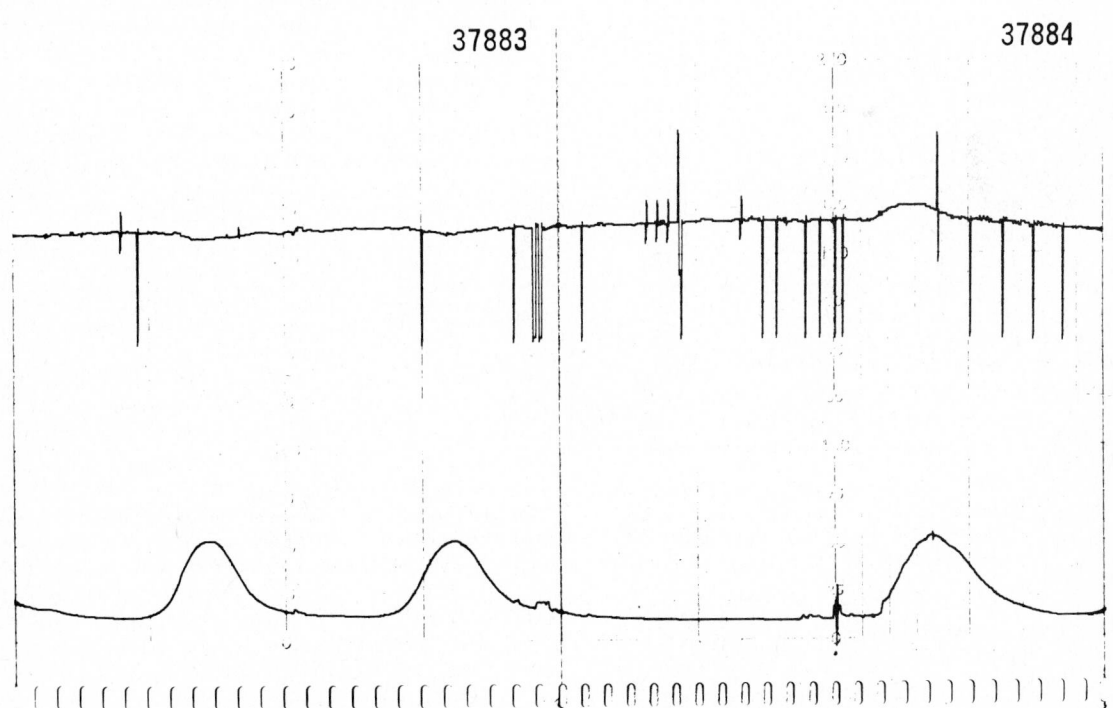

FIG. 11. Record of fetal heart rate and uterine contraction showing decreased baseline variability. Periodic changes are unremarkable (the occasional erratic vertical marks are either artifact or fetal arrhythmia).

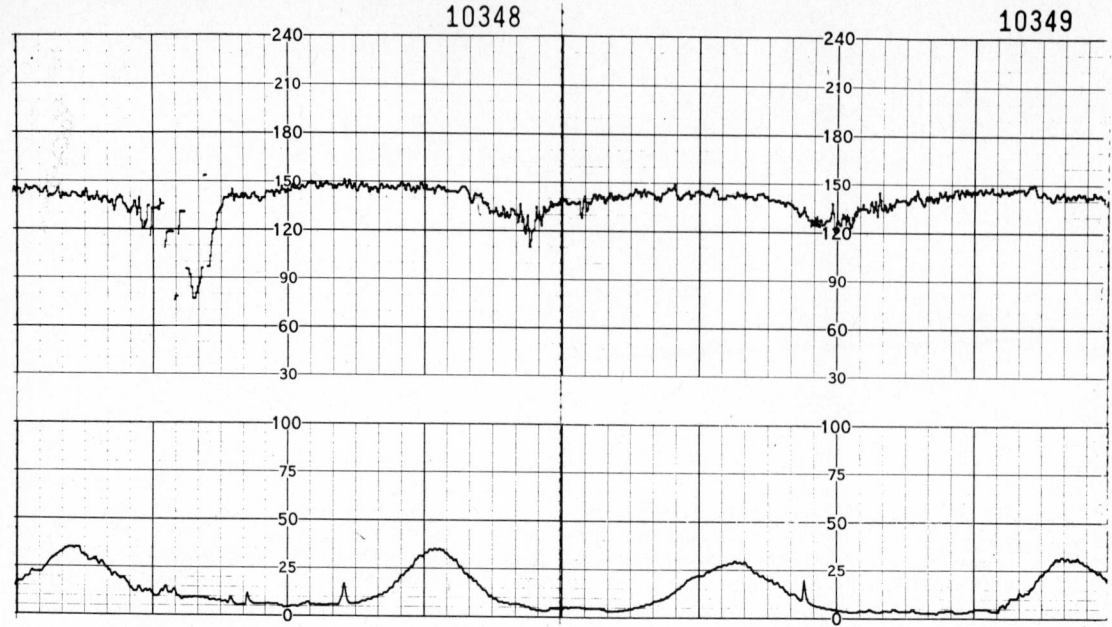

FIG. 12. Record of fetal heart rate and uterine contraction showing persistent late decelerations. This baby was delivered by cesarean section shortly after the record, severely growth-retarded (1700g) at 38 weeks of gestation.

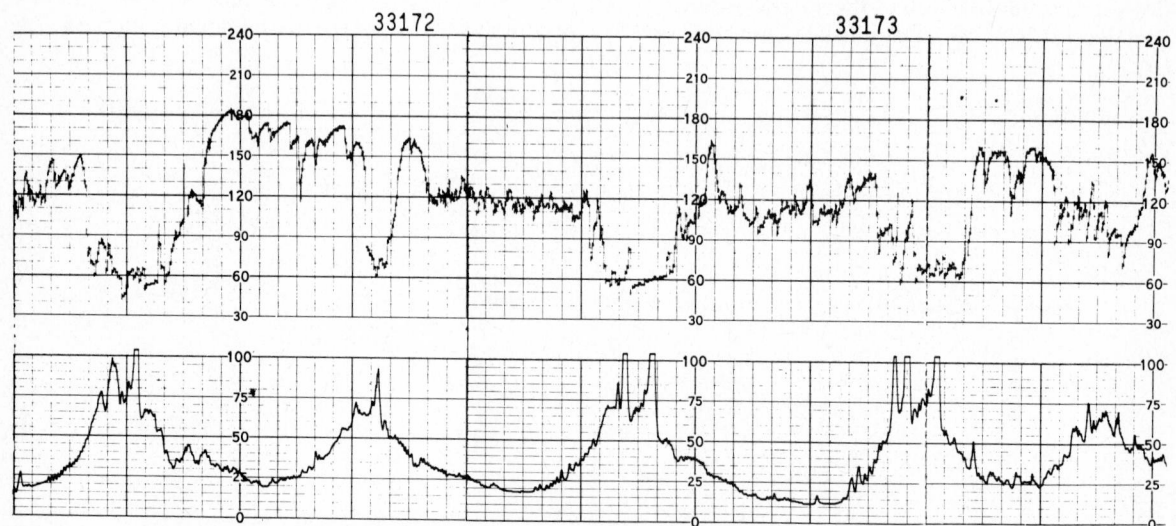

FIG. 13. This record illustrates variable decelerations in the second stage of labor. The transient spikes at the peak of uterine contractions represent maternal pushing efforts. Note that the baseline heart rate is within the normal range, and the baseline variability is normal. This signifies good fetal reserve even in the face of the marked decelerations that occur at the time of the uterine contractions. Shortly after this record a vigorous infant was born.

abolished by alteration of maternal position, and they may be modified by atropine. Their association with fetal depression is in direct proportion to their duration, profundity, and persistency. (Fig. 13).

Acceleration (increases in heart rate) may occur with uterine contractions. They are not generally considered to be associated with fetal depression. Actually, fetal heart rate acceleration, in association with fetal movement, is considered a sign of fetal well-being. Complications of fetal heart rate monitoring have been gratifyingly rare. The most common reported difficulty is mild local infection responsive to topical antibiotics. Rare cases of abscesses requiring drainage and cerebrospinal fluid drainage due to puncture, presumably of a fontanelle, have been reported. Interpretation of the fetal heart rate provides useful information of the presence of fetal asphyxia. In fact, most fetuses that do not show abnormalities of fetal heart rate tracings are born without depression. However, even when abnormalities of fetal heart rate have been present, several infants have not had depression. The presence of these false positives makes it necessary to use an additional technique for evaluation of the fetus. A useful technique is fetal scalp sampling.

Fetal Scalp Sampling

This technique enables the obstetrician to sample blood from the presenting part of the fetus after the membranes have been ruptured (Fig. 14). The fetal scalp is visualized by placing an amnioscope (a long cone-shaped instrument with an attached light source) into the vaginal canal. After cleansing the fetal scalp, a blade attached to a holder is used to make a small stab wound in the scalp. Blood is then collected from a droplet on the surface of the scalp into a capillary tube and analyzed for pH and PCO_2, and base excess can be calculated.

The mean fetal scalp pH early in labor is slightly above 7.30 plus or minus 0.05 (1 SD) and falls by about 0.05 units during labor. Clinical studies have shown that

TABLE 4. Indications for Fetal Blood Sampling

1. Fetal tachycardia
2. Flat baseline
3. Late decelerations
4. Moderate and severe variable decelerations
5. Questionable patterns
6. Certain high-risk categories with probable decreased placental transfer function, eg, intrauterine growth retardation, preeclampsia, diabetes mellitus

pH values below 7.20 are associated with Apgar scores below 7 in the neonate, while pH levels above 7.20 are associated with babies with Apgar scores above 7. However, about 10 percent of fetuses with normal pH levels are born depressed, and about 10 percent of babies with lowered pH levels are vigorous after birth. Those with decreased pH levels who are vigorous at birth are probably influenced by mild maternal metabolic acidosis and equilibration of fixed metabolites across the placenta. Those infants who are born depressed but with normal pH are probably influenced by maternal oversedation or infection, or they may have congenital anomalies. Indications for fetal scalp sampling are summarized in Table 4. Note that the prime use of this technique is to exclude the false positive of continuous fetal heart monitoring.

The use of fetal scalp sampling for determination of blood pH in the management of labor is subject to many qualifying features, and each pH value must be interpreted with due reference to the following considerations: maternal–fetal pH and base excess difference, errors of determination (eg, caput or machine calibration error), stage of labor, relationship of scalp sampling to uterine contractions, transience of the supposed insult causing the fetal acidosis, whether the acidosis is respiratory or metabolic, and influence of any in utero treatment.

Complications of fetal scalp sampling, reportedly less than 1 percent, have largely been hemorrhage and abscess formation. Rare fatalities have occurred in fetuses with blood dyscrasias who continued to bleed in utero after sampling. Occasionally scalp abscesses occur that require incision and drainage.

Although the three techniques for surveillance of the fetus during labor are very useful, they are not completely reliable, since false positive and negative interpretations are encountered. Therefore clinical judgment of the progress of labor and the status of the fetus should also be used in deciding the management of each patient where the exact status of the fetus is uncertain.

INTRAPARTUM FACTORS AFFECTING THE FETUS

Certain types of anesthesia may influence fetal heart rate and acid–base status; epidural and spinal anesthesia may be associated with sympathetic blockade resulting in maternal hypotension, decreased uterine blood flow, and subsequent fetal acidosis, usually of the respiratory type. Several sedatives may decrease the variability of heart rate, and parasympatholytic drugs may increase heart rate and decrease baseline variability. Maternal intravascular volume depletion, which fre-

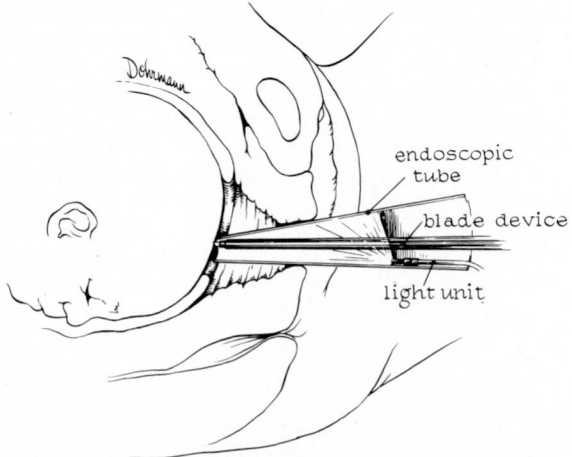

FIG. 14. Schematic representation of the method used to obtain a small sample of blood from the fetal scalp.

quently occurs in severe preeclampsia, may result in fetal respiratory embarrassment due to decreased uterine blood flow; this can be relieved by volume expansion.

In mothers who labor in a supine position, lower body venous return may be occluded by the pregnant uterus and its contents, and the subsequent decreased cardiac output is associated with decreased uterine blood flow with resultant fetal acidosis. This sequence of events can be altered by moving the mother to the lateral recumbent or Trendelenburg position. In the supine position the distal aorta or iliac arteries may be compressed with each uterine contraction (Posiero effect), and this results in a transient decrease in uterine blood flow; this may be modified by altering maternal position.

Uterine contractions are associated with transient decreases in uterine blood flow; this is usually well tolerated by the fetus. However, if the uterine contractions are too frequent or too intense, as with injudicious use of oxytocic agents, the fetus does not have time to recover from the decreased oxygen delivery between the contractions and will become progressively acidotic.

Since the development of the newer methods for monitoring the fetus, it has been possible to document the beneficial effect of certain therapeutic techniques. Table 5 shows the maneuvers that are used for treatment and the possible mechanisms of action of these maneuvers.

The obstetric indications for expediting delivery by cesarean section or rapid vaginal delivery have been altered by fetal monitoring. Expeditious delivery is now carried out for fetal distress that is considered to be nonremediable, as defined by (1) fetal acidosis that is unresponsive to treatment, (2) inability to perform fetal scalp sampling in the presence of persistent abnormal fetal heart rate patterns that cannot be abolished, and (3) episodes of spontaneous and unexplained prolonged fetal bradycardia.

In the ideal perinatal center the pediatrician should be consulted prior to labor and delivery when the fetus is thought to be at risk. This not only assists the obstetrician in knowing how labor and delivery management may affect the neonatal course but also enables the pediatrician to be aware of potential problems. The resuscitation team can be alert to the possibility that urgent treatment may be indicated.

PUERPERIUM

Although several potential complications, both mental and physical, warrant close observation of women in the postpartum period, considerable attention should be directed to the appropriate education of women for their own care and interaction with their babies. This necessitates continued close coordination between obstetric and neonatal physicians and nurses to prevent conflicting approaches to management. The new mother is frequently apprehensive about caring for the newborn child and needs frequent reassurance from her obstetrician, pediatrician, and nurse. Ideally the nurse attending the mother should care for the newborn, rather than having separate maternal and neonatal nurses.

The major obstetric complications are postpartum hemorrhage and endometritis. These may become life-threatening if not dealt with appropriately and promptly. Fever or other indications of puerperal infection merit culturing and a gram stain of the lochia in the endocervical canal. The pediatric staff should be apprised of these investigations.

In the nursing mother milk is usually present in the breasts by the third day after delivery. Several minor problems, such as breast engorgement, cracked and bleeding nipples, and inadequate sucking, can become major problems if not adroitly handled. It is known that the majority of medications ingested by the mother will appear in the breast milk. Unfortunately, little information is available regarding the concentrations of various medications in breast milk. In general, if medications are necessary they should be administered just after the infant has been fed.

It is also necessary to prevent active immunization of the Rh-negative mother if she has delivered an Rh-positive infant. In this instance specific IgG gamma globulin, anti-Rh (D) antibody should be administered. If there has been major fetal–maternal bleeding at the time of delivery, a cross-match of the mother's red cells with the immune globulin solution may show microaggregation. If this occurs, determination of the number of fetal cells in the maternal circulation should be performed to determine the amount of additional immune globulin that is needed to prevent sensitization.

TABLE 5. Treatment of Fetus In Utero

Maneuver	Mechanism
1. Rectify insult	
a. Correct hypotension	Increased uterine blood flow
b. Decrease excess uterine activity	Increased uterine blood flow
2. Change maternal position	Altered placental hemodynamics
a. Lateral	
b. Trendelenburg	
c. Knee–chest	
3. Maternal oxygen administration	Increased oxygen gradient to fetus

References

Freeman RK: The use of the oxytocin challenge test for antepartum clinical evaluation of uteroplacental respiratory function. Am J Obstet Gynecol 121:481, 1975

Kossoff G, Garrett WJ Radovanovich G: Grey scale echography in obstetrics and gynecology. Australas Radiol 18:62, 1974

Milunsky A: Management of the high risk pregnancy. Clin Perinat 1:2, 1974

Nesbitt REL: Perinatal medicine today. Clin Perinat No. 1: 1974

Papiernik E, Kaminski M: Multifactoral study of the risk of prematurity at 32 weeks of gestation. J Perinat Med 2:30, 1974

Queenan JT (ed): The Rh problem. Clin Obstet Gynecol 14:491, 1971

CHAPTER 6

The Newborn Infant

RODERIC H. PHIBBS, *Associate Editor*

Neonatal Mortality and Morbidity. The neonatal period is the first 28 days of life. In terms of health and disease it is the single most important period in all of infancy and childhood, during which the highest mortality occurs. In the past decade neonatal mortality has declined sharply, but it is still 12 per 1000 live births in the United States. Life-time damage from perinatal events is also frequent, with central nervous system injury suffered during labor, delivery, or in the neonatal period, causing a large proportion of the neurologic handicaps that manifest themselves in later childhood, such as cerebral palsy, deafness, and mental retardation.

Abnormalities of birthweight and gestational age are clearly associated with increased neonatal mortality and subsequent morbidity. Karn and Penrose were the first to suggest that deviation from an optimal combination of birthweight and gestational age, at which mortality is lowest, should increase mortality. When mortality is superimposed upon a plot of birthweight and gestational age, this creates a series of concentric rings (Fig. 1), with survival highest in the center or optimal area and decreasing peripherally. Hoffman, Stark, Lundin, and Ashbrook have shown that this relation applies, with considerable variations in the shapes of the rings, to the entire newborn population of the United States. This means that one should consider neonatal mortality in terms of birthweight: gestation group rather than just birthweight or gestation. Table 1 shows such a comparison for some groups of single born infants in California between 1966 and 1970. Note that mortality varies with gestation among infants of the same birthweight and with birthweight among those of the same gestation.

Sex and race are also major determinants of survival. Among infants of comparable weight and gestation, females have a lower mortality than males, and Blacks a lower mortality than Whites. Table 2 shows some premature, low-birthweight groups from California, 1966 through 1970, in which there is a difference between infants of the same sex but different races, and between males and females of the same race. Some of these differences may be due to different rates of functional maturation of certain vital organ systems in

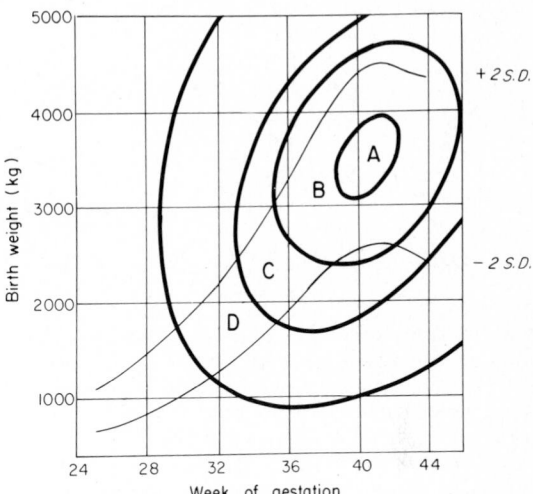

FIG. 1. Birthweight, gestational age, and neonatal mortality. The two thin lines (− 2 and + 2 SD) are the limits of normal birthweight for gestation. Zone A = optimum weight and age for survival (39 to 42 weeks gestation and 3000 to 4000 g birthweight). Mortality is lowest here and increases with deviations in any direction from this optimum. Mortality is greater in zone B than zone A, greater yet in zone C than B, etc.

females compared with males, and in Blacks compared with Whites.

For the entire population, females have a lower neonatal mortality rate than males. On the other hand, Blacks have a higher rate than whites; while small premature Black infants have a lower mortality rate than comparable white babies, more Black babies are born prematurely and with low birthweights. For example, from the same study shown in Tables 1 and 2, the neonatal mortality rate for all single born Black females was 13.6 per 1000, that for single born white females 8.8 per 1000 live births.

TABLE 1. Neonatal Mortality for Single Born Infants of Differing Birth Weights and Gestations

Birthweight (g)	Gestional Age (wk)	Mortality (deaths/1000 births)
1000-1500	28-30	482
1000-1500	30-42	368
1500-2000	30-32	248
1500-2000	28-30	269

Data from Cunningham GC, Hawes WE, Medore C, Norris F, Williams RL: Intrauterine growth and neonatal risk in California, State of California Department of Health, Sacramento.

TABLE 2. Neonatal Mortality for Single-Born Infants at 28 to 30 weeks of Gestation and Weighing 1000 to 1500 g

Race	Sex	Mortality (deaths/1000 births)
Black	Female	305
Black	Male	400
White	Female	457
White	Male	552

Data from Cunningham GC, Hawes WE, Medore C, Norris F, Williams RL: Intrauterine growth and neonatal risk in California, Department of Maternal and Child Health, State of California Department of Health, Sacramento.

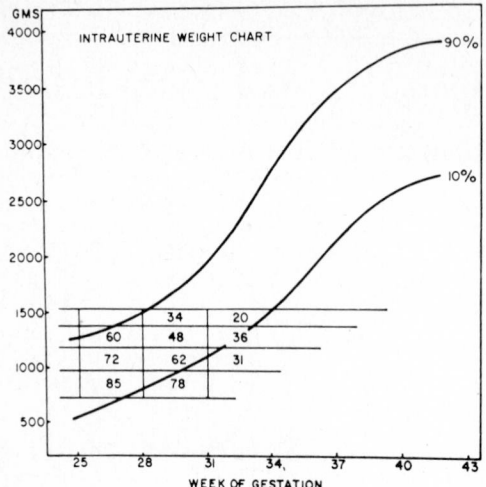

FIG. 2. Percent of moderate to severe handicaps found in a sample of surviving infants with birth weights of 1500 g or less. The outlook for normal development improves with birth weight for a given gestational age and similarly improves with advancing gestational age in any birth weight group. (From Lubchenco, J. Ped., 80:509, 1972.)

The main causes of neonatal death are birth asphyxia, premature birth, hyaline membrane disease (idiopathic respiratory distress syndrome), congenital malformation, infections, and birth trauma from obstetric complications. Death from erythroblastosis was also common until it became a largely preventable disease. Because of variations in the way deaths are reported, it is impossible to define the number of deaths among prematures that were actually due to hyaline membrane

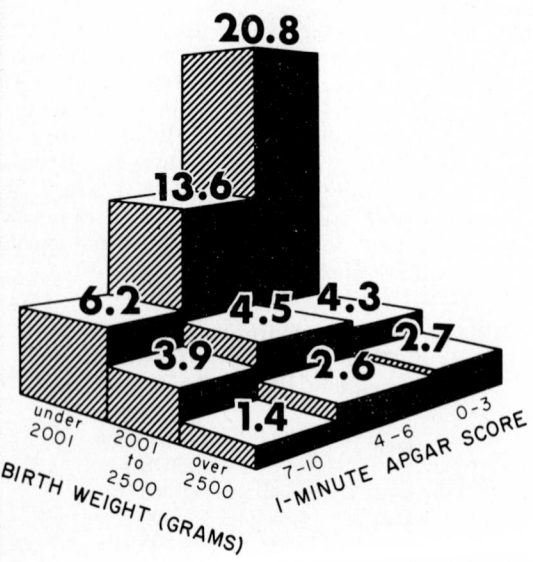

FIG. 3. Correlation between Apgar score (age 1 minute), birth weight, and incidence of neurologic deficit (percent affected) at 12 months of age. (From Collaborative Project for Cerebral Palsy, N.I.H., Bethesda, Maryland.)

disease and its complications or the number of deaths from this disease that were labeled asphyxia. However, as a group, cardiorespiratory failure associated with premature birth, asphyxia, and hyaline membrane disease and its complications accounts for about half of all deaths.

The same processes that are fatal in some infants are responsible for central nervous system injury in others who survive. Thus, infants with abnormalities of birth-weight: gestation who survive the neonatal period have an increased risk of neurologic deficit proportional to the degree of deviation from the optimal (Fig. 2). The presence of cardiopulmonary disease also affects the risk of subsequent neurologic handicaps; the interacting effects of birthweight and birth asphyxia are shown in Figure 3.

THE HIGH-RISK FETUS AND NEWBORN

It is possible to identify before birth or at the time of birth most infants who have a significantly increased risk of neonatal death or serious disease. In addition to assessment of birthweight:gestational age and the degree of intrapartum asphyxia, there are a variety of conditions which can be identified in the pregnant mother that cause an increased risk for the fetus and newborn infant. Some of these are simply indicators of abnormal gestation:birthweight or increased risk of intrapartum asphyxia. Others identify specific processes in the fetus, such as chromosomal anomalies, hemolytic anemia, delayed maturation of the lung, or metabolic derangements which increase the hazard of death and disease within any given birthweight:gestation group (see page 121 for details of high-risk pregnancies). Identification of these cases is of great practical value because the offspring will often benefit from intensive observation beginning during labor and delivery and continuing into the neonatal period. Careful observation allows earlier detection and prevention or treatment of neonatal disease. For example, it is better to prevent hypoglycemia in the infant of a diabetic mother than to allow it to occur and then treat it. This approach of anticipation and prevention is fundamental to the care of the newborn.

Bibliography

Behrman RE, Babson GS, Lessell R: Fetal and neonatal mortality in white middle class infants. Mortality risks by gestational age and weight. Am J Dis Child 121:486, 1971

Bulter NR, Alberman EA: Perinatal Problems. The second report of the 1958 British Perinatal Mortality Survey. London, Livingstone, 1969

Fedrick J, Bulter N: Certain causes of neonatal death. I. Hyaline membranes. Biol Neonate 15:229, 1970

Fedrick J, Bulter N: Certain causes of neonatal death. II. Intraventricular haemorrhage. Biol Neonate 15:257, 1970

Hoffman HJ, Stark CR, Lundin FE, et al.: Obstet Gynecol Surv 29:651, 1974

Karn MN, Penrose LS: Birth weight and gestation time in relation to maternal age, parity and infant survival. Ann Eugen 16:417, 1951

Lubchenco LO, Delivoria-Papadopoulos M, Searls D: Long-term follow-up studies of prematurely born infants. II. Influence of birth weight and gestational age. J Pediatr 81:814, 1972

Naeye RL, Burt LS, Weight DL, et al: Neonatal mortality, the male disadvantage. Pediatrics 48:902, 1971

Wegman ME: Annual summary of vital statistics-1974. Pediatrics 56: 960, 1975

EVALUATION OF THE NEWBORN

RODERIC H. PHIBBS

Assessment, evaluation, and management of the newborn have three general goals. The first is early detection of significant medical problems so that they can be evaluated and treated appropriately. The most serious problems are apparent during the first weeks of life, and most are detectable at or within hours of birth. The second purpose is to protect the newborn from harmful processes to which he is particularly susceptible after birth, such as hypothermia from chilling, or serious infection from exposure to contagious microorganisms. The third is to promote good health by facilitating the normal adaptations to extrauterine life. These range from making certain of effective ventilation of the lungs at birth, establishing adequate nutrition, development of normal mother-infant interactions, to education of the mother to the skills of infant care.

Newborn nurseries employ a set of established routines to ensure attainment of these goals. These vary from one nursery to another in details but follow the principles given in *Recommendations for Hospital Care of Newborn Infants,* which the Committee on the Fetus and Newborn of the American Academy of Pediatrics revises and publishes regularly.

At times these stated goals conflict with one another. When they do, it is important to make the correct compromise between them. A common example of this can occur immediately after birth, when an infant shows mildly abnormal signs, which could signify the onset of very serious disease or could be of no major significance. The uncertainty of a significant problem, plus the desire to promote mother-infant bonding by leaving the two together without producing unnecessary concern in the mother, might favor inaction. However, great harm may be done by delaying the diagnosis and treatment of a serious condition, so that one must act promptly. Except in the most serious situations, however, one can usually permit at least a short period of contact between mother and child but, when this contact is broken prematurely for diagnostic studies or treatment, the reasons must be explained to the mother. Failure to do this can worsen, not prevent, maternal anxiety.

PHYSICAL EXAMINATION

General Principles

Evaluation of the newborn should include a brief examination at birth for life-threatening conditions, a detailed examination within several hours after birth, and repeated evaluations after birth—more frequently during the first 6 hours, less thereafter; and a second detailed examination before discharge.

Several general principles apply to the examination of the newborn.

Usually, the most informative component of the examination is careful inspection. Observe and note all aspects of an infant's appearance and behavior before proceeding with palpation and auscultation.

If one anomaly is present, look for others, because they tend to coexist.

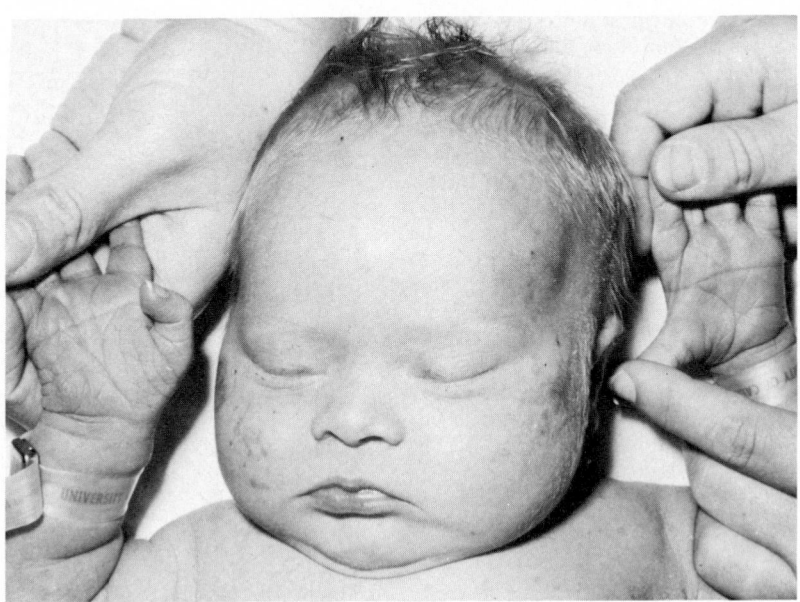

FIG. 4. Down's Syndrome due to Trisomy 21. Note the low nasal bridge, and upward slanted palpebral fissures on the face, Simian creases on palms of hands.

Certain constellations of physical findings and anomalies indicate the presence of specific dysmorphic syndromes, which carry a relatively well-known prognosis. These must be considered in any abnormal-appearing infant. The classic example is the typical features of an infant with Down's syndrome, some of which are shown in Figure 4.

The newborn must be examined specifically for evidence of birth trauma, which is particularly common after breech delivery, shoulder dystocia, and other difficult deliveries. When present, trauma is likely to involve several areas. Therefore, as with anomalies, evidence of trauma in one area demands an especially careful search in another.

Several potential hazards from physical examination must be avoided. These are hypothermia from exposure in a cold room (see section on Thermal Stability, p153), colonization with pathogenic microorganisms transmitted by unwashed hands (or, perhaps more important, suction tubes, etc., that may be reservoirs for bacteria), and physical trauma from rough handling or carelessness.

Examination of the Infant

SIZE AND GESTATIONAL AGE. It is extremely important to make the best possible estimate of an infant's gestational age and to compare several measurements of body size to the range of normal for gestational age. This identifies infants who are at greater than average risk because they are premature and/or undergrown or overgrown for their gestational age. (See p. 173 and p. 175). It also identifies disproportions between various components of body growth; also, the measurements of size form a baseline for future measurement to assess postnatal growth.

Gestational age should be estimated in several ways. Maternal history will provide one estimate but is subject to error, particularly if there was an irregular pattern of menstruation before conception. Physical examination provides additional estimates of gestational age. Neuromuscular behavior provides the best indicator of gestational age; the Section on Neurologic Examination of the Newborn includes a system for making this estimation (p155). Gestational age can also be estimated from the physical characteristics of the skin, hair, external genitalia, ears, and breasts. These differences are described separately at the end of the section on physical examination. Gestation should be estimated by both of these methods to see if the findings coincide with the gestational age estimated from maternal history. If they do not, and maternal history is vague, the age estimated from examination should be used when comparing body size to gestational age. (There are also more involved systems available for estimating gestation from physical findings, for example, the Dubowitz scoring system.)

Soon after birth one should measure and record weight, head circumference, crown-heel length, crown-

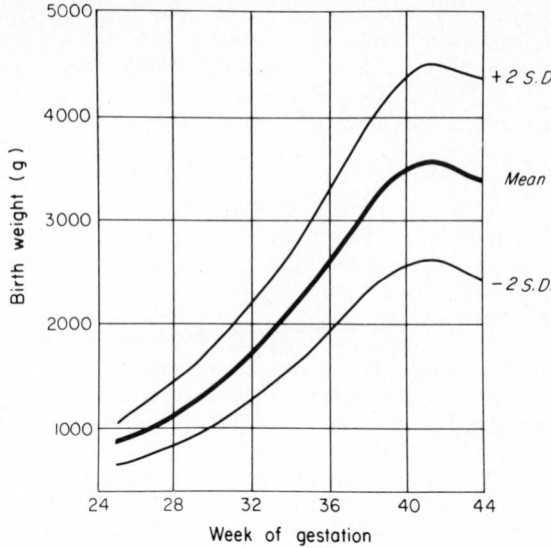

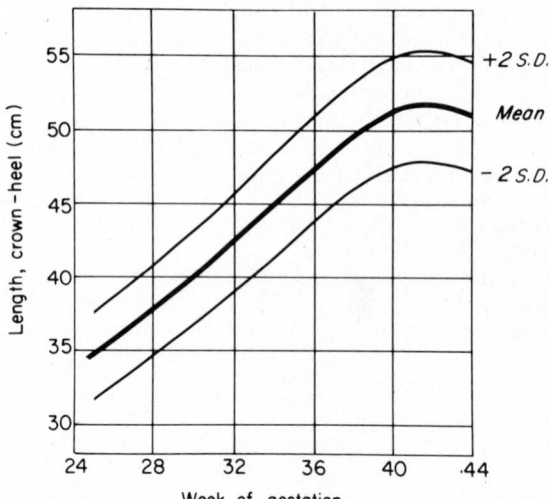

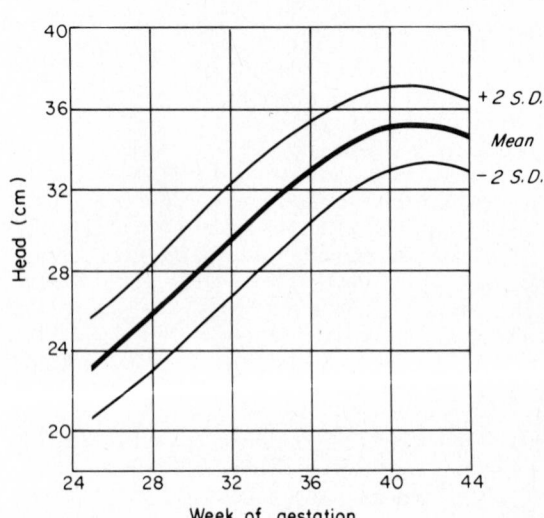

FIG. 5. Intrauterine growth charts. These show the normal values of body weight, length and head circumference for infants born at different gestational ages at sea level (Montreal, Canada). (Redrawn from the data of Usher and McLean: J Pediatr 74:901, 1969).

rump length, and circumferences of chest and abdomen. The first three measurements should be compared with the range of normal for gestational age (Fig. 5), but it is important to use normal values appropriate for geographic location (in North America, normal intrauterine growth varies considerably from one region to another, depending upon the altitude above sea level at which pregnancy and birth occur).

GENERAL INSPECTION. At birth, most newborns cry vigorously, then tend to remain awake for half an hour or more, during which they are extremely active. Their eyes are open, and they move the head from side to side. They make sucking, chewing, swallowing movements, facial grimaces, cry briefly, and have repeated bursts of flexion and extension of the arms and legs. This activity may be continous or interspersed with quiet periods, during which the eyes are open, the head is held in the midline, the arms are flexed, and the legs are partly extended and occasionally crossed. The cry is vigorous and repetitive. A feeble or soft cry is abnormal, as is a high-pitched or shrieking cry; these suggest a neurologic problem. After the first hours of life, the normal term newborn has sleep periods that last 40 or 50 minutes; half of each period is quiet and half is active sleep. (Passive and active muscle tone is discussed in the Section on Neurologic Evaluation, p 156) The complex of irritability and hyperactivity, with sneezing, yawning, profuse sweating, or vomiting suggest withdrawal reaction from maternal/fetal addiction to heroin, morphine, or methadone. Withdrawal signs appear during the first few days after birth in about 75 percent of infants of addicted mothers. Symptoms may appear later and last longer with methadone addiction.

If the examiner gently flexes the elbows, knees, and hips, the limbs will generally tend to fold into a position-of-comfort, and a crying active infant is usually quieted by this posture. Determining the position of comfort of an individual infant is important in assessing the etiology and significance of deformities of the limbs (see below). Figure 6 shows the position-of-comfort for one infant, and illustrates the positional deformities of the limbs in this intrauterine posture.

SKIN. Fine soft lanugo covers the back and dorsal aspects of limbs of the term newborn. Vernix caseosa, a thick white material with the consistency of soft cheese, covers the skin of the 36 to 38 week fetus, but at 40 weeks the amount of this material decreases and is present mainly in the creases of the skin. At term, there is relatively thick subcutaneous tissue, so that the fold of skin over the upper back is usually 0.25 to 0.50 cm thick. The fingernails and toenails are fully formed and extend slightly beyond the tips of the digits. If meconium was passed into the amniotic fluid in utero, this may coat the skin; this is a sign of some fetal distress. If meconium has been in the amniotic fluid for several hours or longer, it will stain the skin, fingernails and toenails, and the umbilical cord with a greenish hue; this is a sign of earlier or more prolonged fetal distress. The postmature infant, ie, from a pregnancy beyond 42 weeks, usually has dry, flaky skin, less than

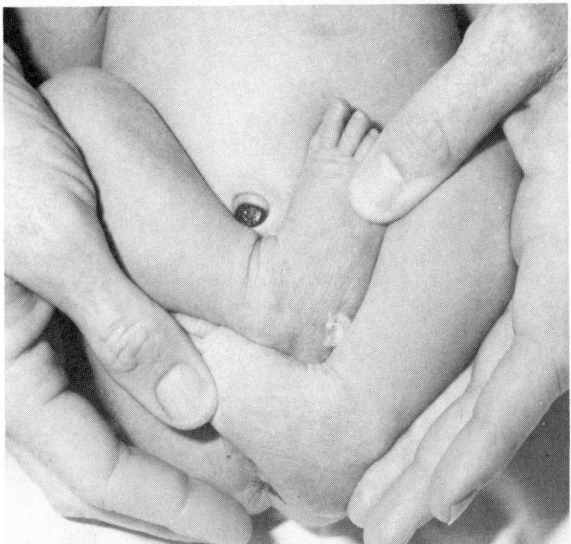

FIG. 6. Position of comfort in a 20-hour-old newborn infant. When placed in this position the infant who had been crying was quiet. The ankles and metatarsals appear to be deformed but all these apparent deformities can be easily corrected with gentle pressure.

normal subcutaneous tissue, long fingernails, and meconium staining of the skin, cord, and nails.

COLOR. The skin of the normal newborn is pink. Pallor may be due to anemia, or to poor peripheral perfusion as occurs with asphyxia, shock, and some congenital heart lesions. With poor perfusion, there is delayed capillary filling of the skin after blanching (generally more than 2 seconds). Pale mottled skin occurs with sepsis or hypothermia. Pallor with a pattern of marbleization occurs with hypothyroidism, but this is rarely detected in the first days. There may be cyanosis of the hands and feet (acrocyanosis), which is normal during the first day. Generalized cyanosis may occur from cardiac or pulmonary disease, hypothermia, or a central nervous system lesion. Plethora may indicate polycythemia.

Ecchymoses generally result from birth trauma, and are often present over the feet, lower limbs, and buttocks following breech delivery. Petechiae over the face after a vertex delivery, or lower limbs after a breech delivery, are usually the result of local vascular stasis from pressure or from compression by an umbilical cord wrapped around the neck. Generalized petechiae suggest a coagulation abnormality. With more severe birth trauma, there is often extensive hemorrhage in the muscles underlying the areas of ecchymotic skin; hemolysis of this extravascular blood may cause severe hyperbilirubinemia.

Most neonatal jaundice, whether physiologic or pathologic (see section on Bilirubin Metabolism, p.1067) is due to an elevated indirect-reacting bilirubin, which gives a yellow-to-orange color to the skin. Elevation of direct-reacting bilirubin gives a yellow-to-green discoloration. It is easier to appreciate the degree of jaundice in a newborn by briefly pressing on the infant's skin with a finger and observing the color in the blanched area. Under normal conditions the degree of hyperbilirubinemia can be estimated roughly from the distribution of the jaundice but not from its intensity. Table 3 shows a simplified version of the system devised by Kramer for this estimation. This system is not a substitute for measurement of serum bilirubin concentration in infants with pathologic processes or even seemingly well infants, but is meant as a guide to indicate when to begin such measurements of bilirubin in otherwise well infants. This system applies only to infants cared for under standard newborn nursery conditions. It does not apply to infants under intensive care nursery conditions, where they are unclothed and often under radiant warmers, nor does it apply to those who have received phototherapy; these conditions make it impossible to estimate bilirubin level from skin color.

TABLE 3. INTENSITY OF JAUNDICE

Zone	Jaundice	Serum Indirect Bilirubin (mg/dl)	
		Average	Maximum
I	Limited to head and neck	6	8
II	Over upper trunk	9	12
III	Over lower trunk, thighs	12	16
IV	Over arms, legs, below knee	15	18
V	Hands, feet	> 15	—

Adopted from Kramer: Am J Dis Child 118-454, 1969

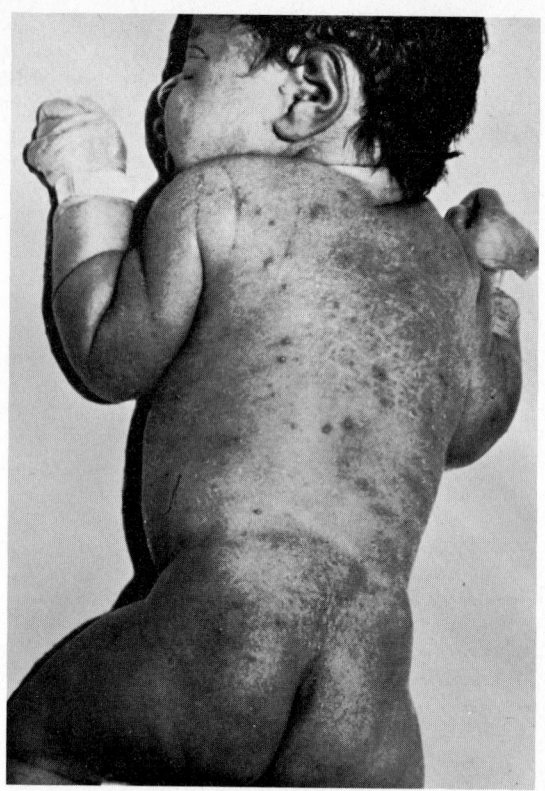

FIG. 7. Erythema toxicum.

Unlike older children or adults, the newborn does not develop detectable scleral icterus until jaundice is severe and indirect bilirubin levels are quite high. The normal newborn commonly develops mild physiologic jaundice at 2 to 4 days of age. Jaundice, which appears during the first 24 hours, is most often due to hemolytic anemia and warrants prompt investigation. The differential diagnosis of neonatal jaundice is extensive and includes many important diseases; it is discussed on p 1067.

RASHES. The normal newborn commonly has some form of benign skin rash. *Milia* are tiny white papules formed at the surface of sebaceous glands, and quite commonly appear over the nose. In *miliaria rubra,* small discrete red lesions develop over obstructed sebaceous glands, usually due to overheating and excessive clothing. In *erythema toxicum* (Fig. 7), there are small vesicles that contain eosinophilic neutrophils. This, and rapid fading, help to distinguish this benign and transient rash from that of serious disease, such as staphylococcal pustules, which usually also have more erythema. Serious systemic infections often present with either a purpuric, maculopapular, or vesicular rash. Some generalized viral infections are characterized by small red papules that contain infiltrations of erythroid cells. With many intrauterine infections there may be thrombocytopenic purpura. *Congenital rubella* often produces a macular purple rash, descriptively called a *blueberry muffin* rash. *Congenital syphilis* may have a red oval maculopapular rash that later becomes brown, or a hemorrhagic vesicular rash; either will commonly involve the palms of the hands and soles of feet. A red maculopapular rash often occurs with *toxoplasmosis. Staphylococcal* disease often presents with pustules from which the organism can be cultured. It may also involve the skin, with extensive bullous lesions due to a toxin elaborated by certain strains of staphylococci, variously called scalded skin syndrome, toxic epidermal necrolysis or, in the older literature, Ritter's disease. In *listeriosis,* there often are purple miliary granulomas of the skin that contain the offending organism, *Listeria monocytogenes.* Cutaneous monoliasis commonly involves the diaper area, producing macerated erythematous skin. This is more common in infants who have received a course of treatment with systemic antibiotics.

Vascular nevi occur in one-third or more of all newborn infants, most often on the forehead, back of the neck, or upper eyelids. They are a deep pink color, generally not very prominent, and tend to fade later in infancy or early childhood. *Strawberry hemangiomas* are more common in premature than in term newborns. In term infants, they may appear as only small pale areas of discoloration that develop into full-blown hemangiomas later in infancy. Sucutaneous *cavernous hemangiomas*

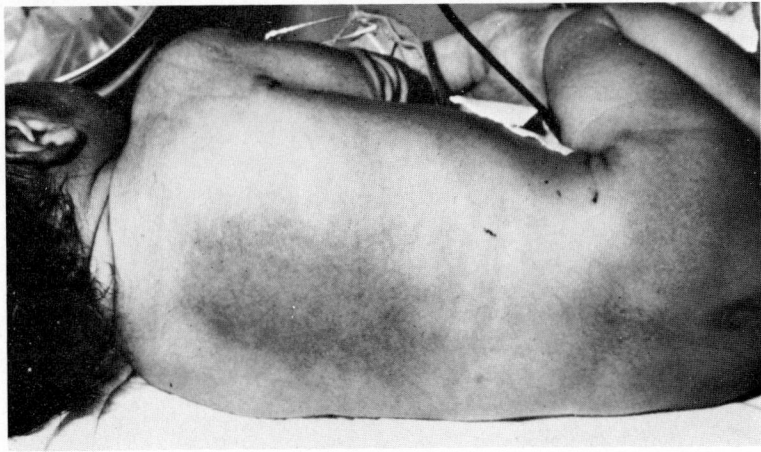

FIG. 8. Mongolian spots.

give a faint red or purple discoloration to the overlying skin.

Mongolian spots (Fig. 8) are dark brown or purple spots, usually over the backs of more darkly pigmented races. *Harlequinism* is a striking transient change in the skin color of the newborn; typically one side of the entire body turns a bright red, the other side is normal or somewhat pale, and the line of demarcation is sharply in the midline. This appears and disappears abruptly, lasts only a few minutes, and may recur. The cause is unknown (instability of the autonomic regulation of peripheral circulation is the suspected cause), and it has no known serious sequelae.

Collodion skin (Fig. 9) is hard shiny skin that gives the appearance of a layer of dried collodion or thin plastic, coating the skin. This becomes brittle and flakes in a few days. Such infants often develop icthyosis later. The severe forms of *epidermolysis bullosa* presents in the newborn as skin that is blistered or eroded on minimal pressure, rubbing, or trauma.

HEAD. After vertex presentation and vaginal delivery of a term or near-term infant, the head shows pronounced effects of labor and delivery. Because of molding, the saggital and lambdoidal sutures are usually overlapped. The bones return to their normal positions during the first few days, so that the sutures are

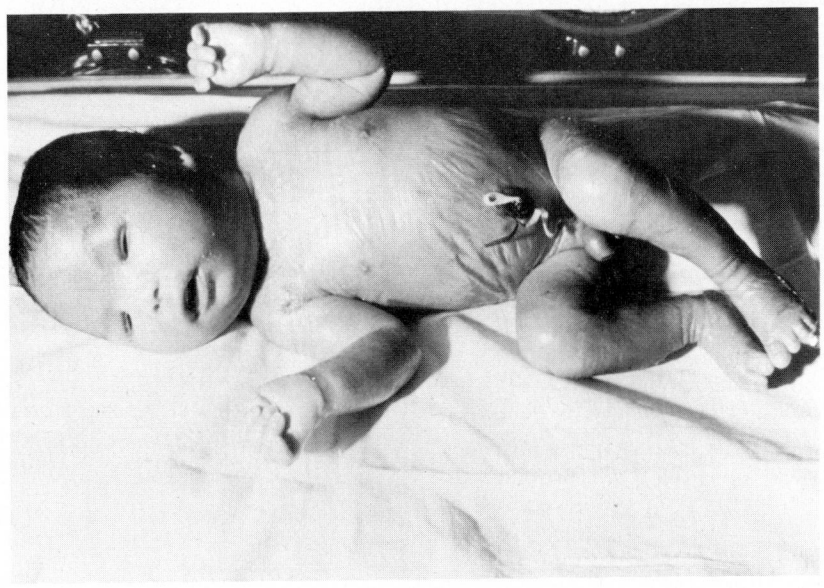

FIG. 9. Collodion skin.

palpable as definite spaces between the edges of the bones, often several millimeters wide. The scalp hair is fine and silky.

Caput succedaneum is edema of the scalp due to local pressure and trauma during labor. With severe trauma, there may be extensive subaponeurotic hemorrhage; with this, the scalp feels more tensely distended than with the usual amount of caput. Hemorrhage can be massive and produce profound shock, most commonly after a difficult delivery and intrapartum asphyxia, and is often accompanied by intracranial hemorrhage and serious brain damage. Other scalp lesions include puncture wounds from intrauterine fetal monitors and sampling sites for fetal blood pH measurements; and small crater-shaped defects that occur with trisomy 13.

Cephalhematomas are subperiosteal hemorrhages secondary to the trauma of labor, usually involving the parietal bones. These are fairly firm, slightly fluctuant masses, usually round, with a palpable rim that gives the impression of a shallow crater in the bone under the mass. These are easily distinguished from caput succedaneum because they do not extend beyond the suture line of the affected bone. Commonly, there are bilateral parietal bone cephalhematomas but they are still palpably distinct from one another. Cephalhematomas will be reabsorbed and should not be aspirated.

THE FACE. The newborn's face often gives the first clue to the presence of one of the dysmorphic syndromes. There may be obvious malformations, such as cleft lip, or underdevelopment of the first arch structures, or the findings may be more subtle. Figure 4 shows the characteristic features of *Down's syndrome.* The main features of the *Pierre Robin syndrome* include a small mandible (micrognathia), a high-arched or cleft palate, and a tongue that is not held forward but falls back into the hypopharynx (glossoptosis) and causes *airway obstruction,* which must be recognized promptly. The obstruction can be relieved with an oral airway, by pulling the tongue forward, or by pulling the mandible forward.

Intrauterine position may produce asymmetry of the face, and pressure on it during labor and delivery may cause a peripheral *facial palsy,* which is mild and usually resolves. This is most obvious during crying. The *zygomatic arch* may also be fractured during labor and delivery; this is detectable by palpation. These complications are more common after forceps delivery. Forceps often leave erythematous marks or bruises on the face, usually in the shape of the forceps blade (Fig. 10). *Horner's syndrome* is obvious on inspection of the face and is usually a consequence of birth trauma to the neck (see Section on the Neck for associated nerve injury, p. 147).

THE EYES. When a newborn is awake and quiet, and his eyes are shaded from bright light, he will generally open them to permit easy inspection. *Congenital microphthalmia* is usually obvious on inspection and palpation. *Congenital glaucoma* presents first as an enlarged cornea followed by its progressive clouding (Fig. 11). Early detection is important in preventing damage

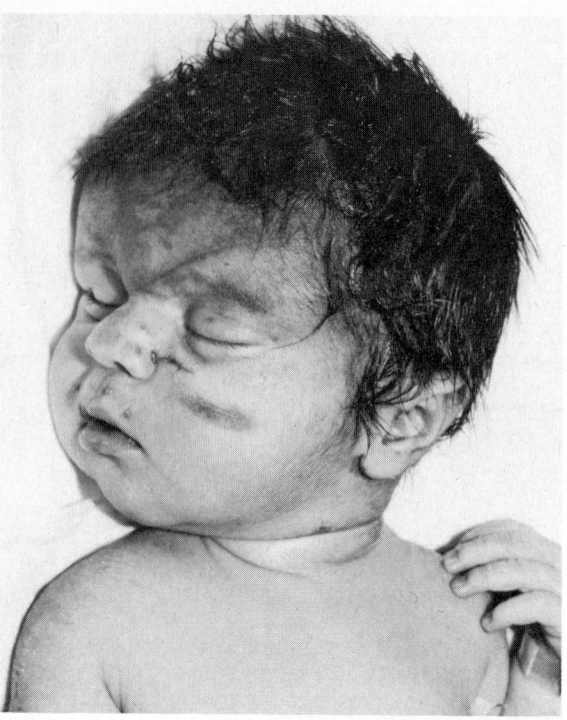

FIG. 10. Forceps marks.

to the eye. A corneal diameter of 11 mm or more is suspect and warrants further investigation.

The conjunctivae are commonly inflamed after instillation of silver nitrate for prophylaxis of gonococcal ophthalmia. This appears rapidly, is often accompanied by a small amount of yellow, sterile discharge on the second day, clears in a few days, and has no serious sequelae. *Gonococcal conjunctivitis* acquired from the birth

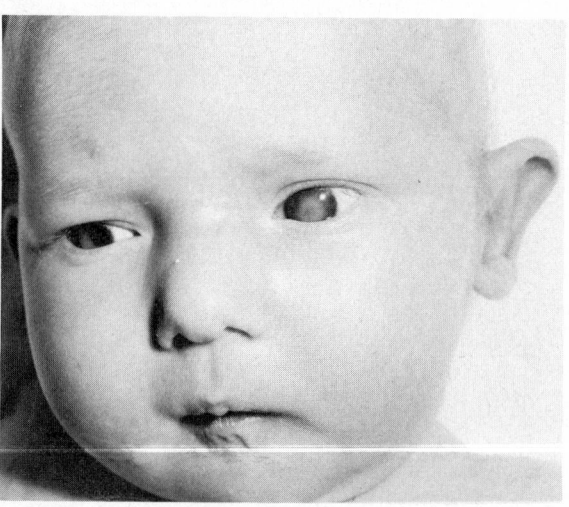

FIG. 11. Glaucoma.

canal progresses rapidly to panophthalmitis, which completely destroys the eye. This infection must be detected and treated promptly. Other common neonatal pathogens, such as *E. coli,* also cause conjunctivitis in the newborn, usually after the first few days. *Inclusion blenorrhea* is a purulent conjunctivitis caused by an organism of the Bedsoniae group, which the infant acquires from the mother's birth canal at delivery. It does not appear until between the end of the first to the third week after birth. These various causes of conjunctivitis must be distinguished from one another by appropriate microbiologic methods.

During ophthalmoscopic examination, it is useful to begin focusing on the anterior of the eye, and then progress back to the retina in order to detect the more anterior lesions, such as cataracts and defects (colobomas) of the iris, which may occur alone but usually as components of various dysmorphic syndromes. The iris, which is usually blue in newborn infants, may have abnormal areas of pigmentation, such as the *Brushfield spots* of Down's syndrome. Generally, it is possible to see the retina but, at the very least, one must see a red reflex, which is the red of the retina seen through the lens. A large cataract will obliterate this. Common areas of minor birth trauma to the eye include edema of the lids and small hemorrhages in the anterior chamber, conjunctivae, or retina. These findings are considered within the range of normal by many physicians because they are common, but they are evidences of birth trauma.

EARS. At term, the ears of the newborn are well formed and contain sufficient cartilage to maintain the normal shape and resist deformation. Malformed auricles or low-set ears are quite common in many dysmorphic syndromes. Small sinuses anterior to the ear are the remnants of the first bronchial cleft. These are relatively common and usually cause no disease. There is a tendency to ignore the tympanic membranes during examination of the newborn infant because they are difficult to see, but this is inappropriate because otitis media does occur in the first days after birth, and can be diagnosed by otoscopic examination. It should always be considered in the child who is suspected of having an infection.

NOSE. Most newborn infants are nose-breathers. If the nose is obstructed, and they are not provoked to cry, most infants will not open their mouths to breathe and may become very hypoxic. Obstructive lesions or foreign bodies in the nose can be lethal. With these, an infant will become cyanotic and have respiratory difficulty, but improves rapidly, whenever stimulated to cry, and will breathe through the mouth but deteriorate again when crying stops. Foreign materials, such as blood, mucus, and meconium must be cleared from the nose at initial evaluation after delivery. Then, it is good practice to pass a soft plastic catheter through each nostril into the oropharynx or stomach, to ensure that the nasal airway is patent. Unilateral or bilateral anatomic obstruction due to *choanal atresia* is rare. Other masses, such as an *encephalocele* protruding into the

nasopharynx, can also cause severe obstruction. Profuse mucopurulent rhinorrhea, which becomes blood-tinged, is likely to be the *rhinitis of congenital syphilis;* there may be accompanying mucocutaneous syphilitic lesions in the mouth. These signs may be present at birth or develop later in the neonatal period.

MOUTH. The mouth of the newborn infant must be examined by both inspection and palpation. Small shiny white masses on the gums, *epithelial pearls,* are common. One or more *incisor teeth* may have erupted, which are often very loose and, whether loose or firm, must usually be removed to facilitate breast feeding. A *ranula* is a relatively common benign cystic mass arising from the floor of the mouth. The tongue is enlarged and protruding in hypothyroidism, Beckwith's syndrome, and in isolated macroglossia. In Down's syndrome, the tongue is protruded, and often makes serpentine tongue movements. The frenulum may be quite short in the newborn, but this rarely interferes with adequate feeding or future function and so does not require surgical treatment. A cleft palate may not be obvious on inspection. The palate must be palpated to rule out a defect. A cleft uvula demands a particularly careful search for a defect in the palate. The palate may be intact but high-arched, with a high vault and sharp curvature in a variety of dysmorphic conditions. The normal newborn will usually suck vigorously, as on a nipple, when one places a finger in his mouth, unless he is sleeping or has been fed recently. With normal effective sucking, the finger is actively drawn into the mouth by the movement of the tongue against the palate in a forward-to-backward motion. This essential function is easily distinguished from simple biting movements, which are ineffective in feeding from the nipple.

NECK. The neck of the newborn appears shorter than that of the older child but has a full range of motion. Limitation of motion suggests an abnormality of the cervical spine. The trachea should be palpable in the midline. Cervical masses, such as a *goiter, cavernous hemangioma,* or *cystic hygroma,* are not only problems in themselves but may compress and obstruct the trachea sufficiently to decrease ventilation. This requires immediate establishment of an adequate airway, usually with endotracheal intubation, with the tip of the endotracheal tube passed well beyond the area of compression. The neck is particularly susceptible to trauma from lateral traction during delivery. This may produce a hematoma of the sternocleidomastoid muscle, which can later fibrose, contract the muscle, and cause *torticollis.* Serious trauma to the neck often involves injury to cervical nerves, which may produce paralysis of the diaphragm, arm, and shoulder muscles (Erb's palsy) or Horner's syndrome. Presence of any one of these warrants a careful search for evidence of the others. *Brachial cleft anomalies* include cysts or sinuses along the anterior edge of the sternocleidomastoid muscle. *Thyroglossal duct cysts* are usually in the ventral midline.

CHEST. The chest of the normal newborn is barrel-shaped. Respiratory excursion is judged easiest in the lateral view of the upper chest because newborn infants breathe principally with their diaphragms. The excursion of the abdominal wall during respiration is also quite prominent. With normal respiration, chest and abdominal wall move together. When the airway is obstructed, or the lungs are stiff, the abdomen appears to enlarge and the chest cage to get smaller with inspiration (paradoxical breathing). The tissue between the ribs may be pulled in during inspiration. These *retractions* are normal during the first few minutes after birth. Thereafter, they are a sign of an abnormal lung, an obstructional airway, or an abnormal chest wall. Mild expiratory grunting and nasal flaring may be normal during the first few minutes after birth, but thereafter signals abnormality of the lung or chest wall. Chest wall respiratory movement should be laterally symmetric. If one side moves less or lags behind the other, this suggests a *pneumothorax,* an elevated paralyzed diaphragm from *phrenic nerve palsy,* or intrathoracic mass—such as herniation of bowel through a *diaphragmatic hernia.* However, absence of such findings does not rule out these lesions. Such lesions may also displace the heart; this can be detected by palpation. *Coughing* in the newborn period is abnormal and usually accompanies interstitial lung disease, such as viral pneumonia. There may be scattered moist rales shortly after birth, presumably due to intra-alveolar lung fluid, but these disappear in a few minutes, and are to be considered abnormal thereafter. Retained lung fluid is more noticeable after cesarean section; large volumes may pour from the mouth when such infants are briefly suspended upside down in the first 15 to 30 minutes after birth. Breath sounds may not be diminished despite marked compression of lung tissue by intrathoracic masses or tension pneumothorax, so that inequality of breath sounds is a valuable sign, but equality of sounds can be misleading.

Prominent bowel sounds heard over the upper chest are another clue to *diaphragmatic hernia.* A murmur extending through systole, and best heard to the left of the sternum in the fourth interspace, is common and is caused by blood flowing through a small *patent ductus arteriosus* (p. 1409). *Premature auricular contractions* are common and apparently not significant. Supraventricular tachycardia, when present, is usually caused by maternal drugs, such as ephedrine, but can be present with myocarditis, or occur spontaneously without evidence of heart disease (p. 1397).

The most common birth injury to the thoracic region is fracture of the clavicles. This is identified by crepitations on rubbing a finger over the length of the clavicle while applying gentle pressure. Supernumerary nipples are a relatively common minor anomaly of the chest wall.

ABDOMEN. The abdomen is normally rather flat in comparison with the chest. An extremely flat or hollow abdomen suggests absence of some of the normal contents, with a *diaphragmatic herniation* of the bowel. Distention suggests dilation of the bowel from functional or anatomic obstruction, accumulation of ascites, blood, or a large mass. Congenital malformations that cause *bowel obstruction* are a relatively common and serious problem; clues to their presence should be sought routinely. Polyhydramnios in the mother or aspiration of more than 20 ml of fluid from the infant's stomach at birth suggests such obstruction.

When a soft plastic catheter is passed through the nose to rule out anatomic airway obstruction, it should then be advanced into the stomach, the contents aspirated, and the volume noted. This should be a routine part of the initial examination in the delivery room. Successful passage of the tube into the stomach suggests, but does not guarantee, that the esophagus is patent.

The common form of *tracheoesophageal fistula* includes proximal esophageal atresia, which does not allow passage of the tube. A small amount of air injected through this catheter, and hearing the resulting noise with a stethoscope on the epigastrium, is usually taken as evidence that the tube has reached the stomach. However, it may still be in the thorax in a blind esophageal pouch with the sounds transmitted over the surface of the chest to the abdomen. If tracheoesophageal fistula is suspected, it is better to pass a catheter with a radiopaque line in it, to check, with a roentgeongram, that it has reached the stomach. Some of the less common forms of tracheoesophageal fistula permit passage of the tube into the stomach.

Vomiting, particularly bile-stained, should suggest bowel obstruction. However, with lower bowel obstructions, vomiting may not occur until late. Absence of passage of any meconium suggests bowel obstruction, but passage of meconium does not rule it out; meconium is commonly passed after birth in infants with small bowel atresia. Peristaltic waves of bowel activity are faintly visible normally over the abdomen. If they are pronounced, this is abnormal. Edema of the abdominal wall occurs with peritonitis.

The *umbilical cord* normally contains two arteries and one vein. The vein is larger than the arteries. The cord should be examined for the presence of these vessels at or soon after birth. A little less than 1 percent of all newborns have only a single umbilical artery; approximately 15 percent of these infants have one or more congenital anomalies, usually involving the neural crest, gastrointestinal, genitourinary, pulmonary, or cardiovascular systems. Among infants with a single umbilical artery who survive the neonatal period, the incidence of serious anomalies later in life is no greater than among infants with two umbilical arteries.

During the first week after birth, the cord dries, becomes yellow, then brown and brittle. Toward the end of the first or during the second week, it usually falls off, releasing a very small amount of opaque yellowish discharge. Occasionally, it remains for several weeks longer. During the first week, a small amount of faint erythema of the skin on the rim of the umbilical stump is common and of no consequence, but more extensive or deep-red erythema, or associated edema, may indicate the onset of omphalitis. This should be considered a serious infection because of the pathway provided by the umbilical vein for spread of the infection into the portal venous sinus in the liver. When this occurs, there often is an erythematous streaking of the skin from the umbilical stump upwards towards the liver.

There is commonly a small defect in the periumbilical musculature of the anterior abdominal wall, which may allow an umbilical hernia. This is rarely, if ever, significant in itself and usually closes as the muscles grow during later infancy and childhood. However, there are several serious defects of the anterior abdominal wall. In an *omphalocele,* some of the abdominal contents pass out through a periumbilical defect in close approximation with the umbilical cord, and the extra-abdominal viscera are covered with fetal amniotic membrane. The extent of the lesion varies widely from one that includes most of the bowel, liver, and spleen at one extreme, to a small bit of peritoneum in the umbilical cord, at the other. The more serious lesion is obvious. The smaller lesion presents a different problem, because a small bit of intestine, extending a short way into the umbilical cord, may not be recognized at birth and can be clamped and cut as the umbilical cord is being tied and cut. *Gastroschisis* results from primary failure of the lateral ventral folds of the developing abdominal wall to close, so that small and large bowel pass out of the abdominal cavity through the defect. Unlike an omphalocele, the herniated bowel is not associated with the umbilical cord and has no covering. Absence of the musculature of the anterior abdominal wall (the so-called *prune belly* infant) is one of the multiple anomalies of Potter's syndrome.

The *liver* is normally palpable 2 to 3 cm below the right costal margin. The liver edge of the normal newborn infant is not sharp and its lower edge may not be felt if palpation is too high or too forceful. The spleen may be palpable 1 cm below the left costal margin. In a variety of pathologic conditions the liver or spleen may be so enlarged that their edges are in the pelvis and may not be recognized by an inexperienced examiner (Fig. 12). The lower edge of the liver may extend down into the lower quadrant of the abdomen on the right side and far over and down into the upper quadrant on the left, where it is often mistaken for an enlarged spleen. A massively enlarged spleen may extend down almost to the iliac crest on the left.

The lower half of each kidney is easily palpable normally. The lower edge is located approximately at the level of the umbilicus about half way between the midline and the side. The right kidney is most easily felt in the supine infant. The examiner flexes the infant's hips with the left hand to relax the abdominal muscles. The right hand is placed, with the palm over the lower right thorax, with fingers extending down over the abdomen, then slowly pressing deeply with the fingers, sweeping them in a cephalad direction. To feel the left kidney, one reverses sides of the baby and the position of the hands. Normally, the palpable portion of the kidney feels as though it is about 2 to 3 cm wide. It is usually possible to distinguish enlarged kidneys, an absent, hypoplastic, horseshoe, or pelvic kidney. Enlarged kidneys may be due to a neoplasm, congenital malforma-

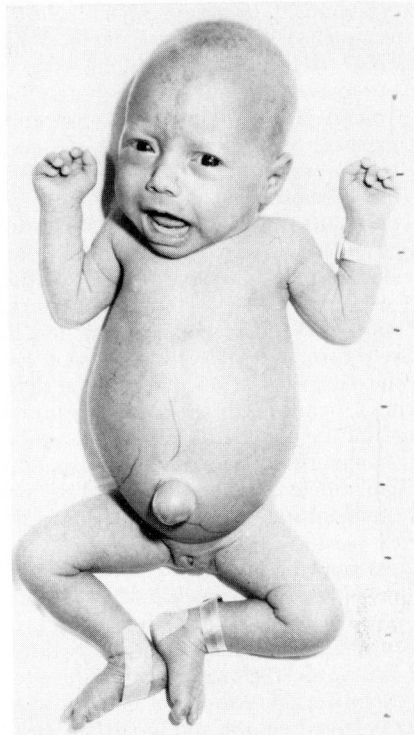

FIG. 12.   Abdominal distention and an umbilical hernia secondary to massive hepatosplenomegaly in an infant recovering from congenital cytomegalovirus infection. The black line on the baby's right side shows the lower edge of the liver, that on the left side below the level of the umbilicus shows the edge of the spleen.

tion, or renal vein thrombosis. They are also often enlarged transiently following a period of severe asphyxia or shock, or in the neonatal hyperviscosity syndrome. Other common masses in the abdomen result from obstruction of the genitourinary system, gastrointestinal tract, or neoplasms.

Serious birth trauma involving the abdomen includes rupture of the spleen, with free blood in the peritoneum; subcapsular hematoma of the liver, which presents as an enlarging liver and elevated right diaphragm; and adrenal hemorrhage, which presents as a discrete palpable mass above the kidney often accompanied by fever. These are usually preceeded by breech delivery and cause shock. With splenic rupture, splenomegaly usually had been present in utero.

EXTERNAL GENITALIA.   The labia minora of the normal newborn girl are quite prominent, meet in the midline, and are completely covered by the labia majora. It is important to identify the urethra, which is normally quite obvious just below the clitoris, and the vagina as distinct orifices; a single orifice or urogenital sinus is abnormal. Normally, white secretions are present in the vagina and on the labia, secondary to fetal stimulation by maternal hormones. These persist a week or more and occasionally are tinged with blood several days after birth. *Hydrometrocolpos* results from an imperforate hymen or from vaginal atresia. While this is most often a serious problem in adolescence when a girl begins to menstruate and there is no pathway for drainage of blood, it can present in the newborn period as a bulging mass protruding through the labia and requires decompression.

The normal newborn male has a penis approximately 3 to 4 cm long and 1 to 1.3 cm wide, and a scrotum that is pigmented and has extensive rugae. Usually the testes are descended into the lower part of the scrotum. *Hydroceles* are quite common at birth, rarely require treatment, and must be distinguished from inguinal hernias that need to be corrected. *Hypospadias* is a very common anomaly, which can vary from a small ventral cleft at the distal end of the penile urethra to a major ventral defect in the length of the penis. Chordee, a ventral bend in the penis, commonly accompanies hypospadias. *Epispadias,* a similar defect on the dorsum of the penis, is much less common, and is considered to be a variant of *extrophy of the bladder.*

Ambiguous genitalia present a common problem in the newborn. Mild masculinization of the female with some enlargement of the clitoris usually can be distinguished from mild feminization of the male with a small penis and hypospadias. However, when the processes are more extensive, the distinction between a female, with a very enlarged clitoris and a partially fused and pigmented labia, and the male, with a very small penis and extensive hypospadias and bifid scrotum, are much less clear (p. 1695).

Trauma to the external genitalia is quite common with breech delivery. In addition to ecchymoses, there may be hemorrhage into testes, scrotum, and pelvic muscles, sometimes to a massive degree. This generally resolves in a few weeks. It is not known whether there are any permanent sequelae in testicular function. Torsion of the testes can occur in the newborn male and is often present at birth, apparently having occurred in utero. The testes are enlarged and firm, with discoloration and induration of the overlying scrotum, but without the vomiting or pain so prominent in such cases in older males.

Imperforate anus is not always obvious on inspection. There may be an imperforate anus with a fistula leading to an opening through the skin of the perineum, ventral to the normal anus, but the fistula will not have the radiating skin creases of a normal anus. There may also be a normal-appearing anal dimple with no opening. Presence of meconium on the perineum and perianal area does not rule out imperforate anus, because this may have passed by way of the skin fistula or via a fistula from the rectum to lower genitourinary tract, which allows meconium to reach the perineum and perianal area. In the male, a fistula allows meconium to appear in the urine.

SPINE.   The spine of the newborn is quite flexible in both the dorsoventral and the lateral axis and restricted movement suggests vertebral anomalies. The entire length of the spine, including the sacrum, should be palpated for bony defects and asymmetries. Midline abnormalities of the skin over the spine, eg, small dimples, tufts of hair, or pilonidal sinuses, may indicate a tract that can allow bacteria on the skin to reach the cerebrospinal fluid. The major neural crest defects of the spine include meningocele, meningomyelocele, and rachischisis. The relatively common tumors of the spine present at birth are teratomas and dermoids.

LIMBS.   Abnormalities of the limbs are quite common in newborn infants. Trauma is common, and approximately 5 percent of all newborn infants have deformities due to positional abnormalities, intrauterine posture, or true malformations (Fig. 13). It is very important to distinguish between joints in one extreme of their normal position and those that are deformed. For example, it is quite common to see feet with ankles extended, rotated inward, or metatarsals deviated medially to give the impression of major structural malformations of foot and ankle. Yet, when the foot is dorsiflexed, one sees that it moves up and down along the axis of the tibia. This shows that the ankle joint is in proper alignment; gentle pressure will untwist the metatarsals so that the foot returns to a normal shape. Usually, if simple manual pressure will correct a deformed joint back to its neutral position and a bit beyond, corrective positioning or simple exercise and stretching will correct the deformity.

About 2 percent of all infants have deformities thought to be due to an intrauterine position that restricted motion and forced the limbs, spine, or face into an abnormal shape. These are proportionally more common among term infants and particularly after prolonged oligohydramnios, presumably because of the greater restrictions in intrauterine motion. Identifying the presumed intrauterine posture by finding the in-

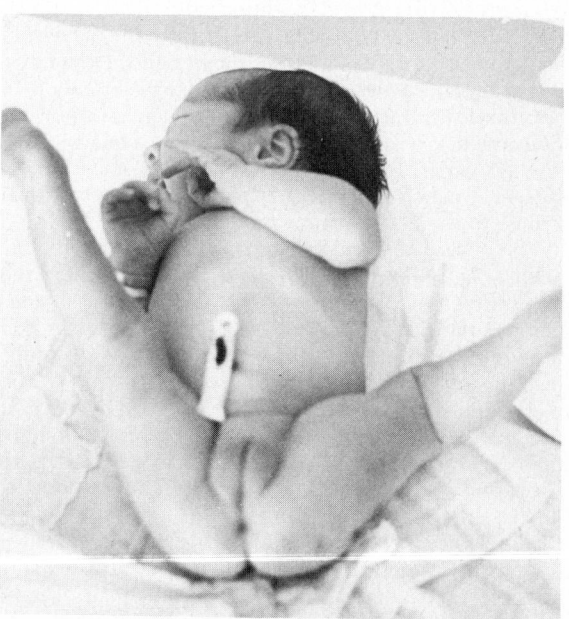

FIG. 13.   Deformities secondary to a frank breech presentation and delivery.

fant's position-of-comfort is very helpful in determining which deformities may be due to this cause. Bands believed to come from the amnion may wrap tightly about a limb and cause a sharp deep circumferential depression. These intrauterine constriction bands may even amputate the digits.

If the hips are flexed to 90°, the legs normally can be abducted until the knees touch the table upon which the infant lies. If this cannot be done, or if the maneuver can only be done on one side, there may be *congenital dislocation of the hip.* In this condition, the head of the femur is displaced posteriorly out of the acetabular fossa. If one hip is dislocated, the affected leg appears shorter and, when viewed from behind, there may be asymmetry of the major gluteal creases. By flexing the hips and palpating the greater trochanters of the femurs one can also detect asymmetry. These signs are not always present and two diagnostic manipulations of the hip joint must be used to be certain there is not a dislocatable hip. These are the Ortolani and the subluxation maneuvers, illustrated and described in detail on p 2029.

With *hemihypertrophy and hemiatrophy* the limbs on one side of the body are noticeably smaller but normally proportioned. With *phocomelia* there is underdevelopment and abnormal shape of the limbs to a variable degree (Fig. 14). The arms may be flipper-like structures with small digits projecting from the end, or there may be no more than a nubbin of tissue at the usual origin of the limb. This was particularly common among infants whose mothers took the drug thalidomide during pregnancy, but it has also occurred spontaneously. The short limbs of *achondroplastic* and *thanatophoric* dwarfs are evident at birth (Fig. 15). Newborns with the severe form of *osteogenesis imperfecta* have limbs that are grosssly deformed by multiple fractures. Newborns with *arthrogryposis multiplex congenita* have severe contractions which involve multiple joints; these cannot be corrected by simple manual pressure.

The most obvious anomalies of the hands and feet are fusions of digits (*syndactyly*) and excess digits (*polydactyly*). The latter may be well-formed extra digits or just small tags of tissue. A number of minor malformations of hands and feet occur in many of the dysmorphic syndromes. Some of the more obvious are the clenched hand, with overriding index finger, the convex or *rocker bottom* foot in Trisomy 18, the widely spaced first and second toes and hands with simian crease, and downward displaced origin of thumbs and underdeveloped incurved little fingers in Down's syndrome (Fig. 4).

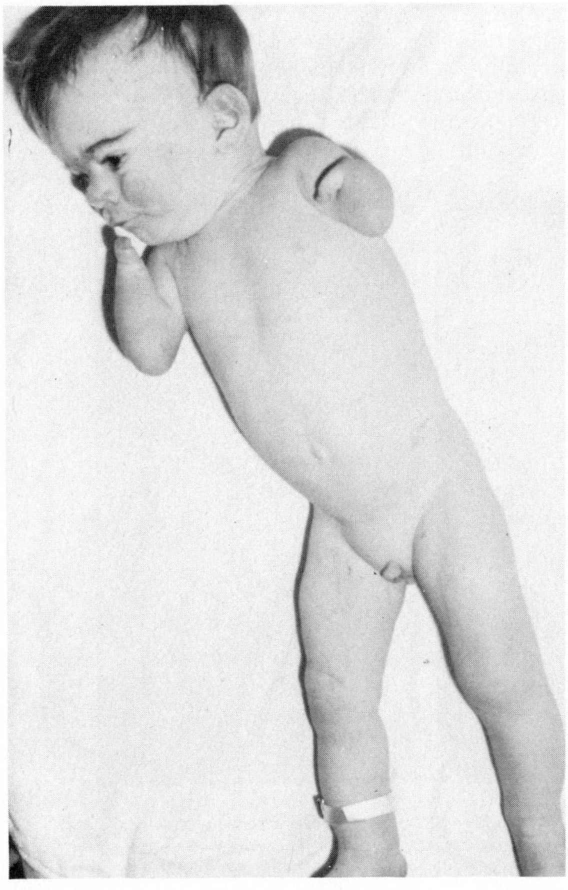

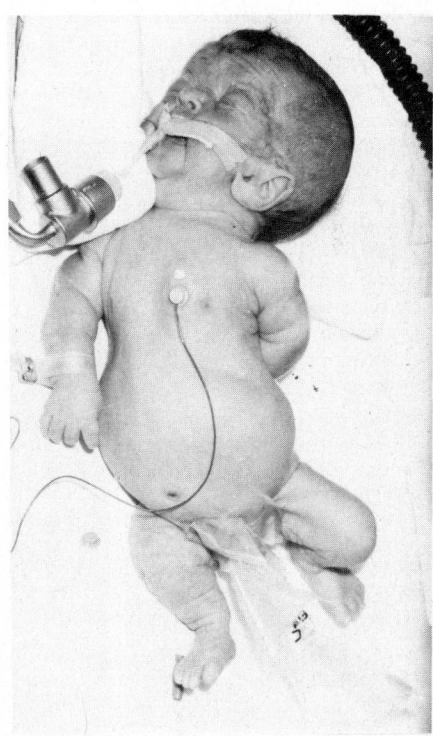

FIG. 15. Achondroplastic dwarf. Note the disproportionately short limbs and large skull. The child was probably a homozygous achondroplastic and had more severe respiratory disease than is usual in achondroplasia (note the endotracheal tube for assisted ventilation).

FIG. 14. Phocomelia.

Common forms of trauma of the limbs include the fractures of the shaft of the femur or humerus and trauma to the cervical nerves causing Erb's palsy, or Klumpke's paralysis of the arm. In Erb's palsy, injury to the 5th and 6th nerves paralyzes the deltoid and upper arm muscles. In Klumpke's paralysis, injury to the seventh and eighth nerves paralyzes the forearm. More extensive injury, which causes complete brachial palsy, is less common. With either fracture or nerve injury, the affected region is immobile. Similar immobility occurs with the pseudoparalysis of congenital syphilis, which involves a bone.

PHYSICAL CHARACTERISTICS OF THE PREMATURE INFANT

General body posture and activity vary with the gestational age of the premature infant. Younger infants lie with limbs unflexed and move about intermittently with flailing movements. Neuromuscular behavior is discussed in detail on p 155.

SKIN.   At 26 to 28 weeks, the skin of the premature infant is deep pink, almost plethoric. There is very little subcutaneous tissue, and the skin folds are only a few millimeters thick. The skin has a translucent, gelatinous appearance, the underlying small vessels are clearly visible, and there is edema over the dorsum of the hands, feet, and anterior tibia. By about 32 weeks, the skin is smoother, thicker, the underlying vessels are seen less

easily, and edema is no longer present. By 36 weeks, it is a light-pink color.

Vernix covers the entire body until 36 to 38 weeks, then decreases. Long and thick lanugo covers the body and face in very premature infants. This diminishes with age, and vanishes from the face and lower back between 32 and 37 weeks. Thereafter it is most prominent over the upper back and disappears completely after term. Meconium staining of the skin is a reliable sign of intrauterine asphyxia only after 32 to 34 weeks gestation. Before that, a fetus does not usually pass meconium when asphyxiated.

HANDS AND FEET.   Before about 32 weeks the fingernails do not reach the ends of the fingertips. The soles of the feet have transverse creases. With increasing gestation, these creases become deeper and cover more of the sole, as shown in Figure 16.

HEAD.   Before 38 weeks, the skull bones are soft and spongy next to the fontanelles. The hair on the scalp is wooly and clumps together before 36 weeks. Eyebrows and lashes are absent before 24 to 27 weeks. The ears of the premature are less well formed and have less supporting cartilage (Fig. 17); before about 32 weeks they are so flexible that when folded forward on itself, the ear will remain in that position. After that time, it will spring back to its normal position.

BREASTS.   The breast nodule is absent before about 36 weeks, and grows in diameter over the next 4 weeks to the 7 to 10 mm size, which is normal for the term infant. Before 34 weeks, the areola and nipple are flat and barely visible. These increase thereafter; and

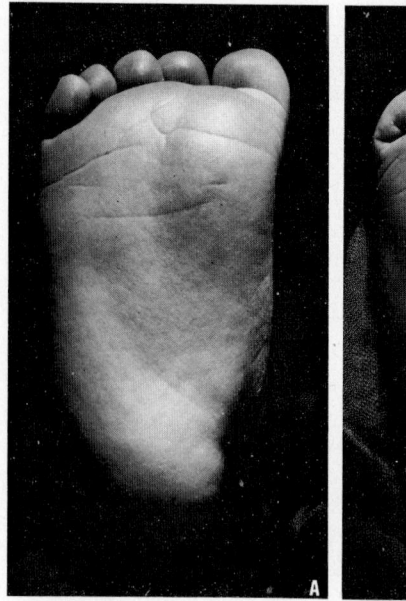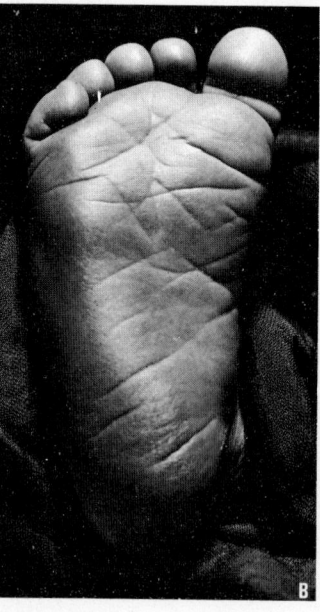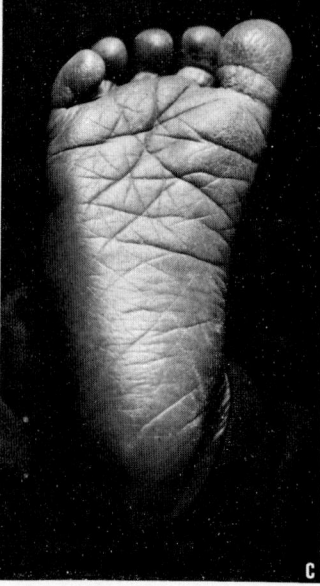

FIG. 16.   A. Foot of an infant of 36 weeks gestational age, showing posterior three-quarters of the sole is smooth. B. Foot of an infant of 38 weeks gestational age, showing some sole creases. C. Foot of an infant of 40 weeks gestational age, showing a complex series of creases extending the whole length of the sole. (From Usher: Pediatr Clin North Am 13:842, 1966).

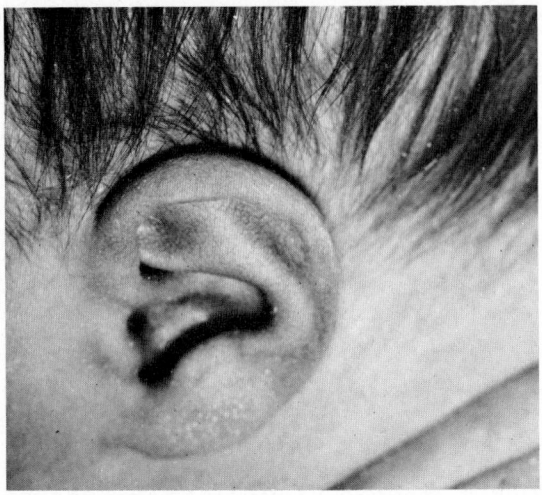 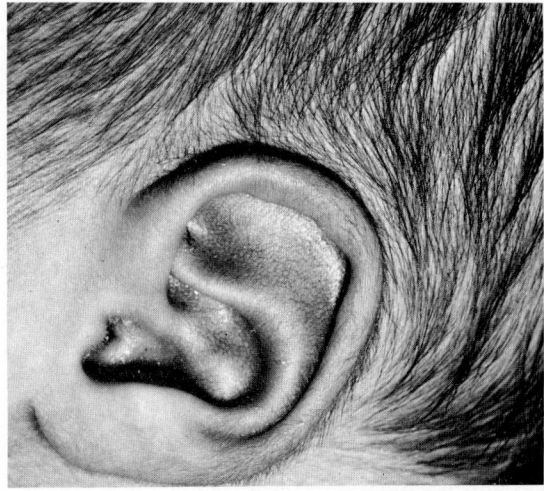

FIG. 17. A. The ear of an infant of 40 weeks gestational age, showing a more rigid earlobe stiffened with cartilage. The hair is rather coarse, each hair being visible separately. B. The ear of an infant of 36 weeks gestational age showing a relatively shapeless, pliable structure with little cartilaginous support. The fineness of the hair can also be seen. (From Usher: Ped. Clin North Am 13:844, 1966.)

the areola becomes stippled and the nipple raises by term.

EXTERNAL GENITALIA. At 29 to 36 weeks gestation, the clitoris and labia minora are very prominent and are not covered by the labia majora, which are widely separated. Later they become partly covered and, by 40 weeks, are completely covered by the labia majora. Before about 36 weeks, the scrotum has few rugae and the testes are high in the scrotum or in the inguinal canal.

Bibliography

Bryan EM, Kohler HG: The missing umbilical artery. Arch Dis Child 49:844, 1974

Dubowitz LMS, Dubowitz V, Goldberg C: Clinical assessment of gestational age in the newborn. J Pediatr 77:1, 1970

Dunn PM: Congenital postural deformities: perinatal associations. Soc Med Proc 65:11, 1972

Popich GA, Smith D: Fontanels, range of normal size. J Pediatr 80:749, 1972

Ralis ZA: Birth trauma to muscles in babies born by breech delivery and its possible fatal consequences. Arch Dis Child 50:4, 1975

Smith D: Recognizable Patterns of Human Malformations. Philadelphia, Saunders 1970

OBSERVATIONS AND CARE
Roderic H. Phibbs

BODY TEMPERATURE. The newborn is likely to lose a great deal of body heat after birth. He remains unclothed much of the time to allow adequate observation. He is usually exposed to a very low ambient temperature in the delivery room, which is often drafty as well, and at birth his skin is covered with amniotic fluid. Thus, he will lose heat by radiation, convection, and evaporation. If measures are not taken to prevent heat loss, body temperature commonly falls to 34C, sometimes lower. The infant responds to this by increasing heat production by catecholamine release, which stimulates metabolism in brown fat. He also attempts to conserve heat by decreasing skin blood flow. The metabolic demands of these responses may double the infant's oxygen consumption. However, hypoxic infants do not respond with any increase in heat production. The response can also be blocked by warming the skin, even though the central body temperature remains subnormal. The stress of this hypothermia significantly worsens the condition of a sick infant.

Usually this problem can be prevented by measures that decrease heat loss. Drying the infant with an absorbant towel immediately after birth, and keeping him wrapped in a warm dry towel or blanket between examinations in the delivery room, will eliminate much of the heat loss. Aluminum foil wrappers designed to enclose the infant's head and body (but not the face) also reduce heat loss. Performing delivery room assessment and resuscitation (if needed) under a radiant warmer also reduces heat loss. However, radiant heaters cannot be used casually. They are capable of causing serious burns of the skin, or overheating the infant; hyperthermia also increases the infant's metabolic requirements and oxygen consumption. The radiant heaters can also cause vasodilation, which may expand vascular capacity and lower arterial blood pressure.

During the first several hours after birth, when the infant undergoes frequent observation, he can be nursed unclothed in an incubator kept at *neutral temperature*. This is the temperature and humidity at which heat loss is minimal and metabolic demands and oxygen consumption are the lowest. For the normal term newborn, this is in the range of 31C to 34C at 50 percent humidity. For a baby clothed, covered with a blanket, and in an open crib, but not exposed to a draft, the temperature is 24C (close to usual room temperature). Alternatively, a radiant warmer can be used, again with the mentioned precautions.

During this period, body temperature should be measured and recorded repeatedly. The relevant temperature is that of the central body or core temperature. Skin temperature may be much lower than this, particularly in a chilled infant in whom skin blood flow will probably be lowered in order to conserve body heat. Rectal temperature is a good indicator of core temperature, but if a firm temperature probe is left in the rectum without constant attention from a nurse, it can perforate the large bowel. Axillary temperature is generally a suitable and safe alternative. The range of normal temperature is 36.5 to 37.2C. When an infant is in an incubator, both the infant's temperature and that of the environment inside the incubator should be monitored and recorded to determine the significance of changes in body temperature. A sudden rise in body temperature can be due to a rise in incubator temperature. But a rise of body temperature above normal, while incubator temperature remains constant, suggests fever and a serious infection.

When an infant is hypothermic, he must be warmed in an incubator or radiant warmer. It is generally best to rewarm at a moderate rate, usually taking 2 to 4 hours to reach normal. Rapid rewarming requires more external heat, which will induce irregular respiration and apnea in premature infants and may be potentially hazardous even in the term newborn. Excessively slow rewarming exaggerates the adverse effects of hypothermia and is accompanied by metabolic acidemia.

CARDIOPULMONARY FUNCTION. Heart rate, blood pressure, respiratory rate, quality of respirations, and color of skin and mucous membranes should be measured or observed and the findings recorded frequently during the first 6 hours after birth when the most threatening cardiopulmonary diseases appear. Thereafter, observations can be less frequent if the infant appears well. In the first 10 minutes after birth, the average heart rate is 160 beats/minute, but it varies from 120 to 200. Thereafter, the average is 120 to 130 (range 90 to 175). The average respiratory rate is 60/minute (range 20 to 100) in the first hour, decreasing to an average of 50 (range 20 to 80) between 2 to 6 hours of age. Respiratory rate varies widely in an individual newborn, and the high upper limits of normal are the highest rates an individual should reach during these variations. An infant with a respiratory rate consistently near the upper limit of normal may be ill. After 6 hours of age, the normal respiratory rate is 30 to 40 (range 20 to 60). The pattern of breathing varies within an individual newborn. Approximately 30 percent of the time the infant has a very regular rhythm, 60 percent of the time it is irregular, and 10 percent of the time there are recurrent brief (about 3-second) pauses.

The range of normal for indirectly measured blood pressure is 65 to 95 mm Hg systolic and 30 to 60 mm Hg diastolic. Pressure varies with birthweight, tending to be higher in heavier babies. Pressure generally falls about 5 mm Hg over the first 1 to 2 hours after birth.

GASTROINTESTINAL FUNCTION. The response of the infant to its first feeding must be observed carefully. Then, such anomalies as tracheoesophageal fistula might become evident. Newborns commonly regurgitate a few milliliters of feeding; vomiting of larger amounts or of bile-stained material suggests disease. During the first days, some infants have large amounts of white mucous material in the stomach, repeatedly regurgitate small amounts, and have difficulty in feeding. Orogastric lavage with saline removes this and improves the infant's feeding. Nutritional intake is measured by the volume of formula taken for bottle-fed babies, and by the change in weight before and after feeding in breast-fed infants. Intake should be noted and recorded.

Passage of meconium usually occurs during the first 6 hours, but may not occur until 24 hours and, rarely, not until 48 hours after birth in a normal infant. The quality of stools during the first week changes from the tarry green-black of meconium, to green, then yellow. The consistency is that of thick or thin paste, and often nonhomogenous, with tiny well-formed particles dispersed in the very loose material. However, normal stools are not watery. During the first week, a newborn infant usually passes three to five stools per day, but may pass up to 10 per day. Breastfed infants tend to have darker yellow or greenish stools, compared with babies who are fed cow's milk formula. Blood in the stools of newborns is commonly maternal blood that was swallowed either at the time of delivery by cesarean section or during breast-feeding, when the mother had a bleeding nipple. This is easily distinguished from the infant's blood by tests that distinguish between adult and fetal hemoglobin.

URINARY FUNCTION. Newborns usually pass urine within 6 hours after birth, often at the time of delivery; however, a few normal infants do not void until 48 hours. A record-keeping system will alert the physician to the infant who has not passed meconium or urine in the normal time.

BODY WEIGHT. The normal newborn loses approximately 5 percent of its birthweight during the first 2 to 4 days and is usually beginning to regain weight before 1 week of age. Weight loss of more than 10 percent is considered abnormal. Length does not change appreciably during this period. Head circumference may decrease by up to 1 cm if a great deal of scalp edema was present at birth and subsided. In many other infants, it increases by 0.5 to 1.0 cm during this time, with relief of the molding that occurred during labor. In others it does not change at all.

TREATMENT OF THE NORMAL NEWBORN INFANT

The only treatment regularly required is prophylaxis to the eyes to prevent gonococcal opthalmia, vitamin K_1 oxide to prevent hemorrhagic disease of the newborn, and care of the umbilicus to prevent its serving as a culture medium for pathogenic microorganisms, the most dangerous of which are clostridia. Cord care is best accomplished by leaving the umbilical cord exposed to air and daily swabbing with alcohol, which dries out the cord so that it becomes a poor culture medium. Never cover it with a moist or airtight dressing. Topical application of antiseptic agents to the cord may reduce colonization, but unless there is an increase in colonization by staphylococci in the nursery, they are usually not necessary.

Newborn infants must be tested for phenylketonuria, preferably 24 hours or more after the onset of feeding. Testing of every infant before discharge from the hospital ensures that all are tested, but such early testing will miss about 10 percent of cases. Routine testing only at a later date (2 to 4 weeks), which would detect the remaining 10 percent, has the disadvantage that many infants might not return for this test and so might not be screened at all.

The time a newborn infant spends in the hospital nursery is not only a period for observation but also for educating the mother. By the time an infant and its mother are discharged, she should have received sufficient practical instruction in caring for her infant so that she is skilled and confident in feeding, bathing, generally caring for her baby and understanding its behavior well enough so that she will not be startled by normal infant behavior. The discharge examination of the infant should be done in the mother's presence, if possible, so she has ample opportunity to question the physician about findings she may think are abnormal. At the time of discharge, there must be definite arrangements for the subsequent well-baby care of the infant. In addition, the mother should be advised that if her infant becomes sick in the near future and she goes to another hospital or doctor for care, the nursery where the baby was cared for after birth must be informed. When a nursery has an outbreak of a serious contagious infection, such as bacterial diarrhea or staphylococcal infection, the first cases often develop signs after discharge and are treated at another facility. Unless the original nursery is informed, there may be a serious delay before they are aware of the problem and take corrective measures.

Bibliography

American Academy of Pediatrics: Recommendations for Hospital Care of Newborn Infants. Evanston, Ill, 1975

Dahm LS, James LS: Newborn temperature and calculated heat loss in the delivery room. Pediatrics 49:504, 1975

Desmond MM, Franklin RR, Vallbona C, Hill RM, Plumb R, Arnold H, Watts J: The clinical behavior of the newlyborn. I. The term baby. J Pediatr 62:307, 1963

Hey E: Thermal neutrality. Br Med Bull 31:69, 1975

Knittle MA, Eitzman DV, Baer H: Role of hand contamination of personnel in the epidemiology of gram-negative nosocomial infections. J Pediatr 86:433, 1975

Motil KJ, Blackburn MG, Pleasure JR: The effects of four different radiant warmer temperature set-points used for rewarming neonates. J Pediatr 85:546, 1974

Stern E, Parmelee AH, Akiyama Y, Schultz MA, Wenner WH: Sleep cycle characteristics in infants. Pediatrics 43:65, 1969

EVALUATION OF THE NEUROMUSCULAR SYSTEM OF THE INFANT

CLAUDINE AMIEL-TISON

GENERAL PRINCIPLES

Neuromuscular evaluation is especially important in the neonatal period. Neurologic behavior varies markedly with gestational age, and its systematic evaluation is the most reliable component of the estimation of gestational age by physical examination. In addition a variety of intrauterine processes may interfere with development of the central nervous system (CNS), and the neurologic assessment of the newborn infant provides the first opportunity to test for these. Also, sick newborn infants are particularly vulnerable to CNS injury, which may cause a permanent handicap in childhood; repeated assessment of neurologic function and development from the neonatal period through the first months of life is important in detecting and evaluating such injuries.

Brain maturation is extremely rapid during the last few months of intrauterine life and in early infancy. As a result, the clinical expression of brain damage in the newborn and the older infant will depend upon the stage of maturation. Brain damage that occurred during the first day of life may not fully express itself until later in infancy. In addition, because normal behavior varies with maturation, one must compare neurologic findings to the normal-for-age in attempting to detect evidence of brain damage.

The first part of this section reviews in detail a method of neuromuscular examination of the newborn, which places particular emphasis upon evaluation of posture, passive and active muscle tone, and the presence of specific reflexes. It outlines the normal findings in newborn infants of differing gestational ages and the changes in findings that occur normally during the first year of life. The second part briefly reviews some of the common abnormal findings in the neonate.

NEUROLOGIC DEVELOPMENT

Cerebral maturation during the last 3 months of fetal life brings about constant modification of muscle tone and of some reflexes. This is the basis of a system whereby the neurologic maturity of the premature infant at different ages can be assessed. In applying this system to small-for-dates babies with type II retardation (see p 173), it has been concluded that brain development during fetal life progresses independent of unfavorable gestational circumstances. Chronic fetal stress is reflected mainly in birth weight and, to a lesser degree, in body length at birth; the brain evolves more in proportion to the gestational age. Thus, an undergrown infant born at 36 weeks of gestation may have a weight which is normal for a 30-week infant and a length normal for 32 weeks but will usually have the neuromuscular behavior of a 36 week infant. The assessment of maturity thus enables intrauterine growth retardation to be recognized.

The main lines of evolution between 28 and 40 weeks gestational age are the progressive increase of tone in flexor muscles, reaching a predominantly flexor posture at 38 to 42 weeks. Muscle tone increases first in the distal segments, proceeds in a caudocephalad direction, and flexor hypertonicity is generalized at term. After birth, passive tone of the flexors remains very strong for the first 3 months, while active tone increases. During the second 3 months, there is a marked diminution of passive tone and further increase in active tone. In the third 3 months passive tone of the flexors decreases further, while extensor tone increases, which is a prerequisite for the infant assuming an upright posture. This assessment does not duplicate the mental and motor scales of infant development.

METHOD OF NEUROLOGIC EXAMINATION

Examination and measurement of the head has already been discussed (p 145). The examination immediately after birth should be followed by a second examination 2 or 3 days later, as the muscle tone changes in the days following birth. The examination should be done when the infant is as wide awake as possible. If he is sleepy, muscle tone becomes much more relaxed and primary reactions are then slow or absent. The best time is about 1 hour prior to a feeding. The state of quiet alertness is essential to obtain most of the responses. Corrected age must be calculated for prematures until the end of the first year.

POSTURE AND SPONTANEOUS ACTIVITY

Spontaneous posture is best appreciated by inspection of the infant while he lies undisturbed.

TONE OF THE NECK EXTENSORS. At all stages of development, when the infant is lying supine in the resting position, the neck is flat, the muscles relaxed, and there is no free space between the neck and the bed. When the neck extensors are hypertonic, the supine infant cannot lie flat and there is a free space between the neck and the bed. This produces a lateral decubitus resting position with the head extended (Fig. 18). This sign may be difficult to interpret in a premature infant with a prominent occiput.

Opisthotonos is hypertonia of the extensor muscles of the spine. The hypertonic muscles arch the back so that the supine infant is unable to lie flat. The extensor muscle contraction sometimes can be provoked in the supine infant by putting the hand behind the neck and lifting, by contact stimulation of these muscles.

HAND CLOSURE. The fists of a newborn are usually closed. However, when the infant is sleeping or very quiet, the hands open and close spontaneously. After 2 months, the hands are open most of the time. After 3 months, the hands are more active. Persistent closure of the hands with the thumb across the palms is abnormal.

Permanent closure of the hands and delayed prehension are abnormal and often coexist with constant abduction of the arms and flexion of the forearms.

ASYMMETRY OF LIMB POSITION. With the head in the axis of the trunk, the posture of the upper and lower extremities should be almost identical. A persistent difference is due to asymmetry in passive tone, unless it can be explained by intrauterine position (see p. 150 Fig. 13).

Facial paralysis is best seen when the infant cries. The affected side of the face is flat and motionless and the eye remains open; on the normal side the lids are closed and the mouth appears to be drawn to the normal side. Passive rotation of the head modifies tone in the limbs; this is the postural asymmetric tonic neck reflex. The arm and leg on the side to which the head is turned become extended, the arm and leg on the other side become more flexed. This reflex is common in the first months after birth.

SPONTANEOUS MOTOR ACTIVITY. Spontaneous motor activity is best evaluated by inspection of the infant while he lies undisturbed. The speed, intensity, and amount of movement vary a great deal in the normal infant and only the most obvious alterations should be considered abnormal. *Incessant tremor* (high frequency, low amplitude) is frequently observed during the first days of life in normal full-term newborn infants who are hungry and crying. It is most readily noted on the extremities and mandible. It is usually abnormal if it occurs during periods of quiet and after the first week. A *burst of clonic movements* (low frequency, high amplitude) is commonly observed as part of the Moro reflex and during spontaneous motor activity in the first hours after birth; these movements are abnormal when they occur frequently or during sleep. *Dyskinetic movements* are sudden extension and pronation of

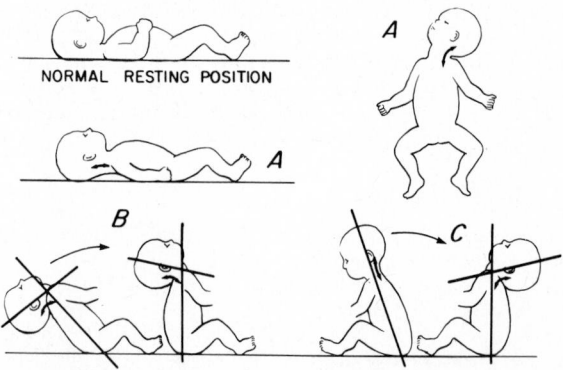

NORMAL RESTING POSITION

A

A

B

C

ABNORMAL HYPERTONIA IN NECK EXTENSORS

FIG. 18. When the neck muscles have normal tone, the supine infant lies flat with no space between neck and surface. When the neck extensors are hypertonic the neck is lifted off the surface and the infant assumes a lateral decubitus posture (A). When the infant with hypertonic neck extensors is lifted from the supine position, the neck remains extended (B) even when the long axis of the body is 90° (C).

the arms, with extension of the leg and foot lasting a few seconds without movement. These are due to transitory contractions of muscle groups and occur spontaneously or can be evoked by examination. They are usually abnormal at all gestational ages. Generalized tonic-clonic seizures are uncommon but, when they occur, the clonic movements are limited to small twitches. More often, a seizure is only tonic, with opisthotonos, extension and elevation of a limb, and/or rotation of the head and eyes. Following these seizures, the infant is hypotonic and has a brief apneic period; these are always abnormal.

Status epilepticus often has a rapid onset and is easy to recognize when clonic movements are present. These occur after prolonged asphyxia and may present as rapidly progressing hypertonia with major clonic movements. Between the fits, disturbances of consciousness and muscle tone persist. More often, seizures are atypical, with such signs as brief hypertonia, chewing movements, or a high-pitched cry. Persistence of coma or erratic and inefficient breathing with apneic episodes should suggest status epilepticus in an infant recovering from birth asphyxia or with birth trauma.

PASSIVE TONE

The examiner can evaluate passive tone by observing and manipulating the infant while he is quiet but not asleep. The resistance of an extremity to these manipulations is measured by noting the angle formed by the movement. During these maneuvers, keep the infant's head in midline position to avoid eliciting the asymmetric tonic neck reflex. The maneuver must be performed slowly and gently, to the point of being uncomfortable. The prematurely born infant is hypotonic and muscle tone increases as gestation advances. Figure 19 shows the changes in passive tone with differing gestational age at birth and Figure 20, the changes from birth through infancy.

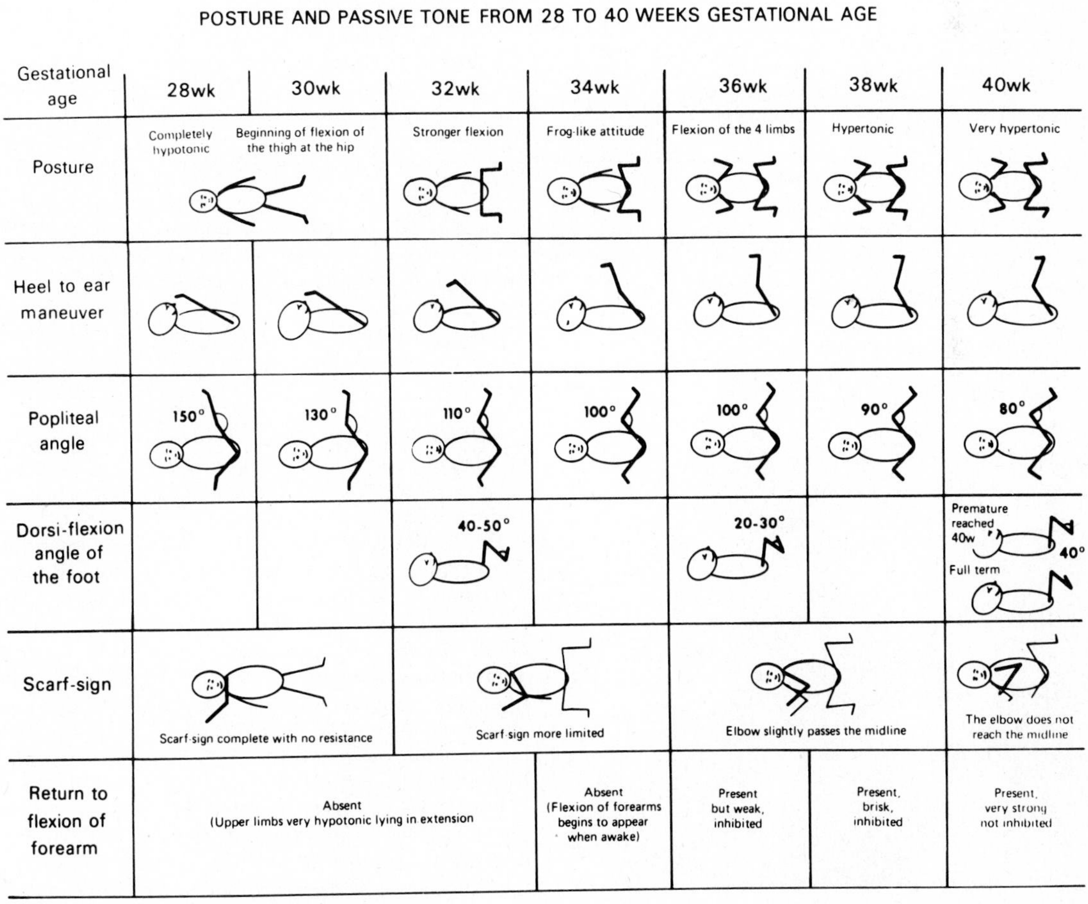

POSTURE AND PASSIVE TONE FROM 28 TO 40 WEEKS GESTATIONAL AGE

Gestational age	28wk	30wk	32wk	34wk	36wk	38wk	40wk
Posture	Completely hypotonic	Beginning of flexion of the thigh at the hip	Stronger flexion	Frog-like attitude	Flexion of the 4 limbs	Hypertonic	Very hypertonic
Heel to ear maneuver							
Popliteal angle	150°	130°	110°	100°	100°	90°	80°
Dorsi-flexion angle of the foot			40-50°		20-30°		Premature reached 40w 40° / Full term
Scarf-sign	Scarf-sign complete with no resistance		Scarf-sign more limited		Elbow slightly passes the midline		The elbow does not reach the midline
Return to flexion of forearm	Absent (Upper limbs very hypotonic lying in extension			Absent (Flexion of forearms begins to appear when awake)	Present but weak, inhibited	Present, brisk, inhibited	Present, very strong not inhibited

FIG. 19. Posture and passive tone from 28 to 40 weeks gestation, indicating the increasing muscle tone in upper and lower extremities which develop with increasing gestational age.

PASSIVE TONE IN THE FIRST YEAR OF LIFE

AGE IN MONTHS	1 2 3	4 5 6	7 8 9	10 11 12
ADDUCTORS ANGLE	40° to 80°	70° to 110°	100° to 140°	130° to 150°
HEEL TO EAR	80° to 100°	90° to 130°	120° to 150°	140° to 170°
POPLITEAL ANGLE	80° to 100°	90° to 120°	110° to 160°	150° to 170°
DORSIFLEXION ANGLE OF THE FOOT	60° 70°	60° 70°	60° 70°	60° 70°
SCARF - SIGN	①	②	③	③
CONSTANT CLOSURE OF THE HANDS	tolerable	no		

FIG. 20. Adductor, hip flexor, popliteal and foot dorsiflex tone during the first year of life. The inner arc and stippled area indicate the minimal angles that are normal. The scarf sign indicates the tone of the shoulder muscles. With the head and chin in the midline, the flexed elbow cannot cross the midline from 1 to 3 months (1), just crosses the midline between 4 and 6 months of age (2), and after 7 months of age can be brought to a position near the lateral border of the body (3).

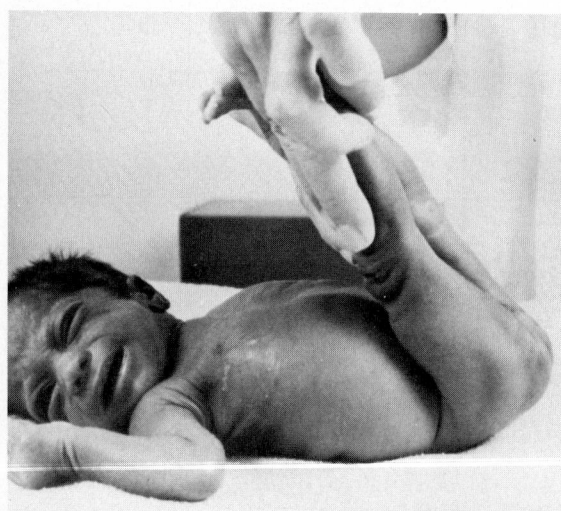

FIG. 21. Heel-to-ear maneuver in a 33-week gestation infant.

ADDUCTOR ANGLE. With the infant lying supine, extend both legs and gently pull them laterally as far as possible. The angle formed by the two legs is the adductor angle.

HEEL-TO-EAR (FIG. 21). With the infant lying flat, lift the legs as far as possible in an attempt to reach the ear with the feet. Record the amplitude of the arc traversed by the legs without lifting the pelvis from the table. If more resistance is felt on one side, the tone is asymmetric. When flexor tone is strong, as in term infants, the popliteal angle is less than 180° during this maneuver. The angle to be measured is the one formed between the table and the infant's heels, not the one formed between the examining table and the thigh.

POPLITEAL ANGLE (FIG. 22). While maintaining the pelvis flat on the table, flex the thigh at the hip to achieve a knee-chest position, then lift the lower segment of the leg and observe the angle between the two legs formed with the thigh, ie, the popliteal angle.

DORSIFLEXION ANGLE. Dorsiflex the foot with the leg extended at the knee, applying pressure

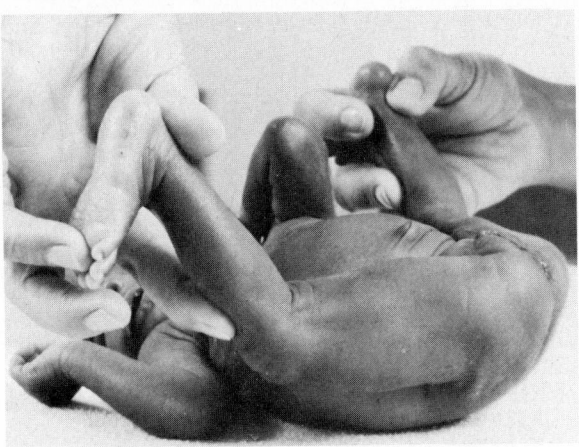

FIG. 22.   Popliteal angle in a 31-week gestation infant.

encircles the neck. The prematurely born infant can assume position (c), the term infant can be moved only to position (a).

FOREARM RECOIL. This can be checked only when the infant is in a spontaneously flexed posture. With the infant supine, fully extend the arm by pulling on the hands, and release; observe how quickly the forearm returns to a position of flexion. If recoil is observed, extend the arms again for 20 to 30 sec, then release them and note if the prolonged extension inhibits the recoil. Recoil increases with increasing gestational age and inhibition disappears.

SQUARE WINDOW ANGLE. Flex the hand on the forearm as much as possible and measure the angle formed between the palm and ventral aspect of the forearm. The angle increases with increasing gestational age.

HAND FLAPPING. When the hand is flapped at the wrist, the amplitude of the movement is symmetrical.

LATERAL ROTATION OF HEAD. Turn the head toward each shoulder, evaluating the resistance of the contralateral muscles. The amplitude of the movement decreases with increasing gestational age and any striking asymmetry is abnormal.

REPEATED VENTRAL FLEXION OF HEAD. After flexing the neck several times, the resistance felt by the examiner normally is unchanged. Increasing resistance after four to five times is abnormal.

VENTRAL FLEXION OF TRUNK. Grasp the flexed legs and pelvis and push them toward the head, flexing the trunk. The amount of flexion decreases with increasing gestational age. It is abnormal if the amplitude is increased such that the knees can be moved quite close to the chin, or decreased so that no flexion at all is achieved.

EXTENSION OF THE TRUNK. Put the infant on his side and, while stabilizing the lumbar spine with one hand, pull both legs backwards with the other hand. The amplitude of this movement is normally very limited (close to zero). It is abnormal if exaggerated such that a dorsal curve is achieved or if the dorsal curve is greater than the curve achieved with ventral flexion.

with the thumb to the sole of the foot. The angle formed by the dorsum of the foot and the anterior aspect of the leg is the dorsiflexion angle. This movement should be carried out twice, first slowly, then quickly. A difference of 10° or more between the slow and the rapid maneuver is abnormal. This angle decreases with increasing gestational age. Unlike most such changes, this represents a decrease in tone (of the posterior muscles of the leg) probably due to stretching by intrauterine posture during the last months of intrauterine life.

FOOT FLAPPING. The foot is flapped at the ankle. The amplitude of the movement imparted should be roughly symmetrical.

SCARF SIGN. The infant's arm can encircle the neck like a scarf. Place the infant in a semireclining position, and use the palm of the hand to support the neck; keep the head straight. Take the infant's hand and try to pull the arm across his chest toward the opposite shoulder, continuing as far posteriorly as possible; observe the position assumed by the elbow in relation to the umbilicus. Three positions are described: (a) the elbow does not reach midline; (b) the elbow passes midline; or (c) there is very ample movement and the arm

TABLE 4. Change in Active Tone from Birth to 1 Year of Age

AGE IN MONTHS	1	2	3	4	5	6	7	8	9	10	11	12
HEAD ERECT AND STEADY		Inconstant						Present				
SITS ALONE MOMENTARILY PULLS TO SITTING POSITION		Absent			Inconstant				Present			
SITS ALONE 30 SECONDS OR MORE		Absent					Inconstant			Present		
STRAIGHTENING WITH LOWER LIMBS AND TRUNK	Present inconstant				Absent			Possible not sustained			Present	

Note: Trunk and leg straightening, which is present at birth, disappears by 3 months and then reappears at 10 months of age.

LATERAL FLEXION OF THE TRUNK. With the infant lying supine, stabilize the flank with one hand and pull the legs to the right, attempting to achieve a bend of the trunk. Repeat on the left side. This movement, depending on the tonicity of contralateral muscles, is normally limited and should be symmetrical.

ACTIVE TONE

The examiner studies active tone when the infant moves spontaneously in response to a given stimulus. The infant must be well enough to allow manipulation of his head and trunk. Figure 23 and Table 4 show the changes in active tone with gestation and with age after birth.

NECK FLEXORS. (Fig. 24) Grasp the shoulders and pull the supine infant to the sitting position while noting the position of the head in relation to the trunk. Somewhat before the vertical position is reached, one can observe that the flexor muscles contract to raise the head. In the full-term infant, extensor and flexor tone is nearly balanced and the head is maintained for about 3 to 5 seconds in the axis of the trunk. The test is abnormal in the term infant if (a) the head, which is

pendulant at first, is pulled passively past the midline and immediately drops forward, or (b) if permanent hypertonicity of neck extensors maintains the head backward and keeps the head from falling downward with gravity at the end of the maneuver.

NECK EXTENSORS. (Fig. 25) With the infant sitting and leaning forward, and the head hanging down on the chest, move the trunk backward and observe the reaction of the head. Before the vertical position is reached, a reaction of the extensors will raise the head in the term infant. It is abnormal if (a) the head, which is pendulant at first, is pulled passively, passes the midline, and drops backward; or (b) if the head, unable to hang on the chest at the beginning of the movement, is maintained strongly by the extensors and passes backward too quickly in such a way that the reaction appears "too good."

SITTING POSITION. With the infant lying on its back, the examiner offers the thumbs and allows the infant to pull himself to a sitting position. With the infant in this position, with legs in semiflexion and spread at an angle of about 50°, the normal term infant can sit without further support for 30 seconds or more. Two abnormal responses may be observed in infants in

ACTIVE TONE FROM 32 TO 40 WEEKS GESTATIONAL AGE

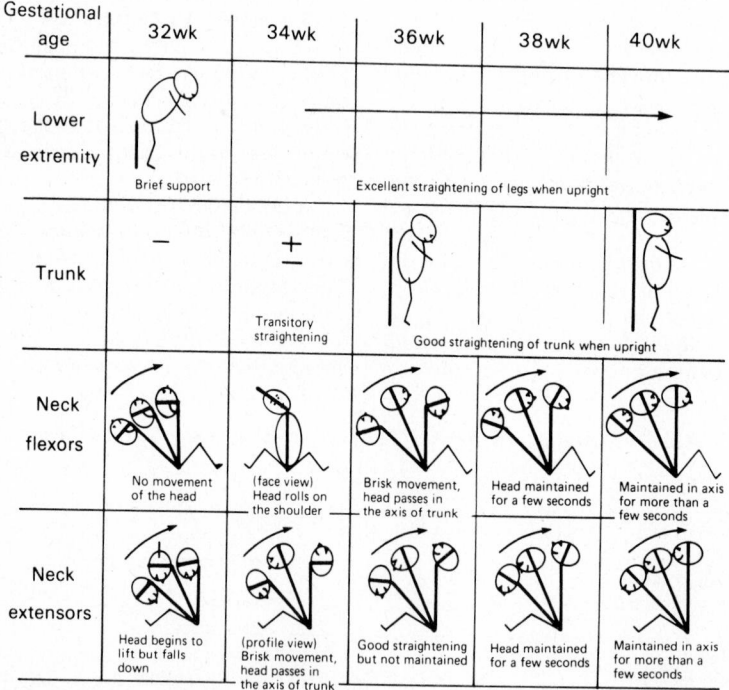

FIG. 23. Change in active muscle tone between 32 and 40 weeks of gestation. At 32 weeks there is only brief leg straightening when the infant is held upright; after 34 weeks leg straightening is excellent and prolonged. From 32 to 38 weeks there is gradual increase in the tone of the neck flexors and at 40 weeks the neck can be maintained in the axis of the trunk while the baby is raised. The neck extensors also gradually increase in tone, their strength being greater than the flexors from 32 to 38 weeks.

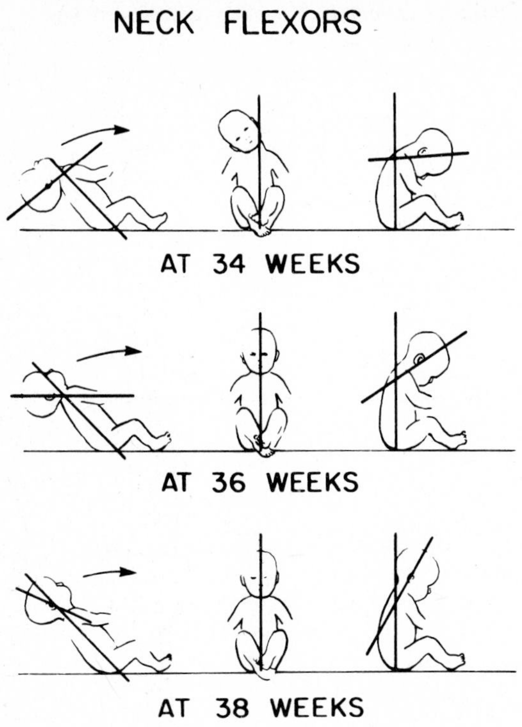

NECK FLEXORS

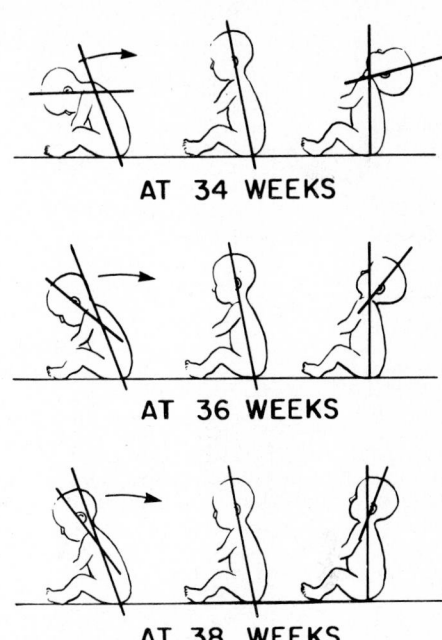

AT 34 WEEKS

AT 36 WEEKS

AT 38 WEEKS

FIG. 24. The neck flexors at three gestational ages showing increasing tone and neck stability.

NECK EXTENSORS

AT 34 WEEKS

AT 36 WEEKS

AT 38 WEEKS

FIG. 25. The neck extensors at three gestational ages showing increasing tone and neck stability.

whom the sitting position cannot be maintained even momentarily: (a) axis is completely hypotonic and the infant leans forward on the knees, or (b) the axis is very rigid and the infant falls backward.

GLOBAL STRAIGHTENING. Hold the infant in a standing posture with the examiner's hands in the axillae, supporting the chest anteriorly so that head and neck are supported, and observe if the legs straighten and the trunk muscles contract to allow the infant to support some of its own weight.

REFLEXES

The newborn infant has many reflexes, but only a few will be discussed. These are outlined and related to gestational age in Table 5; Table 6 shows the changes during infancy.

The examiner evaluates the *sucking reflex* by introducing a finger into the mouth and noting the strength, rhythmicity of sucking, and the synchrony of swallowing. Sucking is weak and asynchronous with swallowing at 28 weeks, is stronger and associated with some swallowing most of the time at 32 weeks, and strong with synchronous swallowing from 34 weeks.

PALMAR GRASP. The examiner inserts an index finger into the hand of the infant from the ulnar side and gently presses against the palmar surface; the palmar stimulation produces a flexion of the fingers onto the stimulating object. If the infant grasps and his hands draw upward, the response to traction spreads to the flexor muscles of the arm so that the normal term infant can be lifted from the bed completely.

MORO REFLEX. Lift the infant's shoulders a few centimeters off the bed by holding both hands in abduction while keeping the back of the head on the bed, then release the hands briskly at the point of maximum abduction. The normal reflex is a brisk abduction of the arms at the shoulder and extension of the forearms at the elbow, followed by adduction of the arms at the shoulder (an embrace) and flexion of the forearms at the elbow. Complete opening of the hands occurs during the first part. Crying is provoked consistently.

CROSSED-EXTENSION REFLEX. Hold one foot in extension and rub the sole. The complete response has three components: (a) extension of the opposite leg after a rapid flexion, or "retreating," (b) adduction of the opposite leg with the foot going toward the stimulated foot, and (c) fanning of the toes. Adduction is the most important component for evaluation of maturation, in which three stages can be described: no tendency to adduction; a tendency to adduct with repeated movements toward the stimulated foot but without reaching it; and complete adduction to the stimulated foot with or without crossing.

AUTOMATIC WALKING. Hold the infant by the trunk and tilt him forward slightly. When the feet contact a solid surface the infant begins to walk.

TABLE 5. The Strength of 6 Reflexes for Infants Between 28 and 40 Weeks Gestational Age

Gestational age(wk)	28	30	32	34	36	38	40
SUCKING REFLEX	Weak and not really synchronized with deglutition		Stronger and better synchronized with deglutition		perfect		
GRASP REFLEX	Present but weak				stronger		excellent
RESPONSE TO TRACTION	absent		Begins to appear	Strong enough to lift part of the body weight		Strong enough to lift all of the body weight	
MORO REFLEX	Weak, obtained just once, incomplete		Complete reflex——➤——➤——➤				
CROSSED EXTENSION	Flexion and extension in a random pattern, purposeless reaction		Good extension but no tendency to adduction		Tendency to adduction but imperfect	Complete response with —Extension —Adduction —Fanning of the toes	
AUTOMATIC WALKING	—	—	Begins tip-toeing with good support on the sole and a righting reaction of the legs for a few seconds	Pretty good. Very fast Tip-toeing		• A premature who has reached 40 weeks. Walks in a toe-heel progression or tip-toes. • A full term newborn of 40w. Walks in a heel-toe progression on the whole sole of the foot.	

TABLE 6. Changes in Reflexes During Infancy.

Reflex	1	2	3	4	5	6	7	8	9	10	11	12
					Age in Months							
ASYMMETRIC TONIC NECK REFLEX		Tolerable						Absent				
AUTONOMIC WALKING	Present	Inconstant						Absent				
PALMAR GRASP	Present											
RESPONSE TO TRACTION		Inconstant						Absent				
MORO REFLEX		Present inconstant						Absent				
LANDAU REFLEX		Absent or Inconstant			Present or not yet					Present		
LATERAL PROPPING REACTION			Absent			Inconstant				Present		
PARACHUTE				Absent		Inconstant					Present	

The asymmetric tonic neck, automatic walking, palmar grasp, and Maro reflex are the primary reflexes. They are abnormal after 4 months of age. The Landau, lateral propping, and parachute are the equilibration reflexes. They should be present by 10 months of age.

ANKLE CLONUS. With the leg relaxed, the infant quiet, and the leg flexed at the hip and knee, rapidly dorsiflex the foot. Ankle clonus consists of a series of rhythmic alternate flexions and extensions of the foot at the ankle. Clonus is abnormal if there are more than 10 beats during the first 3 months after birth, or more than 3 beats after this age.

THE LANDAU REFLEX. While holding the infant in ventral suspension with the head, spine, and legs extended, the examiner flexes the head passively. The reflex is present if the whole body flexes. Normally the reaction is present from the age of 3 months, and in normal infants is always present after 7 months of age.

THE PARACHUTE REACTION. (Fig. 26) Elicit this reflex by suddenly flinging the infant toward the examining table from a position of ventral suspension. The reflex is positive if the arms extend as if to protect himself from falling. This reflex is always present after 9 months of age in normal infants.

THE LATERAL PROPPING REACTION. When the examiner pushes the normal sitting child to one side, the arm on that side extends as if to brace the infant. This response appears between 6 and 8 months.

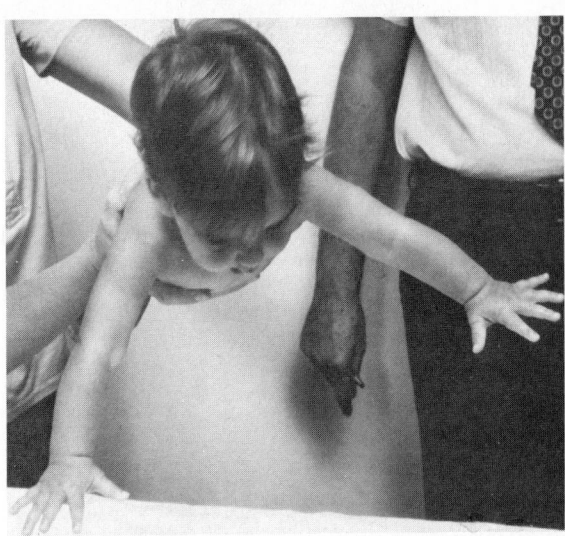

FIG. 26. Parachute reflex in a 10-month-old infant.

SENSORY DEVELOPMENT

There are two simple tests of sensory function:

PURSUIT OF LIGHT. The awake but quiet infant follows a light more readily than an object. The source of light may be a small light or a window with moderate brightness. The normal infant will turn its head toward the light and when the examiner turns its body to either side, the infant's eyes continue to fix on the light.

ACOUSTIC BLINK REFLEX. The normal infant closes his eyes when the examiner claps his hands 30 cm to the side of the ear.

EYES. Downward rotation of the globes, with the pupils partly covered by the lower lids and the sclerae visible above the pupils, is the *setting-sun sign.* It may be constant or elicited in the course of clinical examination. It is abnormal when the levator palpebrae superiori muscles are hypertonic; the lid retraction reveals the upper sclerae and pupil. This is not an isolated finding and is often associated with hyperexcitability. *Marked strabismus* may be convergent or divergent, uni- or bilateral.

SPECIAL STUDIES

The following are useful in evaluating infants with abnormal CNS findings. The *cerebrospinal fluid (CSF)* in otherwise normal infants may be yellowish and have a few hundred red blood cells per cubic millimeter. Less than 20 leukocytes per cubic millimeter and protein of 50 to 130 mg/100 ml is also normal. A *skull roentgenogram* shows the size of the sutures, digital impressions, and in trauma or infection may reveal fractures or periventricular calcifications.

TRANSILLUMINATION. This simple procedure may locate abnormal fluid spaces in the brain. In the normal premature, when a cuffed flashlight is held against the skull, there is a 1 cm halo on the skull around the edge of the light. Transmission of light through a larger area or asymmetrical transillumination is abnormal.

SUBDURAL TAP. Puncture of subdural spaces is mandatory if subdural hemorrhage is suspected or if there is a history of obstetric trauma in an infant with bulging fontanelle, coma, or convulsions from birth. The risk is not negligible; complications include bleeding or infections. *Ventricular taps* are dangerous and there are few indications for the procedure.

ABNORMALITIES OF THE CNS

Precise observation of neurologic signs is the first step in evaluation, but in the neonate, they are influenced by state of arousal, hunger or satiety, and the presence of systemic disease. Thus, initial findings must be used cautiously and follow-up examinations are a necessity. Infants with abnormalities observed throughout the neonatal period are at risk of developing late sequelae. Abnormalities from 1 to 12 months of age are associated with a high incidence of permanent neurologic damage. Abnormalities of the central nervous system are discussed in detail in Chapter 30.

ACUTE PERINATAL BRAIN DAMAGE

Acute brain injury after perinatal stress usually causes a clinical picture that changes rapidly, with progressive improvement and disappearance of initial symptoms. The most common causes of acute pathology are subarachnoid hemorrhages in prematurely born infants and cerebral edema in infants born at term.

Subarachnoid hemorrhage usually occurs in a prematurely born infant who has had asphyxia or birth trauma. These infants have hypertonic muscles, especially the neck extensors; irritability; high-pitched cry; and bloody spinal fluid. Improvement is rapid and by 1 week of age the neurologic abnormalities have usually disappeared. The mild, short course distinguishes these infants from those with large intracranial hemorrhages. When seizures or apnea occur and the above signs persist more than a week, cellular damage to the cerebral cortex probably has occurred or intraventricular or subdural hemorrhages may be present.

Brain edema is the main cause of neurologic abnormality in the mature newborn infant who suffered moderate to severe perinatal asphyxia. These infants are lethargic or irritable, and have decreased reflexes and hypotonic muscles. The cerebrospinal fluid may have an increased protein content, but is otherwise normal.

In both these syndromes, seizures are rare and are more likely to be due to hypoglycemia, hypocalcemia, meningitis, or cerebral necrosis. A detailed discussion of neonatal seizures is presented in Chapter 30.

Fetal Brain Damage

The infant who suffered brain damage earlier in fetal life has a very different pattern from the one with acute perinatal damage in that abnormal neurologic findings change quite slowly after birth.

HYPOTONIA AND HYPERTONIA

GLOBAL ANOMALIES. Abnormality of tone (compared to normal for age) can be generalized (with global hypo- or hypertonia) or limited to specific muscle groups.

Hypertonia of the extensor muscles of neck and spine (see above) is especially important to recognize. Intracranial hypertension, subarachnoid hemorrhage, or meningitis are the usual causes of these findings in the newborn infant.

HEMISYNDROME. Hypo- or hypertonia limited to one side of the body, trunk, or limbs, which produces an asymmetry of tone, is termed a *hemisyndrome*. Occasionally this is the precursor to spastic hemiplegia on the hypertonic side. However, the evolution of most of the hemisyndromes observed in the neonatal period is toward a slow diminution of this isolated asymmetry in passive tone and is without known significance.

Spastic hemiplegia is usually diagnosed between 4 to 6 months of age when the signs become striking: these appear first in the arm, with poor voluntary motility, no prehension, hypertonicity, exaggeration of biceps reflex. The same signs appear a month or so later in the leg.

Spastic diplegia can also be diagnosed with certainty at 4 to 6 months. Most of these infants have been born prematurely. The arms are either normal, or, more often, are used awkwardly and have athetoid movements. There is hypotonia of the neck and trunk. Spas-

ticity develops its full expression during these months, with increasing extensor tone. Infants who have some abnormalities in the first 6 months may improve rapidly between 7 and 8 months of age, and become normal by 1 year. They probably have *minimal brain dysfunction* and are at risk of having learning disorders at 5 to 7 years of age (p. 1764).

DELAYED MOTOR AND MENTAL DEVELOPMENT WITH HYPEREXCITABILITY. These infants continue to have hypertonic legs and the primary reflexes persist. The infants cannot sit, and some develop spastic diplegia a few months later. An infant has definitive *brain damage* or is at *high risk* of having learning problems later in childhood if abnormalities have been observed up to the end of the sixth month or if severe symptoms, such as coma and status epilepticus, have been observed in the neonatal period.

The child is in a *moderate risk* group if abnormalities have completely disappeared by the end of the first 3 months. If an infant is normal at all successive stages of development during the first year, the risk of having a neurologic handicap is extremely low. Even at 1 year of age, the prognosis for an individual child is an approximation. The minor neurologic abnormalities observed during the first year of life most likely indicate minor brain damage, even though the signs will often disappear toward the end of the first year.

Bibliography

Amiel-Tison C: Cerebral damage in full-term new-born. Aetiological factors, neonatal status and long-term follow-up. Biol Neonat 14:234, 1969

Amiel-Tison C: Follow-up of infants presenting neurological abnormalities in the first days of life. In Perinatal Medicine. Bern, Hans Hubert 1972, p 207

Amiel-Tison C: Neurological evaluation of the maturity of newborn infants. Arch Dis Child 43:89, 1968

Amiel-Tison C: Neurologic evaluation of the small neonate, the importance of head straightening reactions. In Gluck L (ed): Modern Perinatal Medicine, Vol 1. Chicago, Year Book Medical Publishers, 1975

Bauer CH, New MI, Miller JM: Cerebrospinal fluid protein values of premature infants. J Pediatr 66:1017, 1965

Bayley N: Bayley scales for infant development. New York, The Psychological Corporation, 1969

Beintema DJ: A neurological study of newborn infants. Clinics in developmental medicine, Vol 28. Spastics International Medical Publications, 1968

Bergstrom AL, Gunther MB, Olow I, Soderling B: Prematurity and pseudoprematurity; studies of the developmental age in underweight newborns. Acta Paediatr 44:519, 1955

Chaplin ER, Schlueter MA, Phibbs RH, et al: Fetal hemoglobin in the diagnosis of subarachnoid hemorrhage. Pediatrics (In press)

Craig WS: Convulsive movements occuring in the first 10 days of life. Arch Dis Child 35:336, August 1960

Cukier F, Amiel-Tison C, Minkowski A: Hyaline membrane disease in the neonates treated with artificial ventilation. Neurological and intellectual sequellae at 2 to 5 years of age. Criti Care Med 2, 265, 1974

Davies DP, Ansari BM, Cooke TJH: Anterior fontanelle size in the neonate. Arch Dis Child 50:81, 1975

Denhoff E, Hainsworth PK, Hainsworth ML: The child at risk for learning disorder, Can he be identified during the first year of life? Clin Pediatr 11:164, 1972

Dreyfus-Brisac C: The bioelectrical development of the central nervous system during early life. In Falkner F (ed): Human Development. Philadelphia, Saunders, 1966

Dreyfus-Brisac C, Monod N: Electroclinical studies of status epilepticus and convulsions in the newborn. In Kellaway P, Petersen I (eds): Neurological and Electroencephalographic Correlative Studies in Infancy. New York, Grune and Stratton, 1964

Drillien CM: Abnormal neurologic signs in the first year of life in low-birthweight infants: Possible prognostic significance. Develop Med Child Neurol 14:575, 1972

Illingworth RS: The Development of the Infant and Young Child, Normal and Abnormal, 5th ed. Edinburgh and London, Churchill Livingstone, 1972

Koroblin R: The relationship between head circumference and the development of communicating hydrocephalus in infants following intraventricular hemorrhage. Pediatrics 56:74, 1975

Minkowski A, Larroche JC, Vignaud J, et al: Development of the Nervous System in Early Life. In Falkner F (ed): Human Development. Philadelphia, Saunders, 1966

Myers RE: Two patterns of perinatal brain damage and their conditions of occurrence. Am J Obstet Gynecol 112:246, 1972

Peiper A: Cerebral function in infancy and childhood. New York, Consultants Bureau, 1963

Prechtl HFR, Beintema D: The neurological examination of full-term newborn infant. Little Club Clin Develop Med No. 12, 1964

Rabe EF: The hypotonic infant. J Pediatr 64:422, 1964

Rose AL, Lombroso CT: A study of clinical, pathological and electroencephalographic features in 137 full-term babies with a long-term follow-up. Pediatrics 45:404, 1970

Saint-Anne Dargassies S: Neurological maturation of the premature infant of 28 to 41 week's gestational age. In Falkner F (ed): Human Development. Philadelphia, Saunders, 1966

Thomas A, Chesni Y, Saint-Anne Dargassies S: The neurological examination of the infant. Little Club Clin Develop Med 1, 1960

Vignaud J: Radiological study of the normal skull in premature and new-born infant. In Falkner R (ed): Human Development. Philadelphia, Saunders, 1966

SUPPORTIVE CARE OF THE PREMATURE AND SICK NEWBORN INFANT

Roderic H. Phibbs

Prematurity

An infant born before 38 weeks gestation is preterm or prematurely born and may have a variety of problems in the neonatal period, which are proportional to the degree of prematurity. Most organ systems are undergoing continued structural and functional development during the last 3 months of intrauterine life. Premature birth requires adaptation to extrauterine life before these organ systems are adequately developed. As a result, such an infant may not be able to maintain his body temperature or to suck and swallow adequate amounts of food. He will become more jaundiced and more susceptible to the neurotoxic effects of unconjugated bilirubin. He also is more likely to have intrapartum asphyxia and respiratory failure after birth because of immature lung structure and function, or poorly developed respiratory control. He may have a widely patent ductus arteriosus with congestive heart failure. Some of these problems require oxygen therapy, but his incompletely developed retinal vessels are more susceptible to the toxic effects of oxygen (retrolental fibro-

plasia). Intraventricular hemorrhage is more common because of structural weaknesses in cerebral blood vessels and abnormalities of coagulation. Premature infants are more susceptible to infections, including acute necrotizing enterocolitis. All of these problems may be viewed as the consequence of temporary inadequacies of development.

Care of the premature infant is largely a matter of helping him compensate for these developmental deficiencies until his organ systems mature. Rather than briefly considering all the diseases and defects of prematurity in this section, these are covered in detail in the chapters dealing with the specific organ systems.

Supportive Care

Some of the aforementioned problems are unique to the premature infant. Most, however, are more common in the premature and may also occur in the full-term infant who is sick with such processes as serious cardiopulmonary disease, sepsis, or from a major congenital malformation or hemolytic disease. All such sick infants are usually cared for together in neonatal intensive care nurseries, so that it is logical to consider their supportive care together. It is estimated that about 60 of every 1000 liveborn infants require such care. The Committee on the Fetus and Newborn of the American Academy of Pediatrics has detailed recommendations on the hospital care of such infants.

OBSERVATIONS. Heart rate, respiratory rate, and blood pressure must be measured frequently in infants with or at risk of cardiopulmonary disease. Heart and respiratory rates are usually monitored by instruments that indicate if either variable exceeds acceptable limits. If an indwelling umbilical arterial catheter is in place, it should be used to measure blood pressure; otherwise an indirect method, such as a Doppler instrument, should be used. Indirect measurement by the

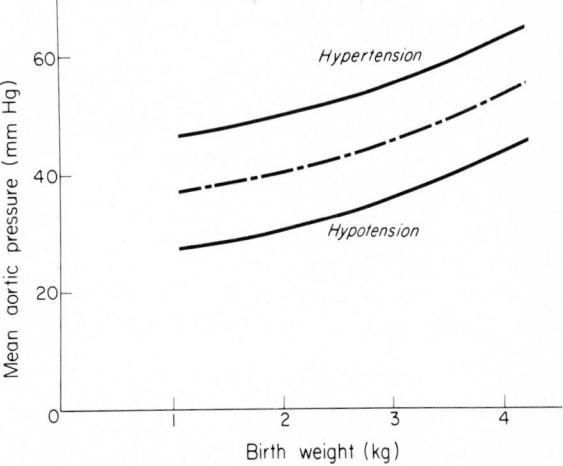

FIG. 27. Range of normal for mean aortic blood pressure for infants of different birth weights. The broken line is the average and the solid lines the upper and lower limits of normal.

flush method is often inaccurate in such infants. The average and range of normal blood pressure varies with birthweight (Fig 27). Intake and output of fluids must be recorded at least daily, and more frequently in critically ill infants. Head circumference should be measured at least weekly and growth compared with the range of normal.

TEMPERATURE. Body temperature must be maintained in the normal range either in an incubator or by radiant heat (see p. 153). The neutral thermal environment for infants in incubators varies both with birthweight and age after birth, as shown in Fig. 28.

FEEDING. Many of these infants cannot suck from a nipple and must be fed by tube. This should be done by an orogastric tube, since a nasogastric tube reduces the diameter of the upper airway by 50 percent and most infants are obligate nasal breathers. The tube must be passed by a skilled person who will not put it down the trachea.

Prematures with small gastric volumes must be given smaller and more frequent feedings (generally every 2 hours). At first they will only accept about 2 ml/kg per feeding. This is then increased by increments of about 1 to 2 ml/kg every feeding, or every other feeding, as tolerated. The volume remaining in the stomach must be checked by aspiration at the start of the next feeding; if the stomach empties completely, the volume of the next feeding can be increased. If not, the residual portion is returned along with enough additional milk to make the volume the same as the previous feeding. Experienced nursery nurses are far more skillful than most

physicians in managing the feeding of such infants, and their opinion should be sought as to whether an infant can tolerate a change in feeding. An increase in the residual volume in the stomach 2 hours after feeding is a nonspecific sign that the infant's condition may have worsened. Sepsis is one of the possible causes.

Some small prematures cannot tolerate such feedings. One reason is that arterial blood oxygen tension falls significantly without any change in carbon dioxide tension, 15 to 30 minutes after gavage feeding. Slow continuous feeding via a catheter left in place in the stomach or duodenum may be needed.

The quality and quantity of infant formula required is discussed on p 202. A premature infant can be breast fed by its mother, who can express her breast milk into a sterile container so it can be given by gavage as long as this route of feeding is required. There are nutritional, immunologic, and emotional advantages to this.

One must not be overzealous in making the small premature infant gain weight rapidly by giving large feedings. If this is done with milk formula of high protein concentration, the excess load of acid may produce a metabolic acidosis (the late metabolic acidosis or feeding acidosis of prematurity). A milk formula with a low solute load will give the infant an excess of water compared to solute; he will handle this by getting rid of the water in the urine but will lose sodium with it and become hyponatremic.

Hypoglycemia is common in the first days after birth in sick and premature infants. Its presence can be detected by testing capillary samples with Dextrostix.

PARENTERAL FLUIDS. Many of these infants require parenteral fluids with electrolytes and glucose when they are too ill to take adequate amounts of gavage. This is particularly true of very premature infants in the first days of life, when the provision of such parenteral fluids will substantially increase survival rate.

Fluid and electrolyte therapy is discussed on p 260; however, there are a few special problems for newborn infants. The amount of water necessary to maintain homeostasis varies, depending upon the rate of insensible water loss, which is governed by the environment. Insensible water loss varies between 25 and 50 ml/kg bodyweight/day in an isolation incubator, with the higher value occurring at lower birth weights. With this, fluid requirements will be 75 to 100 ml/kg/day to maintain a normal urine output (1 to 3 ml/kg/hour). Phototherapy increases insensible water loss and water requirements by about 10 to 20 ml/kg/day. Radiant heaters increase water loss much more, depending upon the particular type of unit used. Some cause insensible water losses as high as 100 ml/kg/day, which increase parenteral fluid requirements into the range of 150 ml/kg/day. The correct fluid requirements for a particular infant can be determined only by close observation of urine output and specific gravity, body weight, and serum electrolyte concentration. The usual type of fluid used is 10 percent glucose with 2–3 mEq/kg/day potassium chloride and 200 mg/kg/day calcium gluconate. The glucose in this solution is usually adequate to prevent hypoglycemia

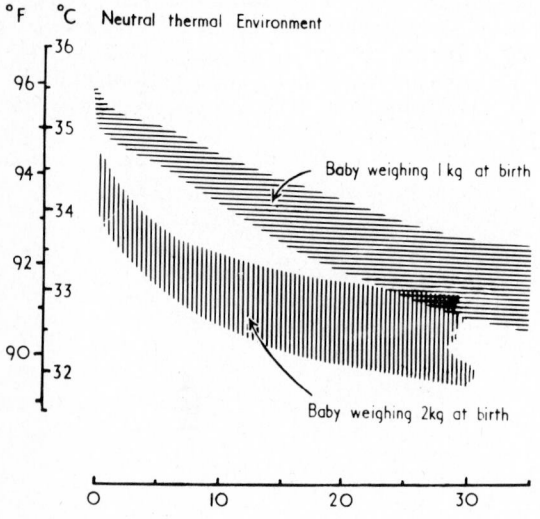

FIG. 28. The neutral operative temperature for a baby lying naked on a warm mattress in draft-free surroundings of moderate humidity (about 50 percent relative humidity) when mean radiant temperature is the same as air temperature. The hatched areas showed the average neutral temperature range for a healthy baby weighing 1 kg (=) and 2 kg (| | |) at birth. (From Hey and Katz: Arch Dis Child 45:328, 1970.)

and, at an infusion rate of 100 ml/kg provides 40 cal/kg/day; however, it presents two problems.

At higher infusion rates, the glucose infused may exceed the glucose utilization rate of the infant, resulting in hyperglycemia, particularly in smaller prematures. For example, a rate of 150 ml/kg/day (which is occasionally needed in a small premature under a radiant warmer) will provide about 10 mg/kg/minute glucose, whereas some very small prematures can utilize only 5 or 6 mg/kg/minute. Hyperglycemia can cause tissue dehydration and an osmotic diuresis from the glucosuria. This requires that the concentration of glucose be lowered.

The other problem occurs when the parenteral infusion is discontinued because the infant can be fed by mouth or by gavage. Abrupt cessation of such a solution will be followed by hypoglycemia. The infusion must be decreased gradually as oral feedings are increased. Blood and urine glucose should be checked regularly while an infant is receiving a glucose infusion and for 12 to 24 hours after it has been stopped.

INFECTION. Premature or sick newborn infants are particularly susceptible to infection, usually from organisms spread by the hands of their attendants or by equipment that acts as a bacterial reservoir. The first line of defense against this is careful hand washing by nursery staff and regular cleaning of equipment. Isolation incubators should be used when practical, although it is difficult to deliver optimal care to the most critically ill infant in an incubator. Isolation incubators filter the air drawn into the unit, not the exhaust, so the unit protects its occupant from the environment but not the reverse. If an infant infected with a contagious disease is put in an incubator, it does not protect other infants in the room. To do that, the others must all be put into incubators.

HYPERBILIRUBINEMIA. This is extremely common in sick newborns and premature infants. One cannot rely upon clinical jaundice to follow the course of hyperbilirubinemia in infants who are unclothed and exposed to radiant heaters. In such critically ill infants bilirubin must be measured repeatedly until it has passed its peak and begins to fall. Diagnosis and management of neonatal jaundice are discussed on p.1077.

VITAMIN K. Usually newborn infants require just a single 1-mg dose of vitamin K to prevent hemorrhagic disease of the newborn; the gastrointestinal tract is colonized with bacteria in the first week after birth and an adequate supply of K will be synthesized thereafter. However, this does not apply for many sick newborn infants who are not fed by mouth and are treated with antibiotics that affect bowel flora. Such an infant requires prophylactic doses of vitamin K (0.5 to 1 mg weekly) for as long as these conditions continue. Larger doses of vitamin K should not be given, as it is potentially toxic.

ANEMIA. Sick newborn infants are often anemic at birth or become so in the first week. Many with severe cardiorespiratory distress have increased red blood cell destruction; frequent sampling of blood also contributes to the problem. Hematocrit must be measured fre-

quently. Severe anemia may require transfusion with packed red cells, which must be crossmatched against the mother just as with blood for exchange transfusion (see p.1141).

OXYGEN THERAPY. Many sick newborn infants require oxygen therapy to relieve hypoxia at some time during their hospitalization. When it is necessary to increase inspired oxygen concentration, it must be administered with great care because a high partial pressure of oxygen (Po_2) in arterial blood in a premature infant is a major factor in the cause of retrolental fibroplasia, a retinal vascular disease that causes blindness (p. 1961).

Susceptibility to retrolental fibroplasia depends upon the state of development of the retinal vasculature and this, in turn, depends upon birthweight and gestation. However there is considerable variability between individuals of comparable gestation. Most cases occur in infants weighing less than 1500 g and it rarely, if ever, occurs in those over 2500 g. Current information suggests that the most susceptible infants can develop this disease when the Po_2 is above 100 torr for as short a period as 2 to 4 hours. Normal infants have a Po_2 of 50 to 90 torr, and sick infants should receive no higher oxygen concentration than that necessary to achieve this normal range. This will vary from individual to individual and from day to day in the same individual depending upon the state of the lungs and circulation. Forty percent O_2 can raise the Po_2 to 250 torr in an infant with normal lungs but 100 percent O_2 may not produce a Po_2 of 50 torr in an infant with severe pulmonary disease.

In infants with moderate or severe cardiopulmonary disease who need treatment with very high concentrations of oxygen or assisted ventilation, arterial blood gas tensions should be measured to detect hypoxia, hyperoxia, and hypercarbia in order to regulate therapy. This applies whether they are prematurely born or term infants. Po_2 also should be measured in premature infants with milder disease who need lower concentrations of oxygen, in order to prevent retrolental fibroplasia. This applies for any infant weighing less than 2500 g or who is below 36 weeks gestation who needs oxygen therapy for more than just a few minutes. Po_2 cannot be estimated from the color of the skin or mucous membranes with sufficient accuracy to prevent injury to the retina.

Oxygen therapy should be adjusted to maintain the Po_2 as nearly as possible between 50 and 90 torr. When the cardiac output and its distribution are normal, this is adequate for tissue oxygenation. Levels below 40 torr are also likely to depress respiration. The frequency of measurements depends upon the stability of the infant's cardiopulmonary status (discussed in sections dealing with specific diseases). Oxygen must be delivered by a system with an oxygen:air blender that reliably delivers any desired oxygen concentration between 21 percent and 100 percent. The actual concentration delivered to the infant's airway must be measured and recorded frequently.

Any prematurely born infant who has received oxygen therapy should have his retinae examined by indirect ophthalmoscopy for retrolental fibroplasia before discharge from the hospital and again in the second or third month after birth.

UMBILICAL VESSEL CATHETERIZATION. Indwelling catheters in premature and other sick newborns usually are passed through the umbilical vessels. They can be used for frequent measurements of cardiorespiratory function, for infusions of drugs, manipulations of blood volumes during resuscitation, and for exchange transfusion. The use of these catheters carries a small but definite risk, and should be limited to situations in which they are essential. They should not be inserted just as a route for parenteral infusions that can just as well be given through a peripheral vein. Careful attention to the anatomic location of the catheter and to the technique for its use will ensure that physiologic measurements are valid and reliable and the complications are kept to a minimum.

Catheterization of the umbilical vein has been common pediatric practice since it was introduced for exchange transfusions three decades ago. A catheter passed through the umbilical vein can end in a variety of locations, many of which are extremely dangerous (Fig. 29). For example, it can go down into the portal vein and obstruct venous return from a segment of bowel, curl up in the portal sinus of the liver and interfere with portal blood flow, go through the ductus venosus, up the inferior vena cava, through the foramen ovale and left atrium, and out into a pulmonary vein. All are dangerous sites for an indwelling catheter. In addition, physiologic measurements made in some of these locations can be very misleading. For example, portal venous pressure is higher than central venous or right atrial pressure and does not reflect the general state of the circulation. Failure to appreciate this can lead to an erroneous diagnosis of a high central venous pressure and congestive heart failure and can result in inappropriate therapy.

Generally, the best location for the umbilical venous catheter tip is the inferior vena cava near the right atrium. This gives a satisfactory measure of central venous pressure. The location of the catheter tip *cannot* be determined by the length of catheter inserted. As soon as the catheter is in place, its location must be checked radiologically. However, it is preferable to use pressure monitoring to determine the location of the catheter tip while it is being inserted. As soon as the catheter is in the vein 2 to 3 cm, it is connected to a pressure transducer and recorder. As the catheter is advanced, the pressure is measured and the pressure changes with respect to respiration are noted. If the tip advances through the ductus venosus into the inferior vena cava and toward the right atrium, both the pressure and the changes in pressure with spontaneous respiration will change as shown in Figure 30. Once localized, the position should be confirmed radiologically.

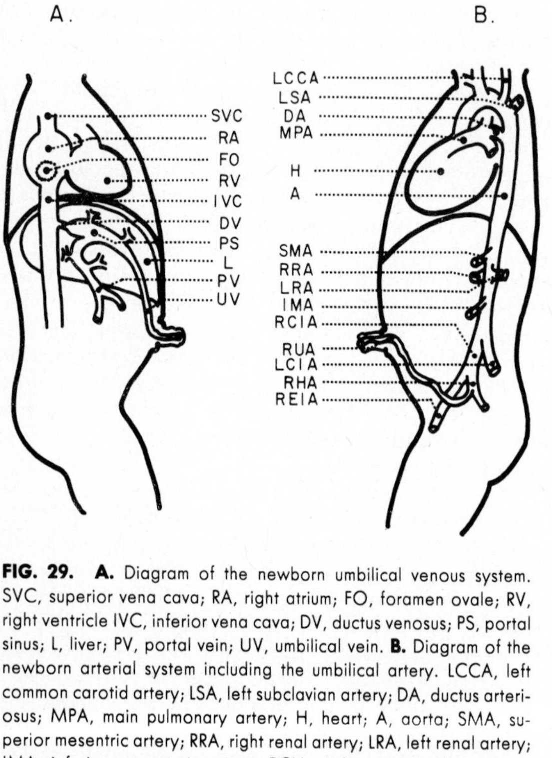

The *umbilical artery* is catheterized when measurements of arterial pressure and arterial blood gas tensions and pH are required. Figure 29B shows that a catheter through one of these vessels usually will pass into the descending aorta. If it is advanced too far up the aorta, it will usually pass through the ductus arteriosus, if patent, into the pulmonary artery. Pressure measurements and blood gas samples from that site will be misleading if this location is not appreciated. Clots can form on both the tip and the sides of this catheter; if they break loose, they may flow into and occlude any artery that originates downstream. Therefore, the catheter tip should be below the origin of the inferior mesenteric artery (at or below the level of the third lumbar vertebra). Tip position should be checked radiologically.

Catheters should be inserted by sterile surgical technique. The catheter should have a single end-hole to minimize clotting in the tip; catheters so designed are available commercially. Figure 31 is a diagram of a complete system for using catheters. Catheters must be kept filled with fluid and free of blood except when removing blood for sampling. As soon as possible after placing the catheter, it should be connected to a parenteral fluid infusion system, and the infant's parenteral fluid needs infused through it with 1 unit heparin added for each milliliter solution.

Major complications from catheters include hemorrhage from disconnected stopcocks, sepsis, air embolism from air injected, or aspiration if the venous catheter is left open to air, vascular spasm of a lower

A.   B.

LCCA
LSA
DA
MPA

SVC
RA
FO
RV
IVC
DV
PS
L
PV
UV

H
A

SMA
RRA
LRA
IMA
RCIA

RUA
LCIA
RHA
REIA

FIG. 29. A. Diagram of the newborn umbilical venous system. SVC, superior vena cava; RA, right atrium; FO, foramen ovale; RV, right ventricle IVC, inferior vena cava; DV, ductus venosus; PS, portal sinus; L, liver; PV, portal vein; UV, umbilical vein. **B.** Diagram of the newborn arterial system including the umbilical artery. LCCA, left common carotid artery; LSA, left subclavian artery; DA, ductus arteriosus; MPA, main pulmonary artery; H, heart; A, aorta; SMA, superior mesenteric artery; RRA, right renal artery; LRA, left renal artery; IMA, inferior mesenteric artery; RCIA, right common iliac artery; RUA, right umbilical artery; LCIA, left common iliac artery; RHA, right hypogastric artery; REIA, right external iliac artery. (From Kitterman, Phibbs and Tooley: Pediatr Clin North Am 17:895, 1970.)

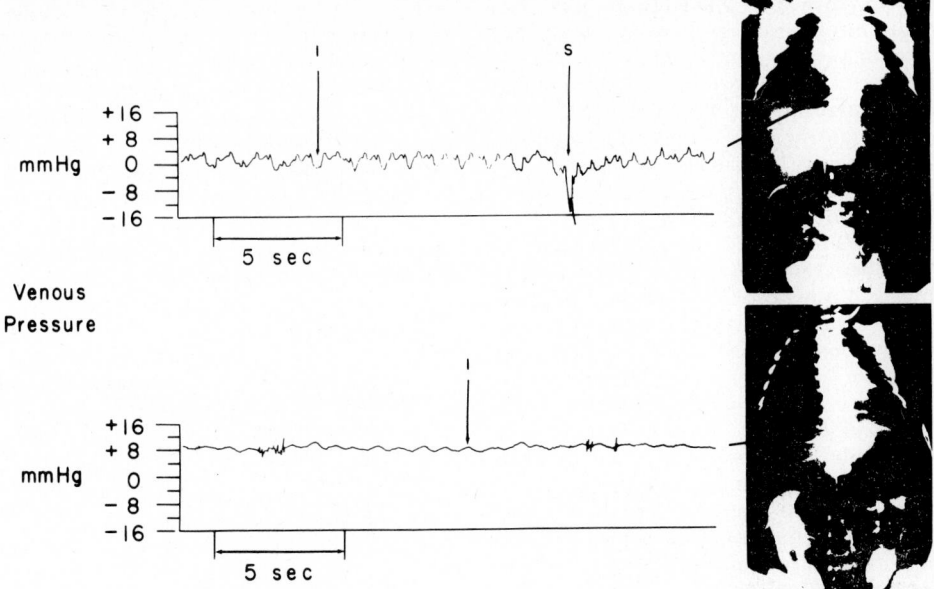

FIG. 30. Differences in venous pressures of a newborn infant and corresponding radiographs when the tip of an umbilical venous catheter is moved from the central venous system to the portal venous system. In the upper film the tip of the catheter lies in the inferior vena cava near the right atrium. The pressure tracing shows venous pressure waves, a negative deflection of more than 4 mm Hg during spontaneous inspiration (I), and a large negative deflection of more than 15 mm Hg during a sigh (S).

In the lower film the catheter had been pulled back through the ductus venosus and the tip lies in the portal system. The portal venous pressure is higher than central venous pressure, there are no venous pressure waves, and there is a small positive deflection during inspiration (I). (From Kitterman, Phibbs, and Tooley: Pediatr Clin North Am 17:901, 1970.)

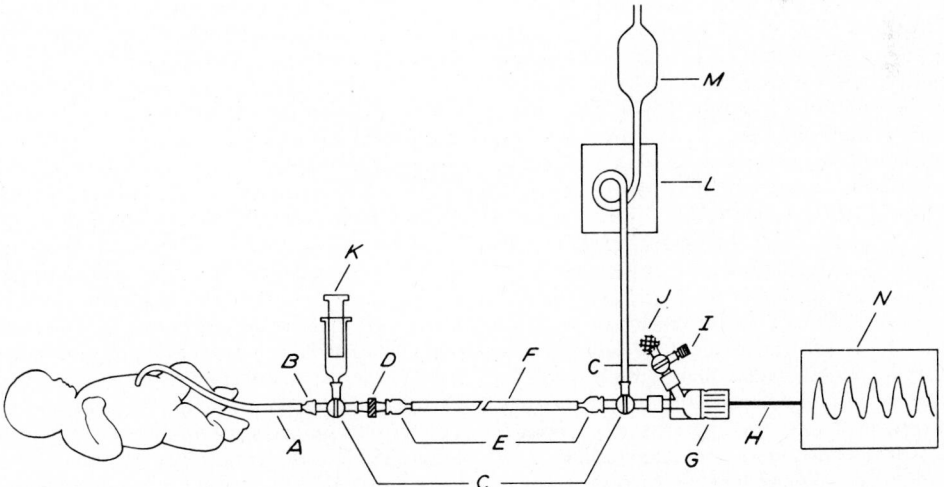

FIG. 31. System for direct measurement of arterial blood pressure in newborn infants. A, No. 5 Fr umbilical artery catheter with single end hole (Argyle) from which the wide proximal end has been cut off to reduce dead space. B, disposable luer stub adaptor, 18-gauge (Intramedic). C, disposable 3-way stopcocks (Pharmaseal). D, luer double male adaptor (B-D). E, 18-gauge blunt needles. F, No. 190 polyethylene tubing, 24 inches long (PE-190). G, pressure transducer (Statham P23D series). H, cable from G to N. I, metal plug adaptor (B-D). J, sterile gauze over opening on three-way stopcock. This is opened to air (after closing system off to infant) in order to obtain a zero pressure baseline for the recording system. K, syringe for flushing system. L, infusion pump. M, parenteral fluid for 8-hour period. N, electronic recorder (Model 7 Polygraph). (From Kitterman, Phibbs, and Tooley: Pediatrics 44:962, 1969.)

limb, and thrombus formation with embolization. Acute necrotizing enterocolitis can result from a misplaced venous catheter that causes venous infarction of a segment of bowel or clot from an arterial catheter too high in the aorta that causes bowel ischemia. One or another of these complications occur in about 5 to 10 percent of all catheterized infants, but can be minimized by careful technique and by removing a catheter at the earliest sign of a serious complication.

TRANSPORT WITHIN THE HOSPITAL. Many sick infants must be taken from the intensive care nursery to other areas of the hospital for special studies or procedures. This creates special hazards for the infant because the movement through hallways or from incubator to procedure table poses special problems, or because he is under the care of medical staff that are not particularly aware of the needs of a sick neonate. Some of the hazards include: (a) hypothermia from drafty hallways, cold procedure rooms, and lack of adequate heating equipment; (b) burns from improperly operated radiant heaters; (c) infection from contaminated equipment; (d) hemorrhage from an intravascular catheter that becomes disconnected or is pulled out; (e) fluid overload from unregulated infusions through intravascular catheters; (f) thrombosis of an indwelling catheter that is left unattended; (g) retrolental fibroplasia from indiscriminate use of oxygen or because some gas delivery systems, including anesthesia machines, are only able to deliver 100 percent oxygen; (h) asphyxia from failure of oxygen or ventilation systems. To prevent such problems, infants should be accompanied by experienced staff from the nursery who will continue to deliver supportive care to the infant while he is out of the nursery.

PARENTS. Intensive care of a small premature or other sick newborn should not totally separate him from his parents. They should be encouraged to come into the nursery to see and touch their baby, in order to promote the emotional bonding that will be necessary for healthy parent-child relations in the future. By supplying breast milk for gavage feedings, a mother can actively contribute in the care of her infant.

DISCHARGE FROM HOSPITAL. When a small premature infant gains sufficient weight, preparations must be made for discharge. The infant must be changed from gavage to nipple feedings, as tolerated. At approximately 1800 to 2000 g weight, he must be given a trial in an open crib to see if he can maintain body temperature outside an incubator. With sicker infants this may have to be delayed until they are larger. During this phase of care, the parents must receive thorough instruction in the care of their infant. This should include practical experience at such procedures as handling, feeding, and bathing the baby.

There is no absolute weight at which a prematurely born infant can be discharged safely. Some healthy vigorous infants can go home when their weight reaches about 2000 g, if the parents are prepared to handle them. Others may have to remain in hospital after they have reached 2500 g, if they are still sick or unstable. No prematurely born infant should go home until he is feeding well, gaining weight, can maintain his body temperature in an open crib, and his parents are prepared to care for him.

After discharge, these infants must continue to be observed. Many become anemic or have an increased risk of neurologic handicaps. Their development should be evaluated repeatedly to detect those specific handicaps that will benefit from remedial therapy. Many of these infants have a mild generalized delay in their neurologic development for the first 2 years of life, but then catch up to normal.

Bibliography

American Academy of Pediatrics: Recommendations for Hospital Care of Newborn Infants. Evanston, Ill, 1975

Hey E: Thermal neutrality. Br Med Bull 31:69, 1975

Kitterman JA, Phibbs RH, Tooley WH: Catheterization of umbilical vessels in newborn infants. Pediatr Clin North Am 17:895, 1970

Roy RN, Sinclair JC: Hydration of the low birth weight infant. Clin Perinatol 2:393, 1975

MULTIPLE BIRTHS
Roderic H. Phibbs

Twins and other multiple-birth infants have a neonatal mortality rate seven times as great as single born infants. Many of their neonatal problems related to abnormalities of birthweight and gestation. Mothers with two or more fetuses characteristically deliver prematurely, so that the infants have the usual risks of prematurity and low birthweight. The limited space available for development of the placentas limits growth so that the average birthweight for multiple births is less than that for single births. Compared to the normal values for single births shown in Figure 5, p 142, the lower limit of normal weight is 300 g less at 34 weeks and 500 g less at 38 weeks in multiple birth.

Competition for the limited space available for placenta development may leave one fetus with far less placenta than its mate(s). This will result in type II intrauterine growth retardation with its associated neonatal problems (see p 173 C-3,) and discordance in body size between the infants at birth. Twins are usually considered discordant if the larger twin's weight is 25 percent greater than that of the smaller twin. It has been suggested that the chronic stress of type II intrauterine growth retardation induces fetal endocrine changes that accelerate maturation of vital organ systems, such as the pulmonary surfactant system, and these same endocrine responses also induce the premature onset of labor. This would work to the advantage of the chronically stressed fetus whose lungs are sufficiently mature to allow survival after premature delivery. However, it would be to the disadvantage of its unstressed mate(s), also born prematurely but without accelerated maturation of the lungs.

Other problems peculiar to twins result from the mechanism of twinning and the types of placentas that develop. "Fraternal" or dizygotic twins result from fertilization and implantation of two separate ova. The two

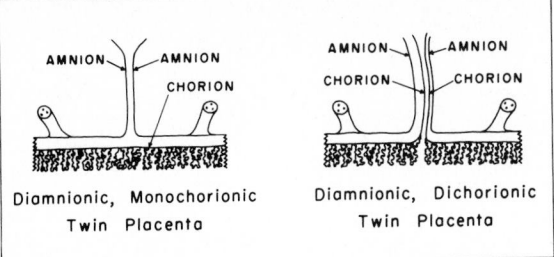

FIG. 32. Diagram of membrane relationship of monochorial twin placenta (left) and dichorial organ (right). The placental surface will not be disrupted when, in monochorial placentas, the amnions are peeled one from the other. A smooth chorionic membrane (Fig. 33) remains on the surface.

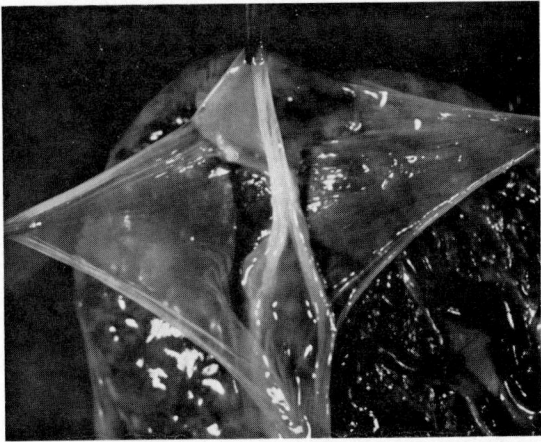

FIG. 33. Diamnionic dichorionic twin placenta. The amnions of the "dividing membranes" are being peeled away from the two chorions which remain in the center. These twins may or may not be dizygous.

resulting blastocytes develop separate placentas, which may or may not be adjacent. If they are close together they may fuse but there will still be two separate chorions producing a dichorionic placenta; they never have a monochrionic placenta. The fetuses may be of the same or opposite sexes. "Identical" or monozygotic twins result when a single fertilized blastocyst splits into two blastocysts. If it occurs after the placenta is formed, there will be just one chorion (monochorionic placenta). If it occurs before implantation, there will then be a dichorionic placenta as with dizygotic twins. Figures 32 and 33 illustrate the differences in these types of placental membranes. Monozygotic twins are of the same sex but need not be completely identical. Mosaicism before the blastocyst splits, or mutations that occur after the split, can cause monozygotic twins to differ.

These facts can be used to help determine the zygosity of twins in most cases:

If the placental is monochorionic they are monozygous

If they are of different sexes, they are dizygous

If they are of the same sex but the placenta is dichorionic, they can be either mono- or dizygous. One then does complete blood grouping; if they are the same in the major blood groups they are monozygous.

The type of placenta markedly affects neonatal mortality which is about three times as great in sets of twins with monochorionic placentas as with sets with dichorionic placentas. In a monochorionic placenta, there may be major anastomoses between the fetal arteries of one fetus and the veins of another, so that one bleeds chronically into the other and produces the "twin-to-twin transfusion syndrome" (Fig. 34).

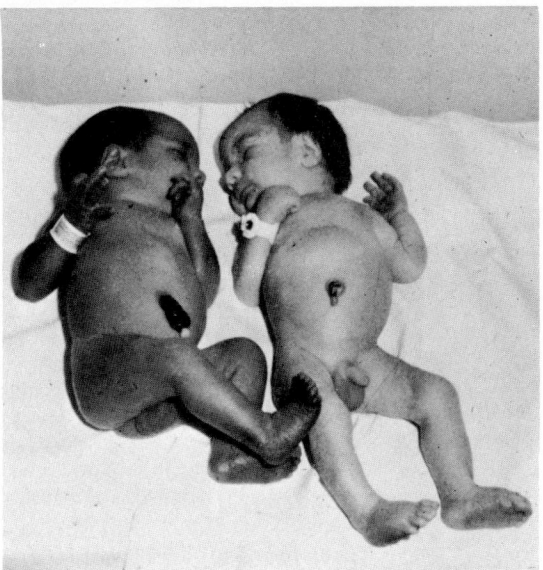

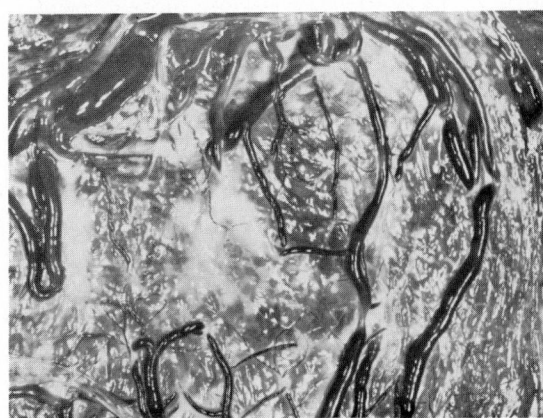

Fig. 34. Monozygous newborn twins with the transfusion syndrome. Severe plethora of twin on left who is also, characteristically, the larger infant. (From Becker and Glass. Am J Dis Child, 106:624, 1963.)

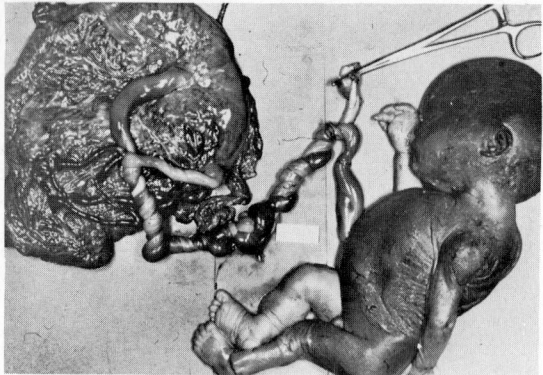

FIG. 35. Monoamnionic twins with one fetus macerated because of entangling and knotting of cords. The survivor, whose cord is clamped, died at age 3 months with extensive cerebral damage, presumably sustained from entangling of cords.

Corner GW: The observed embryology of humam single-ovum twins and other multiple births. Am J Obstet Gynecol 70:933, 1955

Fujikuru T, Froehlick LA: Mental and motor development in monozygotic co-twins with dissimilar birth weight. Pediatrics 53:884, 1974

Ho SK, Wu PYK: Perinatal factors and neonatal morbidity in twin pregnancy. Am J Obstet Gynecol 122:979, 1975

Moore CM, McAdams AJ, Sutherland J: Intrauterine disseminated intravascular coagulation: a syndrome of multiple pregnancy with a dead twin fetus. J Pediatr 74:523, 1969

Naeye RL: Human intrauterine parabiotic syndrome and its complications. N Engl J Med 268:804, 1963

Naeye RL: The fetal and neonatal development of twins. Pediatrics 33:546, 1964

Philip AGS: Fontanel size and epiphyseal ossification in neonatal twins discordant by weight. J Pediatr 86:417, 1975

Potter EL: Twin zygosity and placental form in relation to the outcome of pregnancy. Am J Obstet Gynecol 87:566, 1963

Typically, the donor twin is smaller, perhaps because this drain on its placental circulation causes a situation similar to type II intrauterine growth retardation (p 173); the donor twin is also anemic, unlike the usual type II small for gestational age infant. The recipient is larger, plethoric, and often in cardiorespiratory distress after birth (p. 180). The vasular anastomoses of a monochorionic placenta also allow for a sudden massive twin-to-twin transfusion at delivery from the infant still in utero to the first delivered infant. Here, the problem is sudden overtransfusion, and often acute congestive heart failure results in the recipient. Later on he may also suffer polycythemia as hemoconcentration occurs. The donor may be in acute hemorrhagic shock and will be anemic. In general, the recipient in the twin-to-twin transfusion syndrome has a greater risk of mortality and morbidity than the donor, but both require evaluation and treatment.

With all dichorionic placentas and most monochorionic placentas each fetus is in a separate amniotic sac and there is no chance of their umbilical cords becoming entangled. This can occur in the occasional case of a monochorionic placenta with a single amniotic sac, and perinatal mortality is very high in this group (Fig. 35).

Order of birth is important in multiple births. The firstborn infant has a substantially lower risk of being stillborn, suffering intrapartum asphyxia, or dying in the neonatal period.

Bibliography

Becker AH, Glass H: Twin-to-twin transfusion syndrome. Am J Dis Child 106:624, 1963

Benirschke K, Driscoll SG: The Pathology of the Human Placenta. New York, Springer-Verlag, 1967

Carter CO, VI: Polygenic inheritance and common diseases. Lancet 1:1252, 1969

Chown B, Lewis M, Bowman JM: A pair of newborn human blood chimeric twins. Transfusion 3:494, 1963

SMALL FOR GESTATIONAL AGE (SGA) INFANTS
ANNE H. GASTON

The 7 to 10 percent of infants with a birthweight below 2500 g are not a homogeneous group. They may be small because of premature birth, retarded intrauterine growth, or both. Growth retardation should be diagnosed when an infant's birthweight is more than 2 SD below the expected average weight in relation to gestational age for the same sex and race. They are called infants with intrauterine growth retardation, small for gestational age (SGA), or small-for-dates infants.

There are two main causes for slow intrauterine growth: decreased potential for fetal growth, as with chromosomal abnormalities or intrauterine infection; and restricted potential for growth in an otherwise normal fetus, such as with multiple pregnancies, placental vascular disease, etc. The type of antenatal growth disturbance depends on the time in gestation that the problem begins and on the duration, type, and severity of the insult. Although it has many causes, intrauterine growth failure has three general clinical expressions (Table 7).

Interruption of fetal growth by chromosomal abnormalities or fetal injury between conception and about 24 weeks gestation causes type I intrauterine growth retardation. These infants usually have a decreased number of cells in most organs and a reduced potential for growth. In this type, head growth is often slower than for infants with other causes of growth retardation, and mental retardation is common. Chronic fetal intrauterine malnutrition, beginning between 24 and 32 weeks gestation and associated with material toxemia, hypertension, or renal disease, causes type II intrauterine growth retardation. Placental infarction or maternal hypoxemia after 32 weeks gestation or delayed parturition lead to type III acute fetal malnutrition. Infants with type II and III growth delay have a normal number of cells but these may be of small size; after birth, these infants usually have normal physical growth and intellectual development.

TABLE 7. CAUSES OF 3 TYPES OF SMALL FOR GESTATIONAL AGE INFANTS

Type I—*Early interference with Fetal Growth* **(conception to 24 wk gestation)**

Chromosomal abnormalities, eg, trisomy 21, 13-15, 18
Fetal infection, eg, cytomegalovirus disease, toxoplasmosis, rubella, herpes simples, malaria
Maternal drugs, eg, chronic alcoholism, heroin addiction

Type II— *Chronic Intrauterine Malnutrition* **(24 to 32 wk gestation)**

Inadequate intrauterine space, eg, multiple pregnancy, uterine tumors, uterine anomalies
Placental insufficiency
  Maternal vascular disease, eg, renal disease, essential hypertension, collagen disease, sickle cell disease, toxemia
  Abnormal placentation with decreased placental weight and cellularity
Maternal malnutrition

Type III— *Late Intrauterine Malnutrition* **(after 32 wk gestation)**

Placental infarction or fibrosis
Maternal hypoxemia, eg, high altitude, cyanotic cardiac or pulmonary disease, smoking

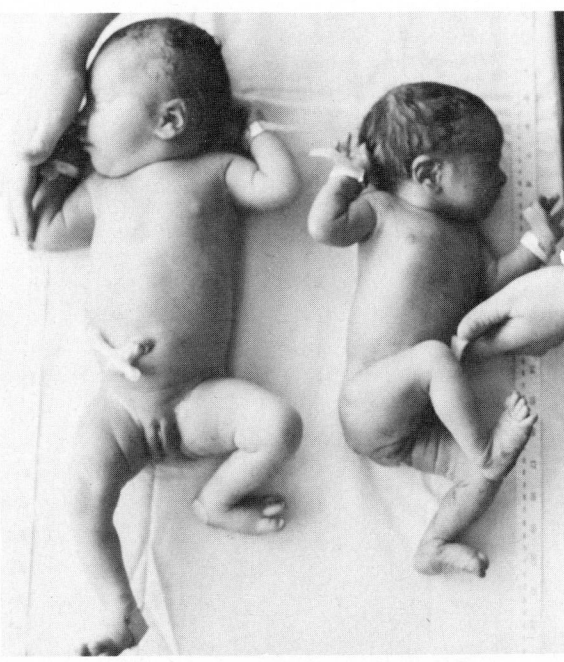

FIG. 36. Twins from a dichorionic pregnancy. The infant on the right weighs 1800 g and is a type II intrauterine growth retarded infant. Note the short arms and legs, the proportionately large head, and wrinkled skin. She has a relatively normal amount of subcutaneous tissue. The twin on the left weighs 3000 g and is of appropriate weight for gestational age.

In some situations, such as rubella infection, both the fetus and placenta fail to grow. In other instances, placental inadequacy limits fetal growth. The discordant twin pregnancy is a striking example of a small placenta associated with an SGA infant. In this condition, there is a marked difference between twins in both placental and fetal size (Fig. 36). The most common placental factors associated with intrauterine growth retardation are those that retard uteroplacental blood flow. These usually produce microscopic changes in the placental circulation. Conspicuous gross lesions, which obliterate part of the placenta (infarct, hemangioma, large thromboses), are infrequent and explain only a few instances of fetal growth retardation.

CLINICAL FINDINGS.   The diagnosis of intrauterine growth retardation can usually be made before birth by history and physical assessment of the fetus, supported by fetal radiography, ultrasonic cephalometry, amniotic fluid analysis for fetal maturity, and urinary estriol measurements. Serial measurements of head size with ultrasound most accurately reflect fetal growth (see p 126 for a discussion of these methods.)

The physical appearance of type I infants is usually characteristic of the specific etiologic factor, eg, rubella, maternal alcoholism, heroin addiction, trisomy syndromes. They are more than 2 SD below the average weight, length, and head circumference for gestational age (Fig. 37). The placenta often appears normal and is appropriate for fetal size. The infant with type II growth retardation is small, with weight and length less than expected. Weight is affected more than length, so that the weight:length ratio is greatly reduced. The head may also be small but usually it is relatively large and close to average for gestational age. There is little subcutaneous fat, and the skin may be loose and thin. Muscle mass is decreased, especially in the buttocks and thighs (Fig. 36). They appear to have an increased risk of infection in infancy and early childhood.

The infant with type III intrauterine growth retardation is underweight but of average length and appears scrawny, suggesting recent weight loss. They often appear alert and anxious (Fig. 38). Scalp hair is sparse and the skin has decreased turgor without lanugo or vernix caseosa and is often meconium-stained and dried and cracked. The skull sutures are widened at birth without increased fontanelle pressure. The umbilical cord is often thin and small. The fingernails and toenails are long. The liver is usually depleted of glycogen. Since the cause of the growth retardation is often inadequate uteroplacental blood flow, labor, and delivery, which produce a further reduction in placental blood flow, may cause severe fetal asphyxia. This stress may be accompanied by passage of meconium which stains the fetus and, if inhaled, may cause meconium pneumonitis (see p 1529).The small amount of liver glycogen is often completely used during labor and delivery so that there is often hypoglycemia in the neonatal period.

Common *laboratory findings* in types II and III SGA infants are hypoglycemia and polycythemia. Hypoglycemia may be severe and occur in the first few hours, or as late as 36 hours after birth. Approximately one-

Birth Weight (grams)

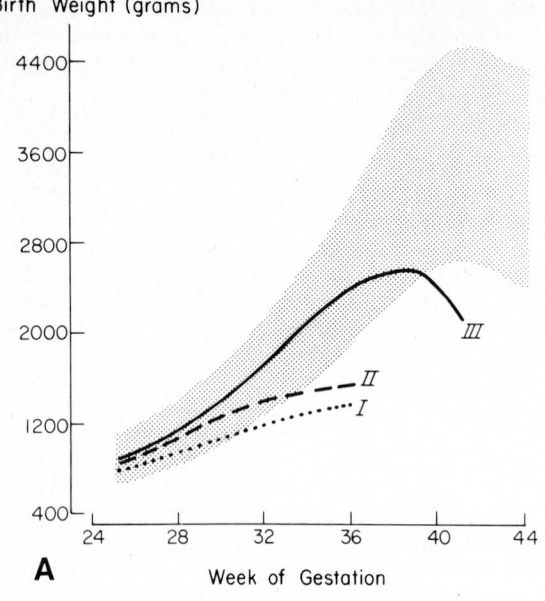

A   Week of Gestation

Length, crown-heel (cm)

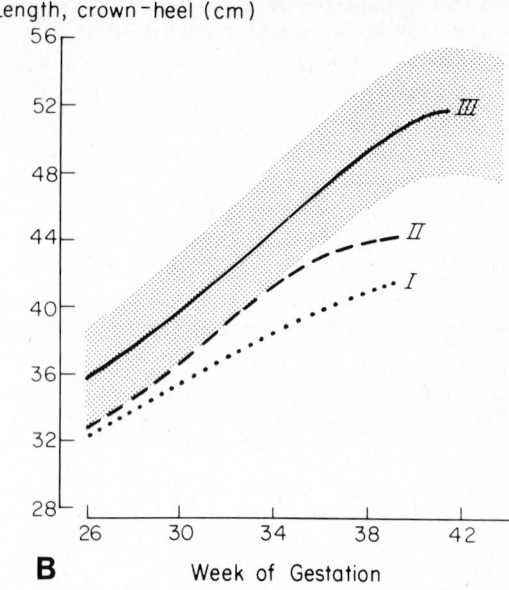

B   Week of Gestation

Head (cm)

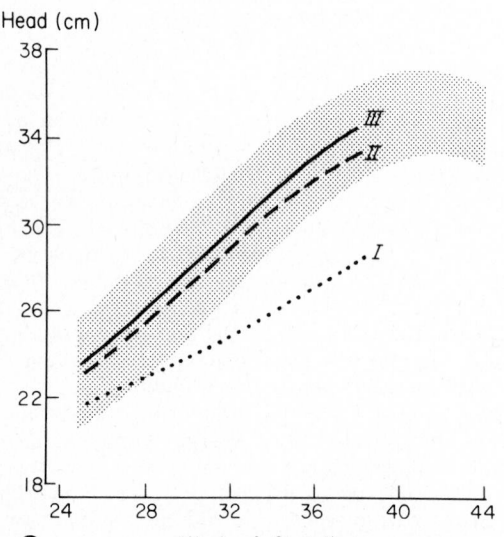

C   Week of Gestation

Fig. 37 A. The stippled area is the range of normal body weights at each gestational age (in utero). The rate of weight gain of the type I infant is slow from early in gestation, and is more than 2 SD below the average at birth, which often occurs before 40 weeks gestation. The rate of weight gain for the type II infant is often normal until the third trimester, when it slows. These infants also frequently deliver before 40 weeks gestation. Weight increases normally in type III infants until late in gestation. Unlike the type I and II infants, they lose weight. Loss of subcutaneous fat allows the skin to hang in loose folds. **B.** The stippled area is the range of normal body length in utero. The rate of linear growth of Type I infants is slow from early in gestation; they are short at birth, which is often prior to 40 weeks gestation. The rate of growth for the type II infant is usually maintained until late in the third trimester, so that if these infants are born before 36 weeks, they may be of normal length. The rate of growth for type III may remain normal throughout gestation. **C.** The stippled area is the range of normal head circumference in utero. Head growth is delayed in type I infants but usually is not far from average for type II infants; type III infants have average head size.

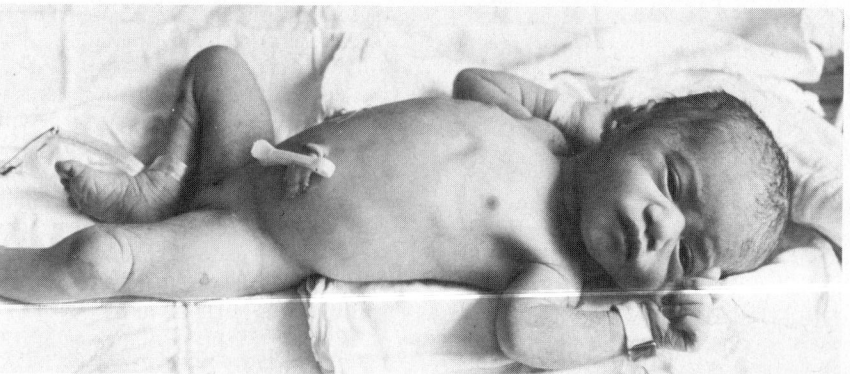

FIG. 38. Type III intrauterine growth retardation. The hands and feet are wrinkled. The extra skinfolds in the legs suggest recent loss of subcutaneous fat. She is long for her weight and is alert.

half of SGA infants have hemoglobin levels above 20 g/dl. Radiographic findings include thymic atrophy and delayed bone development.

TREATMENT. Management of the intrauterine growth-retarded infant begins during labor and delivery. Asphyxia should be diagnosed early and treated. Depression by analgesics should not be allowed to provide additional hazards to the already asphyxiated malnourished fetus. Resuscitation is important, with particular attention to maintenance of body temperature, provision of glucose, and prevention of meconium aspiration. Hyaline membrane disease is uncommon, but pneumothorax and pneumomediastinum frequently occur as complications of meconium pneumonitis. Because hypoglycemia is common, blood glucose should be measured at 2 and 4 hours of age and then every 4 hours. They should be fed at an early age (3 to 4 hours) or be given an infusion of glucose. Since their stomachs are large, they usually eat well and grow rapidly in the postnatal period. Occasional infants with type III intrauterine growth retardation have a "chalasia" syndrome, which requires special care with feeding for the first few weeks after birth. Infants with blood glucose below 30 mg/dl should be given glucose intravenously. The baby's hematocrit should be measured at 2 to 4 hours of age to detect polycythemia which may require treatment by an exchange transfusion with albumin (see p 179) for the management of polycythemia.

PROGNOSIS. The growth potential and neurologic development of SGA infants is related to the type of intrauterine stress. Type I growth-retarded infants often remain small, frequently have congenital abnormalities, and have a high incidence of neurologic and intellectual handicaps. Infants with types II and III growth retardation without intrauterine infection or chromosomal abnormalities, who do not have neonatal asphyxia, prolonged hypoglycemia, or polycythemia, and who grow rapidly after birth, may have a normal potential for ultimate growth and development.

Bibliography

Babson SG, Kangas J: Preschool intelligence of undersized term infants. Am J Dis Child 117:553, 1969

Babson SG: Growth and development of twins dissimilar in size at birth. N Engl J Med 289:937, 1973

Behrman RE, Fisher D, Paton JB, et al: In utero disease and the newborn infant. Adv Pediatr 17:13, 1970

Clifford SH: Postmaturity with placental dysfunction; clinical syndrome and pathologic findings. J Pediatr 44:1, 1954

Gruenwald P: Chronic fetal distress and placental insufficiency. Biol Neonat 5:215, 1963

Gruenwald P: Growth of the human fetus. I. Normal growth and its violation; II. Abnormal growth in twins and infants of mothers with diabetes, hypertension, or isoimmunization. Am J Obstet Gynecol 94:1112; 1120, 1966

Hill DE, Myers RE, Holt AB, et al: Fetal growth retardation produced by experimental placental insufficiency in the rhesus monkey, II. chemical composition of the brain, liver, muscle, and carcass. Biol Neonat 19:68, 1971

Humbert JR: Polycythemia in small for age infants. J Pediatr 75:812, 1969

Kisman LE: Chromosomal abnormalities and intrauterine growth retardation. Pediatr Clin North Am 17:101, 1970

Lubchenko LO, Searles DT, Brazie JV: Neonatal mortality rates; relationship to birth weight and gestational age. J Pediatr 81:814, 1972

Naeye RL, Blanc W, Paul C: Effects of maternal malnutrition on the human fetus. Pediatrics 52:494, 1973

Rosso P, Winick M: Intrauterine growth retardation. A new systemic approach based on the clinical and biochemical characteristics of this condition. J Perinatol Med 2:147, 1974

Sevir JL: Infectious agents and fetal diseases, In Fetal Growth and Development, Waisman M, Kirk-(eds): New York, McGraw Hill, 1970, p 223

Sinclair J, Calderon JS: Low birth weight and postnatal physical development. Develop Med Child Neurol 11:314, 1969

Smith CA: Effect of wartime starvation in Holland upon pregnancy and its product. Am J Obstet Gynecol 53:599, 1947

Warkany J, Monroe BB, Sutherland BS: Intrauterine growth retardation. Am J Dis Child 102:249, 1961

Winick M: Cellular growth of human placenta. III. Intrauterine growth failure. J Pediatr 71:390, 1967

THE OVERGROWN INFANT

Roberta Ballard

The infant whose weight is above the 90th percentile for gestational age presents a number of problems which are as significant as those presented by his intrauterine-growth retarded counterpart (see Fig. 5, p. 142). Some large babies are just constitutionally large. They are usually the offspring of large parents and it is not correct to consider them disproportionately overgrown. Other than complications of delivery due to their very large size, they are at no increased risk of perinatal mortality. The infants of concern are those that are pathologically overgrown. They are not only large but growth and maturation of many organ systems and tissues are abnormal. In some instances, there has been excessive growth at the expense of maturation resulting in immaturity of organ system function. Delayed maturation of the pulmonary surfactant system in infants of diabetic mothers appears to be an example of this.

The most common recognized cause of the large for gestational age infant is maternal diabetes, either gestational or permanent. This occurs even in well controlled maternal diabetes and is believed to be due to increased production of insulin by the fetus in response to intermittent hyperglycemia in the mother. Some infants with cyanotic congenital heart lesions are also overgrown at birth. The mechanism is not clear, but there are some similarities between these and the infants of diabetic mothers, including a tendency to hyperinsulinism. Other infants are overgrown for unexplained reasons, but still have some of the same increased risks of neonatal disease as infants of diabetic mothers. Many large for gestational age infants are both overgrown and prematurely born, which further increases their risk of neonatal mortality and morbidity.

Infant of the Diabetic Mother

Prior to the availability of insulin, women with diabetes seldom produced viable offspring. Even as recently as 1957, total fetal and neonatal wastage, as well as abnormal survivors in infants of diabetic mothers, was reported to be 43 percent compared with 17 per-

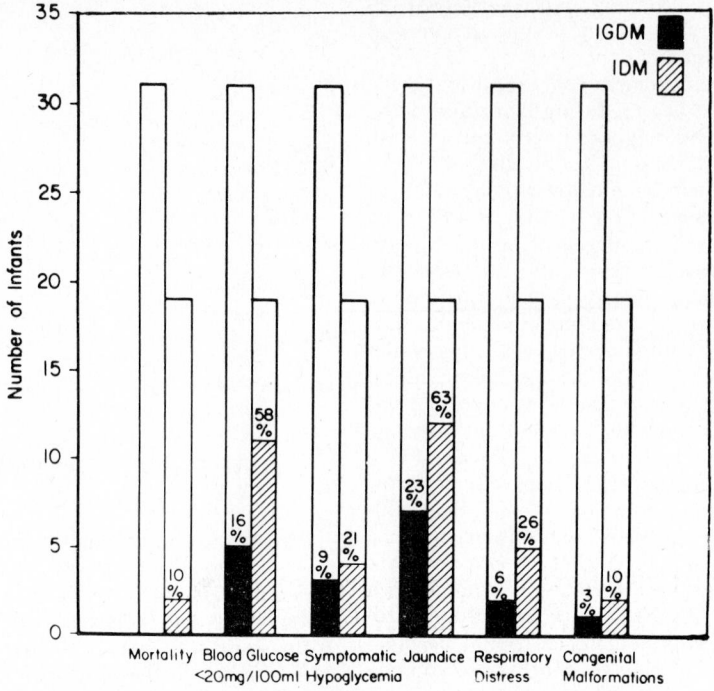

FIG. 39.   Summary for clinical findings for IDM and IGDM. (From Warrner and Cornblath: Am J Dis Child 117:684, 1969.)

TABLE 8. Fetal and Neonatal Wastage in Diabetes Mellitus

	Total No.	Abortions No.	%	Stillbirths No.	%	Neonatal deaths No.	%	Abnormal survivors No.	%
Diabetes	157	17	29.9	18	11.5	13	8.3	6	3.8
Prediabetes	78	16	20.5	4	5.1	1	1.3	2	2.6
Controls	249	31	12.4	3	1.2	9	3.0	1	0.4

From Cornblath, Schwartz: Disorder of Carbohydrate Metabolism in Infancy. Philadelphia, Saunders, 1967, p 58

cent in controls (Table 8). The infants born to mothers with gestational diabetes share in this increased fetal and neonatal wastage. The severity of maternal disease markedly influences both the severity and the character of the fetal and neonatal disease. A mother who is a gestational diabetic or has mild to moderate diabetes will have a large fetus with a large placenta. Such a fetus will have a moderately increased risk of fetal or neonatal death and a greatly increased risk of intrapartum death. The cause of intrauterine death in these large fetuses is unknown. A mother with severe diabetes and severe placental vascular disease will more likely have an undergrown fetus, with risks similar to other type II small for gestational age infants (see p 173) including hypoglycemia, jaundice, respiratory distress, congenital malformations, polycythemia, hypocalcemia, and transient hermaturia (Figs. 39, 40). The most frequent congenital anomalies involve the spine, particularly with the sacral agenesis syndrome; congenital heart disease is also

common. Infants of diabetic mothers were one of the first groups to be clearly identified as needing specialized perinatal care for both the mother and infant. With such care, mortality and morbidity rates have declined significantly during the last 15 years.

Figure 41 shows the striking appearance of a typical large for gestational age infant born to a diabetic mother. These infants present with macrosomia, a cushingoid appearance, plethora, and generalized organomegaly, neurologic immaturity with jitteriness and poor coordination in feeding.

These infants are remarkable not only because like foetal versions of Shadrach, Meshach and Abednego, they emerge at least alive from within the fiery metabolic furnace of diabetes mellitus, but because they resemble one another so closely that they might well be related. They are plump, sleek, liberally coated with vernix caseosa, full-faced and plethoric. The umbilical cord and the placenta share in the gigantism. During the first

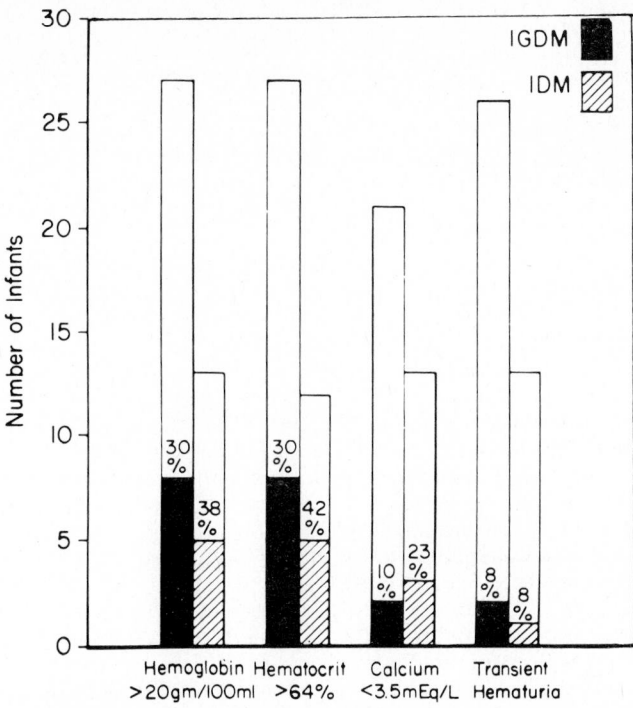

FIG. 40. Summary of laboratory findings for IDM and IGDM. (From Warrner and Cornblath: Am J Dis Child 117:681, 1969.)

24 or more extrauterine hours they lie on their backs, bloated and flushed, their legs flexed and abducted, their lightly closed hands on each side of the head, the abdomen prominent and their respiration sighing. They convey a distinct impression of having had such a surfeit of both food and fluid pressed upon them by an insistent hostess that they desire only peace so that they may recover from their excesses. And on the second day their resentment of the slightest noise improves the analogy while their trembling anxiety seems to speak of intrauterine indiscretions of which we know nothing. (Farquhar)

PRENATAL MANAGEMENT. The care of these infants begins during pregnancy and includes identification and proper management of diabetic mothers (p. 175). In late gestation, the fetus should be evaluated repeatedly, and the risks of continued intrauterine life should be weighed against those of premature delivery, which is often necessary.

MANAGEMENT AT BIRTH. Proper care of the infant of the diabetic mother begins with preparation for the resuscitation of the infant at birth (p 1507). Such infants are premature, often have immature lungs, suffer intrapartum asphyxia, and macrosomia may further complicate the delivery. Even during resuscitation, the possibility of hypoglycemia may be present and blood glucose should be measured repeatedly, beginning immediately after birth. After stabilization, the initial evaluation of the infant should include careful examination for possible congenital defects, particularly skeletal defects or congenital heart disease.

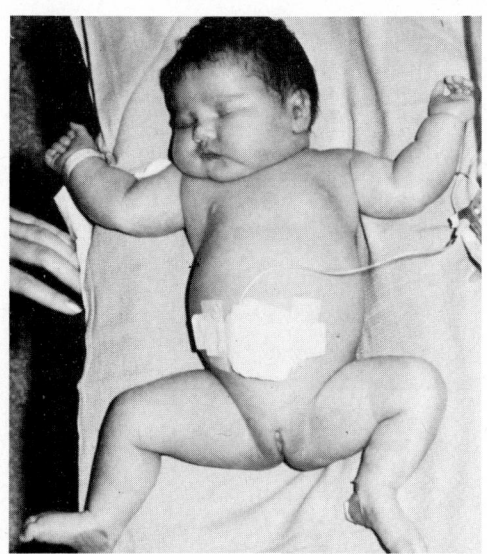

FIG. 41. Infant of a diabetic mother born at 36 weeks of gestation weighing 4400 g.

Hypoglycemia is most likely between 1 and 4 hours after birth. Even though this may be asymptomatic, it must be detected and treated to prevent brain damage. The mechanism of this hypoglycemia, which also occurs to a lesser extent in infants of gestational diabetic mothers, is thought to be a more rapid release of insulin following stimulation, whereas the normal newborn infant has a somewhat sluggish insulin response. In addition, these infants also may have a defect in epinephrine release and, therefore, be less able to mobilize the release of glucose to cope with their hypoglycemic crises. The best treatment is prevention. Sometimes this is possible with early and frequent feedings of glucose water, but usually the severely affected infant requires intravenous glucose beginning with a 10 percent glucose solution at a rate of about 100 ml/kg/day and the adjusting rate or concentration as required to prevent hyper- or hypoglycemia. If hypoglycemia has already occurred it should be treated with intravenous infusions of 10 percent to 15 percent glucose, starting initially with 5 to 10 ml/kg infused over about 10 minutes and followed by infusion of 10 percent glucose. If this is not adequate to stabilize the infant's blood sugar, the concentration should be increased gradually. Bolus infusions of high concentrations of glucose should be avoided, because they are hypertonic, having a sclerosing effect, set off further insulin release, and produce a reactive hypoglycemia, which again requires treatment and makes stabilization of the infant very difficult. Parenteral glucose must never be discontinued abruptly but gradually withdrawn as oral intake is increased (see p 166).

Hypocalcemia is common in these infants, particularly on the second day after birth. Tsang and associates consider that these infants probably suffer from a functional hypoparathyroidism secondary to exposure to increased concentrations of serum-ionized calcium in utero, with suppression of activity of the fetal parathyroid glands. The management of hypocalcemia is usually a simple matter with the use of intravenous or oral calcium gluconate.

HEART FAILURE.   In some infants, the combination of intrapartum asphyxia, hypoglycemia, and hypocalcemia produce myocardial failure. This often mimics, or is superimposed upon, early hyaline membrane disease. It must be treated promptly with simultaneous correction of all the factors that depress myocardial function, viz low PaO_2, low pH, low Ca^{++} and low glucose.

POLYCYTHEMIA.   These infants have increased erythropoiesis and are polycythemic at birth. The blood volume of the prematurely born infant of a diabetic is lower than normal, which might seem incongruous with the polycythemia. However, relatively more of their body is composed of poorly vascularized fat, and since blood volume is expressed as milliliter per kilogram body weight, they probably do not have a blood volume that is low relative to the capacity of their vascular system. Thus, they tend to remain polycythemic after birth and are at risk of all the problems associated with this (see p 179). One such risk is renal vein thrombosis which is particularly common in infants of diabetic mothers.

RESPIRATORY DISTRESS.   Many of the overgrown premature infants have immaturity of the lung and classic hyaline membrane disease; other processes can interact to cause or worsen cardiopulmonary disease. Figure 42 is a schematic illustration of the many

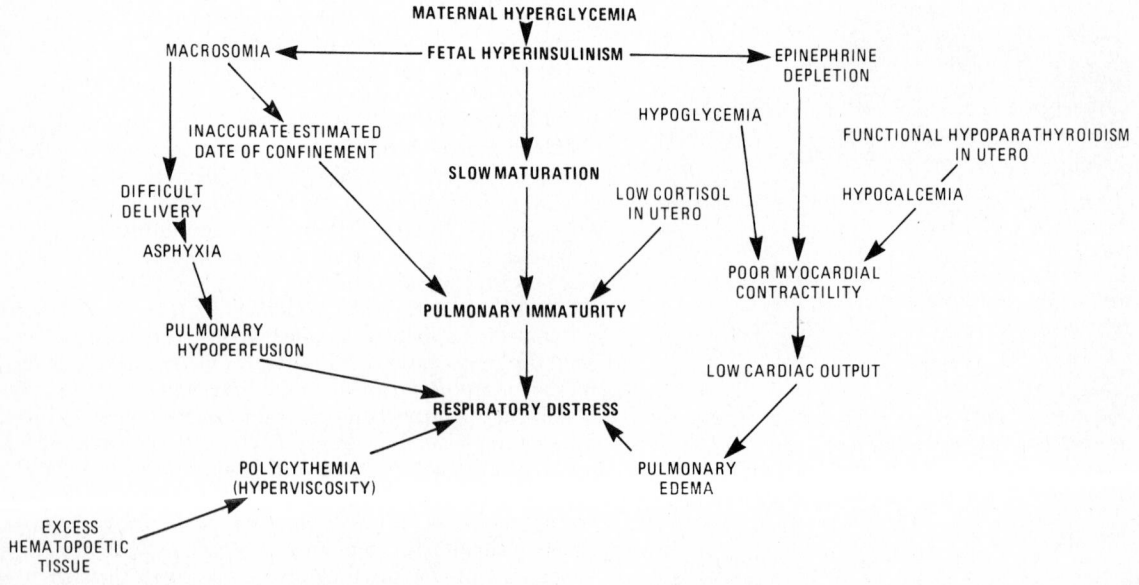

FIG. 42.   Operative processes in infant of the diabetic mother.

factors that may contribute to produce respiratory distress in these infants. Complete care of the infant of the diabetic mother with respiratory distress must take account of all these possibilities.

OUTCOME. From the collaborative study of cerebral palsy, Churchill and associates reported that infants born to mothers who had acetonuria during pregnancy had a significantly lower intellectual development than controls. Priestly found a significant association of increased hypotonia on neurologic examination in newborn infants who had a blood sugar level of less than 10 mg/100 ml. The incidence of eventual diabetes in these infants is not yet known. Velasco showed that glucose tolerance tests were abnormal in many of these children, as long as 2 years after birth. However, the general outlook for infants of diabetic mothers is now quite good, if they receive intensive care extending from early in pregnancy throughout the neonatal course.

Bibliography

Adam PAJ, Schwartz R: Diagnosis and treatment: should oral hypoglycemic agents be used in pediatric and pregnant patients. Pediatrics 42:819, 1968

Avery ME, Oppenheimer EH, Gordon HH: Renal vein thrombosis in newborn infants of diabetic mothers. N Engl J Med 256:1134, 1957

Babson SG, Henderson N, Clark WM: The preschool intelligence of oversized newborns. Pediatrics 44:536, 1969

Battaglia FC, Frazier TM, Hellegers AE: Birth weight, gestational age, and pregnancy outcome, with special reference to high birth weight - low gestational age infant. Pediatrics 37:417, 1966

Churchill JA, Berendes HW, Nemore J: Neuropsychiatric disorders in children of diabetic mothers. Am J Obstet Gynecol 105:257, 1969

Cornblath M, Schwartz R: Disorders of carbohydrate metabolism in infancy, vol. 3, Major Problems in Clinical Pediatrics, WB Saunders, Philadelphia, 1967

Dekaban A, Baird R: Outcome of pregnancy in diabetic women. 1. Fetal wastage, mortality and morbidity in the offspring of diabetic and normal control mothers. J Pediatr 55:563, 1959

Dyson D, Blake M, Cassady G: Amniotic fluid lechithin/sphingomyelin ratio in complicated pregnancies. Am J Obstet Gynecol 122:722, 1975

Klebe JG, Ingomar CJ, Norgaard-Pedersen B: Blood volumes in premature infants of diabetic and non-diabetic mothers, correlated with the time of clamping of the umbilical cord. Acta Paediatr Scand 61:549, 1972

Light IJ, Sutherland JM, Loggie JM, et al: Impaired epinephrine release in hypoglycemic infants of diabetic mothers. N Engl J Med 277:394, 1967

Priestley BL: Neurological assessment of infants of diabetic mothers in the first week of life. Pediatrics 50:578, 1972

Robert MF, Neff RK, Hubbell JP, et al: Association between maternal diabetes and the respiratory-distress syndrome in the newborn. N Engl J Med 294:357, 1976

Tsang RC, Chen I-Wen, Friedman MA, et al: Parathyroid function in infants of diabetic mothers. J Pediatr 86:399, 1975

Velasco MS, Paulsen EP: The response of infants of diabetic women to tolbutamide and leucine at birth, and to glucose and tolbutamide at 2 years of age. Pediatrics 43:546, 1969

Warrner RA, Cornblath M: Infants of gestational diabetic mothers. Am J Dis Child 117:678, 1969

Weiner G: The relationship of birth weight and length of gestation to intellectual development of ages 8 to 10 years. J Pediatr 76:694, 1970

NEONATAL POLYCYTHEMIA
Roderic H. Phibbs

During the first 2 days after birth, some newborn infants have a very high hematocrit and an elevated blood viscosity, which impedes blood flow to tissues and may cause serious, even fatal, disease. This is called neonatal polycythemia or the neonatal hyperviscosity syndrome. It has only recently achieved general recognition as an important clinical entity, and it is not yet clear how frequently it occurs, but it only occurs in a minority of newborns with higher than normal hematocrits.

PATHOPHYSIOLOGY. In experimental animals made acutely polycythemic, blood viscosity rises and, with it, resistance to systemic and pulmonary blood flow. Cardiac output falls and the increased oxygen carrying capacity of the blood is insufficient to offset the decreased flow, so oxygen delivery to tissues decreases. When this experiment was performed in newborn lambs, resistance to blood flow in the pulmonary circulation sometimes exceeded resistance in the systemic circulation; venous blood then flowed from the pulmonary artery through the patent ductus arteriosus into the aorta and worsened the tissue hypoxia. The few comparable observations that have been made in infants with the hyperviscosity syndrome have shown decreased renal function, apparently due to decreased blood flow, high pulmonary artery pressure and right-to-left shunting through the ductus arteriosus and foramen ovale in some cases. When present, these are usually corrected by lowering the hematocrit.

In vitro studies show blood viscosity is affected mainly by red blood cell concentration and by the shear rate during flow. (In a vessel or tube of a constant diameter, shear rate increases with flow.) Figure 43 illustrates these relationships. The abrupt rise in viscosity at

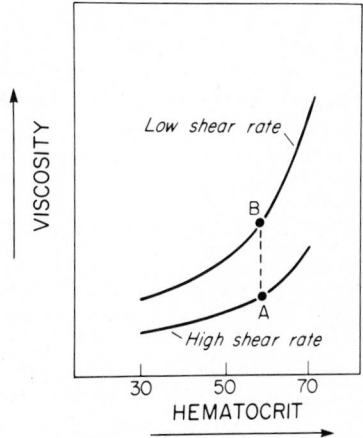

FIG. 43. Effects of hematocrit and shear rate on blood viscosity. Dotted line between A and B illustrates the increase in viscosity that would occur in flowing blood of Hct = 60 percent if flow changed from a high to a low rate.

very low shear rates results from the tendency for red cells to clump together. Plasma proteins, particularly fibrinogen, promote this; high levels of fibrinogen will increase viscosity at low shear rates. At high shear rates, red cell deformability affects viscosity. More rigid cells, such as swollen spherocytic cells, increase viscosity. It is not certain which of these phenomena is more important for blood flow in vessels, but in vivo experiments suggest that general principles do apply, even if in modified form. Resistance to flow increases with increasing hematocrit and also with decreasing flow. These principles are particularly relevant to the clinical syndrome of hyperviscosity. Because several factors may affect viscosity in vivo, it seems unlikely that any one easily measurable variable will consistently identify those infants most likely to develop the syndrome. Because viscosity is shear rate-dependent, any process which suddenly slows blood flow could precipitate disease in an asymptomatic infant with relatively hyperviscous blood or could worsen disease that is already present.

POLYCYTHEMIA. The normal human fetus at term has a higher hematocrit than the adult (see p.1111) and several processes may raise the hematocrit even higher in utero. These include intrauterine growth retardation of the extrinsic variety, in which there is presumed to be chronic hypoxemia, maternal diabetes, twin-to-twin transfusion, maternal-to-fetal transfusion, Down's syndrome, Trisomy D, adrenal hyperplasia, and potentially any of the alpha-chain hemoglobinopathies that produce an increased affinity for oxygen and interfere with the delivery of oxygen to tissue. At the time of delivery, an infant normally receives a transfusion of blood of 5 to 20 ml/kg body weight from the placenta (see p. 844). Over the next 2 to 6 hours, plasma volume decreases and hematocrit rises proportional to the size of this placental transfusion. The hematocrit at the end of that time is the result of the initial hematocrit at birth, plus the volume of the placental transfusion.

CLINICAL FINDINGS. Rarely are signs present at birth. These are usually signs of congestive failure due to a very large transfusion at birth or recent twin-to-twin transfusion, not related to the polycythemia and hyperviscosity, and they respond to phlebotomy. Signs of hyperviscosity usually begin at 2 to 6 hours as hematocrit rises, and almost always before 24 hours of age. The course suggests that normal circulation is maintained for a short time and then obstruction of one or another region of the circulation occurs. Signs vary, depending upon the particular organs suffering underperfusion. The infants appear plethoric, often cyanotic, may have signs of respiratory distress, and often are thought to have cyanotic congenital heart disease. They often have an abnormal cry, appear tremulous and agitated, or depressed, and may feed poorly. In some, these so-called *cerebral* signs progress to convulsions and occasionally to signs of severe brain damage. If the kidneys are involved, they are usually palpably enlarged and there is hematuria and oliguria or anuria. Less often, the gastrointestinal tract is affected with findings of acute necrotizing enterocolitis. The syndrome is more common among small-for-gestational-age infants of mothers with toxemia.

LABORATORY FINDINGS. The infants are all polycythemic, but the level of hematocrit is quite variable. In most reported cases venous hematocrits have been above 68 to 70 percent but a few have had values in the low 60s. Hematocrit often falls after the microcirculation becomes obstructed; some of the reported cases of hyperviscosity syndrome with only mild polycythemia may have had higher hematocrits earlier, which were undetected. Whole blood viscosity is increased at least proportionate to the level of hematocrit; in some infants with abnormally rigid red blood cells, more common in newborns, viscosity may be higher. In these cases, estimates of erythrocyte flexibility, such as rate of filtration through micropores, show the cells are relatively less deformable. Platelet levels are often low, presumably secondary to clotting in obstructed regions of the microcirculation. Measurements of blood gas tensions may show venous admixture which often can be identified, at least in part, as a right-to-left shunt through the ductus arteriosus by simultaneous measurement of PaO_2 above and below the ductus arteriosus (p. 1531). Right-to-left shunt often occurs through the foramen ovale. Often, there is significant hyperbilirubinemia during the first week of age.

COMPLICATIONS. Most of the abnormalities are relieved by reduction of hematocrit, but the common exception is central nervous system pathology. Current experience suggests that many hyperviscous infants with signs of central nervous system injury during the first days of life have more longlasting neural pathology. In those with renal involvement, renal function usually begins to improve before the end of the first week, even in many of the infants with findings suggestive of renal vein thrombosis. There are no data on their renal function later in childhood.

MANAGEMENT. Infants with an increased risk of developing neonatal polycythemia should be observed carefully for evidence of disease during the first day or two after birth, as should any infant with a venous hematocrit consistently greater than 65 percent. Infants with signs that could be due to hyperviscosity should have frequent measurements of hematocrit, and other possible causes of the findings should be ruled out. In evaluating these infants, the capillary blood hematocrit can be used only as a screening measurement because it is almost always higher than that of venous blood, but by a variable amount.

Infants with signs of hyperviscous disease, polycythemia, and no other evident explanation for the findings, should probably have their hematocrits reduced promptly by a small exchange transfusion with plasma or an equivalent fluid. (The limited experience currently available makes a recommendation for any particular program of therapy uncertain, but this is the predominant opinion among authorities on the problem at present.) A satisfactory and readily available solution for exchange is salt-poor albumin added to isotonic saline to give a concentration of albumin equal to 4 g/dl. Sixteen milliliters of standard 25 g/dl commercial preparation of salt-poor albumin combined with 84 ml isotonic saline, gives the desired mixture. The object is to lower the hematocrit to the range of 50 or 55 percent. The volume to be exchanged can be estimated as follows:

$$\frac{Hct_I - Hct_D \times body\ weight\ (kg) \times 90\ ml}{Hct_I} = V$$

Hct_I = infant's present hematocrit
Hct_D = desired hematocrit
V = exchange volume

Either the umbilical artery or vein, or both, must be catheterized in order to reduce hematocrit; these catheters should also be used to monitor the cardiopulmonary status of the infant during the procedure. Reduction of blood volume should be guided by measurements of aortic and/or central venous pressures to avoid overtreatment.

As a general rule, one should not attempt to reduce hematocrit by simple phlebotomy because the effect on hematocrit is too slow and the procedure is potentially dangerous. An abrupt removal of blood will decrease cardiac output and peripheral blood flow. This will decrease shear rate in blood flowing in the peripheral circulation, thereby increasing blood viscosity (Fig. 43), which will worsen, not improve, peripheral circulation. The possible exception to the rule is the infant in overt heart failure in whom phlebotomy may improve cardiac output. On the other hand, reducing blood volume gradually by about 10 ml/kg body weight during the latter part of the exchange transfusion may be beneficial in infants who are polycythemic because of very large placental transfusions. These infants have quite large blood volumes, even after postnatal hemoconcentration. After therapeutic reduction of hematocrit, plasma volume often decreases further and the hematocrit may again rise almost to pretreatment levels; reducing blood volume as hematocrit is reduced prevents this.

As with phlebotomy, any other procedures or condition that lowers cardiac output may aggravate symptoms in an affected infant, or induce hyperviscous disease in an asymptomatic polycythemic infant. Two such conditions, hypoglycemia and hypocalcemia, frequently occur in infants predisposed to neonatal polycythemia and must be watched for and, if possible, prevented.

Several authorities have suggested the possibility of prophylactically reducing the hematocrit of asymptomatic infants with severe polycythemia; suggestions for the level of venous hematocrit which requires treatment vary from 65 to 75 percent. Others suggest the only indications for treatment are the signs of the hyperviscosity syndrome. The argument in favor of prophylaxis is that once central nervous system signs appear, serious damage may already have occurred. The present difficulty with prophylaxis is that most polycythemic infants, even those with a venous hematocrit above 70 percent, do not seem to suffer from it. No study has yet shown the amount of disease that would be prevented and the number of infants that would be unnecessarily treated prophylactically at a given level of polycythemia. If prophylactic reduction of hematocrit is used, current experience suggests it need be used only before 48 hours of age, because polycythemic infants who have not developed any signs of circulatory embarrassment by then appear unlikely to do so thereafter.

Bibliography

Aperia A, Bergqvist G, Broberger O, et al.: Renal function in newborn infants with high hematocrit values before and after isovolemic hemodilution, Acta Paediatr Scand 63:878, 1974

Fouron J-C, Hebert F: Circulatory effects of hematocrit variations in normovolemic newborn lambs. J Pediatr 82:995, 1973

Gross GP, Hathaway WE, McGaughey HR: Hyperviscosity in the neonate. J Pediatr 82:1004, 1973

Leake RD, Thanopoulos B, Nieberg R: Hyperviscosity syndrome associated with necrotizing enterocolitis. Am J Dis Child 129:1192, 1975

Mackintosh TF, Walker CHM: Blood viscosity in the newborn. Arch Dis Child 48:547, 1973

Wells R: Syndromes of hyperviscosity. N Engl J Med 283:183, 1970

NEONATAL SEPSIS
RODERIC H. PHIBBS

Sepsis presents a special set of problems when it occurs in the newborn. The newborn infant has temporary deficiencies in the immunologic system and in leukocyte function (see p 300 and p 1177) which make him particularly vulnerable to such organisms as gramnegative rods and staphylococci that are less of a threat to older individuals. He may be heavily exposed to these organisms in the hospital, either from other infants or bacterial reservoirs on the hands of nursery personnel or equipment. Fetal life, labor, and birth also expose him to such other unusual pathogens as *Listeria monocytogens* or group B *beta hemolytic streptococci* in the birth canal. When sepsis occurs, it often presents with vague and nonspecific physical signs and laboratory diagnosis is equally difficult. Yet, without prompt treatment, it often progresses rapidly to death. (Approximately 40 percent of septic neonates die.)

PREDISPOSING CONDITIONS. Neonatal sepsis occurs in about 0.1 percent of all liveborn infants. It is more common among low birthweight infants, those who have suffered intrapartum asphyxia, and after prolonged rupture of amniotic membranes, particularly if there was amnionitis. Males are more often affected than females. It is also more common among otherwise sick infants who undergo such invasive procedures as surgery or placement of indwelling intravascular catheters.

Physical signs commonly present in sepsis include jaundice, lethargy, a weak cry, respiratory distress, poor feeding, and fever. It had been thought fever was uncommon and that septic infants had either normal or low temperatures. However, if infants are kept in an optimal or near-optimal thermal environment (see p 153) fever is more common, hypothermia is less common and often occurs later when the infant is critically ill. Other less common signs include hepatomegaly or splenomegaly, apnea, cyanosis, vomiting, abdominal distension, diarrhea, irritability, and purpura. In any given case, some of these nonspecific signs could as well be due to a variety of other conditions, such as cardiac anomalies, pulmonary disease, anatomic bowel obstruction, or metabolic abnormalities. Depending upon the site of entry, there may be more specific and localized signs, for example, the periumbilical erythematous streaking of omphalitis, the skin lesions of staphylococcal or pseudomonas infections, or the chest findings in pneumonia.

LABORATORY FINDINGS. A positive blood culture is generally considered to be diagnostic of neonatal sepsis. Unfortunately, a significant number of infants who are later proven septic have had negative cultures. On the other hand, false-positive blood cultures commonly occur from contamination by poor technique in obtaining the sample, or because blood was obtained from the stopcock connection of an indwelling intravascular catheter, which is almost certain to be contaminated. A positive culture is more significant if one is certain that it was drawn properly and contains a single type of organism. (Contaminated specimens often have a mixed growth and sepsis due to two organisms is uncommon.) Other useful cultures include those of urine, cerebrospinal fluid (even in the absence of clear signs of meningitis), and such localized lesions as skin pustules, if present.

Leukocytosis is often present, but can be detected only by comparing the blood cell count to the normal values. These counts have a wide range, which change daily in the first days after birth. Table 9 shows the range of normal for neutrophil counts in term and preterm newborns. Leukopenia is less common and usually occurs later when the infant is critically ill.

TABLE 9. Range of Neutrophil Counts in Peripheral Blood of Normal Term Newborns and Healthy Preterm Newborns During the First 10 Days

Age (day)	Term (per cm)	Preterm (per cm)
Birth	4,000-13,000	2,000-9,000
1	7,000-19,000	2,000-14,000
2	4,000-14,000	2,000-9,000
3	2,000-8,000	2,000-8,000
4–10	2,000-6,000	1,000-7,000

Modified from the data of Xanthou: Arch Dis Child 45:242, 1970

Other laboratory changes that may occur, include hypoglycemia, hyperbilirubinemia—often with an elevation of both direct and indirect reacting bilirubin and thrombocytopenia—with or without other evidence of accelerated intravascular coagulation.

COMPLICATIONS. Approximately one-third of infants with sepsis develop meningitis, the physical signs of which are often no different than those of sepsis. Osteomyelitis is a less common complication. The organisms may also spread to the kidneys or, alternatively, a urinary tract infection may have been the source of sepsis; either possibility warrants examination of the urine. Disseminated intravascular coagulation occurs in neonatal sepsis and, if not present initially, should be looked for during the course of the disease. Shock, presumably due to endotoxin, occurs in neonatal sepsis with either gram-negative rods or gram-positive cocci.

MANAGEMENT. Neonatal sepsis presents a therapeutic dilemma. If one waits until the diagnosis is certain to begin antibiotic treatment, it will be too late to save many septic infants because the disease is so rapidly fatal. Alternatively, if one treats every case of suspected infection as soon as the first suspicious signs appear, most of those treated will not be septic because the early signs are usually nonspecific and appear in so many other conditions. Antibiotic treatment carries a significant risk for newborns so that unnecessary use must be kept to a minimum.

The decision between treating as soon as samples have been obtained for culture and waiting for the results of these cultures is based upon the weight of evidence for infection and the infant's condition. In general terms, treatment should be instituted in the child who is suspected of being septic and is seriously ill with no other obvious cause for the condition, as in the less ill child with several findings suggesting sepsis. The generally well child with only slight evidence of sepsis should not be treated but observed for changes in findings while awaiting the results of the cultures. The actual weighing of evidence in favor of sepsis and the need for immediate treatment can be based only upon the experience and judgment of the individual clinician. There is, as yet, no study that clearly relates quality and quantity of signs with incidence of proven sepsis.

The choice of antibiotics for treatment before results of bacteriologic studies are available depends upon the kinds of organisms usually encountered in the particular nursery and delivery service. This changes both in type of organism and antibiotic sensitivity from nursery to nursery and from year to year. These phenomenona and the basis for a rational choice of drugs, are discussed in Chap 12, p 414.

A special set of problems occurs at the birth of an infant after prolonged (greater than 24 hours) rupture of amniotic membranes. The overall incidence of sepsis after this is approximately 5 percent, so that prolonged rupture of membranes alone warrants only appropriate bacterial cultures and careful observation of the infant. On the other hand, if there is clear evidence of amnionitis, ie, purulent or foul-smelling amniotic fluid or, most important, maternal fever, the chance of neonatal infection is about 50 percent, neonatal mortality is high, and the infant requires prompt antibiotic therapy, even if he appears healthy at birth.

Such tests as examination of the infant's gastric contents for granulocytes or of the amniotic membranes or sections of the umbilical cord for infiltration by granulocytes have been devised to attempt to identify which infants, born after prolonged rupture of membranes, are going to be septic and should be treated at birth. Often all are positive in the absence of demonstrable neonatal sepsis, so that the tests are of limited value for clinical use; various bacterial cultures in this situation are similarly of limited value. Cultures of placenta, amniotic fluid, or the infant's nasopharynx are very often contaminated with vaginal flora. Culture of the infant's external auditory canal is considered to be less susceptible to contamination, but a positive culture does not make the diagnosis of infection, but only suggests the offending organisms if there is an infection. Culture of blood from the umbilical cord is very likely to be contaminated. It may be possible to reduce contamination by double clamping a segment of the cord at delivery, swabbing this with an iodine preparation, and obtaining a specimen of blood by aspiration, from one of the vessels in the segment, with a sterile needle and syringe.

If the physician caring for a mother with prolonged rupture of membranes has begun systemic antibiotic treatment before delivery, the physician carinfor the infant is more or less obligated to continue treatment of the infant until a full course of therapy is completed or there is good evidence that the mother was never infected. There usually is no way to distinguish between a newborn who was infected and successfully but only partially treated in utero and one who was not infected at all.

References

Barbaro CA: Foetal prognosis after spontaneous premature rupture of the membranes. Med J Austral 2:57, 1967

Corrigan JJ: Thrombocytopenia, a laboratory sign of septicemia in infants and children. J Pediatr 85:219, 1974

Dietzman DE, Fischer GW, Schoenknecht FD: Neonatal Escherichia coli septicemia—bacterial counts in blood. J Pediatr 85:128, 1974

Gluck L, Wood HW, Fousek MD: Septicemia in the newborn. Pediatr Clin North Am 13:1131, 1966

Hosmer M, Sprunt K: Screening method for indentification of infected infants following prolonged rupture of amniotic membranes. Pediatrics 49:283, 1972

Pryles CV, Steg NL, Nair S, Gellis SS, Tenny B: A controlled study of the influence on the newborn of prolonged premature rupture of the amniotic membranes and/or infection in the mother. Pediatrics 31:-608, 1968

Wilson HD, Eichenwald HF: Sepsis neonatorum. Pediatr Clin North Am 21:571, 1974

LONG-TERM OUTLOOK FOR HIGH-RISK INFANTS

Jane V. Hunt

Advances in intensive neonatal care have created a new population of survivors who almost certainly would have died before. The subsequent development of these children has been followed at a number of centers, with particular attention to very low birthweight infants and larger newborns with severe respiratory diseases. There has been considerable concern that the marked improvement intensive care has produced in neonatal survival might not be matched by a reduction in neurologic handicaps among survivors.

PREMATURITY. It is now possible to save many infants weighing less than 1500 g and even less than 1000 g. The earliest reports of the later developmental status of small preterm infants were gloomy, but subsequent advances in treatment, notably in feeding, temperature control, and the treatment of respiratory disease have improved the outlook as reflected in several recent studies. The incidence of severe neurologic complications, such as cerebral palsy and frank mental retardation, is decreasing. It still remains to be determined how many of these infants born in the past few years will develop mild disorders in intellectual development in childhood.

Although the incidence of developmental problems is generally correlated with the degree of prematurity, as measured by either gestational age or birthweight, it is also influenced by the causes of prematurity. In a study of 283 children at 1 to 3 years, whose birthweights were under 2000 g, Drillian found that the group who had fetal developmental anomalies had a high risk of moderate or severe developmental handicaps; the group who had adverse factors, such as hypoxia or malnutrition in late pregnancy, had an increased incidence of mild mental retardation or neurologic abnormality; and the group who were "accidentally" delivered prematurely were potentially normal at birth.

The last group may have derived the greatest benefits from intensive neonatal care. The increasing emphasis on fetal care and the monitoring of high-risk pregnancies may bring similar advances to the other categories.

INTRAUTERINE GROWTH RETARDATION. Studies on intellectual development of small-for-gestational-age (SGA) groups have produced variable results. Fitzhardings and Steven, in a study of 96 full-term SGA infants, found that although the average IQ was normal, 50 percent of the boys and 36 percent of the girls were doing poorly in school; there was a higher than normal incidence of mild neurologic signs and speech defects. No association was found between these defects and the degree of intrauterine growth retardation. The average IQ during childhood of SGA infants under 1500 g at birth was normal, but significantly lower than that of the group with birthweights appropriate for dates (Francis-Williams and Davies). Perceptual-motor disabilities and learning disorders were more common in both groups than in the general population. Lubchenco and associates, in a study of infants under 2000 g at birth, found that neurologic and intellectual handicaps were more frequent with lower birthweights, but there was no difference in the incidence in SGA infants and those appropriate for gestational age. They noted, however, that in children who had been larger preterm infants (birthweight more than 2500 g at gestational age less than 38 weeks), there was a relatively high incidence of handicaps.

These varied results suggest that the etiology of the condition, the associated perinatal complications, and neonatal care are all acting to influence outcome.

RESPIRATORY DISEASES OF THE NEWBORN. Problems related to initial resuscitation, apnea, hyaline membrane disease (HMD), and other respiratory distress syndromes are vigorously treated in modern neonatal intensive care units. The status of the survivors is of great interest because of the known associa-

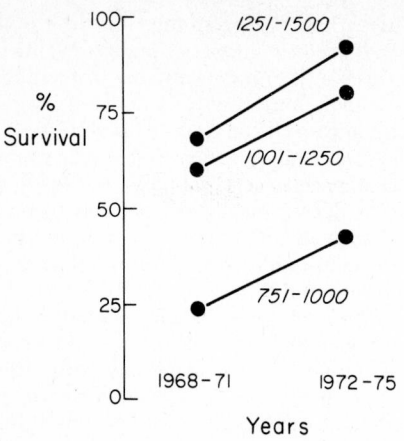

FIG. 44. Change in survival of infants weighing 1500 g or less at birth: born at the University of California, San Francisco between 1965 and 1975.

tion of asphyxia with brain damage and subsequent developmental problems. Also, the association between hyperoxiaand retrolental fibroplasia suggests that all treatment procedures for the newborn must be investigated for potential iatrogenic problems.

The effects of artificial ventilation on the quality of the survivors of respiratory disease have been reported by Stahlman and associates and by Dinwiddie and her coworkers. In both studies no differences in intellectual development were found between those who had been artificially ventilated and those who had not, even though the presumption can be made that those who required ventilation were more seriously ill in the newborn period. However, Stahlman found that a higher percentage of all HMD infants less than 2000 g at birth had intelligence scores below average. Fisch and associates compared the intellectual outcome of survivors of

neonatal respiratory distress syndrome (RDS) and matched controls at 4 years of age and reported that low birthweight and low socioeconomic status were most closely related to poor outcome at this age whereas RDS was not. However, they found an interaction effect between low socioeconomic status and RDS, supporting the conclusions of others that a combination of insults is most detrimental to development.

It appears that the outlook for larger newborns with respiratory disease, who receive intensive neonatal care, including artificial ventilation, is now favorable for normal intellectual development. However, the small preterm infants who have the added complication of respiratory disease continue to be at risk, presumably because of the additive nature of the complications that occur in this group during the newborn period.

CURRENT STATE OF THE PROBLEM. It follows from the preceding discussion that the greatest concern is the intellectual development of very low birth-weight infants (1500 g or less), particularly those with the added stress of respiratory distress. As survival increases among these infants, the incidence of marked handicaps has decreased and the data currently available suggests that the incidence of mild mental retardation and other minor handicaps of intellectual function is also decreasing.

Figure 44 shows the decline in mortality over the years 1965 through 1974 for infants weighing 1500 g or less, born at a representative perinatal intensive care center. Figure 45 shows that during the period when survival increased, the developmental scores at 1 year also increased significantly. Among the more recent survivors, slow development was only slightly more common among those who had hyaline membrane disease than those who did not (Table 10). At 4 years, 50 percent of the infants born 1965-1968 and 70 percent of those born 1969-1972 were entirely normal.

The general outlook for the low birthweight infant has steadily improved, along with advances in newborn

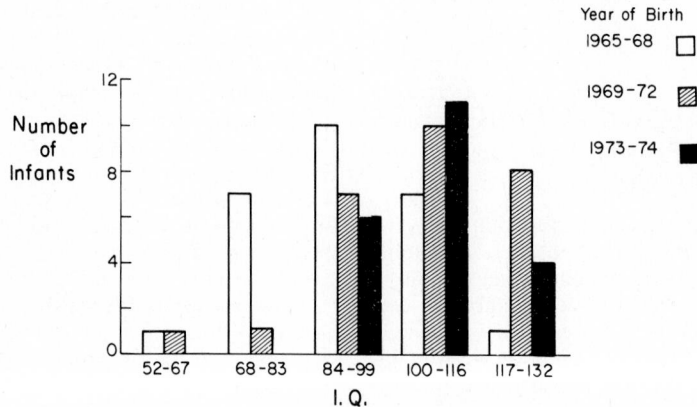

FIG. 45. Distribution of developmental quotients (Cattell and Bayley tests of infant development) of the 66 percent of the survivors from Fig. 44 who were evaluated at one year of age. Note improved performance in the more recent survivors. I.Q.—developmental quotient.

TABLE 10. Developmental status at 1 year of age for 76 infants with birthweight equal to or less than 1500 g, according to presence or absence of clinical respiratory distress syndrome of the newborn (RDS).

Birthdate	No RDS	RDS	Total
1965-68	17	9	26
DQ* below 90	6	6	12
1969-72	16	10	26
DQ* below 90	1	3	4
1973-74	8	13	25
DQ* below 90	0	1	1

*Developmental quotient, adjusted for prematurity from Cattell Scale of Infant Intelligence or Bayley Scales of Infant Development

intensive care. The postnatal environment strongly influences the intellectual development of all children and may be especially important for vulnerable infants, such as those born prematurely or small for gestational age and those who survive respiratory diseases of the newborn. The child who is reared in an advantageous environment may be able to compensate for some initial developmental problems. The disadvantaged child, particularly the child reared in poverty, may fare less well. In fact, socially disadvantaged children are considered a high-risk group in their own right, being at risk for a number of prenatal as well as postnatal environmental conditions that can lead to diminished potential and poor intellectual growth.

References

Cukier F, Amiel-Tison C, Minkowski A: Hyaline membrane disease in ne treated with artificial ventilation: Neurological and intellectual sequelae at two to five years of age. Critical Care Medicine 2:265, 1974

Dinwiddie R, Mellow DH, Donaldson SHC, et al: Quality of survival after artifical ventilation of the newborn. Arch Dis Child 49:703, 1974

Drillian CM: Aetiology and outcome of low-birthweight infants. Develop Med Child Neurol 14:563, 1972

Fisch RO, Bilek MK, Miller LD, et al.: Physical and mental status at 4 years of age of survivors of the respiratory distress syndrome. J Pediatr 86:497, 1975

Fitzhardinge PM, Steven EM: The small-for-date infant. Neurological and intellectual sequelae. Pediatrics 50:50, 1972

Francis-Williams J, Davies PA: Very low birthweight and later intelligence. Develop Med Child Neurol 16:709, 1974

Johnson JD, Malachowski NC, Grobstein R, et al: Prognosis of children surviving with the aid of mechanical ventilation in the newborn period. J Pediatr 84:272, 1974

Luchenco LO, Bard H, Goldman AL, et al: Newborn intensive care and long-term prognosis. Develop Med Child Neurol 16:421, 1974

Stahlman M, Gunnel H, Dolanski E, et al: A six-year follow-up of clinical hyaline membrane disease. Pediatr Clin North Am 20:433, 1973

Stewart AL, Reynolds EOR: Improved prognosis for infants of very low birthweight. Pediatrics 54:724, 1974

CHAPTER 7

Nutrition

LAURENCE FINBERG, *Associate Editor*

Nutrition in its broadest sense determines growth and facilitates metabolic processes. Growing children have exceptional requirements for nutrients; they also are peculiarly vulnerable to disturbances that interfere with their obtaining them. A knowledge of both fundamental principles and practical aspects of nutrition is essential to the physician. This chapter surveys the functions of the essential nutrients and their requirements in health and disease. This section and the next deal with requirements in health. The succeeding sections will discuss diseases that either cause or are the result of nutritional deficiencies.

ENERGY REQUIREMENTS

LAURENCE FINBERG

ENERGY METABOLISM

Like the adult, the child expends energy constantly. Although the process goes on whether he is asleep or awake, it is least rapid during quiet sleep and is far more rapid during periods of muscular activity. To maintain balance, energy must be assimilated from food. The energy value of food is usually expressed in calories, which in considering nutrition refers to kilocalories. When burned in the body, the different foodstuffs have approximately the following energy equivalents: 1 g of fat yields 9 calories; 1 g of protein yields 4 calories; 1 g of carbohydrate yields 4 calories.

The caloric requirements of a growing child may be divided into five categories providing for obligatory losses and for potential energy stored in the course of growth: (1) basal metabolism, (2) bodily activity, (3) growth, (4) caloric loss in the excreta, and (5) specific dynamic action of foods. Efforts have been made to estimate these five components separately, principally by measurement of energy expenditure in a variety of circumstances. The cumbersome methods of direct calorimetry by direct measurement of heat loss have largely been superseded by technically less exacting methods of indirect calorimetry. The subject is confined during relatively short observation periods in a respiration chamber while his oxygen consumption, carbon dioxide and water production, and nitrogen excretion are measured, thus permitting conversion of the chemical reactions involved into equivalent calories. The energy requirements for the various categories are summarized as follows.

BASAL METABOLISM. Basal metabolism refers to the caloric expenditure during rest or sleep; it differs in children from its rate in adults because of the smaller size of the child, which increases heat loss per unit of weight, and because requirements for growth must be included. Basal metabolism is highest during early life when the infant is small and is growing rapidly; it decreases thereafter as size increases and the rate of growth declines. However, it is fairly constant in children of the same age and weight. During the 12 to 18 months following birth, daily basal expenditure averages about 75 calories per kilogram. It then tends to diminish gradually, reaching the adult value of 25 to 30 calories per kilogram by the time growth has ceased. Since most estimates of basal metabolism in infants have been made shortly after feeding, the caloric expenditure measured has also included the specific dynamic action of the food consumed. In the adult, on the other hand, measurements of basal metabolism are commonly made after an overnight fast, so that only maintenance expenditures are measured, and calories for specific dynamic action and growth are excluded.

BODILY ACTIVITY. The great variation in the food consumption of individual children results chiefly from differences in muscular activity. While awake, an infant expends more energy than when asleep, but the magnitude of the increase is highly variable. Vigorous crying may double metabolism temporarily. An average allowance for activity during the first year is 20 calories per kilogram per day. Young or phlegmatic infants may require only half this amount, while unusually active ones may need four times as much. The energy expended in activity by individual children may vary considerably from day to day.

GROWTH. These requirements are variable, since growth is not a constant process. Direct measurements have shown that about 2.5 calories are required for each gram of body weight gained throughout infancy. During the early months of the first year, as much as 15 to 20 calories per kilogram may be stored in the course of rapid normal growth. At the end of the first year the average is about 5 calories per kilogram per day. The amount of energy stored gradually falls in relation to body weight; however, there is a conspicuous but temporary increase during the pubertal growth spurt.

CALORIC LOSS IN THE EXCRETA. On a mixed diet, approximately 10 percent of the intake is normally lost in the excreta, mainly in the form of fat and protein. In infants this amounts to 8 to 11 calories per kilogram per day. In diarrhea and other conditions of disturbed digestion the caloric loss may be greatly increased.

SPECIFIC DYNAMIC ACTION OF FOODS. Specific dynamic action of foods refers to an increase in heat production, which may last 6 to 8 hours, following intake of food. It is most marked after the intake of protein and relatively slight after intake of fat or carbohydrate. The cause of specific dynamic action has been much disputed. It was at one time attributed to expenditures for digestion and absorption, but it is now known to occur after intravenous alimentation. The increased oxidation is not accompanied by an increase in body work; only heat is produced, which is dissipated. According to Krebs and associates, only reactions resulting in the synthesis of adenosine triphosphate (ATP) are capable of performing body work; other oxidations liberate energy in the form of heat. The higher specific dynamic action of protein is attributed to the fact that the combustion of amino acids involves a number of steps that do not lead to the synthesis of ATP; some of these are concerned with the deamination of amino acids and others with the degradation of their carbon skeleton. The measurements of Levine and his associates indicate that on average diets 4 to 8 calories per kilogram are needed to provide for specific dynamic action. On high-protein diets this requirement may be doubled.

The energy requirements during childhood in relation to body weight are shown schematically in Figure 2. There is a gradual decrease in calories per kilogram that continues until about 16 years of age in boys and 13 or 14 years in girls, followed by a more rapid decline to the adult level of 40 to 50 calories per kilogram.

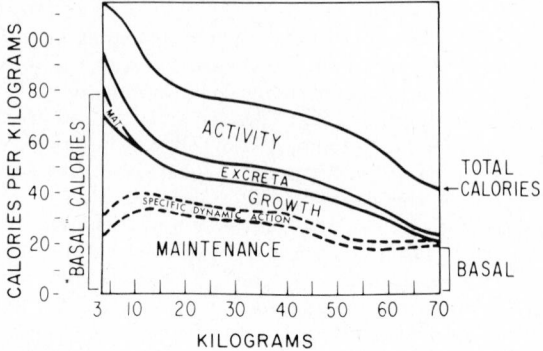

FIG. 2. Daily caloric requirements per kilogram throughout childhood.

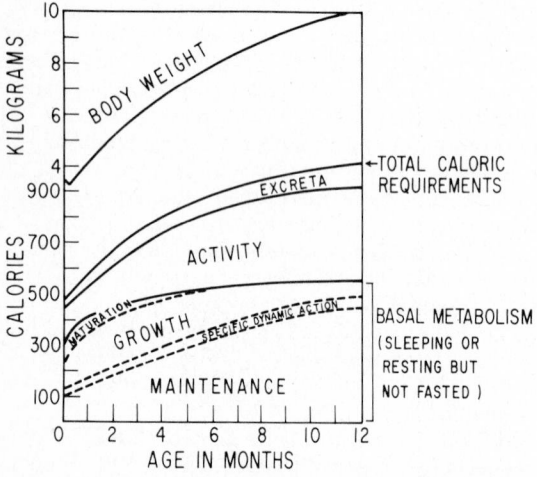

FIG. 1. Daily caloric requirements during the first year of life.

Figure 1 shows the general pattern of the caloric requirements for infants during the first year. During the first week after birth the energy expenditure of an infant is often quite low, especially one who expends a great deal of time sleeping. Moreover, the growth process, which is active in intrauterine life, is temporarily suspended during the period of adjustment to an extrauterine environment. Indeed, during the first 3 days after birth, when the newborn infant takes little food either from breast or from bottle, he is expected to be in negative caloric balance, drawing largely on tissue stores for the energy required for basal metabolic needs and for physical activity. During the second and third weeks after birth the daily caloric requirements rise rapidly to about 100 to 120 per kilogram, after which they fall slowly.

The foregoing data relating caloric requirements to body weight apply only to the *average* child. An obese child has an excess of relatively inert metabolic tissue and consequently needs fewer calories per kilogram than his weight would indicate; conversely, a malnourished child with relatively more active metabolic tissue needs relatively more food. Food requirements in disease vary widely. Although physical activity may be reduced, the basal requirement is increased by fever; in digestive disorders in which considerable portions of food are not absorbed the loss in the excreta may be greatly increased. Often the additional food, although needed, is not tolerated, and the individual must metabolize his body tissues; extra food must be supplied during convalescence to assist him in regaining lost weight.

Figure 3 gives average daily requirements for both sexes from birth to 18 years of age. The caloric requirements during adolescence are greater for both sexes than the standard allowance for adults of moderate activity. During the period of most active growth (14 to 17 years for boys, 12 to 15 years for girls) the amount of food needed to meet caloric requirements is quite large. There are variations due to climate, clothing habits, and activity. An exact estimation of the calories required for any individual child is not possible. The data presented are of value in that they furnish a rough guide as to the amount of food needed. Calculation of the calories enables one to discover whether a child is being grossly underfed or overfed.

PERCENTAGE DISTRIBUTION OF CALORIES. The energy content of a diet may best be expressed in terms of the percentage of calories derived from each of the primary sources of energy—protein, fat, and carbohydrate. Thus, once the optimal (or mini-

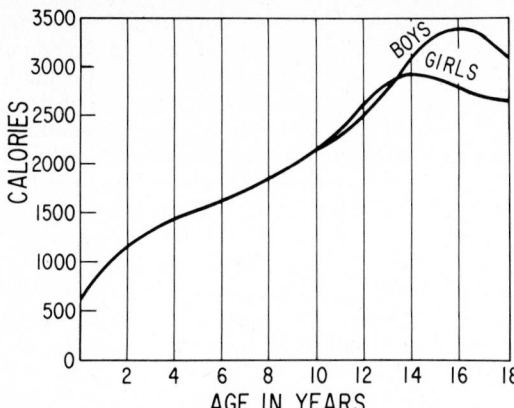

FIG. 3. Total daily calories for both sexes from birth to 18 years of age.

mal) number of calories for intake is decided upon, the distribution allocated to these sources determines their content in the diet. Of the three, only protein seems to have an important minimum. One must recognize the significance of this form of notation, because if the caloric value of a diet should be increased by the addition of carbohydrates, the percentage of protein calories becomes lower and may fall below the minimum (6 to 8 percent), even though the absolute intake stays the same. The consequence will be protein undernutrition. The foregoing example assumes that the higher caloric intake will be absorbed and fully utilized by the subject, thus obligating more amino acids for protein synthesis.

The distribution of calories in breast milk (protein 8 percent, fat 50 percent, carbohydrate 42 percent) has certainly proved to be satisfactory when that food is used. Modified cow's-milk feedings, in which only a little more protein (10 percent of the calories) is given, have been used for many years with success, as have feedings with more protein and less fat (protein 15 percent, fat 35 percent, carbohydrate 50 percent) that have been carried over by tradition from the days when curd indigestion was a problem and when cow's-milk fat was feared.

All diets, for any purpose and for any age, are best understood if analyzed by expression of the primary sources of energy as percentages of the total calories provided. Failure to do so has in the past produced absurd and expensive advice in dietary therapy. Humans can extract energy only from protein, carbohydrate, fat, and ethyl alcohol and their usual degradation molecules. Other species, by virtue of special digestive systems, may derive calories from cellulose and other vegetable substances.

ESSENTIAL HUMAN NUTRIENTS
Laurence Finberg

Until recently it was generally assumed that the vast majority of people in the United States consumed diets of such a varied nature that detailed knowledge of all nutrients required by the growing human being was of only academic interest. Constant changes in eating patterns, with great reliance on manufactured items, and the numerous metabolic disorders becoming subject to dietary management, usually with carefully tailored semipurified diets, have created an awareness of potential and actual deficiencies of micronutrients in medical practice. Although it was recognized that severe malnutrition was prevalent in many parts of the world, it was believed to be a problem of calories, protein, iron, and a few vitamins, notably A and thiamine. We now realize that malnutrition is usually a complex multiple deficiency state and that complete fortification of foods is needed to cope with this problem.

Basic to an appreciation of nutrient requirements and the etiology of deficiency states is an understanding of the relationships between growth and the intakes and expenditures of energy, total nitrogen, essential and semiessential amino acids, essential fatty acids, vitamins, and minerals. Rates of growth and of weight gain, which are not synonymous, are determined primarily by calorie intake. The appetites of infants and children are affected by the caloric density of food, by the content of fat and nitrogen, and by the content and balance among essential amino acids. Small children, over a significant length of time, select diets that are balanced in regard to micronutrients. With the apparent single exception of sodium, however, they will not detect deficiencies of minerals and vitamins, but will continue for a long time to consume diets that may lead to acute clinical deficiency states.

PROTEIN AND AMINO ACIDS
George G. Graham

After oxygen, water, and a source of energy, the nutrients most important for survival are the amino acids. Man, like all monogastric mammals, must consume enough protein to provide nitrogen and some 20 amino acids for the synthesis of new tissue during growth and to replace the nitrogen that is continuously lost from the body even when growth is complete. The ability of a protein to satisfy these requirements is determined primarily by its amino acid composition, for the body is able to synthesize from other compounds only about half of the amino acids needed for tissue protein synthesis; the rest must be provided preformed in the diet, either as the amino acid or in most cases the keto acid, since it is the carbon skeleton that cannot be synthesized. Amino acids that can be synthesized are termed dispensable or nonessential; those that cannot be synthesized are termed indispensable or essential. For man the essential amino acids are valine, leucine, isoleucine, lysine, threonine, tryptophan, phenylalanine, and methionine, and for the young infant, histidine. Two additional amino acids, tryosine and cystine, can only be synthesized from the essential amino acids phenylalanine and methionine, respectively. Since their presence in the diet reduces the need for the precursors, they are commonly called semiessential. Fetuses, small premature infants, and possibly some full-term infants may have a very limited capacity to convert methionine to cysteine and cystine, making these essential amino acids. This classification applies only to dietary requirements for amino acids; they are all equally essential for protein synthesis. The nonessential amino acids can be synthesized by man from organic acids derived from intermediate carbohydrate metabolism, from nitrogen and surplus amino acids, or from such simple compounds as urea.

Many nitrogen-containing nonprotein compounds essential to body function are formed from amino acids; heme, creatine, choline, and glutathione are examples. Tryptophan is the source of the pyridine nucleotides and of serotonin; phenylalanine and tyrosine are precursors of the thyroid hormones, the catecholamines, and melanin; methionine is the most important methyl donor of the body. Amino acids in excess of the needs for synthesis of protein and other compounds are deaminated, primarily in the liver, to yield either ammonia, which is converted to urea and excreted by the kidney, or α-keto acids, which may be used for synthesis of fat, glucose, and other substances. They may also be oxidized to carbon dioxide and water to yield energy in the form of phosphate bonds.

DIGESTIBILITY.   Proteins cannot normally be absorbed intact after the newborn period, but must undergo hydrolysis to oligopeptides and free amino acids. Hydrolysis is initiated in the stomach under the influence of pepsin, which facilitates the splitting of peptide bonds and the formation of shorter polypeptides. The stomach also controls the flow of partially digested food into the intestine, thus preventing overloading of digestion and absorptive capacities. In the intestine the partially digested protein is mixed with pancreatic and intestinal secretions and cells sloughed from the mucosa. It is estimated that these endogenous sources contribute at least as many amino acids as those coming from the dietary protein. Polypeptides undergo further hydrolysis under the influence of proteases and peptidases: trypsin, chymotrypsin, and carboxypeptidases from the pancreas and a mixture of peptidases from the intestine. Intestinal digestion is generally a rapid process.

The apparent digestibility of food protein is estimated by subtracting fecal nitrogen from the amount ingested and expressing the balance as a percentage of intake. For estimates of true digestibility, a correction must be made for endogenous fecal nitrogen (the amount excreted on a protein-free diet). Primarily because of their fiber content, most vegetable proteins are less well digested than those of egg and milk, the common standards of reference. This property adversely affects the net protein utilization of vegetable proteins. However, when the more soluble proteins are isolated, their digestibility closely approximates that of milk or egg protein. It is believed, although not documented, that the various molecular structures of proteins may affect their digestibility and the availability of their amino acids for protein synthesis in the body.

ABSORPTION.   A significant portion of dietary protein is absorbed as oligopeptides. The naturally occurring L-amino acids are transported across the intestinal wall by an active process requiring energy. Different amino acids are transported against concentration gradients at different rates. At high concentrations some compete with others for common transport sites. There is also evidence for individual transport sites, probably of lesser capacity. It is unlikely that such competition is ever of importance in normal individuals, although it may be in some inborn errors of metabolism. For example, the high levels of circulating phenylalanine in phenylketonuria interfere with tryptophan transport.

DISTRIBUTION.   Some amino acids are removed during absorption for the synthesis of intestinal proteins, which have a rapid turnover; others, such as glutamic acid, may be transaminated to alanine, thereby changing their concentrations in the portal vein. However, the pattern of amino acids in the portal blood reaching the liver reflects rather faithfully the pattern in the dietary protein, as the amino acids removed for protein synthesis have a pattern nearly identical to that of the amino acids contributed from endogenous sources.

The liver withdraws amino acids for the synthesis of both liver and plasma proteins and for oxidation of amino acids, particularly of those in surplus, converting the nitrogen to urea. It contributes those that are synthesized, including glycine, serine, alanine, and aspartic and glutamic acids. Despite these alterations, free amino acids in the systemic blood will vary for some time after a meal, according to the dietary pattern. These changes occur sooner and are more marked in the red blood cell, which transports amino acids from the liver to peripheral sites of protein synthesis, particularly muscle. The plasma, which transports amino acids from muscle to liver, has its free amino acid pattern affected later and to a lesser degree, the changes being the result of net difference between synthesis and catabolism. At abnormally high or low levels of protein intake, the plasma pattern is much more affected. Catabolism of excess amino acids is not a very active process; so it is some time before the levels of circulating amino acids return to the basal state. If an essential amino acid is deficient in the diet, its utilization in the intestine, liver, and elsewhere may markedly reduce its level in the systemic circulation, particularly at low levels of protein intake. Even when such an amino acid is not truly deficient, but there is an excess of the remaining essential amino acid, its systemic level is reduced, and the appetite is adversely affected. This last situation is known as amino acid imbalance.

Different tissues incorporate amino acids into protein at different rates. Secretory organs, notably the pancreas and small intestine, have the most rapid rate of uptake, followed by the liver. Muscle does so more slowly, but because it represents such a large fraction of body mass, it accounts for a great proportion of the amino acids utilized.

STORAGE. Unlike the main sources of calories, amino acids are not stored in a readily available form such as glycogen and fat. Body protein content can be increased by high protein intake, but probably no more than 5 percent. This is hardly an efficient store, since it is lost quite rapidly during periods of low intake. Normal body proteins, which are lost first during starvation or low protein consumption and are made up promptly during refeeding, are at times referred to as protein reserves. However, the term labile body proteins seems preferable, since their loss compromises function. These are lost primarily from liver, gastrointestinal tract, pancreas, and kidney. On prolonged depletion, muscle eventually contributes more than the viscera. The amino acids released under these circumstances are reutilized to maintain essential tissues and enzymes, with brain protein and oxidative enzymes particularly well conserved.

When all the necessary amino acids are not available simultaneously in the proper proportions at protein synthetic sites, some portion of those present in relative excess will not be retained, making it inefficient to consume at one meal a protein deficient in an essential amino acid and to compensate for this by consuming the missing amino acid at the next meal. Although energy requirements should be met for most efficient protein utilization, and it is probably preferable for calories to be distributed in a number of spaced meals, it is possible to concentrate all or most of the day's protein intake in one of these meals.

When dietary protein is inadequate, amino acids, coming from proteins that are constantly turning over in most tissues, may be diverted preferentially to tissues of the greatest size and synthesis rate. Such priorities are determined by total caloric intake and homeostatic mechanisms and are regulated by the endocrine and nervous systems through their effects on the transport and enzyme activity.

REQUIREMENTS. Much of the confusion about dietary requirements for nitrogen and essential amino acids can be resolved if it is recognized that these are not absolute for an individual of a given age and size but are determined by the total caloric intake, by the rates of protein synthesis and of growth, and by the physiologic state.

Estimates of the absolute requirement for total nitrogen can be made from data on the amounts required for obligatory urine, stool, and skin losses and data on changes in body composition with age. A general relationship holding for most mammals is the endogenous urinary excretion of 2 mg of nitrogen per basal kilocalorie metabolized. On this basis, assuming a basal expenditure of 60 kcal/kg/day, a 10-kg infant would have a urinary nitrogen loss of 120 mg/kg/day. This figure is approximated when measured urine losses on known protein intakes are extrapolated to a zero intake. On the other hand, when urine losses have been measured on a protein-free diet, these have been of the order of 40 to 60 mg/kg/day. Endogenous fecal nitrogen losses are generally estimated to be about 20 percent of the urine

losses. On protein-free diets they have been reported to be 10 to 20 mg/kg/day. Except under unusual conditions of heavy sweating, skin losses in infants and young children probably do not exceed 10 mg/kg/day. Thus the total obligatory losses of nitrogen lie between 60 and 150 mg/kg/day.

Nitrogen requirements during the first year of life are much higher per unit of body weight than at any other time. Besides rapid growth, with a tripling of body weight, an important process of *chemical maturation* occurs, with a change from approximately 2 percent nitrogen in the full-term newborn to 3 percent at 1 year. The premature infant, starting with a lower weight and lesser percentage of nitrogen, has even greater increments. For the full-term infant normal growth and maturation in the first year represent an average nitrogen requirement of approximately 100 mg/kg/day. Added to the obligatory losses, the total becomes 160 to 250 mg, or roughly 1.0 to 1.6 g of protein per kilogram per day. During the second year the requirements for growth falls to only 20 mg/kg/day for nitrogen, and the total falls to 80 to 170 mg/kg/day. Since chemical maturation is nearly complete in the first 4 months and the rates of weight gain are progressively less during the course of the first year, the requirement of nitrogen is relatively much greater at the beginning than at the end of the first year.

The figures given above assume 100 percent digestibility and utilization of dietary protein. However, this is never the case, even with protein from human breast milk. Although digestibility may be over 95 percent, utilization for protein synthesis is not continuous, not uniform, and not perfectly efficient. In young adults it has been shown that for nitrogen balance to be achieved, 30 percent more of the highest quality dietary protein must be consumed than was estimated from measured losses on a protein-free diet. Although protein synthesis mechanisms are generally responsive to food intake, they have intrinsic rhythms of activity and limits to their capacity. Significant variations in physiologic state, even in quite normal infants, result in periods of poor appetite, increased caloric expenditure, reduced rates of protein synthesis, increased catabolism of protein, and consequent irregularities in the pattern of growth. In order to compensate for these variations in rates of protein utilization, dietary protein intake must of necessity exceed the calculated requirement by a larger amount. Dietary requirements of the highest quality protein, determined from intakes known to be adequate for maximal growth during the first year, have been estimated to average 1.5 g/kg/day, decreasing from approximately 2.2 g at birth to 1.2 g at 1 year; these amounts are as much as 50 percent more than the calculated requirement. Thereafter the dietary requirement of such a protein probably does not exceed 1.0 g/kg/day, even during the growth spurt of adolescence.

The breast-fed infant, or the infant receiving a modified cow's-milk formula at the same level of protein intake, retains approximately 45 percent of the nitrogen intake, an amount very near to that estimated on the thesis of obligatory losses and the requirements for growth and maturation. With increasing age, as other sources of dietary protein gradually replace part or all or the milk protein, digestibility and biologic value become more important, and a correction for these must be made in estimating the requirement.

When we relate the above estimates of dietary protein requirement to those of energy requirements, we can see that approximately 6 to 7 percent of dietary calories must be provided as high-quality protein. This is the range within which the protein/calorie ratio of human breast milk falls. If dietary protein falls below 6 percent of the calorie intake for any length of time, manifestations of inadequacy may appear, even though weight gain to the point of obesity and linear growth continue. This subject is covered further in the section on protein deficiency (p. 211).

Human breast milk, cow's milk, and whole egg proteins, the usual standards of reference, provide approximately 50 percent of their nitrogen as essential and semiessential amino acids. In most vegetable proteins only 32 to 38 percent of the nitrogen is present in this form. It has been shown that the high-quality proteins can have their essential amino acid content diluted with nonessential nitrogen without reducing their utilization by the human infant or child. It has also been shown that well-balanced vegetable proteins can be fed at levels that are critical for milk or egg protein and support equivalent rates of growth. These observations indicate that there is a surplus of essential amino acids in the high-quality animal proteins when they are fed at levels at which total nitrogen is the limiting factor for growth; this surplus is about 20 percent of the amount present. If essential amino acid requirements are estimated on this basis they are similar to the estimates of Holt and Snyderman made from studies with mixtures of pure amino acids. It is now agreed that the pattern of essential amino acids in human breast milk is ideal for the human infant, a revelation that is not too surprising. It is closely approximated by that of whole egg or of cow's milk that has been modified to reduce its content of casein and increase its relative content of lactalbumin and thus approach the proportions in breast milk. As the digestibility of these proteins in high, their net protein utilization is almost identical to that of breast milk.

The contents of essential amino acids in the proteins of common cereals and other vegetable proteins are relatively low, but occasionally there is an unusually high content of one of the essentials. Lysine is markedly deficient in wheat protein. Both lysine and threonine are deficient in rice protein. But in corn, lysine and tryptophan are deficient, and leucine is present in excess. Most legumes have a high protein content, but generally there is a moderate excess of lysine and a marked deficiency of methionine. In commonly consumed mixed diets, such as rice and beans and corn and beans, the high protein and lysine contents of the legumes compensate for their low levels in the cereals. The more generous methionine and cystine contents of the cereals only partially make up for the deficiency in the beans, leaving the sulfur-containing amino acids as the apparently first-limiting item in the diets consumed in most developing countries. In the diets of infants and small children in the same countries, however, the legumes are often not included or are given in very small amounts, leaving lysine as the first-limiting item in their almost exclusively cereal diets. For this reason fish protein concentrates or a variety of soya products (both rich in protein and in lysine) and the synthetic amino acid itself are receiving considerable attention as possible supplements to such diets. Diets based on the most abundant and inexpensive starchy roots and tubers (cassava and sweet potato) are so low in protein that supplementation with a well-balanced protein takes precedence over attempts to correct their specific amino acid deficiencies. Attempts to compensate for this low protein content, or for severe amino acid deficiency, by increasing the total consumption of such items are forestalled by inability to digest the tremendous excess of starch and by the calorie excess, relative to protein, that is automatically created.

The estimates of nitrogen and essential amino acid requirements that have been discussed are based on caloric intakes that support a steady rate of protein synthesis and growth at assumed normal rates. If caloric intake is lower or expenditure is increased, rates of protein synthesis decrease, and so does the requirement. Provision of normal dietary intake of protein under such circumstances results in its partial utilization as a source of energy and excretion of an excess of nitrogen. In the management of renal failure this creates a hazard to health. In such circumstances the provision of essential amino acids or keto acids alone is adequate for a considerable length of time. The accumulated excess of unessential nitrogen in the body, mostly as urea, serves as the nitrogen source for synthesis of the amino group of most of the essentials and all of the nonessentials.

When caloric intake is high, either during rehabilitation from undernutrition or during the accumulation of excess weight, the nitrogen and essential amino acid requirements are higher than usual. If such a relative excess of calories over protein is consumed for more than a few days, signs of protein deficiency will appear (p. 211). With rare exceptions, a diet that provides about 8 percent of calories as high-quality protein will prove adequate at any level of caloric intake and rate of growth. In mixed protein diets, which have poorer digestibility, a lower ratio of essential amino acid to total nitrogen, and a moderate deficiency of one or more essentials, 11 to 15 percent of the total calories as protein is usually adequate. Significant excesses of dietary protein, particularly in situations of limited water intake or excessive insensible losses, commonly result in chronic dehydration and "fever of unknown origin" by virtue of the increase in obligatory renal water excretion.

Natural dietary excesses or deficiencies of amino acids are not known to be of practical significance; the role of excess leucine and relative deficiency of tryptophan in the pathogenesis of pellagra is a possible exception. A specific role for methionine deficiency in hepatic steatosis has been suggested. With these exceptions, no specific lesions of single amino acid deficiency have been documented or are suspected from natural diets. In the management of inborn errors of amino acid metabolism, it is necessary to create borderline deficiency states for the amino acids in question. When these deficiencies become excessive, the manifestations are basically indistinguishable for those of protein deficiency.

If parenteral nutrition is required for a few days in a previously well nourished infant or child, it is seldom necessary to worry about nitrogen and amino acid intakes. It is also unnecessary and injudicious to attempt the provision of normal calorie intake without protein, thus creating an acute protein-deficient state. If parenteral nutrition must be prolonged, or if it is necessary in the severely malnourished, the provision of at least 8 percent of the calories as protein is certainly advisable. Protein hydrolysates or mixtures of synthetic amino acids are superior to intact proteins for parenteral nutrition, since the former are immediately available at the sites of protein synthesis.

FAT

Laurence Finberg

Fat is an integral constituent of all body tissues. The depot fat or adipose tissue serves primarily as an energy reserve and consists almost exclusively of neutral fat. A variable amount of glyceride is present in other tissues, too, but much of their fat is combined as cholesterol esters and phospholipids; other fat complexes include the lipoproteins of the blood and the galactolipids of the brain and other tissues. The depot fat normally constitutes 10 percent or more of the body weight, but in states of inanition it may fall below 1 percent, and in extreme obesity it may exceed 50 percent. Its characteristics are affected by dietary fat. In adults depot fat is relatively unsaturated, having an iodine value between 65 and 80, whereas in the newborn infant it is more saturated, having an iodine value between 30 and 45; the iodine value rises rapidly during the first year. The more saturated fat appears to be less readily mobilized from the depots. The fat pads of the cheeks, the lipid of which remains relatively saturated throughout infancy, show a striking tendency to resist mobilization in inanition. The more saturated character of the fat in the neonatal period may explain the resistance to ketosis in infants.

The tissue lipids are less sensitive than depot fat to alterations in dietary fat. They are always more unsaturated than the ingested fat, and the extent to which they can be depleted in inanition is far more limited.

Fat is readily synthesized from the acetate residues derived from breakdown of carbohydrate and protein. This is true of saturated fats and those with one unsaturated linkage. However, there appears to be difficulty in synthesizing the more highly unsaturated fatty acids (linoleic and arachidonic acids), which are needed by the body in minute amounts. Animal studies have shown that in the absence of these essential fatty acids a characteristic skin disease develops. It is probable that traces of the highly unsaturated fatty acids are essential to man also. However, specific fatty acid deficiency is unlikely to occur in practical dietetics. The level of blood cholesterol is affected by the intake of highly unsaturated fatty acids. The substitution of vegetable fats such as corn oil, safflower oil, and olive oil, which contain a higher proportion of these fatty acids than butter, has a definite depressing effect on the serum cholesterol level, which is taken advantage of in current attempts to prevent atheromatous disease in adults. The importance of including more liberal intakes of these fatty acids in the diet of infants and young children has yet to be shown. It may be mentioned, however, that claims have been made that the seeds of atheromatous disease are planted in early life. Breast milk ordinarily contains more of the essential fatty acids than does cow's milk. However, it seems to result in higher cholesterol levels in the blood, a phenomenon that still cannot be explained.

Infants have been fed for months on virtually fat-free diets without obvious impairment of health, provided fat-soluble vitamins are supplied. The stools may be loose for a time, but this tends to disappear. A tendency toward eczema and asthma has been observed on complete withdrawal of fat from the diet. It is possible that this phenomenon is associated with the increased hydration of the body when carbohydrate is substituted for the fat, a phenomenon discussed below.

Although fat can be withdrawn from the diet without serious consequences, there are good reasons for including it. It is the most concentrated source of energy available and is a vehicle for fat-soluble vitamins. There is some evidence that some fat in the diet improves resistance against infections.

The dangers of a high-fat diet have been greatly overestimated. Ketogenic diets are well tolerated for long periods, barring the development of some intercurrent infection. The view that a high-fat diet per se may lead to fat intolerance does not bear critical analysis; in our experience such disturbances, when seen, can be attributed to factors other than the fat of the diet. There are, however, certain definite indications for reducing the fat intake: (1) certain cases of nausea and vomiting; (2) ketosis, unless induced for therapeutic purposes; (3) lipemia with or without a fatty liver; and (4) lymphatic obstructions leading to chylothorax or chylous ascites. Ketosis occurs when more fat is presented for combustion than can be completely burned; this must be regarded as an unphysiologic state.*

* *The older view that "fats burn in the flame of carbohydrates" and that antiketogenic factors derived from fat and protein are essential to the oxidation of ketone bodies has been reinterpreted. Metabolic products of all three calorigenic foodstuffs enter the citric acid cycle as acetyl CoA, which combines with oxaloacetic acid to form citric acid. Fat, however, enters the cycle only at this point, whereas products of carbohydrate metabolism and those derived from some amino acids can enter the cycle directly at other points. The cycle is thus more readily fed by carbohydrate and protein than by fat and may become overtaxed when supplied only by the acetyl CoA derived from fat, with the result that the ketone bodies accumulate. However, there is a marked ability to adapt to a ketogenic diet, with decreasing quantities of ketones appearing as it is continued.*

Steatorrhea, the loss of an abnormal amount of fat in the stool, has long been regarded as an indication for avoiding fat, a view that is open to question. When fat assimilation is faulty, reducing fat intake will reduce the fecal fat and improve the appearance of the stools. However, it does not follow that fat restriction improves the patient or shortens the disease. Metabolic observations in various types of steatorrhea have shown that the more fat given, the more the patient absorbs, regardless of the loss in the stool, and that there is no resulting washing out of other nutrients or evidence of delayed recovery. This evidence suggests the desirability of liberal fat administration for the sake of maintaining a balanced assimilation of foodstuffs.

Fats differ in their ease of assimilation, depending on their constituent fatty acids. The short-chain fatty acids and those with unsaturated linkages are more readily assimilable. These differences are minimal in the case of the normal infant, but in conditions of steatorrhea, where assimilation is impaired, the substitution of vegetable fats such as corn oil, olive oil, and soybean oil for butter may be of practical value. Fine emulsification of the fat will also aid its assimilation in steatorrhea.

The inhibitory effects of fat on gastric secretion and motility also vary with the composition of the fat, the more readily assimilable fats giving the greater inhibition.

CARBOHYDRATE

Carbohydrate furnishes the most convenient source of energy. Although it is indispensable in the internal economy of the body, carbohydrate is not actually a dietary essential, for it can readily be synthesized from protein and to a considerable extent from fat. The eating habits of Eskimos and other exclusively carnivorous peoples show that a diet containing a minimum of carbohydrate is consistent with health and growth. Infants have been reared successfully on a diet of seal meat chewed by an adult and expectorated into the infant's mouth. The desirability of feeding infants a diet low in carbohydrate, as is the case with unsupplemented cow's milk, has been questioned. That such feedings can be successful is no longer disputed. In older children the influence of high-carbohydrate diets, particularly high-sugar diets, on the development of dental caries appears to be well established.

When an isocaloric shift is made, with carbohydrate calories replacing fat calories, a sudden gain in weight may occur for a few days, after which the previous slope of the weight curve is resumed. The gain in weight is due to water retention accompanied by both extracellular and intracellular electrolyte and some nitrogen. These retained elements are loosely held and are readily lost in the presence of infection or when dietary carbohydrate is replaced by fat. The nitrogen partition in the urine is affected by this dietary shift; on higher fat intake there is an increase in the excretion of total nitrogen and of all nitrogenous substances in the urine except purines, the excretion of which is diminished.

Conversely, on higher carbohydrate intake total nitrogen in the urine falls, although the output of purines rises. The significance of these changes is not entirely clear. Munro has shown that it is the absolute change in carbohydrate intake, rather than change in fat or change in the fat–carbohydrate ratio, that is responsible. Retention of water and electrolytes on high-carbohydrate diets seems to be associated with deposition of glycogen.

Whether resistance to infection can be appreciably altered by a predominance of one or another foodstuff in the diet cannot be answered at the present time. Efforts to reduce the frequency of intercurrent infections in clinically well nourished infants and children by manipulation of the diet have been disappointing.

In infant feeding a carbohydrate supplement is commonly added to cow's milk. Formerly, great importance was attached to the type of carbohydrate used, but it is now realized that differences in behavior of the various carbohydrates are minor and are usually of no importance. The carbohydrates used in infant feeding are described elsewhere (p. 207).

VITAMINS
LAURENCE FINBERG

The term vitamin is applied to a group of organic accessory food factors that must be supplied to the body in small amounts to maintain health. Many vitamins serve as constituents of body enzymes, and all of them may function in this way. A large number of these factors have been described on the basis of observations in experimental animals, but few are of extablished importance in human nutrition. The vitamins important in humans can be classified in three categories: (1) Obligatory vitamins are factors that must always be supplied to maintain health. These include vitamin A (or its carotene equivalent), thiamine, riboflavin, pyridoxine, folic acid, vitamin B_{12}, vitamin C (ascorbic acid), and vitamin D (or its equivalent in ultraviolet radiation). (2) Conditional vitamins are factors needed only in the presence of a deficit of some other nutrient. These are nicotinic acid, choline, and vitamin K. (3) Questionable vitamins are substances concerned in body metabolism that are not yet established as dietary essentials for the *normal human* subject. Until they are shown to be required, exception may be taken to the current practice of designating them as vitamins. Examples are biotin, inositol, pantothenic acid, and vitamin E.

Obligatory Vitamins

Vitamin A, a fat-soluble factor, plays an important part in maintaining the integrity of epithelial structures. It also is a constituent of the visual pigments of the retina. The functional role of vitamin A and the effects of vitamin A deficiency are discussed elsewhere (p. 221).

Thiamine (vitamine B_1), a pyrimidine-thiazole compound, forms the prosthetic group of several respiratory enzymes. A deficiency of thiamine leads to beriberi, which is still an important deficiency disease. In the United States thiamine deficiency is exceedingly rare, being seen only as a result of dietary fads and in alcoholics. Thiamine function and the effects of its deficiency are discussed elsewhere (p. 222).

Riboflavin (vitamin B_2), a greenish yellow pigment that is an alloxazine ribose compound, forms the functional group of a large class of enzymes, the flavoproteins, that are present in every cell. Like thiamine, riboflavin is widely distributed in animal and vegetable foods, and a deficiency becomes possible only when the diet consists largely of refined carbohydrates. Riboflavin deficiency is considered elsewhere (p. 223).

Pyridoxine (vitamin B_6), a methoxy pyridine derivative, is one of the most important cofactors in metabolic reactions. It is the prosthetic group of many enzymes concerned with metabolism of amino acids, proteins, and fat. Because of its wide distribution, pyridoxine deficiency is rarely encountered in man. It has been observed only when some unusual heating procedure has damaged the pyridoxine of the food and in a rare condition known as pyridoxine dependency in which unusually large amounts of this vitamin are required. Pyridoxine deficiency is discussed on (p. 226).

Folic acid (pteroylglutamic acid) is widely distributed in natural foods. It is a constituent of many enzyme systems, notably those concerned with the transfer of single-carbon units. Folic acid deficiency is discussed on page (p. 228).

Vitamin B_{12} (cobalamine), the anti-pernicious-anemia extrinsic factor, is a cobalt porphyrin compound in which the cobalt is linked coordinately to a benzimidazole-ribofuranase-phosphate complex. The terms cobalamin and B_{12} refer to the group as a whole, with its members having individual designations (the cyanide as cyanocobalamin or B_{12a}, the nitrite as nitritocobalamin or B_{12b}, etc). The exact form present in the body is not known, but it appears to be intimately associated with the mitochondria.

Cobalamine is widely distributed in animal tissue but is virtually absent in vegetable products; hence it is sometimes designated the animal growth factor. It is an essential metabolite for all higher animals, but is not necessarily a dietary essential. Herbivorous animals obtain it from bacterial synthesis in the gut. Small amounts are synthesized by intestinal bacteria, but this occurs primarily in the large intestine, from which little is absorbed. Vegetarians who rigorously exclude milk and eggs as well as animal tissues from their diet may, over a period of years, develop evidence of B_{12} deficiency. Thus it seems proper to class B_{12} among the dietary essentials; however, it is of practical importance only to vegetarians and to individuals who lack intrinsic factor and therefore have difficulty absorbing B_{12}.

Absorption of B_{12} from the intestine is dependent on intrinsic factor, a heat-labile enzyme of mucoprotein nature that is defective in pernicious anemia, postgastrectomy anemia, and certain gastrointestinal malformations. Although most patients with pernicious

anemia respond to large doses of oral B_{12}, a few require parenteral therapy.

B_{12} is thought to function in respiratory metabolism. There is evidence that it is concerned with disulfide reductions, with formation of desoxyribose compounds, and with formation of succinate from methyl malonate. Its function is closely related to folic acid, which it may activate; a folic derivative, methyl tetrahydrofolic acid, is frequently found in the urine of untreated patients with pernicious anemia. B_{12} is concerned in some way with the transfer of single-carbon units and with the synthesis of purines and porphyrins. A deficiency of B_{12} induces maturation arrest of the red cells, with macrocytosis and a megaloblastic marrow. The life span of such red cells averages only 60 days. The degenerative changes in the nervous system in B_{12} deficiency have no counterpart in folic acid deficiency.

The administration of B_{12} is indicated in pernicious anemia, fish tapeworm anemia, and postgastrectomy anemia, as well as for complete vegetarians. Reports that it stimulates the growth of premature and malnourished infants have not been substantiated, nor has it proved effective in degenerative disease of the central nervous system, other than that associated with pernicious anemia. The clinical management of pernicious anemia is discussed elsewhere (p. 1126).

Ascorbic acid (vitamin C) is a hexuronic acid of lactone structure. It is a powerful reducing agent known to be involved in collagen synthesis, in utilization of the aromatic amino acids, in the conversion of folic to folinic acid, and in the synthesis of steroids. It is discussed further in connection with scurvy (p. 228) and megaloblastic anemia (p. 1125).

Vitamin D is obligatory because the body has a definite requirement for certain steroids possessing vitamin D activity. This factor is concerned particularly with calcification of the skeleton. The need can be met by providing a vitamin-D containing compound in the diet or by exposure of the body to ultraviolet radiation, which activates a precursor in the skin (7-dehydrocholesterol) and produces a steroid having vitamin D activity. In a sense vitamin D can be regarded as a conditional vitamin, since it is possible to meet the requirements by irradiation alone. By and large, however, we rely on ingested vitamin D to meet the demand, which is greatest in infancy when calcification of the skeleton is proceeding rapidly. The subject is discussed in detail elsewhere (p. 237).

Conditional Vitamins

Nicotinic acid (pyridine-3-carboxylic acid, niacin) has an amide (niacinamide) that is a constituent of the diphospho- and triphospho-pyridine nucleotides (DPN and TPN), the functional groups of a number of important respiratory enzymes. A shortage of this factor is responsible for the development of pellagra (p. 224). Niacin is widely distributed in animal and vegetable foods, but intake is likely to be low when the diet consists predominantly of refined carbohydrates. In the milling of cereals, this factor, like thiamine and riboflavin, is in large part lost. Niacin deficiency is discussed on page 224 .

Choline is a constituent of many important biologic compounds, notably acetylcholine and the lecithin-containing phospholipids. It is intimately concerned with the oxidation of fatty acids, with the turnover of phospholipids, and with fat transport. It also serves as a methyl donor in transmethylation reactions. A deficiency of choline in experimental animals leads to accumulation of fat in the liver, and in the rat it leads to hemorrhagic lesions in the kidney. Although choline is essential in the diet of certain animals, there is good evidence that it can be synthesized in man from methionine. Therefore it cannot be regarded as a human food essential except in states of methionine deficiency. The development of fatty liver in humans does not constitute specific evidence of a deficiency of choline or methionine, for a number of different types of imbalance can produce fatty liver. Administration of choline and methionine is rarely effective in the treatment of fatty liver in humans.

Vitamin K activity is found in a number of quinones, some natural and some synthetic. Vitamin K is a fat-soluble factor, normally present in the body, that is involved in the synthesis of prothrombin and certain other related blood coagulation factors in the liver. It is present in some natural fats, but ordinarily the human requirement is synthesized by the intestinal bacteria. Under exceptional circumstances, however, this synthesis is not adequate, and a deficiency of prothrombin develops. In the first few days of life, before the intestinal bacteria are well established, production of vitamin K in the intestine is limited, and a prolonged prothrombin time is the rule. Only rarely, however, is the degree of deficiency sufficient to lead to hemorrhagic manifestations (p. 1213). Hemorrhagic disease of the newborn is more frequent in premature infants, in whom immaturity of the liver and defective formation of prothrombin from vitamin K play a part. Congenital atresia of the alimentary tract also may be associated with defective synthesis of vitamin K. Prothrombin deficiency is seen in older subjects as a result of liver disease or defective fat absorption in steatorrhea. We have seen it develop following prolonged administration of antibiotics. The administration of vitamin K may be helpful; most authorities recommend its routine administration to all newborn infants, particularly premature infants.

Questionable Vitamins

Biotin appears to function as a constituent of respiratory enzymes. Minute amounts are present in most foods, and animal experiments have shown that it is readily synthesized in adequate amounts by the intestinal bacteria. A deficiency of biotin, which results in a characteristic dermatosis, results only when the biotin so formed is inactivated by eating raw egg white. Egg white contains a protein known as avidin, which combines with biotin and renders it unavailable. Biotin deficiency has been produced experimentally in adult volunteers by a diet containing liberal amounts of raw egg white; it has not been observed in children. The discovery of biotin was followed by a number of uncritical reports of its efficacy in various dermatoses, but these have not been substantiated.

Inositol has an isomer (mesoninositol or muscle sugar) that is closely related to glucose and appears to play an important part in metabolism. It is widely distributed in the body and is found in largest amounts in the heart, brain, and skeletal muscle. In unregulated diabetics and patients receiving glucose infusions there is a marked loss of inositol in the urine. Inositol is a dietary essential for rodents; alopecia develops in its absence. In humans, it appears that inositol can be synthesized.

Pantothenic acid, a compound of β-alanine and dihydroxydimethyl butyric acid, is an integral part of coenzyme A, other constituents being β-mercaptoethylamine, pyrophosphate, and phosphoadenosine. Coenzyme A plays a fundamental part in many metabolic reactions. Its active form, acetyl coenzyme A, is involved in the Krebs cycle, as well as with transfers of two-carbon units generally. It is involved in the synthesis of fats, steroids, and porphyrins and with acetylation and glycine conjugation.

In experimental animals several types of lesions have been produced by diets deficient in pantothenic acid. Dermatitis is prominent in the chick, alopecia is seen in the pig, and gray hair develops in black rats. Anemia, gastrointestinal symptoms, and degenerative changes in the nervous system occur in several species. Rats exhibit gonadal atrophy and adrenal hemorrhages, and there is evidence that they are particularly susceptible to stress; antibody formation may be impaired.

Evidence that humans suffer from pantothenic acid deficiency under natural conditions is only suggestive. The *burning foot syndrome* observed in Japanese war prisoners was reported to respond to the administration of pantothenic acid. It is clear that pantothenic acid is not a human anti-gray-hair factor. A study conducted by Bean on human volunteers showed that rigid exclusion of this compound from the diet, or the administration of an antagonist, led to a variety of symptoms, including fatigue, malaise, nausea and vomiting, abdominal cramps, paresthesias, and muscular incoordination. No evidence has been presented that infants and young children suffer from pantothenic acid deficiency. Pantothenic acid is widely distributed in foods, and the possibility of a deficiency occurring on any natural diet is extremely remote.

Vitamin E, a fat-soluble factor identified as α-tocopherol, is an effective antioxidant. It is a dietary essential for several animal species, but its mechanism of action is not known. In the rabbit, absence of vitamin E gives rise to progressive muscular dystrophy, in the chick a degenerative form of brain disease develops, and in the rat the reproductive organs are affected, with degenerative changes in the testes in the male and resorption of the fetus in the pregnant female. Monkeys develop macrocytic anemia associated with multinucleated megaloblasts. In kwashiorkor patients a similar type of anemia occurs; it responds to vitamin E treatment. The α-tocopheral levels in the blood and tissues can be measured, and there is evidence that it has a role in the human body. Reduced absorption of this factor and lower blood levels have been noted in steatorrhea. György showed that in vitamin-E-deficient animals the red cells were susceptible to hemolysis by hydrogen peroxide. This test has been found by Gordon to be positive in certain premature infants and in patients with cystic fibrosis of the pancreas, and on this basis the administration of vitamin E to such subjects has been recommended. A positive peroxide hemolysis reaction can be reversed by vitamin E administration, but as yet no clinical benefit has been demonstrated. The administration of large amounts of polyunsaturated fat to animals appears to increase their requirements for vitamin E, perhaps because of its antioxidant properties.

In animal nutrition a curious relationship has been demonstrated between vitamin E and the element selenium. Some, but not all, of the manifestation of vitamin E deficiency can be counteracted by trace quantities of selenium in the diet.

Vitamin Supplementation of Human Diets

The discoveries of the various vitamins and the development of simple methods for their manufacture have been followed by their exploitation as food supplements. In the United States this has reached extraordinary proportions. Vitamins have become symbols of health and are ingested in quantities far beyond possible needs. This situation has been brought about by commercial pressures aided by enthusiastic nutrition workers whose attention has been focused on the prevention of deficiency diseases. Skillful advertising, using fear techniques, has created a public demand for vitamins, which in turn brings pressure to bear on the physician. The conscientious physician wishes to make sure that his patients do not suffer from deficiency, but he also feels the obligation to protect them from unnecessary expense and from exploitation of their fear of deficits that they are in no real danger of incurring. The Council on Foods of the American Medical Association has taken the position that administration of accessory factors as such or their incorporation in foods is justified only when a need is demonstrated—a position with which we concur. The effort to render each article of human diet a complete and balanced food, rather than to balance the diet by eating a variety of foods, has little to recommend it. None of the deficiency diseases should be feared with the customary American mixed diets. There is no more justification for giving unnecessary vitamins than for giving unnecessary medication. In both instances there are risks of overdosage that cannot be ignored.

In infants some thought must be given to providing vitamins C and D. Cow's milk, unless reinforced, does not provide enough vitamin D to prevent rickets. Unless he is fed on evaporated milk or fresh milk with added vitamin D, the infant may not receive the 400 international units per day that are normally required during the period of rapid skeletal growth. The rare individual who requires more than this is a medical problem. Hypercalcemia may result from excessive intake or from unusual sensitivity to the action of vitamin D (p. 252).

Vitamin A deficiency is of no concern except in infants who are fed on skim milk. The fat of even half-skimmed milk is ample to meet the infant's needs.

The greatest exploitation has occurred in the case of the B vitamins, for which many unjustifiable claims about health, and particularly mental health, are made. The fact that many of these factors are found together in nature (in yeast and in the germ of cereals) has led to the view that they are functionally related and to their designation as the B complex. This has been interpreted as an indication that a proper balance must be maintained in the intake of these factors.

There appears to be no reason for giving B complex as such. Some of the B factors, as has been pointed out, are readily synthesized and are not needed in the diet. An imbalance caused by administering faulty proportions of the B factors has not been demonstrated. Infants who receive milk and older children on mixed diets are not in danger of acquiring any B deficiency, nor can their health or mentality be improved by supplements of these factors. It is generally admitted that the abolition of pellagra in this country was brought about not by the administration of nicotinic acid but by socioeconomic factors that raised the standard of living in the South and led to a higher tryptophan intake.

WATER AND MINERALS
Laurence Finberg

Water, which constitutes 70 percent of the lean body mass, represents an indispensable and prime constituent of the body. A daily water requirement occurs because of obligatory ongoing losses of water. These losses must occur because (1) energy expended in the form of heat removes water directly through evaporation from skin and lungs, and (2) the energy metabolism producing the heat creates changes in extracellular fluid composition, the adjustment of which obligates loss of water by the kidney. The production and expenditure of heat goes on continuously as the principal mechanism for the maintenance of body temperature within a very narrow range. Most of the bodily energy produced in the resting or basal state goes for this purpose. Clearly, water requirements will vary with the energy produced or, stated in other terms, with the calories metabolized. Hence requirements will be expressed in these terms. Others use the relationships between body surface area and heat loss to express losses as a function of surface area. The concept is similar and for clinical purposes the choice is arbitrary. Inasmuch as the newborn represents an exception to the surface area calculation, and because one may easily memorize a few points on the scale and readily interpolate between them, the caloric expenditure system has a practical advantage. Table 1 permits use of either system and shows the relation-

TABLE 1. Basal Water Requirements in Relation to Age, Weight, and Surface Area

Age	Weight (kg)	Surface Area (M²)	Basal Metabolism (Cal/24 hr)	(Cal/kg/24 hr)	Minimal Basal Water Requirement (ml/24 hr)	(ml/m²/24 hr)	(ml/kg/24 hr)
Newborn	3.3	0.2	150	45	150	750	45
1 wk	3.3	0.2	200	60	200	1,000	60
2 mo	5	0.25	270	54	270	1,080	54
6 mo	8	0.35	400	50	400	1,140	50
12 mo	10	0.45	500	50	500	1,110	50
3 yr	15	0.60	700	47	700	1,170	47
5 yr	20	0.80	900	45	900	1,120	45
8 yr	30	1.05	1,100	37	1,100	1,050	37
13 yr	60	1.70	1,600	27	1,600	840	27

ships. Neither caloric metabolism nor surface area is measured directly; each is estimated from weight and age. At basal conditions, obligatory water losses are approximately as follows:

Insensible (IWL)	45 ml/100 Calories metabolized (skin 30, lungs 15)
Urine	50 ml/100 Calories metabolized
Stool	5 ml/100 Calories metabolized
Total	100 ml/100 Calories metabolized

The Calorie is the kilocalorie. The urine figure assumes no concentration or dilution of solutes by the kidney, and thus a urine osmolality of 300 mOsm/liter. For each 100 Calories metabolized, 12 ml of water are available as "water of oxidation," which reduces the exogenous need. Infants and children on an ordinary diet with ordinary activity expend about 1.5 times the basal energy. Further deviations occur with disease or other pathologic conditions, the most important of which relate to body temperature, activity, and hyperventilation. Total metabolism increases or decreases about 12 percent per degree centigrade change in central body temperature. Activity may increase water loss by about 30 percent, and hyperventilation may triple the loss from the lungs. Other factors such as environmental humidity may play a role. For practical purposes of estimating obligatory water losses, the following four clinical states can be described: (1) basal (as given in Table 1); (2) ordinary diet, activity, and environment (1.5 times basal); (3) unusual fever, activity, or hyperventilation in some combination, but not all maximal (2 times basal); (4) all of the above conditions simultaneously maximal (theoretical only) (3 times basal).

MINERALS

At the present time seven macromineral nutrients are known: sodium, potassium, calcium and magnesium, chloride, phosphorus, and sulfur. The actual minimum requirements of these minerals for growth and maintenance are not known. Table 2 gives retention figures on breast milk and on cow's milk obtained by Swanson. The figures are subject to correction because losses in sweat were not measured. The difference in mineral retention between the two types of feeding is probably exaggerated. As Wallace has pointed out, the errors caused by incomplete collection of excreta and incomplete consumption of food are additive and tend to produce higher apparent retentions on higher intakes. Nevertheless, it seems that chemical maturation, with respect to minerals as well as nitrogen, can be accelerated in infancy by increased intake. Whether this so-called supermineralization of the growing infant is beneficial remains a question.

Essential as the macrominerals are, they are not of practical concern in the feeding of normal infants and children in well-developed countries, since they are adequately supplied by customary food. Deficiencies arise only in pathologic conditions. The chief electrolytes of the body fluids (sodium, potassium, and chloride) have low minimum requirements and wide ranges of acceptable intake. In general, 2 to 3 mEq/100 Calories metabolized represents the midrange for each.

TABLE 2. Retention of Minerals From Milk by Young Infants

	Na	K	Ca	Mg	Cl	P	S	N
Millimoles retained per 24 hr:								
On breast milk	2.4	2.5	1.0	0.3	2.0	1.1	0.45	38.6
On cow's milk	5.2	4.9	5.0	0.7	5.5	3.7	0.27	66.3
Millimoles retained per kilogram increase in body weight:								
On breast milk	104	108	39.6	12.2	88	49.4	19.9	1,690
On cow's milk	205	190	198	28.4	214	145	10.3	2,599

Calcium is required for the formation of bones and teeth; most of it is present in the skeleton. Calcium is also important in blood coagulation and in maintaining the integrity of muscle and nerve. Calcium serves as an activator of important enzymes, including adenosine triphosphatase, succinic dehydrogenase, lipase, and several proteolytic enzymes.

Only a fraction of the calcium intake is absorbed, the variation being from 10 to 40 percent. The amount of calcium that can be excreted in the urine is relatively small, and the body regulates its supply in large part by the amount absorbed; also, a larger fraction is absorbed on a less generous intake. A number of other factors influence calcium absorption. Compounds that form insoluble calcium salts (phosphate, oxalate, phytate) tend to interfere with absorption, while increased acidity of the gut favors it. The introduction of ions that form soluble but poorly dissociated calcium salts (such as citrate, tartrate, and ascorbate) favors absorption. Of far greater importance is the influence of vitamin D and parathyroid hormone.

In the past, considerable emphasis has been placed on maintaining a generous intake of calcium in the diet of growing children, an intake of 1 g/day being widely recommended. It is now realized that this figure is unnecessarily high. In the United States a deficient intake of calcium has not been recognized clinically; rickets and osteomalacia are not due to deficient calcium intake. Even in countries without a dairy industry the diet supplies enough calcium, provided that vitamin D or ultraviolet irradiation is adequate. For the rare infant who must be fed a milk substitute, it is customary to provide as much calcium as is in breast milk, but with this possible exception the intake of calcium need occasion no concern.

Of the small quantity of *magnesium* in the human body, about 70 percent is in the skeleton; a small but relatively constant amount is found in blood plasma and a somewhat larger amount in the tissue cells. In some respects the metabolism of magnesium resembles that of calcium; only a small moiety is absorbed in the intestine, and similar factors influence its absorption. Vitamin D does not appear to exert a controlling influence on magnesium metabolism, but parathyroid hormone influences it to some extent; the administration of parathyroid hormone causes a sharp but very temporary rise in blood magnesium, with increased excretion in the urine, whereas temporary retention of this element follows parathyroidectomy. In experimental animals a deficiency of magnesium leads to erythema of the extremities and to tetany. Magnesium-deficient tetany has also been reported in man.

Magnesium is a constituent of many enzyme systems; it also serves to catalyze various enzyme reactions. Magnesium is in some respects a calcium antagonist. Its administration may cause decalcification of bones and teeth. A similar antagonism is found in the nervous system; an excess of magnesium exerts a sedative action that can be neutralized by calcium. Hibernating animals have been found to have elevated blood magnesium.

About 75 percent of the body *phosphorus* is found in the skeleton, with the remainder consisting largely of organic phosphorus compounds in the cells; the inorganic phosphate of the plasma and interstitial fluids is a small moiety. Among the important organic phorphorus compounds are the nucleoproteins, the phospholipids present in plasma and the compounds concerned in cellular respiration, such as phosphocreatine, adenylic acid, and the adenosine phosphates. Phosphorylation (combination with phosphate) and dephosphorylation (the reverse process) are involved in a large number of metabolic processes, notably those involved in energy transformation. Inorganic phosphates are also important in regulating acid–base equilibrium.

The phosphorus needs of the body can be met entirely by inorganic phosphate in the diet. In milk a large part of the phosphorus is in organic combination as an integral part of the casein molecule combined with the amino acid serine. The requirement for phosphorus is similar to that for calcium during the period of rapid skeletal growth; as the rate of growth diminishes, relatively more phosphorus than calcium is needed for other purposes, and the requirement for phosphorus exceeds that for calcium.

Intestinal absorption of phosphorus is far from complete; as a rule it is between 20 and 50 percent of the quantity ingested. A small portion of the phosphorus ingested in cereals and vegetables is present in the form of phytate and other organic compounds that are poorly assimilated, but the primary factor limiting absorption is the formation of insoluble phosphates, chiefly calcium phosphate and metals. Acidity and the presence of other ions that can combine with calcium (such as oxalates and citrates) tend to promote phosphorus absorption; the reverse is also true. Vitamin D is of far greater importance in promoting phosphorus absorption. The parathyroid hormone has little effect on phosphorus absorption, but increases its excretion in the urine.

Phosphorus deficiency due to inadequate intake has been observed in animals, but whether it occurs in man is questionable. A moderate excess of phosphate in the diet is not harmful, but a great excess of phosphate given by vein may lead to tetany. Retention of phosphate occurs with some types of renal insufficiency, and this may contribute to acidosis. The high concentrations of calcium and phosphorus in the blood that may result from overdosage with vitamin D or with parathyroid hormone may result in pathologic calcification if allowed to persist.

Sulfur is an essential body constituent. It is found in all body proteins in the acids cysteine, cystine, taurine, and methionine. In the form of sulfate it occurs as heparin, as chondroitinsulfuric acid and mucoitinsulfuric acid in the mucoproteins of cartilage and mucus, and in the sulfolipids. Other important compounds are thiamine, lipoic acid, cystathionine, glutathione, and the ergothioneine of the red blood cells. It is an integral part of the coenzyme A molecule, and sulfhydryl groups are concerned with the activities of many enzymes. Sulfur compounds play an important part in the detoxification mechanisms of the body; certain aromatic compounds are excreted as ethereal sulfates, while others are detoxicated by combination with cystine, methionine, or glutathione. There is evidence that the intermediary metabolism of sulfur is greatly disturbed in certain diseases.

The requirement for sulfur can be met only to a limited extent by inorganic sulfates; these can provide for ethereal sulfate formation and for the various sulfate-containing compounds, but not for the amino acid sulfur, the sulfur-containing enzymes, and the other compounds containing reduced sulfur. For these compounds amino acid sulfur is needed. It appears that in man cystine supplies most of the latter needs, the absolute amount of methionine required being small. The small amount of thiamine required must be ingested as such. Although it can be synthesized in the human large intestine from simple sulfur compounds, such thiamine is, by and large, not absorbed.

Specific syndromes of sulfur deficiency are not recognized. In certain parts of the world sulfur amino acids are the limiting factors in the diet, and their lack may cause impaired growth. In experimental animals methionine deficiency will cause fatty liver, but a fatty liver can result from other types of imbalance, and there is little evidence that fatty livers in humans respond to administration of methionine.

Iron forms an integral part of the hemoglobin molecule. It also occurs in other porphyrin compounds, such as myoglobin, catalase, and the cytochrome pigments found in all cells. About 55 percent of the body iron is present as hemoglobin and from 10 to 20 percent as myoglobin; the remainder is in other tissues, either in the form of enzymes or as iron stores. Although the chief function of iron is oxygen transport, it also serves as a stimulus to red cell formation.

The factors controlling iron absorption are incompletely known, but the proportion of ingested iron absorbed appears to be influenced by the need. Usually only about 10 percent of the intake is absorbed, but in states of iron deficiency the proportion may be considerably greater. Inorganic iron is more readily absorbed than organic, and ferrous iron more readily than ferric. Ascorbic acid favors absorption by its reducing action. Iron appears to be absorbed in the form of ferritin, an iron-rich protein. In the blood the iron is reduced, and it circulates mainly in combination with a beta globulin known as transferrin. The iron that is not used is deposited chiefly in the liver and spleen, partly in the form of ferritin and partly as hemosiderin, the latter substance predominating when the stores are very large. Much of the iron liberated from destroyed red cells is reutilized.

A deficiency of iron leads to a hypochromic, microcytic anemia (p. 1119). This is not uncommon in infants fed exclusively on milk beyond the age of 6 or 8 months. The milk-fed infant relies to a considerable extent on stores laid down in the liver in fetal life. Depending on the mother's diet during pregnancy, these may vary from 30 to 500 mg at the time of birth. Premature infants are born with a low store and are particularly susceptible to iron-deficiency anemia. The synthesis of hemoglobin requires other factor besides iron (copper and pyridoxine are two recognized catalysts); but while a deficiency of either of these two factors may procure a hypochromic anemia, such deficiencies are rare, and hypochromic anemia is usually due to iron deficiency.

An excessive intake of iron leads to black stools. In the absence of anemia, only a small amount of ingested iron is absorbed. The indiscriminate use of iron in anemias of all kinds is to be deplored; one must bear in mind that when some other cause is responsible for anemia the administration of iron will lead to its accumulation in the body. Extensive hemosiderin deposits in the liver and spleen may occur after repeated transfusions for some congenital anemias. Acute iron poisoning commonly causes circulatory and cerebral symptoms and in infants may result in death.

During the first 5 to 6 weeks following birth, dietary iron is not readily utilized for hemoglobin formation, and dietary requirement is negligible. Subsequently an intake of 0.3 mg/kg/day appears to be adequate for the early years of life. Thus a child 6 months of age should receive 2.4 mg, and a child 1 year of age should receive 3 mg. A child receiving only milk would get no more than one-half these quantities. The Food and Nutrition Board recommends 1 mg/kg/day for infants, a figure that does not appear to be excessive. Lesser amounts in terms of body weight are recommended for older subjects, the recommendation for adults being 10 mg/day for males and 15 mg for menstruating females.

TRACE ELEMENTS.   Many elements are found in the body in trace amounts. Some of these, such as silicon, boron, aluminium, nickel, arsenic, and lead, have no known physiologic significance, and their occurrence is presumably fortuitous. Other trace elements, such as iodine, copper, manganese, molybdenum, zinc, cobalt, and fluorine, are essential in minute quantities, but these traces are ordinarily found in natural diets, and it is not necessary to make special provision for them. Deficiencies of cobalt, manganese, vanadium, and molybdenum have not been observed in man.

The need for *iodine* for the synthesis of the thyroid hormones thyroxine and triiodothyronine is well established. Lack of this element, even in goitrous districts, rarely manifests itself before puberty. In goitrous regions the use of iodized salt is now so nearly universal that endemic goiter is rare.

Copper is present in minute traces in all cells, the highest concentrations being found in muscle, bone, and liver. The fetal liver contains stores of copper that appear to be of physiologic importance. Copper is a constituent of a number of enzymes, notably respiratory pigments and oxidases of tissues. It is present in the blood mainly as a blue protein complex, ceruloplasmin, the function of which is unknown. There is evidence that copper is needed for hemoglobin synthesis. Exceptional cases of hypochromic anemia have been seen in which infants respond better to copper and iron than to iron alone. Hypocupremia is present in such cases, in contrast to the usual iron-deficiency anemia in which the blood copper is found in excess. It is not clear whether these cases of hypocupremia are due to an unusually low intake or to some metabolic peculiarity. Exact data on the copper requirement in early life are not available. Copper given in moderate excess will cause gastrointestinal disturbance and eventually nervous symptoms. In Wilson's disease there is an accumulation of copper in the tissues that is associated with defective synthesis of ceruloplasmin.

Manganese is found as the metallic complex of the enzyme arginase that is involved in the urea cycle; it is also found in bone phosphatase, leucine aminopeptidase, and several phosphorylating enzymes, as well as in all tissues. In experimental animals manganese deficiency causes interference with growth and reproduction. Manganese deficiency has not been recognized in man.

Zinc is found as the metallic complex of a number of enzymes, among which are carbonic anhydrase, uricase, phosphatases, and carboxypeptidase. Its high concentration in the pancreas is due to its presence in carboxypeptidase. A deficiency of zinc leads to skin lesions and alopecia in animals. Considerable zinc is present in the eye and in normal leukocytes. Leukemic leukocytes, however, contain only about one-tenth of the usual concentrations. Zinc deficiency has been reported from Iran and Egypt as a cause of anemia, dwarfism, and hypogenitalism in male dirt eaters.

Cobalt deficiency has been recognized for years in ruminant animals in Australia and New Zealand as the cause of enzootic marasmus, a condition characterized by progressive anemia, anorexia, and wasting. The ruminant appears to have a peculiar need for this element. That humans also need it to some extent has been established by its presence in vitamine B_{12} (p. 195). Cobalt has been reported to stimulate the formation of erythropoietin.

Molybdenum is one of the most recently established essential trace metals. It occurs as the metal complex of two flavoprotein enzymes—xanthine oxidase and aldehyde oxidase. A molybdenum supplement has been found to catalyze the formation of flavoproteins.

Fluorine is found in low concentration in bones and teeth, particularly in enamel. It appears to be an essential ingredient, in that a deficiency predisposes to dental caries. Minute amounts of fluorine in the drinking water exert a markedly protective effect against caries, and even the local application of fluoride is of some benefit. An excess of flourine in drinking water leads to mottling and discoloration of the enamel, a condition known as fluorosis.

Selenium has not been established as a dietary essential for man, although there is some evidence that it is of nutritive importance in animals and can spare vitamin E in some respects.

Imbalances between the trace elements have been found to be important in animal husbandry and may eventually prove to be of significance in human nutrition. A definite antagonism between copper and molybdenum will interfere with the utilization of copper and lead to copper deficiency; copper in turn will interfere with the absorption of molybdenun. Zinc is known to depress copper absorption, leading to a copper-deficiency anemia. A high calcium intake given to swine may precipitate zinc deficiency. Antagonisms between essential and nonessential trace elements also exist. It appears to be quite as important for the animal organism to maintain homeostasis with these micronutrients as with the macronutrients.

RECOMMENDED DIETARY ALLOWANCES

The modern era of nutrition, with the discovery of the accessory food factors and their corresponding deficiency syndromes, has led to an intensive and laudable effort to eliminate dietary deficiencies. The public as well as dietitians have been educated in regard to deficiencies and their prevention. Standard tables of dietary requirements and recommendations have been developed in many countries. In instances where requirements are not accurately known, a generous figure is supplied to ensure adequacy. Dietary surveys using these standards, but for the most part unaccompanied by physical examinations, have shown a high incidence of dietary deficiency, and corrective measures have been applied on a large scale. The pharmaceutical industry has provided a variety of preparations to meet the daily requirements of the accessory factors, and the food industry has fortified a number of prepared foods with them.

In evaluating the net results of this effort we have on the positive side the almost complete disappearance of vitamin-D-deficiency rickets and scurvy. The disappearance of pellagra is generally attributed to economic factors rather than to nutritional supplementation. On the negative side we have a very considerable expense to the public, a certain amount of poisoning from overdosage, particularly of the fat-soluble vitamins, and much apprehension in regard to deficiencies that are in no sense a menace. It is very difficult to assess the effect of this nutritional "enrichment" upon the changing patterns of disease in the United States. Possible remote effects of overnutrition (with specific nutrients as well as with calories) are now beginning to receive attention.

References

PROTEIN AND AMINO ACIDS

Food and Nutrition Board, National Research Council: Recommended Dietary Allowances, 8th ed. Publication 1694, Washington, DC, National Academy of Sciences, 1974

Graham GG, Placko RP, Acevedot G, Morales E, Cordano A: Lysine enrichment of wheat flour: evaluation in infants. Am J Clin Nutr 22:1459, 1969

Harper AE, Rogers QR: Amino acid imbalance. Proc Nutr Soc 24:173, 1965

Improvement of Protein Nutriture, Washington, DC, National Academy of Sciences, 1974

FAT

Fredrickson DS, Breslow JL: Hyperlipoproteinemia in infants. Ann Rev Med 24:315, 1973

Goldstein JL, et al: J Clin Invest 52:1533, 1973

Hansen AE: Essential fatty acids and human nutrition. Pediatrics 21:494, 1958

CARBOHYDRATES

Calloway DH: Environ Biol. and Med. 1:175, 1971

Caputto R, Barra HS, Cumar FA: Ann Rev Biochem 36:211, 1967

Monro HN: Physiol Rev 31:449, 1951

ENERGY

Finber GL: Amer Dis Child 1976

Powers GF: Am J Dis Child 30:453, 1925

VITAMINS

Vitamin Horm 23:000, 1965

MINERALS

Cheek DB: Human Growth. Philadelphia, Lea & Febiger, 1968

Comar CL, Bronner F (eds): Mineral Metabolism, Vol II, Part B.

Filer, AJ Jr: Nutrition Reviews 29:27, 1971

FEEDING TECHNIQUES AND DIETS
LAURENCE FINBERG

BREAST FEEDING

In many parts of the world the incidence of breast feeding approaches 100 percent. In the United States the incidence is much lower, and there is evidence it is decreasing. Many mothers wish to nurse, and they start out hopefully, but within a few days or weeks some minor difficulty that might have been prevented or corrected causes them to abandon the effort. The lack of hospital personnel interested in and skilled in teaching the technique of breast feeding, and early discharge of the mother and infant from the hospital, are also factors in its declining incidence.

ADVANTAGES. In considering the advantages of breast feeding, a clear distinction needs to be made between *breast milk* and *breast feeding;* the latter is discussed here. The chief advantages of breast feeding are that (1) it is safer, (2) it provides a food that is superior nutritionally, (3) it is more convenient, and (4) it is of psychologic value to the mother and to the infant. The old beliefs that maternal nursing hastened involution of the uterus and improved the shape of the infant's jaw have not been supported by critical evidence.

The relative safety of maternal nursing is important. Maternal antibodies transmitted in milk generally do not survive gastric digestion, although IgA antibody to enterotoxin, present in breast milk of normal mothers, may be a manifestation of natural immunity. But breast milk is relatively free of microorganisms, whereas cow's milk contains large numbers. In addition, the chance for contamination with pathogens is greater with artificial feedings, the latter depending upon the cleanliness of the milk supply and the care with which feedings are prepared. In most regions of the United States the risk is negligible. However, in parts of the world where milk is more likely to be contaminated and where formulas are not carefully prepared, the greater safety of breast feeding is of major importance. The comparative nutritive values of breast milk and cow's milk and the differences between them are discussed on page 366. Most studies have failed to establish a superiority for breast milk. Some mothers consider the convenience of breast feeding one of its major advantages over artificial feeding, which requires preparation and sterilization of formulas. Others object to the fact that breast feeding requires that they give all of the feedings, with the exception of an occasional supplementary bottle. In the United States the advantages of breast feeding are not great in terms of safety, nutritional superiority, or convenience. The possibility that a baby may develop allergy to cow's milk is one important consideration in recommending breast feeding (p. 205). The psychologic benefit of breast feeding is the other important factor. Nursing is emotionally satisfying to many mothers, but this is not valid evidence to support the contention that artificial feeding implies emotional deprivation for the infant. On the other hand, it is possible that the desire and capacity of the mother to nurse her baby successfully may be a manifestation of an attitude favorable for the child's psychologic development.

We believe that the most reasonable approach for the pediatrician is to inquire honestly into the mother's attitude toward breast feeding, to encourage her to do so, and to cooperate in efforts to make the atmosphere in the hospital more conducive to success. On the other hand, the pediatrician should accept the mother's considered decision not to breast-feed her infant and help minimize any feelings of guilt she might have.

CONTRAINDICATIONS. There are times when maternal nursing should not be attempted: (1) No mother who has active clinical tuberculosis should nurse her infant; it exposes the infant to infection. (2) Nursing should seldom be allowed when serious complications have been connected with parturition, such as severe hemorrhage, sepsis, or eclampsia; however, women may recover from these conditions so as to be able to nurse successfully. (3) If the mother is suffering from serious chronic disease or is markedly under nourished, breast feeding is best not attempted. (4) Mastitis is a contraindication for using the affected breast.

SECRETION. The secretion of breast milk commences after parturition; only a few drops may be squeezed from the breasts before delivery. For the first few days the flow is scanty; usually it becomes well established by the third or fourth day, but it may be delayed until the tenth or twelfth day and yet come in abundance. One should not be too ready to decide that there will be no milk, but should persist in stimulating the breasts by suckling the child or by artificial means, such as manual expression or use of an electrical breast pump.

The caloric value of breast milk is about 0.67 calories/ml. On the average, nursing infants consume about 100 to 120 calories per kilogram of body weight per day. The amount of milk varies with the demands of the child in a striking way. Complete emptying of the breast is the strongest stimulus to the production of milk; therefore a hungry infant will soon increase the milk supply. Conversely, when the supply is overabundant, as may happen when the milk first comes in, the breast is incompletely emptied, and within a few days the quantity secreted falls off. The secretion of milk is a somewhat discontinuous process that goes on more actively during periods of actual suckling than in the intervals of rest between nursings. Half of the quantity obtainable from one breast is taken in the first 2 or 3 minutes; after 10 minutes few babies get any milk whatever. Large and vigorous infants obtain more milk than do smaller infants in the average single nursing, whether from one breast or from both.

A mother's ability to nurse her infant is not affected by the season of the year, the parity of the mother, her age, the size of her breasts, antepartum presence of secretion in the breasts, or the return of menstruation. It is affected unfavorably by obesity, by the advent of pregnancy, by the development of infection in the nipple or breast, and by adverse psychologic factors.

COLOSTRUM. The secretions of the early days of lactation, to which the name colostrum has been given, differ quite markedly from the later milk. Colostrum is creamy yellow in color, with a specific gravity of 1.030

and fat than does the later milk. Many of the fat globules are of unusual size, and large numbers of granular cells known as colostrum corpuscles are present. These are four or five times the size of the milk globules, and they are probably mononuclear phagocytes containing numerous fat granules.

The characteristic features of colostrum continue for a period of 5 to 10 days, but it is not until about the end of the first month that the milk assumes its stable or mature character. There is a gradual decrease in protein and minerals and a moderate rise in sugar and fat. When the composition of mature milk is reached, little variation is seen until near the close of lactation.

COMPOSITION. Mature breast milk is similar to cow's milk in appearance; it is sweet to the taste. When it is fresh its pH varies from 6.8 to 7.4, averaging 7.0; specific gravity varies between 1.026 and 1.036. Microscopically there are large numbers of fat globules of variable size, with some granular matter and occasional epithelial cells. Table 3 gives the average composition of the major constituents of mature milk and their common variations in health. The mineral constituents of breast milk are shown in Table 4.

PROTEIN. The total protein of mature milk varies usually from 1.0 to 1.4 percent; in unusual specimens it may vary from 0.3 to 3.5 percent. Protein content is highest in colostrum; after the first month it is relatively constant, but it tends to fall toward the end of lactation. Milk obtained from the early part of each nursing has a somewhat higher protein content than subsequent portions.

The major proteins are casein, α-lactalbumin, and β-lactoglobulin, which are present in the ratio 2:2:1. The preponderance of the whey proteins (albumin and globulin) is in marked contrast to cow's milk, in which most of the protein is casein. It is now known that casein is not a pure protein; it consists of a mixture of at least two and perhaps three distinct entities: α-, β-, and γ-casein. The caseins of human milk have been shown to differ from those of cow's milk, as is also true of the whey proteins. The chief globulins of human milk are a mixture of α- and β-lactoglobulin, of which the latter is by far the larger fraction. Thus far the globulins have not been separated in pure form, although electrophoretic studies indicate that there are at least four components. From the nutritional point of view, whey proteins have been regarded as superior to casein, a view that now seems questionable. Casein is peculiar in that it

TABLE 3. Average Values and Ranges for the Chemical Composition of Mature Milk of Healthy Women

Normal Average and Range (g/100 ml)

Protein	1.1	(0.9–1.6)
Sugar	7.0	(6.5–8.0)
Fat	3.8	(2.0–6.0)
Ash	0.21	(0.15–0.35)
Water	88.0	(87.0–89.0)

to 1.035 and an alkaline reaction (average pH 7.7). It is readily coagulable by heat; sometimes the milk of the first day coagulates spontaneously. It contains more protein than does mature milk (the protein is from 3 to 5 percent), a large part of which consists of globulin. It is also richer in vitamin A activity and in minerals, particularly sodium and potassium. It contains less sugar

TABLE 4. Mineral Constituents of Breast Milk

Period	Total Ash (mg/100 ml)	Na (mEq/liter)	K (mEq/liter)	Ca (mEq/liter)	Mg (mEq/liter)	Cl (mEq/liter)	P (mEq/liter)
Colostrum (1–12 days)	308	14.8	20.0	16.5	2.5	16.3	5.8
Transition (12–30 days)	241	8.3	15.1	14.5	1.3	16.6	5.8
Early mature (1–4 mo)	206	4.8	11.5	17.5	2.1	10.1	4.8
Late mature (4–9 mo)	207	4.3	13.1	16.5	2.1	10.3	4.8
Late milk (10–20 mo)	198	4.3	12.3	14.0	1.7	12.6	4.2

contains a considerable amount of phosphorus in combination with the amino acid serine; it is coagulated by acid or by the enzyme rennin. The difference between the curd of breast milk and that of cow's milk is due chiefly to the greater quantity of casein in the latter.

FAT.   Fat exists as a fine emulsion of particles rarely exceeding 10 μ in diameter. The fat of breast milk consists almost entirely of the neutral fats palmitin, stearin, and olein, with olein predominating; small quantities of free fatty acids and of unsaponifiable matter are present. The fat of breast milk is relatively low in glycerides of the short-chain volatile fatty acids, as compared with the fat of cow's milk. It also commonly contains somewhat more of the polyunsaturated fatty acids. Insull and associates have shown that marked variations in the composition of milk fat occur that depend on the diet of the mother. In general the character of milk fat tends to approach that of dietary fat. The effect of a high-carbohydrate diet is to increase the proportions of lauric and myristic acids and to decrease the proportions of the polyunsaturated fatty acids.

The quantity of fat shows greater variations than the quantity of any of the other constituents. The average is about 3.8 percent, but variations from 2.0 to 6.0 percent are not uncommon. The concentration of fat in breast milk is influenced to some extent by the quantity of fat in the diet, but in part it is a characteristic of the individual mother. The proportion of fat is affected by the time during nursing when the specimen is taken. The first milk drawn may contain only 1 percent fat, while at the end of nursing the last milk to be removed may contain 7 to 8 percent. No analysis is of value unless the specimen comprises practically the whole of the nursing.

SUGAR.   The lactose in milk is in solution. It is more nearly constant than the other ingredients, the usual limits being between 6.5 and 8.0 percent.

MINERALS.   The figures in Table 4 for the mineral constituents of breast milk were obtained by Holt and associates. All of the minerals are present in ample quantities, with the exception of iron, which is present in a concentration of 1.5 to 2.0 mg/ liter.

VITAMINS.   All the known vitamins are present in breast milk, the quantities being greatly influenced by the intake of the mother. Vitamin deficiencies other than vitamin D seldom occur in breast-fed infants in the United States because maternal diets are generally adequate. Without vitamin D prophylaxis, rickets be seen in nursing infants, particularly in those with dark skin or those not exposed to some sunlight.

CONDITIONS AFFECTING COMPOSITION. Diet has little influence on the composition of milk, with the exceptions of vitamins, which are not synthesized in the body, and the character of the fat, which is influenced by the fat of diet. The nursing mother requires more food than the average adult; not only must the calories secreted in the milk (400 to 1,200 per day) be supplied, but a certain amount of energy is consumed in the process of secretion. The water intake must be increased to provide the additional fluid secreted. Apart from this, no change in the usual diet is necessary. The quantity of milk produced is largely independent of the mother's daily fluid intake within wide variations of water consumption.

The use of tobacco, tea, and coffee in moderation is not harmful. Alcohol taken in small amounts does not appear in the milk, but a large intake of alcohol may produce severe toxic symptoms in the infant.

A number of drugs may be eliminated in the milk. Atropine, many of the opium derivatives, mercury, lead, arsenicals, salicyates, iodides, bromides, and some of the alkaloid cathartics have all been found in the milk, sometimes in sufficient quantities to produce symptoms in the nursing child. Barbiturates, sulfonamides, and various antibiotics may also appear in the milk.

The milk of a nursing woman who has become pregnant is generally scanty and poor in fat. The milk of a woman with toxemia of pregnancy may be toxic to the infant.

Occasionally organisms may be found in freshly pumped breast milk; they are chiefly cocci derived from the external milk ducts and are of no importance. In the presence of mastitis, pathogenic bacteria may be found. In septicemia, pathogenic organisms may reach the milk even in the absence of mastitis. Milk obtained from breast-milk dairies contains organisms similar in distribution and quantity to those of cow's milk. Although numerous antibodies have been demonstrated in milk, they apparently do not survive digestion in significant quantities. Allergic phenomena may appear in the nursing infant, presumably as a result of minute quantities of foreign protein transmitted through the milk.

The effects of emotional stresses on the secretion of milk are very striking. Usually, worry, anxiety, fatigue, or any prolonged emotional stress tends to reduce secretion of milk and may arrest it entirely. The psychologic state of the mother, more than any other single factor, appears to determine success or failure in nursing the infant.

ARTIFICIAL FEEDING

The successful feeding of infants demands that the food be digestible, the nutritional requirements be met, and contamination with pathogenic bacteria or other harmful substances be prevented. Since cow's milk, our chief source for infant feeding, is an excellent culture medium, control of milk contamination is essential.

MICROORGANISMS IN MILK.   The bacteriologic control of milk is now a public health problem, with the production and processing of milk sold to the public being regulated by law in most parts of the civilized world. In the United States inspection and testing of cattle have virtually eliminated bovine tuberculosis and have greatly reduced other sources of infection in the animals themselves, especially brucellosis and streptococcal mastitis. Epidemics of milk-borne disease occur from time to time from contamination in handling milk (infections with enteric organisms, streptococci, and staphylococci), but even when these occur infants are seldom affected if terminal sterilization of their food is practiced.

MILK STERILIZATION. Since even the most carefully handled milk occasionally produces disease when fed raw, some form of milk sterilization is now universally employed in feeding infants. Heat sterilization produces a number of changes in the milk aside from destroying the bacteria. The lactalbumin is altered giving the milk a different taste; the casein coagulates in a finer curd, making the milk more digestible. Partial caramelization of the sugar occurs at high temperatures, and there is some destruction of ascorbic acid and thiamine. The nutritional value of the proteins is adversely affected only be severe thermal treatment, which may involve some injury to several amino acids, notably lysine. The extent of these alterations varies with the degree and the duration of thermal treatment.

Pasteurization as generally carried out (holding process, 65 to 68 C for 30 minutes) destroys all pathogenic bacteria and 99 percent of saprophytes. Spores are not destroyed, and unless the milk is kept cool there may be an extensive growth of spore-bearers. In general, pasteurized milk should be kept below 50 F and used not more than 48 hours after delivery. The coagulability and taste of the milk are only minimally affected by pasteurization. About 20 percent of the vitamin C and about 10 percent of the thiamine are destroyed.

In *boiled milk* the taste is further altered, and the curd produced on acidification or after peptic digestion is even finer. About 50 percent of the vitamin C and 30 percent of the thiamine are lost.

Autoclaving milk for 10 minutes at 115 C causes complete destruction of bacteria and spores. The taste is altered considerably, and the milk acquires a slightly yellowish tinge from caramelization of the sugar. The protein is more readily digested, although there is a slight loss of lysine. About 60 percent of the vitamin C and 30 to 50 percent of the thiamine are lost.

Since thiamine is ordinarily present in quantities more than double the minimal requirements, the destruction of this factor by heat need not occasion concern unless the sterilization treatment is unusually severe. The destruction of lysine is negligible. The replacement of vitamin C is, most important, since raw cow's milk contains barely enough to prevent scurvy. All infants fed on sterilized milk must be given a vitamin C supplement.

DIFFERENCES BETWEEN COW'S MILK AND BREAST MILK. Physical differences between cow's milk and breast milk are negligible. The specific gravity of each is between 1.028 and 1.033. The chemical composition of cow's milk varies to some extent with the breed of cow, that of Jerseys and Guernseys being richer in fat than that of Holsteins. In most of the milk marketed, however, the excess fat is removed, with only the legal minimum (usually 3.3 to 3.5 percent) being left. The chief differences between cow's milk and breast milk are shown in Table 5. The proteins of the two milks possess specific antigenic properties, but differences in the characters of the casein coagula are due chiefly to differences in quantity of casein rather than to chemical differences between the two caseins. The assays of the nutritive quality of the protein by Tomarelli and associates showed no differences of statistical significance between the proteins of breast milk and cow's milk. The percentages of essential amino acids in breast milk and cow's milk proteins are quite similar.

The fat of cow's milk differs in some repects from that of breast milk. Differences in the sizes of the fat globules have been described, but in our experience these are inconstant and of no practical importance. Breast milk contains more polyunsaturated fatty acids. Cow's milk always contains a higher proportion of the volatile (short-chain) fatty acids than does breast milk. These

TABLE 5. Average Percentage Composition of Mature Breast Milk and Cow's Milk [a]

Constituents	Breast Milk		Cow's Milk	
Water	87.6		87.2	
Total Solids	12.4		12.8	
Protein	1.0		3.3	
Casein		0.4		2.7
Lactalbumin		0.4		0.4
Lactoglobulin		0.2		0.2
Fat	3.8		3.8[b]	
Lactose	7.0		4.8	
Ash	0.21		0.71	
Sodium		0.015		0.058
Potassium		0.055		0.138
Calcium		0.034		0.126
Magnesium		0.004		0.013
Iron		0.00021		0.00015[c]
Chlorine		0.043		0.100
Phosphorus		0.016		0.099
Sulfur		0.014		0.330
Calories per ounce	22		21[b]	
Calories per 100 ml	71		69[b]	

[a] *From Macy et al: The Composition of Milks.* National Research Council Publication 254, Washington DC, National Academy of Sciences, 1953.
[b] *Much of the milk marketed in the United States contains only the legal minimum of 3.3 to 3.5 percent fat. Its caloric content then averages 20 calories per ounce (66 calories per 100 ml).*
[c] *Consistently higher iron values were reported prior to the introduction of stainless steel dairy equipment.*

TABLE 6. Vitamin Content of 100 ml Breast Milk and Cow's Milk (Fresh)[a]

	Mature Breast Milk	Cow's Milk
Vitamin A	150 USP units	100 USP units
Carotenoids	27 µg	38 µg
B vitamins		
Thiamine	16 µg	42 µg
Riboflavin	43 µg	157 µg
Nicotinic acid	172 µg	85 µg
Pyridoxine	11 µg	48 µg
Pantothenic acid	196 µg	350 µg
Follic acid	0.18 µg	0.23 µg
Choline	9 mg	13 mg
Inositol	39 mg	13 mg
Biotin	0.4 µg	3.5 µg
B_{12}	0.04 µg	0.41 µg
Vitamin C	4.3 mg	1.8 mg
Vitamin D	0.4–10.0 USP units	0.3–4.0 USP units
Vitamin K	26 Dam-Glavind units	100 Dam-Glavind units

[a] From Macy et al: The Composition of Milks. National Research Council Publication, 254, Washington, DC, National Academy of Sciences, 1953.

are formed from carbohydrate rather than from dietary fat and are not appreciably affected by dietary fat intake. The contention that the short-chain fatty acids cause diarrhea is no longer tenable.

The carbohydrates of the two milks (lactose) are identical. As may be seen in Table 5, the common minerals are found in cow's milk in concentrations two to six times as great as in breast milk. Average figures for the vitamin concentrations of the two milks are given in Table 6. The mineral and vitamin concentrations of both milks may be affected by the diet.

MODIFICATION OF COW'S MILK.   Pure cow's milk is not a satisfactory food for many infants. The history of artificial feeding has been one long series of attempts to modify cow's milk to make it more suitable for infants. In modifying milk for infant feeding it is neither possible nor necessary to overcome all the differences between cow's milk and breast milk; in fact, some of the most succesful artifical feedings have differed widely from breast milk in composition. Of prime importance is modification of the character of the casein curd. Unmodified raw cow's milk produces tenacious curds in the stomach; these may give rise to symptoms of indigestion, but more important is the fact that a considerable proportion of the food escapes absorption. Tough beanlike curds that consist of undigested casein and fat are found in the stools. Curd indigestion can be prevented by heating the milk, by diluting it, by adding alkali, by using a protective colloid such as starch or cereal gruel, or by precoagulating the casein into fine curds by careful additon of acid or by fermentation of the milk. It is now common practice to accomplish this by some form of heat treatment. It is also customary to dilute cow's milk; this decreases the protein and fat concentrations of the original milk, with the caloric deficit being made up by adding carbohydrate. The proportions of calories distributed as protein, fat, and carbohydrate in breast milk and in cow's milk, both

unmodified and as commonly fed in formulas, are shown in Table 7.

Carbohydrate may be added in the form of simple sugars or polysaccharides or mixtures of the two. Except in rare instances of disaccharidase deficiency, there is no particular advantage in giving monosaccharides; the normal child is able to invert disaccharides without difficulty. Of the double sugars, lactose would seem the

TABLE 7. Percentage Distribution of Calories

	Protein	Fat	Carbo-hydrate
Breast milk	8	50	42
Cow's milk	20	51	29
Cow's milk (common modifications)[a]	10–15	30–35	50–60

[a] The figures given are only approximate.

logical one to use, since it is the natural carbohydrate of milk. Lactose is relatively expensive and has not been shown to possess any superiority to cane sugar. It ferments somewhat more readily than other disaccharides and has achieved little popularity in infant feeding. Pure maltose is not used for infant feeding. Cane sugar (sucrose) is satisfactory; it is inexpensive and is always available in pure form.

Mixtures of dextrins and maltose have been used widely in infant feeding since their introduction during the last century by Liebig. The claim that the additional time required for their hydrolysis gives better opportunity for absorption is not well supported. They are, however, satisfactory. They have a pleasant taste and may possess some virtue when the time comes for introducing solid foods; being somewhat less sweet than cane sugar, they do not condition the child to a sweet food. Some liquid extracts of malt contain impurities that are somewhat laxative; therefore they are sometimes used in the treatment of constipation. Dextri-Maltose and corn syrup are not laxative for most infants and are widely used for infant feeding.

Diet for Artificial Feeding

Many milk preparations are available for infant feeding. In an earlier era in which symptoms of indigestion were commonly attributed to the food ingested, great efforts were made to control these symptoms by altering the ingredients or the physical state of the formula. It is now appreciated that disturbances of digestion usually originate from other causes; they are largely due to infections, enteric and parenteral. The concern of infant feeding today is not the search for a formula that will arrest symptoms of indigestion, but rather to meet the nutritional requirements of the child.

HOMOGENIZED MILK.   Homogenized milk was introduced in infant feeding to decrease the size of the fat globules in milk as an aid in fat assimilation. That a substantial gain in fat absorption resulted was, however, never conclusively demonstrated. Today milk is homogenized in the course of fortifying it with vitamin D. A secondary gain is the more even distribution of lipid; the fat of homogenized milk does not rise to the surface as cream.

SKIM MILK AND HALF-SKIMMED MILK.   These types of milk came into use when it was noted that there was considerable fat loss in the stools in diarrhea and in certain other states such as prematurity and celiac syndrome. Excessive loss of fat in the stools was attributed to the use of a feeding too rich in lipid. In some quarters this view is still maintained, although it is not easily reconciled with the many observations that have failed to show deleterious clinical effects from feeding fat in steatorrhea and have shown that increasing the fat intake increases fat absorption, despite the absorptive defect. Removal of all or part of the fat greatly increases the solute content of the feeding per calorie, and in infants this may compromise water balance.

HUMANIZED MILKS.   The term humanized milk is applied to a variety of proprietary milk feedings designed to imitate the composition of breast milk and thus differ from cow's milk in one or more of the following respects: lower protein content; lower mineral content, particularly with regard to calcium; substitution of a mixture of vegetable fat (containing more unsaturated fat) for milk fat. Carbohydrate, usually lactose, is added to make up for the reduced protein calories. The need to lower protein content has been questioned, since with heat processing larger amounts of cow's milk protein can be tolerated. The value of reducing the calcium intake is also questionable. Substitution of mixtures of vegetable fat for butterfat ensures in some instances a slightly better fat absorption. In normal infants the difference is negligible, but in cases of steatorrhea the difference may be significant. The effects of polyunsaturated fatty acids in reducing blood cholesterol to keep serum cholesterol at moderate or even low concentrations have attracted attention because of the possibility that over the years arterial atheromatous change may be retarded. The chief value of the humanized milks lies in their convenience and ease of preparation. They are nutritionally adequate foods; a carbohydrate supplement has already been added, and they require only the addition of water.

SPECIAL PRODUCTS.   Several proprietary feedings are available for infants who are allergic to cow's milk, a condition that has been infrequent in our experience. They include goat's milk, the soybean milks (Sobee, Mull-Soy, and Soyalac), meat-base formulas, and an enzymatic digest of casein containing no antigenic protein. There are also several products (eg, Progestimil) in which the nutrients are in their digested forms; thus they present no whole protein molecules. Each of these products has some disadvantage when used as a sole feeding for infants, especially goat's milk and vegetable protein products. The physician should be familiar with these special problems before prescribing such feedings.

CARBOHYDRATE SUPPLEMENTS.   It appears to be immaterial which sugar is given to normal infants as a supplement, except in the presence of disaccharidase deficiency. Starch, too, is well digested after the first few months. In measuring the carbohydrate added the following table may be of value:

APPROXIMATE MEASURES OF DIFFERENT CARBOHYDRATES

Substance	Equivalent
Corn syrup	1½ tbsp = 30 g
Cane sugar	2 tbsp = 26 g
Milk sugar	3 tbsp = 30 g
Dextri-Maltose	4 tbsp = 35 g
Flour, wheat	4 tbsp = 33 g

Dried milk, which now is usually prepared by the spray process, is a virtually sterile product. It does not support bacterial growth and can be kept for some time in opened tins. For this reason it is particularly useful in the absence of refrigeration, and in many countries where refrigeration facilities are limited it is the feeding of choice. The original milk is usually reconstituted by adding one part of the powder to eight parts of water by weight.

Evaporated milk has been subjected to autoclaving and is a sterile product. Its use requires refrigeration facilities, for it is subject to bacterial contamination after a can has been opened. Because of its convenience in preparing feedings, it has become increasingly popular, and it is estimated that currently more than 80 percent of bottle-fed infants in the United States are fed either on evaporated milk or on some prepared milk feeding in evaporated form. Evaporated milk is concentrated 2.25 times, and its composition as marketed is standardized by law:

	Protein (%)	Fat (%)	Carbo-hydrate (%)	Min-eral (%)	Cals (per oz)
Evaporated milk	7	7.85	10	1.6	44
Evaporated milk diluted with equal parts of water	3.5	3.9	5.0	0.8	22
Percentage distribution of calories	20	51	29		

In the processing of both dried and evaporated milks a considerable fraction of the vitamin C is lost and must be replaced. However, heat damage to other vitamins and to protein is minimal.

DIRECTIONS FOR PREPARING FOOD.   If facilities for refrigeration are adequate, all the food needed for 24 hours should be prepared at one time. The appropriate amount of water is placed in a graduated pitcher, and the sugar or other carbohydrate supplement*is added and stirred into solution. The lid of the can of evaporated milk is scalded with hot water and wiped dry with a clean dish towel or paper towel before being opened. After adding the desired amount of evaporated milk, the formula is poured into feeding bottles placed in a rack. Each bottle is capped with a nipple, and the nipple is covered with a protector. The loaded rack is then placed in a covered pail in 2 or 3 inches of water (enough to ensure a free flow of steam for half an hour without risk of its boiling dry) and steam-sterilized for 15 minutes. It is important to wait until steam is escaping freely from the covered pail before starting to count the period of sterilization. The rack is then removed, and the feedings are allowed to cool in room air before being stored in the refrigerator.

When dairy milk is used the bottle should be inverted several times in order to ensure an even distribution of the fat, unless the milk is homogenized. Whole milk feedings, when subjected to terminal sterilization, tend to produce a scum that easily plugs the nipple holes. To prevent this the mixture is boiled in a saucepan for at least a minute and cooled; the scum is removed and the formula poured into scalded or sterilized feeding bot-

*When liquid preparations such as corn syrup are used, their measurement is considerably facilitated by warming.

tles. The bottles are then capped or stoppered with cotton and placed in cold water until quite cool before they are refrigerated.

Terminal sterilization is a traditional procedure in pediatrics and is still generally endorsed by authoritative bodies as a safety measure. However, the need for it has been challenged for those conditions in which the milk supply is beyond question and the water supply meets standard civilian requirements.

DIRECTIONS FOR FEEDING.   It is common practice to warm the food to 100 F by placing the bottle in warm water for a few minutes. The temperature of the milk may be tested by pouring a few drops upon the inner surface of the wrist, where it should feel warm but not hot. However, warming the feeding is not a real necessity, for infants fed cold feedings thrive quite as well. A bottle should not be rewarmed for a second feeding.

Ordinarily an infant should not be more than 20 minutes in taking the food and should not sleep with the nipple in his mouth. The bottle should be placed or held in such a position that the nipple is kept full. At some time during the feeding, and again after it, the infant should be held upright over the nurse's shoulder and patted on the back to allow him to bring up swallowed air.

Feeding During Early Months

The important factor in feeding is the amount of food given in the 24 hours. The number of feedings into which this is divided and the intervals between them are of secondary importance. Infants differ in their response to a schedule. Some do better with relatively large feedings at longer intervals, and others thrive best with smaller feedings given more often; no absolute rule can be laid down. The large majority of healthy infants can readily be trained to take their feedings at 4-hour intervals from the beginning. Fewer feedings each day lessen the labor of the mother or nurse. Schedules suitable for starting normal infants are given in Table 8.

INDICATIONS FOR INCREASING FOOD.   If an infant appears healthy and contented and gains weight regularly, there is no reason to increase his food intake, even if it is providing less than the average caloric requirements. With some placid infants, 80 calories/kg/day seem to be sufficient. The best indications that food

TABLE 8. Food Requirements and Feeding Schedule for Normal Infants

Age	Calories per 24 hr	Milliliters per 24 hr	Ounces per 24 hr	Number of Feedings per 24 hr	Quantity per Feeding (ml)	(oz)
1 month	300–500	450–750	15–25	5 or 6	100–150	3–4.5
2 months	400–580	600–850	20–29	5 or 6	100–180	3.5–6
3 months	480–650	575–1000	24–32	4 or 5	120–220	4–7
4 months	560–700	920–1100	28–35	4 or 5	150–250	5–8
5 months	630–750	1000–1150	31–37[a]	4 or 5	180–250	6–8

[a] It is not advisable to attempt to supply more than about 650 or 700 calories a day as milk formula. When more food is required, other articles should be added to the diet.

should be increased are the weight curve and signs of hunger. The weight curve is important, but one should not be guided by it alone. When it is made the chief concern, there is a temptation to increase the food if the child is not gaining adequately. Gain in weight is seldom continuous; even healthy breast-fed infants may have periods of a week or two during the early months when weight remains stationary. Later there may be even longer periods of stationary weight. Evidences of hunger may be easy to detect, as when an infant finishes his bottle greedily and cries for more or becomes fretful long before his feeding time. At other times it may be difficult to distinguish symptoms of underfeeding from those of indigestion. Crying as a result of hunger may easily be mistaken for colic. Underfeeding may lead to vomiting and even to diarrhea. An infant who remains hungry after finishing his bottle may continue to suck at the nipple and thus swallow considerable air, which may cause regurgitation. So-called starvation diarrhea, seen particularly in small infants who are underfed, consists in the frequent passage of small greenish stools composed of mucus and other secretions. The therapeutic test should be applied if there is any suspicion of underfeeding.

INDICATIONS FOR DECREASING FOOD.   Over feeding may result in loss of appetite; the infant may not finish his bottle. There may be regurgitation after meals if too much food is taken. In the latter event one should not be too ready to conclude that the total daily feeding is too large; it may be that too large a volume is given at one time. Prolonged overfeeding beyond the demands of the appetite is likely to result in digestive disturbances and eventually in failure to gain weight. It is apparent that somewhat similar symptoms may be produced by underfeeding and overfeeding. An examination of the caloric intake will enable one to avoid gross errors in either direction. When the caloric requirements of a particular child have been established empirically, one may make regular increases in the food, as weight is gained, to maintain the caloric intake at the desired level with respect to body weight.

FEEDING BY APPETITE.   The food intake of the breast-fed infant is automatically regulated by appetite. With artificial feeding, apppetite also serves as a useful guide in determining the amount of food required, provided the composition of the formula food is balanced. At each feeding the infant may be offered more formula than is required and allowed to take what he wants within a period of 15 or 20 minutes, the unconsumed excess being then discarded. Although the amount taken at each feeding may vary considerably in the course of a day, as with infants nursed at the breast, the 24-hour intake normally remains quite constant. If the appetite is impaired by illness, such as at the onset of an infection, the consumption of food will be correspondingly reduced, and indigestion resulting from overfeeding will be avoided.

Experience has shown that the more the feeding differs from what may be considered a complete and balanced diet for the infant, the less reliance can be placed upon the appetite. Thus some infants given excessive amounts of fat may become nauseated and refuse food, taking less than their nutritional requirements, while others whose diet is lacking in some essential constituent may develop ravenous appetites and be grossly overfed. Infants given concentrated feedings with inadequate water may take more food than they need in order to satisfy thirst, and conversely, with an over-diluted food, the stomach is likely to be distended and the appetite temporarily satisfied before sufficient food is taken.

COMMON MISTAKES IN INFANT FEEDING.   The mistake is sometimes made of changing feedings too frequently. Before changing an infant's food one should be certain that an indication exists. It is not possible to modify the food in such a way as to relieve every trivial discomfort or disturbance a child may have. Nurses are usually ready to ascribe every slight symptom to the food, particularly if they have strong opinions themselves and are not in full sympathy with the method employed.

It is unwise to make too many changes in the feeding at one time. This does not apply to reductions of food, which must often be made suddenly in acute illness, but rather to increases in the amount of food or the addition of new foods. Changes in both food and feeding schedule should not be made at the same time, nor should more than one article of food be added at a time; otherwise, should untoward results follow, it would be difficult to decide what caused them. Before deciding whether a change of food is beneficial, one should usually allow not less than 3 days to elapse. Another common mistake is the introduction of solid food in quantity with no curtailment of the milk formula. This often results in refusal of food or in vomiting.

INDICATIONS FOR CHANGING FOOD.   In *hot weather* the appetite is often impaired, and a temporary reduction in food intake may be desirable. Since the need for fluid is increased, the volume of the formula should be maintained and additional water given between feedings. A number of other conditions, such as vomiting, diarrhea, constipation, colic, and failure to gain weight, may require changes in feeding. After the age of 3 to 4 months, when additional carbohydrate is provided in the form of cereal, there is no need to add sugar or to otherwise modify the milk; plain boiled milk or diluted evaporated milk may be given.

OTHER FOOD DURING THE FIRST YEAR.   Some form of vitamin D prophylaxis against rickets should be given to all infants after the first week of life. Orange juice or some other antiscorbutic should be given from the second week. One may commence with a teaspoonful a day and rapidly increase the quantity until the juice of one orange is taken per day. Ascorbic acid (25 mg/day) may be given dissolved in water or mixed with one of the feedings.

The time at which solid foods are introduced varies greatly in American practice. As more and more prepared infant foods have become available, the tendency has been to introduce them earlier. They have been successfully fed as early as the first week of life. Competition has developed between mothers and even among physicians in this respect. Granting that solid foods can be fed, if properly subdivided, even to the youngest infants, the question remains whether there is any advantage or disadvantage in doing so.

The reasons given for starting solid foods are two: to provide iron, the one important element in which milk is deficient, and to accustom children to eating the type of food they will subsequently depend upon. There is no advantage in giving iron before the end of the second month, since it is not readily utilized for hemoglobin synthesis before that time. As far as habit is concerned, when solid foods are postponed to beyond 6 months, difficulty may be encountered in getting infants to take them, the difficulty being greater the longer their introduction is postponed. Such difficulties are negligible during most of the first 6 months, and they cannot be said to constitute an argument for introducing solids before the age of 4 months. There are no serious disadvantages to introducing solid foods before 4 months, but more time must be spent in feeding, and some difficulty in handling solid food may be experienced unless the food is placed well toward the back of the mouth.

On the whole, the policy of exclusive milk feedings for the first 3 or 4 months of life appears to have no disadvantages and some distinct advantages from the point of view of convenience. The earlier introduction of solid foods may be regarded as a fad, but in no sense a harmful one.

A great variety of precooked foods for infants is now available. It includes cereals, soups, vegetables, fruits, meat, fish, and egg yolk. For small infants strained (homogenized) fruits, meats, and vegetables are marketed, and for older ones who can do some chewing there are finely chopped ("junior") foods. The order in which these foods are introduced is not a matter of importance. A suggested schedule follows: vitamin D at 1 week; orange juice at 2 weeks; cereal, vegetables, and fruit at 2 to 4 months; meat, fish, or egg at 3 to 5 months; breadstuffs (zwieback, toast, etc) at 5 to 6 months.

New articles of diet should be introduced one at a time; 2 to 3 days should elapse before another addition is made. One should begin with a small quantity of the new food, such as a teaspoonful; it is best given at the beginning of the meal. As each new food is added, the infant will take somewhat less of the old food. It is advisable to reduce the amount of milk offered at the time a solid food is first introduced. As solid foods come to constitute more and milk less of the diet, a variety of solid foods should be given to maintain a balanced diet. Most vegetable proteins are incomplete, and amino acid deficits in one are compensated by others. With increasing dependence on solid foods it becomes easier to adapt an infant to a schedule of three meals a day.

A caution against the early administration of egg to infants is often given, particularly the administration of egg white, on the ground that it may cause allergic symptoms. Some allergists have maintained that early administration of an antigen may induce an allergy that would not otherwise have developed. There is no doubt that hypersensitivity to egg albumin may occur and that it may be extreme, just as it may in the case of the lactalbumin of cow's milk and, less frequently, in the case of wheat or other proteins. Experience with well-defined cases of hypersensitivity indicates that symptoms occur at the first contact with the food, regardless of whether this is early or late, and that decreasing sensitivity appears to result from repeated contact with small doses of the offending antigen rather than from some aging factor. It would thus appear that there is nothing to be gained by deferring contact with egg, and it is no more logical to do so than it would be to defer the administration of cow's milk. The administration of powdered egg yolk, a product marketed for its nonallergic properties, is not altogether without risk, for it has been found difficult with such products to control contamination with *Salmonella* organisms.

During the latter part of the first year the child should become accustomed to a variety of foods and should depend less on milk. *Weaning from the bottle* is a great help in attaining this end. This should be begun by 9 to 10 months; by the end of the first year milk should be taken from a cup. Children who are allowed to continue with the bottle after this time may develop the bottle habit and may refuse solid food as long as the bottle is continued.

Feeding During Second Year

In the second year the diet of a healthy child should be varied and should consist of milk, breadstuffs, farinaceous foods, vegetables, fruit juices or cooked fruit, meat, and eggs. The quantity of milk given need not exceed a pint a day. There is no necessity that a child at this age take milk at all, provided the diet is properly balanced.

It is not possible to prescribe the exact quantities of food to be given. One must rely on the child's appetite, which is a satisfactory guide, particularly if a child feeds himself. The fact that the quantity of food eaten at different times is variable should occasion no concern, for appetite shows considerable variation. Attempts to standardize a child's intake are the cause of many feeding difficulties. Almost invariably the result is loss of appetite and a struggle on the part of parents to make the child eat things it is believed he should have. Cajolery, bribery, and force are useless in such a situation; the child usually enjoys the struggle and the attention he receives. The wisest course is to put before the child a suitable meal and to set a time limit rather than a quantity limit. After 20 or 30 minutes the food should be removed, no matter how little has been eaten. If the audience displays no interest in how little the child eats, with such a regimen it seldom requires more than a few days before normal appetite is reestablished. Children of this age are peculiarly responsive to the emotional circumstances attending the administration of food. Persistant anorexia calls for study of the psychologic, as well as the somatic and dietetic, factors involved.

By the time a child is 18 months old, finely chopped foods can be substituted for the strained infant foods.

It may be advantageous to start the "junior" foods earlier if there is a tendency to constipation. A moderate amount of undigested food in the stool is not an indication for renewed sieving and grinding, but large quantities of unaltered solids may be so. Nuts are prohibited, partly because they are likely to be poorly chewed, but chiefly because of the risk of their being aspirated. The danger of impacted fish bones calls for the avoidance of bony fish. With increasing age of the child, more latitude may be allowed in the child's diet, and children past the age of 2 years may eat any of the usual adult foods according to their taste.

PARENTERAL NUTRITION

In circumstances where oral intake becomes temporarily interdicted for any reason, nutrition may be maintained by parenteral means. If the temporary period lasts no longer than a few days, water, glucose, and electrolytes are the only substances necessary, and these are easily provided through standard intravenous techniques. When a week or more must elapse before oral (or gastrostomy) feeding may be resumed, amino acid hydrolysates in a 5 percent solution plus necessary vitamins may be given to partially offset a catabolic state. For these relatively short periods glucose, water, minerals, and, when indicated, amino acids in amounts adequate to offset losses and spare protein suffice to maintain the patient until ordinary feeding may be resumed.

In special circumstances, such as major small-intestine surgical resection (short bowel syndrome) or other reason for intestinal malfunction, total parenteral nutrition may be accomplished. This requires a carefully devised solution delivering water, calories, protein, or amino acids and the necessary vitamins and minerals, including trace elements. Until recently a practical dilemma often arose: if one infused only solutions isotonic or slightly hypertonic to plasma into veins, the water load became excessive and resulted in either edema or an abnormal urinary output, thus defeating the nutritional intent. On the other hand, if hypertonic solutions were used for long periods, veins became sclerotic, and continuing treatment became impossible. With the availability of less irritating catheters, low-volume delivery, and peristaltic pumps, Dudrick and associates innovated the technique of infusing a hypertonic solution (5 percent amino acid hydrolysate and 15 to 25 percent glucose plus vitamins and electrolytes) directly into a high-flow region of the venous system. While there are problems with maintaining sterility and avoiding catheter clots, the technique can be made to work successfully for periods of many months. Further technical improvement is anticipated. Winters and associates have studied this field thoroughly and have reported good results. However, the procedure remains complex enough that it is still restricted to large centers where the pertinent expertise exists.

References

BREAST FEEDING

Aitkin FC, Hytten FE: comparison ofbreast feeding and artificial feeding. Nutr Abstr Rev 30:341, 1960

Kon SK, Cowie, At. Milk: The Mammary Gland and Its Secretions. New York, Academic, 1961

COW'S MILK

Macy IG, Kelly HJ, Sloan RE: The Composition of Milks. National Research Council Publication 254, Washington, DC, National Academy of Sciences, 1953

McKenzie HA (Ed.): Milk Proteins, Chemistry and Molecular Biology. (2 Vols.), Academic, New York, 1971

Davis CM: Self-selection of diet by newly weaned infants. An experimental study. Am J Dis Child 36:651, 1928

Mellander O, Vahlquist B, Mellbin T, Eklund G: Breast feeding and artificial feeding; a clinical, serological, and biochemical study in 402 infants, with a survey of the litterature. The Norrbotten study. Acta Paediatr Scand [Suppl] 48:116, 1959

Vaughan VC III, Dienst RB, Sheffeld CR, Roberts RW: A study of techniques of formulas for infant feeding. J Pediatr 61:547, 1962

PARENTAL NUTRITION

Dudrick SJ, Wilmore DW, Vars HM, Rhoads JE: Can intravenous feeding as the sole means of nutrition support growth in the child and restore weight loss in an adult?An affifmative answer Ann Surge169:974, 1969

Winters RW (ed.): The Body Fluids in Pediatrics. Boston, Little, Brown, 1973.

Disorders of Nutritional Homeostasis

DEFICIENCIES OF CALORIES AND PROTEIN

GEORGE G. GRAHAM

Significant variations in nutrition during early extrauterine life can result in profound changes that are not easily reversed. Excessive caloric intake may result in a body composition that is different from normal in both cell size and cell number. In addition, there may be major changes in the hormonal mechanisms that control the utilization of nutrients, particularly insulin and growth hormone production. Prolonged undernutrition cannot be presumed to result simply in delayed maturation and growth that are correctable by an optimal diet; physicians must be concerned not only with the heavy death rate from malnutrition but also with possible changes in body composition, performance, and resistance to stress in those who survive malnutrition. The duration and severity of deficits of protein and calories are major determinants of the resulting alterations in rate and nature of growth in the human infant and child.

Prolonged failure to meet basal energy requirements eventually results in cessation of linear growth. At about the same time, cellular multiplication in muscle, fat, and presumably most viscera ceases. There is suggestive evidence for a similar arrest in the central nervous system. Depending on the supply of amino acids and the severity of the caloric deficit, losses of intracellular protein may occur. The clinical picture varies from hypocaloric dwarfism to extreme marasmus. When caloric intake is excessive or adequate, but the supply of essential amino acids and total nitrogen is disproportionately low, or if infection produces intestinal losses or failure or utilization of amino acids, the clinical picture of *kwashiorkor* may occur alone or may be superimposed on that of marasmus. Presumably the caloric intake continues to favor cell multiplication, while protein deficiency results in decreased cell size in muscle and viscera and fat accumulation in hepatic cells.

Hypocaloric dwarfism and marasmus probably represent states of appropriate adaptation to preserve life and facilitate vital functions (particularly those of the central nervous system and liver) at the expense of growth and function in other tissues. Kwashiorkor probably represents failure of adaptation or decompensation of a previously appropriate adaptation. Although considerable overlap exists among hypocaloric dwarfism, marasmus, and kwashiorkor, and most cases have features of deficiencies of both calories and protein, there are distinct differences with regard to age incidence, clinical characteristics, biochemical alterations, response to dietary therapy, and prognosis. Psychosocial dwarfism also deserves special consideration.

HYPOCALORIC DWARFISM

ETIOLOGY AND PATHOGENESIS. Hypocaloric dwarfism, which is very common in the underdeveloped world, also occurs in countries that are well developed medically. Characteristically it results from prolonged consumption of diets low in available energy but balanced in essential amino acids, nitrogen, vitamins, and minerals. In the United States numerous causes have been reported: errors in preparing infant formulas; insistence on breast feeding despite inadequate supplies of milk; insufficient feedings due to intentional or unintentional negligence; intestinal malabsorption; chronic vomiting or regurgitation; anorexia as a result of disease, particularly congenital heart disease; chronic renal insufficiency and chronic infections; impaired utilization of nutrients; and increased caloric expenditure because of infection or metabolic derangement. In the medically underdeveloped world the predominant causes are different: prolonged, inadequate, and unsupplemented breast feeding; excessive dilution of milk; repeated interruptions in normal feeding, usually as a result of frequent infections; and a misguided tendency to withhold food at the slightest provocation.

CLINICAL CHARACTERISTICS. The clinical appearance of the hypocaloric dwarf except for small size, is not striking. As in most cases of malnutrition in early life, the approximately normal "dental age" of the hypocaloric dwarf may be the only clue to true age. Body composition and osseous maturation are appropriate for size rather than for age. Anemia is not promi-

nent, and serum proteins are usually normal, as are the serum concentrations of urea and the plasma amino acids, which reflects the appropriate protein–calorie ratio of the diet.

TREATMENT. Most hypocaloric dwarfs grow at an accelerated rate if they consume ordinary diets with calorie and protein intakes appropriate to their apparent ages and if there is no underlying pathology. Retention of nitrogen and increase in protoplasm are commensurate with those of normal children of similar height and biologic age. Whether they recover their genetic potential depends on the extent of loss of growth potential due to prolonged undernutrition and on the adequacy and duration of rehabilitation.

Some, particularly those whose deprivation began in the neonatal period and who did not grow until the latter part or end of the first year, do not respond well. When caloric intake is increased they may reject or vomit food; alternatively, they may simply become fat. Their linear growth is very slow, with little evidence of catch-up growth, and their nitrogen retention is poor. In these patients it is seldom clear whether some unsuspected intrauterine difficulty or severe prolonged extrauterine caloric deprivation has compromised growth potential.

MARASMUS

ETIOLOGY AND PATHOGENESIS. Infantile marasmus characteristically results from early weaning from the breast, with substitution of grossly inadequate feedings. There is often a high incidence of infectious diarrhea, followed by repeated episodes of starvation in an attempt to control the diarrhea. If breast feeding has been successful for several months before weaning, significant linear growth may have occurred, with a paralleled advance in osseous maturation and growth of brain, lean body mass, supporting tissues, and fat cells. As a result of subsequent starvation, linear growth stops, with a paralled cessation of brain growth, osseous maturation, muscle and fat cell multiplication, and growth of supporting tissues and most visceral tissues. This effect is easily documented in the hair roots, which remain in the resting stage, and in the intestinal mucosal cells, which reveal no mitoses. Very early in starvation most fat cells are depleted, and glycogen stores diminish in muscle and liver. In young infants the fat depots in the cheeks, the so-called sucking pads, are usually conserved. Muscle cells and most visceral cells lose soluble proteins, including many enzymes. Microscopically these tissues are characterized by atrophy, with cardiac muscle less so than skeletal and smooth muscles. Lymphoid tissues suffer early; the thymus, the lymph follicles of the intestine, and the malpighian bodies of the spleen shrink. Cell-mediated responses to infection are apparently impaired. The intestinal mucosa is flattened, and the entire wall becomes paper thin, making biopsy hazardous. The liver usually maintains its structural integrity, altering the direction and magnitude of its functions in order to preserve life. The supporting tissues of the body tend to conserve their structural proteins.

Severe losses of intracellular water may occur, with maintenance or even relative expansion of the extracellular compartment. Wallace aptly described the marasmic infant as "shrinking around his extracellular water." Anemia is usually moderate. Serum albumin levels are normal or slightly reduced, and serum globulins are normal or elevated. No deficiency of the immunoglobulins has been documented. Serum urea is decreased, except when elevated by dehydration. Plasma amino acids may reveal a normal pattern if starvation has been balanced, but as in kwashiorkor, the pattern may be altered if the protein-to-calorie ratio of the diet has been very low; a very low concentration of all the amino acids is seen in some cases.

Fasting blood sugar is normal or low and plasma insulin correspondingly normal or low; free fatty acids are elevated, and growth hormone levels are at the elevated levels seen in normal young infants. There is some impairment of glucose absorption and disappearance after an oral or intravenous load, and there is a markedly decreased insulin release after a variety of stimuli. However, growth hormone levels do not fall promptly after a meal, as they do in normal infants. There is a prompt and efficient fall in free fatty acid levels after a meal, suggesting enhanced insulin sensitivity, possibly the result of the loss of fat stores. There is some evidence of mild hypothyroidism, probably of pituitary origin. Plasma cortisol levels are generally elevated, particularly when severe infection is present. Although plasma aldosterone levels are usually normal, the secretion rate may be elevated. Catecholamine excretion rates are usually low, except when severe infection is present.

In the medically underdeveloped world, particularly in rural areas during famine conditions, it is not unusual to see a similar condition develop in preschool children, school children, and even adults. Many features are different in these older individuals, because much growth has occurred prior to starvation and because of differences in duration of the starvation.

CLINICAL CHARACTERISTICS. The drawn features, wrinkled skin, and hollow temples of the marasmic infant give him the appearance of a very old man. Absence of subcutaneous fat, atrophy of muscles, and potassium deficiency make the skin hang in loose folds (Fig. 4). Bones and joints are prominent, as are the superficial veins. The abdomen is usually scaphoid, but may be distended if diarrhea and potassium deficiency are prominent. Body temperature and blood pressure are usually subnormal, while the pulse rate is quite variable, depending on the presence of associated conditions. Physical activity is almost nil, and the patient's psychologic and social responses are markedly depressed. Pneumonia and pyelonephritis are frequent complications.

TREATMENT. In infantile marasmus response to rehabilitation occurs slowly. If caloric intake is increased rapidly, even with an adequate proportion of protein, severe hypoalbuminemia and sodium retention

with edema frequently develop. Nitrogen retention is poor, and many infants remain in negative balance for many days. If caloric intake is increased cautiously over 1 to 2 weeks there may be initial weight loss and a

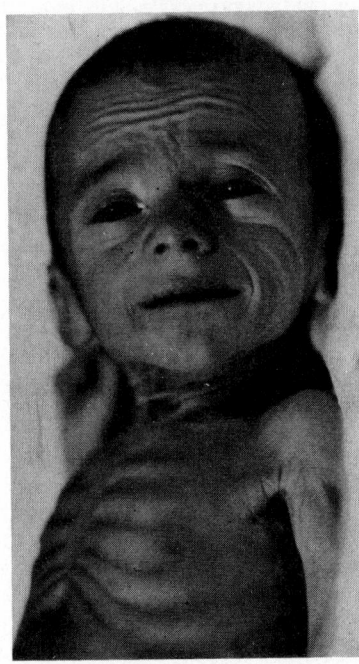

FIG. 4. Marasmus in a patient 7 months of age whose weight is 2,950 g (6 pounds 8 ounces).

moderate fall in serum albumin, along with poor nitrogen retention, but the hazard of sodium retention is less. In a few weeks nitrogen retention improves, serum albumin stabilizes, and rapid weight gain begins, soon followed by accelerated linear growth. Studies done in the course of rehabilitation, however, indicate a persistently decreased muscle cell size and relatively poor increases in intracellular water in young infants.

Glucose absorption and disappearance and free fatty acid levels return to normal fairly rapidly. However, insulin responsiveness is not regained for many weeks in most marasmic infants, which suggests continued sensitivity to insulin. Poor nitrogen retention and slow growth persist in many infants, possibly as a result of the higher concentrations of insulin required for amino acid uptake in muscle. After partial rehabilitation, fasting growth hormone levels and their response to various stimuli are often lower than normal. The levels of adrenocortical hormones return to normal, but thyroid function may continue to be low in some infants.

Reports indicating prompt and avid nitrogen retention and resumption of growth at an accelerated rate usually concern children older than 2 years. In these patients deficits in body length are considerably less severe than deficits in weight, indicating that the malnutrition is of recent onset. In most of them satisfactory nitrogen retention is commonly observed, along with prompt resumption of growth. In younger infants the muscle cell population increases very little during the first 4 months of rehabilitation, whereas in older infants it increases at a relatively rapid rate. Increments in body fat and supporting tissues occur rapidly in both groups when calories are provided in generous amounts. The presence of systemic infection hinders recovery, making the achievement of positive nitrogen balance difficult.

Although intakes of nearly 200 kcal/kg/day are often necessary to establish satisfactory weight gain in young marasmic infants, these levels should be reached gradually and should be maintained only for a relatively short time. When caloric intake is expressed as a function of the expected weight for actual height, and when the possibility of persistent impairment of fat absorption is considered, these intakes do not seem high. There is no prognostic virtue in allowing excessive weight gain, particularly after appropriate weight for height is reached. At this point rehabilitation is far from complete, since muscle mass is still reduced and body fat is now excessive. Nevertheless, caloric intake should be reduced to a level adequate for maintenance of proportional growth; this often occurs voluntarily. At no time should less than 8 percent of calories be provided as high-quality protein. An adequate diet for many months or years is necessary for maximal recovery. When very high caloric intake is necessary, it is preferable to add pure fat and carbohydrate and the appropriate amount of protein to a standard infant formula than to give feedings with high solute loads. When fat malabsorption is present or is anticipated, the additional fat calories may profitably be added in the form of medium-chain triglycerides. The marasmic infant has a reduced glomerular filtration rate and also impaired concentrating and acidifying capacity.

During the initial stages, even when weight is actually being lost rather than gained, correction of the altered body composition is proceeding, and adaptations of growth-regulating mechanisms are being normalized. Early weight gain, if anything, should make the physician suspect water and sodium retention. The most cachectic-looking infant, often mistakenly thought to be dehydrated, may have 80 percent of his body weight as water, a value found in small premature infants.

If manifestations of lactose intolerance develop, a milk substitute of the highest possible quality should be used. In any special formula constructed from individual ingredients, particular attention should be paid to the content of the intracellular cations of potassium and magnesium. As protein is synthesized and cellular composition returns toward normal, these cations are bound in cells, and clinical signs of deficiency may suddenly become apparent. During rehabilitation, deficiencies of other specific nutrients may develop. Clinical vitamin A or folic acid deficiency that is minimal or absent on admission may become quite severe in a few days if an adequate supply is not provided. Iron deficiency will become apparent in a few weeks if an adequate intake is not given. Copper deficiency has also developed during rehabilitation on diets composed exclusively of milk, and it has occasionally been present at the outset of therapy, making absorption of iron from the gut impossible. There is evidence suggestive of both chromium and zinc deficiencies in marasmic infants. Even when no specific deficiencies can be implicated, iron absorption may be very poor, making the use of parenteral iron desirable.

Particular attention must be given to prompt diagnosis and treatment of infection. Many older marasmic infants have tuberculosis, pyelonephritis, or other chronic infections that are often the cause rather than the result of malnutrition. Septicemia due to gram-negative bacteria may develop suddenly in an infant who is seemingly responding well to treatment. Prophylactic use of antibiotics seems, if anything, to increase the incidence. These agents should be used judiciously and only for specific reasons.

The mortality of untreated infantile marasmus probably approaches 100 per cent. Depending on the promptness of diagnosis, the type and extent of any complicating infections, and the degree of sophistication of the treatment facilities, this figure can probably be reduced to below 10 percent. Because of the intense effort and time required, it is almost impossible to treat severely marasmic infants successfully on an outpatient basis; therefore the mortality is much higher in areas without sophisticated hospital facilities. If rehabilitation is not prolonged and if appropriate educational and other changes are not made in the household, the chances of a recurrence or of an early death at home are very high, particularly for those dicharged below 1 year of age.

KWASHIORKOR

ETIOLOGY AND PATHOGENESIS. In many areas of the world there is a significant incidence of kwashiorkor, which was first described in Africa in children weaned after 1 year of age. These children, usually breast-fed successfully for 6 to 18 months, are weaned to diets generous in calories but deficient in nitrogen and in one or more essential amino acids. If previous growth has been satisfactory, if caloric intake is maintained, and if protein deficiency is severe and acute, the manifestations of kwashiorkor may develop rapidly in a child with normal or nearly normal stature and with considerable subcutaneous fat still present. These patients are the so-called sugar babies described in the literature. They experience severe losses of protein, in liver, muscle, and other organs, quite notably in the pancreas. Studies of their intestinal mucosa and hair indicate that cells continue to divide despite the severe shortage of protein. More commonly, kwashiorkor develops over a longer period of time. Linear growth decelerates, and there is loss of body fat and severe loss of muscle and liver protein, with reduced total and circulating albumin. Further deterioration of the protein content and quality of the diet is usually precipitated by episodes of infectious diarrhea or systemic infection. This results in accumulation of liver fat and insidious but sometimes precipitous sodium and water retention. Serum albumin concentration may drop further, often to less than 1 g/100 ml, because of failure of synthesis. Skin and hair changes are usually prominent. Depending on duration and previous nutritional state, loss of fat and muscle wasting are often severe enough to justify the term marasmic kwashiorkor. Sudden access to a more generous caloric intake, or more commonly a severe infection in a marasmic infant, may precipitate hepatic steatosis, hypoalbuminemia, and edema.

Fatal cases of kwashiorkor include these prominent anatomic features: varying degrees of subcutaneous edema, but rarely ascites; atrophy of muscle, especially skeletal muscle, but also smooth muscle and cardiac muscle; atrophic changes in organs with high protein turnover, such as intestinal epithelium and pancreatic acini, in which fibrotic changes have been reported; and varying degrees of hepatic steatosis. In addition, there are characteristic skin lesions and manifestations of complicating infections, notably bronchopneumonia, pyelonephritis, and septicemia. Total body analyses reveal marked deficits of soluble protein and potassium, including potassium deficits in brain tissue.

Estimates of body composition reveal a marked increase in total body water as a percentage of body weight and an increase of extracellular fluid as a fraction of total body water. Despite this alteration, there may be a severe contraction of plasma volume in cases with complicating acute diarrhea. Intracellular fluid is reduced in both absolute and relative terms. Biopsy of the liver reveals increased fat and glycogen and decreased labile protein content, particularly involving enzymes concerned with protein catabolism. In muscle there is a marked decrease in cell size due to loss of water and protein; concentrations of potassium, magnesium, phosphorus, and zinc are decreased, but intracellular sodium is increased. Muscle fat content may be increased. Protein–DNA and RNA–DNA ratios are appreciably reduced. Alterations in intracellular enzymes may occur, as well as reduction in pancreatic exocrine secretion and intestinal disaccharidases.

CLINICAL CHARACTERISTICS. Physical activity is reduced; muscular weakness, apathy, and irritability are prominent. Many of these children remain in a sitting position, even while sleeping. Edema may be gross and generalized (Fig. 5) or slight and localized to the eyelids and feet. Skin changes, when present, are very similar to those of pellagra, but are more extensive. Erythema occurs first, followed by hyperpigmentation, desquamation, depigmentation, and at times ulceration. Picking off the desquamating skin increases the risk of infection. The hair is sparse and fine and breaks or pulls out easily; it is depigmented to a grayish or reddish tint and may be absent over the temples. When adequate dietary protein is provided, newly formed hair is again pigmented, and the discolored portion moves outward. Alternating periods of dietary adequacy and deficiency may result in the so-called flag sign, particularly in long-haired children.

The chronic diarrhea of malnutrition, with frequent small greenish stools, may be complicated by acute infectious diarrhea or disaccharide intolerance, particularly for lactose. In children genetically predisposed to loss of their major lactase activity in childhood, an episode of severe malnutrition may precipitate permanent loss very early. Anorexia may be so severe as to require initial tube feeding, or parenteral feeding if tube feeding is not tolerated. As in marasmus, vitamin and mineral deficiencies may not be apparent, but may develop rapidly during rehabilitation.

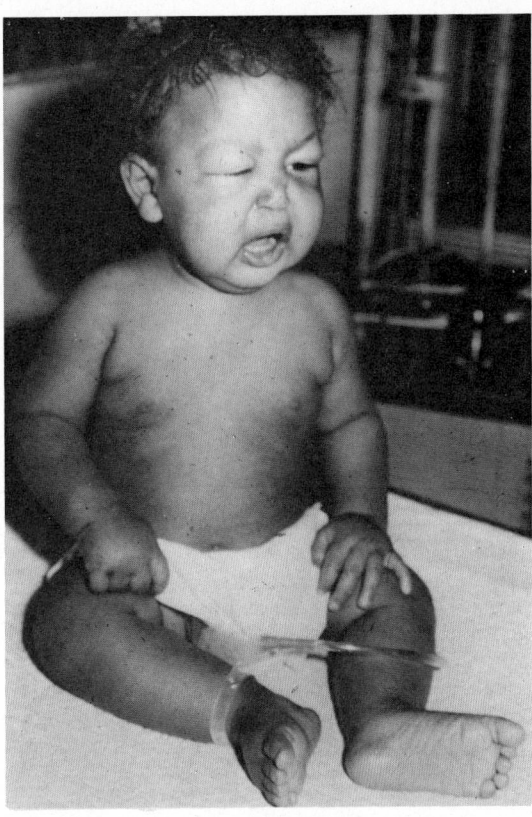

FIG. 5. Marked edema in a patient with kwashiorkor. (From Taitz and Finberg: Am J Dis Child 112:76, 1966.)

Hypoalbuminemia without significant proteinuria immediately distinguishes kwashiorkor from the nephrotic syndrome, which can resemble kwashiorkor. Serum albumin concentration is usually 1.5 to 2.5 g/100 ml, but it may be decreased to below 1 g/100 ml or raised above 3 g/100 ml due to changes in plasma volume. Studies with radioisotopes indicate that plasma albumin levels underestimate the deficit, since extravascular albumin, which normally accounts for 50 percent of the total, is more severely depleted. Despite this, serum albumin levels remain the most reliable clinical indicator of protein deficiency. After 10 to 15 days on a diet in which protein represents less than 6 percent of total calories, most infants and children will suffer a drop of 0.5 to 1.0 g/100 ml in serum albumin level if they continue to gain weight. In kwashiorkor the β globulins and ceruloplasmin may also be reduced. Immunoglobulins are rarely reduced; if they are altered at all they are usually elevated.

Most children with kwashiorkor have characteristic elevations of nonessential plasma amino acids, particularly glycine, alanine, and serine. Most essential amino acids, particularly tyrosine, tryptophan, and the branched-chain amino acids, are severely depressed. These changes are not specific for body protein deficiency, since they also occur in normal infants receiving a low protein diet for 1 to 2 days; they seem merely to indicate dietary protein inadequacy. Typically, there are low levels of serum and urinary urea, as well as serum amylase, lipase, esterase, alkaline phosphatase, and cholinesterase. Serum cholesterol and triglycerides are lowered, but free fatty acids are normal or elevated. A markedly decreased creatinine excretion reflects the reduced muscle mass. Elevated serum bilirubin levels, if present, are due to sepsis or hepatic failure.

Fasting children with kwashiorkor have normal or low blood sugar levels, correspondingly normal or low plasma insulin, and elevated growth hormone levels. There is considerable delay in glucose absorption, a moderately delayed glucose disappearance, and poor or unmeasurable insulin responses to various stimuli, with a delay in suppression of free fatty acid release. Decreased insulin sensitivity is probably the result of severe potassium deficiency and conservation of body fat stores in some children. Growth hormone levels are poorly suppressed by glucose, single amino acids, or a single-protein meal, but they respond well to continued feeding of protein or to infusion of complete amino acid mixtures. Low levels of thyroid hormones are a result of deficient thyroxine-binding globulin, but free thyroxine levels are normal. Aldosterone secretion rates are normal, but plasma concentrations may be elevated. Although cortisol secretion rates are normal, concentrations in plasma are elevated, particularly when severe infection is present. Catecholamine secretion is increased in the presence of severe infection.

Anemia of moderate degree occurs, with normochromia and macrocytosis; severe anemia may occur from chronic blood loss associated with intestinal parasites, particularly hookworm. Deficiencies of protein, folic acid, iron, and copper all play a role in development of anemia. Serum vitamin B_{12} levels are usually elevated. Hypoprothrombinemia secondary to liver involvement and thrombocytopenia due to severe infection may lead to a hemorrhagic tendency.

Severe malnutrition probably does not lead to an increased incidence of infection, but it alters the ability of the child to cope with infection; hence the greater severity and duration of diseases such as upper respiratory infections, diarrheal infections, tuberculosis, and common childhood infections, particularly measles. A generalized fatal form of herpes simplex infection has been reported frequently. Most infections aggravate the malnutrition, leading to a vicious cycle that accounts for the enormous mortality of infants and preschool children in underdeveloped areas.

TREATMENT. Initially, dehydration should be corrected to restore circulation and glomerular filtration. Sodium-containing solutions must be given intravenously, even though there may be a large surplus of sodium and water in the body. Potassium must be added sooner than in the usual case of dehydration, as hypokalemia may be severe and aggravated by hydration, with fatal results; supplementary potassium should be given for about 10 days. It is urgent that protein or amino acids be given immediately, either orally or parenterally or by intragastric tube. However, there is no need for large amounts of protein, which may cause hyperaminoacidemia, aminoaciduria, hypokalemia, hypomagnesemia, hypoglycemia, and severe dehydration after diuresis.

Usually, in the absence of significant infection, provision of a modest supply of high-quality protein, with or without adequate caloric intake, is all that is required. If 2 g of protein and 75 kcal/kg/day are reached after 3 or 4 days and maintained for approximately 20 days, edema will disappear gradually, serum albumin will reach nearly normal levels, and much of the accumulated fat will be cleared from the liver. As much as 65 to 70 percent of ingested nitrogen will be retained. This contrasts with the less than 20 percent retention that occurs in marasmic infants in the first 2 weeks after treatment is started, even when 150 kcal/kg/day are consumed.

Intakes of most vitamins and minerals need not be higher than those appropriate for protein and caloric intakes. Supplementary potassium and therapeutic doses of iron are usually indicated. Routine therapeutic doses of folic acid have been recommended, as have larger doses of vitamin A.

Skin infections and bronchopneumonia are so frequent that antibiotic therapy is probably indicated routinely. Penicillin is usually recommended, since other antibiotics may disturb the precarious balance of intestinal flora and favor the development of gram-negative sepsis, particularly with *Pseudomonas, Proteus,* and pathogenic *Escherichia coli.* Heavy infestation with *Giardia lamblia* may interfere with intestinal absorption and require early treatment; most other parasitic infections can be treated later unless they interfere with recovery.

After partial rehabilitation of children with kwashiorkor, insulin responses are relatively poor for many weeks, but disturbances of glucose absorption and disappearance are no longer seen, free fatty acids are promptly suppressed by meals, and growth hormone levels and responses are normal. Thyroid and adrenal hormone levels also become normal.

Many children recover spontaneously from mild or moderately severe kwashiorkor when their diet or family situation improves; however, they may have repeated seasonal recurrences. Of those that require medical attention, 10 to 40 percent succumb; most deaths during the first 24 hours are due to acute electrolyte disturbances, or to irreversible biochemical changes. During the next 10 days most deaths are due to sepsis. Enthusiastic overtreatment is a great danger.

For every case of marasmus or kwashiorkor there are

probably almost 100 children with more moderate forms of malnutrition and 1,000 children growing at rates below their genetic potential. The problem is socioeconomic rather than medical. Prevention of malnutrition requires the availability of inexpensive and acceptable sources of good-quality protein, improved living conditions, population control, mass education, and adequate health care.

PSYCHOSOCIAL DWARFISM

During the past few years there has been increased recognition in the United States of a condition now usually identified as psychosocial dwarfism or maternal deprivation syndrome.

ETIOLOGY AND PATHOGENESIS. Mothering of children with psychosocial dwarfism has usually been grossly inadequate. They present with severe stunting of linear growth, correspondingly retarded bone age, variations in weight from severe wasting to mild obesity, bizarre eating habits, and prodigious appetites when food is available. Their mothers claim that the prodigious eating is a daily and regular occurrence. A significant difference of opinion exists as to etiology; some believe these children represent examples of prolonged intermittent starvation; others think that there is interference with food utilization or with production of growth hormone . Regardless of etiology, many characteristics distinguish these children from those with other forms of malnutrition.

TREATMENT. If an adequate diet is provided regularly at home or in hospital, the excessive eating soon slows to a normal rate, and prompt acceleration of growth occurs.

GENERAL CONSIDERATIONS

The foregoing discussion might create the impression that children with malnutrition present distinct clinical pictures, but in fact there may be considerable overlap and variation. Older children may become marasmic, and kwashiorkor may occur in infants less than 6 months old. Many children present without visible edema, and yet have fatty livers, hypoalbuminemia, and skin changes. The cause of sodium and water retention is not clear; Hansen has shown that potassium without protein can promote sodium diuresis in many cases of typical kwashiorkor. Loss of potassium or sudden contraction of plasma volume as the result of diarrhea may trigger the development of edema in a severely protein-deficient infant or child. A newborn infant who cannot be fed orally and who is maintained on generous intravenous glucose feedings without protein for more than a few days will develop severe hypoalbuminemia and edema and may develop a fatty liver.

The occurrence of severe marasmus during the first year and kwashiorkor thereafter is probably not due to an age-related difference in response to similar diets. The young infant is more likely to be placed on a near-starvation regime, while the toddler may have access to items rich in calories and poor in protein. The toddler

is also more likely to contract measles and infectious diarrhea, the two most common precipitating causes of kwashiorkor. Even when given identical diets high in calories and low in protein, infants and children may handle them differently. The typical bulkiness and unpalatibility of many such diets, as well as their low protein or specific amino acid content, may decrease appetite and lead gradually to the picture of marasmus. An infection may then precipitate kwashiorkor. Conversely, if generous amounts continue to be consumed for many weeks, the picture of the sugar baby may develop. When sweetened condensed milk was commonly used for infant feeding, such a development was not unusual in prosperous families.

ADAPTATION. Reference has been made to the delicately balanced adaptation to grossly inadequate caloric and protein intakes. Although some of the changes in the pattern of enzymatic activity that help to conserve vital proteins at the expense of expendable tissues have been described, the hormonal and neural mechanisms that bring them about are still not well understood. An understanding of the adaptive responses to severe malnutrition is important in planning programs for rehabilitation and in interpreting their effectiveness. The fact that linear growth continues for some time, despite severe weight loss, suggests that adaptation is not immediate. The age of onset of malnutrition is probably more important than the type of presentation in determining the biochemical and physiologic effects and the rate of recovery. Thus an infant whose growth has been severely restrained from birth will respond initially much like a newborn and require a long period of rehabilitation; one who has grown relatively well for some months and then has suffered a setback is more likely to recover rapidly.

LONG-TERM EFFECTS. In recent years much research effort has been devoted to the study of possible long-term effects of malnutrition in intrauterine and extrauterine life on eventual body size and composition, performance, and particularly intellectual development. Most children who survive severe malnutrition in infancy are stunted in stature and perform poorly in standard tests of intellectual performance. When they have been compared with their siblings who have not experienced acute malnutrition, no differences have been found; this indicates that the deficits may be due to prolonged undernourishment and environmental deprivation, and not to one or more episodes of severe malnutrition.

Animal studies, particularly those in rodents, have produced more suggestive evidence of permanent interference with growth and of behavioral abnormalities following intrauterine or preweaning nutritional deprivation. Studies in pigs and dogs are less impressive, and there have been only limited studies in nonhuman primates.

As physicians responsible for the well-being of children, we should naturally be concerned with the prevention and treatment of all forms of malnutrition. We should not, however, lose sight of the fact that physical and mental development are influenced by the total environment and that food is only one part of it. Long-lasting influences, such as chronic caloric restriction and frequent infections, almost certainly curtail eventual body stature and muscle mass. The environmental requirements for optimal intellectual and behavioral development are less clearly understood, and although adequacy of food may be necessary, an environment with healthy stimulation and learning experiences may be equally important or even more important.

DISORDERS OF LIPID NUTRITION
KAREN KUEHL

In recent years pediatricians have shown renewed interest in lipids and lipid metabolism as epidemiologic and genetic evidence has accumulated linking elevation of serum lipids to premature development of atherosclerosis. Recommendations to the general public to lower dietary cholesterol and saturated fats have provoked controversy and prompted a reexamination of the need for lipids in the diet during childhood.

FAT ABSORPTION. It has been calculated that the diet of the average adult in the United States derives 41 percent of its calories from fats, with an average ratio of polyunsaturated to saturated fat of 0.5:1. The main component of dietary fat is triglyceride (98 percent), with an average cholesterol intake of over 700 mg/day. Most fat calories are derived from the fatty acids, which constitute 95 percent by weight of the triglyceride molecule. The other component of dietary fat is phospholipid. The only essential fat is linoleic acid, which is required for prostaglandin synthesis. Other fatty acids, cholesterol, and phospholipids can be synthesized endogenously as required. The requirement for linoleic acid in infancy is met by a diet in which linoleic acid provides about 4 percent of total caloric requirements.

Fats are emulsified in the duodenum by the mechanical churning action of the gut and by the presence of bile salts. Pancreatic lipase is secreted into the duodenum and hydrolyzes triglycerides to 2-monoglycerides. Bile salts have two other critical roles in absorption of fat besides promoting emulsification; they shift the pH optimum of pancreatic lipase from 8 to 6, which is the pH of the duodenum, and they promote the formation of micelles from bile salts, 2-monoglyceride, fatty acids, cholesterol, and phospholipids. The formation of these micelles, 40 to 50 μ in diameter, greatly increases the surface area of the lipids available for absorption by the intestine. It has been proposed that the intermicrovillus space is of such dimension (500 A) that micelle formation is essential to the penetration of absorbable lipid into this space. However, Dietschy has proposed that the micelle's function is to present a large mass of water-soluble lipid to the rate-limiting layer of unstirred water that must exist in direct opposition to the intestinal brush border. Thus actual absorption of fatty acids monoglycerides, and cholesterol occurs by simple diffusion across the unstirred layer into the intestinal epithelial cell.

Triglycerides containing medium-chain fatty acids (those with less than 12 carbon atoms) are absorbed by a different mechanism; they are absorbed intact and hydrolyzed in the intestinal epithelial cell by a mucosal lipase. The resulting short-chain fatty acids are transported on albumin via the portal vein to the liver. This alternate mechanism for short-chain fatty acid absorption is the basis for the use of medium-chain triglycerides to increase caloric and fat intake in disorders such as pancreatic insufficiency or abetalipoproteinemia in which intestinal absorption of other fats is impaired.

Within the intestinal epithelial cell, 2-monoglycerides plus fatty acids of chain lengths over 12 carbon atoms are resynthesized into triglyceride. This energy-requiring step is thought to be important in giving the organism control over fatty acid composition.

Cholesterol esters in foods are hydrolyzed by an intestinal esterase prior to absorption. Polymerization of this enzyme to its active form requires bile salts. Bile salts are obligatory for the absorption of cholesterol, whereas other detergents (all capable of promoting micelle formation) may replace bile salts in promoting absorption of fatty acids.

Studies of the absorption of dietary cholesterol have led to conflicting results concerning the absolute amount and the percentage of an administered dose that is absorbed. Recent studies have shown that, following a single dose of radioisotopically labeled cholesterol, over a wide range about 45 percent of that administered is absorbed. However, the usual absorption of dietary cholesterol in man is only 200 to 300 mg daily over a wide range of intake; the factors responsible for this relatively stable intake are not clearly understood.

The role of fat intake in increasing cholesterol absorption is related to the formation of micelles. Increased fat intake supplies more monoglyceride and fatty acid for the formation of micelles, which incorporate cholesterol and present it to the intestinal surface. Intestinal cholesterol is absorbed only in the free form and is reesterified within the intestinal epithelial cell prior to secretion as a component of chylomicrons. The cholesterol in the intestine is a mixture of dietary and endogenous cholesterol; the latter is secreted into the duodenum via the bile duct or synthesized by the intestine. Intestinal synthesis of cholesterol is controlled by the concentration of bile salts, and possibly by the amount absorbed from the diet.

Bile acids, which are synthesized from cholesterol in the liver and conjugated with glycine or taurine, are also secreted into the duodenum. All three components (bile salts, dietary cholesterol, and endogenous cholesterol) are partially reabsorbed from the jejunum. Bile salts are largely reabsorbed from the ileum by a process of active transport. The rate of turnover of the exchangeable pool of cholesterol in man, as calculated from fecal losses of neutral steroids and bile salts, is 1 to 2 g daily; thus this much cholesterol must be replaced daily either by synthesis or from the diet.

The intestinal epithelial cell synthesizes triglyceride from absorbed fatty acids and 2-monoglyceride and esterifies the absorbed free cholesterol. These components, as well as phospholipid and small amounts of protein, are assembled into chylomicrons in the endoplasmic reticulum. Intestinal epithelial cells also produce similar particles with a slightly lower triglyceride content known as very low density lipoproteins (VLDL). Transfer of additional proteins, the C proteins, to the VLDL or chylomicrons produced in the intestinal epithelial cells occurs from high-density lipoproteins (HDL) prior to the appearance of the VLDL or chylomicrons in thoracic duct lymph; this transfer is most apparent during fat absorption.

As intestinally produced lipoproteins are discharged from the thoracic duct into the bloodstream, hydrolysis of the triglyceride begins, due to activation of the enzyme lipoprotein lipase. This enzyme is present in serum after heparin infusion and is thought to be localized on the luminal surface of endothelial cells. Activation of the enzyme requires one of the C proteins present in VLDL and HDL. Hydrolysis of the triglyceride releases free fatty acids, which are taken up by adipocytes. Concurrently the C proteins are lost from the lipoprotein particle, resulting in a reduction in size. The chylomicron remnant is taken up in its entirety by the liver. The cholesteryl esters are hydrolyzed, and the cholesterol probably enters the circulation again largely as a component of VLDL of hepatic origin.

FATTY ACIDS. Free fatty acids are transported in blood on albumin, which has many binding sites; two of these have a high affinity for free fatty acids. These free fatty acids supply most of the lipid calories of the diet to the peripheral tissues. Normal serum levels of free fatty acids are low (300 to 700 μEq/liter). However, the half-life of free fatty acid in serum is only 2 to 3 minutes, and up to 25 g of fatty acids can be transported per hour. These free fatty acids are transported from adipose tissue after lipolysis to sites such as heart and muscle, where they can be taken up and used as sources of energy. In the presence of oxygen, fatty acids are catabolized in mitochondria to CO_2 and H_2O via the Krebs cycle after conversion to their acetyl CoA derivatives. Fatty acids that are transported to the liver may be oxidized to ketone bodies or esterified to participate in VLDL formation. Muscle and heart tissues depend on free fatty acids for energy.

LIPOLYSIS. A lipoprotein lipase and a hormone-sensitive lipase are present within the adipose tissue cell. The activity of hormone-sensitive lipase is affected by many hormones, all of which mediate their effects through changes in cellular levels of cyclic AMP. ACTH, glucagon, and catecholamines all increase cyclic AMP levels. Growth hormone, glucocorticoid, thyroxine, and insulin all reduce the activity of hormone-sensitive lipase. Many of the hormones that suppress hormone-sensitive lipase in the adipocyte also stimulate the activity of lipoprotein lipase, which is required for release of free fatty acids from lipoproteins and their incorporation into adipose tissue.

LIPOPROTEINS. The measurable physiologic entities in serum other than free fatty acids are the serum lipoproteins. Recent clinical studies of adults at risk of coronary artery disease have characterized populations according to levels of the various lipoprotein classes rather than total lipid levels. The four lipoprotein classes represent empiric separations of lipid-containing complexes from plasma by sequential adjustment of density with heavy salts. With each density class there may be more than one type of lipoprotein complex. Similarly, in experimental models a particle whose protein composition is characteristic of one density class in the normal may appear in other density classes in an experimentally modified animal. The characteristics of the major lipoproteins are shown in Table 9.

The apoproteins (that is, the lipid-free protein components of serum lipoproteins) are receiving increasing

TABLE 9A. Characteristics of the Major Lipoproteins

	Density	Size (Å)	Electrophoretic Mobility
Chylomicrons	< 0.94	750–10,000	Remain at origin
VLDL	0.94–1.006	300–500	Pre-β
LDL	1.006–1.063	200–220	β
HDL	1.063–1.21	75–100	α_1

TABLE 9B. Compositions of the Lipoprotein Families (Percentage of Dry Weight)

Lipoprotein Constituents	Chylomicrons	VLDL	LDL[a]	HDL
Protein	1–2	10	25	45–55
Triglyceride	80–95	55–65	10	3–8
Unesterified cholesterol	1–3	10	8	3
Esterified cholesterol	2–4	5	37	15
Phospholipids	3–6	15–20	22	30
Carbohydrate	?	< 1	~1	< 1

[a] *LDL is often divided into LDL$_1$, or intermediate-density lipoprotein (density 1.006—1.019) and LDL$_2$ (density 1.019—1.063). Similarly, HDL is divided into HDL$_2$ (isolated between 1.063 and 1.12) and HDL$_3$ (isolated between 1.12 and 1.21).*

attention as awareness of their specific roles in lipoprotein metabolism accumulates. The nomenclature of these apoproteins is based on an initial immunologic assignment to group A, B, or C; they were formerly identified with HDL, with LDL, or with both VLDL and HDL, respectively.

Chylomicrons are secreted by intestinal epithelial cells continuously, but particularly during fat absorption. Some intestinal lipoproteins are the size and density of VLDL and apparently have the same composition as chylomicrons, except that they contain slightly less triglyceride. B protein is required for chylomicron formation, as evidenced by the absence of chylomicron secretion in abetalipoproteinemia. Immunochemical reactions of lipoproteins from intestinal epithelial cells show cross-reactivity with an anti-apo-HDL antibody. Nearly all chylomicron cholesterol is esterified prior to entering the plasma via the thoracic duct lymph. The triglyceride is hydrolyzed in the peripheral capillaries of adipose tissue by lipoprotein lipase, and the fatty acids are taken up into adipose cells; this process requires the presence of insulin. The activity of lipoprotein lipase enzyme is depressed by glucagon· and epinephrine. After hydrolysis of triglyceride, the remnant of the chylomicron is taken up by the liver. The cholesterol esters are hydrolyzed in the liver, and the cholesterol metabolized in the liver forms lipoprotein of membranes.

NORMAL LEVELS OF CHOLESTEROL AND TRIGLYCERIDES. Levels of cholesterol at birth have been of particular interest to investigators attempting to identify familial hypercholesterolemia in children of heterozygotic parents. In newborn infants cholesterol levels are 65 ± 19(SD) mg/100 ml; they increase progressively even within the first 6 months. The usual acceptable levels of cholesterol and triglyceride at various ages are shown in Table 10. It has been suggested that the amount of cholesterol in LDL is a better means of identifying familial hypercholesterolemia; at birth normal cholesterol is 31 ± 6 mg/100 ml.

Clearly some children with increased levels of lipids or lipoproteins have characteristics that are used to identify adults at risk of developing premature atherosclerosis. It would seem likely that if these increases in lipids are genetic they will persist into adult life. The Committee on Nutrition of the American Academy of Pediatrics has recommended cholesterol and triglyceride screening of children who have a first-degree blood relative with a history of myocardial infarction under the age of 50 years. There is as yet no definitive study

to prove that intervention to lower serum lipids in childhood will delay the onset of premature coronary artery disease. However, identification and dietary intervention for children with familial hypercholesterolemia is recommended after 1 year of age by the committee.

There is more disagreement among pediatricians as to the value of dietary modification for the general public, as recommended in 1975 by the Council on Atherosclerosis of the American Heart Association. These recommendations included adjustment of caloric intake to achieve and maintain optimal weight, reduction of daily cholesterol intake to less than 300 mg/day, and change in fat intake such that total fats will provide 35 percent of total calories, to be derived equally from saturated, monounsaturated, and polyunsaturated sources. Pediatricians have expressed concern about the effects of such a dietary modification on development of the central nervous system, the possible hazards of long-term increases in polyunsaturated fat intake, and the possibility of reduced absorption of fat-soluble vitamins. Another concern is based on animal data. Rats that received high-cholesterol diets in infancy responded to later cholesterol challenge with lower serum cholesterol levels than rats who received low-cholesterol diets in infancy. A preliminary study has been done in a small group of children, some of whom were normal and some of whom had familial hypercholesterolemia. One group received low (30 to 50 mg/day) cholesterol intake and a second group received moderate (100 to 200 mg/day) cholesterol intake until the age of 6 months, after which both groups received over 500 mg of cholesterol daily. No difference between the two groups was observed in serum cholesterol levels at 1 year of age. The widespread use of commercially prepared formulas in infant feeding has markedly altered the cholesterol and saturated fat intake of many infants (Table 11). The influence of these diets on future development of atherosclerosis, future response to cholesterol challenge, and effects of high polyunsaturated fatty acid intake in infancy remain to be studied. Specific disorders of lipid metabolism are discussed in Chapter 14.

VITAMIN DEFICIENCY DISEASES

Much of our knowledge of these diseases has been gained from animal experiments, and some of the well-established human deficiencies, such as those of vitamin A, vitamin K, and vitamin B_6, were first recognized in animals. However, the results of animal experiments

TABLE 10. Normal Levels of Cholesterol and Triglyceride at Various Ages Given as Milligrams per 100 Milliliters

Age (years)	Mean and 90% Limits Cholesterol	Triglyceride	VLDL	LDL	Cholesterol in: HDL	HDL
0–19	175 (120–230)	65 (10–140)	5–15	50–120	30–70	30–65
20–29	180 (120–240)	70 (10–140)	5–25	60–170	35–75	35–70
30–39	205 (140–270)	75 (10–150)	5–35	70–190	35–80	30–65
40–49	225 (150–310)	85 (10–160)	5–35	80–190	40–85	30–65
50–59	245 (160–330)	95 (10–190)	10–40	80–210	35–85	30–65

TABLE 11. Comparison of Natural Milks With Formulas That Modify Fat

	Cow's Milk	Breast Milk	Formula 1	Formula 2
Cholesterol (mg/100 ml)	14	20	3.0	1.5
Linoleic acid (g/100 ml)	2.1	10.6	23	35
Fat (g/100 ml)	3.4	4.5	3.7	3.4

must be interpreted with caution, for there are marked species differences in nutritive requirements. The rat, for example, has no difficulty in synthesizing vitamin C. Furthermore, a deficiency of any one factor may give different symptoms in different species. A lack of vitamin E in the rat primarily affects the reproductive system; in the rabbit it produces muscular dystrophy; in the chick it causes encephalomalacia; in the monkey, and perhaps in man also, a specific type of megaloblastic anemia is produced. One cannot assume that the many deficiencies known in experimental animals necessarily have counterparts in man. Human deficiencies also differ from those of experimental animals in that human diets, when defective at all, are likely to be lacking in several factors; the disease pictures are therefore more difficult to separate.

VITAMIN A DEFICIENCY

Donald S. McLaren

Vitamin A deficiency is virtually unknown in North America and Western Europe today, although it is occasionally seen in infants fed skim milk and in malabsorption states. It is, however, widespread throughout most of the developing regions of the world where it is an important cause of blindness. In India, Pakistan, and Southeast Asia it has been estimated that more than 1 percent of all young children are affected.

VITAMIN A AND PROVITAMIN. Vitamin A (retinol) is a colorless, fat-soluble alcohol containing a β-ionone ring and a long aliphatic side chain. It is found in most animal fats (lard excepted), being most abundant in fish liver oils. Two chief forms are known: A_1 predominantly in the livers of saltwater fish, and A_2, in livers of freshwater fish. Four carotenoid pigments of colored vegetables, notably β-carotene, serve as precursors of vitamin A in the diet, with the conversion taking place in the intestinal mucosa. Deficiency occurs if both natural A and carotene are lacking. In general only about one-third of the β-carotene in foodstuffs is available for conversion, and the efficiency of conversion is about 50 percent. Thus 1 μg of β-carotene may be taken to have the same activity as 0.167 μg of retinol.

Preformed vitamin A, or provitamin, is esterified in the small intestine, absorbed by way of the thoracic duct, and transported to the liver, probably attached to β-lipoprotein. Vitamin A deficiency is often associated with protein deficiency. This is believed to result from impairment of transport and possibly storage. In the resting serum almost all of the vitamin is present in the alcohol form.

FUNCTION. The most important function of vitamin A is its role in vision. In the rods of the retina vitamin A, in the form of 11-*cis*-retinol, is bound to a protein opsin to form a photosensitive pigment, rhodopsin (visual purple). When vitamin A is deficient, there is impairment of dark adaptation, and ultimately there is night blindness (nyctalopia). A different pigment containing vitamin A, combined with a different protein, is found in the cones, which function in bright light and in color vision; however, impairment of cone function is less readily demonstrated in vitamin-A-deficient states.

Apart from ocular function, vitamin A appears necessary for the maintenance of epithelial structures—the skin, the mucous membranes, the gastrointestinal tract. It also is necessary for normal growth of bones and teeth. Evidence is accumulating that it exerts a regulatory influence on various membrane systems; in high doses it causes discruption of lysosomes, with release of hydrolytic enzymes. Less well substantiated are suggestions that vitamin A plays a specific role in the biosynthesis of adrenal steroids and in synthesis of mucopolysaccharides.

PATHOLOGY. The effects of deficiency are most conspicuous during periods of active growth. A characteristic change is squamous metaplasia of epithelial tissues. In man this is most conspicuous in the conjunctiva and cornea, although other tissues may be affected. There is no convincing evidence that skeletal deformities or congenital malformations in man can be attributed to deficiency of vitamin A.

PATHOGENESIS. Because of the ability of the liver to store vitamin A, clinical deficiency results only after prolonged depletion. Liver stores must be seriously depleted before serum levels begin to fall, and in turn the concentration in serum must reach a low level before cell function and structure are affected. Quite apart from the diet, important contributing factors to disease are disorders of the alimentary tract affecting absorption of fat, as well as protein malnutrition, which affects its transport and possibly storage.

SYMPTOMS. Vitamin A deficiency can occur at any age, even at birth if the mother is deficient. However, children of 6 months to 4 years are most commonly affected. A defective diet of several weeks is required before symptoms are detected. Night blindness is the earliest symptom of the disease. An ambulant child may be noted to stumble in the dark, but more often this is missed until more serious evidence of eye disease becomes apparent.

As the deficiency state advances, the bulbar conjunctiva becomes xerotic; it becomes dry, thickened, and wrinkled and loses its natural transparency and property of being wetted by tears. Heaping up of desquamated keratinized epithelium close to the limbus may occur, forming a silvery gray plaque with a foamy surface (Bitot's spot); this occurs most commonly on the temporal side.

Conjunctival xerosis is shortly followed by similar changes in the cornea, which loses its luster, becoming dull and hazy. The precorneal film is poorly maintained; when the lids are held apart for about 15 seconds an oil-on-water appearance is seen. The process is still reversible by therapy, but unless it is arrested the keratomalacia proceeds; there may be corneal vascularization, and the stroma may undergo a process of rapid liquefaction known as colliquative necrosis followed by perforation and subsequent rapid destruction of the entire globe.

A follicular hyperkeratotic lesion of the skin known as phrynoderma (Fig. 6) rarely may be caused by vitamin A deficiency. Localized hyperkeratosis can also be caused by vitamin C deficiency, or it may not be related to any dietary deficiency.

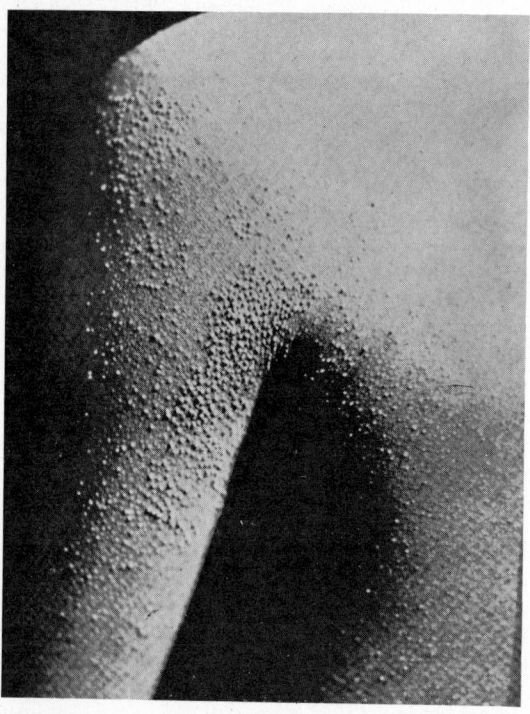

FIG. 6. Hyperkeratosis (phrynoderma) in vitamin A deficiency (From Frazier and Hu: Arch Derm Syph 33:825 1936).

DIAGNOSIS. Special tests exist for measuring dark adaptation, even in infancy, including rod scotometry and electrortinography, but as a rule reliance must be placed on the clinical evaluation of ocular findings, on plasma vitamin A and carotenoid levels, and on responses to therapy. Night blindness is not necessarily due to vitamin A deficiency; other causes

such as retinitis pigmentosa, glaucoma, and high myopia must be ruled out

Plasma levels of vitamin A below 25 international units per milliliter (1 IU=0.33 μg retinol) may be regarded as significantly low, although the average is considerably higher. High carotenoids tend to produce falsely low figures for vitamin A. Significant electroretinographic abnormalities are seen at plasma levels of 20 IU or below. Standards for hepatic stores as studied by liver puncture are still being determined.

TREATMENT. Early diagnosis and prompt and adequate treatment may be sight-saving and, indeed, life-saving. The most severe cases often succumb to complicating infections, perhaps because epithelial barriers are overwhelmed, perhaps because of damage to lysosomes and other membranes.

The symptoms of vitamin A deficiency respond with varying rapidity to treatment. Night blindness may show striking improvement within 1 hour of liberal oral dosage, or improvement may not occur for 2 or 3 weeks. The lesions of xerophthalmia may improve in 2 to 3 days, but 6 to 8 weeks may be required for complete healing. Even if corneal perforation has not occurred, opacities and scars may remain.

Deficiency states usually respond to vitamin A at a dosage of 10,000 IU/kg/day given orally, usually as the palmitate, in a water-dispersible form. Oily preparations are less well absorbed by mouth and are slowly mobilized when given intramuscularly. Larger quantities may be indicated in the presence of a malabsorption syndrome. Intensive therapy should be continued for at least 5 days. Thereafter one may continue daily treatment with a reduced dose (25,000 IU/day). Vitamin A deficiency rarely occurs alone, but is usually associated with protein calorie malnutrition and often with serious infections that require urgent attention.

PROPHYLAXIS. Recommendations very in different countries. Hume and Krebs have demonstrated in experimental studies in adult volunteers that a dose of 1,300 IU/day permits slow recovery from an induced deficiency. Current prophylactic recommendations are usually well above this level. The U.S. Food and Nutrition Board recommends 1,500 IU/day for infants and 3,000 IU/day for adults. American children taking prophylactic vitamin D in the form of fish liver oils and concentrates that also contain vitamin A commonly receive in excess of 6,000 IU/day, and it is not surprising that the American problem in early life is not hypovitaminosis A but *hyper*vitaminosis A. The answer to the prophylaxis of vitamin A deficiency is the same as for all deficiency disease: economic growth and education. Hypervitaminosis A is discussed in detail elsewhere (p. 2023).

THIAMINE DEFICIENCY (BERIBERI)

Beriberi is a disease characterized by organic changes in the nervous system and heart and functional changes in other tissues. It is common in parts of the world where rice occupies a prominent place in the diet. In the United States it is rare, being confined almost exclusively to alcoholics and dietary faddists among adults and to children with chronic digestive disorders. Beriberi may occur at any age, even in nursing infants when the mother's diet is deficient.

Thiamine, a pyrimidine-thiazole compound, is widely distributed in animal and vegetable foods. Although it is present in cereal grains, it is frequently removed in milling; it is only when milled cereals (particularly rice) predominate in the diet that deficiency is likely to be encountered.

Thiamine pyrophosphate constitutes the prosthetic group of three important decarboxylase enzymes. Together with lipoic acid and coenzyme A (CoA) it is concerned with the decarboxylation of pyruvic acid to acetyl CoA, which then enters the citric acid cycle. A second reaction involving thiamine is the oxidative decarboxylation of α-ketoglutaric acid in the citric acid cycle. Thiamine is also a cofactor in the enzyme transketolase, an enzyme concerned in one step of the oxidative pathway of carbohydrate metabolism, the pentose phosphate shunt. In this reaction of oxidative decarboxylation, glucose-6-phosphate is split to form CO_2 and pentose-6-phosphate; the pentose thus formed provides the ribose needed for the formation of nucleic acids and riboflavin. Further degradation of pentose by this same enzyme permits the formation of shorter carbon units. A thiamine-containing enzyme may also be concerned in the oxidation of alcohol.

Thiamine is present in most tissues, the highest concentrations being in liver and heart, followed by brain and muscle. Nervous tissue, unlike other tissues, is incapable of storing thiamine, a fact that may contribute to its vulnerability. In the tissues thiamine is largely in enzyme form, combined with pyrophosphate, magnesium, and protein. Free thiamine is, however, found in the tissues and is excreted in the urine.

PATHOLOGY. Early thiamine deficiency produces no characteristic anatomic changes. In frank beriberi the peripheral nerves and the central nervous system may show myelin degeneration. Degenerative changes have also been observed in hearts of patients with beriberi.

PATHOGENESIS. Thiamine deficiency may develop because of inadequate intake or abnormal loss. Depletion of thiamine may occur in severe and protracted diarrhea. Inadequate intake is not likely to occur in children in the United States.

SYMPTOMS. Apathy, anorexia, and failure to gain weight precede frank manifestations, but neurologic findings may occur with no previous symptoms.

The *neuritis* of thiamine deficiency is in no way characteristic. It is both motor and sensory. The motor and sensory disturbances appear simultaneously, hyperesthesia and areflexia being the earliest neurologic manifestations. In experimental subjects studied in the United States the neuritis that was induced involved the extremities. However, reports from the Orient indicate that the cranial nerves are not infrequently involved; in infants the recurrent laryngeal has been said to be involved, with resulting hoarseness.

Wernicke's syndrome, ophthalmoplegia associated with cerebral disturbances, has been observed in adult alcoholics suffering from thiamine deficiency, but is rare in early life. Convulsions and coma have been observed in infants and young children suffering from beriberi in the Orient.

Thiamine deficiency may cause *edema* unaccompanied by hypoproteinemia or cardiac or renal complications. The edema is often localized, involving an arm, a leg, or one side of the face. Its pathogenesis is not understood.

Cardiac involvement may manifest with tachycardia and progress to cardiac enlargement. The features are similar to those that result from any cause of generalized myocardial failure.

For reasons that are not clear, the manifestations of thiamine deficiency vary greatly in different individuals. One may develop edema, another neuritis, and another cardiac involvement or psychologic disturbance, all maintained under comparable conditions of diet and exercise. The response to therapy in neuritis or myocardial involvement is slow, but anorexia, edema, and neurotic manifestations usually disappear with 24 hours.

DIAGNOSIS. The history may be of help in recognizing thiamine deficiency, but caution is needed in interpreting dietary intake. The diagnosis is often made incorrectly on the basis of an intake below the recommendations of the Food and Nutrition Board, without appreciation of the fact that the recommendations include a generous margin of safety.

Laboratory procedures may be helpful, but they have been infrequently employed. Blood pyruvate level is usually elevated, and blood thiamine level is reduced.

TREATMENT. A dosage of 5 mg/day to an infant and twice that quantity to an adult will correct thiamine deficiency, although the results of damage may persist. There is no evidence that neuritis or carditis, behavior disorders, or loss of appetite (other than that caused by thiamine deficiency) are in any way benefited by the administration of this vitamin.

PROPHYLAXIS. The requirement of thiamine is commonly expressed in milligrams per 1,000 calories in the diet. The minimum requirement 0.14 to 0.20 mg/1,000 calories, which for an infant may be regarded as the total daily requirement. Since thiamine is required primarily for carbohydrate and protein metabolism, fat exerts a sparing effect on thiamine requirement. Thiamine is provided in adequate amounts in most normal diets in the United States. In unusual circumstances supplementation is necessary, such as parenteral feeding for more than a few days.

RIBOFLAVIN DEFICIENCY (ARIBOFLAVINOSIS)

Riboflavin deficiency is rare in the United States, but it still occurs in underdeveloped countries. The clinical picture is characterized by lesions affecting the lips and tongue, the skin, and the eyes. An angular stomatitis (perlèche) is characterized by redness, desquamation, and ulceration with fissures at the mucocutaneous junction. A glossitis, often with a magenta discoloration, has been described, and there may be ulcerative changes with a necrotic exudate. Seborrheic lesions may appear on the face, usually in the nasolabial folds or between the lower lips and chin. The most prominent ocular lesion is a marginal vascularization of the cornea; later there may be cataract formation.

The relationship between these clinical symptoms and the function of riboflavin in the body is not clear. Riboflavin is the prosthetic group of a great many respiratory enzymes—the flavoproteins, which are present in all body cells. The clinical diagnosis is rendered difficult by the fact that none of the symptoms observed in riboflavin deficiency is specific. Angular stomatitis may result from several causes, as may inflammatory lesions of the tongue. The ocular lesions are inconstant and occur in other deficiency states, notably amino acid deficiencies. The clinical diagnosis is based on the combination of these symptoms and the response to riboflavin therapy. It may be confirmed by demonstration of a diminished concentration of riboflavin in the plasma or, preferably, in the red or white blood cells.

There is abundant riboflavin in the diet of the infant and older individuals in the United States, and there is no need for supplementation. In disease states accompanied by loss of weight, a special need for additional riboflavin does not appear to exist. Thus the situation differs from that with certain other vitamins, notably vitamin C, for which there is evidence of an increased need during infections. The daily requirement of the adult for riboflavin, according to Horwitt, is 0.5 to 0.9 mg. Snyderman estimated the requirement of infants to be 0.4 to 0.5 mg/day. Commonly employed milk formulas provide about three times that amount; in breast milk the margin of safety is small but apparently adequate.

NIACIN DEFICIENCY (PELLAGRA)
George G. Graham

A chronic, relapsing generalized disorder popularly characterized by three (or four) d's—dermatitis, diarrhea, dementia (and frequently death)—has been known for over two centuries as pellagra, from the Italian *pelle* (skin) + *agra* (sour). Although it is no longer a major public health problem, pellagra is still seen occasionally in poor, maize-consuming peoples and is particularly frequent among chronic alcoholics; it may also occur in persons with chronic obstructive or absorptive gastrointestinal disorders, in those with malignant carcinoid tumors, and in infants with Hartnup disease, an inborn error of tryptophan metabolism.

ETIOLOGY AND PATHOGENESIS. Goldberger's studies demonstrated conclusively that pellagra was due to an inadequate intake of high-quality protein and most probably to an inadequate intake of the essential amino acid tryptophan. Elvehjem and his associates demonstrated that the vitamin nicotinic acid (niacin) could cure or prevent black tongue, the experimental analogue of pellagra in dogs, as well as the natural disorder in man.

Modern thinking attributes the multiple manifestations of this disorder to a deficiency of the essential coenzymes I and II, niacin adenine dinucleotide (NAD) and niacin adenine dinucleotide phosphate (NADP). These pyridine nucleotides are synthesized directly from dietary niacin or from tryptophan, with niacin or quinolinic acid as intermediates. A generous supply of energy and of the other essential amino acids can divert most of a limited supply of dietary tryptophan to protein synthesis, as well as create an increased requirement for the coenzymes. An excess of leucine in the diet, such as is present in corn, may interfere with tryptophan metabolism, as does a deficiency of pyridoxine.

The hydrogen acceptors NAD and NADP are involved in the conversions of glucose-6-monophosphate to phosphogluconic acid, citric acid to α-ketoglutaric acid, lactic acid to pyruvic acid, alcohol to acetaldehyde, and many other oxidation–reduction reactions.

CLINICAL MANIFESTATIONS. The cutaneous lesions are usually noted first, the characteristic symmetric dermatitis appearing on those parts of the body exposed to sunlight, heat, and other forms of mild trauma. Initially there is an erythema resembling sunburn (or a diaper rash in infants) on the backs of the hands, wrists, forearms, and neck (Casal's necklace), as well as on the faces of both adults and children (Fig. 7). When no exposure to sunlight exists, the lesions may appear first on the elbows, knees, nape of the neck, eyelids, cheeks, perineum, and scrotum. The clearly demarcated affected areas are initially red and infiltrated; they usually itch and burn. In the more acute cases they may progress to vesiculation, cracking, exudation, ulceration, and secondary infection. In the classic chronic case erythema progresses to roughening and keratosis with scaling. In almost all cases a brownish pigmentation develops and in the process of healing peels off, leaving healthy pink skin underneath. If the disease is still active the entire cycle will be repeated, with healing in some areas and simultaneous progression in others.

The mouth may be sore and may show angular stomatitis and cheilosis, possibly due to other associated deficiencies. The tongue may have a raw-beef appearance, being red, swollen, and painful, although usually not depapillated. The rectum and anus are often inflamed as well, with extension to others parts of the digestive tract possibly accounting for the diarrhea and malabsorption that frequently accompany or follow the dermatitis and result in weight loss.

Neurologic manifestations may appear without apparent involvement of the epithelial surface, but they usually follow such involvement. These may be moderate, with some weakness, malaise, anxiety, and depression and a short attention span; or they may be severe, with delirium. In the most chronic forms, amentia, posterolateral cord degeneration, pyramidal signs, and peripheral nerve lesions are also seen. Death may occur suddenly and unexpectedly. Only in the more severe examples of nervous system involvement are permanent residuals likely to be present after proper treatment.

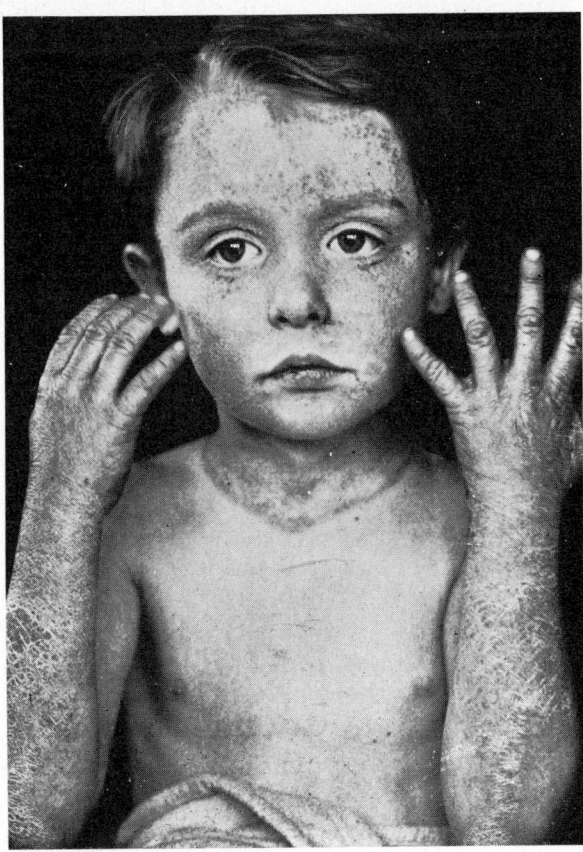

FIG. 7. Pellagra in a 5-year-old boy.

PATHOLOGY. The skin may reveal congestion of papillary blood vessels, edema of the papillae, lymphocytic infiltration of the corium, and most characteristically, notable thickening of the keratinized layer of the epidermis. Lesions of the mucous membranes and intestinal wall, particularly in the colon, resemble those of the skin. Demyelination of the posterolateral columns of the spinal cord and focal demyelination and ganglion cell degeneration of the cerebrum are seen in advanced cases.

LABORATORY FINDINGS. In the urine of adults with pellagra the combined excretion of the two major metabolites of niacin (N_1-methylnicotinamide and its 6-pyridone) is usually less than 2 mg in 24 hours. In milder deficiency states slightly larger amounts are excreted, but they are still below the 5 to 8 mg of N_1-methylnicotinamide and 7 to 10 mg of pyridone of normal subjects on a good diet. Although normal and deficient rates of excretion for infants and children have not been determined accurately, they may be estimated from the relative caloric expenditures. Measurement of one or both metabolites in a 24-or 6-hour urine specimen is the biochemical method most commonly used for diagnosis of pellagra. The plasma tryptophan level is extremely low, even more so than in most cases of kwashiorkor.

DIAGNOSIS. The characteristic skin lesions, with or without digestive and neurologic signs, should suggest the diagnosis, particularly when an abnormal dietary history is elicited or a disease is present that might cause an increased requirement of tryptophan or niacin.

In areas where kwashiorkor is frequent it has been common to attribute its cutaneous manifestations to pellagra, which might well be true. However, the other manifestations of kwashiorkor (depigmentation of the hair, edema, and hypoalbuminemia) are not part of the picture of pellagra. The oral lesions of pellagra, on the other hand, are not usually present in kwashiorkor.

Lesions similar to those of pellagra have developed in infants and children consuming restricted semipurified diets and are believed to be due to complex combined deficiencies of amino acids, vitamins, and trace minerals, particularly zinc. Nontropical sprue may produce skin lesions similar to those of mild pellagra.

When a history of a diet relatively rich in calories, very low in high-quality protein (particularly tryptophan), low in niacin, and relatively high in leucine is elicited, it forms a good basis for the diagnosis. Such a diet, based on maize combined with a generous intake of alcohol, molasses, or sugar, is not uncommon in many parts of the world, including the United States and parts of Western Europe. Rice-based diets are similar, often being lower in tryptophan and niacin than corn-based diets, but they do not often lead to pellagra. This is probably due to the fact that other essential amino acids (particularly leucine) are present in lower concentrations, and less tryptophan goes into protein synthesis, with more being available for conversion to pyridine nucleotides.

TREATMENT. In the acutely ill patient 100 mg of nicotinamide (which lacks the unpleasant side effects of nicotinic acid) given orally or parenterally three or four times daily will promptly relieve most of the manifestations; much smaller dosages of 15 mg daily often are as effective. If a regular and adequate intake of tryptophan in the form of meat, milk, eggs, or another high-quality protein is not provided, high doses of niacin are needed, and prompt relapse will occur when the dose is reduced to prophylactic levels. Experimental evidence suggests that only tryptophan, not niacin, will lead to storage of the pyridine nucleotides.

In milder cases simple curtailment of the excessive caloric intake from alcohol or sugar, or provision of a moderately generous supply of high-quality protein, makes vitamin therapy unnecessary. Attention must be paid to coexisting deficiencies of other vitamins, particularly thiamine, ascorbic acid, and vitamin A.

PREVENTION. Requirements are now commonly expressed in terms of equivalents of milligrams of niacin, calculated from the sum of the nicotinic acid ingested plus 0.017 times tryptophan intake. This calculation is based on the observation that it takes 60 mg of dietary tryptophan to produce the same amount of niacin metabolites in the urine as are produced by 1 mg of niacin.

A diet providing 4.0 mg niacin equivalents per 1,000 kcal is generally pellagrogenic, whereas one providing

4.4 equivalents per 1,000 kcal is protective. Human breast milk provides approximately 8 equivalents per 1,000 kcal. The 1968 recommended daily dietary allowances of the U.S. Food and Nutrition Board for children call for 6.4 to 7.0 equivalents per 1,000 kcal.

VITAMIN B₆ DEFICIENCY
DAVID B. COURSIN

Vitamin B₆ includes the six interconvertible chemical structures pyridoxine, pyridoxamine, and pyridoxal and their respective 5-phosphorylated forms. They are all metabolized through the pyridoxal 5-phosphate pathway, with oxidation to 4-pyridoxic acid, and are excreted in the urine. Pyridoxal 5-phosphate is the most important member of the group; it serves as the coenzyme for numerous enzyme systems that are responsible for the interconversion and metabolism of amino acids, such as transamination, decarboxylation, and desulfuration. In these capacities vitamin B₆ is essential for the metabolism of amino acids, proteins, lipids, and nucleic acids. It also has an important role in the formation of various neurohumors, such as serotonin from tryptophan, and catecholamines, such as norepinephrine and dopamine from tryosine. In addition, it is an integral part of the molecular configuration of phosphorylases A and B that are involved in the first step of glycogen degradation.

These numerous vitamin-B₆-dependent enzyme systems do not have the same binding capacities for pyridoxal 5-phosphate. Therefore, in vitamin B₆ deficiency those with the least capability of retaining the vitamin in the holoenzyme will be most susceptible to its decreased availability. This causes related biochemical and physiologic abnormalities to occur sequentially in accordance with the severity and duration of the deprivation.

Experimental studies with vitamin B₆ deficiency in animals have resulted in reduced fertility, resorption of fetuses, congenital abnormalities, retardation of growth and development, dermatitis, convulsive seizures, reduction of active membrane transport of amino acids, depression of immune responses, oxaluria, and a host of other disorders that reflect the multiplicity of its metabolic roles.

LABORATORY DETERMINATIONS. Vitamin B₆ deficiency can be determined directly by the measurement of its various forms, particularly pyridoxal 5-phosphate in biologic samples. Urinary pyridoxic acid excretion has also been shown to correlate well with decreases in the body stores of the vitamin. Indirect evaluation of deficiency can be made through determination of transaminase activity in serum and red blood cells and by quantification of urinary excretion patterns of metabolites following an L-tryptophan load test of 50 mg/kg to a maximum of 2 g for the adult. Vitamin B₆ deficiency produces abnormalities in the urinary excretion of virtually all of these metabolites, with diagnostically significant changes in kynurenine,

5-hydroxykynurenine, xanthurenic acid, N^1-methylnicotinamide, 2-pyridone, and 5-hydroxyindoleacetic acid. The electroencephalogram is also sensitive to established vitamin B₆ deficiency, with nonspecific, grossly abnormal waveforms that contain alterations in frequency, amplitude, and evoked responses. These abnormal laboratory findings, as well as the clinical symptoms of vitamin B₆ deficiency, are readily corrected with relatively small oral doses (5 to 10 mg) of pyridoxine, thus indicating that the disorders relate specifically to a lack of the coenzyme.

SOURCES AND REQUIREMENTS. Vitamin B₆ is widely distributed in plant and animal food sources, with high concentrations in meat, liver, kidney, whole grains, peanuts, and soybeans. Excessive heating of the vitamin renders it inactive. The general availability of vitamin B₆ in foods is such that a normal individual receiving a well-balanced dietary intake will ingest adequate quantities of the vitamin. Table 12 lists the daily requirements that have been established for various age groups and for pregnant women.

TABLE 12. Estimated Vitamin B₆ Requirements for Various Groups

Group	Amount (mg/day)
Infants	0.10–0.5[a]
Children	0.5–1.5
Adolescents	1.5–2.0
Adults	1.5–2.0
Pregnant women	5.0–10.0

[a] *20 µg/g of protein; these ranges are related to normal ranges of protein intake.*

DEFICIENCY IN MAN. Early observations of vitamin B₆ deficiency in man documented the appearance of dermatitis, cheilosis, glossitis, peripheral neuritis, anemia, and convulsive seizures. In the early 1950s a formula containing 60 µg/liter of vitamin B₆ (compared to 100 µ/liter in human milk) was inadvertently produced by excessive sterilization. Infants maintained on this formula developed hyperactivity, hyperacusis, behavioral changes, and convulsive seizures and had abnormal tryptophan load tests and changes in their electroencephalograms; the symptoms were aggravated by increases in the protein concentration of their diet and were readily corrected by oral administration of 5 to 10 mg of pyridoxine. These studies showed that borderline vitamin B₆ deficiency in man could produce biochemical disturbances in the brain, with derangements of neurophysiologic function. This stimulated widespread interest in the relationship of vitamin B₆ to the central nervous system. To date the pathogenesis of the convulsive seizures has not been completely clarified. One concept that has been explored extensively relates to the reduction of γ-aminobutyric acid in the brain in vitamin B₆ deficiency. The two enzyme systems, requiring pyridoxal 5-phosphate, decarboxylation, and transamination, are involved in γ-aminobutyric acid metabolism and have different affinities for the coenzyme. Therefore, under conditions of deficiency, decarboxylation, with its weaker binding capacity, is unable to function normally. This causes a decrease in the concentration of γ-aminobutyric acid, a lowering of the threshold of central nervous system irritability, and convulsive seizures.

Recent experimental studies on pregnant rats with vitamin B_6 deficiency have demonstrated impaired fetal development. Continuation of the deficiency for even a short time after birth may produce irreversible changes resulting in early death. DiPaolo and associates have shown that intrauterine vitamin B_6 deficiency interferes with renal development; this retardation of maturation causes uremia, lethargy, motor impairment, and tremors after birth and is incompatible with life. While the developing brain of the infant is especially sensitive to vitamin B_6 deficiency, a similar symptom complex of behavioral changes and convulsive disorders has been observed in young adult males. The subjects were maintained on an adequate diet, except for a very low vitamin B_6 content, and within weeks they had developed the same symptoms.

Iatrogenic vitamin B_6 deficiency symptoms in the nervous system may also be produced by a number of drugs such as isonicotinic hydrazide and desoxypyridoxine. The former binds pyridoxal 5-phosphate to render it inactive, while the latter substitutes for pyridoxal 5-phosphate, resulting in inactivation of the holoenzyme complex. In both instances normal vitamin B_6-dependent enzyme activity is decreased. Hence oral prophylactic pyridoxine in doses of 10 to 25 mg/day must be administered in conjunction with these drugs, as well as with others such as penicillamine and cycloserine, which may cause similar effects.

Vitamin B_6 has been used with tremendous doses of INH in cases following attempted suicide; gram-for-gram doses have been effective in preventing convulsions, coma, and death. Vitamin B_6 may also be useful in the treatment of alcoholism. Alcohol may alter vitamin B_6 metabolism and inhibit phosphorylation of pyridoxal, thus reducing its availability as a coenzyme. If so, large doses of vitamin B_6 and even pyridoxal phosphate, per se, may be indicated.

DEPENDENCY. In 1954 an inborn error of vitamin B_6 metabolism was discovered and termed vitamin B_6 dependency. The patient had uncontrolled convulsive seizures shortly after birth and eventually proved to be mentally retarded. Despite a dietary intake of vitamin B_6 in amounts usually considered adequate, daily oral doses of 10 to 25 mg of pyridoxine were necessary to control the seizures; however, mental status did not improve. The tryptophan load test, levels of vitamin B_6, and pyridoxic acid excretion are normal in these individuals.

Vitamin B_6 dependency results from a genetic defect in enzyme systems that require vitamin B_6 and that initiate neurochemical changes in utero. These are evidenced at birth by convulsions and later by mental retardation, unless adequate pyridoxine therapy is instituted soon after birth. It appears that the problem is related to abnormal molecular configuration of the involved apoenzyme, which requires vitamin B_6 in large quantities (5 to 10 times the normal daily requirement) in order to function. Mudd has demonstrated that the genetically abnormal enzyme is operating at only 1 percent of normal activity. Therapy with massive doses of vitamin B_6 increases the activity to 2 percent of normal, a level that permits the system to function adequately.

Homocystinuria, cystathioninuria, and familial xanthurenic-aciduria are other examples of inborn errors of metabolism that result from molecular abnormalities of individual apoenzymes dependent on pyridoxal 5-phosphate (cystathionine synthetase, cystathioninase, and kynureninase, respectively). They also require 10 to 25 mg of pyridoxine daily for normal activity.

In addition to the two clearly defined entities vitamin B_6 deficiency and vitamin B_6 dependency that affect the brain, vitamin B_6 also has been implicated, without any acceptable evidence, in a variety of other central nervous system disorders, such as mongolism, phenylketonuria, and myoclonic epilepsy. Some patients with the latter disorder have been thought to show partial improvement with oral therapy of 100 to 200 mg of pyridoxine daily. A similar experience has been reported in a series of children with a variety of convulsive disorders and mental retardation, abnormal electroencephalograms, and abnormal tryptophan load tests. These patients were found to require doses of pyridoxine in excess of 300 mg/day in order to correct their laboratory findings and to obtain a questionable degree of clinical improvement.

Another form of vitamin B_6 dependency may occur in the hemopoietic system involving enzymes that participated in the normal production of hemoglobin. Patients with this hereditary defect generally develop anemia in early adult life, despite the fact that their diets have contained amounts of vitamin B_6 that are usually adequate. The anemia has been termed pyridoxine-responsive anemia and is different from that resulting from vitamin B_6 deficiency. It is characterized by microcytosis, hypochromia, erythroid hyperplasia of bone marrow, and elevated plasma iron concentration with increased saturation of the total iron-binding capacity of the serum. These manifestations of the genetic defect respond to daily doses of 10 mg of vitamin B_6.

FEMALE HORMONAL ACTIVITY. The hormonal changes that attend menstruation, pregnancy, and the use of anovulatory drugs have been shown to cause abnormal patterns in the tryptophan load test that are indicative of vitamin B_6 deficiency. The nausea and vomiting of the first trimester of pregnancy have been reported in some studies to respond well to pyridoxine, thus indicating that they may relate to a vitamin B_6 deficiency or increased need for the vitamin during that time. Recently studies in patients with toxemia of pregnancy have shown that they have marked decreases in their placental pyridoxal 5-phosphate and pyridoxal phosphokinase. This adds new support to earlier observations of abnormal tryptophan metabolite excretion patterns that suggested marked vitamin B_6 deficiency in such patients. Examination of tryptophan metabolism in subjects receiving anovulatory agents containing estrogen has revealed patterns that are very similar to those seen in pregnancy. These studies suggest that administration of 25 to 40 mg of pyridoxine daily may be indicated in women receiving anovulatory drugs. The early onset of menstruation, the increased occurrence of pregnancy in adolescence, and the widespread use of anovulatory agents in younger age groups all call for an increased awareness of and concern for their potentially important interrelationships with vitamin B_6.

MASSIVE THERAPY. Vitamin B_6 is an outstanding example of a vitamin that in massive doses has a definite pharmacologic effect in specific conditions. Several have been mentioned previously and have been well substantiated with adequate supporting scientific data. This information has been eagerly seized upon by several individuals to support, unjustifiably, the concept of an orthomolecular panacea for a host of medical disorders. Thus very large doses of pyridoxine have been administered to infants, children, and adults suffering from a variety of central nervous system disorders, including hyperkinesis, behavioral abnormalities, convulsive seizures, and mental retardation. Therapy is frequently followed by enthusiastic but vague reports of improvement, with neither sound biochemical data nor adequate documentation of significant changes in behavior and performance. While there may be some merit in the presumed effectiveness of pharmacologic doses of vitamin B_6 in some of these disorders, most of them lack satisfactory substantiation. Furthermore, although toxic and lethal levels of vitamin B_6 have been established in animals, no such studies are available for man. There could be subtle and long-term toxic effects that have not yet been recognized.

Folic Acid Deficiency

That folic acid is an important metabolite has been known for some years, but whether it can be synthesized by the body in adequate quantities has not been determined. Its absence from the diet leads to bone marrow arrest; megaloblastic anemia develops, which may be associated with pancytopenia. However, there is evidence that at least a part of the requirement can be furnished by intestinal bacteria.

Folic acid is widely distributed in nature, notably in green vegetables. Its derivatives, which function as coenzymes in various reactions, are formed from an unstable reduction product, tetrahydrofolic acid, to which various single-carbon groups can be attached; the best known of these is the formyl derivative, known as folinic acid or the citrovorum factor. The requirement of folic acid, ordinarily extremely minute, is considerably affected by factors that convert folic acid into its reduced usable form. Antagonists such as aminopterin and amethopterin prevent this transformation, and ascorbic acid facilitates it; when ascorbic acid is deficient, large amounts of folic acid are needed. Folic acid coen-

zymes are involved in the transfer of single-carbon units —methyl, methylene, methoxy, formyl, and formamino groups. They are also involved in certain steps in the synthesis of purines and porphyrins, in the degradation of histidine, and in the hydroxylation of phenylanine to form tyrosine.

Folic acid deficiency is rarely encountered in children in North America. It has been observed in infants on diets deficient in ascorbic acid; it may result from deficient absorption in diseases of the small bowel or from the use of antifolic compounds in the treatment of leukemia. Occasional instances have been observed after the use of certain anticonvulsive drugs, namely primidone (Mysoline) and diphenylhydantoin (Dilantin). There is now considerable evidence that a folic-acid-deficiency anemia is not an infrequent complication of kwashiorkor, resulting either from a deficient intake of the vitamin or from the presence of some conditioning factor.

Folic acid can induce a hematologic response in various macrocytic anemias of adults, such as pernicious anemia, fish tapeworm anemia, macrocytic anemia of pregnancy, and tropical and nontropical sprue. Its effect in the rare cases of pernicious anemia in children has not been extensively studied, and its use may not be without risk, since despite temporary hematologic remission the nervous lesions associated with pernicious anemia may be made worse.

Folic acid deficiency can be measured by the level of folic acid in the blood; impairment of folic absorption has been determined by measuring the radioactive material in blood following the administration of radioactive folic acid. A simpler useful test of deficiency depends on excretion of an excess of formamino glutamic acid after a histidine load; however, this test, which is also positive in vitamin B_{12} deficiency, is not altogether specific for folic acid deficiency.

Infants may be treated with 1 to 5 mg given orally, although smaller amounts may be effective. In cases of deficiencies induced by antifolic drugs, larger doses may be needed. Folinic acid is more effective in reversing the untoward effects of these drugs.

Vitamin C Deficiency (Scurvy)

Scurvy is a disease caused by prolonged deprivation of ascorbic acid (vitamin C). Although it was known to the ancient Egyptians and has been a familiar scourge of sailors throughout history, infantile scurvy was recognized by Barlow only in 1883. It is still often referred to as Barlow's disease. The most striking manifestations are changes in the bones, leading to pain on motion and a hemorrhagic tendency.

Ascorbic acid is a crystalline compound that is highly soluble in water. It is readily destroyed by boiling, as it is easily oxidized. Ascorbic acid is present in all cells of the body, particularly in metabolically active tissues. High concentrations are found in the retina, in the endocrine glands (particularly the adrenal cortex), in intestinal epithelium, and in leukocytes. It accumulates in sites of connective tissue proliferation, such as in healing wounds. Specific enzyme systems of which ascorbic acid is a cofactor have not been isolated, and what is known of its function is derived from the observed effects of withdrawal and administration. It is a powerful reducing agent and may serve as a regulator of oxidation and reduction in the cells. It protects many enzymes from oxidative damage, among them folic acid reductase, which converts folic to folinic acid and *p*-hydroxyphenylpyruvic oxidase. In ascorbic acid deficiency the tyrosyl compounds *p*-hydroxyphenylpyruvic acid and *p*-hydroxyphenyllactic acid appear in the urine. Ascorbic acid appears to be concerned in the hydroxylation of proline to hydroxyproline, a function in particular demand for connective tissue proliferation. It is also involved in the hydroxylation of tryptophan to form serotonin. It is concerned in some way with absorption of iron and with the formation and degradation of ferritin. It is also involved with cholesterol synthesis, which may be related to its high concentration in the adrenal cortex. Blood cholesterol levels are low in scurvy, and foods that are hypercholesterolemic fail to exhibit their effect until the scurvy is treated. It is of interest that in

several animal species that lack the enzyme gulanolactone oxidase and are hence unable to synthesize ascorbic acid the enzyme is present during embryonic life.

Just how the known chemical functions of the vitamin are related to the anatomic changes resulting from its deficiency is far from clear. The effects of ascorbic acid depletion include defective formation of intercellular cement substance, suspension of collagen production of fibroblasts, hemorrhagic phenomena, and defective formation of bones and teeth.

INCIDENCE. Scurvy is now most frequently seen in infants who have been fed for some months on heated milk formulas without adequate supplements of vitamin C. Healthy infants require 10 mg of ascorbic acid a day, and in the presence of infection double this amount may be required; hence 20 mg per day or more should be provided. Unless the mother's diet is inadequate, breast milk contains 4 to 7 mg/100 ml, which provides adequate protection, since scurvy is seen in breast-fed infants only in the presence of maternal malnutrition. Raw cow's milk contains only about 2 mg/ml (a marginal quantity), one-third to one-half of which is

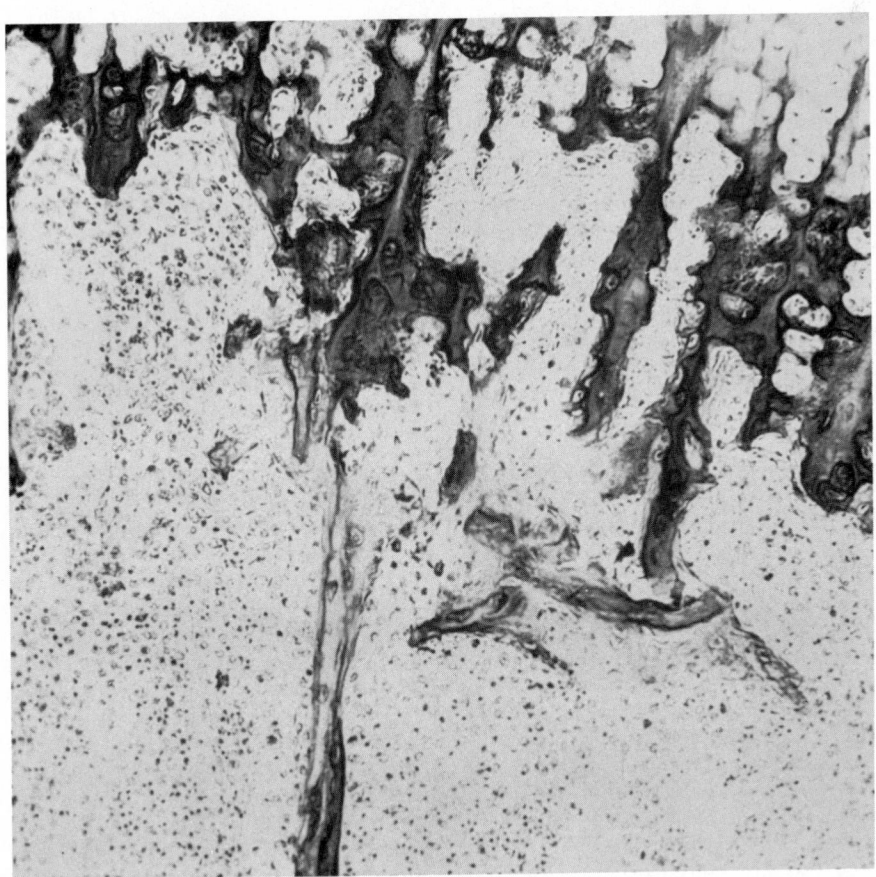

FIG. 8. Zone of preparatory calcification in scurvy. The masses of calcified cartilaginous matrix lying shaftward from the growing cartilage are embedded in "framework marrow," the loose, relatively avascular, cell-poor scorbutic marrow. Several of the matrix elements have been pushed into bizarre alignment; others show fractures, and some of these fractured areas are surrounded by fibrin.

destroyed by the heating to which it is subjected. Scurvy has been seen in children placed on a highly restricted diet for the treatment of allergy.

Most cases of scurvy in the pediatric age group occur between 6 and 15 months of age. The newborn infant usually has a higher concentration of ascorbic acid in plasma at birth than does the mother. Infants rarely suffer complete deprivation of dietary ascorbic acid, and consequently the disease manifests itself slowly. The onset of symptoms is usually delayed from 4 to 9 months after institution of the deficient diet. If the maternal diet is deficient, scurvy may occur in the newborn infant. Scurvy has largely disappeared in the United States, but occasionally it still occurs despite the generally improved understanding of nutritional problems.

PATHOLOGY.   The nature of the pathologic process in scurvy is not clearly understood; the only histologic lesions pathognomonic of scurvy are those found in growing bones and in teeth. The characteristic bone changes are most pronounced in the region where endochondral ossification is proceeding (Fig. 8). The zone of proliferative cartilage becomes inconspicuous, with few mitoses and a disorderly arrangement of the cartilage cell column. In contrast, the amount of cartilage matrix undergoing calcification is abnormally great; at the same time its conversion to bone is impaired, and the brittleness of the large irregular masses of calcified matrix is often reflected in numerous microscopic fractures. Beneath this broad zone of provisional calcification the trabeculae are slender and scarce, and there are few evidences of osteoblastic activity. The marrow between the trabeculae has lost the appearance of normal hematopoietic marrow; it is known as "framework marrow" and consists chiefly of loose embryonic-looking connective tissue, often containing hemorrhages. Periosteal ossification is also inactive, and hemorrhages may be found beneath the periosteum at any part of the shaft between the epiphyseal lines. Epiphyseal separation is common in scurvy, especially in complete degree (infraction). Cleavage usually takes place through the brittle zone of provisional calcification, sometimes with partial detachment of the epiphyseal fragment from the shaft, more often with comminution. The microscopic lesions in the skeleton are widely distributed and are, as a rule, bilaterally symmetric. They are always more intense in places where bone is growing rapidly. Macroscopic subperiosteal hemorrhages are often found (Fig. 9); the most frequent sites are the lower end of the femur, the lower end of the tibia, the upper end of the femur, the bones of the arm (especially the upper end of the humerus), and the skull. Trauma not infrequently plays a part in determining the site of such lesions, as it also does in epiphyseal separation. Scurvy produces characteristic changes in tooth structure identifiable by special techniques.

The buccal lesions are described in the section on symptoms. Among the rare lesions of scurvy may be mentioned hemorrhage into the orbit, giving rise to exophthalmos and sometimes to chemosis and edema of the lids; often there are subconjunctival hemorrhages as well. Visceral lesions are infrequent. There may be

small hemorrhages beneath the pleura, pericardium, and peritoneum; however, hemorrhagic effusions into the serous cavities do not occur. Despite the frequency of microscopic hematuria, the kidneys as a rule show nothing abnormal. The joints usually escape entirely. Cutaneous ecchymoses or hemorrhages in any of the mucous membranes may be seen. Intracranial hemorrhage is rare. The bleeding tendency in scurvy cannot be attributed to any defect of blood coagulation. It is regarded as due to alterations in the blood vessel walls.

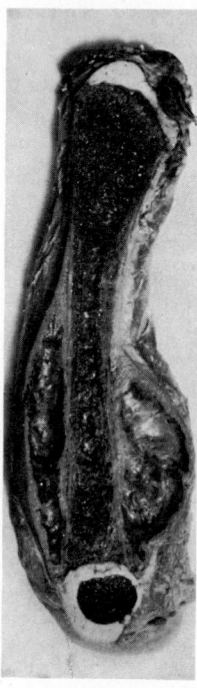

FIG. 9. Femur showing subperiosteal hemorrhages in scurvy of 7 weeks duration.

Other deficiency diseases are not uncommonly associated with scurvy. The presence of rickets complicates the picture in the bones and sometimes makes its interpretation difficult.

SYMPTOMS.   In most cases a period of indisposition, fretfulness, pallor, and loss of appetite precedes the local symptoms. Usually the first symptom to attract attention is tenderness of the legs. This may begin insidiously; at first it may be so slight as to cause the patient to cry only when the diaper is being changed, or there may be a sudden refusal to sit or stand. Hemorrhage in regions other than the lower extremities may mark the onset of the disease. Changes in the arms are commonly found in the early stage, although they are rarely the first feature to attract attention.

The amount of constitutional disturbance is variable. There may be marked fretfulness, poor sleep, pallor, anorexia, and loss of weight; in other cases symptoms of scurvy may continue for several weeks without making any perceptible impression upon the child's nutrition. Pain and disability may come and go. Severe scurvy develops only when the condition is unrecognized and is allowed to progress, or when the diet is completely devoid of ascorbic acid.

In severe cases fever is usually present, the temperature in some instances reaching 38.9 to 39.4 C. Tenderness in the legs becomes constant and is often exquisite, so that any movement or even the slightest touch causes the child to scream with pain or apprehension. The posture is characteristic. There is semiflexion of the thighs and legs and outward rotation of the hips (Fig. 10), the pithed-frog position; the child often lies motionless, and voluntary movements of the extremities cannot be elicited (pseudoparalysis). Disability results chiefly from the pain that motion provokes; when it is marked it usually denotes infraction of an epiphysis. Ecchymoses are occasionally seen about the large joints, and these often suggest that the child has met with an accident. Swelling near the joints, particularly just above the knee, may be so great that the limb is nearly twice the size of its fellow.

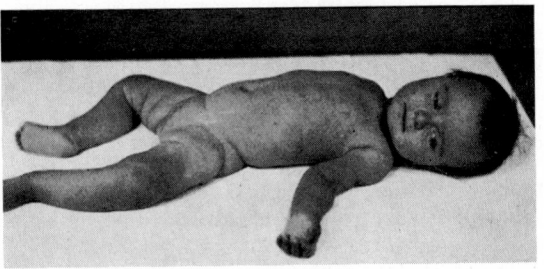

FIG. 10. Scurvy with characteristic posture in an infant 10.5 months old. (From McIntosh: In Brennemann's Practice of Pediatrics, Vol 1, 1959. Courtesy of W. F. Prior Co.)

Evidence of epiphyseal infraction is seen in most of the severe cases, usually unaccompanied by gross displacement. It occurs most frequently either at the lower epiphysis of the femur or tibia or at the upper epiphysis of the humerus; it is often bilateral. Although the condition of the bone is a predisposing factor, relatively mild trauma is usually the immediate cause. Crepitus is obtained only with complete separation and with unwarranted manipulations. The diagnosis can readily be made by roentgenography or from the persistence of local pain more than 3 or 4 days after institution of treatment.

Teeth that have recently erupted or that are about to erupt are often overlaid with redundant, hemorrhagic, or spongy gingiva. Often the gums of the upper jaw alone are involved, those about the upper central incisors being most commonly affected. In the most marked cases the gums may ulcerate, their appearance resembling that of mercurial stomatitis. Pain from sore gums may seriously interfere with the taking of food.

The ribs are commonly involved in scurvy; there is angular mushrooming of the costochondral junctions, with the production of a rosary comparable to that found in rickets. The typical scorbutic rosary is sharper and firmer than its rachitic counterpart and in some instances shows tenderness on pressure, but clinical distinction between the two is not always possible.

Bleeding may occur from almost any of the mucous membranes; the hemorrhages are generally small but may be repeated frequently. Hematemesis is rare, as also is the passage of recognizable blood by rectum, but occult blood can often be demonstrated in the stools. Microscopic hematuria occurs in about 33 percent of cases; gross hematuria is less common. In some patients with blood in the urine, albumin and casts are present, thus suggesting the diagnosis of hemorrhagic nephritis; the abnormal findings disappear shortly after treatment is started.

Petechiae and ecchymoses in the skin may be found in the vicinity of the gross bone lesions; widespread petechial eruptions are sometimes seen. If there is a superimposed skin disease associated with scurvy, such as measles, varicella, or furunculosis, the lesions are usually hemorrhagic. Other changes in the skin are seldom encountered in infants, but are seen with increasing frequency after 2 to 3 years even in mild cases. The earliest sign noted in experimentally induced human scurvy is a follicular hyperkeratosis indistinguishable from that associated with vitamin A deficiency. Follicular hyperkeratosis in children is more often due to deficiency of ascorbic acid than to deficiency of vitamin A.

The blood picture in early scurvy may be normal, despite the presence of pallor. A macrocytic anemia appears quite commonly, and in many instances it has been shown to result from a double deficiency of folic acid and ascorbic acid. In the presence of an abundance of vitamin C in the diet, only a small amount of folic acid is needed, whereas when folic acid is abundant little or no vitamin C is required to prevent anemia. Folic acid in massive doses will reduce the tyrosyl derivatives in the urine of scorbutic patients. Scurvy causes no characteristic changes in the leukocytes. Serum calcium and inorganic phosphorus concentrations are normal. The serum alkaline phosphatase activity is usually depressed. A recent study by Hoad and associates has revealed that in experimental scurvy in man the manifestations of Sjögren's syndrome appear along with the better known scorbutic symptoms and signs, thus suggesting a common pathway for the action of ascorbic acid and the as yet unknown pathogenesis of a form of rheumatoid arthritis.

ROENTGENOGRAPHIC APPEARANCES. There are three features characteristic of early scurvy (Fig. 11): (1) There is a ground-glass appearance of the shaft due to atrophy of the trabeculae. The cortex is usually thinned out, and next to the epiphyseal line it may consist of a thin streak or may even vanish. (2) A broadened epiphyseal line (the zone of provisional calcification of cartilage matrix) is conspicuous, particularly at the lower end of the femur and at both ends of the tibia; it may be finely irregular. (3) Beneath the

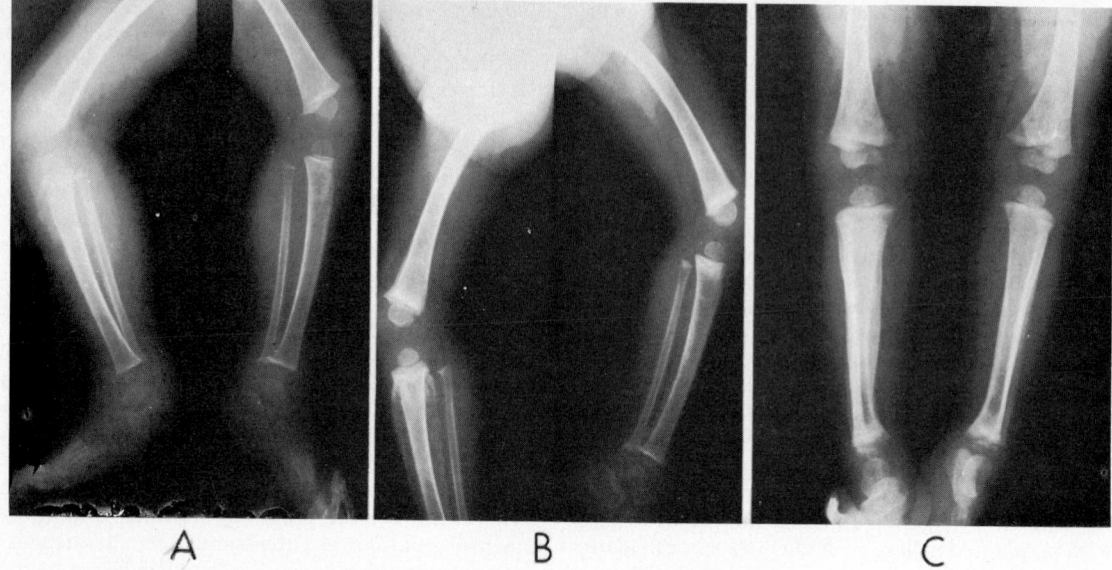

FIG. 11. Advanced scorbutic changes in a 16-month-old infant. A. The leg exhibits severe osteoporosis, with lucent centers of both epiphysis and shaft. The cortical bone is thinner. The proximal tibia shows a transverse lucent line under the epiphyseal plate, known as the scurvy line. Fractures are present in the metaphyseal ends of the long bones, with exhibition of the "corner sign" seen best in the proximal fibula. There is periosteal elevation and beginning periosteal new bone production best demonstrated in the distal femur. B. After 2 weeks of therapy there is healing, with remineralization and calcification of subperiosteal hematomata along the shafts. C. After 12 weeks there is further healing, with ossification of the hematomata.

broad epiphyseal line is a *zone of rarefaction* corresponding to the regions of greatest trabecular attrition (the scurvy line). This zone is often narrow and difficult to detect in early scurvy. The first two of these diagnostic features can be observed in the epiphyseal centers of ossification: the ground-glass appearance, with trabecular atrophy within the center, and the dense epiphyseal line apearing as a ring surrounding the epiphyseal center, most dense on the side toward the bone itself.

Displacement of the epiphysis is indicated by faulty alignment of the epiphyseal line with the shaft of the bone. Partial separation of the epiphysis commonly occurs without displacement. This appears as a crack separating the epiphyseal line from the shaft and extending part way across the width of the bone. After hemorrhage has occurred, the first evidences of calcification in the elevated periosteum are seen as spurs of newly formed bone attached to the epiphyseal line, pointing toward the shaft of the bone.

As scurvy heals the sites of subperiosteal hemorrhage take on a striking appearance. New bone is laid down in periosteum that has been detached from the underlying shaft, so that in the course of 1 or 2 weeks the full extent of periosteal stripping is dramatically revealed. Later, as the hematoma resorbs, the shell of a new bone contracts and becomes more dense. Where considerable epiphyseal displacement has taken place, the restitution of normal contour may require as long as a year.

DIAGNOSIS. The diagnosis of scurvy seldom presents difficulty; the essential features are age incidence, extreme tenderness of the legs, spongy swollen gums, swelling near the large joints, a tendency to hemorrhages, and usually a history of prolonged use of heated or canned milk.

Disability resulting from trauma alone seldom has the symmetric distribution of scorbutic manifestations. Cases with pseudoparalysis may be mistaken for poliomyelitis. Hyperesthesia is rarely as marked in poliomyelitis as in scurvy, and painful stimulation of the extremities will usually indicate that actual paralysis is not present. The locomotor disability of scurvy may suggest rheumatic fever, but the resemblance is only superficial. In cases with high fever, scurvy may be mistaken for acute suppurative arthritis or osteomyelitis. The radiographic picture of infantile cortical hyperostosis bears some resemblance to that of gross scorbutic lesions in the healing stage, but other evidence of scurvy is lacking.

The osteochondritis of early congenital syphilis has many clinical and radiographic features in common with scurvy. However, syphilitic osteochondritis is found at an early age, almost always less than 4 months, while scurvy characteristically occurs after the age of 4 months.

Hematemesis from scurvy has led to a mistaken diagnosis of peptic ulcer; loss of blood from the intestine may suggest intussusception. When hemorrhagic manifestations are absent, confirmatory evidence of scurvy may be obtained by the Rumpel-Leede phenomenon or other tests of capillary fragility.

The biochemical tests used in diagnosis include measurement of ascorbic acid in plasma, load tests in which plasma concentration or urinary excretion is followed after a specific load, measurement of ascorbic acid in the buffy coat of centrifuged blood, and a functional test based on the urinary excretion of certain tyrosine metabolites after administration of tyrosine.In normal subjects on a generous intake, ascorbic acid levels in the plasma usually range from 0.5 to 1.5 mg/100 ml. In frank scurvy the concentration is usually zero. The plasma level is affected by recent intake: sudden withdrawal of the vitamin will cause the plasma concentration to fall to zero in a few weeks, although months may elapse before symptoms are detectable; conversely, administration of ascorbic acid to a depleted subject will raise the plasma level before the needs of the body have been met. Similar criticism applies to load tests in which a standard load is given to a child. A rise in plasma ascorbic acid concentration and in subsequent urinary output of the vitamin indicates that the stores are virtually filled, whereas failure to demonstrate a rise indicates that the stores are incompletely filled. In a scorbutic patient the daily oral administration of 200 mg of ascorbic acid may fail to evoke a distinct rise in the urinary level for 3 or 4 days, while in an adequately nourished subject the urine gives a strongly positive test within 24 hours.

More closely correlated with symptoms is the ascorbic acid content of the buffy coat. In normal subjects the concentration is about 30 mg/100 ml. On withdrawal of vitamin C from the diet the level falls at a fairly constant rate, reaching zero after about 4 months of depletion. Clinical manifestations of scurvy are usually detectable when ascorbic acid cannot be found in the leukocyte-platelet layer.

A simple and sensitive test for scurvy is the functional test based on excretion of the so-called tyrosyl compounds *p*-hydroxyphenylpyruvic acid and *p*-hydroxyphenyllactic acid after administration of tyrosine itself or after a protein-containing meal. These acids are readily detected in the urine by the Millon reagent. In the normal subject tyrosyluria is absent, whereas in scurvy it is constantly present. Another functional test devised by Gabuzda and associates consists in the administration of a test dose of folic acid. Its conversion to folinic acid is impaired in scurvy.

PROPHYLAXIS AND TREATMENT. To prevent the development of scurvy, every infant receiving boiled, pasteurized, dried, or evaporated milk should be given antiscorbutic food as early as the first 2 weeks. Orange juice is convenient; one teaspoonful daily should be given at first, and the amount should be rapidly increased to the juice of one orange daily. Most canned and frozen orange juice preparations provide an adequate source of vitamin C. Pure ascorbic acid is easy to administer; it may be given by itself, 25 or 50 mg being dissolved in a small amount of water and fed by spoon, or the tablet may be crushed and dropped into a feeding just before the bottle is offered, or it may be included in a polyvitamin supplement. One should not attempt to mix the day's dose of ascorbic acid in with the 24-hour feeding, lest the greater part of it be destroyed by oxidation. All fresh fruits have antiscorbutic properties, and the ascorbic acid content of vegetables is not as a rule completely destroyed in cooking. Consequently, by the time a child is taking a varied diet, there is no necessity to give ascorbic acid.

In treatment of frank scurvy large doses of vitamin C are required, and pure ascorbic acid in daily amounts of 500 or even 1,000 mg may be used to supplement the diet. The total requirement for replenishment of the depleted stores is often as much as 2 g; the entire quantity needed for maximal healing over a period of 8 days may be administered at one time. Oral administration is ordinarily preferable to parenteral injection; with intravenous injection large amounts are lost in the urine. Orange juice and other natural sources of the vitamin will generally effect equally rapid symptomatic improvement.

COURSE AND PROGNOSIS. Fatal scurvy is now rarely seen. It is only in neglected cases with severe malnutrition or other complications that the prognosis is doubtful. Secondary infections, like pneumonia, may cause death. The results of treatment are usually prompt. Within the first 24 hours improvement in disposition and appetite is evident, and there is prompt disappearance of tenderness from the extremities. Persistence of tenderness suggests separation of an epiphysis. Microscopic hematuria may persist for as long as 2 weeks, but large hemorrhages from the kidney or gastrointestinal tract usually cease promptly. Fever seldom persists more than 2 or 3 days.

Repair of the bone lesions begins at once, although a week or more is required before radiologic improvement can be detected. One of the earliest changes seen is new calcification as periosteal bone production is resumed. The elevated periosteum gradually contracts as the hemorrhage beneath it is absorbed. Even after marked displacement of an epiphysis the alignment between the shaft and the epiphyseal fragment is gradually restored with growth of the bone. Roentgenologic evidences of scurvy may be recognizable years later in the form of a prominent transverse line buried in the shaft, which once represented the broad epiphyseal line of acute scurvy; the circular or oval area of rarefied trabecular bone that once comprised the scorbutic center of ossification may persist, buried in the middle of a center that has grown much larger (Fig. 11C). Permanent deformities resulting from scurvy have not been observed.

References

DEFICIENCIES OF CALORIES AND PROTEIN

Bradfield RB, Cordano A, Graham GG: Hair-root adaptation to marasmus in Andean Indian children. Lancet 2:1395, 1969

Cheek DB, Hill DE, Cordano A, Graham GG: Malnutrition in infancy: changes in muscle and adipose tissue before and after rehabilitation. Pediatr Res 4:135, 1970

Dean RFA: Kwashiorkor. *In* Gairdner D (ed): Recent Advances in Pediatrics. London, JA Churchill, 1965

Graham GG: The later growth of malnourished infants. Effects of age, severity and subsequent diet. In McCance RA, Widdowson EM (eds): Calorie Deficiencies and Protein Deficiencies. London, JA Churchill, 1968, p 301

————: Cordano A, Blizzard RM, and Cheek DB: Infantile malnutrition: Changes in body composition during rehabilitation. Pediat. Res. 3:579, 1969

Snyderman SE, Holt LE Jr, Norton PM, Roitman E, Phansalkar SV: The plasma aminogram. I. Influence of the level of protein intake and a comparison of whole protein and amino acid diets. Pediat. Res. 2:131, 1968

Winick M, Mayer KK, Harris RC: Malnutrition and environmental enrichment by early adoption. Science 190:1173, 1975

DISORDERS OF LIPID NUTRITION

American Academy of Pediatrics, Committee on Nutrition: Childhood diet and coronary heart disease, Pediatrics, 49:305, 1972

Blumenthal S, Jesse MJ: Atherosclerosis: a pediatric problem? Cardiovasc Clin 4:11, 1972

Childhood Diet and Coronary Heart Disease Committee on Nutrition, American Academy of Pediatrics: Pediatrics 49:305, 1972

Dietschy JM, Wilson JD: Regulation of cholesterol metabolism. N Engl J Med 282:1128, 1179, 1241, 1970

Frederickson D, Levy R, Lees R: Fat transport in lipo proteins. N Engl J Med 276:32, 94, 148, 215, 273, 1967

Glueck CJ, Fallat RW, Tsang R: Hypercholesterolemia and hypertriglyceridemia in children. Am J Dis Child 128:569, 1974

Goldstein JL, Schrott HG, Hazzard WR, Bierman EL, Motulsky AG: J Clin Invest 52:1533, 1973Tôx6

Hamilton RL: Synthesis and secretion of plasma lipoproteins. Adv Exp Med Biol 26:7, 1972

Johnston JM: Mechanisms of fat absorption. In Code CF, Heidel W (eds): Handbook of Physiology, Vol 3, Section 6. Washington, DC, American Physiological Society, 1968

Primary prevention of the atherosclerotic diseases: a report of the atherosclerosis study group and the epidemiology study group. Circulation 42:A55, 1970

VITAMIN A DEFICIENCY

Hodges RE, Kolder H: In Bieri JG (ed): Summary of proceedings, Workshop on Biochemical and Clinical Criteria for Determining Human Vitamin A Nutriture. Washington, DC, National Academy of Sciences, 1971, p 10

Hume EM, Krebs HA: Vitamin A requirement of human adults. An experimental study of vitamin A deprivation in man. Special Report 264. London, Medical Research Council, 1949

McLaren DS: Malnutrition and the Eye. New York, Academic, 1963

———— Shirajian E, Tchalian M, Khoury G: Xerophthalmia in Jordan: Am J Clin Nutr 17:117, 1965

————: Oomen HAPC, Escapini H: Ocular manifestations of vitamin A deficiency in man. Bull WHO 34:357, 1966

Moore T: Vitamin A. Amsterdam, Elsevier, 1957

Vaughan DG: Xerophthalmia. Arch Ophthalmol 51:789, 1954

Wald G: The visual function of vitamin A. In: Vitamins and Hormones. New York, Academic, 18:417, 1960

THIAMINE DEFICIENCY

Andrews VL: Infantile beriberi. Philippine J Sci Sect B 7:67, 1912

Brin M: Erythrocyte as a biopsy tissue in the functional evaluation of vitamin adequacy. JAMA 187:762, 1964, also correspondence: J Nutr 86:319, 1965

Burch HB, et al: Nutrition survey and tests in Bataan, Philippines. J Nutr 42:9, 1950

Davis RA, Wolf A: Infantile beriberi associated with Wernicke's encephalopathy. Pediatrics 21:409, 1958

Holt LE Jr: The thiamine requirement of man. Fed Proc 3:171, 1944

————: Najjar VA: The clinical diagnosis of deficiencies of thiamine, riboflavin and niacin. Lancet 63:11, 1943

———— Nemis RL, Snyderman SE, Albanese AA, Ketron KC, Guy LP et al : The thiamine requirement of the normal infant. I. Nutrition 37:53, 1949

Kinney TD, Follis RH Jr (eds): Conference on Beriberi, Sponsored by World Health Organization and Other Organizations. Fed Proc 17 (Suppl 2):3, 1958

RIBOFLAVIN DEFICIENCY

Foy H: Effect of riboflavin deficiency on bone marrow function and protein metabolism of baboons. Br J Nutr 18:307, 1964

Hills OW: Clinical aspects of dietary depletion of riboflavin. Arch Intern Med 87:682, 1951

Holt LE Jr: Studies of B Vitamin Requirements of Infants. Currents in Nutrition. New York, National Vitamin Foundation, 1950

Horwitt MK, Hills OW, Havey CC, Lieberte, E, Steinberg DL : Effects of dietary depletion of riboflavin. J Nutr 39:357, 1949

———— Harvey CC, Hills OW, Liebert E : Correlation of urinary excretion of riboflavin with dietary intake and symptoms of ariboflavinosis. J Nutr 41:247, 1950

Sebrell WH, Butler RE: Riboflavin deficiency in man: preliminary note, Publ Health Rep 53:2282, 1938

Snyderman SE, Kotron KC, Burch HB, Lowry OH, Bessey OA, Guy LP, Holt LE : The minimum riboflavin requirement of the infant. J Nutr 39:219, 1949

Sydenstricker VP: The clinical manifestations if nicotinic acid and riboflavin deficiency. Ann Intern Med 14:1499, 1941

NIACIN DEFICIENCY

Goldsmith GA: Niacin: antipellagra factor, hypocholesterolemic agent. JAMA 194:167, 1965

Krehl WA, Teply LJ, Sarma PS, Elvehjem CA: Growth-retarding effect of corn in nicotinic acid-low rations and its counteraction by tryptophane. Science 101-489, 1945

Nishizuka Y, Hayaishi O: Studies on the biosynthesis of nicotinamide-adenine-dinucleotide. J Biol Chem 238:3369, 1963

Truswell AS, Hansen JDL, Wannenburg P: Plasma tryptophan and other amino acids in pellagra. Am J Clin Nutr 21:1314, 1968

VITAMIN B$_6$ DEFICIENCY

Baker EM, Canham JE, Nunes WT, Sauberlich, HE, McDowell ME: Vitamin B$_6$ requirements for adult men. Am J Clin. Nutr. 15:59, 1964

DiPaolo RV, Caviness VS Jr, Kanfer JN: Delayed maturation of the renal cortex in the vitamin B$_6$ deficient newborn rat. Pediatr Res 8:546, 1974

Harris RS, Wool IG (eds): International Symposium on Vitamin B$_6$ Vitamins and Hormones, Vol 22. New York, Academic, 1964, p 359

Kelsall MA (ed: Vitamin B$_6$ in metabolism of the nervous system. Ann NY Acad Sci 166:1, 1969

————: Report of the Committee on Nutrition. American Academy of Pediatrics. Vitamin B$_6$ requirements in man. Pediatric. 38:1068, 1966

Mudd SH: Pyridoxine-responsive genetic disease. Fed Proc 30:970, 1971

Sebrell WH Jr, Harris RS (eds): The Vitamins, Vol 2, 2nd ed. New York, Academic, 1968, p 1

FOLIC ACID DEFICIENCY

Baugh CM, Krumdieck CL, Baker HJ, Butterworth CE Jr: Studies on the absorption and metabolism of folic acid. I. Folate absorption in the dog after exposure of isolated segments to synthetic pteroylpolyglutamates of various chain lengths. J Clin Invest 50:2009, 1971

Vilter RW: Folic acid. *In* Wohl MG, Goodhart RS (eds): Modern Nutrition in Health and Disease, 3rd ed. Philadelphia, Lea & Febiger, 1964, p 409

Zalusky R, Hebert V: Failure of formamino glutamic acid (FIGLU) excretion to distinguish vitamin B_{12} deficiency from nutritional folic acid deficiency. J Clin Invest 40:1091, 1961

VITAMIN C DEFICIENCY

Barlow T: On cases described as "acute rickets" which are probably a combination of scurvy and rickets, scurvy being an essential and rickets a variable element. Medico-Chirurgical Tr 66:159, 1883; reprinted Arch Dis Child 10:223, 1935

Barnes MJ, Kodicek E: Biological hydroxylations and ascorbic acid with special regard to collagen metabolism. Vitam Horm 30:1, 1972

Crandon JH, Lund CC, Dill DB: Experimental human scurvy. N Engl J Med 22:353, 1940

Dogramaci I: Scurvy; a survey of 241 cases. N Engl J Med 235:185, 1946

Fabro S, Rinaldini LM: Loss of ascorbic acid synthesis in embryonic development. Dev Biol 11:468, 1965

Follis RH Jr, Park EA, Jackson D: The prevalence of scurvy at autopsy during the first 2 years of age. Bull Johns Hopkins Hosp 87:569, 1950

Gabuzda GJ, Phillips GB, Schilling RF, Davidson CS: Metabolism of pteroylglutamic acid and citrovorum factor in patients with scurvy. J Clin Invest 31:756, 1952

Harper AE: The recommended dietary allowances for ascorbic acid. In: Second Conference on Vitamin C. New York, New York Academy of Sciences, 1975

Hoad J, Burns CA, Hodges RE: Sjögren's syndrome in scurvy. N Engl J Med 282:1120, 1970

Jackson D, Park EA: Congenital scurvy: a case report. J Pediatr 7:741, 1935

McIntosh R: Infantile scurvy (Barlow's disease). In: Brennemann's Practice of Pediatrics, Vol I. Hagerstown, Md WF Prior, 1959, chap 35

Morris JE, Harpur ER, Goldbloom A: The metabolism of /-tyrosine in infantile scurvy. J Clin Invest 29:325, 1950

Park EA, Guild HG, Jackson D, Bond M: The recognition of scurvy with especial reference to the early x-ray changes. Arch Dis Child 10:265, 1935

Tolbert BM, et al: Chemistry and metabolism of ascorbic acid and ascorbate sulfate. In: Second Conference on Vitamin C. New York, New York Academy of Sciences, 1975

VITAMIN D AND THE METABOLISM OF CALCIUM, PHOSPHATE, AND BONE

HAROLD E. HARRISON

Bone is a complex solid system made up of an organic fibrillar matrix into which is incorporated a hard crystalline mineral. This provides the combination of tensile strength and compressive strength that makes bone an excellent structural material for support of body weight and muscle pull. In addition, there is a cellular component, for bone is a growing, living tissue that remodels and reshapes itself by reaction to the forces acting upon it. The bone cells not only function to alter the size and shape of the bone, but by their metabolic activity they alter the rate of formation and dissolution of bone crystals. The skeleton thus can serve as a reservoir of calcium, magnesium, phosphate, and carbonate ions, which through the influence of bone cell activity and in response to the composition of extracellular fluid can help to maintain stable concentrations of these ions in the body fluids.

Disorders of bone structure can result from (1) abnormalities of ionic composition of the extracellular fluid that directly influence the mineral phase of the bone, (2) disorders of the organic matrix, the collagen and protein–polysaccharide complex, and (3) abnormalities of bone cell metabolism. In the first category are the various forms of hypophosphatemic rickets, whether due to vitamin D deficiency or specific abnormalities of renal tubular transport of phosphate. In the second group are diseases such as osteogenesis imperfecta and scurvy in which collagen formation is impaired. Copper deficiency may cause rarefaction of bone by impairment of collagen formation, and abnormalities of mucopolysaccharide metabolism also lead to structural changes, as in Hurler's syndrome. Metaphyseal dysostosis is also probably a disorder of bone matrix. Under abnormalities of bone cell metabolism can be grouped such disorders as hyperparathyroidism, hypoparathyroidism, hypophosphatasia, and possibly osteopetrosis, as well as the many disorders in which growth is disturbed.

Three ions (calcium, phosphate, and magnesium) have in common the fact that a large proportion of the body content of each of these minerals is sequestered in the solid state in bone, and there is an interrelationship between the homeostasis of these ions and bone growth and structure.

Calcium is the most abundant mineral in the body, but only a minute fraction of the calcium is in solution in the body fluids. Most of it is present as a crystalline deposit in the skeletal matrix. It has been estimated that the total calcium content of the body of the newborn infant is about 20,000 mg, but the calcium in solution in the body fluids of the infant is calculated to be not more than 160 mg, less than 1 percent of the total. Each day during the first year of life more than 160 mg of calcium can be deposited in the skeleton, so that in early infancy the calcium added to bone in 1 day may equal the total amount in solution in the body fluids. This indicates the extent of the turnover of extraskeletal calcium in the body during this period. The relatively large store of calcium in bone is available to the body if calcium intake is reduced, so that normally the serum calcium does not fall below physiologic limits even on low intakes. However, hypocalcemia or hypercalcemia can occur in the face of apparently normal bone stores of calcium, since the deposition of calcium in bone or dissolution of calcium from bone is not simply a matter of chemical solubility but also requires metabolic activity of bone cells for transport of calcium into and out of the bone. Vitamin D and parathyroid hormone stimulate the metabolic activity of bone cells so as to increase the dissolution of bone mineral and matrix at the surface of these cells. The hormone calcitonin, on the other hand, apparently inhibits this function of bone cells, thus leading to reduction of bone mineral solubilization and to hypocalcemia. Calcitonin is probably of secondary importance in calcium homeostasis in the mammal. The other tissue that plays a major role in the regulation of calcium metabolism is the intestinal mucosa. The absorption of calcium is dependent in part on the calcium intake and other factors in the diet, but the efficiency of calcium absorption is variable and is influenced by vitamin D, by the age of the subject (being greater in the young growing subject), and by other factors such as cortisol. Kidney function plays a lesser role in the control of serum calcium levels, in contrast to its major role in regulation of the concentrations of other ions in the body fluids. Renal tubular reabsorption of calcium is ordinarily fairly complete, and urinary calcium is usually less than 5 percent of that filtered. If the calcium load presented to the kidney is too great, renal injury may result due to hypercalciuria and precipitation of calcium in tubules and peritubular spaces or in the outflow tract. In addition, hypercalcemia produces renal vasoconstriction and glomerular damage. The important control of serum calcium levels is accomplished by intestinal absorption of calcium and by the balance between the uptake of calcium by the skeleton and the feedback of calcium from the skeleton into the body fluids.

The concentration of calcium ion in extracellular fluid is of physiologic importance in systems other than those concerned with bone mineral deposition and resorption. Calcium ions participate in the reactions leading to fibrin formation; they are essential in the maintenance of rhythmic cardiac muscle contraction, in the sequence of skeletal muscle contraction and relaxation, and in the initiation and transmission of the electrical impulse in nerve cells and fibers. For many of these functions the concentration of calcium ion required is so low that these processes continue despite considerable reduction of extracellular calcium ion concentration. Tetany (ie, increased excitability of the nervous system) results when the ionized calcium is decreased to about half the normal value. Changes in cardiac muscle function also may occur at this stage, as shown by a prolonged Q-T interval in the electrocardiogram, and in rare instances by partial heart block. Cardiac arrhythmia associated with hypocalcemia can be accentuated by an increase in extracellular potassium.

Determination of the calcium ion concentration of serum is possible by use of a calcium ion electrode, but this is not a convenient method for the clinical laboratory, which usually determines only the total serum calcium. This includes the undissociated calcium proteinate and the small amount of calcium chelated with citrate and other organic acids. At normal levels of serum protein about 45 percent of the total calcium in serum is bound to protein, chiefly albumin, and this fraction of protein-bound, nondiffusible, undissociated calcium is proportional to the concentration of serum protein. The total serum calcium can be reduced to 7.5 mg/100 ml in the hypoalbuminemic patient or elevated slightly above 11 mg/100 ml in a dehydrated patient with increased serum albumin concentration without

charges in the ionized calcium level. The total serum calcium concentration under physiologic conditions is approximately the same in the growing child as in the adult (10.0 $\pm$ 0.5 mg/100 ml).

The *plasma inorganic phosphate* is almost entirely in the ionized diffusible form, although a small fraction of bound phosphate, presumably an undissociated calcium-phosphate-protein complex, is present in hyperphosphatemic states. The concentration of intracellular phosphate is much greater than that in the extracellular fluid, but it is chiefly present as organic phosphoric esters. Intestinal uptake of phosphate, formation and resorption of the bone salt, and movement of phosphate into and out of cells Vôx are all factors in the control of plasma inorganic phosphate concentrations; the cells of the renal tubules provide a major homeostatic function by regulating phosphate excretion in urine. If serum inorganic phosphate concentration is 5 mg/100 ml and glomerular filtration rate is 70 ml/min or approximately 100 liters/24 hours, the phosphate in glomerular filtrate is 5,000 mg/24 hours, which is greatly in excess of the amount available from the diet. Most of this phosphate must be retrieved by the renal tubules if body phosphate content is to be maintained and increased. If renal tubular reabsorption of phosphate is reduced by injury to tubule cells or action of regulatory mechanisms, serum inorganic phosphate will fall until the filtered phosphate is reduced to amounts that are within the capacity of the renal tubular reabsorptive capacity. Conversely, if glomerular filtration is reduced and renal tubular uptake of phosphate persists, the serum inorganic phosphate concentration will rise until a balance is again achieved. Thus renal hypophosphatemia or hyperphosphatemia may result from imbalance of glomerular filtration rate and rate of renal tubular reabsorption of phosphate. Depression of the glomerular filtration rate to less than 20 percent of the normal value will be associated with a rise of serum inorganic phosphate unless the intake or intestinal absorption of phosphate is severely limited. The normal range of serum phosphate concentration varies with age and growth phase, as shown in Table 13. The differences between the values in infants and adults depend on the relative magnitudes of tubular reabsorption of phosphate and glomerular filtration rates at different ages. Pituitary growth hormone increases tubular transport of phosphate independently of parathyroid hormone. The effects of parathyroid hormone and vitamin D on serum phosphate concentration are discussed on pages 237 and 238 , respectively.

Acute hypophosphatemia can occur during periods

TABLE 13. Variation of Serum Phosphate and Magnesium With Age[a]

Age Group	Phosphate (mg/100 ml)	Magnesium (mg/100 ml)
Premature infants	7.9 $\pm$ 0.28	1.70 $\pm$ 0.10
Newborns, full-term	6.1 $\pm$ 0.33	1.81 $\pm$ 0.06
1–10 years	4.6 $\pm$ 0.16	2.25 $\pm$ 0.07
Adults	3.5 $\pm$ 0.19	2.41 $\pm$ 0.05

[a] *From unpublished data of H. E. Harrison, M.D. All values are means $\pm$ SE of means.*

of starvation, as in patients with severe infections or other disturbances who are being maintained on intravenous fluids; cell phosphate is maintained at the expense of extracellular phosphate under these conditions. Administration of glucose leads to uptake of phosphate by the cell, causing further depression of serum phosphate, which persists if no phosphate is available from the diet. This phenomenon is seen in the subject with diabetic ketosis treated with glucose and insulin. Although the serum inorganic phosphate may drop to exceedingly low levels, there is no evidence of physiologic abnormality directly associated with transient hypophosphatemia. Incorporation of inorganic phosphate into intravenous solutions has been recommended, but there is no proof of the need or value of such addition, unless patients are maintained for many days on intravenous nutrients. Prolonged symptomatic hypophosphatemia has been found in patients on intravenous hyperalimentation with glucose and amino acid solutions deficient in phosphate. Chronic hypophosphatemia is of major physiologic significance, since the rate of crystallization of bone mineral in matrix is dependent upon the concentration of inorganic phosphate. The crystalline phase of bone mineral is hydroxyapatite, with the basic formula $Ca_{10}(PO_4)_6(OH)_2$. The formation of bone mineral depends not only on the concentration of Ga^{++} but also on the concentration of inorganic phosphate (P_1). Formation of bone mineral can occur only when the product $Ca^{++} \times P_i$ is sufficiently high to permit crystallization of hydroxyapatite from the extracellular fluid on a template provided by the organic matrix of cartilage or bone. Thus a high concentration of P_i favors the movement of Ca^{++} into the solid phase, while a low concentration of P_i keeps the Ca^{++} in the body fluids. Chronic hypophosphatemia can result from inadequate intake of phosphate, as in intravenous alimentation, and also from renal tubular defects resulting in excessive phosphate wastage in urine, or from impaired absorption of phosphate. Iatrogenic hypophosphatemia has been observed to result from excessive intake of antacids containing aluminum hydroxide. Insoluble aluminum phosphate forms in the intestinal contents and prevents absorption of phosphate. This form of hypophosphatemia, as well as that due to intravenous alimentation, has been associated with muscle weakness and increased rate of red blood cell disappearance.

Magnesium, like phosphate, is an important intracellular solute as well as a component of the insoluble bone crystal. About 40 percent of body magnesium is in tissue cells, and about 60 percent is in bone mineral. Intracellular magnesium is an indispensable cofactor of cell enzyme systems and is not readily released to maintain serum magnesium concentrations, so that skeletal magnesium is the important buffer that releases or takes up magnesium in response to changes in extracellular concentration of this ion. About two-thirds of the plasma magnesium is ionized, and the remainder is protein-bound. The total serum magnesium concentration in normal subjects ranges between 1.8 and 2.5 mg/100 ml. Levels are somewhat lower in infants than in adults

(Table 13). The evidence suggests that bone magnesium is present at the surface of the bone crystal as carbonate and citrate and that bone magnesium is in equilibrium with extracellular Mg^{++} ion concentrations.

RICKETS AND OSTEOMALACIA

Rickets and osteomalacia are disorders of bone mineralization in which osteoblastic activity and production of bone matrix continue but in which there is a lag in the rate of mineralization of the matrix, so that accumulation of unmineralized matrix results. Rickets is the process in growing bone, whereas osteomalacia is the same physiologic disturbance in bone that is no longer growing in length but is still undergoing remodeling. The most important physiologic basis of rickets and osteomalacia is a deficiency of inorganic phosphate in the extracellular fluids, with or without an associated deficiency of calcium.

Vitamin D Metabolism and Physiology

Vitamin D is a generic term for a group of steroids, the most important of which are cholecalciferol (vitamin D_3) and ergocalciferol (vitamin D_2). The natural source of vitamin D for the human is the cholecalciferol produced in the skin following exposure to the ultraviolet radiation of sunshine, which activates the skin 7-dehydrocholesterol. The conversion of ergosterol to vitamin D_2 by similar ultraviolet radiation is the source of the relatively inexpensive vitamin D available in enriched milk and vitamin concentrations. Neither cow's milk nor breast milk ordinarily contains appreciable quantities of vitamin D (Table 14), which explains the high incidence

TABLE 14. Amounts of Vitamin D Available in Foods

Breast milk	0–10 IU/100 ml
Cow's milk	0.3–4 IU/100 ml
Butter	35 IU/100 g
Egg yolk	25 IU/average yolk
Calf liver	15 IU/100 g
Herring	1,500 IU/100 g
Mackerel	1,800 IU/100 g
Salmon, canned	300 IU/100 g
Tuna, canned	250 IU/100 g
Sardines, canned	600 IU/100 g
Cod liver oil	175 IU/100 g

of rickets that was at one time encountered in infants living in climatic conditions in which there was little exposure to sunshine. Rickets has become a rare disease in those areas in which oral administration of vitamin D, usually in the form of enriched milk, has effectively eliminated the dependence of the infant on sunshine.

Vitamin D, whether endogenously produced cholecalciferol or ingested cholecalciferol or ergocalciferol,

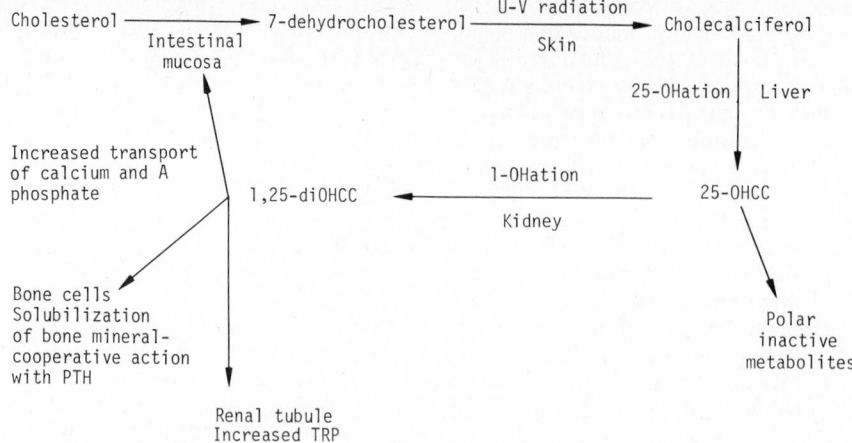

FIG. 12. Vitamin D cycle: metabolism of vitamin D to active metabolite, 1,25-dihydroxycholecalciferol (1,25-diOHCC).

undergoes a metabolic transformation before it is physiologically active (Fig. 12). The first step is hydroxylation at the 25 carbon in the side chain, resulting in 25-hydroxy vitamin D. In the rat, and very likely in man, this hydroxylation occurs chiefly if not exclusively in the liver. The 25-hydroxy compound is then the substrate of a kidney mitochondrial system that adds a hydroxyl group at the 1 carbon position in the A ring to form 1,25-dihydroxy vitamin D, which is the active physiologic agent. This operates on intestinal mucosal transport of calcium and phosphate and on renal tubular transport of phosphate; in cooperation with parathyroid hormone it operates on bone cell metabolism, leading to solubilization of bone mineral and release of calcium and phosphate into extracellular fluid.

The physiologic justification for this metabolic cycle appears to be that it permits regulation of rates at a number of steps controlling the concentration of the final active product, 1,25-dihydroxy vitamin D, and thus the role of this compound in calcium homeostasis. The 25-hydroxylation in the liver cell is controlled to some extent by product concentration and 1-hydroxylation is controlled in the kidney by parathyroid hormone, either directly or through tissue phosphate or calcium concentration. Stimulation of 1-hydroxylation by parathyroid hormone permits adaptation to a low-calcium diet by increase of parathyroid hormone output, resulting in an increase of the concentration of 1,25-dihydroxy vitamin D in plasma at a constant intake of vitamin D or constant exposure of skin to sunshine. Control at two stages of the rate of formation of 1,25-dihydroxy vitamin D presumably prevents vitamin D toxicity in individuals heavily exposed to sunshine and still permits adequate vitamin D activity with relatively limited exposure. Another control mechanism not shown in this cycle is skin pigmentation, which absorbs the energy of ultraviolet light before it reaches the 7-dehydrocholesterol in the deeper layers of the skin. This is presumably the cause of the increased susceptibility of dark-skinned individuals to vitamin D deficiency when dietary sources are limited and exposure to sunshine must be relied upon. The control mechanisms fail, unfortunately, when a large excess of vitamin D is taken orally. It may be that at high concentrations of unmetabolized vitamin D or of 25-hydroxy vitamin D or both the negative feedback on their physiologic activity through serum Ca^{++} concentration and parathyroid hormone output is not the controlling factor for regulation of the concentration of 1,25-dihydroxy vitamin D.

On the basis of our current knowledge, the various forms of rickets can be divided into two main groups: those in which there is some interference in the metabolic cycle of vitamin D leading to a diminished concentration of the active compound, 1,25-dihydroxy vitamin

TABLE 15. Classification of Varieties of Rickets and Osteomalacia on Basis of Deficiency of Active Vitamin D Metabolite or Hypophosphatemia Due to Defect of Renal Tubular Reabsorption of Phosphate (Target Cell Abnormality)

Deficiency of Active Vitamin D Metabolite	Target Cell Abnormality
Vitamin D deficiency	Fanconi syndrome
Absence of sunshine	Cystinosis
Dietary lack	Tyrosinosis
Vitamin D malabsorption	Other causes
Liver disease	Renal tubular acidosis
Anticonvulsant drugs	Genetic primary hypophosphatemia
Renal disease	
Vitamin D dependency	Hypophosphatemia with
(1-hydroxylation	nonendocrine tumors
abnormality)	

D, and those due to an abnormality of the target cells responsible for calcium and phosphate homeostasis such that normal concentrations of these ions cannot be maintained. The only target cell abnormality thus far demonstrated involves the mechanism for retrieval of phosphate from glomerular filtrate by the renal tubule cell. This defect in tubular reabsorption results in renal hypophosphatemia. In the first group, lack of the active vitamin D compound causes impaired calcium absorption from the intestine, hypocalcemia, and attempted compensation by secondary hyperparathyroidism, which may not be adequate to correct the hypocalcemia. In the second group, hypocalcemia and secondary hyperparathyroidism are not present, and the rickets is predominantly a phosphate-deficiency phenomenon. The various clinical entities of these two groups are listed in Table 15.

Rickets Due to Deficiency of Active Vitamin D Metabolite

The active vitamin D compound is required for the efficient absorption of calcium and phosphate from the intestine and also for the efficient conservation of phosphate by the renal tubule. The latter action is probably both a direct effect of vitamin D and an indirect action resulting from suppression of output of parathyroid hormone. The net result of lack of vitamin D is a decrease in the concentration of both calcium ion and phosphate ion in extracellular fluids, so that the ionic concentrations are inadequate for mineralization of bone matrix. The deficiency of phosphate ion is the more critical, and if the hypophosphatemia is severe the serum calcium ion concentration may remain in the normal range because of markedly decreased uptake of calcium phosphate by bone. A secondary effect of the deficiencies of calcium and phosphate is an overproliferation of osteoblasts, possibly in response to the deformation produced in the structurally weak bone. The elevated alkaline phosphatase activity in serum in vitamin D deficiency represents release of this enzyme from the osteoblasts. An additional manifestation of vitamin D deficiency is a generalized amino-aciduria due to abnormality of renal tubular reabsorption of amino acids. This renal amino-aciduria resembles that found in the renal tubular injury of cystine storage disease, lead poisoning, or Wilson's disease. It has been suggested that the amino-aciduria of vitamin D deficiency is a manifestation of excess parathyroid hormone secretion.

The hypocalcemia of vitamin D deficiency is due not only to poor absorption of calcium from the intestine but also to failure of response of the bone cells to parathyroid hormone. There is experimental evidence that the full expression of the action of parathyroid hormone does not occur in the vitamin-D-deficient subject. In chronic vitamin-D-deficiency rickets hypocalcemia becomes less pronounced as the serum inorganic phosphate levels decrease to very low levels. However, a febrile illness or starvation with liberation of tissue phosphate and consequent increase of extracellular phosphate can precipitate hypocalcemia in the rachitic child. This mechanism explains the frequent association of tetany with infections in the days when vitamin-D-deficiency rickets was common.

PATHOLOGY. The morphologic changes in the rachitic bones have been described in detail by Park and by Follis. Normally, at the epiphyses of the growing long bones there is proliferation and maturation of the cartilage cells. The columns of cartilage cells are surrounded by matrix in which mineral is deposited, resulting in a uniform zone of calcified cartilage at the junction of the bone and cartilage. Capillaries from the bony side invade the degenerating cartilage cells, forming tunnels in the calcified matrix; osteoblasts that penetrate along with the capillaries deposit osteoid (ie, the organic matrix of bone). The osteoid is in turn mineralized as the calcified cartilage matrix is reabsorbed. Thus there is an orderly deposition of layer upon layer of new bone, with continous resorption and remodeling of the bone until the final stable structure is achieved. In rickets the sequence of events is disturbed, starting with failure of calcification of the cartilage matrix. The capillaries invade the degenerating cartilage in a highly haphazard and irregular pattern, and proliferating osteoblasts form osteoid, which accumulates without being mineralized. A broad zone of proliferative cartilage and osteoid develops in which bone mineral is irregularly deposited. This rachitic intermediate zone or metaphysis is a bulky mass consisting of cartilage, invading blood vessels, osteoblast, fibroblasts, and marrow elements (Fig. 13). Islands of uncalcified cartilage covered with osteoid are found instead of the regular arrangement of chondro-osseous trabeculae. This rachitic intermediate zone does not have the rigidity of the normal bone–cartilage junction. It is compressed and deformed by pressure and extends laterally, producing knobby ends of bones that are characteristic of rickets. Much of the deformity of the long bones in rickets can be explained by the bending and twisting of the yielding rachitic metaphysis. The angulation of the lower end of the tibia, for example, results from posterior displacement of the epiphysis by muscle pull because of lack of structural resistance of the rachitic intermediate zone. In the shaft the bone trabeculae are covered with layers of unmineralized osteoid. The volume of bone is reduced, while there is an increased volume of uncalcified organic matrix. Poorly mineralized layers of osteoid are also deposited subperiosteally. The bone shaft lacks rigidity and is bent by muscle pull or weight bearing, and in severe rickets it may be easily fractured. As the process becomes chronic, however, the bone shaft becomes considerably thickened by deposition of excessive matrix with partial mineralization. The failure of mineralization of the organic matrix is also seen in the membranous bone of the skull, the pelvis, and the bodies of the vertebrae, causing the characteristic coarse, almost cystic, structure of these bones.

ROENTGENOGRAPHIC FINDINGS. The structural abnormalities of bone that can readily be detected by roentgenogram are relatively late changes, and the

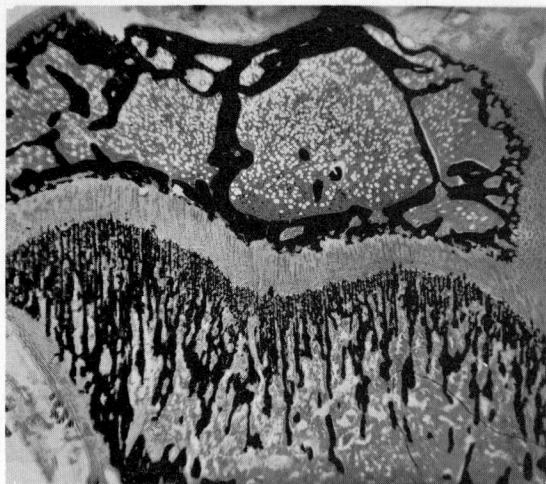 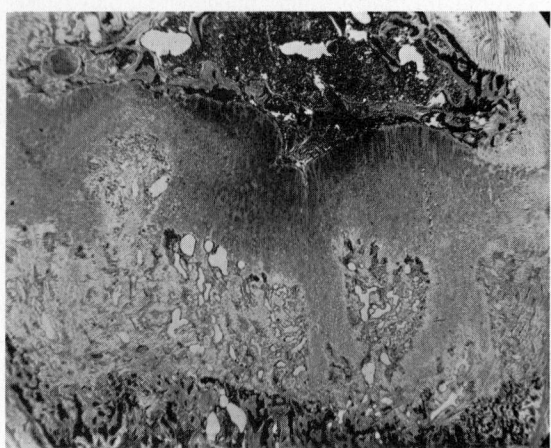

FIG. 13. Morphology of rachitic intermediate zone as seen in experimentally induced rickets in rat. The sections are stained by the von Kossa method, which stains the bone mineral black. Left: tibia of normal rat. The narrow regular zone of cartilage separating the epiphyseal plate of metaphysis from the center of ossification in the epiphysis is well demonstrated. The cartilage plate is composed of orderly rows of cartilage cell embedded in the matrix, and the epiphyseal plate is formed by a regular band of calcified matrix. Right: tibia of rachitic rat. The broad, irregular, rachitic intermediate zone is composed of degenerating cartilage, islands of capillaries, osteoblasts, and unmineralized osteoid. At the bottom the bony trabeculae forming the irregular epiphyseal margin of the metaphysis are seen.

histologic and biochemical disorders of rickets may exist before there is visible change in the gross bone structure. Among the roentgenographic changes are the following: increased width of the uncalcified portion of the bone between the center of ossification in the epiphyses and the end of the bony metaphysis; irregularity of the epiphyseal plate and its distortion by pressure, so that there is cupping of the ends of the bone, with projection of processes of mineralized tissue into the rachitic intermediate zone forming spurs and an irregular fringe effect; coarse trabecular structure of the shaft of the bone due to the increased volume of nonmineralized matrixes surrounding the trabeculae; and often a layer of poorly mineralized matrix beneath the periosteum, producing the effect of apparent separation of the periosteum from the underlying cortex. These manifestations and the roentgenographic pattern that appears when healing and mineralization of the osteoid occurs are shown in Figure 14. When healing occurs the new bone is laid down in a more orderly pattern than that of the disorganized structure of rachitic bone, and the demarcation between new normal bone and old rachitic bone may be present for some time after healing seemingly has been completed. In advanced cases bending and angulation of the long bones may be visualized. Marked thickening of the bone can result from overproliferation of osteoid, especially along the concave aspect of the tibia in chronic rickets, in which periods of partial healing and progression of the active rachitic changes may alternate. In cases of acute severe rickets, greenstick fractures may be present.

Nutritional Vitamin D Deficiency

Vitamin D deficiency has its genesis in the first few months of life, but considerable time is required before the skeletal changes are sufficiently advanced to result in visible deformity. The biochemical changes, however, may be present after a few months of deprivation of vitamin D. Hypocalcemic tetany on a rachitic basis may occur as early as 2 to 3 months of age, particularly in prematurely born infants. A few instances of so-called congenital rickets have been reported. These infants were born of mothers with osteomalacia who were themselves vitamin-D-deficient because of both dietary deprivation and lack of exposure to sunshine. However, under ordinary living conditions pregnant women receive enough vitamin D, either in foods or vitamin supplements or by exposure to sunlight, to provide adequate stores of vitamin D for the fetus. Therefore the newborn infant has some reserves of vitamin D that may maintain adequate function for several months, despite lack of dietary intake from birth.

At present, most instances of nutritional vitamin D deficiency in the United States occur in babies who have been breast-fed for the first year, but who have not received vitamin D supplements because of the mothers' mistaken notion that breast milk is adequate to meet all nutritional requirements of the infant. The vitamin D content of nonenriched cow's milk is also inadequate, but most infants fed on cow's milk mixtures now receive milk enriched with vitamin D, as evaporated milk, enriched homogenized milk, or prepared infant feeding mixtures, all of which have added vitamin

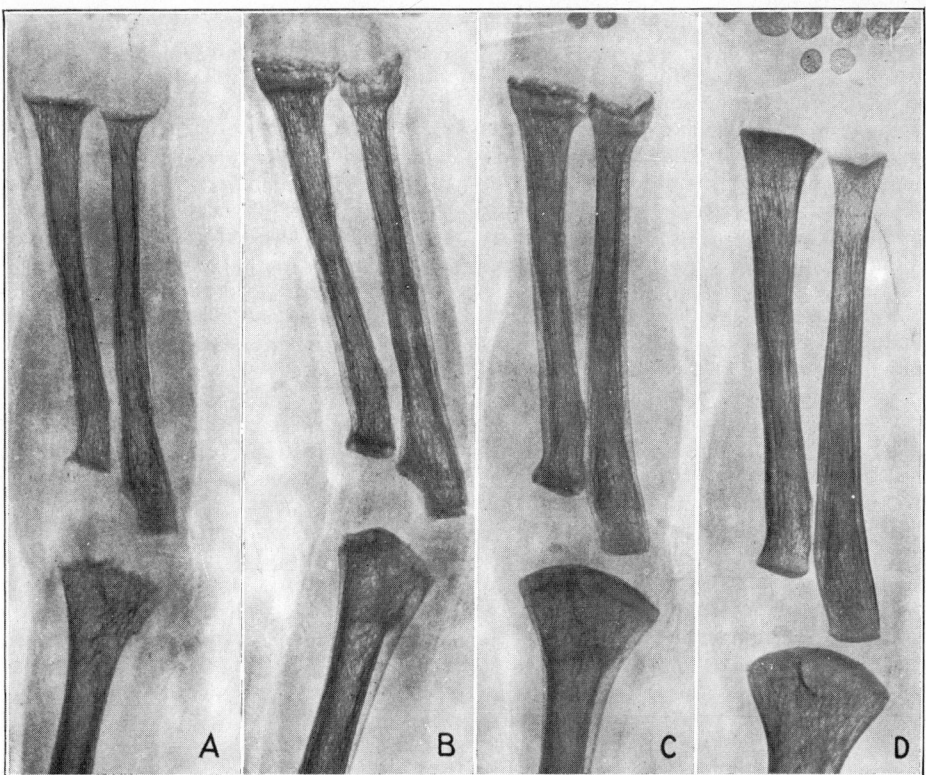

FIG. 14. Roentgen-ray appearance of bones in advanced rickets, showing typical healing. A. Active rickets. B. Healing in progress after 27 days of treatment, showing new line of calcification in metaphyses. C. Healing after 34 days of treatment, showing dense lines of calcification and increase in periosteal calcification. D. Complete healing after 3 months. (From Special Report Series No. 77, Medical Research Council, London, 1923. By permission of Her Majesty's Stationery Office.)

D. An increased incidence of vitamin D deficiency is now being encountered in a population in which there is strict adherence to a form of vegetarianism in which all foods of animal origin are proscribed except human milk.

On occasion the diagnosis of rickets is made incidentally when affected infants are seen because of pneumonia or other infections. The febrile illness may precipitate hypocalcemic tetany with convulsive seizures as the presenting manifestation, or the early deformities of rickets may be noted on examination in the absence of specific complaints. In some instances radiographs of the chest may reveal enough of the bony structure of the humeri to suggest the diagnosis of rickets.

One of the early signs of rickets in the infant under 6 months of age is craniotabes; this results from thinning of the inner tables of the skull by pressure of the intracranial contents, with failure of remineralization, and is usually most pronounced in the posterolateral portions of the skull. The thin skull bone can be indented like a Ping-Pong ball by pressure of the finger, snapping back when the pressure is released. Rachitic craniotabes must be differentiated from physiologic craniotabes, which is usually limited to the bone close to the suture lines, particularly the lambdoidal suture, and is more likely to be found in infants under 3 months of age. Rachitic craniotabes can be more extensive and is present in somewhat older infants. As rickets becomes more chronic the skull bones become thicker, and the frontal and parietal bosses become prominent. Growth of the skull bones is delayed, so that the fontanelle and suture closures are delayed.

The rachitic rosary is produced by swelling of the rachitic intermediate zone at the junction of the costal cartilage and the calcified portion of the rib. When it is extensive it can be seen as well as felt. Slight prominence of the costochondral functions can be felt in normal infants during the first year of life, and a tentative diagnosis of rickets made on this basis alone may not be supported when biochemical or roentgenographic studies are made. In the later stage of rickets the chest deformity is more pronounced, with pulling in of the costal cartilages and protrusion of the sternum, producing pigeon-breast deformity. The lower portion of the rib cage is also flared out, and a depression is produced by the pull of the diaphragm on the yielding rib structure (Harrison's groove). If the rachitic process progresses without treatment, deformity of the vertebral bodies results with scoliosis.

The deformities of the long bones are initially knobby, with prominence of the epiphyses particularly at the wrists and the ankles. The increased width of the proliferative cartilage separating the epiphyseal centers of ossification from the shaft of the bone may produce a characteristic abnormality of certain epiphyses, such as those of the malleoli, giving the impression of a double epiphysis on palpation. Before weight bearing occurs the lower end of the tibia may show angulation due to posterior displacement of the distal epiphysis by a strong pull of the gastrocnemius-soleus muscle group. This angulation is aggravated by the posture of sitting with legs crossed. When weight bearing occurs the femora show lateral bowing, with either genu valgum or genu varum deformity. In addition, bowing and medial torsion of the tibia can occur, so that the femora are externally rotated to keep the feet from toeing in. This causes instability of the hip joints, with a resulting waddling gait. A waddling gait may also result from a coxa vara deformity. Deformities of the pelvis also occur in rickets, and in the past these were responsible for serious problems of dystocia in women who had rickets in infancy. Severe vitamin D deficiency can interfere with growth of the tooth buds, so that delayed appearance of the deciduous teeth may result and the enamel may be hypoplastic when the teeth finally appear. Another manifestation of severe rickets is poor muscle tone. Abdominal distension, lordosis, and difficulty in walking may result from this as well as from the skeletal deformity. These major deformities are now rare, except in cases of rickets not responsive to ordinary vitamin D therapy.

VITAMIN D REQUIREMENTS. The vitamin D requirements of infants and children are satisfied by a daily intake of 400 IU, either as ergocalciferol (vitamin D_2) or cholecalciferol (vitamin D_3). Evaporated milk and the various modified milk preparations for infant feeding are fortified with vitamin D_2 in the amount of 400 IU per can or per equivalent of a quart of whole cow's milk. Homogenized, vitamin-D-enriched pasteurized milk also contains 400 IU of vitamin D_2 per quart. Infants fed these cow's milk preparations usually consume a quart of milk or its equivalent daily by 2 months of age and will therefore receive the required 400 IU.- The prematurely born infant is an exception in this regard since his caloric and milk intakes will be much less than those of the full-term infant for several months. These infants should be given a vitamin D supplement in addition to the vitamin D supplied by milk, so that the total intake is at least 400 IU daily; however, it is not necessary to give premature infants larger amounts of vitamin D than full-term infants. It is important that the breast-fed infant also receive a vitamin D preparation supplying 400 IU daily.

In some parts of Europe the practice of giving young infants a single large dose of vitamin D, usually 500,000 IU, has been recommended. Since vitamin D is slowly inactivated or excreted, this dose will provide protective levels for 3 to 6 months, making it unnecessary to give daily doses of vitamin D. The danger of such a regimen is that these large loads may be complemented by vitamin D in other foods resulting in hypervitaminosis D. The use of prophylactic doses of vitamin D greatly in excess of 400 IU/day should be discouraged. In eagerness to prevent rickets and promote growth, multivitamin preparations or vitamin D concentrates providing several thousand units of vitamin D per day sometimes have been prescribed. Although there is considerable variation in tolerance to vitamin D, some children develop evidences of hypervitaminosis D on daily doses that are only moderately in excess of the usual requirement. The entity known as idiopathic hypercalcemia (p. 252). may possibly represent hypervitaminosis D due to accumulation of vitamin D from doses of only a few thousand units per day.

VITAMIN D-DEFICIENCY RICKETS. Vitamin D-deficiency rickets can be treated with doses of vitamin D of 10,000 IU/day for 30 to 60 days. This dosage can be given in the form of vitamin D_2 in propylene glycol (Drisdol), which is miscible in milk, orange juice, and other fluids, or as an irradiated ergosterol concentrate in oil, which can be given by dropper. An alternative method of treatment is to give a single massive dose of vitamin D of 600,000 IU. For this purpose a vitamin D concentrate in oil is required, since the propylene glycol solution is too dilute and the large volume of solvent could produce serious side effects, particularly depression and stupor. One advantage of treatment by a single large dose is that the earliest evidence of recovery (elevation of the serum phosphorus level) may be seen within a few days, thus providing assurance that the problem is not one of increased requirement for vitamin D, which would necessitate further study of the underlying problem. Another indication for the use of a large dose is hypocalcemia due to vitamin D deficiency. If a single large dose of vitamin D is given, calcium homeostasis is restored much more rapidly than with moderate daily doses; the period during which there is danger of hypocalcemic tetany is thereby reduced. If this complication of rickets does occur it can be treated by intravenous injection of calcium as a 10 percent solution of calcium gluconate; 5 to 10 ml are injected slowly, with monitoring of the heart rate, because too rapid an elevation of plasma calcium causes bradycardia and even cardiac arrest.

IMPAIRED INTESTINAL ABSORPTION OF VITAMIN D. Vitamin D-deficiency rickets may develop in infants as the result of defective intestinal absorption of vitamin D, despite ordinarily adequate dietary intakes. A variety of disturbances of fat absorption with increased fecal fat loss may be associated with failure of vitamin D absorption. We have observed two male siblings who developed rickets along with signs of vitamin D deficiency at the end of the first year of life; both had increased loss of fat in the stool, possibly because of a congenital defect of lipase activity. However, in infants with cystic fibrosis vitamin D deficiency is rare, despite the disturbance of lipolysis and fat absorption. Exclusion of bile from the intestinal tract, as in biliary atresia, also is a cause of malabsorption of vitamin D.

Rickets due to Impaired Metabolism of Vitamin D

RICKETS ASSOCIATED WITH LIVER DISEASE. Rickets has occurred in young infants with infectious hepatitis. This was once thought to be due to impaired vitamin D absorption, but the newer knowledge of vitamin D metabolism indicates that impaired formation of the active metabolite 25-hydroxy vitamin D is responsible. This is of interest because it appears that relatively mild liver disease may cause early rickets in young infants.

RICKETS ASSOCIATED WITH ANTICONVULSIVE DRUG THERAPY. Rickets and osteomalacia have been seen in patients with chronic seizure disorder receiving anticonvulsive drugs, particularly combinations of diphenylhydantoin and phenobarbital. It is thought that these drugs induce hepatic enzymes that metabolize 25-hydroxy vitamin D to more polar metabolites, thus reducing its availability as a substrate for 1-hydroxylation in the kidney and resulting in a deficiency of 1,25-dihydroxy vitamin D. Although hypocalcemia, hypophosphatemia, rickets, and osteomalacia may occur in patients on anticonvulsive drugs, they are rare. This is probably explained by the fact that vitamin D supplies are more than adequate in most cases to offset diversion of part of the 25-hydroxy vitamin D. The extra vitamin D requirement of children on anticonvulsive drugs is about 3,000 IU/week.

VITAMIN D-DEPENDENT RICKETS. It has long been recognized that occasionally a child will require much more vitamin D than the standard 400 IU daily to prevent rickets. Prader reported several cases in which there was a familial occurrence, with a genetic pattern indicating transmission as an autosomal recessive. These patients develop later rickets (beyond the first year of life) with characteristic deformities and radiographic changes. Serum calcium concentration is frequently reduced, and tetany may ocur. The serum phosphate concentration is reduced, but not as uniformly or as strikingly as in primary hypophosphatemic rickets. Like patients with ordinary vitamin D deficiency, children with vitamin D-dependent rickets show generalized renal amino-aciduria; this is another feature differentiating it from primary hypophosphatemia, in which amino-aciduria does not occur. Vitamin D-dependent rickets is treated with vitamin D in doses appropriate for each individual. Some patients respond to 5,000 to 15,000 IU/day, but others need more. With adequate amounts of vitamin D, serum calcium and phosphate concentrations return to normal, and renal amino-aciduria disappears. Normal alkaline phosphatase levels are restored, and radiographic evidence of healing occurs. Vitamin D treatment must be continued to maintain normal values, or a relapse will result. The metabolic defect is thought to be an abnormality or deficiency of the kidney enzyme causing inadequate 1-hydroxylation of 25-hydroxy vitamin D. A few patients have been treated successfully with 1 to 3 μg daily of 1 α-hydroxycholecalciferol or 1,25-dihydroxycholecalciferol. These compounds are presently available only for investigational use.

Another type of increased vitamin D requirement occurs sporadically; it is more gradual in onset, and manifestations may not appear until later childhood, when bone pain and limitation of activity because of pain on weight bearing are noted. Serum calcium and phosphorus levels are reduced, but hypocalcemia is not consistent; alkaline phosphatase activity in serum is elevated. The roentgenographic findings are those of osteomalacia and hyperparathyroidism, with the latter sometimes predominant (Fig. 15). On bone biopsy the histologic features of osteitis fibrosa cystica may be present, as well as those of osteomalacia. The condition is assumed to be due to a block in the metabolic cycle of vitamin D, with secondary hyperparathyroidism that has become predominant. Treatment consists of vitamin D in amounts necessary to restore normal serum calcium and phosphorus levels; 25,000 to 50,000 IU/day may be required. Renal osteodystrophy, the bone disease associated with severe renal insufficiency, also represents secondary hyperparathyroidism associated with chronic 1,25-dihydroxy vitamin D deficiency; it is discussed on page 246.

Hypophosphatemia of Renal Tubular Origin With Associated Rickets

Impairment of renal tubular reabsorption of phosphate due to intrinsic defects of renal tubular metabolism or to toxic injuries of renal tubule cells causes renal hypophosphatemia. The deficiency of inorganic phosphate in extracellular fluids then results in a reduced rate of deposition of bone mineral in matrix and consequent rickets. The forms of hypophosphatemic rickets not due to deficiency of the active vitamin D metabolite (1,25-dihydroxy vitamin D) may be classified under the headings of primary hypophosphatemia, acquired vitamin-D-resistant rickets, renal tubular acidosis, and the Fanconi syndrome.

PRIMARY HYPOPHOSPHATEMIA. Primary hypophosphatemia, or familial vitamin D-resistant rickets, is the result of a hereditary metabolic defect that involves the phosphate transport system of the renal tubules and possibly that of the intestine, so that severe hypophosphatemia results despite vitamin D therapy. It is possible that interference with calcium transport also may be present, but this is responsive to large doses of vitamin D. The defect usually is inherited as a dominant characteristic, so that it may be traced through successive generations and may involve one or more siblings. In most families the inheritance is through a gene on the X chromosome, so that the heterozygous females frequently have a milder disease than the hemizygous males. The severity of the physiologic and pathologic changes may be variable, and the defect may not be recognized in some members of the family unless they are carefully studied. Hypophosphatemia and short stature may be the only findings. The hereditary pattern of an autosomal recessive gene may also occur; sporadic

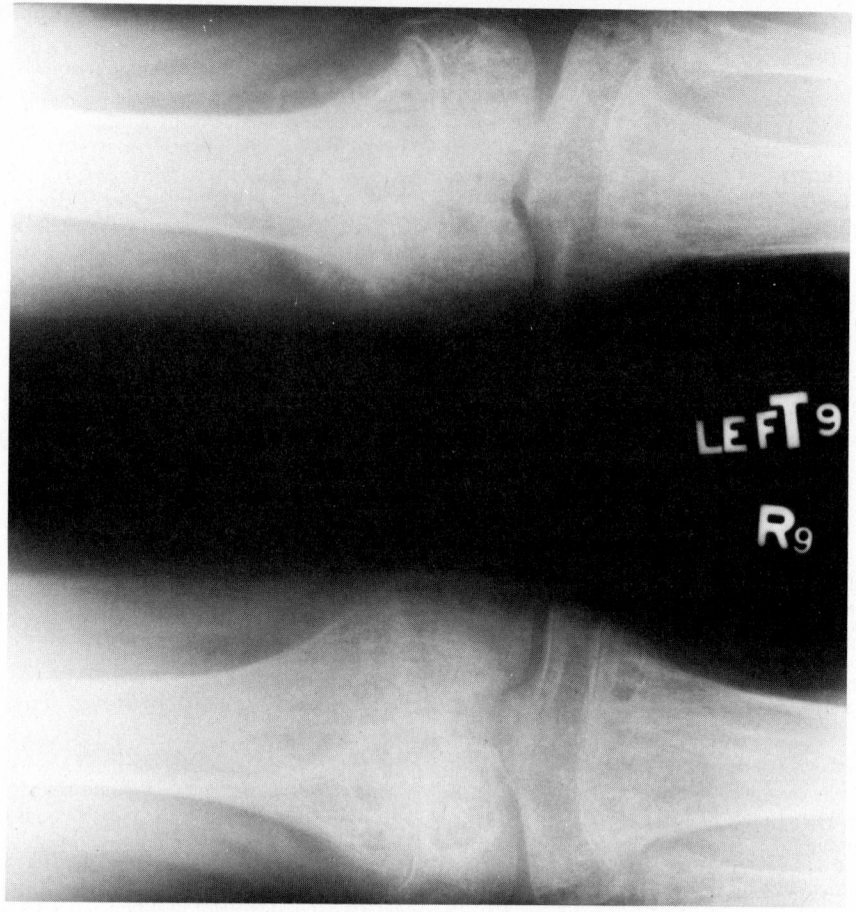

FIG. 15. Roentgenographic changes of secondary hyperparathyroidism presented by 15-year-old male with long-standing increased requirement of vitamin D and reduction of serum calcium and phosphate concentrations on ordinary intake of vitamin D. These changes were reversed by vitamin D treatment.

cases have been reported with no apparent hereditary basis. The marked hypophosphatemia is associated with normal serum calcium and moderately elevated alkaline phosphatase levels; a defect of phosphate and calcium absorption is present, so that stool calcium and phosphate levels are high and urinary calcium excretion is decreased. Administration of large doses of vitamin D increases calcium and phosphate absorption from the intestine, so that serum calcium levels may be abnormally high while phosphate concentrations remain low. In children with ordinary rickets serum phosphorus rapidly becomes normal with small doses of vitamin D. The fundamental defect in resistant rickets is impairment of renal tubular reabsorption of phosphate; renal amino-aciduria is not a feature of this type of rickets. Vitamin D metabolism is normal; thus treatment with 1,25 dihydroxycholecalciferol has not corrected the renal hypophosphatemia.

The clinical picture is variable; retardation of growth precedes the appearance of obvious bony deformities, but may not be seen until the age of 6 to 18 months. Short stature and the progressive skeletal changes of rickets after the first year in children who have received vitamin D or who have been exposed to sunshine should suggest this syndrome. The roentgenographic changes are those of chronic rickets modified by retardation of bone growth. (Fig. 16).

In the past, treatment with large amounts of vitamin D has resulted in renal injury due to hypervitaminosis D. The therapy currently recommended is to add large amounts of phosphate to the diet in an effort to increase serum phosphate concentration and hasten healing. Phosphate intake of 1.5 to 2.0 g/day as phosphorus, added in divided doses to the ordinary diet as sodium and potassium phosphate, is necessary. Some patients develop abdominal discomfort and diarrhea, but by gradual increase of dose it may be tolerated. In order to avoid a high intake of sodium, we have used a potassium phosphate mixture (Neutra-Phos-K).

With high-phosphate feeding, calcium absorption is

reduced and secondary hyperparathyroidism may develop unless calcium absorption is maintained by increased dosage of vitamin D or dihydrotachysterol. We prefer to use dihydrotachysterol because in pharmacologic doses it increases calcium absorption from the intestine but has a shorter biologic half-life than vitamin D, and thus there is less danger of cumulative effect with hypercalcemia. Doses of 0.2 to 1 mg/day of dihydrotachysterol have been adequate in most patients. An equivalent effect can be obtained with vitamin D (25,000 to 100,000 IU/day). The effectiveness is assessed from 24-hour urinary excretion of calcium: if intestinal absorption of calcium is inadequate, urinary calcium is less than 25 mg/day; with adequate doses of dihydrotachysterol or vitamin D, urinary calcium excretion rises. Urinary calcium excretion of more than 150 mg/day is a signal to reduce dosage. Serum calcium concentrations should be monitored to avoid hypercalcemia. Although postabsorptive serum phosphorus remains low, serum phosphorus rises after each dose to levels sufficient to initiate deposition of calcium phosphate in the matrix of cartilage and bone. Following

cessation of growth, treatment may be discontinued; however, some patients in the third and fourth decades have developed osteomalacia and arthritis resulting from abnormal bone structure and joint deformation requiring continuation of therapy.

Some patients have been treated with dihydrotachysterol without phosphate supplement in doses of 1 to 2 mg/day. Calcium and phosphorus levels in serum and calcium excretion in urine should be monitored weekly for the first 2 to 3 months. Subsequently, every 3 to 6 months a 12-hour or 24-hour urine specimen should be analyzed for calcium and creatinine. When the ratio of calcium/creatinine is below 0.4, toxicity is not present.

If treatment is instituted early, deformities and marked stunting of growth can be prevented; however, growth retardation is usually not completely overcome. If the diagnosis is not made until the age of 2 years, significant deformities may have developed, and healing may be so slow that these deformities may progress. Lateral and anteroposterior bowing of the femora with genu valgum and anterior bowing and medial torsion of the tibiae may cause serious disability and require or-

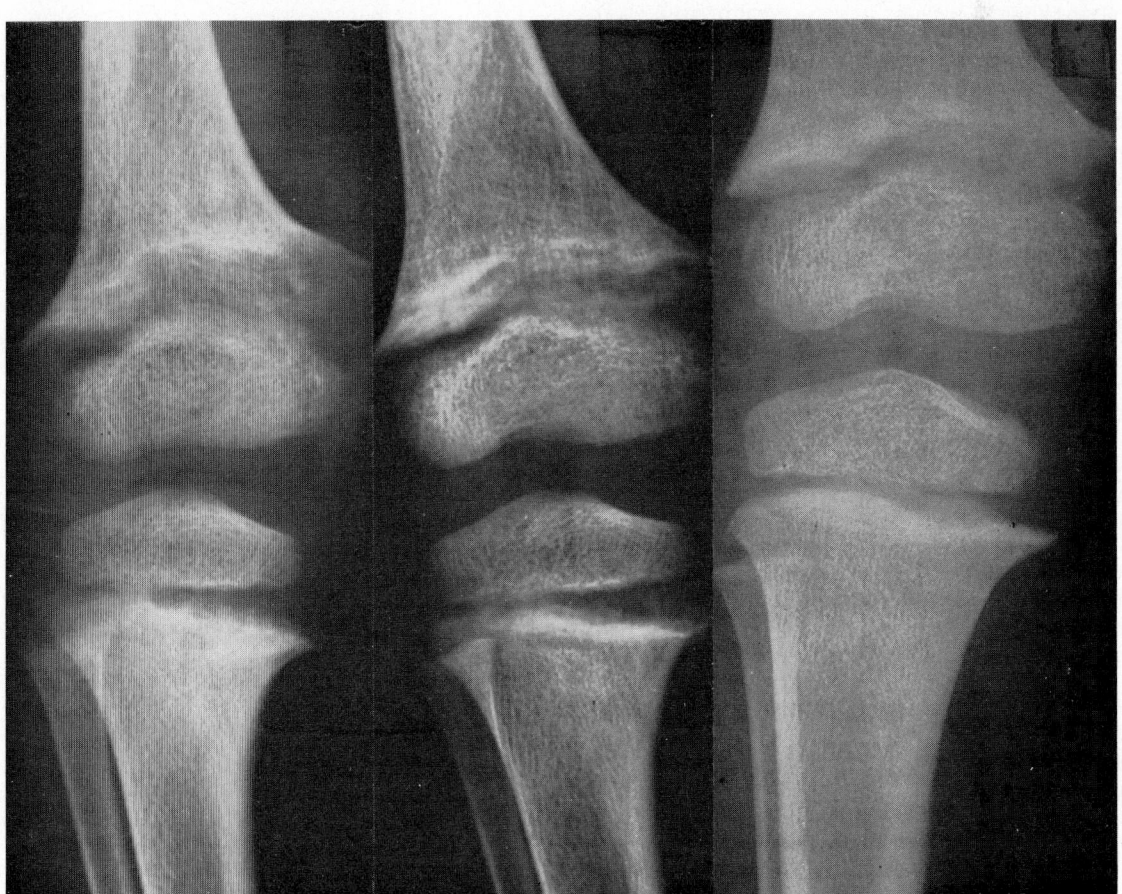

FIG. 16. Roentgenographic findings in 3-year-old patient with primary hypophosphatemia. A. Before treatment. B. Following 4 months of treatment. C. Following 10 months of treatment. The treatment in this case consisted of dihydrotachysterol without added phosphate. (From Harrison and Harrison: Clin Orthop 33:147, 1964.)

thopedic intervention. Radiographic evidence of healing of rickets should be obtained before any surgery. Vitamin D should be discontinued several weeks prior to and subsequent to osteotomy, since if it is continued during the period of immobilization, acute hypercalcemia and hypercalciuria may occur.

HYPOPHOSPHATEMIC VITAMIN D-RESIST-ANT RICKETS IN LATER CHILDHOOD. This is a rare condition in which no metabolic defect is evident during infancy and childhood. During later childhood or early adult life, bone and joint pain, swelling of joints, especially the knees and ankles, and difficulty in walking develop. Severe muscle weakness may occur, and this may be so marked as to suggest a diagnosis of progressive muscular dystrophy. Generalized osteomalacia occurs, and irregularities of the metaphyseal ends of the bones are seen on radiologic examination. Severe deformities of spine and extremities may result. This syndrome is similar to hereditary hypophosphatemia in that the serum calcium concentrations are in the low normal range, 9 to 10 mg/100 ml, while the serum phosphorus levels are reduced, often below 2 mg/100 ml. Serum alkaline phosphatase activity is moderately elevated. Balance studies reveal poor intestinal absorption of calcium and reduced excretion of calcium in urine. Intestinal absorption of phosphate also is diminished, but renal clearances of phosphate are high despite the extremely low serum phosphorus levels, indicating a renal tubular defect in phosphate reabsorption.

It is now recognized that some of these patients have connective tissue tumors that may possibly secrete a phosphaturic principal other than parathyroid hormone. In addition, these patients may show hyperglycinuria or renal glycosuria. The tumors may be within the skeleton, resembling nonossifying fibromas, or they may be extraskeletal, in deep subcutaneous tissue or in unusual locations such as the nasal septum or pharyngeal wall. Histologically they are of mesenchymal origin, but they have been variously diagnosed as ossifying hemangiomas, neurinomas, or pericytomas. Strenuous efforts should be made to find such tumors in patients with acquired hypophosphatemia, since removal of the tumor results in dramatic improvements. If a tumor cannot be found and removed, the treatment of these patients is similar to that of patients with familial hypophosphatemic vitamin-D-resistant rickets.

RENAL TUBULAR ACIDOSIS WITH RICKETS AND OSTEOMALACIA. This syndrome is probably an inborn error or renal tubule cell metabolism. In most reported cases there has been no familial occurrence, but the condition has occurred in siblings, thus suggesting inheritance as an autosomal dominant trait. The biochemical disturbances are discussed on page 237. Treatment with alkalinizing solutions corrects the acidosis and allows healing of rickets without administration of large amounts of vitamin D.

FANCONI SYNDROME. The term Fanconi syndrome has been applied to a group of conditions characterized by renal glycosuria, renal amino-aciduria, and hypophosphatemia, with associated rickets and osteomalacia. This combination suggests proximal renal tubular dysfunction; the renal tubular injury may result from several congenital or acquired causes   (p. 237). The hypophosphatemia and the rickets can be treated with administration of vitamin D in doses of 25,000 to 50,000 IU/day or more; correction of acidosis is also important.

Intrinsic Disorders of Bone That Resemble Rickets

Abnormalities of bone metabolism may result in defective formation of bone and cartilage matrix in which bone mineral fails to deposit normally despite normal serum concentrations of calcium and phosphorus. Two such diseases that may be confused with rickets because of similar skeletal deformities and radiographic changes are hypophosphatasia and metaphyseal dysostosis.

HYPOPHOSPHATASIA. Hypophosphatasia is a hereditary disease transmitted by an autosomal recessive gene. In the homozygote, tissue and serum alkaline phosphatase activities are markedly reduced. Serum phosphorus levels are normal; serum calcium levels may be normal, but sometimes they are elevated as high as 12 to 15 mg/100 ml. Radiographs show marked disorganization of mineralization at the ends of the shafts (Fig. 17). Abnormalities of dentition and skull growth, with premature fusion of the cranial sutures, may occur. Spontaneous improvement tends to occur with growth. Cortisol therapy has been reported to improve calcification of the bones.

METAPHYSEAL   DYSOSTOSIS. Metaphyseal dysostosis is a rare disorder, presumably of congenital origin, associated with progressive deformities of the long bones that mimic the deformities of chronic rickets. The radiographs resemble those of primary hypophosphatemic   vitamin-D-resistant   rickets.   Serum calcium, phosphorus, and alkaline phosphatase concentrations are normal, and phosphate or vitamin D therapy is ineffective. The bony lesions are progressive, and severe deformity may result. Pathologically there is an excess of nonmineralized osteoid, but the underlying defect of the matrix is unkown. There is no known treatment, but osteotomy may be necessary to correct severe deformities of the lower extremities.

PARATHYROID GLANDS
Harold E. Harrison

The parathyroid glands arise from the third and fourth pharyngeal pouches as the four glands that are usually embedded in the capsule of the thyroid. There may be more than four glands, and one or more may be found in the thymus gland or in aberrant locations in the neck. Histologically there are two major cell types: the chief cell and the oxyphilic cell, the latter not ordinarily being seen until after puberty. During hyperplasia of the parathyroids a highly vacuolated variant of the chief cell (the wasserhelle or water-clear cell) may predominate. The glands synthesize a polypeptide molecule of about 9,500 daltons molecular weight (proparathyroid hormone) that is converted into the active circulating hormone by the splitting off of six amino acids. This molecule subsequently undergoes degradation, with formation of smaller fragments that

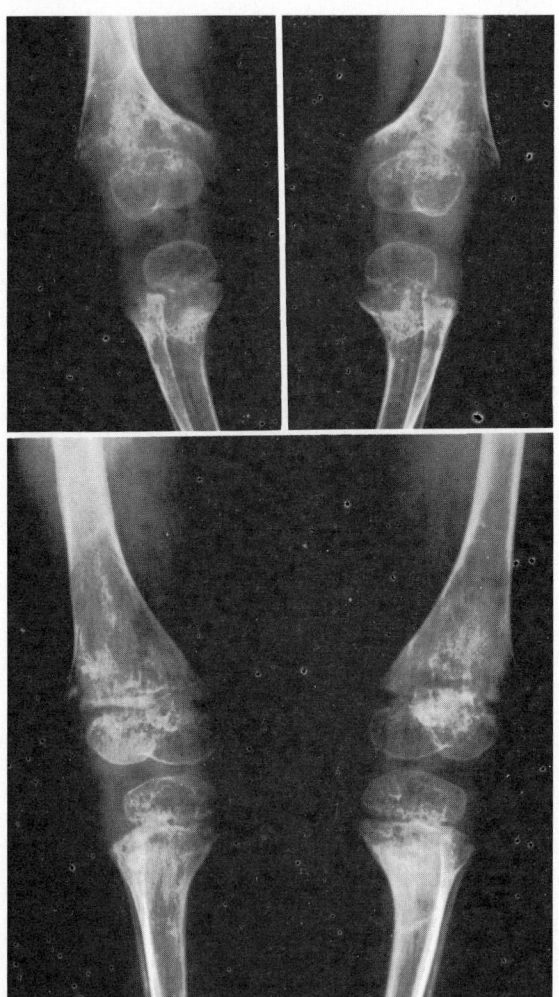

FIG. 17. Hypophosphatasia shown in roentgenograms of knees. Top: age 2 years 2 months. Bottom: age 4 years 10 months.

may or may not have physiologic activity. Because of the multiplicity of polypeptides circulating, the immunoassay of parathyroid hormone may give variable results, depending upon which molecules the particular antibody recognizes. The value of the measurement of immunoreactive parathyroid hormone (IPTH) will be discussed later.

Parathyroid hormone has at least three functions: (1) alteration of bone cell development and metabolism, with resulting increased solubilization of bone mineral

and concomitant dissolution of bone matrix causing resorption of bone and liberation of the ions Ca^{++} and HPO_4^- into extracellular fluid due to an action on both osteocytes and osteoclasts; (2) inhibition of net tubular reabsorption of phosphate, thus increasing renal clearance of a phosphate; (3) stimulation of conversion of 25-hydroxy vitamin D to 1,25-dihydroxy vitamin D in the kidney. This last action may explain the effect of parathyroid hormone in increasing calcium and phosphate absorption by the intestine, although the possibility of a direct action on intestinal transport remains. The actions on bone cells and renal tubules have been shown to be mediated by increased concentrations of cyclic AMP resulting from stimulation of adenylcyclase in cell membranes; in the kidney this is associated with increased cyclic AMP excretion in urine. The net result of increased parathyroid hormone secretion is to increase the entrance of $Ca++$ and HPO_4^- into extracellular fluids; however, only the concentration of calcium ions increases. The concentration of HPO_4^- decreases because of the phosphaturia resulting from reduced tubular reabsorption. The rate of parathyroid hormone secretion is controlled by the concentrations of Ca^{++} and Mg^{++} in the fluid surrounding the cells; a deficiency of either stimulates secretion and an excess inhibits it. A marked deficiency of Mg^{++} causes failure of parathyroid gland function, with inadequate secretion of hormone as well as possible refractoriness of bone cells to the hormone.

Hypoparathyroidism

TRANSIENT PHYSIOLOGIC HYPOPARATHYROIDISM. In the early postnatal period the parathyroid glands are relatively unresponsive, as manifested by lack of increase of parathyroid hormone concentration in response to reduced serum calcium ion concentration. This may be due to suppression of parathyroid gland function during fetal life by the relatively high concentration of calcium ion in fetal plasma resulting from transplacental transfer of calcium ion and possibly the physiologic hyperparathyroidism of the last trimester of pregnancy. Initially there may also be a partial target cell unresponsiveness to parathyroid hormone action. This hypofunction of parathyroid glands can result in neonatal hypocalcemia, either within the first 36 to 48 hours following birth or several days or weeks after feeding with high-phosphate milk.

The factors predisposing to early hypocalcemia are prematurity, asphyxia, acidosis, difficult and prolonged labor, and neonatal metabolic abnormalities due to maternal diabetes. The common factor may be increased metabolism and breakdown of cell organic phosphate with release of inorganic phosphate into extracellular fluid. The phosphate combines with Ca^{++}, thus decreasing calcium ion concentration. Inadequate parathyroid gland response results in a lack of compensation and a progressive decrease of Ca^{++}. The usual manifestations are increased excitability of the nervous system, with muscle hypertonicity, laryngospasm, and convulsions; hypocalcemia is probably the most common single cause of convulsions in the neonatal period. Some infants may present primarily with apneic episodes and marked lethargy, rather than hyperexcitability. The diagnosis is made by determination of serum calcium; usually total serum calcium (ie, protein-bound calcium, filterable calcium complexes, and ionic calcium) is measured. At present, calcium ion concentrations, using a Ca^{++} electrode, are not generally determined. If the total serum calcium is reduced below 7.5 mg/100 ml a reduction of calcium ion is possible, and if symptoms are present then treatment should be started. This consists of slow intravenous injection of 2ml/kg of 10 percent calcium gluconate; it is given with constant monitoring of heart rate, since a rapid infusion may cause bradycardia and even cardiac arrest. The dose may be repeated in 6 hours, or calcium gluconate (4 to 6 ml/kg/24 hours) may be given by constant infusion. Symptoms may not recur after this initial course; if hypocalcemia persists it can be treated by the regime given below for late hypocalcemia. Prematurely born infants often show continued hypocalcemia for several weeks, and it may possibly contribute to respiratory difficulties.

Late or postfeeding hypocalcemia of the newborn appears after several days of feeding in otherwise healthy, full-term infants and is related to phosphate intake. It is rare in breast-fed infants, since breast milk has a phosphorus content of 150 to 175 mg/liter, in contrast to the 1,000 mg/liter of cow's milk. The high intake of phosphorus, together with a low rate of glomerular filtration, leads to an increased concentration of serum phosphorus, with resultant reduction of ionized calcium. Symptoms may occur within 4 to 5 days, or they may occur only after several weeks. Initial symptoms are poor feeding, vomiting, and cyanotic spells followed by recurrent tonic and clonic convulsions; sudden onset of convulsions may be the first sign. Some infants present with lethargy and are suspected of having infection; serum levels of calcium and phosphorus should be measured in cases of suspected neonatal infection. Reduction of ionized calcium alters the electrical activity of the heart, producing a prolongation of the Q-T interval. Occasionally bradycardia and heart block may occur (p. 1402).

The principles of treatment are to reduce serum phosphate levels by sequestration of phosphate in the intestine, thus preventing its absorption, and to increase absorption of calcium from the intestine. This can be accomplished simply by adding a calcium salt to the diet so that calcium is in great excess, which results in precipitation of calcium phosphate in the gut; a ratio of calcium to phosphorus of 4:1 by weight provides a sufficient excess of calcium. In the infant calcium lactate and calcium gluconate are most suitable, since they are soluble in milk and do not produce gastrointestinal irritation or metabolic disturbances. Syrup of Neo-Calglucon is a palatable but expensive preparation of calcium gluconogalactogluconate; it contains a high concentration of sucrose, which may cause diarrhea in the newborn. For this reason we do not recommend its use. If the infant is receiving a cow's milk feeding providing

500 mg of phosphorus and 600 mg of calcium, an additonal 1,400 mg of calcium would have to be added to give a calcium-to-phosphorus ratio of 4:1. This would be supplied by 11 g of calcium lactate powder; feeding of only 2 to 3 g of calcium lactate, as is sometimes done, would be without benefit. With treatment, serum calcium concentrations can rise to values above normal as serum phosphorus is decreased. This does not indicate recovery of parathyroid function, since the serum calcium concentration may fall again when calcium supplement is withdrawn and serum phosphorus concentration rises. The elevation of the serum calcium concentration above normal is probably due to lack of removal of absorbed calcium by the bone when concentrations of extracellular phosphate are low. This can easily be corrected by reducing the extra calcium supplement so that serum phosphorus concentration rises sufficiently to prevent hypercalcemia. It is of interest that serum magnesium concentrations are inversely related to serum phosphate. In transient physiologic hypoparathyroidism of the infant, treatment may be needed only for 7 to 10 days or for as long as 4 to 6 weeks.

Emergency treatment of convulsions or laryngospasm may be needed. The convulsions of hypocalcemia are relatively refractory to the usual anticonvulsive agents, phenobarbital and diphenylhydantoin. Intravenous calcium gluconate should be given in the dosage mentioned previously.

PERSISTENT HYPOPARATHYROIDISM. Congenital absence of the parathyroids may be seen in conjunction with failure of thymus development (DiGeorge syndrome) or without abnormality of the thymus. The initial presentation of this condition may resemble that of transitory physiologic hypoparathyroidism. Suspicion of a more severe deficiency of parathyroid function will arise because of poor response to therapy with calcium, with persistence of hypocalcemia. Determination of immunoreactive parathyroid hormone (IPTH) should be of value, since the concentrations should be undetectable. If thymatic aplasia is also present the immunologic abnormalities consequent to the lack of this organ will be present (p. 316).

In later infancy and childhood idiopathic hypoparathyroidism may occur, presumably due to disappearance of parathyroid function. It is currently thought that the major cause is autoimmunity, and antibodies against parathyroid tissue may be demonstrated. Autoimmune parathyroid disease may be associated with more widespread autoimmune injury to other secretory cells, including adrenal cortex and gastric mucosa; parathyroid insufficiency thus may be complicated by adrenal insufficiency and pernicious anemia. These autoimmune diseases of the endocrine system can have a genetic basis, which is particularly evident in the combination of hypoparathyroidism and adrenal insufficiency, a familial autosomal recessive disorder. The chronic hypocalcemia of parathyroid insufficiency is associated with metabolic abnormalities of ectodermal tissue, manifesting as alopecia, abnormal pitting and ridging of fingernails, and cataracts. The ectodermal changes may be present in patients without the nervous system manifestations of hypocalcemia; children with ectodermal defects, particularly cataracts, should have determinations of serum calcium. The skin and nails are susceptible to infection with *Candida,* which causes intractable moniliasis; this is particularly severe in patients with combined hypoparathyroidism and hypoadrenalism, and death from systemic moniliasis has been reported. Another manifestation whose pathogenesis is uncertain is perivascular calcification in the basal ganglion area of the brain.

In hypoparathyroidism total serum calcium concentration is usually less than 7.5 mg/100 ml. Serum phosphorus concentration may be as high as 10 to 12 mg/100 ml in the hypoparathyroid infant and 5 to 6 mg/100ml in the hypoparathyroid adult; serum magnesium concentration is also frequently reduced. Levels of alkaline phosphatase are usually normal, but may be somewhat increased in the infant. Bone radiographs are normal. Infants and young children often present with generalized convulsions that may be precipitated by fever but that are usually repetitive. Electroencephalographic tracings may be indistinguishable from those of the grand mal seizures of idiopathic epilepsy; thus serum calcium and phosphorus levels should be measured in all cases of convulsions. Older patients may develop chronic tetany with hyperexcitability of the peripheral nervous system. The motor manifestations are muscle spasm causing laryngospasm and carpopedal spasm, in which the hands and feet are extended and adducted. The motor nerves can be stimulated by tapping. If the facial nerve is tapped anterior to the parotid, a muscle contraction of the orbicularis oris or oculi is obtained (Chvostek's sign). Tapping of the peroneal nerve behind the head of the fibula produces the peroneal sign (dorsiflexion and external rotation of the foot). The motor nerves also have a lowered threshold to electric excitation (Erb's sign), or to ischemia produced by interruption of arterial circulation for a few minutes (Trousseau's sign). The sensory manifestations are numbness and paresthesias of the extremities. Incomplete hypoparathyroidism can result from inadvertent parathyroidectomy or injury to the vascular supply of the parathyroids during subtotal thyroidectomy.

TREATMENT. Incomplete hypoparathyroidism in older children and adults following thyroidectomy sometimes can be treated by large amounts of calcium in the diet to sequester phosphate in the gut and prevent its absorption. This requires 2 to 5 g of calcium given as capsules or as a 10 percent suspension of calcium carbonate, which contains 40 percent calcium. Calcium lactate can be used, but much larger amounts are required to supply an equivalent quantity of calcium. In the complete absence of parathyroid hormone, large amounts of vitamin D or vitamin D-like steroids such as dihydrotachysterol are needed to increase calcium absorption from the gut and to increase solubilization of vone mineral by stimulation of bone cell metabolism. Pharmacologic amounts of vitamin D given chronically also reduce tubular reabsorption of phosphate. Prolonged treatment with vitamin D steroids will reduce serum phosphorus concentrations to some extent and also raise serum calcium. Vitamin D or dihydrotachysterol can be combined with calcium carbonate or calcium lactate, but it is usually possible to maintain serum calcium concentrations in children with vitamin D alone.

Dihydrotachysterol is more potent than vitamin D as a pharmacologic substitute for parathyroid hormone; its chief advantage is its more rapid inactivation in the body, thus making cumulative toxicity less likely than with vitamin D. In infants and young children the dose of dihydrotachysterol is usually 0.1 to 0.5 mg/day, and in older children and adults it is 0.5 to 1.0 mg/day. The dose is adjusted to maintain the serum calcium concentration in the low normal range of 8.5 to 10 mg/100 ml. A rise of serum calcium concentration above 10.5 mg/100 ml calls for temporary discontinuance of treatment and resumption at a lower dosage after serum calcium concentrations have decreased. If vitamin D_2 (ergocalciferol) is used rather than dihydrotachysterol, the corresponding doses in infants and children are 15,000 to 50,000 IU/day (0.38 to 1.25 mg) and 50,000 to 150,000 IU/day in adults (1.25 to 3.75 mg). Patients receiving more than 100,000 IU/day are at risk of becoming hypercalcemic, and since vitamin D is so slowly inactivated and eliminated from the body, once toxic effects occur it may be necessary to discontinue treatment for months before serum calcium concentrations begin to fall.

Sudden onset of hypercalcemia in a patient with idiopathic hypoparathyroidism who has been controlled for some time on a stable dose of dihydrotachysterol or vitamin D should cause one to consider the possibility that adrenal insufficiency has developed. Cortisol antagonizes the action of vitamin D on intestinal absorption of calcium, and a sudden decrease of cortisol secretion can result in rapid increase of serum calcium concentration. These patients are difficult to treat.

Refractoriness to vitamin D or dihydrotachysterol can develop in hypoparathyroid patients who initially responded satisfactorily; this refractoriness may be overcome by changing the steroid, but sometimes huge doses of either steroid may be relatively ineffective. This may be associated with marked steatorrhea, a rare complication of hypoparathyroidism; the steatorrhea diminishes if serum calcium is increased. A low-fat diet or substitution of medium-chain triglycerides for part of the dietary fat, addition of calcium carbonate to the diet, and addition of dihydrotachysterol in amounts of 5 to 10 mg/day may break the vicious cycle, with return of more normal responsiveness. Magnesium chloride in doses of 2 to 4 mEq/kg/day has been used to try to improve steroid responsiveness.

Because of the newly recognized role of parathyroid hormone in controlling the rate of conversion of 25-hydroxy vitamin D to the active vitamin D metabolite (1,25-dihydroxy vitamin D), the latter compound and another synthetic vitamin D derivative (1α-hydroxy vitamin D) have been used experimentally in the treatment of hypoparathyroidism. Preliminary evidence indicates that these compounds are much more potent than either vitamin D or dihydrotachysterol and may be the drugs of choice.

PSEUDOHYPOPARATHYROIDISM. Pseudohypoparathyroidism is a genetically determined abnormality of response to parathyroid hormone in which the hormone fails to activate specific adenylcyclase in kidney and bone. There is therefore no phosphaturic response to parathyroid extract nor an elevation of serum calcium concentration. In addition to the refractoriness of the target cell to parathyroid hormone, these patients have an abnormality of growth that is independent of hypocalcemia. They are short and stocky and have round faces and short pudgy hands and feet. A characteristic abnormality is growth failure of the fourth and fifth metacarpals and metatarsals, so that the fourth and fifth fingers and toes are strikingly short. When the hands are clenched no knuckles are evident at the ends of the fourth and fifth metacarpals, since they are so short. Mental retardation of modest degree is usually present. Intracranial calcification and periarticular subcutaneous calcification is more prominent than in patients with hypoparathyroidism. Family studies suggest a dominant mode of genetic inheritance. Individuals have been described who have characteristic morphologic changes, but normal serum calcium and phosphorus concentrations, a condition termed pseudo-pseudohypoparathyroidism. Treatment of the hypocalcemia is the same as in idiopathic hypoparathyroidism.

HYPOPARATHYROIDISM AND MAGNESIUM DEFICIENCY. Hypomagnesemia can be seen in infants with transient physiologic hypoparathyroidism secondary to the marked hyperphosphatemia that is also present in these patients; it is corrected by reduction of serum phosphate by addition of calcium salts to the feeding. However, there are rare instances of primary hypomagnesemia due to a defect of intestinal absorption of magnesium; these patients have secondary hypocalcemia that is not corrected until serum magnesium is increased by intramuscular injection of magnesium sulfate or feeding of a magnesium salt such as magnesium chloride. In primary hypomagnesemia there is secondary hypoparathyroidism because of the need for magnesium for normal secretory activity by the parathyroids. Secondary hypoparathyroidism can also result from the magnesium deficiency of chronic intestinal malabsorption, as seen in Crohn's disease or in patients who have had surgical removal of a considerable portion of the small intestine. Hypomagnesemia, with or without hypocalcemia, can cause tetany and convulsions and should be suspected if the reduction of serum calcium concentration does not seem great enough to account for the severity of the manifestations, or if the hypocalcemia is not corrected by the treatment previously outlined in the section on hypoparathyroidism. Serum magnesium concentrations below 1.0 mg/100 ml (0.8 mEq/liter) indicate the possibility of primary hypomagnesemia. The initial therapy can be intramuscular injection of magnesium sulfate (0.2 ml/kg of 50 percent $MgSO_4 \cdot 12H_2O$), which should raise the serum

magnesium concentration into the physiologic range. If renal function is normal the serum magnesium concentration will return to pretreatment levels in 4 to 6 hours, so that repeated injections must be given to maintain normal concentrations. For chronic treatment oral magnesium as magnesium chloride, citrate, or lactate (2 to 4 mEq/kg/day) in divided doses can be used.

Hyperparathyroidism

Primary hyperparathyroidism is rare during childhood. It is usually due to genetically determined hyperplasia of the parathyroids. There have been several reports of an autosomal recessive inheritance of parathyroid hyperplasia with onset in infancy; there are also families in which parathyroid hyperplasia is transmitted as an autosomal dominant and is often associated with other endocrinopathies of the thyroid and adrenal glands and pancreas (multiple endocrine neoplasia, type I). Although it is genetically determined, the manifestations may not appear until adult life; however, asymptomatic children of affected adults may show hypercalcemia and hypophosphatemia. As in adults, an adenoma of a single parathyroid may also occur.

The manifestations of hyperparathyroidism result from (1) systemic effects of hypercalcemia (anorexia, constipation, failure to thrive, polyuria, lethargy, and with marked hypercalcemia, stupor, and death), (2) demineralization of bone, with pathologic fractures and deformities, and (3) renal damage due to calcinosis or stone formation with obstruction and infection. Most infants with congenital hyperplasia of the parathyroids show the systemic symptoms of hypercalcemia. Renal calculi are rare as a presenting manifestation in childhood.

Hyperparathyroidism is diagnosed primarily from elevation of total serum calcium levels. The upper limit of normal depends on the method used, but with standard atomic absorption spectrophotometry, values consistently above 11 mg/100 ml are abnormal. Serum phosphorus concentrations are reduced, usually below 4 mg/100 ml. Alkaline phosphatase activities are not consistently elevated; high alkaline phosphatase usually indicates disease. Bone destruction may occur; the mildest form is generalized demineralization; more severe changes include subperiosteal erosion, particularly in the phalanges, metacarpals, and lateral portions of the clavicle. Destructive changes at the growing ends of the long bones also occur, as well as patchy demineralization of the membranous bones of the skull. Other causes of hypercalcemia, such as hypervitaminosis D and idiopathic hypercalcemia, are usually not associated with reduction of serum phosphorus concentrations. Hypercalcemia due to sarcoid is extremely rare in childhood but may be suspected if serum globulin is markedly increased and there is other evidence of sarcoidosis.

Determination of immunoreactive parathyroid hormone (IPTH) can be of value in the differential diagnosis. If the disorder is due to hypervitaminosis D or increased sensitivity to vitamin D (idiopathic hypercalcemia or sarcoidosis), the IPTH levels are very low, whereas in hyperparathyroidism they are either elevated or at the upper limits of normal and are thus relatively high in relation to high serum calcium concentrations. Because of heterogeneity of the parathyroid hormone (PTH) polypeptides in plasma and differences in their recognition by different immune sera, results of IPTH levels from different laboratories are not the same. There is also a diurnal variation in serum PTH concentration; determinations should be made at a uniform time, preferably by a single laboratory; they should also be interpreted in relation to the serum calcium concentration determined at the same time. An additional differential diagnostic procedure is the use of suppressive doses of adrenocorticoids, cortisol, prednisone, or dexamethasone. The hypercalcemia of hypervitaminosis D, idiopathic hypercalcemia, tumors, or sarcoid usually responds to a 10-day course of adrenocorticoids, whereas that of hyperparathyroidism is ordinarily refractory.

Acute hypercalcemia is treated by maintenance of hy-

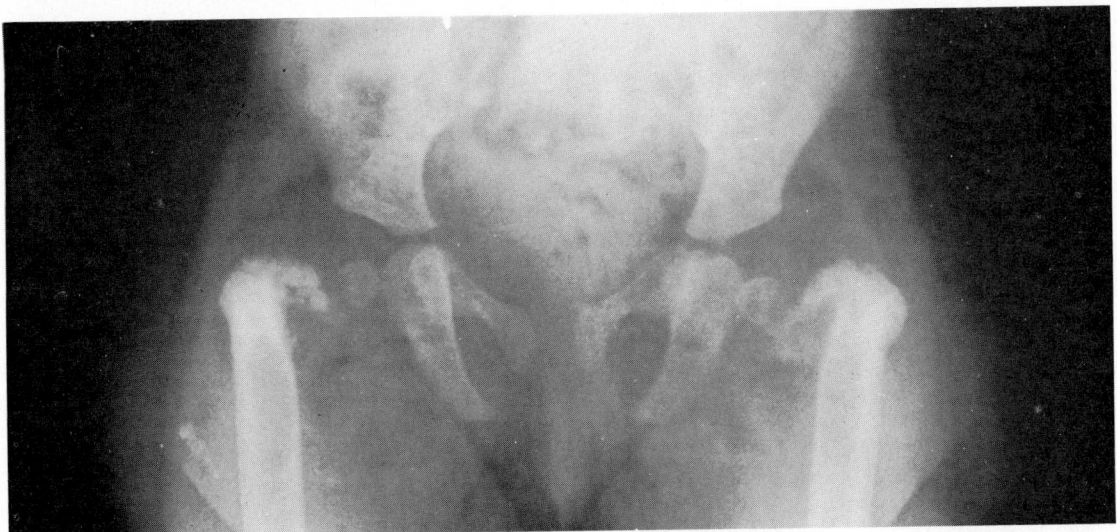

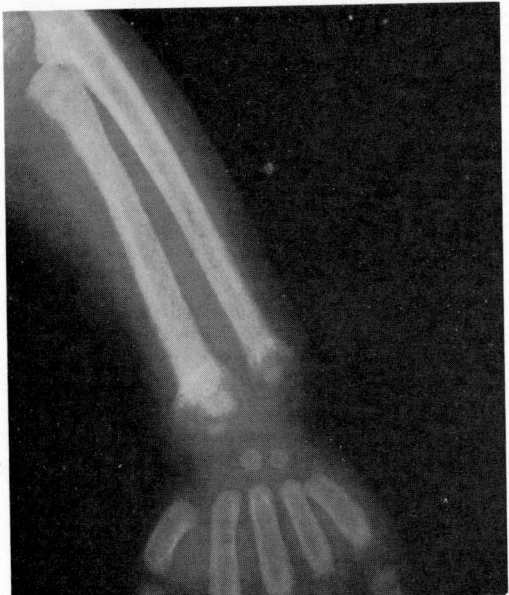 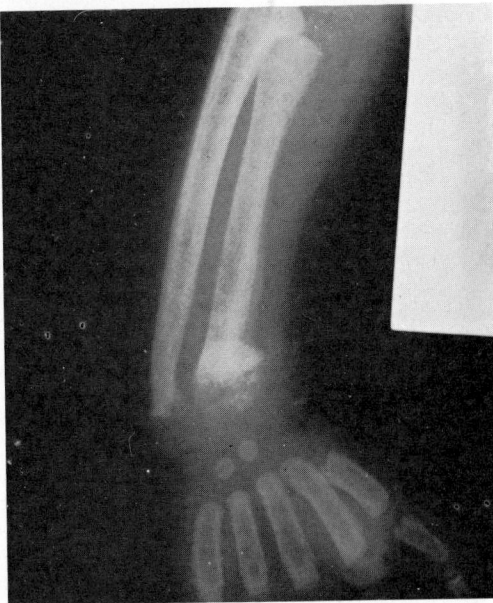

FIG. 18. Bone changes in secondary hyperparathyroidism. This child with congenital hypoplasia of both kidneys developed an extraordinary degree of secondary hyperparathyroidism with marked subperiosteal erosion and destruction of the femoral necks and the distal ends of the radii. These lesions healed following treatment with calcium salts and dihydrotachysterol, as outlined in the text.

dration and production of natriuresis and calciuresis. These effects can be achieved by the intravenous injection of a natriuretic such as furosemide or ethacrynic acid, with replacement of the sodium and potassium lost in the urine. Thiazide diuretics cannot be used for this purpose, since they cause increased tubular reabsorption of calcium and reduction of urine calcium excretion. Following emergency treatment of the acute hypercalcemia, the chronic hypercalcemia can only be treated adequately by parathyroidectomy. In adults, hypercalcemia and hypophosphatemia of hyperparathyroidism have been ameliorated by oral intake of phosphate salts equivalent to 2 g or more of phosphorus daily; this treatment has not been evaluated in children. Treatment by parathyroidectomy is complicated by the fact that usually the chief cell hyperplasia involves all the parathyroids; partial parathyroidectomy, with removal of three of the four glands, has been unsuccessful in many of these patients. Total parathyroidectomy results in subsequent hypoparathyroidism, which must be treated for the remainder of the child's life. After parathyroidectomy a rapid drop in serum calcium concentration with tetany can supervene; serum calcium should be monitored and intravenous calcium gluconate given if the calcium concentration decreases rapidly. After total parathyroidectomy treatment with oral dihydrotachysterol or vitamin D may be necessary.

Secondary hyperparathyroidism (renal osteodystrophy): Secondary parathyroid hyperplasia and hypersecretion are induced by elevation of serum phosphate and lowering of serum calcium ion concentrations. In renal insufficiency with marked reduction of glomerular filtration rate, serum phosphate levels are markedly elevated. The serum calcium concentrations are reduced due to decreased intestinal absorption of calcium as well as to lessened solubility of calcium in the presence of phosphate excess. The resulting parathyroid hyperfunction does not necessarily restore normal levels of calcium ion or phosphate, but produces osteitis fibrosa and bone demineralization. Low serum calcium concentration is in part due to calcium malabsorption. Patients with renal insufficiency show a resistance to the normal physiologic action of vitamin D on intestinal calcium absorption. The elevated serum phosphate concentrations are also responsible for reduction of serum calcium levels by the reprecipitation of calcium phosphate in soft tissues as well as bone. The bone lesions are more complex than those of primary hyperparathyroidism, and histologic evidences of rickets and osteomalacia, as well as osteitis fibrosa, are seen. On radiographic examination both the changes of rickets at the ends of the long bones and the subperiosteal erosions of hyperparathyroidism are seen (Fig. 18). The rachitic changes have been variously ascribed to chronic acidosis, to low calcium ion concentrations, or to some hypothetical disturbance of bone matrix resulting in inhibition of calcification. Despite the hypocalcemia, metastatic calcification may be found in blood vessels and subcutaneous tissue in patients with marked hyperphosphatemia.

The renal lesion causing the osteodystrophy may be hypoplasia of the kidneys, obstructive uropathy, chronic pyelonephritis, or chronic diffuse glomerulonephritis, but slow progression is necessary so that the skeletal changes become manifest before the metabolic disturbances of renal insufficiency are incompatible with growth. In the advanced stages, dwarfism, anemia, and chronic acidosis are seen, along with deformities of weight-bearing bones that cause joint pain and interfere with gait.

Improvement may be obtained by the combination of a high-calcium, low-phosphate diet and vitamin D or dihydrotachysterol. It is usually necessary to reduce the absorption of dietary phosphate with calcium carbonate or lactate (p. 248) or with aluminum hydroxide suspension, which precipitates phosphate in the intestinal lumen. Excessive vitamin D or dihyrotachysterol will enhance metastatic calcification, so that treatment must be followed by careful monitoring of serum calcium levels and radiographic examinations of bones and soft tissues. Metastatic calcification will be lessened if the absorption of phosphate is reduced. If treatment is started early the skeletal manifestations may be prevented. Even when the skeletal changes are marked, as in Figure 18, they can sometimes be reversed by treatment. In some individuals treatment is ineffective, and it has been suggested that the parathyroids have become independent of control by calcium ion concentration and behave like primary hyperplastic glands. Following successful renal homotransplantation, the biochemical changes of primary hyperparathyroidism may be reversed. However, in some cases they may continue or even develop further if overt hypercalcemia has been prevented by the high plasma phosphate accompanying renal failure. If there is persistent evidence of failure of feedback control of parathyroid secretion, with progression of bone disease, parathyroidectomy is indicated.

IDIOPATHIC HYPERCALCEMIA

Idiopathic hypercalcemia of infancy is a condition in which serum calcium concentrations of 12 mg/100 ml or greater occur without obvious cause. It has been suggested that this disorder represents an unusual sensitivity to amounts of vitamin D that would not be toxic to most infants. Certain features of the disease, such as low birth weight, abnormalities of facial structure, and defects of the heart and great vessels, suggest that the disorder has its onset in intrauterine life.

The disease presents insidiously, with anorexia, irritability, vomiting, constipation, and growth failure in the first few months after birth. Slow motor development and mental retardation are frequent findings. The so-called elfin facies, with depressed nasal bridge, prominent upper lip, receding mandible, high narrow palate, and low-set ears, is characteristic. In later childhood dental malocclusion, hypoplasia, and caries are common. In the severe forms renal calcinosis and insufficiency develop, with hypertension, proteinuria, and microscopic hematuria. Abnormalities of the great vessels, particularly supravalvular aortic stenosis and peripheral pulmonary artery stenosis, may be an integral part of the syndrome. Radiographs show increased density of the base of the skull and the metaphyseal ends of the long bones. There are no changes indicative of hyperparathyroidism, but submetaphyseal rarefaction similar to that seen in hypervitaminosis D has been reported. Serum phosphorus levels are normal, unless there is renal insufficiency.

Idiopathic hypercalcemia can be differentiated from hyperparathyroidism by the absence of hypophosphatemia, by the radiographic findings, and by the clinical picture, particularly the characteristic facies and cardiac lesions, if they are present. In idiopathic hypercalcemia serum calcium concentrations almost invariably return to normal following 7 to 10 days of treatment with cortisol or prednisone, whereas the hypercalcemia of hyperparathyroidism is usually refractory. Some individuals demonstrate poor growth, mental retardation, suggestive facies, and the vascular lesions of supravalvular aortic stenosis and/or peripheral pulmonic stenosis, but consistently normal serum calcium levels. The possibility that hypercalcemia was present in the early evolution of the disorder has been suggested, and this has been reinforced by evidences of renal calcinosis in some cases.

Idiopathic hypercalcemia is treated by feeding a very low calcium diet and eliminating vitamin D intake. A low-calcium feeding mixture for infants can be prepared using strained meats as the source of protein, with addition of carbohydrates and vegetable oil. All milk preparations are eliminated. If the hypercalcemia does not respond within 2 weeks of the institution of dietary measures, or if manifestations of hypercalcemia are marked, prednisone should be administered. Adrenocorticoid therapy can be tapered rapidly after 4 to 6 weeks if the serum calcium concentration has returned to normal; the low-calcium diet is continued. The patient can then be tested at intervals to see if the calcium intake can be increased; when addition of calcium to the food does not cause elevation of serum calcium concentrations, the child can resume a standard diet. After recovery, vitamin D does not cause an exacerbation.

References

VITAMIN D METABOLISM AND PHYSIOLOGY

DeLuca HF: Vitamin D: the vitamin and the hormone. Fed Proc 33:2211, 1974

Fraser D, Kooh SW, Scriver CR: Hyperparathyroidism as the cause of hyperaminoaciduria and phosphaturia in human vitamin D deficiency. Pediat Res 1:425, 1967

Harrison HE: Vitamin D and calcium and phosphate transport. Pediatrics 25:531, 1961

Rasmussen H, Bordier P: The Physiological and Cellular Basis of Metabolic Bone Disease. Baltimore, Williams & Wilkins, 1974

NUTRITIONAL VITAMIN D DEFICIENCY

Committee on Nutrition, American Academy of Pediatrics: The prophylactic requirement and the toxicity of vitamin D. Pediatrics 31:512, 1963

Dent CE, Richens A, Rowe DJF, Stamp TCB: Osteomalacia with long term anticonvulsant therapy in epilepsy. Br Med J 4:69, 1970

Fraser D, Kooh SW, Kind HP, Holick MF, DeLuca HF: Pathogenesis of hereditary vitamin D-dependent rickets. An inborn error of vitamin D metabolism involving defective conversion of 25-hydroxyvitamin D to 1-25-dihydroxyvitamin D. N Engl J Med 289:817, 1973

Scriver CR: Vitamin D dependency. Pediatrics 45:361, 1970

HYPOPHOSPHATEMIA OF RENAL TUBULAR ORIGIN WITH ASSOCIATED RICKETS

Albright F, Burnett CH, Parson W, Reifenstein EC Jr, Roos A: Osteomalacia and late rickets: the various etiologies met in the United States with emphasis on that resulting from a special form of renal acidosis; the therapeutic indications for each etiological sub-group and the relationship between osteomalacia and Milkman's syndrome. Medicine 25:399, 1946

Harrison HE, Harrison HC: Hereditary Metabolic bone disease. Clin Orthop 33:147, 1964

————The Fanconi syndrome. J Chronic Dis 7:346, 1958

Salassa RM, Jowsey J, Arnaud CD: Hypophosphatemic osteomalacia associated with non-endocrine tumors. N Engl J Med 283:65, 1972

HYPOPARATHYROIDISM

Albright F, Burnett CH, Smith PH, Parson W: Pseudohypoparathyroidism: an example of the "Seabright-Bantam syndrome": report of three cases. Endocrinology 30:922, 1942

Bakwin H: Tetany in newborn infants. Am J Dis Child 54:1211, 1937

Dent CE, Morgans ME, Harper CM, Philpot GR, Trotler WR: Insensitivity to vitamin D developing during the treatment of post-operative tetany. Its specificity as regards the form of vitamin D taken. Lancet 2:687, 1955

Gardner LI: Tetany and parathyroid hyperplasia in the newborn infant: influence of dietary phosphate load. Pediatrics 9:534, 1962

Harrison HE: Hypoparathyroidism. Modern Treatment 7:636, 1970

————Lifshitz F, Blizzard RM: Comparison between crystalline dihydrotachysterol and calciferol in patients requiring pharmacologic vitamin D therapy. N Engl J Med 276:894, 1967

Suh SM, Tashjian AH, Matsuo N, Parkinson DK, Fraser D: Pathogenesis of hypocalcemia in primary hypomagnesemia; normal end-organ responsiveness to parathyroid hormone, impaired parathyroid gland function. J Clin Invest 52:153, 1973

Sutphin W, Albright F, McCune DJ: Five cases (three in siblings) of idiopathic hypoparathyroidism associated with moniliasis. J Clin Endocrinol 3:625, 1943

Tsang RC, Light LJ, Sutherland JM, Kleinman LI: Possible pathogenic factors in neonatal hypocalcemia of prematurity. J Pediatr 82:423, 1973

PRIMARY HYPERPARATHYROIDISM

Anderson J, Harper C, Dent CE, Philpot GR: Effect of cortisone on calcium metabolism in sarcoidosis with hypercalcemia. Lancet 2:720, 1954

Cutler RE, Reiss E, Ackerman LV: Familial hyperparathyroidism. A kindred involving eleven cases with a discussion of primary giant cell hyperplasia. N Engl J Med 270:859, 1964

Goldbloom RB, Gills DA, Prasad M: Hereditary parathyroid hyperplasia: a surgical emergency of early infancy. Pediatrics 49:514, 1971

Hillman DA, Scriver CR, Pedris S, Shragovitch I: Neonatal familial primary hyperparathyroidism. N Engl J Med 270:483, 1964

Lowe KG, Henderson JL, Park WW, McGreal DA: The idiopathic hypercalcemia syndromes of infancy. Lancet 2:101, 1954

Nolan RB, Hayles AB, Woolner LB: Adenoma of parathyroid gland in children: report of case and brief review of literature. Am J Dis Child 22:622, 1960

SECONDARY HYPERPARATHYROIDISM

Bricker NS, Slatopolsky E, Reiss E, Avioli LV: Calcium, phosphorus and bone in renal disease and transplant. Arch Intern Med 123:543, 1969

Castleman B, Mallory TB: Parathyroid hyperplasia in chronic renal insufficiency. Am J Pathol 12:553, 1937

DeLuca HF: The kidney as an endocrine organ involved in the function of vitamin D. Am J Med 58:39, 1975

Follis RH Jr: Renal rickets and osteitis fibrosa in children and adolescents. Bull Johns Hopkins Hosp 87:593, 1950

Gill G, Pallota J, Kashgarian M, Kessner D, Epstein FH: Physiologic studies in renal osteodystrophy treated by subtotal parathyroidectomy. Am J Med 46:930, 1969

Stanbury SW: Calcium and phosphate metabolism in renal failure. In Straus MB, Welt LG (eds): Diseases of the Kidney. Boston, Little, Brown, 1971, p 305

IDIOPATHIC HYPERCALCEMIA

American Academy of Pediatrics, Committee on Nutrition: The relation between infantile hypercalcemia and vitamin D—public health implications in North America. Pediatrics 40:1050, 1967

Bonham Carter RE, Sutliffe J: A syndrome of multiple arterial stenosis in association with the severe form of idiopathic hypercalcemia. Arch Dis Child 39:418, 1964

Garcia RG, Friedman WF, Kaback MM, Rowe RD: Idiopathic hypercalcemia and supravalvular aortic stenosis. Documentation of a new syndrome. N Engl J Med 271:117, 1964

Lightwood R, Stapleton T: Idiopathic hypercalcemia in infants. Lancet 2:255, 1953

OBESITY

Elsa Proehl Paulsen

There are good reasons for those concerned with the well-being of children to be interested in the problem of obesity. Fat children suffer from the contemptuous attitudes of their peers and frequently their parents. As a result, lifelong feelings of inadequacy may be generated. Physical limitations imposed by their size and embarrassment over their appearance serve to deny them many pleasant and healthful activities of childhood. Furthermore, obesity continues into adult life in more than 80 percent of overweight children. Epidemiologic studies in adults have shown a significant correlation between marked obesity and mortality attributed to cardiovascular disease and diabetes. Unfortunately the long-term treatment of obesity in children, as in adults, has generally ended in failure. If progress is to be made in lessening the prevalence of this disorder, increased emphasis must be placed upon prevention.

Obesity, defined as a marked increase of body fat, is easily recognized. It is more difficult to assess its severity and especially to interpret lesser degrees of excess weight. An increase in lean body mass (LBM) rather than fat may account for increased weight; LBM may vary considerably in children of the same height. Also, data in weight tables drawn from selected ethnic and socioeconomic groups are not universally applicable, since such weights are by definition normative and not necessarily desirable weights. The average or "normal" weights of adults in the United States have increased significantly over the past 30 years. A similar trend toward increased weight has been noted in children (Fig. 19). Whether these increases in mean weight during the growing period will eventually contribute to health problems in adult life poses an important question. Even with their limitations, height–weight tables are adequate for estimating excessive overweight. Children whose weights are 10 to 20 percent above the mean for

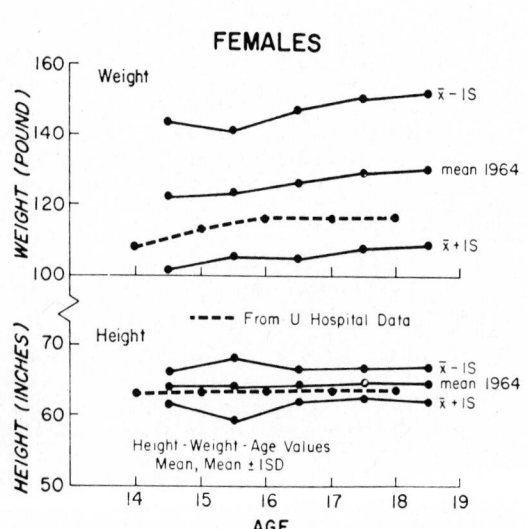

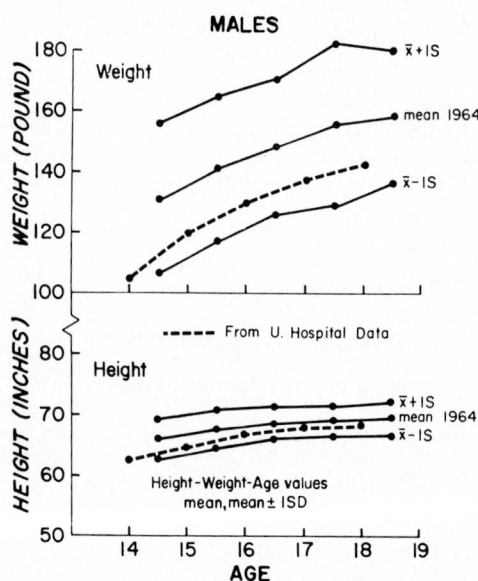

FIG. 19. Comparison of heights and weights of Iowa teenagers obtained in 1964 (solid lines) with those published in 1943 (dash line), taken from University Hospital data, widely known as the Iowa Norms. (From Hodges and Krehl: Am J Clin Nutr 17:200, 1965.)

their height and age are defined as markedly over-weight; those with weights greater than 20 percent above the mean are defined as obese.

INCIDENCE.   A survey of 300 normal infants up to 1 year of age by Shukla and associates in England revealed an incidence of infantile obesity of 16.7 percent and an incidence of overweight of 27.7 percent. No such data are available among infants in the United States. Surveys in high school students in various parts of the United States indicate rates of obesity ranging from 10 to 30 percent. Differences in cultural, social, and economic backgrounds of the children probably account for much of the variation. It has been shown that birth weights of children who later become obese do not differ significantly from those of children whose later weights are normal. However, in Eid's study in Sheffield, England, infants who had excessive weight gain during the first 6 months had a much higher incidence of overweight at 6 to 8 years. Similarly, Heald noted that mean weight was significantly greater at 1 year in girls who were obese at 15 years than it was in girls who were of normal weight at 15 years. Mossberg indicates that there are two peaks of onset of childhood obesity: from birth to 4 years and from 7 to 11 years.

ETIOLOGY

GENETIC FACTORS.   Evidence from studies of twins shows that genetic factors play a role in the development of obesity in children. Newman and associates found a high correlation for weight between monozygotic twins but not between disygotic twins or between siblings at comparable ages; this correlation was not affected by having the twins reared in different environments. Seltzer and Mayer found that obesity occurred significantly more often in adolescent girls with endomorphic body type than in those with mesomorphic or ectomorphic body types. This further supports a genetic determinant in obesity, since the hereditary nature of body build is fairly well documented.

ENERGY BALANCE.   Factors that control the balance between caloric intake and energy expenditure and lead to maintenance of or deviation from normal weight remain poorly understood. The human (unlike the rat) is unable to detect the correct energy imbalance over the short period of a day. Several studies confirm that a caloric imbalance requires more than a week to be restored. Humans also are incapable of maintaining body weight within very narrow limits, although it is obvious that a control system operates in most people to prevent *excessive* weight gains. This is readily appreciated from the fact that an energy excess of only 50 calories/day would lead to a gain of an extra 6 pounds in 1 year. Thus severe obesity can develop with a positive energy balance that cannot be measured by present techniques.

Energy intake of normal subjects of the same age and activity level may vary as much as twofold, and it bears no consistent relationship to body weight. There is no indication that all obese subjects eat significantly more than persons of normal weight, and some eat less. Excessive caloric intake remains one of the causes of obesity, although it is often impossible to demonstrate this in any one individual, given the wide range of normal variability.

The regulation of food intake is influenced by many factors that begin early in life. Family eating patterns and attitudes about food, socioeconomic factors, peer group pressures, television commercials, and school lunches of varying nutritional value all help to set patterns of food choice and levels of caloric intake in the growing child. Teaching programs in nutrition are generally inadequate from grade school through medical school, and this apathetic view is reflected in far greater increases in weight than in height over the past 30 years in the vast majority of children in the United States.

Subcortical influences on feeding behavior emanate from two centers in the hypothalamus: a satiety center and a feeding center. Some years ago destructive lesions in the rat resulting in marked obesity appeared to fix the site of the satiety center in the ventromedial nucleus (VMN); however, using more precise methods, Gold has shown that obesity results from destruction of the nearby *ventral noradrenergic bundle.* The centers respond to the physiologic cues of hunger and satiety, but the mechanisms have not been delineated. Mayer has postulated the presence of receptors sensitive to changes in glucose utilization within the cells, whereas Kennedy has proposed a feedback mechanism sensitive to the stores of body fat. The centers do not allow normal or obese subjects on a regular diet to detect sudden and rather substantial increases or decreases of calories. Their importance seems to lie in appreciating extremes of intake, and they appear to play a minor role in influencing eating behavior and development of obesity.

Psychologic factors play an important role in determining food intake, and they begin to exert their influence early in life. The passage of time reinforces their influence, making it increasingly difficult to alter attitudes about food and patterns of eating. Psychologic factors are probably the most important explanation for perpetuation of childhood obesity into adulthood.

An individual's energy output is determined by metabolic costs at rest and during eating and exercising. At rest, protein turnover, synthesis of new tissues, maintenance of body temperature, and other autonomic functions constitute the major expenditures. Resting metabolic rate rises following a meal, and it is unrelated to the muscular activity of digestion. The thermic effect of food (specific dynamic action) follows both protein and carbohydrate intake and is quantitatively similar in normal, lean, and fat persons. During periods of caloric restriction and weight loss, resting metabolic rate falls. Its fall is greater than can be accounted for by tissue loss, and on refeeding it rises before body weight increases. These changes suggest that tissue metabolic activity is altered to resist body weight change, undernutrition leading to conservation of energy and overnutrition to increased energy loss. Thus subjects on a fixed low caloric intake lose weight gradually, a clinical finding that is discouraging to the dieter.

The hypothesis that overnutrition leads to increased energy losses in the form of heat is termed thermogenesis and is a disputed concept. However, there is evidence to suggest that weight gain following overnutrition varies considerably, and this cannot be accounted for by differences in energy expenditure. Biochemical evidence to support the concept has been found in increased activity of mitochondrial α-glycerophosphate dehydrogenase of adipose cells after overnutrition. This enzyme operates in the α-glycerophosphate cycle that shuttles hydrogen from NADH in the cytoplasm to the flavoprotein FAD in the mitochondria. Thus α-glycerophosphate is diverted from forming triglyceride into a less efficient pathway, and the excess energy is released as heat. Galton and Bray have found this enzyme to be abnormally low in adipose cells of severely obese humans; they also have found that after calories are restricted the levels are reduced even further.

Energy expenditure during physical exercise is a relatively small part of total daily output, unless the exercise is vigorous and prolonged. The fact that obese children are thus relatively unimportant as a cause of their obesity. Caloric expenditure per hour in sedentary activities is about 40 calories; during normal walking it is 100 to 150 calories, for brisk walking 250 calories, and for swimming or tennis 300 to 700 calories.

ADIPOSE TISSUE

BODY COMPOSITION.   Body fat is estimated by two techniques: (1) anthropometric evaluation estimates subcutaneous fat by skin fold thicknesses, various body circumferences, or thickness of tissue measured from radiograms or ultrasound; (2) measurement of total body fat may be made either directly by estimation of specific gravity by underwater weighing or helium displacement or indirectly by measuring lean body mass (LBM) using deuterium to measure total body water or by taking whole-body counts of naturally occurring radioactive potassium (^{40}K); subtracting LBM from body weight will thus approximate body fat.

Studies of development of fat stores in normal children have shown that there are two periods of relative increase in body fat. One begins shortly after birth and becomes maximal between 6 and 18 months; it is similar in both sexes, although girls have proportionately more fat at all ages. There is then a regression of fat relative to the increases in bone and muscle in both sexes. At about 8 years the amount of body fat again increases; boys have increases in LMB that exceed those in body fat, with resultant decreases in percentage of body fat; girls develop absolute and relative increases in body fat during adolescence.

In obese children the acceleration in weight gain resulting in overweight and eventual obesity coincides with the normal periods of accelerated fat deposition. Forbes found that obese children could be separated into two groups (1) those with increased LBM, who were overweight from birth and who tended to have increased stature and advanced bone age; (2) those with normal LBM, who had average heights and normal bone age. The latter group had become obese later in childhood.

ADIPOSE CELLS.   Adipose cells increase in number until puberty, when adult values are reached. Brooks and associates have found that all obese children have increased cell size, but those already obese by 1 year of age also have marked increases in cell *number*. Children with onset of obesity in later childhood have cell numbers that in the majority fall within two standard deviations of the normal mean. Obese adults also fall into two populations: (1) those with an increase in cell size, whose obesity began in adulthood, and (2) those with increase in cell size and number, whose obesity dates from childhood.

Weight loss at any age beyond 1 year results in decreased cell size, but not in decreased total cell number; it is not known whether this is true in obese infants under 1 year. Important questions to be resolved are whether cell number is under environmental or genetic control or both, whether the rate of multiplication can be arrested prior to achievement of the adult number, and whether hyperplastic cells differ metabolically from normal cells when they are depleted of their fat.

METABOLISM.   The body's major energy stores reside in adipose tissue because of its mass and its high caloric density. Adipose tissue is not inert, undergoes constant change; its volume depends on the equilibrium between deposition and mobilization of triglyceride, the storage form of fat. It has generally been thought that adipose tissue in obese individuals has sluggish metabolism. Recent studies with radioactive-labeled compounds reveal that metabolic activity of adipose tissue is increased in obese adults.

Triglycerides, which consist of a molecule of glycerol with three long-chain fatty acids, are formed and deposited in the adipocyte by incorporation of preformed lipids (both those from the diet and those synthesized in the liver) and de novo synthesis from glucose within the cell. Preformed lipids are hydrolyzed at the cell wall by lipoprotein lipase, and only the free fatty acids (FFA) enter the cell, where along with fatty acids formed in situ they are esterified with α-glycerophosphate, the activated form of glycerol. Glycerol formed during lipolysis cannot be reutilized, so that its active form must be synthesized from glucose within the cell. Therefore, since glucose cannot be derived through gluconeogenesis in adipose cells and glycogen stores are small, the rate of glucose uptake by the cell is one of the major regulators of triglyceride synthesis.

Triglyceride formation is also regulated by the rates of glucose utilization in the various metabolic pathways operative in the fat cell. In addition to entering the glycolytic pathway and serving as a source of α-glycerophosphate and of acetyl CoA for fatty acid synthesis, glucose enters the pentose or hexose monophosphate pathway. This metabolic pathway is very active in fat cells and is important as the source for nucleotides

(TPNH, NADH$_2$) used as cofactors in the synthesis of triglycerides.

Triglycerides are hydrolyzed by a hormone-sensitive lipase distinct from lipoprotein lipase. The FFA may be reesterified or may enter the circulation bound to albumin. They serve two functions: they are a primary source of the energy requirements of skeletal muscle, liver, and heart, and they serve as regulatory factors, primarily in the liver but also in muscle and adipose cells. By influencing certain enzyme reactions, FFA in the liver can stimulate gluconeogenesis and increase ketone formation. In muscle they interfere with glucose utilization. In the adipose cell, through a feedback mechanism, they inhibit further free fatty acid release.

In obese subjects fasted overnight, FFA are elevated well above normal. In such subjects one would anticipate an exaggeration of their metabolic influences. Indeed, Shreeve and associates have shown a twofold increase above normal in ^{14}C-glucose production from labeled pyruvate in obese adults fasted overnight. The utilization of the increased glucose entering the circulation is impaired in the muscle cells because of the high levels of FFA; the increased glucose is taken up by the adipose cells and stored as fat.

Obese subjects have been reported to have impaired fat mobilization; this is based on the findings of lower than normal plasma FFA levels after prolonged fasting or exercise, decreased arteriovenous differences of plasma FFA after a brief fast, and resistance to the development of ketonemia after fasts of varying lengths. However, Nestel and Whyte have questioned these findings. They found that turnover rates of plasma FFA, expressed in relation to body surface area, were 25 percent greater in obese subjects than in nonobese subjects. For a given plasma FFA concentration the turnover rate was greater in obese subjects and was significantly correlated with plasma FFA level and with fat mass. Obese subjects also had higher turnover rates of triglycerides than the nonobese, and these correlated with the elevated plasma triglyceride levels. Thus there is evidence of increased metabolic activity in adipose tissue of obese individuals: *increased* mobilization of free fatty acids countered by *increased* triglyceride formation.

REGULATORY FACTORS

NERVOUS SYSTEM. The hypothalamus can influence glucose and lipid metabolism by affecting release of certain hormones. Stimulation of the medial hypothalamus, or sympathetic area, can elicit secretion of catecholamines.

ENDOCRINE HORMONES. Insulin is the major regulator of body fat stores because it not only stimulates synthesis but inhibits lipolysis of triglycerides. It acts by enhancing glucose entry into the adipose cells as well as muscle cells and FFA entry by maintaining the enzyme lipoprotein lipase; it appears to facilitate enzyme reactions of phosphorylated glucose, leading to triglyceride synthesis within the cell; and it inhibits the hormone-sensitive lipase that hydrolyzes triglycerides.

In both male and female rats estrogens act synergisti-

cally with insulin in stimulating the synthesis of lipids from glucose. Such synergism, if present in humans, would explain the normally accelerated deposition of fat during adolescence. Lipolysis can be induced in man by numerous hormones, including cathecholamines, growth hormone, glucagon, cortisol, thyroxine, TSH, ACTH, and secretin. The lipolytic hormones are believed to act by enhancing formation of cyclic adenosine 3',5'-monophosphate (cyclic AMP) from ATP. Cyclic AMP catalyzes the conversion of inactive lipase to its active form. Abnormalities in plasma levels of some of the lipolytic hormones (growth hormone, cortisol, and glucagon) have been found in obese children and adults. Also, growth hormone levels are reduced in the fasting state, and diurnal variation is suppressed; responses to insulin-induced hypoglycemia, arginine, exercise, and prolonged fasting are poor or absent. In experimental animals impaired growth hormone secretion is an early feature of obesity. In addition to its lipolytic activity, growth hormone can block fat synthesis in the adipose cell by inhibiting glucose oxidation and FFA synthesis.

There is no evidence of decreased thyroid function in uncomplicated obesity. Blood levels of protein-bound iodine are normal, and studies with radioisotope-labeled thyroxine reveal no evidence of defective peripheral utilization. In studies where, in addition to caloric restriction, desiccated thyroid was administered to obese subjects and to myxedematous patients, weight loss was observed in both groups. However, densitometric studies revealed that the loss was predominately from LBM. Therefore, thyroid medication is contraindicated as a therapeutic measure to stimulate weight loss in obesity.

EXPERIMENTAL OBESITY

MAN. Sims and his colleagues have provided important insights into obesity by inducing weight increases of 15 to 30 percent in lean male volunteers by overfeeding with a normally constituted diet. It was difficult to induce obesity; several volunteers who ingested their normal caloric intakes while following their usual daily routines for 3 to 5 months increased their weights by only 10 to 12 percent, and others failed to gain at all. As weight increased they developed an aversion to breakfast, but they also developed sensations of hunger between meals, even though caloric intakes were as high as 10,000 calories/day. The metabolic and endocrine abnormalities seen in spontaneously obese subjects were induced in those volunteers who did become obese. The endocrine abnormalities observed in spontaneously obese subjects thus appear to be secondary to the obese state.

A finding in experimental obesity in mice is particularly relevant to obese human subjects. When weight is reduced in genetically obese mice by starvation, and they are then fed ad libitum, they return to their exact prestarvation weights. Such observations have been reported in obese adults who achieved weight losses they were unable to sustain. These findings suggest individual limits to weight gain that may relate to the number of adipose cells, to their capacity to hypertrophy, and perhaps to an abnormal avidity for lipid storage.

Risks of Obesity

Efforts to lose weight consume time, money, and energy; they are frustrating to all concerned and are usually unrewarding. Therefore a realistic appraisal is needed of the health risks that face overweight and obese children, not only in childhood but also in their adult years. The psychologic risk in childhood far outweighs the medical risk, and it results from the cultural view of obesity as unhealthy and unsightly. In projective tests given to obese adolescent girls, Monello and associates noted that girls have intense feelings of discrimination and the character traits of passivity, withdrawal, expectation of rejection by peers, and marked signs of self-rejection. Stunkard and Mendelson found that adults whose obesity began in the adolescent period often had poor self-images and tended to consider their obesity causally related to failures and disappointments.

The serious medical risks of obesity are in the adult years, but they have not been adequately studied. Abraham and associates examined the incidence of diabetes, hypertensive vascular disease (HVD), arteriosclerotic heart disease (ASHD), and cardiovascular renal disease (CVRD) in a group of white males 30 to 40 years of age whose weights at 9 to 13 years of age were on record. The risk for all conditions other than CVRD was greater in those who were very obese as children (weight > 20 percent above average). It is interesting that there was a high risk for HVD and CVRD in those adults who had become overweight after being underweight as children. Adult obesity also carries an increased risk for diabetes, but as was shown by O'Sullivan, this is important only in individuals with a diabetic family history.

Many of the problems confronting the obese subject are simply the result of an exaggerated mechanical load. Exertion or respiratory infections may lead to severe respiratory distress. In extreme obesity, decreased ventilation with accumulation of carbon dioxide may lead to apneic spells, lethargy, and somnolence, a clinical state referred to as the Pickwickian syndrome.

Obese children often have itching, inflammation, and furuncles in moist skin folds and on the inner aspects of the thighs. Adolescent girls may develop menstrual irregularities. As in adults, obese children may have impaired glucose tolerance; in one study the incidence of significant impairment was 23 percent. Reduction of weight to normal may result in disappearance of the hyperglycemia.

Differential Diagnosis

Lesions invading the hypothalamus such as craniopharyngiomas, tumors of the pituitary, or cysts (as in Fröhlich's syndrome) can cause obesity. The sexual in-

fantilism, growth retardation, and diabetes insipidus that sometimes accompany the obesity in these conditions are due to invasion of the pituitary. Obesity also occurs in the Laurence-Moon-Biedl syndrome. Prader and associates have described a syndrome of obesity, muscular hypotonia, hypogenitalism, hypogonadism, mental retardation, and occasionally asymptomatic hyperglycemia. Fasting hyperlipogenesis, a defect described in obese hyperglycemic mice, has also been observed in these patients.

The distinction between the rare case of Cushing's syndrome in children and uncomplicated obesity may be difficult; however, several important differences are noteworthy. In Cushing's syndrome the distribution of fat is truncal, linear growth is impaired, and osteoporosis and hypertension are present. In uncomplicated obesity the distribution of fat is generalized, growth is normal or accelerated, and osteoporosis and hypertension are absent. It should be appreciated that falsely high blood pressure readings are recorded commonly when the arm is obese. The increased urinary 17-hydroxycorticoids or 17-ketogenic steroids frequently seen in the obese can be suppressed by amounts of dexamethasone that do not suppress the increases in Cushing's syndrome. In patients with Cushing's disease, but not in other obese patients, the diurnal variation in plasma cortisol concentration disappears.

Adolescent girls with generalized obesity, mild or moderate hirsutism, and amenorrhea or menstrual irregulatiries should be evaluated for possible endocrine dysfunction. Several types of ovarian dysfunction, such as the Stein-Leventhal syndrome, may be present with this triad.

Treatment

Emphasis should be placed on prevention of obesity, since attempts at treament often are unsuccessful. The need for educating the general public in good nutrition is apparent, since trends toward increased weight for age and height are significant among all ages. It remains to be determined if changes in infant feeding practices, such as early addition of cereal and provision of large amounts of calories, may cause the increased cell numbers noted in subjects whose obesity began in childhood and whether such increased cell numbers generate a propensity to obesity. Obese individuals from families in which there is a high incidence of hypertensive vascular disease and diabetes should be particularly attentive to following good habits of nutrition, and the pediatrician should be concerned about proper weight increases in all infants and children.

The decision to undertake treatment of an obese child rests on many factors, the most important being the degree of patient and parent cooperation. However, a concerted effort should be made in all instances in which risks such as serious obesity-related psychologic problems, hypertension, or abnormal carbohydrate tolerance are present in the patient or in close family members.

A primary goal in a reducing program is to effect a

permanent change in eating pattern. The child as well as the family must be involved in the educational process of learning what good nutrition is; they must practice it together, and in various ways the family must aid the child who is trying to lose weight. These are some simple suggestions: keep high-calorie foods off the menu and out of the house; keep food out of sight; limit eating to one room and restrict eating to mealtimes; give smaller portions so two may be had; have older children keep a daily calories count; don't rush through meals, but eat slowly; have low-calorie snacks available after school; encourage exercise to keep thoughts diverted from food. Have the child keep a weight graph (record weight each morning after voiding); have short-term goals and give rewards appropriately. The physician should explain that weight losses in the first week will be greater than those that follow. This is due to losses from the glycogen pool, which has a high content of water (70 percent). Adipose tissue, with its lower water content (20 percent) and higher caloric density, is lost more slowly and with greater effort. In addition, as noted earlier, the resting metabolic rate decreases with calorie restriction.

The diet should contain the total protein requirement for normal growth, with caloric restriction being entirely in fats and carbohydrates. There is no evidence that the composition of the diet will enhance weight loss, but a high-protein diet is more satisfying than one high in carbohydrate. The caloric content should be equal to or slightly below the child's requirement to maintain ideal weight. Greater restrictions are unrealistic unless carried out in a hospital. Total fasting, sharply curtailed intake, or surgical bypass are absolutely contraindicated in the growing child. Ideally the initial phase of the program should be carried out in a supervised setting where the child and parents can learn the procedures and restrictions of the diet that must be carried out at home if success is to be expected.

EXERCISE. Daily exercise in any form for at least 1 hour is desirable to establish a life style that will not encourage increasing obesity. The child should be encouraged in a variety of sports, especially those he can continue into adulthood. Members of the family should join the youngster in these activities to encourage regularity of performance.

MEDICATIONS. Thyroid treatment is not indicated unless there are clinical and laboratory data clearly documenting a state of hypothyroidism. The use of anorexigenic drugs is not encouraged; at best, they are effective for only brief periods of a few months. Also, drugs may interfere with the problem of meeting caloric balance realistically.

PSYCHOLOGIC SUPPORT. The obese child under treatment should be seen often by the physician for encouragement and praise. The physician should elicit cooperation from the whole family. An obese parent, especially, should be encouraged to lose weight along with the child. A nagging battle between child and parent should be avoided, and although it is often difficult for parents, the adolescent should be given major responsibility for the treatment program. Attention to the cosmetic features of obesity often provides motivation to the adolescent. In the majority of patients, little more than a holding operation can be effected, rarely a cure. However, even this is encouraging, and the patient should never be treated harshly or abandoned for failure to lose weight. Current evidence suggests that some features of the problem may well be beyond the patient's control.

While the struggle against established obesity often fails because of the multiplicity of interrelated known and unknown factors, the occasional success and the support provided make the effort worthwhile. In the area of prevention, and during the early development of obesity, the clinician may play a very important part in preserving later health.

References

Abraham S, Collins G, Nardseick M: Relationship of childhood weight status to morbidity in adults. Public Health Rep 86:273, 1971

Brook CGD, Lloyd JK, Wolf OH: Relation between age of onset of obesity and size and number of adipose cells. Br Med J 2:25, 1972

Clayton RN, Grossman L, Mayeda TK, Gold RM: Hypothalamic obesity: the myth of the ventromedial nucleus. Science 182:448, 1973

Eid EE: Follow-up study of physical growth of children who had excessive weight gain in first six months of life. Br Med J 2:74, 1970

Forbes GB: Growth of the lean body mass during childhood and adolescence. J Pediatr, 64:822, 1964

———: Lean body mass and fat in obese children. Pediatrics 34:308, 1964

Galton DJ: The Human Adipose Cell. London, Butterworth, 1971

Garrow JS: Energy Balance and Obesity in Man. New York, American Elsevier, 1974

Goodman HM: Growth hormone and the metabolism of carbohydrate and lipid in adipose tissue. Ann NY Acad Sci 148:419, 1968

Heald FP, Hollander RJ: The relationship between obesity in adolescence and early growth. J Pediatr 67:35, 1965

Hodges RE, Krehl WA: Nutritional status of teenagers in Iowa. Am J Clin Nutr 17:200, 1965

Keys A, Aravanis C, Blackburn H, van Buchem FSP, Buzina R, Djordjevic BS, et al: Coronary heart disease: overweight and obesity as risk factors. Ann Intern Med 77:15, 1972

Knittle JL: Obesity in childhood: a problem in adipose tissue cellular development. J Pediatr 81: 1048, 1972

Mann GV: The influence of obesity on health. N Engl J Med 291:178, 226, 1974

Mayer J: Some aspects of the problem of regulation of food intake and obesity. N Engl J Med 274:610, 662, 722, 1966

National Center for Health Statistics: Public Health Services, 1970, 1973. Series 11, Numbers 104 and 124. Washington, DC, US Department of Health, Education and Welfare, 1970, 1973

O'Sullivan JB: Population retested for diabetes after 17 years: new prevalence study in Oxford, Massachusetts. Diabetologia 5:211, 1969.

Paulsen EP, Richenderfer L, Ginsberg-Fellner F: Plasma glucose, free fatty acids, and immunoreactive insulin in 66 obese children. Diabetes 17:261, 1968

Salans LB, Cushman SW, Weisman RE: Studies of human adipose tissue. J Clin Invest 52:929, 1973

Shreeve WW, Hoshi M, Oji N, Shigeta Y, and Abe H: Insulin and the utilization of carbohydrates in obesity. Am J Clin Nutr 21:1404, 1968

Shukla A, Forsyth HA, Anderson CM, Marwah SM: Infantile overnutrition in the first year of life: a field study in Dudley, Worcestershire. Br Med J 4:507, 1972

Sims EA, Goldman RF, Gluck CM, Horton ES, Kelleher PC, Rowe DW:

Experimental obesity in man. Trans Assoc Am Physicians 81:153, 1968

Stunkard A, Mendelson M: Disturbances in body image of some obese persons. J Am Diet Assoc 38:328, 1961

Winick M (ed): Symposium on Childhood Obesity. Current Concepts in Nutrition. New York, Wiley (in press)

WATER AND ELECTROLYTE PHYSIOLOGY

LAURENCE FINBERG

Water, the major constituent of the body, comprises 70 percent of the fat-free mass; it serves as the solvent for cell solids and as the transport medium among cells, tissues, and organs. Water has the largest daily turnover of any body component and serves as the solvent for wastes; in addition it plays a crucial role in body heat regulation. In this section normal and abnormal water and electrolyte physiology will be discussed in terms of body composition, obligatory expenditure and requirement of water, and pathogenesis of dehydration.

BODY WATER COMPOSITION

Part of the body water is within cells; together with the dissolved solute, this is termed intracellular fluid (ICF). Water outside of cells has a different solute composition and is termed extracellular fluid (ECF). These two compartments, representing the major anatomic and functional divisions of water in the body, undergo changes during early development. At birth the ECF constitutes about 30 percent of the lean body mass, falling to about 25 percent at a few months of age and to about 20 percent by the end of puberty. Conversely, the ICF increases from about 38 percent to 45 percent and then to 50 percent of the lean body mass during these periods of development. The electrolyte composition may best be shown by diagrams such as those devised by Gamble, now called Gamblegrams (Fig. 20). These diagrams emphasize electroneutrality and indicate the usefulness of reporting concentrations in milliequivalents per liter. Since the major ionic constituents (Na^+, K^+, Cl^-, and HCO_3^-) are univalent, milliequivalence and milliosmolality are almost the same for the three fluids of greatest physiologic interest: the ICF, the ECF, and a subcompartment of the ECF, the blood plasma.

Water molecules and most ions diffuse freely across the cell membranes that separate the compartments. The distinctive compositions of ICF and ECF result from an energy-dependent process that exludes Na^+ from the cells—at least relatively so from muscle cells, the most numerous in the body. The remaining differences are attributable to two factors: the impermeability of cell membranes to protein and some other large cellular anions and the absence of osmotic concentration gradients because of the rapid and free passage of water between compartments.

The ECF itself has several components; in addition to the interstitial water there are several specialized sub-

components, including tendon water, ocular, synovial, and cerebrospinal fluids, and most important blood plasma, which accounts for about a quarter of the ECF or 6 percent of the body weight (Fig. 20). The plasma remains confined to the vascular space in spite of the free permeability of the capillary and the elevated hy-

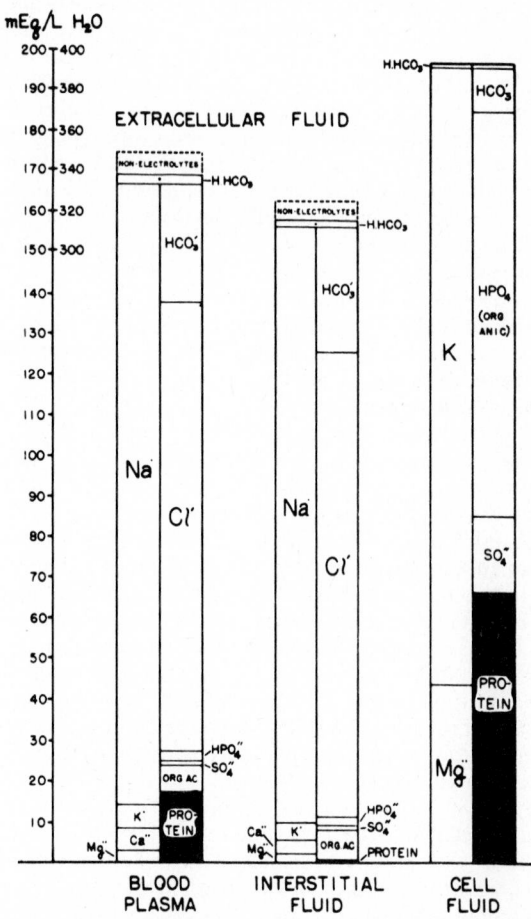

FIG. 20. Diagrams comparing the composition of plasma, interstitial fluid, and ICF. While there are differences in total electrical charge owing to differing quantities of multivalent ions, the osmolal concentrations are obligatorily identical. (Reprinted by permission of the publishers from James L. Gamble: *Chemical Anatomy, Physiology, and Pathology of Extracellular Fluid.* Cambridge, Mass., Harvard University Press, copyright 1942 by J. L. Gamble; 1947, 1954 by the President and Fellows of Harvard College.)

drostatic pressure at the arterial end. Starling's analysis first made it clear that the hydrostatic pressure is offset by the relative impermeability of the plasma proteins, especially albumin, and that the plasma volume is dynamically preserved as the blood streams through the capillary bed.

Thus plasma volume, as a fraction of the ECF, depends primarily on the amount of protein within the vascular space. Since the protein acts as an anion, a

Gibbs-Donnan equilibrium applies to concentration differences of solutes between plasma and interstitial fluid. Since plasma volume has crucial significance to circulation, and preservation of circulation remains a prime consideration in problems of hydration, the chemical anatomy and the mechanism of partition of the ECF into plasma and interstitial fluid have major clinical relevance. Accordingly, the albumin content of plasma determines one of the most important aspects of water physiology.

Sodium and its accompanying anions do not diffuse into or out of the cerebrospinal fluid (CSF) and ocular fluid as rapidly as water. Hence, when sodium concentration in the ECF undergoes rapid change, a volume change occurs temporarily in the CSF until a new steady state develops some hours later. In this sense, whenever the osmolal concentration of ECF varies rapidly, the entire CNS may be thought of as analogous to a single large cell bathed in it. The water content of the CNS (ICF and ECF plus CSF) will either shrink with hypernatremia or expand with hyponatremia when either disturbance occurs rapidly. Thus rapid infusion of 5 percent glucose in water will cause swelling of the brain, which in some clinical circumstances may be deleterious.

CHEMICAL HOMEOSTASIS

In addition to diffusion, osmosis, and selective permeability or extrusion, there are other processes operating to maintain constancy of composition of body fluids. The most important of these is hydrogen ion metabolism, which is regulated principally by the lungs and kidneys. Despite the fact that H^+ appears in minute concentration (nanomolar), a very narrow pH range must be maintained for life processes to proceed. Accordingly, acid–base homeostasis depends on the presence of buffer systems, principally bicarbonate–carbonic acid, that afford maximum resistance to change at pH 7.4. The mathematic statement of this buffering system may be summarized by the Henderson-Hasselbalch equation:

$$pH = pK' + \log \frac{(HCO_3^-)}{(H_2CO_3)}$$

The value for pK' in biologic fluids is 6.1, and H_2CO_3 may be expressed as the partial pressure of Co_2 in millimeters of mercury multiplied by the solubility constant 0.03. The equation then becomes

$$pH = 6.1 + \log \frac{(HCO_3^-)}{Pco_2 \times 0.03}$$

Then at physiologic pH

$$7.4 = 6.1 + \log \frac{(HCO_3^-)}{Pco_2 \times 0.03}$$

or $\log \dfrac{(HCO_3^-)}{Pco_2 \times 0.03} = 1.3$

Antolig 1.3 = 20; so a buffer ratio of 20:1 defines a normal pH. The chemical relationship among the reactants may be expressed as

$$H^+ + HCO_3^- \overset{\text{carbonic}}{\underset{\text{anhydrase}}{\rightleftharpoons}} H_2CO_3 \rightleftharpoons H_2O + CO_2 \uparrow$$

These interrelationships determine for the most part what happens to pH when there is an increased production of H^+, a loss of HCO_3^-, or a retention or excessive elimination of CO_2. Primary charges in H^+ or HCO_3^- are termed metabolic, whereas primary changes in CO_2 are respiratory. Any change in one of the reactants results in a change in the other two, which affects the buffer ratio HCO_3^-/CO_2 in such a way as to minimize change in pH. When pH in blood falls below the normal range, an acidemia is said to be present. Conversely a rise in pH is termed alkalemia. A change initiated by the addition of acid (H^+) or the loss of base, (HCO_3^-) reduces the numerator of the buffer ratio. However, induced hyperventilation will then bring about a corresponding change in the denominator (CO_2). When the ratio is preserved with the reactants in lower absolute concentrations, the pH remains normal and the result is called acidosis; similarly the opposite change is termed alkalosis. The terms metabolic and respiratory denote respective changes from metabolic or respiratory abnormalities, whether primary or compensatory. In this system of nomenclature only a change in pH receives the suffix -emia, but a metabolic acidemia will usually be accompanied by a partially compensatory reduction in Pco_2, so that the disturbance has a respiratory component.

To assist in assessing the components separately, Sigaard-Anderson has introduced the term base excess to represent the metabolic component of a hydrogen ion disturbance when the Pco_2 has been mathematically adjusted to a normal value of 40 mm Hg. This quantity represents the amount per liter of strong acid (H^+) or strong base (OH^-) theoretically necessary to titrate the blood back to a normal pH. This number value, while not a biologic entity, provides a simple quantitative assessment of the metabolic side of a disturbance of the hydrogen ion steady state.

The foregoing discussion ignores, for purposes of simplicity, the role of hemoglobin and other buffers that play lesser but not insignificant roles in acid–based adjustments. Also ignored are such factors as the effects of rate of change, the role of the skeleton, and many other contributing systems. For a more detailed discussion the reader is referred to the specialized Refer-

TABLE 16. Approximate Basal Water Requirements in Relation to Age, Weight, and Surface Area[a]

Age	Weight (kg)	Surface Area (m²)	Minimal Basal Water Requirement		
			(ml/kg) (or cal/kg)	(ml/m²)	(ml/24 hr)
Newborn	2.5–4	0.2–0.23	50	750	125–200
1 week–6 months	3.0–8	0.2–0.35	65–70	1000–1100	200–520
6–12 months	8.0–12	0.35–0.45	50–60	1000–1050	500–600
12–24 months	10–15	0.45–0.60	45–50	1000–1050	500–750

[a] From Finberg: Pediatrics 45:1029, 1970.

ences. A consideration of the four types of disturbance follows. Each of them, when present, will almost always be accompanied by some degree of compensation.

METABOLIC ACIDOSIS. Metabolic acidosis may result from a primary increase in H^+ (such as accumulation of increased amounts of keto acids in diabetes, starvation, or salicylate intoxication) or from a primary loss of base (HCO_3^-) in the stool or urine. It also results when the kidney fails to excrete the normal amount of nonvolatile acid substances produced during metabolism of protein, chiefly acid sulfates and phosphates. Also tissue hypoxia leads to excess release of acid metabolites from anaerobic glycolysis or dying cells. The physiologic compensation for metabolic acidosis is hyperventilation, which by reducing the Pco_2 maintains the buffer ratio closer to 20:1.

METABOLIC ALKALOSIS. Metabolic alkalosis results from primary loss of H^+ (for example, from loss of gastric secretion without pancreatic secretion) or from administration of base. The vomiting of infantile pyloric stenosis is the classic example in pediatrics. Compensation for metabolic alkalosis is by hypoventilation, which raises the Pco_2; however, it is limited by the resulting hypoxia.

RESPIRATORY ACIDOSIS. Respiratory acidosis results from hypoventilation causing primary CO_2 retention. When the patient is breathing air, hypoxia necessarily also occurs, leading by way of disturbed metabolism to a metabolic acidosis as well. Partial compensation occurs through renal excretion of H^+.

RESPIRATORY ALKALOSIS. Respiratory alkalosis, a primary reduction in CO_2, results from hyperventilation and may be compensated by renal excretion of base as bicarbonate.

The preceding discussion has outlined only the main elements of the whole complex problem of electrolyte and H^+ homeostasis. For most clinical problems this knowledge will suffice, largely because several body organs function vigorously to maintain the status quo. These include the lungs, the kidneys, and the adrenal cortices. The lungs excrete CO_2 directly, which chemically includes an ion of acid (H^+) and of base (HCO_3^-), and thus they control directly the partial pressure of the gas (Pco_2). As previously indicated, the kidney excretes the nonvolatile acid in the urine through a series of equisitely adjusted mechanisms. The kidney also maintains ECF composition by excretion or retention of water, Na^+, K^+, CL^-, HCO_3^-, and diva-

lent ions, in addition to excreting organic substances. The adrenal and posterior pituitary add a fine regulatory control on the kidney for the excretion of water and electrolytes.

MAINTENANCE REQUIREMENTS

Water needs arise from ongoing expenditure of energy; this occurs at a high rate in mammals, primarily to produce the heat necessary to maintain body temperature. Thus water needs relate to caloric expenditure, which depends in part on the relationship between mass and surface area. The two most commonly used reference points are calories expended and surface area; Table 16 shows their relationship to age and weight, both of which are available. Basal values may be extrapolated when necessary by the rule of thumb that under ordinary ward conditions water needs are approximately 1.5 times basal requirements.

Physiologic water expenditures are as follows:

Skin and lungs	45 ml/100 cal metabolized
Urine (at 300 mOsm/liter)	50 ml/100 cal metabolized
Stool	5 ml/100 cal metabolized
Total	100 ml/100 cal metabolized

The expenditure of 100 calories produces 12 ml of water, so that the net requirement is 88 ml/100 cal. It should be emphasized that while deficits of water are usually estimated as a direct proportion of mass, maintenance requirements for water are related to energy expenditure, which is not a linear function of mass.

Sodium requirements are very low, but with intact renal function the range of tolerance is very broad. Potassium is less well conserved and must be provided more liberally; however, with renal insufficiency and oliguria, K^+ concentration in ECF may rise quickly to dangerous levels. Both of these cations may be safely administered for maintenance in amounts of 2 to 3 mEq/100 calories metabolized.

PATHOGENESIS OF DEHYDRATION

Dehydration may best be considered clinically in terms of disturbances in the following five categories: volume, osmolality, H^+ status, ICF ion deficits, and ECF–skeleton steady state. Table 17 lists these factors, with a brief outline of clinical and laboratory highlights.

TABLE 17. Clinical Appraisal of Problems of Hydration[a, b]

Point of Appraisal	Clinical Symptoms and Signs	Laboratory Determination of Greatest Value
1. Volume	Circulatory impairment Skin changes Eye and fontanelle changes Oliguria	Body weight Urea N in serum

2. Osmolality	For hypernatremia:
	  CNS signs
	  disturbance of consciousness
	  hypertonicity of muscles
	  increased reflexes
	  Marked thirst
	  "Inapparent dehydration" with good
	circulation for degree of loss
	For hyponatremia:
	  There occurs an exaggeration of the
	signs listed under Volume
		Na^+ in serum

3. Hydrogen ion status	Hyperpnea in acidosis	CO_2 content (HCO_3-) in serum or pH and P_{CO_2}
4. Intracellular ion deficits	Abdominal distension Muscle weakness Diminished reflexes	K^+ in serum (limited use) Electrocardiogram
5. Calcium homeostasis	Tetany Convulsions	Ca^{++} in serum (complex interpretation) Electrocardiogram

[a] *From Finberg: Pediatrics 45:1029, 1970.*

[b] *In this table only the symptoms and signs of dehydration have been given. A companion group of signs for the corresponding disturbances of overhydration has been omitted for simplicity. The same points of appraisal and the same laboratory examinations may be advantageously used.*

In the present discussion physiologic principles will be stressed; in the following section these are applied to diarrheal disease of infancy.

VOLUME. In most dehydrated states body water and solute are lost together in approximately physiologic proportion, the net loss being the total loss minus whatever intake has been maintained. The effect of such loss first becomes clinically manifest when plasma volume drops to the level where the circulation is impaired. Once this has occurred the whole process becomes accelerated, and the situation becomes dangerous. Although subjective evidence of dehydration occurs early, objective evidences such as tachycardia and dryness of skin and mucous membranes often do not appear until about 5 percent of the body weight has been lost over a very short time. When 10 percent weight loss has occurred rapidly without change in osmolality, circulation becomes significantly impaired and shock occurs. Slightly more loss, up to 15 percent of weight in a day, may be irreversible.

OSMOLALITY. The importance of osmolality derives from the division of the body water into compartments. The principal physiologic role of NaCl appears to be the partition of body water into its two main spaces, ECF and ICF. The body content of sodium (other than skeletal) and its accompanying anions, chiefly chloride, essentially determine the relative volume of water in the two compartments. For a given volume of body water, a higher sodium content will mean more ECF volume and correspondingly less ICF volume. Thus high sodium content with volume loss

produces cellular desiccation. Conversely, low sodium content with a deficit of water volume produces proportionately greater ECF loss. These two disturbances have been designated hypernatremic dehydration and hyponatremic dehydration, respectively.

Hypernatremic dehydration may be deceptive clinically because of the relatively greater preservation of the circulation. However, because of several factors the CNS shows disproportionate insult from hypernatremia. First, the nature of sodium and water transport into the CNS interstitium and CSF results in brain shrinkage and sometimes hemorrhage. The bleeding occurs secondary to capillary rupture after dilation because of negative pressure when the shrinking brain pulls away from the rigid cranium. Thrombosis may in turn follow hemorrhage. Second, "idiogenic osmols" arise within body cells, including the brain, and this phenomenon may produce disturbances of neurologic function (at least its occurrence and the disturbances are associated). Finally, disturbances of calcium homeostasis with hypocalcemia occur during hypernatremic dehydration when potassium has been lost. Potassium losses are often large, and replacement of this ion seems to facilitate ICF repair.

Experience has made it clear that the twin danger in treating hypernatremic dehydration are (1) too rapid an infusion of dilute solution, leading to brain swelling and convulsions, and (2) too much sodium in the repair solution, enhancing CNS hemorrhage or resulting in generalized edema. Two important principles of management would appear to be gradual replacement of deficit when shock is absent and generous provision of potassium when high urine output makes this safe.

Hyponatremic states may be symptomatic, with diminished body water volume, as in Addison's disease or following loss of gastrointestinal fluid with replacement of volume but not of electrolyte. On the other hand, in conditions such as K^+ deficiency or impairment of renal water excretion, the hyponatremia is more likely to be asymptomatic because the ECF volume is normal. Under these circumstances ICF volume is increased, as is total body water.

In calculating requirements for therapeutic correction of symptomatic hyponatremic states, it must be realized that NaCl will be distributed osmotically throughout total body water, not the ECF alone, because water moves freely by osmosis to dilute administered solute. To avoid overhydration the salt should be administered as a hypertonic solution (0.5- to 1-M) in amounts estimated from a space distribution equal to about 70 percent of the lean body mass. For example, the amount required to raise the Na^+ concentration 20mEq/liter in a 10-kg child would be $10 \times 0.7 \times 20 = 140$ mEq, which is equal to 140 ml of 1-M NaCl. For safety, only one-half the calculated amount should be given rapidly, the other half being given a few hours later after the patient's condition has been reassessed and electrolyte levels have been measured again, if possible.

HYDROGEN ION STATUS. Disturbances of H^+ steady state in dehydration are usually secondary to one or more of the following: circulatory failure with tissue hypoxia or diminished renal function, starvation with ketosis, or specific losses of acid or base. When volume and osmolality are adequately restored, the kidneys and lungs will usually adjust the H^+ disturbances as long as neither renal nor pulmonary disease accompanies the disorder. When indicated, base may be given as bicarbonate, lactate, or acetate. Similarly, H^+ may be given as NH_4^+ salts, although this rarely proves necessary. In maintenance solutions the neutral chloride ion should account for about three-quarters of the anion, the remaining quarter being a base such as lactate.

Consideration of the distribution space for administered bicarbonate would require a complex analysis beyond the scope of this discussion. For clinical purposes one-third of the body weight can be taken as the immediate or short-term (a few hours) distribution space, with about double this quantity for the long-term distribution. When an anion base such as bicarbonate or lactate is given, there must be an accompanying cation, usually Na^+. Care must be taken not to impose a sudden osmolal burden, shifting body water suddenly from the brain to the ECF. A dose of up to 3 mEq/kg of weight has been shown to be safe, whereas more than 9 mEq/kg in a 12-hour period produces risk of brain injury.

Administration of bicarbonate will not only increase the HCO_3^-, but because of mass action the CO_2 (H_2CO_3) concentration will also rise. CO_2 diffuses more rapidly than HCO_3^- through body spaces. Hence in the CSF the CO_2 rise precedes the HCO_3^- rise; pH in CSF

therefore falls while pH in plasma is rising. The effect is short-lived, and its clinical importance has not been demonstrated for changes produced by small bicarbonate infusions, but there is a suggestion that larger dosages, greater than 5 mEq/kg, may be dangerous.

INTRACELLULAR POTASSIUM ION LOSSES. In many clinical varieties of dehydration, potassium will be lost from the cellular water. Frequently this loss remains masked until ECF solute and volume have been restored. At that time clinical evidences of K^+ loss may appear, including muscle weakness, ileus, abdominal distension, and sometimes electrocardiographic changes. Because K^+ replacement to cells must take place through the ECF, the rate must be carefully watched to prevent toxicity. A safe daily dosage when urine volume has become normal is 3 mEq/kg/24 hours. The concentration of potassium in intravenous solutions should not be higher than 40 mEq/liter.

EXTRACELLULAR   FLUID–SKELETON STEADY STATE. In a number of circumstances of dehydration, calcium levels in the ECF may fall. Renal impairment with phosphate retention, rapid dilution of body fluids, and sudden change in pH may all encourage hypocalcemia and tetany. Hypernatremic dehydration particularly precipitates hypocalcemia by a mechanism distinct from those mentioned, but apparently only when there is a concomitant deficit of potassium. Any of these hypocalcemic states may readily be treated by 10 ml of 10 percent calcium gluconate per 500 ml of infused solution.

References

Darrow; DC: The significance of body size. Am. J Dis Child 98:416, 1959

———— A Guide to Learning Fluid Therapy. Springfield, Ill, Charles C Thomas, 1964

Dell RB: In Winters RW (ed): The Body Fluids in Pediatrics. Boston, Little, Brown, 1973, p 23

Finberg L: Hypernatremic dehydration. Adv Pediatr 16:325, 1969

————: The management of the critically ill child with dehydration secondary to diarrhea. Pediatrics 45: 1029, 1970

Holliday M, Segar WE: Maintenance need for water in parenteral fluid therapy. Pediatrics 19:823, 1957

Sigaard-Anderson, O: Acid-base Status of the Blood, 3rd ed. Baltimore, Williams & Wilkins, 1965

Winters RW (ed): The Body Fluids in Pediatrics. Boston, Little, Brown, 1973, pp 46, 95, 113

DEHYDRATION AND ENTERIC DISEASE
Laurence Finberg

Dehydration commonly results from the vomiting and diarrhea associated with gastrointestinal disease. Many of the principles of treatment of fluid and electrolyte disturbance originated from study of these disorders. For this reason the principles discussed earlier in this chapter will now be applied to the management of infantile diarrheal disease. Similar concepts may be applied to dehydrated states arising from other causes.

Correction of the physiologic disturbances that accompany diarrhea and vomiting is of primary importance to the outcome. Vomiting often represents an early manifestation of the response to the infection or to abnormal water loss. Anorexia may be an even earlier symptom, and interference with intake hastens the appearance of serious functional disturbances involved in the pathogenesis of dehydration, such as loss of body water volume, changes in body fluid osmolality, disturbance of homeostasis, loss of intracellular ions, and disturbance of calcium homeostasis. Each of these disturbances must be appraised and considered in evolving a therapeutic plan. In addition, attention must be given to clinical indications of disturbances requiring supportive therapy.

Empirical observation has indicated that when diarrheal disease occurs in breast-fed infants, removal of the infant from the breast is rarely, if ever, necessary. There must be an early decision concerning the need for vigorous parenteral therapy requiring hospitalization. In North America and other areas where severe malnutrition has become rare and where *Shigella* bacilli and *Vibrio* cholerae are not encountered, the need for such treatment arises primarily in the patient whose oral intake has been markedly reduced, usually by persistent vomiting. Consideration of the intake needed merely to offset normal ongoing water losses makes it clear that in the presence of abnormal water loss without replacement the body weight may be reduced by 10 percent in only a few hours. Correction of dehydration requires an estimate of the extent of the physiologic disturbances, which may be considered in five major categories:

VOLUME. First the volume of deficit already incurred must be estimated. A careful history will usually reveal gradual cessation of intake. The objective physical findings of dehydration first appear when about 5 percent of the body weight has been lost within a 24-hour period. Experience clearly justifies the clinical maxim that changes in body weight as great as 1 percent or more between two measurements within 24 hours may be considered to be loss or gain of water. At about 5 percent rapid weight loss the clinical manifestations include dryness of mucous membranes and skin, mild tachycardia, and oliguria. When about 10 percent weight loss has occurred the signs are more ominous and, except when hypernatremia is present, are predominantly circulatory, since the losses are principally at the expense of the extracellular fluid (ECF). Tachycardia has by this time become pronounced, skin and membranes are very dry, and oliguria may be approaching anuria. The fontanelle, if open, will be palpably depressed, and the eyeballs will also be sunken into their sockets. The skin will show loss of elasticity and turgor. Owing to the nature of the subcutaneous tissue in the abnormal wall of infants, the abdominal skin remains in folds when gently pinched, and the color (blood) returns slowly to the compressed skin. The extremities will show mottling, and the distal portions will be cool to the touch. The infant frequently displays apathy and mild somnolence. When 15 percent of weight has been lost rapidly, a nearly moribund state of circulatory collapse will be present, frequently irreversible. Between each pair of landmarks the clinician may reasonably interpolate the estimated percentage of

weight loss. The degree of accompanying undernutrition, when present, may modify the clinical picture.

Weight, the most important measurement, should be determined with precision, since the admission weight will be the baseline for gauging success during the critical period of management. The level of urea nitrogen in serum provides a rough guide to the accuracy of the estimated circulatory disturbance. Repair of total volume and distribution of water between compartments are the two most important clinical determinants for successful therapy.

OSMOLALITY. Measurement of sodium concentration in infants with diarrhea has shown that in about 65 to 75 percent the sodium concentration in serum is in the normal range, the infants being isonatremic; about 10 percent are hyponatremic and from 15 to 25 percent hypernatremic. The importance of considering osmolality as reflected by the sodium concentration stems from its effect on the distribution of body water. In hypernatremic dehydrated states partial preservation of ECF occurs at the expense of the intracellular fluid (ICF), and as a result the circulation remains relatively intact.

Assessment of *hypernatremia* from the clinical history and physical findings alone cannot be accurate, but the experienced clinician can frequently suspect significant degrees of it. The clinical history almost always reveals an abrupt interruption in fluid intake, preceded occasionally by a high-solute feeding. Skim milk with a high solute load per calorie, concentrated evaporated milk mixtures, or improperly made solutions of water, salt, and sugar have often been incriminated. Serious salt poisoning has resulted from the error of mistaking salt for sugar. Anything that predisposes to excessive loss of water without proportionate solute loss may contribute to the background history. Persistent high fever, hyperventilation, and low humidity have all been contributory factors. Young infants whose surface areas are large relative to their weights are especially susceptible.

The physical presentation of these infants will depend on the severity of the volume loss, the degree of hypernatremia, and the rate of occurrence of the dehydration. The earliest recognition of hypernatremia from physical findings usually occurs when an infant has lost about 10 percent of body weight. Unlike the previous description, this infant will have a relatively intact circulation. The skin usually has a velvety sheen, and the abdominal wall sometimes has a doughy consistency. High fever, which is often present, may be a result as well as a cause of dehydration. Typically these infants display a peculiar combination of lethargy when undisturbed and marked irritability when mildly stimulated. They will scream with a high-pitched cry and tremble, only to slide back into somnolence when the stimulus is withdrawn. If the process is detected early there may be evidence of avid thirst. The neurologic signs usually progress in roughly the following manner: hypertonicity of muscles in the extremities and mild nuchal rigidity, markedly active deep tendon reflexes, twitching of muscle groups, and generalized tremulousness; finally, either total obtundation of sensorium or convulsions or both appear. The convulsions may be either focal or generalized.

Hyponatremia during dehydration occurs only when a high intake of water has been maintained without sufficient solutes. Giving large amounts of water or tea as the only oral intake, or parenteral glucose water with insufficient sodium, is the usual cause. In hyponatremic dehydration there is a greater proportion of ECF depletion per degree of volume deficit. Thus circulatory embarrassment appears with a relatively small degree of deficit and quickly becomes profound, making evident the need for additional sodium in therapy.

HYDROGEN ION HOMEOSTASIS. In diarrheal disease of infancy a metabolic acidosis or acidemia usually develops as a result of three separate disturbances. First, stool losses usually contain more bicarbonate than body fluids, the source of the base being the digestive fluids. Since stool pH results in part from bacterial action in the gut in fermenting organic substrates, an acid stool may appear even though excess base is being lost from the body. Second, the partial starvation and dehydration that accompany diarrhea give rise to ketosis and increased lactic acid production, thus increasing the nonvolatile hydrogen load. Finally, disturbance in renal function, particularly reduced glomerular filtration rate, impairs the capacity of the kidney to excrete the nonvolatile acids. The last factor is the limiting one in the interrelated processes. Consequently, whenever rates of glomerular filtration and urine flow can be reestablished quickly by proper adjustments of the vascular volume and the distribution of body water, the acidosis quickly recedes. If the process is very severe or if lasting renal impairment exists, correction of acidemia may require administration of base.

The only reliable physical sign of acidosis is hyperpnea, which may be less apparent in young infants than in older children. The usual laboratory measurement for assessing acidosis has been the CO_2 content of the plasma, which approximates the HCO_3^- concentration. In recent years improved instrumentation has made it possible to measure arterial pH values and Pco_2 and to evaluate the acid–base disturbance more completely. In most instances of diarrheal disease, correction of acidosis will be accomplished principally by the kidney.

INTRACELLULAR LOSSES. Careful studies of infants with diarrheal disease by Darrow, and later by Cooke and Darrow, have shown that potassium losses of 8 to 12 mEq/kg play an important part in the disability of these patients, particularly during the recovery period. Physical signs of potassium deficiency include abdominal distension, muscular weakness, and diminished reflexes. The electrocardiogram may show evidences of K^+ deficiency as well. Levels of K^+ in serum must be interpreted carefully, since they may be normal or even high during periods of oliguria even in the presence of severe deficiency in total body potassium. Improving hydration and correcting the acidosis, if it is present, unmasks the K^+ deficiency both clinically and biochemically. At this point CO_2 content tends to be high. Once urine output is assured, K^+ should be given

routinely to infants with dehydration secondary to diarrhea.

CALCIUM HOMEOSTASIS. Disturbances in calcium homeostasis are not common. The problem is almost invariably hypocalcemia, which occurs more often in hypernatremic dehydration, although rarely to a level where tetany occurs. However, the presence of phosphate retention and the occurrence during therapy of rapid dilution and increasing pH may aggravate the situation and produce symptoms. Values for serum Ca^{++} can be interpreted more fully if serum phosphate, protein, and pH determinations are also made.

IMPLEMENTATION OF FLUID THERAPY

The quantity and composition of the hydrating fluids should be selected on the basis of the needs of the individual patient. The volume of water to be administered in 24 hours should represent the volume of the estimated deficit, the estimated usual maintenance water (calculated as 1.5 times the basal requirement), and additions for any ongoing abnormal losses. When hypernatremia is suspected or diagnosed, the volume to replace the deficit should be distributed over 48 hours rather than included in the first 24 hours of therapy.

If the usual isonatremic type of dehydration is present, the sodium content allocated to the deficit fraction should approximate ECF water, or about 150 mEq/liter. No sodium need be added to this figure on the first day. Thus the maintenance fraction of the allocated water should contain glucose to combat starvation and ketosis, but no electrolytes. Potassium should be added after urine output is established. The anions for the Na^+ and K^+ should be Cl^- (75 percent) and base (25 percent) as bicarbonate, lactate, or acetate. In patients with very severe acidemia, some additional base should be given as bicarbonate. The infant who has lost 10 percent of his body mass will thus require 100 ml/kg of deficit water and 15 mEq/kg of deficit sodium (one-half and two-thirds of these, respectively, if he is hypernatremic), plus about an equal volume of maintenance water with glucose to which approximately 3 mEq of K^+ per kilogram will be added when it is safe to do so.

Although fluids may be given by other routes, continuous intravenous infusion should be used whenever possible in the early treatment of severe dehydration. The phases of treatment may be designated as emergency, repletion, early recovery, and resumption of nutrition. Unless near-fatal undernutrition exists as a concomitant, there is no need to increase stool losses by oral administration of protein, fat, or even large amounts of glucose. Thus a brief period of 6 to 24 hours of fasting and thirsting, followed by a gradual buildup of nutrient, will be anticipated.

EMERGENCY. The objectives during this phase, (to restore circulation and renal function), are achieved through rapid intravenous infusion of sufficient solution to restore vascular volume. The amount depends on the choice of solution. Whole blood, single-donor plasma, and 5 percent albumin (in doses of 20 ml/kg of body weight*) all have the advantage over noncolloid solutions of producing a more prolonged expansion of the vascular system. They may be followed by a similarly rapid infusion of 10 percent glucose in water, which will hasten urine output and provide glucose to starving cells. The lack of immediate availability, the expense, and the possibility of reactions or hepatitis are disadvantages to the use of blood or its derivatives. A solution of 10 percent glucose with 75 mEq of Na^+ (55 Cl^- and 20 HCO_3 $-$) per liter in a dose of 40 ml/kg given in 15 to 30 minutes has been equally successful. This phase is omitted in infants with hypernatremia, who are less likely to have circulatory impairment from volume depletion. However, if such a patient does present with even mild shock, either albumin or plasma should be given promptly, since life processes must take priority over the slight risk of further increasing the sodium content.

REPLETION. The repletion phase follows the emergency treatment and generally lasts about 6 to 8 hours. The calculated amounts of water and salt remaining are given moderately rapidly by intravenous infusion. K^+ is withheld until urine formation has been observed. The volume given in this phase plus that already given will equal approximately the estimated deficit. However, the repletion will still be incomplete because of ongoing losses, normal and possibly abnormal.

EARLY RECOVERY. The third phase lasts until the end of the first 24 hours. The remainder of the calculated fluid is given, plus any additions for abnormal losses. In this phase fluids may be given by mouth, using, if preferred, a glucose-electrolyte mixture. An example of a suitable solution would be one containing: 3.5% glucose, Na^+ 30–50 mEq/liter, K^+, 20 mEq/liter, Cl^- 20–50 mEq/liter, and a base (eg citrate, lactate, acetate), 20–30 mEq/liter. By the end of 24 hours the patient should have gained 8 to 9 percent in weight. If the change in weight is significantly less or more, the situation should be reanalyzed.

Hypernatremic patients should be treated more slowly, omitting the rapid phase and expanding the total time for repletion to 48 hours. In addition, calcium gluconate (10 ml of a 10 percent solution) should be added to each 500 ml of infusion, and the K^+ content of the fluid should be maximal (40 mEq/liter) once urine output has been established. These measures en-

hance cellular hydration and protect against changes in CSF pressure.

EARLY CONVALESCENCE. Milk feedings should be resumed gradually, substituting about 20 percent of the day's volume with a glucose-electrolyte mixture. The glucose concentration should be about 5 percent, and the sodium and potassium contents should provide 2 to 3 mEq of each ion per 100 ml of water. Too rapid a resumption of calories increases stool osmolality, which with impaired absorption often causes abnormal stool water loss. Some infants have a transient intestinal lactase deficiency lasting up to a few months, making a lactase-free feeding desirable during this period. A protein hydrolysate with glucose as the carbohydrate has been used successfully in this circumstance. In some centers such a preparation is used routinely for a few weeks for infants who are more seriously ill in an attempt to avoid a relapse.

SEQUELAE

The question of ultimate growth in infants who have had long-term diarrhea has been discussed in the section of malnutrition, with which diarrhea (infectious and noninfectious) is so clearly related. Permanent neurologic damage, primarily following hypernatremic dehydration, represents an added hazard for these patients. One careful series indicated an 8 percent mortality and an 8 percent rate of permanent cerebral sequelae. Precise data from prospective studies comparing hypernatremic dehydration with simple dehydration of diarrheal disease are not available, but it seems likely that the serious residual damage, presumably due to hemorrhage, is severalfold higher in the hypernatremic group. Whether adjusted therapy following its recognition improves this situation also remains unknown, but recent experience justifies hope that improvement will result.

For convenience, the weight used may be the dehydrated weight. To offset this "error" the water of oxidation may be ignored.

References

Cooke RE: Contributions of the laboratory to the practical management of disorders of body water and electrolytes. Pediatrics 16:555, 1955

Darrow DC, Pratt EL, Flett J JR, Gamble AH, Wiese HF: Disturbances of water and electrolytes in infantile diarrhea. Pediatrics 3:129, 1949

Dell RB: In Winters RW (ed): The Body Fluids in Pediatrics. Boston, Little, Brown, 1973, p 134

Finberg L: Hypernatremic dehydration. Adv Pediatr 16:325, 1969

———: Diarrheal dehydration. In Winters RW (ed): The Body Fluids in Pediatrics. Boston, Little, Brown, 1973, p 349

Govan CD, Darrow, DC: The use of potassium chloride in the treatment of the dehydration of diarrhea in infants. J Pediatr 28:541, 1946

Macauly D, Watson M: Hypernatremia in infants as a cause of brain damage. Arch Dis Child, 42:485, 1967

CHAPTER 8

Genetic Principles In Pediatrics

HAROLD M. NITOWSKY, *Associate Editor*

The extent of human diversity is readily apparent to the pediatrician because he deals with children who normally differ in their physical, physiologic, and behavior attributes and in their rates of development of these characteristics. Such diversity is manifest not only in health but also in individual variation in susceptibility and reaction to disease. Clearly some of these differences can be attributed, at least in part, to environmental circumstances. However, they also reflect inborn or genetic differences, for with the exception of monozygotic twins, no two individuals are exactly alike in genetic endowment.

Advances in our knowledge of human genetic disease have been dependent principally on developments in three related disciplines: *Population genetics* deals with the study of the distribution of specific genes in different populations and the impact that such genes have on maintenance of gene frequency, natural selection, and evolution. *Cytogenetics* is concerned with the location and organization of the genetic material on the chromosomes and the genetic aberrations associated with morphologic or numeric abnormalities of these structures. *Biochemical genetics* deals with the chemical identity of the gene and its product and the mechanisms by which the information coded in the genes regulates cellular metabolism. Although for many years man was regarded as an unsuitable subject for genetic study, recent contributions to the broad discipline from studies of human inborn metabolic disorders and chromosome abnormalities seem to emphasize that for some studies of genetic mechanism or gene action man is a unique subject for genetic investigation.

MOLECULAR GENETICS

HAROLD M. NITOWSKY

In the development of the concept of the fundamental unit of heredity, three basic properties were ascribed to the gene: it had to have a specific function in the cell, it had to be capable of exact self-replication in order to preserve this functional specificity from one generation to the next, and it had to be susceptible to sudden change or mutation at some finite frequency so that new genes differing in function could arise and thereby permit evolution of living forms. Classic genetic studies have elucidated how genes are arrayed in a linear order on the chromosome, how they are transmitted to an individual from his parents via the ovum and sperm so that they are present in pairs, and how, because of alterations arising from mutation, multiple forms of a gene, or alleles, can occupy a particular gene locus.

Major advances in molecular genetics in recent decades have provided insight into the basis for these unique properties of the gene. The discovery that the chemical bearer of the genetic code is deoxyribonucleic acid (DNA) and the elucidation of the molecular structure of this substance have provided insight into the basis and mechanism for gene specificity, gene mutation, and gene replication. Insight into the mechanism of gene action has come with the unraveling of the genetic code and the recognition that the primary biochemical role of DNA in the cell is to direct the synthesis of enzymes and other proteins.

The DNA molecule is made up of two very long polynucleotide chains coiled around a common axis to form a double helix. The regular alternation of phosphate and sugar groups forms the backbone of the DNA chain. A nitrogenous base consisting of a purine (adenine or guanine) or a pyrimidine (thymine or cytosine) is attached to each sugar group and projects inward from the chain. The two chains are held together by hydrogen bonding between the pairs of bases projecting at the same level from each chain. Because of their molecular structure there are certain restrictions in hydrogen bonding in the DNA chains, so that adenine pairs with thymine, and guanine with cytosine.

A gene can be regarded as a segment of DNA containing several hundred or thousand base pairs. Since variations in the linear sequence of base pairs along the chain can occur, a great many different permutations are possible, each of which is structurally and therefore functionally unique. Because of the restrictions in pairing, the sequence of bases in one chain fixes the sequence of bases in the other. Replication of the DNA can occur by the unwinding and separation of the chains and the re-formation on each chain of a DNA molecule with a complementary base sequence. Gene mutations can be envisaged as the consequence of an alteration of the base pair sequence of the particular gene, reflecting perhaps the change of only one base for another in the sequence. Other more drastic changes of the DNA, such as the deletion or duplication of base sequences, also can result in mutation.

The phenotype of the organism can be attributed, in the final analysis, to the distinctive activities and properties of a complex of different enzymes and other proteins synthesized in the cells. By their action these proteins define and control the complex pattern of metabolic and developmental processes that characterizes the individual. Proteins are composed of one or more polypeptide chains that are made up of long strings of amino acids linked by peptide bonds in a specific linear order. There are 20 different amino

TABLE 1. The Genetic Code

Second Nucleotide

First Nucleotide	A or U			G or C			T or A			C or G			Third Nucleotide
A or *U*	**AAA** *UUU*			**AGA** *UCU*			**ATA** *UAU*			**ACA** *UGU*			A or *U*
	AAG *UUC*	Phe		**AGG** *UCC*			**ATG** *UAC*	Tyr		**ACG** *UGC*	Cys		G or *C*
	AAT *UUA*			**AGT** *UCA*	Ser		**ATT** *UAA*			**ACT** *UGA*	Stop		T or *A*
	AAC *UUG*	Leu		**AGC** *UCG*			**ATC** *UAG*	Stop		**ACC** *UGG*	Trp		C or *G*
G or *C*	**GAA** *CUU*			**GGA** *CCU*			**GTA** *CAU*			**GCA** *CGU*			A or *U*
	GAG *CUC*			**GGG** *CCC*			**GTG** *CAC*	His		**GCG** *CGC*			G or *C*
	GAT *CUA*	Leu		**GGT** *CCA*	Pro		**GTT** *CAA*			**GCT** *CGA*	Arg		T or *A*
	GAC *CUG*			**GGC** *CCG*			**GTC** *CAG*	Gln		**GCC** *CGG*			C or *G*
T or *A*	**TAA** *AUU*			**TGA** *ACU*			**TTA** AAU			**TCA** *AGU*			A or *U*
	TAG *AUC*	Ile		**TGG** *ACC*			**TTG** *AAC*	Asn		**TCG** *AGC*	Ser		G or *C*
	TAT *AUA*			**TGT** *ACA*	Thr		**TTT** *AAA*			**TCT** *AGA*	Arg		T or *A*
	TAC *AUG*	Met		**TGC** *ACG*			**TTC** *AAG*	Lys		**TCC** *AGG*			C or *G*
C or *G*	**CAA** *GUU*			**CGA** *GCU*			**CTA** *GAU*			**CCA** *GGU*			A or *U*
	CAG *GUC*			**CGG** *GCC*			**CTG** *GAC*	Asp		**CCG** *GGC*			G or *C*
	CAT *GUA*	Val		**CGT** *GCA*	Ala		**CTT** *GAA*			**CCT** *GGA*	Gly		T or *A*
	CAC *GUG*			**CGC** *GCG*			**CTC** *GAG*	Glu		**CCC** *GGG*			C or *G*

The DNA codons appear in boldface type; the complementary RNA codons are in italics. A = adenine, C = cytosine, G = guanine, T = thymine. "Stop" represents nonsense triplets that appear to designate termination.

acids, so that with sequences of 100 to 500 amino acids, the number of possible structures is large. The folding of the polypeptide chain, which results in a three-dimensional structure with characteristic properties and functional activity, depends on the linear sequence of amino acids.

Studies with microorganisms and other systems have shown that the sequence of amino acids in the polypeptide chain is determined by the sequence of base pairs in a given gene and that each amino acid is specified by a sequence of three consecutive nonoverlapping bases. Studies of the genetic code, which appears to have universal biologic application, have shown that the four characteristic bases of the DNA chain can occur in 64 different triplet sequences, and each of 61 of these triplets specifies one of 20 amino acids (Table 1). The excess number of triplets in relation to the number of amino acids indicates the presence of degeneracy of the code, in that a particular amino acid may be coded by two or more different base triplets.

Several types of ribonucleic acid (RNA) molecules are involved in the translation of the base sequence in the DNA into the corresponding sequence of amino acids in a polypeptide chain. The first involves the formation of an RNA chain that is complementary in base sequence to one of the separate DNA chains. Similar base pairing restrictions apply, except for the substitution of uracil for thymine. This RNA strand, known as messenger RNA (mRNA), separates from the DNA and passes out of the cell nucleus to the ribosomes in the cytoplasm, which are the site of protein synthesis. Amino acids attached to another species of RNA molecule, known as transfer RNA (tRNA), are incorporated into a polypeptide chain in a sequence specified by the mRNA template. The tRNA molecules are relatively small and occur as a series of distinct forms, each specific for a particular amino acid by virtue of the presence in the polynucleotide sequence of a base triplet complementary to a base triplet in mRNA that codes for the

amino acids. The polypeptide chain is made sequentially, one amino acid being added at a time, starting from the amino terminal end. Thus the information coded in the genes serves as a blueprint for the structure of all the cellular enzymes and other proteins. In addition to specifying structure, genes appear to be concerned in regulating synthesis of proteins, although the mechanism for such regulation remains to be elucidated for multicellular organisms.

MUTATION. Mutation, or change in the genetic material, can readily be understood in terms of alteration of the base sequence of the DNA. When the term is used without further specification, it usually refers to a point mutation, or a change in a single base with substitution of one for another. Thus a change in DNA from CTT to CAT (Table 1) causes a substitution of valine for glutamic acid in the polypeptide chain, an alteration that occurs in the beta chain of sickle hemoglobin (p. 1149).

A second class of mutation is that resulting from nonhomologous pairing and unequal crossing-over, as depicted schematically in Figure 1. During the meiotic process in gametogenesis, homologous chromosomes

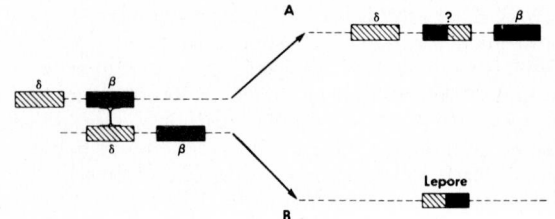

FIG. 1. Mutation as a result of nonhomologous pairing and unequal crossing-over. In A, gene duplication occurs from crossing-over between B and S genes. In B, a fusion gene occurs from crossing-over within a gene, a process presumed to have produced the gene for Lepore hemoglobin.

pair, but if the matching is not precise, unequal crossing-over occurs. The result is either duplication or deletion of genetic material. Gene duplication has been demonstrated as an important factor in evolution. The separate genes that specify the various polypeptide chains of hemoglobin (the beta chain of hemoglobin A, the delta chain of hemoglobin A_2, the gamma chain of hemoglobin F, and the alpha chains of all these hemoglobins), as well as the single polypeptide chain of myoglobin, appear to have evolved from a primordial common ancestral gene through the process of gene duplication and subsequent independent mutation of the separate genes.

Nonhomologous pairing with unequal crossing-over also can cause deletion of part of a gene or part of two contiguous genes. Study of the amino acid sequence in some abnormal hemoglobins suggests that this was the type of mutation responsible for the altered protein. Hemoglobin Lepore (p. 1157) is presumed to be an example of a mutation due to unequal crossing-over. The genes for the beta and delta chains of hemoglobin are probably contiguous. In a person with hemoglobin Lepore, the normal beta and delta chains are replaced by a polypeptide chain that has the structure of the delta chain at one end and of the beta chain at the other. As shown in Figure 1, a fusion gene specifying a hybrid polypeptide chain of this type could have arisen by unequal crossing-over.

A third class of mutation is that resulting in gross chromosomal abnormalities. This class includes abnormalities of chromosome number as a result of errors in chromosome segregation during mitosis or meiosis and abnormalities of chromosome structure (eg, chromosomal deletions, translocations, or inversions) as a result of chromosome breakage.

In general, mutations that represent a change in the genetic material are likely to be deleterious in terms of selection and evolution. Reliable estimates of spontaneous mutation rates have been obtained with microorganisms. These rates can be increased by such factors as ionizing radiation, certain chemicals, and an increase in temperature. On the other hand, precise estimates of mutation rates in man are difficult to obtain. The figures of 1 to 5 mutations per 100,000 loci per generation are frequently cited and have been derived, at least in part, from studies of dominantly inherited pathologic traits. It has been estimated that each person carries a genetic load of four or more mutant genes, which would be lethal in the homozygous state. Increases in the number of undesirable recessive genes caused by mutation may persist for many generations before being expressed in a homozygote.

Only those mutations that occur in the genetic material of the gametes will lead to heritable changes. Mutations involving somatic cells will be transmitted to the descendants of that cell, but not to subsequent generations of individuals. However, to the extent that such alterations may be associated with some forms of neoplastic disease, they may be considered a form of lethal mutation.

References

Hood LE, Wilson JH, Wood WB: Molecular Biology of Eukaryotic Cells. Menlo Park, Calif, WA Benjamin, 1975

Ingram VM: Biosynthesis of Macromolecules, 2nd ed. Menlo Park, Calif, WA Benjamin, 1971

Stent GS: Molecular Genetics. San Francisco, WH Freeman, 1971

Watson JD: Molecular Biology of the Gene, 2nd ed. New York, WA Benjamin, 1970

GENETIC DISEASE IN FAMILIES AND POPULATIONS

Helen M. Ranney

In the somatic cells of man and other diploid organisms, autosomes (all chromosomes except the sex chromosomes are autosomes) are found in pairs, one of each pair being from each parent. Consequently somatic cells contain two genes at each locus, which may in some examples be two base sequences responsible for the manufacture of autosomally controlled proteins. The term locus refers to any particular region on the chromosome that is occupied by a given gene. Alleles are alternate forms of genes that could occupy a given locus. Although two genes for each autosomal trait will be present in any individual, several alleles may be present in a group of individuals. For example, in the ABO blood group system an individual may have any two genes (eg, AA or AO or AB) but not, of course, three genes, although the allelic genes A, B, and O are present in a population. If the two genes are identical (ie, AA) the individual is homozygous for that factor; if the two genes differ (eg, AO or AB) the individual is heterozygous.

STUDIES OF FAMILIES

Much of our knowledge of human heredity is derived from studies of the patterns of inheritance of certain characteristics or diseases. In these patterns (an example of which is illustrated in Figure 2) the proband (propositus, index case) is indicated by an arrow, males by squares.

AUTOSOMAL DOMINANT INHERITANCE. If the characteristic or disease in question is manifest in the individual heterozygous for that gene (ie, if a single dose of the gene results in manifestations) then that character is *dominant,* and the gene itself is (more conveniently than correctly) referred to as dominant. In autosomal dominant inheritance the trait will be found in one parent (of either sex) and in half the sons and half the daughters of an affected individual. This is the expected result of a mating in which a parent passes either the normal or the mutant gene to the offspring and the corresponding gene derived from the other parent is normal. The offspring who have the abnormal gene will manifest the trait, and the remainder (one half) will be normal. The homozygous state for many diseases that exhibit a dominant mode of inheritance is not known; many are probably lethal before birth. When a disease

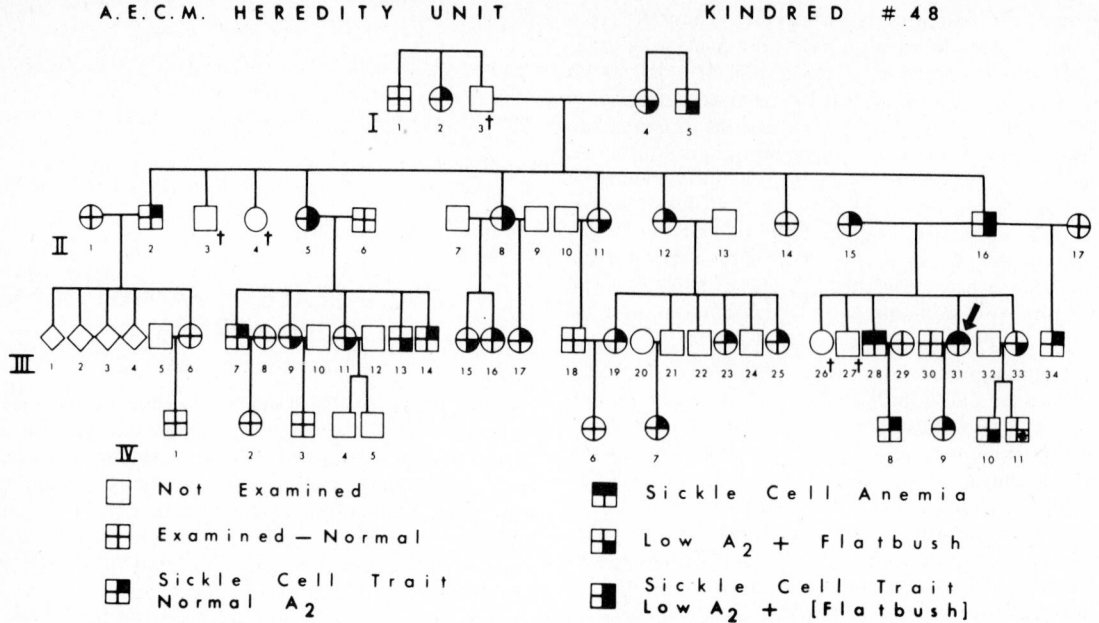

FIG. 2. Pedigree of a family in which three individuals (II-5, II-8, and II-16) were heterozygous for both a β-chain hemoglobin abnormality (Hb S) and a δ-chain variant (Hb Flatbush). (For technical reasons, presence of Hb Flatbush in the presence of Hb S had to be inferred from the accompanying depression of Hb A_2.) Note that the offspring of these three individuals had either Hb S or Hb Flatbush. Also, from studies of generation 1, the genes for S and Flatbush would be expected to be in repulsion in II-5, II-8, and II-16.

is determined by a dominant gene, the disease is not usually encountered in offspring of unaffected individuals, and only occasionally is a skipping of generations observed. In these circumstances the apparently unaffected parent may have minimal or even undetectable evidence of the presence of the gene in question. When more sophisticated laboratory techniques are utilized, manifestations of the gene can frequently be detected in such phenotypically apparently normal parents. For example, when the apparently unaffected sibling of a patient with hereditary spherocytosis (HS) has a child with HS, the autohemolysis test may disclose a previously undetected erythrocyte defect in the parent.

AUTOSOMAL RECESSIVE INHERITANCE. Whereas in autosomal dominant inheritance the trait or disorder is the result of a single abnormal gene, the designation *recessive* implies that both genes must be abnormal for the appearance of clinical manifestations. While the heterozygote is symptomatic in diseases that are determined by dominant genes, only the homozygote is symptomatic in the case of recessive genes. Since the heterozygous state for recessives does not generally result in readily detectable clinical manifestations, the patterns of inheritance of autosomal recessives have certain distinguishing features: the parents, both heterozygous, are generally clinically normal; the disease affects both sexes equally, and sibships in which more than one child is affected are frequent; particularly in the case of rare recessive traits, a high incidence of consanguinity is observed in parents; affected patients

who marry normal persons usually have only normal offspring; if both parents have the same recessive disease, all their offspring will be affected. Thus in the usual pedigree in which the parents are heterozygotes, one-fourth of the offspring inherit the abnormal genetic factor from each parent and are affected, one-half are heterozygotes like the parents, and one-fourth are normal. In considering expected ratios (such as one-half affected offspring of a parent with a dominant trait, or one-fourth affected offspring of matings of individuals heterozygous for a recessive trait) it should be emphasized that the ratios are theoretical and that families in which no individual has been affected will not be detected. In studies of small families that have been identified by the presence of an affected individual, inclusion of the probands will result in higher ratios than those predicted.

The distinction between dominant and recessive traits is useful, but it is to some extent arbitrary. Heterozygous carriers of many recessive diseases can be recognized by appropriate tests and are therefore distinguishable from normals. For example, the heterozygote for sickle cell trait is readily recognized, although serious manifestations generally occur only in homozygotes with sickle cell anemia.

X-LINKED INHERITANCE. The differences in the sex chromosomes (XX for females and XY for males) provide the basis for characteristic patterns of inheritance for genes carried on the X chromosome. The traits determined by genes carried on the X chromosome may be either recessive or dominant in the female, but in the male, who has only one X chromosome, the trait will always be expressed. Alternatively stated, a female may be heterozygous or homozygous for an X-linked gene, but the male can only be hemizygous; and X-linked genes that are recessive in females will consequently have clinical manifestations in males. In large pedigrees the pattern of inheritance may suggest X linkage, dominant or recessive, since the trait will *not* be transmitted from father to son. When the X-linked trait is a rare recessive, the affected individuals will be males who are related to each other through females. In pedigrees of serious X-linked recessive disorders such as hemophilia, the affected males may not survive to have children. The history of disease in maternal uncles and in the sisters' male children should be sought in possible X-linked disorders.

Recessive X-linked disorders are occasionally found in females who are homozygous for the disorder. Instances of homozygosity in females will, of course, be observed if the abnormal gene is common in the population (as in glucose-6-phosphate dehydrogenase deficiency in blacks) or if consanguineous matings have occurred in the pedigree. The heterozygous female (the carrier in the case of recessives) transmits the abnormal gene to one-half of her sons and one-half of her daughters. The hemizygous male transmits the gene to all of his daughters and none of his sons. The homozygous female transmits a single abnormal gene to all of her sons, as well as her daughters (who will be affected if the trait is dominant and will be carriers if the trait is recessive). An unaffected male in a family with an X-linked disorder will not transmit the disorder to any of his children.

LYON HYPOTHESIS. Although many genes are known to be carried on the X chromosome, the X-linked gene products, such as antihemophilia factor (AHF) or glucose-6-phosphate dehydrogenase (G6PD), do not show significant quantitative differences between normal males (with one X) and females (with two X's). Furthermore, there is a wide range of expression in the heterozygous female carriers for X-linked diseases: some carriers of hemophilia have no demonstrable deficiency of AHF, while others have intermediate levels. In 1961 Lyon suggested that one X chromosome in each cell of the female is randomly inactivated in early embryogenesis and that the descendants of each cell may carry the same pattern of inactivation. Thus each cell of the female would contain only one active X chromosome, and the levels of X-linked gene products would be the same in normal individuals of either sex. If random inactivation occurred when only a few cells were present, then in some heterozygous carriers for AHF more normal than abnormal X chromosomes would be inactivated, and consequently decreased levels of AHF might be observed.

SEX INFLUENCE ON AUTOSOMAL INHERITANCE. Certain traits are genetically determined by autosomal factors but have different manifestations in males and females. The most frequently cited example is pattern baldness, which is determined by an autosomal gene; it behaves as a dominant in men and as a recessive in women. Distinction between sex influence and X linkage may be difficult in small pedigrees that do not include significant numbers of father–son relationships. If a sex-influenced disorder results in infertility of affected males, the distinction between autosomal dominant and X-linked recessive inheritance may not be possible.

ALLELISM, INDEPENDENT ASSORTMENT, AND LINKAGE. While alleles appear to segregate as the chromosome number is reduced by half at meiosis, certain genes, as Mendel originally observed, assort independently. The most informative pedigrees concerning allelism versus independent assortment of two genetic factors include two (or preferably more) offspring of a parent who is heterozygous for both traits under investigation and a parent who has neither trait, ie, the parental mating is a test cross. Examples of the inheritance of human hemoglobins serve to illustrate the differences. Hemoglobins S and C, both β-chain abnormalities, behave as alleles and segregate as indicated in Figure 3. Each child of a parent with sickle

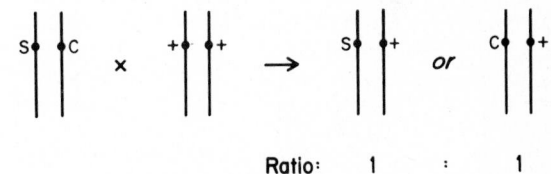

Ratio:　1　:　1

FIG. 3. Segregation of allelic genes for Hb S and Hb C. Vertical bars indicate portions of chromosome. Note that none of the offspring has either parental genotype. Studies of offspring of a test cross ie., marriage of heterozygote for two abnormal traits to a normal) are very useful for this type of analysis.

cell/hemoglobin C disease will have either S trait or C trait, but no child will inherit both S and C or both normal hemoglobin genes.

Certain other abnormal hemoglobins are abnormal in the α polypeptide chain. Individuals with variants in both the α and β chains have been described (such individuals have four major hemoglobin components), and the composition of the hemoglobin of their offspring provides evidence for independent assortment (Fig. 4). From examination of Figures 3 and 4 it is obvious that when the genes are allelic only two types of offspring result from a test cross, but if the two genes assort independently four types of offspring may occur.

In some recessive diseases the demonstration of independent assortment may disclose that different genetic factors underlie what appears to be phenotypically the same disease. Thus if two parents who appear to have the same recessive disorder (and would therefore be homozygous) have normal children, the inference that the parents do not have the same abnormal gene despite similar clinical manifestations is a good one. Ideas concerning allelism of certain genes determining proteins can be deduced from studies of protein structure. Alterations in a single polypeptide will probably

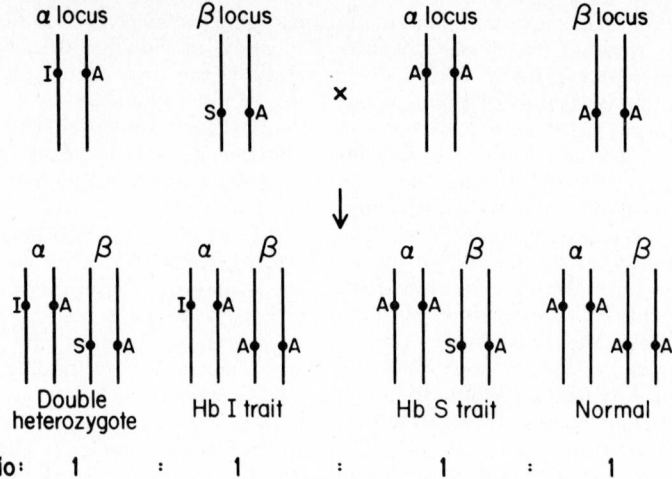

FIG. 4. Independent assortment of α- and β-chain loci appears in offspring. Note that four types of offspring may be observed from a test cross. Sufficient data are not available for choosing either independent assortment or linkage as the determining factor for the α and β Hb loci in humans.

be determined by alleles, as in the β polypeptide chain of hemoglobin. Nonallelic genes would be expected to control different polypeptides or proteins.

While in Figure 4 the α and β loci of hemoglobin are depicted on separate chromosome pairs, the available data would also be compatible with their presence on a single chromosome, but separated by a considerable distance. In the latter circumstance the presence of parental genotypes (normal and double heterozygous) in the offspring would result from crossing-over. Each chromosome must carry many genes, and when two genes are very near each other on the chromosome the likelihood of crossing-over is small. Thus by family studies of traits in humans it may not be possible to distinguish allelism from close linkage. (Differences in gene products may be used to favor linkage over allelism). When genes are located farther apart on the same chromosome, the chances of crossing-over during meiosis increase; as a result of crossing-over the genes on opposite members of a chromosome pair in the parent will lie on the same chromosome in the gamete. (The importance of crossing-over for rearrangement of genes should be recalled: it results in the transmission of genes from both grandparents on the same chromosome.) If the genes lie sufficiently far apart on the same chromosome, crossing-over may be so frequent that pedigree data will suggest independent assortment. For demonstration of linkage, then, the loci must be at a distance sufficiently small that the recombinant types are encountered less frequently than in the 1:1:1:1 ratios that would result from independent assortment.

As a result of crossing-over, genes that were originally in the *trans-* position (linked in repulsion) come to lie on the same chromosome in the *cis-* position (linked in coupling). The results of a test cross for two traits in the *cis-* position will differ from the results if the genes are in the *trans-* position. A theoretical example of studies of linkage in the *trans-* position is depicted in Figure

5 (top). If two factors A and B (whose corresponding normal alleles are a and b) are observed to segregate in the offspring of the mating AaBb × aabb in the ratios Aabb (40) + aaBb (40) + AaBb (10) + aabb (10), the genes for A and B are neither independent nor allelic. The less frequent types (AaBb and aabb) are the recombinants that result from crossing-over. Linkage and the relative distances between loci can be deduced from such pedigree data: the proportion of recombinants increases with the distance between loci. In the third type of offspring in the example of Figure 5 (top), genes A and B have come to lie on the same chromosome and are linked in coupling. Note in Figure 5 (bottom) that a test cross for linkage in coupling will result in predominantly parental types (AaBb or aabb) in the offspring. Whether linkage is in coupling or in repulsion can usually be established from studies of the parents of the double heterozygotes.

Data regarding autosomal linkage from studies of pedigrees are difficult to obtain. The ABO locus and the locus for the nail-patella syndrome are linked; one type of hereditary elliptocytosis and the Rh locus are linked, as are the Lutheran blood group and secretor loci. From Figure 2 it is clear that the loci for the δ chain of hemoglobin A₂ and the β chain of hemoglobin A are linked. A large number of linked genes on the autosomes have been identified by studies of somatic cell hybrids.

X LINKAGE. The mapping of the X chromosome is a great deal easier than the mapping of autosomes, since the fact that the genes are on the same chromosome is usually established from the pedigree. The occurrence of traits in the sons of mothers heterozygous for the two X-linked defects yields the necessary information; the father is irrelevant to the study since he transmits X-linked factors only to his daughters. Whether the X-linked traits were in repulsion or in coupling in the mother can be determined from studies of

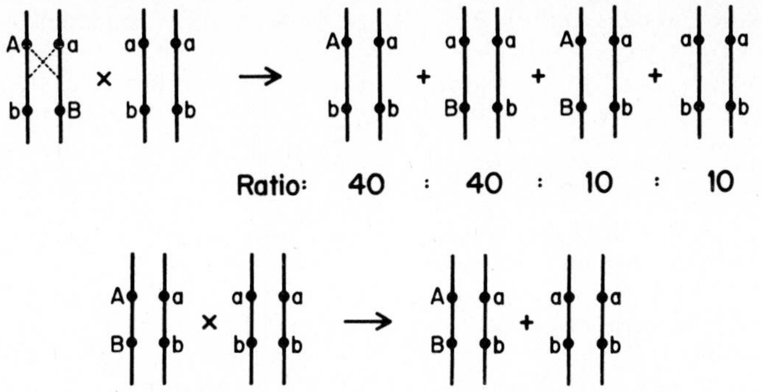

FIG. 5. *Top.* Linkage and crossing-over. Genes A and B are linked in repulsion. Test cross yields four classes of offspring, of which the last two are recombinants resulting from crossing-over (indicated by dotted lines). Fewer of the offspring will be found in recombinant than in nonrecombinant classes. With linkage in repulsion, most offspring receive either A or B and do not resemble parents. Chances for crossing-over increase as the chromosome segment separating the two genes becomes larger. *Bottom.* Offspring of test cross of individuals in third group of offspring at top of figure, in whom A and B are linked in coupling. Note that offspring have phenotypes like parents (AB/ab or ab/ab) in this case. Possible recombinant types are not given in this diagram.

her father. Studies of X-linked genetic factors have been summarized by McKusick in a tentative map of the X chromosome: loci for Xg blood groups, G6PD, color blindness (deutan), and hemophilia appear to occur in that order.

BLOOD TYPE AND DISEASE.   In recent years the incidence of certain diseases has been noted to be greater in people with certain blood types. For example, duodenal ulcer is more common in people with blood type O than in those with blood type A. Such association is not based on genetic linkage; in large populations (as a result of crossing-over) genetic linkage is usually demonstrated for *loci* rather than for specific genes. The physiologic basis of association of disease with blood types is not understood.

MULTIFACTORIAL TRAITS.   While most of the traits that have been studied intensively from the biochemical standpoint are determined by single genes, numerous common traits are determined by several genes. Many of these multifactorial or quantitative traits, such as stature, skin color, and intelligence, are greatly influenced by environment. One of the outstanding features of multifactorial traits is the continuous distribution that is observed when the trait is measured in a large population. Such a continuous distribution contrasts with the discontinuous curves observed when unifactorial traits are studied, for in the latter case values may correspond closely to normal, homozygous, and in some cases heterozygous states. Statistical approaches to the evaluation of multifactorial traits are based on observations of resemblances among relatives.

Twin Studies

Studies of traits of monozygotic and dizygotic twins have long been used in distinguishing the effects of heredity and environment. Definitive interpretation of zygosity may not be easy. Determinations of genetic markers (eg, blood groups, red cell and serum proteins,

and enzymes) can establish dizygosity, but definitive proof of monozygosity rests on tests for these markers and on acceptance of skin grafts between the two individuals, or on studies of the fetal membranes if they are available. All monochorionic twins are monozygotic, but some monozygotic twins will have two chorions and even two placentas. Twin studies in which the occurrence of a given trait in monozygotic twins is compared with that in dizygotic twins are valuable in analysis of some genetic problems.

Population Genetics

Some of the concepts of population genetics facilitate appreciation of the genetic aspects of disease. The number of loci available for a gene and its allele will, in a population of diploid organisms, be twice the number of individuals. In systems in which two or more different gene products can be detected, as in the MN blood groups or the hemoglobins, gene frequency can be determined by a simple count. For example, in a population of 10,000 that includes 1,400 individuals with sickle cell trait, 50 individuals with sickle cell anemia (homozygous for Hb S without other β-chain abnormalities), and 8,550 individuals with normal hemoglobin, the gene frequency is as follows:

$$\text{Hb S} \quad \frac{1,400 + (2 \times 50)}{20,000 \text{ (total no. of genes)}} = 0.075$$

$$\text{Hb A} \quad \frac{1,400 + (2 \times 8,550)}{20,000} = 0.925$$

The Hardy-Weinberg law indicates that the genetic structure of a large, stable, randomly mating population will be constant in successive generations. Observations on gene and genotype frequencies are useful in deciding about the equilibrium of a population. The gene frequency of a given trait is the proportion of the loci in a population occupied by that gene; hence the sum of the frequencies of all the alleles for a given locus will be unity. If p designates the frequency of Hb β^A and q designates that of Hb β^S ($p + q = 1$), the observed value of either p or q may be used to calculate the chances that an individual will have two β^A genes (p^2) or two β^S genes (q^2) or be heterozygous ($2pq$). In the example cited, gene frequency for Hb S and Hb A was determined by simple counting; calculation of expected genotype frequencies from values of p or q may indicate a significant departure from equilibrium, ie, the observed frequency of one genotype may be quite different from that expected from gene frequency. For example, if 9 (instead of 50) patients with sickle cell anemia, 1,400 with sickle cell trait, and 8,591 with normal hemoglobin had been observed in the population of 10,000, the value for q (Hb β^S) from counting would be 0.0709, and its value by calculation from q^2 (9/10,000) would be 0.03. This population, with frequencies of 14 percent sickle cell trait and about 0.1 percent sickle cell anemia, would not be in equilibrium. Mutation, losses of homozygotes, immigration, and nonrandom mating will all obviously disturb the equilibrium, but in the absence of such factors gene frequency will remain stable from generation to generation.

In addition to appraisal of the equilibrium of a population, calculations based on the binomial or Hardy-Weinberg law find extensive use in studies of recessive diseases. If q^2 represents the incidence of a recessively determined disease (eg, 1/10,000), then the gene frequency q will be $\sqrt{1/10,000} = 1/100$. Since $p + q = 1$, the incidence of the remaining genotypes can be calculated: $p^2 = (99/100)^2 = 98.01$ percent (normals); $2pq = 2 \times 1/100 \times 99/100 = 1.98$ percent (heterozygotes). Such arithmetic demonstrates the strikingly high incidence of carriers for rare recessive disorders.

The unusual frequencies of certain traits (or diseases) in a population derived from a small ancestral group is explained by genetic drift. McKusick has shown that in certain Pennsylvania Amish who are descended from a few immigrants the incidence of a very rare recessively determined disease (dwarfism-polydactyly) suggests a carrier (heterozygote) rate of about 13 percent in that population. One of the small group of original Amish émigrés must have been a carrier for this gene, and its present high incidence represents the result of genetic drift. Genetic drift obviously will occur largely in small populations that for geographic or social reasons tend to marry within the group (isolates).

POLYMORPHISM. Traits that exist in a population in two or more discontinuous forms are said to be polymorphic. Sex and eye color are examples of polymorphism. When genes result in genetic death (ie, failure of the individual to reproduce at the usual rate), as in sickle cell anemia, a gradual loss of these genes from the population under study results. To maintain a polymorphism for deleterious genes, replacement of the genes lost by death of homozygotes is necessary. Obviously, different mechanisms might exist for such replenishment: the mutation rate might be high enough to maintain the gene frequency, families in which losses of homozygotes have occurred might deliberately have more children to make up for the losses, or there might

be some selective advantage of heterozygotes over normal homozygotes. The latter mechanism, called balanced polymorphism, has been invoked to explain the high incidence of sickle cell trait in certain areas of Africa where homozygotes for hemoglobin S surely have a low reproduction rate. There is evidence to suggest that in these areas children with sickle cell trait are more resistant to fatal cerebral malaria than are children with normal hemoglobin. Thus the genes for Hb S lost in patients with sickle cell anemia are balanced by the loss of genes for Hb A in malaria, and a high incidence of Hb S trait is preserved. It seems probable that balanced polymorphism on the basis of selective advantage of the heterozygote explains the persistence of many genes that result in genetic death in affected homozygotes. However, in the majority of instances the specific advantage conferred by heterozygosity remains to be clarified.

CONSANGUINITY. The known increase in frequency of recessive diseases in the offspring of consanguineous marriages lends support to the notion that such marriages are not desirable. Each individual may be presumed to carry several deleterious recessive genes that will not be expressed in his offspring unless his marital partner carries the same genes. The chance that the offspring of two related parents will be homozygous for a given gene increases with the degree of relationship and is expressed as the coefficient of inbreeding (F). Values for F are ⅛ for offspring of uncle–niece marriage and 1/16 for children of first cousins. In families in which a rare recessive disease has been observed, the chances that a child will be affected are obviously greatly increased by consanguinity of the parents. However, despite the sound theoretic objection to consanguineous marriages, most of the offspring of first-cousin marriages in families lacking a history of recessive disease are healthy, a fact that may help alleviate the panic that sweeps some families when first-cousin marriages are announced.

References

Baglioni C: The fusion of two peptide chains in hemoglobin Lepore and its interpretation as a genetic deletion. Proc Natl Acad Sci USA 48:1880, 1962

Court Brown WM: Human Population Cytogenetics. Amsterdam, North-Holland, 1967

Harris H: The Principles of Human Biochemical Genetics, 2nd ed. New York, American Elsevier, 1975

Kirkman HN, Riley HD, Crowell BB: Different enzymic expressions of mutants of human glucose-6-phosphate dehydrogenase. Proc Natl Acad Sci USA 46:938, 1960

Lyon MF: Gene action in the X-chromosome of the mouse (Mus musculus L). Nature 190:372, 1961

McKusick VA: Human Genetics, 2nd ed. Englewood Cliffs, NJ, Prentice-Hall, 1969

————: Mendelian Inheritance in Man. Catalogs of Autosomal Dominant, Autosomal Recessive and X-Linked Phenotypes, 4th ed. Baltimore, Johns Hopkins Univ Press, 1975

Perutz MF, Lehmann H: Molecular pathology of human hemoglobin. Nature 219:902, 1968

Thompson JS, Thompson MW: Genetics in Medicine, 2nd ed. Philadelphia, WB Saunders, 1973

DEVELOPMENTAL GENETICS

S. Gluecksohn-Waelsch

All biologic form and function, including processes of development, are under genetic control; the field that deals with the mechanisms by which genes act in development and differentiation is known as developmental genetics.

CHROMOSOMES AND DEVELOPMENT.

Chromosomes, the carriers of genes, control development, and normal development requires a full set of chromosomes. The role of genes during development extends from control of protein and enzyme structure and synthesis to all phases of morphogenesis. Throughout development there appears to be a well-determined temporal and spatial pattern that underlies the sequential activation of different genes in differentiating cells, tissues, and organs. Moreover, the reaction of the developing organism to a variety of noxious agents is also under genetic control, and susceptibility and resistance to teratogenic agents vary depending on the presence of different genes. Among the external agents causing chromosomal abnormalities are viruses, chemicals, and ionizing radiation. Quantitative estimates yield a figure of 0.25 percent as the overall incidence of chromosomal abnormalities responsible for congenital defects at birth in the general population. When anomalies of number and structure are included, the overall incidence of chromosomal abnormalities that are severe enough to cause prenatal death becomes considerably higher; it is estimated to be more than 5 percent. The diversity of biochemical and metabolic processes and the interaction of cells, tissues, and organs with each other account for the fact that a mutational change of a single gene may lead to a multiplicity of manifestations. A better understanding of the mechanisms of the genetic control of all aspects of development is an important prerequisite for possible prevention and control of abnormalities of development.

SINGLE GENES AFFECTING DEVELOPMENT.

A considerable proportion of single gene mutations, autosomal as well as sex-linked, produce effects clearly manifest at birth, in the form of either morphologic or metabolic abnormalities. The analysis of mechanisms by which these gene-controlled disturbances arise requires observations of sequential stages of development and experimental procedures that are not applicable to humans. However, experimental material is available for study in the large variety of mutations in other mammals, particularly the laboratory mouse; studies of these mutants have revealed mechanisms of gene-controlled abnormal development that may apply to similar conditions in man.

Congenital renal agenesis and dysplasia may be caused by mutant genes in both man and mouse. It has been shown in the mouse that inductive interaction between ureteric bud and metanephrogenic mesenchyme normally required for kidney morphogenesis fails to occur in mutant embryos. The reason for this failure to interact seems to lie in general growth retardation that affects the two primordia differentially. Therefore the ureteric bud, which is retarded in its growth, does not reach the metanephrogenic mesenchyme when the latter is ready to react to the inductive stimulus with further differentiation into secretory tubules. The effects of this mutation on temporal and integrative aspects of kidney differentiation clearly indicate that genes normally control these phases of differentiation.

PLEIOTROPIC EFFECTS.

Developmental studies of mutant gene effects are particularly valuable when single mutations appear to cause multiple defects, a phenomenon referred to as pleiotropy. The mutations causing macrocytic anemia in the mouse are also responsible for abnormalities involving hair pigment and the gonads. The mutation causing kidney agenesis produces skeletal anomalies as well. Human congenital defects due to the action of pleiotropic genes include, among many others, acrocephalosyndactyly with malformations of skull and extremities; osteogenesis imperfecta with brittle bones, blue sclerae, and otosclerosis; and Marfan's syndrome with anomalies of the eye, the skeleton, and the cardiovascular system. In this developmental analysis of pleiotropic effects caused by a single gene mutation, attempts are made to find the earliest and most immediate defect that could be responsible for all subsequent anomalies. As a result of such studies, a so-called pedigree of causes may be constructed where the original cause is the immediate effect of the mutant gene and all others arise from it secondarily. However, in the majority of cases it has not been possible to fit all pleiotropic effects into such pedigrees with ease. A good example is offered by the mutations that simultaneously cause abnormalities of erythropoiesis, gonadal development, and pigmentation. In spite of careful studies it has not been possible to establish a series of sequential effects connecting the three developmental systems so that the abnormality of one might be responsible for the abnormalities affecting the others, as should be the case in a typical pedigree of causes. It may be assumed that three closely linked genes (rather than one gene) enclosed in a deletion are the cause of the abnormalities of the three systems. However, since one series of alleles at the W locus, and another independent gene (S1) causes the same associated anomalies in the mouse, this explanation of a deletion of three closely linked factors is unlikely. The observations of the pleiotropic effects indicate a close developmental relationship between the three systems, the nature of which remains to be demonstrated.

PENETRANCE AND EXPRESSIVITY.

The genetic concepts of penetrance and expressivity have strong developmental implications. A dominant mutation with *reduced penetrance* is defined as one that manifests itself in only a certain proportion of heterozygotes. This reduced penetrance may be due to various causes, such as the protection that other genes or the maternal environment provide for at least a proportion of embryos to prevent the potential damage inflicted upon them by the mutant gene. *Expressivity* refers to the degree of manifestation of a gene; a gene may have slight and hardly noticeable effects, or it may cause defects of considerable scope. Clinically, variable expressivity of a gene results in a disease state of greater or lesser severity. Mechanisms similar to those described for penetrance that are operating during prenatal life may be responsible for the observed variations of gene expressivity.

PRENATAL RESISTANCE AND SUSCEPTIBILITY. Genes are involved in the control of resistance and susceptibility to a variety of agents during prenatal development. In mice, genetic analysis has revealed genetic control of periods of susceptibility of embryos to several teratogens, such as those causing cleft palate. The different gene-controlled sensitive periods are responsible for the different effects of identical teratogens in genetically different animals. It is known that the palate of the mouth forms as the result of fusion of the palatal shelves. It has been shown that closure of the palate normally occurs at different times of development in different strains of mice. Those strains in which closure occurs early are less susceptible to the effects of teratogens than are those strains where closure occurs late. Therefore gene-determined differences in the temporal pattern of a developmental process may serve to explain differences in resistance and susceptibility to teratogens of different inbred strains of mice.

LETHAL GENES. Genes causing prenatal or perinatal death in mammals are referred to as lethal genes. These have played a prominent role in the analysis of mammalian development and differentiation because of their particularly drastic and thus easily recognizable effects. Considerable proportions of prenatal and perinatal deaths in man are likely to be due to lethal genes that interfere with normal development and differentiation.

PHENOCOPIES. The phocomelia mutation in the mouse is of particular significance because it produces a phenotype that bears a close resemblance to the abnormalities of limb development observed in so-called thalidomide babies. A similarity of a phenotype caused by environmental agents to one resulting from the effects of deleterious genes is implied in the term phenocopy. Identical phenotypes may owe their existence to a variety of causes of genetic or environmental nature. Cleft palate, for example, may be due to the effect of different genes and may also result from the exposure of the pregnant mother to teratogenic agents. Renal agenesis in the mouse may result from different mutant genes. Nervous system abnormalities, such as anencephaly, may raise from the action of dominant or recessive genes; they may also result from maternal exposure to radiation during gestation. Similarly, vitamin deficiencies of the mother during gestation may lead to developmental defects indistinguishable from those caused by certain mutant genes. An important point in considering congenital defects is that the phenotype in itself does not reflect a specific genotype or a particular etiologic agent; also, different genotypes may produce similar or identical phenotypes. The developing mammalian embryo appears to be limited in the number of ways in which it may react to a variety of abnormal stimuli stemming from the action of genes or environmental factors.

INBORN ERRORS OF METABOLISM. Developmental genetics encompasses not only morphologic but also biochemical and metabolic aspects of development and their genetic control. A large proportion of genetically caused inborn errors of metabolism have their earliest effects during embryonic stages despite the homeostatic action of the maternal environment. In man the etiology of inborn errors of metabolism with their frequent pleiotropic effects is usually throught to lie in mutations of structural genes for the respective enzymes. The model system of the radiation-induced albino alleles in mice reveals mechanisms of causation of biochemical errors that may well include morphogenetic and ultrastructural attributes. Thus not only may morphogenesis be affected secondarily by genetically caused metabolic errors, it may in turn be a causative factor in the origin of errors of metabolism. The mutual interdependence of enzyme differentiation and morphogenesis is a concept that must be kept in mind in the consideration of problems of inborn errors of metabolism.

GENETIC CONTROL OF DIFFERENTIATION. Another aspect of developmental genetics is concerned with the role of genes in the control and regulation of *differentiation.* The complexity of organization of the mammalian organism requires a large number of regulatory and controlling functions. These are carried out by corresponding genes and also by genes involved in synthesis of enzymes and proteins. The great increase of DNA content in cells of higher organisms as compared with those of bacteria has been interpreted as possibly reflecting the need for a large variety of controlling elements in complex processes of morphogenesis.

Determination. One of the most puzzling problems of differentiation is that of determination. At a certain stage of development the multitude of developmental potentialities of a particular cell is narrowed down until the cell is channeled into one specific developmental pathway. Thus the cell has become determined to differentiate into one type only, such as nerve or cartilage or muscle cell. This process of determination does not seem to involve a change in the cell's genetic makeup. Not much is known about the specific role of genes in determination; terms such as *derepression* or *repression* of genes are descriptive rather than analytic.

Among the questions to be answered is that of the reversibility of determination. Is a cell or tissue that has been determined to give rise to a certain cell or tissue type (for example, nervous tissue) capable, under the appropriate conditions, of differentiating into a totally different cell type, such as muscle? In transplantation experiments in *Drosophila,* Hadorn was able to demonstrate that determination may be reversed. He showed that under certain experimental conditions tissues already determined to form leg structures, for example, could be made to differentiate into head structures. This phenomenon has been called transdetermination. Its discovery and its interpretation for the role and state of genes in differentiation represent significant progress in modern developmental genetics.

Nuclear Transplantation. The question of gene activation and inactivation during development, and of the extent to which such inactivation is reversible, has been the subject of another important experimental approach, namely that of nuclear transplantation. These experiments have emphasized the effect of cytoplasmic factors on the pattern of gene activity in the nucleus. The mechanisms of differentiation and determination have been shown to involve significant nuclear–cytoplasmic interactions.

CHIMERAS. In recent years a powerful new method has been developed for the study of gene effects, gene control, and gene interactions during development: the successful fusion of late cleavage stages or of morulae of mouse embryos of different genotypes. The fusion products are cultured for a day and subsequently transferred to the uterus of a female made pseudopregnant by mating with a vasectomized male. Surviving embryos are tetraparental chimeras. Over a period of years various developmental processes and their genetic control in mammals have been studied with this method: differentiation of somites, muscle, skeleton, hair, pigmentation, and sensory organs, as well as abnormalities of hematopoiesis, hereditary retinal degeneration, sex development and hermaphroditism, and the ontology of the immune system.

References

Davidson EH: Gene Activity in Early Development. New York, Academic, 1968

Erickson RP, Gluecksohn-Waelsch S, Corti CF: Glucose-6-phosphatase deficiency caused by radiation-induced alleles at the albino locus in the mouse. Proc Natl Acad Sci USA 59:437, 1968

Fraser FC: Some genetic aspects of teratology. In Wilson JG, Warkany J (eds): Teratology, Principles and Techniques. Chicago, Univ Chicago Press, 1965, p 21

Gardner RL, Lyon MF: X chromosome inactivation studied by injection of a single cell into the mouse blastocyst. Nature 231:385, 1971

Gluecksohn-Waelsch S: Lethal genes and analysis of differentiation. Science 142:1269, 1963

————: Erickson RP: The T-locus of the mouse: implications for mechanisms of development. In Moscona AA, Monroy A (eds): Current Topics in Developmental Biology, Vol V. New York, Academic, 1970

Gurdon JB: Nuclear transplantation and the control of gene activity in animal development. Proc R Soc Lond [Biol] 176:303, 1970

Hadorn E: Dynamics of determination. In Locke M (ed): Major Problems on Developmental Biology. New York, Academic, p 85, 1966

Lyon M: Gene action in the X-chromosome of the mouse (Mus musculus L.). Nature 190:373, 1961

Mintz B: Gene control of mammalian differentiation. Ann Rev Genet 8:411, 1974

Saxen L, Rapola J: Congenital Defects, New York, Holt, Rinehart & Winston, 1969

HUMAN CYTOGENETICS

ARTHUR ROBINSON AND DAVID C. PEAKMAN

A new era in human cytogenetics began in 1956 with the discovery by Tjio and Levan that the chromosome number in man is 46, that human somatic cells contain 23 pairs of chromosomes (the diploid number), and that the germ cells have 23 chromosomes, one member of each pair (the haploid number). The field developed very rapidly during the next 20 years to become an important part of medicine in general and pediatrics in particular. At least 0.5 percent of live-born infants have a gross chromosomal aberration, often associated with serious disease.

Since chromosomes can be delineated only during mitosis, it is important to examine human material containing many cells in a dividing state. Although this condition exists to some degree in bone marrow, this tissue is not readily available for routine biopsy. Therefore in order to collect and examine many mitoses it is necessary to utilize tissue culture techniques to stimulate rapid in vitro growth of more accessible tissue such as lymphocytes obtained from peripheral blood and fibroblasts obtained from skin biopsy. For appropriate indications such as prenatal diagnosis, cells obtained from amniotic fluid are cultured. Bone marrow biopsies can be examined directly or after 24 hours of culture if there are insufficient numbers of dividing cells in the original specimens.

The method and period of culture vary with the tissue sampled. However, the shortest possible period of culture is desirable in order to approximate in vivo conditions and to mitigate the environmental effects of the culture system on the chromosome constitution of the cells. Specimens of peripheral blood are most frequently used; they require a relatively short period of culture (60 to 72 hours). Lymphocytes are unique in requiring a mitogenic agent to stimulate them to undergo cell division. Although there are a variety of mitogens, the one used most widely is the plant protein phytohemagglutin (PHA). This nonspecific mitogen is added to a sample of blood that has been suspended in a culture medium. After 3 days of in vitro cultivation colchicine or its analogue colcemide is added to suppress spindle formation, permitting the collection of dividing cells with contracted chromosomes characteristic of the metaphase portion of the mitotic cycle. A hypotonic solution is added to swell the cells and separate the chromosomes from eath other. The preparations are then fixed, spread on microscope slides, and stained with appropriate stains. Fibroblast and amniotic cell cultures do not require a mitogenic agent, but longer periods of culture (about 3 weeks) are necessary in order to obtain a sufficient number of cells for analysis. In a variety of myeloproliferative diseases such as leukemia, cytologic studies may be carried out by culturing peripheral blood samples for 24 hours in the absence of any mitogenic agent.

CHROMOSOME IDENTIFICATION. The system for numbering and ordering the chromosomes according to size and arm ratio that was adopted by an international study group in 1960 has been modified by new staining techniques that permit unequivocal identification of each chromosome in the human karyotype. These methods utilize the fluorescent dye, quinacrine, or the nucleoprotein Giemsa stain. They produce a pattern of bands along the length of the chromsome that is unique to each homologous pair and permits precise identification of each chromosome pair. It also facilitates identification of structural rearrangements of the chromosome (deletions, duplications, translocations, inversions, isochromosomes). Although there are a variety of techniques available, the Q (quinacrine) and G (Giemsa trypsin) banding methods are the ones employed most widely. R banding produces bands that are the reverse of G bands. C (centromere) bands stain constitutive heterochromatin in the region of the centromere or primary constriction of the chromosome.

The chromosomes are numbered consecutively according to a descending order of size, the one exception being that chromsome 21 is in reality slightly smaller than chromosome 22. However, since the former was found to be trisomic in Down's syndrome (mongolism) and was originally labeled 21, it was decided to retain this designation. The chromosomes also can be classified into seven groups (A to G) according to size, and within each group homologous pairs can be identified by their unique banding patterns. Chromosomes also can be described by the location of their centromeres as metacentric (numbers 1, 3, 19, and 20), submetacentric (numbers 2, 4 to 12, and 16 to 18), or acrocentric (numbers 13 to 15, 21, 22, and Y). The acrocentric chromosomes, except for the Y, frequently have small satellites at the ends of their short arms (Fig. 6).

Structural variations have been observed in the human karyotype; these can appear as elongation of the centromere regions of chromosomes numbers 1, 9, and 16, enlargement of satellites of any of the acrocentric chromosomes, variation in the length of the long arm of the Y chromosome, and pericentric inversions, especially of chromosome 9. Additional markers can be found with quinacrine staining, such as intense fluores-

cence of the centromere of chromosome 3 and marked fluorescence of some of the satellites. Characteristically the long arm of the Y chromosome fluoresces more intensely than any other chromosome segment, but occasionally (in about 1 in 1,000 males) the Y chromosome is small and nonfluorescent. These structural variations are frequently inherited, and they can be utilized as chromosome markers to determine the parental origin of the chromosome (Fig. 7). A variation in chromosome number has been observed frequently in the cells of older individuals. Women over 55 years of age tend to lose an X chromosome, and men over 65 years of age tend to lose a Y chromosome from many of their cells.

CHROMOSOME NOMENCLATURE. International conferences have been held on four occasions since 1960 (the most recent at Paris in 1971) (Fig. 6) to establish and revise the system of nomenclature for describing chromosomes. The pairs of autosomes (nonsex chromosomes) are identified by the numbers 1 through 22 and the sex chromosomes by X and Y. According to the convention adopted a karyotype is described by noting in order the number of chromosomes, the sex chromosome constitution, and any abnormality, including additional, missing, or abnormal chromosomes. For example, the karyotype of a female infant with Down's syndrome is designated 47,XX,+21. Structural changes are designated by single letters or abbreviations as follows: p = short arm of chromosome, q = long arm of chromosome, del = deletion, t = translocation, r = ring chromosome, i = isochromosome, inv = inversion. A plus or minus sign

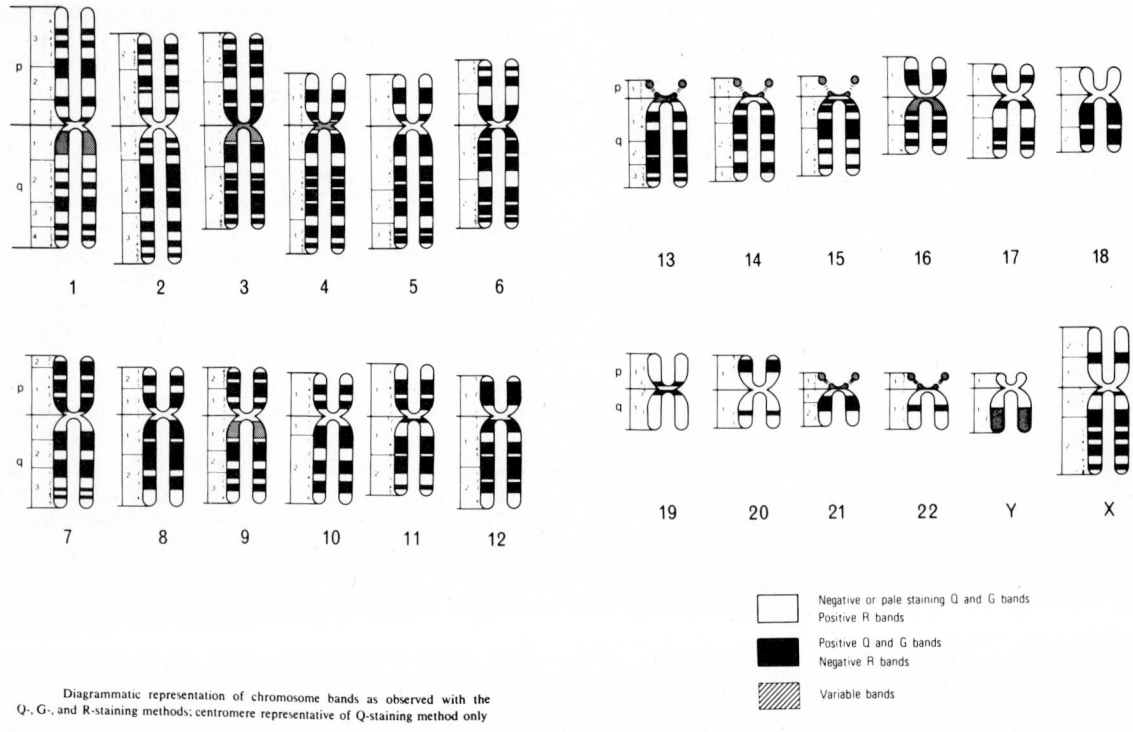

Negative or pale staining Q and G bands
Positive R bands

Positive Q and G bands
Negative R bands

Variable bands

Diagrammatic representation of chromosome bands as observed with the Q-, G-, and R-staining methods; centromere representative of Q-staining method only

FIG. 6. Chromosome identification (Paris conference, 1971). (From Birth Defects 14:271, 1971.)

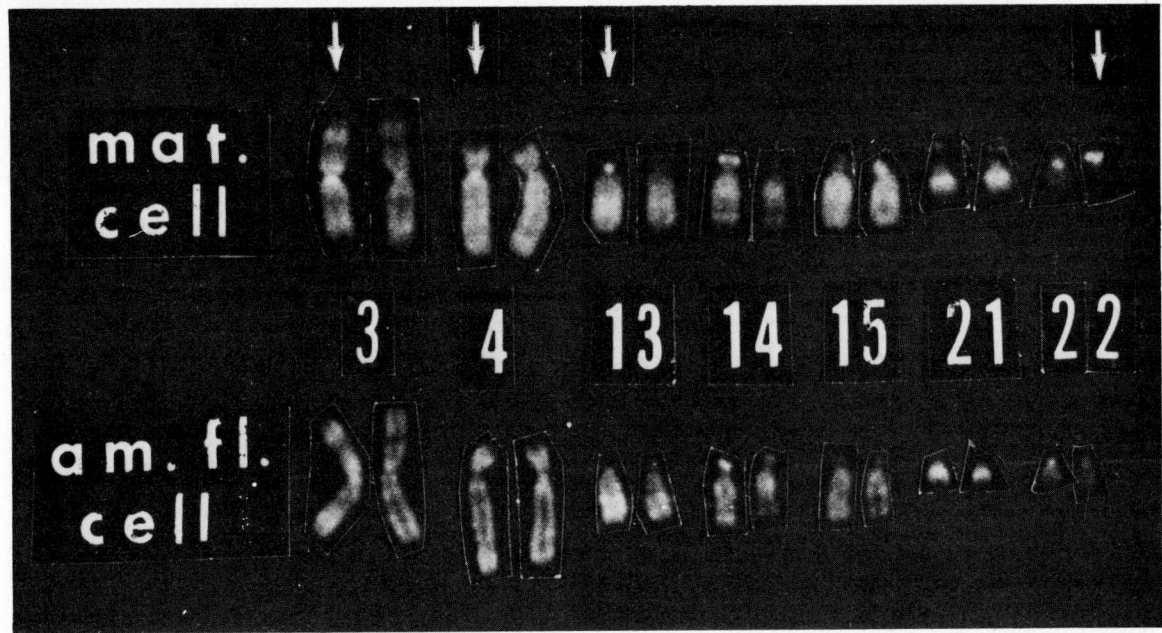

FIG. 7. Demonstration of the use of Q polymorphisms to identify differences between maternal cells and cells derived from amniotic fluid. The arrows designate chromosomes in the maternal complement that have a polymorphism not present in the amniotic fluid cell complement.

used after the chromosome indicates an increase or decrease in length of the particular segment. Some examples follow:

46,XY,18q− describes a karyotype where material has been deleted from the long arm of chromosome 18.

46,XY,del(18)(q21) is a more precise description of a similar deletion where the break point has been identified by means of a banding technique as being at band 21 on the long arm of chromosome 18.

45,XX,t(14;21)(p11;q11) describes a karyotype in which there is a balanced translocation involving the long arms of two acrocentric chromosomes (a number 14 and a number 21), the break points being located close to the centromere on the short arm of chromosome 14 and the long arm of chromosome 21 (Fig. 8).

46,XY,−14,+t(14;21)(p11;q11) describes a karyotype in which the same translocation is present but is in the unbalanced state, resulting in a trisomy for the long arm of chromosome 21.

46,XX,t(1;19)(q12;p13) describes a karyotype in which there is a reciprocal translocation involving an exchange between the long arm of chromosome 1 and the short arm of chromosome 19 (Fig. 9).

CHROMOSOME ABNORMALITIES. Abnormalities of the chromosome complement may involve either a change in chromosome number or a change in the structure of one or more of the chromosomes. A cell with twice the chromosome number of the haploid set is called diploid. Cells with a chromosome number that is an integral multiple of the haploid set greater than two are polyploid. Cells with an abnormal number of chromosomes that are not polyploid are aneuploid. This is usually due to a missing chromosome (chromo-

some monosomy) or to an extra chromosome, in which case there are three homologues of a given chromosome (chromosome trisomy).

Aneuploidy is usually attributed to nondisjunction,

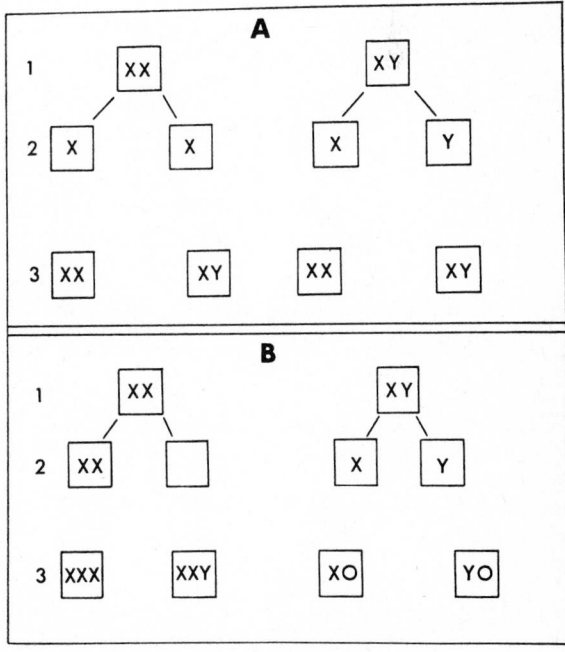

FIG. 8. Karyotype demonstrating a translocation involving chromosomes 14 and 21: 45,XY,t(14;21)(p11;q11).

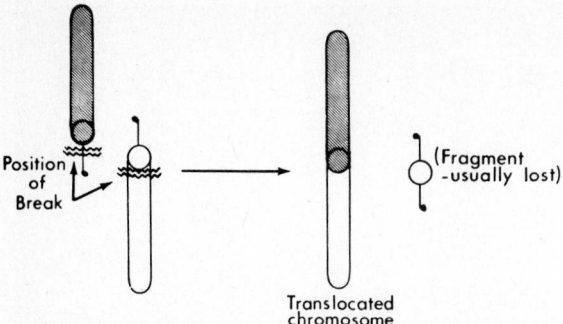

Position of Break

(Fragment -usually lost)

Translocated chromosome

Reciprocal translocation between two non-homologous satellited chromosomes.

FIG. 9. Karyotype demonstrating a balanced translocation involving the long arm of chromosome 1 and the short arm of chromosome 19: 46,XX,t(1;19)(q12;p13).

which is a failure of normal division of chromosomes so they are distributed unequally between the two daughter cells. This may occur during meiotic division of the gametes (in either the first or second division) or during the early mitotic cleavage stages of the fertilized egg, as a postzygotic phenomenon. In the former case two types of gametes are formed: those that lack a chromosome and those with an extra chromosome. When one

of these is involved in fertilization the resulting zygote will be either monosomic or trisomic for the particular chromosome (Fig. 10). When postzygotic nondisjunction occurs, the resulting individual may have chromosome mosaicism, in which there are two or more cell populations differing in chromosomal constitution. The phenotype of such a person depends on which chromosome is involved and the time in embryonic development when nondisjunction occurred. Mosaicism may also be due to chromosome lag, the failure of a chromosome to migrate during anaphase to one pole of the dividing cell, which results in its subsequent loss.

Structural abnormalities result from chromosomal breaks with or without abnormal rejoining of the damaged ends; these may result in deletions, isochromosomes, ring chromosomes, or translocations. Deletions are such as occur in 5p— or cri du chat syndrome. Isochromosomes result from misdivision of the centromere, which divides transversely rather than vertically. The result is an abnormal metacentric chromosome with either two long arms or two short arms. A person with an isochromosome becomes trisomic for the arm that constitutes the isochromosome and monosomic for the one that is missing. Thus females with an isochromosome of the long arm of the X are monosomic for the short arm and have Turner's syndrome: 46,Xi(Xq). Ring chromosomes are found when the two ends of a chromosome break off and the two

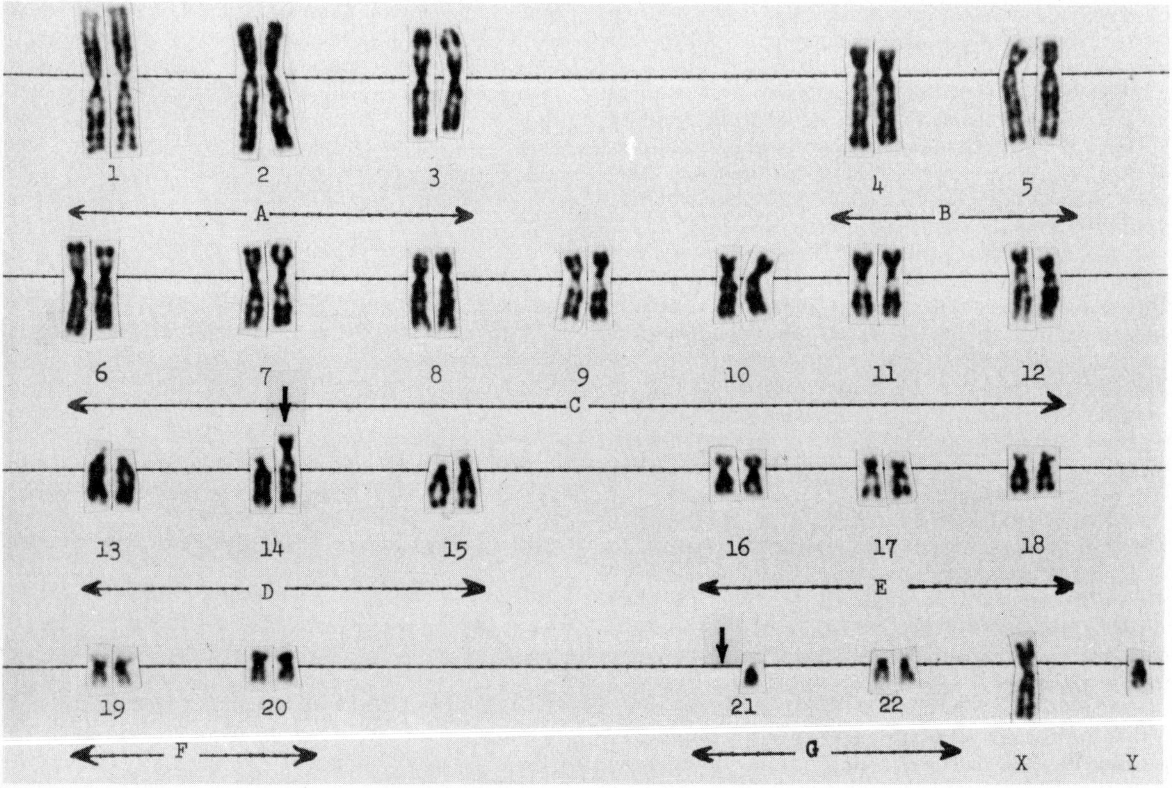

1 2 3 4 5

A B

6 7 8 9 10 11 12

C

13 14 15 16 17 18

D E

19 20 21 22 X Y

F G

FIG. 10. Diagrammatic representation of normal sex chromosome disjunction (A) and sex chromosome nondisjunction (B) with resultant aneuploidy in the fertilized zygotes.

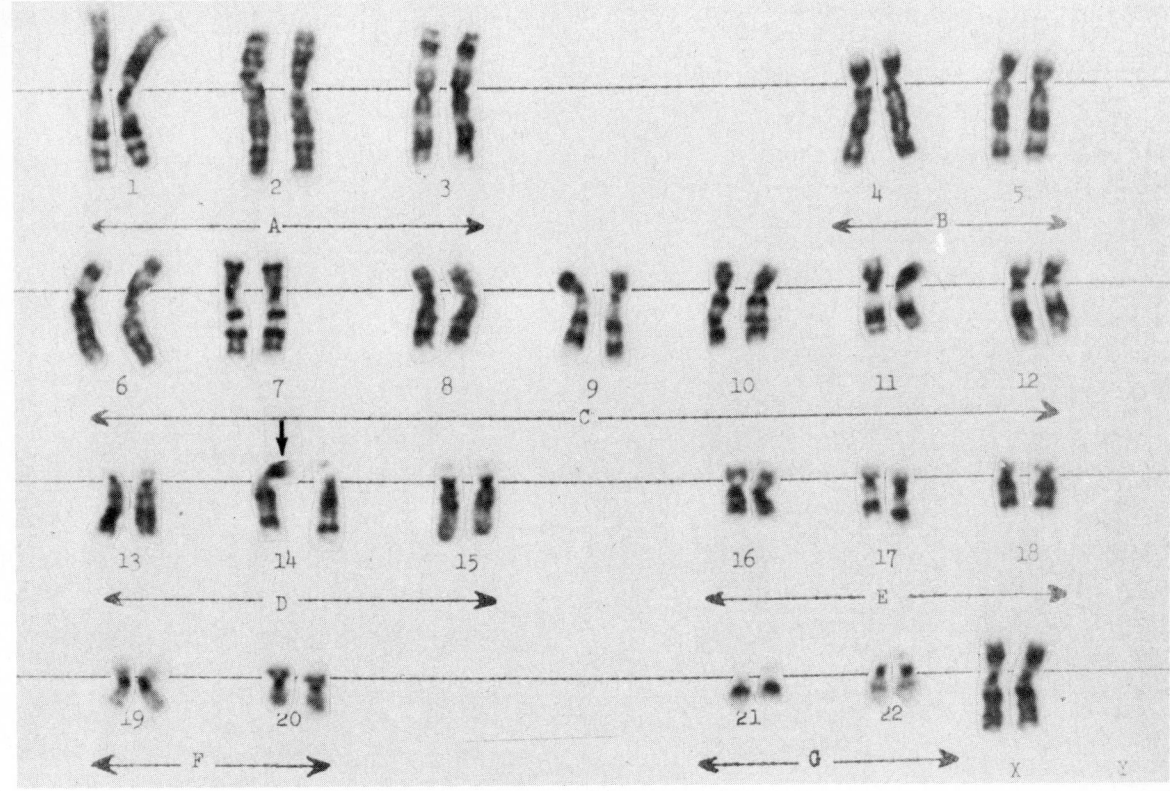

FIG. 11. Diagrammatic representation of a robertsonian (centric fusion) translocation.

remaining "sticky" ends adhere. This has been described for chromosome 18 (among others) and results in a phenotype similar to that of the 18q— syndrome. A ring X chromosome (46,XXr) has occasionally been observed in patients with Turner's syndrome. The translocation type of structural abnormality results from the breakage of two nonhomologous chromosomes, with rejoining of the broken pieces in new ways. When this occurs without significant loss of chromosome material the translocation is described as balanced, and the individual is phenotypically normal. One type of translocation, the Robertsonian or centric fusion, occurs with breakage near the centromere of two nonhomologous acrocentric chromosomes, with the long arms joining to form a large chromosome with virtually all the genetic material intact; the reciprocal small metacentric chromosome representing the short arms is usually lost (Fig. 11). Since this loss generally has no clinical effect, even though the karyotype now has only 45 chromosomes, it is assumed that this portion of the genome carries little if any important genetic information. When a germ cell with one of these chromosome translocations is involved in a fertilization, the resulting zygote may be genetically balanced or unbalanced. In the case of a reciprocal translocation, the unbalanced zygote resulting from inheritance of only one of the translocation chromosomes from a balanced parent will have partial trisomy or partial monosomy, depending on the amount and distribution of chromosome material in-

volved (duplication-deficiency syndrome). In the case of a parent with a Robertsonian translocation, the progeny may have 45 chromosomes with a balanced translocation carrier state resembling that of the parent (Fig. 8), 46 chromosomes with the translocation chromosome and an extra copy of one of the autosomes (the unbalanced condition) (Fig. 12), or 46 chromosomes with a normal chromosome complement. Apparently 50 percent or more of the germ cells of a translocation carrier are chromosomally normal, and if these are involved in formation of the conceptus, these progeny will have a normal karyotype. Whenever an individual is identified as having a translocation (balanced or unbalanced) it is essential to examine close family relatives, since they have a greater chance of being carriers of the balanced translocation and of having abnormal children with unbalanced karyotypes. Amniocentesis for intrauterine diagnosis of a fetus with a chromosome abnormality may aid couples who face such a risk.

ETIOLOGY OF CHROMOSOMAL ABNORMALITIES. Little is known about the etiology of nondisjunction, which is presumed to be the most frequent cause of numerical chromosomal abnormalities. The incidence of progeny with autosomal trisomy has been observed to increase in frequency with maternal age. This maternal age effect may be related to the fact that the full complement of oocytes present in the ovaries at birth is arrested in prophase of the first meiotic division, and further meotic division is continued only at a time

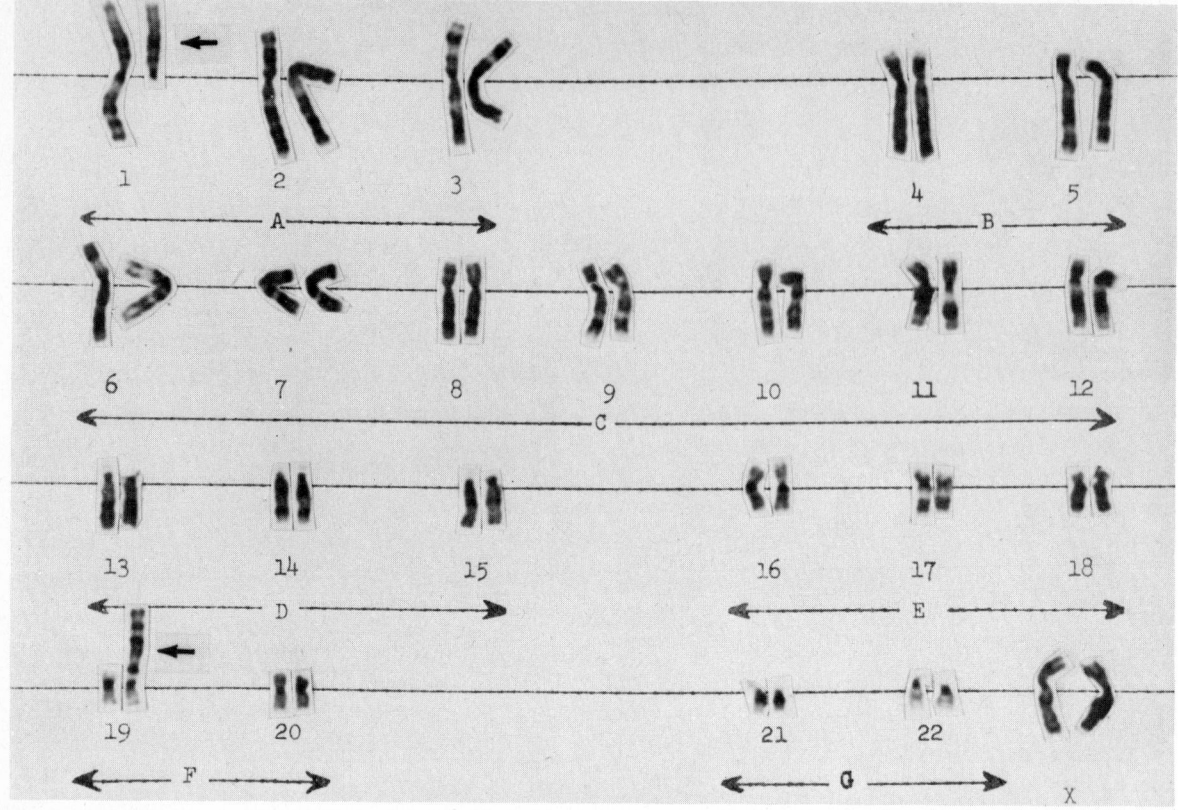

FIG. 12. Karyotype demonstrating an unbalanced translocation resulting in chromosome 21 being present in the trisomic state: 46,XX,−14,+t(14;21)(p11;q11).

of ovulation, which may occur 40 years later. It has been postulated that these older oocytes are more susceptible to nondisjunction. In contrast, paternal age appears to have no effect on the occurrence of nondisjunction, possibly because spermatogenesis begins only after puberty and mature sperm develop in 70 days after meiosis begins during the reproductive period of the male.

Another factor believed to increase the risk of nondisjunction is ionizing radiation. Several studies have shown that mothers of children with trisomy 21 (Down's syndrome) have a history of significantly higher exposure to ionizing radiation than those in comparison groups. In addition, exposure of mammalian cells in culture to small doses of x-ray increases the number of cells with aneuploidy, reflecting an abnormality of mitosis. Elevated titers of thyroid autoantibodies in serum have been reported in patients with a variety of conditions associated with aneuploidy, especially those with Down's syndrome; elevated titers have also been observed in their mothers and other close relatives. Several epidemiologic studies have revealed newborn infants with chromosomal abnormalities in a clustering that resembles the temporal variation of infectious disease. Therefore the suggestion has been made that viral infection in individuals predisposed to autoimmune disease may increase the risk of meiotic nondisjunction. Genes predisposing to nondisjunction have been dem-

onstrated in animal models. Similar genetic determinants may occur in man, which may explain the reported occurrence of multiple instances of aneuploidy within a family.

Epidemiologic studies on the incidence of abnormalities involving the sex chromosomes and the incidence of chromosome 21 in newborns strongly suggest that nonrandom environmental causes of nondisjunction do exist, some of which are seasonal in their occurrence. Similarly, a variety of factors have been implicated in the production of chromosomal breaks that result in the various structural chromosomal abnormalities that have been described. Thus some viral infections, including measles and hepatitis, have been shown to produce chromosome breaks, both in vivo and in vitro. At least three recessively inherited genetic diseases (Fanconi's anemia, Bloom's syndrome, and ataxia-telangiectasia) have been associated with an increased tendency for chromosome breakage. Interestingly, individuals with these diseases also have an increased susceptibility to neoplasia. Ionizing radiation, even in the small doses associated with diagnostic radiographs, also breaks chromosomes. In these cases there is a marked tendency toward abnormal rehealing.

Finally, a variety of chemical agents, including known carcinogens, produce chromosome breakage. As yet there is no conclusive evidence that hallucinogens (such as LSD) or tranquilizers (which may produce an increased number of chromosome breaks) have any adverse genetic effects. Indeed, in the absence of translocations of deletions occurring in the gametes involved in conception, the biologic significance of an increased incidence of chromosome breaks in cells undergoing mitosis remains unknown.

CLINICAL ABNORMALITIES. The brain and the gonads are two organ systems that are very sensitive to chromosome imbalance. As a result, mental retardation and sterility are frequent abnormalities in individuals with chromosomal aberrations. In general, the developing organism suffers greater pathologic disturbances from abnormalities involving the autosomes than the sex chromosomes. This difference may be due to the fact that in the cells of the female only one X chromosome normally is genetically active, with the other being inactivated (Lyonization). In contrast, there is no comparable mechanism for genetic inactivation of any of the autosomes. In addition, when one of two X chromosomes is abnormal, it is generally the abnormal one that is inactivated. Diploid cells require at least one normal X to be viable. Studies of chromosome abnormalities associated with early spontaneous abortions indicate that monosomy and trisomy for the larger autosomes are lethal conditions.

CHROMOSOMES AND FETAL WASTAGE. An important finding in cytologic studies of spontaneous abortions is that abnormalities of the chromosomes are a major cause of fetal wastage. It has been estimated that 5 to 10 percent of human conceptions have abnormal chromosomes. The majority of these (at least 95 percent) are spontaneously aborted. Between 30 and 50 percent of first- and second-trimester spontaneous abortions are found to have chromosomal abnormalities, the higher figure occurring during the first 2 months of pregnancy. Numerical chromosomal abnormalities account for the vast majority of chromosomal aberrations among spontaneous abortions, with only 3 percent being due to translocations. For the most part, these findings were obtained prior to use of the banding techniques, and additional abnormalities due to small deletions and translocations undoubtedly have been missed.

Abnormalities of each of the 23 pairs of chromosomes have been found in spontaneous abortuses. Monsomy X is the most frequent abnormality, accounting for 20 percent of the total. Autosomal trisomies account for 40 percent of the abnormalities, with trisomy 16 being the most frequent. Triploidy is another frequent finding, especially in hydatidiform moles. In a WHO report on 1,400 spontaneous abortuses, chromosome abnormalities were found in 80 percent of abnormal fetuses and in only 7 percent of phenotypically normal fetuses. A recent study by Boué and Boué suggests that if a woman has a spontaneous abortion with a chromosomal abnormality there is an increased likelihood of finding a chromosomal abnormality if she has a second spontaneous abortion. The abnormality in the second abortus will not necessarily be the same as that found in the first. If confirmed, these findings may be of importance in genetic counseling.

SEX CHROMOSOMES. In humans the male is heterogametic in that he produces two kinds of sperm (X-containing and Y-containing). Unlike the situation in *Drosophila,* in which the fly with only one X (the XO pattern) is male, in man the Y chromosome is necessary for maleness. Although no genes have been definitely located on the Y chromosome, there is evidence suggesting that a locus on the short arm of the Y regulates the development of the testis. Moreover, recent studies suggest that one or more histocompatibility genes are also located on the Y. On the other hand, at least 95 genetic loci have been assigned to the X chromosome, although very few of them have anything to do with sex determination.

SEX CHROMATIN. Unlike the determination of the full chromosome complement, which requires study of mitotic cells, the sex chromosome complement can be determined by examination of interphase cells. This procedure is carried out by examining buccal cells obtained by scraping the inside of the cheek and placing the cells on a microscope slide. The cells can be stained with one of a variety of nucleoprotein stains and checked for the presence of X chromatin bodies (Barr bodies) using bright-field microscopy. These densely stained planoconvex chromatin masses are approximately 1 μ in diameter and are usually located at the periphery of the nucleus. According to the X chromatin rule the number of Barr bodies present in a cell is one less than the number of X chromosomes; ie, one Barr body = two X chromosomes, two Barr bodies = three X chromosomes. A normal female will have a single Barr body in 20 to 40 percent of the nuclei of cells obtained from buccal smear, whereas a normal male with a single X chromosome and a Y chromosome will have nuclei without any typical Barr bodies. In a normal female the proportion of X chromatin-positive nuclei varies with the tissue samples, amnionic membrane having more than 90 percent Barr-positive nuclei.

Since the introduction of fluorescent dyes it has become possible to demonstrate the presence of a Y chromosome in interphase cells by examination of the preparations with fluorescence microscopy. The Y chromatin body appears as a small bright mass (representing the intensely fluorescent long arm of the Y chromosome) that can usually be observed in the majority of cell nuclei (Fig. 13). In about 1 in 1,000 males the distal part of the long arm of the Y is absent, and no Y chromatin mass is demonstrable. By the combination of X and Y chromatin staining techniques it is possible to determine the sex chromosome complement of an individual using relatively simple and rapid procedures. Examination of buccal smears for X and Y chromatin constitution is only a screening procedure. Such examinations in which the sex chromatin constitution and phenotype of the patient do not agree or in which abnormal numbers of sex chromatin bodies are found should always be confirmed by chromosome analysis.

DISORDERS ASSOCIATED WITH SEX CHROMOSOME ABNORMALITIES. About 0.25 percent of all newborn infants have abnormalities of the sex chromosomes. Although most of these infants ap-

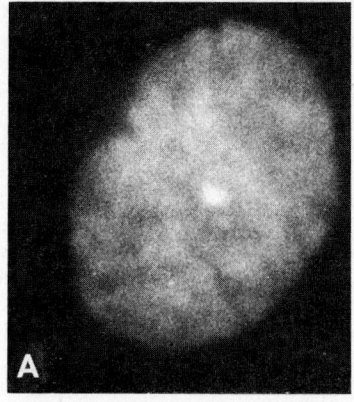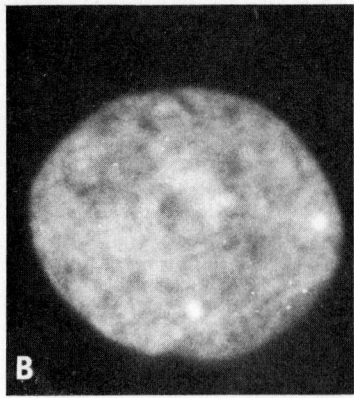

FIG. 13.　Cells from buccal smear preparations demonstrating (A) the single fluorescent Y body associated with an XY sex chromosome complement and (B) the double fluorescent Y bodies associated with an XYY complement.

pear normal at birth, they can be identified by examination of their sex chromatin status.

Turner's Syndrome.　Turner's syndrome (45,X) is one of the few sex chromosome abnormalities that can be diagnosed in the newborn from clinical manifestations. In our series of 20,000 female newborns the incidence of this disorder was about 1 in 3,000, although others have found a significantly lower frequency (1 in 5,000). These figures do not include many of the individuals with 45,X/46,XX mosaicism or those with partial deletion of an X: 46,XXp−, 46,XXq−, 46,Xi(Xq), or 46,Xi(Xp). In our experience 45,X mosaicism occurs with an incidence of 1 in 1,500. Only 1 in 40 conceptuses with a 45,X karyotype survives to birth, making the overall incidence of 45,X conceptions as high as 1 in 75. Some of the characteristic signs and symptoms of Turner's syndrome in order of their frequency are listed in Table 2. Females with 45,X chromosomes are

TABLE 2. Clinical Findings in Turner's Syndrome in Order of Decreasing Frequency

Short stature
Gonadal dysgenesis (usually streak gonads)
Primary amenorrhea and infertility
Sexual infantilism in adults
Broad chest with wide-spaced nipples
Congenital lymphedema (especially of dorsum of hands and feet)
Low posterior hairline
Cubitus valgus
Webbing of neck
Narrow, hyperconvex, deep-set nails
Renal anomalies, especially horseshoe kidney
Coarctation of the aorta
Excessive pigmented nevi

negative for X chromatin and Y chromatin, and hence their karyotypes can be surmised by examination of a buccal smear. However, any abnormality should be confirmed by chromosome analysis. Those patients with the phenotype of Turner's syndrome and an isochromosome of the long arm of the X chromosome, 46,Xi(Xq), are X-chromatin-positive.

The diagnosis of this disorder should be suspected and a buccal smear should be examined in a newborn female with any of the following findings: congenital lymphedema (this usually recedes during infancy), webbing of the neck (or excess loose skin in the posterior neck), coarctation of the aorta (suspected because of inability to palpate a femoral arterial pulse in the groin). A buccal smear should be part of the work-up of any femal child with short stature. Mental retardation is not characteristic of this syndrome, being present in less than 10 percent, although visual motor perceptual problems are often present. The likelihood of school difficulties, the marked shortness (final height may be about 147 cm), and the prospect of sterility present psychologic problems requiring sensitive handling by the pediatrician. Intravenous pleiography and evaluation of renal function are indicated. At the appropriate time in adolescence, cyclic hormone therapy should be started in order to produce development of secondary sex characteristic (p. 1705). Some authors have recommended use of small doses of androgens at about 10 years of age to increase height. Milder forms of the phenotype can be seen with X chromosome mosaicism. There is no maternal age effect in the occurrence of this condition as there is with the various trisomy syndromes.

Klinefelter's Syndrome.　The symptom complex of Klinefelter's syndrome occurs in males with a 47,XXY karyotype. Some individuals with this abnormal karyotype do not have the manifestations of the syndrome. Since most boys with a 47,XXY karyotype do not have signs and symptoms of Klinefelter's syndrome, it is inappropriate to designate them as having the syndrome. Signs of the abnormality, as listed in Table 3, usually develop in later life. The frequency of male newborns with a 47,XXY karyotype has varied between 1 in 600 and 1 in 800 in various studies. Mosaics have milder symptoms. The presence of X and Y chromatin bodies on buccal smear strongly suggests a 47,XXY kayotype, and chromosome analysis for confirmation of the diagnosis is indicated. In these patients urinary gonadotropins become abnormally elevated at puberty and

TABLE 3. Signs and Symptoms in Klinefelter's Syndrome

Micro-orchidism, azoospermia, and sterility, consistently present
Gynecomastia
Generally tall with a eunuchoid build
Diminished I.Q., usually mild
Diminished facial hair
Occasionally antisocial personality and/or emotional disturbances

remain so in adulthood. Histologically the testis is characterized by hyalinization and atrophy of the seminiferous tubules, with clumps of Leydig cells interspersed between them. Some of these abnormalities have been found in the gonads of infants and children with a 47,XXY karyotype.

Rarely, males may have a 48,XXXY or a 49,XXXXY karyotype. These individuals are usually more severely mentally retarded and are more likely to have other congenital malformations. The greater the number of X chromosomes an individual has, the more severe are the abnormalities. Males with a 49,XXXXY karyotype differ from patients with Klinefelter's syndrome in being short rather than tall.

XYY Male. It is inappropriate to describe individuals with a 47,XYY karyotype as having the XYY syndrome, since the symptomatology of these males varies greatly, some being quite normal. The term is stigmatizing because of the suggestion that males with this abnormality are destined to become criminals. The most characteristic finding is increased height (over 183 cm). Other physical findings include acne, tremor of the hands, and genital abnormalities. Various personality characteristics have been noted that can be generally described as diminished tolerance for frustration. However, there is inadequate information to predict that a newborn with a 47,XYY karyotype will have some of the abnormalities noted. The incidence of the 47,XXY karyotype in the male newborn population is roughly 1 in 1,000, whereas the prevalence in mental and penal institutions is four to five times higher. It is important to accumulate further data to determine the frequency of behavior problems in children with this karyotype and to identify those at risk for behavior problems in later life, so that early therapy can be instituted.

Trisomy X. The incidence of the trisomy X (47,XXX) abnormality in female newborns is about 0.12 percent; the prevalence appears to be as much as four times greater among retarded adult females. Women with this karyotype vary greatly in their phenotypes and may be normal or may present with underdevelopment of secondary sex characteristics, primary or secondary amenorrhea, and mild mental retardation. For this reason the outcome in a newborn with a 47,XXX karyotype currently cannot be predicted. Females with 48,XXXX or 49,XXXXX chromosomal constitutions are much rarer and are more severely affected. Less frequent sex chromosome abnormalities are listed in Table 4.

DISORDERS ASSOCIATED WITH AUTOSOMAL ABNORMALITIES.

In general, these abnormalities are associated with more serious clinical disorders. With the advent of modern banding techniques they have been found to be more common than abnormalities of the sex chromosomes. The most serious forms are the trisomies involving entire chromosomes, which are characterized by low birth weight, marked mental retardation, and multiple malformations. The partial trisomies and monosomies and mosaics are usually less serious. Monosomy of an autosome, with rare exception, does not result in a viable infant. The most common viable trisomies involve chromosomes 21, 18, and 13, although on rare occasions patients with trisomy for chromosomes 22 or 8 have been reported. Mosaicism for trisomy 8 has recently been reported to be fairly common. An acquired autosomal lesion is the Ph[1] chromosome discussed later.

Down's Syndrome. The abnormal karyotype in Down's syndrome (p. 1777) may be of three general types: trisomy 21, which occurs in 95 percent of affected individuals; unbalanced Robertsonian translocations involving chromosome 21, which occurs in 4 percent of affected persons, either t(14q,21q), t(21q,22q), or t(21q,21q); or trisomy 21 mosaicism, which occurs in the remaining 1 percent. Rarely, t(15q,21q) translocation trisomies have been reported. For approximately half the patients with an unbalanced translocation, one of the parents (usually the mother) has a chromosome number of 45 and is a carrier of a balanced translocation. Most of these inherited forms of Down's syndrome

TABLE 4. Other Diseases of Sex Chromosomes

Chromosomal Disorder	Karyotype	Prominent Characteristics
Klinefelter's variants	48,XXXY, 49,XXXXY	More severe mental retardations, radioulnar synostosis, congenital heart disease
XX male	46,XX	Similar to Klinefelter's or partial feminization; occasionally a true hermaphrodite
Mixed gonadal dysgenesis (male pseudohermaphrodite)	45,X/46,XY mosaicism	Some of the findings present in Turner's syndrome with infantile female secondary sex characteristics and variable degree of masculinization; tendency to develop gonadoblastomas
Male pseudohermaphrodite; testicular feminizing syndrome	46,XY	Tall, well-feminized, sterile female with testes; a sex-linked recessive gene defect where there is lack of end organ response to dihydro-testosterone, the active metabolite of testosterone
True hermaphrodite	46,XX, 46,XY, 46,XX/46,XY	Ovum on one side, testis on other, or ovotestes on one or both sides; varying degrees of abnormal sex phenotype
Polysomy X	48,XXX, 49,XXXX	No typical syndrome; increased risk of mental retardation, emotional disturbances, and sterility

TABLE 5. Autosomal Trisomies

Disease	Major Clinical Features	Laboratory Features
Down's syndrome	Mental retardation, short stature, characteristic facies, flat occiput, flat nasal bridge, epicanthal folds, oblique palpebral fissues, congenital heart disease, transverse palmar crease, abnormal dermatoglyphics, increased incidence of leukemia	Abnormal karyotype: trisomy 21, trisomy 21 mosaicism, tranlocation trisomy with centric fusion 14/21, 21/21, 21/22
Trisomy 18 (Edwards syndrome)	Mental retardation, failure to thrive, hypertonicity, prominent occiput, micrognathia, low-set ears, congenital heart disease, renal abnormalities, flexion deformities of fingers, rocker-bottom feet, cleft lip$\pm$ palate, abnormal dermatoglyphics (simple arches on fingers); death within 2 years	Trisomy 18, occasionally an unbalanced translocation involving 18
Trisomy 13 (Patau syndrome)	Mental retardation, failure to thrive, sloping forehead and microcephaly, anophthalmia, colobomas, capillary hemangiomas, cleft lip and palate, apneic spells, deafness, polydactyly, congenital heart disease, polycystic kidneys, cryptorchidism or bicornuate uterus; death usually during the first year	Trisomy 13, occasional mosaic, rarely a 13/13 translocation; abnormal lobulation and multiple projections on neutrophils are often present; fetal hemoglobin is elevated, and Gower embryonic hemoglobin is often present

involve the t(14q,21q) translocation; only 5 percent of the t(21q,22q) patients have a carrier parent.

The clinical features (Table 5) are the same in all forms of trisomy 21, although the mosaics (eg, 46,XY/47,XY,+21) may present with less severe abnormalities. Some of them, with a low ratio of abnormal to normal cells, are phenotypically normal. It is important to determine the karyotypes of affected individuals and their parents for the purpose of genetic counseling. Down's syndrome is the most common autosomal abnormality seen in live-born infants; the incidence is about 1 in 600 births. Recent data suggest that the overall incidence may have decreased to about 1 in 900 in the Western world. This change is probably related to a shift in the distribution of maternal ages to younger age groups. Whereas 10 to 13 percent of pregnant women in England and the United States were over 35 years old several decades ago, more recently this figure has dropped to 3.5 to 4.5 percent. Mothers of children with Down's syndrome fall into two groups: the maternal- age-dependent group (about 34 years) whose children have trisomy 21 and the maternal-age-independent group (26 to 28 years) whose children have either trisomy 21 or one of the translocation trisomies.

Patients with Down's syndrome have a good prognosis for life (life expectancy of 30 to 50 years) with modern therapy to treat the complications of congenital heart disease and leukemia. They are more susceptible to infection and tend to age more rapidly. Females are fertile and run a risk of approximately 50 percent of having similarly affected offspring. Males are generally sterile. Management includes supportive care and prevention of complications. A program for active stimulation of infants and special schooling may help affected children achieve their maximum potential. The average I.Q. is about 50, with a wide range of variation.

The recurrence risk for this condition following the birth of an affected child has been derived from empirical risk data, and the best estimates of recurrence risk for trisomy 21 (both parents with a normal karyotype) have been derived from experience with women having amniocentesis for intrauterine diagnosis of another affected child. The data suggest that the recurrence risk

may be as high as 1 to 3 percent. Mothers who carry a balanced translocation (14/21 or 21/22) have a 10 to 15 percent risk of recurrence. Fathers who have a 14/21 or 21/22 balanced translocation are less likely to have affected children, the risk being less than 5 percent but probably greater than 1 percent. Those rare unfortunates (mothers or fathers) carrying a 21/21 translocation are doomed to have only children with Down's syndrome. The risk for affected children in the maternal-age-dependent group has also been arrived at by intrauterine diagnosis; for women of maternal age 35 to 39 years it is about 2 percent, and for women 40 to 45 years of age it is about 4 percent. These figures may be

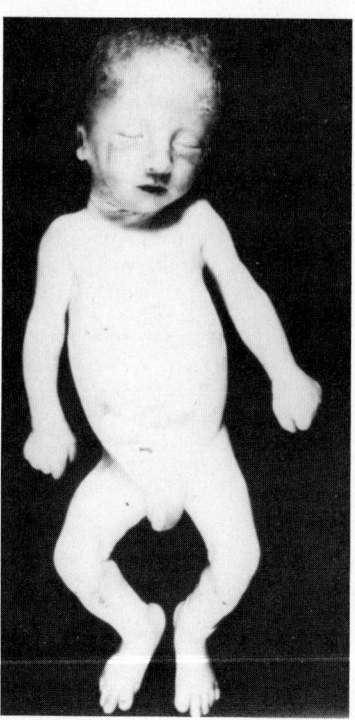

FIG. 14.   Newborn demonstrating features of trisomy 18. (Courtesy of Dr. Harold Nitowsky.)

modified as experience with intrauterine diagnosis accumulates. They are higher than previous data obtained on newborns and may reflect the possibility that some fetuses with trisomy 21 diagnosed in utero do not survive to term.

Trisomy 18. Trisomy 18 (Edwards syndrome) (Fig. 14) occurs with an incidence of approximately 1 in 4,-500 live births. The prognosis for postnatal survival is poor in comparison with Down's syndrome. Developmental retardation is severe, and death usually occurs during the first 2 years of life. The symptoms are very characteristic, and the diagnosis can usually be suspected on physical examination (Table 5). Treatment is limited to supportive care. On occasion it is important to decide soon after birth how extensive and elaborate the approach to therapy should be. A rapid confirmation of the suspected diagnosis can be arrived at by direct examination of mitotic figures obtained from bone marrow.

Trisomy 13. Banding patterns have helped to clarify the fact that the condition formerly called trisomy D is actually trisomy 13 (Patau syndrome) (Fig. 15). Triso-

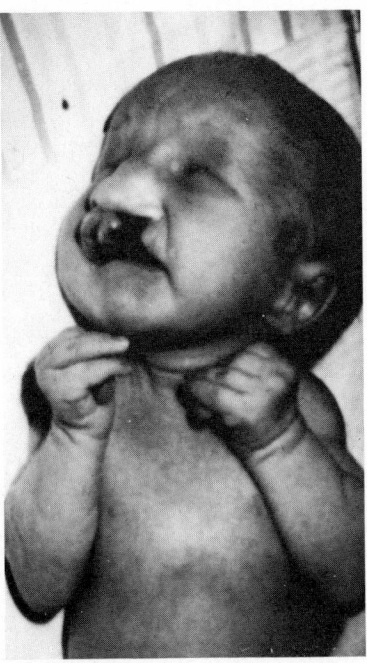

FIG. 15. Newborn demonstrating features of trisomy 13. (Courtesy of Dr. Harold Nitowsky.)

mies of the other two chromosomes in the D group (14 and 15) have not been found in live-born infants. There is some overlap in the clinical signs of this syndrome (Table 5) with those of trisomy 18. Nevertheless, in these patients the clinical picture is generally quite distinct, with sloping forehead, microphthalmia, hemangioma of the forehead, severe cleft lip and palate, apneic spells, flexion deformities of the fingers, and generalized hypotonia. The incidence of trisomy 13 at birth has been estimated at about 1 in 5,000. Death usually oc-

curs during the first 6 months of life and always by 2 years of age. A characteristic postmortem finding is an abnormal segmentation of the forebrain, which is subsumed by the term holoprosencephaly.

Deletion Syndromes. Although autosomal monosomies are usually lethal in man, partial monosomies are not, and several typical syndromes caused by this type of abnormality have now been described (Table 6). The

TABLE 6. Deletion Syndromes

Karyotype	Major Clinical Features
46,XY(XX),4p—	Severe mental retardation, microcephaly, epicanthi, coloboma, beaked nose, cleft palate, micrognathia, inguinal hernia, hypospadias, growth deficiency of prenatal onset
46,XY(XX),5p—	Severe mental retardation catlike cry (in infancy), microcephaly, round facies, low-set ears, inguinal hernia, short metacarpals, hypotonia, strabismus
46,XY(XX),18p—	Variable mental retardation, micrognathia, flat nasal bridge, low-set and large ears, short hands
46,XY(XX),18q—	Mental retardation, microcephaly, midfacial dysmorphism, prominent antihelix, atretic ear canals, carp-shaped mouth, cryptorchidism, long tapering fingers, often absence of IgA
46,XY(XX),13q—	Mental retardation, failure to thrive, microcephaly, hypertelorism, ptosis, microphthalmia and colobomata, hypoplastic or absent thumbs, occasional retinoblastoma, congenital heart disease, genitourinary abnormalities

best known is the cri du chat syndrome (5p—), so named because the cry of the affected infant is high-pitched and resembles that of a kitten. Occasionally the same phenotype has been produced by a ring chromosome 5. Parents of these children sometimes have a balanced reciprocal translocation.

NEW CHROMOSOMAL SYNDROMES. Recently, various new syndromes have been described that reflect the advent of chromosome banding methods and the ability to identify unusual structural rearrangements. In general, these new syndromes comprise a group with more subtle chromosome defects in which one of the parents may have a balanced translocation. Amniocentesis and prenatal diagnosis make it possible to prevent the birth of subsequent progeny with similar chromosome lesions. Although there is much overlap in the findings of the various syndromes, there are recurring clinical findings that suggest chromosomal disease. These include failure to thrive, mental retardation, cleft lip and/or cleft palate, congenital heart disease, presence of a third fontanelle, abnormal dermatoglyphics, single flexion crease on the fifth finger, and genital abnormalities. Mental retardation, plus any one or two of these, in the absence of other diagnoses indicates the need for chromosome analysis. In several of these new syndromes too few cases have been described to be certain that the chromosomal lesion is the cause of the syndrome. A few of the more firmly established ones are listed in Table 7.

CHROMOSOMES AND NEOPLASIA. One of the unanswered questions in human cytogenetics is the relationship of chromosome abnormalities to the etiology

TABLE 7. New Chromosomal Syndromes

Karyotype	Major Clinical Manifestations
4p+ (partial trisomy of short arm of 4)	Severe psychomotor and growth retardation, microcephaly, prominent glabella, rounded nose, large tongue, prominent jaw abnormal vertebrae and pelvis hypoplastic ribs
Trisomy 8 mosaicism	Mild to moderate mental retardation, strabismus, large ears, upturned nose, thick everted lower lip, high arched palate, micrognathia, vertebral anomalies, genitourinary anomalies, thick bulging skin with deep furrows especially on hands and feet, restricted movement of some small and large joints; absence of patellae is very characteristic
21q—	Mental and motor retardation, hypertonia antimongoloid slant, cleft palate, large external auditory canals and hypospadias
Partial trisomy 22 (22q+)	Coloboma (cat eye), anal atresia, severe mental retardation, hypertelorism, antimongoloid slant, abnormal ears, genitourinary anomalies, and congenital heart disease
Trisomy 22	Same as above; add microcephaly, cleft palate, micrognathia, low-set nipples

of neoplasia. With the application of the newer banding techniques to chromosome studies of cancer cells, it has become apparent that chromosome rearrangements occur more commonly in these cells than had previously been realized. In addition, patients with inherited diseases that are associated with chromosome instability (namely, Bloom's syndrome, Fanconi's anemia, ataxia-telangiectasia, and xeroderma pigmentosum) have a very high risk of malignancy. Since the chromosome instability in these diseases precedes, often by many years, the appearance of malignancy, it is reasonable to consider the possibility of a cause-and-effect relationship between these phenomena. Karyotypes from affected patients (especially with the first three diseases) show a high frequency of metaphases with broken chromosomes and rearrangements. Recently, increased sister chromatid exchange has been demonstrated in patients with Bloom's syndrome, but not with Fanconi's anemia. Patients with xeroderma pigmentosum show a defect of the mechanism for repair of DNA replication following ultraviolet irradiation.

The one consistent chromosome anomaly present in a malignancy occurs in chronic myelogenous leukemia (CML). At least 90 percent of patients with this disorder show a deletion of the long arm of chromosome 22

(Ph[1] chromosome). Banding studies have shown that the missing fragment generally is translocation to one of the chromosomes of the C group, usually to the long arm of chromosome 9. Of particular interest has been the demonstration that cells containing the Ph[1] chromosome constitute a clone, having all descended from a single cell. When the condition of a patient with CML deteriorates and acute leukemia develops, not infrequently two or three Ph[1] chromosomes, as well as other changes, can be seen in the metaphase spread. In fact, the presence of two or three Ph[1] chromosomes may presage the progression of leukemia from the chronic to the acute stage.

Trisomy of chromosomes 8 or 9 (Fig. 16) and

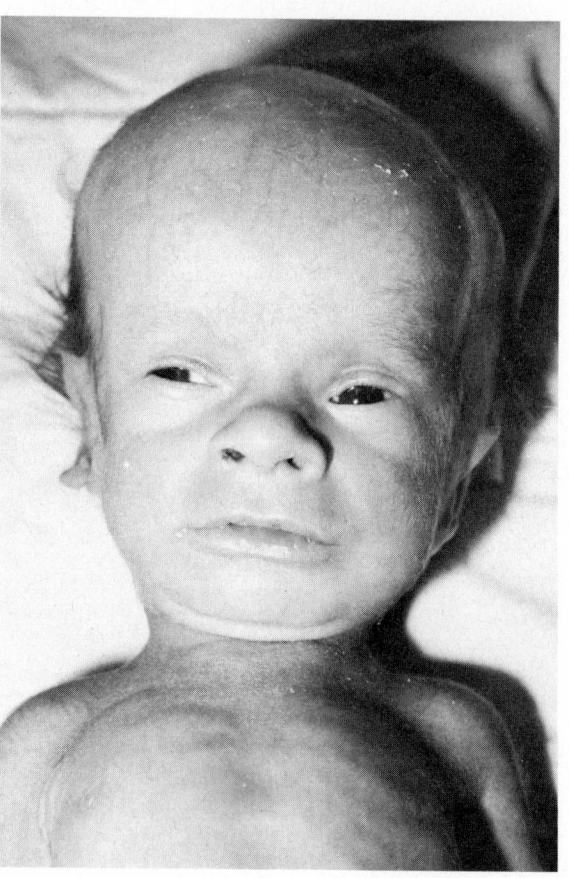

FIG. 16. Infant demonstrating facies of trisomy 8 mosaicism. (Courtesy of Dr. Arnold Greensher.)

monosomy of chromosome 7 have been reported in bone marrow cells of some patients with acute leukemia and occasionally in preleukemic conditions. In trisomy 21 (Down's syndrome) the risk for developing leukemia is about 1 percent, approximately 30 times greater than in the general population. Leukemia is also reported to occur more often in patients with other types of aneuploidy, such as 47,XXY (Klinefelter's syndrome).

In summary, chromosome abnormalities are often present in human neoplasms. Furthermore, there is suggestive evidence that, at least in one kind of malignancy (leukemia), a chromosomal abnormality antedates the malignancy.

References

Bergsma D: Birth Defects Atlas and Compendium. Baltimore, Williams & Wilkins, 1973

Boué J, Boué A, Lazar P, Gueguen S: Outcome of pregnancies following a spontaneous abortion with chromosomal anomalies. Am J Obstet Gynecol 116:806, 1973

Carr D: Chromosomes and abortion. In Harris H, Hirschhorn K (eds): Advances in Human Genetics. New York, Plenum, 1971

German J: Chromosomes and Cancer. New York, Wiley, 1974

Hamerton J: Human Cytogenetics, Vols I and II. New York, Academic, 1971

Lewandowski R, Yunis J: New chromosomal syndromes. Am J Dis Child 129:515, 1975

Miller O, Miller D, Warburton D: Application of new staining techniques to the study of human chromosomes. In Steinberg A, Bearn A (eds): Progress in Medical Genetics—IX. New York, Grune & Stratton, 1973

Standardization in Human Cytogenetics. Paris Conference 1971. Birth Defects Orig. Art. Sec. VII: 7, 1972

Tjio JH, Levan A: Chromosome number of man. Hereditas 42:1, 1956

Yunis J: Human Chromosome Methodology. New York, Academic, 1974

DERMATOGLYPHIC ANALYSIS

Harold M. Nitowsky

Epidermal ridges on the volar aspects of the hands and feet form a variety of pattern configurations termed *dermatoglyphics.* Although the ridge configurations are altered in characteristic ways in a variety of disorders, these alterations have seldom been pathognomonic for a particular condition. Rather, they simply provide additional data that when viewed in relation to the total pattern of malformation may enhance the clinician's capacity to arrive at a specific overall diagnosis.

Ridges develop in relation to volar pads. The latter appear at about the sixth week of gestation and attain maximal size by the 12th to 13th weeks. At that time patches of elevated ridges become evident and grow and coalesce as the volar pads regress. By the fourth month of fetal life the epidermal ridges are well developed. Palmar creases develop during the second and third months of intrauterine life. Once completed, the epidermal ridges and palmar creases remain unchanged, except in size, for life. Although genetic factors play an important role in determining ridge configurations, nongenetic factors may exert an influence as well. Variability of patterns is sufficiently great that no two individuals have identical ridge patterns. Dermatoglyphic patterns may be classified into various groups as follows:

Finger Patterns. Finger patterns may be divided into arches, loops, and whorls, as illustrated diagrammatically in Figure 17. Triradii occur at the juncture of three sets of converging ridges. In the *arch* pattern the ridges

enter from one side and flow to the other side. The features that characterize a *loop* include a triradius, at least one recurring ridge, and a ridge count of at least one across a recurring ridge. If the ridges enter and leave from the ulnar side, an ulnar loop is formed; if they enter and leave from the radial side, a radial loop results. *Whorls* have at least two triradii and may consist of a spiral or ellipse pattern in the simple whorl or two interlocking loops in the double whorl.

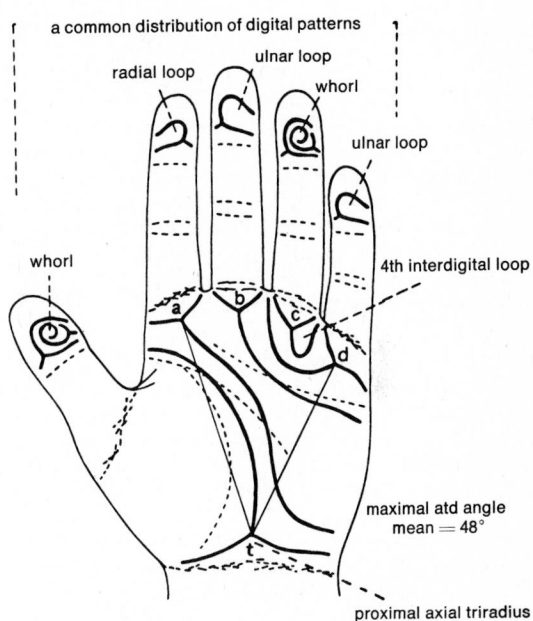

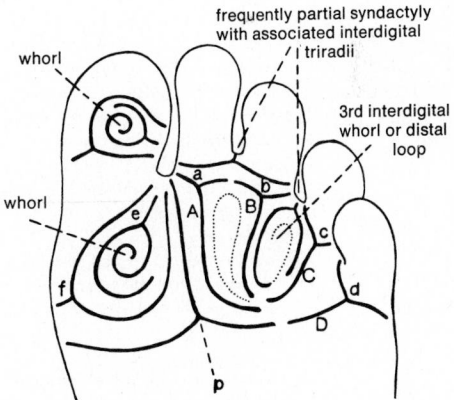

FIG. 17. Diagram of palm and sole showing pattern areas, triradii, and finger pattern types. The solid lines and dotted lines denote the dermal ridge configurations, and the dashes within the palm represent the creases.

Finger Ridge Count. A ridge count is obtained from the number of ridges crossed by a line from the triradius to the core of the pattern. The total finger ridge count averages 145 in males and 127 in females.

Palmar Patterns. The palmar area is divided into various zones within which a pattern may or may not be present. These areas include the hypothenar, thenar, and interdigital areas. Triradii are found normally beneath each finger and in the axial line of the palm. The distal triradii are called *a, b, c,* and *d* from index to little finger, respectively. The axial triradius is called *t* and is usually not more than 10 percent of the distance between the distal crease of the wrist and the proximal crease of the middle finger. However, the axial triradius may be displaced distally toward the ulnar or toward the radial border of the palm. More than one axial triradius may be present.

Palmar Creases. Normally, two deep transverse creases are found on the palm, but occasionally only one is present. A single palmar crease, called a simian line, and a single phalangeal flexion crease may be found in certain clinical disorders.

Foot Patterns. On the foot the ridge patterns on the hallucal area and on the great toe are classified as arches, loops, and whorls. An open field in the hallucal area simply means a relative lack of complexity in patterning and thereby implies a low surface contour at the time ridges developed. The hallucal area of the sole usually has a loop or whorl pattern; a lack of such pattern is unusual in the normal. It is found in about half the patients with Down's syndrome and as an occasional feature in other disorders. A summary of some aberrant patterns and unusual frequency or distribution of dermatoglyphic patterns in several chromosomal disorders is presented in Table 8.

TABLE 8. Dermatoglyphic Findings in Some Chromosomal Disorders

Clinical Disorder	Dermatoglyphic Abnormalities
Down's syndrome (mongolism, trisomy 21)	Excess ulnar loops, radial loops increased on fourth and fifth digits, increased *atd* angle, simian line, single flexion crease on fifth digit
Trisomy E (trisomy 18)	Excess arches on digits (usually more than 6), single flexion crease on digits, simian line
Trisomy D (trisomy 13)	Increased *atd* angle, simian line, arch fibular or arch fibular S pattern on hallucal area
Turner's syndrome (XO gonadal dysgenesis and cytologic variants)	Increased whorls on fingers, increased *atd* angle, S hypothenar pattern, increased *a-b* ridge count
Klinefelter's syndrome (XXY and cytologic	Loops with low ridge counts on digits, excess arches on fingers
Cri du chat (5p—)	Increased *atd* angle, simian line

GENETIC COUNSELING
HAROLD M. NITOWSKY

In the majority of instances genetic counseling is concerned with advising patients on the risks of recurrence of hereditary disorders in future progeny. It is therefore indirectly involved with the prevention of these disorders. In addition to discussing recurrence risks, the genetic counselor must explain, as simply as possible, the nature of the disorder and the meaning of the term genetic. Moreover, he must dispel the feelings of guilt that parents often experience after having a child with a genetic abnormality, and he must provide appropriate advice and support as the occasion demands.

In considering human disease as part of a broad spectrum, one finds at one extreme the conditions that are entirely genetic in causation and at the other extreme the nutritional deficiencies and infectious diseases that are almost entirely due to environmental factors. Between the two extremes are many relatively common conditions, such as diabetes mellitus and certain congenital malformations, in which both genetic and environmental factors are involved. Disorders that are entirely genetic in etiology either are chromosomal abnormalities or are due to single gene mutations (unifactorial). The latter are individually rare, the mode of inheritance is simple (dominant, recessive, or X-linked), and the chances of recurrence are high (greater than 1 in 10). Conditions that etiologically are partly genetic are generally due to interaction between many genes and the environment (multifactorial). These disorders are common, the mode of inheritance is complex, and the chances of recurrence are usually low (less than 1 in 10).

Before providing genetic advice it is essential to investigate the family pedigree; at the minimum this should include information about the health of all first-degree relatives, ie, parents, siblings, and children of the person seeking such advice. If the disorder is not severe it may be possible to trace it back through several generations. On the other hand, if the condition is severe, affected individuals may not have survived to have children and to transmit the disease to subsequent generations. In such cases the affected individual is sporadic, being the only person in the family with the defect, which is usually the result of a new mutation.

SINGLE GENE MUTATIONS. *Autosomal dominant* traits affect both males and females and often show great variation in expressivity (p. 272). For example, in a patient with osteogenesis imperfecta the only manifestation of the disease may be blue sclerae, whereas other individuals, even in the same family, can be very severely affected with multiple fractures. Sometimes the gene may not express itself at all, in which case it is said to be nonpenetrant. This phenomenon may explain apparent skipped generations in certain pedigrees. On the other hand, careful examination often shows that the skipped individual has definite although mild manifestations, representing a forme fruste of the disorder. Careful clinical examination of both apparently healthy parents of a child with an autosomal dominant disorder is therefore essential before the possibility of a new mutation can be considered.

If an individual with an autosomal dominant anomaly marries a normal person, on the average, half their children will be affected. Some autosomal genes are expressed more frequently in one sex than in the other. This is referred to as sex-influenced inheritance. For example, hemochromatosis is much more common in males than in females, who often do not develop symptoms until after menopause.

Autosomal recessive traits also affect both sexes, and since only homozygotes manifest the disorder, the heterozygous parents are unaffected. On the average, 1 in 4 offsping of two heterozygotes has the abnormal trait. Unlike the situation with an autosomal dominant trait, it is generally impossible to trace the disease through several generations. All the affected individuals in a family are usually in one sibship. The parents of a child with a rare recessive disorder are often related, since relatives are more likely to have inherited the same gene from a common ancestor. The rarer a disorder the higher the incidence of consanguinity. However, the fact that in a particular family the parents are not related does not preclude the condition from being recessively inherited. On average, 1 in 4 of the offspring of two heterozygotes is affected.

An X-linked recessive trait is one that is due to a mutant gene on the X chromosome. Hemizygous males (with the mutant gene on their single X chromosome) are affected, but heterozygous females (carriers) are usually normal. Diseases inherited in this manner are transmitted by healthy female carriers and by affected males if the disorder is not severe or is treatable. All the daughters of an affected male will be carriers, and all his sons will be normal. In severe X-linked disorders, such as Duchenne's muscular dystrophy, affected males do not survive to have children, and the disorder is transmitted by female carriers. In the case of a woman who is a carrier of Duchenne's muscular dystrophy, half her sons will be affected and half her daughters will be carriers.

Quite often in serious X-linked conditions there is only one affected male in a family. Such a sporadic case may be the result of a new mutation in the X chromosome that is inherited from the mother. However, there is also the possibility that the mother might be a carrier, the mutant gene by chance not having been transmitted to any of her male relatives but inherited only through the female line, perhaps for several generations.

MULTIFACTORIAL INHERITANCE.

There are many fairly common conditions in which there is a definite familial tendency, the proportion of affected relatives being greater than in the general population. However, the proportion of affected relatives is often of the order of 5 percent and therefore much less than would be expected for single gene mutations. Although the low familial incidence in some of these conditions has been ascribed to genes being incompletely penetrant, this explanation is unsatisfactory. It is much more likely that such conditions are caused by many genes and the effects of environment, or the so-called multifactorial inheritance.

In multifactorial inheritance it may be assumed that there is some hypothetic underlying attribute that is related to the causation of the disease. This is referred to as the individual's liability, which includes not only his genetic predisposition but also the environmental circumstances that render him more or less likely to develop the disease in question. Further, it may be assumed that the curve of liability has a normal distribution in both the general population and in relatives, but the curve for the latter is shifted to the right. In the general population the proportion of individuals above the threshold for manifestation of the disorder constitutes the population incidence. Among relatives the proportion above the threshold is the familial incidence. This model has been applied to measurable characteristics (such as stature and intelligence) and has also been used to explain the familial incidence of such conditions as diabetes mellitus, congenital pyloric stenosis, cleft lip with and without cleft palate, anencephaly and spina bifida, clubfoot, and congenital dislocation of the hip.

In conditions in which the inheritance is believed to be multifactorial, there are several consequences of the model depicted. The incidence will be greatest among the relatives of more severely affected individuals, because they presumably are more extreme deviants along the curve of liability. By similar reasoning it would also be expected that the incidence among siblings born subsequent to the index case would be greater the more affected relatives there were in the family. In spina bifida, for example, after the birth of a single affected child the incidence among subsequent siblings is approximately 4 percent; but it is 10 percent after the birth of two affected children, and evidence suggests the risk is higher still if another close relative is also affected.

RECURRENCE RISK. Estimation of the risk of recurrence in the individual case depends on a precise diagnosis and an established etiology. Before giving genetic counseling, a careful clinical examination and investigation of the affected individual are essential. In order to arrive at the correct diagnosis it may be necessary to refer to death certificates and autopsy and biopsy reports. It may also be necessary to examine the parents or other relatives in certain situations. Without such information it may not be possible to give reliable genetic advice.

In establishing the etiology the pedigree should include information on the health of at least all first-degree relatives, consanguinity, abortions, maternal exposure to radiation, drugs and infections during pregnancy, and details of any birth trauma. Finally, the possibility of genetic heterogeneity must always be considered. The literature should be searched for information on this point and on the relative frequencies of the various modes of inheritance. When the precise diagnosis is known and the mode of inheritance is clearly established, genetic couneling is usually straightforward and is based on expected mendelian ratios. However, in the case of autosomal recessive conditions, an individual (whether homozygous or heterozygous) is unlikely to have affected children unless the spouse also carries the same mutant gene, which is unlikely if the condition is rare.

In fairly common conditions in which genetic factors appear to play a part but where there is no simple mode of inheritance, the risks of recurrence are based on the observed frequencies of the conditions among relatives

TABLE 9. Empiric Risks for Some Common Disorders

Disorder	Incidence (%)	Sex Ratio M:F	Normal Parents Having a Second Affected Child (%)	Affected Parent Having an Affected Child (%)	Affected Parent Having a Second Affected Child (%)
Anencephaly	0.20	1:2	2	—	—
Cleft palate only	0.04	2:3	2	7	15
Cleft lip ± cleft palate	0.10	3:2	4	4	12
Clubfoot	0.10	2:1	3	3	10
Congenital heart disease (all types)	0.60	—	1–4	1–4	—
Pyloric stenosis	0.30	5:1			
male index			2	4	13
female index			10	17	38
Spina bifida	0.30	2:3	4	—	—

of affected individuals, so-called empiric risks. Many of these conditions are probably heterogeneous; they include disorders of various causation. Empiric risk figures are therefore unsatisfactory, as they merely represent an average figure for any one condition. A list of empiric risk figures for some common disorders is shown in Table 9. If a genetic etiology for a particular condition has not been established, and yet the family history clearly suggests a particular mode of inheritance, then genetic counseling should be based on the family history, since this condition may represent a unique situation.

In general, trisomy 21 (Down's syndrome), trisomy 13, trisomy 18, and other chromosomal abnormalities are usually the result of errors in meiosis during gametogenesis, and the chances of recurrence are small. However, if one of the parents happens to be a mosaic or carries a balanced translocation, the situation is different. If one of the parents is a mosaic it may be very difficult to give reliable genetic advice, because it is impossible to estimate what proportion of the parental gonadal tissue is normal. If one of the parents carries a translocation, genetic counseling depends on the cytogenetic findings and the sex of the carrier parent.

A common problem arises when healthy parents have a child with a particular disorder or abnormality and there is no history on either side of the family of anyone similarly affected. There are several possible explanations for such a situation. First, the disorder may be a phenocopy, perhaps due to maternal exposure during pregnancy. Second, it may be due to a chromosome abnormality, but apart from Down's syndrome, most disorders associated with specific chromosome abnormalities are very rare, and the chances of recurrence are small. A third possibility is that of a new autosomal dominant mutation, in which case there is little chance of recurrence in subsequent children. This is a distinct possibility if the condition is known to be inherited as an autosomal dominant, if it is always fully penetrant, and if on examination both parents are found to be unaffected. Fourth, it might be an autosomal recessive disorder. Evidence in favor of this etiology would be

parental consanguinity or the demonstration that both parents are heterozygotes by an appropriate biochemical or other type of test. Finally, it could represent an X-linked recessive disorder. It is important to recognize this possibility, because an unaffected sister might then be a carrier. Clinical evidence might suggest this mode of inheritance. It might also be possible to demonstrate a biochemical or other abnormality in the mother but not in the father, which would suggest that the disorder was X-linked.

PRENATAL DIAGNOSIS. Amniocentesis for prenatal diagnosis of fetal genetic abnormalities has added a new dimension to the prediction of risks for inheritance of genetic disorders. Heretofore the genetic counselor has estimated the risks for occurrence of a genetic abnormality in future progeny from an analysis of the family history, information about the mode of genetic transmission of the disorder, and other data. Now, however, amniocentesis permits evaluation of the status of each fetus, independently and with relative certainty for a broad spectrum of genetic abnormalities. As a result of the liberalization of abortion laws and the development of safe and accurate techniques for prenatal diagnosis, selective termination of pregnancy if the fetus is affected can be offered as a means to prevent the birth of an infant with a condition that is lethal or that may result in irremediable mental or physical handicaps. However, since many types of fetal abnormalities cannot be diagnosed by currently available methods, amniocentesis offers no guarantee that the infant will be free of all possible abnormalities.

Various techniques have been developed for detecting abnormalities in the human fetus in utero (Table 10). These may conveniently be divided into those that study the fetus directly and those that study the fetus indirectly from changes in the mother's urine or blood. Some techniques for studying the fetus directly include radiography for skeletal abnormalities, amniography and fetography for soft tissue abnormalities, sonography, and fetal electrocardiography. However, these techniques may be of limited value in early pregnancy. Biopsy of membranes, placenta, and fetus is still at the

TABLE 10. Techniques for Antenatal Diagnosis

Direct (fetal)
  Radiography
    Skeletal
    Soft tissue (amniography, fetography)
  Electrocardiography
  Sonography
  Biopsy
    Membranes
    Placenta
    Fetus
  Fetoscopy
  Amniocentesis
Indirect (maternal)
  Urine
  Blood

experimental stage, as is direct visualization of the fetus (fetoscopy), which may prove particularly valuable in the antenatal diagnosis of certain congenital abnormalities.

The usual approach to antenatal diagnosis of genetic disease is the study of amniotic fluid and its contained cells. Amniotic fluid cells are of fetal origin, being largely derived from the surface layers of the fetal skin but with contributions from other sources such as the buccal mucosa and amnion. The origin of the amniotic fluid itself is more complex and depends on the stage of gestation. Specimens of amniotic fluid are generally obtained by aspiration through the abdominal wall (transabdominal amniocentesis). This technique is carried out after the 14th week of gestation when the uterus rises above the symphysis pubis and the volume of amniotic fluid is large enough to sample safely. Experience indicates that the transabdominal approach is a relatively safe technique that entails little risk to the mother (such as hemorrhage or infection) or to the fetus (precipitation of abortion, trauma). The findings of a collaborative study sponsored by the National Institute of Child Health and Human Development indicate that the overall risk of amniocentesis is less than 0.5 percent.

Uncultured amniotic fluid cells have been used for biochemical and histologic studies, but these methods are probably too unreliable for diagnosing most biochemical disorders in utero or too nonspecific to be of value. The main use of uncultured cells is for sex prediction based on sex chromatin and fluorescence studies. From the former the number of X chromosomes can be determined, and from the latter the number of Y chromosomes. However, there are limitations to these techniques, so that it is important to confirm the findings by chromosome studies on cultured cells.

The main indications for chromosome studies on cultured amniotic fluid cells are in families where one of the parents is a mosaic or carries a translocation that in the unbalanced state may cause severe physical or mental abnormality, or because of increased maternal age, since the latter is associated with an increased fetal risk of trisomy 21, trisomy 13, trisomy 18, and Klinefelter's syndrome. The main application of chromosome stud-

ies of amniotic cell cultures has been in the antenatal diagnosis of Down's syndrome. Because of the increased risk of trisomy 21 with maternal age (as high as 1 in 60 over age 40), it has been recommended that amniocentesis be offered to all pregnant women over 35 years of age.

There are several pitfalls and limitations of antenatal chromosome studies. One of the most serious problems is the possible misinterpretation of a karyotype that morphologically appears normal, but contains a chromosome rearrangement that may be associated with severe physical or mental abnormality. In general, if both products of a reciprocal translocation cannot be recognized in one of the parents, then antenatal chromosome studies are probably not justified in a pregnancy at risk. However, these difficulties are less likely with the newly introduced staining techniques that permit precise identification not only of individual chromosomes but also of structural rearrangements of the chromosomes.

An important development in recent years has been the use of cultured amniotic fluid cells for the antenatal diagnosis of inherited biochemical disorders. This usually involves the demonstration of reduced activity of a particular enzyme in cell extracts. Many enzyme activities have been demonstrated in cultured amniotic fluid cells, and therefore genetic disorders associated with deficiency of these enzymes have been diagnosed or are potentially diagnosable in utero (Table 11). Unfortunately it is not yet possible to diagnose cystic fibrosis of the pancreas prenatally, as it is one of the most common inherited metabolic disorders. On a worldwide basis sickle cell anemia is probably the most common serious genetic disorder affecting man. Until recently it was believed that hemoglobin β-chain synthesis was not switched on until around the time of birth, and therefore there seemed little prospect of being able to diagnose sickle cell anemia in utero. However, recent studies have shown that β-chain synthesis begins in early fetal life, and provided the technical difficulties of obtaining specimens of fetal blood can be overcome, it may soon be possible to diagnose sickle cell anemia in utero. It is likely that during the next few years there will be a substantial increase in the number of inherited metabolic disorders that can be diagnosed antenatally.

An important prerequisite of using cultured amniotic fluid cells for biochemical diagnosis is the establishment of reliable control values for enzymes in normal amniotic fluid cells. Recent observations suggest that cultures of amniotic fluid cells consist of cells with different biochemical properties and morphologic characteristics. The implication of these studies is that it is essential to establish normal biochemical properties for each cell type if an accurate antenatal diagnosis of a disorder is to be made. Another important problem is the effect culture conditions may have on enzyme levels. Cells usually have to be cultured for several weeks before there is sufficient material on which to base a diagnosis. During this period cells may undergo changes with concomitant alterations in enzyme levels. Further, the levels of a number of enzymes have been shown to vary

TABLE 11. Hereditary Biochemical Disorders That Have Been or Are Diagnosable In Utero

Enzyme	Disorder
Hexosaminidase A	Tay-Sachs disease
α-1,4-glucosidase	Pompe's disease
Acid phosphatase	Acid phosphatase deficiency
α-galactosidase	Fabry's syndrome
Sphingomyelinase	Niemann-Pick disease
Hypoxanthine guanine phosphoribosyl trans-ferase	Lesch-Nyhan syndrome
Arylsulfatase A	Metachromatic leukodystrophy
β-galactosidase	Generalized gangliosidosis
Branched-chain keto acid decarboxylase	Maple syrup urine disease
Gal-1-phosphate uridyl transferase	Galactosemia
Cystathionine synthetase	Homocystinuria
$^{35}SO_4$ uptake	Hunter/Hurler syndromes
Cystine accumulation	Cystinosis
Glucocerebrosidase	Gaucher's disease
Amylo-1,6-glucosidase	Forbes disease
Amylo-(1, 4 1, 6)-transglucosidase	Andersen's syndrome
Ornithine transaminase	Hyperornithinemia
Argininosuccinase	Argininosuccinic-aciduria
Histidase	Histidenemia
G6PD	G6PD deficiency
Endonuclease	Xeroderma pigmentosum
Valine transaminase	Hypervalinemia
Cystathioninase	Cystathioninuria
Phytanic acid oxidase	Refsum's disease
Ornithine carbamyltransferase	Hyperammonemia
Arginase	Argininemia
Fucosidase	Fucosidosis
α-Mannosidase	Mannosidosis

during the cycle of cell growth in culture. Accordingly, control material ideally should be amniotic fluid cells from normal fetuses of comparable gestational age that have been grown in culture for approximately the same length of time, in the same medium, and under identical conditions and then harvested at the same stage in the growth cycle as amniotic fluid cells from a fetus at risk.

Biochemical analysis of supernatant amniotic fluid as a means of diagnosing genetic disease in utero would have considerable advantage over methods that depend on study of cultured amniotic fluid cells, which is technically difficult and requires several weeks before results can be obtained. However, the former approach is likely to be of value only in those metabolic disorders that are associated with changes in urinary composition (since amniotic fluid is largely derived from fetal urine after the first trimester) and that are not diet-dependent.

Genetic abnormalities not associated with any specific biochemical or chromosomal abnormality present a problem in antenatal diagnosis. However, in certain congenital abnormalities, and particularly in CNS malformations such as spina bifida and anencephaly, changes occur in the biochemical composition of amniotic fluid that are of value in antenatal diagnosis. Thus there is a significant increase in the level of α-feto-protein in amniotic fluid in more than 90 percent of fetuses with anencephaly or open neural tube defects.

For some fetal genetic disorders not associated with any biochemical or chromosome abnormality, genetic linkage may be helpful for prenatal diagnosis. The underlying principle is that the loci for a marker trait and the particular disorder in question should be closely linked on the same chromosome and therefore should be likely to segregate together in a particular family, and the marker trait should be detectable in amniotic fluid or its contained cells. Two such linkages have been described: the loci for G6PD and hemophilia A and the loci for ABH-secretor status and myotonic dystrophy. Since the loci for G6PD and hemophilia A are closely linked on the X chromosome and since the G6PD phenotype can be determined in amniotic fluid cells, this may be valuable in the antenatal diagnosis of hemophilia in populations where G6PD variants are common. Second, the loci for secretor status and myotonic dystrophy are within measurable distance of each other, and the secretor status of the fetus can be determined from amniotic fluid in early pregnancy.

Not all clinics or hospitals are equipped to carry out diagnostic amniocentesis and the culture of amniotic fluid cells in situations where there is a high or clear-cut risk for a fetal disorder. Since cultures of amniotic cells can be grown several days after the procedure, if properly handled, it may be preferable to develop selected centers for these studies. Future application of amniocentesis in pregnancies at risk for chromosome or biochemical abnormalities may require the mobilization of laboratory resources on a regional or national basis to permit the most efficient delivery of optimal services at the lowest possible cost.

GENETIC ADVICE. Factors that influence the parents' decisions whether they will accept the risk of having an affected child include the severity of the abnormality, whether there is an effective treatment, statistical risk, and their religious attitudes, socioeconomic status, and education. The genetic counselor usually does not try to influence the parents' decision, although when the risks involved are high, advice in regard to family limitation may be indicated.

Contraception is not the only course of action open to parents faced with this problem. Other alternatives include sterilization or artifical insemination (if the father is affected). Following the liberalization of abortion laws, termination of pregnancy is another possibility if the mother becomes pregnant with substantial risk of serious abnormality. Selective abortion has also become a possibility whereby a pregnancy may be terminated when it is known that the fetus is abnormal.

There is ample evidence to suggest that a significant number of persons in the population are at high risk of having a child with a serious hereditary disorder and are unaware of the fact. In the past the finding of such individuals has often been a matter of chance, depending largely on the awareness of their physician. Therefore there may be justification for setting up genetic registers in which families at high risk are recorded, so that individuals in these families can be followed up and given appropriate counseling when they reach child-bearing age.

In giving genetic advice it is not sufficient merely to quote risk figures; insofar as is posible the nature and cause of the disease should be explained to the parents. Feelings of guilt and misconceptions about etiology should be removed. Other problems may also have to be discussed, including child adoption, abortion, sterilization, and perhaps even artificial insemination. Since the consequences of genetic counseling can be profound and far-reaching, such advice should never be given lightly. It involves not only familiarity with the medical and genetic aspects of hereditary disease but also an awareness of the serious personal problems that are often involved.

References

Carter CO: The inheritance of common congenital malformations. Prog Med Genet 4:59, 1965

Emery AEH: Antenatal diagnosis: limitations and future prospects. Birth Defects Orig. Art. Sec. X: 289, 1974 Nat. Sci. Foundation

Fraser FC: Current issues in medical genetics: genetic counseling. Am J Hum Genet 26:636, 1974

McKusick VA: Mendelian Inheritance in Man, 4th ed. Baltimore, Johns Hopkins Univ Press, 1975

Nadler HL:,Prenatal detection of genetic disorders. In Harris H, Hirschhorn K (eds): Advances in Human Genetics, Vol 3. New York, Plenum, 1972, p 1

Nitowsky HM, Legum CL: Genetic counseling: general principles and clinical applications. Schulman I. (ed): Advances in Pediatrics, Vol 18. Chicago, Year Book, 1971, p 13

Roberts JAF: Genetic prognosis. Br Med J 1:587, 1962

CHAPTER 9

Immunologic Disorders of Childhood

Diane W. Wara and Arthur J. Ammann

From the moment an infant leaves the sterile environment of the uterus, it is continually assaulted by foreign antigens in the form of microbial agents (bacteria, viruses, fungi, and protozoa) and inert agents inhaled from the atmosphere or ingested during feeding. The function of the immune system is to prevent or retard the local establishment or systemic dissemination of these agents; in addition the immune system acts to prevent the development of autoimmune disease and malignancy. The immune system is composed of four primary components. The first, antibody-mediated immunity, carries out its function by means of immunoglobulins in the secretions, plasma, and interstitial spaces. The second, cell-mediated immunity, carries out its function by means of lymphocytes in the blood and peripheral lymphoid tissue. The third, the phagocytic system, consists of a variety of mononuclear and polymorphonuclear cells within the blood and in the tissues engaged in the ingestion and killing of microorganisms.

The fourth component, the complement system, acts synergistically with the remainder of the immune system to enhance resistance to microbial infection.

ANTIBODY-MEDIATED IMMUNITY

The development of competent immunity probably follows the division of stem cells into at least three populations (Fig. 1). The stem cell in the chicken may come under the influence of the bursa of Fabricius; although there is no direct evidence in man for the existence of an equivalent organ, several investigators feel that the tonsils, adenoids, Peyer's patches, and appendix collectively form the bursa equivalent, while others think that this function resides in the bone marrow. The cells that come under the influence of the bursa equivalent circulate in the peripheral blood and in lymphoid tissue and are referred to as B cells. Between 20 and 30 percent of the total peripheral blood lymphocytes can be specifically identified as B lym-

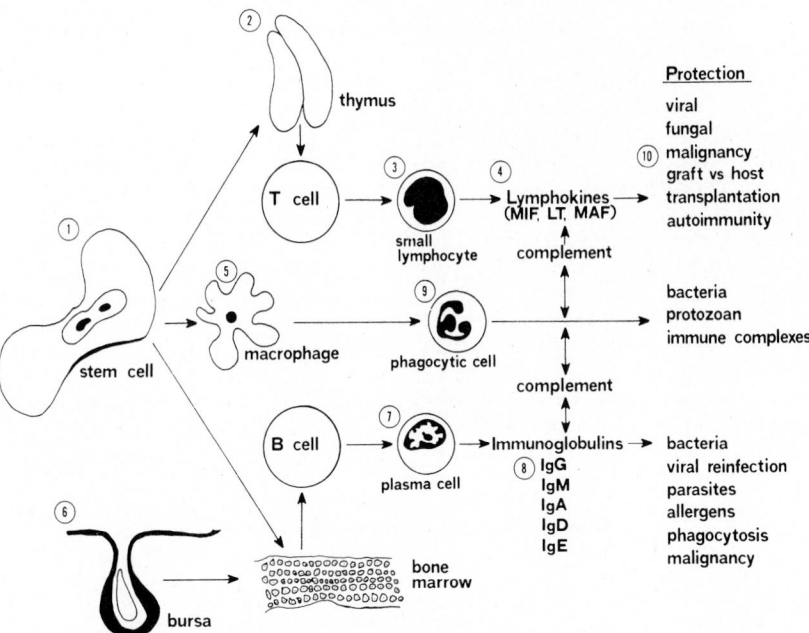

FIG. 1. Physiology of immunity. Schematic representation of development of immune system. The numbers refer to known defects in the development of immunity: 1. Severe combined immunodeficiency; 2. DiGeorge syndrome; 3. Thymic hypoplasia with abnormal immunoglobulin synthesis; 4. Chronic mucocutaneous candidiasis; 5. Wiskott-Aldrich syndrome; 6. Congenital hypogammaglobulinemia; 7. Acquired hypogammaglobulinemia; 8. Selective IgA deficiency; 9. Chronic granulomatous disease; 10. Malignancy.

phocytes, which have on their surface membranes immunoglobulin, immunoglobulin-like receptors, and/or receptors for the complement components. B cells may be present in two forms; studies have shown that B lymphocytes can transform into plasma cells, which then are capable of synthesizing and secreting specific antibodies. The function of peripheral blood B cells is probably to recognize specific antibody, which is subsequently distributed systemically.

It is thought that each B cell produces a highly specific antibody molecule. All the antibody molecules taken collectively are termed immunoglobulins. This large array of individual antibody molecules can be divided into various immunoglobulin classes and subclasses according to different molecular structures and antigenic qualities. Each immunoglobulin is composed of two heavy chains and two light chains linked together by disulfide bonds. The ability to identify separate immunoglobulin classes resides in the Fc (crystallizable) portion of the heavy chain of the molecule. This portion of the molecule has a relatively constant amino acid sequence within each immunoglobulin class, which allows for the separation of immunoglobulins into five distinct classes. The Fab portion of the molecule also determines the specific function of the various immunoglobulin classes, such as placental passage and complement fixation. The Fab portion of the immunoglobulin molecule is composed of both heavy and light chains. This portion has a highly variable amino acid sequence that permits the diversification necessary for combination with multiple antigens.

The separation of immunoglobulins into five distinct classes has resulted in the isolation and subsequent definition of unique characteristics and specific functions of each class (Table 1). Immunoglobulin G comprises 70 to 80 percent of the total immunoglobulins; it is distributed intravascularly and throughout the interstitial spaces and has a molecular weight of approximately 150,000 daltons. The mean adult concentration is 1,200 mg/dl; however, values in children must be compared with the norms for their ages (Table 2). IgG can be divided into four subclasses; most of the subclasses both bind complement and are transferred across the placenta from the maternal circulation to the fetus. The majority of antibody directed against virus, bacteria, and fungi is of the IgG class. IgG may also be considered the memory antibody, as it has the capacity to persist for long periods of time following antigenic stimulation. Antibodies that form following densensitization for allergies or that form in association with certain malignancies may have the capability of blocking certain biologic functions. Frequently these antibodies are in the IgG class.

Immunoglobulin M comprises 5 to 10 percent of the total immunoglobulins under normal circumstances and has a molecular weight of 900,000 daltons. The mean adult concentration is 150 mg/dl. IgM forms rapidly following primary antigenic stimulation and is maintained in the intravascular space. Newborns do not normally have IgM present in the cord blood, as IgM does not cross the placenta and usually is not synthesized in large amounts in utero. Elevated IgM in cord blood or in blood obtained during the newborn period may be taken as evidence of premature synthesis of antibody; it frequently represents a response to either intrauterine or neonatal infection. The majority of antibodies formed against polysaccharides and against gram-negative bacterial antigens are of the IgM class. The spleen may play an important role in the production of IgM antibody, and this may account for a portion of the increased susceptibility to infection following splenectomy.

Immunoglobulin A comprises 10 to 15 percent of the total immunoglobulins; it has a molecular weight of approximately 180,000 daltons and is contained primarily in the secretions and in the intravascular space. The mean adult concentration of IgA is 300 mg/dl in the serum. Immunoglobulin A does not cross the placenta and does not bind complement; it is thought to be effective in providing local immunity. There has been adequate documentation that local infection with viral agents can be prevented by this form of immunoglobulin. Secretory IgA is found in colostrum and in breast milk in concentrations 10 to 100 times that found in serum.

Little is known concerning the function of immunoglobulin D. It is present in the serum in low amounts, usually less than 1 percent of the total immunoglobulin. Mean adult serum concentration is 3 mg/dl; the molecular weight of IgD is 180,000 daltons. Antibody activity against a variety of microbial agents has been demonstrated, but as yet there is no conclusive evidence that IgD has a unique function. Recently IgD has been demonstrated on the surface of certain malignant cells, and it has been suggested that IgD may indicate the presence of undifferentiated or "primitive" cells.

Immunoglobulin E is present in the serum in the lowest concentration, comprising less than 0.01 percent

TABLE 1. Properties of Immunoglobulins

	IgG	IgM	IgA	IgD	IgE
Monomer units	1	5	1–3	1	1
Molecular weight (daltons)	150,000	900,000	180,000–500,000	180,000	200,000
Serum concentration, adult mean (mg/dl)	1,200	150	300	3	0.03
Biologic half-life (days)	25	5	7	2.8	2.3
Active placental transfer	+	+	—	—	—
Binds complement	+	+	—	—	—

TABLE 2. Normal Values for Immunoglobulins at Various Ages[a]

AGE[b]	IgG (mg/dl)	IgA (mg/dl)	IgM (mg/dl)
Newborn	600–1670	0–5	6–15
1–3 months	218–610	20–53	11–51
4–6 months	228–636	27–72	25–60
7–9 months	292–816	27–73	12–124
10–18 months	383–1070	27–169	28–113
2 years	423–1184	35–222	32–131
3 years	477–1334	40–251	28–113
4–5 years	540–1500	48–336	20–106
6–8 years	571–1700	52–535	28–112
14 years	570–1570	86–544	33–135
Adult	635–1775	106–668	37–154

[a] *From Buckley et al: Pediatrics 41:600, 1968.*
[b] *Difference in immunoglobulin levels as reported by different authors based on the use of different reference antigens.*

of the total immunoglobulins. The mean adult concentration is 0.03 mg/dl; the molecular weight is approximately 200,000 daltons. IgE is present in the plasma, but can be quantitated only by sensitive techniques such as radioimmunoassay. In the tissue, IgE is bound to mast cells, and in the peripheral circulation it is bound to basophils. When cell-bound IgE combines with specific antigens, a variety of pharmocologic agents are released. Histamine, slow-reacting substance of anaphylaxis (SRS-A), and eosinophilic chemotactic factor have been identified as substances released following antigenic combination with cell-bound IgE. These agents subsequently produce physiologic effects that result in clinical allergic symptomatology (p. 331).

Severe deficiency of antibody-mediated immunity is characterized by total absence of all immunoglobulin classes. The spectrum of antibody-deficiency syndromes, however, can vary from complete absence of immunoglobulins to absence of a single immunoglobulin class. Rarely an individual may have normal levels of all immunoglobulins but will not respond with an increase in functional antibody titer following specific immunization.

In general the development of specific antibodies in response to antigenic challenge is considered a beneficial effect. However, in certain circumstances the development of antibody can result in acute or chronic disease. The development of IgE antibody may prevent specific local damage caused by foreign antigens inhaled into the lung or ingested into the intestinal tract; alternatively, IgE antibodies may induce severe asthma or gastrointestinal tract symptoms. Antibody that does not differentiate between "self" and "nonself" antigen may result in the development of autoimmune disease. The chronic production of antibody in inappropriate amounts may result in circulating immune complexes, which then can be deposited in the kidney and produce acute or chronic nephritis. Malignant proliferation of a clone of antibody-producing cells, termed myeloma, can occur following the uncontrolled production of antibody. Although such malignancies are rare in children, the presence of chronic intrauterine infection such as syphilis or toxoplasmosis may result in the production of myeloma-like antibody. Antibody may also block beneficial effects, such as the cellular destruction of malignant cells.

CELL-MEDIATED IMMUNITY

The differentiation of stem cells into a population of competent mediators of cellular immunity occurs in the thymus gland. It has been demonstrated in various animal species that stem cells migrate to the thymus and are subsequently distributed throughout the lymphoreticular system. The maturation of stem cells into mature T cells may occur either as a result of direct contact with the epithelial portion of the thymus or by means of a hormonal "induction." Several thymic humoral factors have been identified, including thymosin, thymic humoral factor, and thymopoietin. These substances have not been completely characterized, but they would appear to be distinct biochemically and functionally, thus suggesting that the thymus may elaborate several humoral factors.

Thymectomy studies in newborn animals clearly demonstrate the necessity of the thymus for maintenance of normal immunologic function. In general, neonatal thymectomy results in a wasting syndrome, with early death of the animal. If the thymectomy is delayed until adult life, less profound effects result. In man, ablation of the thymus by irradiation or thymectomy has not resulted in significant alteration of immunologic function. Removal of the gland is probably incomplete and thus allows for some degree of thymic regeneration. Additionally, it is known that cellular immunity is well established in the human fetus by 20 weeks of gestation and that the thymus is capable of generating long-lived lymphocytes that may survive for many years. At birth, cells from the thymus of the infant have already been distributed as competent T cells throughout the peripheral bloodstream and the lymphoreticular system.

The majority of peripheral blood lymphocytes of normal infants and children are T cells. These thymus-derived lymphocytes can be identified by their ability to form rosettes with sheep erythrocytes in vitro. A specific antigenic marker, such as the theta antigen found on mouse T cells, is not present on human cells. As a result it has been difficult to identify the specific location of T cells in tissues in man. Histologic studies of lymphoid material obtained from patients with thymic deficiency indicate that collections of T cells occur in specific locations such as the periarteriolar area of the spleen and the so-called T-cell-dependent areas of the lymph nodes. These are located in the paracortical and perifollicular regions of the lymph nodes.

Cell-mediated immunity is important in protection against viral, fungal, and protozoan infections, as well as against malignancy and autoimmune disease. There is now evidence in animal models and in man that more than one population of thymus-derived lymphocytes exist. Specifically in man, a subpopulation of T cells probably supplies suppressor cell function, helping the body to distinguish self antigens from nonself antigens and acting to regulate other immune functions.

Once a T cell has become sensitized to a specific antigen, it will react to that antigen on second exposure either by going into blast transformation or by releasing a variety of substances termed lymphokines. Sensitized lymphocytes that react to foreign antigen by blast transformation may have direct cytotoxic effects on other cells and thus act to control the replication and dissemination of foreign antigens such as those present on malignant cells. T cells are responsible for the rejection of foreign grafts such as skin, heart, or kidney. A sensitized T cell reacts on reexposure to a specific antigen by the release of lymphokines. Lymphokines may act in a variety of ways to amplify the immunologic reactivity to foreign antigen. Certain lymphokines have been identified and studied in detail. Migration-inhibition factor (MIF) is released from lymphocytes following exposure to antigen, and in vitro it prevents the migration of macrophages away from the sensitized lymphocytes and foreign antigen. It is postulated that the in vivo function of MIF may be to concentrate macrophages in areas of infection. Lymphocytes may also release interferon on exposure to mitogens or specific antigens. Transfer factor may also be a T cell product that serves to regulate the responses of lymphocytes to specific antigens. Transfer factor is a low-molecular-weight substance (2,-000 to 3,000 daltons) obtained from normal lymphocytes. It is believed to have the capability of transferring specific cell-mediated immunity from a donor to a normal recipient. Evidence has recently been obtained that transfer factor may contain RNA components.

In addition to the specific functions carried out by T cells alone, T cells appear to be necessary for normal antibody production by B lymphocytes. T–B cell interaction may result from direct cell contact, or T cells may elaborate humoral factors necessary for B cell function. The means by which T cells are capable of recognizing specific antigens are not clear. Currently there is considerable controversy as to whether T cells have immunoglobulin receptors on their surfaces similar to those of B cells. Some investigators think that T cells have 7S IgM-like receptors, while others have theorized that T cells have the capability of concentrating antigen on their surfaces.

As in antibody-mediated immunity, not all cell-mediated immune function is beneficial. Excessive sensitization and the subsequent release of lymphokines may result in severe local and systemic reactions, eg, poison oak dermatitis and farmer's lung. In other instances individuals may become sensitized to common environmental agents such as *Aspergillus*, which then results in chronic lung disease.

PHAGOCYTOSIS

Phagocytosis is the process by which cells ingest replicating and nonreplicating agents encountered in the environment in order to contain or destroy them. A characteristic common to cells engaged in phagocytosis is the high intracellular content of granules that contain hydrolytic enzymes associated with lysosomes. Neutrophils are the primary circulating phagocyte, while macrophages are phagocytic cells that reside in the tissue. Monocytes are derived from the bone marrow; subsequently they may differentiate into tissue macrophages.

In order for phagocytes to perform their role, they must be produced in adequate numbers and mobilized at the appropriate time. The normal individual produces an estimated 120 billion neutrophils each day; the half-life of a neutrophil is short (6 to 7 hours). Mobilization of phagocytes is either by means of random movement or by specific movement toward an area of inflammation (chemotaxis). A normal phagocytic cell responds to chemotactic factors from certain bacteria by mobilization toward the factors. Chemotactic factors are released from bacteria following activation of the complement system.

Phagocytes possess a selective ability to recognize foreign antigens. The mechanism for this form of recognition is not completely known, but it involves both specific antibody formation and phagocytic activity. Prior to phagocytosis foreign antigens such as bacteria must interact with serum proteins. The preparation of bacteria for phagocytosis is termed opsonization. Opsonins are composed primarily of immunoglobulins of the IgG class. Normal opsonic activity will not occur without both the Fab and the Fc portions of the immunoglobulin molecule. The Fab portion adheres to the bacteria, while the Fc portion adheres to receptors on phagocytic cells. Bacteria may also activate the complement pathway to enhance the deposition of fragments of C3, which then attach to specific complement receptors on phagocytic cells. The phagocytic cell recognition of an opsonized particle as foreign depends on the presence of receptor molecules on the surface of the phagocytic cell and on the appropriate opsonization of the foreign particle.

Following the interaction between a foreign antigen and a phagocytic cell, the phagocytic cell forms pseudopodia, which surround the particle and fuse on the distal side. The particle is thus encased in a phagocytic vacuole or phagosome. Ingestion of the foreign particle is an active process requiring ATP, glycolysis, glycogenolysis, and oxidative phosphorylation. Agents that increase intracellular levels of cyclic AMP or inhibit glycolysis decrease phagocytosis; an example of such an agent is the steroid, prednisone.

Following the phagocytosis of opsonized foreign particles, cytoplasmic organelles fuse with the membrane of the phagosome and then degranulate. The granules contain enzymes that act with other cell metabolites to destroy the foreign particle. Compounds that increase cyclic AMP levels impair the process of degranulation, while compounds that increase cyclic GMP levels enhance degranulation.

Following the ingestion of foreign particles by phagocytic cells, there is a rapid increase in oxygen consumption and hydrogen peroxide production and a 10-fold increase in the oxidation of glucose through the hexose monophosphate shunt. The enzymatic basis of this oxidative burst remains controversial. Two oxidases specifically involved in human neutrophils have been identified: NADPH oxidase and NADH oxidase. The enzymes reduce oxygen to a superoxide anion. The anion may then spontaneously or enzymatically be reduced to hydrogen peroxide, or it may react with previously formed hydrogen peroxide to yield reactive hydroxyl radicals. Hydrogen peroxide can then enter the cytoplasm of the cells. The hydrogen peroxide–myeloperoxidase–halide system is the most important of the neutrophil bactericidal systems. Iodide is the most potent of the halides. Iodination of bacterial cell walls occurs when iodide is employed in a cell-free system with myeloperoxidase and hydrogen peroxide. Iodination and superoxide generation may be important for optimal bactericidal activity within the phagocyte.

A variety of nonspecific microbicidal systems is known to exist in neutrophils. Certain bacteria, such as pneumococci, may be killed by alterations in the pH within a phagocytic vacuole. Cationic proteins with selective bactericidal activity against certain gram-negative and gram-postive organisms have been identified. Lactoferrin has bacteriostatic properties, and lysozymes are capable of hydrolyzing the mucopolysaccharides of bacterial cell walls.

Although the hydrogen peroxide–myeloperoxidase–halide system has been best defined in circulating neutrophils, it is probable that tissue macrophages function in a similar manner. Tissue macrophages reside in the spleen, lymph nodes, bone marrow, and pulmonary alveolar system. The liver sinusoids contain a type of macrophage termed a Kupffer cell. The ingestion and destruction of foreign antigens by tissue macrophages are most likely of as much importance as the function of circulating neutrophils. Monocytes, although they may differentiate into tissue macrophages, probably have additional functions in the immune system.

COMPLEMENT

The complement system consists of nine serum factors that act sequentially to amplify the effect of anti-

body-mediated immunity, cell-mediated immunity, and phagocytosis (Fig. 2). The molecular weights of these nine factors vary from 79,000 to 400,000 daltons. The serum concentrations vary from approximately 150 mg/dl (C3) to nanogram amounts. The first component of complement (C1) can be divided into three subcomponents, C1q, C1r, and C1s, which are activated sequentially. C1s binds to C4, and an additional enzymatic site is uncovered on C1 that effects the cleavage of C2. One of the fragments (C2a) combines with a fragment of C4 (C4b) to form C3 convertase. If C3 is available it is split by C3 convertase into two fragments, C3a and C3b. C3b is responsible for the cleavage of C5. When C5 combines with C6 and C7, an active complex is formed, which then interacts with C8 and C9, carrying out the final steps of the complement sequence and allowing for lysis of the antigen-antibody-complement complex.

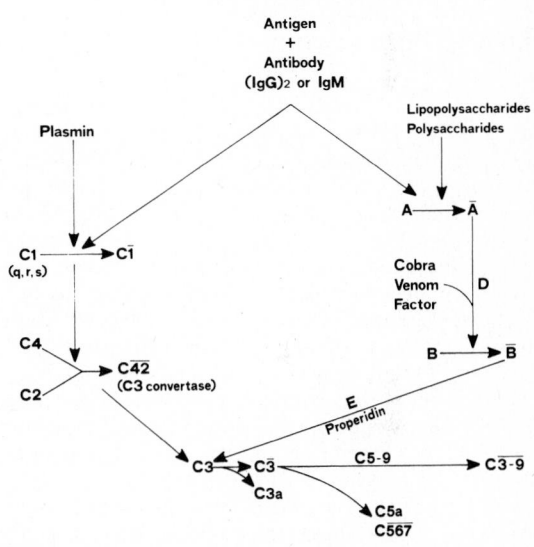

FIG. 2. Schematic representation of the complement system in man.

An alternate pathway for the activation of complement components exists. Properdin and factor B can bypass the initial three components of complement (C1, C4, and C2) and activate C3 directly. C3 can be activated directly by antigen–antibody complexes or by polysaccharide. Nonimmunologic mechanisms are capable of activating the entire pathway. Trypsin, lysosomal enzymes, and bacterial proteases can activate the complement system. Plasmin, an active protein in the clotting mechanism, is capable of activating C1. Inhibitors of complement activation are present at C1 (C1 esterase inhibitor), C3, and C5.

Complement has numerous biologic effects. The binding of complement to specific antibodies of the IgG and IgM classes involves the complement system in the antibody-mediated immune mechanism. Phagocytosis of foreign particles is facilitated by their opsonization by both complement and specific antibody. Phagocytic cells have binding sites for C3 that may add to the adherence between antigen-antibody-complement complexes and phagocytes. Two complement factors (C3a and C5a) effect smooth muscle contraction and are termed anaphylatoxins. Additionally, these same two factors have chemotactic activity. C567 as a unit has strong chemotactic activity. A split product of C4 may act to neutralize viruses independent of other immune mechanisms.

As in antibody-mediated and cell-mediated immunity, not all complement reactions are beneficial. The anaphylatoxins may produce systemic reactions in a nonspecific manner similar to those associated with specific allergies. The adherence of complement (in addition to antibody) to certain cells may result in their lysis, as in Coombs-positive hemolytic anemia. Circulating antigen-antibody-complement complexes may deposit in the kidney and initiate immune-complex disease.

CLINICAL PRESENTATION

Since genetic factors are operative in many immunodeficiency disorders, the majority of patients are infants and children with increased susceptibility to infection early in life. It is estimated that children with primary deficiencies of their antibody-mediated immune system comprise 50 to 75 percent of all cases of primary immunodeficiency. The exact incidence in the general population remains unknown, but it has been estimated to be approximately 1 case per 100,000 population. This statistic excludes patients with selective IgA deficiency, the incidence of which may be as high as 1 in 400. Patients with combined antibody and cellular immunodeficiency comprise approximately 25 percent, and all of the other immunodeficiency disorders account for the remaining 75 percent.

In the absence of a constellation of specific clinical symptoms or signs suggesting immunodeficiency, such as is found in ataxia-telangiectasia, it may be difficult to determine when an immunologic evaluation should be initiated. However, there are numerous suggestive signs and symptoms that may help the clinician (Table 3). The number of infections that a "normal" child may experience before the physician should consider an immunologic evaluation is difficult to determine, but certain factors should be viewed with suspicion: repeated upper respiratory tract infections and/or pneumonia in an infant less than 3 months of age; repeated infections in an infant under 9 months of age who has had relatively little exposure to infectious agents, such as an only child; repeated infections that result in unusual complications such as chronically draining ears, bronchiectasis, chronic diarrhea, or secondary infection such as candidiasis; and continual infections without periods of good health between illnesses in a child of any age. Infants with immunodeficiency frequently are chronically ill and thus fail to thrive. Alternatively, a physician may elect to delay an evaluation for immunodeficiency if repeated respiratory infections are associated with a strong family history of allergy, if the child is one of many siblings, or if he is attending nursery school for the first time.

TABLE 3. Clinical Features Associated With Immunodeficiency[a]

A. Features frequently present and highly suspicious:
  1. Chronic infection
  2. Recurrent infection (greater than expected)
  3. Unusual infecting agents
  4. Incomplete clearing between episodes of infection or incomplete response to treatment

B. Features frequently present and moderately suspicious:
  1. Skin rash (eczema, *Candida,* etc)
  2. Diarrhea (chronic)
  3. Growth failure
  4. Hepatosplenomegaly
  5. Recurrent abscesses
  6. Recurrent osteomyelitis

C. Features associated with specific immunodeficiency disorders:
  1. Ataxia
  2. Telangiectasia
  3. Short-limbed dwarfism
  4. Cartilage-hair hypoplasia
  5. Idiopathic endocrinopathy
  6. Partial albinism
  7. Thrombocytopenia
  8. Eczema
  9. Tetany

[a] *From Ammann and Wara: Curr Probl Pediatr 5:11, 1975.*

The presence of unusual or opportunistic organisms such as *Pneumocystis carinii, Aspergillus,* or *Serratia marcescens* suggests a diagnosis of primary immunodeficiency. Recurrent infection with microbial agents such as pneumococcus or *Haemophilus influenzae* suggests immunodeficiency disease. Chronic *Candida* infection, especially when resistant to therapy, may indicate the presence of cellular immunodeficiency. A phagocytic defect may be present when children are infected with microbial agents of normally low pathogenicity such as *Staphylococcus albus* or *Serratia marcescens.*

Patients with immunodeficiency disorders may develop infections in unusual locations. Chronic nail or mouth infections with *Candida* or liver abscess or osteomyelitis without an antecedent cause may be the initial manifestation of immunodeficiency. Unusual complications of routine events may be the initial presentation. Frequently children with severe cellular immunodeficiencies develop progressive illness following immunization, and more recently paralytic poliomyelitis and progressive encephalitis have been reported following immunization with attenuated live polio virus.

Abnormal physical findings associated with immunodeficiency disorders may be found in any organ system (details of specific syndromes will be discussed under individual disorders). Patients with immunodeficiencies generally appear chronically ill, pale, and irritable; they may have decreased subcutaneous fat and distended abdomens. Dermatologic manifestations may include chronic eczema, vitiligo, recurrent skin abscesses, and frequent maculopapular rashes. Conjunctivitis is frequently present. *Candida* infections of the mucous membrane and mouth ulcers may be present. Cheilosis is common. Sinopulmonary infection is found early in patients with immunodeficiency, but radiologic changes are not specific. Cervical lymph nodes and tonsils may be absent in spite of recurrent throat infections; alternatively, the lymph nodes may be enlarged or suppurative. Gastrointestinal involvement is frequent in children with immunodeficiency, and diarrhea is a primary symptom. The liver and spleen are frequently enlarged. Joint and bone involvement have been described in a variety of diseases. An arthritis similar to that seen in patients with rheumatoid arthritis has been described in patients with hypogammaglobulinemia. Neurologic abnormalities may include slow development, residual effects of meningitis or encephalitis, or ataxia.

The type of infection may suggest which portion of the immune system might be deficient. Defective antibody immunity is associated with recurrent bacterial infection. Recurrent viral infection may also occur, but it is not usually overwhelming. Abnormalities of cellular immunity are frequently associated with increased susceptibility to viral, fungal, and protozoan infections, with an increased incidence of both malignancy and autoimmune disease. Defective phagocytosis is usually associated with recurrent bacterial infection resulting in chronic lung disease and chronic abscess formation. Recurrent bacterial infection and autoimmune disorders occur with complement deficiencies.

LABORATORY STUDIES

The laboratory studies that will be discussed are organized into two groups: screening tests and tests capable of establishing a definitive diagnosis. Screening tests are readily available and can be obtained through community laboratories. Complex studies are available at most major medical centers. Definitive tests that allow one to establish a specific diagnosis should always include evaluation of two aspects of the immune system: the quantity of cells or cell product that is present and the quality or function of the cell being evaluated.

INITIAL SCREENING EVALUATION (TABLE 4). Antibody-mediated immunity is intact if immunoglobulins (IgG, IgM, and IgA) are quantitatively normal and if specific antibody formation can be documented. Quantitation of serum IgG, IgM, and IgA is performed by radial diffusion in agar with appropriate standards; the accuracy of this method is 10 to 15 percent, and therefore values must be at least two standard deviations from the mean before they can be considered abnormal. The method cannot be used to detect IgE, which is present in small amounts and therefore is detected only by a more sensitive assay such as radioimmunoassay. IgG deficiency should be considered only if values are below 200 mg/dl. Deficiency of IgM and IgA

should not be diagnosed unless values are below 10 mg/dl. Values should always be compared to those for normals of comparable ages (Table 2).

In rare instances patients may have quantitatively normal immunoglobulins that do not function. In order to demonstrate intact antibody-mediated immunity in a patient, the physician must demonstrate both quantitatively normal immunoglobulins and an ability of the

TABLE 4. Initial Screening Evaluation

Antibody-mediated immunity
  Quantitative immunoglobulins: measures IgG, IgM, IgA
  Schick test: measures specific IgG antibody response
  Isohemagglutinin titer (anti-A and anti-B): measures IgM function

Cell-mediated immunity
  White blood cell count with differential: measures total lymphocytes
  Delayed hypersensitivity skin tests: measures specific T cell response to antigens

Phagocytosis
  White blood cell count with differential: measures total neutrophils
  Nitroblue tetrazolium (NBT) dye test: measures neutrophil metabolic function

Complement
  C3 and hemolytic complement quantitation: quantitates complement activity

patient to mount a specific antibody response. Normal infants and children who have been immunized with diphtheria-pertussis-tetanus (DPT) vaccine have adequate levels of antibody against diphtheria toxin. The antibody will neutralize diphtheria toxin, and no reaction will be observed following skin testing with Schick reagent. If the patients have received gamma globulin within 30 days of testing, or if infants still have maternal antibodies (up to 6 months of age), a nonreactive Schick test may falsely indicate the presence of actively synthesized antibody. The presence of isohemagglutinins (greater than 1:4 after 1 year of age) may be used to evalute antibody formation. Isohemagglutinins normally develop by age 1 year as a result of the cross-reaction between polysaccharides of *Escherichia coli* that colonize the gut and red blood cell antigens A and B. The study is not valid in individuals who have received gamma globulin or in infants who still have maternal antibody. The production of other specific antibodies, such as to typhoid or pneumococcus, may be measured if appropriate exposure has been documented or if immunization has been performed. It is important to emphasize that if a patient is suspected of having an immunodeficiency disorder, no live or attenuated virus immunization should be performed in an attempt to document specific antibody production. Cases of paralytic poliomyelitis have been described in immunodeficient infants who have received attenuated polio vaccine. Only highly purified nonreplicating immunizing agents should be used for testing of immunodeficient individuals.

Cellular immunity is usually intact if the total lymphocyte count at any age is greater than 1,200/mm^3 and if a positive delayed hypersensitivity skin test can be demonstrated. The patient with a total lymphocyte count of less than 1,200/mm^3 should be suspected of having defective cell-mediated immunity; however, lymphopenia may also be secondary to immunosuppressive agents, malignancy, autoimmune disease, or viral infection. Although a depressed total lymphocyte count is useful for the screening of both primary and secondary immunodeficiency, the total lymphocyte count may on occasion be normal or even elevated in patients with severe cellular immunodeficiency. In this instance, while lymphocytes are normal in number, they are not necessarily functioning cells.

The application of specific antigens by intradermal injection may result in the expression of competent cell-mediated immunity as evidenced by induration and erythema at the skin test site 24 to 48 hours following the injection. The usual battery of skin tests used in the pediatric population consists of *Candida* (Dermatophytin O), PPD, streptokinase-streptodornase (Varidase diluted to 40 units/ml of streptokinase and 1 unit/ml of streptodornase), mumps antigen, and in selected geographic areas either histoplasmosis or coccidioidomycosis. All antigens are injected intradermally in a volume of 0.1 ml. In order for these tests to be valid, several requirements must be fulfilled. The examiner must be certain of the activity of the antigen. The delayed hypersensitivity skin test should be read at both 24- and 48-hour intervals. Occasionally individuals who have large amounts of circulating antibody may develop an Arthus-like reaction 6 to 8 hours following injection of the antigen; this may be confused with a delayed hypersensitivity reaction. Skin tests are of value only when previous exposure to the antigen can be documented. A negative skin test may mean either lack of appropriate exposure or lack of normal immunity. In spite of the above precautions, a positive delayed hypersensitivity skin test provides extremely useful information about specific immunity.

The presence of a thymic shadow on a chest radiograph of a newborn infant makes the diagnosis of defective cellular immunity highly unlikely. The procedure in older children is less useful, as the thymus is difficult to visualize beyond 1 year of age. The thymus may become significantly reduced in size if the individual has undergone severe stress, and it may not be visualized on either anteroposterior or lateral views of the chest even during the newborn period.

Screening tests for a phagocytic disorder of the granulocytes include the total leukocyte count, the differential count, and the morphologic appearance of the cells. Neutropenia is significant when the neutrophil count (percentage of neutrophils times total white blood cell count) is less than 1,200/mm^3; if neutropenia persists it should be further investigated by bone marrow aspiration. Occasionally the total neutrophil count may be suppressed as a result of severe infection such as staphylococcal septicemia. Neutropenia is seen following viral infection, but is more frequently a result of drug reactions or the use of immunosuppressive agents. In the neonatal period neutropenia may be the result of autoantibody or isoantibody that has been transferred placentally from the maternal circulation; in this case the antibody is formed against the infant's white blood cells, which then are destroyed. The rare Chediak-Higashi syndrome can be diagnosed when giant granules are observed in the cytoplasm of peripheral blood leukocytes seen on routine Wright stain smears. Absence of the spleen is suggested by the finding of Howell-Jolly bodies in peripheral red blood cells and should be suspected if a patient has repeated episodes of sepsis that are otherwise unexplained.

The most common immunodeficiency involving phagocytosis is chronic granulomatous disease (CGD). A normal nitroblue tetrazolium test (NBT) essentially excludes this diagnosis. NBT is normally a colorless compound that is reduced by metabolically activated neutrophils to a dark blue insoluble substance. Neutrophils containing reduced NBT (blue compound) are termed NBT-positive cells. More than 6 percent of neutrophils are spontaneously NBT-postive cells. A much higher percentage of neutrophils are NBT-positive when they are obtained from patients with active bacterial infection or when the test is performed following the exposure of the patient's leukocytes to solid particles or endotoxin along with the dye in vitro; stimulation of neutrophil metabolism results in more than 60 percent of the cells becoming NBT-positive. In patients with CGD the neutrophils remain NBT-negative.

Complement and opsonic function should be evaluated in patients with recurrent infections in which antibody, cellular, and phagocytic immunity are normal. Screening tests include the assay of the third component of complement (C3) and the total hemolytic complement activity (CH$_{50}$). C3 is present in the serum in the largest quantity of any of the components; it can easily be measured by single radial diffusion and generally reflects the total complement activity. Total serum complement activity is best assessed by measurement of CH$_{50}$; this is performed by evaluating the degree of hemolysis of sheep erythrocytes by antibody when test serum is used as a complement source. Since there is a wide range of normal values for this test, each laboratory must establish its own normal levels. Decreased CH$_{50}$ may represent decreased production of any of the complement components, increased catabolism of any of the complement components, or utilization of complement in immune-complex disease.

DEFINITIVE EVALUATION OF ANTIBODY-MEDIATED IMMUNITY. If screening tests indicate that a patient may have deficient antibody-mediated immunity, several tests are available for further evaluation of this system (Table 5). Although myelomas are extremely rare in children, if a patient has selective elevation of a single immunoglobulin class, protein electrophoresis may be of benefit in detecting "M proteins."

If the diagnosis of hypogammaglobulinemia is established by total quantitative immunoglobulins (igG, igM, and igA) of less than 250 mg/dl, quantitation of peripheral blood B lymphocytes may be helpful in differentiating congenital from acquired disease. Lymphocytes in the peripheral blood may be identified specifically as B cells by the presence of immunoglobulin receptors on their surface. This test utilizing immunofluorescence

TABLE 5. Evaluation of Antibody-Mediated Immunity

Test	Comment
Protein electrophoresis	Use only to diagnose hypogammaglobulinemia or to evaluate for an M protein
Immunoglobulin quantitation	Best procedure for quantitation of IgG, IgM, IgA, and IgD
Radioimmunoassay	IgE quantitation; not generally available
Schick test	DPT immunization must be complete; use to evaluate IgG function
Isohemagglutinins	Use to evaluate IgM function; titer > 1:4 after 1 year of age
Specific antibody response	Use to evaluate immunoglobulin function; tetanus, diphtheria, typhoid, etc; do not immunize with live virus if immunodeficiency is suspected
B cell quantitation	Measurement of number of circulating B cells; normal is 20 to 30 percent

is available in specialized laboratories. Patients with acquired hypogammaglobulinemia usually have normal numbers of peripheral blood lymphocytes that stain for immunoglobulins; in congenital hypogammaglobulinemia there are no cells that stain for immunoglobulin. It was previously thought that biopsies were of value in patients with immunodeficiencies, especially if the diagnosis was equivocal. However, present laboratory technology is sufficiently sophisticated to provide the information necessary for specific diagnosis and avoid the necessity of biopsy.

DEFINITIVE EVALUATION OF CELL-MEDIATED IMMUNITY.   If screening studies indicate that cellular immunodeficiency may be present, additional quantitation of circulating T lymphocytes and evaluation of their function should be obtained (Table 6). Because approximately 70 percent of the circulating blood lymphocytes are T cells, the total lymphocyte count represents primarily T cells rather than B cells.

However, specific quantitation of T cells may be performed in vitro. Thymus-derived lymphocytes have the special property of permitting the in vitro binding of sheep erythrocytes to their surface membranes; they are then termed T cell rosettes. T cell rosettes do not measure a particular function of thymus derived cells but merely indicate their quantitative presence. Severely depressed levels of T cell rosettes (less than 20 percent) are seen in cellular immunodeficiency disorders. Depression of T cell rosettes has also been reported in patients with acute and chronic viral infections, malignancy, and autoimmune disease. Elevated levels of T cell rosettes have been described in patients with infectious mononucleosis.

The function of peripheral blood lymphocytes can be evaluated in vitro by isolating the patients's lymphocytes and exposing them in culture to a variety of mitogens, specific antigens, and foreign cells. Animal and human studies indicate that phytohemagglutinin (PHA) is a specific mitogen for thymus-derived lymphocytes and tests the effector function of lymphocytes by measuring their ability to transform into blast cells. Defective lymphocyte transformation is usually seen in

TABLE 6. Evaluation of Cell-Mediated Immunity

Test	Comment
Total lymphocyte count	Normal at any age > 1,200/mm³
Delayed hypersensitivity test	Use to evaluate specific immunity to antigens; suggest *Candida*, mumps, PPD, and SKSD (streptokinase-streptodornase 4 µg/0.1 ml)
Lymphocyte response to mitogens, (PHA), antigens, and allogeneic cells (MLC)	Use to evaluate T cell function; results expressed as stimulated counts divided by resting counts, equals stimulation index
T cell rosettes	Use to quantitate the number of circulating T cells; normal > 60 percent
Migration-inhibition factor	Use to evaluate lymphokine released from sensitized lymphocytes, which causes inhibition of macrophage migration

severe forms of cellular immunodeficiency disease. Chronic or debilitating disease may result in depressed lymphocyte transformation, but absent transformation is usually seen only in congenital cellular immunodeficiency. Increased lymphocyte transformation has been observed in patients who have received multiple blood transfusions, in some normal newborns, and in allergic individuals. Their cells may be "turned on" by foreign antigen stimulation in vivo.

In addition to the stimulation of isolated peripheral blood lymphocytes by PHA, lymphocytes can be stimulated by a specific antigen to which they have been previously exposed. This study appears to be more sensitive than delayed hypersensitivity skin tests in determining previous exposure and normal reactivity to an antigen. Thus a patient who is suspected of having normal cellular immunity to a particular antigen but who has a negative delayed hypersensitivity skin test to that antigen may demonstrate blast transformation of lymphocytes when they are exposed in vitro to an antigen such as *Candida.*

The ability of lymphocytes to recognize foreign cells can be tested in lymphocyte culture by mixing the patient's lymphocytes with foreign lymphocytes. Peripheral blood lymphocytes are isolated both from the patient and from a histoincompatible (immunologically nonidentical) donor. The histoincompatible cells act as a stimulus to cause normal thymus-derived lymphocytes to divide. Because both patient and donor cells are mixed together in the same test tube, division of the donor cells must be blocked. This is accomplished by treating the donor lymphocytes with either mitomycin C or irradiation.

In all instances—stimulation of isolated lymphocytes by mitogen (PHA), foreign antigen, or histoincompatible lymphocytes—the ability of the patient's cells to respond is measured by the uptake of radioactively labeled material following a suitable incubation time. The uptake of radioactive material by the patient's stimulated cells is compared to the uptake of radioactive material by the patient's nonstimulated cells; the two numbers are divided and a stimulation index is obtained. Because of variations between laboratories, normal values for each of these studies must be obtained from each laboratory

T cells, following exposure to specific antigens or mitogens, have the capacity to release lymphokines that may act in a specific manner or may recruit other mediators of immunity. Migration-inhibition factor (MIF) has been partially characterized and is known to be released in vitro following exposure of sensitized lymphocytes to antigens. MIF prevents the migration of macrophages from an area surrounding lymphocytes in the presence of antigen. MIF is felt to correlate with delayed hypersensitivity and lymphocyte stimulation by specific antigen.

In the past, rate of skin graft rejection was utilized to evaluate delayed hypersensitivity. However, because of its complexity, because of the fact that it frequently results in intense sensitization to histocompatibility antigens, and because of the increased sophistication of laboratory tests, the evaluation of skin graft rejection is rarely necessary at the present time.

DEFINITIVE EVALUATION OF PHAGOCYTOSIS. If screening tests for defective phagocytosis indicate a possible abnormality, further evaluation is indicated (Table 7). When a patient is suspected of having either chronic granulomatous disease or a killing defect for a particular organism, bacterial and fungal killing curves may be performed in specialized laboratories. The test is performed by incubating the patient's peripheral leukocytes with a predetermined number of organisms; optimally the patient's cells are incubated with an organism with which he has been infected previously. The intracellular killing of these organisms by the patient's cells is compared to the killing of organisms by cells obtained from a normal individual. Patients with chronic granulomatous disease may fail to kill the ingested organisms or may kill them more slowly than normal.

TABLE 7. Evaluation of Phagocytosis

Test	Comment
Quantitative nitroblue tetrazolium (NBT)	Use for diagnosis of chronic granulomatous disease and for detection of carrier state
Quantitative killing curve	Use for diagnosis of chronic granulomatous disease; can be performed using organisms isolated from individual
Chemotaxis	Abnormal in a variety of disorders associated with frequent bacterial infection; does not provide a specific diagnosis; performed using a Boyden chamber utilizing a microscopic or radioactive technique; Rebuck window provides a qualitative result
Random migration	Abnormal in lazy leukocyte syndrome; tests nonchemotactic migration of leukocytes
Cotton-wool, glass-wool adherence	Abnormal in several disorders associated with recurrent bacterial infection; does not provide a specific diagnosis

Chemotaxis is the specific migration of phagocytic cells toward an agent. Migration can be measured in several manners. The skin window technique (Rebuck) is a relatively simple procedure that measures leukocyte mobility and provides qualitative information. The skin is abraded, a glass cover slip is placed over the abraded area for varying periods of time, and the numbers and types of cells that migrate into the area and adhere to the glass cover slip are then determined. Recently the Boyden chamber has been utilized to measure cellular chemotaxis. Phagocytic cells are placed on one side of a Millipore filter and a chemotactic source on the other; the number of cells that migrate through the filter toward the source is then determined. The random migration of cells can be evaluated by placing the buffy coat (white blood cells) of the peripheral blood in an upright capillary tube and measuring the distance of random migration over a specific time. The ability of peripheral leukocytes to adhere to cotton-wool or glass-wool columns has also been used to detect defects in phagocytosis. Disorders detected by these methods appear to be rare, and the clinical usefulness of these tests has not been fully determined.

DEFINITIVE EVALUATION OF COMPLEMENT. If either C3 or hemolytic complement is abnormal and a patient is suspected of having a complement deficiency, individual complement components can be measured by specialized laboratories (Table 8). C5 dysfunction, which is a disorder associated

TABLE 8. Evaluation of Complement

Test	Comment
C1q, C1r, C1s	Deficient in disorders associated with recurrent bacterial infection and autoimmunelike disease
C3	Decreased in specific disorders associated with recurrent bacterial infection
C4	Decreased in disorders associated with immune-complex formation (eg, SLE); also decreased in hereditary angioneurotic edema
C5	Associated with Leiner's disease; present in normal amounts but functionally abnormal

with recurrent infections, resembles Leiner's disease. Patients with this disorder have normal levels of C5, but C5 functions abnormally. Assay for C5 dysfunction is performed only in specialized laboratories.

DISORDERS OF ANTIBODY-MEDIATED IMMUNITY

Hypogammaglobulinemia

Hypogammaglobulinemia is present when the total immunoglobulins are less than 250 mg/dl (IgG is usually less than 200 mg/dl). Major aspects of cellular immunity are intact in patients with uncomplicated hypogammaglobulinemia. Four major groups of hypogammaglobulienmia exist: congenital, acquired, transient, and secondary.

PATHOGENESIS. The bursa of Fabricius is an organ associated with the gastrointestinal tract in the avian species and has been shown to be necessary for immunoglobulin production. In patients with congenital hypogammaglobulinemia it is thought that stem cells have not come under the influence of the mammalian equivalent of the bursa. The bursa equivalent has not been definitely identified in man, but it may be either

the microenvironment of the bone marrow or certain tissues associated with the gastrointestinal tract, such as the appendix, tonsils, and adenoids. Patients with congenital hypogammaglobulinemia usually lack plasma cells in the tissue and identifiable B cells in the peripheral blood. Patients with transient or acquired hypogammaglobulinemia may have normal numbers of circulating B cells, thus suggesting that congenital hypogammaglobulinemia results from an absence of B cells, while acquired hypogammaglobulinemia results from a failure of B cells to synthesize and/or release immunoglobulins. Recently it has been shown that certain patients with acquired hypogammaglobulinemia have suppressor cells that are capable of turning off in vitro production by normal cells.

Transient hypogammaglobulinemia may be a result of delayed production of immunoglobulin; it is an extension of the normal physiologic hypogammaglobulinemia that occurs in all infants. There is some evidence that transient hypogammaglobulinemia may be related to maternal isoimmunization against fetal immunoglobulin antigens in a manner analogous to Rh immunization.

Secondary hypogammaglobulinemia is most frequent in protein-losing states such as the nephrotic syndrome and protein-losing enteropathy. In both of these disorders the serum albumin is always reduced first.

CLINICAL MANIFESTATIONS. The age at onset of clinical symptoms in infants with congenital hypogammaglobulinemia is related to a number of variables: levels of passively transferred maternal immunoglobulin, exposure to microbial agents, antibiotic treatment of infections, and availability of medical care. Infants with congenital hypogammaglobulinemia usually become symptomatic at about 5 months of age, when passively transferred immunoglobulins are at the lowest level; however, serious infection does not necessarily follow. If treatment of infection is prompt or if exposure to microbial agents is minimal, then increased numbers of infections or significant infection may not occur for months or even years.

Infants with transient hypogammaglobulinemia may present with a clinical picture identical to that of congenital hypogammaglobulinemia but improve spontaneously in a period of 3 to 4 months, while infants with congenital hypogammaglobulinemia remain symptomatic until specific therapy is instituted.

Patients with any form of hypogammaglobulinemia experience recurrent and/or severe infections with certain organisms such as pneumococcus and *Haemophilus influenzae*. Recurrent otitis media, pneumonia, and meningitis are the most common infections, and frequently they fail to respond to standard treatment. Patients do not have intervals of clinical well-being between episodes of acute infection. Occasionally, even with appropriate therapy, chronic otitis media or chronic lung disease develop. In some instances the initial symptoms in acquired hypogammaglobulinemia are related to malabsorption rather than infection; the patient may develop a celiac-like syndrome with severe diarrhea and weight loss. The parasite *Giardia lamblia* frequently causes malabsorption. Other symptoms develop after long-standing hypogammaglobulinemia: abnormal dental decay, dental abscesses, conjunctivitis, recurrent skin infection, and eczematoid skin lesions. A picture like that of rheumatoid arthritis has been described in patients with hypogammaglobulinemia; it may appear in both untreated and treated patients or in patients receiving inadequate amounts of gamma globulin.

DIAGNOSIS. Hypogammaglobulinemia may be diagnosed when total serum immunoglobulins are at a level of less than 250 mg/dl (IgG is usually less than 200 mg/dl). Usually all five classes of immunoglobulins are diminished. Although protein electrophoresis may be used to establish a diagnosis, specific immunoglobulin quantitation is recommended in all cases, as exact values are frequently necessary to differentiate the various forms of hypogammaglobulinemia and to follow the course of the patient. A diagnosis of congenital hypogammaglobulinemia cannot be made with certainty until a child is older than 18 months. At 18 months an infant with transient hypogammaglobulinemia will usually spontaneously begin to produce immunoglobulins. The presence of low levels of IgG (less than 200 mg/dl) in association with significant levels of IgM and IgA (greater than 20 mg/dl) makes the diagnosis of congenital hypogammaglobulinemia less likely than that of transient hypogammaglobulinemia. Immunoglobulin values should be repeated at 3-month intervals until the patient is older than 18 months. If IgG, IgM, and/or IgA values are increasing, then transient hypogammaglobulinemia is a likely diagnosis. If the patient is receiving gamma globulin therapy, then IgM and IgA levels may be followed sequentially, as commercial gamma globulin does not contain significant amounts of these immunoglobulins. In patients with significant recurrent infections, one should not hesitate to repeat immunoglobulin quantitation at 6-month intervals if initial values are at borderline low levels. Occasionally patients with acquired hypogammaglobulinemia become symptomatic prior to developing abnormal immunoglobulin values; repeat measurement 3 to 6 months later usually establishes the diagnosis. Patients with secondary hypogammaglobulinemia may have low IgG values, but they also tend to have normal values of the high-molecular-weight immunoglobulins, particularly IgM. Serum albumin levels are useful in differentiating secondary hypogammaglobulinemia due to a protein loss, as a decrease in serum albumin precedes the decrease in immunoglobulins in both the nephrotic syndrome and in protein-losing enteropathy. Difficulty in diagnosis may be encountered in patients with congenital or acquired hypogammaglobulinemia who develop severe diarrhea and malabsorption.

Immunoglobulin values alone are usually sufficient to establish a diagnosis of hypogammaglobulinemia. However, if values are borderline low, or if transient hypogammaglobulinemia is suspected, documentation of the lack of specific antibody response following immunization may be necessary. In the past the Schick test, following DPT immunization, was utilized, but Schick test material is no longer readily available. A patient suspected of having an immunodeficiency disorder should not be immunized with live viral agents for diagnosis or for therapy. The antibody response is therefore best quantitated following immunization with killed agents such as tetanus and diphtheria.

Patients with the various forms of hypogammaglobulinemia generally have intact cell-mediated immunity. As patients become older they may acquire defects in cell-mediated immunity. This is seen more frequently in individuals with adult variable-onset hypogammaglobulinemia than in patients with congenital hypogammaglobulinemia.

Patients with hypogammaglobulinemia should be evaluated for associated disorders. *Giardia lamblia* is frequently the cause of malabsorption; the diagnosis of *Giardia* is best made by appropriate pathologic stains of specimens from the upper gastrointestinal tract obtained by biopsy. Other causes of malabsorption such as lactose intolerance or celiac disease may be diagnosed by appropriate tolerance tests. Sequential pulmonary function studies are important in assessing the adequacy of treatment in controlling chronic lung disease.

Immunoglobulin values should be obtained in all family members. Occasionally hypogammaglobulinemia or selective IgA deficiency may be found in relatively asymptomatic individuals.

TREATMENT. Gamma globulin treatment provides adequate replacement therapy to prevent life-threatening illness. Commercial gamma globulin contains primarily IgG, with only trace amounts of IgA and IgM. Small amounts of IgD and IgE are also present. The specific antibody activity of gamma globulin preparations varies from donor to donor. Gamma globulin pooled from multiple donors is highly effective in preventing the majority of common infections. Various regimens have been devised for the use of gamma globulin in treating hypogammaglobulinemia. Our preference is to begin with a dose of 0.2 ml/kg as a single intramuscular injection. Following this starting dose the amount of gamma globulin administered should be governed by two factors: the quantity that can be tolerated by the patient and the dose necessary to control infection. Initially a single monthly injection is usually sufficient and will result in the prevention of systemic infections such as pneumonia, meningitis, and otitis media. A gradual increase in dose by 1 to 2 ml per injection per month may be necessary if the initial dose is not effective. If the intramuscular injection of gamma globulin on a monthly basis becomes uncomfortable for the patient, or if additional gamma globulin therapy is necessary, the total dose can be divided into two equal injections given at the same time. Additional increases can be accomplished by administering the gammaglobulin at biweekly or weekly intervals without decreasing the efficacy of therapy. Rarely, anaphylactoid reactions occur following gamma globulin injection. These are not true allergic reactions, but usually result from the formation of aggregates in the gamma globulin preparation with subsequent systemic distribution.

The aggregates and reaction can be eliminated by ultracentrifugation of the gamma globulin prior to administration. Alternatively, a different gamma globulin preparation may be used.

If the maximum amounts of gamma globulin do not adequately control recurrent infection, regular intravenous infusion of fresh frozen plasma may be added to the treatment regimen. One unit of fresh frozen plasma may be administered monthly between the ages of 1.5 and 14 years. Patients older than 14 years may be given two units monthly. Under 1.5 years of age, 10 ml/kg is an adequate dose. Fresh frozen plasma and gamma globulin can be given on a monthly basis, with each administered at alternate 2-week intervals. Although fresh frozen plasma contains significant amounts of IgM and IgA, whereas gamma globulin contains only trace amounts, the short half-life of both IgM and IgA results in an insignificant increase in their levels in serum following the plasma infusion. Nevertheless, significant benefit may be achieved by the addition of fresh frozen plasma in a patient who is not completely controlled by gamma globulin alone.

Selected antibiotics used on an intermittent or continuous basis may improve control of infection. Broad-spectrum antibiotics are most useful, especially those that are effective against *Haemophilus influenzae* and pneumococcus. In spite of adequate replacement therapy with gamma globulin and plasma and maximum use of antibiotics, chronic pulmonary disease may appear. The use of pulmonary physical therapy should be taught to parents and used intensively during acute respiratory infections. Continuous physical therapy is necessary once chronic lung disease develops. Chronic otitis media may be associated with subsequent hearing loss.

PROGNOSIS. Patients with uncomplicated hypogammaglobulinemia can survive to the third or fourth decade without serious physical handicap. Chronic lung disease appears to develop in some patients despite what appears to be adequate gamma globulin therapy. The addition of fresh frozen plasma and antibiotic therapy may decrease the number of individuals developing this complication, but long-term studies are not yet available. Patients with hypogammaglobulinemia have an increased incidence of malignancy, although it is not as great as in patients with ataxia-telangiectasia or the Wiskott-Aldrich syndrome. Patients with adult variable-onset hypogammaglobulinemia may develop a thymoma and should have yearly chest radiographs as part of their regular evaluations.

Selective IgA Deficiency

Patients with selective IgA deficiency have less than 5 mg/dl of serum IgA and normal or increased levels of other immunoglobulins. The majority have absent secretory IgA. Cell-mediated immunity is usually intact.

PATHOGENESIS. The disorder occurs as frequently as 1 in 400 individuals and appears to be inherited as an autosomal recessive or dominant. All studies to date indicate that patients with selective IgA deficiency have some IgA in the serum, although the amounts detected may be quite small. The majority have absence of IgA in the secretions, with normal amounts of secretory or transport piece; rarely, they may have normal levels of IgA in the secretions. Others may have increased amounts of low-molecular-weight IgM. These observations may explain some of the variability in clinical symptoms seen in these patients. Usually there are normal numbers of peripheral blood lymphocytes bearing IgA receptors, which suggests that selective deficiency may be a result of an absence of secretion of IgA by B cells. Cell-mediated immunity is usually intact.

CLINICAL MANIFESTATIONS. Patients with selective IgA deficiency have an increased incidence of allergy, sinopulmonary infection, gastrointestinal tract disease, and autoimmune disease. The age of onset of symptoms may vary considerably and may be related to compensatory mechanisms and/or environmental factors.

DIAGNOSIS. The diagnosis of selective IgA deficiency can be made by quantitation of immunoglobulins. Less than 5 mg/dl of serum IgA is found in most patients; 98 percent of patients also have absent salivary IgA. In the serum, IgA and IgM may be elevated; IgE is usually normal. Selective IgA deficiency is frequently associated with other abnormalities such as the presence of low-molecular-weight IgM (7S) and abnormal ratios of immunoglobulin light chains. Autoantibody and antibody to bovine milk are found with an increased frequency. As the patients lack serum IgA, they are capable of making antibodies against IgA, and some of these individuals have experienced anaphylactic reactions following the infusion of blood products containing IgA. Antibodies against IgG (rheumatoid factor) and IgM may also be present. Recently some patients with selective IgA deficiency have been found to have depressed T cell interferon production. This may be an additional variable determining susceptibility to infection.

Other disorders associated with IgA deficiency and depressed cell-mediated immunity should be excluded when evaluating a patient found to have absent IgA. One such disorder is ataxia-telangiectasia, an immunodeficiency disorder associated with more severe clinical and laboratory abnormalities.

TREATMENT. Gamma globulin should not be used for treatment of patients with selective IgA deficiency, as they are capable of making normal antibodies in other immunoglobulin classes. These patients may form anti-IgA following exposure to IgA contained in gamma globulin. They then become susceptible to an anaphylactic reaction following blood transfusion. There appears to be a decrease in the number and severity of sinopulmonary infections in some patients who are treated with broad-spectrum antibiotics at the onset of respiratory illness. Patients with selective IgA deficiency should be followed closely for the development of autoimmune disease. Associated diseases, such as celiac disease or asthma, should be treated in the same manner as in individuals with normal IgA. If patients require blood, only packed washed red blood cells should be used. Some blood banks have available IgA-deficient donors who can be used for cross-matching with IgA-deficient recipients; the possibility of an anaphylactic reaction following blood transfusion is then avoided.

PROGNOSIS.   Long-term survival to the fifth and sixth decade has been described. Recurrent sinopulmonary infection may diminish with age. Generally, the prognosis for patients with selective IgA deficiency, unassociated with any other disorder, appears to be good.

SELECTIVE IGM DEFICIENCY.   Selective IgM deficiency is a rare disorder associated with absent (less than 5 mg/dl) IgM, normal levels of other immunoglobulins, and normal cell-mediated immunity.

PATHOGENESIS.   Patients with selective IgM deficiency have not been studied in sufficient detail to allow speculation concerning possible etiologies.

DIAGNOSIS.   Quantitative immunoglobulins, with levels of IgM of less than 5 mg/dl, establish the diagnosis. Other immunoglobulins and studies of cell-mediated immunity are usually normal. Immunodeficiency disorders associated with depressed levels of IgM and abnormalities of cell-mediated immunity should be excluded, eg, Wiskott-Aldrich syndrome.

CLINICAL FEATURES.   Patients with selective IgM deficiency have a marked susceptibility to infection with polysaccharide-containing organisms such as pneumococcus and *Haemophilus influenzae.* The clinical course is similar to that of infants who have been splenectomized.

TREATMENT.   Too few patients have been evaluated to provide definitive conclusions regarding treatment. However, it would appear appropriate, in view of the peculiar susceptibility of these patients to certain bacteria, to treat them with ampicillin; this could be given on a continuous basis or, as in patients following splenectomy, instituted at the time of any acute illness.

PROGNOSIS.   The prognosis appears to be extremely variable. Individual case reports indicate that overwhelming infection from polysaccharide-containing organisms is a frequent cause of death.

CELLULAR IMMUNODEFICIENCY DISORDERS

Severe Combined Immunodeficiency Disease

Severe combined immunodeficiency disease (SCID) is characterized by complete absence of both antibody-mediated and cell-mediated immunity. The term severe is used to distinguish this form of immunodeficiency from other syndromes in which partial defects in both antibody-mediated and cell-mediated immunity are present; these latter disorders are termed combined immunodeficiency. Older usage employed the terms Swiss-type lymphopenic agammaglobulinemia and sex-linked lymphopenic agammaglobulinemia to describe this disorder. The terms autosomal or sex-linked are used to differentiate the two forms of inheritance.

PATHOGENESIS.   Two alternative concepts may explain the dual system abnormality found in SCID. The most popular theory attributes the combined immunodeficiency to a defective stem cell population. The absence of an appropriately dividing stem cell would result in a lack of cells capable of migrating to the thymus and bursa equivalent. The lack of lymphoid tissue and the thymic aplasia found in these patients would therefore be secondary to an absent migration of stem cells to the appropriate organ capable of modifying stem cells into immunocompetent T and B cells. Support for this concept was obtained following the successful reconstitution of both T and B cells with a bone marrow transplantation in a patient with SCID; following this, the appearance of a thymus gland as demonstrated radiologically and normal architectural appearance of lymphoid tissue were described.

An alternative theory suggests that the defect lies primarily in the organs responsible for the development of competent T and B cells. Stem cells may be present, but cannot develop into immunocompetent cells without the presence of a normal thymus and bursa equivalent. Under these circumstances it is postulated that a bone marrow transplant is successful because it provides a source of immunocompetent T and B cells that have already been acted upon by the thymus and bursa equivalent of the donor.

With discovery of certain enzyme deficiencies associated with combined immunodeficiency disease, it is possible that the basic defect in some patients with SCID might also be related to an enzymatic abnormality as yet undiscovered (p. 315).

CLINICAL FEATURES.   Infants with SCID usually become ill early in life and succumb to overwhelming infection before 1 year of age. These patients are susceptible to a wide variety of infections caused by viruses, bacteria, fungi, or protozoa. Because maternal antibody is insufficient to completely protect these infants, they usually become symptomatic within the first 3 months of life. Viral infections may be acquired naturally or may occur as a result of immunization with attenuated viral vaccines; cytomegalovirus is a frequent cause of pneumonia. Following oral polio immunization, polio virus may be cultured from the stool for a period of months. Several patients have succumbed from progressive polio virus infection of the central nervous system following immunization; others have died with disseminated vaccinia following smallpox immunization.

A variety of severe bacterial infections may occur. The administration of gamma globulin will protect against infection by certain organisms, but not others. Thus an infant may be protected against pneumococcus and *Haemophilus influenzae* but remain susceptible to infection with gram-negative organisms such as *Pseudomonas* and *Escherichia coli,* which are frequent causes of death.

Of the fungal infections, chronic *Candida* appears to occur most often; extensive oral involvement may result in esophageal erosions and/or vocal cord involvement manifested by a hoarse voice. Chronic diarrhea may also result from intestinal mucosal involvement.

Pneumocystis carinii is the most common protozoan infection and causes progressive pneumonitis. The infection may be present for months, producing only low-grade fever and chronic cough. Rapid acceleration may occur at any time, resulting in more typical manifestations of the disease, including cyanosis, rapid respirations, and a normal-sounding chest with a severely abnormal chest radiograph. Although various diagnostic measures have been used to make an early diagnosis of *P. carinii* pneumonia, an open lung biopsy is usually necessary. Prompt institution of therapy is necessary if the infant is to survive.

Patients with SCID are totally lacking in cell-mediated immunity and thus are susceptible to the graft-versus-host reaction (p. 322). This may appear following the infusion of any blood product containing viable lymphocytes. Since the initial signs and symptoms appear 7 to 20 days after the infusion, a diagnosis is not always made. Initial clinical findings may mimic a viral infection and include skin rash, hepatosplenomegaly, and fever. In addition, the presence of a graft-versus-host reaction increases the susceptibility of the infant to infection, and the infant may succumb to overwhelming disease before a diagnosis is established. It is sometimes difficult to evaluate infants with SCID who have an established maternal–fetal graft-versus-host reaction, as chronic changes may mimic other conditions such as Letterer-Siwe disease or acrodermatitis enteropathica.

DIAGNOSIS. An early diagnosis of SCID is necessary if the infant is to survive until definitive therapy can be instituted. Defective cell-mediated immunity can be diagnosed at the time of birth if the disorder is suspected, eg, from a positive family history. Although lymphopenia is frequently present, it is not always found and therefore cannot be relied upon as a screening procedure. A diagnosis of defective cell-mediated immunity is established by demonstrating decreased numbers of T lymphocytes (usually less than 10 percent T cell rosettes) and lack of in vitro lymphocyte response to mitogens and to allogeneic cells in mixed lymphocyte culture. These defects persist throughout the life of the infant.

Documentation of defective antibody-mediated immunity during infancy is difficult. Normal infants have only small amounts of serum IgM and IgA, and the presence of normal amounts of IgG is merely an indication of placental passage of IgG. Active immunization of an infant suspected of having SCID can be performed; however, it has recently been appreciated that many normal infants fail to respond to a variety of antigens. On occasion an indirect approach to the evaluation of antibody-mediated immunity may be utilized. Most infants with the capability of snythesizing antibodies will respond to chronic or recurrent infections by producing significant amounts of IgM and IgA early in life. An infant who has experienced chronic infection but who lacks IgM and IgA probably has hypogammaglobulinemia. Because of these diagnostic difficulties, however, absence of antibody-mediated immunity cannot be documented with certainty until the infant reaches the age of about 5 months.

Additional studies may assist in establishing a diagnosis. Bone marrow aspiration may reveal the absence of plasma cells. Lymph node biopsy usually reveals hypocellularity, absence of germinal centers, and lack of corticomedullary differentiation. Rectal biopsy usually shows a lack of lymphoid tissue and absence of plasma cells. Skin tests for delayed hypersensitivity are of value in older children, but may be negative in normal infants and therefore are of little assistance in the documentation of deficient cell-mediated immunity during infancy. Skin grafts are not recommended, as they may sensitize the individual to histocompatibility antigens.

TREATMENT. Treatment of the underlying antibody and ceullular immunodeficiency is best accomplished utilizing histocompatible bone marrow transplantation. Because of the genetics of histocompatibility antigens, donors are best found among the siblings of the patient. The general requirement for a compatible donor for bone marrow transplantation is identity at all four HLA loci and nonreactivity of the donor against the recipient in mixed lymphocyte culture. Recently it has been found that successful bone marrow transplantation can be performed between HLA-nonidentical individuals who are identical at the mixed lymphocyte culture (MLC) locus. However, this is very rare, and only a few successful transplantations have been performed in HLA-nonidentical individuals. Once a compatible donor has been obtained, the technique of bone marrow transplantation is relatively easy. Two methods have been utilized: intravenous infusion of filtered bone marrow and intraperitoneal injection. There are advocates for each procedure, and both appear to be successful. In spite of careful matching at the HLA and MLC loci, most patients experience a mild graft-versus-host reaction following transplantation. The patient who received the first successful bone marrow transplant has now survived 10 years following the initial therapy, and more than 40 successful transplantations have been performed since that time.

In the absence of a compatible donor for bone marrow transplantation, there is no completely satisfactory approach to therapy. Transplantation of fetal tissue has had limited success. Several patients have survived fetal liver transplantations for prolonged periods of time; others have received transplantations of fetal thymus, and there are at least two long-term survivors (more than 3 years). Fetal thymus transplantation has resulted in T cell reconstitution without any evidence of B cell immunity. The patients are treated with gamma globulin to provide passive antibody. Another approach to therapy has involved maintenance of the patient in a sterile atmosphere for prolonged periods of time. This is of little value in patients who already have experienced recurrent infections.

When administering any blood product containing potentially viable lymphocytes, irradiation of the blood product with 3,000 to 6,000 rad is suggested, as this will eliminate all viable cells and avoid the complication of graft-versus-host reaction. Once a graft-versus-host reaction has become established, no currently utilized program has been effective in eliminating the reaction. Steroids and immunosuppressive agents, as well as antilymphocyte globulin, have been used; but a continuous downhill course usually occurs, and the patient may expire from complications of the graft-versus-host reaction, such as infection.

PROGNOSIS. In the absence of a histocompatible bone marrow transplant, the prognosis for patients with SCID is extremely poor. The majority of patients die before the age of 1 year from chronic or acute infection; a few have survived beyond 3 years. One of these has been kept in a germ-free environment, and two others have received fetal thymus transplants.

Cellular Immunodeficiency with Abnormal Immunoglobulin Synthesis (Nezelof Syndrome)

Nezelof syndrome is a primary immunodeficiency disease characterized by varying degrees of cellular immunodeficiency and normal or nearly normal immunoglobulin levels, with absent or minimal specific antibody production. This disorder affects both males and females.

PATHOGENESIS. A genetic basis for this disorder, with an autosomal recessive inheritance pattern, is suggested by the occurrence of the disease in both male and female siblings. However, patients without positive family histories have been described. The inclusion of a variety of immunodeficiency disorders in this category may be somewhat arbitrary. Since patients have abnormalities of both antibody-mediated and cell-mediated immunity, they have combined immunodeficiency. Many earlier reports of so-called Nezelof syndrome have lacked adequate studies of cell-mediated immunity; it is not certain that all cases were identical.

Several alternative explanations exist for the pathogenesis of this syndrome. It is possible that a defective stem cell would result in the absence of both cellular and antibody-mediated immunity. However, it is more likely that the thymus gland is abnormal and does not allow for maturation of T lymphocytes. The ability of fetal thymus transplants to reconstitute the immune function in some patients argues for the latter possibility. It appears that prior to reconstitution the deficient cell-mediated immunity results in diminished or absent T–B cell cooperation, which is necessary for the production of specific antibody. In addition the preservation of the plasma cell series argues for an intact B cell system and therefore an intact stem cell system. Recent evidence that a thymic humoral factor, thymosin, is capable of reconstituting cell-mediated immunity to varying degrees in different patients suggests that the thymic defect in some patients may be a lack of production or secretion of thymic humoral factors.

Since the age of onset both of documented cellular immunodeficiency and of clinical manifestations varies from infancy to as late as 3 to 4 years, and since the response to specific therapy such as fetal thymus transplantation varies among patients, it is most likely that the diagnosis of Nezelof syndrome contains within it a variety of disorders yet to be defined. The late onset of severe recurrent infection in a subgroup of these patients and the documentation that cellular immune

function may diminish with time suggest that in some patients thymic attrition occurs; the cause of this attrition remains unknown.

The pathologic findings in patients with this disease parallel the clinical and immunologic observations. Postmortem findings may include a small dysplastic thymus that consists of epithelial cells and mesenchyme without lymphocytes or typical Hassall's corpuscles. The thymus-dependent areas of the lymph nodes and spleen are depleted; cells of the plasma cell series are preserved.

CLINICAL MANIFESTATIONS. In contrast to patients with SCID, patients with thymic hypoplasia may have an onset of symptoms varying in severity in infancy or only after several years. Recurrent pneumonia, frequent otitis media and upper respiratory tract infections, severe diarrhea, and sepsis are usual findings. The infections are similar to those encountered in patients with SCID.

When infections become chronic, or if diarrhea occurs, the children fail to thrive. Physical examination reveals evidence of chronic infection. Tonsils and lymph nodes may be either absent or enlarged. Many patients succumb within a year of diagnosis, but some have survived beyond 5 years. When death occurs it is usually due to overwhelming sepsis.

DIAGNOSIS. Studies of antibody-mediated immunity are usually abnormal. Infants may have a deficiency or an elevation of one or more immunoglobulins. However, panhypogammaglobulinemia is rarely present. A specific antibody response to injected antigens is either diminished or absent. Some patients have a nonreactive Schick test following immunization with diphtheria-pertussis-tetanus or a normal titer of isohemagglutinins, suggesting that at one time they were capable of producing specific antibody. However, when patients are immunized with a specific antigen such as keyhole limpet hemocyanin or pneumococcal polysaccharide, a deficient antibody response is noted.

Variable deficiencies of cell-mediated immunity are found. Lymphopenia is the most characteristic finding, and delayed hypersensitivity skin tests are usually negative. In vitro lymphocyte responses to mitogens, specific antigens, or allogeneic cells, as well as T cell rosettes, may all be abnormal, or only a single test may be abnormal. A thymic shadow is generally absent on chest radiography. The lymphoid architecture, especially of the thymus-dependent areas, is abnormal.

TREATMENT. Therapy directed against specific infectious disease present in the infant may permit the child to survive until specific immunotherapy can be instituted. Gamma globulin injections or fresh frozen plasma infusions may be of value if the patient is unable to produce specific antibody, in spite of normal gamma globulin levels.

Reconstitution of cell-mediated immunity has been attempted by various methods. Experience with histocompatible bone marrow transplantation in such patients is limited. Recently transfer factor has been given with some success. Other patients have been reconstituted successfully with fetal thymus transplants. Reconstitution of cell-mediated immunity following fetal thymus transplantation occurs within weeks; it generally is transient, requiring additional transplants, and has not been associated with either graft-versus-host reactions or HLA chimerism. The mechanism of reconstitution in these patients is most likely related to the release of thymic humoral factors by the fetal thymus gland and maturation of the patient's circulating prethymic or thymic cells by these factors. Recently partial reconstitution of cell-mediated immunity in selected patients with this diagnosis has been accomplished by repeated injections of a thymic humoral factor termed thymosin.

PROGNOSIS. Because of the heterogeneity both of the immune defects and of the clinical severity of disease in patients with this diagnosis, the long-term prognosis varies. However, the predominant pattern is that of early onset, severe progressive infections, and death within several years following diagnosis. The longest known survivor of this disease died at 16 years with chronic lung disease and cor pulmonale.

Combined Immunodeficiency Disease Associated With Adenosine Deaminase or Nucleoside Phosphorylase Deficiency

Combined immunodeficiency disease associated with enzyme deficiency is characterized by autosomal recessive inheritance and varying degrees of antibody and cellular immunodeficiency. Infants may present with clinical and laboratory findings identical to those in patients with well-defined SCID or with a disease similar to the Nezelof syndrome.

PATHOGENESIS. The association between inherited adenosine deaminase deficiency and combined immunodeficiency in more than 15 patients, and between inherited nucleoside phosphorylase deficiency and cellular immunodeficiency in 1 patient, suggests but does not prove that enzymatic deficiencies are related etiologically to immunodeficiency disease. Both adenosine deaminase and nucleoside phosphorylase are necessary for the normal catabolism of the purine adenosine. The enzyme adenosine deaminase catalyzes the conversion of adenosine to inosine, while the enzyme nucleoside phosphorylase catalyzes the conversion of inosine to hypoxanthine. The precise mechanism underlying the effect of adenosine deaminase deficiency or nucleoside phosphorylase deficiency on the immune response is unknown. It has been suggested that pyrimidine "starvation" secondary to the accumulation of adenine nucleotides as a result of adenosine deaminase deficiency may be related to the immunodeficiency. Others postulate a more direct suppressive effect on lymphocyte function caused by elevated intracellular levels of cyclic AMP. Similarly, a blockade in inosine (adenosine) metabolism because of a specific enzyme deficiency may lead to accumulation of metabolic intermediates, which then would be capable of interfering either with nucleic acid metabolism or with more specialized cell function.

Recent evidence strengthens the probability of a causal relationship between the enzyme deficiencies and the immunodeficiencies observed in these children. A patient with SCID and adenosine deaminase deficiency was given frozen irradiated erythrocytes as a source of adenosine deaminase. The patient's red blood cell adenosine deaminase increased, and in vitro lymphocyte responses to phytohemagglutinin and allogeneic cells became normal 7 days after transfusion. The peripheral blood absolute lymphocyte count became normal, and a thymic shadow appeared on a chest radiograph. The duration of this apparent restoration of immunity remains to be determined.

The pathologic examination of thymus glands obtained from infants with combined immunodeficiency and adenosine deaminase deficiency, regardless of the severity of their cellular immunodeficiency disease, is striking. Hassall's corpuscles are present, and thymic epithelium is differentiated; this is in marked contrast with their absence in the classic combined immunodeficiency disease. A possible interpretation of these findings is that immunologic attrition began after lymphoid cells had already populated the thymus. If this interpetation is correct, infants with adenosine deaminase deficiency may be capable of maturing stem cells initially. This process may be arrested later, either because of a shortage of the enzyme or because of the eventual loss of maternal enzyme that had previously crossed the placenta and made the intrauterine environment of those infants suitable for T and B cell differentiation.

CLINICAL MANIFESTATIONS. Patients with either SCID or the Nezelof syndrome and associated absence of adenosine deaminase present in a similar manner. There is marked variability in the age of onset, the severity of symptoms, and the eventual age of death in children with adenosine deaminase deficiency and immunodeficiency. A small group of patients have absent cell-mediated immunity and antibody-mediated immunity; the majority of infants in this group have radiologic skeletal abnormalities, including concavity and flaring of anterior ribs, abnormal bony pelvis, abnormal contour and articulation of posterior ribs and transverse processes, platyspondylisis and thick growth-arrest lines. Infants with adenosine deaminase deficiency but with a syndrome similar to the Nezelof syndrome do not have the associated radiologic findings.

A single patient with cellular immunodeficiency, quantitatively normal immunoglobulins, a normal ability to form antibody in response to specific antigen, and absence of nucleoside phosphorylase has been identified. This patient was initially diagnosed as having a modified type of Diamond-Blackfan syndrome, because of persistent anemia with a hypoplastic bone marrow, and has had recurrent upper respiratory tract infections, otitis media, pneumonia, and diarrhea from birth.

DIAGNOSIS. Patients suspected of having combined immunodeficiency (either severe or variable) should be evaluated as outlined under laboratory studies. Infants with this syndrome have a significant lymphopenia, an absence of or marked decrease in all parameters of cell-mediated immunity, and variable deficiencies of antibody-mediated immunity. Immunoglobulin levels may be markedly depressed, normal, or elevated. Patients may either produce specific antibody following antigen stimulation or have no response. Quantitation of red blood cell enzymes, including adenosine deaminase and nucleoside phosphorylase, will establish their lack in patients with this syndrome.

TREATMENT. Ideally, therapy for patients with immunodeficiency disease and an associated enzyme defect would be replacement of the specific enzyme. This approach has been reported successful in a single patient with SCID and adenosine deaminase deficiency, who received frozen irradiated erythrocytes. Other approaches to therapy are similar to those suggested for patients with SCID or the Nezelof syndrome without an associated enzyme defect. Several patients have received successful bone marrow transplants.

PROGNOSIS. Prognosis appears to be related to the age of onset of infections, the age of diagnosis of immunodeficiency, and the severity of infection; those with early onset of infection, and for whom there is no therapy available, appear to have as poor a prognosis as infants with immunodeficiency but with normal enzyme function.

Thymic Hypoplasia With Hypocalcemia (DiGeorge Syndrome)

Children with thymic hypoplasia have congenital tetany, abnormal facies, congenital heart disease, and an increased susceptibility to infection. The disease is characterized pathologically by the absence or hypoplasia of both the thymus and parathyroid glands. Both males and females are affected, and the mode of inheritance is unknown.

PATHOGENESIS. Both the thymus and parathyroid glands develop following epithelial evaginations of the third and fourth pharyngeal pouches during the sixth to eighth week of intrauterine life. By the twelfth week the thymus gland has migrated caudally to its permanent position in the anterior mediastinum. During the same time period certain aortic arch structures develop from the same pharyngeal pouches, and the philtrum of the lip and the ear tubercle differentiate. At this critical time of development it is most likely that some event occurs that interferes with pharyngeal pouch development or evagination, resulting in the abnormalities described. Abnormal development of the thymus gland can result in either complete or partial lack of the thymus, or an abnormal location of the gland.

The fetal thymus gland is essential for the development of competent cell-mediated immunity, as it most likely serves to mature stem cells into competent T lymphocytes; if it is lacking or abnormal, a partial or complete deficiency in cellular immunity occurs.

CLINICAL MANIFESTATIONS. Newborn infants generally present with congenital heart disease and/or hypocalcemia that is resistant to traditional treatment and may result in tetany during the first hours of life. Facies are characterized by an antimongoloid slant of the eyes,

hypertelorism, a carp shaped mouth, notched ear pinnae, and micrognathia. If the infants survive the newborn period, recurrent infection, chronic candidiasis, and diarrhea occur. The infants fail to thrive and are susceptible to sudden death.

DIAGNOSIS. The diagnosis of the DiGeorge syndrome is made in an infant with neonatal hypocalcemia, aortic arch abnormalities, and abnormal facies by documenting abnormal cellular immune function. Quantitative immunoglobulins are usually normal, but antibody response following antigenic challenge may be diminished. Cellular immune function, when evaluated during the neonatal period, may be absent or relatively normal; the percentage of thymus-derived lymphocytes as determined by T cell rosettes is usually depressed. Cellular immune function, if normal during the neonatal period, may become abnormal during infancy. Infants with variants of the DiGeorge syndrome have been described, with mild immunologic defects or with the spontaneous return of cell-mediated immune function.

TREATMENT. Treatment during the neonatal period is directed toward control of the hypoparathyroidism and surgical correction of the aortic arch abnormalities. If a cellular immune defect is documented, fetal thymus transplantation is recommended. Reconstitution of cell-mediated immunity in patients with the DiGeorge syndrome following fetal thymus transplantation occurs rapidly (within 8 hours). Thus far it appears to be complete and permanent and is not associated with graft-versus-host reactions or HLA chimerism; therefore it is most likely mediated by a thymic humoral factor.

PROGNOSIS. If an infant survives the newborn period and has a reparable cardiac anomaly, the prognosis is related to the immunocompetence. Cellular immunity may be completely reconstituted by a fetal thymus transplant, and long-term survivors have been reported following this procedure. Alternatively, an infant may have only a partial thymic defect that either may correct spontaneously or may not result in significant infectious complications.

OTHER DISORDERS WITH ABNORMAL CELLULAR IMMUNE FUNCTION

Wiskott-Aldrich Syndrome

The Wiskott-Aldrich syndrome is a sex-linked recessive disorder characterized by thrombocytopenia, eczema, recurrent infection, and an inability to form specific antibody to polysaccharide antigens. Varying defects in cell-mediated immunity and deficient antibody response to antigens other than polysaccharide have been described.

PATHOGENESIS. Because of the number of abnormalities associated with the Wiskott-Aldrich syndrome, it is difficult to postulate a single pathogenic mechanism. Early in the disease thrombocytopenia with subsequent bleeding is responsible for the morbidity and mortality. Initially thrombocytopenia was thought to be a result of a defect in platelet production or release. However, bone marrow aspirates obtained from patients with thrombocytopenia secondary to the Wiskott-Aldrich syndrome are normal; but platelet size and survival are decreased. It has been suggested that the alpha granules of platelets, as well as the alpha granules of macrophages, are metabolically defective in these patients; this might explain both the decreased platelet survival and the inability of patients to respond to immunization with specific antigens by antibody production. A second feature is the inability to respond to polysaccharide antigens with specific antibody formation. It has been postulated that this specific lack of response is due to defective macrophage processing of polysaccharide. Alternatively, abnormal lymphocyte–macrophage interaction has been proposed. However, at least with in vitro studies, it has been impossible to improve cell function by mixing macrophages obtained from normal donors with cells from patients with the Wiskott-Aldrich syndrome. It has also been postulated that macrophages from patients with the Wiskott-Aldrich syndrome lack normal surface receptors for IgG and/or IgM. Regardless of the specific mechanism underlying the inability to respond to polysaccharide antigen with the production of specific antibody, the result of this deficiency are an abnormal immunoglobulin pattern. Early in life, quantitative immunoglobulins may be normal. However, as sequential immunoglobulin levels are obtained, quantitatively, serum IgM fails to increase. Isohemagglutinins are either depressed or absent. Infection by polysaccharide-containing organisms is a persistent clinical problem early in life.

Patients with the Wiskott-Aldrich syndrome have normal plasma cells, normal thymus glands, and normal lymph node morphology early in life. However, as they age immunologic attrition occurs and eventually results in the loss of antibody-mediated and cell-mediated immune function. Thus in many instances, when an infant is diagnosed early in life, evaluation of the child's cellular immune function yields normal results. As the child ages a profound cellular immunodeficiency occurs. It has been suggested that the immunologic attrition is related to the patient's inability to process polysaccharide antigens; the inability to handle antigens might result in disruption of normal lymphoid tissue. If lymph nodes and/or thymus glands are evaluated histologically late in the course of the disease, they may show marked depletion of lymphoid elements and abnormal architecture. As the severity of immunologic abnormalities increases, the patients become susceptible to infection with *P. carinii* and herpes simplex and neoplasia.

Incomplete forms of the disease have been reported. Patients with thrombocytopenia, low isohemagglutinins, and increased serum IgA, but no history of recurrent infection or eczema, have been described. An adult patient with the clinical triad of the Wiskott-Aldrich syndrome, but with less severe immunologic abnormalities and a relatively benign clinical course, has been reported.

CLINICAL MANIFESTATIONS. The earliest manifestations, usually occurring during the newborn period, are petechiae and bleeding secondary to thrombocyto-

penia. Subsequently bleeding from the gastrointestinal tract following a viral illness may occur. Severe and recurrent infection by polysaccharide-containing organisms usually occurs after 5 months of age. As patients become older, bleeding becomes less frequent, and eczema and recurrent infection becomes more severe.

Eczema, when it is present, has the characteristic distribution of allergic eczema; however, as the child ages the eczema may become more extensive and often is superinfected. Hepatosplenomegaly may develop as the child grows older. Chronic pulmonary disease, sinusitis, and chronic otitis media occur. As cellular immune function decreases, an increased incidence of viral and protozoal infections has been noted, as well as an increased incidence in malignancy and autoimmune disease. Herpetic lesions may be present on the skin. Chronic herpetic infection of the eye may lead to blepharoconjunctivitis and chronic keratitis. In about 20 percent of cases ocular complications are present. Malignancy is generally lymphoreticular and occurs in the central nervous system and/or abdomen. Monoclonal gammopathies, autoimmune hemolytic anemia, and arthritis have been described in patients with this syndrome.

DIAGNOSIS. The diagnosis of Wiskott-Aldrich syndrome can usually be made during the neonatal period, since thrombocytopenia is present at birth. Patients are unable to make antibodies following immunization with polysaccharide antigens. Characteristically, isohemagglutinins are absent, serum IgM is low, and IgA and IgE are elevated. As the patients become older, they fail to make antibodies to other antigens and begin to demonstrate progressively more severe defects in cell-mediated immunity.

TREATMENT. Early in life, bleeding difficulties secondary to thrombocytopenia are major clinical management problems. Splenectomy is contraindicated in patients with a diagnosis of Wiskott-Aldrich syndrome and has been associated with a more fulminant course and early death from septicemia. Steroids have been utilized in an attempt to increase the platelet count, but they have not proved successful and may enhance susceptibility to infection. Topical treatment of chronic eczema with local steroids is useful.

When patients survive the neonatal period, overwhelming infection becomes the main cause of death. Aggressive and early antibiotic treatment is indicated and should be directed primarily against pneumococcus, meningococcus, and *Haemophilus influenzae*. Gamma globulin and/or fresh frozen plasma infusions have been used.

Transfer factor therapy has been beneficial in some patients and has led to subsequent decrease in the number of recurrent infections and improvement in the eczema. Previously negative skin tests have been converted to positive, and MIF has been produced by the patient's cells. However, no change in lymphocyte function has been noted, and no change in the platelet count has followed therapy. The effect of transfer factor in this syndrome may be related to the degree of immunologic deficiency at the time of treatment; it is most likely that the successful use of transfer factors requires the presence of a responsive lymphocyte population. Complications of transfer factor therapy have been reported; they include nephrotic syndrome and Coombs-positive hemolytic anemia.

A single patient with the Wiskott-Aldrich syndrome was treated by bone marrow transplantation following immunosuppression. The patient's cell-mediated immunity was partially reconstituted, and a decrease in clinical symptoms occurred, but platelet levels remained depressed.

PROGNOSIS. Patients with the Wiskott-Aldrich syndrome who die in infancy usually die with massive bleeding episodes secondary to thrombocytopenia. The average age at death is about 4 years. With increasing age, mortality generally results either from severe overwhelming infection or from development of malignancy. The oldest known survivor is now 16 years old.

Immunodeficiency With Ataxia-Telangiectasia

Immunodeficiency with ataxia-telangiectasia (p. 0000) is inherited as an autosomal recessive disorder and is characterized by progressive onset of ataxia, telangiectasia, and variable immunodeficiency that may involve both antibody-mediated and cell-mediated immunity.

PATHOGENESIS. Immunodeficiency with ataxia-telangiectasia is typically associated with variable onset of clinical symptomatology and definite progression of the disease with time. Any theory concerning the etiology of this disorder must therefore take into account the progressive deterioration of the patient as well as the multiple system involvement.

Studies in these patients have shown thymic abnormalities consisting of loss of corticomedullary differentiation, lack of Hassall's corpuscles, and generalized hypoplasia. Lymph node architecture is abnormal and usually is associated with lymphocyte depletion and diminished follicle formation. A majority of patients also have gonadal abnormalities consisting of gonadal dysgenesis and testicular atrophy. Telangiectatic blood vessels have been described in the skin and lung. A defect in embryogenesis of mesenchyme has been postulated as the mechanism resulting in these multiple defects. Although this theory might explain the thymic defect and the telangiectasia, it would not explain the consistent involvement of the central nervous system wherein the lesions are degenerative in nature and are not related to blood vessel abnormalities.

The involvement of both endocrine organs and the thymus could be related to a deficiency in tropic hormones. This possibility is supported by the observation that some patients have lesions in the anterior pituitary and hypothalamus. However, detailed endocrinologic evaluation has demonstrated only elevated follicle-stimulating hormone (FSH) and 17-ketosteroid values in the urine.

An increased incidence of autoantibodies has been described; it is possible that an underlying autoimmune disease exists in these patients, with gradual loss of both thymic and endocrine organ function. However, no autoantibody directed against central nervous system tissue has been described, and this theory does not provide adequate explanation for the progressive ataxia that is present in all patients.

A slowly progressive viral infection may be responsible for the gradual deterioration of the patient. An underlying immunodeficiency (primary defect) could predispose the patient to chronic viral infection and attrition of immunologic function.

The variable, progressive deterioration of immunologic function in ataxia-telangiectasia can best be explained by a process of immunologic attrition, as has been observed in other immunodeficiency disorders. The precise etiology of immunologic attrition is not known, but it appears to be a fairly constant feature of ataxia-telangiectasia, the Wiskott-Aldrich syndrome, and other immunodeficiency diseases such as adult variable-onset hypogammaglobulinemia. When studied initially, patients with ataxia-telangiectasia may have normal antibody-mediated immunity and normal cell-mediated immunity; with time, there may be a gradual loss of antibody responsiveness to specific antigens, as well as selective loss of various immunoglobulins. Cellular immunity may show mild dysfunction initially, and then with time marked abnormalities may occur. It could be postulated that the gradual loss of immunologic function is related to repeated infection and premature exhaustion of the immune system. Alternatively, it is possible that patients with ataxia-telangiectasia have only a limited amount of competent immunity, which becomes exhausted with time and leads to increased susceptibility to infection.

CLINICAL MANIFESTATIONS. Each of the primary clinical manifestations (ataxia, telangiectasia, recurrent sinopulmonary tract infection) is independently variable in appearance and progression. Ataxia may be manifested as soon as the infant begins to sit, or it may be delayed for 6 to 8 years. When ataxia is the only manifestation of the disease, the patient may require several years of evaluation before the diagnosis can be made. As the ataxia progresses there is irregularity of gait, slurred speech, and development of variable choreoathetoid or ticlike movements. Typically the eye movements are irregular, resulting in a dysconjugate gaze. Late in the course of the disease, extrapyramidal and posterior column signs may appear. At this point reflexes are diminished and muscle weakness is prominent. Sensory involvement can occur, although this is extremely rare.

Telangiectasia usually appears later than ataxia and may be delayed until beyond 6 years of age. Initially the telangiectasia occurs on the bulbar conjunctivae. As this progresses, telangiectasia may be found on the lateral aspect of the nose, on the ear lobes, and in the antecubital and popliteal areas.

Recurrent sinopulmonary tract infections are a prominent feature of ataxia-telangiectasia. Patients may present with recurrent sinopulmonary tract infection or may not experience infection until well beyond the second decade of life. In the majority of individuals, however, ataxia and recurrent sinopulmonary infection are present simultaneously, and the presence of ataxia-telangiectasia should be suspected.

DIAGNOSIS. If a patient presents with ataxia, telangiectasia, and recurrent sinopulmonary tract infection, a diagnosis can be established on a clinical basis. However, since a period of 4 to 6 years may elapse before the complete syndrome is present, additional studies may be required to make an early diagnosis. Most commonly the antibody-mediated immunity consists of a selective absence of IgA, with a deficiency of IgA and IgE as the second most frequent abnormality. In some patients the immunoglobulins may be normal or elevated, or various combinations of elevated and depressed levels of the five immunoglobulin classes may occur. Variable degrees of deficiency in antibody response to specific antigens have been described. In addition, there is a high incidence of a variety of autoantibodies.

Studies of cell-mediated immunity indicate a deficiency in about 60 percent of patients. This can be demonstrated by negative results in delayed hypersensitivity skin tests and depressed response of isolated peripheral lymphocytes to phytohemagglutinin, allogeneic cells, and specific antigens. Depressed numbers of circulating thymus-derived lymphocytes have been observed, as measured by T cell rosettes.

Older patients have been shown to have diminished 17-ketosteroid excretion in the urine associated with elevated levels of FSH. An unusual form of diabetes with relative insulin resistance has been described. Liver function studies have been abnormal in numerous patients. Anti-smooth-muscle and antimitochondrial antibodies that are known to be associated with chronic active hepatitis have been described. Pneumoencephalograms have demonstrated dilatation of the ventricular system and diffuse cerebral atrophy. Electromyograms have shown fibrillation potentials indicative of anterior horn cell disease. No consistent patterns have been observed with electroencephalograms. Elevation of α-fetoprotein has been described in the majority of patients.

Pathologic examinations of tissues have shown abnormalities in multiple systems. In the central nervous system there is a loss of Purkinje and granular cell layers in the cerebellum—evidence of anterior horn cell degeneration, demyelination of the posterior columns, and degenerative changes in the hypothalamus and pituitary. Examination of immunologic tissue usually reveals atrophy of the thymus, which lacks corticomedullary differentiation and Hassall's corpuscles. The lymph nodes are usually small, with depleted thymus-dependent and thymus-independent areas.

Numerous malignancies have been described in patients with ataxia-telangiectasia: lymphosarcoma (the most common), leukemia, adenocarcinoma, dysgerminoma, and medulloblastoma.

TREATMENT. No specific treatment is available to halt the progression of the disease. Symptomatic treatment has provided relief from sinopulmonary tract infection. Broad-spectrum antibiotics may be used on an intermittent or continuous basis to assist in the control of recurrent or chronic sinopulmonary tract infection. Although there are no well-documented studies on the use of gamma globulin therapy in these patients, its use in those patients who have extremely low levels of immunoglobulins and/or who fail to make antibodies following antigenic stimulation would appear logical. Monthly fresh frozen plasma infusion has been used to treat a number of patients with this disorder, but no controlled studies have been reported.

Other attempts at immunotherapy have been made, but the numbers of patients treated have been too small to provide definite conclusions regarding efficacy. Some patients have received fetal thymus transplants, followed by improvement in cellular immunity. Transfer factor has been given to a number of patients, but no beneficial effect has been documented. Transplantation of histocompatible bone marrow would theoretically provide reconstitution of both antibody-mediated and cell-mediated immunity. However, as many patients with ataxia-telangiectasia have some degree of cell-mediated immunity, it would be necessary to provide immunosuppression prior to performing transplantation; such attempts have not yet been made.

Standard treatment cannot be used in the management of malignancies in patients with ataxia-telangiectasia. The patients are extremely sensitive to immunosuppressive regimens; even small doses of radiation therapy and/or chemotherapeutic agents may result in severe reactions and early death. Malignancies must therefore be treated cautiously, using small doses initially with frequent determination of tumor response before increasing dosages.

PROGNOSIS. The variability in onset and progression of the disease makes it impossible to provide an accurate prognosis in an individual patient. Life expectancy may range from several years following onset of symptoms to as long as 40 years. Similarly, there may be rapid clinical deterioration, and the patient may become a complete invalid after several years of symptoms or may be able to function normally in school well into teenage years. It appears that the rate of clinical deterioration may be related to the degree of immunodeficiency; those patients with severe abnormalities of both antibody-mediated and cell-mediated immunity develop recurrent infection, with rapid progression of the disease.

Chronic Mucocutaneous Candidiasis

Chronic mucocutaneous candidiasis is characterized by persistent *Candida* infection that involves the skin, mucous membranes, and/or nails. It is frequently associated with idiopathic endocrinopathy. This disorder occurs in both males and females.

PATHOGENESIS. The basic defect is unknown. As in other immunodeficiency disorders, such as ataxiatelangiectasia and the Wiskott-Aldrich syndrome, there may be variable onset of symptoms. In some patients the idiopathic endocrinopathy may precede the *Candida* infection by as long as 10 to 12 years, while in others chronic *Candida* may be the first presentation. Initially it was felt by some investigators that chronic *Candida* infection was secondary to hypoparathyroidism with hypocalcemia. However, the *Candida* may be present for years without evidence of abnormal parathyroid function.

Idiopathic endocrinopathy is most frequently associated with autoantibodies directed against the endocrine organ involved. In some cases the autoantibody may be found prior to diminished endocrine organ function. As the endocrinopathy progresses the autoantibody may disappear. This observation has led to the postulate that the autoantibody is an indicator of organ destruction rather than the cause of the organ pathology.

Chronic *Candida* infection can usually be related to an abnormality in cell-mediated immunity. The majority of patients have negative delayed hypersensitivity skin tests to *Candida* in the face of severe candidiasis; others may have an inability to produce MIF when their lymphocytes are exposed to *Candida* antigen. Other patients have a more severe defect, with an inability of their lymphocytes to transform when exposed to *Candida* antigen in culture. Although these observations offer an explanation for the chronic *Candida* infection, it is difficult to postulate that a basic defect in cell-mediated immunity can predispose to the development of endocrine organ destruction.

One theory that attempts to provide a unifying hypothesis for both the defective cellular immunity and the endocrinopathy suggests that autoimmunity is the basis for the entire disorder. The thymus is considered an endocrine organ with hormonal production. A basic defect in cellular immunity present in these patients could then result in the development of autoantibodies against target organs. The variable nature of the disease would be dependent on the onset and severity of the destructive process mediated by autoantibody.

CLINICAL FEATURES. Chronic *Candida* infection is most commonly present in the oral cavity. In older females severe vaginal candidiasis may be present. The *Candida* may also involve fingernails and toenails and in severe forms may be present on the skin of the face, hands, and feet. Frequently this takes the form of granulomatous lesions in a "stocking and glove" distribution; in this form there are usually clear areas of demarcation between involved and uninvolved skin.

Other manifestations of the disease relate to associated endocrinopathies. Patients may present with pigmentation secondary to Addison's disease or tetany secondary to hypoparathyroidism and hypocalcemia. Hypothyroidism, diabetes, and pernicious anemia occur less frequently than Addison's disease and hypoparathyroidism.

In most instances the chronic *Candida* infection remains localized to mucous membranes, and dissemination to blood, lungs, and other organs is not observed. Other infections have been described. Relatively severe viral infections may precede the onset of endocrinopathy, and acute or chronic hepatitis has been noted. Late in the course of the disease, patients may have difficulty with recurrent respiratory tract infections, and occasionally infection with other organisms has been described (*Trichophyton rubrum*, *Epidermophyton floccosum*, and *Mycobacterium*).

There is an increased incidence of psychiatric disorders in patients with chronic candidiasis. It is difficult to attribute this abnormality to any one etiology, as these individuals have severe, long-standing disfiguring disease as well as multiple endocrine aberrations that may well result in psychiatric difficulties.

DIAGNOSIS. A diagnosis of chronic mucocutaneous candidiasis can usually be made on the basis of clinical presentation. The distribution of the chronic *Candida* infection is typical, and the disorder is relatively resistant to treatment. It is important, however, to be certain that the patient does not have any other immunodeficiency disorders associated with chronic *Candida* infection. The DiGeorge syndrome, ataxia-telangiectasia, and SCID should be excluded. Most of the patients with these disorders present at an earlier age than do patients with chronic mucocutaneous candidiasis, and these disorders are associated with laboratory abnormalities that are much more extensive than those found in chronic mucocutaneous candidiasis.

Patients with chronic mucocutaneous candidiasis usually have intact antibody-mediated immunity, with high titers of antibody to *Candida* and elevated immunoglobulin levels. The response to immunization with a variety of antigens is normal. Studies of cell-mediated immunity reveal a normal response of isolated peripheral lymphocytes to foreign cells and to mitogens. An occasional patient may not respond to phytohemagglutinin. About 50 percent of the patients have a diminished response of isolated lymphocytes to *Candida* antigen, and the majority have abnormal delayed hypersensitivity to *Candida* antigen. In most instances this correlates with a diminished MIF response to *Candida* antigen in vitro.

Once a diagnosis of chronic mucocutaneous candidiasis has been established, the patient should receive a complete endocrinologic evaluation, including investigation of adrenal, pituitary, thyroid, gonadal, pancreas, and parathyroid functions. Patients should then be followed yearly, and studies should be repeated if any suspicious symptoms arise. It is important to realize that the disease is progressive and that the majority of patients will eventually develop an endocrinopathy. Patients who present initially with an endocrinopathy should be completely evaluated for additional endocrinologic defects, as well as for the presence of cellular immunodeficiency.

TREATMENT. Initially patients may respond to the treatment of *Candida* infection consisting in application of local antifungal agents such as nystatin, amphotericin B, and miconazol, but usually these agents ultimately fail to control the infection. In severe cases the most successful treatment has been the use of intravenous amphotericin B combined with the administration of transfer factor obtained from a delayed hypersensitivity *Candida*-positive donor; repeated courses of therapy may be necessary. The success of this treatment does not appear to be dependent on the degree of immunodeficiency. Some individuals may respond to relatively low doses of amphotericin B given on a regular basis. Unmatched lymphocyte infusions have been used by some investigators; however, this has the potential of producing a graft-versus-host reaction and is not recommended. Fetal thymus transplantation has been attempted in several patients, with some success. Immunotherapy has no effect on the progressive development of endocrinopathies. These must be treated individually with replacement therapy.

PROGNOSIS.   Patients with chronic mucocutaneous candidiasis usually do not die from systemic infection. They may survive for prolonged periods of time, well into the second or third decade. If there is an associated endocrinopathy, they are more difficult to manage, and sudden death from unsuspected adrenal insufficiency may occur. Patients rarely survive beyond the third decade, and death is usually a result of hepatic or endocrine failure.

Immunodeficiency With Short-Limbed Dwarfism

Immunodeficiency with short-limbed dwarfism has been associated with three major forms of immunologic aberration: defective antibody-mediated and cell-mediated immunity, defective cell-mediated immunity alone, or defective antibody-mediated immunity alone. One of these forms (deficiency of cell-mediated immunity with short-limbed dwarfism) may be associated with cartilage-hair hypoplasia. The disorder affects both males and females.

PATHOGENESIS.   A unifying hypothesis is not available to adequately explain the association between immunodeficiency, short-limbed dwarfism, and cartilage-hair hypoplasia. Although the immunodeficiency may vary from complete absence of both B and T cell immunity to partial absence of cellular or antibody-mediated immunity, the clinical and radiologic features of short-limbed dwarfism remain constant. The disorder may be suspected at the time of birth from characteristic clinical features and confirmed by radiologic findings. However, short-limbed dwarfism and cartilage-hair hypoplasia can occur without any evidence of immunodeficiency, which suggests that the immunodeficiency and skeletal abnormalies are inherited in an independent manner.

DIAGNOSIS.   The various forms of immunodeficiency associated with short-limbed dwarfism are similar to those entities not associated with skeletal abnormalities. In the form associated with combined immunodeficiency, cell-mediated immunity is completely absent, with lymphopenia commonly present as

well as a lack of response of peripheral blood lymphocytes to mitogens. At autopsy an absence of lymphoid tissue and a hypoplastic thymus have been described. Antibody-mediated immunity is usually absent, as evidenced by hypogammaglobulinemia and a lack of antibody production following specific immunization.

In the form of short-limbed dwarfism associated with an isolated defect in cell-mediated immunity, there are several unique features present. Laboratory studies indicate a more severe immunodeficiency than that suggested by clinical observation of susceptibility to infection. Lymphopenia is usually present, and the peripheral blood lymphocytes are unresponsive to mitogens. In some patients the lymphoctyes do not respond to allogeneic cells. Despite these rather severe generalized defects in cell-mediated immunity, the patients seem to survive most infections, including viral illness, without complications. However, when exposed to varicella or when immunized with smallpox, they develop progressive and fatal disease. The lymphocytes also fail to respond with increased transformation to varicella and smallpox viruses. In contrast to the specific and generalized deficiency of cell-mediated immunity present in these patients, antibody-mediated immunity is usually normal, with normal levels of immunoglobulins and normal antibody formation against varicella.

Only two patients with short-limbed dwarfism and antibody immunodeficiency have been described. Total hypogammaglobulinemia was present in both patients (male and female siblings), while cell-mediated immunity as assayed by lymphocyte response to mitogens and allogeneic cells was normal.

Several radiologic abnormalities are characteristic of these patients, including scalloping, irregular sclerosis, and cystic areas of the metaphyseal portions of the bones; the skull and spine are usually normal. A paucity of cartilage cells and a failure of orderly columnar architecture is observed on microscopic examination of bone. In those patients in whom cartilage-hair hypoplasia is found, the hair has a reduced diameter (usually less than 0.048 mm), with a lack of central pigment core. Typically, therefore, the hair is thin and light in color. In a few patients with short-limbed dwarfism, cartilage-hair hypoplasia, and defective cell-mediated immunity, congenital megacolon has been reported. Radiologic and biopsy findings confirmed the diagnosis of aganglionic megacolon.

CLINICAL FINDINGS.   Clinical features are largely dependent on the associated immunodeficiency. Patients with combined immunodeficiency present with severe bacterial and fungal infections, and all cases have had a fatal outcome. Those with defective cell-mediated immunity are uniquely susceptible to varicella infection and progressive vaccinia following smallpox immunization; if exposure to these two viral agents is avoided, they may survive up to four decades. Individuals with short-limbed dwarfism and defective antibody-mediated immunity are susceptible to bacterial infections and progressive lung disease.

Other clinical manifestations relate to the presence of

short-limbed dwarfism; initially some patients were reported as having achondroplasia because of generalized short stature, but the clinical features are distinct from those of achondroplasia. Patients with short-limbed dwarfism have a normal head circumference, short and pudgy hands, and short fingernails that are normal in width; in some the joints are loose and there is limitation of elbow extention. There may be a redundancy of skin folds surrounding the neck and extremities; this is usually apparent at birth and disappears as the infant grows. When cartilage-hair hypoplasia is present, the scalp hair is sparse, and the eyebrows and eyelashes have a light color and fine texture.

TREATMENT.   Treatment of the various forms of immunodeficiency associated with short-limbed dwarfism is similar to that of immunodeficiency diseases unassociated with skeletal abnormalities. Patients with combined immunodeficiency disease theoretically could receive histocompatible bone marrow transplants. To date no successful bone marrow transplantations have been performed, and the majority have expired by 1 year of age with either infection or graft-versus-host disease. The lack of successful transplantations relates to the lack of histocompatible donors. Individuals with cellular immunodeficiency appear to handle the majority of infections quite well, with the exception of varicella and vaccinia. These patients might also benefit from bone marrow transplantation if histocompatible donors are available. One patient, who had progressive vaccinia, was treated with fetal thymus transplants and subsequently received a successful bone marrow transplant. Patients with short-limbed dwarfism and defective antibody-mediated immunity are treated in the same manner as those with hypogammaglobulinemia.

PROGNOSIS.   The prognosis is dependent upon the associated immunologic aberration. No patients with combined immunodeficiency and short-limbed dwarfism have survived beyond 1 year of age. Patients with short-limbed dwarfism and defective cell-mediated immunity have survived beyond 40 years of age. Survival is related to exposure to varicella and smallpox immunization. Of the two patients reported with defective antibody-mediated immunity and short-limbed dwarfism, one expired during childhood with overwhelming sepsis. The other is alive with chronic lung disease and repeated sinopulmonary tract infections.

OTHER CELLULAR IMMUNODEFICIENCY DISORDERS

Immunologic Attrition Disease (Acquired Immunodeficiency)

There are several reports of patients who for a variety of reasons have been studied immunologically and have been found to have normal antibody and cell-mediated immunity. As some of these patients have been followed, there has been simultaneously an increase in their susceptibility to infection and a decrease in their immunologic function. This decrease in immunity may occur over a period of months or years. Once attrition begins, the disorder usually progresses to a fatal outcome.

Immunologic attrition may also occur in other well-defined immunodeficiency disorders, such as in patients with ataxia-telangiectasia and the Wiskott-Aldrich syndrome. The etiology of immunologic attrition is not known. It has been postulated that certain infectious agents may be lymphotropic and cause sudden and severe depletion of cellular immunity. In some cases it is possible that patients are endowed with a limited amount of competent immunologic tissue, which becomes "stressed" with repeated infections and results in gradual loss of remaining immunity.

Episodic Lymphopenia With Lymphocytotoxin (Immunologic Amnesia)

A number of patients have been reported who have had lymphopenia associated with a lymphocytotoxin. The clinical course of these patients is characterized by recurrent infection, eczema, and impaired cell-mediated and antibody-mediated immunity. It is not clear whether this disorder is distinct from other immunodeficiency diseases associated with recurrent viral infection. Lymphocytotoxins have been reported in a variety of viral illnesses, including infectious mononucleosis, rubella, and measles, as well as following immunization with viral vaccines and in patients with autoimmune disease. Their presence in a patient with antibody and cellular immunodeficiency may therefore reflect only the increased susceptibility to viral infection with the production of lymphocytotoxins and subsequent lymphopenia. The episodic nature of the disorder may be a consequence of the episodic nature of recurrent infections in patients with immunodeficiency disease.

Graft-Versus-Host Disease

Patients who develop graft-versus-host reactions (GVHR) are incapable of rejecting foreign incompetent cells that are histoincompatible with their own. The requirements for a GVHR are cellular immunocompetence (graft), cellular immunodeficiency (host), and histocompatibility differences between graft and host.

PATHOGENESIS.   Following the infusion of immunocompetent cells into a host with cellular immunodeficiency, a proliferation period is required before signs and symptoms appear. The reaction occurs as the donor's cells attack the patient's tissues (ie, skin, gastrointestinal tract, lung, kidney, and central nervous system). All of the host cells have antigens that are recognized as foreign by the graft cells. The source of immunocompetent donor cells may be blood transfusions, exchange transfusions, fresh plasma, maternal cells, or attempts at immunotherapy (eg, bone marrow, fetal liver, or fetal thymus transplantation).

CLINICAL FEATURES.   Two major forms of GVHR exist: acute and chronic. The acute form occurs 7 to 30 days following the infusion of immunocompetent cells. The first clinical feature is a maculopapular rash, followed by hepatosplenomegaly, diarrhea, and tachypnea. There is a fulminant, acute form of GVHR that presents as toxic epidermal necrolysis. The chronic form is associated with hyperkeratotic, scaling skin rash, hepatosplenomegaly, hair loss, chronic diarrhea, and wasting. This latter form may be confused with Histiocytosis X. Certain features of chronic GVHR also resemble acrodermatitis enteropathica.

DIAGNOSIS. The presence of characteristic physical findings in an immunodeficient patient with a history of having received immunocompetent cells 7 to 30 days previously strongly suggests the diagnosis of GVHR. A skin biopsy may be diagnostic in the chronic form of the disease, the features include dyskeratosis, parakeratosis, and mononuclear cell infiltration of the epidermis. A definitive diagnosis can be established by demonstrating cell chimerism in the patient. Sex chromosome or HLA chimerism may be utilized. In cases of therapeutic transplantation of immunocompetent cells, where transplanted cells have identical histocompatibility antigens, other genetic markers may be required (eg, isoenzymes).

TREATMENT. Prevention of GVHR is essential, because treatment of an established GVHR is ineffective. Steroids, immunosuppressive drugs, and antilymphocyte serum have all been used, but at best they only postpone the inevitable progression of GVHR. However, GVHR may be prevented entirely by irradiation of all blood containing viable white cells with 3,000 to 6,000 rad.

PROGNOSIS. Patients with GVHR appear to have increased susceptibility to infection, even exceeding that related to their underlying disease. Thus patients with GVHR die from overwhelming infection. Rarely patients may develop a chronic GVHR involving the skin, liver, gastrointestinal tract, and/or lung; they may survive for periods ranging from months to years.

PHAGOCYTIC AND GRANULOCYTIC DISORDERS

Neutropenia

Neutropenia (p. 1179) exists when the number of circulating neutrophils is below 1,200/mm^3. Most of the causes of neutropenia remain unknown. In some instances it may be due to an isoimmune phenomenon following placental passage of antibodies directed against an infant's neutrophils. In general, patients with an uncomplicated neutropenia have a good prognosis, perhaps because they are able to mobilize monocytes in a compensatory manner. Infections may be frequent, but they are generally not severe. Patients with neutropenia may have recurrent aphthous ulcers and/or stomatitis. Disorders that are associated with neutropenia, as well as depressed numbers of mononuclear cells, are usually also associated with more severe infections. The pancytopenias of bone marrow failure and drug-induced agranulocytosis are invariably fatal.

Splenic Deficiency Disorders

An increased susceptibility to infection with polysaccharide-containing organisms is seen in patients following splenectomy at any age (p. 1196); however, the most important prognostic factors appear to be the age of the patient at the time of splenectomy, the presence of an adequate number of opsonins in the form of antibody (specifically IgM), and absence of an additional disorder that could compromise immune function. The young animal, who has not yet formed specific antibody, is dependent on the spleen for containment of rapidly multiplying organisms such as pneumococci, *Haemophilus influenzae,* and meningococci. In man, in the absence of adequate levels of antibody, the spleen assumes primary importance in the prevention of overwhelming infection from these same organisms. Increased amounts of specific IgM antibody form against these organisms as an infant is exposed with increasing age. The specific IgM antibody provides a second barrier against rapid multiplication of organisms. The susceptibility of older individuals to overwhelming infection following splenectomy generally requires the presence of an additional immunologic defect. Thus patients with sickle cell disease who have a defect in the alternate complement pathway in addition to autosplenectomy have an increased susceptibility to infection at any age. Patients who have had splenectomy for staging of Hodgkin's disease may be unable to form antibody or may have defective cell-mediated immunity, in addition to the splenectomy. Splenectomy in patients with the Wiskott-Aldrich syndrome is uniformly fatal. The treatment of patients who have had splenectomy is not uniformly agreed upon. However, infants who have been splenectomized probably should receive prophylactic antibiotics until about 3 years of age, when the susceptibility to infection decreases. The antibiotics that have been suggested vary, but ampicillin appears to be the best choice. In the future many patients will probably receive immunization with purified polysaccharide vaccines.

Tuftsin Deficiency

Tuftsin deficiency is a familial lack of a phagocytosis-stimulating tetrapeptide that is cleaved from a parent immunoglobulin molecule in the spleen. The deficiency has been described in two families. Tuftsin appears to be absent in splenectomized patients. The disorder is associated with both local and systemic severe bacterial infections. Determination of tuftsin levels in specialized laboratories establishes the diagnosis. Gamma globulin is administered routinely, and acute bacterial infections are treated with appropriate antibiotics.

Lazy Leukocyte Syndrome

The lazy leukocyte syndrome is a defective phagocytic response to normal chemotactic stimuli and is associated with severe recurrent infection and neutropenia. Both males and females are affected. The patients are unable to mobilize a normal store of polymorphonuclear cells to the peripheral bloodstream, which results in inadequate phagocytosis in vivo. Humoral and cellular immunity are normal, as is in vitro leukocyte phagocytosis and bacterial killing. The syndrome is associated with recurrent low-grade fevers, gingivitis, stomatitis, and otitis media. Clinical toxicity and fever are frequently mild or absent during documented infection. Patients are apparently unable to mobilize a normal store of neutrophils, as demonstrated by abnormal in vivo inflammatory response measured by skin window or Rebuck window technique, with no polymorphonuclear cells migrating to the abraded area; also, stimulation of the marginal pool of polymorphonuclear cells by the administration of epinephrine is abnormal, and stimulation of the marginal pool of neutrophils by the administration of endotoxin is abnormal. In vitro evaluation of both chemotaxis and random neutrophil migration is abnormal. Specific infections are treated with antibiotics. The prognosis remains unknown.

Chronic Granulomatous Disease

Chronic granulomatous disease (CGD) is an inherited defect of white cell bactericidal function. The killing of certain microbial agents is abnormal and results in recurrent infection. The syndrome is most often inherited as a sex-linked recessive trait; however, several females have been described with CGD.

PATHOGENESIS. Patients with CGD have polymorphonuclear leukocytes with normal phagocytosis but defective bactericidal function. In patients with CGD 80 to 90 percent of bacteria remain viable inside the leukocyte after 120 minutes of incubation in vitro whereas in normal persons less than 1 percent remain viable. In addition to an abnormality of polymorphonuclear leukocyte function, there is some evidence of abnormal function of eosinophils and mononuclear phagocytic cells.

The basic defect in leukocytes of patients with CGD is deficient respiratory oxidative metabolic activity. The neutrophils do not respond to the phagocytosis of particles or bacteria with increased hexose monophosphate shunt activity, increased oxygen consumption, or increased hydrogen peroxide production. As has been discussed, hydrogen peroxide in association with myeloperoxidase and a halide has potent bactericidal activity. Lack of hydrogen peroxide most likely results in the killing defect documented in patients with this disease. The lack of production of free hydrogen radicals and hydrogen peroxide is a result of an enzyme deficiency (NADP oxidase or NADPH oxidase) in males. It has been postulated that females with a similar disease lack glutathione peroxidase. Patients with CGD have a remarkable lack of infections due to bacteria that contain hydrogen peroxide (those bacteria lacking a catalase), such as streptococci or pneumococci. These organisms supply their own hydrogen peroxide to the patient's white cells and are killed normally by chronic granulomatous disease neutrophils, thus acting in a suicidal manner.

It has recently been demonstrated that superoxide (designated O_2^-), a product of conversion of oxygen to hydrogen peroxide, may be a potent bactericidal factor. Since there is very little increased oxygen consumption during phagocytosis in patients with CGD, superoxide is not produced. This defect may add to the defective production of hydrogen peroxide in limiting bacterial killing.

CLINICAL MANIFESTATIONS. CGD is inherited primarily as a sex-linked recessive trait, but recently an autosomal recessive form of the disease has been described. Children with the disease generally present with recurrent infection during the early months of life, but they may be entirely well until teenage years. The infected lesions are primarily in anatomic sites that receive constant challenge by large numbers of bacteria. Regional adenopathy occurs frequently in the cervical and inguinal areas; following incision and drainage of these areas, healing occurs slowly. Hepatosplenomegaly is a common finding and may be associated with multiple liver abscesses. Pulmonary disease generally presents acutely; pneumonia may be fatal if the etiologic agent is not identified rapidly and appropriate therapy instituted. Other presenting symptoms may include osteomyelitis, persistent diarrhea, perianal abscess, and ulcerative stomatitis. Patients with CGD often present with infection caused by unusual bacteria. The isolation of *Staphylococcus epidermidis*, *Serratia marcescens*, *Candida*, or *Aspergillus* from an osteomyelitic or pulmonary infection should alert the physician to the possibility of CGD.

DIAGNOSIS. All studies of antibody-mediated and cell-mediated immunity are normal. A screening procedure for diagnosis is the quantitative nitroblue tetrazolium dye test; if a patient has CGD his cells will not reduce dye from white to blue. The diagnosis may be established by performing a bacterial killing curve with the patient's cells and an organism isolated from infection in the patient; if CGD is present the patient's cells will not kill the bacteria at a normal rate. In many laboratories oxygen consumption and bacterial iodination are used as additional diagnostic studies. Phagocytic cells obtained from the mothers of affected males with CGD may display intermediate defects in bacterial killing. These studies are useful for detecting the carrier state in female adult relatives as well as female siblings of the patient; however, if the studies are normal the possibility of the carrier state cannot be eliminated.

TREATMENT. Treatment of this disorder has not been entirely successful, although earlier diagnosis and more aggressive therapy have resulted in a considerable improvement in prognosis. Currently patients with this disorder are surviving into and beyond teenage years. The single most important factor in management of patients with CGD is the prompt diagnosis of the microbial agent responsible for an acute infection. Most of the bacterial agents to which these patients are susceptible respond to prompt treatment with appropriate antibiotics. *Aspergillus* is the most difficult organism to treat, and in most instances it must be treated with intravenous amphotericin B for prolonged periods. Therapy with continous antibiotics has been attempted, primarily with sulfisoxazole (Gantrisin). More recently, rifampin has been used in the treatment of a single patient with CGD. The basis for the use of these antibiotics has been the in vitro demonstration of improved killing of microorganisms in the presence of the drugs by leukocytes isolated from patients with CGD. There are insufficient clinical studies at present to determine whether this approach to therapy will improve prognosis. An experimental approach to therapy has included infusion of granulocytes obtained from a normal person and administered to the patient during an acute infection. However, because of the difficulties of obtaining large numbers of granulocytes, their short half-life, and the relative expense of this procedure, insufficient experience is available to document specific benefit.

Chediak-Higashi Syndrome

The Chediak-Higashi syndrome (p. 1928) is an autosomal recessive disorder associated with severe bacterial infection, partial oculocutaneous albinism, and giant cytoplasmic granules in many cells including the peripheral blood leukocytes. Recurrent bacterial infections, partial albinism, hepatosplenomegaly, and central nervous system abnormalities are consistent clinical findings. There is a high incidence of lymphoreticular malignancy. The characteristic giant cytoplasmic granular inclusions can be observed in the polymorphonuclear cells of a routinuely stained peripheral blood smear under ordinary light microscopy. Defects in neutrophil chemotaxis, as well as abnormal intracellular killing of organisms, have been described in patients with this disorder. In contrast with chronic granulomatous disease, there is abnormal killing of streptococci and pneumococci, as well as staphylococci and *Serratia marcescens*. The killing of organisms is not absent, but is delayed. Treatment is directed toward appropriate therapy with antibiotics for specific infection. The prognosis is generally poor, as most patients die during childhood; however, several survivors have been reported in the third decade.

Glucose-6-phosphate Dehydrogenase Deficiency

Both males and females have been described with complete absence of leukocyte glucose-6-phosphate dehydrogenase activity (p. 1928). Patients with absent glucose-6-phosphate dehydrogenase have deficient cellular NADH and NADPH; therefore, in spite of normal oxidase activity, there is little hexose monophosphate shunt activity, and little hydrogen peroxide is produced. The bactericidal deficiency is similar to that found in patients with chronic granulomatous disease. Patients may have a clinical presentation similar to that seen in males with CGD. One patient has been described who had an absence of the enzyme in red blood cells and presented with chronic nonspherocytic hemolytic anemia. Phagocytosis of microbial agents is normal, but killing is abnormal. The defect is similar to that found

in CGD. A diagnosis of leukocyte glucose-6-phosphate dehydrogenase deficiency is established by demonstrating absence of the enzyme in the appropriate cells. Treatment is similar to that of CGD, as patients are susceptible to the same organisms.

DISORDERS OF THE COMPLEMENT SYSTEM

Hereditary Angioneurotic Edema

Hereditary angioneurotic edema (HANE) is a rare condition inherited as an autosomal dominant and characterized by episodic but self-limited circumscribed edema of the subcutaneous tissues, skin, and mucous membranes of the gastrointestinal or upper respiratory tract.

PATHOGENESIS. C1 esterase inhibitor normally acts to regulate C1 activation; uncontrolled C1 activity may result in activation of the entire sequence of complement components. Patients with HANE have either a deficiency of functioning C1 esterase inhibitor or normal amounts of nonfunctioning inhibitor. In the first type, secondary to decreased synthesis, the quantity of inhibitor is reduced when measured both enzymatically and antigenically. In the second type, synthesis is normal; levels measured antigenically are normal, but the levels measured enzymatically are low.

Plasma obtained from patients with HANE during an attack of angioedema provokes increased capillary permeability when injected intradermally into the patient's own skin. The lesion produced in the skin involves interendothelial cell gaps in the postcapillary venule, extravasation of vascular contents, and some degranulation of mast cells. However, the lesion can neither be prevented nor reversed with antihistamines. Plasma obtained from patients with documented HANE during an asymptomatic period does not evoke the same response. The permeability factor generated in plasma during an acute attack is a peptide; it is not blocked by antihistamine, and it has some characteristics of a kinin, but is not identical to bradykinin. Presently it is thought that this peptide is derived from C2, following activation of the complement complex, because of lack of C1 esterase inhibitor. However, other biochemical events may be involved in the formation of the angioedema that characterizes this syndrome.

CLINICAL MANIFESTATIONS. The onset of symptoms in patients with HANE is usually in infancy or childhood. Affected individuals are subject to sudden attacks of circumscribed subcutaneous edema. The swelling may be severe enough to cause disfigurement of the affected part, but it is a noninflammatory edema—nonpitting, nonpruritic, and painless. The areas that are generally affected are the skin of the extremities or face and the mucous membranes of the gastrointestinal tract, pharynx, or larynx. Involvement of the gastrointestinal tract mucous membrane leads to attacks of colicky abdominal pain associated with vomiting and occasional diarrhea; the severity of symptoms has occasionally led to surgical intervention. Laryngeal edema may lead to obstruction and necessitate a tracheostomy. It is relatively common to find one type of attack preceding by 2 or 3 weeks the development of a full clinical picture; patients with acute intermittent abdominal pain may, on occasion, prove to have classic HANE. Acute attacks usually last 1 to 4 days and may be separated by periods of remission ranging from days to years. Generally the cause of an individual episode of edema is obscure. Exercise, extremes of temperature, emotional trauma, physical trauma, and menses have been associated with the onset of episodes of angioedema. The frequency and severity of the attacks usually increase at adolescence and subside during the fifth to sixth decades.

DIAGNOSIS.   During an acute episode of HANE, a patient's serum will contain decreased amounts of hemolytic complement and the complement components C2 and C4. However, during periods of remission, hemolytic complement and C2 are normal; C4 remains decreased because of increased catabolism. During acute attacks and during remissions the serum levels of C3 remain relatively normal. Thus in patients suspected of having HANE, decreased serum C4 confirms the diagnosis. C1 esterase inhibitor can be quantitated by immunochemical means, but about 15 percent of all patients with HANE have a biologically inactive form of C1 esterase inhibitor that is immunochemically identical with the normal. In these patients the electrophoretic mobility of the molecule is abnormal. Other variations have been noted, and the specific diagnosis of C1 esterase inhibitor abnormalities by laboratory means is often difficult.

TREATMENT.   Acute attacks of HANE have been treated by attempts to replace the missing inhibitor. Prevention of the attacks may best be achieved by preventing the consumption of inhibitor. Infusions of fresh frozen plasma (assumed to contain the missing inhibitor) have been reported to be successful in treating acute episodes of HANE. Epinephrine is occasionally useful in controlling swelling. The intravenous administration of diuretics is helpful in halting the progression of angiodema. Tracheostomy should be performed immediately in patients with laryngeal obstruction.

Periods of remission are reported to be prolonged by prophylactic use of an antifibrinolytic agent, ϵ-aminocaproic acid (EACA); it apparently acts by sparing the consumption of C1 esterase inhibitor. However, the side effects of prolonged administration are considerable, and they limit its usefulness. Tranexamic acid, an analogue of EACA, has been found to have fewer side effects and equal effectiveness.

In addition to administering appropriate therapy, the physician can increase the patient's awareness of his disease. The symptoms associated with HANE are benign, except for upper airway edema, which is life-threatening. With any sign of laryngeal involvement, the patient should seek medical help.

PROGNOSIS.   The long-term prognosis for patients with this disorder remains unknown with the currently available therapy.

Familial C5 Dysfunction

In familial C5 dysfunction a genetic defect resulting in C5 dysfunction, severe seborrheic dermatitis, diarrhea, and sepsis has been described. The entity resembles Leiner's disease. The exact mode of transmission is unclear; both males and females are affected. C5, when quantitated immunochemically, is normal in patients with this disorder; however, it is dysfunctional and is ineffective as a chemotactic stimulus. Patients with this disorder fail to thrive; they have severe seborrheic dermatitis, diarrhea, and recurrent sepsis due primarily to staphylococci and gram-negative enteric bacilli. Children with familial C5 dysfunction may have leukocytosis and hypergammaglobulinemia. A defect in the phagocytosis of baker's yeast particles, which is corrected when C5 is added, has been demonstrated. Fresh plasma infusions (presumed to contain functioning C5) are an effective form of therapy. Fresh frozen plasma is unlikely to contain adequate amounts of C5 activity to effect clinical improvement. However, since patients with C5 dysfunction have clinical symptomatology in common with patients who have deficient cell-mediated immunity, it is essential that a specific diagnosis be made. Normal cellular immunity should be demonstrated in these patients before fresh plasma is used as therapy, since the potential of inducing a graft-versus-host reaction with infusions of fresh blood products exists if deficient cellular immunity is present. If the diagnosis of C5 dysfunction is made, antibiotic therapy directed toward staphylococci and gram-negative bacteria is indicated, in addition to fresh plasma. The prognosis in this disorder is not known. Without treatment the mortality rate appears to be higher than 50 percent.

C1q, C1r, C1s, and C2 Deficiencies

C1q, C1r, C1s, and C2 deficiencies are inherited defects of individual complement components affecting both males and females. Each deficiency may be associated with a syndrome similar to systemic lupus erythematosus (SLE) and an increased susceptibility to bacterial infection. The defects can be detected by quantitation of individual complement components, which is usually performed only in specialized laboratories. Total hemolytic complement determination may be used as a screening procedure, and levels are usually low. Treatment of the SLE-like syndrome is identical to that for the disease when it is not associated with a complement deficiency. Congenital deficiency of complement components should be differentiated from low complement secondary to immune-complex deposition in patients with SLE; treatment of the SLE-like syndrome with prednisone and/or immunosuppressants will not alter complement values if a complement deficiency is associated with the underlying disease. In these patients parameters other than complement should be used to monitor therapy. There is no treatment for the specific complement abnormalities.

C3 Deficiency

C3 deficiency is a rare disorder secondary to hypercatabolism and/or hyposynthesis. Recurrent infections, including pneumonia, otitis media, and sinusitis, have been described. Decreased levels of C3 are diagnostic of this deficiency. Acute infections are treated with antibiotics. In one patient the effects of an infusion of 500 ml of normal plasma were dramatic; it resulted in complete or partial restoration of all complement-mediated functions for up to 17 days. Patients with C3 hypercatabolism have increased serum levels of C3 inactivator.

References

Ament ME, Ochs HD: Gastrointestinal manifestations of chronic granulomatous disease. N Engl J Med 288:382, 1973

Ammann AJ, Hong R: Selective IgA deficiency: report of 30 cases and a review of the literature. Medicine 50:223, 1971

————Sutliff W, Millinchick E: Antibody mediated immunodeficiency in short-limbed dwarfism. J Pediatr 84:200, 1974

August CS, Rosen FS, Filler RM, et al: Implantation of fetal thymus, restoring immunological competence in a patient with thymic aplasia (DiGeorge syndrome). Lancet 2:1210, 1968

Beck P, Wills D, Davies GT, Lachmann PJ, Sussman MA: A family study of hereditary angioneurotic oedema. Q J Med 17:317, 1973

Cleveland WW, Fogel BJ, Brown W, et al: Fetal thymic transplant in a case of DiGeorge syndrome. Lancet 2:1211, 1968

Cooper MD, Chase HP, Lowman JT, Krivit W, Good RA: Wiskott-Aldrich syndrome: immunologic deficiency disease involving the afferent limb of immunity. Am J Med 44:499, 1968

Davis SD, Antibody deficiency diseases. In Stiehm ER, Fulginiti VA (eds): Immunologic Disorders in Infants and Children. Philadelphia, WB Saunders, 1973, p 184

Dennehy JJ: Hereditary angineurotic edema. Ann Intern Med 73:55, 1970

Fraley EE, Feldman BH: Renal hypertension. N Engl J Med 287:550, 1972

Gatti RA, Meuwissen HJ, Allen HD, Hong R, Good RA: Immunologic reconstitution of sex-linked lymphopenic immunological deficiency. Lancet 2:1366, 1968

Giblett ER, Ammann AJ, Wara DW, Sandman R, Diamond LK: Nucleoside-phosphorylase deficiency in a child with severely defective T-cell immunity and normal B-cell immunity. Lancet 1:1010, 1975

Gold SB, Hanes DM, Stites DP, Fudenberg HH: Abnormal kinetics of degranulation in chronic granulomatous disease. N Engl J Med 291:332, 1974

Greaves MF, Owen JJT, Raff MC: T and B Lymphocytes. Origins, Properties and Roles in Immune Responses. Amsterdam, Excerpta Medica, New York, American Elsevier, 1974

Hitzig WH: Congenital thymic and lymphocytic deficiency disorders. In Stiehm ER, Fulginiti VA (eds): Immunologic Disorders in Infants and Children. Philadelphia, WB Saunders, 1973, p 215

Johnston RB Jr, McMurry JS: Chronic familial granulomatosis. Am J Dis Child 114:370, 1967

Kirkpatrick CH, Rich RR, Bennett JE: Chronic mucocutaneous candidiasis: model-building in cellular immunity. Ann Intern Med 74:955, 1971

Klebanoff SJ: Antimicrobial mechanisms in neutrophilic polymorphonuclear leukocytes. Semin Hematol 12:117, 1975

Lawlor GJ, Ammann AJ, Wright WC Jr, et al: The syndrome of cellular immunodeficiency with immunoglobulins. J Pediatr 84:183, 1974

Meuwissen HJ, Pollara B, Pickering RJ, et al: Combined immunodeficiency disease associated with adenosine deaminase deficiency. J Pediatr 86:169, 1975

Miller ME, Nilsson UR: A familial deficiency of the phagocytosis-enhancing activity of serum related to a dysfunction of the fifth component of complement (C5). N Engl J Med 282:354, 1970

Peterson RDA, Cooper MD, Good RA: Lymphoid tissue abnormalities associated with ataxia-telangiectasia. Am J Med 41:342, 1966

Roitt I: Essential Immunology, 2nd ed. Oxford, Blackwell Scientific, 1974

Ruddy S, Gigli I, Austen KF: The complement system of man (first of four parts). N Engl J Med 287:489, 1972

————Gigli I, Austen KF: The complement system of man (third of four parts). N Engl J Med 287:592, 1972

————Gigli I, Austen KF: The complement system of man (fourth of four parts). N Engl J Med 287:642, 1972

Senn HJ, Jungi WF: Neutrophil migration in health and disease. Semin Hematol 12:27, 1975

Sheffer AL, Austen KF, Rosen FS: Tranexamic acid therapy in hereditary angioneurotic edema. N Engl J Med 287:452, 1972

Stossel TP: Phagocytosis: recognition and ingestion. Semin Hematol 12:83, 1975

Vyas GN, Stites D, Brecher G (eds): Laboratory Diagnosis of Immunologic Disorders. New York, Grune & Stratton, 1974

Walker WA, Hong R: Immunology of the gastrointestinal tract: part I. J Pediatr 83:517, 1973

————Hong R: Immunology of the gastrointestinal tract: part II. J Pediatr 83:711, 1973

CHAPTER 10

Allergy

Oscar Lee Frick

INTRODUCTION

In 1880 Blackley had discovered that grass pollen could cause his attacks of hay fever; when he applied rye grass pollen to an abraded area of his skin, local urticaria and intense itching occurred in a wheal-and-flare pattern. He also utilized exposed glass slides for making pollen counts. In 1911 Noon discovered that repeated injections of grass pollen extracts could protect patients with hay fever; this protection was found by Cooke and associates in 1935 to be due to protecting or blocking antibodies. In 1919 Ramirez accidentally found that a normal person who received a blood transfusion from a horse-asthmatic individual also developed asthma upon exposure to horses; thus the allergic reactivity had been passively transferred by blood. In 1921 Prausnitz and Küstner demonstrated such passive transfer experimentally; subsequently this became known as the Prausnitz-Küstner (PK) reaction, which they believed to be caused by a skin-sensitizing antibody or reagin. Reaginic antibody was identified as a new immunoglobulin E (or IgE) by the Ishizakas in 1966. Von Pirquet's concept of allergy included a wide range of hypersensitivity phenomena. Coca, however, limited the concept of allergy to the usual human allergic diseases of asthma, hay fever, and eczema by employing the term atopy (strange disease); this implied a hereditary component and immediate reactivity. For many years the allergist restricted his practice to these states, but the recent recognition of multiple kinds of immune responses to an antigenic stimulus has again broadened the concept of clincial allergy to the original von Pirquet definition.

Medical and Economic Significance of Allergic Diseases

The NIH estimates that 31 million Americans (15 percent of the population) suffer from some form of allergic disease. Although deaths from allergic disease are relatively few (4,000 deaths from asthma and 300 from anaphylaxis per year in the United States), the major impact of these diseases is in chronic disability and discomfort and loss of time from work and school. Currently 8.6 million Americans are handicapped by asthma, and about 14 million either are or have been afflicted. Thus allergic disease, including asthma, ranks as the third most frequent chronic disease in the United States, behind only heart disease and mental illness and ahead of cancer.

Among children under 15 years of age, 2 million have asthma and about 250,000 are rendered invalid with intractable asthma that is unresponsive to medical treatment. The 1964 United States National Health Survey indicated that asthma accounted for 23 percent of absenteeism from school and for 33 percent of all chronic diseases in children under 17 years of age. The obvious educational deprivation of these 2 million asthmatic children is compounded by partial loss of hearing in children with chronically blocked noses and ears because of allergy, so that another 2.5 million children cannot learn efficiently.

The economic impact of these diseases on a family was studied in 21 families in California; the study indicated that caring for an asthmatic child or children in a family costs from 2 to 30 percent of the annual family income. As for adults, the National Health Survey of 1964 indicated that on a "daily average" 25,400 persons were absent from work because of chronic allergic conditions and that the total number of work days lost was 6.24 million. Hospitalization figures show that in 1968 there were 134,000 patients with asthma and allergy, with 8.3 days average stay in the hospital, with an annual hospitalization cost of $62 million. Thus, in terms of human suffering and economic impact, allergic disease is one of the major chronic illnesses in the country, affecting both young and old.

Classification of Hypersensitivity Reactions

Formerly, classification of hypersensitivity was as either immediate or delayed reactivity that depended primarily on time and was synonymous with either antibody-mediated reactions or cellular immune reactions. In 1963 Gell and Coombs introduced a more useful classification of hypersensitivity that has gained worldwide acceptance.

TYPE I (ANAPHYLACTIC-ATOPIC) REACTION. Upon first exposure to an antigen, the animal or individual responds by forming antibody that may be any one of the five classes IgG, IgM, IgA, IgD, or IgE. Such antibodies are either "fixed" to certain target cells, such as mast cells or basophils in various organ tissues, or "complexed" with antigen on or near the surface of such target cells. Combination of antigen with tissue-fixed antibodies results in a surface activation of an enzymatic pathway, or cascade, which leads to the dissolution or expulsion of mast cell granules and release of their chemical contents, such as histamine, heparin, slow-reacting substance of anaphylaxis (SRS-A), and kinins. These potent inflammatory chemicals affect adjacent tissue cells and cause such phenomena as smooth muscle contraction in the bronchus, leakage of capillary endothelial cells, and stimulation of mucus-secreting cells. They are responsible for the symptoms of anaphylaxis and atopy (or allergy) in man.

Anaphylaxis is a universal phenomenon in almost all animals and man and may be caused by any antibody class, especially by IgG, IgE, and occasionally IgM. Under proper conditions all members of a species can be anaphylactically sensitized, so that they will react with anaphylaxis characteristic for that species upon exposure to antigen. Anaphylactic antibodies may be homocytotropic, such as IgE and IgG, which when passively transferred into another member of the same species sensitize the recipient for anaphylaxis. Heterocytotropic antibodies of IgG or IgM class may passively sensitize the skin of other species, eg, rabbit or mouse IgG in guinea-pig skin, the classic test for passive cutaneous anaphylaxis (PCA).

Atopic sensitization appears to occur only in certain individuals of a species who have a genetic predisposition for sensitization to certain antigens. Thus in man, atopic or allergic sensitization occurs in certain families predominantly, although isolated atopic individuals without a family history have been found. It has recently been recognized that some individuals have immune-response genes to certain antigens in man and animals that are related to the tissue transplantation antigens.

Clinical examples of type I hypersensitivity in man are anaphylaxis to penicillin and other drugs, allergy (eg, hay fever, asthma, eczema), and anaphylactoid reactions caused by aggregated gamma globulin injection.

TYPE II (CYTOLYTIC OR CYTOTOXIC) REACTION. Antibodies of the IgM or IgG class are usually involved with activation of complement components leading to cytolysis. The antigen is usually the target cell itself or a drug or other chemical attached either by absorption or by chemical bonding to the cell's surface. Cells may be foreign to the host or may be altered in such a way that the host recognizes the cells as being foreign and responds by making antibody to such cells. Upon subsequent exposure of such a sensitized animal or individual to the drug, chemical, or altered cells, an antibody reaction will occur on the cell surface, which leads to the activation of the complement cascade that results in lysis or death of the target cell. Clinical examples of cytolytic reactions are hemolytic anemia secondary to penicillin-sensitizing red cells and agranulo-cytosis or thrombocytopenia secondary to drug attachment to leukocytes or platelets. Many kinds of autoimmune reactions are probably of this type, wherein a normal body constituent is altered and thus is recognized as foreign by the host, which tries to use an immunologic means of getting rid of such foreign body constituents.

TYPE III (ARTHUS OR TOXIC-COMPLEX) REACTIONS. Neither antigen nor antibody is coupled to a target cell surface. Rather, complexes of free antigen and antibody are circulating; either they form microprecipitates in vessels or tissue fluids or they are free in antigen-excess toxic-complex form. In the Arthus reaction antigen and IgG or IgM antibody at optimal proportions form microprecipitates in capillaries. Such complexes activate the C5, C6, and C7 components of the complement cascade that are chemotactic for leukocytes. Neutrophils ingest the antigen–antibody complexes and release their granule contents, which destroy the capillary basement membrane and thus cause edema and other inflammatory changes. Occlusion of capillaries by masses of immune complexes and neutrophils causes ischemia and necrosis of the region; the skin has the classic lesion found in the Arthus reaction. Similar pathology occurs in the kidney in toxic-complex-induced acute glomerulonephritis of the lumpy-bumpy type. In serum sickness, complexes of IgG or IgM antibody and antigen are in the zone of antigen excess in small complexes having a composition of three antigens and two antibodies, or slightly larger. Such complexes cause smooth muscle contraction and leakage of the vascular endothelium in the skin, joints, and kidney. As soon as the antigen disappears and complexes form either at equivalence or in antibody excess, the symptoms of serum sickness disappear. Many drug reactions, such as that from penicillin, are of this serum-sickness type.

TYPE IV (CELLULAR IMMUNE OR DELAYED HYPERSENSITIVITY) REACTIONS. In type IV reactions serum antibodies are not involved, and delayed hypersensitivity cannot be passively transferred with serum; however, passive transfer of sensitized lymphocytes causes cellular immune responses in the recipient upon contact with the antigen. Such sensitized lymphocyte–antigen reactions cause release of lymphokines, eg, migration-inhibition factor (MIF), lymphotoxin, macrophage-activation factor (MAF), interferon, and many others. Lymphokines exert their activities on other adjacent cells, which then take part in the inflammatory response. For example, antigen-activated sensitized lymphocytes release MIF, which causes circulating monocytes to become activated into macrophages that are concentrated in the area and leave the circulation to enter the adjacent tissues for the inflammatory response. Clinical examples of cellular immune responses are the tuberculin reaction, contact dermatitis, heterograft or homograft rejection, and tumor dissolution by sensitized lymphocytes.

The Gell and Coombs classification of hypersensitivities is most useful in thinking about mechanisms of hypersensitivity. However, one must keep in mind that antigens rarely give rise to a single type of immune response and that several types of hypersensitivity may coexist or follow in succession upon exposure to a certain antigen. For example, degradation of penicillin can cause hypersensitivity reactions of all four types, eg, anaphylaxis by IgE antibodies, hemolytic anemia by IgG action on red cells, serum sickness by IgM toxic complexes, and interstitial nephritis by sensitized lymphocytes in the kidney. While one type of hypersensitivity pattern may dominate the clinical picture, other types of hypersensitivity may complicate the pathophysiology and possibly the treatment.

Atopy

IMMUNOLOGY. In genetically predisposed individuals, exposure to certain kinds of antigens, called allergens, causes the induction of IgE antibodies. Allergens are peculiar antigens in that they are glycoproteins whose molecular weights range from 10,000 to 40,000 daltons, they are generally highly polar and rich in sulfur-containing amino acids, and they can immunize in minute amounts. For example, during an entire ragweed pollen season a patient with ragweed hay fever is exposed to only nanogram amounts of ragweed antigen E (the major ragweed allergen) (Fig. 1). The allergen usually enters by a natural portal such as the respiratory passages, the alimentary tract, or the skin. IgE-forming lymphocytes and plasma cells are found in highest concentrations lining the respiratory and alimentary tracts; few are found in the conventional lymph nodes or in circulating blood. An individual who has been induced to form IgE antibodies that enter the circulation and then fix to basophils and tissue mast cells is considered to be allergically sensitized. Upon such an individual's next exposure to the allergen by any route, the antigen (Fig. 2) will enter the tissue fluids and circulation and find its way to the IgE-sensitized target cells. As a result of antigen combining with two tissue-fixed IgE molecules, a physical distortion of the IgE occurs at the mast cell surface; this leads to activation of an enzymatic cascade similar to the complement cascade (both of which start with a C1 esterase) and culminates with the dissolution of the mast cell granules and release of their contents, such as histamine, SRS-A, bradykinin, and eosinophil chemotactic factor of anaphylaxis (ECF-A). Released histamine causes contraction of adjacent smooth muscles (especially in the bronchi), capillary permeability between the endothelial cells with leakage of intravascular fluids into the tissues, edema, and stimulation of mucous glands and cells that results in mucus accumulation. SRS-A causes marked prolonged smooth muscle constriction (lasting for hours) and is the principal mediator of asthmatic bronchial constric-

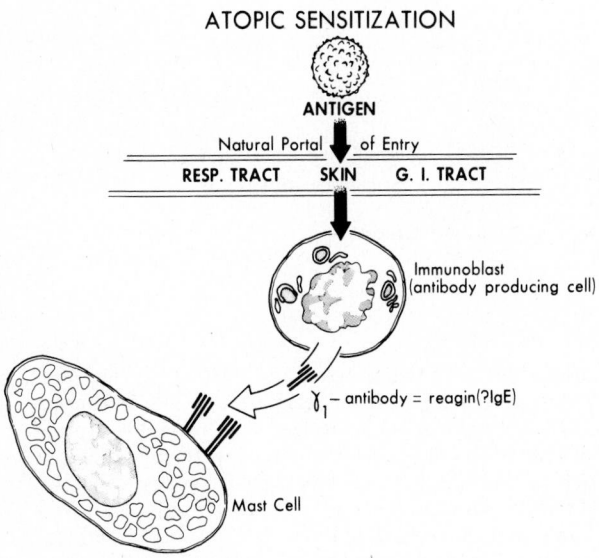

FIG. 1. Atopic Sensitization.

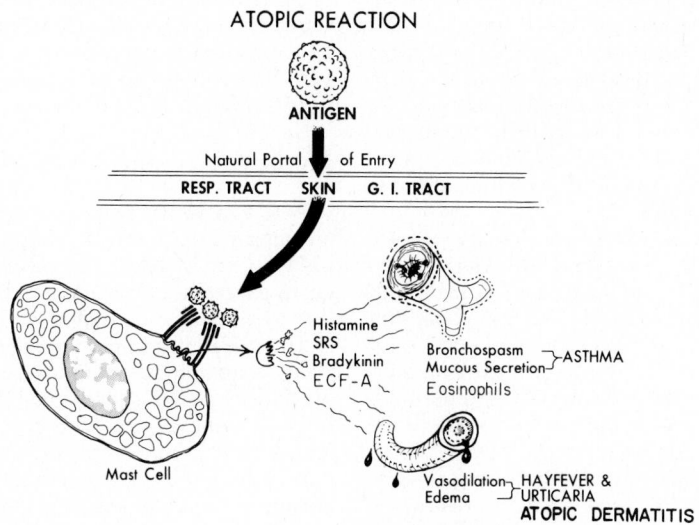

FIG. 2. Atopic Reaction.

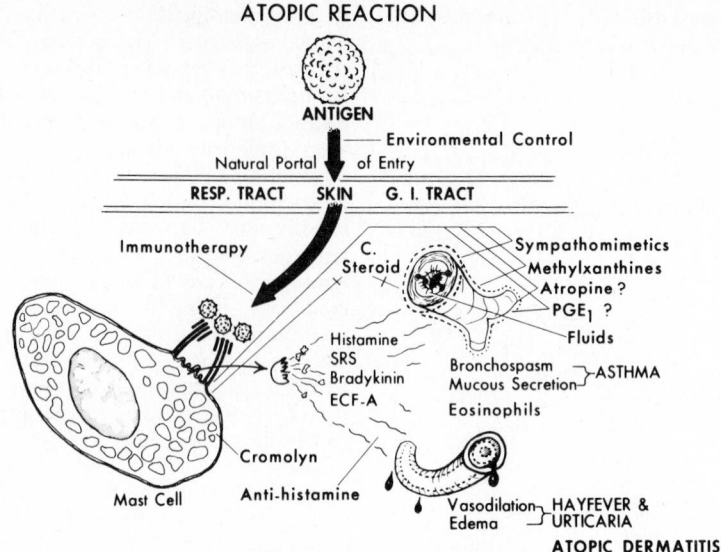

FIG. 3.   Therapeutic measures to interrupt the atopic reaction.

tion. Bradykinin causes smooth muscle constriction, edema, and mucus secretion. ECF-A causes eosinophils to be attracted to the inflammatory area; eosinophils ingest antigen–antibody complexes and probably destroy or inactivate them. Furthermore, the eosinophils contain a natural antihistaminic compound and arylsulfatase that cleaves the SRS-A molecule into inactive fragments. Thus eosinophils appear to exert a negative-feedback control on the allergic inflammatory reaction.

The treatment of allergic disorders has been directed toward interrupting this pathway of immunologic and pharmacologic mechanisms by attacking at various points with immunotherapy and drugs (Fig. 3). The primary avenue of attack is identification of the allergen for that patient and elimination of sources of the allergen. While this approach is reasonably successful for some allergens, for others (such as pollens, molds, and environmental factors) complete elimination is not possible, and the pathogenic mechanisms are subject to attack farther down the line.

Immunotherapy, or hyposensitizing injections for hay fever and asthma, was introduced by Noon in 1911 and has been quite successful for many patients. Elucidation of the mechanism of protection has come only recently (Fig. 4). Injection of an allergen subcutaneously allows the antigen to be taken up by the regional lymph nodes; this gives rise to an IgG or IgM antibody response, thus circumventing the IgE-forming cells lining the respiratory and alimentary tracts. These IgG and IgM antibodies have a blocking or neutralizing capacity that intercepts allergen on subsequent exposure and neutralizes the antigen in the circulation or tissues. Such antigen-blocking (IgG- or IgM-blocking) antibody

complexes are phagocytized and destroyed, thus preventing the antigen from reaching the IgE antibodies fixed to the surfaces of mast cells and basophils. If sufficient blocking antibodies are present, all the antigen is neutralized, and the allergic reaction will not occur. However, clinically a large dose of allergen can overwhelm the blocking antibodies, and some allergen may get through this defense to react with IgE antibodies on mast cells, thus resulting in a reduced allergic reaction. In clinical practice correlation of symptomatic improvement with titers of blocking antibody is excellent in some patients, but in the majority such correlation is relatively poor, which indicates that other mechanisms are operating in many patients.

It has recently been shown that immunotherapy causes a fall in IgE antibodies.

PATHOPHYSIOLOGY

With von Behring's discovery in 1890 that an animal antiserum to diphtheria toxin could be used successfully to cure a child of dread diphtheria, immunology changed from a laboratory curiosity to a practical science for understanding and treating diseases in man. During the next decades investigators around the world used immunologic methods to discover antisera to other diseases and toxins. In 1901 Richet and Portier, in an attempt to find a prophylactic antiserum against toxins from marine creatures, discovered that some immunizations could be harmful. Dogs injected with sea anemone toxin had a mild reaction on their first exposure, but upon a subsequent injection of that toxin they developed shock, and some succumbed instead of being

IMMUNIZATION TREATMENT

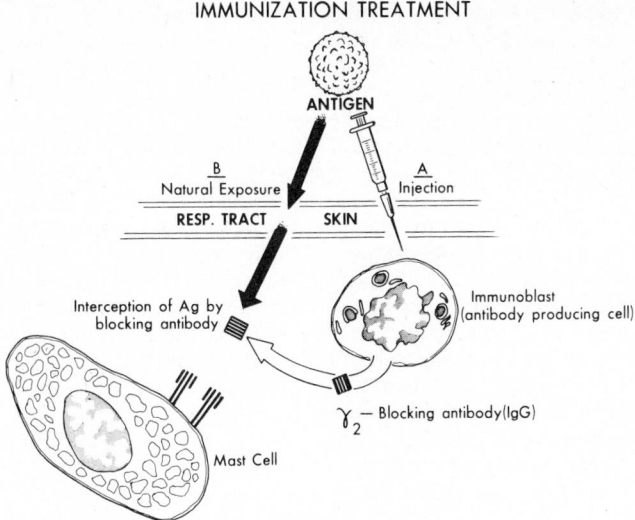

FIG. 4. Immunization treatment: production of IgG-blocking antibodies.

protected. They termed this anaphylaxis or antiphylaxis, in that such immunized animals were hypersensitive to the toxin, which was harmful to the animal.

Von Pirquet proposed the term allergy, or changed reactivity, wherein "allos" implied a deviation from the behavior of the normal individual. He restricted use of the term immunity to those processes in which the introduction of a foreign substance into an organism caused no clinically evident reaction, whereas an allergy was a change in such a reaction behavior. He defined an allergen as an antigen that led to the production of antibodies that caused supersensitivity. He included among allergens the agents of infectious diseases, the poisons of mosquitoes and bees, the pollens causing hay fever, the urticaria-producing substances of strawberries and crabs, and other organic substances.

Following the lead of Theobold Smith, who described asphyxial anaphylactic shock in guinea pigs, Meltzer suggested that "asthmatics are individuals who are sensitized to a specific substance, and the attack of asthma sets in whenever they are intoxicated by that substance." In 1911 Dale and Laidlaw identified histamine (β-aminoethylimidazole) as a smooth muscle contracting material that was released as a result of anaphylactic shock, and they suggested that it was the mediator of such reactions to that allergen, over a period of months or years, probably by a mechanism of induced immunologic tolerance. In many patients there is good correlation of reduction in IgE antibody titer and symptomatic improvement, but this is not universal. Both May and Levy have demonstrated a "nonspecific desensitization" of the target basophils following immunotherapy. For example, a patient with hay fever symptoms from both ragweed and *Alternaria*

mold was treated with only ragweed extract for several months, following which leukocyte histamine release with both ragweed and *Alternaria* was decreased significantly. Furthermore, his cells failed to release histamine with anti-IgE serum, indicating that a nonspecific desensitization of histamine release from his basophils had occurred. In Levy's study in children the best correlation with symptomatic improvement occurred with this desensitization of the basophils; therefore in certain patients protection by immunotherapy may involve primarily one pathway, but protection by the other mechanisms may also contribute. Thus the protective effect of immunotherapy may be a mosaic of three or perhaps even more mechanisms of action.

AUTONOMIC NERVOUS SYSTEM IN ALLERGIC PATHOPHYSIOLOGY. It has been recognized for decades that patients with asthma have hyperirritable airways, or "twitchy lungs," and that patients with atopic dermatitis have itchy skins with abnormal vasomotor skin reflexes, eg, the delayed blanch reflex. In 1967 Szentivanyi proposed the β-adrenergic blockade theory of asthma in which he postulated an autonomic imbalance in the bronchi. In order to maintain normal bronchial tone, or homeostasis, there are opposing autonomic nervous system interactions. Parasympathetic stimulation through the vagus, mediated by acetylcholine, causes bronchial smooth muscle constriction. Szentivanyi observed in guinea pigs that ablation of the posterior hypothalamus (source of the parasympathetic nuclei) prevented anaphylactic bronchospasm and death in sensitized animals, while ablation of the anterior hypothalamus (source of the sympathetic nuclei) caused an increase in anaphylactic bronchospasm and death. Sympathetic stimulation caused bronchial smooth muscle relaxation mediated by epinephrine. Therefore the bronchial smooth muscle tone is maintained by alternating stimulation of the parasympathetic (constricting) and sympathetic (dilating) nervous systems. The term cholinergic may be used to denote the parasympathetic nervous system and the term adrenergic to denote the sympathetic nervous system.

The β-adrenergic blockade theory of asthma postulates that the allergic individual has a quantitatively weak adrenergic response and therefore an impaired bronchial relaxation control. Szentivanyi suggested there was a genetic quantitative or qualitative deficiency in epinephrine effect of the bronchial smooth muscles. As a result there is a normal cholinergic or bronchoconstrictive response and an impaired β-adrenergic or bronchodilating response that cause an irritable bronchus or one that goes into spasm with only slight stimuli and failure of the homeostatic bronchodilating response.

Irritant receptors in the bronchi just below the epithelial surface have been demonstrated by Widdicombe. The afferent fibers of these irritant receptors are carried by the vagus nerve to the hypothalamus, where they synapse with efferent vagal fibers and then return to the bronchial smooth muscles. Gold et al demonstrated that antigen-induced bronchoconstriction in "asthmatic" dogs was reversible within 1 sec by atropine or rapid cooling of the vagus; subsequent warming of the vagus caused a return of bronchospasm. Furthermore, antigen placed into one bronchus caused reflex bronchospasm in both bronchi; this could be interrupted by atropine or by cooling the ipsilateral vagus. These studies indicate a reflex parasympathetic arc involving irritant receptors in the bronchi and smooth muscle constriction in the bronchi. Inhalation of allergens in bronchial provocation tests caused increased airway resistance that could be prevented or reversed by administration of atropine intravenously or by aerosol in allergic human subjects.

In addition to the autonomic nervous controls involving afferent and efferent nerves, there are pharmacochemical controls of the end-organ cells that modulate the degree of allergic responsiveness. This is at the level of the "second messenger" in cells that involves cyclic 3′,5′-adenosine monophosphate (cyclic AMP) and cyclic 3′,5′-guanosine monophosphate (cyclic GMP) and their antagonistic or balancing reactions. The yin-yang theory of hormonal control by opposing or reciprocal actions of cyclic AMP and cyclic GMP has been proposed by Goldberg. In allergic reactions the modulating effect of a balance between cyclic AMP and cyclic GMP has been demonstrated for the release of mediators (Fig. 5) from the target mast cells and basophils and the bronchial smooth muscle cells in asthmatic individuals and probably the epidermal c.

Sutherland proposed the second-messenger concept in which he found that a hormone (the first messenger) reacted with a receptor unit on the cell surface or membrane of the responding cell. This membrane contained an enzyme, adenylate cyclase, that was activated by the first-messenger hormone. Intracellular adenosine triphosphate (ATP) was converted by active adenylate cyclase to cyclic AMP; this induced the cell enzymes to perform the cell's physiologic function. For example, in a liver cell cyclic AMP activated a kinase-kinase enzyme to activate a phosphokinase that in turn activated phosphorylase A, an inactive enzyme, into phosphorylase B, an active enzyme; this converted glucose-6-phosphate into glucose-1-phosphate, culminating in the glucose metabolic pathway for the conversion of glycogen through glucose into carbon dioxide, energy, and water. Cyclic AMP was inactivated by phosphodiesterase to 5′-AMP.

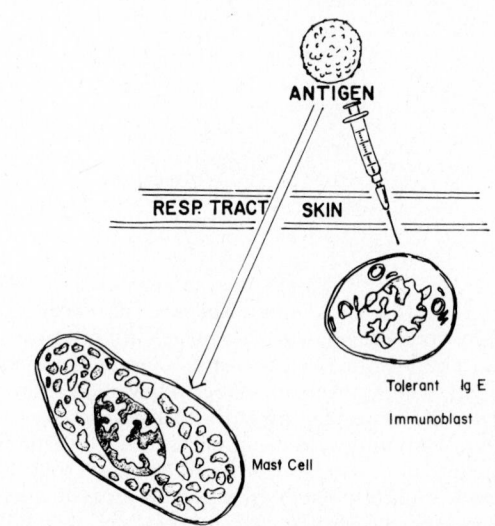

FIG. 5. Yin-yang balance between the β-adrenergic system and the cholinergic–α-adrenergic system on mast cell mediator release and smooth muscle action. (Adapted from Goldberg: Hospital Pract 9:127, 1974.)

Epinephrine converts inactive adenylate cyclase to its active form, which catalyzes the formation of cyclic AMP from ATP. Corticosteroid hormones reinforce this action of epinephrine in forming increased amounts of cyclic AMP. Methylxanthine drugs such as theophylline, theobromine, and caffeine inactivate phosphodiesterase, thus preventing the metabolic breakdown of cyclic AMP and causing high intracellular concentrations of cyclic AMP.

The amount of histamine released from blood basophils from ragweed-allergic individuals with ragweed antigen is inhibited or reduced in the presence of epinephrine and/or theophylline. Minute doses of each drug are ineffective in inhibiting histamine release when administered separately, but when administered together the same doses markedly inhibit histamine release. This synergism between epinephrine and other β-adrenergic drugs and theophylline in the control of asthma has been known for many decades and is widely utilized in the treatment of asthma. Subsequently the release of SRS-A and ECF-A, as well as histamine, from allergically sensitized mast cells of the lung (from a preparation of sensitized, chopped human lung fragments) has been shown to be modulated by drugs that influence the level of cyclic AMP and cyclic GMP.

Orange and associates have shown that the β-adrenergic agonists epinephrine and isoproterenol inhibit the release of histamine, SRS-A, and ECF-A from lung mast cells, whereas α-adrenergic stimulation by norepinephrine enhances the release of these mediators. Further enhancement of histamine release occurs with administration of the β-adrenergic blocker propranolol along with norepinephrine. On the other hand, administration of the α-adrenergic blocker phentolamine with the β-adrenergic agonist isoproterenol markedly inhibits the release of mediators. Coffey and associates have suggested that the α-adrenergic receptor is the enzyme ATPase that competes with adenylate cyclase for ATP. Activation of ATPase converts ATP directly to its inactive 5'-AMP form without intermediary cyclic AMP formation, thus circumventing smooth muscle relaxation.

Robison and associates have demonstrated that cyclic AMP causes a relaxation of bronchial smooth muscles. Epinephrine converts inactive adenylate cyclase into active adenylate cyclase; this in turn catalyzes the conversion of ATP to cyclic AMP, causes bronchial smooth muscle relaxation—an effect of practical importance in the management of asthma. Similarly, theophylline, which inactivates cyclic AMP metabolic degradation, causes a rise in smooth muscle cyclic AMP and bronchial smooth muscle relaxation. It is not yet known whether α-adrenergic receptors actually exist in human bronchial smooth muscle.

The β-adrenergic system has two sets of receptors: (1) the β_1 receptor that controls heart rate and force of contraction, lipolysis, and free fatty acid level in the blood and (2) the β_2 receptor that controls vascular, bronchial, and uterine smooth muscle relaxation, glycogenolysis, and blood glucose concentration. Both receptors are blocked by propranolol, but only β_1 receptors are blocked by practolol and only β_2 receptors are blocked by butoxamine. Recently several specific β_2-adrenergic agonist drugs have been developed (salbutamol, metaproterenol, and terbutaline); they have little or no β_1 function. Such drugs are finding clinical usefulness in the treatment of asthma, especially in treatment of adults with cardiac problems, because they produce primarily smooth muscle relaxation and inhibition of mediator release, with little cardiac acceleration or arrhythmia.

Smith and Parker have shown that both mixed leukocytes (presumably basophils) and lymphocytes of patients with severe chronic asthma have a slightly decreased amount of total cyclic AMP and that exposure of such cells to isoproterenol causes no rise in cyclic AMP. Such cells from patients with hay fever, as well as from nonallergic individuals, exhibit a fourfold rise in cyclic AMP with similar doses of isoproterenol. This would indicate a decreased responsiveness of cells of asthmatic individuals to β-adrenergic agonists. That this effect is not limited to circulating blood cells has been shown by Lockey, who has found that asthmatic individuals given epinephrine have an abnormally low rise in blood glucose and free fatty acids, when compared to normal nonallergic individuals. Furthermore, Ouellette and Reed have shown that influenza vaccine further impairs the rise in blood glucose and free fatty acids after epinephrine administration, indicating that this virus infection further aggravates the β-adrenergic blockade of asthma. It has been suggested that other virus infections, especially membrane-binding ones such as respiratory syncytial virus, herpes simplex, and possibly lymphocytic choriomeningitis virus and *Mycoplasma,* increase β-adrenergic blockade and therefore aggravate or augment the release of histamine under appropriate circumstances.

Adenylate cyclase in the membrane of basophils has three different receptors that when stimulated can independently cause a rise in intracellular cyclic AMP. Such cells, in the presence of propanolol, which blocks the β-adrenergic effect of isoproteronol, can still respond to prostaglandin E_1 or E_2 and/or histamine per se to cause a rise in intracellular cyclic AMP and inhibit further histamine release (Fig. 6). The histamine receptor for adenylate cyclase activation is not inhibited by conventional antihistamines such as mepyramine, a so-called H-1 antagonist, but is blocked by burimamide, an H-2 histamine antagonist, which indicates that the H-2 receptor is responsible for histamine activation of adenylate cyclase and the rise in intracellular cyclic AMP that in turn inhibits further histamine release. Therefore histamine itself exerts a feedback control on further release of histamine from basophils and presumably mast cells. Similarly, prostaglandin E_1 or E_2 in the presence of both propanolol and burimamide can activate adenylate cyclase to cause a rise in intracellular cyclic AMP and inhibit the release of histamine. If, indeed, the basic defect in asthma, or especially in status asthmaticus, is a failure of the β-adrenergic receptor to respond to epinephrine, adenylate cyclase may still be stimulated by giving prostaglandin E_1 or E_2 to cause a rise in cyclic AMP and inhibit mediator release and presumably also to cause smooth muscle relaxation. Such an approach with prostaglandin E_1 in the treatment of status asthmaticus is currently under investigation.

Cholinergic modulation of the asthmatic response at the cellular level involves cyclic GMP. Acetylcholine, the cholinergic agonist, acts upon the cholinergic cell receptor (which has recently been identified as "guanylate cyclase") that apparently occurs in both the cell membrane and the cell substance and is thereby activated to convert guanyl triphosphate (GTP) to cyclic GMP, which in turn is metabolized by a phosphodiesterase into an inactive 5'-GMP form (Fig. 6). Cyclic GMP causes an augmentation of release of histamine, SRS-A, and ECF-A from mast cells and also causes constriction of bronchial smooth muscles, both of which mech-

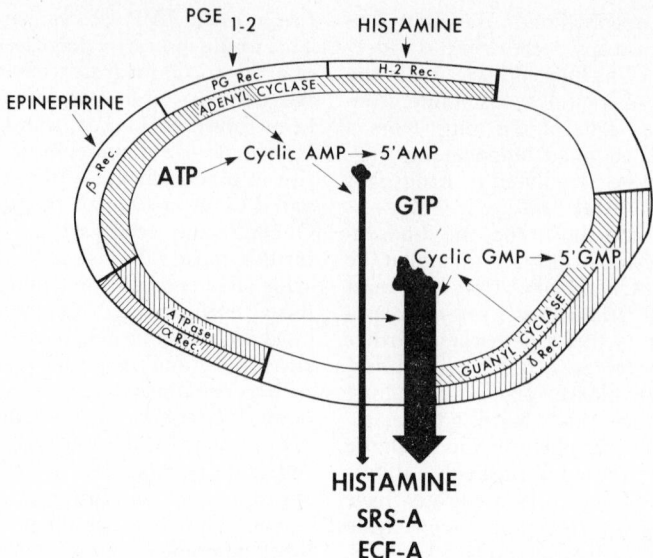

FIG. 6. Three adenylcyclase receptors and one guanylcyclase receptor in mast cells that modulate mediator release. (Adapted from Bourne et al: J Immunol 108:695, 1972.)

anisms are involved in the pathophysiology of asthma. In vitro experiments with sensitized chopped human lung fragments have shown that methacholine (Mecholyl) and carbachol simulate the effect of acetylcholine with a greatly prolonged effect. In fact, inhalation of minute doses of methacholine has been used clinically to demonstrate the hyperirritability of the bronchi in asthmatic patients.

Therefore the cholinergic cellular modulation of allergic responsiveness complements the α-adrenergic stimulus for increased histamine or mediator release and bronchial smooth muscle contraction that is especially prominent in allergic individuals. This is opposed by the β-adrenergic agonists epinephrine and isoproterenol and their newer analogues by raising cyclic AMP and inhibiting mediator release from mast cells, thereby causing bronchial smooth muscle relaxation (Fig. 6).

It has been proposed that the basic defect in asthma is a genetic defect in adenylate cyclase or cyclic AMP, with a resultant failure in the homeostatic negative-feedback control, thus shutting off mediator release, as well as failure of homeostatic bronchial smooth muscle relaxation. Others suggest that the problem in asthma is overactivity or hyperactivity of the cholinergic system that can be treated only with cholinergic antagonists such as atropine or newer atropinelike agents, eg, methylatropine. Whether all asthmatic individuals have the same basic mechanism in impaired autonomic controls or whether in some individuals the problem is primarily β-adrenergic blockade and in others cholinergic hyperactivity remains to be elucidated. Or perhaps it is a combination of both.

Szentivanyi has observed that mice immunized with conventional antigens respond with IgG or IgM antibodies; however, mice treated with *Bordetella pertussis* vaccine, which causes a β-adrenergic blockade, respond strongly to the same antigens with a homocytotropic, or IgE-like, antibody. This suggests that β-adrenergic blockade causes a shift in the immunoglobulin class of responding antibody from the conventional IgG and IgM classes to IgE reaginic class. It is possible that an analogous situation occurs in allergic man, where the predominant response is IgE reaginic antibodies to many allergens. Lymphocyte formation and antibody formation are under similar β-adrenergic and cholinergic controls; the production of IgE antibody by allergic individuals may be caused by an imbalance in the cyclic AMP–cyclic GMP system.

Atopic dermatitis, with its thickened, lichenified skin and abnormal dermal vascular responses, may be caused by a similar imbalance in the adrenergic–cholinergic controls. Studies of mitotic rates in epidermis from normal and atopic individuals have shown that inhibition of mitosis appears to be a function of the β-adrenergic system. The mitotic rate of epidermal cells from nonallergic individuals is markedly inhibited by β-adrenergic stimulation. However, in both involved and uninvolved skin from patients with atopic dermatitis, the mitotic rate is augmented by β-adrenergic stimulation. Similarly, in patients with psoriasis an increase in mitotic rate of the basal cells of the epidermis is characteristically seen and accounts for the thick skin lesions; the mitotic rate in cultures of skin cells from psoriatic patients is increased by epinephrine. Experimental evidence suggests that a β-adrenergic blockade mechanism operates in the skin of patients with atopic dermatitis and psoriasis. In each of these conditions this suggests the operation of a β-adrenergic blockade that fails to cause a feedback-inhibition control on the rate of mitosis of skin cells.

The concept that autonomic imbalance exists in allergic individuals has not yet been conclusively demonstrated. Studies should be conducted in infants or in individuals in whom chronic drug administration has not influenced autonomic balance control.

References

Avner SE: β-adrenergic bronchodilators. Pediatr Clin North Am 22:129, 1975

Bourne HR, Lichtenstein LM, Melmon KL: Pharmacologic control of allergic histamine release in vitro: evidence for an inhibitory role of 3'5'-adenosine monophosphate in human leukocytes. J Immunol 108:695, 1972

Cooke RA, Barnard J, Hebald S, Stull A: Serological evidence of immunity with coexisting sensitization in a type of human allergy (hayfever). J Exp Med 62:733, 1935

Davis DJ: NIAID initiatives in allergy research. J Allergy Clin Immunol 49:323, 1972

Gell PGH, Coombs RRA, (eds): Clinical Aspects of Immunology, 2nd ed. Oxford, Blackwell, 1969, p 575

Gold WM, Kessler GF, Yu, DYC: Role of the vagus nerve in experimental asthma in allergic dogs. J Appl Physiol 33:719, 1972

Goldberg ND: Cyclic nucleotides and cell function. Hospital Pract 9:127, 1974

Ishizaka K, Ishizaka T: Physiochemical properties of reaginic antibody. J Allergy 37:169, 1966

Kaliner M, Orange RP, Austen KF: Immunologic release of histamine and SRS-A from human lung. IV. Enhancement by cholinergic and α-adrenergic stimulation. J Exp Med 136:556, 1972

Kay AB, Austen KF: The IgE-mediated release of an eosinophil leukocyte chemotactic factor from human lung. J Immunol 107:899, 1971

Lands AM, Arnold A, McAuliff JP, Ludena FP, Brown TG Jr: Differentiation of receptor systems activated by sympathomimetic amines. Nature (Lond) 214:597, 1967

Levy DA: Manipulation of the immune response to antigen in the management of atopic disease in man. In Ishizaka K, Dayton D (eds): The Biological Role of the IgE System. Bethesda, USDHEW, 1974, p 239

Noon L: Prophylactic inoculation against hayfever. Lancet 1:1572, 1911

Orange RP, Austen WG, Austen KF: Immunologic release of histamine and SRS-A from human lung. I. Modulation by agents influencing cellular levels of cyclic 3'5'-adenosine monophosphate. J Exp Med, 134:1365, 1971

————— Murphey RC, Austen KF: Inactivation of SRS-A by arylsulfatases. J Immunol 113:316, 1974

Ouellette JJ, Reed CE: Increased response of asthmatic subjects to methacholine after influenza vaccine. J Allergy 36:558, 1965

Parker CD, Bilbo RE, Reed CE: Methacholine aerosol as test for bronchial asthma. Arch Intern Med 115:452, 1965

Prausnitz C, Küstner H: Studien über Überempfindlichkeit. Centralbl für Bakteriol (1 Abt Orig) 86:160, 1921

Richet C, Portier P: De l'action anaphylactique de certains venins. Compt Rend Soc de Biol 54:170, 1902

Smith JW, Steiner AL, Parker CW: Human lymphocyte metabolism. Effects of cyclic and noncyclic nucleotides on stimulation by phytohemagglutinin. J Clin Invest 50:441, 1971

Stanworth DR: Allergy structure and function. In Immediate Hypersensitivity. Amsterdam, North Holland, 1973 p 127

Sutherland EW, Robison GA: The role of cyclic 3'5'-AMP in responses to catecholamines and other hormones. Pharmacol Rev 18:145, 1966

Szentivanyi A: The β-adrenergic theory of the atopic abnormality in bronchial asthma. J Allergy 42:203, 1968

Von Pirquet C: Allergie. Munch Med Wochenschr 53:1457, 1906

Yu DYC, Galant SP, Gold WM: The role of the parasympathetic nervous system in human asthma: inhibition of antigen-induced bronchoconstriction by atropine in asthmatic patients. J Appl Physiol 32:823, 1972

GENETICS OF ATOPY

It was known to the ancients (as reported by Maimonides in his *Treatise on Asthma* in 1190 A.D.) that asthma occurred in succeeding generations. The first extensive study of heredity in asthma was by Cooke and Vander Veer, who found that 48 percent (244/504) of their allergic patients had an immediate family history of allergy, while only 12 percent of a comparable nonallergic group had such a family history. Sixty-eight percent of individuals with a bilateral family history of allergy developed allergy before age 10, while 51 percent with a unilateral family history and 38 percent with no immediate family history had allergic symptoms. They tried to fit this to a mendelian simple recessive pattern. Subsequent studies have shown the genetic pattern of allergy to be more complex. Schwartz studied the pedigrees of 191 patients with asthma and found the trait in each generation; this suggested a dominant inheritance with incomplete (approximately 40 percent) penetrance. Van Arsdel and Motulsky found a 16.7 percent incidence of asthma or hay fever in 5,800 college students; 58 percent of allergic and 22 percent of nonallergic students had a positive family history of allergy. They stated that when both parents were allergic, 58.1 percent of the offspring were also affected. With one affected parent, 38.4 percent of the children showed allergy. When both parents were normal, only 12.5 percent of the offspring were allergic. They concluded that genetic factors and not merely chance accounted for these percentages and that the inheritance could be explained either by incompletely recessive genes or by a polygenic system for allergy. The theory of the polygenic system is currently favored by geneticists.

Some strains of guineas pigs respond with antibody formation to injections of a particular antigen, while other strains do not respond. McDevitt and Chinitz discovered in mice an association between histocompatibility antigens (H-2) in cells and the ability to respond to a particular antigen; they called this an immune-response (Ir) gene. Some strains of mice fail to make IgG or IgE antibodies to small doses of ovomucoid or penicillin, whereas other strains have high titers of such antibodies. With ovalbumin the mouse strain responses are reversed. Thus an immune response to low doses of a particular antigen is related to H-2 genes.

An entirely different genetic factor may be noted in certain mouse strains immunized with various doses of multiple antigens. All strains make IgG antibodies, but some strains (of the same H-2 allotype) make no IgE antibodies. Other strains make a great deal of IgE antibody—apparently they have an H-2-related IgE locus. Therefore mice have at least two independent sets of genetic controls for IgE antibody production to various antigens.

A ragweed hay fever haplotype has been noted in family studies. In one study in a particular allergic family, most of the ragweed-sensitive individuals had the same HL-A haplotype; this occurred in 20 of 26 family members (77 percent), while no ragweed hay fever occurred in family members with other haplotypes (none of 20). The hay fever haplotype was different in different families.

Total serum IgE level also appears to be under separate genetic control, because monozygotic twins have almost identical concentrations, while dizygotic twins and siblings are quite different. Bronchial hyperreactivity to methacholine and to exercise also appears to be transmitted genetically.

In summary, genetic factors in allergy are complex and involve at least three or more gene loci. However, by employing HL-A typing in a newborn infant born into an allergic family and comparing HL-A antigens with those of other allergic family members, it may be possible to predict if such an infant will be susceptible to allergy.

References

Benacerraf B, McDevitt HO: Histocompatibility-linked immune response genes. Science 175:273, 1972

Cooke RA, Vander Veer A Jr: Human sensitization. J Immunol 1:201, 1916

Levine BB: Genetic controls on reagin production. In Goodfriend L, Sehon AH, Orange RP (eds): Mechanisms of Allergy. New York, Marcel Dekker, 1973, p 97

Schwartz M: Allergy. In Sorsby A (ed): Clinical Genetics. London, Butterworth, 1953, p 551

Van Arsdel WT, Motulsky AG: Frequency and hereditability of asthma and allergic rhinitis in college students. Acta Genet 9:101, 1959

DIAGNOSTIC EVALUATION

The major objectives of the medical history are to determine whether the child has an allergic disease and to discover the factors that contribute to the occurrence of symptoms. The child should be actively involved in the history-taking process and not merely a bystander. A spontaneous account of the symptomatology and events as related by the child, and subsequently by the parents, gives the most accurate picture.

History of Specific Allergen Exposure

A description of the detailed course of the illness is the most important part of the allergy history. The traditional questions of reporting (When? Where? What? How?) apply also to the taking of an allergic history. Under the heading of when, the date of onset of the first symptoms of the disease should be as accurate as possible, the month perhaps placed by proximity to a holiday, in order to try to determine a seasonal onset that might coincide with certain seasonally airborne allergens. A description of springtime onset is not sufficient. The trees in an area pollinate, according to their species, at fairly definite times each year, and a particular tree pollen etiology may be established by careful questioning. This leads to the question of where an attack may have occurred, such as in a dusty or even mildewed basement or playroom, as contrasted to the upholstered living room or bedroom areas. Next should follow particular questions of what and how in regard to specific allergens. Questions about the major allergens such as animal dander, house dust, molds, and certain foods and medications may help to establish an etiologic diagnosis.

Some physicians use a printed environmental survey form to cover all the commonly suspected allergens and to make sure that none are missed. This is often best done by allowing the patient to take the form home and consult with the other members of the family. In addition to the symptoms involved in the chief complaint, a specific history of common allergic symptoms should be detailed; for example, urticaria, itching, and other rashes are suspect. Nasal itching, sneezing, rhinorrhea, eye irritation or tearing, intermittent hearing loss, recurrent ear infection, wheezing, cough, dyspnea, exercise-induced coughing, nocturnal wheezing, gastrointestinal upsets, diarrhea, vomiting, headaches, urinary frequency, and enuresis may be caused by allergies. It is important to know whether corticosteroids have been used; even though corticosteroids may have been absent from therapy for a year, there still may be manifestations of adrenal suppression that require further burst steroid therapy in acute stress situations, such as a severe infection or even surgery.

The family history or the familial association of allergic diathesis has been employed for more than a century. One is primarily interested in such a history in the parents, siblings, and grandparents. A family pedigree drawing may be useful as a review of the family situation with respect to allergy. A systemic review should be taken of each patient, because allergic manifestations can involve any system of the body.

Physical Examination

The facial appearance of a child may indicate allergy, especially with chronic nasal obstruction. Such children often have periorbital edema and bluish discoloration, the so-called allergic "shiner," resulting from venous obstruction secondary to nasal congestion. Mouth breathing is also secondary to chronic nasal obstruction. There may be a long face with high cheekbones, a high arched palate with a marked overbite, and other orthodontic abnormalities resulting from nasal obstruction. The nasal mucosa has characteristic grayish color and watery discharge. Tenderness of the paranasal sinuses and their transillumination may be helpful in diagnosis.

Inspection of the chest may reveal the increased anterior/posterior diameter of chronic asthma from hyperinflation, which may be substantiated by percussion and by diaphragmatic motion on deep inspiration and expiration. Asthmatic wheezing may be readily apparent, but minimal wheezing may be seen on forced expiration or following exercise. Finger clubbing, edema of the extremities, and cyanosis should be noted; they might tend to exclude asthma and suggest cystic fibrosis as a possibility. Skin rashes, especially in certain distributions of the flexural creases, may suggest atopic dermatitis.

Laboratory Studies

Eosinophilia is common in allergy; it ranges from 3 to 10 percent, although it may occasionally be higher, especially in an infectious situation in asthma. Eosinophilia greater than 25 percent is rarely seen in allergy and may suggest parasitic or more serious autoimmune disease, such as periarteritis nodosa. Urinalyses and blood chemistries are usually normal in allergic individuals. A routine chest x-ray should be obtained in all children with asthma to exclude other chest diseases causing bronchial obstruction.

Pulmonary Function Tests (See Chap. 28)

A preliminary or screening assessment of lung function can be obtained in the physician's office with relatively simple and inexpensive equipment. These include measurements of air flow; if air flow is impaired, measurements can reflect the degree of airway resistance that is the cardinal lesion in asthma. This increased airway resistance is caused by narrowing of the air passages from spasm of the bronchial smooth muscle, mucosal edema, and mucus plugging. Such increases in airway resistance are also found in emphysema, chronic bronchitis, and cystic fibrosis. However, in these diseases the changes are fairly constant, whereas in asthma they are intermittent. At times, airway resistance in asthma may even be normal by several pulmonary function measurement techniques. In fact, a cardinal diagnostic method in the differential diagnosis of asthma is the reversal of increased airway resistance by administration of inhaled or ingested bronchodilator medication. It has been estimated that the asthmatic's work of breathing at rest may be increased from 5 to 25 times normal. It had been thought that in asthma there was complete reversal of impaired airway resistance at times of freedom between attacks and with the use of bronchodilator therapy; this appears to be the case as measured by relatively crude pulmonary function measures. But with the new, more sophisticated measurements of airway resistance, it has become apparent that there is rarely complete normalization of air flow in a chronic asthmatic between attacks. This probably reflects a rapid clearing of the upper or major airways, where airflow is measured by the relatively crude tests. But the smaller airways still may have considerable mucus plugging for weeks after an asthmatic attack, and air flow in small airways is measured by the newer tests or adaptations of spirometry, such as the maximal midexpiratory flow rate (MMFR).

The most simple pulmonary function test is the match test, in which a lighted match is held 6 inches from the patient's mouth and he is asked to blow out the match without pursing his lips. A peak expiratory flow rate meter (PEFR) is a versatile field device for screening air flow measurement. A small flowmeter measuring up to 100 liters/minute is suitable for smaller, cooperative children; for older children and adults a 1,000-liters/minute regular model is suitable. This test measures the flow rate at the steepest point of the expiratory spirogram. Chai and associates observed that in children who were monitored four times a day by peak flow measurements, a significant fall in flow rate preceded an asthma attack by many hours; thus a fall in the flow rate could be used as a sign to increase bronchodilator treatment.

The forced vital capacity or forced expiratory volume (FEV) is measured with a simple spirometer, which records the tidal volume breathing and inspiratory and expiratory volumes and their rates of flow. Tables of normal values for lung volumes and flow rates in children have been published by Polgar and Promadhat. The FEV_1 is the volume of air expelled in 1 sec; in mild asthma forced vital capacity may be normal, but 5 to 10 sec or more may be needed to complete expiration. Both the vital capacity and the PEFR are effort-dependent. Practice and patience are necessary, as well as some explanation, especially with smaller children who are often not cooperative.

Inhalation Provocation Tests

Changes in the pulmonary function tests FEV_1, MMFR, and PEFR in an asthmatic child by inhalation of graded amounts of suspected allergen are widely used in Europe for the specific diagnosis of asthma. In fact, in Scandinavia no child is given immunotherapy with an allergen that has not caused a bronchospasm on inhalation provocation. Such tests are usually done on an inpatient basis, because while the initial reaction (within minutes) is usually what one is interested in, there may be secondary or delayed bronchospasm to these allergens that can occur 6 to 12 hours after the challenge. Because of the economic considerations of hospitalization, such inhalation provocation tests are not widely performed on asthmatic patients in the United States.

The methacholine inhalation challenge test, as described by Parker, is used in some clinics to test bronchial lability for the differential diagnosis of asthma. In the tests by Parker and associates, one to five inhalations of methacholine (25 mg/ml) caused less than a 30 percent decrease in FEV_1 in normal children and less than a 10 percent decrease in FEV_1 in normal adults. In asthmatics, however, one to five inhalations of methacholine (0.5 mg/ml or 5 mg/ml) consistently produced more than a 20 percent decrease in FEV_1. Mild induced episodes of bronchospasm subsided spontaneously within a few minutes to an hour, but they were usually terminated with an aerosol of isoproterenol (5 mg/ml) immediately after conclusion of the test. There have been no delayed reactions to methacholine as with inhaled allergens; the methacholine test can be used safely in an outpatient service. Recently, inhalation provocation tests for nasal function have been devised that utilize special devices for measuring nasal surface or nasal air pressure.

Ophthalmic Testing

Ophthalmic testing is occasionally used as a specific provocation test. Dried allergen about the size of a pinhead is placed in the conjunctival sac. Within 20 minutes the conjunctiva becomes reddened, with lacrimation, itching, and rhinitis; this can be terminated with epinephrine eye drops. If no reaction has occurred within 20 minutes, the eye may be washed with normal saline and the procedure repeated with another suspected allergen. This test is time consuming and inconvenient and is not commonly performed.

Allergens

Allergens are antigens that give rise to IgE antibody formation in susceptible allergic individuals. They are usually protein in nature, but they sometimes contain large or predominant amounts of carbohydrate. The allergens purified today generally are in the molecular weight range of 10,000 to 40,000 daltons. They have an unusually high percentage of polar amino acids and sulfur-containing amino acids (methionine and cystine) that cause cross-linking. Several antigens have been highly purified, eg, ragweed antigens E and K, which comprise 95 percent of the ragweed allergenic activity. The majority of ragweed-allergic patients (75 percent) react with antigen E and another 10 percent with antigen K exclusively, but there is reaction to both antigens in most patients. Codfish muscle, animal dander, and grass pollen allergens are also available in a highly purified state. Allergenic extracts are generally watersoluble and are prepared by first defatting the allergen by ether extraction. No adequate standardization of potency has yet been developed.

Allergy Skin Testing

Skin tests in which a small amount of the suspected allergen is either scratched into or injected into the superficial layers of the skin have been used for over a century for specific diagnosis of suspected allergen. Within minutes a localized wheal-and-flare reaction occurs that may last 30 to 60 minutes and is accompanied by itching. Several methods of skin testing are regularly employed: scratch, prick, intradermal injection, and passive transfer.

In the scratch method a deep scratch is made into the skin, usually of the back or upper arm; one scratch is made for each allergen to be tested. A scratch deep enough to incise the epidermis, but not deep enough to draw blood, about 0.5 cm long is made. A drop of allergen solution is placed on the scratch and rubbed in,

with the scratch slightly pulled open by pressure. The scratch test should be read in 20 to 30 minutes, to allow for full development. In the prick method a darning needle tip is pricked through a drop of allergen solution into the skin. For the scratch and prick methods the most concentrated allergen solutions available are used, eg, 5 or 10 percent pollen extracts in 50 percent glycerin preservative. If a marked reaction begins to appear within minutes, the allergen extract can be washed out to prevent further exposure to that allergen at that site. The scratch and prick methods have the advantage of greater diagnostic specificity and safety because the reacting allergen can be removed.

For intradermal (intracutaneous) skin tests, dilutions of allergenic extracts of 1:1,000 and 1:100 weight by volume are generally used. From a 1-ml tuberculin-syringe with a No. 26 or 27 needle, 0.02 to 0.05 ml is injected into the superficial skin of the upper or lower arm (occasionally the thigh) at intervals of 1 cm or more. In a child, from 12 to 20 intradermal skin tests can be done at one sitting. A wheal-and-flare reaction is observed and graded after 10 to 20 minutes. If the test with 1:1,000 allergen is negative, a 1:100 diluted allergen is subsequently tested. The chief advantage of an intradermal skin test is its greater sensitivity and precise end-point titration of that sensitivity. A major disadvantage is that once the material has been injected it cannot be removed if a large local reaction or even systemic symptoms occur. Therefore constitutional reactions with this method are more common than with the scratch and prick methods. Intradermal tests should be done only on the extremities, so that if a constitutional reaction does occur a tourniquet can be placed proximal to the test site to slow down the absorption of the allergen.

Passive transfer or Prausnitz-Küstner (PK) skin tests have some distinct advantages. In some patients dermographia interferes with scratch or intradermal skin testing, in that all the sites tested become positive. Also, in children with extensive eczema with no skin sites suitable for testing, or in children who are uncooperative to skin testing, the PK test can be performed on another nonallergic individual with serum from the patient.

For the PK test the patient's blood is drawn aseptically as for a blood culture. After clotting, the serum is removed and cultured for sterility. Into 20 to 60 sites in the skin of the back or the arm of the recipient (a nonallergenic parent or relative) are placed 0.1-ml aliquots of the patient's serum. These sites are marked with indelible ink. After 24 to 48 hours, which is enough time for the patient's IgE antibodies to fix to the recipient's skin, the sites are injected with 1:100 or 1:1,000 (wt/vol) allergenic extracts. Within 10 to 30 minutes a typical wheal-and-flare reaction will occur at any recipient skin site injected with allergen to which the patient is allergic. The passively transferred IgE antibodies persist up to 6 weeks in the recipient's skin, but they do not transfer the clinical allergy to that subject. As controls, the allergens to be tested must also be injected into the recipient at sites that have not been passively transferred, to make sure that the recipient himself is not allergic to these materials. The major disadvantage to this method is the danger of passively transferring serum hepatitis from the patient to the recipient; therefore the serum to be injected is routinely screened for Australia antigen, and the recipients are usually members of the patient's own household who would already have had a similar exposure to hepatitis.

Radioallergosorbent Test (RAST)

For specific IgE antibodies the amount of antibody to a specific allergen in a patient's serum can be tested using small aliquots for each allergen (Fig. 7). In the laboratory the allergen is coupled to an insoluble immunosorbent such as cyanogen bromide-activated cellulose particles or filter paper disks. Such allergen-coated disks are reacted with the patient's serum, which contains IgE antibody to that allergen, and they adsorb to the sorbent. Subsequently radioiodinated (^{125}I) antihuman IgE serum made in rabbit or goat is reacted with the sorbent. The sorbent is thoroughly washed free of other antibodies and serum components and counted in a gamma counter; the ^{125}I adsorbed to the sorbent is a quantitative measure of the amount of specific IgE antibodies to that allergen. Currently there is available commercially a panel of about 50 allergens for which RAST can be performed, requiring 5 to 10 ml of serum; but the test is still quite expensive and the results somewhat variable.

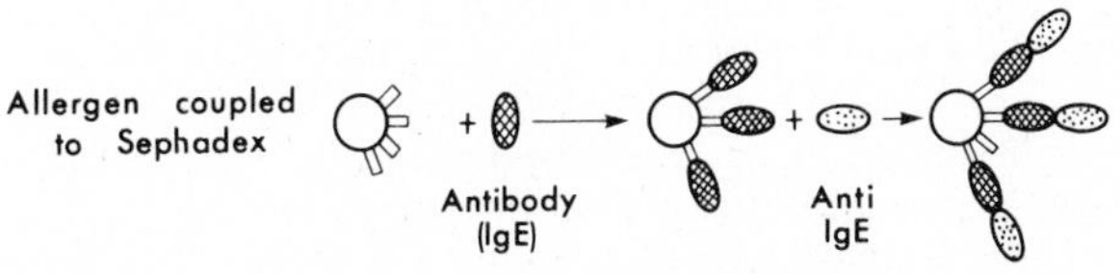

FIG. 7. Outline of the major steps in the radioallergosorbent test (RAST) for specific IgE antibodies. (Adapted from Stanworth: In Immediate Hypersensitivity, 1973. Courtesy of North Holland Publishing.)

Histamine Release from Leukocytes

Specific allergen-induced release of histamine from buffy coat basophils from allergic patients is another means of in vitro testing of allergic reactivity that is finding clinical application (Fig. 8). Heparinized patient's blood (10 to 20 ml) is allowed to settle with Dextran. Red cells are removed and leukocytes are washed, counted, and resuspended in a buffer solution. After addition of the allergen and incubation for 20 to 30 minutes, histamine is released from the leukocytes if the patient is allergic to that allergen. The quantity of histamine released is measured by either spectrofluorometry, bioassay, or ^{14}C-labeled histamine enzyme assay, all of which can measure nanograms of histamine. It is also possible to passively sensitize leuko-

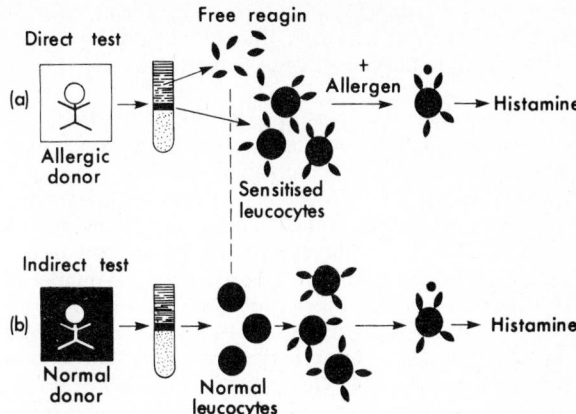

FIG. 8. Outline of major steps in the direct (a) and indirect (b) leukocyte histamine release assay. (Adapted from Stanworth: In Immediate Hypersensitivity, 1973. Courtesy of North Holland Publishing.)

cytes of a nonallergic individual with serum from an allergic patient; then the test is carried out as described. Currently this test is time-consuming and expensive and impractical for routine clinical use.

Eosinophil Count

In allergic rhinitis, from 20 to 30 percent eosinophils up to 70 to 90 percent may be observed in an irregular distribution in nasal mucus. In infectious sinusitis many bacteria and neutrophils are visible with relatively rare eosinophils. In vasomotor rhinitis one sees mostly epithelial cells, much mucus, and relatively few neutrophils or eosinophils.

Skin Window Eosinophil Response

The anterior surface of the forearm is scrubbed with iodine and alcohol and dried. Skin is abraded to the prickle cell layer. One drop of suspected allergen is dropped on the abraded area, which is then covered with a glass slide 30 mm square. Micropore tape and elastic bandage secure the windows. After 24 hours the slides are removed and examined for eosinophils. The control window (prepared using saline) usually contains less than 2 percent eosinophils. A positive test window has a 3 percent increase in eosinophils, or greater.

Environmental Control

Removal of sources of household inhalant allergens is the single most effective diagnostic and therapeutic measure in the management of allergic diseases. House dust control measures are described below. Obviously, improvement in allergic symptoms upon removal of a feather pillow from a feather-sensitive child constitutes a good diagnostic test and treatment. Similarly, symptomatic improvement upon removal of a household pet, such as a cat, dog, guinea pig, or rabbit, confirms the specific diagnosis of dander hypersensitivity.

Food elimination diets are diagnostic methods for establishing specific foods as causes of symptoms; they are discussed later with the subject of food allergy.

HOUSE DUST ALLERGY. More effective than any other procedure in relieving the symptoms due to house dust is the removal of its various sources in the home. The bedroom, particularly, must be made as dust-free as possible. More time is spent breathing the air of this room than any other. In fact, a child spends close to 12 out of 24 hours in this one room. Since much of the other half of the child's life is spent out of doors or at school, where there is no contact with house dust, the problem centers largely on the bedroom.

The chief sources of house dust are mattresses, box springs, upholstered-furniture, pillows, and stuffed toys containing kapok or cotton linters. These two substances and a tiny mite that they harbor are the most important contributors to house dust. The mite can also be found on the mattress surface and the bed frame and under the bed.

Woolen rugs, hair pads, feathers, down, and the hair, dander, and saliva of pets can also be troublesome additions to house dust. Dust particles float in the air and are not easily visible, except when a shaft of sunlight happens to reveal them. When breathed into the nose of a house-dust-sensitive patient, these particles can cause swelling of the mucous membrane, mucus production, and nasal discharge, ie, nasal allergy. In the lung the same process may cause asthma. House dust is related to lint and to what is in the vacuum cleaner or carpet sweeper, but has nothing to do with dirt or soil. Such outside dust is not usually allergenic.

In preparing a dust-controlled bedroom the following steps should be taken:

1. The bed should have a simple metal or wooden frame. An upholstered couch or sofa or headboard will not do. If a second bed is in the room, it must also be prepared as will be described, even though it is not in use.

2. The mattress should be made of either rubber, polyurethane foam, or other synthetic material. Otherwise it must be encased in a recommended encasing,* not an ordinary plastic one, since they usually develop splits. If a box spring is used, it also must be encased if it contains felted cotton, linters, or kapok. If the mattress rests on a pallet (plywood covered by a little upholstery), remove the upholstery and place the encased mattress on the bare plywood.

3. Remove all upholstered furniture, stuffed toys, and feather or kapok pillows from the room. Rubber pillows or those stuffed with Dacron or other synthetic fiber should be used on the bed and need not be encased. A toy stuffed with similar material may also be in the room.

* *Obtainable through Allergen-Proof Encasing, 1450 E. 363rd St., Eastlake, Ohio 44094; in Canada, 325 Devonshire, Windsor, Ontario.*

4. Cotton, rayon, or synthetic fiber blankets are best, but woolen blankets are usually also tolerated. They may be used unless otherwise directed. Woolen rugs and hair rugpads are apt to be more troublesome. As soon as possible they should be replaced with linoleum or small washable cotton mats. Cotton or synthetic fiber rugs and rubber rugpads are more difficult to keep clean but are also permitted.

5. Comforters or quilts, if used, must be stuffed with Dacron or some other synthetic fiber, not kapok or cotton.

6. Close and then *permanently seal* all furnace pipe outlets leading into the room. Otherwise the room will become filled with dust-laden air during the operation of the furnace. An electric heater may be used to heat the room if necessary.

7. Remove heavy drapes and other dust catchers. The entire room should have a thorough initial cleaning from top to bottom. Include the moldings, lights, shelves, closets, and walls. Then keep the room dust-free with thorough weekly cleaning. Especially vacuum the mattress surface, the bed frame, and under the bed.

8. Do not allow the patient to nap or sleep elsewhere unless the bed has been prepared as above. A couch, sofa, or upholstered headboard cannot be properly encased and is therefore not permitted. If the patient is confined to bed by illness, do not bring in extra kapok or feather pillows. He should remain in his own dust-free bedroom, not move to his parent's bedroom or a livingroom sofa. When he travels, remember to take along his own pillow or an encasing.

9. The child's playroom should be as dust-free as his bedroom.

If a child is allergic to a pet, it is essential that it not be allowed in the house. If he is not allergic to the pet, it should be kept out of his bedroom, or even better out of the house, since otherwise the likelihood of his becoming sensitized is greatly increased.

The improvement that follows attention to house dust in the bedroom can, if necessary, be increased by changes along similar lines in other rooms frequented by the child. Feather or kapok pillows and old upholstered furniture may be especially troublesome. *The above precautions should be continued for many years even though symptoms are absent.*

References

Bullock JD, Bodenbender JG, Deamer WC, Frick OL: Skin window eosinophil response in house dust allergy. J Allergy 48:153, 1971

Gleich GJ, Larson JB, Jones RT, Baer H: Measurement of potency of allergy extracts by their inhibitory capacities in the radioallergensorbent test. J Allergy Clin Immunol 53:158, 1974

Jones RS: Assessment of respiratory function in the asthmatic child. Br J Med 2:972, 1966

King TP, Norman PS, Lichtenstein LM: Isolation and characterization of allergens from ragweed pollen. IV. Biochemistry 6:1992, 1967

Lichtenstein LM, Norman PS, Winkenwerder WL: Clinical and in vitro studies on the role of immunotherapy in ragweed hayfever. Am J Med 44:514, 1968

McFadden ER Jr: The chronicity of acute attacks of asthma—mechanical and therapeutic implications. J Allergy Clin Immunol 56:18, 1975

Parker CD, Bilbo RE, Reed CE: Methacholine aerosol as test for bronchial asthma. Arch Intern Med 115:452, 1965

Polgar CG, Promadhat V: Pulmonary Function Testing in Children: Techniques and Standards. Philadelphia, WB Saunders, 1971, p 87

Wide L, Bennich H, Johansson SGO: Diagnosis of allergy by an in vitro test for allergen antibodies. Lancet 2:1105, 1967

Wright BM, McKerrow CB: Maximum expiratory flow rate as a measure of ventilatory capacity. Br Med J 2:1041, 1959

ALLERGIC RHINITIS

Allergic rhinitis is the simplest and most clear-cut form of allergy. When it is due to a specific pollen like ragweed, it is used as the clinical experimental model of allergic disease for the testing of new pharmacologic and other modalities of treatment. Allergic rhinitis may be seasonal (hay fever) or perennial or a mixture of the two. It affects 10 percent of the population.

The nose has three primary functions: to filter large particles from the air and to warm and moisten the air, as well as the olfactory or smell function. Nasal linings are under autonomic nervous control, with the sympathetics causing constriction and cooling, while cholinergics cause vasodilatation and warming. In patients with allergic rhinitis, recumbency increases nasal congestion because of hydrostatic pressure increase; exercise causes nasal vasoconstriction.

The mechanism of allergic rhinitis is well understood, and it serves as a model for allergic diseases in general. An allergen such as a pollen grain enters the nasal passages; the allergen is extracted by the nasal mucus and absorbed. In the nasal submucosa mast cells coated with IgE antibodies react with the absorbed allergen to cause the release of mediators, such as histamine, SRS-A, and ECF-A. These cause increased vascular permeability, itching and mucus secretion, and eosinophil infiltration into the area. Histamine appears to be the main mediator, in that many of the effects can be blocked by prior treatment with antihistaminic drugs, although their effect is not complete. Histologically there is marked edema of the nasal mucosa connective tissue, with large numbers of eosinophils and prominent mucosal goblet cells. The basement membrane is thickened. However, Connell found destruction of the basement membrane during the pollen season and suggested that the increased permeability allowed more allergen to reach the subepithelial mast cells, thus aggravating the clinical picture. He termed this heightened sensitivity the priming effect. It took several months for these damaged basement membranes to heal, after which the membranes became less sensitive to the pollens.

The symptoms of allergic rhinitis include itching and sneezing, increased nasal congestion or stuffiness, and a clear watery discharge. These nasal symptoms are associated with itching of the soft palate and the eyes, with excessive tearing and conjunctival injection. There is frequently a nasal quality to the speech; the child may have a postnasal drip that causes him to cough or to develop hoarseness and morning nausea. Sleep may be disturbed, with mouth breathing, snoring, and an occasional complaint of sore throat in the morning. The child may have peculiar mannerisms to relieve the nasal itching, eg, nose rubbing, the "allergic salute" in which the nose is rubbed upward with the palm of the hand, or unusual grimacing. If the symptoms are severe there may be associated systemic symptoms such as fatigue, irritability, depression or malaise, anorexia, or abdominal discomfort, which may have been the origin of the term hay fever, although there is no actual change in temperature. Children may also complain of itching in the ear, or "popping" as the Eustachian tube becomes edematous and intermittently blocked.

On physical examination the nasal mucosa is usually pale or bluish and swollen; there may be a profuse, watery discharge that may excoriate the skin of the upper lip. If there is concomitant infection the nasal discharge may be yellowish or greenish, in which case the nasal mucosa would appear red and injected. The conjunctivae may be red and the eyelids swollen, with excessive tearing. There is often a typical allergic facies in such a child, with pale skin suggesting anemia and allergic "shiners" caused by marked infraorbital edema. Across the lower third of the nose a transverse nasal crease may be observed from repeated allergic salutes; this takes about 2 years to develop. The tonsils and adenoids are frequently markedly enlarged, and in children with a previous tonsillectomy and adenoidectomy the adenoids will be seen to have grown back, sometimes with a string of mucus attached. The maxillary sinuses may be tender from secondary infection. The eardrums may appear congested, with absent landmarks due to secondary secretory otitis (p. 969). Cervical lymph nodes are not generally enlarged unless there has been secondary infection.

Allergens Associated with Allergic Rhinitis

The clinical picture of allergic rhinitis may occur only in certain seasons due to pollens or mold spores in the air, or it may be perennial due to a daily inhalant exposure such as house dust or animal dander. Plants pollinate at definite seasons that vary with regional location. Plants that pollinate primarily by wind currents disseminate huge amounts of light-weight pollen into the air. Such plants rarely have colored flowers. Plants with flowers usually pollinate via insects, and the color and perfume are required to attract the insects; their pollen is heavy and sticky, to stick to the insect bodies, and thus their pollens rarely cause allergic rhinitis. Wind-borne grass and weed pollens may carry for many miles; thus pollen exposure in a certain locale may be impossible to avoid.

Tree pollens are generally heavier and do not carry as far; therefore the trees in the immediate surroundings are of more allergenic importance to the patient.

Mold spores of saprophytic fungi occur in seasons when there is decaying vegetation and proper moisture conditions, such as in the spring and late fall. In areas of grain harvest, *Alternaria* and *Hormodendrum* predominate on the harvested grain in autumn; thus the mold season follows the ragweed season in the Midwest. The mold-sensitive patient may experience symptoms in places of high mold concentrations, such as barns with mold growing on hay, damp basements, and on a lawn after mowing because of mold growing in the soil underneath the grass, although the patient may not be grass-pollen-sensitive.

House dust is a major inhalant antigen that comes from decaying vegetable or animal matter, commonly from mattresses, upholstery, and rugs. A predominant major antigen in house dust is the house dust mite, *Dermatophagoides pteronyssinus* and *farinae,* which live on moist human scales and are found most commonly in bedding. Mites grow optimally at 80 percent humidity and 25 C temperature, but they can flourish over a wide range of humidity and temperature.

Animal antigens are of special importance for children because of their close contact with pets. Most important are the antigens in the animal dander from epithelial shedding and saliva, especially from dogs and cats. The insoluble nature of animal hair makes this a rather poor antigen, but the dander proteins from skin and secretions are most important. These may become a major component of house dust in a home with pets. All fur- or feather-bearing pets such as guinea pigs, rabbits, hamsters, gerbils, rats, mice, and birds are sources of such problems. Once a child becomes sensitive to the dander of one animal, he is apparently much more liable to become sensitive to danders of other animals. This is seen in experimental laboratory workers who, as a result of an occupational exposure to such animals, may develop respiratory allergy that can preclude them from continuing their work. Often such persons have a childhood history of cat or dog sensitivity. Cat, horse, and guinea-pig danders are highly allergenic, often causing 4+ skin tests. However, a 1+ skin test result to dog dander in a family where there is a dog is of much more significance than a 4+ cat dander test in a family where there is no cat. This point must be emphasized to patients and their families.

Foods can sometimes cause respiratory allergic symptoms and should be checked for if pollens, house dust, animal danders, and molds do not appear to be implicated in the patient's problems. There may be nonspecific nasal irritants such as tobacco smoke, perfumes, and newspaper ink that trigger nasal congestion and sneezing and are interpreted by allergic patients to be specific allergens.

Diagnosis

A history of the typical symptoms, seasonal relationships, and exposures to the possible precipitating antigens is the most important diagnostic measure. Examination of the nose during symptoms shows the clear watery discharge and pale, bluish, edematous mucosa that confirms the historical findings. A nasal smear may be markedly positive for eosinophils, but these may be obscured by secondary invasion of neutro-

phils during infection. Blood eosinophilia may range from 300 to 800 eosinophils per cubic millimeter or 4 to 11 percent of the differential. Skin tests by both scratch and intradermal methods with a panel of pollens, household inhalants, animal danders, and molds are generally useful in defining the specific allergens. Positive skin tests must be correlated with the history to sort out which ones are relevant to the patient's problem. Some physicians suggest confirmatory conjunctival tests with suspected allergen, but these are difficult to do in children; others advocate nasal inhalation challenge with suspected allergen to confirm the skin tests. However, the priming effect (or lack of it) may influence such nasal provocative tests. Recently, RAST and leukocyte histamine release tests have been introduced as confirmatory in vitro tests to substantiate the significance of positive skin tests. These offer a potent addition to specific allergic diagnosis.

Differential Diagnosis

Noisy breathing and excessive nasal discharge may be due to obstruction such as those caused by choanal atresia, congential syphilis, or foreign objects in the nostrils. Toddlers and school age children may have recurrent upper respiratory infections, but in these children an allergic mechanism should be sought for and ruled out if possible. Some children with cystic fibrosis have nasal obstruction, purulent discharge, and mouth breathing, and children with immunodeficiency diseases may have recurrent upper respiratory infections, usually with a purulent yellowish or greenish nasal discharge. Children with IgA deficiency with impairment of the local mucosal defense may have recurrent bacterial infections in the nose, ears, and sinuses. In older children tumors such as nasal pharyngeal angiofibroma and adenopapillomas of the larynx should be ruled out. Nasal mastocytosis occasionally occurs wherein there is easy lability of mast cells and an increased number of such cells that discharge upon minimal external stimuli. Chronic rhinitis may be complicated by chronic use of nose drops of the decongestant sympathomimetic type.

Complications

Complications of chronic allergic rhinitis may be recurrent infections of the nose, ears, and sinuses secondary to blockage of the orifices caused by edema. Chronic occlusion of the venous sinuses of the nose may lead to secondary changes resulting in the typical allergic facies, with a high palate and orthodontic deformities. These may be aggravated by chronic finger sucking as the child tries to relieve his palatal itching. Nasal speech and possible serous otitis with damping of the hearing often results in speech problems. The child never hears sounds correctly and cannot phonate properly, and therefore he learns incorrectly. He may never understand the complete meaning of words, and this may retard his school progress. With proper allergic therapy these conditions may sometimes be reversed.

Treatment

Children with mild seasonal rhinitis over a limited period and children with occasional intermittent acute symptoms from exposure to danders, house dust, or molds in certain situations, as well as children with mild nonprogressive perennial symptoms, may be treated with antihistamic drugs. Often an antihistaminic may be effective for several weeks or months and then appear to lose its effectiveness. Switching to another antihistaminic will often relieve symptoms. The physician should become familiar with at least one of each major group of antihistamines, such as the ethanolamines (diphenhydramine, Benadryl), the ethylenediamines (tripelennamine, Pyribenzamine), each 0.5 mg/kg, and the alkylamines (chlorpheniramine, Chlor-Trimeton), 0.1 mg/kg. Antihistamines may have side effects such as drowsiness or depression that may limit their usefulness in children because of the resultant lack of concentration and difficulty with school work. Sometimes switching to an antihistamine of a different class will give better results. A patient with severe allergic rhinitis may continue to have symptoms even when taking antihistamines, because the concentration in the tissues may be insufficient to counter all the histamine and other mediators locally released by the antigen–antibody reaction.

The α-adrenergic sympathomimetic drugs, especially phenylephrine (Neo-Synephrine) (0.25 mg/kg), cause vasoconstriction of the mucosal vessels and are useful in short-term treatment of allergic rhinitis and vasomotor rhinitis. However, there is considerable rebound, and chronic use of these agents leads to rhinitis medicamentosa. Oral use of α-adrenergic sympathomimetics is considerably less efficient; however, they are commonly combined with antihistamines, often in a timed-release capsule.

Cromolyn sodium prevents the release of mediators from mast cells. In Europe, variable results have been reported with cromolyn in the treatment of seasonal allergic rhinitis. A commercial nasal inhaler for cromolyn powder is reported to be quite successful. Trials in the United States are not sufficiently far along to recommend this product.

Topical nasal corticosteroids such as aerosolized dexamethasone are useful for allergic rhinitis. Very small amounts of corticosteroids are needed for this local control, and fewer side effects occur than with systemic steroids. They have been used for relatively short pollen seasons, such as at the height of the ragweed season in the eastern United States. However, long-term use in chronic rhinitis should be discouraged, especially in children, because systemic absorption of dexamethasone can cause adrenal suppression. Beclomethasone and flunisolide, which are not as readily absorbed, have been successful in controlling allergic rhinitis as well as asthma. Oral corticosteroids produce dramatic results in acute episodes of allergic rhinitis, but its mild symptoms do not warrant chronic use of such systemic corticosteroid because of their possible side effects. They are not viewed as appropriate therapy.

Immunotherapy with appropriate allergens that by history and skin tests are important for the patient's allergic symptoms is the only true prophylactic measure available for treatment of this condition, other than allergen removal. Immunotherapy with adequate dosage is often quite successful in children with allergic rhinitis. We aim for a full pollen season with no symptoms; attainment of this goal often occurs within 3 years of instituting perennial therapy. For short pollen seasons, such as ragweed in the eastern United States, preseasonal therapy is more commonly practiced: injections for 2 months before the pollen season and continuing during the pollen season, then injections ceasing with the first frost.

The most difficult problem for the pediatrician in managing allergic rhinitis is to know when he can follow the child with antihistaminics and vasoconstrictors and when a more complete allergic work-up is required. Boyden has suggested that children in the following categories be worked up more intensively for allergy and that subsequent food and inhalant elimination and hyposensitization should supplement symptomatic medication: (1) infants with allergic rhinitis who have frequent colds and otitis media as complications; often such children respond well to certain food elimination diets and prophylactic environmental control, even though allergy skin tests may be negative; (2) children with seasonal hay fever that is not easily controlled with short courses of antihistamines, who become drowsy, or who require frequent changes of antihistamines; (3) children who experience increased symptoms each year or who develop perennial symptoms; (4) children with seasonal hay fever who develop asthma or early signs of wheezing and cough; and (5) older children with perennial nasal allergy, complaints of sinus problems, or constant colds. Such children may in addition have marked inhalant allergy and multiple food allergies; they may have trouble concentrating in school; they may be hyperactive or sluggish and have irritable dispositions. They may develop nasal polyps in adolescence, if their conditions go uncontrolled. Immunotherapy and a food elimination diet may be helpful in such situations.

Prognosis

Immunotherapy may take several years to effect definite improvement or clearing of the allergic rhinitis. Rackemann found that in hay fever patients treated preseasonally with ragweed extract, if it was begun during childhood, 20 percent were cured by the age of 25 years; but in the majority of patients symptoms recurred at least in mild degree until age 50 or older. In a 5-year study of farm children with allergic rhinitis, Smith found that less than 10 percent were symptom-free, 80 percent had moderate rhinitis, and 15 percent had severe rhinitis. In a similar study of grade school students, Freeman and Johnson found that after 4 years 20 percent had cleared and 25 percent had become worse. However, it is extremely rare for a patient with allergic rhinitis who has been treated with immunotherapy to develop asthma after 6 to 12 months of treatment. This is the most powerful argument for immunotherapy in the treatment of allergic rhinitis. It has been estimated by allergists in private practice that from 22 to 75 percent of children with allergic rhinitis, if untreated, subsequently go on to develop asthma. However, in several epidemiologic studies only 3 to 5 percent of such children on immunotherapy develop asthma during the period of the study. Allergists probably see the more highly allergic patients and the more severe cases of hay fever, and these are more likely to develop asthma.

References

Boyden MS: Nasal Allergy. In Speer F, Dockhorn RJ (eds): Allergy and Immunology in Childhood. Springfield, Ill, Charles C Thomas, 1973 p 501

Connell JT: Quantitative intranasal pollen challenge. III. The priming effect in allergic rhinitis. J Allergy 43:33, 1969

Gibson CJ, Maberly DJ, Lal S, Ali MM, Butter AG: Double-blind crossover trial comparing nasal beclomethasone diprioprionate and placebo in perennial rhinitis. Br Med J 4:503, 1974

Miyamoto T: Purification and characterization of allergens: house dust. In Yamamura Y, et al (eds): Allergology. Amsterdam, Excerpta Medica, 1974.

Rackemann F, Edwards M: Asthma in children. A followup study of 688 patients after an interval of 20 years. N Engl J Med 246:858, 1952

Voorhorst R, Spieksma FTM, Varekamp H: House-Dust Atopy and the House-Dust Mite. Leiden, Stafleu's Scientific, 1969

BRONCHIAL ASTHMA (See Chap. 28)

Asthma has been defined as recurrent episodes of wheezing or dyspnea characterized by a significant increase in resistance to air flow. Either spontaneously or following treatment, periods of complete or almost complete freedom from symptoms may occur, accompanied by a substantial decrease in resistance to air flow.

Symptoms and Signs

Asthma usually manifests as attacks of increasing severity of airway obstruction that may, in milder form, be only some chest tightening or cough and prolonged expiration. As the attack worsens, wheezing and prolonged expiration increase, and rhonchi become audible, with increasing cough and sputum. Dyspnea may become apparent, accompanied by hyperinflation, inspiratory wheezing, and use of accessory muscles of respiration. The patient usually becomes apprehensive, restless, anxious, and fatigued. As he proceeds into respiratory failure, the wheezing may become less audible, and there may be decreased breath sounds that may be misinterpreted as improvement in the patient's status, when in reality the condition may proceed rapidly to fatality.

Between attacks the patient may appear symptomatically to be quite well; this is characteristic of the reversibility of asthma. Pulmonary function tests that measure

the resistance of large airways may be completely normal in the free interval between attacks; however, it is now being recognized with more sophisticated pulmonary function tests, especially those that measure small-airway resistance, that there is some impairment between attacks. Mucous plugs may be expelled from the large airways promptly following medication for an attack, but the minute mucus plugs in the smaller bronchi may take many weeks to clear. Asthma may be classified into various types, such as extrinsic, intrinsic, mixed, exercise-induced, and aspirin-sensitive types.

Extrinsic asthma is the type most commonly seen in children; it represents the classic form of type I immediate hypersensitivity in which allergens give rise to IgE antibodies that in turn react on the surface of mast cells to cause the release of mediators such as histamine and SRS-A to cause bronchospasm, bronchial mucosal edema, and excessive bronchial mucus secretion. The common allergens are pollens, house dust, animal danders, molds, and foods, the last more commonly in children. This type of asthma usually starts in childhood or in the young adult years and may last throughout life or may abate in the later years or decades.

Intrinsic asthma is more commonly seen in adults. Attacks of intrinsic asthma are usually associated with infections; there is often copious mucus, especially of the purulent type. IgE antibodies are not readily demonstrable, and there is little correlation with skin tests and known allergens; however, many of these patients have high total IgE levels, which might indicate allergy to some as yet unknown antigens, possibly some bacteria or viruses. Pure intrinsic asthma is rather rare in children, although there are some who have attacks only with respiratory infection. This is more common in the infantile and early toddler years and generally has a good prognosis when no other IgE-mediated allergy is demonstrable. Such infants are often diagnosed as having "asthmatic bronchitis" or "bronchiolitis." This has recently been associated with virus infections, such as respiratory syncytial virus and parainfluenza virus infection, and possibly *Mycoplasma*. Intrinsic asthma generally does not respond well to immunotherapy, and corticosteroids are often necessary for control.

Mixed asthma is more common in children in whom there is an infectious component, especially as a trigger mechanism that is superimposed on an extrinsic IgE-mediated allergy. This situation may persist into adulthood.

Exercise-induced asthma occurs in a small group of children and adults who have asthma after running or heavy exercise. Immediate bronchodilation may develop and last several minutes, but if exercise is continued there is progressively increased airway resistance that impairs the efficiency of the patient's performance. In many cases sufficient adrenalin may be produced during exercise to counter the bronchoconstriction, but upon conclusion of the exercise, severe bronchospasm may occur within 5 minutes. IgE antibodies are not demonstrable in these patients. Curiously, however, cromolyn sodium appears to be quite effective in controlling exercise-induced symptoms; this may implicate histamine and mast cells in the pathogenesis. Some patients have extremely hyperreactive airways, possibly due to a cholinergic–adrenergic imbalance with markedly active irritant receptors. Attacks are triggered by nonallergic stimuli such as weather or temperature changes, by smog or air pollutants, by strong fumes such as paint or gasoline, or by emotional disturbances. These patients are especially sensitive to the methacholine inhalation challenge test.

Aspirin asthma is a particularly severe form of intrinsic asthma that usually occurs in the middle or late decades and is only rarely seen in children. It is often associated in the triad of severe asthma, nasal polyposis, and aspirin sensitivity. Within minutes to several hours after aspirin ingestion, such patients experience severe rhinorrhea, followed by flushing, wheezing, dyspnea, and cyanosis within minutes, and occasionally vomiting or nausea. This form of asthma carries a high degree of mortality in older adults. The mechanism is unknown, but may be pharmacologic rather than immunologic.

Pathology

Following death from status asthmaticus, the pathologic findings are characteristic. The lungs are hyperinflated and pale in color; the surface may have emphysematous blebs, and occasionally even a tear may be seen if a pneumothorax has occurred. On the cut surface numerous mucous plugs exude from the bronchi; entire casts may be extruded with gentle pressure. On microscopic examination the most striking feature is the thickening of the basement membrane and the convolutions in the epithelial surface secondary to spasm of the hypertrophied smooth muscles surrounding the bronchi. Heavy mucus with some plugs may be obvious, and there is often eosinophilic infiltration of the submucosa. In patients who die from status asthmaticus there is a reduction in the number of mast cells in the bronchi. This suggests degranulation of the mast cells during the attack of status asthmaticus.

Diagnosis

The history is the chief tool for diagnosing the typical asthmatic attack. Initially a patient may experience nasal symptoms such as itching, sneezing, or rhinorrhea and conjunctival itching; subsequently he may develop some tickling in this throat, mild cough, and tightening of his chest. The coughing increases and wheezing becomes apparent. The child is more comfortable sitting up leaning forward; he may develop grunting respiration and occasionally chest or abdominal pain. The child is usually pale, but cyanosis occurs only in severe attacks. With coughing, vomiting may occur, and sometimes this clears sufficient tracheal and bronchial mucus that the attack may abate temporarily.

On physical examination the chest is hyperinflated and hyperresonant to percussion. There are prominent expiratory wheezes, and as the attack progresses inspiratory wheezes develop. Musical rales may appear later, and areas of atelectasis and pneumonia may cause percussion dullness. The nose and eyes are often injected and have watery discharge. The child is pale, has a rapid respiratory rate, and is restless; as the attack continues, panic may even take over, with superimposed hyperventilation compounding the attack. As the attack proceeds and the child tires and enters respiratory failure, cyanosis increases rapidly, but the breath sounds and wheezing may abate somewhat. In fact, a silent chest may be a most grave sign. With treatment, as the attack subsides and the color improves, the wheezing may actually increase temporarily, as the air is getting through to formerly closed segments of lung.

Between attacks the child may appear normal, although the chest may have an increased anteroposterior diameter if he has chronic asthma. On auscultation the lungs may sound quite clear, although on deep expiration some rhonchi may be heard. A child with chronic asthma may have growth retardation, even if he is not on corticosteroids, because this chronic illness interferes with nutrition and appetite.

Laboratory Studies

During an attack the chest roentgenogram shows overinflation, with flat diaphragms and hyperlucency of the lung fields. There may be patchy areas of infiltrate or atelectasis secondary to mucus plugging of small or medium airways; on occasion, an entire lobe is collapsed with density. Between attacks the x-ray may show only increased bronchial markings and some hyperlucency. As a complication, pneumomediastinum or pneumothorax may occur during an attack. Air may dissect along the perivascular sheaths toward the hilar regions and substernally, and up into the neck in pneumomediastinum; or a peripheral air sac may rupture with a pneumothorax, causing lung compression. The white count is normal, but a leukocytosis may be present during the attack. An eosinophilia of 5 to 20 percent may be present in quiescent or active asthma.

Lung function studies are not often possible during an attack; however, some children can be followed with a peak expiratory flow rate (PEFR), and the course of therapy may thus be monitored. Following the attack the pulmonary function studies as described earlier will give valuable information as to the child's respiratory status. In the discussion on treatment of status asthmaticus, the blood gases will be further discussed.

In all children with chronic pulmonary problems, a sweat chloride test should be performed to rule out cystic fibrosis, which can masquerade as asthma or other respiratory illnesses. There have been reports of elevated sweat chlorides in some patients with asthma, and some studies indicate that children with cystic fibrosis more often have the complication of asthma than is the case in the general population. The relationship between these two illnesses is still under study.

Differential Diagnosis

In infants and toddlers the chief differential with wheezing is bronchiolitis, which in many instances may go on to develop into asthma; this accounts for the intermediate term asthmatic bronchiolitis. There may be a prodrome of fever, cough, and malaise, with subsequent wheezing that is often inspiratory and does not respond to epinephrine injection. Rales and rhonchi are prominent, although the respiratory distress may not be as severe. There is usually a leukocytosis with bacterial origin or a lyphocytosis with viral origin. Eosinophils are not prominent in either the blood or nasal smear. These attacks are usually viral in origin, especially respiratory syncytial virus, parainfluenza virus, and *Mycoplasma pneumoniae*, although they may be complicated by *Haemophilus influenzae* and pneumococci that may lead to pneumonia. For the young child with recurrent episodes of bronchiolitis or frequent respiratory tract infections, a search for inhalant and food sensitivities should be made, as well as an evelution of immune status, especially for IgA deficiencies. Croup (laryngotracheobronchitis) may be associated with wheezing, but more commonly there is an inspiratory stridor, a barking cough and hoarseness, and often a prominent red epiglottis from which *Haemophilus influenzae* may be isolated, although it is more commonly of viral origin.

Cystic fibrosis must be excluded in any child who has recurrent respiratory infection. A sweat chloride of greater than 60 mEq/liter and a sodium greater than 70 mEq/liter are diagnostic of cystic fibrosis (p. 995).

A foreign body in the trachea, bronchi, or esophagus that causes bronchial compression may cause wheezing and chronic respiratory distress. Usually the symptoms are quite constant, and epinephrine fails to relieve the problem. If the object is radiopaque, an x-ray can locate the foreign body and determine its nature. Children often, however, aspirate nonopaque foreign bodies such as peanuts, beans, or plastic that are not readily visible on x-ray exam but may show a shift of the heart and mediastinum away from the obstructed side.

Heart disease or vascular rings can compress the trachea or bronchi sufficiently to cause wheezing that is generally constant and is not relieved by epinephrine. Tracheal and esophageal compression may cause choking and cyanosis (especially when feeding), dyspnea, stridor, and difficulty in swallowing. X-ray examination showing the air outline of the trachea may show compression of the esophagus, as may a barium swallow; this should point in the direction of such a vascular anomaly.

In children, other obstructions of the respiratory tract may occur, such as laryngeal or bronchial stenosis; they may be congenital or occasionally may be due to burns, such as with lye. Furthermore, neoplasms in the mediastinum and enlarged mediastinal lymph nodes, possibly secondary to tuberculosis, may encroach upon the trachea and bronchi and cause wheezing.

Immunodeficiency diseases with recurrent respiratory infections associated with coughing and wheezing should be ruled out with quantitative determination of immunoglobulin levels and an assessment of cellular immune status.

Hypersensitivity pneumonitis is more common in adults, especially from occupation exposure to inhaled organic dusts and proteins, eg, farmer's lung from moldy hay, bagassosis from sugar cane residue, and conjunctivitis from *Bacillus subtilis* found in detergent manufacture. However, such diseases are being recognized in children more often; one of the first described was pigeon-breeder's disease. The disease often presents with wheezing and coughing that simulate asthma; but it usually includes fever and malaise, and if it is chronic it may include weight loss, clubbing, and even cyanosis. Parakeets or canaries in a household provide sufficient bird protein to cause inhalation hypersensitivity and give an insidious slow form of this illness. It is associated with precipitating antibodies to bird proteins and also a cellular immune component. Avoidance of the offending antigen, once it is discovered, usually results in reversal of the condition, which may be aided by corticosteroid therapy.

Complications

STATUS ASTHMATICUS. By definition, an attack of asthma that does not respond to three consecutive injections of epinephrine 1:1,000 subcutaneously constitutes status asthmaticus, which generally requires hospitalization. The patient is anxious, pale, and restless and has severe wheezing and often cyanosis. Vomiting and abdominal pain and distension may occur. Dehydration may result from lack of fluid intake, perspiration, and vomiting. In a severe asthma attack there is initial respiratory alkalemia from hyperventilation. With increasing respiratory difficulty, CO_2 retention and respiratory acidemia occur; later metabolic acidemia is superimposed as lactic acid and ketones accumulate from starvation and muscular effort. Ultimately respiratory failure develops, breath sounds decrease, and extreme restlessness occurs, later to be superseded by stupor, unconsciousness, and death. Changes in blood gases reflect the clinical course. In the early stages $PaCO_2$ may be decreased due to hyperventilation, with pH normal or slightly increased. PaO_2 may be slightly reduced. With progression, $PaCO_2$ rises, pH falls, and PaO_2 is reduced. Respiratory failure occurs when the $PaCO_2$ reaches 75 to 80 mm Hg or more, or the pH is less than 7.2, at which point emergency measures such as intubation and assisted ventilation must be taken.

As bronchi become plugged with mucus, patchy or lobular atelectasis may ensue, with an increase in arteriovenous pulmonary shunting. In one study the normal shunting was less than 7 percent in normal patients, whereas in patients with atelectasis there was a mean of 17 percent shunting.

With moderate asthma attacks pulmonary vascular resistance and pulmonary artery pressure increase slightly. Secondary to the blood gas changes in status asthmaticus, marked pulmonary vasoconstriction with right heart enlargement may occur. Cardiac arrhythmias may occur as a result of catecholamine treatment, and even ventricular fibrillation may occur.

PNEUMOMEDIASTINUM AND PNEUMO-THORAX. Pneumomediastinum and pneumothorax are occasional serious complications of an asthma attack that usually occur in older children with severe chronic asthma. The sudden onset of severe air hunger, marked anxiety, and restlessness, with a hard brassy cough and chest or neck pain, should make one suspect this complication. Chest pain is usually not associated with an asthma attack; thus the presence of pain should alert one to the possibility of pneumomediastinum. Physical signs are absence of cardiac dullness from overlying air, subcutaneous crepitus, especially in the neck region, and increasing cyanosis. Occasionally a crunching sound is heard in synchrony with the heartbeat. There is apparently little relationship between the occurrence of pneumomediastinum and pneumothorax and the prognosis of asthma.

A chest roentgenogram confirms the diagnosis. In the anteroposterior view, air in the mediastinum may outline the medial borders of the lungs and the lateral borders of the heart and thymus. The air column may be seen in the fascial planes and subcutaneous areas of the neck in the prevertebral area. On lateral view, air may be seen in the anterior mediastinum displacing the heart and thymus backward. However, in this view mediastinal air may be confused with air in the pleural space and air in the distended lungs. In pneumothorax the pleural air may be generalized or localized, compressing the adjacent lung. A check-valve obstruction in the pleural opening may cause increased intrapleural pressure that can, if severe enough, further compress the lung and displace the heart and mediastinum to the opposite side. The pleural air shadow of uniform diminished density surrounds the collapsed opaque lung.

ATELECTASIS. In an asthma attack the thick, tenacious mucous hypersecretion results in multiple plugs of large, small, and medium airways, with collapse of the lung segment distal to the plug. Larger bronchi or even lobar bronchi may be obstructed, resulting in collapse of a whole lobule or even lobe with shift of the mediastinum.

PNEUMONIA. Atelectatic lung segments are open to bacterial infection and pneumonia; thus fever, purulent sputum, and wet sticky rales, with an increase in neutrophils on the blood and sputum smears, are signs of pneumonia. A chest roentgenogram should confirm the diagnosis, and the organism may be cultured from the sputum and treated appropriately with antibiotics.

RIGHT MIDDLE LUNG SYNDROME AND BRONCHIECTASIS. Recurrent atelectasis of the right middle lobe occurs because of the acute "takeoff" angle of the right middle lobe bronchus that makes this lobe particularly susceptible to mucus plugging during an asthma attack. A child with recurrent asthma, severe coughing and wheezing, and rales over the right lateral and posterior lung field should have a chest film, in which right middle lobe consolidation may be apparent with compensatory hyperinflation of the other two right lobes. Repeated infection of the atelectatic lung segments, especially the right middle lobe, often leads to chronic infection and saccular bronchiectasis that may be amenable only to surgical correction.

Treatment

The goal of treatment is the immediate and sustained reversal of bronchial smooth muscle spasm and reduction of bronchial mucosal edema and mucous secretion. Bronchodilators should be used early in the course of an attack, and these should be supplemented with general support measures such as oxygen and hydration, as well as reassurance to the patient.

EPINEPHRINE. Aqueous epinephrine 1:1,000, 0.01 ml/kg (0.3 ml/m^2) subcutaneously up to a maximal dose of 0.2 ml, promptly relaxes the bronchial smooth muscles, within minutes after subcutaneous injection and within 15 sec after aerosol inhalation. Epinephrine also stimulates α-adrenergic receptors, which constrict bronchial vessels, resulting in reduction of mucosal edema and possibly less mucus secretion. Most attacks of asthma will subside with the first epinephrine injection, but this dose may be repeated twice at 20-minute intervals and, if necessary, in 3 to 4 hours. Further repeated rapid injections of epinephrine may result in overdosage, with vomiting, pallor, headaches, sweating, arrhythmias, and eventually death by pulmonary edema from increased pulmonary capillary filtration pressure. Furthermore, subarachnoid hemorrage and hemiplegia have been reported from sudden hypertension.

SUSTAINED-ACTION SYMPATHOMIMETICS. Sus-Phrine (epinephrine 1:200 in thioglycollate) is a slowly absorbed suspension that acts over 6 to 12 hours. A dose of 0.005 ml/kg (0.125 ml/m^2) every 8 to 12 hours subcutaneously is useful for sustained action in children in whom there is immediate but unsustained effectiveness of aqueous epinephrine. About 25 percent of the epinephrine in Sus-Phrine is absorbed within minutes, and the rest is released slowly over a period of hours. Epinephrine in oil is now rarely used in pediatric practice. Terbutaline (Bricanyl), 0.25 mg by subcutaneous injection, has been approved for children over 12 years of age in the United States and is used routinely in younger children in Europe. This is primarily a β_2-adrenergic agonist that relieves bronchospasm dramatically but does not have the cardiostimulatory and vascular effects of epinephrine. It has a peak action within minutes, but lasts for 2 to 6 hours; it may replace epinephrine as the drug of choice in an asthma attack. Disadvantages of terbutaline are that it lacks α-adrenergic effect and there is little reduction of bronchial mucosal edema. Sulbutamol, another β_2-adrenergic agonist, has also been used in Europe for prolonged action, but it is not yet available in the United States.

ETHYLNOREPINEPHRINE. Ethylnorepinephrine (Bronkephrine), 0.02 ml/kg (0.5 ml/m^2) subcutaneously, is helpful in a child who is unable to tolerate epinephrine because of headaches, vomiting, or tachycardia. It can be used in the presence of hypertension, because it decreases the diastolic pressure, although there is a transient rise in systolic pressure. It can be repeated in 4 hours.

ISOPROTERENOL. This strong β-adrenergic agonist is used mostly as an inhalation aerosol but is also effective by the sublingual, intravenous, and rectal routes. It is rapidly absorbed from mucosal surfaces and lasts about 30 minutes, but it is rapidly inactivated in the sputum, thus making exact sublingual dosage difficult to determine in children. Isoproterenol 1:200 is aerosolized by pump nebulizers or positive-pressure ventilators such as the Maximist, Bird, or Bennett. The dosage of four drops in 2 ml normal saline for nebulization may be repeated every 4 to 6 hours.

Inhalers in which isoproterenol (0.075 mg) is delivered with each inhalation of Freon-propelled gas are rapidly effective and widely used in adults, but they are easily subject to abuse and are not advised for children. Overuse of inhaled isoproterenol may cause marked rebound bronchospasm that is refractory to other forms of treatment, the so-called locked lung syndrome. In such patients the bronchospasm improves only upon discontinuance of the use of inhaled isoproterenol.

Sudden death from cardiac arrest has repeatedly been observed in hypoxic patients given both isoproterenol and epinephrine. Patients have been found dead, still clutching the nebulizer. It has been suspected that there is an incompatibility of epinephrine and isoproterenol in patients with limited cardiac reserve, and in several cases death has been attributed to ventricular fibrillation.

Intravenous isoproterenol for severe status asthmaticus has dramatically reduced the number of such patients who require intubation and mechanical ventilation. An intravenous solution of isoproterenol, 10 μg/ml (0.5 mg Isuprel in 50 ml fluid), is given with a slow-infusion pump with an initial starting dose of 0.1 μg/kg/minute and increased at a rate of 0.1 μg/kg/minute every 15 minutes, as determined by Paco$_2$. Isoproterenol is increased until the Paco$_2$ begins to drop, or until there are changes in the heart rate or rhythm, which are being continuously monitored. Persistent arrhythmias or heart rate above 200 beats per minute are contraindications to the continuation of intravenous isoproterenol. Isoproterenol is most useful in children, in whom there is less likelihood of arrhythmias than in adults. Arterial blood gases are essential for monitoring the drug dosage, and it should be administered only where continuous cardiac monitoring is possible in an intensive care unit. Its mechanism of action appears to involve both its β_2-adrenergic activity as a bronchodilator and its β_1 action as a cardiac stimulant and pulmonary arterial vasodilator.

METHYLXANTHINES. Theophylline, theobromine, and caffeine block phosphodiesterases, especially those that catabolize cyclic AMP; this causes a cellular rise in cyclic AMP that in turn causes bronchial smooth muscle relaxation and inhibition of mediator release from the mast cells. Aminophylline (theophylline and ethylenediamine), in addition to being a bronchodilator, also decreases pulmonary vascular resistance and

increases renal blood flow and cardiac output. Intravenous aminophylline (4 mg/kg) may be given over a 30-minute period every 6 hours. With the currently increased availability of rapid assays of serum aminophylline concentrations and monitoring of theophylline blood levels, much higher doses may be given to reach the therapeutic levels of between 10 and 20 μg/ml. Since aminophylline is degraded at variable rates in different individuals, monitoring of plasma levels is desirable, if not mandatory. In some children 7 to 8 mg/kg are required to achieve a plasma concentration of 10 μg/ml or greater. In others, 4 mg/kg cause very high or toxic levels of 25 to 35 μg/ml, with vomiting, cardiac arrhythmias and arrest, hyperirritability, and convulsions. We anticipate that soon routine monitoring of intravenous aminophylline with plasma levels will become imperative. When a severely asthmatic child presents at an emergency room, it must be determined what his aminophylline intake has been over the previous 24 hours, so as to avoid overdosage and toxicity. Aminophylline is absorbed rapidly from the rectum and can be used in doses of 6 mg/kg every 6 hours. Suppositories are not recommended because absorption is variable.

DYPHYLLINE. Dyphylline (Neothylline), 250 mg/ml, is a soluble neutral derivative of theophylline for relatively painless intramuscular use. It has been effective as a singular injection of 4 mg/kg in children where intravenous infusion was not practical or necessary.

CORTICOSTEROIDS. Corticosteroids are useful in severe asthma; their effect is to reverse tissue damage and relieve inflammation. Steroids may reinforce the action of catecholamines by increasing cyclic AMP level, causing bronchorelaxation, but other mechanisms such as increasing vascular integrity and decreasing fibroblast proliferation are probably more important, because response to steroids occurs only 12 to 36 hours after administration. The usual suppressive dose of prednisone is 20 to 80 mg/day (2 mg/kg/24 hours); this can be lowered by 5 to 10 mg/day to a maintenance dosage of 5 to 10 mg. Although high initial doses may be required, we try to limit the duration to 7 to 10 days to prevent the serious adrenal insufficiency that occurs with prolonged corticosteroid administration. If a child has had corticosteroids during the previous year, it is imperative to again give steroids during severe asthma attacks, especially with status asthmaticus, or if other stressful situations are encountered such as major surgery or severe infection. Hydrocortisone (Solu-Cortef) 4 mg/kg intravenously every 2 to 4 hours or methylprednisolone (Solu-Medrol) 2 mg/kg at similar intervals will result in more rapid corticosteroid effect within 8 to 12 hours. If there is a family history of diabetes mellitus or if there has been exposure to tuberculosis, smallpox, or varicella, steroids may be used, but with great caution.

ATROPINE. The vagus nerve is the most powerful contributor to bronchospasm through cholinergic stimulation; this is blocked by atropine and other muscarinic drugs. Until the 1930s atropine was used, often with dramatic results. However, atropine fell into disrepute because a number of deaths occurred that were thought to be related to drying of bronchial mucous secretions by atropine. Recently there has been renewed interest in atropine, especially in its aerosolized form, for the reversal of bronchospasm of asthma. Because atropine action is short, prolonged-action forms are being developed, such as methylatropine and SCH-1000, which may soon find increasing topical usage for the treatment of asthma.

ANTIBIOTICS. Unless there are areas of atelectasis or consolidation, or yellowish or greenish mucus, we withhold antibiotic therapy. Fever and leukocytosis are not reliable indications of infection, as they occur with severe asthma alone. If infection does occur, the choice of antibiotics depends upon the type of suspected organism; for pneumococci, streptococci, and *H. influenzae* we prefer ampicillin or tetracycline.

SEDATIVES. Anxiety and irritability may be symptoms of hypoxia in asthma, as well as emotional distress; oxygen inhalation is indicated if hypoxia is present. Sedatives that depress the respiratory center and drive should be avoided, as they mask the signs of impending respiratory failure. Morphine and Demerol are contraindicated, except in those children who have been intubated and are on assisted ventilation. Ataractics, such as thorazine and hydroxyzine, have some mucus drying action and may occasionally be beneficial through their atropinelike activity. Chloral hydrate, 15 mg/kg every 6 hours, may occasionally be helpful.

IPECAC. In some instances induction of vomiting may dislodge mucous plugs during an acute attack; thus 5 ml of syrup of ipecac may be given and may be repeated once in 15 minutes, but no more than two doses should be given.

FLUIDS AND ELECTROLYTES. If an asthma attack is severe and prolonged, significant dehydration may occur from poor fluid intake and fluid loss from hyperventilation, perspiration, and vomiting. Simple fluid replacement with intravenous glucose and saline or water may give immediate results in the control of asthma. If acidemia is present, intravenous sodium bicarbonate, 2 mEq/kg by rapid infusion over 20 to 30 minutes, may produce dramatic effects; an additional 2 mEq/kg may be given over the next 2 hours, following which blood gases should be monitored hourly.

OXYGEN. Hypoxia is frequently noted during severe asthma; it is manifested by dyspnea, anxiety, and cyanosis. Rapid relief can often by obtained with oxygen administered by a plastic nasal cannula or Eliott-type open face mask at flow rates of 6 to 10 liters/minute. The inspired oxygen concentration achieved is variable, but usually these methods produce inspired oxygen concentrations of 35 to 40 percent. Arterial blood gases should be monitored hourly during severe status asthmaticus and several times a day as the patient is improving. Mist therapy was once used universally to liquefy airway secretions and mobilize mucus; however, it is now apparent that most of the fluid administered by nebulizer is absorbed in the laryngotracheal area and does not reach the bronchi to liquefy the mucus. Recently more reliance has been placed upon intravenous fluids and less upon mist therapy; however, mist reduces the water loss from hyperventilation in acute asthma and thus still has some therapeutic use.

The clinical criteria of respiratory failure proposed by Downes and associates are severe inspiratory retractions to absence of inspiratory breath sounds, generalized muscle weakness, decreased level of consciousness and response to pain, cyanosis in 40 percent inspired oxygen concentration. These are grave signs in status asthmaticus and require intubation and assisted ventilation. This program of therapy is outlined on p. 1550.

Management of Complications

In pneumomediastinum and pneumothorax treatment is directed toward relief of the asthma; intermittent positive-pressure breathing is contraindicated. Therapeutic response of the asthma to medication stops the flow of air into the mediastinum and permits absorption of the air over about 7 to 10 days. With conservative therapy almost all patients recover without complications. Occasionally extensive pneumonia or bilateral pneumothorax may complicate the picture. Tracheotomy has been used in such failures to reduce the dead space and facilitate tracheobronchial aspiration. In patients with tension pneumothorax, insertion of a water-sealed intercostal tube may be necessary.

Aminophylline poisoning may occasionally complicate treatment of asthma, resulting in vomiting (especially of blood or coffee-colored material), central nervous system irritability, convulsions, and cardiac arrhythmias and distress. Treatment consists of general supportive measures such as intravenous fluids and oxygen; occasionally short-acting barbiturates may be required to counter central nervous system irritability.

General Daily Management of Asthma

Between attacks the child with asthma may feel perfectly well and have no symptoms or signs. However, mucous plugs in the small bronchi may not clear for several weeks after a severe attack. With recently developed tests for small-airway function, it is apparent that even asymptomatic patients with asthma have significant impairment of pulmonary function. Some children may have continuity signs such as mild cough, especially at night, or cough and dyspnea on exertion, especially with running. Consequently bronchodilator medications formerly given for symptomatic treatment are now more commonly prescribed on a regular basis. Combination bronchodilators, including ephedrine hydrochloride 24 mg, theophylline 130 mg, and phenobarbital 8 mg or hydroxyzine hydrochloride 10 mg, are still being widely used. There is considerable controversy regarding the use of combination medications. Marked synergism appears to exist between catecholamines and methylxanthines in low dosage. However, the efficacy of ephedrine has been questioned, and it has been suggested that theophylline is the main effective ingredient in the combinations. It has further been suggested that ephedrine should not be used because it causes irritability.

Theophylline for oral use is available alone or in combination in about 20 preparations on the American market. The amount of theophylline base varies greatly in different preparations; thus it is important to know the actual amount of the base when prescribing. The effective plasma level of 10 to 20 μg/ml is usually achieved with a dose of 3 to 5 mg/kg every 6 to 8 hours in children or 125 mg qid in adults. The dose is variable, since theophylline degradation is quite different in different individuals, and the optimal dose must be determined.

The sympathomimetic ephedrine has been used in China for more than 5,000 years; it has a sustained action stimulating both α- and β-adrenergic receptors. It is effective in controlling mild asthma in a dosage of 0.5 mg/kg every 4 hours. The usual schoolchild dose is 12 mg every 6 hours for both prevention and control of mild bronchospasm. Because ephedrine causes emotional irritability and occasional insomnia from its stimulating action on the central nervous system (CNS), a barbiturate, hydroxyzine, or antihistamine is added to counter this irritability effect.

New β_2-adrenergic sympathomimetics have recently been introduced in the United States. These agents have prolonged action over 4 to 6 hours promoting bronchodilatation with minimal CNS-stimulating and cardiac actions. The resorcinol metaproterenol (Alupent), 1.3 to 2.6 mg/kg, is effective and is well tolerated in children. Alupent is available in 20-mg tablets and as a syrup at 10 mg per teaspoon. Another resorcinol with a tertiary butyl group, terbutaline (Bricanyl or Brethine), has a more potent effect on bronchial muscle and a less active effect on heart muscle than metaproterenol; it has a long action of about 6 hours and minimal side effects.

Another group of derivatives with potent β_2-adrenergic activity are the saligenins, one of which (salbutamol) is about to be licensed in the United States. Given intravenously in animals, salbutamol is 20 times more effective than metaproterenol in preventing bronchospasm, which makes it nearly as effective as isoproterenol but much longer lasting. The oral dose in adults is about 2 to 5 mg, following which bronchodilatation occurs in about 15 minutes, reaches its maximum in 1 or 2 hours, and lasts 4 to 6 hours. Another saligenin, salmefamol, has action similar to that of salbutamol, but has an even longer duration of action of 6 to 8 hours. These newer sympathomimetics are also effective by aerosol administration and are available as metered-dose nebulizers; however, because of their ease of administration and long duration of action, overdosage from overuse is a major danger, especially in children, and nebulizars cannot be recommended in children at this time.

In children with severe chronic asthma, Chai found that when he monitored the peak expiratory flow rate (PEFR) with a Wright peak-flow meter four times a day a significant fall in the PEFR occurred several hours before an attack. When this fall was noted, he promptly increased the bronchodilator medication and was able to keep the children relatively free of attacks for many months. Although Chai's study was conducted in a residential home for asthmatic children, we have been successful in similarly monitoring PEFR in such children at home with a Wright peak-flow meter purchased by the parents (about $200): with a 10 percent or greater fall in the PEFR, the dose of bronchodilators has been increased, and attacks of asthma appear to have been aborted.

Cromolyn sodium (Intal, Aarane) was licensed in the United States in 1973, but it has had prior extensive use in Europe since 1967. Its mode of action is unique in that it prevents the release of mediators from tissue mast cells, probably by stabilizing lysosomal membranes. Cromolyn has been highly effective in certain cases of extrinsic asthma, especially in children, in which allergen, IgE antibodies, and mediators are involved. It is also quite effective in exercise-induced asthma, but the mechanism of its action in such cases is unknown. It is less effective in infectious or intrinsic asthma, which may be primarily cholinergically mediated in adults and in some children. Curiously, it has been effective in some cases of interstitial alveolitis involving IgE, IgG, and cellular immunity; it is presumed that its action is to inhibit the initial IgE response that triggers the secondary immune reactions.

Cromolyn sodium is inactivated rapidly in liquid form; therefore it is administered as an inhaled powder by a specially constructed Spinhaler that disperses the fine powder that the patient inhales on deep inspiration. After inhaling, the breath is held for about 15 sec to coat the respiratory passages before exhaling. Inhalations are repeated until the powder in the capsule is used, usually about 5 to 6 breaths in children. The usual dose is four capsules of 20 mg each inhaled at about 6-hour intervals. The upper dosage limit of cromolyn has not yet been determined in man. Cromolyn is a prophylactic drug in asthma; it is not a bronchodilator once an attack has started. Cromolyn is rarely effective on the first or second day of administration, but requires several days to a week to exert its full effect. Changes in pulmonary function tests may be somewhat erratic; some patients have marked clinical improvement with little pulmonary change, while others have dramatic improvement in both.

In some children inhalation of any powder, including cromolyn, may be irritating and may set off a coughing attack that makes the drug's administration difficult. Although isoproterenol aerosols are not usually advised in children, we recommend one or two inhalations of isoproterenol 5 minutes prior to cromolyn to produce bronchodilatation that counteracts powder-induced bronchoconstriction caused by cromolyn. Isoproterenol is not regularly required, but in some cases it makes the administration of cromolyn practical. In a number of studies in children in American clinics, there was improvement of 80 percent or more in the test groups over the placebo groups. Such improvement holds over many months and even years when the child responds to cromolyn, as long as it is continued.

Thus far, in 8 years of clinical application, cromolyn has been found to be remarkably free of side effects or toxicity. Occasional instances of nasal congestion and transient rashes have occurred, but these have disappeared when cromolyn has been discontinued. In our studies, Addis counts, which have been performed routinely over 3 years, have all been normal. Some of the most dramatic effects of cromolyn have been in steroid-dependent children with severe chronic asthma, in whom it has been possible to markedly reduce or suspend the steroids. Cromolyn has also been found to be useful in patients who know they will be exposed to a known allergen over a short period of time, eg, the ragweed pollen season for 6 weeks. In these circumstances cromolyn is started 2 weeks before the expected pollen season, is continued through that season, and is then discontinued. It must be emphasized that cromolyn is not a panacea but is a useful adjunct to conventional antiasthmatic therapy. We have reserved cromolyn therapy for those asthmatic children who do not respond adequately to other measures and who ordinarily would require corticosteroids: when a trial of cromolyn is instituted before starting corticosteroid therapy, it may be found that in some children who formerly would have required corticosteroids, cromolyn is successful.

The therapeutic indications for the use of corticosteroids in asthma recommended by Siegel are severe acute allergic reactions, self-limiting allergic entities such as seasonal pollen asthma, reactions like serum sickness when the corticosteroid is given only for short periods of about 7 days, severe chronic allergy that incapacitates the patient, any stress (such as surgery) in a patient who has had corticosteroid therapy during the previous year, and coexisting disease (such as a surgical procedure) that necessitates control of the asthma before its own treatment.

Because of the high incidence of side effects and potentialy serious hazards, corticosteroids are avoided in children whenever possible. If hormone therapy is necessary, the lowest possible dosage over the shortest period of time is used. Caution should be exercised in administering steroids to children with diabetes or a family history of diabetes and to children with chronic infections, hypertension, or cardiovascular disease. Steroids may have serious adverse effects on almost any organ system, and if any serious complications occur, treatment should be stopped. Certain complications are frequent and mild and are considered to be tolerable. These are edema, facial plethora, weight gain, cushingoid appearance, acne, skin striae, hypertrichosis, insomnia, headache, and leg cramps.

In asthma, especially in children, usually relatively low doses of corticosteriods will suffice to control the serious symptoms. Hydrocortisone and cortisone have considerable mineralocorticoid effects with fluid retention, and therefore increased potassium and decreased sodium intake are necessary. Newer steroids such as triamcinolone have considerable propensity to produce muscle myopathy, while dexamethasone greatly stimulates the appetite; they are often avoided in children. These also significantly suppress growth in children because of their cumulative effects. The shorter-acting corticosteroids prednisone and prednisolone are most commonly used in children.

An asthma-suppressive dose of prednisone or prednisolone is usually about 2 mg/kg per 24 hours; however, the dose of corticosteroid should be adjusted, depending on the severity of the symptoms. Once suppression of the allergic symptoms has occurred, the dose can rapidly be tapered over several days to a week to a maintenance dose of prednisone of 5 to 15 mg/day. If symptoms continue to be suppressed for several days to a week, an alternate-day regimen of prednisone or prednisolone may be started, giving twice the former daily dose on alternate mornings. With this approach steroids can be administered to children with severe asthma for prolonged periods, even years, without significant adrenal suppression or inhibition of growth. On a long-term regimen of corticosteroids, the growth rate must be monitored carefully; blood pressure should also be measured regularly and urinalysis performed. In a child on long-term corticosteroid therapy, it is prudent to have a periodic evaluation of the hypothalamic-pituitary-adrenal axis. If stimulation of the adrenal by ACTH does not induce an increase in plasma cortisol or urinary steroids, severe renal suppression may be inferred. Other tests such as metapyrone or insulin responses may provide evidence of adrenal suppression at an earlier stage (p. 1625).

Recently several topical steroids have been introduced for treatment of asthma by the inhalation route. Beclomethasone has had extensive trials in England; it is characterized by its low systemic absorption. One puff of the nebulizer introduces 50 μg of beclomethasone dipropionate, and the recommended dose is 100 to 800 μg/day divided into four doses. When inhaled doses to control asthma have exceeded 2 mg/day, impairment of the pituitary-adrenal function has been demonstrated. In numerous studies patients switched from oral corticosteroids to beclomethasone have been able to reduce significantly or even give up the oral steroids. Topical administration is not practicable in the treatment of status asthmaticus.

Antihistamines are usually ineffective in relieving symptoms in most asthmatic patients. In certain patients with asthma, antihistamines may be helpful, although the mechanism of action is unknown. If conventional bronchodilators are ineffective, a short trial of antihistamines may be indicated.

References

Aaronson DW: Asthma, General Concepts. In Patterson R (ed): Allergic Diseases, Diagnosis and Management. Philadelphia, JB Lippincott, 1972

Avner SE: β-adrenergic bronchodilators. Pediatr Clin North Am 22:129, 1975

Barboriak JJ, Sosman AJ, Reed CE: Serological studies in pigeon breeder's disease. J Lab Clin Med 65:600, 1965

Bernstein TL, Siegel SC, Brandon MJ, et al: A controlled study of cromolyn sodium sponsored by the Drug Committee of the American Academy of Allergy. J Allergy Clin Immunol 50:235, 1972

Bierman CW: Pneumomediastinum and pneumothorax complicating asthma in children. Am J Dis Child 114:42, 1967

———— Pierson WE: The pharmacologic management of status asthmaticus in children. Pediatrics 54:245, 1974

Connell JJ: Asthmatic deaths. Role of the mast cells. JAMA 215:769, 1971

Cox JSG: Disodium cromoglycate. Mode of action and its possible relevance to the clinical use of the drug. Br J Dis Chest 65:189, 1971

Ellis EF, Eddy ED: Anhydrous theophylline equivalence of commercial theophylline formulations. J Allergy Clin Immunol 53:116, 1974

Godfrey S: Exercise-induced asthma—clinical, physiological, and therapeutic implications. J Allergy Clin Immunol 56:1, 1975

———— The place of a new aerosol steroid, beclomethasone dipropionate, in the management of childhood asthma. Pediatr Clin North Am 22:147, 1975

Huber HL, Koessler KK: The pathology of bronchial asthma. Arch Intern Med 30:689, 1922

Maselli R, Casal GL, Ellis EF: Pharmacologic effects of intravenously administered aminophylline in asthmatic children. J Pediatr 76:777, 1970

Reisman RE: Asthma induced by adrenergic aerosols. J Allergy 46:153, 1970

Siegel SC: Corticosteroids and ACTH in the management of the atopic child. Pediatr Clin North Am 16:287, 1975

Yu D, Galant S, Gold WM: Inhibition of antigen-induced bronchoconstriction by atropine in asthmatic patients. J Appl Physiol 32:828, 1972

ATOPIC DERMATITIS AND ECZEMA (See p. 354)

The association of asthma with skin rashes was noted as early as 1607 by Helmont, but by the late 1800s there was mass confusion concerning the terminology for different kinds of dermatitis, some associated with asthma and rhinitis. However, in 1892 Besnier described a severe itching rash with an autonomic nervous component associated with asthma and hay fever; this syndrome has been called Besnier's prurigo in Europe and atopic dermatitis in the United States. Atopic dermatitis in its acute phase is vesicular, with edema among the epithelial cells of the epidermis; the term eczema has been applied. Subsequently the term infantile eczema has been used synonymously with the term atopic dermatitis.

The incidence of atopic dermatitis is difficult to determine because it is frequently confused with other forms of dermatitis; however, it is known to occur in greater frequency in colder climates, especially in Scandinavia and among Orientals. The condition is common in infants, with a rapid decline after the age of 3 years, but it persists into adult life in mild form in about one-third of patients. In Stifler's 21-year follow-up study of infantile eczema, 50 percent of patients subsequently developed hay fever and 20 percent asthma.

Pathology

The epidermis is characterized by hyperplasia, acanthosis, and intracellular and intercellular edema (spongiosis). The normal undulating rete ridges extending into the corium of the basal layer are flattened, presumably by filling with rapidly proliferating cells. The keratinocytes are enlarged and swollen; some are damaged and show phagolysosomes. Cytoplasmic tonofibrils that make keratin are aggregated into irregular runs or enlarged keratohyaline granules. Basal layer cells have increased ribosomal activity. It appears that keratinization is unable to keep up with rapid cell proliferation.

The corium shows deep vascular dilation, with surrounding cellular infiltrate composed mostly of small lymphocytes and monocyte macrophages with collections of eosinophils and some basophils. The pathologic picture is similar to that of contact dermatitis, although atopic dermatitis has somewhat more intercellular edema (spongiosis) and eosinophil accumulation.

Pathophysiology

A severe itching dermatitis has long been recognized as an accompaniment in patients with hay fever and asthma, or in family members. Commonly such patients have infantile eczema that clears at about the age of 2 years, to be followed shortly by asthma that continues through adolescence and clears, but they develop allergic rhinitis in adulthood. Such patients have positive skin tests, and recently very high levels of serum IgE have been observed in patients with atopic dermatitis (in fact, much higher levels of IgE than in asthma or hay fever). However, immunotherapy and conventional pharmacologic methods of controlling allergic reactions, such as antihistamines and sympathomimetics, generally have been unsuccessful in alleviating atopic dermatitis lesions.

Brocq first suggested that these patients may have abnormal neural control of the skin; he named the condition neurodermatitis. In 1952 Eyster observed abnormal physiologic responses, such as white dermographia, to stimuli in the skin of patients with atopic dermatitis. When stroked with a blunt point, such patients initially developed the normal red line, which was replaced in 15 sec by an abnormal larger white line and blanching surrounded by a red flare, but no whealing. Lobitz and Campbell observed that the normal axon reflex flare following acetylcholine intradermal injection was followed by blanching; this delayed blanch could be blocked by atropine but not by procaine, and it occurred in 70 percent of their patients with atopic dermatitis. They suggested that atopic dermatitis patients have a vasoconstrictor response to acetylcholine, in contrast to the normal vasodilator response. West noted that 40 percent of symptom-free relatives of patients with atopic dermatitis had the delayed blanch response to intradermal acetylcholine, thus suggesting a genetic aberration.

Davis and Lawler observed dilated capillaries and edema at the site of acetylcholine injection, and Ramsay found that acetylcholine caused a high skin blood flow from vasodilatation, with edema resulting later. Thus it appears that acetylcholine causes vasodilatation in normal skin and atopic dermatitis skin but that the latter has overreactive skin vessels that produce a delayed blanch from edema, which obscures the dilated capillaries. Patients with atopic dermatitis also have an overreaction of sweat glands to acetylcholine.

The threshold of itching is markedly reduced in patients with atopic eczema. Itching and scratching appear to be important to pathogenesis, in that patients with severe atopic eczema who have become paraplegic have had clearing of the dermatitis below the spinal cord lesion, while it has continued as before in areas above the lesion. Similarly, a child with severe atopic eczema who was bandaged on one side had complete clearing of the dermatitis on the bandaged side, while on the free side the rash continued as before. Itching is due to a direct stimulation of nerve endings rather than to a vascular response, and it is not affected by acetylcholine or catecholamines. Histamine and proteolytic enzymes activated from cell dissolution appear to be involved in initiating itching.

As mentioned previously (p. 347), autonomic imbalance in the lung may be the basis for the mechanism of asthma. A similar autonomic imbalance in the blood vessels, sweat glands, and basal cells of the epidermis may account for the symptoms of atopic dermatitis. Hemels has suggested that patients with atopic eczema have minimal β-adrenergic control of the skin, since β-adrenergic blockade, which normally increases sweat output, has no effect in atopic patients.

Smith has shown that mitosis and cellular immunity appear to be affected by agents that control cyclic AMP content in cells. Carr and Reed have shown that β-adrenergic agents stimulate DNA in cultured normal epidermal cells but not in those taken from affected or unaffected areas of the skin from atopic eczema patients. They concluded that such epidermal cells were insensitive to β-adrenergic stimulation and suggested that the acanthosis in atopic eczema is due to failure of the β-adrenergic system to inhibit epidermal cell mitosis.

Recent evidence suggests that patients with atopic dermatitis have a decrease in cellular immunity associated with high IgE levels in the serum.

Clinical Symptoms and Signs

The first manifestation of allergy, especially if there is a positive family history, is commonly infantile eczema that usually begins at about 3 months of age but can occur earlier. Erythematous patches, papules, and vesicles that apparently itch first appear on the cheeks and the diaper area. These rapidly break down and ooze and then may become crusted; the lesions may rapidly spread to the chin, forehead, scalp, trunk, and extremities. An especially severe form is atopic erythroderma, in which the whole body skin is fiery red and thickened with scaling and exfoliation. There is apparently intense itching, as the infant is continually rubbing, and is unable to lie still; this often interferes with feeding, and the infant's nutrition may suffer. Secondary infection is common, with enlarged generalized lymph nodes. The hands and feet are usually cold. Some infants may start with a papular eruption on the scalp that develops the usual oily and scaly features of cradle cap or seborrheic dermatitis; later the typical dry, atopic vesiculopapular appearance of atopic dermatitis develops. Circumoral erythema and papular eruption associated with drooling may precede eczema.

Over a period of many months or at about the second year of life the dermatitis may clear, even completely, and never recur. In some infants the ingestion of certain foods appears to be associated with an exacerbation of symptoms, but this usually disappears after the second year. Some children, however, continue to have moderate to severe eczema until adolescence. The rashes are usually confined to the areas of creases, the flexor surfaces of the limbs such as the antecubital fossae, popliteal spaces, wrists and ankles, the neck under the chin, and especially behind the ears (the latter site is often the only residual site remaining on an otherwise clear skin). In older children the rash is usually papular and dry, but there is still intense itching with visible scratch marks. The skin is usually lichenified, thick, and scaly, with the normal dermal lines markedly accentuated into a mosaic. The severe itching may become acute at night, resulting in chronic loss of sleep with irritability and often behavior problems. Below the eyes there may be a prominent extra skin fold, and the hairs of the eyebrows may be rubbed away.

Vascular responses may be altered, particularly to temperature changes. The hands and feet tend to be cold, and they warm slowly when reheated; the bluish feet of atopic erythroderma are an extreme form of this abnormal vascular response. In contrast, the antecubital and popliteal regions cool more slowly than normal and rapidly vasodilate on warming, with increased perspiration.

At puberty, many adolescents will lose their atopic dermatitis, but in some it will persist in the childhood flexural pattern into adulthood. Commonly there are acute exacerbations during periods of emotional stress and during the menstrual period. Thus in adults the term neurodermatitis is often substituted for the term atopic dermatitis, although it is fundamentally a continuing manifestation of the same process.

Climate may markedly affect the course of dermatitis; sweating appears to cause acute exacerbation. During the colder seasons in which warmer, often wool, clothing is worn, there is increased sweating of the flexures and worsening of the rash. Direct contact with the minute stiff hairs of wool causes marked increases in itching and in the lesions. In cold climates with dry heating, there is a further drying of an already dry skin with exacerbation. During the summer months when less clothing is worn and the skin is open to sunshine, there is often dramatic clearing of the eczema; however, in hot, humid climates that cause heavy perspiration and also prevent its evaporation, there is often marked exacerbation of the lesions.

Laboratory Diagnosis

Eosinophilia is a prominent feature, often 20 percent or more; total leukocyte count is often elevated from secondary infection. Serum IgE level is usually high; levels of 1,000 ng/ml or higher are common. Serum IgM may also be elevated secondary to the recurrent or chronic skin infections, although IgG and IgA are usually normal.

Acetylcholine (1 mg) injected intradermally in nonallergic individuals causes redness within minutes that lasts about 15 to 20 minutes; in patients with atopic dermatitis, and in many other nondermatitic allergic persons, the initial redness after acetylcholine is superseded by blanching in 3 to 5 minutes and a wheal, often with pseudopods, that may last for 1 hour.

Skin tests for allergens may be markedly positive, but due to the extreme irritability of the skin they may or may not be clinically significant. In cases of severe atopic dermatitis lesions covering most of the body, it may not be possible to accomplish satisfactory skin testing.

Differential Diagnosis

Atopic dermatitis should be differentiated from seborrheic dermatitis, Leiner's disease, Ritter's disease, *Candida* infections, Wiskott-Aldrich syndrome, Letterer-Siwe disease, and pityriasis rosea (Chap. 17). Control of the secondary infection often leads to a marked subsidence in the eczema lesions.

VIRUS INFECTIONS OF THE SKIN. Less common, but much more serious, are pox virus infections such as vaccinia and herpesvirus that can lead to generalized viral infection over the whole skin, but especially severe at sites of atopic dermatitis. There is often generalized systemic infection involving internal organ systems and the central nervous system; encephalitis may be fatal.

ECZEMA VACCINATUM. Eczema vaccinatum is a generalized skin and systemic infection with vaccinia virus that is likely to occur in children with atopic dermatitis who are vaccinated or who come in contact with a recently vaccinated individual. Therefore smallpox vaccination should not be given to any patient or any member of that patient's family until at least 1 year after all the atopic dermatitis lesions have completely cleared. Eczema vaccinatum is characterized by an exaggerated local vaccination lesion; this spreads to other areas of atopic dermatitis. Regional lymph nodes are markedly enlarged and may ulcerate, as may the primary skin areas. Necrosis and massive loss of tissue may follow the ulceration. There is often accompanying fever, dehydration, and generalized toxicity. Central nervous system involvement may lead to convulsions, confusion, coma, and death. A 12 to 30 percent mortality rate has been reported. The recent availability of human vaccinia immunoglobulin, given in a dose of 0.6 ml/kg intramuscularly, has markedly reduced the mortality and morbidity from this serious condition. Methisazone may be of use in arresting the disease progress. Patients with atopic dermatitis who are returning to the United States from abroad need no longer be vaccinated if they have a statement from a physician stating its contraindication.

ECZEMA HERPETICUM. Herpes simplex causes a generalized systemic virus infection similar to that of eczema vaccinatum; it extensively involves the skin in all the areas of atopic dermatitis; this is referred to as Kaposi's varicelliform eruption. There may be high fever, dehydration, and systemic involvement of the internal organs and the central nervous system, with convulsions, coma, and death. Commonly a child with atopic dermatitis will be kissed by someone with a herpes simplex lesion on the lips or mouth; therefore the parents should be warned against such contacts by the child with atopic dermatitis.

MOLLUSCUM CONTAGIOSUM. Molluscum contagiosum is normally a mild pox virus skin infection. However, in patients with atopic dermatitis there may be a generalized systemic molluscum contagiosum that resembles the aforementioned vaccinia and herpes complications.

CONTACT DERMATITIS. Contact dermatitis, an iatrogenic complication of atopic dermatitis, may develop from topical medications such as neomycin and parabens that are so often used in dermatologic creams and ointments. These are potent sensitizers, especially if repeatedly applied to open or weeping skin lesions.

CATARACTS. In patients with atopic dermatitis, cataracts may form quite early, often in the third decade of life, but rarely in children. The cataract has a dense subcapsular plaque with radiating fibers; it occurs first centrally in the pupil and spreads to the periphery of the lens.

SUDDEN DEATH. Although sudden death was once common in children hospitalized for treatment of severe atopic dermatitis, it is rare since antibiotics have been available. It presumably was due to overwhelming infection.

Treatment

Treatment of atopic dermatitis involves topical therapy, general symptomatic treatment, and specific therapy if indicated. Topical therapy is the same as in general dermatologic management. Wet dressings are applied to open, weeping lesions with boiled water, saline, or a mild antiseptic such as Burow's solution (aluminum acetate 1:10 to 1:40). Dressings should be removed for about 11 hours a day to prevent skin maceration. Systemic antibiotic therapy is given if the lesions are infected. Topical corticosteroids are used after the acute weeping is controlled. Lotions or creams are used for moist lesions, whereas ointments are used on dry skin. Considerable systemic absorption may occur, especially of the newer fluorinated corticosteroids such as triamcinolone and dexamethasone. Fluorinated steroids with lower systemic absorption have been developed, such as fluocinolone (Synalar), flurandrenolone (Cordran), betamethasone (Celestone), betamethasone valerate (Valisone), and fluocinonide (Lidex). These are used as 0.01, 0.05, and up to 0.2 percent ointments and creams. The effectiveness may be increased by intermittent use of occlusive dressings, such as Saran Wrap, during the night, or for limited times during the day. Because of the systemic absorption of topical steroids, the adrenal function should be monitored. Crude coal tar ointments (3 to 5 percent) applied every 12 hours may be effective, but they are messy and stain clothing. Water-soluble nonstaining light tar preparations such as 3 percent liquor carbonis detergens (LCD) are cleaner but less effective. Coal tar baths (30 ml of LCD in a bathtub of water) may relieve itching. Drying of the skin should be avoided, as it leads to excessive itching. Therapy is directed toward keeping the skin soft and moist. In the Scholtz treatment, bathing in water is restricted to once weekly, and the skin is cleaned with cetyl alcohol (Cetaphil lotion) at least twice a day. Control of the itching and scratching is most important. Use of cotton stockings and mittens has been successful in preventing scratching during sleep. Cutting the fingernails and smoothing them daily with an emery board may help to avoid some of the trauma of scratching. Sedatives, antipruritics, and tranquilizers have been used with varying success. Cornstarch or oatmeal baths (Aveeno), 2 cups per tub, may relieve itching.

Generally, the use of systemic corticosteroids is avoided but in acute situations that require hospitalization, a course of corticosteroid therapy for 1 week may be useful. In those cases corticosteroids are used as in status asthmaticus (p. 348), with high initial doses for 3 days, and tapering over the next 4 to 5 days.

TABLE 1. Basic Elimination Diet

Diet for:

This diet excludes all cereals (wheat, corn, oats, rice, barley, and rye). It also excludes milk, egg, chocolate, cola, nuts, citrus fruits, spices, pepper, and, in fact, everything not mentioned below.

Foods allowed:

Bread and bakery products: Those made from lima beans, soybeans, or potato, and their combinations: may also be flavored with vanilla or the fruits allowed.

Starches: tapioca, potato (fried, baked, mashed, boiled, or hash brown), yams, and sweet potato.

Vegetables: string beans, carrots, beets, squash, spinach, celery, Swiss chard, onion, lettuce, avocado, cauliflower, artichokes, asparagus, lima beans, soybeans.

Fruits: plum, prune, apricot, pear, fig, date, peach, pineapple, persimmon, strawberry, raspberry, and their juices and jams, rhubarb.

Meat or poultry: fish, lamb (leg, stew, roast, chops), beef (ground, roast, steak, stew), turkey, chicken, and bacon.

Desserts: fruits (stewed, fresh, dried, canned), any artificially flavored Jell-O, gelatin, popsicle (except orange); tapioca may be mixed with the fruit and sweetened with sugar and vanilla.

Soup: chicken, turkey, beef, and lamb, thickened with tapioca, if desired.

Gravy: chicken or beef, thickened with potato flour.

Butter and oils: may have butter and margarin, Crisco, Wesson oil, and other vegetable oils and peanut oil.

Other: brown and white sugar, maple sugar, vanilla, salt, maple syrup, white vinegar, sunflower seed, and pine nuts.

Specific Treatment

In infants and toddlers, certain foods, particularly egg, wheat, and milk, may be suspected of contributing to the eczema, but a specific food allergen rarely can be found. If a role for a food is strongly suspected, a trial elimination diet for 4 weeks each may implicate one of them as the offending agent. Foods that give positive skin test reactions may be suspected and may also be eliminated from the diet for a 4-week trial. If specific elimination diets do not improve the condition, a simple basic elimination diet consisting of only one food in each major category may be tried (Table 1). This should be continued only for 3 to 4 weeks to estimate its usefulness, and children should not be kept on such restricted diets over a period of months. Mineral and vitamin supplements must be added. Specific inhalant allergens, such as the sources of house dust, animals, feathers, and kapok, should be removed.

Specific immunotherapy for atopic dermatitis is generally unsuccessful. The usual doses of extract of inhalants or pollens produce acute flareups of the lesions. The psychologic effect of atopic dermatitis must also be considered. These infants and children are often unattractive in appearance and may be subconsciously rejected by the parents, which can have serious repercussions. Children may also be rejected by their peers, and during adolescence the disfiguring lesions of atopic dermatitis may seriously affect the child's social and sexual contacts, thus leading to considerable psychologic disturbance. Atopic dermatitis is a long-term, often lifelong, problem with which the patient must learn to live.

References

Carr R, Reed CE: Effect of catecholamines on DNA synthesis in epidermis from normal subjects and patients with atopic eczema. J Allergy Clin Immunol 51:255, 1973

Davis MJ, Lawler JC: Observations on the delayed blanch phenomenon in atopic subjects. J Invest Dermatol 30:127, 1958

Lobitz WC, Campbell CJ: Physiologic studies in atopic dermatitis (disseminated neurodermatitis). I. The local cutaneous response to intradermally injected acetylcholine and epinephrine. AMA Arch Dermatol Syph 67:575, 1953

McGeady SJ, Buckley RH: Studies of cell-mediated immune function in atopic eczema. J Allergy Clin Immunol 53:72, 1974

Prose PH: Pathologic changes in eczema. J Pediatr 66:178, 1965

Ramsay C: Vascular changes accompanying white dermographism and delayed blanch in atopic dermatitis. Br J Dermatol 81:37, 1969

Rostenberg A Jr, Solomon LM: Atopic dermatitis and infantile eczema. In Samter M (ed): Immunological Diseases. Boston, Little, Brown, 1971, p 920

Scholtz JR: Management of atopic dermatitis. Calif Med 102:210, 1965

Smith JW, Steiner AL, Parker CD: Human lymphocyte metabolism; effects of cyclic and non-cyclic nucleotides on stimulation by phytohemagglutinin. J Clin Invest 50:442, 1971

Stifler WC: A 21 year followup of infantile eczema. J Pediatr 66:166, 1965

Sulzberger MB: Atopic dermatitis. In Fitzpatrick TB (ed): Dermatology in General Medicine. New York, McGraw-Hill, 1971, p 680

URTICARIA AND ANGIOEDEMA

Urticaria is characterized by itching skin reactions with redness and central edema, which may be localized or generalized. It may involve mucous surfaces, including the tongue, epiglottis, and larynx, and can be life-threatening from asphyxia. In children, acute isolated episodes are most frequent. Chronic urticaria lasting weeks to months and even years is usually generalized and is much more common in adults, especially women.

Angioedema is a much larger lesion of local or generalized swelling, often involving the lips, eyes, ears, and limbs in a brawny induration that may itch but is more often painful. The larynx can be involved and cause asphyxia.

Histamine is the primary mediator of urticaria or hives; presumably this comes from tissue mast cells or circulating basophils. Although histamine is probably also involved in angioedema, the main mediator appears to be bradykinin, which causes pain as well as itching. Other mediators, such as prostaglandin E_1, cause strong cutaneous vasodilatation in man, but little itching. The slow-reacting substance of anaphylaxis (SRS-A) and serotonin increase vascular permeability in animals, but their role in man has not been substantiated. Cholinergic stimulation with acetylcholine causes some forms of physical urticaria, although it may act through histamine release. Activation of complement by either the direct or alternate pathway causes release of the complement peptides C3a and C5a, which are known as anaphylatoxins and cause release of histamine from mast cells. Histamine appears to be the primary mediator and may activate other mediator systems in the pathogenesis of urticaria.

Immunologic mechanisms account for only a quarter or less of cases of chronic urticaria. Gell and Coombs have classified them as type I, anaphylactic; type II, cytotoxic; and type III, antigen–antibody complex syndromes. The type I anaphylactic mechanism involves the traditional allergies to foods, parasites, pollens, and *Hymenoptera,* to which IgE antibodies are formed that attach to mast cells; upon subsequent exposure of the mast cells to antigen the mast cells release histamine, thus causing the urticarial lesion. In the type II mechanism cellular antigens, such as mismatched erythrocytes in transfusion reactions, react with IgG or IgM antibodies that activate complement components and release anaphylatoxins C3a and C5a, which release histamine from mast cells. In type III, antigen–antibody complexes are formed from drug–protein interactions where IgG antibodies activate complement C3a and C5a, with histamine release from mast cells. Certain drugs and chemicals act directly as liberators of histamine from mast cells. These include antibiotics, thiamine, d-tubocurare, quinidine, morphine, cocaine, surfactants such as Tween 20 and bile salts, and certain foods such as strawberries, shellfish, and citrus fruits. They may act directly on C3 to produce anaphylatoxin, which acts on mast cells to release histamine. Physical agents (such as cold, heat and sunlight, and vibration) and neurogenic stimulation (such as heat and emotional upsets) may act through acetylcholine to release mediators from mast cells. Host factors, such as the status of the autonomic balance between the cholinergic and the α- and β-adrenergic systems, make the blood vessels more or less susceptible to the effects of any of the above mechanisms. Factors affecting endocrine status, such as menopause, diabetes mellitus, menstruation, and myxedema, all potentiate the histamine release mechanisms. The actual importance of anaphylatoxins in the release of histamine in man is still unresolved.

Diagnostic Investigation

Patients should be advised of the difficulty in arriving at a specific etiologic diagnosis, but they should be reassured that the condition is self-limiting, although it may take months or even several years to abate. Often the patient will be able to identify the offending circumstance or material.

It is usually impossible to suggest a cause from the appearance of the urticarial lesion, but some lesions are fairly characteristic: dermographia has wheals along the lines of scratches, or pressure friction from clothing; in papular urticaria in children, persistent lesions last several days and are caused by insect bites, such as by fleas, bedbugs, and mites; cholinergic urticaria has small, central wheals of 1 to 3 mm with a large surrounding erythema; urticaria pigmentosa is common in children and has pigmented macules or papules (rubbing such lesions causes urticaria); yellow urticaria may occur in hepatitis, often before jaundice is manifest, and is due to bile salt irritation.

Specific classes of agents should be considered as possible etiologic factors. Drugs and chemicals are most commonly involved; penicillin and its derivatives are responsible for about a quarter of these cases. Other drugs include aspirin and various vaccines. Various infections may be responsible; parasitic infestation is commonly associated with urticaria and causes marked eosinophilia and high IgE levels in serum. In children, acute viral infections may be associated with hives, especially mononucleosis, coxsackie infections, and hepatitis. Foods such as seafood, fresh berries, and citrus may act as histamine liberators; fish, nuts, peanuts, and eggs cause IgE antibody reactions. In chronic urticaria food allergy is more difficult to implicate. Skin tests may be useful in the acute kind, but they are rarely helpful in chronic cases. Inhalants such as pollens, animal danders, and fish odors may cause urticaria in patients with other forms of respiratory allergy. Urticaria may be a prominent feature of insect stings and bites, especially in children. Contactants from plants such as nettles, from marine creatures such as the Portuguese man-of-war and sea nettles, and from various insects and arthropods such as caterpillars, beetles, tarantulas, spiders, and moths may also be responsible.

In children, physical factors, particularly cold exposure, are often common causes. Exposure to cold apparently causes a change in a skin protein that is recognized as foreign by the host, thus causing the formation of antibody. Such cold sensitivity can be passively transferred to a normal individual. If there is a massive, sudden exposure to cold (eg, plunging into a cold swimming pool), massive urticaria with marked vascular leakage and shock can result in death from drowning. When an ice cube or a tube of cold water is placed on the skin for 2 to 5 minutes and the skin is then reheated, a wheal and erythema will occur at the point of cold contact. Urticaria may also be secondary to cryoglobulinemia, cryofibrinogenemia, or cold hemolysin, particularly in adults with infectious or connective tissue disease. Heat may cause urticaria, especially of the cholinergic kind, with small lesions and large flares. Solar or light urticaria may occur upon exposure to light of different wavelengths. Urticaria may occur in association with systemic diseases, especially in adults, as a result of vasculitis occurring secondary to systemic lupus erythematosus, scleroderma, and dermatomyositis. Psychogenic factors may be associated with transient urticaria, especially in children. Continued emotional stress may be responsible for chronic urticaria, eg, in families where there is parental discord or there are school or work problems.

Treatment

If no cause for his symptoms can be found, the patient will require much reassurance and symptomatic therapy. Usually antihistamines give the best relief, especially those with sedative effects that can be given at bedtime. The antihistamines act specifically to counter histamine, but they may be as effective as antipruritics and local anesthetics. Cyproheptadine (Periactin) is apparently most effective in cold urticaria. Recently hydroxyzine (Atarax and Vistaril) has been used for both its antihistaminic and tranquilizing effects. Sympathomimetics, such as ephedrine and epinephrine, are very effective for relief of urticaria. In acute, severe urticaria, particularly with angioedema, if the voice thickens or respiratory difficulty develops, indicating laryngeal edema and obstruction, epinephrine subcutaneously is mandatory; tracheotomy or intubation may be required. Corticosteroids are rarely used in chronic urticaria, but in an extreme state they may produce temporary remission if given for a short course. In a self-limited illness such as serum sickness, with severe urticaria and neurologic involvement, systemic corticosteroids may be beneficial. Immunotherapy has generally been unsuccessful, except in the case of *Hymenoptera* sensitivity. Occasionally patients with cold urticaria may be desensitized by exposure to water whose temperature is gradually decreased each day. Generally, the results have not been encouraging.

References

Bokisch VA, Müller-Eberhard HJ: Anaphylatoxin inactivator of human plasma; its isolation and characterization as a carboxy peptidase. J Clin Invest 49:2427, 1970

Mathews KP: A current view of urticaria. Med Clin North Am 58:185, 1974

Thompson JS: Urticaria and angioedema. Ann Intern Med 69:361, 1968

CONTACT DERMATITIS

Contact dermatitis is the most common form of allergic dermatitis in children and adults; it is allergic under the broad definition of hypersensitivity, being of the Gell and Coombs type IV delayed hypersensitivity or cellular immune reaction. It occurs by contact with allergen, which may be only the simple haptenic portion, such as a simple chemical or metal that comes in contact with the skin. The chemical hapten reacts with a skin constituent, probably a skin protein, that then forms a "foreign" immunogen that sensitizes lymphocytes. Upon subsequent exposure to the haptene, chemical, or allergen, sensitized lymphocytes react and transform to large lymphocytes; they then release mediators or lymphokines such as migration-inhibition factor (MIF) and chemotactic factors for other cells such as lymphocytes, macrophages, and basophils. When MIF is released into the small vessels of the skin, it causes monocytes to slow down and accumulate in the area. These become activated (or "angry") to become macrophages, which invade the local tissue and release lysosomes and their enzymatic contents, causing marked local inflammation. The relatively few sensitized lymphocytes release chemotactic factors that immobilize and accumulate nonsensitized host lymphocytes in the area of inflammation. Only about 1 or 2 percent of the lymphocytes in a contact dermatitic lesion are specifically sensitized to the allergen. Recently basophils have been shown to accumulate in areas of contact dermatitis, and histamine released from them may cause skin edema. Serum antibodies are not involved in these reactions, and the lesions of contact dermatitis cannot be passively transferred with serum, although they can be passively transferred with sensitized lymphocytes.

Atopic individuals are not more susceptible to contact dermatitis than is the general population. In fact, there are several recent reports that poison ivy and poison oak reactions may occur less frequently in atopic individuals than in nonallergic persons. The only exception to this generalization is that patients with chronic atopic dermatitis to whom potent sensitizing drugs such as neomycin and parabens have been applied frequently may have an increased contact sensitivity to these agents by virtue of their frequent iatrogenic exposure.

Clinical

The skin area exposed to the contactant allergen may appear normal for 12 to 24 hours after contact; the area then becomes reddened and indurated from intradermal edema. Vesicles appear. The vessels leak fluid, crust over, and finally heal after about a week. Especially sensitive are exposed areas such as the eyes, ears, neck, face, and hands; but any part of the skin in contact with the allergen may be involved. The distribution of the rash may give important clues to the source of the offending allergen.

Patch Test

The test materials are placed on a small gauze pad or filter paper covered with adhesive tape and aligned in rows on areas of uninvolved skin, preferably on the back. The skin is washed with alcohol or acetone and allowed to dry before the patches are applied. Powdered materials are suspended in saline and applied to the gauze. Recently several commercial screening patch sets have become available. Open testing may be used for irritating materials that should not be enclosed, such as perfumes and toiletries. After 48 to 72 hours the adhesive patches are removed, and 20 minutes later the sites are examined for vesicles, redness, and induration. Several control patch tests should be placed, as some patients are sensitive to the adhesive materials. If a strong irritation to any one patch occurs before 48 hours, it should be removed. The positive test sites will subside in a few days; this may be hastened by local applications of corticosteroid cream. Patients on corticosteroid therapy may have suppressed, delayed skin tests.

Treatment

Topical therapy of open weeping, itching, and inflamed lesions is best accomplished with wet compresses with saline, water, or Burow's solution (1:20). Upon subsidence of the acute lesion, topical corticosteroids, such as 0.5 percent hydrocortisone ointment, or 0.01 to 0.05 percent fluorinated corticosteroids, such as betamethasone valerate (Valisone), are applied. If the lesions are extensive and the patient is in marked discomfort, systemic corticosteroids may be used for 5 to 7 days, with relatively high doses for the first 3 days, then tapering off rapidly. As a result of scratching, secondary infection may occur; it should be treated with oral antibiotics. Topical antibiotics are contraindicated because of their high sensitizing capacity.

Specific Therapy or Prophylaxis

Recognition of the offending agent is still the best prophylaxis. Children should be taught to recognize and avoid poison ivy and oak. Specific hyposensitization for poison ivy has been generally unsuccessful. Recently an experimental preparation of purified urushiol catechol has been reported to be more successful than previous preparations. Side effects of hyposensitization include fever, dermatitic eruption, stomatitis, pruritus ani, and urticaria. Therefore we feel that hyposensitization is still experimental and is not recommended for the treatment of children at this time.

References

Dvorak HF, Simpson BA, Bask RC, Leskowitz S: Cutaneous basophil hypersensitivity. III. Participation of the basophil in hypersensitivity to antigen-antibody complexes, delayed hypersensitivity and contact allergy. J Immunol 107:138, 1971

Epstein WL, Baer H, Dawson CR, Khurana RG: Poison oak hyposensitization. Evaluation of purified urushiol. Arch Dermatol 109:356, 1974

Jones HE: Allergic contact sensitivity in atopic dermatitis. Arch Dermatol 107:217, 1973

Sulzberger MB, Wolf J, Witten VH, Kopf AW: Dermatology: Diagnosis and Treatment, 2nd ed. Chicago, Year Book, 1961

ANAPHYLAXIS

Anaphylaxis was the first allergic reaction recognized. It was described by Richet and Portier in 1902. Anaphylaxis occurs within minutes of exposure to allergen; in man it may lead to respiratory obstruction and arrest and/or circulatory collapse and death within 30 minutes. The degree of reaction may vary widely, from a mild itching and urticaria to death. About 500 fatalities from anaphylaxis occur annually in the United States.

The antigen may be injected and rapidly absorbed, with symptoms starting within 20 to 30 sec; or it may be ingested or inhaled, in which case it must be absorbed, and the reaction may occur within 1 to 5 minutes. Anaphylaxis has been caused in man by a number of substances, including proteins, chemical haptenes used as drugs, and polysaccharides. Materials implicated include stinging insect venoms, pollen or other allergen extracts, heterologous serum, enzymes and hormones, haptenic drugs such as penicillin or its analogues, other antibiotics, procaine, salicylates, and dextrans. Ingestion of foods, especially nuts, egg, legumes, citrus, fish and shellfish, and inhalation of the products of cooking fish or roasting nuts, as well as wheat and buckwheat in bakers, have been observed to cause anaphylaxis. Physical allergy such as cold urticaria may cause anaphylaxis from sudden immersion of the patient in cold water. Intramuscular injection of aggregated human gamma globulin from a preparation that has been standing for some weeks has resulted in fatal anaphylaxis. Rupture of a hydatid cyst may cause anaphylaxis from massive release of antigen in a sensitized individual.

The clinical presentation may begin with mild local or generalized itching or burning of the skin, flushing, sweating, apprehension, a mild irritative cough, pallor and hypertension, nausea and vomiting. Symptoms progress rapidly to involve, in man, four major organ systems: the skin (angioedema); the gastrointestinal tract (abdominal pain, vomiting, and diarrhea); the respiratory tract (chest tightness or pain, wheezing, dyspnea, cyanosis); and the cardiovascular system (rapid and weak pulse, unconsciousness, collapse, arrhythmia, cardiac arrest). Death may occur within 10 minutes.

The mechanism of anaphylaxis is a type I IgE antibody-mediated reaction in which the allergen combines with IgE antibody on the surface of mast cells, causing release of mediators, primarily histamine and bradykinin. These cause increased capillary and venous permeability, resulting in tissue edema, especially of the epiglottis and larynx in man; loss of intravascular fluid, causing vascular collapse or systemic shock; and smooth muscle contraction of the bronchial and urinary tracts, causing bronchospasm, vomiting, abdominal pain, and bowel and urinary incontinence.

Treatment

ACUTE EMERGENCY. Steps to follow are: (1) keep calm, to avoid panic in the patient and in your aides; start treatment promptly; do not wait for mild symptoms to subside. (2) Administer epinephrine hydrochloride (adrenalin) 1:1,000 in a dose of 0.2 to 0.5 ml intramuscularly (or subcutaneously) into the limb opposite the antigen injection site; massage the area to promote absorption. (3) Apply a tourniquet proximal to the antigen injection site and inject epinephrine hydrochloride 1:1,000 in a dose of 0.2 ml locally into the site to slow absorption of the antigen. (4) Lay the patient flat with his feet elevated, and keep him warm with a blanket. If respiratory difficulty occurs, his head and chest may be elevated slightly. (5) Inject diphenhydramine hydrochloride (Benadryl), 20 to 30 mg intramuscularly, to competitively inhibit the effect of further histamine release (it will not counter the effects of histamine already released). Other injectable antihistamines may be used, eg, chlorpheniramine maleate (Chlor-Trimeton), 10 mg intramuscularly, or promethazine hydrochloride (Phenergan), 25 mg intramuscularly. (6) Administer oxygen by mask or nasal catheter; if the airway becomes obstructed from epiglottic or laryngeal edema, endotracheal intubation or tracheostomy may be necessary. (7) Start an intravenous infusion. If shock symptoms are present, a reduction may be required. Start with normal saline, but change as quickly as possible to a colloid such as 6 percent dextran, 5 percent human serum albumin or plasma, 500 to 1,000 ml, to restore intravascular volume; then administer intravenous diphenhydramine hydrochloride, 1 mg/kg (up to 50 mg in older children or adults). (8) Check the patient's systolic pressure. If it is normal or systolic pressure is higher than 60 mm Hg, and if respiratory difficulty continues, administer intravenous aminophylline, 250 to 500 mg (or 3 mg/kg) slowly over a period of 10 minutes (since aminophylline is also a vasodilator, too rapid administration may aggravate vascular collapse). If the blood pressure is very low, with a systolic level less than 40 mm Hg, give catecholamines intravenously. Usually vasoconstrictors have been recommended. Norepinephrine may be given slowly by pump infusion or by drip in doses of 0.1 up to 0.5 μg/kg/minute. Metaraminol (Aramine) and phenylephrine (Neo-Synephrine) are also α-adrenergic agonists that have been used to produce vasoconstriction. More recently, in treatment of endotoxic and traumatic shock, the use of α-adrenergic drugs has been questioned. Isoproterenol hydrochloride (Isuprel) has been used to increase cardiac output and peripheral blood flow. It is infused intravenously in doses of 0.1 to 0.25 μg/kg/minute. Dopamine has also been effective. The value of these β-adrenergic agents in anaphylactic shock has not been adequately evaluated. (9) If the reaction is severe and the hypotension or respiratory obstruction is not responding to treatment, hydrocortisone sodium succinate (Solu-Cortef), 50 to 100 mg, or dexamethasone sodium phosphate (Decadron), 4 to 8 mg, may be added to the intravenous drip. Corticosteroids may bring about slow improvement, but they

TABLE 2. Drugs and Equipment for an Anaphylactic Emergency Tray

Drugs

Epinephrine hydrochloride solution 1:1,000, 1-ml ampules or 10-ml vials

Antihistamines for injection:
Diphenhydramine hydrochloride (Benadryl), 10-ml vial (10 mg/ml) or 1-ml ampule (50 mg/ml)
Chlorpheniramine maleate (Chlor-Trimeton), 1-ml ampule or 10-ml vial (both 10 mg/ml)
Promethazine hydrochloride (Phenergan), 1-ml ampule or 10-ml vial (both 25 mg/ml)

Parenteral fluids:
Normal saline or 5 percent dextrose in saline or distilled water (refrigeration unnecessary)
Salt-poor normal serum albumin (human), 25 percent 20 ml, or 6 percent dextran in saline or in 5 percent distilled water (refrigeration unnecessary)

Aminophylline, 250 mg in 10-ml ampule

Metaraminol bitartrate (Aramine), ampules or vials (10 mg/ml)

Soluble corticosteroid for parenteral use:
Hydrocortisone sodium succinate (Solu-Cortef), vial (100 mg/ml)
Dexamethasone sodium phosphate (Decadron), 1-ml and 5-ml vials (4 mg/ml)

Equipment

Tourniquet
Endotracheal tubes, several sizes for children
Tracheostomy set and surgical instruments for a cutdown
Suction apparatus
Syringes, several 1-ml tuberculin and several larger, 5 to 10 ml
Hypodermic needles, several No. 20 or 22 and several No. 25 or 27

are not emergency drugs in acute anaphylaxis. Wasting time to find a vein for hydrocortisone administration and omitting epinephrine has been fatal in some cases of anaphylaxis. In the presence of cardiac arrest, resuscitation measures as outlined previously (p. 1499) will have to be instituted.

PRECAUTIONS. Any physician or dentist giving a large number of injections, especially allergists, pediatricians, and anesthesiologists, would be wise to have an emergency tray containing the equipment and drugs listed in Table 2 for treating anaphylaxis. This should be checked regularly.

PREVENTION. A good history is most important, especially regarding any previous reactions following ingestion or injection of a drug or biological. Medic-Alert cards indicating the drug involved should be carried by such persons. Since most anaphylactic reactions are iatrogenic, no unnecessary medications should be given. Individuals with a personal family history of allergy have an unusual capacity to form IgE antibodies, which are involved in anaphylaxis; and they have an increased incidence or greater intensity of such reactions than do nonallergic individuals.

INSECT STINGS

Hymenoptera stings cause about 40 fatalities annually in the United States, which is only a small fraction of the thousands of allergic reactions to these stings each year.

Honeybees cause the most insect stings because of their close association with man in beekeeping. Stings by bumblebees, wasps, yellow jackets, and hornets may also produce allergic reactions. Their venoms are a mixture of potent pharmacologic proteins (eg, honeybee venom consists of histamines, phospholipase A and B, mellitin, apamine, lecithinase, hyaluronidase, and vanillylmandelic acid). However, the primary allergen in honeybee venom is phospholipase A, which accounts for more than 90 percent of the allergic reactivity.

CLINICAL REACTIONS. There may be merely a puncture and slight erythema lasting only a few minutes. This is common in beekeepers who have been stung repeatedly and presumably have developed natural immunity to the venom. Lack of exposure for several weeks results in increased reactivity on renewed exposure. In others, mild local reactions are common, with erythema and painful swelling, which lasts several hours. More severe local reactions may involve swelling of an entire limb, but no generalized signs. Wasps and hornets are scavengers and may inject bacteria along with venom, causing cellulitis that may require antibiotic therapy. Immediate systemic allergic reactions may occur, with a local wheal and flare, generalized itching, and massive urticaria. In more severe reactions, within a few minutes there may be sneezing, coughing, tightness of the chest or throat, wheezing and asphyxia, and signs of circulatory impairment, with pallor, rapid pulse, hypotension, anxiety, and collapse. Loss of consciousness and death may occur in 5 to 30 minutes. There may be delayed vascular reactions that resemble serum sickness, with urticaria, polyarthralgia, lymphadenopathy, and fever that may start 7 to 10 days after the sting and gradually subside within a week. An overwhelming number of stings may cause severe intestinal symptoms, edema, fever, headache, drowsiness, and convulsions; these may not be allergic, but rather a reaction to the large amount of injected venom.

DIAGNOSIS. The nature of the stinging insect is usually not known or only suspected. If a stinger is noted, the insect was a honeybee or a bumblebee; absence of a stinger usually indicates a yellow jacket, wasp, or hornet sting. Specific immunotherapy in the past consisted of a mixture of all four *Hymenoptera* antigens. Recent evidence indicates that specific venom therapy is more effective, and thus identification of the stinging insect is desirable.

SKIN TESTS. Extracts of whole-body homogenates of the specific insects are diluted to concentrations of 1 in 10 million or 1 in 1 million for intradermal or scratch skin testing, and repeat tests are made every 10 minutes with 10-fold increases in concentration until there is a definite wheal (5 mm) and flare. The tests should be performed carefully, and an anaphylaxis treatment tray should be at hand. Skin tests should be delayed 1 to 2 weeks after a sting, since tachyphylaxis may occur. The newer in vitro diagnostic tests (RAST and leukocyte histamine release) may avoid the risk of skin testing and may become routine diagnostic tests for insect sting hypersensitivity.

TREATMENT. Treatment of the systemic allergic reaction is the same as for generalized anaphylaxis (p. 361). Delayed reactions similar to serum sickness may be treated with corticosteroids and antihistamines for 7 to 10 days. Local reactions may require cold compresses, and local urticaria may be helped by an antihistaminic.

SPECIFIC IMMUNOTHERAPY. Because of difficulty in identifying the species of the stinging insect, a mixture of whole-body extracts (homogenates) from all four major *Hymenoptera* species has been used. One starts with an extract dilution one-tenth of the dose that gives a threshold skin reaction. This is increased by 50 percent in volume once or twice a week until a 1:100 or 1:10 extract is tolerated. This approach has usually decreased the severity of response to subsequent stings, but many untreated individuals also have less response. Some individuals who did not improve after whole-body extract treatment have responded to treatment with pure venom. The measurement of specific IgE antibodies to specific venoms by RAST and leukocyte histamine release has made definitive diagnosis and specific treatment more feasible. Phospholipase A is the principal allergen in bee venom, and immunotherapy with phospholipase A seems more promising than treatment with bee whole-body extract. It is hoped that with more specific therapy, a greater fall in IgE antibodies will be achieved, with increasing production of IgG-blocking antibodies.

NONSPECIFIC PROPHYLACTIC MEASURES. Such patients should be provided with an anaphylaxis kit, which is commercially available. It includes epinephrine in a plastic syringe in a fixed dose that can be given with little difficulty, a tourniquet, and an oral antihistamine. Such patients should have a Medic-Alert card indicating insect hypersensitivity.

References

Austen KF: Systemic anaphylaxis in man. JAMA 192:108, 1965

Barnard JH: Studies of 400 hymenoptera sting deaths in the United States. J Allergy Clin Immunol 52:259, 1973

Barr SE: Allergy to hymenoptera stings—review of the world literature 1953–1970. Ann Allergy 29:49, 1971

Frick OL: Anaphylaxis. In Gellis SS, Kagan BM (eds): Current Pediatric Therapy, Vol 4. Philadelphia, WB Saunders, 1970, p 934

Reisman RE, Arbesman CE: Stinging insect allergy, current concepts and problems. Pediatr Clin North Am 22:185, 1975

Sobotka A, Franklin R, Valentine M, Adkinson NF, Lichtenstein LM: Honeybee venom. Phospholipase A as the major allergen. J Allergy Clin Immunol 53:103, 1974

Yocum MW, Johnstone DE, Condemi JJ: Leukocyte histamine release in hymenoptera-allergic patients. J Allergy Clin Immunol 52:265, 1973

SERUM SICKNESS

Serum sickness (toxic complex disease) is a type III Gell and Coombs hypersensitivity state that was quite common when heterologous animal antiserum was used to treat infectious diseases such as diphtheria, tetanus, and pneumococcal and meningococcal infections. With the advent of antibiotics, antiserum therapy diminished greatly. However, animal antisera are still used for the treatment of snake and arthropod venom poisoning, rabies, botulism, diphtheria, and gas gangrene, as well as in transplantation immunity with ALG (antilymphocyte globulin) or ATG (antithymocyte globulin). Symptoms like those of serum sickness from drug allergies such as penicillin and its derivatives are more frequent now.

The pathogenesis of serum sickness has been demonstrated in experimental animals. In one study, following an injection of radionuclide-labeled antigen, serum antigen concentration fell rapidly initially from equilibration with tissues; there was then gradual clearance of antigen lasting about 6 days, followed by a sudden clearing of antigen at 12 to 14 days. During this time there was no free antibody in the serum, but when antigen disappeared from the serum, serum antibody levels rose rapidly and reached a peak in the next 5 to 6 days. The symptoms of serum sickness and the lesions (arteritis, splenic inflammation, and glomerulonephritis) appeared during the time of rapid clearance of antigen from the circulation. Antigen–antibody complexes in antigen excess were observed in the serum at the time of increasing serum sickness symptoms and pathology. As soon as all the antigen disappeared from the circulation, antigen–antibody complex proportions became equivalent, at which time the symptoms and pathology of serum sickness began to clear. Therefore it appeared that antigen–antibody complexes in the region of antigen excess were toxic for those tissues involved in serum sickness.

Histologic sections of the glomeruli, spleen, and arteries from animals and also patients with serum sickness show, with fluorescence labeling, deposits of antigen, gamma globulin (IgG and IgM), and complement (C3) localized at or near the basement membranes. In the kidney these take on a lumpy-bumpy pattern on the side of the basement membrane away from the vessel lumen and are enclosed by the foot processes of the epithelial cells. Similar lesions are seen in poststreptococcal glomerulonephritis. The incidence of serum sickness increases directly with the amount of foreign serum injected. Formerly, when 100 ml or more of foreign serum was given, about 90 percent of patients developed the syndrome, whereas only about 10 percent reacted from 10 ml of serum. The current use of "despeciated" serum globulin, which has been subjected to peptic digestion, has further reduced the incidence of serum sickness.

Serum sickness symptoms usually begin 7 to 12 days (but may occur at 5 to 20 days) after the serum injection. If the patient has previously received the same type of foreign serum, an accelerated reaction may occur after 1 to 5 days. Local irritation and itching at the injection site may occur first, followed by a generalized itchy urticarial or angioedematous rash. The rash may be maculopapular and erythematous and sometimes purpuric; typical erythema multiforme may occur. There usually is fever of moderate degree, with headache and general malaise. Arthralgia occurs in half the patients, and inflammatory effusions may occur in several joints. Generalized lymphadenopathy that may be painful usually occurs in the regional nodes but may become generalized. The spleen is often enlarged and may be tender. Nausea, vomiting, and abdominal pain may occur. Generalized edema and weight gain are frequent. Rarely, peripheral neuropathy and even the Guillain-Barré syndrome may be encountered. Central nervous involvement has occurred, with optic neuritis, transient hemiplegia, and coma. As in experimental animals, transient renal disease and arteritis may be evident, and coronary artery involvement may be evidenced by electrocardiographic changes.

On laboratory examination the leukocyte count may be normal or slightly elevated, and eosinophilia is common late in the disease. Occasionally there are atypical lymphocytes or circulating plasmacytes and a slightly elevated sedimentation rate. The differential diagnosis includes infectious mononucleosis, rheumatic fever, and glomerulonephritis.

The course of serum sickness is variable, ranging from a few days of urticaria to 1 to 2 weeks of severe illness with marked itching and joint pains and occasional laryngeal obstruction. The Guillain-Barré syndrome and other neurologic complications may last several months, but recovery is usually complete. In rare instances of death, inflammatory changes in the blood vessels, kidneys, liver, adrenals, and myocardium have been noted.

Treatment

Because the illness is self-limiting, the main objective is symptomatic relief until the process subsides. Because urticaria, angioedema, and arthralgia are usually the main complaints, antihistamines, epinephrine, tranquilizers, and sedatives are used extensively. Aspirin may be useful for the fever and arthralgia. Depending upon the severity of the patient's symptomatology, a course of 5 to 7 days of systemic corticosteroids is indicated. High doses of corticosteroids are indicated for neurologic involvement. After recovery, active immunization for tetanus should be given so that antiserum will not be required again.

References

Arbesman CE, Hyman I, Dauzier G, Kantor SZ: Immunologic studies of a Guillain-Barré syndrome following tetanus antitoxin. NY State J Med 58:2647, 1958

————Kantor SZ, Rose NR, Witebsky E: Serum sickness: serologic studies following prophylactic tetanus anti-toxin. J Allergy 31:257, 1960

Dixon FJ, Vazquez JJ, Weigle WO, Cochrane CG: Immunology and pathogenesis of experimental serum sickness. In Lawrence HS (ed): Cellular and Humoral Aspects of Hypersensitivity States. New York, Hoeber, 1959, p 354

Germuth FG: Comparative histologic and immunologic study in rabbits of induced hypersensitivity of the serum sickness type. J Exp Med 97:257, 1953

DRUG ALLERGIES

Most drugs are simple organic chemicals of low molecular weight, and thus they are not immunogenic; however, during their metabolism, especially by the liver, active groups may be formed that couple readily with serum albumin and globulins, or with erythrocytes and platelets. These normal body constitutents coupled with a foreign chemical are recognized as foreign materials by the body's immunologic defense mechanisms. Lymphocytes become sensitized, and some convert to antibody-producing plasma cells against the autologous protein with the attached drug. These antibodies may be in the IgE, IgG, IgM, or IgA classes, and cellular immune responses may occur. An individual so sensitized may on a future exposure to the drug react directly with the drug itself, or with the drug conjugated onto a body protein. Any of the four types of hypersensitivity responses may occur (p. 329).

Since the liver has only about 10 major pathways to detoxify chemicals, for which liver microsome enzymes are required (eg, *O*-dealkylation, *N*-hydroxylation, deamination, hydroxylation of aromatic rings), a limited number of possible conjugates can be formed; thus a certain degree of immunologic cross-reactivity among drugs may be noted. Biologicals, which are proteins or carbohydrates, may be immunogenic in their own right, particularly the hormones such as insulin and corticotropin (ACTH). Being of high molecular weight, biologicals are immunogenic per se.

In penicillin allergy, several metabolic pathways are clinically important; the minor metabolic pathway is responsible for most anaphylactic reactions. Rashes and symptoms like those of serum sickness are caused by IgE antibodies to major pathway products. Acute hemolytic anemia has been reported in some patients receiving high doses of intravenous penicillin (40 million units daily) for treatment of infectious endocarditis. With large amounts of penicillin, the membranes of many erythrocytes become coated with penicillin G and are recognized as being foreign, which leads to formation of IgG and IgM antibodies that react with the red cells and cause lysis.

The major penicilloyl determinant causes the formation of IgG antibodies in recently treated patients, concomitant with IgE antibody production. The IgG antibodies appear to act as blocking antibodies and prevent IgE-mediated anaphylactic reactions. Because large amounts of antigen are required for the formation of IgG antibodies, blocking antibodies to minor determinants do not occur. This may explain the development of anaphylactic reactions with the minor determinants.

Diagnosis of Penicillin Allergy

Many individuals develop a rash or other reactions during infections in which penicillin has been administered; these patients are often labeled as being penicillin-allergic. Several immunologic studies have shown that only about 10 percent of such patients have penicil-

lin antibodies. This would suggest that most so-called penicillin reactions are secondary to the infection or possibly to other drugs. A diagnostic skin test for penicillin allergy has been developed using penicilloyl polylysine (PPL) that produces a wheal and flare in patients with IgE antibodies to the major determinant (Kremers Urban Co., Milwaukee, Wisc.). Polylysine has been coupled with minor penamaldyl-penicillamine to make minor determinant skin test materials. These are not commercially available, but they are useful for detecting IgE antibodies that may lead to anaphylactic reactions from penicillin.

Treatment of Penicillin Reactions

If a patient has had a previous penicillin reaction, non-penicillin-related antibiotic should be chosen. If penicillin is clearly the drug of choice, such as in group A β-hemolytic streptococcal endocarditis, it may be administered under controlled circumstances, as shown by Levine and Bierman. If both the major determinant and minor determinant skin tests are negative, penicillin G can be given without incident. If the major determinant skin test is positive and the minor determinant skin test negative, maculopapular rash or serum sickness is likely to occur; in such patients concomitant corticosteroid therapy may be indicated. If the major determinant skin test is negative and the minor test positive, anaphylaxis is likely. Severe anaphylaxis can be avoided by pretreating with high doses of antihistamines (diphenhydramine) and corticosteroids, with epinephrine at hand.

So-called aspirin allergy is a major problem, especially in adults, but there is little evidence that this is an immunologic reaction. The acetyl derivative of salicylates appears to be involved, because aspirin-sensitive patients can often tolerate other forms of salicylates but occasionally have reactions with other acetylated compounds. The adult syndrome of asthma that begins in middle age, aspirin sensitivity, and nasal polyps is not associated with antibodies to aspirin. Although aspirin sensitivity has been reported in children, it is rare. Desensitization or immunotherapy to drugs is not practical and has met with little success. There are reports of successful immunotherapy with the protein antigens, such as insulin or corticotropin. For insulin hypersensitivity, changing from pig insulin to insulin from another species such as cow has occasionally been successful.

Anaphylactic reactions to human gamma globulin are usually due to aggregates of gamma globulin in a bottle that has been allowed to sit for some time. Upon intramuscular injection of such gamma globulin, there may be some inadvertent intravenous injection of some of these aggregates, which release anaphylatoxins from complement activation; these cause the release of histamine and anaphylactic symptoms. It is therefore best to use fresh gamma globulin preparations, and they may be centrifuged at high speed to remove a major portion of aggregates. Recently, "despeciated" gamma globulin treated with enzymatic digestion has offered a new approach to intravenous gamma globulin therapy, although it is still experimental.

Anaphylaxis to gamma globulin has also occurred from Gm groups, which are genetic markers (Gm) on immunoglobulins, mostly on IgG, analogous to blood groups on erythrocytes. If a patient lacks a particular marker and is repeatedly transfused with IgG with that marker, antibody to that Gm marker develops. Upon further transfusion of mismatched IgG, anaphylaxis or a transfusion reaction may occur, but they are rare. Problems arise more commonly in IgA-deficient or IgA-absent individuals who receive repeated transfusions of plasma that contains IgA. IgA is recognized as a foreign protein and stimulates production of anaphylactic antibodies. Upon subsequent administration of IgA, anaphylaxis may occur. An IgA-deficient patient should receive either packed red cells for transfusion or transfusion from another IgA-negative individual.

References

Bierman CW, Van Arsdel PP Jr: Penicillin allergy in children: the role of immunological tests in its diagnosis. J Allergy 43:267, 1969

Ellis EF, Henney C: Adverse reactions following administration of human gamma-globulin. J Allergy 43:45, 1969

Gell PCH, Coombs RRA: Clinical Aspects of Immunology, 2nd ed. Oxford, Blackwell, 1968, p 575

Levine B: Immunologic mechanisms of penicillin allergy. N Engl J Med 275:1115, 1966

——Zolov DM: Prediction of penicillin allergy by immunological tests. J Allergy 43:231, 1969

Samter M: The pathogenesis of reactions to drugs. In Serafini U (ed): New Concepts in Allergy and Clinical Immunology. Amsterdam, Excerpta Medica, 1971, p 191

——Beers RF: Concerning the nature of intolerance to aspirin. J Allergy 40:281, 1967

Vyas GN, Perkins HA, Fudenberg HH: Anaphylactoid transfusion reactions associated with anti-IgA. Lancet 2:312, 1968

CHRONIC SEROUS OTITIS MEDIA

This may be defined as impaired hearing due to prolonged accumulation of fluid behind a tympanic membrane for a period of at least 6 weeks. Normal transmission of sound depends on air in the middle ear and equalization of pressure on both sides of the eardrum. Following infections, fluid accumulates in the middle ear; such fluid is purulent if it is from bacteria and serous or clear if it is from viruses. Mechanical obstruction causes transudation of plasma; if it is of allergic origin the fluid is usually serous. Politzer suggested that blockage of the eustachian tube was followed by rapid absorption of air, leaving a vacuum in the middle ear that causes transudation of plasma fluids into the middle ear cavity. Cilia beating toward the blocked eustachian tube orifices also force air out, adding to the vacuum. Otologists report that serous otitis is the most common pediatric problem they encounter.

The incidence of serous otitis appears to be increasing; many causes have been suggested. Suehs felt that inadequate antibiotic therapy for infected otitis media aborted the infection before suppuration could occur,

and chronic serous discharge resulted. However, not all patients with serous otitis have had antibiotic therapy. Otologists have suggested that insufficiently frequent myringotomies and incomplete adenoidectomies may account for this increasing incidence.

Allergists have observed that the pseudostratified columnar ciliated epithelium lining the eustachian tube and middle ear is similar to that in the nose, trachea, and bronchi. They suggest that the middle ear is merely an extension of the nasal cavity and should also be subject to allergic reactions. A high incidence of allergy has been reported in children with recurrent secretory otitis.

Pathophysiology

The eustachian tube opens frequently, upon swallowing, permitting the air pressures on both sides of the eardrum to remain equal. The moist mucous inner surfaces of the eustachian tube stick together; the resulting surface tension is overcome by swallowing, which momentarily opens the tube and admits air. Infectious or allergic inflammation causes edema and may produce mechanical obstruction; this causes a negative pressure that may lead to transudation of plasma. It is possible that increased protein concentration of the fluid increases osmotic pressure and attracts additional fluid into the ear.

In children, and especially infants, the eustachian tube is short and wide and runs horizontally from the pharynx to the middle ear, permitting easy access to fluid from the pharynx to the middle ear. In later childhood the tube elongates and slopes downward about 45 degrees from the middle ear, permitting middle ear drainage; thus young children are more likely to develop middle ear infection from the nasal pharynx.

The eustachian tube is lined with ciliated pseudostratified columnar cells interspersed with goblet cells. The tympanic cavity is lined with clumps of ciliated cells in islands surrounded by flat nonciliated cells, but near the ciliated islands are raised nonciliated cells that appear to be secretory. Lim has classified chronic otitis media into mucoid and serous types. In the mucoid type there is a great increase in goblet cells; the lamina propria is rich in plasma cells and lymphocytes. The fluid or "glue" exudate is rich in secretory elements and breakdown products of pus cells, which favors a postinfective origin for the mucoid type. On the other hand, in the serous type the eustachian tube mucosa has much intercellular edema in the epithelial and connective tissue layers, with marked infiltrates of macrophages, lymphocytes, and plasma cells. This is similar to the pathology in allergic inflammation of the bronchial and nasal mucosa, although eosinophils are not common in serous otitis. The eustachian tube and hypotympanum are rich in mast cells that are a source of histamine. Experimentally the eustachian tube responds to histamine with swelling, which can be lessened by antihistamine therapy. Epinephrine and α-adrenergic stimulating drugs can constrict capillaries and open the tubes, while cholinergic and β-adrenergic drugs increase the swelling and close the lumen. Autonomic nervous controls thus may affect the eustachian tube.

Several studies have shown that serum protein, gamma globulin, and IgE levels in middle ear fluid are similar to those in plasma, thus suggesting that it is a transudate. It has been suggested that serous otitis media is not an allergic disease, but that in about one-third of patients with chronic recurrent serous otitis media edema of the eustachian tube and nasal pharynx occurs secondary to allergy. This results in eustachian tube dysfunction and causes middle ear disease.

Clinical Findings

The primary symptom is hearing loss, which may be insidious and discovered only on routine audiogram screening; it may be transient and fluctuate with periods of normal hearing. This tends to minimize the concern of the parents and the physician. Although the drum may appear normal or bulging, it is usually retracted, with a prominent short process of the malleus. It is often dull and may be pink, gray, slightly yellow or amber, or blue. A fluid level or air bubbles may be visible. Pathognomonic of secretory otitis is a chalky white handle of the malleus. Mobility of the drum may be impaired when it is examined by the pneumatic otoscope.

A conductive type of hearing loss due to middle ear fluid may be diagnosed with tuning forks; the low tones, at frequencies of 256 and 512 Hz, are usually lost first. On audiometry, a hearing loss of 15 decibels in at least two frequencies is considered significant. Because of its insidious nature, the hearing loss may persist for months or years, and there may be speech or learning impairment due to the child's inability to hear words correctly and understand their meaning. In some children the defects may be so severe that the child is considered mentally retarded.

Allergic Diagnosis

A history of allergy was noted in 40 percent of parents of children with apparently allergic serous otitis. Eosinophilia of 10 percent or more in a nasal smear suggests allergy. Immediate skin tests may be useful if an inhalant or pollen sensitivity is suspected. Skin tests for foods are generally unsatisfactory, and elimination and provocation diets may prove useful for such a diagnosis. The elimination of milk, chocolate, corn, wheat, and eggs has often proved useful in alleviating food-induced serous otitis.

Treatment

Ventilation of the middle ear may succeed, with decongestants such as phenylephrine hydrochloride (Neo-Synephrine) topically, or oral phenylephrine or ephedrine, and antihistaminics. Ventilation maneuvers, such as the Valsalva maneuver or politzerization, may be therapeutically useful. Air displaces fluid and de-creases fluid accumulation. Any infection should be controlled with antibiotic therapy.

Repeated myringotomies to remove fluid in patients not responding to medical treatment are advocated by some otologists. Prolonged ventilation of the middle ear has been attempted by placing plastic tubes through the tympanic membranes, but the lumen usually plugs; if the maneuver is successful it is usually due to air leakage around the tube. Adenoidectomy may be successful in many patients where decongestants, myringotomies, and tubings have not helped.

Immunotherapy

If the occurrence of serous otitis is seasonal, a pollen may be suspected, in which case immunotherapy may be effective. For allergy to house dust or animal danders, removal of the allergen is more important than immunotherapy. For a food allergen, elimination is the only satisfactory treatment. In children with recurrent serous otitis who had had repeated adenoidectomies and tube placings without success, Lecks found that two-thirds responded to allergic management, eg, environmental control, food elimination, and/or immunotherapy.

Medical treatment with vasoconstrictors, antihistamines, and ventilation techniques helps about half the patients with serous otitis; in about 20 percent the origin may be allergic, and these are helped by antiallergic therapy. Surgical intervention with myringotomies, placing of tubes, and adenoidectomies may be helpful in the recalcitrant chronic cases.

References

Fernandez AA, McGovern JP: Secretory otitis media in allergic infants and children. South Med J 58:581, 1965

Hussl B, Lim D: Experimental middle ear effusions: an immunofluorescent study. Ann Otol Rhinol Laryngol 83:332, 1974

Lecks HI: Allergic aspects of serous otitis media in childhood. NY State J Med 61:2737, 1961

Reisman RE, Bernstein J: Allergy and secretory otitis media. Clinical and immunologic studies. Pediatr Clin North Am 22:251, 1975

Suehs OW: Secretory otitis media. Laryngoscope 62:998, 1952

Whitcomb NJ: Allergy therapy in serous otitis media associated with allergic rhinitis. Ann Allergy 23:232, 1965

FOOD ALLERGY

Numerous adverse reactions to ingestion of foods have been described, beginning in the time of Hippocrates. May cautions that not all such reactions are allergic, but may be due to enzyme deficiencies, toxicity in food, drugs, antibiotic contaminants, bacteria or their by-products, or additives. The term allergic should be reserved for immunologic reactions of one of the four types of hypersensitivity that involve IgE, IgG, IgM, or IgA antibodies or cellular immune reactions.

Immediate anaphylactic reactions to foods are IgE-mediated. Fish, nuts, eggs, legumes (peanuts and beans), and shellfish are common allergens for such reactions. Immediate skin tests are positive with the suspected allergen, and passive transfer with serum is positive; in fact, the original Prausnitz-Küstner (PK) passive transfer study was accomplished with fish antigen. IgE antibodies may be detected in vitro by RAST and by leukocyte histamine release. Allergens may be rapidly absorbed through the intestinal mucosa into the circulation. Following passive transfer of allergic serum into the skin of a normal recipient, ingestion of the suspected allergen results in a positive skin test within 15 to 60 minutes; the antigen may be intact protein or an antigenic product of its digestion. The intestinal mucosa is rich in IgE-forming plasma cells, which probably are the origin of the anaphylactic antibodies to food proteins. The clinical model of anaphylaxis to foods parallels that of ragweed-induced hay fever. In addition to anaphylactic shock from certain foods, less severe reactions such as rhinitis, asthma, urticaria, and abdominal pain or vomiting may occur within minutes; these are also associated with IgE antibodies.

Similar allergic symptoms may occur only a few hours after ingestion of a particular food and may last for days. In a study of delayed-onset food allergy, we demonstrated positive skin tests only rarely, and leukocyte histamine release with the suspected allergen in 30 percent. The symptomatology in these patients improved markedly upon food elimination. Later we demonstrated a specific leukocyte migration-inhibition factor to milk or corn proteins from lymphocytes in about half of these patients; all had IgG antibodies to many foods. These findings suggest that other immunologic mechanisms may be involved in delayed-onset food allergy. These may be Arthus-type immune complexes of IgG or IgM antibodies, or reactions like that of serum sickness, or true cellular immune reactions or tuberculin-like reactions. Malabsorption syndromes such as celiac disease or nontropical sprue are associated with elevated, specific IgA antibodies to wheat and milk proteins in the serum. These IgA antibodies may replace the function of IgE antibodies in the pathogenesis of malabsorption syndrome or protein-losing enteropathies. Saperstein found that sera of milk-allergic patients often gave positive guinea-pig passive cutaneous anaphylaxis (PCA) tests with milk proteins; guinea-pig PCA tests with human sera are positive only with IgG antibodies, which may indicate an immune complex mechanism. Therefore delayed-onset food allergy may involve immune reactions other than those mediated by IgE.

Buckley and Dees observed that children lacking IgA commonly had circulating precipitating antibodies (IgG) to food proteins, such as milk and egg; they suggested that secretory IgA in the intestines prevented immunologically, the absorption of whole undigested proteins and that if the IgA barrier was missing such protein antigens were absorbed by the intestine and taken up by the lymphatics to regional nodes where other antibodies were stimulated. It is possible that the frequent occurrence of food allergies in infants is related to slow development of the secretory IgA barrier; once the IgA barrier develops fully at about 1 year of age, the incidence of food allergy diminishes markedly.

Clinical Findings

Almost all systems of the body may be involved in adverse reactions to foods. Most common are the respiratory tract (with rhinitis, cough and wheeze, and less commonly laryngeal edema), the gastrointestinal tract (with nausea and vomiting, abdominal pain, diarrhea, constipation, malabsorption, and protein-losing enteropathy), the skin (with urticaria, eczema, and maculopapular and other rashes, vascular collapse or shock), the genitourinary tract (with frequency and urgency, burning, enuresis, proteinuria, and vaginitis). Central nervous system involvement causes intermittent headaches and convulsions and the tension fatigue syndrome in which apathy and lassitude alternate with irritability and restlessness and personality changes. The incidence of reactions to food varies widely; various reports claim that 0.3 to 7 percent of individuals are allergic to cow's milk. Based on this, breast feeding should be encouraged for the first 6 months of life, and introduction of new foods should be limited until the IgA barrier develops.

Diagnosis

The history is especially important in establishing the diagnosis of food allergy, with special attention being given to correlation of onset of symptoms with ingestion of a particular food. With the anaphylactic type of reaction, these events are usually obvious to the patient. In these cases in vivo skin testing should be avoided, as it may provoke anaphylaxis. If necessary, confirmation may be obtained with the in vitro RAST or leukocyte histamine release tests. The history is not as useful in delayed-onset food allergy; a dietary diary may be helpful. If any foods are suspect, a trial elimination diet should alleviate the symptoms, with reintroduction of the food provoking them. In those instances in which a specific food cannot be incriminated, several forms of elimination diets have been proposed. In children, the common food allergens are cow's milk, eggs, chocolate, cereals such as corn and wheat, legumes (peanuts, beans, soybeans), oranges, fish, beef, and chicken. We have found that diets eliminating milk and chocolate or corn and wheat will improve the symptoms in about 80 percent of food-allergic children. At the beginning of an elimination diet trial, we make a symptom and medication score with which to compare the clinical course while on elimination diets. The diet should have at least a 3-week and preferably a 6-week trial, because it may take a week for the body to rid itself of traces of an offending food allergen. If improvement occurs, the suspected offender is reintroduced cautiously in an attempt to provoke the symptoms. It may take several weeks before sufficient antibody is reformed to cause symptoms. If elimination of the four main offending foods is not successful, we resort to a more drastic basic elimination diet consisting of a few simple foods (Table

1). To this basic elimination diet, a new food class is added every 4 days until the offending food is identified or until the case for food allergy is insupportable. Another cardinal caution that must be emphasized is to use the elimination diet trial only for a predetermined time; do not permit an elimination diet that is inconclusive to run on for months.

Because successful elimination diet trials require a great deal of parental cooperation and sophistication, alternative diagnostic methods for food allergy have been sought, thus far with little consistent success. Skin tests with food extracts appear to be generally unreliable, in that there are numerous irritative positive reactions; also, negative skin tests occur frequently when the diagnosis of a food allergen has been established by elimination diet. There may be many reasons for this discrepancy. Usually, food testing extracts are prepared from fresh uncooked foods; cooking may denature the allergen so that there may be a false positive test with the raw food. On the other hand, certain foods become allergenic only after cooking; enzymatic digestion of the food may produce new allergens. Skin tests show only IgE antibodies, not those of other immunoglobulin classes nor sensitized lymphocytes. In spite of this, Goldman showed that carefully performed skin tests with milk proteins were positive in about 60 percent of allergic children, but only 6 percent of nonallergic children.

X-ray studies with suspected allergenic food mixed with barium for gastrointestinal examination may show changes such as gastric retention, hypermotility, or abnormal segmentation of the small intestine or bowel. These examinations are cumbersome and expensive and are not indicated, as only one food can be tested at a time.

Fecal or rectal swab eosinophilia, or blood eosinophilia, may suggest a food allergen reaction. Currently a number of specific immunologic tests are being evaluated for diagnosis of food allergy, eg, RAST, leukocyte histamine release test, and lymphocyte transformation test.

References

Buckley RH, Dees SC: Correlation of milk precipitins with IgA deficiency. N Engl J Med 281:465, 1969

Galant SP, Bullock J, Frick OL: An immunological approach to the diagnosis of food sensitivity. Clin Allergy 3:363, 1973

Gerrard JW, MacKenzie JWA, Goluboff N, Garson JZ, Maringas CS: Cow's milk allergy: prevalence and manifestations in an unselected series of newborns. Acta Paediatr Scand [Suppl 1] 1973, p 234

Golbert TM, Patterson R, Pruzansky JJ: Systemic allergic reactions to ingested antigens. J Allergy 44:96, 1969

Goldman AS, Sellars WA, Halpern SR, et al: Milk allergy. II. Skin testing of allergic and normal children with purified milk proteins. Pediatrics 32:572, 1963

Hoffman DR, Haddad ZH: Diagnosis of IgE-mediated reactions to food antigens by radioimmunoassay. J Allergy Clin Immunol 54:165, 1974

Liu HY, Tsao MU, Moore B, Giday Z: Bovine milk protein-induced intestinal malabsorption of lactose and fat in infants. Gastroenterology 54:27, 1967

May CD: Food allergy. In Fomon SJ (ed): Infant Nutrition. Philadelphia, WB Saunders, 1974, p 435

Rowe AH: Elimination Diets and the Patient's Allergies, 2nd ed. Philadelphia, Lea & Febiger, 1944, p 156

Saperstein S, Anderson DW Jr, Goldman AS, Kniker WT: Milk allergy. III. Immunological studies with sera from allergic and normal children. Pediatrics 32:580, 1963

GASTROINTESTINAL ALLERGY

Anaphylaxis in many species is accompanied by symptoms of gastrointestinal distress. Thus it is expected that the gastrointestinal tract may respond to either direct or indirect antigen exposure in an allergic individual. Although foods are the most common source of gastrointestinal symptoms, food allergy is not limited to this organ system; the respiratory, urinary, and central nervous systems can respond to food allergens. Furthermore, some patients have nausea, vomiting, and diarrhea after exposure to inhaled allergens; 90 percent of inhaled pollen lands in the stomach and 10 percent or less in the bronchi. Indirect gastrointestinal allergy may be part of a systemic allergic reaction to inhaled or injected allergens, eg, anaphylaxis, generalized urticaria.

The lamina propria of the intestine is rich in plasma cells and forms all the immunoglobulins, but in particular IgA and IgE in a ratio of about 100 to 1; both are considered to be secretory immunoglobulins. IgA antibody newly formed by the plasma cells traverses the mucosal epithelial cells that produce secretory-piece protein and forms a complex of secretory IgA consisting of two IgA monomers held together with one molecule of secretory piece. The piece covers the hinge region of the IgA monomer, protecting this vulnerable portion from digestive enzyme attack; secretory IgA functions as an efficient antibody in the presence of trypsin and pepsin, which digest other proteins. Some IgA, without the secretory piece, is absorbed into the circulation. IgE antibody is vulnerable to tryptic digestion, but less so than IgG and IgM antibodies.

A teleologic explanation for the normal functional role of IgE antibodies is offered in its defensive role against parasitic infections. Both plasma and intestinal IgE levels are elevated in nematode and some protozoan infections. In several animal species the young are readily infected with roundworms that are cleared after several weeks by the self-cure phenomenon associated with a rise in IgE and IgG antibodies to that parasite. IgE antibody in the intestinal mucosa reacts with parasitic antigen to cause the release of histamine; this causes intestinal vasodilatation and leakage of plasma that is rich in IgG antiparasite antibodies. Such IgG antibodies agglutinate on the surface of the parasite, starve it, and aid in its destruction by macrophages.

Clinical Findings

Symptoms and signs of gastrointestinal responses to antigens occur along the entire tract, from the mouth to the anus.

MOUTH. The lips may be inflamed and the corners of the mouth cracked from contact sensitization to chemicals or foods, especially lipstick in older girls. In infants, circumoral or chin eczema may follow contact with irritant foods such as oranges, carrots, tomatoes, and spinach. The lips and buccal mucosa may be very swollen after ingestion of small amounts of certain foods (eg, eggs, fish, and nuts), and there may be associated urticaria and swelling of the tongue and laryngeal tissues, which could be life-threatening. Hypersensitivity stomatitis occurs from contact sensitivity to dental materials. Aphthous stomatitis (canker sores) may be caused by some foods, especially chocolate, nuts, and citric and acetic acids.

STOMACH. Nausea, vomiting, and anorexia may have an allergic origin. In some infants, pylorospasm caused by cow's milk may be so intense as to cause projectile vomiting, so that pyloric stenosis is diagnosed and surgically corrected. Changing to a soy or Nutramigen formula may sometimes relieve such pylorospasm. Acute attacks of nausea and vomiting that occur in cyclic fashion in older children have been attributed to "abdominal migraine." They have a sudden onset, last several days, and recur at weekly or monthly intervals. Vomiting may be severe, and headache, diarrhea, and abdominal pain are often associated. Elimination of certain foods may control these cyclic episodes in some children, thus suggesting an allergic origin.

INTESTINE. Abdominal pain from intestinal distension and hyperperistalsis may be of allergic origin. Infantile colic is commonly attributed to cow's milk and is found especially where there have been frequent changes of formula. Often there is a dramatic alleviation of colic after changing to a non-cow's-milk formula, such as soybean, meat base, or protein hydrolysate formulae.

COLON. Diarrhea that results from irritability and hypermotility of the colon has multiple causes including allergy. Infantile diarrhea with loose greenish or mucousy stools is sometimes relieved by changing from a cow's-milk formula to one of soybean or meat base or by removing or changing cereals. In older children with irritable colon or mucous colitis, diarrhea and mucus in the stool are usually attributed to psychologic causes; however, it may coexist with asthma and improve after elimination of certain foods from the diet. Therefore Vaughan has suggested a basic similarity between asthma and mucous colitis, in that both are characterized by smooth muscle spasm and increased secretion of mucus.

Although intestinal bleeding is rare in children, it has been associated with milk-induced diarrhea, protein loss, and coproantibodies of IgA type to milk proteins that clear on removal of milk from the diet; this suggests an Arthus-type mechanism. A similar Arthus-type mechanism may operate in anaphylactoid purpura (Schönlein-Henoch purpura), which involves the skin, gastrointestinal tract, joints, and kidney in a syndrome that resembles severe continuing serum sickness.

ANUS. Pruritus ani may be caused by eggs, tomatoes, potatoes, wheat, and buckwheat, which suggests food allergy. Occasionally hay fever patients are affected similarly during the pollen season by swallowed pollen that is eliminated through the rectum.

References

Gerrard JW: Gastrointestinal allergy in infants. In Speer F, Dockhorn RJ (eds): Allergy and Immunology in Children. Springfield, Ill, Charles C Thomas, 1973, p 570

Jones VE, Ogilvie BM: Protective immunity to Nippostronglus brasiliensis: the sequence of events which expels worms from the rat intestine. Immunology 20:549, 1971

Katz J, Spiro HM, Herskovic T: Milk-precipitating substance in the stool in gastrointestinal sensitivity. N Engl J Med 278:1191, 1968

Minor JD, Frick OL: Leukocyte inhibition factor (LIF) production in "delayed onset food allergy." J Allergy Clin Immunol 55:88, 1975

Tada T, Ishizaka K: Distribution of γE-forming cells in lymphoid tissues of the human and monkey. J Immunol 104:377, 1970

Tomasi F: Distribution and synthesis of human secretory components. In Dayton D, Small P, et al (eds): The Secretory Immunologic System. Bethesda, National Institute of Child Health and Human Development, 1971, p 41

Wilson JF, Heiner DC, Lahey ME: Milk-induced gastrointestinal bleeding in infants with hypochronic microcytic anemia. JAMA 189:568, 1964

NEUROLOGIC ALLERGIES

Although recurrent headaches are common in children, the incidence of migraine headaches has been estimated at only about 5 percent. There are many causes of headache; after organic causes have been excluded, there are many children with unexplained recurrent headaches that have been termed migraine or allergic headache. Whether these are truly immunologic in origin remains to be proved; in some children, removal of specific allergens from the environment or diet is associated with improvement. In older children and adults, classic migraine with an aura, nausea, and vomiting is less amenable to allergy treatment.

Headache is generally thought to result from cranial vessel constriction and subsequent vasodilatation that stretches pain fibers. The vessels respond readily to epinephrine and norepinephrine with vasoconstriction; they dilate with histamine, serotonin, and kinins, which are known mediators of allergic responses. It is therefore conceivable that perivascular mast cells containing histamine, serotonin, and kinins could be sensitized with IgE or IgG antibodies and release their mediators upon contact with antigen, causing cranial symptoms.

Clinical Findings

Most children with such headaches indicate the forehead or area above one eye, or temple, as the involved area, with other areas rarely involved. The headache is commonly associated with dizziness, nausea, anorexia, photophobia, blurred vision, and occasionally vomiting. In a study of 143 patients presenting with migraine headaches, Speer reported that 20 percent of these were children. He found that inhalants such as molds and house dust were often incriminated and that marked improvement occurred with environmental control measures and immunotherapy. Foods, especially milk, chocolate, and corn, were also a factor in most of these children.

References

Bille B: Migraine in school children. Acta Paediatr Scand [Suppl 136] 51:151, 1962

Speer F: Allergic migraine. In Speer F, Dockhorn RJ (eds): Allergy and Immunology in Childhood. Springfield, Ill, Charles C Thomas, 1973, p 628

TENSION FATIGUE SYNDROME

Fatigue, irritability, inner tension, and awkwardness were associated with chronic rhinitis and headaches by Baker in 1898, even before allergies had been established as clinical entities. Rowe subsequently called attention to "allergic toxemia" in patients with hay fever and asthma that he felt was due to certain foods and was amenable to elimination diet control. In 1954 Speer suggested the term allergic tension fatigue syndrome for the diffuse symptoms and signs commonly found in allergic individuals.

Clinical Findings

The syndrome presents with alternating periods of tension and fatigue, which may occur within a few hours or a day, but the swings in mood may last several days to weeks. The tension fatigue syndrome appears to be an accentuation of a normal pattern of mood changes. Tension is manifested by hyperkinesis, with clumsiness, overreactivity, manual control problems, inability to relax, hyperesthesia with irritability, insomnia, photophobia, and hypersensitivity to noise. The fatigue phase has a motor component of tiredness and sluggishness and a sensory component of torpor and generalized muscle achiness. Various organ systems are involved, especially the respiratory tract, the nose with nasal stuffiness, sneezing, or itching that results in venous congestion manifesting signs of infraorbital circles (allergic "shiners") and edema. Coughing and wheezing are sometimes associated. There is usually pallor of the skin, especially of the face, and increased sweating. Abdominal pains, headache, and muscle pains are common; enuresis occurs frequently. In more severe forms, central nervous involvement may cause mental depression, irrational behavior, paranoid ideas, inability to concentrate, and nervous tics. In children, behavior disturbance and school problems may be the presenting complaint. The allergist may see the patient because of the common respiratory complaints.

In our study of 94 children with tension fatigue syndrome related to food sensitivity, the most common signs and symptoms in order of frequency were respiratory tract allergy, allergic rhinitis and asthma, abdominal discomfort, headaches, tenseness and irritability, facial pallor with infraorbital circles, tiredness and easy fatigability, and musculoskeletal pain. The pathophysiology is completely unknown, and this syndrome is difficult for physicians to recognize or even to accept as real. However, allergists have observed that elimination of certain foods, or occasionally a particular inhalant, may cause dramatic improvement within a few weeks; this is maintained until the food or inhalant is reintroduced, at which time the syndrome recurs.

Pathophysiology

Our attempts at immunologic documentation have been negative; we were unable to demonstrate IgE antibodies to common foods by skin tests, leukocyte histamine release, RAST, or cellular immunity (MIF production). The generalized systemic nature of the symptomatology suggests a generalized vascular response, possibly with edema, which might occur from allergic mediators such as histamine, bradykinin, serotonin, and possibly tyramine. In recent studies on migraine headaches, increased circulatory serotonin has been shown to occur in the preheadache phase and drop sharply with the onset of pain. An injection of reserpine drops blood serotonin and precipitates a migraine headache in susceptible subjects. A serotonin antagonist, methysergide, is the only effective prophylactic drug for migraine. The brain is the serotonin repository in man. Tyrosine is the source of the vasoactive amine tyramine that is metabolized by monoamine oxidases (MAO) to inactive hydroxyphenylacetic acid (HPAA). MAO inhibitor drugs block the enzymatic deamination of tyramine; this accumulates in the blood and acts as a toxic vasoactive amine, causing hypertension and headache of the migraine type. It was observed that certain patients taking MAO inhibitor drugs developed migraine headaches when eating foods high in tyramine or tyrosine-containing foods. Reducing the amounts of such foods or eliminating the inhibitor drugs relieved the migraine headaches; therefore it is conceivable, but not proved, that the vasoactive amines serotonin and tyramine might be involved in the pathogenesis of the tension fatigue syndrome. Both chocolate and cheese are rich in tyramine and are involved in migraine headaches and commonly cause the symptoms of tension fatigue syndrome.

Diagnosis

If there are sufficient clinical symptoms and signs to make one suspect the presence of the tension fatigue syndrome, and if other organic causes have been ruled out, a food elimination diet trial may be started. In our clinic the majority of children respond favorably to a milk- and dairy-product-free and chocolate-free diet over 4 to 6 weeks. Subsequently a provocative reintroduction of milk products, and possibly later chocolate, should recreate the symptoms in order to convince the patients, parents, and physician of the necessity to resume elimination of the offending foods. If there is no change on the milk and chocolate elimination diet, elimination of wheat and eggs is next tried. Although foods appear to cause the symptoms in the vast majority of cases of tension fatigue syndrome, a possible inhalant allergy should not be overlooked.

Treatment

If a diagnostic trial elimination diet is successful, and especially if provocative reintroduction of the food causes symptoms to return, long-term elimination of the offending foods is indicated. It is our practice to eliminate such a food for a least a year before attempting another provocative test.

References

Galant S, Bullock JD, Frick OL: An immunological approach to the diagnosis of food sensitivity. Clin Allergy 3:363, 1973

Speer F: Allergic tension-fatigue syndrome in children. Ann Allergy 12:168, 1954

Tretyakora KA, Fets AN: Total blood serotonin concentration in patients with migraine during and between attacks. Hemicrania 1:14, 1970

Urinary Allergies

The urinary tract ductal system is lined with smooth muscle and has a cuboid epithelium; there is a rich submucosal vascular supply and mast cells. Since it is a secretory surface, there are many plasma cells that secrete IgA and IgE, in similarity to those in the respiratory and gastrointestinal tract mucosa. Therefore one would expect that the urinary tract mucosa could respond to allergens in a type I anaphylactic or atopic response. Although this has not been widely reported, there are sporadic observations of urinary symptoms in patients with hay fever and asthma; frequently, urinary symptoms are worse during a specific pollen season. Furthermore, anaphylaxis in animals and in man has both urinary and fecal incontinence as a major component; this indicates that the bladder smooth muscle can partake of an immune reaction.

Clinical Findings

ENURESIS. An association of frequent urinary infections and allergic respiratory and gastrointestinal problems has been reported repeatedly. Dietary elimination regimens may improve the symptoms of enuresis, and the cholinergic blocking agent imipramine is very effective in many children. In enuretic children on imipramine therapy, there is an increase in bladder capacity, with a clinical improvement in the enuresis; this may be due to relaxation of chronically spastic bladder smooth muscles. Gerrard suggests that elimination of food allergens in some children with enuresis will remove the antigenic load that may be inducing the bladder muscle spasm. Crook reported that recurrent cystitis and vulvovaginitis in girls, and burning on urination and tugging on the penis in boys, were associated with food sensitivity and occasionally with inhalant allergy. The common foods were milk, corn, chocolate, citrus, and food colorings, the removal of which improved the symptomatology. Although more objective evidence of the association or reaginic antibodies with enuresis and bladder allergy is needed, the possibility of such a relationship should be kept in mind by any physician treating children.

ORTHOSTATIC ALBUMINURIA. Matsumura and associates studied 16 children with orthostatic albuminuria for evidence of food allergy. The majority had other associated symptoms, such as dizziness, fatigue, weakness, discomfort, and pallor. Removal of a suspected food from the diet caused a prompt clearing of the albuminuria, and reintroduction of the food caused its return. Milk was the predominant offending allergen, occuring in 12 of the 16 patients, whereas egg and soybean were implicated in the other cases.

NEPHROTIC SYNDROME. Seasonal nephrotic syndrome has been reported occasionally, and Reeves found a marked rise in IgE, particularly pollen-specific IgE, during the attacks in two patients. The syndrome has also occurred following bee stings.

Allergic antibodies have been associated with only a few cases of seasonal nephrotic syndrome; whether this association is pure coincidence, or the allergic attack is sufficiently stressful to initiate nephrotic symptoms, or there is truly an IgE antibody reaction occuring in the kidney in nephrosis awaits further investigation.

References

Esperanca M, Gerrard JW: Nocturnal enuresis. Comparison of the effect of imipramine and dietary restriction on bladder capacity. Can Med Assoc J 101:721, 1969

Gerrard JW, Jones B, Shokier MK, Zaleski A: Allergy and urinary tract infections. Is there an association? Pediatrics 48:995, 1971

Hardwicke J, Soothill JF, Squire JR, Holti G: Nephrotic syndrome with pollen hypersensitivity. Lancet 1:500, 1959

Matsumura T, Kuruome T, Fukushima I: Significance of food allergy in the etiology of orthostatic albuminuria. J Asthma Res 3:325, 1966

Reeves WG, Cameron JS, Johansson SGO, et al: Seasonal nephrotic syndrome. Description and immunological findings. Clin Allergy 5:121, 1975

Wittig HJ, Goldman AS: Nephrotic syndrome associated with inhaled allergens. Lancet 1:542, 1970

CHAPTER 11

Collagen Vascular Diseases (Rheumatic Diseases)

Arthur J. Ammann and Diane W. Wara

The rheumatic diseases discussed in this chapter are all chronic diseases that have in common inflammatory changes of the connective tissue throughout the body. Included for specific discussion are juvenile rheumatoid arthritis, systemic lupus erythematosus, dermatomyositis, scleroderma, necrotizing arteritis (Schönlein-Henoch purpura, polyarteritis, Wegener's granulomatosis, giant cell arteritis), Sjögren's syndrome, and rheumatic fever. In general the etiologies of these disorders remain unknown, and specific laboratory and clinical diagnostic criteria are lacking. However, each disease usually presents as a distinct entity. For example, chronic arthritis is associated with rheumatoid arthritis, inflammation of the muscle is associated with dermatomyositis, and renal disease is associated with systemic lupus erythematosus. But since each of these diseases can affect almost any organ in the body, specific diagnosis in a particular patient may be difficult, and the diseases in fact represent a broad spectrum of clinical entities.

Although the underlying etiology of each disease remains obscure, most investigators feel that autoimmune phenomena are involved. Unusual responses by the body to infection, to stress, or to hormonal changes that result in the production of antibody against the self are probably present in each disease entity; that is, a child would develop antibody against his own cell nuclei in systemic lupus erythematosus or against thyroid in thyroiditis. It is not clear, however, whether the production of autoantibody is directly related to the initiation of disease in each disorder or whether in some instances the onset of disease and alteration of tissue may actually precede and stimulate the development of autoantibodies. Further, in some instances the production of autoantibody may be an appropriate response of the immune system to an insult by foreign antigen such as a viral agent. Patients with polyarteritis appropriately form antibody to hepatitis-associated antigen (HB-Ag), which may be localized along the elastic membrane of arterial walls. Subsequent interaction of antigen (HB-Ag), antibody, and complement may lead to the pathologic changes characteristic of the disease.

It is now thought that, in addition to the development of antibodies, thymus-derived lymphocytes (T cells) may be involved in the pathology of autoimmune disease. Lymphocytes, in addition to antibodies, may attack one's own cells. Cellular sensitization has recently been demonstrated in patients with dermatomyositis and polymyositis. In this sense the concept of autoimmune disease has broadened in recent years to include both the antibody and cellular immune systems. In normal children and adults a portion of the thymus-derived lymphocyte population also acts to protect the body against the development of autoantibodies. The exact malfunction that results in the production of autoantibodies or cell sensitization and thus in the development of collagen vascular disease remains unknown.

JUVENILE RHEUMATOID ARTHRITIS

Juvenile rheumatoid arthritis (JRA) is a chronic inflammatory disease that always involves the joints, but may produce extensive connective tissue and visceral lesions.

ETIOLOGY. The etiology of JRA and the mechanisms that are responsible for the chronic joint disease remain unknown. No autoantibody specific for the disease has been documented. Although both chronic infection and underlying immunodeficiency disease have been hypothesized, neither is well substantiated. A genetic predisposition to develop JRA probably exists. An increased prevalence of histocompatibility antigen B27 has been found in adult patients with rheumatoid arthritis; 42 percent of 26 patients with this disease were found to have B27, in contrast to 6 percent of normal controls. Other studies have not demonstrated any significant association between JRA and histocompatibility antigens.

In spite of years of intensive research, it has not been possible to isolate a microorganism thought to be specifically related to the onset of rheumatoid arthritis. Various organisms that have been evaluated in the past include streptococci, *Mycoplasma,* and viruses. At the present time the most speculation concerns viruses; however, electron micrographs of synovial fluid have failed to demonstrate viral particles, and such agents have not been recovered from joints with disease.

Although it has been impossible to document an underlying immunodeficiency disease as the primary cause of rheumatoid arthritis, there is a large aggregate of evidence that points to a major role for immunologic reactivity in the perpetuation of rheumatoid inflammation. Unidentified initiating factors probably stimulate a synovitis that serves to trigger the local synthesis of IgG and rheumatoid factor (IgM anti-IgG) by plasma cells within the joint. The antigen–antibody aggregates then activate the complement sequence, which is followed by depletion of hemolytic complement activity in the synovial fluid in the presence of normal serum levels of complement. Activation of the complement sequence leads to generation of several biologically active materials that attract polymorphonuclear leukocytes into the joint cavity, where they phagocytize the immune complexes, thus leading to the formation of the rheumatoid arthritis (RA) cells. The neutrophils, following phagocytosis, are stimulated to discharge hydrolases from lysosomal granules. These enzymes, in addition to increased amounts of fibrinogen, are thought to initiate the destructive changes characteristic of rheumatoid joint disease.

CLINICAL FEATURES.   JRA is arbitrarily defined as beginning before the age of 16 years. It is slightly more common in females than in males and is said to affect as many as 250,000 children in the United States. Although JRA may begin at any age, an increased incidence of onset generally occurs from 1 to 3 years of age and later from 8 to 12 years of age. Approximately 20 percent of the children have acute systemic JRA, which is characterized by febrile onset, variable joint manifestations, rash, generalized lymphadenopathy, and splenomegaly, occasionally by cardiac disease and liver disease, and rarely by gastrointestinal tract disease. This form of JRA is commonly termed Still's disease. Other children with JRA have primarily arthritis that is present at the onset of illness. In 30 percent of cases only a single joint, usually the knee, is involved; in 50 percent multiple joints are involved. The disease is termed polyarticular if more than four joints are involved and pauciarticular if fewer than four joints are affected. Although all children with JRA have arthritis, children with systemic JRA, monoarticular or pauciarticular JRA, and polyarticular JRA differ in clinical presentation, systemic complications, laboratory studies, and prognosis. Therefore each type will be discussed separately.

JRA that presents in systemic form typically begins with fever characterized by daily temperature elevations to 39 C or higher with a rapid return to normal or even subnormal levels. The elevated temperatures usually occur in the evening and are frequently preceded by chills. The rash seen in these children is characteristic: salmon-colored morbilliform rash, often with central clearing, may occur anywhere on the body. The rash is fleeting and occurs at the time of temperature elevation; it may be associated with pruritus. Hepatosplenomegaly occurs in approximately one-third of these children; even fewer have transient abnormal liver function tests and abnormal liver biopsies. Pleuritis, pericarditis, and interstitial lung infiltrates occur rarely. All the patients with systemic JRA also have joint involvement, although early systemic disease is often much more severe than the arthritis and may precede the arthritis by as much as 6 months. The systemic disease is not usually a cause of permanent illness; however, chronic arthritis with joint disability does develop in a significant number of these patients.

Children with monoarticular or pauciarticular arthritis characteristically have joint involvement most fre-quently in the knees, ankles, and elbows; the small joints of the hand are conspicuously spared. Painless swelling of the joint is common in a patient with monoarticular onset; this should not detract from a proper diagnosis. Although fatigue and low-grade fevers are occasionally seen, the only significant systemic manifestation observed in this form of JRA is iridocyclitis, which has been said to occur in as many as 25 percent of these children. Eye disease can be present without eye pain, redness, or other clinical signs; it may be present without active arthritis. Because the eye disease is a result of inflammation that cannot be visualized by routine ophthalmologic examination, slit-lamp examination is imperative in these children. Current recommendations are that slit-lamp examination be performed every 3 months from the time of diagnosis until the child is 19 years old. The eventual outcome for patients with iridocyclitis, in spite of vigorous therapy, may be blindness.

Polyarticular JRA is characterized by arthritis of multiple joints, including the fingers and toes. Systemic manifestations are rare. The onset of the disease may be slow, and joint involvement initially may be manifested only by stiffness and swelling. Severe pain, erythema, and warmth are unusual. Limitation of motion of the involved joints occurs early in the disease and may be associated with synovial thickening. Joint involvement is usually symmetric, and the large joint may be involved first. Iridocyclitis is extremely rare in this form of the disease.

LABORATORY STUDIES.   No single laboratory test will confirm the diagnosis of JRA (Table 1). Routine laboratory studies such as complete blood count and erythrocyte sedimentation rate are frequently normal in patients with monoarticular, pauciarticular, or polyarticular arthritis. However, the complete white blood cell count may be helpful, because counts up to 100,000/mm^3, of which 90 percent are neutrophils, are found in patients with infectious arthritis, whereas white blood cell counts in patients with rheumatoid arthritis are usually between 15,000 and 25,000/mm^3 with 50 to 90 percent neutrophils. The majority of children with acute systemic JRA have elevated white blood cell counts (12,000 to 50,000/mm^3) during active disease and elevated erythrocyte sedimentation rates. Patients with systemic lupus erythematosus and joint involvement usually have leukopenia. Rheumatoid factor is rarely positive in children with JRA, except in the pauciarticular form, where it may be positive in up to 15 percent of patients. Antinuclear antibody (ANA) may be positive; if so it is often positive in a speckled pattern that may be seen on immunofluorescence and may be associated with elevated antibodies to extractable nuclear antigen. It is now thought that if a child has monoarticular or pauciarticular arthritis and a positive ANA the likelihood of that child eventually developing eye disease is increased. A diagnosis of JRA in a patient with a positive rheumatoid factor and positive ANA should be made with caution, as these tests are more frequently positive in patients with systemic lu-

Table 1. Laboratory Differentiation of Diseases Related to Collagen Vascular Disease

Studies	SLE	Rheumatoid Arthritis	Rheumatic Fever	Chronic Active Hepatitis
Total WBC counts	Frequently decreased	Frequently increased	Normal to increased	Usually normal
Coombs' test	Frequently positive	Rarely positive	Negative	Rarely positive
Urinalysis	Frequently abnormal	Normal	Normal	Rarely abnormal
C3 and/or CH$_{50}$	Frequently decreased	Normal to elevated	Usually normal	Rarely decreased
Autoantibody				
ANA	Positive (high titer)	Rarely positive (low titer)	Negative	Rarely positive (low titer)
LE prep	Frequently positive	Negative	Negative	Rarely positive
Anti-DNA	Fequently positive (high titer)	Positive (low titer)	Negative	May be positive (low titer)
Anti-smooth-muscle	Negative	Negative	Negative	Positive

pus erythematosus. In difficult cases, antibodies to DNA may be obtained. High titers occur in patients with systemic lupus erythematosus, but not in patients with JRA.

TREATMENT. Effective management of patients with JRA begins with early diagnosis. Aspirin is the preferred drug for therapy (a total of 80 to 130mg/kg body weight per day divided into 4 to 6 doses). The more frequent and higher doses are usually reserved for children with more severe disease. Serum salicylate levels should be maintained between 20 and 30 mg/dl; levels should be obtained just prior to the next dose of aspirin. Gastric irritation may be reduced by using enteric-coated aspirin or choline salicylate. Treatment should be continued for 1 year beyond any indication of active disease and should be reinstituted if necessary. If aspirin is not effective in treating the systemic disease in children with an acute febrile onset, prednisone may be initiated for a brief period. It is unwise to continue long-term prednisone therapy in children with JRA; although it is effective in controlling the disease, the side effects are great. Side effects include aseptic necrosis, vertebral collapse, and growth retardation, in addition to those that might be expected from the underlying disease. Physical therapy is essential in preventing long-term disability. A physical therapist may teach the parents of the patient a program of regular daily exercises that can be performed in the home. Exercises should aim to maintain strength and joint mobility. Recreation and sports also can help to achieve these goals.

In addition, as has been emphasized previously, ophthalmologic slit-lamp examinations are imperative in children with monoarticular or pauciarticular JRA, since the most devastating long-term effect of this form of JRA is iridocyclitis.

PROGNOSIS. When diagnosis of JRA is made early in the course of the disease, long-term prognosis is excellent. Children with systemic manifestations of the disease usually do not have ongoing systemic illness; however, chronic arthritis with joint disability does develop in a number of these patients. If a child with monoarticular or pauciarticular JRA does not develop eye disease, has well-controlled acute joint disease, and has maintained the full range of motion of all joints through vigorous physical therapy, then by age 19 or 20 years the disease generally becomes quiescent, and the patient may be expected to lead a completely normal life. Because limitation of joint movement occurs relatively early in the history of polyarticular JRA, physical therapy should be rapidly initiated. Again, with the use of aspirin in conjunction with physical therapy, the long-term prognosis for a normal adult life is excellent.

SYSTEMIC LUPUS ERYTHEMATOSUS

Systemic lupus erythematosus (SLE) is a nonmalignant self-perpetuating disease in which there is multisystem involvement, with certain organs more frequently affected than others. The disease may be mild and limited to a single organ, or it may be severe with diffuse and rapid progression. SLE can be diagnosed by evaluation of the clinical presentation in association with the presence of certain autoantibodies that are characteristic of the disease.

ETIOLOGY. Children with SLE are presumed to have a genetic predisposition for the development of characteristic autoantibodies that are associated with the disease. Many of the autoantibodies determine the clinical manifestations of SLE in a particular patient. Anemia may be the result of a Coombs-positive hemolytic process; thrombocytopenia may result from autoantibodies directed against platelets; lymphopenia may result from autoantibodies against lymphocytes. In most instances, however, the abnormal antibodies do not directly result in specific organ destruction. Rather, it is likely that the major manifestations of SLE are a result of immune-complex deposition (antigen, antibody, complement) in various organs. Disease activity in SLE is greatest when antibodies to antinuclear factors (ANA) are highest and serum complement levels are lowest, suggesting again that the production of characteristic lesions is a result of the combination of an antigen, an antibody, and complement.

Initial support for theories of a genetic predisposition for the disease was obtained from studies of an experimental animal model, the NZB/NZW mouse. The NZB mouse may develop an SLE-like syndrome; crossing NZB and NZW mice results in hybrids with a high incidence of an SLE-like disorder. It was postulated that a genetic mechanism was operative, but the events that triggered the onset of SLE were not clear. Laboratory investigation demonstrated that the autoimmune phenomenon occurring in the NZB/NZW hybrids was virtually identical to that found in humans with SLE. In mice the presence of viral particles was demonstrated prior to the onset of disease, thus indicating a possible viral induction of SLE. Further, in the mouse model an early abnormality in both the cell-mediated and the antibody-mediated immune systems was demonstrated; a deficiency of thymus-derived suppressor cells was postulated. A suppressor cell deficiency might result in the lack of tolerance to certain antigens and the subsequent overproduction of autoantibody.

A genetic influence on the development of SLE is also suggested from studies in humans. SLE has been found in at least five pairs of identical twins. Family members of patients with SLE have an increased incidence of hypergammaglobulinemia, rheumatoid factor, ANA, and other autoimmune diseases such as rheumatoid arthritis, Sjögren's syndrome, and scleroderma.

Infection results in clinical exacerbation of SLE, thus providing further evidence that infection may be a trigger mechanism in individuals genetically predisposed to the disease; however, the precise infecting agent has not been identified. Patients with SLE have reticular tubular structures on electron micrographs of kidney biopsies and in peripheral blood lymphocytes. This is thought by some investigators to be additional evidence for a viral etiology comparable to the persistent viral particles found in the NZB/NZW mouse model. In several studies elevated titers of antibody to specific viral agents, including rubella, *Mycoplasma,* and streptococcal antigens, have been found in sera from patients with SLE. However, in all SLE sera there is a diffuse elevation of immunoglobulins that probably represents nonspecific elevation of antibody titers to various infecting agents.

Certain drug reactions have been associated with SLE-like syndromes, including clinical disease and laboratory abnormalities similar to those found in patients who spontaneously develop SLE. Many drugs have been implicated, but the most common are hydralazine, procaine amide, and anticonvulsants. In adults the incidence of SLE-like syndromes and autoantibody formation following procaine amide therapy may be extremely high, thus suggesting that this drug has a propensity to produce a reversible SLE-like syndrome rather than to uncover an underlying lupus diathesis in a genetically predisposed patient. In children, however, the incidence of an SLE-like syndrome following drug therapy seems to be much rarer, and some patients reported to have drug-induced SLE have been found later to have developed SLE spontaneously.

The primary pathologic alterations of SLE consist of fibrinoid deposition and lupus erythematosus (LE) bodies. Fibrinoid is an eosinophilic material that is deposited along connective tissue fibers and in blood vessels; however, it is not diagnostic of SLE and can be found in other disorders. LE bodies are round, oval, or spindle-shaped formations approximately the size of a cell nucleus and are usually found in tissues at peripheral areas of necrosis where nuclei are undergoing pyknosis or karyorrhexis. LE bodies probably represent the in vivo counterpart of the in vitro LE phenomenon. Microscopic changes characteristic of SLE may be found in the skin, heart, spleen, choroid plexus, and kidney. Immunohistochemical studies invariably demonstrate the presence of immunoglobulin and complement in a lumpy-bumpy pattern characteristic of immune-complex deposition. In the skin, immune-complex deposition may be found at the dermal–epidermal junctions in both clinically affected and unaffected areas. The nephritis produced by immune-complex deposition can be divided into three distinct forms: *focal proliferative,* characterized by focal lesions involving some but not all gomeruli; *diffuse proliferative,* involving nearly all glomeruli, with major changes producing irregular endothelial and mesangial cell proliferation, irregular thickening of capillary loops, increased basement-membrane-like material, infiltration by neutrophils, and obliteration of capillary lumens; and *membranous,* involving uniform thickening of glomerular loops, with virtually no increased cellularity.

The variation of type and severity of organ involvement in patients with SLE poses some difficulty in postulating a basic immunopathologic mechanism for the disease. Variation may be partially explained on the basis of different degrees of immune-complex (antigen, antibody, complement) formation. Insoluble complexes are rapidly cleared by the reticuloendothelial system. Antigen must be present in slight excess in order to form soluble immune complexes, which subsequently are deposited in affected organs. An individual may form lesser amounts of antibody, resulting in a greater degree of soluble immune complex in the circulation with subsequent deposition in involved organs. Variation in severity may also be related to the ability of antibody to fix complement, which is dependent on the class of immunoglobulin. Certain individuals who do not have renal disease have been shown to have antibody against nuclear factors composed primarily of non-complement-fixing immunoglobulin. In addition, the type of autoantibody formed determines the clinical manifestations of disease. In the mixed collagen vascular syndrome, an SLE-like disease, individuals have high titers of antibody to ribonuclease-sensitive extractable nuclear antigen (ENA). Although these individuals also have antibody against other nuclear factors, they do not have typical manifestations of SLE, and they have a much lower incidence of severe renal disease.

CLINICAL FEATURES. The female:male ratio is 8:1. SLE may present at virtually any age; the youngest recorded patients have had onset of symptoms prior to 1 year of age. Neonatal SLE has not been reported, although infants born to mothers with SLE may have transient skin manifestations of the disease.

The two primary clinical manifestations of SLE are skin rash and arthritis. The characteristic butterfly rash appears to be sunlight-sensitive and may exacerbate during viral infection or emotional stress. A variety of other skin lesions often are present and can be found on the palms of the hands and soles of the feet. They have a vasculitis-like appearance, with intense erythema that blanches under pressure. Mucous membrane involvement occurs, with lesions having a vasculitis-like or lichen-planus-like appearance. Skin manifestations of SLE without systemic disease (discoid lupus) are extremely rare in children. Rheumatoid nodules have been described in patients with SLE, and on biopsy they appear identical to those found in other rheumatic disorders. A prominent indicator of disease activity is hair loss; hair may also become dry and brittle. Joint symptomatology is a prominent feature of SLE. Arthralgia is invariably present and may be associated with fusiform swelling of the fingers. Severe arthritis is present only infrequently, and deforming arthritis is rare.

The extent of renal involvement varies, but is the main factor in determining the ultimate prognosis in a patient with SLE. Nephritis is the most common presentation of kidney involvement; however, on occasion a patient may present with the nephrotic syndrome. The degree of kidney involvement is difficult to assess without a kidney biopsy. There are many instances of normal urinary sediment and normal kidney function associated with a kidney biopsy showing the presence of moderate immunoglobulin and complement deposition. Hypertension is usually not present at the time of diagnosis, but it appears to develop as the renal disease progresses. Various forms of cardiac involvement may occur: tachycardia, cardiomegaly, congestive heart failure, pericardial effusion, and heart murmurs have all been described. Endocardial involvement may occur, resulting in formation of small flat vegetations, most commonly on the mitral valves. On occasion an erroneous diagnosis of rheumatic fever has been made. The lung may be involved more frequently than was previously appreciated. Pleural effusions and a diffuse increase in bronchiovascular markings may be present. On careful questioning the patient may be found to have dyspnea on exertion or nonspecific fatigue that improves when therapy is instituted. Hepatosplenomegaly and lymphadenopathy may occur. The liver may be extensively involved, with diffuse abnor-

malities of liver function and jaundice. Under such circumstances it may be difficult to distinguish the patient with SLE and liver involvement from the patient with chronic active hepatitis and joint symptomatology, except by laboratory studies. Mild gastrointestinal tract symptoms are common; abdominal pain occurs during active disease and may be related to serositis or pancreatitis.

Peripheral blood vessels may be severely involved. Raynaud's phenomenon is a common complaint and is invariably associated with the presence of cryoglobulins in the serum. Central nervous system manifestations may occur; personality disorders are frequent, and patients may present with overt pyschoses or seizures. It is occasionally difficult to differentiate between central nervous system abnormalities resulting from active SLE and those resulting from steroid treatment. In general, central nervous system involvement secondary to SLE is associated with other clinical and laboratory evidence of active disease.

Avascular bone necrosis has been described in SLE, but many of the reported cases have occurred in patients on steroid therapy; thus steroids have been implicated in the etiology of this complication. The mechanism is not known, but the disorder is usually self-limiting. Surgical treatment is sometimes necessary. Diffuse muscle weakness may occur and may result from myositis or steroid myopathy.

Eye involvement in SLE may consist of conjunctivitis or hemorrhagic lesions secondary to hypertension or vasculitis. Other eye complications such as cataracts are primarily related to drug therapy. Uveitis and episcleritis are rare in children.

An SLE-like syndrome termed mixed collagen vascular disease recently has been described. Patients with this disorder may present with clinical features of a variety of autoimmune disorders: marked muscle weakness in a distribution similar to that found in dermatomyositis, Raynaud's phenomenon, difficulty in swallowing, sclerodermatous skin changes, and marked arthritis. Renal involvement is rare in this disorder, and the prognosis appears to be much better than that in SLE. The disorder can be distinguished from SLE by the finding of high titers of ribonuclease-sensitive ENA antibody.

A variety of SLE-like disorders have been described in association with congenital deficiencies of the complement components C1q, C1r, C1s, and C2. Clinical manifestations of SLE, including renal involvement, appear to be relatively mild in these individuals, perhaps because the deficiency of complement protects against immune-complex formation. However, these patients appear to be more susceptible to recurrent bacterial infection than patients with uncomplicated SLE; this is probably a direct consequence of the associated complement deficiency.

DIAGNOSIS. The diagnosis of SLE can usually be made on a clinical basis with confirmation by laboratory studies. In unusual cases where the clinical manifestations of SLE are similar to those of other diseases, such as rheumatic fever or chronic active hepatitis, or where patients present with a single manifestation such as thrombocytopenia, the diagnosis may rest on laboratory tests rather than clinical evidence. An early diagnosis of SLE is extremely important, as it may prevent potential complications of the disease or subsequent presentation with more severe manifestations as a result of delayed treatment.

The antinuclear antibody (ANA) is the single most readily available and important test for the diagnosis of SLE. In a patient not on treatment, the ANA is positive in virtually 100 percent of patients with active disease. Initiation of immunosuppressive therapy prior to testing may result in a negative antinuclear factor lasting for periods of weeks or months. The identification of ANA indicates the presence of antibody against double- or single-stranded DNA, RNA, or ENA. In most laboratories the antinuclear factor is determined by an immunofluorescence technique that utilizes animal or human cells as a substrate, the patient's sera containing antibody to substrate nuclei and fluorescein-labeled anti-IgG. Some laboratories may titer the antibody or may report various patterns of immunoglobulin deposition in cell nuclei, such as homogeneous, speckled, and shaggy. Titers of ANA, the various patterns, and the immunoglobulin class do not necessarily correlate with the severity or type of clinical presentation. A possible exception is the identification of a speckled antinuclear pattern that is seen more frequently in the mixed collagen vascular disease syndrome associated with anti-ENA. Since the ANA is a sensitive indicator of SLE, one should be cautious about making a diagnosis of SLE in the absence of a positive ANA. Although the sensitivity of the ANA for the diagnosis of SLE is high, it is not specific for the diagnosis; a positive test may be present in other disorders such as chronic active hepatitis, Sjögren's syndrome, and rarely JRA.

The LE preparation is less frequently positive in children with SLE than in adults. However, a positive LE prep is more specific for the diagnosis of SLE than is a positive ANA test. Rarely, patients with chronic active hepatitis may have a positive LE prep. During the active phase of this disease, anti-smooth-muscle and antimitochondrial antibodies may also be positive and should serve to distinguish this disorder from SLE with liver involvement.

Anti-DNA antibodies combine the sensitivity of the antinuclear factor with the specificity of the LE prep. Almost without exception, patients with SLE have high titers of antibody against DNA. Some laboratories report results as antibodies against both double-stranded (native) DNA and single-stranded (denatured) DNA. Low titers of antibody to DNA may be found in other autoimmune diseases. High titers of ribonuclease-sensitive antibody to ENA are found in the disorder of mixed collagen vascular disease. This study is not yet available in most laboratories.

Serum complement studies are valuable for determining the severity, progression, and control of disease. Several complement factors can be measured in a quantitative manner. The most readily available measurement of complement is C3 quantitation. The hemolytic complement (CH50) is a sensitive indicator of complement consumption, and it decreases rapidly as disease becomes active. It does not measure a specific complement component. Serum C4 quantitation has also been found useful. There is some indication that quantitation of C4 in the cerebrospinal fluid will assist in the diagnosis of central nervous system involvement resulting from active SLE. C4 levels are low in the cerebrospinal fluid when central nervous system dysfunction is due to lupus, and they are normal when involvement is due to drugs or other causes. As ANA and anti-DNA antibodies may revert to normal shortly after institution of therapy, the study of complement components in a serial manner may greatly assist in the management of patients with SLE.

Kidney function must be monitored closely. The urine sediment, serum creatinine, creatinine clearance, and Addis count are useful indicators of the severity of kidney involvement. In addition, patients with active renal disease and SLE excrete increased quantities of urine light chains (immunoglobulin light chains) because of failure of the proximal tubules to reabsorb light chains at a normal rate. Serial quantitation of urine light chains is helpful in following disease activity in the kidneys. There is not complete agreement on the necessity of kidney biopsy when the initial diagnosis of SLE is made. However, it is important to realize that the kidney can be involved with immune-complex deposition in the absence of any abnormality of creatinine clearance or of urine sediment. It may be useful, therefore, to obtain biopsy information to ascertain the extent of renal involvement, as this information may influence the choice of therapy.

Nonspecific laboratory abnormalities occur frequently in SLE. The sedimentation rate is usually markedly elevated, but may be normal or reduced. Serum immunoglobulins are diffusely elevated. Serum complement and serum haptoglobin may be increased. Because of the nonspecific elevation of many serum components, it is important to obtain a baseline evaluation in patients with SLE. A patient who is thought to have hemolytic anemia may have a presumed normal haptoglobin value if only a single determination is available. However, serial studies may indicate that the "normal" value is in fact reduced when compared to a previously elevated value.

TREATMENT. Treatment regimens vary considerably. There is not complete agreement as to which drugs should be used, the doses that should be given, or the duration of therapy necessary for control of the disease. Most authors agree that early and aggressive treatment has resulted in considerable improvement in the ultimate prognosis of patients with SLE. Cautious monitoring of drug therapy and reassessment of clinical laboratory status is essential, because overtreatment can result in severe immunosuppression and increased susceptibility to infection, which may be fatal.

Rarely, patients with isolated arthritis, normal serum complement levels, and no evidence of renal disease may be managed with aspirin alone. However, steroids are the mainstay of treatment for patients with SLE.

Recommendations vary from a starting dose of 0.5, to 2 mg/kg/day of prednisone or equivalent steroid. We prefer to individualize the dose with the severity of the disease as evidenced by clinical manifestations and laboratory abnormalities. If the dosage is not adequate it is increased to a maximum of 2 mg/kg/day of prednisone or equivalent. We do not recommend alternate-day steroid therapy in the treatment of patients with SLE. Patients are maintained on the lowest daily dose of steroid that will control clinical and laboratory abnormalities. All patients are followed at regular intervals, even when they are clinically well. If laboratory studies on two successive occasions indicate an exacerbation of the disease (elevated anti-DNA titer, low serum complement value), the steroids are increased by 5 to 10 mg/day until the abnormalities are corrected. At this point steroids are again tapered to maintenance dosages. Only rarely may patients with SLE be managed without steroid therapy.

Immunosuppressive agents such as cyclophosphamide, azathioprine, and chlorambucil have been used to assist in the control of SLE when high doses of steroids are ineffective. Occasionally patients will have severe side effects from steroids even in low doses. The addition of an immunosuppressive agent may permit control of the disease with the use of lower doses of steroid.

We prefer chlorambucil at a starting dosage of 2 mg/day in patients over 3 years of age and 1 mg/day in patients under 3 years of age. Patients are treated to the point of leukopenia (white cells less than 3,000/mm^3) by increasing the dose by 1 to 2 mg each day at 3-day intervals. Once leukopenia occurs, the dose is reduced by 1 to 2 mg each day to a maintenance dose. Patients should be warned of the side effects of all immunosuppressive agents, which include increased susceptibility to infection and possible future sterility. All patients on combined steroid and immunosuppressive therapy must be observed cautiously for subtle evidence of infection. Toxoplasmosis, *Pneumocystis carinii, Aspergillus,* and other fungal infections occur frequently. As most of these infections can now be treated, an early diagnosis is important.

Patients who have severe arthritis may benefit by the addition of salicylates to the treatment regimen in doses similar to those used in patients with rheumatoid arthritis (80 mg/kg/day). Skin manifestations of SLE frequently respond to the addition of hydroxychloroquine to the regimen. The recommended dosage is 5 to 7 mg/kg/day. Hydroxychloroquine only infrequently causes ocular abnormalities; however, the patient should be examined by an ophthalmologist every 6 months while on treatment. Side effects other than ocular changes include bleaching of the hair and pigmentation of the skin.

Certain factors such as infection, emotional trauma, menarche, and/or menses and exposure to sunlight may result in exacerbation of well-controlled SLE. Minor exacerbations respond readily to small, brief increases in steroid therapy. Patients may be partially protected from the effects of sunlight by clothing and the use of topical sunscreens such as Pabafilm.

PROGNOSIS. The prognosis in SLE has greatly improved in recent years. Sensitive laboratory studies have resulted in earlier diagnosis of the disease, which has resulted in prompt treatment and easier control. The mortality in SLE is determined primarily by two factors: the extent of renal involvement and the degree of immunosuppression resulting from therapy. The two primary causes of death in SLE are renal failure and death from opportunistic infection. It is therefore essential that patients be followed closely and that the amount of medication they receive be adequate to prevent progression of renal disease but not result in severe immunosuppression. The long-term risks of prolonged immunosuppressive therapy are not fully known at this time. Theoretically, prolonged immunosuppression might result in an increased incidence of malignancy. As studies relating to the early diagnosis and long-term treatment of patients with SLE become available, the ultimate prognosis of this disease will become known.

DERMATOMYOSITIS AND POLYMYOSITIS

Polymyositis is characterized by nonspecific inflammation and degeneration of skeletal muscle and skin. When the myopathy of polymyositis is associated with a characteristic skin rash, the diagnosis of dermatomyositis may be made.

ETIOLOGY. The etiology of dermatomyositis is unknown; although it is generally grouped with collagen vascular disorders because of certain clinical and laboratory similarities, documentation of an autoimmune etiology is not complete.

Antibody-mediated immunity and cell-mediated immunity have been investigated in patients with dermatomyositis and polymyositis. Antimyosin antibodies have been demonstrated in these disorders, but they are also found in other dystrophic and neurogenic processes. These autoantibodies are not cytotoxic to muscle cells. Studies utilizing immunofluorescence techniques have shown that IgG, IgM, and C3 are deposited in blood vessel walls in patients with active polymyositis and dermatomyositis. Recently developed techniques have permitted the investigation of cellular sensitization in these patients. Specific sensitization of peripheral blood lymphocytes to muscle antigen in patients with dermatomyositis has been demonstrated using peripheral blood lymphocyte transformation with muscle antigens, lymphocyte cytotoxicity of muscle in culture, and a leukocyte migration test in the presence of muscle antigen. These studies indicate that cellular autoimmunity may result in the development of dermatomyositis.

Some reports have also suggested a possible viral etiology of dermatomyositis. Viral particles have been observed on electron micrographs of biopsied muscle. There is also clinical suggestion of an association between the onset of dermatomyositis and certain viral infections.

The overall incidence of malignant tumors in adults with dermatomyositis is 15 to 20 percent. Many varieties have been identified, including carcinoma of the breast, stomach, lung, ovary, gallbladder, kidney, and uterus, as well as lymphoma and thymoma. Dermatomyositis may antedate the onset of tumor by months or years, and frequently the disease may improve with removal of the tumor. No precise relationship between dermatomyositis and malignancy has been proven, and this association in children is extremely rare.

CLINICAL FEATURES.   The disease may have its onset from infancy through adulthood. Incidence is approximately equal in males and females; in some series there is a slight preponderance of females. The onset is usually insidious, with symptomatology occurring 2 to 8 weeks before medical attention is sought. Muscle weakness is usually the primary complaint, with the proximal limb and trunk muscles being most severely involved; the affected muscles are weak and may be indurated and tender. Distal muscle strength and deep tendon reflexes are maintained in most instances. Muscle atrophy does not occur until very late in the course of the illness.

Dermatologic manifestations consist of a lilac discoloration of the eyelids (heliotrope) often associated with periorbital edema. Ocassionally the periorbital edema may be the initial presenting feature. Characteristically there is a scaly, erythematous dermatitis over the dorsum of the hands covering the metacarpophalangeal and proximal interphalangeal joints. The rash may be present on the knees, elbows, and medial malleoli, as well as the face and neck. The rash resembles a traumatic lesion, and when it is present only over the knuckles it may be mistaken for a repeated abrasion. The rash is considered by some to be pathognomonic of dermatomyositis.

Subcutaneous or periarticular calcifications occasionally occur. The deposits may be isolated small nodules that will produce breakdown of overlying skin. The appearance of calcification may be a good sign and herald the end of active disease. Respiratory problems resulting from involvement of the diaphragm may occur. Palatal weakness, dysphagia, and small-bowel hypomotility have also been observed; anal and bladder sphincter abnormalities are rare. Cardiac arrhythmias and heart block have been reported.

Generalized lymphadenopathy, splenomegaly, and Raynaud's phenomenon are occasionally present. Arthralgia may be found, but overt arthritis is rare. In general, the association of muscle weakness with skin rash and multiple organ involvement should alert one to diagnostic possibilities other than dermatomyositis.

DIAGNOSIS.   Five major criteria can be used to diagnose dermatomyositis in childhood. The first is the presence of progressive symmetric weakness of the limb-girdle muscles and anterior neck flexors. Second, there is evidence of necrosis of type I and type II muscle fibers. Biopsy specimens of clinically affected muscle demonstrate variation in fiber size, perivascular inflammatory infiltrate, regeneration of muscle fibers, with basophilia, large vesicular sarcolemmal nuclei, and prominent nucleoli. The third criterion is an elevation of skeletal muscle enzymes in the serum. Creatine phos-

phokinase is the most useful enzyme to follow during treatment. Frequently aldolase, glutamic oxaloacetic or pyruvic transaminase, and lactate dehydrogenase are also elevated. The fourth important finding relates to the electromyographic analysis of muscle function. In dermatomyositis the abnormalities that have been described consist of fibrillations, positive sharp waves, and bizarre high-frequency repetitive discharges. The final important sign is the characteristic heliotrope rash with periorbital edema and a scaling erythematous dermatitis. Patients may present with only one of the above features. Dermatomyositis has been diagnosed in the absence of an abnormal muscle biopsy, in the absence of electromyographic abnormalities, and in the absence of serum enzyme elevations. When muscle atrophy is extensive, or after long-standing disease, the enzymes may be normal even in the presence of active myositis.

A number of disorders are frequently confused with dermatomyositis. Patients are occasionally misdiagnosed as having muscular dystrophy, a disorder in which serum enzymes may also be elevated. Central nervous system or peripheral neurologic disease may also be associated with muscle weakness. Certain infections such as trichinosis, schistosomiasis, and toxoplasmosis have been associated with myositis. Endocrinopathies such as thyrotoxicosis, myxedema, Cushing's syndrome, and myasthenia gravis have been reported to occur in association with polymyositis. The use of penicillamine has been reported to result in myositis.

TREATMENT.   Although spontaneous remissions and exacerbations may occur, dermatomyositis and polymyositis will usually respond to steroid therapy if patients are treated early and aggressively. There is recent evidence that prognosis is directly related to the rapidity of diagnosis and treatment with prednisone at a dose of 1 to 2 mg/kg/24 hours. Treatment should be continued until symptoms improve and serum enzymes return to normal. Steroids then can be tapered gradually to a dose required to maintain normal muscle function and normal enzyme levels. Rapid tapering of prednisone should be avoided, as this may result in reappearance of symptoms and elevation of enzymes. Immunosuppressive agents (methotrexate) have been used in some patients resistant to steroids, but experience in children is limited. During the acute phase of the disease, when there may be respiratory and swallowing difficulties, close observation for the development of pneumonia is suggested. Active physical therapy and postural drainage are also recommended.

PROGNOSIS.   Several recent studies have suggested that prompt diagnosis and treatment will result in an improved prognosis. The majority of children may have complete recovery with little or no residual dysfunction. A few individuals may have late progression of dermatomyositis; death is usually a result of respiratory complications.

SCLERODERMA

Scleroderma is a disorder of unknown etiology with generalized involvement of connective tissue. In addition to inflammatory, fibrotic, and degenerative changes in the connective tissue, vascular lesions are present in the skin, synovium, and internal organs such as the esophagus, heart, lung, and kidney. Scleroderma that is limited to cutaneous involvement (morphea) is more common in children than is the systemic disease.

CLINICAL FEATURES. Both systemic scleroderma and morphea are more common in females than in males. Onset of the disease may be at any time during childhood. In most cases Raynaud's phenomenon, gradual swelling of the distal portions of the extremities, joint complaints, or a gradual thickening and tightening of the skin are the initial complaints. Frequently these symptoms persist for 2 years or more prior to diagnosis.

Early in the disease the skin becomes edematous and the fingers may be swollen. Gradually the edema is replaced by thickening of the skin. In the diffuse systemic form of the disease this induration is generally symmetric, but in the more limited form (morphea) it may be confined to patchy areas. As the changes progress they are occasionally accompanied by hyperpigmentation, telangiectasia, or subcutaneous calcification. Raynaud's phenomenon is produced by paroxysmal vasospasm of the fingers and is present in about 90 percent of patients with systemic scleroderma. Angiography of the digital arteries of patients with Raynaud's phenomenon and scleroderma has demonstrated narrowing and/or obliteration of these vessels. Although complaints of joint pain are frequent and polyarthralgia is often diagnosed, objective evidence of arthritis is rare. Joint stiffness affects primarily the fingers, wrists, knees, and ankles. Muscle weakness and atrophy may occur in as many as one-third of children with systemic scleroderma, but they do not progress and are not associated with pain; these are common findings in children with dermatomyositis, and they serve to differentiate the two disorders.

The disease may involve internal organ systems more often than specific complaints would indicate. Esophageal dysfunction is present in approximately 90 percent of adults with systemic scleroderma and is probably the most common manifestation of internal involvement. Roentgenographic abnormalities generally demonstrate diminution of peristaltic activity of the lower portion of the esophagus. Most patients develop pulmonary disease with interstitial and alveolar fibrosis. Although chest radiographs in children are generally normal, pulmonary function tests are often abnormal. Cardiac disease is less common, but myocardial fibrosis with involvement of the small coronary arteries may lead to left ventricular failure. Renal disease is relatively rare during childhood, but if it develops it is a major cause of death. Malignant arterial hypertension is associated with rapidly progressive and irreversible renal insufficiency.

DIAGNOSIS. No single laboratory study will confirm the diagnosis of scleroderma. Rather, the clinical picture is characteristic in both morphea and progressive systemic sclerosis. The routine laboratory studies tend to be normal. In children, rheumatoid factor and the LE phenomenon are generally negative. Anti-DNA antibodies and ANA may be positive, but the titers are lower than those usually found in patients with SLE. Hypergammaglobulinemia may be present.

Roentgenographic abnormalities of the esophagus are present in more than 50 percent of children with scleroderma. Obstructive arterial disease can be demonstrated by arteriography in more than 95 percent of those with Raynaud's phenomenon.

TREATMENT. Because systemic scleroderma is rare in childhood and progresses slowly, the efficacy of treatment is unknown. Many therapeutic agents have been tried without clear-cut benefit. These include corticosteroids, salicylates, D-penicillamine, chloroquine, and P-aminobenzoic acid. Vigorous physical therapy early in the disease is thought by most clinicians to be important in the prevention of contractures secondary to severe cutaneous scleroderma.

PROGNOSIS. When scleroderma is limited to cutaneous involvement, the prognosis is generally excellent. Active disease may arrest over a period of months to years. However, the long-term prognosis for children with systemic scleroderma is less well defined. The extent of renal involvement, pulmonary disease, or cardiac disease probably dictates the long-term prognosis.

NECROTIZING ARTERITIS

A group of clinical syndromes are characterized by inflammation of the blood vessels, primarily of medium- or small-caliber arteries, and by clinical symptoms that reflect the location and severity of vascular involvement. When the blood vessels involved are small and nonmuscular, the disease takes the clinical form of Schönlein-Henoch syndrome (anaphylactoid purpura). When larger muscular arteries are involved, the clinical syndrome is termed polyarteritis; variants of this syndrome have been described, including hypersensitivity angiitis, Wegener's granulomatosis, giant cell arteritis, and Takayasu's arteritis (pulseless disease). Inflammation of the blood vessels is also found in other well-characterized autoimmune diseases, including SLE, rheumatoid arthritis, rheumatic fever, and dermatomyositis.

ETIOLOGY. The etiology of these disorders remains unknown. Circumstantial evidence has associated the vascular lesions found in these disorders with allergy, prior infection, and autoimmune phenomena. Animals given large doses of foreign protein have developed diffuse vasculitis. The vasculitis is characterized by immune-complex deposition of the foreign antigen and antibody in vessel walls. In the animal model complement is activated, resulting in a series of events leading to increased vascular permeability, chemotaxis of polymorphonuclear leukocytes, and basement membrane damage. In some patients with necrotizing vasculitis pathologic features have been present that have been similar to these experimental findings. However, the presence of complement and immunoglobulin deposition in these disorders is not a consistent finding, and thus the precise cause of these clinical syndromes remains unknown. Recently hepatitis-associated antigen (Australia antigen) has been demonstrated along the elastic membrane of arterial walls in about one-third of patients with polyarteritis. In addition, immunoglobulin and complement have been identified. These findings suggest an infectious etiology in some cases of polyarteritis. Histologic and clinical features serve to separate the various disorders in this section.

The onset of clinical symptomatology in the various disorders may be acute or insidious. No typical clinical syndrome can be described. Patients may present with fevers of unknown origin, abdominal pain, bronchial asthma or pneumonia, renal disease, cardiac failure, myalgia, peripheral neuropathy, or intractable headaches. Usually a diagnosis of multiple system disease is suggested because of a combination of features. Laboratory findings that are common include leukocytosis, eosinophilia, abnormal urine sediment, and elevated erythrocyte sedimentation rate. Angiography occasionally demonstrates dilatation of the involved arteries. However, biopsy of clinically involved organs remains the principal means of establishing the diagnosis of all these entities except Schönlein-Henoch purpura.

Schönlein-Henoch Purpura

The clinical syndrome of Schönlein-Henoch vasculitis includes nonthrombocytopenic purpura, arthralgia or mild arthritis, renal disease, abdominal pain, and gastrointestinal hemorrhage. The disease occurs primarily in children. The skin lesion, which is not always classic purpura, is the most characteristic sign; the visceral lesions are more difficult to diagnose, but result in serious complications. A widespread angiitis involving small arterioles and capillaries of all affected organs, including the synovium, is the basic pathologic lesion. A perivascular infiltrate with polymorphonuclear leukocytes is present along with endothelial cell swelling and leukocyte platelet thrombi. Children with this syndrome have been found to have increased levels of serum IgA. In addition, IgA deposition has been demonstrated in cutaneous blood vessel walls and in kidney mesangium. Findings characteristic of glomerulonephritis are found on kidney biopsy when renal involvement is present. In addition to deposition of IgA in the mesangial areas, C3 and properdin are present in capillary walls, and deposits of fibrinogen are found in the epithelial crescents.

Although many patients with this disease give a history of previous respiratory tract infection, evidence for a relationship between streptococcal infection and onset of Schönlein-Henoch purpura is not conclusive. Hypersensitivity to various foods and drugs has also been implicated, but again the evidence is not conclusive.

The onset of the disease may be acute, with the simultaneous appearance of several manifestations, or it may be insidious, with the appearance of different manifestations over a period of weeks. Skin lesions are the hallmark of the disease and are present in all patients with this diagnosis; whether visceral manifestations may be present in the absence of the rash is unknown. Skin lesions usually appear first on the lower extremities, but they generally involve the buttocks and less frequently the upper extremities, trunk, and face. The classic lesion begins as an erythematous maculopapule that blanches on pressure but later becomes petechial or purpuric. The purpuric areas generally are raised; they change from red to purple in color, then become rusty, and eventually fade, occasionally leaving a small scar. The skin lesions generally appear in crops and at any time are usually at the same state of maturity. Other skin lesions may be present, including erythema multiforme and erythema nodosum. Approximately two-thirds of affected children have arthritis. The most commonly involved joints are the knees and ankles; joint symptoms usually resolve after a few days, and residual deformity is rare. About two-thirds of affected children have gastrointestinal symptoms at some point in the course of their disease. Colic and abdominal pains, frequently associated with vomiting and gross or occult blood in the stools, may occur. Failure to recognize the syndrome of Schönlein-Henoch vasculitis may result in an unnecessary laparotomy because of the sudden onset of acute abdominal pain. Rarely, intussusception, obstruction or bowel infarction, and perforation occur. Renal involvement is potentially the most serious manifestation of the disease and may occur in 25 to 50 percent of children during the acute phase. The first sign of renal disease is generally hematuria; moderate azotemia and hypertension may follow. Although most children with renal disease recover, some continue to have abnormal urinary sediment, and a few develop chronic renal disease and renal failure that necessitates transplantation.

There is no specific therapy for this disease. If gastrointestinal symptoms are present during the acute phase, prednisone may often bring dramatic improvement. Steroids do not seem to affect renal involvement. Therapy of chronic nephritis with immunosuppressive agents remains experimental.

Polyarteritis

In the syndrome of polyarteritis the muscular arteries are primarily involved. In the same patient, arteries may show varying stages of acute and healing lesions. Thrombosis and segmental (fibrinoid) necrosis of blood vessels is observed. The inflammatory reaction is composed primarily of neutrophils. Blood vessels along the mesentery of the gastrointestinal tract, liver, kidney, pancreas, and muscles may be involved. Coronary artery involvement appears to be common in the infantile presentation of this disorder. Local evidence of uterine, epididymal, testicular, skin, and brain involvement has been described. Clinical manifestations of polyarteritis are variable and nonspecific. Prolonged or intermittent fever is common, and various rashes have been described, including maculopapular erythema, erythema multiforme, and urticaria. Conjunctivitis, rhinorrhea, and other respiratory symptoms are commonly present.

Infants and children may present with congestive heart failure and/or complaints related to the presence of hypertension. Rarely, gangrene of the extremities may be observed as an initial symptom. When the kidney is involved, renal failure may be the presenting abnormality. The long-term prognosis, if this disease is diagnosed during childhood, is poor; death may occur from renal failure, cardiac failure, or severe gastrointestinal or central nervous system disease. Preliminary evidence indicates that corticosteroids may suppress the acute clinical manifestations of the disease and improve long-term prognosis. Prolonged therapy may be required.

Hypersensitivity Angiitis

Hypersensitivity angiitis results from the inflammation of arteries, arterioles, and venules. Patients presenting with this disorder frequently have an allergic history. Initial symptomatology may be diffuse and may include arthralgias, purpura, and evidence of renal disease.

Wegener's Granulomatosis

Wegener's granulomatosis is characterized by widespread vasculitis involving both arteries and veins. Granulomatous necrosis may be present in the upper and lower respiratory tract, and vasculitis may involve both arteries and veins of the lungs and kidneys. The disorder has been described in an infant 3 months of age, but is more frequent in the third and fourth decades of life. The most common presenting complaint is a sense of discomfort around the nose and sinuses. This may progress to rhinorrhea and nasal mucosal ulceration. Pulmonary symptoms such as cough, hemoptysis, and pleuritic pain are frequent. Fever, anorexia, malaise, or weight loss, although nonspecific, may be the primary reason the patient seeks medical attention. In approximately one-third of cases peripheral manifestations are found that include arthritis, arthralgia, skin ulceration, serous otitis media, conjunctivitis, corneal ulceration, and necrogranulomatous hepatitis. The heart may be involved, with granulomatous inflammation of muscle and vessels leading to arrhythmias. Although the kidney is involved in over 80 percent of cases, major clinical abnormalities are rarely present early in the disease, and hypertension secondary to kidney involvement is unusual. However, the development of renal involvement usually includes microscopic hematuria, and kidney disease generally progresses rapidly. The long-term prognosis in patients with this disorder is generally considered to be poorer than the prognosis in other types of arteritis. Corticosteroid therapy has been attempted, but is usually unsuccessful. Complete clinical remission in a limited number of cases has occurred following therapy with alkylating agents or other immunosuppressive drugs; with the early use of these agents the long-term prognosis of this disease may change.

Giant Cell Arteritis

The arteritis found in patients with giant cell arteritis is of a more limited form than that seen in other diseases in this category. Segmental vascular changes are present; they consist of infiltration with inflammatory cells, the presence of giant cells, and intimal proliferation with vascular occlusion with or without thrombosis. Lesions are usually localized in cranial arteries, ophthalmic, temporal, and brachiocephalic arteries, and the thoracic and abdominal aorta. The more limited involvement of specific arteries in this disease accounts for the more limited clinical presentation. Systemic symptoms such as fever, sweats, anorexia, fatigue, headache, abdominal pain, myalgia, and arthralgia may be found in patients with giant cell arteritis. Cardiac involvement may occur and may result in manifestations similar to those of rheumatic fever. Painful nodules may be present in the scalp, and tenderness and thickening of the temporal artery may be observed. Corticosteroids are very effective in the treatment of giant cell arteritis, and their efficacy in the prevention of blindness is well known

Takayasu's Arteritis

Patients with Takayasu's arteritis (pulseless disease) may have clinical and laboratory features that are similar to those of giant cell arteritis. The thoracic aorta and the proximal segments of its large branches are most frequently involved in an indolent inflammatory reaction that leads to narrowing and obliteration of the vessels; the abdominal aorta and its branches are less frequently involved. Histologically there is a focal or diffuse inflammatory reaction consisting of round cell infiltration in the media and adventitia. Disruption of the elastic laminae is seen in association with degeneration of the media and proliferation of the fibrous tissue. Giant cells may be seen. Extensive calcification may occur. Dilatation of the aorta may lead to aortic insufficiency or aneurysmal dilatation with the formation of collateral circulation. The disease affects females more frequently than males. Manifestations of Takayasu's disease are related to arterial obstruction. Transient visual disturbances, vertigo and syncopal attacks, intermittent angina attacks, and hypertension may occur. Arterial disease is indicated by loss of pulsations, local tenderness, bruits, and Raynaud's phenomenon. Generalized symptoms such as fever, polyarthralgia, polyarthritis, and muscle soreness are observed. During the early stages of the disease corticosteroids may induce a rapid remission, and pulsations may return. In the chronic phase intravascular thrombosis may be prevented by the use of anticoagulants. Arterial grafts have been inserted in some patients when well-defined segments of large vessels have been occluded.

SJÖGREN'S SYNDROME

Sjögren's syndrome is characterized by a chronic inflammatory state resulting in decreased lacrimal and salivary gland secretion (sicca complex). The diminished secretions result in keratoconjunctivitis sicca and xerostomia. Approximately 50 percent of patients with Sjögren's syndrome have rheumatoid arthritis.

ETIOLOGY.   The etiology of Sjögren's syndrome is not known. The clinical and pathologic features are similar to those of other collagen vascular diseases; there is a high degree of association between Sjögren's syndrome and rheumatoid arthritis; some patients may have features of SLE, polyarteritis, or polymyositis.

Pathologic features consist primarily of alterations in the parotid and lacrimal glands. Focal ectasia and intraductal proliferation of epithelial and myoepithelial cells are observed. The lobules of the glands are infiltrated with mature-appearing lymphocytes. Within the lobules of the parotid or lacrimal glands, acinar atrophy with lymphoid replacement may occur. A similar process may involve the smaller salivary glands and glands responsible for secretions in the upper gastrointestinal and respiratory tracts. It is possible that this hyposecretion in the tracheobronchial tree results in poor bronchial drainage and secondary infection, thus accounting for the pulmonary infiltrates frequently encountered in patients with Sjögren's syndrome. The pancreas is only infrequently involved and rarely accounts for significant clinical abnormalities.

CLINICAL FEATURES.   Over 90 percent of patients with Sjögren's syndrome are female, with a mean age of 50 years at the time the initial diagnosis is made. The disease has been reported in patients as young as 5 years of age, but it is extremely rare in the pediatric population. Patients generally present with established rheumatoid arthritis and a history of slowly developing sicca complex; those who are otherwise well may rapidly develop severe oral and ocular dryness accompanied by episodic parotitis. Salivary insufficiency causes difficulty in chewing, swallowing, and phonating, adherence of foods to mucosal surfaces, ulcers of the mucous membranes, lips, and tongue, and markedly increased incidence of dental caries. The extreme oral dryness may require frequent ingestion of liquids, and patients may find it necessary to moisten the oral mucosa repeatedly with fluid. Dryness of the nasopharynx may lead to epistaxis, hoarseness, and recurrent otitis media. The parotid gland enlargement is often recurrent and symmetric and is accompanied by erythema, tenderness, and fever; rapid fluctuation in gland size may be observed.

Patients with keratoconjunctivitis sicca may have burning sensations, inability to produce tears in response to emotion or local irritants, sensations of foreign bodies in the eyes, gritty or sandy sensations, photosensitivity, eye fatigue, accumulation of thick ropy strands at the inner canthus, and film that interferes with vision.

Raynaud's phenomenon is present in 20 percent of these patients. Some may present with or may develop nonthrombocytopenic purpura, usually accompanied by hypergammaglobulinemia; the latter may be associated with renal tubular acidosis. Hepatosplenomegaly, chronic active hepatitis, acute pancreatitis, acute celiac disease, and gastric achlorhydria are additional findings in some patients. A number of different malignancies have been reported, including pseudolymphoma with pulmonary lymphoid infiltration, reticulum cell sarcoma, and primary macroglobulinemia. Other clinical symptoms are related to associated disorders such as rheumatoid arthritis, SLE, or polymyositis.

LABORATORY STUDIES.   Nonspecific anemia, leukopenia, elevated sedimentation rate, and hypergammaglobulinemia may be present. A variety of autoantibodies may be positive, thus resulting in confusion in diagnosis. In most series over 90 percent of patients have positive rheumatoid factors in high titers. Antinuclear factor is present in 70 percent, and over 15 percent have positive LE cells. The Coombs' test is frequently positive. Certain autoantibodies appear to be more specific for Sjögren's syndrome. The majority of patients have anti-salivary-duct antibody, which can be demonstrated by immunofluorescence or other antibody techniques. Antithyroglobulin antibodies may be found in those patients who have associated chronic thyroiditis (about 5 percent).

Studies are available to determine the degree of lacrimal and parotid gland involvement. The Schirmer filter paper test is a semiquantitative measure of tear formation. Through the use of rose bengal dye and biomicroscopy of the eye, grossly visible or microscopic abnormalities of the bulbar conjunctiva or cornea may be observed. Salivary scintigraphy may be used to determine the uptake, concentration, and excretion by the major salivary glands of intravenously injected radioactive material. Biopsy of the minor salivary glands in the lower lip will demonstrate significant lymphoid infiltration characteristic of Sjögren's syndrome.

TREATMENT.   Patients may have long-standing Sjögren's syndrome without severe complications. Treatment generally is symptomatic, and patients may devise their own techniques for keeping mucous membranes moist. Eye complications may be prevented by the use of 0.5 percent methyl cellulose eye drops. Steroids and immunosuppressive agents can be used if life-threatening complications occur. Steroids should not be used to treat hypergammaglobulinemia or purpura, as symptoms may become more severe following therapy.

PROGNOSIS.   Sjögren's syndrome carries a high morbidity, with complications relating primarily to mucous membrane discomfort and ocular difficulties. The long-term prognosis is related to associated disorders such as SLE, rheumatoid arthritis, polymyositis, and/or the development of malignancy.

RHEUMATIC FEVER

Rheumatic fever is an inflammatory disease that is usually a sequel to infection with group A streptococci and affects the heart, joints, central nervous system, and subcutaneous tissue.

ETIOLOGY.   Abundant clinical and laboratory data support the concept of an etiologic relationship between infection with group A streptococci and subsequent development or exacerbation of rheumatic fever.

These can be summarized as follows: primary and secondary attacks of rheumatic fever can be prevented by treatment and/or eradication of streptococcal infections; preceding streptococcal infection can be documented in virtually all cases of acute rheumatic fever by the presence of increased titers of antibody to streptococcal antigens; a large number of clinical and epidemiologic studies show an association between the incidence of group A streptococcal infection and rheumatic fever; group A streptococcal antigens have been shown in the laboratory to cross-react with sarcolemma and subsarcolemma sarcoplasm of cardiac myofibers; the sera of patients with rheumatic fever and rheumatic heart disease contain antibodies that react with both streptococcal antigens and cardiac antigens.

The means by which cardiac damage occurs in rheumatic fever are probably related to immunopathologic destruction of muscle. Studies performed on cardiac tissue taken from children who have died following fulminant acute rheumatic fever show deposition in the myocardium of complement, IgG, IgM, and IgA. Although these studies suggest an active immunopathologic mechanism for cardiac damage, they do not determine whether specific antibody results in cardiac damage or whether the production of antibody reactive with cardiac antigen follows cardiac destruction.

Pathologic changes in rheumatic fever are found throughout the body, occurring primarily in connective tissue and around small blood vessels. The most characteristic lesion, considered to be pathognomonic of rheumatic fever, is the Aschoff body, which consists of an inflammatory lesion associated with swelling and fragmentation of collagen fibers and alterations in the staining characteristics of connective tissue. Endocarditis produces a verrucose valvulitis that may heal with fibrous thickening and adhesions of valve commissures and chordae tendineae, resulting in variable degrees of valvular stenosis and insufficency. Impairment of the function of the mitral and aortic valves occurs most commonly; the tricuspid is affected less frequently, and the pulmonary valve is rarely damaged.

Pathologic changes in the joints consist primarily of exudative changes with edema of synovial membranes, focal necrosis in the joint capsule, edema and inflammation in periarticular tissue, and joint effusion. In contrast to the situation with the heart, pathologic changes in the joints are completely reversible. Subcutaneous nodules that are seen during the acute phase of the disease resemble Aschoff bodies and are composed of granulomas with localized areas of fibrinoid swelling of collagen and perivascular infiltration with large cells, pale nuclei, and prominent nucleoli. "Rheumatic pneumonia" consists of exudative and inflammatory changes without Aschoff bodies. The pathologic changes that occur in patients with chorea are not consistent, and little postmortem information is available, since patients with active chorea rarely die.

An individual propensity to develop rheumatic fever is suggested by several epidemiologic studies. Rheumatic fever occurs in 3 percent of patients who carry an infecting strain for more than 3 weeks following con-

valescence whereas an incidence of only 0.3 percent is found in those individuals carrying the organism for less than 3 weeks. Individuals who have increases in antistreptolysin O titers greater than 250 units/ml following streptococcal infection have a 5 percent incidence of rheumatic fever, while less than 1 percent of those with increases of less than 100 units/ml develop the disease. Patients with streptococcal infections and a history of previous rheumatic fever have a 5 to 50 percent greater incidence of rheumatic fever than patients with no prior history of the disease; this tendency declines with age. Environmental factors (latitude, altitude, humidity), economic factors, and age appear to influence the incidence of rheumatic fever; this is probably because the same factors influence the incidence of streptococcal infection.

CLINICAL FEATURES. Many of the clinical manifestations of rheumatic fever occur in other collagen vascular disorders. A patient presenting with cardiac, joint, and dermatologic abnormalities should be evaluated for rheumatic fever, rheumatoid arthritis, and SLE (Table 1). The diagnosis of any one of these disorders can be made only by a complete clinical and laboratory evaluation of all three.

The major clinical manifestations of rheumatic fever include carditis, polyarthritis, chorea, subcutaneous nodules, and erythema marginatum (Table 2). If all of

TABLE 2. Abbreviated Jones Criteria for Guidance in Diagnosis of Rheumatic Fever[a]

Major manifestations
1. Carditis
   a. Murmur
   b. Cardiomegaly
   c. Pericarditis
   d. Congestive heart failure
2. Polyarthritis
3. Chorea
4. Erythema marginatum
5. Subcutaneous nodules

Minor manifestations
1. Clinical
   a. History of previous rheumatic fever
   b. Arthralgia
   c. Fever
2. Laboratory
   a. Increased ESR, C-reactive protein, WBC count, anemia
   b. Prolonged P-R and Q-T intervals on EKG

Supportive evidence
1. Recent scarlet fever
2. Throat culture positive for group A streptococci
3. Increased ASO or other streptococcal antibodies

[a] *The presence of two major manifestations or one major and 2 minor manifestations with supportive evidence of recent streptococcal infection indicates a high probability of rheumatic fever.*

these manifestations are present simultaneously, then few errors in diagnosis are made. Frequently, however, the patient presents with only one or two clinical manifestations of the disease.

In classic rheumatic fever there is an *acute migratory*

polyarthritis that is associated with a febrile illness. In general the larger joints of the extremities are affected, but arthritis may occur in the hands, feet, spine, and other joints such as the temporomandibular and sternoclavicular joints. The joint effusions that occur do not persist. Usually, as pain and effusion subside in one joint, another becomes involved, but several joints may be involved simultaneously. The Jones criteria for the diagnosis of rheumatic fever (Table 2) state that the arthritis should involve two or more joints, should be associated with at least two minor manifestations such as fever and elevated sedimentation rate, and should be associated with an elevated antibody titer to one of the streptococcal antigens.

The majority of patients with *rheumatic carditis* do not have symptoms referable to the heart. When signs and symptoms do occur, they may be mild, such as tachycardia disproportionate to the degree of fever, or they may be severe and result in congestive heart failure. Carditis may be manifested by tachycardia, a gallop rhythm, heart sounds with a "tic-tac" quality or arrhythmias. Dropped beats with varying degrees of heart block are associated with prolongation of the conduction time. Prolongation of the P-R interval and other electrocardiographic changes are common in rheumatic fever and do not constitute acceptable criteria for the diagnosis of rheumatic carditis. Pericarditis may appear suddenly and may be associated with precordial pain, a friction rub, or a striking increase in heart size. More commonly, however, patients with pericarditis remain asymptomatic, and an increase in heart size is detected on routine roentgenograms. A definite clinical diagnosis of cardiac involvement can be made only if one or more of the following are found: (1) pericardial friction rub or effusion; (2) an increase in heart size shown by roentgenogram; (3) the appearance of, or change in the character of, organic heart murmurs. The most frequent murmur encountered in rheumatic fever is an apical systolic murmur indicative of mitral regurgitation. In acute rheumatic fever with mitral regurgitation, the third heart sound is frequently accentuated, resulting in a prediastolic gallop rhythm. With severe mitral regurgitation, the third heart sound may be followed by or be replaced by a low-pitched mid-diastolic rumble. This murmur may occur in other forms of acute carditis as well as in severe anemias. The murmur of aortic regurgitation is the second most common murmur heard in patients with rheumatic fever. Death may occur during the acute phase of carditis or following clinical recovery; permanent cardiac damage may result in long-term disability, usually due to mitral or aortic valvular insufficiency and/or stenosis.

Subcutaneous nodules occur as painless small (0.5 to 1 cm) swellings over bony prominences, primarily over the extensor tendons of the hands, feet, elbows, scalp, scapulae, and vertebrae. Nodules tend to occur in crops and may persist for days to months after the onset of acute rheumatic fever. Subcutaneous nodules are not specific for rheumatic fever and may occur in rheumatoid arthritis as well as SLE.

Chorea is characterized by sudden, aimless, irregular movements of the extremities frequently associated with emotional instability and muscle weakness. The onset may be gradual, with complaints that the child is nervous. The patient may become clumsy and may stumble, fall, or drop objects. Facial grimacing and various speech disorders occur. As the chorea becomes more severe, the irregular jerking movements become sufficently violent to produce injuries occasionally. Muscle weakness may also be profound. Most of the choreiform movements subside during sleep and are exaggerated by emotions. Characteristically, if the patient is asked to extend the arms, hands, and fingers, flexion of the wrists and hyperextension of the metacarpophalangeal joints are observed. The pronator sign may be elicited: following raising of the arms above the head there is gradual pronation of the hands (apposition of the dorsal aspects of the hands). Other signs consist of an inability to hold the tongue still when it is protruded and spasmodic contractions of the hands when the patient intentionally grips objects or the examiner's hand.

Erythema marginatum, the characteristic rash associated with rheumatic fever, consists of an evanescent, pink, erythematous macula, often with a clear center and serpiginous outline. The rash is transient, migratory, and nonpruritic; it blanches with pressure and is found primarily on the trunk and proximal extremities.

Other clinical features of rheumatic fever, the so-called minor Jones criteria (Table 2), are of little value in assisting in a diagnosis. Fever may be variable and may persist for weeks. Arthralgia is frequently present, but in the absence of objective migratory polyarthritis this symptom does not assume major diagnostic importance.

LABORATORY EVALUATION. The erythrocyte sedimentation rate and C-reactive protein are almost always elevated in patients with acute rheumatic fever. The values are influenced by previous salicylate or steroid therapy, by the extent of anemia, and by the degree of congestive heart failure. These observations, in addition to the fact that these studies may be abnormal in virtually any other inflammatory state, indicate that they are of little value for the specific diagnosis of acute rheumatic fever. Similarly, the electrocardiographic abnormalities of a prolonged P-R interval, although present in over 20 percent of patients, lack specificity. Leukopenia or urinalysis abnormalities probably do not occur in rheumatic fever, and their presence in a patient with joint and cardiac abnormalities would be suggestive of SLE.

The isolation of group A streptococci from a patient suspected of having acute rheumatic fever provides strong evidence for the diagnosis. Interpretations must be made cautiously, however, as a significant number of normal children may be carriers of streptococci. The failure to isolate streptococci from patients with known rheumatic fever may be related to prior antibiotic therapy, to the presence of only small numbers of organisms, or to inadequate cultures.

Probably the most specific and most reliable proof of

a previous streptococcal infection can be obtained from studies of serum antibody titers against the organism. A rising antibody titer to specific streptococcal antigens is of greater significance than a single elevated value. However, if the patient presents more than 2 months following acute streptococcal infection, antibody titers may be declining or may be low. This occurs most frequently in patients whose initial or only manifestation of rheumatic fever is carditis or chorea. The most widely used serologic test is antibody formation against streptolysin O (ASO). Titers of at least 333 units in children and 250 units in adults are considered elevated. Other antibody tests that are available are antideoxyribonucleotidase B (anti-DNase B), antihyaluronidase (AH), antistreptokinase (ASK), and antinicotinamide-adenine dinucleotidase (anti-NADase). A twofold rise in titer to one or more of the above antigens can be demonstrated in virtually all cases of acute or recurrent rheumatic fever if serum samples are obtained within 2 months of the streptococcal infection. Antibodies directed against the sarcolemmal sarcoplasma of cardiac myofibers are found in patients with rheumatic carditis, but this study is not generally available and may be positive in disorders other than rheumatic fever that are associated with cardiac damage. Patients who present with fever, rash, arthritis, or carditis should have studies performed to exclude abnormalities associated with SLE and rheumatoid arthritis. These include antinuclear antibodies, LE prep, anti-DNA titers, and rheumatoid factor.

TREATMENT. In a patient who has been diagnosed as having acute rheumatic fever, a course of penicillin should be given even if cultures for group A streptococci are negative. Either 1.2 million units of benzathine pencillin G given as a single intramuscular injection or 600,000 units of procaine penicillin G given as a daily injection for 10 days is effective therapy. Erythromycin in a dose of 1g orally for 10 days may be substituted for penicillin in those individuals who are allergic to penicillin. Prophylaxis against recurrent rheumatic fever should be instituted immediately following acute therapy. The most effective prophylaxis consists of 1.2 million units of benzathine penicillin G given as a monthly injection. Alternative therapy consists of either 200,000 units of penicillin given orally twice each day or 1g of sulfadiazine given orally once each day. The optimal duration of prophylaxis is uncertain, and the safest recommendation would be to continue therapy indefinitely.

Salicylates and steroids are of value in controlling the acute clinical manifestations of rheumatic fever. Steroids are most effective as anti-inflammatory agents and may bring the patient under control more quickly; prednisone is utilized in a dose of 1 to 2 mg/kg/day. There continues to be controversy as to whether steroids, when started early in mild carditis, can prevent or reduce ultimate cardiac damage. Studies of patients with moderate to severe carditis treated with salicylates or steroids have failed to demonstrate any superiority of either drug in modifying the duration of acute disease or residual heart damage after 5 years of follow-up. Patients with rheumatic fever who develop congestive

heart failure should be treated with steroids rather than salicylates because of their more prompt effect. Although digitalis may fail to significantly benefit the patient with severe myocarditis, it is frequently successful in the control of congestive heart failure in patients with valvular insufficiency. Digitalis should be started cautiously, because toxic manifestations occur with relatively small doses when acute myocarditis is present (p. 1481).

Salicylates alone are used by most physicians to treat patients with acute rheumatic fever uncomplicated by carditis, since the prognosis in this group of patients is excellent. Acetylsalicylic acid is usually used, in a dose of 70 to 150 mg/kg/day. The duration of treatment is related to the course and severity of the disease. The minimum period is usually 6 weeks. When steroids or salicylates are discontinued, the dose should be reduced gradually over a period of 4 to 6 weeks. If rebound occurs, reinstitution of full therapy for an additional 4 to 6 weeks may be necessary.

Specific treatment for chorea is not available. In general, reduction in physical and mental stress is advisable, with institution of adequate protective measures to prevent self-injury during severe episodes. Occasionally, in very severe cases, steroids have been helpful.

PROGNOSIS. Approximately 75 percent of patients with acute rheumatic fever are well after 6 weeks, and less than 5 percent are symptomatic beyond 6 months. Individuals with chorea or intractable carditis account for the latter group. Recurrent rheumatic fever does not occur in the absence of recurrent infection when more than 8 weeks has elapsed following withdrawal of steroids or salicylates. Up to 70 percent of patients who develop carditis during the initial episode of acute rheumatic fever recover without any residual evidence of heart disease. If significant murmurs do not develop within 6 months of the onset of acute rheumatic fever, it is highly unlikely that heart disease will appear, in the absence of recurrences. Evidence of permanent cardiac damage is greater in those patients who have experienced severe carditis during acute rheumatic fever. Approximately 70 percent of the patients who experience congestive heart failure and pericarditis during acute rheumatic fever develop evidence of permanent heart disease, versus 20 percent of patients with only mild carditis during the acute disease. In individual patients the clinical course during recurrent episodes of rheumatic fever tends to be similar to that seen during the initial acute episode. Patients with recurrent rheumatic fever appear to have a greater incidence of permanent heart damage following carditis than do patients having only a single episode.

References

JUVENILE RHEUMATOID ARTHRITIS

Bernstein B, Takahasai M, Hanson V: Cardiac involvement in juvenile rheumatoid arthritis. Pediatrics 85:313, 1974

Calabro JJ: Chronic iridocyclitis in juvenile rheumatoid arthritis. Arthritis Rheum 13:406, 1970

——— Marchesano JM: The early natural history of juvenile rheumatoid arthritis: a ten year follow up study of 100 cases. Med Clin North Am 52:567, 1968

Kornreich H, Malouf NM, Hanson V: Acute hepatic dysfunction in juvenile rheumatoid arthritis. J Pediatr 79:27, 1971

Lindsley CB, Schaller JB: Arthritis associated with inflammatory bowel disease in children. J Pediatr 84:16, 1974

Schaller J, Wedgwood R: Juvenile rheumatoid arthritis: a review. Pediatrics 50:940, 1970

SYSTEMIC LUPUS ERYTHEMATOSUS

Drinkard JP, Stanley TM, Dornfield L, et al: Azathioprine and prednisone in the treatment of adults with lupus nephritis. Medicine 49:411, 1970

Kellum RE, Haserick JR: Systemic lupus erythematosus: a statistical evaluation of mortality on a consecutive series of 299 patients. Arch Intern Med 113:200, 1964

Melsin AG, Rothfield N: Systemic lupus erythematosus in childhood: analysis of 42 cases with comparative data on 200 adults followed concurrently. Pediatrics 42:37, 1968

DERMATOMYOSITIS AND POLYMYOSITIS

Bitum S, Daeschner CW, Travis LB, Dodge WF, Hopps HC: Dermatomyositis. J Pediatr 64:101, 1964

Miller JJ: Late progression in dermatomyositis in children. J Pediatr 83:543, 1973

Peter JB, Bohan A: Polymyositis and Dermatomyositis. N Engl J Med 292:344, 1975

Sullivan DB, Cassidy JT, Petty RE, Burt A: Progress in childhood dermatomyositis. J Pediatr 80:555, 1972

SCLERODERMA

Bluestone R, MacMahon M, Dawson JM: Systemic sclerosis and small bowel involvement. gut 10:185, 1969

Dabich L, Sullivan D, Cassidy J: Scleroderma in the child. J Pediatr 85:770, 1974

Dubois EL, Chandor S, Friou G, Bischel M: Progressive systemic sclerosis (PSS) and localized scleroderma (morphea) with positive LE cell test and unusual manifestations compatible with systemic lupus erythematosus (SLE). Medicine, 50:199, 1971

Medsger TA, Jr, Masi A, Rodnan G, Beredek TG, Robinson H: Factors affecting survivorship with systemic sclerosis (scleroderma). A life analysis of 309 patients. Ann Intern Med, 75:369, 1971

NECROTIZING ARTERITIS

Fronhert PP, Sheps SG: Long term followup study of periarteritis nodosa. J Med 43:2, 1967

Gocke DJ, Konrad HSU, Morgan C, et al: Association between polyarteritis and Australia antigen. Lancet 2:1149, 1970

Nakao K, Ikeda M, Kimata S, et al: Takayasu's arthritis: clinical report of 84 cases and immunologic studies of seven cases. Circulation 35:1141, 1967

Roberts FB, Feterman GH: Polyarteritis nodosa in infancy. J Pediatr 63:519, 1963

SJÖGREN'S SYNDROME

Anderson LG, Cummings N, Asofsky R, et al: Salivary gland immunoglobulin and rheumatoid factor synthesis in Sjögren's syndrome: natural history and response to treatment. Am J Med 53:456, 1972

Cummings NA, Schall G, Asofsky R, Anderson LG, Talal N: Sjögren's syndrome—newer aspects of research, diagnosis and therapy. Ann Intern Med 75:937, 1971

Shearn MA: Sjögren's Syndrome. Philadelphia, WB Saunders, 1971

RHEUMATIC FEVER

Feinstein AR, Spagnulo M, Wood H, et al: Rheumatic fever in childhood and adolescents: long term epidemiologic study of subsequent prophylaxis: streptococcal infections and clinical sequelae. Ann Intern Med 60:86, 1964

Kuttner AG, Doyle E, Walsh Z, et al: Comparison of prednisone and aspirin therapy on incidence of residual rheumatoid heart disease. N Eng J Med 262:895, 1960

Spagnulo M, Pasternack B, Taranta A: Risk of rheumatic fever recurrences after streptococcal infections: prospective study of clinical and social factors. N Engl J Med 285:641, 1971

Spence J, Hill B, Bywaters EGL, et al: The evolution of rheumatic heart disease in children: five year report of a cooperative clinical trial of ACTH, cortisone, aspirin. Circulation 22:503, 1960

Stollerman GH: Factors determining attack rate of rheumatic fever. JAMA 177:823, 1961

Taranta A, Uhr JW: Post-streptococcal disease. In Samter M (ed): Immunological Diseases. Boston, Little, Brown, 1971, p 601

CHAPTER 12

Bacterial and Viral Infections

DAVID H. CARVER AND HORACE L. HODES, *Associate Editors*

Bacterial Diseases

BACTERIAL STRUCTURE AND PHYSIOLOGY

PATRICK A. MURPHY

Bacteria have several structural and physiologic features that are of direct medical interest. Some of these features account for the ability of the bacterial organism to evade the host defenses and are essential for its survival within the host tissues. When a single such feature is essential to the survival of a bacterium, specific antibody developed in the host tissue either naturally or following artificial immunization may provide effective immunity. Toxins and extracellular enzymes may account for much or all of the pathology found in disease; again, effective immunity can often be induced.

The *capsule* of a bacterium is of great importance in its pathogenicity because this is the surface with which phagocytic cells must interact. In most pathogenic species of bacteria the inner components show little variation between strains, but the outer layer exists in multiple forms that are unrelated antigenically. A typical example is the pneumococcus, which has 82 distinct types of capsule. The virulence of pneumococcal strains can be clearly related both to the chemical structure of their capsules and to the amount of capsule each organism carries. During the course of infection with pneumococci, anticapsular antibody is synthesized; it opsonizes the organisms so that they can be phagocytosed and destroyed. Recurrent infection with the same strain is rare and suggests a defect in antibody synthesis, but there is little serologic cross-reactivity between strains, so that experience with one strain is no defense against infection with another. The K antigens of gram-negative bacilli may serve a similar function; there is a marked association of *Escherichia coli* type K1 with neonatal meningitis, and most strains of *E. coli* from urinary tract infections have generous amounts of K antigen. Capsules are clearly related to virulence in *Klebsiella,* and the pathogenicity of *Pseudomonas aeruginosa* is partly dependent on its slime layer.

We have no clear idea how capsules inhibit phagocytosis; they are usually nonirritant by themselves, and they are also nontoxic to internal organs such as the liver. Organisms that produce no extracellular toxins or enzymes characteristically produce spreading infection with much edema and very little tissue damage. A good example is pneumococcal pneumonia, which usually consolidates a whole lobe of the lung and yet almost never causes scarring or abscess formation.

The *cell wall* has a complex structure and shows fundamental differences between gram-positive and gram-negative bacteria. In virtually all organisms (except mycoplasmas and certain halophils) the basal layer is a mucopeptide that provides structural rigidity and supports the cell membrane against the internal osmotic pressure. Gram-positive organisms usually have another polymer, teichoic acid, covalently bonded to the mucopeptide. Different species of gram-positive organisms have their own special additions to this basic structure. The mucopeptide layer of many gram-positive organisms is toxic when injected into animals. Thus streptococcal mucopeptide causes chronic dermal inflammation when injected subcutaneously into rabbits, and injections into joints produce arthritis. Intravenous injection produces myocarditis, although the lesions do not resemble those of rheumatic fever. These phenomena probably are of pathogenetic significance, because bacterial cell walls are broken down with difficulty in mammalian tissues and tend to persist for a long time.

Because mammalian cells do not possess a wall, there is no structural component in the human that corresponds to the mucopeptide of bacteria. Several antibiotics work by inhibiting the synthesis of mucopeptide. The most important are the penicillins and cephalosporins, which inhibit the final cross-linking reaction; cycloserine inhibits the incorporation of D-alanine, and vancomycin inhibits the incorporation of the cell wall monomer. Organisms deprived of their cell wall by any of these antibiotics form osmotically sensitive variations that soon burst unless the medium is hypertonic. If the organisms are prevented from growing, lysis does not occur, and they survive in a dormant state. Clinically the most important application of this fact is in the treatment of abscesses, empyemas, osteomyelitis, and similar infections. Many of the organisms in these situations are growing very slowly, if at all, and consequently they are not killed by penicillin and similar antibiotics even if they are fully sensitive in vitro.

The cell wall teichoic acids are not toxic, but they are immunogenic, and high titers of antibody to them develop in patients with chronic staphylococcal infections, especially endocarditis. It is possible that they may potentiate the toxicity and immunogenicity of the mucopeptide. It is known that high levels of cell-mediated immunity to staphylococcal cell walls exist in most humans. This immunity is thought to explain the pronounced tendency to localization and necrosis in staphylococcal infections. Delayed hypersensitivity reactions in man and animals can be elicited more efficiently by complexes of mucopeptide and teichoic acid than by mucopeptide alone. Teichoic acid itself does not cause a reaction.

In noncapsulated organisms the cell wall is the outer surface, and there is often a component that serves the same antiphagocytic function as the capsule. Thus there are over 60 types of M protein in streptococci and over 30 types of agglutinogen in staphylococci. The functions of other components such as the streptococcal T and R proteins, the pneumococcal C substance and M protein, and the staphylococcal bound coagulase are undefined. However, specific cell wall components include phage receptors and bacteriocin receptors, both of which may be useful in epidemiologic analysis. *Staphylococcus aureus* cell walls contain protein A, which reacts with the Fc portion of all normal IgG molecules, which makes any type of serologic analysis very difficult; the cells agglutinate and the bound IgG fixes complement. This is why *S. aureus* is usually classified by phage typing.

A function whose importance is only just becoming appreciated is the capacity of bacteria to adhere to the surface of cells in their preferred habitat. In order to maintain itself in the throat, streptococci must be able to bind the epithelial cells, so that they will not be washed away and swallowed. Virulent streptococci bind tightly to pharyngeal cells, while avirulent ones do not. Furthermore, if a virulent strain loses its M protein it loses the capacity to adhere. Stripping off the M protein with trypsin or covering it with specific antibody likewise abolishes adhesion. This evidence suggests that M protein is the responsible factor.

The gram-negative cell wall has a basal layer of mucopeptide, but there are no teichoic acids. Covalently bonded to the mucopeptide is a specific lipoprotein that rises vertically from the bacterial surface and terminates in a hydrophobic lipid moiety. This is embedded in a second membrane layer composed of phospholipid and protein similar to, but not identical with, those of the true cell membrane. Between the mucopeptide layer and the outer membrane is a space called the periplasmic space, which is of great importance to the economy of the organism. Degradative enzymes of many types are bound or physically trapped in this space, and substrates diffusing through the outer membrane are broken down into monomers that can then be absorbed into the cell proper. It is thought that this feature is responsible for the ability of gram-negative organisms to live in the most diverse habitats and to survive a variety of toxic substances.

The *outer membrane* holds digestive enzymes and their products near the cell, so that they are not wasted by diffusing away. This means that very dilute solutions can be colonized and also that a very wide range of carbon sources can be assimilated, since the cell needs only a few permease systems to transport carbohydrate or other monomers into the cytoplasm. Depending on the strain of microbe, the outer membrane may exclude a whole variety of toxic substances. These properties

explain why gram-negative organisms are so successful in colonizing taps, sinks, respirator nebulizers, intravenous fluids, local anesthetics and other injectables, and solutions intended to sterilize cystoscopes and similar equipment. Species that are predominantly sensitive to antibiotics and disinfectants do not survive well in hospitals and tend to be replaced either by resistant variants of the same species or by different species altogether. This ubiquity in the hospital environment, coupled with resistance to disinfectants and antibiotics, explains why we are currently plagued by infections with gram-negative organisms never previously regarded as pathogenic, such as *Serratia marcescens, Providencia stuartii,* and *Pseudomonas cepacia.*

Most of the outer membrane is composed of phospholipid and protein, but a very important component is the lipopolysaccharide, also called *endotoxin.* This substance is composed of a glycophospholipid (lipid A) covalently linked to a core region of about eight individual sugar residues that in turn is linked to a chain of repeating sugar units. Lipid A is incorporated into the outer membrane, presumably by hydrophobic bonding. Endotoxin has a wide range of actions in the body. As far as the organism is concerned, endotoxin contributes significantly to the barrier function of the outer membrane. Rough mutants that have lost the ability to add on the repeating carbohydrate chains show susceptibility to antibiotics that were formerly excluded and to lysozyme, a neutrophil granule enzyme that hydrolyzes the basal mucopeptide. Also, periplasmic enzymes leak away during growth.

As far as the host is concerned, endotoxin is one of the main surface antigens of gram-negative organisms; the O antigen is simply the repeating carbohydrate unit discussed earlier. Enterobacteria that contain many repeating units in their endotoxins are much less susceptible to lysis by antibody and complement, apparently because the reaction occurs at the end of the long chains and little complement binds to the vulnerable outer membrane. They are also resistant to phagocytosis.

Endotoxins are very irritant molecules. Lipid A appears to be toxic in its own right, without any immunologic component. It activates the Hageman factor and hence leads to the release of plasma kinins. The clotting sequence may also be activated, and large doses of endotoxin promote a consumption coagulopathy with secondary fibrinolysis. Platelets and neutrophils are clumped, and subsequently various vasoactive substances and proteolytic enzymes are released. Neutrophils also liberate a small protein (leukocyte pyrogen) that acts on anterior hypothalamic nuclei to cause fever. In addition to all these effects, endotoxin fixes complement directly via the alternate pathway, giving rise to the binding of C3 and later components, with the liberation of anaphylatoxins and chemotactic factors. Since most normal sera contain antibody against O antigens, complement may also be fixed by the classic pathway. Endotoxin produces local inflammation when injected into the skin and produces fever and variable degrees of disseminated intravascular coagulation when injected intravenously. The most spectacular example of the latter is the generalized Shwartzman phenomenon. Large doses of endotoxin produce hypotension and death in shock. The O antigens of gram-negative bacteria exist in many variants. In the salmonellae these varieties are regarded as different species; in the escherichiae and klebsiellae they are not. Each variant requires the host to make a different antibody, thus contributing to the survival of the organisms.

As in gram-positive bacteria, the "social functions" of the organism are mediated by specific features of its outer surface. Receptors for phages, colicins, and mating must all exist. Certain enterobacteria such as shigellae and salmonellae depend for their pathogenicity on the ability to bind to and penetrate epithelial cells. The nature of the binding site is unknown, but since avirulent strains can arise as the result of a single mutation, presumably a specific receptor is involved. Antibody against the endotoxin prevents binding, and the presence of secretory IgA antibody correlates well with resistance to disease in both man and animals. Again, this does not mean that the endotoxin itself is the receptor, because the antiendotoxin antibody might interfere with receptor function by steric hindrance. Nonpenetrating avirulent mutants retain their O antigens.

The *cell membrane* is of less direct medical interest than the cell wall. It is not exposed, and so it has little influence on pathogenicity or immunity, and it is too similar to mammalian cell membranes to allow much selectivity of drug action. Many antibiotics such as gramicidin and tyrothricin have ring structures with hydrophobic exteriors and hydrophilic interiors; when they insert into the membrane, a direct communication is opened between the inside and outside of the cell. All these antibiotics are too toxic for clinical use. Polymyxin B probably acts in a similar manner, but its neurotoxicity, ototoxicity, and renal toxicity have rendered it all but obsolete. The cell membranes of all gram-positive organisms contain teichoic acid; this is covalently bound to membrane lipid. The teichoic acid/lipid complex can be transferred from organisms to erythrocytes and from there to the surfaces of tissue cells. It has been suggested that this may supply a mechanism for the sensitization that occurs in rheumatic fever.

Internal components of bacteria may contribute to the pathogenesis of disease when the organisms are broken up, but we know very little about this. However, there are some well-known differences between bacterial and mammalian intermediary metabolism that allow an opportunity for effective antibiotic action. Enzymes in a biosynthetic pathway are a favorite target, but blockage of only one step can often be overcome by accumulation of precursors or by the use of alternative pathways. A better approach is to block the same pathway in two different places. Trimethoprim inhibits bacterial dihydrofolate reductase about 20,000 times more efficiently than it inhibits the mammalian enzyme. When trimethoprim is used in conjunction with a sulfonamide that blocks folic acid synthesis, most organisms are unable to grow.

There are major differences between mammalian and bacterial *ribosomes*. Many valuable antibiotics, including the aminoglycosides, chloramphenicol, tetracycline, erythromycin, and lincomycin, inhibit bacterial ribosomal function. The aminoglycosides bind so tightly that their action is essentially irreversible and the organism is killed. The others are usually bacteriostatic. Mitochondrial ribosomes are similar to bacterial ribosomes and are also susceptible to these antibiotics; however, permeability barriers prevent the antibiotics from reaching them in vivo. For example, streptomycin does not enter cells at all; chloramphenicol enters cells but is excluded from mitochondria.

An increasing clinical problem is *antibiotic resistance,* and organisms have many ways of achieving this. The simplest is to modify a target enzyme so that it still binds the natural substrate but no longer binds the inhibitor; this is the usual basis of sulfonamide resistance in grampositive organisms. In gram-negative organisms there is a change in permeability of the outer membrane such that sulfonamide is no longer admitted. Clinically, by far the most important mechanism is for the organism to synthesize an enzyme that can destroy the antibiotic activity. Penicillinases hydrolyze a crucial link in the molecule; other antibiotics are often inhibited by substitution with an acetyl, phosphoryl, or adenylyl group. These latter require intracellular cofactors such as ATP and CoA, and the enzymes are therefore intracellular. Since the cell wall cross-linking reaction that is inhibited by penicillin occurs extracellularly, penicillinase is of use to the organism only when secreted extracellularly or into the periplasmic space. The synthesis of a new enzyme is not an event that can occur by mutation; a new gene must be supplied. In the laboratory, resistant variants can be produced by successive mutations in the gene for a preexisting enzyme. This type of resistance develops slowly, and chromosomal genes are not usually responsible for the development of clinically significant antibiotic resistance. Rather, genes responsible for antibiotic resistance are usually carried on plasmids—small self-replicating pieces of DNA usually about 1 or 2 percent of the size of the chromosome.

Plasmids can exist and replicate as independent entities in the cytoplasm; however, some plasmids can also insert into the chromosome of the bacterium. Plasmids that have the ability to insert into and detach from the host chromosome are called *episomes.* An inserted episome is replicated with the host chromosome, and thus it will be transmitted to all the daughter cells. It may also be transmitted to new cells by whatever means the host cell uses for exchanging genetic information— mating, transformation, or transduction. Plasmids also have independent methods of ensuring their transfer to a new host. Some, like the resistance transfer factors of gram-negative bacilli, code for a special conjugation apparatus; others, such as the plasmids responsible for penicillin resistance in *S. aureus,* are dependent for their transmission on a phage.

In the absence of antibiotics, organisms carrying plasmids are rare, but owing to the enormous rate of replication of bacteria, the few resistant forms can rapidly multiply and dominate the population once antibiotics are used. It has been shown that this is the usual mechanism in any individual patient; however, over longer periods of time enteric bacteria may transmit resistance transfer factors across species lines, so that an organism formerly completely susceptible to an antibiotic may become almost totally resistant. Once plasmids have become widely disseminated in a population of organisms, resistance may continue for a long time even in the absence of the antibiotic. This is why over half of community-acquired staphylococcal infections are now due to penicillin-resistant organisms.

Some bacteria are able to form *spores* that can survive for long periods under conditions where the vegetative organisms would not. A number of diverse clinical infections can be related to spore-forming organisms. Botulism from inadequately sterilized food, gas gangrene and tetanus from contamination of wounds by soil, and woolsorters' disease (pulmonary anthrax) are examples. Inefficient autoclaves occasionally allow clostridial spores to survive, and gas gangrene and tetanus may follow surgical operations.

Many organisms secrete into the medium soluble substances that contribute to disease. The simplest examples are those where the organism forms a single well-defined *toxin* that can be clearly related to the pathologic changes found in the disease. Botulism and staphylococcal food poisoning appear to be straightforward intoxications, in which disease is clearly related to the amount of toxin ingested. Diseases such as diphtheria and tetanus, where the organism must establish a foothold in the tissues, are not so simple. Diphtheria toxin blocks protein synthesis by inactivating the translocation enzyme EF2. Tetanus toxin blocks the action of the inhibitory transmitter on spinal cord motor neurons. In both cases the clinical features of the disease are clearly explained by intoxication. However, spores of *Clostridium tetani* cannot germinate at the oxidation–reduction potential found in normal tissue, and the disease can develop only if some other factor depletes the local oxygen supply. Experimentally this may be done by causing necrosis of muscle with one of a number of irritants; by interfering with the local blood supply, or by simultaneous infection with some oxygen-consuming organism. Clinically tetanus is a complication of dirty wounds containing foreign material. In the case of diphtheria, only about 10 percent of children infected with the bacillus develop clinical diphtheria, and in most epidemics only about 10 percent of clinical cases have resulted in death. The causes of this varied response to infection remain obscure, but presumably they reflect the fact that diphtheria bacilli often can establish residence in the throat without invading tissue and that those organisms that do succeed in invading tissue do not always produce enough toxin to cause cardiac failure.

From the practical point of view this hardly matters; the toxin is responsible for the pathology, and immunization against the toxin prevents disease. If the same toxin is made by all strains of the organism, the disease can essentially be wiped out by immunizing all children against it. Some diseases, such as botulism, are too rare to make this worthwhile. Others, such as cholera, can be adequately prevented in other ways. Even in communities where sanitation is defective and is likely to remain so, immunization against cholera is not yet feasible, because the toxin has only recently been purified and adequate clinical trials of the vaccine have not yet been conducted. If multiple toxins exist, immunization is more difficult. Both staphylococcal and *Clostridium perfringens* food poisoning could theoretically be prevented by immunization with mixed toxoids, but both diseases are relatively trivial; so in practice we rely on the proper handling of food for their prevention.

Most bacteria do not secrete toxins that produce pathology at a distance from the organisms. However, a variety of soluble substances are excreted into the medium that may produce tissue damage in the immediate environment, may contribute to the inflammatory response, or may protect the bacteria from phagocytes. Most of these substances are *bacterial enzymes* that can damage living tissue—proteinases and other hydrolytic enzymes. Substances whose modes of action are not (or were not) understood, but that lyse or otherwise damage cells, are called toxins. Examples are streptolysin O and the staphylococcal α toxin. Substances that specifically lyse polymorphs are known as leukocidins; the Panton-Valentine toxin of *S. aureus* is the best known. It has not been possible to show that any one of these substances is all-important to the pathogenesis of disease; specifically, immunization against them has not been clinically effective. Nonetheless, their properties are very suggestive. The *S. aureus* α toxin, for example, produces intense vascular spasm and dermonecrosis that results in a lesion resembling a boil.

Other substances secreted into the medium by organisms are of importance to the inflammation the organisms induce. It has only recently been realized that even during exponential growth substantial quantities of wall components such as mucopeptide and teichoic acids are released in soluble form; as already mentioned, these are irritant. Almost all bacteria liberate chemotactic factors into the medium that attract neutrophils; in general, these are small proteins or polypeptides in the 3,000- to 6,000-dalton range. In turn, neutrophils that have phagocytosed organisms liberate substances that attract more neutrophils, so that the inflammatory response is self-perpetuating as long as any extracellular organisms remain.

Some organisms secrete substances that enable them to avoid phagocytosis. The pneumococcus continually sheds the outer layer of its capsule, presumably taking with it whatever opsonins might have attached. Perhaps the reason that no one of these short-range toxins and enzymes seems to be essential to pathogenicity is because there are so many of them. The staphylococci, for example, produce the α toxin, three other hemolysins, the Panton-Valentine leukocidin, coagulase, lipase, hyaluronidase, DNAse, a protease, and protein A. In addition, some organisms survive phagocytosis, and the local necrosis is compounded by established delayed hypersensitivity in most people.

Perhpas *P. aeruginosa* is the best example of an invasive organism whose properties can be used to explain features seen in infected tissues. *Pseudomonas* produces a number of extracellular proteases that collectively break down proteins, including collagen, and cause hemorrhagic lesions when injected into the skin. A phospholipase produced by the organism kills cells by destroying their membranes. This is of interest in two connections: the organism produces much more of it in diabetic serum than in normal serum, which perhaps may explain the susceptibility of diabetics to malignant otitis externa and other gangrenous *Pseudomonas* infections: it also is highly active against pulmonary surfactant and may be partially responsible for the grim prognosis of *Pseudomonas* pneumonia. These bacterial products may explain local manifestations of *Pseudomonas* infection, but they do not account for death from *Pseudomonas* bacteremia. This appears to be due to a protein exotoxin that causes only edema when injected into the skin. Intravenous injection of exotoxin into mice or rabbits leads to leukopenia, acidosis, shock, and eventual circulatory collapse. At autopsy there is necrosis of hepatocytes and renal tubular cells, and there is widespread edema in the organs, including the lungs. All these are features of lethal *Pseudomonas* infection in man.

Immunity to pyogenic bacteria should theoretically be easy to achieve, but it is difficult in practice. Survival of bacteria in tissue is largely dependent on avoiding phagocytosis; the overwhelming majority of organisms taken up by cells are destroyed. Antibody directed against the outer layer enhances phagocytosis and is usually protective against infection; the difficulty lies in the multiplicity of types. In closed populations, where only a few types are causing trouble, immunization may be effective.

Another situation in which immunization against bacterial surface antigens probably will be useful is in patients who have a gross defect in host defenses, where infection by a specific organism that is difficult to control by other methods is prevalent. Both burned patients and leukemic patients are susceptible to *P. aeruginosa* infections. In burned patients very successful results have been obtained by active immunization with *Pseudomonas* endotoxin, because antibody against this surface antigen enhances phagocytosis and protects against infection. The only problem is that other organisms move into the vacuum, and currently *P. stuartii* sepsis is the most common cause of death on wards where immunization against *Pseudomonas* is practiced. In leukemics the results have been less successful, apparently because both the disease and its treatment prevent the patient from mounting an immune response. Leukemics are also susceptible to infection with enterobacteria, and here again an immunologic approach shows promise.

Most bacteria either have structural components that are irritant or secrete soluble substances with toxic or enzymatic activity, and these, coupled with the host response, can reasonably explain the local lesions. The pneumococcus, which does not produce such substances, causes a bland edematous type of inflamma-

tion. Then why does the pneumococcus destroy joints, and why are pneumococcal meningitis and endocarditis lethal? A number of explanations have been offered. The first was metabolic competition for nutrients such as oxygen or glucose, and the second was poisoning of tissue by products of bacterial metabolism such as lactic acid. However, calculations for all reasonable bacterial population densities show that these factors are insignificant compared to the normal metabolic turnover of mammalian cells. For example, the fall in CSF glucose in meningitis cannot be attributed to its use by the bacteria. It also seems unlikely that competition for some special nutrient such as an amino acid or pyrimidine base can be significant. A more useful explanation of the local damage in joints and other closed cavities may be that the organisms usually attain a high population density, are in the stationary phase of growth, and consequently expose the tissue to irritant components that are hidden by the capsule in the exponential phase. Two mechanisms for this are known to exist: the pneumococcal capsule becomes defective in the stationary phase, so that the cell wall components such as mucopeptide are uncovered; in addition, the pneumococcus possesses autolytic enzymes that produce bacterial lysis soon after growth ceases, so that the tissue is exposed to internal components and cell wall fragments. All normal people above the age of 2 years have established cell-mediated immunity to pneumococcal nucleoproteins, and thus the local inflammation is enhanced by acquired immunity. Presumably, much of the damage is actually mediated by destructive enzymes released from the lysosomes of neutrophils and macrophages that are attracted into the area. In pneumococcal endocarditis, which paradoxically is acute and ulcerative and rapidly leads to valve perforation, there is heavy infiltration of the valve by neutrophils. The bacteria are enmeshed in fibrin and platelets and do not usually reach the valve surface.

The cause of death in most bacteremias is not known. The possibility of toxins secreted only in vivo should not be dismissed lightly. The *Pseudomonas* lethal toxin was only recently discovered; previously it was not found because it is destroyed in vitro by the proteases also secreted by the organism.

Endotoxin promotes disseminated intravascular coagulation, activation of the complement cascade, and liberation of kinins. The dominant feature in shock due to gram-negative bacteremia is spasm of small blood vessels with tissue anoxia, apparently because endotoxin sensitizes the arterioles to catecholamines. Fluid is lost from the circulation by vomiting and diarrhea (also effects of endotoxin) and by loss into inflamed tissue, as well as generally through the anoxic leaky capillaries. The lowered intravascular volume then promotes further vasoconstriction. The resultant systemic acidosis produces generalized malfunction of tissues, including the heart, and may contribute to a cycle in which cardiac failure leads to more tissue anoxia, and so on. The renal failure, hepatic failure, and mental confusion so characteristic of advanced gram-negative sepsis can all be explained as the consequence of anoxia and acidosis, although there may be specific effects as well.

Lysosomal enzymes from phagocytes, both neutrophils and macrophages, are known to mediate several types of experimental local inflammation. Systemic injection of leukocyte granules can cause disseminated intravascular coagulation, plugging of pulmonary capillaries with masses of neutrophils and platelets, and eventually death in shock. Certain features of infections are known to be mediated by small proteins liberated from phagocytes; they include fever, the sequestering of iron and zinc in the reticuloendothelial system, and the synthesis of the acute phase reactant proteins by the liver. (During inflammation of any type the liver synthesizes increased quantities of α_2-globulins, specifically fibrinogen, ceruloplasmin, and C-reactive protein. The raised fibrinogen is responsible for the elevated erythrocyte sedimentation rate.) There are no data on the systemic release of toxic substances from phagocytes in natural infections, but the idea is not implausible. There are a number of studies that show elevated serum levels of lysosomal enzymes such as β-glucuronidase and muramidase in experimental infections and endotoxin poisoning. Also in experimental infections the lysosomes of liver cells were more fragile than normal, and the quantity of non-membrane-bound lysosomal enzymes in liver tissue was increased.

It is possible that nontoxic bacterial products cause death by acting as antigens. Experimentally, death may be caused in animals by inducing anaphylactic hypersensitivity, serum sickness, or delayed hypersensitivity. Anaphylaxis is probably not important in most bacterial infections, because the bacterial population builds up gradually, usually over many days, and desensitization would be expected. Furthermore, edema and urticaria are uncommon in bacterial infections. Some features of bacterial disease are undoubtedly due to serum-sickness-type lesions caused by antigen–antibody complexes. However, it is quite difficult to kill an animal quickly with serum sickness, and in human bacteremias it has been found that arthritis, skin rashes, enlarged lymph nodes, nephritis, and arteritic lesions are exceptional. The best candidate would appear to be delayed hypersensitivity, or cell-mediated immunity (CMI). Normal people show delayed reactions when injected intradermally with a wide variety of dead bacteria. The responsible antigens would appear to be the internal components, which, as mentioned earlier, are relatively stable. Thus infection with an pneumococcus would be expected to establish CMI to all pneumococci, and similarly for other species of bacteria. There is in the normal human population established CMI to many bacteria, and it is known that injection of a large quantity of an antigen to which there is established delayed hypersensitivity can cause rapid death. As regards humans, no more can be said, but an old forgotten experiment of Lindgren may be of interest: Normal guinea pigs were injected intrathecally with dead pneumococci. They flourished. The experiment was then repeated using guinea pigs that had been sensitized to the pneumococcus; it gave positive delayed reactions in the skin. Many

of them died within 24 hours, and all of them showed acute sterile meningitis at autopsy.

References

Clowes RC: Molecular structure of bacterial plasmids. Bacteriol Rev 36:361, 1972

Costerton JW, Ingram JM, Cheng K-J: Structure and function of the cell envelope of gram negative bacteria. Bacteriol Rev 38:87, 1974

Hitchings GH, Burchall JJ: Inhibition of folate biosynthesis. Adv Enzymol 27:417, 1965

Knox KW, Wicken AJ: Immunological properties of teichoic acids. Bacteriol Rev 37:215, 1973

Liu PV: Extracellular toxins of Pseudomonas aeruginosa. J Infect Dis 130 [Suppl]:94, 1974

Luderitz O, Galanos C, Lehman V, et al: Lipid A: chemical structure and biological activity. J Infect Dis 128 [Suppl]:17, 1973

McCarty M: The streptococcal cell wall. Harvey Lect 65:73, 1971

Smith H: Biochemical challenge of microbial pathogenicity. Bacteriol Rev 32:164, 1968

ANTIBACTERIAL DRUG THERAPY
DAVID H. SMITH and PIERCE GARDNER

Analyses of pediatric practices in the United States have revealed that up to 75 percent of all children seen as outpatients by a physician have an infection and that approximately one-third of such visits result in the prescription of one or more antibacterial drugs. The physician must therefore be familiar with the body of knowledge that has developed over the past three decades regarding the interactions of drugs and bacteria, the undesired side effects of antibiotic therapy, and the host factors important to optimal results of such therapy. In this section we have summarized the current status of antibiotic therapy of acute pyogenic bacterial diseases in infants and children. The specific diseases are discussed in other sections of this chapter.

PRINCIPLES OF ANTIBACTERIAL THERAPY

Before therapy is initiated, cultures and smears (if feasible) of infected fluid or tissue should be obtained. Single cultures suffice for many infections, but multiple cultures should be obtained in infections such as subacute endocarditis in which the cultured material may contain small concentrations of bacteria. In order to realize the potential of the diagnostic bacteriology laboratory, cultures must be collected properly and delivered promptly to the laboratory, accompanied by pertinent clinical information. Blood and urine cultures are often contaminated due to inadequate preparation of the skin or the genitalia. Intravenous catheters and needles are so commonly colonized by bacteria that blood cultures should be obtained only at a separate venipuncture. Anaerobic bacteria, which commonly cause abscesses in deep tissues such as brain, liver, or lung, may be killed by oxygen within minutes; thus they may not be isolated unless the specimen is promptly placed under anaerobic conditions. Gonococci are so sensitive to environmental factors that inoculation of transport culture medium at the bedside significantly increases isolation rates.

Clinical information provides the basis for the selection of media and the duration of incubation required for isolation of fastidious or unusual organisms (eg, *Bordetella pertussis, Brucella, Francisella*). Even though bacteria may not be isolated from cultures obtained after onset of appropriate antibiotic therapy, the yield of positive cultures warrants their collection, particularly in patients with continued evidence of systemic infection. Gram-stained smears of infected materials often provide the first clue to the identity of the infecting agent and may be useful in the evaluation of the relative numbers of the different bacteria in mixed infections. In patients who have received prior antibiotic therapy or who have rapidly progressive infections, such as myonecrosis caused by *C. perfringens,* the gram-stained smear is often the laboratory test on which initial therapeutic decisions are based. In the examination of purulent specimens a technically acceptable preparation is one in which the nuclei of the polymorphonuclear leukocytes are pink (not blue). The most common error in the preparation of gram-stained smears is inadequate decolorization (commonly associated with smears that are too thick), which often results in the interpretation of precipitated Gram's stain as gram-positive cocci.

When the clinical situation dictates that antibacterial therapy be started before culture results are available, an effective choice of drugs can usually be made on the basis of gram-stained smears of the infected materials, the bacteria most likely to be involved in the disease process (Table 1), the probable antibiotic sensitivities of the suspected pathogens, and the pharmacologic properties of the drugs.

Specific therapy directed against the presumed or identified pathogen is generally preferable to broad-spectrum shotgun therapy. Treatment with a single antibiotic is generally preferred. Combinations of antibiotics may be used for synergistic activity or when mixed infections exist. Combinations are also commonly used to treat critically ill patients thought to have a septic disease prior to the laboratory identification of the causative bacteria and to prevent the emergence of bacteria resistant to a single antibiotic, as in tuberculosis. Deterrents to the use of multiple antibiotics include possible antagonism and increased risk of side effects and superinfection. Antagonistic effects of combinations of certain antibiotics with bactericidal and with bacteriostatic actions can be demonstrated in experimental models and have been observed in certain clinical studies. Although the importance of these observations to individual cases remains undefined, it seems reasonable to use combinations of antibiotics that do not exhibit in vitro antagonism whenever possible. Bactericidal antibiotics may have advantages over bacteriostatic drugs in patients with impaired host defenses (eg, gamma globulin deficiencies, leukocyte deficiencies or dysfunctions), in immunosuppressed patients, and in infections in which host defenses play a minimal role in the elimination of the causative bacteria, as in bacterial endocarditis.

The pharmacology and toxicology of the antibacterial agents must be considered in the choice of therapy. Properties such as diffusion into the site of infection or route of excretion may be important determinants of the outcome of the prescribed therapy. Lack of awareness of common or serious side effects of antibiotics may result in needless compromise of the function of the eighth cranial nerve, kidneys, or liver, as well as other deleterious effects. When organs important to drug excretion are functionally impaired, alteration of dosage is often necessary.

Superinfection occurs most commonly in association with broad-spectrum antibiotic therapy. Therefore an effective antibiotic with a narrow spectrum of activity is preferable to an antibiotic or a combination of antibiotics with a broader spectrum, provided that factors such as toxicity and pharmacologic properties are comparable. For example, penicillin G or V should be used in preference to ampicillin for infections caused by susceptible bacteria. An adequate dose should be given by an appropriate route for a duration sufficient for the purpose of the therapy. The primary goal of penicillin therapy for group A streptococcal pharyngitis is prevention of rheumatic fever. Therefore therapy should be continued for 10 days, despite the usual prompt resolution of acute symptoms. The route of administration depends on the clinical situation: a parenteral route is recommended for the patient with vomiting; intravenous administration is required for patients in shock or when high peak serum levels of antibiotic are advantageous (eg, bacterial meningitis, endocarditis). Antimicrobial drugs do not obviate the need for correction of abnormalities in respiration, oxygenation, blood volume, and fluid and electrolyte status. Likewise, certain infections such as abscesses and gas gangrene cannot be cured without surgery.

The evaluation of the efficacy of the selected therapy depends primarily on the response of the patient and secondarily on laboratory data. Accurate appraisal of antibiotic resistance requires standardized laboratory methods and may not always correlate with the clinical response. Bacterial resistance to antibiotics is generally relative, and thus resistant bacteria may be eliminated from organs with unusually high concentrations of antibiotics, such as organs of excretion. Furthermore, in vitro resistance to the polymyxins, sulfonamides, and trimethoprim is often difficult to assess accurately. Therefore, if a patient with a non-life-threatening infection is responding satisfactorily, therapy need not be changed because the causative bacteria is resistant by tests to the drug being administered.

It is useful to measure the antibiotic concentrations in serum or appropriate body fluids on one or more days early in the clinical course of certain major infections caused by staphylococci, group D streptococci, and enteric bacilli. When practical, specimens should be obtained at the times at which highest and lowest antibiotic concentrations are anticipated. These data can then be used to determine the kinetics of antibiotic excretion. Peak serum concentrations in excess of 10 times the bactericidal concentration are associated with the best clinical response.

TABLE 1. Microorganisms Most Likely to Cause Infection in Children*

Skin and Subcutaneous Tissues
Skin infections
1. Dermatophytoses
2. *Staphylococcus aureus*
3. *Streptococcus pyogenes* (group A)
4. *Haemophilus influnzae*
5. *Neisseria gonorrhoeae*
Burns
1. *Staphylococcus aureus*
2. *Pseudomonas aeruginosa*
3. *Proteus species*
4. *Streptococcus pyogenes* (group A)
Wound infections
1. *Staphylococcus aureus*
2. *Escherichia coli* (or other gram-negative rods)
3. Anaerobic streptococci
4. *Streptococcus pyogenes* (group A)
5. *Clostridium*

Eyes
Cornea and conjunctiva
1. Viruses (herpes simplex and adenoviruses most common)
2. *Chlamydia:* trachoma, inclusion conjunctivitis
3. *Diplococcus pneumoniae*
4. *Staphylococcus aureus*
5. *Haemophilus influenzae*
6. Coliform bacilli
7. *Haemophilus aegypticus*
8. *Neisseria gonorrhoeae* (newborns)

Nasal Mucous Membrane
1. Viruses
2. *Staphylococcus aureus*
3. *Diplococcus pneumoniae*
4. *Treponema pallidum* (newborns)

Sinuses
1. *Diplococcus pneumoniae*
2. *Staphylococcus aureus*
3. *Haemophilus influenzae*
4. *Klebsiella-Aerobacter*
5. *Streptococcus pyogenes* (group A)

Ear
Auditory canal
1. *Staphylococcus aureus*
2. *Streptococcus pyogenes* (group A)
3. *Pseudomonas aeruginosa* (chronic)
Middle Ear
1. *Diplococcus pneumoniae*
2. *Haemophilus influenzae*
3. *Staphylococcus aureus*
4. *Streptococcus pyogenes* (group A)
5. *Pseudomonas aeruginosa* (chronic)
6. *Proteus specres* (chronic)

Mouth
1. Herpesviruses
2. *Candida albicans*
3. Fusospirochetes (Vincent's infection)

Throat
1. Viruses
2. *Streptococcus pyogenes* (group A)
3. Fusospirochetes (Vincent's infection)
4. *Candida albicans*
5. *Corynebacterium diphtheriae*

Trachea and Bronchi
1. Viruses
2. *Diplococcus pneumoniae*
3. *Haemophilus influenzae*

Pleura
1. *Staphylococcus aureus*
2. *Diplococcus pneumoniae*
3. *Haemophilus influenzae*
4. *Mycobacterium tuberculosis*
5. Anaerobic streptococci
6. *Streptococcus pyogenes* (group A)

Lungs
Pneumonia
1. Viruses
2. *Diplococcus pneumoniae*
3. *Mycoplasma pneumoniae*
4. *Haemophilus influenzae*
5. *Klebsiella-Aerobacter*
6. *Staphylococcus aureus*
7. *Mycobacterium tuberculosis*
8. *Streptococcus pyogenes* (group A)
Abscess
1. *Staphylococcus aureus*
2. *Diplococcus pneumoniae*
3. *Bacteriodes*
4. Fusospirochetes (Vincent's infection)
5. Anaerobic streptococci
6. *Klebsiella-Aerobacter*

Enteric Tract
1. Viruses
2. *Staphylococcus aureus* (food poisoning)
3. *Escherichia coli*
4. *Salmonella species*
5. *Shigella species*
6. *Staphylococcus aureus* (enterocolitis)
7. *Pseudomonas aeruginosa* (enterocolitis)

* Adapted from Med Lett Drugs Ther Handbook of Antimicrobial Therapy, p. 8, revised edition 1976.

TABLE 1. Microorganisms Most Likely to Cause Infection in Children (cont.)

Liver and Biliary Tract
1. *Escherichia coli*
2. *Klebsiella-Aerobacter*
3. *Proteus species*
4. *Bacteriodes*
5. *Salmonella species*

Urethra
1. *Neisseria gonorrhoeae*
2. *Mycoplasma*
3. *Mima*
4. *Treponema pallidum*

Female Genital Tract
Vagina
1. *Neisseria gonorrhoeae*
2. Herpes virus
3. *Candida albicans*
4. *Streptococcus pyogenes* (group A)
5. *Treponema pallidum*

Bladder, Ureters, and Kidneys
1. *Escherichia coli* (or other
   9 gram-negative rods)
2. *Streptococcus pyogenes* (group D)
3. *Staphylococcus aureus*
   (after surgery)

Central Nervous System
Meninges
1. Viruses
2. *Haemophilus influenzae*
3. *Diplococcus pneumoniae*
4. *Neisseria meningitidis*
5. *E. coli* or other coliform bacilli
   (perinatal period)
6. *Streptococcus pyogenes* (group B)
   (perinatal period)
7. *Staphylococcus aureus*
   (after surgery)
8. *Mycobacterium tuberculosis*
9. *Cryptococcus neoformans*
10. *Listeria monocytogenes*
    (newborns, immunosupressed individuals)
11. *Coccidioides immitis* (in endemic areas)
Abscess
1. *Bacteroides*
2. Anaerobic streptococci
3. *Staphylococcus aureus*

Bones (Osteomyelitis)
1. *Staphylococcus aureus*
2. *Salmonella species*
3. *Mycobacterium tuberculosis*
4. *Streptococcus pyogenes* (group A)

Joints
1. *Staphylococcus aureus*
2. *Haemophilus influenzae*
3. *Streptococcus pyogenes* (group A)
4. Gram-negative rods
5. *Neisseria gonorrhoeae*

Endocardium
1. *Streptococcus viridans*
2. *Staphylococcus aureus*
3. Anaerobic streptococci
4. *Streptococcus pyogenes* (group D)

Pericardium
1. Viruses
2. *Staphylococcus aureus*
3. *Diplococcus pneumoniae*
4. *Streptococci* (all groups)
5. *Mycobacterium tuberculosis*
6. *Neisseria meningitidis*
7. *Haemophilus influenzae*

Blood (Septicemia)
Newborn infants
1. *Escherichia coli* (or other
   coliform bacilli)
2. *Staphylococcus aureus*
3. *Streptococcus pyogenes* (group B)
Children
1. *Haeomophilus influenzae*
2. *Neisseria meningitidis*
3. *Staphylococcus aureus*
4. *Diplococcus pneumoniae*
5. *Escherichia coli* (or other
   coliform bacilli)

Peritoneum
1. *Escherichia coli* (or other
   gram-negative rods)
2. *Streptococcus pyogenes* (group D)
3. Diplococcus pneumoniae
4. *Bacteroides* (or other
   gram-negative rods)
5. Anaerobic streptococci
6. Clostridium

When appropriate antibiotic therapy fails, reassessment and intensification of diagnostic efforts are indicated. Common reasons for failures of therapy include misdiagnosis of viral infections and failure to take prescribed oral medications. Unusual persistence of respiratory or urinary tract infections should lead to a search for structural abnormalities or foreign bodies. Repeat cultures may indicate superinfection or alteration of the antibiotic sensitivity pattern of the original etiologic bacteria. Unusual bacterial forms such as L forms rarely cause the persistence of infections.

The prophylactic use of antibiotics is most likely to succeed when directed against a specific organism, such as penicillin versus group A streptococci or gonococcus. Prophylaxis against infections caused by mixed or unknown bacteria is rarely successful, and it carries the risks of superinfection, toxicity, and allergy.

The public health aspects of antimicrobial therapy should be considered by the prescribing physician. The use of antibiotics not only affects the bacterial ecology of the individual patient but also may affect that of the hospital or community by creating a selective force favoring the emergence of drug-resistant bacteria. The potential effectiveness of the antibiotic armamentarium for the treatment of future infections may thereby be reduced.

MECHANISMS OF ACTION OF ANTIMICROBIAL DRUGS

The clinical efficacy of an antibacterial drug depends on its ability to inhibit bacteria at concentrations that are not toxic for mammalian cells. This selective toxicity is achieved by taking advantage of differences in the biochemistry of the parasite and the host. Rapid expansion of knowledge in the field of cell biology has defined certain of these differences and has resulted in a better understanding of the biochemical basis for the action of many antimicrobial drugs. A summary of the current understanding of the mechanism of action of certain of the commonly used antimicrobial drugs is presented in order to illustrate certain principles for the proper clinical use of these agents.

AGENTS AFFECTING BACTERIAL WALLS. The wall confers on bacteria their characteristic shape, their resistance to osmotic and mechanical trauma, and part of their pathogenicity. Because of the high osmotic pressure of bacterial cytoplasm, cell-wall-deficient bacteria (L forms) lyse in isotonic media but not in hypertonic media. The walls of all bacteria, including spirochetes and actinomycetes, contain a network of polymers of alternating units of *N*-acetylglucosamine and *N*-acetylmuramic acid that are cross-linked by polypeptides. This peptidoglycan and many of its constituents are unique to bacteria. This complex polymer is synthesized in several stages. Disaccharide polypeptide precursors of peptidoglycan are synthesized in the cytoplasm and then transferred to a lipid carrier that transports them across the protoplasmic membrane to the growing end of the peptidoglycan where the polypeptide side chains are polymerized by a transpeptidation reaction. The peptidoglycan layer is generally covered by additional macromolecular polymers that are exposed to the environment and that provide immunologic specificity. In gram-positive bacteria these surface polymers include teichoic acids, carbohydrates (eg the group-specific antigens of streptococci), and polypeptides (eg the M proteins of group A streptococci). Exterior to the peptidoglycan of gram-negative bacteria is a lipopolysaccharide polymer composed of an interior lipid attached to an exterior polysaccharide. The core of this polysaccharide is thought to be uniform for each major group of the *Enterobacteriaceae;* the exterior side chains vary in composition, conferring the O antigen specificity. Some gram-negative bacteria have surface carbohydrate capsules or polypeptide polymers. The outer layers of the bacterial wall are not so critical for structure as peptidoglycan, but they play a major role in the cell's pathogenicity, either by direct toxicity (eg, the lipopolysaccharide layer) or by protecting the bacterium from phagocytosis or immune lysis.

Penicillin inhibits the transpeptidation reaction and certain other enzymes involved in the structure of peptidoglycan; therefore treated sensitive bacteria produce defective walls. The semisynthetic penicillins and the structurally related cephalosporins have similar actions. These mechanisms and the specificity of peptidoglycan for bacterial cells explain the remarkable tolerance of man for penicillin and the spectrum of inhibited microorganisms: effectiveness that differs only quantitatively against gram-negative and gram-positive bacteria, spirochetes, and actinomycetes, but no activity against cell-wall-deficient bacteria, *Mycoplasma, Chlamydia, Rickettsia,* fungi, protozoa, and viruses. Bacitracin specifically inhibits peptidoglycan synthesis by reducing the availability of the lipid carrier that transports the disaccharide pentapeptide subunits across the cell membrane. Vancomycin blocks the wall acceptor of these subunits and thereby inhibits peptidoglycan synthesis. Since dormant bacteria do not produce cell wall, antibiotics affecting wall synthesis are active only against growing bacteria.

AGENTS AFFECTING BACTERIAL MEMBRANE. The cytoplasmic membrane lies immediately inside the bacterial wall. It retains required intracellular metabolites and is the site of systems that transport out waste products and externalize macromolecules, exoenzymes, and wall and capsule precursors. The membrane also contains many transport systems for the active uptake of nutrients and salts that permit the bacterial cell to scavenge efficiently and to maintain a relatively constant intracellular ionic composition independent of extracellular concentrations. Bacteria do not possess mitochondria; their electron transport systems are located in the membrane. Because of the importance of membrane functions, damage to it is generally irreversible and lethal.

The bacterial membrane is composed of about 40 percent lipid, 60 percent protein, and small amounts of carbohydrate. Membranes of different bacteria are antigenically distinct. The composition of the bacterial membrane differs notably from that of mammalian cells by the absence of sterols and by the types of phosphatides in the lipids. Polymyxin B and colistin (polymyxin E) contain methyloctanoic acid and a basic cyclic polypeptide. These groups give these antibiotics the surface-active properties of a cationic detergent. The polymyxins destroy the bacterial membrane, presumably by binding to its lipids, and rapidly kill resting and growing bacteria. The toxic effect of the drug on certain mammalian tissues (renal, neurologic) may reflect that the involved cells share with sensitive bacteria the membrane binding sites for these drugs.

AGENTS AFFECTING NUCLEIC ACID SYNTHESIS. Bacteria do not possess a nuclear membrane, but their single chromosome (a single, closed circular molecule of DNA) is intimately related to the cytoplasmic membrane. The components of bacterial DNA and RNA are universal to all cells. It is not surprising, therefore, that few drugs have been found that selectively inhibit bacterial nucleic acid synthesis. Nalidixic acid selectively inhibits the polymerization of bacterial DNA, but its precise mechanism of action has not been defined. Rifamycin selectively inhibits bacterial RNA synthesis by its effect on the DNA-dependent RNA polymerase, an activity that provides the most direct evidence that the RNA polymerase of bacteria differs significantly from that of mammalian cells.

AGENTS AFFECTING PROTEIN SYNTHESIS. Proteins are synthesized by a complex series of reactions in which the nucleotide sequence of the gene being translated is ultimately encoded into a specific sequence of amino acids. A single molecule of mRNA carrying the genetic information complexes with several ribosomes. Each trinucleotide codon in the mRNA specifies the binding of a certain tRNA, to which is linked a specific amino acid (aa-tRNA) by pairing with a complementary sequence. This recognition step occurs at a site (A) on the ribosome. The bound tRNA is then moved to an adjacent ribosomal site (P) (translocation), with the mRNA moving coordinately to expose the next trinucleotide. After a new aa-tRNA enters the recognition site at (A), the amino acid of the complex at P is enzymatically transferred back to that at A (peptidyl transfer). The free tRNA left at P is released as the cycle is repeated. When the mRNA is completely read, the completed polypeptide is released and the ribosomal mRNA complex disrupted (a matter of seconds in bacteria growing at 37 C).

The aminoglycoside antibiotics (streptomycin, neomycin, kanamycin, gentamicin) bind irreversibly to individual structural proteins of the smaller of the two ribosomal subunits, and in so doing they presumably distort binding site A. They therefore block recognition or provoke errors in the binding between mRNA and the tRNA of incoming aa-tRNA. Such misreading facilitates the incorporation of genetically inaccurate amino acids into the growing polypeptide and hence the synthesis of faulty protein. This binding also promotes the release of ribosomes from polysomes and blocks the

formation of polysome precursors—actions that are responsible for the lethal activity of these agents. The tetracyclines bind to the smaller subunit of the ribosome, thereby reversibly inhibiting the binding of aa-tRNA to the A site. Chloramphenicol, lincomycin, and erythromycin compete for reversible binding on the larger ribosomal subunit. The first two of these agents block the binding of peptidyl-tRNA complexes at P and thus peptidyl transfer. Erythromycin also blocks the P site, inhibiting peptidyl transfer and translocation. These mechanisms account for the observations that cross-resistance between certain of these drugs is common, their antibacterial effects are generally not additive or synergistic, and they may inhibit the growth of cell-wall-deficient bacteria.

The protein synthetic schema described for bacteria is shared, at least in part, by many other types of cells; hence certain antibacterial agents inhibit *Chlamydia,* *Rickettsia,* and *Mycoplasma.* However, the protein synthetic system of mammalian cells is relatively insensitive to antibacterial drugs. Chloramphenicol inhibits the protein synthesis and terminal respiration of isolated mitochondria, but the biologic importance of these effects and their relation to the inhibition by chloramphenicol of human bone marrow are not known. Similarly, it is not known if the toxic effects for man of the aminoglycosides and tetracyclines are due directly to their effects on the ribosome.

AGENTS AFFECTING INTERMEDIARY METABOLISM. Intermediary metabolism includes those reactions that produce energy or macromolecular precursors. The discovery of the antibacterial activity of sulfonamides and the recognition that they compete with *p*-aminobenzoic acid (PABA) prompted the synthesis and testing of the antibacterial activity of thousands of analogues of essential metabolites. Unfortunately, only a few agents have been found that possess the selective toxicity required of a clinically useful antimicrobial drug. PABA is a precursor of folic acid, which is a cofactor in the transfer of single carbon fragments from serine to methionine, purines, and thymine. Because of their structural similarity to PABA, all sulfonamides competitively inhibit the enzyme that produces dihydrofolate. They compete as a substrate for the enzyme and are converted into a faulty product that further inhibits folate-dependent reactions. Trimethoprim, a pyrimidine analogue, acts at a subsequent step in folic acid metabolism, inhibiting the enzyme that reduces dihydrofolate to tetrahydrofolate. The combination of trimethoprim and a sulfonamide is synergistic for a wide spectrum of bacteria.

The selective toxicity of the sulfonamides depends on the requirement of mammalian cells for exogenous folate, the inability of all clinically important bacteria to utilize exogenous folate (presumably because of impermeability), and a concentration of single carbon metabolites in body fluids that is generally too low to reverse the effect of the concentrations of sulfonamide attainable during therapy. Mammalian cells also utilize the enzyme attacked by trimethoprim; the selective toxicity of the drug resides in its 60,000-fold greater affinity for the bacterial enzyme. The clinical uses of sulfonamides and trimethoprim are affected by these molecular phenomena: The drugs have a wide spectrum because almost all bacteria require endogenous folate. All sulfonamides inhibit the same reaction, and therefore mutant bacteria whose affected enzymes are resistant to any given sulfonamide preparation are resistant to all others. Since the growth of treated sensitive cells continues until intracellular folate is depleted, the inhibition effected by these drugs is not rapid. The high concentrations of single carbon metabolites in sites of extensive tissue destruction (abscesses, burns) reduce the therapeutic efficacy of these drugs. The toxicity of the sulfonamides for man cannot be related to their metabolic effects, but is due to their insolubility or host hypersensitivity. Trimethoprim may occasionally affect mammalian cells, particularly in the presence of depleted folate stores.

GENERAL COMMENTS. Antimicrobial agents that irreversibly inhibit bacteria at effective concentrations are defined as bactericidal, while the inhibition caused by a bacteriostatic agent is reversed when the agent is removed from the environment. This distinction is not absolute, however, for bactericidal antibiotics have no lethal effect at subinhibitory concentrations, while bacteria inhibited for long periods by bacteriostatic drugs may not survive. Furthermore, these definitions have been derived from in vitro studies and do not take into account host defenses.

That antibiotics in combination may not be more effective than a single agent is supported by considerable experimental and clinical experience. As noted earlier, a bacterium whose protein synthesis has been stopped at one step is generally not further inhibited by another drug inhibiting a subsequent reaction in the sequence. Similarly, two types of inhibitors of mucopeptide synthesis are no more effective against susceptible bacteria than one. On the other hand, the combination of trimethoprim and a sulfonamide (which inhibit distinct sequential enzymes involved in folic acid synthesis) is synergistic for a wide spectrum of bacteria. Since inhibitors of mucopeptide synthesis and the aminoglycoside antibiotics kill only growing bacteria, stopping protein synthesis with tetracycline or chloramphenicol prevents or stops the lethal action of the former drugs. On the other hand, the penicillin-induced damage of the cell wall may facilitate the uptake of aminoglycoside antibiotics. The lethal actions of penicillins and aminoglycosides in combination are therefore often synergistic. Therefore knowledge of the mechanisms of action of the antimicrobial drugs provides guidelines for decisions on the effectiveness of multiple drugs; however, clinical situations must be evaluated individually.

RESISTANCE TO ANTIMICROBIAL AGENTS

BIOCHEMICAL BASIS OF DRUG RESISTANCE. At least four mechanisms exist whereby bacteria may be resistant to an antibiotic: (1) The antibiotic target may be insensitive to the drug. (2) The target may be sensitive, but the cell envelope may be impermeable to the drug. Most gram-negative bacilli, for example, are not affected by several thousand times the concentration of erythromycin that inhibits gram-positive bacteria. In contrast, envelope-deficient derivatives of many resistant gram-negative bacilli are inhibited by fractions of the concentrations required to inhibit the parent strain. The pattern of bacterial susceptibilities to various penicillins is based in large part on selective permeability of the bacterial envelope. (3) The bacteria may produce an enzyme that inactivates the drug. The β-lactamase that cleaves the β-lactam ring of penicillin is the best known example of this mechanism. However, enzymes that specifically inactivate streptomycin, spectinomycin, kanamycin, neomycin, gentamicin, or chloramphenicol by conjugating phosphate, adenylate, or acetate groups to the drugs are commonly the basis for the respective resistances. (4) Certain phenotypic (or environmental) phenomena may affect drug susceptibility. All antibacterial drugs, with the exception of the polymyxins, affect only growing bacteria; thus bacteria in nutritionally deficient media are drug-resistant. Since aminoglycosides have little or no effect on bacteria growing anaerobically, sensitive (facultative anaerobic) bacteria are protected when shifted from an aerobic to an anaerobic environment. The activity of certain antibiotics is dramatically influenced by pH: the increased activity of erythromycin and the aminoglycoside antibiotics at an alkaline pH has clinical importance in the treatment of urinary tract infections. Ionic composition and concentration affect the potency of many antibiotics.

GENETIC BASIS OF DRUG RESISTANCE. The bacterial chromosome contains a few thousand genes, each of which mediates the synthesis of a single protein. A spontaneous alteration in the chemical composition of a gene (a mutation) may prevent the synthesis of the gene product or alter its composition so that its function is affected. A mutation of the gene or genes mediating the synthesis of the (macromolecular) target of an antibiotic may render that bacterium drug-resistant. At cell division the chromosome, including the mutant gene, is replicated and segregated into each of the two daughter bacteria. Although a spontaneous mutation occurs only once in every 10^6 to 10^8 cell divisions, these rare resistant bacteria gain ascendancy when sensitive bacteria are inhibited by an antibiotic. This mechanism of mutation and selection is the genetic basis for antibiotic resistance mediated by the bacterial chromosome. Critical laboratory studies have indicated that spontaneous mutations affecting different genes usually occur independently and at the same relative frequency. Thus resistance (via mutation) to two drugs with different mechanisms of action occurs once in every 10^{12} to 10^{16} generations; resistance to three agents occurs once in 10^{18} to 10^{24} generations. Since multiple mutations are so rare, the use of multiple agents is successful in the prevention of the emergence of resistant strains during long-term therapy of a disease caused by bacteria whose antibiotic resistance is mediated only by mutation (eg, tuberculosis).

The prevalence in hospitals of bacteria resistant to

multiple antibiotics, particularly *S. aureus* and enteric bacilli, is much higher than would be predicted if these resistances were due to mutation. Furthermore, the observations that bacteria of different genera (eg, *E. coli* and *Shigella*) with identical patterns of multiple drug resistance can be recovered from the stool of one individual cannot easily be explained by the theory of mutation and selection. These observations have now been found to be due in large part to self-replicating extrachromosomal genetic elements denoted variously as plasmids, episomes, or R (resistance) factors that may contain one gene or multiple genes mediating individual drug resistances. These factors replicate and segregate in daughter bacteria at cell division and can also be transferred between bacteria, either by viruses (*transduction*) or in the case of enteric bacteria by direct cell contact (*conjugation*). The drug-resistant plasmids of *S. aureus* cannot be transmitted to other genera of bacteria, whereas those of gram-negative bacilli can be transferred among all species of enteric bacteria. The experimental transfer of R factors by transduction is about 10^{-2} to 10^{-5} as efficient as conjugation, which may affect 1 in every 10^2 to 10^3 bacteria under ideal circumstances. Interbacterial transfer by either mechanism and the expression of R factor resistance are completed in less than one cell division (as short a time as 30 minutes). Certain practical questions about R factors remain to be answered, but existing data indicate that they are widespread and commonly mediate the drug resistances of *S. aureus,* group D streptococci, H. influenzae and enteric bacilli isolated from clinical specimens.

TESTING DRUG RESISTANCE. In an attempt to predict the clinical efficacy of antimicrobial agents, bacteria isolated from sites of infection are tested for antibiotic susceptibility in vitro. The original technique for the quantitation of antibiotic sensitivity utilizes tubes of broth containing serial dilutions of drug inoculated with a constant concentration of bacteria and observed for the lowest drug concentration that prevents growth (*minimal inhibitory concentration*) and kills the bacteria, determined by subculture (*minimal bactericidal concentration*). The results usually correlate with the clinical efficacy of the tested drugs. Resistance is also assessed by spreading bacteria on solid medium containing different concentrations of antibiotics and observing the presence of growth after incubation. However, these methods are not used routinely in most laboratories because of the number of procedures and the cost.

In the most commonly used method, filter paper disks impregnated with antibiotic are placed on a lawn of bacteria spread on the surface of nutrient agar. After an appropriate period of incubation the diameter of inhibited bacterial growth is measured and compared to standards. This method is convenient, but accurate interpretation requires the use of properly prepared plates of Mueller-Hinton medium, rigid control of the quantity of bacteria plated and the concentration of drug in the disk, accurate measurement of the zone of inhibited growth, and comparison of this zone to those of bacteria whose drug susceptibility has been documented previously by the tube dilution method. When these standards are met, the results of this diffusion method correlate well with clinical experiences.

It should be emphasized that drug sensitivities need not be performed routinely on all bacterial isolates. Such tests are rarely if ever required for such agents as pneumococci and group A streptococci, which show little variation of drug sensitivity patterns. Isolates from voided urine should be tested only if significant numbers of bacteria in pure or repeated cultures are found. However, any growth from percutaneous aspirates of the bladder is significant. Drug sensitivity tests for anaerobic bacteria have not been as well standardized as have those for aerobic bacteria, and therefore their relationship to clinical experiences is less well defined. Sensitivity tests should be routinely performed on *S. aureus,* group D streptococci, *Neisseria,* and enteric bacteria isolated from infected sites. In cases of endocarditis, life-threatening infections, or infections caused by unusual bacteria, antibiotic sensitivity tests should be performed by the more accurate tube dilution assay.

ASSAYS OF ANTIBIOTIC CONCENTRATIONS

The increasing need to treat patients with impaired liver or renal function with relatively toxic antibiotics and the realization that antibiotic excretion is highly individualized have emphasized the need to quantitate antibiotic concentrations in body fluids. The most readily available assays are functionally identical to the methods used to assess bacterial resistance. Test specimens are serially diluted in broth, inoculated with a standard suspension of bacteria, and incubated; subsequent growth is compared to standards. This method can provide very useful information, particularly when total antibiotic activity against the bacteria causing the disease is measured. Its limitations include the requirements for a modest volume of test specimen, an overnight incubation, inaccuracy of up to 100 percent, and the need for different test bacteria if the concentrations of multiple antibiotics are to be assayed simultaneously.

Antibiotics can also be assayed by *plate methods* in which the test fluid is inoculated on a filter paper disk that is then placed on a lawn of test bacteria, the subsequent zones of inhibited bacterial growth being compared to those produced by known quantities of antibiotic. Although this assay can be performed in 4 to 7 hours, it retains the other disadvantages of microbiologic methods. Accordingly, enzymatic and radioimmunoassay methods that are rapid, that are antibiotic-specific, and that require minute volumes of specimen have been developed.

The *enzymatic methods* employ antibiotic-inactivating enzymes produced by R factors. They appear to be the most accurate of the antibiotic assays, but at present they require radioactive substrates and are available only for aminoglycoside antibiotics. Experience with radioimmunoassay for gentamicin is accumulating. It seems reasonable that ongoing experience will soon define the optimal methods for antibiotic assay, as well as the indications for their use.

ANTIMICROBIAL AGENTS

Narrow-Spectrum Agents

PENICILLIN. The penicillin antibiotics remain the drugs of choice for most infections due to gram-positive cocci, gram-positive bacilli, *Neisseria,* and spirochetes. In addition, they are effective against some gram-negative rods and many anaerobic bacteria. The wide variety of preparations allows the physician to individualize therapy, but it also requires an awareness of pharmacologic differences such as absorption, peak blood concentrations, rates of renal clearance, and protein binding.

ORAL PENICILLIN. Penicillin G (benzylpenicillin) is inexpensive and has been used successfully for many years, but it is acid-labile and is absorbed poorly when given with food. Penicillin V and phenethicillin are relatively acid-resistant and are absorbed from a full stomach, although higher blood levels are achieved when they are given 1 hour before or 2 hours after meals.

PARENTERAL PENICILLIN G. The various parenteral penicillin preparations produce widely differing peak blood levels and durations of activity. To attain high blood levels rapidly, aqueous penicillin must be used. The rapid excretion of aqueous penicillin in children beyond infancy with normal renal function requires that it be administered frequently (usually every 2 to 4 hours) for optimal therapy. Aqueous penicillin G is prepared as a potassium or sodium salt. One million units contain approximately 1.7 mEq of cation (usually potassium), which must be taken into consideration when large doses are administered to patients with poor renal function or electrolyte disorders.

Procaine penicillin is absorbed slowly, which usually results in low serum concentrations; therefore it should be used only in infections caused by highly susceptible organisms, such as pneumococci or group A streptococci. Benzathine penicillin produces blood concentrations of less than 0.1 IU/ml for as long as 3 to 4 weeks. Therefore it is used only against group A streptococci for prophylaxis of patients with rheumatic heart disease or in epidemic situations or therapeutically when adherence to a program of oral penicillin seems questionable or improbable.

β-LACTAMASE-RESISTANT PENICILLINS. Semisynthetic β-lactamase-resistant penicillin analogues are used primarily to treat infections caused by *S. aureus* that are resistant to penicillin G (β-lactamase producers). All are significantly less potent than benzylpenicillin against other microorganisms. The available preparations differ considerably in properties such as protein binding and in vitro effectiveness, but none has clearly established clinical superiority. The emergence of *S. aureus* isolates that are resistant to all these penicillins (and to the cephalosporins) has become a serious problem in Europe and has been reported in the United States.

Methicillin. Methicillin is the least thoroughly protein-bound (20 percent) of the semisynthetic penicil-
lins. It is less potent against most bacteria by in vitro testing than other β-lactamase-resistant penicillins. Because of its instability in an acid medium, no oral preparation is available.

Oxacillin. Oxacillin is more active than methicillin against penicillin-resistant *S. aureus* in vitro, but it is more thoroughly protein-bound (80 to 90 percent). Although oxacillin is acid-stable, blood levels following oral administration are markedly diminished by food in the stomach, and oxacillin should in general be reserved for parenteral use.

Nafcillin. Nafcillin shares with oxacillin the properties of marked activity against *S. aureus* in vitro and a high degree of protein binding. Of the semisynthetic penicillins, nafcillin has the greatest activity against gram-positive organisms other than *S. aureus.* The drug is concentrated in the biliary tract. Although nafcillin is acid-stable, absorption from the gastrointestinal tract is not reliable, and parenteral administration is advised.

Cloxacillin and Dicloxacillin. Cloxacillin and dicloxacillin are absorbed significantly better from the gastrointestinal tract than are the other β-lactamase-resistant penicillins; therefore they are the oral preparations of choice in this category.

"BROAD-SPECTRUM" PENICILLINS.

Ampicillin. The penicillin analogue ampicillin affects the same spectrum of gram-positive bacteria as benzylpenicillin. In addition, it has activity against *Haemophilus influenzae* and most *E. coli, Proteus mirabilis, Shigella,* and *Salmonella.* Hetacillin is a more expensive analogue that is rapidly broken down into ampicillin in the blood; therefore it should not be considered a separate drug. Ampicillin has been the antibiotic recommended most frequently in the therapy of bacterial meningitis of unknown origin in the toddler, and it is the preferred agent in the treatment of infections caused by *H. influenzae, Shigella,* and enterococci. Recent documentation of *H. influenzae* and *Shigella* resitant to ampicillin means that such infections can no longer automatically be treated with ampicillin. Many authorities recommend that all systemic infections believed to be caused by *H. influenzae* be treated with chloramphenicol until the organism is shown to be sensitive to ampicillin. Due to the high concentrations achieved in bile, ampicillin has been used in biliary tract infections caused by susceptible organisms (including *Salmonella*). Because of its limited gram-negative spectrum and its susceptibility to β-lactamase, ampicillin should not be used alone in the treatment of sepsis of undefined etiology and should not be used to treat infections due to penicillin-resistant *S. aureus.* The maculopapular rash that commonly occurs during ampicillin therapy (especially in patients with infectious mononucleosis) usually does not indicate true penicillin allergy and should not preclude future use of penicillin.

Amoxicillin. Amoxicillin has the same antibacterial spectrum as ampicillin, and like ampicillin it is susceptible to β-lactamase activity. It is better absorbed from the gastrointestinal tract and is claimed to cause less diarrhea. Amoxicillin, unlike ampicillin, is not effective in the treatment of even sensitive *Shigella* infections, possibly because of decreased concentrations in the large bowel resulting in greater proximal absorption.

Carbenicillin.   In high concentration, carbenicillin is effective against many strains of *P. aeruginosa* and *Proteus,* as well as the usual penicillin spectrum. High concentrations appear in the urinary tract, and best results with carbenicillin have been in the treatment of urinary tract infections. Success has been variably reported in the treatment of *Pseudomonas* pneumonia and septicemia in leukopenic patients. Highly resistant strains of *Pseudomonas* may emerge during therapy. Synergistic antibacterial activity of carbenicillin and gentamicin has been demonstrated against most *Pseudomonas* isolates, and these drugs used together probably represent the most effective antibiotic therapy for severe *Pseudomonas* infections. Carbenicillin and gentamicin should never be mixed together in the same intravenous bottle, since they react chemically and become inactivated.

Carbenicillin is destroyed by penicillinase. Its activity is increased at acid pH. Because carbenicillin is a disodium molecule and is used in very high doses, the sodium administered (about 6 mEq/g) must be considered in order to avoid overload. In addition to the parenteral form, an oral preparation for use only in urinary tract infections is available.

ADVERSE REACTIONS.   Hypersensitivity to the penicillins is common with all preparations. Because all penicillins share the same basic chemical structure, patients with hypersensitivity to one preparation may react to any of the others. However, sensitivity only to a specific penicillin has been described. Immediate reactions include anaphylaxis, angioneurotic edema, and urticaria. Therapeutic measures include prompt administration of epinephrine, maintenance of the airway, and support of the cardiovascular system. Delayed reactions include fever, eosinophilia, serum sickness, a variety of dermatologic conditions (ranging from a slight rash to exfoliative dermatitis), and occasional autoimmune phenomena such as vasculitis and Coombs-positive hemolytic anemia. Interstitial nephritis is a rare complication of therapy with semisynthetic penicillins, especially methicillin. Abnormally high central nervous system concentrations produced by high serum concentrations, such as by maximum-dose therapy in patients with marginal renal function or by erroneous intrathecal doses, may cause myoclonic jerks and convulsions. Although several skin test reagents have been developed to detect penicillin allergy, only penicilloyl polylysine has been licensed. Thus a careful history of atopic reactions and previous adverse response to penicillins remains the single most important method of preventing hypersensitivity reactions.

ERYTHROMYCIN.   The clinical efficacy of erythromycin is restricted to infections caused by gram-positive organisms, spirochetes, *Mycoplasma pneumoniae, Neisseria meningitidis, B. pertussis* and some rickettsia. Most *S. aureus* currently isolated are sensitive to erythromycin, but resistance may develop rapidly during therapy. The drug diffuses well throughout most body fluids. Differences exist in the absorption and blood levels attained by the numerous erythromycin formulations currently available for oral administration, but no one preparation has established clinical superiority. Among the oral preparations, erythromycin estolate yields the highest blood levels, but its use may be associated with cholestatic hepatitis, especially when administered for a prolonged period of time. Gastrointestinal upset is common, and rash is a rare occurrence. Parenteral preparations are available but are seldom used because large volumes must be administered to obtain adequate dosage by the intramuscular route and phlebitis frequently complicates intravenous use. Erythromycin is used most commonly for *Mycoplasma* infections and as an alternative drug in patients allergic to penicillin.

LINCOMYCIN AND CLINDAMYCIN.   Lincomycin and clindamycin are similar to erythromycin in absorption, distribution, and spectrum, except that they are not as active against *Neisseria* or *Mycoplasma.* Clindamycin is also active against anaerobic bacteria, including *Bacteroides,* anaerobic streptococci, and some clostridia, and it has emerged as a first-line drug for severe infections caused by these bacteria. These antibiotics do not penetrate into the cerebrospinal fluid, and thus they cannot be used for central nervous system infections. Some studies suggest, but do not prove, special effectiveness in the therapy of chronic osteomyelitis. Diarrhea and gastrointestinal upset are common. Clindamycin has been associated with severe colitis, including rare fatalities. While this complication has been observed most commonly in adults, the use of clindamycin should be restricted, at present, only to life-threatening infections caused by anaerobic bacteria. Uncommon complications include cholestatic jaundice, neutropenia, rash, and cardiac arrhythmias with rapid intravenous infusion.

VANCOMYCIN.   Vancomycin is bactericidal for virtually all clinical isolates of gram-positive bacteria. It is not absorbed from the gastrointestinal tract, and its administration by the intramuscular route is too painful; therefore it is only given intravenously. Its use is further limited by other side effects, which include ototoxicity, nephrotoxicity, rashes, fever, and phlebitis. Because of its antibacterial effectiveness, Vancomycin is often recommended for severe infections caused by enterococci in patients allergic to penicillin. It is the most potent antibiotic active against methicillin-resistant *S. aureus.* Oral administration is often recommended for staphylococcal enterocolitis.

BACITRACIN.   Bacitracin is a polypeptide antibiotic effective against almost all gram-positive bacteria. Significant nephrotoxicity and hypersensitivity reactions have caused bacitracin to be largely supplanted by less toxic drugs in the systemic treatment of infections. Bacitracin is poorly absorbed when used topically or administered orally. Therefore it is used primarily in the topical treatment of localized infections, particularly those caused by *S. aureus.*

Intermediate-Spectrum Agents

CEPHALOSPORINS. Cephalosporins are similar to penicillin in chemical structure and mechanism of action. They are effective against most gram-positive cocci, including β-lactamase-producing *S. aureus,* but they are less active against enterococci. In addition, the cephalosporins are bactericidal for most strains of *Klebsiella, P. mirabilis, E. coli, Salmonella,* and *Shigella* at concentrations that can be achieved in vivo. However, the concentration of drug required to kill gram-negative bacilli is usually significantly higher than that required to kill gram-positive organisms.

Adverse reactions are similar to those manifested to penicillin. Although most patients with penicillin allergy tolerate cephalosporins well, a small but definite risk of cross-sensitivity exists. Patients receiving cephalosporins commonly develop a positive Coombs test, but hemolytic anemia is rare. *Cephalothin,* which must be administered parenterally, is irritating, and phlebitis is common with its intravenous use. *Cephaloridine,* an intramuscular preparation, is well tolerated, but is associated with renal toxicity in high doses. *Cefazolin,* a newer preparation available for both intravenous and intramuscular use, produces higher peak serum levels than other cephalosporins; it is more potent against *E. coli* and is reported to cause less phlebitis and little nephrotoxicity. Oral preparations include *cephaloglycin,* which is approved only for urinary tract infections because poor blood concentrations are achieved, and *cephalexin,* an alternative to penicillins in the treatment of soft tissue infections due to gram-positive cocci and an agent that is active against certain urinary tract infections.

The cephalosporins are used primarily to treat patients with infections caused by penicillin-resistant *S. aureus* or sensitive enteric bacilli. Since many gram-negative bacteria are resistant to these drugs, they cannot be expected to give broad-spectrum coverage in gram-negative sepsis caused by an unknown organism. Although potent in vitro, they are rarely effective against *Salmonella* and *Shigella* infections. These drugs have not been effective in treating bacterial meningitis, presumably because of the high degree of protein binding and poor cerebrospinal fluid penetration.

SULFONAMIDES. Although sulfonamides show in vitro effectiveness against a wide variety of organisms, including the common gram-positive cocci, many enteric bacilli, *H. influenzae, Nocardia,* and some *Chlamydia,* their clinical effectiveness is much more limited. Current major uses include treatment of urinary tract infections caused by *E. coli* and (in combination with penicillin) treatment of otitis media. The prophylactic ingestion of sulfonamides prevents group A streptococcal infections, and they can be used for this purpose in patients with a history of rheumatic fever. Sulfonamides do not prevent postinfectious complications of established group A streptococcal infection, and therefore they should not be used to treat such infections. Sulfonamides that are poorly absorbed from the gastrointestinal tract have been used primarily in patients undergoing bowel surgery or in patients with ulcerative colitis. Although sulfonamides usually eradicate sensitive meningococci from the nasopharynx and have therefore been used for prophylaxis, a high percentage of strains causing disease in this and other countries in the 1970s are highly resistant to sulfonamides. Because certain products of tissue necrosis interfere with the action of sulfonamides, these drugs should be used primarily in infections with minimal suppuration.

The use of sulfonamides has been associated with a wide variety of adverse drug reactions. Of these, mild hypersensitivity reactions (rash, fever) are the most common, although hepatitis, vasculitis, bone marrow depression, and Stevens-Johnson syndrome may occur. Sulfonamides are among the drugs that may produce hemolytic anemia in patients with G6PD deficiency. Nephrotoxicity is now rare, owing to the use of more soluble sulfonamides (eg, sulfisoxazole, trisulfapyrimidines). Since sulfonamides compete with bilirubin for albumin binding sites, their use should be avoided in neonates in order to avoid the risk of kernicterus.

STREPTOMYCIN. Streptomycin has variable effectiveness against the common enteric bacilli and *H. influenzae.* Even when used against a bacterium that is sensitive to the drug by in vitro tests, streptomycin should not be used alone because of the rapid development of high-level resistance during therapy. Anaerobic gram-negative bacilli (the most numerous organisms in the bowel flora) and clostridia are resistant to streptomycin and other aminoglycoside antibiotics (kanamycin, gentamicin), and therefore the common use of these drugs to treat anaerobic infections following peritoneal soilage is questionable. In vitro synergism with penicillin against sensitive enterococci has been demonstrated, and endocarditis caused by such bacteria should be treated with this combination of antibiotics. Because the activity of streptomycin is greatly increased at alkaline pH, urine should be alkalinized for maximum effect in urinary tract infections. Streptomycin remains an effective first-line drug in the treatment of tuberculosis, but it should always be used with another antituberculous agent. It is used with tetracyclines to treat brucellosis and plague.

KANAMYCIN. Kanamycin is effective against most Enterobacteriaceae. *Pseudomonas* and *Bacteroides* are generally resistant. Kanamycin was introduced as an antistaphylococcal drug and remains an effective second-line drug against most strains of *S. aureus.* It also is active against *Mycobacterium tuberculosis.* As with all the aminoglycoside antibiotics, it is poorly absorbed from the gastrointestinal tract and thus is administered by either the intramuscular or the intravenous route. Kanamycin is most commonly used to treat sepsis of unknown etiology and infections caused by susceptible gram-negative bacilli, particularly in infants and young children. The incidence of resistant Enterobacteriaceae has become a problem in certain nurseries.

Minor hypersensitivity reactions (rash, eosinophilia, fever) may occur at any dose. However, serious adverse reactions (renal failure and irreversible deafness) are dose-related and are usually avoidable if the daily dosage is limited to 15 mg/kg body weight and the duration of therapy does not exceed 10 to 14 days in patients with normal renal function. These reactions are rare in young children. Renal function and auditory acuity (especially high-frequency) should be monitored closely in patients receiving prolonged courses. Rarely, neuromuscular block with respiratory paralysis has been reported when kanamycin has been administered to patients by the intraperitoneal or the intravenous route. Neostigmine and calcium gluconate have been reported to reverse this complication. In situations in which toxic levels of kanamycin are present, prompt reduction of blood levels can be achieved by either peritoneal dialysis or hemodialysis.

NEOMYCIN AND PAROMOMYCIN. Neomycin and paromomycin are similar to kanamycin in structure, action, and antibacterial spectrum, but they are rarely used parenterally due to a high incidence of nephrotoxicity and ototoxicity. They are poorly absorbed from the gastrointestinal tract; therefore their primary use has been in oral treatment of gastrointestinal pathogens (eg, infant diarrhea due to sensitive enteropathogenic *E. coli*) and in suppression of bowel flora. Malabsorption and intercurrent staphylococcal enterocolitis may complicate the oral use of these drugs. Absorption through wounds irrigated with neomycin may result in toxic blood levels, particularly in patients with renal failure.

NITROFURANTOIN. Nitrofurantoin, an oral agent, inhibits most common gram-positive and gram-negative pathogens (except *Pseudomonas*). The prompt renal excretion of nitrofurantoin produces adequate urine levels but negligible blood levels. Therefore its use is limited to treating urinary tract infections, where it is used most commonly for suppression of infection rather than for therapy of acute disease. Gastrointestinal upset and abdominal cramping are common side effects. Nitrofurantoin macrocrystals may produce greater tissue levels of drug and cause less gastrointestinal upset. Other adverse reactions include rashes, peripheral neuropathy, allergic pneumonitis, and hemolytic anemia in patients who are G6PD-deficient. Nitrofurantoin should not be administered to the newborn because it competes with bilirubin for binding to albumin. *Nitrofurazone*, another furan derivative, is widely used as a topical antibacterial agent, especially in burn patients.

POLYMYXINS B AND E. Polymyxin B and polymyxin E (colistimethate sodium) are essentially interchangeable when dosage is adjusted. They are effective against virtually all *Pseudomonas* and common Enterobacteriaceae (except *Proteus* and *Serratia*). *Bacteroides* species and the gram-positive bacteria are resistant. The polymyxins are poorly absorbed from the gastrointestinal tract; they penetrate tissues poorly and do not enter the cerebrospinal fluid. These drugs are used primarily to treat known *Pseudomonas* infections and gram-negative sepsis when *Pseudomonas* is suspected. Results of therapy of soft tissue infections outside the urinary tract have been variable. Oral preparations have been used successfully to treat gastroenteritis caused by enteropathic *E. coli*. Both polymyxin B and colistimethate sodium are excreted in the urine and are nephrotoxic. Patients treated systemically should be monitored closely for abnormalities of urine sediment or renal function while receiving these agents. Minor neurologic complaints (circumoral paresthesias, mild ataxia) are common. Rarely, high blood levels of these drugs may result in neuromuscular block with weakness and respiratory insufficiency.

GENTAMICIN. The aminoglycoside antibiotic gentamicin is active against *S. aureus* and most common aerobic gram-negative bacilli, including *Pseudomonas*. It is not effective against anaerobic organisms and certain enterococci. Like other aminoglycoside drugs, gentamicin is poorly absorbed from the intestinal tract and thus is administered systemically. Gentamicin has become the antibiotic most commonly employed in the therapy of gram-negative sepsis of unknown etiology and severe infections due to *Pseudomonas, Serratia,* and kanamycin-resistant enteric bacilli. Where the drug has been used extensively the occurrence of gentamicin-resistant enteric bacilli has been reported.

Adverse drug reactions are similar to those with other aminoglycosides. Ototoxicity (vestibular greater than cochlear) and nephrotoxicity are probably dose-related and require that auditory and renal function be monitored during therapy. Serum levels vary with age due to differences in the volume of distribution. The dose should be adjusted accordingly: newborn to 5 years - 2.5 mg/kg; 5 to 10 years - 2.0 mg/kg; older than 10 years - 1.5 mg/kg. Gentamicin is given on a q8h schedule after the first week of life, when it is given q12h (see Newborn Infants). Serum levels following standard doses are highly individualized, and they should be assayed in critical situations. An early theory that gentamicin competes with bilirubin for albumin binding and therefore should not be used in newborn infants has been disproved.

TOBRAMYCIN. The aminoglycoside tobramycin has virtually the same pharmacokinetics and antibacterial spectrum as gentamicin, but it is more active in vitro against *P. aeruginosa* and less active against *S. marcescens* and *Providencia* species. Some, but not all, gentamicin-resistant strains of *Pseudomonas* are susceptible to tobramycin. As with other aminoglycosides, tobramycin has little or no activity against anaerobic organisms. Initial clinical studies suggest that tobramycin is as effective as, and no more toxic than, other aminoglycosides. Overuse of this drug will promote the emergence of R-factor-mediated resistance. Therefore tobramycin should be reserved for the treatment of *Pseudomonas* infections or other infections in which the organism is resistant to other aminoglycosides. The important adverse reactions appear to be similar in frequency and magnitude to those of gentamicin. Curarelike neuromuscular block following high doses has been observed in animals.

As with gentamicin and kanamycin, serum levels of tobramycin should be monitored when possible, since individual variation in dose response is common and the margin between therapeutic levels (4 to 8 µg/ml) and toxic levels is small. If excessive serum concentrations occur in patients unable to excrete the drug due to renal failure, dialysis should be considered (hemodialysis is more effective than peritoneal dialysis). Monitoring of renal, auditory, and vestibular functions is advisable, especially in patients receiving more than 10 days of therapy or with preexisting renal disease. Minor hypersensitivity reactions (eosinophilia, rash, or fever) may occur.

NALIDIXIC ACID. Nalidixic acid is an oral agent that is bactericidal for most commonly isolated aerobic gram-negative bacilli, but not *Pseudomonas.* It is not effective against gram-positive organisms. It is absorbed well from the gastrointestinal tract, but serum and tissue levels of the drug are variable. Since it is concentrated in the urine, it is used only to treat urinary tract infections. Bacteria with high levels of resistance to nalidixic acid are often isolated during therapy. Common adverse reactions from nalidixic acid include gastrointestinal upset and allergic responses (rash, fever, eosinophilia). Occasionally, neurologic complaints including headache, dizziness, psychosis, and convulsions have been reported. These problems have limited its use in pediatric practice.

Broad-Spectrum Agents

TRIMETHOPRIM-SULFAMETHOXAZOLE.
This fixed drug combination (80 mg of trimethoprim, 400 mg of sulfamethoxazole) has antibacterial synergy in vitro against virtually all the common enteric bacilli (except *Pseudomonas*), *S. aureus, H. influenzae, Neisseria gonorrhoeae, Brucella, Nocardia,* and some isolates of enterococcus. Recent clinical studies have demonstrated efficacy against *Pneumocystis carinii.* An expanding literature from Western Europe suggests that this drug combination is effective in a variety of infections, including urinary tract infections, certain cases of typhoid fever, gonorrhea, and respiratory tract infections caused by pneumococci and *H. influenzae.* This combination has no role in the treatment of infections caused by sulfonamide-resistant bacteria. Furthermore, toxicity and cost do not recommend it as a penicillin substitute. Thus the role of this agent in pediatric practice remains to be defined. At this time it is approved for use in the United States only for chronic urinary tract infections in children older than 12 years and *Pneumocystis carinii* pneumonia.

Adverse reactions are similar to those listed for sulfonamides. The incidence of rashes has been reported to be as high as 5 percent. Hematologic side effects might be expected because of their association with sulfonamides and the antifolate activity of trimethoprim. Leukopenia, thrombocytopenia, agranulocytosis, and aplastic anemia have been reported, but their incidence is unknown. Folate-deficient anemia is not uncommon, and it may be severe, especially in patients with marginal or depleted folate stores.

METHENAMINE. Methenamine has little native antibacterial activity, but at a pH of less than 5.5 it hydrolyzes to produce formaldehyde and mandelic acid. Therefore its use is limited to the treatment of chronic urinary tract infections, in which it acts as a surface antiseptic agent. In patients receiving methenamine the urinary pH must be monitored with indicator paper, and acidifying agents such as ascorbic acid, methionine, ammonium chloride, or acid ash diet may be required to maintain acidity. If the urine is not sufficiently acidified or if the infection is due to a urea-splitting organism such as *Proteus,* the drug is usually ineffective. Patients cannot be treated simultaneously with methenamine and sulfonamides because they react chemically and form a precipitate in the urine. Adverse drug reactions are uncommon, but they may consist of mild gastrointestinal upset, hematuria, and rarely ataxia. Metabolic acidosis from the acidifying agents may occur in patients with impaired renal function.

CHLORAMPHENICOL. Chloramphenicol affects most common gram-negative bacilli, including *H. influenzae* and anaerobic bacilli (but not *Pseudomonas*), and most gram-positive organisms, including *S. aureus.* It is also effective against many *Rickettsia,* the *Chlamydia,* and *Treponema pallidum.* Chloramphenicol is well absorbed from the gastrointestinal tract and diffuses well into tissues and the cerebrospinal fluid. It can be administered orally or intravenously.

Restriction of the use of chloramphenicol has been urged because of the rare but potentially fatal occurrence of aplastic anemia (estimated at 1 in 30,000). This idiosyncratic reaction is not dose-related. Therefore, as alternative antibiotics have been developed, the indications for chloramphenicol have diminished. However, it remains the drug of choice in severe *Salmonella* disease and in certain rickettsial diseases. Because of its ready diffusion into the brain and its effectiveness against anaerobic bacteria, chloramphenicol is recommended by most physicians for treatment of brain abscesses. Other indications for chloramphenicol include initial treatment of bacterial meningitis in areas in which ampicillin-resistant *H. influenzae* is common (recent recommendations are discussed under ampicillin), treatment of meningitis in patients allergic to penicillin, and treatment of infections caused by anaerobic organisms. Other adverse reactions associated with chloramphenicol are dose-related and reversible. They include interference with iron metabolism, as manifested by increased serum iron and decreased iron binding capacity, vacuolization of erythrocyte precursors in bone marrow, decreased circulating reticulocyte count, anemia, and leukopenia.

Chloramphenicol is conjugated in the liver with glucuronide and subsequently excreted in the urine. Because the glucuronide transferase system is not fully developed in premature infants, the administration of chloramphenicol may produce excessive blood concentrations, resulting in the "gray baby" syndrome. This shocklike syndrome may result in death unless the condition is recognized and the drug discontinued. Other rare reactions include optic neuritis and peripheral neuritis.

TETRACYCLINES. The antibacterial spectrum of the tetracyclines is broad but variable. They are moderately effective against the common gram-negative rods, except *Proteus* and *Pseudomonas.* Recently their effectiveness against anaerobic organisms (*Bacteriodes, Clostridium*) has not been uniform. Resistance is common among staphylococcal and streptococcal isolates. Tetracyclines are used to treat *M. pneumoniae, Rickettsia,* and *Chlamydia* infections and *H. influenzae* infections of the respiratory tract in older children. In addition, they are used in the treatment of acne, brucellosis, plague, leptospirosis and cholera and as an alternative to penicillin in gonorrhea and syphilis. They may be preferred for the treatment of certain urinary tract infections. *Doxycycline* is the tetracycline of choice in patients with renal failure, since dosage adjustment is not necessary. *Minocycline,* although effective in the treatment of meningococcal carriers, is no longer recommended because of the unacceptable incidence of vestibular toxicity.

Adverse reactions of a wide variety have been associated with the tetracyclines, including gastrointestinal reactions, superinfection, dermatologic reactions, and pseudotumor cerebri. Permanent binding of tetracycline to calcium may produce a dose-related brownish discoloration of the teeth when the drug is administered during the period of dental calcification (from the fifth month of gestation to approximately 8 years of age).

Although their pharmacologic properties may differ, the numerous preparations of tetracyclines have approximately the same clinical efficacy, except as noted. The increasing prevalence of resistant strains of common pathogenic bacteria, the introduction of alternative antibiotics, and an increased awareness of the toxic side effects have led to less frequent use of the tetracyclines in pediatric infections.

Intravenous Administration

The intravenous route is commonly used to administer antibiotics to hospitalized patients: it is mandatory for treating patients in shock and is preferred when high blood levels are important (eg, in meningitis, endocarditis, osteomyelitis) or when altered hemostasis precludes intramuscular injections. Factors to be considered when drugs are administered intravenously include the following:

Stability in Solution. The stability of the drug in solution may be influenced by the pH, the concentration of drug, and the type of intravenous solution. Aminoglycosides, chloramphenicol, lincomycin, cephalothin, penicillin G, carbenicillin, and nafcillin are stable for 24 hours at room temperature in 5 percent dextrose and 0.9 percent NaCl. Ampicillin, oxacillin, methicillin, and erythromycin lactobionate are stable for periods of 4 to 8 hours, but bottles should not be kept at room temperature for prolonged intervals.

Incompatibilities. The list of incompatibilities of drugs in intravenous solutions has expanded dramatically during the last few years and includes virtually all antimicrobial drugs (see *Medical Letter on Drugs and Therapeutics,* January 1974). In general, it is preferable to mix each antibiotic in a separate bottle and administer it at the appropriate interval by a piggyback arrangement.

Continuous Versus Intermittent Doses. Although laboratory studies indicate that bacterial killing by intermittent administration of antibiotics is superior to that by continuous therapy, there is no convincing clinical evidence to show that one method is preferable. When using drugs that are unstable or when high peak levels are desirable because of infection in poorly accessible tissue, intermittent therapy (at intervals appropriate to the excretion pattern of the drug) is preferable to continuous therapy.

Intravenous Devices. Infections associated with intravenous catheters are a significant cause of hospital-acquired infection and mortality. Rates of infection with needles (especially scalp vein needles) are lower than with plastic catheters. Reduction of intravenous catheter infection has been dramatic when the following steps have been observed: Carefully prepare the skin with iodine solutions followed by alcohol rinses. The iodine wash must dry to produce maximum antibacterial effects. Inspect the catheter site at least twice daily and remove it if phlebitis or intravenous malfunction is present. Remove all catheters within 72 hours of insertion unless there are compelling reasons for continued use of the same intravenous site. The use of an antibacterial ointment at the site of entry may reduce the rate of infection in cutdowns.

Microorganisms and Particular Infections

The choice of antibiotics in the initial therapy of severe infections and the choice of bacteriologic media and culturing techniques presupposes some knowledge of the bacterial pathogens most likely to cause certain types of infections. The causative pathogen of some infections, such as erysipelas caused by group A streptococci, can be predicted with a high degree of accuracy on the basis of the clinical presentation. In other infections such as wounds or pneumonia the etiologic agent is more difficult to predict on clinical grounds, and the initial choice of therapy becomes a statistical guess based on the data available (gram-stained smear and clinical features) and knowledge of the common offending pathogens together with their antibiotic sensitivity patterns. A list of common infections and the most frequently associated pathogens is presented in Table 1.

Choice of Agents

Once a bacterial pathogen is known or suspected, the choice of antibiotic is dependent on those factors discussed earlier. These factors include the antibiotic sensitivities of the pathogen, the pharmacologic and toxic properties of the drug, the presence of altered hepatic or renal function, a history of allergy, and the location of the infection. It is important to tabulate at regular intervals the antibiotic sensitivity patterns of common bacterial pathogens (particularly gram-negative bacilli and *S. aureus*) isolated in each hospital, since these patterns may vary widely from hospital to hospital or at different times within the same institution. Suggestions regarding the choice of antibacterial agents usually effective against particular pathogens are offered in Table 2.

PROPHYLACTIC USE OF AGENTS

The early success of antibacterial drugs in therapy of bacterial infections led to the optimistic hope that their prophylactic administration to patients at high risk of developing infections because of increased exposure or increased host susceptibility would prevent bacterial disease. Unfortunately, attempts at prophylaxis against a broad spectrum of bacteria for prolonged periods generally have not been successful; they carry the risk

of adverse drug reactions and superinfection. In general, prophylaxis is most likely to be successful when a specific drug is directed against a specific organism.

Certain situations in which prophylactic administration of antimicrobial agents appears to be useful are listed in Table 3. Other situations in which the efficacy of prophylactic antimicrobial agents is less clear have been omitted from Table 3. These include premature rupture of membranes, prolonged labor, exchange transfusion, open heart surgery, prolonged neurosurgical or orthopedic operations, and preoperative bowel flora preparation. While antimicrobial agents are commonly used in these situations, controlled studies are few, and a wide range of opinion exists regarding their efficacy.

TABLE 2. Choice of Antimicrobial Agents*

Organism	Drug	Infection	Dose (per kg per day)
Gram-positive cocci			
1. *Diplococcus pneumoniae*	Penicillin G (alt. erythromycin, cephalosporins)	Pneumonia	25,000 IU
		Soft tissue (empyema)	100,000 IU
		Meningitis	250,000 IU
2. *Staphylococcus aureus* (penicillin-sensitive)	Penicillin G	Abscess	25,000 IU
		Pneumonia	100,000 IU
		Severe infection	250,000 IU
3. *Staphylococcus aureus* (penicillin-resistant)	β-lactamase-resistant penicillin (alt. cephalosporins, erythromycin, Vancomycin)	Mild infection	25–50 mg (dicloxacillin)
		Severe infection	300 mg (methicillin) 200–300 mg (oxacillin)
4. *Staphylococcus albus*	Penicillin G (alt. chloramphenicol)	Meningitis, severe infection	250,000 IU
5. *Streptococcus pyogenes* group A†	Penicillin G (alt. see 1)	Pharyngitis	25,000 IU
		Cellulitis, pneumonia	25,000–50,000 IU
		Empyema, bacteremia	100,000 IU
6. *Streptococcus pyogenes* group B	Penicillin G	Meningitis, septicemia	100,000 IU
7. *Streptococcus pyogenes* group D	Penicillin G plus Gentamicin Ampicillin	Subacute Endocarditis (treat 4–6 weeks) Urinary tract infection	250,000 IU 5 mg 50–100 mg
8. *Streptococcus viridans*	Penicillin G (alt. see 1) plus streptomycin	Subacute endocarditis (treat 4 weeks, use streptomycin for 2 weeks)	250,000 IU 20 mg
Gram-positive bacilli			
1. *Clostridium perfringens*	Penicillin G (alt. chloramphenicol)	Gas gangrene‡	250,000 IU
2. *Clostridium tetani*	Penicillin G (alt. tetracycline, erythromycin	Tetanus§	250,000 IU
3. *Corynebacterium diphtheria*	Penicillin G (alt. erythromycin)	Diphtheria‖	25,000 IU
4. *Listeria monocytogenes*	Ampicillin (alt. tetracycline, chloramphenicol)	Meningitis	150–300 mg
Gram-negative cocci			
1. *Neisseria gonorrhoeae*	Penicillin G	Gonorrhea	4.8 million IU (total dose) males or females
	Spectinomycin		30 mg/kg males, 60 mg/kg females
	Tetracycline Ampicillin (plus probenecid)		30 mg/kg for 5 days 40 mg/kg after probenecid 15 mg/kg
	Penicillin G	Systemic infection	100,000 IU
2. *Neisseria meningitidis*	Penicillin G (alt. ampicillin chloramphenicol, erythromycin)	Meningitis, septicemia	250,000 IU

TABLE 2. Choice of Antimicrobial Agents* (cont.)

Organism	Drug	Infection	Dose (per kg per day)
Gram-negative bacilli			
1. Anaerobic enteric bacilli (*Bacteroides* etc)	(a) Penicillin (b) Clindamycin (alt. chloramphenicol, tetracycline)	Abscess	(a) 100,000 IU (b) 20–40 mg
2. *Bordetella pertussis*	Erythromycin	Pertussis	40 mg
3. *Brucella* species	Tetracycline plus Streptomycin (alt. chloramphenicol)	Brucellosis	30 mg 20–40 mg
4. *Enterobacter-Serratia*	Gentamicin (alt. kanamycin, chloramphenicol, tetracycline, colistin)	Systemic infection	5–7.5 mg
5. *Escherichia coli*	(a) Sulfisoxazole (alt. trisulfaprymidines) (b) Ampicillin	Urinary tract infection	(a) 50–150 mg (b) 50–100 mg
	(a) Ampicillin (b) Cephalothin (c) Kanamycin (d) Gentamicin (e) Chloramphenicol	Systemic infection	(a) 200–300 mg (b) up to 250 mg (c) 15 mg (d) 5–7.5 mg (e) 100 mg
	(a) Neomycin (b) Colistin sulfate	Gastroenteritis	(a) 50–100 mg (b) 15–20 mg
6. *Francisella tularensis*	Streptomycin	Tularemia	20–40 mg
7. HB organisms	Chloramphenicol (alt. tetracycline, ampicillin)	Abscess	100 mg
8. *Haemophilus influenzae*	(a) Chloramphenicol (b) Ampicillin	Meningitis, systemic infection	(a) 100 mg (b) 150–300 mg
	(a) Ampicillin (b) Penicillin G plus (c) Sulfisoxazole	Otitis	(a) 50–100 mg (b) 25,000 IU penicillin, (c) 100 mg
9. *Klebsiella* species	(a) Kanamycin (alt. gentamicin, colistin) (b) Cephalothin	Systemic infection	(a) 15 mg (b) 250 mg
10. *Mima-Moraxella-Herellea*	Gentamicin (alt. chloramphenicol, tetracyclines)	Systemic infection	5–7.5 mg
11. *Proteus mirabilis*	Ampicillin (alt. cephalothin, kanamycin, chloramphenicol)	Urinary tract infection	50–100 mg
12. *Proteus* (indole-positive) species	Kanamycin (alt. gentamicin, tetracycline, chloramphenicol, carbenicillin)	Urinary tract infection	15 mg
13. *Pseudomonas aeruginosa*	Gentamicin plus Carbenicillin (alt. polymyxin B, colistin)	Systemic infection	15 mg 400 mg
14. *Salmonella* species	Chloramphenicol (alt. ampicillin, trimethoprim-sulfamethoxazole)	Systemic infection	100 mg
15. *Shigella* species	Ampicillin (alt. tetracycline, sulfonamide)	Enterocolitis	50–100 mg
16. *Vibrio cholera*	Tetracycline	Cholera	30 mg
17. *Yersinia pestis*	Tetracycline plus Streptomycin	Plague	30 mg 15–30 mg
Spirochetes			
1. *Leptospira* species	Penicillin G	Meningitis, septicemia	100–150,000 IU
2. *Treponema pallidum*	Penicillin G	Congenital syphilis	50,000 IU
	(a) Penicillin G (b) Benzathine penicillin (alt. tetracycline)	Venereal disease	(a) 100,000 IU (for 10 days) (b) 24 million IU (given once)
	Penicillin G	Neurosyphilis	100,000 IU (for 21 days)

* Intended as rough guidelines only.
† Always treat for 10 days to prevent postinfectious sequelae.
‡ Efficacy of antitoxin (horse) is debatable.
§ Also use human antitoxin 250 IU.
∥ Also use horse antitoxin, 20,000–80,000 IU.
Adapted from Med Lett Drugs Ther, Handbook of Antimicrobial Therapy, revised edition 1974 p. 16

TABLE 3. Some Situations in Which Prophylactic Antimicrobial Drugs May Be Useful

Infection	Drug	Dose
1. Group A streptococcal infections in patients with rheumatic heart disease	Penicillin (alt. sulfonamide, erythromycin)	(a) 200,000 IU penicillin G bid, po (b) 600,000–900,000 IU benzathine penicillin G im q 3–4 weeks
2. Meningococcal infection	Rifampin (alt. sulfonamide	10–20 mg/kg/day
3. Syphilis exposure (adolescent)	Penicillin if bacteria are sensitive)	2.4 million IU procaine benzathine penicillin G im (test VDRL q 3 months for 1 year)
4. Gonorrhea exposure (adolescent)	Penicillin (alt. spectinomycin, ampicillin tetracycline)	4.8 million IU procaine penicillin im (test VDRL q 3 months for 1 year)
5. Gonococcal ophthalmia	Silver nitrate	1 drop 1% solution each eye
6. Prevention of bacterial endocarditis following manipulative procedures in patients with rheumatic heart disease		
(a) *Streptococcus viridans*	(a) Penicillin	(a) 25,000 IU/kg aqueous and 25,000 IU/kg of procaine penicillin 1 hour before; 25,000 IU/kg procaine penicillin daily x 2 after dental extraction
(b) Enterococcus	(b) Penicillin and streptomycin	(b) Same as above plus streptomycin 15 mg/kg 1 hour before and bid for 2 days after urinary tract manipulation or abdominal surgery
7. Tuberculosis (any child with positive PPD reaction)	Isoniazid	10 mg/kg each day for at least 12 months
8. Diphtheria (exposed susceptible)	Penicillin G Diphtheria toxoid	600,000–2,000,000 IU for 7–10 days 0.5 ml im
9. Pertussis (exposed susceptible)	Erythromycin	30–50 mg/kg/day x 10 days
10. Enteropathic *E. coli* in newborn infants	Neomycin	50–100 mg/kg/day po
11. Grossly contaminated injury, including bites	Penicillin Tetanus toxoid Soap and water Antibacterial ointment	50,000 IU/kg/day 0.5 ml im (when indicated) Plenty Topical ointment to entry site
12. Intravenous polyethylene catheter (cut down) (avoid when possible)		

SPECIAL SITUATIONS

IMPAIRED KIDNEY FUNCTION. Since most antimicrobial agents or their metabolites are excreted by the kidneys, modification of dosage is frequently necessary in patients with impaired kidney function. Information on which to base recommendations is incomplete, and the modifications suggested in Table 4 are intended as general guidelines only. Drugs that are nephrotoxic and are excreted by the kidneys may result in a cycle of deteriorating kidney function and increasing blood levels of drug if close supervision is not maintained. All patients receiving nephrotoxic drugs should be monitored at frequent intervals for abnormalities of urine sediment and alteration of kidney function. Serum concentrations of antibiotics should be measured when assay systems are available. Until firmer guidelines can be established, it seems wise to avoid toxic drugs excreted by the kidneys when alternative choices exist, use nephrotoxic drugs for as short a period as is consistent with good therapy, and use short-acting preparations when a choice exists.

IMPAIRED LIVER FUNCTIONS. The liver and bile collecting systems can affect antimicrobial agents in a variety of ways. Drugs may be concentrated in the gallbladder where levels may be several hundred times the serum concentration. Drugs may be modified or conjugated in the liver, which often results in changes in physical properties such as solubility or biologic properties such as antimicrobial action or toxicity. Many drugs excreted by the liver are reabsorbed in the small bowel (enterohepatic circulation) and subsequently excreted in the urine. The liver serves as the primary route of excretion or degradation for a small

TABLE 4. Modification of Antibiotic Dosage in Renal Disease*

Antibiotic	Major Excretory Route	Dosage Modification
I. Little or no change		None
Cloxacillin, dicloxacillin[‡]	Kidney (liver)	
Chloramphenicol[†]	Liver	
Doxycycline[#]	Liver	
Erythromycin[†]	Liver	
Oxacillin,[†] nafcillin[†]	Kidney (liver)	
Penicillin[†] (low dose)	Kidney	
II. Minor alteration		In anuric patient give full dose on first day followed by half dose thereafter
Amphotericin B	Liver and kidney	
Ampicillin[§]	Kidney (liver)	
Carbenicillin[‡§]	Kidney (liver)	
Cephalothin,[†§] cephalexin[§]	Kidney and liver	
Lincomycin,[†] clindamycin	Liver and kidney	
Methicillin[†]	Kidney (liver)	
Penicillin G[†] (high dose)	Kidney	
III. Moderate alteration		1. Severe azotemia: ½ dose q day
Tetracycline[†#]	Kidney	2. Anuria: ½ dose q 3 days
Chlortetracycline[†#]	Liver	
IV. Major alteration		1. Normal or slightly reduced dose if CrCl > 30 ml/min and BUN < 50
Cephaloridine[‡§]	Kidney	
Colistin[†]	Kidney	2. Half dose q day if CrCl 10–30 ml/min and BUN > 50
Gentamicin[‡§∥]	Kidney	
Tobramycin[∥]	Kindey	3. Half dose q 2–3 days if CrCl < 10 ml/min or BUN > 80
5-fluorocytosine[∥]	Kidney	
Kanamycin[‡∥]	Kidney	
Polymyxin B[†]	Kidney	
Steptomycin[‡∥]	Kidney	
Vancomycin[†]	Kidney	

V. Renal insufficiency is a relative contraindication to the use of the following drugs:
(1) nitrofurantoin drugs, (2) naladixic acid, (3) absorbable sulfonamides (including trimethoprim-sulfamethoxazole), (4) methenamine mandelate, and (5) tetracyclines other than doxycycline

* With some general rules of thumb based on fragmentary evidence.
† Not appreciably removed by dialysis.
‡ Significant removal by peritoneal dialysis.
§ Significant removal by hemodialysis: 15–25% AV difference.
∥ Significant removal by hemodialysis: 25% AV difference.
Doxycycline is the tetracycline preparation of choice in renal failure.

but important group of drugs (Table 4). Studies of antibiotic toxicity have generally been conducted in animals and healthy humans, and it is therefore difficult to offer concrete guidelines for dosage regimes in humans with impaired liver function. Only minor amounts of cephalosporins and semisynthetic penicillins are excreted in the liver; therefore alteration of dosage is necessary only in severe liver diseases. Erythromycin and lincomycin are relatively nontoxic at high levels, but since they are excreted primarily in bile, modification of dosage is advisable in patients with liver failure. Erythromycin estolate has been associated with cholestatic hepatitis and probably should be avoided in this setting. Chloramphenicol dosage should be reduced in patients with liver disease, since the reversible bone marrow toxicity appears to be related to the serum levels of free (unconjugated) drug. Because of the small but definite hepatic toxicity of sulfonamides, these drugs are best avoided in liver disease. All the tetracycline preparations are concentrated in the liver and bile, although there is marked variation with regard to subsequent excretion in feces and urine. Chlortetracycline and doxycycline are the most dependent on hepatic excretion and should be avoided in liver disease. Other tetracyclines are excreted primarily in the urine, but since severe dose-related hepatic toxicity may occur, tetracyclines should be used with caution and at low doses in patients with liver disease.

PREMATURE OR NEWBORN INFANTS. In choosing antimicrobial agents for premature or newborn infants it is important to recognize that liver function and kidney function are not fully developed in the neonate. Failure of infants to conjugate chloramphenicol with glucuronides may lead to accumulation of toxic serum levels and result in peripheral vascular collapse ("gray baby" syndrome). Sulfonamides compete with bilirubin for albumin binding sites and thereby increase the risk of kernicterus. Immaturity of renal tubular function in newborns prolongs the half-life of the penicillins and cephalosporins. Therefore the dosage and frequency of administration should be reduced during the first weeks of life. High doses of penicillin in the newborn may result in central nervous system irritation, with mycoclonic jerks and convulsions.

Excretion of aminoglycosides (eg, gentamicin) is prolonged during the first week of life, regardless of gestational age. Doses of gentamicin, for example, should therefore be given at 12 hour rather than 8 hour intervals during the first week.Young children, in general, appear to be relatively spared from the ototoxic and nephrotoxic effects of the aminoglycoside antibiotics (streptomycin, kanamycin, and gentamicin). The recent report that gentamicin competes with bilirubin for albumin binding appears to be an artifact; this drug is therefore an appropriate choice for indicated infections of the newborn infant.

Bibliography

Brande AI: Antimicrobial drug therapy. W.B. Saunders Company. Phil, 1976.

Franklin TJ, Snow GA: Biochemistry of antimicrobial action. Chapman and Hall Ltd., London, United Kingdom, 1975.

Gardner P, Provine HT: Manual of acute bacterial infections. Little Brown and Co. Boston, Mass 1975.

McCracken GH, Eichenwald HF: Antimicrobial therapy. J. Pediatr. 85:-297-312, 415-456, 1975.

INFECTION OF IMMUNOSUPPRESSED HOST

WALTER T. HUGHES

The infections that supervene in patients who are receiving immunosuppressive therapy or who suffer from primary or secondary immunodeficiency disorders are sufficiently different from those acquired by otherwise normal children to merit separate consideration. Through these compromised patients one can best appreciate the importance of intact host defense mechanisms in coping with the myriad microorganisms in the environment. The ability to maintain a disease-free state depends on the integrity of various components that function to prevent invasion of the host by microbial agents. These components include anatomic barriers such as skin and mucous membranes, opsonins, phagocytes, complement activity, humoral and secretory antibodies, cellular immunity, interferon production, and proper ecologic balance of the microbial flora. If one or more of these factors is functioning improperly, the host becomes more susceptible to infection. Since the vast majority of organisms immediately available to the compromised host are the commensal or saprophytic microbes of the exogenous or endogenous flora, these opportunistic organisms account for most of the serious infections in the immunosupressed patient. Although a number of entities such as sickle cell anemia, cystic fibrosis, diabetes mellitus, burns, and surgical asplenia are associated with susceptibility to specific infections, consideration will be given here only to those conditions creating extreme susceptibility to serious infections.

UNDERLYING CAUSES. Malignancies. In children with cancer the risk for infection varies considerably with the type of neoplasm. Infections are more frequent and severe in patients with generalized lymphoproliferative malignancies, such as leukemia or lymphoma, than in those with solid neoplasms, such as Wilms' tumor or Ewing's sarcoma. Impaired cell-mediated immunity, humoral antibody response, quantitative or qualitative phagocyte deficits, low serum complement levels, or decreased interferon production have been associated with various types of cancer. Obstructive and ulcerative tumor lesions provide sites for infection.

Aplastic Anemia, Congenital and Acquired Neutropenias. Patients with aplastic anemia or congenital or acquired neutropenias acquire infection because of an inadequate number of phagocytic granulocytes.

Chronic Granulomatous Disease. Children with chronic granulomatous disease are especially susceptible to infection from staphylococci, certain gram-negative bacilli, and *Candida* species. The phagocytes ingest but are unable to kill certain bacteria and fungi because of inability to generate hydrogen peroxide, thus compromising the myeloperoxidase-hydrogen peroxide-halide system.

Immunosuppressive Drugs. Corticosteroids alter humoral and cellular immune responses, diminish phagocytosis and neutrophil migration, and stabilize the lysosomal membranes. Azathioprine impairs the primary and secondary immune responses and cellular immunity and causes leukopenia. Cyclophosphamide, 6-mercaptopurine, and methotrexate can impair humoral antibody response and may cause leukopenia.

X-irradiation. Immunosuppressive doses of x-irradiation affect both cellular immunity and immunoglobulin production.

Immune Deficiency Disorders. The immune deficiency disorders are discussed in Chapter 9.

Kwashiorkor. Children with severe protein calorie malnutrition are at high risk for opportunistic infections such as gram-negative bacillary sepsis, fungal infections, generalized herpes simplex infection, and cytomegalic inclusion cell disease. Although it is not thoroughly established, it is believed that impaired cell-mediated immune response and possibly humoral immunity may be affected.

CAUSATIVE AGENTS. The organisms that account for over 95 percent of the serious infections in the immunosuppressed host are listed in Table 5 and are rated as to the relative frequency with which they occur. These organisms represent predominantly the normal

TABLE 5. Causative Agents of Serious Infections in Immunosuppressed Patients

Relative Frequency Encountered	Organisms			
	Bacteria	**Fungi**	**Viruses**	**Other**
Frequent	*Pseudomonas aeroginosa, E. coli, Proteus* species *Klebsiella-Enterobacter Serratia, Staphylococcus aureus*	*Candida albicans, Aspergillus* species, *Cryptococcus neoformans*	Varicella zoster, Herpesvirus hominis, Cytomegalovirus, Hepatitis A and B	*Toxoplasma gondii, Pneumocystis carinii*
Infrequent	*Pseudomonas* and other species, *Bacteroides* species, *Staphylococcus epidermidis*, Enterococci, Streptococci, *S. pneumoniae, Clostridium* species, *Salmonella* species	Candida and other species, Rhizopus, species, Mucor species	Epstein-Barr virus, Measles	*Nocardia asteroides, Mycoplasma*
Rare	*Citrobacter, Flavobacterium,* Hemophilus species, *Hafnia, Aeromonas hydrophila,* Herellea-Mimeae tribe, *Bacillus* species, Corynebacteria, *Listeria monocytogenes, Mycobacterium tuberculosis*	*Histoplasma capsulatum, Blastomyces dermatitidis, Coccidioides immitis*	Vaccinia	

microbial flora of the intestinal tract, oral cavity, and skin, or they may occur as latent organisms in healthy individuals. It is on this premise that new problems in clinical microbiology and infectious diseases are emerging wherein the traditional terms virulence, avirulence, pathogenic, and nonpathogenic are not meaningful. Attention must now be directed to the status of the host and all organisms in its approximate environment. No organism isolated from blood, bone marrow, cerebrospinal fluid, or biopsy specimens can be discounted as a contaminant without careful correlation with the clinical evaluation. The significance of such isolates must be made by the clinician, not the bacteriologist in the laboratory.

CLINICAL MANIFESTATIONS. Significant infection rarely occurs in the absence of any sign or symptom. Fever is the hallmark of infection and is seldom abated by immunosuppressive drugs. Fever must be considered to be of infectious etiology until proven otherwise. The extent and pattern of the febrile response is of no diagnostic significance.

The immunosuppressed patient is usually unable to localize infection at the portal of entry; therefore the expected signs and symptoms of a specific infection may not occur. The child with agranulocytosis may respond to a staphylococcal skin infection by vesicle formation rather than by a purulent abscess; he may respond to *Diplococcus pneumoniae* with diffuse pneumonitis rather than lobar pneumonia. With bacterial meningitis, signs of meningeal irritation and neutrophils in the spinal fluid may be absent. However, in the immunosuppressed child the skin lesions caused by varicella zoster virus, herpesvirus hominis, and *P. aeruginosa* are usually sufficiently characteristic to make a reliable presumptive diagnosis. Anorectal lesions are usually caused by gram-negative enteric bacilli. Bacterial sepsis presents with fever, but jaundice, abdominal pain, lethargy, petechiae, and erythematous macules may occur. Careful search for anal, oral, infusion-site, finger-prick, paronychial, and ulcerative skin lesions should be made to locate a portal of entry for bacteria.

Fever, tachypnea, flaring of the nasal alae, intercostal retraction, and absence of rales associated with bilateral diffuse alveolar disease demonstrated by roentgenography strongly suggest *Pneumocystis carinii* pneumonitis. The diagnosis can be established only by the identification of the causative agent in material obtained by lung aspirate or biopsy. Other causes of diffuse pneumonitis are cytomegalovirus, E.B. virus, varicella zoster virus, mycoplasmas, adenovirus, measles virus, herpesvirus hominis, *Toxoplasma gondii,* and in some instances bacteria or fungi.

MANAGEMENT. For specific treatment see the specific disease entities described in other chapters.

General Principles. A few axioms can be set forth for the management of the immunosuppressed host: (1) Consider fever to be a sign of infection unless proven otherwise. (2) Granulocytopenia with an absolute neutrophil count of 1,000/mm³ or less renders the individual highly susceptible to bacterial infection. (3) Consider any organism to be a potential pathogen. Instruct the laboratory to identify all isolates and not to make decisions as to which isolates are contaminants and which are normal flora. (4) When the causative agent for an infection is identified, continue surveillance for mixed or sequential infections. (5) Withhold or modify immunosuppressive therapy during the infection if the status of the primary disease permits. (6) Administer immune serum globulin (human) (ISG) if hypogammaglobulinemia or agammaglobulinemia exists. There is no other indication where the use of ISG during the acute infection is of proven value. (7) Antibiotics, preferably bactericidal, should be administered *intravenously* in maximum dosage immediately after the diagnosis or presumptive diagnosis of systemic bacterial infection. (8) Monitor patients for toxicity and adverse side effects of antimicrobial agents. The efficacy of granulocyte transfusions for neutropenic patients with infection has not been firmly established, and little work has been done to evaluate the use of leukocyte transfer factor in the immunosuppressed host during times of life-threatening infection.

Preventing Infection. Instruct parents and children on increased susceptibility to infection. Have them report early signs and symptoms of infection, follow basic principles of good hygiene, avoid contact with individuals with even minor contagious infections, and avoid prolonged exposure to large groups of people. Although live-virus vaccines such as measles, mumps, rubella, and smallpox should never be given, the diphtheria, pertussis, and tetanus immunizations can be given if indicated. Influenza vaccine is indicated in some patients where an immune response can be expected. Passive immunization with immune serum globulin is given after exposure to measles and infectious hepatitis type A, and specific hyperimmune globulin preparations are given to susceptible individuals after exposure to varicella or vaccinia. Protected environments using "life island" or laminar-flow rooms may offer some benefit to certain patients, but thorough evaluation of these systems with children has not been reported.

References

Anderson RJ, Schafer LA, Olin DB, Eickhoff TC: Infectious risk factors in the immunosuppressed host. Am J Med 54:453, 1973

Hughes WT, Feldman S, Cox F: Infectious diseases in children with cancer. Pediatr Clin North Am 21:583, 1974

Merigan TC, Stevens DA: Viral infections in man associated with acquired immunological deficiency states. Fed Proc 30:1858, 1971

Rodriguez V, Burgess M, Bodey GP: Management of fever of unknown origin in patients with neoplasms and neutropenia. Cancer 32:1007, 1973

NEONATAL SEPTICEMIA AND MENINGITIS

GEORGE H. MCCRACKEN, JR.

Although systemic bacterial infections in the newborn are uncommon, their occurrence results in significant mortality and long-term morbidity. The etiologic agents of neonatal septicemia and meningitis have changed during the past several decades. This is due in part to unexplained alterations in the epidemiologic characteristics of specific bacterial agents, to increased use of broad-spectrum antibiotics during the perinatal period, and to the use of complex resuscitation and respiratory apparatuses that act as fomites for nosocomial infection. It is imperative that physicians be aware of these broad changes in etiologic agents and of the historical experience within a specific nursery in order to diagnose infection promptly and initiate appropriate antimicrobial therapy. The incidence of sepsis neonatorum is approximately 1 case per 1,000 live full-term births and 1 case per 250 live premature births. Neonatal meningitis occurs in approximately 1 case per 2,500 live births. These incidence rates vary from nursery to nursery and depend in part on the conditions predisposing to infection.

PREDISPOSING FACTORS. Sex, prematurity, and specific prenatal complications predispose to neonatal infections. Postnatally acquired bacterial diseases occur more commonly in males. An important exception is the early onset form of group B streptococcal septicemia, which is seen with equal frequency in males and females. Complications arising during pregnancy, particularly during the process of delivery, increase the incidence of neonatal septicemia and meningitis. Fetal distress manifested as passage of meconium and abnormal fetal heart tones and rate is frequently associated with infantile infections. Toxemia of pregnancy, precipitous delivery, abruptio, and many other obstetric complications place the infant at high risk. Prolonged rupture of fetal membranes is usually considered a risk factor. However, other events associated with ruptured fetal membranes, such as chorioamnionitis, maternal fever, and prematurity, most likely play the more significant role in predisposing to infection. It is important to emphasize that even in the setting of documented maternal infection neonatal disease is uncommon.

Over the past 5 years ventilatory equipment and monitoring devices have made it possible to treat severely ill infants more effectively. However, these apparatuses have acted as fomites for relatively nonpathogenic organisms ("water bugs") that may cause nosocomial disease. The frequency of these infections varies, and they are usually sporadic. It may be difficult to recognize these opportunistic infections because of the severe underlying illnesses requiring intensive therapy and the frequent use of antimicrobial agents in these infants.

ETIOLOGY.   The major organisms responsible for neonatal bacterial diseases have changed during the past decades. Group A β-hemolytic streptococci were most common in the 1930s and early 1940s and were replaced by coliform organisms in the late 1940s and 1950s. In the late 1950s and early 1960s coagulase-positive *Staphylococcus aureus* caused significant neonatal disease. Group B β-hemolytic streptococci and coliforms, particularly *Escherichia coli,* have been the most common causative organisms during the past decade. Familiarity with the past experience of a given nursery or intensive care unit is invaluable in guiding selection of antimicrobial therapy for suspected bacterial disease. A recent survey of 12 North American hospitals showed that the group β streptococci and *E. coli* accounted for approximately 70 percent of all cases of neonatal meningitis. *Listeria monocytogenes* contributed an additional 5 percent of cases. The mean incidence rates of group B streptococcal and *E. coli* diseases at Parkland Memorial Hospital in Dallas from 1969 through 1973 were 1.35 (0.59 to 2.44) cases and 0.69 (0.44 to 0.95) cases per 1,000 deliveries, respectively.

EPIDEMIOLOGY AND PATHOGENESIS.   Until recently little was known about the epidemiology and pathogenesis of neonatal bacterial infections, particularly those caused by the two most common etiologic agents (group B streptococci and *E. coli*). Recent evidence strongly suggests that the majority of neonatal streptococcal and coliform infections are transmitted vertically from mother to infant. The streptococcal organisms of group B_{III} are the agents most frequently associated with early and late-onset meningitis, while B_{II} and B_{Ia} organisms are the major causes of early onset septicemia. These latter organisms normally reside in the genital tract of healthy females, and asymptomatic vaginal infection rates of pregnant women range from 5 to 30 percent. Although most infants born to culture-positive mothers are colonized with the identical group B organism, less than 1 percent of these infants develop disease.

While *E. coli* has been recognized for several decades as a significant cause of neonatal disease, investigations of the serotypes involved or of the epidemiologic factors leading to neonatal disease have never been undertaken. The recent finding that 80 percent of *E. coli* strains causing neonatal meningitis possess a specific capsular polysaccharide (K1 antigen) has provided a convenient laboratory beginning for epidemiologic and pathogenetic studies. Current evidence indicates that this capsular K1 antigen, either alone or in association with specific somatic antigens, confers virulence to these organisms. K1 antigen is associated with approximately 40 percent of *E. coli* strains causing neonatal septicemia, with 19 percent of strains causing pyelonephritis, and with only 10 percent of strains causing septicemia in adults. Animal studies have documented the

virulence of K1-bearing strains and have shown that pretreatment with specific K1 antiserum prevents the lethal effect in mice. The outcome of neonatal meningitis is directly correlated with the presence, concentration, and persistence of K1 antigen in cerebrospinal fluid and blood of these infants.

The *E. coli* K1 strains are common inhabitants of the gastrointestinal tract of healthy babies, children, and adults. Approximately 20 percent of neonates, 30 percent of children, and 50 percent of women during the childbearing years yield *E. coli* K1 strains on rectal culture. Approximately two-thirds of babies born to culture-positive women will themselves be colonized. Conversely, 80 percent of colonized babies have mothers with identical K1 strains in their rectums. These *E. coli* K1 organisms do not appear to cause gastrointestinal disease. Current studies are under way to evaluate the role of specific anticapsular antibody in protection and recovery from disease.

CLINICAL FEATURES.   Most infants with septicemia and/or meningitis present clinically with nonspecific signs and symptoms that are usually first detected by the nurse or mother rather than by the physician. The most common early manifestations of illness are altered temperature, lethargy or irritability, and poor feeding. Temperature elevation above 38 C is significant in newborn babies. Signs and symptoms in some infants may suggest respiratory disease (tachypnea and cyanosis) or gastrointestinal disease (vomiting, abdominal distension, and diarrhea). Seizures are commonly observed and may be a result of direct central nervous system inflammation or may be associated with hypoglycemia or hypocalcemia. A bulging fontanelle is usually a late clinical sign, and Kernig and Brudzinski signs and stiff neck are unusual. Hepatosplenomegaly, jaundice, and petechiae are classic signs of neonatal infection, but they represent late manifestations.

DIAGNOSIS.   Although it is tempting to recommend a work-up for septicemia and meningitis in all infants with nonspecific clinical signs and symptoms, this is both impractical and unnecessary in many cases. A complete history and physical examination coupled with clinical experience are the best guides in determining the extent of work-up. If doubt exists, a blood culture and complete cerebrospinal fluid examination should be obtained.

During the past decade several screening tests have been described that are purported to aid the physician in making the diagnosis of neonatal infection. Although a few of these tests are helpful in identifying the high-risk infant, the diagnosis of septicemia or meningitis can be made only by recovery of the organism from blood or cerebrospinal fluid cultures. It is frequently helpful to obtain cultures of other sites prior to initiating antimicrobial therapy. For example, percutaneous bladder aspiration of urine for culture may be helpful in identifying the urinary tract as the primary focus of infection. Nasopharyngeal, skin, and rectal cultures are usually positive in the early septicemic form of listeriosis and group B streptococcal disease.

The peripheral white blood cell count is difficult to interpret in newborn infants. Total white cell counts of 20,000 to 30,000/mm^3 may be seen in healthy neonates. Absolute band-form counts may be elevated early in bacterial infections, but leukocytosis with predominance of juvenile forms may also be observed in infants with congenital viral infections. Tests for C-reactive protein, erythrocyte sedimentation rate, histology of umbilical cord sections, and smear of the gastric aspirate for polymorphonuclear cells have all been recommended for identification of infants with systemic bacterial disease. Although some of these laboratory tests have been positively correlated with neonatal infection, their success in identifying such infants varies among institutions.

The unstimulated nitroblue tetrazolium test to differentiate viral from bacterial disease has been used in older infants and children with variable success. Because the percentage of polymorphonuclear cells that reduce dye is elevated in healthy neonates, this test has not been useful in diagnosing bacterial disease. However, recent evidence suggests that the nitroblue tetrazolium test may be significantly reduced in neonates with bacterial disease, presumably due to a toxic effect on leukocytes. Elevated serum macroglobulin values are not observed early in the course of postnatally acquired bacterial diseases.

The diagnosis of purulent meningitis can be made with certainty only by isolation of the offending pathogen from cerebrospinal fluid cultures. A number of screening tests for diagnosing bacterial meningitis have been described, but most are nonspecific and have not been adequately evaluated in neonates. Two tests deserve mention. The first is the detection of specific capsular polysaccharide antigen in cerebrospinal fluid using countercurrent immunoelectrophoresis; *E. coli* K1, *Diplococcus pneumoniae, Neisseria meningitidis,* and *Haemophilus influenzae* antigens have been measured by this method in spinal fluid specimens. The second test involves assay of spinal fluid endotoxin by the *Limulus* lysate test. This method is applicable only to meningitis caused by gram-negative organisms, and it has not been adequately evaluated in neonates.

PATHOLOGY.   The histopathologic description of neonatal bacterial infections is obtained from postmortem examinations and therefore is not representative of the full spectrum of these diseases. Studies of the fulminant, early onset form of group B streptococcal disease have shown primarily a bronchopneumonia and shock without histologic evidence of meningeal involvement. The most consistent findings at necropsy of babies dying of meningitis are a purulent exudate of the subarachnoid space (meninges) and of the ependymal surfaces of the ventricles, a noninfectious encephalopathy, and vascular inflammation. The inflammatory responses of neonates are similar to those observed in adults with meningitis, with the exception that babies have a sparsity of plasma cells and lymphocytes during the subacute stage of meningeal reaction. Hydrocephalus can be demonstrated in approximately half of the autopsied infants, and many have the communicating type. Subdural effusions occur rarely in neonates, but this complication of meningitis is common in infants 3 to 12 months of age. Varying degrees of phlebitis and arteritis of intracranial vessels can be found in all infants dying of meningitis. Thrombophlebitis with occlusion of veins may occur in the subependymal zones.

SPECIFIC DISEASES.   Group B Streptococcal Illness.   The group B streptococci are the most frequent gram-positive bacteria causing neonatal meningitis. This organism produces a spectrum of illness ranging from asymptomatic bacteremia to fulminant septicemia and meningitis. Less common manifestations of group B disease are septic arthritis (particularly of the hip), osteomyelitis, pneumonia with empyema, cellulitis, sinusitis, otitis media, and conjunctivitis. Early recognition of these unusual presentations of this disease has important epidemiologic and therapeutic implications. Septicemia and meningitis are the most common and serious forms of neonatal group B streptococcal illness. The acute septicemic form of disease has its onset within the first 12 hours after birth and presents as acute respiratory distress with or without shock. Chest radiography usually reveals aspiration pneumonitis. The pathogenesis of this form of disease is most likely on the basis of aspiration of infected amniotic fluid or cervical secretions at the time of delivery. Cultures from multiple sites on the newborn baby yield the organism, thus indicating generalized colonization of the infant prior to or at the time of delivery. The mortality rate in this fulminant disease is 50 to 80 percent. Pneumonitis is the primary finding on pathologic examination, and postmortem cultures of lung, blood, and cerebrospinal fluid yield the pathogen. However, histologic evidence of meningitis is usually lacking. The delayed meningitic form of disease presents at approximately 2 to 12 weeks of life and is indistinguishable from other forms of purulent meningitis. The mortality rate in group B streptococcal meningitis is 20 to 40 percent.

Staphylococcal Disease.   The phage group I *S. aureus* that was common in the late 1950s is still present in some nurseries and occasionally causes serious systemic neonatal disease. The pathogenicity of this organism is based on its ability to invade skin and the musculoskeletal system and produce furuncles, breast abscesses, and osteomyelitis. Septicemia is usually secondary to local invasion. When *S. aureus* is recovered from blood cultures of neonates, a careful search should be made for the primary focus. More recently, phage group II coagulase-positive staphylococci have emerged as a common cause of neonatal infection. Although this organism may be invasive, pathogenicity depends primarily upon production of an exotoxin (exfolitin). Clinical disease may take one of several forms, including bullous impetigo, toxic epidermal necrolysis, Ritter's disease, and nonstreptococcal scarlatina. Collectively these diseases have been referred to as the expanded scalded skin syndrome. The initial finding in Ritter's disease is generalized erythema associated with edema and tenderness. After several days a distinctive desquamation of large sheets of epidermis occurs that is distinguished from the fine desquamation observed in the second and third weeks of streptococcal scarlet fever. Large flaccid bullae are commonly noted in Ritter's disease; after being ruptured they leave a tender, weeping, erythematous base. The infant may appear toxic with the generalized form of disease.

E. coli Disease.   *E. coli* is the most common gram-negative pathogen in neonates, and it accounts for approximately 70 percent of all cases of meningitis caused by enteric bacilli. Clinical illness and routine laboratory findings of *E. coli* disease are indistinguishable from the other causes of neonatal meningitis, with the exception of the time necessary to sterilize cerebrospinal fluid culture. Whereas spinal fluid cultures from infants with gram-positive meningitis are usually sterile within the first 24 hours of therapy, the average duration of positive spinal fluid cultures in meningitis caused by enteric organisms is 3 to 4 days. In some infants sterilization may take 7 to 10 days. The duration of positive spinal fluid cultures is directly correlated with outcome. The disparity in the time necessary to sterilize spinal fluid cultures is unexplained, but may relate to difficulty in achieving spinal fluid antibiotic concentrations that are consistently greater than the minimal inhibitory concentration for the pathogen. It is common to identify microorganisms in the meningeal exudate of infants dying with meningitis due to gram-negative pathogens and to detect capsular K1 antigen in brain tissue of infants with *E. coli* K1 meningitis many days after administration of seemingly effective antibiotics. The mortality rate of *E. coli* meningitis is approximately 20 to 30 percent and in some areas may be as high as 50 to 60 percent.

Listeria monocytogenes.   The pathogenesis and the clinical features of diseases caused by *L. monocytogenes* are similar to those of group B streptococci. A fulminant disseminated form of disease appears during the first several days of life. The pathogen is acquired transplacentally, and many organ systems are involved. Cultures from multiple sites yield the organism. The infant frequently presents with hypothermia, lethargy, and poor feeding. A characteristic rash consisting of small erythematous papules scattered primarily on the trunk may be observed in some infants. Chest radiographs reveal a granulomatous type of infiltrate in some patients, and hepatosplenomegaly is common.

A delayed form of neonatal listeriosis occurs in the second week through fifth week of life and involves primarily the meninges. The clinical presentation is indistinguishable from that of delayed group B streptococcal disease. One distinctive feature is the mononuclear cellular response in the spinal fluid of these patients, as compared with the predominance of polymorphonuclear cells observed in most other forms of purulent meningitis. It is frequently difficult to identify the small slender gram-positive rods on stained smears of cerebrospinal fluid. The bacteriology laboratory should be alerted to the possibility that *Listeria* is the pathogen, because these organisms are frequently misinterpreted as diphtheroids and are discarded.

THERAPY.   Rational use of antibiotics requires an understanding of the neonate's constantly changing physiologic and metabolic processes, which profoundly affect the pharmacokinetic properties of antimicrobial agents. It is no longer satisfactory to fractionate adult dosages of antibiotics and administer them to newborns and young infants. The dosage schedules outlined in Table 6 are designed for neonates and are based on clinical pharmacologic studies performed in newborn infants. When these drugs are used for treatment of septicemia and meningitis, it is advisable to monitor serum and cerebrospinal fluid concentrations, because there are considerable variations in these levels among patients. In addition, it is recommended that repeat blood and cerebrospinal fluid cultures be obtained 24 to 36 hours after initiation of therapy in order to document bacteriologic cure. Persistence of positive blood cultures should alert the physician to the possibilities that the pathogen is resistant to the drugs employed or that sequestered sites of infection exist that are not amenable to antimicrobial therapy alone. For example, renal parenchymal infection secondary to an obstructive lesion requires drainage as well as antibiotic therapy.

TABLE 6. Dosage Schedule for Antibiotics Used Parenterally for Therapy of Neonatal Septicemia and Meningitis

| Drug | Disease | Daily Dosage (Number of Divided Doses) | |
		Infants < 1 Week of Age	Infants 1 to 4 Weeks of Age
Crystalline penicillin G	Septicemia	50,000 IU/kg (2)	75,000 IU/kg (3)
	Meningitis	100,000 IU/kg (2)	100,000–150,000 IU/kg (3)
Ampicillin	Septicemia	50 mg/kg (2)	100–150 mg/kg (3)
	Meningitis	100 mg/kg (2)	200 mg/kg (3)
Carbenicillin	Septicemia and meningitis	225–300 mg/kg (3 or 4)	400 mg/kg (4)
Methicillin	Septicemia	50 mg/kg (2)	150–200 mg/kg (3)
	Meningitis	100 mg/kg (2)	200–300 mg/kg (3)
Kanamycin	Septicemia and meningitis	10–20 mg/kg (1 or 2)*	20–30 mg/kg (2 or 3)
Gentamicin	Septicemia and meningitis	5 mg/kg (2)	7.5 mg/kg (3)

See text for specific dosage recommendations.

Initial therapy of sepsis neonatorum before identification of the pathogen should include a penicillin and an aminoglycoside. We prefer ampicillin or carbenicillin and either kanamycin or gentamicin. The advantages of these two penicillin analogues over the parent compound (penicillin G) is their activity against *Listeria*, the enterococci, and many *E. coli* strains. Kanamycin is the preferred aminoglycoside drug for susceptible coliform bacteria because there is extensive clinical experience with this drug in neonates. Recent studies have demonstrated that more than 90 percent of *E. coli* strains from nurseries previously experiencing kanamycin resistance are again susceptible to this drug. If kanamycin is used, it may be preferable to combine it with carbenicillin in order to achieve effective activity against *Pseudomonas*. Pharmacologic studies have shown that the dosage of kanamycin should be increased in order to consistently attain peak serum concentrations in the therapeutic range (15 to 25 μg/ml). The revised kanamycin dosage is 10 mg/kg administered intramuscularly every 12 hours to all neonates, with two exceptions. First, infants 1 to 3 days of age with birth weights below 2,000 g should be given the 10 mg/kg dose once daily. After the infant has reached 4 days of age the dose should be given every 12 hours. The second exception involves infants 7 days of age and older who weighed 2,000 g or more at birth. These babies should receive 10 mg/kg administered intramuscularly every 8 hours. Gentamicin has been used safely and effectively for the treatment of neonatal bacterial diseases. In order to preserve its effectiveness, this drug should be reserved for therapy of infections caused by kanamycin-resistant coliforms and by *Pseudomonas* species. Ampicillin is the penicillin analogue preferred for combination with gentamicin, unless *Pseudomonas* infection is suspected.

The drugs used for initial therapy of neonatal meningitis are the same as for sepsis neonatorum, but the recommended dosages are larger for penicillin, ampicillin, and methicillin (Table 6). The efficacy of intrathecal therapy in neonatal meningitis has never been established. The Cooperative Neonatal Meningitis Study Group was established in 1971 to evaluate the role of intrathecal gentamicin in this disease. Analysis of the first 110 patients in the study has demonstrated no clear differences in mortality rate or in incidence of long-term neurologic sequelae between parenteral therapy alone or parenteral plus intrathecal therapy.

Once the specific pathogen of neonatal septicemia and meningitis has been identified and susceptibility studies are available, the most appropriate drug or drugs should be used. Generally, crystalline pencillin G is recommended for group B streptococci, ampicillin for *L. monocytogenes*, methicillin for penicillin-resistant *S. aureus*, kanamycin or gentamicin alone or in combination with carbenicillin or ampicillin for enteric bacilli, and carbenicillin for indole-positive *Proteus* species. Ampicillin with or without gentamicin is the preferred therapy for enterococcal disease. Carbenicillin with or without the addition of gentamicin is the preferred therapy for *Pseudomonas* disease of neonates.

Guidelines for determining duration of therapy during the neonatal period are often lacking because objective evidence of illness may be minimal. In the absence of deep tissue involvement or abscess formation, therapy for sepsis neonatorum is usually continued for 5 to 7 days after clinical improvement. Therapy for meningitis is continued for a minimum of 2 weeks after sterilization of cerebrospinal fluid cultures. From a practical standpoint, this amounts to 2 weeks of therapy for meningitis caused by gram-positive organisms and a minimum of 3 weeks of therapy for meningitis caused by gram-negative pathogens.

Attention to general supportive therapy is of utmost importance in caring for infants with meningitis. Disturbances of fluid and electrolyte balance are common, particularly in the first several days of illness when inappropriate antidiuretic hormone secretion may lead to fluid retention and hyponatremia. Ventilatory assistance is frequently necessary, and blood pressure should be carefully monitored. During the course of illness, hemoglobin and hematocrit values should be checked frequently, because infection may exaggerate and prolong the anemias of infancy, particularly in premature infants. Some authorities recommend transfusion with fresh whole blood as a means of providing nonspecific factors of host resistance.

References

Franciosa RA, Knostman JD, Zimmerman RA: Group B streptococcal neonatal and infant infections. J Pediatr 82:707, 1973

Hood M: Listeriosis as an infection of pregnancy manifested in the newborn. Pediatrics 27:390, 1961

Howard JB, McCracken GH: The spectrum of group B streptococcal infections in infancy. Am J Dis Child 128:815, 1974

——— McCracken GH: Reappraisal of kanamycin usage in neonates. J Pediatr 86:949, 1975

McCracken GH: Pharmacological basis for antimicrobial therapy in newborn infants. Am J Dis Child 128:407, 1974

——— The rate of bacteriologic response to antimicrobial therapy in neonatal meningitis. Am J Dis Child 123:547, 1972

——— Shinefield HR: Changes in the pattern of neonatal septicemia and meningitis. Am J Dis Child 112:33, 1966

——— Sarff LD, Glode MP, et al: Relation between Escherichia coli K1 capsular polysaccharide antigen and clinical outcome in neonatal meningitis. Lancet 2:246, 1974

Melish ME, Glasgow LA: Staphylococcal scalded skin syndrome: the expanded clinical syndrome. J Pediatr 78:958, 1971

Overall JC: Neonatal bacterial meningitis. J Pediatr 76:499, 1970

Robbins JB, McCracken GH, Gotschlich EC, et al: Escherichia coli K1 capsular polysaccharide associated with neonatal meningitis. N Engl J Med 290:1216, 1974

BACTERIAL MENINGITIS
ARNOLD H. EINHORN

Inflammation of the meninges may follow the invasion of the spinal fluid by any of a wide range of infectious agents. All varieties of bacterial meningitis occur more frequently in infants and children than in adults. Only bacterial infection due to pyogenic organisms will be discussed here. Tuberculous meningitis will be described separately (p. 468). Although mortality rates have been altered dramatically as a result of the introduction of antibacterial therapy, pyogenic meningitides are still among the most serious infections encountered in pediatrics.

The proportions of cases due to the different organisms vary from year to year; there are also considerable geographic differences. In the absence of meningococcus epidemics, bacterial meningitis in infants and children is due predominantly to *Haemophilus influenzae*. Next in frequency are those cases caused by *Diplococcus pneumoniae* and *Neisseria meningitidis*. In the first month of life gram-negative bacilli of enteric origin are more common; among the latter, *Escherichia coli* (K1 capsular antigen) holds first place. *Pseudomonas aeruginosa* and *Proteus* meningitides, although in general less common, are no longer exceptional. Staphylococcal meningitis is very rare, even in the newborn period. Group B β-hemolytic streptococci can cause an appreciable percentage of meningitis in the neonatal period, and group A β-hemolytic streptococci may cause meningitis at any age. Isolated instances of meningitis due to *Listeria monocytogenes* have also been reported in the neonatal period; the morphologic similarity of these gram-positive rod-shaped bacteria to nonpathogenic diphtheroids may constitute a difficulty in bacteriologic diagnosis. There have been increasing reports of meningeal infections involving two or more organisms simultaneously. These *mixed* bacterial meningitides have their highest incidence in young infants. In approximately 15 to 20 percent of patients whose cerebrospinal findings indicate the presence of pyogenic meningitis it is not possible to demonstrate any etiologic agent. Some of these may represent *sympathetic* meningitis; in others the organism probably has been suppressed by treatment administered earlier.

By and large, the clinical picture, pathologic lesions, and prognosis in pyogenic meningitis depend more on the age of the patient, the duration of infection, and the kind of treatment the patient has received than on the etiologic agent. Therefore pyogenic meningitis will be discussed as a syndrome, with the peculiar features of specific infections being pointed out where necessary.

PATHOLOGY. The typical pathologic picture of the patient who dies from pyogenic meningitis is today seen only in those who receive inadequate or late treatment. The reader is referred to texts on pathology for the great variety of lesions that may be found in the untreated disease. The pathologic lesions that concern us here are those found early in the infection. It is important to recognize the clinical signs they produce and to define their causes while they are still reversible.

The common varieties of bacterial meningitis most often evolve from a metastatic lesion seeded during bacteremia, although they may result from an extension from a purulent regional focus such as otitis media, mastoiditis, or sinusitis. There is reason to believe that endothelial damage of cerebral vessels precedes meningitis caused by meningococcus or *H. influenzae* and that the degree of vascular damage determines whether the patient will exhibit signs of encephalitis in addition to signs of meningitis. Thrombosis of small cerebral as well as meningeal vessels is found in some cases. In general, pneumococcal or *E. coli* meningitis of infants also appears to evolve from a metastatic lesion. However, staphylococcal meningitis is often secondary to a contiguous focus in all age groups. In the older child, as in the adult, meningitis caused by pneumococcus type III or β-hemolytic streptococci is most frequently due to extension from a neighboring infection. Regardless of whether meningitis evolves from a metastatic lesion or from a neighboring focus, a respiratory infection nearly always initiates the process. In general, a febrile upper respiratory infection is followed by bacteremia of varying duration before invasion of the spinal fluid.

CLINICAL FEATURES. Since survival in pyogenic meningitis and residual sequelae depend not only on appropriate therapy but also on early institution of treatment, the importance of early recognition of the meningeal infection cannot be overstressed.

In older children headache and photophobia are often presenting complaints. Fever, vomiting (often projectile in type), and convulsions are common symptoms. In some instances persistent fever may be the only objective sign of illness. If the meningitis is not recognized and antibiotics are given in doses inadequate for elimination of the infectious agent, most of the signs of meningeal inflammation and of increased intracranial pressure will be masked. These symptoms and signs may also be absent in fulminant disease.

In untreated patients older than 6 or 7 months clinical signs of early meningeal inflammation are easily detected. These consist of hyperesthesia, pain and resistance on flexion of the neck, and positive Kernig and Brudzinski signs. Except for transient delirium, the sensorium is clear at the onset. In young infants nuchal rigidity is most often absent, and the only specific feature of meningitis may be increased tension or bulging of the anterior fontanelle due to increased intracranial pressure.

The elevation of intracranial pressure in acute meningitis is partly due to impaired circulation of cerebrospinal fluid by purulent material, to cerbral edema, and probably to accrued cerebrospinal fluid production secondary to inflammation. In spite of the increased intracranial pressure, papilledema is rare early in the course of pyogenic meningitis. Blurring of the disk margins may be seen, but without definite edema. Whenever papilledema is present early in the course of acute bacterial meningitis, the existence of an associated intracranial complication should be suspected, such as subdural empyema, brain abscess, or sinus thrombosis. Because of the heightened intracranial pressure, it is well to measure the cerebrospinal fluid pressure carefully when performing a lumbar puncture in meningitis and to remove the fluid very slowly using a small-gauge needle in order to minimize the danger of brainstem and temporal lobe herniation.

Petechial or purpuric lesions are most commonly present in meningococcal infection, but they can be associated with sepsis and meningitis due to any other organisms. They have no particular characteristic distribution and are occasionally bullous or necrotic. In severe meningococcal infections with bacteremia, petechial lesions may appear, and symptoms of shock (Waterhouse-Friderichsen syndrome) may develop with alarming rapidity before clincial signs of meningitis are detectable. There is reason to believe that these patients suffer from widespread effects of the bacterial endotoxins and diffuse intravascular coagulation.

In the young infant less than 6 months of age, particularly in infants 2 or 3 months of age or less, the clinical diagnosis of early meningitis may be a major problem. The clinical signs of meningeal irritation that are relied on in older subjects may not be found until the meningitis is well advanced; thus different criteria must be used. In infants *2 or 3 months of age or more*, fever is almost always present. Distension of the fontanelle, if present, is a valuable sign. If the fontanelle is too small or if dehydration prevents development of fullness of the fontanelle, other manifestations should serve to arouse suspicion: unexplained fever, projectile vomiting, alternating drowsiness and irritability, a vacant stare, a high-pitched cry, and sometimes the presence of cranial bruits. In infants less than 2 or 3 months of age fever is often absent. Hypothermia, cyanosis, jaundice, poor feeding, poor activity, irregular breathing, and unusual jitteriness or drowsiness are the signs that may point to meningitis. Sudden enlargement of the head over a 24-hour period may also constitute an important clue. Because early recognition of meningitis in the young infant is so difficult, it is recommended that the spinal fluid be examined in all young infants with unexplained fever and in infants less than 3 months of age who have any unusual symptom of illness.

The severity of the meningeal infection and of the accompanying cerebral involvement correlate fairly closely with the rapidity of progression of symptoms following onset. Convulsions, stupor, or coma appearing within the first 24 hours, often accompanied by high fever, indicate a serious infection. In view of the frequent association of convulsions with the onset of meningitis, a lumbar puncture should be performed in all patients with febrile convulsions occurring for the first time. The cerebrospinal fluid, when first examined, may show a very low sugar concentration of less than 15 mg/100 ml and numerous organisms on direct smear. Complete recovery may ensue if adequate therapy is applied immediately, even though the course during treatment may be alarming and marked by irritative phenomena or localized cerebral dysfunction such as hemiplegia or facial paralysis. In uncomplicated meningitis focal cerebral signs and seizures that appear early can be related to cortical necrosis or occlusive phlebitis or arteritis. In most patients the sensorium clears markedly within 24 hours after institution of treatment, organisms are promptly eliminated from the spinal fluid, and the sugar concentration rises significantly.

Persistence of fever, stupor, and focal signs of cerebral irritation such as involuntary muscle movements and localized muscle weakness are not incompatible with eventual full recovery. In general, however, the longer such signs last the more unfavorable the outlook. Prominent and persisting focal cerebral signs always raise the question of an associated focal process such as subdural effusion, subdural empyema, brain abscess, or cerebral embolism produced by a bacterial endocarditis. Occasionally a patient with meningitis caused by *H. influenzae* progesses rapidly downhill despite early therapy, with the cause of death remaining obscure even after autopsy.

ETIOLOGIC DIAGNOSIS. CLINICAL CLUES. Bacteriologic identification of the organism causing meningitis is essential in order to select optimal therapy. It has been mentioned previously that the clinical signs depend more on the stage and severity of the meningitis, the child's age, and the amount of treatment given than on the type of infectious agent. However, certain clinical features may suggest the nature of the infectious agent.

H. influenzae type B meningitis is unusual in infants less than 2 months old. Its incidence is highest during the remainder of infancy and in early childhood; it declines to very low levels in the preschool and school-age child. In the United States *H. influenzae* is by far the most common etiologic agent responsible for bacterial meningitis in children between 6 months and 3 years of age. In almost all cases the *H. influenzae* strains are type B. The majority of patients with *E. coli, Pseudomonas,* or *Salmonella* meningitis are less than 1 month of age. Enteric bacteria cause meningitis so rarely in older children that a congenital dermal sinus or immunologic defect should be suspected. Meningitis due to *Staphylococcus aureus,* a rare form of bacterial meningitis confined mostly to the neonatal period, may also be associated with communicating dermal sinuses or may follow neurosurgical procedures.

Most infants who develop *D. pneumoniae* meningitis are between 3 and 6 months of age. The older child who, without sickle cell disease or head trauma, develops pneumococcal (especially type III) or hemolytic streptococcal meningitis is usually found to have purulent otitis media, mastoiditis, or lobar pneumonia. *D. pneumoniae* is the organism involved at any age in recurrent meningitides that result from basal skull fractures, particularly those with fractures of the cribriform plate of the ethmoid. There is also a higher incidence of pneumococcal meningitis in infants and children with sickle cell anemia.

Petechial skin lesions suggest *N. meningitidis,* although not all children with this variety of meningitis have petechiae. The association of petechiae and purulent meningitis is by no means diagnostic of meningococcal disease only, for they can occur, although less commonly, with sepsis due to other organisms.

Swelling of one or several joints, particularly the small joints of the hands or feet, may be associated early in the disease with the invasion of the bloodstream by *N. meningitidis* or *H. influenzae.* In meningococcal meningitis a sterile effusion develops occasionally in a single large joint late in the course of the illness. However, purulent arthritides can occur, although rarely, as a sep-

TABLE 7. Differential Diagnostic Features of Cerebrospinal Fluid in Meningitis

Type of Meningitis	Cell Count	Predominant Cytology	Chemistry	
			Sugar	Protein
Sympathetic	Low	Polymorphonuclear	Normal	+
Pyogenic	High	Polymorphonuclear	Low*	+ + + +
Tuberculosis	Moderate to high	Mononuclear	Low	+ to + + + +
Lead encephalitis	Low	Mononuclear	Normal	+ + to + + + +
Viral meningitis	Low to moderate	Mononuclear†	Normal	+ to + + +

* *May be normal or only slightly reduced in early mild pyogenic meningitis.*
† *An early polymorphonuclear reaction is not uncommon.*

ticemic complication of any form of bacterial meningitis.

LABORATORY FINDINGS.   Only by examination of the cerebrospinal fluid can a definitive diagnosis of the meningitis be established and the etiologic agent identified. Cultures of blood and spinal fluid must also be obtained before antimicrobial therapy is instituted in any patient suspected of having meningitis. If petechiae are present, gram-stained smears of the scrapings from these lesions will frequently provide the bacteriologic diagnosis.

Specific differences in the spinal fluid cytology, in the number of cells, and in the concentration of sugar and protein characteristic of the various types of central nervous system infections are outlined in Table 7. A mononuclear cell response and normal concentration of sugar suggest a viral infection. In viral meningitides the spinal fluid cells are predominantly mononuclear within 24 to 48 hours after the onset of illness, although a transient polymorphonuclear preponderance is commonly seen at the early stage of aseptic meningitis. In lead encephalitis the findings are not unlike those seen in some viral infections. When the concentration of protein is normal or only slightly elevated, lead encephalitis is less likely. The decreased spinal fluid sugar of 40 mg/100 ml, or less than one-half the blood sugar, distinguishes tuberculous meningitis from viral infections and lead encephalopathy. In any patient with a positive skin reaction to tuberculin who shows an increased number of cells with mononuclear predominance and an abnormally low concentration of sugar in the spinal fluid, treatment for tuberculous meningitis is indicated after collection of appropriate fluids for culture. In sympathetic meningitis, which is an inflammatory reaction produced by a contiguous infection such as mastoiditis or sinusitis without invasion of the spinal fluid, there may be a mild polymorphonuclear reaction and a slight protein elevation, while the sugar remains normal and the fluid sterile. In mild pyogenic meningitis the findings may be identical except for the growth of bacteria on culture of spinal fluid and occasionally the documentation of bacteria on smear.

Every effort should be exerted toward an immediate bacteriologic identification whenever there is a predominance of polymorphonuclear cells and a decrease in the sugar concentration in the spinal fluid of

a patient. Organisms may be sufficiently numerous to be seen on microscopic examination of a gram-stained smear of the spinal fluid or in the sediment after centrifugation. The morphology of the bacteria on a direct smear with methylene blue, and by Gram's method if possible, provides important clues. In the case of *H. influenzae*, meningococci, and pneumococci, immediate proof can be obtained by demonstration of capsular swelling on exposure of the organism to type-specific antibody. Thus in the presence of gram-negative pleomorphic rods that suggest *H. influenzae* the capsular swelling test confirms this impression and immediately excludes other gram-negative bacilli such as *E. coli, Salmonella*, and *Pseudomonas*.

The concentration of sugar in the spinal fluid* serves

* *Rapid semiquantitative screening tests for estimating the approximate concentration of spinal fluid sugar are valuable diagnostic aids in emergency situations. They are simple and are quickly performed and require only minute amounts of fluid:*

1. Screening test using Benedict's solution: 1 ml of qualitative Benedict's solution is placed in each of a series of six tubes 75 × 12 mm in size. The following volumes (ml) of spinal fluid are added to tubes 1 through 5: 0.05, 0.1, 0.15, 0.20, and 0.25. The sixth tube serves as control. The tubes are immersed in a boiling water bath for 10 minutes, after which the degree of reduction (presence of yellow pigment, varying from green to orange) is read in a bright light. The sugar concentration may then be estimated as shown:

Tube No.	CSF Vol. (ml)	Reduction of Benedict's Solution				
1	0.05	+	0	0	0	0	0
2	0.1	+	+	0	0	0	0
3	0.15	+	+	+	0	0	0
4	0.2	+	+	+	+	0	0
5	0.25	+	+	+	+	+	0
6	0.00	0	0	0	0	0	0
Sugar concentration (mg/100ml)		> 50	40–50	30–40	20–30	10–20	< 15

2. Screening test using rapid enzyme strips: this procedure, developed by Cornblath and his group, is a modification of the standard reagent strip (Dextrostix) technique. With the aid of a microbulb, one drop of spinal fluid is applied to the reactive end of a reagent strip, allowed to stand for 3 minutes, and then washed off with 5–N sodium hydroxide (20 percent NaOH). The orange color that develops is compared to a color chart prepared from plasma standards of known glucose concentrations. The color change produced is permanent, and the reagent strip can be made part of the hospital record.

as a major guide in differentiating bacterial and viral infections. It also offers a good index of the severity of infection and the response to treatment: the lower the concentration the more severe the infection. However, in mild pyogenic meningitis spinal fluid sugar may be only slightly decreased or even normal. In overwhelming pneumococcal infection of the newborn, organisms may be present with neither cellular response nor decrease in glucose. On the other hand, there have been reports of lowered spinal fluid sugar in mumps meningoencephalitis.

In patients who respond to therapy, recovery from infection is accompanied by a prompt rise in the concentration of sugar to normal levels. However, in some young infants the sugar may not respond in this fashion; although the culture of the spinal fluid may be found to be sterile within 24 hours after therapy is started, the sugar concentration may continue below normal for several weeks or even longer. The blood sugar level is normal in these infants, and when the blood sugar is raised by intravenous injection of glucose the spinal fluid sugar concentration measured at varying intervals thereafter show some rise, but does not return to normal levels. These findings suggest that the infection has injured the transport mechanism. The cause for the low spinal fluid sugar in bacterial meningitis was initially attributed to utilization of glucose by the bacteria. This explanation is no longer accepted. On the basis of experimental data it has been postulated that the low spinal fluid sugar in bacterial meningitis results from a combination of increased cerebral glucose utilization secondary to increased glycolysis and a defective glucose transport mechanism.

CSF IN PARTIALLY TREATED BACTERIAL MENINGITIS. Antimicrobial therapy before diagnostic lumbar puncture may significantly alter the CSF findings and make it difficult to distinguish pyogenic from aseptic meningitis, especially if small doses have been given. As a rule, pretreatment with nonmeningitic doses of antibiotics does not affect all components of the CSF simultaneously. However, ranges of CSF cytology, sugar, and protein sometimes overlap sufficiently to make absolute certitude impossible. Several procedures have been developed that may be diagnostically helpful in such instances. Determination of CSF lactic dehydrogenase activity and isoenzyme analysis permit differentiation of bacterial and nonbacterial central nervous system infections even after pretreatment with antibiotics. The *Limulus* lysate test is said to be a reliable method to establish the bacterial etiology of a questionable spinal fluid. Finally, data have been presented suggesting that specific capsular antigen of *H. influenzae* type B, *D. pneumoniae*, and *N. meningitidis* can be identified by countercurrent immunoelectrophoresis (CIE), even when only minute amounts are present. The latter test is specific and inexpensive and is easy to perform, but it requires high titer of specific antisera.

TREATMENT. The application of the following principles will increase the probability of complete recovery in patients suffering from the common varieties of pyogenic meningitis: (1) prompt identification of the infecting organism, (2) early intravenous administration of antibacterial therapy, (3) adoption of a therapeutic program designed for both rapid destruction of bacteria and suppression of emergence of resistant strains, (4) avoidance of toxic therapeutic agents, and

TABLE 8. Recommended Treatment for Pyogenic Meningitis

Organism	Drug	Initial Dose	Maintenance
Undetermined etiology	Chloramphenicol succinate and	25 mg/kg, iv	100 mg/kg/day, iv, divided into 3 to 4 doses
> 2 months of age	Sodium penicillin G	100,000 IU/kg, iv	300,000 IU/kg/day, iv, in 6 divided doses; duration of therapy 10 to 14 days
< 2 months of age	Gentamicin and	2 mg/kg, iv or im	7.5 mg/kg/day in 4 divided doses
	Ampicillin	150 mg/kg iv	400 mg/kg/day in 6 divided doses
Haemophilus influenzae	Chloramphenicol succinate	Premature: 10 mg/kg, iv

Full term < 1 week: 10 mg/kg, iv
Others: 25 mg/kg, iv | Premature infants (and full-term infants < 1 week old): 25 mg/kg/day, iv, in 3 divided doses
Full-term infants 1–4 weeks old: 75 mg/kg/day, iv, in 3 divided doses
> 4 weeks: 100 mg/kg/day, iv, in 3 divided doses; duration of therapy 10 to 14 days |
| *Neisseria meningitidis* | Penicillin | Sodium penicillin G: 100,000 IU/kg, iv | Sodium penicillin G: 300,000 IU/kg/day, iv, divided into 6 doses; duration of therapy 7 days |
| *Diplococcus pneumoniae* or β-hemolytic streptococci, group A or group B | Penicillin | Sodium penicillin G: 100,000 IU/kg, iv | Sodium penicillin G: 300,000 IU/kg/day, iv, divided into 6 doses; duration of therapy at least 10 days after spinal fluid is sterile and patient is clinically well |

TABLE 8. Recommended Treatment for Pyogenic Meningitis (cont.)

Organism	Drug	Initial Dose	Maintenance
Escherichia coli	Gentamicin	2 mg/kg, iv and intrathecally or into ventricle* (in 0.85% NaCl solution): < 2 years: 1.0 mg; > 2 years: 2.0 mg	7.5 mg/kg/day, iv, in 4 divided doses; intrathecal or intraventricular dose: once daily for first 3 days, then once every other day;* duration of therapy: iv therapy is continued at least 14 days after child is clinically well and spinal fluid is normal, except for moderate lymphocytosis
Staphylococcus aureus	(a) Methicillin and (b) Penicillin	(a) Methicillin: 150 mg/kg, iv in 3–4 ml/kg of saline over 30 minutes and (b) Sodium penicillin G: iv in 30 minutes in 50 ml/m² of saline < 1 year: 100,000 IU/kg 1–6 years: 1,200,000 IU 6–12 years: 2,500,000 IU	(a) Methicillin: iv: 400 mg/kg/day in 6 divided doses for a minimum of 14 days after spinal fluid is sterile; po: cloxacillin, 300 mg/kg in 4 divided doses for 14 days more or (b) Sodium penicillin G if organism is sensitive to penicillin: iv: Dosage same as for *N. meningitidis*; duration: 14 days after spinal fluid is sterile, then if all clinical signs of disease have been absent for several days change to: po: penicillin V for 14 days more: < 12 years: 90,000 IU/kg/24 hours, given in 6 divided doses; > 12 years: 6,000,000 IU/24 hours, given in 6 divided doses, duration of therapy minimum 28 days
Salmonella	Chloramphenicol	Chloramphenicol succinate: premature and full-term infant < 1 week old: 10 mg/kg, iv; all others: 25 mg/kg, iv	Chloramphenicol succinate: iv: premature infant and full-term infant < 1 week old: 25 mg/kg/day, iv in 3 divided doses; full-term infant 1–4 weeks old: 75 mg/kg/day, iv, in 3 divided doses; 4 weeks old: 100 mg/kg/day, iv, in 3 divided doses; duration of iv therapy: at least 14 days after spinal fluid is sterile.
Pseudomonas aeruginosa (Bacillus pyocyaneus)	Gentamicin	Gentamicin: iv: 2.5 mg/kg; intrathecally or into ventricle (in 0.85% NaCl solution): < 2 years: 1.0 mg; > 2 years: 2.0 mg	Gentamicin: iv: 7.5 mg/kg/day in 4 divided doses; intrathecally or into ventricle: (in 0.85% NaCl solution): < 2 years: 1.0 mg/day > 2 years: 2.0 mg/day; duration of therapy: iv or im antibiotics are continued 14 days minimum after child is clinically well and spinal fluid is normal (except for moderate lymphocytosis); intrathecal therapy is given once daily for 3 days, then every other day until spinal fluid is normal

* It is not clear that intrathecal therapy has improved outcome. It has recently been shown that intrathecal administration does not permit the drug to enter the ventricular system, and death due to ventriculitis may result. Hence some authors now place antibiotic directly into a ventricle; results seem to be improved by this procedure.

(5) recognition and treatment of hyponatremia. Dosage and route of administration must be planned to attain maximal effective concentrations in the spinal fluid as promptly as possible and to maintain these levels until viable organisms are eliminated. Antibiotics such as penicillin G, the semisynthetic penicillins including ampicillin and kanamycin, diffuse poorly into the spinal fluid if the meninges are intact. Passage of most antibiotics with a high blood-brain barrier (ie, those that cross the blood-brain barrier with difficulty) becomes significantly greater when the meninges are inflamed. In the case of penicillin, because of its relatively low toxicity, the limited diffusion can be overcome by using very large doses intravenously. A daily dose of 200,000 to 400,000 IU/kg body weight is required. Under these circumstances the concentration of the antimicrobial agent in the spinal fluid becomes bactericidal for organisms such as pneumococci, meningococci, and hemolytic streptococci.

The therapeutic programs that may be used for the most frequently occurring varieties of pyogenic meningitis are outlined in Table 8. It is often impossible, even for a competent microbiologist, to identify the etiologic agent by direct microscopic examination of the spinal fluid. Since the pathogenic organism can be identified with absolute certainty only by culture, the initial therapeutic program in meningeal infections should be one that is as effective as possible against *all* the most common etiologic agents. Such a treatment regimen is outlined under the heading Undetermined Etiology in Table 8. Once the culture demonstrates the causative organism, the therapeutic program can be adjusted accordingly. Otherwise the initial therapy is continued.

All patients with pyogenic meningitis are best treated with antibacterial agents *by continued intravenous route* for at least 10 to 14 days—longer if the patient remains febrile or even mildly symptomatic. Treatment of meningococcal meningitis can be discontinued earlier, usually after 7 days if the patient is clinically well and the spinal fluid is completely normal.

During the past few years strains of *H. influenzae* type B that are resistant to ampicillin have been isolated from blood and spinal fluid of children with meningitis; such organisms have been reported from at least 26 states (June, 1975). The percentage of the strains of *H. influenzae* that are resistant to ampicillin is not known, but the result of treating such a strain with ampicillin would be so disastrous that this drug should not be used for initial treatment of *H. influenzae*. It is therefore necessary to start therapy with chloramphenicol (100 mg/kg/day in four divided doses), to which no *H. influenzae* strains have been found to be resistant, until there is proof beyond any doubt that *H. influenzae* is sensitive to ampicillin.

The *intrathecal route* is seldom needed. The intravenous administration of appropriate antibiotics at dosages that are both safe and effective permits adequate concentrations to be attained within the cerebrospinal fluid within 1 hour after institution of therapy. Intrathecal administration of antibiotics is used by some pediatricians in treating meningitis due to *E. coli, P. aeruginosa*, and other enteric organisms, but it is difficult to determine the value of this procedure.

The effectiveness of antimicrobial therapy will be reflected in the findings of the spinal fluid collected 24 hours following institution of therapy. With good response to treatment the spinal fluid should be bacteriologically negative on direct stained smear and on culture; the glucose content should be increased, and the cytology should show a marked shift from polymorphonuclear to mononuclear predominance. Total cell count and protein concentration may show initial rises. A repeat lumbar puncture after 24 hours of therapy is desirable in all instances where the initial response to treatment is not satisfactorily dramatic. We strongly recommend that in every patient with pyogenic meningitis the spinal fluid be examined again on the day therapy is discontinued. Treatment should not be terminated unless the spinal fluid findings are negative, except for the persistence of a lymphocyte count of less than 20/mm^3.

HYPONATREMIA. Severe hyponatremia accompanied by symptoms and signs of water intoxication may develop in the course of acute infections of the central nervous system. The hyponatremia of meningitis appears to be the result of inappropriate antidiuretic hormone secretion with ensuing water retention and to some extent losses of sodium in the urine. To prevent water intoxication, limitation of fluid intake during the acute phase of the illness is mandatory. Both the antibiotics and the daily requirements in electrolytes should be given in the smallest total amount of water possible. A total daily intake of approximately 1,000 to 1,200 ml/m^2 appears to be both safe and adequate. To achieve simultaneously the desired fluid restriction and the sodium intake required, the antibiotics administered intravenously may be dissolved in a mixture consisting of equal parts of 0.166-M sodium bicarbonate or lactate, normal saline, and 10 percent glucose. Subsequently the sodium content of the solution may be reduced by using 1 part 0.166-M sodium lactate, 2 parts normal saline, and 3 parts 10 percent glucose. In the presence of severe symptoms of water intoxication, especially when convulsions occur, the patient requires treatment with hypertonic fluids: administration of approximately 3 mEq of sodium chloride per kilogram, or 0.6 ml of 3 percent NaCl solution per kilogram, given over a period of 2 hours appears to be both safe and effective.

SHOCK. Adrenal corticosteroids have been advocated as adjuncts to the antibacterial treatment of bacterial meningitis. Controlled trials with both small and large doses of corticosteroid have failed to demonstrate any significant benificial effect of steroid therapy. When shock is present, hydrocortisone in large doses should be given intravenously in combination with plasma. This recommendation is not based on the belief that meningococcemia and other severe bacterial infections cause a decrease in adrenal corticosteroid production; in fact, available data indicate that patients with severe and even fulminant meningococcemia, but without adrenal hemorrhage, may have normal or high levels of cortisol in the blood. Migeon has shown that fulminant meningococcemia with adrenal hemorrhage results in failure of adrenal function, and he has concluded that such patients may require hormonal replacement therapy.

Shock due to bacterial endotoxins is due primarily to adverse effects on the circulation, with intravascular coagulation playing a role in some cases. These endotoxins produce at first prolonged vasoconstriction of arteries, arterioles, veins, venules, and capillaries. Vasodilation of arteries, arterioles, capillaries, and venules follows; the veins remain constricted. Blood pressure falls and blood flow to vital organs is diminished. Venous return to the heart is reduced, and cardiac output falls. Fluid goes from the capillaries into the tissues, decreasing the volume of circulating blood. When shock is severe or prolonged, it may become irreversible.

Results of experimental data in animals and reports of beneficial effects in humans suggest that hydrocortisone in large doses of 25 to 50 mg/kg given intravenously in a single injection counteracts the vasoconstricting effects of the endotoxin and effectively relieves the shock. This therapy may be repeated in 1 or 2 hours, if indicated. Epinephrine and norepinephrine are contraindicated in the treatment of endotoxic shock, since they only add to the vasoconstriction and decreased blood flow.

ADDITIONAL THERAPEUTIC MEASURES. Antipyretic medications are usually unnecessary. For marked hyperpyrexia, sponging with tepid water will help to reduce the body temperature. In the acutely ill patient excessive temperature elevations may be forestalled by maintaining the patient in a cooled croupette tent.

The effect produced by intravenous mannitol, or dexamethasone on the brain swelling of purulent meningitis is in general not as impressive as when the cerebral edema is associated with brain tumor, toxic encephalopathy, or cerebral trauma. However, dramatic improvement has occurred on occasion after administration of mannitol in meningitis. Consequently the use of mannitol is warranted in instances where the cerebral edema is progressing rapidly with signs of impending brainstem herniation, manifested by fixed pupils, disappearance of the doll's eyes phenomenon, decerebrate posturing or total flaccidity, and deteriorating respirations. This osmotic agent may be given intravenously over a 30-minute period: as a 10 to 15 percent solution at 1.0 to 2.0 g/kg body weight. Less rebound occurs with mannitol than with urea. If dexamethasone is used the dose is initially 0.2 to 0.4 mg/kg intravenously, followed by 0.1 to 0.2 mg/kg intramuscularly every 6 hours.

Heparin therapy has been recommended for the treatment of diffuse intravascular clotting associated with fulminant meningococcemia. The results have not been as encouraging as originally hoped, and its use has been abandoned pending further studies.

Convulsions, which frequently complicate the course of pyogenic meningitis, must be treated with appropriate anticonvulsive therapy (p. 1848) and careful positioning of the patient to prevent aspiration. Phenobarbital alone or in combination with diphenylhydantoin, diphenylhydantoin alone, rectal paraldehyde, or Valium is usually effective in controlling the seizures. Once controlled, diphenylhydantoin should be continued by oral or intramuscular route throughout the entire illness.

In infants and children who appear seriously ill, we institute anticonvulsive therapy from the time of admission as a preventive measure. After an initial dose of phenobarbital combined with diphenylhydantoin, each at a dose of 5 mg/kg, the patient is continued on maintenance therapy with diphenylhydantoin alone, as during the acute phase of the illness. Whenever seizures appear during the course of the meningitis, water intoxication and subdural effusion should be suspected, and subdural taps are advisable, even on the first hospital day.

SUBDURAL EFFUSIONS COMPLICATING MENINGITIS. The frequency of subdural effusions in the course of pyogenic meningitis was first pointed out by McKay and associates. Subsequent investigators have confirmed the high incidence of this complication, approaching 50 percent in young infants in whom the subdural space is explored routinely. Recovery of 2 ml or more of xanthochromic fluid with a protein content exceeding by 40 mg that of the spinal fluid is considered to indicate subdural effusion. The subdural fluid may be sterile and indistinguishable from that found in the later stages of a chronic subdural hematoma or it may be purulent and yield on culture the same organism responsible for the meningitis.

Subdural effusions, which are extremely rare in meningococcal meningitis, most commonly accompany meningeal infections due to *H. influenzae* and *D. pneumoniae*. In several of our own patients with pyogenic meningitis, subdural empyema was present at the time of onset or within hours after the onset of symptoms. In all instances except one the patients were infants less than 4 months of age; organisms involved were, in order of frequency: *D. pneumoniae*, *Salmonella*, and β-hemolytic *Streptococcus*. Antibiotic levels determined on all fluids collected from the effusions consistently showed satisfactory levels.

The part played by subdural fluid collections in producing irreversible cerebral damage is a matter that has stimulated great interest. Clinical signs of cortical injury can be found in children in whom no subdural fluid has been found. The majority of patients in whom an abnormal volume of subdural fluid is obtained have no clinical signs of cerebral damage. They may show only prolongation of the febrile state, irritability, and failure to take adequate food, especially fluids, and some are troubled by repeated vomiting. Because of unwillingness to perform a burr hole operation as a routine procedure, the incidence of subdural fluid collections in children older than 1 year is not well established.

Any of the following signs or symptoms occuring in a patient with purulent meningitis is an indication to perform a subdural tap for the presence of fluid in the subdural space: a marked bulging of the fontanelle persisting after lumbar puncture; failure to show good clinical response despite 48 to 72 hours of adequate antimicrobial therapy; the presence of an area of erythema, edema, and local heat involving the region of the anterior fontanelle that may indicate a purulent subdural effusion; convulsions at any time in the course of meningitis; persistent vomiting recurring after initial clinical improvement; disturbances in auditory acuity; or changes in the optic disks. A rapid increase of head circumference on repeated measurements constitutes a highly suggestive clue, especially if associated with persistent or recurrent intracranial bruits. Transillumination of the skull, echoencephalography, electroencephalography, radionuclide imaging (using technetium) and computer-assisted-tomography (CAT scan) may be helpful in establishing the diagnosis.

Treatment consists of subdural taps through the coronal sutures, repeated on alternate days for 3 to 4 weeks. In the majority of cases the fluid ceases to reaccumulate, and no further treatment is necessary. If the fluid persists for a 3- to 4-week period despite repeated subdural paracentesis, surgical exploration may be indicated for possible removal of a membrane enclosing the subdural fluid.

PROGNOSIS. Prior to 1936, when the first sulfonamides became available, the most common varieties of meningeal infections were fatal, with the exception of meningococcal meningitis. Advances in antibacterial therapy have made possible the survival and complete recovery of a large proportion of affected children. Overall fatality rates range from 10 to 15 percent. Of the common types of purulent meningitides, *H. influenzae* infections in infants more than 1 year of age show the lowest fatality rate; mortality in influenzal meningitis occurs mainly in infants under 1 year of age. In pneumococcal meningitis the death rate exceeds 25 percent in infants under 1 year; it is lower in older infants and in children, but higher than in patients of a similar age group with *H. influenzae* meningitis. In meningococcal meningitis the highest mortality occurs in children with fulminant meningococcemia. The Waterhouse-Friderichsen syndrome is responsible for a 20 percent fatality rate in meningococcus infections. Mortality rates and subsequent disabilities are highest in the small infant; more than 65 percent of infants 1 month of age or less who develop pyogenic meningitis die. The higher porportion of deaths in those varieties of meningitides that are due to organisms other than *N. meningitidis, H. influenzae,* and *D. pneumoniae* is in part a reflection of the high incidence of such infections in very young infants in whom the diagnosis has been delayed.

Accurate estimates of residual handicaps following pyogenic meningitis are not readily available, and the relative frequency with which these handicaps may be anticipated has not been well defined. At least 10 to 15 percent of the surviving patients show persistent neurologic sequelae, including cerebral damage, hydrocephalus, motor deficits, spastic hemiplegia, visual or auditory impairment, vestibular damage, seizure states, mental retardation, hyperactivity, and inability to learn. Hydrocephalus, a dreaded complication due to inflammatory obstruction of the various pathways of cerebrospinal fluid circulation, is encountered primarily in young infants in whom the infection is detected late, at a far-advanced stage of infection. The majority of children with neurologic sequelae are left with significant intellectual impairment; sometimes manifestations of residual damage are subtle and may consist of mild cerebral dysfunction, specific learning disabilities, and behavior problems.

An estimate of the fatality rate and the sequelae of *H. influenzae* meningitis was published by Mortimer in 1973. He estimated that there are about 10,000 cases of *H. influenzae* meningitis in the United States annually. About 8 percent of these patients die, a loss of 800 lives each year. Furthermore, about 35 percent of the approximately 9,200 survivors (some 3,200 children) of an attack of *H. influenzae* meningitis are incapacitated for life or have serious and permanent sensory or neuromotor residua.

PROPHYLAXIS OF HOUSEHOLD CONTACTS.
Prophylactic chemotherapy is not required for household contacts of patients with meningitis due to *D. pneumoniae.* In the usual circumstances this is also true for contacts of infants and young children with *H. influenzae* meningitis. However, co-primary and secondary cases of meningitis are not uncommon among household contacts of patients with meningococcal meningitis. In one epidemic of type A meningococcal meningitis 11 percent of cases were found to be co-primary or secondary household contact cases. Furthermore, the percentage of carriers of virulent meningococci in the family of a patient with meningitis is very high. For these reasons prophylactic treatment of all household contacts would seem to be warranted. Sulfonamides were very effective for this purpose before the emergence of strains of meningococci that are resistant to these drugs. At present they cannot be relied upon to prevent meningococcal infection or meningitis, unless it is known that the infecting organism is sensitive to sulfonamides. Rifampin alone or rifampin combined with minocycline has been used for reducing the nasal carrier rate with very good results. In one series a combination of the two drugs reduced the nasal carrier rate to zero, and this rate persisted for at least 2 weeks after the drugs were discontinued. However, both these drugs may produce toxic symptoms (especiallly minocycline), and there is not sufficient proof of their effectiveness in preventing meningitis among exposed children to judge their true value for this purpose. In fact, at least one case of failure of rifampin to prevent meningococcal meningitis has been reported. Oxytetracyclines, erythromycin, and ampicillin are not effective as prophylactic agents against meningococcal disease. Also, secondary cases of meningococcal meningitis occurred in families who received phenoxymethylpenicillin or benzylpenicillin orally for 4 days.

If it is known with certainty that the infecting meningococcus is sensitive, sulfonamide prophylaxis is the method of choice. It is clear that when penicillin G is given in small doses prophylactically it does not effectively prevent meningitis. However, it is a most effective curative drug when given in therapeutic dosage for a sufficient time. For this reason, when sulfonamide sensitivity has not been proved, the method recommended to prevent meningogoccal meningitis in family contacts is to use therapeutic doses of orally administered penicillin for 7 days. For an adolescent we give a daily dose of 8 to 10 million IU of penicillin G for 7 days. For younger children the dose is scaled down in proportion to body weight. If it is not possible to give a proportional oral dose of penicillin to a small child, procaine penicillin G may be given by intramuscular injection twice daily for a minimum of 5 days. An infant should receive 150,000 IU twice daily and older children 300,000 to 600,000 IU every 12 hours. The alternative procedure is to observe the exposed child at frequent intervals and to treat the child at once if any symptoms or signs suggestive of meningococcemia or meningitis develop.

School contacts of a patient with meningococcal meningitis ordinarily do not require antibacterial therapy. However, in epidemic situations such therapy may be indicated; the same considerations apply to physicians and nurses treating patients with meningococcal disease.

ACTIVE IMMUNIZATION. Vaccines have recently been licensed against diseases caused by *N. meningitidis* serogroups A and C, prepared either as monovalent or bivalent antigens. The antigens consist of purified bacterial cell wall polysaccharides. Adverse reactions are mild and infrequent. The duration of immunity conferred by these vaccines is still unknown, and the vaccine does not appear to be effective in children less than 2 years of age. In the United States these vaccines have been used chiefly in military populations. As more information accumulates, use of these vaccines may increase in an effort to control outbreaks of disease caused by *N. meningitidis* serogroups A and C and for persons traveling into epidemic areas. Vaccines may also prove to be useful in conjunction with chemoprophylaxis for household contacts of a patient with meningococcal meningitis. At present, release of these vaccines for epidemic control requires consultation with the Center for Disease Control in Atlanta, Georgia.

Because of the serious nature of *H. influenzae* meningitis, clinical trials are now under way that are testing two methods of active immunization of very young infants. Two vaccination methods are being studied. David H. Smith and colleagues are immunizing children by intramuscular injection of polyribophosphate, the capsular antigen of *H. influenzae* type B. John H. Robbins and associates are attempting to produce active and permanent protection against *H. influenzae* meningitis by feeding children strains of *E. coli* organisms that have antigens that react with antibodies made against the capsular carbohydrate antigen of type B *H. influenzae*. If these nonpathogenic *E. coli* establish themselves in the intestine, it is very likely that they will induce antibodies that will be effective against the capsular antigen of type B *H. influenzae*.

References

Barrett FF, Eardley WA, Yow MD, Leverett HA: Ampicillin in suppurative meningitis. J Pediatr 69:343, 1966

Balagtos RC, Levin S, Nelson KE, Gotoff S: Secondary and prolonged fevers in bacterial meningitis. J Pediatr 77:957, 1970

Bell WE, McCormick WF: Neurologic Infections in Children. Philadelphia, WB Saunders, 1975

Bland RD, Lister RC, Ries JP: Cerebrospinal fluid lactic acid level and pH in meningitis. Am J Dis Child 128:151, 1974

Center for Disease Control: Morbidity and mortality. Weekly report for week ending June 14, 1975. Atlanta, CDC. 24:205, 1975

Coonrod JD, Rytel MW: Determination of aetiology of bacterial meningitis by counter-immunoelectrophoresis. Lancet 1:1154, 1972

Dodge PR, Swartz MN: Bacterial meningitis. A review of selected aspects: II. Special neurologic problems, postmeningitic complications and clinicopathological correlations. N Engl J Med 272:954, 1003, 1965

Eickholf TC, Finland M: Changing susceptibility of meningococci to antimicrobial agents. N Engl J Med 272:395, 1965

Fine RN, Kurtz HM, Krieger G: Hemophilus influenzae type A meningitis. J Pediatr 70:962, 1967

Gitlin D: Pathogenesis of subdural collections of fluid. Pediatrics 16:354, 1955

Haggerty RJ, Ziai M: Acute bacterial meningitis. Adv Pediatr 13:129, 1964

Hitchcock E, Andreadis A: Subdural empyema: a review of 29 cases. J Neurol Neurosurg Psychiatry 27:422, 1964

Ingram DL, Anderson P, Smith DH: Countercurrent immunoelectrophoresis in the diagnosis of systemic diseases caused by Hemophilus influenzae type b. Pediatrics 81:1156, 1972

Lazarus JM, Sellers DP, Marine WM: Brief recordings: Meningitis due to the group B beta-hemolytic streptococcus. N Engl J Med 272:146, 1965

Leedom JM, Ivler D, Mathies AW: Importance of sulfadiazine resistance in meningococcal disease in civilians. N Engl J Med 273:1395, 1965

Lewin EB: Partially treated meningitis. Am J Dis Child 128:145, 1974

Mace JW, Peters ER, Mathies Jr. AW: Cranial bruits in purulent meningitis in childhood. N Engl J Med 278:1420, 1968

Mangos JA, Lobeck CC: Sustained hyponatremia in nervous system infections. Pediatrics 34:503, 1964

McCracken GH, Eichenwald HF: Antimicrobial therapy. J Pediatr 85:297, 451, 1974

McGee EE, Canthen JC, Brackett CE: Meningitis following acute traumatic cerebrospinal fistula. J Neurosurg 33:312, 1970

Menkes JH: Causes for low spinal fluid sugar in bacterial meningitis: another look. Pediatrics 44:1, 1969

Migeon CJ Kenny FM, Hung W: Adrenal function in meningitis. Pediatrics 40:163, 1967

Mortimer EA Jr: Immunization against Hemophilus influenzae. Pediatrics 52:633, 1973

Murray JD, Fleming PC, Anglin CS: Acute bacterial meningitis in childhood. Clin Pediatr 11:455, 1972

Nachum R, Lipsey A, Siegel SE: Rapid detection of gram-negative bacterial meningitis by the Limulus lysate test. N Engl J Med 289:931, 1973

Overall JC: Neonatal bacterial meningitis. J Pediatr 76:499, 1970

Robinson MG, Watson RJ: Pneumococcal meningitis in sickle-cell anemia. N Engl J Med 274:1006, 1966

Smith DH, Peter G, Ingram DL: Responses of children immunized with the capsular polysaccharide of Hemophilus influenzae Type b. Pediatrics 52:637, 1973

Smith M: Acute bacterial meningitis. Pediatrics 17:285, 1956

Stiehm ER: Factors in the prognosis of meningococcal infections. J Pediatr 68:457, 1966

——— Neonatal meningococcal meningitis. J Pediatr 68:654, 1966

Swartz MN, Dodge PR: Bacterial meningitis—a review of selected aspects. I. General clinical features, special problems and unusual meningeal reactions mimicking bacterial meningitis. N Engl J Med 272:725, 779, 842, 898, 1965

Wehrle PF, Mathies AW, Leedom JM: Acute bacterial meningitis. In Smith CA (ed): The Critically Ill Child. Philadelphia, WB Saunders, 1975

Whitecar JP: Recurrent pneumococcal meningitis. N Engl J Med 274:1285, 1966

Williams RDB: Alterations in glucose transport mechanism in patients with complications of bacterial meningitis. Pediatrics 34:491, 1964

BOTULISM

ALEX J. STEIGMAN

Botulism results from the ingestion of foods in which *Clostridium botulinum* has grown and produced a deadly neurotoxin. Although it is an intoxication rather than an infectious disease, outbreaks of varying size are the rule rather than the exception. Because prompt recognition of this uncommon disorder may be life-saving, constant awareness of the threat of botulism is mandatory. Circumscribed outbreaks within a family unit or its neighbors usually result from foods improperly prepared in the home. Common home-prepared foods, as well as such exotica as fermented beaver tail and seal meat in Alaska, have caused this disease. A wide variety of commercially prepared foods have produced scattered cases. *Wound botulism* is a problem in which neurophysiologic disturbances and clinical symptoms are similar to those of botulism by ingestion. However, the appearance of symptoms may be delayed for several days or a week or more after the injury. Crushing injuries, compound fractures, and similar injuries occurring where contamination with anaerobes in the soil is possible should especially be suspected.

ORGANISM AND TOXIN. *C. botulinum* is an anaerobic or microaerophilic gram-positive spore-producing rod. Its worldwide natural habitat is soil, both inland and at the shores of bodies of fresh or salt water. *C. botulinum* is classified into types A, B, C, D, E, and F according to the immunologic specificities of the toxins each produces. Man is affected principally by types A, B, and E and more rarely by type F. The toxic effects arise at the myoneural junction, presumably by preventing the release of acetylcholine from the demyelinated ends of cholinergic nerves. Peripheral adrenergic nerves are not affected. There is no known pharmacologic antagonist. Type-specific or polyvalent therapeutic antitoxin is the only available direct antagonist for the toxins.

The spores can survive cold temperatures for some months and can withstand boiling for several hours; they can be destroyed at 120 C in 30 minutes. When spores germinate they produce toxin over a wide range of temperatures, extending as low as 6 C. Optimum production of toxin occurs at about 30 C. Once toxin is formed it is relatively thermolabile; it can be inactivated in food if boiled (100 C) for 10 minutes or heated at 80 C for 30 minutes. A pentavalent toxoid can be prepared for active immunization of individuals at high risk, such as special laboratory workers engaged in germ-warfare projects. There is no cross-protection among the several types. On recovery from botulism, patients are again fully susceptible to the disease, since botulism is an intoxication rather than an infection.

FOOD SOURCES. Fruits, vegetables, meats, freshwater and saltwater fish, and the products derived from these foods, whether prepared at home or commercially, have all been involved. These foods that have caused botulism have variously been prepared as soups, juices, pickles, salads, stews, or meat or fish pastes or spreads; they may have been smoked, salted, spiced, air dried, cured by hanging, or vacuum packed in cellophane bags. These foods need not have been stored for long periods in order to cause botulism; rapid toxin formation may occur in fresh fruits and gutted fish exposed to insufficient heat and provided with vacuum or anaerobic conditions. The spores may survive several hours at 100 C; there is some variation in strains. Generally speaking, outbreaks due to home-prepared items are restricted to the family and neighbors. Contaminated commercially prepared foods marketed on a large scale by modern distribution methods have caused scattered outbreaks. The common source may go unrecognized for a time, with tragic delay in establishing treatment and control. Unfortunately, the foods involved often have not undergone accompanying proteolytic changes from other bacteria; consequently they may have no offensive taste or odor to serve as a warning or as a clue when a mysterious illness appears in a family or group. It may take the illness of a second or third patient in an outbreak to raise the suspicion of botulism.

CLINICAL OUTCOME. The clinical outcome in exposed persons depends on several factors, including the amount of ingested toxin, the speed of onset of symptoms, the serotype of *C. botulinum* toxin involved, and especially the promptness of diagnosis and treatment. Not all persons react similarly to the ingestion of a given amount of toxin, which may be because of the amount of trypsin in the stomach and the pH of the stomach at the time of ingestion. In experimental animals the effects of type E toxin have been shown to be markedly potentiated in the presence of trypsin and a slightly acid pH. Also, there may be genetically determined biochemical differences among individuals in the effects of toxin on the myoneural junction.

CLINICAL PICTURE. Several hours to several days may elapse after ingestion of toxin before symptoms appear. In wound botulism there may be a delay ranging from days to a week or more. Symptoms due to failure of acetycholine release at the myoneural junctions include nausea, vomiting, blurred vision, lassitude, vertigo, diplopia, dry mouth, and abdominal fullness. Unexplained cranial nerve weakness should arouse immediate suspicion. With progression there is weakness and paralysis leading to dysphonia, dysphagia, urinary retention, and labored breathing. On physical examination patients are usually afebrile and mentally alert, and deep tendon reflexes are preserved despite the weakness. The pupils are large and respond sluggishly. The mouth and tongue are dry; the abdomen is distended. Objective sensory disturbance does not occur.

AIDS TO DIAGNOSIS. Blood counts, urinalyses, chemical examination of the blood and spinal fluid, and cultures of stools or gastric contents are not helpful in diagnosis. Toxin may be demonstrable in the patient's blood. When suspected foods are still available, mouse inoculation under appropriate conditions may verify existence of the toxin and its specific type. It is also possible to identify *C. botulinum* from the suspected food or wound by anaerobic culture. The chief aid to diagnosis is awareness of the fact that the patient is in a suitable setting for botulism. In locally confined outbreaks, knowledge of the patient's having attended a wedding, party, or picnic, together with knowledge of a similar mysterious illness in an index case, helps to sound the alarm. Poliomyelitis, tick-bite paralysis, myasthenia gravis, accidental ingestion of psychotropic medication by toddlers, small bowel obstruction, labyrinthitis, behavior disturbances attributed to the animation and excitement of a party or celebration, and other mistaken diagnoses have understandably been considered in the first patient in an outbreak of botulism.

MANAGEMENT.   The chief purpose of therapy is to avoid respiratory failure. Emergency facilities must be at hand for tracheostomy or tracheal intubation, together with mechanically assisted ventilation, which should be used before there are signs of advanced fatigue or exhaustion. Because some toxin may remain unabsorbed in the bowel, cleaning enemas are recommended. Antitoxin to be given intravenously should be obtained as rapidly as possible. Ideally, antitoxin specific for the toxin type involved should be given; however, the type is seldom known initially. When a mass-produced commercial product is suspected, steps should be taken to advise the public and to impound the product. Suspicious wounds should be surgically explored. For some time it was believed that only types A and B occurred with any degree of frequency in the United States, but types E and F have also been encountered.

Bivalent (A and B) botulism antitoxin is prepared by Lederle Laboratories, whose regional distribution centers can expedite delivery. Monovalent (E) antitoxin prepared by Connaught Laboratories in Canada is licensed for use in the United States and may be obtained at all times by telephoning the Center for Disease Control in Atlanta, Georgia: (404) 633-3311 or (404) 633-2176. Polyvalent (ABEF) antitoxin is prepared in Denmark by the State Serum Institute. Although it is not licensed for use in the United States, a supply is on hand at the Center for Disease Control. Since these antitoxins are of equine origin, preliminary skin tests for sensitivity are essential. Sensitive individuals must be desensitized prior to therapy. A single large intravenous dose is recommended rather than several daily doses. The dose for the bivalent and polyvalent antitoxins is 100,000 IU or more and for the monovalent type E, 10,000 to 20,000 IU.

References

Center for Disease Control: Botulism in the United States, 1899–1973. Handbook for Epidemiologists, Clinicians, and Laboratory Workers Atlanta, CDC, 1974
Center for Disease Control: Surveillance summary of Botulism USA, 1974. Morbidity and Mortality Weekly Report, Atlanta, CDC. 24:39, 1975

BRUCELLOSIS
James B. Brayton

Brucellosis is an infectious disease due to organisms belonging to the genus *Brucella* that are transmitted to man from animals. Brucellosis in man may be acute or chronic and may be caused by any of four species of *Brucella.* Swine, cattle, goats, sheep, and dogs are the most frequent sources of infection. Strains of *Brucella* have been isolated from deer, elk, moose, water buffalo, camel, bison, fowl, jackrabbit, ground squirrel, squirrel, wild rat, and field mouse. Infection in man may also occur without clinical illness.

In the latter part of the nineteenth century the febrile illness brucellosis was a puzzlement to the British military medical personnel stationed in the Mediterranean area. It appeared to be different from malaria or typhoid fever. Marston, a Royal Army surgeon, presented a report of his illness in 1863 that was an accurate clinical description of brucellosis. Sir David Bruce described the etiologic agent in 1887. Bang, in Denmark, reported in 1897 the recovery of another species, *B. abortus,* from aborting sows. The classic monograph, "Mediterranean, Malta or Undulant Fever," by Hughes, appeared in 1897. The epidemiology of brucellosis on the island of Malta was clearly defined by the reports of the Mediterranean Fever Commission issued between 1905 and 1907.

ETIOLOGY.   Brucellae are small gram-negative coccobacilli that are nonmotile and do not form spores. The four species described in human infections are *B. suis* (swine), *B. melitensis* (goats), *B. abortus* (cattle), and *B. canis* (dogs). Differentiation of the four species is based on biochemical reactions, serologic tests, and resistance of the organisms to the bacteriostatic actions of various dyes.

EPIDEMIOLOGY.   The natural reservoir of brucellosis is in domestic animals, especially swine, cattle, goats, and dogs. In animals the brucellae tend to localize more abundantly in the mammary gland and in the pregnant uterus. Large numbers of organisms may be shed in the milk of apparently healthy animals for months or years, and the disease may produce abortions in pregnant animals. Man contracts the disease by direct contact with infected animals or with contaminated secretions and excretions. Epidemiologic evidence has been presented that suggests infection by the aerosol route. Human infection also occurs through ingestion of raw milk, and cheese produced from unpasteurized milk has been linked to human illness. Canine infections with *B. canis* were first reported in 1966 and have subsequently been recognized as being widespread in the United States, particularly in field dogs. Two *B. canis* human infections were reported in 1973. Because *B. canis* antibody does not react with the *B. abortus* antigen used in febrile agglutinin testing, the incidence of human *B. canis* may be higher than the reported infections would indicate.

In 1973 there were 168 human cases of brucellosis reported to the Center for Disease Control; 31 percent of these patients reported contact with swine, 26 percent with cattle, and 26 percent with either swine or cattle. In 20 percent of the cases the most probable source of infection was considered to be ingestion of unpasteurized dairy products, the majority of which originated outside the United States. Brucellosis is still primarily an occupational disease of abattoir workers, livestock handlers, and veterinarians. One must also consider the ingestion of foreign dairy products and association with canine pets when considering the diagnosis of brucellosis.

The role of the brucellae as a cause of abortions in humans is unclear. Poole reported a case of a pregnant woman who contracted acute brucellosis (diagnosed by serologic methods) and subsequently aborted spontaneously; *B. abortus* was isolated from the amniotic fluid. Sarram studied 51 women with second-trimester abortion in a brucellosis-endemic area of Iran. Six of these women showed clinical and laboratory signs of brucellosis. In five of the six cases placental and/or fetal materials obtained from the products of abortion were culture-positive for *B. melitensis*.

PATHOGENESIS. The brucellae organisms are obligate intracellular parasites. After they enter the body they are phagocytized by monocytes and leukocytes, in which they multiply. The organisms are then disseminated to the reticuloendothelial system where they may persist for several months. They tend to localize particularly in the lymph nodes, bone marrow, spleen, and liver. Formation of tubercules or granulomas may occur, with foreign body giant cells and Langhans' giant cells. Sometimes the brucellae induce necrosis of tissues, and small abscesses may be seen. However, caseation is not a feature of brucellosis. Chronic brucellosis may involve the genitourinary organs, skin, brain, and kidneys.

CLINICAL FEATURES. The incubation period is usually between 5 and 30 days, but occasionally it may be as long as 6 months. Brucellosis may have an abrupt onset with chills, fever, and sweats; more characteristically the disease begins insidiously with vague symptoms. Table 9 lists the major symptoms of 146 cases in the United States during 1973. Contrary to classic descriptions, the temperature curve does not usually demonstrate the remittent or undulating type of fever. Fever, lymphadenopathy, splenomegaly, and hepatomegaly are the most consistent physical findings. Usually the total leukocyte count is normal or slightly depressed, and there is a relative lymphocytosis. In chronic brucellosis the findings may be localized to the long bones, genitalia, vertebral column, liver, spleen, or skin.

DIAGNOSIS. A history of animal contact or ingestion of unpasteurized dairy products may suggest brucellosis. Of the serologic tests, the standard tube agglutination test yields the most standardized results and is easily performed. A titer of 1:160 or higher is indicative of infection. Cross-reactions occur with *Francisella tularensis;* so both tests should be performed. Usually the titer to the infecting agent is higher. Vaccination against *Vibrio cholerae* may produce brucellae agglutination titers of 1:160 or higher up to 1 year following immunization. The definitive laboratory test for confirming a clinical diagnosis of brucellosis is a positive culture. The *Brucella* skin test offers no advantage

in the diagnosis of acute infections. The skin test itself may cause a fourfold rise in the agglutination titer. The skin test is most helpful in surveys to detect previous exposure to Brucella antigen after the agglutination test has become negative. This skin test remains positive long after exposure to the brucellae. The differential

TABLE 9. Human Brucellosis by Major Symptoms (146 Cases, United States, 1973)*

Symptom	Cases	Percentage
Fever		
Intermittent	110	75.3
Constant	17	11.7
Not specified	11	7.5
Total	138	94.5
Chills	103	70.5
Weakness	99	67.8
Body aches	98	67.1
Sweating	94	64.4
Malaise	88	60.3
Headache	76	52.1
Weight loss	69	47.3
Anorexia	62	42.5

* Includes confirmed and presumptive cases; adapted from Center for Disease Control: Burcellosis Surveillance. Washington DC, US DHEW, March, 1975, p 10.

diagnosis would include diseases associated with lymphadenopathy, lymphocytosis, hepatosplenomegaly, and granuloma. Lymphoma, tuberculosis, infectious mononucleosis, and toxoplasmosis should be considered.

PROGNOSIS. The mortality in 160 patients followed by Buchanan between 1960 and 1970 was nil; likewise, the complication rate was low (0.6 percent). He attributes these favorable findings to early diagnosis and treatment. Relapses of clinical illness do occur.

TREATMENT. Tetracyclines for 21 days in standard oral dosages are recommended. If relapse occurs, another 21-day course of oral tetracyclines with intramuscular streptomycin at 15 to 30 mg/kg/day is suggested. This daily dosage of streptomycin should be divided into two equal doses and given every 12 hours. The trimethoprim-sulfamethoxazole combination has also been shown to be clinically effective in acute brucellosis. Caution is advised when contemplating using the aforementioned drugs during pregnancy. Steroids may be necessary at the onset of therapy to reduce the risk of a Herxheimer reaction.

Avoidance of animal contacts and exposure to brucellae are important in prevention. Likewise, elimination of animal reservoirs and immunization among the natural animal reservoirs are essential. Avoidance of ingestion of unpasteurized dairy products is also important. The significance of canine brucellosis for human infections has not yet been established.

References

Buchanan TM, Faber LC, Feldman RA: Brucellosis in the United States, 1960–1972: an abattoir-associated disease. Clinical features and therapy. Medicine 53:403, 1974

Center for Disease Control: Brucellosis surveillance. Washington DC, US DHEW, 1975, p 10

Daikos GK, Papapolyzos N, Marketos N, et al: Trimethoprim-sulfamethoxazole in brucellosis. J Infect Dis 128 [Suppl]:S731, 1973

Robertson L, Farrell ID, Hinchliffe PM: The sensitivity of brucella abortus to chemotherapeutic agents. J Med Microbiol 6:549, 1973

Serram M, Feiz J, Foruzandeh M, Gazanfarpour P: Intrauterine fetal infection with brucella melitensis as a possible cause of second-trimester abortion. Am J Obstet Gynecol 119:657, 1974

White PC, Baker EF, Roth AJ, Williams WJ, Stephens TS: Brucellosis in a Virginia meat-packing plant. Arch Environ Health 28:263, 1974

CHOLERA

CHARLES C. J. CARPENTER

Cholera is an acute illness caused by an enterotoxin elaborated by *Vibrio cholerae* that have colonized the small bowel. In its most severe form there is rapid loss of fluid and electrolytes from the gastrointestinal tract that results in hypovolemic shock and metabolic acidosis; if it is left untreated it can cause death.

ETIOLOGY. *V. cholerae* are short, curved gram-negative rods readily seen in gram-stained smears of the watery excreta of patients with cholera. Rapid presumptive diagnosis can be made either by fluorescence microscopy using fluorescein-labeled type-specific antibody or by a *Vibrio* immobilization test employing dark-field or phase microscopy and type-specific sera. *V. cholerae* grow rapidly on a number of selective media, including bile salt agar, glycerin/tellurite/taurocholate agar, and thiosulfate/citrate/bile salt/sucrose (TCBS) agar. On TCBS agar, vibrios can be distinguished from other enteric organisms by a distinct opaque yellow appearance. Distinction between the two major serotypes, Inaba and Ogawa, is made by slide agglutination with type-specific antisera. Identification of the El Tor biotype is important for epidemiologic purposes; it is distinguished from the classic biotype by its resistance to polymyxin B, by its resistance to Mukerjee's choleraphage type IV, and by causing hemolysis of sheep erythrocytes.

EPIDEMIOLOGY. For the past two centuries cholera has been endemic in the delta of the Ganges River, with annual epidemics in major population centers in West Bengal and Bangladesh. The disease has made periodic incursions into other portions of southern Asia and Southeast Asia and has given rise to seven major pandemics since 1832. Unlike its predecessors, the most recent pandemic (1962–1974) has thus far failed to reach the Western Hemisphere. Man is the only documented natural host and victim of *V. cholerae*, although a carrier state in other species remains a possibility. Several major epidemics have been waterborne, and water appears to play the major role in transmission of *V. cholerae* in endemic rural areas. However, during major epidemics, direct contamination of food with infected excreta may also be important. Individuals with mild or asymptomatic infections (contact carriers) play a major role in dissemination of epidemic disease. With infection by the El Tor *V. cholerae* biotype, which is responsible for the current pandemic spread of the disease, the ratio of asymptomatic infection to clinical disease may be higher than 10 to 1. A prolonged gall bladder carrier state may develop in 3 to 5 percent of adult patients convalescing from cholera, but this has never been observed in the pediatric age group. In the cholera-endemic areas of Bangladesh and West Bengal, cholera is predominantly a disease of children; attack rates are 10-fold greater in individuals below the age of 10 years than in those over the age of 20 years.

PATHOGENESIS AND PATHOLOGY. All signs, symptoms, and metabolic derangements in cholera result from the rapid loss of fluid and electrolytes from the gut. These losses result from increased secretion of isotonic fluids by all segments of the small bowel. The increased electrolyte secretion is caused by a heat-labile protein enterotoxin (molecular weight 84,000 daltons) that is elaborated by pathogenic strains of *V. cholerae*. The enterotoxin exerts its characteristic effect on electrolyte secretion without causing morphologic damage to the gut mucosa. The only consistent pathologic alterations in the gut during cholera are slight edema of the lamina propria and moderate dilatation of capillaries and lymphatics in the tips of villi. The cholera enterotoxin rapidly binds to the gut epithelial mucosal cells and causes, after a lag period of about 30 minutes, a prolonged increase in mucosal adenylcyclase activity. The resulting increase in intracellular cyclic adenosine 3',5'-monophosphate causes secretion of isotonic fluid by all segments of the small bowel. Precise studies have demonstrated that the pediatric cholera stool has sodium and chloride concentrations significantly less than those of plasma, a bicarbonate concentration approximately twice that of plasma, and a potassium concentration four to eight times that of plasma. The loss of large quantities of intestinal fluids thus leads to severe extracellular fluid depletion, with resultant hypovolemic shock, base deficit acidosis, and progressive potassium depletion. The cholera vibrios do not invade any tissue, nor has the enterotoxin been shown in the naturally occurring disease to have a direct effect on any organ other than the small intestine.

CLINICAL MANIFESTATIONS. The clinical onset of cholera is generally abrupt, painless, watery diarrhea. In severe cases 10 percent of the body weight may be lost within a few hours, leading rapidly to profound shock. At varying intervals after onset of diarrhea, vomiting may ensue; this is characteristically effortless and is not preceded by nausea. In the more severe cases muscle cramps are almost invariably present and commonly involve the calves. When first seen by the physician, the child who is severely ill with cholera is cyanotic and has sunken eyes and cheeks, scaphoid abdomen, poor skin turgor, and thready or absent peripheral pulses. The voice is high-pitched or inaudible; the vital signs include tachycardia, tachypnea, and low or unobtainable blood pressure. There may be either low-grade fever or slight hypothermia. The heart sounds are distant and often inaudible, and bowel sounds are usually hypoactive. Alterations in mental status are variable; the child often remains oriented, although apathetic, even in the face of severe hypovolemic shock. In all epidemics there are large numbers of mild cases in which fluid loss from the gut is not severe enough to require hospitalization. There are even larger numbers of completely asymptomatic people who transiently excrete *V. cholerae.*

Loss of fluid and electrolytes continues for 1 to 7 days, and subsequent manifestations depend on the adequacy of replacement therapy. With prompt fluid and electrolyte repletion, physiologic recovery is remarkably rapid and uniform despite continuing voluminous diarrhea. If therapy is inadequate the mortality rate in hospitalized cases may exceed 50 percent. The important causes of death are hypovolemic shock, uncompensated metabolic acidosis, and uremia. When renal failure occurs, the characteristic pathologic findings are those of acute tubular necrosis secondary to prolonged hypotension.

DIAGNOSIS. In endemic or epidemic areas the working diagnosis of cholera should be made on the basis of the clinical picture; fluid and electrolyte replacement therapy should be instituted immediately. Although a choleralike illness may be caused by microorganisms other than *V. cholerae,* the resulting physiologic and metabolic abnormalities are the same, so that identical intravenous and/or oral electrolyte therapy should be used in all such cases. Diagnostic culture techniques are relatively simple. A reliable and practical method consists of direct plating of feces on TCBS agar. Typical opaque yellow colonies appear in 18 hours. Final identification requires agglutination with group- and type-specific antisera and demonstration of characteristic biochemical reactions. Rapid tentative diagnosis may be made by direct observation of the characteristic rapid motility of the comma-shaped bacilli in fresh feces by dark-field microscopy. Group- and type-specific antisera will immobilize homologous strains and clearly distinguish them from other vibrios.

PROGNOSIS. With adequate therapy the mortality rate approaches zero. Largely because of the mechanical problems inherent in the administration of large amounts of fluid to small children, there is still a mortality rate of 1 to 2 percent in pediatric cases despite the best currently available therapy.

TREATMENT. Since all known signs, symptoms, and metabolic abnormalitites in cholera result directly from the fluid and electrolyte loss from the gut, the primary therapeutic principle is prompt replacement of the fluid and electrolyte losses. In addition, since eradication of *V. cholerae* from the gut reduces fluid losses by 50 to 70 percent in the average cholera case, antimicrobial therapy (with tetracycline, chloramphenicol, or furazolidone) is also an important part of therapy.

Several solutions have been widely and successfully used for the initial rehydration and for maintenance of electrolyte balance in children. Complications resulting from inappropriate hydration therapy, which will be discussed below, can be successfully prevented if the treatment is closely supervised by trained medical or paramedical personnel. An effective single intravenous replacement solution is NAMRU-2 solution, which contains the following concentrations of solutes: sodium, 90 mEq/liter, chloride 64 mEq/liter, potassium 15 mEq/liter, bicarbonate 45 mEq/liter (as acetate), calcium, 2 mEq/liter, magnesium 2 mEq/liter, and glucose 20 g/liter. This solution supplies adequate free water in addition to appropriate quantities of electrolytes. It also contains enough glucose to prevent the hypoglycemia that occasionally occurs in children with cholera. Trials with this solution have demonstrated its effectiveness in maintaining electrolyte balance. The most commonly available commercial solution for replacement of fluid loss in cholera is lactated Ringer's solution. When this solution is used in the treatment of cholera, both potassium and glucose supplementation should be given by mouth.

Determination of the appropriate volume and rate of fluid administration is of critical importance. As in adult patients, fluid requirements for children may be estimated clinically. For clinical evaluation the following guidelines are useful. Mild dehydration (slightly decreased skin turgor and tachycardia, but good peripheral pulse and normal sensorium) indicates an isotonic fluid deficit of about 5 percent of body weight. With moderate dehydration (marked decrease in skin turgor, tachycardia and hypotension, but normal sensorium) the fluid deficit is 6 to 10 percent of body weight. Severe dehydration (the above signs plus cyanosis, stupor or coma, and lack of peripheral pulses) is associated with a fluid deficit exceeding 10 percent of body weight. The initial estimated fluid deficit should be administered within 2 to 4 hours after initiation of therapy. The rate of infusion must be closely monitored to prevent overhydration, for the survival of the child with cholera is more dependent on continued close supervision than on the precise composition of the intravenous fluid. Attention must be directed especially to maintenance of adequate hydration (whether judged by clinical or laboratory parameters), to avoidance of overhydration (determined by auscultation of lungs and inspection of neck venous filling), and to providing free water, as needed, by the oral route (generally the patient's own thirst mechanism is a good guide to oral water requirements).

Complications are both more common and more serious in children that in adults. The most serious include pulmonary edema (often with superimposed pneumonia), stupor, coma and convulsions, and cardiac arrhythmias. Pulmonary edema may result from too rapid administration of the required intravenous fluids in the presence of severe metabolic acidosis and/or from administration of excessive quantities of intravenous fluids. Severe metabolic acidosis causes a shift of intravascular fluid from the systemic to the pulmonary circulation. Rapid administration of intravenous fluids before the metabolic acidosis has been corrected may cause pulmonary edema even in the absence of overt overhydration. Even after correction of acidosis, pulmonary edema occasionally occurs in children with cholera as the result of injudicious administration of too large a volume of intravenous fluids. Whereas they are exceedingly rare in adult cholera patients, stupor, coma, and convulsions may occur in up to 10 percent of small children. These central nervous system manifestations sometimes result from hypoglycemia, which can be avoided by intravenous administration of glucose. They may also be due to electrolyte imbalance or to cerebral edema related to overhydration.

The mean potassium concentration in the stools of children with cholera is higher than that of adults. The physiologic consequences of potassium depletion are more serious in the child than in the adult cholera patient. Serious arrhythmias, hypotension, and even cardiac arrest may occur in children with degrees of potassium depletion (15 to 20 percent of total body potassium) that are generally tolerated by the adult. Since the potassium deficit is rarely severe at the time the child arrives at a treatment center, the hypokalemia can be avoided by intravenous or oral administration of adequate quantities of potassium.

Oral replacement of water and electrolytes is consistently effective in children who are alert and able to retain fluids administered by mouth. Oral treatment has greatly reduced mortality from cholera during the most recent pandemic. A solution containing glucose 20 g/liter, sodium bicarbonate 4 g/liter, sodium chloride 4 g/liter, and potassium chloride 1.5 g/liter has proved to be consistently effective. This solution, administered orally at a rate equal to stool losses, can be given to mild cholera cases throughout the course of illness, and it is also satisfactory in the more severe cases once the hypovolemic shock has been corrected by initial rapid intravenous fluid therapy. Successful management of the child with oral therapy requires just as close supervision as does management with intravenous solutions, with careful monitoring of pulse, skin turgor, and neck veins. Supplemental intravenous fluids must be administered whenever clinical signs of saline depletion recur.

Immunization with two injections of the standard commercial vaccine (containing 10 billion killed *V. cholerae* per milliliter) provides significant (60 to 70 percent) protection to children for the relatively short period of 4 to 6 months. At present, careful hygiene is the only sure protection against cholera.

References

Carpenter CCJ, Greenough WB, Gordon RS: Pathogenesis and patho-physiology of cholera. In Barua D, Burrows W (eds): Cholera. Philadelphia, WB Saunders, 1974

Guttman RA, Dratz DJ, Whalen GE, Watten RH: Double blind fluid therapy evaluation in pediatric cholera. Pediatrics 44:922, 1969

Lindenbaum J, Akbar R, Gordon RS, et al: Cholera in children. Lancet 1:1066, 1966

Mahalanabis D, Choudhuri AB, Bagehi NG, Bhattacharya AK, Simpson TW: Oral fluid therapy of cholera among Bangladesh refugees. Johns Hopkins Med J 132:97, 1973

Mahalanabis D, Watten RH, Wallace CK: Clinical aspects and management of pediatric cholera. In Barua D, Burrows W (eds): Cholera. Philadelphia, WB Saunders, 1974

Mosley WH: The role of immunity in cholera. A review of epidemiological and serological studies. Tex Rep Biol Med 27:227, 1969

Pierce NF, Sack RB, Mitra RC, et al: Replacement of water and electrolyte losses in cholera by an oral glucose-electrolyte solution. Ann Intern Med 70:1173, 1969

DIPHTHERIA

HORACE L. HODES

Diphtheria is a specific infectious disease caused by a toxin-producing organism, *Corynebacterium diphtheriae* (Klebs-Löffler bacillus). It is characterized by membranous inflammation of the upper respiratory passages and degenerative changes in the viscera and nervous system, the latter caused by the toxin.

ETIOLOGY. The morphology and growth characteristics of *C. diphtheriae* are described in works on bacteriology. Only strains that produce the specific exotoxin are virulent and capable of producing the disease. It has been shown that avirulent strains can be converted into virulent toxin producers when exposed to bacteriophages associated with toxin-producing strains.

EPIDEMIOLOGY. The disease is transmitted by direct contact with diseased persons or healthy carriers. Individuals with pharyngeal diphtheria are more of a menace than those with laryngeal disease. The morbidity and mortality from diphtheria began to decline in the United States around 1900, following the introduction of diphtheria antitoxin. This decline was accelerated in the late 1920s with the introduction of programs of active immunization. In Baltimore, for example the diphtheria rate was 260 per 100,000 in 1900, 124 per 100,000 in 1925, and zero in 1960. Natural changes in bacteria–host relationships have probably contributed to this result.

PATHOLOGY. Pseudomembranous lesions are commonly found on the mucous membrane of the pharynx, tonsils, and uvula, less frequently in the nose, larynx and lower respiratory tract. Occasionally the process extends to the middle ear or to the esophagus and stomach; it may also involve the skin or the mucosa of the genital organs. The pseudomembrane consists of necrotic epithelium embedded in inflammatory exudate that has coagulated on the surface. Inflammatory changes are found in the surviving underlying epithelium and may extend into the submucosa, where hemorrhagic manifestations may occur. The bacilli remain in these surface lesions; only exceptionally do they invade deeper structures, and even more rarely do they cause bacteremia. Toxin, however, is absorbed from the local lesion, causing damage in distant organs and tissues.

Myocarditis is a common lesion, the changes being degenerative rather than inflammatory. They vary from simple cloudy swelling with loss of striations in the muscle fibers to well-defined foci of hyaline degeneration, often accompanied by fatty degeneration. Minute hemorrhages may be present, and in some cases there is an accompanying round cell infiltration. The conducting system is frequently involved. The liver cells show degenerative changes at autopsy; there may be scattered areas of focal necrosis. Hepatic function may be impaired to some extent. The kidneys commonly show cloudy swelling, with swollen granular epithelial cells of the convoluted tubules. Exceptionally there may be a well-marked interstitial nephritis with extensive accumulation of mononuclear cells between the tubules. Glomerular nephritis is almost unknown. Lesions in the adrenal cortex similar to those present in meningococcemia are often found in fatal cases. Degenerative changes in the nervous system occur in nearly all fatal cases. In the cord they are seen in the ganglion cells of the anterior horns and in the posterior root ganglia. The cranial nerves and their centers may be affected; however, the cortex is spared. Other lesions encountered are degenerative changes in the spleen and lymph nodes; there may be subcapsular hemorrhages. Subcutaneous hemorrhages are not infrequent. At times the hemorrhagic tendency may be attributed to thrombocytopenia, but in other cases the cause appears to be vascular.

SYMPTOMS. The incubation period of diphtheria is usually between 2 and 5 days. The onset is often insidious, with mild sore throat and only moderate fever. The throat, at first only red, soon exhibits a gray or white deposit on the tonsils or the pillars. This patch may spread, or multiple patches may coalesce to form a membrane that may cover the tonsils, the soft palate, and the uvula. The grayish white membrane is adherent and cannot readily be removed by a swab; its borders are usually sharply defined. The cervical lymph nodes usually show some swelling.

The onset may be more abrupt, with higher fever and more marked constitutional symptoms, or a mild case may progress insidiously to a more severe one. The process may spread until it involves a large part of the pharyngeal surface, with extension into the nose or downward into the larynx. In other cases the nasal or laryngeal diphtheria occurs without obvious involvement of the pharynx. Primary nasal diphtheria is seen particularly in infants and very young children; it may be very mild, the only sign being a bloody nasal discharge and excoriation about the nostrils. Laryngeal diphtheria at the onset is indistinguishable from other forms of acute laryngitis. A steady progression of symptoms, with increasing stridor, dyspnea, and cyanosis, indicates that the process is not a simple viral laryngitis.

In the average case of mild or moderate severity the process tends to subside spontaneously, usually by the fifth or sixth day. The membrane begins to loosen and separate; with its disappearance the local symptoms abate rapidly: the discharge ceases, the lymph nodes decrease in size, and deglutition and breathing become normal. With antitoxin the process subsides more rapidly. Constitutional symptoms may outlast the local manifestations, and late complications may be seen even in a relatively mild case.

In some cases the disease runs a much more malignant course than that described, with a high fatality rate. The symptoms are severe from the outset. The membrane usually covers the entire pharynx, often extending to the nose and the middle ear, and occasionally spreading to the buccal cavity. There is great swelling of the tonsils and uvula, and it is often impossible to obtain a view of the pharynx. Sometimes the inflammation is of a necrotic character, and there may be extensive sloughing of the tonsils, the uvula, or the soft palate. The nasal discharge is generally abundant and often offensive in odor. There is marked swelling of the cervical lymph nodes and frequently extensive infiltration of the cellular tissue of the neck, so that the head is thrown back to relieve pressure upon the larynx and trachea. The swelling sometimes forms a distinct collar, reaching from ear to ear and filling out the whole space beneath the jaw (bull neck). Pressure on the jugular veins leads to congestion of the face. The temperature is usually high; it follows no regular course, but generally fluctuates widely from 102 to 106 F. In some cases, however, it may never be above 101 F. The pulse is weak, rapid, and compressible. The peripheral circulation is poor, and the extremities are often cold; there is striking muscular weakness, and both vomiting and diarrhea are frequent. There may be excitement, restlessness, and active delirium, or dullness, apathy, and stupor. The urine contains albumin and casts but rarely blood. Nervous symptoms are prominent in these cases. Death generally occurs while the local disease is at its height and may result from respiratory obstruction or from circulatory failure.

COMPLICATIONS. *Myocardial involvement* is demonstrable in about 50 percent of patients with diphtheria when frequent electrocardiographic records are made. It is more likely to occur in the severe forms, particularly those with bull neck. It may develop as early as the second day or as late as 6 weeks after onset. In fatal cases it usually develops early. A change in the quality of the first sound is the first physical sign. The sound becomes fainter, and the muscular element is lost, the persistent valvular element giving rise to a tick-tack quality. The first heart sound may be replaced by a blowing murmur, and cardiac enlargement may be demonstrable. Nearly any form of arrhythmia may be noted—extrasystoles, dropped beats, and tachycardia. Abnormal electrocardiographic findings ordinarily have little clinical significance unless accompanied by clinical signs. This is particularly true of elevation of the S-T segment. On the other hand, prolongation of the P-R interval, ectopic beats, and heart block may be considered definitive indications of myocardial disease.

Cardiac failure may be heralded by a worsening of the

quality of the heart sounds, by enlargement of the liver, or by rales at the lung bases. There may be abdominal pain and vomiting. Venous pressure is elevated, and circulation time is prolonged. There may be evidences of peripheral circulatory collapse; the blood pressure falls abruptly, there is pallor, and the extremities are cold. Death may follow quickly. In such patients Rich and Hodes observed severe degenerative changes in the adrenal cortex, changes that were not conspicuous in patients dying in cardiac failure without evidences of shock.

Some form of *paralysis* occurs in 10 to 20 percent of all patients with diphtheria. It may occur even after a mild attack, although it is more common in severe cases. The muscles of the palate are the first and often the only ones to suffer; less frequently the muscles of accommodation, the extraocular muscles, the pharynx, the diaphragm, and the muscles of the extremities are involved. The intercostals are sometimes affected. Palatal paralysis is revealed by a nasal quality to the voice and regurgitation of fluids through the nose. The more severe the attack and the longer antitoxin is delayed, the earlier and more widespread the paralysis is likely to be. In severe cases it develops by the fifth or sixth day. In other instances paralysis may develop as late as the sixth week, particularly paralysis of the extremities. Disability from diphtheritic paralysis may be extreme. The patient may not be able to swallow or raise his head; he may require a respirator. Fortunately it is rarely prolonged for more than 10 days, even in the most severe cases, and recovery is usually complete.

LABORATORY FINDINGS. The blood commonly shows a leukocytosis proportional to the severity of the attack, but in the most severe cases there is sometimes leukopenia. Immature granulocytes may be present. A moderate hypoplastic anemia is common, and it may persist into convalescence. Thrombocytopenia occurs in some cases. Changes in the spinal fluid are found in a few instances of diphtheritic paralysis; there may be an elevated protein content and some increase in mononuclear cells.

DIAGNOSIS. Reliance cannot be placed on a direct stained smear for identification of diphtheria bacilli. With proper media (Löffler's, blood agar, or medium containing potassium tellurite), cultivation of diphtheria bacilli offers little difficulty early in the disease; however, repeated cultures are necessary in some cases. Microscopically, with fluorescence antibody technique, the diagnosis can be made more rapidly, and a higher percentage of positive cultures can be obtained. Cultures should always be made before antibiotics are given, for penicillin, tetracyclines, and erythromycin may interfere with the growth of *C. diphtheriae*. All positive cultures should be tested for virulence. The recovery of β-hemolytic streptococci from a culture does not rule out the diagnosis of diphtheria, for in our experience these are found in about 30 percent of cases of diphtheria.

There is nothing specific about the appearance of the throat in diphtheria, and several other conditions may give rise to pseudomembranous inflammations that may be clinically indistinguishable from it, including infectious mononucleosis, toxoplasmosis, streptoccocal pharyngitis, moniliasis, and infection with Vincent's organisms. If serious doubt exists it is always safer to assume that diphtheria is present and to treat with antitoxin. However, a few points of clinical difference may be mentioned. The membrane in diphtheria tends to be darker and grayer in color and more fibrous in appearance than in the other conditions mentioned; it tends to be more firmly attached to the underlying mucosa, and when it is pulled away bleeding is more likely to occur. It usually begins on the tonsils, spreading toward the uvula. Knowledge of the patient's immune status may be of help; a recent immunization or booster injection with diphtheria toxoid makes the diagnosis of diphtheria less likely.

Laryngeal and tracheobronchial diphtheria must be differentiated from other forms of croup (p. 434). Membrane is found on the tonsils or pharynx in about 85 percent of these cases; in its absence the diagnosis may be difficult. Clinical differentiation cannot definitely be made between diphtheria and laryngotracheobronchitis caused by streptococci, *H. influenzae,* or viruses. The onset of laryngitis caused by *H. influenzae* is often extremely abrupt, with epiglottitis being intense. However, again, when there is doubt about the diagnosis it is wise to assume that one is dealing with diphtheria.

TREATMENT. Diphtheria antitoxin should be administered as promptly as possible, following a skin or conjunctival test for sensitivity to horse serum. Antitoxin is capable of neutralizing only that toxin that is free in the circulation; it has no effect on toxin that has become attached to cells (a process that takes place rapidly). It should be given in a single injection, the dose depending on the severity of the case. In mild and moderately severe cases we inject 40,000 IU intramuscularly, regardless of the age or weight of the patient. Patients with severe pharyngeal diphtheria or with laryngeal diphtheria receive 40,000 IU intravenously in addition to 40,000 IU intramuscularly. When given intravenously, the antitoxin should be diluted 1:20 in isotonic sodium chloride solution and administered at a rate not exceeding 1 ml/minute.

Some patients who recover from diphtheria after treatment with antitoxin are found to have a positive Schick reaction. For this reason many physicians give diphtheria toxoid as well as antitoxin to all patients with diphtheria. The first dose of toxoid may be injected at the end of the first week of illness, with the second and third doses 1 and 2 months later.

Penicillin exerts a definite action against diphtheria bacilli, but antitoxin must always be given in addition. Penicillin is useful in two additional ways: it is effective against the streptococci that frequently are secondary invaders, and it decreases the number of persons who remain carriers after recovery. Aqueous procaine penicillin, 300,000 IU, should be given intramuscularly daily to small children; twice this dosage should be given to larger children. Erythromycin at a dosage of 20 mg/kg/day may be used for children who are sensitive to penicillin, since this antibiotic acts in a similar manner against *C. diphtheriae* and streptococci. Antibiotics should be continued for 7 to 10 days. It should be reemphasized that antibiotics must never be used as a substitute for diphtheria antitoxin, but in conjunction with it.

General Measures. All patients with diphtheria should be confined to bed and should remain there until it is certain that all danger of cardiac damage has passed. During the first 2 weeks of illness the patient should be kept flat in bed, and all exertion should be avoided. Patients suffering from diphtheria frequently have low blood sugar levels. For this reason the diet should be high in carbohydrate. During the acute stage of the disease a liquid diet containing fruit juices, sweetened cocoa, and milk is most satisfactory. Patients with bull neck diphtheria, who are often unable to swallow, should receive intravenous injections of dextrose solutions in order to maintain a normal blood sugar concentration.

Treatment of Complications. With laryngeal diphtheria considerable benefit may be obtained from the use of a nebulizer or a steam tent in which oxygen as well as moisture are supplied. Experience and expert judgment are required in the matter of intervention to relieve an obstructed airway. One of the best indices is the patient's ability to rest quietly and to sleep. The degree of restlessness and distress, the amount of inspiratory retraction, the presence of cyanosis, and changes in arterial blood gases and pH are the criteria to be watched closely. Cyanosis, a sharp rise in blood carbon dioxide tension, and a decrease in arterial blood pH demands immediate intervention. Tracheotomy is now the procedure generally employed; it should be performed under local anesthesia. It by-passes the laryngeal obstruction and permits removal of membrane from the trachea and bronchi.

Myocarditis requires absolute rest; the patient should not be permitted to move about in bed or feed himself. He should not sit up to use a bedpan or for any other reason. Digitalization is indicated for all patients who show clinical or electrocardiographic evidence of moderately severe myocarditis, even if compensated. With decompensation the treatment is similar to that described elsewhere for cardiac insufficiency (p. 1480). Circulatory collapse requires intravenous administration of plasma or blood and drugs to elevate the blood pressure; cortisone may be helpful. There is no specific treatment for paralysis. When this involves the muscles of deglutition, gavage with a polyethylene tube is indicated.

Treatment of Carriers. Some patients continue to harbor organisms for weeks or months after recovery. They should be given a course of penicillin: 300,000 to 600,000 IU of procaine penicillin daily for 10 days. If bacilli are still present in the nose or throat, erythromycin (20 mg/kg/day) should be given for 1 week. If this fails, tonsillectomy and adenoidectomy may be considered, but they should not be carried out until 3 months after the acute attack. Antitoxin is without value in the treatment of carriers.

PROGNOSIS. The outcome in a given case depends on several factors—the age of the patient, the location and extent of the membrane, the strain of the organism, and the promptness with which antitoxin is administered. The risk is greatest in younger children, particularly those with laryngeal involvement. Patients with extensive membranes and with bull neck appearance within 48 hours after onset have in our experience had a fatality rate around 30 percent. With clear-cut myocarditis the fatality rate is equally high, and with shock the outcome is nearly always fatal. The importance of early antitoxin therapy is shown by the data in Table 10.

PROPHYLAXIS. Patients should be quarantined until two or three successive negative cultures are obtained 1 week after discontinuance of antibiotics. All family members and those who have had close contact with a patient should have nose and throat cultures; if the cultures are positive, they should be treated as de-

TABLE 10. Influence of Time of Injection of Antitoxin on Mortality in Diphtheria*

Time of Injection After Onset	Patients	Deaths	Fatality Rate (%)
1st day	355	1	0.27
2nd day	1,018	17	1.67
3rd day	1,509	57	3.77
4th day	720	82	11.39
Later	469	119	25.37
Total	4,071	276	6.77

* Data courtesy of Health Department, Chicago, Illinois.

scribed for carriers. Exposed children, if unimmunized, should be given a 7-day course of penicillin (300,000 to 600,000 IU procaine penicillin by intramuscular injection daily), and active immunization should be started. Previously immunized children should be given a booster injection.

IMMUNITY. Immunity may be measured by the Schick test or the Moloney test. *The Schick* I test demonstrates the presence or absence of circulating antitoxin sufficient to neutralize a test dose of toxin injected into the skin. Test material (0.1 ml containing 1/50 MLD toxin) is injected intradermally, and simultaneously a control injection is made using Schick test material heated to 60 C for 15 minutes to destroy the toxin. In the nonimmune individual a positive reaction (erythema 5 mm in diameter) develops at the test site within 48 hours. It reaches a peak in 4 to 7 days and then subsides, leaving a pigmented spot that may persist for weeks. No reaction ordinarily occurs at the control site. Occasionally a subject is sensitive to the peptone of the test injection and exhibits a false-positive test at the control area that usually appears within 24 hours and does not persist. A positive Schick test indicates susceptibility to diphtheria; an individual whose reaction is negative may be regarded as immune.

The Moloney test consists of an intradermal injection of diphtheria toxoid (0.1 ml of a 1:100 dilution of fluid toxoid). A positive reaction (erythema developing in 18 to 24 hours) denotes allergy to products of the diphtheria bacillus and indicates immunity on a nonantitoxic basis. A positive reaction is rare in very young children, but it becomes more frequent with advancing age. A positive Moloney reaction may be regarded as evidence of immunity to diphtheria. Individuals with a positive Moloney test will react with constitutional symptoms following the usual injection of toxoid. Since older children are often Moloney-positive, the Moloney test should be employed before giving toxoid to children more than 8 years of age.

Active Immunization. Although many infants are protected during the first few months of life by antitoxin received from the mother transplacentally, this is not always the case, and it is currently recommended to start immunization at the age of 1.5 to 2 months. Diphtheria toxoid (alum-precipitated or adsorbed on aluminum phosphate or aluminum hydroxide) is the product of choice. It may be given alone or with pertussis vaccine and tetanus toxoid (DPT). An initial course of three injections of DPT given a month apart in early infancy is a commonly recommended procedure. An appreciable number of infants lose their immunity within a year, as measured by a return to a positive Schick test. By the end of 3 years this number is large enough to be significant. For this reason booster injections of DPT should be given at 15 months and at 3 years of age. DPT is also given at 4 to 6 years of age. At 12 years of age injections of combined "diphtheria and tetanus toxoid for adult use" is recommended. This preparation contains a maximum of 2 Lf of diphtheria toxoid, which is less than one-tenth of the amount which is in preparations used for infants. The "adult type" toxoid causes little or no reaction even in patients who have a positive Moloney reaction.

References

Belsey MA, Belsey TM, Sinclair M, Roder MR, Le Blanc Dr: Corynebacterium diphtheriae skin infections in Alabama and Louisiana. Factors in epidemiology of diphtheria. N Engl J Med 280:135, 1969

Bundesen HN, Fishbein WI, White JL: Diphtheria immunity in Chicago. JAMA 112:1919, 1939

Freeman VJ: Studies on virulence of bacteriophage-infected strains of C. diphtheriae. J Bacteriol 61:675, 1951

Frost WH: Papers of Wade Hampton Frost, MD. *In* Maxey KF, (ed): A Contribution to Epidemiological Method. London, Commonwealth Fund, 1941

Harding ME: The Circulatory Failure of Diphtheria. London, Univ London Press, 1920

Hodes HL: Diphtheria. *In* Reimann HA (ed): Treatment in General Medicine. Philadelphia, FA Davis, 1947

Pappenheimer AM Jr: The diphtheria bacilli and the diphtheroids. *In* Dubos RJ (ed): Bacterial and Mycotic Infections of Man, 3rd ed. Philadelphia, JB Lippincott, 1958

Report of the Committee on the Control of Infectious Diseases. Evanston, Ill, American Academy of Pediatrics, 1974

Rich AR: A peculiar type of adrenal cortical damage associated with acute infections, and its possible relation to circulatory collapse. Bull Johns Hopkins Hosp 74:1, 1944

Rolleston JD: Diphtheritic paralysis. Arch Pediatr 30:335, 1913.

GONOCOCCAL INFECTIONS
E. Richard Moxon

During the last two decades there has been a relentless increase in the incidence of infections due to *Neisseria gonorrhoeae* in the United States. The current annual rate exceeds 300 cases per 100,000 population, with an absolute increase as well as a relative increase in gonococcal infections among adolescents. Of the more than 700,000 cases reported yearly, 25 percent occur in young adults less than 20 years of age, of which 1 to 2 percent are in children less than 14 years of age. These facts emphasize the importance of gonococcal infections in the young. Recognition and management of childhood gonococcal infections demand the careful attention of pediatricians and related health workers. The epidemiologic and sometimes legal proceedings resulting from this diagnosis demand a meticulous teamwork approach if optimal management as well as limitation of disease spread are to be achieved.

Man is the sole reservoir from which the gonococcus spreads to other susceptible persons. Among adults, approximately 80 percent of females and 25 percent of males infected with *N. gonorrhoeae* are asymptomatic. (Similar data for children are not available since pelvic examination is not a routine part of the evaluation of pediatric patients.) This reservoir of undetected infection poses a major obstacle to disease control.

Most cases of gonorrhea are acquired through a sexual relationship with an infected person. Newborn infants may be infected following exposure to the infected birth canal. An unusual epidemic in an institution occurred following the use of contaminated rectal thermometers. In rare cases intimate contact with infected persons, particularly under conditions of poor hygiene and overcrowding, may also result in nonvenereal spread of gonorrhea. Gonococcal infections of young children resulting from sexual abuse are frequently not properly classified without exhaustive interviewing of the family and other potential contacts. The child with gonorrhea may be the index case that provides an indication of infection in other members of the family or circle of friends. The techniques of investigation and interview in such situations require a delicate combination of thoroughness and tact, since hostility and alienation of a family are all too easily aroused. Such cases may uncover instances of child abuse, sexual exploitation, or assault. On the other hand, false accusation or failure to recognize the subtle distinctions between sexual experimentation and unlawful sexual exploitation may result in much turmoil and distress for both the physician and patient.

N. gonorrhoeae is a gram-negative diplococcus. Smears typically reveal paired bacterial cells that are kidney-shaped, with their concave sides adjacent. As with other members of the same genus, this bacterium is fastidious in its nutritional demands. This fact accounts in part for the somewhat limited ability of the gonococcus to survive outside of its natural breeding ground and host (man). Gonococci grow optimally if freshly plated on prewarmed media under aerobic conditions and incubated in the presence of 4 to 10 percent CO_2 at 35 to 36 C. Chocolate agar is a satisfactory growth medium, but cultures obtained from mucosal surfaces may include a variety of other organisms capable of overgrowing or inhibiting growth of *N. gonorrhoeae*. Thus a selective medium, such as that devised by Thayer and Martin, can be extremely advantageous. This medium is enriched with antibiotics (Vancomycin, colistimethate, and neomycin) to inhibit growth of other organisms. Another variant is Transgrow medium, which consists of Thayer-Martin medium enriched with 10 percent CO_2, additional nutrients, and trimethoprim lactate; it has proved most useful for mail-in cultures.

Colonies of *N. gonorrhoeae* are oxidase-positive and turn pink and then purple when incubated in the presence of 1 percent tetramethylparaphenyldiamine hydrochloride. However, this latter characteristic is shared by other saprophytic microorganisms found in human genital secretions. Additional bacteriologic confirmation of the identity of *N. gonorrhoeae* can be obtained using sugar reactions, since it ferments glucose but not sucrose and maltose. Examination of suitable smears treated with antiserum conjugated with fluorescein dye is also of proven usefulness. Under appropriate conditions of growth, four morphologically distinct colonies of *N. gonorrhoeae* can be identified (types I, II, III, and IV). Types I and II predominate in cultures obtained from sites of recent infection. This is of interest since these two types (but not types III and IV) produce infection when inoculated experimentally into volunteers. Types I and II also possess pili; these filamentous structures project from the bacterial cell surface and appear to facilitate attachment of gonococci to mucosal cell surfaces. The chemical structure of these pili is currently the subject of investigation and may provide a basis for serologic testing for the presence of gonococcal infection.

PATHOGENESIS. The gonococcus has a predilection for infecting mucosal surfaces lined by columnar, as opposed to stratified, epithelium. Thus the urethra, cervix, rectum, vagina, and oropharynx of the infant and young child are favored sites of initial colonization. Local factors (for example, the pH of vaginal mucus and the thickness of the mucosa) are important modifiers in determining susceptibility to infection. Bacterial pili probably play a significant role in effecting adhesion between the host and bacterial cell surfaces. In the absence of such firm attachment, gonococci would be dislodged by secretions or by the force of the urinary stream. Following this initial phase of colonization, the bacteria penetrate into the subepithelial tissues where multiplication takes place. This phase of the infection has not been well studied. The typical inflammatory response is attributed to the effect of endotoxin, which stimulates the production of exudate and a polymorphonuclear leukocyte response. Spread of *N. gonorrhoeae* from the initial locus of infection occurs by contiguous, lymphatic, or hematogenous routes, and in the female spread occurs from the endocervix to the internal pelvic organs. Involvement of Bartholin's glands and other perineal glands and their ducts is common, but the uterine cavity is usually spared. When untreated, tubo-ovarian infection may result in abscess formation, scarring, and interference with reproductive functions. In addition to being a site of primary infection, the anorectal tissues are frequently involved by spread from a genitourinary site of infection. In the male, urethral involvement may lead to infection of the seminal vesicles, epididymis, and prostate. Abscess formation and scarring may cause sterility. Hematogenous spread of gonococci can follow infection of genitourinary or extragenital tissues, although such infections are uncommon. The structures most commonly involved following hematogenous spread are synovial joints, skin, and more rarely meninges and endocardium. Even more rarely, liver, muscle, bone, lung, and myocardium have been involved.

IMMUNOLOGY. Infection with *N. gonorrhoeae* is associated with production of local and systemic antibody as well as cell-mediated responses. The significance of this immunologic activity is not well understood, and it is generally accepted that prior infection does not confer protective immunity against subsequent exposure. Precise information regarding the chemical composition of the gonococcal cell and its component membranes is lacking.

CLINICAL MANIFESTATIONS. The incubation period of gonorrheal infection is varied, but symptoms usually appear within 1 week of infection. In males the majority of infected individuals present with urethritis. This has been described at all ages, beginning with the newborn. Most gonococcal infections in the mature female are asymptomatic, but there may be thick purulent cervical or urethral discharge. Detailed descriptions of the classic signs and symptoms can be found in appropriate texts on adult medicine. However, the following types of gonococcal infection are of particular relevance to the pediatrician and child health worker.

LOCALIZED INFECTIONS. Gonococcal Ophthalmia. Gonococcal ophthalmia may occur at any age, but it notoriously afflicts the newborn infant who is infected by contact with gonococci from the birth canal. One or both eyes may be infected. Instillation of 1 percent silver nitrate solution to all newborns shortly after birth has greatly reduced the number of cases of gonococcal ophthalmia neonatorum. Nevertheless, despite its proven value, failure of silver nitrate prophylaxis does occur. The appearance of a purulent or serosanguinous discharge, typically some 2 to 7 days after delivery, should prompt careful evaluation of a gram-stained smear and culture for the presence of *N. gonorrhoeae.* Purulent discharge occurring within 48 hours of birth is most often the result of chemical conjunctivitis, and during the second week it is very likely to be caused by inclusion blenorrhea. Edema, congestion of lids and conjunctiva, periorbital swelling, and adherence of eyelashes to one another because of purulent exudate comprise the typical clinical picture of gonococcal ophthalmia. A gram-stained smear of the exudate shows an abundance of polymorphonuclear leukocytes, some containing intracellular diplococci. If it is not treated spontaneous recovery may occur, but permanent damage such as iridocyclitis, and corneal ulceration occurs in about one-third of untreated cases. In view of the serious consequences of gonococcal ophthalmitis, treatment should be commenced as early as feasible, based on the results of a gram-stain smear, without awaiting cultural confirmation.

Vulvovaginitis and Urethritis. Approximately one-fifth of all cases of vulvovaginitis in preadolescent girls are caused by infection with *N. gonorrhoeae.* Before puberty the vaginal mucosa is more susceptible to infection than it is in the mature female. The majority of gonococcal infections in young girls less than 9 years of age result from sexual abuse by an infected adult or adolescent. After the age of 10 years increasing numbers of such infections result from voluntary participation in sexual activity. Typically, girls with vulvovaginitis present with thick green or creamy vaginal discharge that is voluminous. However, asymptomatic cases have been described in which signs are absent or minimal, consisting of labial erythema and scanty secretions. The incidence of cases is unknown, since examination of the perineum in young girls is usually omitted unless there are specific complaints. Since the endocervical glands in the prepubertal female are not developed, spread to the fallopian tubes and upper genital tract occurs infrequently. However, tubal infection or peritonitis is a recognized complication in approximately 6 percent of untreated cases. Septic complications, such as arthritis, have also been reported. Gonorrheal infections in preadolescent males usually present as urethritis or sterile pyuria and may be otherwise asymptomatic. Penile abscesses and epididymitis may complicate untreated cases.

DISSEMINATED INFECTIONS. Disseminated disease has increased proportionately with the rising incidence of gonococcal infections, but it constitutes only 0.1 to 0.3 percent of the more than 300 cases per 100,000 population reported annually. Hematogenous spread of gonococci may originate from local infections at sites such as the eyes, oropharynx, skin, rectum, and genitourinary tract and may occur at any age; but there is a predisposition to dissemination during the neonatal period, during pregnancy, and at the time of menses, as well as in drug users and in patients with accompanying liver disease. Disseminated infection is strikingly fre-quent among asymptomatic female carriers. There is an increased risk of disseminated gonococcemia in the neonatal period, particularly of arthritis and meningitis. In one study orogastric cultures of newborn infants showed approximately 2.5 percent to be colonized with gonococci, representing 20 percent of infants born to mothers known to be infected prior to delivery. Although none had positive blood culture, 10 of these 13 neonates with positive orogastric cultures fared poorly and manifested nonspecific signs of neonatal sepsis. The seriousness of untreated gonococcemia in neonates was well documented in a nursery epidemic occurring in Philadelphia in 1927. Fifty-three of 67 infants infected with *N. gonorrhoeae* had arthritis, of which 25 percent had residual joint problems 3 years later.

Arthritis and tenosynovitis are the most common manifestations of disseminated gonorrhea in adolescents and adults. During the phase of bacteremia a migratory polyarthritis is typical. All joints may be affected, but knees, ankles, and wrists prevail. Accompanying skin lesions are common and consist of clusters of erythematous or hemorrhagic lesions about 2 mm in diameter whose centers are gray and black because of necrosis or hemorrhage or both. Skin lesions are found most frequently on the extremities, clustered around joints. At the time of bacteremia, cultures of joint fluid are rarely positive, but later there may be localization of bacteria to one or more joints, at which time there may be purulent effusion containing viable gonococci.

More than 30 cases of gonococcal meningitis have been reported among newborn infants and adults. It may present as a typical pyogenic meningitis, but frequently the simultaneous presence of urethritis, arthritis, or cutaneous lesions affords clues as to its etiology. Incorrect identification of the organism isolated from cerebrospinal fluid, resulting in an inaccurate bacteriologic diagnosis, is not an infrequent occurrence. Thus a review of 500 assumed meningococcal isolates sent to the NIH for grouping revealed that 10 were in fact *N. gonorrhoeae.*

DIAGNOSIS. In cases of gonococcal ophthalmia, vulvovaginitis, and urethritis, examination of a stained smear of the purulent discharge will usually reveal intracellular gram-negative diplococci. Although this finding is virtually diagnostic, confirmatory cultures are important for precise bacteriologic identification, especially for medicolegal purposes. In females, symptomatology is usually insufficient evidence for presumptive diagnosis, and gram-stained smears of secretions from the vagina or endocervix are frequently negative. The presence of nonpathogenic *Neisseria* species (eg, *N. sicca, N. subflora*) may on rare occasions result in false-positive smears. Thus at present the diagnosis of gonorrhea in females is best accomplished by culture. Specimens collected from both the endocervical canal and the rectum should be cultured.

Diagnosis of disseminated disease is difficult, since cultures of blood, joint fluid, or skin lesions show growth of gonococci in less than one-third of patients; even under optimal circumstances in which all three tissues are cultured less than 50 percent of cases are

TABLE 11. Recommended Treatment for Childhood Gonococcal Infections*

Form of Disease		Hospitalization	Drug	Daily Dosage	Route of Administration	Duration of Treatment
Neonatal	Ophthalmia	Yes	ACPG[†]	50,000 IU/kg in 2–3 doses	iv	7 days
	Disseminated infection	Yes	ACPG	75,000–100,000 IU/kg in 4 doses	iv	10 days
Prepubertal	Vulvovaginitis or Urethritis (uncomplicated)	No	APPG plus Probenecid	75,000–100,000 IU/kg 25 mg/kg	im oral	Single dose
	Vulvovaginitis or Urethritis (complicated)	Yes	ACPG or APPG	75,000–100,000 IU/kg in 4 doses 75,000–100,000 IU/kg	iv im	7 days
Alternative regimes in case of allergy or treatment failure						
Age < 6 years						
	Uncomplicated	No	Erythromycin	40 mg/kg in 4 doses	oral	7 days
	Complicated	Yes	Cephalothin	60–80 mg/kg in 4 doses	iv	7 days
Age > 6 years						
	Uncomplicated	No	Tetracycline	40–60 mg/kg in 4 doses	oral	7 days
	Complicated	Yes	Tetracycline	40–60 mg/kg in 4 doses	iv	7 days

* Adapted from USPHS Publication 97–796, 1974.
† ACPG = aqueous crystalline penicillin G; APPG = aqueous procaine penicillin G.

confirmed bacteriologically. However, a technique utilizing a fluorescein-labeled antibody has resulted in a correct diagnosis in 88 percent of 16 patients in one reported series.

TREATMENT. In order to be successful, drugs administered to patients with gonorrhea should attain bactericidal concentrations for an adequate time (12 to 18 hours). They should be inexpensive and free from unwanted side effects and should be rapidly eliminated, so as to minimize emergence of resistant strains. Finally, the drug should cure (not mask) incubating syphilis, and it should do so administered as a single dose. Long-acting penicillins, although effective against syphilis, attain insufficiently high concentrations for the treatment of gonorrhea. Current therapeutic recommendations for treatment of gonorrhea in childhood are summarized in Table 11.

References

Barrett-Connor E: Gonorrhea. Curr Probl Pediatr 3:1, 1973

Branch G, Paxton R: A study of gonococcal infections among infants and children. Public Health Rep 80:347, 1965

Cooperman MB: Gonococcus arthritis in infancy; clinical study of 44 cases. Am J Dis Child 33:932, 1927

Grossman M, Drutz DJ: Venereal disease in children. Adv Pediatr 21:97, 1974 Schulman I, ed.

Handsfield HH, Hodson WA, Holmes KK: Neonatal gonococcal infection: I. Orogastric contamination with Neisseria gonorrhoeae. JAMA 225:697, 1973

Litt IF, Edberg SC, Finberg L: Medical progress. Gonorrhea in children and adolescents; a current review. J Pediatr 85:595, 1974

Nazarian LF: The current prevalence of gonococcal infections in children. Pediatr 39:372, 1967

HAEMOPHILUS INFLUENZAE INFECTIONS

DAVID N. SMITH AND JOHN ROBBINS

Bacteria of the genus *Haemophilus* were first recovered by Pfeiffer in 1892 from the sputum of individuals afflicted during an influenza pandemic. The requirement that blood be present for growth of the bacteria and the presumption that these bacteria caused the pandemic prompted the designation *Haemophilus influenzae*. Subsequently other bacterial species have been designated as members of the genus *Haemophilus* on the basis of similar morphology and physiology: they are small, pleomorphic, gram-negative bacilli that are strict parasites; they require enriched media containing blood or certain derivatives for growth (Table 12); and they are facultatively aerobic, nonmotile, and non-spore-forming. Most *Haemophilus* species infect only man, and all of these are found in the respiratory tract, with the exception of *H. ducreyi*, which causes chancroid. Most species are not pathogenic for their host. *H. influenzae* is the most important of the human species that cause respiratory tract and invasive diseases (eg, meningitis, bacteremia, epiglottitis, cellulitis, and pyarthrosis). Accordingly, this discussion will focus primarily on this species.

BACTERIOLOGY *H. influenzae* is distinguished from other bacteria by its morphology and its growth requirements (Table 12). This organism may exist with or without a capsular polysaccharide. Colonies of nonencapsulated isolates are usually 0.5 to 1.5 mm in

TABLE 12. Properties of *Haemophilus* Species

Species	Normal Host	Normal Habitat	Growth Factor Requirement X	V	Hemolysis
H. influenzae	Man	URT*	+	+	−
H. parainfluenzae	Man	URT	−	+	−
H. aegypticus	Man	URT, eye	+	+	−
H. hemolyticus	Man	URT	+	+	+
H. parahemolyticus	Man	URT	−	+	+
H. ducreyi	Man	Genital	+	−	+
H. suis	Swine	URT	+	+	
H. ovis	Sheep	URT			
H. gallinarum	Fowl	URT	+	+	
H. hemoglobinophilus	Dog	Genital	+	−	−

* URT = upper respiratory tract.

diameter after overnight incubation on enriched solid medium, and they appear rough or granular. Colonies of encapsulated isolates are usually 3 to 4 mm in diameter and initially appear mucoid or glistening; subsequent excretion of capsular polymer (not autolysis) results in an umbilicated appearance. Colonies grown on enriched media appear microscopically as relatively uniform, small coccobacilli (1 μ × 0.3 μ); under less than optimal conditions *H. influenzae* often grow as long filaments or short chains. Counterstaining with the safranin red dye used in Gram's stain may be variable. *H. influenzae* in clinical specimens are therefore frequently misdiagnosed as pneumococci, *Neisseria,* or enteric bacilli. Visualization of the refractile capsule is often possible and can be enhanced by reaction with specific anticapsular antibody (quellung reaction).

H. influenzae require a heat-labile V factor and a heat-stable X factor found in erythrocytes for *aerobic* growth. The former factor can be replaced by coenzyme I (DPN), coenzyme II (TPN), or nicotinamide nucleoside; this last factor can be replaced by hematin. *H. influenzae* do not require hematin for *anaerobic* growth, apparently because heme-containing enzymes are needed only for aerobic respiration. *H. parainfluenzae* never require hematin. Since this metabolic requirement is the primary basis for the laboratory differentiation of the two species, confusion may arise if *H. influenzae* are grown anaerobically (eg, following stab inoculation under the surface of solid medium). Fermentation reactions and tests of other metabolic activities are variable and are not useful in identification. The capacity of most *H. influenzae* to convert tryptophan to indole results in a characteristic odor.

H. influenzae will grow in any enriched nonselective liquid or solid medium supplemented with the required nutrients. They will usually grow on standard blood-containing media, but optimal growth is realized if the erythrocytes are disrupted during preparation of the medium by heat (chocolate or Levinthal medium) or enzymes (Fildes medium) to release the growth factors. Excessive heat destroys the required V factor; commercial media must therefore be quality controlled before use in diagnostic laboratories. Medium prepared with enriched broth supplemented by sterile DPN and hema-

tin obviates this problem. Growth requirements are determined by inoculation of specifically deficient media or observation of growth around filter paper disks impregnated with either DPN or heme. "Satellism" in the hemolytic area around colonies of *Staphylococcus aureus* growing on solid blood agar is often used to identify *H. influenzae.* Since some strains are said to grow best in 5 to 10 percent carbon dioxide, it is standard practice to incubate specimens suspected of containing *H. influenzae* in a candle jar or an incubator purged with carbon dioxide. Routine subculture at 24 hours obviates the inhibition of growth observed in many primary blood cultures. *H. influenzae* lose viability rapidly on drying, heating, and suspension in buffers without added protein; clinical specimens should therefore be transported and inoculated onto appropriate culture media without delay.

The surface structures of *H. influenzae* are primary in its pathogenicity and immunogenicity. The structure and composition of the outer membrane are similar to those of other gram-negative bacilli. The membrane contains a lipopolysaccharide cell wall (endotoxin) with its terminal carbohydrate O antigens and a number of poorly defined immunogenic proteins. Small percentages of natural isolates are encapsulated. Pittman demonstrated six antigenically distinguishable capsular types and designated them a through f. Subsequently

TABLE 13. Serologic Antigens of *H. influenzae* Capsular Polysaccharides

Type	Sugar	PO$_4$	Acetyl
a	Glucose	+	−
b	Ribose, ribitol	+	−
c	Galactose	+	−
d	Hexose	−	−
e	Hexosamine	−	+
f	Galactosamine	+	+

each of these polymers was found to be a complex carbohydrate whose composition has been described (Table 13). The type b capsular polymer is unique among this genus in containing pentose sugars: ribose and, as recently described, ribitol phosphate (hence its designation PRP). Strains with decreased or absent capsular antigen arise spontaneously from encapsulated strains. Although this variation was originally described as S → R, recent observations suggest that the terminology of May is more appropriate: M (fully encapsulated) → S (partially encapsulated) → R (nonencapsulated). The genetic basis of this variation and the natural existence of its converse (R → S → M) remain undescribed. Alexander demonstrated that DNA purified from an M strain could transform an R strain to the serotype of the donor M strain; she also documented the possible co-production of two capsular antigens following transformation of one M type with DNA from a second type. Transformation of *H. influenzae* in the host has not been studied, but the recent demonstration of pneumococcal transformation in experimentally infected mice supports that possibility. Transformations between *H. aegypticus* and *H. influenzae* and between *H. influenzae* and *H. parainfluenzae* demonstrate the close genetic relationships of these species.

H. influenzae type b releases its capsular antigen (PRP) during growth in vitro and in the host. PRP can be identified with specific antiserum by several techniques, the most sensitive of which are countercurrent electrophoresis, agglutination of latex particles to which antibody is nonspecifically adsorbed, and inhibition of binding of radioactive PRP. The type A, B, and C capsules share antigenic determinants with certain pneumococcal capsules, while the type B capsule is immunologically cross-reactive with the capsules of certain species of bacilli, diphtheroids, lactobacilli, *S. aureus*, *S. epidermidis*, streptococci, *Escherichia coli*, and *Pseudomonas*. *H. influenzae* in clinical specimens and cultures can be identified and typed by the quellung reaction, by agglutination, or by direct immunofluorescence with antisera produced by organisms of specific capsular types. The accuracy of serologic diagnosis depends on the test employed, the experience of the observer, and the potency and purity of the typing sera; false-negative reactions (antibody titer too low) and false-positive reactions (serum contains antibody to outer membrane or capsular antigens shared with other bacteria) are not uncommon.

EPIDEMIOLOGY.   *H. influenzae* are found only in man, primarily in the upper respiratory tract. They can be recovered from nasopharyngeal cultures of up to 80 percent of healthy individuals. At least 50 percent of children have at least one *H. influenzae* infection during their first year of life, and essentially all are infected by 3 years of age. Asymptomatic nasopharyngeal infection may last days to a few months; it is not eradicated by systemic antibody activity and may not be eliminated by antibiotic therapy adequate to cure type B meningitis. Of the isolated strains, up to 25 percent are encapsulated, one-half of which are type B. *H. influenzae* diseases occur worldwide and for the most part are endemic. Unusually high attack rates of meningitis occur in certain communities, and multiple cases occur in up to 3 percent of affected families. Available data indicate that *H. influenzae* type b meningitis occurs unusually frequently among impoverished, rural, and black individuals; children with sickle cell disease also appear to have an increased susceptibility.

Local respiratory tract disease is relatively independent of the age of the host, but systemic *H. influenzae* diseases have a marked age relationship: newborns, older children, and adults are rarely affected. Of children with *H. influenzae* bacteremia without focus and those with *H. influenzae* cellulitis, most are younger than 2 years of age; of those with meningitis, 40 percent are 3 to 24 months of age; most of those afflicted with epiglottitis and pneumonia are 2 to 5 years of age. About 60 percent of children with invasive diseases are boys. In temperate climates most cases occur during the winter months.

Considerable evidence indicates that the prevalence and incidence of systemic *H. influenzae* type B diseases have increased over the past 45 years. Thus the percentage of acute bacterial meningitis due to *H. influenzae* has increased about twofold to approximately 60 percent; the current incidence is 35 to 50 cases per 100,000 children per year for children under 5 years of age in the United States. The basis for this increase is not understood. Improved diagnostic laboratories and diminution in the prevalence of protective antibody due to excessive use of antibiotics have been implicated. On the other hand, there has been no significant change in the percentage of cases of acute bacterial meningitis due to *H. influenzae;* such a change should have occurred with improved diagnostic facilities. There is no meaningful basis for comparing surveys of the current and previous prevalence of specific antibody activity (see below). However, it is significant that the age-related incidence of *H. influenzae* type B meningitis is the same today as 30 years ago. The possibility that this increase in *H. influenzae* type B disease has resulted from a change in the antigenic composition and/or virulence of the organisms is being studied.

PATHOGENICITY.   Occasionally, asymptomatic nasopharyngeal infection by nonencapsulated or encapsulated strains develops into symptomatic disease that may spread contiguously to involve the sinuses, middle ear, or bronchi. Encapsulated strains may invade local tissues and cause epiglottitis, pneumonia, pericarditis, or facial cellulitis, or they may enter the bloodstream and produce metastatic disease in the meninges or joints. At least 95 percent of invasive strains are type b. *H. influenzae* endotoxin inhibits respiratory cilia in vitro, but the possibility that this phenomenon plays a role in disease has not been studied in the host. No evidence suggests the existence of a pathogenic extracellular toxin or enzyme. That synergy between *H. influenzae* and certain respiratory viruses may be important in the initiation of colonization or production of local respiratory disease is supported by studies in experimental models and by the significant frequency of coisolation of such agents during surveillance studies of young children.

The pathogenicity of invasive diseases is related to the age of the host and the presence of type b capsule. The age-related susceptibility to *H. influenzae* type B meningitis and its inverse correlation to circulating specific antibody were first reported in 1932. The possibility of additional age-related factors has been suggested by observations made with an experimental model of this disease. When rats inoculated intranasally with *H. influenzae* type B are colonized, they may develop nasopharyngitis and subsequently bacteremia, meningitis, and pyarthrosis. Meningitis does not develop without bacteremia. Furthermore, in a colony of nonimmune animals susceptibility to meningitis is inversely related to age: infant rats are susceptible, while weanling and adults animals are resistant to the disease. The primacy of the capsule in the pathogenicity of type B strains is indicated by the excessive prevalence of this capsular type among cases of systemic disease as compared to its prevalence in nature, the antiphagocytic effect of the capsule in vitro and in experimentally infected animals, the pathogenicity of type B (but nonencapsulated) strains, for experimentally infected animals, and the protective activity of anticapsular antibody in the experimental model.

IMMUNITY. The classic study of Fothergill and Wright strongly indicated that antibody to the capsular antigen plays a primary role in host immunity to *H. influenzae* type B. The protective role of systemic antibody has been further documented by the resistance provided experimental animals by minute quantities of anticapsular antibody, the beneficial results of rabbit antibacterial serum in therapy of meningitis, and the efficacy of prophylactic gamma globulin for boys with X-linked agammaglobulinemia, who are unusually susceptible to diseases produced by this organism. A relatively high percentage of healthy adults and older children have been reported to have no antibody activity detectable by hemagglutination or bactericidal assays. Therefore the possibility of a change in the prevalence of antibody activity during the 44 years since the Fothergill-Wright study has been raised. The limited numbers of individuals, particularly adults, examined in the original study and the differences in laboratory methods make it impossible to compare the results of such serologic surveys. Furthermore, other recent studies, especially those employing a radioimmunoassay of antibody activity that is 50 to 100 times more sensitive than other techniques, have demonstrated type-specific antibody activity in nearly all older children, adults, and newborn infants. It is therefore likely that many of the differences in the results of serologic surveys are due to technical factors.

Studies of patients recovering from systemic *H. influenzae* type B disease and those immunized with a purified capsular immunogen have revealed a marked age relationship to anticapsular antibody: infants respond infrequently and with poor responses; younger children have intermediate reactivity; older children and adults develop marked responses that cannot be boosted further. The level of detectable antibody activity following disease is further complicated by antigenemia, which may last from days to weeks, is more common and prolonged in infants, and is inversely related to the timing and quantity of the subsequent antibody response. A few children have been observed who have failed to produce anticapsular antibody detectable by radioimmunoassay following systemic disease and who have subsequently developed a second distinct episode of type B invasive disease. Although these children appear to have been immunologically paralyzed for periods ranging up to months, all who have been studied to date have subsequently raised anticapsular antibody activity. These observations indicate the need for further research and for close follow-up of young children recuperating from invasive *H. influenzae* type B disease. Individuals recuperating from *H. influenzae* type B epiglottitis were found in one study to have higher anti-PRP titers than those recovering from *H. influenzae* type B meningitis, even when the data were corrected for age differences. Those recuperating from epiglottitis had significant differences in the composition of certain erythrocyte and lymphocyte antigens when compared to healthy blood donors or to those who have had *H. influenzae* type B meningitis; children recovering from *H. influenzae* type B meningitis also differed significantly from healthy individuals in certain lymphocyte surface antigens. Although these data suggest that production of anti-PRP antibody and/or development of certain *H. influenzae* type B diseases may have a genetic basis, further evaluation of this concept is required.

Antibody to *H. influenzae* type B can develop after infection with bacteria carrying an immunologically cross-reactive capsule. Such antibody is bacteriolytic in the presence of complement in vitro and protects animals from an experimental challenge with *H. influenzae* type B. Antibody activity bactericidal for *H. influenzae* type B can also be directed to outer membrane proteins, and such activity is widely distributed among adults. The protective nature of these antibodies, their distribution among infants and children, and the basis for their stimulation are under study. The possibility that host immunity to *H. influenzae* type B results from a composite of antibody activities that are directed to each of several *H. influenzae* surface antigens and are stimulated by infection with any of several different types of bacteria seems plausible.

DISEASES. *H. influenzae* can cause local respiratory tract or invasive diseases. A recent 1-year survey of children hospitalized in Denver, Colorado, revealed that *H. influenzae* was the most common cause of bacteremic disease and that 54 percent of the affected children had meningitis, 14 percent had pneumonia (4 percent with pericarditis), 11 percent had bacteremia without focus, 11 percent had facial cellulitis, 10 percent had epiglottitis, and 1 percent had pyarthrosis.

Meningitis. The signs and symptoms of *H. influenzae* meningitis depend on the child's age and the time during the course of the disease at which he is examined. Most children have a preceding upper respiratory tract infection, some with focal disease such as otitis media. Fever, anorexia, vomiting, and a significant alteration in cerebral function (eg, irritability, listlessness, or convulsions) are commonly observed. Older children may complain of headache and stiff neck. Examination usually reveals a child in acute distress with tachycardia, tachypnea, fever, positive Brudzinski and/or Kernig signs, and, if younger, a full or bulging fontanelle. The signs and symptoms may be less well defined in younger children. For example, crying during diapering or while being held may be the only indication of spinal cord irritation. The results of lumbar puncture will determine the diagnosis. There should be little reluctance to perform this procedure, since the diagnosis depends on the findings. Therapeutic results correlate inversely with the time required to make the diagnosis and institute appropriate therapy. There is little risk associated with performance of lumbar puncture, except for children with closed fontanelles who have increased intracranial pressure from other intracerebral disease. Further considerations of acute bacterial meningitis are presented elsewhere.

Pneumonia. *H. influenzae* may cause either bronchopneumonia or lobar pneumonia; approximately one-half of the latter group of patients have associated empyema. Occasionally the pneumonic disease may spread to produce a purulent pericarditis. The differential diagnosis of *H. influenzae* bronchopneumonia includes other bacterial, viral, and mycoplasmic etiologies; lobar disease, particularly that with pleural involvement, is most often confused with pneumococcal or *S. aureus* disease.

Epiglottitis. Epiglottitis produces a brief and violent disease with acute onset of fever (usually 102 to 105 F), sore throat, dysphagia, and general malaise. The dysphagia leads to puddling of oropharyngeal secretions. Respiratory distress develops and is characterized by tachypnea, stridor, supraclavicular and subcostal retractions, and a sitting position with the chin extended, which is taken unconsciously to increase the diameter of the airway. If cough is present it is hoarse and relatively mild for the degree of respiratory distress. The child usually refuses fluids or food and becomes apprehensive. Increasing airway obstruction is accompanied by increasing hypoxia and attendant neurologic signs: apprehension, followed by restlessness, increasing irritability, and if the hypoxia is severe, coma. The rapidity of the progression of symptoms is dramatic; over one-half of these patients require hospitalization and airway intubation within 12 hours after the initial onset of their symptoms.

Examination usually reveals an acutely ill, toxic child with obvious upper respiratory obstruction and often hypoxia or cyanosis and varying degrees of neurologic dysfunction. Cervical adenitis or pneumonia are present in 20 percent of cases. Meningitis can also be present, but it is rare. The epiglottitis is markedly edematous and erythematous and occludes the airway as a ball valve in proportion to the swelling. Since examination may traumatize the epiglottis and thereby enhance the edema and reduce the airway, it should be performed by very experienced personnel in a setting in which tracheal intubation can be performed immediately (preferably in an operating room). Radiography of the lateral neck may aid in the diagnosis; but it cannot replace local inspection, and it may consume critical time.

There are no other diseases that produce this constellation of signs and symptoms. Problems in differential diagnosis arise from confusion with viral croup and, if late in the course, other causes of coma that are accompanied by increased respiratory effort. Children with viral croup have a more protracted, milder disease, often in the setting of an outbreak of respiratory illness in the family characterized by low-grade temperature, hoarseness, stridor, and a repetitious, barking, nonproductive cough. Examination of the epiglottis is diagnostic. A question of intracranial disease (meningitis, brain abscess, tumor, hemorrhage, and metabolic causes of coma such as diabetic acidosis) may be raised in cases of epiglottitis that has progressed to severe hypoxia. Since a patent airway is critical to the survival and the neurologic function of the individual with epiglottitis, and since tests to prove other diagnoses take considerable time (often in areas of the hospital in which emergency care is difficult), examination of the epiglottitis must be performed *initially* in all such cases.

Bacteremia of Unknown Origin. Acutely ill children of 6 to 36 months of age with temperatures higher than 39C and nonspecific symptoms such as vomiting, irritability, coryza, rhinorrhea, myalgia, and elevated peripheral neutrophil counts may have bacteremia. Most cases are caused by pneumococci, but *H. influenzae* is the second most common etiologic agent. Diagnosis is made from the blood culture, and it often surprises the examining physician. Such children often respond to therapy without evidence of localized disease; others develop clinically evident sinusitis, meningitis, pneumonia, or septic arthritis subsequent to their positive blood cultures.

Cellulitis. *H. influenzae* can cause a cellulitis that is characterized by a raised, warm, tender area of distinctive reddish blue hue, usually on the cheek, or less commonly periorbital in location. The child is usually moderately febrile and toxic and has a history of preceding rhinorrhea and fever. *H. influenzae* cellulitis on the limbs and hands has been seen, but very rarely. The distinctive color, location, and clinical course suggest the etiology, but streptococcal or staphylococcal causes must be distinguished.

Pyarthrosis. Characteristically the child with *H. influenzae* arthritis has had a preceding upper respiratory illness; he then becomes acutely ill and toxic, and it is observed that he guards and does not move one limb. Examination reveals limited motion of the involved joint, which is usually a large or weight-bearing joint. Multiple joint involvement is uncommon. Evidence of local inflammation (heat, swelling, tenderness on motion) is usually evident. Radiographs demonstrate joint effusion and local inflammation (loss of characteristic tissue planes), but no abnormalities in the long bones. The other major cause of this disease (*S. aureus*) usually affects older children (over 2 years of age) and commonly produces osteomyelitis, which is exceedingly rare with *H. influenzae.*

Local Respiratory Tract Diseases. The nasopharyngitis, sinusitis, and otitis media caused by *H. influenzae* cannot be distinguished clinically from those due to other causes. Acute pharyngitis is only rarely caused by this organism. Chronic bronchitis (particularly in debilitated hosts, including agammaglobulinemic individuals and in the young child with cystic fibrosis) is commonly due to *H. influenzae.*

DIAGNOSIS. Pyarthrosis in a child under 2 years of age, facial cellulitis, and epiglottitis can generally be diagnosed as being caused by *H. influenzae* type B on a statistical basis; for this organism causes more than 80 percent of the cases of these diseases. However, confirmation of the etiologic diagnosis in these and other diseases requires microbiologic studies, for there is no definitive clinical basis for distinguishing the causative microorganism. Available methods include identification of bacteria or bacterial products by stain or immunologic techniques and recovery of viable bacteria. The accuracy of the laboratory diagnosis depends on the technique employed, the site of origin of the positive specimen, and the timing of the specimen collection in relation to the course of the disease and antibiotic therapy. Gram stains of infected body fluids (eg, cerebrospinal, joint) correlate with culture results in 70 percent of cases. Of the rest of culture-positive specimens, 15 percent have negative smears, while another 15 percent have misinterpreted smears. Methylene blue stains of such specimens generally yield similar results. Results with quellung reactions are generally less accurate, but are related to the experience of the observer.

The capsular PRP of type B strains can be detected in either the serum or CSF of 90 percent of children with meningitis by countercurrent electrophoresis. Despite the relatively widespread distribution of immunologically cross-reactive antigens among bacteria in nature, false-positive reactions are unusual. Latex agglutination detects the antigen in a higher percentage of such specimens, but special techniques must be employed to eliminate a 10 percent rate of nonspecific false-positive results. It is anticipated that reagents for these tests will soon be available commercially. Inhibition of binding of radiolabeled antigen is the most sensitive and accurate technique for detecting PRP, but this procedure is performed in only a few research laboratories. PRP can often be detected in infected pericardial fluid (pericarditis) or joint fluid (septic arthritis), but it is found infrequently in the serum of children with epiglottitis, presumably because of the fulminant course of this disease and the time required for antigen release from the invasive bacteria. Antigen and nonviable bacteria often persist following the sterilization of an infected body fluid by antibiotic therapy. For example, up to 20 percent of treated children with meningitis have detectable antigen in sterile serum or spinal fluid. Thus antigen detection is often helpful in diagnosing children with meningitis who have previously received antibiotics. Recent evidence indicates that both the concentration of PRP in serum or spinal fluid at onset of definitive therapy for meningitis and the duration of antigenemia provide prognostic information regarding the clinical course of the child.

Positive nasopharyngeal cultures are not very meaningful because of the high carrier rate of *H. influenzae* in healthy individuals. Positive cultures of blood and spinal, joint, pericardial, pleural, and tissue fluids are diagnostic. To prove that *H. influenzae* is the cause of otitis media would require culture of middle ear exudate. Such a definitive diagnosis is rarely needed, and tympanocentesis can be recommended only in complicated cases as therapy. Recovery of *H. influenzae* in pure or predominant culture in a sputum or tracheal aspirate is strong evidence of an etiologic role in bronchitis or pneumonia, particularly if the specimen also contains polymorphonuclear leukocytes. Needle aspiration of the edge of the site of cellulitis or of diseased lung markedly increases the rate of diagnosis and is recommended in very sick or complicated patients. Cultures of the inflamed epiglottis are generally positive, but as noted above they should be taken only when an airway can be guaranteed. Prior to the start of antibiotic therapy, blood cultures are positive in up to 90 percent of all children with pneumonia, septic arthritis, facial cellulitis, epiglottitis, and meningitis caused by *H. influenzae.* Even if antibiotic therapy has been initiated, the yield is sufficiently great to recommend that blood cultures be taken from all such patients.

Invasive *H. influenzae* type B diseases are usually associated with peripheral leukocytosis and meningitis with a significant normocytic anemia of unknown etiology. However, these findings are not diagnostic. Infected body fluids generally have decreased glucose and increased protein concentrations and excessive numbers of polymorphonuclear leukocytes. The spinal fluid of children with acute bacterial meningitis (including *H. influenzae*) almost uniformly contains excessive concentrations of lactate and often of tissue enzymes (eg, lysozyme, glutamic oxaloacetic transaminase). Such determinations can be useful in distinguishing bacterial from viral meningitis, but they have no role in determining the etiologic bacteria. Children with invasive *H. influenzae* diseases have no diagnostic or consistent changes in serum chemical or protein constituents.

THERAPY. If not treated, systemic *H. influenzae* diseases, particularly meningitis and epiglottitis, have a very high if not uniform mortality. Chloramphenicol therapy provides adequate concentration of joint and cerebrospinal fluids and produces excellent results. The potential toxicity of chloramphenicol and the excellent results obtained with ampicillin therapy prompted the widespread acceptance of this latter agent as the antibiotic of choice for *H. influenzae* diseases. Although *H. influenzae* were uniformly sensitive in the past, strains of type B organisms resistant to several times the concentration of ampicillin attainable in body fluids with optimal therapy have recently been recovered. These strains owe their resistance to a plasmid-mediated β-lactamase; they are equally pathogenic and transmissable as sensitive strains, and they are not eliminated by ampicillin therapy. Such strains are widely distributed, and at the end of 1975 they comprised 5 to 10 percent of all type B strains isolated in the eastern United States. Ampicillin resistance now exists among nonencapsulated strains as well, but with a lower incidence. Ampicillin resistance can be determined by standard tube dilution of agar diffusion assays of antibiotic activity or by a direct test for β-lactamase activity, which can be easier, more direct, and quicker.

It is now recommended that all systemic diseases that are potentially the *H. influenzae* in origin be treated with chloramphenicol until such time as the *H. influenzae* strain is proved to be sensitive to ampicillin. Chloramphenicol dosage should be 100 mg/kg/day given intravenously in four divided doses at 6-hour intervals. Because chloramphenicol is considered to be less than optimal therapy for pneumococcal meningitis, penicillin should be added to the chloramphenicol therapy if any question of pneumococcal disease cannot be eliminated. If the etiologic strain is sensitive, ampicillin should be given intravenously at 300 to 400 mg/kg/day at 4-hour intervals. The duration of therapy depends on the disease and the status of the individual patient. All systemic diseases should be treated intravenously, at least until cultures of the infected area are sterile and the patient is afebrile and without evidence of active infection for 3 to 5 days. In the case of meningitis, a normal spinal fluid profile, particularly absence of polymorphonuclear leukocytes, is sought before stopping therapy. Thus most children with meningitis require 10 to 14 days of therapy. However, a small percentage of children, particularly those under 1 year of age, continue to have abnormally low CSF glucose concentrations beyond the expected duration. If this is associated with a continued polymorphonuclear response in the cerebrospinal fluid, continued therapy is indicated until focal intracranial infection can be eliminated by appropriate radiologic studies (eg, technetium imaging and computer-assisted tomography) and by subdural taps. Prolonged hypoglycorrhachia often reflects a severe infectious insult to the glucose transport mechanism of the blood-brain barrier; as an isolated phenomenon it may not require prolonged antibiotic therapy.

Children with meningitis caused by sensitive strains occasionally do not completely clear their disease with ampicillin therapy, but develop new symptoms and findings in their cerebrospinal fluid following the cessation of therapy. Such therapeutic failures are often associated with therapy that has been too brief or given at too low a dosage or by a route other than intravenously. In other cases the circumstances suggest loculated disease that was not completely eradicated by acceptable therapy. Retreatment is indicated according to the above guidelines. Chloramphenicol is commonly recommended for second treatments, primarily because of its greater penetrability into the spinal fluid and the usual restoration of normal barriers to ampicillin diffusion at this stage in the disease. However, retreatment with ampicillin can be successful.

Children with endocarditis or pericarditis should re-

ceive 4 to 6 weeks of intravenous therapy. Ampicillin and chloramphenicol diffuse well into inflamed joint spaces; thus there is no indication for local instillation of antibiotics. Children with bronchitis and otitis media may be treated orally with ampicillin in doses of 50 to 100 mg/kg/day in four divided doses until their symptoms are alleviated, plus 3 to 4 days; hence the usual total course is 7 to 10 days.

H. influenzae type B resistant to chloramphenicol have not been recovered in the United States, but unpublished observations in European centers in 1975 have revealed strains bearing plasmids mediating resistance to chloramphenicol and/or tetracycline. Although the distribution and pathogenicity of these strains are not yet defined, it seems prudent to test the sensitivity of strains when the results of chloramphenicol therapy appear disappointing.

Antibiotic therapy is only one facet of the management of the child with an *H. influenzae* disease. Those with meningitis require careful evaluation of their airway, consideration of oxygen therapy and transfusion, vigorous treatment of shock and intravascular coagulation, conservative fluid replacement, anticonvulsive therapy, and medical management of cerebral edema (p. 1819). Guarantee of the airway is critical to the child with epiglottitis. Abundant evidence indicates that drug therapy (eg, steroids, vaporized racemic epinephrine) plays a secondary and unproven role in this quest; therefore either tracheostomy or tracheal intubation is uniformly recommended. The choice between these two procedures depends on the experience and skill of the physician, the age of the child, the severity of the symptoms, and the availability of nursing supervision. The small size of the infant trachea and its peculiar location in the neck of a chubby infant have led to tragedies in the performance of a tracheostomy, especially by inexperienced surgeons. Therefore, under no circumstances should a tracheostomy be performed on a child with epiglottitis until the trachea has been intubated. Cool moist air at high humidity supplemented by oxygen as needed is an important adjunct to management. Mild sedation may be beneficial if apprehension is significant. Parenteral fluids are generally required to maintain fluid and electrolyte balance without disturbing the child. Infected joint fluid should be aspirated from the child with septic arthritis to reduce the pressure and to eliminate toxic substances that may adversely affect the metabolism of the joint cartilage. Repeated aspirations may be needed, but installation of a surgical drain is rarely required in *H. influenzae* disease.

PROGNOSIS.   The prognosis of *H. influenzae* diseases treated appropriately depends on the organ involvement. Even with optimal therapy the mortality rate in meningitis and epiglottitis is 5 to 10 percent. Mortality is greatest among infants younger than 1 year of age and those who are not brought to medical attention until their disease is well established. Up to 40 percent of children with *H. influenzae* meningitis have significant sequelae, the most frequent of which are seizures, hearing deficits, motor disabilities, decreased intellectual activity, and emotional disability. Unfortunately, definitive diagnosis of postmeningitic neurologic sequelae is often not possible for weeks to months; the hospital discharge diagnoses of both normal and abnormal states are often disproved. Continued long-term evaluation is therefore required.

Children who recover from pyarthrosis, cellulitis, and bronchopneumonia have no sequelae. Nearly all those with empyema and pericarditis are also completely cured, but rarely a child may require surgical decortication of constrictive fibrotic adhesions. Children with acute otitis media do well, but the child with recurrent otitis media must be examined carefully for a possible hearing deficit, which in turn can be primary in speech and learning problems. Bronchitis is often difficult to eradicate, usually because of the primary disease of the host; it can progress to bronchiectasis and serious chronic pulmonary disease and dysfunction.

PREVENTION. Although secondary cases of invasive *H. influenzae* diseases occur at significantly increased rates among siblings of patients with the primary diseases, no successful prophylaxis exists at present. Antibiotic therapy sufficient to cure meningitis often does not eliminate nasopharyngeal infection, and no evidence indicates that such therapy will eliminate the risk of subsequent invasive disease. Parents of children with systemic *H. influenzae* disease should therefore be advised of the potential risk, and symptomatic siblings of patients should be examined without delay.

Several considerations argue for active immunization against *H. influenzae* type B: the incidence rates of systemic diseases, particularly meningitis, have been increasing for 45 years; therapy is now complicated by the increasing prevalence of strains resistant to preferred antibiotics; the mortality rate for meningitis has remained constant at about 5 to 10 percent for the past 25 years; children recovering from meningitis face an unacceptably high incidence of significant neurologic damage; incidence and mortality rates of meningitis now equal or exceed those that were observed for several other infectious diseases (eg, pertussis, tetanus, poliomyelitis, rubeola) prior to the introduction of active immunization for them. Because of the primacy of the type B capsule in pathogenicity and the therapeutic efficacy of anticapsular serum, attention has focused initially on a vaccine composed of purified capsular PRP. This vaccine has been found to be nontoxic and immunogenic for older children and adults. The frequency and titer of vaccine-induced antibody response correlate inversely with the age of the child; children under 2 years of age respond infrequently and with low titers. Recent data suggest that this vaccine protects children older than 2 years from meningitis but that it is not effective for younger children. Therefore new approaches have been initiated to develop an effective agent for active immunization, particularly of younger children. Oral ingestion of nonpathogenic species of *E. coli* that have a capsule immunologically cross-reactive with PRP is being evaluated. Also under study is a less purified vaccine in which a native outer membrane complex of lipopolysaccharide-protein-PRP of *H. influenzae* type B is conserved. Both approaches promote protective antibody in experimental animals, but immunogenicity and efficacy in children of the most susceptible ages remain to be proved.

OTHER HUMAN *HAEMOPHILUS* SPECIES. *H. parainfluenzae* has nonencapsulated and encapsulated strains (Table 12). It is a common inhabitant of the normal nasopharyngeal flora and may cause local respiratory tract disease, but only very rarely is it invasive. Many strains identified initially as *H. parainfluenzae* in systemic lesions are subsequently found to be *H. influenzae. H. aegypticus* (Koch-Weeks bacillus) causes purulent conjunctivitis, particularly among children. *H. ducreyi* causes chancroid, a venereal disease that is characterized by a 1- to 2-week incubation, from one to five low centrally ulcerating lesions of 2 to 20 mm that are erythematous out of proportion to induration (ie, soft chancre), and regional lymphadenitis. The diagnosis is suggested by microscopic examination of fresh smears and is proved by culture. *H. hemolyticus* and *parahemolyticus* are common nonpathogenic residents of the upper respiratory tract.

References

Alexander HE: Treatment of type b Hemophilus influenzae meningitis. J Ped itar 25:517, 1944

American Academy of Pediatrics Committee on Infectious Diseases: Ampicillin-resistant strains of Hemophilus influenzae type B. Pediatr 55:145, 1975

Bradshaw MW, Schneerson R, Parke JC Jr, Robbins JB: Bacterial antigens cross-reactive with the capsular polysaccharide of Hemophilus influenzae b. Lancet 1:1095, 1971

Fothergill LD, Wright J: Influenzal meningitis: relation of age incidence to bactericidal power of blood against causal organism. J Immunol 24:273, 1933

Fraser DW, Darby CP, Koehler RE, Jacobs CF, Feldman RA: Risk factors in bacterial meningitis: Charleston, South Carolina. J Infect Dis 127:271, 1973

May JR: Colonial morphology, antigens and pathogenicity of Haemophilus influenzae. Sci Basis Med 1967, 3:211

Moxon ER, Smith AL, Averill R, Smith DH: Haemophilus influenzae meningitis in infant rats after intranasal inoculation. J Infect Dis 129:154, 1974

Pittman M: Variation and type specificity in the bacterial species Hemophilus influenzae. J Exp Med 53:471, 1931

Robbins JB, Schneerson R, Argaman M, Handzel ZT: Haemophilus influenzae type b: disease and immunity in humans. Ann Intern Med 78:259, 1973

Schneerson R, Robbins J: Induction of serum Haemophilus influenzae type b capsular antibodies in adult volunteers fed cross-reacting Escherichia coli 075:K 100:H5. N Engl J Med 292:1093, 1975

Smith DH, Ingram DL, Smith AL, Gilles F, Bresnan MJ: Bacterial meningitis. A symposium. Pediatr 52:586, 1973

——— Peter G, Ingram DL, et al: Responses of children immunized with the capsular polysaccharide of Hemophilus influenzae type b. Pediatr 52:637, 1973

Smith EWP Jr, Haynes RE: Changing incidence of Hemophilus influenzae meningitis. Pediatrics 50:723, 1972

Todd JK, Bruhn FW: Severe Haemophilus influenzae infections. Am J Dis Child 129:607, 1975

Turk DC, May JR: Haemophilus influenzae. Its Clinical Importance. London, English Universities Press, 1967

LEPTOSPIROSIS

MICHAEL KATZ

Leptospirosis is a multisystem disease that was described under a variety of clinical syndromes before the discovery of the etiologic agent unified these syndromes into one disease. Thus, such conditions as Weil's disease, swamp fever, and field fever in Europe, 7-day fever (nanukayami) or autumnal fever (hasami-Netsu) in Japan, cane-field fever in Australia, and bushy creek fever and Fort Bragg fever in the United States are now known to have resulted from leptospiral infections. The original opinion that only rodents acted as hosts for *Leptospira* has now been abandoned in the face of ample epidemiologic evidence that swine, cattle, and dogs also serve as reservoirs. Although at least a dozen species of *Leptospira* are known to infect man, only three do so with any frequency: *L. icterohaemorrhagiae* (from the rat), *L. pomona* (from swine), and *L. canicola* (from cattle and dogs). Leptospirosis was once thought to be more common in Europe and Asia than in the United States, but there is no evidence that this is so; apparently many cases of leptospirosis have been unrecognized. Among 318 cases of definite leptospirosis recorded by the Center for Disease Control, only 54 (17 percent) were recognized as leptospirosis at the time of initial evaluation by a physician. It is quite likely that many cases go unrecorded.

The reservoir animals retain leptospires in the renal tubules and shed large numbers of them in their urine for months after the infection. Man becomes infected through contact with animal urine, either directly, or secondarily through contaminated soil or water. *Leptospira* are very sensitive to acid pH and will perish in acid in a few hours, but in an alkaline or a neutral medium they will persist for weeks, provided the temperature is above 22°C. Thus during the warm seasons stagnant waters and moist soil are common sources of the infection. Infection can be acquired through cut or abraded skin, or in the case of immersion, through respiratory or conjunctival epithelium. It is doubtful that the gastrointestinal tract is a route of infection in view of the sensitivity of the *Leptospira* to acid pH.

CLINICAL MANIFESTATIONS. Clinical manifestations vary somewhat with the infecting species. *L. canicola* and *L. pomona* tend to cause less severe disease than *L. icterohaemorrhagiae.* In general, leptospirosis is a biphasic disease that develops after a median incubation period of 1 week, but with a range of 2 to 20 days. The first phase, lasting for 4 to 7 days, is the septicemic stage. It is characterized by fever, headache, myalgia, and gastrointestinal disturbances such as abdominal pain, nausea, and vomiting. Physical examination in this stage usually reveals an acutely ill patient who may be confused or delirious. Conjunctivitis, pharyngeal injection, lymphadenopathy, hepatosplenomegaly, macular exanthem, and icterus may be seen. During this stage the patient will have leptospiremia and proteinuria. The fever ends by lysis, and the patient may remain asymptomatic and comfortable for 1 to 3 days, at which time the second phase of the disease will occur. This stage will begin with meningitis, which may be subclinical, and with fever, which may be of lower grade than during the first stage. Some patients may be asymptomatic during the second stage. Physical examination may reveal uveitis and focal neurologic signs. The results of lumbar puncture will show aseptic meningitis. During this stage the patient no longer has leptospiremia, but now has leptospiruria. Since antileptospiral antibodies are present during this stage, the second stage is sometimes defined as the immune stage.

Some 10 percent of patients develop a severe form of this disease characterized by prolonged fever, jaundice, azotemia, hemorrhage, vascular collapse, and altered state of consciousness. The same biphasic pattern of the disease can be seen in this severe manifestation of leptospirosis, but the severity of symptoms and their prolongation may last well into the second stage and obscure the signs that mark the end of the first stage. Careful monitoring of temperature may reveal a reduction or even disappearance of fever for a day or so. The pathogenesis of this severe manifestation of leptospirosis is not clearly understood, but it has been suggested that it may be due to a toxin elaborated by the microorganism. Although such a toxin has not been demonstrated unequivocally in human infection, a toxic effect of mouse plasma derived from infected animals has been demonstrated in uninfected recipients. Moreover, there has been evidence of an in vitro cytopathic effect of such plasma on tissue cultures. At the opposite end of the spectrum are the inapparent infections, as demonstrated by the presence of antileptospiral antibodies in individuals who do not have the clinical disease. However, such instances are thought to be rare.

DIAGNOSIS. Clinical diagnosis of leptospirosis must obviously be considered in patients with aseptic meningitis, hepatitis, influenza, and fever of undetermined origin. The definitive diagnosis can be established only by demonstration of leptospires in the blood or urine of patients, either by culture or by inoculation into guinea pigs, hamsters, or mice. A microagglutinin test will detect antibodies, which begin to appear between 6 and 12 days after the infection and reach their peak in 1 month. A rise in titer, or seroconversion, is the indirect indication of acute leptospirosis.

PROGNOSIS. The prognosis depends on two principal factors: the virulence of the infecting organism and the age of the patient. In anicteric leptospirosis death is virtually unknown. On the other hand, the classic Weil's disease caused by the more virulent organisms has a definite risk of death. In a series reported by McCrumb the death rate for 244 patients was 0.8 percent, but it was 19 percent for those who had developed jaundice. Similar death rates of jaundiced patients have been reported in other series. Mortality tends to be higher in older adults than in children.

TREATMENT. Although claims of effectiveness of penicillin or the tetracyclines have been made, especially if these drugs are administered early in the infection, there is no evidence that antimicrobial therapy affects the natural course of this disease. At the present time there is no vaccine effective against leptospirosis.

References

Barkin RM, Glosser JW: Leptospirosis, an epidemic in children. Am J Epidemiol 98:184, 1973

Edwards GA, Domm BM: Human leptospirosis. Medicine 39:117, 1960

Knight LL, Miller NG, White RJ: Cytotoxic factor in the blood and plasma of animals during leptospirosis. Infect Immun 8:401, 1973

Leptospirosis Survey in the United States 1970. Morbidity Mortality 20:460, 1971

McCrumb FR Jr, Stockard JL, Robinson L, et al: Leptospirosis in Malaya. I. Sporadic cases among military and civilian personnel. Am J Trop Med Hyg 6:238, 1957

Memoranda: Research Needs in Leptospirosis. Bull WHO 47:113, 1972

MENINGOCOCCAL INFECTIONS
ELI GOLD AND DAN M. GRANOFF

Meningococci continue to cause serious disease throughout the world. Epidemics have recently been reported from such scattered geographic regions and diverse socioeconomic settings as Brazil, the Middle East, and Finland. Although similar epidemics have not occurred in the United States since the 1940s, isolated outbreaks in this country continue to pose a problem, particularly among high-risk populations such as military recruits and young children. In 1963 it was first recognized that many of the strains of meningococci causing disease in this country and throughout the world were resistant to sulfonamides. The problem of sulfonamide-resistant meningococci has persisted, but fortunately patients infected with such strains respond well to penicillin. A major problem is our inability to eliminate the sulfonamide-resistant organisms in healthy carriers; penicillin is ineffective, and minocycline and rifampin have been tried for this purpose, but there appears to be no completely effective drug available.

Meningococci (*Neisseria meningitidis*) are fastidious gram-negative endotoxin-containing organisms that have some of the traits of gram-positive organisms. They inhabit the respiratory tract, from which they may be disseminated via the bloodstream; they have a spectrum of antibiotic sensitivity similar to that of pneumococci, streptococci, and some staphylococci. *N. meningitidis* are extremely labile organisms and are rapidly inactivated outside the body by drying, heat, or contact with germicides. Smears of pus taken from infected sites characteristically contain large numbers of intracellular gram negative biscuit-shaped diplococci. The organism has rather simple nutritional requirements, but is susceptible to the toxic effect of amino acids and many other constituents of media.

Growth of the organism is best on an enriched medium such as chocolate or Mueller-Hinton agar in an atmosphere of 2 to 20 percent carbon dioxide obtained by using a candle jar or carbon dioxide incubator. When a selective medium is desirable, Thayer-Martin agar, developed for the isolation of the gonococcus, may also be used for isolating meningococci. Typical colonies grown on transparent medium are smooth glistening tear drops that contain cytochrome oxidase. Testing for this uncommon enzyme provides a rapid means for the presumptive identification of members of the *Neisseria* genus. Classic strains ferment dextrose and maltose, but atypical variants recently isolated from children may also ferment lactose.

The meningococci have classically been divided into four groups (A, B, C, and D) on the basis of specific serologic reactions. Additional groups known as X, Y, Z, and A4317 have also been described, and some of the strains previously thought to be nontypable can be identified as belonging to one of these new groups. The serologic subgroups of meningococci have considerable epidemiologic and immunologic importance. They serve as specific markers for studying outbreaks and transmission of disease; they are also important in the current efforts being made toward development of specific meningococcal vaccines.

EPIDEMIOLOGY. The annual rate of reported meningococcal infection in the United States had been relatively constant for 5 years, but it declined in 1972 and 1973 from 1.2 to 0.66 per 100,000 population. The incidence varies in different regions of the country, with higher rates being reported from the Southeast. More cases occur in late winter and early spring than in summer and early fall. Cases among military personnel have usually accounted for 10 percent of the total, but these have also shown a significant decrease. Whether the lowered rate in this group is related to the recent widespread use of serotype C meningococcal vaccine in military personnel remains to be ascertained. Meningococcal infection is properly included among the large group of childhood diseases, since it has its highest incidence rate among infants and young children. One-third of all cases in the United States occur in children less than 5 years of age, and the highest specific rate is in the group less than 1 year of age. A secondary increase in incidence has been found in the group 15 to 24 years of age, but thereafter the incidence falls to insignificant levels.

Major epidemics of meningococcal disease prior to 1963 were caused by group A strains; only sporadic or small outbreaks were caused by serotypes B or C. In the past several years, however, group A organisms have accounted for only 2 percent of meningococcal isolates submitted to the National Communicable Disease Center. Groups B and C, and more recently group Y organisms, are now the predominant serotypes associated with severe clinical disease. Concurrent with the observed change in distribution of serotypes has been a modest but perceptible decline in the prevalence of sulfonamide-resistant strains. Approximately 15 percent of group B isolates and 80 percent of group C strains are resistant to sulfadiazine (1.0 mg/ml or more), while group Y organisms, which are responsible for nearly 15 percent of recently reported illnesses, are for the most part sensitive to the sulfonamides.

PATHOGENESIS. Meningococci are transmitted from person to person by droplet spread, as are many other agents that inhabit the respiratory tract. Infection of a susceptible host is followed by a period during which meningococci multiply in the nasopharynx, but development of overt disease is uncommon. The carrier rate for meningococci averages 10 percent, but only about 1 in 10,000 individuals colonized by meningococci develops a significant illness. In these vulnerable few the host is apparently unable to limit the growth and dissemination of the organism, and bacteremia with or without meningitis results.

Immunity to meningococcal disease is closely related to the presence of bactericidal antibodies. In the newborn these are acquired transplacentally, and they protect most infants during the first few months of life, after which there is a reciprocal relationship between presence of antibody and incidence of infection. Natural immunity may be initiated following subclinical infection with a group-specific strain; more commonly it may derive from asymptomatic nasopharyngeal carriage of atypical nontypable meningococci or other bacteria possessing cross-reacting antigens. Thus as children become older the proportion with immunity increases, and the incidence rate of meningococcal infection diminishes. In the vulnerable individual bacteremia may follow nasopharyngeal infection as the primary systemic event. Meningococci are deposited throughout the body, but they appear to have a particular predilection for the meninges and skin. The other major clinical manifestations of generalized meningococcal infection are bleeding and shock produced by the action of endotoxin on the endothelium of small vessels.

CLINICAL DISEASE AND DIFFERENTIAL DIAGNOSIS. The dominant features of meningococcal disease are fever, rash, and meningitis. In approximately one-half of all patients typical petechiae or larger purpuric lesions appear, usually most apparent on the chest, upper arms, and axilla. Maculopapular rashes are also common and may occur in the absence of petechiae.

The most common presentation of meningococcal infection is *acute bacterial meningitis*. Older children typically have abrupt onset of fever, headache, irritability, and lethargy, but hyperactivity, delirium, or complaints of aching all over are not uncommon. Nuchal rigidity is a prominent sign except in young infants, where fever, poor feeding, vomiting, and lethargy are often the presenting complaints. A bulging fontanelle may be the other major clue indicating infection of the central nervous system. Suspicion of meningitis, especially if supported by evidence of meningeal irritation, is an indication for immediate lumbar puncture. Cerebrospinal fluid should be removed slowly through a small needle in sufficient quantity for smear, culture, cell count, and sugar and protein determinations. Measurement of pressure is often also helpful. The typical cerebrospinal fluid findings are an increase in white blood cell count with a predominance of polymorphonuclear leukocytes (from 100 to several thousand cells per cubic millimeter), a decrease in spinal fluid sugar as manifested either by an absolute level of 40 mg/100 ml or less or by a level less than two-thirds of the blood sugar level, an elevated protein, and/or positive smear or culture. Occasionally a positive culture is obtained from a cerebrospinal fluid with few or no cells, but ordinarily the high cell count, low sugar, and elevated protein make it easy to distinguish bacterial meningitis from viral aseptic meningitis. Both countercurrent immunoelectrophoresis and *Limulus* lysate assay (which would detect any endotoxin and not specifically the meningococcus), if available, can be of help in supporting the diagnosis of meningococcal infection in atypical or complicated cases. Petechial rash is more likely to occur with meningococcal infection than with *H. influenzae* or pneumococci, but if a definite bacteriologic diagnosis cannot be made, treatment with ampicillin (in portions of the country where *H. influenzae* are not resistant) or chloramphenicol combined with penicillin (which covers all three of these possibilities) should be instituted. Modifications of drug therapy can be made when culture results are available.

The range of other clinical manifestations that may result from the meningococcus is equaled by that of few organisms. In the fulminant form of disease meningitis may be absent, but signs and symptoms of septic shock, often heralded by a spreading hemorrhagic rash, may progress rapidly and lead to death within a period of hours. In other patients the onset of illness may be insidious, accompanied only by low-grade fever, arthralgia, and an evanescent rash. These manifestations may disappear spontaneously over a period of a few days or may progress to an illness of greater intensity. Rarely a chronic form of meningococcemia occurs that produces intermittent fever, chills, joint pains, and petechial or maculopapular eruption that persists for several days. Patients with this form of disease often initially have good health between episodes, but over a period of months of recurring episodes they gradually show clinical deterioration: enlargement of the spleen occurs, and endocarditis, meningitis, or death may supervene at any time.

A common problem is differentiating streptococcal infection with petechiae from acute meningococcemia, especially when sore throat and adenopathy are not present. Rarely, other bacterial infections such as typhoid fever, bacterial endocarditis, or systemic gonococcal infections may also mimic the presentation of meningococcal disease. Other clinical entities that may cause diagnostic perplexity are viral illnesses, particularly enteroviruses such as echovirus 9 or coxsackievirus A9, atypical measles, and rickettsial diseases such as Rocky Mountain spotted fever or endemic typhus. In the majority of such patients a careful appraisal of the clinical, laboratory, and epidemiologic data associated with illness will usually lead to the correct diagnosis. However, when uncertainty exists and meningococcemia is suspected, it is prudent to obtain bacterial, viral, and other appropriate studies and begin antimicrobial therapy.

TREATMENT. In the preantibiotic era the mortality rate for meningococcal meningitis varied from 15 to 85 percent, depending on the particular outbreak and the age group affected. The death rate among young infants was 90 percent. The development of type-specific antiserum shortly after the turn of the century reduced the risk of death to about 30 percent; this figure fell to 12 to 15 percent with the advent of sulfonamides, but this is where it has remained. The availability of antibiotics, sophisticated fluid therapy, steroids, and other pharmacologic agents has not resulted in a further significant reduction in the mortality rate from meningococcal disease.

The diagnosis of meningococcemia with or without meningitis calls for prompt administration of appropriate antimicrobial therapy. Penicillin is the drug of choice. Treatment with ampicillin, or chloramphenicol combined with penicillin, may also be used if the etiology of the bacterial meningitis is uncertain. Therapy should be given by the intravenous route (100,000 to 400,000 IU/kg/day divided into three or four hourly doses), and in the uncomplicated disease it should be continued for 7 days. Intravenous chloramphenicol is the desired therapy in patients suspected of having penicillin allergy. Cephalosporin are not effective for treating such infections and should not be used.

Most patients with meningococcal infection whose illness is diagnosed promptly and who have the benefit of treatment with a proper antibiotic recover and suffer no apparent residual effect. Those whose illness is not recognized or who do not receive adequate antibiotic therapy may have a prolonged course, with thrombosis of cerebral vessels, infarction of brain, and permanent central nervous system damage. The major fear with meningococcal infection is shock, usually accompanied by extensive purpura and followed by death (Waterhouse-Friderichsen syndrome). The precise mechanism of endotoxin shock in man is not clear, nor is it known whether fulminant shock and intravascular coagulation, which frequently occur together, are independent or related phenomena. Studies of endotoxin shock in different animals conducted by different workers provide conflicting ideas as to what happens in man, and it is difficult to decide what specific therapeutic approaches are indicated in the human patient. There is no convincing evidence at this time that the use of steroids (in either physiologic or pharmacologic dosage), heparin, or vasodilators has improved the prognosis of endotoxin shock. The administration of vasoconstrictors may be harmful. Patients with meningococcal infection should be treated with antibiotics and appropriate intravenous fluids. Vital signs, especially blood pressure, should be monitored, and if hypotension develops an immediate attempt should be made to maintain blood volume.

Occasionally a patient may also have myocarditis as a consequence of meningococcal infection. In this clinical setting caution should be exercised in regard to overzealous volume expansion, since it may carry with it the risk of cardiac decompensation. Monitoring the central venous pressure in such an individual may also be useful, and treatment with rapid-acting digitalis preparations should be instituted at the first signs of congestive heart failure.

Hydrocortisone in large doses (40 to 50 mg/kg) administered intravenously and repeated every 30 to 60 minutes for three to four doses has been advocated for patients with severe meningococcemia, mostly on the basis of theoretical indications; clinical experience with its use shows neither clear-cut benefit nor evidence of harm. Vasodilators such as isoproterenol or phenoxybenzamine have been shown to be of value in the management of shock in laboratory animals, but no one has had sufficient success in the treatment of meningococcal shock with these agents to recommend their general use. The occurrence of intravascular coagulation with severe bleeding into skin and viscera appears to be more common in patients with high initial levels of circulating meningococcal polysaccharide antigen, and it is associated with a decrease in components of the intravascular clotting reaction, ie, platelets, factors V and VIII, prothrombin, and fibrinogen. These observations have been the basis for attempts to treat intravascular coagulation with heparin, but again the results have been variable. Coagulation defects may be brought under control by this therapy, but unfortunately this does not necessarily ensure patient survival. It may be reasonable, in centers where adequate facilities are available, to measure clotting factors in patients with meningococcal shock and initiate treatment with heparin when there is evidence of intravascular coagulation and depletion of coagulation factors. Heparin may be given intravenously in a dose of 1 mg/kg (100 IU) every 4 hours as needed to maintain the clotting time at 20 to 30 minutes until coagulation factors return to normal levels.

Subdural effusions may occur following meningococcal meningitis, and they should be considered in any patient with an atypical course characterized by persistent fever, bulging fontanelle, lethargy, vomiting, or neurologic signs. Increasing head size or translucent areas in the temporal portion visible by transillumination of the infant skull are presumptive signs of subdural effusions. Arthritis or cutaneous vasculitis may present 3 to 4 days after initiation of therapy, especially in adults. Circulating and localized antigen–antibody complexes have been detected in such patients, suggesting that allergy to meningococcal antigen may be an explanation for these phenomena. It should be noted that there are reports in the literature concerning the isolation of meningococci from the joints of patients with arthritis. Another delayed manifestation of meningococcal disease is pericarditis, with or without effusion, which may appear during the second week of illness heralded by fever, tachycardia, and signs of cardiac enlargement. In contrast to the pericarditis that may be present at the onset of illness, bacterial cultures in the delayed-onset variety are nearly always sterile. Nevertheless, pericardiocentesis should be promptly performed if active infection is suspected or if the patient develops signs of cardiac tamponade.

PROPHYLAXIS. The changes in the sulfonamide sensitivity patterns of the meningococci have removed an effective tool for eliminating carriers and protecting those who come in contact with patients. Penicillin and related drugs that are highly effective for treating systemic meningococcal infections do not eliminate the carrier state. However, two newly licensed drugs (minocycline and rifampin) have been tested in adults and found to be of use in eradicating carriage of meningococci. Unfortunately there is little experience with these agents in children, and so their general use in these patients cannot be recommended.

The probability of meningococcal disease occurring among close associates of a patient is difficult to determine, but it is clearly greater than among the population as a whole. The use of prophylactic chemotherapy for close contacts of patients is at present controversial. Many physicians do not recommend any form of prophylaxis unless the organism is known to be sulfonamide-sensitive. Others prescribe sulfonamide prophylaxis even though there is an approximately 50 percent probability that the causative agent will be sulfonamide-resistant. Penicillin in large parenteral doses is advised by some authorities; they argue that suppression of the meningococci may interfere with disease production even though the bacteria are not eliminated. The approach has not been adequately evaluated. Close surveillance of all contacts is obviously required to identify any secondary cases rapidly, regardless of what drugs may be administered.

Vaccines prepared from purified meningococcal polysaccharides (groups A and C) appear to be nontoxic. Unfortunately, as immunizing agents they appear to be least effective in the infant less than 1 year of age. Preliminary reports of vaccine trials indicate that 3-month-old infants respond weakly but consistently to group C antigen and weakly and inconsistently to group A antigen. Booster injections of the group C polysaccharide result in decreased antibody production as compared to primary immunization at the same age; however, booster injections at 18 months of age with the group A polysaccharide produce a higher antibody titer than primary immunization at that age. The implication of these observations is that group A vaccine may be administered to an infant 7 months of age (for example) with the expectation of a modest antibody response that will increase further following a booster shot at the age of 1 year. However, group C vaccine not only provokes a poor antibody response in the child less than 1 year of age but also does not have the potential to produce a booster response when administered a second time some months later. Meningococcal vaccine may be useful only in the child more than 1 year of age.

References

Devine LF, Hannah JM, Hagerman CR, et al: Minocycline and rifampin: proposed treatment regimen for the elimination of meningococci from the nasopharynges of healthy carriers. Milit Med 138:20, 1973

Goldschneider I, Lepow ML, Gotschlich EC: Immunogenicity of the group A and group C meningococcal polysaccharides in children. J Infect Dis 125:509, 1972

Gotschlich EC, Goldschneider I, Artenstein MS: Human immunity to the meningococcus. J Exp Med 129:1385, 1969

Greenwood BM, Whittle HC, Dominic-Rajkovic O: Counter-current immunoelectrophoresis in the diagnosis of meningococcal infections. Lancet 2:519, 1971

Hathaway WE: Heparin therapy in acute meningococcemia. J Pediatr 82:900, 1973

Hodes HL: Care of critically ill child: endotoxin shock. Pediatr 44:248, 1969

Nachum R, Lipsey A, Siegel SE: Rapid detection of gram-negative bacterial meningitis by the Limulus lysate test. N Engl J Med 289:931, 1973

Wiggins GL, Hollis DG, Weaver R: Prevalence of serogroups and sulfonamide resistance of meningococci from the civilian population in the United States, 1964–1970. Am J Public Health 63:59, 1973

MYCOPLASMA INFECTIONS
WALTER L. HENLEY

Mycoplasma, originally known as pleuropneumonia-like organisms (PPLO), are the smallest known microorganisms able to reproduce in a cell-free medium. They are 125 to 250 mμ in size and resemble L forms of bacteria, to which they may be related. The mycoplasma lack cell walls and require sterols and protein for growth in colonies of characteristic morphology. They do not stain with Gram's stain due to the absence of cell walls, but they appear as small pleomorphic cocci or short rods or hollow ring forms with Giemsa staining. Several members of the genus *Mycoplasma* have been implicated in human disease. They can be differentiated antigenically by agglutination, hemagglutination inhibition, and immunofluorescence. Complement fixation yields cross-reactions among the mycoplasma. The most specific tests for their identification require antibody to inhibit their metabolism and growth. *M. pneumoniae* causes primary atypical pneumonia and is the most important member of the genus. It can absorb and lyse certain types of erythrocytes within 24 to 48 hours, and primary atypical pneumonia is often accompanied by the production of cold hemagglutinins. *M. hominis* has been recovered from the mouth and urogenital tract. It has caused pelvic abscess and has been found in the bone marrow of patients with leukemia. Experimental intranasal inoculation has produced exudative pharyngitis and tonsillitis in man. *M. orale* types I, II, and III, *M. salivarium,* and *M. fermentans* can also be recovered from the mouth. The species known as the *T strains of Mycoplasma* have been recovered from the urogenital tracts of patients with urethritis and vaginitis, as well as from normal individuals. Their recovery is not proof of their etiologic status unless accompanied by a significant rise in specific antibody. However, there is strong epidemiologic evidence in the demonstration of the microorganism in a man following coitus with an infected woman and isolation of T strains from both partners. *M. hominis* and T strains have been cultured from maternal blood and fetal tissue. Rarely the newborn may be infected with an organism acquired during passage through the birth canal. Isolation of the microorganism must be associated with specific antibody rise to prove infection, since the microorganism is a frequent contaminant of solid and liquid media. The species *M. hominis* has also been isolated from healthy individuals and occasionally from patients with pneumonia. An increase in the isolation of the mycoplasma from patients with leukemia or patients on immunosuppressive therapy raises the possibility of latent infection.

M. PNEUMONIAE INFECTION. With the introduction of antibiotics it was noted that some patients with pneumonia did not show an immediate favorable response to chemotherapy. At first they were thought to have viral pneumonia, but some responded to tetracycline and streptomycin. They had a rise in hemagglutinins, which agglutinated human group O erythrocytes at 0 to 4 C but not at 37 C. Some patients also had agglutinins to an α-hemolytic *Streptococcus* known as *Streptococcus* MG. In 1944 Eaton and associates isolated an agent that could be propagated in eggs and produced pneumonia in animals. In 1962 Chanock and associates cultured the agent on cell-free agar medium. The microorganism could be stained with fluorescein-conjugated antibody obtained from the convalescent sera of patients. It was identified as one of the mycoplasma and named *M. pneumoniae*.

EPIDEMIOLOGY. *M. pneumoniae* can cause pneumonia in any age group, but it most commonly affects adolescents and young adults. The true extent of infection is not known, since isolation of *M. pneumoniae* is usually attempted only in patients with pulmonary infiltrates. Prospective studies have shown that infection is widespread and that the microorganism can cause upper respiratory infection, bronchitis, and otitis media. The prevalence of infection varies from year to year, with incidence lowest in the summer. Infection spreads mostly readily on close contact within families, in day-care centers and schools, and among military recruits.

CLINICAL DISEASE. Atypical pneumonia may be produced by various microorganisms. If bacterial infection has been ruled out, viral pneumonias must be considered in the differential diagnosis. The incubation period for *M. pneumoniae* pneumonia ranges from 10 to 20 days. The symptoms may be those of upper respiratory disease with or without cough. Fever, chills, malaise, headache, anorexia, and abdominal pain, as well as conjunctivitis, have been described. Symptomatology is generally greater in patients with pneumonia. The radiographic evidence of pulmonary infiltration is often striking, although there may be few findings on physical examination. Younger children usually exhibit less distress, but the disease may mimic bronchiolitis, and the cough may be paroxysmal, as in pertussis. Younger children have been reported to be susceptible to recurrent infection. Children with sickle cell disease are susceptible to more severe disease with multiple pulmonary infiltrates and pleural effusion.

PHYSICAL EXAMINATION. The child usually appears less ill than the fever indicates. There may be rhinitis, pharyngeal erythema, enlarged submandibular and cervical lymph nodes, otitis media, and conjunctivitis. Rhonchi may be heard, as well as rales associated with dullness to percussion and decreased breath sounds in the same areas. Pleural friction rub is uncommon. Respiratory and pulse rates rise, depending on the extent of pulmonary involvement and temperature elevation. Dyspnea and cyanosis are rare. The cough is dry initially; sputum containing pus, desquamated cells, and the microorganisms appears during the course in the patient ill with pneumonia.

LABORATORY FINDINGS. The leukocyte count usually shows no significant change, whereas the erythrocyte sedimentation rate rises. Children with sickle cell disease often show leukocytosis without an elevated erythrocyte sedimentation rate. After 10 to 20 days there is usually a rise in complement-fixing, fluorescent, and growth-inhibiting antibodies. At that time the appearance of cold hemagglutinins can be detected in approximately half the patients, while *Streptococcus* MG agglutinins are found in a smaller percentage.

RADIOGRAPHIC FINDINGS. Radiographs show infiltration that appears to fan from the hilum to the periphery and is usually confined to one lobe. Occasionally more than one lobe is involved, and rarely there is massive pulmonary involvement with pleural effusion. Lesions that resemble miliary granuloma are even more unusual. There are increased bronchovascular markings due to peribronchial inflammation, bronchial and bronchiolar infiltration, and vascular engorgement. Spotty areas of atelectasis may be seen.

DIAGNOSIS. The diagnosis is made by isolating *M. pneumoniae* from the nasopharynx and sputum on special medium containing serum and yeast extract with penicillin and thallium acetate to inhibit contaminating bacteria (thallium acetate, however, is lethal to T strains). A rise in one of the antibodies against the isolated microorganism must be demonstrated during convalescence. The differential diagnosis includes all microorganisms (bacterial, viral, or rickettsial) that can produce upper and lower respiratory tract infection. It is rarely necessary to consider hypersensitivity pneumonias or parasitic etiology in the differential diagnosis. If bacterial infection has been ruled out, the agents that must be considered in the differential diagnosis include adenovirus, influenza, parainfluenza, and psittacosis virus. Pneumonia caused by respiratory syncytial virus and *M. pneumoniae* almost always occurs in different age groups. Atypical pneumonia can result from infection with *Coxiella burnetii* (Q fever), but less often than from infection with *M. pneumonia*. The rises in cold hemagglutinins and *Streptococcus* MG agglutinins are of some diagnostic value, but they can also be induced by microorganisms other than *M. pneumoniae*, so that a rise in growth-inhibiting antibody or one of the other antibodies is necessary for definitive diagnosis, particularly if the agent has not been isolated. Similarly, a rise in antibody to one of the other microorganisms listed tends to exclude the diagnosis.

COURSE AND COMPLICATIONS. The disease usually lasts 1 to 2 weeks. In patients with pulmonary infiltrates the radiographic findings may persist twice as long. The illness is prolonged in the small proportion of patients who suffer massive pulmonary involvement and/or pleural effusion such as is seen in children with sickle cell disease. Complications (reported because of relative infrequency) include meningitis, meningoencephalitis, acute cerebellar ataxia, Guillain-Barré syndrome, hepatitis, erythema multiforme, hemolytic anemia, intravascular coagulation, myocarditis, pericarditis, renal failure, and fatal infection.

TREATMENT. Erythromycin (50 mg/kg/day in four oral doses for 1 or 2 weeks) is the antibiotic of choice because of its narrow antimicrobial spectrum. Tetracycline is effective, but it has undesirable side effects on children with developing dentition and on gastrointestinal flora. Similarly, the aminoglycosides have been reported to be effective, but they are ototoxic and alter the gastrointestinal flora. Although there is improvement with the antibiotic, the microorganism is not always eradicated; it may be isolated on culture as the patient appears convalescent. Penicillin is ineffective because of the lack of cell walls in the mycoplasma.

Inhalation of humid air is important in order to avoid accumulation of thick mucus; it is the cornerstone of therapy. Decongestants are of little value, and expectorant medication is rarely useful in older children. Dehydration should be prevented by liquid intake. Intravenous fluids may be required in small children or in children with dyspnea due to severe disease. Oxygen inhalation is needed only in the rare patient with respiratory decompensation. Antipyretics may be required in patients with high fever. Convalescent care is necessary in a previously ill child; the duration depends on the severity of the illness.

PREVENTION. An elevated antibody titer protects patients against reinfection; children have occasionally shown a fall in antibody titer with recurrent infection. The role of cell-mediated immunity in prevention is not yet clear. Experimental infection has produced coryza or pneumonia in 75 percent of controls; 90 percent of volunteers with elevated antibody levels were protected. An experimental vaccine has been shown to be effective, but no commercial vaccine is currently available, nor is it needed at present for general immunization of children.

References

Denny FW, Clyde WA Jr, Glazen WP: Mycoplasma pneumoniae disease: clinical spectrum, pathophysiology, epidemiology and control. J Infect Dis 123:74, 1971

Fernald GW, Collier AM, Clyde WA Jr: Respiratory infections due to Mycoplasma pneumoniae in infants and children. Pediatr 55:327, 1975

Grix A, Giammona ST: Pneumonitis with pleural effusion in children due to Mycoplasma pneumoniae. Ann Rev Respir Dis 109:665, 1975

McCarty M: Bacterial and mycotic infections. In Davis BD, Dulbecco R, Eisen HN, Ginsberg HS, Wood WB (eds): Microbiology, 2nd ed. Hagerstown, Md, Harper & Row, 1973, p 929

Murray HW, Masur H, Senterfit LB, Roberts RB: The protean manifestations of Mycoplasma pneumoniae infections in adults. Am J Med 58:229, 1975

Shulman ST, Bartlett J, Clyde WA Jr, Ayoub EM: The unusual severity of Mycoplasma pneumonia in children with sickle cell disease. N Engl J Med 287:164, 1972

PERTUSSIS, PERTUSSIS SYNDROME, AND PARAPERTUSSIS

James D. Connor

PERTUSSIS

Pertussis is an acute disease of the respiratory tract usually characterized by progressive, repetitive paroxysmal coughing, mild systemic complaints, and lymphocytosis. The hallmark of the clinical disease is an inspiratory whoop; for that reason it is commonly referred to as whooping cough. Pertussis occurs throughout the world in immunized and unimmunized populations, usually causing sharp outbreaks or epidemics of disease in cycles of 2 to 4 years. The disease is caused by infection with minute bacilli known as *Bordetella pertussis*, which were first isolated from children with the disease by Bordet and Gengou in 1906. Although infection may occur at any age, the clinical disease is most frequently recognized in older infants and children with typical paroxysms and the characteristic inspiratory whoop. The morbidity is associated with the severity of coughing paroxysms and is especially marked in infants under 1 year of age. The incidence has continued to decline throughout the era of active immunization. The mortality rate has also declined markedly in both the immunized and the unimmunized populations in the highly developed countries.

ETIOLOGY. *B. pertussis* was originally known as the Bordet-Gengou *Bacillus* and was then assigned to the genus *Haemophilus* along with *Haemophilus influenzae*. After it was recognized that the pertussis bacillus did not require X and V factors for growth, a separate genus (*Bordetella*) was identified; it now also includes *B. parapertussis* and *B. bronchiseptica* (formerly *Brucella bronchiseptica*). Growth of pertussis bacilli utilizing optimal liquid or semisolid medium results in a highly uniform minute coccobacillary appearance of the organisms, which are approximately $0.5~\mu$ in length and faintly eosinophilic after Gram's stain. The bacilli are nonmotile and encapsulated. After initial isolation, when grown under less than optimal conditions, pleomorphism will develop, including long rod forms mixed with coccoid and ovoid organisms. The change in appearance of the bacilli is accompanied by defective antigenic structure and includes loss of the protective antigen that induces protection in animals and in humans. The bacilli carry various other antigens including agglutinogens, which provide means of identification of different antigenic types among the genus *Bordetella* and which are used to identify individual clinical strains of *B. pertussis*. Eldering and Kendrick identified agglutinogen types 1 through 6 among various strains of *B. pertussis*, types 2, 3, and 5 being major agglutinogens and 4 and 6 being minor. Type 7 is common to the genus; type 12 is species-specific for *B. bronchiseptica* and type 14 for *B. parapertussis*. Therefore, using adsorbed immune serum it is possible to differentiate antigenically between the three members of the genus by agglutination. Although there are common antigens among the genus, no cross-immunity has been recognized. Other antigens of *B.*

pertussis include heat-labile and heat-stable toxins, histamine sensitizing factor, hemagglutinins, and lymphocyte-promoting factor. The last is the factor responsible for a characteristic lymphocytosis that appears during the paroxysmal-stage disease or after immunization with whole killed bacillary vaccine. It may be induced specifically in laboratory animals by injection of the factor isolated from whole bacilli. It is not apparent which of these antigens (if any) play a role in the pathogenesis of disease.

INCIDENCE. In relatively isolated unimmunized populations pertussis occurs in sharp outbreaks and epidemics. During epidemics the incidence of the characteristic acute disease is highest among infants and young children. This age group is at risk from lack of exposure, having been born after the preceding epidemic. In this group the primary attack rate may be as high as 40 to 60 percent, with a secondary attack rate among family members of 70 to 90 percent. Among the immunized the attack rate varies between 16 and 50 percent, for various countries, probably depending on manner of surveillance, potency of vaccine, and age of the immunized. When outbreaks occurring among highly immunized populations are carefully studied, very young infants, as well as older children and adults may comprise the majority of cases, since older infants and younger children recently immunized have relatively greater protection. There is no recognized carrier state; infant cases considered index cases in families may actually occur as a result of unrecognized introduction of the infection by an infected adult member. The manner in which the endemic reservoir of infection is maintained has yet to be determined. The disease usually occurs in late spring or summer and persists throughout the fall and into early winter. Outbreaks among susceptible hospital personnel may be particularly inconvenient, and they have been known to jeopardize critically needed health care services.

The mortality rate has fallen remarkably over the last three decades, even among the youngest infants, in which it has always been the highest. Elimination of protein calorie malnutrition as a commonly occurring disease may be the most important reason for the decline. Since antibiotics are not effective in reducing the morbidity of the primary disease and are not effective in shortening the course, a primary effect on mortality is unlikely. However, secondary complications of any infectious nature, such as bacterial pneumonia, probably have been controlled by antibiotics. Primary nursing care and supportive measures may also be responsible for reduced mortality.

The reduction in incidence of the disease clearly began before introduction of general immunization programs in this country, but certainly the wide use of potent killed bacillary vaccines has in part been responsible for a continuing fall in incidence. However, other factors also may play an important role through introduction of a bias in reporting; that is, most general diagnostic laboratories have never developed the methods necessary for isolating and identifying *B. pertussis*, and young graduating physicians may not have had experience with the clinical disease. Therefore the diagnosis goes unconfirmed and may go unreported. The low incidence reported at present among highly immunized populations is unlikely to fall further unless effective means of immunizing those under 3 to 4 months of age and susceptible adults are found.

The greatest morbidity of the disease is due to repetitive paroxysmal coughing that is inexorable, fatiguing, and at times pernicious. In the very young, individual paroxysms may present with frightening signs of hypoxia (cyanosis), asphyxia (paleness, limpness, posttussive cyanosis), recurrent vomiting, and overt signs of mucous impaction of trachea or larynx and thus require intensive supportive care. The minimal duration of this degree of care is usually 5 to 7 days in moderate or severe cases with frequent paroxysmal attacks. A minority of patients may require acute care for longer periods. As frequency, duration, and severity of attacks decrease, the morbidity is recognized only during an attack; during the most severe period fatigue, weakness, pallor, anorexia, and somnolence may characterize the interval between paroxysms. Following the early paroxysmal stage, nighttime attacks may continue to occur over a prolonged period, sometimes for 1 to 5 months following the acute illness, with significant disruption of rest patterns of adult members of the household. The period of greatest frequency of recovery of bacilli from the nasopharynx of infected individuals is during the catarrhal (preparoxysmal) stage and early paroxysmal stage. This correlates with the period of highest communicability; in rare cases it is possible to transmit the infection during the later stages and to isolate bacilli for prolonged periods.

Prior to the period of increased frequency of international travel, isolated populations such as are found in the Faroe Islands and in Iceland responded to pertussis infection with isolated epidemics occurring at intervals of 5 to 7 years, with no cases between epidemics. The infection reached all susceptibles within a moderate period (usually about 1 year) and then disappeared until a new generation of susceptibles developed and reintroduction was accomplished. With the new ease of movement within urban societies and across international boundaries, the characteristic of the epidemic has changed to that of waves that occur on a base of relative subepidemic or endemic proportion. Thus it is likely that cases will occur throughout a given outbreak period with a high order of relative frequency, then subside to a lower endemic frequency and recur each year seasonally.

Susceptibility to the disease is found during the early weeks or months of life, thus attesting to the lack of protection provided by maternally transmitted antibody and also predicting the ineffectiveness of biologic means of inducing passive protection. In comparison to the character of most childhood infections, the mortality of pertussis is significantly higher among females than among males at all ages. At one time 90 percent of cases with characteristic clinical disease occurred in children under the age of 9 years. In recent years there has been a considerable shift downward in age, with a predominance of cases occurring among the very young in whom immunization was missed or was incomplete. In most recent outbreaks in the United States the great majority of cases have occurred in those under 5 years of age, and more than 50 percent have occurred in the group less than 1 year of age. In other countries where general immunization is practiced most cases also occur within the first 10 years of life, and a majority within the first 5 years. The morbidity rate (cases reported per 100,000 population) has continued to decline throughout most of the world; in the United States it had declined to 4.2 cases per 100,000 population by 1970. In other countries with general immunization practice the morbidity rate is also declining; however, in some countries it still reaches above 80 per 100,000 population. These differences probably relate to the extent of saturation of the susceptible population with effective vaccines and to the reliability of vaccines. In countries yet to establish effective vaccine programs, the morbidity rate varies from 100 to 500 per 100,000 population.

The mortality rate among immunized and unimmunized has continued to decline more rapidly than the morbidity rate. The decline in mortality is probably related to adequate nutrition, literacy rate, and accessibility of acute medical care. The case fatality ratio in the United States for all cases fell to 0.3 percent or less during the 1960s and may in the 1970s be below 0.1 percent. In some countries in Eastern Europe, as well as in Western Europe, England, and Scandinavia, the mortality has reached a nadir, with no calculable rate. Thus various factors have provided satisfactory solutions to the problem of mortality in those countries; the incidence of the disease may not decline further until more effective means of inducing and maintaining immunity are found. In contrast, in Central America, the case fatality ratio was 18 percent in the 1960s, and it continues to be high in other countries where the populations are predominantly rural, where the literacy rates are low, and where accessibility to acute medical care is limited.

CLINICAL SYNDROME. The clinical syndrome of pertussis has been divided into several stages, beginning with the early and most communicable period called the catarrhal or preparoxysmal stage. The *catarrhal stage* begins at the end of the incubation period, or about 5 to 10 days after positive contact has been established. Generally the manifestations are those of any beginning upper respiratory infection, with irritation of the mucous membranes, hacking cough, and fever. The duration of the catarrhal stage is usually 7 to 10 days, and it is generally not recognized as pertussis. The *paroxysmal stage* begins at the end of the catarrhal stage; if there was fever during the catarrhal stage it usually subsides. The disease usually is first recognized during the paroxysmal stage. Particularly in older infants and children this stage is marked by crescendo development of inexorable paroxysmal coughing. Ultimately the paroxysms may come with any stimulus (eg, speech, swallowing, movement, tracheal pressure) and with increasing frequency, severity, and duration as the paroxysmal stage progresses. Each paroxysm may consist of several bouts separated by momentary intervals insufficient for inspiration, until hypoxia and partial asphyxia occur. The terminus of the paroxysmal episode may be marked by a massive single inspiratory stroke causing the whoop of inspiratory stridor. During severe paroxysms the patient may become plethoric or cyanotic, with bulging eyes and anxious or frantic countenance; it may appear that the patient's life is threatened. After severe episodes the immediate post-tussive period may be marked by apparent respiratory arrest. In infants the post-tussive period may also be marked by a state of exhaustion and lethargy during which usual environmental stimuli fail to bring about a typical response. In the most severely affected infants this state may merge into the next paroxysm with awakening. Vomiting is frequently associated with the end of a paroxysm. Paroxysmal coughing may last from 7 days to a month and may vary from mild uncomplicated episodes to severe protracted episodes requiring hospitalization and acute supportive care. In unusual cases the paroxysms may continue to develop for 2 to 5 months, especially at night. Infants, particularly those under 6 months of age, may not develop typical paroxysms and thus may go undiagnosed. The typical whoop may not be a part of the clinical syndrome in young infants; instead, recurrent periods of apparent strangling and asphyxia may characterize the disease, thus leading to a variety of presumptive diagnoses other than pertussis.

In a majority of cases (estimated to be 80 percent in unimmunized older infants and children) there are characteristic hematologic findings that develop during the paroxysmal stage and are helpful in making the diagnosis; these are the appearance of hyperleukocytosis and lymphocytosis in peripheral blood. The total white blood cell count may rise to greater than $100,000/mm^3$; commonly the count is in the range of $25,000$ to $40,000/mm^3$, with a predominance of small mature lymphocytes in the differential analysis. These cells appear in the circulation as a result of discharge of the marginal pool under the influence of the lymphocyte promoting factor of *B. pertussis*. Again, the finding of hyperleukocytosis may not be present in infants under 6 months of age who have the disease; however, relative lymphocytosis usually is present. The *convalescent stage* is usually characterized by a return to normal activity and development, without complications. In a majority of patients immunity is conferred by a single attack.

Complications. These are steadily declining among infants and children in highly developed countries. The former observation of bronchiectasis is no longer part of the total morbidity of pertussis in the United States. Likewise, it is very uncommon to observe central nervous system complications, such as seizures or encephalopathy, even in severe outbreaks. Less serious complications include epistaxis (nosebleed) and hemorrhage into soft tissues about the eyes and into the conjunctivae due to intense venous pressure accompanying paroxysms. Occasionally hemorrhage from the tracheobronchial tract may accompany or follow the paroxysm; usually these hemorrhagic episodes do not result in serious complication or marked blood loss. Rarely, intracranial hemorrhage may occur accompanied by signs of neurologic damage; the symptoms and signs of intracranial hemorrhage commonly resolve during the decline of the paroxysmal stage. At one time otitis media and purulent pneumonia were recognized as being important and frequent complications of pertussis; the use of antibiotics to eradicate *B. pertussis* from the tracheobronchial tree is probably responsible for the disappearance of these complications. Other mechanical complications include anal prolapse, hernia, and trauma to the frenum of the tongue.

The differential diagnosis includes other infections giving rise to tracheobronchial lymphadenopathy, a foreign body in the bronchial airway, necrotizing bronchiolitis caused by adenovirus, interstitial pneumonitis caused by respiratory syncytial virus and parainfluenza virus, and *H. influenzae* type B bronchitis; any of these may cause a cough of paroxysmal nature. Some of the viral infections result in frequent vomiting with the paroxysms. Both *B. parapertussis* and *B. bronchiseptica* infections may cause a mild clinical syndrome indistinguishable from mild to moderate pertussis.

PATHOLOGY. From pathologic examination of tissues from the lungs of infants and children dying of pertussis or its complications it is evident that there are three types of lesions that predominate in the respiratory tract. In early paroxysmal and midparoxysmal stages of the disease peribronchitis and peribronchiolitis may develop, consisting of moderate to dense accumulations of round cells infiltrating the supporting tissues of smaller bronchi and bronchioles. These cells include lymphocytes, mast cells, and plasmocytes. At this stage or a later stage of the disease endobronchiolitis and endobronchitis may also be found; these lesions consist of damage to the respiratory membrane, with accumulation of debris within the lumen, along with infiltration of the wall by mononuclear cells. Clusters of bacilli may be found on the ciliated epithelial cells or mixed with debris, but they are not found in peribronchial tissues. Atelectasis may also be present. In prolonged or severe disease alveolar lesions consisting of thickening of the wall, mononuclear cell infiltration, and accumulation of fibrinous debris have also been described. Peribronchial lymphadenopathy commonly accompanies the peribronchial lesion. A late pathologic change consists of dysplasia of the bronchial epithelium, with replacement of columnar by squamous cells in a thickened membrane. Although the pathology of the disease is well established, the pathogenesis of the changes has not been determined. During infection, bacterial replication is essentially confined to the respiratory mucous membrane, without bacillemia. However, as exemplified by induction of lymphocytosis by the lymphocyte promoting factor, antigenemia undoubtedly occurs; thus the immune response of the host is probably generated through both local and humoral mechanisms.

IMMUNITY. Immunity probably is conferred through a variety of host factors, none of which has been identified as being of singular importance in solid protection. Agglutinins correlate with the immune state when present in high serum concentrations after immunization or after unrecognized infection; immunity may be present in the absence of serum agglutinins. Bactericidal antibody develops after animal infection or immunization with pertussis strains without protective antigen. Antihemagglutinin antibody and complement-fixing antibody, when present in high serum concentrations, also correlate with protective immunity; as with agglutinins, their absence does not necessarily signify susceptibility to infection. The greatest correlation with protective immunity lies with the mouse-protective antibody, which is determined in a biologic test where administration of convalescent serum provides the mouse protection against a lethal intracerebral infection initiated with a mouse-virulent strain of pertussis. However, the presence of protective antibody in serum is predictive of immunity only after active infection or intensive (complete) immunization. In the latter case immunity wanes rapidly, so that adults or children 5 years or more away from the last immunizing injection are liable to an attack rate of 35 to 95 percent when exposed in families in which there is an index case. On the other hand, naturally acquired immunity is highly effective, with an estimated recurrence rate of approximately 2 percent. Undoubtedly there are factors of importance other than protective antibody, and these are probably present on surface membranes as well as at the initial site of infection within the respiratory tract. Enhanced phagocytosis is characteristic of immune serum; antiadherence factors also are present. These and other factors may have an effect that limits or controls the loci of early infection. When inflammation develops at the site of infection on the respiratory membrane, the organisms may then be exposed to immune serum containing protective antibody and to the action of complement-dependent bactericidal antibody. Much work must be done before any clear definition of immunity to pertussis is available.

LABORATORY DIAGNOSIS. The medium and the principles that are important in the isolation and identification of *B. pertussis* were originally described by Bordet and Gengou. Bordet-Gengou (B-G) culture medium, with minor modifications, is still preferred in the diagnostic laboratory. Commercial preparations from which final complete medium is prepared are usually satisfactory; such medium, when properly prepared, adequately stored, and appropriately used, will result in frequent isolations of *B. pertussis* from nasopharyngeal swabs of individuals with clinical disease. The isolation rate depends on using a concentration of whole blood in the final medium higher than that usually utilized in diagnostic bacteriology. For that reason, 20 to 30 percent whole defibrinated sheep blood is incorporated in appropriately prepared Bordet-Gengou medium. The medium may be stored in sealed plastic sleeves for 2 weeks or longer and remain adequate for isolation, so long as the agar surface is glistening, moist, and cherry red when used.

Incubation should be in a humidified environment at 35 C for 5 to 7 days. Minute milky white convex colonies may be found as early as 72 hours of incubation or as late as 5 to 6 days. The frequency of isolation may be improved by streaking two B-G plates, with one containing 0.25 IU of penicillin G per milliliter of agar and the other plate containing no penicillin. Some strains are sensitive to penicillin G even at this level; overgrowth of nasopharyngeal microflora may be controlled by this concentration of penicillin G. The appearance of *B. pertussis* on gram-staining a single colony from the isolation plate is characteristically that of minute, lightly staining gram-negative coccoid and ovoid bacteria. In cases where the medium is inadequately prepared, pleomorphism may be noted, with long rod forms mixed with coccobacillary forms. Final identification is established by antigenic means. Macroscopic agglutination occurs when a moderate suspension of bacteria is mixed with specific immune serum against *B. pertussis*. The suspension is prepared by swabbing the surface of a plate where there is confluent growth and immersing the swab in several drops of saline on a glass slide or plate; serum is then diluted and added to the slide suspension. With slow agitation and mixing, agglutination occurs in 5 to 10 minutes. Macroscopic agglutination firmly establishes a final identification of the *Bordetella* genus. A similar slide preparation from a suspension (air-dried and reacted with fluorescein-conjugated specific immune globulin derived from immune serum) will show bright specific fluorescence under the ultraviolet microscope. The diagnostic immunofluorescence method is rapid and provides immediate final identification of nasopharyngeal infection. Differentiation of *B. pertussis* and *B. parapertussis* can be made by using commercially prepared immunoflourescence reagents against each; intense fluorescence with the *B. pertussis* globulin conjugate usually indicates that the isolated bacilli are *B. pertussis*, although rarely *B. parapertussis* are found (1 to 10 percent of cases in the United States).

The immunofluorescence technique can also be used to obtain an immediate specific diagnosis by examining N-P swabs for *B. pertussis*. Nasopharyngeal swabs are used to make several smears on clean glass slides. After air-drying, the immunofluorescence globulin reagent is applied to the smears, and the excess stain is removed by appropriate washing. Under the ultraviolet microscope the minute coccoid or ovoid bacteria in a diagnostic smear will be highly fluorescent. Properly applied, the direct immunofluorescence method will result in a frequency of bacteriologic diagnosis equaling that of the culture method or exceeding it. By either method, study of unimmunized cases in the paroxysmal stage of the disease should result in a specific diagnosis with a frequency of 70 to 90 percent. In contact cases and immunized cases a laboratory diagnosis is established less frequently.

Differentiation by bacteriologic characteristics is also practical. In contrast to *B. pertussis*, both *B. parapertussis* and *B. bronchiseptica* will form colonies on diffusion agar,

without blood, during subcultivation. *B. parapertussis* colonies have a characteristic light chocolate pigment, whereas *B. pertussis* colonies remain pearly white. Biochemical differences are also found among the species and may also be used in differentiation.

None of the serologic methods used to make a retrospective diagnosis of pertussis is in general use. The agglutination test has been the most widely applied serologic procedure; however, it has been utilized most commonly in evaluating responses to immunization, not to the natural infection, since the agglutinating antibody may be absent in human or animal serum that has protective antibody. Thus, after natural infections in infants, agglutinins may be present in only 30 to 50 percent, in contrast to the protective antibody present in 90 to 100 percent.

Recently a gel precipitin method has been developed that is simple and inexpensive; in agar it demonstrates precipitating antibody against extracted *B. pertussis* antigens. Betweeen 80 and 90 percent of patients with the clinical syndrome develop gel precipitins during convalescence; 25 to 30 percent of immunized cases also develop these antibodies. The gel precipitin test may have application to the routine diagnosis of an infection in an unimmunized patient or to the identification of an outbreak. In the latter case it has been found that 80 to 90 percent of clinical cases will have precipitin antibody in convalescent serum, as contrasted to 25 to 30 percent of newborns and immunized children and adults without illness.

TREATMENT. Small infants markedly affected by frequent paroxysms, especially when they are complicated by post-tussive exhaustion and spells of unresponsiveness, should be hospitalized for supportive care. In infants who have been well nourished and who are well developed the height of the paroxysmal stage may be reached and passed in a period of 5 to 7 days, and the need for hospitalization then declines. Intravenous hydration is required infrequently. Oxygenation is usually not a requirement, since during a paroxysm the inspiratory volume is ineffective and between paroxysms the respiratory exchange is adequate. When seizures develop they may be repetitive, requiring both anticonvulsive therapy and strong supportive measures. In the most severe case in infants, respiratory arrest of a transient type may occur following extensive paroxysms and may require resuscitation. Endotracheal suction by a direct or indirect method is infrequently required, since compacted endobronchial mucus is usually expelled at the terminus of a paroxysm. However, during episodes of post-tussive cyanosis, moderate suctioning may be required to remove incompletely expelled mucus from the upper airway as well as the trachea. Antitussive medications are to be avoided, as well as heavy sedation.

Malnourishment may develop in severe prolonged cases due to exhaustion, lack of intake, and frequent vomiting. Small repetitive feedings are usually tolerated immediately after a paroxysm (or after vomiting), when the cough reflex is suppressed. Likewise, a feeding may be repeated directly after loss of the previous meal. In the hospital strict isolation is required to reduce contact with susceptible children, visiting adults, and hospital employees.

As measured by clinical response, the benefit of antibiotic chemotherapy has never been proved in comparison to placebo controls. However, erythromycin for 5 to 7 days in appropriate dosage will eradicate infection on the tracheobronchial membrane and reduce contact spread of the infection. Ampicillin has been recommended, but in some cases pure cultures of pertussis bacilli have been found on nasopharyngeal swabs after ampicillin therapy. Several reports show modification of the clinical course of pertussis after corticosteroid therapy, as compared to placebo controls. Therefore in severe cases cortisone at an appropriate pharmacologic dosage for 5 to 7 days may prove to be of benefit. Corticosteroids are not recommended for mild or moderate cases. Like antibiotics, pertussis hyperimmune globulin has not proved to be effective when used during the paroxysmal stage. Nevertheless, some physicians recommend hyperimmune globulin for severely affected infants under 6 months of age, since earlier studies reported moderate benefit.

IMMUNIZATION. The standard method of active immunization against pertussis utilizes three primary injections of a highly concentrated suspension of killed whole *B. pertussis* organisms in a repository vehicle combined with diphtheria and tetanus toxoids (DPT). Slow absorption from the repository injection site provides an adjuvant effect on immune response; thus the combined form of immunization against the three diseases is preferable to injections of solitary antigens. Since there is no effective immunity against pertussis in the newborn period, immunization is started as soon as the immune response mounted by the infant is adequate to provide protection. For this reason the primary injection series usually begins at 2 to 3 months of age and is completed by 4 to 5 months of age. Immunity against pertussis is not developed until some time after the second injection; the magnitude of protection is extended by the third injection. In order to further extend protection, a booster is given at 1 year of age and is repeated one or two times before school age is reached. Most estimates of protection after full immunization have been derived from studies of immunized children who have had intimate contact with the naturally occurring disease; such studies indicate that pertussis may develop in 12 to 50 percent of immunized children. The greatest protection is observed during the first 36 months after completion of the series or after a booster. Immunity wanes remarkably after 3 years. Lambert's study of an epidemic in Kent County, Michigan, concluded that 7 years after the last immunization the attack rate was 47 percent and after 12 years or more the rate was 95 percent among contacts exposed to index cases in families.

Up to 25 percent of infants receiving second or third injection of DPT vaccine may have a local or systemic response, or both, consisting of swelling and tenderness at the injection site and moderate fever beginning 12 to 24 hours after injection and declining sharply within 24 hours. Earlier in the vaccine era, evidence of encephalitis following second or third injections of DPT in infants was seen with a frequency of 1 case per 200,-000 vaccine doses; however, this complication is now rare, occurring with a frequency in this country of less than 1 case in 1 million doses. Latest statistics comparing morbidity of immunization and morbidity of disease continue to demonstrate the benefit of general immunization against pertussis.

Another type of pertussis vaccine is commercially available; it contains a soluble protective antigen derived from *B. pertussis* combined with diphtheria and tetanus toxoids. This vaccine also induces mouse-protective antibody and agglutinins in recipients; however, field comparison of its protective value with that of standard killed bacillary vaccine has not been required by licensing agencies.

A vaccine booster injection may suffice to establish immunity in a previously immunized family contact. However, active immunization during the incubation period or during active disease is neither effective nor desirable. The effectiveness of commercially prepared hyperimmune globulin in preventing pertussis in contacts has not been proved. However, it is not infrequently used in attempted prophylaxis, particularly in small infants where the risk of moderate or severe morbidity is high. Chemoprophylaxis should be attempted in infant or child contacts, preferably using erythromycin for 5 to 7 days. If the disease does not develop after the full incubation period, the exposed individual should then be immunized appropriately. Disease in exposed adults is usually moderate, and it may be mild or uncharacteristic. Since the attack rate is very high in adults of families with index cases, it may be appropriate in the future to consider prophylactic treatment and immunization of the older age group as well as infants and children.

PERTUSSIS SYNDROME

Pertussis syndrome is the title given to a syndrome that is clinically indistinguishable from pertussis, but in which no evidence of infection with *B. pertussis* or *B. parapertussis* can be detected, while evidence of other infectious agents, including viruses, can be demonstrated. Pertussis syndrome is relatively new terminology, first occurring in the 1960s and frequently being used in the last 10 years. *Adenoviruses* are the infectious agents most frequently associated with pertussis syndrome; types 1, 2, 3, 5, and 6 have been isolated from nasopharyngeal and pharyngeal swabs, and some of these serotypes have been isolated from urine and stools of patients during the paroxysmal stage. Likewise, rises in viral antibody have been demonstrated in convalescent serum. Evidence of adenoviral infection in infants and children with the syndrome exceeds the combined rate of viral isolation and serologic titer rise in a matched control population, thus indicating a strong association between the viral infection and the disease. However, there is a paradox involved: among those patients in whom a bacteriologic diagnosis of pertussis infection can be established there also is a marked increase in the relative frequency of adenoviral infection. In addition, the frequency of pertussis antibody rise occurring in those with demonstrable viral infection is high, thus further indicating an association between the viral infection and infection with pertussis bacilli. Recent reports correlate with observations made earlier in the century by pathologists who frequently found intranuclear inclusions in the lungs of patients dying of pertussis. To date, no proof exists of a solitary viral infection causing the typical pertussis syndrome, since animals infected with adenoviruses fail to produce a pertussis syndrome, as do the secretions of patients after passage through bacterial filters. Neither is there enough evidence, based on reports to date, to exclude adenoviruses as the causes of endemic or sporadic cases. However, it is clear that the relative frequency of adenoviral infection among bacteriologically proven cases is very high. In the combined infection it is yet to be determined whether the viral infection is reactivated from a latent state or whether host susceptibility for one or the other is enhanced by a primary agent.

PARAPERTUSSIS

Parapertussis is an acute disease of the respiratory tract caused by infection with *B. parapertussis.* The characteristics of the clinical syndrome are indistinguishable from those of a mild or moderate case of pertussis. The frequency of the disease is approximately 2 to 10 percent that of pertussis, and during an outbreak the diagnosis is evident clinically in only 5 percent of those carrying an infection. *B. parapertussis* are coccobacillary gram-negative nonmotile bacilli that on primary isolation are usually indistinguishable from *B. pertussis;* they were first described by Eldering and Kendrick in the United States in 1937 and later during the same year by Bradford and Slavin, who brought attention to pigment changes that are useful in the laboratory differentiation of *B. parapertussis* and *B. pertussis.* On Bordet-Gengou medium the growth of colonies of *B. parapertussis* is more rapid than that of *B. pertussis,* but otherwise the colonies may be entirely characteristic of the latter until a pigment change occurs that lends a light chocolate hue to the colonies of parapertussis bacilli. Transfer to regular infusion agar usually may be accomplished from the isolation plate, and this quickly serves to distinguish it from *B. pertussis. B. parapertussis* shares antigens (agglutinogens) with both *B. pertussis* and *B. bronchiseptica* and will react lightly with immunofluorescent serum against *B. pertussis* because of antigen or antigens common to both.

The incidence of parapertussis is estimated to be 2 to 10 percent that of pertussis. The disease, in Denmark, occurs in 4-year cycles, with a distinct wave or outbreak occurring in between pertussis outbreaks and rising above endemic disease in an urban environment. As with pertussis, it is assumed that the most contagious period is during the catarrhal stage, prior to the occurrence of paroxysms. The morbidity of a single case can be that of moderately severe pertussis; however, it is

commonly mild. Mortality is certainly rare; however, fatal cases have been reported in which *B. parapertussis* was isolated from the trachea at postmortem examination. In recognized cases the clinical syndrome is usually that of mild pertussis. Most of the cases go unrecognized, even during an outbreak, for the clinical visibility of the disease is low in comparison to pertussis. Occasionally more severe cases occur and are often diagnosed as pertussis. It is presumed that the infection proceeds in the same manner as with pertussis, but it is more difficult to distinguish clearly separate stages, since the total period of the clinical disease is usually shorter and the severity is less than in pertussis. However, when paroxysms develop they are characteristically those of pertussis, and typical whoops may be heard.

The pathology of parapertussis in the human has not been well described because of the mildness of the disease; however, in animals mononuclear cell inflammation surrounding and within bronchi and bronchioles closely resembles pertussis pathology. There is no cross-immunity between parapertussis and pertussis. As with pertussis, the immunity following disease is solid, and a second attack is rare. Immunization against pertussis does not protect against parapertussis. The disease is not preventable by any currently available means. Treatment is usually not required, although in moderately severe cases supportive care may be justified.

References

PERTUSSIS

Aftandelians R, Connor JD: Immunologic studies of pertussis. Development of precipitins. J Pediatr 83:206, 1973

Barnhard HJ, Kniker WT: Roentgen findings in pertussis. Am J Roentgenol Radium Ther Nucl Med 84:445, 1960

Bradford WL, Day E, Bery GP: Improvement of the nasopharyngeal swab method of diagnosis in pertussis by the use of penicillin. Am J Public Health 36:468, 1946

Brooksaler F, Nelson JD: A re-appraisal and report of 190 confirmed cases. Am J Dis Child 114:389, 1967

Buchanan TM, Broohn GF: Pertussis in the US. J Infect Dis 122:123, 1970

Eldering G, Hornbeck C, Baker J: Serological study of Bordetella pertussis and related species. J Bacteriol 74:133, 1957

Felton HM: Pertussis: current status of prevention and treatment. Pediatr Clin North Am 4:271, 1957

Holwerda J, Eldering GD: Culture and fluorescent antibody methods in diagnosis of whooping cough. J Bacteriol 86:449, 1963

Jernelius H: Pertussis with pulmonary complications: A follow-up study. Acta Paediatr Scand 53:247, 1964

Kurt TL, Yeager AS, Guerette S, Dunlop S: Spread of pertussis by hospital staff. JAMA 221:264, 1972

Miller JJ Jr, Leach CW, Saito TM, et al: Comparison of the nasopharyngeal swab and the cough plate in the diagnosis of whooping cough and Hemophilus pertussis carriers. Am J Public Health 33:839, 1943

Munoz JJ: Symposium on relationship of structure of microorganisms to the immunological properties. I. Immunological and other biological activities of Bordetella pertussis antigens. Bacteriol Rev 27:325, 1963

Pittman M: Bordetella pertussis—bacterial and host factors in the pathogenesis and prevention of whooping cough. In Infectious Agents and Host Reactions. Mudd, S (ed) Philadelphia, WB Saunders, 1970, p 239

Preston NW, Stanbridge TN: Efficacy of pertussis vaccines: a brighter horizon. Br Med J 3:448, 1972

Ross CA, Calder MC, Cruickshank R, et al: Diagnosis of whooping cough: comparison of serological tests with isolation of Bordetella pertussis. A combined Scottish study. Br Med J 4:637, 1970

Welsh JD, Denny WF, Bird RM: The incidence and significance of the leukemoid reaction in patients hospitalized with pertussis. South Med J 52:643, 1959

White R, Finberg L, Tramer A: The modern morbidity of pertussis in infants. Pediatrics 33:705, 1964

Zamora AF, Chiozza A, Alonso AT: Complications of whooping cough in 500 cases. Rev Assoc Med Argent 76:121, 1962

PERTUSSIS SYNDROME

Collier AM, Connor JD, Irving WR Jr: Generalized type 5 adenovirus infection associated with the pertussis syndrome. J Pediatr 69:1073, 1966

Connor JD: Evidence for an etiological role of adenoviral infection in pertussis syndrome. N Engl J Med 283:390, 1970

McCordock HA, Smith MG: Intranuclear inclusions: incidence and possible significance in whooping cough and in variety of other conditions. Am J Dis Child 47:771, 1934

Nelson KF, Gavitt F, Batt MD, Kallick CA, Reddi KT, et al: The role of adenoviruses in the pertussis syndrome. J Pediatr 86:335, 1975

Olson LD, Miller G, Hanshaw JB: Acute infectious lymphocytosis presenting as a pertussis-like illness; its association with adenovirus type 12. Lancet 1:200, 1964

PARAPERTUSSIS

Bradford WL, Slavin B: An organism resembling Hemophilus pertussis: with special reference to color changes produced by its growth upon certain media. Am J Public Health 27:1277, 1937

———— Parapertussis. Lancet 75:232, 1955

Eldering G, Kendrick PL: Incidence of parapertussis in Grand Rapids area as indicated by 16 years' experience with diagnostic cultures. Am J Public Health 42:27, 1952

Lautrop H: Epidemics of parapertussis. Lancet 1:1195, 1971

Miller JJ Jr, Saito TM, Silverberg RJ: Parapertussis: clinical and serological observations. J Pediatr 19:229, 1941

Zuelzer WW, Wheeler WE: Parapertussis pneumonia. Report of 2 fatal cases. J Pediatr 29:493, 1946

RAT-BITE FEVER

William L. Bradford

Two quite distinct infections may be conveyed by the bite of the rat, but they have only minor differences in symptomatology. One of these diseases, caused by *Spirillum minus*, is known as *sodoku*. Although it is relatively common in Japan, it appears to be an infrequent cause of rat-bite fever in the United States. More common in this country are infections due to a pleomorphic bacillus known as *Streptobacillus moniliformis*. This latter organism is occasionally acquired by means other than a rat bite, as in the milk-borne epidemic observed in Haverhill, Massachusetts, that was traced to a cow thought to have been bitten on the teat by a rat. Failure to differentiate between infections caused by these two agents has caused considerable confusion in the literature.

SPIRILLUM MINUS INFECTION. A few well-authenticated cases of rat-bite fever caused by *Spirillum minus* have occurred in children in this country. The infection is characterized by a relatively long incubation period (1 to 3 weeks), after which the wound, having healed, exhibits a return of erythema, induration, and tenderness; often there is evidence of lymphadenitis. As the infection becomes generalized, intermittent fever, chills, and a rash develop. The febrile periods are fairly regular, with the temperature often reaching 104 F, lasting for a day or two, and then being followed by a period of several afebrile days. The rash is generalized and maculopapular; it tends to appear with the febrile periods and disappear between them, and the wound likewise flares up at these times. Muscle pain is common during the acute phase, but joint symptoms are exceptional.

The disease runs a relapsing course, with the febrile episodes gradually becoming less severe and less frequent until eventually in the course of several weeks the fever subsides. Anemia develops in some cases, and a moderate leukocytosis is not uncommon. A false-positive Wassermann test is commonly obtained. The diagnosis can be established by growing the organisms in blood culture, by dark-field examination of lesions, and by animal inoculation. Guinea pigs or white mice inoculated in the groin or genitals will develop chancrelike lesions in which the organism can be identified; it can also be recovered from the blood and peritoneal fluid. It has characteristic morphologic features. Since laboratory mice and guinea pigs may harbor these organisms spontaneously, the animals inoculated should be studied first to make sure that their blood is free from organisms.

STREPTOBACILLUS MONILIFORMIS INFECTION. Infections caused by *Streptobacillus moniliformis* are characterized by a shorter incubation period (usually less than 1 week), by less evidence of reaction around the bite, and usually by absence of lymphadenitis. Intermittent fever and rash are seen, with the eruption being maculopapular or occasionally urticarial. The febrile periods are less regular than in the spirillar disease. Upper respiratory symptoms are sometimes present, and at times abscesses may develop in various parts of the body. The most common difference is the development of arthritis in the majority of cases. The small joints of the extremities are often involved. The leukocyte count usually exceeds that seen in sodoku, often reaching 20,000 or even 30,000/mm^3. A false-positive Wassermann reaction is occasionally encountered. Although fatalities have occurred, the disease tends to subside spontaneously in the great majority of cases, even without specific treatment. Periarteritis nodosa has been observed as a rare complication

Laboratory verification of the diagnosis depends on cultivation of the organism from the blood or joint fluid or on demonstration of agglutinins in the serum. Special culture media are required, as well as familiarity with the characteristics of the organism, which may exist in two different forms: the typical streptobacillary form consisting of long filaments that tend to fragment and that show peculiar nodular excrescences and a more resistant vegetative form known as L, which consists of minute granules capable of passing a Berkefeld filter.

This latter form is closely related to a group of organisms that cause pleuropneumonia in mice.

TREATMENT.   The drug of choice for both varieties of rat-bite fever is penicillin. Moderate dosage will suffice for cure in cases of short duration, but in those that have run a prolonged course because of failure to be recognized, high dosage is required. In a few refractory cases addition of a tetracycline has eliminated the organisms.

References

Adams JM, Carpenter CM: Symposium on unusual infections in childhood; rat-bite fevers. Pediatr Clin North Am 2:101, 1955

Brown TM, Nunemaker JC: Rat-bite fever; a review of the American cases with re-evaluation of etiology; report of cases. Bull Johns Hopkins Hosp 70:201, 1942

Place EH, Sutton LE Jr: Erythema arthriticum epidemicum (Haverhill fever). Arch Intern Med 54:659, 1934

Prouty M, Schafer EL: Periarteritis nodosa associated with rat-bite fever due to Streptobacillus moniliforms (erythema arthriticum epidemicum). J Pediatr 36:605, 1950

Schwartzman G, Florman AL, Bass MH, Karelitz S, Richtberg D: Repeated recovery of a spirillum by blood culture from two children with prolonged and recurrent fevers. Pediatr 8:227, 1951

Watkins CG: Rat-bite fever. J Pediatr 28:429, 1946

TUBERCULOSIS

DEXTER S.Y. SETO AND RICHARD M. HELLER

Tuberculosis is an infectious disease of man caused by mammalian tubercle bacilli (*Mycobacterium tuberculosis, M. bovis*) or rarely *M. avium*. For centuries it has been recognized as a widespread and serious clinical entity and a major cause of death and prolonged disability throughout the world.

EPIDEMIOLOGY

In the United States tuberculosis is still a leading cause of death among infectious diseases, despite its steadily declining incidence. The Center for Disease Control in Atlanta, Georgia, reported 30,273 new cases and 3,600 deaths in 1974 for rates of 14.3 new cases and 1.8 deaths per 100,000 population. These rates are 46 percent and 58 percent lower than the respective rates in 1964. The prevalence of positive tuberculin skin tests, based on a 0.2 percent rate of reactors among 6-year-old children entering school and a 0.7 percent rate among adolescents, also represents a decline for both age groups of about 75 percent since 1964.

Evidence for the incidence of tuberculosis is based on surveys using tuberculin tests, radiography, clinical recognition of the disease, reports to health agencies, and examination of autopsy material. The data indicate that the infection is most heavily concentrated in metropolitan urban centers, where significant percentages of the population live in circumstances such as poverty that favor transmission of the disease. Tuberculosis in the United States is now predominantly a disease of the elderly, with about three-fourths of the newly reported cases coming from a reservoir of people who have positive tuberculin tests as the sole manifestation of their infection. These represent endogenous reactivation or exacerbation of infections that occurred many years ago. The favorable trend that has consistently been recorded over the years can only partially be attributed to therapy, since improvement in the tuberculosis picture had been occurring even before the development of effective chemotherapy. However, the rate of decline has been least in the pediatric group. Children are infected by adults, and as long as the disease persists in adults, susceptible children will continue to become infected. In addition to known cases of tuberculosis, additional numbers of unidentified cases exist that are unknown even to the sufferers themselves. These cases are largely responsible for the new infections. The importance of undiagnosed and unreported cases of tuberculosis is reflected in the fact that each year about 1,800 cases of tuberculosis are first detected following death.

When a person with active pulmonary disease coughs or sneezes, minute droplets of varying sizes are dispersed in the air. The quantity of tubercle bacilli discharged into the environment depends on the number of organisms in the sputum, the amount and characteristics of the sputum, the type and frequency of cough, and the degree to which the patient covers up the cough or sneeze. Inhalation of the bacilli-laden droplet nuclei and their implantation on lung tissue are necessary for transmission of infection. The particle must be of a size less than $5.0\ \mu$ to gain access to the alveoli. Larger inhaled particles that carry tubercle bacilli are stopped in the nasal and upper respiratory tract and eliminated. Evidence suggests that tubercle bacilli lodged on fomites, linen, furniture, and books do not constitute a significant infection hazard. Most of them are killed through drying, heat, and sunlight. Dried secretions are very difficult to fragment and suspend in air, and even if airborne particles do arise from surfaces they are usually too large to reach the lung. Almost all primary complexes occur in the lungs as a result of droplet transmission. Infrequently, ingested bacilli may cause a primary focus is the intestinal tract, tonsil, or mucous membranes of the mouth. Other unusual primary lesions in the skin or conjunctiva are due to local infection. In areas where bovine tuberculosis is still prevalent, infection with bovine bacilli by drinking contaminated milk may produce the primary lesion in the nasopharynx or intestinal tract.

The chance of a child contracting the infection from an adult with acute disease depends on the degree of sputum infection, the length and frequency of contact, and the other circumstances surrounding the contact. The incidence of infection in contacts increases significantly if the index case is sputum-positive. The infecting person may be a family member, relative, visitor, babysitter, or teacher. Epidemics in schools are initially characterized by the finding of a number of recently infected children within a short period of time. It becomes increasingly evident as the risk of exogenous tuberculous infection falls that the frequency of tuberculosis in any age group in adult life is a measure of the degree to which that group is exposed to tuberculosis and the incidence of primary infection during childhood. The key to control of tuberculosis in children is early detection of adult cases followed by appropriate treatment.

BACTERIAL PROPERTIES

The mycobacteria are classified as a genus (*Mycobacterium*) of the family Mycobacteriaceae in the order Actinomycetales. All mycobacteria have the property of acid-fastness, resisting decoloration by acidified organic solvents. Mycobacteria range from widespread innocuous inhabitants of soil and water to organisms that are responsible for human diseases. The agents of human tuberculosis are *M. tuberculosis* and the closely related *M. bovis. M. avium,* the agent of avian tuberculosis, occasionally causes disease in man.

The tubercle bacilli are curved rods about 2 to 4 μ long and 0.2 to 0.5 μ wide. They are obligate aerobes and can grow in simple synthetic media with glycerol or other compounds as the carbon source and ammonium salts as the nitrogen source. Growth of tubercle bacilli is characteristically slow, the shortest doubling time in rich medium being about 12 hours. For this reason egg yolk has been a prominent constituent of enriched media, since mycobacteria have a nutritional preference for lipids. The organisms grow best between 37 C and 41 C; they have a characteristic colony morphology, they lack pigmentation, and they react to neutral red. Virulent strains grow on the surface of liquid or on solid media as intertwining serpentine cords, and they possess catalase and peroxidase activity.

Polysaccharide is a major component of tubercle bacilli that exists in chemical union with lipid in the cell wall. The most striking feature of the composition is the very high lipid content, which amounts to 20 to 40 percent of the dry weight. The lipid-rich cell wall accounts for the hydrophobic property, acid-fastness, relative impermeability, and resistance to the bactericidal action of antibodies and complement. Among the lipids and fatty acids unique to the cell walls of mycobacteria are true waxes, glycolipids, and mycolic acids. A mycoside of high molecular weight, wax D in water-and-oil emulsion, enhances the antigenicity of a variety of added substances. The crude phosphatide fraction evokes a cellular response resembling tubercle formation, including caseation necrosis. The protein component produces delayed-type hypersensitivity reactions in tuberculin-sensitized animals.

IMMUNITY

The cutaneous inoculation of tubercle bacilli into an uninfected guinea pig causes an indolent local reaction followed by marked multiplication of the bacilli and dissemination, but a similar inoculation in a previously infected animal produces only an acute local reaction without multiplication of bacilli and dissemination. This is the classic demonstration of the Koch phenomenon, which represents cell-mediated immunity to the tubercle bacilli.

The immunity is mediated by thymus-derived small lymphocytes and is manifested by a high degree of resistance to tubercle bacilli and a delayed type of hypersensitivity to tuberculin. When the sensitized lymphocytes are stimulated by antigens of the tubercle bacilli, products of activated lymphocytes or lymphokines are produced that alter macrophage activity. The activated macrophages show accelerated metabolism, increased lysosomal granules, and increased enzyme and bactericidal activity in which there is enhancement of intracellular killing of tubercle bacilli. This enhanced activity of altered macrophages is nonspecific, since similar activated macrophages can be obtained from animals infected with various other bacteria, such as *Listeria monocytogenes.* However, its induction is specific since only lymphocytes modified by specific interaction with the infecting organism can induce the change in the macrophages.

The delayed type of hypersensitivity is also mediated by one of the products of the activated lymphocytes and is expressed as a cutaneous reaction to tuberculin that occurs in 48 to 72 hours. The hypersensitivity develops 4 to 8 weeks following tuberculosis infection and generally is permanent, except in early therapy where reactivity occasionally disappears. This suggests that persistence of tubercle bacilli in dormant foci is necessary for permanent reactions. Although antibodies to the various components of tubercle bacilli are generally found in low titers in tuberculous individuals, they have no prognostic value with respect to the course of the disease.

PREDISPOSING FACTORS

Among persons infected with tuberculosis only a small proportion develop overt disease. The transition from infection to mild or serious disease depends on various factors besides the presence of tubercle bacilli. The importance of genetic factors in host resistance has been definitely established experimentally in inbred lines of rabbits. In man there is epidemiologic evidence that suggests there are racial differences in resistance that may be associated with different lengths of exposure of the race to the selective pressures of a tuberculous environment. In the United States the incidence of tuberculosis and the ratio of deaths to cases are especially high among American Indians, Eskimos, and Blacks. However, this evidence is only circumstantial, since the differences may well be due to environmental factors such as poor socioeconomic conditions rather than to specific factors of native susceptibility.

The significance of hormonal factors is suggested by variations in resistance with age and sex. Tuberculosis is likely to be severe in infants because of a delay in development of resistance. The severity of disease decreases between 5 and 12 years of age, with susceptibility rapidly increasing at adolescence. In young adults tuberculosis is more frequent in females, which may be attributed to metabolic changes that occur in puberty.

Among the metabolic diseases, diabetes mellitus is frequently complicated by tuberculosis. The only occupations that are directly associated with lowered resistance to tuberculosis involve workers who are exposed to silica dust that is in a finely divided state and in high concentration. Although many intercurrent infections decrease the tuberculin reaction, only measles (rubeola) has been incriminated in lowering resistance to tuberculosis. The skin reactivity to tuberculin disappears in the preeruption stage of measles and does not reappear for 2 to 3 weeks, but it is not known whether there is a relation between the change in skin sensitivity and the increase in susceptibility.

PATHOGENESIS

In a tuberculous infection the primary complex consists of the local disease at the portal of entry of tubercle bacilli and in the regional lymph nodes that drain the area of the primary focus. The infection may occur anywhere in the body, but the lung is the most common site in human beings. After inhalation of tubercle bacilli there is multiplication of bacilli in the pulmonary parenchyma, with a response of inflammatory exudate consisting of polymorphonuclear leukocytes. Almost simultaneously some of the bacilli are carried from the site of inoculation through the lymphatic system to the regional group of lymph nodes that drain the area in which the primary focus is located. Replacement of leukocytes by macrophages forming a loose focus of infiltrated tissue begins during the second day and persists for 6 to 12 days or more. The infiltrating macrophages become progressively more compact and finally tend to elongate and partially fuse together to form the typical epithelioid cell tubercle. As the tubercle bacilli multiply a change occurs in the reaction to the bacilli and their metabolic products. Hypersensitivity develops in the host after 4 to 8 weeks, and the cutaneous reaction to tuberculin becomes positive. Necrosis of the central portion of the lesion occurs and persists as a yellowish cheesy mass called caseous material. As acquired resistance and hypersensitivity develop, the lesion becomes walled off by the deposition of collagen by fibrocytes and the formation of a capsule. During the following months the tuberculous lesion frequently heals by resolution (with a return to normal), by fibrosis, or by calcification in 6 months to several years.

The nodal component of the primary complex shows less tendency to heal completely than the parenchymal focus. Even after calcification has occurred, caseation and viable tubercle bacilli may persist for years. The lymph nodes are an important factor in the progression of primary disease, since they have a tendency to enlarge and soften. They may then encroach upon or invade adjacent viscera such as the bronchi, blood vessels, pericardium, or esophagus.

During the early stage of infection at the portal of entry, before hypersensitivity develops, a small number of tubercle bacilli reach the bloodstream via the lymphatic system and regional nodes. This sporadic dissemination tends to cease after acquired resistance is established. Some tubercle bacilli that disseminate are killed without establishing any focus of infection. Others progress at varying rates into sites of active disease. They may regress and completely heal or they may remain quiescent, containing viable tubercle bacilli that may resume their activity many years after the onset of the primary infection.

The risks in primary tuberculosis for both local and hematogenous complications are influenced by a number of factors that include natural resistance, dose and virulence of the infecting tubercle bacilli, presence of intercurrent disease, age, stress, nutrition, and organ susceptibility. These complications occur in a sequence over a period of time, and they have been formalized into a timetable of complications. The greatest risk for progression of the primary complex, with extension of parenchymal disease and occurrence of meningitis and miliary tuberculosis, is in the first 12 months after primary infection. Age is an important factor in that for all children infected under 5 years of age the risk for developing meningitis or miliary disease in 12 months is 4 percent, which decreases between 5 and 10 years of age and then increases again at puberty. Skeletal lesions appear in 2 to 3 years. Renal and skin lesions occur very late and are rarely seen before 5 years after infection.

CLINICAL SPECTRUM

All clinical tuberculosis proceeds from the first primary infection, in some cases immediately (as in infants and adolescents) but most often after a variable period of latency. In a few persons, especially adolescents, reactivation produces a pattern of chronic or adult-type pulmonary tuberculosis. It is a generalized disease of lifelong duration that may affect every system and may present itself in different ways. But because it is most frequently produced by airborne infections, pulmonary disease predominates.

PRIMARY TUBERCULOSIS.   Pulmonary Tuberculosis.   Primary tuberculosis is the disease produced by the first infection with tubercle bacilli and includes the *primary complex* (parenchymal lesion and regional lymph node) and direct progression of its components. The incubation period is from 2 to 8 weeks, during which time the skin is nonreactive to tuberculin. The usual mode of onset is insidious, and except for the anorexia and inactivity that may accompany a low-grade fever, all of which are nonspecific, there are no other associated symptoms. At the end of the incubation period, delayed hypersensitivity becomes manifest as a positive tuberculin skin reaction, at times accompanied by fever of short duration and erythema nodosum. Radiographic signs frequently appear at this time, even though there may be an absence of respiratory symptoms (Fig. 1). In the majority of cases primary infections are innocuous; healing then proceeds, with calcification of the *Ghon complex* sometimes occurring as early as 6 months, but

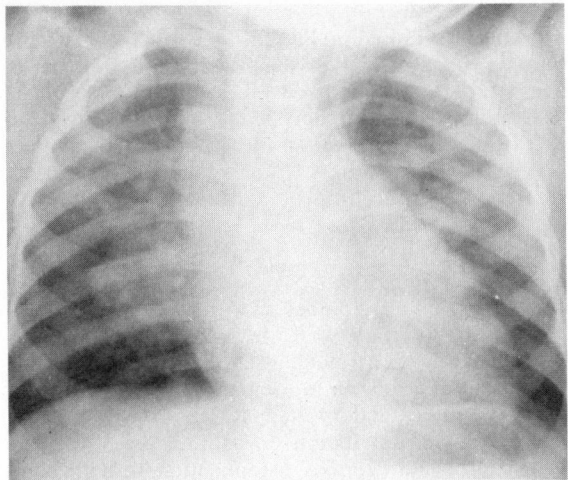

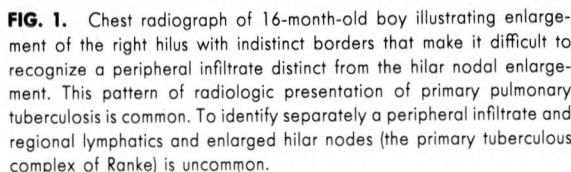

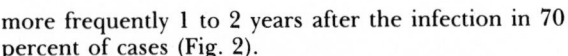

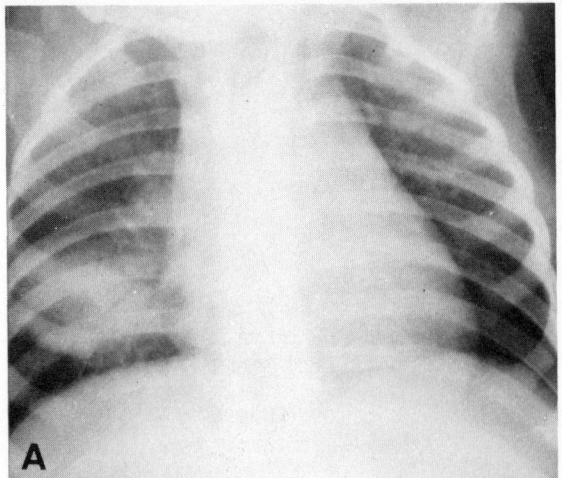

FIG. 1. Chest radiograph of 16-month-old boy illustrating enlargement of the right hilus with indistinct borders that make it difficult to recognize a peripheral infiltrate distinct from the hilar nodal enlargement. This pattern of radiologic presentation of primary pulmonary tuberculosis is common. To identify separately a peripheral infiltrate and regional lymphatics and enlarged hilar nodes (the primary tuberculous complex of Ranke) is uncommon.

more frequently 1 to 2 years after the infection in 70 percent of cases (Fig. 2).

Locally Progressive Primary Pulmonary Tuberculosis. At times the pulmonary component of the primary complex does not follow the usual benign course, but progresses locally. The onset is acute, with the parenchymal focus progressing to bronchopneumonia or lobar pneumonia. The area of caseation enlarges and eventually sloughs its necrotic contents into the adjacent bronchi, disseminating the infection and producing new areas of pneumonia. An open cavity may result and may be viewed radiographically within the primary focus. Factors that favor persistence of cavities are the rigidity of the fibrous wall and the elastic tension of the surrounding tissue. Tension cavities may develop because of a valve-type mechanism at the bronchial communication that may allow air to enter but not escape. Cavity closure may result by contraction of the fibrous capsule, by cicatricial narrowing and closure of the bronchial lumen, and by intrabronchial mucous plugging that allows the lumen to fill with exudate and the remaining air to resorb. Open healing of the cavity may occur, with absorption of caseous material, leaving a space lined by scar tissue that forms a capsule. The most frequent symptoms are cough, fever, and night sweats. Expectoration of sputum and hemoptysis are usually associated with advanced disease and the development of a cavity or ulceration of a bronchus. Abnormal physical signs in the lungs consist mainly of rales, dullness, and diminished breath sounds.

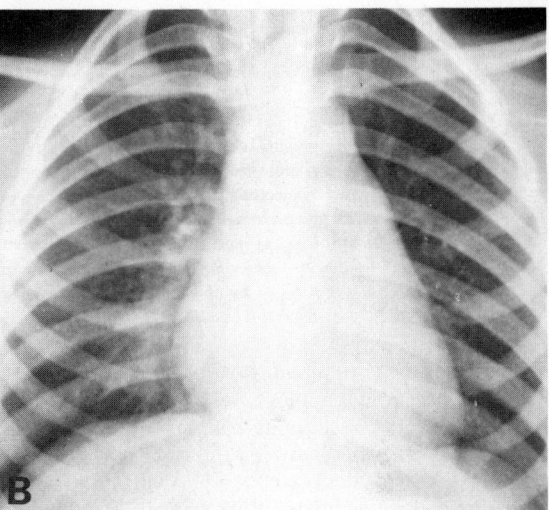

FIG. 2. A. Radiographic appearance of primary tuberculosis in a 6-year-old boy. Note peripheral infiltrate and right hilar enlargement. **B.** After antituberculous therapy for 2 years, calcification in the right hilum is seen. There is still a small area of increased radiodensity in the right lower lobe, probably a fibrotic scar.

Tracheobronchial Lymph Node and Endobronchial Disease

Involvement of a bronchial wall by an enlarging adjacent lymph node is a common complication of the primary complex; it occurs with a frequency of 5 to 20 percent in primary tuberculosis. As part of the Ghon complex, the lymph nodes that drain the primary focus become infected and consequently enlarged. Because these nodes are situated in the acute angles of the branching bronchi, there is distortion and compression of the bronchial lumen. This is a segmental lesion that shows as an opacity occupying the area of a pulmonary segment or a lobe (Fig. 3).

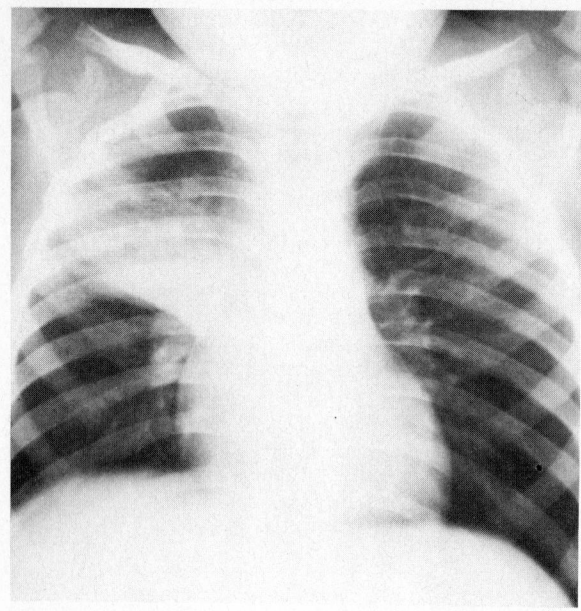

FIG. 3. This 18-month-old girl with known tuberculous exposure developed an upper respiratory infection. A PPD was positive, and this radiograph showed partial atelectasis of the right upper lobe and the suggestion of right hilar and paratracheal lymph node enlargement. Endoscopy confirmed narrowing of the right upper lobe bronchus that was thought to be due to tuberculous involvement of the bronchus, although extrinsic compression by enlarged nodes could not be excluded.

Endobronchial tuberculosis develops when the lymph node becomes adherent to an adjacent bronchus and pressure is exerted on its wall. Perforation follows, and a fistula is formed between the node and the bronchus, with the exuded caseous material being free to disseminate the infection to other segments of the lung. The frequency of development of a segmental lesion is related to the age of the child, with the risk in infants being substantial because of the narrower bronchi. The time of onset is usually the first 6 months of infection, when lymphadenitis is most active.

In the early stage of bronchial disease there are usually no symptoms. Atelectasis may develop silently. When coughing progresses it often becomes brassy and paroxysmal. Wheezing may be heard because of narrowing of the bronchial lumen. In endobronchial involvement there is a variation in the duration of the lesion, as demonstrated by bronchoscopy, from several months to a year. Bronchiectasis occurs in about 60 percent of patients, but this condition usually causes no clinical problem. Abnormal bronchograms are seen, but symptoms of illness and secondary bacterial infections rarely occur.

Therapy should include isoniazid at a dosage of 10 to 20 mg/kg/day and either ethambutol (15 to 25 mg/kg/day) or p-aminosalicylic acid (PAS) (200 to 300 mg/kg/day). Treatment does not prevent the anatomic changes that occur in the bronchi and parenchyma. It confines the infection within the involved segment and prevents dissemination. Prednisone (1 to 2 mg/kg/day) should be used as adjunct therapy. In order to be effective, steroids must be used early in the course of the disease, with response occurring after the drug has been used for 3 to 4 weeks. Although they shorten the period of obstruction, it is not clear that steroids decrease the complications of bronchiectasis.

Pleural Effusion

Pleurisy with effusion occurs with a frequency of 5 to 35 percent, the highest incidence being in the young adult; it is infrequent in children under 6 years of age. Pleurisy usually is seen in the first 6 to 12 months following infection, and it is most frequently an extension of a subpleural tuberculous focus. Less often it occurs as part of a hematogenous dissemination, with the pleural lesions being of hematogenous origin. Although the effusions are usually unilateral, bilateral involvement occurring either simultaneously or successively is seen in 4 percent of children with pleurisy.

The clinical course may vary from mild illness with slight malaise, cough, fever, and weight loss to illness with acute onset with chills and pleuritic pain. Chest pain or discomfort, if present at the onset, may disappear, with accumulation of a significant amount of fluid. Large amounts of fluid may cause respiratory distress. Physical examination usually reveals dullness to percussion and lack of breath sounds. Egophony may be present over the upper level of the fluid. The duration of the problem varies. In some cases the effusion is transient, lasting only a few days, but more typically it subsides gradually over a period of several months. The prognosis is good in children, in whom the development of pleurisy does not increase the risk of subsequent complications of tuberculosis. This is in marked contrast to adults, where 50 percent of pleural effusions are associated with chronic pulmonary tuberculosis.

The diagnosis is established by examination of the pleural fluid, which is usually clear and rarely hemorrhagic; protein content is increased, cell (lymphocyte) count is greater than 1,000/mm^3, and glucose level is less than 30 mg/100 ml. Tubercle bacilli are cultured in 50 percent of cases. Needle biopsy of the parietal pleura shows typical tubercles in about 60 percent of cases, and frequently tubercle bacilli are seen on microscopic examination and are grown in culture. In half of the needle biopsies where nonspecific histologic reactions are seen, a diagnosis of tuberculous pleurisy may be established by an open biopsy of the pleura.

Therapy should include isoniazid (10 to 20 mg/kg/day) and either ethambutol (15 to 25 mg/kg/day) or p-aminosalicylic acid (200 to 300 mg/kg/day). Treatment shortens the acute phase of the illness, hastens absorption of the pleural fluid, and reduces the risk of further local or hematogenous complications. Steroids may be used as supplementary therapy; they have been shown to increase the rate of absorption of the pleural fluid. Prednisone (1 to 2 mg/kg/day) should be used for 3 to 4 weeks if there is significant effusion. Once the initial diagnosis has been made, repeated thoracocentesis and drainage of the effusion are not necessary, since these procedures do not make any difference in immediate or ultimate prognosis.

Chronic Pulmonary Tuberculosis

Chronic pulmonary tuberculosis is often referred to as adult-type or reinfection tuberculosis; it represents endogenous reinfection from a source of tubercle bacilli previously established in the body. Pulmonary sources include the original parenchymal focus, regional lymph node, and Simon foci, which are apical seedings established during the early bacillemia from the primary focus. Chronic pulmonary tuberculosis usually remains a pulmonary disease, in contrast to primary tuberculosis, which may be an initial phase of a systemic disease. This difference is based on the fact that the tissues are sensitized to tuberculin in chronic pulmonary disease. This condition tends to evoke an accelerated reaction that localizes the tubercle bacilli and prevents progression by the lymphatics.

The risk of developing chronic pulmonary tuberculosis is greatest during adolescence; it is most likely to occur in children who experienced their first infections when they were more than 7 years of age. The initial lesion is a small area of pneumonia that may progress to caseation and liquefaction, thereby producing a cavity. The clinical picture is that of respiratory infection with dyspnea, malaise, cough, and fever. As the disease advances the amount of sputum increases; hemoptysis may occur, and the patient may appear to be chronically ill with weight loss.

Hematogenous Tuberculosis. There are three types of hematogenous spread: an occult dissemination that may later produce clinical manifestations, a single generalized process that causes acute miliary disease, and a repeated or protracted spread. The clinical picture that results from this varies and is dependent on the quantity of tubercle bacilli and their toxic products, frequency of dissemination, host factors, and susceptibility of the target organs.

Occult Hematogenous Tuberculosis. Early in the course of the initial infection, before hypersensitivity to tuberculin is developed, there is dissemination of a small quantity of tubercle bacilli through the lymphohematogenous route. Although the bacilli may seed any organ of the body, the apices of the lungs, spleen, and superficial lymph nodes are most commonly involved. Suitable conditions that help establish a sentinel focus include host factors, especially age, and inherent resistance of the viscera. Clinical evidence of this transient spread may occasionally be noted 2 to 3 months after the infection, with enlargement of the spleen and liver or superficial lymph nodes that lasts for several weeks.

Protracted Hematogenous Tuberculosis. Protracted hematogenous tuberculosis is an early complication of primary tuberculosis, and it was once responsible for 15 percent of deaths of untreated children. It is caused by repeated release of varying quantities of tubercle bacilli whenever a caseous focus erodes the wall of a blood vessel. Occasionally it may occur later in the course of primary tuberculosis, when the disseminating lesion is a chronic focus in lymph nodes or other organs. The result of protracted dissemination may be an acute illness or a prolonged one, as metastases continue to develop into foci of acute disease.

The earliest symptom is a high fever that may be persistent or intermittent. The repetition of the seeding is often manifested by the appearance of successive crops of papulonecrotic tuberculides in association with enlargement of the spleen, liver, and all the superficial and deep lymph nodes. The skeletal system is often involved, with several bones and joints being affected. Pulmonary lesions seldom develop early, but later lesions of various sizes appear and progress to diffuse pulmonary disease. The prognosis is very good following treatment, which is similar to that for acute miliary tuberculosis.

Acute Miliary Tuberculosis. Miliary tuberculosis is an early complication of primary tuberculosis; it usually occurs within the first 6 weeks after onset and is most likely to affect infants and young children. The pathologic picture is caused by a massive invasion of the bloodstream by tubercle bacilli from a caseating focus that has eroded a blood vessel. The tubercle bacilli become lodged in small capillaries and form tubercles of uniform size, which may vary from 2 mm (the size of a millet seed) to larger lesions. Despite the variable size of the lesion, the clinical picture is usually constant.

The onset of miliary tuberculosis may be insidious, with anorexia, weight loss, and low-grade fever. Radiographic evidence of primary pulmonary disease is frequently seen. Usually a sudden rise in temperature to 39 C or 40 C, which may be persistent or intermittent, indicates the onset of complications. Definite mottling on chest radiography follows febrile onset after 1 to 2 weeks. Although the child may appear acutely ill, there are very few respiratory signs and symptoms. Subsequently, respiratory distress and cyanosis appear. Accompanying findings include hepatosplenomegaly and lymphadenopathy in 50 percent of patients. Choroidal tubercles that usually appear several weeks after the onset of illness are found in varying frequencies in generalized dissemination (13 to 87 percent). In about one-third of cases meningitis is found. Radiography demonstrates that throughout the lungs there is uniform distribution of tubercles, which appear as a generalized mottling (Fig. 4).

The diagnosis of protracted hematogenous tuberculosis should be considered in any child with a fever of unknown origin, and it is a potential complication in untreated primary tuberculosis. Ten percent of patients may have a negative tuberculin test. The chest radiograph is characteristic enough to make a presumptive diagnosis with compatible epidemiologic and clinical findings. Liver biopsy or bone marrow aspiration for

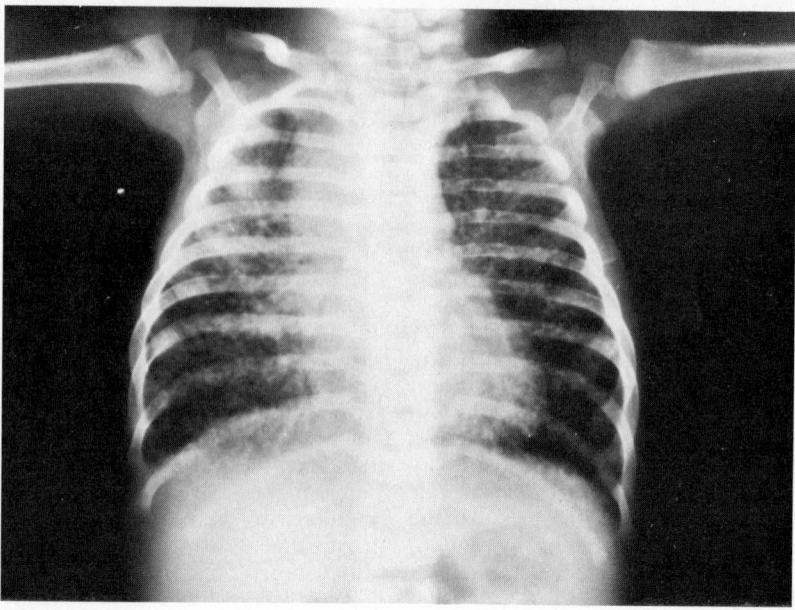

FIG. 4. This 5-month-old boy was seen because of irritability and chronically ill appearance. Chest radiography shows hematogenous dissemination of tuberculosis (miliary pattern), possibly from a right upper lobe primary focus. There are enlarged right paratracheal and hilar nodes.

bacteriologic and histologic examination may help in achieving a rapid diagnosis.

Therapy of miliary tuberculosis should include a three-drug regimen of isoniazid, rifampin, and either ethambutol or streptomycin. The dosage of isoniazid is 15 to 20 mg/kg/day. Rifampin is given at a dosage of 20 mg/kg/day, and streptomycin dosage is 40 mg/kg/day, with a maximum daily dose of 1 g. Streptomycin should be used for 1 to 3 months, or until the patient has responded and is stable. Rifampin should be used for 3 to 6 months. After the patient is stable, the daily dose of isoniazid should be reduced (10 mg/kg); combined therapy of isoniazid and ethambutol should be continued for 24 months. Prednisone (1 to 2 mg/kg/day) should be used if there is toxicity or respiratory distress. Lumbar puncture should be performed at weekly intervals as long as clinical signs persist because of the persistent threat of meningitis.

Treated miliary tuberculosis responds slowly, with fever subsiding in 2 to 3 weeks. Resolution of the chest radiogram occurs in 5 to 13 weeks, with calcification being rare. Whereas in the preantibiotic era miliary tuberculosis was usually fatal, the prognosis today is very good. Most treated patients recover fully if they are not moribund when first seen. Even after therapy is discontinued children should remain under observation, because the extensive dissemination may have caused dormant foci that may later recur as active lesions.

EXTRAPULMONARY TUBERCULOSIS. TUBERCULOUS MENINGITIS. Meningitis is the most serious complication of tuberculosis. Before the development of effective therapy it was nearly always fatal. It is an early complication of primary tuberculosis, usually developing within 12 months of infection and most frequently affecting children under 5 years of age.

The *pathogenesis* is based on a metastatic caseous lesion being formed in the cerebral cortex during the early occult hematogenous dissemination of the primary infection. As the lesion increases in size it reaches the overlying meninges and then infects the subarachnoid space. This concept is supported by pathologic findings showing focal cortical lesions communicating with the meninges. Tuberculous meningitis is always a meningoencephalitis. The site of greatest involvement of the meninges is around the brainstem. By virtue of its anatomic distribution the exudate commonly causes paresis of the third and sixth cranial nerves and obstruction of the basal cisterns, which often results in hydrocephalus. Arteritis also commonly causes occlusion of vessels and infarction of brain tissue. Depending on the extent of the lesions, this may result in varied neurologic deficits. The accumulation of exudate and its subsequent organization, as well as arteritis, infarction, and cerebral edema, all contribute to the clinical manifestations.

The *signs* and *symptoms* can be related to the pathologic changes, and a clinical classification of severity has been found to be useful in assessing prognosis. The onset is insidious, with fever always present, but the fever is of a low grade at first. Intermittent vomiting is present in half of the cases. The most striking symptom is apathy, which parents describe as either a general lack of interest or drowsiness. Irritability, anorexia, and intermittent headaches are frequent. Sudden onset of convulsions is seen in 20 percent of cases, most frequently in children under 2 years of age.

The *course* of meningitis may be divided into three stages. The initial stage of general nonspecific symptoms lasts from 1 to 2 weeks, during which time the patient is fully conscious and shows no focal neurologic signs. The second stage may start suddenly, with drowsiness, nuchal rigidity, positive Kernig and Brudzinski signs, and increased deep tendon reflexes. Occasionally there may be sudden onset of ptosis or internal strabismus. In those patients who have little or no evidence of meningeal irritation, other signs of encephalitis are seen, including disorientation, slurred speech, athetoid movements of the extremities, and peripheral tremors. In the third stage of meningitis the patients are unresponsive and exhibit opisthotonos, decerebrate rigidity, irregular respirations, hemiplegia or paraplegia, and frequently signs of increased intracranial pressure.

The diagnosis is established by examining the cerebrospinal fluid (CSF). The white blood cell count ranges from 10 to 350 cells/mm^3. Although the cells are predominantly lymphocytes, early counts may show a predominance of polymorphonuclear leukocytes, occasionally being as high as 1,000 cells/mm^3. The glucose level is normal early, but it tends to decrease (below 40 mg/100 ml) as the disease progresses (second and third stages). The protein level is usually elevated (above 40 mg/100 ml) and continues to increase. Levels over 300 mg/100 ml are found in advanced disease, and sudden increases to over 1 g/100 ml are usually associated with obstruction of the flow of CSF. The chloride content is frequently below normal. Because of the high protein levels, the CSF develops a pellicle on standing that may contain tubercle bacilli. Tubercle bacilli are cultured in about 50 percent of cases.

The tuberculin test is positive in 90 percent of patients, with anergy being found in late and terminal cases. A presumptive diagnosis of tuberculous meningitis can be made in the absence of a positive tuberculin test if there is epidemiologic evidence of tuberculosis and the characteristic CSF findings are present. Evidence of tuberculosis on chest radiography has been reported to be present in 42 to 90 percent of patients.

Specific therapy includes a three-drug regimen of isoniazid (15 to 20 mg/kg/day), rifampin (20 mg/kg/day), and either ethambutol (15 to 25 mg/kg/day) or streptomycin (40 mg/kg/day, with a maximum daily dose of 1 g). Streptomycin should be used for 1 to 3 months, or until the patient has responded and is stable. Rifampin should be used for 3 to 6 months. After the patient is stable the daily dose of isoniazid should be reduced to 10 mg/kg, with combined therapy of isoniazid and ethambutol being continued for 24 months. Prednisone (1 to 2 mg/kg/day) should be added in advanced stages of meningitis or when there is evidence of CSF obstruction (rapidly increasing CSF protein). The use of steroids may lower mortality, but late morbidity may be more frequent in the survivors.

There is a close correlation between the *prognosis* and the stage of the disease in which treatment is begun. Nearly all children treated during the first stage of tuberculous meningitis survive without any significant sequelae. If severe neurologic findings are already present when therapy is started, the prognosis must be guarded, since mortality and morbidity are increased at this stage. Complications include hydrocephalus, deafness, paralysis, and developmental retardation. The clinical response to therapy is slow and is usually manifested as a stable course without further progression during the first several weeks, followed by a gradual improvement clinically. The CSF response is also slow, with the glucose level rarely returning to normal before several weeks and the pleocytosis and elevated protein frequently taking several months.

SKELETAL TUBERCULOSIS.   Skeletal tuberculosis usually results from hematogenous dissemination of tubercle bacilli early in the course of the primary infection. Occasionally lesions of the spine and thoracic cage may develop from drainage from contiguous caseous lymph nodes. Bone and joint manifestations develop over a variable time period after the initial infection, frequently within 1 year. Presently, about 1 percent of patients hospitalized with tuberculosis have skeletal complications. The most common site of tuberculous bone involvement is the spine; such involvement occurs in about one-third of patients, most frequently in the thoracic region. Next in frequency is the hip, and then the knee, with dactylitis of the hands and feet being an infrequent complication. Any bone may become infected, and multiple bone lesions are seen in disseminated forms of tuberculosis. Functional use and age appear to influence the site of the disease. In infants who do not stand or walk, spondylitis is unusual. Dactylitis occurs almost solely in infants, probably because of the greater vascularity of the bones.

The pathologic process usually begins in the metaphyseal portions of the epiphyses because of the rich blood supply. As the lesion progresses, granulation tissue and caseation develop; they destroy bone both by pressure necrosis and by direct infection. The lesion progresses by cortical destruction and by formation of cold abscesses, which develop as the necrotic process invades the surrounding tissue. The destruction may involve only the bone, but often it extends through the epiphysis into the capsule of the joint.

Tuberculosis of Spine   In tuberculosis of the spine (*Pott's disease*) the common site of spinal involvement is the vertebral body, which undergoes progressive destruction. With continued weight bearing, vertebral collapse results, which may produce a kyphotic deformity (gibbus). Early invasion of the disk space occurs when there is involvement of the anterior superior or epiphyseal vertebral region. Paravertebral abscesses occur late in the course of the disease and are observed in about 75 percent of patients. They often extend beneath the anterior longitudinal ligament and may dissect considerable distances along fascial planes, presenting as relatively asymptomatic cold abscesses or draining sinuses.

The pathologic changes produced in the vertebrae form the basis for the usual signs and symptoms of tuberculosis of the spine. Rigidity of the spine is due to muscular spasm, which results from an effort to mini-

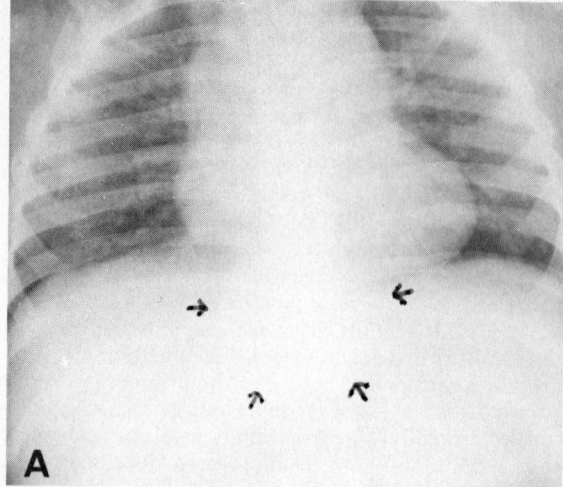

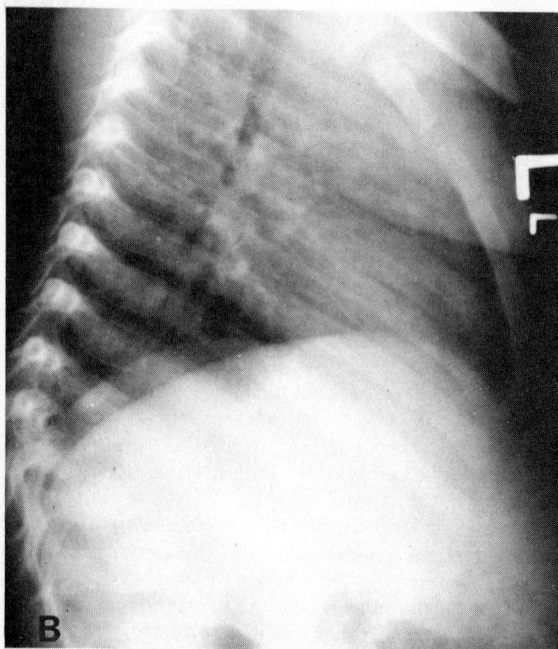

FIG. 5. A. This 26-month-old boy was well until 3 months prior to admission, when he developed difficulty in rising from the sitting position. Two months later he became markedly kyphotic and was unable to walk. This radiograph shows a paraspinal mass between T-9 and T-11, largely on the right side. **B.** Lateral view demonstrates moderate destruction of the ninth, but more severe destruction of the tenth and eleventh, thoracic vertebral bodies. At surgery a large vertebral and paravertebral abscess containing 80 ml of pus was evacuated. An intervertebral disk was found floating in the pus.

mize pain by immobilization. Characteristic positions result from attempts to relieve pressure. The early symptoms of night cries and restlessness are explained by the pain, which is felt when the protective spasm is relaxed during sleep. Referred pain caused by radiculitis is often intermittent and varies according to the site of the disease. Motor paralysis due to pressure on the spinal cord by paraspinal abscess may precede the de-

velopment of a spinal deformity. The earliest sign of spinal cord compression is usually clonus, followed by a positive Babinski sign, reflex changes, and progressive sensory and motor loss.

In cervical spondylitis, pains are usually referred to the axilla, neck, and arms. The most frequent evidence of muscle spasm is torticollis. The child favors a position of supporting his head and chin with his hands, and he may cry when he is jarred. Deformity of the spine is usually seen when disease is evident radiographically. Early evidence of a cervical lesion may be a cold abscess in the retropharyngeal space, in the neck, or the supraclavicular spaces.

When the thoracic vertebrae are involved the referred pain may be sternal or intercostal. The patient maintains an erect posture when standing, avoids bending over, and moves very slowly in rising, sitting, or lying down. In midthoracic lesions bony deformity is frequently the first evidence of tuberculosis (Fig. 5). Signs of spinal cord pressure are rare in thoracic disease, especially in lower thoracic lesions. Cold abscesses arising from the upper thoracic vertebrae occasionally may rupture into the pleura and appear as pulmonary lesions on radiography.

Lumbar spondylitis causes a posture that features a stiff back and a widened gait. Referred pain in one leg and a limp are frequently the first symptoms. When paralysis occurs the sphincters may also be involved. When cold abscesses are due to disease of the lower thoracic or lumbar vertebrae, they frequently develop in the sheath of the psoas muscle and may point to the iliac fossa, gluteal folds, or the inguinal region.

Dactylitis. Dactylitis occurs mainly in infants and young children, probably because of the greater vascularity of the bones at that age. The basic pathology is a tuberculous endarteritis. The earliest abnormal sign is thickening of the bone, which may be painless. As the swelling progresses, the overlying skin becomes thin and glossy. Radiographs show cystic bone destruction (Fig. 6). Although there may be significant swelling, especially after a cold abscess has formed, healing frequently takes place with little deformity.

Tuberculosis of Other Bones. Any bone may be infected in tuberculosis, but usually there is evidence of infection elsewhere in the body. The lesions may involve the shafts of long bones, appearing as destruction or rarely as periostitis on radiographs. Multiple lesions are frequently seen in disseminated disease. Pain is the most frequent complaint, or there may be painless swelling either over the site of the bone lesion or far removed from it.

Tuberculosis of Joints. Pain is a prominent symptom in joint disease, and it is usually local, except in disease of the hip joint, where it may be referred to other areas. In the early stages of joint disease, pain is due to intraarticular tension, but later it is due to destruction of tissue. Another common early symptom, stiffness, is caused by a decrease in the synovial fluid because of the tuberculous infection. This is most marked in the morning, and it diminishes as the day progresses because the amount of joint fluid increases with motion. Because of pain, which is usually increased by motion, and stiffness,

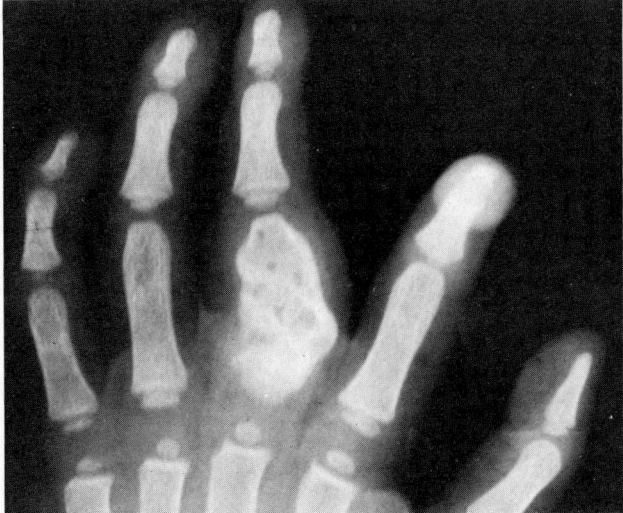

FIG. 6. Radiograph of the fingers of a 2-year-old girl with deformity and cystic rarefaction of the proximal phalanx of the third finger of the left hand. These changes characterize tuberculous dactylitis or spina ventosa.

there is limitation of the degree of motion in the affected joint, which may be manifested by a limp or a failure to execute fine motions. The joint is usually held in a flexion position, which minimizes tension. As with bone involvement, relaxation of muscular spasm results in pain and disturbance in sleep. Usually some degree of swelling is present, and it may be accompanied by muscular atrophy. Tuberculous joint disease is much more frequent in the lower than in the upper extremities, with the hips and knees being involved most frequently.

The possibility of skeletal tuberculosis should be considered whenever bone or joint symptoms occur in a patient who has tuberculosis or who has had it in the past. Failure to react to tuberculin will exclude tuberculosis if anergy can be ruled out. Tubercle bacilli may often be demonstrated in joint fluid on culture. Biopsy of the synovial membrane or bone lesion, especially the vertebrae, for culture, smear, and histologic study is helpful.

Antituberculous drugs have greatly improved prognosis by shortening the chronic course of skeletal disease and by permitting drainage of cold abscesses when necessary without creation of chronic sinus tracts. They also permit the safe use of diagnostic procedures such as biopsy and joint aspiration. Isoniazid at a daily dosage of 20 mg/kg should be used until the patient is stable; then the dosage should be reduced to 10 mg/kg daily. Isoniazid and either ethambutol (15 to 25 mg/kg/day) or *p*-aminosalicylic acid (200 to 300 mg/kg/day) shoud be given for 2 years. Rifampin (20 mg/kg/day) may be added for 3 to 6 months if the skeletal lesions are extensive, as in Pott's disease. Immobilization of the involved region by bed rest, brace, or plaster cast is important. Traction overcomes flexion or adduction deformities in the extremities. Weight bearing on the affected bone is best avoided in the early stages. Subsequently, limited non-weight-bearing exercises are of value to decrease muscle atrophy and prevent contractions. Surgery may be indicated for removal of a tuberculous focus or abscess and for stabi-

lization of diseased joints to prevent deformity. Synovectomies may be useful in aiding the eradication of persistent joint disease. In vertebral tuberculosis, cord compression and paraplegia demand prompt surgical decompression. Drainage of abscesses and spinal fusion for stability may also be necessary.

TUBERCULOSIS OF SUPERFICIAL LYMPH NODES. Superficial lymphadenitis is an early complication of primary tuberculosis; it occurs with a frequency of 3 to 5 percent. In most instances adenitis is an early hematogenous complication occurring in the first 6 months after infection. Occasionally a group of superficial nodes may become infected from direct lymphatic drainage from an extrapulmonary primary focus such as the skin. Infrequently the infected node does not quickly develop into a focus of active disease, but viable tubercle bacilli persist. In these instances the first evidence of disease in the lymph nodes may occur years after the initial infection. The most frequent sites infected are cervical, axillary, and inguinal nodes.

In the early stages the lymph nodes are firm, discrete, and not tender. Adenitis may present in several ways. The most frequent clinical situation is a gradual development of a painless enlargement of the infected node over a period of several weeks. Infrequently there may be a rapid onset, with sudden enlargement of the node and a clinical picture of toxicity. With this acute reaction, early abscess is the rule. Another way of presenting is reactivation of an old infection. There may be painless enlargement of the node, with a history of previous swelling in the same place, or there may be a small hard mass that suddenly begins to enlarge.

In the majority of cases untreated tuberculous adenitis undergoes spontaneous softening within 6 to 12 months. As necrosis and caseation occur, the capsule of the node may rupture so that adjacent nodes become adherent to each other and to the overlying skin, which appears thin, shiny, and erythematous. If rupture occurs through the skin, a sinus tract will develop.

The diagnosis should be suspected in any patient with enlargement of superficial lymph nodes. The most frequent problem in the differential diagnosis of tuberculous cervical adenitis is with infections caused by the atypical or unclassified mycobacteria. The distinguishing features of tuberculous cervical adenitis are a family history of contact with tuberculosis, positive chest radiograph, multiple groups of infected nodes, and differential skin testing results using purified protein derivative (PPD-S) and atypical mycobacterial antigens that show a larger reaction to PPD-S.

The initial treatment should include antibiotics such as penicillin because of the possibility of a pyogenic infection. Antituberculous therapy may be started simultaneously or after several weeks. Treatment should consist of isoniazid (10 mg/kg/day) combined with either ethambutol (15 to 25 mg/kg/day) or p–aminosalicylic acid (200 to 300 mg/kg/day) for 12 to 18 months. If the lymph nodes are freely movable, even if they are markedly enlarged, drug therapy alone may effect a cure. If caseation necrosis occurs (most likely in several months), surgical excision of the node is advised. Needle aspiration or incision and drainage should be avoided because of the possible complication of a sinus tract. During surgery careful attention should be given to removal of all necrotic tissue and to closure of the wound with healthy skin.

URINARY TRACT TUBERCULOSIS. Tuberculosis of the kidney begins with hematogenous dissemination of the tubercle bacilli to the renal cortex during the early phase of the initial infection. This is regarded as a late complication, because the interval between primary infection and renal disease is usually 4 years or more. As the latent foci begin to progress, caseation necrosis destroys the renal parenchyma with fistulous tracts developing and leading into the renal pelvis. The infection may spread through the ureter into the bladder and in males to the prostate and epididymis. Since tubercle bacilli cannot pass through an intact nephron, baciIluria indicates a focus of active disease.

In the early stages of renal disease there are usually no symptoms. The infection is first suggested by persistent pyuria from which no bacteria can be cultured. Proteinuria and microscopic hematuria are also found. Secondary involvement of the bladder may cause frequency, urgency, and sometimes hematuria. Epididymitis may be the first indication of disease. The urine culture is usually positive for tubercle bacilli. A urologic investigation is necessary to define the extent of the lesions. The earliest changes are usually in the upper and lower renal calyces, with the appearance of irregularities due to erosion of the parenchyma. Cavities are seen in advanced disease. When urinary symptoms are present, cystoscopy is indicated.

Treatment with antituberculous drugs should be for 2 years. If the intravenous pyelogram (IVP) is normal, isoniazid (10 mg/kg/day) and either ethambutol (15 to 25 mg/kg/day) or p–aminosalicylic acid (200 to 300 mg/kg/day) should be used. If the IVP is abnormal, initial therapy should include isoniazid, rifampin (20 mg/kg/day), and ethambutol. Rifampin should be continued until urine cultures are negative for 6 months;

then isoniazid and ethambutol should be continued for the remainder of treatment. Because ureteral stricture may appear during therapy and cause hydronephrosis an IVP and cystoscopy should be performed every 6 months during active treatment and annually thereafter for a 10-year period.

SKIN TUBERCULOSIS. Cutaneous infections are caused either by direct contact with tubercle bacilli, with the disease being localized, or by hematogenous dissemination, in which the skin lesions are often scattered.

Localized Cutaneous Tuberculosis. Common sites for inoculation with tubercle bacilli include the lower extremities and the face. Usually there is a small wound that apparently heals, but later the wound breaks down and is accompanied by painless swelling of the regional lymph nodes. The diagnosis is often missed because the lesion at the site of entry may be insignificant.

Scrofuloderma. Scrofuloderma is usually due to a focus of acute tuberculosis in lymph nodes or in the skeletal system that progresses to involve the overlying skin. As the skin becomes attached to the underlying mass, rupture occurs and a sinus tract develops. Tubercle bacilli can frequently be seen in the discharge from these lesions. The skin becomes infected with tubercle bacilli and heals by the formation of scar tissue. Scrofulodermas are seen most frequently on the face and neck, usually secondary to tuberculous cervical adenitis.

Lupus Vulgaris. Lupus vulgaris, which appears as an erythematous cluster of nodules, is rare in children and in many instances probably represents a residual stage of scrofuloderma.

Verruca Cutis. Verruca cutis consists of small painless nodules that occasionally are accompanied by regional adenitis. This usually represents a local cutaneous superinfection of tubercle bacilli in a tuberculous patient.

Papulonecrotic Tuberculids. Papulonecrotic tuberculids are due to hematogenous dissemination and are therefore of significant diagnostic value. They are seen in all stages of development and include vesicles, pustules, and dried umbilicated lesions and actually represent miliary tubercles. Other cutaneous lesions that are variations of tuberculids are lichen scrofulosorum, which is a collection of indolent inflammatory papules, and erythema induratum, which consists of deep ulcerations surrounded by induration appearing on the posterior aspect of the lower leg.

Erythema Nodosum. Erythema nodosum is probably due to a local hypersensitivity reaction to tuberculin. It is characterized by fever and painful reddish or violaceous nodules (1 to 3 cm) usually located on the anterior surface of the tibia and the extensor surface of the forearms. These lesions do not contain tubercle bacilli. Erythema nodosum is not pathognomonic of tuberculosis; it also occurs in association with a number of other complications, such as streptococcal infections, coccidioidomycosis, and sarcoidosis.

OCULAR TUBERCULOSIS. Ocular tuberculosis may be due to primary infection, but it is more frequently due to hematogenous dissemination. *Primary tuberculosis of the conjunctiva* is caused by direct inoculation of tubercle bacilli. The lesions are yellowish gray nodules that often coalesce to form an ulcer. Enlargement of the preauricular node occurs and may persist even after the conjunctivitis subsides. Other ocular lesions include those involving the uveal tract and the retina, which are more frequent in adults. *Tubercles of the choroid* are seen in varying frequency in miliary disease. *Phlyctenular conjunctivitis* represents hypersensitivity to tuberculin and is characterized by small grayish gelatinous nodules on the limbus. Since they frequently develop after a severe reaction to a tuberculin test, caution should be taken in testing individuals who may be highly sensitive to tuberculin.

TUBERCULOSIS OF HEART AND PERICARDIUM. Pericarditis is the most frequent of the cardiac lesions, but even this is a rare complication of tuberculosis. The route of infection is through the bloodstream or by direct spread from adjacent caseous lymph nodes. Since the pericardial lesion that develops is not specific clinically, diagnosis can be made only by culture of pericardial fluid, which is only infrequently positive, or by tissue biopsy. Constrictive pericarditis may occur if treatment is delayed or inadequate, and this usually requires surgical decortication.

ABDOMINAL TUBERCULOSIS Gastrointestinal infection usually is an enteritis involving the jejunum and ileum and may be a sequel of advanced pulmonary disease in which there is superinfection of the mucosa by swallowed tubercle bacilli. In the past a frequent cause was bovine tuberculosis contained in unpasteurized milk. The lesions of *tuberculous enteritis* develop into shallow ulcers that are responsible for the symptoms of pain, diarrhea, constipation, and weight loss.

Infection of abdominal lymph nodes may be part of a primary complex or the result of hematogenous spread. The course of these nodes is similar to that of tuberculous nodes elsewhere. They enlarge and become adherent to the visceral peritoneum and may encroach on the intestinal tract, producing varying degrees of obstruction.

Peritonitis that complicates tuberculosis may be of several types. Generalized peritonitis is part of a hematogenous dissemination. Localized or plastic peritonitis may be due to direct extension from lymph node infection, or it may originate from tuberculous salpingitis. Usually the lymph nodes, peritoneum, and omentum are matted together and may be palpated as an irregular mass. Peritonitis may occur with an effusion; it may represent either direct extension from a primary intestinal focus or a hematogenous infection. The onset of ascites is frequently accompanied by fever. The rapid accumulation of fluid and the abdominal discomfort suggest the diagnosis, which is confirmed by paracentesis and examination of the fluid.

Infections of the spleen and liver may occur during occult or generalized hematogenous dissemination, but they rarely exist as solitary lesions. In acute miliary tuberculosis a diagnosis may often be established by a needle biopsy of the liver with culture and histologic examination in patients who are tuberculin-negative.

TUBERCULOSIS OF MOUTH AND UPPER RESPIRATORY TRACT. *Tuberculosis of the tonsils, adenoids, buccal mucosa, and larynx* may result from hematogenous seeding, from direct contact with tubercle bacilli as in a primary infection, or from direct contact with infectious sputum of patients who have chronic pulmonary disease. Symptoms vary with the site of the disease. Thus granulomatous ulcerations of the mouth may cause pain and dysphagia, and hoarseness may occur when lesions are present in the larynx.

Infection of the middle ear and mastoids may result from hematogenous spread or from tubercle bacilli entering the middle ear from infected adenoids and the nasopharynx during coughing or sneezing. Characteristically there is no pain, and perforation of the tympanic membrane may occur with serous or purulent discharge from which tubercle bacilli can be cultured. Frequent complications include facial paralysis, labyrinthitis, and deafness. Extension to the mastoid cells frequently occurs, with very little pain as mastoiditis develops. The complication commonly requires surgery for removal of necrotic bone.

TUBERCULOSIS OF ENDOCRINE AND EXOCRINE GLANDS. Isolated infections in all the endocrine glands and several exocrine glands (lacrimal, salivary, and mammary) have been reported; they may represent direct progression from contiguous areas of tuberculosis or hematogenous spread. The latter type of infection is most frequent in the adrenal glands, where it represents a late stage of tuberculosis, since the average interval between initial infection and the onset of Addison's disease is 15 years.

CONGENITAL TUBERCULOSIS. Congenital tuberculosis may occur when a pregnant woman has advanced tuberculosis, either miliary or cavitary disease, during which there is dissemination of tubercle bacilli and infection of the placenta. The subsequent manner of spread from the placenta determines the site of the primary complex. Tubercle bacilli transmitted through the placenta become lodged in the liver. When the lesion in the placenta becomes ulcerative, inhalation or ingestion of infected amniotic fluid produces lesions in the lungs or digestive tract. The prognosis of intrauterine infection is usually serious, with death occurring either in utero or within 5 weeks after birth with manifestations of generalized infection. The criteria for congenital tuberculosis include the following: establishment of the tuberculous nature of the infection; determination of whether the primary complex is in the fetal liver; in the absence of a primary complex in the fetal liver, an onset of tuberculosis at birth or within a few days; definite exclusion of extrauterine infection.

In the therapeutic approach to an infant born of a mother with tuberculosis, factors that should be considered are the activity of maternal disease and its treatment, the likelihood of a congenital infection, and the therapy or prophylaxis for the infant. Environmental considerations are important, since infants have become infected with tuberculosis even though their mothers have had minimal disease and have been separated from them immediately after birth. This suggests that someone else in the environment was the probable source of infection.

Mother with Untreated Advanced Pulmonary Disease. Maternal isolation and separation should be effected immediately after birth and continued until the disease is not contagious. The infant should have a tuberculin test and chest radiograph. If there is no evidence of tuberculosis, isoniazid (5 to 10 mg/kg/day) should be given for 3 months, after which the tuberculin test should be repeated. Isoniazid should be continued for 1 year if the tuberculin test is positive, or discontinued if it is negative. BCG vaccine may be used if there is a high-risk environment for tuberculosis when isoniazid is stopped.

Mother on Therapy for Pulmonary Tuberculosis. Maternal isolation and separation should be immediate and should be continued until the disease is not contagious. Under these circumstances the maternal risk to the infant is negligible, and the infant may be given a repeat tuberculin test in 3 months. If the family environment is thought to carry a high risk for tuberculosis, BCG vaccine may be used—but not until the tuberculin test has been repeated at 3 months. Earlier use of the vaccine will confuse the interpretation of the tuberculin test.

Mother with Treated or Untreated Inactive Tuberculosis. No separation or isolation of the mother is necessary. The infant requires no therapy or prophylaxis, but a tuberculin test should be given at intervals of 3 to 6 months for the first year. The mother should be followed with postpartum chest radiographs at 6-month intervals because of the risk of reactivation of tuberculosis, especially if her disease was inactive for less than 5 years. If the follow-up of the infant is uncertain, BCG vaccine should be used.

DIAGNOSTIC METHODS

HISTORY. A history of exposure to another patient with tuberculosis may frequently suggest the diagnosis if the patient's clinical manifestations are compatible with the disease.

TUBERCULIN TEST. The tuberculin test is based on the fact that infection with *M. tuberculosis* produces a specific sensitivity to certain products of the organism that are contained in culture extracts. The intradermal injection of tuberculin in sensitized individuals induces an area of induration with erythema that varies in size and intensity according to the amount of tuberculin injected and the individual's sensitivity. Two preparations of tuberculin are presently used. Old tuberculin (OT) is made by heat-sterilizing and filtering cultures of tubercle bacilli and evaporating the bacilli-free filtrate to one-tenth its original volume. Purified protein derivative (PPD) consists of the active protein substance obtained from filtrates of autoclaved cultures of tubercle bacilli that have been grown on a synthetic medium and then extracted either by trichloroacetic acid or neutral ammonium sulfate precipitation. PPD is preferred because its strength is standardized, and more uniform results are obtained. Presently, a polysorbate (Tween 80) is added to PPD in order to reduce the adsorption of tuberculin to plastic and glass surfaces; it is then referred to as stabilized tuberculin. A reference tuberculin (PPD-S) was adopted by the World Health Organization in 1952 as the international standard mammalian PPD tuberculin.

Three techniques of applying the tuberculin test are generally used. The intradermal (Mantoux) test is performed by the intradermal injection of 0.1 ml of the desired concentration of tuberculin (Table 14). The standard dose that should be used is PPD intermediate (5 TU). First-strength PPD (1 TU) should be used in any individual suspected of being highly sensitive to tuberculin. Second-strength PPD (250 TU) is of value in excluding a diagnosis of tuberculosis with a negative reaction. A positive reaction is less helpful in supporting the diagnosis because of false-positive reactions due to cross-reactions with atypical mycobacteria. One TU detects 95 percent and 5 TU detects 99 percent of those infected with tuberculosis. The jet injection method uses a jet gun to deliver 5 TU of PPD intradermally under high pressure. Multiple-puncture tests use a skin puncture technique, either by an application with points on which tuberculin is dried (tine test) or by puncturing through a film of liquid tuberculin. Although there is generally good correlation of results between the multiple-puncture and Mantoux tests, because of the small percentage of false positives and false negatives, tine tests should be used for large-scale screening rather than in making specific diagnoses.

The tests should be read in 72 hours. For the Mantoux test the transverse diameter of induration should

TABLE 14. Approximate Tuberculin Equivalents*

Test Strength	Tuberculin Units (TU)	PPD (mg/dose)	OT Dilution	OT (mg/dose)
First	1	0.00002	1:10,000	0.01
Intermediate	5	0.0001	1:2,000	0.05
Second	250	0.005	1:100	1.0

* Adapted from Diagnostic Standards and Classification of Tuberculosis. Courtesy of the National Tuberculosis and Respiratory Disease Association, New York, N.Y., 1969.

be measured. Erythema without induration is not significant. Induration of 10 mm or more is a positive test; induration of 5 to 9 mm is a doubtful reaction and may reflect cross-sensitivity to atypical mycobacteria. However, if the patient has had close contact with a person who has tuberculosis or if the patient has radiographic or clinical evidence of disease, he should be managed as a positive reactor even if the reaction is between 5 and 9 mm. A reaction of less than 4 mm induration is negative. In measuring the multiple-puncture tests (tine), the diameter of the largest single reaction of induration should be used. If the reaction consists of discrete papules, the diameters of separate areas of induration should not be added. Induration of 5 mm or more is a positive test; induration of 2 to 4 mm is a doubtful reaction. These tests should be confirmed by a Mantoux test.

A positive tuberculin test demonstrates that infection is present, but it does not prove the presence of active disease. Sensitivity requires 4 to 8 weeks to develop and tends to persist. It may wane in the elderly or if treatment is given in the early stages of infection. Sensitivity to tuberculin may be decreased by measles, rubella, and varicella, and it may remain suppressed for a number of weeks after these illnesses. Vaccination with measles and yellow fever vaccines has a similar effect. Overwhelming tuberculosis, sarcoidosis, or administration of steroids also may suppress the tuberculin test. Repeated testing of the uninfected individual does not sensitize to tuberculin, but it may have a booster effect in individuals who have low degrees of sensitivity due to heterologous mycobacterial antigens.

LABORATORY DIAGNOSIS. A tentative diagnosis of tuberculosis is usually made by demonstrating acid-fast bacilli in smears of sputum or other clinical specimens using acid-fast stains such as the Ziehl-Neelsen stain. Some laboratories favor a rapid screening method using fluorescent dyes, such as auramine or auramine and rhodamine. The material still should be cultured because of the relative insensitivity of acid-fast stains in detecting tuberculosis and because it is necessary to grow the organisms so that they may be characterized, especially regarding drug sensitivity.

Secretions from the lungs may be obtained by expectoration, laryngeal swab, saline vapor, tracheal suction, bronchoscopy, or gastric lavage. In children, since sputum is rarely produced, gastric lavage is the method most frequently used for collection of specimens. A plastic disposable gastric tube is introduced through a nostril into the stomach, aided by swallowing motions. The gastric contents are aspirated and collected. Sterile water (20 to 50 ml) is inserted through the tube, and the gastric contents are aspirated and pooled. Gastric lavage should be done on three consecutive days, early in the morning with the patient fasting and recumbent. Once peristalsis is activated, the yield of positive cultures decreases significantly. For this reason gastric lavage cannot be done on an ambulatory basis. Direct examination of gastric washings is misleading because nonpathogenic acid-fast bacilli may normally be found.

Only about one-fourth to one-third of gastric lavages of children suspected of having tuberculosis have positive cultures. The clinical specimens are concentrated and digested, usually with sodium hydroxide, and inoculated onto culture media, such as buffered egg-potato medium (Löwenstein-Jensen) or Middlebrook oleic acid agar. A positive culture usually grows out in 4 to 8 weeks.

CONTROL OF TUBERCULOSIS

Control of tuberculosis is based primarily on drug therapy, both for treatment and for prevention of the disease. Proper use of drugs requires a basic knowledge of the natural history of tuberculosis, information about drug toxicity, and knowledge of the factors that affect the response of the tubercle bacilli to them. Several new drugs have recently been introduced, and better means of utilizing all available drugs based on these considerations have been established.

ANTITUBERCULOUS DRUGS. Antituberculous drugs have been divided into two groups. First-line drugs are those most commonly used for initial treatment, and second-line drugs are usually used when drug resistance or drug intolerance or toxicity is encountered. For children, the drugs of the first-line group include isoniazid, *p*-aminosalicylic acid, ethambutol, streptomycin, and rifampin.

Isoniazid. Isoniazid (INH) is a synthetically produced drug that is the most potent and most valuable single drug in the treatment of tuberculosis. When it is administered orally a plasma concentration 20 to 80 times the usual level required to inhibit the growth of tubercle bacilli (0.02 to 0.05 μg/ml) may be reached within several hours, with high concentrations persisting for 6 to 8 hours in plasma and sputum. INH penetrates readily into the cerebrospinal fluid, even in the absence of inflammation, and into caseous tissue, where it is fully active in the pH range of inflamed tissues. It is partially conjugated in the liver to an acetylated inactive, nontoxic form. The rate and degree of acetylation are genetically determined. Both free and acetylated forms of the drug are excreted in the urine.

The principal side effects of INH are peripheral neuritis and hepatitis. Peripheral neuritis results from competitive inhibition of pyridoxine metabolism. This is more likely to occur at higher dose levels of INH (> 10 mg/kg/day) in alcoholics and individuals with poor nutrition. This is rarely a problem in children, although precautions must be taken during adolescence or when the total daily dose of INH exceeds 300 mg. In those situations where pyridoxine deficiency is a problem, pyridoxine (10 mg for each 100 mg of INH) should be used daily.

INH hepatitis has received considerable attention because of its disturbingly high rate of occurrence, and INH has caused death among patients receiving the drug for prophylaxis. Transient elevation of liver enzymes has been documented in 10 percent of patients, all asymptomatic. In most instances enzyme levels return to normal, without withdrawal of the drug. The rate of overt clinical hepatitis is close to 1 percent, with frequency variations depending on age. It is rare in individuals under 20 years of age. The observed frequency in other age groups is as follows: age 20 to 34, up to 0.3 percent; age 35 to 49, up to 1.2 percent; over age 50, up to 2.3 percent. It is not recommended that patients taking INH be followed by repeated liver function tests unless there is a previous history of liver disease or predisposition to the development of liver disease. Careful questioning about symptoms should be done monthly, with warnings to report such symptoms promptly. Other infrequent side effects are convulsions, psychoses, loss of memory, allergic manifestations, and a lupuslike syndrome, with arthritis and the presence of antinuclear factor.

For prophylaxis the recommended dosage of INH is 10 mg/kg/day, with a maximum of 300 mg/day. In clinical disease, depending on the severity, INH may be given at a dosage of 20 mg/kg/day, with a maximum of 500 mg/day. When clinical improvement and stability are observed, the dosage should be reduced to the lower recommended dosage previously described in the sections dealing with the various clinical forms of tuberculosis. INH is available in tablets of 50 mg and 100 mg and in flavored syrup at 10 mg/ml. A parenteral preparation is also available.

Ethambutol. Ethambutol is an odorless water-soluble compound with very effective antituberculous activity. It is rapidly absorbed from the gastrointestinal tract and is excreted in the urine, mainly with its form unchanged. At the recommended dosage of 15 to 25 mg/kg/day, peak serum levels of 3 to 5 μg/ml that are bacteriostatic for tubercle bacilli are quickly reached. The only important toxic effect is a retrobulbar neuritis that results in loss of visual acuity, defects in visual fields, and inability to distinguish between the colors red and green. Fortunately the visual changes are completely reversible. This side effect should be monitored by monthly studies of visual acuity and visual fields and tests for green color vision. The drug should be discontinued if there is more than a two-line loss of visual acuity as measured on a Snellen eye chart, if there is contraction of visual fields, or if there is loss of green color vision.

Ethambutol is a very effective drug when used in combination with other drugs, and it is well tolerated, with minimal toxicity. Because of this it has largely replaced *p*-aminosalicylic acid in the treatment of tuberculosis. Unfortunately, the inability to monitor in children the toxic effect of retrobulbar neuritis by the required visual exams limits its use in young children. In fact, the package brochure accompanying the drug advises against its use in children. Despite this limitation, ethambutol should be used in those clinical situations that require a second drug, providing reliable examinations can be done. The recommended dosage is 25 mg/kg/day for 6 to 8 weeks, followed by a reduction to 15 mg/kg/day. The drug is supplied in 100- and 400-mg tablets.

Para-aminosalicylic acid. The bacteriostatic drug *p*-aminosalicylic acid (PAS) has a lower potency than the other first-line drugs. However, it remains important because of its capacity to delay bacillary resistance when used in combined therapy. PAS also increases the amount of free INH in the blood because it competes for acetylation in the liver. PAS is readily absorbed from the gastrointestinal tract, with recommended dosages giving a peak concentration of 5 to 10 mg/100 ml of serum in 2 hours. It diffuses to some extent into serous surfaces and reaches the cerebrospinal fluid in small amounts. It is conjugated in the liver and excreted in the urine in this form.

Gastrointestinal disturbances are the principal side effects, but leukopenia, hepatitis, fever, rashes, and lymphadenopathy also have been described. Toxic reactions of a hypersensitivity type occur in 6 percent of patients. PAS is used in combination therapy, but because of its side effects it is being replaced by ethambutol. The recommended dosage is 0.2 g to 0.3 g/kg/day. It is supplied in 0.5-g and 1-g tablets.

Streptomycin. Streptomycin was the first effective antituberculous drug. It is given intramuscularly and is rapidly absorbed into the bloodstream, reaching peak levels that are 50 to 100 times more than the minimal inhibitory concentration of 0.2 μg/ml. It diffuses readily into the pleural fluid, but does not diffuse into the cerebrospinal fluid unless there is inflammation of the meninges. Streptomycin is largely excreted in the urine, with an 80 percent recovery within 24 hours.

The principal toxic effect is eighth nerve damage, mainly of the vestibular branch, resulting in vertigo and ataxia that is usually permanent. Hearing loss is less common and usually affects the high-frequency range before the lower frequencies are affected. Children readily adjust to vestibular defect with minimal difficulty. At current dosage schedules, hearing defects are rare in children. Other infrequent side effects include fever, dermatitis, and agranulocytosis.

Streptomycin is administered by intramuscular injection at a dosage of 30 to 40 mg/kg once daily, with a maximum dose of 1 g. Because of rapid development of resistance to streptomycin it is never used alone, but is given in combination with other drugs. It is usually used for 2 to 3 months, until clinical improvement and stability occur; then it is discontinued, being replaced when necessary by a drug that may be given orally. Following the recently proven efficacy of rifampin, which for the first time affords superior oral regimens, the use of streptomycin is becoming very limited.

Rifampin. Rifampin is a semisynthetic drug derived from *streptomyces mediterranei* that has wide antimicrobial activity against viruses, bacteria, and mycobacteria. It is absorbed readily from the gastrointestinal tract after oral administration, with peak concentrations of 6 to 32 μg/ml (MIC for *M. tuberculosis,* 0.5 μg/ml) occurring in 3 hours. Rifampin readily diffuses to all tissues and body fluids, including the cerebrospinal fluid; it is excreted primarily through the biliary tract and kidneys.

Rifampin has been hailed as the most effective antituberculous drug since isoniazid. The properties that make it an excellent drug include high peak levels, long duration of activity, and experimental antituberculous activity in mice equal to that of isoniazid. Also of great importance is the fact that natural resistance of tubercle bacilli to rifampin is found less frequently than resistance to isoniazid (rifampin, 1 in 10^6 to 10^8; isoniazid, 1 in 10^4 to 10^6). Clinical studies have clearly justified the predictions of the efficacy of rifampin. Multiple-drug-resistant far-advanced tuberculosis can be brought to culture conversion and quiescent status in 70 percent of cases with drug regimens that include rifampin. With rifampin and isoniazid, for the first time a two-drug oral regimen that is relatively nontoxic and is easy to take has resulted in sputum conversion that is superior to that previously obtained only with three-drug regimens.

The place of rifampin in treatment includes retreatment, drug-resistant problems, and serious life-threatening situations; however, its role in the initial treatment of tuberculosis is unclear and is being evaluated to see if it offers any advantage over other drugs. The possible advantages of either decreasing relapse rate or shortening the duration of therapy would justify its routine use despite its high cost (at least $500 per year compared to $2.50 per year for isoniazid). Rifampin is relatively nontoxic, with the principal side effect being hepatitis, which occurs with a frequency of 1 percent. Hepatitis seems to be more common in patients who are treated with the combination of rifampin and isoniazid. Gastrointestinal disturbances, rashes, reversible leukopenia, and elevation of blood urea nitrogen have been reported. In children rifampin is recommended for retreatment, drug-resistant tuberculosis, and serious diseases such as miliary tuberculosis, meningitis, and extensive renal and skeletal tuberculosis. It should be used in combination therapy for 3 to 6 months and then discontinued. Since data for the administration of this drug in the United States are limited, package brochures advise against its use in children. However, there is ample evidence of its clinical value in children in Europe. The suggested dosage is 20 mg/kg/day (maximum 600 mg). Rifampin is supplied in 300-mg capsules.

Other Drugs. The remaining antituberculous drugs are used entirely for retreatment or in children whose disease is complicated by drug resistance. Ethionamide is moderately effective, but its use is restricted by gastrointestinal toxicity and hepatotoxicity. Kanamycin and viomycin are administered intramuscularly, but both are ototoxic and nephrotoxic. Pyrazinamide is given orally; it is moderately effective but is hepatotoxic. Cycloserine is given orally and is moderately effective, but it is toxic for the central nervous system.

PREVENTION. **Chemoprophylaxis.** The basis for preventive therapy is, in reality, treatment of clinically inapparent infections, which are thus prevented from developing into progressive tuberculosis. Extensive trials conducted by the U.S. Public Health Service show a consistent reduction of morbidity in treated groups. The protection afforded by 1 year of preventive therapy for those at risk of developing tuberculous disease continues for at least 6 years after the therapy has been stopped. The long-term effect on late reactivity is as yet unknown. Since more than three-fourths of the active cases of tuberculosis today come from a reservoir of asymptomatic tuberculin-positive individuals, the chemoprophylaxis program has been very effective in reducing the incidence of disease. In children chemoprophylaxis has been effective in reducing extrapulmonary as well as pulmonary manifestations of tuberculosis, especially in those under 4 year of age.

Isoniazid is used alone for chemoprophylaxis at a dosage of 10 mg/kg/day (maximum 300 mg) for 1 year. Currently no other drug has been demonstrated to be effective for preventive therapy. The dose recommended for its use is based on a comparison of the risk of hepatic injury with the benefit of preventive therapy. Besides this consideration, priorities for chemoprophylaxis must take into account the ease of identifying and supervising persons for whom preventive therapy is indicated and their likelihood of infecting others. Since the risk of hepatitis is rare in the group under 20 years of age, isoniazid should probably be used for all children who are tuberculin reactors as well as for recent converters.

The following groups, for whom chemoprophylaxis is recommended, are listed in order of priority: (1) Household members and other close associates of persons with recently diagnosed tuberculous disease. The risk of being infected and of developing disease is 2.5 percent for the first year. However, the risk of developing disease is 5 percent for those already infected (tuberculin-positive) at the time of initial examination. Those contacts who have negative tuberculin tests should receive preventive therapy for 3 months and be tested again. If they are then tuberculin-positive, therapy should be continued for 12 months; but if the Mantoux test is negative and exposure has ended, preventive therapy may be discontinued. (2) Persons with a positive tuberculin skin test and a chest radiograph consistent with nonprogressive tuberculous disease in whom there are neither positive bacteriologic findings nor a history of adequate therapy. The rate of reactivation has been observed to be between 1 and 4.5 percent per year. (3) Newly infected persons. The risk is about 5 percent during the first year after infection. The term newly infected person should be applied only to those who have had a tuberculin skin test conversion within the previous 2 years. Since there are so many variations in the Mantoux test, a converter should be defined as a person whose tuberculin skin test has increased by at least 6 mm from less than 10 mm induration to greater than 10 mm. (4) Positive tuberculin skin reactors in special clinical situations. These situations and conditions increase the risk of developing tuberculous disease and require preventive therapy in those who are infected: steroid therapy; immunosuppressive therapy; hematologic and reticuloendothelial diseases, such as leukemia and lymphoma; diabetes mellitus; silicosis; postgastrectomy states. (5) Other positive reactors. Preventive therapy is mandatory for positive reactors through age 6 years and is highly recommended to age

35 years. Among persons under 35 years of age who are tuberculin reactors, the benefit of isoniazid therapy clearly outweighs the risk of hepatitis. Among positive tuberculin reactors above 35 years of age with normal chest radiographs the risk of hepatitis precludes the routine use of preventive therapy, unless one of the additional risk factors listed above is present. The members of this group should be considered on an individual basis in situations where there is a likelihood of serious consequences to contacts who may become infected. Examples are persons who live in a closed environment or who work with children.

Before chemoprophylaxis with isoniazid is started, screening procedures should be carried out. Contraindication to the use of isoniazid are previous isoniazid-associated hepatitis, severe adverse reactions to isoniazid, and any acute liver disease. Situations in which there is no contraindication, but in which special attention is indicated, include the following: concurrent use of any other drug; use of diphenylhydantoin in which a reduction in dosage is necessary because isoniazid may decrease the excretion of diphenylhydantoin; use of alcohol, which may be associated with a higher incidence of isoniazid hepatitis; current chronic liver disease; previous history of side effects possibly (but not definitely) related to isoniazid; pregnancy. Although no harmful effects to the fetus caused by isoniazid have been documented, preventive therapy generally should be started after delivery.

Routine monitoring by repeat liver function tests is not useful in predicting hepatitis and should therefore not be done except in patients who have a history of liver disease or who are predisposed to its development. Otherwise, patients should be questioned monthly for signs and symptoms of hepatic injury and should be advised that if any of these develop they should discontinue the drug and report for evaluation.

Vaccination.   Bacillus Calmette-Guérin (BCG) was derived from a strain of *M. bovis* attenuated through years of serial passage in culture at the Pasteur Institute in Lille, France. There are many BCG vaccines available in the world today; they are all derived from the original strain, but they vary in antigenicity and efficacy. Their variations probably have resulted from genetic changes and differences in techniques of production, methods and routes of vaccine administration, and characteristics of the populations and environments in which the vaccines have been studied. Earlier controlled trials of liquid vaccines prepared from different BCG strains showed protection ranging from 0 to 80 percent. The vaccines now available in the United States differ from those used in earlier clinical trials in that many culture passages have since taken place and there have been various modifications in methods of preparation and preservation. Current vaccines are freeze-dried, and although their efficacy has not been directly demonstrated, they can be inferred to have an efficacy of approximately 75 percent.

BCG has been associated with adverse reactions, including localized ulceration, lymphadenitis, osteomyelitis, lupoid reactions, and disseminated infection and death, but only in children with impaired immune responses. In countries such as the United States where the incidence of tuberculosis is low, tuberculosis can be better controlled by modern methods of case detection, chemotherapy, and preventive treatment. Under certain circumstances BCG vaccine may be useful. It may be used in individuals who are not infected with tuberculosis and who fit into the following categories: (1) those who are at risk of repeated exposure to persistently untreated or ineffectively treated pulmonary tuberculosis such as infants of mothers with tuberculosis; (2) those members of well-defined groups with excessive rates of new infections despite the usual surveillance and treatment programs, such as alcoholics, drug addicts, and migrants, who usually do not have a regular source of health care.

Vaccination should be performed only in those who are skin-test-negative to 5 TU of tuberculin PPD. Vaccination may be carried out by oral administration, subcutaneous injection, or multiple skin puncture, or by the preferred route of intradermal injection. The usual dose is 0.1 mg in 0.1 ml intradermally, which produces a skin reaction in 2 to 3 weeks featuring a papule that vesiculates and heals with a small scar. A repeat tuberculin skin test should be given in 2 to 3 months, with a positive reaction implying resistance. If the skin test is negative, repeat vaccination is necessary. Ideally the patient should be removed from contact with tuberculosis until his tuberculin skin test becomes positive.

The disadvantage of BCG is the hypersensitivity to tuberculin that it produces, which may cancel the value of tuberculin testing for the diagnosis of tuberculosis. The degree and duration of BCG-induced tuberculin reactions vary with the type and preparation used. If one uses 5 TU of tuberculin (PPD intermediate) and defines the reaction as 10 mm induration (minimum reaction for diagnosis), the reaction induced by BCG infrequently exceeds 12 mm and usually is transient, gradually declining until within a few years it usually is less than 10 mm. It is recommended that those who are vaccinated be retested with tuberculin periodically, with the reaction being recorded, so that comparisons can be made that will be helpful in differentiating subsequent changes.

TREATMENT. General Management.   When the diagnosis of tuberculosis is established in a child, the immediate family and close contacts should all be tested with tuberculin skin tests and chest radiographs. Children with asymptomatic primary tuberculosis may be treated and followed in the clinic. Most children with symptomatic primary tuberculosis, even though it is minimal to moderate in extent, probably should be admitted to the hospital, for several reasons: to take cultures (gastric cultures are invalid on an ambulatory basis), to observe the patient for drug tolerance, to prevent contagion, to establish a proper relationship with the family and impress on them the potential gravity of the disease (which may minimize problems of compliance), and to provide time to screen household contacts for susceptibility. Fortunately, most childhood tuberculosis, with the exception of chronic pulmonary and

TABLE 15. Treatment for Complications of Tuberculosis

Type	Drug	Daily Dose	Duration
Miliary tuberculosis	Isoniazid	20 mg/kg	Initial 4–6 weeks
		10 mg/kg	2 years
	Ethambutol*	15–25 mg/kg	2 years
	and		
	Rifampin	20 mg/kg	3–6 months
	or		
	Isoniazid	20 mg/kg	Initial 4–6 weeks
		10 mg/kg	2 years
	Rifampin	20 mg/kg	3–6 months
	and		
	Streptomycin	20–40 mg/kg	1–3 months, until patient stabilized
	Ethambutol*	15–25 mg/kg	Added for duration of therapy when streptomycin stopped
Tuberculous meningitis		Same as above	
Skeletal tuberculosis		Same as above	
Renal tuberculosis			
IVP abnormal		Same as above	
IVP normal	Isoniazid	10 mg/kg	2 years
	Ethambutol*	15–25 mg/kg	2 years

* If visual exams cannot reliably be performed, PAS (200 to 300 mg/kg) should be substituted. Adult doses INH 300 mg/day, Rifampin 600 mg/day, Streptomycin 1.5–2.0 g/day.

cavitary disease, is usually noncontagious if the patients are asymptomatic and minimally contagious if pulmonary lesions and symptoms are present. Since sputum production and cough are minimal and antituberculous drugs are very effective in quickly reducing infectivity, most uncomplicated cases should probably be isolated for about 1 week. Chronic pulmonary and cavitary tuberculosis should be managed in isolation and followed by sputum smears and cultures.

Specific Therapy. The object of specific therapy is to arrest the progress of the disease as rapidly as possible by preventing the multiplication of tubercle bacilli. This is accomplished by using a combination of the best available drugs, which also delays the emergence of bacillary resistance. However, there are some limitations to therapy that are based on the nature of the tuberculous lesions, which tend to create certain environmental conditions that protect the tubercle bacilli from host defenses. These conditions also promote a metabolically inactive state in the organisms that protects them from the action of antituberculous drugs. Since all tubercle bacilli are not eradicated, natural host defenses are relied on in rendering the disease inactive.

The first-line drugs from which combination regimens are chosen include isoniazid, *p*-aminosalicylic acid (PAS), ethambutol, streptomycin, and rifampin. These drugs must be used for 18 to 24 months to effect a cure. They can all be given in a single daily dose rather than divided doses without sacrificing any therapeutic effect; however, PAS should be administered in three or four divided doses to reduce gastrointestinal side effects. Chemoprophylaxis is usually the only situation in which one drug is used alone in therapy: isoniazid (10 mg/kg/day) is used for 1 year. In minimal to moderately advanced uncomplicated primary disease, as well as in chronic tuberculosis, isoniazid (10 mg/dg/day) is used

with either ethambutol (15 to 25 mg/kg/day) or PAS (200 to 300 mg/kg/day) for 18 to 24 months. Ethambutol is preferable, providing that monthly visual exams can always be performed. Otherwise, PAS should be used.

Most complications of tuberculosis, especially the disseminated forms of the disease, should be treated initially with a combination of three drugs (Table 15). Even though there is no evidence that the addition of a third drug offers any advantage as long as two of the drugs are isoniazid and rifampin, the addition would seem justified in a serious life-threatening or potentially crippling disease where drug sensitivities are unknown.

Steroids have been used in supplementary therapy for some forms of tuberculosis (Table 16). Although these drugs are known to suppress the tuberculin skin test and to cause exacerbation and dissemination of untreated tuberculosis, they are tolerated well as long as antituberculous drugs are used simultaneously. The usual regimen is prednisone (1 to 2 mg/kg) or an equivalent dosage of hydrocortisone parenterally. They

TABLE 16. Indications for Steroid Therapy

Type	Indication
Endobronchial tuberculosis	Obstruction from endobronchial lesion or nodes compressing a bronchus
Pleural effusion	Significant effusion
Miliary tuberculosis	Toxicity and respiratory distress
Tuberculous meningitis	Neurologic signs, actual or impending block of cerebrospinal fluid
Pericarditis	Acute inflammation and effusion

are used for periods of 4 to 8 weeks, until signs of improvement have occurred, and then gradually tapered.

References

GENERAL

Gerbeaux J: Primary Tuberculosis in Childhood. Springfield, Ill, Charles C Thomas, 1970

Lincoln EM, Sewell EM: Tuberculosis in Children. New York, McGraw-Hill, 1963

Miller FJW, Seal RME, Taylor MD: Tuberculosis in Children. Boston, Little, Brown, 1963

EPIDEMIOLOGY

Gunnels JJ, Bates JH, Swindoll H: Infectiousness of culture positive tuberculosis patients on chemotherapy. Am Rev Respir Dis 105:989, 1972

Horwitz O, Palmer CE: Epidemiological basis of tuberculosis eradication. Dynamics of tuberculosis morbidity and mortality. Bull WHO 30:609, 1964

Houk VM, Baker JH, Sorensen K, Kent DC: The epidemiology of tuberculosis infection in a closed environment. Arch Environ Health 16:26, 1968

Lincoln EM: Epidemics of tuberculosis. Adv Tuberc Res 14:157, 1965

Louden RG, Spohn SK: Cough frequency and infectivity in patients with pulmonary tuberculosis. Am Rev Respir Dis 99:109, 1969

O'Grady F, Riley RL: Experimental airborne tuberculosis. Adv Tuberc Res 12:150, 1963

Riley RL: The J Burns Amberson lecture. Aerial dissemination of pulmonary tuberculosis. Am Rev Tuberc 76:931, 1957

———— Mills CC, O'Grady F, Sultan LO, Wittstadt F, Sivpuri DN: Infectiousness of air from a tuberculosis ward. Am Rev Respir Dis 85:511, 1962

IMMUNITY

Kallmann FJ, Reisner D: Twin studies on genetic variations in resistance to tuberculosis. J Hered 34:269, 1943

Lurie MB: Resistance to Tuberculosis. Experimental Studies in Native and Acquired Defensive Mechanisms. Cambridge, Harvard Univ Press, 1965

Mackaness GB: The Adaptive Transfer of Acquired Cellular Resistance, Rational Therapy and Control of Tuberculosis. Gainesville, Univ Florida Press, 1970

———— The immunological basis of acquired cellular resistance. J Exp Med 120:105, 1964

Myers JA, Bearman JE, Dixon HG: Natural history of tuberculosis in the human body. VIII. Prognosis among tuberculin reactor girls and boys of thirteen to seventeen years. Am Rev Respir Dis 91:896, 1965

PATHOGENESIS

Gerbeaux J: Primary Tuberculosis in Childhood. Springfield, Ill, Charles C Thomas, 1970

Lincoln EM, Sewell EM: Tuberculosis in Children. New York, McGraw-Hill, 1963

Miller FJW, Seal RME, Taylor MD: Tuberculosis in Children. Boston, Little, Brown, 1963

Rich AR: The Pathogenesis of Tuberculosis, 2nd ed. Springfield, Ill, Charles C Thomas, 1951

Wallgran A: The time-table of tuberculosis. Tubercle 28:245, 1948

PULMONARY TUBERCULOSIS

Bentley FJ, Grzybowski S, Benjamin B: Tuberculosis in Childhood and Adolescence with Special Reference to the Pulmonary Forms of the Disease. London, National Association for Prevention of Tuberculosis, 1954

Lincoln EM: Course and prognosis of tuberculosis in children. Am J Med 9:623, 1950

———— Gilbert L, Morales SM: Chronic pulmonary tuberculosis in individuals with known previous primary tuberculosis. Dis Chest 38:473, 1960

PLEURAL EFFUSION

American Thoracic Society: Therapy of pleural effusion. A statement by the Committee on Therapy. Am Rev Respir Dis 97:479, 1968

Arrington CW, Hawkins JA, Reichert J, Hopeman AR: Management of undiagnosed pleural effusions in positive tuberculin reactors. Am Rev Respir Dis 93:587, 1966

Feller J, Porter M: Physiologic studies of the sequelae of tuberculous pleural effusion in children treated with anti-microbial drugs and prednisone. Am Rev Respir Dis 88:181, 1963

Lincoln EM, Davies PA, Bovornkitti S: Tuberculous pleurisy with effusion in children: a study of 202 children with particular reference to prognosis. Am Rev Tuberc 77:271, 1958

Roper WH, Waring JJ: Primary serofibrinous pleural effusion in military personnel. Am Rev Tuberc 71:616, 1955

Scharer L, McClement JH: Isolation of tubercle bacilli from needle biopsy specimens of parenteral pleura. Am Rev Respir Dis 97:466, 1968

ENDOBRONCHIAL TUBERCULOSIS

Giammona ST, Poole CA, Zelkowitz P, Skrovan C: Massive lymphadenopathy in primary pulmonary tuberculosis in children. Am Rev Respir Dis 100:480, 1969

Lincoln EM, Harris LC, Bovornkitti S, Carretero RW: Endobronchial tuberculosis in children: a study of 156 patients. Am Rev Tuberc 77:39, 1958

Morrison JB: Natural history of segmental lesions in primary pulmonary tuberculosis. Arch Dis Child 48:90, 1973

Nemir RL, Cardona J, Vaziri F, Toledo R: Prednisone as an adjunct in the chemotherapy of lymph node–bronchial tuberculosis in childhood. Am Rev Respir Dis 95:402, 1967

Weber AL, Bird KT, Janower ML: Primary tuberculosis in childhood with particular emphasis on changes affecting the tracheobronchial tree. Am J Roentgenol Radium Ther Nucl Med 103:123, 1968

MILIARY TUBERCULOSIS

Heinle EW Jr, Jensen WN, Westerman MP: Diagnostic usefulness of marrow biopsy in disseminated tuberculosis. Am Rev Respir Dis 91:701, 1965

Lincoln EM, Hould F: Results of specific treatment of miliary tuberculosis in children; a follow-up study of 63 patients treated with antimicrobial agents. N Engl J Med 261:113, 1959

Minit P: Miliary tuberculosis in chemotherapy era. Medicine 51:139, 1972

TUBERCULOUS MENINGITIS

Lincoln EM: Tuberculous meningitis in children with special reference to serous meningitis. I. Tuberculous meningitis. Am Rev Tuberc 56:75, 1947

———— Tuberculous meningitis in children with special reference to serous meningitis. II. Serous tuberculous meningitis. Am Rev Tuberc 56:95, 1947

———— Sordillo SVR, Davies PA: Tuberculous meningitis in children: a review of 167 untreated and 74 treated patients with special reference to early diagnosis. J Pediatr 57:807, 1960

Lorber J: The results of treatment of 549 cases of tuberculous meningitis. Am Rev Tuberc 69:13, 1954

O'Toole RD, Thornton GF, Mukherjee MK, Math RL: Dexamethasone in tuberculous meningitis. Ann Intern Med 70:39, 1969

Sumaya CV, Simek M, Smith MHD, et al: Tuberculous meningitis in children during the isoniazid era. J Pediatr 87:43, 1975

Todd RM, Neville JG: The sequelae of tuberculous meningitis. Arch Dis Child 39:213, 1964

Udami PM, Rarekh UC, Dastur DK: Neurological and related syndromes in CNS tuberculosis: clinical features and pathogenesis. J Neurol Sci 14:341, 1971

Wasz-Hockert O, Donner M, Miettinen P, et al: Late prognosis in tuberculous meningitis. Acta Paediatr [Suppl] 51:141, 1962

Zarabi M, Sane S, Gerdanig BR: The chest roentgenogram in the early diagnosis of tuberculous meningitis in children. Am J Dis Child 121:389, 1971

SKELETAL TUBERCULOSIS

American Thoracic Society, Committee on Therapy, Subcommittee on Surgery: Present status of skeletal tuberculosis. Am Rev Respir Dis 88:272, 1963

Bosworth DM: Modern concepts of treatment of tuberculosis of bones and joints. Ann NY Acad Sci 106:98, 1963

Davidson PT, Horowitz I: Skeletal tuberculosis. Am J Med 48:77, 1970

Hunt DD: Problems in diagnosis of osteoarticular tuberculosis. JAMA 190:95, 1964

Jones WC, Miller WE: Skeletal tuberculosis. South Med J 57:964, 1963

Milgram L: Skeletal tuberculosis in children treated for primary and miliary tuberculosis. Am Rev Tuberc 75:897, 1957

Walker GF: Failure of early recognition of skeletal tuberculosis. Br Med J 1:682, 1968

TUBERCULOSIS OF SUPERFICIAL LYMPH NODES

Black BG, Chapman JS: Cervical adenitis in children due to human and unclassified mycobacteria. Pediatrics 33: 887, 1964

Davis SD, Cornstock GW: Mycobaterical cervical adenitis in children. J Pediatr 58:771, 1961

Miller FJW, Seal RME, Taylor MD: Tuberculosis in Children. Boston, Little, Brown, 1963

URINARY TRACT TUBERCULOSIS

American Thoracic Society, Committee on Therapy: The present status of genitourinary tuberculosis. Am Rev Respir Dis 92:505, 1965

Ehrlich RM Lattimer JK: Urogenital tuberculosis in children. J Urol 105:461, 1971

Lattimer JK, Boyes T: Renal tuberculosis in children. Pediatrics 22:1193, 1958

CONGENITAL TUBERCULOSIS

Avery ME, Wolfsdorf J: Diagnosis and treatment: infants of tuberculous mothers. Pediatrics 42:519, 1968

Kendig EL Jr: The place of BCG vaccine in the management of infants born of tuberculous mothers. N Eng J Med 21:520, 1969

——— Prognosis of infants born of tuberculous mothers. Pediatrics 26:-97, 1960

Light IJ, Saidlemon M, Sutherland JM: Management of newborns after nursery exposure to tuberculosis. Am Rev Respir Dis 109:415, 1974

Pridie RB, Stradling P: Management of pulmonary tuberculosis during pregnancy. Br Med J 2:78, 1961

DIAGNOSTIC METHODS

Brody J, Overfield J, Hammes LM: Depression of the tuberculin reaction by viral vaccines. N Engl J Med 271:1294, 1964

Diagnostic Standards and Classification of Tuberculosis. New York, National Tuberculosis Association, 1974

Edwards PQ, Edwards LB: Story of the tuberculin test from an epidemiologic viewpoint. Am Rev Respir Dis [Suppl] 81:1-47, 1960

Landi S, Held HR, Tseng MC: Disparity of potency between stabilized and nonstabilized dilute tuberculin solutions. Am Rev Respir Dis 104:385, 1971

Palmer CE, Edwards LB: Tuberculin test in restrospect and prospect. Arch Environ Health 15:792, 1967

——— Edwards LB, Hopwood L, Edwards PQ: Experimental and epidemiologic basis for the interpretation of tuberculin sensitivity. J Pediatr 55:413, 1959

Rosenthal SR: The disk-tine tuberculin test (dried tuberculin disposable unit). JAMA 177:452, 1961

Seibert FB, Dufour EH: Comparison between the international standard tuberculins, PPD-S and old tuberculin. Am Rev Tuberc 69:585, 1954

Starr S, Berkovich S: Effects of measles, gamma-globulin modified measles and vaccine measles on the tuberculin test. N Engl J Med 270:386, 1964

PREVENTION

American Thoracic Society, Committee on Therapy, National Tuberculosis and Respiratory Disease Association, Center for Disease Control: Joint statement on the preventive treatment of tuberculosis. Am Rev Respir Dis 110:371, 1974

Comstock GW: Isoniazid prophylaxis in an undeveloped area. Am Rev Respir Dis 86:810, 1962

Ferebee SH: Controlled chemoprophylaxis trials in tuberculosis. A general review. Adv Tuberc Res 17:28, 1970

——— Mount FW: Tuberculosis morbidity in a controlled trial of the prophylatic use of isoniazid among household contacts. Am Rev Respir Dis 85:490, 1962

Fine MH, Furcolow ML, Chick EW, Baumer DS, Arik M: Tuberculin skin test reactions. Effects of revised classification on comparative evaluations. Rev Respir Dis 106:752, 1972

Lifschitz M: The value of the tuberculin skin test as a screening test for tuberculosis among BCG vaccinated children. Pediatrics 36:624, 1965

Mount FW, Ferebee SH: Preventive effects of isoniazid in the treatment of primary tuberculosis in children. N Engl J Med 265:713, 1961

Recommendation of the Public Health Service Advisory Committee on Immunization Practices: BCG Vaccines. Morbidity and Mortality, Weekly Report 24:69. Atlanta, Center for Disease Control, 1975

Rosenthal SR, Loewinsohn E, Graham ML, et al: BCG vaccination against tuberculosis in Chicago: a twenty year study statistically analyzed. Pediatrics 28:622, 1961

Smith DW: Why not vaccinate against tuberculosis. Ann Intern Med 72:419, 1970

Tuberculosis Vaccines Clinical Trials Committee, Medical Research Council: BCG and vole bacillus vaccine in the prevention of tuberculosis in adolescents, second report. Br Med J 2:379, 1959

TREATMENT

American Thoracic Society, Ad Hoc Committee on the Treatment of Tuberculosis in Children: The treatment of tuberculosis in children. Am Rev Respir Dis 99:304, 1969

American Thoracic Society, Committee on Therapy: Treatment of drug resistant tuberculosis. Am Rev Respir Dis 94:125, 1966

American Thoracic Society: Preventive treatment in tuberculosis. A statement by the Committee on Therapy. Am Rev Respir Dis 91:297, 1965

Dieu JC, Adenis-Lamarre F, Bitar M, et al: Rifampin in the treatment of lymph node and pulmonary involvement of primary tuberculosis in infants and children. Rev Tuberc Pneumol (Paris) 34:320, 1970

Doster B, Murray FJ, Newman R: Ethambutol in the initial treatment of pulmonary tuberculosis. Am Rev Respir Dis 107:177, 1973

Kendig EL Jr, Brummen DL: Tuberculosis. In Kagan BM (ed): Antimicrobial Therapy. Philadelphia, WB Saunders, 1974

Lincoln EM, Vera-Cruz PG: Progress in treatment of tuberculosis: results of antimicrobial therapy in a group of 420 children with tuberculosis. Pediatr 25:1035, 1960

Maddrey WC, Boitnott JK: Isoniazid hepatitis. Ann Intern Med 79:1, 1973

Mitti V, Catena E, Delli Veneri F, DeMichell G, Mana A: Rifampin in association with isoniazid, streptomycin and ethambutol, respectively in the initial treatment of pulmonary tuberculosis. Am Rev Respir Dis 103:329, 1971

Newman R, Doster B, Murray FJ, Ferebee S: Rifampin in initial treatment of pulmonary tuberculosis. Am Rev Respir Dis 103:461, 1971

Raleigh JW: Rifampin in treatment of advanced pulmonary tuberculosis. Report of a V.A. cooperative pilot study. Am Rev Respir Dis 105:397, 1972

Steiner M, Cosio A: Primary tuberculosis in children. Incidence of primary drug-resistant disease in 332 children observed between the years 1961 and 1964 at the Kings County Medical Center of Brooklyn. N Eng J Med 274:755, 1966

Wolinsky E: New anti-tuberculosis drugs and concepts of prophylaxis. Med Clin North Am 58:697, 1974

MISCELLANEOUS

Cawson RA: Tuberculosis of the mouth and throat with special reference to the incidence and management since the introduction of chemotherapy. Br J Dis Chest 54:40, 1960

Hageman JH, D'Esopo MD, Glenn WWL: Tuberculosis of the pericardium. N Engl J Med 270:327, 1964

Massaro D, Katz S, Sachs M: Choroidal tubercles. Ann Intern Med 60:231, 1964

Okel BB, McLean RL: Tuberculous peritonitis in the chemotherapy era. South Med J 55:156, 1962

Philip RN, Comstock GW, Shelton JH: Phlyctenular keratoconjunctivitis among Eskimos in southwestern Alaska. I. Epidemiologic characteristics. Am Rev Respir Dis 91:171, 1965

Ustvedt HJ: The position of suprarenal tuberculosis in the time-table of tuberculosis. Acta Tuberc Scand [Suppl] 21:102, 1949

DISEASES CAUSED BY OTHER MYCOBACTERIA

EMANUEL WOLINSKY

From 1 to 5 percent of cases of granulomatous disease that are apparently tuberculous in origin are caused by mycobacteria other than mammalian tubercle bacilli. In adults the most common manifestation of these infections is chronic pulmonary disease, but in children they usually involve the cervical lymph nodes and the skin. Isolated instances of disseminated or pulmonary disease in children have been reported, but they are very rare.

BACTERIOLOGY. *Mycobacterium tuberculosis* and *M. bovis* are known as the mammalian tubercle bacilli. The other mycobacteria associated with disease in man are the following: *M. leprae* is the agent of leprosy. *M. avium* (the avian tubercle bacillus) rarely causes disease in man in the United States, but there have been many case reports from England, the Scandinavian countries, and other parts of Europe. The cervical lymph nodes have been the sites of involvement in most of such cases involving children. *M. kansasii* are slow-growing organisms that demonstrate a yellow pigment only after exposure to light. This species causes much of the adult human mycobacterial disease throughout the world that is not due to mammalian tubercle bacilli. *M. marinum*

causes a tuberculosislike disease in fish and superficial skin infection in man. The organisms grow best at 30 C to 33 C and are pigmented yellow only after light exposure. *M. ulcerans* is the cause of severe ulceration of the skin and subcutaneous tissues, mainly in Australia, Africa, and Malaysia. The bacilli grow very slowly, and only at 32 C to 33 C. *M. intracellularis* (also known as Battey bacilli) are slow-growing, essentially nonpigmented bacilli resembling *M. avium.* Some prefer to call them *M. avium-intracellularis* or simply the *M. avium* complex. These organisms are the major cause of nontuberculous mycobacterial disease in the southeastern United States, Australia, Japan, and other parts of the world and are commonly found in the soil. *M. scrofulaceum* produce smooth yellow orange colonies and should be differentiated from two other scotochromogenic species not ordinarily associated with disease in man: *M. gordonae* and *M. flavescens. M. scrofulaceum* is rarely associated with adult pulmonary disease, but it is the most common agent of mycobacterial lymphadenitis in children. Soil and water harbor large numbers of scotochromogenic mycobacteria, especially *M. gordonae. M. fortuitum-chelonei* grow rapidly and on ordinary culture medium; they are found in abundance in soil and dust and rarely cause disease in immunocompetent individuals. They may be the cause of injection site abscesses and lymphadenitis in children. Three other species have been described recently: *M. xenopi, M. szulgai,* and *M. simiae.* Their roles as agents of disease in children remain to be elucidated.

CLINICAL CONSIDERATIONS. *Lymphadenitis* is the most common childhood disease associated with these mycobacteria. In most areas of the United States at the present time, granulomatous adenitis in children is more likely to be due to infection with other mycobacteria than to infection with *M. tuberculosis* or *M. bovis.* The involved nodes are usually submandibular and unilateral, although they may be seen in other locations such as the femoral, inguinal, epitrochlear, and mediastinal regions. Systemic indications of infection are usually lacking. The nodes tend to soften and break down more rapidly than tuberculous nodes, and once drainage starts it usually continues for many weeks or months despite chemotherapy. The reason for the lack of response is the natural resistance of most of these strains to the available antituberculosis drugs, including rifampin. An exception is *M. kansasii,* which is usually sensitive to rifampin and only moderately resistant to isoniazid.

Nontuberculous mycobacterial adenitis has been described in children ranging in age from 10 months to 13 years, but it is most often seen in the preschool period. There is usually no history of tuberculosis in the family and no evidence of disease elsewhere in the body. The chest radiograph is, as a rule, negative. The PPD tuberculin skin test is likely to be weakly positive because of cross-sensitivity, but the reaction to tuberculin derived from the homologous organism is usually greater than the reaction to standard tuberculin. When the reaction to 5 TU of PPD is negative or doubtful, a skin test with 250 TU will usually clarify the situation. It will almost always be strongly positive. The histologic appearance of the diseased tissue may be the same as that seen in ordinary tuberculosis, or it may reveal a dimorphic reaction similar to that seen in cat-scratch disease. The etiologic agent is most often *M. scrofulaceum.* Strains of *M. kansasii, M. avium* complex, *M. fortuitum,* and other species may also cause the disease, especially in geographic locations where a certain species is known to be prevalent in the environment, eg, *M. avium* complex in Georgia.

The treatment of choice is complete excision. Should the node be too large or fluctuant when first seen, incision and drainage may be advisable until the lesion is small enough to be excised. Sometimes the node will recede spontaneously, and continued observation without surgery may be considered when the diagnosis is not in question. Needle aspiration for diagnostic purposes may be useful in selected cases. Drug therapy is of questionable benefit, since most of the strains are quite resistant to available drugs. However, *M. kansasii* infection may respond to the combination of rifampin, isoniazid, and ethambutol. Complete healing usually occurs, and late relapse has not been seen in our series.

According to our present knowledge the infection is not communicable, and these children do not need to be isolated or labeled as tuberculous. They should not be subjected to unnecessary prolonged courses of drugs and to the ostracism that may accompany the diagnosis of tuberculosis. Since the skin reaction to tuberculin may persist for many years, even after excision of the involved nodes, this disease probably accounts for some of the false-positive skin reactions to PPD in patients who do not have tuberculosis. One should avoid the inclusion of these children in prophylactic chemotherapy programs as recent tuberculin converters or preschoolers with positive reactions.

The definitive procedure for establishing the diagnosis is recovery and identification of mycobacteria from cultures of material obtained by aspiration or at surgery. Strong suspicion of the correct diagnosis should be raised by the unilateral submandibular location, lack of disease elsewhere, negative chest radiography, lack of exposure to tuberculosis, lack of response to penicillin or to antituberculosis drugs, and weak skin test reaction to 5 TU of PPD.

Swimming pool granuloma is a benign self-limited skin disease consisting of ulcerating papules, usually at the sites of minor abrasions received while swimming in contaminated pools. The causative organism, *M. marinum,* may be cultured from skin and from the water in the pool. The lesions appear 2 to 3 weeks after infection and usually heal slowly after several months, leaving a scar. A large outbreak of the disease involving about 300 individuals, many of them children, occurred in Colorado in 1959. Sporotrichosislike suppuration of the skin may also be seen in *M. marinum* infections.This type is usually acquired as a result of a minor injury to a hand in contact with a home aquarium. Either type of infection may result in a long-lasting skin hypersensitivity to tuberculin. *M. marinum* is relatively resistant to isoniazid and *p*-aminosalicylic acid, but it is sensitive to ethambutol and rifampin. These last two drugs, in combination, may be used if treatment is deemed necessary.

A few cases of fatal *disseminated mycobacterial disease* in children have been reported; these infections were caused by *M. kansasii, M. scrofulaceum,* or one of the members of the *M. avium* complex. In addition, there have been a few reports of pulmonary disease in children in which *M. kansasii* or *M. scrofulaceum* seemed to be playing a role. For disseminated disease or severe disease other than accessible lymphadenitis, drug treatment may be attempted based on the identity of the infecting organism and its in vitro drug sensitivity pattern. *M. kansasii* infections will usually respond well to a three-drug regimen of isoniazid, rifampin, and ethambutol. For the mycobacteria that are more drug-resistant, a four-drug regimen including the three oral drugs already mentioned plus daily intramuscular administration of streptomycin or kanamycin must be used.

References

Adams RM, Remington JS, Steinberg J, Seibert JS: Tropical fish aquariums; a source of Mycobacterium marinum infections resembling sporotrichosis. JAMA 211:457, 1970

Bialkin G, Pollak A, Weil AJ: Pulmonary infection with Mycobacterium kansasii. Am J Dis Child 101:739, 1961

Black BG, Chapman JS: Cervical adenitis in children due to human and unclassified mycobacteria. Pediatr 33:887, 1964

Davis SD, Comstock GW: Mycobacterial cervical adenitis in children. J Pediatr 58:771, 1961

Kendig EL Jr: Unclassified mycobacteria in children. Am J Dis Child 101:749, 1961

Krieger I, Hahne OH, Whitten CF: Atypical mycobacteria as a probable cause of chronic bone disease. J Pediatr 65:340, 1964

Kubin M, Kruml J, Horak Z, Lukavsky J, Vanek C: Pulmonary and nonpulmonary disease in humans due to avian mycobacteria. I. Clinical and epidemiologic analysis of nine cases observed in Czechoslovakia. Am Rev Respir Dis 94:20, 1966

Mollohan CS, Romer MS: Public health significance of swimming pool granuloma. Am J Public Health 51:883, 1961

Reid JD, Wolinsky E: Histopathology of lymphadenitis caused by atypical mycobacteria. Am Rev Respir Dis 99:8, 1969

Runyon EH: Adv in Tuberc Res, 14:235, 1965

Smith DH, Doherty RA, DeLemos RA: Unclassified mycobacterial infection and disease in children residing in Massachusetts. J Pediatr 67:759, 1965

Wolinsky E: Nontuberculous mycobacterial infections of man. Med Clin North Am 58:639, 1974

Gomez F, Zimpfer F: Sporotrichoid Mycobacterium marinum infection treated with rifampin-ethambutol. Am Rev Respir Dis 105:964, 1972

Yakovac WC, Baker R, Sweigert C, Hope JW: Fatal disseminated osteomyelitis due to an anonymous Mycobacterium. J Pediatr 59:909, 1961

TULAREMIA

Crystie C. Halsted

EPIDEMIOLOGY. Tularemia (rabbit fever, deer fly fever), an uncommon infectious disease of children, is a zoonosis that primarily affects lagomorphs (hares and rabbits) and rodents (muskrats, beavers, squirrels, voles). Variable susceptibility and sensitivity to tularemia occur among vertebrates. Hares and rabbits are very susceptible and sensitive to the effects of the infection, while dogs, cats, and horses have lowered susceptibility and sensitivity. Thus animals capable of transmitting infection to man may not be clinically ill. A number of arthropod vectors are important in the transmission of tularemia from animal to animal and also from animal to man. Common vectors in the United States are ticks (*Dermacentor andersoni,* the wood tick, *Dermacentor variabilis,* the dog tick, *Amblyomma americanum,* the Lone Star tick) and the deer fly (*Chrysops discalis*). Less common vectors are fleas, mosquitoes, and lice. Transovarian transmission of tularemia in ticks, which was previously believed to represent an efficient means of preserving the organism in nature, has not been confirmed by more recent investigations. Man, who is an accidental host, acquires infection by direct exposure to tissues and secretions of infected animals or from the bites of vectors. Animal contact sources besides the rabbit include deer, coyotes, foxes, muskrats, woodchucks, opposums, sheep, squirrels, skunks, and rats. Infection may also be acquired by way of contaminated water or aerosols or ingestion of inadequately cooked infected meat. Water may become contaminated by the excreta and carcasses of diseased animals, including birds, and tularemia organisms can survive in water and mud. Under cold and subfreezing conditions, survival of organisms on straw and in rabbit carcasses has been noted for as long as 2 years. Aerosol infection is especially important as the source of laboratory-acquired disease. Infection occasionally arises as a result of contact with an animal that has recently preyed upon or pawed another animal harboring tularemia. Transmission of tularemia from man to man has not been reported.

Tularemia exists throughout North America and parts of Europe and Asia. It has been a reportable disease in the United States since 1927. A steady decline in incidence has been noted since 1939. In 1973 the reported incidence in the United States was 0.75 cases per 1 million persons, which is less than 200 cases per year. The true incidence of tularemia is difficult to establish because of failure of diagnosis in mild or asymptomatic infection and the variable symptomatology associated with the disease.

Most cases occur in adult males, thus reflecting the increased exposure of this group. Children of both sexes and women appear to be equally susceptible when adequately exposed. While conditions favoring exposure are found most often in rural areas, infection may also occur sporadically in suburban and urban settings. The seasonal incidence of tularemia varies and is dependent on the route of transmission, Mountain and Pacific regions report an increase in cases during summer and fall related to vector-borne infection. East North Central, east South Central, and South Atlantic states report an increase in cases in winter, which appears to be related to contact with wild rabbits.

BACTERIOLOGY. *Francisella tularensis,* the organism causing tularemia, is a small gram-negative nonmotile pleomorphic coccobacillus. The name derived in part from the site of its original isolation in Tulare County, California, where McCoy, in 1911, retrieved it from ground squirrels suffering a plaguelike disease. Appropriate bacteriologic classification of this organism has been the subject of controversy. Recently it has been reclassified from the genus *Pasteurella* to the genus *Francisella.* The latter term was adopted in honor of Dr. Edward Francis, who in the 1920s described the human infection, labeled the disease tularemia, noted the similarities between the rodent-borne disease in California and the deer-fly-borne disease in Utah, and in other ways added to our information about tularemia.

Francisella tularensis requires special enriched medium (blood-cystine-dextrose agar) for its isolation. It is highly infectious for laboratory personnel, and significant morbidity and death have occurred from isolation attempts. Currently in the United States two different strains of *F. tularensis* are recognized; they differ in virulence, biochemical reactions, and epidemiologic patterns, although they are serologically homogenous. Jellison type A strains are highly virulent for man and rabbit; they ferment glycerol and possess citrulline ureidase activity. Such strains are associated with the classic tick-borne tularemia of the rabbit. Jellison type B strains are associated with milder disease in man; they are avirulent for the rabbit, they fail to ferment glycerol, and they lack citrulline ureidase activity. These strains are associated with water-borne infections of rodents. Type B strains appear to be similar to palearctic strains responsible for tularemia in Europe, where the disease is less severe than the usual rabbit-associated tularemia that occurs in the United States.

CLINICAL CONSIDERATIONS. The clinical manifestations of tularemia in man vary with the strain of the infecting organism and the route of infection. A given strain may also be associated with a spectrum of illness varying from asymptomatic infection to severe disease. Several clinical forms of tularemia are recognized, and they are categorized as ulceroglandular, pneumonic, oropharyngeal or pharyngotonsillar, glandular, and oculoglandular. *Ulceroglandular disease* is the most common form, and it occurs when organisms gain entry through the skin. An ability of the organism to penetrate apparently intact skin has been reported, but entry by way of unnoticed tiny cracks or fissures or through openings of dermal appendages such as hair follicles may also explain entry through the skin. Local replication of organisms at the entry site results in the formation of an erythematous macule that becomes indurated and finally undergoes central necrosis over a period of 48 to 96 hours. Regional lymph nodes enlarge, and some may become fluctuant and drain spontaneously in the course of illness. Fever, which is persistent and may reach 104 F to 106 F, begins coincidentally with the development of the local lesion. In the absence of specific treatment, the fever, adenopathy, ulcer, and associated systemic symptoms persist for as long as 2 to 4 weeks. Persistent bacteremia is associated with more severe infections, and seeding of other organs and lymph nodes may occur. The *pneumonic form* of tularemia results from bacteremic spread to lungs, which may derive from all varieties of infection and from alveolar localization of infected aerosols. High bacterial counts in tissues and blood of infected animals provide an opportunity for generation of infected aerosols during the skinning and evisceration of animals. The presenting complaints in the pneumonic form of disease, whether it be primary and a result of aerosol spread or secondary and related to bacteremic spread, are often nonspecific; they include fever, chills, headache, myalgia, nausea, and vomiting. Indications of pulmonary involvement may be minimal, although cough, pleuritic chest pain, and dyspnea are occasionally reported. There is no uniform radiographic picture, and the following patterns are reported in association with tularemia: miliary, hilar adenopathy, bronchopneumonia, pneumonitis, lobar consolidation, abscess formation, and pleural effusion. The oval density pattern originally described as characteristic of tularemic pneumonia is present in only a few patients with pulmonary involvement. *Oropharyngeal tularemia* results from ingestion of contaminated material and presents as an acute tonsillitis associated with cervical adenitis. The pharynx and tonsils may become covered with a gray white necrotic membrane, and ulceration in the oropharynx may also be present. The *glandular form* of tularemia arises from bacteremic spread of *F. tularensis,* with prominent involvement of lymph nodes. In this type the portal of entry is unknown or is so insignificantly involved that it is unrecognized. *Oculoglandular disease* occurs from conjunctival inoculation of organisms by aerosol, splashing of contaminated fluids, or direct contact with contaminated fingers or hands. Pain, itching, and photophobia are seen, accompanied by congestion, lacrimation, and mucopurulent discharge. Regional lymph nodes, especially the preauricular nodes, enlarge and may suppurate. Serious ocular complications may ensue occasionally in untreated patients. *Typhoidal tularemia,* in which fever, malaise, myalgia, and headache predominate, was once believed to be a consequence of enteric infection. Studies in volunteers have recently shown that man is relatively unsusceptible to tularemia on peroral exposure, and they raise questions about this route of infection in typhoidal disease. Another explanation offered for this form of disease is that infected aerosols are created during mastication of contaminated meat and are localized to the respiratory tract, from which organisms may reach the bloodstream via hilar lymphatics. In all forms of tularemia, and especially in patients who are more severely affected, fever, malaise, myalgia, and headache may persist for a month. Prolonged convalescence associated with weakness that lasts for several weeks, episodically recurring fever, and persistent adenopathy has been described.

PATHOLOGY. Pathologically, the lesion in all forms of tularemia consists of focal accumulation of inflammatory cells: polymorphs, mononuclear cells, and histiocytes. These foci may go on to develop liquefaction necrosis. In the subacute and healing stages mononuclear cells and fibroblasts predominate. Infection of experimental animals shows the same pathologic lesion as that seen in man. Studies on the pathogenesis of tularemia indicate that the presence of specific delayed hypersensitivity, rather than serum antibody, is important in the elimination of *F. tularensis* by the host. In this respect *F.tularensis* resembles other intracellular facultative organisms such as *Listeria monocytogenes.*

DIAGNOSIS. The diagnosis of tularemia is not difficult when there is a history of contact with an appropriate animal or vector and the patient has ulceroglandular disease. Unfortunately, such history is often not volunteered by the patient and is not solicited by the physician until after the diagnosis is established, often inadvertently by some other means. Lack of familiarity with the clinical presentations of tularemia results in failure to include this disease in the differential diagnosis of unexplained fever and pneumonia. Because of its many clinical forms, tularemia can be confused with many other illnesses, including cat-scratch fever, sporotrichosis, infectious mononucleosis, streptococcal pharyngitis, toxoplasmosis, diphtheria, typhoid, brucellosis, rat-bite fever, plague, Q fever, psittacosis, *Mycoplasma* infection, lymphoma, and Hodgkins disease. *F. tularensis* can be cultured from blood, sputum, exudates, and gastric washings in the early phase of illness if proper medium is inoculated, thus establishing the diagnosis. Isolation of the organism may also be accomplished by intraperitoneal injection of appropriate specimens into guinea pigs and mice. These animals die 7 to 10 days after inoculation, and the organism may then be subcultured from the blood or spleen. Because of the hazards of infection to laboratory workers, all attempts to isolate *F. tularensis* should involve experienced personnel who follow precisely the recommendations for handling this organism. The diagnosis of most tularemia infections is made by serologic means rather than by isolating the organism. A reliable *serum agglutination reaction* is available. Significant titers (1:80 to 1:160) appear during the second week of illness and reach levels as high as 1:10,240 in the fourth through sixth weeks of illness. The titer may remain elevated for a month after infection, but it subsequently falls, so that years after infection no detectable titer remains. A fourfold rise in agglutination titer is indicative of recent infection. Unfortunately such agglutination reactions are not positive in the initial 7 to 10 days of illness. An additional difficulty with the agglutination test for tularemia is that sera from patients with brucellosis may show cross-reactions. Tularemia may be distinguished serologically from brucellosis by the fact that the agglutination titer is higher with the homologous antigen. Serologic cross-reactions do not occur between *Yersinia pestis* and *F. tularensis,* although the clinical manifestations of the diseases caused by these organisms may be similar.

A *skin test* exists that is sensitive and specific for tularemia and has the advantage of being positive earlier in the course of the illness than agglutination reactions. It detects delayed hypersensitivity to *F. tularensis.* It also remains positive after agglutinins have disappeared. Unlike the *Brucella* skin test, it does not induce agglutinins in skin-tested individuals. It has been extensively tested by the U.S. Public Health Service, but unfortunately it is not commercially available. There are no other laboratory findings that are helpful in establishing the diagnosis. The white blood cell count is often normal, although leukocytosis has occasionally been reported. C-reactive protein and erythrocyte sedimentation rate are elevated during the acute illness.

PROGNOSIS.   Infection with *F.tularensis* that is left untreated is associated with an estimated 5 percent mortality in ulceroglandular disease. The mortality increases to 30 percent when pneumonia is present with any form of disease. These mortality figures probably represent estimates for the more virulent type A disease. Mortality figures for the less virulent type B disease are probably less. One bout of infection usually confers lifelong immunity.

THERAPY.   Treatment with an appropriate antibiotic results in prompt defervescence of symptoms, with a much shortened course of illness. Streptomycin is presently the drug of choice; it is given at a dosage 30 to 40 mg/kg/day in two divided doses for 3 days, followed by 20 mg/kg/day for an additional 3 days. Tetracycline and chloramphenicol have been shown to be beneficial in treatment of tularemia infection, but such treatment may be associated with failure to eradicate the organism and relapse of the disease when the drug is stopped. Other aminoglycosides (kanamycin and gentamicin) have been reported to be effective in isolated cases.

PREVENTION.   Prevention of tularemia is accomplished by avoiding contact with rabbits and rodents, in whom the frequency of tularemia infection is significant. The interstate transport of wild rabbit meat should be prohibited. Carcasses of wild animals should not be handled directly. Protective clothing and other precautions against bites of ticks and deer flies can decrease vector-borne disease. While tularemia may occur in several members of a family, these cases arise as a result of simultaneous exposure and not by case-to-case spread of disease. Since man-to-man transmission has not been documented, there appears to be no need to isolate hospitalized patients. An effective immunogenic attenuated live vaccine is available for use by persons having unavoidable exposure to tularemia. The killed vaccine has been shown to afford inadequate protection. Further study of the ecology of tularemia may result in recommendations for better control of this zoonosis.

References

Bloom ME, Shearer WT, Barton LL, Mallinckrodt E: Oculo-glandular tularemia in an inner city child. Pediatr 51:564, 1973

Boyce JM: Recent trends in the epidemiology of tularemia in the United States. J Infect Dis 31:197, 1975

Buchannan TM, Brooks GF, Brachman, PS: The tularemia skin test. Ann Intern Med 74:336, 1971

Claflin JL, Larson, CL: Infection—immunity in tularemia: specificity of cellular immunity. Infect Immun 5:311, 1972

Hopla CL: The ecology of tularemia. Adv Vet Sci Comp Med 18:25, 1974

Hornick RB: Tularemia. In: Infectious Diseases. Hoeprich PD (ed), Hagerstown, Md, Harper & Row, 1972

———— Tularemia epidemic: 1968. Correspondence. N Engl J Med 280:1310, 1969

Levy HB, Webb CH, Wilkinson JD: Tularemia as a pediatric problem. Pediatr 6:113, 1950

Miller RP, Bates JH: Pleuropulmonary tularemia: Am Rev Respir Dis 99:31, 1969

Overholt EL, Tigertt WD, Kadull PJ, Ward MK, Charkas ND: An analysis of forty-two cases of laboratory acquired tularemia. Am J Med 30:785, 1961

Schricker RL, Eigelsbach HT, Mitten JK Hall WC: Pathogenesis of tularemia in monkeys aerogenically exposed to Francisella tularensis 425. Infect Immun 5:734, 1972

Young LS, Bicknell DS, Archer BG, Clinton JM, Leavens LJ: Tularemia epidemic: Vermont 1968. N Engl J Med 280:1253, 1969

SALMONELLA, SHIGELLA, AND ENTEROPATHOGENIC *E. COLI* INFECTIONS

ERWIN NETER

SALMONELLA INFECTIONS

Bacteria of the genus *Salmonella* produce a variety of clinical symptoms ranging from the inapparent infection of a carrier through mild gastroenteritis, food poisoning, suppurative lesions, and *Salmonella* fever to typhoid fever. The genus *Salmonella* is comprised of more than 1,400 serotypes. The group as a whole is characterized as follows: the organisms are gram-negative motile bacteria that produce acid or acid and gas from glucose and other substances but do not ferment sucrose, lactose, salicin, or raffinose; they do not produce urease, nor do they liquefy gelatin; they decarboxylate lysine, arginine, and ornithine. Aberrant strains are only rarely encountered. The genus is subdivided largely on the basis of the antigenic structures of its members. It is the O antigen, a heat-stable lipopolysaccharide, that characterizes the serogroup (A, B, C, etc), and the members of each group are further subdivided into serotypes on the basis of the heat-labile H or flagellar antigens. Most strains are biphasic and produce flagellar antigens of two kinds. According to the most recent classification, three species are recognized, namely *S. typhi* (or *S. typhosa*), *S. choleraesuis*, and *S. enteritidis*. The last species includes all other serotypes.

Certain strains contain yet another antigen, the Vi antigen. Although named virulence (Vi) antigen, its relationship to the pathogenesis of salmonellosis in man has not been elucidated. Bacteriophages are Vi-specific and can be used in differentiation of types. Infections with *S. typhosa*, *S. paratyphi* A, *S. schottmülleri* (*S. paratyphi* B), and *S. hirschfeldii* (*S. paratyphi* C) are confined almost exclusively to man. A few other host-adapted serotypes, such as *S. pullorum* and *S. gallinarum*, cause disease in animals and only rarely in man. Most other salmonellae are harbored widely among rodents, swine, and other mammals, as well as in birds; they may invade the eggs of ducks and hens and have been responsible for widespread infection in man through contaminated egg powder prepared for human consumption.

The more important serotypes in human disease, exclusive of *S. typhosa*, are *S typhimurium, S. montevideo, S. newport, S. oranienburg, S. schottmülleri, S. bareilly, S. enteritidis, S. choleraesuis,* and *S. derby.* Serotypes such as *S. paratyphi* A are only rarely encountered. The relative frequencies of certain serotypes differ in relation to the type of infection, such as gastroenteritis versus *Salmonella* fever and septicemia. For example, in one large series (MacCready and associates) *S. typhimurium* was responsible for approximately 79 percent of cases of gastroenteritis and only 4 percent of cases of systemic infection; in contrast, the respective figures for *S. choleraesuis* were 26 percent and 56 percent. In addition, among all recognized cases of salmonellosis, the numbers and proportions caused by individual types vary in different localities and from one period to another. Nevertheless, *S. typhimurium* has been the most frequently isolated serotype in the past in most parts of the world. Although the number of serotypes is increasing, it should be kept in mind that only a few account for the majority of human infections. Thus, based on data from the National Communicable Disease Center, 50 serotypes have accounted for approximately 91 percent of some 19,000 isolates from man. Typhoid fever is no longer as great a public health problem in the United States as are the other salmonelloses.

Salmonellosis

Strictly speaking, the term salmonellosis includes typhoid fever as well as infection by all other types of salmonellae. By custom, however, typhoid fever is discussed as a separate entity (p. 488); the term salmonellosis will be used here to refer to infections caused by salmonellae other than *S. typhi.*

EPIDEMIOLOGY. Infection is acquired by ingestion of the bacteria. These may be in food or water supplies that have become contaminated from the droppings of infected animals or by food handlers who are carriers. The disease also may be acquired more directly from a human carrier or from patients with mild or severe gastroenteritis by contact via hands or handled objects. Intensive family studies of children with clinical salmonellosis have brought to light the frequent occurrence of subclinical or mild intestinal infections of mothers and other children in the household, often preceding a more serious clinical infection in infants or younger siblings. Human-to-human (fecal–oral) infection is frequent in sporadic infections of young children. The meat of an infected animal may also contain the organisms, as may the eggs of infected fowl, notably hens and ducks. In 1952 large numbers of cases were traced to egg powder contaminated with *S. montevideo.* An outbreak of *S. derby* infection among patients and employees of 53 hospitals in 13 states occurred in 1963 that probably was due to contaminated raw or undercooked eggs. Secondary infections arising from carriers and patients with mild infections played a significant role. A nursery epidemic has been described that was traced to contamination of the water in the trap of a resuscitating apparatus. More recently, a widespread waterborne *S. typhimurium* outbreak involving 18,000 of 120,000 residents occurred in California. It has been shown that more than half of the patients convalescent from salmonellae infections excrete the organisms in the fourth week, and 10 percent excrete them as late as 12 weeks, while 7 percent were still carriers after a year. Infants are more likely to remain carriers than are older children.

PATHOLOGY. Little is known of the pathologic anatomy of salmonellae infections other than typhoid fever. In the rare fatal cases of enteric fever caused, for example, by *S. schottmülleri* or *S. choleraesuis,* the lesions found in the intestine at postmortem examination resemble those seen in infection with *S. typhi,* except for being generally milder.

SYMPTOMS. Four general classes of clinical infection are encountered: enteric fevers of protracted type resembling typhoid fever; acute gastroenteritis or so-called food poisoning; a localizing infection in which, following a bacteremic phase that is often unrecognized, foci of active disease become manifest in the form of meningitis, osteomyelitis, urinary tract infection, etc; subclinical or inapparent infection.

Salmonella Fevers. The symptoms of the septicemic infections caused by *S. paratyphi,* by *S. schottmülleri,* and occasionally by other nontyphoid salmonellae cannot clearly be differentiated clinically from those of typhoid fever. The patient may have fever for several days without localizing signs or symptoms to suggest the diagnosis. At times *rose spots* appear, the spleen may become palpable, and leukopenia may be present. Constipation is somewhat more common than diarrhea, and anorexia may be severe. The duration of the febrile stage tends to be shorter than in typhoid fever, lasting from 1 to 3 weeks, and the patient may never appear seriously ill. Relapse is exceedingly rare, and complications such as perforation of the gut are almost unknown. Of all the clinical forms of infection produced by nontyphoid salmonellae, enteric fever is the most uncommon.

Gastroenteritic Type. In only a small percentage of infants and children with diarrheal disease from all causes is the illness due to salmonellae. Conversely, of all salmonellae infections, gastroenteritis (including food poisoning) is by far the most common clinical entity. The incubation period may be as short as a few hours or as long as 3 days. The number of stools passed in 24 hours may be anywhere from 4 to 20 or more, and the degrees of associated anorexia, nausea, vomiting, and abdominal pain are variable. In only a small proportion is blood or pus found in the fecal discharges, either grossly or on microscopic examination. Fever, when present, is usually greatest at onset; it seldom persists more than a few days. Dehydration, acidosis, and a shocklike state may ensue unless appropriate measures are taken promptly to forestall water and electrolyte imbalance. The picture of toxemia with vasomotor collapse that is occasionally encountered has also been attributed to endotoxin produced as a result of rapid multiplication of the organisms in the intestine. In the great majority of cases symptoms subside spontaneously within 2 to 4 days. Numerically the gastroenteritic type of salmonellae infection predominates in early life, especially in infants, and the organism most frequently found responsible is *S. typhimurium*. Intestinal infection may occasionally lead to the development of appendicitis.

Localized Infections.   Metastatic infection caused by salmonellae may follow the septicemia of the typhoidal form of the disease; it also may complicate a comparatively mild illness clinically indistinguishable from a digestive upset, or it may appear in the absence of any recognizable preceding symptoms. Among these distant localizations, arthritis is the most common, but osteomyelitis, pyelonephritis, cystitis, meningitis, endocarditis, and soft tissue abscesses have also been reported. Patients with sickle cell disease seem to be particularly susceptible to *Salmonella* osteomyelitis.

Inapparent Infections.   There are suggestions that subclinical infections with salmonellae are more common than is generally supposed. They are usually discovered in the course of epidemiologic surveys instituted following identification of an index case in a household, hospital ward, or other relatively closed population group. Positive stool cultures or significantly high serum agglutinin titers may be obtained in symptom-free subjects who have been exposed to an infected patient or who have consumed contaminated food. The duration of the carrier state bears little relation to the severity of symptoms at the time of the initial infection.

DIAGNOSIS.   Salmonellosis should be considered in any obscure febrile disease and in every case of diarrhea, with or without vomiting. Among young subjects isolated cases without any clue as to the source of infection are more frequent than those in which there is a history of a number of persons becoming sick after partaking of some common food.

The laboratory diagnosis rests on the recovery and proper identification of the pathogen from suitable materials. Salmonellae are isolated from rectal swabs or stool specimens in patients with gastroenteritis or food poisoning; the pathogen may also be recovered from the contaminated food in the latter instance. Depending on the particular localized lesion, pus, spinal fluid, or urine should be cultured. Salmonellae are identified on the basis of motility, biochemical activity, and antigenic structure. Serogroup determination by means of appropriate commercially available group-specific antisera can be accomplished in most hospital laboratories. For final serotyping the strains may have to be forwarded to special centers such as state laboratories. In some patients, particularly those with *Salmonella* fever, a specific antibody response to the pathogen can be demonstrated, thus aiding in the etiologic diagnosis. Antibody studies on patients with gastroenteritis or food poisoning are not done on a routine basis.

PROGNOSIS.   The prognosis of salmonellosis depends on the localization of the infection, the age of the patient, and the presence or absence of underlying disease. In otherwise healthy infants and children, *Salmonella* gastroenteritis has a favorable prognosis. The outlook is more guarded when infection occurs in premature infants or in subjects with underlying diseases, such as malignancy, or when the infection is systemic in nature. In a series of 2,625 cases analyzed by MacCready and associates during a 16-year period, including patients of all ages, the overall case fatality rate was 1.4 percent. In *S. choleraesuis* infections the case fatality rate was 16.1 percent; for *S. enteritidis*, 4.8 percent. In contrast, the case fatality rate for typhoid fever in the same population was 8.0 percent. Meningitis, although a rare complication of salmonellosis, carries a serious risk to life. Clearly, fatality rates are substantially lower if special efforts are made to include subclinical and mild infections.

TREATMENT.   In temperate climates the common varieties of salmonellae infections in children are dealt with by the host defenses so effectively that by the time the etiologic agent is identified the patient is usually on the way to recovery. Chloramphenicol or ampicillin may be used for the treatment of *Salmonella* fever, septicemia, and serious suppurative infections. The relative values of these and certain other drugs have not been definitely established. There is convincing evidence that antibiotics are not effective, either clinically or bacteriologically, in the treatment of *Salmonella* gastroenteritis. In addition, studies have shown that after antibiotic therapy the carrier state is prolonged. For these reasons antibiotics are not indicated for the therapy of *Salmonella* gastroenteritis in otherwise healthy children, nor should they be used routinely for the treatment of carriers. Recent observations suggest that trimethoprim-sulfamethoxazole may be effective in the treatment of *Salmonella* carriers and in treating gastroenteritis.

PREVENTION.   Measures for the control of salmonellosis of man include the following: appropriate water sanitation and food hygiene, control of such materials as fish meal, proper handling and cooking of potentially contaminated foods, isolation of patients with salmonellosis when admitted to hospitals, proper handling of contaminated discharges, strict enforcement of aseptic techniques, and continuing education regarding fecal–oral spread of infection. Specific immunization against *Salmonella* fever due to *S. paratyphi* A and B has been utilized for years, but there is no evidence of its efficacy. Furthermore, such immunization cannot provide significant protection against infection by many other salmonellae. The triple vaccine, which also contains typhoid bacilli, is not recommended.

Typhoid Fever

Typhoid fever is caused by *S. typhi*, which shares its O antigen with other members of group D; but the combination of O and flagellar antigens makes it antigenically unique. In addition, strains of *S. typhi* may contain Vi antigen, whose presence renders the microorganisms inagglutinable or poorly agglutinable by the corresponding O antibodies. *S. typhi* also differs from most other salmonellae in certain biochemical activities: characteristically only acid, and not gas, is produced from a variety of substrates, such as glucose, whereas the vast majority of other salmonellae produce both acid and gas. Antigenically homogeneous strains of *S. typhi* can be divided into various phage types, depending on susceptibility to standardized phages. Identification of the phage types of isolated strains aids materially in epidemic investigations.

In the past there were frequent serious epidemics of typhoid fever, but today in the developed countries typhoid fever has been strikingly controlled. Nonetheless, occasionally outbreaks do occur, such as the epidemics at Zermatt, Switzerland, and at Aberdeen, Scotland. Such unusual epidemics as the large-scale outbreaks of the past were due to contaminated water or food. The few sporadic cases seen in this country usually can be traced to a carrier.

It is important to keep in mind that bacteremia occurs early in typhoid fever; this initial bacteremic phase leads to localization of the pathogen in the intestine, skin, and elsewhere. For these reasons the blood culture usually is negative during the third week, in spite of septic temperatures.

PATHOLOGY. In general, the lesions in a young patient resemble those in an adult, except in severity. The ileum and upper colon often show only moderate congestion of the mucous membrane, with swelling of Peyer's patches, solitary lymphoid follicles, and mesenteric lymph nodes; ulcers, when present, are seldom large or deep. The spleen is usually enlarged. Lesions are rarely found in the heart, kidneys, or liver.

SYMPTOMS. In the older child the history, physical signs, and course are not significantly different from these features in the adult; but in general the disease is milder, its duration is shorter, and complications are infrequent. In infants the signs of illness are usually so nonspecific that the diagnosis of typhoid fever is seldom entertained; the first clue is usually provided by growth of the organisms in blood culture. The disease in infants is generally even milder than in children of school age. The onset is usually gradual, with headache, malaise, anorexia, and fever that rises in a steplike manner in 4 to 7 days to about 104 F. The pulse remains comparatively slow. Diarrhea may be present, usually alternating with constipation and being associated with abdominal distension and tenderness. Rose-colored spots over the abdomen, splenomegaly, and delirium or stupor are less common than in the adult with typhoid fever, but they do occur. At all ages, except in infancy, leukopenia and low red cell sedimentation rate are uniform features. In the infant and the child less than 2 years of age, leukocytosis is frequent and may be as high as 20,000 to 25,000 cells/mm³; rose spots are very rare. The onset can be quite sudden, often with convulsions. Pyogenic infection may in rare instances localize in the urinary tract, the central nervous system, the bones and joints, or elsewhere.

DIAGNOSIS. The definitive diagnosis of typhoid fever is established by the isolation and identification of *S. typhi* from the blood during the first week or 10 days of illness and/or from the feces after the first stage of the illness. In some patients the pathogen is also present in the urine and in respiratory secretions. Occasionally it can be isolated from the rose spots. The

diagnosis on immunologic grounds can be made by the demonstration of a specific antibody response (Widal test). Rises of the corresponding O and H antibodies, or high titers of these antibodies, provide strongly suggestive evidence of *S. typhi* infection. It must be emphasized that increased H titers and normal O titers are seen in subjects after immunization with typhoid vaccine. Also, high O titers and normal *S. typhi* H titers are encountered in patients with *Salmonella* group D infection other than *S. typhi*. Carriers, who excrete *S. typhi* in the feces and frequently harbor the pathogen in the biliary system, often have elevated titers of Vi antibodies.

TREATMENT. Therapy of *S. typhi* infections in infants and children is governed by the same principles used in treating typhoid fever in adults. The problem of nutritional wasting, which is potentially severe, has been eliminated by liberal feeding early in the disease and by treatment of dehydration and electrolyte imbalance with parenteral injections.

Either ampicillin or chloramphenicol may be used for specific therapy. The former drug is preferred by some physicians, not because of its superior effectiveness but because of the serious complications that rarely are associated with the latter drug. Chloramphenicol is highly effective at a daily dosage of 50 to 100 mg/kg of body weight given intravenously in four equally spaced doses. Oral medication should be used as soon as possible. Even though bacteremia uniformly disappears within 12 hours after institution of this regimen, the patient seldom shows improvement for at least 2 days. In adults with marked toxemia, adrenocorticosteroid therapy combined with chloramphenicol causes dramatic improvement within 24 hours. No evidence of harm from steroids has been encountered when they are given for only 4 or 5 days, by which time chloramphenicol has taken effect.

The duration of chloramphenicol therapy needed to prevent recrudescence is about 3 weeks, although many patients are cured after only 10 days. When the carrier state has developed, chloramphenicol alone will not eliminate organisms from the intestinal tract. Ampicillin (75 to 100 mg/kg/day) in three or four divided doses for 3 to 6 weeks is sometimes effective in the treatment of carriers.

Chloramphenicol has greatly reduced the fatality rate of typhoid fever, which in treated cases is now approximately 2 percent. In the Aberdeen typhoid outbreak, involving a total of 507 patients of whom 86 were children, not a single death occurred among the latter. Recently, in both adults and children, it was shown that orally administered trimethoprim-sulfamethoxazole and amoxicillin were effective in the treatment of chloramphenicol-resistant and chloramphenicol-sensitive *S. typhi* infections. These new approaches are particularly important in dealing with antibiotic-resistant strains such as have been encountered in Mexico.

PROPHYLAXIS. The prevention of typhoid fever outbreaks requires proper water sanitation, food hygiene, and prevention of dissemination of the pathogen from carriers and patients. Every effort must be made to identify carriers. Such individuals must not be employed as food handlers, and the regulations in force regarding typhoid carriers must be carefully followed. Treatment of carriers by means of antibiotics has not yielded uniformly favorable results. Recent observations suggest that trimethoprim-sulfamethoxazole may be effective in the treatment of typhoid carriers. Further studies are needed to evaluate this drug regimen.

Personal protection against typhoid fever may be accomplished by active immunization. Although typhoid vaccine has been used for decades, only recently has its efficacy been established in controlled field studies. It has been shown that the phenol vaccine is superior to the alcohol vaccine, although both are substantially effective. More recent investigations suggest that the acetone vaccine may be even better. Routine vaccination against typhoid fever is not recommended for children living in countries where epidemics are rare. Safe travel to other countries in which typhoid fever is still prevalent can be accomplished by immunization with a potent vaccine according to the following schedule. For children over 10 years of age two subcutaneous injections of 0.5 ml, separated by 4 weeks or more, are recommended; for children between the ages of 6 months and 10 years 0.25 ml should be used instead of 0.5 ml. If immunity has to be established more rapidly, three injections at the same doses at weekly intervals can be used. Under conditions of repeated or continued exposure, booster doses should be given at least every 3 years. Even if the interval is longer than 3 years after effective primary immunization, the single booster dose is probably adequate. Instead of subcutaneous injection of the booster dose, 0.1 ml of the vaccine may be given intradermally over the deltoid area.

SHIGELLOSIS

Dysentery, an infectious disease involving primarily the colon, may be caused by *Entamoeba histolytica* (amebic dysentery) or by members of the genus *Shigella* (bacillary dysentery). This section deals only with shigellosis. Only rarely are shigellae responsible for extraintestinal infections.

ETIOLOGY.   Dysentery occurs with special frequency in summer and early autumn, but sporadic cases are seen at all seasons. The disease is more common in warm than in cold climates, and both the morbidity and mortality rates vary inversely with the standards of home hygiene of a given geographic area. Dysentery is apt to be prevalent in communities in which facilities for refrigeration of food are inadequate. Although shigellosis occurs in individuals of all ages, for unexplained reasons it is surprisingly rare in infants under the age of 3 months.

The genus *Shigella* is divided into four major groups: *S. dysenteriae, S. flexneri, S. boydii,* and *S. sonnei.* In turn, the *S. dysenteriae* group comprises 7 members, the *S. flexneri* group 12 members, and the *S. boydii* 7 members. Only the Shiga bacillus, which belongs to the *S. dysenteriae* group, produces an exotoxin. In the past the greater severity of Shiga bacillus infection was ascribed to this toxin. In recent times, however, these infections have not differed substantially from those caused by other shigellae, and the role of this toxin in the pathogenesis of shigellosis remains obscure. In certain countries of the world, such as Japan, *S. flexneri* predominates; in other countries, such as England and the United States, *S. sonnei* is the organism most frequently encountered. All shigellae may cause both sporadic and epidemic dysentery in man. The members of the alkalescens-dispar group, which are no longer included within the genus *Shigella,* generally do not cause dysentery and certainly are not responsible for epidemics. On the other hand, these organisms may produce extraintestinal infections such as those of the urinary tract.

EPIDEMIOLOGY.   The infection is believed to enter the body through the alimentary tract in all cases. Although dogs, particularly puppies, are susceptible to inoculation and sometimes exhibit the disease spontaneously, the important reservoir of the infection is man. Contamination of a food supply occasionally occurs on a large scale; a number of milkborne and some waterborne epidemics have been described, but these are rare. The housefly may play an important part in disseminating the disease, as was shown by the observations of Lyon in West Virginia. Most isolated cases are caused by carriers, often adults, who may never have manifested symptoms but who may have suffered from a very mild, transient diarrhea that attracted little attention. Between 2 and 3 percent of infected individuals carry the organism for more than 3 months. Subclinical infection occurs more frequently than is generally recognized. On rare occasions shigellae may be transmitted from the mother to the newborn infant during delivery. The incubation period is usually 2 or 3 days, although it may vary from 12 hours to 8 days.

PATHOLOGY.   In fatal cases the disease involves primarily the colon. The cecum and first portion of the ascending colon and the sigmoid are more commonly involved than the transverse portion. In less than half the cases the ileum is also affected, usually for a distance of about 50 cm, and the lesion here is always less advanced than in the colon.

There is at first a diffuse inflammation of the mucosa, which is swollen and reddened, without any tendency toward localization in the lymphoid structures. The vessels are dilated, and punctate hemorrhages are present. The secretion of mucus is increased. At this time microscopic sections show hyperemia and infiltration of the mucosa and submucosa with inflammatory cells, both polymorphonuclear leukocytes and mononuclear cells. The crypts often contain leukocytic exudate. The submucosa is usually slightly edematous.

As the process advances the more prominent portions of the mucosal folds are found to be more deeply reddened, and flecks of yellow opaque membrane appear to become confluent along the crests of the transverse folds. In a longitudinal direction the more flattened strips of mucosa produced by the Taeniae are more conspicuously affected than the pouches between them. The formation of opaque, dry, yellowish membranes may extend to involve the whole mucosal surface in diffuse fashion, but usually it sloughs away in smaller or larger portions to produce irregular shallow ulcers. The whole intestinal wall is thickened and stiffened; swelling of the submucosa is obvious on cross section. Microscopically the membrane is made up of fibrin, debris of cells of the exudate, and necrotic mucosa. It may involve only the superficial layers, leaving the deeper portions of the crypts intact, or it may involve the whole mucosa. There are hemorrhages into the underlying tissues, which, although not yet necrotic, are infiltrated with inflammatory cells—polymorphonuclear leukocytes and mononuclear cells. The inflammatory reaction in the submucosa is much more marked than in the early stages. Ulceration usually stops at the submucosa, but the muscularis mucosae may be destroyed, and sometimes the muscular layers are exposed. Perforation is very uncommon. Ulceration is usually not pronounced before the second or third week.

In more protracted cases the ulcers are lined by a pink satinlike membrane that is sometimes difficult to distinguish from mucosa, and in section this is found to be composed of a layer of granulation tissue densely infiltrated with mononuclear cells. Plasma cells are often quite conspicuous. New growth of epithelium can be seen at the margins of the ulcers.

SYMPTOMS. Bacillary dysentery may be clinically indistinguishable from nonspecific diarrhea. The stools are loose for only a few days, fever is slight or absent, the appetite is scarcely affected, and the child hardly seems ill. In other cases the constitutional disturbance is equally mild, but the stools contain mucus with streaks of blood. Careful bacteriologic studies applied to an entire community without regard to individual complaints have suggested that mild cases may actually outnumber those that are clinically more conspicuous.

In cases of moderate severity, in which clinical recognition is more likely, the onset is usually sudden, often with fever, vomiting, anorexia, and abdominal pain. Diarrhea promptly appears, and frequent thin green or yellow stools that contain undigested food are passed. Later the discharges contain blood and mucus and are often preceded by intestinal cramps and accompanied by tenesmus. With persistent anorexia the stools contain less and less food residue and consist mainly of bile-stained exudate; they may number 20 or 30 a day. The mucus may be clear and jellylike, or it may be mixed with pus and bile-stained flecks. Blood may be seen in almost every stool, usually streaking the mucus, but rarely in clots. These stools are almost odorless, having a faint musty smell rather than a fecal smell. Prolapse of the rectum is frequent and may occur with nearly every stool. For the first 24 hours the temperature is usually high, from 102 F to 104 F; thereafter it commonly ranges from 99 F to 102 F. Vomiting is seldom troublesome after the first day, and adbominal distension is exceptional either at the onset or later. The loss of water and electrolytes is often very great in the early stages and may lead to severe dehydration, with prostration, sunken eyes, dryness of mucous membranes, and sores on the lips and teeth. Acidosis may develop rapidly; indeed, the first few hours of an attack

of dysentery may be most critical. Leukocytosis may be present, although it seldom exceeds 15,000 cells/mm^3. The duration of acute symptoms varies. The first sign of improvement is generally the disappearance of blood from the stools, which at the same time become less frequent, and the pain and tenesmus cease. Defervescence and recovery of appetite usually precede the return of entirely normal stools. Convalescence is often slow, and it may be weeks before the lost weight and strength are regained. In some cases the intestine remains hyperirritable for months after an attack, during which time minor dietary indiscretions may lead to a recurrence of diarrhea, with mucus in the stools but without demonstrable dysentery organisms.

In the past, fatality rates from shigellosis were high, and in many underdeveloped countries this is so even today. Fatal dysentery is encountered only rarely in developed countries. Serious infection may develop in patients with underlying diseases. In the United States fatal outcome of shigellosis is rare. In one epidemic studied extensively in western New York only one death occurred among more than 200 patients. The fatal case was that of a patient with leukemia under treatment with corticoid hormone who contracted a *Shigella* infection.

COMPLICATIONS. Major complicatons are those accompanying endotoxic shock with circulatory collapse. In children convulsive seizures are not infrequent. Other complications have decreased in number and severity since sulfonamides and antibiotics came into general use. Invasion of the bloodstream and metastatic complications caused by dysentery bacilli themselves are very exceptional. There is no evidence available to indicate that shigellosis is related etiologically to ulcerative colitis.

DIAGNOSIS. Proctoscopic examination may disclose congestion and edema of the mucous membrane indicating actual enteritis. The involved mucosa bleeds readily. In more severe cases a fibrinous membrane may be found, or ulcers ranging in size from follicular to 1 or 2 cm in diameter may be seen. The absence of lesions in proctoscopic examination does not, of course, exclude bacillary dysentery.

Accurate diagnosis depends on bacteriologic evidence. In any case of diarrhea the stools should be carefully inspected for flecks of blood or streaks of pus, and suspicious material should be examined under the microscope. Appreciable numbers of polymorphonuclear leukocytes are found in almost all cases of dysentery, as well as in *Salmonella* enteritis. When both pus and blood are present there is strong probability that either *Shigella* or *Salmonella* infection is the cause, although amebic colitis cannot be excluded without additional evidence.

Bacteriologic examination of freshly passed feces or material obtained on rectal swabs usually results in recovery of the shigellae. In some cases two or more cultures may be required. The pathogen is identified on the basis of morphologic characteristics, biochemical activities, and antigenic structure. Group-specific and type-specific *Shigella* antisera are available for identification. Since shigellae as a rule do not invade the bloodstream, blood cultures play no role in diagnosis. Diagnostic tests for demonstration of antibody responses of patients are not available for routine purposes, although they may be of considerable help in epidemiologic studies.

PROPHYLAXIS. In hospitals patients with shigellosis should be under enteric precautions to prevent infection of other subjects. For the protection of household contacts the features to be stressed are the careful washing of hands, terminal sterilization of formulas for infants, adequate refrigeration of food, and protection from flies. Vaccines for active immunization are not available. Prevention of community outbreaks requires appropriate water sanitation, food hygiene, and other measures effective in prevention of dissemination of enteric pathogens.

TREATMENT. Proper control of dehydration, including restoration of lost electrolytes, is usually the most immediate concern in the treatment of dysentery. This has been discussed elsewhere (p. 264). Numerous antibacterial agents have been used in the treatment of shigellosis, including streptomycin, the tetracylines, chloramphenicol, polymyxin B, colistin, furazolidone, and ampicillin. Ampicillin is the drug of choice of many physicians. According to recent observations, trimethoprim-sulfamethoxazole may be effective, and it may find a place in the treatment of shigellosis due to ampicillin-resistant strains. Since the susceptibility of shigellae to these drugs differs substantially in various localities and at various times, it is strongly recommended, notably when shigellosis is prevalent in a community, to determine the in vitro susceptibility of the pathogens as a guide to clinical therapy. In view of the frequently mild course of shigellosis that is seen in children at the present time, clinical evaluation of the relative merits of various chemotherapeutic agents presents difficulties. Certain patients become carriers even after a course of chemotherapy. Only under unusual circumstances should further treatment be given in an attempt to eradicate the carrier state.

In considering diet for patients with shigellae infections, the character of the stools should not be used to indicate the condition of the patient's digestion. His diarrhea may be only the result of the inflammatory process. The appetite is usually an excellent guide to follow. Residue should be avoided, but other dietary restrictions are not needed. Adsorbents such as kaolin and pectin have not impressed us with their usefulness. The same may be said of carob flour. Raw fruits have been widely recommended, and except for citrus fruits they are well tolerated; but they appear to have no specific virtue. The appetite may totally fail in prolonged febrile cases, even after subsidence of the fever in patients who are very weak. Transfusion may be of help. Since vitamin deficiencies, notably those of the B group, are likely to be seen in protracted cases, a supplement that provides for these factors as well as for vitamin C should always be given.

Opium may be of help when there is pain, tenesmus, and great frequency of stools. The dose should be regulated by the severity of these symptoms. The deodorized tincture (laudanum) and paregoric are, we believe, preferable to other preparations. Repeated small doses are better than a single large dose. Severe tenesmus, when associated with prolapse of the rectum, is sometimes effectively relieved by a suppository containing benzocaine.

ENTEROPATHOGENIC *E. COLI* ENTERITIS

ETIOLOGY. Some 50 years ago the German pediatrician Adam presented evidence of the association between certain biochemically characterized strains of *Escherichia coli* and diarrheal disease of infants. During the 1940s and 1950s antigenically identified serotypes of *E. coli* were related to serious outbreaks of diarrheal disease among newborn infants. On epidemiologic grounds, as well as on the basis of a few volunteer studies of the effectiveness of certain antibiotics in therapy and prophylaxis and the specific antibody responses of some of these patients, these serotypes were considered as probable etiologic agents and were referred to as enteropathogenic. In addition to their presence in epidemics, these strains were also encountered in sporadic cases. Age was a particularly striking determinant of the disease, since clinical illness was far more commonly encountered in young infants than in older children and adults. Among the more than 140 serogroups of *E. coli*, the following have been associated with enteritis of infants and young children: O26:B6, O55:B5, O86:B7, O111:B4, O112:B11, O119:B14, O124:B17, O125:B15, O126:B16, O127:B8, and O128:B12. These serotypes of *E. coli* are only very rarely encountered in extraintestinal infections (a feature worthy of future studies). For unexplained reasons, *E. coli* O55:B5, O111:B4, and O127:B8 were encountered more frequently in epidemics than *E. coli* O26:B6. Without question, diarrheal disease associated with these serotypes has become much milder in recent years. Clearly the antigens characterizing these serotypes are not responsible for the disease, and its pathogenesis has remained unexplained.

With the identification of a powerful enterotoxin produced by *Vibrio cholerae*, which is responsible for the diarrheal features of cholera, the question arose whether enterotoxins might also explain disease associated with *E. coli* in animals and man. Recent intensive studies have identified two toxins produced by *E. coli,* one being heat-labile and antigenically related to the enterotoxin of *V. cholerae* and the other being heat-stable. Strains of *E. coli* may produce both or only one of these toxins, and these strains are referred to as enterotoxic *E. coli* (EEC). Strains of *E. coli* may have local tissue-invasive properties and may be referred to as enteroinvasive. Such strains have been isolated from adults and children, including patients with traveler's diarrhea. Whether the strains encountered during the epidemics of three decades ago produced enterotoxin and/or had enteroinvasive capacity is not known. However, it is known that enterotoxin information is not directly associated with the O and K antigens of enteropathogenic strains, a feature that is not surprising in view of the fact that enterotoxin production is plasmid-dependent. Further studies are needed before the role of enterotoxin-producing and enteroinvasive strains of *E. coli* in diarrheal disease of various age groups can be elucidated. Attention should be called to the significant recent advances in the area of viral enteritis made by Hamilton and associates (see References).

EPIDEMIOLOGY. It is thought that in the majority of epidemics studied in recent years the causative agent has been transferred from infant to infant by contact with hands, linen, or equipment—in other words, by some error in nursery technique. It is important to keep in mind that infants with EEC enteritis frequently shed extraordinarily large numbers of pathogens in the feces. Occasionally adults, including nurses, are fecal carriers of EEC or other pathogens and thus may serve as a source of infection of newborn infants. Transmission of EEC, salmonellae, and shigellae from mother to child during delivery may result in infection of the newborn infant, who in turn may transmit the infection to others in the nursery. The importance of airborne transmission of the infection has not been satisfactorily evaluated, but it is currently believed to be minor.

PATHOLOGY. No specific pathologic changes are found. The intestinal mucosa is congested but shows no ulceration, and there may be evidences of parenchymatous degeneration or secondary infection in other organs.

SYMPTOMS. The incubation period is usually short and may in some instances be a matter of only a few hours, with diarrhea being the first symptom. Fever is not striking at the onset and may be absent in mild cases; in severe cases the temperature may rise rapidly as the condition progresses. Leukocytosis is not characteristic. The stools are watery; they contain neither blood nor pus and, as a rule, little mucus. The discharges may be very frequent and may be passed with considerable force. The appetite is lost, and often there is vomiting. Loss of weight may be precipitous, and serious dehydration may develop rapidly. The mucous membranes are dry, and the pharynx and tongue are often fiery red; however, the bacteriology of the respiratory tract is not abnormal. Death may occur within a few days, with acidosis and dehydration, or after some weeks of progressive nutritional failure. As a rule, however, symptoms abate gradually, and the infant eventually resumes his growth. The principal complications are secondary infections, chiefly of the respiratory or urinary tract, the meninges, or the skin. Unless effective chemotherapy is utilized, recurrence of EEC enteritis is not infrequent. Permanent residua are scarcely ever encountered.

PROGNOSIS. Case fatality rates in individual epidemics vary greatly, but they have tended in recent years to average less than 5 percent. Not for years has an epidemic been reported in this country with as high a mortality as 50 percent. In a widespread community outbreak of enteritis due to *E. coli* O111:B4 reported by Kessner and associates, the fatality rate for neonates

was 16 percent, and the rate for the entire population 5.9 percent.

DIAGNOSIS. Except during epidemics, an etiologic diagnosis in individual cases cannot be established on clinical grounds alone. Therefore it is essential that isolation and identification of the pathogen be performed by the appropriate laboratory methods. The fluorescence antibody technique makes possible rapid presumptive identification of EEC. Unfortunately, at this time identification of enterotoxic and enteroinvasive strains of *E. coli* is not possible in most clinical laboratories. Identification of the serologically characterized enteropathogenic strains may no longer be indicated in the absence of outbreaks of the disease.

PROPHYLAXIS. It is imperative to diagnose infectious enteritis of the newborn without delay and to take steps for the prevention and control of epidemics. Appropriate chemotherapy of infected infants, chemoprophylaxis of exposed individuals, and proper aseptic technique are required. It may be necessary to close the nursery to further admissions until the last infant has been discharged and the nursery has been disinfected. It is important that the hospital be notified promptly if infectious enteritis develops in infants shortly after they are discharged from a nursery. Attention should also be called to the appropriate reporting of cases to health departments, according to existing laws and regulations. The fact that several large hospital services have been entirely free from such epidemics over a period of several years may probably be ascribed to careful attention to routine procedures of nursing care and to preparation and administration of feedings (in which terminal sterilization of formulas is believed to play a significant part). In addition, poorly understood changes in virulence of enteropathogenic strains may have played a significant role.

TREATMENT. Numerous antibacterial agents have been used for oral treatment and prophylaxis of bacterial enteritis of newborns and older infants, including neomycin, polymyxin B, colistin, ampicillin, and others. Chemotherapy is more often indicated in infections of the newborn than in those of older children. Since strains of EEC, and of other bacterial pathogens as well, are occasionally resistant to one or more antibacterial agents, in vitro susceptibility tests should be carried out, notably during epidemics, as a guide to clinical chemotherapy. An antigen has recently been prepared for possible use in the prophylaxis of this infection and is under clinical trial. The role of locally produced antibodies (notably IgA) in immunity remains to be explored. The possible usefulness of antienterotoxin and enterotoxoid remains to be determined. Nonspecific treatment differs in no essential way from that for diarrhea in infants (p. 991).

References

SALMONELLA INFECTIONS

Abrams IF, Cochran WD, Holmes LB, Marsh EB, Moore JW: A Salmonella newport outbreak in a premature nursery with a one-year follow-up. Effect of ampicillin following bacteriologic failure of response to kanamycin. Pediatr 37:616, 1966

Aserkoff B, Bennett JV: Effect of antibiotic therapy in acute salmonellosis on the fecal excretion of salmonellae. N Engl J Med 281:636, 1969

Bate JG, James U: Salmonella typhimurium infection dust-borne in a children's ward. Lancet, 2:713, 1958

Black PH, Kunz LJ, Swartz MN: Salmonellosis—a review of some unusual aspects. N Engl J Med 262:811, 864, 921, 1960

Cherubin CE, Fodor T, Denmark LI, et al: Symptoms, septicemia and death in salmonellosis. Am J Epidemiol 90:285, 1969

Clementi KJ: Treatment of Salmonella carriers with trimethoprim-sulfamethoxazole. Can Med Assoc J 112:28S, 1975

Clyde WA Jr: Salmonellosis in infants and children; a study of 100 cases. Pediatr 19:175, 1957

Collins RN, Treger MD, Goldsby JB, et al: Interstate outbreak of Salmonella newbrunswick infection traced to powdered milk. JAMA 203:838, 1968

Eisenberg GM, Brodsky L, Weiss W, Flippin HF: Clinical and microbiological aspects of salmonellosis. Am J Med Sci 235:497, 1958

Galloway H, Clark NS, Blackhall M: Paediatric aspects of the Aberdeen typhoid outbreak. Arch Dis Child 41:63, 1966

Geddes AM: Trimethoprim-sulfamethoxazole in the treatment of gastrointestinal infections, including enteric fever and typhoid carriers. Can Med Assoc J 112: 35S, 1975

Gilman RH, Terminel M, Levine MM, et al: Comparison of trimethoprim-sulfamethoxazole and amoxicillin in therapy of chloramphenicol-resistant and chloramphenicol-sensitive typhoid fever. J Infect Dis 132:630, 1975

Han T, Sokal JE, Neter E: Salmonellosis in disseminated malignant diseases. A seven-year review (1959–1965). N Engl J Med 276:1045, 1967

Hook EW: Salmonellosis: certain factors influencing the interaction of Salmonella and the human host. Bull NY Acad Med 37:499, 1961 (second series)

———— Campbell CG, Weens HS, Cooper GR: Salmonella osteomyelitis in patients with sickle cell anemia. N Engl J Med 257:403, 1957

Hughes JG, Carroll DS: Salmonella osteomyelitis complicating sickle-cell disease. Pediatrics 19:184, 1957

MacCready RA, Reardon JP, Saphra I: Salmonellosis in Massachusetts; a sixteen-year experience. N Engl J Med 256:1121, 1957

Marx MB: The effect of interspecies contact upon diarrhea morbidity and salmonellosis in children. J Infect Dis 120:202, 1969

Neter E, Drislane AM, Harris AH, Jansen GT: Diagnosis of clinical and subclinical salmonellosis by means of serologic hemagglutination test. N Engl J Med 261:1162, 1959

Philbrook FR, MacCready RA, Van Roekel H, et al: Salmonellosis spread by a dietary supplement of avian source. N Engl J Med 263:713, 1960

Robertson RP, Wahab MFA, Raasch FO: Evaluation of chloramphenicol and ampicillin in salmonella enteric fever. N Engl J Med 278:171, 1968

Rosenstein BJ: Salmonellosis in infants and children. Epidemiologic and therapeutic considerations. J Pediatr 70:1, 1967

———— Shigella and Salmonella enteritis in infants and children. Bull Johns Hopkins Hosp 115:407, 1964

Salmonella infections. Med Lett Drugs Ther 10:50, 1968

Sanders E, Sweeney FJ Jr, Friedman EA, et al: An outbreak of hospital-associated infections due to Salmonella derby. JAMA 186:984, 1963

Schroeder SA, Aserkoff B, Brachman PS: Epidemic salmonellosis in hospitals and institutions. N Engl J Med 279:674, 1968

Simon HJ, Miller RC: Ampicillin in the treatment of chronic typhoid carriers. Report on fifteen treated cases and a review of the literature. N Engl J Med 274:807, 1966

Watt J, Wegman ME, Brown OW, et al: Salmonellosis in a premature nursery unaccompanied by a diarrheal disease. Pediatr 22:689, 1958

Whitby JMF: Ampicillin in treatment of Salmonella typhi carriers. Lancet 2:71, 1964

SHIGELLOSIS

Bibile SW, Cooray MPM, Balasubramaniam K, Gulasekaram J: Comparative trial of drugs in bacillary dysentery. J Trop Med Hyg 64:300, 1961

De La Torre JA, Olarte J, Joachin A: Treatment of shigellosis with tetracycline in infants under 2 years of age. Pediatr 23:1136, 1959

Diarrhea caused by Shigella. Med Lett Drugs Ther 10:38, 1968

DuPont HL, Hornick RB, Dawkins AT, Snyder MJ, Formal SB: The response of man to virulent Shigella flexneri 2a. J Infect Dis 119:296, 1969

Eichner ER, Gangarosa EJ, Goldsby JB: The current status of shigellosis in the United States. Am J Public Health 58:753, 1968

Fischler E, Wallis K: Investigation of drug sensitivity in Shigella and its correlation with in vivo sensitivity. Ann Paediatr 201:49, 1963

Freitag JL: A water-borne outbreak of dysentery. Health News 37:4, 1960

Gerstmann PE, LaVeck GD: Shigellosis: mass drug therapy in an institutional setting. Am J Public Health 53:266, 1963

Gordon JE, Ascoli W, Pierce V, Guzman MA, Mata LJ: Studies of diarrheal disease in Central America. VI. An epidemic of diarrhea in a Guatemalan highland village, with a component due to Shigella dysenteriae, type 1. Am J Trop Med Hyg 14:404, 1965

Greenberg M, Frant S, Shapiro R: Bacillary dysentery acquired at birth. J Pediatr 17:363, 1940

Haltalin KC: Neonatal shigellosis. Report of 16 cases and review of the literature. Am J Dis Child 114:603, 1967

———— Nelson JD, Hinton LV, Kusmiesz HT, Sladoje M: Comparison of orally absorbable and nonabsorbable antibiotics in shigellosis. A double blind study with ampicillin and neomycin. J Pediatr 72:708, 1968

———— Nelson JD, Kusmiesz HT, Hinton LV: Comparison of intramuscular and oral ampicillin therapy for shigellosis. J Pediatr 73:617, 1968

———— Nelson JD, Ring R, Sladoje M, Hinton LV: Double-blind treatment study of shigellosis comparing ampicillin, sulfadiazine, and placebo. J Pediatr 70:970, 1967

Jao RL, Jackson GG: Asymptomatic urinary-tract infection with Shigella sonnei in a chronic fecal carrier. N Engl J Med 268:1165, 1963

Marks MI: Pharmacokinetics and efficacy of trimethoprim-sulfamethoxazole in the treatment of gastroenteritis in children. Can Med Assoc J 112:32S, 1975

Mata LJ, Urrutia JJ, Garcia B, Fernandez R, Behar M: Shigella infection in breast fed Guatemalan Indian neonates. Am J Dis Child 117:142, 1969

Mitsuhashi S: Review: the R factors. J Infect Dis 119:89, 1969

Moorhead PJ, Parry HE: Treatment of sonne dysentery. Br Med J 2:913, 1965

Neter E: Shigella sonnei infection at term and its transfer to newborn. Obstet Gynecal 17:517, 1961

———— Epidemiologic and immunologic studies of Shigella sonnei dysentery. Am J Public Health 52:61, 1962

———— Harris AH, Drislane AM: Comparative study of hemagglutination and agglutination tests for the determination of the antibody response of patients with S. sonnei dysentery. Am J Clin Pathol 37:239, 1962

Reller LB, Gangarosa EJ, Brachman PS: Shigellosis in the United States: five-year review of nationwide surveillance, 1964–1968. Am J Epidemiol 91:161, 1970

Salzman TC, Scher CD, Moss R: Shigellae with transferable drug resistance: outbreak in a nursery for premature infants. J Pediatr 71:21, 1967

ENTEROPATHOGENIC E. COLI ENTERITIS

Baker JA, Neter E (eds): Epidemic and endemic diarrheal diseases of the infant. Ann NY Acad Sci 66:3, 1956

Behbehani AM, Wenner HA: Infantile diarrhea. A study of the etiologic role of viruses. Am J Dis Child 111:623, 1966

Danielsson D, Laurell G: The fluorescent antibody technique in the diagnosis of enteropathogenic Escherichia coli, with special reference to sensitivity and specificity. Acta Pathol Microbiol Scand 76:601, 1969

Ewing WH: Sources of Escherichia coli cultures that belonged to O antigen groups associated with infantile diarrheal disease. J Infect Dis 110:114, 1962

Gorbach SL, Khurana CM: Toxigenic Escherichia coli. A cause of infantile diarrhea in Chicago. N Engl J Med 287:791, 1972

Gordon JE: Acute diarrheal disease. Am J Med Sci 248:345, 1964

Hamilton JR, Gall DG, Kerzner B, Butler DG, Middleton PJ: Recent developments in viral gastroenteritis. Pediatr Clin North Am 22:747, 1975

Hodes HL: The etiology of infantile diarrhea. In Levine SZ (ed) Adv Pediatr Vol 8. Chicago, Year Book, 1956, p. 13

Kalser MH, Cohen R, Arteaga I, et al: Normal viral and bacterial flora of the human small and large intestine. New Engl J Med 274:500, 558, 1966

Kessner DM, Shaughnessy HJ, Googins J, et al: An extensive community outbreak of diarrhea due to enteropathogenic Escherichia coli O111:B4. I. Epidemiologic studies. Am J Hygiene 76:27, 1962

Neter E: Enteritis due to enteropathogenic Escherichia coli. J Pediatr 55:223, 1959

——— Enteropathogenicity of Escherichia coli. Am J Dis Child 129:666, 1975

Olarte J, Galindo E, Joachin A: Sensitivity of Salmonella, Shigella, and enteropathogenic Escherichia coli species to cephalothin, ampicillin, chloramphenicol, and tetracycline. Antimicrob Agents Chemother 1962, p 787

——— Epidemic diarrhea in premature infants. Etiological significance of a newly recognized type of Escherichia coli (O142:K86(B):H6). Am J Dis Child 109:436, 1965

Rudoy RC, Nelson JD: Enteroinvasive and enterotoxigenic Escherichia coli. Am J Dis Child 129:668, 1975

Sack RB: Human diarrheal disease caused by enterotoxigenic Escherichia coli. Ann Rev Microbial 29:333, 1975

Stulberg CS, Zuelzer WW, Nolke AC, Thompson AL: Escherichia coli O127:B$_8$, a pathogenic strain causing infantile diarrhea. Am J Dis Child 90:125, 1955

Wachsmuth IK, Stamm WE, McGowan JE Jr: Prevalence of toxigenic and invasive strains of Escherichia coli in a hospital population. J Infect Dis 132:601, 1975

Yow MD: Antibiotic management of acute infectious gastroenteritis of infancy. Pediatr Clin North Am 10:163, 1963

STAPHYLOCOCCAL COLONIZATION

Henry R. Shinefield

Although staphylococcal disease occurs in all age groups, the most serious manifestations of illness caused by *Staphylococcus aureus* are seen in the newborn baby or in infants and children with altered host resistance.

INFANT COLONIZATION. Several facts about the dynamics of infant colonization with *S. aureus* are now clear: the nares and umbilicus of the infant are colonized shortly after birth; the major sources of infection are the nursery personnel, with the attendant's hands being the most important source of infant contamination; fewer than 10 *S. aureus* cells will initiate umbilical colonization in 50 percent of newborns, while approximately 250 organisms will achieve a similar effect on the nasal mucosa. Combinations of factors probably account for the fact that the colonization rate of 4- to 5-day-old infants in a given nursery may vary from 10 to 90 percent, despite no obvious changes in personnel, environment, or nursery techniques. The umbilicus is usually colonized before the nares, and the incidence of colonization is higher among males than females. By the time the infant is 4 to 8 weeks old the colonization rate of the umbilicus approaches zero, while nasal colonization after the first year of life is in the adult range of 20 to 40 percent.

NURSERY INFECTION. The aim in all programs for control of staphylococcal disease in the newborn is to prevent colonization of the neonate with virulent strains of staphylococci. General clinical experience and controlled investigations have proved that such protection cannot be achieved by strict asepsis on the part of nursery personnel, by vigorous environmental control including the use of ultraviolet lights, or by utilization of a rooming-in program for the newborn. As a last resort in some outbreaks nurseries have been closed, but even this has not curtailed epidemics in all instances.

Washing with hexachlorophene soon after birth and daily thereafter has been suggested to control colonization. This technique has been associated with a diminution of staphylococcal skin colonization and skin lesions, but it has had little or no effect on nasal colonization; also, it has not been effective in controlling *S. aureus* colonization when it is initiated during the height of an epidemic.

A method successfully employed by the author, as well as by others, to terminate colonization of premature and full-term infants with virulent *S. aureus* during nursery epidemics utilizes the phenomenon of bacterial interference. Artificial colonization of the nares and umbilicus of newborn infants with a selected strain of *S. aureus* of low virulence within the first 2 hours after birth results in prompt termination of nursery outbreaks of infection and disease caused by hospital strains of *S. aureus*. Artificial colonization of newborns is at present indicated only during epidemics when both the staphylococcal colonization and disease rates of infants are high; routine colonization of all infants in nonepidemic periods is not recommended.

All individuals with staphylococcal lesions should be excluded from the nursery and obstetric area. The asymptomatic nasal carrier should also be removed from contact with the newborn infant when it is ascertained that the *S. aureus* strain carried is the same as the one causing trouble in newborns. Carriers of strains that are not contributory to infant disease need not be excluded from contact with newborns. Many of the nursery attendants who are carriers of epidemic strains of *S. aureus* are transient carriers; they lose their colonization when they are removed from the nursery or when the predominant nursery strain infecting infants is deliberately changed.

It is possible to eliminate nasal carriage from permanent carriers of *S. aureus* for short periods of time with the use of a variety of antibiotic regimens. Following cessation of antibiotics, return of the resident strain may be prevented in about 60 to 80 percent of cases by deliberate recolonization with a selected less virulent strain of *S. aureus*. If only antibiotics are used, the resident strain can be detected in the nares of 60 to 70 percent of treated individuals within 2 to 4 weeks after therapy is stopped. A surveillance program of periodic infant and attendant cultures in the nursery may be helpful in early detection of epidemics of *S. aureus*.

DISEASE IN NEWBORN.   Staphylococcal disease rates in infants depend more on the strain of *Staphylococcus* than on the incidence of colonization. Colonization with "wild" or nonepidemic strain of *S. aureus* is associated with disease rates of about 5 percent, while colonization with virulent hospital strains, usually strains in phage group 1, may result in disease rates approaching 70 percent. Epidemics of bullous impetigo (Ritter's disease) have been caused only by strains in phage group 2. A specific toxin responsible for this manifestation of staphylococcal disease has been isolated from this group of staphylococci.

Although skin lesions may be seen while the baby is in the nursery, serious staphylococcal disease stemming from colonization of the newborn is most common when the infant is between 3 weeks and 6 months of age. Therefore an accurate determination of the incidence of nursery-acquired infection requires surveillance outside the hospital, which can be done by a telephone survey.

Aside from impetigo, illnesses in infants associated with *S. aureus* include septicemia, osteomyelitis, pneumonia, localized boils, meningitis, and mastitis. Staphylococcal disease also may be transmitted from the infant to the family in the form of maternal mastitis or furunculosis, which may then be traded within a family for periods as long as 6 or 7 years.

DISEASE IN OLDER INFANTS AND CHILDREN.   Aside from the newborn, the infants and children usually afflicted with severe staphylococcal infections are those individuals who have deficiencies in host resistance, such as leukemia or other malignancies, cystic fibrosis, systemic collagen disease, or agammaglobulinemia. Included in this group with so-called altered host states are infants and children who have been subjected to cardiac or neurosurgical procedures, as well as those who have been treated for a long period of time with multiple or broad-spectrum antibiotic agents. Manifestations of staphylococcal disease in this group of individuals include septicemia with widespread metastatic lesions, staphylococcal pneumonia, endocarditis, enterocolitis, meningitis, and brain abscess. These syndromes are discussed in detail elsewhere.

An interesting feature of staphylococcal disease that follows cardiac or neurosurgical procedures (particularly those requiring rubber or plastic tubes) is the high proportion of strains of staphylococci that are coagulase-negative; although these organisms are usually saprophytic, the ability of coagulase-negative strains of staphylococci to produce disease in these circumstances as well as in the newborn is well documented. In otherwise healthy children, furunculosis, cellulitis, and osteomyelitis are the most common manifestations of staphylococcal disease.

TREATMENT.   In general, therapy for staphylococcal disease should consist of a sound antimicrobial regimen coupled with surgery when indicated. Some staphylococcal infections that occasionally occur, especially minor skin infections such as folliculitis, require no treatment at all in most cases. Established abscesses with localized collections of pus should be drained; the method may range from incision and drainage of a skin abscess to closed underwater drainage of a pleural empyema cavity.

The selection of a drug and the route of administration in therapy of staphylococcal disease is influenced by the age of the patient, the severity of the illness, and the probable antibiotic resistance of the *Staphylococcus*. Illness caused by *S. aureus* that develops in hospitalized patients and in infants recently discharged from the hospital or their contacts must be assumed to be caused by hospital strains of *S. aureus*, ie, strains that produce penicillinase and are therefore resistant to penicillin.

Bactericidal drugs administered systemically should be used in the treatment of serious staphylococcal disease. If the organism is sensitive to benzylpenicillin (penicillin G), this is still the drug of choice. When the disease is associated with hospital strains of staphylococci, the semisynthetic pencillinase-resistant penicillins are the drugs of choice. If the patient is allergic to penicillin or one of its semisynthetic derivatives, cephalothin (Keflin) may be used in the treatment of serious staphylococcal disease. However, it is becoming increasingly apparent that some of the patients allergic to penicillin are also allergic to cephalothin. Gentamicin may also prove to be useful in treatment of patients allergic to penicillin. Oral administration of any antimicrobial agent in the treatment of serious staphylococcal disease is not recommended because of the unpredictable absorption, the care required to ensure administration on an empty stomach, and the necessity for monitoring serum levels.

In the treatment of moderate staphylococcal disease, oral medication may be used. Penicillin G or phenoxypenicillins are the drugs of choice if the organism is penicillin-sensitive. Erythromycin or lincomycin may be used if the patient is allergic to penicillin. If the organism is penicillin-resistant the oral preparations of the semisynthetic penicillins (oxacillin, cloxacillin, or dicloxacillin) should be used.

Individuals and families with chronic recurrent furunculosis may be protected from lesions by artificial nasal colonization with a strain of *S. aureus* of low virulence (strain 502-A). This regimen includes a period of local and systemic antibiotic treatment prior to colonization.

Nonspecific agents used in the therapy of disease associated with *S. aureus* include various vaccines, toxoids, gamma globulin, and bacteriophage. In controlled observations there has been no good evidence that any of these substances is of significant value in the treatment of staphylococcal disease.

References

Boris M, Shinefield HR, Romano P, McCarthy DP, Florman AL: Bacterial interference. Protection against recurrent intrafamilial staphylococcal disease. Am J Dis Child 115:521, 1968

Gezon HM, Thompson DJ, Rogers KD, Hatch TF, Taylor PM: Hexachlorophene bathing in early infancy. Effect on staphylococcal disease and infection. N Engl J Med 270:379, 1964

Hurst V: Colonization in the newborn. In Maibach HA, Hildick-Smith G (eds): Skin Bacteria and Their Role in Infection. New York, McGraw-Hill, 1965, p 127

Light IJ, Sutherland JM, Schott EE: Control of a staphylococcal outbreak in a nursery, use of bacterial interference. JAMA 193:699, 1965

Melish ME, Glasgow LA: The staphylococcal scalded-skin syndrome. Development of an experimental model. N Engl J Med 282:1114, 1970

Schaffer TE, Baldwin JN, Wheeler WE: Staphylococcal infections in nurseries. Adv Pediatr 10:243, 1958

Shinefield HR, Ribble JC, Boris M, Sutherland JM: The Ohio epidemic. Am J Dis Child 105:655, 1963

——— Ribble JC, Eichenwald HF, Boris M, Sutherland JM: Bacterial inference. In Maibach HA, Hildick-Smith G (eds): Skin Bacteria and Their Role in Infection. New York, McGraw-Hill, 1965, p 235

——— Ribble JC: Current aspects of infections and diseases related to staphylococcus aureus. Ann Rev Med 16:263, 1965

STAPHYLOCOCCAL ENTEROCOLITIS AND FOOD POISONING

ALEX J. STEIGMAN

STAPHYLOCOCCAL ENTEROCOLITIS

Staphylococcal enterocolitis (pseudomembranous enterocolitis) is a serious condition that fortunately is rarely seen in children. Its most frequent occurrence is in adults being prepared for or convalescing from intestinal surgery. Multiple cleansing enemas and the use of antimicrobial agents, especially orally, may so reduce the content of gram-negative organisms that intestinal overgrowth with coagulase-positive *S. aureus* occasionally results.

A distended tender abdomen, fever, vomiting, diarrhea, dehydration, and shock may occur very abruptly. Large shreds of small and large intestine appear in the stools. Treatment must be prompt and vigorous (as for cholera), with vast amounts of fluid and electrolyte replacement being monitored closely by frequent laboratory assistance. Therapy for bacterial shock, including corticosteroids, is warranted. Vancomycin may be given orally, since it inhibits staphylococci without further reducing the content of gram-negative bacteria.

The necrotizing enterocolitis of infancy, such as may be seen in Hirschsprung's disease, is also a severe condition, but it is quite a different disease. One might expect staphylococcal enterocolitis to develop in certain other children, such as those with cystic fibrosis who have been taking oral antibiotics for extended periods, those with hepatic failure who are being treated with colonic irrigations and oral antibiotics, and infants and children undergoing extensive intestinal resections for various reasons. However, for the most part children seem to be largely unaffected by this very serious condition.

STAPHYLOCOCCAL FOOD POISONING

In the United States nearly 40 percent of all patients reported with acute food poisoning are of school age. Cases are most commonly due to ingestion of preformed, thermostable staphylococcal enterotoxins. When investigation is thorough the same phage types of coagulase-positive *S. aureus* are recovered from the responsible food and from nose and hands of persons who have been involved in its preparation. The clinical picture results from direct intoxication rather than infection and is due to enterotoxin A more often than enterotoxins B or D. Phage types implicated include 6/47/53/54/75/83a, 53/83/85/86, 6/47/53/85, and 54/75/77.

School cafeterias, restaurants, picnics, and parties usually set the stage for outbreaks. Meats, poultry, fish, salads, and custards are the usual culprits when prepared in bulk and set aside to be cooled and reheated prior to serving. There is some individual variation in response to a given amount of tainted food ingested. From 25 percent to almost 100 percent of exposed persons may show symptoms. The responsible foods are not putrefied and have neither bad taste nor odor. Between 1 and 7 hours, but usually after about 4 hours, symptoms appear as follows: increased salivation; nausea; vomiting and retching; midabdominal colicky pain, *not* as a rule radiating to the right lower quadrant; sweating and prostration, sometimes progressing to shock; muscle aching; headache. There is no fever, and the accompanying diarrhea is relatively mild or in some instances absent.

Fatality is virtually unknown in staphylococcal food poisoning, but the abrupt distress and prostration are very considerable, especially in school populations. Parenteral fluid administration may be necessary for the sickest children for 12 to 24 hours, but rarely longer. Cathartics should *not* be given; any attempt to speed exit of the toxin is in vain. Patients may resume oral intake at their own discretion. There are no known sequelae; no resistance to subsequent exposure is gained.

References

Silverman SJ, Knott AR, Howard M: Rapid sensitive assay for staphylococcal enterotoxin and a comparison of serological methods. Appl Microbiol 16:1019, 1968

Terplan K, Paine JR, Shefer J, Egan R, Lansky H: Fulminating gastroenteritis caused by Staphylococcus: its apparent connection with antibiotic medication. Gastroenterology 24:476, 1953

STREPTOCOCCAL INFECTIONS

GROUP A β-HEMOLYTIC STREPTOCOCCI
MILTON MARKOWITZ

Group A β-hemolytic streptococci are a frequent cause of illness in children. The more typical infections due to these bacteria include pharyngotonsillitis, scarlet fever, and the skin diseases impetigo and erysipelas. These infections are important in children because of the morbidity associated with them and their suppurative complications and because of the potential seriousness of their nonsuppurative sequelae (rheumatic fever and acute glomerulonephritis). Many of the complications of streptococcal infections can be prevented by accurate diagnosis and adequate therapy.

BIOLOGY AND IMMUNOLOGY. Streptococci are gram-positive organisms that tend to grow in chains. They are broadly classified by their reactions on mammalian blood cells. The clear zone of hemolysis surrounding colonies grown on mammalian blood agar distinguishes β-hemolytic streptococci from the α (green or partial hemolysis) and γ (nonhemolytic) species.

The β-hemolytic streptococci can be divided into a number of groups based on a specific carbohydrate antigen (C carbohydrate substance) in the cell wall. Eighteen distinct serologic groups have been recognized, and these groups have been designated by the letters A, B, C, etc. The serologic method of Lancefield is precise, but it is not feasible as a rapid diagnostic test. Group A organisms can be identified more rapidly by using appropriate fluorescein-conjugated antiserum. Group A strains can also be distinguished from other groups by differences in sensitivity to bacitracin. A bacitracin disk containing 0.02 units placed on the primary blood agar plate will inhibit growth of most group A strains, while those organisms that are not of group A are generally resistant to this antibiotic. This simple screening procedure is adaptable to use in routine laboratory and office practice.

Human infections are caused chiefly by group A organisms, and it is the only group involved in initiating rheumatic fever and acute glomerulonephritis. Group B streptococci have been identified as a cause of neonatal sepsis and meningitis. Mild pharyngitis may sometimes be due to group C or group G organisms. These groups are also frequently found in the pharynx of the healthy carrier. Group D (enterococci) strains are associated with sepsis of the newborn, genitourinary infections, and bacterial endocarditis. The other groups may cause serious disease, but they rarely occur in children.

The group A streptococcal cell wall contains a protein layer made up of the M, T, and R proteins. Of these, the M protein is the most important constituent. It is an immunologically specific antigen, and with antisera containing specific M antibody it is possible to subdivide group A streptococci into more than 50 distinct types. The identification of M serotypes has provided a valuable tool for epidemiologic investigation. For example, studies of this nature have shown that certain types (nephritogenic types), notably type 12, are more frequently associated with outbreaks of glomerulonephritis than are other types.

Strains containing M protein resist phagocytosis by human leukocytes, and a relationship between streptococcal M protein content and virulence has been demonstrated. Antibodies to M protein form the basis for human streptococcal immunity. This antigen stimulates production of type-specific antibodies that protect against infection with a homologous type but confer no immunity against other M types. Thus multiple streptococcal infections due to different types are the rule, and immunity is acquired only over a period of many years.

The T protein is also an immunologically distinct antigen that can be used to type streptococci. Typing by T agglutination is useful for identifying organisms not typable by the M protein precipitin method. In general, streptococci isolated from skin lesions can be typed only by the T agglutination technique. Studies of streptococcal skin infections have shown that they are caused chiefly by a few special types.

Group A streptococci secrete a large variety of enzymes and toxins (extracellular substances). With the exception of erythrogenic toxin, the roles of these substances in human disease are unknown. Erythrogenic toxin is responsible for the rash of scarlet fever. Streptococci vary in their ability to elaborate toxin, and it has been shown that streptococci infected with bacteriophage are good producers of erythrogenic toxin. Erythrogenic toxin stimulates the formation of antitoxin antibodies, which provide immunity against the scarlatiniform rash but not against streptococcal infections. However, since all toxins are not serologically identical, a second attack of scarlet fever may sometimes occur.

Many of the other extracellular substances are also antigenic and stimulate antibodies in man. Measurement of these antibodies is extremely useful as evidence of a recent streptococcal infection. The test for antibodies against streptolysin O (antistreptolysin O or ASO) is well standardized and is the most commonly performed streptococcal antibody determination. It is elevated in 70 to 80 percent of patients following untreated streptococcal infection.

EPIDEMIOLOGY. Streptococcal infections occur during all seasons and in all climates. However, pharyngeal infections are most common in the northern regions of the United States during the winter and early spring months. On the other hand, skin infections occur more frequently during the summer months, when abrasions and insect bites are likely to occur; streptococcal pyoderma is also prevalent in the southern parts of the country.

Streptococcal infections are uncommon in children under 2 years of age, although nursery epidemics have been described. The incidence is highest in young school-age children, chiefly because the school is an important locus for spread. Transmission usually occurs at school or in the home following direct contact with airborne droplets from the respiratory tracts of symptomatic or asymptomatic individuals. The recently infected, untreated respiratory tract carrier is the most dangerous and most common source of spread. However, transmission may occur via other carrier sites, including skin lesions, fingernails, and even the perianal region. These reservoirs may play an important role in disseminating streptococcal impetigo. Spread by contaminated food is occasionally a cause of explosive outbreaks of pharyngitis.

Multiple cases in a family are common. The risk to child contacts in the same household varies from 20 to 50 percent, depending on the virulence of the organism, the degree of crowding, and other factors. Streptococci may spread through the family over a period of several weeks, but most of the acquisitions among contacts occur within a few days after the index case has been identified. While adults in the family are much less likely to acquire streptococci, studies have shown that as many as 15 percent of mothers may harbor the organism. For reasons that are not at all clear, some families appear particularly prone to streptococcal infections.

CLINICAL MANIFESTATIONS. PHARYNGITIS. The signs and symptoms of streptococcal pharyngitis vary greatly. The infection may go unrecognized because of the paucity of constitutional or localizing symptoms, or the patient may be extremely toxic. In the latter situation there is a rapid onset of high fever accompanied by malaise, headache, sore throat, and severe pain on swallowing. Vomiting and abdominal pain may be prominent symptoms at the onset, suggesting a gastroenteritis. Coryza, hoarseness, cough, and diarrhea are uncommon. Examination of the pharynx and tonsils in the classic picture reveals one or more of the following findings: beefy redness of the pharyngeal tissues, edema of the uvula, flecks or confluent exudate on the tonsils, and petechiae on the soft palate. The anterior cervical glands are enlarged and tender. Skin petechiae are not uncommon, and a frank scarlatiniform rash may be present.

The diagnosis of a streptococcal illness can be made with fair certainty on the basis of clinical findings alone only when a characteristic rash is present. In the absence of a rash, the diagnosis can be strongly suspected if the pharyngeal findings are typical, especially when exudate is present. The findings are generally less characteristic in patients without tonsils, and in a significant number of patients the pharynx shows a variable degree of redness without any of the other features noted above. Furthermore, pharyngeal exudate in children under 3 years of age is more often associated with viral infection than with streptococcal infection. Indeed, streptococcal illness in young children is atypical and is usually characterized by anorexia, low-grade fever, and purulent nasal discharge with excoriations around the nares.

It is apparent, therefore, that streptococcal respiratory disease can present with various clinical pictures, and it is often difficult to distinguish between viral and streptococcal pharyngitis. An awareness of the current epidemiology of infections in the family or in the community can be helpful. However, the diagnosis can be made with assurance only by bacteriologic means. The throat culture is a simple and accurate method to confirm the diagnosis. Many communities have laboratories that process cultures sent in by mail. Some physicians have found it expedient to use a small office incubator and commercially available selective medium (sheep blood agar) that simplifies identification of β-hemolytic streptococci.

SCARLET FEVER. Scarlet fever is a streptococcal illness associated with a characteristic rash. It is due to an infection with erythrogenic toxin-producing group A streptococci in individuals who do not have antitoxin antibodies. It is now encountered less commonly than in the past, but the incidence is cyclic, depending on the prevalence of toxin-producing strains and the immune status of the population. The modes of transmission, age distribution, and other epidemiologic features are otherwise similar to those of streptococcal pharyngitis.

Prior to 1940 scarlet fever often presented as a particularly virulent form of streptococcal disease with marked toxic manifestations and a high incidence of septicemia and suppurative complications. At the present time the disease is much milder, probably because antimicrobial agents abort the illness, although a change in virulence of the organisms may be playing a role.

The rash appears within 24 to 48 hours after onset of symptoms, although it may be present with the first signs of illness. It often begins around the neck and spreads over the trunk and extremities. It is a diffuse, finely papular, erythematous eruption producing a bright red discoloration of the skin, which blanches on pressure. It is often more intense along the creases of the elbows, axillae, and groin. The skin has a goose-pimple appearance and feels rough to the touch. The face is usually spared, and there may be pallor around the mouth. After 3 to 4 days the rash begins to fade and is followed by a furfuraceous desquamation over the trunk and frank peeling of the skin around the fingertips.

In addition to the findings noted in streptococcal pharyngitis, there are punctate erythematous lesions on the palate and on the surrounding mucous membranes. The tongue is coated and the papillae are swollen. Following desquamation the reddened papillae are prominent, giving the tongue a strawberry appearance.

The typical case of scarlet fever is not difficult to diagnose. However, the milder form with equivocal pharyngeal findings can be confused with rubella, exanthema subitum, and drug eruptions. Staphylococcal infections are occasionally associated with a scarlatiniform rash. A history of recent exposure to a streptococcal infection is helpful. Isolation of the β-hemolytic streptococci from the nasopharynx will confirm the diagnosis in doubtful cases. If the patient is seen several days after the onset, peeling around the fingers should arouse suspicion of a recent attack of scarlet fever.

PYODERMA. Streptococcal pyoderma or impetigo is a superficial infection of the skin that appears first as a discrete papulovesicular lesion surrounded by a localized area of redness. The vesicles rapidly become purulent and covered with a thick, confluent, amber-colored crust that gives the appearance of having been applied to the skin. The lesions may occur anywhere, but are more common on the face and extremities. If untreated, they run a chronic course spreading to other parts of the body. Regional lymphadenitis is common. The chronic form may involve the deeper layers of the skin, causing a condition known as ecthyma, but a concomitant deep-seated cellulitis rarely occurs.

Streptococcal impetigo is generally not accompanied by fever or other systemic reactions. Impetiginized excoriations around the nares or the earlobes are seen with active streptococcal infections of the nasopharynx or with purulent otitis media. However, impetigo is not usually associated with an overt streptococcal infection of the upper respiratory tract. Furthermore, streptococci can be isolated from the pharynx in only a minority of cases of streptococcal impetigo. For these reasons the concept that the respiratory tract is the primary source of infection in streptococcal impetigo has been questioned, and the evidence now suggests that infections can spread to other individuals directly from the skin lesions. Multiple cases in the same family are common.

It may be difficult to distinguish clinically between streptococcal and staphylococcal impetigo. The latter lesions are more often bullous; they have a thinner crust and occur more commonly in neonates and young infants. In older children mixed infections are common. At times staphylococci overgrow the culture and obscure the presence of streptococci. However, careful bacteriologic studies have shown that streptococci are found with or without staphylococci in as many as 80 percent of children with impetigo. It would seem prudent, therefore, to treat impetigo in older children as a streptococcal infection.

ERYSIPELAS. Erysipelas is an acute streptococcal infection involving the deeper layers of the skin and the underlying connective tissue. It is rarely seen in infants and children at the present time. The skin over the affected area is swollen, red, and very tender. Superficial blebs may be present. The most characteristic finding is the sharply defined, slightly elevated border. At times reddish streaks of lymphangitis project out from the margins of the lesion. A septic fever and other signs of infection are present. The characteristic skin lesion distinguishes this condition from other bacterial causes of cellulitis. Staphylococci, a common cause of cellulitis, produce a diffuse brawny inflammation without a sharply demarcated border. However, other bacteria may sometimes cause erysipelaslike lesions. Cultures obtained by needle puncture of the inflamed area will usually reveal the etiologic agent.

COMPLICATIONS. In the untreated or inadequately treated patient with streptococcal pharyngitis the acute phase of the illness usually subsides within several days, but the child may continue for some weeks to feel below par, with loss of appetite, pallor, fatigability, and low-grade fever. In such patients the pharynx and tonsils may show residual signs of infection along with slightly enlarged and tender anterior cervical lymph glands. The pharyngeal culture will usually demonstrate a moderately heavy growth of β-hemolytic streptococci. Antimicrobial therapy generally results in marked improvement.

Suppurative complications from the spread of streptococci to adjacent structures were very common before antibiotics became available; they usually made their appearance within a week after onset of the pharyngitis. Cervical adenitis, otitis media, mastoiditis, and sinusitis still occur in children in whom the primary illness has gone unnoticed or in whom treatment of the pharyngitis has been inadequate. Such patients are also vulnerable to serious metastatic infections involving the meninges, bones, or joints. The diagnosis is made by isolating β-hemolytic streptococci from the bloodstream or from the site of the localized abscess. Intensive antimicrobial therapy is indicated.

The nonsuppurative sequelae (rheumatic fever and acute glomerulonephritis) are well-recognized complications of streptococcal infections, although the pathogenetic mechanisms are still poorly understood. The latent period between the infection and the onset of these complications varies from 1 to 2 weeks for glomerulonephritis and from 2 to 4 weeks for rheumatic fever. There is also a difference in the relationship of these sequelae to the site of the streptococcal infection. Glomerulonephritis can follow group A streptococcal infections of either the pharynx or the skin, whereas rheumatic fever is a sequel of a pharyngeal infection and rarely if ever follows pyoderma. The attack rate of rheumatic fever following untreated streptococcal pharyngitis varies from 0.3 to 3 percent, the higher incidence occurring during some of the epidemic outbreaks of streptococcal infections. There is no known relationship between the M serotype causing a streptococcal pharyngitis and the occurrence of rheumatic fever, although the possibility of rheumatogenic strains cannot be excluded. On the other hand, acute glomerulonephritis occurs more commonly after pharyngeal infections with certain M serotypes, particularly type 12 but also types 49, 1, and 4. Recent evidence also indicates that nephritis after pyoderma is more common following skin infections with a few serotypes. However, the types associated with pyoderma and nephritis (types 2, 55, and 57) differ from the nephritogenic types found in the upper respiratory tract. The incidence of acute glomerulonephritis varies with the prevalence of nephritogenic strains in the community. In outbreaks associated with nephritogenic strains in the pharynx or in skin lesions the incidence of nephritis varies from 10 to 15 percent.

TREATMENT. Streptococcal infections should be treated with sufficient antibiotic therapy to eradicate the organisms. Treatment that accomplishes this goal will diminish the spread to family and school contacts, virtually prevent all suppurative complications, and minimize the chance of developing nonsuppurative complications, especially rheumatic fever.

The indications for treating patients with scarlet fever or with the classic features of streptococcal infections are usually straightforward, and therapy is warranted prior to bacteriologic confirmation. In less typical cases it is desirable to withhold treatment until the bacteriologic findings are known. This approach is feasible if the laboratory report can be made available within 24 to 48 hours. It may not always be possible to distinguish the true streptococcal infection from an intercurrent illness in a patient who happens to be carrying β-hemolytic streptococci in his pharynx. The number of colonies in the throat culture may be helpful, since there are usually numerous colonies, and rarely fewer than 10, in patients with streptococcal infection. If the organisms are not group A streptococci, it is likely that the patient is a carrier. It has been suggested that certain group A infections are relatively benign, rarely lead to complications, and therefore may not require vigorous therapy. There are no absolute criteria for selecting such cases, and one should be aware that in at least one-third of patients with rheumatic fever the preceding streptococcal infection is subclinical in nature.

Group A streptococci are exquisitely sensitive to penicillin, and resistant strains have never been encountered. Penicillin is therefore the drug of choice for pharyngeal and skin infections as well as for the suppurative complications. The type of penicillin used and the route of administration are not nearly as important as the duration of treatment. A therapeutic level for a minimum period of 10 days is necessary to eradicate the organisms in most patients. Oral penicillin in doses of 800,000 to 1.2 million IU daily for 10 days is a satisfactory form of treatment. If penicillin G is used, it must be administered either before or 2 hours after meals. Phenoxymethylpenicillin may be given without regard to food. The newer penicillins (dicloxacillin, nafcillin, and ampicillin) offer no advantage over the less expensive penicillins in therapy of streptococcal infections. The major problem with all forms of oral therapy is the risk that the drug will be discontinued before the 10-day course has been completed, chiefly because the child usually appears to have recovered in 3 or 4 days. Therefore when oral treatment is prescribed the necessity of completing a full course of therapy must be emphasized. If the parents seem unlikely to comply because of family disorganization, difficulties in comprehension, or for other reasons, parenteral therapy is indicated. A single intramuscular injection of 600,000 to 1.2 million IU of benzathine penicillin G is the most efficacious and often the most practical method of treatment. Its only disadvantage is soreness around the site of injection that may last for several days. The local reaction is diminished when benzathine penicillin G is combined with procaine penicillin G. However, when this combination is used in a single injection, one must be certain that an adequate amount of benzathine penicillin G is administered.

From 10 to 15 percent of patients treated with a full course of penicillin continue to harbor β-hemolytic streptococci. The reasons for these bacteriologic failures are not clear. It has been suggested that penicillinase-producing staphylococci in the pharynx may interfere with the action of penicillin, but if this does occur it is not the cause of most failures. Indeed, the use of penicillin active against both streptococci and staphylococci does not seem to reduce the incidence of bacteriologic relapses. Not infrequently the pharyngeal culture following treatment shows β-hemolytic streptococci that prove not to be group A organisms and need be no cause for concern. However, if group A streptococci do persist, a second course of penicillin, preferably with benzathine penicillin, should be given. There is some evidence to suggest that lincomycin may be more effective than penicillin for such patients, but this observation needs to be confirmed.

There are occasions when streptococci persist even after several courses of antibiotics. Organisms can be carried for months without any evidence of illness. Such individuals are not likely to develop complications. They are lightly colonized and are not dangerous to others. The carrier state may also aid in the development of type-specific immunity. When signs of illness do reappear, it is almost always due to an infection with a new serotype. Some individuals are especially prone to recurrent streptococcal infections, and in such patients the tonsils are often incriminated as a source of the difficulty. There is some evidence that tonsillectomy reduces the frequency of streptococcal infections, although this may be more apparent than real, since it is easier to culture streptococci from patients with tonsils. While repeated proved streptococcal infections of the tonsils may be an indication for removal, the age of the child as well as other factors must be taken into consideration.

There is the additional problem of treating a patient who is allergic to penicillin. The sulfonamides should not be used, since they suppress but do not eradicate the streptococci. Since from 30 to 40 percent of group A streptococci are resistant to tetracycline, it also should not be employed. Erythromycin or lincomycin are satisfactory drugs for patients allergic to penicillin. Although strains of group A streptococci resistant to these drugs have been reported, the possibility of encountering such a strain is rare at the present time. The dosage for erythromycin or lincomycin is 25 mg/kg/day for 10 days.

Systemic penicillin therapy is indicated for streptococcal pyoderma. A possible exception is the patient seen early with very few lesions that clear rapidly following removal of the crusts and cleansing of the affected areas with hexachlorophene soap. If the lesions persist, spread, or recur, antibiotic therapy should be started. Ointments containing bacitracin or neomycin fail to eradicate the streptococci in a significant number of patients. Penicillin orally or an injection of benzathine penicillin G is effective for streptococcal pyoderma regardless of whether staphylococci are also present. The question of whether penicillin therapy reduces the incidence of nephritis following pyoderma cannot be answered at the present time.

Complete isolation of patients with streptococcal infections is not warranted. There is a rapid decrease in the number of organisms after 3 days of adequate treatment, and children can usually return to school within 5 days. However, since it is necessary to maintain a therapeutic drug level for 10 days for maximum eradication of the organisms, if oral agents are used medication must be continued while the child attends school. As a matter of convenience the full daily requirement of oral penicillin can be given in two divided doses during the later stage of treatment. The use of a single injection of benzathine penicillin G obviates the need for maintaining treatment after the patient returns to school.

PREVENTION. The only specific indication for the long-term use of antibiotics to prevent streptococcal infections is for patients who have had an attack of acute rheumatic fever. Prevention can be accomplished by monthly injections of 1.2 million IU of benzathine penicillin G, 200,000 IU of oral penicillin twice a day, or 0.5 to 1.0 g of sulfadiazine daily. While the last drug should not be used for the treatment of streptococcal infection, it is an effective prophylactic agent.

The frequency with which streptococcal infections spread to other members of the family raises the question of prophylaxis for household contacts. The use of small prophylactic doses of penicillin or another antimicrobial agent is unwise, since individuals already infected will be undertreated. An alternative method of treating the entire family with therapeutic doses for 10 days is expensive, and in families under good medical supervision it is probably unwarranted. However, the incidence of positive cultures in members of families living in crowded quarters may be as high as 50 percent, and since these families do not usually have easy access to medical care, treatment of the entire family at the time the index case is identified may be justified. A more desirable approach is to culture all members of the family within a few days after the first case is discovered and treat the individuals with positive cultures as well as those who subsequently show evidence of clinical infection. This approach should always be used when a patient with acute glomerulonephritis is identified, since multiple cases in one family may occur.

Apart from rheumatic fever prophylaxis and the prevention of intrafamily spread, the ability to prevent streptococcal infections is very limited at the present time. Mass prophylaxis is generally not feasible except during epidemics in military populations and occasionally during large outbreaks in schools. The possibility of a streptococcal vaccine offers the promise of a more biologic and more easily applied method than is presently available. The M protein antigen involved in streptococcal immunity has been purified and has been shown to induce antibodies in human volunteers. The ideal vaccine would need to contain purified M antigens of more than 50 serotypes, a seemingly insurmountable problem. However, since most streptococcal infections are caused by a relatively small number of types, an effective vaccine against prevalent strains may be feasible. The question of complete safety has not been fully resolved and will not be until the relationships of streptococcal substances such as M protein to human disease have been elucidated. Until a better method for preventing streptococcal infections becomes available, the proper management of these infections is the surest way to minimize the incidence of complications.

References

Breese BB: Beta hemolytic streptococcal infections in children. Pediatr Clin North Am 7:843, 1960

Dillon HC: Group A type 12 streptococcal infection in a newborn nursery. Am J Dis Child 112:177, 1966

Eickoff TC, Klein JO, Daly K, Ingall D, Finland M: Neonatal sepsis and other infections due to group B beta-hemolytic streptococci. N Engl J Med 271:1221, 1964

Lancefield RC: Current knowledge of type-specific M antigens of group A streptococci. J Immunol 89:307, 1962

McCarty M: The hemolytic streptococci. In Dubos RJ, Hirsch JB (eds): Bacterial and Mycotic Infections of Man. Philadelphia, JB Lippincott, 1965

Maxted WR: The use of bacitracin for identifying group A hemolytic streptococci. J Clin Pathol 6:224, 1953

Quie PG, Pierce HC, Wannamaker LW: Influence of penicillin-producing staphylococci on the eradication of group A streptococci from the upper respiratory tract by penicillin treatment. Pediatr 37:467, 1966

Rammelkamp CH Jr: Epidemiology of streptococcal infections. Harvey Lect 51:113, 1957

Rosenstein BJ, Markowitz M, Goldstein E, Kramer I, O'Mansky B, Seidel H: Factors involved in treatment failures following oral penicillin therapy of streptococcal pharyngitis. J Pediatr 73:513, 1968

Sanders E, Foster MT, Scott D: Group A beta-hemolytic streptococci resistant to erythromycin and lincomycin. N Engl J Med 278:1221, 1964

Stollerman GH: Prospects for a vaccine against group A streptococci: the problem of the immunology of M proteins. Arthritis Rheum 10:245, 1967

Wannamaker LW: Differences between streptococcal infections of the throat and of the skin. N Engl J Med 282:23, 78, 1970

GROUP B β-HEMOLYTIC STREPTOCOCCI

ALEX J. STEIGMAN

The group B β-hemolytic *Streptococcus* (GBS) is now recognized as an important pathogen, especially in early life. GBS has been known in the past as an inhabitant of the adult female urogenital system and the urethra of male consorts. The incidence of this generally silent infection in women varies; it has been observed in many parts of the world.

CLINICAL CONSIDERATIONS. Newborn infants may have simple colonizations of GBS, or they may have very serious consequences. Different forms of GBS disease are observed, with distinctive clinical epidemiologic and bacteriologic findings.

Immediate Perinatal Period. If infection occurs during labor and delivery there may result in the newborn infant an overwhelming pneumonia and septicemia that may be accompanied by meningitis. Maternal factors predisposing to greater severity of disease include premature labor, prolonged rupture of membranes, chorioamnionitis, and maternal perinatal fever. Under these circumstances a rapidly downhill clinical course occurs, fatal within 24 to 48 hours. The acute respiratory distress, especially in low-birth-weight infants, may erroneously be ascribed to the respiratory distress syndrome. The abrupt onset of respiratory symptoms and shock soon after delivery suggests that intrauterine infection with rapid multiplication of the organism may have begun prior to the onset of labor. The reported mortality rate is 50 to 60 percent in this form of GBS disease.

Delayed-Onset Disease with Meningitis. Normal newborn infants, at an interval of 1 week to several months after delivery, may develop septicemia with acute pyogenic meningitis due to GBS. The onset may be insidious for 1 to 2 days. The disease responds to penicillin therapy; nevertheless, the mortality approximates 15 to 20 percent, and neurologic and mental abnormalities following recovery are not rare. Less frequent manifestations of GBS disease in young infants include osteomyelitis, otitis media and impetigo neonatorum.

BACTERIOLOGY. The specificity of the Lancefield groups of β-hemolytic streptococci is due to different specific capsular polysaccarides (C substances). There are four subtypes of GBS (Ia, Ib, II, and III); the specificity of each is determined by an additional capsular polysaccharide (S substances). This is unlike the case with the better-known group A β-hemolytic streptococci, in which the subtypes owe their specificities to a protein M substance.

Many institutions are not in a position to distinguish by specific serologic tests among the letter-designated groups of β-hemolytic streptococci. On the basis of resistance to bacitracin, disk cultures are often reported presumptively as being β-hemolytic *Streptococcus* not group A. When the source of such a specimen is a newborn or a very young infant (blood, cerebrospinal fluid, umbilical, throat, skin), or the specimen is from the maternal urethra or vagina, the likelihood of GBS should immediately be entertained. Additional indirect confirmatory tests generally available are a rapid test for hydrolysis of sodium hippurate, bacitracin susceptibility, and tolerance to 6.5 percent sodium chloride broth. Subtyping of GBS strains requires referral to specific study centers.

EPIDEMIOLOGY AND DISEASE CONTROL. The primary reservoir of GBS infection without disease is the female urogenital system (urethra and vagina principally); hospital personnel appear to represent an additional source of infection. Mothers may remain carriers for a long time with not only positive genital and rectal cultures but also positive throat and skin cultures.

The carrier state in colonized babies and adults is difficult to eradicate, despite the ready susceptibility of GBS to penicillin. Infants may be infected by mothers or hospital attendants in the early days of life or by parents and others in the next weeks or months at home. Babies successfully treated for meningitis with penicillin may continue to harbor GBS in their alimentary tracts. The ability of this organism to persist on mucous surfaces, despite penicillin therapy, creates an important problem of control, which is similar to the problem with *Niesseria meningitidis*. Investigations of humoral and cellular immune reactions of the host have not yet clarified the nature of this serious disease, whose

increasing incidence is not due merely to improved recognition. It is considered possible that some mothers have only a surface infection and therefore develop no circulating immunoglobulin GBS antibodies that might help alleviate the clinical picture of acute early-onset disease.

In terms of maternal-to-infant infection, the GBS situation is more complex and serious than is gonococcal infection. Some authorities believe that primary prevention requires prepartum and/or intrapartum cultures, with immediate use of penicillin in the mother and newborn for those found infected. This will not eradicate the carrier state or colonization, but it may decrease the incidence of early-onset, severe, often fatal neonatal disease. The infants who develop delayed-onset disease with meningitis and/or other clinical manifestations are equally perplexing: one must consider whether clinically silent colonization at birth has been activated by some intercurrent environmental event, or whether transmission of infection has occurred some days or weeks later at home.

Reference

Baker CJ, Barrett FF: Transmission of group B streptocci among parturient women and their neonates. J Pediatr 83:919, 1973

SYPHILIS
Laurence Finberg

Syphilis is an infectious disease with both acute and chronically relapsing phases. The causative organism becomes widely disseminated, and the resultant pathology may have a direct or indirect effect on every organ and tissue of the body. Long clinically latent periods are common. In temperate climates and in highly developed societies, the principal mode of transmission of the disease is through sexual contact. In addition, infants may be infected prior to birth—a form of the disease called prenatal or congenital syphilis. Although the term congenital is inaccurate, it is so widely accepted that it is used here interchangeably with prenatal as signifying syphilis acquired in utero or at birth.

The tropical diseases yaws and pinta and the condition known as endemic syphilis (sometimes given such local names as bejel in the Middle East and njovera or dichuchwa in parts of Africa) are closely related and probably are clinical variants of syphilis. The variations probably result from environmental factors of climate and culture and possibly also from genetic differences in parasite or host or both. In these conditions, seen mostly in children, spread takes place through nonsexual direct bodily contact.

In the United States the present reported incidence of syphilis exceeds 25,000 new infectious cases per year. The estimated actual incidence is in excess of 60,000. The occurrence of the disease, which had declined sharply following the introduction of penicillin (from over 100,000 reported infectious cases in 1947 to a low of 6,250 in 1957), has thus shown a marked increase.

Prenatal (congenital) syphilis reported among infants under 1 year of age has doubled in incidence during the past decade. Since the disease is both preventable and effectively treatable, the public health significance is apparent.

ETIOLOGY.   Syphilis is caused by an anaerobic spirochetal organism, *Treponema pallidum.* The organism varies from 4 to 10 μ in length and usually consists of from 6 to 14 coils. The causative treponemas of yaws and pinta, although given different species names (*T. pertenue* and *T. carateum*), are morphologically and otherwise indistinguishable from *T. pallidum.* Identification of the living organism is accomplished by dark-field microscopy of a preparation of the serous discharge from gently abraded lesions. A scraping of the moist umbilical cord of an infected infant provides a suitable preparation for finding the spirochetes. The presence of the organism in tissue is demonstrated by Levaditi (silver) stains. *T. pallidum* is destroyed by temperatures over 40 C and does not multiply at temperatures below 30 C. The organism cannot survive even for a few minutes without moisture; it is this characteristic, plus the anaerobic requirement, that makes transmission by fomites nearly impossible.

TRANSMISSION OF PRENATAL SYPHILIS.   As already noted, syphilis is usually transmitted venereally. Since infection results in a bacteremia, the disease may also be transmitted via the bloodstream across the placenta from mother to fetus. Ample evidence strongly suggests that this event does not result in infection during the first half of pregnancy. From the fifth lunar month until termination of pregnancy, a mother may transmit the disease to her infant during periods of spirochetemia. Should the mother remain untreated she may continue to infect successive infants over a number of years. During the early months of the illness in the untreated mother the probability is about 95 percent that the infant will acquire the disease in utero. With the passage of years the probability diminishes. How many years a mother may remain infectious from the original illness cannot be stated with certainty, because superinfection cannot be excluded in those instances where pregnancies separated by 20 years have produced syphilitic infants. Third-generation syphilis, which undoubtedly has occurred, must be subject to the same reservation. The phenomenon of diminution of severity of infection in succeeding pregnancies (Kassowitz's law) probably illustrates decreasing infective doses. The most severely infected fetus becomes a macerated stillborn with disseminated tissue damage; the least affected will be asymptomatic at birth; in between is the symptomatic syphilitic infant who has an increased chance of being born prematurely.

INFECTIOUSNESS OF ACUTE FORM.   Any moist lesions on the maternal skin or mucous membrane may be infectious on intimate contact, so that the birth process itself may be a time of acquisition of disease. Similarly, moist lesions, including nasal secretions, of an infected infant are infectious, but the contact must be rather intimate. Thus while care in handling infants with open lesions is needed, there is no airborne spread. The only caution required is that those whose hands might ordinarily touch the moist lesions or secretions be alert to avoid contact with open lesions or wear protective gloves. Twenty-four hours after appropriate therapy with penicillin, patients are noninfectious.

PATHOGENESIS AND NATURAL COURSE. Syphilis in the early stages is a relapsing, intermittently infectious process. In the acquired form there may be a *primary or chancre stage*, with a lesion at the point of entry and in regional lymph nodes. This phase, which is often omitted even in older individuals, does not occur in the prenatal variety.

The early disease, which is characterized by intermittent hematogenous dissemination, causes symmetric and pervasive involvement of body tissues. After a time the chronic lesions may develop in localized foci in almost any tissue. Late lesions tend to be asymmetric, to involve marked tissue reaction, and to be noninfectious. Pathologic studies illustrate this distinction, showing primarily round cell infiltration and subacute inflammation in early disease and a granulomatous process with marked tissue necrosis and scarring in the late form.

The general types of pathology described may occur in any organ or tissue, making possible an extraordinarily large number of clinical variants. The disease occurring in infancy and early childhood has several pathologic features distinguishing it from disease acquired in later life. A severely affected fetus shows some unique features, including interstitial fibrosis of the liver, spleen, and sometimes other organs and a *pneumonia alba* consisting of increased connective tissue infiltrating the lung. Another difference is the rarity of cardiovascular involvement in the childhood disease, contrasted with an incidence of 15 percent, most commonly aortitis, in adults. This difference, apparently attributable to developmental factors, seems to hold in children for both the congenital disease and that acquired prior to puberty.

Another major difference is the occurrence of the *stigmata* of congenital syphilis. These lesions are the results of precisely timed damage to developing tissue during the early phase of the disease, with manifestations becoming visible only later in life. They are of three kinds: scarring of tissue that is affected early, such as the lips and nose; destructive lesions to tissues such as teeth that do not erupt until late childhood; tissue alteration leading to allergic-type lesions such as interstitial keratitis. These stigmas, while characteristic of congenital syphilis, are in fact nonspecific and can be imitated, although rarely, by other disease processes.

The natural course of untreated syphilitic illness in the adult has been well described in a very careful epidemiologic study carried out in Oslo over an extended period of time. Approximately 50 percent of patients, one-half of whom were seropositive, had no long-term ill-effects. Roughly another quarter of the patients had late benign manifestations, such as gummas or liver involvement. The final 25 percent had one of the more severe late forms (cardiovascular syphilis or neurosyphilis). Most, but not all, of the late forms are seropositive.

No comparable data are available for childhood syphilis; moreover many severely infected infants succumb or are stillborn, making the comparison more difficult. However, if one removes the cardiovascular complications and makes allowance for the early mortality in the infantile group, clinical experience suggests that the course of untreated syphilis in children is similar to that of acquired syphilis in adults.

IMMUNOLOGY AND SERODIAGNOSIS. The antibody response to syphilitic infection has been widely studied but remains imperfectly understood. The infection confers good immunity against symptomatic reinfection if the original process is not treated during the first few years. During the early years of the disease, while humoral antibody titers are high, living organisms persist and may be recovered. Even many years later the organisms may be recovered, although the tissues appear altered in such a way that a new infection may not be acquired. Following adequate treatment early in the disease, reinfection occurs readily, with the clinical course duplicating that of the original infection.

There are both nonspecific antibodies (reagin) and specific antibodies (*Treponema*-immobilizing) that appear in response to syphilitic infection. Both appear in the adult; they are IgM and IgG in size. Maternal IgG may be transmitted to the fetus across the placenta, so that maternal antibody (reagin and specific) may appear in both infected and noninfected newborns. The neonate is relatively incapable of manufacturing IgG, but he may make his own IgM antibody. Recently Alford and associates demonstrated the presence of an IgM-fluorescent treponemal antibody in the serum of newborn infants. This test permits a specific serologic laboratory diagnosis to be made during the first days of life. It is important that the test for specific IgM be performed by expert laboratories, since studies have shown that many routine laboratories are reporting false-positives for this test.

The nonspecific antibody is also found in response to other diseases, which may be divided into three categories useful in differential diagnosis. First, in other treponemal diseases, such as yaws and pinta, the titers of non-specific antibodies are similar to those in syphilis, and indeed the significance is probably identical; for these conditions the specific antibody response is also similar if not identical. Second, certain chronic diseases, especially leprosy, result in reagin production in moderately high titer; this point must be remembered in those areas where leprosy is prevalent. Finally, a large variety of infections and connective tissue diseases may produce a lower titer of reagin, the biologic false-positive. Those of special importance to the pediatrician are infectious mononucleosis, vaccinia, chickenpox, and lupus erythematosus. A number of mild viral infections may also result in an increased titer of reagin. For acute infections the phenomenon is transitory, and in all of these instances the titers are low and seldom exceed a dilution of 1:16.

Despite these limitations, reagin tests (serologic tests for syphilis, STS) remain a useful and valuable tool in the diagnosis of syphilis because of speed and ease of determination. The VDRL (Venereal Disease Research Laboratories) test and some of its modifications providing rapid determination give a high degree of sensitivity. The specificity requires interpretation by the clinician, occasionally reinforced by confirmatory use of the more cumbersome and expensive specific tests such as the treponema immobilization test (TPI). Thus far, none of the specific tests has been adapted to a sensitive form that is at once technically rapid, reliable, and inexpensive, although because of its specificity the TPI has great value in resolving diagnostic problems.

The STS commonly performed fall into two technical categories: those typified by the Wassermann and Kolmer, which use the technique of complement fixation, and those typified by the Kahn, Eagle, Mazzini, and VDRL, which measure flocculation. The flocculation technique is simpler and faster and hence is more widely used for sera. *Quantitative titration* of these antibodies is possible and very useful, both for diagnostic differentiation and for following patients, since in early disease the antibody disappears over a period of a few months following therapy. Measurement of antibody in cerebrospinal fluid requires a complement-fixation method.

When a flocculation test is performed on any serum that may have a high titer, it is important to run a *high-dilution specimen* as well as the standard dilution during the initial screening process. Occasionally a high level of antibody may inhibit flocculation in the standard dilution and be interpreted as a negative test (the prozone phenomenon); this phenomenon is encountered commonly during early syphilis in infants.

The antibody transferred from mother to fetus transplacentally (7S) will produce a positive STS in the infant. The titer may be equal to but not higher than the mother's. The TPI antibody behaves similarly. Both disappear from the infant following a logarithmic curve, being unmeasurable in most infants at 8 weeks and in all at 12 weeks of age. Most infected infants have very little of their own (19S) antibody at birth (about one-third are seronegative, having neither passive nor active antibody), but invariably some is produced by 8 weeks of age. The two titer curves, one falling and one rising, merge to produce a single resultant with a variety of possible configurations. Using standard serologic procedures, interpretation of diagnostic significance may in some instances be made only after 8 or 12 weeks of age, although usually an earlier decision may be reached even without supporting clinical data. If adequate treatment is given early in the disease, the STS titer begins to fall within 4 weeks. From the foregoing facts one may appreciate the difficulties in interpreting, for clinical purposes, serologic data on an asymptomatic seropositive infant who has received penicillin.

EARLY CONGENITAL (PRENATAL) SYPHILIS. As already indicated, the most severely infected infants are stillborn. Most live-born syphilic infants have no visible lesions at birth. When lesions are present they are most commonly on the skin and in the bones. In the first week of life syphilis may produce a bullous lesion of the skin on the palms and soles. This almost pathognomonic lesion, although quite uncommon, has importance, because no other syphilitic skin lesion at any age forms bullae or vesicles. The more usual pattern of skin involvement is a diffuse, symmetric, copper-colored maculopapular rash that is most intense on the face, palms, and soles. It is an infiltrative type of lesion that when gently scraped with a scalpel will yield serum teeming with treponemas. If left untreated, about 90 percent of syphilitic infants will eventually have some kind of skin lesion. Many varieties of papular skin rashes may occur and recur over the next months with a high predilection for mucocutaneous sites, oral and anal. Perioral lesions may result in scarring, with fissures that persist. The recurrences become progressively less symmetric with time. The perianal condylomatous lesion (condyloma latum) so commonly seen in adults is also seen in infancy (Fig. 7).

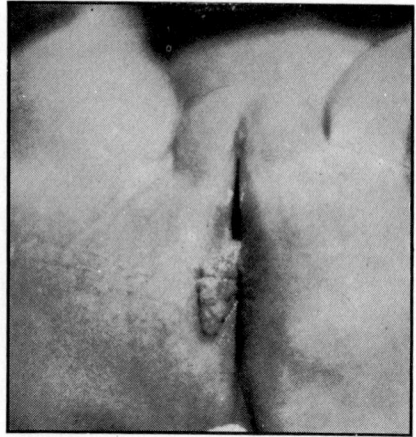

FIG. 7.   Syphilitic condyloma of an infant 9 months of age.

A rather characteristic mucous membrane lesion of infants having no counterpart in the adult is *snuffles*, a rhinitis producing a serous discharge that frequently becomes secondarily infected. The lesion may extend to the nasal cartilage and cause sufficient damage to result in *saddle nose deformity*.

The disease produces widespread lesions in the skeleton, resulting in quite characteristic radiographs that reveal osteochondritis at metaphyseal plates, a generalized symmetric periosteal elevation, and symmetrically occurring osteomyelitic lesions. The humerus is the most commonly involved bone, with the tibia next; indeed, if other bones are involved, these two are almost sure to be involved as well. Wimberger described a bilateral motheaten appearance of the medial aspects of the proximal tibia that is highly characteristic of congenital syphilis. Over 90 percent of infants with manifest congenital syphilis show skeletal lesions similar to

those just described. They have their onset typically between 1 and 3 months of age, and the process is usually self-limited, with healing occurring spontaneously over the next few months; the rate of healing is not noticeably affected by treatment. Radiographic findings usually disappear by 5 months of age. Only rarely will these skeletal lesions remain active and cause permanent damage.

The bone lesions are often asymptomatic. Occasionally, perhaps because of secondary trauma, there is pain, often manifested by a pseudoparalysis that may be unilateral, involving either an arm or a leg, as first described by Parrot. Later in infancy there may be recurring isolated bone lesions; dactylitis, frequently asymmetric, is a typical example.

Jaundice as a manifestation of syphilitic hepatitis sometimes appears early in congenital syphilis. This lesion does clear faster and more surely with treatment. Other viscera are involved less commonly. Splenomegaly and generalized lymphadenopathy are frequent manifestations of the early systemic illness. The epitrochlear nodes commonly enlarge as a part of this phenomenon. Palpation of these nodes therefore may provide or heighten clinical suspicion of syphilis; this sign remains useful throughout early childhood. Involvement of the kidney, when present, takes the form of a glomerular nephritis which presents as a nephrotic syndrome. Syphilitic etiology represents almost half of all instances of nephrotic syndrome under six months of age.

Invasion of the central nervous system is common during early congenital syphilis, although it is usually asymptomatic. Examination of the cerebrospinal fluid will frequently reveal pleocytosis and an elevated protein content. This early invasion may be regarded as a part of the early disease for which no additional treatment is needed. All patients treated for syphilis should have a spinal fluid examination 6 months to 2 years later, at which time any abnormality traceable to syphilis provides indication for retreatment.

The serologic titer in all forms of congenital syphilis is high during the first 2 years and is reversible by treatment.

LATE CONGENITAL SYPHILIS.   The diagnosis of late congenital syphilis may be suspected from the stigmata, from the presence of continued active disease, or from a persistenly positive STS in an asymptomatic child. As already pointed out, the stigmata represents the end stage of an early lesion. The most common and most typical of the stigmata are *Hutchinson's teeth*. The lesion, the first of Hutchinson's triad, refers to the upper central incisors of the second dentition. Deciduous teeth often normally exhibit the characteristics caused by syphilis in the permanent teeth. Hutchinson's teeth are screwdriver- or peg-shaped and sometimes notched (Fig. 8). Frequently teeth other than the central incisors are also peg-shaped. Molars may have extra cusps that are poorly formed and crumble under normal use. All syphilitic teeth demonstrate deficient enamel and decay more readily than normal. The Hutchinson incisor is visible by radiography in its preeruptive site from about

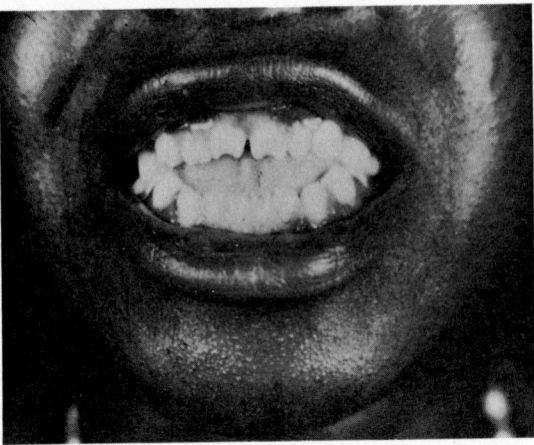
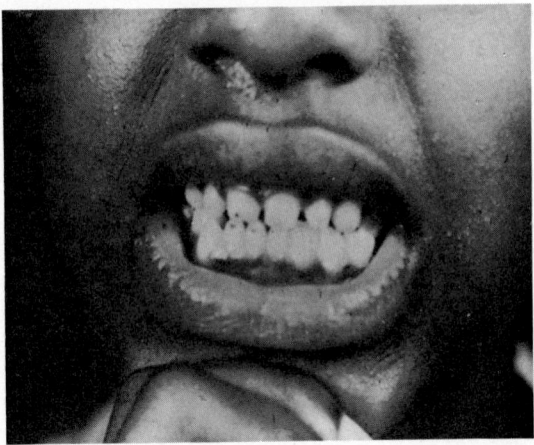

FIG. 8. Two common clinical variations of Hutchinson's teeth.

1 year of age. The scars of perioral lesions give rise to the fissuring called *rhagades,* another inactive end result of an early lesion (Fig. 9).

Examples of late congenital syphilis representing an active tissue response to earlier sensitization are interstitial keratitis, eighth nerve deafness, and *Clutton's joints.* The first two of these form the remaining members of Hutchinson's triad. However, since deafness is quite rare, the original triad itself is rare; Clutton's joints are a more common manifestation.

Interstitial keratitis has its onset between 3 and 20 years of age (most commonly between 6 and 14). It is an intense inflammatory vascular infiltration of the cornea accompanied by an iritis, which may be followed by a dense cicatricial scar producing blindness (Fig. 10). Although usually bilateral, it may appear in one eye before the other, and one side may be much more seriously affected. The lesion is not related to any other syphilitic activity, and it is not prevented by treatment given after the first year of disease; it is not benefited by specific antiluetic therapy; patients may even be seronegative. The condition is a potential cause (and at one time a common cause) of blindness. Early stages are characterized by marked photophobia, lacrimation, and a hazy appearance of the cornea. Later, as the acute inflammation subsides, scarring occurs.

Clutton's joints are symmetric synovial effusions,

FIG. 9. Syphilitic facies showing rhagades.

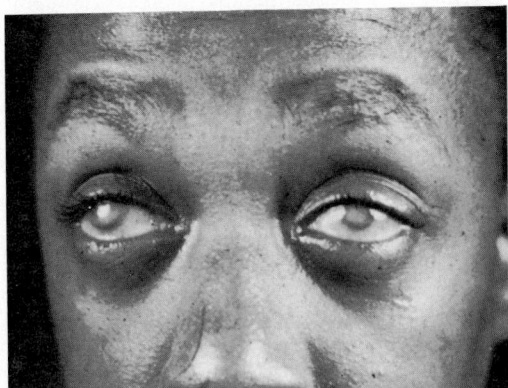

FIG. 10. Syphilitic interstitial keratitis showing acute inflammation.

usually of the knees, that are sometimes painless but more often warm and painful. The process tends to be self-limited and benign. This manifestation, too, is unrelated to active syphilis and unresponsive to specific therapy.

Among active forms of late disease are gummas and osteitis, which are among the late benign syphilitic lesions. The palate and nasal septum are predilectional sites for destructive gummas, with saddle nose and perforated palatal deformities possible end results. Persistent periostitis gives rise to thickened clavicles and to a usually asymmetric *saber shin*.

A more important form of active late syphilis is that involving the central nervous system, with the most common type being meningovascular. Paresis, a more pontentially dangerous form of central nervous system syphilis, occurs in juveniles and may be detected in a preparetic state by examination of the CSF. The examination shows complement-fixing antibody, pleocytosis, and elevation of protein concentration. If untreated, parenchymal involvement may be severe and eventually irreversible. Juvenile tabes rarely occurs.

Any form of late congenital syphilis may have become spontaneously seronegative by the time the disease is recognized. Paradoxically, some patients become serofast, signifying an indefinitely high serologic titer unresponsive to treatment, even though therapy is otherwise successful. Paresis and active gummas are almost always found in seropositive patients with late congenital syphilis.

SYPHILIS ACQUIRED IN CHILDHOOD.   The disease may be and has been acquired by sexual contact at any age after birth. The clinical and pathologic characteristics in children with acquired syphilis are similar to those of the disease in adults, except that children acquiring syphilis do not develop late cardiovascular lesions. Early skin lesions frequently take a serpiginous form, especially on darkly pigmented skin. Late skin lesions are often corymbiferous in distribution. Epitrochlear adenopathy is again a common clinical feature. When the disease is acquired after the early months of life, the stigmata, including interstitial keratitis, do not appear in later life.

TREATMENT.   Syphilitic infection is exceedingly responsive to penicillin therapy. Thus far, no naturally occurring resistant organisms have been described. Either a low continuous blood level or a high intermittent blood level for 7 to 10 days almost uniformly removes *T. pallidum* from the body. The fetus may be successfully treated in utero via medication given to the mother. Here a high blood level in the mother is necessary to assure adequate transplacental levels in the fetus.

The neonate may be successfully treated by a dose of 50,000 to 100,000 IU of penicillin G per kilogram of body weight. Either intermittent divided doses of aqueous penicillin or a single repository dose have been recommended in the past. Kaplan and McCracken have raised the question whether benzathine penicillin G should be discontinued in treatment of congenital syphilis and treatment be confined either to aqueous penicillin G or (as a second choice) procaine penicillin. They base this recommendation on the lack of penicillin activity in 3 of 4 cerebrospinal fluid specimens following injection with benzathine penicillin.

A troublesome pediatric problem is the proper management of a seropositive, asymptomatic newborn. Ideally one should not treat the baby until sufficient follow-up time has permitted distinction between passive transfer of antibody and manufacture of antibody. In practice, fear that follow-up will be unsuccessful or that an extremely precarious medical situation (as in the small premature) may deteriorate has led to treatment by presumptive diagnosis. The use of penicillin treatment for a nonsyphilitic infection has sometimes made it necessary to assume that syphilis was also present, without adequate proof. The important principle in any of these situations is to ensure adequacy of dosage and later follow-up.

Infants usually demonstrate a *Herxheimer reaction* that takes the form of a short, sharp febrile spike about 6 to 8 hours after the first dose of penicillin. This event is without danger and may even be helpful as a diagnostic aid when one decides to treat presumptively, since its occurrence indicates syphilitic infection.

For treatment given during the first few months of life, complete success is the rule. There is no lasting damage, nor are there sequelae of neurosyphilis and interstitial keratitis. The serologic titer as customarily measured gradually falls to zero. When treatment is delayed beyond 1 or 2 years the stigmata, including interstitial keratitis, may occur. Late symptomatic neurosyphilis will not occur if treatment and retreatment are continued until the CSF is free of cells and the protein concentration falls to normal prior to the onset of symptoms. The clearing of the CSF of cells should occur within 3 months of treatment; failure constitutes indication for retreatment.

The treatment of late congenital syphilis should be undertaken if no prior treatment has been given or if evidence of activity is present. Herxheimer reactions occur about 25 percent of the time in active disease, and again they are not deleterious. Previous comments about the use of spinal fluid cell counts as a measure of activity also apply here; neurosyphilis has not been observed subsequently in patients whose CSF was negative 5 years after therapy.

The allergic or hypersensitive manifestations of late congenital syphilis respond better to nonspecific therapy. In particular, interstitial keratitis is very responsive to topical corticosteroids instilled in the eye 4 to 6 times a day until symptoms disappear. The results are quite dramatic, and scarring with blindness appears to be preventable by this means. Clutton's joints are symptomatically relieved by systemic steroids, and eighth nerve deafness has been reported to have also benefited from this treatment.

Serologic titer is not affected by treatment of late congenital syphilis, but follows a natural course toward either seronegativity or serofastness.

Although heavy metals and antibiotics other than

penicillin have known antisyphilitic properties, they are all so inferior to penicillin that their use cannot be recommended.

References

Alford CA Jr, Polt SS, Cassady GE, Straumfjord JV, Remington JS: γM-Fluorescent treponemal antibody in the diagnosis of congenital syphilis. N Eng J Med 280:1086, 1969

Davis BD, Moore DH, Kabat EA, Harris A: Electrophoretic, ultracentrifugal, and immunochemical studies on Wassermann antibody. J Immunol 50:1, 1945

Fiumara NJ: Acquired syphilis in three patients with congenital syphilis. N. Eng. J.Med. 290:1119, 1974

Kaplan JM, McCracken Jr GH: Clinical Pharmacology of benzathine penicillin G in neonates with regard to its recommended use in congenital syphilis. J. Pediatr 82:1069, 1973

McDonald R, Wiggelinkhuizen J, and Kaschula ROC: The nephrotic syndrome in very young infants. Amer J Dis Child 122:507, 1971

Nelson RA Jr, Mayer MM: Immobilization of Treponema pallidum in vitro by antibody produced in syphilitic infection. J Exp Med 89:369, 1949

Oppenheimer, EH and Hardy, JB: Congenital syphilis in the newborn infant: clinical and pathological observations in recent cases. Johns Hopkins Med. J.129:63-82, August, 1971

Rein GR, Reyn A: Serology of treponematoses. Bull WHO 14:193, 1956

Schroeter, AL, Lucas, JB, Price, EV, and Falcone, VH: Treatment for early syphilis and reactivity of serologic tests. JAMA 221 (5): 471, 1972

Stokes JH, Beerman H, Ingraham NR Jr: Modern Clinical Syphilology, 3rd ed. Philadelphia, WB Saunders, 1944

Thomas EW: Syphilis: Its Course and Management. New York, Macmillan 1949

Youmans JB: Syphilis and other venereal diseases. Med Clin North Am 48(573), May 1964

TETANUS

Edward L. Pratt

Tetanus (lockjaw) is an acute infection caused by *Clostridium tetani*, the tetanus bacillus, which was discovered bu Nicolaier in 1884. The disease is characterized by stiffness of the skeletal muscles of any part of the body (particularly the muscles of the jaw), by tonic spasms, and by convulsions. The symptoms are due to a powerful exotoxin that affects the neuromuscular end plates and the motor nuclei of the central nervous system. Infection is acquired almost invariably from contamination of a wound.

ETIOLOGY. The tetanus bacillus is an anaerobic spore-bearing organism. It is widely distributed in the soil in many parts of the world. The bacillus is normally present in the intestines of horses, cattle, and other herbivora and is found at times in man. From 2 to 30 percent of normal adults harbor this organism, the highest proportion being found in agricultural communities. The bacillus produces two soluble toxins (tetanolysin and tetanospasmin), the former an unstable hemolytic substance that apparently plays little part in the pathology of the disease. Tetanospasmin, the substance usually meant when tenanus toxin is spoken of, produces the convulsions and the stiffness of muscles. It has a peculiar affinity for nervous tissue. Unlike many other toxins it does not produce reddening of the skin. A number of subgroups of the bacilli have been identified, but the toxins they produce are identical.

IMMUNITY. All ages are susceptible to tetanus, presumably equally so. Protection is afforded only by active or passive immunization. Although some immunity appears to be conferred by an attack, this is very transient. Instances of relapse and second attacks, although rare, have been reported.

INCIDENCE. The incidence of tetanus reflects the geographic distribution of the organisms, the standards of cleanliness, and the awareness of the risk from contaminated wounds. Although tetanus of the newborn has been practically eliminated from cities in this country, it is still common elsewhere due to the practice of applying animal excreta to the umbilical stump for hemostasis. The increasing use of prophylaxis in connection with wounds of all kinds and widespread use of active immunization in recent years have greatly reduced the incidence in children. Legislation restricting the sale of fireworks has eliminated that menace in many states. In many large pediatric hospitals scarcely one case a year is now seen.

PATHOGENESIS. Tetanus may occur even though no portal of entry can be found; this was the case in 29 percent of a group of patients treated at the Children's Hospital in Boston. A wound that is apparently of little consequence often serves as a portal. The injuries most likely to lead to tetanus are puncture wounds, which provide ideal anaerobic conditions, and burns and crushing wounds, which involve necrosis of tissue and become contaminated with dirt. Blank-cartridge wounds have been a common cause, with the wadding carrying the organism. A considerable number of cases have been caused by infected vaccines, sera, or catgut. It is a mistake to suppose that tetanus bacilli are confined to the soil; the spores are readily spread by birds or insects. We know of an instance in which a splinter in the nose, acquired in the top of a tree, led to tenanus. It has followed the stings of bees and wasps.

The bacilli themselves are confined to the primary wound, where they proliferate and produce toxin. The manner in which the toxin is distributed through the body is still subject to some dispute. According to Abel and his collaborators, some of it diffuses from the nidus in the wound to the surrounding muscles, but the greater part is taken up in the the circulation and is thus distributed to the tissues. Other investigators believe that tetanus toxin travels along axis cylinders to reach the spinal cord and medulla. Action of toxin at the myoneural junctions is responsible for the stiffness of muscles that forms a conspicuous feature of the symptomatology; the toxin's action in the central nervous system lowers the threshold of reflexes in which the lower motor neurons are involved and induces susceptibility to reflex spasms and convulsions. Toxin combines firmly with nerve tissue, and once symptoms have set in it cannot readily be detached by antitoxin, however administered. On the other hand, toxin free in the circulating blood can be neutralized by antitoxin. If the patient survives, eventual recovery is complete.

Two clinical forms of tetanus are seen: generalized tetanus and local tetanus, the former the result of widespread distribution of toxin, the latter caused by local distribution of toxin in the vicinity of the portal of entry. The two forms may be combined. In children local tetanus is distinctly rare. The stiffness may make its first appearance in a single group of muscles, such as those of the jaw, the muscles of deglutition, or muscles in other parts of the body.

PATHOLOGY. There are no characteristic morphologic changes produced by tetanus. In some fatal cases cerebral edema has been found, and there may be various lesions secondary to the violent spasms, such as hemorrhage in muscles or even rupture of skeletal muscles and compression fractures of vertebral bodies.

SYMPTOMS. Symptoms usually begin between 5 and 12 days after infection, although the incubation period may be considerably longer than this or, in the most serious cases, as short as 1 to 2 days. The local wound shows nothing peculiar, and the symptoms are essentially the same no matter where the wound is located. The onset is generally insidious, with gradually increasing stiffness of muscles, particularly those of the neck and jaw. Within 24 hours the disease is generally fully developed; the stiffness of the jaw and neck is then very marked, swallowing may be difficult, and other parts of the body musculature become involved. The spasms of tetanus are quite characersitic. Cutaneous, auditory, or visual stimulation and attempts at voluntary motion initiate paroxysmal contraction of the muscles of the body as a whole that lasts for 5 or 10 sec. During the spasm the body becomes as rigid as a board; the head is retracted, the back arched in opisthotonos, the legs and feet extended, the arms outstretched with fists clenched and thumbs adducted. The jaws are immobile, and the face assumes a peculiar, fixed expression known as the *risus sardonicus*. The eyebrows are raised, the palpebral fissures narrowed, the angles of the mouth drawn downward and outward, and the upper lip pressed firmly against the teeth. Consciousness is not lost; often the patient is very apprehensive.

At first these spasms are infrequent; there is complete relaxation between them, and they occasion little discomfort. As the disease progresses they become more numerous and prolonged and may be painful; often they are initiated by the slightest stimulus. Relaxation between the seizures is then only partial, with a considerable degree of rigidity persisting. The paroxysms may affect the respiratory muscles or those of the larynx, with fatal results. The posture often gives little idea of the intensity of the contractions, for opposing muscle groups are equally involved. Partial or complete relaxation occurs during sleep or with anesthesia, and sedatives may afford some relief. Spasm of the sphincters with retention of urine is common. Sweating is sometimes very marked; fever is moderate or absent. The blood count and spinal fluid show no constant changes.

A number of our cases have not conformed to the typical picture just described. Trismus, although usually present sooner or later, was the first symptom in only 6 of 22 cases. In others the symptoms were first noted in the neck, the back, the extremities, or the abdominal muscles. In some cases pain was severe from the outset; in others the only complaint was stiffness. The location of these initial symptoms bore no relation to that of the injury. In five instances the onset was with general convulsions.

The duration of tetanus in fatal cases is seldom more than 3 or 4 days, and it may be less than 24 hours; on the other hand we have known a patient to die in convulsions as late as 12 days, at a time when recovery seemed well under way. Death usually results from respiratory failure, the temperature sometimes showing an abrupt terminal rise. Patients who recover seldom have much fever; after several days the paroxysms gradually decrease in frequency and the muscular rigidity diminishes, although several weeks may elapse before they disappear entirely. Trismus is often the last symptom to disappear.

DIAGNOSIS. There are few diseases with which tetanus is apt to be confused. The history of a wound, the onset with trismus, the facial expression, and the spasm accentuated by external stimuli are quite characteristic. In the neonatal period intracranial injuries or developmental defects of the brain may produce comparable symptoms, but after the first few weeks of life it is most unusual for convulsions to be provoked by external stimuli, save in tenanus. Strychnine poisoning may simulate tetanus; however, trismus is rare, and persistent rigidity between paroxysms is not present, although the contraction resulting from external stimulation may last many seconds. Meningitis may be difficult to rule out without lumbar puncture. We have seen cases of serum sickness accompanied by arthralgia of the temporomandibular joint in which for a while tetanus was suspected. The differentiation from rabies is discussed with that condition.

Apical abscesses of the molar teeth and peritonsillar or retropharyngeal abscesses may lead to trismus, but the generalized increase in muscle tone and risus sardonicus are not present. Ingestion of tranquilizers and antiemetics, particularly the phenothiazine derivatives, may lead to muscle spasms that are easily confused with tetanus. The history of availability or ingestion of such medicines, plus the lack of a more or less symmetric increase in muscle tone and the presence of a positive urine test for such drugs, should clarify the diagnosis.

Local tetanus should be thought of when stiffness of muscles and irritability to local mechanical stimuli develop in the neighborhood of a wound, particularly a compound fracture that has been put up in traction-suspension. Immobilization favors the development of local tetanus by slowing the lymph flow, and infected bone may harbor tetanus bacilli for a long time, permitting toxin to be formed many weeks after the original prophylactic injection of antitoxin.

PROPHYLAXIS. The ideal agent for *passive immunization* for children with tetanus-prone injuries who have not been actively immunized and have not had a tetanus booster within the past 10 years, or in whom the status of immunity against tetanus is unknown, is 250 units of human tetanus immune globulin intramuscularly. Tetanus antitoxin from human serum eliminates the danger of foreign-serum reactions, provides protective levels of circulating antibodies for 3 or 4 weeks, and interferes less than does antitoxin from animal serum with the immune response to fluid tetanus toxoid. In highly contaminated wounds with extensive tissue necrosis, twice the dose of human serum tetanus antitoxin should be given. If tetanus antitoxin from human serum cannot he obtained, the subcutaneous or intramuscular injection of 5,000 American units of antitoxin prepared in horses (or cows) may be given after all precautions, including scratch, intradermal, and ophthalmic tests for serum hypersensitivity, have been carried out. Every child given passive immunization should be started on and followed through a complete course of basic active immunization against tetanus, so that passive immunization becomes truly a once-in-a-lifetime procedure. An initial dose of fluid tenanus toxoid should be given at another site in another syringe at the same time the antitoxin is given.

Active immunization against tetanus is one of the most highly successful immunization procedures available. Every infant should receive three injections of DPT (combined tetanus toxoid, diphtheria toxoid, and pertussis vaccine), 0.5 ml each, at intervals of 4 to 6 weeks or more, starting at 2 to 4 months of age, followed by a booster at 15 to 18 months and another booster at about 4–6 years of age . After that, boosters of tetanus-diphtheria toxoid of the adult type should be given every 10 years throughout life.

All physicians should attempt to detect nonimmunized children and adults and urge active immunization plus a regular schedule of boosters. Ideal opportunities for doing this occur when patients appear for an injury, for checkups, and for immunizations for travel. Patients should have records of the status of their immunizations so that confusion will not exist. The U.S. Public Health Service Advisory Committee on Immunization has stated that a review of tetanus in the United States in recent years has failed to reveal documented cases occurring in individuals with adequate primary immunization. Available evidence shows antitoxin persisting at protective levels for at least 5 years after four doses of tetanus toxoid. Ability to react promptly to booster injections persists for a longer time. In wound management it is therefore unnecessary to use booster injections more often than every 5 years. For persons whose immunizations are still incomplete following wound management, the remainder of the recommended series should be given. Severe injuries or those heavily contaminated or with large necrotic areas or accompanied by extensive blood loss may require both a booster of toxoid and 250 units of human tetanus immune globulin in a different site from a different syringe, even though the patient was previously actively immunized.

TREATMENT. The management of tetanus should be governed by three basic considerations: prevention of additional toxin reaching the central nervous system, control of life-endangering spasms while oxygenation and hydration are maintained, and elimination of therapeutic risks. The expected value of any measure must be balanced against any disturbance it may cause the patient.

Tetanus antitoxin in sufficient quantity will prevent toxin as yet unbound from reaching the central nervous system. The proof of this statement has been irrefutably demonstrated by the thousands of patients with contiminated wounds protected from tetanus by adequate passive immunization. The dose of antitoxin should be gauged by the severity of the disease and not by the size of the patient. Human antitoxin, if available, in doses of 3,000 to 6,000 units, always intramuscularly, is adequate according to the information available to date. If equine or bovine antitoxin must be used, clinical and immunologic data indicate that 20,000 to 60,000 American units are sufficient in clinical tetanus. Highly purified antitoxin and all precautions against sensitivity and thermal reactions should be employed. In mild cases the intramuscular route, being the safest, is preferred. In severe cases one-third may be given intravenously and the rest intramuscularly. Intrathecal antitoxin can produce severe and at times fatal reactions, and the evidence that this route is more effective than the others has not been clearly demonstrated in patients.

It is essential that injuries receive proper surgical care, but mutilating operations undertaken merely because the lesion may be the site of elaboration of toxin are not indicated. Penicillin and other antibiotics used in the control of ordinary wound infection will not neutralize tetanus toxin.

The ideal agent for control of spasms without depression of vital functions or other toxic effects has not yet been discovered. In mild and moderately severe cases sedation with paraldehyde or secobarbital sodium may be satisfactory. In more severe cases meprobamate at a dosage of 80 to 100 mg intramuscularly every 3 to 4 hours for neonates and up to 300 mg per dose for children, may be tried and, if necessary, supplemented by chlorpromazine, 0.5 mg/kg body weight. Sedation, particularly the use of muscle relaxants (phenoxypropanediol, mephenesin, or methocarbamol), should be a collaborative effort with a skilled anesthesiologist whenever possible. In severe cases effective anticonvulsive sedation can be maintained only by continuous intravenous administration or 0.4 percent solution of pentobarbital (4 g of powdered barbiturate added to 1 liter of 5 percent glucose in water). The rate of flow must be constantly supervised and should be adjusted to maintain the patient at the level where he has no spasms when left undisturbed, but will respond with increased muscle tone if stimulated. Anesthesia should not be so light as to permit spasms to interfere with respirations nor so deep as to cause respiratory depression. A tracheotomy is essential. Theoretically curare and similar muscle relaxing agents should be ideal for controlling spasms, but their use in tetanus should be attempted only by skilled personnel with the equipment necessary to combat respiratory depression or paralysis and to manage excessive secretions in the respiratory passages. Meperidine (Demerol) is the drug of choice for relief of pain.

Maintenance of oxygenation is of prime importance. One must prevent the accumulation of secretions in the pharynx and the tracheobronchial tree, control spasms of the pharynx and glottis or respiratory muscles, and avoid respiratory depression. Tracheostomy is the only adequate method of dealing with trancheobronchial obstruction and is essential for laryngeal or pharyngeal spasms. It should be performed early whenever indicated. In newborns tracheostomies are unsatisfactory and dangerous. For these patients endotracheal tubes are preferred to tracheostomies to provide an adequate airway. A dependable apparatus for giving oxygen under controlled positive pressure should always be at the bedside. An efficient mechanical respirator should be available if possible.

Satisfactory hydration can be maintained by giving enough fluid intravenously to cover the expenditures from the lungs, skin, and kidneys. The concentration of glucose and of electrolytes in the hydrating fluid should be determined from estimates of requirements (p. 260). Small plastic tubes have lessened the irritation of tube feeding, but they should be used with special caution during the first week, when severe spasms often follow any manipulation. Because of the risk of aspiration of food or gastric contents, resumption of oral feeding should not be hurried.

A darkened, noise-free environment, gentle skillful nursing, and clear accurate records of the amounts, frequency, and effects of the drugs administered are invaluable.

PROGNOSIS.   Tetanus is relatively simple to prevent, but its treatment is still unsatisfactory. The overall mortality remains between 30 and 50 percent, in spite of all therapeutic measures. The most accurate indication of prognosis in an individual patient may be judged by a composite of the following clinical features listed in the order of their importance: the period of time from the onset of first symptoms recognized by the patient until generalized spasms occur; the length of the incubation period; the severity of symptoms in the patient at the time of admission. When progression of symptoms has been longer than 60 hours, with the incubation period over 8 to 10 days, appropriate management should lead to recovery. Most patients who survive 10 days of symptoms eventually recover completely. The disease leaves no sequelae.

Every patient with clinical tetanus should have, before discharge, films of the spine to detect crushing of the bodies of the thoracic or lumbar vertebrae, since these occur in a majority of the severe cases. Following recovery from clinical tetanus the physician must accept the responsibility of seeing to it that the patient is actively immunized against tetanus, because tetanus is a nonimmunizing disease. Instances have been reported of motor paralysis following antitoxin given for either therapeutic or prophylactic purposes.

References

American Academy of Pediatrics: Report of the Committee on the Control of Infectious Diseases, 15th ed. Evanston, Ill, 1974

Earle AM, Mellon WL: Tetanus neonatorum: a report of thirty-two cases. Am J Trop Med Hyg 7:315, 1958

Howard FH, DeVere W: Intramuscular meprobamate in the treatment of tetanus in infants and children. J Pediatr 60:421, 1962

Human antitoxin in prophylaxis and treatment of tetanus. Med Lett Drugs Ther 7:13, 1965

Jenkins MT, Luhn NR: Active management of tetanus, based on experiences of an anaesthesiology department. Anesthesiology 23:690, 1962

Lafoere FM, Lowell SY, Bennett JV: Tetanus in the United States 1965–1966. N Eng J Med 280:564, 1969

McComb JA: The prophylactic dose of homologous tetanus antitoxin. N Engl J Med 270:175, 1964

Margileth AM, Shaul JF, Love J: The status of immunization in 1963. Med Clin North Am 43:1393, 1963

Peebles TC, Levine L, Eldred MC, Edsall G: Tetanus-Toxoid Emergency Boosters. N Engl J Med 280:575, 1969

Pratt EL: Clinical tetanus; a study of 56 cases with special reference to methods of prevention and a plan for evaluating treatment. JAMA 129:1243, 1945

Skudder PA, McCarroll JR: Current status of tetanus control. Importance of human tetanus-immune globulin. JAMA 188:625, 1964

Viral Infections

VIRAL REPLICATION

KENNETH BERNS

Viruses constitute a particular challenge to medicine. The ability to prevent some viral infections by vaccination is of long standing. However, in many other infections such as the common cold or influenza the multiplicity of immunizations that would be required for protection effectively precludes this route. In these cases, and in the cases of viral infections too rare to warrant the dangers inherent in mass vaccination programs, it would be preferable to be able to identify the agent and subsequently to treat in a specific manner. However, specific antiviral therapy has proved difficult to achieve. In contrast to bacteria, which conduct their own metabolism that differs in many respects from that of mammalian cells and thus offers specific therapeutic targets, viruses are obligate intracellular parasites that use most of the cell's own metabolic machinery. Thus specific therapeutic targets in viral infections are much more limited, and the potential for therapeutic toxicity is correspondingly greater. In order to design specific antiviral drugs rationally, a detailed knowledge of the mechanism of viral infection at the molecular level is necessary. Those reactions that are discovered to differ in infected cells as compared with uninfected cells will thus constitute specific targets for potential antiviral therapy.

Two major factors have been responsible for our ability to obtain increased information concerning animal virus multiplication. The first is the ability to maintain animal cells in tissue culture. Although studies with whole animals have led to important findings concerning the pathogenesis of viral infections and the ability of the host to respond, tissue culture provides an opportunity to study infection at the cellular and molecular level by establishing critical variables required for an understanding of events at the molecular level. A second important factor has been the knowledge obtained from studies using bacteria and bacterial viruses. The basic assumption of molecular biology is that, although details may vary from species to species, events at the molecular level obey many if not all of the same rules regardless of the species concerned.

There are three potential phases in the life cycle of a virus. The present-day classification of viruses is based on the structure of the virus in the extracellular phase. However, by definition, viruses must replicate intracellularly (ie, they are obligate intracellular parasites); this is the second phase. A third phase in the life cycle of many viruses is the establishment of the stable association between the viral genome and the host cell in which replication of the viral genome is coordinated with that of the host, but no complete viruses are formed. In some cases the viral genome is actually inserted into the host genome (eg, the RNA tumor viruses). Previously, many viruses were classified by the species they infected and the symptoms, such as infection, they produced. However, careful study has shown that many closely related viruses are capable of infecting more than one species and can produce a variety of symptoms depending on the specific circumstances of the infection. Viruses are now classified according to the structure of the virion, as determined by physical, chemical, and immunologic techniques. The major aspects of virion structure that are considered in classification are whether the genome is DNA or RNA, the physical structure of the genome, the presence or absence of a lipid envelope, the size, the presence of specific enzymes associated with the virion, and the presence of common antigens. Thus, for example, the paramyxoviruses are closely related by the above criteria, although some (eg, parainfluenza) cause superficial respiratory disease, while others (eg, mumps) result in systemic infections.

Study of the structure of the virion often will yield insight into potential mechanisms of intracellular viral replication. The virion is the product of such replication; thus any models of viral multiplication must be able to account for the known properties of the virion. Basically a virus is a piece of nucleic acid containing genetic information that in the extracellular or virus-particle phase is surrounded by a protective coat of protein. The protein and nucleic acid constitute the nucleocapsid, which in some cases is in turn surrounded by a lipid-containing membrane.

There are tremendous variations in the chemical and physical properties of the nucleic acid genomes that have been isolated from different types of virus particles. In some cases the genome is DNA, ranging in molecular weight from 1.4×10^6 daltons (parvoviruses) to 125×10^6 daltons (poxviruses). The DNA may be a single strand (parvoviruses) or a Watson-Crick double helix (adenovirus). It may also be linear (pox-

viruses) or circular (papovaviruses) in form. The genomes of DNA viruses have one property in common: each is a single DNA molecule. Other viruses have RNA genomes. The variation in molecular weight for RNA genomes seems to be more limited, ranging from 2×10^6 (picornaviruses) to 12×10^6 (reovirus). Again the genome may be a single strand of RNA (myxoviruses) or double-stranded (reovirus). RNA virus genomes seem to share one characteristic: they are all linear. However, in contradistinction to the DNA virus genomes, some of the RNA virus genomes are segmented, being composed of more than one piece of RNA (influenza, reovirus).

In the virus particle the viral nucleic acid is surrounded by the capsid, a layer composed of repeating protein subunits. The capsid proteins appear to be primarily structural in nature, without significant enzymatic activity. However, there is considerable evidence of specific enzymes contained within the capsid. The most prominent class of enzymes to be described are the polymerases, enzymes that synthesize nucleic acids. Polymerases require a nucleic acid template, which they use to synthesize a polynucleotide chain containing a complementary necleotide sequence (a complementary nucleotide sequence contains the base adenine in place of thymine, guanine in place of cytosine, and vice versa). Virus-particle-associated polymerases have been described that synthesize RNA using RNA as a template (myxoviruses) or DNA as a template (poxviruses). Likewise DNA polymerases may use either DNA (hepatitis B virus) or RNA (RNA tumor viruses) as a template. As described in a subsequent section, the presence of a virion-associated polymerase can be closely correlated to specific aspects of the multiplication of the virus in question. Some viruses do not have and do not require virus-particle-associated polymerases in order to replicate (eg, adenovirus, poliovirus).

The envelope that surrounds some types of virus particles (eg, herpesviruses, myxoviruses) is a lipid bilayer. In the electron miscroscope it is easy to visualize spikes or projections from many of these envelopes; the most thoroughly studied are those of the myxoviruses. The spikes are glycoproteins (proteins with associated sugars attached) with specific biologic activities. In the case of the myxoviruses, one type of spike is a neuraminidase, an enzyme that cleaves a terminal neuraminic acid residue from a polysaccharide. A second type of spike is a hemagglutinin, which attaches to specific glycoprotein receptors on the cell surface.

Because the study of animal virus genetics is in its infancy, it is difficult to assess which of the components of the virion are determined by the genetic information contained within the viral nucleic acid genome. Clearly the nucleic acid is virus-specific. The best conclusion at the present time is that all or most of the proteins in the virion are determined by the viral genome while lipid components (the envolope) and sugar components (attached to the spikes projecting from the envelope) are determined by the genetic information in the DNA of the host. Table 17 lists the characteristics of human viruses.

TABLE 17. Characteristics of Human Viruses

Family	DNA/RNA	Virion Polymerase	Envelope	Replication Site	Examples of Human Pathogens
DNA viruses					
Adeno	DS	—	—	N	Adenovirus
Papova	DS	—	—	N	Progressive multifocal leukoencephalopathy
Pox	DS	RNA	+	C	Smallpox, vaccinia
Herpes	DS	—	+	N	Herpes simplex, varicella zoster, cytomegalovirus, Epstein-Barr
Parvo	SS	—	—	N	Adeno-associated virus
Hepatitis B	DS	DNA	+	?	Hepatitis B
RNA viruses					
Picorna	SS	—	—	C	Poliovirus, echovirus, coxsackievirus, rhinovirus
Reo	DS	RNA	—	C	Reovirus
Orthormyxo	SS	RNA	+	N?	Influenza
Paramyxo	SS	RNA	+	C	Parainfluenza, rubeola, mumps; respiratory syncytial?
Rhabdo	SS	RNA	+	C	Rabies
Toga	SS	—	+	C	Group A + B arboviruses + rubella?
Arena	SS	?	+	C	Lassa, lymphocytic choriomeningitis
Corona	SS	?	+	C	Human respiratory gastroenteritis
Bunyamwera	SS	?	+	C	Arboviruses
Leuko	SS	DNA	+	N	RNA tumor virus; human?

In order to infect a cell the virus first must be able to attach to the cell and then penetrate the cytoplasmic membrane. Some viruses seem to be able to attach to and penetrate almost all cells (adeno-associated virus); others are species-specific (poliovirus), and still others are not only species-specific but also tissue-specific (the vaccine strains of poliovirus). The details of attachment that have been determined are quite sparse, but a well-studied example is the myxovirus hemagglutinin that projects from the virus envelope and can attach to specific glycoprotein receptors on the surfaces of susceptible cells.

The mechanism of penetration is a subject of controversy. All viruses seem capable of being taken up by susceptible cells by means of viropexis, a process equivalent to phagocytosis. However, this results in the virus still being contained within a cytoplasmic vesicle lined by cytoplasmic membrane. Two potentially different mechanisms of viral penetration of the cytoplasmic membrane have been observed in the electron microscope. Nonenveloped virus (adenovirus) has been observed to pass directly through the membrane. In the case of enveloped viruses (eg, myxovirus) the envelope may fuse with the cytoplasmic membrane, leading to the release directly of the protein/nucleic acid portion of the virus (the nucleocapsid) into the cytoplasm of the cell.

Once inside the cell the virus can then begin the actual process of multiplication. The first step is at least a partial uncoating of the viral genome by stripping away some or all of the protein of the nucleocapsid. Most of this is apparently done by proteolytic enzymes already present within the cell. In at least one case, that of the poxviruses, the synthesis of new proteins coded for by the virus is required to complete the process.

The location in the cell where uncoating takes place depends in part on where the genome replicates. Most DNA viruses (parvovirus, papovavirus, adenovirus, herpesvirus) replicate their genomes in the nucleus, but some, such as poxviruses, replicate the genome in the cytoplasm. In contrast, most RNA viruses replicate their RNA in the cytoplasm; but there are exceptions, such as RNA tumor viruses and possibly influenza virus. The location of genome replication and the type of genome to be replicated help to determine the source of polymerases and other enzymes used for this purpose. Those DNA viruses that replicate in the nucleus can use the normal cellular enzymes involved in host DNA synthesis (although there may be some modification of these). However, the poxviruses, which replicate their DNA in the cytoplasm, are physically separated from the appropriate cellular enzymes and so must cause the synthesis of virus-coded enzymes in order for DNA replication to occur. Those reactions requiring use of an

RNA template (RNA-dependent RNA synthesis and RNA-dependent DNA synthesis) do not normally occur in eukaryotic cells, and thus all RNA viruses must provide their own enzymes for genome replication. In some cases, as noted above, these are brought in with the virion, and in others they are synthesized de novo.

The dogma of molecular biology states that messenger RNA is the intermediary that transmits the genetic information contained in DNA to the synthetic machinery of the ribosomes where the information is translated into proteins. In the case of DNA viruses there are two stages of messenger RNA synthesis during the course of infection. Prior to DNA replication only those sections of the genome that are related to the synthesis of enzymes required for DNA replication are transcribed into messenger RNA. This is termed early messenger RNA. Once DNA replication starts, those portions of the DNA that code for the structural proteins of the virion and any enzymes necessary for virion assembly are also transcribed to form late messenger RNA. Apparently the early messenger RNA continues to be synthesized late into infection.

With RNA viruses RNA serves the function of DNA. In some cases the RNA in the virion can also serve directly as the messenger RNA, so that once this RNA is uncoated it can attach directly to ribosomes and direct the synthesis of viral proteins (poliovirus). However, with other RNA viruses (myxovirus) the messenger RNA is the complement of the RNA strand in the virion, and thus this type of virion presents a paradox. To produce virus-specific proteins a virus-specific messenger RNA must be synthesized; yet to produce the viral messenger RNA a virus-specific protein (the RNA-dependent RNA polymerase) is required. The solution of this seeming parodox is quite straightforward. These are the virions (eg, myxovirus, rhabdovirus) that contain and bring into the cell an RNA-dependent RNA polymerase that can produce the messenger RNA once uncoating of the virion has proceeded to the appropriate stage.

Various aspects of viral multiplication are discussed in the sections on specific infections.

ANTIVIRAL THERAPY. It is evident that significant numbers of the events involved in viral infections are unique and thus are potential therapeutic targets. In spite of this, antiviral therapy is in its infancy, and in only a few instances has it appeared at all promising. An ideal therapy would be to prevent viral entry into the cell. An example of a drug reported to do so is amantadine hydrochloride, which prevents intracellular penetration by influenza A. To be effective, however, amantadine must be administered prophylactically, a handicap that, in addition to its side effects, has restricted its usefulness. More success has been achieved with metabolic analogues that interfere with viral DNA synthesis. The role of analogues of DNA components, including idoxuridine, cytosine arabinoside, and adenine arabinoside, in herpesvirus infections is discussed elsewhere (p. 531).

N-methylisatin 3-thiosemicarbazone (Marboran) has been reported to be effective when used prophylacti-cally in smallpox contacts, although other reports have questioned its value. The mechanism of action of this drug has been determined in vitro to involve a block in viral protein synthesis. Late viral messenger RNA cannot attach to ribosomes and thus is not translated into protein.

Other drugs that have been tried clinically appear to involve more risk for the patient than for the virus. Although there are few drugs available now, potential therapeutic targets are known against which future drugs may be developed. High on the list would be viral polymerases that are different from any existing in normal cells. These would include the RNA-dependent RNA polymerases required by all RNA viruses except RNA tumor viruses and the reverse transcriptase of the RNA tumor viruses. Several rifampicin and streptovaricin derivatives have been reported to inhibit reverse transcriptase in vitro and cell transformation and tumor formation in experimental animals. Another potential target would be assembly of the virus particle.

A therapeutic agent of great potential is interferon, a cellular protein induced by virus infection. Released extracellularly, it has the ability to protect cells against subsequent infection. Interferon is not virus-specific, ie, interferon produced in response to infection by one type of virus will protect cells against infection by almost any other virus. However, interferon is species-specific, so that human interferon will not protect cells of other species and vice versa. The mechanism of protection is uncertain; it seems to involve the selective block of viral protein synthesis as opposed to normal cellular protein synthesis. Unfortunately, clinical trials with interferon or with drugs known to induce endogenous interferon production have so far proved to be disappointing. In spite of the slow progress in antiviral therapy, studies on the molecular basis of viral multiplication have greatly increased our understanding of the process and should promote greater success in this area in the future.

CAT-SCRATCH DISEASE

ANDREW M. MARGILETH

Cat-scratch disease, or CSD (benign nonbacterial lymphadenitis, inoculation lymphoreticulosis), is a nonfatal systemic illness characterized by tender regional lymphadenopathy frequently accompanied by a primary skin lesion and a history of contact with (and usually a scratch from) a cat. The natural course of the disease is for the enlarged node to persist for 1 to 2 months in a generally healthy child, followed by gradual spontaneous resolution.

EPIDEMIOLOGY. Over 1,400 patients have been reported since the first description of CSD by Debré in 1950. An estimated 2,000 unreported cases occur annually in the United States; about 80 percent occur in patients under 20 years of age. The disease is worldwide and occurs in all races; the sexes are affected equally. In temperate zones most cases have occurred during fall and winter. Several house and city epidemics have been recorded.

ETIOLOGY. Although it is unidentified, the etiologic agent is probably a virus, since careful studies have excluded aerobic and anaerobic bacteria, mycobacteria, mycoplasma, and fungi. In one unconfirmed study sections of infected monkey and human lymph nodes showed intracellular and extracellular granules that appeared identical to elementary bodies of psittacosis. In another study herpeslike virus particles have been found in the cell cytoplasm of biopsied human lymph nodes. During the acute illness CSD patients have a transient state of lymphocyte unresponsiveness similar to that noted in patients with a variety of illnesses caused by viruses and mycoplasma.

The mode of transmission is well known. The illness usually follows a scratch or a lick from a kitten or cat (70 percent). Rarely it has occurred following a dog or monkey bite or a scratch from a thorn, wood splinter, or codfish bone. Contact with cats occurs in about 90 percent of those afflicted. An inoculation site may be found in 55 to 96 percent of patients. The disease has been transmitted to man, monkey, and Hartley guinea pigs; regional lymphadenopathy has been produced in each species following an intradermal injection of material aspirated from suppurative lymph nodes of patients. No cats studied have shown evidence of illness, and attempts to isolate virus from cat saliva or claws have been unsuccessful. Apparently the cat acts as a mechanical vector for the causative agent, since cats do not react to skin tests with cat-scratch antigen.

PATHOLOGY. Biopsied lymph nodes may show distinct but nonspecific stages: reticulum cell hyperplasia followed by tuberclelike granulomata, then multiple microabscesses, and ultimately frank abscess formation. Consequently a presumptive histopathologic diagnosis of tularemia, brucellosis, tuberculosis, or sarcoidosis might be considered.

CLINICAL MANIFESTATIONS. The patient generally does not appear to be ill in spite of the impressive degree of lymphadenopathy; however, malaise, fever, and flulike symptoms may be present initially. From 3 to 10 days elapse from the scratch or contact until a primary skin papule or pustule forms; occasionally unilateral conjunctival granulomas occur. An inoculation site (a scratch or a primary lesion or both) may be detected in 55 to 96 percent of patients, depending on how carefully the child is examined and the time of the initial examination. Most primary lesions persist for 1 to 3 weeks, some for 6 to 7 weeks. Regional lymphadenopathy develops about 2 weeks (range 3 to 50 days) after the scratch. The enlarged node or nodes are invariably tender for the first 1 or 2 weeks and are commonly found in the head, neck, or axilla. Epitrochlear, inguinal, femoral, or popliteal areas are involved less frequently; involvement of multiple sites occurs in 6 to 10 percent of patients. In the majority of cases the node size varies from 1 to 6 cm, and the enlargement persists for 2 to 3 months. In a very few patients lymphadenopathy has persisted for 6 to 24 months. Suppuration of

nodes occurs in about one-fourth of patients referred to hospitals, but it is seen less commonly (10 percent) in office practice. In 300 cases observed by the author, no clinical signs other than lymphadenopathy occurred in about one-third. About one-third had fever ranging from 38 C to 41 C and usually lasting for 5 to 9 days but sometimes up to 1 month; 40 percent of these patients had malaise or a flulike syndrome generally lasting about 4 days but occasionally as long as 3 weeks. Various exanthemata, including maculopapular, petechial, erythema nodosum, or multiform types, have been reported in about 4 percent of patients. The rash usually lasts 4 to 9 days.

Unusual clinical manifestations have included the oculoglandular syndrome of Parinaud, encephalitis, thrombocytopenic purpura, osteomyelitis, and primary atypical pneumonia. CSD should always be considered in any patient with an ocular lesion and parotid area swelling due to preauricular lymphadenopathy (Fig. 11).

Children with central nervous system involvement may develop encephalopathy, meningitis, radiculitis, polyneuritis, or myelitis with paraplegia. The onset of neurologic symptoms is usually sudden and accompanied by fever; it occurs within 1 to 6 weeks of the onset of adenopathy. The frequency of major symptoms and signs found in 41 cases with central nervous system involvement was coma or convulsions in two-thirds, neurologic abnormalities in one-fourth, and lethargy or confusion or both in one-sixth. In 12 of 22 patients with central nervous system involvement, pleocytosis or elevated protein or both were detected. Electroencephalograms are abnormal in the majority of these patients. Severe manifestations have lasted for 1 to 2 weeks, with gradual recovery to normal status in 1 to 6 months in most patients. Recovery from thrombocytopenic purpura, osteomyelitis, pneumonitis, and Parinaud's syndrome has been complete.

LABORATORY DATA. Laboratory tests are not diagnostic, but eosinophilia is reported in 8 to 43 percent of patients. Initially the number of polymorphonuclear cells may be increased, with a mild leukocytosis. The sedimentation rate is usually elevated during the first few weeks of adenopathy, thus suggesting inflammatory lymphadenitis.

SKIN TESTS. A skin test using cat-scratch (CS) antigen is positive in 90 percent of patients who are clinically suspected of having CSD and have had cat scratches and/or contact. A negative skin test often occurs if the duration of illness is less than 3 or 4 weeks, and about 10 percent of patients with typical CSD will have negative skin tests with 1 or 2 different antigens. The positive reaction consists of a wheal or papule with 5 mm or more of induration, with or without erythema, occurring 48 to 72 hours after intradermal inoculation of 0.1 ml of antigen. Induration may persist for 5 to 6 days or longer. A positive test may be obtained for years after an episode of CSD. False-positive reactions have been reported in veterinarians, healthy persons, and family contacts; the overall incidence is only 5 percent. Thus the limit of confidence for a positive reaction is

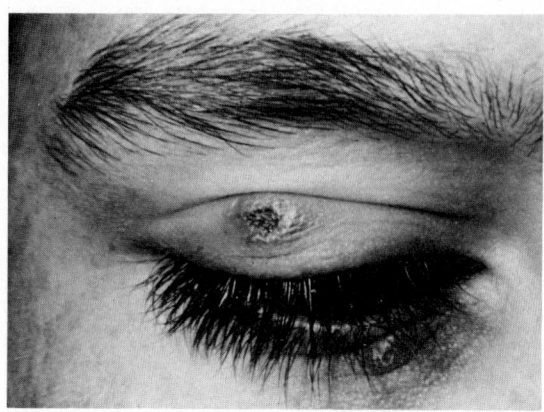
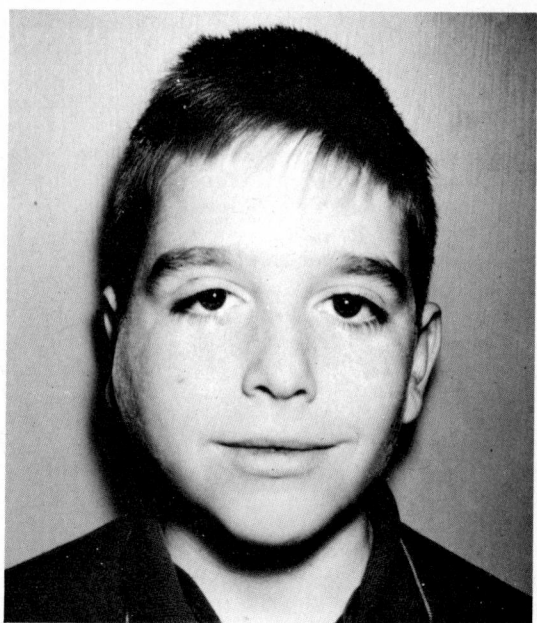

FIG. 11. Oculoglandular syndrome in a 12-year-old boy with crusted upper and lower eyelid pustules (left) for 2 months and multiple preauricular lymph node involvement (right) due to cat-scratch disease. Lymphadenopathy persisted for 7 months in spite of four aspirations of sterile pus.

about 95 percent. Repeated skin testing with CS antigen in the same patients has not produced positive reactions. Skin tests with atypical mycobacterial antigens have rarely been positive in most patients with CSD; 3 of our 230 patients with CSD tested with atypical mycobacterial antigens had positive reactions to PPD.

ANTIGEN PREPARATION. Since CS antigen is not available commercially, all aspirated pus should be saved as a source of CS antigen. The pus is immediately diluted (1:4) with normal saline solution, cultured for fungi, aerobic and anaerobic bacteria, and mycobacteria, and heated for 10 to 24 hours at 60 C on each of three consecutive days to destroy hepatitis virus, if it is present. After 8 to 10 weeks, if all cultures are negative, the material is ready for use in skin testing. No preservative is added; however, all antigens should be stored at temperatures below 0 C. Antigens prepared in this manner have been used for skin testing for 5 years without loss of activity.

DIAGNOSIS. Regional lymphadenopathy must be present during the course of the disease. Three of the four following manifestations would confirm the diagnosis in a typical case, whereas all four would be necessary in an atypical case: a history of animal (usually cat) contact or presence of a scratch or a primary lesion; aspiration of sterile pus from the node (a presumptive diagnostic test for CSD) or negative laboratory studies excluding other etiologic possibilities; a positive skin test to CS antigen (5 percent false-positives occur; use of only one antigen may give a false-negative result in 10 to 20 percent of patients); and node biopsy showing histopathology consistent with CSD. If a negative skin test is found to one or two different CS antigens applied simultaneously and again 4 weeks later, and if other studies are negative, a biopsy must be considered to rule out a benign tumor or lymphoma. The presence of tenderness favors adenopathy due to cat scratch or a pyogenic or mycobacterial adenopathy rather than a tumor.

DIFFERENTIAL DIAGNOSIS. CSD should be considered in all patients with persistent or chronic lymphadenopathy, since it is the most common cause of regional lymphadenitis in children or adolescents. Other less common causes are lymphogranuloma venereum, typical or atypical tuberculosis, bacterial adenitis, tularemia, brucellosis, histoplasmosis, coccidioidomycosis, sarcoidosis, toxoplasmosis, infectious mononucleosis, and benign or malignant tumors. In atypical forms of CSD one must consider benign recurrent parotid lymphosialoadenopathy, Parinaud's oculoglandular disease, encephalitis, pneumonia, thrombocytopenic purpura, erythema nodosum, and osteomyelitis, as well as fluctuant lymphadenopathy simulating cystic hygroma or a thyroglossal duct cyst.

TREATMENT. In the majority of patients no active therapy is needed. The best therapy is reassurance that the adenopathy is benign and that it will probably subside spontaneously within 1 to 2 months. Thus management consists of reassurance, analgesics for pain, and aspiration if suppuration occurs. Lack of response to antimicrobials is the rule, and a therapeutic trial of an antibiotic is not recommended. In the child whose node suppurates, needle aspiration, usually performed without local anesthesia, is preferred to incision and drainage. An 18- or 20-guage needle is inserted through normal skin at the base of the mass in order to avoid a chronic sinus tract in the event that a tuberculous lesion is present. Aspiration provides material for skin test antigen, relieves painful adenopathy, and the patient usually becomes symptom-free within 24 to 48 hours. If fluid reaccumulates, reaspiration may be needed. Application of moist soaks to the primary lesion may effect drainage and shorten the duration of lymphadenopathy. The efficacy of steroid therapy in CSD is questionable, and its use seems unjustified. Excisional biopsy of the node is rarely done, but it may occasionally be necessary because of persistent pain or for diagnostic purposes.

PREVENTION.   Because of increasing numbers of pets in the home (50 million cats in the United States), CSD will be difficult to prevent. Disposal of the suspect cat is not recommended, since the cat involved is invariably well and less than 10 percent of family members scratched by the same cat develop CSD. The patient with CSD does not require isolation or quarantine, as there is no evidence of disease spread from man to man.

PROGNOSIS.   The prognosis is excellent; lymphadenopathy usually regresses spontaneously in 2 months. One attack appears to confer lifelong immunity. Complications and sequelae are almost nonexistent and have not been reported in typical cases. In 1 patient with encephalopathy death apparently occurred during treatment of continued seizures with hypothermia. A rare case has been reported where the patient had chronic adenopathy for 2 years. Only 2 patients have had a recurrence of the same adenopathy after an interval as long as 3 years.

References

Altman RP, Margileth AM: Cervical lymphadenopathy from atypical mycobacteria—diagnosis and surgical treatment. J Pediatr Surg 10: 419, 1975

Lyon LW: Neurologic manifestation of cat-scratch disease. Case report and review of literature. Arch Neurol 25:23, 1971

Margileth AM: Cat-scratch disease in 65 patients: evaluation of cat scratch skin test antigen in 109 subjects. Clin Proc Child Hosp DC 27:213, 1971

Schulkind ML, Ayoub EM: Cell-mediated immunity in cat-scratch disease. J Pediatr 85:199, 1974

CHICKENPOX

PHILIP A. BRUNELL and SAUL KRUGMAN

Chickenpox (varicella) is a relatively benign acute contagious disease characterized by a generalized vesicular eruption and mild constitutional symptoms.

ETIOLOGY.   Chickenpox is caused by varicella zoster (V-Z) virus. This virus is a member of the herpesvirus group, rather than the poxvirus group as the name chickenpox might imply. Varicella has been transmitted experimentally to man by inoculation of vesicular fluid

obtained from patients with either zoster (p. 520) or varicella. V-Z virus can be isolated in cultures of human cells from young vesicles but not from respiratory secretions. Virus in vesicular fluid has been shown by electron microscopy to be spherical and to have two concentric outer membranes. It measures approximately 200 mμ in diameter. Complement-fixing antibody can be demonstrated in sera obtained as early as 7 days after onset of disease. Antigen for this test can be prepared from virus obtained from patients with zoster or with varicella.

EPIDEMIOLOGY.   Varicella is predominantly a disease of childhood, with the highest incidence in patients 2 to 8 years of age, but it has occurred at all ages, from the newborn period to the ninth decade of life. Both sexes and all races are equally susceptible. In temperate climates there is usually a higher incidence during the winter and spring months.

Chickenpox is highly contagious and is comparable to measles in this respect. The primary attack rate following household exposure has been estimated to be 87 percent. Subclinical infection rarely if ever occurs. Infection is spread chiefly by direct contact with patients who have varicella or zoster. Under hospital ward conditions the disease may be spread by indirect contact if adequate isolation technique is not practiced. Otherwise, it is only rarely contracted through the medium of a third person. Transmission via the airborne route is also possible and has received much emphasis in recent years. However, in our experience the airborne mode of transmission has played an insignificant role in the dissemination of infection.

The crusts, unlike those of smallpox, do not contain viable virus. The period of contagiousness probably extends from 1 day before to 5 days following the onset of rash. The incubation period ranges from 11 to 20 days, but is usually about 14 days.

IMMUNITY.   One attack of varicella usually confers a lifelong immunity to the disease; second attacks have been reported but are very rare. We have occasionally seen a relapse shortly after recovery from an attack. Although maternal varicella antibody is transplanted across the placenta when pregnant women get varicella, it is uncertain whether women who had varicella in childhood transfer their immunity to their fetuses. The rarity of the disease in the first 3 months of life suggests that the newborn infant possesses a transient immunity; on the other hand, infants born of mothers who have had varicella have developed the disease in the newborn period. Chickenpox during the first 10 days after birth may result in disseminated infection with a fatal outcome.

PATHOLOGY.   The initial lesion is a macule that develops first into a papule and then into a vesicle occupying chiefly the prickle cell layer of the skin. The roof of the vesicle is formed by the stratum corneum and lucidum and the base by the deeper prickle cell layer. According to Unna, a reticulating liquefaction in a few prickle cells initiates the process of vesiculation. Ballooning degeneration takes place in the cells of the vesicle, forming giant cells that can be identified in scrapings of the base of the vesicle. The pathologic lesion is characterized by eosinophilic Cowdry type A intranuclear inclusions.

Postmortem examination of infants who have died of varicella reveals characteristic cellular changes in the esophagus, pancreas, liver, renal pelves, ureters, bladder, and adrenal glands. The lesions, including the intranuclear inclusions, are similar to those seen in the skin. Autopsy reports of adults with primary varicella pneumonia have described changes consistent with a viral pneumonia. The cellular exudate consists chiefly of large mononuclear cells, while polymorphonuclear cells and bacteria are scarce. Typical type A intranuclear inclusion bodies characteristic of chickenpox may be found in the alveolar septal cells.

SYMPTOMS.   Symptoms prior to the appearance of the rash are mild or absent. A rash first appears on the scalp, face, or trunk. The majority of lesions progress rapidly from macule to papule to vesicle with a surrounding erythema. This red areola is most distinct at the time of the fully formed vesicle and fades as the latter dries. Occasionally lesions are seen in which a vesicle is not surrounded by a red areola. The process of drying begins at the center; this causes a slight depression, giving the vesicle an umbilicated appearance. As the lesion dries and the areola fades, a crust forms that falls off in about 5 to 20 days, depending on the depth to which the skin has been involved.

The lesions appear in crops over a period of 3 to 5 days; they involve the scalp, face, trunk, and extremities. The distribution of the lesions is predominantly centripetal, the greater concentration of the lesions being on the trunk rather than on the extremities. Vesicles also develop on the mucous membranes of the mouth, most commonly over the palate. They rupture rapidly, so that the lesion presents as a shallow ulcer grossly indistinguishable from that of herpetic stomatitis. The palpebral conjunctiva, pharynx, larynx, and trachea may also be involved.

The most striking manifestation of the eruption is the presence of lesions in all stages in any one general area. Macules, papules, vesicles, and crusts are present in close proximity. The pocks are usually most abundant over the back and shoulders. In mild cases there may be little or no fever, with only a few scattered lesions. In an average case the temperature ranges from 38.5 C to 39 C. In severe cases the entire body is covered with innumerable lesions, and the patient is acutely ill with a temperature of 40 C to 40.5 C. The fever gradually subsides as the crops of lesions cease to appear and the vesicles begin to dry and become crusted. There is no significant change in the number and type of blood cells.

Varicella, like many other viral infections, is much more severe in adults than in children. In our experience primary varicella pneumonia is not an uncommon manifestation of the disease in the older age group. The respiratory symptoms may be minimal or very marked, with cough, severe dyspnea, cyanosis, hemoptysis, and varying degrees of prostration. These symptoms usually appear during the first week of the illness and are more apt to be associated with an extensive skin eruption. Physical examination of the chest reveals a paucity of signs. Radiographs show diffuse nodular infiltrations throughout both lung fields that clear slowly in the course of 2 to 6 weeks. During a 6-month period 10 of 30 adults with varicella presented clinical and radiographic evidence of primary varicella pneumonia.

Recent prospective studies suggest that pneumonia may be less common in adults with varicella than our experience with hospitalized cases might indicate. Of 114 military personnel with varicella, it was found that only 4 percent had clinical signs and 16 percent had radiographic evidence of pulmonary involvement. Adults with varicella pneumonia may also have myocarditis, hepatitis, nephritis, and bleeding manifestations.

COMPLICATIONS.   Complications are not common in children. However, in one large series reported by Bullowa and Wishik, 5.2 percent of cases presented some type of complication. Secondary infection of the local skin lesions with staphylococci may cause impetigo, furuncles, cellulitis, erysipelas, or conjunctivitis. Septicemia, suppurative arthritis, osteomyelitis, and acute glomerulonephritis may be sequelae to the local skin complications. Primary varicella pneumonia may be complicated by pleurisy with effusion and mediastinal emphysema.

Encephalitis, a rare complication of chickenpox, is similar to postmeasles and postvaccinal encephalitis, both pathologically and clinically, except for the frequent cerebellar signs seen with chickenpox encephalitis. It is discussed elsewhere (p. 1877). Other neurological complications reported include transverse myelitis, peripheral neuritis, and optic neuritis.

An unusual and fatal course has been described by Haggerty and Eley in a scattered group of 12 children who contracted varicella while on cortisone therapy. The fulminating infection was usually hemorrhagic, ending in death within a few days. In these patients the daily dose of cortisone varied from 25 to 499 mg and had been given over periods ranging from a few days to 2 months before the development of varicella. The patients' ages ranged between 11 months and 8 years. Steroid therapy was being given for rheumatic fever, for various blood dyscrasias, or for asthma.

A report by Wright and associates calls attention to severe hypoglycemia as a complication of varicella. Three infants 3 to 6 months of age developed hypoglycemia with intractable seizures between the fourth and sixth posteruptive days and died within 24 hours. Spinal fluid sugar concentration in all three cases was below 11 mg/100 ml. Occasionally bullous or purpuric skin lesions may be seen in the course of varicella. Varicella has been reported as one of the more frequent viruses associated with Reye's syndrome (p. 1099).

DIAGNOSIS.   Varicella usually poses no problem in diagnosis. One can usually elicit a history of contact about 2 weeks prior to the onset. The illness produces few systemic signs and often no prodromal symptoms. The primary skin lesion is a vesicle, but lesions in various stages of development—macules, papules, vesicles, and crusts—are present at the same time. The lesions are most numerous on the trunk and relatively sparse on the extremities.

The problem of differentiating varicella from smallpox occasionally arises. In smallpox the constitutional symptoms that precede the eruption are severe, whereas with varicella the patient is most acutely ill at the height of his rash. The lesions of smallpox are all of uniform age and size in any one general area; they take from 5 to 6 days to develop and are deeper than the lesions of varicella, usually with a central umbilication. The eruption of smallpox is usually centrifugal; that is, the concentration of lesions on the face, hands, and feet tends to be greater than on the trunk. The vesicular fluid of chickenpox does not produce lesions on a rabbit's cornea nor on the chorioallantoic membrane of a chick embryo. The vesicular fluid from smallpox lesions can also be used as antigen for a specific smallpox complement fixation test. And finally, a smear prepared from the base of a vesicle and treated with Giemsa's stain reveals the presence of tremendously enlarged giant epithelial cells and intranuclear inclusions in varicella, herpes simplex, and herpes zoster, but not in smallpox. Modified smallpox may be clinically indistinguishable from varicella. Under these circumstances the diagnosis can be clarified by laboratory procedures.

Bullous impetigo may occasionally be difficult to differentiate from varicella. In rickettsialpox, vesicular lesions are superimposed on a firm papule. The eruption is usually preceded by a febrile illness with grippe-like symptoms. An eschar is present at the site of the mite bite. Rickettsialpox and generalized herpes simplex can be differentiated from varicella by laboratory tests. Pemphigus, dermatitis herpetiformis, and drug eruptions may occasionally cause problems in differential diagnosis. Hemorrhagic chickenpox may be confused with meningococcemia or with hemorrhagic smallpox. Insect bites and papular urticaria may also be mistaken for the early stage of varicella.

TREATMENT. In general, isolation and quarantine in the home are unnecessary. Chickenpox is usually spread before it is clinically manifest; it is usually very benign and is one of those inevitable diseases of childhood. Even in institutions quarantine is of questionable value.

Regular preparations of gamma globulin do not prevent the occurrence of chickenpox. However, Ross's data suggest that extremely large doses of gamma globulin used prophylactically may reduce the number of lesions and hence the general severity of varicella in family contacts. A gamma globulin preparation obtained from the serum of patients convalescent from herpes zoster has been found to be effective in preventing chickenpox in household contacts. To be effective the preparation must be given within 3 days after exposure. The convalescent zoster globulin is not yet commercially available, but it should become so within the next year. Prophylaxis is recommended for children who are likely to experience severe disease. These include children under 1 month of age, those who are under treatment with steroids, and those with malignant diseases. The same is true for patients receiving immunosuppressive therapy. In the face of a known exposure or an epidemic, steroids should not be prescribed for susceptible individuals unless absolutely necessary in an emergency situation. If exposed to varicella, susceptible patients on long-term steroid therapy should have the steroid dosage lowered to a maintenance level.

Washing with soap will not spread the virus and may decrease the chances of bacterial infection. Bathing in a bath containing starch will provide temporary relief of itching. Calamine lotion is also used to relieve itching. Since scratching of lesions by children is inevitable, fingernails should be trimmed.

Herpes Zoster

Herpes zoster is caused by the V-Z (varicella zoster) virus and occurs when patients who have previously had chickenpox have reactivation of virus believed to be latent in neural tissue. The painful vesicular lesions follow a dermatome distribution. It is particularly common in patients with deficient immunologic function such as those with malignancies. However, it is also seen in otherwise normal people. Susceptible individuals exposed to patients with herpes zoster will develop chickenpox since zoster patients are contagious and the V-Z virus causes both chickenpox and zoster.

References

Armstrong RW, Gurwith MJ, Waddell D, Merigan TC: Cutaneous interferon production in patients with Hodgkin's disease and other cancers infected with varicella or vaccinia. N Engl J Med 283:1182, 1970

Brunell PA, Gershon AA: Passive immunization against varicella-zoster infections and other modes of therapy. J Infect Dis 127:415, 1973
———— Gershon AA, Hughes WT, Riley HD Jr, Smith J: Prevention of varicella in high risk children: a collaborative study. Pediatrics 50:718, 1972

Feldman S, Hughes WT, Daniel CB: Varicella in children with cancer: seventy-seven cases. Pediatrics 56:388, 1975

Srabstein JC, Morris N, Larke RPB, et al: Is there a congenital varicella syndrome? J Pediatr 84:239, 1974

CYTOMEGALOVIRUS INFECTIONS
JAMES B. HANSHAW

Cytomegalic inclusion disease (CID), generalized salivary gland virus disease, cytomegaly, and inclusion disease are synonyms for an illness caused by cytomegalovirus infection. Although frequently an inapparent infection it may be a cause of fetal encephalitis, with damage to the developing central nervous system. Disease also occurs in patients on immunosuppressive therapy and others subject to opportunistic infections. The virus has been associated with a mononucleosislike illness in previously well patients and in individuals receiving transfusions of blood.

ETIOLOGY. Cytomegalovirus infection is caused by a species-specific agent with the physiochemical and electron microscopic characteristics of a herpesvirus. In 1955 it was isolated in human fibroblastic tissue culture from infants with CID as well as from adenoid tissue of school-age children. A cytopathic effect was noted in vitro that was characterized by large intranuclear inclusions. The propagation of the virus provided the basis for development of specific serologic tests.

EPIDEMIOLOGY. The distribution of cytomegalovirus infection is ubiquitous. The prevalence of complement-fixing antibodies is especially high in communities where there is crowding and where living conditions are substandard. Approximately 50 percent of women in the childbearing age group are seropositive, the range being from 20 to 90 percent. Approximately 4 percent of pregnant women excrete the virus in the urine, and it can be isolated from the cervix of another 10 to 15 percent. In the several studies that have been done in this country and in the United Kingdom, 0.5 to 1.2 percent of newborns are virus-positive. Thus cytomegalovirus is the most common of the human fetal infections. In some countries infection occurs in the majority of infants during the first year of life. In the United States complement-fixing antibody is present in 2 to 15 percent of infants from 6 to 24 months of age.

PATHOGENESIS AND PATHOLOGY. Cytomegalovirus apparently does not induce a highly communicable infection. A substantial number of individuals remain susceptible to the infection in adult life. The virus has been isolated from saliva, breast milk, urine, cervical secretions, semen, feces, the upper respiratory tract, and circulating leukocytes. Virus is probably transferred by intimate contact with an infected individual or by infusion of blood from an asymptomatic blood donor. Nursing personnel working on infant wards and newborn nurseries do not have a higher prevalence of complement-fixing antibody than women in the general population. There is evidence that the placenta itself is infected prior to transmission to the fetus.

The *symptomatic* newborn is rarely without neutralizing, complement-fixing, and immunofluorescent IgM antibodies in the cord serum. The presence of specific IgM antibody is of value in differentiating maternal from fetal antibody because of the failure of maternal IgM antibody to pass the placental barrier. Antibody in the serum of the congenitally infected infant does not prevent the persistence of virus excretion for years after birth. The precise mechanism of this remarkable chronicity is not known.

Among adults with renal transplants receiving immunosuppressive therapy, over 90 percent develop active cytomegalovirus infection if they have cytomegalovirus antibody prior to surgery. Approximately half of seronegative patients subsequently become infected on immunosuppressive therapy. Cytomegalovirus infection tends to be focal in character, with spread of the virus from cell to cell. Infected cells may be greatly enlarged and contain eosinophilic intranuclear and basophilic cytoplasmic inclusions.

CONGENITAL INFECTION. CLINICAL MANIFESTATIONS. Approximately 95 percent of infected infants are asymptomatic. The clinical manifestations encountered most frequently among *symptomatic* newborns are, in order of decreasing frequency, hepatosplenomegaly, jaundice, purpura, microcephaly, chorioretinitis, and paraventricular cerebral calcifications. Any one of these signs may occur alone. A petechial rash on the first day after birth is suggestive of cytomegalovirus infection. Often the only physical finding is a general failure to thrive or increased irritability. Some infants have repeated respiratory infections.

The frequency of various congenital abnormalities in infants with CID is increased; these include clubfoot, inguinal hernia, strabismus, high-arched palate, microcephaly, and deafness. There are several reports of associated congenital heart disease, but the etiologic relationship of these abnormalities to the infection has not been established.

The major complications of congenital cytomegalovirus infection are sequelae involving the central nervous system. There is little evidence that extraneural involvement of viscera such as the liver, spleen, kidney, or lungs results in any permanent damage to these organs. Blindness is associated with macular chorioretinitis or optic atrophy. Unilateral or bilateral deafness may be complete or may be limited to the higher frequencies. Spastic quadriplegia or hypotonia are common manifestations in severely affected infants. Psychomotor function may range from a vegetative state with no meaningful communication to milder abnormalities with minimal effect on speech, behavior, and motor coordination.

DIAGNOSIS. The diagnosis of congenital infection is usually not suspected at birth because of the high proportion of asymptomatic infections. The presence of infection (not necessarily disease) can be established by virus isolation in human fibroblastic tissue culture from the urine, blood, upper respiratory tract, or biopsy material, by demonstration of cytomegalovirus IgM antibody in the cord or neonatal serum, by persistent cytomegalovirus complement-fixing or hemagglutination-inhibiting antibody beyond 6 months of age, or by demonstration of large nuclear inclusion-bearing cells in the urine sediment at birth.

DIFFERENTIAL DIAGNOSIS. Toxoplasmosis. Cytomegalovirus infection resembles toxoplasmosis in striking detail. However, toxoplasmosis is more likely to be associated with microphthalmia, *scattered* cerebral calcifications, hydrocephalus, and chorioretinitis. The demonstration of specific *Toxoplasma* antibody titers persisting beyond 6 months of age or the presence of *Toxoplasma* IgM antibody in early infancy strongly suggest congenital infection.

Rubella. Congenital cytomegalovirus and congenital rubella may be difficult to distinguish in the neonatal period. Both can be associated with a purpuric rash, jaundice, microcephaly, and deafness. However, the presence of central cataracts is strong presumptive evidence of rubella. If these are associated with a congenital heart lesion, the probability of rubella is high. Specific laboratory tests for rubella virus or rubella IgM antibody or serial hemagglutination-inhibiting antibody tests are required for a definitive diagnosis.

Herpesvirus Hominis. Herpesvirus hominis (herpes simplex) infection is usually transmitted to the infant during labor and has its onset in the second week after birth. The disease is often fulminant in character and may present as a meningoencephalitis, pneumonitis, or undiagnosed vesicular rash. The virus is readily isolated from vesicular lesions.

Bacterial Sepsis. Infants with bacterial sepsis usually are more lethargic than infants with CID, and they rarely have a petechial rash. Although the diagnosis rests on a positive blood culture, the decision to treat with antibiotics must be made on the basis of early clinical findings.

PROGNOSIS. The prognosis in congenital infection must be guarded in an infant with symptoms at birth. Approximately 75 percent usually have some central nervous system sequelae. Although asymptomatic infants discovered on routine surveys have a more favorable outlook, there is preliminary evidence that approximately 30 to 40 percent of infants with cytomegalovirus IgM in the cord serum have detectable central nervous system sequelae 5 years after birth. Deafness may not become apparent until the second year of life. The absence of cytomegalovirus IgM antibody in the cord serum and a birth weight above 3,000 g are favorable prognostic signs.

ACQUIRED INFECTION. Cytomegalovirus acquired in infancy and early childhood is usually inapparent, although occasionally respiratory symptoms with pneumonia, paroxysmal cough, petechial rash, hepatomegaly, and splenomegaly may occur. Central nervous system disease due to infection acquired after birth has not been demonstrated, although there are reports of associated myoclonic seizures in infants and infectious polyneuritis in adults. Chorioretinitis has been described rarely following acquired infection.

Hepatomegaly and mildly abnormal liver function tests are found in well individuals excreting cytomegalovirus in the urine and also in patients with cytomegalovirus (CMV) mononucleosis. The latter patients may experience malaise, fever, chills, myalgia, sore throat, headache, anorexia, and abdominal pain. On physical examination, pharyngeal edema without exudate, lymphadenopathy, and splenomegaly may be present. Atypical lymphocytosis is common. Some patients have maculopapular rashes, especially if ampicillin is administered. Abnormal serologic reactions including cold agglutinins, antinuclear antibody, and cryoimmunoglobulins have been described. A similar illness has been noted in patients 2 to 4 weeks after receiving blood transfusions. This condition, referred to as post-transfusion mononucleosis, is clinically similar to CMV mononucleosis. Acquired cytomegalovirus infection has also been associated with autoimmune hemolytic disease, ulcerative lesions of the gastrointestinal tract, post-transplantation pneumonia, and thrombocytopenic purpura.

There is equivocal evidence that the mild liver dysfunction associated with acquired cytomegalovirus infection is capable of progressing to chronic hepatitis, granulomatous hepatitis, or cirrhosis of the liver. Children with chronic hepatitis or chronic liver disease may have a higher prevalence of active infection, but the relationship of this infection to the pathogenesis of chronic liver disease is uncertain. For the majority of cytomegalovirus infections acquired after birth, recovery occurs without significant complications. The symptoms of CMV mononucleosis may persist for 5 to 10 months after the onset of the disease.

The diagnosis of acquired cytomegalovirus infection in a patient with mononucleosislike symptoms can be established by virus isolation as described above. Isolation of cytomegalovirus from peripheral leukocytes has been reported in this syndrome. Serologic determinations, such as the presence of specific immunofluorescent IgM antibody or a fourfold rise or decline in complement-fixing antibody, must be interpreted with more caution than in the newborn period because of cross-reactions with other cell-associated herpesviruses and a tendency for complement-fixing antibody to fluctuate widely in normal subjects. Patients with CMV mononucleosis are always heterophile-antibody-negative.

CMV mononucleosis may be difficult to distinguish from heterophile-antibody-negative infectious mononucleosis, since both conditions occur in young adults, have atypical lymphocytosis, anginal symptoms, abnormal liver function tests, splenomegaly, and fever. In addition, the cytomegalovirus IgM (FA) test is positive in cytomegalovirus and infectious mononucleosis, presumably because Epstein-Barr virus (EBV) and cytomegalovirus share common antigens. A patient with CMV mononucleosis usually has virus in the urine, upper respiratory tract, and peripheral leukocytes. EBV antibody can be measured by an indirect immunofluorescence technique. The complement fixation tests for EBV and cytomegalovirus are specific for each agent.

A jaundiced patient with CMV mononucleosis may clinically resemble one with infectious or serum hepatitis. A serum glutamic oxaloacetic transaminase level above 800 units is unusual for cytomegalovirus infections at any age and common in icteric infectious hepatitis. Both conditions may be associated with atypical lymphocytosis. Jaundice in an adult is far less common in cytomegalovirus infection than in infections with other hepatitis viruses. A history of recent contact with a jaundiced person is strong evidence in favor of infectious hepatitis. Serum hepatitis antigen may be detected in the serum of many patients with serum hepatitis. The presence of generalized adenopathy and splenomegaly is more likely to be associated with mononucleosis than with disease due to either the infectious hepatitis virus or the serum hepatitis virus.

Although acquired cytomegalovirus infections are usually benign, they may be life-threatening in a patient subject to opportunistic infection. Progressive pneumonitis, hemolytic anemia, purpura, gastrointestinal ulceration, hepatitis, pericarditis, and encephalitis have been described in such individuals.

TREATMENT. There is no satisfactory treatment for cytomegalovirus infections. The use of corticosteroids, gamma globulin, and antiviral drugs, such as deoxyuridine, floxuridine, cytosine arabinoside, and adenine arabinoside has variously been reported to have equivocal, beneficial, or no effect on the clinical course. These reports are difficult to evaluate because of the small numbers of individuals treated, the multiple factors operating simultaneously, and the variability of virus excretion in individuals tested at different times.

PREVENTION. It is not possible to prevent cytomegalovirus infection at the present time. Handwashing and gown technique should be used by individuals working with patients with known cytomegalovirus infection in a hospital setting. Usually this is ineffectual because of the difficulty the physician has in making the diagnosis. Almost everyone in a given population will acquire cytomegalovirus at some time in life. The possibility of preventing natural infection by the use of a live vaccine is under active investigation.

References

Benyesh-Melnick M: Cytomegaloviruses. In Lennette EH, Schmidt NJ (eds): Diagnostic Procedures for Viral and Rickettsial Infections, 4th ed. New York, American Public Health Association, 1969, p 701

Hanshaw JB: Congenital cytomegalovirus infection: fifteen year perspective. J Infect Dis 123:555, 1971

Plummer G: Cytomegaloviruses in man and animals. In Melnick JL (ed): Progress in Medical Virology. Basel, Karger, 1973, p 92

Weller TH: The cytomegaloviruses: ubiquitous agents with protean clinical manifestations. N Engl J Med 285:203, 267, 1971

EXANTHEMA SUBITUM

Philip A. Brunell and Saul Krugman

Exanthema subitum was well described by Zahorsky in 1913 under the name of roseola infantum. Later it was given the name exanthema subitum by Veeder and Hempelmann. Although long ignored outside of North America or regarded as an atypical form of one of the other familiar eruptions, especially rubella, it has been reported from various parts of the world and now seems to be recognized with increasing frequency.

Circumstantial evidence indicates that the infection is caused by a filterable virus. No organism is consistently recovered, and the course of the disease is uninfluenced by antibacterial therapy. Intramuscular injection of blood or serum taken from patients at the height of the fever has produced a similar illness in 3 of 14 recipients, with fever developing in 6 to 9 days, an eruption appearing following defervescence at 9 to 12 days, and associated neutropenia and relative lymphocytosis. Comparable transmission experiments suggest that the etiologic agent is also present in the patient's nasopharyngeal secretions. However, efforts to propagate it in tissue culture have thus far been unsuccessful.

About 80 percent of cases occur between the ages of 6 and 18 months, and most cases occur before the age of 3 years. There is no sex predilection. The disease may be found at any time of year, although peaks of incidence in May and October have been reported. The great majority of cases occur sporadically; even when no attempt is made to isolate the patient, transmission of the disease to siblings and other close contacts is decidedly rare, and institutional epidemics are almost unknown. Nevertheless, in urban life the probability that any individual infant will acquire the disease is relatively strong. In Rochester, New York, Breese found that about 16 percent of infants followed closely from the time of birth developed exanthema subitum by the age of 1 year. The rarity of cases after early childhood and the comparative lack of susceptibility of infants during their first 6 months of life suggest that virtually all adults have developed a lasting active immunity as a result of previous infection and that the mother transfers temporary immunity passively to her offspring. Nothing is known of the pathologic anatomy of exanthema subitum beyond its clinical manifestations.

The onset is acute, with fever that may reach 39.5 C to 40.5 C and occasionally with initial convulsions. Although irritability, drowsiness, anorexia, and often mild catarrhal symptoms are present, a striking feature of the disease is that the patient does not seem as ill as the height of his fever might lead one to expect. After 2 to 4 days of fever the temperature falls by rapid lysis, and coincidentally with defervescence the rash makes its appearance. It is macular or maculopapular in type, looking not unlike that of rubella; it affects principally the trunk, neck, and retroauricular region, largely sparing the face and extremities. Itching, if present at all, is mild. After a few hours the eruption begins to fade, and within 2 to 3 days it has usually disappeared, leaving neither pigmentation nor desquamation. Enlargement of lymph nodes, especially of the occipital and postauricular groups, is commonly present at the height of the rash. Mild leukocytosis may accompany the onset of fever, but characteristically the granulocyte count decreases promptly, leading to leukopenia with relative lymphocytosis by the second or third day. Systemic symptoms usually disappear with defervescence. In a small fraction of cases the eruption appears before the temperature has completed its return to normal. In others the febrile stage is prolonged to 5 or 6 days.

Exanthema subitum is distinguished from rubella by the height and duration of fever preceding the appearance of the eruption. It is differentiated from measles by the absence of Koplik's spots, lacrimation, and coryza, as well as by the fact that the patient is afebrile or nearly so at the height of the rash. An eruption accompanying infectious mononucleosis or some of the enterovirus infections may cause difficulty until appropriate laboratory studies have been made. Echovirus 16 and coxsackievirus B5 may cause an illness accompanied by a rash that resembles roseola. Some patients ill with these viruses develop the rash after defervescence. In an infant or young child under treatment with a sulfonamide or penicillin, drug sensitivity may be wrongly inferred when a rash appears. Treatment is purely symptomatic.

Complications are exceedingly rare, although the incidence of central nervous system involvement appears to be higher than can be accounted for simply by febrile convulsions. Stupor and coma have been described at the height of the febrile stage; some patients have shown prolonged or repeated seizures, stiff neck, increased intracranial pressure, and rarely a mononuclear pleocytosis in the cerebrospinal fluid suggestive of encephalopathy. Many children showing these signs have recovered completely; others have been left with residua—hemiparesis, epilepsy, intellectual impairment, and sometimes cerebral atrophy demonstrable by pneumoencephalography. The pathogenesis of such complications is not well understood. Some may result from cerebral anoxia secondary to prolonged generalized convulsions at the height of the infection; others suggest direct invasion of the central nervous system, presumably by the virus that causes the disease. A guarded prognosis must be given when conspicuous nervous symptoms accompany the febrile stage.

References

Berenberg W, Wright S, Janeway CA: Roseola infantum (exanthem subitum). N Engl J Med 241:253, 1949

Breese BB Jr: Roseola infantum (exanthem subitum). NY State J Med 41:1854, 1941

Burnstine RC, Paine RS: Residual encephalopathy following roseola infantum. Am J Dis Child 98:144, 1959

Clemens HH: Exanthem subitum (roseola infantum); report of eighty cases. J Pediatr 26:66, 1945

Hellström B, Vahlquist B: Experimental inoculation of roseola infantum. Acta Paediatr 40:189, 1951

Kempe CH, Shaw EB, Jackson JR, Silver HK: Studies on the etiology of exanthema subitum (roseola infantum) J Pediatr 37:561, 1950

Letchner A: Roseola infantum; a review of fifty cases. Lancet 2:1163, 1955

Veeder BS, Hempelmann TC: A febrile exanthem occurring in childhood (exanthem subitum). JAMA 77:1787, 1921

Zahorsky J: Roseola infantum. JAMA 61:1446, 1913

VIRAL GASTROENTERITIS

HORACE L. HODES

In the late 1930s several studies of outbreaks of diarrhea in hospital nurseries suggested that viruses might cause gastroenteritis. By 1940 several viral causes of gastroenteritis in animals (calves, cats, mice) had been discovered. In 1942 Light and Hodes isolated a filterable virus from newborn infants ill with diarrhea in a Baltimore hospital. This virus caused diarrhea in young calves and could be passaged readily from one calf to another in series. Infants developed neutralizing antibodies against the virus during convalescence from the gastroenteritis. The virus was not found in unaffected infants, and such infants had no antibodies against the virus.

ROTAVIRUS DIARRHEA. In 1973 Bishop and associates observed virus particles in 6 of 9 biopsy specimens of duodenum obtained from children with acute gastroenteritis in Melbourne, and Flewett and associates reported from England that a high percentage of infants and children under 5 years of age with gastroenteritis were excreting, in their stools, the virus described by Bishop. The virus resembled the reoviruses, but it has been shown to belong to a new group of viruses, which probably will be officially named the rotaviruses because they have the appearance on electron microscopy of a double-rimmed wheel. The rotavirus that causes diarrhea is 67 nm in diameter; its nucleic acid is a double-stranded RNA, arranged in 11 segments (reoviruses contain double-stranded RNA in 10 segments).

Rotavirus is probably the most common cause of diarrhea of infants and young children, at least in developed countries. Although rotavirus infection of adults is common, it very rarely causes gastroenteritis. Rotavirus diarrhea is more common in winter than in summer, although it occurs throughout the year. The incubation period is 24 to 72 hours. Vomiting is a prominent symptom; the disease may be severe, and fatalities among infants have been reported. The virus causes a sharp decrease in disaccharidase secretion in the intestine. Diagnosis of rotavirus infection may be made by finding the characteristic virus particles in suspensions of stool examined by electron microscopy.

NORWALK VIRUS DIARRHEA. Kapikian and associates isolated a virus that commonly causes epidemic gastroenteritis among adults as well as children. This virus was first isolated from a man with gastroenteritis during a diarrhea outbreak in Norwalk, Ohio. It is a small virus (27 nm in diameter) that has been classified with the parvoviruses. It has been cultivated in organ cultures of human fetal intestine, and it has caused gastroenteritis in a human volunteer. The Norwalk virus usually causes mild gastroenteritis. Parvoviruses have been found in the feces of neonates and may cause gastroenteritis in the first weeks after birth.

OTHER VIRUSES. It is also now apparent that coronaviruses cause diarrhea among children as well as among adults; they have been shown to be associated with diarrhea in India and in West Africa. Also, three outbreaks of diarrhea apparently due to a coronavirus have been reported from Bristol, England. A number of enteroviruses have been proposed as etiologic agents of gastroenteritis; it is very probable that these viruses do sometimes cause diarrhea. However, because enteroviruses are found so frequently in the intestinal tract of normal children, it is difficult, on epidemiologic grounds, to determine their importance in causing gastroenteritis.

TREATMENT. There is no specific treatment for any of the viral agents described. Prompt treatment with fluid and electrolytes should be instituted when dehydration is present, and it should be kept in mind that fatalities in young infants have been observed. Furthermore, rotaviruses have been shown to cause disaccharidase deficiency, and the possibility of prolonged deficiency should be kept in mind.

References

Bishop RF, Davidson GP, Holmes IH, Ruck BJ: Virus particles in epithelial cells of duodenal mucosa from children with acute non-bacterial gastroenteritis. Lancet 1:1281, 1973

Davidson GP, Bishop RF, Townley RRW, Holmes IH, Ruck BJ: Importance of a new virus in acute sporadic enteritis in children. Lancet 1:242, 1975

Flewett TH, Bryden AS, Davies H: Virus particles in gastroenteritis. Lancet 4:1497, 1973

Kapikian A, Wyatt RG, Dolin R, et al: Visualization by immune electron-microscopy of a 27-nm particle associated with acute infectious nonbacterial gastroenteritis. J Virol 10:1075, 1972

Light JS, Hodes HL: Studies on epidemic diarrhea of the new-born; isolation of a filtrable agent causing diarrhea in calves. Am J Public Health 33:1451, 1943

—— Hodes HL: Isolation from cases of infantile diarrhea of a filtrable agent causing diarrhea in calves. J Exp Med 90:113, 1949

VIRAL HEPATITIS

James W. Mosley

The term viral hepatitis defines a clinical and pathologic entity caused by at least two agents that otherwise differ virologically, immunologically, and epidemiologically. The nosologic terms used earlier (infectious hepatitis and serum hepatitis) have been replaced by type A hepatitis and type B hepatitis. Both forms can be transmitted by contact, and both can be transmitted by percutaneous introduction.

Laboratory procedures for specific diagnosis of type A hepatitis are limited to a few research centers. Specific techniques for diagnosis of type B hepatitis are generally available in all hospitals and clinics. The test for hepatitis B surface antigen should be used routinely in the evaluation of all cases of suspected viral hepatitis, even in children, regardless of epidemiologic background. Prior to the availability of specific tests for hepatitis A and B viruses, there were epidemiologic data suggesting that the syndrome of viral hepatitis could be mimicked occasionally by other known agents and also regularly produced by viruses not previously identified. The ability to diagnose type A and type B hepatitis has resulted in a group of cases to which the designation non-A/non-B has temporarily been applied.

CLINICAL PICTURE. The onset of viral hepatitis in children is often abrupt. Typically the child becomes sufficiently ill within a period of 12 to 24 hours to curb activities spontaneously. Less frequently the onset is gradual, over a period of several days, with tiredness and poor appetite being the only complaints. Other common symptoms during the preicteric phase of the illness include fretfulness and irritability, headache, lack of appetite, nausea, vomiting, generalized aching, and right upper quadrant or epigastric discomfort. Constipation and diarrhea occur occasionally and with equal frequency. A slight nasal discharge or mild sore throat may occur in 10 to 20 percent of children. Fever in the range of 37.5 C to 38.0 C is moderately frequent; higher levels are seen occasionally.

After 3 to 7 days of such symptoms the urine becomes brown because of the excretion of bilirubin. This finding is often the first clue to the diagnosis of viral hepatitis; it is followed at 1 day to several days by detectable conjunctival jaundice and then generalized jaundice. In a large percentage of icteric cases, excretion of bilirubin into the gastrointestinal tract is sufficiently reduced to result in white or gray stools. The icteric phase of the illness may last from a few days to several weeks. It is seldom more prolonged than 10 days in children.

It should be emphasized that viral hepatitis is a generalized disease. The nausea and vomiting may be related, at least in part, to the occurrence of gastritis and duodenitis. Hemolytic anemia (especially in children with glucose-6-phosphate dehydrogenase deficiency) and thrombocytopenia have been described; carditis also occurs in severe cases. However, except for the gastrointestinal symptoms, these manifestations rarely cause clinical concern.

A number of children will experience anicteric hepatitis. Diagnosis is usually made only when the illness follows exposure to a known source of infection, such as a jaundiced sibling or some suspected common source or mechanism of infection. Symptoms in anicteric hepatitis have approximately the same frequency as in the preicteric phase of icteric disease, but they are milder and of briefer duration. Icteric relapse is a relatively rare event.

In addition to icteric and anicteric illnesses, the agents of viral hepatitis can produce asymptomatic infections. Such infections have usually been detected from serial determinations of laboratory tests for hepatic dysfunction when there was known exposure. The frequency with which abnormal results are found depends on the sensitivity of the particular test used and the frequency with which the child is tested. Infections are now also known to occur with hepatitis B virus, in which even serial biochemical tests show no deviation; it is probable that such nonhepatitic infections will be documented for hepatitis A virus and any newly recognized agents.

Rarely, a child with icteric hepatitis may progress to massive necrosis of hepatic parenchymal cells, with the clinical picture of acute hepatic failure. Although this complication can occur early in the course of the disease, it usually supervenes after 5 to 15 days in the icteric phase. Initially, drowsiness returns, sometimes accompanied by irritability and inappropriate verbal responses. Asterixis is often elicited (stages I and II). If the child progresses into steadily deeper obtundation (stage III) and unresponsiveness even to painful stimuli (stage IV), the prognosis is very poor. As a herald to obtundation, hyperexcitation with shouting, screaming, and wild movements may be seen. A case fatality rate among children with acute hepatic failure of 59 percent in two recent series is only modestly better than that of 67 to 80 percent seen in adults. However, if recovery occurs it is usually without sequelae.

BIOCHEMICAL INDICES. Reliance for the diagnosis of hepatitis (ie, hepatic necrosis and inflammation) is placed on the so-called liver function tests. These are more accurately described as indices of hepatic dysfunction. One must recognize also that to a greater or lesser extent they are all nonspecific for any form of liver disease; none is diagnostic of viral hepatitis. In general, these tests can be placed in one of three broad categories: those in which release of enzymes by damaged hepatic cells, and possibly an increased rate of synthesis, results in an increase of enzymatic activities in serum; those in which there is decreased excretion of various substances into the bile, especially bilirubin and sulfobromophthalein; those that measure decreased rates of proteins synthesized in the liver (eg, clotting components other than factor VIII).

In the average case in pediatric practice, laboratory tests are most helpful in the preicteric stage, when the diagnosis is not clear (p. 1092). At that time the most useful are the serum alanine and aspartate aminotransferases (SGPT and SGOT, respectively) assays and a test for bilirubin in the urine. Of these, the alanine aminotransferase is the most sensitive, but a semiquantitative test for bilirubinuria can be easily performed in the physician's office. If the latter is positive and the history is otherwise compatible, the child can usually be considered to have viral hepatitis.

Once the diagnosis is established, laboratory tests are usually needed only in patients sufficiently ill to require hospitalization. To follow the course of the illness, the prothrombin time is the most meaningful measurement in terms of severity and prognosis. There is usually no point in determining sulfobromophthalein retention in a patient who is icteric or has an elevated serum bilirubin; either of the latter findings is already sufficient indication of decreased hepatic excretory capacity. In addition, severe allergic reactions to this dye sometimes occur. Neither the height of the serum aminotransferase activity nor that of the serum bilirubin correlates well with the severity of illness. In addition, serum enzyme levels may remain elevated for varying periods in convalescence. Unless accompanied by other findings, they do not indicate clinically significant persistence of infection.

DIFFERENTIAL DIAGNOSIS.   Excluding newborns, viral hepatitis is by far the most common cause of jaundice in infants and children in the United States. However, there are other causes that must be considered in every patient, even in an epidemic setting. Among adolescents, infectious mononucleosis frequently produces a subclinical hepatitis and occasionally jaundice. The occurrence of pharyngitis sufficiently severe for the patient to complain of it spontaneously is suggestive of mononucleosis rather than viral hepatitis. Pronounced lymphadenopathy and splenomegaly are also more suggestive of infectious mononucleosis. Atypical lymphocytes occur in both diseases, as well as in a number of other viral infections; however, a finding of more than 10 percent atypical lymphocytes suggests infectious mononucleosis. The heterophil titer is occasionally elevated in viral hepatitis, and appropriate absorption studies should be carried out if an abnormal result is obtained. A jaundiced patient with cytomegalovirus mononucleosis may clinically resemble one with hepatitis A or B. An SGOT level above 800 units is unusual in the former and common in the latter. Generalized lymphadenopathy and splenomegaly, which are common in cytomegalovirus mononucleosis, aid clinically in the differential diagnosis, since they are less common in viral hepatitis.

A history of exposure to a jaundiced dog is of concern in a jaundiced child only when the canine illness is leptospiral, especially that form due to *Leptospira icterohaemorrhagiae*. Contact with urine from an infected dog can result in transmission to members of the family. Conjunctival suffusion, leukocytosis, proteinuria, pyuria, and frank meningitis are all suggestive of this diagnosis. Canine viral hepatitis is not responsible for clinically recognized human infections.

Other causes of jaundice in children include hemolytic anemia and cholelithiasis. The latter is most frequently seen in children with familial hemolytic disorders. In a child severe vomiting, obtundation, and elevated serum aminotransferase activity, Reye's syndrome must be considered, in addition to fulminant viral hepatitis. The occurrence of an elevated creatine phosphokinase level (indicating muscle involvement), a normal or mildly elevated bilirubin, and a prothrombin time greater than 20 percent of the control value are all indicative of Reye's syndrome, rather than encephalopathy due to fulminant viral hepatitis.

MANAGEMENT.   There is no specific treatment for viral hepatitis. Several studies have shown that the important measures in promoting rapid convalescence are adequate rest when the patient feels ill and maintenance of a good caloric intake. These measures can usually be provided at home, unless conditions there are unsatisfactory or the disease is of greater severity than usual. In general, parents may be encouraged to keep the patient in bed during the acute phase of the illness, certainly so long as the child stays there willingly. As he begins to feel better and desires increased activity (which may coincide with the appearance of jaundice), quiet activities indoors should be allowed. He should remain away from school until jaundice has disappeared, although infectivity with hepatitis A is lost soon after onset of the icteric phase. Even a mildly icteric child is regarded as a menace to the health of the community and creates a clamor for widespread administration of immune globulin.

The total caloric intake appears to be the most significant factor in promoting recovery. Recommendations for high-protein and low-fat diets were based on outmoded pathophysiologic concepts and have no place in modern practice. The patient's appetite is often better in the morning than later in the day, and administration of a large share of the day's calories at breakfast is helpful when anorexia or nausea is still a problem. Supplemental administration of the B vitamins is frequently recommended, although their value has not been demonstrated. A decreased prothrombin time is usually not corrected by administration of vitamin K. The defect is in hepatic synthesis of clotting factors rather than in absorption of vitamin K, unless the jaundice has been of long duration. Antibiotics are of no value in treatment, and routine administration of corticosteroids is to be strongly discouraged.

Progression to hepatic precoma or coma is a matter of serious concern. The child or adolescent should be hospitalized immediately for evaluation if drowsiness *after* onset of jaundice is reported by a parent. Restriction of protein, administration of nonabsorbable antibiotics to reduce ammonia production by intestinal bacteria, and supplemental feeding with glucose by nasogastric tube or intraveneously are employed as treatment. Administration of a corticosteroid in large doses is traditional, but its value is very doubtful. Exchange transfusion, plasmapheresis, cross-circulation to a liver preparation, and total-body washout are not of benefit, nor is the use of specific antibody administered as hyperimmune plasma or globulin.

Some improvement in prognosis in recent years is entirely attributable to better supportive care, including acid–base and fluid balance and management of respiratory and cardiac irregularity and arrest. Therefore the child should be in an intensive care unit where proper equipment and trained personnel are available for such emergencies. If the hands are washed after patient contact and sterilization of equipment is practiced, the patient with fulminant viral hepatitis poses no likely hazard to personnel or to other patients in the unit.

TYPE A HEPATITIS. Hepatitis A virus has not been demonstrated to replicate in any cell culture system, but at least two species of nonhuman primates are susceptible to infection, and electron microscopy has opened the way to detection of both viruslike particles and antibodies to one or more of the components of the virus. Hepatitis A virus has tentatively been classified as belonging to the enterovirus group on the basis of its size, a cytoplasmic localization of the particle in hepatic parenchymal cells, heat stability at 60 C for 1 hour, ether stability, acid stability, and reactions compatible with RNA content.

Epidemiology. The incubation period of type A hepatitis has been documented to range from 15 to 48 days, with 30 days more common. The incubation period is probably related in part to the size of the inoculum, but it is not influenced by the route of infection. The agent is in blood in the latter part of the incubation period and the early phase of the acute illness. Experimental studies have not demonstrated infectivity after the first few days of the icteric phase, and chronic viremia is not known to occur. The virus is excreted in the feces from as early as 2 weeks prior to onset until the early part of the icteric phase. Chronic intestinal shedding does not appear to be epidemiologically significant in most circumstances. Therefore hepatitis A virus is ecologically dependent on serial propagation in humans; no reservoir is known.

Type A hepatitis is most commonly transmitted from person to person, especially among children of school age. A history of exposure to a jaundiced person from 2 to 6 weeks prior to onset of symptoms can be obtained in 20 to 40 percent of pediatric cases. However, even in a communitywide epidemic, prior exposure is not recognized by the majority of patients, for whom the source of infection is presumed to be persons with anicteric illnesses and inapparent infections. Type A hepatitis transmitted from person to person is a cyclic disease with periodic rises and falls in incidence. However, in the United States and some western European countries the long-term trend since the late 1940s has been downward. Sporadic cases occur between epidemics, especially in larger cities where there is a population of sufficient size to maintain the chain of infection. During the course of an epidemic the spread of the disease is relatively slow, with cases building up over a period of several months.

In addition to transmission from person to person, type A hepatitis may be spread through fecal contamination of water or food. It is, in fact, the only enterovirus for which transmission by a common vehicle is well accepted. A common-vehicle epidemic is most often recognized when a large number of cases occur in a period of 2 to 4 weeks. Waterborne disease most often results from private supplies with inadequate safeguards. However, institutional, camp, and municipal supplies have become contaminated and have caused large-scale epidemics. When waterborne transmission occurs, cases among adults usually outnumber those among children. This is presumably due to a lower proportion of subclinical cases in adults. Acquisition of type A hepatitis by swimming or accidental immersion in contaminated water has not been documented.

Food can also serve as a vehicle for infection. The frequency with which epidemics traceable to food have been recognized has increased in recent years, presumably as a result of greater alertness. Most of the recognized epidemics have taken place in schools or other institutions in which a population eating in a particular cafeteria or other facility has remained together throughout the incubation period. Additional epidemics probably go unrecognized because the population is not so localized or because questioning is not sufficiently detailed to point to exposure at a particular place. In some instances a person assisting in food preparation has had a recognizable illness at an appropriate interval before the beginning of the epidemic; otherwise, inapparent infection in a foodhandler is assumed. Contamination of a food at its source is known only with raw shellfish, although frozen strawberries have been suspected.

Careful questioning with regard to all exposures is worthwhile; the existence of a large-scale common-vehicle epidemic has on a number of occasions been recognized first from the history of a particular exposure given by a few patients seen in close proximity. In addition, all cases should be reported to the health department, as routine investigation for potential vehicles is now practiced by many city and county health departments.

Special Clinical Features. The onset is more abrupt in type A than in type B hepatitis, and fever is more frequent. Among young children the ratio of inapparent to clinically diagnosable cases is probably lower for type A than for type B hepatitis. The fatality rate in clinically apparent cases is very low in the pediatric and adolescent age groups.

Prevention. Normal immune globulin (ie, IgG derived from donors unselected on the basis of prior experience with viral hepatitis) continues to be effective in small doses, probably because of the extent of prior experience among adults in the general population. If the incidence of type A hepatitis continues to decline, selection of donor units found to contain antibody may become necessary. Under any circumstances, standardization of antihepatitis A content seems likely in the next several years.

Most cases occurring in susceptible family members have their onset more than 2 weeks after that of the index case. This lag usually allows enough time for immune globulin to be administered to other family members relatively early in the incubation period. The sooner immune globulin is administered, the more effective it appears to be. For persons with a known exposure, a single injection of 0.02 to 0.04 ml/kg body weight provides adequate protection. In practice, administration of 1 ml for children weighing less than 50 kg and 2 ml for all other persons is a convenient approach.

It has been demonstrated that many household contacts to whom immune globulin has been administered have had changes in liver function indicative of inapparent infection. It is probable, therefore, that immune globulin prevents clinical disease but not infection among most exposed family members. There is no evidence that subsequent development of active immunity is impaired. Because a child can be spared an illness of 1 to 3 weeks duration by giving him immune globulin, there is no reason to withhold this material when household exposure occurs. It is also worthwhile to immunize passively adult members of the household regardless of their age, despite the fact that the secondary attack rate in adults is lower. When the disease does occur in adults, it is often more severe. It is probable that most of those who are susceptible are already infected by the time the nature of the illness is recognized. Therefore there is no point in isolating ill persons from other members of the family; reliance should be placed on passive immunization.

Concern has often been expressed that administration of immune globulin to exposed individuals facilitates the spread of type A hepatitis by permitting persons excreting the virus to remain ambulatory. In several situations it has been found that administration of immune globulin to half of the population was sufficient to curtail transmission of the agent to those not receiving such protection. This suggests that persons experiencing inapparent infection as a result of having received immune globulin do not usually serve as a source for others. Accordingly, there is no reason to restrict activities of persons who have been exposed and have received immune globulin as prophylaxis. Until hepatitis A virus can be grown in a cell culture system, there is no prospect for a vaccine for active immunization.

TYPE B HEPATITIS. The hepatitis B virus is a DNA virus not yet characterized sufficiently to be assigned to any genus. The virion itself is 42 nm in diameter, with a 27-nm core produced in the nucleus of the hepatic parenchymal cell. Antigens (a, d or y, w or r, and perhaps others) of the protein coat are added after migration of the nucleoprotein core into the cytoplasm; the mechanism of release from the cell after the virion is covered is not yet known. Diagnostically the most important fact is that the coat or surface proteins are produced in great excess over the quantity required to cover the cores, and this surplus is released into serum as cylindrical and spherical particles. It is the great excess of viral antigen that permitted its fortuitous discovery by a precipitin line on double diffusion in an Ouchterlony system.

Serologic Diagnosis.   The a surface antigen is common to all strains of hepatitis B virus thus far described, and it occurs on the surfaces of all three types of particles. Usually only one of the determinants in each of the d,y and w,r pairs occurs, so that subtypes are distinguishable on the basis of combinations (adw, adr, ayw, ayr). Such subtyping can be useful epidemiologically.

The term hepatitis B surface antigen (HB_sAg) may be considered as applying to either the a component common to all strains (comparable to the Australia antigen as originally described) or the combination of all surface antigens contributing to particle detectability. The test for HB_sAg is commonly available in hospital laboratories and is the basis for screening blood donors for the carrier state. It becomes positive 1 to 2 months prior to onset of symptoms, before any abnormality in serum enzymes is detectable. It is positive at the onset of jaundice in 70 to 80 percent of cases and remains positive into convalescence in 40 to 50 percent. HB_sAg positivity is also an index of the carrier state, which supervenes in 5 to 10 percent of overt cases and in larger proportions of some special groups. The corresponding antibody (anti-HB_s) does not become detectable until 1 month to several months after HB_sAg disappears. Therefore it is not very useful clinically, but it can be helpful in special situations in documenting HB_sAg-negative cases suspected of being type B disease. Tests for core antigen (HB_cAg), the corresponding antibody (anti-HB_c), and virus-induced DNA polymerase are at present research procedures without immediate clinical applicability.

The test for HB_sAg should be routine in the work-up of patients with illnesses compatible with viral hepatitis. A positive test that becomes negative in convalescence is diagnostic of type B hepatitis. A persistently positive test is presumptive evidence, the probability being inversely proportional to the carrier rate in the population from which the patient comes. Persistent positivity is also compatible with an interposed episode due to another agent infecting a carrier.

Epidemiology.   The epidemiologic concept of type B hepatitis has changed drastically as a result of the ability to detect chronic infection by the hepatitis B virus. Far from being an agent found largely in developed countries and dependent on modern medical procedures for transmission, it occurs worldwide; high prevalences have been found in a variety of remote, relatively isolated populations. Hepatitis B virus maintains itself in a reservoir of human carriers and is transmitted by a wide variety of mechanisms.

The extent of the carrier reservoir differs widely among populations, with a genetic predisposition to the carrier state being one possible explanation for the variation. However, other factors must influence its occurrence, because there is a similar propensity to chronic hepatitis B infection among diverse groups with certain medical problems; these include the mentally retarded regardless of etiology (although the predisposition seems to be highest in Down's syndrome), patients with severe renal disease of any etiology requiring long-term hemodialysis, and patients with hematogenic malignancies. Although patients in some of these groups have impaired immunologic defenses, others have no demonstrable defect, despite intensive search with sophisticated techniques. In contrast to many viral illnesses (such as measles and varicella) that are more severe in patients who are immunologically compromised, hepatitis B virus characteristically causes milder illness or is subclinical. However, congenital or acquired hypogammaglobulinemia is an exception; type B hepatitis in these patients usually has a fatal outcome.

During the latter part of the incubation period, during acute infection, and in chronic infection the virus can be detected in saliva (probably as a result of transudation in crevicular fluid at the gingival margins), urine, semen, menstrual blood, breast milk, articular fluid, and ascitic fluid. Early claims for its presence in feces were based on nonspecific reactions; antigenic and structural integrity are rapidly lost in the presence of intestinal and bacterial enzymes. The risk of clinical or subclinical infection in any population depends on the extent of the carrier reservoir, the opportunities for percutaneous transfer, and socioeconomic and behavior characteristics permitting oral–oral transfer and venereal transmission.

The mechanisms of infection are extremely varied. The most efficient is the transfer of blood from one individual to another, by transfusion or through contaminated instruments. Any implement that breaks the skin of two successive persons without sterilization has the potential for transmitting type B hepatitis. This includes needles and syringes, whether used licitly by health-care professionals or illicitly for self-injection of psychotropic drugs. Also to be considered among pediatric cases are ear-piercing and acupuncture. Oral–oral transmission among children is probably due in large part to shared food items and to the placing of objects contaminated by saliva in the mouth. Biting by infected persons can also result in infection. Among adolescents, sexual contact may be important. Another mechanism of particular interest and concern to the pediatrician is vertical transmission from the acutely or chronically infected mother to the fetus or neonate. Specific serologic testing indicates that no more than 15 percent of cases of overt viral hepatitis in children in the United States is due to type B hepatitis, and the same appears to be true in many other countries. Nonetheless, testing for hepatitis B surface antigen is still appropriate in all cases because clues to etiology from epidemiologic evidence are not necessarily reliable.

Special Clinical Features. Contrary to previous assumptions, the ratio of subclinical to clinical infection appears to be much higher in type B than in type A hepatitis. Other features include a higher proportion with gradual rather than abrupt onset and occurrences of urticarial rashes and joint manifestations. Among adults the case fatality rate is also higher than for type A disease, a feature not verified for children. Hepatitis B infection has been associated with and is presumably a cause of polyarteritis and glomerulonephritis due to formation of immune complexes. Chronic infection may be associated with (1) no manifestation other than antigenemia, (2) mild abnormalities in serum enzyme levels but no clinically significant compromise of hepatic function, or (3) chronic active hepatitis leading to cirrrhosis and death. Chronic infection also appears to predispose to hepatocellular carcinoma.

Prevention. Screening of all blood donors for HB_sAg is now required in the United States and in several other countries. In conjunction with a sensitive radioimmunoassay technique, this measure has reduced the incidence of transfusion-associated type B hepatitis. HB_sAg-negative blood occasionally results in type B disease in recipients, probably due to low levels of coat proteins in relation to numbers of infectious virions produced. The main risk in transfusion-associated hepatitis is the way the donor is recruited; the risk of infection from blood from collecting agencies that pay some or all of their donors is as much as 10-fold higher than that from blood collected by banks relying on voluntary contributions.

When plasma from individual donors is pooled, a single donation from a carrier contaminates all of the units derived from that pool. Therefore the risk from pooled products is greatly enhanced. Regardless of the method of treatment, pooled plasma is no longer used in the United States because of its hazards. Partial fractionation to remove the components that coagulate when plasma is heated at 60 C for 10 hours results in a plasma protein fraction that is safe, as is serum albumin similarly heated. Both derivatives serve the same purpose as pooled plasma and have the advantage of safety. The immune globulin fraction is safe without heat treatment.

The pooled derivates presently in use that can still cause type B hepatitis are the concentrates of clotting factors. Cryoprecipitate preparations from small pools are preferable to the commercially prepared concentrates made from very large pools of plasma from paid donors. Fresh frozen (single-unit) plasma is preferable to either from the standpoint of hepatitis, unless the patient has antibodies to hepatitis B virus.

Viral hepatitis transmitted by unsterile instruments is entirely preventable. Syringes, needles, and other equipment that break the skin or mucous membranes should be sterilized by one of three means: boiling for 30 minutes, autoclaving at 15 pounds of pressure for 30 minutes, or sterilizing in dry heat at 160 C for 1 hour. Ethylene oxide sterilization of items that cannot be heated is also effective, but the need to monitor its effectiveness makes it less suitable for the practitioner's office than for the hospital.

The greatest problem in prevention at the present time is in dealing with subjects exposed to a carrier in the household. Epidemiologic studies indicate that, except for spouses, the short-term risk of transmission within 6 to 12 months is low, but the long-term risk is high. By testing all family members for hepatitis B surface antigen *and* antibody, presumed susceptibles can be identified. If all members have already experienced infection, no problem exists. In general, restrictions and precautions other than strictly separate use of items such as toothbrushes and razors are probably ineffective and inadvisable for psychological reasons.

Hepatitis B immune globulin, prepared from plasma known to contain antibodies to components of hepatitis B virus, has been found in some situations to protect against exposure to type B hepatitis. The range of indications for use of this material and the appropriate dose remain to be determined.

Normal immune serum globulin has been tried in the prevention of type B disease, but results have been irregular and unpredictable. Recent lots seem more likely to have some effect against exposures to small inocula than those used in the past. Antibody levels are higher, probably due in part to a wider experience of the American donor population with type B disease during the epidemic that has been in progress since 1967. More important, the present ability to detect carriers eliminates units with high concentrations of viral antigens in the plasma pools from which lots of normal globulin are prepared. In the past, such units must have combined with hepatitis B virus antibodies and lowered their titers in the IgG fraction.

If hepatits B immune globulin is not available, normal globulin may be tried for intimate contacts of acute cases and noncontinuous percutaneous exposures to carriers. The appropriate dose is unknown, but it would seem reasonable to administer 0.1 to 0.2 ml/kg body weight as soon as possible after exposure, and again 30 days later. An attempt at prophylaxis is not needed in a child who has household contact with an acute case in either a parent or a sibling, since the secondary attack rate is very low in the United States under these circumstances. Continuous household exposure to a carrier, such as a parent undergoing long-term hemodialysis, cannot be approached practically by continued administration of normal globulin. Even though the agent has not been propagated in cell cultures, a killed-virus vaccine for active immunization against type B hepatitis is theoretically possible because the appropriate viral antigens can be harvested from the plasma of carriers. Candidate vaccines are now being prepared, but 5 to 10 years may be required to evaluate immunogenicity, safety, and effectiveness.

OTHER HEPATITIS VIRUSES.   The evidence for agents causing human hepatitis other than hepatitis A virus, hepatitis B virus, and the occasionally hepaticomimetic agents (eg, Epstein-Barr virus, cytomegalovirus) is derived from two sets of observations made almost entirely in adults. If transfusion-associated hepatitis were due only to hepatitis A and B viruses, one would expect a bimodal distribution of incubation periods, with its trough in the interval between 45 and 49 days after blood administration. Instead, one finds a unimo-

dal curve with a peak at that point, which suggests an additional agent with a modal incubation period of 45 to 49 days. This inference has recently been strengthened by negative tests for both hepatitis A and B viruses in most of those cases that have occurred since testing of donors for hepatitis B surface antigen became routine. Since 1956 there have been reported instances of persons (usually individuals abusing drugs with shared injection equipment) who have had three separate attacks of acute viral hepatitis, and recently four separate episodes have been described. Serologic testing has demonstrated that these extra episodes cannot be attributed to repeated infection by hepatitis A or B viruses nor to other agents likely to be hepaticomimetic. Therefore there may be as many as two new (previously unrecognized) agents. Their role in the pediatric age group remains to be determined.

VIRAL HEPATITIS IN PREGNANCY.   It seems likely that viral hepatitis in pregnancy, due to any of the agents regularly producing it, is no more serious than in the nongravid woman and does not increase fetal risk. Follow-up of children born to mothers who have experienced viral hepatitis at any time in pregnancy has not indicated an increased frequency of congenital abnormalities of any type. Therefore the occurrence of viral hepatitis during pregnancy is not an indication for interruption from the standpoint of either mother or fetus. Neonatal viral hepatitis is discussed elsewhere (p. 1085).

References

Brzosko WJ, Krawczyński K, Nazarewicz T, Morzycka M, Nowoslawski A: Glomerulonephritis associated with hepatitis-B surface antigen immune complexes in children. Lancet 2:477, 1974

Dietzman DE, Matthew EB, Madden DL, et al: The occurrence of epidemic infectious hepatitis in chronic carriers of Australia antigen. J Pediatr 80:577, 1972

Dupuy JM, Frommel D, Alagille D: Severe viral hepatitis type B in infancy. Lancet 1:191, 1975

Kattamis CA, Demetrios D, Matsaniotis NS: Australia antigen and neonatal hepatitis syndrome. Pediatrics 54:157, 1974

—— Tjortjatou F: The hemolytic process of viral hepatitis in children with normal or deficient glucose-6-phosphate dehydrogenase activity. J Pediatr 77:422, 1970

Krugman S, Giles JP: Viral hepatitis, type B (MS-2 strain): further observations on natural history and prevention. N Engl J Med 288:755, 1973

Litt IF, Cohen MI: The drug-using adolescent as a pediatric patient. J Pediatr 77:195, 1970

Provost PJ, Wolanski BS, Miller WJ, et al: Physical, chemical and morphologic dimensions of human hepatitis A virus strain CR 326. Proc Soc Exp Biol Med 148:532, 1975

Reisler DM, Strong WB, Mosley JW: Transaminase levels in the post convalescent phase of infectious hepatitis. JAMA 202:37, 1967

Schweitzer IL, Mosley, JW, Ashcavai M, Edwards VM, Overby LB: Factors influencing neonatal infection by hepatitis B virus. Gastroenterology 65:277, 1973

Szmuness W, Prince AM, Hirsch RL, Brotman B: Familial clustering of hepatitis B infection. N Engl J Med 289:1162, 1973

Villarejos VM, Visoná KA, Gutiérrez A, Rodríquez A: Role of saliva, urine, and feces in the transmission of type B hepatitis. N Engl J Med 291:1375, 1974

HERPES SIMPLEX VIRUS INFECTIONS

ANDRE J. NAHMIAS AND M. OUSAMA TOMEH

Herpes simplex viruses (HSV) are among the most common infectious agents affecting individuals in the pediatric age group. HSV belong to a family of DNA viruses that includes, besides the other human viruses (cytomegalovirus, varicella zoster, and Epstein-Barr virus), over 60 other viruses infecting many species ranging from fungi to man. All HSV have the capacity to persist throughout the life of the host, which provides them a great evolutionary survival advantage; however, for man this property is responsible for the clinical problem of recurrent infections. There are at least two distinct serotypes of HSV (HSV-1 and HSV-2), and they have different modes of transmission. HSV-1 is transmitted chiefly via a nongenital route, whereas HSV-2 is most often transmitted venereally or from a mother's genital infection to the newborn. The mode of spread of each of the two virus types is reflected by its relative prevalence at different ages and by its pattern of clinical distribution within the host. Thus HSV-1 infections occur most frequently during childhood and usually affect body sites above the waist (mouth, lips, eyes, face). HSV-2 infections, on the other hand, occur most often during adolescence and young adulthood and involve body sites below the waist (genitalia, buttocks, thighs). The majority of infections in newborns, which can involve external as well as internal sites, are also caused by HSV-2.

Although infections in individuals without prior exposure to either virus type (primary infections) may often be subclinical, they tend to cause more severe clinical manifestations than infections occurring in individuals previously exposed to HSV. The clinical manifestations caused by either virus may also be more severe in certain types of hosts (such as the newborn or immunocompromised patient) and with involvement of certain sites (such as the central nervous system).

VIROLOGY. HSV consist of four major components: a centrally located core surrounded by three concentric structures (the capsid, the tegument, and the envelope). The core contains DNA coiled around proteins arranged in the form of a barbell. The icosahedral capsid contains 162 capsomeres and measures about 100 nm. Between the capsid and the envelope is the tegument, composed of fibrilous material. The envelope, derived from nuclear and occasionally other cell membranes, gives the complete virus particle a diameter of 150 to 200 nm. The lipid composition of the envelope makes the virus particularly susceptible to ether and other lipid solvents.

The proteins on the envelope of the virus are very similar to those found on the membranes of infected cells; thus immune mechanisms can operate not only on the virus itself but also on cells infected by the virus. Antibodies alone, for instance, are incapable of inhibiting cell-to-cell spread of the virus; together with complement or with mononuclear cells (K cells), antibodies can lyse HSV-infected cells in vitro. There are at least 49 proteins specified by the virus, of which about 33 are found in the virion. Variations in the proteins within strains of either type of HSV may influence immune responses and serodiagnosis. The DNA of HSV-1 and HSV-2 is a linear double-stranded molecule with a molecular weight of 99 ± 5 million daltons. About half of the HSV-1 and HSV-2 DNA sequences are homologous, and the guanine + cytosine content of the DNA of the two types varies by 2 moles/dl (Table 18).

HSV-1 and HSV-2 have a wide in vitro and in vivo host spectrum, being capable of infecting a large variety of cell cultures of human or animal origin and a great number of experimental animals, including nonhuman primates. Variability in the in vitro or in vivo behavior of the two virus types can be demonstrated in some of these systems (Table 18). In humans, including newborns, either HSV type appears to be capable of infecting any body site, if it can be transmitted to that site by external or internal spread.

It has long been appreciated that recrudescences occur in individuals with circulating HSV antibodies. Although the possibility of low-level virus multiplication around the site of involvement cannot be completely ruled out as a possible mechanism for viral persistence,

TABLE 18. Differences Between Herpes Simplex Viruses (HSV) Types 1 and 2*

Characteristic	HSV–1	HSV–2
Clinical	Infects primarily nongenital sites	Infects primarily genital sites
Epidemiologic	Transmission primarily via nongenital route	Transmission primarily via genital route (venereal or mother-to-newborn)
Biochemical: DNA guanine + cytosine (moles/dl)	67	69
Homology of viral DNA	About 50%	About 50%
Biologic:		
Chick embryo (chorioallantoic membrane)	Small pocks	Large pocks
Mice (genital or intramuscular inoculation)	Less neurotropic	More neurotropic
Tissue culture cells	Differences between the two virus types in their ability to propagate, their cytopathic characteristics, or plaque size in certain cell culture lines	

* Adapted from Nahmias and Roizman: N Engl J Med 289:667, 719, 781, 1973.

the best evidence at present favors latency of the virus in a noninfectious form in the sensory ganglia. This conclusion is supported by extensive experimental data in mice, rabbits, and humans. Infectious virus cannot be demonstrated in sensory ganglia; however, using special cultivation methods of the ganglia, infectious virus can be reactivated within several days or weeks. Oncogenic potential of HSV in animals has recently been demonstrated. Together with epidemiologic and other approaches linking HSV to human cancers, particularly cancer of the cervix, these findings raise questions about the possible risk of some of the preventive and therapeutic modalities discussed below.

EPIDEMIOLOGY.   Humans with either primary or recurrent infections are the only natural source of HSV. No natural animal source has been recognized, but individuals exposed to macaque monkeys may acquire a simian B herpesvirus infection of the central nervous system that is clinically similar to HSV encephalitis.

Individuals with clinical or subclinical HSV infections can transmit the virus directly to others by close personal contact, such as kissing, wrestling, or sexual intercourse. Spread of virus by saliva is exemplified by cases of herpetic paronychia in medical or dental personnel who handle the infected oral cavities of patients or contaminated catheters. This mode of viral transmission makes HSV a potential nosocomial infection and may account for the occasional outbreaks of HSV infection in families and in orphanages and other closed populations. Airborne transmission by air droplets or skin squames can also be inferred from some clinical and epidemiologic observations.

Genital HSV-2 and less commonly genital HSV-1 infection in pregnant women has been found to be the major source of virus for the newborn. The genital infection in the mother may have been acquired from sexual contact prior to pregnancy. However, the acquisition of the virus by a pregnant woman late in pregnancy from a male with penile herpes, with subsequent genital transmission to the infant at delivery, has been well documented. Most infected infants will have acquired the herpesvirus around the time of delivery on passage through the infected birth canal or when membranes have been ruptured for over 4 hours. Transplacental transmission, which has been well documented with HSV experimental infection of animals, has been suggested by a few cases of infants with chronic central nervous system or ocular manifestations detected soon after birth. The transmission of HSV to the newborn postnatally from other infected newborns, nursery personnel, or family contacts has not been well substantiated, despite the fact that at least 1 percent of nursery personnel show evidence of clinical or subclinical HSV infection.

HSV neonatal infections have been estimated to range from 1 in 30,000 to 1 in 3,500 deliveries. These infections are more common in premature infants than in full-term infants. Neonatal herpes is also most often noted in infants born to primigravid mothers. Several seroepidemiologic studies have demonstrated that the prevalence of HSV infection is closely related to socioeconomic conditions and to sexual mores. Thus about half of 5-year-old children and two-thirds of adolescents of lower socioeconomic groups have HSV-1 antibodies. The frequency of HSV-1 antibodies in higher socioeconomic groups is approximately half of these figures. HSV-2 antibodies begin to be detected around the age of 14 years; approximately 15 percent of adolescents who begin sexual activity at an early age will possess such antibodies.

The incubation period for neonates with herpetic infection or for older individuals with either primary HSV-1 or HSV-2 infections ranges from 2 to 20 days, with an average of 6 days. The incubation period for encephalitis, which is more difficult to assess, is probably longer.

PATHOGENESIS AND IMMUNITY.   Primary HSV-1 and HSV-2 infections are often clinically inapparent in both children and older individuals, partly because the more common primary sites of infection, such as the mouth or cervix, are not readily visible. When infection occurs in persons who have had no previous contact with HSV, symptoms and signs of illness (when they are manifest) are more severe than in individuals who have acquired antibodies to either HSV-1 or HSV-2 or both. In primary infections fever is generally higher, and lesions are more extensive and of longer duration. Also, constitutional symptoms are more severe, and local adenopathy is more pronounced.

Primary HSV infections are particularly severe in certain types of patients: these include severely malnourished children, those with associated measles, patients with severe burns or chronic skin disorders (such as eczema), individuals receiving immunosuppressive therapy, patients with cancers (particularly of the lymphohematopoietic organs), and children with certain forms of immune deficiency (such as the Wiskott-Aldrich syndrome). In such individuals, as in the newborn, the virus may disseminate to internal organs. The pathogenesis of primary HSV infection has been defined most thoroughly in severely malnourished children. In such cases, as a result of the initial replication of virus at the portal of entry, there is a primary viremia resulting in involvement of certain susceptible organ sites. A secondary viremia then ensues, with further dissemination to visceral organs and more extensive damage. Thus the clinical spectrum may differ, depending on which organ sites are involved and the amount of cellular damage in these organs.

In the noncompromised host, recovery of virus from the blood or peripheral leukocytes has been infrequent. It is therefore not clear at present whether HSV affects areas other than the local site and regional lymph nodes. However, the recovery of HSV-2 from peripheral blood leukocytes and from the cerebrospinal fluid of patients with meningitis suggests that blood dissemination may occur more commonly than was previously realized. Several human and experimental animal observations suggest that HSV may spread neurogenically when encephalitis occurs in otherwise normal individuals. Viral spread from superficial areas of skin to deeper layers may be prevented by the meshwork of connective tissue fibers, because of their size and also because of the possible effects of the negative electric charge on the virus of acid mucopolysaccharides in connective tissues. The pathogenesis of the deeper ocular manifestations associated with HSV has been attributed either to direct viral involvement or to a hypersensitivity reaction.

The pathogenesis of the disseminated forms of neonatal herpes occurring in infants without transplacentally acquired antibodies appears to be similar to that of primary herpes in the severely malnourished child, although the brain is involved much more often in the newborn. Direct neurogenic spread to the brain, and possibly to the retina, appears to occur also in newborns.

In individuals with primary HSV infection, humoral antibodies usually can be detected within 1 to 3 weeks by a variety of neutralization, complement-fixation, complement-mediated cytolysis, antibody-mediated mononuclear cell cytolysis, or passive hemagglutination tests. With special serologic methods it is also possible to demonstrate an early rise of IgM antibodies to HSV, followed by IgA and IgG antibodies. In the newborn, IgM antibodies to HSV can usually be detected within 1 to 4 weeks after birth and are present for 6 months or more. In addition to the humoral response, a cell-mediated response occurs within 1 to 2 weeks after onset of infection in both man and experimental animals. Individuals with serum neutralizing antibodies will usually demonstrate also a delayed hypersensitivity skin test response to HSV antigens. It is not yet clear which of these humoral or cellular factors operate in curtailing the virus in a primary infection or in a newborn who has no antibodies.

Although HSV-1 or HSV-2 infections in individuals with prior HSV-1 and/or HSV-2 infections tend to be less severe clinically than primary infections, in compromised hosts such infections tend to be more extensive and chronic. HSV encephalitis, which was formerly believed to occur only in association with a primary infection, has now been documented in individuals with prior HSV infection. Similarly, although newborns with maternal HSV antibodies originally were believed to be protected from acquiring HSV infections, several cases of neonatal herpetic disease, including fatalities, have been recorded in such infants.

In recurrent HSV infections all individuals appear to possess neutralizing antibodies in varying titers, and usually these do not rise after a recurrence. However, it appears that clinically apparent or inapparent recurrences might be necessary to maintain the neutralizing titer at constant levels in the serum. There are also individuals with frequent herpetic recurrences who possess persistent levels of IgG, IgA, and IgM antibodies to HSV in their serum and who may demonstrate a significant boost in titer of antibodies of the various immunoglobulin classes after a recurrence. Individuals with recurrences also demonstrate positive responses in a variety of in vitro cell-mediated assays. Preliminary data suggest that depression in certain lymphokines (eg, macrophage inhibitory factor, interferon or leukocyte inhibitory factor) may be correlated with increased predilection to HSV recurrences.

In vitro studies indicate that both nonspecific and specific mechanisms are involved in stopping the cell-to-cell spread of HSV, since neutralizing antibodies alone cannot prevent this type of viral spread. In addition, in vitro observations indicate that neutralizing antibodies are unable to inactivate large amounts of extracellular virus and may operate together with complement or with nonimmune or immune mononuclear cells (K cells) in lysing HSV-infected cells.

CLINICAL MANIFESTATIONS. The clinical spectrum of HSV-1 and HSV-2 infection varies in several important respects according to whether the host is a newborn or a normal or compromised child or adolescent. Thus, whereas asymptomatic HSV infections in the newborn appear to be infrequent, they are common in older individuals. Although neonatal herpes is very often serious, resulting in a high fatality rate or sequelae in survivors, the large majority of cases of HSV infections (other than those of the brain) occurring in normal children and adolescents are of mild to moderate severity. Only in the compromised older individual does the severity of the infection occasionally approach that found in the newborn. A third point of difference is that the majority of neonatal infections are caused by HSV-2, whereas, except for venereally transmitted infections in children and adolescents, all other infections are primarily caused by HSV-1.

CHILD AND ADOLESCENT. Mouth. The oral cavity is by far the most common site of HSV infection in children, with the peak incidence occurring in children 1 to 5 years of age. Although the majority of such infections are stated to be subclinical, careful clinical observations may detect a few oral ulcers. The severity of the clinically apparent infection varies, as do the sites of the oral lesions. Thus one or more of the following sites may be affected: buccal mucosa, tongue, palate and fauces. The gums may also be inflamed and bleed readily. Cervical adenopathy is often present; the temperature is usually around 39 C but may be as high as 41.1 C. Excessive salivation may result from pain on swallowing and feeding and even fluid intake may be painful. Hospitalization for fluid and electrolyte therapy may be indicated in severe cases. The oral lesions and clinical symptoms usually resolve within 10 days. Occasionally herpetic infection of other sites such as the face or eyes may accompany the oral lesions, and finger-suckers or cuticle-biters in particular may develop concomitant infections of the fingers. Encephalitis is a very infrequent complication.

In normal children no significant sequelae occur other than for those individuals destined to have recurrent infections. Although herpetic recurrences are infrequent as a cause of lesions in the mouth itself, virus is not infrequently cultured from the oral cavity of individuals with no apparent clinical lesions. In the compromised host, as in the newborn, oral infections may extend to involve the esophagus or lungs and may disseminate to the liver and other visceral organs.

Oral infections are almost always caused by HSV-1; however, oral–genital sexual practices may cause HSV-2 infection of the oral cavity, either with no evidence of disease or with clinically apparent lesions. Oral herpetic infections are usually readily diagnosed clinically. However, if the lesions are present only on the fauces, they may be confused with herpangina and less often with group A streptococcal infection, infectious mononucleosis, and diphtheria. When the herpetic oral lesions are more widespread, they may be misdiagnosed as hand-foot-and-mouth disease (coxsackievirus A disease), Vincent's angina, moniliasis, and the stomatitis associated with trauma or Stevens-Johnson syndrome. In some patients, particularly those receiving immunosuppressive therapy, oral herpes is very often confused with the stomatitis associated with drugs. One of the most common misdiagnoses is made in cases with recurrent oral ulcers that are presumed to be of herpetic origin. However, the large majority of such patients have canker sores or aphthous stomatitis that are nonherpetic in etiology.

Lips. The lips are the most common site for herpetic recurrences due to HSV-1 (cold sores, fever blisters), but they are infrequently the site of primary infection. Although most HSV oral infections occur in early childhood, recurrent labial herpes is not as frequent in children as in adults, and the frequency of recurrence varies greatly from individual to individual. It is not uncommon for febrile illnesses to trigger a recurrence that tends to extend beyond the lips to the face and neck. Labial recurrences usually involve the same or very close sites, but on occasion they involve the contralateral side of the lips and other areas of the face. Labial herpes begins with a burning sensation or itching for 1 to 2 days prior to appearance of lesions. Despite the prodromal symptoms, on occasion some individuals may not develop any herpetic lesion, or the lesion may be aborted and a typical vesicle will not develop. In the compromised host the lips and adjacent facial areas may be involved for prolonged periods. Labial herpes is unlikely to be misdiagnosed, although occasionally the lip lesions may be mistaken for herpes zoster, aberrant vaccinia, and even staphylococcal pustules.

Skin. Primary and recurrent HSV infections may cause skin vesicles and ulcers on almost any part of the body, including face, hands, and feet. Obvious trauma to the skin is occasionally found. Primary skin infections may be accompanied by deep burning pain, edema, lymphangitis, lymphadenopathy, and fever. The vesicles in primary or recurrent infections may appear singly or in clusters; they tend to become pustular, crust over, and heal within 1 week, usually leaving no scars. The skin lesions can occasionally assume a zosteriform distribution and may be severe and of prolonged duration in individuals compromised by certain cancers or immunosuppressive therapy.

Four new forms of skin involvement associated with HSV infection have been described in recent years. The first, herpetic paronychia of the fingers occurring in medical or dental personnel, has been mentioned earlier. Such finger lesions are often very painful and easily confused with bacterial infections. However, herpetic paronychia does not require surgical drainage, which can prolong the healing time beyond the usual 2 to 3 weeks. A second type of HSV skin infection that has recently been described is herpes gladiatorum, a HSV infection that occurs in wrestlers. Such infections develop in skin areas abraded during the course of a wrestling match after contact with an individual with either an inapparent or clinically apparent HSV infection. The third new type of HSV infection occurs in patients with severe burns. In such individuals the disease may be particularly severe, as it may be associated with herpetic pneumonia and disseminated infection. The fourth new type of skin lesion associated with either primary or recurrent HSV infection is erythema multiforme, which has been noted with gingivostomatitis, genital herpetic infection, and labial herpes. The lesions of erythema multiforme may recur with every recrudescence of the herpetic infection. They can also be induced by inactivated herpesvirus preparations, which suggests that they are due to hypersensitivity reaction to viral antigens.

A severe form of skin HSV infection is eczema herpeticum, which occurs in individuals with preexisting chronic skin conditions. This entity, a form of Kaposi's varicelliform eruption, is seen most frequently in children with atopic eczema and occasionally in those with diaper rash. It may also be observed in children with the Wiskott-Aldrich syndrome. Eczema herpeticum is most often caused by a primary HSV infection, but it may occur as a recurrent infection either in eczematous skin areas or in intact skin after the eczema has cleared. There is usually prodromal fever, followed by the appearance of crops of vesicles; the vesicles may then umbilicate and become pustular, confluent, and hemorrhagic. In severe cases large areas of skin are affected, leading to marked losses of proteins and fluids. The virus usually remains localized to the skin, but on occasion it may disseminate to the visceral organs or to the brain. A mortality of about 5 percent is due either to such viral dissemination or to bacterial superinfection.

HSV infections of the skin are sometimes difficult to diagnose, particularly when the patient is not seen until the lesions have become crusted or pustular, or when the affected skin area is denuded. In such cases the herpetic infection may be confused with bacterial or fungal infection or with allergic dermatitis or insect bites. When HSV skin lesions assume a zosteriform distribution they are readily mistaken for herpes zoster, although the diagnosis of recurrent herpes zoster should always raise the question of HSV. Eczema herpeticum is most difficult to differentiate from eczema vaccinatum or eczema coxsackium associated with hand-foot-and-mouth disease. It also may be misinterpreted as increased severity of the underlying skin disorder or as a bacterial or fungal infection.

Eyes. Herpetic involvement of the eye is of particular medical concern because it may cause loss of vision. Primary infections may be accompanied by conjunctivitis and tender preauricular nodes, with or without associated keratitis. Conjunctivitis is also occasionally noted with recurrent infection, but the most common recurrent form is herpetic keratitis. This entity is readily diagnosed clinically because of the characteristic dendritic, branched, flourescent-staining corneal ulcers. Herpetic vesicles are occasionally present concomitantly on the eyelid or on other parts of the face or in the mouth. A history of trauma to the eye may occasionally be elicited. Recurrent keratitis is usually unilateral, but about 5 percent of cases may have bilateral involvement; recurrences within 2 years are seen in at least one-quarter of patients. Deeper ocular involvement, including stromal keratitis and iridocyclitis, occurs occasionally. Corticosteroids in the absence of antiviral drugs should be avoided in ocular herpes, as they have been implicated in contributing to deeper ocular involvement, including perforation of the globe.

Urogenital Tract. Infection of sites in the urogenital tract by HSV is of particular concern to the pediatrician for several reasons. First, it is now apparent that genital herpetic infection is a common venereal disease and that at least one-third of these infections occur in individuals 18 years old or younger. It has been observed in even younger girls who were sexually molested. Occasional genital infections, for example in a 3-year-old male, are autoinfections from concomitantly infected sites, such as the mouth. Second, the fetus and newborn may be infected secondary to genital HSV during pregnancy. Finally, there is the possible relationship between genital herpetic infection and cervical cancer.

About 90 percent of urogenital infections are caused by HSV-2, although some of the HSV-1 infections may result from oral–genital contact. Herpetic infections were originally considered to involve only the external genital sites in the male and female; hence the term herpes progenitalis (which should be abandoned). However, it is now appreciated that the most common site of involvement in females is the cervix (the vagina being less commonly infected) and that infections of the prostate or seminal vesicles can occur in males. In addition, the virus may infect the urethra, bladder, and anorectal area in both sexes.

Approximately 25 to 30 percent of genital infections are primary, in which case symptoms tend to be more severe, with fever, constitutional signs, pelvic or sciatic pain, regional adenopathy, and dysuria. The vulvar, penile, or perineal lesions demonstrate characteristic vesicles that are usually multiple. However, herpetic infections of the cervix are more difficult to diagnose clinically, since the large majority do not demonstrate any lesions suggestive of herpes. Urogenital infections in individuals with prior experience with either HSV-1 or HSV-2 will usually be less severe than primary infections. However, recurrent infections may also be accompanied by pain and dysuria, and especially with frequent recurrences the problem may be psychologically incapacitating.

The complications of genital herpetic infections include meningitis, radiculitis, myelitis, urethral stricture, labial fusion, and bacterial or mycotic superinfection. The herpetic lesions may be confused with the lesions associated with other venereal diseases, particularly chancroid and less often syphilis and lymphogranuloma venereum. At least 10 percent of cases of genital herpes occur in individuals with some other venereal disease such as gonorrhea. Other less common problems in differential diagnosis are genital involvement by varicella zoster, diphtheria, Vincent's angina, impetigo, and the recurrent ulcers associated with canker sores in the mouth.

Nervous System. HSV infections have been associated with a variety of neurologic manifestations, including encephalitis, meningitis, radiculitis, and myelitis. Evidence for the role of the viruses in Bell's palsy and in chronic neurologic and psychiatric disorders is much more tenuous. Almost all of the isolates from the brain of individuals beyond the newborn age group have been HSV-1. This virus has very infrequently been isolated from the cerebrospinal fluid (CSF) of patients with HSV encephalitis. On the other hand, HSV-2 has frequently been associated with CSF pleocytosis and with several cases of meningitis, and the virus is more readily recoverable from the CSF than is HSV-1 Herpes simplex virus encephalitis is also discussed elsewhere (p. 1875).

The diagnosis of HSV involvement of the nervous system is very difficult to make on clinical grounds alone. Unlike the situation with the newborn, in whom the concomitant findings of visible herpetic lesions and encephalitis make the diagnosis of HSV encephalitis almost certain, similar findings in older individuals are not diagnostic; the reason is that herpetic recurrences may be triggered by febrile illnesses or diseases of the central nervous system of nonherpetic etiology. HSV encephalitis must be differentiated from encephalitis due to other causes, both infectious and noninfectious. It must also be differentiated from other causes of localized brain masses, such as tumors or brain abscesses. Brain biopsy is the only certain way to diagnose HSV encephalitis. It is also difficult to differentiate HSV meningitis from the multitude of other causes of the aseptic meningitis syndrome. The association of a clinically evident genital herpetic infection would strongly suggest this diagnosis. Since cases of HSV meningitis are primarily caused by HSV-2, this disease is rarely found in children, but it may be encountered in adolescents and in immunologically compromised individuals.

IMMUNOLOGICALLY COMPROMISED HOST. HSV infection may cause severe localized disease or disseminated infection in immunologically impaired persons, including individuals with certain cancers such as Hodgkin's disease and other lymphomas, patients undergoing immunosuppressive therapy, and children with certain immunologic deficiencies. Severe herpetic disease also occurs in patients with chronic skin conditions and severe burns. The basic defect common to all these conditions has not been ascertained, although a common denominator may be a defect in cellular immunity. Disseminated herpetic disease, which occurs in severely malnourished children in developing countries, has not been reported in this country except occasionally in association with measles or pertussis. Clinical signs of disseminated infection may be nonspecific, such as poor feeding and poor weight gain; they may also include jaundice, hepatosplenomegaly, pneumonitis, and abnormal CNS findings. Hypotension may develop, with a rapid deterioration and a fatal outcome. The diagnosis is usually difficult to make in such cases, but it should be suspected in compromised individuals, particularly if clinically visible herpetic lesions are noted.

FETUS AND NEWBORN.   The clinical spectrum and outcome of neonatal herpetic infection, as noted in 298 published or personally studied cases, are presented in Table 19. Unlike neonatal cytomegalovirus infection, which is most often asymptomatic, intensive virologic studies to detect subclinical HSV cases have been generally unrewarding. However, clinical manifestations of HSV infections among infants in the first month of life may often be missed or misdiagnosed.

Separation of cases into various groups of disseminated or localized infections is important for several reasons, one being the possible pathogenetic mode of viral spread. Thus in disseminated cases with evidence of visceral organ involvement, the virus must have reached these organs via the blood. In such cases the brain may demonstrate no histopathologic changes, the virus may not be recoverable, or the virus may be recovered from the brain in the absence of demonstrable histopathologic findings. Furthermore, virus can usually be isolated from the CSF in neonatal cases of encephalitis with visceral organ involvement. The absence of clinical or laboratory evidence of visceral organ involvement in some of the cases of neonatal herpetic encephalitis and the frequent inability to isolate virus from the CSF, as noted in cases of encephalitis in older individuals, suggest that the virus may be neurologically transmitted to the brain.

Another important reason for classifying cases of neonatal herpes into different groups is related to prognosis, which is much worse in disseminated cases than in those with localized disease other than in the CNS. It must be emphasized that it is not possible in any one case to determine whether skin or throat infection will remain localized or be manifest later as disseminated disease and/or encephalitis, since about half of such cases will develop progressive disease. It should also be stressed that the true prognosis may not be reflected in the figures given in Table 19, since in most reported cases follow-up of surviving infected infants was often inadequate.

The disseminated form of HSV infection affects primarily the liver and the adrenals, but many other organs are also commonly involved, including the spleen, brain, trachea, lungs, esophagus, stomach, kidneys, pancreas, heart, and bone marrow. Initial indications of illness may appear at birth or only after 21 days postnatally, the average being 6 days. Nonspecific constitutional signs are most frequent, including hypoactivity, vomiting, respiratory difficulty, and occasionally fever. External signs suggestive of herpetic infection, such as skin vesicles, are absent in more than half of the cases. The infants may demonstrate hepatosplenomegaly, jaundice with direct hyperbilirubinemia, bleeding diathesis, and CNS abnormalities, including convulsions. The course of disseminated infection is generally stormy with rapid deterioration. Shock and disseminated intravascular coagulation may occur terminally. A few survivors with no apparent sequelae have been recorded, but in general this form of herpetic disease has a very grave prognosis.

The eye can be the primary and only site of HSV involvement, or it can be associated with local CNS or disseminated infections. One or both eyes may be involved by conjunctivitis, keratitis, or chorioretinitis, either alone or in combination. The sequelae comprise residual corneal scars, chorioretinitis leading occasionally to blindness, or cataracts, in which case HSV can be isolated from the lens.

The newborn may demonstrate only skin lesions,

TABLE 19. Clinical Spectrum and Outcome of Neonatal Herpes Simplex Infection*

| Clinical Groups | No. Cases | Outcome in Infant | | |
| | | Died | Survived | |
			With Sequelae	Without Apparent Sequelae
Disseminated				
Without CNS involvement	98	90	1	7
With CNS involvement	96	68	15	13
Localized[†]				
CNS	51	19	24	8
Eye	15	0	6	9
Skin	33	1	8	24
Oral cavity	3	0	0	3
Asymptomatic	2	0	0	2
Total	298	178	54	66

* From Nahmias et al: In Krugman S, Gershon A (eds): Infections of the Fetus and Newborn Infant, 1975. Courtesy of The National Foundation–March of Dimes.
† Classified according to major site of involvement in cases where more than one site is infected.

without evidence of associated ocular, CNS, or disseminated involvement. The skin lesions are characteristically vesicular, but rapid ulceration and skin denudation may confuse the diagnosis. The skin lesions can appear on any part of the body at varying times. They are more likely to be in the perianal region in the case of breech deliveries, and they are often found on the head in case of cephalic deliveries or when the virus is introduced with a fetal monitor. The skin vesicles in localized cases or in survivors of disseminated infections can recur repeatedly over the following years, occurring not only at the site of original involvement but also in previously unaffected skin areas. Other skin manifestations of neonatal HSV include an exanthem that appears as red patches on the first day after birth, a generalized erythematous macular exanthem noted early, and petechiae that are noted later in infants with disseminated infection. Erythema multiforme has also been recorded in one case. Although the majority of infants with local skin infections survive with no apparent sequelae, a few cases have been found later to demonstrate psychomotor retardation or chorioretinitis. These observations point to the need for careful neurologic and ophthalmologic examinations and follow-up studies in all such cases. Very few cases have so far been reported of infections of the oral cavity only or with subclinical infections. These infants appear to have survived without sequelae.

A few cases of neonatal herpes have been suspected within the first 24 hours of life because of the appearance of visible lesions in that period. Although such cases provide evidence of an intrauterine infection, they do not prove a transplacental infection. In most such cases membranes have been ruptured for prolonged periods, indicating an ascending infection. Reports of infants who demonstrate microcephaly or chorioretinitis within the first few days of life are more suggestive of a transplacentally transmitted infection.

Neonatal herpes may be suspected if the mother has had genital herpes during pregnancy. The diagnosis is particularly likely when visible lesions of the skin or oral cavity are present or when characteristic herpetic keratitis is visualized. The skin lesions are not uncommonly erroneously diagnosed as being due to bacterial infections, and they may also be misdiagnosed as herpes zoster or varicella. However, this entity in newborns is most unusual in the absence of maternal infection with varicella zoster virus during pregnancy. It is particularly difficult to diagnose HSV infection clinically in infants with chorioretinitis, CNS findings, or disseminated disease. In such cases the differential diagnosis with infections caused by toxoplasmosis, rubella virus, and cytomegalovirus is very difficult without laboratory aids. For this reason we have grouped these infections into the TORCH complex of perinatal infections (TOxoplasmosis, Rubella, Cytomegalovirus Herpes).

LABORATORY DIAGNOSIS. Herpetic gingivostomatitis, labial herpes, herpetic keratitis, and some forms of cutaneous and genital herpes can usually be diagnosed clinically, although these herpetic diseases may be mistaken for other infectious and noninfectious entities. The diagnosis of the various forms of herpetic infection in the newborn and severe infections such as encephalitis or disseminated disease in the normal or immunologically compromised individual requires specific laboratory aids, particularly when therapy is contemplated.

Morphologic Aids. The intranuclear inclusions and multinucleated giant cells that are seen in Papanicolaou-stained smears of cells obtained by scraping the base of herpetic vesicles or ulcers of the skin or mouth or by scraping the conjunctiva or cornea are characteristic of herpesviruses, including HSV and varicella zoster viruses. The intranuclear inclusions are less readily apparent in Wright-stained or Giemsa-stained smears. In most instances there is little problem in differentiating clinically between HSV and varicella zoster infection. However, the inclusions in urinary cells make it difficult to distinguish HSV from cytomegalovirus infection. Papanicolaou smears of the cervix are particularly helpful to detect subclinical herpetic cervicitis in adolescent girls. The morphologic findings in this genital site have been found to be specific for HSV and to be about two-thirds as sensitive as virologic methods.

Biopsy or autopsy material should be fixed preferably in Bouin's fixative rather than formalin in order to enhance the demonstration of the characteristic inclusions and giant cells. Such material obtained from the brain or various other organs has been particularly useful in the diagnosis of suspected neonatal herpes. It should be appreciated that multinucleated cells can be produced by nonherpetic diseases and that intranuclear inclusions in the brain may be observed with subacute sclerosing encephalitis or simian herpes B and varicella zoster encephalitis. More specific virologic assays are therefore required for definitive diagnosis.

Virologic Aids. Clinical specimens for virus isolation should either be processed as rapidly as possible or frozen at -70 C until processed. It is better to keep the specimen for a few hours at 4 C icebox temperature than in the -15 C freezing compartment. The recent development of a transport medium (Leibovitz-Emory) has facilitated the problem of shipment of clinical specimens, since the swab with which the specimen is obtained, when placed in this medium, can be stored and shipped at ambient temperature.

Virus can readily be isolated in a number of tissue culture systems, and almost pathognomonic cytopathic effects can be detected as rapidly as a bacterial culture, usually within 1 to 3 days. Specific identification of HSV and its antigenic types can then be made by neutralization or immunofluorescence techniques; the latter can be used for rapid identification and direct typing of herpes simplex in clinical specimens. Immunofluorescence tests are particularly helpful in the diagnosis of HSV in brain biopsies of patients with encephalitis, and they are now under study for detection of HSV antigens in CSF leukocytes. In addition, HSV can be demonstrated in vesicular fluid and biopsy or autopsy specimens by the use of electron microscopic techniques, which reveal enveloped or nonenveloped virus particles. The morphologic appearance of HSV by this technique cannot be distinguished from that observed in other herpesviruses, such as cytomegalovirus or varicella zoster virus. The virus can be distinguished as HSV by the use of HSV antibodies labeled specifically with ferritin or horseradish peroxidase.

Serologic Tests.   Many serologic assays can be used to demonstrate HSV antibodies, including neutralization, complement fixation, passive hemagglutination, complement-mediated cytolysis, and indirect fluorescence antibody tests. A primary infection is suggested by the finding of a fourfold or greater rise in titer between the acute serum and the convalescent serum obtained 1 week or more later. Since such a titer rise may be observed with recurrent infections, the distinction between primary and recurrent infection is occasionally difficult. For seroepidemiologic surveys, neutralization assays have proved to be more sensitive than complement fixation tests.

The HSV antibody type (type 1 and/or 2) can be determined by more specialized serologic procedures like microneutralization, kinetic neutralization, multiplicity analysis, and inhibition passive hemagglutination tests. Since there is partial crossing between the two HSV types, some sera, particularly those from individuals who have experienced both types of infections, may be difficult to characterize. This problem may be alleviated once type-specific antigens for each of the two virus types are purified.

Indirect immunofluorescence tests have recently been developed to detect HSV antibodies in the IgM, IgG, and IgA classes of immunoglobulins. Thus IgM HSV antibodies can be used to diagnose neonatal herpes in patients with no characteristic findings in the eyes, throat, or skin. Such IgM antibodies usually appear within 1 to 4 weeks after birth and persist for at least 6 months. The detection of IgM or IgA antibodies in the serum of older individuals unfortunately cannot be used to differentiate a primary from a recurrent HSV infection, since such antibodies occasionally can be found in recurrent cases. The appearance of IgM, IgA, or IgG HSV antibodies in the CSF is also not diagnostic of HSV encephalitis, since occasionally these antibodies may be transuded into the CSF from the blood in patients with CNS disease due to other causes such as tuberculous meningitis. A similar problem is encountered if passive hemagglutination tests are applied to the CSF of patients suspected of having encephalitis. However, the major difficulty is that detectable CSF HSV antibodies may not appear for some time after onset of HSV encephalitis.

In vitro assays for cell-mediated immunity to HSV are still in the research stage, but they may prove to be useful in diagnosis or in demonstration of individuals more prone to HSV recurrences. Positive skin tests of delayed hypersensitivity can be elicited with inactivated HSV preparations that correlate well with the presence of serum neutralization antibodies. Such HSV skin test materials are not available for clinical use.

PREVENTION AND TREATMENT.   Preventive measures for the milder forms of herpetic disease in normal individuals are not practical at present. However, contact with individuals with overt herpetic lesions should be avoided in certain groups of compromised hosts, including children with chronic skin diseases, severe burns, or immunologic defects or those on immunosuppressive therapy. Despite such precautions, patients may become infected with virus from persons with subclinical infections. Protective gloves should be worn by hospital personnel caring for patients with overt herpetic infections. This measure is particularly warranted for the prevention of herpetic paronychia in personnel using suction catheters.

Men with penile herpetic lesions should be cautioned to avoid sexual intercourse with women who are pregnant, particularly during the third trimester, because of the potential of the mother for acquiring an infection close to the time of delivery that can be transmitted to the newborn. Controlled studies have not yet been done to evaluate whether neonatal herpes can be prevented by performance of a cesarean section in women acquiring genital herpes close to the time of delivery. Current information suggests that at least 50 percent of newborns delivered vaginally will become infected and that the risk that infected infants will be severely damaged or killed by the herpetic infection is quite high. It appears that a cesarean section performed more than 6 hours after rupture of membranes would not be successful in protecting the newborn, since the opportunity for an ascending viral infection would be great. Amniocentesis in women with genital herpes aorund the time of delivery should also be considered. If HSV is detected in the amniotic fluid, it is doubtful that abdominal delivery would be helpful. Individualization of each case and close communication between obstetrician and pediatrician are mandatory.

Mild cases of gingivostomatitis require no therapy except the maintenance of proper oral hygiene and, in case of pain, the application of a topical anesthetic. In severe cases fluid and electrolyte therapy may be needed. Herpetic infections of the lips, skin, and genitalia will also usually require no specific therapy. Analgesic ointments may relieve pruritus and burning, and antibacterial ointments may prevent secondary infection. Topical idoxuridine (IDU) has been used for these conditions, but its effectiveness has been questioned by controlled studies. IDU in higher concentration combined with dimethyl sulfoxide (DMSO) is reported to be more effective than IDU alone; however, DMSO is approved only for investigative studies in the United States.

Consultation with an ophthalmologist is advisable for children with ocular herpes. For superficial corneal infections, topical IDU, as a solution or as an ointment, is applied to the eye at frequent intervals. Such treatment is usually effective, but recurrences are not prevented. It appears that the antiviral drug adenine arabinoside (Ara-A) is as effective as IDU for topical therapy and may be particularly useful in cases of IDU-resistant HSV ocular infections. Because ocular herpes can be worsened by the use of corticosteroids, these drugs should be avoided, except if combined with antiviral drugs for the treatment of stromal keratitis. The use of corticosteroids in cases of HSV encephalitis has not been well evaluated.

Systemic administration of IDU and several other antiviral drugs has been used to a limited extent in the treatment of HSV encephalitis, neonatal herpes, and severe HSV infection in compromised hosts. These drugs, which (like IDU) all interfere with viral DNA synthesis, include Ara-A and cytosine arabinoside (Ara-C). All of them have potential toxic effects, especially on the hematopoietic system; they may also be immunosuppressive. Because of their great toxicity, IDU and Ara-C are generally no longer recommended for systemic use. Ara-A appears less likely to cause fever. In addition, unlike the other two drugs, Ara-A is metabolized to its hypoxanthine derivative, which retains antiviral activity. Close monitoring of hematopoietic, liver, and kidney function is required. The effectiveness of any antiviral drug is difficult to evaluate, since some untreated patients with severe forms of HSV infection have survived with no ill-effects, whereas other patients have died in spite of therapy. Controlled studies that are currently under way should allow determination of the true efficacy and the toxic effects of Ara-A. The mechanisms responsible for protection of the host from severe HSV disease and for the frequency of recurrences are still incompletely understood. In addition, many specific and nonspecific measures, such as hyperthermia, macrophage activators, interferon or interferon stimulants, transfer factor, or HSV antibodies, await evaluation. The efficacy of other older approaches is also still unestablished. Thus many types of immunizing agents have been used for treatment of recurrent herpes. The oldest method was autoimmunization, whereby virus from a recurrent site was applied to another site. Recurrences on the new site occurred on occasion, and this approach is no longer used. Although repeated smallpox vaccination is still being done, control studies have not demonstrated any real effectiveness. In addition, severe vaccinia reactions have been reported in some compromised hosts treated in this manner.

Inactivated HSV-1 or HSV-2 vaccines have also been used for several years, but their efficacy has not been evaluated. A more recent approach involving the application of a vital dye, such as neutral red or proflavine, followed by exposure to light, for the treatment and prevention of recurrent herpetic lesions also awaits evaluation. The possible relation of HSV to human cancer and the in vitro ability of inactivated HSV to cause neoplastic transformation encourage caution in the use of either inactivated HSV vaccines or vital dye treatment.

It should also be noted that certain patients, such as those with eczema herpeticum and neonatal infection, are prone to secondary bacterial infection requiring use of antibacterial therapy. Careful fluid, electrolyte, and blood monitoring may also be indicated, as well as measures to combat shock and disseminated intravascular coagulation.

INFECTIOUS MONONUCLEOSIS

WARREN A. ANDIMAN AND GEORGE MILLER

Infectious mononucleosis (Pfeiffer's disease, glandular fever) is an acute infectious disease caused by the Epstein-Barr virus (EBV). It is generally a benign, self-limited illness whose major diagnostic features are fever, lymphadenopathy, sore throat, and lymphocytosis with atypical lymphocytes. The presence of heterophile antibodies with a characteristic absorption pattern is diagnostic, but heterophile antibodies are not invariably detected in childhood mononucleosis.

ETIOLOGY. EBV is a herpesvirus first detected by electron microscopy in cell cultures derived from Burkitt lymphomas. The virus is lymphotropic for B lymphocytes, and in the laboratory EBV has only been cultivated thus far in lymphocytes of man and certain nonhuman primates. The causal relationship between EBV and mononucleosis was first suspected when a laboratory technician working with Burkitt lymphoma cells developed mononucleosis and concomitantly developed antibodies to EBV antigens present in the cultured lymphoma cells. A large body of evidence now implicates EBV as the etiologic agent of mononucleosis. Antibodies to a number of EBV-associated antigens are absent prior to mononucleosis, but they appear during the course of the disease and persist thereafter, probably for life. Only persons without EBV antibodies are susceptible to the disease; conversely, EBV antibodies confer immunity to mononucleosis. Included among the antibody responses to EBV during mononucleosis are specific IgM antibodies, which suggests that the infection is primary. EBV can regularly be recovered from the peripheral blood of patients with acute mononucleosis, as well as from subjects with a past history of the disease. The virus is also present in the oropharyngeal secretions in 80 to 90 percent of acute cases. Oropharyngeal excretion of EBV continues for many months after mononucleosis.

Certain aspects of the disease, including lymphoproliferation and heterophile antibody responses, have been reproduced in nonhuman primates following inoculation with EBV. EBV has the interesting biologic property of causing lymphocytes to grow continuously in cell culture, and this property may in part be responsible for the pathogenesis of the disease.

EPIDEMIOLOGY. One must be careful to distinguish between the epidemiology of EBV infection and the epidemiology of the disease mononucleosis. EBV infections are most often acquired in childhood, usually without clinically recognizable symptoms. Between ages 2 and 6 years there is a rapid increase in the prevalence of antibody-positive children; a second wave of seroconversion begins at 11 years of age. Socioeconomic factors and hygienic environment influence the age at which infection is acquired. In lower socioeconomic groups approximately 80 percent of children have antibody by the age of 6 years. In developing countries 95 percent of children are EBV-antibody-positive by this age. By contrast, in higher socioeconomic classes 40 to 50 percent of adolescents entering college are EBV-seropositive. The disease mononucleosis occurs during infection in adolescence and early adulthood. On the basis of prospective surveys the ratio of apparent to inapparent EBV infections is between 1:2 and 1:4 in the college-age group. In a college population about 10 percent of susceptibles become infected each year.

Epidemiologic and laboratory evidence suggests that transmission of EBV occurs via oropharyngeal excretion and close personal contact such as kissing and other means of salivary exchange. The role that urinary or fecal excretion of the virus may play in transmission is not known. Rare instances of post-transfusion heterophile-positive mononucleosis due to parenteral transmission of EBV have been documented. Transplacental or intrauterine infections, in contrast to the other herpesvirus infections, have not yet been recognized. Since oropharyngeal excretion of EBV occurs in 15 to 20 percent of the general population for prolonged periods after mononucleosis, it is likely that a silent viral carrier state provides the main reservoir of infection. Studies of families and of students in college dormitories indicate that mononucleosis does not spread primarily from case to case, for secondary attack rates are generally low. An unanswered question is why EBV infections are so highly communicable in young people and less so later in life. It is likely that, following the initial infection, EBV persists for life and may be periodically reactivated; but the role of reactivated virus in the genesis of disease or in transmission has not yet been clarified.

PATHOLOGY. Since mononucleosis is generally benign, anatomic studies have been limited to excised lymph nodes and liver biopsies; only rarely has autopsy material been examined. The major systems involved are the lymph nodes, peripheral blood, spleen, liver, and much less often the heart, lungs, kidneys, and central nervous system.

In severe cases the lymph nodes and spleen become soft, fleshy, and hyperemic. Marked cellular infiltration with atypical mononuclear cells causes blurring of lymph node architecture. However, the capsule and perinodal fat are not invaded. Nodal medullarry histology may suggest leukemia. Cells resembling the Reed-Sternberg giant cells of Hodgkin's disease have been found in mononucleosis nodes. The splenic trabeculae and capsule become thinned because of cellular infiltrates in the splenic pulp. Extensive involvement of the lymph tissue of the naso-oropharynx is common.

The liver is subject to three main forms of pathology: portal exudates consisting almost entirely of mononuclear cells, invasion of the sinusoids by these same cells, and less frequently, areas of focal parenchymal necrosis filled with mononuclear cells. The histology may be difficult to distinguish from that of infectious hepatitis. Electron microscopic studies reveal essentially normal hepatocyte structure, with the exception of dilated endoplasmic reticulum, a finding also characteristic of infectious hepatitis. No virus particles are seen within the liver.

The central nervous system is subject to congestion, edema, and perivascular mononuclear infiltration in the leptomeninges, as well as in the brain substance proper. Myocarditis, interstitial pneumonitis, and glomerulonephritis have been described.

CLINICAL MANIFESTATIONS. Although the clinical manifestations of mononucleosis have sometimes been described as protean, the principal signs and symptoms of the disease in the older child, adolescent, or young adult are remarkably consistent. The incubation period is 30 to 50 days, based on contact studies in West Point cadets and on the few cases of heterophil-positive mononucleosis that have occurred following blood transfusion. There is a prodromal period of 3 to 5 days marked by mild symptoms of headache, malaise, and fatigue. *Sore throat* occurs during the first week of illness and is present in over 80 percent of cases. There is hyperplasia of all the lymphoid tissue in the oropharynx; the tonsils in particular are markedly enlarged and covered with shaggy gray exudate. The uvula and soft palate have a gelatinous appearance and during the first week are sometimes showered with fine petechiae. In about 30 percent of cases of mononucleosis the throat culture is positive for β-hemolytic streptococci. *Fever,* with temperature elevations of 39.5 C or higher in the more severe cases, lasts for about 10 days and then falls gradually by lysis over an additional 7 to 10 days. In some cases low-grade fever lasts for several weeks.

Generalized *lymphadenopathy* of gradual onset is characteristic. The anterior and posterior cervical chains are involved most commonly, but axillary, epitrochlear, inguinal, mediastinal, and mesenteric adenopathy are also found. The nodes are usually single, 2 to 4 cm in diameter, not matted, firm, and moderately tender. Splenomegaly is observed in approximately one-half of patients during the second and third week of illness. Splenic rupture is rare, but is a potentially serious complication of the disease. Hepatomegaly and liver tenderness are found in about 10 percent of patients; jaundice is detected in less than 5 percent. However, the majority of patients have elevated levels of SGOT and serum LDH that persist from weeks to months after the disease. Chronic liver disease has not been described as a sequela.

A maculopapular rash occurs in about 5 percent of cases. For unknown reasons, a high proportion of patients with mononucleosis given ampicillin develop a rash. Urticarial, bullous, hemorrhagic, and scarlatiniform rashes have also been described. Bilateral supraorbital edema may be an early sign in the disease. Pneumonia and rarely pleural effusion are seen. The radiographic findings are similar to those of atypical pneumonia. Several central nervous system syndromes have been described in association with mononucleosis.

They include aseptic meningitis, encephalitis, acute psychosis, coma, transverse myelitis, acute cerebellar syndrome, and infectious polyneuritis. Complete recovery from CNS involvement is usual, but serious sequelae such as paralysis of limbs or respiratory muscles occur in rare instances.

In the toddler and young child, infection with EBV is rarely accompanied by the classic picture of mononucleosis; instead, the infection is usually clinically silent. There may be a much milder form of mononucleosis consisting of pharyngitis, low-grade fever lasting less than 1 week, slight hepatosplenomegaly, and rash. Even when the classic picture of mononucleosis is present in the young child, the heterophil agglutination is sometimes not detected. The reasons for the differing responses of young children and older children to EBV infection are not known.

LABORATORY DIAGNOSIS. Hematologic findings. During the first week of illness the total leukocyte count may be normal or there may be leukopenia due to granulocytopenia. By the second to third week leukocytosis is found, usually between 10,000 and 20,000 cells/mm^3, but occasionally as high as 50,000 cells/mm^3. There is absolute lymphocytosis; usually more than 50 percent of peripheral leukocytes are lymphocytes, of which 10 to 20 percent or more are atypical lymphocytes. Recent studies indicate that the increase in lymphocytes is due to both B and T cells. The atypical lymphocyte, or Downey cell, has a higher cytoplasm-to-nucleus ratio than a normal lymphocyte. The nucleus has coarse chromatin, and occasionally nucleoli are seen. Some atypical cells are in DNA synthesis, as indicated by uptake of ^{3}H-thymidine. The cytoplasm of the atypical cell is more basophilic and vacuolated than normal. The exact relationship of the atypical lymphocyte to the EBV-infected cell is not known, but it is unlikely that many of the atypical cells are virocytes. Hemolytic anemia, sometimes due to autoantibodies, is found rarely in mononucleosis. Thrombocytopenia, usually without bleeding, is also recognized during the early weeks of the disease.

Heterophile antibodies. The sera of most, but not all, mononucleosis patients contain an agglutinin for sheep erythrocytes. This antibody, an IgM moiety, appears usually during the first or second week of illness, and titers slowly decline over a period of 3 to 6 months. The height of the heterophile antibody titer is not related to clinical severity or to the degree of atypical lymphocytosis. Heterophile antibodies do not cross-react with any known EBV-associated antigens, and the manner in which EBV infection induces heterophile antibodies is not known. Heterophile antibodies found in mononucleosis sera can be differentiated from sheep cell agglutinins found in sera of some normal persons and in sera of patients with serum sickness on the basis of differential absorption with crude antigens prepared from guinea-pig kidney or bovine erythrocytes (Table 20). The titer of heterophile antibody in mononucleosis sera is not significantly reduced by absorption by guinea-pig kidney, but it is completely absorbed by beef erythrocytes. Serum sickness agglutinins are absorbed

TABLE 20. Differential Absorption of Heterophile Antibodies

Serum	Agglutination of Sheep Red Cells After Absorption With:	
	Guinea-Pig Kidney	Beef Red Blood Cells
Normal (Forssman)	−	+
Infectious mononucleosis	+	−
Serum sickness	−	−

by both antigens, whereas Forssman antibodies are only absorbed by guinea-pig kidney. A heterophil titer of 1:40 or greater following absorption with guinea-pig kidney is considered diagnostic of mononucleosis.

Several rapid slide tests or spot tests have become available in recent years to expedite the diagnosis. Most of these are based on the agglutination of formalin-stabilized horse red blood cells by heterophile-antibody-positive sera. The differential absorption with guinea-pig kidney and beef red blood cells is included in some of these procedures. Although these spot tests have the advantage of great rapidity and ease of performance, false-positive reactions have been reported in the hands of the technically inexperienced.

During acute mononucleosis there is a marked increase in the total serum IgM and, to a lesser extent, IgG. Many abnormal immunologic reactivities have been detected in mononucleosis sera, including antibodies that agglutinate erythrocytes in the cold, antibodies directed against other erythrocyte antigens, and transient positive serologic tests for rheumatoid factor and for syphilis.

Specific Anti-EBV Responses. Antibodies to several EBV antigens are absent before mononucleosis; they appear during the course of the disease and persist for years thereafter. Some antibodies, such as those directed against viral capsid antigens, are already at maximum titer (1:40 to 1:320) when the diagnosis of mononucleosis is entertained; therefore diagnostic antibody titer rises against this antigen cannot usually be demonstrated. However, other species of antibody, including complement-fixing antibody and antibody directed against the EBV nuclear antigen, appear more slowly, and increases in antibody titer can be shown between acute and convalescent specimens. A test for IgM directed against viral capsid antigen as an index of recent infection appears to hold promise, for the presence of specific anti-EBV IgM correlates well with the presence of heterophile antibodies.

DIFFERENTIAL DIAGNOSIS. In the early stages of the disease when sore throat with exudative tonsillitis predominates, it is difficult to distinguish infectious mononucleosis (im) from streptococcal infection, diphtheria, and other types of exudative viral tonsillitis. The results of the throat culture and the ultimate appearance of atypical lymphocytes and a positive heterophil test clarify the diagnosis.

The hematologic abnormalities and the lymphadenopathy and splenomegaly may raise the possibility of lymphoma. The heterophile antibody test is very useful here in the differential diagnosis. Ultimately study of bone marrow or lymph node morphology may be required. There does not appear to be any etiologic association of EBV with acute lymphoblastic leukemia, for mononucleosis has been described as an intercurrent infection during acute leukemia. Several cases of lymphoma following classic mononucleosis have been described, but there does not seem to be any clearly defined risk of development of lymphoma in patients with mononucleosis.

A heterophil-negative mononucleosis syndrome can be caused by cytomegalovirus (CMV) (p. 520). The characteristics of CMV mononucleosis are atypical lymphocytosis, fever, splenomegaly, and hepatomegaly. Sore throat, tonsillar exudate, and cervical adenopathy are usually not present. CMV mononucleosis is most often recognized following transfusion of fresh blood (postperfusion syndrome). The diagnosis of CMV mononucleosis is made by recovery of the virus from the urine and peripheral blood leukocytes and by demonstrating antibody rises to the virus.

Infectious hepatitis is frequently confused with mononucleosis accompanied by jaundice. The distinguishing features are the absence of the marked pharyngeal syndrome and the absence of heterophils in hepatitis. Atypical lymphocytes are found transiently early in hepatitis, but they are not associated with absolute lymphocytosis.

Acquired toxoplasmosis is associated with fever, lymphadenopathy, lymphocytosis with atypical lymphocytes, and a protracted course. There is often an associated pneumonitis. A definitive diagnosis is made by isolation of *Toxoplasma gondii* and by specific serologic tests such as fluorescence antibody.

The early stages of rubella may be impossible to distinguish from IM, since cervical adenopathy, fever, malaise, and atypical lymphocytes are present. The rash of rubella is invariably on the face, whereas the rash of mononucleosis is usually found on the trunk and extremities. The increase of atypical and total lymphocytes in the second week of illness distinguishes IM from rubella.

In acute infectious lymphocytosis and in the pertussis syndromes there is absolute lymphocytosis, but it consists of small mature lymphocytes. Adenopathy and splenomegaly are not characteristic of acute lymphocytosis.

When neurologic features of IM predominate and precede the more classic findings of the disease, the diagnosis of infectious polyneuritis (Guillain-Barré), aseptic meningitis, or meningoencephalitis may be made. The presence of heterophile antibodies and the peripheral blood picture help clarify the diagnosis when they become manifest.

TREATMENT.   The treatment of IM is directed toward supportive symptomatic relief. No specific chemotherapeutic agent is available. Aspirin and saline gargles ease the pain associated with the pharyngitis. Codeine may be necessary for short-term relief of severe tonsillitis and lymphadenitis. Corticosteroids have been used to ameliorate the symptoms of severe pharyngeal edema and toxemia as well as to treat the complications of hemolytic anemia, thrombocytopenia, and central nervous system involvement. Hepatic function and the heterophile titer are not altered by use of steroids. Corticosteroids should not be used routinely in mononucleosis. If used for airway obstruction, for example, the total course need not exceed 7 days.

Activity should be determined by the severity of symptoms. Complete bed rest is usually unnecessary. Vigorous sports and contact activities should be avoided in the presence of splenic enlargement. Penicillin or other antibiotics should be used only when concurrent throat cultures are positive for β-hemolytic streptococci. Ampicillin should be avoided, when possible, because of its frequent association with skin rash in this disease.

PROGNOSIS.   The outcome is generally excellent, even in cases where the symptoms of malaise and lassitude persist for long periods. Recently, however, several *fatal* cases of mononucleosis have been reported in one family in which there appears to be a genetic defect in immunologic response to EBV infection. Significant morbidity is associated with the rare occurrence of splenic rupture, infectious polyneuritis, laryngeal edema, nasopharyngeal hemorrhage, and myocarditis.

References

Bar RS, Deher CJ, Clausen KP, et al: Fatal infectious mononucleosis in a family. N Engl J Med 290:363, 1974

Evans AS, Niederman JC, McCollum RW: Seroepidemiologic studies of infectious mononucleosis with EB virus. N Engl J Med 279:1121, 1968

Henle G, Henle W, Diehl V: Relation of Burkitt's tumor-associated herpes-type virus to infectious mononucleosis. Proc Natl Acad Sci USA 59:94, 1968

——— Henle W, Horwitz CA: Antibodies to Epstein-Barr virus-associated nuclear antigen in infectious mononucleosis. J Infect Dis 130:231, 1974

Hoagland RJ: Infectious Mononucleosis. New York, Grune & Stratton, 1967

Mangi RJ, Niederman JC, Kelleher JE, et al: Depression of cell-mediated immunity during acute infectious mononucleosis. N Engl J Med 291:1149, 1974

Miller G, Niederman JC, Andrews LL: Prolonged oropharyngeal excretion of Epstein-Barr virus after infectious mononucleosis. N Engl J Med 228:229, 1973

——— Shope T, Heston L, et al: Prospective study of Epstein-Barr virus infections in acute lymphoblastic leukemia of childhood. J Pediatr 80:932, 1972

VIRAL RESPIRATORY INFECTIONS
DAVID S. HODES

Acute respiratory diseases are the most common ailments with which practicing pediatricians have to deal, and it has become apparent in recent years that viruses are the most frequent etiologic agents. Viruses are exclusively the cause of the common cold syndrome; they also play a prominent role in the production of pharyngitis. It is less generally recognized that viruses are the major cause of lower respiratory tract illness (LRI-disease at or below the level of the epiglottis) as well as upper respiratory illness (URI) in children. A number of well-controlled epidemiologic studies have indicated that viruses play a more prominent role in primary LRI than in LRI that develops as a complication of other illnesses.

The common cold, marked by rhinitis and subjective or objective evidence of pharyngeal involvement, is produced in children by primary infection with the many types of rhinoviruses, enteroviruses, and adenoviruses; the coronaviruses also may play a role. In children beyond the first few years of life the common cold can also be produced by reinfection with respiratory syncytial virus and the parainfluenza viruses. Several viral infections of the pharynx produce characteristic pathology. The herpangina syndrome produced by some enteroviruses, the stomatitis produced by herpes simplex virus, and the tonsillopharyngitis produced by the Epstein-Barr (infectious mononucleosis) virus are discussed elsewhere. Pharyngitis combined with conjunctivitis (pharyngoconjunctival fever) is caused by a number of adenovirus types.

Classification of lower repiratory tract viral syndromes is more complicated, since the affected organs are not readily available for casual inspection. Denny and associates have offered the following definitions of the lower respiratory tract illnesses (LRI): *Croup:* hoarseness with barking cough with or without inspiratory stridor. *Tracheobronchitis:* deep cough with rhonchi audible in the larger air passages. *Bronchiolitis:* expiratory wheezing, often with evidence of air trapping. *Pneumonia:* fine rales or evidence of consolidation. The incidence of LRI is very high throughout the pediatric age group, ranging from 30 illnesses per 100 children per year during the first year of life to 6 per 100 in adolescents. Altogether, a great number of viruses can be recovered by swabbing the throats of patients with LRI, and in general these viruses cannot be recovered from healthy control subjects. The viruses include respiratory syncytial virus, parainfluenza viruses, influenza viruses types A and B, adenoviruses, rhinoviruses, and occasionally enteroviruses. The number of possible offending serotypes is well over 100.

Despite the large number of potential viral pathogens, there is a marked preponderance of three particular agents: respiratory syncytial virus and parainfluenza viruses types 1 and 3 (para 1 and para 3). These agents account for about 70 percent of all virus isolations. When viral isolates are correlated with syndromes, different patterns of association of agent and illness can be delineated. Respiratory syncytial virus is, in cases of primary infection, an agent with a distinct predilection for the lower respiratory tract, accounting for almost 40 percent of all viral isolates obtained from children with bronchiolitis and pneumonia. In patients who are ill enough to require hospitalization, even higher percentages are obtained; nearly 70 percent recovery of the virus has been reported when special care is used in culturing in the epidemic situation. Para 1, by contrast, seems to have an affinity for laryngeal tissue, being im-

plicated in nearly half the cases of croup from which a virus is isolated. Para 3 seems equally prone to cause croup, bronchitis, bronchiolitis, or pneumonia.

RESPIRATORY SYNCYTIAL VIRUS

VIROLOGY.   Respiratory syncytial virus (RSV) was first isolated in 1956 by Morris and Blount, who recovered the agent from a chimpanzee with coryza. The virus was first associated with pediatric respiratory disease in 1957 by Chanock, who suggested the currently accepted name because of the characteristic syncytial cytopathic effects the virus causes in tissue culture. Virologic studies have shown that RSV is an enveloped, RNA-containing virus. Two forms, presumably biologically equivalent, can be distinguished morphologically: a spherical form with a diameter of about 110 nm and a long filamentous form measuring up to 2,000 nm. The viral envelope is marked by spikelike projections 10 to 15 nm in length, while the nucleocapsid reveals helical symmetry. From its morphologic appearance, from what is known of its biochemical characteristics, and from the syncytia it forms in cell monolayers, RSV would be classified in the paramyxovirus group along with mumps, measles, and the parainfluenza viruses. However, viral taxonomists have been reluctant to make this classification, since the RSV nucleocapsid has certain subtle morphologic differences from the paramyxoviruses and since RSV, unlike the paramyxoviruses, lacks both a hemagglutinin and a neuraminidase. It is likely that RSV will be classified in a separate virus group along with pneumonia virus of mice. Biochemical characterization of the structural components of RSV and of the events of its growth cycle has been hindered by the lability of the agent and by the relatively low concentrations of the virus that can be grown in tissue culture. The work that has been done suggests parallels with the paramyxoviruses. The virus matures by budding from the infected cell surface, although the bulk of the infectivity remains cell-associated. Although there is some indication that slight serologic differences may occur among different strains of RSV, these differences have never been shown to be of significance clinically, and for practical purposes the virus is thought of as having a single serotype. RSV produces coryza in chimpanzees. It replicates in the respiratory tracts of a number of small laboratory animals, but does not produce clinical disease in these species.

EPIDEMIOLOGY.   RSV has worldwide distribution, and it is difficult to find seronegative individuals beyond the toddler age group in almost any population. Several long-term epidemologic studies have demonstrated that RSV is the most important viral respiratory pathogen of infancy and early childhood. The peak incidence of disease occurs in the first year of life, with most serious illness occurring within the first 6 months. Long-term surveillance has indicated that RSV produces yearly epidemics in the late winter and early spring: January through April in the Northern Hemisphere, July through October in the Southern Hemisphere. Isolation of the virus in other months is sporadic and rare. Among seriously ill patients, boys outnumber girls by a ratio of nearly 2 to 1.

PATHOGENESIS. RSV is extremely important as a cause of bronchiolitis and pneumonia in young infants. Initial infection leads to replication of the virus in the oropharynx and nasopharynx. In young infants the infection frequently spreads to the bronchi and bronchioles. In patients who come to autopsy, necrotizing lesions of bronchial and bronchiolar epithelium and peribronchiolar infiltration with lymphocytes are found. The bronchioles are occluded by mucus, fibrin, and cellular debris. There is evidence of air trapping with alveolar enlargement. Sometimes pneumonitis and patchy atelectasis and emphysema are present. There is a mononuclear cell inflammation of the alveoli, small bronchioles, alveolar ducts, and interstitium. Cytoplasmic inclusion bodies have been noted, but syncytial formation has not been found. RSV is unusual in that it causes serious disease (pneumonia and bronchiolitis) principally in children younger than 6 months of age. For many viruses, infants in this age group are protected by passively transferred serum maternal antibody; in the case of RSV, serum maternal antibody provides no protection. Some authors have even postulated that in the absence of secretory antibody, local or systemic cellular immunity, or other unknown factors, serum antibody (either of maternal origin or induced by vaccination) may lead to exacerbation of RSV infections and produce the characteristic pathology of bronchiolitis and pneumonia. Supporting this concept is the experience with intramuscularly administered inactivated RSV vaccines: Children who received such immunization developed brisk serum antibody responses, but on a subsequent natural exposure to RSV some experienced unusually severe illness. In such children RSV bronchiolitis occurred through the toddler age group, suggesting a pathologic role for serum antibody and giving evidence that physical size of the bronchioles alone is not the explanation for the usual increased severity of disease in young infants. It has been postulated that antigen–antibody complexes in the lungs may be the cause of severe RSV disease, but such complexes have not been demonstrated, and serum complement is not depressed in the acute states of illness. It is conceivable that maternally derived serum antibody serves to depress the infant's own immune responses in some fashion, thus leading to increased viral proliferation and more severe disease. In any case, immunity to RSV is transient and imperfect, and seropositive adult volunteers are readily reinfected. However, the illness produced is generally a trivial URI.

There is considerable interest in the relationship of RSV bronchiolitis and the subsequent occurrence of chronic asthma. Some short-term studies have indicated that evidence of atopy is found in infants who experience bronchiolitis outside of the epidemic situation and not associated with RSV, but not in infants acquiring RSV bronchiolitis in the course of the annual RSV epidemic. However, in a long-term follow-up study in Australia, Rooney and Wilson found that some 40 percent of infants with proven RSV bronchiolitis developed repeated wheezing attacks later in life. It would seem unlikely that RSV is a cause of the atopic condition, but very likely that the agent is a potent stimulant of wheezing in the asthma-prone individual. There is evidence that reinfection with RSV frequently triggers wheezing attacks in children with chronic asthma.

Studies from hospital epidemics indicate that the incubation period of RSV-induced respiratory diseases is about 4 to 8 days. Viruses can be detected in respiratory secretion up to 5 days before the onset of symptoms and for at least 7 days thereafter. Person-to-person spread of RSV is extremely effective; in some outbreaks 90 percent of exposed population showed evidence of infection.

CLINICAL FEATURES. RSV bronchiolitis is marked by initial symptoms indistinguishable from those of the common cold: the infant may show a nasal discharge and cough, and there may be mild fever. Within 1 to 2 days the breathing becomes more labored, and temperature elevation is evident. Substernal and intercostal retractions are noted during inspiration. The chest is hyperexpanded and hyperresonant, giving evidence of air trapping. The expiratory phase is prolonged, and expiratory wheezes are heard; rales may or may not be present. Radiographs of the lungs reveal hyperexpansion, increased bronchial markings, and sometimes areas of atelectasis, although the last are usually too small to detect. If the disease is severe, cyanosis and prostration occur. The respirations become more rapid and shallow. With increasingly severe exhaustion, the infant may die. Estimates of the case fatality rate range from less than 1 percent to 5 percent. Full recovery may take about 2 weeks.

The distinction between RSV bronchiolitis and pneumonia is often arbitrary. Frequently the bronchiolitic syndrome is marked by evidence of alveolar involvement, such as rales and the presence of patchy infiltration on radiography. RSV pneumonia may also occur in the absence of any bronchiolitic manifestation such as wheezing. This condition also is most common in young infants. The symptoms are not distinguishable from those seen in many other virus pneumonias. Cough, fever, and malaise may occur. In younger infants the presence of pulmonary disease is sometimes not suspected. The temperature may be either normal or elevated. Rales are heard irregularly, and the chest radiograph reveals patchy areas of consolidation that may be shifting. The pneumonia generally resolves spontaneously in the course of a few weeks, but fulminant cases leading to death do occur.

SPECIFIC LABORATORY DIAGNOSIS. Isolation of RSV may be accomplished by inoculating nasopharyngeal, nasal, or oropharyngeal material onto tissue culture. Human cells (HEp-2 and HeLa) are the most satisfactory. Since RSV is quite labile at room temperature, great care must be exercised to inoculate the material promptly. Under proper conditions virus growth may be detected by the appearance of syncytial cytopathic effects in from 3 to 14 days. Viral isolates may be identified by use of specific antisera, but when such sera are not available the identity of the virus may be determined presumptively by hemadsorption of the infected monolayer with guinea-pig red blood cells. An agent producing syncytial cytopathic effects in HEp-2 or HeLa cells that does not hemagglutinate is, by presumption, RSV. Diagnosis of RSV infection can also be made in some laboratories by treating cells obtained by scraping the pharyngeal mucosa using immunofluorescence techniques.

RSV infection induces rises in both complement-fixing (CF) and neutralizing antibodies. However, in young infants (the population most often affected by severe disease) the CF response is likely to be blunted, and the neutralization test is difficult to interpret when not performed expertly. Therefore virus isolation is of particular importance.

TREATMENT. Most cases of RSV bronchiolitis and pneumonia are mild and self-limited. However, because of the severe nature of the occasional case, the pediatrician should be aware of two principles in treating the disease: First, RSV bronchiolitis generally reaches its peak severity in 48 to 72 hours. Therefore an infant seen after this time may be presumed to be on the road to recovery. Second, CO_2 retention may be presumed to begin when the respiratory rate surpasses 60 per minute. Infants exhibiting such rates must be considered in danger. Using these guidelines, decisions for or against hospital admission are made more readily. In doubtful cases a brief admission for observation is advisable and, in the opinion of many, mandatory in infants under 6 months of age.

Treatment of bronchiolitis is symptomatic. Oxygen administration can be beneficial in severe cases along with maintenance of hydration by means of intravenous fluids, if necessary. Sedation may be of use, but restlessness may be a sign of early hypoxemia, and a diagnostic sign is lost when it is masked. Bronchodilators are of no value. Controlled clinical trials have not demonstrated any beneficial effect of adrenocorticosteroids.

The association of clinical bronchiolitis with *Haemophilus influenzae* was made in one study, but it has never been confirmed. However, initial treatment of patients with ampicillin has become so ingrained that it seems pointless to argue against it. But a plea can be made to stop treatment if nasopharyngeal cultures for *H. influenzae* are negative.

PROPHYLAXIS. Inactivated RSV vaccines produce exaggerated disease in vaccinees exposed to natural RSV infections. Since natural reinfection with RSV is the rule rather than the exception, it seems unlikely that any vaccine could eliminate all RSV disease. However, it is hoped that live attenuated vaccines will be developed that can prevent the development of serious disease in infants under the age of 6 months. Such attenuated vaccines might induce resistance closely akin to that protecting older children from serious illness. Attenuated mutants that are temperature-sensitive appear to offer particular advantage. These agents can replicate in the cooler upper airways and give rise to both local and systemic antibody and/or cellular immune responses. Being temperature-sensitive and unable to replicate at the higher temperature of the lung, they should not have the capacity to produce lower airway disease. One temperature-sensitive mutant strain has been evaluated as a possible vaccine and found to be unsatisfactory because it produced respiratory illness of an unacceptable severity. Other strains are currently under investigation.

PARAINFLUENZA VIRUSES

VIROLOGY. The human parainfluenza viruses are members of the paramyxovirus group; they show close resemblance to animal paramyxoviruses (Newcastle disease virus, Sendai virus, simian virus 5) in morphology and properties, as well as considerable serologic cross-reactivity with animal agents serologically (eg, parainfluenza type 1 and Sendai virus). The parainfluenza viruses are large (150 to 200 nm) enveloped viruses containing single-stranded RNA. The nucleocapsid exhibits helical symmetry, and the viral envelope is covered with spikelike projections. If analogy can be made with the animal paramyxoviruses, these spikes contain two viral glycopeptides. The larger of these probably contains both the viral hemagglutinin and the neuraminidase activator, while the smaller may be responsible for hemolytic and cell-fusion-promoting properties. A polypeptide associated with the envelope and a nucleoprotein are also found. The intracellular biochemical events that occur when human parainfluenza viruses infect cell monolayers have yet to be elucidated. However, Sendai virus has been studied extensively. In the case of this agent the viral RNA is apparently transcribed into messenger RNA of lower molecular weight. From these are generated the virus polypeptides that are then assembled into mature viruses at the cell surface. Virus matures by budding from the cell surface, although most of the infectivity remains cell-associated.

The human parainfluenza viruses include at least four serotypes (1 to 4). Each of these serotypes has a type-specific hemagglutinin (HA) antigen and a type-specific CF antigen. The former antigens are associated with the viral envelope and the latter, which are nonsedimenting, with the nucleocapsid. There is no antigen common to all the parainfluenza viruses of man, but reinfection with one parainfluenza virus serotype (particularly type 3) can lead to heterotypic serologic responses to the other types. Clinical mumps infection leads to heterotypic responses to the parainfluenza viruses in a significant percentage of cases. There is considerable cross-reaction between type 1 and the rodent Sendai virus, but the two are distinguishable. Infection of the hamster with para 1 virus results in homotypic antibody only; infection with Sendai virus results in the formation of antibody reactive with both Sendai and para 1 virus. Two subtypes of para 4, A and B, have been described.

EPIDEMIOLOGY. Types 1, 2, and 3 are the agents that have an important clinical impact in man, especially types 1 and 3. Longitudinal surveys have revealed that para 1 virus is responsible for large outbreaks of croup that occur biennially in the fall months. Para 2 virus is responsible for smaller biennial fall outbreaks of croup occurring in the year when para 1 virus is absent from the community. Para 3 virus is usually endemic in the community and can present at any time of the year, causing disease of the small airways.

As with RSV, serious parainfluenza virus disease is concentrated in the youngest age groups. Para 1 infection occurs in the first year of life, but there is less of a tendency for children under the age of 6 months to be infected than is the case with RSV. The incidence of infection is highest in the second and third years of life, the most important years for croup. Serious para 1 disease is about twice as common in boys as in girls. Para 2 epidemiology is less well worked out than that of para 1, since the virus is far less common. However, it would appear from limited data that there are close parallels with para 1. Significant para 3 disease is also essentially limited to children under the age of 5 years and has been found to cause disease in the first 6 months of life. The virus is highly infectious and is capable of producing epidemics in closed populations on occasion.

PATHOGENESIS.   As with RSV, initial viral replication is in the pharynx. Subsequently there is spread to the lower tract, where viral proliferation in the epithelial mucous glands causes cell degeneration and subsequent inflammation. Available data indicate that, as in the case of RSV, local rather than systemic humoral immunity provides the most important defense against serious infection. It has been shown, for example, that when adult volunteers are challenged with parainfluenza viruses the intensity of subsequent virus shedding correlates inversely with the level of nasal-secretion antibody, but not with the level of serum antibody. Further, trials with inactivated parainfluenza vaccines that produced brisk serum antibody responses when injected have failed to demonstrate any protective effect against natural virus infection. Immunity to parainfluenza viruses is, at best, incomplete, since adult volunteers with positive serum antibody titers presumably acquired via natural infection can readily be infected, with the production of URI symptoms. Studies of hospital epidemics indicate a high attack rate and implicate shedding of virus before the appearance of symptoms.

CLINICAL FEATURES.   The clinical presentation of a child with para-1-induced croup is ushered in by a URI of several days' duration, followed by hoarseness, a croupy cough, and inspiratory stridor. With increasing respiratory stress the child may become restless and may prefer to lie down. Retractions are evident in the more severe cases. There may be pharyngeal hyperemia. In most cases the temperature is elevated, usually being between 37.8 C and 40 C. White cell counts average around 12,000 to 14,000, with a slight predominance of polymorphonuclear granulocytes. It is generally believed that viral croup syndromes are associated with lower fever and leukocyte counts and have a more insidious onset and produce less prostration

than the epiglottiditis due to *H. influenzae*. In the latter condition the diagnosis can be made by the discovery of the cherry-red epiglottis on physical examination or swelling of the epiglottis as demonstrated by a lateral radiograph of the upper airways. The distinguishing characteristics of diphtheritic croup are discussed on page 1556. The bronchiolitic and pneumonitic syndromes produced by parainfluenza viruses are not clinically distinguishable from those produced by RSV.

SPECIFIC LABORATORY DIAGNOSES.   Para 1 may be recovered from nasal or oropharyngeal swabs taken within a few days after the onset of symptoms. Primary monkey kidney cells and human embryonic kidney cells will support the growth of para 1, but the development of cytopathic effects is not common. The virus can be detected in 3 to 4 days by hemadsorption of guinea-pig red cells that is blocked by specific antiserum. The patient's serum will show a rise in complement-fixing or hemagglutination-inhibition (HAI) titer. Similar procedures apply to the diagnosis of disease caused by para 2, although here serial passage in tissue culture is more likely to result in the appearance of syncytial CPE. Para 3 may show stringy CPE in primary kidney cultures, but this is often not apparent in the first passage. Adaptation to HEp-2 or HeLa cells results in the production of dramatic syncytia. Sera may be examined for rises in HAI, CF, or neutralization titers, but it must be recalled that in older individuals reinfection can take place despite the presence of systemic antibody. Since all the parainfluenza viruses are quite labile, the inoculation of fresh specimens is of the utmost importance. Bedside inoculation is most advantageous. If transport medium must be used, the inclusion of 5 percent protein will enhance virus stability.

TREATMENT.   Treatment of parainfluenza infections of the respiratory tract is basically supportive, but there are special considerations in the case of croup. When there is difficulty in distinguishing viral croup from that produced by *H. influenzae,* some authors have seen no objection to treatment with ampicillin. However, the possibility that epiglottiditis could be caused by the emerging ampicillin-resistant strains of this organism would seem to dictate the use of chloramphenicol, and the potential danger of this agent must be considered. Supportive measures include the inhalation of moist air or oxygen. Sedatives must be used with great care because these drugs may hide the restlessness that accompanies impending respiratory failure. In severe cases, tracheostomy may be life-saving, and it is imperative that an experienced surgical team be alerted early in the course of hospital management. The role of steroids and other emergency modalities is discussed more fully elsewhere (p. 1577).

PROPHYLAXIS.   As noted above, inactivated parainfluenza vaccines have been produced. These are strongly antigenic, but they have been shown to be ineffective in preventing disease. Current research efforts are aimed at developing temperature-sensitive live attenuated parainfluenza vaccines similar to those being developed for RSV. As yet, attempts to induce such agents have not been successful.

INFLUENZA VIRUSES

VIROLOGY. The influenza viruses are members of the orthomyxovirus group. The spherical influenza virion consists of an outer lipoprotein envelope surrounding central nucleocapsid material. The overall diameter of the spherical virion is about 100 to 120 nm. Filamentous forms also occur. The envelope is uniformly studded with spikelike projections that protrude from the lipid moiety on its outer surface. These projections measure some 10 to 15 nm in length and have been found to be glycopeptides that contain the biologically and pathologically significant properties of the virus. The spikes are of two varieties: one is associated with the hemagglutinin (HA) and the other with the neuraminidase (NA) activities of the virion. The inner surface of the envelope consists of the nonglycosylated viral membrane protein (M). The ribonucleoprotein (RNP) core consists of single-stranded RNA closely associated with a nucleoprotein (NP) and two other high-molecular-weight proteins (P_1 and P_2). The RNP exhibits helical symmetry.

In the past 5 years a great deal of information has been amassed concerning both the viral polypeptides and the viral RNA. It now appears that the hemagglutinin spike is a dimer (150,000 daltons) of two noncovalently linked glycopeptides designated HA (75,000 to 80,000 daltons). HA can be cleaved (at least when the virus is grown in certain cell systems) into two smaller glycopeptides HA_1 and HA_2. These are apparently held together by disulfide bonds. HA_1 has a molecular weight of 50,000 to 60,000 daltons and is more heavily glycosylated than HA_2, which has a molecular weight of 20,000 to 30,000 daltons. HA_2 appears to be located proximally on the HA spike and is closely associated with the envelope, while HA_1 is distal. The neuraminidase spike probably consists of a tetramer (220,000 to 250,000 daltons) of four glycopeptides (60,000 to 65,000 daltons) designated NA. This tetramer seems to be the active viral neuraminidase.

The membrane protein, or M, has a molecular weight of 21,000 to 27,000 daltons. It is the most abundant protein in the virion and accounts for fully one-third of the viral mass. The nucleoprotein (NP) has a molecular weight of 53,000 to 60,000 daltons, while P_1 and P_2, which are present only in small amounts, are in the range of 81,000 to 94,000 daltons. These latter two polypeptides have been suggested as the enzymes that catalyze viral RNA synthesis (RNA polymerases).

The influenza virus RNA has a molecular weight of nearly 5 million daltons. However, it is now clear that this total genetic information is divided into six or seven smaller and loosely linked molecular units that range in size from 350,000 to 1 million daltons. While the precise chemical forces that bind the smaller RNA units to each other and to the NP to form the RNP are not known, it is clear that the segmented nature of the influenza genome allows for exchange of the units when two different influenza virions infect the same cell (genetic recombination). This property, perhaps unique among the pathogenic RNA viruses of man, has great

significance for the epidemiology of influenza and profound significance for the problem that the control of pandemic influenza presents.

The sometimes confusing taxonomy of the influenza viruses is best understood in relationship to the viral polypeptides. The grossest classification of the agents is that of type specificity, and this is based on the antigenic properties of the internal polypeptides NP and M. On the basis of the antigenic properties of these peptides, as demonstrated by CF reactions, the influenza viruses are divided into three types: A, B, and C. In most laboratories today antibody to the NP antigen (sometimes identified as soluble antigen, S) is the basis of the CF test and of virus typing. In addition to type-specific antigens, influenza viruses also possess strain-specific antigens. These reside in the HA and NA moieties, and their serology has been worked out most elaborately in the influenza A agents. Currently strains of influenza A viruses are identified according to the nature of the strain's HA and NA antigens. A standard nomenclature has been devised.

The first well characterized human influenza A virus was isolated in 1933. Previously known simply as influenza AO, it is most conveniently identified by its HA and NA antigens, which have been designated H0N1. Subsequent antigenic changes, which presumably arise by genetic alteration, have led to evolution of new influenza A strains. Thus the 1968 Hong Kong strain is characterized by the antigens H3N2. Less marked antigen variations can be identified by a title. Thus the current England influenza strain, which arose in 1972, shows minor neuraminidase variations from the Hong Kong strain and is designated H3Ñ2. In effect, major alteration in the surface antigens of influenza A introduces a new virulent virus into the environment, since antibody against previous antigens will not be protective to the host. Consequently there is little hope that influenza A pandemics can be prevented by a simple program of childhood vaccination.

It is also possible to achieve some degree of strain characterization for influenza B viruses, but the considerable immunologic cross-reaction and the systematization achieved with influenza A has not been possible. Influenza C has not been studied definitively. The biochemical studies outlined above have all been performed on strains of influenza A.

EPIDEMIOLOGY. Winter epidemics of influenza A occur every 2 to 3 years as minor antigenic shifts in the viral surface antigens appear. In interepidemic winters smaller outbreaks occur involving new young susceptibles and those who have escaped the previous epidemic. The spread of the virus becomes almost universal in this manner, and the intensity of epidemics is heightened by the short incubation period of 1 to 2 days and the fact that the illnesses are generally mild and the victims frequently continue at work or at school. Within a few years the majority of the population, including children, will have acquired antibody. At varying intervals major antigenic shifts occur. These events result in radical alteration of the HA or NA antigens and render antibody to previous antigens nonprotective. Worldwide pandemics associated with considerable excess mortality then ensue. Isolation of human influenza A virus occurred in 1933. This virus, designated A (H0N1), was prevalent until 1947, when antigenic shift occurred, giving rise to influenza A (H1N1). This agent produced a series of epidemics until 1957, when simultaneous changes in both the HA and NA antigens produced influenza A (H2N2, Asian). Since individuals possessing antibody to the H1N1 antigens were unprotected from infection, a large pandemic occurred. In 1968 further alteration in the HA resulted in A (H3N2, Hong Kong), which caused another pandemic. There were slight alterations in the NA antigen that produced A (H3N̄2, London) in 1972, with an increase in number and severity of cases, but the outbreak did not reach pandemic proportions.

The antigenic alteration in influenza is, of course, an expression of genetic alteration of the viral RNA. Since the influenza RNA is for practical purposes broken into segments, it is possible that genetic material can be easily exchanged when two different influenza virions infect a single cell. It has been suggested that the new influenza strains arise by recombination of genetic material from human influenza viruses with genetic material from animal influenza viruses (for example, influenza viruses affect fowl, pigs, and horses). Genetic recombination with the eventual production of new strains might arise in these hosts. One unexplained phenomenon is the universal disappearance of old strains when new ones appear. Influenza B viruses also show periodic epidemics, but the biology of these agents is not as well understood as that of influenza A. Influenza C apparently makes little clinical impact.

PATHOGENESIS. Influenza infection is initated by virus inoculation in the upper or lower airways, usually by virus-containing droplets. As with other respiratory viral infections, the course is principally determined by the presence or absence of specific secretory IgA antibody. Mucus also contains certain glycopeptides that tend to inhibit viral attachment to the cells of the respiratory mucosa. However, the glycopeptides can be inactivated by viral NA if this enzyme is not neutralized by specific antibody of the host. Uninhibited virus attaches to the respiratory epithelium by reaction of its surface spikes with cell membrane receptors. This step can be blocked by local antibody. Antibody to the HA of the virus is apparently most important in controlling infection, but antibody to the NA also has an important role. In successful infection, virus begins to replicate in the respiratory epithelium; it is then shed into the respiratory secretions and local spread ensues. The eventual result is death of the epithelium with desquamation. The entire airway from pharynx to alveoli may be involved. In the majority of cases the infection does not reach extreme severity because it is limited by inflammation, diffusion of serum antibody through the damaged epithelium, and perhaps also by interferon.

Although there have been a few reports of the isolation of viable, replicating influenza virus from a variety of human tissues, the agent remains for practical purposes limited to the respiratory tract. Viremia (blood-borne dissemination of viable virus) is extremely rare. By contrast, it seems likely that viral antigen is disseminated by the bloodstream, resulting in the formation of antigen–antibody complexes and producing the familiar systemic manifestation of the disease. Damage to the respiratory epithelium induced by influenza impairs clearance of bacteria; as a result, superinfection is frequent, pneumococci and *Staphylococcus aureus* being common offenders.

CLINICAL FEATURES. The incubation period of influenza is short, generally 1 to 3 days, in keeping with the highly localized nature of its replication. There is often a hacking cough, but the most dramatic symptoms are sudden chills and fever with headache, myalgia, malaise, and prostration. The eyes may be painful. Later, with advancing epithelial destruction, varying degrees of rhinitis may appear. Fever may reach 40 C. Physical findings in the typical case are few. There may be signs of pharyngeal and conjunctival infection, but examination of the lungs is generally negative in the uncomplicated case, and positive chest radiographs are the exception rather than the rule. Other laboratory studies are usually within normal limits, with the exception of elevation of the sedimentation rate.

In most cases there are no complications, and recovery occurs after a few days. In pandemic years, however, severe illness is more likely to occur. When pneumonia complicates the picture, it usually occurs after 5 to 7 days of illness, although it is occasionally seen as early as the second day. Symptoms include severe dyspnea, cyanosis, and the production of small amounts of bloody sputum. The physical findings in the lungs are seldom impressive. Localized pneumonia is often caused by secondary bacterial infection with pneumococci and *S. aureus* being frequent offenders. Bilateral or diffuse pneumonia is strongly suggestive of primary hemorrhagic viral pneumonia.

It is quite possible that the clinical picture of influenza illness will vary with antigenic drift. The Hong Kong pandemic of 1968 was associated with severe croup in children that frequently required tracheostomy. Cardiac and neurologic manifestations have been associated with influenza infection, but these are very rare.

SPECIFIC LABORATORY DIAGNOSIS. The most satisfactory means of diagnosis is isolation of the virus. Material obtained by throat swab is incubated in certain tissue culture systems or in embryonated chicken eggs. Virus growth can be detected after 2 to 3 days by hemadsorption or, on occasion, by production of cell destruction. Rapid diagnosis may be achieved by adding fluorescent antiinfluenza serum to nasal smears. This immunofluorescence technique is most likely to be successful when it is done early in the illness.

Influenza infection can also be diagnosed by demonstration of rises in CF, HAI, or neutralizing antibody titers. The measurement of neutralizing antibody titers is cumbersome and time-consuming. HAI systems are frequently employed and are strain-specific for the hemagglutinin; however, they are complicated by nonspecific inhibitors that require heat inactivation or other treatment for their removal. CF tests done with crude antigen preparation are not strain-specific, but this problem can be avoided by using the virus hemagglutinin as the antigen instead of a crude antigen preparation.

TREATMENT. The treatment of uncomplicated influenza is symptomatic. The use of prophylactic antibiotics to prevent bacterial superinfection is not recommended. If pneumonia does supervene, attempts to detect the presence of bacterial superinfection should be carried out vigorously. Sputum, throat, and blood should all be cultured and smears examined. Diagnostic lung puncture may be of value. If these efforts are fruitless, particularly in the face of focal pneumonia, an agent active against both pneumococci and *S. aureus* should be given. The administration of humidified oxygen is required in severe cases. When the pneumonia is so severe that the patient's life is threatened, assisted ventilation may be necessary.

PROPHYLAXIS. Currently available influenza vaccines are prepared by formalin inactivation of the extraembryonic fluids of virus-infected chick embryos. Considerable purification of this material can be obtained by use of the zonal ultracentrifuge. Vaccines that are now being manufactured are prepared from one serotype of influenza A (H3N2) and one serotype of influenza B. The vaccine is administered subcutaneously and is generally given only to children who are at particular risk because of compromised cardiopulmonary status or other problems. Patients with rheumatic heart disease, chronic pulmonary disease (including cystic fibrosis), and diabetes are frequently given the vaccine on a routine basis. Two doses are given in the initial immunization procedure against a given strain, with subsequent yearly boosters, usually in the fall. Current influenza vaccines are immunogenic and are capable of reducing the attack rate from the vaccine-strain virus by about 60 percent.

Despite the efficacy of presently available vaccines, many problems in influenza prophylaxis remain. First, antigenic variation is a constant problem. When new strains arise, new vaccines must be generated, tested, and distributed with dispatch in order to ward off pandemics. The technical problems involved are numerous. A second problem is that of adverse reactions. With earlier vaccines, some 15 percent of vaccinees experienced fever, pain, and erythema at the injection site and systemic myalgias. With today's more highly purified preparations this rate has been reduced fourfold. This problem may be further alleviated by the use of subunit vaccines, which are pure preparations of surface antigens. These vaccines are apparently without side effects and are also more highly antigenic than inactivated whole-virus vaccines. A third defect of contemporary procedures is their failure to stimulate the local secretory immune system of the respiratory tract when parenteral inactivated vaccines are used. The most promising approach toward overcoming this problem seems to be the development of attenuated mutants. Temperature-sensitive attenuated mutants offer the same advantages with influenza viruses as they do with other respiratory agents. Moreover, by taking advantage of the capacity of influenza for genetic recombination, it has been possible to transfer the temperature-sensitive attenuation characteristic from one strain of influenza virus to another. This virologic genetic engineering gives rise to the possibility of quickly developing attenuated mutant variants when new, potentially pandemic strains arise. The attenuation "gene" would simply be introduced into the new strain by genetic recombination, and the resultant attenuated virus would be used as a vaccine.

Several other approaches to influenza control are being explored. Amantadine hydrochloride has been shown to be effective in preventing influenza infection if given before virus exposure. In addition, there is probably a slight therapeutic effect after infection is established. Amantadine may prove to be a useful adjunct to influenza prevention. However, there is danger of CNS toxicity if the recommended doses are exceeded, and the bulk of the clinical experience has involved adults. Results so far obtained with interferon inducers and with locally applied interferon are not very dramatic.

ADENOVIRUSES

The adenoviruses were originally discovered by Rowe in 1953, when he and his colleagues noted cytopathic effects in cell cultures of explanted human adenoids. The agents were subsequently found to cause latent infections in the tonsils and adenoids of most children, being recoverable from the explanted tissue but not by direct culture of throat swab material or inoculation of macerated tissue onto cell culture in the usual fashion. The viruses are nonenveloped DNA viruses that are icosahedral in shape and measure 70 to 80 nm in diameter. The icosahedron is made up of 252 morphologic subunits or capsomers, 240 of which are known as lexons, hollow hexagons each having six adjoining neighbors. The remaining 12 capsomers are pentonic, located at the vertices of the icosahedron and having five neighbors. From each penton extends a fiber 10 to 25 nm long tipped with a terminal knob. The viruses thus have the appearance of a space satellite with extending antennae. There are 31 recognized human adenovirus serotypes.

Adenovirus infection usually begins in the pharynx or conjunctiva, with the small intestine occasionally being the colonized site. In general the virus remains quite localized, and the incubation period of any induced illness is therefore short, usually less than 1 week. Regional lymph nodes are invaded, and latent infection of the tonsils and adenoids is established. This is of no apparent consequence. The virus may be excreted in the feces long after recovery from illness and long after virus shedding from the pharynx has ceased.

A number of disease entities have been associated with adenoviruses, but their impact is probably less than is commonly assumed. The adenoviruses account for 5 to 7 percent of respiratory illnesses in children, although the infection rates may vary considerably. Great care must be taken in evaluating the association of adenoviruses with disease entities, since some 2 to 3 percent of children without acute disease may shed adenoviruses in the pharynx, and shedding in stool is even more common. Nonetheless, long-term longitudinal studies, such as those of Brandt and associates, have demonstrated statistically significant differences between the rates of isolation of certain adenovirus serotypes in patients ill with respiratory diseases and the rates of isolation from matched controls.

The following syndromes seem clearly associated with adenovirus infection. First, adenovirus types 4 and 7 are a significant cause of upper respiratory disease, predominantly in the military population. Types 1, 2, 3, 5, 6, and 21 have also been implicated. The typical clinical picture includes sore throat, headache, fever, cervical lymphadenopathy, and malaise. Occasionally pneumonia with an interstitial radiographic pattern supervenes. Very rarely such illness is devastating, particularly when types 2, 4, 7, and 21 are involved. Epidemic keratoconjunctivitis (shipyard eye) has been linked with type 8. Pharyngoconjunctival fever, a combination of fever, conjunctivitis, and pharyngitis most commonly seen in young children, can be caused by types 3 and 7.

A number of other syndromes have been associated with adenovirus infection, including neonatal sepsis, nephritis, CNS infections, and hemorrhagic cystitis. The precise significance of these associations is not known. Considerable interest has recently been centered on the association of adenoviruses with a pertussislike syndrome. Since *Bordetella pertussis* as well as an adenovirus is frequently isolated in these patients, the exact roles being played by adenoviruses in producing disease is uncertain.

Adenoviruses can be cultured from either throat or rectal swab material. Human embryonic kidney is generally regarded as the best cell system, although continuous human cell lines are quite satisfactory. Primary isolation may take up to 3 weeks. CF antibodies may be measured in the serum.

There is no known specific treatment for adenovirus diseases, although live virus vaccines for types 4 and 7 have been used successfully in military settings. Certain types of adenovirus are oncogenic in hamsters and provide an important tool for cancer research. However, there is no indication that the agents are oncogenic in man.

RHINOVIRUSES

Rhinoviruses are small (20 to 30 nm), nonenveloped, icosahedral, RNA-containing viruses. They are grouped with the enteroviruses to form the picornavirus family, but are distinguished from the enteroviruses by their acid lability and slightly greater buoyant density in cesium chloride. Most have limited ability to replicate at normal human body temperatures. This trait usually confines them to the cooler upper respiratory passages. Their acid lability precludes gastrointestinal invasion.

There are at least 90 different human rhinovirus serotypes.

The association of rhinoviruses with the common cold is well known. The prevalence of rhinovirus is greatest during the fall months. Rhinoviruses probably cause colds more frequently in adults than they do among the pediatric population, although they are an important cause of colds in children. Children occasionally develop rhinovirus lower respiratory infections including croup, bronchitis, bronchiolitis, and pneumonia. The occurrence of such infections in adults is decidedly unusual. As with other respiratory viruses, secretory antibody appears to be more important than serum antibody in preventing disease.

The clinical picture of rhinovirus disease calls for little comment. Coryza, cough, and sore throat are seen, usually without fever. Rhinoviruses apparently have little tendency to cause pharyngeal exudates or cervical lymphadenopathy. No specific treatment is available. Because of the numerous serotypes capable of causing disease and because of the uncertainties concerning the long-term persistence of even naturally acquired type-specific immunity, the control of rhinovirus infection by means of vaccines must be considered to be a distant possibility.

CORONAVIRUSES

The coronaviruses are enveloped, pleomorphic, RNA-containing viruses that measure about 120 nm in diameter. The surface is marked by petallike, narrow-based projections measuring 15 to 20 nm in length. Several different strains have been identified. The growth of coronaviruses in tissue culture is limited, and organ culture using explants of human embryonic trachea or nasal epithelium is sometimes necessary. Blind passage in human diploid cells is sometimes used. Serologic studies are generally the most useful for diagnostic and epidemiologic purposes.

Clinically, coronaviruses appear capable of causing the common cold. Perhaps 3 to 5 percent of such illnesses in man are attributable to these agents, and the proportion may be greater in seasons of high coronavirus prevalence. Coronavirus infections appear to be the most common in the winter months; coronavirus epidemics have occurred. There are hints from some laboratories that the viruses may occasionally cause lower respiratory tract disease in infants, but further studies are required to clarify this matter.

References

GENERAL

Cherry JD. Newer respiratory viruses: their role in respiratory illnesses of children. Adv Pediatr 20:225, 1973

Glezen WP, Denny FW: Epidemiology of lower respiratory disease in children. N Engl J Med 288:498, 1973

RESPIRATORY SYNCYTIAL VIRUS

Brandt CD, Kim HW, Arrobio JO, et al: Epidemiology of respiratory syncytial virus infection in Washington, DC. III. Composite analysis of eleven consecutive yearly epidemics. Am J Epidemiol 98:355, 1973

Chanock RM, Kapikian AZ, Mille J, Kim HW, Parrott RH: Influence of immunologic factors in respiratory syncytial virus disease. Arch Environ Health 21:347, 1970

Ditchburn RK, McQuillin J, Gardner PS, Court SDM: Respiratory syncytial virus in hospital cross-infection. Br Med J 3:671, 1971

Hall CB, Douglas RG Jr: Clinically useful method for isolation of respiratory syncytial virus. J Infect Dis 131:1, 1975

Kim HW, Arrobio JO, Brandt CD, et al: Safety and antigenicity of temperature sensitive (TS) mutant respiratory syncytial virus (RSV) in infants and children. Pediatrics 52:56, 1973

McIntosh K, Arbeter AM, Stahl MK, et al: Attenuated respiratory syncytial virus vaccines in asthmatic children. Pediatr Res 8:289, 1974

Parrott RH, Kim HW, Arrobio JO, et al: Epidemiology of respiratory syncytial virus infection in Washington, DC. II. Infection and disease with respect to age, immunologic status, race and sex. Am J Epidemiol 98:289, 1973

Rooney JC, Williams HE: The relationship between proved viral bronchiolitis and subsequent wheezing. J Pediatr 79:744, 1971

PARAINFLUENZA VIRUSES

Brandt CD: Parainfluenza virus epidemiology. Pediatr Res 8:422, 1974

Fulginiti VA, Eller JJ, Sieber OF, et al: Respiratory virus immunization. I. Field trial of two inactivated respiratory virus vaccines; an aqueous trivalent parainfluenza virus vaccine and an alum-precipitated respiratory syncytial virus vaccine. Am J Epidemiol 89:435, 1969

Kingsbury DW: Paramyxovirus replication. Curr Top Microbiol Immunol 59:1, 1973

Smith CB, Bellanti JA, Chanock RM: Immunoglobulins in serum and nasal secretions following infection with type 1 parainfluenza virus and injection of inactivated vaccines. J Immunol 99:133, 1967

——— Purcell RH, Bellanti JA, Chanock RM: Protective effect of antibody to parainfluenza type 1 virus. N Engl J Med 275:1145, 1966

Vargosko AJ, Chanock RM, Huebner RJ, et al: Association of type 2 hemadsorption (parainfluenza 1) virus and Asian influenza A virus with infectious croup. N Engl J Med 261:1, 1959

INFLUENZA VIRUSES

Compans RW, Klenk HD, Caliguiri LA, Choppin PW: Influenza virus proteins. I. Analysis of polypeptides of the virion and identification of spike glycoproteins. Virology 42:880, 1970

Eickhoff TC: Committee on immunization against influenza: rationale and recommendations. J Infect Dis 123:446, 1971

Fox JC, Kilbourne ED: Epidemiology of influenza. Summary of Influenza Workshop, IV. J Infect Dis 128:361, 1973

Hill DA, Baron S, Perkins JC, et al: Evaluation of an interferon inducer in viral respiratory disease. JAMA 219:1179, 1972

Hornick RB, Togo Y, Mahler S, Iezzone D: Evaluation of amantadine hydrochloride in the treatment of A2 influenzal disease. WHO Bull 41:671, 1969

Howard JB, McCracken GH Jr, Luby JP: Influenza A2 virus as a cause of croup requiring tracheostomy. J Pediatr 81:1148, 1972

Kilbourne EC, Butler WL, Rossen RD: Specific immunity in influenza. Summary of Influenza Workshop, III. J Infect Dis 127:220, 1973

Merigan TC, Reed SE, Hall TS, Tyrrel DAJ: Inhibition of respiratory virus infection by locally applied interferon. Lancet 1:563, 1973

Murphy BR, Chalhub EG, Nusinoff SR, Chanock RM: Temperature-sensitive mutants of influenza virus. II. Attenuation of TS recombinants for man. J Infect Dis 126:170, 1972

Ruben FL, Jackson GG: A new subunit influenza vaccine: acceptability compared with standard vaccines and effect of dose on antigenicity. J Infect Dis 125:656, 1972

Schultze IL: the structure of influenza virus. II. A model based on the morphology and composition of subviral particles. Virology 47:181, 1972

Smith JWG: Vaccination in the control of influenza. Lancet 2:330, 1974

Webster RG, Campbell CH, Granoff A: The in vivo production of "new" influenza viruses. III. Isolation of recombinant influenza viruses under simulated conditions of natural transmission. Virology 51:149, 1973

ADENOVIRUSES

Brandt CD, Kim HW, Vargosko AJ, et al: Infections in 18,000 infants and children in a controlled study of respiratory tract disease. I. Adenovirus pathogenicity in relation to serologic type and illness syndrome. Am J Epidemiol 90:484, 1969

Connor JD: Evidence for an etiological role of adenoviral infection in the pertussis syndrome. N Engl J Med 283:390, 1970

Dudding BA, Wagner SC, Zeller JA, et al: Fatal pneumonia associated with adenovirus type 7 in three military trainees. N Engl J Med 288:1289, 1972

Nelson KE, Gavitt F, Batt MD, et al: The role of adenoviruses in the pertussis syndrome. J Pediatr 86:335, 1975

RHINOVIRUSES

Andrewes CH: Rhinoviruses and the common cold. Ann Rev Med 17:361, 1966

Stott EJ, Killington RA: Rhinoviruses. Ann Rev Microbiol 26:503, 1972

CORONAVIRUSES

McIntosh K, Chao RK, Krause HE, et al: Coronavirus infection in acute lower respiratory tract disease of infants. J Infect Dis 130:502, 1974

——— Kapikian AZ, Turner HC, et al: Seroepidemiologic studies of coronavirus infection in adults and children. Am J Epidemiol 91:595, 1970

LYMPHOCYTIC CHORIOMENINGITIS

Alfred L. Florman

Lymphocytic choriomeningitis, a form of benign lymphocytic meningitis, is caused by a specific virus that was first encountered by Armstrong and Lillie in 1933 while studying St. Louis encephalitis. Two years later Rivers and Scott proved that the virus is pathogenic for man, producing a meningitis or mild encephalitic syndrome; soon afterward, reports of cases in children began to appear. The name is derived from the marked involvement of the choroid plexus when monkeys are infected with this virus. Although accurate identification of the infection has been possible for several years, the number of recognized cases remains rather small, and their distribution is primarily in large cities. To some extent this is due to the fact that appropriate steps are not always taken for identification of the virus in suspected cases. Except for a single instance, reported by Komrower and associates from Manchester, England, in which the infection appeared to be transmitted from mother to fetus in utero, the disease seems not to be communicable from man to man. While a wide variety of animals are susceptible, the great reservoir of the infection is located in ordinary house mice; in five of six attempts made, Armstrong and Lillie recovered the virus from mice trapped in the households of infected patients. Since a history of handling mice or of other direct contact is missing in the great majority of instances of proved infection, indirect transmission has been postulated, as by inhalation of desiccated mouse excreta or by some insect vector. The fact that the disease seldom occurs in midsummer would tend to exonerate mosquitoes and ordinary house flies.

In children, meningitis is the most important manifestation of the infection. Some cases are limited to a grippelike illness without meningitic symptoms, and immunologic studies indicate that inapparent infection may occur in childhood as well as at older ages. However, pneumonic and bizarre neurologic syndromes, some of them fatal, such as are occasionally encountered among adults, have not been reported in children. The pathology of the disease, as it affects children, can therefore not be accurately described.

As a rule the onset of symptoms is abrupt, with fever, malaise, restlessness, loss of appetite, headache, occasionally with drowsiness or even stupor, vomiting, photophobia, and abdominal pain. The temperature is usually 38 C to 39 C but may reach 40.5 C. Neck rigidity and Kernig and Brudzinski signs are generally found, increasing the suspicion of bacterial meningitis and leading to diagnostic lumbar puncture. This procedure not infrequently makes the patient feel better, with less headache and general distress. Although the patient may seem quite ill for 2 or 3 days, improvement progresses rapidly, and most children are afebrile and apparently well at the end of a week. Except for a few reported instances of pneumonia there have been no complications and no residua.

The spinal fluid at the height of symptoms is under increased pressure and contains from 100 to 2,000 cells/mm³, which are almost all lymphocytes. Its protein concentration is usually somewhat increased, but sugar and chloride values are normal. Pleocytosis commonly outlasts the fever, but there may be a late increase in spinal fluid protein, so that in convalescence its concentration may be out of proportion to the number of cells. False-positive serologic tests for syphilis have been reported in the spinal fluid of these patients. The sedimentation rate of the blood and the leukocyte count are usually unchanged.

Differentiation from bacterial meningitis is usually made quite readily from the findings in the spinal fluid. On the other hand, the conditions that may cause a mononuclear pleocytosis with normal concentration of sugar include mumps, poliomyelitis, coxsackievirus and herpesvirus infections, various specific and nonspecific forms of encephalitis, infectious mononucleosis, syphilis, leptospirosis, lymphogranuloma venereum, lead poisoning, and even certain tumors. Every effort should be made to obtain satisfactory evidence of etiology. At the height of the disease the virus is present in the blood as well as in the cerebrospinal fluid; even after defervescence, as long as pleocytosis remains, it may be recovered from the latter source by inoculation of susceptible animals, eg, mice and guinea pigs. Retrospective identification of the infecting agent may be made by demonstrating a rise in the patient's serum titer of complement-fixing or neutralizing antibodies a few weeks after onset.

Treatment is symptomatic. Premature resumption of activity may result in prolongation of headache and malaise.

References

Cole GA, Gilden DH, Monjan AA, Nathanson N: Lymphocytic choriomeningitis virus: pathogenesis of acute central nervous system disease. Proc Soc Exp Biol Med 30:1831, 1971

Emmons RW, et al: Follow-up on hamster-associated LCM infection—United States. Morbidity Mortality 23:110, 1974

Hotchin J, Sikora E, Kinch W, Hinman A, Woodall J: Lymphocytic choriomeningitis in a hamster colony causes infection of hospital personnel. Science 185:1173, 1974

MEASLES
SAMUEL L. KATZ

Measles (rubeola, morbilli) has been for centuries one of the most common communicable diseases. A striking reduction in reported cases of the disease first began in the United States with the licensure in 1963 of measles virus vaccines, and similar decreases in incidence have occurred in other nations where these vaccines have been utilized. However, it is important that physicians retain their familiarity with the disease and its complications. The cardinal manifestations have varied little, although changes in environmental hygiene and sanitation, as well as improved host nutrition, have attenuated the overall clinical picture among many populations. Recurrent epidemics, with great severity and serious complications still occur in economically and medically underdeveloped countries. Alterations in the basic properties and behavior of the virus itself have not been substantiated.

VIROLOGY. Measles is a paramyxovirus. It has many close similarities to canine distemper and rinderpest (cattle plague) viruses. Its internal component of ribonucleic acid (RNA) within a helical protein capsid is enclosed by an outer membrane of lipid and protein. The virus hemagglutinates only primate erythrocytes (simian most effectively) and does not have a neuraminidase. Electron photomicrographs demonstrate virons that are roughly circular or oval and average 1,200 to 1,400 Å in diameter. In general the virus is markedly heat-labile, but it remains very well preserved for long periods at low temperatures. It is rapidly inactivated by ultraviolet light and other forms of radiation, by proteolytic enzymes such as trypsin, and by chemical agents including ether, acetone, and formalin. Measles virus propagates in a large variety of both primary cell cultures and stable lines; the former generally are most sensitive in attempts to recover the agent from patients; successful propagation in the latter cultures usually requires a period of laboratory adaptation. Cells of human and simian origin seem most reliable for initial isolation of virus, but after varying numbers of serial passages it will multiply readily in cultures prepared from cells of other species. The growth rate in vitro is less rapid than that of many other agents; infective virus is released by budding slowly from intact cells until they lose their integrity, releasing the major portion of cell-associated virus.

The morphologic changes induced in cell cultures by measles virus are characterized by the formation of large, multinucleate giant cells or syncytia and by the appearance of eosinophilic inclusions that are seen in both the nuclei and cytoplasm when infected cells are stained. A second cytopathic effect is the change of affected polygonal cells to spindle or stellate form. Of particular note is the marked similarity of these syncytia and inclusions induced in vitro to the multinucleate giant cells with inclusions that are observed in histologic specimens prepared from many tissues of patients with measles.

Antibodies appear in the serum after 12 to 15 days following infection of man or experimental animals. They specifically neutralize viral infectivity, fix complement with viral antigen, and inhibit viral hemagglutination and hemolysis. No evidence has been found of significant variation among measles strains isolated during the past 19 years. This homogeneity correlates with the extreme rarity of second attacks of the disease. The sharing of some antigens and other properties with canine distemper and bovine rinderpest viruses remains principally of evolutionary interest; it has no significance in the protection of man against measles. However, the reverse phenomenon has been demonstrated, in that measles protects some animals against infection with rinderpest and canine distemper viruses.

PATHOLOGY. The cellular reaction is predominantly a monocytic one. Widespread lymphoid hyperplasia in adenoids, tonsils, thymus, spleen, Peyer's patches, appendix, and lymph nodes is characteristic; within these reaction foci, the large, multinucleate giant cells are found. Inclusion-bearing cells also abound in the trachea, bronchi, and bronchioles. With involvement of the mucosal lining of these respiratory passages, the affected epithelium is sloughed into the lumen along with macrophages, mucus, and cellular debris. Squamous metaplasia of bronchial mucosa follows. A pronounced peribronchial mononuclear exudate extends to varying degrees in an interstitial pattern, and macrophages appear in alveolar walls.

In the skin, early hyaline necrosis of epidermal cells is followed by perivascular exudation of serum, proliferation of endothelial cells, and necrosis of epithelial elements. Destruction of hair follicles and sebaceous glands may occur in the affected area, and a late perivascular lymphoid cuffing of small vessels has been reported. The buccal area lesions (Koplik's spots) develop as a focal necrosis of the basal epithelium of the submucous glands, with round cell collections and formation of vesicles.

Late in the course of the disease, up to 70 percent of peripheral leukocytes may show chromosomal breakage for a short time. Although their significance has not been determined, similar alterations of chromosomes have been found in the course of other viral infections.

When encephalomyelitis follows measles, a striking perivascular demyelination occurs predominantly in white matter but also in deeper cortical layers. Perivascular cuffing by microglial cells, lymphocytes, and plasma cells is apparent around small veins, in which the endothelial cells are swollen. The neuropathologic findings of subacute sclerosing panencephalitis (SSPE)

are described elsewhere (p. 1880), but their hallmark is the presence of inclusion bodies in neuronal and glial cells.

PATHOGENESIS. Although all the events comprising the complete pathogenesis are still not known, it is possible to construct a reliable outline by correlating virologic and histologic data with clinical events. Infection is initiated when a susceptible individual receives, either directly by inhalation into the upper respiratory tract or indirectly via the conjunctival sac, virus-laden droplets discharged from the nasopharyngeal secretions of a measles patient. At the portal of entry a short period of local viral multiplication and limited spread ensues, followed by a brief, low-titer, primary viremia that distributes the agent to distant sites, where virus replicates actively in lymphoid tissues. A prolonged secondary viremia of higher titer occurs, associated with the onset of the clinical prodromata and the widespread dissemination of virus. From that time (about 9 or 10 days after the initial exposure) until the beginning of rash, virus can be detected throughout the body, especially in the respiratory tract and in lymphoid tissues; it can also be recovered from the nasopharyngeal secretions, urine, and blood. The patient is most highly communicable to others during this 5- to 6-day period. With the onset of rash (about 14 days after initial infection) viral replication diminishes, and by 16 days it is difficult to recover virus except from the urine, where it may persist for an additional several days. Coincident with the appearance of exanthem is the detection in serum of circulating measles antibodies found in nearly 100 percent of patients by the second day of rash. Striking clinical improvement begins at this time, interrupted a few days later in a varying number of patients by secondary illness caused by bacteria that have migrated across the damaged respiratory tract lining. Sinusitis, otitis media, and bronchopneumonia develop more readily where edema, exudation, and lymphoid hyperplasia have produced local obstruction and the loss of ciliated epithelium has compromised normal defense mechanisms.

Central nervous system (CNS) involvement is most likely a result of viral invasion of the CNS during the secondary viremia. As many as 10 percent of patients develop a significant cerebrospinal fluid (CSF) pleocytosis, and 50 percent show electroencephalographic aberrations at the peak of illness. However, only 0.1 percent develop signs and symptoms of encephalomyelitis. It has not been possible to recover virus from CSF or CNS tissue of these patients. The CNS abnormalities appear several days after the acute illness, when serum antibody abounds and infectious virus is no longer detectable at sites where it was plentiful earlier. Recovery of measles virus from CNS tissues of SSPE patients many years after primary measles infection has emphasized the need for further clarification of the interactions of this virus and the CNS, both acutely and chronically. SSPE may be labeled a slow measles virus encephalitis.

EPIDEMIOLOGY. In most countries measles was a disease of early childhood, with peak incidence among youngsters of preschool and early school age. The very high attack rate among exposed susceptibles resulted in a periodicity of epidemics at intervals of 2 or 3 years, when a new crop of susceptibles had arisen. In crowded urban areas, the 1- to 5-year-old group showed the highest incidence, while the age distribution shifted to 5- to 10-year-olds in suburban or rural areas, where exposure was postponed until school attendance began. Late winter and early spring, in temperate zones, were the usual seasons for outbreaks. Nearly 100 percent of young adults have had measles or measles vaccine, but a rare individual may escape the disease in childhood only to acquire it in the third decade or later when exposed to infected children.

The epidemiology in isolated island or other remote population groups is quite different. Under such circumstances, many years elapse between outbreaks, allowing the accumulation of a large population of susceptibles of all ages. An explosive and severe epidemic results if the virus is inadvertently reintroduced into the community by a traveler who arrives while incubating measles. The usual period of infectivity ranges from 6 or 7 days prior to the appearance of rash through the second or third day of the exanthem. This correlates with the time of laboratory-detectable viral shedding. Coughing and sneezing during the catarrhal period enchance the spread of droplet infection, the principal mode of contagion. The relative lability of virus on exposure to light, drying, and heat limits its duration of infectivity and precludes transmission by an immune individual or by fomites. Man is the only known natural host, but other primates (especially Old World monkeys) are susceptible and may develop disease when intimately exposed to infected children or after deliberate laboratory infection. There are no known insect vectors.

IMMUNITY. A single attack of measles confers lifelong immunity. The immune individual whose serum antibody titer has diminished to low or even undetectable levels may occasionally show a rapid, anamnestic antibody rise after exposure or inoculation, but this occurs in the absence of any symptoms or signs of infection and without detectable virus shedding. Vaccination with live attenuated measles vaccines confers comparable lasting immunity; inactivated antigens have produced only a transient protective effect for 6 to 18 months.

When measles has been modified or aborted by the administration of immune gamma globulin early in the incubation period, the immunologic outcome is variable. In general a durable immunity may follow the development of modified overt disease. The complete absence of any clinical manifestations usually coincides with a transient protective effect followed by a return to the fully susceptible state after the degradation of the passively acquired antibody in the ensuing 6 to 8 weeks. A small number of exceptions have been observed in which overt, modified disease was later followed by a return to full susceptibility; conversely, the complete prevention of detectable illness permitted subclinical infection and a permanent immunity. For any individual

patient the immunologic status following globulin-altered infection can be determined only by measuring circulating measles-specific antibodies. Such an antibody test should be delayed until 6 to 8 weeks after globulin administration.

Since the virus-neutralizing antibodies are among those immunoglobulins that cross the placenta readily, infants born to mothers immune to measles are protected against infection during their first 6 or 7 months after birth. With the catabolism of maternal antibody, babies become increasingly susceptible in the second half of their first year and may, on exposure, develop disease of varying severity. Those with modified or occult illnesses are thought to be examples of partial protection by residual transplacentally acquired antibody. The infant of the rare mother who has never had measles or vaccine is susceptible at birth and may acquire the infection at any time postnatally. Studies of secretory antibody in the IgA component of respiratory tract secretions have demonstrated the presence of measles-specific antibodies following natural infection or live attenuated vaccine, but not after inactivated antigens.

CLINICAL PICTURE. In most cases the signs and symptoms of measles are highly characteristic, and their time of appearance and sequence after infection are consistent. Approximately 10 days after exposure, fever and malaise first signal the onset of illness. Cough, coryza, and conjunctivitis (the three Cs) begin by the eleventh day. A gradual worsening of these catarrhal symptoms accompanies a steady rise in fever over the next 4 days. Two days prior to the appearance of exanthem, Koplik's spots, the classic enanthem, develop. With the onset of rash 14 days after infection, the clinical picture attains its maximal severity, reaching a peak that coincides with involvement of the entire body by the eruption on its second to fourth days. Constitutional symptoms throughout this 10-day period vary, but headache, abdominal pain, vomiting, diarrhea, and myalagia are frequent complaints. Fever reaching 40.5 C or 41.1 C, often accompanied by chills, is not unusal when the rash is most florid. Febrile seizures may occur in children predisposed to them.

There is nothing unique about the coryza, which is characterized by nasal congestion, runny nose, and sneezing. The conjunctivitis causes edema of the lids, increased lacrimation, and frequently photophobia. Sharply demarcated, transverse, linear injection of the lower lid margins, called Stimson's line, is present before the more generalized conjunctival inflammation obscures it. The hacking cough is distressing, with a progressive increase in frequency and severity throughout the prodromal period. With the abrupt fall in temperature, after rash has covered the entire body, the catarrhal symptoms subside dramatically, except that the cough persists for another 7 to 10 days.

Koplik's spots, pathognomonic of measles, appear 24 to 48 hours before the exanthem. They consist of a bluish white dot, about 1 mm in diameter, surrounded by a rose-red areola. They tend to appear first on the buccal mucosa opposite the lower molars. Best seen in bright daylight, they are discrete and few in number initially, but within 1 day they increase rapidly and may spread to cover the entire buccal and some of the labial mucosa. At their peak they are also seen on the lacrimal caruncle and have been described on the mucous membranes of the vagina and rectum. With the onset of rash they fade, and by the second day of the eruption they frequently have disappeared. A nonspecific enanthem with red macular palatal lesions may precede the Koplik's spots and remain after the latter have faded.

Rash commences as discrete, irregular, erythematous macules behind the ears, on the neck, and along the hairline. As it progresses caudad over the ensuing 24 hours to involve the face, trunk, and arms, careful palpation reveals a papular component. Involvement of the legs and feet by the end of the second or early in the third day finds the lesions on the cheeks already coalescent; in severe cases confluent areas of rash also appear on the trunk and extremities. The skin becomes edematous and the face swollen. Although the exanthem ordinarily blanches with pressure, a fine petechial component is often present but may not be appreciated until fading of the acute redness has left a faint brown discoloration. The exanthem fades slowly, in the same order of progression as its initial appearance; this process usually begins by the third or fourth day after onset. Subsidence of the florid eruption is followed by a fine, furfuraceous desquamation that may be overlooked. Among children with protein deficiency the desquamation is far more extensive and may be complicated by multiple pyogenic skin abscesses. Uncommonly, measles rash may have a pruritic element.

The marked generalized lymphadenopathy and splenomegaly that arise early in the course of the acute illness may persist for several weeks. High fever at the peak of illness may be accompanied in some children by marked irritability, somnolence, or a state of delirium; these are transient manifestations and resolve dramatically with the disappearance of pyrexia. They do not correlate with the occurrence of subsequent CNS complications. Black measles, a severe form of the disease with a generalized hemorrhagic rash, bleeding from the nose, mouth, and gastrointestinal tract, and marked systemic toxicity, is rarely seen; it was reported more frequently by authors in the past. Perhaps it included some features of disseminated intravascular coagulation.

DIAGNOSIS. The regular sequence of prodome, Koplik's spots, and generalized rash permit a clinical diagnosis with a high degree of reliability. Except under unusual circumstances where definite confirmation is required, virus isolation in cell cultures or demonstration of an antibody rise is unnecessary. Of the available serologic tests, the measles hemagglutination-inhibition (HI) antibody determination is the most practical, combining ease and rapidity of performance with specificity and reliability of response. Within 1 to 2 days of the onset of rash, serum antibodies to the various measles antigens are detectable; they increase rapidly thereafter to reach peak titers in the next 2 to 4 weeks. Complement-fixing antibodies may then gradually diminish over a period of years, while virus-neutralizing

and HI antibodies persist indefinitely after an initial drop during the 2 to 6 months following their attainment of maximal titers.

Cytologic techniques for the demonstration of multinucleate giant cells in nasal secretions during the prodromal period and for the detection of inclusion-bearing cells in the urine, either at the time rash appears or soon after, have been helpful diagnostically. The material is stained best by the Papanicolaou technique, but Wright's stain has proved satisfactory for the nasal smears. A more reliable and specific test has been examination of urinary sediments for cells containing measles antigen that can be labeled by fluorescent antibodies. Less specific laboratory support is found in the low white blood cell count with an absolute neutropenia and marked lymphopenia in the prodromal period and during the rash.

The differential diagnosis includes rubella, infectious mononucleosis, roseola, scarlet fever, typhus, Rocky Mountain spotted fever, enterovirus or adenovirus exanthemata, and rashes due to drug sensitivity (especially barbiturates, hydantoins, penicillins, and sulfonamides). Koplik's spots are said to be pathognomonic of measles; somewhat similar buccal mucosal lesions may rarely accompany coxsackievirus A9 infections. The latter occur without prodromata or exanthem. Rubella is a far milder illness, without cough and with distinctive lymphadenopathy usually restricted to the posterior cervical, suboccipital, and postauricular nodes. Roseola (exanthema subitum) has an entirely different sequence, since the rash first appears after the fever has subsided. The peripheral blood count and smear in infectious mononucleosis contrast strikingly with the leukopenia of measles.

COMPLICATIONS. A wide variety of complications may be observed during the acute stage of measles or shortly thereafter. The greatest number occur in the respiratory tract; other sites are also involved, although less commonly. They are listed in Table 21 by probable etiology. Complications attributable to the initial measles virus infection are due to exaggerated or abnormal patterns of response. The widespread destruction of cells lining the respiratory tract and the accompanying reactive inflammation produce the usual catarrhal stage of measles. In the proper anatomic setting, and with only a moderate enhancement of these responses, severe laryngotracheobronchitis (croup) or bronchiolitis may result; the former may cause sufficient airway obstruction to require tracheostomy, especially in children less than 3 years of age. In infants, only a moderate increase of local secretions and edema of the bronchiolar walls is necessary to produce wheezing, dyspnea, retractions, cyanosis, hyperresonance on percussion of the chest, and diffuse fine rales on auscultation. This latter picture does not differ from that of bronchiolitis due to respiratory syncytial or other viruses.

An extremely rare but almost uniformly fatal interstitial pneumonia (giant cell pneumonia) has been noted in immunocompromised children who develop a progressive, persistent measles virus infection without

TABLE 21. Complications of Measels Virus Infection

Viral	Bacterial	Uncertain Etiology
Laryngotracheobronchitis	Otitis media	Thrombocytopenic purpura
Bronchiolitis	Sinusitis	Depression of delayed
Pneumonitis	Mastoiditis	cutaneous hypersensitivity
Keratoconjunctivitis	Pneumonia	Effects on underlying disease:
Myocarditis	Noma	Tuberculosis
Mesenteric adenitis–appendicitis	Furunculosis	Cystic fibrosis
Interstitial (giant cell) pneumonia		Malnutrition
Encephalomyelitis		Nephrotic syndrome
Subacute sclerosing panencephalitis (slow measles encephalitis)		

the typical exanthem and with a unique failure to form measles-specific antibodies. To date, nearly all patients who have been studied with giant cell pneumonia have had some severe underlying disorder, such as leukemia, Letterer-Siwe disease, or severe combined immunodeficiency. The radiographic picture reveals a marked, interstitial pattern emanating from both hilar regions. Measles virus can be recovered repeatedly from sputum or nasopharyngeal swabs, and typical giant cells are seen when respiratory tract secretions are stained. Attempts to prevent this complication or to treat it with exceedingly large volumes of immune globulin or measles-convalescent plasma have rarely been successful.

A benign, asymptomatic keratoconjunctivitis accompanies measles but leaves no sequelae. It is of particular interest because of its persistence for periods as long as 4 months after the acute illness. The lesions can be visualized only by slit-lamp biomicroscopy; they are said to be distinct from those caused by other agents. Myocarditis has been reported; it is a very rare complication of little clinical significance. Transient electrocardiographic abnormalities commonly occur during measles. The diffuse lymphadenopathy that accompanies measles involves the mesenteric nodes and is thought to cause the abdominal pain of varying severity that commonly occurs. Symptoms and signs identical with those of acute appendicitis may result. Surgical intervention during the prodromal period has occurred sufficiently often to familiarize the pathologist with measles appendicitis, characterized by obliteration of the appendiceal lumen by lymphoid hyperplasia and by the presence of typical giant cells in the mucosa.

Complications of bacterial origin result principally from invasion of pyogenic organisms into areas where lining cells have been damaged by the virus. Otitis media and bronchopneumonia are the most common; they may be due to β-hemolytic streptococci, pneumococci, *H. influenzae* type B, or staphylococci. The peribronchitis and interstitial pneumonitis seen in nearly all measles patients are viral in etiology and resolve rapidly with the development of generalized rash and the subsidence of fever. A second fever spike, or failure of the initial one to drop after the eruption has reached its peak, suggests the presence of secondary bacterial infection. The appearance of a peripheral leukocytosis

with a shift to the left is confirmatory. If physical findings are not sufficiently revealing, a chest radiograph may disclose bronchopneumonia or a segmental or lobar involvement. Smears and cultures of sputum, tracheal aspirates, pleural fluid, blood, or other appropriate materials will assist immeasurably in establishing the etiology and will permit selection of a proper antimicrobial agent. Attempts at prevention of secondary bacterial complications by giving prophylactic antibiotics during the catarrhal stage of measles have been unsuccessful and are injudicious. Aside from failing to decrease the incidence of these infections, such indiscriminate use of antimicrobials tends to diminish those organisms that are susceptible to their effects, so that later complications result from invasion by more resistant bacteria or fungi that have flourished in the altered milieu.

In areas where protein deficiency is a childhood problem, measles is accompanied by a higher rate of bacterial complications. In addition, manifestations such as noma and furunculosis, rarely seen in well-nourished children, may occur. Among children who acquire measles in their early years and who are also heavily parasitized by helminths and enteropathogenic bacteria, the vomiting and diarrhea that may normally accompany the illness are more virulent and may precipitate dehydration, acidosis, and frank kwashiorkor. The high morbidity and mortality rates from measles reported from some nations in Latin America, Africa, and Asia seem best explained by the young ages of the patients, these severe complications, and the unavailability of prompt therapy.

Of those syndromes that may follow measles, the most dreaded are the various CNS complications. By far the most common is encephalomyelitis (p.1876), but toxic encephalopathy, retrobulbar neuritis, thrombophlebitis of cerebral veins. hemiplegias from vascular infarction, and ascending paralysis with polyneuropathy have all been reported. There is much speculation about their etiology; the hypothesis favored until recently invoked a hypersensitivity type of response similar to that found in experimental allergic encephalomyelitis. Evidence against the possibility that encephalomyelitis is due to a direct invasion of the brain by the virus were the following observations: failure to recover virus in cell cultures from either CSF or CNS tissue of patients, the usual delay in onset of symptoms until several days after appearance of detectable circulating measles antibodies, and an inability to reproduce the syndromes in susceptible monkeys inoculated with measles virus intracerebrally, intraspinally, and cisternally. However, the high incidence of abnormal electroencephalograms recorded in measles patients who have no CNS signs or symptoms during the acute stage, as well as the description of rare giant cells in sections of CNS tissue from encephalitis patients, remain unexplained. Coupled with the isolations of measles viruses from CNS tissue of SSPE patients, these features call for a reexamination of the pathogenesis of all measles–CNS interactions. A cellular cocultivation technique to isolate measles virus from brain tissue obtained post mortem from an adult who died 6 weeks after the onset of acute measles encephalitis has been reported.

With the exception of toxic encephalopathy, which appears with striking rapidity at the peak of fever and rash, the other more common CNS manifestations become apparent after the acute illness, following a period of improvement lasting 2 days or more. Seizures, altered states of consciousness, and sudden lapse into coma frequently mark the onset of encephalomyelitis. The patient's fever returns, and there is a marked peripheral leukocytosis. The CSF findings and laboratory determinations, as well as the subsequent clinical course, are indistinguishable from those of other postinfectious encephalitides. All patients show striking electroencephalographic changes. The incidence of overt encephalomyelitis appears to be about 0.1 percent. Mortality figures range from 10 to 25 percent, and significant sequelae in the motor, intellectual, sensorial, or emotional spheres are said to occur in 20 to 50 percent of those who survive. The use of corticosteroid therapy has not altered these grim figures. Treatment consists of good nursing care, with reduction of extreme pyrexia, control of seizures, maintenance of a clear airway, fluid and electrolyte replacement, and nutritional supplementation if the period of coma is prolonged.

During the early viremic phase of measles there is a constant thrombocytopenia of insufficient magnitude to cause spontaneous bleeding, but it may reflect megakaryocytic damage by the virus. Another unexplained postinfectious complication that is rarer, thrombocytopenic purpura, appears 4 to 14 days after the rash and may produce marked skin purpura, genitourinary and gastrointestinal bleeding, and epistaxis. In contrast to their lack of efficacy in the CNS syndromes, corticosteroids produce prompt relief, with cessation of bleeding and steady return of platelet counts to normal. This response reinforces the concept that this complication may also be some form of autoimmune phenomenon.

The deleterious effects that measles may exert on some underlying disorders are incompletely understood. Reactivation or exacerbation of tuberculosis during measles has been repeatedly documented in outbreaks among populations with a high incidence of tuberculosis and in hospitals where tuberculous children have resided. One contributing cellular immune deficit is the loss of delayed cutaneous hypersensitivity to tuberculoprotein (and other antigens) that occurs with measles and persists for several weeks thereafter, so that a previously positive reactor may give a negative skin test. The striking damage to respiratory tract epithelium and interstitial tissues, coupled with the negative nitrogen balance occurring during acute measles, may partially explain the deterioration noted in some patients with cystic fibrosis who undergo unmodified measles. Infants with dietary protein deficiency may lapse into frank kwashiorkor during measles. This stems from a combination of decreased oral intake, increased gastrointestinal losses (due to vomiting and/or diarrhea), and the negative nitrogen balance of the infection. In contrast to these undesirable side effects, measles may sometimes induce a diuresis in children with refractory nephrotic syndrome.

Since measles remains a disease of infancy and childhood in most populations, it is uncommon to encounter a susceptible woman who acquires the infection during pregnancy. Data collected from outbreaks among isolated communities involving susceptibles of all ages have shown that gestational measles frequently induced premature delivery, stillbirth, or abortion, but was not associated with an increased incidence of congenital malformation.

TREATMENT. Except for general supportive measures, there is no therapy for the patient with uncomplicated measles. Bed rest, avoidance of bright light if there is marked photophobia, encouragement of fluid intake, and the judicious use of antipyretics for high fever and suppressants for distressing cough may be beneficial symptomatically. Provisions for high humidity and, when indicated, increased oxygen concentration offer some added relief to infants with severe croup or bronchiolitis. More specific measures such as the use of proper antimicrobials should be employed in the treatment of secondary bacterial complications.

PROPHYLAXIS. PASSIVE IMMUNIZATION. Human immune (gamma) globulin given soon after exposure can alter the clinical course and the antigenic effects of measles virus infection. The resultant immunity, after a modifying dose of globulin, is usually of lasting duration, while the immunity that follows a preventive dose is most often transient, with return of susceptibility after 4 to 8 weeks. If exposed to measles, a susceptible child should promptly be given globulin, 0.25 ml/kg body weight, to prevent measles. The globulin must be administered intramuscularly as soon after exposure as possible. If more than 6 days have elapsed, one cannot rely on globulin either to prevent or to modify the illness. Patients with globulin-modified measles display great variations in clinical course, with prolongation of the incubation period and varying expression of signs and symptoms, but they do remain a source of potential contagion to their contacts. Because of its transitory nature, passive protection should always be followed in 8 weeks by active immunization.

Dosages of globulin as large as 1.0 ml/kg or transfusions of correspondingly large volumes of convalescent plasma have been advocated for exposed susceptible children with lymphoma, leukemia, disseminated malignancy, or other conditions characterized by depression of cell-mediated immunity because of their predisposition to develop giant cell pneumonia. Unfortunately the results of such seroprophylaxis have been unpredictable and variable. The most reliable protection for such high-risk patients is careful attention to active measles immunization of their siblings, classmates, and other regular contacts. The likelihood of exposure to "wild" measles is thereby markedly reduced.

ACTIVE IMMUNIZATION.   Subsequent to the licensure of attenuated measles virus vaccines in March, 1963, vigorous programs of immunization against measles were conducted in this country and elsewhere. As a result, in the 1970s there have been fewer than 40,000 measles cases reported annually in the United States, in contrast to numbers estimated in excess of 1 million each year prior to vaccine availability. The availability of safe, effective means for inducing active immunity that appears comparable to that afforded by the natural, more virulent disease has distinct advantages over passive methods. The attenuated vaccines provide an infection that is noncommunicable. Rather than depending on capricious exposure to the natural disease, the optimal time and method for use of vaccine can be selected for any child. The secondary bacterial infections and neurologic complications that accompany natural or even modified measles do not follow attenuated vaccines. The prophylactic efficacy of live vaccines properly administered approaches 95 percent, whereas the long-term protection after modification or prevention with globulin is erratic.

Over the past 12 years more than 60 million children have received live measles vaccines in this country. Several types have been used. With the original Edmonston B vaccines, globulin was used at the discretion of the physician to provide an even milder clinical response. If concomitant administration of globulin was desired, it was given intramuscularly at a different site and in a separate syringe to prevent any direct neutralization of the attenuated virus. The further-attenuated vaccines evoke reactions similar to those noted after injection of chick cell Edmonston B with globulin. Continued surveillance of children who received live vaccines 12 to 15 years ago reveals the persistence of antibody and protective effect comparable to those that follow natural measles. The febrile responses that occur in 5 to 15 percent of children induce surprisingly little discomfort, toxicity, or disability. A modified exanthem of varying extent may occur after the fever, but it is observed in less than 5 percent of the inoculated children.

Formalin-inactivated measles virus vaccines were initially prepared and used in the mid-1960s to a limited extent. Among the disadvantages were the requirement for three monthly injections to stimulate seroconversion, as well as the rapid disappearance of detectable antibody over the succeeding 6 to 18 months, with reemergence of susceptibility to measles. Because of these objections, their use was later restricted to chil-

dren for whom the live vaccine might carry some enhanced risk. Additionally, schedules were studied in which two or three monthly doses of killed vaccine were followed by an injection of the live attenuated virus. The stated objective was to reduce to an absolute minimum any clinical reactivity of the live vaccine; this effect was achieved, but the procedure was cumbersome and costly, requiring a succession of visits to the physician or clinic. Another unfavorable feature of this schedule was the observation that as many as 25 to 50 percent of children immunized in this fashion developed fever and marked local reactions, with pain, heat, erythema, and induration 2 to 5 days after the last injection. These adverse responses were self-limited and seemed to represent a form of delayed hypersensitivity reaction.

By 1967 a more serious syndrome had been observed in children exposed to natural measles several years after immunization with killed vaccine alone. An atypical form of measles developed in these partially immune children. It was characterized by very high fevers, edema of the extremities, pneumonitis, and a hemorrhagic and/or urticarial rash most prominent on the extremities. The reports of such cases were sufficient to discourage any further use of inactivated measles antigens, and they are no longer available in this country. Some of the manifestations of the atypical illness strongly suggested a hypersensitivity phenomenon, the pathogenesis of which may have interesting relationships to other combinations of inactivated and live virus antigens (p. 561) that have proved deleterious. Because of these unfavorable results, inactivated measles vaccines were withdrawn from use in the United States. Studies with more highly purified viral antigens have been continued in West Germany.

To ensure the maximum 95 to 98 percent rate of seroconversion, live vaccines should not ordinarily be used for infants before 12 months of age. However, they may be administered as early as 6 months of age if the likelihood of exposure is greater than usual. If given at such an early age, their immunogenicity may be obviated by residual maternal antibody. In the rare instance of a baby born to a mother who is herself still susceptible to measles, successful use of attenuated virus is possible at any time but is inadvisable prior to 3 months of age. Somewhat analogous to the effect of transplacental antibody, but less prolonged, is the interference with vaccination that will result from recent administration of immune (gamma) globulin or blood transfusion from an immune donor. Depending on the dose administered, immunization should be postponed for 6 to 12 weeks to allow degradation of the exogenous antibody.

Through careful formulation, polyvalent active attenuated vaccines have been prepared combining measles, rubella, and mumps viruses. These have been found safe and efficacious and have resulted in reduced costs and fewer visits to physician or clinic for immunization. As a result they have generally replaced the earlier monovalent vaccines. The overall performance record of measles vaccine remains reliable. In the face of local outbreaks of measles among clusters of unimmunized susceptible children, a few vaccinated children have developed modified or frank disease. Epidemiologic investigations have revealed a consistent prophylactic efficacy of greater than 90 percent among properly immunized populations. Some breakthroughs have been traced to improper storage of vaccine, so that virus was subjected to the deleterious effects of heat and/or light. Measles vaccine virus, like its most virulent progenitor, may diminish cutaneous delayed hypersensitivity reactions to tuberculoprotein. For this reason a tuberculin test to ensure its reliability should be applied before or at the same time vaccine is administered. If it is delayed until after vaccine, a variable period of 2 to 8 weeks may elapse before return of full responsiveness to the skin test. Legitimate concerns about the CNS interactions of measles virus have been extrapolated from reactions that accompany natural infection. Careful surveillance of vaccine recipients for acute CNS involvement has failed to reveal sequelae within 30 days of administration at a level above the incidence of acute CNS dysfunctions in a similar control group followed for the same period of time without vaccine. The association of SSPE with natural measles as a slow virus CNS infection has led to a review of the measles experience of nearly 400 SSPE patients diagnosed from 1964 to 1974. Among this group there were approximately 30 patients whose only known exposure to measles virus was to the attenuated variant. Until the host factors responsible for the development of SSPE have been elucidated, it is not possible to offer comment other than the reassurance that reported cases of SSPE have markedly diminished since the widespread use of measles vaccine.

Measles immunization has now taken its place in the ideal preventive medicine program for every infant. For the unusual adult who has had neither measles nor immunization against it, live vaccine is safe, effective, and urgently indicated to prevent a disease that is even more debilitating than in childhood. Continuing surveillance will be required to provide additional data on possible sequelae of vaccination and on the efficacy of national and international programs to achieve widespread protection against measles and its complications.

References

Babbott FL Jr, Gordon JE: Modern measles. Am J Med Sci 228:334, 1954

Burgasov PN, Andzaparidze OG, Popov VF: The status of measles after five years of mass vaccination in the USSR. WHO Bull 49:571, 1973

Cherry JD, Feigin RD, Shackelford PG, Hinthorn DR, Schmidt RR: A clinical and serologic study of 103 children with measles vaccine failure. J Pediatr 82:802, 1973

Enders JF, Katz SL, Milovanovic MV, Holloway A: Studies on an attenuated measles-virus vaccine. I. Development and preparation of the vaccine. N Engl J Med 263:153, 1960

Linnemann CC Jr: Measles vaccine: immunity, reinfection and revaccination. Am J Epidemiol 97:365, 1973

Nader PR, Horwitz MS, Rousseau J: Atypical exanthem following exposure to natural measles: eleven cases in children previously innoculated with killed vaccine. J Pediatr 72:22, 1968

Panum PL: Observations made during the epidemic of measles on the Faroe Islands in the year 1846. In Roueche B (ed): Curiosities of Medicine, New York, Berkley, 1964

Schaffner W, Schluederberg AES, Byrne EB: Clinical epidemiology of measles in a highly immunized population. N Engl J Med 279:783, 1968

Sever JL, Krebs H, Ley A, Barbosa LH, Rubinstein D: Diagnosis of subacute panencephalitis. The value and availability of measles antibody determinations. JAMA 228:604, 1974

TerMeulen V, Muller D, Kackell Y, Katz M: Isolation of infectious measles virus in measles encephalitis. Lancet 2:1172, 1972

MUMPS

Sydney S. Gellis

Mumps (epidemic parotitis) is an acute, contagious, generalized viral infection characterized by swelling and tenderness of the parotid gland and sometimes the other salivary glands. Involvement of the testes in males who have reached puberty is frequent. Involvement of the central nervous system also occurs not infrequently, and either orchitis or meningoencephalitis may occur in the absence of salivary gland swelling.

ETIOLOGY. The contagious character of mumps was noted by Hippocrates in the fifth century B.C. Although a viral etiology was long suspected, it was first established in 1918 by Wollstein, who transferred the disease to cats by injection of filtered saliva. In 1934 Johnson and Goodpasture transferred it to monkeys; in 1945 Habel, and shortly afterward Levens and Enders, successfully established the growth of the virus in chick embryos. Since then vaccines against the disease, skin tests employing attenuated virus, and complement-fixation and neutralization tests have been developed.

Intimate contact is usually required to communicate the disease, with spread occurring through droplets of saliva in which virus is carried. According to Enders, a patient may become contagious about 48 hours before swelling of the parotid is noted. It is impossible to fix with certainty the duration of the communicable period; the virus has been demonstrated in the saliva of patients as late as the sixth day of parotitis. Most public health authorities require isolation until all swelling has disappeared and until any complications have cleared.

It appears definitely established that patients with meningoencephalitis without parotitis may transmit the infection to contacts who subsequently develop parotitis. Mumps is endemic at all times; epidemics of the disease occur most frequently in the winter and spring months. The communicability of mumps is less than that of measles, chickenpox, or whooping cough, although the occurrence of mumps meningoencephalitis or orchitis without parotitis and the probable occurrence of subclinical parotitis suggest that the disease is more communicable than previously believed. The average incubation period is 18 days, but the range is said to extend from 8 to 37 days. The shortest interval observed by Enders has been 14 days and the longest 25 days.

Immunity following an attack of mumps is lifelong. Most cases of second and third attacks of so-called mumps have probably been confused with recurrent nonepidemic parotitis, which is frequently allergic in origin. The use of complement-fixation and neutralization tests will help distinguish this disease from mumps.

Individuals of all ages are susceptible to mumps. The majority of cases occur in children between the ages of 5 and 15 years. Transplacental immunity probably accounts for the infrequency of mumps in the first 6 months after birth. However, the disease has been observed in an infant 1 day old whose mother had mumps at the time of delivery. The oldest patient on record was a 99-year-old male.

PATHOLOGY. The most striking change in the salivary glands consists of edema. Minute hemorrhages may be found in the capsule, and there is intense hyperemia throughout the gland. The acinar cells show varying degrees of necrosis and infiltration with mononuclear cells; the walls of the salivary ducts are swollen, with resulting obstruction to the ducts. Subsequently the acinar cells regenerate; at no time is there any preponderance of polymorphonuclear cells, and fibrosis does not occur during healing.

SYMPTOMS. In the milder cases the local symptoms are the first to attract attention; in more severe cases there are frequently prodromal symptoms of 12 to 48 hours' duration: anorexia, headache, vomiting, pains in the back and limbs, and fever. The initial temperature in a mild attack is 37 C to 38 C; in more severe attacks the fever may range from 39C to 40 C.

Of the local symptoms, pain, which is referred to the posterior part of the jaw just below the ear, usually precedes the swelling of the salivary glands; it is increased by movement of the jaws and by pressure. Sour foods or liquids may increase the pain, although this finding is relatively infrequent in children and is not reliable as a diagnostic aid. The swelling may begin simultaneously in both parotids, but more frequently one side is involved 1 or 2 days in advance of the other. It usually reaches its maximum on the third day, remains stationary for 2 or 3 days, and then subsides gradually. The degree of swelling varies with the severity of the attack. When it is marked, the patient may be so changed in appearance as to be almost unrecognizable. The swelling fills the lateral region of the neck between the jaw and the sternomastoid muscle and extends forward on the face to the zygomatic arch, so that the center of the tumor is usually the lobe of the ear. Characteristically the lobe of the ear is pushed upward and outward by the swelling. The other salivary glands may swell simultaneously with the parotids or several days later, even after the parotid tumor has disappeared. Occasionally swelling of the submaxillary or sublingual glands occurs before that of the parotids, and in rare instances these may be the only glands affected. When the submaxillary gland is involved, the swelling also extends downward to include the neck. Involvement of the sublingual gland is accompanied by swelling below the tip of the chin and to one side or the other of the midline. The skin over the swollen glands retains a normal color but may become tense and shiny.

In the large series of cases studied by McGuinness and Gall, 70 percent showed enlargement of both parotids.

The papilla at the mouth of Stensen's duct or Wharton's duct may be reddened and somewhat swollen. This is not a reliable sign, since in many children the duct openings may normally have such an appearance. Since salivary secretion may be considerably diminished, dryness of the mouth may add to the patient's discomfort. Exceptionally, distressing salivation occurs.

The constitutional symptoms of mumps usually last from 3 to 5 days; the swelling continues about a week longer. In more severe cases swelling may continue for 10 to 14 days.

Since mumps is considered a generalized disease, *meningoencephalitis* cannot strictly be regarded as a complication. It is described in detail elsewhere (p. 1875). Other types of nervous system involvement that may occur in mumps consist of tranverse myelitis, ascending paralysis, hemiplegia, optic neuritis, and eighth nerve deafness. Of these, deafness is the most common; it is estimated that in 5 percent of the institutionalized deaf in this country the deafness was due to mumps.

Orchitis is rare in childhood: among 230 cases of mumps it was seen in only 10 boys, all of them over 12 years of age. A report by Connolly suggesting that orchitis in infants and children is more common than was generally thought requires confirmation. When orchitis occurs it is generally toward the end of the first week or the beginning of the second week; it is usually accompanied by fever, chills, and testicular swelling. The involvement is almost always unilateral. Just as meningoencephalitis may occur in the absence of apparent parotitis, so may orchitis make its appearance as the sole manifestation of mumps. The swelling and inflammation usually last from 4 to 7 days and may be followed by atrophy.

Involvement of the ovaries in adult females is not uncommon, having been estimated to occur in 5 percent of cases. Inflammations of the thyroid gland, thymus, breasts, lacrimal glands, and prostate have been reported, but they are quite uncommon. Pancreatitis may occur toward the end of the first week of mumps; it is usually sudden in onset, with severe nausea and vomiting, epigastric pain, and tenderness. Pancreatitis occurs much less frequently in children than in adults. Recent studies of the possible relationship of mumps infection to endocardial fibroelastosis have yielded variable results, and the relationship cannot be said to be established and acceptable.

Myocarditis may result from mumps; electrocardiographic changes resembling those of rheumatic carditis have been reported. No symptoms are noted, but the sedimentation rate may be elevated for a considerable period. Rarely, hepatitis or nephritis may occur in the course of mumps. Pitting edema of the soft tissues overlying the sternum develops not infrequently, particularly if both parotids are greatly swollen or both submaxillary glands are involved.

LABORATORY TESTS. The white blood cell count in mumps parotitis is usually normal or slightly low, with a relative lymphocytosis. The count becomes higher with an increase in polymorphonuclear leukocytes in the presence of meningoencephalitis or orchitis.

The complement-fixation test developed by Enders and Kane has proved to be a reliable method for detecting antibody rise during convalescence from mumps. Henle has devised a special method of complement fixation using different antigen components from virus grown in chick embryos—the V (virus) antigen and the S (soluble) antigen, which is separable from the virus by ultracentrifugation. The S antibodies reach a high titer relatively quickly. The V antibodies develop later and persist for years, whereas the S antibodies usually disappear 6 to 12 months after the acute infection. Such tests have proved most helpful in diagnosis of mumps meningoencephalitis or orchitis in the absence of parotitis.

Skin tests employing virus grown in chick embryos and inactivated by heat, ultraviolet light, or formalin have been standardized by several different investigators. These tests are carried out in a manner similar to the tuberculin test and give rise to erythema and induration if antibody is present. The erythema or induration should be more than 10 mm in diameter at the end of 48 hours in order to be considered positive. However, the commercially available mumps skin test antigens give misleading results and cannot be used to determine the state of immunity of exposed adults.

Virus neutralization tests involve inoculation of chick embryos and virus–serum dilution mixtures after incubation, harvesting of chick embryo materials, and testing for evidence of virus multiplication by complement fixation against a known positive mumps serum. The neutralization tests have been employed less extensively than complement-fixation tests; neutralization antibody titer has been shown to be elevated early in the course of mumps. When low titers are found the likelihood of development of orchitis appears to be increased.

An elevation of serum or urine amylase is nearly always present in the first week of parotitis. This increase usually disappears by the end of the second week. There is some evidence that the increase is due only to inflammation of the parotid glands and that involvement of the other salivary glands or the testes has no effect on amylase levels. Therefore a rise in amylase does not necessarily reflect pancreatitis, although pancreatitis may occur.

PROPHYLAXIS. The relatively benign course of mumps in children as compared with that in adults argues for deliberate exposure to the disease during childhood. Active immunization against mumps is now feasible. An effective live attenuated mumps virus vaccine grown in chick embryo cell cultures is commercially available. After subcutaneous injection of the recommended dose (0.5 ml) of the vaccine, antibody against mumps virus appears in more than 95 percent of subjects. The vaccine has not caused fever or other clinical symptoms. The persistence of antibody following vaccination has not yet been determined, but excellent protection against contracting mumps has been demonstrated for over 2 years. Because of the uncertainty of the duration of the immunity afforded, and because mumps is not a serious disease in children before puberty, the Committee on Infectious Diseases of the American Academy of Pediatrics recommends that vaccine be given mainly to children approaching puberty, to adolescents, and to adult males who have no knowledge of having had mumps. There is no known contraindication to vaccination of young children, except that revaccination before puberty may prove to be necessary.

It is recommended that children under 1 year of age not be given mumps vaccine. Furthermore, it should not be given to children who are allergic to egg proteins, to any person suffering from an illness that alters resistance to infection, or to any person taking a drug that has the same effect.

There is no evidence that convalescent serum or hyperimmune serum globulin (human) is of value in protecting exposed susceptible persons. The same is true of inactivated mumps vaccines. The value of vaccination with live attenuated vaccine for protection of susceptible adults and pubescent and adolescent children who have been exposed to mumps is not known, but there is no contradiction to its use in this circumstance. The vaccination might protect against subsequent exposure if the exposure under consideration failed to cause infection.

TREATMENT. If the patient is only mildly ill, insistence on bed rest does not appear necessary; the severely ill patient will prefer to remain in bed. There is no evidence that continued activity by adults with the disease increases the danger of orchitis. Some patients obtain comfort from warm applications to the parotid areas; others prefer cold. Aspirin gives some relief, especially with regard to general malaise. Most young children with the disease continue on their regular diet with amazingly little discomfort. Diethylstilbestrol has been recommended for the prevention of orchitis in adults with mumps; it is of doubtful value.

There is no treatment for mumps meningoencephalitis. Repeated lumbar punctures may afford some patients considerable relief from headache, nausea, and vomiting.

References

Brickman A, Brunell PA: Susceptibility of medical students to mumps: comparison of serum neutralizing antibody and skin test. Pediatrics 48:447, 1971

Kilham L, Margolis G: Induction of congenital hydrocephalus in hamsters with attenuated and natural strains of mumps virus. J Infect Dis 132:462, 1975

Levitt LP, Rich TA, Kinde SW, et al: Central nervous system mumps: a review of 64 cases. Neurology 20:829, 1970

Sults HA, Hart BA, Zielezny M, Schlesinger ER: Is mumps virus an etiologic factor in juvenile diabetes mellitus? J Pediatr 86:654,1975

Yamauchi T, St Geme JW, Oh W, Davis CWC: The biological and biochemical pathogenesis of mumps virus-induced embryonic growth retardation. Pediatr Res 9:30, 1975

PICORNAVIRUSES AND POLIOMYELITIS

EDWARD C. CURNEN, JR.

Picornavirus is a term introduced in 1962 by an international study group as a new name for a large family of viruses with similar properties that may have had a common phylogenetic origin. The word means small (pico) ribonucleic acid (RNA) virus. The picornaviruses include two major categories, those of human origin and those of lower animals:

A. Picornaviruses of human origin
1. Enteroviruses
   a. Polioviruses
   b. Coxsackieviruses A
   c. Coxscackieviruses B
   d. Echoviruses
2. Rhinoviruses
3. Unclassified
B. Picornaviruses of lower animals

Enteroviruses have their natural habitat in the alimentary tract. They include the polioviruses, the coxsackieviruses groups A and B, and the echoviruses (enteric cytopathogenic human orphanviruses). Rhinoviruses (p. 558) are recovered mainly from the upper respiratory passages of man. Newly discovered strains of picornaviruses from human sources are designated as unclassified until further identification permits permanent assignment to an appropriate subgroup. Viruses with similar properties recovered from lower animals are also classified as picornaviruses.

Picornaviruses are relatively small, of the order of 15 to 30 mμ in diameter; they have an RNA core and no lipid component, as indicated by resistance to inactivation by ether. The infective particles have been postulated to be constructed according to the principles of cubic symmetry, with an inner RNA core surrounded by a small number, perhaps 32, of regularly arranged protein subunits. Infection has been induced with RNA extracted from representative polioviruses, coxsackieviruses A and B, and echoviruses. Viral activity is well preserved at −70 C to −20 C. Thermostability varies under different conditions, but probably all picornaviruses are inactivated by heating at 60 C to 65 C for 30 minutes. In contrast to enteroviruses, rhinoviruses are unstable at low pH in the range of 3 to 5.

Picornaviruses of human origin appear to be pathogenic in nature only for man, although many induce infection and disease when introduced experimentally into laboratory animals. Conversely, it has not been shown that picornaviruses of animals are significantly related to disease in man. Enteroviruses are recovered from the oropharynx, but more copiously and for longer periods from the feces. On the other hand, rhinoviruses are commonly recovered from the nose and throat and are detected only rarely in the feces.

Picornaviruses of man, with the exception of a few coxsackievirus A types, can be propagated in tissue cultures of various primate cells. Cultivation in cells of other animals has been less successful. Unlike enteroviruses, which multiply readily at 36 C to 37 C, rhinoviruses grow best in rolled cultures at 33 C, a temperature approximating that of the human naso-pharynx. Growth of picornaviruses appears to occur exclusively in the cytoplasm and with many but not all virus types it is associated with characteristic cellular damage or cytopathic effect (CPE). Interference has been noted between different enteroviruses as well as between members of this group and other viruses.

The antigenic properties of picornaviruses have been determined by a variety of techniques, but mainly by neutralization tests in experimental animals or by tissue cultures and complement-fixation tests. Although some cross-relationships have been noted within subgroups, identification of more than 90 specific serotypes has been reliably established. Three types of poliovirus are recognized. The coxsackieviruses A include 23 types, numbered 1 to 24, type 23 being identical with echovirus 9. There are 6 coxsackieviruses B. The echoviruses number more than 30 types, although type 10 has been reclassified as a reovirus and type 28 as a rhinovirus. The rhinoviruses are represented by at least 30 well-established types, and evidence for the existence of more than twice that number has been reported. Infection of man by a picornavirus usually is followed by the appearance of homologous antibody.

CHARACTERISTICS OF ENTEROVIRUSES

In addition to having the characteristic properties of all picornaviruses, enteroviruses have other features in common. Serologic surveys for detection of antibody in various population groups have indicated that experience with these agents is not only ubiquitous but also cumulative. In temperate zones enteroviruses and associated disorders occur mainly during summer and fall; in tropical areas they may be encountered throughout the year. With the exception of coxsackievirus A21 (Coe), infection is more common among children than adults.

In areas of poor socioeconomic conditions where hygienic conditions are poor, enteroviruses excreted in feces are distributed rapidly and at an early age. Although flies have been found to harbor enteroviruses in nature and experimentally, the importance of flies in trasmission has not been determined. The extent to which respiratory secretions account for dissemination of infection by enteroviruses is also not known. As the oropharynx is a common portal for both alimentary and respiratory tracts, it is difficult to determine by which of these routes virus is seeded or whether pharyngitis and tonsillitis represent enteric or respiratory infections.

Enteroviruses have been associated with a varied and ever increasing number of clinical disorders. Current classifications of the enteroviruses and the associated forms of human disease that appear to be induced by them are indicated in Table 22. It is evident that a single virus may have the capacity to induce more than one form of illness and that each clinical syndrome may be caused by any one of several different viruses.

POLIOMYELITIS

DOROTHY M. HORSTMANN

Poliomyelitis (infantile paralysis) is an acute viral infection in which only a small percentage of those in-

TABLE 22. Classification of Enteroviruses and Associated Illnesses

Enteroviruses	
Poliomyelitis (3 types)	Paralytic poliomyelitis (mild to severe)
	Polioencephalitis
	Cerebellar ataxia
	Nonparalytic poliomyelitis
	Abortive poliomyelitis, pharyngitis, or undifferentiated febrile disorder
Coxsackieviruses A (23 types)	Aseptic meningits (epidemic, types 7, 9; sporadic, many types)
	Paralysis (types 4, 7, 9)
	Encephalitis (types 2, 5, 6, 7, 9)
	Ataxia (types 4, 9)
	Guillain-Barré syndrome (types 2, 5, 6, 9)
	Herpangina (types 1–6, 8, 10, 22)
	Lymphonodular pharyngitis (type 10)
	Acute respiratory illness (types 9, 21, 24 in addition to herpanginal strains); pharyngitis or undifferentiated febrile disorder (many types)
	Exanthem (types 2, 4, 5, 9, 16)
	Hepatitis (types 4, 9, 10)
Coxsackieviruses B (6 types)	Aseptic meningitis (types 1–6)
	Paralysis (types 1–5)
	Encephalitis (types 1, 2, 3, 5)
	Epidemic myalgia (types 1–5)
	Encephalomyocarditis in early infancy (types 1–5)
	Myocarditis and/or pericarditis (types 1–5)
	Exanthem (types 1, 3, 4, 5)
	Orchitis (types 1–5)
	Hepatitis (type 5)
	Acute respiratory illness, pharyngitis, or undifferentiated febrile disorder (types 1–5)
Echoviruses (30 types)	Aseptic meningitis (types 1–7, 9, 11–23, 25, 30, 31)
	Paralysis (types 1, 2, 4, 6, 7, 9, 11, 16, 18, 30)
	Encephalitis (types 2, 3, 4, 6 7, 9, 11, 14, 18, 19)
	Guillain-Barré syndrome (types 6, 22)
	Ataxia (type 9)
	Exanthem (types 1–7, 9, 11, 14, 16, 18, 19)
	Diarrhea (types 11, 14, 18)
	Acute respiratory illnesses, pharyngitis, or undifferentiated febrile disorder (types 1, 3, 6, 11, 19, 20, and others)

fected develop the characteristic clinical picture of fever, headache, vomiting, stiff neck and back, and sometimes flaccid paralysis of various muscle groups. More often it presents as a mild nonspecific febrile illness, or the infection remains completely asymptomatic. It is prone to appear in epidemic form, particularly in the summer. The disease has apparently been known since earliest times, but the first description appeared at the end of the eighteenth century in Michael Underwood's textbook on diseases of children. Not until the late nineteenth century did epidemics begin to appear. These increased in frequency and severity in certain parts of the world until the mid-1950s, when prophylactic immunization was introduced. In countries in which vaccination has been widely used, there has been a dramatic decline in incidence of the disease.

ETIOLOGY. The viral etiology of poliomyelitis was discovered by Landsteiner in 1908. At present the polioviruses are classified as members of the enterovirus family and share the physical and chemical characteristics of this subgroup of picornaviruses.

Three distinct serotypes are recognized, type I being the one most commonly associated with epidemics. There is some sharing of antigens, particularly between types II and I, and some degree of cross-protection is indicated by both experimental and epidemiologic data.

The polioviruses induce paralytic disease in monkeys and chimpanzees, and some strains, particularly of type II, also infect mice. The discovery by Enders, Weller, and Robbins in 1949 that polioviruses will grow in tissue cultures of nonneural primate cells is a landmark of modern medicine and has had far-reaching implications for virology in general.

EPIDEMIOLOGY. The principles of the epidemiology of poliomyelitis were first worked out by the Swedish investigator Wickman, who published his monograph on the subject in 1908, the same year that isolation of the virus was reported by Landsteiner. Subsequent investigations proved that infections with polioviruses are common, but that disease is relatively rare except in epidemics, and even then the ratio of inapparent infections to clinical cases is probably more than 100 to 1 (Fig. 12). There is a marked seasonal

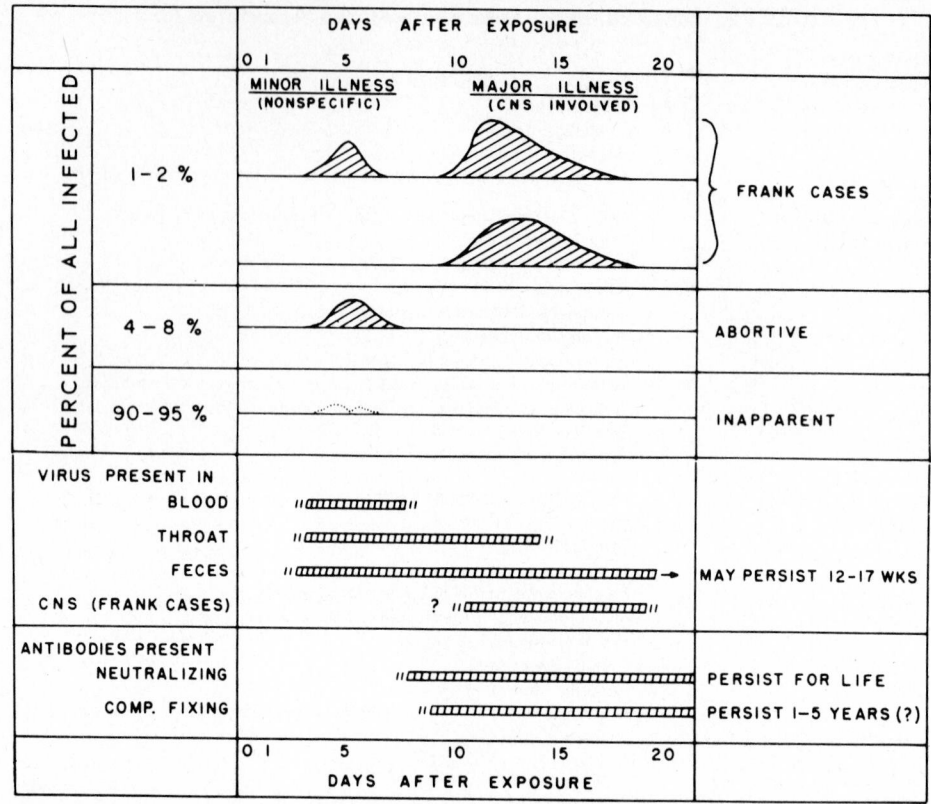

FIG. 12. Schematic diagram of the clinical and subclinical forms of poliomyelitis, showing presence of virus and antibodies in relation to the development and subsidence of infection. [Adapted from Bodian and Horstmann: In Horsfall and Tamm (eds): Viral and Rickettsial Infections of Man, 4th ed, 1965. Courtesy of J. B. Lippincott.]

incidence of the disease in temperate climates, with sharp increases in summer and fall; in tropical areas infection and disease tend to occur throughout the year.

Poliomyelitis has been both endemic and epidemic in all parts of the world. The age group attacked in endemic poliomyelitis and in early outbreaks is the youngest; 90 percent of paralytic cases are in children under 5 years of age. Once epidemics appear, they tend to recur, and after a few years increasing proportions of cases occur in older children and young adults. This evolution of the epidemic disease has been correlated with changes in sanitary environment: in populations living under poor conditions of sanitation and hygiene the viruses are widely disseminated, infection (largely inapparent) and immunity are acquired in the first few years of life, there are no epidemics, and sporadic cases are confined to the infantile age group. With economic development and improved sanitation and hygiene, exposure and infection are delayed; the number of susceptibles builds up, and unless prophylactic vaccination is carried out, an epidemic may result when a virulent strain is introduced. The introduction of both inactivated and live attenuated oral vaccines has had a marked impact on the incidence of the disease in parts of the world where they have been used extensively.

Virtual control of paralytic poliomyelitis has been achieved in large geographic areas, but in others, particularly tropical ones, first epidemics are still appearing.

Mode of Spread. Polioviruses are spread primarily by human association, and the healthy carrier is as infectious as the frank case. Young children form the bulk of susceptibles in any population and are the most effective spreaders of the virus. During active infection, virus is present in the throat and intestinal excreta; whether transmission is from the pharynx of one person to the oropharynx of another or whether the fecal–oropharingeal circuit is the major one seems to depend on the epidemiologic circumstances. There is evidence that in populations with high standards of hygiene, pharyngeal spread is the more important, particularly during epidemics. In contrast, in populations living under conditions of poor sanitation, where fecal contamination is apt to be extensive, the fecal–oropharingeal route is of greater importance and accounts for the high rate of poliovirus circulation among young children. In the family setting both routes may be well traveled, particularly if there is a child under 2 years of age; regardless of socioeconomic level, a young child can be regarded as creating a microclimate of poor sanitation.

PATHOGENESIS. Figure 12 correlates the pathogenesis of infection with the clinical course. Poliovirus enters the body by way of the oropharynx and is implanted in the walls of the pharynx and the intestinal tract, where primary multiplication occurs, presumably in lymphatic tissue and/or mucosal epithelial cells. From 3 to 5 days after exposure, virus is present in the throat, blood, and feces. This may be accompanied by symptoms of the so-called minor illness, or the infection may be completely asymptomatic. In either event the sites of viral multiplication at this stage appear to be the intestinal tract, the lymph nodes, and viscera such as liver and spleen. In the majority of infections this constitutes the entire course, and only in very few is there further progression and involvement of the CNS. The period of viremia that precedes CNS involvement lasts several days and disappears as antibodies develop. Invasion of the CNS is thought to be by way of the bloodstream, although experiments in monkeys and chimpanzees indicate that poliovirus can travel along neural pathways, and it is possible that this occurs in the natural infection under certain circumstances.

PATHOLOGY. The characteristic lesions of poliomyelitis are in the gray matter of the spinal cord, the medulla, the precentral gyrus of the cerebral cortex, and the deep nuclei of the cerebellum. Neuronal necrosis, chromatolysis, neuronophagia, and outfall of cells occur. Focal and diffuse infiltration of leukocytes and perivascular cuffing are found in areas of neuronal damage. Besides CNS lesions, hyperplasia of lymph nodes is often observed, and in some cases myocarditis is present.

CLINICAL MANIFESTATIONS. The clinical manifestations of poliomyelitis range from nonspecific minor illness to severe paralytic disease. The proportion of frank cases that can be diagnosed on clinical grounds alone is estimated to be not more than 1 or 2 percent of infections occurring during an epidemic and may be considerably less under endemic conditions. Figure 12 illustrates the relative frequency of the several forms: the frank case (paralytic or nonparalytic), the abortive or minor illness, and the completely inapparent infection.

PREDISPOSING FACTORS. Factors that determine which expression the infection will take in a given individual are not completely understood. They include the nature of the infecting strain (whether it is highly virulent), age of the patient (older individuals being more likely to develop severe paralysis), and probably the virus dosage. Other factors are recognized as predisposing to the paralytic form: *Tonsillectomy:* If tonsillectomy is performed at a time when an individual has an inapparent infection and harbors poliovirus in his throat, bulbar poliomyelitis follows within 7 to 14 days in a considerable proportion of instances. There is also evidence that those whose tonsils have been removed at any time in the past are more susceptible to the bulbar form of the disease than are those with intact tonsils. *Pregnancy:* Pregnant women have a higher incidence than do nonpregnant women of the same age, presuma-

bly due in part to hormonal factors but also to the generally greater exposure of pregnant women to young children. *Recent inoculations:* Injections of diphtheria toxoid, pertussis vaccine, tetanus toxoid, or any combination of these three within 1 month (usually 8 to 17 days) prior to onset are associated with a higher incidence of paralysis. Following DPT immunization there is definite correlation between the site of injection and the site of paralysis. However, the extra risk of poliomyelitis from injections is apparently small, particularly in children under 1 year of age, and it is negligible in those under 6 months. *Physical exertion and trauma:* Both trauma and physical exertion around the time of onset of the preparalytic phase have been shown to increase the likelihood of severe paralysis, particularly in adults.

INCUBATION PERIOD. The range of the incubation period is considered to be 5 to 35 days, with an average of 7 to 10 days from the time of exposure to the onset of CNS signs. The interval encompassing exposure, viral implantation in the alimentary tract, and the minor illness phase is considerably shorter (2 to 3 days). Investigations with attenuated strains indicate that viral multiplication and excretion may occur in vaccinees within 24 hours, and contact infections may appear as soon as 3 days later.

SYMPTOMS AND SIGNS. Two basic patterns of clinical response are recognized, the *minor illness,* or abortive type, and the *major illness.* The minor illness (first phase), estimated to account for 80 to 90 percent of infections with any clinical signs, may be so mild as to be unnoticed. Usually there are slight fever, malaise, headache, sore throat, and sometimes vomiting, lasting 24 to 72 hours. The physical examination and spinal fluid are normal and indication of CNS involvement is lacking. There is no more to the entire disease in most instances, and because of its nonspecific character it cannot be diagnosed clinically. In a few patients, symptoms recur after several days of well-being (the biphasic course), and the major illness (second phase) appears. More commonly, particularly in older children and adults, the major illness begins without a previous minor illness, with fever, headache, stiff neck, stiff back, muscle pain and tenderness, and sometimes hyperesthesias and paresthesias. In paralytic cases, weakness of various muscles and loss of superficial and deep tendon reflexes occur. The site of paralysis depends on the location of lesions in the spinal cord or medulla. In the bulbar form the cranial nerve nuclei are involved, with resulting paralysis of the pharyngeal, laryngeal, facial, and other muscles innervated by the cranial nerves. Difficulty in swallowing, nasal regurgitation, and nasal voice are early signs of bulbar poliomyelitis. Occasionally the clinical picture is dominated by encephalitic signs.

The influence of age on the clinical manifestations is marked. In the childhood form of the disease the biphasic course is more common, the onset of symptoms of the major illness is sudden, fever is high, and the preparalytic phase is short, with paralysis often developing as the temperature falls and when the child begins to feel better. In the adult form of the disease the onset is gradual, with a long prodromal period lasting up to a week and with little fever; however, in contrast to the pattern in children, pain, either superficial or deep, is a prominent symptom. The type and severity of paralysis also vary in relation to age. Except for infants under 1 year of age, who tend to have predominantly spinal paralytic disease with high fatality rates, the disease is less severe in children than in young adults. This is evidenced by the greater frequency of quadriplegia, respiratory paralysis, and death in groups over 15 years of age. However, bulbar paralysis without spinal involvement is more common in children. A difference in sex incidence of paralytic poliomyelitis is also related to age. Up to 15 years of age, males outnumber females approximately 2 to 1, whereas in young adults there is a slight excess among females.

PHYSICAL FINDINGS.   The patient with the minor illness syndrome reveals no abnormalities except listlessness, fever, and some redness of the pharynx. In *nonparalytic poliomyelitis* the clinical findings are similar to those in aseptic meningitis associated with other enteroviruses, the severity of the illness tending to increase with the age of the patient. The temperature is elevated, and there is neck and sometimes back stiffness, but the patient does not appear to be as ill as one with bacterial meningitis.

In the preparalytic phase of *paralytic poliomyelitis* the findings are similar to those in the nonparalytic phase; but often the patient appears more acutely ill. His face is flushed even though the temperature is not high, and not infrequently he appears anxious, tremulous, and emotionally overwrought. Nuchal rigidity may be minimal and apparent only in the last degree of neck flexion. Stiffness of the back, tightness of the hamstrings, and stiffness, spasm, and tightness of other muscle groups may be present. The reflexes are normal and active early in the course; Kernig and Brudzinski signs are sometimes positive. A few hours before onset of paralysis there is often a loss or diminution of superficial abdominal and spinal reflexes, as well as hyperactivity of the deep reflexes and fasciculation of muscle groups. The site of the reflex changes and of fasciculation frequently heralds the site of paralysis. As weakness progresses, deep reflexes disappear; with widespread paralysis, all reflexes, superficial and deep, may be lost.

TYPES OF PARALYSIS.   In general, cases are defined as paralytic only if muscle weakness persists beyond 2 or 3 weeks. Localization and degree of paralysis depend on the site and concentration of neuronal lesions. A given number of destroyed nerve cells scattered over a wide area of the cord may produce no muscle weakness, while destruction of the same number concentrated in the anterior horn area supplying a given muscle may result in complete paralysis of that muscle. Cases are classified anatomically as *spinal* if weakness is limited to muscles supplied by motor neurons in the cord or *bulbar* if the cranial nerve nuclei or medullary centers are involved. A combination of the two forms, *bulbospinal,* beginning with paralysis of the legs and ascending to

involve abdominal and thoracic muscles of respiration, arms, and finally medullary centers and cranial nerve nuclei, occurs in the most severe cases, particularly in adults. Rarely the clinical picture is predominantly one of encephalitis or acute cerebellar ataxia.

In the *spinal* paralytic form asymmetric involvement is characteristic. When the cervical cord is affected, weakness of the muscles of the shoulder girdle, arms, neck, and diaphragm and intercostals may appear. Lumbar cord involvement is reflected in paralysis of the muscles of the abdomen, back, and legs. The legs are more frequently affected than the arms, especially in young children. Paralysis of the bladder and urinary retention are seen in cases with weakness of the lower extremities, particularly in adults, and more commonly in men than in women.

In *bulbar* poliomyelitis the cranial nerve nuclei are most commonly attacked, then the respiratory centers in the medulla, and least often medullary vasomotor centers. The tenth cranial nerve nuclei are involved most often, resulting in paralysis of the pharynx, the soft palate, and the vocal cords. Nasal voice, hoarseness, increased accumulation of secretions in the oropharynx, difficulty in swallowing and regurgitation of fluids through the nose may develop. Paralysis of the facial nerve is also observed frequently. Less often, ocular palsies, pupillary disturbances, and weakness of muscles supplied by the fifth cranial nerve are noted.

In *spinal* poliomyelitis respiratory failure results from weakness or paralysis of the intercostals, diaphragm, and abdominal muscles. One or both sides of the thorax and/or diaphragm may be affected, and accessory respiratory muscles in the neck and the alae nasi may come into action. Weakness of abdominal muscles results in difficulty in coughing and consequently difficulty in bringing up mucous secretions. As respiratory failure progresses, apprehension, changes in the sensorium, and cyanosis appear; respiration becomes more and more shallow, but a regular rhythm is maintained. In *bulbar poliomyelitis* respiratory failure is a result of involvement of the respiratory center in the medulla or of paralysis of the pharyngeal muscles, with obstruction of the airway by pooled secretions; commonly a combination of these is present. Early signs of inadequate ventilation are irregularities in depth and rhythm of respirations, increased restlessness, anxiety, inability to sleep, rapid pulse rate, and rising blood pressure; all of these signs may develop before cyanosis appears. At times respiratory failure occurs with alarming suddenness and progresses rapidly, with lengthening periods of apnea, Cheyne-Stokes respiration, mental confusion, and sometimes delirium. In addition there may be signs of circulatory collapse due to vasomotor center involvement. In this situation the face has a dusky, flushed appearance, and the lips are cherry red. The pulse is rapid (150 to 200 per minute), often irregular, and difficult to palpate. The blood pressure is usually elevated, and the pulse pressure drops; shock and pulmonary edema add to the problems of respiratory failure in this often fatal form of the disease. Circulatory disturbances arise frequently in the course of severe, life-threatening paralytic poliomyelitis and are associated with high mortality rates. Myocardial failure may be secondary to pulmonary complications, hypoxia, or electrolyte imbalance; in some cases signs of acute myocarditis develop, accompanied by typical ECG changes.

LABORATORY DIAGNOSIS. The blood shows no characteristic abnormalities. Moderate leukocytosis is not uncommon in the acute febrile stage. Spinal fluid findings are of considerable diagnostic aid in the major illness. An elevated cell count (above 8 to 10 cells/mm^3) is characteristic; the usual range is 20 to 300, but occasionally it may be as high as 1,000 or more. During the first few hours after onset of CNS signs, polymorphonuclear leukocytes predominate, but this is followed by a prompt shift, so that approximately 90 percent of the cells are lymphocytes. In a small proportion of cases there is no increase in cells, and the CSF may remain normal even in the presence of severe paralysis. The CSF sugar content is not altered; the protein may be slightly elevated early in the course, rising gradually to moderate levels by the second and third weeks and returning to normal by the sixth week.

Virus isolation is the method of choice in confirming the diagnosis; the earlier the specimens are taken, the greater the chance of success. Tissue cultures of a variety of primate cells, either continuous line or primary outgrowth, are highly sensitive test systems. The virus is present in the throat during the acute phase of illness, and it is shed in the feces for several weeks and occasionally for months (Fig. 12).

Neutralization and complement fixation (CF) are the commonly used serologic tests for the diagnosis of poliovirus infections. As shown in Figure 12, neutralizing and CF antibodies appear early in the course of the *disease,* which is relatively late in the course of *infection.* As in other systems, a fourfold or greater rise in titer between the acute and convalescent specimens is diagnostic. Since a considerable number of patients already have high, even maximum, levels of antibody at the time of admission to the hospital, it is possible to demonstrate significant rises in not more than 50 percent of cases.

DIFFERENTIAL DIAGNOSIS. In the presence of an epidemic in which there are many paralytic cases, the *abortive* form and *nonparalytic poliomyelitis* can be suspected on the basis of epidemiologic evidence. However, an etiologic diagnosis can be made only in the laboratory, for these syndromes can be induced by a variety of other agents. The clinical findings in aseptic meningitis due to polioviruses do not differ significantly from those in aseptic meningitis associated with coxsackieviruses and echoviruses, mumps, herpesvirus, lymphocytic choriomeningitis, and leptospirosis. *Paralytic poliomyelitis* is usually not difficult to recognize, but it is increasingly evident that other enteroviruses are also capable of inducing a clinical pattern indistinguishable from poliomyelitis. However, polioviruses still account for the majority of cases of paralysis, particularly those with severe involvement, while transient mild weakness is more characteristic of infections associated with coxsackieviruses and echoviruses. Epidemic pleurodynia may resemble poliomyelitis very closely, especially when chest pain is accompanied by transient weakness of the diaphragm and involvement of the limbs. In geographic areas where arbovirus infections occur, diseases due to those agents must be considered. They are more apt to present predominantly an encephalitic picture; limb paralysis, when it occurs, tends to be spastic rather than flaccid. Other diseases to be ruled out include meningoencephalitis due to mumps or herpesvirus, postexanthematous encephalitis, shoulder girdle neuritis, Bell's palsy, infectious polyneuritis (Guillain-Barré syndrome), tuberculous meningitis, brain abscess, acute rheumatic fever, acute osteomyelitis and in some situations hysteria.

TREATMENT. There is no specific treatment. The course of the disease is not altered by antimicrobial drugs, convalescent serum, or gamma globulin. Medical management consists of supportive therapy appropriate to any acute infection and anticipation and handling of complications.

General Measures. Patients with either the abortive or the mild nonparalytic form require no treatment other than bed rest at home for the duration of fever. In the more severely affected hospitalized patient mild analgesics are indicated for relief of headache and discomfort. Protection of the patient from undue activity in the early phase of the major illness is an important prophylactic measure. The treatment of paralytic poliomyelitis often requires the combined efforts of the pediatrician, orthopedist, and specialist in physical medicine. In the acute febrile stage, efforts are directed toward making the patient as comfortable as possible, maintaining his fluid and electrolyte balance, and protecting any weakened muscles. Pain and spasm of muscles may be relieved by intermittent application of moist hot packs for 20-minute periods several times daily.

As long as the fever persists there is likelihood of extension of paralysis, and close observation is necessary to detect complications demanding active measures. Problems that may arise include respiratory failure, circulatory disturbances, abdominal distension, urinary retention, and bacterial infection.

Respiratory Failure. The management of the acutely ill patient with respiratory failure poses a complex and often rapidly changing series of problems that may severely tax the ingenuity and judgment of the physician, even if he is experienced in handling such cases. If severe impairment of respiratory muscle function alone is present, the tank respirator is indicated. It should be used when signs of respiratory decompensation are progressive and the vital capacity reaches less than 50 percent of normal. For children, respiratory rates up to 30 with pressures of $+3$ to -12 or -15 are recommended, and for adults rates of 18 with pressures of $+3$ to -18, but these must be adjusted to the individual case, taking care to avoid underventilation or overventilation. Weaning from the tank respirator should begin within several days. The chest (cuirass) respirator and the rocking bed are useful adjuncts during the weaning period, but they are inadequate for handling the acute stage of respiratory failure.

In bulbar cases with central respiratory failure and obstruction due to pooling of bronchotracheal secretions, continuous oxygen inhalation, postural drainage, and removal of secretions with a suction apparatus generally suffice. If these measures fail to keep the airway clear, a high tracheostomy is indicated. This procedure is also necessary if abductor paralysis of the vocal cords develops or if there are repeated bouts of pulmonary atelectasis requiring tracheal aspiration and bronchoscopy. Adequately humidified oxygen is given through the tracheostomy tube in concentrations of 40 to 60 percent, although emergencies may necessitate 100 percent for brief periods. Positive-pressure respiration through a cuffed tracheostomy tube may be substituted for the tank respirator in patients requiring artificial respiration. The tank respirator is contraindicated in bulbar poliomyelitis unless a tracheostomy has been performed so that adequate suctioning of secretions can be carried out.

Bladder Paralysis. A parasympathetic drug such as Urecholine is useful in inducing voiding. If the patient fails to respond, a second dose may be given before resorting to catheterization. Bladder paralysis usually lasts only a few days, and an indwelling catheter is rarely necessary.

Infection. Patients with respiratory problems, especially if tracheostomy has been performed, are particularly subject to pneumonia; urinary tract infections are not uncommon in those requiring repeated catheterization. The incidence of such infection is not reduced by prophylactic use of antimicrobials, and this practice is contraindicated because it favors the emergence of drug-resistant organisms. Once infection develops, appropriate therapy should be given based on the nature and sensitivity of the infecting agent, as in other similar infections.

Convalescent Care. Convalescent care is largely a matter of physical therapy and should begin soon after the acute phase has subsided, with gentle passive movements progressing to active exercises as strength improves. Attention to the many emotional problems of the patient faced with some degree of disability is of major importance.

PROGNOSIS. Complete recovery is usual in nonparalytic poliomyelitis and in cases with slight muscle weakness. If paralysis is present, recovery of muscle function continues for a period of approximately 18 months to 2 years. However, 60 percent of the ultimate improvement is achieved by the end of 3 months, and 80 percent by 6 months. The final result depends on the extent of nerve cell damage. Some muscles may show no recovery or may never improve beyond 10 percent of normal function, while others recover normal strength.

The death rate from paralytic poliomyelitis has been reduced in recent years due to improved techniques in handling respiratory failure, which is responsible for most of the deaths in both the bulbar and spinal paralytic forms of the disease. Overall mortality at present is estimated to be about 4 percent, but it is as high as 10 percent in severe epidemics involving older age groups.

PREVENTION. Poliomyelitis is now a preventable disease, and immunization is indicated for all children. Two types of vaccine are available: one is a formalin-inactivated preparation (Salk) that is given by injection, and the other is a live attenuated virus vaccine (Sabin) administered orally. Passive immunization with gamma globulin is of uncertain value at best and is not recommended.

INACTIVATED PREPARATION. Following the introduction of inactivated poliovirus vaccine by Salk in 1955, the incidence of paralytic poliomyelitis declined sharply to less than 10 percent of former rates in countries where it was used extensively. The effectiveness of the vaccine depends on the stimulation of antibodies that are capable of neutralizing the virus, presumably blocking it in blood and tissues, and thus preventing invasion of the CNS and paralytic disease. However, antibodies derived *only* from such vaccination do not significantly inhibit viral multiplication in the intestinal tract, although they have a suppressive effect on multiplication in the pharynx.

A basic course of immunization with inactivated vaccine requires four doses, the first three at monthly intervals and the fourth 6 to 12 months later. The vaccine is given in 1-ml amounts subcutaneously. For infants the schedule is integrated with other immunizations (p. 55); quadruple vaccines (DPT and poliomyelitis) are available. For maintenance of adequate antibody levels, repeated yearly booster doses are recommended.

Inactivated vaccine has proved safe and effective; it is stable on storage in refrigerator, and it causes remarkably few side effects. Sensitization to foreign protein and penicillin has not been significant. Yet in spite of its good record, certain problems remain that make it a less effective immunizing agent than the oral live attenuated virus vaccine. The problems include the rapid falloff of antibody levels in infants and young children who have never experienced natural infection, the occurrence of epidemics in certain well-vaccinated areas (with 20 to 30 percent of the paralytic cases being in individuals who have received three or more doses), the difficulty of reaching a high percentage of young children with four or more doses of a vaccine that has to be injected, and the need for repeated booster injections over the years to maintain adequate antibody levels.

LIVE ATTENUATED VIRUS VACCINE (SABIN). Oral vaccine possesses certain advantages that make it the optimum form of immunization to protect the individual and the community from paralytic poliomyelitis: It simulates natural infection; in addition to antibody conversion, it induces a state of relative resistance of the intestinal tract to reinfection. In a well-immunized community this provides a potent barrier to invasion by wild polioviruses. There are indications that antibodies induced by oral vaccine persist for years, thus obviating the need for repeated booster doses. The vaccine induces infection and immunity rapidly, even in the youngest age groups. It is thus effective in stopping epidemics if given to a large enough segment of the susceptible population. Ease of administration favors a high acceptance rate and is a particular advantage in communitywide programs. Some 350 million persons in various parts of the world have now been immunized, and the results attest to the safety and effectiveness of the vaccine. Since the vaccine induces an actual infection, there is a certain amount of contact spread, particularly among young children. This is limited, however, and there is no evidence that it results in harmful effects (except for very rare cases of paralytic disease in contacts of vaccines); some view it as an advantage, for it increases the number of persons immunized. Last year 6 cases of paralytic poliomyelitis occured in the U.S. with four of these either in vaccines or contacts of vaccines. This compares very favorably with the 55,000 cases of paralytic poliomyelitis in the U.S. which occured in a single year prior to the use of the poliovirus vaccines.

The vaccine is available in a trivalent form or as monovalent preparations of each of the three types. There is an increasing tendency to use the trivalent form because of its logistic advantages. Optimum use of the vaccine involves a communitywide immunization program in which infants over 2 months of age, children, and young adults are covered; this is followed by a continuous program of immunization of infants and preschool children who enter the community. In all types of programs the main target is the preschool group, for such young children form the bulk of susceptibles in any population and are the chief spreaders of wild polioviruses.

Individuals with immunodeficiency should not be given live poliovirus vaccine. Paralytic disease has occured when vaccine had been given with B cell abnormalities.

Primary Immunization of Infants. Either monovalent or trivalent vaccines may be used. The first dose is generally given at approximately 2 months of age. If monovalent vaccines are used, they should be given in the order type I, type III, type II at 6- to 8-week intervals. If trivalent vaccine is given, three doses are recommended. Whether monovalent or trivalent is used in the primary course, a fourth dose, consisting of trivalent vaccine, should be given to infants at 12 to 15 months of age.

Primary Immunization of Other Preschool Children. The procedure may conform to that outlined for infants, with the exception that the fourth dose may be omitted, or the primary course may consist of two doses at 6- to 8-week intervals followed by a third dose approximately 1 year later.

Primary Immunization of All Others. If monovalent vaccines are used, they should be given in the order type I, type III, type II. If trivalent vaccine is given, two doses 6 to 8 weeks apart are satisfactory.

Immunization of All Children on Entering School. A single dose of trivalent vaccine is regarded as desirable on entrance to school for all children who have previously been immunized with oral vaccine. This is designed to fill in any antibody gaps resulting from the occasional failure to achieve a vaccine take with one or another type during the primary course of immunization. If the child has never received oral vaccine, a full course using monovalent or trivalent vaccine should be given.

Procedure for Partially Immunized Children. Oral vaccine may be ineffective if the complete series is not given. Persons who at some time have had a partial or complete series of injections of the inactivated vaccine (Salk) should receive a complete series of oral vaccine in either monovalent or trivalent form, as outlined above. After the full series of the oral form has been completed, no further injections of inactivated vaccine nor doses of oral vaccine need be given.

Immunization in the Presence of an Epidemic. The virus type responsible should be identified and the corresponding monovalent vaccine offered on a communitywide basis as quickly as possible. All age groups from 2 months up should be included.

The ultimate control of poliomyelitis in well-immunized populations has become a realizable goal since the introduction of oral vaccine. The marked decline in reported cases in the United States reflects the greatly reduced circulation of wild polioviruses. This in turn makes widespread vaccination of young children born into the community of greatest importance, since they are largely deprived of opportunities for acquiring natural immunizing infections. Failure to protect such children could result in the buildup of a susceptible population in which epidemics might reappear should a virulent poliovirus strain be introduced.

COXSACKIEVIRUSES

EDWARD C. CURNEN, JR.

ETIOLOGY. Coxsackieviruses have the capacity to induce fatal disease in suckling mice or hamsters. The name is derived from the town of Coxsackie, New York, where strains were first encountered in 1947 by Dalldorf and Sickles. Dalldorf classified coxsackieviruses into two groups based on the histopathologic changes observed in suckling mice. In these animals group A viruses induce flaccid paralysis and widespread necrosis of striated muscle without lesions elsewhere. Group B viruses cause spastic paralysis and disseminated disease characterized by focal myositis and, in addition, necrosis of fat, myocarditis, encephalomyelitis, hepatitis, and pancreatitis, the last produced by some strains in mature as well as in suckling mice.

Coxsackieviruses are among the smallest that affect man. Estimates based on filtration, centrifugation, and electron microscopy indicate that these viruses are spherical particles approximately 28 mμ in diameter and remarkably uniform in size. Coxsackieviruses are unusually stable. Infected materials can be preserved for long periods in glycerin or frozen at -20 C to -70 C and can be kept for many days at room temperature without significant loss of viral activity.

At present, 23 types of group A, designated A1 to A24 excluding A23 (now classified as echovirus 9), and 6 types of group B, designated B1 to B6, are recognized. They can be identified and differentiated by neutralization and complement-fixation tests with specific immune sera prepared in animals, as well as by determinations of active immunity. Tests dependent on hemagglutination can also be carried out with the coxsackieviruses that possess this property (A7, A20, A21, A24, B1, B3, B5). Circulating antibodies can usually be detected in the human or animal host within 2 weeks of infection or onset of symptoms.

Coxsackieviruses have been studied less extensively in laboratory animals other than the mouse. Strains of A7, A14, and group B viruses have been found occasionally to induce poliomyelitislike lesions in monkeys. These and other coxsackieviruses cause mild or clinically inapparent infections in monkeys and chimpanzees. Only two types (A2 and A8) have multiplied in chick embryos and two types (A2 and A4) in cultures of chick cells. Strains of all six group B viruses propagate readily in monkey kidney and various human cell cultures, and all but a few group A types (A1, A4, A5, A6, A19, A22) have been grown in human amnion cells. Strains of coxsackievirus B have been observed to have an oncolytic effect after serial passage through HeLa tumors in rats.

EPIDEMIOLOGY. Coxsackieviruses have been encountered in populated areas throughout the world. Like other enteroviruses they have been recovered most commonly from human feces and pharyngeal swabbings, and also from sewage and flies. Strains of all group B serotypes and of many group A viruses have been recovered from cerebrospinal fluid of patients with viral meningitis. Recovery of a coxsackievirus during life from blood, urine, or other sources has not been common. Virus in relatively high titer has been found in the brain, myocardium, and other organs of newborn infants and rarely of older persons after death. Coxsackieviruses have been recovered from individuals of both sexes and different races, more frequently from children than from adults. No natural nonhuman reservoirs of infection have been found.

Some coxsackieviruses cause epidemics of human disease at unpredictable intervals. At least nine group A viruses may cause herpangina, and group B viruses (B1 to B5) have caused outbreaks of epidemic myalgia. All six group B viruses can also induce meningoencephalitis, sometimes in association with epidemic myalgia; these agents are now recognized as important etiologic agents of the aseptic meningitis syndrome. Strains of group B and A7 and A9 coxsackievirus have been associated with and are thought to be responsible for paralysis in some patients. Group B viruses may also cause generalized infection with encephalitis, myocarditis, and hepatitis in newborn infants similar to that produced experimentally in suckling mice. Transmission may be from mother to fetus in utero or from mother to infant postpartum, as well as from one infant to others in the nursery. Myocarditis and pericarditis in older children and adults have also been attributed to group B coxsackieviruses; in a few instances group A viruses have been implicated on the basis of uncertain evidence. Hepatitis has also been reported in older patients infected with coxsackievirus B5. Coxsackievirus A10 has been recovered from the stools of hepatitis patients and contacts. Acute illnesses have been associated with exanthems in epidemics of infection with coxsackieviruses A9 and A16 and in sporadic distribution with coxsackieviruses A2, A4, A5, B1, B3, B4, and B5.

The etiologic relationship of coxsackieviruses to other illnesses with which they have been found to be associated has not been so clearly established and in many instances has probably been fortuitous. This relationship is particularly likely for group A viruses, which have been encountered much more frequently than group B viruses in stools from healthy persons and from patients with poliomyelitis or other concurrent but apparently unrelated illnesses. The absence of reports of successive infections with strains of a single type of coxsackievirus supports other indications that immunity to infection by a coxsackievirus is type-specific and relatively enduring. The incubation period of infection by coxsackieviruses may range from 1 to 14 days, but is usually shorter, with a mean of 3 to 5 days. The spread of infection by coxsackieviruses is similar to that by polioviruses, with communicability especially high in the home environment.

CLINICAL DISORDERS. ASEPTIC MENINGITIS. Aseptic meningitis can be induced by any one of a large number of viruses. All of the group B and 16 different group A coxsackieviruses have been recovered from sporadic cases; group B and A7 and A9 viruses have been associated with epidemics. All of the group B viruses and at least 12 group A types have been recovered from spinal fluid.

Clinical features of aseptic meningitis attributable to a coxsackievirus are not distinctive. The onset may be sudden or gradual. Approximately half the cases exhibit a prodromal stage during which viremia has occasionally been detected. Anorexia, nausea, fever, headache, and abdominal pain are common complaints before the onset of meningeal signs. Later, more severe headache, drowsiness, vomiting, and discomfort or stiffness of the neck or back appear. The temperature may rise to 40 C and usually subsides within 10 days. On examination, hyperemia of the pharynx, occasionally with discrete ulcers of the mucous membrane, and resistance to nuchal flexion may be detected. Kernig and Brudzinski signs are likely to be demonstrable; tendon reflexes are usually normal.

The white blood cell count is generally normal. The leukocytes of the cerebrospinal fluid are increased in number, usually to about 500 cells/mm^3, but occasionally as high as 2,000. Although mononuclear cells are more numerous, initially the proportion of polymorphonuclear cells may be as high as 50 percent. The levels of sugar and protein in the fluid are normal.

Except in young infants with generalized infection, the course is usually benign. Although rash, muscular weakness, or persistent myalgia may be present, they are not characteristic features.

PARALYSIS AND OTHER NEUROLOGIC DISORDERS. Paralysis, encephalitis, and infectious neuronitis are relatively rare in association with coxsackieviruses. Paralytic illnesses have been observed in patients infected with coxsackievirus A4, A7, A9 and B1 to B5. In most instances paralysis has been mild and transitory. Excluding newborns with generalized infection, encephalitis has been found in association with only coxsackieviruses A2, A5, A6, A7, A9, B1, B2, B3, and B5. Coxsackieviruses A4 and A9 have been recovered from fecal specimens of patients with ataxia, and A2, A5, A6, and A9 have been encountered sporadically in patients with Guillain-Barré syndrome.

EPIDEMIC MYALGIA.   Epidemic myalgia (pleurodynia, Bornholm disease) was apparently first recognized by Finsen, who observed epidemics in 1856 and 1863 in Iceland. One name derives from the classic description by Sylvest, a Danish physician who studied an outbreak on the island of Bornholm. Coxsackieviruses B1 to B5 have been associated with epidemics of this disorder, and their role as etiologic agents is now generally recognized.

Epidemic myalgia has occurred in outbreaks throughout the world, with the highest incidence in the summer and fall. Several members of a family may be affected, each with somewhat different symptoms. The incubation period is commonly 2 to 4 days. Fever and pain usually develop suddenly, sometimes following vague prodromal symptoms. The characteristic feature is muscular pain, sometimes excruciatingly severe, typically located in the chest or upper abdomen, occasionally elsewhere. Pain in the lower abdomen may simulate that of an acute surgical condition. Tenderness or swelling may be detected at the site of pain. Headache is a frequently associated complaint, and occasionally stiffness of the neck is present. Splenomegaly is uncommon. Clinical laboratory findings are usually normal. The temperature often reaches 40 C and persists for a period ranging from 3 to 9 days. In approximately 25 percent of cases the course of the symptoms and fever is diphasic. Meningitis, pleurisy, pericarditis, and in mature males, orchitis are infrequent complications.

ENCEPHALOMYOCARDITIS OF NEWBORNS.   Strains of group B coxsackievirus may cause acute, generalized, and sometimes fatal intrauterine or neonatal infection in newborn infants. Gear in South Africa first called attention to this association. Severe illness appears suddenly at any time during early infancy, sometimes a few hours or days after a brief episode of mild diarrhea. Cases have occurred when epidemic myalgia or aseptic meningitis attributable to the homologous group B coxsackievirus was present in the vicinity, and also following an acute febrile illness of a mother at about the time of delivery. In affected infants, hypothermia or fever, with elevations of temperature to 40 C, anorexia, tachycardia, cyanosis, icterus, pallor, cardiomegaly, hepatomegaly, electrocardiographic signs of myocarditis, and development of circulatory collapse are characteristic features. Examination of the cerebrospinal fluid may reveal xanthochromia, pleocytosis, and an elevated level of protein. The course may be rapidly fatal or may lead to complete recovery. In fatal cases virus has been recovered from the brain and spinal cord as well as from the myocardium and other organs. Postmortem examinations have revealed lesions in the brain, heart, liver, and other organs resembling those seen in experimentally infected newborn mice.

ACUTE MYOCARDITIS OR PERICARDITIS.   The occurrence of myocarditis or pericarditis in older children and adults infected with a coxsackievirus of group B or less frequently of group A has also been reported. In rare instances the virus has been recovered from pericardial fluid or, in fatal cases, from the myocardium. The etiologic role of these and other viruses in surviving patients with acute cardiac disorders has not been established.

HERPANGINA.   Huebner and associates first demonstrated the etiologic role of six different group A coxsackieviruses in relation to an acute self-limited febrile illness affecting mainly children during the summer months and characterized by distinctive faucial lesions. They pointed out that a similar clinical entity had been described in 1924 by Zahorsky and named by him herpangina. This disorder has now been etiologically associated with nine group A coxsackieviruses (A1 to A6, A8, A10, and A22).

Characteristically the illness is initiated by an abrupt elevation in temperature that ranges to 40.6 C and lasts from 1 to 4 days. Anorexia, dysphagia, and vomiting are frequently present, and patients over 2 years of age complain of sore throat. Headache and abdominal pain are also common symptoms. The pharynx is usually hyperemic, and frequently, although not invariably, one or more discrete grayish vesicles averaging 1 to 2 mm in diameter (or at a later stage shallow ulcers surrounded by a read areola) may be seen. These are commonly located on the fauces, soft palate, and uvula, less frequently elsewhere in the oropharynx, but not characteristically on the pharyngeal, gingival, or buccal mucosa. The lesions disappear within a few days after the temperature returns to normal. Recovery is usually uncomplicated, although associated esophagitis, genital ulceration, and parotitis have been reported. In typical cases the clinical laboratory findings are normal.

ACUTE LYMPHONODULAR PHARYNGITIS.   Acute lymphonodular pharyngitis is a self-limited febrile disorder similar to herpangina that was observed in an epidemic associated with coxsackievirus A10. Examination revealed small white or yellowish nodular lesions of the uvula, anterior pillars, and posterior pharynx that healed without ulceration. The acute course of illness resembled that of herpangina.

FEVER WITH LYMPHADENITIS.   Coxsackieviruses A5 and A6 were observed in Africa associated with a disorder resembling glandular fever. The illness was characterized by an abrupt onset, with fever and tender swollen lymph nodes; stiffness of the neck and splenomegaly were noted in a few instances. The fever subsided in 4 to 10 days.

HAND-FOOT-AND-MOUTH DISEASE.   Coxsackieviruses A5 or A16 have been recovered from infants and children with a syndrome called hand-foot-and-mouth disease characterized by vesicular and ulcerative lesions in the mouth and maculopapular rash and vesicles on the hands and feet. In some cases a transient erythematous rash has been seen on the buttocks as well as the extremities. The course is acute and usually self-limited, although four fatal cases in infants infected with coxsackievirus A16 have been reported.

EXANTHEMA. In addition to the maculopapular and vesicular skin lesions observed in some cases of infection with coxsackieviruses A5 and A16, rashes occasionally have been reported in association with other types of coxsackieviruses A and B. These are generally maculopapular, although vesicles and urticaria or petechiae have been seen in some cases of infection with coxsackieviruses A9, B3, and B5.

HEPATITIS. Evidence of hepatic disease in newborn infants with generalized infection by a coxsackievirus B is well documented. There are indications that other coxsackieviruses may affect the liver in older subjects. Coxsackieviruses A10 and B5 have been encountered in outbreaks of mild hepatic disorder, and coxsackieviruses A4 and A9 have been recovered respectively from the blood and from the liver postmortem in individual patients with signs of hepatitis.

ACUTE RESPIRATORY ILLNESS AND OTHER UNDIFFEREN-TIATED DISORDERS. In addition to herpagina and other illnesses characterized by pharyngitis, coxsackieviruses A have been found in association with acute respiratory illnesses, including both undifferentiated and recognizable forms. A strain of A24 virus (Pett) was recovered from the feces of children during an institutional outbreak of respiratory disease. Strains of A21 virus (Coe) have been encountered repeatedly in outbreaks of acute respiratory infection, mainly among military recruits, and they have been shown to cause common colds or mild febrile upper respiratory illness in human volunteers. In an outbreak of illness among infants and children attributed to infection with coxsackievirus A9, three had pneumonia, and the virus was recovered from the liver and lung of one who died.

Infection with each one of the coxsackieviruses B has produced a varied spectrum of clinical manifestations in the community and often within a single family. Sore throat or other respiratory symptoms may occur during the prodromal stage in patients with aseptic meningitis or pleurodynia, and they may be the only features of illness in other members of the household. Coxsackieviruses B of several serotypes have been encountered in outbreaks of febrile respiratory illness in families, camps, and institutions. Coxsackieviruses B3 and B5 were found in association with prevalent respiratory disease among infants and children during serial long-term studies in an orphanage. Coxsackieviruses B have also been recovered occasionally from patients with croup, bronchiolitis, vesicular pharyngitis, pneumonia, and pleurisy, but they are not considered to be major causes of these clinical entities. On the other hand, mild respiratory illnesses are probably frequently attributable to coxsackieviruses B, especially during the summer and fall.

DIAGNOSIS. Diagnosis of infection by a coxsackievirus may be suggested by the clinical and epidemi-ologic findings and can be verified in the laboratory by isolation of the virus and demonstration of a related increase in specific neutralizing antibodies. Tissue culture techniques have supplemented but not replaced the use of suckling mice for these purposes. Rises in titer of complement-fixing antibodies against heterologous as well as homologous coxsackieviruses occur in human serum following infection by these agents; hence determinations by this technique are of limited diagnostic value. It should be emphasized that *infection* by a coxsackievirus can be demonstrated by laboratory methods alone, but diagnosis of *disease* caused by one of these agents requires careful correlation of supporting clinical, epidemiologic, and laboratory evidence.

Differentiation of aseptic meningitis caused by a coxsackievirus from bacterial meningitis, leptospirosis, space-occupying lesions, or infections of the central nervous system caused by other viruses such as poliomyelitis, mumps, lymphocytic choriomeningitis, equine encephalitis, and echovirus or herpes simplex virus is often indicated by clinical and epidemiologic evidence and can usually be verified in the laboratory.

Recovery of a coxsackievirus from cerebrospinal fluid collected during the acute stage of illness is positive diagnostic evidence. When both a coxsackievirus and another viral agent, especially a poliovirus or echovirus, are isolated simultaneously from a patient, it may be difficult to determine the relative etiologic significance of each virus. Paralysis caused by an enterovirus other than a poliovirus has been encountered occasionally in individual patients, but, with the possible exception of coxsackievirus A7, not in epidemic distribution. On the basis of present knowledge it seems reasonable for the clinician to attribute flaccid paralysis without associated loss of sensation occurring in the course of acute febrile illness to infection by a poliomyelitis virus, unless supporting evidence is convincing that another agent is responsible.

Myalgia attributable to group B coxsackieviruses has to be differentiated from other causes of thoracic and abdominal pain. In epidemic myalgia the pain may suggest pleurisy or an abdominal emergency, but radiographs of the chest rarely reveal pleural or pulmonary involvement. Consideration of epidemic myalgia, particularly during the season of prevalence or in the presence of a local outbreak, may avert unnecessary surgery. Orchitis complicating epidemic myalgia or aseptic meningitis must be differentiated from mumps.

Herpangina in the community is suggested by its occurrence in seasonal outbreaks, and in individual patients it is suggested by the presence of discrete vesicular or ulcerative lesions characteristically located on the anterior pillars of the tonsils, the soft palate, uvula, or tonsils. In this respect the lesions are usually distinctive and differ from those attributable to herpes simplex virus. The latter may occur in the faucial areas, but are generally distributed more diffusely in the gingival and buccal mucosa on mucocutaneous borders and skin. Occasionally lesions similar to those of herpangina are seen in patients infected with coxsackievirus B or echoviruses. The enanthems of other bacterial and viral diseases, moniliasis, infectious mononucleosis, blood dyscrasias, deficiency diseases, and heavy-metal poisoning are unlikely to be confused.

Myocarditis in the newborn attributable to a group B coxsackievirus is suggested by tachycardia, signs of myocarditis, and circulatory collapse occurring during the neonatal period. The diagnosis is particularly likely if epidemic myalgia is prevalent in the vicinity or if the mother has an acute illness that could be attributable to infection by the same virus. This disorder must be differentiated from congenital heart disease and other neonatal anomalies or infections. In older patients, carditis attributable to a coxsackievirus may be difficult to distinguish from other forms of acute cardiac disease.

Knowledge of the clinical manifestitations of infection by coxsackieviruses is still incomplete. The possibility of infection by one of these agents should therefore be considered in any case of unexplained illness occurring in characteristic epidemiologic circumstances.

PROGNOSIS. Complete recovery from disease caused by coxsackieviruses can usually be expected, except in newborn infants, in whom infection with a group B virus may prove fatal.

TREATMENT AND CONTROL MEASURES. No form of therapy is known that acts directly on coxsackieviruses. At present, treatment is entirely supportive and symptomatic. Specific measures to control infection by these viruses are not available.

ECHOVIRUSES

EDWARD C. CURNEN, JR.

The development of tissue culture techniques for the recovery of viruses from the alimentary tract led to the discovery of a hitherto unrecognized group of viruses, some of which were promptly shown to cause human disease. These agents are designated echoviruses (enteric cytopathogenic human orphan viruses).

ETIOLOGY. The echoviruses characteristically induce cytopathic effects (CPE) in cultures of human and simian cells. When grown in susceptible cells under agar, they produce areas of necrosis or plaques that have characteristics sufficiently distinctive to aid in identification. In general, echoviruses do not induce overt disease in monkeys or suckling mice. Echovirus 9, however, following passage in tissue culture, induces lesions in suckling mice similar to those resulting from infection by coxsackieviruses A. Moreover, some echoviruses have been found experimentally to cause neuronal changes in monkeys; paralysis has been observed with types 7 and 14, and meningitis has been established in these animals with types 6 and 16. Chimpanzees, when infected with echoviruses 4 and 6, excrete the homologous agent and develop antibodies against it without exhibiting clinical evidence of disease. Different cell systems in tissue culture and renal cells from different species of monkey vary in their susceptibility to echoviruses. Little is known concerning the

histopathology resulting from infection by echoviruses in man, as few fatalities have been recorded. A virus later identified as echovirus 2 was the only agent recovered by Steigman and associates from the spinal cord of a child who died of a disease that clinically and pathologically resembled bulbar poliomyelitis.

Thirty different antigenic types of echovirus, numbered 1 to 33, have now been identified serologically, utilizing neutralization and complement-fixation techniques and, where possible, hemagglutination tests. Types 1 and 8 are now considered as type 1. Types 10 and 28 have been reclassified as reovirus and rhinovirus, respectively. Within certain types, especially types 4 and 6, striking differences between strains have been observed. Although slight antigenic relationships with other enteroviruses have been suggested, the echoviruses appear to be distinct entities within the family of enteroviruses and clearly distinguishable from other known viral agents that affect man. It is noteworthy, however, that viruses similar to echoviruses have been encountered, apparently as natural parasites, in monkeys, cattle, and swine.

Echoviruses are relatively small particles, similar not only in size but also in other physical characteristics to coxsackieviruses and polioviruses. Interference between echoviruses and active poliomyelitis vaccine viruses has been demonstrated in man. In the laboratory, interference between echoviruses and other viruses has been observed, thus providing, in the case of rubella virus, a technique for detection.

EPIDEMIOLOGY. Echoviruses have been detected in many parts of the world, both by recovery of virus and by demonstration of specific antibodies. Infection by these agents has occurred more commonly in warm seasons and in poorer socioeconomic conditions, and more frequently in children than in adults. Virus has been recovered more readily from feces than from the oropharynx or other sources, although in patients with meningeal involvement virus may also be found in the cerebrospinal fluid. At different times and in quite widely separated localities, epidemics of aseptic meningitis have been caused by echoviruses types 4, 6, 9, 11, 16, and 30. In individual cases meningeal involvement has been attributed to a total of 24 types. Strains of at least 17 echovirus types have been recovered from cerebrospinal fluid. An exanthem has been encountered in association with infection by 13 types of echoviruses. Some patients infected with type 9 or, infrequently, with type 4 virus had both aseptic meningitis and an exanthem during the course of illness. Patients infected with type 16 virus have shown either rash or meningeal involvement, but to date these features have not been reported together in the same individual. Whenever aseptic meningitis attributable to one of these viruses has been epidemic, other instances of both less severe and inapparent infections by the same agent have also been found to be prevalent in the vicinity. The high attack rate and rapid dissemination of these viruses within families indicate both a high degree of communicability and a relatively short incubation period.

CLINICAL DISORDERS. ASEPTIC MENINGITIS. The onset is usually abrupt, with headache, often localized as retrobulbar, being the most frequent and severe symptom. Fever and stiffness of the neck or back are almost invariably present. Myalgia may be a complaint in more than 50 percent of cases. In many patients with meningitis attributable to echovirus type 9, and occasionally in patients infected with a type 4 virus, a fine, sometimes morbilliform, maculopapular, erythematous exanthem appears during the acute phase of illness, distributed most commonly on the face and upper portion of the trunk. Lymphoid hyperplasia in the posterior pharynx and occasionally ulcerations of the oral mucosa resembling those of herpangina may be seen during infection with some of the echoviruses, including types 6 and 16. Cervical or generalized lymphadenopathy may be present. The course is usually benign, with fever lasting for about a week and malaise persisting sometimes for several weeks.

Patients with aseptic meningitis usually have total leukocyte counts of the cerebrospinal fluid below 500 cells/mm^3; in patients with type 9 infection, however, the counts frequently exceed 1,000. Polymorphonuclear forms are present in the cerebrospinal fluid early in the course of illness and, except with type 4 infections, may initially exceed 50 percent; eventually the cells are predominantly lymphocytic. The protein content of the fluid is normal or slightly elevated; the sugar content is characteristically normal. The white blood cell count is usually normal. Most patients recover completely, but in some cases disability may be protracted for weeks or months, and minor subjective or neuromuscular complaints may persist even longer.

PARALYSIS AND OTHER NEUROLOGIC DISORDERS. Muscular weakness and paralysis associated with alteration of reflexes similar to those in poliomyelitis have been observed in patients with meningeal involvement infected with at least 10 types of echovirus, and fatal cases of infection with types 2, 6, 7, and 11 have been recorded. The findings indicate that some of these agents induce poliomyelitislike neuropathy in man.

Encephalitis has been reported in association with 10 types of echovirus, but the clinical pattern has been diverse and the evidence for an etiologic relationship has been inconsistent. Similarly, the etiologic significance of echoviruses 6 and 22 in patients with Guillain-Barré syndrome remains uncertain. Cerebellar ataxia has been observed in patients infected with echovirus 9.

EXANTHEM. Maculopapular exanthems have been recognized as a characteristic feature of infection with types 4, 9, and 16 echoviruses. Rashes have been especially common in association with epidemics of type 9 infection in patients with and in those without meningeal involvement. A rash (Boston exanthem) has also been a conspicuous feature in outbreaks of a mild febrile illness caused by strains of virus related to or identical with echovirus 16.

Rashes have been observed in association with 10 other echoviruses; they appear to be more common in infants and children than in adults. Most frequently the exanthems have been maculopapular, but vesicles, urticaria, and petechiae have also been described.

DIARRHEA. The association of certain echoviruses, particularly types 11, 14, and 18, with diarrheal disease in infants and children has been observed, and an etiologic relationship have been suggested.

ACUTE RESPIRATORY ILLNESS. A number of echoviruses have been associated with acute respiratory illnesses. Echovirus 11 (U or Uppsala virus) was recovered in Sweden from children with nondiphtheritic croup; it was also found in children and adults with acute respiratory infections, and it induced brief febrile illnesses in experimentally infected human subjects. Echovirus 6 has been recovered from patients with mild illnesses during epidemics of meningitis attributable to this agent and from children and adults with pharyngitis and conjunctivitis in Japan. Among infants in a Japanese institution, echovirus 1 was reported to be associated with upper respiratory infection, diarrhea, and a rubellalike rash. A diagnosis of pneumonia was made in some cases during an epidemic of infection with echovirus 9. Echovirus 19 has been encountered in infants and children with mild respiratory disease and has been recovered in a fatal case during an outbreak of severe respiratory disease in premature infants. Echovirus 20 has been found in infants with minor respiratory disorders and diarrhea. Volunteers experimentally infected with this agent developed fever, pharyngitis, and, in two instances, coryza. Echoviruses, however, do not appear to be of major importance in the causation of respiratory disease.

DIAGNOSIS. As with other enteroviruses, diagnosis of *infection* by an echovirus can be confirmed in the laboratory, but diagnosis of *disease* can be established only by careful correlation of associated clinical, epidemiologic, and laboratory evidence. All of the echoviruses are cytopathogenic and can be identified by neutralization tests with specific immune serum in cultures of renal cells from rhesus monkeys. The presence of infection may be demonstrated by the detection of virus specimens from the patient and by the demonstration of a related antibody response in the patient's serum of fourfold or greater magnitude. Because of considerable antigenic variation among strains of certain types, particularly types 1, 3, 4, 5, 6, and 9, so-called prime strains and specific antisera may be required for serologic identification.

Aseptic meningitis caused by an echovirus must be distinguished from that attributable to a different virus, especially another enterovirus or mumps virus. In patients with a rash or lymphadenopathy, infectious mononucleosis, leptospirosis, and meningoccal or rickettsial infection may have to be considered. The cerebrospinal fluid findings are usually similar to those in other enteroviral infections. In patients infected with type 9, however, the leukocyte count in the spinal fluid may exceed 1,000 cells/mm^3 and may be predominantly polymorphonuclear, suggesting a bacterial meningitis. Recovery of virus from the cerebrospinal fluid provides the most convincing confirmation of the diagnosis of meningitis attributable to an echovirus.

In patients with rash and without meningitis, rubella may be suspected. Exanthematous disorders associated with echovirus 9 or 16 (Boston exanthem) can be differentiated from rubella by the shorter incubation period of 3 to 8 days, the absence of suboccipital adenopathy, and the usually different seasonal incidence. Supporting evidence of infection with echovirus may be provided by the laboratory.

In patients with diarrhea and other minor illnesses, the presence of associated infection with an echovirus may suggest a causal relationship, but this is difficult to establish.

PROGNOSIS. Infections with an echovirus are usually benign and self-limited. Patients with involvement of the central nervous system may occasionally develop paralysis or encephalitis, which in rare instances can be fatal.

TREATMENT AND CONTROL MEASURES. No therapy is known that directly affects any of the enteroviruses. Treatment is entirely supportive and symptomatic. Specific measures to control infection by echoviruses are not available.

References

POLIOMYELITIS

Deforest A, et al: The effect of breast-feeding on the antibody response of infants to trivalent oral poliovirus vaccine. J Pediatr 83:93, 1973

Miller DA, Miller OJ, Dev VG, Hashmi S, Tantravahi R: Human chromosome 19 carries a poliovirus receptor gene. Cell 1:167, 1974

Miller LW, McGowan JE, Leffingwell LM: Poliomyelitis in a high risk population: do we need to immunize the newborn? Pediatrics 49:532, 1972

Rousseau WE, Noble GR, Tegtmeier GE, Jordan MC, Chin TDY: Persistence of poliovirus neutralizing antibodies eight years after immunization with live, attenuated-virus vaccine. N Engl J Med 289:1357, 1973

Wyatt HV: Hypothesis: poliomyelitis in hypogammaglobulinemics. J Infect Dis 128:802, 1973

COXSACKIEVIRUSES

Coleman TJ, Gamble DR, Taylor KW: Diabetes in mice after coxsackie B₄ virus infection. Br Med J 3:25, 1973

Tang TT, Sedmak GV, Siegesmund KA, McCreadie SR: Chronic myopathy associated with coxsackievirus type A9. N Engl J Med 292:608, 1975

Tindall JP, Callaway JL: Hand-foot-and-mouth disease—it's more common than you think. Am J Dis Child 124:372, 1972

ECHOVIRUSES

Philip AGS, Larson EJ: Overwhelming neonatal infection with ECHO 19 virus. J Pediatr 82:391, 1973

RABIES

JAMES B. BRAYTON

Rabies is an acute viral disease of the central nervous sytem that is characterized by encephalomyelitis. It is usually transmitted by bites of dogs, cats, bats, and wild animals. The disease is characterized by restlessness, excitation, and severe intermittent spasms of the larynx and pharynx, especially on sight of food or water. The latter symptom accounts for the synonym hydrophobia. Following the period of excitation, generalized paralysis occurs, and death follows in a few days.

Rabies has been prevalent since antiquity; it was described by Democritus in 500 B.C. and by Aristotle in 322 B.C. Celsus, in A.D. 100, recognized the association of a bite with the transmission of rabies and was the first to recommend cauterization of the bite wounds.Galen, in A.D. 200, advised surgical excision of the wound site. Transmission by saliva was reported in 1804 by Zinke. In 1881 Pasteur demonstrated that virus was present in the saliva and the central nervous sytem of the rabid dog. In 1885 Pasteur modified the pathogenicity of the rabies virus and produced a vaccine from infected nerve tissue of rabbits. In 1908 Fermi discovered that by inactivating the virus-infected nerve tissue with phenol he could still produce an effective vaccine. In 1903 Negri demonstrated that inclusion bodies were present in this disease, and this became a valuable diagnostic tool. In 1921 Haupt found that vampire bats could become symptomless carriers of rabies virus. Up to the present time, various modifications of nerve tissue vaccines have been made, and now much of the postexposure prophylactic vaccine used in humans is made in duck embryo.

ETIOLOGY. Rabies fixed virus has been estimated from filtration to be from 100 to 150 mμ in diameter; it is not readily filterable. Electron microscopy shows that rabies virus looks like a bullet and has a symmetric structure somewhat like a beehive. Rabies is an RNA virus and is classfied on a morphological basis by the WHO Expert Committee on Rabies as a rhabdovirus. It is resistant to phenol, antibiotics, and commonly used skin antiseptics, with the exception of benzalkonium chloride and other quaternary ammonium compounds. Rabies virus is quickly destroyed by ultraviolet light, sunlight, strong acids, and alkali. Aqueous suspensions of rabies virus are inactivated in 30 minutes at temperatures of 54 C to 56 C. Infectivity may persist for years if the virus is desiccated and kept in a frozen state at 4 C.

EPIDEMIOLOGY. Rabies virus has an extensive host range, infecting all warm-blooded animals experimentally. Virus can be recovered from the central nervous system, saliva, urine, milk, lymph, and blood. Natural reservoirs of rabies can be divided into two categories: the sylvatic (existing in wild animals) and the domestic, with the dog being the most important. The domestic category used to be the most important, with dogs, cats, and farm animals being primarily involved. However, in the United States and other developed countries, canine rabies has decreased in incidence due to more stringent control of dogs and widely used vaccination programs. Wild carnivorous animals are now the most frequent source of rabies infection for man.

Seventy-nine percent of all confirmed animal rabies cases in 1973 occurred in wildlife; skunks, foxes, bats, and raccoons are the primary reservoirs. Rabies is not endemic in rodents. The incidence of rabies in bats, including fruit-eating bats, in the United States has markedly increased in the last decade; 45 states reported confirmed cases of rabies in bats during 1973. Although bat rabies accounts for only 15 percent of the reported wildlife rabies, since 1970 bat-associated rabies has been the most frequent source of human infection in the United States. At times bats seem to tolerate infection with rabies virus better than other animals; they become asymptomatic carriers and live and remain infectious for long periods of time.

Rabies is enzootic in all continents except Australia and Antarctica. Some of the large islands are rabies-free, such as Britain, Hawaii, Cyprus, and New Zealand. Compared with many other diseases on a global scale, human deaths and animal losses from rabies may not be striking, but they are significant. Kaplan estimates that 700,000 to 1 million people are subject annually to a vaccination regime that sometimes causes serious side effects. Yearly human rabies deaths throughout the world are estimated to be in the thousands. Rabies may occur in any climate or season, and susceptibility does not seem to vary with age, sex, or race. The incidence of rabies infection is highest in children, probably because of their friendliness toward animals and their inability to defend themselves. The attack rate in persons bitten by rabid animals is difficult to estimate; it depends on the location of the wound, the depth of the bite, the presence of saliva infected with virus, and the protection afforded by clothing. Veeraraghaven reported that the attack rate in persons bitten by proved rabid animals in India from 1946 to 1962 was 8.4 percent in those individuals who were given a complete course of nervous tissue antirabies vaccine, as compared to 50 percent in those persons who were not vaccinated.

PATHOGENESIS Bite wounds usually introduce the virus in infective saliva. Occasionally licks may introduce the virus on abrasions, but the virus will not be introduced through intact skin. The virus travels centripetally via the peripheral nerves at an estimated rate of 3 mm/hour toward the central nervous system. In the case of canine rabies it should be noted that saliva is not infectious earlier than 5 days prior to the onset of symptoms in the dog. The principal pathologic changes of rabies infection are generally confined to the central nervous sytem; they consist of neuronal necrosis and nonsuppurative encephalitis. They are most pronounced in the thalamus, hypothalamus, substantia nigra, pons, and medulla. The spinal cord and sympathetic ganglia may also show similar changes. The most distinctive feature of rabies infection is the presence of the pathognomonic Negri bodies. These specific inclusion bodies are found in the cytoplasm of neurons and consist of acidophilic structures.

When the salivary glands are infected, degeneration of the acinar epithelial cells and a mononuclear infiltrate in the interstitial tissue may be seen. The lacrimal glands, the pancreas, and the tubular epithelium of the kidney may also show similar focal degeneration. The lymph nodes show a toxic degeneration. A specific diagnosis of rabies cannot be made, pathologically, if Negri bodies are not found in the neurons of the central nervous system, as the rest of the pathologic picture may be compatible with other viral encephalitides.

CLINICAL FEATURES. The incubation period ranges from 8 days to 1 year; it is usually 1 to 2 months. It is likely to be short following severe lacerations of the head and neck. The clinical course may be divided into three progressive phases: the prodromal phase, the excitation phase, and the terminal or paralytic phase. The prodromal phase may begin with pain and numbness at the site of the wound. Fever, irritability, headaches, restlessness, perspiration, and insomnia may follow.

The excitation phase appears rapidly; there is much apprehension and even terror. Twitching, delirium, meningismus, and mild convulsive movements are seen. One of the outstanding clinical features is related to swallowing. When attempting to swallow food or liquid, painful violent spasms of the larynx and pharynx may occur. Later, just the sound, smell, or sight of liquid may precipitate these violent spasms. During these periods cyanosis may be present. Choking and aspiration are quite common. The temperature is elevated (39.5 C to 40.5 C), and generalized convulsions may occur. Maniacal behavior such as tearing of the clothes and bedding often occurs. However, biting and fighting is quite rare in human rabies. Intermittent periods of relative calm ensue, during which the patient is often quite lucid.

The paralytic phase appears with progressive paralysis, cessation of spasms, and coma, with death following shortly. Occasionally, progressive ascending paralysis may be the predominant symptom, this type of rabies being known as the dumb type. Human-to-human exposure must be considered, and isolation procedures should be undertaken to protect hospital personnel caring for patients with rabies. Ceseghino cites an instance where 36 hospital employees caring for a child with rabies required duck embryo vaccination. Death in man usually ensues within 1 week after the onset of symptoms.

The white blood cell count ranges between 20,000 and 30,000 cells/mm^3, with a polymorphonuclear leukocytosis. The cerebrospinal fluid is usually clear, with normal or slightly increased pressure. Occasionally there is a mild pleocytosis consisting mostly of mononuclear cells ranging between 30 and 100 cells/mm^3. The urine may show albumin, acetone, hyaline casts, and reducing substances.

DIAGNOSIS. When classic symptoms are present and there is a history of an animal bite, the differential diagnosis is not difficult. Careful questioning should be carried out regarding animal bites and/or association with a rabid animal, even months before symptoms appear. Tetanus should be considered in the differential diagnosis. Symptoms of trismus and muscle spasms in tetanus are usually persistent, whereas they are intermittent in rabies. In other forms of viral encephalitides convulsions usually occur earlier than in rabies. Strychnine and other ingestions, as well as poliomyelitis, can usually be ruled out by a careful history. Isolation of virus from the saliva, cerebrospinal fluid, lacrimal secretions, nasal secretions, and urine should be attempted, but negative results should not be considered definite, since the virus is secreted intermittently from these sites. Occasionally, rising serum neutralization titers may be seen in patients with a prolonged clinical course.

After death, fluorescent antibody examination of brain tissue is fast, reliable, and accurate if carried out properly. Microscopic examination of brain tissue for Negri bodies is also reliable and accurate, but it takes several days. Mouse inoculations of brain tissue suspensions also require several days, but they allow isolation of the virus.

PROGNOSIS.   The only known recovery from human rabies was reported recently by Hattwick.

CONTROL.   Measures for controlling canine rabies include quarantine of susceptible dogs for the latency period of the disease, elimination of stray dogs, and vaccination of pets with live virus. The *Revised Compendium of Animal Rabies Vaccines* developed by the National Research Council lists the vaccines available in the United States for animals and gives recommendations as to their appropriate use. No vaccine is currently licensed for use in wildlife. In the event that it is necessary to vaccinate wildlife, only inactivated vaccines should be used. Local and state regulations are necessary in order to have an effective, uniform control program. Two large metropolitan areas of the United States, where there has been no confirmed rabies in indigenous dogs and cats for many years, consider themselves rabies-free for dogs and cats. The pets in these metropolitan areas who inflict bites are observed for 10 days, but antirabies treatment for bitten people is discouraged except in unusual cases. International cooperation is also necessary to prevent introduction of this disease into rabies-free areas.

Sylvatic rabies is harder to control, but poisoning, hunting, and trapping programs are of use in certain circumstances. Rabies in bats throughout the world still remains the most perplexing problem in overall control.

TREATMENT.   Rational treatment can be carried out only when the following factors are considered: (1) Species of the biting animal: carnivorous animals, such as skunks, foxes, coyotes, wolves, raccoons, dogs, and cats are most likely to be infectious; farm animals, squirrels, opossums, weasles, muskrats, and mongooses may occasionally be infectious. Of course, bats should be highly suspected. Bites of rodents seldom require treatment. (2) Circumstances of the biting incident: An unprovoked attack is more likely to occur with a rabid animal, as contrasted to the provoked attack that may ensue when children tease or bother pets while they are feeding. (3) Extent and location of the bite: Severe exposures are multiple wounds, deeply penetrating wounds, or any bite on the head, neck, hands, or fingers. Mild exposures are scratches, licks, and single lacerations on the body, except the head, neck, hands, or feet. Open wounds or abrasions could be contaminated with infected saliva by licking. Inhalation of aerosolized rabies virus has been associated with the death of a laboratory worker. (4) Vaccination status of the biting animals: Adult animals properly immunized

have only a minimal chance of developing rabies and transmitting it. It should be noted that live virus vaccines should be given only to the recommended species. Other species of animals may be more susceptible, and if they are given the wrong live vaccine they may develop a clinical case of rabies. (5) Presence of rabies in the region: Provided that adequate surveillance and laboratory facilities exist in an area, it is most important to know if rabies exists in the region and in what species. This type of information usually can be provided by local public health officials. (6) Surveillance of biting animals: Dogs and cats that bite humans should be confined and observed by a veterinarian for at least 5 days and preferably 7 to 10 days. Illness in the biting animal should be reported to the local health officials and the patient's private physician immediately. If an animal must be killed to be captured, it should be done in a manner so as not to traumatize the head. Likewise, if the animal dies the head should be shipped under refrigeration to a competent laboratory for diagnosis. For wildlife under suspicion, the animal should be killed and its head submitted for laboratory examination.

POSTEXPOSURE PROPHYLAXIS.   (1) Local treatment of the wound: Immediately the wound should be copiously flushed with water or soap and water. After removing all traces of soap the wound should be flushed with a quaternary ammonium compound; one that is widely available is benzalkonium chloride (Zephiran). Soap will inactivate these compounds. Primary closure or suturing of the wound is not recommended. Control of bacterial infections and tetanus prophylaxis should be carried out. (2) Table 23 is a guide to a specific systemic postexposure treatment developed by the Advisory Committee on Immunization Practices. If passive immunization is indicated, hyperimmune equine serum should be given as soon as possible, preferably within 24 hours after the bite. A portion of the serum should be infiltrated around the wound site and the rest given intramuscularly. The recommended dose is 40 IU/kg. Allergic reactions and serum sickness are common with this biologic; thus a careful history of previous allergy should be taken, and skin or eye testing should be done for hypersensitivity. A hyperimmune rabies immune globulin (HRIG) obtained from adult human volunteers is now available and should eliminate the problem of serum sickness. The recommended dose of HRIG is 20 IU/kg. A portion should be used to infiltrate the wound and the rest given intramuscularly. In general, hyperimmune serum is recommended for all bites by animals in which rabies cannot be excluded and for nonbite exposures from animals proven rabid or strongly suspected of being rabid.

Active immunization in the United States in now predominantly with the duck embryo vaccine (DEV), which is prepared by inoculating embryonated duck eggs with fixed virus that is inactivated with β-propiolactone. Nerve tissue vaccine (NTV) previously was used. This vaccine was prepared from infected rabbit brain tissue and inactivated with phenol or ultraviolet light. Both vaccines are comparatively effective. During 1957–1967, treatment failures in the United States were

TABLE 23. Postexposure Antirabies Guide [†]

Animal	Condition at Time of Attack	Treatment Bite[‡]	Nonbite[‡]
Wild			
Skunk			
Fox	Regard as rabid	S + V[1]	S + V[1]
Raccoon			
Bat			
Domestic			
Dog	Healthy	None[2]	None[2]
	Escaped (unknown)	S + V	V[3]
Cat	Rabid	S + V[1]	S + V[1]

Adapted from: Morbidity and Mortality Weekly Reports 21 (Suppl 25):17, 1972.

[†] These recommendations are only a guide. They should be used in conjunction with knowledge of the animal species involved, circumstances of the bite or other exposure, vaccination status of the animal, and presence of rabies in the region.

[‡] See text definitions.

-V= Rabies vaccine.

S= Antirabies serum.

[1] = Discontinue vaccine if fluorescent antibody tests of animal killed at time of attack are negative.

[2] = Begin S + V at first sign of rabies in biting dog or cat during holding period (10 days).

[3] = 14 doses of DEV.

1 in 24,500 for DEV-treated persons and 1 in 19,600 for NTV-treated persons. DEV is widely used because it is relatively free of neurologic complications such as polyneuritis, ascending paralysis, and meningoencephalitis, which have been problems with the NTV. Clinical trials are now being carried out with promising inactivated tissue culture vaccines that are not yet released for general use.

DEV is administered subcutaneously, giving daily 1-ml doses for 14 days, usually varying the injection site on the abdomen. In severe exposures or exposures involving wild animals, two injections per day for the first 7 days and one daily injection for the next 7 days are recommended. If the biting animal is healthy 5 days after the exposure, the vaccine may be discontinued. The daily dosage is the same for adults and children. If hyperimmune serum is given, the initial course should be followed at 10 and 20 days with booster doses of DEV.

Major complications associated with DEV are rare, but local reactions are common; they include pain (100 percent), erythema (97 percent) and pruritus (13 percent). Systemic symptoms such as fever, malaise, and myalgia occur in about 33 percent of recipients, and adenopathy in 15 percent. Anaphylaxis is seen in less than 1 percent of recipients and usually occurs during the first five daily doses in persons sensitized with other vaccines containing avian tissue. Skin testing for hypersensitivity should be done before administering the first dose of vaccine. If anaphylaxis, dyspnea, or urticaria develop, antihistamines, epinephrine, oxygen, and steroids should be immediately available. Steroids should be used with caution, as impairment of vaccine antibody responses with ACTH and cortisone in animals has been reported. If serious allergic reactions occur with DEV, then the NTV should be used. Central nervous system reactions to DEV are rare, but they do occur.

Between 1958 and 1971 an estimated 434,000 individuals received DEV; there were 13 reports of transverse myelitis, peripheral or cranial neuropathy, or encephalopathy. When meningeal or paralytic reactions develop, vaccination should be discontinued.

PREEXPOSURE VACCINATION.   Preexposure vaccination can be performed with DEV in high-risk groups such as veterinarians, biologists, ecologists, and animal handlers. Two 1-ml injections should be given subcutaneously in the deltoid region 1 month apart, followed by a booster in 6 months. Boosters should be given every 2 to 3 years thereafter. Levels of serum neutralization antibodies should be determined 1 month after the first booster injection. When an immunized person with previously demonstrated antibodies has a mild exposure, one booster dose of DEV should be given. If the exposure has been severe, five daily doses should be given, followed by a booster in 20 days. If it is not known that a previously immunized person has rabies antibodies, then a complete DEV series should be given.

References

Cereghino JJ, Osterud HT, Pinnas JL, Holmes MA: Rabies: a ra e disease but a serious pediatric problem. Pediatrics 45:839, 1970

Corey L, Hattwick MAW: Treatment of persons exposed to rabies. JAMA 232:272, 1975

Hattwick MAW, Rubin RH, Music S, et al: Post-exposure rabies prophylaxis with human rabies immune globulin. JAMA 227:407, 1974

——— Weis TT, Stechschulte CJ, Baer GM, Gregg MB: Recovery from rabies, a case report. Ann Intern Med 76:931, 1972

Kaplan MM: Epidemiology of rabies. Nature 221:421, 1969

Morbidity and Mortality Weekly Report 24:82, 1975

Public Health Service Advisory Committee on Immunization Practices: Rabies Prophylaxis. Morbidity and Mortality Weekly Reports 21 (Suppl 25):17, 1972

Rubin RH, Hattwick MAW, Jones S, Gregg MB, Schwartz VD: Adverse reactions to duck embryo vaccine, range and incidence. Ann Intern Med 78:643, 1973

Veeraraghaven NI: Rabies. A. The Value of 5 Percent Sample Vaccine in Human Treatment—Comparative Mortality Among the Treated and Untreated. Annual Report of the Director, 1962, and Scientific Report, 1963, the Pasteur Institute of Southern India Coonoor. Madras, India, Diocesan Press, 1964, p 33

WHO Expert Committee on Rabies: Sixth Report, WHO Technical Report Series No 321. Geneva, WHO, 1973

Winkler WG, Fashinell TR, Leffingwell L, Howard P, Conomy JP: Airborne rabies transmission in a laboratory worker. JAMA 226:1219, 1973

Zoonoses Surveillance: Annual Rabies Summary, 1973. Atlanta, Center for Disease Control, 1973

RUBELLA

Louis Z. Cooper

Postnatal Rubella

Rubella (German measles, 3-day measles) is the mildest of the common viral exanthems of childhood. It is an endemic and epidemic illness, apparently worldwide in distribution, that is characterized by a generalized maculopapular rash and postauricular and suboccipital lymphadenopathy. Fever and constitutional complaints are typically mild, and complications are uncommon. Rubella is a disease of major significance because of the high incidence of congenital defects in children whose mothers are infected during early pregnancy. Typical anomalies caused by this congenital infection are known collectively as the rubella syndrome. Deafness, congenital heart diseases, cataracts, and retardation are the most common of these defects.

Rubella was first described in the English literature by Maton, who in 1815 pointed out the features that distinguish it from scarlet fever and measles (rubeola). In 1866 Veale coined the "short and euphonious" name rubella as a substitute for Rotheln, a term then favored in Germany.

Rubella attracted little attention until 1941, when Norman Gregg, an Australian ophthalmologist, reported 68 cases of congenital cataract in infants whose mothers had had rubella during early pregnancy in the severe epidemic of 1940. He also pointed out that low birth weight, high incidence of congenital heart disease, and high mortality rate characterize the infant with severe congenital rubella. Many investigators subsequently confirmed and extended Gregg's pioneering observations.

The primary obstacle to diagnosis and control of rubella was overcome in 1962 when two independent groups simultaneously described the isolation of rubella virus in tissue culture and procedures for determination of specific rubella-neutralizing antibody in the serum. In 1964 the largest epidemic of rubella in at least 30 years swept across the United States. The magnitude of this epidemic, combined with the availability of specific diagnostic tools and the efforts of many investigators, produced an almost explosive expansion in our knowledge of rubella and the hazards of rubella acquired in utero and dramatized the need for adequate control measures. After extensive field trials, live attenuated rubella virus vaccine was licensed in 1969; it is hoped that this has been accomplished in time to prevent future epidemics and eventually to provide a solution to the rubella problem.

ETIOLOGY.   Rubella virus has certain features that suggest a relationship to the arbovirus group. Its pleomorphic appearance in electron micrographs has not been established with certainty. Initial estimates of particle size ranging between 100 and 300 mμ have been revised to 500 to 750 mμ by Best and associates. The virus is thermolabile; inactivation is rapid at 37 C and at room temperature. However, it can be stored for short periods at -20 C and is relatively stable for months at -60 C. Hemagglutination and complement-fixation antigens have been prepared in several tissue culture cell systems and serve as the basis for practical serologic tests. The virus is destroyed by exposure to ether, chloroform, cesium chloride, and sodium deoxycholate, but replication is not prevented by idoxuridine. Adamantine hydrochloride prevents growth in tissue culture, but has no effect on rubella infection in man. Rubella appears to be both antigenically stable and distinct from all other known viruses.

EPIDEMIOLOGY.   Although rubella occurs in all areas of the world, variations in epidemiologic patterns have been described from country to country. In the past these differences have been obscured by difficulty in clinical diagnosis and the significant, apparently variable, incidence of subclinical infection. With the impetus provided by development of effective rubella vaccines and the availability of a practical serologic test (the rubella hemagglutination-inhibition antibody test), recent studies have documented these differences. Prior to widespread use of rubella vaccines in 1969 in the continental United States, rubella occurred primarily in children during the elementary school years (the first group experience) and during high school. A small but significant minority did not become infected until early adulthood. Rubella was a noticeable inconvenience when infection spread through military recruit centers and universities, and it created a major problem among young women in early pregnancy.

Rubella remains an endemic illness in the United States, with a seasonal peak in the late winter and spring. Its greatest impact has resulted from epidemics that in the past occurred at 6- to 9-year intervals. In 1964 in New York City the last severe nationwide pandemic produced a 10-fold increase in reported cases over the mean for the previous 10 years. Fetal mortality, in association with congenital infection, were correspondingly high. Following vaccine licensure and widespread use among children ages 1 to 12 years (approximately 60 million doses in 1969–1976), the reported incidence of rubella has been at an all time low. Although the disease continues to occur in children and young adults, small outbreaks have been confined essentially to unimmunized populations (for example, in high school classes rather than in the elementary schools). The long-term epidemiologic effects of widespread immunization remain to be seen.

Serologic studies have demonstrated that approximately 75 to 90 percent of adult Americans have had rubella in the past. This immunity status is essentially the same in those with and those without clinical histories of the disease. Suceptibility to rubella is much more common (approaching 50 percent) among young adults living in Puerto Rico and Hawaii. In contrast, on the island of Taiwan, where pandemics occur at approximately 10-year intervals, rubella susceptibility among adults is a rarity. Protection of young infants by transplacentally acquired rubella-specific antibody occurs in direct proportion to the immunity status of women of childbearing age.

The immunity that persists after clinical or inapparent rubella is protective against another episode of the disease. Although heavy reexposure may provoke an anamnestic type of antibody response, there is no evidence at this time that reinfection can contribute to the chain of transmission or that fetal damage can occur if reinfection takes place during early pregnancy.

COMMUNICABILITY.   Infection is usually by airborne spread of infected droplets. Patients are most contagious for a few days before, during, and after the onset of rash, although virus may be present in pharyngeal secretions for as long as 1 week before and 2 weeks after the onset of rash. The patient with subclinical infection is also a source of rubella virus. Although shared eating utensils have been shown to transmit rubella, direct person-to-person contact appears to be the usual mode of spread because of the relative instability of rubella virus. Persons who are immune to rubella have never been shown to carry the virus from an infected patient to a susceptible one. Infection acquired postnatally does not produce a chronic carrier state. In contrast, congenital rubella is characterized by chronic infection that may persist for months after birth. These infants are a particular hazard for hospital personnel.

Rubella is less highly contagious than measles. In both experimental and natural settings relatively brief exposure of a group of susceptible children to a child with rubella produces variable results ranging from clinical and inapparent infection in some children to no infection in others. This unpredictability is one reason rubella parties for exposure of young girls in the past met with little general enthusiasm. The prevalence of rubella in a somewhat older age group than measles also has been interpreted as evidence that rubella is less contagious than measles.

CLINICAL   MANIFESTATIONS.   The   clinical manifestations of rubella present a spectrum of disease ranging from totally inapparent infection to a characteristic pattern of adenopathy, rash, and low-grade fever. The incubation period is from 14 to 21 days. A typical clinical course begins with adenopathy involving primarily the postauricular, occipital, and posterior cervical nodes,which may be slightly painful and moderately tender. Although these symptoms usually clear promptly as the rash fades, the nodes may remain palpable for several weeks. Adolescents and adults may complain of malaise, headache, a low-grade fever, sore throat, and mild coryza during a 1- to 5-day prodromal period that frequently accompanies the onset of adenopathy. In young children the mild prodrome is usually overlooked.

The rubella rash is variable and has no feature that is indisputably diagnostic. It may be no more than a transient blush, but classically it persists for 2 to 3 days in a pattern that has been called kaleidoscopic because of its changing appearance. Initially small, irregular pink macules begin on the face and spread rapidly (usually within 24 hours) to the neck, trunk, arms, and ultimately the legs. By the next day these lesions may have coalesced, developed a maculopapular component, and become quite scarlatiniform. The face frequently is clearing by the time a full-blown rash is seen on the lower legs, where coalescence is uncommon. Desquamation is rare.

An enanthem (described by Forchheimer in 1898) consisting of punctate or slightly larger red spots on the soft palate may be present during the late prodrome and early rash phase. These lesions are not pathognomonic of rubella. Scarlet fever, infectious mononucleosis, measles, and other viral exanthems may be accompanied by similar palatal lesions.

Fever is uncommonly as high as 39 C to 39.5 C, but it may be absent in children. The illness is characteristically associated with little or no debility in children and even in many young adults.

Polyarthralgia and polyarthritis are such common manifestations of rubella among women as to be considered a typical manifestation of the disease. Joint involvement is less common in men and is uncommon in children. Symptoms most typically appear with the rash or within several days after its onset, but rarely they may precede the onset of rash by several days. Involvement, which is frequently symmetric, may range from subjective morning stiffness to full-blown arthritis characterized by swelling, redness, tenderness, and effusion. Objective signs and severe symptoms usually clear within several days to 2 weeks, but rarely may persist several months. The proximal interphalangeal joints are affected most frequently, and (in the order of decreasing frequency) the metacarpophalangeal joints, wrists, elbows, knees, ankles, feet, shoulders, and spine may be involved.

Paresthesia, most typically numbness and tingling or "pins and needles," often accompanies and may outlast the joint symptoms. This may be caused by compression of the median nerve in the carpal tunnel, presumably due to synovitis in the area under the volar carpal ligaments.

Although there are striking similarities between rubella arthritis and early acute rheumatoid arthritis, the critical difference is in the course and subsequent outcome. Joint manifestations in rubella are transient and produce no deformity. There is no evidence that rubella causes or contributes to development of any form of chronic arthritis.

COMPLICATIONS.   Encephalitis.   Postinfectious encephalitis, clinically indistinguishable from that following measles or varicella, is a rare but serious complication of rubella. However, it is less frequent (1 case per 5,000 is the highest estimate) than postmeasles encephalitis (1 case per 800 to 1,000). Symptoms and signs of central nervous system involvement usually develop 2 to 4 days after the onset of rash. Autopsies in fatal cases have revealed severe nonspecific neuronal degenerative changes without demyelinization and with minimal perivascular infiltration.

Rubella virus has never been isolated from cerebrospinal fluid or brain in cases of postinfectious encephalitis. The fact that the onset of symptoms coincides with the appearance of rubella antibody in the serum has encouraged speculation that this complication may have an immunologic component.

Thrombocytopenic Purpura. Many patients have slight but definite decreases in their platelet counts during the course of uncomplicated rubella. This thrombocytopenia, which usually occurs within 1 week after the onset of rash, is rarely severe and symptomatic. Presenting complaints usually include purpura, epistaxis, bleeding from the gums, hematuria, and gastrointestinal bleeding. Splenomegaly is not present. Abnormal capillary fragility also contributes to the problem of hemostasis. Megakaryocytes are present in normal numbers, but platelet formation is rarely seen, a pattern similar to that commonly observed in idiopathic thrombocytopenic purpura. Prognosis is generally excellent, but fatalities due to uncontrolled central nervous system hemorrhage do occur rarely. Most patients become symptom-free within 2 weeks, in association with return of platelet counts to normal levels. Rarely, patients are plagued by asymptomatic thrombocytopenia that persists for months. It is common practice to institute steroid therapy for symptomatic cases and to utilize platelet transfusion and fresh whole blood when necessary.

LABORATORY STUDY. Diagnosis of rubella can be confirmed only by virus isolation or demonstration of rising titers of rubella antibody in the serum. Although virus isolation is frequently impractical because of expense and the relative lability of rubella virus, serologic testing utilizing improved standardized techniques should be available for rational diagnosis and management.

Certain basic features of virus excretion and antibody response must be understood if these tools are to be used effectively: (1) Rubella virus may be cultured from the pharynx and serum as early as 1 week before the onset of rash. Virus is promptly cleared from the serum after the rash appears, but persists in pharyngeal secretions usually for several days after the rash and uncommonly for as long as 2 weeks (Fig. 13). Urine and stool are unreliable sources of rubella virus. (2) Rubella antibody may be measured in a variety of test systems based on neutralization, hemagglutination inhibition (HI), complement fixation (CF), immunofluorescence (FA), and immunodiffusion and precipitation. Most of these techniques are appropriate only for research laboratories. However, the rubella HI antibody test standardized by the Center for Disease Control (CDC Standard Rubella HI Antibody Test) is a rapid, sensitive, economical, and reliable procedure well suited for general clinical use. In certain circumstances the CF test can provide important additional information and serve as a useful backup for the HI test.

The patterns of HI, CF, and neutralizing antibody responses during rubella are also illustrated in Figure 13. Absence of rubella HI or neutralizing antibody at the time of exposure indicates susceptibility to rubella.

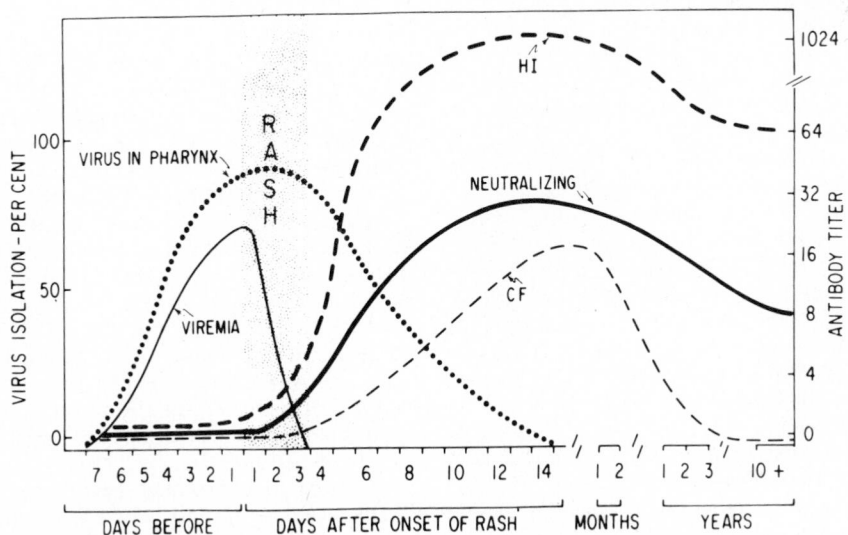

FIG. 13. Schematic illustration of the natural history of rubella demonstrating the pattern of viremia, virus excretion in the pharynx, and development and persistence of HI, neutralizing, and CF antibody. (Adapted from Cooper and Krugman: *Ophthalmol* 77:434, 1967.)

This is not necessarily true of CF antibody, which usually does not persist for years after infection. The presence of antibody at exposure confirms past rubella infection (or rubella vaccination), indicates protection from another episode of the disease, and in the pregnant woman obviates the fear of rubella-induced congenital malformation. The presence of low levels of these antibodies does not necessarily provide protection against subclinical reinfection. Fortunately the characteristics and implications of reinfection appear to be quite distinct from primary rubella, as will be detailed.

In patients with clinical rubella, HI and neutralizing antibodies are detectable within 24 to 48 hours after onset of the rash, and peak titers are reached within 6 to 12 days. In most laboratories rubella HI titers attain peak levels that are 10- to 100-fold greater than neutralizing antibody titers. In subclinical rubella (primary rubella without rash) HI and neutralizing antibodies usually reach detectable levels 14 to 21 days after exposure, a time that corresponds to the onset of rash in clinical disease. The initial immunoglobulin is rubella-specific IgM. However, this response is a transient one, and rubella IgG becomes the predominant antibody usually before peak titers are reached.

Following reexposure to rubella, a person with a low level of antibody (from the past rubella or vaccination) may experience an anamnestic response. This reinfection phenomenon appears to be more common among persons with vaccine-induced immunity than with immunity as a consequence of unattenuated or natural rubella. There is no evidence at this time that the reinfected person is a significant source of contagion for others or that the fetus is at risk when this event occurs during early pregnancy.

The CF antibody response after rubella infection is slower than the HI response. Therefore it is sometimes possible to demonstrate a diagnostic rise in CF antibody with paired sera that would not show such a rise in HI antibody. In spite of this delayed response, often it is not possible to confirm unequivocally the diagnosis of recent rubella when the first blood specimen is obtained more than 1 week after the rash.

The neutralizing, θ-precipitin, and FA antibody responses are similar to the HI response, but titers are consistently lower. The t-precipitin response, like that of CF antibody, is delayed and transient.

The hemogram frequently is characterized by a mild leukopenia with a relative lymphocytosis that may include a few atypical cells. The platelet count frequently falls slightly, but severe thrombocytopenia is uncommon. Serologic tests for rheumatoid factor may be positive in patients with rubella arthritis. In general, the incidence of positive tests has paralleled the sensitivity of the test used and has been inversely proportional to its selectivity or discrimination.

DIFFERENTIAL DIAGNOSIS. Rubella should not be confused with measles. The typical measles prodrome, the prominent cough, conjunctivitis, Koplik's spots, and the general severity of the disease distinguish measles from rubella. Even mild scarlet fever is associated with more fever, pharyngitis, and anterior cervical adenopathy than is usually seen in rubella. (The characteristic scarlet fever rash is described elsewhere in this chapter.) A leukocytosis, a positive culture of group A streptococci, and a rise in antistreptolysin O titer help in diagnosing scarlet fever. In infectious mononucleosis the pharyngitis, generalized adenopathy, and splenomegaly are more prominent than in rubella, and the rash is less prominent. A marked atypical lymphocytosis and positive heterophile antibody titer and Epstein-Barr virus antibody titer support the diagnosis of infectious mononucleosis.

Exanthema subitum (roseola) occurs in younger children (6 months to 3 years.) Characteristically, several days of high fever and defervescence precede the onset of a rash. No such clearcut pattern exists for erythema infectiosum. The lacy appearance of the rash, its prominence on the extremities more than the trunk, bright red raised rash on the face, and slightly more prolonged duration of this illness are said to distinguish it from rubella. Unfortunately, the etiologic agents responsible for these latter exanthems are still unidentified.

The greatest difficulty in diagnosis is produced by mild exanthematous illnesses occurring during interepidemic years. These may be caused by known agents, such as representatives of the enterovirus or adenovirus groups, or by agents as yet unknown. In the absence of epidemiologic clues, typical clinical pattern, or virologic study, unequivocal diagnoses are impossible in these cases.

PREVENTION AND THERAPY. The available information suggests that in the United States widespread use of rubella vaccines (approximately 60 million doses since 1969) is preventing epidemics and protecting vaccine recipients from disease. This has been accomplished using two strains of attenuated rubella virus (HPV-77 and Cendehill strains). The HPV-77DE$_5$ rubella virus vaccine is prepared in duck embryo cell culture (DE$_5$) after attenuation during 77 passages in African green monkey kidney cells (HPV-77). Another HPV-77 derivative (HPV-77DK$_{12}$) prepared in dog kidney cells (DK$_{12}$) has been withdrawn from the market because it was more likely to produce joint reactions. The Cendehill strain vaccine was attenuated and prepared in rabbit kidney cells.

Another strain of attenuated rubella virus, RA27/3, has been licensed and used widely in Western Europe. This vaccine, isolated initially from an infected fetus, was attenuated and is prepared in human diploid fibroblasts. RA27/3 vaccine has been administered by nasal droplet as well as by subcutaneous inoculation. Licensure in the United States (expected in 1976) will be for subcutaneous administration, with the same indications and precautions applied to HPV-77DE$_5$ and Cendehill vaccines.

All three strains of attenuated virus vaccines (HPV-77DE$_5$, Cendehill, and RA27/3) are highly immunogenic, producing seroconversion in more than 95 percent of susceptible vaccinees. They rarely produce rash or fever, but they do cause transient shedding of small quantities of vaccine virus from pharyngeal secretions. Nevertheless, for practical purposes the vaccines are not contagious. Susceptible vaccinees also experience transient low-grade viremia. Inadvertent vaccination of rubella-susceptible women during early pregnancy has led to fetal infection. Small quantities of virus have been detected in numerous organs from fetuses obtained at therapeutic abortion. At this time, no children have been born with birth defects attributable to inadvertent vaccination during pregnancy. Nevertheless, the teratogenic potential of rubella vaccines remains an open question.

There are some differences in frequency of reactions and immunogenicity among the three vaccines. For unknown reasons, although each of the rubella vaccines rarely causes other signs or symptoms of rubella, they are all capable of provoking arthralgia, arthritis, and paresthesias indistinguishable from natural rubella. As with natural (unattenuated) rubella, these complaints are common among women and relatively uncommon in children. The HPV-77DK$_{12}$ dog kidney preparation yielded the highest serum antibody titers, but it was also most likely to provide these reactions. Since no significant advantages could be documented for this vaccine, it is no longer available for use. Differences in reactogenicity among the other vaccine strains have not been documented unequivocally.

Live attenuated rubella virus vaccine is recommended for all boys and girls between 1 year of age and puberty. Widespread use of vaccine in children should protect them, eliminate the reservoir responsible for epidemic rubella, and markedly decrease the likelihood of rubella exposure for susceptible women in early pregnancy. Postpubertal females should be vaccinated only after determination of rubella susceptibility by HI antibody test and assurance that they are not pregnant and that the risk of pregnancy is essentially nil for at least 2 months after vaccination. Pregnant women should not be immunized, but should be tested for rubella susceptibility. The immediate post partum period is an excellent time to vaccinate susceptible women.

Careful studies of immunity to rubella following vaccination have demonstrated that after sufficient exposure vaccinees may be reinfected. As with reinfection following natural rubella, this phenomenon is characterized by an anamnestic or booster type antibody response and transient low-level pharyngeal shedding of virus. Viremia has not been detected. Additional studies will be required before current expectations can be confirmed that reinfection is not contagious and cannot lead to fetal infection.

In this regard, the RA27/3 strain of vaccine appears to have certain theoretical advantages compared to HPV-77 and Cendehill vaccines. Immunization with RA27/3 strain is more likely to stimulate production of nasal secretory and immunoprecipitin antibodies. These antibodies are invariably detectable after natural infection. Their role in rubella immunity remains to be clarified.

The use of gamma globulin (commercially available human immunoglobulin) in prophylaxis of rubella during pregnancy is still a controversial issue. When administered in large quantities (0.15 to 0.25 ml/kg) before or shortly after exposure, the incidence of subclinical infection is increased and perhaps the rate of infection is decreased. However, gamma globulin does not prevent rubella or congenital rubella in a predictable or reliable fashion. Recently, experimental lots of gamma globulin prepared from donors with high titers of rubella antibody (rubella immune globulin) have been shown to prevent detectable viremia, if not infection, when administered shortly after volunteers were challenged with rubella virus. Rubella immune globulin may eventually be useful in special circumstances, such as following exposure of those susceptible pregnant women for whom therapeutic abortion would be unacceptable.

There is no specific chemotherapy for rubella, and no symptomatic measures are necessary for this mild illness in most instances. Aspirin is of value in management of the constitutional complaints and arthritis that are more frequently seen among adults. It is the consensus that corticosteroids are indicated for severe thrombocytopenic purpura. There is no evidence that the steroids are of benefit in rubella encephalitis.

CONGENITAL RUBELLA

Rubella during early pregnancy frequently results in fetal infection, which may be chronic and may produce a spectrum of congenital illness known as the rubella syndrome.

PATHOGENESIS. The mechanisms responsible for the unique teratogenic potential of rubella are not known, although many steps in the sequence of maternal–fetal infection have been well documented.

Maternal viremia may persist for 1 week before the onset of rash and may lead to placental infection. In early pregnancy this infection does not persist in maternal placental tissue (the decidua), but does persist in the chorionic villi. Fetal viremia then may produce disseminated fetal infection. Timing is of great importance. Organogenesis occurs during the second week through the sixth week after conception, so that infection is a maximum hazard to the heart and eyes at that time. During the second trimester of pregnancy, as the fetus develops increasing immunologic competence (eg, the presence of plasma cells and ability to produce IgM), it no longer seems susceptible to the chronic infection that is characteristic of intrauterine rubella during the early weeks. In contrast to the situation that occurs with thalidomide or radiation, where a single exposure during early pregnancy exerts its effects at that time only, the available evidence suggests that chronic infection contributes to the acute illness seen in the newborn period (eg, bone lesions, hepatitis, and purpura) and to the progressive psychomotor retardation observed occasionally during infancy.

Two mechanisms play important roles in rubella embryopathy. The most obvious is the ability of rubella virus to provoke an inflammatory response in certain organs. The more specialized mechanism has been elucidated in tissue culture studies and confirmed by clinical observation. Only a small number of cells (1 in 1,000 to 1 in 250,000) are infected in utero. Daughter cells from these clones are characterized by slower growth and limited doubling potential. At autopsy, infants with congenital rubella have hypoplasia or undergrowth of certain target organs; ie, these organs have a subnormal number of cells. The key to the teratogenicity of rubella virus may ultimately be found in a molecular explanation of its ability to inhibit multiplication of human cells.

EPIDEMIOLOGY AND RISK.   In urban areas of the United States, approximately 20 percent of women of childbearing age are susceptible to rubella. Prospective data from the Collaborative Perinatal Research Study indicate that 3.6 percent of pregnant women had rubella in the 1964 epidemic, in contrast to an infection rate of 0.1 to 0.2 percent in the interepidemic years. Although definitive information concerning the risk of serious malformations following maternal rubella is difficult to obtain, and experience has varied even in prospective studies, the hazard is clearly maximal during the first 8 weeks of pregnancy, when it probably exceeds 50 percent. Risk of serious abnormality appears to decrease progressively thereafter, with 20 percent a conservative estimate for the ninth week through the sixteenth week. In our experience, the risk is minimal later in the second trimester and nil thereafter.

Spontaneous and therapeutic abortions contribute significantly to the mortality in congenital rubella. In a prospective study of the 1964 epidemic by Siegal, Fuerst, and Peress, fully 75 percent of 333 pregnancies complicated by rubella in the first trimester did not go to term. Specifically, 213 (64 percent) were terminated electively, and 38 (32 percent) of the remaining 120 aborted spontaneously.

CLINICAL MANIFESTATIONS.   The consequences of rubella in utero are varied and unpredictable. Spontaneous abortion, stillbirth, live birth with anomalies (single or in combination), and normal infants are represented in this spectrum. Virtually every organ may be involved, either transiently, progressively, or permanently. It is beyond the scope of this text to describe in detail this wide range of rubella-associated disease, but because of their frequency, certain manifestations will be explored in greater depth.

Neonatal Manifestations.   During the newborn period congenital rubella may be manifested by a number of acute conditions that are self-limiting in those infants who survive. Neonatal thrombocytopenic purpura, characterized by a variable number of red-purple macular "blueberry muffin" lesions, is the most common and striking of these manifestations (Fig. 14). It is usually associated with a high incidence of other transient lesions, such as radiolucencies in the metaphyseal portion of the long bones, hepatosplenomegaly, hepatitis, hemolytic anemia, and bulging anterior fontanelle with or without pleocytosis in the cerebrospinal fluid. This clinical picture represents the most severe evidence of congenital infection. Low birth weight, congenital heart disease, cataracts, deafness, and retardation with and without microcephaly frequently accompany the transient lesions and contribute to a poor prognosis. The mortality rate in one group of 58 infants with purpura exceeded 35 percent in follow-up through the first year of life.

Cardiac Defects.   Congenital heart disease may not be detected for days after birth. Patent ductus arteriosus,

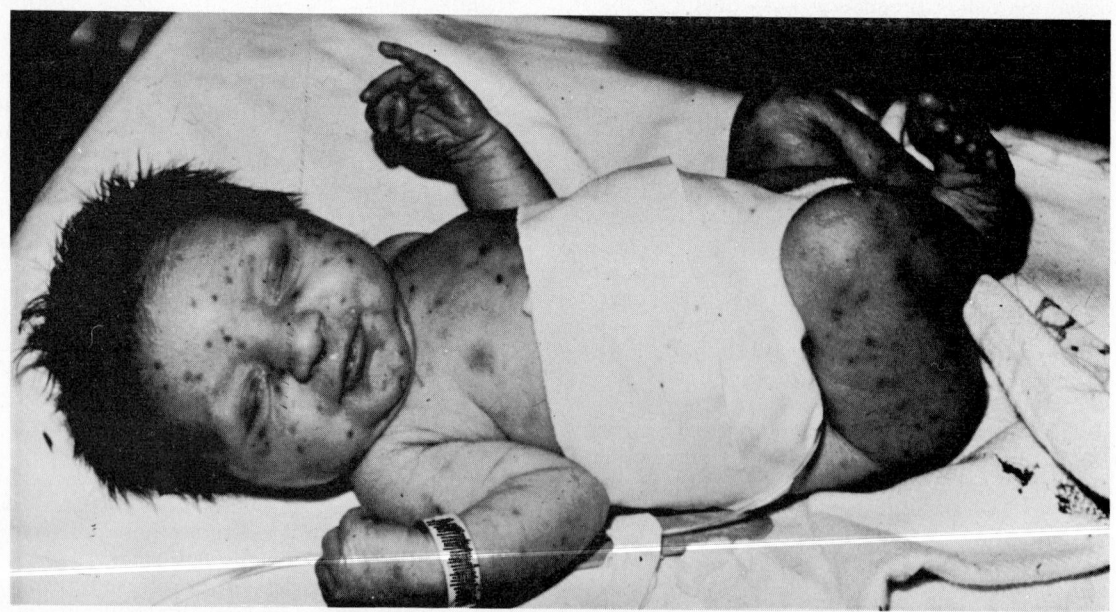

FIG. 14.   "Blueberry muffin" lesions; thrombocytopenic purpura due to congenital rubella.

with or without stenosis of the pulmonary artery or its branches, and atrial and ventricular septal defects are the most common lesions, but more complex structural defects are not rare. Although many infants tolerate the cardiac defects well, others have developed congestive failure in the first months of life. The poor outcome in the group with congestive failure contributes significantly to the high mortality rate.

Hearing Loss. Deafness due to congenital rubella may be severe or mild, bilateral or unilateral. It is permanent and is generally thought to be of the sensory type caused by damage of the organ of Corti, although defects in the middle ear structures have been reported. Mild or unilateral hearing loss frequently escapes detection unless children are studied longitudinally by audiometric testing. By the same token, it is clear that many children have communication disorders that are central in origin and that may be confused with sensorineural deafness. Deafness and communication disorders may be the only overt manifestions of congenital rubella, especially if maternal infection occurs after the first 8 weeks of pregnancy.

Eye Defects. The most characteristic ocular anomaly is a pearly nuclear cataract that may be unilateral or bilateral; it is frequently associated with microphthalmia. The lesion may be absent at birth or so small that it may not be detected without careful ophthalmoscopic examination (using the +8 lens held 6 to 8 inches from the eye).

Congenital glaucoma, which may be present at birth or may develop during infancy, is clinically indistinguishable from hereditary infantile glaucoma. The cornea is enlarged and hazy, the anterior chamber is deep, and ocular tension, measured under anesthesia, is increased. Rubella glaucoma is a true phenocopy. It is important to distinguish this disease from corneal clouding, which is self-limited and is also seen during the newborn period in infants without congenital rubella. The glaucoma may require prompt surgical intervention; no therapy is necessary for transient corneal clouding.

Retinopathy, characterized by discrete, patchy black pigmentation, quite variable in size and location, is probably the most common ocular manifestation of congenital rubella. There is no evidence that this anomaly of the pigment epithelium of the retina interferes with vision. However, recognition of this lesion is a valuable aid in the diagnosis of congenital rubella.

Developmental and Neurologic Defects. Rubella in utero frequently is pathogenic for the central nervous system. This neurovirulence of rubella virus has been confirmed by histopathologic and virus studies among autopsied infants, a high frequency of cerebrospinal fluid abnormalities including positive virus isolation among surviving infants, and a broad spectrum of developmental and neurologic defects.

Delayed psychomotor development during infancy is a hallmark of congenital rubella, even among many children who eventually do well. This severe early lag corresponds temporally to the period of active clinical encephalitis that has been well characterized by Desmond and her colleagues. The most common consequence of the permanent brain damage from this encephalitis is mental retardation, ranging from mild to profound. Behavior disturbances and manifestations of minimal cerebral dysfunction are also common. Less common are severe spastic diplegia and autism. Communication disorders of central origin, masquerading as deafness, have been mentioned previously. The combination of cognitive and behavior deficits with auditory and visual impairment frequently is severe enough to require residential placement.

Progressive rubella panencephalitis, a severe progressive neurologic deterioration beginning during the second decade of life, has been described recently as a rare complication of congenital rubella. Intellectual deterioration, myoclonus, ataxia, and seizures have progressed to death over the course of several years. High rubella antibody titers in serum and cerebrospinal fluid, elevated spinal fluid protein and gamma globulin levels, histopathologic changes of progressive panencephalitis, and isolation of rubella virus from brain biopsy after repeated serial passage and co-cultivation techniques add to the obvious parallel between this condition and the subacute sclerosing panencephalitis that is a rare and late sequela of measles.

TEMPORAL RELATIONSHIPS. Cardiac defects, cataracts, and glaucoma occur predominantly after maternal rubella during the first 2 months of pregnancy. Hearing loss and neurologic manifestations may follow maternal infection any time during the first and, less commonly, through the second trimester. The transient manifestations of congenital rubella seen in newborn infants are most common after early maternal infection, but they are observed occasionally after infection beginning in the third month.

LABORATORY STUDY. **Virus Isolation.** The infant with congenital rubella may remain chronically infected for months after birth. Virus has been cultured from pharyngeal secretions, urine, cerebrospinal fluid, and virtually every organ. Certain damaged organs may be more highly infected than those that are normal. The incidence of virus shedding decreases with advancing age, as seen in Figure 15. Isolation of virus from the blood is rare and probably occurs only in infants who cannot produce antibodies.

Immune Response. Newborn infants with congenital rubella have serum rubella antibody titers comparable to those observed in their mothers. Much of this antibody is transplacentally acquired IgG, but the presence of rubella-specific IgM reflects in utero antibody production by the fetus and, when present, is diagnostic of congenital rubella. In all but rare infants, by the end of 1 year IgG is usually the dominant rubella antibody. Detectable levels of HI or neutralizing antibody persist for years in most children. However, a minority, despite congenital infection, have declining titers of HI antibody beginning during the second year of life. By age 5 years approximately 20 percent of children with this disease have undetectable levels of antibody. Loss of

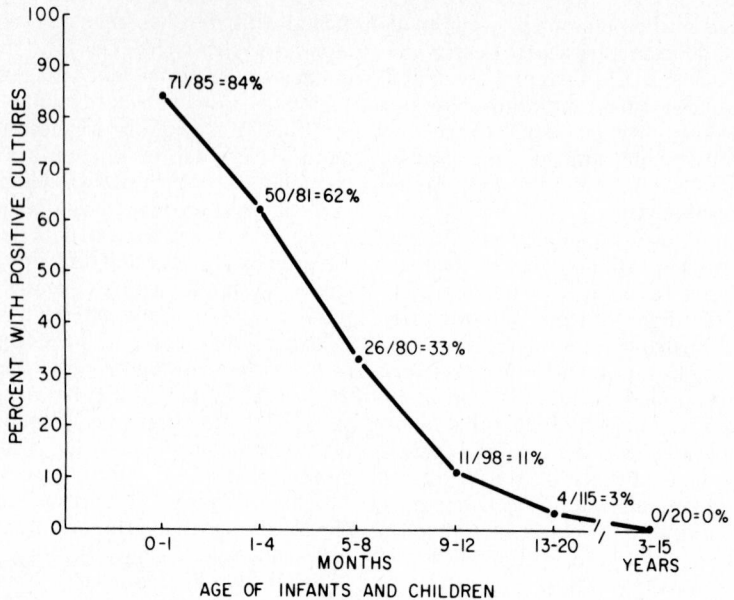

FIG. 15.   Incidence of rubella virus isolation in infants with congenital rubella correlated with age at which cultures were obtained. The denominator indicates the number of infants with positive virus isolation. (From Cooper and Krugman: *Arch Ophthalmol* 77:434, 1967.)

antibody cannot be correlated with severity of clinical disease. For purposes of diagnosis the presence of rubella antibody that persists in infancy beyond age 6 months without evidence of postnatal infection essentially confirms the diagnosis of congenital rubella. In our experience the diagnosis may also be confirmed among children age 3 years and older whose HI antibody has declined to undetectable levels by administration of rubella vaccine. In contrast to more than 95 percent of normal rubella seronegative children who develop good levels of antibody after vaccination, the seronegative child with congenital rubella rarely responds (eg, only 2 of 21 such children had antibody boost to barely detectable levels).

Most infants with congenital rubella are no longer shedding virus and have a normal pattern of serum immunoglobulin at age 1 year. Rare infants, however, have persistent severe dysglobulinemia characterized by low levels of IgG with or without elevation of IgM. This may be associated with persistent infection and other evidence of altered immune response. Although evidence has been presented that lymphocytes from infants with congenital rubella failed to respond in vitro to the mitogenic stimulation of phytohemagglutinin and had an increased number of chromosomal gaps and breaks, further studies have not confirmed these observations.

Other Laboratory Study.   Since multisystem disease is common, many tests not involving the virus laboratory may be abnormal. A listing is beyond the scope of this text.

PROGNOSIS.   In a large group of infants with neonatal thrombocytopenic purpura, the mortality exceeded 35 percent after the first year of follow-up; this was not usually due to bleeding but to sepsis, congestive heart failure, and general debility. Overall mortality in a group with various abnormalities due to rubella was approximately 10 percent. Mortality is greatest during the first 6 months of life. The long-term outlook for many infants with severe cardiovascular disease and severe growth and psychomotor retardation is guarded. However, a surprising number of children with multisystem involvement make excellent adjustments over the years. The prognosis for a normal life is excellent for children with only minor defects, and Menser, Dods, and Harley have emphasized that the developmental potential of many patients has been significantly underestimated during their preschool years.

DIFFERENTIAL DIAGNOSIS.   Certain transient features of congenital rubella such as neonatal thrombocytopenic purpura, hepatosplenomegaly, hepatitis, and x-ray defects of the long bones are similar to those observed with other congenital infections such as cytomegalovirus, toxoplasmosis, and syphilis. Association with other evidence of rubella teratology such as cataracts, glaucoma, and typical cardiac defects or a positive maternal history of rubella frequently simplifies the differential diagnosis. Confirmation depends on specific laboratory tests, which are becoming available in many areas.

MANAGEMENT.   Infants with congenital rubella may be contagious as long as they are shedding this virus in their pharyngeal secretions. This problem is greatest during early infancy (Fig. 15). In general, infants who carry rubella for longer periods are the ones more severely damaged and retarded in growth and development, but in the absence of laboratory facilities one can only speculate about the probability that a given infant is contagious.

As in postnatal rubella, there is no specific therapy for congenital rubella. Since any organ system may be involved by this infection, consultation with other specialists should be sought when abnormalities are first suspected. A well-coordinated aggressive effort to deliver early comprehensive service to the infant with congenital rubella and his family can make an enormous difference in the ultimate life style of the entire family constellation. The importance of early detection of auditory and visual impairment and incorporation of adequate educational therapy including parent education and counseling cannot be overemphasized. Referral to centers with particular interest in congenital rubella is advisable whenever practical.

References

Best JM, Banatvola JE, Almeida JD, Waterson AP: Morphological characteristics of rubella virus. Lancet 2:237, 1967

Brody JA, Sever JL, Schiff GM: Prevention of rubella by gamma globulin during an epidemic in Barrow, Alaska in 1964. N Engl J Med 272:127, 1965

Green RH, Balsamo MR, Giles JP, Krugman S, Mirick GS: Studies of the natural history and prevention of rubella. Am J Dis Child 110:348, 1965

Gregg NM: Congenital cataract following German measles in the mother. Trans Ophthalmol Soc Aust 3:35, 1942

Horstmann DM, Liebhaber H, Le Bouvier GL, Rosenberg DA, Halstead SB: Rubella: reinfection of vaccinated and naturally immune persons exposed in an epidemic. N Engl J Med 283:771, 1970

Kenny FM, Michaels RH, Davis C: Rubella encephalopathy. Am J Dis Child 110:374, 1965

Menser MA, Dods L, Harley JD: A twenty-five year follow-up of congenital rubella. Lancet 2:1347, 1967

Naeye RL, Blanc W: Pathogenesis of congenital rubella JAMA 194:1277, 1965

Parkman PD, Buescher EL, Artenstein MS: Recovery of rubella virus from army recruits. Proc Soc Exp Biol Med 111:225, 1962

———— Meyer HM Jr, Kirschstein RL, Hopps HE: Development of a live attenuated rubella virus. N Engl J Med 275:569, 1966

Plotkin SA, Boue AM, Boue JG: The in vitro growth of rubella virus in human embryo cells. Am J Epidemiol 81:71, 1965

Proceedings of the International Conference on Rubella Immunization, 1969. Am J Dis Child 118:1, 1969

Rawls WE, Desmyter J, Melnick JL: Serologic diagnosis and fetal involvement in maternal rubella. JAMA 203:627, 1968

Rubella Symposium Issue. Am J Dis Child 110:345, 1965

Sever JL, Schiff GM, Huebner RJ: Frequency of rubella antibody among pregnant women and other human and animal populations. Obstet Gynecol 23:153, 1964

Siegal M, Fuerst HT, Peress NS: Fetal mortality in maternal rubella: results of a prospective study from 1957–1964. Am J Obstet Gynecol 96:247, 1966

Stewart GL, Parkman PD, Hopps HE, Douglas RD, Meyer HM Jr: Development of a rubella virus hemagglutination inhibition test. N Engl J Med 276:554, 1967

Townsend JJ, Baringer JR, Wolensky JS, et al: Progressive rubella panencephalitis: late onset after congenital rubella. N Engl J Med 292:990, 1975

Weil ML, Itabashi HH, Cremer NE, et al: Chronic progressive panencephalitis due to rubella virus simulating SSPE. N Engl J Med 292:994, 1975

SMALLPOX
C. HENRY KEMPE

Smallpox (variola major and variola minor) is an acute, highly contagious exanthematous disease caused by a specific filterable virus and characterized by a 3-day preeruptive febrile period that is followed by a generalized eruption. It is a disease of great antiquity known to have been endemic in Asia and Africa for many centuries before its introduction into Europe by the Saracens in the Middle Ages. Brought to America by the Spanish explorers, it soon devastated the native Indian population. During the seventeenth and eighteenth centuries smallpox was the most deadly epidemic disease in Europe and America; but following Jenner's demonstration in 1798 of the value of cowpox as a preventive of smallpox, and the subsequent popularization of vaccination, the incidence of variola major has been dramatically reduced. Outbreaks still occur sporadically through importation of virus from endemic centers in Southeast Asia, Central Africa, and Central and South America. The world's total incidence is about 400,000 cases annually.

A milder type of smallpox (variola minor) appeared with the Brazil epidemic of 1910, to which the name alastrim was given. Smallpox occurring in a partially immune subject produces another mild form, often referred to as varioloid.

ETIOLOGY. Variola virus is comparatively large, having a diameter of about 200 mμ. When viewed through the light microscope its particles are barely discernible and appear spherical in shape, but studies with the electron microscope show single elements to be shaped like bricks, with central circular, denser areas. The central body, which contains deoxyribonucleic acid, has certain characteristics of a nucleus. Variola virus appears to be indistinguishable from vaccinia virus, both in appearance and in its chemical constituents. It withstands drying for many months, even when kept at room temperature. Anaerobic conditions favor survival.

Smallpox occurs more commonly in the colder months of the winter and spring than in summer. While susceptibility is universal, there being no natural immunity, the disease does not have the epidemic potential of either chickenpox or measles. The number of vaccinated individuals in the community seems to determine the spread of the virus in a given outbreak. During the incubation period exposed persons are not infectious, but with the onset of the fever that heralds viremia, the possibility of transmission of the disease by way of secretions of the nose and throat can be assumed. Virus has been demonstrated in the saliva on the first day of the skin rash. In cases of hemorrhagic smallpox the patient may be infectious throughout the febrile period.

Infection probably spreads from the mouth and upper respiratory tract in the preeruptive stages; later the skin lesions contribute the bulk of infectious particles to the patient's environment. Spread of infection is sometimes indirect; infected cotton or bed linen has been responsible for secondary cases not in direct contact with patients.

PATHOLOGY. The site of entry of the virus is believed to be the mucous membrane of the upper respiratory tract. The site of viral multiplication during the 12-day incubation period is not known, but the patient is not infectious. It is likely that primary multiplication of smallpox virus occurs early in the lymphoid tissue of the respiratory tract; a transient primary viremia then occurs, which results in infection of the cells of the reticuloendothelial system and further multiplication of the virus within these cells. The onset of the febrile illness occurs with the liberation of virus particles from the cells of the reticuloendothelial system and heralds the secondary and more severe viremia. This secondary viremia is also short-lived, because while virus can sometimes be isolated from the patient's blood during the first 40 hours of the clinical illness, it is usually not found in the blood after the second day of fever except in patients who are destined to die. Lesions that later appear in the skin and mucous membranes undoubtedly result from dissemination of the virus at this time.

The earliest pathologic change seen on histologic examination is dilatation of the blood vessels in the corium and edema of the papillary body, followed by perivascular concentration of mononuclear cells. Epithelial cells of the malpighian layer swell and undergo degeneration. Fluid collects and a loculated vesicle is formed. There then occurs a migration of mononuclear and polymorphonuclear cells from the engorged capillaries of the corium to the damaged epithelial layers to form a pustule. In cases of hemorrhagic smallpox there is extensive hemorrhage in the dermis, and the overlying epithelial cells may show necrosis. As the pustules dry, scabs form that consist of cellular exudate and necrotic epithelium, under which new epithelium grows in from the sides. The peripheral blood shows initial leukopenia with relative lymphocytosis. As secondary infection of pustules occurs, leukocytosis follows.

In patients who die during the early stages of the disease, the lungs frequently show pneumonic exudate, and hemorrhages are found in the alveoli. Hemorrhages may also be found in the submucosa of the intestinal tract, and focal areas of round cell infiltration may be seen in all other organs. In cases of hemorrhagic smallpox, extensive petechial hemorrhages may be seen in all organs.

Cytoplasmic inclusion bodies (Guarnieri bodies) are seen in the skin lesions of smallpox. These are generally eosinophilic; they have a granular appearance with an irregular outline and may be as large as the nucleus.

SYMPTOMS. The incubation period averages 12 days, with a range of 10 to 16 days. The onset of illness is abrupt and is characterized by high fever (to 40 C) accompanied by delirium, toxemia, headache, backache, and vomiting. The child is apprehensive and appears severely ill. The preeruptive febrile period generally lasts 3 days, the exanthem appearing toward the end of the third or the beginning of the fourth day, usually after appreciable symptomatic improvement. The eruption has a typical centrifugal distribution, being more marked on face, forearms, hands, legs, and feet than on the trunk. It quickly progresses through the papular and vesicular stages to the pustular stage. Characteristically, in each skin area affected, lesions tend to be at the same stage of development. Promptly after the appearance of the rash the child may feel better, and the temperature may drop slightly. Lesions are commonly seen on the mucous membranes of the mouth and throat, but these do not go on to pustulation. The pustular stage, occurring within a few hours of the vesicular eruption, usually begins on the fifth day of disease and is frequently accompanied by a secondary fever and a rise in leukocyte count. Pustules usually dry after 8 to 10 days and form scabs that drop off in the course of the next 3 weeks.

A direct relationship exists between the nature and extent of the rash and the severity of the disease. Thus a partially immune child may have a mild febrile illness that never progresses to eruption (*variola sine eruptione*). Modified cases of smallpox in vaccinated children, or in young infants who have acquired transplacental passive immunity, may have only a few discrete lesions. In other cases the eruption may be profuse or even confluent. In hemorrhagic smallpox, lesions generally do not progress beyond the papular or vesicular stage, and extensive bleeding occurs into the lesions as well as elsewhere.

Infants with smallpox commonly experience febrile convulsions, vomiting, and diarrhea in the preeruptive phase. The fever generally remains high as the eruption appears, usually for 2 days rather than for 3 days after the onset of the illness.

The preeruptive stage of variola minor (alastrim) may simulate that of variola major, but is usually much less severe. It is presumably due to an attenuated strain of virus. The distribution and course of the eruption are the same, but the rash is generally much more mild, and secondary fever is uncommon. The disease is indistinguishable from mild cases of variola major in well-vaccinated children. The two types of disease are entirely distinct, and an outbreak of variola minor (alastrim) never gives rise to cases of variola major. The two types may exist simultaneously as two spontaneous outbreaks, as in Detroit in 1924.

COMPLICATIONS. Pyogenic infections of the skin and joints as well as osteomyelitis occur frequently unless antibacterial prophylaxis is employed. While accompanying pneumonitis is probably evidence of variola virus multiplication, secondary bacterial pneumonia can occur late in the pustular stage. Blindness may result from corneal lesions. A demyelinating encephalitis and peripheral neuritis may also occur.

DIAGNOSIS. In the presence of an epidemic, smallpox may be diagnosed with relative ease in the preeruptive febrile stage, with accuracy by blood tests, and with strong probability on clinical evidence alone. At the very onset of an epidemic or in a sporadic case, a mistaken diagnosis of influenza or dengue is commonly entertained in older children, while in infants or small children any infectious disease may be suspected.

Occasionally a severe case of varicella causes difficulty, but a careful search will usually reveal lesions of different ages. Eczema vaccinatum may suggest smallpox if a history of vaccination or of contact with a successfully vaccinated person is not obtained.

When a typical eruption occurs in a subject whose disease has not been modified by active or passive immunity, the diagnosis of smallpox presents no great difficulty. In these circumstances the steps required to prevent spread of infection should be taken promptly without waiting for results of laboratory tests.

There are three main diagnostic tests available, each of which has special value, depending on the stage of disease and the type of specimen that can be obtained: (1) Smears on clean glass slides from scrapings of the bases of smallpox lesions can be examined microscopically for virus elementary bodies. A positive answer may be obtained within 1 hour. (2) Complement-fixation tests can be used in two ways: to detect the presence of free antigen (virus) in the patient's blood in the preeruptive febrile stage of the disease or in the skin lesions from the earliest time of their appearance until the last scabs fall off; to detect antibodies in the patient's serum. Results are available in 24 hours. (3) Virus isolation is relatively easy on the chorioallantoic membrane of the embryonated egg, utilizing the patient's blood in the first 2 or 3 days of illness (preeruptive phase) or material from skin lesions (eruptive or scabbing phase). Virus isolation is the most conclusive test, but results are not obtainable for 72 hours.

Collection of Specimens

Blood: Collect 5 ml of venous blood. Allow it to clot and separate the serum under sterile conditions. Freeze both serum and clot separately for shipment to the laboratory. Smears: Scrape the bases of several lesions with a sharp blade onto clean glass slides and allow them to dry. Smears are of particular value in the papulovesicular phase of the eruption. Vesicle or pustule fluid: Aspirate several vesicles or pustules, utilizing a tuberculin syringe with a small needle. After obtaining approximately 0.2 ml of fluid, place both the syringe and the needle, together with the contents, in a large tube. Seal securely, wrap, and forward, preferable refrigerated with solid carbon dioxide, to the laboratory. All specimens must be careful labeled "Caution! Contains material from suspected smallpox patient. Vaccinate all persons in contact with this material."

PROGNOSIS. Case fatality rates vary directly with the severity of illness. Hemorrhagic smallpox tends to be fatal in more than 98 percent of cases, confluent smallpox in 50 percent, and discrete smallpox in less than 8 percent. While the average case fatality rate of variola major continues to be about 30 percent, that of variola minor is less than 1 percent.

TREATMENT. There is no specific antibiotic therapy for smallpox. However, penicillin and the broad-spectrum antibiotics are highly effective in preventing secondary bacterial complications that frequently occur during and after the pustular phase of the disease. Procaine penicillin, 600,000 IU/day intramuscularly, or one of the tetracyclines in doses ranging from 25 to 50 mg/kg/day intramuscularly is indicated.

Hyperimmune vaccinal gamma globulin produced from the serum of recently vaccinated adults has been shown to be effective in the modification of smallpox in children known to have been exposed to the disease, provided it is given before the onset of fever. No observations are available on the use of hyperimmune vaccinal gamma globulin in the therapy of early smallpox.

N-methylisatin 3-thiosemicarbazone (Marboran) is now under trial as a therapeutic agent in the early stages of smallpox. Another thiosemicarbazone, 4-bromo-3-methylisothiozole-5-carboxaldehyde-thiosemicarbazone, is also being tested. There is some slight indication that the latter drug may decrease the mortality rate in severe smallpox in vaccinated patients.

In serious cases of smallpox in children, severe dehydration may result from the pain associated with swallowing. Intravenous fluid therapy may be difficult in the face of massive skin involvement. Increased fluid requirements are, of course, associated with any febrile illness, and fluid loss from skin lesions may be considerable. Oliguria and renal insufficiency may become irreversible. Early use of intensive parenteral fluid therapy or of gastric feeding through a polyethylene tube holds promise. Baths and local applications to the skin are to be discouraged. It is important, however, to attempt to clean the eyes with warm normal saline solution in order to prevent matting and to decrease the chance of permanent involvement of the cornea. In severe confluent smallpox and in hemorrhagic smallpox, shocklike states have been observed frequently; plasma, hydrocortisone, or prednisone may be of value in management of the most critical phase. Oxygen and, when indicated, digitalis are of considerable help.

PROPHYLAXIS. The general measures to be taken on the discovery of a case of smallpox include immediate vaccination of contacts, removal of the patient to an isolation hospital, and prompt revaccination of all hospital personnel. Some sanitary codes require that the patient's house be disinfected. All contacts of the patient during the infective period of the disease must be closely supervised for 16 days. Detailed inquiry into the source of infection may result in the discovery of a mild or atypical primary case and the subsequent discovery of other secondary cases. The immediate use of laboratory aids may be of value in identifying doubtful cases.

Active immunization of close contacts, by vaccination after exposure, generally will not protect from the disease; many fatal infections have occurred in individuals successfully vaccinated 9 days before the onset of illness. However, vaccinia immune gamma globulin prepared from the serum of recently vaccinated adults and injected intramuscularly into household contacts of smallpox patients may provide protection. Vaccinia immune gamma globulin administered soon after known exposure provides passive immunity some time prior to the viremia that signals the onset of clinical disease.

Vaccinia immune gamma globulin is given intramuscularly in a single dose of 0.12 to 0.24 ml/kg body weight. Requests for the globulin can be made at any hour to regional consultants for the Center for Disease Control. These consultants are authorized to release vaccinia immune globulin. If the regional consultant is not known, the information may be obtained by calling the Center for Disease Control, Atlanta, Georgia (day: 404-633-3311; night: 404-633-2176). The globulin may also be obtained commercially from Hyland Laboratories, Costa Mesa, California (714-540-5000). The vaccinia immune gamma globulin should be given 12 to 24 hours after the person exposed to smallpox is vaccinated.

Marboran has been shown to greatly reduce the incidence of smallpox after exposure to the disease. This is true when the drug is used alone or in conjunction with vaccination. Among more than 1,100 household contacts who were given Marboran by mouth, only three mild cases of smallpox occurred. In a control group similar in number, age, and percentage vaccinated after exposure to smallpox, there were 78 cases of smallpox and 12 deaths. The drug was shown to be effective even when given more than 6 days after contact with a smallpox patient. For prophylaxis, Marboran is given in doses of 1.5 to 3.0 g twice a day for 4 days. It very frequently causes vomiting, and an antiemetic should be used with it.

Immunity to smallpox is possible only in the presence of antibody, either acquired passively from the maternal circulation in infants less than 6 months of age or developed actively following smallpox vaccination or recovery from smallpox. In highly endemic areas, such successful vaccination confers solid immunity for approximately 1 year. Partial immunity may be conferred for many years, but in the presence of virulent smallpox yearly vaccination is required.

VACCINIA. Smallpox vaccine commonly in use is prepared from the vaccinia lesions on the skin of inoculated calves or sheep or from the allantoic membranes of chick embryos. All currently used smallpox vaccine contains infective virus, and all successful vaccinations are deliberately induced mild viral infections. It is thought that within 1 year after primary vaccination the risk of an attack is 0.001 the risk in the unvaccinated, within 3 years it is 0.005, within 10 years it is 0.125, and within 20 years it is 0.5. After 20 years there is little if any protection from clinical infections. However, the mortality in smallpox patients successfully vaccinated many years before is less than in the unvaccinated. There is no question that regular revaccination induces a high degree of immunity even to very massive exposure to the disease. Mass vaccination in the remaining endemic areas in Asia and Africa will in time reduce the susceptible population below that necessary to permit the survival of the pathogenic virus.

VACCINATION PROGRAM. The U. S. Public Health Advisory Committee on Immunization Practices, supported by the Committee on Infectious Diseases of the American Academy of Pediatrics, has concluded that nonselective smallpox vaccination of the public is no longer justifiable and has recommended discontinuation of routine and compulsory smallpox vaccination in the United States:

"The policy of nonselective vaccination for protection against smallpox began when smallpox was widespread and uncontrolled. Under those conditions, it was a rational, necessary procedure, and legal regulations were passed to ensure vaccination of the public.

"Today, nonselective vaccination against smallpox unnecessarily exposes a large segment of the United States public to the risk of complications resulting from vaccination—a risk greater than the probability of their contracting the disease.

"The probability of contracting smallpox in the United States today is extremely low and continues to decrease. There has not been a documented case of this disease in the United States since 1949, and importation is the only way in which smallpox could occur in this country. Importation is unlikely because worldwide eradication efforts have brought about a significant decrease in the number of cases of smallpox and in the number of smallpox-endemic areas. In this country, there is a national surveillance system to identify suspect cases. Upon confirmation of a suspect case, there are efficient emergency procedures for managing the case and contacts and preventing spread of the disease. For most people in the United States, the probability of contracting smallpox is so small that the risk of complications from vaccination outweighs the benefits derived from it. For this reason, nonselective vaccination of the public is no longer justifiable. Vaccination should routinely be required only of people at special risk: travelers to and from countries where smallpox is still endemic and health services personnel who come into contact with patients."

CONTRAINDICATIONS TO VACCINATION. We now recommend that routine vaccination of children not be carried out in the United States. At present (1976) smallpox is endemic in only one country, Ethiopia, and it is expected that the worldwide eradication of smallpox will occur in the near future. However, proof of vaccination within the past 3 years is required for travelers entering some countries. There continues to be a need, therefore, to emphasize and to observe scrupulously the contraindications to vaccination.

Primary routine vaccination is generally contraindicated in patients with failure to thrive, dysgammaglobulinemia, blood dyscrasias, eczema or other dermatitides, and radiation or other immunosuppressive therapy, as well as in those exposed to infectious diseases. Vaccination is also contraindicated in unvaccinated siblings of children with eczema. In the eczematous child, vaccination can safely be carried out with attenuated vaccine or under the cover of vaccinia immune gamma globulin during a period when the skin is relatively clear. If vaccination is carried out under these circumstances, it will spare the child the danger of acquiring accidental infection from a sibling or playmate at a time when he is not properly protected.

In adults, vaccination or revaccination is fraught with danger for patients with neoplastic diseases, including

Hodgkin's disease, lymphomas, and other conditions involving the prolonged use of corticosteroids, nitrogen mustard, or radiation therapy.

In view of the new recommendations of the USPHS, travel to nonepidemic areas outside the United States by a person who has an absolute contraindication such as eczema or a neoplastic disease should no longer present a problem, since smallpox vaccination would not be required on reentering the country. If such a person must travel to an endemic area, the use of vaccinia immune gamma globulin or chemoprophylaxis with Marboran should be considered so as to provide temporary protection and act as a substitute for the use of vaccination with live vaccinia virus.

VACCINATION TECHNIQUES. To minimize the risk of unnecessary complications, the following practices are recommended:

Age. In nonendemic areas, primary vaccination is best carried out when the child is between 1 and 2 years of age. There are no conclusive data indicating the exact period when complication rates are minimal. Transplacental maternal immunity may modify early primary vaccination and, in endemic areas, make it desirable to vaccinate in the first month of life, provided the mother has been vaccinated. Vaccination of newborn infants has been carried out without complications. However, in such cases in endemic areas, revaccination should be carried out after an interval of 6 months. If primary vaccination is delayed for several months, children who are at increased risk, such as those suffering from the Swiss type of agammaglobulinemia, will have been readily identified by their clinical course and will therefore not become casualties of smallpox vaccination.

Site. Primary vaccination and revaccination are best performed on the outer aspects of the upper arm, over the insertion of the deltoid muscle, or behind the midline. Reactions are less likely to be severe on the upper arm than on the lower extremities or other parts of the body. With proper technique, resultant scars are small and unobtrusive.

Preparation of Site. With a clean skin, the best preparation is none at all. Chemical skin cleansers may leave a residue that contains virus-inactivating material, while vigorous physical cleansing of the site may create minute abrasions that then can become the site of secondary vaccinia eruptions, with resultant involvement of a comparatively large skin area.

Technique. Regardless of age, routine primary vaccination should be carried out with no more than two or three pressures being made with the side of a needle. These pressure points should be in as close proximity as possible, and carried out only at one site. With the highly potent vaccines currently in use, more numerous pressures are not necessary and should not be utilized in a nonimmune individual. When children or adults are to be revaccinated after a lapse of more than 5 years, the same small number of pressures should be used. For revaccination within a 5 year period, in individuals known to have had a major reaction, the full complement of 30 strokes can safely be used.

Reaction. The terminology for the reactions after vaccination or revaccination should follow that recommended by the Expert Committee on Smallpox of the World Health Organization. A successful primary vaccination is one that on examination after 7 to 10 days presents a typical Jennerian vesicle. If this is not present, vaccination must be repeated with fresh vaccine, applying a few more strokes of the needle. The successful revaccination is one that on examination 1 week (6 to 10 days) later shows a vesicular or pustular lesion, or an area of definite palpable induration and congestion surrounding a central lesion; this lesion may be a scab or an ulcer. These reactions are termed *major reactions;* all others should be called *equivocal reactions*. A major reaction indicates viral multiplication with consequent development of immunity. An equivocal reaction may merely represent an allergic response, which could be elicited by inactive vaccine or poor technique in someone who had been sensitized by earlier vaccination, or the equivocal reaction may result from sufficient immunity to prevent viral multiplication. Since the allergic response cannot be readily differentiated from the one due to true immunity, another vaccination should be performed using a different lot of vaccine if there is the possibility that it is of weak potency, and the procedure should be completed with an additional number of pressures. The site should be examined 1 week later, and if the result is again equivocal, revaccination should be repeated using a full 30 pressures as recommended by Leake. For the sake of expediency, an equivocal reaction to revaccination with a minimal insertion may be followed by vaccination at two sites, not less than 2 inches apart, using known potent vaccine. This method will make a third return unnecessary in almost all instances.

In summary, successful smallpox vaccination consists of the production of a major reaction. When potent vaccine and good technique are used, the repeated inability to produce a major reaction can be assumed to be due to solid immunity from previous immunization.

Frequency. Revaccination is essential to reinforce the immunity conferred by previous vaccination. This not only maintains a high level of immunity against smallpox but minimizes the risk of complications on revaccination. To maintain adequate immunity against smallpox, revaccination should be carried out at approximately 5-year intervals. Those at some increased risk, such as hospital personnel and public health personnel, members of the armed forces, and those working at port or airline offices, as well as shipping personnel, should be revaccinated at least once every 3 years. When exposure to smallpox is probable, by travel or residence in a smallpox-endemic area, annual revaccination is desirable.

Complications. The true rate of complications in the United States is not known and is confused by the inclusion of more severe primary reactions among the complications. Complications are not reportable diseases through any of the usual state health department methods. Life-threatening complications of primary vaccination include eczema vaccinatum, postvaccinal encephalitis, and vaccinia gangrenosa (progressive vaccinia). The principal danger after revaccination is vaccinia gangrenosa, a condition in which the impairment of the patient's immune mechanism permits the continuing multiplication of the vaccinia virus. Vaccinia gangrenosa is seen in seemingly normal individuals as well as those suffering from dysgammaglobulinemia, Hodgkin's disease, leukemia, blood dyscrasias, and other conditions in which steroid therapy or ionizing irradiation have been administered therapeutically. The presence of these conditions is an absolute contraindication to vaccination. Human vaccinial immune globulin (VIG) has frequently been shown to be effective in the prevention and treatment of eczema vaccinatum and has also been used extensively in the treatment of other complications, where it also produces a significant reduction in mortality. VIG reduces the incidence of postvaccinal encephalitis. Of 106,674 recruits of the Royal Netherlands Army, 53,630 received hyperimmune vaccinia immune gamma globulin, while the remaining 53,044 received a placebo. In the gamma-globulin-treated group, 3 cases of postvaccinal encephalitis occurred, as against 13 in the control group, with one fatality occurring in each group. Gamma globulin failed to have a major effect on the severity and duration of the encephalitis produced by the vaccination, and it was not effective in treatment. There is evidence that transplacental maternal immunity is also effective in modifying the course of primary vaccination; significant reactions are rarely reported in the very young infant whose mother has been vaccinated in the past. In cases of vaccinia gangrenosa, the simultaneous use of vaccinia immune globulin and Marboran appears to be of value. The therapeutic dose of the drug is 200 mg/kg orally initially, followed by 50 mg/kg every 6 hours for 3 days. After a rest of 3 days, another 3-day course may be required.

Adequate early treatment of the complications of smallpox vaccination can materially reduce the morbidity and mortality. Through the Center for Disease Control, experts are available for telephone consultation. When such consultation is used in conjunction with VIG and chemotherapeutic agents, effective diagnostic and therapeutic aids are available for all.

CONCLUSIONS.   We in the United States are now in an interim period in regard to smallpox prophylaxis. Whereas the areas of the globe where smallpox is endemic are gradually being diminished, there is an increased chance of exposure as a result of increasing travel to and from smallpox-endemic regions. A number of changes in vaccination practice are indicated to avoid unnecessary complications. Reducing the risk of vaccinia complications by a more gentle vaccination technique and the recognition (and legal acceptance) of additional medical contraindications will help to eliminate many of the opportunities for complications to develop. It is likely that either modified live vaccinia virus or a killed product will soon be available for prevaccination in an effort to make possible safe immunization of those who require it.

References

SMALLPOX

Public Health Service Advisory Committee on Immunization Practices: Smallpox vaccination of hospital and health personnel. Morbidity Mortality 25:9, 1976

VACCINIA

Krugman S, Katz S: Smallpox vaccination. N Engl J Med 281:1241, 1969

Lane JM, Millar HD: Routine childhood vaccination against smallpox reconsidered. N Engl J Med 281:1220, 1969

——— et al: Complications of smallpox vaccination. N Engl J Med 281:1201, 1969

ORNITHOSIS, LYMPHOGRANULOMA, TRACHOMA, AND INCLUSION CONJUNCTIVITIS

The agents that cause this group of diseases belong to a single genus, *Chlamydia* (formerly called Bedsoniae), and they are more closely related to bacteria than to viruses. They are obligate intracellular parasites that have enzymes to synthesize proteins and nucleic acids. The chlamydiae have a common morphology and a common family antigen. Multiplication occurs by binary fission. In infected tissues they produce intracytoplasmic aggregates or elementary bodies, which are sometimes visible by light microscopy when stained with Giemsa or other basophilic dyes. Unlike most viruses, they are susceptible in vitro to sulfonamides, penicillin, tetracyclines, and other antibiotics, although the responses of patients with clinical disease are not always dramatic. Infection can be transmitted to animals experimentally, and the chlamydiae can be grown in the yolk sac of chick embryo.

ORNITHOSIS

Ornithosis was originally called psittacosis when its transmission to man from psittacine birds, chiefly parrots, parakeets, and lovebrids, was established. Subsequently the avian reservoir was found to be much larger, including pigeons, doves, chickens, turkeys, and pheasants. The bird that transmits the infection may be ill or may have an inapparent infection without recognizable symptoms. Close contact, as with a household pet, can often be established. Cases of ornithosis have been reported from all parts of the world, and all age groups are believed susceptible. Since the disease is not universally reportable, its exact incidence and distribution are not accurately known, but as many as 444 cases have been recorded in a single year from all parts of the United States. The disease, besides being an occupational hazard of commercial bird handlers, is also at time responsible for localized household epidemics. Direct transmission of the infection from man to man appears to be possible. Serologic evidence strongly suggests that in some instances infection produces negligible symptoms.

In fatal cases the principal lesions are found in the lungs. There is patchy bronchopneumonia, sometimes with moderately large confluent areas of consolidation. Lymphocytes, histiocytes, and plasma cells predominate in the exudate, although polymorphonuclear cells may be found as well. Bacterial infection may be superimposed. Pleural effusion, splenic enlargement, and meningitis have been described.

The symptoms of ornithosis are those of a respiratory infection with a bothersome dry cough usually accompanied by weakness and anorexia out of proportion to the fever, which is often mild. Splenomegaly may be found. More rarely, jaundice, convulsions, meningitic signs, and abdominal pain have been described. The leukocyte count is either normal or low. Radiographs of the lungs frequently show faint and poorly localized shadows suggesting parenchymal involvement, less often a clearcut picture of pneumonia or pleural effusion. The patient responds little, if at all, to antibacterial therapy. Active illness lasts from a few days to 3 or 4 weeks.

History of contact with a sick bird, perhaps a household pet or an unexpectedly friendly pigeon, provides an important diagnostic lead, although in many cases this information is lacking. Clear proof of the diagnosis during life may be obtained by recovery of the agent from the patient's blood after inoculation into the yolk sac of a chick embryo or by demonstration of a rise in titer of complement-fixing antibody during an interval of 2 to 6 weeks. In some cases in which verification of the diagnosis is sought late in the course, after the organism is no longer in the blood, a high initial titer followed 6 months or so later by a fall may be taken as strongly suggestive of an attack of ornithosis. In fatal cases the agent is usually recoverable from pulmonary tissue.

Tetracycline is probably the most effective drug for the treatment of ornithosis. It should be continued for at least 10 days after the temperature returns to normal in order to minimize the danger of relapse.

Fatalities are rare in childhood. Convalescence is sometimes prolonged. Late residua have not been described.

LYMPHOGRANULOMA

Lymphogranuloma venereum (lymphogranuloma inguinale) is occasionally seen in young children, who may acquire it by direct transmission from an infected adult. The primary lesion consists of a vesicle and subsequent ulcer, both of which are usually missed entirely, enlargement of lymph nodes being the first feature to attract attention. The nodes of the groin are commonly involved, although nodes in other areas, such as the neck, may be the only ones noticed to be enlarged. In some cases neither the initial ulcer nor lymphadenopathy is observed, residual scarring being responsible for the first symptoms; in these cases the most common syndrome is lower bowel obstruction from rectal stricture.

The lesion in biopsied material consists of a chronic inflammatory reaction in the involved lymph nodes and surrounding structures. There is conspicuous infiltration of cellular tissue with lymphocytes, histiocytes, and plasma cells; granulocytes, including eosinophils, and giant cells may also be found. Bacteria are absent, but basophilic cytoplasmic inclusions within macrophages may be seen, sometimes in the form of the fine granules, at other times as rounded masses as large as the nucleus or even larger.

Involved lymph nodes are sometimes painful as well as tender, and in the course of enlargement they tend to adhere both to each other and to the overlying skin. Suppuration may occur, with discharge and sinus formation; however, as a rule the nodes change but little in consistency, remaining firm and gradually becoming less tender. In the early stages there may be some fever and malaise, but in general the systemic symptoms are mild. Scarlatiniform eruptions and erythema nodosum have been described, and splenic enlargement and generalized lymphadenopathy may be observed. Meningitic symptoms are seen in some cases, but rarely is any change found in the cerebrospinal fluid. The organisms may be detected in the blood.

The agent may be recovered throughout most of the course of the infection. Almost equally strong proof of etiology is provided by demonstrating a fourfold or greater rise in titer of complement-fixing antibody between acute-phase serum sample and convalescent-phase sample. The antigen generally used is grown in chick embryo tissue culture. Demonstration of antibody at a level of 1:32 or greater, even without subsequent rise in titer, is almost equally significant. The Frei test, a skin test made originally with heat-killed material obtained from a bubo, but now more commonly with tissue culture antigen, is carried out by intracutaneous injection and is read in much the same manner as a tuberculin test. When positive, it supports the clinical diagnosis of lymphogranuloma venereum. However, a negative test may be obtained both early and late in the disease at a time when the complement-fixing antibody is readily demonstrable and even while organisms are in the blood, a circumstance that detracts greatly from the value of the Frei test. Adrenocorticosteroids have been shown to suppress a positive test.

Differential diagnosis of chronic focal lymphadenopathy must include, in addition to lymphogranuloma venereum, chronic pyogenic bacterial infection, tuberculosis, tularemia, cat-scratch disease, and lymphoma or other neoplasm. Lymphogranuloma must be considered in all cases of rectal stricture.

Treatment, as in ornithosis, consists in administration of full doses of a sulfonamide, pencillin, or tetracycline or some combination of them. Excision of lymph nodes has been employed, but it should not be necessary. Rectal stricture may respond to carefully graduated dilation.

TRACHOMA AND INCLUSION CONJUNCTIVITIS

The trachoma and inclusion conjunctivitis (blennorrhea) agents are classified as members of the psittacosis group because they share morphologic and biologic characteristics, as well as the group antigen, with other members of the group. The TRIC (trachoma inclusion conjunctivitis) agents can be grown in the yolk sacs of embryonated eggs.

Trachoma infects many inhabitants of Africa and Asia. In the United States it is endemic in Indian reservations. Trachoma infection is limited to the eye. In endemic areas, agents shed from the eyes of active patients cause infection in early childhood that progresses slowly toward blindness. Initial manifestations include conjunctival hyperemia, follicular hypertrophy, lacrimation, and discharge from the eye. Inward curvature of the eyelids and lashes, conjunctival scarring, and corneal vascularization and opacification occur later. Either topical tetracycline therapy or systemic sulfonamides instituted early in the course of infection can cure trachoma infections and lead to complete healing. Conjunctival scarring and corneal vascularization and opacification are not reversible.

The inclusion conjunctivitis agent resides in the genital tract (cervix and urethra) of adults, and newborns are infected at the time of birth. The manifestations in newborns consist of an acute purulent conjunctivitis that occurs between 5 and 17 days after birth. Without therapy the disease progresses for 1 to 2 weeks and then gradually subsides over 3 to 6 months. The disease leaves no residual scarring, and corneal vascularization and opacification do not occur. The infection responds to topical therapy and tetracyclines. Adults can acquire a follicular nonpurulent conjunctivitis from swimming pools contaminated with genital secretions. Although the untreated infection can persist for months, it leaves without any residua. As in the newborn, topical tetracycline therapy quickly eliminates the infection.

References

ORNITHOSIS

Berman S, et al: Ornithosis in infancy. Pediatrics 15:752, 1955

Breton A, Gaudier B, Ponté C: L'ornithose-psittacose en pathologie infantile. Arch Fr Pediatr 17:879, 1960

Christensen PM: Ornithosis; a study of virus and antigen. Acta Pathol Microbiol Scand [Suppl] 118:1, 1957

Gordon FB, Harper IA, Quan AL, et al: Detection of Chlamydia (Bedsonia) in certain infections of man. J Infect Dis 120:451, 1968

Wang SP, Grayson JT: Classification of TRIC and related strains with micro immunofluorescence. In Nichols RL (ed): Trachoma and Related Disorders Caused by Chlamydial Agents. Princeton, Excepta Medica, 1971

LYMPHOGRANULOMA

Banov L Jr: Rectal lesions of lymphogranuloma venereum in children; review of the literature and report of a case in a ten-year-old boy with rectal stricture. Am J Dis Child 83:660, 1952

Favre M, Hellerström S: The epidemiology, aetiology and prophylaxis of lymphogranuloma inguinale. Acta Derm Venereol [Suppl 30] (Stockh) 34:1, 1954

Greaves AB, Taggart SR: Serology, Frei reaction, and epidemiology of lymphogranuloma venereum. Am J Syph 37:273, 1953

Levy H: Lymphogranuloma venereum in children. J Pediatr 11:812, 1937

Roth D, Schulick R: Isolated cervical lymphogranuloma venereum in a child. Pediatrics 8:489, 1951

SLOW VIRUS INFECTIONS
MICHAEL KATZ

Conventionally, virus infections have been considered to produce acute diseases with defined incubation periods of several days to several weeks and a rapid course terminating in either good health or death. Rarely such acute viral infections leave lifelong sequelae, such as deafness after mumps or paralysis after poliomyelitis. The concept of slow virus infections is relatively new, having been first proposed in 1954 by Bjorn Sigurdson in Iceland. In its current version this concept holds that there are host–virus interactions that develop on a time scale of years rather than weeks. The host suffers no disease during the very long incubation period, but once the disease has developed its course is relatively rapid and usually fatal. Their long course distinguish slow virus infections from chronic infections that are characterized by remissions and exacerbations.

According to Sigurdson's postulate, all of the stages of virus–cell interactions known to take place in the conventional infections also occur in the slow infections; only the time scale is stretched. Although this conception may not be entirely correct, there is at present no definitive explanation of the pathogenesis of slow virus infections that would apply in all instances. Thus the primary factors unifying these infections are the extraordinarily long incubation period and the almost invariable course of relentless deterioration usually leading to death.

Currently, slow virus infections are divided into those caused by unconventional and conventional agents. Among the first are the so-called spongiform encephalopathies. These diseases have incubation periods in experimental animals ranging between 18 months and 4 years. Their pathologic hallmark is vacuolization of the gray matter, resulting in status spongiosus; they are remarkably free of inflammatory reactions. Although the agents themselves have not been isolated, infection can be achieved by inoculation of tissue homogenates of the affected animals into other animals. Experimental studies, based on in vivo infection, have revealed that the infectious agents are quite resistant to physical modalities such as heat and radiation and to chemical agents such as fat solvents and proteolytic and nucleolytic enzymes. The agents are also quite small, the estimated size ranging from 27 nm to 7nm. They are thought to contain small quantities of nucleic acids tightly bound to cell membranes, which protects the nucleic acids from damage. The major example of a spongiform encephalopathy is scrapie in sheep. The only two human diseases in this category are kuru and Creutzfeldt-Jakob disease, which are quite rare.

Kuru has been known to occur only in the highlands of New Guinea, in the Fore people, among whom the disease is endemic. Until the mid-1960s kuru in adults showed predominance among women; children of both sexes were equally affected. Recently the incidence of kuru has been on the decrease, and the sex differential has virtually disappeared.

The earliest symptom of kuru is unsteadiness of gait, which evolves into ataxia. There are also personality changes leading to euphoria in some victims. Ultimately the victim becomes unable to walk and simply lies down and awaits death. Most victims of kuru die within 6 months of the onset of first symptoms, succumbing usually to secondary causes such as pneumonia. Few laboratory tests have been carried out on the afflicted individuals. Notably, the cerebrospinal fluid is normal. Primary pathologic changes are limited to gray matter, which shows astrocytosis, loss of neurons, and the vacuolization mentioned above.

The mode of transmission is uncertain, but it has been possible to transmit kuru experimentally to chimpanzees by inoculating them with brain homogenates of kuru victims. Intracerebral and extracerebral parenteral inoculation resulted in kuru after an incubation period ranging between 18 months and 4 years. In a transmission from chimpanzee to chimpanzee the incubation period was shortened in some instances to less than a year. It has been possible to transmit this disease to other simian hosts. Transmission through the oral route has not been successful. In view of its transmission by inoculation, it is possible that kuru in its natural setting has been transmitted during the process of ritual cannibalism, but probably only through contact of abraded skin with the diseased tissues rather than through ingestion. The relationship to cannibalism is supported circumstantially by the concomitant decrease in kuru with the decrease in cannibalism.

Creutzfeldt-Jakob disease has a worldwide distribution, but it is rare. It has not been described in children. Pathologically it resembles kuru and like kuru it has been transmitted to chimpanzees. There is no known therapy for either of these two diseases.

Slow virus infections due to conventional viruses probably result from an unusual host–virus relationship; thus they may be a consequence of an ineffective host response to the infectious organism. Tolerance of the infection may result either because it occurred at a time when the host was temporarily immunoincompetent or because of a genetically dependent specific immunoincompetence of a particular host. On the other hand it is possible that the agents, although conventional, may have become altered either before or during the process of the infection. They may therefore be different in some respect and thus be capable of developing a defective infection that is primarily intracellular and persistent, despite the presence of adequate immunologic host defense mechanisms. The defect may depend on development of defective interfering particles or on a fortuitous infection with a temperature-sensitive mutant that may be prevented from normal replication at the body temperature of the host.

Two human diseases have been attributed to such slow infections with conventional agents: subacute sclerosing panencephalitis (SSPE) and progressive multifocal leukoencephalopathy (PML). Isolation of viruses in vitro from patients with these diseases has been difficult and has depended on laborious rescue of the agents from the tissues of the patients. This has been accomplished by establishment of cell cultures from these tissues and by co-cultivation of them with human or simian tissue culture lines.

SSPE is a disease of children and young adults with an incidence of approximately 0.1/100,000. It has an insidious onset, with gradual impairment of the intellect and unusual behavior. Seizures begin early and are typically myoclonic. These evolve into sustained myoclonic seizures; the patient lapses into coma and becomes spastic and decorticate. The electroencephalogram has a characteristic burst-suppression pattern. Cerebrospinal fluid has increased concentration of gamma globulin. Death often is a result of an intercurrent bacterial infection. The course is variable in length, but most patients die within 2 years of the onset of their first symptoms. Rare long-term remissions have been reported. There is a strong etiologic association of SSPE with measles virus. All patients have elevated titers of serum and cerebrospinal fluid measles antibodies.

The histologic picture of the affected brain and spinal cord shows involvement of both gray and white matter, with perivascular cuffing, gliosis, and RNA-containing intranuclear inclusion bodies in the neurons and oligodendroglial cells. There is a substantial loss of neurons. Electron microscopic studies reveal nuclear and cytoplasmic accumulation of structures resembling nucleocapsids of a paramyxovirus. In a number of cases a measles-like virus has been rescued from explants of SSPE brain tissues. SSPE affects predominantly boys. Epidemiologic studies have shown that SSPE patients tend to have had measles early in life, before the age of 2 years.

It has not been possible to identify a definitive immune defect in SSPE patients, although specific failure of cell-mediated immunity and the presence of a circulating inhibitor of cell-mediated immunity have been suggested by several studies. On the other hand, viruses isolated from SSPE patients can be distinguished by their in vitro behavior from standard measles viruses, but not sufficiently so to consider them different viruses. The distinctions that have been observed may well have resulted from their prolonged residence in and adaptation to the brain tissue, which may have rendered them neurotropic. At the present time pathogenesis of SSPE remains obscure. There is no effective therapy.

PML is a rare degenerative demyelinating disease of the brain characterized by the development of bizarre giant astrocytes. It occurs usually in debilitated patients who are affected by a multisystem disease such as a lymphoma and who are therefore immunoincompetent. PML has been invariably fatal. It has not been reported in children. In all instances when the affected brain tissue has been examined under the electron microscope it was noted to contain structures resembling papovaviruses. Recently papovaviruses have been rescued from brain tissues of patients with PML. There have been no cases of PML among children.

Many diseases are candidates for consideration as slow virus infections, most prominently multiple sclerosis (MS). Viral etiology of MS has been postulated on epidemiologic grounds, and serologic studies have suggested an association between MS and measles and vaccinia viruses; however, these associations remain inconclusive. Although consistent isolations of viruses from MS brains have not been achieved, isolation of a parainfluenza 1 virus from two human patients with MS has been reported; its etiologic relationship to the basic disease is yet to be established.

There have been speculations on a priori grounds that epilepsia partialis continua, Alzheimer's disease, and some collagen diseases, notably lupus erythematosus, may also be examples of slow virus infections.

References

Gibbs CJ Jr, Gajdusek DC: Biology of kuru and Creutzfeldt-Jakob diseases. In Zeman W, Lennette E (eds): Slow Virus Diseases. Baltimore, Williams & Wilkins, 1974

Hotchin J (ed): Slow Virus Diseases. Prog in Med Virol, 18:1-350, 1974

——— Persistent and Slow Virus Infections. Monographs in Virology, Vol 3. Basel, Karger, 1971

Hunter GD: Scrapie, a prototype slow virus infection. J Infect Dis 125: 427, 1972

Katz M: Measles and central nervous system diseases; a critical appraisal. Med Microbiol Immunol 160:247, 1974

Koprowski H, Meulen V ter: Multiple sclerosis and parainfluenza 1 virus. J Neurol 208:175, 1975

Meulen V ter: Pathogenic aspects of measles virus infections. Med Microbiol Immunol 160:165, 1974

———Katz M, Müller D: Subacute sclerosing panencephalitis, a review. Curr Top Microbiol Immunol 57:1, 1972

Preble OT, Youngner J: Temperature sensitive viruses and the etiology of chronic and inapparent infections. J Infect Dis 131:467, 1975

Sell KW, Ahmed A, Strong DM: Plasma and spinal fluid blocking factor in SSPE. N Engl J Med 288:215, 1973

Weiner LP, Narayan O: Progressive multifocal leukoencephalopathy. In Thomas RA, Green JR (eds): Advances in Neurology. New York, Raven, 1974

Wolfgram F, Ellison GW, Stevens JG, Andrews TM: Multiple Sclerosis; Immunology, Virology, and Ultrastructure. UCLA Forum in Medical Sciences, No 16. New York, Academic, 1972

HUMAN RICKETTSIOSES

HERBERT L. DUPONT AND LARRY K. PICKERING

Rickettsiae are similar in size and morphologic structure to bacteria; they resemble this group of microorganisms also in that they divide by binary fission, they contain RNA and DNA, and their growth in vivo is inhibited by broad-spectrum antibiotics. However, rickettsiae are so fastidious that growth requirements are met only by an intracellular milieu. They can be propagated by inoculation into susceptible animals such as the guinea pig, mouse, and chick embryo. However, because of their high infectivity, cultivation in the laboratory is hazardous to exposed personnel. Rickettsiae appear as pleomorphic coccobacilli and are either purple or pink with Giemsa or Macchiavello stains. They are spread by blood-sucking insects, including lice, fleas, mites, and ticks.

Human rickettsioses, with the exception of Q fever, are primarily arthropod-borne diseases characterized by high fever and generalized rash. The most constant and outstanding clinical feature of rickettsial infection is an intense headache that usually is frontal or generalized and often is associated with retroorbital pain and photophobia. Rickettsial diseases are separated into four groups on the basis of epidemiologic, clinical, and serologic characteristics. Table 24 compares the various factors that characterize the important rickettsial diseases in man.

The pathologic lesion of the exanthematous arthropod-borne rickettsioses includes generalized involvement of small blood vessels observed especially in the skin, subcutaneous tissue, and central nervous system. The principal vascular changes consist of endothelial swelling and perivascular infiltration of mononuclear cells, plasma cells, and macrophages. In general the symptomatology correlates with the degree and location of vascular involvement. Q fever differs from other rickettsial diseases in that the usual mode of spread is through inhalation of the causative agent. Cutaneous involvement is not apparent, and disease generally is confined to the lungs and liver. Ticks are infected naturally, but they probably are not important vectors in the transmission of Q fever.

In the early 1900s Felix isolated a strain of *Proteus vulgaris* (OX-19) from the urine of a patient with typhus fever that was antigenically similar to *Rickettsia prowazekii*. The patient studied had high titers of OX-19 agglutinins. Such OX-19 antibodies are found uniformly in patients with epidemic or endemic (murine) typhus and Rocky Mountain spotted fever. Other *Proteus* strains have been related antigenically to the etiologic agents of scrub typhus (OX-K) and Rocky Mountain spotted fever (OX-2). *Proteus* agglutinins usually peak in titer after the second week of illness and fall to insignificant levels within 3 months following illness. Sera of patients with Q fever and rickettsialpox do not agglutinate the *Proteus* antigens used in the Weil-Felix reaction. Specific serologic reactions using rickettsial antigens in complement-fixation, agglutination, or neutralization tests are more reliable than the Weil-Felix reaction, since they identify the specific rickettsial infection. Complement-fixing antibodies may persist in low titers for a decade or more after a rickettsial infection.

The tetracycline antibiotics and chloramphenicol are very effective in the treatment of patients with rickettsial diseases. In scrub typhus, defervescence is dramatic within 24 hours; it is less rapid in patients with Rocky Mountain spotted fever and typhus fever. Relapses occur only if antibiotics are given very early in illness, prior to the fourth febrile day.

Tetracycline and chloramphenicol are rickettsiostatic drugs that suppress but do not destroy the organisms. It remains for the immune processes of the host to finally eradicate the infection. Also, these organisms

TABLE 24. Human Rickettsioses

	Typhus		Spotted Fever Group		Tsutsugamushi Fever	Q Fever
Disease	Epidemic typhus	Murine typhus	Rocky Mountain spotted fever	Rickettsialpox	Scrub typhus	Q fever
Rickettsia	*R. prowazekii*	*R. mooseri*	*R. rickettsii*	*R. akari*	*R. tsutsugamushi*	*Coxiella burnetii*
Arthropod vector	body louse	rat flea	tick	mouse mite	trombiculid mites	tick
Animal reservoir	man	rat	tick, small animals	house mouse	small rodents	cattle, sheep, goats, ticks (?)
Seasonal occurrence	Winter–Spring	Summer–Fall	Spring–Summer	Spring–Summer	Hot, rainy seasons (Summer)	Variable
Incubation period	7–14 days	7–12 days	2–14 days	2–7 days	10–18 days	9–21 days
Cutaneous manifestations	Spreads peripherally	Spreads peripherally	Spreads centrally, palms & soles	Initial lesion, generalized vesicles	Initial lesion, spreads peripherally	No rash
Mortality — Untreated	2–40% (depends on age)	2%	10–40%	0%	1–60% (depends on population)	< 1%
Treated	< 1%	0%	1–10%	0%	< 1%	0%
Weil-Felix reaction	OX=19	OX=19	OX=19 OX=2	None	OX=K	None
Complement fixation	Specific	Specific	Specific	Specific	None	Specific
Killed	Attenuates disease	Available, not adequately tested	Attenuates disease	None	Not available	Effective, high local reactivity
Live	Promising	None	None	None	None	Promising

Row-group labels (left margin): Epidemiology, Clinical, Serology, Vaccine

may remain intracellularly viable for years in various body tissues. Viable pathogenic rickettsiae have been isolated from the lymph nodes of patients convalescent from scrub typhus, epidemic typhus, and Rocky Mountain spotted fever. In the case of louse-borne (epidemic) typhus, recrudescence can result decades following symptomatic infection, which is known as Brill-Zinsser disease. General discussions of differential diagnosis and treatment are given in the sections dealing with specific rickettsial infections.

TYPHUS FEVERS

The three major diseases in this group are epidemic or louse-borne typhus, endemic or murine typhus, and Brill-Zinsser disease. The diseases show similar clinical characteristics, which makes differentiation difficult in the individual case. Louse-borne epidemic typhus is the most serious of the diseases and differs from the others in overall severity, including frequency of complications and case fatality rate. The three illnesses are characterized by high fever, skin eruption, and generalized vascular involvement. Except for the skin lesion, no finding is typical. Inflammatory lesions of small blood vessels occur in many organs of the body, including the skin, brain, spinal cord, heart, liver, kidneys, and spleen. Invasion of vascular endothelium may result in formation of mural thrombi, and areas of skin necrosis over pressure points or symmetric gangrene of the extremities may rarely be seen. The etiologic agents of epidemic and endemic typhus are antigenically similar, and cross-reaction occurs with *Proteus* or rickettsial complement-fixation and agglutination tests. They usually can be distinguished by specific complement-fixation and agglutination tests and by the inability of the etiologic agent of epidemic typhus (*R. prowazekii*) to produce a scrotal reaction in guinea pigs (tunical vaginalis inflammation).

The differential diagnosis of typhus fever includes the other rickettsial diseases, meningococcemia, rubeola, typhoid fever, malaria, acquired toxoplasmosis, smallpox, coxsackievirus and echovirus infections, and leptospirosis.

Epidemic Typhus

EPIDEMIOLOGY. The last recorded outbreak of epidemic or louse-borne typhus in the United States was in 1920 and 1921 among inhabitants of an Indian reservation in the Southwest. While an occasional case of laboratory- or hospital-acquired infection may occur (usually as an airborne infection), most commonly the disease is transmitted to man by systemic introduction of infected louse feces through an abrasion in the skin. Unlike other rickettsial diseases, man is the reservoir of *R. prowazekii.* The body louse and occasionally the head louse are infected by feeding on a person with rickettsemia. Rickettsiae multiply within cells lining the alimentary tract of the louse and are eliminated in feces. The cycle is continued by fecal contamination of a newly susceptible individual. Infected material may gain entrance into the body through an abrasion or perforation of the skin. Other routes include the upper respiratory tract by inhalation of dried infected louse excreta and the conjunctival sac through direct contamination. Infected lice usually die within a week after they become infected. They are adapted to humans and will inhabit the linings and crevices of clothing. Sharing of lice with others occurs frequently in congested populations in close contact.

CLINICAL FEATURES. The incubation period of louse-borne typhus is 7 to 14 days and is shortened (as with other rickettsial diseases) by a large infectious dose. The illness begins suddenly, with initial symptoms of malaise, prostration, and chills, followed shortly thereafter by intense headache and high temperatures that invariably rise to 39.5 C or higher by 48 hours of illness and persist for 12 to 18 days in untreated uncomplicated cases. Several diseases, such as epidemic typhus, murine typhus, Rocky Mountain spotted fever, malignant tertian malaria, leptospirosis, typhoid fever, brucellosis, and lobar pneumonia, are characterized by persistently elevated temperature.

Between the third day and seventh day of disease, a faint rose-colored cutaneous eruption develops. Initially the skin lesions are macular and faintly papular, with variation in size (2 to 4 mm in diameter) and indefinite borders that fade on pressure. Within 24 to 48 hours the lesions become dark red and no longer blanch on pressure. The eruption appears initially on the chest, flanks, and inner arm surfaces and then often spreads to the lower arms, buttocks, and thighs. The face, palms, and soles rarely are involved, in contrast to the distribution of rash in patients with Rocky Mountain spotted fever. During the course of severe infection the macules develop into petechiae and larger ecchymoses or coalesce to form large hemorrhagic areas and necrotic lesions, particularly in those areas where there is pressure.

The mortality rate in untreated patients ranges from 2 to 40 percent, depending on the age and underlying health of the infected individual. Mortality rates increase with age. The illness is more difficult to recognize in children because of fewer constitutional symptoms and a sparse rash. The severity of the infection relates to the degree of generalized vascular involvement. Hypotension, oliguria with azotemia, and stupor leading to coma may occur in a child with widespread untreated infection. Superimposed bacterial complications that prolong morbidity and increase fatality include bronchopneumonia, parotitis, otitis media, and systemic abscesses.

Early in the illness leukopenia with a relative lymphocytosis is common. Elevated leukocyte counts occur during the second or third week in untreated patients. Other common abnormalities are normocytic anemia, microscopic hematuria, hyponatremia, hypochloremia, albminuria, hypoalbuminemia, and azotemia in severely ill patients. The confirmatory laboratory findings are the demonstration of a fourfold or greater rise in antibody titers for *Proteus* OX-19 and specific rickettsial complement-fixation antigens that occur 1 to 3 weeks after the onset of illness. Rickettsial agglutinins, neutralizing antibodies, and antibodies to an erythrocyte-sensitizing substance (ESS) are specialized serologic tests ordinarily not available.

CONTROL. The control of epidemic typhus includes destruction of lice through use of residual insecticides and disinfection of bedding and clothing laden with infected louse feces. Early identification and isolation of patients and institution of treatment with effective antibiotics plus vaccination of susceptible persons are important measures. The available vaccine is a killed, formalin-treated rickettsial suspension cultured in chick embryo yolk sacs. It confers limited, rather than absolute, immunity. It does significantly reduce mortality and morbidity. Of greater promise is a live vaccine prepared from the attenuated E strain of *R. prowazekii* isolated initially in Madrid in 1941. Results of a recent field trial conducted during an epidemic show this vaccine to be effective. Most convalescent patients are immune to subsequent attacks of either epidemic or murine typhus fever, although there are relatively rare instances of recurrence (Brill-Zinsser disease).

Brill-Zinsser Disease

In 1910 Brill described patients in New York City whose disease clinically resembled classic typhus fever; after examination of epidemiologic and immunologic data, Zinsser correctly postulated that the disease was a recrudescence of Old World typhus. Most patients with Brill-Zinsser disease have had attacks of typhus fever in endemic centers of Europe or other countries in early life. During the recurrent illness, which is less severe, the serologic response and characteristics of the rickettsial illness resemble a mild form of louse-borne typhus. It is presumed that the rickettsiae persist in the tissues of the host for years and under appropriate stress result in illness. Fever persists for 8 to 12 days, the rash is pink and macular, and death is unusual. Complement-fixing antibodies of the 7S type appear on about the third febrile day and reach high titers. Two differences in the serologic response of Brill-Zinsser disease when compared to the primary attack of epidemic typhus include an earlier rise in specific antibodies (due to prior sensitization of antibody-producing cells) and the absence of rise in agglutinins to *Proteus* antigens (ie, negative Weil-Felix reaction).

Murine (Endemic) Typhus

EPIDEMIOLOGY. Unlike louse-borne typhus, endemic or murine typhus occurs annually in the United States. The disease usually occurs in the southeastern coastal states, with a high incidence in Texas. Port cities with heavy rat infestations are favored sites. Murine typhus, primarily an infection of rats, is caused by *R. mooseri*. Transmission occurs from rat to rat via the flea (*Xenopsylla cheopis*) and by the rat louse. Neither the rodent nor flea succumbs to the infection, and rickettsiae remain viable and virulent in the rat flea for 5 weeks

or more. There is no transovarian transmission of rickettsiae by fleas or lice. Man acquires endemic typhus when bitten by an infected flea or through inhalation of infected flea excreta. The infection may occur naturally in domestic cats, with spread to humans by cat fleas.

CLINICAL FEATURES. The incubation period ranges from 7 to 12 days. Prodromal symptoms include headache, myalgia, arthralgia, and backache, followed by gradually increasing temperature that may reach 41.2 C in children and last 2 weeks in untreated patients. On the fifth to eighth day of illness, a cutaneous eruption occurs. As in epidemic typhus, the rash first appears on the trunk and spreads peripherally, rarely involving the face, palms, or soles. Initially the skin lesion is dull, red, and macular, becoming papular as it matures. In contrast to epidemic typhus, the exanthem does not usually become purpuric, and it lasts only a few days in most cases. Twenty percent of children do not have a prominent rash. Central nervous system symptoms and peripheral vascular collapse are uncommon in this form of typhus fever, except in the elderly. Murine typhus is usually mild to moderately severe, with a mortality rate in the untreated of about 2 percent. Differentiation from epidemic typhus depends on the demonstration of specific complement-fixing antibodies or agglutinins using purified antigens. *Proteus* OX-19 agglutinins are elaborated in patients with either murine or epidemic typhus.

CONTROL. Control of endemic typhus usually requires elimination of the rat reservoir, while insecticide spraying of rat burrows is effective in controlling the flea. A killed *R. mooseri* vaccine is protective in animals and is recommended only for laboratory personnel working with the causative agent. Patients convalescent from murine typhus fever are solidly immune to epidemic typhus and vice versa.

SPOTTED FEVER GROUP

The spotted fever group contains at least eight antigenically related rickettsiae, of which five cause human disease. Rickettsiae are classified into subgroups according to the results of species-specific complement-fixation testing in mice, cross-immunity studies in inoculated guinea pigs, and mouse toxin neutralization tests.

The Rocky Mountain spotted fever caused by *R. rickettsii* is identical with São Paulo typhus, which occurs in South America, particularly in Brazil. In the Mediterranean countries, fievre boutonneuse or Marseilles fever caused by *R. conorii* differs in that primary eschar or ulcer with adjacent adenitis often develops at the site of the initial tick bite. The exanthem in such patients is characteristically reddish and papular. Immunologically related strains of rickettsiae cause tick-borne typhus in Africa, India, Russia, and other countries. They are identified as Siberian tick typhus (*R. siberica*), South African tick-bite fever (*R. conorii*), North Queensland tick typhus (*R. australis*), and rickettsialpox (*R. akari*).

Rocky Mountain Spotted Fever

EPIDEMIOLOGY. Rocky Mountain spotted fever was initially identified as black measles by the residents of the Snake River Valley of Idaho and was first recorded by Wood in 1896. Ricketts, working in the Bitter Root Valley of Montana, proved that the disease was transmitted by ticks. Wolbach's classic studies of the pathology of the disease and the causative agent were published in 1919. The early association of this disease with the Rocky Mountain states led to general acceptance of the name of the disease. However, the disease occurs throughout the United States, with two major endemic regions, ie, three Rocky Mountain states (Colorado, Montana, and Wyoming) and three South Atlantic states (Maryland, Virginia, and North Carolina). Although spotted fever was first identified in the Rocky Mountain area, more than half of the reported cases occur annually east of the Mississippi River.

Woodsmen and laborers who are exposed in rural endemic foci such as fields and forests are at risk of infection. Children become infected during picnics and occasionally when pet dogs harbor infected ticks. Infection usually results from a tick bite or occasionally from abrasions in the skin that become contaminated with infected tick feces or tissue juices. Infection rarely may result from autoinoculation or aerosolization of infectious inocula by laboratory personnel. Ricketts demonstrated that adult female ticks harbor pathogenic rickettsiae throughout their lifespan of several years. Rickettsiae may be found in all stages of the tick and can be transmitted during copulation or transovarially. Hence they serve as both vector and major reservoir. Small animals such as squirrels, rabbits, puppies, chipmunks, rats, mice, and weasels experience mild infections but are not important as agent reservoirs. Five species of ticks serve as vectors of *R. rickettsii*. The western American or Rocky Mountain wood tick (*Dermacentor andersoni*) ranges into the midwest. The eastern wood tick or the American dog tick (*D. variabilis*) and the Lone Star tick (*Amblyomma americanum*) serve as vectors in the middle Atlantic and south central portions of the United States. *D. parumapertus* and *Haemaphysalis leporispalustris* serve as reservoirs of the rickettsial agent in nature; yet they rarely bite man. In some localities when cases are reported 3 percent of ticks are infected, although the usual incidence is less than 0.1 percent. Rickettsiae are introduced into human skin via infected salivary gland secretions or feces. Infected ticks that have hibernated during winter must ingest a blood meal and reactivate the virulence of the rickettsiae before human infection occurs. Ticks are most active as disease vectors from April to September; they hibernate in the earth during winter.

CLINICAL FEATURES. Rocky Mountain spotted fever is a generalized infection of unusual severity occurring in scattered areas of the United States. Often the disease is not diagnosed due to its infrequency and lack of physician awareness of the epidemiology and clinical features. A history of a tick bite is elicited in about 80 percent of patients. The remaining patients generally report an exposure to tick-infested woods or dogs. The incubation period ranges from 2 to 14 days, averaging about 7 days. Large infectious doses of rickettsiae are associated with short incubation periods and more serious infections.

Illness usually begins with nonspecific manifestations of headache, photophobia, chills, fever, myalgia, arthralgia, and anorexia. Fever appears abruptly and quickly reaches 39.5 C to 40.5 C. Higher temperatures are characteristic of illness in children. A cutaneous eruption appears on the second to fourth days of illness. The initial lesions consist of pink irregular macules that occur initially on ankles or feet or on the flexor surfaces of the wrists, arms, or hands. The lesions blanch on pressure. It is possible to better visualize the characteristic exanthem by soaking the extremity with a warm water or alcohol compress, preferably in the afternoon, when the temperature is usually higher. Soon the lesions spread to the trunk and face. Within 1 to 3 days the skin lesions assume a darker purpuric hue and fail to fade on pressure (Fig. 16). As the illness progresses the lesions coalesce to form large areas of ecchymosis. Necrosis and gangrene of the extremities may occur, particularly in patients with vascular collapse. Mucous membranes of the oral cavity, pharynx, eye, and genitalia may be involved. Pressure applied to an extremity with a tourniquet or sphygmomanometer may evoke petechiae (Rumpel-Leede phenomenon). Hepatomegaly and altered liver function commonly occur. The spleen is palpable in 50 percent of patients.

The exanthem is evidence of vasculitis involving small vessels. Rickettsiae invade and proliferate in endothelial cells, leading to swelling of the endothelium of capillaries, venules, and arterioles. Occassionally, large vessels are involved. *R. rickettsii* characteristically multiply in cell nuclei as well as in the cytoplasm. The media of vessels often show extensive changes, and a surrounding mononuclear infiltrate is characteristic. Blood extravasates into the tissue immediately adjacent to involved vessels. Interference with arterial blood supply through thrombosis may lead to ischemic changes, especially in the skin where necrosis and gangrene may result. In severely ill patients microinfarcts appear throughout the central nervous system, heart, lungs, liver, kidneys, or other tissues. Central nervous system involvement is greater in patients with Rocky Mountain spotted fever than in other rickettsial diseases. It may simulate meningitis, encephalitis, or convulsive disorders. Headache is almost always present, the sensorium is clouded, and convulsions may occur. Deafness is common in severe cases and usually abates, as do the other neurologic manifestations, weeks later. Generally, those patients with an extensive, widespread exanthem are more seriously ill than patients with a sparse rash. Electroencephalograms taken a year or more after infection have shown minor changes in some patients in spite of the absence of neurologic signs.

During the second week of illness in untreated patients, peripheral vascular collapse, azotemia, electrolyte disturbances, pneumonia, and pyogenic complications occur. Thrombocytopenia is commonly found in Rocky Mountain spotted fever and is due to peripheral sequestration or an injury to platelets. Far less frequently a consumption coagulopathy occurs with associated depression of fibrinogen and clotting factors V and VIII. Occasionally the vitamin-K-dependent clotting factors (II, VII, IX, X) may be depressed because of altered liver function. The cerebrospinal fluid is generally clear, with normal or slightly elevated pressure; the protein may be minimally elevated, the sugar is normal, and a lymphocytic pleocytosis (10 to 200 cells/mm^3) may be seen.

The differential diagnosis of Rocky Mountain spotted fever once the rash has appeared includes rubeola, typhus fever (epidemic and endemic), scrub typhus, meningococcemia, "sepsis," typhoid fever, rat-bite fever, leptospirosis, and enteroviral infection when accompanied by a rash.

Rickettsemia extends into the middle of the second week of illness. Male guinea pigs may be infected by intraperitoneal injection of 4.0 ml of whole blood or emulsified blood clot. The animal develops fever and scrotal swelling, with redness and hemorrhagic necrosis. Smears of the inflamed tunica vaginalis often show rickettsiae.

The Weil-Felix reaction with the *Proteus* OX-19 strain is invariably positive; a titer of 1:160 or higher is diagnostic. Agglutinin titers for *Proteus* OX-19 and OX-2 occur in patients with Rocky Mountain spotted fever; occasionally the OX-2 titer exceeds that of the OX-19. The complement-fixation test with rickettsial antigens is diagnostic, with a fourfold rise in serum titer usually to 1:16 or higher during the second and third febrile weeks. Such antibodies persist for at least 8 years or more in low titers; *Proteus* agglutinins disappear within several months.

The mortality rate in untreated patients ranges from 10 to 40 percent, increasing significantly with lack of adequate therapy and age. In all rickettsioses, including Rocky Mountain spotted fever, children have a good prognosis. Yet it is erroneous to infer that children suffer mild infections, since mortality rates of 20 percent occur in children. Frequently the illness is mistaken for rubeola or another illness, and tetracycline or chloramphenicol is not given until the pathophysiologic changes have progressed to a critical point. Available antibiotics and use of measures to support the circulatory system could virtually eliminate fatality.

CONTROL. It is impractical to attempt eradication of *R. rickettsii* because of its established reservoir in ticks. Man acquires infection from the tick, which must be attached several hours before infection occurs. Children should be examined carefully after exposure in fields or wooded terrain. Ticks should be removed with forceps by gentle traction, and crushing of the arthropod should be avoided. Tick tissue juices and feces are laden with rickettsiae that are highly infectious and can lead to infection through a local abrasion. The site of tick attachment should be washed with soap and water and compressed with an alcohol sponge.

There are two types of vaccines. A phenol formalin-

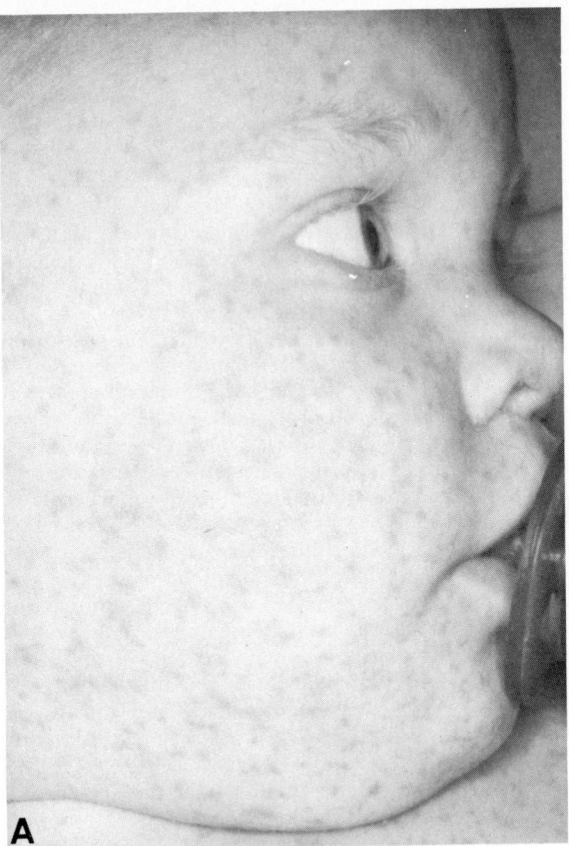

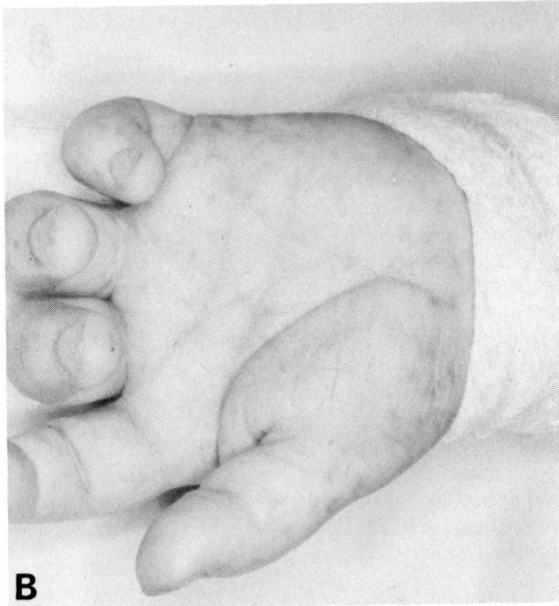

FIG. 16. Two-year-old white male with confirmed Rocky Mountain spotted fever **A.** Generalized petechial eruption that began on the extremities and became most pronounced over the trunk, face, and upper extremities, can be noted. The child is in the second week of illness. **B.** Petechial rash involving the palms.

killed preparation obtained from infected tick tissues was developed in the early 1920s. The current commercially available vaccine is an inactivated suspension of rickettsiae cultivated in yolk sacs of embryonated eggs. Both vaccines produce immunity in guinea pigs. Field studies have shown some protective value of the tick vaccine, while the commercially available chick tissue vaccine has been shown to impart a similar degree of immunity in experimental animal models. Recent studies of Rocky Mountain spotted fever in volunteers have shown that neither vaccine affords a high order of protection against contracting the disease. Yet the illness in vaccinated volunteers is milder and responds rapidly to specific antibiotic treatment, and the vaccine probably should be given to laboratory personnel working with *R. rickettsii.*

Rickettsialpox

R. akari, the cause of rickettsialpox, is antigenically related to the etiologic agent of Rocky Mountain spotted fever. The disease was identified initially in 1946 during an outbreak among apartment tenants in New York City. The illness resembled adult chickenpox, and a newly identified rickettsial organism was isolated.

EPIDEMIOLOGY. House mice harbor *R. akari,* which are transmitted to man by mites. This mild illness occurs in persons who live in congested urban centers.

CLINICAL FEATURES. The incubation period ranges from 2 to 7 days following attachment of an infected mite. In 90 percent of cases an initial lesion (site of mite bite) occurs as a firm red papule 0.5 to 2.0 cm in diameter. The center ulcerates, leaving a crusted eschar that may persist several weeks. The initial lesion is not painful, nor does it itch. The illness is characterized by fever, chills, headache, and a sparse papulovesicular eruption. Within 1 to 3 days after the onset of fever, scattered erythematous macules and papules develop, showing no characteristic distribution. The skin lesions enlarge, become more papular, and then form vesicles resembling the eruption of varicella. Within a week the eruption disappears without scarring. The disease seldom lasts longer than 10 days. Complications and fatalities are rare. The exanthem differs from varicella in that the lesions are deeply seated and randomly distributed and are associated with an initial eschar. Several disorders that also resemble rickettsialpox are primary herpetic infection of the skin, generalized vaccinia, mild smallpox, and *Mycoplasma* infection.

CONTROL. Effective control measures include eradication of rodent reservoirs and use of miticidal chemicals. There is no vaccine.

SCRUB TYPHUS

EPIDEMIOLOGY. Scrub typhus or tsutsugamushi fever is of significant importance to those traveling to endemic rural and jungle areas of Asia and the Southwest Pacific. Historically scrub typhus has been an important disease among military populations stationed in these areas. The causative rickettsiae, *R. tsutsugamushi* or *R. orientalis,* are transmitted to man by the larval or chigger stage of trombiculid mites. The reservoir includes the mite vector (infection can be transovarially acquired) as well as rats and other rodents. Scrub typhus occurs in persons whose occupations expose them to infected mites.

CLINICAL FEATURES. The incubation period is usually 10 to 18 days. Initially a cutaneous lesion appears at the site of mite attachment, most commonly in the covered moist portions of the body such as the perineum, scrotum, buttocks, or axilla. The lesion begins as an asymptomatic pink papule and increases in size, with central necrosis forming a black scab 4 to 8 mm in diameter. The eschar may be noted at the onset of clinical signs or 3 to 5 days prior to fever and other manifestations. The primary lesion is not painful and does not itch. Diffuse tender adenopathy, more marked in the areas of the eschar, commonly occurs. Onset of illness is abrupt, with chills, fever, headache, and prostration. By the end of the first febrile week a maculopapular eruption develops on the chest and abdomen and gradually spreads to involve the entire body. The hands and face are usually spared. In untreated cases, hematologic abnormalities, pneumonia, encephalitis, or cardiac involvement may develop during the second week of illness; each is associated with a poor prognosis.

During the second week of illness the Weil-Felix reaction is often positive for the *Proteus* OX-K strain and negative for *Proteus* OX-19 and OX-2. The differential diagnosis includes typhoid fever, dengue, typhus fevers, malaria, and leptospirosis. Between 24 and 36 hours after institution of chloramphenicol or tetracycline the toxic signs abate, the patient becomes afebrile, and rash and eschar regress. Patients with scrub typhus respond to antibiotic therapy more promptly than do those with the other rickettsial infections. The mortality rate is negligible in treated individuals.

CONTROL. Infected mites are implanted firmly in endemic areas. Miticidal chemicals impregnated in clothing, insect repellents applied to exposed skin, and widespread use of insecticides are effective control measures for persons exposed. It is advisable to wear protective clothing when in endemic areas. In unusual situations it may be advisable to administer antibiotics prophylactically. Chloramphenicol has been given in 3-g single doses every 5 days for 7 doses and has prevented clinical infection. In these field studies there was no evidence of blood dyscrasia or bone marrow depression secondary to the chloramphenicol. Longer-acting antibiotics such as doxycycline are now being appraised.

Q FEVER

Q fever is caused by inhalation of *Coxiella burnetii.* The causative agent is unlike other rickettsiae in that it is highly resistant to wide temperature changes, desiccation, and chemical agents, it does not cause a cutaneous eruption after producing illness in humans, and it does not elicit X agglutinins of the Weil-Felix reaction. Illness is characterized by headache, fever, and respiratory and hepatic signs.

EPIDEMIOLOGY. The agent resides in ticks that may serve as vectors in spreading infection to animals and rarely man. *C. burnetii* commonly produces asymptomatic infection in cows, goats, and sheep. Infected animals shed rickettsiae in their milk and feces, and placentae may be heavily infected. The organism is hardy; it withstands drying and wide temperature changes and has been recovered from ambient air in the vicinity of infected animals. Human infection usually follows occupational exposure to infected livestock, with inhalation of infected dust from exposure to hides or the highly infectious products of conception. A single organism may cause clinical infection, yet man-to-man transmission surprisingly is rare.

CLINICAL FEATURES. Between 9 and 21 days after exposure, illness occurs suddenly, with chills, fever, malaise, and intense headache. Soon after the onset a nonproductive cough commonly develops. Pulmonary rales are frequently audible; yet they are less impressive than the chest radiograph, which reveals patchy consolidation or nodular infiltrates. In patients with Q fever, respiratory manifestations usually predominate; but in some individuals hepatic involvement overshadows pulmonary findings, which may be absent. Such liver involvement suggests infectious hepatitis or an acute abdominal infection. Q fever may masquerade as abacterial endocarditis, pericarditis, myocarditis, aseptic meningitis, encephalitis, or obscure fever. Occasionally the illness mimics infectious mononucleosis. Q fever should be suspected in a patient with "atypical pneumonia" or "infectious hepatitis." When the primary manifestations suggest pulmonary involvement, other illnesses to consider are primary atypical pneumonia, viral and bacterial pneumonia, psittacosis, influenza, and tularemia.

During the acute illness there may be wide swings in temperature, which may reach 40.5 C, with a gradual defervescence after 5 to 15 days. Severe complications are unusual, and mortality is rare. Pulmonary involvement consists of patchy interstitial pneumonitis containing fibrin and mononuclear exudate. The alveolar walls and ducts as well as terminal bronchioles are infiltrated by large mononuclear cells. Liver involvement is common and consists of focal necrosis with infiltration of round cells and eosinophils and granuloma formation.

The diagnosis of Q fever generally is established by documenting a fourfold or greater rise in complement-fixing antibodies during infection. In certain centers the causative agent may be demonstrated using the fluorescent antibody technique, which employs a labeled antibody directed against *C. burnetii*. As with the other rickettsiae, the etiologic agent can be isolated from blood or other body tissues by inoculation of guinea pigs, although this is not routinely done because of the hazards to laboratory personnel.

CONTROL. Most infections occur through direct or indirect contact with livestock. Since infection in livestock is of no consequence economically, eradication of this reservoir has not been undertaken. Whether long-term therapy with antibiotics placed in animal feed would be effective is unknown. Effective killed Q fever vaccine made from phase I antigen is available. This vaccine causes significant local reactivity and sterile abscesses, particularly after booster doses. A live attenuated strain of *C. burnetii* is used in the Soviet Union and is under study in the United States.

DIFFERENTIAL DIAGNOSIS OF RICKETTSIAL INFECTIONS

Early in the infection, before the rash has appeared, differentiation of rickettsial infection from other febrile illnesses is difficult. A history of a recent tick bite is helpful. The rash of meningococcemia resembles Rocky Mountain spotted fever; yet the lesions are tender and generally develop earlier in the infection. Gram-negative cocci can be identified on staining of material from a petechial lesion in meningococcemia, and the causative agent can be cultured from the site. The rash of rickettsioses occurs on about the fourth day of disease and gradually becomes petechial.

In the authors' experience, Rocky Mountain spotted fever is most often mistaken for rubeola. In measles the prodromal period is characterized by fever, respiratory symptoms, Koplik's spots, and rash that begins on the face and neck and spreads to the trunk. Petechial lesions are uncommon. The rose spots of typhoid fever appear usually on the lower chest or abdomen and remain delicate, without hemorrhagic character. The rash of infectious mononucleosis is usually morbilliform on the trunk and rarely becomes petechial.

Murine typhus is a milder disease than louse-borne typhus or Rocky Mountain spotted fever. Its rash is less extensive, nonpurpuric, and nonconfluent, and vascular complications are uncommon. Differentiation of rickettsial infections often must await results of specific serologic tests. The rash of Rocky Mountain spotted fever begins on the periphery of the body, while the rash of classical and endemic typhus is generally noted initially in the axillary folds and on the trunk, only later extending peripherally. Louse-borne typhus is not recognized in the United States except in the form of recurrent typhus fever (Brill-Zinsser disease). Rickettsialpox is differentiated from Rocky Mountain spotted fever by the initial lesion, the relative mildness of the illness, and the early vesiculation of the rash. The Weil-Felix reaction is positive in Rocky Mountain spotted fever and in epidemic and murine typhus, but it is negative in rickettsialpox and Q fever.

TREATMENT OF RICKETTSIOSES

All rickettsial infections respond to early therapy with either tetracycline or chloramphenicol. The dose of either drug for children is 50 to 100 mg/kg/24 hours (orally in divided doses) for 5 days. If parenteral therapy is necessary, chloramphenicol is the preferred drug; it should be given intravenously in the same dosage outlined above. Due to the occasional occurrence of hepatic toxicity with intravenous tetracycline, if this agent is to be employed intravenously the dose should be reduced to 15 mg/kg/24 hours. In each rickettsial disease, therapy can be discontinued once the temperature has returned to normal for 24 hours, but therapy should be continued for at least 5 days. Relapses generally occur only in those individuals treated during the first several days of fever. Such early treatment usually occurs in laboratory-acquired infections, when a diagnosis can be readily made. In instances when early therapy is instituted, a short second course of antibiotic treatment might be utilized after an interval of 5 days without treatment, although this has not been shown to be superior to a continual 2-week course of therapy. If a relapse occurs, another 5-day course of antibiotics should be given. There is no evidence that rickettsiae develop resistance to the drug. Antibiotic therapy, while usually unnecessary, will shorten the duration of rickettsialpox. Q fever is readily controlled by specific therapy, and relapses do not occur.

General and Ancillary Supportive Treatment

In spite of specific therapeutic effects, there are certain limitations of presently utilized regimens. Fever persists from 2 to 4 days following the initiation of appropriate antibiotic therapy (tetracycline or chloramphenicol). Headache and other manifestations of toxemia may persist for variable periods after the institution of treatment. In seriously ill patients, vascular collapse leading to shock, necrosis of the skin and other tissues, cerebral edema, and azotemia are complications that may arise. A reduction of total blood volume is sometimes found. The fundamental mechanisms leading to tissue alterations and toxemia are unknown. Early in the course of the infection, both nitrogen and sodium are excreted in the urine, creating a state of negative nitrogen balance and hyponatremia. The most important reason for the continuing negative nitrogen balance in patients with infections is lack of sufficient protein intake to supply body demands. A general diet providing 3 to 5 g of protein per kilogram of normal body weight in addition to adequate carbohydrates will supply the patient nutritionally if he is able to eat; otherwise, parenteral amino acid solutions can be utilized for protein supplementation.

One of the most striking findings seen in children seriously ill with a rickettsial disease is hyponatremia. Depressed levels of serum sodium in addition to depressed serum chloride levels have been noted to occur in many other infectious diseases, in addition to the massive potassium losses that can occur in patients with severe acute infections. Because of the generalized derangement of cellular function in these patients, as well as the common finding of inappropriate antidiuretic hormone secretion, injudicious use of fluids and saline actually may be harmful. Using parenteral fluids containing 3 percent saline, or rapid administration of any parenteral fluid, is contraindicated unless the patient appears in shock. If shock should occur, blood transfusions, parenteral administration of preformed protein supplements such as albumin, and judicious use of a plasma expander may have a favorable effect on the impending circulatory collapse. If renal shutdown and uremia occur, overloading the circulation with protein supplements and fluids is to be avoided. Clinical judgment and frequent laboratory determinations of hemoglobin, hematocrit, electrolytes, and plasma proteins will govern the tempo with which corrective measures are employed. The volume of fluid given should be based on the child's weight or surface area. If parenteral fluids are administered too rapidly or in too large an amount, additional tissue and cerebral edema may occur and may greatly increase the load on a weakened myocardium.

Adrenal cortical hormones may be utilized for their antitoxemic effects. The most striking clinical effects are alleviation of headache, earlier defervescence, dissipation of toxemia, and return of appetite. Hormone treatment exerts an ameliorating effect on toxemia in patients with Rocky Mountain spotted fever and typhus fever when used in conjunction with antibiotics. Steroids are unnecessary in the routine case, but are of practical value in patients first observed late in the course of illness, when supplemental antitoxemia measures can be life-saving.

There is evidence, with all rickettsial diseases, that following infection, in spite of antibiotic therapy, rickettsiae may persist in tissues and theoretically may reactivate following the use of corticosteroids or ionizing radiation, which lower host resistance. Perhaps there is a Brill-Zinsser form of recrudescence for each of the rickettsial diseases other than epidemic typhus fever.

References

Harrell GT: Rocky Mountain spotted fever. Medicine 28:333, 1949

Hattwick MAW, Peters AH, Gregg MB, Hanson B: Surveillance of Rocky Mountain spotted fever. JAMA 225:1338, 1973

Haynes RE, Sanders DY, Cramblett HG: Rocky Mountain spotted fever in children. J Pediatr 76:685, 1970

Hazard GW, et al: Rocky Mountain spotted fever in the eastern United States. Thirteen cases from the Cape Cod area of Massachusetts. N Engl J Med 280:57, 1969

Older JJ: The epidemiology of murine typhus in Texas, 1969. JAMA 214:2011, 1970

Ormsbee RA: Q fever rickettsia. In Horsfall FL Jr, Tamm I (eds): Viral and Rickettsial Infections of Man. Philadelphia, JB Lippincott, 1965, p 1144

Schachter J, Sung M, Meyer KF: Potential danger of Q fever in a university hospital environment. J Infect Dis 123:301, 1971

Smadel JE: Status of the rickettsioses in the United States. Ann Intern Med 51:421, 1959

——— Elisberg BL: Scrub typhus rickettsiae. In Horsfall FL Jr, Tamm I (eds): Viral and Rickettsial Infections of Man. Philadelphia, JB Lippincott, 1965 p 1130

Snyder JC: Typhus fever rickettsiae. In Horsfall FL Jr, Tamm I (eds): Viral and Rickettsial Infections of Man. Philadelphia, JB Lippincott, 1965, p 1059

Torres J, Humphreys E, Bisno AL: Rocky Mountain spotted fever in the Mid-South. Arch Intern Med 132:340, 1973

Woodward TE, Jackson EB: Spotted fever rickettsiae. In Horsfall FL Jr, Tamm I (eds): Viral and Rickettsial Infections of Man. Philadelphia, JB Lippincott, 1965, p 1095

HEMORRHAGIC FEVERS

Heinz F. Eichenwald and Vu van Dzi

The terms hemorrhagic, virus hemorrhagic, and epidemic hemorrhagic fevers are used more or less interchangeably to describe a large number of separate entities occurring in many parts of the world caused by a variety of related as well as unrelated etiologic agents. Many of these diseases have been studied incompletely clinically, virologically, or epidemiologically; little is known of some of them aside from their occurrence. Most are transmitted to man by arthropods (eg, Southeast Asian hemorrhagic fever) and others by arachnids such as ticks and mites (Omsk fever, Korean hemorrhagic fever); still others may have no vector, but are perhaps acquired from close contact with rodent reservoirs (Bolivian hemorrhagic fever). In general the infections transmitted by arachnids are localized in occurrence and tend to affect adults more than children, while those acquired from mosquitoes are found over larger areas and usually cause more illness in the pediatric age group.

It is difficult to classify the different entities in any systematic or logical manner; thus it has become customary to identify each disease by its principal geographic location. From a strictly clinical standpoint, it is possible to divide the hemorrhagic fevers loosely into those that are or are not accompanied by renal involvement.

Hemorrhagic Fevers with Renal Syndrome

The prototype for this group of diseases is Korean hemorrhagic fever, more properly called Far Eastern hemorrhagic fever. Similar diseases occur in Siberia, European Russia, the Balkans, and Czechoslovakia. These illnesses are generally arachnid-borne; some are transmitted by mites, others by chiggers, and others perhaps by fleas. A variety of small rodents serve as reservoirs. Far Eastern hemorrhagic fever is primarily a disease of adults; the few children that have been affected have generally experienced a rather mild disease.

CLINICAL MANIFESTATIONS. Illness begins abruptly, with a febrile phase and chills, followed by lethargy and prostration. Generalized myalgias, headache, and abdominal pain commonly occur. A characteristic marked facial flush precedes the appearance of fine petechiae, which often occur initially on the soft palate and conjuntivae and later about the axilla and in skin areas subject to pressure or trauma. The febrile phase is further characterized by a rapid decline of blood platelet levels associated with increased capillary fragility. On the third to fifth days intense proteinuria occurs abruptly, and the hematocrit rises. The patient complains of intense thirst, but when fluids are administered his discomfort is increased and edema may result.

During the last day of the febrile phase (about 5 to 7 days after onset) hypotension or shock may occur, progressing on occasion to confusion and delirium. Massive proteinuria continues, blood urea nitrogen levels rise, and urine specific gravity falls. Toward the end of this phase, ecchymosis, hemoptysis, hematemesis, melena, and hematuria may occur. As the patient's arterial pressure returns to normal, he enters an oliguric phase; blood urea nitrogen levels increase very rapidly, and a variety of electrolyte disturbances may be found. A peculiar hypervolemic syndrome commonly occurs, characterized by hypotension and distension of superficial veins, but without increased intravenous pressure or congestive heart failure. Further hemorrhagic manifestations often are noted at this time. The oliguric phase usually persists 3 to 5 days and is followed by a diuretic phase lasting from a few days to several weeks and marked by fairly rapid improvement in renal function. A diuresis of from 3 to 8 liters/day may occur suddenly, and the patient may again develop shock. Survivors then enter the convalescent phase, which may last several weeks, with gradual improvement in proteinuria and nitrogen retention.

PATHOLOGY. Histologically the disease presents several distinctive features. Gelatinous protein-rich massive retroperitoneal edema is found in patients succumbing during the hypotensive phase. The kidneys are diffusely involved; lesions consist of areas of necrosis in the medullary pyramids. Microscopically, glomeruli and convoluted tubules are usually unaffected, but engorged vessels and extravasated blood are found around the loops of Henle and collecting tubules, with hemorrhage in the junctional zone. In addition, there is extensive necrosis of tubular epithelium and rupture of many tubules. In other organs there is similar evidence of widespread capillary damage manifested by dilation and rupture with extravasation of erythrocytes.

THERAPY. Treatment is supportive and symptomatic. No known drug favorably affects the course of the disease. Fluid intake should be restricted during the febrile phase; shock is treated in the usual manner. In severe cases of shock the slow infusion of salt-poor albumin appears beneficial, and continuous administration of pressor drugs is perhaps helpful. During the oliguric and diuretic phases, water and electrolyte balance should be carefully maintained; during oliguria, therapy is that for acute renal failure.

PROGNOSIS. Patients treated by the various techniques of modern medical care experience a mortality rate of about 5 percent; those cared for in their primitive villages by traditional methods die only slightly more frequently.

HEMORRHAGIC FEVERS WITHOUT RENAL SYNDROME

This group of diseases is generally caused by arboviruses; most are transmitted by mosquitoes, although a few are mite- or tick-borne. The best studied and thus prototypic illness is Southeast Asian (Thai) hemorrhagic fever, which possesses an unusual epidemiology and certain distinctive clinical features.

EPIDEMIOLOGY. All four types of dengue virus have been recovered from patients with this disease, although type 4 would appear to be uncommonly involved. Chikungunya virus also has been incriminated in the etiology of the disease; the frequency of occurrence of this type of arbovirus seems to vary from outbreak to outbreak. In any event, diseases caused by the dengue viruses or Chikungunya agent are clinically indistinguishable.

The disease characteristically occurs in sharp epidemics affecting large numbers of individuals over a period of relatively few weeks. Despite the high prevalence in many parts of the world of the causative viruses and their vectors, the occurrence of this type of hemorrhagic fever is limited to Southeast Asia. Furthermore, the disease is found only among certain groups of indigenous children, with Caucasians being affected very rarely, if at all, although the latter group frequently develops classic dengue fever following infection. The age distribution is quite limited; few cases of hemorrhagic fever are found in patients older than 9 years of age. Furthermore, the disease occurs most commonly among urban dwellers and is rare in small rural villages, even though dengue fever is highly prevalent in adults and children residing in these latter areas.

The mosquito *Aedes aegypti* is the principal vector, transmitting the virus from human to human. No animal or avian reservoir has been identified. As a general rule the disease is most prevalent during the rainy season when mosquitoes are abundant; in Thailand, for example, cases tend to cluster in the months from June to October.

PATHOGENESIS. It was demonstrated a number of years ago that Thai hemorrhagic fever is associated with secondary, heterologous dengue virus infection, a finding that suggests the possibility that immunopathologic processes determine whether infection with one of these viruses results in benign dengue or in hemorrhagic fever. Circulating antigen–antibody complexes may occur in this disease, because high levels of both antibody and infectious virus are present in the serum early in the course of the illness. More recent studies have demonstrated marked depression in complement components, especially C3; and it has been shown that both the classic and alternate complement pathways are activated, with reduction of C4 and C3 proactivator levels in most patients. In fact, the level of depression of C3 can be correlated with the severity of disease. The fairly consistent findings of low platelet counts, lowered fibrinogen levels, presence of circulating fibrin split products, and reduced Hageman factor suggest that disseminated intravascular coagulation is part of the hemorrhagic shock syndrome. Since complement has been shown to be capable of initiating blood coagulation through the platelets, it is possible that the intravascular coagulation in dengue hemorrhagic fever may also be a consequence of intravascular complement activation.

CLINICAL MANIFESTATIONS. The onset of the illness is usually sudden, with high fever often accompanied by chills and nearly always by severe headache. Drowsiness and restlessness are common. The patient may complain of severe aches in his joints and muscles, especially in the lower extremities, back, shoulder girdles, and retro-orbital region. Gastrointestinal symptoms (nausea and vomiting, 70 percent, abdominal pain, 40 percent) are common. Respiratory symptoms and signs consist of cough and pharyngitis and occur in nearly half of the patients; radiographically, about two-thirds of these have evidence of diffuse interstitial pneumonia, with some developing a pleural effusion that usually consists of varying quantities of slightly turbid, yellowish fluid. By the third day of illness, hepatomegaly is apparent in the majority of patients.

In about 20 percent of children a generalized maculopapular eruption appears during the first 2 to 3 days of illness, often fading rapidly; but it may then be followed by a petechial rash. More commonly, petechiae may occur without any preceding skin manifestations. Purpura develops at some time during the course of the illness in nearly every patient, often associated with hematemesis, epistaxis, or melena. A peculiar shocklike state with hypotension and cold cyanotic extremities but a warm flushed body occurs during the third to fifth day in 30 to 40 percent of children. Convulsions during this stage signal a grave prognosis. After 5 to 7 days the patient begins to improve, often with dramatic suddenness, and he rapidly returns to his former state of health.

LABORATORY. A consistent finding is profound thrombocytopenia during the first 2 to 3 days of illness that reaches its lowest levels at about the fifth day. Counts may remain low for 1 to 5 days, rarely longer, and then return rapidly to normal. As mentioned earlier, there are alterations in serum complement component levels, and various laboratory studies may suggest the presence of disseminated intravascular coagulation. No other consistent hematologic findings occur. Transient transaminase elevations are sometimes encountered and are probably related to liver disease. Urine changes are limited to the occasional finding of albuminuria.

PATHOLOGY. Aside from scattered areas of hemorrhage, the only consistent pathologic findings are seen in the lungs, liver, and spleen. The lungs are involved by an interstitial pneumonia with scattered histiocytes in the alveoli. The liver parenchyma is swollen with collections of fatty material in hepatic cells and occasional areas of lymphocytic infiltration. The malpighian corpuscles of the spleen reveal the most specific changes: granulomatous lesions with clumps of monocytoid cells with abundant cytoplasm occasionally fused into a syncytium.

THERAPY.   Therapy is symptomatic and supportive. The administration of oxygen is indicated in patients with extensive pulmonary involvement and dyspnea. Shock is treated in the usual manner with intravenous fluids, plasma, plasma expanders, etc. Hematocrit determinations are useful to detect early signs of hemoconcentration, which usually precedes circulatory failure in these patients, and this simple procedure can also be used to monitor the effects of administered fluids. With prolonged shock, metabolic acidosis may develop; it should be corrected with sodium bicarbonate. Some highly agitated patients may need sedation; chloral hydrate orally or rectally appears safe and effective. Blood transfusions are indicated only in children with severe bleeding such as hematemesis and melena. While the use of glucocorticoids has been advocated, there is no evidence that these hormones favorably affect the course of the illness, reduce bleeding, or hasten the return of normal platelet counts.

Similarly, the infusion of heparin to counteract intravascular coagulation has not been shown to be beneficial in this disease.

PROGNOSIS.   Mortality rates appear to vary somewhat from outbreak to outbreak, but the overall death rate is approximately 15 percent; it is higher in infants under 1 year of age. With appropriate treatment of shock, a rate below 5 percent has been achieved. It has repeatedly been noted that children treated by practitioners of oriental medicine prior to hospitalization have unusually high death rates, which may possibly be related to the use of toxic herbal medications.

References

Gajdusek DC: Virus hemorrhagic fever. J Pediatr 60:841, 1962

Nelson ER: Hemorrhagic fever in children in Thailand. J Pediatr 56:101, 1960

Pathogenic mechanisms in dengue hemorrhagic fever: report of an international collaborative study. WHO Bull 48:117, 1973

Powell GM: Clinical manifestations of epidemic hemorrhagic fever. JAMA 151:1261, 1953

CHAPTER 13

Mycotic and Parasitic Diseases

MURRAY WITTNER

MYCOTIC AND MYCOTIC-LIKE DISEASES

ACTINOMYCOSIS

Human actinomycosis is caused by the ray fungus, *Actinomyces israelii,* which produces an indolent granulomatous suppurative infection. *Actinomyces* is not infrequently found in buccal smears and tonsillar exudate from healthy individuals. Infection is thought to be caused by traumatic introduction of the patient's own flora into his tissues. Actinomycetes are not true fungi. Human actinomycosis is included in this section because the clinical course and pathology of this infection closely resemble those of many of the mycotic diseases. *A. israelii* is encountered throughout the world. It is a gram-positive, anaerobic, branching, filamentous actinomycetes bacterium that has not been isolated from any source in nature other than the mucous membranes, oral cavity, gastrointestinal tract, carious teeth, and tonsils of man.

CLINICAL FEATURES. There are three principal clinical forms: the oral or facial (cervicofacial), pulmonary, and abdominal. Each of these is slowly progressive, producing at times remarkably little local or systemic disability. In the *oral* type, which carries the best prognosis, a hard swelling may form at the root of a carious tooth or around the site of a dental extraction. It usually causes little pain, but it gradually enlarges, often producing marked deformity. The overlying skin becomes shiny and purple, and spontaneous discharge of thin exudate may occur either externally or within the buccal cavity, often persisting for weeks.

Pulmonary actinomycosis sometimes follows aspiration of a foreign body; at other times it develops insidiously. Pneumonia, which is at first acute, fails to resolve. Cough and mild fever persist, and the patient's condition gradually worsens. There may be little expectoration, and physical signs are those of a consolidated lung. The involved region may become secondarily infected, with production of foul sputum and clinical evidence of bronchiectasis. Septic fever often develops as the diseased area extends. Unless rapid death supervenes, the thoracic wall is eventually eroded, and characteristic pus containing sulfur granules is either discharged or aspirated from a subcutaneous abscess.

Abdominal actinomycosis begins most frequently in the appendix, as a complication of a perforating gastrointestinal ulcer or following penetration of the mucosa of the colon by a sharp object such as a knife, ingested bone, or gunshot wound. Differentiation from pyogenic appendicitis, salpingitis, cholecystitis, cystitis,

or pyelonephritis is possible only after exploratory laparotomy, unless the abscesses rupture onto the surface of the body and produce a typical draining sinus from which the organisms can be recovered. The initial symptoms are insidious and are related to the organ involved. As the disease progresses, local granulomatous lesions form; they may spread to involved associated tissue including bone, liver, gallbladder, or ovaries. The spine and ribs are rather frequently involved, either by metastatic hematogenous spread or by direct extension from a pulmonary or abdominal focus. Areas of bone destruction seen on radiography usually reveal a proliferative periosteal reaction as well. In time the infection tends to extend to the surface, but not necessarily over the site of the deep lesion.

DIAGNOSIS. Actinomycosis may be suspected when an indolent inflammatory lesion is shown not to be caused by tuberculosis, which is far more common. Lesions about the jaw are usually mistaken for chronic pyogenic infection or tumor. On radiography, all these lesions resemble tuberculosis, except for their unusual locations, such as the shaft of a rib or lamina of a vertebra. Exudate or aspirated material should be carefully examined for sulfur granules. These are yellowish gray masses up to 5 mm in diameter that are colonies of organisms. On a slide preparation they show the gram-positive mycelial filaments in characteristic radial arrangements at the margin of a central gram-negative zone. However, bacteria such as *Staphylococcus aureus* can form similar granules. Actinomycetes are easily cultivated in thioglycolate semisolid medium, below the surface, provided the inoculum does not contain secondary invaders. To obtain pure cultures from contaminated sources, brain-heart infusion glucose blood agar is seeded and incubated anaerobically. In the presence of active infection, serum agglutinins may reach high titers.

TREATMENT. The success of penicillin in the treatment of actinomycosis has greatly improved the once grave prognosis of this disease. Penicillin therapy for 30 to 45 days should be followed by wide surgical excision of the lesions, with the surgical wound packed open for drainage. Following surgery, intramuscular penicillin is given in daily doses of from 2 to 5 million IU for 12 to 18 months. In severe cases 12 million IU of intramuscular penicillin per day or 10 to 20 million IU per day given intravenously may be necessary. In cases where treatment with penicillin fails or cannot be tolerated, antibiotics such as chloramphenicol, streptomycin, tetracycline, and sulfonamides may be used. Amphotericin B, nystatin, and griseofulvin do not inhibit *A. israelii* and are not recommended for therapy.

NOCARDIOSIS

Nocardiosis is the result of an acute or chronic suppurative (usually primary) pulmonary infection by *Nocardia asteroides* that occasionally spreads to a variety of sites by hematogenous dissemination. The bacterium *N. asteroides* is a pathogenic, aerobic, gram-positive, weakly acid-fast, branched filamentous actinomycetes having filaments or hyphae rarely exceeding 1 μ in diameter. The organism is a widespread soil saprophyte. It frequently causes an opportunistic infection in individuals with severe underlying disease, particulary if they are receiving immunosuppressive therapy. Nocardiosis may accompany other opportunistic mycotic infections in the same clinical setting.

CLINICAL FEATURES. Pulmonary nocardiosis is most frequently encountered as a single lesion, but it may occur as a widely disseminated infection resembling miliary tuberculosis; there may be consolidating or cavitary lesions. The infection is often associated with fever, night sweats, pleuritic pain, weight loss, malaise, and a productive cough containing a moderate amount of purulent sputum. Metastatic lesions to the brain are common, and they often present with headache, nausea, and vomiting. Skin and subcutaneous lesions are frequent and are presumably the results of hematogenous spread or direct suppurative extension through the chest wall, in similarity to the sinus tracts seen in actinomycosis. However, if sulfur granules are present in nocardiosis they are small (< 1 mm); they are composed of loosely interwoven filaments and are weakly acid-fast. Renal lesions are not rare, and endocarditis has been reported.

DIAGNOSIS. Sputum and other exudates should always be examined using Gram's stain and modified acid-fast stains. In addition, direct culture of these exudates without antibiotics is recommended. Biopsy material should be stained by special methods for bacteria, such as the Brown and Bren and a modified Fite stain (acid-fast). Serology or skin testing for nocardiosis is generally not available.

THERAPY. Therapy consists of prolonged courses of a sulfonamide in conjunction with ampicillin. Recent reports advocate the use of trimethoprim-sulfamethoxazole, especially in central nervous system involvement. This combination rapidly passes the blood-brain barrier in effective concentrations. In addition, all lesions, wherever possible, must be incised and drained.

ASPERGILLOSIS

Aspergillosis is a mycotic disease that may be caused by any of several species of *Aspergillus. A. fumigatus* has been implicated in most of the disseminated and pulmonary infections. On occasion, noninvading spherical colonies or fungus balls caused by *A. niger* have been isolated from bronchiectatic sacs. Numerous species of *Aspergillus* flourish throughout the world, often growing as saprophytes on decaying vegetation. It is therefore reasonable to expect that human exposure to spores of potentially pathogenic species, especially *A. fumigatus,* is far more frequent than is reflected in the relatively few clinical cases of disseminated and pulmonary aspergillosis. Although primary aspergillosis has been reported in the absence of such factors as underlying disease, prolonged antibiotic administration, or corticosteroid therapy, such an occurrence is so unusual that intensive investigation for the existence of a predisposing condition should be undertaken. Moreover, occupational exposure to large numbers of spores among bird handlers, fur cleaners, and farmers is usually associated with severe pulmonary hypersensitivity symptoms, termed farmer's lung, rather than with deep-seated infections. Allergic aspergillosis may cause rhinitis, dyspnea, and productive cough. Pulmonary infiltrates may be detected, and *Aspergillus* may be isolated from nasal and/or bronchial exudates. However, tissue invasion is unusual. It is believed that IgE antibodies are an important factor in these complaints.

CLINICAL FEATURES. Pulmonary aspergillosis is most frequently a complication of an underlying pulmonary disease such as tuberculosis, bronchiectasis, abscess, pneumonia, or carcinoma. The mycotic infection may be highly virulent and unrelenting, spreading from the bronchi to the parenchyma as necrotizing pneumonia that may eventually cavitate. Fever, moderate to severe hemoptysis, and a productive cough with purulent sputum in which hyphae may be seen are frequent manifestations. Radiographic findings may be characteristic if fungus balls (aspergilloma) are present. Dissemination to the brain, heart, kidneys, bone, and skin may occur in a small number of cases. Aspergillosis is unusual in infants and children, most cases having been associated with prematurity, pneumonia, and antibiotic or steroid therapy.

PATHOLOGY. The hyphae may proliferate throughout the pulmonary tissues; after invading blood vessels they may result in widespread hematogenous dissemination. The fungus may proliferate on walls of tuberculous cavities or may produce granulomatous lesions with radial proliferation of hyphae. In the areas of necrotizing pneumonia, hyphae can often be identified by use of hematoxylin and eosin. Occasionally it may be necessary to resort to special stains in order to identify typical mycelial structure. In histopathologic sections the hyphae are 3 to 4 μ in diameter. They are septate and reveal dichotomous branching. The septa are readily identified in sections stained with the Gridley (periodic acid Schiff) technique. In disseminated disease the lesions appear as acute pyogenic abscesses, and the symptoms depend on the organs invaded. Brain, kidney, and myocardium are the most frequent sites of metastatic growth.

DIAGNOSIS. Direct examination of sputum for hyphal elements is often rewarding, but the significance of the positive examination must be viewed with caution. Even repeated positive preparations may only signify the presence of the fungus growing as a harmless saprophyte. Radiographic evidence along with the direct examination may provide stronger support for the diagnosis. Sputum and bronchial aspirates should be cultured at room temperature with antibiotic on Sabouraud's medium.

THERAPY. Few strains of *Aspergillus* respond to 5-fluorocytosine. However, amphotericin B has been successful in doses of 15 to 45 mg/kg. Response may be less than desired in those patients in whom there has been vascular invasion with infarction and necrosis. Such lesions should be surgically excised. Similarly, localized lesions (or aspergillomas) should also be removed surgically. Antibiotic therapy is usually ineffective.

BLASTOMYCOSIS

North American blastomycosis (Gilchrist's disease) is caused by the fungus *Blastomyces dermatitidis*. With few exceptions it has been regarded as a disease limited to the United States and Canada, where the prevalence is greatest in the Mississippi Valley and the southeastern states. However, there have been cases of blastomycosis reported from Mexico, Venezuela, and various parts of Africa, such as Tunisia, Tanzania, and the Republic of South Africa. Although cases usually occur sporadically and affect adults with outdoor occupations, a small epidemic was reported in 1955 in which 6 of the 11 cases occurred in children, the youngest being 6 months of age. Current evidence indicates close resemblances between the clinical patterns of blastomycosis and other deep mycoses, notably coccidioidomycosis and histoplasmosis.

CLINICAL FEATURES. It is now apparent that the lungs are frequently the portal of entry for *B. dermatitidis*, which results in a primary pulmonary form of the disease. At the present time little is known of so-called inapparent or subclinical cases of pulmonary blastomycosis such as are recognized in coccidioidomycosis. In the clinically apparent primary cases the onset is insidious, resembling a mild respiratory infection accompanied by low-grade fever, chest pain, and nonproductive cough. As the symptoms gradually increase in severity, night sweats, high spiking fevers, hemoptysis, weakness, anorexia, and weight loss are evident. Severe *primary pulmonary blastomycosis* is difficult to differentiate from active tuberculosis. Radiographic studies of the chest may show extensive involvement of mediastinal nodes. Occasionally there is evidence of extensive pulmonary miliary disease; death may follow while the disease is still confined to the lungs or the patient may recover slowly. More frequently, however, extrapulmonary dissemination occurs.

Disseminated blastomycosis is the result of hematogenous spread of the infection from the lungs to other areas of the body. Most frequently the disease involves the cutaneous and subcutaneous tissues, as well as bone, central nervous system, and urogenital tract. In contradistinction to South American blastomycosis, the gastrointestinal tract is usually spared. Granulomatous lesions of the liver and spleen are found in over 40 percent of disseminated cases. The kidneys, prostate, epididymis, bladder, and testes are often involved, causing dysuria, pyuria, and hematuria.

Chronic cutaneous blastomycosis follows hematogenous spread from primary pulmonary infection. It is the most common form of North American blastomycosis and is the initial presenting complaint of most patients. The skin lesions initially appear as benign, papulopustular nodules that enlarge peripherally to form elevated, ulcerating, and verrucous granulomas. As the lesion extends at its periphery, the central area heals, leaving a soft atrophic scar. *Primary cutaneous blastomycosis* is an unusual form of the disease resulting from inoculation of *B. dermatitidis* into the skin. A papule forms at the inoculation site, followed by an ascending lymphangitis and lymphadenopathy of the affected limbs, closely mimicking the clinical picture of sporotrichosis. In those cases that have been described, all patients recovered without developing the chronic cutaneous form or dissemination.

DIAGNOSIS. Clinical diagnosis must be confirmed by laboratory studies. These include microscopic examination of smears, scrapings, aspirates, sputum, and bronchoscopic washings for the presence of the characteristic yeastlike cells. This material should also be spread on the surface of Sabouraud's agar slants and incubated at room temperature or 30 C. The yeast phase may be obtained in culture by inoculating glucose blood agar medium and incubating at 37 C. Usually the blastomycin skin and complement-fixation tests are positive except in recently infected individuals. Since cross-reactions between North American blastomycosis and histoplasmosis are not uncommon, a single serologic examination must be interpreted with caution. However, serial serologic determinations obtained during acute, convalescent, and recovery phases are most specific. Most authorities regard a heightened intracutaneous test of the delayed hypersensitivity type (and a low or absent titer in a complement-fixation test) as indicative of a favorable prognosis; a high complement-fixation titer has usually been correlated with extensive and often fatal disease. Apparently less than 50 percent of the sera from persons with proven blastomycosis gives a positive complement-fixation test. Thus a negative reaction has little value and does not exclude the presence of active disease. The prognosis for life in chronic cutaneous blastomycosis is generally good; however, healing does not usually take place without appropriate therapy.

TREATMENT. Untreated widely disseminated disease always has a poor prognosis. The aromatic diamidines stilbamidine and hydroxystilbami dine have been used with moderate success in many cutaneous cases, but they have not been useful in the serious disseminated form, especially when immunologic resistance is low. Excellent results have been obtained with the use of amphotericin B, although internal lesions do not seem to respond as well, skin lesions heal promptly, with up to 80 percent cures. It is notable that cases that have failed to respond to previous therapy are now being successfully treated with amphotericin B (p. 617).

COCCIDIOIDOMYCOSIS

Coccidioidomycosis (San Joaquin Valley fever) is a mycotic infection caused by the fungus *Coccidioides immitis*. Two general forms of the disease are recognized in man: a nonfatal, self-limited primary infection, usually of the respiratory tract, that may be acute, subacute, or asymptomatic; a secondary, often fatal, granulomatous form of a chronic and progressive nature. In the acute primary respiratory form the infection occurs almost exclusively by inhalation of airborne dust containing arthrospores of *C. immitis*. Coccidioidomycosis, therefore, is not contagious, and sources of infection are usually exogenous. It has repeatedly been demonstrated that soil is the natural habitat of *C. immitis*, and from such soil sources the fungus enters the lungs and causes primary pulmonary infection. As may be expected, the incidence increases sharply in the dry late summer months, and measures that effectively diminish dust have been shown to reduce markedly the incidence of infection.

Even though the first case of coccidioidomycosis was reported in Argentina, practically all of the subsequent cases have been recorded in the United States. Endemic areas exist in the western United States (particularly the southern half of California, southern Arizona, western and southern Texas, and New Mexico) in the northern states of Mexico, and in the Gran Chaco region of South America. Occasionally cases have been reported from Venezuela and Central America and possibly from Russia. In arid regions the peak incidence of acute infection occurs during the hot summer and autumn months when dusty field work is in progress. Infections have occurred in tourists simply passing through endemic areas during the hot, dry summer season. Cattle, sheep, dogs, and wild rodents in these areas are infected. The disease has been found in dogs in nonendemic areas, as in Iowa, Kansas, and the province of Quebec. In highly endemic areas 70 to 90 percent of long-time residents have been infected; as many as 50 percent of susceptible individuals may become infected following residence of 6 months in an endemic area, with the highest incidence usually occurring in the dusty summer and fall months. In endemic areas of California the incidence of positive coccidiodin skin tests increases from 17 percent in children residing in the area for 1 year or less to 77 percent for those living in the area for 10 years or more. Thus, where the population is stable the disease is predominantly a childhood infection. As measured by skin tests, no sex difference is present for the acute form of the disease. However, because erythema nodosum is more common in females, particularly at puberty, the acute form with erythema nodosum tends to be seen more often in girls.

Age does not appear to be a factor in susceptibility to infection; a fatal pulmonary form in a 3-week-old infant has been reported.Primary pulmonary disease can occur at all ages, although extrapulmonary spread and pulmonary cavitation appear to be less common in children than in adults. Among patients with the granulomatous form of the disease, males predominate, although less strikingly among children than among adults. The progressive form occurs in about 1 percent of clinically manifest infections in white males and in a much higher proportion in blacks and Filipinos. The primary infection, if it does not lead to dissemination, establishes a strong and lasting immunity.

PRIMARY FORM. In about 60 percent of cases no symptoms are present, and evidence of the existing infection is confined to the positive coccidioidin skin test. In the remaining 40 percent of cases symptoms of the acute primary infection occur from 10 days to 4 weeks (usually 10 to 14 days) following infection with arthrospores. Most of these cases are associated with mild symptoms resembling a cold or influenza. However, in a small minority of patients the primary attack may be most severe, with fever, dry cough, malaise, muscular pains, backache, headache, sore throat, and marked anorexia. A nonproductive cough, occasionally blood-streaked sputum, or frank hemoptysis may occur, suggesting pulmonary cavitation. Pleuritic pains are present in about one-third of cases. During the initial phase of the disease an erythematous rash may appear on the trunk, often extending over the entire body. When accompanied by sore throat and constitutional symptoms, the infection may be confused with scarlet fever or measles. Occasionally the rash may be vesicular and resemble varicella. Arthralgia, particularly of the knees and ankles, may be present. Conjunctivitis is commonly observed. The symptoms subside in about 1 week, in most cases without sequelae. In about 10 percent of clinically apparent cases the fever recurs after about 3 to 18 days, and erythema nodosum develops. Raised erythematous, roughly circular, tender nodules appear on the anterior tibial surfaces and not infrequently on the lateral surfaces of the thighs, hips, and buttocks, as well as the extensor surfaces of the arms, forearms, and elbows. These later become purplish, then brown, disappearing in about 1 to 3 weeks. Patients manifesting erythema nodosum are not likely to experience the disseminated chronic form of the disease.

Physical examination of the lungs reveals little of significance. Occasionally a friction rub, a pleural effusion, or fine crackling rales can be demonstrated. Radiography reveals soft patches of density extending out from the hilum, peribronchial thickening, peripheral or interlobar pleural effusions, and hilar adenopathy. In 2 to 8 percent of the clinically apparent cases cavities develop, usually solitary (90 percent), either within or outside of the pneumonic patch. Cavities usually disappear a few weeks after the acute symptoms have subsided. Occasionally an unusually large cavity may persist and remain unchanged for months or even years in an otherwise symptomless patient. Persistence of a cavity is not in itself an expression of the chronic disseminated form of the disease. Calcification occurs in healing primary pulmonary lesions as well as in hilar nodes. The radiographic changes are similar to, if not indistinguishable from, those of tuberculosis. Although a cutaneous lesion may be the first indication of infection, it usually indicates dissemination from a previously unrecognized primary pulmonary focus.

DISSEMINATED FORM. The disseminated or progressive form of coccidioidomycosis (coccidioidal granuloma), which fortunately is rare, occurs more frequently in dark-skinned races. Dissemination of the infection usually takes place within 6 months after the acute illness, but may follow the acute illness without free interval. After 1 year dissemination is unlikely. Progressive invasive granulomatous lesions may occur in the lungs, lymph nodes, bones, joints, skin, or meninges. Pulmonary lesions consist of pneumonic areas, cavitation, pleural effusion, or numerous discrete miliary lesions or abscesses. Bronchial adenopathy is present. Osteomyelitis, periostitis, and arthritis are common. The skin lesions usually begin as painless small nodules that gradually enlarge, suppurate, ulcerate, and then become encrusted. They occur most frequently on the scalp, forehead, nose, face, lips, supraclavicular region, thorax, hand and forearm, and leg and foot. In children from 1 months to 6 years of age, complaints referrable to the skeleton and soft tissues are more frequently encountered than are respiratory symptoms. In older children respiratory complaints predominate. Meningitis is more common in children, and unless early vigorous treatment is initiated, it is invariably fatal. The course of the granulomatous form of the disease is less prolonged in children.

DIAGNOSIS. While the clinical or epidemiologic history may arouse suspicion of the disease, a positive diagnosis of coccidioidomycosis may be made by the proper use of the coccidioidin skin test, a precipitin test, a specific complement-fixation test, identification of *C. immitis* by culture or animal inoculation, and histologic demonstration of characteristic double refractile spherules in biopsy material.

In positive reactors, 0.1 ml of a 1:100 dilution of coccidiodin injected intracutaneously produces induration greater than 5 mm in diameter when the test is read at 24 and 48 hours. An initial negative test during the acute illness followed by a positive reaction by the fourth week is diagnostic. A greater dilution should be used for patients with erythema nodosum, since they may be hyper-reactive. A negative coccidioidin test in a patient with erythema nodosum usually eliminates the possibility of coccidioidomycosis. In disseminated or extrapulmonary granulomatous forms there may be no reaction to even undiluted coccidioidin. Injection of coccidioidin for skin testing does not stimulate antibody production and therefore does not interfere with subsequent dermal or serologic tests. Reactors to histoplasmin may also react slightly to high concentrations of coccidioidin, and tests must be interpreted with caution.

Diagnostic humoral antibodies develop more slowly than does skin reactivity in the uncomplicated acute respiratory form of the disease. Precipitins are present in 50 percent of cases in the first week and 90 percent by the third week; they frequently decline after the third week of the disease, but occasionally persist for about 4 months. Complement-fixing antibodies appear after the first week of the disease and usually decline in the second month, but the complement-fixation reaction may persist for several years. Unusually high titers often correlate with the severity of the disease or with the presence of the disseminated progressive form. A rising complement-fixing serum titer is evidence of impending dissemination, a titer of 1:16 or higher being almost always indicative of disseminated disease. Negative serologic tests virtually rule out the chronic disseminated form of the disease. Generally, serologic tests are positive when the skin test is positive and vice versa. The demonstration of antibodies against *C. immitis* is of particular diagnostic value in patients with clinical evidence of dissemination in whom the skin test is negative.

The organisms may be found in the sputum, in cultured gastric washings, in purulent exudates of lesions, and in centrifuged sediment obtained from cerebrospinal, peritoneal, or pleural fluid. Direct microscopic examination of a cover slip preparation is inaccurate. Suspicious cultures should always be confirmed by animal inoculation. Intraperitoneal inoculation of white mice or intratesticular inoculation of guinea pigs results in pure suspensions of the organisms for culture. The organisms may be cultivated easily, but unusual care in the handling of infected material should be exercised, since the arthrospores are so light and easily broken away from the spore-bearing stalk that a mere puff of wind or breath can release a cloud of spores from a culture and carry them for considerable distances. All nonimmune persons are then in danger of becoming infected by inhaling the spores; infections have often occurred in this way, and on occasion they have been fatal.

In tissue sections the sporangium can be recognized as a double refractile spherical body that contains endospores and shows no budding. There is often a marked leukocytosis with a shift to the left. Occasionally a striking eosinophilia may be present, erroneously suggesting the presence of Löffler's syndrome. The spinal fluid in 75 percent of cases of meningitis contains complement-fixing antibodies. A "paretic" colloidal gold curve may be found.

TREATMENT. Primary coccidioidomycosis requires no therapy, since it is a self-limited disease. However, until amphotericin B was introduced the disseminated form had a fatality rate of about 50 percent, despite all available therapy. Oral and intramuscular administration of this antibiotic appear to be of little value. Intravenous administration of the drug should be employed in maximally tolerated doses daily or on alternate days until signs of the infection are eradicated. Such treatment is indicated in patients with disseminated infection or threatened dissemination or those with extending or exacerbating chronic pulmonary disease; it should also be given to individuals having persistent fever with malaise associated with pulmonary involvement and hilar adenopathy. Coccidioidal meningitis, which is usually fatal within 1 year if untreated, appears to be definitely improved by amphotericin B administration via combined intravenous and intrathecal or intraventricular routes. Dosage and length of therapy are discussed under cryptococcosis (p. 618).

HISTOPLASMOSIS

Histoplasmosis (Darling's disease) is an intracellular infection caused by the dimorphic fungus *Histoplasma capsulatum*. The disease occurs throughout the world and affects all age groups. The highest incidences of severe or fatal illness are in infancy and again in old age. Histoplasmosis was first described by Darling in 1905 from three fatal cases in Panama. However, almost four decades passed before the notion was dispelled that histoplasmosis was usually a fatal infection. Epidemiologic studies demonstrated frequent positive dermal reaction to histoplasmin, an antigen prepared from cultures of *H. capsulatum*. The widespread incidence of positive reaction, especially in the eastern central United States, provided important evidence of a widespread benign or inapparent form of the disease. Subsequently direct confirmatory evidence was obtained. It is erroneous to regard histoplasmosis as a disease of the central United States, since it is as common on the East Coast as in the Mississippi Valley.

H. capsulatum has been isolated from soil, usually near old chicken coops, bat caves, and barnyards where it has been enriched with decayed manure. Focal outbreaks of histoplasmosis have been reported in families, children, or other individiduals who have been playing in or cleaning out old abandoned chicken houses or visiting caves inhabited by bats. *Histoplasma* can be isolated in soil under trees in which starlings and other birds roost, and this mechanism may be responsible for urban transmission.

In soil, or in the laboratory at room temperature, employing Sabouraud's culture medium, *H. capsulatum* exhibits typical mycelial growth. Early aerial growth is white and cottony, later turning light tan to brown. Microscopic examination reveals branching septate hyphae-bearing oval microconidia 2 to 4 μ in diameter. As the culture matures, rounding macroconidia 8 to 14 μ are found; these are adorned with evenly spaced appendages that stain intensely for mucopolysaccharide. If inhaled or inoculated, spores promptly transform into typical yeast forms and reproduce intracellularly as oval budding yeasts 2 to 4 μ in diameter possessing a distinct capsule. The yeast phase can be reproduced in the laboratory if mycelial elements are transferred into enrichment medium and grown at 37 C.

PATHOGENESIS AND PATHOLOGY. There is considerable evidence to suggest that in the vast majority of cases the respiratory tract is the usual portal of entry. Primary ulcerative lesions of the skin, the mucous membranes of the mouth, the nasopharynx, and

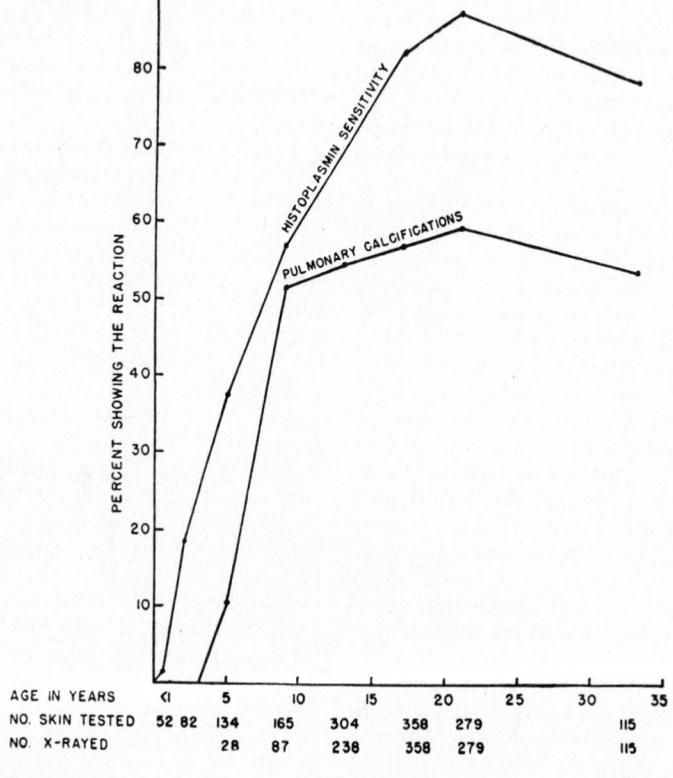

FIG. 1. Prevalence of histoplasmin sensitivity and pulmonary calcifications according to age in an area in which histoplasmosis is highly endemic.

the intestinal mucosa have been described. Such lesions may disseminate or remain localized to the region involved. The organism is generally found within macrophages and other cells of the reticuloendothelial system. The primary pulmonary complex of histoplasmosis closely resembles that of tuberculosis, consisting of single or multiple small subpleural lesions with lymphatic spread to regional hilar lymph nodes. Central caseous necrosis with epithelioid and Langhans-type giant cells are often seen. These lesions frequently heal with calcification. In hematogenous dissemination the lungs almost always show miliary tubercles, as do the spleen, liver, lymph nodes, and bone marrow. All tissues and organs may be involved with the exception of cartilage and cortical bone.

CLINICAL ASPECTS.   The clinical spectrum of histoplasmosis extends from inapparent or asymptomatic infection to fatal fulminant disease. Several clinical types have been suggested: primary acute form; severe disseminated form; chronic cavitary form; mucocutaneous form.

Primary Acute Form.   The primary acute form of histoplasmosis is usually a mild, or more often an asymptomatic, inapparent pulmonary infection in which the aspirated organisms stimulate the formation of one or more subpleural tubercles. As in primary pulmonary tuberculosis, macrophages laden with organisms travel along lymphatics to regional peribronchial and hilar nodes where secondary tubercles are formed. A significant proportion of these calcify and can be detected by chest radiography. The histoplasmin skin test turns positive about 3 to 5 weeks after infection. Figure 1 illustrates the relationship of histoplasmin sensitivity to pulmonary calcifications and their frequency in an area of high endemic frequency. Occasionally there may be large numbers of calcified scars. At times multiple lesions may be seen by radiography throughout the lung fields; they may persist for months or more before disappearing.

In symptomatic cases that are demonstrated to be histoplasmosis by subsequent positive conversion of the histoplasmin skin test in the absence of a positive tuberculin test, the most frequent pulmonary symptoms are nonproductive cough, shortness of breath, chest pain, hoarseness, and cyanosis. Fever, night sweats, arthralgias, and weight loss are commonly seen. During this acute stage erythema nodosum may be observed. Exposure to large numbers of organisms, as when children play in caves containing bat guano rich in *H. capsulatum*, may result in a severe and sometimes fatal

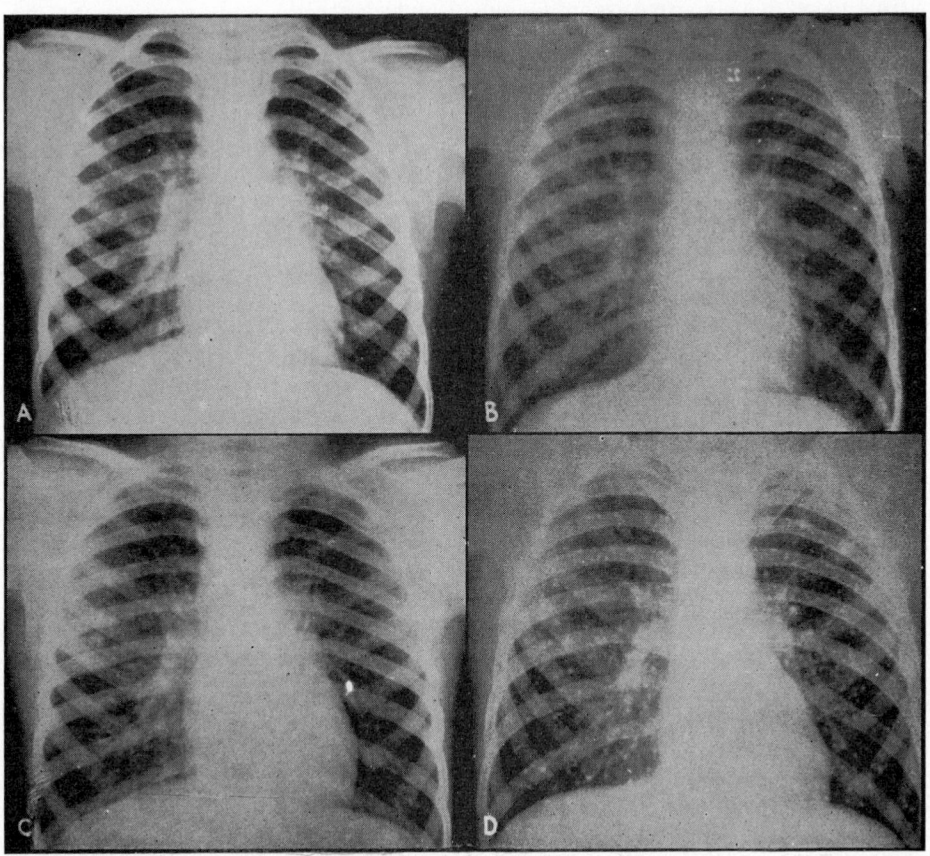

FIG. 2.   Development of pulmonary calcification in a case of severe nonprogressive histoplasmosis. *A.* January 1947. *B.* August 1949, at the time of the patient's hospital observation; *C.* November 1950. *D.* September 1961.

pulmonary infection that may or may not have disseminated. Usually, however, these patients recover, and the myriad pulmonary tubercles eventually calcify (Fig. 2). The frequent finding of calcified splenic tubercles in individuals with no clinical history of histoplasmosis suggests that asymptomatic hematogenous dissemination may frequently occur. In mild self-limited attacks no specific antifungal therapy is indicated.

Severe Disseminated Form. The severe disseminated form of histoplasmosis occurs more frequently in infants, young children, and elderly debilitated patients. While pulmonary symptoms may be inconspicuous, fever, hepatosplenomegaly, anemia, leukopenia, weight loss, and generalized lymphadenopathy may dominate the picture. Signs and symptoms can be those of endocarditis, meningitis, or adrenal insufficiency; gastrointestinal involvement may be manifested by diarrhea. Pneumonitis is not infrequent. Lesions of the skin and mucous membranes of the mouth are common in young patients. Severe anemia, thrombocytopenia, leukopenia can occur, as well as purpura, ecchymosis, and gastrointestinal hemorrhage in the late or terminal stages.

Once the diagnosis of disseminated histoplasmosis is suspected, it should not be difficult to obtain cultural confirmation from blood, bone marrow aspiration, or biopsy of lymph node, liver, spleen, or ulcer. Cultures of blood and bone marrow will be positive in about half the cases. The histoplasmin skin test in disseminated disease may remain negative in about 50 percent of cases, although the complement-fixation test usually, but not always, turns positive. Recent studies have pointed out that subsequent to a single positive histoplasmin skin test, complement-fixing antibody titers of up to 1:256 have developed in 7 to 12 healthy persons. These titers have persisted for months. Therefore, if complement fixation is to be done after skin testing, yeast-phase antigens should be used. The value of the histoplasmin skin test is limited in disseminated disease. Conversion from negative to positive during acute illness is regarded as significant; a positive reaction in a young child is highly suggestive of active disease. In older individuals, however, it can only be interpreted as indicative of previous infection.

Serologic evidence can be the major factor in establishing a diagnosis of histoplasmosis. These data may be obtained by complement fixation, immunodiffusion, or latex agglutination, usually in combination. If the complement-fixation test is employed it is essential to use both intact yeast-form cells and soluble mycelial filtrate antigens (histoplasmin), since the use of only one antigen does not provide adequate diagnostic coverage, inasmuch as patients with known disease may react only to one or the other of these antigens. While titers of up to 1:16 can only be considered presumptive evidence, titers of 1:32 or greater are highly suggestive. However, a fourfold rise or fall in titer is of even greater importance in the diagnosis. Other serologic tests, such as immunodiffusion and latex agglutination, may also be useful as screening methods in the detection of histoplasmosis.

Chronic Cavitary Form. Chronic cavitary pulmonary histoplasmosis is seen most frequently in adults. Radiographically and symptomatically it closely resembles cavitary tuberculosis. This type of histoplasmosis represents disseminated disease and has a poor prognosis. These patients may demonstrate any of the severe manifestations of disseminated histoplasmosis, and if they remain untreated they usually die.

Mucocutaneous Form. Mucocutaneous histoplasmosis may be due to hematogenous dissemination during a primary pulmonary infection or may occur following reactivation. Spread may also occur from an active extrapulmonary site. Cutaneous and mucocutaneous lesions have been noted in nearly half the reported cases of histoplasmosis and may appear as ulcerations and granulomas of the oral mucosa, papules, plaques, abscesses, or impetiginous zones. It is not uncommon to isolate organisms from these mucocutaneous lesions. On occasion, subcutaneous nodules, perforated nasal septum, peritonsillar abscess, and rectal ulcers have been recorded.

Primary cutaneous histoplasmosis has been described, and the criteria for such a diagnosis include: a history of inoculation with subsequent formation of a skin lesion within several weeks at the point of trauma, evidence that the wound contained the fungus, regional lymphadenopathy and lymphadenitis, no history of previous infection, and conversion of the skin test from negative to positive and a rising serologic titer.

TREATMENT. Amphotericin B is the agent of choice for the treatment of disseminated histoplasmosis. The decision whether to use this drug depends on the type of disease present. Most infections are either asymptomatic or self-limited, and only occasional primary infections may be so severe as to require therapy. However, chronic pulmonary and disseminated histoplasmosis usually require therapy. Both the chronic progressive pulmonary form and the disseminated form should receive a total course of 30 to 35 mg/kg of amphotericin B at 1.0 to 1.5 kg/day. Surgery is of no greater benefit than drug therapy alone. In disseminated histoplasmosis, patients should receive 25 to 35 mg/kg amphotericin B. All patients with disseminated disease should have an evaluation of their adrenal cortical activity in order that corticosteroid replacement can be provided if adrenal cortical insufficiency has occurred.

CRYPTOCOCCOSIS

Cryptococcosis (torulosis) is a cosmopolitan mycotic disease caused by a yeastlike fungus, *Cryptococcus neoformans*. With few exceptions it is conceded by most workers that avian excrement (particularly that of pigeons) is the primary source of *C. neoformans* and that the occasional recovery from soil that has been reported depends on previous contamination with avian feces. *C. neoformans* is a spherical cell that reproduces by budding and varies widely in size, from 4 to 20 μ in diameter. It is surrounded by a mucopolysaccharide capsule that, depending on the strain, varies in thickness from almost undetectable to nearly twice the diameter of the cell. Cryptococcosis is seen most frequently in individuals with serious underlying disease such as leukemia, lymphosarcoma, Hodgkin's disease, diabetes mellitus, or in those receiving long-term steroid or immunosuppressive therapy.

CLINICAL ASPECTS. Infection usually is acquired by inhalation of the organisms. Disease may remain localized to the pulmonary parenchyma, and subsequently hematogenous dissemination may occur to any organ of the body. Central nervous system involvement is particularly common, and cryptococcal meningitis is regarded as the most frequent cause of mycotic meningitis. Recent evidence would suggest that pulmonary cryptococcal infection may be common and asymptomatic, in similarity to primary pulmonary tuberculosis.

Pulmonary Cryptococcosis. Pulmonary infection may be clinically asymptomatic and may be discovered as a solitary nodule only by chance during radiography. However, pulmonary disease can be clinically apparent, with cough that is frequently productive of mucoid sputum, chest pain, fever, weight loss, occasionally hemoptysis, and night sweats. Single or multiple cavitary lesions, often bilateral, containing mucoid material may arise with or without symptoms. These lesions may persist for some time and subsequently heal spontaneously without drug therapy or dissemination to the central nervous system. However, lesions may be infiltrative and diffuse. Discovery of *Cryptococcus* in sputum usually is regarded as clear-cut evidence of pulmonary cryptococcosis, although there is evidence that a carrier state may exist.

Cerebral Cryptococcosis. Dissemination to the central nervous system results in signs and symptoms typical of meningitis, cerebral abscess, or tumor. These may include headache, nausea, vomiting, vertigo, low-grade fever, nuchal rigidity, positive Kernig and Brudzinski signs, papilledema, and increased spinal fluid pressure. Examination of the spinal fluid may reveal lymphocytosis, elevated protein, and reduced glucose. While untreated disease usually is fatal in 3 to 6 months, indolent cryptococcal meningitis may linger for years. Fulminant cases that are fatal in a few weeks also may occur.

DIAGNOSIS AND PREVENTION. The demonstration of budding organisms in India ink preparations of the spinal fluid establishes the diagnosis. Isolation of cryptococci from multiple blood cultures is highly suggestive of disseminated disease, especially in a compromised host. Therefore, therapy should be promptly initiated. *C. neoformans* is readily cultured on Sabouraud's dextrose agar at 37 C, but not at 44 C. Supplementary media are especially useful, but it should be remembered that cryptococci are inhibited by cycloheximide. An especially useful differential medium is commonly termed birdseed agar. This medium contains a chemical found in the common birdseed *Guizotia abyssinica* that causes cryptococci colonies to develop a characteristic brown pigment that is catalyzed by a phenol oxidase.

Recent results of serodiagnosis of cryptococcosis have resulted in the development of several diagnostically and prognostically useful tests. A latex agglutination test appears to be most useful for detecting cryptococcal meningitis. The test is performed on any of the patient's body fluids. An indirect fluorescent antibody (IFA) test appears to be valuable, as does a conventional slide agglutination test. However, a charcoal particle test appears to be more sensitive than the whole-cell agglutination test, but not as specific. The most effective measure for preventing cryptococcosis would be to reduce wild pigeon flocks. Handlers of pigeons can also be protected by using a solution of sodium hydroxide and lime in and around pigeon coops; this seems to destroy *C. neoformans* effectively.

TREATMENT. While treatment of focal pulmonary lesions is by surgical excision, cryptococcal meningitis is treated with amphotericin B. The relapse rate with amphotericin is about 25 to 30 percent; however, cryptococcal meningitis was almost always fatal prior to this drug. Amphotericin B is also the drug of choice for the treatment of blastomycosis, disseminated coccidioidomycosis, disseminated histoplasmosis, and systemic candidiasis. It is not without a number of undesirable and sometimes imposing side effects. These include fever, chills, headache, nausea, vomiting, anorexia, phlebitis, anemia, hypokalemia, and azotemia. Amphotericin is poorly absorbed from the gastrointestinal tract and therefore is usually administered intravenously. Since it is excreted slowly by the kidneys, it need not be administered more than once a day. Administration on alternate days also provides therapeutic blood levels and is tolerated far better by the patient. Therapy is begun with a dose of 0.25 mg/kg and is gradually increased, while the patient is carefully observed for signs of drug toxicity. Renal function is monitored by blood urea nitrogen determination by serum creatinine level and creatinine clearance, and by the appearance in the urine of erythrocytes, leukocytes, albumin, or granular or cellular casts. As long as the patient is tolerating the dosage, it may be increased up to a daily maximum of 1 mg/kg, but in no instance should it be higher than 1.5 mg/kg. Therapy usually spans a period of about 10 weeks or more, with the total adult dose usually being between 2 and 4 g. If relapse should occur, treatment should be reinstituted. Thrombophlebitis at the intravenous site may be a serious technical impediment to prolonged intravenous therapy, especially in children.

Renal toxicity caused by amphotericin B has been extensively studied. It has been shown that patients may develop a renal tubular acidosis syndrome and that urinary excretion of potassium may result in serious hypokalemia. It is important, therefore, that patients receive potassium replacement. Similarly, citrate may be of value in reducing the likelihood of renal calcinosis, which is a frequent complication of amphotericin B therapy.

5-Fluorocytosine is a new oral antifungal agent related to the antimetabolite 5-fluorouracil. It appears to be much less toxic than amphotericin B, and it has in vivo and in vitro activity against *C. neoformans*, *Candida* species, and *Torulopsis glabrata*. Unlike amphotericin, it does not seem to be useful against *Histoplasma*, *Blastomyces*, and *Coccidioides*. Patients with candidal septicemia, cryptococcal meningitis, and cryptococcal pulmonary disease have been treated with 5-fluorocytosine with variable success. In candidiasis it is essential that drug susceptibility tests be carried out prior to and during therapy, since about half the *Candida* strains, and especially species other than *C. albicans,* are resistant to 5-fluorocytosine. Nevertheless, a significant number of reports have indicated therapeutic success with this drug, including cases where amphotericin had failed. Results in cryptococcosis are less impressive, indicating the emergence of resistance during therapy. Further studies are necessary to ascertain the efficacy of combined drug therapy. The dosage of 5- fluorocytosine is 150 mg/kg daily for 2 to 6 weeks, depending on response. Since the drug is excreted primarily in the urine, blood levels should be monitored in those patients with renal insufficiency. Inasmuch as pancytopenia and other blood dyscrasias have been noted, it is recommended that during therapy white blood cell counts and hematocrits be checked twice weekly.

PHYCOMYCOSIS

Phycomycosis (mucormycosis) is a collective term applied to mycotic infections most often caused by species of *Absidia, Mucor, Rhizopus,* and *Basidiobolus.* These fungi are found normally throughout the world, occurring as saprophytes in decaying vegetation, fruits, and feces of herbivores. Similarly, phycomycosis has been reported from all parts of the world, but especially in persons with uncontrolled diabetes mellitus, in those with debilitating and/or terminal disease, and as a complication of steroid or immunosuppressive therapy.

CLINICAL DISEASE.   Increasing awareness of the clinical setting in which phycomycosis may occur probably accounts for part of the increased incidence of antemortem diagnoses. The triad of diabetic acidosis, facial or orbital cellulitis, and meningoencephalitis is well documented. Pulmonary involvement is not uncommon. It may cause a severe necrotizing pneumonitis with multiple foci of pulmonary infarction. This is attributed to the characteristic invasion of blood vessels by hyphae resulting in vasculitis and thrombosis. Central nervous system involvement usually is by direct extension from orbital or paranasal sinus infection. Invasion of any portion of the gastrointestinal tract may occur. Signs and symptoms are variable and may include diarrhea, pain, melena, hematemesis, and peritonitis.

DIAGNOSIS.   The diagnosis of phycomycosis should be entertained in debilitated patients in whom progressive fulminating sinusitis, orbital cellulitis, or pneumonitis occurs. Histopathologic diagnosis is relatively clear-cut, with the finding of very broad, rarely septate, haphazardly branched hyphae that deeply stain with ordinary hematoxylin. The hyphae are much broader than those seen in aspergillosis.

TREATMENT.   Amphotericin B is the drug of choice (p. 927). Correction of diabetic acidosis, if present, is important, since recent studies have suggested that diabetics (and especially those in acidosis) have impaired polymorphonuclear leukocyte mobilization.

CANDIDIASIS

Candidiasis is a fungus infection caused by yeastlike fungi of the genus *Candida. C. albicans* has been implicated in the overwhelming number of cases, but other species of *Candida,* given the opportunity, may also cause severe illness. (Previously the causative organism was known as *Monilia,* and therefore the disease was termed moniliasis.) *Candida* are frequently isolated from individuals in whom they do not seem to be causing disease. Typically they can be found in sputum, feces, vaginal secretion, and mouth, but rarely on normal skin. Factors that predispose to production of superficial or deep-seated disease by *Candida* are not precisely known. However, it is recognized that individuals with endocrine disorders such as diabetes mellitus, hypoparathyroidism, hypoadrenalism, and hypothyroidism, those with various blood dyscrasias such as leukemia and agranulocytosis, those with malignant states and malnutrition, and those receiving antibiotic, steroid, or immunosuppressive therapy are more frequently found with candidiasis than are individuals enjoying normal health. Occasionally, direct inoculation of organisms by drug addicts who are otherwise healthy has resulted in fatal *Candida* endocarditis. Although disseminated candidiasis in the newborn period has been reported, it is far more common to encounter oral lesions, ie, thrush (p. 885) , together with lesions of the perianal and diaper areas (p. 617). Generally these children are otherwise healthy; however, some may be premature. *C. albicans* found in skin, sputum, urine, and feces usually appears as rounded or oval budding cells, or blastospores, about 3 to 6 μ in diameter. These tend to elongate and form pseudohyphae. In deep-seated infections pseudohyphae may be the form most easily recognized, although blastospores, if looked for, usually will be found.

There has been increasing clinical awareness of *deep-seated candidiasis,* as well as increased incidence. Moreover, it has become clear that other species of *Candida* besides *C. albicans* are opportunistic pathogenic organisms, and their recovery from patient material must not be dismissed routinely as nonpathogenic contamination. Other than *C. albicans,* the most frequently identified species have been *C. tropicalis, C. parapsilosis, C. guilliermondi,* and *C. krusei.*

Candidiasis of the alimentary canal may occur at any age, although it is more common in infancy and in the elderly, often following oral candidiasis. Vomiting is the outstanding symptom of *Candida* esophagitis and is often exacerbated by feeding. Diarrhea and dehydration are frequent accompaniments. The distal third of the esophagus is most often involved.

Intestinal candidiasis has been reported with increasing frequency, and it is often related to antibiotic and steroid therapy. Enteritis is characterized by increasingly frequent loose bowel movements, abdominal discomfort, and rectal pain occasionally accompanied by mucosal bleeding. Sigmoidoscopic or macroscopic examination may reveal multiple gray brown plaques that may be covered with friable membrane. Microscopic examination usually reveals both pseudohyphae and yeast forms. Granulocyte response is variable. The presence of mycelial elements in the bowel has been interpreted to mean mucosal invasion, whereas the predominance of yeasts or blastospores has been regarded as nonpathogenic or saprophytic existence.

Candidiasis of the urinary tract may cause cystitis or pyelonephritis, the latter being the result either of local spread from the bladder or of hematogenous seeding in disseminated candidiasis. While urinary tract disease can be particularly difficult to detect, in several recent studies the demonstration of *Candida* by careful catheterization or suprapubic tap, taken together with elevated urinary protein and leukocytes, has been regarded as highly suggestive of invasive bladder and /or renal disease. Although present techniques for the diagnosis of upper urinary tract infection are inadequate, repeated isolation of the organism together with clinical and laboratory evidence of infection demands serious consideration of the etiologic role of *Candida.*

Pulmonary candidiasis is quite rare, despite the frequency with which the organism is isolated from sputum. *Candida* bronchitis, on the other hand, is relatively common, apparently occurring by direct spread from the oral cavity and oropharynx.

Systemic and disseminated *Candida* infections have been increasing, most notably in individuals undergoing therapy for acute leukemia, although a few cases have been reported in otherwise seemingly normal individuals. The majority of these cases appear to be the result of direct inoculation into the bloodstream during long-term intravenous therapy. While spontaneous recovery from candidemia can occur on removal of the source of infection, serious complications such as candidal meningitis, pyelonephritis, or endocarditis may intervene. *Candida* endocarditis resembles subacute bacterial endocarditis. Typically, large friable vegetations occur that tend to embolize to large vessels of the extremities, head, and kidney. Blood cultures positive for *Candida* are usually obtained. Despite therapy, the prognosis for this complication of candidiasis is almost uniformly poor.

DIAGNOSIS. Establishing a definitive diagnosis of candidiasis may be an extremely difficult exercise. Recognition of organisms isolated from human material is less troublesome than interpretation of their significance. Many workers regard the predominance of mycelial or M forms as a reliable indication of a pathogenic infection with *C. albicans.* The trouble with this is that other species of *Candida* do not form pseudohyphae as readily or to the same degree as *C. albicans,* but may still be pathogenic. Evidence has been obtained indicating increased invasiveness with transformation from yeast (Y forms) to pseudohyphal growth. Therefore it is important to collect and examine clinical material immediately, since the presence of protein often stimulates Y-to-M transformation and can lead to serious misinterpretation.

Intradermal or complement-fixation tests generally are not helpful in determining invasive disease, since many normal individuals will be positive reactors.

Precipitating antibodies against cytoplasmic candidal antigens is a reasonably specific index of candidiasis. Agglutination, latex agglutination, and immunodiffusion tests are also important tools for the diagnosis of systemic candidiasis. The latex test has greater sensitivity than the immunodiffusion, but there have been reports of cross-reaction in patients with cryptococcosis and tuberculosis. Rising precipitin or agglutinin titers are believed to be reliable indices of visceral disease. The latex agglutination test also has prognostic value in monitoring the progress of infection during therapy. It is important to reemphasize that one should *not* disregard recovery in blood cultures of so-called nonpathogenic yeasts without careful patient evaluation and subsequent negative cultures. Demonstration of *Candida* species in biopsy material should be supported,where possible, with cultural identification.

TREATMENT. Alimentary tract infection can be treated with 500,000 units of mycostatin administered orally four times daily for 1 week. If antibacterial therapy is implicated in the overgrowth of *Candida,* it should be withheld. Systemic or disseminated candidiasis is treated with amphotericin B or 5- fluorocytosine. Unfortunately candidal endocarditis does not respond as well as other forms of systemic candidiasis to amphotericin therapy. It is believed the large, bulky vegetations preclude the drug's reaching and therefore inhibiting the organisms. Following surgical removal of valvular vegetations, a clinical cure of candidal endocarditis has been reported. This may indicate the heroic measures that may be necessary to save life in candidal endocarditis.

PROGNOSIS. The outlook for recovery from alimentary tract infection is excellent if treatment is instituted promptly. The prognosis in systemic candidiasis is always guarded, even with amphotericin therapy. Endocarditis has an ominous outlook, being almost uniformly fatal despite amphotericin or surgical therapy.

References

GENERAL

Abernathy RS: Treatment of systemic mycoses. Medicine 52:385, 1973
Conant NF, Smith DT, Baker RD, Calloway JL: Manual of Clinical Mycology, 3rd ed. Philadelphia, WB Saunders, 1971, p 755
Douglas JB, Healy JK: Nephrotoxic effects of amphotericin B, including renal tubular acidosis. Am J Med 46:154, 1969
Drutz D, Spickard A, A Rogers D, Koenig MG: Treatment of disseminated mycotic infections: A new approach to amphotericin B therapy. Am J Med 45:405, 1968
Emmons CW, Binford CH, Utz JP: Medical Mycology, 2nd ed. Philadelphia, Lea & Febiger, 1970
Fetter BF, Klintworth G, Hendry W: Mycoses of the Central Nervous System. Baltimore, Williams & Wilkins, p 214, 1967
Hildick-Smith G, Blank H, Sarkany I: Fungus Diseases and Their Treatment. Boston, Little, Brown, 1964, p 494
Lennette E, Spaulding EH, Truant J: Manual of Clinical Microbiology, 2nd ed. Washington, DC, American Society for Microbiology, 1974
Wilson JW, Plunkett OA: The Fungous Diseases of Man. Berkely, Univ California Press, 1965
Wolstenholme GEW, Porter R: Systemic Mycoses, Ciba Foundation Symposium. Boston, Little, Brown, 1967

ACTINOMYCOSIS

Dundon S, Byrnes CK: Pulmonary actinomycosis in childhood. J Irish Med Assoc 52:26, 1963

Paul FM: Two cases of thoracic actinomycosis in children. Arch Dis Child 37:276, 1963

Peabody JW, Jr, Seabury JH: Actinomycosis and nocardiosis: a review of basic differences in therapy. Am J Med 28:99, 1960

Spilsbury BW, Johnstone FR: The clinical course of actinomycotic infections: 14 cases. Can J Surg 5:33, 1962

NOCARDIOSIS

Adams AR, Jackson JM, Scopa J, Lane GK, Wilson R: Nocardiosis: diagnosis and management with a report of three cases. Med J Aust 1:669, 1971

Maderazo E, Quintiliani R: Treatment of nocardial infection with trimethoprim and sulfamethoxazole. Am J Med 57:671, 1974

ASPERGILLOSIS

Aslam PA, Eastridge CE, Hughes FA Jr: Aspergillosis of the lung—an eighteen year experience. Chest 59:28, 1971

Blattner RJ: Pulmonary aspergillosis in children. J Pediatr 70:139, 1967

Finegold SM, Drake W, Murray JF: Aspergillosis: a review and report of twelve cases. Am J Med 27:463, 1959

Hughes W: Generalized aspergillosis. Am J Dis Child 112:262, 1966

Luke J, Bolande LRP, Gross S: Generalized aspergillosis and aspergillus endocarditis in infancy. Pediatrics 31:115, 1963

Mahvi T, Webb HM, Dixon CD, Boone JA: Systemic aspergillosis caused by Aspergillus niger after open-heart surgery. JAMA 203:520, 1968

Young RC, Bennett JE, Vogel CL, Carbone PP, Vita TT: Aspergillosis: the spectrum of disease in 98 patients. Medicine (Baltimore) 49:147, 1970

Vedder JS, Schorr WF: Primary disseminated pulmonary aspergillosis with metastatic skin nodules. JAMA 209:1191, 1969

BLASTOMYCOSIS

Chuck EW: Blastomycosis—the enigma of systemic mycoses. Chest 60:2, 1971

Furcolow M, Balows A, Menges RW, Pickar D, McClellan JT, Sahba A: Blastomycosis JAMA 198:115, 1968

Gephard MC, Hanlon TJ: Blastomycosis. Arch Dermatol 84:660, 1961

Turner DJ, Wadlington WB: Blastomycosis in childhood: treatment with amphotericin B and a review of the literature. J Pediatr 75:708, 1969

COCCIDIOIDOMYCOSIS

Ajello L: Coccidioidomycosis, Symposium, 2nd ed. Tucson, Univ Arizona Press, 1967

Drips W Jr, Smith CE: Epidemiology of coccidioidomycosis: a contemporary military experience. JAMA 190:1010, 1964

Sarosi G, Parker J, Tosh F: Pulmonary coccidioidomycosis. N Engl J Med 283:326, 1970

Winn WA: Recent advances in the therapy of coccidioidomycosis. In Dalldorf G (ed): Fungi and Fungous Diseases. Springfield, Ill, Charles C Thomas, 1962, p 315

——— Primary cutaneous coccidioidomycosis. Re-evaluation of its potentiality based on study of three new cases. Arch Dermatol 92:221, 1965

Winter B, Villaveces J, Spector M: Coccidioidomycosis accompanied by acute tracheal obstruction in a child. JAMA 195:1001, 1966

Ziering WH, Rockas HR: Long-term treatment with amphotericin B of disseminated disease in a three-month-old baby. Am J Dis Child 108:454, 1964

HISTOPLASMOSIS

Christie A: Histoplasmosis and pulmonary calcification; geographic distribution. Am J Trop Med Hyg 31:742, 1951

——— Peterson JC: Pulmonary calcification in negative reactors to tuberculin. Am J Public Health 35:1131, 1945

——— Peterson JC: Histoplasmin sensitivity. J Pediatr 29:417, 1946

Emmons CW: Histoplasmosis: animal reservoirs and other sources in nature of the pathogenic fungus, Histoplasma. Am J Public Health 40:436, 1950

Friedman JL, Baum GL, Schwarz J: Primary pulmonary histoplasmosis: associated pericardial and mediastinal manifestations. Am J Dis Child 109:298, 1965

Furcolow ML, Mantz HL, Lewis I: The roentgenographic appearance of persistent pulmonary infiltrates associated with sensitivity to histoplasmin. Public Health Rep 62:1711, 1947

Parker J, Sarosi G, Doto I, Bailey R, Tosh F: Treatment of chronic pulmonary histoplasmosis. N Engl J Med 283:225, 1970

Schwarz J, Baum GL: The history of histoplasmosis from 1906 to 1956. N Engl J Med 256:253, 1957

Sutliff W: Histoplasmosis cooperative study. V. Amphotericin B dosage for chronic pulmonary histoplasmosis. Am Rev Respir Dis 105:60, 1972

Tesh RB, Schacklette MH, Diercks FH, Hirschl D: Histoplasmosis in children. Pediatrics 33:894, 1964

Vanek J, Schwartz J: The gamut of histoplasmosis. Am J Med 50:89, 1971

CRYPTOCOCCOSIS

Campbell GD: Primary pulmonary cryptococcosis. Am Rev Respir Dis 94:236, 1966

Lewis JL, Rabinovich S: The wide spectrum of cryptococcal infection. Am J Med 53:315, 1972

Littman ML, Walter JE: Cryptococcosis: current status. Am J Med 45:922, 1968

Randall RE Jr, Stacy WK, Toone EC, et al: Cryptococcal pyelonephritis. N Engl J Med 279:60, 1968

Salyer WR, Salyer DC, Baker RD: Primary complex of Cryptococcus and pulmonary lymph nodes. J Infect Dis 130:74, 1974

Siewers CMF, Cramblett HG: Cryptococcosis (torulosis) in children. Pediatrics 34:393, 1964

PHYCOMYCOSIS

Abramson E, Wilson D, Arky RA: Rhinocerebral phycomycosis in association with diabetic ketoacidosis. Report of two cases and a review of clinical and experimental experience with amphotericin B therapy. Ann Intern Med 66:735, 1967

Straatsma BR, Zimmerman LE, Gass JDM: Phycomycosis: A clinicopathologic study of fifty-one cases. Lab Invest 11:1018, 1962

CANDIDIASIS

Androile VT, Kravetz HM, Roberts WC, Utz JP: Candida endocarditis, clinical and pathologic studies. Am J Med 32:251, 1962

Eras P, Goldstein M, Sherlock P: Candida infection of the gastrointestinal tract. Medicine, 51:367, 1972

Kauffman C, Tan JS: Torulopsis glabrata renal infection. Am J Med 57:217, 1974

Kozinn P, Taschdjian CL, Seelig MS, Caroline L, Teitler A: Diagnosis and therapy of systemic candidiasis. Sabouraudia 7:98, 1969

Toala P, Schroeder S, Daly A, Finland M: Candida at Boston City Hospital. Arch Intern Med 126:983, 1970

Winner HI, Hurley R: Symposium on Candida Infections. London. E&S Livingstone, 1966, p 249

——— Candida Albicans. Boston, Little, Brown, 1964

Parasitic Diseases

Parasitic diseases are caused by helminths, protozoans, and arthropods. The organisms included within this restricted definition afflict more than half the world's population; the conditions they cause often result in chronic debilitating disease and death. Parasitic infections are more frequently encountered in tropical and subtropical areas, where they constitute the leading cause of serious infectious diseases. A warm and moist climate, poor sanitation, low socioeconomic status, and inadequate diet are among the important factors contributing to the prevalence of parasitic deseases in these areas. Many diseases that were previously regarded as tropical diseases are in reality cosmopolitan. The rise in immigration from tropical and subtropical areas and the advent of worldwide tourism have contributed to the increasing incidence of parasitism in temperate climates.

Children are infected with parasites more frequently than adults, primarily because of the infant's oral behavior and his inability to ward off the bite of an arthropod vector. Furthermore, during the first decade of life there is greater morbidity and mortality from parasitic infection as a consequence of the lack of acquired humoral and tissue immunity in the young host. In Southeast Asia, for example, malaria still remains a leading cause of infant mortality.

HELMINTHIC DISEASES

The word helminth derives from the Greek; it means worm and is usually used to refer to five phyla: the roundworms (phylum Nematoda), flukes and tapeworms (phylum Platyhelminthes), the leeches (class Hirudinea, phylum Annelida), and two other phyla of little medical interest, the Acanthocephala and Nematomorpha. Diseases caused by helminths are summarized in Table 1.

Diseases Caused by Nematodes

The nematodes (roundworms) are cylindrical, unsegmented, elongated white organisms. The parasitic species infecting man may range from a fraction of a millimeter to well over a meter in length. The female is usually larger than the male, in some species by almost 1,000-fold. The nematode integument consists of a tough, resistant, relatively impermeable, noncellular outer cuticle secreted by an immediately underlying epithelial layer, the hypodermis. The cuticle may be smooth, striated, or adorned with spines. Suspended within the pseudocoelom or body cavity are a complete digestive tract, primitive excretory and nervous systems, and a highly developed reproductive system. The daily egg-laying capacity of some species may exceed a quarter of a million. It is understandable that these parasites have thrived so successfully throughout the warm moist areas of the world.

Nematodes have four larval stages, with a molt separating each; on emerging from the final molt there is a fifth stage, the immature adult. Depending on the species, the initial molt may occur within the ovum (*Trichuris, Ascaris*), in the soil as free-living larvae (*Necator, Ancylosioma*), or in an intermediate host (*Wuchereria, Loa*). The final molts then occur in the definitive host. The mode of entry into the final host may be by inges-

tion of infective ova (*Ascaris, Enterobius*), by penetration of the skin by infective larvae (*Necator, Strongyloides*), or by inoculation of the larvae by an insect bite (*Filaria*).

Ascariasis

Ascariasis is caused by infection with the giant intestinal roundworm *Ascaris lumbricoides*. The ancient Greeks and Romans singled out this worm as the most common intestinal parasite, and it remains the most frequently encountered and widely distributed helminth to this day. Stoll has estimated a world incidence of 644 million individuals, with 3 million infected in North America alone. It is the largest intestinal roundworm commonly infecting man; females measure 20 to 40 cm, males 15 to 30 cm; the female contains as many as 27 million eggs at one time and may lay approximately 200,000 eggs a day. These broadly ovoid eggs are 45 to 75 μ in length and 35 to 50 μ wide (Fig. 3). The fertilized egg consists of a remarkably impervious thin inner shell, a thick transparent midlayer, and the characteristic, often bile-stained, mamillated outer shell. Unfertilized eggs are broader and longer (about 90 μ by 45 μ) and usually lack the albuminoid mamillated outer coat.

The eggs, which are passed in the feces, continue their development and become infective after the first-stage larva molts within the egg. The eggs are remarkably resistant to drying, low temperatures, and many chemicals. Development may be as rapid as several weeks, but in adverse situations it can be delayed for extended periods, only to resume when suitable conditions return. Children often infect themselves and others by playing in the same areas where they eliminate their wastes. In regions where human wastes are used as fertilizer, as in the Orient, *Ascaris* infection is especially frequent.

Eggs containing the infective second-stage larvae never hatch in the soil. However, when ingested and stimulated by enzymes in the duodenum, the larvae emerge actively from a small tear in the weakened egg shell, quickly traverse the intestinal mucosa, and enter the mesenteric lymphatics and venules. They then enter the portal circulation and reach the pulmonary vascular bed, where they usually perforate the alveolar endothelium and epithelium to enter the alveolar space. They molt twice, and by the tenth day fourth-stage larvae ascend the respiratory tree to the epiglottis and are swallowed (Fig. 4). The vast majority of ascarids finally settle in the jejunum. Following a fourth and final molt, copulation occurs, and mature females begin ovipositing in 2 to 2.5 months.

PATHOLOGY.   As with many of the helminthic diseases, the pathology found during the initial or larval migrating stages is quite distinct from that caused by adult worms. Intestinal penetration and migration through the liver are usually of little pathologic importance. However, invasion of the respiratory system by migrating larvae results in alveolar hemorrhages, and pulmonary damage can be extensive, especially if there are large numbers of larvae migrating. In young children *Ascaris* pneumonia (Löffler's pneumonia) may be particularly serious and may result in confluent bron-

TABLE 1. Human Parasitic Infections: Helminthes

Disease	Parasite	Location in Man	Transmission	Typical Clinical Findings	Diagnosis	Treatment	Age Incidence
NEMATODES							
Ascariasis	*Ascaris lumbricoides*	Adult: small intestine; larvae: lung	Ingestion of eggs from soil or food	Vague abdominal distress, nervousness, cough during lung stage	Eggs in feces	Piperazine, pyrantel, mebendazole	Most prevalent 2–14 years
Visceral larva migrans	*Toxocara canis, T. cati*	Liver, lung, kidneys, heart, brain, eye, striated muscle	Ingestion of eggs from soil	Hepatomegaly, eosinophilia, fever, hyperglobulinemia, geophagy	Clinical or biopsy	Thiabendazole (?)	2–15 years
Enterobiasis	*Enterobius vermicularis*	Ileocecal region	Ingestion of eggs	Perianal pruritus	Scotch tape swab	Piperazine, pyrantel mebendazole	Most prevalent 5–14 years; sharpest increase 2–5 years
Trichuriasis	*Trichuris trichiura*	Ileocecal region	Ingestion of eggs from soil or food	Generally slight abdominal discomfort	Eggs in feces	Mebendazole, hexylresorcinol	Most prevalent 5–10 years; heaviest infection 5 years
Hookworm	*Ancylostoma duodenale, Necator americanus*	Small intestine	Larva penetrates skin	Abdominal pain and anemia	Eggs in feces	Pyrantel, mebendazole	Infancy to peak incidence at 16–30 years
Cutaneous larva migrans	*Ancylostoma braziliense, A. caninum*	Skin	Larva penetrates skin	Pruritus; inflammatory serpiginous skin lesions	Physical exam	Freezing or thiabendazole, mebendazole	Beyond infancy, sharpest increase 2–5 years with peak at 5–14 years
Strongyloidiasis	*Strongyloides stercoralis*	Small intestine	Larva penetrates skin	Diarrhea, abdominal discomfort	Larvae in feces	Thiabendazole	Children and adults, especially in childrens' institutions
Trichinosis	*Trichinella spiralis*	Early: small intestinal wall; late: striated muscle cysts	Ingestion of cysts in pork	Early: diarrhea, fever, eosinophilia, orbital edema; late: muscle pain	Skin test, biopsy	Cortisone early + thiabendazole	All age groups, usually above 2 years
Bancroft's filariasis	*Wuchereria bancrofti*	Lymphatics, lymph nodes	Mosquito inoculation of larvae	Lymphangitis, fever, lymphedema	Microfilariae in blood (8:00 P.M. to 2:00 A.M. in nocturnal forms), serologic tests	Diethylcarbamazine, surgery	Infection begins in infancy; disease seen in adolescents and adults
Malayan filariasis	*Brugia malayi*	Lymphatics, lymph nodes	Mosquito inoculation of larvae	Lymphangitis, lymphadenitis lymphedema	Microfilariae in peripheral blood smear, serologic tests	Diethylcarbamazine, surgery	Infection begins in infancy; disease seen in adolescents and adults
Onchocerciasis	*Onchocerca volvulus*	Subcutaneous tissue	Inoculation of larvae by black fly (*Simulium*)	Subcutaneous nodules, blindness	Microfilariae in skin biopsy	Excision of nodules, diethylcarbamazine + suramin	In Central and South America frequent in children less than 10 years; in Africa more often in children older than 10 years

Disease	Organism	Location	Mode of infection	Symptoms	Diagnosis	Treatment	Age group
Loaiasis	*Loa loa*	Subcutaneous tissues	Inoculation of larvae by deer flies (*Chrysops*)	Fugitive swelling and inflammation	Microfilariae in peripheral blood smear in daytime	Excision of worm, diethylcarbamazine	Older children and adults
Dracontiasis	*Dracunculus medinensis*	Subcutaneous tissues	Ingestion of water flea (cyclops)	Cutaneous ulcer, subcutaneous tunnels	Physical examination	Removal of worm, niridazole	Children after weaning (2–3 years)
TREMATODES							
Schistosomiasis	*Schistosoma mansoni*	Venules of large intestine	Cercariae penetrate skin	Early: fever, dysentery; late: hepatic insufficiency	Eggs in feces, rectal biopsy, liver biopsy	Stibophen, Miracil D, antimony dimercaptosuccinate	Especially in children 4 years of age and over
	S. japonicum	Venules of small intestine	Cercariae penetrate skin	Early: fever, GI complaints; late: hepatic insufficiency	Eggs in feces, liver biopsy, rectal biopsy	Tartar emetic, stibophen	
	S. haematobium	Venules of urinary bladder	Cercariae penetrate skin	Early: fever (esp. white child), urticaria, cough; late: urinary tract problems	Eggs in urine, cystoscopic examination	Stibophen, miracil D, tartar emetic, niridazole antimony dimercaptosuccinate	
Fascioliasis	*Fasciola hepatica*	Biliary ducts	Ingestion of metacercariae on vegetation	Biliary tract symptoms	Eggs in feces or duodenal aspirate	Emetine, bithionol	Older children, adolescents, and especially adults
Clonorchiasis	*Clonorchis sinensis*	Biliary ducts	Ingestion of metacercariae of freshwater fish	Biliary tract symptoms	Eggs in feces or duodenal aspirate	Chloroquine, dehydroemetine	Frequent reinfection beginning early childhood; disease in later adulthood
Fasciolopsiasis	*Fasciolopsis buski*	Small intestine	Ingestion of metacercariae on aquatic vegetation	Diarrhea, abdominal pain	Eggs in feces	Hexylresorcinol, tetrachloroethylene	Young children and adults in the first decade disease most severe
Paragonimiasis	*Paragonimus westermani*	Lung	Ingestion of metacercariae from crabs and crayfish	Rusty or blood-streaked sputum, fever	Eggs in sputum or feces	Bithionol, chloroquine	Infection often acquired during first decade
CESTODES							
Diphyllobothriasis	*Diphyllobothrium latum*	Small intestine	Ingestion of plerocercoid larva in fish	Usually asymptomatic; rarely, pernicious anemia or abdominal discomfort	Eggs in feces	Yomesan, paromomycin	Occasional cases in childhood
Sparganosis	*Spirometra* species	Subcutaneous and muscle tissues	Ingestion of larvae or application of infected meat poultices	Fever, hypersensitivity reactions, pain and induration	Biopsy	Excision	All age groups

TABLE 1. Human Parasitic Infections: Helminthes (cont.)

Disease	Parasite	Location in Man	Transmission	Typical Clinical Findings	Diagnosis	Treatment	Age Incidence
CESTODES (cont.)							
Taeniasis	*Taenia solium*	Small intestine	Ingestion of cysticerci in pork	Usually asymptomatic; occasional abdominal discomfort	Eggs in feces and gravid proglottids with 7–13 uterine branches	Yomesan, paromomycin	Gradual increase above the age of 2 years
Cysticercosis	*Cysticercus cellulosae*	Muscle, central nervous system, eye	Ingestion of eggs in swine feces	Neurologic, visual symptoms	Radiography	Excision	Gradual increase above the age of 2 years
Taeniasis	*Taenia saginata*	Small intestine	Ingestion of cysticerci in beef	Usually asymptomatic; occasional abdominal upset or toxic symptoms	Eggs in feces and gravid proglottids with more than 15 uterine branches	Yomesan, paromomycin	Gradual increase above the age of 2 years
Hymenolepiasis	*Hymenolepis nana*	Small intestine	Ingestion of eggs from human feces	Abdominal discomfort	Eggs in feces	Yomesan, paromomycin	Children 2–15 years
	Hymenolepis diminuta	Small intestine	Accidental ingestion, insects infected with cysts	Usually asymptomatic	Eggs in feces	Yomesan, paromomycin	Almost exclusively in children under 3 years
Hydatid disease	*Echinococcus granulosus*	Liver, lung, central nervous system	Ingestion of eggs from dog feces	Often asymptomatic, signs of intracranial pressure, cough, intraabdominal mass	Physical exam, radiography, serology	Surgical removal	Infection acquired in infancy, childhood
Dipylidiasis	*Dipylidium caninum*	Small intestine	Ingestion of cysticerci in flea	Vague abdominal complaints	Eggs or proglottids in feces	Yomesan, paromomycin	Almost exclusively in children and infants

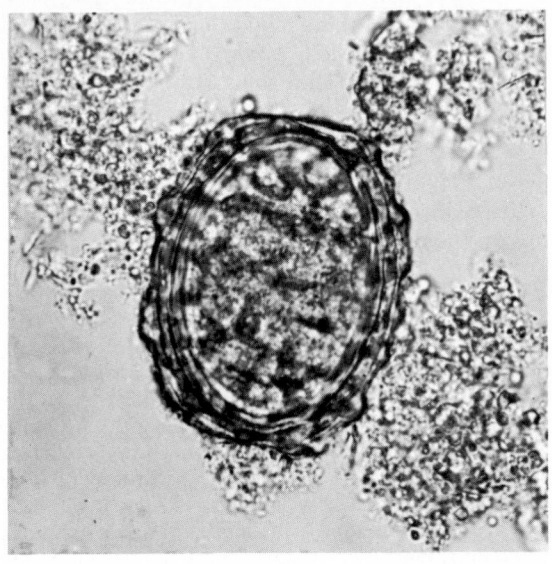
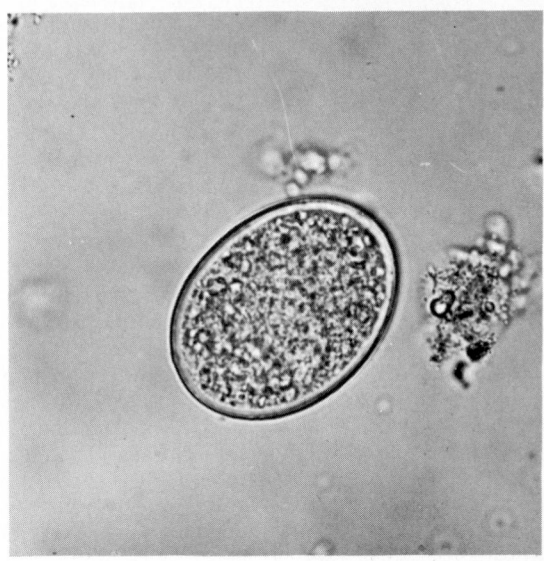

A   B

FIG. 3. *Ascaris lumbricoides* (×448). A. Typical egg passed in fresh feces. B. Decorticate ovum.

chopneumonia, in which the alveoli are filled with red blood cells, eosinophils, fibrin, and polymorphonuclear leukocytes. Larvae occasionally may traverse the pulmonary circulation and produce serious lesions in the eye, central nervous system, and kidney. Thus larval ascariasis can, on occasion, resemble visceral larva migrans. There may be slight pathologic manifestations or none at all, with a small number of adult worms in the jejunum. Heavy infections, especially in children, may necessitate surgical intervention as a result of intestinal obstruction or occasionally perforation. Rarely, ascarids may migrate into the biliary and pancreatic ducts, causing jaundice or acute pancreatitis.

SYMPTOMS. During the period of larval invasion and migration, cough, dyspnea, fever (39.5 C to 40.5 C), rales, and dullness to percussion of the chest may be evident. Hemoptysis may occur, and larvae may be found in the sputum. Radiographic evidence of consolidation and widening of the pulmonary hilum may be seen, and a markedly elevated eosinophil count is often found (Löffler's syndrome). During this phase other manifestations of hypersensitivity, such as urticaria, are frequently encountered in individuals who are repeatedly infected. Among young children, pulmonary ascariasis may have a fatal termination in about 0.2 percent of cases. Allergic manifestations such as bronchial asthma and urticaria may persist until the infection is eliminated.

Adult worms in the small intestine, unless they are numerous, are generally associated with few symptoms. They are presumed to subsist on semidigested food in the lumen, although there are occasional reports of erythrocyte digestion. The most frequently noted symptoms in children are vague epigastric pains, nausea, vomiting, and anorexia. At times, severe, intermittent,

colicky abdominal pain may be the result of partial intestinal obstruction. The more serious problems encountered with *Ascaris* infection result from migration of adult worms into the bile and pancreatic ducts and com-

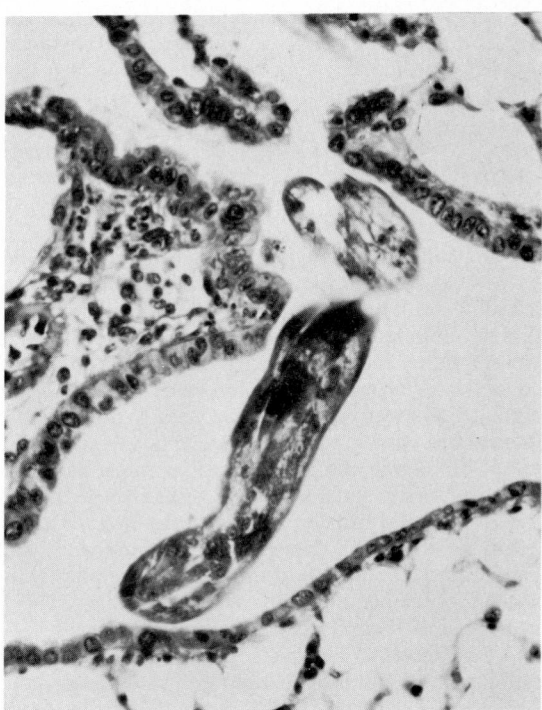

FIG. 4. *Ascaris* larvae in the lung of an experimental animal (×320).

plete intestinal obstruction. These complications may follow tetrachlorethylene therapy for concurrent hookworm disease or may occur in debilitating illness when the environment becomes unsuitable for the worms' requirements. Worms may occasionally migrate cephalad and emerge through the mouth or nose or migrate posteriorly and pass per rectum. These dramatic events cause a great deal of alarm in the patients and parents.

DIAGNOSIS. Generally the diagnosis is established by finding and identifying eggs in the feces. Occasionally an adult worm is passed, or worms may be outlined with contrast medium during the course of a radiographic examination.

TREATMENT. The drug of choice for eliminating the adult worm is piperazine citrate (Antepar), which is available as a syrup or tablet. The daily dosage for patients weighing up to 30 pounds is 1 g; 30 to 50 pounds, 2 g; 50 to 100 pounds, 3 g; over 100 pounds, 3.5 g.Therapy is given daily for two consecutive days. In severe cases it may be repeated after 1 week. Pyrantel pamoate may also be used, 11 mg/kg (maximum 1 g) in a single dose. Mebendazole is also very effective, 100 mg twice daily for 3 days, but it is contraindicated in pregnancy, since it traverses the placenta. Larvae are not affected by any anthelmintics employed for therapy. Intestinal obstruction often responds to medical management consisting of duodenal suction, parenteral fluids, electrolyte correction, and instillation of piperazine into the duodenal tube. If this fails, surgical intervention is required to remove the obstructing worms. No special effort should be made to remove all the worms in the intestinal tract. Individuals tolerate this infection quite well unless large numbers of larvae are migrating through the lungs or intestinal obstruction intervenes. Sanitary disposal of wastes, proper cooking of foods grown in night soil, and education (especially of children) would go a long way to decrease the incidence of ascariasis.

Visceral Larva Migrans

Young children are frequently abnormal hosts of the dog ascarid *Toxocara canis* and occasionally of the cat ascarid *T. cati*. The worms are unable to complete their usual development in the human host, and they provoke a severe tissue reaction causing considerable damage and at times acute disease. Infected dogs seed the neighborhood with eggs, which proceed to develop into infective ova containing second-stage larvae. When ingested, the larvae hatch in the upper intestinal tract, penetrate the intestinal wall, gain access to the mesenteric vessels, and usually migrate to the liver, less frequently to the lungs, kidneys, heart, brain, eye, and striated muscle. Small children are most frequently infected, presumably as a result of their promiscuity with dirt as well as their close association with pets.

PATHOLOGY. Lesions are necrotizing or granulomatous and heavily infiltrated with eosinophils. The larvae eventually are encapsulated by a dense fibrous wall and die. The liver is most frequently found to contain these tiny, gray white granulomatous nodules. The retina and vitreous are occasionally invaded, sometimes leading to blindness.

SYMPTOMS. In mild infections the disease can be virtually asymptomatic, eosinophilia being the only clue. However, the most characteristic clinical picture, especially in a small child, is hepatomegaly, eosinophilia, fever, cough, and wheezing. On occasion, neurologic signs or impairment of vision may be the only manifestation of the infection. Pulmonary embarrassment can at times be severe. Hyperglobulinemia is often found. Geophagia is commonly reported in a large percentage of infected children.

DIAGNOSIS. Although diagnosis is usually made on clinical grounds, liver biopsy provides the best opportunity to make a definitive diagnosis. Serologic methods are not entirely reliable, since cross-reactions with many nematodes may occur. However, recent studies indicate that the bentonite flocculation and/or indirect hemagglutination tests may be sufficiently specific, especially if differential absorption of *Ascaris* antibody is carried out prior to running the reaction with *Toxocara* antigen. As with several other helminthic infections, markedly elevated anti-hemagglutinin A titers have been reported to be associated with visceral larva migrans infection.

TREATMENT. Although thiabendazole has been advocated as specific therapy for this infection, it is uncertain whether this compound alters the course of the disease. Similarly, it is not yet clear if steroid therapy is helpful in severe cases. In most cases the prognosis is quite favorable. However, if the infection is heavy, or if larvae invade critical foci the outcome can be serious or even fatal. Periodic eradication of *Toxocara* infection in household pets by anthelmintics and keeping children away from areas such as sandboxes in which dogs (and especially cats) defecate may also be helpful.

Enterobiasis

Enterobiasis is caused by the pinworm *Enterobius vermicularis*. Although pinworm infection is worldwide, it is more common in temperate climates where children are more heavily clothed and are in closer association with one another. Pinworms infect people in all socioeconomic levels, but residents of institutions or dormitories and family groups are more often affected; children are more susceptible than adults.

Adult worms are small, yellow white, and elongated; typically they inhabit the appendix, cecum, and nearby areas of ileum and ascending colon. Females are 8 to 13 mm long and males 2 to 5 mm. The distended uterus may contain as many as 17,000 eggs, many of which are deposited on the perianal and perineal skin by the migrating gravid female. At room temperature in humid conditions the ova will survive 2 to 3 weeks, resisting destruction by the usual household disinfectants. They are light and will float in air, especially when bed linens or clothes are cast off, thereupon being ingested or inhaled and later swallowed. Frequently the external migration of the gravid female is associated with intense perianal pruritus and scratching, so that anus-to-finger-to-mouth transmission is most common. Retroinfection may also occur when larvae of deposited eggs hatch and migrate back into the intestine, developing to maturity in 2 to 2.5 weeks. Embryonated eggs, when deposited, usually require but a few hours to become infective; and if they are swallowed the larvae escape in the duodenum and develop to maturity in the cecal area within 2 to 6 weeks.

PATHOLOGY.   The majority of infections are without significant pathologic lesions. The intense pruritus ani may provoke such severe scratching that local bleeding, secondary pyogenic infection, and lichenification may result. Whether pinworms are a primary cause of appendicitis remains unsettled. Most pathologists consider their presence in an acutely inflamed appendix an unimportant incidental finding (Fig. 5). In young females the adult worms have been known

ing in young girls may lead to vaginitis and frequent masturbation. Eosinophilia seldom accompanies the infection.

DIAGNOSIS.   Nocturnal perianal pruritus in children strongly suggests pinworm infection. Small, creamy white worms often may be found if examination of the perianal region is made when the child is awakened by itching. Inasmuch as ova are seen infrequently in the stools, the Scotch tape swab technique (NIH swab) is the diagnostic method of choice. A 2.5 inch (6-cm) piece of Scotch tape is folded with its sticky side out over the end of a wooden tongue blade. It is firmly applied against either side of the perianal region. Next, the tape is placed sticky side down on a microscope slide and is examined directly for pinworm ova (Fig. 6). It is

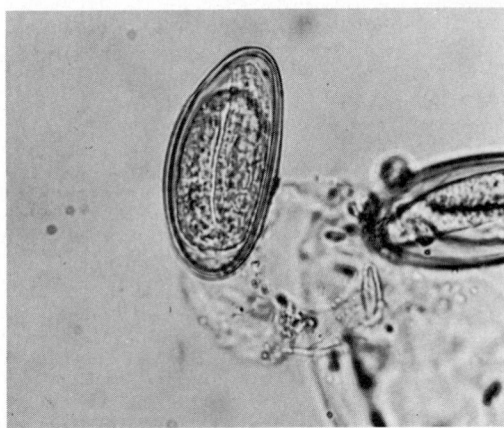

FIG. 6.   Eggs of pinworm on Scotch tape preparation ($\times$448).

preferable to take the swabs in the morning immediately before the patient gets out of bed, and certainly before bathing. One swab on each of three consecutive days is usually sufficient to detect the eggs.

TREATMENT.   There are several preparations that are excellent for treatment of enterobiasis: pyrantel pamoate, 11 mg/kg (maximum 1 g) once a day for 3 days, or mebendazole one dose of 100 mg for 1 day. Piperazine compounds, which are highly effective, are best taken in the morning before breakfast for seven consecutive days. The daily dose of piperazine citrate for patients weighing up to 15 pounds is 250 mg; 16 to 30 pounds, 500 mg; 31 to 60 pounds, 1 g; over 60 pounds, 2 g.

Usually the prognosis is good, with few or no serious side effects. Since transmission and reinfection occur so readily, eradication is difficult, and the physician often elects to treat the entire family simultaneously. Vigorous hygienic measures should also be instituted. Daily baths, frequent washing of hands, laundering and boiling of bedsheets, underwear, and nightclothes, and vigorous vacuum cleaning all help to control reinfection. In the author's experience, a second course of therapy 3 weeks after completion of the first has resulted in nearly 100 percent cure. Personal cleanliness is probably the most effective means of prevention. Fingernails

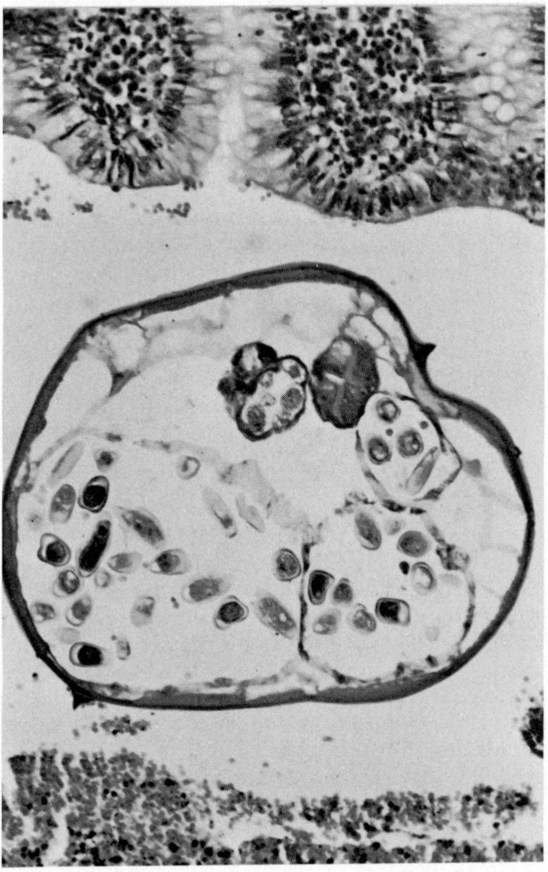

FIG. 5.   Cross section of a female pinworm (*Enterobius vermicularis*) in the lumen of the appendix ($\times$140).

to migrate into the vagina, uterus, and fallopian tubes, being encapsulated finally in the peritoneal cavity. In several instances a chronic granulomatous salpingitis or endometritis has been reported as a result of these ectopic adult worms.

SYMPTOMS.   Pruritus ani, most often intense at night, may awaken the child or cause restless sleep. The child may become irritable and nervous. Perianal itch-should be cut short and hands washed frequently and vigorously. Infected children should sleep alone and wear tight-fitting pajamas. The bedclothes and linens should be boiled daily. However, it is nearly impossible to control dust-borne infective eggs.

Trichuriasis

Trichuriasis is produced by the whipworm *Trichuris trichiura.* This nematode is quite distinctive, having an attenuated whiplike anterior and a broader, fleshier posterior portion. The males are from 3 to 4.5 cm in length with a coiled posterior end; the females are from 3.5 to 5 cm with a blunt posterior end. The eggs are typically barrel-shaped, about 50 by 22 μ; they are usually bile-stained, the ends containing unstained polar plugs (Fig. 7). Adult worms live in the cecum, with their

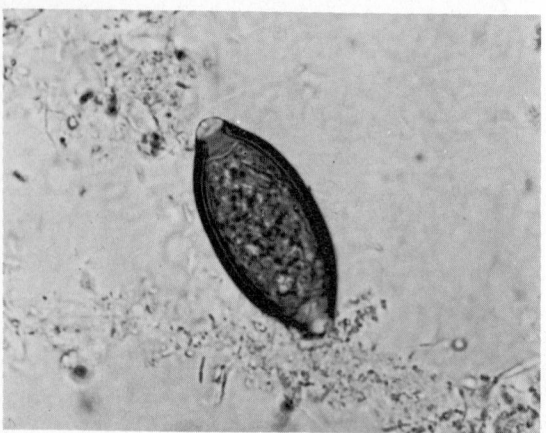

FIG. 7. Egg of the whipworm (*Trichuris trichiura*) in feces ($\times$ 280).

anterior portions buried in the mucosa. Occasionally the appendix and other portions of the large intestine are infected. The female lays large numbers of eggs each day that pass out in feces. After 2 to 4 weeks in warm, shady, moist soil, an infective-stage larva is present within the ovum. When ingested, the larva hatches in the upper small intestine, temporarily penetrates the crypts of Lieberkühn, where it feeds and develops, and then slowly makes its way to the cecal region, becoming a mature egg-laying adult in about 1 to 3 months. Whipworm infection is cosmopolitan, but is far more common in warm moist regions. The prevalence of infection is highest in children 5 to 15 years of age due to their relaxed hygienic habits. Contaminated food and water may be a source of infection as well.

PATHOLOGY. The worm produces a small inflammatory focus at the site of attachment to the intestinal mucosa and ingests whole blood as a part of its diet. Heavy infections may be associated with superficial mucosal erosions, colitis, and in young children, rectal prolapse. Individuals on marginal diets who have heavy whipworm infections may also develop a microcytic hypochromic anemia due to relentless chronic blood loss. Eosinophilia up to 25 percent can be found.

SYMPTOMS. Light infections are usually without clinical manifestations; occasionally there may be complaints of anorexia, insomnia, or vague abdominal pain. In moderate uncomplicated clinical infections, abdominal pain (often localized to the right lower quadrant), flatulence, fever of 37 C to 38.5 C, nausea and vomiting, weight loss, and pruritus are the most frequent complaints. Heavy infections may be accompanied by diarrhea, tenesmus, blood-streaked stools, and rectal prolapse. Without laboratory stool examinations, trichuriasis is difficult to differentiate from other intestinal nematode infections. Concentration techniques readily reveal the characteristic ova.

TREATMENT. Mebendazole 100 mg twice a day for 3 days is highly effective in curing *Trichuris* infection. This drug may be repeated after 1 week if necessary. Personal cleanliness, such as the washing of dirty hands, and sanitary waste disposal would essentially eliminate trichuriasis. In light infections prognosis is excellent. However, heavy infections can lead to serious complications unless the worms are eliminated.

Hookworm Disease

Since ancient times hookworm infection has been one of the major diseases of mankind. It currently infects an estimated one-fourth of the world's population. *Necator americanus,* so-called American hookworm, is the prevailing species in the southern United States and most of the warm areas of the world. *Ancylostoma duodenale,* the so-called Old World hookworm, is primarily a parasite of the Mediterranean basin, northern India, north China, Japan, and the west coast of South America. It accounts for approximately 15 percent of the world's hookworm infections.

Hookworms are about 1 cm long and 0.3 to 0.4 cm in greatest breadth, males being slightly smaller than females. They range from creamy to gray white and possess a distinctive oral or buccal capsule containing cutting plates in *Necator* and two pairs of upper teeth in *Ancylostoma.* The posterior tip of the male forms a distinctive broad, transparent umbrellalike copulatory bursa. Adult hookworms reside in the upper portions of the small intestine attached to the mucosa by their buccal capsules (Fig. 8). A mature female lays thousands of eggs daily; the eggs are about 68 by 38 μ and of similar appearance in both species. Usually the eggs have reached the two- to eight-cell stage when seen in the stool, although later stages may be found if passage is delayed because of constipation (Fig. 9).

If the eggs are deposited in warm, moist, sandy, shady soil they develop rapidly, so that characteristic first-stage rhabditoid larvae hatch within 1 to 2 days. Growth is rapid, and a molt occurs after 3 days of feeding on bacteria and fecal debris. The second-stage larvae continue to feed and grow, so that by the fifth to tenth day a second molt results in nonfeeding, filariform third-stage infective larvae. These are negatively geotropic and tend to rise to the top level of the moist soil, where they remain awaiting contact with human skin. They actively penetrate the skin, usually of the interdigital spaces of the bare feet, enter subcutaneous capillaries,

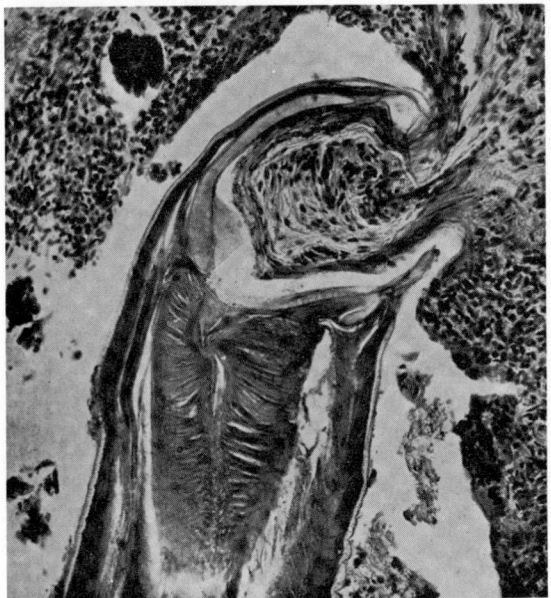

FIG. 8. Hookworm attached to intestinal wall. (From Hunter, Frye, and Swartzwelder: *Manual of Tropical Medicine,* 4th ed, 1966. Courtesy of W. B. Saunders.

and are carried to the lungs, where they penetrate the capillaries and enter the alveoli. The larvae next ascend the respiratory tree and are swallowed. During the latter period they undergo a third molt, forming a temporary buccal capsule by which they attach to the intestinal villi. After the fourth and final molt they feed and grow to maturity, with their eggs appearing in the feces about 5 to 6 weeks after infection. While accidental ingestion of infective-stage larvae of *A. duodenale* will result in direct development of mature adults, migration through the lungs by *N. americanus* seems to be indispensable.

PATHOLOGY. Larvae of *Necator* often produce extensive subcutaneous damage beneath the site of invasion; together with pyogenic bacteria carried in with the invading larvae, they may cause a papulovesicular lesion that later ulcerates and eventually clears in about 10 to 14 days. Lobular pulmonary consolidation is distinctly uncommon during the lung phase. The important abnormality is a microcytic hypochromic anemia resulting from continuous sucking of the host's blood. It has been estimated that each worm may take in, and partially utilize, about 0.5 ml of blood a day. Blood loss of this magnitude may be well compensated if the worm burden is small in an otherwise healthy, well-nourished individual.

SYMPTOMS. Ground itch is associated with the initial larval skin invasion by *Necator*. During the course of the initial infection there may be cough, low-grade fever, acute abdominal disturbances, intermittent diarrhea, and a markedly elevated eosinophilia. As the disease becomes chronic, even with frequent reinfection, the symptoms depend primarily on the individual's diet, state of health, and acquired immunity. Therefore patients with comparable worm burdens may be either symptomatic or relatively asymptomatic, the latter complaining only of vague abdominal discomfort. Similarly, anemia may be completely compensated by adequate diet, or the patient may complain of weakness, dizziness, and weight loss. As the worm burden increases there may be palpitations, tachycardia, and edema associated with either hypoproteinemia and/or congestive heart failure. In children, physical and sexual development may be retarded. Pica and geophagia are often seen among infected children. If poor nutrition is corrected and specific anthelmintic therapy is provided, recovery is usual.

DIAGNOSIS. Definitive diagnosis requires identification of the eggs in the feces. Occasionally rhabditoid larvae may be found in stools and must be differentiated from rhabditoid larvae of *Strongyloides stercoralis,* which possess a much shorter buccal chamber.

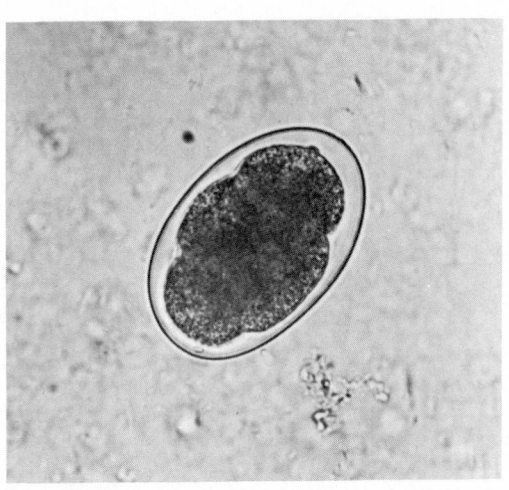
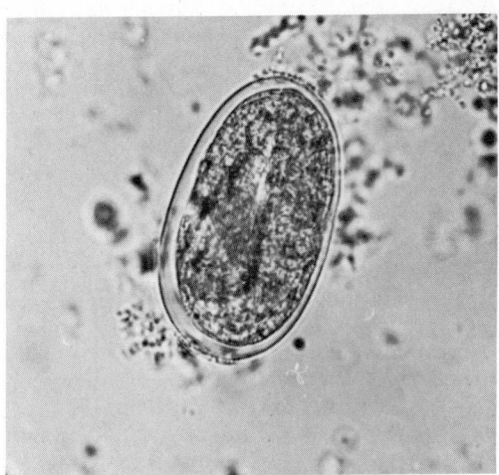

FIG. 9. Hookworm (*Necator americanus*) eggs recovered from feces (× 448). *A.* Typical 4-cell stage. *B.* Developing motile larva.

In tropical areas, of course, infection with both of these worms is frequently encountered. The ova of *Trichostrongylus orientalis* also must be differentiated from those of hookworm. The clinical picture of hookworm usually is not sufficiently distinctive to rely on clinical impression alone.

TREATMENT. Pyrantel pamoate, 11 mg/kg (maximum 1 g) per day for up to 3 days, is highly efficacious. Mebendazole, 100 mg twice a day for 3 days, is also excellent for the treatment of either *Ancylostoma* or *Necator*. The control of hookworm infection depends on education of individuals in rural communities. Sanitary disposal of feces and the wearing of shoes have had a marked effect in reduction of infection in the southern United States. Improvement in the nutritional status of infected individuals often will alleviate all clinical signs of infection.

Cutaneous Larva Migrans

Creeping eruption, or cutaneous larva migrans, is caused most frequently by infection with the filariform larvae of *Ancylostoma braziliense*, which ordinarily infect dogs and cats, although other species of larval hookworms such as *A. caninum*, *N. americanus*, and *Uncinaria stenocephala* have been incriminated. *S. stercoralis* occasionally causes a similar picture. In Southeast Asia the larvae of *Gnathostoma spinigerum* may cause creeping eruption, as may the larvae of the horse bot fly *Gasterophilus*. These larvae migrate in the stratum germinativum, creating serpiginous dermal tunnels with marked erythema and pruritus. Secondary bacterial infection is common. The larvae may wander in the skin for several weeks or months, but they generally fail to gain access to the circulation.

Creeping eruption is frequently encountered in the southern United States, especially in the summer and fall months, in bathers, workmen, and children who have been exposed to moist, sandy soil contaminated with dog and cat feces. Generally the infection is self-limited and requires no treatment. In persistent or severe infections, topical therapy by freezing with ethyl chloride has been used with varying success. Recent reports suggest thiabendazole, 25 mg/kg twice a day for 3 to 4 days, may be helpful. Topical application of a 10 percent aqueous suspension of thiabendazole has been advocated. Mebendazole has also been reported useful in this condition. Periodic anthelmintic therapy of dogs and cats should help reduce exposure to these worms.

Strongyloidiasis

S. stercoralis is the etiologic agent of strongyloidiasis. The disease is primarily one of warm areas and is found sporadically in temperate climates. The parasitic female is an extremely small (2.2 by 0.04 mm), nearly transparent thin worm; hence the name threadworm. She resides buried in the mucosa of the upper small intestine, feeding and depositing eggs. Rhabditoid larvae hatch within the tissues and penetrate the mucosa to enter the lumen; these usually pass out with the feces (Fig. 10).

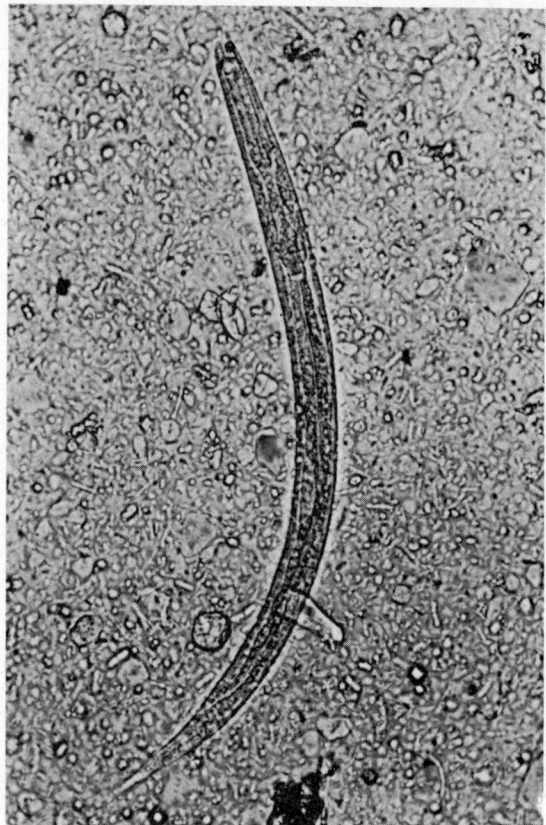

FIG. 10. Rhabditoid larva of *strongyloides stercoralis* passed in feces (×280).

After being deposited in the soil, the larvae develop into infective-stage filariform larvae either directly or indirectly after one or more intervening free-living generations. In warm and very moist soil with organic debris, free-living generations develop within 24 to 36 hours into sexually mature males and females that mate and lay eggs.

Rhabditoid larvae that hatch in the soil may repeat the free-living cycle indefinitely, or they may molt, producing filariform infective-stage larvae. On contact they penetrate the skin, enter a subcutaneous capillary, and are carried to the lungs. There they penetrate the capillary wall and enter alveoli, where they molt several times to become adolescent worms. They next ascend the respiratory tree and are swallowed, then invading the intestinal mucosa. It is not entirely clear where copulation occurs, or if parthenogenesis is the rule. Parasitic males have not been unequivocally identified in this species. If rhabditoid larvae molt in the intestinal lumen while passing down the bowel and become infective filariform larvae, autoinfection may occur. Filariform larvae may invade the mucosa of the ileum or large bowel, enter portal vessels to be carried to the lungs, and finally journey to the intestine to mature within the mucosa. Occasionally they pass out in the stool and penetrate the perianal skin, causing autoinfection or cutaneous larva migrans. Therefore, it is entirely possible that a relatively minor infection may become moderate to severe, and individuals may maintain their infection indefinitely without further outside reinfection. The incidence of strongyloidiasis increases above 5 years of age and is especially common in mental institutions, orphanages, and prisons.

PATHOLOGY. Soon after the larvae penetrate the skin, pruritic erythematous blotches and papules appear. Giant urticarial lesions are seen in previously sensitized individuals. Serious pulmonary involvement is not often encountered, although there are occasional reports of transient patchy pneumonitis associated with marked eosinophilia (Löffler's syndrome). The principal lesion is found in the upper portions of the small intestine, where injury to the mucosa by both adults and migrating larvae may cause a severe duodenitis and jejunitis, with marked eosinophilic and mononuclear cell infiltration. In heavy infections granulomatous inflammation and mucosal necrosis are extensive, leading to eventual fibrous scarring.

SYMPTOMS. The initial larval invasion of the skin is accompanied by pruritus, and the pulmonary phase is often associated with a dry cough. Although mild infections may be entirely asymptomatic, a heavier worm burden is often accompanied by nausea, vomiting, epigastric pain, weakness, and mucous diarrhea, which may be exhausting and unrelenting. A spruelike syndrome has been reported. Eosinophilia is nearly a constant finding with this infection, although it usually declines somewhat with chronicity. Untreated *Strongyloides* infection may last a lifetime, which presumably is due to the internal autoinfective cycle that maintains the infection within the host. It is not uncommon that such individuals will complain only of midepigastric distress that is relieved by food, milk, or antacids. Such symptoms often evoke the diagnosis of peptic ulcer disease, and these patients are treated for many years as ulcer patients. The presence of eosinophilia together with ulcer symptomatology should raise one's suspicion of strongyloidiasis. Recently a number of cases of fatal, overwhelming, disseminated strongyloidiasis have been reported. These cases involved compromised or debilitated hosts who had been immunosuppressed for a variety of reasons, such as during therapy for Hodgkin's disease, malignant lymphoma, renal transplantation, nephrotic syndrome, leprosy, and severe hepatic disease. Thus pulmonary infiltrates and rising eosinophilia while on steroid therapy should alert one to the possibility of disseminated strongyloidiasis.

DIAGNOSIS. The presence of rhabditoid larvae in the stool is diagnostic. Care must be taken to distinguish the larvae of *Strongyloides* from those of hookworm, *Trichostrongylus,* and some other nonparasitic, fecal-inhabiting nematode larvae. In pulmonary involvement, examination of the sputum may reveal the larvae. On occasion it may be necessary to aspirate and examine duodenal contents in order to find larvae.

TREATMENT. Thiabendazole, 25 mg/kg twice a day for 2 to 3 days, is the drug of choice. Side effects such as anorexia, dizziness, nausea, and vomiting are common. Diarrhea, pruritus, epigastric distress, and drowsiness may occasionally occur. Thiabendazole therapy has been associated rarely with hyperglycemia, rash, leukopenia, hypotension, and bradycardia. Generally the prognosis is good, except in heavy untreated cases. Absence of eosinophilia and the presence of leukopenia are regarded as poor prognostic signs. All individuals found to harbor this infection should receive therapy, inasmuch as fatal disseminated strongyloidiasis can occur in the elderly, in the debilitated, and in individuals who may be undergoing therapy with steroids or other immunosuppressive agents. Just as in hookworm infections, individuals should be cautioned against walking barefoot. Sanitary waste disposal coupled with education are most essential for control of this disease.

Trichinosis

Infection with *Trichinella spiralis* is found in most parts of the world in which raw or insufficiently cooked pork is consumed. Therefore trichinosis is comparatively common in the United States, Mexico, and Europe and relatively unimportant in predominantly Moslem and Hindu countries. When an individual ingests meat infected with *Trichinella* cysts, larvae excyst in the duodenum, invade the mucosa of the small intestine, and in 5 to 7 days develop into tiny adults. After fertilization the female continues to grow and may burrow deeply into the intestinal wall, where she begins to deposit larvae that invade the intestinal lymphatics and venules. About 1,000 to 1,500 larvae are discharged each day throughout the 1 to 4 months of life of the adult. By the second week larvae are migrating throughout the body, and by the third week encystment in striated muscle is in progress. Here the larvae may remain viable for years, but usually they succumb within 6 to 9 months, slowly calcifying.

Although human infection with these worms is a developmental blind alley, the disease is naturally perpetuated by cannibalistic rats. Pigs, bears, and other flesh-eating animals may be secondarily infected. Pigs fed unsterilized infected garbage are probably the main source of trichinous meat in the eastern United States. From time to time home-cooked sausage serves as the nidus of family, neighborhood, or church epidemics. Ingestion of contaminated hamburger is another common source of infection. The current meat-packing practices in the United States generally result in dispersing and diluting infected meat, so that most infected individuals develop either mild or asymptomatic disease.

PATHOLOGY. During the initial or intestinal stage of the disease there may be some petechiae and minor mucosal bleeding. The main lesions are found in striated muscle, where there is fiber hypertrophy, edema, and degeneration. An acute interstitial inflammatory exudate is commonly seen. Eventually the larvae become entombed in an ovoid cyst (Fig. 11). Although larvae do not encyst in the heart, their presence during migration often results in an acute myocarditis. Inva-

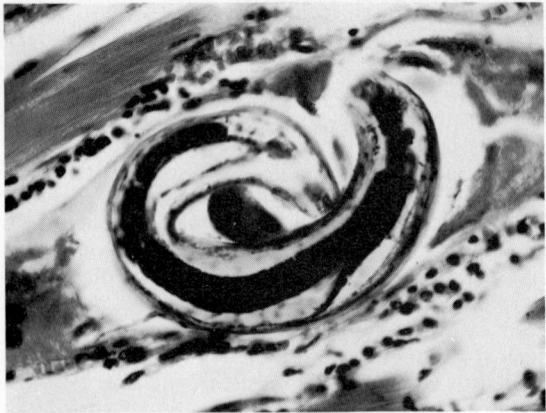

FIG. 11.   Encysting larva of *Trichinella spiralis* in deltoid muscle. An acute inflammatory infiltrate is present about the fragmented muscle (×448).

sion of the central nervous system may provoke a non-suppurative meningitis or granulomatous inflammatory changes in the basal ganglia, medulla, and cerebellum. Eosinophilia may reach 90 percent during the height of larval invasion.

SYMPTOMS.   Clinical symptoms depend primarily on the number of worms ingested at any one time, as well as the number of larvae produced and the sites of invasion. During the intestinal phase invading larvae and adult worms often cause acute gastrointestinal symptoms, including nausea, vomiting, and diarrhea, as well as fever, diaphoresis, and urticaria. When larvae enter the general circulation, new symptoms may occur, so that edema of the eyelids and face, splinter hemorrhages of the nailbeds, fever, and cardiac and respiratory symptoms may become evident. Severe tenderness, pain, and spasm occur during the period of muscle invasion. Cardiac failure and death can occur at this time. Central nervous system symptoms include headache, stiff neck, and psychoses. Ocular involvement, especially periorbital edema and chemosis, is most typical and suggestive of the diagnosis. In patients surviving the period of muscular invasion, muscular tenderness is all that remains; it gradually diminishes after about 12 to 18 months. Unless the infection is heavy, patients ordinarily do well.

DIAGNOSIS.   Early diagnosis is difficult, unless one can elicit a history of eating raw or partially cooked pork. The presence of similar symptoms in members of the same family is often suggestive; however, other infections such as staphylococcal or salmonella food poisoning, shigellosis, and amebiasis must be considered. Eosinophilia, periorbital edema, and splinter nail hemorrhages are most characteristic. At a later stage, biopsy of the deltoid, biceps, or gastrocnemius muscles can provide the definitive diagnosis. The latex flocculation test becomes positive in 17 to 21 days, and the complement-fixation tests become positive after 3 and 4 weeks; these provide strong evidence for the diagnosis. In light infections muscle biopsy is often unrewarding, while serologic tests are diagnositc.

TREATMENT.   Recent clinical trial suggests that thiabendazole, 25 mg/kg twice a day for 5 to 7 days, may be an effective remedy during the intestinal phase. It is not clear whether it is of benefit during the circulating or encysting stages. In human infections, administration of adrenocorticosteroids during the period of larval invasion of the general circulation has been reported to reduce the febrile period and the total duration of illness. In experimental studies, however, adrenocorticosteroids have caused a fourfold increase in invading larvae. They have also suppressed immune reactions, favoring secondary infection.

Since infection is primarily the result of eating raw or partially cooked pork and pork products, the disease can be prevented by thoroughly cooking the meat at 55 C to 58 C for 1 hour. The thermal death point of the encysted larvae is from 62 C to 70 C. Furthermore, larvae of *Trichinella* are killed by freezing for 36 hours at −27 C, 24 hours at −30 C, or 40 minutes at −35 C. The United States government does not inspect meat for infection by this worm; therefore proper education in the preparation of pork and pork products is necessary. Boiling garbage before it is fed to hogs also will help to reduce the incidence of infection.

Dracontiasis

The guinea worm, *Dracunculus medinensis,* known since antiquity as the fiery serpent, is found in Asia, Africa, and a few isolated regions in the Western Hemisphere. The female worm, averaging about 1 m in length by 1 to 2 mm in diameter, usually lives in the subcutaneous tissues of the distal portions of the arms and legs. There a papule that forms near the anterior portion of the work vesiculates and ruptures, leaving an ulcer (Fig. 12). When the extremity is placed in water, a loop of the worm's uterus prolapses into the ulcer and freely discharges motile larvae into the water. This will recur each time the extremity is immersed, until the uterus is emptied and the adult worm dies, usually after several weeks. Thereafter, the larvae are ingested and mature in freshwater copepods of the genus *Cyclops.* When an individual drinks contaminated water, infective larvae are set free; they penetrate the intestinal wall and usually migrate to the retroperitoneal tissues, where they require about 8 to 12 months to mature. The female then migrates to the skin of an extremity in order to discharge her brood. The fate of the adult male worm is unknown. In endemic areas infection begins in childhood, and individuals are reinfected repeatedly throughout life. Infection is uncommon before the age of 3 years, since young children and infants are breastfed and seldom drink infected pond or well water.

The presence of the worms in the deep tissues is usually without side effects. Migration to the skin is signaled by manifestations of severe hypersensitivity, such as urticaria, pruritus, erythema, and on occasion dyspnea and a shocklike state. The skin ulcers are seen most commonly on the ankle or between the metatarsal bones, although they have been described in almost all locations. A mild to moderate eosinophilia usually accompanies the infection. Secondary infection of

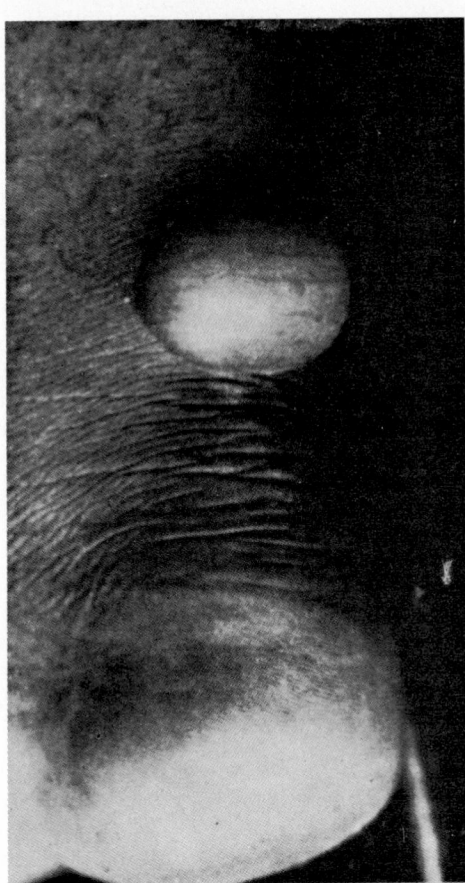

FIG. 12. Blister caused by the presence of the female guinea worm (*Dracunculus medinensis*) in the underlying skin. [From Basu: In Rab and Smith (eds): Clinical Surgery, Vol. 8, 1965. Courtesy of Butterworth.]

the ulcer and worm tract may provoke fibroblastic proliferation that can result in contractures of the involved joint.

Diagnosis can be made only at the time the skin ulcer appears or if the outline of the adult worm can be seen beneath the skin. Surgical removal of the worm is frequently advocated. The time-honored native method of gradually rolling the worm onto a stick, a few centimeters a day, is as much used today as in ancient times (Fig. 13). Severe inflammation and necrosis usually follow if the worm is torn during removal. Therefore the worm is killed by local infiltration with acriflavine or mercuric bichloride before removal is attempted. Oral prophylactic diethylcarbamazine has been advocated to prevent development of adult worms. Niridazole (Ambilhar) has been shown to be remarkably efficacious for the treatment of individuals infected with adult guinea worms. The recommended dosage is 25 mg/kg day (maximum 1.5 g/day) in 2 divided doses for 7 days.

Bancroft's Filariasis

Wuchereria bancrofti, the filarial worm responsible for Bancroft's filariasis, is a creamy white threadlike nema-

tode. The adults invade and live coiled together in the lymphatics and lymph nodes, attaining considerable length; males reach 4 cm, females 8 to 10 cm. The gravid females discharge motile sheathed embryos (microfilariae) that invade and circulate in the blood of their definitive host. If a suitable mosquito ingests microfilariae with a blood meal, larval development proceeds through a series of molts within the insect's thoracic muscles. After 2 weeks infective third-stage filariform larvae have developed; they migrate to the mouth parts of the mosquito and enter the skin when the mosquito next bites. The larvae invade peripheral lymphatics, continue their development to adulthood, and copulate, with microfilariae generally appearing in the peripheral blood in about a year.

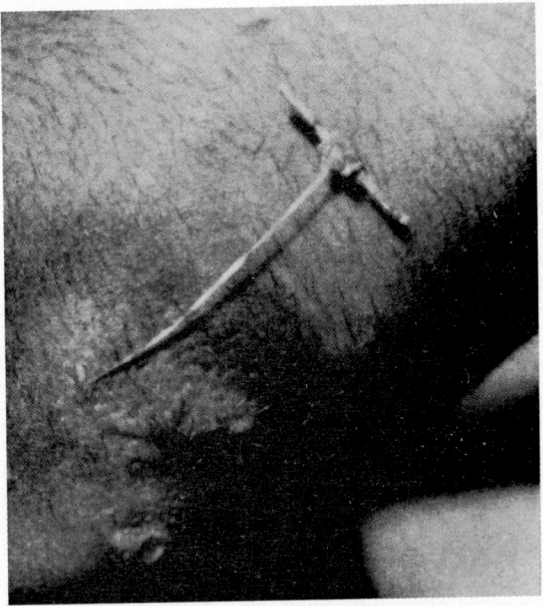

FIG. 13. The guinea worm is extricated from the elbow, several centimeters a day, by winding upon a stick. [From Basu: In Rab and Smith (eds): Clinical Surgery, vol. 8, 1965. Courtesy of Butterworth.]

Although man is the only known definitive host for Bancroft's filariae, there are many species of *Culex*, *Aedes*, and *Anopheles* mosquitoes that are natural vectors. The infection is found throughout all tropical and semitropical areas of the world. In endemic zones the incidence gradually increases with age, but infection begins early in childhood. In some Pacific islands, where a third of the population over 5 years of age may be infected, the disease may not be evident until many years have elapsed and repeated infections have occurred.

PATHOLOGY. Living and dead adult worms provoke a severe lymphangitis wherever they lodge in the body. In the vicinity of the worm there occurs a perilymphangitic reaction composed of numerous eosinophils, plasma cells, macrophages, and foreign body giant cells, as well as an obliterative endolymphangitis due to reticuloendothelial cell proliferation. Lymphatic channels are eventually obliterated, being replaced by fibrous or hyalinized scar tissue. Sometimes worms calcify. Nevertheless, their presence acts as a persistent inflammatory focus, often called the focal point of O'Connor. Lymph flow improves between attacks as inflammation subsides. Repeated bouts of elevated lymphatic pressure with compensatory dilatation, varices, and collateralization finally lead to almost total obstruction as fibrosis becomes widespread. If obstruction occurs in areas of loose connective tissue, such as the retroperitoneum, spermatic cord, and mesentery, lymphatic varicosities result. If obstruction involves afferent lymphatics of more compact connective tissue, such as in the lower extremities, lymphedema and elephantiasis are seen.

SYMPTOMS.   Acute symptoms are not usually observed in endemic areas, inasmuch as infection has usually been acquired repeatedly since infancy. Newcomers to these areas, however, may show the acute disease, which usually begins with fever and a painful descending lymphangitis, funiculitis, or lymphadenitis. Other symptoms such as urticaria, erythema, fugitive swellings, and eosinophilia are frequently encountered. These attacks can recur for several months. The disease eventually passes to a chronic stage, indicated by lymphadenopathy, usually of the inguinal region. Lymphatic obstruction may finally lead to elephantiasis of various body members. Chyluria may occur if, as a result of retroperitoneal obstruction, distal lymphatic vessels rupture into the bladder, ureter, or kidneys.

DIAGNOSIS.   Diagnosis is made by detecting microfilariae in the peripheral blood. Hematologic examination should be done between 8:00 P.M. and 2:00 A.M. in those areas were microfilarial nocturnal periodicity occurs. Serologic or intracutaneous tests employing *Dirofilaria immitis* antigen can be most helpful during the biologic incubation period when microfilariae are not being produced. Lymph node biopsy may reveal the worms. If the worms are not found, the histologic features are often suggestive.

TREATMENT.   Diethylcarbamazine (Hetrazan) quickly clears the blood of microfilariae. Evidence is not clear-cut as to whether this compound kills the adult worms or sterilizes the female. The dosage is 2 mg/kg three times a day, after meals, for at least 3 weeks. During therapy, mild allergic manifestations are frequently encountered, such as fever, rash, and headache. Enlarged elephantoid limbs often respond to conservative management such as rest, elevation, and tight bandaging or stockings. Surgical intervention may be required in advanced disease. It is often necessary to treat recurrent bacterial cellulitis or lymphangitis with the appropriate antibiotics for mixed streptococcal-staphylococcal infections. Prognosis is generally good if repeated infections can be avoided. The transmission of Bancroft's filariasis can be controlled by mosquito eradication. Since diethylcarbamazine prophylaxis reduces the number of microfilariae in the blood, the opportunity for transmission of the infection is greatly reduced.

Malayan Filariasis

Brugia (Wuchereria) malayi is an important filarial disease of man throughout Southeast Asia, Ceylon, southern India, Korea, and China; it produces lymphangitis, eosinophilia, and elephantiasis. Treatment is similar to that for *W. bancrofti.*

Onchocerciasis

Onchocerca volvulus is a filarial worm that causes blinding filariasis. The adult worms are found coiled in subcutaneous nodules. Adult females shed microfilariae that unsheath immediately. These rarely enter the bloodstream, but usually migrate in subcutaneous and cutaneous tissue (Fig. 14), sometimes entering the conjunctiva. Species of the black fly *Simulium* are the intermediate hosts in which larval development occurs. The fly transmits the infective stage on taking its next meal.

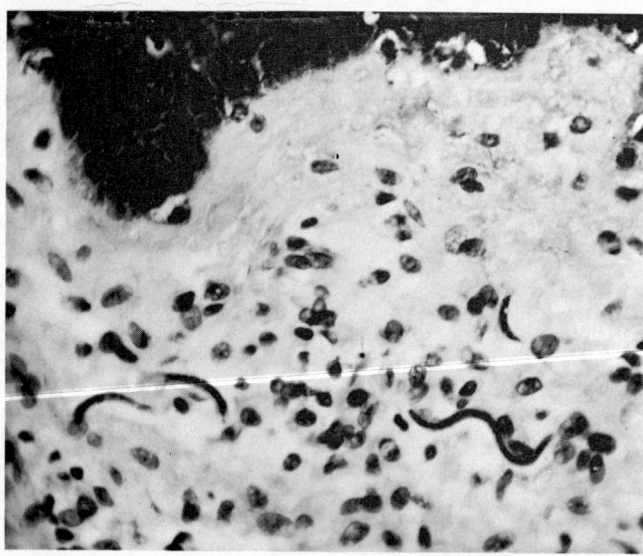

FIG. 14.   Microfilariae of *Onchocerca volvulus* in subcutaneous tissues.

Onchocerciasis is found extensively in West and Central Africa and scattered in certain districts in Central and South America and southern Mexico. In Central America onchocerciasis is limited to the highlands of Guatemala along fast-flowing river beds and streams, where black flies prevail. Although infection of children under 10 years of age is less common in Africa, children in Central America are often found with tumors of the scalp and shoulders.

A fibrous tumor forms about the developing adult worms. These tumors are quite common in the scalp and shoulders of Guatemalan children and about the pelvis in Africans. Ocular manifestations are associated with migrating microfilariae invading the cornea, orbit, and optic disk, resulting in photophobia, iridocyclitis, retinitis, and choroiditis. Vision, at first impaired, may be totally lost with invasion of the optic nerve. It is not entirely clear whether the ocular manifestations are a result of hypersensitivity to the microfilariae and their products or to direct injury by the invading worms.

Skin lesions (onchodermatitis) are not uncommon. Initially they are associated with pruritus and often are accompanied by a papular eruption. It is believed that macular dyspigmentation (hyperpigmented spots with central depigmented zones) is a complication of the early infection. These lesions may persist for weeks or years and are believed to be the result of an allergic reaction to the microfilaria in the skin. The next stage of onchodermatitis is characterized by thickening due to intradermal edema. In Central America patients may develop an erysipeloidlike lesion involving the face and upper trunk. Eventually many patients, especially in Africa, develop lichenification or thickening of the skin, especially over the buttocks and thighs. Finally the involved skin becomes atrophic or presbydermic, with loss of elasticity, giving the patient a prematurely aged appearance. This loss of dermal elasticity is believed to be responsible for the development of pseudoadenolymphocele, or hanging groin, as described by Nelson. Needle aspiration of a nodule and examination for microfilariae, or biopsy of the top layer of epidermis, can often provide absolute diagnosis.

Excision of all nodules, followed by therapy with diethylcarbamazine, is probably the best procedure to prevent or minimize ocular and other allergic manifestations. The recommended dosage is 0.1 mg/kg daily for 2 to 3 weeks. Allergic symptoms can be controlled with antihistamines or steroids. Suramin may also be employed in combination with diethylcarbamazine. A trial dose of 5 mg/kg should first be employed, followed by a dose of 20 mg/kg 5 days later. The same dose should be given every 5 to 7 days until a total of 10 doses have been administered. If ocular manifestations do not develop, the prognosis is generally good. Elimination of the intermediate host and surgical excision of tumors as soon as they appear reduces the possibility of further transmission.

Loaiasis

Loaiasis is caused by the African eyeworm *Loa loa.* It is confined to an extensive area of the western and midcentral portions of Africa, where an estimated 13 million people are infected. The worm is transmitted with the bite of tabanid flies, members of the genus *Chrysops.* The adult worms live and migrate through subcutaneous tissues, often causing a transient inflammatory reaction termed fugitive swelling. It is not uncommon for the adults to wander under the conjunctiva, causing some consternation but little damage. Sheathed microfilariae are found in the peripheral blood during the day (there is diurnal periodicity). Allergic manifestations, such as giant urticaria, fever, and a markedly elevated eosinophilia of 50 to 80 percent may occur. Surgical removal of the adults from subcutaneous sites such as the back, breast, groin, anterior chamber of the eye, or bridge of the nose effects a complete cure. Although therapy with diethylcarbamazine is highly effective, it should not be undertaken without careful observation for serious allergic reactions. Antihistamines or steroid hormones may be used as an adjunct to specific drug therapy. The recommended dosage of diethylcarbamazine is 2 mg/kg three times a day for 19 days. It is not necessary to remove the dead worms; they will be absorbed in about 2 weeks. Loaiasis can best be prevented by insect control measures and by treatment of existing infection, which diminishes the incidence of microfilariae.

DISEASES CAUSED BY TREMATODES

The trematodes (flukes) are exclusively parasitic flatworms that are leaflike, bilaterally symmetric, and lacking in a body cavity. All flukes that infect man have rather complex life histories, during which there may be a succession of intermediate hosts in which multiplication takes place. Sexual reproduction occurs in the final host, man. Adult flukes possess an outer noncellular cuticle that may exhibit spines, tubercles, or hooks. They all possess a ventral sucker or acetabulum for holding their position, as well as an anterior muscular oral sucker that leads to a simple digestive tract. Whereas their excretory, nervous, and circulatory systems are rather primitive, they have highly specialized organs for reproduction. All the trematodes that infect man, other than the blood flukes (*Schistosoma*), are monoecious (hermaphrodites).

Trematode eggs shed in the final host pass to the outside in either feces (*Schistosoma, Clonorchis, Fasciola*), urine (*Schistosoma haematobium*), or sputum (*Paragonimus*). A ciliated larva, the miracidium, emerges from the egg either before or after ingestion by a snail and usually becomes a saclike structure termed a first-generation sporocyst. The latter develops large numbers of reproductive cells that form either second-generation sporocysts (*Schistosoma*) or rediae (*Clonorchis, Fasciola, Paragonimus*), in which proliferate other germinal cells that develop into cercariae. These escape from the snail and by swimming or crawling make their way to another host. Most digenetic trematodes encyst in or on a second intermediate host, such as a fish (*Clonorchis*), crab, or crayfish (*Paragonimus*) or vegetation (*Fasciola*), as metacercariae. The cercariae in the schistosomes actively penetrate their final host and develop to maturity, whereas metacercariae are consumed by the final host and excyst before maturing.

Schistosomiasis

The blood flukes, *S. mansoni, S. japonicum,* and *S. haematobium,* have supplanted malaria as the chief world health problem. These worms are widely distributed, *S. mansoni* being found in Africa, Puerto Rico, Venezuela, Brazil, Surinam, many of the West Indies islands, Israel, and Arabia. *S. haematobium* is widespread in Africa, the Near East, Iran, Iraq, southern Portugal, and a small area of western India. *S. japonicum* is limited to China, several foci in Japan, the Celebes, Thailand, and the Philippine Islands.

The blood flukes are morphologically similar, but there are distinctive differences. The broader, robust males are characteristically found embracing the longer (10 to 26 mm) slender females within a gynecophoric canal during copulation and the ensuing oviposition. Typically the sexually mature forms of *S. mansoni* are found in the mesenteric venules of the colon and those of *S. japonicum* in the venules of the small intestine; adults of *S. haematobium* are found predominantly in the urine, but ova of the other species are generally recovered in the feces. The eggs, which are fully mature when passed in feces or urine, are readily distinguished by their distinctive lateral or terminal spines (Fig. 15). After dilution of the excreta in water, a free-swimming ciliated miracidium hatches. It penetrates a snail and rapidly undergoes metamorphosis and growth into a saclike first-generation sporocyst. The latter produces and liberates hundreds of second-generation sporocysts, each in turn producing myriad fork-tailed cercariae that subsequently are shed into water. It is not unusual for a single miracidium ultimately to produce thousands of cercariae. On contact, cercariae quickly penetrate the skin of the bather, shed their tails, and enter the venous circulation. After a brief period in the pulmonary circulation, many schistosomules make their way to the intrahepatic portal vessels where they settle down, feeding on blood, growing to maturity, pairing and mating. In several weeks they again take up their journey; they leave the intrahepatic veins and migrate retrograde to their respective sites in intestinal or vesicle venules and begin ovipositing. Eggs first appear in feces in 6 to 8 weeks in *S. mansoni* infections and in 4 to 6 weeks for *S. japonicum;* they appear in urine in *S. haematobium* infections in 10 to 14 weeks.

PATHOLOGY. The important pathologic lesions are caused by deposition of eggs in the tissues. There are always minute petechiae at the site of cercarial invasion. Small pulmonary infiltrates composed of eosinophils, neutrophils, and petechial hemorrhages may be found as the larvae (schistosomules) continue their migration. The deposition of eggs in the intestine provokes severe granulomatous inflammation, with pseudotubercle formation and fibroblastic proliferation. The affected intestinal wall may become thickened, fibrotic, and rigid. Eggs that are swept back into and lodge in the liver cause pseudotubercles and periportal fibrosis (Symmer's pipestem fibrosis) (Fig. 16).

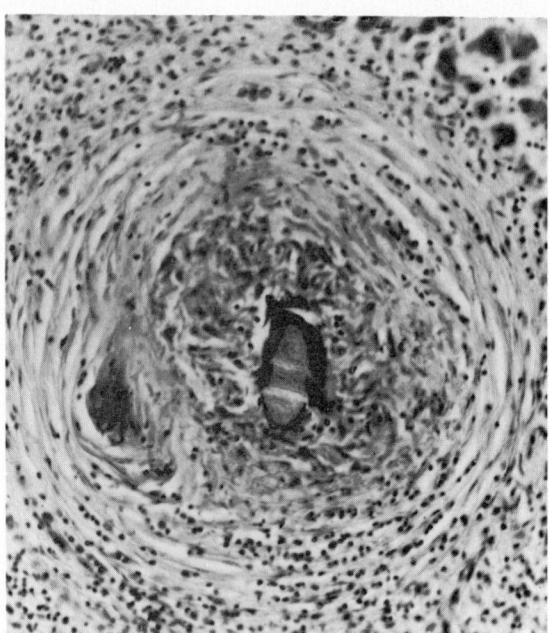

FIG. 16. Periportal fibrosis and pseudotubercle surrounding an ovum in Manson's schistosomiasis. Acid-fast stain (×140).

Fibrocongestive splenomegaly may result from presinusoidal portal hypertension; collateral venous channels may become prominent, with the development of coronary and esophageal varices. Eggs may embolize the lungs, causing endarteritis and periarteritis with formation of angiomatoid bodies and pseudotubercles. Rarely, ova reaching the central nervous system may cause granulomas and pseudotubercles.

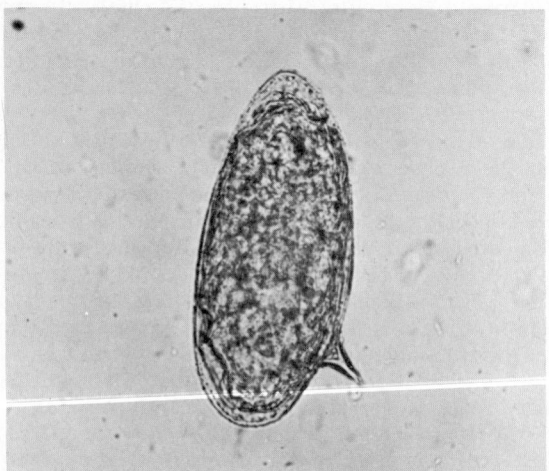

FIG. 15. *Schistosoma mansoni* egg recovered in feces (×448).

Eggs deposited in the vesical venules pass into the urinary bladder, which may undergo mucosal hyperplasia and severe inflammation. Papillomas are commonly found; intramural fibrosis with calcification about the eggs often follows. As egg laying proceeds the urethra and ureters are often involved in a proliferative fibrotic reaction, leading to elephantiasis of the penis and scrotum, hydronephrosis, and pyelonephritis. Bladder carcinoma is frequently associated with long-standing *S. haematobium* infection, especially in Egypt. Present epidemiologic evidence strongly supports schistosomal etiology of this neoplasm.

SYMPTOMS. Cercarial penetration of the skin is often accompanied by intense itching (kabure itch) and urticarial rash and occasionally by vesiculation. Other manifestations are usually absent until the parasites have reached the portal system. Children will occasionally have fever, eosinophilia, and enlarged tender liver and spleen. Schistosomal fever (Katayama disease) or acute schistosomiasis may appear 4 to 10 weeks after exposure and is characterized by intermittent bouts of chills, fever, and sweating, often misdiagnosed as malaria. Severe constitutional signs, epigastric pain, and schistosomal dysentery, with blood and mucus in the feces, are virtually constant features of acute *S. mansoni* infection. Lymphadenopathy, splenomegaly, tender enlarged liver, arthralgia, urticaria, periorbital edema, and eosinophilia of 20 to 60 percent are frequent manifestations. Liver function tests are usually normal, although a positive cephalin flocculation test and some increase in bromsulphalein retention may be recognized. Hypergammaglobulinemia is often pronounced. Despite the absence of eggs in stool or urine during this early stage, there is much evidence to suggest that these acute symptoms are a result of hypersensitivity to the ova and their miracidial secretions. The acute symptoms generally subside within 1 year or 18 months, but intermittent bouts of diarrhea and constipation can persist.

Severe cicatrization of the bowel wall can produce intestinal obstruction. Massive splenomegaly, portal hypertension, and venous collateralization may appear, but hepatic failure usually does not occur until very late. Leukopenia, thrombocytopenia, or pancytopenia may be seen as a result of hypersplenism. Pulmonary lesions are less frequent and are rarely serious. In older children, dyspnea, cough, precordial pain, and occasionally hemoptysis and congestive failure are associated with pulmonary hypertension culminating in cor pulmonale. Since *S. japonicum* is a more prolific egg-layer than either of the other species, serious disease may occur with fewer worms, and the infection tends to be more severe, especially in children. Periportal fibrosis is an earlier manifestation. Initially, infection with *S. haematobium* may cause painless hematuria, but as cicatrization of the bladder wall proceeds, dysuria, frequency, and urgency are frequently present. Ureteral colic often accompanies ureteral fibrosis. *S. japonicum* has been responsible for most of the cases involving the central nervous system, causing the sudden onset of severe headache, seizures, and some-

times coma. Eggs embolizing to the spinal cord may evoke symptoms of transverse myelitis.

DIAGNOSIS. Identification of eggs that have been recovered in stool or urine or obtained by rectal or bladder biopsy provides the specific diagnosis. Direct examination of material biopsied from rectum or bladder and pressed between two glass microscope slides constitutes the best and swiftest method for making the diagnosis. Liver biopsy is often helpful in identifying ova. Skin tests are useful in adults, but have been less so in children. Cross-reactions with trichinosis must be excluded. The complement-fixation test becomes positive early in the infection, but the titer falls with chronicity. The circumoval precipitin test, which is specific, can be used as a guide in evaluating therapy; it becomes negative about 6 months after therapeutic cure. For the individual patient immunologic methods are not suitable for making a diagnosis of schistosomiasis. It is essential that schistosome eggs be found in stools, urine, or biopsy specimen in order to establish the definitive diagnosis.

TREATMENT. Specific drug therapy can be helpful if implemented before irreparable intestinal and hepatic damage has occurred. General supportive therapy, such as supplemental food and vitamins, should also be provided. In advanced disease the toxicity of the usual chemotherapeutic agents may be life-threatening, especially when liver damage is already widespread. It is therefore essential to ascertain that a patient harbors living adult worms before instituting therapy. This can readily be accomplished by performing a hatch test or by examining the egg under reduced light to observe flagellar movement of miracidial flame cells.

In patients under 16 years of age lucanthone (Miracil D) has been employed extensively for the treatment of *S. mansoni* and *S. haematobium* infections. The recommended dosage is 5 mg/kg three times daily for seven consecutive days. Side effects such as dizziness, nystagmus, nausea, and vomiting may occur. The skin may become transiently yellow. Severe side effects, including mental aberration, confusion, and agitation, are seen in adults taking lucanthone.

Niridazole (Ambilhar) has been shown in extensive trials to be effective against both *S. haematobium* and *S. mansoni.* However, its toxicity may limit its usefulness. At present stibophen (Fuadin) remains the drug of choice for *S. haematobium* and (in patients over 16 years of age) for *S. mansoni* infections. Stibophen is supplied in ampules containing 5 ml of a 6.3 percent solution or a total of 315 mg of drug (42.5 mg antimony). It is administered intramuscularly, 1.5 ml the first day, 3.5 ml the second day, 5.0 ml the third day, and 5 ml every other day for 18 more injections (a total of 100 ml or 6.3 g Fuadin or 0.85 g antimony). Children weighing less than 50 kg usually receive two-thirds to three-quarters this dosage, and treatment is started with 0.75 to 1 ml and increased to 4 ml. Infants less than 1 year of age are given one-half this dosage. Treatment may be repeated after 4 months. Toxicity is not a frequent problem. Nausea, vomiting, diarrhea, and arthralgias may occur; if they are severe the daily dosage should be reduced and the treatment period extended. Serious renal, hepatic, and/or cardiac disease may contraindicate stibophen therapy. Antimony dimercaptosuccinate (Astiban) is as effective as stibophen and has the same side effects. *S. japonicum* infection responds best to therapy with tartar emetic (potassium antimony tartrate).

Hycanthone, a hydroxymethyl derivative of lucanthone, has been used extensively in Africa, the Caribbean islands, and South America. It is given in a single intramuscular injection. A number of serious drawbacks that probably limit its usefulness have been reported. The drug may cause acute or subacute massive hepatic necrosis, and it has been reported to be a powerful mutagenic agent. Experimental studies suggest that hycanthone may arrest ovipositing for a number of months, only to have it resume at a later date. Therapeutic success is usually measured by the absence of viable ova in follow-up stool examination after 3, 6, and 12 months.

In those individuals with portal hypertension who have had an episode of bleeding from ruptured esophageal varices, portacaval, splenorenal, or split shunts are advocated. It is important that drug therapy be instituted and completed prior to shunt surgery; otherwise increased seeding of the lungs with schistosome eggs will occur with secondary, rapidly developing pulmonary hypertension. Postshunt drug therapy can cause a sudden shift or embolization of a large quantitiy of adult worms to the lungs, with serious consequences.

The prognosis is most favorable in early or light infections with *S. mansoni* and *S. japonicum* if treatment is provided. In heavy or late infections, with severe hepatic and intestinal disease, the outlook is serious; death may result from bleeding esophageal varices, hepatic failure, or intercurrent infection. Similarly, the prognosis is good in light and early infections with *S. haematobium* that are treated early. In advanced urogenital tract disease pyogenic infection is difficult to control, making the outlook very poor.

Although control of schistosomiasis seems possible on theoretical grounds, little progress has occurred. The infection has been increasing and spreading throughout the world. In some areas almost 100 percent of the population over 2 years of age is infected. Previously noninfected areas have recently become endemic, and the large migration of Puerto Ricans to the continental United States has made schistosomiasis a major disease in New York and several other large cities. In endemic areas children acquire the infection almost as soon as they can walk and wade in water in which they urinate and defecate. Presumably destruction of the molluscan host would prevent further development of the disease, but such control measures have been only temporarily effective. Mass chemotherapy has had only fair to moderate success, since there has been a high rate of reinfection. Although improved sanitary waste disposal would help to control spread of schistosomiasis, education of the general population and provision of controlled swimming facilities may ultimately lead to eradication of this disease.

Schistosomal Dermatitis

Swimmer's, clam digger's, or collector's itch is caused by cercariae of various species of avian and mammalian blood flukes. The infection is acquired by campers and bathers both in freshwater lakes and along the east and west coasts of the United States. The cercariae are liberated by snails and enter the skin. In a few moments an intense pruritus is followed by urticariform rash. These subside shortly, leaving a small macule, only to be followed in several hours by severe itching, edema, and papules that may persist for several weeks. The initial exposure is relatively symptom-free, but with repeated exposure the reaction becomes more severe. Most of the cercariae are trapped and die in the upper portions of the dermis, many never getting beyond the prickle-cell layer of the epidermis.

The diagnosis is usually made from the history and the presence of skin lesions. Bathing areas can be freed of this menace by destroying the snails or the food they require. Rubbing the skin dry with a towel, or the application of rubbing alcohol immediately on leaving the water, may be effective in preventing infection. Antihistamines such as trimeprazine or diphenhydramine have been used with varying degrees of success in ameliorating the pruritus.

Paragonimiasis

Paragonimus westermani, the Oriental lung fluke, is widespread throughout most of the Far East, parts of Africa, and South America, The adult flukes usually live encapsulated in the lung and are about 1 cm long by 0.5 cm wide. The golden brown oval eggs have an obvious cap (operculum) and measure about 100 by 55 μ. They are deposited in the lung and then coughed up and expectorated or swallowed and passed in the feces. After several weeks of development in water, a miracidium hatches and enters a snail. A few weeks later sporocysts and rediae are produced. Cercariae are soon released that invade crayfish or crabs, encysting in muscle and viscera. After a person ingests infected crayfish, the metacercariae excyst in the duodenum, penetrate the intestinal wall, and migrate in the peritoneal cavity through the diaphragm and into the pleural cavity and lungs. They develop to maturity in lung tissue, where their presence stimulates pronounced fibroblastic encapsulation. Their presence in extrapulmonary tissue, especially brain, may give rise to bizarre neurologic symptoms. In nature there are many wild animals such as tigers and other cats, foxes, dogs, and pigs that may serve as definitive hosts for this trematode.

Infection usually is acquired by eating poorly cooked or pickled crab and crayfish. In some areas children are as frequently infected as are adults, and the incidence in females is far greater than in males. An oriental custom of treating measles, whooping cough, and diarrhea with the juice of freshly crushed crabs accounts for the large number of pediatric infections.

PATHOLOGY. The parasitized lung may possess small fibrotic nodules, which in man usually contain a single worm. These cysts are closer to the pleural surface and are fitted with a brown gelatinous material. Following death of the worm, pulmonary cysts shrink and become densely fibrotic, occasionally calcifying. Cerebral involvement is due to invasion by adult forms or migrating metacercariae. A severe meningoencephalitis or cerebral abscess may result. Parasites form nodules in other locations such as the omentum, pericardium, liver, spleen, and subcutaneous regions.

SYMPTOMS. Pulmonary symptoms may first be noted after about 3 months or longer, although the only evidence of infection may be persistent fever. Rust brown sputum is copiously produced; frank hemoptysis, pain, and dyspnea are also common. Since the pulmonary cysts are in open contact with bronchioles, sputum usually contains eggs. With central nervous system invasion, headache, seizures, hemiplegia, and visual impairment may occur. Eosinophilia is usual. Intestinal involvement may cause only vague abdominal symptoms or at times bloody diarrhea with mucus.

DIAGNOSIS. The clinical symptoms may require differentiation from tuberculosis, bronchiectasis, schistosomiasis, amebiasis, and brain tumor. The definitive diagnosis is made by finding the eggs in sputum or feces. In children, who usually swallow their bronchial secretions, it is more frequent to find ova in the feces.

TREATMENT. Until recently there had been no satisfactory therapy for paragonimiasis. Emetine alone or combined with sulfonamides has been used with equivocal results. Early infections have been reported to respond satisfactorily to chloroquine. Bithionol taken orally at a dosage of 30–50 mg /kg every other day until 10 to 15 doses are administered has had excellent results, with no relapses a year after treatment. Surgical excision of cerebral lesions is indicated. In light infection, or if the worms do not settle in some critical focus, the prognosis is good. Avoiding the consumption of uncooked and pickled crabs and crayfish, together with an intensive educational campaign, is the best means of preventing this disease.

Clonorchiasis

The Chinese liver fluke, *Clonorchis sinensis*, is found throughout most of eastern Asia. It is a moderate-size worm (10 to 25 mm by 3 to 5 mm) that lives in the biliary passages of man, although it occasionally invades the pancreatic duct. Its eggs (29 by 16 μ) are most distinctive, possessing a prominent operculum. They are discharged into the bile ducts and passed out in the feces; they hatch after ingestion by snails, in which sporocysts and rediae develop. Cercariae eventually escape from the snails and encyst under the scales or in the flesh of freshwater fish. If the uncooked infected fish is eaten, the metacercariae excyst in the duodenum, enter the common bile duct, and migrate to the intrahepatic biliary radicals, where they mature in about 3 to 5 weeks. Infection with *Clonorchis* is common wherever uncooked fish is eaten. Although it is not unusual for young children to consume raw fish and acquire the infection, the disease is usually the result of cumulative infection during a lifetime of enjoying this delicacy. The incidence is quite low under 5 years of age, but it gradually increases with age. Metacercariae are quite resistant to refrigeration, brine, vinegar, and spices.

PATHOLOGY. The presence of the worms in the distal bile passages provokes ductal epithelial hyperplasia, fibroblastic proliferation of the wall, and periductal fibrosis with infiltration of neutrophils, eosinophils, lymphocytes, and plasma cells. In heavy infection, hepatic damage can be severe, leading to the development of extensive periportal fibrosis. Hepatomas are frequently encountered in severely diseased livers. Worms also seem to act as a nidus for stone formation.

SYMPTOMS. Depending on the number of infecting worms, the disease may be asymptomatic or may present as complete biliary obstruction. There may be an enlarged tender liver and recurrent bouts of chills and fever. In later years signs of recurrent cholecystitis and biliary obstruction appear. It is not unusual for an infection with hundreds of worms to be active for 20 years or more with little or no serious side effects. Recovery of eggs in the stools or duodenal aspirate will provide the definitive diagnosis.

TREATMENT. Although no reliable therapy is available, chloroquine has been recommended. Patients often require several courses of therapy before a cure is effected. The recommended dose is 300 to 600 mg of chloroquine base a day until the patient has taken a total of about 15 g (base). Secondary suppurative cholangitis should be treated with appropriate antibiotics, and surgical intervention may be indicated for biliary obstruction. In light infections the outlook usually is good. Avoiding raw fish is probably the best means of reducing infection. Since human feces are used to fertilize fish ponds in which carp are being raised, composting feces before use decreases the spread of clonorchiasis.

Fascioliasis

Fasciola hepatica, the sheep liver fluke, is found wherever sheep are raised. It is common in many areas of the United States, South and Central America, Europe, Cuba, Africa, and Hawaii. Children and adults are sporadically infected, although sheep and cattle are probably the natural definitive hosts. *Fasciola* is a large (30 by 13 mm) leaflike worm that lives in the biliary passages. Large (140 by 75 μ) immature bile-stained eggs are shed into the proximal biliary ducts and passed out with feces into water, where they develop. A miracidium hatches and penetrates a snail. The sporocysts produce first-generation rediae. Second-generation rediae and then cercariae are formed. These emerge from the snail and usually encyst on aquatic vegetation, such as watercress. If infected vegetation is consumed, the metacercariae excyst in the duodenum, penetrate the intestinal wall, migrate through the peritoneum, penetrate Glisson's capsule and hepatic parenchyma, and settle and mature in the biliary ducts. The presence of the flukes in the biliary passages stimulates ductal epithelial proliferation and periductal fibrosis, with associated inflammatory cells. Eosinophilia may exceed 80 percent.

Patients often present with right upper quadrant pain, fever, dyspnea, and hepatomegaly. In light infections, however, the initial period of invasion is often asymptomatic. After the flukes have settled in the biliary ducts, fever, hepatomegaly, urticaria, biliary colic, and occasionally jaundice, intermittent diarrhea, weight loss, and generalized wasting occur. Eosinophilia is a constant finding. Children are more severely affected. Ingestion of infected raw sheep and goat livers in countries of the Middle East may cause pharyngeal infection called *halzoun*. The young flukes may migrate into the fossa of Rosenmüller and invade the eustachian tube or may cause fatal obstruction of the larynx and trachea. Definitive diagnosis is made by recovering the eggs from the stool or duodenal aspirate.

Early infections are apparently benefited by intramuscular emetine therapy, 1 mg/kg (maximum 65 mg daily) for 10 to 12 days. Bithionol has also been used successfully at a daily dosage of 30 mg/kg for 20 days. The outlook is serious in all but light infections. Education of individuals living in endemic areas to avoid consuming uncooked green vegetables, especially watercress, would probably eradicate fascioliasis as a human disease.

Fasciolopsiasis

In Asia and the Southwest Pacific, *Fasciolopsis buski* is one of the more frequently encountered intestinal flukes of man and swine. The worm is quite large (20 to 75 mm by 8 to 20 mm) and is found attached to the wall of the upper small intestine. Eggs are passed continuously in the feces and cannot be distinguished from those of *Fasciola hepatica*. Development is similar to that of *Fasciola*, with cercariae encysting on the bulb of the water chestnut as well as other aquatic vegetation. Infection occurs by accidental ingestion of the metacercariae. Excystation occurs in the duodenum, where they attach to the wall and develop to maturity. The worms produce severe ulcerative lesions at their sites of mucosal attachment and sometimes intestinal obstruction.

In children the toxic and allergic manifestations are striking. Edema, mucous diarrhea, malabsorption, and generalized wasting occur. Heavy infections in childhood often reveal anasarca and ascites. Intoxication and severe prostration may end fatally if treatment is not initiated. Eosinophilia is always present. Definitive diagnosis is made by finding the eggs in the stools and by clinical history. Fascioliasis must be excluded. Light infections that are treated have a good prognosis.

Several anthelmintics are used for fasciolopsiasis. Hexylresorcinol at a dosage of 400 mg orally from 1 to 7 years of age and 1 g at 13 years of age and over yields relatively high cure rates. Tetrachloroethylene, 0.25 ml per year of age, can also be used. However, hexylresorcinol is less toxic and is therefore preferred. Peeling or immersion of vegetables in boiling water for a few seconds will prevent infection.

DISEASES CAUSED BY CESTODES

The cestodes are exclusively parasitic flatworms, generally referred to as tapeworms. The adult worms typically have a scolex or head that may possess suckers and/or hooklets and serves as an organ for attachment. The distal portion of the scolex is termed the neck, which is the growth zone of the tapeworm, so that segments or proglottides closest to the neck are most immature. Those farther down the chain are mature, and the most distal group consists of gravid proglottides. Each mature proglottid possesses at least one complete, highly organized male and female reproductive tract. A digestive tract is usually absent, food being absorbed directly through the worm's integument. The nervous and excretory systems are poorly developed. With the single exception of *Hymenolepis nana*, tapeworms that infect man require one or more intermediate hosts to complete their life cycles. Adult cestode infections may persist for years, depriving the host of important nutriment. However, the larval infection often produces the more serious and sometimes fatal disease.

Taeniasis

The pork tapeworm, *Taenia solium,* and the beef tapeworm, *T. saginata,* are the common tapeworms of man. The disease has been known since ancient times and is found wherever insufficiently cooked pork or beef is consumed. Infection with the pork tapeworm has become rather uncommon in the United States, although it remains an important disease in Mexico and parts of South America. Generally, beef tapeworm infection is more prevalent.

The adult worms live in the upper small intestine, *T. solium* measuring 2 to 8 m and *T. saginata* 3 to 10 m or more. The scolex of the pork tapeworm, distinguished by having a crown or rostellum that contains a double row of hooklets, is said to be armed. The scolex of *T. saginata* is without hooks and therefore unarmed. The gravid uterus holds tens of thousands of eggs; each contains a mature six-hooked (hexacanth) embryo termed an oncosphere. The eggs are 30 to 40 μ in diameter and are similar in all members of the *Taenia* group. If the eggs are ingested by a suitable intermediate host, such as swine (*T. solium*) or cattle (*T. saginata*), the embryo is liberated. It penetrates the intestinal wall and enters the bloodstream. In the case of *T. solium* it may invade all the tissues of the body, where it develops into a cysticercus or bladder worm. Cysticerci are ellipsoidal, white, translucent cysts into which the scolex is inverted. The cysticercus is dissolved when the infected pork is consumed. Next, the scolex evaginates, attaching to the intestinal wall; it rapidly develops into an adult tapeworm. The cysticerci of *T. saginata* generally invade and develop in skeletal muscle; otherwise the life history is similar to that of *T. solium*.

PATHOLOGY.   The adult worm seldom produces important lesions, although it may occasionally cause intestinal obstruction in children because of its huge size. If the eggs of *T. solium* are ingested, the larval stage may develop in every tissue of the body, a condition termed cysticercosis cellulosae. The consequence of this infection depends on the organ invaded. The larvae generally cause an inflammatory infiltrate of eosinophils, plasma cells, neutrophils, and lymphocytes with eventual necrosis and fibrosis and calcification of the parasite. Human cysticercosis by *T. saginata* almost never occurs, only three authenticated cases having been reported in the world literature.

SYMPTOMS. The presence of adult *T. solium* usually causes little more than vague abdominal distress, perhaps alternating bouts of constipation and diarrhea. The symptoms in children, however, are often more pronounced. The huge adults of *T. saginata* are more likely to evoke severe hunger pains, weight loss, and epigastric pain, symptoms that may resemble peptic ulcer. It is not unusual for patients to report they can feel the worm moving. Eosinophilia may reach 55 percent. Neurologic complaints such as paresthesias, diplopia, and occasionally epileptiform seizures presumably result from absorption of neurotoxic material of helminthic origin. The presence of cysticerci in muscle is generally of little consequence. However, cerebral cysticercosis (Fig. 17) often provokes serious signs and

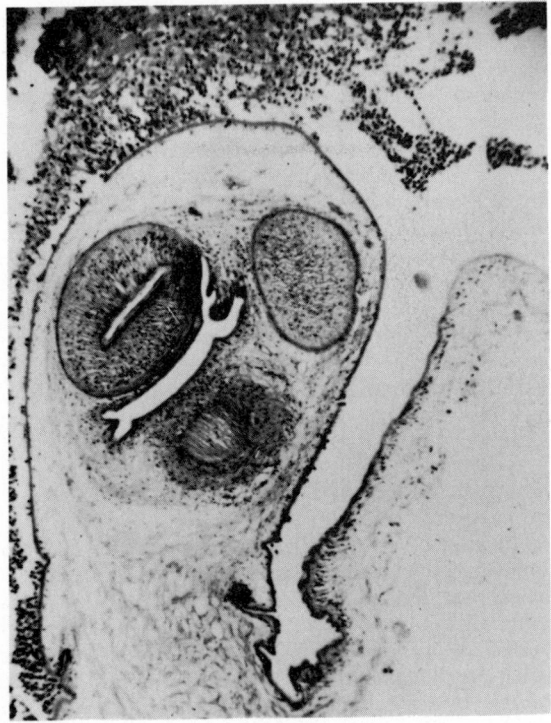

FIG. 17. Cysticercosis cellulosae of the brain discovered at autopsy.

symptoms that may mimic cerebral neoplasm. Headache, changes in behavior pattern, and jacksonian type seizures are common. Invasion of the orbit may cause pain and blurring, flashing, or loss of vision.

DIAGNOSIS. Since identification of the eggs is not specific, the definitive diagnosis is made by finding the proglottides in feces. Gravid segments of *T. solium* have 7 to 12 primary uterine lateral branches, whereas *T. saginata* have 15 or more. Radiographic examination of

muscle or brain may suggest the diagnosis if the cysticerci have calcified. Biopsy is required to diagnose cysticercosis. Intestinal infection has an excellent outlook, but cysticercosis can be most serious. In the brain or heart the prognosis is grave, although cerebral lesions have been successfully excised.

TREATMENT. Until recently quinacrine (Atabrine) was the drug of choice for the treatment of *T. solium.* The usual method of treatment is as follows: (1) Bland, liquid diet the day prior to treatment. (2) A sodium sulfate purge in the evening and a cleansing enema in the morning prior to administration of the drug. (3) Quinacrine is given in the morning on an empty stomach, according to the following schedule: body weight 40 to 75 pounds, 400 mg total; 76 to 100 pounds, 600 mg total; over 100 pounds, 600 mg total (adult dose). In young children a 100-mg tablet is given every 5 minutes along with a 250-mg sodium bicarbonate tablet. In older children two quinacrine tablets may be administered every 5 minutes until the total dose is given. Nausea and vomiting should be anticipated and avoided. Prochlorperazine (Compazine) can be administered an hour before drug therapy: 0.16 mg/kg orally or 0.08 mg/kg intramuscularly. (4) A saline purge is given several hours after therapy.

Recently the aminoglycoside paromomycin (Humatin) has been shown to be effective in tapeworm infections. It is given to children with *Taenia* or *Diphyllobothrium* infections as a single oral dose of 75 mg/kg after a light morning meal. Patients with *T. solium* infections are sedated with prochlorperazine prior to therapy and then given a mild purgative (Phospho-Soda) several hours after receiving paromomycin.

Several other drugs have been used in the treatment of taeniasis with excellent results. One of these, niclosamide (Yomesan), is recommended as the drug of choice for the treatment of *T. saginata, Diphyllobothrium latum,* and *Hymenolepis nana* infections. The following dosage schedules are suggested for *T. saginata* and *D. latum:* children weighing 25 to 75 pounds: 2 tablets (1 g) chewed thoroughly in a single dose; children weighing more than 75 pounds: 3 tablets (1.5 g) chewed thoroughly in a single dose; adults: 4 tablets (2 g) chewed thoroughly in a single dose. No special dietary restrictions are necessary before or after treatment with Yomesan. The best time to take the drug is after a light meal with a few sips of water. Yomesan is not yet recommended for children under 2 years of age or for pregnant women. Treatment of cysticercosis is surgical removal whenever possible.

Taeniasis can be prevented by thorough cooking of pork or beef. Refrigeration of beef at −10 C for 5 days and pork for 4 days, or heating at 72 C for 5 minutes, will usually kill all cysticerci. Since cysticercosis may be acquired from contaminated food or water, sanitary waste disposal would eliminate this route of infection. Personal cleanliness by individuals harboring the adult worm would prevent hand-to-mouth infection. Care to avoid regurgitation of gravid proglottides and the subsequent release of eggs during therapy for the adult worm should prevent autoinfection.

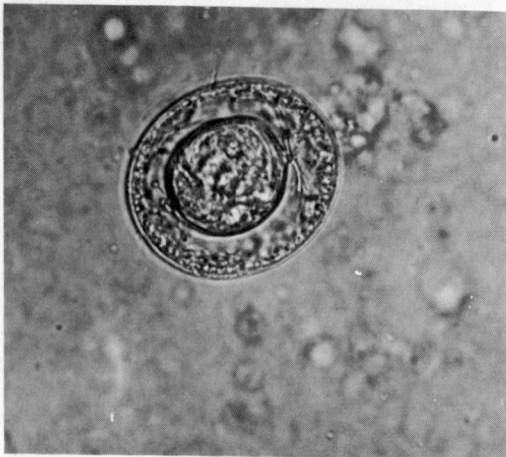
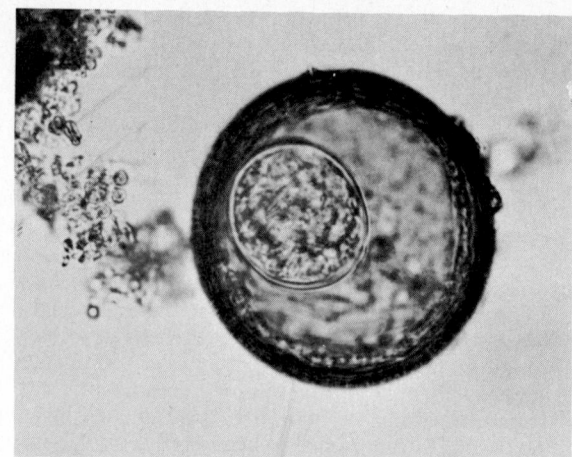

FIG. 18. *Left.* Hymenolepis nana egg recovered from feces. Note polar filaments (×448). *Right.* Hymenolepis diminuta ovum. Polar filaments are absent, and it is larger than *H. nana* (×448).

Hymenolepiasis

The dwarf tapeworm, *Hymenolepis nana,* is found in most warm regions of the world. It is the most common tapeworm infection in the southeastern United States and Latin America. The adult is only 0.5 cm in length and is attached to the mucosa of the ileum by a scolex that possesses four suckers and a retractable armed rostellum. The entire worm usually contains about 200 proglottides. The gravid uterus holds about 100 to 200 mature eggs 30 to 60 μ in diameter (Fig. 18). No intermediate host is required to complete the life cycle. The eggs are passed in the feces and ingested by a new or the same host (autoinfection). The embryo or oncosphere hatches and penetrates a villus, where it becomes a larva or cercocyst. The larva emerges from the tissue and attaches to the intestinal mucosa by its scolex. In 2 to 3 weeks the new worm is producing eggs. There is evidence that hyperinfection can occur when eggs liberated in the small intestine hatch and immediately penetrate a villus to undergo a new cycle. As a result of hyperinfection, children may harbor many hundreds or thousands of adult worms. Experimental evidence suggests that certain strains of *H. nana* undergo larval development in various fleas and mealworms. Subsequently these larvae have developed to adults in mice. At the present time human infection with murine strains is most unusual. A closely related species, *H. diminuta,* which commonly parasitizes the rat and mouse, infrequently infects man. Most of the 200 reported human cases have been in children under 3 years of age. Development of this tapeworm requires an intermediate host. Presumably, infected rat fleas (*Nosopsyllus, Xenopsylla*) and mealworms (*Tenebrio*) are accidentally ingested, and the mature adults develop in about 3 weeks. Since *H. nana* is usually transmitted directly, it often infects entire families and institutions, children being most heavily infected.

Little direct damage is done by the worms. In moderate to heavy infections, headache, dizziness, intermit-tent diarrhea, and abdominal cramps are sometimes noted. Slight eosinophilia is usual. Definitive diagnosis is made by identifying characteristic eggs in the stool.

Niclosamide (Yomesan) therapy has been used with excellent results. The following schedule is recommended: children weighing 25 to 75 pounds: on the first day, 2 tablets (1 g) chewed thoroughly, then 1 tablet (0.5 g) daily for the subsequent 5 to 7 days; children weighing more than 75 pounds: on the first day, 3 tablets (1.5 g) chewed thoroughly, then 2 tablets (1 g) daily for the subsequent 5 to 7 days; adults: 4 tablets (2 g) chewed thoroughly in a single dose each day for 5 to 7 days. Paromomycin therapy has been employed successfully by administering 45 mg/kg daily for 5 to 7 days. Mild diarrhea often accompanies this regime, but it stops once therapy is concluded.

Dipylidiasis

The dog tapeworm, *Dipylidium caninum,* is an occasional parasite in the small intestine of humans. The majority of infections occur in children under 8 years, but many in infants under 6 months of age. The ova of *Dipylidium* are ingested by the larval dog or cat flea, in which they become cysticercoid larvae. A child becomes infected by accidental ingestion of the infected flea. Infection is often asymptomatic, although some children experience vague intestinal disturbances. Allergic manifestations have been reported. Intestinal obstruction has been a rare complication. Treatment is the same as described for taeniasis. Periodic treatment of pets for tapeworm infection will control spread of this infection.

Diphyllobothriasis

Diphyllobothrium latum, the fish tapeworm, is a frequent human parasite in many of the lake regions of Europe, northern Minnesota, Michigan, and the adjacent regions of Canada. It is also found in Chile, Argentina, parts of China, and Africa. The Scandinavian custom of eating various delicacies made with raw fish and the practice of tasting raw fish when preparing gefilte fish are some of the common means of infection.

The adult tapeworm lives in the small intestine, where it may attain a size of over 10 m; it consists of about 3,000 proglottides. The scolex has a pair of sucking grooves (bothria) by which it holds to the mucosa. The gravid uterus expels its eggs in bursts through a uterine pore into the intestinal lumen, and the ova are evacuated in the feces. The operculate eggs, measuring about 66 by 44 μ (Fig. 19), require about 2 weeks to

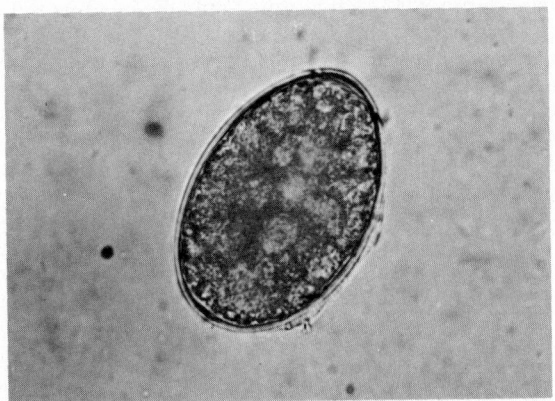

FIG. 19. Operculate egg of fish tapeworm (*Diphyllobothrium latum*) recovered in feces (×448).

develop in the water. A free-swimming ciliated embryo (coracidium) hatches and is ingested by a copepod (class Crustacea, phylum Arthropoda) in which it develops into a procercoid larva. When the infected copepod is eaten by a freshwater fish the procercoid larva invades the muscle, where it grows into a plerocercoid or sparganum larva. Usually the first fish is prey for larger fish, such as salmon, pike, perch, and trout, and the larva again invades the muscle of the second fish. If the fish is consumed raw or inadequately cooked, the plerocercoid larva develops into a mature adult in about 5 weeks.

The presence of this parasite in the small intestine is frequently cited as a cause of a profound macrocytic anemia resembling pernicious anemia. It has now been demonstrated convincingly that the worm deprives its host of vitamin B_{12}. Intestinal obstruction, as a result of infection with this huge worm, has been reported. It is unusual for patients to have any serious complaints. Eosinophilia and leukocytosis are evident.

Discovery of the characteristic operculate eggs in the stool provides the specific diagnosis. In the absence of anemia, the prognosis is excellent. With elimination of the worm and treatment of the anemia with vitamin B_{12}, the outlook is similarly good. Treatment of fish tapeworm is the same as that described for taeniasis. Careful cooking of freshwater fish would eliminate all possibility of human infection. Sanitary sewage disposal would prevent viable eggs from reaching the intermedi-

ate host. Sale of fish originating in heavily infested lakes should be regulated. Freezing at −10 C for 24 hours will kill the larvae.

On occasion, larvae of tapeworm species closely related to *D. latum, Spirometra,* have been found in human subcutaneous and muscle tissues. This condition is called sparganosis. The application of raw meat poultices to the eye, as well as accidental ingestion of infected copepods, is believed responsible for these infections. Ocular sparganosis may cause serious impairment of vision. Surgical removal of these worms is usually advocated.

Echinococcosis

Hydatid disease is the result of human infection with the larval stage of a dog tapeworm, *Echinococcus granulosus.* Similarly, the larval stage of *E. multilocularis,* a tapeworm of foxes and dogs and their relatives, may occasionally cause alveolar hydatid disease. Sheep- and cattle-raising areas throughout the world are the most heavily parasitized regions. Most cases in the United States are found in immigrants from endemic areas such as Italy, Greece, and Syria. However, there have been a number of autochthonous cases reported from various parts of the United States. Basque sheep farmers who have settled in California have shown a high incidence of infection, as have sheep ranchers in several areas in Utah. A sylvatic cycle has been reported in the north central United States, Canada, and Alaska and has been responsible for sporadic human cases. The wolf and coyote act as definitive hosts and caribou and moose as intermediate hosts. When hunters kill moose or caribou they often feed the infected offal to their dogs, who then become definitive hosts and may transmit the infection to household members, especially children.

Most hydatid cyst infections are acquired in childhood and are attributed to close and unhygienic association with canine pets. The latter are the optimal definitive hosts, and humans serve as relatively uncommon, but suitable, intermediate hosts. Frequent natural reservoirs of hydatid cysts other than cattle and sheep include goats, camels, monkeys, reindeer, and moose.

The adult worm consists of a scolex and usually one immature, one mature, and one gravid proglottid (Fig. 20). They live attached to the villi of the dog's small intestine. The eggs or gravid proglottides are passed in the feces. When they are swallowed an embryo hatches in the duodenum, penetrates the intestinal wall, and enters the bloodstream. Most of the larvae lodge in the liver (48 to 70 percent); some settle in the lungs (15 to 29 percent); and a few make their way to various other foci throughout the body. Many larvae are destroyed by the host. However, the survivors begin to develop into expanding cysts that after 5 to 6 months are about 10 mm in diameter. The cyst wall is differentiated into an inner cellular germinal layer and an outer noncellular friable laminated portion. Brood capsules, in which scolices may develop, bud off from the germinal layer. The brood capsule and its scolices are called hydatid sand (Fig. 21). When this unilocular hydatid cyst is consumed

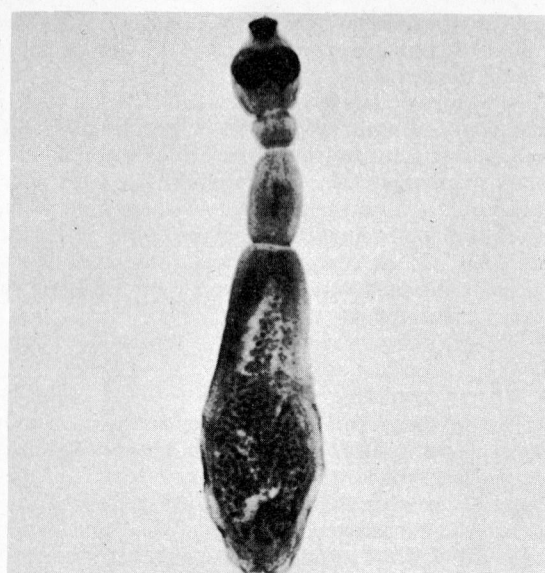

FIG. 20. *Echinococcus granulosus,* entire worm (×28).

by a suitable definitive host, adult tapeworms develop in the small intestine. The growth pattern of unilocular hydatid cysts in bone is quite different from that in liver or lung. The hyaline outer wall is poorly developed, and the germinal membrane proliferates over the bony spicules, destroying bone tissue in its wake.

PATHOLOGY. The presence of the cyst in parenchymal tissue stimulates an encapsulating inflammatory and fibroblastic reaction. These expanding cysts may cause important destruction of hepatic and pulmonary tissues. Moreover, the fluid within the friable cyst may leak into surrounding tissue, causing a severe hypersensitivity reaction, sometimes culminating in fatal anaphylactic shock. At other times the leaking cyst may seed hydatid sand over the peritoneum or lung, resulting in the development of multiple cysts. A single unilocular cyst may grow to such huge proportions that it impairs hepatic function or obstructs major biliary ducts. Cerebral hydatid cysts usually destroy nervous tissue by slow expansion, while pulmonary cysts are usually well encapsulated, but may rupture and drain into the bronchi and be coughed up. Osseous involvement results in progressive rarefaction of the bone and subsequent collapse. Calcified old hydatid cysts often

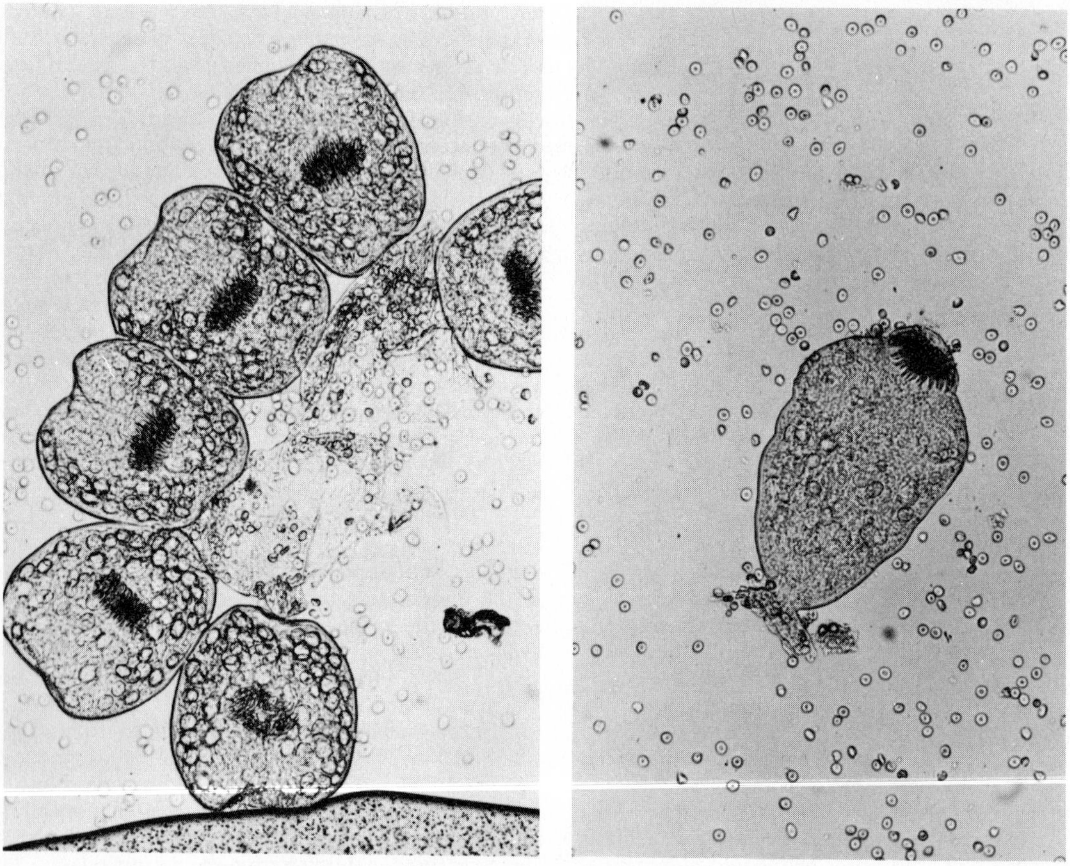

FIG. 21. Hydatid sand. *Left.* Scolices invaginated into cyst membrane (×140). *Right.* Evaginated scolex with hooklets; stalk is present by which the scolex is continuous with the germinal epithelium (×140).

are found by radiography or as incidental autopsy findings.

SYMPTOMS. If the cysts develop in a particularly vital area, symptoms appear early. However, hepatic involvement is often without symptoms, and the cysts may become so huge as to be a physical burden. Pulmonary involvement may cause dyspnea, hemoptysis, and chest pain. It is not unusual for this disease to lie dormant 20 to 30 years before the onset of any symptoms. Hypergammaglobulinemia and eosinophilia are often present, and if leakage of hydatid fluid occurs, eosinophilia may rise dramatically.

DIAGNOSIS. Relatively specific serologic tests are currently available. The hemagglutination, bentonite flocculation, and complement-fixation tests are all reliable. The Casoni skin test may be performed with some measure of confidence if proper controls are carried out. Finding the scolices, brood capsules, or daughter cysts in aspirated hydatid fluid obtained at surgery will provide the definitive laboratory diagnosis. Percutaneous aspiration of the cyst is dangerous and should not be attempted. Hepatic calcification aids in localization of a lesion but is not pathognomonic. A radiographic liver scan may be helpful in detecting the lesion and should be part of the work-up in suspected cases. If the cyst is not located in a vital position, patients will live for prolonged periods. If it is accessible to excision, the outlook is favorable.

TREATMENT. Surgical removal is advocated for all accessible cysts. The cyst wall is usually approached carefully, entered with a needle, and aspirated. The same volume of hypertonic saline (30%) is returned to the cyst to sterilize its contents before enucleation is attempted. Recently, various hydatid antigens have been employed in an attempt to cure the infection. Although desensitization and general improvement may occur, they are not often curative. No chemotherapy is available currently. Dogs should be prevented from eating sheep carcasses, which should be buried or burned. Periodic anthelmintic treatment of dogs is advocated.

Multilocular Hydatid Disease

Alveolar hydatid infection caused by larval *E. multilocularis* in humans consists of irregular, usually empty cavities with wrinkled hyaline membranes, little fluid, and few if any scolices. The hyalinized walls are generally scanty, and the inner germinal membrane tends to proliferate. These irregular noncircumscribed growths are not usually operable; therefore these infections always have a grave prognosis.

References

GENERAL

Basu AK: Tropical surgery. In Rab C, Smith R (eds): Clinical Surgery, Vol 8. Washington DC, Butterworth, 1965

Belding DL: Textbook of Parasitology, 3rd ed. New York, Appleton-Century-Crofts, 1965

Brown HW: Basic Clinical Parasitology, 3rd ed. New York, Appleton-Century-Crofts, 1969

Faust EC, Russell PF, Jung RC: Craig and Faust's Clinical Parasitology, 8th ed. Philadelphia, Lea & Febiger, 1970

Goodman LS, Gilman A: The Pharmacological Basis of Therapeutics, 5th ed. New York, Macmillan, 1975

Hunter GW, Frye WW, Swartzwelder JC: A Manual of Tropical Medicine, 4th ed. Philadelphia, WB Saunders, 1966

Jelliffe DB: Child Health in the Tropics, A Practical Handbook for Medical and Paramedical Personnel, 2nd ed. London, Edward Arnold, 1964

Kagan IG, Norman L: Serodiagnosis of parasitic diseases. In Lennette E, Spaulding E, Truant J (eds.): Manual of Clinical Microbiology, 2nd ed. Washington, DC, American Society of Microbiology, 1974, p 645

Kudo RR: Protozoology, 5th ed. Springfield, Ill, Charles C Thomas, 1966

Maegraith BG, Gilles HM (eds): Management and Treatment of Tropical Diseases. Oxford, Blackwell Scientific, 1971

Van Der Hoeden J (ed): Zoonoses. Amsterdam, Elsevier, 1964

Von Brand T: Biochemistry of Parasites, 2nd ed. New York, Academic, 1974

Woodruff AW: Pathogenicity of intestinal helminthic infections. Trans R Soc Trop Med Hyg 59:585, 1965

NEMATODES

Anast BP, Birch CL: Strongyloidiasis. Strongyloides stercoralis: report of 62 cases. J Am Med Wom Assoc 18:623, 1963

Babich D: Strongyloidiasis. A report on twenty cases. Ethiop Med J 4:57, 1965

Beaver PC, Snyder CH, Carrera GM, Dent JH, Lafferty JW: Chronic eosinophilia due to visceral larva migrans. Pediatrics 9:7, 1952

Braun RC: Hookworm anemia in a neonate. Ghana Med J 4:169, 1965

Brown RE: Neurological manifestations associated with ascariasis. Trop Geogr Med 17:121, 1965

Danaraj TJ, Pacheco G, Shanmigaratnam K, Beaver PC: The etiology and pathology of eosinophilic lung (tropical eosinophilia). Am J Trop Med Hyg 15:183, 1966

Duke BOL: Studies on the chemoprophylaxis of loaiasis. II. Observations on diethylcarbamazine citrate (Banocide) as a prophylactic in man. Am Trop Med Parasitol 57:82, 1963

Edeson JFB, Wilson T: The epidemiology of filariasis due to Wuchereria bancrofti Brugia malayi. Annu Rev Entomol 9:245, 1964

Foy H, Nelson GS: Helminths in the etiology of anemia in the tropics, with special reference to hookworms and schistosomes. *Exp Parasitol 14:240, 1963*

Gilbert MG, Carbonnell ML: Pancreatitis in childhood associated with ascariasis. Pediatrics 33:589, 1964

Hawking F: Advances in filariasis especially concerning periodicity of microfilariae. Trans R Soc Trop Med Hyg 59:9, 1965

Hogan MJ, Kimura SJ, Spencer WH: Visceral larva migrans and peripheral retinitis. JAMA 194:1345, 1965

Huntley CE, Costas MC, Lyerly A: Visceral larva migrans syndrome: clinical characteristics and immunologic studies in 51 patients. Pediatrics 36:523, 1965

Jaggi OP: Pulmonary manifestations of intestinal ascariasis in children. J Assoc Physicians India 13:803, 1965

Layrisse M, Roche M: The relation between anemia and hookworm infection. Results of surveys of rural Venezuelan population. Am J Hygiene 79:279, 1964

Lee DL: The Physiology of Nematodes. London, Oliver and Boyd, 1965

Mehrotra MP, Malavuja US: Single dose treatment of hookworm disease with bephenium hydroxynaphthoate. Indian J Med Sci 17:930, 1963

Most H: Trichinellosis in the United States. Changing epidemiology during past 25 years. JAMA 193:871, 1965

Nelson GS: Onchocerciasis. Adv Parasitol 8:173, 1970

TREMATODES

Aréan VM: Schistosomiasis. A clinicopathologic evaluation. In Sommers SC (ed): Pathology Annual, Vol 1. New York, Appleton-Century-Crofts, 1966, p 68

Cook JA, Woodstock L, Jordan P: Two-year follow-up of Hycanthone-treated schistosomiasis mansoni patients in St Lucia. Am J Trop Med Hyg 23:910, 1974

Cort WW: Studies on schistosome dermatitis. Am J Hygiene 52:251, 1950

Diaconita G, Goldis G: Investigations on pathomorphology and pathogenesis of pulmonary paragonimiasis. Acta Tuberc Scand 44:51, 1964

Dusek J, Kubasta M, Kodousek R, Kubastova B: Needle biopsy of the liver in schistosomiasis mansoni: the value of histological examination. J Trop Med Hyg 68:189, 1965

Einhorn AH, Fritsch A, Dwork KG, Shookhoff HB: Schistosoma mansoni infection in children—treatment with lucanthone hydrochloride (Nilodin). Am J Dis Child 104:30, 1962

Fripp PJ: Bilharziasis and bladder cancer. Br J Cancer. 19:292, 1965

Gelfand M, Gilles HM: Filling defects of the bladder on intravenous pyelography in children passing schistosome ova in the urine. J Trop Med Hyg 69:4, 1966

Gibson JB, Sun T: Chinese liver fluke—Clonorchis sinensis—its occurrence in Hong Kong. Bull Int Acad Pathol 60:94, 1965

Kloetzel K: Natural history and prognosis of splenomegaly in schistosomiasis mansoni. Am J Trop Med Hyg 13:541, 1964

Lees REM: Lucanthone hydrochloride in the treatment of Schistosoma mansoni infection. Trans R Soc Trop Med Hyg 60:233, 1966

Pantelouris EM: The Common Liver Fluke, Fasciola Hepatica L. London, Pergamon, 1965

Sadun E, Maiphoon C: Studies on the epidemiology of the human intestinal fluke, Fasciolopsis buski (Lankester) in central Thailand. Am J Trop Med Hyg 2:1070, 1953

Schacher JF, Khalel GM, Salman S: A field study of halzoun (parasitic pharyngitis) in Lebanon. J Trop Med Hyg 68:226, 1965

Stauber LA: Swimmer's itch in New Jersey. J Parasitol 44:108, 1958

Wang C, Liu J, Chang T, Miao H: The clinical manifestations and bithionol therapy of paragonimiasis in Szechuan province. Chin Med J 83:163, 1964

Warren KS: The immunopathogenesis of schistosomiasis: a multidisciplinary approach. Trans R Soc Trop Med Hyg 66:417, 1972

Yokogawa S, Cort WW, Yokogawa M: Paragonimus and paragonimiasis. Exp Parasitol 10:81, 1960

CESTODES

Dixon HBF, Lipscomb FM: Cysticercosis—an analysis and follow-up of 450 cases. Med Res Counc Spec Rep Ser (Lond) No 299, 1961

Echinococcosis. WHO Bull 39:1, 1968

Heinz HJ, Klintworth GK: Cysticercosis in the aetiology of epilepsy. S Afr J Med Sci 30:32, 1965

LaFond DJ, Thatcher DS, Handeyside RG: Alveolar hydatid disease. JAMA 186:35, 1963

Seftel HC, Heinz HJ: Treatment of human tapeworm infections with yomesan—single dose treatment in non-fasting subjects. S Afr Med J 38:263, 1964

Swartzwelder JC, Beaver PC, Hood MW: Sparganosis in southern United States. Am J Trop Med Hyg 13:43, 1964

Tanowitz HB, Wittner M: Paromomycin in the treatment of Diphyllobothrium latum infection. J Trop Med Hyg 76:151, 1973

Vachier E, Hillman DC: Solitary pulmonary hydatid cyst. Report of a case and discussion of its differential diagnosis. Pediatrics 35:699, 1965

Von Bonsdorff B: Dyphyllobothrium latum as a cause of pernicious anemia. Exp Parasitol 5:207, 1956

Wittner M, Tanowitz H: Paromomycin therapy of human cestodiasis with special reference to hymenolepiasis. Am J Trop Med Hyg 20:433, 1971

Yokogawa M, Hoshimura H: Treatment of Hymenolepis nana in children with cestocide Bayer 2353 (Yomesan). Jap J Parasitol 11:387, 1962

PROTOZOAN DISEASES

Representatives of each major group of the phylum Protozoa cause serious human disease. As unicellular or acellular organisms, the Protozoa may be distinguished from all other phyla of the animal kingdom. Their diversity of size, shape, mode of reproduction, and environmental adaptation is without parallel. Many of the important protozoan diseases summarized in Table 2 will be considered in this section.

Amebiasis

HOWARD B. SHOOKHOFF (REVISED BY MURRAY WITTNER)

Amebiasis is the condition caused by infection with *Entamoeba histolytica* or *Dientamoeba fragilis*. *E. histolytica*, as its name implies, is capable of penetrating and destroying tissues. Infection may extend to the liver and occasionally to other organs. *D. fragilis* has not been proved to be invasive, but it does produce symptoms. Its effects are limited to the colon. *E. histolytica* is a protozoan varying from about 10 to 35 μ in diameter. The infection is transmitted by resistant cysts that vary in size from 5 to 20 μ. The nucleus typically shows a fine regular peripheral chromatin and a small, usually central, karyosome. The trophozoite is characterized by a progressing flowing motility. The cyst is identified in its early stages by the presence of rod-shaped refractile chromatoid bars and when mature by the presence of two pairs of typical nuclei. *D. fragilis* has no known cyst form. The trophozoite is usually small, averaging 8 to 10 μ in diameter. Among the identifying characteristics is the presence of pointed or leaf-shaped pseudopods. Most of the organisms have two nuclei. This parasite is often overlooked because of its small size. It can be found only in freshly passed stools. Recent studies have shown that *D. fragilis* is not an ameba, but belongs taxonomically among the *Trichomonas* flagellates. For the present, however, *Dientamoeba* will be retained in this section.

PATHOLOGY. The most frequent site of lesions is the cecum in *E. histolytica* infections, but any or all parts of the colon, including the appendix, may be involved. Occasionally the process involves the terminal portion of the ileum. The parasite evokes little cellular reaction when it invades the tissues of the colon. It causes lysis with edema and produces ulcers of varying size, usually extending into the submucosa. The mucosa between the ulcers is usually normal, although in a few cases there is diffuse inflammation resembling that of non-specific ulcerative colitis. In severe infections the ulcers may extend to the peritoneal surface with perforation. Healing of ulcers rarely produces gross scarring.

Abscesses of the liver due to *E. histolytica* may be single or multiple, and most usually occur in the right lobe. The process is one of liquefaction necrosis, and the contents typically have a red brown color. It is not true pus. As in the colon, *E. histolytica* evokes little cellular reaction. The parasites are found in the wall of the abscess; they are difficult to find in the necrotic contents. Rarely, *E. histolytica* produces abscesses in the lung and brain and granulomatous processes in the skin and colon. The pathology of *D. fragilis* infections is not well known. There have been no fatalities. Since there is no tissue invasion, there are no ulcers and no metastatic complications.

TABLE 2. Human Parasitic Infections: Protozoa

Disease	Parasite	Location in Man	Transmission	Typical Clinical Findings	Diagnosis	Treatment	Age Incidence
Malaria malignant tertian benign tertian quartan oval	*Plasmodium falciparum* *P. vivax* *P. malariae* *P. ovale*	Intraerythrocytic	Sporozoites inoculated by female *Anopheles* mosquito	Fever, splenomegaly, anemia	Parasites in peripheral blood smear	Chloroquine, pyrimethamine, quinine Chloroquine, primaquine	Peak incidence in first decade of life
Toxoplasmosis	*Toxoplasma gondii*	Central nervous system, lung, heart	Transplacental, insufficiently cooked meats; cat litter	Chorioretinitis, hydrocephalus, seizures	Radiography (cerebral calcification), serologic	Pyrimethamine, sulfonamides, spiramycin	Congenital and post natal; incidence rises with age
Amebiasis	*Entamoeba histolytica*	Large intestine, liver	Ingestion of cysts in water and food	Diarrhea, abdominal distress dysentery	Trophozoites or cysts in feces	Intestinal: metronidazole, diodoquin, paromomycin; Extraintestinal: metronidazole, chloroquine, dehydroemetine	Varies with sanitation; common in children's institutions
Dientamebiasis	*Dientamoeba fragilis*	Large intestine	Ingestion of trophozoites	Diarrhea	Trophozoites in feces	Diodoquin, paromomycin	Higher incidence in institutions
Balantidiasis	*Balantidium coli*	Large intestine	Ingestion of cysts in water or food	Mild to severe diarrhea or dysentery	Trophozoites or cysts in feces	Tetracyclines, diodoquin, paromomycin	Poor sanitation and close institutional contact
Giardiasis	*Giardia intestinalis*	Small intestine	Ingestion of cysts in water or food	Mucous diarrhea, abdominal distress, spruelike symptoms	Trophozoites and cysts in feces	Quinacrine, metronidazole	Most common in children, especially in institutions
Trichomonas vaginitis	*Trichomonas vaginalis*	Vagina, urethra, prostate	Sexual contact; occasionally unsanitary bathing facilities	Vaginal discharge, pruritus, burning sensation	Trophozoites in vaginal or prostatic secretions	Metronidazole	Uncommon in preadolescent males and females

647

TABLE 2. Human Parasitic Infections: Protozoa (cont.)

Disease	Parasite	Location in Man	Transmission	Typical Clinical Findings	Diagnosis	Treatment	Age Incidence
Chagas' disease	*Trypanosoma cruzi*	Early: peripheral blood; late: intracellular, heart, GI tract, CNS, etc	Trypanosomal forms enter skin or mucous membranes in feces of kissing bug (*Triatoma*)	Edema, myocarditis, neurologic symptoms, Romaña's sign, megaesophagus, megacolon	Early: trypanosomes in peripheral blood; late: xenodiagnosis serologic tests	Bayer 7602, Altafur	Peak incidence in children 2–3 years
African sleeping sickness	*T. gambiense* *T. rhodesiense*	Blood, lymphatics, spinal fluid	Through skin by bite of tstse fly (*Glossina*)	Fever, lymphadenopathy, meningoencephalitis	Trypanosomes in peripheral blood smear, lymph node aspirate, spinal fluid	Blood infection: suramin or pentamidine; CNS infection: tryparsamide, melarsoprol	Usually in 20–30-year age group; more frequent in children during epidemics
Leishmaniasis kala-azar	*Leishmania donovani*	Within histiocytes and macrophages of spleen, liver, GI tract	Through skin, usually bite of sandfly (Phlebotomus)	Fever, hepatomegaly, malaise, bleeding diathesis	Bone marrow aspiration, liver biopsy	Ethylstibamine, hydroxystilbamidine	Frequent in infants, adolescents
cutaneous oriental sore	*L. tropica*	Within histiocytes and macrophages in skin	Through skin, usually bite of sandfly (*Phlebotomus*)	Skin ulcer of exposed areas, ulceration of naso-oral mucosa, erosion of external ear	Smear and culture from ulcer scraping	Pentostam, dry ice, stibophen, Berberine sulfate	All ages and sexes; custom to give immunizing lesion
mucocutaneous	*L. brazillensis*	Within histiocytes and macrophages in skin and mucous membranes				Pentostam, chloroquine, amphotericin B	Varies with region; in some more than 75% infection in children
Pneumocystis pneumonia	*Pneumocystis carinii*	Pulmonary alveolar cells and in alveolar exudate	Prematurity, contact, immunosuppression	Dyspnea, cough, fever	Sputum examination and open pleural biopsy	Pentamidine isethionate, hydroxystilbamidine, pyrimethamine + sulfadiazine	Especially in first 6 months of life; premature infants

PATHOGENESIS. Transmission of amebiasis due to *E. histolytica* results from ingestion of cysts in food, on fingers, or on other objects directly contaminated with human feces. Particularly vulnerable are institutionalized children with severe psychiatric disturbance or mental retardation and children brought up in environments devoid of sanitary facilities where the soil near dwellings is contaminated with dejecta. More normal persons living in environments with adequate sanitary controls may be infected by ingestion of raw vegetables grown in fecally contaminated soil. Food and dishes may be contaminated by infected food handlers who fail to wash their hands effectively. Infection may also occur from improperly protected water supply or from ice produced under unsanitary conditions. After cysts are ingested, the wall is weakened by digestive enzymes. Trophozoites emerge from the cysts and attack the wall of the colon. The presence of intestinal bacteria is essential to production of lesions. The mode of transmission of *D. fragilis,* which has no known cyst form, is unknown.

EPIDEMIOLOGY. Amebiasis is by no means a tropical disease; it occurs all over the world. In general the prevalence of the infection varies inversely with the degree of sanitation. Where there is virtually no sanitary control of the environment or in institutions where patients cannot be kept clean, the rate of infection may exceed 70 percent. Poor sanitation is not limited to warm areas of the earth; in areas with permafrost it is difficult to establish satisfactory drainage, and amebiasis has been found prevalent in some Eskimo populations. The first case of amebic dysentery ever recognized occurred in Leningrad in the colder fringe of the temperate zone. Amebiasis is usually less common in children than in adults, but there is no inherent immunity. Amebic dysentery has been described during the first weeks of life. Such cases are rare, however, since many children are fairly well protected from peroral infection during their early months. Amebic infections, once acquired, tend to persist. In areas where sanitation is poor, there is a gradual increase in childhood infection during the first 15 years of life. Epidemics of amebiasis occur occasionally and are usually related to some gross defect in the water supply system.

SYMPTOMS. Of all persons infected with pathogenic amebae, only a small proportion have severe symptoms at any one time. Many more have mild symptoms, and probably half or more are asymptomatic. These are often called carriers, but the term is misleading because they may subsequently develop mild or severe symptoms. Illness due to amebiasis usually has a subacute or chronic course. An acute onset is uncommon. The symptoms are frequently intermittent rather than continuous.

Severe cases are characterized by marked diarrhea, often with blood and mucus in the stools. It is not uncommon for patients to have tenesmus, with the evacuation consisting of several drops of bright red blood-stained mucus. Direct microscopic examination of such a specimen usually reveals enormous numbers of large erythrophagous trophozoites. Abdominal pain often accompanies the diarrhea, but it is not necessarily severe. Appetite is usually diminished, and nausea may be present, but vomiting occurs infrequently. Fever and leukocytosis are sometimes present. If the febrile reaction is marked, it raises the suspicion of a liver abscess. In these severe cases sigmoidoscopy often shows abnormalities. Usually these consist of discrete ulcerations separated by a normal mucosa, but occasionally a diffusely inflamed friable mucous membrane indistinguishable from that of nonspecific ulcerative colitis is found. Barium enema may be negative, or there may be areas of spasm, especially in the cecum, which may be contracted and irregular. Occasionally, there is evidence of ulceration, and rarely a localized tumorlike process called ameboma is seen in the cecum or other portion of the colon.

The majority of patients with clinical disease have mild symptoms. In adults these are of two types—gastrointestinal and constitutional. Aside from diarrhea, gastrointestinal symptoms are usually vague. Abdominal pain may occur, but more often there is ill-defined distress or abdominal distension. Constitutional symptoms include fatigue, low-grade fever, and backache or other vague somatic aching that is often not sufficiently severe to lead to medical consultation. Children are less likely to be articulate about such complaints. A common clinical picture is recurrent mild diarrhea with poor appetite, pallor, sometimes mild fever, and some retardation of growth. Nausea may occur but vomiting is uncommon. The liver is often palpable and sensitive, although actual abscess is relatively rare. There may be diffuse abdominal tenderness. In these relatively mild cases sigmoidoscopy usually shows no abnormalities. Blood count, erythrocyte sedimentation rate, and liver function tests are usually normal. Amebiasis should be suspected in any child with vague persistent or recurrent illness associated with gastrointestinal symptoms.

DIAGNOSIS. The clinical manifestations of intestinal amebiasis are not diagnostic. Even in those few cases with typical ulcerations seen through the sigmoidoscope the diagnosis should be confirmed by the identification of the parasites in the stool or in scrapings from the ulcers. Identification of amebae requires considerable experience, and errors are frequent unless the technician has received special training. Furthermore, specimens must be obtained under proper conditions. The most useful specimen is a freshly passed diarrheal stool, which should be examined for trophozoites within 20 to 30 minutes in warm physiologic saline solution. If blood-streaked mucus is present, this is the most likely portion of the stool to show parasites.

In the absence of diarrhea a cathartic should be administered. For children over the age of 6 years, saline laxatives such as the mixture of sodium phosphate and sodium acid phosphate marketed as Fleet's Phospho-Soda can be used. The average dose is 25 ml of the solution, and it is made more acceptable by administering a carbonated soft drink as a chaser. In younger children milk of magnesia given the night before the examination is usually more acceptable and more effective. The dose is from 10 to 20 ml, depending on the size of the child. Any other laxative that is not oily and that can be expected to produce a partially liquid stool may be used. If the specimen cannot be examined promptly, it may be preserved in a polyvinyl alcohol mixture and stained and examined at a later convenient time. This method is slightly less satisfactory than the fresh examination, since light infections may be missed. Cysts are not regularly preserved by this method. Examination of nondiarrheal stools or stools that are not fresh is by no means useless. In *E. histolytica* infections, if cysts are present, they persist for many hours or several days unless the specimen is allowed to dry out. If only a few cysts are present, they may be uncovered by concentration methods. Occasionally trophozoites can be found in formed stools if they are examined fresh.

The finding of amebic cysts or trophozoites by a reliable observer is definitive. A negative report on a formed specimen, or a specimen that is diarrheal but is not examined promptly cannot rule out the presence of such an infection. The yield of positive findings in freshly passed diarrheal stools is about four times that for casual specimens in *E. histolytica* infections. With *D. fragilis* the fresh specimen is mandatory. The parasite is often difficult to stain in preserved preparations. The presence of cysts does not indicate an inactive infection or a carrier state. Either form of the parasite is diagnostic of infection. Cultivation of the stool for amebae is generally much less successful than direct examination. It has some value as a supplementary method in cases in which the diagnostic characteristics of amebae found on direct examination are not definitive.

Various serologic methods are currently available that must be performed in specialized laboratories, but they are frequently negative in intestinal amebiasis. The complement-fixation test has generally been superseded by the indirect hemagglutination (IHA), gel diffusion, or indirect fluorescent antibody (IFA) techniques. The sensitivity of each test varies with the type of infection. In patients with acute amebic dysentery, sensitivity of these tests is less than in extraintestinal disease. The least sensitivity is found in asymptomatic states. Using the IHA technique in amebic liver abscess has yielded very high diagnostic accuracy (up to 100 percent); in acute amebic dysentery the IHA test is only slightly less specific. The greatest difficulty is encountered in the asymptomatic carrier of *E. histolytica* cysts. Immunofluorescence tests appear to be about as sensitive as the IHA, but specificity is somewhat less.

COMPLICATIONS. *Liver abscess* is the most frequent complication of amebiasis. Although the infection must gain entrance through the colon, it may occur in the absence of amebic colitis or a history suggestive of prior involvement of the colon. While less frequent in children than in adults, it is not as exceptional as was thought in earlier years. If the diagnosis is not made, it may be fatal. The common clinical manifestations are fever, enlargement and tenderness of the liver, polymorphonuclear leukocytosis, and anemia. The liver enlargement is usually manifest on abdominal palpation, and it is not infrequently possible to outline a distinct mass within the enlarged liver. Radiographic examination of the chest may show upward displacement of the

right leaf of the diaphragm, which if it occurs in the absence of palpable enlargement is of great diagnostic importance. There may also be evidence of consolidation at the base of the right lung or a right pleural effusion or both. Children who are old enough usually complain of upper abdominal pain. At times pain is referred to the right shoulder or to the right lower quadrant of the abdomen.

Liver function tests are usually normal, with the exception of the serum alkaline phosphatase, which is elevated in one-third of cases in adults. Such elevation may be difficult to interpret in children. The leukocyte count may be normal, but marked elevation of the erythrocyte sedimentation rate is a constant finding.

The diagnosis of amebic liver abscess is supported by the finding of *E. histolytica* in the stools. However, in most reported series this is stated to occur only in a minority of cases. One may suspect that the use of post-cathartic specimens might well yield a higher proportion of positive results. Serologic tests are almost always positive and should be obtained without delay. If pus is aspirated from the liver it may have the typical red brown color, but just as often it is yellow or gray green. Absence of bacteria on smear and culture is strongly suggestive of an amebic etiology of the abscess. Amebae are often not found on direct examination of aspirated pus, but they may be found more easily if the pus is liquefied with a streptokinase-streptodornase mixture and the resulting sediment carefully examined. If surgical drainage has been performed, the pus escaping after the first day is very likely to show amebae, provided no specific therapy has been given, since it comes from the wall of the abscess.

Valuable indirect evidence of liver abscess may be obtained by scanning of the liver following administration of an appropriate radiolabeled substance. It must be emphasized that neither routine aspiration nor surgical drainage is recommended in most cases of suspected liver abscess. The safest procedure is to give specific therapy and observe the response. If the abscess is amebic, results are usually dramatic. If there is no response within 3 or 4 days, aspiration of surgical drainage is indicated. There may be a bacterial abscess, a secondarily infected amebic abscess, or a nonsuppurative lesion.

Amebic abscess of the lung is usually secondary to abscess of the liver, although a few primary cases have been reported. *Amebic abscess of the brain* is extremely rare and is usually secondary to liver abscess. *Ameba cutis* is usually secondary to perforation of the abdominal wall following rupture of an adjacent anterior amebic hepatic abscess. It also may occur as a result of perforation of the rectum, with a fistula sinus extending from the perirectal tissue to the perineal skin, or as a perianal extension of amebic colitis. These lesions are extremely painful and are prone to secondary bacterial infection.

Ameboma (amebic granuloma) is a granulomatous tumorlike mass that occasionally develops in the large intestine and may clinically and radiographically mimic carcinoma of the bowel. This lesion often consists of a granulomatous, fibrous, edematous mass that encroaches on the bowel lumen and may give the signs and symptoms of obstruction. Eosinophils are seen in the inflammatory necrotic central zone, along with a few amebae. These patients often have peripheral eosinophilia.

TREATMENT. In children with asymptomatic *intestinal amebiasis,* treatment with diiodohydroxyquin (Diodoquin) alone is usually sufficient. The dose is 0.325 g (one-half tablet) three times a day for 20 days in children weighing less than 20 kg; from 20 to 39 kg the dose should be 0.65 g twice a day; for children 40 kg and over, 0.65 g three times a day. When there are definite symptoms, such as recurrent diarrhea or abdominal pain, metronidazole, 15 mg/kg three times a day for 1 week to 10 days, should be used together with a luminal amebicide such as Diodoquin. Alternatively, tetracycline at a dosage of 0.25 g four times a day for 5 days should be given to children 20 kg or more in weight, preceding or simultaneously with the Diodoquin. For children less than 20 kg the dosage of tetracycline should be 0.25 g three times a day. In cases of severe dysenteric amebiasis, therapy should be initiated with metronidazole and Diodoquin as described above. If therapeutic response is not evident in 48 to 72 hours, it may become necessary to employ an alternative amebicide, dehydroemetine, which is administered by deep subcutaneous injection, 1 to 1.5 mg/kg daily (120 mg maximum) for not more than 5 days. Often the dysentery will be controlled after two or three injections. At this point dehydroemetine should be discontinued and metronidazole-Diodoquin treatment instituted. An alternative to metronidazole is tetracycline, 250 mg four times a day for children 20 kg or more; for those less than 20 kg the dosage of tetracycline should be 250 mg three times a day. It should be recognized that dehydroemetine, like emetine, is a highly effective tissue amebicide with no luminal activity. Both of these alkaloids are highly toxic and may cause vomiting, abdominal pain, severe myalgia, tachycardia, hypotension, and profound EKG abnormalities, including fatal arrhythmias. They should be avoided in children as well as in patients with renal, cardiac, or muscle disease unless all other amebicides fail.

Most cases of *liver abscess* will respond dramatically to metronidazole therapy in the dosage described above. Thus metronidazole should be instituted immediately. Similarly, most abscesses will yield to chloroquine therapy. The total dosage of chloroquine phosphate should be 200 mg/kg, with a maximum of 10 g. The usual daily dose is 5 mg/kg twice a day, the maximum individual dose being 250 mg. Many believe that chloroquine should be combined with dehydroemetine. The authors feel that the best procedure is to give dehydroemetine as suggested for severe dysentery and to discontinue it as soon as a clear clinical response has occurred. At that time chloroquine treatment should be instituted. In all cases, following the chloroquine, tetracycline and Diodoquin should be given. In a small minority of cases aspiration or surgical drainage will be required. Incomplete resolution of the abscess is indicated by persistence or recurrence of fever, by persistence of leukocytosis, or by a persistently elevated erythrocyte sedimentation rate. The patient should not be dismissed from follow-up until temperature and leukocyte count have remained normal for at least 2 weeks after metronidazole or chloroquine therapy has been completed and the sedimentation rate has shown progressive decrease toward normal. If dehydroemetine therapy is elected, then careful monitoring of the patient's heart and blood pressure is indicated. Recent reports have implicated metronidazole as a carcinogenic agent in laboratory animals and in mutagenicity testing in Salmonella. These data suggest prudence in using this drug when alternative therapy may be available.

Skin granuloma requires dehydroemetine in the dosages already indicated. Metronidazole can be used.

Warm stool examinations should be negative at approximately 1, 3, and 6 months after completion of all treatment before the child is discharged from observation. If the treatment outlined above for intestinal amebiasis should fail, there are a number of other agents that can be substituted for Diodoquin. One of the most effective is paromomycin (Humatin). The dosage should be 25 mg/kg/day in two or three divided doses for 5 days.

Primary Amebic Meningoencephalitis

In 1958 Culbertson reported that previously unsuspected free-living, soil-inhabiting amebae could invade the central nervous system and cause fatal meningoencephalitis. Within a few years a number of reports appeared from various parts of the world essentially confirming this observation. The organism isolated from pathologic lesions has been identified as *Naegleria gruberi.* However, other reports have described other species of free-living amebae, ie, *Acanthamoeba* and *Hartmanella* species. At present it is not entirely clear whether all these species may be implicated or just *Naegleria gruberi.* Unambiguous identification of these organisms is not routine; they should be referred to a qualified protozoologist for confirmation.

Significantly, in almost every case of primary amebic meningoencephalitis a recent history of swimming in fresh or brackish water has been obtained. In one instance, however, recent extraction of two maxillary molars had occurred. It is believed the amebae gain access to the body through the nasal mucosa. Moreover, Culbertson has been able to produce the disease in mice by instilling *Naegleria* or *Acanthamoeba* into the nares of mice.

With but a single exception, all cases have occurred in young, previously healthy individuals between the ages of 8 and 27 years. The onset of symptoms usually has been abrupt and has been fatal within 1 to 2 days. A fulminant course marked by severe headache, nausea, vomiting, and rapidly deepening coma has been reported. Cerebrospinal fluid examination may reveal large numbers of neutrophils; sugar may be low or normal and protein elevated. Erythrocytes may be found. Microscopic examination of fresh cerebrospinal fluid under high magnification on a warm stage may reveal motile amebae.

Most histopathologic studies have shown severe lytic necrosis and hemorrhage along the base of the brain in the regions of the olfactory bulbs and cerebellum; organisms, although difficult to discern, can be identified under high magnification with ordinary staining methods. Isolation of amebae from liver, spleen, and lung in one case and the presence of myocarditis in several other cases suggest that dissemination may occur. At present it is not entirely certain whether the portal of entry is always by way of the nasal mucosa, cribriform plate, and then into the neural tissue, since experimental infections may also result in severe hemorrhagic pneumonia.

Naegleria infection does not seem to respond to the usual antiprotozoal drugs. However, there is a single report in which early diagnosis of *Naegleria* infection was successfully treated with amphotericin B by both systemic and intracisternal administration.

Malaria

Malaria is a disease of man and other vertebrates caused by sporozoa of the genus *Plasmodium*. The disease has been known since antiquity. Hippocrates, who studied in Egypt, unmistakably described the various forms of malaria. Long before the etiology of malaria was discovered by Laveran at the end of the nineteenth century it was clear that malaria was related to the emanations of the swamps; thus the name malaria. At present there are four species of *Plasmodium* recognized as the usual etiologic agents of human malaria: *P. falciparum, P. vivax, P. malariae,* and *P. ovale.* Recently some cases of naturally acquired simian malaria have been reported; it is not clear how widespread this may be. However the discovery was not unexpected, inasmuch as it is well known that other simian malarias can be successfully transmitted to man by artificial means.

Until recently malaria was the most important parasitic disease of man (schistosomiasis now occupies the position); it infects an estimated 100 million individuals throughout the world and accounts for just under 1 million deaths annually. It is found, with few exceptions, throughout the tropical and subtropical zones and parts of the temperate zones, wherever a suitable species of anopheline mosquito exists. However, over the past two decades extensive malaria eradication programs have been responsible for eliminating or reducing this disease in many endemic areas of the world. Moreover, with widespread low-priced travel becoming commonplace, it is essential to consider malaria in those individuals who have returned from malarious regions.

In order to successfully complete its life cycle, *Plasmodium* requires an alternation of a vertebrate host in whom schizogony occurs with a female anopheline mosquito in whom sporogony takes place. Studies by Fairly during World War II demonstrated that within 1 hour of an infective mosquito bite sporozoites disappear from the circulation. The mystery of their disappearance was finally solved when it was found that on leaving the circulation the sporozoites invaded hepatic parenchymal cells and underwent repeated nuclear divisions, producing as the end product of schizogony many thousands of merozoites. The parasitized host cell next ruptures, releasing these merozoites, many of which are phagocytized by the host, although others enter another hepatic cell to initiate schizogony anew. During this pre-erythrocytic cycle the patient's blood is free of parasites, and he cannot transmit the disease (ie, this is the prepatent period). As this period ends, merozoites leave the liver and invade red blood cells, initiating the erythrocytic cycle. Within the parasitized erythrocytes, schizogony is repeated regularly, releasing new groups of merozoites into the bloodstream. After a period of time some merozoites invade red cells, and rather than undergo schizogony they develop into macrogametocytes or microgametocytes. These subsequently must be ingested by a suitable mosquito in order to undergo further development. Merozoites formed as a result of the initial or primary pre-erythrocytic cycle in *P. falciparum* apparently differ from those of the other three species; they do not reinvade liver cells, but enter the circulation and invade erythrocytes. Thus, unlike the other three species of human *Plasmodium, P. falciparum* does not maintain both exoerythrocytic and erythrocytic cycles simultaneously. This distinction is of the utmost importance with regard to therapy and is probably the basis for relapse in *P. vivax* and *P. ovale* infections.

Shortly after a suitable anopheline mosquito ingests gametocytes together with her blood meal, the male or microgametocyte forms 6 to 8 microgametes (exflagellation). Similarly, the female or macrogametocyte undergoes maturation to become a gamete, and fertilization takes place with fusion of the microgamete and macrogamete. During the next 12 to 24 hours the resulting zygote elongates and becomes a motile ookinete, which actively penetrates the epithelial cell brush border of the midgut and comes to rest on the inner aspect of the peritrophic membrane of the mosquito's stomach. Here development proceeds as the zygote becomes a rounded, enlarged oocyst in which sporogony occurs, resulting in thousands of sporozoites. Subsequently the mature oocyst ruptures, liberating huge numbers of sporozoites into the mosquito's hemocoel. These invade all the insect's tissues, many reaching the salivary glands. Thus, when the mosquito next feeds, infective sporozoites are inoculated into the human host; depending on climatic conditions and other host factors the mosquito cycle takes 7 to 20 days or longer.

PATHOLOGY. Other than destruction of a few liver cells there is little evidence to suggest that significant pathologic damage can be attributed to the preerythrocytic or exoerythrocytic stages. However, the invasion and cyclical destruction of erythrocytes and progressive increase of peripheral parasitemia is in part responsible for a developing anemia of varying severity that usually depends on the plasmodial species involved. The observations of Kitchen suggest that *P. vivax* invades reticulocytes, *P. malariae* prefers mature erythrocytes, and *P. falciparum* has no preference. This may in part account for the greater parasitemia often encountered in *P. falciparum* malaria. Erythrocyte destruction is enhanced by erythrophagocytosis of non-parasitized cells. Nevertheless, it is most unusual to obtain evidence of red cell sensitization by either direct or indirect Coombs test. During acute episodes the hematocrit and hemoglobin determinations are reduced; reticulocytosis is usually present, and bone marrow aspiration reveals erythroid hyperplasia. There may be moderate leukocytosis, although leukopenia and thrombocytopenia are also frequently encountered early in the acute episode.

With increased destruction of erythrocytes, malarial pigment (hemozoin), as well as hemosiderin, cell debris, and merozoites, may stimulate reticuloendothelial activity. The viscera, including the brain, may take on a slate gray to black appearance as a result of sequestered malarial pigment.

The spleen may enlarge during an acute attack. At this time the capsule is thin and easily torn, and the pulp is diffluent. After many years the capsule becomes thickened and the pulp fibrous. Splenomegaly is then irreversible. Splenic enlargement is so typical that palpation has been used for epidemiologic purposes to determine indices of prevalence, distribution, and intensity of malaria. Hepatomegaly is also common. Kupffer cells are filled with brown to black hemozoin and parenchymal cells with yellow hemosiderin. There may be centrilobular necrosis that may be related to hypoxemia. Liver function usually is not seriously impaired, although there may be increases in conjugated bilirubin, SGOT/SGPT, and BSP retention. Serum albumin may decrease, and there is almost always an absolute increase in serum globulins.

For many years it has been recognized that erythrocytes infected with *P. falciparum* become sequestered in visceral capillaries where schizogony takes place. Recent experimental evidence has shown changes in the cell membrane of erythrocytes parasitized by late-stage trophozoites and schizonts. It is believed that these alterations are responsible for the tendency of these cells to clump and adhere to capillary endothelium. Thus capillary occlusion, or decreased flow, appears to be responsible for the hypoxemic lesions that may be found especially in the brain and gastrointestinal tract. Lesions resembling those of glomerulonephritis have been reported most frequently, although not exclusively, in children with *P. malariae* infection.

The development of immunity to malaria involves both humoral and cellular mechanisms. Increased phagocytic activity, hyperplasia of reticuloendothelial components, and the appearance of high titers of strain-specific protective antibodies in serum are important features of the immune response. In endemic or hyperendemic regions infants are born with passive immunity to malaria as a result of placental transfer of protective IgG antibodies. During the first few years of life repeated infection and active disease may result in acquired active immunity. Such immunity may keep individuals relatively free of clinical attack even in the presence of significant parasitemia. Serum gamma globulin levels become markedly increased with the development of immunity. Moreover, inoculation of hyperimmune globulin has been shown to prevent or diminish an acute malaria attack. During an acute episode the levels of circulating complement fall, and antigen-antibody-complement complexes have been localized by immunofluorescence techniques to the glomerular basement membrane of the kidney. Whether these findings can be implicated in the nephrotic syndrome of *P. malariae* is not entirely clear.

The role of fixed macrophages in malaria as an expression of cell-mediated immunity is highly suggestive. A number of studies have shown that a large portion of the normal circulating erythrocyte population, as well as platelets, may be engulfed by activated macrophages in the spleen, liver, and marrow, significantly contributing to the anemia. Whether this represents macrophage activation by lymphocyte products or a nonspecific host hyperphagocytic state is not settled. Therefore it seems likely that the enhanced host phagocytic activity is responsible for the frequent pathologic findings in malaria of hepatosplenomegaly, anemia, and thrombocytopenia.

CLINICAL ASPECTS. Older children and adults may exhibit the typical clinical picture of malaria characterized by intermittent febrile episodes, anemia, and splenomegaly. The incubation period (interval from infectious mosquito bite to symptoms) in the nonimmune subject varies widely, depending on the species and strain of *Plasmodium* (*P. falciparum*, 9 to 14 days; *P. ovale*, 16 to 18 days; *P. malariae*, 18 to 40 days; *P. vivax*, 12 to 17 days). However, certain strains of *P. vivax* may have incubation periods of 6 to 12 months or more, and following the discontinuance of suppressant drugs, *P. malariae* and *P. ovale* can exhibit delayed primary attacks of several years.

The initial or primary attack often is heralded by a short prodromal period of several days to a week and consists of irregular fevers, anorexia, chilliness, arthralgias, abdominal discomfort, and mild diarrhea. This is followed by the primary attack that lasts several weeks, during which there are recurring intermittent paroxysms classically consisting of four more or less distinct stages: shaking chills, high fever, drenching sweats, and an apyretic period. The paroxysms recur at approximately 48-hour intervals with *P. vivax*, *P. ovale*, and *P. falciparum* (tertian fevers); *P. malariae* recurs every 72 hours (quartan fever). Since the paroxysm coincides with rupture of infected erythrocytes and release of merozoites, pigment, and cell debris into the circulation, many workers have come to regard this as a cause-and-effect relationship. Acute splenic enlargement is often associated with left upper quadrant pain. Usually renal and hepatic function remain unimpaired. *P. falciparum*, or malignant tertian malaria, accounts for most of the severe or pernicious complications and nearly all the deaths.

A wide range of symptoms referable to central nervous system involvement may be seen, presumably related to those areas of the brain in which capillary occlusion and/or hypoxemia have occurred. The onset of cerebral malaria may appear unheralded and may occur when the parasitemia is low or high. Nevertheless, it should be emphasized that the degree of parasitemia is most often correlated with a fatal outcome in *P. falciparum* malaria. Meningeal signs are especially common in children, but examination of the cerebrospinal fluid usually is normal. Alternatively, severe gastrointestinal, cardiovascular, respiratory, or urogenital symptoms can dominate the picture and may have a fatal termination. Glomerulonephritis associated with *P. malariae* usually has a poor prognosis.

The natural history of untreated malaria is such that clinical attacks or relapses become less frequent, and after a variable period the infection disappears. *P. falciparum* infection lasts about 9 months to 1 year and *P. vivax* 1 to 8 years, but *P. malariae* can persist for decades as a latent infection, and relapses have occurred after 30 years. While congenital malaria undoubtedly occurs in endemic areas, it is a rare event. In most instances the mother acquired the disease during pregnancy. This may result in fatal termination of the pregnancy, or the child may develop malaria early in the perinatal period.

During the first few years of life the acute disease may be unlike malaria as seen in adults. The child is restless, dull, and irritable, with little or no appetite. Abdominal pain and vomiting are frequent. The liver and spleen are enlarged; temperature may range from 38.5 C to 41 C and may be continuous, remittent, or intermittent. Typical paroxysms seldom occur. If untreated, the child's condition may worsen and he may die, or the acute symptoms may gradually abate, passing into a stage of chronic malaria. The spleen may become exceedingly large, extending into the pelvis; it is liable to spontaneous or traumatic rupture. Some children develop malarial cachexia, which usually has a fatal outcome.

Considerable evidence has been accumulated indicating that individuals with abnormal hemoglobins, especially sickle cell trait, have fewer parasites and milder disease than those with normal hemoglobin. Individuals with erythrocyte glucose-6-phosphate dehydrogenase deficiency are said to be similarly disposed. Epidemiologic studies from Africa seem to implicate malaria as an important factor in the etiology of Burkitt's lymphoma. It is presumed that continuous stimulation of the lymphoid system in chronic malaria increases its susceptibility to neoplastic transformation by Epstein-Barr virus.

DIAGNOSIS. The definitive diagnosis of malaria is made by microscopic identification of the organisms on stained thin and thick blood smears. It is important to examine thick films, since they provide a higher concentration of parasites, which is indispensable when parasitemia is low or thin films are negative. Preferably, the blood smear should be stained with Giemsa's stain, although Wright's stain can be used. Since parasites are continuously present in peripheral red blood cells during schizogony, blood can be taken and examined at any time with *P. vivax*, *P. ovale*, and *P. malariae* infections. In *P. falciparum* infections, however, only rings may be present immediately after the fever peaks. If symptoms have been present for 7 to 9 days, usually gametocytes will be present in the peripheral blood, and species identification can readily be made. The fluorescent antibody technique yields excellent results as a specific diagnostic test if it is available. However, it should not be used as the basis to initiate drug therapy, since titers may remain elevated for a considerable period after cure.

TREATMENT. The management of malaria demands prompt chemotherapy, but also the patient must be given supportive care while being kept under careful observation. It is essential, especially in *P. falciparum* malaria, to assess the parasitemia frequently by examination of blood smears three to four times daily. Fatalities rise dramatically when the parasitemia exceeds $100,000/mm^3$; thus patient management must be guided by this criterion.

Antimalarial chemotherapy is outlined in Table 3. Treatment of the acute attack is aimed at destroying erythrocytic stages of the parasite as rapidly as possible. For this purpose chloroquine is the drug of choice; it is a powerful schizonticidal 4-aminoquinoline that may be administered by the oral route or, if necessary, by the intramuscular route. Clinical and parasitic response can usually be detected in 72 hours, although it may take another 72 hours for all signs and symptoms to subside. Gametocytes of *P. falciparum* will often be detected for several weeks thereafter.

Certain strains of *P. falciparum* from Southeast Asia and parts of Central and South America have been found resistant to therapeutic doses of chloroquine. Quinine should be employed when resistance is encountered. It is preferable to use oral quinine, but in serious situations, or if vomiting intervenes, it may be given by the intravenous route. Toxicity to quinine can develop rapidly if renal function is impaired. The use of quinine alone is often associated with a significant recrudescence rate, which can be reduced appreciably by also giving an absorbable sulfa drug such as sulfadiazine, 100 mg/kg/day in four divided doses for 5 days (2 g maximum), and pyrimethamine, 1 mg/kg in two divided doses daily for 3 days (maximum 25 mg twice a day for 3 days).

Primaquine should be given for the eradication of persisting hepatic (exoerythrocytic) stages of *P. vivax*, *P. ovale*, and *P. malariae*. It is unnecessary, however, for *P. falciparum* malaria, since secondary exoerythrocytic forms apparently are not formed. Similarly, it is unnecessary in the treatment of transfusion malaria, since erythrocytic forms do not establish an exoerythrocytic cycle. Primaquine may cause hemolysis in individuals with glucose-6-phosphate dehydrogenase deficiency. In high doses it may cause hemolytic anemia, methemoglobinemia, and leukopenia. It should not be used concurrently with quinacrine (Atabrine), quinine, or sulfonamides.

Chemoprophylaxis with chloroquine is highly effective and will suppress all clinical activity of the disease except for resistant strains of *P. falciparum*. However, it is important to realize that prophylaxis with chloroquine does not prevent infection; it only destroys erythrocytic stages. Hepatic or exoerythrocytic stages

TABLE 3. Summary of Clinical Use of Chloroquine, Quinine, and Primaquine in Malaria

Clinical Situation	Drug and Usual Preparation	Route of Administration	Dose as Active Base or as Salt	Dosage and Schedule of Administration
Clinical attack	Chloroquine phosphate, UPS XVII*	Oral	Base	0 hours, 10 mg/kg; 6 hours, 5 mg/kg; 24 hours, 5 mg/kg; 48 hours, 5 mg/kg
	Quinine sulfate, USP XV† +	Oral	Salt	20–30 mg/kg/day divided into 3 doses for 7–10 days
	Pyrimethamine +	Oral	Base	1 mg/kg daily for 3 days in 2 divided doses (see text)
	Sulfadiazide	Oral		100 mg/kg day divided in 4 doses for 5 days (see text)
Emergency requirement for parenteral route	Chloroquine dihydrochloride‡	Intramuscular	Base	5 mg/kg, may be repeated once in 24-hour period
	Quinine hydrochloride, USP XV§	Intravenous	Salt	10 mg/kg well diluted in saline over 1-hour period, may be repeated twice in 24-hour period
Eradication, exoerythrocytic stage	Primaquine phosphate, USP XVII″	Oral	Base	0.3 mg/kg once a day for 14 days
Personal prophylactic suppression	Chloroquine phosphate, USP XVII#	Oral	Base	5 mg/kg once a week

* *Drug of choice; maximal initial dose 600 mg of the base.*
† *For use only in case of resistance to chloroquine and other antimalarials; maximal total daily dose 2 g.*
‡ *Use oral route as soon as possible; maximal single dose 300 mg of the base.*
§ *Use oral route as soon as possible; maximal single dose 650 mg.*
″ *Do not use concurrently with quinacrine or sulfonamides; discontinue if evidence of hemolysis; maximal single dose 15 mg of the base.*
Start 1 week before and continue 1 month after being in malarious area; maximal single dose 300 mg of the base.

remain unaffected, and clinical disease may become evident once prophylaxis is discontinued. Therefore on leaving a malarious area it is essential to initiate primaquine therapy before suppression with chloroquine is discontinued (Table 3).

The transfusion of whole blood or plasma has increasingly become recognized as a means of acquiring malaria. Similarly, drug addiction or the use of unclean hypodermic needles has been implicated as a means of transmitting the disease. With this means of infection the incubation period is usually short, generally depending on the number of parasites transmitted with the donor's blood. Malaria acquired as a result of blood transfusion can be an especially hazardous complication in view of the perilous condition of the patient requiring a blood transfusion and the difficulty in making the diagnosis of malaria for an unsuspecting physician, especially in nonmalarious areas.

African Trypanosomiasis

Two types of African trypanosomiasis are recognized: Gambian or mid-African and Rhodesian or East African sleeping sickness. They are similar protozoan diseases caused by the hemoflagellates *Trypanosoma gambiense* and *T. rhodesiense*, and occur only in those areas of central, west, and east Africa in which various species of *Glossina*, the tsetse fly, are found. *T. gambiense* and *T. rhodesiense* are pleomorphic flagellates varying from 15 to 30 μ in length by 1.5 to 3.5 μ in breadth. In Giemsa-stained blood smears they may appear long and slender, with an undulating membrane and free anterior flagellum, or short and broad without a free flagellum. There are no intracellular forms, but at various stages of the disease they may be found in the peripheral blood, lymphatics, lymph nodes, cerebrospinal fluid, and neural tissue. The two species are morphologically indistinguishable, but they maintain separate biologic characteristics in cross-inoculation experiments.

Outside of man there is no important reservoir host for *T. gambiense*, while *T. rhodesiense* is found naturally infecting wild game animals. In the tsetse fly trypanosomes undergo cyclic development; multiplying in the midgut and hindgut and migrating anteriorly they occupy the salivary glands and ducts, becoming infective about 15 to 35 days after the infecting blood meal. Metacyclic infective forms are inoculated into the bite wound when the tsetse fly next feeds. Although all age groups are susceptible to infection, the factors that influence human prevalence rest largely on occupational exposure to suitable tsetse flies and involve their breeding and feeding habits. Thus young adult males are found to be most frequently infected. During epidemics, when all age groups are infected, mechanical transmission may occur. Congenital transmission has been reported, but it must be very unusual.

PATHOLOGY. Within a few days after the bite an elevated, firm, erythematous nodule appears at the site of the wound; it may subside in several weeks or go on to ulcerate. At this time organisms may be found in the peripheral blood, and the initial symptoms of the acute disease may appear. These include irregular spiking fever, rash, arthralgias, headache, and facial edema and may persist for weeks or months, after which lymphadenitis becomes apparent. The superficial nodes are especially evident, such as the posterior cervical chain (Winterbottom's sign). During the many months of lymphatic involvement these tissues may become acellular and fibrotic. In about a year the disease enters a chronic stage, with signs and symptoms of central nervous system involvement. Trypanosomes are found in cerebrospinal fluid, in the subarachnoid space, and in brain substance. Meningoencephalitis and myelitis are evident. The meninges are thickened, and within the brain substance there is perivascular cuffing with lymphocytes and plasma cells. Foci of trypanosomes can be found in the brain tissue surrounded by microglial cells and macrophages. Neuronal degeneration and softening occur in the late stages.

Neurologic symptoms become the most prominent features of the disease. The patient becomes listless, melancholic, and lethargic, with slurring speech and tremors of the tongue and limbs. These finally merge into a deepening sleep from which it becomes ever more difficult to rouse the victim. Patients usually die either of malnutrition, malaria, dysentery, or other intercurrent infection. The course of East African sleeping sickness can be fulminant and therefore accelerated. If untreated, it usually terminates fatally in 8 to 12 months. Pathologic changes in the central nervous system are not as pronounced or as extensive as those found in mid-African sleeping sickness.

DIAGNOSIS. Definitive diagnosis is made by finding trypanosomes in blood and bone marrow smears, in lymph node aspirates in early or acute disease, and in cerebrospinal fluid in late or chronic disease. It is essential to employ both thick and thin blood smears, as well as to examine the buffy coat from 10 to 20 ml of citrated whole blood or the sediment from 5 ml of centrifuged cerebrospinal fluid. Culture and/or animal inoculation are sometimes the only successful means of obtaining a diagnosis; the fluorescent antibody test may prove useful.

TREATMENT. In its early stages African trypanosomiasis yields far more readily to therapy than in the late chronic CNS stage. Prior to CNS disease, suramin (Naphuride) is the drug of choice. Although it is of low toxicity, it is excreted almost entirely by the kidneys and may cause significant renal damage. Urinalysis should be done the day following administration of each dose of suramin to assure there is no evidence of renal damage. Therapy must be discontinued if albuminuria and/or granular casts appear. Suramin is given intravenously every 4 to 6 days. It is dissolved in

10 ml of sterile distilled water. The initial test dose is 300 to 500 mg; the subsequent adult dose is 1 g until a total of 10 g is administered. Even though suramin does not cross the blood-brain barrier, intrathecal administration should not be attempted.

Pentamidine is an effective alternative drug for the treatment of early African trypanosomiasis. It is given as an intramuscular injection of 4 mg/kg of the base daily or every other day for a total of 5 to 10 injections. Pentamidine is dissolved in no more than 3 ml of distilled water. The course may be repeated after 1 week. Patients should receive this drug while lying down, since transient hypotensive episodes, palpitations, and vertigo are not uncommon. It is contraindicated in renal disease.

In chronic or late-stage disease, tryparsamide (Fourneau 270), a pentavalent arsenical, is used in Gambian but not Rhodesian trypanosomiasis. It is administered intravenously, freshly dissolved in 10 ml of sterile distilled water once each week. The dosage is 40 to 50 mg/kg. Ten to 15 injections should be given (the initial dose should be reduced and subsequent injections increased gradually up to the maximum of 40 to 50 mg/kg). A 1-month rest period is necessary before repeating the course. Although acute toxicity is not a frequent problem, tryparsamide may cause optic atrophy, dermatitis, and any of the other well-known side effects of arsenicals. The onset of ophthalmologic disturbances demands immediate cessation of tryparsamide therapy.

Melarsoprol (Arsobal) is a compound consisting of the trivalent arsenical melarsen oxide and BAL. It is considered more effective than tryparsamide for the treatment of CNS trypanosomiasis and more effective against *T. rhodesiense*. It is administered in the hospital as a 5 percent solution in propylene glycol. The recommended dose is 3.6 mg/kg intravenously on each of four consecutive days. The course of therapy should be repeated after 1 week. Neither renal nor optic nerve toxicity is observed with this drug, but arsenic toxicity can be a problem.

If therapy is initiated prior to significant central nervous system involvement, the outcome is usually favorable. Untreated infections often end fatally. With few exceptions, control of the vector has proved to be a difficult if not impossible task. Prevention of tsetse fly bites and chemoprophylaxis may be the best means of eliminating the disease from an area. Both suramin and pentamidine have proved to be excellent in this regard.

American Trypanosomiasis

Chagas' disease is caused by the hemoflagellate *Trypanosoma cruzi*, which was first discovered in 1911 in the blood of a serious ill, wasted Brazilian child suffering from fever, lymphadenopathy, and anemia. The disease is limited to the Western Hemisphere, being prevalent in South and Central America and Mexico. There have been two autochthonous cases reported from the United States. *T. cruzi* is a pleomorphic spindle-shaped organism 15 to 20 μ long with a central nucleus, undulating membrane, and single flagellum

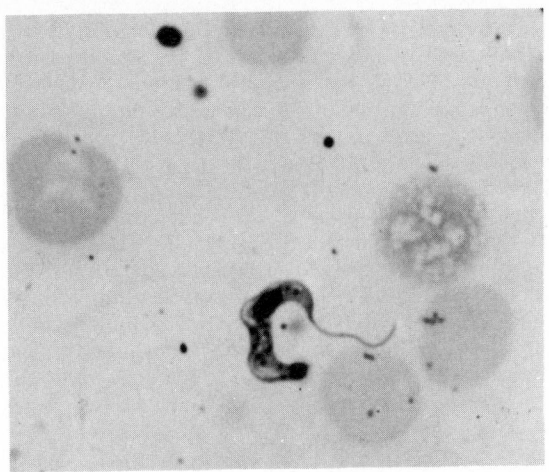

FIG. 22. *Trypanosoma cruzi* in the peripheral blood (×1,277).

(Fig. 22). In man or other mammals it has an intracellular phase in which the trypanosomal form undergoes profound morphologic changes to assume a leishmanial (amastigote) form that is but 2 to 4 μ in diameter and is without a flagellum.

Other than man, various domesticated and wild animals serve as excellent reservoir hosts. Armadillos and opossums are commonly infected throughout the endemic zones. In Maryland, Georgia, and Florida many raccoons are naturally infected. Recent studies have demonstrated naturally infected reduviid bugs in many parts of the southwestern United States and California. Usually the infection is acquired when the organisms are deposited on the skin along with the feces of biting reduviid bugs (*Rhodnius, Panstrongylus, Triatoma*). The bite, which is commonly at the mucocutaneous junction of the lips or eyes, can be either extremely painful or painless, depending on the vector; and the flagellates are introduced into the bite wound by rubbing or scratching, or they may traverse adjacent intact mucous membranes. Chagas' disease is far more common in children than in adults. Nearly 80 percent of patients are under 21 years of age, with the disease being most frequent in infants between 2 months and 2 years of age.

PATHOLOGY. The primary or initial lesion (chagoma) is caused by invasion of histiocytes, fat cells, and other subcutaneous tissues of the bite area. The intracellular leishmanial (amastigote) forms proliferate rapidly, destroying host cells and quickly reinvading others. This pattern stimulates a marked inflammatory process that appears on the skin as a firm red nodule. As infection disseminates from the bite area, a gelatinous edema spreads along subcutaneous, fascial, and muscular planes. Lymphatic invasion with histiocytic proliferation and granulomatous lymphadenitis may cause regional lymphatic obstruction. Invasion and destruction of myocardial fibers is almost invariably found (Fig. 23) and is accompanied by a diffuse inflammatory exudate. Fibrinous pericarditis and pericardial effusion are nearly constant findings. Mild endocardial and subendocardial involvement is usually present. After many years, diffuse hypertrophy, focal fibrosis resembling ischemic changes, and scattered inflammatory infiltrates are found. Organisms may or may not be evident.

Gastrointestinal invasion, with destruction of muscle and ganglion cells, may cause megacolon and megaesophagus, although other tubular organs may also be affected. Central nervous system disease is characterized by invasion of neuroglial cells and by scattered glial nodules in the gray and white matter. Neuronal degeneration as well as perivascular and meningeal cellular infiltrates are commonly encountered.

Trypanosomes ordinarily cannot be found in the peripheral blood more than 30 or 40 days after the initial infection. Furthermore, reproduction does not occur in the trypanosomal stages; therefore most of the widespread manifestations of Chagas' disease must be attributed to the leishmanial (amastigote) or intracellular stage of the infection. Mechanisms of immunity in Chagas' disease have not been as well studied as in other protozoan infections. Asymptomatic infections are known to exist, since humoral antibodies can be detected. It is conjectural whether this represents acquired resistance to a pathogenic strain or immunity

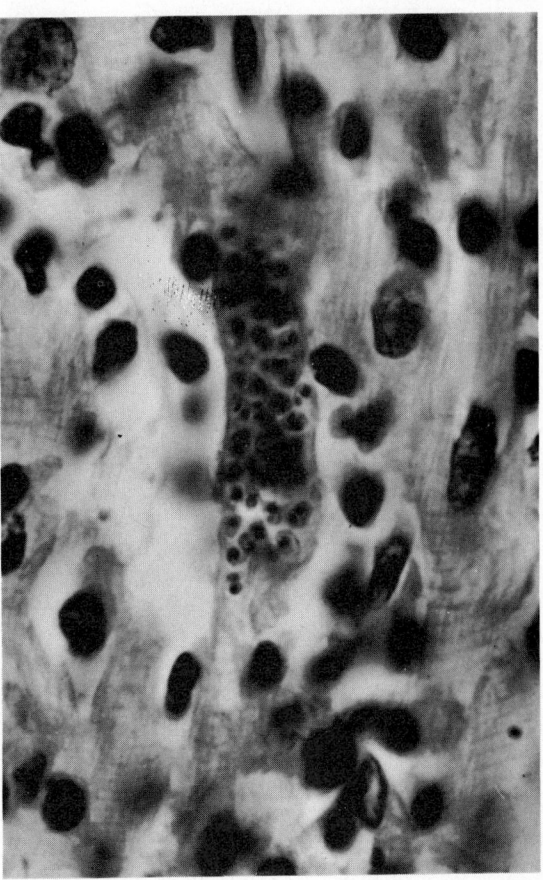

FIG. 23. Leishmanial forms of *Tryponosoma cruzi* in the myocardium (×1,277).

resulting from a previous infection with a nonvirulent strain. It is generally conceded that circulating antibodies, at least those that are measured, do not confer protection. That cellular immunity plays an important role in Chagas' disease is suggested by a number of animal studies in which neonatal thymectomy or administration of antilymphocyte serum has resulted in significantly increased parasitemia and mortality. Moreover, the passive transfer of spleen cells from immune animals has conferred protection.

SYMPTOMS. In children the onset of the disease is characterized by intermittent daily fever, followed by generalized nonpitting edema and unilateral palpebral edema (Romaña's sign). Lymphadenopathy, hepatosplenomegaly, urticaria, signs of meningeal irritation, various behavior problems, and focal neurologic symptoms may be part of the clinical picture. Acute chagasic myocarditis may be accompanied by premature ventricular contractions, atrial fibrillation, partial or complete heart block, or progressive congestive failure. Usually the cardiac symptoms abate, leaving little early evidence of residual disease, although recent studies have suggested that myocardial destruction may continue to smolder for many years and lead to severe heart disease in 20 to 30 years. Evidence of persisting parasite infection in long-standing chagasic heart disease is scanty, and many authors regard chronic myocarditis to be the result of cytotoxic interaction of *T. cruzi*-sensitized lymphocytes with nonparasitized heart cells as a result of a crossreacting common antigen of both the heart and parasite. However, on clinical grounds it is extremely difficult to differentiate coronary heart disease in older patients or rheumatic heart disease in younger patients from chagasic heart disease. Residual neurologic symptoms, such as focal or generalized seizures and behavior disorders, may occur.

DIAGNOSIS. Definitive diagnosis depends on demonstration of the parasite in the blood or tissues. It must be emphasized that examination of the peripheral blood is of value only during the initial acute disease or during chronic exacerbation. Animal inoculation with blood from a patient will often aid in the diagnosis. Liver biopsy, bone marrow aspiration, or splenic puncture will often provide the answer. At times, xenodiagnosis may be the only means by which organisms can be found: laboratory-reared reduviid bugs are permitted to feed on the patient or his fresh blood and are then allowed to feed on uninfected guinea pigs. The latter are examined for trypanosomes after about 45 days.

Serologic tests can be useful during various stages of the disease. The precipitin test may be positive during the acute episode, while the complement-fixation test (Machado-Guerreiro test) is useful for diagnosis of chronic disease. The fluorescent antibody and indirect hemagglutination tests are becoming valuable diagnostic tools for the diagnosis of Chagas' disease.

TREATMENT. Supportive therapy is all that is currently available during the chronic stages of the disease. In the acute phase Bayer 7602, a 4-aminoquinoline compound, has been advocated, since it clears the blood of trypanosomal forms. However, it is ineffective against the tissue stages. Recently, *l*-furaltadone (Al-

tafur) has been used in oral doses of 30 mg/kg/day for 15 days, followed by 10 mg/kg/day for 3 months. This compound also appears to be active only against the trypanosomal forms. The outlook is serious in children during the acute illness. It is especially grave when neurologic symptoms dominate the picture. Chagasic heart disease is currently believed to be far more widespread than previously suspected. The prognosis is also poor once symptoms of cardiac failure appear. Residual spraying with DDT, dieldrin, or gamma benzene hexachloride (BHC) is an effective means of killing reduviid bugs. Education of individuals in the community in the habits of kissing bugs and their relationship to Chagas' disease is the most important facet of long-term control.

Visceral Leishmaniasis

There are three generally recognized species of *Leishmania* that infect man. Although they are morphologically indistinguishable, their serologic reactions, geographic distributions, and clinical manifestations are sufficiently distinctive to separate them. However, in some areas overlapping characteristics are so prevalent that some workers, notably Alder, regard the three species as a complex with strain and racial intergrades. Leishmanial organisms exist in mammalian tissues as small intracellular oval bodies 2 to 4 μ in diameter without a free flagellum. In the sandfly (*Phlebotomus*) the oval body elongates (15 to 20 μ) and extends a single anterior flagellum (leptomonad or promastigote form).

Kala-azar or visceral leishmaniasis is caused by *Leishmania donovani*, American or mucocutaneous leishmaniasis is caused by *L. braziliensis*, and oriental sore or cutaneous leishmaniasis is the result of infection with *L. tropica*. These organisms live and proliferate in the cytoplasm of reticuloendothelial cells, eventually destroying them. When sandflies bite an infected individual the ingested leishmanial (amastigote) forms are transformed in the insect's intestine into leptomonad (promastigote) forms. From the midgut enormous numbers of organisms produced by longitudinal binary fission migrate to the insect's buccal cavity to be inoculated during the next blood meal.

Visceral leishmaniasis is found in Asia, the Middle East, Africa, southern Europe (Mediterranean littoral), and South and Central America. The disease appears to exist in at least two epidemiologic forms: (1) A Mediterranean type affects young children (1 to 4 years of age) and also dogs or feral animals. This type extends from the Mediterranean through central Asia into China; it is also present in parts of South America. (2) An Indian type predominates in children between 5 and 15 years of age; dogs are not important reservoir hosts. In East Africa the disease is in some ways similar to the Indian type, except that the disease is not often found in children, but in the elderly. Some investigators regard the East African form as separate from the Indian type.

PATHOLOGY. The principal pathologic lesions are a result of reticuloendothelial cell hyperplasia, especially in the spleen and liver. Later the marrow and lymph nodes are filled with infected macrophages, and concomitant leukopenia and anemia develop. Similarly, the kidneys may be filled with infected macrophages, and invasion of submucosal and mucosal macrophages in the intestine sometimes is associated with severe ulceration.

The immunologic response to *L. donovani* is imperfectly understood. At the bite wound a small dermal lesion may develop; the parasites, initially localized in dermal macrophages, disseminate within these macrophages to the spleen, liver, bone marrow, and lymph nodes predominantly. Within these organs generalized lymphocytogenesis and histiocytogenesis occur, resulting in hepatosplenomegaly. Massive hyperglobulinemia is found, but this outpouring of humoral antibody appears to be nonspecific and is nonprotective. As the lymphoid organs and marrow are crowded out by macrophages, lymphocytopenia and/or pancytopenia may occur. Resistance to visceral leishmaniasis is essentially absent once the infection has visceralized. However, after chemotherapeutic cure an acquired immunity emerges; delayed hypersensitivity, as demonstrated by the Montenegro skin test, becomes evident. Moreover, concomitant with chemical cure and the appearance of delayed hypersensitivity, hypergammaglobulinemia abates. Usually the immunity to visceral leishmaniasis is complete and longlasting following chemotherapeutic cure. However, relapse, as seen in post-kala-azar dermal leishmanoid or East African kala-azar, is characterized by delayed hypersensitivity, dermal localization of parasites, and moderate hypergammaglobulinemia. It is of interest that while macrophage activation has resulted in enhanced phagocytosis of parasites, macrophages remain unable to kill parasites. The appearance of dermal delayed hypersensitivity at the time acquired immunity appears suggests that cell-mediated immunity plays an important role in protection. Further work on the immunology of visceral leishmaniasis is needed.

SYMPTOMS. Infantile kala-azar may begin either suddenly, with high fever and vomiting, or insidiously, with irregular daily fever, anorexia, weight loss, lassitude, and pallor. Purpura, cyanosis, severe anemia, diarrhea, and splenomegaly are also seen. A general bleeding diathesis often becomes evident shortly before death. After several months patients usually die if the disease is untreated. In less fulminating cases the clinical course is more protracted, usually ending fatally after 1 or 2 years.

In older children the disease tends to assume a more chronic course, with marked emaciation, edema, brittle hair, massive splenomegaly, and dusky slate-gray complexion (kala-azar is also called black sickness). Hyperglobulinemia, leukopenia, and anemia are typically found. As a result of the patient's general debility, death often results from such intercurrent infections as pneumonia, amebic or bacillary dysentery, and malaria.

Post-kala-azar dermal leishmanoid is a common complication of Indian and East African kala-azar. It is characterized by the appearance of hypopigmented, erythematous, or nodular lesions of the skin of the face, chest, neck, and buttocks. The lesions are believed to represent a modified form of *L. donovani* infection in which the parasites no longer are able to invade the viscera and are localized to the skin. This change in tissue tropism of *L. donovani* is not understood; it usually appears either spontaneously or more commonly after inadequate therapy.

DIAGNOSIS. Kala-azar is diagnosed by finding the organisms in stained smears of peripheral blood or bone marrow. Cultures of the blood or marrow on NNN medium are most useful. Splenic puncture and liver biopsy usually are the most rewarding procedures, but they are not without serious hazard in individuals with a bleeding diathesis. The Sia water test is usually positive, but it is not specific, since it only indicates elevated serum globulin. Fluorescent antibody and indirect hemagglutination tests are more specific but may not be readily available. The Montenegro or leishmanin skin test, which is negative during acute infection, becomes positive during the latter part of therapy. Untreated kala-azar is fatal in 75 to 85 percent of infantile cases and 90 to 95 percent of adult cases. Properly treated, 85 to 95 percent of cases can be cured.

TREATMENT. Kala-azar usually responds to treatment with pentavalent antimonials such as pentostam. Ethylstibamine (Neostibosan) has been most effective. Children usually are given an initial intramuscular dose of 250 mg, followed by eight daily doses of 300 mg until a total of 2.65 g has been administered. Generally the number of doses has to be increased for Chinese, Mediterranean, and African cases, since they are more resistant to therapy. In the antimony-resistant cases, stilbamidine or hydroxystilbamidine has been employed with excellent results. It is given very slowly intravenously on alternate days until the maximum dose of 10 injections of 3 mg/kg each has been given. Therapy is repeated 2 weeks later. The initial doses are usually reduced to test for sensitivity. Epinephrine should be available. Trigeminal neuropathy may follow stilbamidine therapy and can persist for years; however, hydroxystilbamidine therapy is reported to be free of this complication.

There are many aspects to the control of leishmaniasis. Sandflies (*Phlebotomus*) can readily be eliminated by residual spraying with DDT. Since sandflies ordinarily do not fly very high, sleeping quarters should be above ground level. Animal reservoirs, such as infected dogs, should be destroyed. Early therapy will prevent family and neighborhood transmission.

Cutaneous Leishmaniasis

Cutaneous leishmaniasis is found throughout the Middle East, along the Mediterranean basin and islands, in East and West Africa, India and southwest Asia, South and Central America, and southern Mexico. In man, infection by *L. tropica* produces self-limited skin ulcers with parasites situated in macrophages in and about the lesions. These hemoflagellates almost never visceralize in man. In many areas dogs or rodents are found naturally infected and are believed to be natural reservoirs of infection. As with visceral leishmaniasis, various species of sandflies transmit the infection, although contact transmission is possible and is the basis of the long-standing practice in middle and central Asia of immunizing inoculations, ie, "vaccination" to prevent possible disfigurement by a natural infection.

Old World leishmaniasis, or oriental sore, is often classified as wet or dry type. The wet or rural form is believed to be transmitted by *L. tropica* major and is found chiefly in various rodents on the edges of deserts. The dry or urban form is preponderantly anthropronotic; it is caused by *L. tropica* minor and is transmitted by sandflies that frequently feed on humans and occasionally dogs. The dry form of oriental sore is characterized by a long incubation period, long duration of active infection, and large numbers of parasites present in the dermis. The moist type, by contrast, has a relatively short incubation period, with rapid healing and a paucity of parasites in the skin.

The disease usually begins with a small red vesicular lesion, the skin of which dries, encrusts, and drops off, revealing a shallow ulcer. The ulcer progressively enlarges and characteristically has raised, sharp indurated margins. Healing usually takes place in 3 to 18 months, often leaving an obvious depressed scar. However, it is not uncommon for single or multiple papules to heal directly without extensive ulceration.

The epidemiology and etiology of American cutaneous leishmaniasis has become an extremely complex subject. In South and Central America it is evident that there are many varieties of leishmaniasis, the mucocutaneous form (espundia) being but one of these. In contrast to Old World cutaneous leishmaniasis, American cutaneous disease is closely tied to the forests of South and Central America, and each variety has its own distinct epidemiology and pathologic picture; descriptions of several of these follow:

Chiclero ulcer, which is found in Mexico, Guatemala, and Honduras, is believed to be caused by *L. mexicana* and is seen most frequently as an occupational disease of forest workers such as those who cut mahogany and collect chicle gum. It is a zoonotic disease of several sylvatic arboreal rodents. The chiclero ulcer is most often seen as a chronic disfiguring disease of the ear that may persist for many years. The infection never metastasizes to mucous membrane. Organisms are difficult to find in the lesion. The Montenegro or leishmanin skin test is usually positive.

Pian-bois, of Venezuela and French Guiana, is manifested by scattered open weeping ulcers. There have been reports of metastases to mucous membranes in a small percentage of cases.

Leishmaniasis tegumentaria diffusa is ascribed to *L. pifanoi* and is encountered on the northwest coast of Brazil and Venezuela. Large, heavily parasitized dermal plaques or nodules are present. Infected cells can be isolated from the blood, but visceral lesions are not encountered. The Montenegro skin test is negative. A number of authors have likened tegumentaria diffusa to lepromatous leprosy, and similarly it is believed to be the result of anergy or failure of cell-mediated immunity. In the Ethiopian form of this disease humoral antibodies are present.

Mucocutaneous leishmaniasis is caused by *L. braziliensis* and is the classically described form of American leishmaniasis that causes espundia. It is found in Brazil, Peru, Ecuador, Chile, Bolivia, and Paraguay east of the Andes. It is estimated that nasal involvement may occur in up to 80 percent of infections, with up to 30 percent that eventually mutilate the mucous membrane of the mouth, nose, palate, larynx, and trachea. These cases are eventually fatal due to intervening sepsis. The mucous membrane lesions usually appear several years after a cutaneous ulcer has healed. Once mucous membrane involvement occurs, the infection is highly resistant to chemotherapy.

Uta, caused by *L. peruana,* is found high in the Andes of Peru and Boliva. The disease is relatively mild, with few cases involving mucous membranes. Dogs are found as natural reservoirs of this infection.

DIAGNOSIS. In the cutaneous forms of leishmaniasis, microscopic examination of tissue obtained from the edge of the ulcer or inoculation of some of the material into NNN medium usually will confirm the diagnosis. Mucocutaneous leishmaniasis has an excellent outlook if treated before metastatic lesions to mucous membranes appear; otherwise the outlook is poor, since these lesions are often refractory to therapy. Uncomplicated *L. tropica* always responds well to therapy.

THERAPY. Therapy for early mucocutaneous leishmaniasis is the same as for oriental sore. If few ulcers are present they are treated by local infiltration with various antimonial compounds such as stibophen (Fuadin); carbon dioxide snow or electrocoagulation can also be used. Systemic treatment with pentostam, a pentavalent antimonial, has also been instituted in order to prevent the development of secondary (metastatic) cutaneous or mucocutaneous lesions. The latter are often resistant to therapy and may require many courses of retreatment. Amphotericin B currently is being used for the treatment of mucocutaneous lesions. Despite serious side effects, this drug seems to be effective in cases otherwise drug-resistant.

Giardiasis

Giardia intestinalis (G. lamblia) is the most frequently diagnosed intestinal flagellate of man. It is found in most areas of the world, but it is more prevalent in warmer regions. *Giardia* lives in the duodenum and jejunum and has both trophic and cystic stages. It is about 10 to 20 μ long by 5 to 15 μ wide and has four pairs of flagella and two nuclei. The trophozoite (motile stage) usually is found in liquid stools, whereas the cyst (8 to 10 μ by 7 to 10 μ) appears in formed feces. Transmission is believed to be accomplished by ingestion of the cysts, probably following direct close contact, as in pinworm disease (p. 626), although contaminated food and water may also be a source of infection. Giardiasis is much more common in children than in adults; it is also common among inmates of institutions and in orphanages. Occasionally epidemics have been reported. Individuals with IgA deficiency are frequently infected with *Giardia*.

In heavy infections it is not unusual for patients to have vague upper abdominal discomfort, mucous diarrhea, flatulence, and steatorrhea. In children the manifestations can be more pronounced, with celiac or spruelike symptoms. Direct examination of the diarrheic stool will usually reveal motile trophozoites. Cysts can readily be found in formed stools by direct examination and concentration methods.

The infection yields readily to quinacrine therapy. The recommended dosage is 2 mg/kg orally three times a day, after meals, for 5 days, with a maximum total daily dose of 300 mg. Giardiasis has also been treated successfully with metronidazole (Flagyl), given for 5 days in divided doses after meals as follows: for children under 2 years of age, 125 mg; 2 to 4 years, 250 mg; 5 to 8 years, 375 mg; 9 years and over, 500 mg. Metronidazole has been reported to be carcinogenic in animals. Its use for the treatment of giardiasis should be discouraged unless no other therapy is effective in symtomatic cases.

Balantidiasis

Balantidium coli is the only common parasitic ciliate and the largest protozoan parasite of man. The motile or trophozoite form is from 50 to 200 μ long and 40 to 70 μ wide. Its surface is covered with cilia, and a prominent groove, the cytostome, is present anteriorly. When stained, a large bean-shaped macronucleus and smaller micronucleus are evident. Although swine and various primates are commonly infected with an organism morphologically indistinguishable from *B. coli*, it has been found extremely difficult to infect man with porcine or simian forms. It appears that the disease is transmitted from man to man by contact and poor sanitation. Therefore it is not surprising to find an increased prevalence of this infection in mental institutions, prisons, and orphanages. The ciliates are found in the large intestine, where they usually invade the mucosa and produce ulcers similar to those caused by *Entamoeba histolytica*. Rarely, intestinal perforation or extraintestinal invasion may occur.

Although asymptomatic infection is common, it may be associated with mild to fulminant symptoms consisting of diarrhea or dysentery. The disease often resembles amebiasis, from which it must be differentiated. In asymptomatic cases spontaneous cure is not unusual. Treatment with Carbarsone or Diodoquin has been successful. Recently, oral tetracycline, 20 mg/kg three times a day (maximum of 2 g daily), has given satisfactory results.

Toxoplasmosis

Toxoplasmosis is a protozoan infection of humans and other mammals with *Toxoplasma gondii,* an obligate intracellular protozoan parasite recently shown to belong to the class Sporozoa and to have coccidian affinities with an enteroepithelial cycle and oocyst production in cats and other felines. Although many species of *Toxoplasma* have been described since Nicolle and Manceaux established the genus for the organism they observed in the gondi, a North African rodent, all appear to be but a single species. In 1923 Jankü made the first report of human *Toxoplasma* infection (eye). However, 30 years elapsed before Wolfe and associates isolated the organism from infants who had died of encephalitis. As more case reports appeared it became evident that toxoplasmosis was widespread and could be acquired in utero as well as postnatally. Furthermore, as serologic methods were developed, it became clear that most human infection was inapparent or were associated with only minor symptoms.

ETIOLOGY.   *Toxoplasma* has been shown convincingly to be a coccidian parasite of cats and other felines. In the intestinal epithelium of cats a sexual cycle takes place that leads to the formation of oocysts, which are passed in the cat's feces and undergo sporulation in the soil or cat litter by initially forming two sporocysts, each of which forms four sporozoites. Sporogony takes from 1 to 5 days, depending on temperatures. Ingestion of this infective oocyst by nonfeline mammals or birds results in widespread infection of host tissues by intracellular reproduction of trophozoites. After a period of rapid reproduction, trophozoites (tachyzoites) accumulate in cysts, where the rate of reproduction declines. Tissue cysts may finally contain hundreds of trophozoites (bradyzoites) most frequently located in the brain, heart, and skeletal muscle cells. These cysts, which may persist for years or for the life of the host, are surrounded by a tough, argyrophilic, PAS-positive cyst wall. Following human ingestion of tissue cysts contained in rare or uncooked meat, trophozoites are released; they may reside briefly in the intestinal epithelium before they disseminate throughout the body and reproduce in many cell types, it is therefore possible for infection to be acquired by ingestion of infective oocysts in the soil or cat litter, by ingestion of tissue cysts in rare or raw meat, or by congenital transmission during acute infection during pregnancy.

Morphologic studies of *T. gondii* trophozoites in peritoneal exudate or tissue culture have demonstrated that it is crescentic, measuring 4 to 7 μ by 2 to 4 μ (Fig 24); it appears to divide by a process termed en-

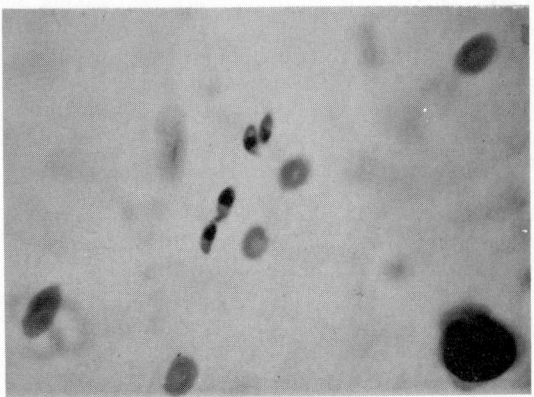

FIG. 24. Extracellular *Toxoplasma* in mouse peritoneal fluid stained by Wright's method.

dodyogeny rather than by longitudinal binary fission. Masses of organisms may be seen within the cytoplasm of host cells, superficially resembling *Leishmania* or *Histoplasma*. Electron photomicrographs reveal rather elaborate, highly specialized organelles, clearly confirming the sporozoan affinities of these organisms.

The intracellular proliferative forms can be found in almost every type of tissue cell other than non-nucleated erythrocytes. When an infected cell is overcrowded with parasites it ruptures, and the liberated parasites penetrate other cells. Groups of toxoplasmas surrounded by a limiting membrane are found in host tissue (Fig. 25).

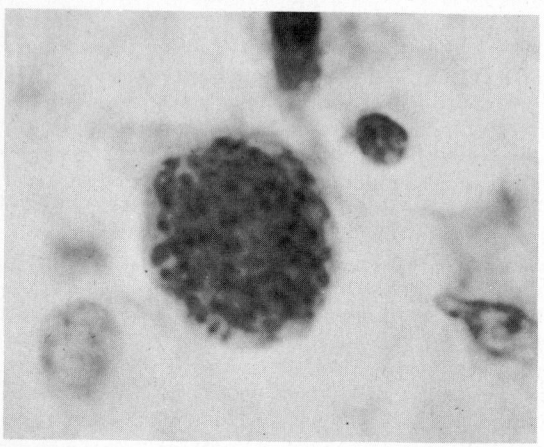

FIG. 25. Cyst containing large numbers of *Toxoplasma* in subcortical area of 9-month-old infant.

Previously it was believed that the membrane was primarily derived from the host, and therefore these structures were called pseudocysts. However, ultrastructural studies have demonstrated that this membrane is derived primarily from the parasite; thus the structure is a true cyst. *Toxoplasma* can be transmitted experimentally to numerous mammals and birds, and large numbers of naturally infected animals have been found, including dogs, rodents, chickens, pigeons, and ducks.

EPIDEMIOLOGY. Congenital or transplacental transmission of toxoplasmosis has been clearly established. Generally, transmission occurs only if the primary infection occurs during pregnancy. Evidence seems reasonably clear that the fetus is at greatest risk during the first and second trimesters. The notion that toxoplasmosis gives rise to habitual abortion is no longer regarded as valid by most workers in the field. That postnatal or acquired toxoplasmosis can be transmitted to humans by carnivorism has been established by numerous observations, most notably in France, where the eating of raw or rare meat is a tradition, and in the United States, where a group of Cornell University medical students acquired the infection following ingestion of rare hamburger.

The main difficulty in understanding the worldwide distribution of toxoplasmosis and its customary occurrence in herbivores as well as vegetarians was explained by the studies of Hutchison, who in 1965 discovered fecal transmission of *Toxoplasma* in cats. Finally, there have been recent reports of transmission of *Toxoplasma* to immunosuppressed hosts following organ transplantation or blood transfusion.

There are many surveys that show that the incidence of infection increases with age, but the rate of increase differs depending on the population and its eating habits and the locality studied. Areas in which climatic factors such as moisture and warmth favor viability of *Toxoplasma* oocysts demonstrate the highest prevalence of *Toxoplasma* antibodies. In the United States it has been shown that the yearly antibody acquisition rate is 0.5 to 1 percent; the rate for children is lower than for adults.

While circulating antibody with accessory factor will kill extracellular toxoplasmas, intracellular forms are protected. Experimental studies indicate that cell-mediated immunity has an important role in toxoplasmosis. Many varieties of antibodies have been studied in humans infected with *Toxoplasma.* The dye test antibody, which has been studied the longest appears identical to the antibody measured in the indirect fluorescent antibody (IFA) test; they appear simultaneously and persist for about the same period. Complement-fixing antibodies appear about 14 to 21 days after infection and are short-lived, persisting in man for a month to several years. The indirect hemagglutination antibody (IHA) titers generally agree with those of the IFA and dye tests. However, important differences have been described, as patients with acute toxoplasmosis have an earlier rise in the dye test and IFA titers than the IHA. Moreover, the hemagglutination antibodies tend to persist longer. It has also been reported that in congenital toxoplasmosis the IHA test may remain negative for months after birth. Therefore, it is clear that the IHA procedure cannot be substituted for the IFA or dye test in suspected cases of congenital or acquired acute toxoplasmosis.

PATHOLOGY. The pathologic lesions may be widespread, affecting many organs and tissues. In congenital disease neurologic and ocular lesions are generally more common than in acquired disease. In congenital toxoplasmosis focal disseminated areas of necrosis and miliary granulomatous inflammation are found. The periventricular and aqueductal tissue of the brain may be particularly affected. Many yellow soft areas are seen in the cortex, basal ganglia, medulla, and leptomeninges (Fig 26).

Calcification, microcephalus, and hydrocephalus are all common sequelae. *Toxoplasma* cysts may persist for years without provoking cellular reaction. Chorioretinal lesions are a result of necrosis and subsequent gliosis. The older yellow white lesions are fibrotic scars of the destroyed retina. In extraneural sites lymph node hyperplasia and focal necrosis are common. Pulmonary involvement usually consists of parasitized alveolar cells in areas of interstitial pneumonia. Proliferation of organisms in the myocardium, hepatic parenchyma,

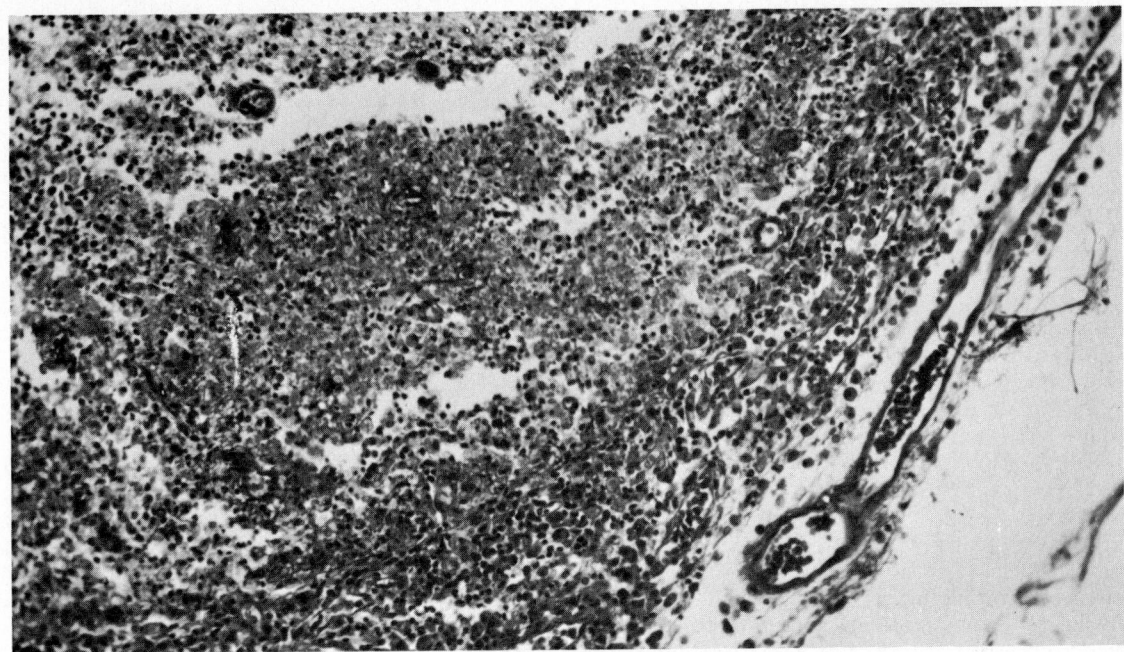

FIG. 26. Active *Toxoplasma* lesion in the brainstem of a 3-day-old infant.

spleen, and adrenals is commonly associated with focal necrosis.

SYMPTOMS. Serologic evidence strongly suggests that most human and other animal infections are inapparent and asymptomatic. Acute infection acquired immediately before or during pregnancy may cause fetal infection, and the disease may present as a severe fulminating, rapidly fatal infection. The factors that determine this spectrum are only partially known, but they are believed to be related to host immunity, virulence of the infecting strain, and size of the inoculum.

In *acute congenital toxoplasmosis* the infant may be severely jaundiced, with a maculopapular rash, thrombocytopenic purpura, and hepatosplenomegaly, Seizures, opisthotonos, and chorioretinitis also occur. Spinal fluid may contain increased protein and cells. These children usually die in the first month of life. The majority of survivors have severe mental retardation, complete or partial blindness, and psychomotor disturbances (p. 1773). *Subacute congenital disease* often is not observed until some time after birth, when intracerebral calcification, chorioretinitis, hydrocephalus (sometimes progressive), and psychomotor disturbances are found (Fig. 27).

Acquired toxoplasmosis is usually asymptomatic. Moreover, it is now clear that there are at least three main clinical types. The incubation period of these varieties is unknown. The acute acquired form is a fulminating disease with an erythematous rash, fever, malaise, myositis, dyspnea, acute myocarditis, and encephalitis. Fatal outcome is common. Fortunately this form of toxoplasmosis is extremely rare. A subacute glandular form is characterized by generalized lymphadenopathy, with or without fever. It is often mistaken for infectious

mononucleosis, and the heterophile antibody test is negative. Recovery usually occurs slowly over a period of several months. Chronic toxoplasmosis develops in those individuals who become immune. Cysts remain viable in tissues for years without stimulating an inflammatory response. However, periodically a cyst may rup-

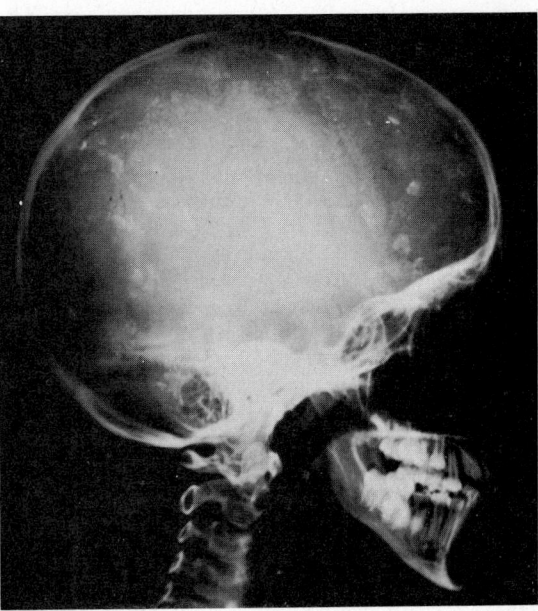

FIG. 27. Disseminated calcific deposits in the brain of a 6-year-old child with proven congenital toxoplasmosis.

ture, usually followed by a brisk inflammatory reaction and destruction of the released bradyzoites. Ocular lesions are formed in the retina with secondary involvement of the choroid. Such lesions may be small and remain inactive, or cysts may rupture and cause additional inflammatory scarring. While *Toxoplasma* retinochoroiditis is usually a self-limited disease, occasionally it may become progressive and threaten vision. As discussed earlier, when immunity is suppressed, whether by disease, drug, or radiation therapy, chronic toxoplasmosis may reactivate and acute disease may occur.

DIAGNOSIS.   It is rather unusual to isolate the organisms from the blood or spinal fluid. Therefore diagnosis usually rests on serologic evidence. The Sabin-Feldman dye test depends on the rationale that living *T. gondii* incubated with immune serum in the presence of fresh normal activator serum loses its ability to be stained with an alkaline solution of methylene blue. The test becomes positive 1 to 3 weeks after infection; the titer increases for many months, gradually declining over a period of 5 years or more. It may remain positive for life. The significance of low titers is not entirely clear. According to Feldman, while titers of 1:4 are probably significant, as well as reproducible, he usually considers titers of 1:8 or 1:16 positive in population studies. However, rising titers in serum specimens taken 2 weeks apart are indicative of recently acquired infection. Stable titers indicate only that the patient has had the infection. The IFA test, as discussed previously, is replacing the dye test, since it is easily performed and seems to be measuring the same antibody.

The complement-fixation test is used as an adjunct to the dye or IFA tests. It is useful to indicate active disease, a titer of 1:8 being significant. A toxoplasmin skin test is available, but it is of questionable aid in a single situation. The hemagglutination test appears to be an excellent test. Its limitations are discussed above. Remington has described an IgM fluorescent antibody test to aid in the diagnosis of congenital toxoplasmosis. Congenital infections in human infants have both IgG and IgM antibodies, but an uninfected child born to a mother with *Toxoplasma* antibody has only IgG. Presumably IgM does not pass an intact placenta.

Other than the relatively few severe neonatal cases, the disease is usually mild and carries a favorable prognosis. Rehabilitation of handicapped children may improve the prognosis in those in whom neurologic lesions remain. Maternal infection acquired before pregnancy has occurred does not present a risk to the fetus, provided the mother has dye test antibodies. Infection acquired during pregnancy carries a high risk to the developing fetus. However, future pregnancies usually are assumed to be without risk.

TREATMENT.   Chemotherapy is based on the experimental evidence in mice and tissue culture that pyrimethamine (Daraprim) and sulfonamides have marked synergistic activity against *Toxoplasma* organisms. Infants with active disease should be treated in the hope of arresting the process. Acquired cases should probably be treated; however, the benefit of therapy is difficult to assess since spontaneous remission is so frequent. Patients on immunosuppressive therapy having

toxoplasmosis, those with *Toxoplasma* meningitis, or those with ocular manifestations when macular damage appears likely should also receive chemotherapy.

Recommendations for infants are sulfadiazine 100 mg/kg daily in divided doses and pyrimethamine 1 mg/kg daily after a loading dose of 2 mg/kg daily for 3 days. Adults should receive sulfadiazine 3 g daily with 50 mg pyrimethamine daily for the first 3 days, then 25 mg thereafter. (Older children receive half this dose.) Treatment should continue for 4 weeks. It is important to monitor the leukocyte and platelet counts twice weekly. Folinic acid should be given during therapy in order to prevent leukopenia and thrombocytopenia. Recent studies suggest that the antibiotic spiramycin, 2 to 3 g in four divided daily doses for 3 weeks, is an effective antitoxoplasmosis agent. It is not generally available in the United States.

Several simple measures can be suggested to prevent toxoplasmosis. Eating raw or rare meats should be avoided. Infected meat or eggs can be made safe by thoroughly heating to at least 60 C. Individuals who handle raw meat should wash their hands carefully thereafter. It has been shown that smoking, curing in brine, and freezing at −40 C for 9 days will kill the bradyzoites in pork. A typical home freezer is not a certain method of killing the cysts.

Since cats are the important source of oocysts, it is important to recognize where the various sources of infection might be. As cats defecate in loose soil and sand, it is important to protect children from these sites. Cat litter should not be handled by vulnerable pregnant women without disposable gloves. Young domestic cats that are fed raw meat, which is often contaminated, may be an important source of human infection. The handling of this raw meat by pet owners has been suggested as perhaps a more important source of infection than oocysts discharged by cats. Household cats that are not permitted to roam and are fed only dry, canned, or cooked food have little opportunity to become infected. However, their feces should be discarded every day before the oocysts have had a chance to sporulate (1 to 5 days) and become infective. Cat feces should be buried or flushed down a toilet.

PNEUMOCYSTIS PNEUMONIA   In 1912 Delanoe and Delanoe described cysts from the lungs of rats infected with *Trypanosoma lewisi* and termed them *Pneumocystis carinii*. These organisms previously had been observed by Chagas in 1909 in guinea pigs infected with *T. cruzi* and by Carini in 1910 in rats also infected with *T. lewisi*. However, it was not until 1942 that human infection was described by van der Meer and Brug in two infants and an adult. The association of *Pneumocystis* with interstitial plasma cell pneumonia was first reported in premature infants by Vanek in 1951 in central Europe. Shortly thereafter it became apparent that the disease was worldwide, often occurring in institutional epidemics.

The taxonomic status of *Pneumocystis carinii* has not been resolved; ultrastructural studies fail to support those who believe this organism is a protozoan with close sporozoan affinities. It resembles no other protozoan similarly studied. Some expert protozoologists now believe *Pneumocystis* is not a protozoan, but rather a fungus. Similarly, many mycologists deny the fungal affinities of *pneumocystis.*

Although *interstitial plasma cell pneumonia* has been reported most often in premature or term infants during the first 4 months of life, sporadic cases are seen in older children and adults. Leukemia, lymphoma, hypogammaglobulinemia, and other severe debilitating diseases have often been associated with this infection. More recently, *Pneumocystis* pneumonia has been reported in a large group of patients receiving immunosuppressive therapy.

In smears of pulmonary exudate or in tissue sections, oval to round extracellular organisms that resemble cysts about 8 to 12 μ in diameter are found. These questionable cysts are intensely argyrophilic with Gomori's methenamine silver technique. Otherwise, in ordinary hematoxylin and eosin sections they are obscured by the characteristic foamy alveolar exudate (Fig. 28). Intracellular forms that may be schizonts are sometimes seen in alveolar lining cells.

The lungs postmortem are gray to pink, voluminous, firm, and airless. Alveoli are filled with a foamy eosinophilic material in which octonucleate cysts may be found. The alveolar septa are thickened and infiltrated with lymphocytes, monocytes, and sometimes plasma cells; neutrophils are notably absent. The onset of the disease may be slow and insidious. Cough, tachypnea, and cyanosis are often seen. Radiologic findings are not characteristic. In some instances marked respiratory distress does not appear until several days prior to death. In nonfatal illness the recovery may take many weeks. Infant mortality is reported to vary from 10 to 50 percent, with an average of about 40 percent. Since most cases in older children and adults have been associated with usually fatal underlying disease, prognosis is grave.

Until recently all treatment of *Pneumocystis* pneumonia had been unsuccessful; however, several antiprotozoan compounds have been reported to be of benefit in a limited number of cases. Intramuscular pentamidine isothionate and intravenous hydroxystilbamidine have given satisfactory results. The dosage of each is 4 mg/kg for 10 to 12 days. Currently, trimethoprim 20 mg/kg/day and sulfomethoxazale 100 mg/kg/day in 4 doses for 14 days are regarded the treatment of choice. Gamma globulin is also administered if there is coexisting hypogammaglobulinemia. Megaloblastic bone marrow changes should be anticipated as a serious complication of drug therapy. Pyrimethamine and sulfadiazine have been suggested to be useful in therapy. Frequent sputum examination and percutaneous or open lung biopsy have been advocated, since early diagnosis may be life-saving.

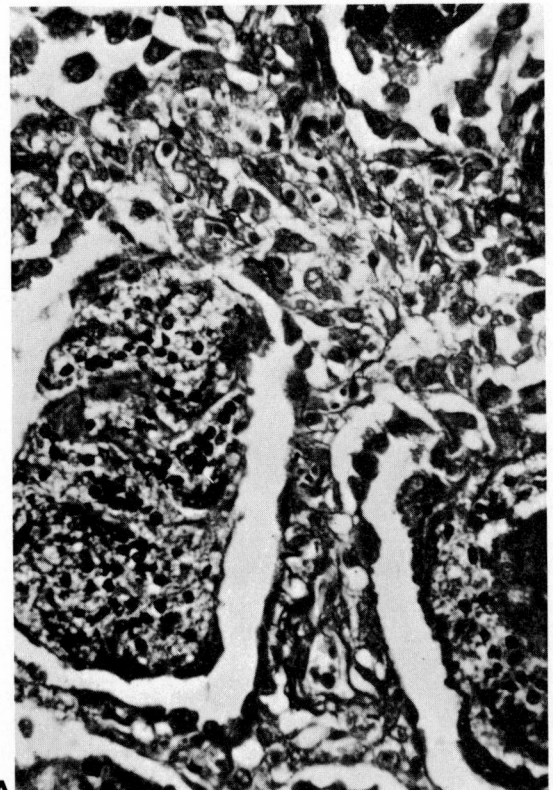 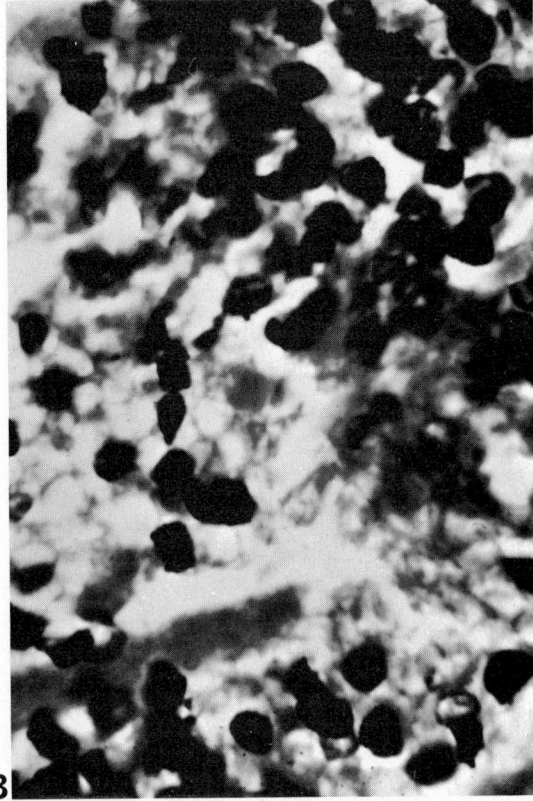

FIG. 28. *Pneumocystis carinii* pneumonia. *A.* Within the foamy alveolar exudate are small, intensely argyrophilic cysts demonstrated by the Gomori methenamine silver technique ($\times$280). *B.* Cysts of *Pneumocystis* under higher magnification from the same case as *A.* ($\times$1,260).

References

AMEBIASIS

Adi FC: Clinical features of hepatic amoebiasis (a review of 120 cases). W Afr Med J 14(NS): 181, 1965

——— Amoebiasis: WHO Tech Rep Ser No 421, 1969

Datta DV, Singh SA, Chkuttani PN: Treatment of amebic liver abscess with emetine hydrochloride, niridazole and metronidazole. A control clinical trial. Am J Trop Med Hyg 23:586, 1974

Dorrough RL: Amebic liver abscess. South Med J 60:305, 1967

Healy GR: Use of and limitations to the indirect hemagglutination test in the diagnosis of intestinal amebiasis. Health Lab Sci 5:174, 1968

——— Laboratory Diagnosis of Amebiasis. Bull NY Acad Med 47:478, 1971

Powell SJ, McLeod I, Wilmot AJ, Elsdon-Dew R: Metronidazole in amoebic dysentery and amoebic liver abscess. Lancet 2:1329, 1966

Tanowitz HB, Wittner M, Rosenbaum RM, Kress Y: In vitro studies on the differential toxicity of metronidazole in protozoa and mammalian cells. Ann Trop Med Parasit 69:19, 1975

MALARIA

Berberian DA: Recent advances in malariology. Am J Med 46:96, 1969

Brooks MH, Kiel FW, Sheehy TW, Barry KG: Acute pulmonary edema in Falciparum malaria. N Engl J Med 279:732, 1968

Bruce-Chwatt LJ: Malaria and blackwater fever. In Diseases of Children in the Subtropics and Tropics. London, Edward Arnold, 1958

Einhorn NH, Tomlinson WJ: Estivoautumnal (P. falciparum) malaria, a survey of 493 cases of infection with P. falciparum in children. Am J Dis Child 72:137, 1946

Hendricksen RG: Quartan malarial nephrotic syndrome. Lancet 1:1143, 1972

Kagan IG: Seroepidemiology and serologic diagnosis. Exp Parasit 311:-126, 1972

McGregor IA: Immunology of malarial infections and its possible consequences. Br Med Bull 28:22, 1972

Powell RD: The chemotherapy of malaria. Clin Pharmacol Ther 7:48, 1966

Resistance of Malaria parasites to Drugs. WHO Tech Rep Ser No 296, 1965

Russell PF, West LS, Manwell RD, Macdonald G: Practical Malariology, 2nd ed. London, Oxford Univ Press, 1963

Wilcox A: Manual for the Microscopical Diagnosis of Malaria in Man, 1960 ed. Washington, DC, USPHS, US Government Printing Office, 1960

GENERAL

Adler S: Immunology of leishmaniasis. Isr J Med Sci 1:9, 1965

Allibone EC, Goldie W, Marmion BP: Pneumocystis carinii pneumonia and progressive vaccinia in siblings. Arch Dis Child 39:26, 1964

Blattner R: Pneumocystis carinii infection: treatment with pentamidine isothionate. J Pediatr 67:332, 1965

Burke BA, Good RA: Pneumocystis carinii infection. Medicine 52:23, 1973

Comparative studies of American and African trypanosomiasis. WHO Tech Rep Ser No 411, 1969

Cortner JA: Giardiasis, a cause of celiac syndrome. Am J Dis Child 98:311, 1959

Desmonts G, Couvreur J: Congenital toxoplasmosis. A prospective study of 378 pregnancies. N Engl J Med 290:1110, 1974

De Vita V, Emmer T, Levine A, Jacobs B, Berard C: Pneumocystis carinii pneumonia. Successful diagnosis and treatment of two patients with associated malignant processes. N Engl J Med 280:287, 1969

Duma RJ, Ferrell HW, Nelson EC, Jones MM: Primary amebic meningo-encephalitis. N Engl J Med 281:1315, 1969

Esterly JA, Warner NE: Pneumocystis carinii pneumonia. Twelve cases in patients with neoplastic lymphoreticular disease. Arch Pathol 80:433, 1965

Feldman HA: Toxoplasmosis. N Engl J Med 279:1370, 1431, 1968

Frenkel JK, Dubey JP, Miller NL: Toxoplasma gondii: fecal forms separated from eggs of the nematode Toxocara cati. Science 164:432, 1969

——— Toxoplasma in and around us. Bioscience 23:343, 1973

Glasser L, Delta BG: Congenital toxoplasmosis with placental infection in monozygotic twins. Pediatrics 35:276, 1965

Hawking F: Recent work on Trypanosoma cruzi in Brazil and Central America. J Trop Med Hyg 67:211, 1964

Kean BH, Kimball AC, Christenson WN: An epidemic of acute toxoplasmosis. JAMA 208:1002, 1969

Mauel, Behun R: Cell-mediated and humoral immunity to protozoan infections. Transplant Rev 19:121, 1972

Moore GT, Cross WM, McGuire D, et al: Epidemic giardiasis at a ski resort. N Engl J Med 281:402, 1969

Neal RA, Garnham PCC, Cohen S: Immunization against protozoal diseases. Br Med Bull 25:194, 1969

Remington JS, Miller M, Brownlee I: IgM antibodies in acute toxoplasmosis. I. Diagnostic significance in congenital cases and method for their rapid demonstration. Pediatrics 41:1082, 1968

Ryckman RE, Ryckman AE, Folkes DL, Robb PL, Olsen LE: Epizootiology of Trypanosoma cruzi in southwestern North America. J Med Entomol 2:87, 1965

Smith E, Gaspar IA: Pentamidine treatment of Pneumocystis carinii pneumonia. Am J Med 44:626, 1968

Western K, Perera D, Schultz M: Pentamidine isethionate in the treatment of Pneumocystis carinii pneumonia. Ann Intern Med 73:695, 1970

DISEASES CAUSED BY ARTHROPODS

Arthropods (phylum Arthropoda) are of medical importance as causal agents of disease in themselves, as obligatory intermediate hosts, and as mechanical vectors of innumerable disease-producing organisms. Included among the medically important arthropods are the true insects, centipedes, scorpions, spiders, ticks, mites, and various *Crustacea*, including crabs, crayfish, and copepods. As direct agents of disease or human annoyance, arthropods may cause (1) *serious envenomization*, which may be hemolytic, hemorrhagic, neurotoxic, or vesicating; (2) *dermatitis*, which is the result of either bites or direct skin invasion; (3) *myiasis*, which is due to invasion of organs or tissues by dipterous (true fly) larvae; (4) *allergy or hypersensitivity*, which is often a result of certain insect stings or bites; (5) Entomophobia or psychoneurotic behavior in the presence of real or imaginary bugs.

Hymenopterous Disease

The sting of a bee or wasp is accompanied by the introduction of venom, which in nonsensitized individuals usually causes pain, induration, and redness that lasts several hours. The more important reactions in allergic individuals are discussed elsewhere (p. 361). The sting of the fire ant (*Solenopsis*) results in an initial flare and wheal that later vesiculates. In several days to a week the pustule ruptures, encrusts, and forms a scar. Local application of ice or other soothing lotion to the area is all that is required. The harvester ants,

Pogonomyronex, readily attack man and give a painful sting. Severe and fatal reactions in farm animals have been reported. Fortunately this is quite rare in humans.

Arachnidism

The arachnids are a large group (class Arachnida) of arthropods; they include the spiders, scorpions, mites, and ticks.

LATRODECTISM. Contrary to common belief, most spiders are harmless and shy. There are several spiders that can cause serious and sometimes fatal envenomization if they are provoked. Most notable is the bite of the female black widow spider (*Latrodectus mactans*), which often is not felt and resembles a pinprick. At the point of the bite there may be slight swelling and twin minute red spots. Immediately after the attack lymphatic absorption of the toxin begins, as the patient experiences local sharp, throbbing pain that increases in intensity for several hours, by which time vascular spread has occurred. Symptoms are most severe and usually include diaphoresis, nausea, vomiting, hypertension, and intense agonizing spasms, especially of the abdominal muscles. Spasticity of other muscle groups depends on the area of the bite. Severely affected individuals develop profound shock, delirium, and coma, with death occuring in 4 to 5 percent of these. Usually, however, the symptoms regress and the victim recovers.

The symptoms are generally more severe in children than in adults, and treatment should be initiated as soon as possible with 10 percent calcium gluconate or methocarbamol (Robaxin) as muscle relaxants. Antivenin should be given by intramuscular injection; it is usually effective within 30 minutes. If necessary it may be repeated within 1 or 2 hours. Tourniquets or other procedures suggested for snakebites are ineffective. The bite of the brown spider, *Loxosceles reclusa,* is discussed elsewhere.

SCORPIONS. The scorpion has stingers at the terminal portion of its abdomen that it uses to strike its victim swiftly and repeatedly. There are many dangerous species that accidentally sting humans, children being especially vulnerable. Most deaths are seen in children under 4 years of age. In Mexico, for example, where scorpions have been responsible for 82 percent of 24,627 deaths from poisonous animals over a 10-year period, more than 80 percent of these fatalities have occurred in children under 5 years of age and 94 percent in those under 10 years of age.

There are two types of scorpion venom: a relatively harmless local cytotoxic material and the often fatal neurotoxic venom that also has hemolytic and cytolytic properties. There is an immediate sharp pain as a result of the sting, which is often followed by numbness or drowsiness and peculiar itching sensations about the nose, mouth, and throat. There may be salivation, diaphoresis, nausea, vomiting, fever, spasm of muscles of mastication, and dyskinetic movements of the extremities. After a short while salivation decreases, objects appear dim, strong light becomes painful, and strabismus is often pronounced. Pulmonary and gastrointestinal hemorrhage may occur, and generalized convulsions appear. These increase in severity, lasting several hours or until death. Generally it is regarded as a good prognostic sign if the patient survives 3 hours.

Treatment should be initiated as soon as possible, especially in children. Specific antiscorpion serum is generally available in those areas in which these dangerous animals exist. A tourniquet should be applied above the wound and an ice pack placed on the area to delay absorption. Morphine is contraindicated. Convulsions may be controlled with large doses of phenobarbital.

MITES AND TICKS. The larvae of the North American chigger mite or red bug (*Eutrombicula alfreddugèsi*) may cause severe, almost intolerable itching followed by wheals and pustules. Children are especially sensitive. Treatment includes bathing the affected area with alcohol, and relief of itching can be obtained with topical anesthetics, such as the following mixture; 5 percent benzocaine, 2 percent methylsalicylate, 0.5 percent salicylic acid, 73 percent ethyl alcohol, and 19.5 percent water. Quotane ointment, a commercial preparation, is most useful. Diethyltoluamide is an excellent chigger repellent.

Scabies is caused by the itch mite, *Sarcoptes scabiei,* and is found in lower socioeconomic groups whose personal hygiene is often substandard. Most infestations are transmitted by personal contact in bed. The female mite enters the thin skin between the fingers, in the popliteal and antecubital fossae, and on the penis and breast. Initially the infestation is undetected, but after a month or so allergic manifestations appear as an intense vesiculopapular rash. In infants it may assume a more bullous appearance, especially on the face. The female mites may burrow several centimeters into the stratum corneum, and as a result of severe excoriation secondary pyogenic infection often complicates the disease. Treatment is usually initiated with a prolonged warm bath or soak in order to soften the skin and open the tunnels. A cream base containing 1 percent gamma benzene hexachloride (BHC) is applied over the entire body, and after 24 hours a cleansing bath is taken. This treatment kills both mites and eggs; therefore, a second application is usually unnecessary.

The bite of a tick can be extremely painful and can be associated with febrile symptoms. On occasion the feeding female tick, especially in young children, causes a progressive ascending flaccid motor and sensory paralysis. Envenomization by the engorging tick is believed responsible. Prompt recovery usually follows removal of the offending organisms; however, death by respiratory failure may occur if they are permitted to remain. Removal is best accomplished by gently pulling the tick off with the fingers. If sterile instruments are available they may be employed to apply gentle traction on the tick, after which the point of a needle or scalpel is slipped under the mouth parts. The tick will then come loose with a minimum of tissue. It is essential to inspect the tick to ensure that it has been removed intact (ie, with the mouth parts); otherwise a tick granuloma of the skin will ensue. The area should be cleansed with antiseptic. Various repellents, such as dimethyl phthalate or diethyltoluamide, are effective when impregnated in clothing.

Insect Bites

The bites of many insects (class Hexapoda) such as mosquitoes, bedbugs, fleas, and lice affect individuals differently. Some react with severe inflammatory manifestations; others seem completely oblivious. Contact with blister beetles may cause severe vesication. Many caterpillars (larvae of butterflies and moths) possess so-called urticarial hairs that cause severe dermatitis on contact with the skin. The sting of certain caterpillars is often followed by severe pain, fever, nausea, vomiting, and in young children temporary paralysis that subsides as the local lesion heals. The female chigoe flea (*Tunga penetrans*) burrows into and is almost completely enveloped by the host's skin. Usually it penetrates between the toes or on the soles of the feet, creating nodular ulcerated swellings. Frequent washing with dilute Lysol or surgical removal and antiseptic dressings are necessary to obtain satisfactory healing.

Human infestation with lice usually is limited to three organisms: the head louse (*Pediculus humanus* var. *capitis*), the body louse (*P. humanus* var. *corporis*), and the crab louse (*Phthirus pubis*). Skin lesions caused by these insects are discussed elsewhere (p. 887). Pruritus, most intense at night, usually leads to loss of sleep, irritability, and general depression. Pediculosis is transmitted by personal contact under crowded and unsanitary conditions, often in cold climates. The head louse is especially prevalent in children with long hair. It may become epidemic in dormitories or institutions. Fortunately, the crab louse is not usually encountered in the pediatric age group. Lice can be readily eliminated by showering and the topical application of 1 percent benzene hexachloride either as lotion, ointment, or shampoo. It may be necessary to repeat treatment. On occasion a resistant infestation may require 2 percent piperonyl butoxide with 0.2 percent pyrethrins or 0.03 percent cupric oleate.

Centipedes

Centipedes (class Chilopoda) are provided with powerful poisonous claws with which they attack and kill their prey. Although they are greatly feared, the bite is no more severe than the sting of a honeybee. The pain diminishes rapidly and usually requires no therapy. Remington has reported only a single death (a 7-year-old child) from the bite of a centipede.

Myiasis

The invasion of organs and tissues by fly maggots (larvae of order Diptera) is termed myiasis. When maggot infestations are caused by species that usually are scavengers or saprophagous, the condition is termed accidental myiasis. If the maggot is of a necrophagous or facultative sarcophagous species, it is called a semi-specific myiasis; infestations caused by obligatory sarcophagous species are then termed obligate myiases.

Accidental myiasis is usually the result of ingestion of fly eggs in food or water. These infestations are transitory, larvae being passed in the stool without incident. On rare occasions stubborn intestinal myiasis may result. Urinary myiasis has been reported, probably as the result of flies depositing their eggs about the external urethral orifice, especially in warm weather when people sleep without covers. The larvae presumably hatch and migrate into the urethra. Symptoms can be severe, with pain, blood, purulent discharge, dysuria, and frequency.

Various *semiobligate myiases* are caused by flesh flies (*Sarcophaga*) or blowflies (*Calliphora, Phaenicia*) when the adults oviposit in or about open wounds. Severe damage can result from these infestations, which usually afflict helpless infants or the seriously injured. Cutaneous myiasis resembling furuncles may be caused by larvae of *Wohlfahrtia*.

Obligate myiasis, caused by the primary screwworms (*Callitroga*), may cause severe, sometimes fatal, suppurative nasopharyngeal and otic infestations. These flies are attracted to open wounds or nasal secretions in which they ovipost. *Hypoderma*, the eel fly, often attacks man, with children being infested far more often than adults. The larvae actively penetrate the skin and wander for months (larva migrans), causing severe pain, cramps, and general malaise. The human botfly, *Dematobia hominis*, deposits her eggs on the bodies of other blood-sucking flies that in turn drop the eggs on the human skin. Larvae hatch and actively penetrate the skin, producing a large tumorous nodule in which they reside. After about 6 weeks they leave the host and drop to the ground; they then enter the soil, where they pupate.

Children can be protected from myiasis by proper screening or netting. Dipterous infestations should be treated promptly by debridement or curetting, followed by topical antibiotic therapy with bacitracin, polymyxin, or neomycin and sterile dressing.

References

Bettini S: Epidemiology of latrodectism. Toxicon 2:93, 1964

Buxton PA: The Louse. London, Edward Arnold, 1939

Frazier CA: Allergic reactions to insect stings: a review of 180 cases. South Med J 57:1028, 1964

Fuller HS: Medical and veterinary acarology. Ann Rev Entomol 1:347, 1956

Herms WB, James MT: Medical Entomology, 5th ed. New York, Macmillian, 1961

Horen WP: Arachnidism in the United States. JAMA 185:839, 1963

Horsfall WR: Medical Entomology: Arthropods and Human Disease. New York, Ronald Press, 1962

Jung RC, Derbes VJ, Burch AD: Skin response to solenamine, a hemolytic component of fire-ant venom. Dermatol Int 2:241, 1963

Keegan HL, Macfarlane WV (eds): Poisonous Animals and Noxious Plants of the Pacific Region. New York, Pergamon, 1963

Marinkelle CJ, Stalinke HL: Toxicological and clinical studies on Centruroides margaritatus (Vervais), a common scorpion in western Colombia. J Med Entomol 2:197, 1965

McMillan CW, Purcell WR: Hazards to health: the puss caterpillar, alias woolly slug. N Engl J Med 271:147, 1964

Miller DG: Massive anaphylaxis from bee stings. In Buckley E, Porges N (eds): Venoms. Washington, DC, Am Assoc Adv Sci Publ No 44, 1959, p 117

Mueller HL: Further experiences with severe allergic reactions to insect stings. N Engl J Med 261:374, 1959

Remington CL: The bite and habits of a giant centipede (Scolopendra subspinipes) in the Philippine Islands. Am J Trop Med Hyg 30:453, 1950

Rose I: A review of tick paralysis. J Can Med Assoc 70:175, 1954

Stalinke HL: Scorpions, rev ed. Tempe, Ariz, Poisonous Animals Research Laboratory, Arizona State Univ, 1956

Symes CB, Muirhead-Thompson RC, Busvine JR: Insect Control in Public Health. Amsterdam, Elsevier, 1962

Zinsser H: Rats, Lice, and History. Boston, Little, Brown, 1935

Zumpt F: Myiasis in Man and Animal in the Old World. A Textbook for Physicians, Veterinarians, and Zoologists. London, Butterworth, 1965

CHAPTER 14

Anomalies of Metabolism

Harold M. Nitowsky, *Associate Editor*

BIOCHEMICAL ASPECTS OF GENE ACTION

Harold M. Nitowsky

The term *inborn error of metabolism,* which was introduced by Garrod at the turn of the century, has been applied to a group of genetically determined biochemical disorders that are caused by specific congenital defects in structure or function of protein molecules. Many of the inborn metabolic errors have significant clinical and pathologic consequences that are the direct results of the biochemical disorder. However, the importance of these disease entities goes beyond their immediate relevance to clinical medicine. Studies of specific inborn metabolic errors have been instrumental in elucidating normal biochemical pathways, in establishing the structure and function of various types of macromolecules, and in illuminating genetic concepts and mechanisms. Thus, the definitions of the enzymatic defects in phenylketonuria, albinism, and alkaptonuria have provided important information about the pathways of aromatic amino acid metabolism. Similarly, studies of hemoglobin variants have provided insight into the structure and function of the normal hemoglobin molecule.

Since the primary amino acid sequence of proteins is dependent on the nucleotide sequence of the gene that codes for the polypeptide, variations in protein structure or function are the overt manifestations of gene mutation. Many mutations are easily detected by virtue of the chemical or clinical disturbance resulting from the altered protein. On the other hand, an even greater number of mutations may remain inapparent because the changes in the protein either lead to no significant functional disturbance or are lethal and therefore may never be observed.

Mutations not only affect the primary structure of the protein but also influence the rate of synthesis of a protein and hence its concentration in the cell. In microorganisms there is ample evidence for control or regulator genes that modulate the rate of synthesis of polypeptides by acting on the specific structural genes. Theoretically, mutations involving regulator gene loci may produce effects that are indistinguishable from those involving structural gene loci by controlling the quantitative expression of structural genes and their products. Such mutations might be expected to yield a wide range of effects, from complete cessation of synthesis of a specific protein to markedly exaggerated production. The change from production of fetal to adult type of hemoglobin, the induction of enzymes in response to hormones or chemical agents, and the mechanisms inherent in cellular differentiation suggest that regulator genes exist in man and other higher organisms. However, there is inadequate evidence to support the contention that any of the inborn errors of metabolism results from mutations involving regulator gene loci rather than structural gene loci. In virtually every instance where such a mechanism has been postulated to account for diminished enzyme activity, isolation and purification of the enzyme have revealed a structural alteration leading to diminished substrate affinity, altered catabolic rate, or some other change accounting for loss of activity. Even increased enzyme activity, such as that of hepatic δ-aminolevulinic acid synthetase in acute intermittent porphyria, may reflect a structural rather than a regulator gene mutation. Such structural alterations may be associated with enhanced affinity or stability of the protein and therefore greater activity.

Although Garrod stressed enzymatic defects that produce a block in an anabolic or catabolic pathway, inborn errors have been described for all types of protein. Mutations have been described that affect functions of cell membranes in the intestine, kidney, and other organs that lead to diminution in the transport of sugars, amino acids, phosphate, vitamins, cations, and water. These mutations may reflect either alteration or absence of a specific membrane carrier protein or *permease* or of an abnormality in the membrane receptor sites for hormones or other mediators. Other mutations involve serum proteins, such as albumin or the immunoglobulins. As with all the inborn errors, such abnormalities may have important clinical consequences or none at all. Thus the immunoglobulin deficiency syndromes may lead to considerable morbidity and early death, whereas variations involving serum transferrins have no obvious deleterious effects.

The majority of the inborn errors are characterized by a decrease in or an absence of activity of an intracellular enzyme. The loss of enzyme function in many of these disorders may be produced by complete cessation of enzyme synthesis or by production of a mutant protein that has lost the ability to carry out its usual function. Although it is difficult to distinguish between these possibilities, immunochemical studies have been useful as a means of differentiating between lack of synthesis and formation of an antigenically similar but functionless cross-reacting material (CRM). An example of this phenomenon in man comes from studies of recessively inherited isolated growth hormone deficiency, in which some patients demonstrate a CRM-positive material that appears to be ineffective biologically.

Other inborn errors, as exemplified by citrullinemia,

are characterized by only a partial loss of enzyme activity, reflecting a decreased affinity of the enzyme for its substrate. Similarly, in other inborn errors such as cystathioninuria the mutant enzyme binds necessary cofactors abnormally and thus shows decreased activity. In such instances enzyme activity may be restored to nearly normal levels in vivo as well as in vitro in the presence of high coenzyme concentrations.

The mutant enzyme or protein may be unstable and may show an accelerated rate of destruction in vivo. This mechanism accounts for diminished enzyme activity in some forms of G6PD deficiency. Still another mechanism of reduced enzyme activity may involve a change in subunit interaction or aggregation as a result of an alteration of one of the component polypeptide subunits.

GENETIC HETEROGENEITY

A specific clinical or biochemical phenotype may be produced by more than a single genotype. The term genetic heterogeneity is used to describe this phenomenon. Recent studies have shown that genetic heterogeneity exists for many inborn errors of metabolism. Indeed, this is not surprising in view of the findings with the many hemoglobin variants. There is a growing body of evidence that the single amino acid substitutions, deletions, duplications, and other alterations that have been described for the hemoglobin molecule also apply to other protein types, including enzymes and serum proteins. Genetic heterogeneity may result from allelic mutations (more than one mutation at a single locus) or nonallelic mutations (involving different loci). The presence of such heterogeneity may be demonstrated by genetic, clinical, and chemical investigations. Differences in the mode of inheritance per se have indicated heterogeneity in certain phenotypically similar disorders, as in the case of the Hurler and Hunter syndromes. In other instances variations in the manifestation of the defect in the heterozygote have revealed genetic heterogeneity. Such findings in studies of families with cystinuria have led to the conclusion that the disorder results from at least three different allelic mutations. In other instances, discovery of separate specific biochemical steps in a complex metabolic pathway has led to evidence of genetic heterogeneity. For example, elucidation of the separate pathways for glycogen synthesis and degradation led to the recognition of several different enzyme defects and distinguishable disorders that can result in the common end point of excessive glycogen accumulation in the liver. The identification of genetic heterogeneity has clinical as well as genetic significance. The recognition of transient elevation of blood phenylalanine in the newborn infant as an entity distinct from phenylketonuria has obvious therapeutic implications, as well as important ramifications for family planning and genetic counseling.

CONSEQUENCES OF ENZYME DEFECTS

The effect of a given genetic alteration on cellular metabolism in the inborn errors will depend on the function of the mutant protein and the severity of the defect. It is possible, however, to make certain generalizations about the consequences of these defects in terms of a hypothetical metabolic process, as shown in Figure 1.

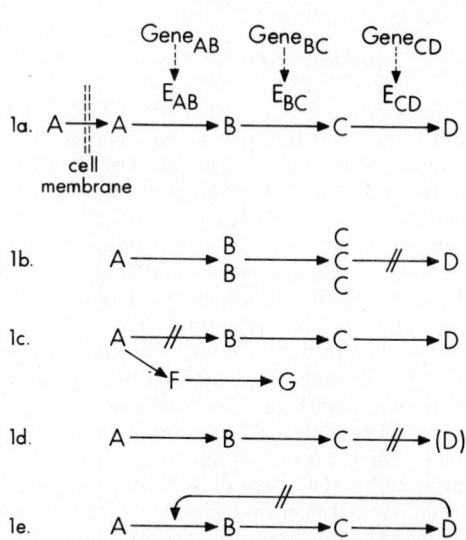

FIG. 1.   Schematic representation of biochemical sequence, where A, B, C, D = substrate and products of major pathway; F, G = products of alternate pathway; E_{AB}, E_{BC}, E_{CD} = enzymes catalyzing conversion of A to B, B to C, and C to D.

Precursor deficiency (Fig. 1a).   If the specific transport system for substance A into the cell is defective, the intracellular concentration of A may be so low that enzyme AB will not be saturated with its substrate. This could slow the entire reaction sequence and result in inadequate formation of B, C, and D. In Hartnup disease, intestinal transport of tryptophan is defective. Since tryptophan is an important precursor of intracellular nicotinamide, patients with this disorder may exhibit cerebellar ataxia, a characteristic dermatitis, and other signs of nicotinamide deficiency.

Precursor accumulation (Fig. 1b).   A defect in enzymes AB, BC, or CD might lead to intracellular accumulation of the immediate or remote precursor of the reaction. The marked increase in blood galactose levels in patients with a galactokinase deficiency is an example of such a disturbance. In homocystinuria, on the other hand, in addition to homocystine, the immediate precursor of the blocked reaction, methionine, a remote precursor, accumulates as well.

Alternate pathway utilization (Fig. 1c).   If conversion of substance A to substance B is impaired by a defect in enzyme AB, an accessory pathway to F and G may become prominent. Thus in phenylketonuria, absence of phenylalanine hydroxylase activity leads to overproduction and excretion in the urine of phenylpyruvic, phenyllactic, and phenylacetic acids, compounds that are ordinarily not detected in the blood or urine.

Product deficit (Fig. 1d).   If product D is the physiologically active product of the reaction sequence, a block at any one of the steps prior to D may result in inadequate formation of D. Thus in albinism, melanin is not formed because of a lack of tyrosinase activity.

Absence of feedback control (Fig. 1e).   The end product of the reaction sequence, D, may regulate the activity of the first enzyme in the biosynthetic pathway, enzyme AB. This phenomenon of end product or feedback inhibition has been studied intensively in microbial systems. Several inborn errors of metabolism in man are associated with abnormalities in feedback regulation, although the biochemical events involved are not well understood. Thus in the Lesch-Nyhan syndrome a defect in hypoxanthine guanine phosphoribosyl transferase results in failure to regulate de novo synthesis of uric acid and leads to marked overproduction of this end product.

Inborn errors of metabolism may have their important clinical effects in almost any body system, and many will be described in the sections of this book devoted to specific organ systems. Thus the hemoglobinopathies (p. 1148), disorders of the clotting mechanism (p. 1209), disorders of pigment metabolism (p. 756), defects of hormone synthesis (p. 1599), defects of vitamin metabolism (p. 220), defects of intestinal digestion (p. 1002), and defects of mineral metabolism (p. 237) are discussed elsewhere. The following sections are devoted to metabolic and transport disturbances involving amino acids, purines and pyrimidines, carbohydrates, lipids, porphyrins, and serum proteins.

References

Bondy PK, Rosenberg LE (eds): Duncan's Diseases of Metabolism, 7th ed. Philadelphia, WB Saunders 1974

Harris H: The Principles of Human Biochemical Genetics, 2nd ed. Amsterdam, North Holland, 1975

Stanbury JB, Wyngaarden JB, Frederickson DS (eds): The Metabolic Basis of Inherited Disease, 3rd ed. New York, McGraw-Hill, 1971

Amino Acids, Purines, and Pyrimidines

Disorders of metabolism of purines and amino acids are among the classic inborn errors of metabolism. Gout has been known since Hippocrates, and it was with the study of disorders of amino acid metabolism that Garrod introduced the inborn errors of metabolism to the world and opened up the field of human biochemical genetics. This area of genetic disease has also continued to produce new or previously unrecognized diseases. Rates of discovery show no signs of slackening.

DISORDERS OF AMINO ACID METABOLISM

William L. Nyhan

The diseases of amino acid metabolism present with a wide variety of clinical manifestations. Some of this variety is indicated in Table 1, in which the disorders of amino acid metabolism and some of their major manifestations have been summarized. Many of these abnormalities interfere with the development of the central nervous system and thus lead to mental retardation. On the other hand, some are associated with no abnormality of intelligence, which suggests that other inborn errors of metabolism may occur in populations of children with normal mentality who have never been screened. Another population in which metabolic disease should be sought is that group of infants who are very ill in the newborn period. Increasing numbers of metabolic disorders are now known to produce severe illness and death very early in life. Obviously such infants may die undiagnosed, with their disease remaining undiscovered. A listing of some of these diseases is given in Table 2. Diagnosis and early management are especially important, as these diseases that present with overwhelming illness early in life do not necessarily lead

to mental retardation. Exchange transfusion or dialysis may be life-saving at the time of initial diagnosis early in infancy. The most common of the inborn errors of amino acid metabolism is phenylketonuria. All of the others appear to be relatively rare.

PHENYLKETONURIA

Phenylketonuria is a genetically determined disorder of metabolism in which phenylalanine cannot be converted to tyrosine (Fig. 2) and phenylpyruvic acid is excreted in the urine. Since the advent of programs in which entire populations of newborn infants are screened for the presence of phenylalanine in the blood in concentrations higher than 6 mg/dl, it has become evident that there are varieties of phenylalaninemias, or hyperphenylalaninemias, in addition to what has come to be known as classic phenylketonuria.

CLINICAL FINDINGS.   In classic phenylketonuria the most important clinical characteristic is mental retardation. Most untreated patients have severe degrees of mental retardation, with intelligence quotients under 30. However, a few untreated phenylketonuric individuals with borderline intelligence have been observed. Phenylketonuric infants appear normal at birth, but early symptoms occur in over one-half of them. Vomiting has been severe enough to lead to surgery for pyloric stenosis. Irritability, an eczematoid rash, or a peculiar odor may also be present in the early months. The characteristic smell of phenylketonuric patients has been described as mousey, wolflike, musty, or barny and has been correlated with the excretion of phenylacetic acid in the urine. General physical development is usually normal, and these are often good-looking children. They are fair-haired, fair-skinned, and blue-eyed in over 90 percent of cases, but dark skin, hair, or

TABLE 1. Inborn Errors of Amino Acid Metabolism

Disorder	Enzyme Defect*	Manifestations
Phenylketonuria	Phenylalanine hydroxylase	Blond hair, blue eyes, eczema, $FeCl_3$, mental retardation
Tyrosinosis (Medes)		Urinary reducing substance
Tyrosinosis	p-Hydroxyphenylpyruvic acid oxidase	Hepatic cirrhosis, renal Fanconi syndrome
Alkaptonuria	Homogentisic acid oxidase	Dark urine, reducing substance, ochronosis, arthritis
Albinism	Tyrosinase (melanocyte granules)	Lack of pigment (local or universal), skin, hair, and eyes
Histidinemia	Histidase	Speech retardation, $FeCl_3$, may have mental retardation
Isovaleric-acidemia		Mental retardation, odor, convulsions, coma, death[†]
Maple syrup urine disease	Branched-chain keto acid decarboxylase	Urinary odor, coma, flaccidity, opisthotonos
Hypervalinemia	Valine transaminase	Mental retardation, death[†]
Propionic-acidemia	Propionyl CoA carboxylase	Recurrent vomiting and ketosis, thrombocytopenia, neutropenia, osteoporosis, mental retardation, death[†]
α-Methyl-β-hydroxy butyric-aciduria	α-Methylacetoacetyl CoA thiolase	Intermittent acidosis, ketosis, hyperglycinemia syndrome, mental retardation
β-Methylcrotonyl glycinuria	β-Methylcrotonyl CoA carboxylase	Failure to thrive, dermatitis, ketosis, acidosis, death[†]
Methylmalonic-acidemia	Methylmalonyl CoA isomerase	As in propionic-acidemia
Nonketotic hyperglycinemia		Convulsions, cerebral palsy, mental retardation, death[†]
Oxalosis	Glyoxylate carboligase	Renal calculi, renal failure
Hyperprolinemia	Proline oxidase, Δ'-pyrroline-5-carboxylic acid dehydrogenase.	Nephropathy, deafness, mental retardation
Hydroxyprolinemia	Hydroxyproline oxidase	Small kidneys, hematuria, mental retardation
Pyroglutamic-acidemia		Chronic acidosis, ataxia, mental retardation
Argininosuccinic-aciduria	Argininosuccinase	Trichorrhexis nodosa, seizures, mental retardation
Citrullinemia	Argininosuccinate synthetase	Mental retardation, death[†]
Hyperammonemia	Carbamyl phosphate synthetase, ornithine transcarbamylase	Episodic coma, mental retardation
Hyperlysinemia	Lysine α-ketoglutarate reductase	Convulsions, hypotonia, growth retardation
Cystathioninuria	Cystathionase	Mental retardation; may be normal
Homocystinuria	Cystathionine synthase	Ectopia lentis, thromboembolism, failure to thrive, mental retardation
Sarcosinemia		Mental retardation, vomiting, failure to thrive

*In each instance it is recognized that there may be heterogeneity in which multiple forms of a defective enzyme may lead to different phenotypic manifestations. For instance, in the decarboxylation of the branched-chain keto acids a complete deficiency leads to classic maple syrup urine disease; a different level of defect leads to a milder disease known as branched-chain keto-aciduria. In this table only one form has been listed.
† The disorders designated as causing death are those in which a rapid fulminating course often complicates early infancy.

TABLE 2. Inborn Errors of Metabolism That May Lead to Overwhelming Illness or Death in Early Infancy

Disorder	Procedures for Screening or Otherwise Suspecting the Disease*
Citrullinemia	Blood ammonia; urine amino acids; urine orotic acid
Isovaleric-acidemia	Smell; thin-layer chromatography for isovaleryl glycine
Ketotic hyperglycinemia	Ketonuria; serum or urine glycine; serum propionic acid; urine methylcitrate
Maple syrup urine disease	Smell; paper chromatography of branched-chain amino acids; 2,4-dinitrophenylhydrazine test
Methylmalonic-acidemia	Ketonuria; methylmalonic acid in urine or blood; methylcitrate in urine
Propionic-acidemia	Serum or urine glycine

All of these procedures should be followed where there are positive results by definitive quantitative assays.

irrides do not exclude the diagnosis. Eczematoid dermatitis occurs in about one-fourth of the patients. Widely spaced incisor teeth, pes planus, partial syndactyly, epicanthus, and microcephaly are less common manifestations.

Neurologic findings are not prominent. One-third of the patients have none, while minimal signs, such as hyperactivity of the deep tendon reflexes or mildly hypertonic muscles, occur in another one-third. More severely involved patients may have full-blown manifestations of spastic cerebral palsy. Purposeless hand posturing, rhythmic rocking, and tremors of the hands may occur. Hyperkinetic activity, uncontrollable temper, and other behavior problems are common. Seizures occur in about one-fourth of the patients, predominantly in those most severely retarded; electroencephalographic abnormalities have been described in approximately 80 percent. The pneumoencephalogram may reveal cortical atrophy.

Autopsy reports are scarce, but lack of myelinization in the central nervous system resembling Schilder's leukodystrophy may be seen if histologic studies are carried out in childhood. The absence of these findings

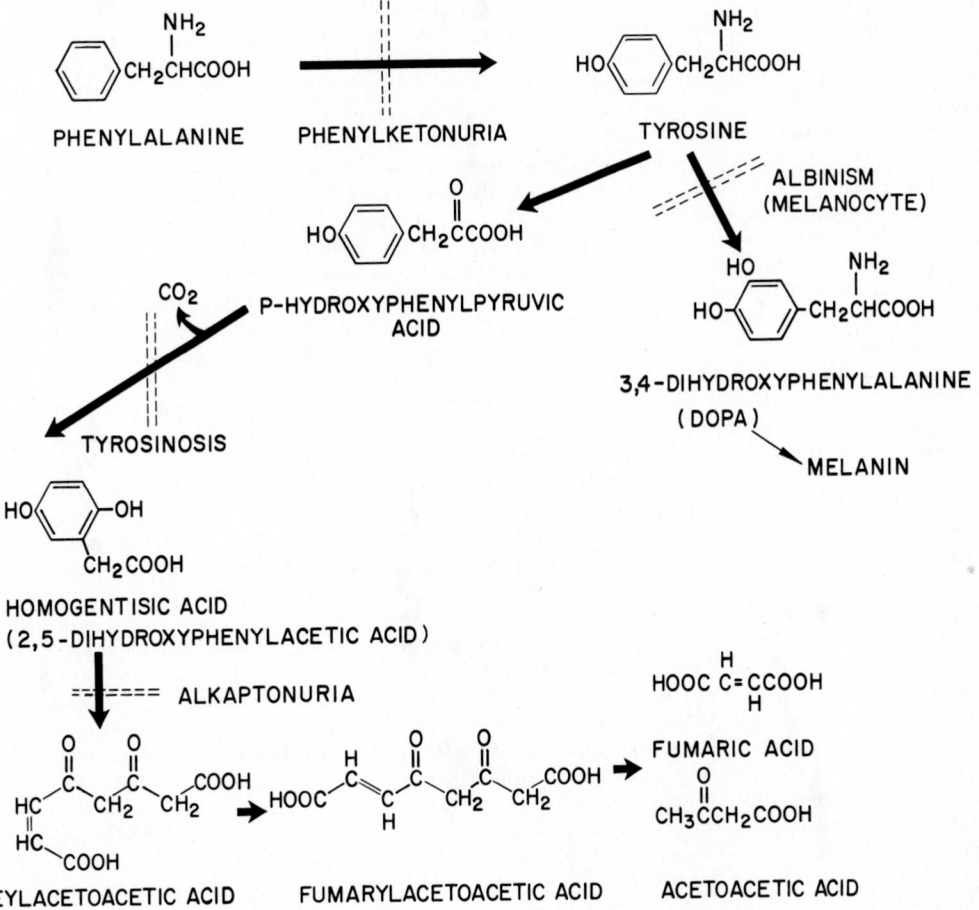

FIG. 2. Metabolism of phenylalanine and tyrosine. Sites of metabolic blocks in alkaptonuria, albinism, phenylketonuria, and tyrosinosis are indicated.

in patients studied after 21 years of age suggests that the formation of myelin is delayed or inhibited by the chemical abnormality, which is consistent with the idea that the manifestations of phenylketonuria are those of an intoxication. This concept is strengthened by the documentation of severe mental retardation resulting from intrauterine development in a phenylketonuric mother. The children with this intrauterine syndrome are, of course, heterozygotes, but the degree of retardation observed has been greater than that of the homozygotic mother

BIOCHEMICAL FINDINGS. Phenylalanine (Fig. 2) is normally converted to tyrosine in the first step of its oxidative metabolism. The tyrosine formed is then oxidized, ultimately forming acetoacetate and fumarate, which are readily converted to carbon dioxide and water. The fundamental defect in phenylketonuria is the absence of phenylalanine hydroxylase. This enzyme is composed of two distinct protein fractions, a labile fraction found only in liver and a stable fraction that is widely distributed in mammalian tissues. It is the labile fraction that is lacking in phenylketonuria.

In the presence of a block in phenylalanine hydroxylase, tyrosine becomes an essential amino acid, and alternate pathways are used to metabolize phenylalanine. Phenylalanine is converted by transamination to phenylpyruvic acid and is further reduced to phenyllactic acid or decarboxylated to phenylacetic acid, which may be conjugated to form phenylacetyl glutamine. Conversion to o-hydroxyphenylacetic acid probably follows the formation of o-tyrosine. In phenylketonuria, phenylalanine and these metabolic products accumulate in body fluids. These compounds are not abnormal metabolites, but normal metabolites in abnormal amounts. Plasma phenylalanine concentrations range from 6 to 80 mg/dl in patients with phenylketonuria, in contrast to values approximating 1 mg/dl in controls. Most patients with classic phenylketonuria have concentrations well over 30 mg/dl throughout infancy. There is a roughly linear relationship between levels of phenylalanine in the blood and urinary excretion of phenylpyruvic acid.

There are a number of secondary effects of the accumulation of phenylalanine and its metabolites. Decreased pigmentation has been related to the inhibition of tyrosinase by phenylalanine. Decreased levels of 5-hydroxytryptamine (serotonin) in phenylketonuric patients appear to follow the inhibition of 5-hydroxytrytophan decarboxylase by phenylpyruvic, phenyllactic, and phenylacetic acids. Similarly, there are decreased amounts of epinephrine, norepinephrine, and dopamine, presumably due to an inhibition of dopamine decarboxylase. The metabolites that accumulate in phenylketonuria also inhibit glutamic acid decarboxylase in brain and would thus be expected to inhibit the formation of γ-aminobutyric acid.

GENETICS. Phenylketonuria occurs in 1 of every 10,000 to 20,000 persons. It is equally represented in the two sexes. It is transmitted as an autosomal recessive characteristic. Many heterozygotes may be recognized by the measurement of plasma concentrations of phenylalanine and tyrosine after oral loading with phenylalanine, but there is overlap with the normal population, and a normal phenylalanine tolerance curve does not exclude heterozygosity.

THERAPY. Successful prevention of the clinical manifestations of the disease by restriction of dietary intake of phenylalanine has provided strong support for the concept that the clinical disease is an intoxication produced by the abnormal chemical milieu in which these patients must live and develop. Preparations such as Lofenalac make long-term treatment economically feasible and palatable. Dietary therapy readily lowers levels of phenylalanine in the blood; concomitantly, phenylpyruvic acid and its metabolic products disappear. Blood levels of serotonin rise. Clinical improvement in neurologic findings, in behavior, and in electroencephalograms is observed. Eczematoid lesions heal, and increase in pigmentation occurs. Patients tolerate the diet well. However, restriction of phenylalanine can be too great; under these circumstances tissue breakdown occurs and levels of phenylalanine increase. Hypoglycemic convulsions have been observed, with at least one fatality. These complications should not occur with careful observation of patients receiving the diets and regular determination of levels of phenylalanine in the plasma. At the same time it should be pointed out that the management of infant on a low-phenylalanine diet is not easy. It should certainly never be undertaken in a baby who does not have phenylketonuria. Furthermore, phenylketonuric infants often vomit or refuse feedings. Infections may complicate the metabolic state. Management should probably be under the direction of someone with experience with these problems and laboratory facilities for routine accurate determination of the serum phenylalanine concentrations. It has not always been recognized that all infants, including those with phenylketonuria, require a certain amount of phenylalanine. These minimal essential quantities are known and should be employed in management.

The major criterion of whether dietary therapy is worth undertaking is its effect on mental capacity. The fine points on this subject are now under cooperative study in the United States. In general, the diet is effective in preventing mental deficiency as well as neurologic abnormalities if it is started in the first weeks of life. Treatment of patients for the first time after the age of 3 years is without effect on mental development. Therapy may sometimes be of use in the clinical management of older patients because of beneficial effects on eczema, seizures, or uncontrollable behavior, even in the absence of effects on intelligence; but the major indication for treatment is preventive therapy for infants. A loss of 5 I.Q. units for each 10 weeks that treatment is delayed has been calculated. This figure is only approximate, but it provides a strong argument for early diagnosis and early institution of dietary therapy.

DIAGNOSIS AND SCREENING. It has now become routine in the United States and most of the developed countries of the world to test all newborn infants for phenylketonuria as early as possible. Urine tests are of limited value for this purpose, for phenylpyruvic acid is not detected until plasma phenylalanine levels exceed 15 to 20 mg/dl and may be absent from the urine of phenylketonuric patients for 1 to 2 months. Current screening procedures employ an assay for the concentration of phenylalanine in a drop of blood spotted on a piece of filter paper. The most common is an inhibition assay that depends on the competitive inhibition of *Bacillus subtilis* by the phenylalanine analogue β-2-thienylalanine. If a blood sample contains more than a certain concentration of phenylalanine, inhibition is overcome and the organism grows. Accumulating experience indicates it to be an effective method of detecting individuals with levels of phenylalanine over 6 mg/dl, at which level the test is considered positive. There are variations in the rate at which levels of phenylalanine rise in phenylketonuric babies, particularly if there are inadequacies in early protein intake. Since infants leave newborn nurseries very early, screening programs should make provisions for additional determinations in the first weeks of life if all hyperphenylalaninemic infants are to be detected. Once the physician is confronted with a positive screening test, he must then make a diagnosis, and this may not be easy.

It is not yet always possible to distinguish reliably and early among all the types of hyperphenylalaninemia. Furthermore, this may never be possible in day-to-day clinical practice in a disease in which the enzyme and its defect are restricted to the liver, preventing ready assessment of the primary molecular expression of the abnormal gene. Nevertheless, it has been determined how to sort out those infants who do or do not require dietary treatment.

The first step in diagnosis is quantitative analysis of the concentrations of phenylalanine and tyrosine in the blood. Most infants turned up in the screening programs simply have delayed maturation of amino-acid-metabolizing enzymes, and their tyrosine concentrations are very high. These infants can then be excluded and followed expectantly. The patient with classic phenylketonuria generally has a very rapid rise in serum concentration of phenylalanine on a normal diet, to levels well over 30 mg/dl, and the concentration of tyrosine is low. Regardless of concentration, we prefer to hospitalize infants with elevations of serum phenylalanine without tyrosine in order to study their serum phenylalanine while they are receiving a known daily intake of this amino acid and to examine fresh urine for the excretion of the metabolites phenylpyruvic acid and o-hydroxyphenylacetic acid. We initiate dietary therapy in patients who excrete these metabolites and who have high concentrations of phenylalanine in the blood.

When the babies are 3 to 4 months old we readmit them to the hospital and challenge with a 3-day phenylalanine load. A diet consisting of 24 ounces of evaporated milk diluted 1:1 with water provides a phenylalanine load of 180 mg/kg for the average baby at this age. On this amount of dietary phenylalanine an infant with classic phenylketonuria will experience a steady rise in serum concentration to a level over 30 mg/dl. Metabolites will appear in the urine. Challenge

of an older infant can be carried out using phenylalanine (180 mg/kg) added directly to the usual diet. These methods reliably distinguish patients with hyperphenylalaninemia who do not need treatment from patients with phenylketonuria who do.

TYROSINOSIS

Tyrosinemias are much more common than phenylalaninemias. In addition to the tyrosinemias that result from delayed maturation of tyrosine-metabolizing enzymes and are particularly common in premature infants, tyrosinemia occurs in scurvy and many forms of liver disease. Three disorders are included under the term tyrosinosis.

In the form first described, tyrosinosis is an extremely rare metabolic disorder characterized by excretion of *p*-hydroxyphenylpyruvic acid in the urine. There are probably no clinical manifestations of this metabolic abnormality, although the patient initially described had myasthenia gravis. These patients have a reducing reaction to the urine that is due to excretion of *p*-hydroxyphenylpyruvic acid. Patients with liver disease excrete abnormal quantities of this keto acid, but levels found in tyrosinosis have been nearly 10 times the highest values observed in liver disease. The metabolic abnormality of tyrosinosis could result from a deficiency of *p*-hydroxyphenylpyruvic acid oxidase (Fig. 2). Exogenously administered homogentisic acid is metabolized normally. The oxidation of *p*-hydroxyphenylpyruvic acid to homogentisic acid requires ascorbic acid. The increased excretion of tyrosine and *p*-hydroxyphenylpyruvate that occurs in scurvy and in prematurity can be reversed by administration of vitamin C.

A much more common form of tyrosinosis is manifested by abnormalities in hepatic and renal function. Symptoms may begin early in infancy with an acute rapid course to demise, or they may progress more chronically. Although the disease has been described in two forms, acute and chronic, both have occurred in the same family, indicating that a single disease is involved. Most patients have presented with failure to thrive and have been found to have hepatosplenomegaly. The livers of these patients are cirrhotic, and icterus, ascites, and hemorrhage often ensue. They also develop a renal tubular acidosis of the Fanconi type, with glycosuria, hyperphosphaturia, and generalized amino-aciduria. Associated with systemic acidosis, hypophosphatemia, and typical radiographic changes is clinical rickets. Mental retardation has not been observed with regularity. A few patients have been found to have hepatomas at autopsy.

Biochemical alterations include elevated concentrations of tyrosine in plasma, usually in the range of 3 to 12 mg/dl, and the excretion of tyrosyl compounds in the urine. Of these compounds, *p*-hydroxyphenyllactic acid is the most prominent, and *p*-hydroxyphenylpyruvic acid and *p*-hydroxyphenylacetic acid are also formed in appreciable quantities. Methionine concentrations in the plasma are also usually elevated. Hypoglycemia may occur with liver failure. Coagulation defects are common. Study of the enzymes of liver obtained at biopsy have indicated a deficiency of *p*-hydroxyphenylpyruvic acid oxidase, but it has not been established that this is the primary expression of the abnormal gene.

Genetic transmission appears to be autosomal recessive. A particularly high frequency (0.67/1,000 births) has been observed in a French Canadian isolate. Frequency data are not available for other populations.

Treatment has been undertaken with diets low in both phenylalanine and tyrosine. Some patients have responded quite favorably in both clinical and chemical features of the disease. Others have not.

Another form of tyrosinemia has been described in which the activity of tyrosine aminotransferase is deficient in the soluble cytoplasm of the liver. None of the patients with this disorder has had any evidence of hepatic or renal damage. One patient described in detail had multiple congenital anomalies and severe mental retardation and exhibited self-mutilative behavior. He had corneal ulcers early in life and erythematous papular lesions on the palms and soles. Plasma concentrations of tyrosine ranged from 20 to 60 mg/dl. A number of metabolites, including *p*-hydroxyphenylpyruvic acid, *p*-hydroxyphenyllactic acid, *p*-hydroxyphenylacetic acid, and *N*-acetyl tyrosine, were present in large amounts in the urine.

Five other patients have been reported. All of them have had marked retardation of mental development. A number have had corneal ulcers and lesions on the palms and soles that were either erythematous or keratotic.

Tyrosine aminotransferase is found in the mitochondria and in the cytoplasm. The mitochondrial enzyme is normal in these patients. Only the cytoplasmic enzyme is deficient.

ALKAPTONURIA

Alkaptonuria results from a defect in the enzyme homogentisic acid oxidase. It is characterized by a dark color of the urine. In this disorder fresh urine appears normal, but on standing and particularly after alkalinization, oxidation of homogentisic acid proceeds, and a dark brown or black pigment appears in the urine. This should permit the condition to be recognized very early in life, but the diagnosis is usually first made in adult life during routine urinalysis or during investigation of arthritis. The urine also gives a positive test for reducing substance and a positive ferric chloride test. Testing for glucose with glucose oxidase sticks is negative. Alkaptonuria may be demonstrated by exposing undeveloped photographic film, which is immediately blackened by the urine.

Persons with this condition are usually asymptomatic in childhood. After the third decade, deposition of brownish or bluish pigment is seen, particularly in the ears and sclerae. The deposition of pigment, which may be extensive in fibrous tissues, is referred to as ochronosis. Ochronotic arthritis occurs later. Symptoms may resemble those of rheumatoid arthritis or osteoarthritis. Some degree of limitation of motion is usually seen, and complete ankylosis is common. Degeneration in the intervertebral disks may be striking. The condition is inherited as a mendelian recessive characteristic.

Homogentisic acid is a colorless compound that is readily transformed on standing to a black pigment. Although homogentisic acid is excreted in large quantities in the urine, levels of the compound in blood are not detectable. Normal individuals given homogentisic acid metabolize it completely, but alkaptonuric persons excrete it nearly quantitatively. This disorder is a classic model for the so-called no-threshold metabolic disorders, in which, in spite of a metabolic block due to an absence of an enzyme, accumulation of metabolic intermediates behind the block is observable only on analysis of the urine.

The suggestion by Garrod that the disorder results from absence in the liver of the enzyme that catalyzes the oxidation of homogentisic acid (Fig. 2) marked the birth of the one-gene-one-enzyme hypothesis and was a watershed in biochemical genetics. This concept was confirmed by La Du and associates, who found the enzyme catalyzing the conversion of homogentisic acid to maleylacetoacetate to be absent in biopsied liver from an alkaptonuric patient.

ALBINISM

Albinism is an inherited metabolic defect confined to the pigment cell, the melanocyte, in which this cell cannot form melanin. Albinism occurs in fish, birds, and mammals and in all races of man. Universal albinism, in which melanin is absent from the pigment cells of the skin, hair, and retina, is readily recognized. A variety of localized forms occur in which the defect may be confined to an area of skin, to the eyes, or to a white forelock of hair. The skin in universal albinism is milk white; the hair is white or yellow and in Caucasians is very fine. The iris is generally blue. The pupil is red in children, but it usually becomes black in adulthood. Photophobia is characteristic, as is horizontal nystagmus. Visual acuity is nearly always decreased. The skin is sensitive to light, and these patients have a propensity to develop skin cancers.

Universal albinism is inherited as a mendelian recessive characteristic, although more than one gene produces the disorder. Normally pigmented children have occurred in a family in which both parents were albinos. Localized forms of albinism may be inherited as dominant, recessive, or (as in the case of ocular albinism) sex-linked characteristics. A few patients have been reported in which universal albinism has been associated with prolonged bleeding time and peculiar pigmented reticuloendothelial cells in the marrow, lymph nodes, and liver.

The relationship of the formation of melanin to the metabolism of phenylalanine and tyrosine is indicated in Figure 2. Melanin is a polymer that exists in nature with a high molecular weight. It is a brown or black insoluble material contained in the melanin granules of the melanocytes, where the entire transformation from tyrosine takes place. These granules can be demonstrated with the electron microscope and have been shown to be present, but without melanin, in albinism. The enzyme tyrosinase is a copper-containing oxidase that catalyzes the first two steps in the conversion of tyrosine to melanin. The first step (conversion of tyrosine to 3,4-dihydroxyphenylalanine) is the limiting step, for the second step and most of the rest of melanogenesis may occur nonenzymatically. Tyrosinase has been demonstrated in tissues radioautographically by a method in which ^{14}C-labeled tyrosine is converted to melanin and has been shown to be absent in the usual form of albinism.

Tyrosinase can be demonstrated by incubating hair roots with tyrosine. It is now clear that there are tyrosinase-positive as well as tyrosinase-negative forms of universal albinism. The tyrosinase-positive patients have creamy rather than milk white skin; the hair may be yellow, and it tends to darken with age. These patients have severe visual defects, but less so than tyrosinase-negative albinos, most of whom are ultimately legally blind.

HISTIDINEMIA

Histidinemia is a disorder of intermediary metabolism in which large amounts of histidine are found in blood and urine. The condition must be included in the differential diagnosis of phenylketonuria, for the urine is positive when examined with ferric chloride. The condition may occur without clinical manifestations, but more than half of these patients have speech retardation. Mental retardation and growth retardation have also been observed in individual patients. Relatively fair hair and blue eyes have been common.

Histidine is normally converted by histidase to urocanic acid, which is further metabolized to formiminoglutamic acid and ultimately to glutamic acid. In histidinemia elevated concentrations of histidine have been demonstrated in the plasma, urine, and cerebrospinal fluid. Imidazolepyruvic, imidazolelactic, and imidazoleacetic acids are excreted in the urine, and imidazolepyruvic acid is responsible for the positive ferric chloride test. Many patients also have elevations of alanine in the plasma.

Deficiency of histidase has been demonstrated by direct assay of the enzyme in skin. When histidine cannot be converted to urocanic acid, it is converted to imidazolepyruvic acid and its derivatives, much as phenylalanine is metabolized in phenylketonuria.

MAPLE SYRUP URINE DISEASE

In maple syrup urine disease (branched-chain ketoaciduria) the major cerebral symptoms appear very rapidly in the newborn period, and there is an odor of the urine reminiscent of maple syrup. The branched-chain amino acids leucine, isoleucine, and valine are present in high concentration in the blood and urine, and the keto acid analogues are found in the urine.

CLINICAL FINDINGS. Infants with maple syrup urine disease appear well at birth. In the typical case symptoms begin at 3 to 5 days after birth and progress rapidly to death within 2 to 4 weeks. Early manifestations of the disease may be feeding difficulty, irregular respirations, or progressive loss of the Moro reflex. Characteristically these patients develop convulsions, opisthotonos, and generalized muscular rigidity with or without intermittent flaccidity. In most patients death has occurred early in infancy following the development of decerebrate rigidity. Severe hypoglycemia has occasionally been observed. Slight cortical atrophy has been seen on pneumoencephalography. In patients surviving past the first year, defective myelinization similar to that of phenylketonuria has been reported.

A few patients have been described in whom milder forms of the disease have occurred with characteristic biochemical abnormalities. The condition in these patients is known as intermittent branched-chain aminoaciduria and appears to represent a distinct alteration at the same locus as that of classic maple syrup urine disease. Ataxia and repeated episodes of lethargy progressing to coma have been seen without mental retardation. These episodes have been induced by infection and by surgery with anesthesia, and they have responded to removal of milk from the diet and substitution of parenteral fluid therapy.

A disorder of branched-chain keto acid decarboxylation has been described by Scriver and associates in which abnormal accumulation of amino acids in blood is completely reversed by administration of thiamine. The patient described was retarded and had an abnormal electroencephalogram, but had not had any of the life-threatening crises typical of maple syrup urine disease. The therapeutic dose of thiamine hydrochloride was 10 mg/day.

The feature that permits any form of branched-chain keto-aciduria to be distinguished from other cerebral degenerative diseases of infancy is the characteristic maple-syrup odor of the urine, skin, or hair. It may smell to some like caramel, and it has been likened to the smell of an oast house. The odor may become evident after 1 or 2 days of life and may persist thereafter, but considerable variation in intensity has been observed, and in some specimens the odor cannot be detected. Freezing the urine intensifies the odor in an oil at the top of the specimen. Keto acids may be recognized in the urine by the yellow precipitate that forms on the addition of 2,4-dinitrophenylhydrazine. These diseases all appear to be transmitted as autosomal recessives.

BIOCHEMICAL ABNORMALITIES. Maple syrup urine disease is caused by an abnormality in metabolism of branched-chain amino acids. Increased quantities of leucine, isoleucine, and valine are found in the plasma and urine.

The catabolism of leucine and the other branched-chain amino acids is initiated by deamination to the keto acids, α-ketoisocaproic acid, and the corresponding derivatives of isoleucine and valine. This is followed by decarboxylation to coenzyme A (CoA) derivatives, in similar fashion to the decarboxylation of α-ketoglutarate to succinyl CoA.

The presence of the keto acid derivatives of leucine, isoleucine, and valine in the urine and the absence of the decarboxylation products suggest that the block is in the oxidative decarboxylation of the keto acids. This can be demonstrated in leukocytes or in fibroblasts in culture. Patients with the classic disease are unable to convert ^{14}C-labeled leucine to [14]CO_2, a conversion that is readily made in control infants. The oxidation of α-ketoisocaproic acid to CO_2 is similarly deficient. In patients with intermittent branched-chain keto-aciduria there is a partial defect in this decarboxylation process. In thiamine-responsive patients, treatment with thiamine permits oxidative decarboxylation of leucine at a rate 40 percent of normal.

THERAPY. Success in the dietary therapy of phenylketonuria provided a model for the treatment of other metabolic disorders. Furthermore, the metabolites that accumulate in branched-chain keto-aciduria have been shown to inhibit the formation of γ-aminobutyric acid in vitro. Experience has now been accumulated in maple syrup urine disease with prolonged use of a synthetic diet made up of individual amino acids in which the intakes of leucine, isoleucine, and valine are closely controlled. Concentrations of the branched-chain amino acids in plasma can in this way be maintained within normal limits. As one might imagine, therapy is very difficult and may require prolonged hospitalization; most patients will have had permanent brain damage before treatment is started. Experience with siblings of previous patients, in whom very early diagnosis is possible, and with at least 1 patient detected by a neonatal screening program indicates that a normal I.Q. may be achieved.

HYPERVALINEMIA

Hypervalinemia has thus far been observed in a single patient in Japan. The patient was retarded both mentally and physically, and he was hyperkinetic. Vomiting and difficulty with feeding were prominent findings early in infancy. He was treated for a time with a diet low in valine. There was concomitant lowering of the concentration of valine in plasma improvement in weight gain, and reduction of vomiting and hyperactivity.

The plasma concentration of valine was as high as 10 mg/dl, and there was increased excretion in the urine. A defect has been documented in the leukocyte in the transamination of valine.

PROPIONIC-ACIDEMIA

Propionic-acidemia (ketotic hyperglycinemia syndrome) is a disorder of branched-chain amino acid metabolism in which elevated concentrations of propionate are found in body fluids. These patients also have elevated concentrations of glycine. A number of disorders of amino acid metabolism present with abnormal concentrations of glycine in the blood, urine, and cerebrospinal fluid. These include nonketotic hyperglycinemia, propionic-acidemia, and methylmalonic-aciduria. Isovaleric-acidemia may also present with hyperglycinemia. All of these disorders present clinically with overwhelming illness in early infancy. Patients with propionic-acidemia and methylmalonic-acidemia have what has been called the ketotic hyperglycinemia syndrome.

This syndrome is characterized by recurrent episodes of metabolic acidosis, and massive ketosis, similar to those observed in diabetic coma. These patients may also have neutropenia, thrombocytopenia, and osteoporosis severe enough to lead to pathologic fracture. Mental retardation occurs, except in cases of early diagnosis and effective dietary therapy. Symptoms have begun as early at 18 hours after birth, with vomiting, acidosis, and ketonuria. Death has occurred in intractable acidosis, and it seems probable that other patients may have died unrecognized early in life. Convulsive seizures and electroencephalographic abnormalities may be found. The disease appears to be transmitted as an autosomal recessive.

The diagnosis can be suspected clinically. It should be documented chemically by quantitative assay of the concentrations of propionate and glycine in plasma. Examination of the urine by paper chromatography may be helpful, but the amounts of glycine excreted in normal urine are large, and a prominent glycine spot is commonly encountered. It is therefore easy to overlook hyperglycinuria with the methods commonly used in screening the urine for amino acids. Plasma glycine concentrations in this condition are often as high as 10 times those of controls. Even in the presence of hyperglycinemia the diagnosis requires demonstration of increased quantities of propionate in the blood by gas–liquid chromatography.

These patients excrete a number of distinctive metabolites in the urine, and their presence may indicate the diagnosis. Probably the most unusual of these metabolites is methylcitrate. Others are hydroxypropionate, tiglate, tiglyl glycine, and propionyl glycine. Restriction of dietary intake of protein in these patients has long been known to reduce the frequency and severity of attacks of ketosis and acidosis. Ketosis was later found to be produced by administration of leucine, isoleucine, threonine, valine, or methionine. Attacks also develop in association with infection, and elevated concentrations of leucine and valine have been observed in the plasma during such episodes. These observations led to an understanding of the area of the metabolic defect. There is no longer any reason to subject an infant to such a challenge, which could be dangerous, for the site of the molecular defect can be assessed. The defect is in the enzyme propionyl CoA carboxylase, which catalyzes the formation of methylmalonyl CoA from propionyl CoA (Fig. 3). This defect explains the intolerance of these patients for isoleucine, methionine, valine, and threonine, for they are all metabolized through this pathway. The defect can be demonstrated in leukocytes and in cultured fibroblasts and amniotic fluid cells.

Diets in which very small amounts of protein (0.5 g/kg/day) are supplemented with amino acids other than those listed above appear to be tolerated by pa-

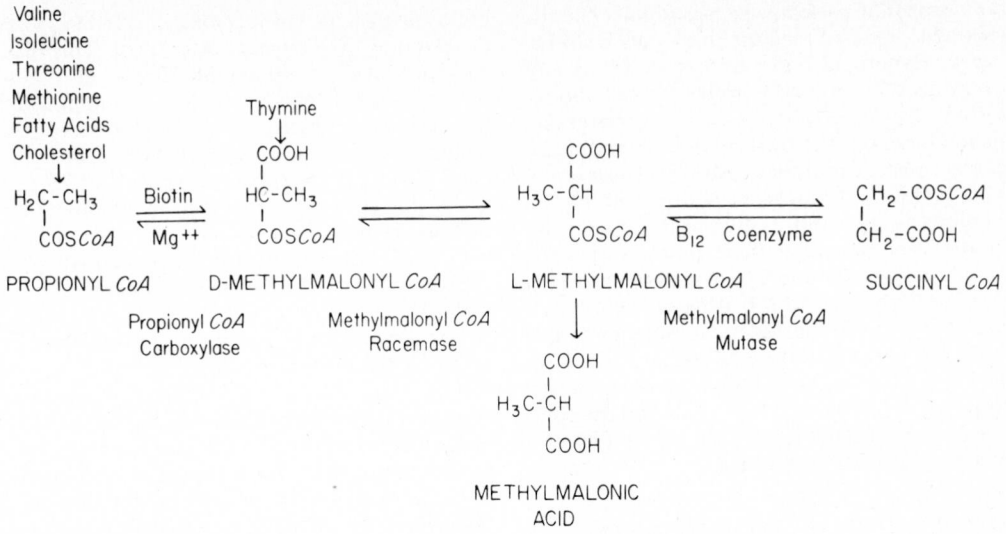

FIG. 3.   Site of the defect in methylmalonic-acidemia. Metabolism of propionic acid.

tients with the disease. At least 2 infants have now been diagnosed early in infancy and raised according to these dietary principles. Both have reached the age of 6 years, and they appear to have normal intelligence.

METHYLMALONIC-ACIDEMIA

At least three different disorders present as methyl-malonic-acidemia. They have clinical manifestations similar to those of the ketotic hyperglycinemia syndrome. Episodes of keto-acidosis may begin very early in life. They may lead to coma and death. Neutropenia is a prominent manifestation, and thrombocytopenia may occur. These patients usually have osteoporosis. Mental retardation has regularly been observed in surviving patients. Infections are common and they may precipitate life-threatening keto-acidosis. Some patients have had chronic monilial infection. The red cells are normal, and there is no megaloblastosis. Growth retardation is striking. Convulsions and abnormalities of the electroencephalogram have been observed.

Methylmalonic acid is found in elevated concentrations in the plasma. Levels of about 10 mg/dl are common. Urinary excretion of methylmalonic acid may exceed 500 mg/day. This compound is not normally detectable in blood or urine. In patients it has also been found in the cerebrospinal fluid and in tissues obtained post mortem. Increased amounts of glycine are found in blood and urine, but in contrast to the situation with methylmalonic acid, they correlate poorly with the clinical status of the patient. Concentrations of vitamin B_{12} in the blood are normal.

Methylmalonic acid is normally formed from methyl-malonyl CoA, which is a product of the propionyl CoA carboxylase reaction (Fig. 3). Methylmalonyl CoA occurs in two isomeric forms that are interconverted by a racemase. One form is converted by methylmalonyl CoA mutase to succinyl CoA, which can then be metabolized through the citric acid cycle. This pathway is a branch point in the metabolism of amino acids, fats, and carbohydrates. The amino acids isoleucine, valine, methionine, and threonine are catabolized along this pathway, and they are all precursors of methylmalonic acid in man. A defect in methylmalonyl CoA mutase has been suggested by the occurrence of methylmalonic acid in the urine. Furthermore, propionic acid oxidation is defective in vivo, in leukocytes, and in cultured fibroblasts. Methylmalonic acid oxidation is also impaired. Succinate oxidation is normal. The mutase enzyme has a vitamin B_{12} coenzyme.

Patients have been treated with vitamin B_{12} in large doses. Some have responded and some have not, thus delineating two forms of the disease. Patients who do not respond to vitamin B_{12} may be successfully treated with diets low in threonine, isoleucine, valine, and methionine. In a third form of methylmalonic-acidemia increased quantities of homocystine and cystathionine have been found in the urine. The single patient with this form was found to have a defect in the activity of tetrahydrofolate methyltransferase, and the data indicate a defect in the accumulation of coenzymatically active derivatives of vitamin B_{12}. The individuals responsive to vitamin B_{12}, who have no problem with sulfur amino acid metabolism, have a defect in the conversion of vitamin B_{12} to deoxyadenosyl vitamin B_{12}.

β-METHYLCROTONYL GLYCINURIA

Two patients have been described in whom large amounts of β-methylcrotonyl glycine and β-hydroxy-isovaleric acid have been found in the urine. In the patient described by Eldjarn and associates the parents were first cousins. The patient, who was reported at the age of 4 months, had had feeding difficulties from the second week. Hypotonia and retarded development were soon evident. Deep tendon reflexes were absent. The patient described by Gompertz and associates had persistent vomiting, ketosis, and acidosis. An erythematous rash was resistant to topical therapy. This patient has a dramatic clinical response to therapy with biotin. The skin lesions disappeared, as did the abnormal compounds in the urine; with time these returned, but the clinical manifestations did not. These patients excreted β-methylcrotonyl glycine and β-hydroxyisovaleric acid in the urine. The patient reported by Gompertz was also found to excrete tiglyl glycine and appeared to have defects in the carboxylation of both β-methylcrotonyl coenzyme (CoA) and propionyl CoA. This and the clinical response in the patient suggest the possibility of a defect in the metabolism of biotin.

α-METHYL-β-HYDROXYBUTYRIC-ACIDURIA

α-Methyl-β-hydroxybutyric-aciduria is a disorder of isoleucine metabolism that has been reported in 4 patients. The patient of Daum and associates was first admitted in coma following an upper respiratory infection. He was found to have severe metabolic acidosis. Thereafter he had multiple episodes of recurrent ketosis and acidosis. The second patient had had a sister who had died at 12 months of age in a similar episode. The patient was studied at 4 years of age because of vomiting and ketonuria. She had normal mental development, but her older brother, who had the same disease, was retarded.

These patients were all typical examples of the ketotic hyperglycinemia syndrome. However, the concentration of glycine in the blood was never elevated. In contrast, the patient of Keating and associates had the ketotic hyperglycinemia syndrome in its complete expression. In addition to recurrent episodes of ketosis and acidosis, this patient was operated on for pyloric stenosis. She also had neutropenia, thrombocytopenia, and osteoporosis. Large amounts of glycine were found in her blood and urine.

α-Methyl-β-hydroxybutyric acid and α-methylacetoacetic acid were found in the urine of these patients. Chemical identification was confirmed by mass spectrometry. Isoleucine was converted imperfectly to carbon dioxide, while labeled propionate and methylmalonate were oxidized normally in the fibroblast. These observations suggest that the defect in these patients is in the β-ketothiolase that converts α-methylacetoacetyl CoA to propionyl CoA and acetyl CoA.

NONKETOTIC HYPERGLYCINEMIA

Patients with nonketotic hyperglycinemia have all had severe seizure disorders. One patient had almost continuous status epilepticus for much of his first year of life. Convulsions and irritability, or lethargy have been observed in the first days after birth. This disease can also produce overwhelming illness in the neonatal period. Death in the first year is common. All patients that have been described in detail have had very severe mental retardation. In most there was little functional cortical activity. Two had microcephaly. Hypertonicity and hypotonicity have been observed, often in the same patient. Hyperreflexia is the rule. Porencephaly and ventricular dilatation have been seen on pneumoencephalography. The electroencephalograms were abnormal.

Concentrations in plasma of glycine have been elevated. A range of about 5 to 12 mg/dl has been observed. The amounts of glycine in the urine and cerebrospinal fluid have also been increased. This disorder was originally described as hyperglycinemia with hypo-oxaluria, but it is now apparent that hypo-oxaluria is not a regular concomitant of this disease. Neutropenia has been observed in only 1 patient. None has had ketoacidosis. On the other hand, respiratory acidosis has been observed at times of extreme illness. A defect has been found in vivo in the conversion of carbon 1 of glycine to CO_2 and of carbon 2 of glycine to carbon 3 of serine. This would be consistent with a defect in an enzyme catalyzing the conversion of glycine to CO_2 and hydroxymethylte-trahydrofolic acid. This is known as the glycine cleavage enzyme.

SARCOSINEMIA

Sarcosine is the N-methyl derivative of glycine. It is formed from dimethylglycine, which may be a product of betaine or choline. Sarcosine is not normally present in the blood in amounts sufficient to be detected. The same is true of the urine, although occasionally sarcosinuria is found after the ingestion of lobster or certain other foods. Seven patients have been reported with sarcosinemia. Three have had subnormal intelligence. The others have had shortness of stature. Sarcosine concentrations in the blood have ranged from 0.5 to 6.8 mg/dl . Urinary excretion of sarcosine has been as high as 168 mg/24 hours in a patient less than 1 year of age and 500 mg/24 hours in a 2-year-old. A deficiency of hepatic sarcosine dehydrogenase has been postulated; however, data on this question are not clear.

HYPEROXALURIA AND OXALOSIS

Primary hyperoxaluria is a metabolic disorder in which large amounts of oxalate are excreted in the urine, leading to calcium oxalate lithiasis and nephrocalcinosis. When extrarenal deposits of calcium oxalate ensue, the condition is known as oxalosis. There have been reports of 20 to 30 patients, in most of whom the diagnosis was not established during life. Early onset of symptoms such as urolithiasis, hematuria, passage of calculi, and colic, as well as nephrocalcinosis, urinary tract infections, and extrarenal deposits, is sufficiently characteristic to warrant investigation for the presence of oxalate in the urine. Renal failure is common; the mean age at death in 16 cases has been 4 years. Attempts at treatment have not been effective. Most instances of the disease have been isolated cases, but the disease is probably caused by a rare recessive gene. Four affected siblings have been reported, as well as one set of identical twins.

Oxalic acid is a dicarboxylic acid that forms a calcium salt of very low solubility. It may be formed from glyoxylic acid, which may be formed from glycine or glycolic acid. It may also be a metabolite of ascorbic acid. In patients with hyperoxaluria the levels of oxalate excretion may approximate 30 times those of control subjects. It is clear that the oxalate found in the urine is of endogenous origin and that glycine is a precursor. Isotope-labeled glycine is rapidly converted to urinary oxalate, but the proportions of oxalate made from glycine are the same in patients and controls. A rate of conversion of injected ^{14}C-glyoxylate to respiratory CO_2 in patients that is only 20 percent that of controls would appear to localize the site of the defect to the metabolism of glyoxylic acid. There is a carboligase enzyme that catalyzes the reaction of glyoxylate and α-ketoglutarate to α-hydroxy-β-ketoadipate and is present in the soluble and mitochondrial portions of the cell. It has been reported that the soluble but not the mitochondrial enzyme is low in activity in the liver of oxaluric patients.

Treatment of this disorder has been unsatisfactory. Reports of successful management of oxalosis with calcium carbimide, which might be expected to inhibit glyoxylate formation by tying up glycoaldehyde, have not been confirmed. Renal transplantation has been unsuccessful because oxalate has been deposited in the transplanted kidney.

HYPERPROLINEMIA AND HYDROXYPROLINEMIA

Hyperprolinemia was first recognized in a family in which cerebral dysfunction, renal anomalies, nephropathy, and deafness occurred in various members. The initial patient was a male infant who presented at 2 years of age with congenital renal hypoplasia, deafness, convulsions, and mental retardation. He was found to have hyperprolinemia, as were three female siblings who had electroencephalographic abnormalities. One of the siblings had renal hypoplasia, nerve deafness, hematuria, and electroencephalographic abnormality. Neither her proline levels nor those of the father were abnormal. Hematuria and deafness occurred frequently in the mother's family in a pattern suggesting dominant inheritance.

In affected persons concentrations of proline in plasma were between 7.8 and 20.1 mg/dl. Proline was not elevated in the cerebrospinal fluid. Proline and hydroxyproline, which are not found in the urine after the neonatal period, were prominent; in some instances glycine excretion was increased. It was found that infusion of proline into normal adults produced a hydroxyprolinuria and glycinuria, as well as prolinuria,

indicating that the urinary findings are secondary to a basic defect in the metabolism of proline.

Hydroxyprolinemia has been described in a mentally retarded girl who also had increased numbers of leukocytes and erythrocytes in the urine and who showed small kidneys radiographically. Shortness of stature was also observed. Her mother was also mentally retarded, but had no hydroxyproline abnormality. Thus both hyperprolinemia and hydroxyprolinemia have been associated with mental retardation and with nephropathy. In involved families, members with the metabolic abnormality have had no clinical defect, and vice versa. Therefore it remains possible that these abnormalities of amino acid metabolism are simply biochemical phenotypes without clinical disease.

Free hydroxyproline was first observed on a routine paper chromatogram. Quantitative assay indicated markedly elevated quantities of hydroxyproline in the blood and urine. Interestingly, the amounts of glycine and proline in the urine were normal. It is now known that there are two forms of hyperprolinemia: type I, in which there is a deficiency of proline oxidase, and type II, in which the next enzyme on the degradative pathway, Δ'-pyrroline-5-carboxylic acid dehydrogenase is deficient. In hydroxyprolinuria a defect in hydroxyproline oxidase has been observed.

CYSTATHIONINURIA

Cystathioninuria is a rare metabolic disorder first reported in two adults with mental deficiency. It has also been observed in patients with thrombocytopenia and endocrinopathy, as well as in individuals with no disease. Possibly the biochemical defect is coincidental, but most patients have had some clinical abnormality. The first two patients described were 64 and 44 years of age when it was recognized. Developmental retardation was present from birth. One was otherwise normal except for talipes calcaneovalgus. The other had acromegaly, small ears, deafness, and facial clefts. Abnormal amino-aciduria has generally been found in the course of routine screening. Cystathioninuria also occurs in a secondary fashion in patients with neuroblastoma or hepatoma or in galactosemia or other forms of hepatocellular disease.

Cystathionine is an intermediate in the formation of cysteine and homoserine from methionine and serine. Cystathionine is normally cleaved to form cysteine and α-ketobutyrate. The compound is not usually found in the urine, but in these patients as much as 500 to 1,300 mg may be excreted each day. Cystathionine is not usually detected in blood. Administration of methionine leads to an increase in cystathionine excretion. Pyridoxine (vitamin B_6) may lead to a decrease. High doses (5 to 10 mg/kg/day) of vitamin B_6 have been used to maintain blood and urine cystathionine concentrations near zero. The enzyme cystathionase has been found to be defective in the liver of patients with cystathioninuria, and the in vitro addition of large amounts of pyridoxine has corrected the defect. Thus the abnormality appears to be in the enzyme structure responsible for binding of the coenzyme.

The disorder is transmitted as an autosomal recessive disease. Small but abnormal quantities of cystathionine, which may be found in the urine of heterozygotes, may be increased by oral administration of methionine.

Homocystinuria

Homocystinuria is a disorder in metabolism of the sulfur-containing amino acids. It is the second most common inherited disorder of amino acid metabolism; the first, phenylketonuria, is much more common. Homocystinuria is especially prevalent in Ireland, where a frequency of 0.7 per 100,000 population has been estimated.

Most patients described have been mentally retarded. Many have had marked failure to thrive. They have been thin and hypertonic, and they have died before 1 year of age. Less severely affected patients have had mental retardation without systemic disease. Ectopia lentis is the most characteristic feature of the disease. It may be the only manifestation of disease. Cataracts have also been seen, as well as glaucoma. The hair is usually fair and sparse, the complexion fair, and the eyes blue. A malar flush and livido reticularis are characteristic. Most patients have had osteoporosis and skeletal abnormalities, such as genu valgum, pes cavus, or pectus excavatum or carinatum. Most have had osteoporosis. Patients are frail and thin. They have been mistaken for patients with Marfan's syndrome and vice versa. However, in homocystinuria the joints tend to be limited in mobility rather than hypermobile.

Spontaneous thromboembolic phenomena, both arterial and venous, have been prominent in homocystinuria. They have often been the cause of death in the disease. Occlusion of coronary, renal, or cerebral arteries or veins may lead to major complications such as hemiplegia or renal hypertension, as well as death. Pulmonary embolism is a frequent terminal complication. Many have convulsions, and the electroencephalogram is usually abnormal. Classic tests of clotting function have been normal, but platelets from these patients have shown unusual adhesiveness. Furthermore, the addition of homocystine to normal blood causes the platelets to become sticky.

Homocystine is an intermediate in the metabolism of methionine that is not detected in the usual assays of amino acids in body fluids. After the conversion of methionine to S-adenosylmethionine, demethylation yields S-adenosylhomocysteine, which is cleaved to homocysteine. This compound is normally combined with serine in the presence of cystathionine synthase to form cystathionine. Free homocysteine condenses to form the disulfide homocystine, as does cysteine to form cystine.

The presence of homocystine in the urine may be the only readily detectable abnormality in these patients, but the compound should be detectable in the blood, and levels of methionine are usually elevated. The amounts of homocystine in the urine of these patients usually exceed 20 mg/day and can be increased by oral administration of methionine. The mixed disulfide of cysteine and homocysteine is also present in the urine. Screening of urine for the presence of homocystine can be carried out by the addition of nitroprusside following treatment with cyanide.

The enzymatic defect in the most common form of homocystinuria involves cystathionine synthase. This is consistent with an absence of cystathionine in the brain. The enzyme defect can be demonstrated using biopsied liver or cultured fibroblasts or amniotic fluid cells. The disorder is transmitted as an autosomal recessive trait. Heterozygotes have reduced levels of activity of cystathione synthase.

Experience with treatment has provided the first evidence of genetic heterogeneity in homocystinuria, for some patients respond to the administration of large doses (100 to 500 mg/day) of pyridoxine and some do not. Patients who respond to pyridoxine should be treated with this vitamin. Those who do not respond to pyridoxine may be treated with a diet in which methionine is restricted and a supplement of cystine is added. There is accumulating evidence for clinical benefit from each of these forms of therapy.

Homocystinuria may result from defects other than that of cystathionine synthase. The disorder in which homocystinuria coexists with cystathioninuria and methylmalonic-aciduria tends to lead to overwhelming illness and death early in life, as does the usual form of methylmalonic-aciduria. Four patients have been described with this disorder. Enzyme assay in these patients reveals abnormally low activity of N^5-methyltetrahydrofolate homocysteine methyltransferase. In this reaction 5-methyltetrahydrofolate is demethylated to tetrahydrofolate, yielding the methyl group for the conversion of homocysteine to methionine. In this group of patients the activity of the enzyme can be restored to normal in vitro by the addition of methyl vitamin B_{12}. These data indicate that the defect is not in the apoenzyme of the methyltransferase. Furthermore, fibroblasts derived from these patients cannot convert hydroxy vitamin B_{12} to methyl vitamin B_{12}. It is deoxyadenosyl vitamin B_{12} that serves as cofactor for methylmalonyl CoA mutase, and these fibroblasts are also unable to convert hydroxy vitamin B_{12} to deoxyadenosyl vitamin B_{12}. The underlying defect is probably in the uptake or reduction of vitamin B_{12}.

A different form of abberant vitamin B_{12} metabolism leads to homocystinuria because of the role of vitamin B_{12} in the activity of methyltransferase. These patients have a familial selective vitamin B_{12} malabsorption. They have megaloblastic anemia, and they excrete methylmalonic acid as well as homocystine. All of these findings disappear on treatment with parenteral vitamin B_{12}.

Three patients have been described in whom homocystinuria was due to deficiency of $N^{5,10}$-methylenetetrahydrofolate reductase. These patients have 10 times the normal concentration of methionine and normal concentrations of vitamin B_{12}. They do not have methylmalonic-aciduria. Study of cultured fibroblasts has revealed the defect in $N^{5,10}$-methylenetetrahydrofolate reductase. This leads to a deficiency in methyltetrahydrofolate, which is the methyl donor in the methyltransferase reaction that converts homocysteine to methionine.

UREA CYCLE DISORDERS

Argininosuccinic-aciduria

Argininosuccinic-aciduria is one of a group of metabolic defects involving enzymes of the urea cycle. Twenty-five patients have been reported, and two clinical forms have been distinguished. One is a neonatal form that leads to early death from overwhelming illness. Two patients with this disease have been reported. In the late-onset form, most patients have been severely mentally retarded, with generalized seizures and electroencephalographic abnormalities. Ataxia has been common, and hepatomegaly is another regular feature. A certain number of these patients have had short brittle hair that seldom needed cutting and was diagnosed as trichorrhexis nodosa. The biochemical findings of the disease occur in patients in whom mental retardation is only mild and there are no other abnormalities.

Argininosuccinic acid is an intermediate in the urea cycle. It is formed from citrulline and aspartic acid and is not normally found in body fluids. Argininosuccinic-aciduria represents a failure in the cleavage of this compound to arginine and fumaric acid, which is catalyzed by argininosuccinase. This enzyme is defective in argininosuccinic-aciduria. Correlation of the severity of the clinical disease and molecular abnormality has not yet been made.

Low plasma concentrations of argininosuccinic acid and its very high urinary excretion in this condition are consistent with very efficient renal clearance. For these reasons this and similar conditions have been called no-threshold amino-acidurias. This is to distinguish these metabolic disorders from disorders of transport, in which an amino acid occurs in the urine without elevation in plasma concentrations. High concentrations of argininosuccinic acid are found in the cerebrospinal fluid. Therefore, it has been suggested that the enzyme defect is present in the brain and that argininosuccinic acid produced in the brain may produce cerebral symptoms. Disruption in the urea cycle is indicated by the fact that these patients develop postprandial elevations of blood ammonia and signs of ammonia toxicity. Dietary protein restriction has been employed in treatment.

Citrullinemia

Citrullinemia is a disorder of urea cycle metabolism that was originally recognized through screening surveys of the urine of mentally retarded children for amino acids. It is now apparent that there are at least three forms of citrullinemia, and there is good correlation between the severity of the clinical disease and the nature of the molecular defect.

The acute neonatal form of citrullinemia has been reported in 5 patients, and we have seen 2 other patients. Most diseases that present with acute overwhelming illness in the neonatal period are probably much more common than reports in the literature would suggest. Of these 7 patients, all but 1 patient died at less than 1 week of age. The picture is that of death in coma with respiratory arrest. Blood concentrations of ammonia are very high.

Patients with the second form of citrullinemia have episodic vomiting and postabsorptive elevation in blood ammonia. Severe vomiting, coma, and seizures may develop. Usually there is severe mental retardation (I.Q. values less than 40), as well as microcephaly.

The third form of citrullinemia has been reported in only 1 patient, a boy who may be clinically normal. He was admitted to hospital because of aspiration and tachypnea, and he was found to have citrullinemia on a routine screen. There was no hyperammonemia, even postprandially.

As in the case of argininosuccinic-aciduria, urea excretion may be normal in this condition, but 1 patient had persistently low blood urea nitrogen. The metabolic block in this disease is in the formation of argininosuccinic acid from citrulline. Argininosuccinic acid synthetase has been found to be deficient in liver and in fibroblasts cultured from the skin. The disorder is inherited as as an autosomal recessive. The parents of the first patient were first cousins. Molecular heterogeneity is evident in the levels of activity of argininosuccinic acid synthetase, but it is virtually absent in patients with the acute neonatal form and is considerably greater in the third or benign form.

Carbamyl Phosphate Synthetase Deficiency

The first step at which a defect in the urea cycle leads to hyperammonemia is that of carbamyl phosphate synthetase. This enzyme catalyzes the formation of carbamyl phosphate from NH_4^+ and HCO_3^- and thus provides a branch point to pyrimidine biosynthesis as well as urea synthesis. Clinical manifestations are those of ammonia intoxication. Episodic vomiting, lethargy, and stupor or coma may be seen as early as 10 days after birth. Most patients who have been described have been mentally retarded. Convulsions have been reported. Elevated concentrations of ammonia are found in the blood and cerebrospinal fluid. Assay of the enzyme requires liver tissue.

Ornithine Transcarbamylase Deficiency

Carbamyl phosphate reacts with ornithine in the presence of ornithine transcarbamylase to form citrulline. Assay of this enzyme also requires liver. A number of patients have been described with deficiency of this enzyme. The gene is on the X chromosome. Involved males have usually died in the newborn period. Symptoms have begun with vomiting and lethargy and progressed to coma. Activity of the enzyme in liver has been less than 2 percent of normal. Female patients have had a more indolent disorder leading to mental retardation. Episodic vomiting, hypotonia, and lethargy have been prominent. Some have had seizures. Concentrations of ammonia are elevated, and increased amounts of orotic acid are found in the urine.

ARGININEMIA

Three patients with argininemia have been described. They presented, like other patients with hyperammonemia, with vomiting and retardation of mental and motor development. One had a spastic tetraparesis, two had seizures, and one had an abnormal electroencephalogram. Hepatomegaly was observed, as were abnormalities of liver function tests. The blood ammonia was markedly elevated both in the fasting state and postprandially. In the urine there was a cystinurialike pattern in which excretions of cystine, lysine, and ornithine were elevated, as well as that of arginine. Citrulline was also excreted in abnormal quantities. The concentration of arginine in the plasma was 6 to 15 times normal. The cerebrospinal fluid concentration was also increased. Arginase assays were performed on the erythrocytes of the patients, and the activity was greatly reduced or unmeasurable. The activity of the enzyme in liver has not been assayed.

ORNITHINEMIA

Two types of ornithinemia have been reported. In the first, mental retardation, prolonged icterus, and electroencephalographic abnormalities are associated with increased concentrations of ornithine in the blood. There is a generalized amino-aciduria, but no hyperammonemia or homocitrullinuria. The activity of hepatic ornithine keto acid transaminase (OKT) is deficient. In the second there is mental retardation, ataxia, and hyperammonemia. Ornithinemia is associated with homocitrullinuria. The activity of OKT in fibroblasts is normal. OKT catalyzes the conversion of ornithine and an α-keto acid, such as α-ketoglutarate, to pyrroline carboxylate and an amino acid such as glutamate.

HYPERLYSINEMIA

A number of different inborn errors of metabolism present with elevated concentrations of lysine in the blood. One of these is due to a deficiency of lysine: α-ketoglutarate reductase. The first child described had mental retardation and delayed physical development, but subsequently 2 children were mentally and physically normal. Consanguinity has been observed. Concentrations of lysine in the blood are elevated, with levels generally exceeding 10 mg/dl. The product of the reductase enzyme is saccharopine. This pathway is the major route of lysine catabolism. The enzyme defect is demonstrable in cultured fibroblasts. Saccharopinuria has been found in 2 patients as a result of routine screening of mentally retarded individuals. Plasma lysine has been elevated in both. It seems likely that this abnormality is due to a defect in saccharopine dehydrogenase.

An alternate pathway for the catabolism of lysine is through pipecolic acid. A patient was described who appeared to have a defect in this pathway because large amounts of pipecolic acid were found in the plasma and urine. Concentrations of lysine were not elevated. This child died of a progressive neurologic disease associated with hepatomegaly.

Another disorder has been described under the heading of lysine intolerance in which the subject has episodic ammonia intoxication and coma. Such a patient would be clinically indistinguishable from those described under hyperammonemia. Patients described from Finland as having familial protein intolerance all had hyperammonemia and hyperlysinuria.

β-ALANINE ABNORMALITIES

Hyper-β-Alaninemia and Carnosinemia

Hyper-β-alaninemia has been reported in a single infant who died very early in life; the symptoms were neonatal somnolence, hypotonia, and intermittent seizures that could not be controlled with the usual anticonvulsive therapy. Deep tendon reflexes were depressed. β-Alanine was found to be elevated in the blood, urine, and cerebrospinal fluid. Large amounts of taurine and β-aminoisobutyric acid were also found in the urine. γ-Aminobutyric acid was present in the plasma, urine, and cerebrospinal fluid. The concentration of γ-aminobutyric acid in brain tissue obtained post mortem was markedly increased.

Carnosine is the dipeptide of β-alanine and histidine. It is normally present in high concentrations in muscle and is thus a common dietary constituent. It is not normally found in the blood. Seven patients have been reported with carnosinemia. Five of them have had progressive neurologic degeneration with onset early in infancy. They have also had seizures and electroencephalographic abnormalities. However, 2 patients have been described with the biochemical abnormality but without clinical manifestations of abnormality. Carnosinase activity is normally present in the serum. It is absent in patients with carnosinemia.

Carnosinemia should be distinguished from normal dietary carnosinuria. Patients with carnosinemia have persistent carnosinuria while receiving a diet free of carnosine. They do not have 1-methylhistidine in the urine. Normal individuals receiving a meal rich in protein such as white meat of chicken excrete anserine and β-alanyl-1-methylhistidine, and the urine always contains 1-methylhistidine.

PYROGLUTAMIC-ACIDEMIA

Pyroglutamic-acidemia was first described by Eldjarn and associates in Norway in 1970. A second patient was observed in Sweden. The condition is of special interest because of the possibility that this compound is an index of the operation of a γ-glutamyl cycle involved in the transport of amino acids in the kidney.

Metabolic acidosis is a consistent feature of this disorder. In the first patient this was first observed at the age of 16 years, just before he was to be operated on for a hiatal hernia. It became life-threatening in the postoperative period. Over a 3-year period of study he was admitted to hospital five times, always revealing a chronic acidosis, without acute exacerbations. The second patient developed a severe metabolic acidosis on the third day of life. This was correctable with NaHCO₃. She had exacerbations of acidosis whenever alkali thereapy was discontinued. This patient had no other abnormalities. By 14 months of age her physical and intellectual development had been normal. The first patient was mentally retarded. He was also spastic and had an intention tremor and an ataxic gait. At the age of 16 years he began to have episodes of violent vomiting. It is not clear that any of his clinical manifestations are related to his pyroglutamic acidemia.

Pyroglutamic acid is 2-pyrrolidone-5-carboxylic acid. It has been known as a cyclized condensatin product of glutamic acid, forming regularly with the loss of a molecule of water when glutamic acid is heated to 150 C to 160 C. Glutamine cyclizes readily to pyroglutamic acid in aqueous solutions at physiologic pH. The compound does not react with Ninhydrin; therefore it is not detectable using routine methods of screening the urine for amino acids. It has been found using gas–liquid chromatography.

The first patient excreted 30 to 40 g of pyroglutamate in the urine in 24 hours. Blood serum concentrations were as high as 50 to 60 mg/dl or 4 to 5 mEq/liter. This would account for the acidosis. In the second patient 6 to 7 g of pyroglutamate were excreted each day in the urine.

The kidney appears to be the site of formation of pyroglutamate. A relationship has been suspected between renal ammonia production and pyroglutamate formation. It is generally accepted that the amide nitrogen of glutamine is the source of renal NH_4^+. Spontaneous deamination of glutamine in aqueous solutions yields predominantly pyroglutamate, not glutamate. Furthermore, there is generally a close parallelism in patients with pyroglutamic-aciduria between the amounts of pyroglutamate and ammonia in the urine.

Pyroglutamate can be formed in the enzymatic hydrolysis of γ-glutamyl peptides. The γ-glutamyl transport theory postulates that free amino acids are normally taken up from the glomerular filtrate as it passes by the proximal tubular cell by the formation of γ-glutamyl amino acid dipeptides in a transpeptidase-catalyzed reaction in which the γ-glutamyl moiety is supplied by glutathione (γ-glutamylcysteinyl glycine). This dipeptide then is the intracellular transport form of the amino acid. It is in turn released by the γ-glutamyl cyclotransferase reaction that yields the original free amino acid and pyroglutamate out of the γ-glutamyl moiety.

References

PHENYLKETONURIA

Guthrie R, Susi A: A simple phenylalanine method for detecting phenylketonuria in large populations of newborn infants. Pediatrics 32:338, 1963

Jervis GA: Phenylpyruvic oligophrenia deficiency of phenylalanine-oxidizing system. Proc Soc Exp Biol Med 82:514, 1953

Koch R, Blaskovics M, Wenz E, Fishler K, Schaeffler G: Phenylalaninemia and phenylketonuria. In Nyhan WL (ed): Heritable Disorders of Amino Acid Metabolism. New York, Wiley, 1974, p 109

Shear CS, Wellman NS, Nyhan WL: Phenylketonuria: experience with diagnosis and management. In Nyhan WL (ed): Heritable Disorders of Amino Acid Metabolism. New York, Wiley, 1974 p 141

TYROSINOSIS

Buist NRM, Kennaway NG, Fellman JH: Disorders of tyrosine metabolism. In Nyhan WL (ed): Heritable Disorders of Amino Acid Metabolism. New York, Wiley, 1974, p 160

Medes G: A new error of tyrosine metabolism: tyrosinosis. The intermediary metabolism of tyrosine and phenylalanine. Biochem J 26:917, 1932

ALKAPTONURIA

Garrod AE: The incidence of alkaptonuria: a study in chemical individuality. Lancet 2:1616, 1902

La Du BN, Zannoni VA, Laster L, Seegmiller JE: The nature of the defect in tyrosine metabolism in alcaptonuria. J Biol Chem 230:251, 1968

ALBINISM

Fitzpatrick TB: Albinism. In Stanbury JB, Wyngaarden JB, Fredrickson DS (eds): The Metabolic Basis of Inherited Disease. New York, McGraw-Hill, 1960, p 428

Witkop CJ Jr, White JG, King RA: Oculocutaneous albinism. In Nyhan WL (ed): Heritable Disorders of Amino Acid Metabolism. New York, Wiley, 1974, p 177

HISTIDINEMIA

Ghadimi H, Zischka R: Histidinemia. In Nyhan WL (ed): Amino Acid Metabolism and Genetic Variation. New York, McGraw-Hill, 1967, p 133

La Du BN, Howell RR, Jacoby GA, Seegmiller JE, Zannoni VG: The enzymatic defect in histidinemia. Biochem Biophys Res Commun 7:-398, 1962

MAPLE SYRUP URINE DISEASE

Dancis J, Hutzler J, Rokkones T: Intermittent branched chain ketoaciduria: variant of maple syrup urine disease. N Engl J Med 276:84, 1967

Goedde HW, Keller W: Metabolic pathways in maple syrup urine disease. In Nyhan WL (ed): Amino Acid Metabolism and Genetic Variation. New York, McGraw-Hill, 1967, p 191

Menkes JH, Hurst PL, Craig JM: A new syndrome: progressive familial infantile cerebral dysfunction associated with an unusual urinary substance. Pediatrics 14:462, 1954

Schulman JD, Lustberg TJ, Kennedy JL, Museles M, Seegmiller JE: A new variant of maple syrup urine disease (branched-chain ketoaciduria). Am J Med 49:118, 1970

Scriver CR, Mackenzie S, Clow CL, Delvin E: Thiamine-responsive maple syrup urine disease. Lancet 1:310, 1971

HYPERVALINEMIA

Dancis J, Hutzler J, Tada K, et al: Hypervalinemia: a defect in valine transamination. Pediatrics 39:813, 1967

PROPIONIC-ACIDEMIA

Ando T, Nyhan WL: Propionic acidemia and the ketotic hyperglycinemia syndrome. In Nyhan WL (ed): Heritable Disorders of Amino Acid Metabolism. New York, Wiley, 1974, p 37

Childs B, Nyhan WL, Borden M, Bard L, Cooke RE: Idiopathic hyperglycinemia and hyperglycinuria, a new disorder of amino acid metabolism. I. Pediatrics 27:522, 1961

METHYLMALONIC-ACIDEMIA

Morrow G III: Methylmalonic acidemia. In Nyhan WL (ed): Heritable Disorders of Amino Acid Metabolism. New York, Wiley, 1974, p 61

Nyhan WL, Fawcett N, Ando T, Rennert OM., Julius RL: Response to dietary therapy in B_{12} unresponsive methylmalonic acidemia. Pediatrics 51:539, 1973

Rosenberg LE, Lilljequist AC, Hsia YE: Methylmalonic aciduria. N Engl J Med 278:1319, 1968

Stokke O, Eldjarn L, Norum KR, Steen-Johnson J, Halvorsen S: Methylmalonic acidemia: a new inborn error of metabolism which may cause fatal acidosis in the neonatal period. Scand J Clin Lab Invest 20:313, 1967

OTHER DISORDERS OF BRANCHED-CHAIN AMINO ACID METABOLISM

Daum RS, Scriver CR, Mamer OA, et al: An inherited disorder of leucine catabolism causing accumulation of α-methyl-β-hydroxybutyrate, and intermittent metabolic acidosis. Pediatr Res 7:149, 1973

Eldjarn L, Jellum E, Stokke O, Pande H, Waaler PE: β-Hydroxyisovaleric aciduria and β-methylcrotonylglycinuria: a newborn error of metabolism. Lancet 2:521, 1970

Gompertz D, Draffan GH: The identification of tiglylglycine in the urine of a child with β-methyl-crotonylglycinuria. Clin Chim Acta 37:405, 1972

Hillman RE, Keating JP, Beta-ketothiolase deficiency as a cause of the "ketotic hyperglycinemia syndrome." Pediatrics 53:221, 1974

Keating JP, Feigin RD, Tenenbaum SM, Hillman RE: Hyperglycinemia with ketosis due to a defect in isoleucine metabolism: a preliminary report. Pediatrics 50:890, 1972

NONKETOTIC HYPERGLYCINEMIA

Ando T, Nyhan WL, Gerritsen T, et al: Metabolism of glycine in the nonketotic form of hyperglycinemia. Pediatr Res 2:254, 1968

Gerritsen T, Kaveggia E, Waisman HA: A new type of idiopathic hyperglycinemia with hypo-oxalauria. Pediatrics 36:882, 1965

Ziter FA, Bray PF, Madsen JA, Nyhan WL: The clinical findings in a patient with nonketotic hyperglycinemia. Pediatr Res 2:250, 1968

SARCOSINEMIA

Gerritsen T, Waisman HA: Hypersarcosinemia. An inborn error of metabolism. N Engl J Med 275:66, 1966

Scott CR: Sarcosinemia. In Nyhan WL (ed): Heritable Disorders of Amino Acid Metabolism. New York, Wiley, 1974. p 324

HYPEROXALURIA

Elder TD, Wyngaarden JB: the biosynthesis and turnover of oxalate in normal and hyperoxaluric subjects. J Clin Invest 39:1337, 1960

Smith LH Jr, Williams HE: Hyperoxaluria (glycolic-aciduria). In Nyhan WL (ed): Amino Acid Metabolism and Genetic Variation. New York McGraw-Hill, 1967, p 239

Solomons CC, Goodman SI, Riley CM: Calcium carbimide in the treatment of primary hyperoxaluria. N Engl J Med 276:207, 1967

HYPERPROLINEMIA AND HYDROXYPROLINEMIA

Efron ML, Bixby EM, Pryles CV: Hydroxyprolinemia II.A rare metabolic disease due to a deficiency of the enzyme hydroxyproline oxidase. N Engl J Med 272:1299, 1965

Pelkonen R, Kivirikko KI: Hydroxyprolinemia. An apparently harmless familial metabolic disorder. N Engl J Med 283:451, 1970

Shafer IA, Scriver CR, Efron ML: Familial hyperprolinemia, cerebral dysfunction and renal anomalies occurring in a family with hereditary nephropathy and deafness. N Engl J Med 267:51, 1962

CYSTATHIONINURIA

Frimpter GW: Cystathioninuria: nature of the defect. Science 149:1095, 1965

————— Haymovitz A, Horwith M: Cystathioninuria. N Engl J Med 268:333, 1963

Scott CR, Dassell SW, Clark SH, Chiang-Teng C, Swedberg KR: Cystathioninemia: a benign condition. J Pediatr 76:571, 1970

HOMOCYSTINURIA

Barber GW, Spaeth GE: The successful treatment of homocystinuria with pyridoxine. J Pediatr 76:463, 1969

Carson NAJ, Cusworth DC, Dent CE, et al: Homocystinuria: a new inborn error of metabolism associated with mental deficiency. Arch Dis Child 38:425, 1963

Mudd SH: Homocystinuria and homocysteine metabolism: selected aspects. In Nyhan WL (ed): Heritable Disorders of Amino Acid Metabolism. New York, Wiley, 1974, p 429

Perry TL: Homocystinuria. In Nyhan WL (ed): Heritable Disorders of Amino Acid Metabolism. New York, Wiley, 1974, p 395

UREA CYCLE DISORDERS

Bachmann C: Urea cycle. In Nyhan WL (ed): Heritable Disorders of Amino Acid Metabolism. New York, Wiley, 1974, p 361

Morrow G III, Barness LA, Efron ML: Citrullinemia with defective urea production. Pediatrics 40:565, 1967

Westall RG: Argininosuccinic aciduria: identification and reactions of the abnormal metabolite in a newly described form of mental disease, with some preliminary metabolic studies. Biochem J 77:135, 1960

ARGININEMIA

Tergeggen HG, Lavinha F, Colombo JP, Van Sande M, Lowenthal A: Familial hyperargininemia. J Genet Hum 20: 69, 1972

ORNITHINEMIA

Kekomäki MP, Raiba NCR, Bickel H: Ornithine-ketoacid aminotransferase in human liver with reference to patients with hyperornithinaemia and familial protein intolerance. Clin Chim Acta 23:203, 1969

Shih VE, Efron ML, Moser HW: Hyperornithinemia, hyperammonemia, and homocitrullinuria. A new disorder of amino acid metabolism associated with myoclonic seizures and mental retardation. Am J Dis Child 117:83, 1969

————— Schulman JD: Ornithine-ketoacid transaminase activity in human skin and amniotic fluid cell culture. Clin Chim Acta 27:73, 1970

HYPERLYSINEMIA

Colombo JP, Richterich R, Donath A, Spahr A, Rossi E: Congenital lysine intolerance with periodic ammonia intoxication. Lancet 1:1014, 1964

Dancis J: Abnormalities in the degradation of lysine. In Nyhan WL (ed): Heritable Disorders of Amino Acid Metabolism. New York, Wiley, 1974, p 387

β-ALANINE ABNORMALITIES

Perry TL: Carnosinemia. In Nyhan WL (ed): Heritable Disorders of Amino Acid Metabolism. New York, Wiley, 1974, p 293

Scriver CR, Pueschel S, Davies E: Hyper-β-alanemia associated with β-aminoaciduria and γ-aminobutyric aciduria, somnolence and seizures. N Engl J Med 274:636, 1966

PYROGLUTAMIC-ACIDEMIA

Eldjarn L, Jellum E, Stokke O: Pyroglutamic acidemia. In Nyhan WL (ed): Heritable Disorders of Amino Acid Metabolism. New York, Wiley, 1974, p 479

Jellum E, Kluge T, Borresen HC, Stokke O, Eldjarn L: Pyroglutamic aciduria, a new inborn error of metabolism. Scand J Clin Lab Invest 26:327, 1970

Orlowski M, Meister A: The γ-glutamyl cycle: a possible transport system for amino acids. Proc Natl Acad Sci USA 67:1248, 1970

DISORDERS OF AMINO ACID TRANSPORT

WILLIAM L. NYHAN

HARTNUP DISEASE

Hartnup disease is an unusual disorder in which the transport of certain amino acids, including tryptophan is abnormal in the intestine and in the renal tubule. It was named for the first family described, in which 4 of the 8 children of parents who were first cousins were affected. The constant feature of the disease is an amino-aciduria of characteristic pattern.

Clinical characteristics are intermittent and variable. Affected siblings in the original family did not develop clinical manifestations until 6 to 8 years of age. Patients have appeared to develop pellagra, with a red scaly eruption on the exposed skin. Photosensitivity is present, and therefore manifestations in the skin are related to exposure and dosage of ultraviolet radiation. In addition, patients have cerebellar ataxia that occurs in attacks of variable severity, but the effects are completely reversible. Other patients have had attacks of collapsing or fainting or severe headache or psychiatric abnormalities similar to those observed in pellagra. Mental retardation is common but not uniform, and deterioration has not been documented. Attacks have been precipitated by infection, sulfonamide therapy, and dietary inadequacy. Genetic analysis suggests transmission as an autosomal recessive characteristic. Cases have been reported very infrequently in North America; this may reflect a degree of protection against clinical symptoms by a generally very adequate diet.

Patients may be recognized, even in the absence of symptomatology, by the amino-aciduria. It is renal in type, and plasma concentrations of amino acids are normal or somewhat decreased. The following amino acids are excreted in 5 to 10 times the usual amounts: threonine, serine, asparagine, glutamine, alanine, valine, isoleucine, leucine, tyrosine, phenylalanine, histidine, and tryptophan. This is a large group of amino acids, but the pattern is striking. It differs from the commonly encountered generalized amino-aciduria in that excretions of glycine, glutamic acid, and lysine are normal and that there is no free proline or hydroxyproline in the urine. The dibasic amino acids arginine and ornithine are excluded, as is lysine. The urine in this condition is also characterized by the presence of a number of indolic derivatives of tryptophan. Indican (indoxyl sulfate), indolylacetic acid, indolylacetylglutamine, and

breakdown products of indolylpyruvic acid are readily recognized using paper chromatography. On the other hand, normal products of tryptophan metabolism such as kynurenine and nicotinic acid are found in reduced amounts. These patients respond to an oral load of tryptophan with abnormally increased excretion of indican and indolic acids. Tryptophan loading after sterilization of the intestinal flora with antibiotics results in a small increase in indole excretion in control subjects, while patients with Hartnup disease have virtually no increase, and unabsorbed trytophan accumulates in the feces. These observations indicate that there is a defect in the absorption of tryptophan in the cells of the intestine as well as in the kidney. The idoles found in the urine in this disease are secondary to the action of intestinal bacteria on unabsorbed tryptophan.

Most patients have been treated with nicotinamide. It is not certain that improvements observed in cutaneous and neurologic manifestations with treatment were not spontaneous, but treatment is recommended, as is good general protein nutrition.

CYSTINURIA

Cystinuria is an inherited defect in renal tubular function in which the reabsorption of cystine, lysine, aginine, and ornithine is impaired. The abnormality is of clinical significance because of the isolubility of cystine, which forms stones when it is present in the urine in high concentration. The excretion of the other three amino acids does not influence the health of the patient.

Patients with cystinuria generally develop calculi some time before the age of 30 years. Some have large numbers of calculi that require surgical removal for relief of colic or obstruction. Repeated infections of the urinary tract and renal failure are common. The stones are aggregations of cystine that vary from tiny sands or gravel to staghorn calculi filling the renal pelvis or huge calculi of the bladder. Pure cystine crystals are radiolucent, but a variable calcium content provides opacity in many stones. These patients do not have symptoms other than those resulting from stone formation. Statistically, groups of patients with cystinuria are shorter in stature than others. They should be distinguished from patients with cystinosis, in whom the Lignac-de Toni-Fanconi syndrome of glycosuria, generalized amino-aciduria, phosphaturia, and renal rickets is associated with deposits of cystine in tissues such as the kidney, cornea, and bone marrow. Such patients do not have abnormal amounts of cystine in the urine.

In cystinuria the concentrations of cystine and the other amino acids in the blood are not elevated. The clearances of cystine, lysine, arginine, and ornithine are markedly elevated. That of cystine approximates the glomerular filtration rate. These amino acids compete for a common tubular transport mechanism, and infusion of lysine in control individuals results in an increase in excretion of the other three amino acids, while in cystinuric individuals lysine infusion does not alter the excretion of the other three, thus indicating that they are already being excreted maximally. Evidence has been obtained that, as in Hartnup disease, there is also a disorder of intestinal absorption in some patients with cystinuria that involves the amino acids cystine, lysine, arginine, and ornithine. Inefficiently absorbed lysine, arginine, and ornithine are converted by intestinal bacteria to the diamines cadaverine and putrescine, which may be detected in the urine as well as in the feces.

Genetic studies indicate that there are at least three forms of cystinuria in which the homozygotes are clinically indistinguishable. They are now designated types I, II, and III. In type I the heterozygotes are detectable only by studies of intestinal transport of cystine or the dibasic amino acids. This is the most common form, accounting for almost two-thirds of all carriers. Type I homozygotes, of course, also have the intestinal transport defect. In types II and III the heterozygotes excrete increased amounts of cystine and lysine in the urine. Excretion of arginine and ornithine may also be increased. Type II differs from type III in that an oral load of cystine appears not to be absorbed into the blood, and lysine transport is altered in intestinal cells in vitro. The three genes are allelic, and double heterozygotes have been observed who carry two different abnormal genes and thus have clinical manifestations of homozygous cystinuria.

Cystinuria is relatively common, occurring about once in every 20,000 live births. The condition can be screened for as in homocystinuria using the simple cyanide nitroprusside test. Confirmation of the diagnosis requires a quantitative assay of cystine content.

Treatment of cystinuria is aimed at prevention of urinary lithiasis. Stones are regularly seen when cystine concentrations are over 300 mg/liter, which occur with excretions of over 250 mg of cystine per gram of creatinine. Crystallization and stone formation can be minimized by increasing urine volumes or by increasing cystine solubility. However, very large amounts of oral fluids are required. Alkalinization can markedly promote the solubility of cystine, but the effect is small until the urine pH is over 7.6, which is not readily achieved physiologically. Systematic drinking of water through the night is essential for maintenance of adequate urine volumes, but in practice very few adults and almost no children will drink enough to prevent stones. Therefore penicillamine therapy has brought about a real advance in the management of this disease. Penicillamine forms a mixed disulfide with cysteine that is considerably more soluble than cystine. The addition of this compound to readily crystallizing cystinuric urine prevents crystallization. Similarly, oral administration of penicillamine to crystinuric patients is capable of reducing cystine contents in the urine to levels at which stones should not form. This type of therapy requires careful quantitative monitoring of cystine excretion and its concentration in urine if success is to be achieved.

Two conditions that relate to cystinuria are currently known as hyperdibasicamino-aciduria and hypercystinuria. In the former the dibasic amino acids lysine, ornithine, and arginine are excreted in large amounts because of a renal tubular absorptive defect, but cystine excretion is normal. Lysine transport in the intestine also appears to be abnormal. The trait is inherited as a dominant and appears to have no clinical manifestations. In the other condition, cystine is excreted in the urine in increased amounts due to a specific tubular transport defect, while excretion of the dibasic amino acids is normal. The amounts of cystine in the urine in this condition are only 25 percent of those found in cystinuria. Clinical manifestations have not been observed, but the disorder has been observed in only one family. The existence of these two conditions indicates that more than one transport system is involved in the excretion of cystine and the dibasic amino acids. Anyone with large amounts of cystine in the urine is in danger of developing calculi.

IMINOGLYCINURIA

Renal iminoglycinuria appears to be a benign chemical abnormality without clinical manifestations. Its occurrence has provided interesting information on human renal tubular transport. In this situation there is selective impairment in the shared transport system for proline, hydroxyproline, and glycine. Net renal tubular reabsorption of the imino acids is about 80 percent of normal, and that of glycine is about 60 percent of normal. An intestinal transport defect for the same amino acids has been observed in some families but not in others.

In most heterozygotes there is impaired renal tubular transport of glycine. Thus these individuals may present with tubular hyperglycinuria. It is thought that this accounts for patients with glycinuria reported as having a dominantly inherited condition. On the other hand, some heterozygotes may be silent (that is, they may have no glycinuria). These observations and those of intestinal transport suggest that there is more than one allelic mutation responsible for iminoglycinuria.

References

HARTNUP DISEASE

Baron DN, Dent CE, Harris H, Hart EW, Jepson JB: Hereditary pellagra-like skin rash with temporary cerebellar ataxia, constant renal amino-aciduria, and other bizarre biochemical features. Lancet 2:-421, 1956

Milen MD, Crawford MC, Girao CB, Loughridge L: The metabolic abnormality of Hartnup disease. Biochem J 72:30P, 1959

Scriver CR: Hartnup disease. A genetic modification of intestinal and renal transport of certain neutral alpha-amino acids. N Engl J Med 273:530, 1965

CYSTINURIA

Crawhall JC: Cystinuria—Diagnosis and treatment. In Nyhan WL (ed): Heritable Disorders of Amino Acid Metabolism. New York, Wiley, 1974, p 593

——— Scowen EF, Watts RWE: Effect of penicillamine on cystinuria. Br Med J 1:588, 1963

Harris H, Robson EB: Cystinuria. Am J Med 28:774, 1957

Rosenberg LE: Genetic heterogeneity in cystinuria. In Nyhan WL (ed): Amino Acid Metabolism and Genetic Variation. New York, McGraw-Hill, 1967, p 341

IMINOGLYCINURIA

Rosenberg LF, Durant JL, Elsas LJ: Familial glycinuria. An inborn error of renal tubular transport. N Engl J Med 278:1407, 1968

Scriver CR: Renal tubular transport of proline, hydroxyproline and glycine: III. Genetic basis for more than one mode of uptake in human kidney. J Clin Invest 47:823, 1968

———— Bergeron M: Amino acid transport in kidney. The use of mutation to dissect membrane and transepithelial transport. In Nyhan WL (ed): Heritable Disorders of Amino Acid Metabolism. New York, Wiley, 1974, 515

ANOMALIES OF PURINE AND PYRIMIDINE METABOLISM

William L. Nyhan

Hyperuricemia

Primary gout (hyperuricemia) has been recognized since antiquity as a genetically determined disorder in which increased concentrations of uric acid are found in the blood. It is now clear that populations of hyperuricemic patients are quite heterogeneous. The numbers and types of these disorders are just beginning to be defined.

Hyperuricemia may or may not be associated at any period of life with clinical manifestations such as acute gouty arthritis, tophaceous accumulations of uric acid in and around joints and elsewhere, urinary calculi or crystalluria, and progressive renal failure. It may be that primary gout is renal in etiology as well as metabolic (Table 3). In addition, secondary gout may occur in association with conditions in which large numbers of cells are being broken down, especially in leukemia and its treatment and in conditions in which there is chronic glomerular insufficiency. Uric acid levels in the blood may also be secondarily raised by compounds that compete with uric acid for renal tubular secretion, such as

TABLE 3. Types of Hyperuricemia

Primary	
Metabolic:	overproduction
Renal:	diminished clearance
Secondary	
Cell turnover:	leukemia, polycythemia vera, hemolytic anemia
Renal:	glomerular insufficiency
Pharmacologic:	block urate secretion, chlorthiazide and other diuretics, lactic acid

Any condition that produces hyperuricemia may lead to all the clinical manifestations of gout if it is sufficiently prolonged.

chlorthiazide. Lactic acid accumulating endogenously in metabolic disease may also produce this effect. Elevations of uric acid in the blood have been found in glycogen storage disease due to glucose-6-phosphatase deficiency, and clinical gout has been reported in patients with this disease. Hyperuricemia has also been reported in association with diabetic ketoacidosis, pregnancy, obesity and its treatment with total starvation, hypercholesterolemia, hypoparathyroidism, and psoriasis. Concentrations of uric acid in Down's syndrome may be somewhat higher than in control children. Gout of any type is rare in childhood, and even apparently clear examples of secondary gout in children should be investigated for the presence of a primary inherited disorder.

Primary gout is predominantly a disease of the adult male, occurring in the female after menopause. Hyperuricemia is found in approximately 25 percent of the relatives of gouty individuals. Among these individuals it generally develops in the male after 16 years of age. Occurrence in a teenage male appears to represent the occasional early manifestation of a particularly severe case of gout. In the earlier literature only 17 patients less than 10 years of age with gout had been reported. In this group male predominance was not as striking as in older individuals, nor was the predilection for disease in the lower extremities and the great toe. The early occurrence of tophi, deformities, and renal failure has been striking. Severe gout has usually been a prominent feature in other members of the family. It is probable that all of these patients have had hyperuricemia on the basis of overproduction of uric acid, but only a few have been studied from this point of view. In a patient in whose family severe early gout was common, excessive quantities of uric acid were excreted in the urine as early as 3 months of age, and he converted considerably more ^{15}N-labeled glycine to uric acid than did controls.

Lesch-Nyhan Syndrome

Another type of hyperuricemia in childhood was defined in 1964 in association with a disorder of the central nervous system. This syndrome is relatively more common. Information has been obtained on well over 100 patients, and a number have been reported in the literature. As the pathogenesis of this problem has become clearer, other forms of hyperuricemia have been recognized in children, and certain subgroups of gout in adults have been defined.

The cardinal clinical features of this syndrome are mental retardation of major proportions, cerebral palsy, choreoathetosis, and self-destructive biting (Fig. 4). The biting is not associated with anesthesia. It can be inhibited only by firm physical restraint. Most of the patients have destroyed parts of their lips, and some have partially amputated fingers. Manifestations like those of gout in adults have included hyperuricemia, acute arthritis, hematuria, urinary obstruction associated with crystalluria and calculi, and tophi. Adults with gout have been subclassified on the basis of whether they excrete increased amounts of uric acid in the urine. Patients excreting more than 600 mg of uric acid per day are termed hyperexcretors, while nonhyperexcretors with gout often excrete less uric acid than controls. Children with the Lesch-Nyhan syndrome generally excrete over 600 mg/day. Relative to body weight, control children excrete approximately 10

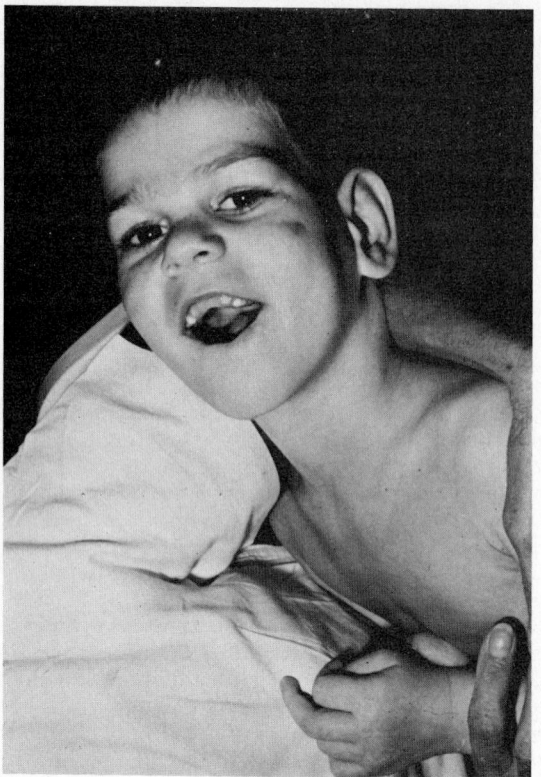

FIG. 4. Hyperuricemia and complete deficiency of the enzyme HGPRT in a 5-year-old boy. He had mental retardation and athetoid cerebral palsy. Self-mutilation is evident in the bitten lower lip.

mg/kg/day, while patients excrete over 40 mg/kg/day. Another way to express urinary excretion is in terms of the excretion of creatinine. These patients usually excrete 3 to 4 mg of uric acid per milligram of creatinine, while in control individuals this ratio is less than one. Overproduction of uric acid is striking. This has been most accurately studied by determining the conversion of isotope-labeled glycine to uric acid. Among adults with overproduction gout, approximately twice as much glycine is converted to uric acid as in controls. These patients have been found to convert 20 times as much glycine to uric acid as controls, and this represents overproduction of uric acid from glycine greater than any previously recorded.

The disease is transmitted as an X-linked recessive characteristic. The primary expression of the abnormal gene is in the activity of the enzyme hypoxanthine guanine phosphoribosyl transferase (HGPRT), which catalyzes the reaction of these purines with phosphoribosyl pyrophosphate to form their respective nucleotides inosinic acid and guanylic acid.

The activity of the enzyme in these patients is too low to be distinguished from zero in the erythrocytes. The enzyme is apparently present in all tissues of the body. Thus the defect can be detected in cultivated fibroblasts and in cells obtained at amniocentesis, and prenatal diagnosis can be made. Female heterozygotes have been shown to have two cell populations, which is definitive confirmation of the Lyon hypothesis of X inactivation. However, the blood of the female carrier is always normal in enzyme activity. The female carrier can be detected most readily by examination of enzyme activity in hair roots.

The treatment of gout in the adult has depended on the use of uricosuric agents. In childhood one would expect most hyperuricemic patients to have increased urinary urate. The use of uricosuric agents in patients of this sort is contraindicated and may lead to acute failure. Dietary therapy has little to recommend it. The treatment of acute gouty arthritis is with colchicine, which must nearly always be given at a dosage sufficient to produce diarrhea in order to terminate an acute attack.

The development of allopurinol for the treatment of hyperuricemia is a significant therapeutic advance. This agent, hydroxypyrazolopyrimidine, depends on the inhibition of xanthine oxidase for the lowering of uric acid concentrations in blood and urine. Side effects are extremely rare, and it is highly effective in treating those aspects of gout or hyperuricemia (arthritis, nephropathy, and tophi) that are caused by uric acid. Treatment with allopurinol has no effect on the cerebral manifestations of hyperuricemic children.

Other Hyperuricemias

It is now apparent that there are a number of different X-linked defects in the enzyme HGPRT. Partial deficiencies account for a certain number of adults with overproduction gout. Children have been observed in whom partial defects in this enzyme have led to renal stone disease, but without abnormalities of the central nervous system.

Other hyperuricemias have begun to be recognized in childhood in which there is overproduction of uric acid but no abnormality in activity of HGPRT. One of these patients also had mild mental retardation, failure to cry with tears, and behavior suggestive of autism.

XANTHINURIA

Xanthinuria is a rarely encountered metabolic disorder in which large amounts of xanthine are excreted in the urine. It may occur without any clinical manifestations, although it was initially recognized in a 4-year-old girl with urinary xanthine calculi and attendant signs of hematuria, frequency, and nonopaque filling defects on pyelography. On the other hand, most individuals in whom xanthine stones are found do not have this disorder. Patients with xanthinuria do not have elevated concentrations of xanthine in the blood. The condition may be diagnosed by the presence of abnormally low concentrations of uric acid in the serum.

Xanthine is the immediate precursor of uric acid. It is formed normally from guanine through the action of guanase, and from hypoxanthine via xanthine oxidase.

Xanthine oxidase is an enzyme of very general substrate specificity that is also responsible for the conversion of xanthine to uric acid. It is found in liver, milk, and intestinal mucosa. Studies carried out on biopsy material from a patient and controls have indicated that this enzyme is deficient in xanthinuria.

The differential diagnosis of hypouricemia includes disorders such as Wilson's disease and the Fanconi syndrome in which renal abnormalities result in inefficient renal tubular reabsorption. This is the defect in the Dalmation dog, where uric acid is cleared at the rate of glomerular filtration. A similar anomaly has been reported in a healthy young man. Treatment of xanthinuria involves the promotion of solution of xanthine in the urine by increasing fluid intake and by alkali therapy.

OROTIC-ACIDURIA

Orotic-aciduria is an inherited disorder of pyrimidine metabolism. It has been studied in detail in a single patient who died of overwhelming varicella at 2.5 years of age. However, extensive studies have been carried out on the family, and they have served to establish genetic transmission as an autosomal recessive characteristic and to localize the metabolic defect. Furthermore, iatrogenic orotic-aciduria has been observed to be a regular concomitant of cancer chemotherapy with 6-azauridine.

Orotic-aciduria is characterized clinically by megaloblastic anemia that is resistant to therapy with vitamin B_{12}, folic acid, or ascorbic acid. Leukopenia, retarded growth, and blue sclerae are also noted. A devastating response to what is usually mild infection is often seen in megaloblastic anemias of early life. The feature that led to the recognition of the condition was crystalluria; crystals precipitated on standing at room temperature, and they were particularly prominent at times of acute illness when the patient reduced his fluid intake. Urethral and ureteral obstruction has been observed on the basis of precipitated crystals.

The biosynthesis of pyrimidines begins with carbamyl phosphate (the compound involved in formation of citrulline from ornithine) and aspartic acid (which yields carbamylaspartic acid). Ring closure to dihydro-orotic acid is followed by oxidation to orotic acid. Orotic acid is converted to its ribonucleotide (orotidylic acid) via the enzyme orotidylic pyrophosphorylase. Orotidylic acid is converted in the presence of orotidylic decarboxylase to uridylic acid, which can then be incorporated into the nucleic acids or transformed to other pyrimidine nucleotides. Orotidylic acid is also readily dephosphorylased to its riboside orotidine. Patients treated with 6-azauridine excrete large amounts of both orotic acid and orotidine in the urine, which is consistent with the action of the drug as a competitive inhibitor of orotidylic decarboxylase. In congenital orotic-aciduria, only orotic acid is found in excess in the urine. Enzymatic studies carried out on the parents of the first patient indicated reduced activities of both orotidylic acid decarboxylase and orotidylic pyrophosphorylase.

These studies have been traced through four generations of this family, establishing an autosomal recessive mode of transmission. Erythrocytes, liver tissue, and fibroblasts of homozygotes have now been shown to be deficient in the activity of both enzymes.

A therapeutic approach to this condition has been successfully made by replacement of the missing nucleotide or its precursor. Excellent remission has been obtained with a mixture of the pyrimidine nucleotides cytidylic acid and uridylic acid. Hematologic response has been accompanied by weight gain for the first time in 18 months and marked improvement in activity and development. Concomitantly, the amounts of orotic acid in the urine have decreased, an effect that suggests a negative-feedback effect of the nucleotides on earlier steps in pyrimidine biosynthesis. Preparations of nucleotides are not well tolerated by mouth. However, the response to oral uridine is equally as good, and it is readily tolerated. Patients with the disease have now been successfully maintained on this therapy for long periods of time.

β-AMINOISOBUTYRIC-ACIDURIA

The excretion of large amounts of β-aminoisobutyric acid in the urine appears to be not a disease but rather a laboratory curiosity and an example of human variation that may be under genetic control. This compound is a breakdown product of the DNA pyrimidine thymine, which may also be formed from valine. Since it reacts with ninhydrin, it may be found in the urine in the course of analysis for amino acids. β-Aminoisobutyric-aciduria may be found as a genetic trait or in conditions such as leukemia, where its presence may reflect increased breakdown of cellular nucleic acids. The genetic trait is inherited as a recessive characteristic. It occurs in about 10 percent of Caucasians, 20 percent of black Americans, and as many as 40 percent of Orientals and American Indians.

References

HYPERURICEMIA

Francke U, Bakay B, Nyhan WL: Detection of heterozygous carriers of the Lesch-Nyhan syndrome by electrophoresis of hair root lysates. J Pediatr 82:472, 1973

Kogut MD, Donnell GN, Nyhan WL, Sweetman L: Disorder of purine metabolism due to partial deficiency of hypoxanthine guanine phosphoribosyl transferase. Am J Med 48:148, 1970

Lesch M, Nyhan WL: A familial disorder of uric acid metabolism and central nervous system function. Am J Med 36:561, 1964

Nyhan WL, James JA, Teberg AJ, Sweetman L, Nelson LG: A new disorder of purine metabolism with behavioral manifestations. J Pediatr 74:20, 1969

The Lesch-Nyhan syndrome. In Creger WP (ed): Annual Review of Medicine, Vol 24. Palo Alto, Annual Reviews, 1973, p 41

Rosenthal IM, Gaballah S, Rafelson MD Jr: Gout in infancy manifested by renal failure. Pediatrics 33:251, 1964

Seegmiller JE, Rosenbloom FM, Kelley WN: Enzyme defect associated with a sex-linked human neurological disorder and excessive purine synthesis. Science 155:1682, 1967

XANTHINURIA

Watts RWE, Engelman K, Klinenberg JR, Seegmiller JE, Sjöersdma A: Enzyme defect in a case of xanthinuria. Nature 201:395, 1964

OROTIC-ACIDURIA

Fallon HJ, Smith LH, Graham JB, Burnett CH: A genetic study of hereditary orotic aciduria. N Engl J Med 270:878, 1964

Huguley CM Jr, Bain JA, Rivers SL, Scoggins RB: Refractory megaloblastic anemia associated with excretion of orotic acid. Blood 14:615, 1959

Smith LH Jr, Huguley CM Jr, Bain JA: Hereditary orotic aciduria. In Stanbury JB, Wyngaarden JB, Fredrickson DS (eds): The Metabolic Basis of Inherited Disease. New York, McGraw-Hill, 1972, p 1003

Carbohydrates

James B. Sidbury, Jr.

A discussion of carbohydrate metabolism must consider dietary intake, transport, assimilation, storage, and mobilization of the sugars. In the liver, cells not only take glucose from the surrounding media but also return it for regulation of its concentration in the media (interstitial fluid and blood). The liver mobilizes glucose in response to specific hormones. The deposition of glucose into glycogen is affected by glucose concentration and certain hormones, such as insulin and hydrocortisone. Fatty acid metabolism is intimately related to and in part is regulated by carbohydrate metabolism. Similarly, certain amino acids are considered gluconeogenic because through transamination and a series of enzymatic steps they are able to form glucose and glycogen. Figure 5 shows the interrelationships among these intermediates. We are only just beginning to understand some of the controlling systems. They are complex and involve several different mechanisms, such as hormonal stimulation or inhibition and feedback control, whereby one of the intermediates of a series of reactions inhibits an earlier step in the series when the latter reactant has reached a certain concentration. Each enzyme protein, and hence enzyme activity, is under genetic control. Mutations can and do occur, resulting in an absence, a decreased amount, or an alteration of the activity of the affected enzyme protein, which may then give rise to an abnormal function and a recognizable alteration that we call a disease. More often than not the disease we recognize (phenotype) is not a direct reflection of the altered or absent protein function but rather is due to other enzyme systems that have been secondarily altered by the primary event. The study of these genetic metabolic abnormalities can yield considerable information about normal metabolic interrelationships.

The clinician is faced with many problems in diagnosing and treating patients with these conditions. The proper tests must be performed to reveal the abnormality. The information is then used to supply the missing substance when possible (such as insulin in diabetes), to design a diet that bypasses the defective system (as with galactose in galactosemia), or to provide an agent that will in some way overcome the failure of regulation (such as ACTH and cortisone in some patients with hypoglycemia).

DIABETES MELLITUS

William B. Weil, Jr. and Arthur F. Kohrman

Diabetes mellitus is a chronic disease, usually familial in origin, in which the basic lesion is unknown. It is thought that the fundamental genetic abnormality is present from conception, despite the variable time of clinical onset in childhood or adult life. The disease, when clinically apparent, is seen initially as a complex disturbance in carbohydrate utilization; later, most patients show abnormalities of the vascular system. The onset, extent, and sites of vascular damage are highly variable in different patients. The prevalence of diabetes mellitus in children under 15 years of age is estimated to be 40 cases per 100,000 population in the United States. The incidence of this disease in children is of the order of 10,000 new cases each year in the United States.

GENETICS. Most geneticists agree that there is a strong genetic predisposition that contributes to the clinical expression of diabetes, but that specific environmental factors such as infectious agents, diet, and life patterns are important in triggering development of a clinically recognizable disorder. Recent studies indicate quite clearly that the genetic component is itself heterogeneous and suggest that there are multiple distinct entities that are manifest as clinical diabetes.

Classic evidence for a heritable component in diabetes rests primarily on observation of a threefold increase in risk of diabetes among first-degree relatives of known diabetics and on a concordance of 48 percent reported for diabetes among monozygotic twins, as opposed to 8 percent concordance with dizygotic twins. Autosomal recessive inheritance has been suggested by many investigators, but the reported low incidence of clinical diabetes among offsprings of two diabetic parents is inconsistent with simple recessive transmission. In studies utilizing either abnormal glucose tolerance or loss of the initial peak of glucose-stimulated insulin secretion as biochemical markers, some investigators have found virtually 100 percent concordance in monozygotic twins or, when modified for age and rate of appearance of biochemical abnormality, have predicted that 100 percent of offspring of conjugal diabetics would eventually develop glucose intolerance. While these findings are seemingly compatible with autosomal recessive inheritance, they are not inconsistent with polygenic or heterogeneous modes of transmission. Those individuals who actually manifest clinical diabetes at any given time represent only a proportion of individuals who, by virtue of their genotype, are at risk for developing the disorder. As a result, distinguishing between as yet unaffected but genotypically susceptible individuals and genetically unaffected individuals is impossible. Consequently it is also impossible to distin-

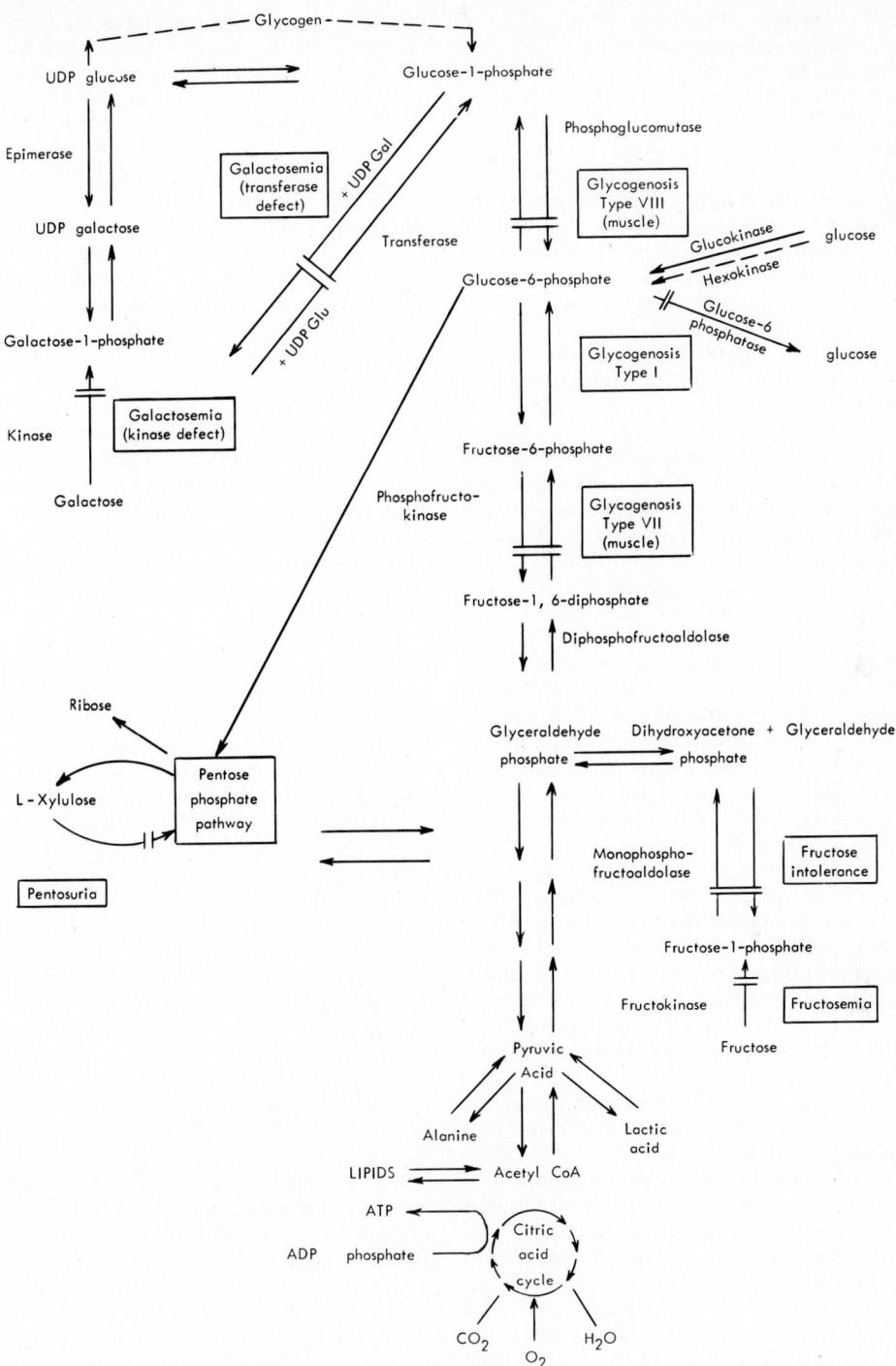

FIG. 5. Pathways of carbohydrate metabolism.

guish autosomal recessive inheritance from polygenic inheritance on the basis of population studies alone.

Several recent investigations indicate that in certain families the adult-onset type of diabetes appearing in adolescence or childhood may be inherited as an autosomal dominant. Several four-generation families are included in these studies with consistent parent-to-child transmission in which all affected offspring have an affected parent and in which approximately 50 percent of appropriate offspring are affected. Additionally, an antagonist to insulin action has been identified in some kindreds, and when it is present it appears to be inherited in an autosomal dominant fashion.

The most prevalent forms of diabetes mellitus may be due to polygenic inheritance in which alleles at an undetermined number of loci may, because of their combined actions, induce a genetic predisposition to diabetes. Interaction of an appropriate genotype with one or several environmental factors such as diet, viral agents, pregnancy, or stress would then lead to clinical symptomatology. In this model the stronger the genetic predisposition, the smaller the environmental component required to produce actual disease. The converse would also be true. Recent studies suggesting that some cases of the juvenile-onset type of diabetes follow viral illness are compatible with this hypothesis. A polygenic model is also quite consistent with the unimodal distribution of values for glucose tolerance in the total population and with the low incidence of diabetes among offspring of conjugal diabetics. Furthermore, the clinical and physiologic variability in the expression of diabetes in relatively inbred ethnic populations circumstantially supports the polygenic model. Strong positive evidence for polygenic inheritance will require the identification of specific enzyme alterations in carbohydrate metabolism among diabetics. By analogy to gout, another broadly defined, widespread, and genetically heterogeneous disorder of metabolism for which multiple specific enzyme alterations have now been defined, it can be inferred that both polygenic inheritance and genetic heterogeneity are reasonable hypotheses in diabetes.

Several methodologic problems contribute to the difficulty of studying hereditary factors in diabetes. For example, although diabetes is clinically quite variable, most population studies of genetic factors operative in diabetes have considered it to be a single disorder; thus new data must now be collected in which specific subpopulations are described. Second, the primary lesions giving rise to clinical diabetes are not known; the observable derangements in carbohydrate metabolism may be several steps removed from the primary metabolic defect or defects. The absence of specific primary biochemical markers and the consequent reliance on a complex metabolic phenomenon for case identification (glucose intolerance) make genetic analysis nearly impossible. Recent reports indicate that certain histocompatibility antigens in the HL-A system (HL-A8 and W15) are present in a significantly higher proportion of insulin-dependent diabetics than in either nondiabetic or insulin-independent diabetics. Further studies may demonstrate that these antigens are markers for juvenile-type diabetes or that they identify a genotype with increased susceptibility to specific environmental factors important in the etiology and pathogenesis of diabetes.

Genetic counseling of families at risk for diabetes should probably proceed very cautiously until more is known. In families with clearly autosomal dominant patterns of inheritance, appropriate figures can be given immediately. However, in view of the statistic data presently available, the World Health Organization's suggestion that known diabetics should not marry one another seems unreasonable.

ETIOLOGY.   The fundamental lesion might reside in the peripheral (extrapancreatic) body tissues or in the pancreas or in both. In the juvenile, particularly, we are limited in our understanding of the pathogenesis of diabetes because of our scarce and fragmentary knowledge concerning the natural history of the biochemical changes that precede frank clinical diabetes. There have been experimental observations to support a variety of interpretations, and only general approaches can be discussed here.

A primary insensitivity to insulin action in the peripheral muscle and adipose tissue might initially force elevated insulin secretion for maintenance of normoglycemia, with ultimate exhaustion of pancreatic beta cell secretory capacity. It is possible to postulate a model in which peripheral factors leading to insulin resistance and pancreatic factors (possibly genetically determined) that set limits on the ability of the pancreas to respond to increased demands for insulin secretion might combine to produce the clinical diabetic state in the face of a variety of simultaneous environmental stresses. Among the findings that suggest a significant role for peripheral factors is the increased requirement of insulin for normoglycemia in both chemical and clinical diabetics that fluctuates significantly with the degree of obesity; in some juvenile as well as adult chemical diabetics, glucose intolerance can be markedly moderated if not completely ameliorated by weight reduction. On the other hand, evidence for reduced capacity for insulin secretion is found in asymptomatic patients with glucose intolerance but without frank clinical diabetes (so-called chemical diabetes). In these patients, both juvenile and adult, delays in insulin secretion in response to glucose load have been demonstrated. Some investigators have also reported absence of the first of the two peaks of insulin secretion that normally follow a glucose load in chemical diabetics. These observations could be combined in a conceptual synthesis that could account for many of the variations seen in clinical severity, age of onset, and genetic heterogeneity described previously.

The presence of serum antagonists to insulin or specific antibodies that might reduce the effectiveness of circulating insulin could constitute another possible stimulus to abnormal demands on the pancreas for insulin secretion. Similarly, the diabetogenic actions of growth hormone and adrenal corticosteroids might contribute to a peripheral demand for insulin secretion by stimulation of lipolysis and hepatic gluconeogenesis. Indeed, some investigators suggest a major role for growth hormone in the initiation of the sequence of events leading to clinical diabetes.

Recently much attention has been focused on proinsulin, a precursor of insulin in the process of its synthesis in the pancreatic islets. However, most studies show that levels of proinsulin and insulin are generally parallel, and no convincing evidence has been brought forth to suggest that the proinsulin molecule or its various fragments or other abnormalities of insulin synthesis play a role in the pathogenesis of diabetes mellitus.

Apparent clustering of cases of juvenile diabetes mellitus following outbreaks of various viral diseases has been reported. It has been suggested that virus infection of the pancreas may provide a specific etiology for diabetes in a small number of cases. Whether these agents would operate alone or become environmental insults to provoke the clinical appearance of diabetes in a genetically predisposed individual remains speculative. Autoimmunity has also been implicated in the etiology of diabetes in a small number of children. The evidence is circumstantial and arises from the observation that circulating antibodies to endocrine (thyroid, adrenal, and parathyroid) and gastric tissues are found in increased frequency in children with diabetes. While it is generally observed that children with diabetes treated with exogenous insulin almost uniformly develop circulating antibodies to insulin, these have not been demonstrated in new untreated diabetics and thus are not likely to be involved in the etiology of diabetes. Recently, specific antibodies to pancreatic islet cells have been demonstrated by immunofluorescence techniques in a large proportion of patients with previously untreated juvenile-onset diabetes. Whether these antibodies are related to the pathogenesis of juvenile diabetes or represent another early manifestation of the disease is unknown at present.

There has been much interest in a possible role for glucagon, the pancreatic alpha cell secretion, in the pathogenesis of the diabetic syndrome. Following development of a reliable radioimmunoassay for glucagon, it became clear that increased levels in serum are present in most, if not all, untreated diabetic subjects. More recently, strong evidence has been introduced to implicate glucagon in a significant role in the pathogenesis of the keto-acidotic manifestations of untreated diabetes mellitus. Thus the concept of the diabetes syndrome as the absence of insulin secretion alone becomes even less tenable.

PATHOLOGY. Despite the incontrovertible evidence that both juvenile-onset and adult-onset diabetes are associated with islet beta cell dysfunction, no consistent morphologic islet cell pathology has yet been demonstrated that can be implicated as a causal or primary defect. Among the major histopathologic changes of the pancreas, hyalinization of the islets of Langerhans is perhaps the most typical lesion described. The reported prevalence of hyalinization appears to be related to the age of the patients studied; it is rarely present in juvenile diabetics. The presence of hyaline does not appear to be related to either the duration or the severity of the diabetic state. In addition, a significant number of nondiabetic individuals develop hyalinization of their islets as they get older. The reported incidence of hyaline in nondiabetic populations over 50 years of age varies from 10 to 16.6 percent. The hyaline material found within islets has the histochemical and ultrastructural characteristics of amyloid. It has been reported that the amyloid within islets will bind fluorescein-labeled insulin, thus suggesting that the amyloid may be composed, at least in part, of an antibody to insulin.

Fibrosis of the exocrine and endocrine pancreas is seen in both adult-onset and juvenile diabetes. In one series interacinar fibrosis was found in 60 percent of adult-onset diabetics and in 40 percent of matched controls. In the same series intrainsular pericapillary fibrosis was less common but more specific, being present in 19 percent of diabetics but only 7 percent of controls. Some degree of fibrosis is not uncommon in most cases of juvenile diabetes.

Several authors have reported that in comparison to nondiabetics there is an absolute reduction of approximately 50 percent in islet cell mass in juvenile diabetics because of a reduction in beta cells. The reduction in islet cell mass is three times greater in young patients with chronic diabetes than in those dying within the first 8 weeks of their disease. Using differential granule stains, complete or partial degranulation in all juvenile diabetics under the age of 20 years has been noted in one series. In addition, beta cell degranulation is present in 80 percent of patients between 20 and 40 years of age, in 50 percent of those between 40 and 60 years, and in 33 percent of those over 60 years. There is generally good agreement between these findings and the amount of extractable insulin present in the pancreas in diabetics of various ages.

Finally, a rare inflammatory lesion of islets has been described in children and young adults with a history of fulminant diabetic coma, presumably precipitated by infection in a patient with no previous history of diabetes. The islets of Langerhans are infiltrated by lymphocytes and on occasion by monocytes and neutrophils. Diminution of beta cell granulation and vacuolization has been described in association with the inflammatory infiltrate. An autoimmune or an infectious etiology has been postulated for this lesion, but direct evidence is lacking.

The vascular and neural complications of diabetes mellitus, which are usually seen in long-standing cases but occasionally in juveniles, are accompanied by characteristic lesions of the retina, the kidney, the peripheral nerves, and the large and small blood vessels of the entire body. A description of these complications and their progression is beyond the scope of this chapter; appropriate references are cited. The relationship of the time of onset and severity of these lesions to degree of control of blood sugar levels remains a lively controversy with obvious implications for the general approach to clinical management adopted by each physician.

Of considerable controversy are the electron microscopic observations of thickening of the basement membrane of small vessels in peripheral muscle of prediabetic individuals who have neither hyperglycemia nor glucose intolerance. Those observations raise the question that the terminal vascular phenomena heretofore considered to be complications of long-standing diabetes may actually be independent expressions of another, more basic lesion. However, other evidence disputes these findings and relates the extent of the basement membrane thickening to the duration and severity of the carbohydrate intolerance.

PATHOPHYSIOLOGY. Whatever the basic abnormality in diabetes mellitus, the clinically apparent metabolic disturbances can be related to three general alterations: reduced entry of glucose into the cell, which leads to unavailability of carbohydrate as a substrate for energy needs, and utilization by the cell of alternate substrates, namely, fatty acids derived from adipose stores and amino acids from body protein. Alterations in carbohydrate metabolism include accumulation of ingested carbohydrate in the blood, increased glycogenolysis, reduction of hepatic glycogen synthesis, and increased gluconeogenesis from amino acids.

Fat is the alternate substrate first utilized when carbohydrate is unavailable. The result of increased fatty acid oxidation is increased production of acetyl CoA and subsequent accumulation of the by-products of acetyl CoA metabolism: acetone, acetoacetic acid, and β-hydroxybutyric acid. This process is enhanced by the increased lipolysis seen in the absence of insulin. In the normal individual the ketone substances can be used as sources of energy, primarily in muscle, but in the untreated diabetic they accumulate faster than they are utilized. The result is elevated ketone levels in the serum and urine.

Since the keto acids have a lower effective pK′ than bicarbonate, the major extracellular buffer, bicarbonate, is converted to carbonic acid and water with elevation of H^+ in the body fluids; the ketones are excreted as salts. These processes contribute to the excessive cation losses (sodium and potassium) in the urine and the large obligatory water loss resulting from the osmotic diuresis due to hyperglycemia and glycosuria. The result of these events is the complex of hyperglycemia, ketonemia, acidemia, glycosuria, ketonuria, and severe dehydration characteristically seen in the diabetic with untreated keto-acidosis.

Elevated serum cholesterol is another result of increased acetyl CoA production. Lipolysis is very active in the untreated diabetic, and serum triglyceride and free fatty acid levels are also high. The utilization of protein to supply amino acids for gluconeogenesis is coupled with decreased rates of protein synthesis. These factors combine to produce the weight loss, diminished rate of growth, and cachexia frequently seen in the untreated juvenile diabetic patient.

JUVENILE DIABETES MELLITUS. A diabetic state has been recognized in the immediate neonatal period; it appears to be a transitory and self-limited process without known cause, and only occasionally does it require insulin. However, cases of permanent diabetes mellitus have been reported beginning in the first 6 months after birth. Marked differences exist in the manifestations of this disease in children and adults. Because of these differences, which are summarized in Table 4, the approach to diagnosis and treatment is altered in a way appropriate to the age group involved.

PREDIABETES AND SUBCLINICAL DIABETES. Prediabetes refers to that period of life from conception until the first abnormalities in carbohydrate metabolism can be detected in a future diabetic. There is evidence to suggest that during this period, in some cases, biochemical abnormalitites may exist in the absence of clinical signs and may be demonstrable by means of special testing. It is also at this stage that the earliest changes in the vascular system have been detected. By definition, the ordinary fasting blood sugar, glucose tolerance test, and cortisone-stressed glucose tolerance test are all normal in the prediabetic stage.

The second stage of this disease has been termed subclinical diabetes and represents the period during which carbohydrate metabolism may be grossly abnormal only in the presence of infection or other stressful situations such as surgery or trauma. Similarly, the cortisone-stressed glucose tolerance test will be abnormal during this period, whereas the fasting sugar and glucose tolerance test in the absence of stress will remain normal. The child will be asymptomatic, and the presence of carbohydrate intolerance is usually noted accidentally. Urinalysis performed during an acute illness or following trauma or surgery may be reported as indicating the presence of glucose in the urine. Immediate investigation with an oral glucose tolerance test will usually reveal an abnormality in carbohydrate metabolism. A short period later the test will revert to normal. The durations of the prediabetic and subclinical stages are unknown, and individuals may remain in one or the other of these stages throughout childhood. It is even conceivable that some individuals may live a full lifetime in one of these stages of diabetes without ever developing clinically apparent diabetes.

The use of oral hypoglycemic agents has been advocated for children in this stage in an attempt to postpone the onset of overt diabetes. One might argue that the use of such agents could actually hasten the appearance of the clinical state by further stressing the already incompetent and presumably deteriorating mechanisms of insulin secretion. In addition, the results of a long-term study of the oral agents in adults have raised questions about their efficacy and caused very serious concern about their safety. The use of these agents, therefore, is generally considered to be contraindicated and, despite controversy, should remain so until more is known concerning the etiology and natural history of the diabetic state.

LATENT DIABETES. The third state in the progression of the diabetic state has been termed latent or chemical

TABLE 4. Comparison of Juvenile and Adult-Onset Forms of Diabetes Mellitus

Characteristic	Juvenile	Adult-Onset
Onset	Rapid, obvious	Slow, insidious
Obesity	No role	Predisposing factor
Dietary treatment alone	Not adequate	Possible in one-half of cases
Use of oral hypoglycemic agents	Contraindicated	Probably not indicated
Need for insulin	Universal	Present in one-half of cases
Hypoglycemia and keto-acidosis	Common	Uncommon
Symptomatic degenerative vascular changes	After adolescence	May be present at time of diagnosis

diabetes. This period is characterized by a persistently abnormal glucose tolerance test but normal fasting blood sugars. There are elevated blood sugar levels and glycosuria following meals. From retrospective evaluation it would appear that this stage of diabetes is relatively brief in children, lasting from several days to several months. However, it is becoming increasingly obvious that with meticulous testing there are significant numbers of children in whom these changes of latent diabetes can be demonstrated. The number varies from study to study, but up to one-third of the siblings of diabetic children have been reported to show changes in glucose tolerance. Presently available data indicate that less than 10 percent of the siblings of juvenile diabetics who require insulin become frankly diabetic themselves, thus indicating that there is a significant population of children who show chemical changes of latent diabetes without clinical manifestations. The old belief that the period of latent diabetes, if detectable, was relatively brief in children must therefore undergo revision. Since there is no way of determining which of the children with latent diabetes will become overtly diabetic, or on what timetable, mass screening of juveniles is not advised, although future studies may reveal a particular high-risk population for whom screening would be indicated. Postprandial hypoglycemic episodes may occur periodically in this stage prior to the onset of overt diabetes as a premonitory indication of overt diabetes.

OVERT DIABETES. Overt clinical diabetes mellitus usually appears abruptly in children, and the transition from the latent to the overt stage is often accompanied by some stress such as infection or emotional upset. The pattern of the age of onset of overt diabetes in children suggests several factors that may be important in precipitating the transition to this stage; 20 to 25 percent of children with diabetes develop the disease between 5 and 10 years of age, and an additional 40 percent between 10 and 15 years of age. In addition to the increased incidence with each 5-year age increment, there are several peak years of incidence in childhood, the two most readily recognized being approximately 6 and 12 years of age, corresponding to the beginning of the school years and the beginning of adolescence.

DIAGNOSIS. Diagnosis of diabetes mellitus in young people is usually simple and straightforward.

Characteristically the transition from the latent to the overtly diabetic state occurs rapidly and dramatically. The classic symptoms of polyuria, polydipsia, and polyphagia are prominent and occur in at least three-fourths of the cases. Polyuria is frequently manifest by nocturia or by some change in previously established patterns of urination, such as onset of enuresis. Weight loss or failure to gain weight is the next most common complaint.

Other manifestations frequently encountered are fatigability and lethargy. On occasion the preliminary symptoms are so mild that they are relatively unnoticed by the family, and the presenting complaints may be abdominal pains and vomiting characteristic of ketosis, increased respiratory effort resulting from acidosis, or the decreasing state of consciousness of diabetic coma (Fig. 6).

The more advanced the diabetic state when first seen, the simpler it is to arrive at the proper diagnosis. If the patient has hyperglycemia, glucosuria, ketonuria, and metabolic acidosis, there are few conditions other than diabetes that could produce these findings. In the less severe states it becomes increasingly difficult to make the diagnosis with certainty. Abnormal elevation of blood sugar values is essential for the diagnosis of untreated diabetes mellitus, but glucosuria with normoglycemia may occur with renal glycosuria and in metabolic disturbances associated with other alterations in the renal tubular handling of glucose.

In the presence of borderline or equivocal laboratory findings, in the absence of ketonuria, and when a classic history is lacking, definitive therapy should be withheld until the diagnosis is clearly established. The patient whose values are not clearly abnormal is likely to be in a subclinical or latent diabetic stage that has been exacerbated by a recent stressful situation. It is difficult to determine if or when such an individual is going to become frankly diabetic. Until more information is available about the natural course of these early stages of diabetes in children, it is well not to treat with hypoglycemic agents. If such a child is going to become frankly diabetic, there is no known harm in procrastinating until more obvious findings are present. The difficulty in choosing this course is in communication with the family. A thorough explanation of the implications inherent in a diagnosis of diabetes mellitus will usually

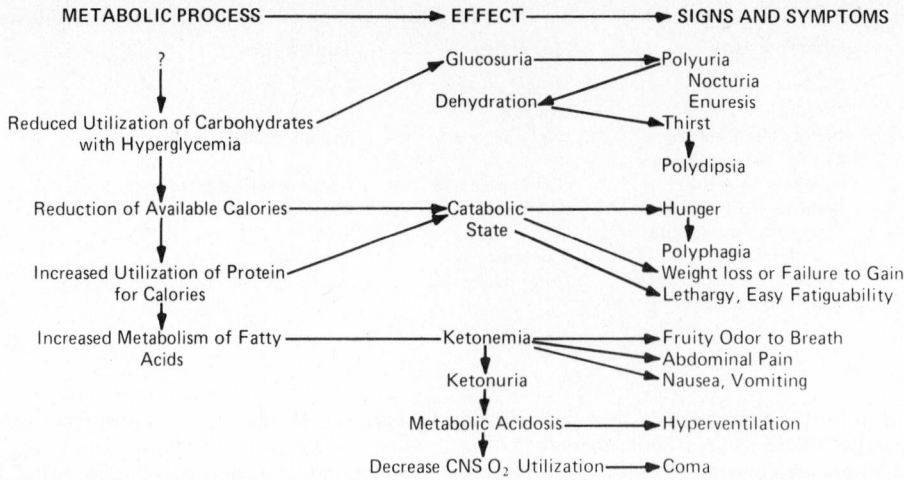

FIG. 6. Mechanisms by which disturbed metabolic processes produce signs and symptoms of diabetes mellitus.

convince the family that one should have a very clear picture of the diagnosis before proceeding with treatment.

Although hospitalization is usually indicated when diabetes mellitus is the likely diagnosis, there are a few circumstances in which it may be appropriate to establish the diagnosis and begin treatment on an ambulatory basis. An example would be in a child with hyperglycemia and glucosuria, but no ketosis or acidosis, in a stable and intelligent family that is already familiar with the disease process. In the presence of glucosuria and ketonuria, and obviously in the patient with acidosis and coma, hospitalization should be immediate. Unsuspected acidosis may already be present or acidosis may develop in a matter of hours in any child with glucosuria and ketonuria. Once symptoms are present, the course may become rapidly progressive, and treatment should be begun as soon as the diagnosis is established.

Severity of Initial Illness. The symptoms with which the child presents will be directly related to the degree and duration of metabolic derangement at the time of admission. One can arbitrarily divide the degree of severity into four classes. The first class, in which hyperglycemia and glucosuria are present, will be associated with symptoms such as polyuria, polydipsia, polyphagia, weight loss, and easy fatigability. The second state is that with hyperglycemia, glucosuria, ketonemia, and ketonuria; additional findings may include abdominal pain, anorexia, vomiting, and dehydration. The third clinical state is characterized by the added element of acidosis. Such patients will have hyperventilation, dyspnea, and exhaustion as prominent complaints. At the fourth level of severity children demonstrate hyperglycemia, ketosis, acidosis, and an altered state of consciousness, which may proceed to coma and may be the most important element.

In diabetic keto-acidosis the laboratory values that prove useful include blood glucose and serum acetone,

carbon dioxide content, PCO_2, pH, sodium, and potassium. Of interest, but not generally of immediate value, are serum cholesterol, total lipids, blood urea nitrogen and/or creatinine, serum calcium, and serum phosphorus. To a considerable extent the serum sodium concentration tends to fall with elevation of the blood sugar. In general, an increase of 180 mg/dl in blood glucose will be associated with a decrease of 5 mEq/liter in serum sodium. This relationship is generally based on osmotic equalities, but it may be modified by other physiologic variables.

In the presence of the marked lipemia occasionally seen in untreated diabetics, the levels of all serum electrolytes may appear falsely low due to displacement of the aqueous phase by the lipids contained in the serum. A condition known as hyperosmolar coma occurs rarely in children, but more often in adults. In this state, serum Na^+ concentration may be normal, with very high blood sugar values, thus producing a marked increase in serum osmolarity. It is important to recognize this condition to avoid giving glucose in the initial intravenous fluids. In hyperosmolar coma, ketonemia and ketonuria may paradoxically be absent. Failure to recognize the entity of nonketotic hyperosmolar coma may result in serious delays in diagnosis and in initiation of appropriate therapy. Children with diabetic keto-acidosis are almost always potassium-depleted when first seen. Although initial serum potassium values may be low, normal, or elevated, potassium therapy should be started early.

Infection is often a precipitating agent in any abrupt change in the course of the diabetic state, and procedures necessary to detect infection should always be considered. Leukocytosis itself does not indicate the presence of infection, since white blood cell counts of 20,000 to 30,000 cells/mm³ may occur without infection in diabetic keto-acidosis. If infection is suspected and appropriate cultures have been taken, antibiotic therapy should be instituted.

Among many variables tested, serum ketone levels, measured as acetone, correlate best with survival. In addition, the appropriate serum acetone determination is especially useful in the initial hours of treatment of diabetic acidosis. This procedure can easily be carried out at the bedside, without special technical help or equipment. It is performed as described in Table 5.

TABLE 5. Serum Acetone Determination

Draw blood; after clotting, separate serum (table-top centrifuge)
Add one drop serum to each of 4 to 10 small test tubes
Add tap water: 1 drop to first tube (1:2), 2 drops to second tube (1:3), 3 drops to third tube (1:4), then serial dilutions from 1:4 to 1:8, 1:16, 1:32
Test each tube with Ketostix or Clinistix or Acetest tablet
Record highest dilution that gives faintest purple color (ie, 1:2, 1:3, 1:4, etc)

Laboratory Diagnosis. In juveniles the diagnosis of diabetes mellitus can usually be made without resorting to glucose tolerance tests. Normal values for blood glucose are relatively constant, and the presence of a fasting blood glucose level above 110 mg/dl or a 2-hour postprandial glucose level above 140 mg/dl or a 3-hour level above 120 mg/dl is sufficient evidence for the presumptive diagnosis of diabetes mellitus; one or more of these findings are usually present. Similarly, an elevated blood glucose value accompanied by polyuria and glucosuria are usually sufficient to make the diagnosis of diabetes mellitus and should be the signal for careful observation and prompt initiation of therapy.

The uses of glucose tolerance testing are limited, in general, to two situations: (1) There may be transient glycosuria in a child under stress, such as with fever or following a surgical procedure; the stressful situation may, in fact, provide the opportunity for the detection of chemical diabetes in that child, and it is generally recommended that such transient glycosuria be followed by careful glucose tolerance testing after the child has recovered from the acute incident. (2) There are families in which diabetes has been diagnosed and in which there will be an advantage in identifying other members of the family with glucose intolerance or chemical diabetes. However, as discussed earlier, this type of screening, even within a family, is controversial, and one must weigh carefully the relative value of the information to be gained against the uncertainty and anxiety almost certain to occur in the family in which chemical diabetes is identified.

The factors normally affecting insulin secretion and the elements involved in the general metabolic handling of a glucose load are multiple and extremely complex in their interrelationships. Even though there are severe limitations and many potential sources for error, a well-performed oral glucose tolerance test, in a properly prepared subject, provides the best general information about the overall state of carbohydrate tolerance in most circumstances. The cortisone-stressed glucose tolerance test, primarily a research procedure, may provide a means of detecting subclinical diabetes. The intravenous glucose tolerance test is a more specific measure of the factors that affect peripheral uptake of glucose and the variables related to liver function, but it does not provide an estimate of the state of the normal stimuli for insulin secretion that arise in the gastrointestinal tract.

The variables that can influence the performance and interpretation of oral glucose tolerance tests can be divided into three categories: First, there are significant differences between normal levels of glucose determined on plasma and on whole blood. Similarly, different values will arise from the different chemical methods used for glucose estimation. It is thus necessary to clearly ascertain the normal values and methods used in the laboratory at hand. A second factor is concerned with the administration of the glucose load itself; a variety of commercial glucose preparations or substitutes may be obtained that are intended to make a more palatable substance for administration. However, like the 20 percent aqueous glucose solution usually used, these may provoke nausea and in some cases vomiting. Nausea delays gastric emptying and may result in spurious abnormalities of the curve of glucose tolerance. It is necessary that the oral glucose load be standardized; current recommendations are for 1.75 g/kg, up to a maximum of 100 g. Some investigators have used larger amounts of glucose (up to 2.5 g/kg) in children under 3 years of age. Glucose tolerance tests may be affected by variations in the patient. There are differences in the normal standards for glucose tolerance testing with age, although these are not great. In addition, patients with intercurrent infection or with transient endocrine stress may also show temporary abnormalities of glucose tolerance. The dietary state of the patient is also significant; if there has been a temporary or long-standing dietary insufficiency, especially of carbohydrate, a diabetic type of glucose tolerance curve may be seen in individuals who will show a completely normal pattern when well nourished. Finally, it must be remembered that there is a great multiplicity of factors, known and unknown, involved in insulin secretion. These include humoral, gastrointestinal, neural, and psychologic variables. An abnormality of any of these may produce abnormal glucose tolerance tests that must be repeated when the patient has returned to a more normal state. Although normal values for each laboratory should be established, the values in Table 6 can be used as general guidelines to the normal limits

TABLE 6. Glucose Tolerance Standards*

Time (min)	Mean Blood Glucose (mg/dl)	+/- 2 SD
0	80	100
30	140	210
60	120	180
120	100	140
180	75	120
240	80	110

Adapted from Drash: J Pediatr 78:919, 1971.

for oral glucose tolerance testing in children. These are derived from a group of children between the ages of 4 and 16 years using glucose oxidase reagents.

INITIAL MANAGEMENT. The severity of the diabetic state at the time of admission will determine the approach to therapy. Appropriate treatment should be given for infection or for shock if they are present. The approach to insulin therapy that follows is relatively aggressive. Recent investigations indicate that equally good results are obtained with considerably less insulin given by continuous infusion at a rate of 0.1 unit/kg/hour. Further experience may show that the continuous infusion technique is optimal. However, the long-term success of the aggressive approach to initial management, in terms of both mortality rate and rate of recovery, justifies presenting it here.

The newly diagnosed keto-acidotic child with diabetes usually requires relatively high doses of regular insulin during the early phases of treatment. In these patients there may be relative resistance to the effects of insulin in promoting glucose uptake, due possibly to a combination of the effects of acidemia, ketonemia, and lipemia on the action of insulin and the antagonistic effects of high levels of growth hormone, catecholamines, and corticosteroids that are present. However, the relative resistance to insulin diminishes rapidly with correction of the basic metabolic disorder. The treatment of diabetic keto-acidosis includes four substances: insulin, glucose, salts, and fluids. The typical course of the patient in response to adequate therapy is shown in Figure 7. Children with previously treated diabetes mellitus may not require the same vigorous approach to insulin therapy. No more than half the amount of insulin calculated as follows should be given as the initial injection in the previously treated diabetic child, and individual evaluation must determine subsequent insulin dosage.

Insulin. The amount of regular insulin administered initially is based on the child's condition when he arrives at the hospital. Four clinical states of severity can be defined, and regular insulin is given correspondingly in a dose of 1, 2, 3, or 4 units/kg body weight. The first state, requiring 1 unit/kg, is defined as the presence of glucosuria alone. The second state is characterized by the presence of glucosuria plus ketonuria; the third, as glucosuria, ketonuria, and acidosis, defined by a serum carbon dioxide content of less than 15 mEq/liter and/or an arterial blood pH of less than 7.30 (venous blood pH < 7.25). Acidosis of significant degree can usually be judged clinically by the presence of Kussmaul respirations. The fourth state, requiring 4 units/kg, involves the presence of glucosuria, ketonuria, acidosis, and a decrease in level of consciousness. The entire amount of insulin is given subcutaneously unless there is evidence of actual or impending peripheral vascular collapse. In such a situation the initial dose insulin is given intravenously (Table 7).

The initial dose of insulin is followed in 3 to 4 hours with a second dose, the size of which is based on the change in serum acetone. If the serum acetone has risen in the intervening 3 to 4 hours, the amount of insulin given is twice that of the initial amount. If the serum acetone is unchanged, the initial amount of insulin is repeated. In most situations the serum acetone has fallen from its initial value, and one-half the initial dose is given at this time. The same schedule is used for the insulin dosage given 6 to 8 hours after therapy is begun. (The initial insulin dosage is used as the reference point for these calculations.)

The fourth administration of insulin will be given at approximately 12 hours after therapy is begun. At this time the serum acetone should be considerably lower, and the blood glucose should have fallen to values approaching normal. The urinary glucose will also have decreased. The amounts of insulin given at this time and at 18 hours are based on the degree of glucosuria and ketonuria. An empirical rule that is usually satisfactory is to give 5 units of insulin for each + of urinary sugar (measured with Benedict's solution or Clinitest tablets), 5 additional units in the presence of detectable ketonuria, and 10 additional units if the ketonuria remains 4 +. For children under 5 years of age the amount of insulin for the fourth and fifth injections should be halved.

Glucose. The amount of glucose to be administered during the initial hours of therapy has been the subject of considerable controversy. During the first few hours of treatment there is undoubtedly sufficient glucose in the body stores to meet most requirements, but it is unable to enter cells for utilization. Additional large amounts of carbohydrate given before cellular glucose uptake has been restored may have deleterious effects. Serious hyperosmolarity with neurologic sequellae may occur; in addition, the excess unusable glucose will be excreted and will accentuate the osmotic diuresis, adding further to fluid and electrolyte losses, especially losses of potassium. However, because of the need to maintain isotonicity of the intravenous fluids, 2.5 percent glucose can be given safely during the early hours of therapy.

As soon as the urine glucose begins to fall below 4 +

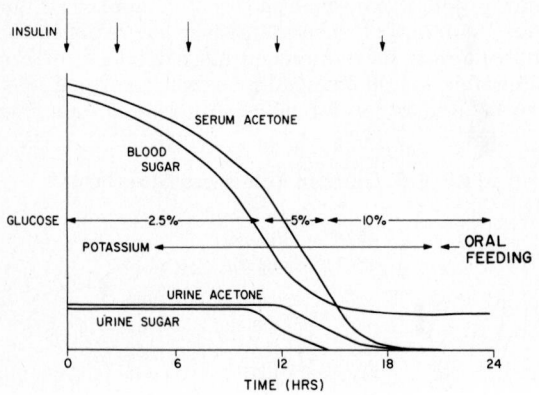

FIG. 7. Typical course of first day's treatment.

TABLE 7. Diabetes Diagnosed in an 8-Year-Old Child*

	Glucosuria	Glucosuria Ketonuria	Glucosuria Ketonuria Acidosis	Glucosuria Ketonuria Acidosis Coma
Initial treatment				
Insulin	1 u/kg = 25 u (sc) Oral, ad lib	2 u/kg = 50 u (sc) iv	3 u/kg = 75 u (sc) iv	4 u/kg = 100 u (sc) iv (initial push of 10 ml/kg = 250 ml)
Fluids				
Maintenance		65 ml/kg = 1700 ml/d	75 ml/kg = 2000 ml/d	75 ml/kg = 2000 ml/d
Repair		50 ml/kg = 1300 ml/d	75 ml/kg = 2000 ml/d	75 ml/kg = 2000 ml/d
Total		115 ml/kg = 3000 ml/d	150 ml/kg = 4000 ml/d	150 ml/kg = 4000 ml/d
Rate		185 ml/hr × 8 hr; 95 ml/hr × 16 hr	250 ml/hr × 8 hr; 125 ml/hr × 16 hr	
Composition		Na^+ = 75 mEq/liter, Cl^- = 75 mEq/liter	Na^+ = 50 mEq/liter, Cl^- = 50 mEq/liter, HCO^- = 25 mEq/liter	Na^+ = 50 mEq/liter, K^+ = 50 mEq/liter, Cl^- = 25 mEq/liter, HCO_3^- = 25 mEq/liter, glucose = 2.5%
Treatment after 4 hr				
Insulin (serum acetone falling)		25 u (sc)	35 u (sc)	50 u (sc)
Fluids				
Composition			Na^+ = 50 mEq/liter, K^+ = 25 mEq/liter, Cl^- = 50 mEq/liter, HCO_3^- = 25 mEq/liter, glucose = 2.5%	
Treatment after 8 hr				
Insulin (serum acetone falling)		25 u (sc)	35 u (sc)	50 u (sc)
Fluids (blood sugar ≦ 300 mg/dl)				
Composition			Increase glucose to 5%	
Treatment after 12 hr				
Insulin (urine sugar 3+, acetone 4+, blood sugar ≦ 250 mg/dl)		25 u (sc)	25 u (sc)	25 u (sc)
Fluids				
Treatment after 16 hr				
Insulin (urine sugar 1+, acetone 2+)		10 u (sc)	10 u (sc)	10 u (sc)
Fluids				
Composition			Increase glucose 10%	

*26 kg, 130 cm, 1 m^2.

or the blood glucose is approaching 200 mg/dl, it is necessary to supplement available carbohydrate by increasing the glucose in the infusion to 5 percent. Once the urine glucose becomes 1+ or negative, or the blood glucose is less than 180 mg/dl, the infused glucose is increased to 10 percent. These amounts will provide sufficient substrate so that additional insulin can be given to restore metabolism to normal; this in turn will promote the correction of the ketosis and acidosis. Usually, after 18 to 24 hours of treatment, high-carbohydrate clear fluids may be given orally. As the oral feedings become adequate, the intravenous fluids may be discontinued, usually between 24 and 36 hours after the onset of therapy.

Fluids and Electrolytes. All fluids are initially given intravenously, and nothing is given by mouth for 18 to 24 hours. The quantity of parenteral fluid required during the treatment of diabetic acidosis can be calculated in the same manner as in any situation requiring parenteral fluids. A common error, however, is failure to recognize the large urinary volume and the increased rate of insensible water loss that may occur during the first 8 to 12 hours of treatment. Failure to provide an increase in the maintenance fluid requirements to meet these losses can result in a much slower rate of rehydration. During the second 12-hour period of treatment maintenance fluid requirements will decrease toward those expected for a child of that size.

Generally, half of the calculated 24-hour fluid volume is given in the first 8 hours. A useful solution for initial treatment contains 75 mEq/liter of Na^+, 50 mEq/liter of Cl^-, and 25 mEq/liter of HCO_3^- or lactate. Although there is a theoretic objection to the use of lactate instead of bicarbonate, extensive clinical experience suggests that the danger is more theoretic than real. Thus a commonly used commercially available fluid for initial treatment is half-strength lactated Ringer's solution in 2.5 percent dextrose.

Additional sodium bicarbonate is indicated in those situations where it is judged that the respiratory center may fail due to the excessive stimulation of an extreme degree of metabolic acidosis (e.g., arterial pH below 6.95). Within a few hours, if urinary output is adequate and serum potassium is normal or low, potassium replacement therapy should be started, changing the composition of electrolytes in the infusion to Na^+ 50 mEq/liter, K^+ 25 mEq/liter, Cl^- 50 mEq/liter, and HCO_3^- or lactate 25 mEq/liter. The treatment program is summarized in Table 7.

The greatest cause of mortality and serious morbidity during the acute management of diabetes presently relates to failure to recognize the magnitude of whole-body potassium losses in the keto-acidotic child. The use of the electrocardiogram with the observation of T wave changes is an effective way of monitoring changes in serum potassium levels. The T wave is best monitored in limb lead 2, where increased height and peaking are characteristic of elevated serum K^+ and isoelectric or negative T waves are indicative of hypokalemia. Therapy for keto-acidosis occurring in a child

previously diagnosed and treated will be similar to that in the untreated diabetic.

TREATMENT ON SECOND DAY. During the second day of therapy the child should be on oral feedings. He should receive approximately four injections of regular crystalline insulin during the 24-hour period. The amount of insulin to be given before each meal and at approximately 10:00 P.M. can be judged as in the previous 12 hours: 5 units of regular insulin for each + of urinary glucose, 5 units for slight acetone, and 10 units for 4+ acetone. These first-voided urines (see below) are obtained prior to each meal and prior to 10:00 P.M. At 10:00 P.M. the amount of insulin given is calculated by assigning 2.5 units per +.

In some cases during the period from 18 to 48 hours after treatment is begun hyperglycemia and glucosuria will disappear in spite of infusion of hypertonic glucose. Under these circumstances insulin should be withheld until hyperglycemia or glucosuria reappears. An alternative approach on the second day of treatment is to assume that the child will require approximately 1.5 units/kg/day and to provide this amount, giving one-third before breakfast, one-fourth before lunch, one-fourth before supper, and one-sixth at bedtime.

LATER TREATMENT. The philosophy of management that one adopts after the first few days will to a great extent determine much of the therapy from that time on. At one end of the therapeutic scale there is the concept that normoglycemia and absence of glucosuria are the ideal standards of control. In this concept hyperglycemia is felt to have a profound influence on the subsequent development of the degenerative complications of this disease. Adherents to this concept believe that individuals with proper training and supervision can maintain a state of normoglycemia without undue difficulty and without occurrence of hypoglycemic reactions. At the other end of the therapeutic scale there are physicians who believe that the degree of glucosuria is of little consequence and that therapy should be constituted so that the patient is free of ketonuria and overt symptoms. These physicians believe that the control of carbohydrate metabolism will have essentially no effect on the ultimate vascular degenerative phenomena.

A middle course, which is subscribed to by the majority of physicians, sets as its goal the achievement of the least hyperglycemia and the least glucosuria that are compatible with a relatively normal everyday life and with the greatest freedom from hypoglycemic reactions. With this program it is usually possible to achieve reasonable control of carbohydrate metabolism with a single injection of insulin given prior to breakfast each day or with two injections per day, one before breakfast and one before supper. There is an increasing tendency in the United States to favor two injections per day.

From the amount of insulin required during the second 24-hour period, one can judge relatively accurately the daily insulin requirement for the next few weeks. In general, the total daily requirement will be equivalent to 1 to 2 units/kg/day. An insulin mixture can be started on this basis on either the third or fourth day (see below) using the total requirement of the second day as a starting point.

Insulin. Three major types of insulin are now available: short-acting (regular, crystalline, and semilente); intermediate (NPH, lente, and globin); and long-acting (protamine zinc and ultralente). The curves of activity of these insulins are shown in Figure 8.

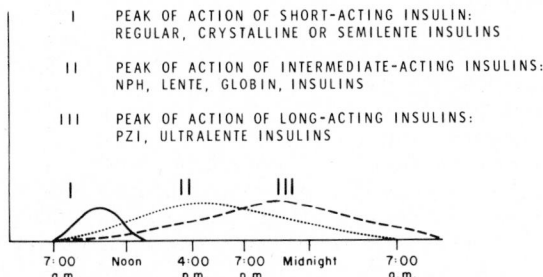

I	PEAK OF ACTION OF SHORT-ACTING INSULIN: REGULAR, CRYSTALLINE OR SEMILENTE INSULINS
II	PEAK OF ACTION OF INTERMEDIATE-ACTING INSULINS: NPH, LENTE, GLOBIN, INSULINS
III	PEAK OF ACTION OF LONG-ACTING INSULINS: PZI, ULTRALENTE INSULINS

FIG. 8. Curves of activity of various forms of insulin.

Although there are occasional instances requiring unusual dosage forms and combinations, the physician is well advised to select one of the common mixtures and to use this with the majority of patients. The most common insulin mixture today is a combination of an intermediate insulin (such as NPH or lente) and a short-acting insulin (such as regular insulin) mixed in the same syringe. These are usually given in the ratio 3:1 or 4:1 (intermediate:regular), in keeping with their relative duration of action (18 to 24 hours:6 hours). If two injections per day are to be used, a common approach is to use a 2:1 mixture (2 intermediate, 1 short) prior to breakfast and half that total as an intermediate insulin prior to supper. Two injections per day are particularly useful when nocturnal–early morning glucosuria significantly exceeds afternoon–early evening glucosuria. It is also often helpful in controlling late morning glucosuria to avoid giving large amounts of short-acting insulin prior to breakfast. There are essentially no circumstances in which long-acting insulins (protamine zinc or ultralente) can be recommended for use in young children with diabetes. The risk of undetected hypoglycemic episodes occurring in the middle of the night is very high when long-acting insulins are used.

Insulin is now provided in a standard U100 form (100 units/ml), and appropriate U100 disposable syringes are used. A special pediatric U100 syringe of smaller total volume and wider unit divisions is now available for children taking less than 20 units per injection. All diabetics should be managed with U100 insulin and the appropriate syringe to avoid the problems resulting from confusion between the previous U40 and U80 strengths.

Diet. During the period of hospitalization, regulation of dietary intake aids in the approximation of the daily insulin requirement. It is assumed that after discharge the average child will receive a reasonable diet at home, and such a diet may be prescribed under hospital conditions. The total calories required can be approximated by the use of tables or one of several simple formulas given in Table 8. The diet should be divided to give approximately one-fourth of the calories at each meal, one-eighth at a midafternoon feeding, and one-eighth at a bedtime feeding.

TABLE 8. Diet calculations: Daily Calories

1. 1,000 calories, plus 100 times age in years = total daily calories
   or
2. 90, minus 3 times age in years = calories/kg/day
   Calories/kg times weight (kg) = total daily calories

Example:
   8-year-old child, weight 28 kg
      1,000 + 8 (100) = 1,800 calories/day
         or
      90 − 3(8) = 66 calories/kg
      66 × 28 = 1,848 calories/day
Approximate distribution for 50% carbohydrate, 30% fat, 20% protein:
      225 g carbohydrate (50% of 1,800 = 900 calories) (900 ÷ 4 = 225 g)
      60 g fat (30% of 1,800 = 540 calories) (540 ÷ 9 = 60 g)
      90 g protein (20% of 1,800 = 360 calories) (360 ÷ 4 = 90 g)

Although it is wise to prescribe a specific diet in the hospital where activity and emotional state are relatively constant, this is generally not the situation at home. Therefore, it is important that the dietician or the individual working with the child and family on home management understand this distinction. Since the general diet eaten by American children approximates 50 percent of the calories from carbohydrate, 30 percent from fat, and 20 percent from protein, it is reasonable to utilize the same composition in the hospital (Table 8). Such a diet is also now considered appropriate by many nutritionists for children in general, including those with diabetes. In keeping with the concept that a self-selected diet is most appropriate at home, the dietician should help the child and family understand how the individual patterns of the family members either are or could be made to be compatible with an appropriate nutrient intake for the child. In addition, as with any family seeking dietary guidance, it is reasonable to suggest reduction of saturated fats and cholesterol in the entire family diet. The goal is to have the child with diabetes eating the same foods as the family, and in a quantity sufficient to satisfy hunger.

Control. Control of the diabetic state during this first week of therapy is judged on the patient's general condition and on the measurement of the amount of glucose in the urine. Urinary glucose, when measured quantitatively, is a reasonable integrated measure of the above-normal fluctuation in the blood glucose. Urine collections are divided into three portions. The first collection is made between 7:00 A.M. and 1:00 P.M., the second from 1:00 P.M. until 7:00 P.M., the third from

7:00 P.M. until 7:00 A.M. The first period corresponds to the duration of action of regular insulin, and the second period corresponds to the hours covering the maximum action of intermediate insulin; the overnight collection reveals to some extent whether a second injection of intermediate-acting insulin is required prior to the evening meal. Control is considered adequate when the glucose in the total 24-hour urine is equivalent to 5 percent or less of the total ingested calories (grams of glucose × 4 calories/g); control is excellent when this can be reduced to less than 2.5 percent.

After the child is home, control is assessed using several factors: urinary glucose in a 24-hour urine (criteria are the same as in the above paragraph); freedom from hypoglycemic episodes; growth in height and weight consistent for age-specific standards, allowing for previously established constitutional characteristics; emotional well-being of the child and family. Following the initial 7 to 10 days of therapy, edema of the lower extremities may occur abruptly in some patients. The pathophysiology is not clear, but it has been considered to be similar to the edema occasionally seen when starved individuals resume feeding. No specific therapy is indicated, as the process is self-limited.

PATIENT AND FAMILY EDUCATION. The educational program for the family is equal in importance to the medical management of the patient and should go hand in hand with the treatment and education of the child. Since adequate education of the family plays a major role in the ultimate success of management of the child on an ambulatory basis, the instructional process will be discussed in some detail. The in-hospital education programs for diabetic children should be tailored to their needs and should be appropriate to their age and experience. Often children with diabetes are placed into classes with adults with far-advanced or crippling complications; in such a situation the psychologic effects can be catastrophic.

Initial Explanation. During the first day of hospitalization a preliminary discussion with the family is indicated. The ability of the child and the family to comprehend and incorporate educational programs during the initial few days of hospitalization may be limited by their state of adjustment, and the pace and content of instruction must be individually tailored. Confirmation of the diagnosis should be explained to the family, and a general description should be given of what diabetes mellitus is. It is usually wise to state that the disease is familial and that a predisposition must have come from both sides of the family, even though no family history may be apparent in either parental line at the time.

Parents often feel guilt that their child's diabetes may be the result of errors in dietary supervision, discipline, or other child-rearing practices. Such parents should be clearly told that the presence of the disease was determined at conception and that the onset of clinical diabetes is not known to be related to any single extrinsic factor of that sort. The family should be reassured that the child can lead a near-normal life under proper medical management.

Later one can explain in a systematic way the various facets of carbohydrate metabolism and the management of diabetes that will enable the family to work intelligently with the physician. It is useful to schedule a series of daily 1 hour conferences with the parents to cover specific topics each day and to allow time for the family to raise questions. Each day it is wise to summarize the discussion of the previous day and to assess their understanding of what has already been presented.

Educational Information. The discussion with the family can be divided into four major topics: The family should receive detailed clarification about factors that tend to raise the level of *blood sugar* (primarily food, emotional tension, and infections) and about those that lower the level of blood sugar (primarily insulin and exercise). In the discussion concerning food an important point to raise is that the body has the ability to break foods down to small units and to rebuild these into any one of the major nutritional components (carbohydrates, proteins, or fats). Consequently all foods have a tendency to raise the level of blood sugar, although at different rates; for example, glucose raises the level of blood sugar more quickly than starches and proteins. Since it is impossible to constantly regulate all the variables involved in the control of blood sugar, it seems impractical to attempt to rigidly control anything other than the insulin administration. Day-to-day variation in the amount of exercise and in the emotional state of a child can be compensated for by the resultant variation in the child's natural inclination and needs for food. These natural drives control appetite as well in the adequately treated diabetic as in the normal child, so that growth in height and weight usually proceeds smoothly and proportionately. With this reasoning the child with diabetes is allowed to set his own level of caloric intake and to adjust this level, with supervision, from meal to meal and day to day. However, the parents should understand the general range of average total calories appropriate for the child's age, size, and growth status, so that gross overnutrition or undernutrition can be recognized. The only external control generally necessary is a moderate restriction in intake of simple carbohydrates. The explanation given to the family for this limitation is that with the loss of the fine regulation of insulin release in diabetics, sudden loads of glucose are not utilized and are consequently wasted in the urine. It is also important to indicate the significance of sugar in the urine, as it reflects changes in the blood sugar, and to clarify the difference between instantaneous measurement of sugar in the blood and the summation of blood sugars as represented by the amounts of sugar in the first-voided and second-voided urine specimens.

Information on the subject of *hypoglycemia* includes the origin of the symptoms in hypoglycemia on the basis of the norepinephrine response and the lack of glucose for brain metabolism, with a description of the progression of the signs and symptoms of hypoglycemia: hunger, irritability, jitteriness, sweating, somnolence, confusion, staggering, decreased awareness, and finally coma and convulsions. The uniqueness of each child's symptom pattern must be emphasized. The somewhat self-limited aspect of the hypoglycemic convulsion should be mentioned. The treatment of hypoglycemia with oral or parenteral glucose and the possible use of glucagon injections should be discussed. More important, stress should be placed on the prevention of hypoglycemia by knowledge of the periods when it is most likely to occur and recognition of its earliest symptomatology.

Mechanisms for the development of *hyperglycemia, ketosis, acidosis,* and *coma,* as well as their signs, symptoms, treatment, and prevention, should be clarified; particular attention should be called to the difference between hypoglycemia (rapid onset and relatively frequent occurrence) and hyperglycemia and ketosis (slower onset and the possibility of intervening therapy). At this point it is often wise to discuss the natural course of the illness in the child given appropriate treatment. The sudden onset of the so-called honeymoon period 2 to 6 weeks after treatment has begun should be introduced. The reduction in insulin requirement to less than 0.5 unit/kg/day and the relative freedom from glucosuria, hypoglycemia, and ketosis should be emphasized. The prompt recognition of the beginning of this period must be stressed so that the parents can be prepared to reduce the daily insulin rapidly (about one-third of the total amount per day). The gradual increase in insulin requirement that follows the honeymoon period (2 to 24 months) should be explained in terms of an expected failure of endogenous insulin production. The variations in insulin requirements with overall activity patterns, the increase with adolescence, and the stabilization after growth has ceased all need to be mentioned. The family may wish to discuss some aspects of adult life at this time, but this can be deferred to a later date if they desire; topics to be included are childbearing, vocational planning, long-term complications, and life expectancy. Specific vocational counseling and genetic counseling may be helpful at a later date.

The practicalities of *management,* including discussion of the various kinds of insulins (e.g., the short-, intermediate-, and long-action insulins) and the role of insulin mixtures, should be discussed. The storage of insulin and the maintenance of the insulin in current use at room temperature should be clarified. Injection techniques should be discussed in detail, including a plan for rotation of injection sites on a regular basis. The disposable needle and syringe can be recommended. Finally, the role of the so-called self-regulated diet should be stressed. Participation of the entire family in the diet and the importance of midafternoon and prebedtime feedings and their composition should be emphasized.

It is also well to point out differences between the manifestations of diabetes in adults and children and to indicate that the vascular complications of adults are not a problem during childhood. Foot care, cuts, bruises, broken bones, and related phenomena are of no more consequence in the child with diabetes than they are in nondiabetic children, unless secondary infection occurs; then the emphasis should be on the way the infection may temporarily increase the insulin requirement and on the fact that diabetes was not the cause of the infection.

As much of this information as possible should be shared with the child. If possible, a dietician who understands the concept of a self-regulatory diet, a nurse, and a social worker should be included in the educational process, but the majority of it is best handled by the physician, or by a specially trained diabetes health specialist who is able to work with the total problem.

At some time between the establishment of a diagnosis of diabetes in a child and that child's marriage, genetic counseling is appropriate. Depending on the sophistication of the patient, one may discuss the problem as one similar to a recessive trait, or one may wish to go into greater detail and bring out the role that unknown environmental factors may play in determining the phenotype that results from a variety of possible genotypes. In any case, it is reasonable to state that if the individual with diabetes marries another person with diabetes their children will have somewhat less than the theoretic risk of 100 percent of developing diabetes. If the individual marries a carrier, the risk of children eventually developing diabetes is no greater than 50 percent and probably somewhat less. If the marital partner is not diabetic, but the actual genetic status is unknown, the risk of a child from such a marriage developing diabetes is probably less than 1 in 8.

Family Reaction.   During the early discussions with the family and in their subsequent visits it will be apparent that at least four stages exist in the family's acceptance of this disease. In the initial stage of disbelief, the family may make statements such as "It can't be true" and "I'm sure the doctor will find that there's something else wrong." This stage usually lasts 1 or 2 days, but it may on occasion be very prolonged. The second stage of acceptance is an intellectual one in which the family understands the problem but is not yet emotionally ready to accept the total picture. The duration of this intellectual acceptance may vary from a week to a year or more in some families. Eventually the family develops an emotional acceptance in which it can freely discuss the problems involved in this disease with the physician, the child, and other medical personnel. The fourth and final stage is social acceptance; it occurs when the family has intellectually and emotionally accepted the disease and can accept it on a social level as well. In this stage the family is comfortable in discussing the problem with those individuals in the child's environment, such as teachers, neighbors, and others who need to have some knowledge of the child's condition for proper supervision. The stage of total acceptance may appear as early as 1 to 2 months after diagnosis in some families, but it may take as long as 5 to 10 years in others.

Preparation for Home Care.   By the time the child is regulated on an intermediate insulin or insulin mixture and the family is adequately educated for home care, one or both parents should have had the opportunity to give several insulin injections under supervision and should feel relatively comfortable doing this. The parents should also have accurately tested a number of urine specimens for sugar and acetone. The urine sugar should be measured using Benedict's solution, Clinitest tablets, or Dextrostix paper strips. The Clinitest method is preferred by the authors. The older child can perform a number of these activities himself. It is our strong belief, however, that children should not be pushed or forced into giving their own insulin injections, although they might well be taught this technique for use in special situations.

EXTENDED CARE.   The care of children with diabetes mellitus can be handled extremely well in the office of any physician who is willing to accept the child's abnormality of carbohydrate metabolism as only one of a number of aspects of a total problem. Assessment of the overall management of these children must include consideration of social and emotional health as well as evaluation of carbohydrate metabolism.

Initial Home Care.   Following discharge from the hospital, it is wise to have the parent call the physician for several mornings prior to giving the insulin injection in order to discuss the results of the previous day's urinalyses and the insulin dose for that day. In this way final control of the insulin requirement can be achieved at home in the child's more natural surroundings.

Changing Insulin Requirements.   Initially the insulin dose will generally average approximately 1 to 2 units/kg, but there is wide individual variation in insulin requirements at all stages. This insulin requirement will persist for a period of approximately 2 to 6 weeks following the initiation of therapy (Fig. 9). The child's urine and blood glucose values will usually then de-

crease rapidly, and hypoglycemia may occur. The family should already be aware that the insulin requirement may drop precipitously over a period of 2 to 5 days, and in about 5 percent of newly diagnosed children may actually go to zero at this time. If the family and the child have been adequately prepared, it is preferable not to discontinue insulin injections even if the child remains aglycosuric during this period. For the majority of children the insulin requirement will fall to less than 0.5 unit/kg. During this honeymoon period there appears to be a temporary reestablishment of minimal insulin secretion. The child's condition will then remain relatively stable during a period varying from 2 months to 2 years. The number of hypoglycemic reactions and the tendency to ketosis and acidosis will greatly diminish.

The inevitable increase in insulin requirement may be gradual or abrupt and may occur in association with a traumatic episode or infection. The final insulin dosage will approach a value of 1 unit/kg/day and will remain in that range throughout the remainder of the child's life. There is great individual variation, however, and the range is wide.

Evaluation of Carbohydrate Metabolism.   The level of blood glucose will be affected not only by the amount of insulin administered but by multiple variables that include food intake, amount of physical activity, and emotional state of the child. The result of these multiple factors is that blood glucose levels vary greatly during a 24-hour period, and this variation may often occur quite rapidly. As a consequence, single blood glucose determinations are of limited value in attempting to evaluate control of carbohydrate metabolism through

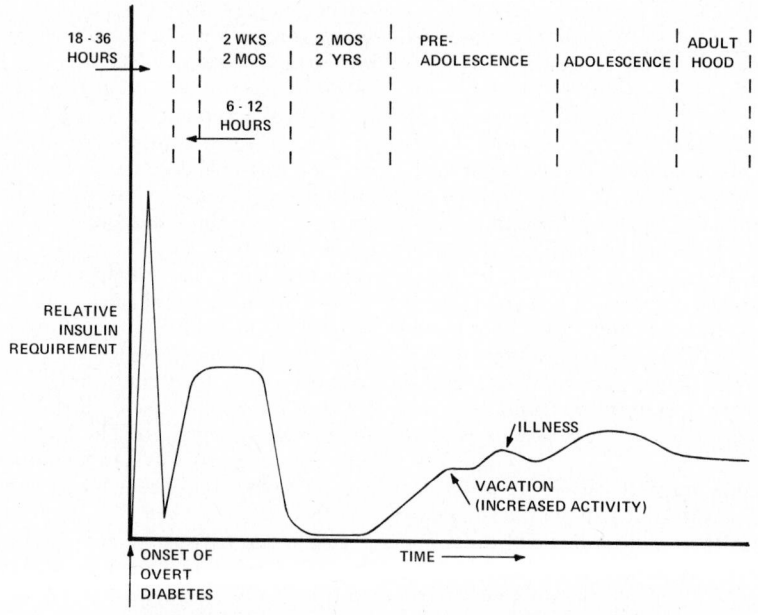

FIG. 9.   Typical natural course of juvenile diabetes mellitus.

the day. However, since most children have a relatively normal renal threshold for glucose, the amount of glucose in the urine is proportional to the time and degree of elevation of blood glucose above 180 mg/dl. Therefore evaluation of carbohydrate metabolism on an ambulatory basis may be accomplished by a combination of occasional 24-hour urine glucose determinations (every 2 to 4 months) and the daily testing of single specimens in the home. About once a year, or whenever control of glucosuria becomes a problem, a divided 24-hour collection should be done to ascertain if the mixture being used is in the correct proportion. When considering a change from one injection per day to two per day, a divided 24-hour urine is also most helpful in evaluating such a change. For most children, examination of the urine glucose prior to breakfast and prior to the evening meal will suffice for daily testing at home.

Two alternatives exist regarding the collection of daily urine specimens: The *first voiding* obtained may be examined, or the bladder may be emptied and a second specimen may be collected a few minutes later. The first urine voided on arising reflects blood glucose variation during most of the night, whereas the sample obtained by a *second voiding* will reflect the blood glucose as it exists at that time. Similarly, in the afternoon the first specimen obtained prior to the evening meal will reflect blood glucose levels during much of the afternoon, and a second specimen will reflect the blood glucose level for the few minutes prior to its being obtained. In general, one is more interested in the longer period of time, so that the first specimen obtained in the morning and the first specimen obtained in the late afternoon are more useful for overall evaluation purposes.

Although urinalyses for glucose are valuable for assessment of control of carbohydrate metabolism, several difficulties occur. It is not uncommon to find glucose in the urine in the presence of hypoglycemia. This occurs when insulin activity and exercise combine to lower the blood glucose relatively suddenly to hypoglycemic levels, while the bladder contains urine that was formed during previous periods of hyperglycemia. In this circumstance the more recently formed glucose-free urine only partially dilutes the urine that contains glucose, and thus the overall specimen is positive for glucose. This sort of problem has led many physicians and families to abandon the urine sugar method because of presumed unreliability. When hypoglycemia is suspected, a second-voided urine obtained a few minutes after the bladder has been previously emptied is useful for evaluating the symptomatology.

Another problem with single urine specimens is that without a knowledge of volume and without a precise determination of the amount of glucose in the urine the total carbohydrate balance during a 24-hour period is unknown. As a result, a 4+ urine glucose may be associated with good control in one child and extremely poor control in another. Since the ordinary urine test gives a 4+ reading for glucose concentrations of 2 percent *or greater,* a persistent 4+ throughout the day could represent as little as 20 g of glucose in a 1,000-ml 24-hour urine volume (which is generally considered ade-

quate control) or more than 150 g in a 24-hour urine that had a volume of 3,000 ml. Usually, as the urinary glucose concentration approaches 5 percent the volume of urine increases markedly. The recent 2-drop test using Clinitest tablets obviates some of the previous problems, since a 4+ reaction becomes equivalent to 5 percent glucose. However, the daily pattern of urine testing tends to reflect a relatively consistent pattern of control for that particular child. Therefore, a quantitative measure of 24-hour urinary carbohydrate compared with the findings of the daily urine tests provides better evaluation of the daily changes. It is easy to obtain a 24-hour urine specimen in the home, to preserve it with thymol crystals, to have the family measure and record the total volume, and to mail an aliquot to the physician for evaluation.

Reasonable control, which can be obtained with most preadolescent children, becomes more difficult during adolescence. In essence, the aim in the regulation of carbohydrate metabolism is to achieve the minimum amount of carbohydrate in the urine (and the most nearly normal blood glucose); however, total absence of glucosuria cannot often be maintained without risk of hypoglycemic reactions, and the amount of glucosuria sought should be the minimum that avoids hypoglycemic reactions and permits a life style compatible with normal physical and emotional growth.

Problems of undernutrition and overnutrition in children with diabetes are generally managed as they are in nondiabetic children. An exception is the child who has had prolonged periods of inadequate amounts of insulin concomitant with long-standing insufficient dietary intake. This combination results in stunted growth due to the catabolic tendency of the inadequately treated diabetic state and in development of a massively enlarged liver with marked fatty infiltration. This complex has been termed the *Mauriac syndrome* and is treated by providing more adequate insulin therapy and a sufficient diet. The growth retardation, if it has been sufficiently prolonged, may never be fully corrected.

A more common problem is the child treated with excessive insulin who overeats in response to frequent hypoglycemia and whose blood sugar frequently vacillates between hypoglycemia and hyperglycemia. In such patients, insulin dosage may be raised by the physician or family to very high levels in small increments in an attempt to render the patient aglycosuric. The result is transient hypoglycemia followed by increased appetite and intake of food; these in turn produce more glycosuria, and the cycle is then repeated with an elevation of insulin dosage. In such a stepwise fashion huge insulin doses can be reached and fairly well tolerated. This situation, often called the *Somogyi phenomenon,* is responsible for much of the so-called brittleness of the juvenile diabetic. A clue to the diagnosis of this situation may be the periodic occurrence of hypoglycemia or aglycosuria in a patient who is receiving excessive doses of insulin and is usually spilling sugar and showing great fluctuations in blood sugar level. In such a child, reduction in insulin dosage results in less hypoglycemia, less hunger, lowered caloric intake, and then decreased hyperglycemia. However, such reduction may have to be done extremely slowly to avoid ketosis.

One of the most common reasons for addition of incremental doses of insulin is the attempt on the part of the physician or parent to counteract the appearance of small amounts of acetone in the morning. It must be remembered that a significant number of nondiabetic children have acetonuria following an overnight fast as a normal occurrence and that specific changes in insulin dose in response to transient acetonuria that is present in the morning but disappears during the course of the day are not necessary.

Activity.   Since activity and insulin requirement vary inversely, the insulin requirement will tend to decrease with the onset of increased activity of summer vacation, and the reverse will occur in the fall. On the other hand, because of the vagaries in every child's day it is impractical to attempt to adjust insulin daily on the basis of expected activity. This kind of daily fluctuation is best countered by allowing the child's appetite to coordinate activity and dietary intake.

Intercurrent Illness.   There is no way to predict whether the child's insulin requirement will rise or fall with an infection. With the increased rate of metabolism usually associated with infection and fever there will be increased caloric utilization, and the insulin requirement will rise. However, with infections that are marked by severe anorexia or vomiting the food intake may fall sharply and the insulin requirement may decrease somewhat.

A satisfactory approach during a period of illness is to use regular insulin and to give the child four injections a day, based on that child's usual requirements. The amount of each injection should be modified during the course of the day in accordance with dietary intake and urine testing. One begins such a day by giving one-third of the previous total daily dosage as a single injection of regular insulin before breakfast. The situation is assessed again at midday; if the child is eating but does not have excessive ketonuria and glycosuria, one-fourth of the total day's requirement is given at this time. However, if the child has eaten poorly and the urine sugar is negative, this dose of insulin is omitted. If, on the other hand, the child has eaten but the urine is positive for sugar and acetone, the noon dose of insulin may be increased to twice the estimated amount. This same evaluation is carried out in the evening, and the dose of insulin is prescribed in the same way. Before sleep, the same procedure is followed, and the estimated dose at this time is one-sixth of the total daily dose.

The important adjunct to insulin during a period of illness is caloric intake. Since the child will utilize calories whether he is eating or not, some insulin will always be required. If medically indicated, it is reasonable in an ill child with diabetes to restrict oral intake to clear fluids high in carbohydrate. However, with a flexible insulin program, any type of intake, as well as fasting for a period of 6 to 12 hours, is entirely compatible with home care. The early use of such a flexible program in an illness will frequently prevent the complications of hypoglycemia or acidosis that otherwise might appear.

Family Relationships.   The regulation of the carbohydrate metabolism of diabetic children requires relatively little of a physician's time. Considerably more time should be devoted to dealing with the child's anxieties and concerns about diabetes and with the parent's attitudes and concerns about the child and about themselves. Early in the illness the physician normally works primarily with one parent, and the parents work more closely with the child than does the physician. Nevertheless, the relationships between the parents, between the child and both parents, and between the diabetic child and brothers and sisters all play a role in the overall success of the management of the patient.

The interaction between the disease and family relationships will relate to the age of the diabetic child. Prior to adolescence the child's dependence on the parents may be increased by the physical bonds necessitated by the care of the diabetic state, especially if the parents are overprotective. In adolescence these same factors may increase the tension in the conflict over independence and dependence that is characteristic of this age. These reactions may result in an overly dependent preadolescent and an extremely rebellious adolescent.

The occurrence of diabetes in a child may also alter the relationships between the parents and the nondiabetic siblings. These well children may resent the child with diabetes because of the real or imagined added attention he receives. The well children may also become hostile or overly solicitous because of guilt toward the child with diabetes. In addition, the well children may reject the parents, demand increased attention from them, or overreact to the attention or lack of attention they receive.

It is obvious from experience with the evaluation of difficult management problems that each of the family interrelationships can at times produce considerable instability in the program to establish relatively normal carbohydrate metabolism. But the majority of problems are centered around the parent-child relationship, and it is this area that needs to be examined first when difficulties in diabetic management are encountered. However, one will often have to examine *each* of the relationships and include the child's relationships with peers and the school situation before entirely clarifying a problem. In these situations the assistance of a social worker may be quite valuable.

With time the physician–child relationship should become dominant so far as the care of the diabetic state is concerned. It is a mistake, however, to move too rapidly toward this state. The technical ability and intelligence of many children make it possible for them to give their own insulin and to assume the entire management of their care at a very early age. Because of this possibility there has been a tendency for physicians to feel that this seeming independence is a sign of maturity and is something to be sought. However, the preadolescent child's personality is often not equipped to handle these serious responsibilities, although intellectual ability is sufficient. Although children may well wish to learn how to give their own insulin in order to spend the night with a friend, it should not be assumed that they should routinely administer such a potentially dangerous medication.

Adolescence.   Adolescents are often in rebellion against the restraining persons, problems, and forces around them. Therefore adolescence is not the time for the physician or family to emphasize the restrictive aspects of diabetes; rather, it is the time when the physician should be willing to accept the vagaries in diabetic management that occur and to express an understanding of the influences that have led to these irregularities.

The tendency of adolescents to eat irregularly, to consume large quantities of carbohydrates, and to keep irregular hours is well known and well understood in the nondiabetic child. The intense desire of the adolescent with diabetes to conform to this pattern should be given serious consideration in management. A period of erratic and unpredictable behavior at this age does not necessarily predict such a pattern in adult life. The physician's role is to help the adolescents understand why they are trying to deny the existence of diabetes by omitting insulin, by eating irregularly, or by refusing to test urine. The physician should not use punitive measures to try to correct this behavior. To help the parents of the adolescent with diabetes to understand and share in such an approach is another important task of the physician.

Finally, it should be noted that during adolescence there will likely be another period of relatively rapid increase in insulin requirement. This requirement will often exceed the 1 unit/kg average that has been the pattern until this time. However, following the turmoil and rapid growth of adolescence, the insulin requirement will generally decrease and stabilize for the remaining years of care.

Summer Camps.   Concern with emotional needs leads many families and physicians to consider summer camps for children with diabetes. These camps fall into two types. In the first category the camp is visualized as a medical facility in which to teach the child how to cope with problems of diabetes and how to survive as an independent person. In such a camp emphasis is placed on learning to give one's own insulin and to select one's own diet and on teaching the children the basic physiology of carbohydrate metabolism and the manifestations of hypoglycemia and keto-acidosis. A primary goal of such a camp is to increase the child's fund of knowledge about diabetes during the time as a camper. It is apparent that such activities, which possibly are appropriate to children 14 years of age and older, are much less so to younger children.

The other camp philosophy is to provide a summer recreational experience for a child that will encourage a concept of self as a near-normal individual who can partake in ordinary children's activities comfortably without fear. The care of the diabetic state is as unobtrusive as possible; the goal is to provide the child with a happy and educational experience in terms of play, sports, and group living. The fact that such a camp segregates children with diabetes from other children

tends to negate the concept of normality. However, in the first few years of overt diabetes, particularly from ages 7 to 10, children with diabetes need assurance that they have the ability to function in a camp situation without parental support, before being ready to participate in regular camp activity with nondiabetic children. Such reassurance is occasionally necessary in older children as well.

The adolescent will have quite individual needs that will depend on the duration of the disease as well as the individual level of adjustment. Many of these children will do better in a regular summer camp for several years.

OTHER DRUGS.   Despite claims to the contrary, it would appear that the oral hypoglycemic agents have no role in the treatment of juvenile diabetes. The apparent effect of these compounds in supplementing or even completely replacing insulin during the early periods of juvenile diabetes is transient, and they offer no protection against keto-acidosis. In addition, serious concerns have arisen concerning the long-range effects of the oral hypoglycemic agents on the cardiovascular system. Therefore it would appear advisable to eliminate these compounds from management programs for the child with diabetes.

Recent evidence has indicated that the thiazide compounds have a hyperglycemic action. Although this is not a contraindication to their use in appropriate situations requiring a diuretic, one should be aware that they have a tendency to raise the blood glucose in some children with diabetes.

The adrenal glucocorticoids are also diabetogenic, and their use in the child with diabetes mellitus will frequently lead to an increase in the insulin requirement. Much has been written about the problem of steroid diabetes and whether a permanent diabetic state can be induced with these compounds. It would appear that transient diabetes mellitus can be induced in some individuals with corticosteroids, and in a few of these permanent diabetes will result. However, it may be that this action occurs only in those individuals who are in a subclinical or latent diabetic state prior to the onset of steroid therapy; the steroid may then act as a precipitating factor, as described in the section on the natural course of the disease.

Glucagon, another hyperglycemic agent, has been proposed in the management of hypoglycemic reactions of insulin-treated diabetic patients. This compound, obtained from the alpha cells of the islets of Langerhans, acts on the phosphorylase system to increase the conversion of glycogen to glucose. The advantage of glucagon over epinephrine (which is also glycogenolytic) for the treatment of hypoglycemia is the absence of sympathomimetic activity. We generally recommend that families keep several ampules of glucagon in the home for treatment of hypoglycemia when oral intake is not possible or appropriate.

It has been suggested that somatostatin, the somatotrophin-release-inhibiting factor, may find a role in the management of diabetes because of its capacity to suppress glucagon secretion. Recent research indicates that suppression of glucagon may ameliorate the severity of the keto-acidotic manifestations of diabetes. At the present time, however, somatostatin is a research tool only. A problem with its future use is its profound inhibition of growth hormone secretion, which will probably limit the ultimate use of somatostatin in children.

PROGNOSIS. Mortality from diabetes mellitus during childhood has become minimal. However, deaths do occur from massive overdosage of insulin, or more rarely with severe keto-acidosis. The single variable that correlates with mortality in keto-acidosis is the duration of the process. This fact emphasizes the need for prompt diagnosis and institution of therapy when keto-acidosis occurs.

The ultimate outcome for the child with diabetes mellitus remains obscure. Although it is dangerous to predict the prognosis for children developing diabetes today from retrospective data on children who developed the disease 20 to 40 years ago, certain generalizations may be valid. For adults whose disease began 30 to 40 years ago the prognosis has been poor, since up to 90 percent of these indivudials have developed disabling and frequently fatal degenerative vascular complications. The vascular complications consist of small vessel changes termed microangiopathy that are characteristic of diabetes mellitus and atherosclerosis of the larger vessels that is similar to that process in other situations. The microangiopathies are the major problem for the child, as they tend to manifest themselves as neuropathies, retinal disease leading to blindness, and renal disease leading to renal failure. These problems may begin clinically in the second decade of life, but more frequently they appear in the third and fourth decades, often when the individual is in midcareer and has a family with young children. On the average, death occurs in affected individuals around the age of 50 years. It is of interest, however, that in most long-term series as least 10 percent of affected children remain free of these complications well into adult life.

References

Drash A: Diabetes mellitus in childhood: a review. J Pediatr 78:919, 1971

Gepts W: Pathology of islet tissue in human diabetes. In Steiner DF, Freinkel N (eds): Handbook of Physiology, Vol 1. Washington, DC, American Physiological Society, 1972, p 289

Gerich JE, Lorenzi M, Bier DM, et al: Prevention of human diabetic ketoacidosis by somatostatin: evidence for an essential role of glucagon. N Engl J Med 292:985, 1975

Jackson R, Guthrie RA, Guthrie DW, Waiches HM: The definition of chemical diabetes in children. Metabolism 22:229, 1973

Knowles HC Jr, Guest GM, Lampe J, Kessler M, Skillman TG: The course of juvenile diabetes treated with unmeasured diet. Diabetes 14:239, 1965

Muller WA, Faloona GR, Unger RH: Hyperglucagonemia in diabetic ketoacidosis: its prevalence and significance. Am J Med 54:52, 1973

Reaven G, Oletsky J, Farquhar J: Does hyperglycemia or hyperinsulinemia characterize the patient with chemical diabetes? Lancet 1:1247, 1972

Renold AE, Stauffacher W, Cahill G: Diabetes mellitus. In Stanbury JB, Wyngaarden JB, Frederickson DS (eds): The Metabolic Basis of Inherited Disease, 3rd ed. New York, McGraw-Hill, 1972, p. 83

Rosenbloom AL: The natural history of diabetes mellitus. Public Health Review 2:115, 1973

——— Criteria for interpretation of the oral glucose tolerance tests in children and insulin responses with normal and abnormal tolerance. Metabolism 22:301, 1973

Somogyi M: Exacerbation of diabetes by excess insulin action. Am J Med 26:1, 1959

The University Group Diabetes Program: A study of the effect of hypoglycemic agents on vascular complications in patients with adult-onset diabetes. Diabetes 19[Suppl 2]:747, 1970

Weil WB: Juvenile diabetes mellitus. N Engl J Med 278:829, 1968

White P, Graham C: The child with diabetes. In Marble A, White P, Bradley R, Kroll L (eds): Joslin's Diabetes Mellitus. Philadelphia, Lea & Febiger, 1971

Williamson JR, Vogler NJ, Kilo C: Microvascular disease in diabetes. Med Clin North Am 55:847, 1971

MELLITURIA

GEORGE N. DONNELL AND WILLIAM B. BERGREN

Mellituria (the presence of a sugar in the urine) may result from a variety of causes, including increased ingestion, altered gastrointestinal absorption, interference in the metabolism of a particular sugar, or defects in renal tubular transport. Mellituria may be missed on routine examination. Since the glucose oxidase test is specific for glucose, more general methods should be employed to detect other sugars.

Small amounts of sugars of dietary origin (sucrose, lactose, galactose, fructose) may appear in the urine of the newborn or premature infant. Varying amounts of these sugars may also be found in the urine of some patients with sepsis, gastrointestinal disease, or impaired liver function. Normal individuals sometimes excrete lactose or sucrose following increased intake of these sugars. Lactosuria is not uncommon during the last trimester of pregnancy and lactation.

Altered carbohydrate metabolism may lead to increased blood levels and overflow into the urine, as in diabetes mellitus, galactosemia, and fructosuria. On the other hand, glycosuria may occur in the absence of hyperglycemia in entities characterized by defective renal tubular reabsorption. This form of renal glycosuria occurs in patients with cystinosis and Wilson's disease and following exposure to certain drugs and heavy metals. Primary renal glycosuria and the glycosurias associated with various renal tubular disorders are discussed elsewhere (p. 1300). The present discussion is limited to melliturias resulting from disorders of sugar metabolism.

GALACTOSE METABOLISM

The term galactosemia denotes the presence of elevated levels of galactose in the blood, and it is generally employed to describe the genetic disorder in which activity of the enzyme galactose-1-phosphate uridyl transferase (transferase) is deficient. Elevation of blood galactose is also found in galactokinase deficiency.

Consequently it is preferable to designate galactosemia on the basis of the specific enzyme involved.

The principal dietary source of galactose is the disaccharide lactose in milk. Lactose is enzymatically hydrolyzed in the intestine to its corresponding monosaccharides (galactose and glucose). Galactose can be utilized both for energy and for the synthesis of galactose-containing cell components. It enters the mainstream of energy-producing metabolism via conversion to glucose by a pathway in which three enzymatic reactions are involved (Fig. 5). Functional impairment of any one of these reactions effectively blocks galactose utilization.

The first reaction results in phosphorylation of galactose to galactose-1-phosphate catalyzed by galactokinase in the presence of adenosine triphosphate (ATP) and magnesium ion. In the second step there is an exchange of galactose-1-phosphate for the glucose-1-phosphate moiety of uridine diphosphate glucose (UDPG), resulting in the formation of UDP galactose (UDP Gal) and release of glucose-1-phosphate. This reaction is catalyzed by the enzyme transferase. Finally UDP Gal is transformed to UDPG by the enzyme UDP galactose-4'-epimerase, a reversible reaction that involves the interconversion of galactose and glucose. UDP Gal is the starting point for synthesis of many of the vital galactose-containing compounds of the body. In the absence of dietary galactose, or if a block in the pathway of galactose metabolism exists, synthesis of UDP Gal (from UDPG) can occur by reversal of the epimerase reaction.

In addition to the major metabolic pathway, a number of minor pathways have been described, but the significance of these routes for the disposition of galactose is not clear. However, the reduction of free galactose to the sugar alcohol galactitol by the enzyme aldose reductase is important in the pathogenesis of cataracts in galactosemia.

Galactokinase Deficiency

Galactokinase deficiency was first reported in 1965 by Gitzelmann. Although other manifestations have been described, the only consistent clinical finding is lenticular cataract. The disorder is transmitted as an autosomal recessive abnormality. Both males and females have been found to be affected. Carrier parents have intermediate levels of erythrocyte galactokinase activity. The estimated incidence, based on heterozygote detection, is 1 in 40,000 to 1 in 50,000.

The defect is in the first step of galactose metabolism. Consequently galactose accumulates, but not galactose-1-phosphate. Galactosuria and galactosemia are present. Galactitol in the urine is a consequence of galactose accumulation, and the formation of galactitol in the lens leads to the formation of cataracts.

Early recognition of this disease is difficult because of the lack of systemic symptoms. The lenticular cataracts may not become evident until they are advanced. Postnatal screening for this disorder is not yet generally practiced. However, the routine examination of urine for reducing sugar early in infancy can provide a clue to the presence of the disorder.

Treatment of the galactokinase defect includes exclusion of galactose and lactose from the diet; the diet is identical to that employed for galactosemia due to transferase deficiency. The long-term outcome is not known, but on theoretic grounds progression of cataracts should be preventable. It has been suggested by Monteleone and Beutler that there is an increased incidence of cataracts in heterozygotes for galactokinase deficiency. This has not been proven, but it raises the question of the need for treatment of known carriers to prevent cataracts. Restriction of dietary galactose for a heterozygote mother during pregnancy may be advisable.

Galactosemia

Galactosemia involves the second step of the galactose metabolic pathway, in which activity of the enzyme galactose-1-phosphate uridyl transferase (transferase) is lacking.

CLINICAL MANIFESTATIONS. The infant with galactosemia usually appears normal at birth, and the clinical manifestations occur after the start of milk feeding. There is early evidence of liver involvement, and hepatomegaly is the most constant physical finding. Jaundice is frequent, and it persists in varying degrees until institution of diet therapy. Weight loss occurs as a result of vomiting and occasionally diarrhea. Lethargy and hypotonia are frequent. The clinical course of some infants is fulminant, and death may occur early from inanition, infection, or hepatic failure. Severe infection often is a complication of the disease and is a frequent cause of death in the untreated infant. The diagnosis of galactosemia should always be considered in an infant suspected of sepsis. In some patients cataracts may be noted as early as a few days of age, but because of the difficulty in detecting small lenticular opacities in the young infant, most are not diagnosed until later.

Clinical manifestations may vary in degree. Most infants have severe symptoms, and prompt treatment is urgent. In the untreated patient who survives beyond infancy, physical development is unsatisfactory, and there is a high risk of mental retardation. Specific neurologic abnormalities are infrequent, although convulsions have been described. Nonspecific abnormalities have been observed in electroencephalograms.

In a small number of mild cases the diagnosis may be overlooked for weeks or months. In some of these patients, the presence of a transferase defect is uncertain. However, vague digestive difficulties, retarded physical and mental development, cataracts, and perhaps intolerance to milk should suggest the possibility of galactosemia. This suspicion is strengthened if mellituria and proteinuria are found.

PATHOPHYSIOLOGY. It is recognized that galactose metabolites accumulate in tissues, but the basis for the clinical manifestations remains unclear. It has been postulated that these result from the inhibition by galactose-1-phosphate of a variety of enzyme systems.

There are no specific histologic alterations in the brain to account for the mental retardation. Changes in the liver in the untreated patient vary with age and severity of the disease. The prominent feature in the young severely ill infant is a marked fatty change of the liver, which may result in part from starvation and infection. In untreated infants cirrhosis may develop. A frequent histologic finding in the liver of young infants is a rosettelike arrangement of liver cells about dilated canaliculi filled with bile pigment. This finding should suggest galactosemia, but it is not restricted to this disease.

Although the pathogenesis of liver damage is unclear, it is doubtful that free galactose or galactitol is responsible, since liver involvement is not found in patients with galactokinase deficiency. The conventional tests for liver function are usually abnormal. The bilirubin levels usually are moderately elevated, with a variable ratio of indirect and direct forms. Retention of bilirubin may result from injury to hepatic cells by metabolites of galactose. Edema and ascites are present in about 15 percent of untreated children, due in part to malnutrition and in part to liver dysfunction. Another sign of liver involvement is hypoprothrombinemia. All patients appear to have some renal involvement. Proteinuria and generalized amino-aciduria can be demonstrated, and these abnormalities disappear after institution of treatment. Cataracts have been ascribed to the formation and accumulation of galactitol in the lens.

DIAGNOSIS. Although a presumptive diagnosis of galactosemia can be made on clinical grounds, laboratory confirmation is essential. The presence of galactose and protein in the urine of a symptomatic patient depends on continued ingestion of galactose. However, the presence of galactose in the urine is not in itself diagnostic. The galactose tolerance test is not specific and may be hazardous to the affected infant by inducing hypoglycemia and hypokalemia. Confirmation of diagnosis depends on assay of transferase activity in erythrocyte lysates. In the affected individual, erythrocyte transferase activity is entirely or almost entirely absent. Measurement of the galactose-1-phosphate content of erythrocytes may be a useful adjunct to diagnosis and may be useful for monitoring therapy.

Programs to screen newborn infants for galactosemia have been instituted in many areas. Two methods are in general use, but neither provides a sufficient basis for a definitive diagnosis. False-positive findings are not uncommon, particularly among genetic variants with reduced transferase activity. One screening test involves a microbiologic assay (Guthrie) and is dependent on the presence of galactose in the blood sample. Consequently both kinase and transferase defects may give a positive result. The other test (Beutler) detects only transferase deficiency. Transferase is present in cultured amniotic cells from the normal fetus, and prenatal detection of transferase deficiency is feasible.

TREATMENT. Treatment includes elimination of galactose or lactose from the diet and must be initiated as soon as possible in order to avoid the accumulation of galactose metabolites in tissues. The deficient enzyme cannot be replaced, and dietary measures offer an effective alternative. Clinical manifestations subside after restriction of galactose intake. Avoidance of foods containing galactose (milk and foods containing milk products) is the basis for a galactose-restricted diet. Casein hydrolysates, meat-based preparations, and soybean formulas may be employed as milk substitutes. Galactose-containing oligosaccharides are known to be present in some foods, especially legumes, but these compounds are not digested in the intestinal tract.

As the child grows older, solid foods may be added. Particular care must be taken to avoid commercial food products containing lactose as an additive, and food labels must be examined carefully. Any product containing milk, lactose, casein, whey, dry milk solids, or curds should be avoided. Nutritional adequacy of the diet must not be overlooked. A calcium supplement may be required, and adequate intake of other minerals and vitamins is necessary. Problems in aherence to the diet may occur because of inadequate supervision by the parent or because of intake of foodstuffs with unsuspected galactose content. Education of the parent and child, together with careful interim dietary histories, may be helpful in identifying any problems. Rigid exclusion of dietary galactose during the first year of life is essential. There are differences of opinion about the duration of a restricted dietary regimen. Since amelioration of the metabolic defect has not been demonstrated, it is our policy to restrict intake of milk throughout life. However, at the time affected children enter school they are permitted to eat breads, sauces, and other prepared foods that may contain small amounts of milk products.

PROGNOSIS. Dietary treatment of the infant with galactosemia is essential. Most of the clinical features are reversed following therapy. Jaundice disappears in a few days, and weight gain is restored in 1 to 2 weeks. Although there is a rapid decrease in liver size, in some patients it does not return to normal for several months. Cataracts may improve, but residual lesions may persist indefinitely. A normal growth pattern can be achieved on dietary therapy. The long-term effects on intellectual status are difficult to assess, but several studies indicate that treated patients, as a group, achieve at least low-normal intelligence scores. Most untreated patients develop mental retardation. The outcome is better with early treatment, but there are reports of apparently successful results when treatment is delayed as late as 1 year of age. Visual motor problems, which are common even in treated galactosemic children, may be responsible for learning difficulties. Recognition and provision for special assistance may facilitate adjustment to school.

GENETICS. Galactosemia is inherited as an autosomal recessive disorder, with the carrier having half-normal erythrocyte transferase activity. The incidence of the disease is estimated as 1 in 60,000, although this is only an approximation because of the occurrence of genetic variants in the population.

There are at least two known genetic variants of transferase that are not associated with clinical manifestations (Duarte and Los Angeles). The Duarte transferase variant differs from the normal enzyme in that it has a lower activity and a different electrophoretic mobility on starch gel. This variant occurs commonly, with a carrier frequency of about 12 percent. Homozygotes for the Duarte variant have half-normal erythrocyte transferase activity and may be indistinguishable from galactosemia heterozygotes. However, the Duarte variant can be distinguished by gel electrophoresis, and the combination of enzyme activity and electrophoretic mobility provides a means for distinguishing this genetic variant. The second variant (Los Angeles) is characterized by normal to increased activity and a different electrophoretic pattern.

It now has been shown that most patients with clinical galactosemia have a mutant transferase in which alteration in the protein structure has resulted in loss of enzyme activity. It appears that the mutation is not identical in all affected individuals. One family showed a transferase with altered electrophoretic mobility; in another an unstable transferase was demonstrated.

FRUCTOSE METABOLISM

Fructose is an important source of dietary carbohydrate. It is a component of the disaccharide sucrose, and it also occurs in fruits and vegetables as the free monosaccharide. Certain oligosaccharides such as raffinose and stachyose contain fructose, but these sugars are not utilized by humans. There are two principal pathways by which fructose is metabolized in man (Fig. 5). In the liver, fructose is phosphorylated to fructose-1-phosphate in the presence of ATP and the enzyme fructokinase. This enzyme also has been demonstrated in kidney and intestinal mucosa. In muscle and adipose tissue, fructose is phosphorylated by hexokinase to fructose-6-phosphate. The principal disorders of fructose metabolism are essential fructosuria and hereditary fructose intolerance.

Essential Fructosuria

Essential fructosuria is a rare benign abnormality that is transmitted as an autosomal recessive trait. The incidence in the general population is estimated as approximately 1 in 130,000. Because individuals with essential fructosuria are asymptomatic, recognition is difficult; thus the incidence is probably higher. The diagnosis is made by finding a reducing sugar in the urine that is confirmed as fructose by chromatography. The urine is abnormal only after ingestion of foods containing fructose or sucrose. With fructose loading tests, abnormally high levels of blood fructose are found. The enzyme defect involves a deficiency of liver fructokinase. No treatment is necessary.

Hereditary Fructose Intolerance

Hereditary fructose intolerance (HFI) is an inborn error of fructose metabolism due to a deficiency of hepatic aldolase. This enzyme catalyzes the conversion of fructose-1-phosphate to glyceraldehyde and acetone phosphate, as well as the conversion of fructose-1,6-diphosphate to glyceraldehyde-3-phosphate and acetone phosphate. In patients with HFI the activity of liver aldolase is reduced to between 10 and 50 percent of normal with fructose-1,6-diphosphate and to less than 10 percent with fructose-1-phosphate.

CLINICAL FINDINGS. Individuals with HFI are symptomatic when fructose is ingested in the diet. Ingestion of fructose-containing foods results in hypoglycemia, which manifests as tremors, disorientation, vomiting, and if it is servere, convulsions and coma. Chronic ingestion of fructose during infancy may also result in clinical findings similar to those of galactosemia, including failure to thrive, hepatomegaly, vomiting, jaundice, hyperbilirubinemia, proteinuria, and amino-aciduria. If fructose-containing foods are continued the infant may die. In contrast to the infant with galactosemia, the infant with HFI who is breast-fed remains symptom-free.

In some patients gastrointestinal symptoms predominate, while in others hypoglycemia is the major abnormality. Symptomatology tends to be severe in infants and milder in older individuals. This may be due to the strong aversion that usually develops in the older child for sweets, fruits, and other foods containing fructose. This also may explain why patients with HFI tend to have a minimum of caries.

PATHOPHYSIOLOGY. The primary enzymatic deficiency in HFI is a marked reduction of activity in liver fructose-1-phosphate aldolase. The hypoglycemia that occurs is thought to be due to impaired glycogenolysis or gluconeogenesis, and not to hyperinsulinism. The biochemical consequences of the enzyme deficiency include decreases in intracellular ATP and inorganic phosphate. There is secondary inhibition of fructokinase, phosphorylase, and the residual hepatic aldolase activity. Evidence for the inhibitory effect of fructose-1-phosphate in HFI patients is supported by the demonstration that neither glucagon nor adrenalin produces hyperglycemia following fructose ingestion. Chronic fructose ingestion in affected infants may lead to liver involvement, which is reflected by hepatomegaly that is due in part to an accumulation of lipids. Serum transaminase (SGOT) levels may be increased. Histologic examination of the liver has shown lesions of early cirrhosis.

DIAGNOSIS. Although the diagnosis of HFI is often suggested by the patient's history, it should be confirmed by laboratory tests. The significant abnormal laboratory findings include hypoglycemia, fructosuria, and amino-aciduria. Blood fructose may or may not be elevated. The administration of fructose orally (0.25 g/kg) or intravenously results in a precipitous and prolonged fall in blood glucose and in serum phosphorus, together with an elevation of serum uric acid levels. A fall in serum potassium levels is a variable finding. Blood fructose may remain high for an extended period, and fructose may be found in the urine. During the course of the test the induced hypoglycemia may become severe, and glucose administration may be necessary.

TREATMENT.   Treatment of the acute symptoms involves the correction of hypoglycemia by intravenous administration of glucose-containing solutions. Long-term therapy of this condition is accomplished by avoiding foods that contain fructose and sucrose. As a rule the prognosis for treated patients is very good. Hereditary fructose intolerance appears to be inherited as an autosomal recessive abnormality. However, a dominant pattern of inheritance has also been described and has raised the possibility of at least two genetic forms of the disorder. It is not possible at the present time to detect persons heterozygous for the abnormality.

PENTOSE METABOLISM

In the urine of normal individuals, small amounts of arabinose, xylose, and ribose may be found, as well as trace amounts of xylulose and ribulose. Ribosuria (D-ribose) has been demonstrated in some patients with muscular dystrophy. The only condition in which there is a marked excretion of pentose is essential pentosuria.

Essential Pentosuria

Essential pentosuria is a benign disorder that principally affects Jews and is inherited as an autosomal recessive abnormality. The urine contains L-xylulose that is excreted in increased amounts due to a block in conversion of xylulose to xylitol in the uronic acid pathway. The condition usually is discovered accidentally, and no treatment is required.

A number of drugs are known to increase the rate at which glucose enters the uronic acid pathways; aminopyrine and antipyrine have been reported to increase the excretion of L-xylulose in pentosuric subjects. It has been reported that the heterozygote for essential pentosuria can be identified by use of a glucoronolactone loading test.

References

Hsia DYY (ed): Galactosemia. Springfield, Ill, Charles C Thomas, 1968

Kalckar HM, Kinoshita JH, Donnell GN: Galactosemia: biochemistry, genetics, pathophysiology and developmental aspects. In Gaull GE (ed): Biology of Brain Dysfunction, Vol 1. New York Plenum Press, 1973, p 31

Herman RH, Zakin D: Fructose metabolism. Am J Clin Nutr 21:245, 315, 516, 693, 778, 1968

Hiatt HH: Pentosuria. In Stanbury JB, Wyngaarden JB, Frederickson DS (eds): The Metabolic Basis of Inherited Disease, 3rd ed. New York, McGraw-Hill, 1972, p 119

HYPOGLYCEMIA

ANTHONY S. PAGLIARA

GLUCOSE HOMEOSTASIS

Hypoglycemia in children is a common clinical finding and is associated with a wide variety of disorders. In the fasted individual the maintenance of a normal blood glucose level is dependent on (1) an adequate supply of endogenous gluconeogenic substrates (ie, amino acids, glycerol, and lactate), (2) functionally intact hepatic glycogenolytic and gluconeogenic enzyme systems, and (3) a normal endocrine system for integrating and modulating these two processes. The adult human being is capable of maintaining a normal blood glucose level even when totally deprived of calories for weeks or, in the case of obese subjects, for months. In contrast, the normal neonate and child exhibit a progressive fall in blood glucose to hypoglycemic levels when fasted for even short periods (eg, 24 to 48 hours). The reasons for this difference between the immature and adult human being are not clear, but it is obvious that the young individual, when fasting, is unable to supply sufficient glucose to meet the obligatory demands of the body for this sugar. In the immediate postprandial period (ie, 4 to 8 hours), glucose supply is derived primarily from hepatic glycogen stores, whereas with prolonged fasting the organism must depend on de novo synthesis of glucose (ie, gluconeogenesis).

Recent studies in man and laboratory animals and studies with in vitro liver perfusion preparations have demonstrated that the availability of an adequate supply of gluconeogenic substrates is a rate-limiting factor for gluconeogenesis. Both in vivo and in vitro studies further indicate that the gluconeogenic amino acids play the dominant quantitative role as glucose precursors. When livers from fasted rats are perfused with mixtures of lactate, glycerol, and amino acids in physiologic concentrations, over 50 percent of the glucose formed is derived from the amino acids. In the fasting adult man approximately 50 percent of net glucose production is derived from amino acid precursors, 30 percent from lactate (ie, Cori cycle), and 10 percent from glycerol (ie, lipolysis) (Fig. 10). Of the various gluconeogenic amino acids, alanine is quantitatively by far the most important. Transhepatic catheterization studies in human beings indicate that in excess of 50 percent of the glucose derived from gluconeogenic amino acids is formed from alanine; furthermore, the plasma alanine level exhibits the most precipitous fall of all amino acids during fasting in both adults and children. Correspondingly, during fasting, alanine constitutes the predominant amino acid mobilized from skeletal muscle (ie, the major protein reservoir and largest metabolic mass in the body). In the immediate postprandial period (12 to 14 hours) approximately 40 percent of total amino acid efflux from muscle is in the form of alanine, and approximately 20 percent is alanine after prolonged starvation (4 to 6 weeks). On the basis of these studies the existence of an alanine–glucose cycle has been proposed (analogous to the Cori cycle involving lactate) in which alanine represents the transport form of carbon and nitrogen derived from skeletal muscle metabolism that is converted to glucose and urea in the liver. The control mechanisms for this cycle have not been elucidated, but they are thought to be in part hormonally mediated. Since alanine constitutes only 6 to 7 percent of the

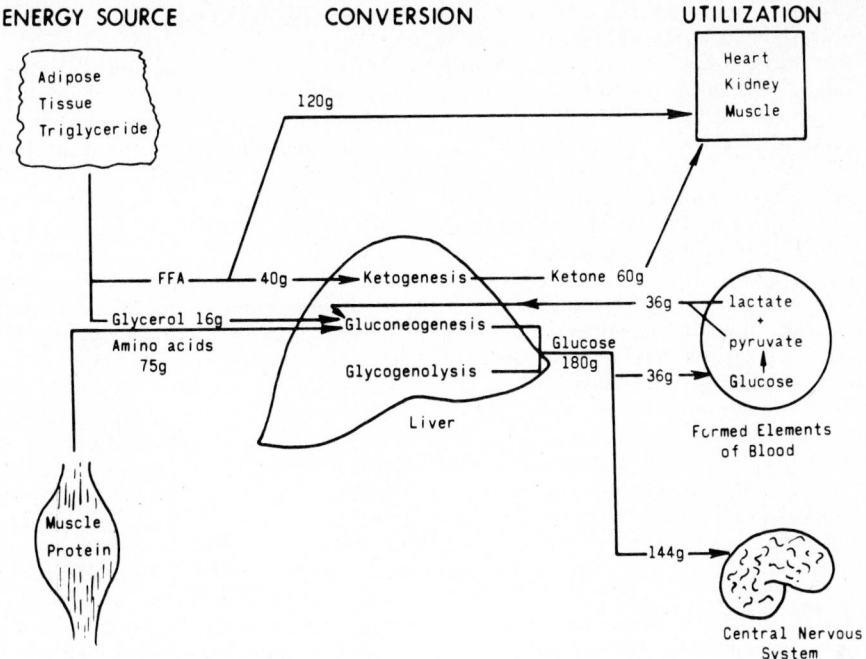

FIG. 10. Schematic representation of fuel metabolism in normal fasted man illustrating the energy sources (triglyceride, protein, glycogen, and lactate) and their hepatic conversion and peripheral tissue utilization. (Adapted from Cahill: *N Engl J Med* (282:668, 1970.)

amino acid composition of skeletal muscle protein, it seems likely that the major portion of alanine efflux represents alanine synthesized by the transamination of pyruvate derived by the oxidative deamination of gluconeogenic amino acids entering the Krebs cycle.

Glutamine is another important potential gluconeogenic substrate, and it represents a significant portion of the total amino acid efflux from the skeletal muscle during fasting. Its quantitative contribution to hepatic gluconeogenesis has not been as clearly defined as has that of alanine, and its role as a major substrate for renal gluconeogenesis in the acutely fasted state has not been elucidated. Marliss and associates have demonstrated that muscle is a major source of glutamine synthesis in man and that the splanchnic bed is a site of its removal. Further, it has been demonstrated that the intestinal tract rather than the liver is the site of splanchnic glutamine uptake, and it has been suggested that glutamine is not an important endogenous substrate for hepatic gluconeogenesis.

In the basal postabsorptive state a typical 70-g adult has a caloric requirement of 1,600 to 1,800 calories per day. Most of these calories are supplied by free fatty acids derived from lipolysis of triglycerides stored in the adipose tissue. However, this adult also exhibits an obligatory daily requirement for glucose approximating 150 to 180 g. Since the glycogen stores in liver (Table 9) are able to meet only 40 to 50 percent of this requirement, the individual rapidly becomes dependent on gluconeogenesis to maintain an adequate supply of glu-

cose. Although the total glycogen content of muscle is significantly greater than that of liver (Table 9), this glycogen moiety is not readily mobilized except by strenuous physical work or anoxia. Since approximately 50 percent of de novo glucose production is derived from protein sources, it is obvious that the protein stores of the body would be rapidly depleted by prolonged fasting if the adult continued to require 2 to 2.5 g of glucose per kilogram of body weight per day. For example, a 70-kg man would lose 75 g of protein per day (representing about 600 g of muscle mass) or 4.2 kg of muscle mass per week. Since adults are capable of sustaining total caloric deprivation for prolonged periods of time, it is obvious that adaptive mechanisms must supervene to prevent the inanition and death that would rapidly occur due to loss of functional and structural protein secondary to the glucose demands of the organism. The only known source for net de novo glu-

TABLE 9. Fuel Stores of a 70-kg Man

Fuel	Amount (kg)	Calories
Fat (adipose tissue)	15	141,000
Protein (muscle)	6	24,000
Glycogen (muscle)	0.150	600
Glycogen (liver)	0.075	300
Total		165,900

Adapted from Cahill: N Engl J Med 282:668, 1970.

cose synthesis is protein (net conversion of fat to glucose requires a dicarboxylic acid cycle that is not present in mammals); thus it seems obvious that the only
feasible conservation mechanism involves a decrease in
the glucose requirements of the organism.

It is well recognized that the brain, the formed elements of the blood, and the renal and adrenal medullae
have obligate requirements for glucose as their source
of energy (Fig. 10). Indeed, in the case of the red blood
cell mass the absence of mitochondria makes this tissue
totally dependent on glycolysis as a source of energy.
Since approximately 80 percent of the total basal glucose requirement of the individual is represented by the
metabolism of the central nervous system, the only
adaptation that the organism could make that would
significantly reduce glucose requirements would be in
this tissue. The brain can adapt during fasting to the
utilization of ketone bodies; indeed, it derives over half
of its energy from the oxidation of ketones under these
conditions. This adaptation results in a marked decrease in the demand for de novo glucose synthesis and
consequently permits the organism to conserve its vital
protein stores.

It becomes evident from the above considerations
that the newborn infant and young child are at a precarious balance between their obligatory glucose requirements and their ability to maintain this supply during
caloric deprivation. Specific measurements of glucose
requirements in the young child are lacking, but on the
basis of animal studies it would appear that they are
twofold to threefold greater than in the adult. Despite
this increase, the glycogen stores of the liver are sufficient to meet these demands for at least 8 to 12 hours.
After 24 to 36 hours the young child is totally dependent on gluconeogenesis for his glucose supply; this is
clinically evident in many by a poor glycemic response
to glucagon under these circumstances. One factor that
probably contributes to the high glucose requirement
of the young child is the relative increase of brain mass
to total body mass in this age group. However, there is
not complete agreement that the glucose requirements
of the neonate and young child per kilogram of body
weight are significantly greater than those of the adult.
Even if the glucose requirements were the same, the
immature individual is still less able to defend his blood
glucose, since his gluconeogenic potential may be significantly less than that of his adult counterpart. Since
over 50 percent of de novo glucose production is
derived from protein stores, and the protein mass of the
newborn infant and young child relative to total body
mass is significantly smaller than in the adult, the ability
to mobilize an adequate supply of endogenous
gluconeogenics substrate may be compromised in the
infant and child.

In a later section (p. 725) the key enzymes involved
in glycogen degradation and synthesis and gluconeogenesis are discussed. Although it has been well documented that the kidney is capable of gluconeogenesis,
studies in adult human beings indicate that the net glucose contribution of this organ is relatively small until
after very prolonged periods of fasting.

ENDOCRINE SYSTEM

Insulin is the predominant hormone regulating the
blood glucose level, since it is the only hormone whose
direct action is to decrease the influx of glucose and
acelerate the efflux of glucose from the vascular space.
Insulin stimulates the transmembrane movement of
glucose into skeletal and cardiac muscle and adipose
tissue and the conversion of glucose to glycogen and
triglyceride, as well as the intracellular transport of
amino acids in these tissues and their incorporation into
protein. At even low concentrations insulin is a potent
inhibitor of adipose tissue lipolysis. The net effect of
these actions on peripheral tissues is to accelerate glucose disappearance from the blood and decrease the
supply of gluconeogenic substrates (ie, glycerol and
amino acids) presented to the liver. In concert with
these peripheral actions, insulin stimulates hepatic
glycogen synthesis, impairs glycogenolysis, and
markedly depresses hepatic gluconeogenesis. Current
information suggests that these hepatic effects reflect an
action of the hormone on the adenyl cyclase–cyclic nucleotide phosphodiesterase system, resulting in a decrease in cellular concentration of cyclic adenosine
monophosphate. This action would result in activation
of glycogen synthetase, inhibition of the phosphorylase
system, and an ultimate decrease in the levels of
gluconeogenic enzymes.

It is now recognized that the pancreatic arterial glucose level is not the only determinant of insulin release
and that hormone secretion is influenced by a variety of
nutritional and hormonal factors. A number of amino
acids are capable of either directly stimulating insulin
release from the beta cell or potentiating the effect of
glucose on hormone secretion. Furthermore, oral
ingestion of protein and glucose provokes the secretion
of enteric factors that themselves stimulate insulin release. Under normal circumstances insulin secretion is
primarily observed only during periods of nutrient
ingestion; only minimal quantities need be secreted
during fasting to prevent the development of unre-
strained ketoacidosis. In all species thus far examined,
plasma insulin falls to very low levels during caloric
restriction; values below 5 to 10 μunits/ml are routinely
noted in the human being under these circumstances. Consequently insulin levels greater than 5 to 10
μunits/ml in association with blood glucose levels below 50 mg/dl are distinctly abnormal. The peripheral
plasma level of the hormone will be significantly lower
than in the portal vein, reflecting both transhepatic removal (approximately 50 percent of a physiologic load
is removed in one transhepatic passage) and dilution in
the total vascular space. Nevertheless, in the few studies
reported of simultaneous measurements of insulin in
portal and peripheral venous blood, the peripheral values have parallelled the concurrent portal ones.

Opposed to the hypoglycemic effects of insulin are
the actions of adrenocorticotropic hormone (ACTH),
cortisol, glucagon, epinephrine, and growth hormone.
The net effect of these hormones is to increase the
ambient blood glucose level by the following mech-

anisms: inhibiting glucose uptake by muscle (ie, epinephrine, cortisol, and growth hormone), increasing endogenous gluconeogenic amino acid supply by mobilization from muscle (ie, cortisone), activating lipolysis and providing increased free fatty acids as a source of energy and glycerol for gluconeogenesis (ie, epinephrine, glucagon, growth hormone, ACTH, and cortisol), inhibiting insulin secretion from the pancreas (ie, epinephrine), acute activation of glycogenolytic and gluconeogenic enzymes (ie, epinephrine and glucagon), and chronic induction of gluconeogenic enzyme synthesis (eg, glucagon and cortisol).

DEFINITION AND SYMPTOMS OF HYPOGLYCEMIA

Children are usually symptomatic when the true blood glucose reaches a concentration of approximately 40 mg/dl. Symptoms are frequently absent despite extremely low blood glucose levels in newborn infants. Cornblath and Schwartz have suggested that blood sugar levels less than 30 mg/dl in the full-term neonate and less than 20 mg/dl in the premature or small-for-gestational-age (SGA) infant should define hypoglycemia in this age group.

Two factors that are frequently overlooked when interpreting glucose concentrations are the analytic method used and whether blood or serum (plasma) is being examined. Since the water content of whole blood is approximately 15 percent less than that of serum, and since glucose is not completely equilibrated between red cell water and serum, serum or plasma glucose levels will be approximately 15 percent higher than whole blood values. A larger number of chemical and enzymatic methods are currently in use for the determination of glucose. The enzymatic methods using glucose oxidase or a combination of hexokinase and glucose-6-phosphate dehydrogenase specifically measure glucose. On the other hand, a variety of reducing methods are not as specific for glucose and therefore may occasionally give falsely elevated glucose levels in the newborn infant.

The clinical symptomatology associated with a rapid and acute fall in blood glucose reflects primarily excessive epinephrine secretion (ie, sweating, weakness, tachycardia, nervousness, and hunger). If the hypoglycemia is not relieved, manifestations of cerebral dysfunction such as headache, irritability, mental confusion, psychotic behavior, seizures, and coma become progressively more prominent. With frequent or prolonged episodes of hypoglycemia, permanent central nervous system dysfunction may result. As mentioned previously hypoglycemic symptoms in the neonatal period are either less obvious or absent, and they may be completely overlooked.

HYPOGLYCEMIC SYNDROMES

The hypoglycemic syndromes have been divided arbitrarily into two main groups: transient neonatal hypoglycemia and hypoglycemia of infancy and childhood (Table 10). The vast majority of neonates developing hypoglycemia in the first 24 hours after birth will have either a prenatal history (ie, mothers with diabetes or toxemia) or physical findings (ie, small for gestational age or prematurity) that identify them as high-risk infants. Although the hypoglycemia occurring in most newborn infants remits spontaneously within hours to days of diagnosis, it is important to recognize that chronic hypoglycemia in these infants can occur soon after birth and can be due to well-defined hepatic enzyme defects, endocrine deficiencies, or persistent hyperinsulinism.

TABLE 10. Classification of Hypoglycemia

Neonatal hypoglycemia
  Hypoglycemia associated with SGA infants
  Transient hyperinsulinemia of newborns
    Infant of diabetic mother
    Erythroblastosis fetalis
    Beckwith-Wiedemann syndrome
  Other factors associated with neonatal hypoglycemia
    Bacterial sepsis
    Hypoxemia
    Miscellaneous
Hypoglycemia of infancy and childhood
  Hyperinsulinism
  Substrate-limited hypoglycemia
    Ketotic hypoglycemia
    Hypoglycemia associated with endocrine deficiencies
  Hepatic enzyme deficiencies
    Glycogen storage diseases
      Glucose-6-phosphatase
      Amylo-1,6-glucosidase
      Defects of phosphorylase enzyme system
    Fructose-1,6-diphosphatase deficiency
    Glycogen synthetase deficiency
    Galactose-1-phosphate uridyl transferase deficiency
    Fructose-1-phosphate aldolase deficiency
  Maple syrup urine disease
  Reye's syndrome
  Drug-induced hypoglycemia
    Ethyl alcohol
    Salicylates and related compounds
    Oral hypoglycemic agents

Neonatal Hypoglycemia

Glucose is rapidly transported across the placenta; thus the fetal plasma glucose level closely approximates the maternal concentration. Consequently the fetus during gestation is not dependent on its own gluconeogenic capacity, since it is constantly being supplied with a glucose infusion from maternal sources. In this context one would anticipate that the gluconeogenic mechanisms (eg, hepatic gluconeogenic enzymes, transaminases, and protein catabolic systems) in placentates would not be fully developed until near or soon after parturition. Although very little is known about the time of induction of the hepatic gluconeogenic enzymes in the human fetus, in vitro perfusions with radioisotope-labeled precursors and in vitro studies with fetal liver slices have clearly demonstrated that in the experimental animal fetus gluconeogenesis is either absent or markedly depressed. Measurements of the levels of specific gluconeogenic enzymes have shown considerable species variation, but in general they have confirmed the conclusion that certain key rate-limiting enzyme activities are low near the time of parturition and do not reach full activity until several hours to days after delivery. Detailed information concerning the maturation of the hepatic gluconeogenic enzymes in human beings is essential if we are to understand fully the various pathogenic mechanisms responsible for the development of transient hypoglycemia of the newborn infant.

From the point of view of glucose homeostasis and energy requirements, it is rather surprising that in highly developed countries the neonate immediately following delivery is placed in a position of being fully dependent on his own resources, whereas in less sophisticated societies he is supported by being put immediately to the breast. The normal healthy newborn infant does have adequate stores of fat and glycogen to sustain a short period of caloric deprivation and appears to be capable of mobilizing these substrates as energy sources. For example, within a few hours after delivery the plasma free fatty acids are elevated, and glucagon evokes a glycemic response. However, glycogen stores are limited, and within a short period of time the neonate becomes dependent on gluconeogenesis as the sole mechanism for meeting the obligate glucose requirements of the central nervous system and other glucose-dependent tissues. Despite these considerations, it has been a common practice to withhold feeding of normal neonates for 12 hours, and even longer periods of caloric deprivation have been suggested in the past for low-birth-weight infants to avoid the problem of aspiration.

Throughout gestation the normal fetus is exposed to an ambient plasma glucose level similar to that of the mother. There is no a priori reason to believe that on delivery the glucose-dependent tissues of the neonate are more tolerant to low glucose supply than those of the adult. Indeed, the very opposite seems more likely, since many critical structures have yet to reach maturation. In this context it is difficult to accept current definitions of significant hypoglycemia, ie, the presence of at least two sequential blood glucose values under 30 mg/dl during the first 72 hours of life and 40 mg/dl thereafter in the full-size infant born at term, and under 20 mg/dl in the infant of low birth weight.

The definition of hypoglycemia in the low-birth-weight neonate within the first 72 hours of life is based on neonates who had prolonged periods of caloric deprivation, who by definition were abnormal (premature and small for gestational age), and who would appear to have had defects in gluconeogenesis. Although the value of < 20 mg/dl represents the lower limit of two standard deviations from the mean glucose concentration in the low-birth-weight infants studied, this value does not represent the normal, much less the ideal, blood glucose concentration, since it is derived from an abnormal population. In addition, brain damage has been reported in infants with blood glucose levels less than 30 mg/dl. Evaluations of premature infants breast-fed immediately after birth demonstrated that the lowest mean plasma glucose value was 54 mg/dl, which occurred at 36 hours.

Although it is well documented that the nadir of blood glucose frequently occurs within 2 to 3 hours following birth, this should not be construed as being either the normal or a desirable concentration for later hours of life. Until further studies relating to the effect of early feeding on the blood glucose concentration have been performed, it may be advisable to try to maintain the plasma glucose concentration above 40 mg/dl in all neonates.

HYPOGLYCEMIA ASSOCIATED WITH SGA INFANTS. Infants whose weights are below the 10th percentile for gestational age have been found to have an increased risk of transient neonatal hypoglycemia. These infants have been termed intrauterine-growth-retarded or SGA infants. The cause of the growth retardation is not clear, but it may be related to placental insufficiency; however, chromosomal defects and congenital viral syndromes have been implicated.

Lubchenco and Bard have shown that the risk for development of blood sugar levels less than 30 mg/dl in the SGA infant is best correlated with the degree of maturation of the infant, ie, the incidence of hypoglycemia was 67 percent in premature, 25 percent in term, and 18 percent in post-term SGA infants. The factor predisposing these infants to the development of hypoglycemia could theoretically be a defect in any one of the essential requirements for the maintenance of normal glucose homeostasis, including integrity of the hepatic gluconeogenic and glycogenolytic pathways, sufficient endogenous gluconeogenic substrate, and appropriate hormonal secretion to modulate the first two processes.

Various studies have demonstrated elevated plasma concentrations of growth hormone and cortisol in low-birth-weight infants. Therefore it must be concluded that the pituitary gland and the pituitary adrenal axis are responding appropriately in the early hours of life. Insulin has been implicated in a variety of specific clinical and pathologic disorders in the newborn, but hyperinsulinemia has not been found in these infants. It has recently been demonstrated that these infants have a hyperglucagonemic response to alanine infusion, which is evidence against glucagon insufficiency being the etiology of the hypoglycemia. In regard to substrate availability, there are insufficient data for any general conclusions regarding formation or utilization of free fatty acids, glycerol, and ketone bodies during the first 24 hours after birth.

Hyperlactatemia and hyperalaninemia are well established findings in patients with defects in hepatic gluconeogenesis, either congenital (ie, glucose-6-phosphatase or fructose-1,6-diphosphatase deficiencies) or acquired (ie, lactic-acidemia). Both hyperalaninemia and hypoglycemia have been observed within a few hours after birth in SGA infants of hypertensive mothers. Also, hyperlactatemia and hyperamino-acidemia are present in the SGA infant. Figure 11 compares the plasma glucose, alanine, blood lactate, and pyruvate in full-term and SGA infants from birth through the first 24 hours. The persistence of hyperlactatemia and hyperalaninemia is most compatible with a defect in gluconeogenesis compromising the ability of the infant to utilize gluconeogenic substrates entering at or below pyruvate. With decreased hepatic gluconeogenesis a larger proportion of hepatic glucose release must be derived from stored glycogen, which may result in rapid depletion and would explain the poor glycemic re-

sponses observed in these infants on challenge with glucagon.

Hypoglycemia develops in only 40 to 50 percent of SGA infants. Significant inverse correlations of plasma glucose and lactate and of glucose and alanine support a causative relationship between gluconeogenic substrates and the plasma glucose concentration. These observations, together with the pattern of other potential gluconeogenic amino acids and the inability of the SGA infant to utilize administered alanine as a gluconeogenic substrate during the first day after birth as compared to normal infants, are strong evidence for a transient defect in hepatic gluconeogenesis.

TRANSIENT HYPERINSULINEMIA OF NEWBORNS. Hyperinsulinemia has been documented in infants of mothers with various forms of diabetes mellitus (ie, chemical, clinically overt, and insulin-requiring). Although there is technical difficulty in documenting hyperinsulinemia in the newborn of the insulin-requiring mother because of intereference of insulin antibodies in the radioimmunoassay, on postmortem examination marked hyperplasia of the beta cells and high contents of insulin in the islet cells are seen. Infants with erythroblastosis fetalis also have a high incidence of hypoglycemia that is secondary to hyperinsulinemia. Beta cell hyperplasia also has been found at postmortem examination in these infants. In the offspring of diabetic mothers beta cell hyperplasia is considered to be secondary to the chronic hyperglycemia resulting from the elevated maternal blood glucose level; no etiology is apparent in the erythroblastotic infant.

In addition, beta cell hyperplasia has been observed in Beckwith-Wiedemann syndrome, a disorder characterized by macroglossia, omphalocele, hyperplastic visceromegaly, and frequently hypoglycemia. The hypoglycemia, when it occurs in these patients, is profound, but it spontaneously improves over the first few days after birth. Hyperinsulinemia and elevated insulin-like activity have been documented in a number of these infants. Any newborn with macroglossia and/or exomphalos should be followed prospectively for the development of hypoglycemia so that prompt therapy can be instituted to minimize the central nervous system dysfunction frequently observed with this disorder.

OTHER FACTORS ASSOCIATED WITH NEONATAL HYPOGLYCEMIA. Neonatal bacterial sepsis is associated with hypoglycemia and accelerated rates of glucose disappearance following intravenous glucose administration. Whether the hypoglycemia is secondary to poor antecedent caloric intake or to the effects of circulating endotoxins on glucose homeostatic mechanisms has not been established. In support of this latter possibility, hypoglycemia has been observed in adults with gram-negative bacteremia, and in animal studies gram-negative infection and exogenously administered endotoxins have been associated with hypoglycemia, hepatic glycogen depletion, and decreased rates of gluconeogenesis.

Neonatal hypoxemia frequently is associated with

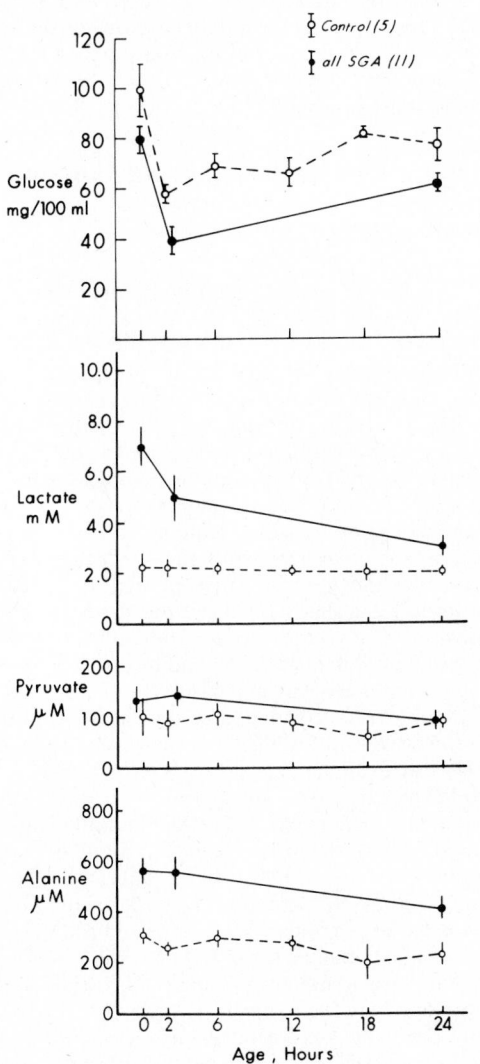

FIG. 11. Plasma glucose, blood lactate, blood pyruvate, and plasma alanine concentrations of normal and SGA infants during the first 24 hours of life (mean ± SEM). (From 0000: N Engl J Med 291:322, 1974.)

hypoglycemia in the early hours after birth. In neonatal animal studies it has been observed that tissue oxygenation is a prerequisite for the establishment of hepatic gluconeogenesis. Therefore, under the stress of difficient tissue oxygenation, hepatic glycogen stores would be rapidly depleted, and with a superimposed functional defect in gluconeogenesis, hypoglycemia could ensue. In addition, children with chronic hypoxemia secondary to cyanotic congenital heart disease are generally growth-retarded and can develop fasting hypoglycemia. Whether their hypoglycemia is secondary to inadequate caloric intake, and therefore is substrate-mediated, or whether it is the result of defective hepatic gluconeogenesis remains to be determined.

Hypoglycemia has also been reported in infants born to toxemic mothers, and it has occurred in association with hypothermia in the newborn infant. In the latter situation cause and effect are not clear, since hypothermia is a common finding in adults with hypoglycemia. Hypoglycemia in the neonate in association with hypothermia may well be related to more rapid utilization of endogenous glycogen stores in the face of decreased ability to perform gluconeogenesis. Infants have also been described with severe unresponsive hypoglycemia in whom alpha cells were reported to be absent from the pancreas. With the advent of the glucagon immunoassay, techniques are now available to document a deficiency of this glucoregulatory hormone.

The time at which the neonate is begun on a feeding schedule varies. Most nurseries tend to have a fixed program in which the initial feeding consists of 5 percent glucose at 4 to 12 hours after delivery in the normal neonate and even sooner in the premature or SGA infant. Five percent glucose (6.6 calories/ounce) is a poor nutritional substitute for human colostrum, which contains 6.4 percent lactose, 3 percent lipid, 2 to 3 percent protein, and 18 calories/ounce. It has frequently been argued that 5 percent glucose is safer than milk as an initial feeding should aspiration occur. However, studies in newborn rabbits have revealed no pathologic differences 24 hours after intratracheal instillation of either 5 percent glucose or a formula feeding.

It is advisable to monitor the blood glucose level of all high-risk infants (ie, SGA infants, premature infants, infants of diabetic mothers, etc) at 1- to 2-hour intervals with Dextrostix. Since variable and inconsistent results are frequently observed with this method at low blood glucose concentrations, test results with Dextrostix are frequently compared with plasma glucose values determined by reliable laboratory methods. If the blood glucose level with this method is 45 mg/dl or less, a blood specimen should be obtained for measurement of glucose by the glucose oxidase method, and the infant should be started immediately on a feeding of 5 percent glucose followed subsequently at 2- to 3-hour intervals with standard formula feedings. Throughout this time the blood glucose level should be monitored before each feeding; in the large majority of instances, adequate glucose concentrations are maintained by this practice. However, if the plasma glucose value remains

below 40 mg/dl by specific measurement, an intravenous infusion of 10 to 25 percent glucose can be given. Although specific rates of glucose administration have been suggested, the variability in requirement between patients is so great that the rate of administration should be individualized, and the patient should be given an amount of glucose that will maintained his plasma glucose above 40 mg/dl. This approach to therapy requires frequent monitoring of the blood glucose and close observation of the volume of fluid being administered. On rare occasions hypoglycemia persists despite this infusion, and then cortisone acetate should be administered intramuscularly at 8-hour intervals (total dose 5 mg/kg body weight per day). On this regimen the blood glucose level is readily stabilized in the vast majority of infants. Usually the intravenous infusion of glucose can be tapered after 48 hours and cortisone acetate therapy gradually eliminated during the subsequent 4 to 5 days. If hypoglycemia persists for more than 72 hours on this regimen, other causes for the disorder must be sought.

Hypoglycemia of Infancy and Childhood

Hyperinsulinism

In 1954 McQuarrie described recurrent hypoglycemia in a group of children whose symptoms usually appeared before 2 years of age and who exhibited a natural tendency to spontaneous remission with advancing age; they demonstrated a uniformly favorable response to treatment with ACTH or cortisone. He thought that this condition represented a single clinical syndrome that he called idiopathic hypoglycemia. Two years later Cochran and associates reported that a high-protein diet increased the frequency of hypoglycemic attacks in some of these children; they suggested that leucine was the specific cause of hypoglycemia. DiGeorge and Auerbach reviewed the cases of leucine-sensitive hypoglycemia up to 1960 and noted that approximately 33 percent of patients with idiopathic hypoglycemia were leucine-sensitive and about 50 percent demonstrated evidence of beta cell hyperplasia. With the advent of the insulin imunoassay it was demonstrated that the leucine-sensitive hypoglycemic child exhibited an excessive insulin secretory response to this amino acid. Furthermore, many of the nonleucine-sensitive individuals diagnosed as having idiopathic hypoglycemia were also noted to have abnormally elevated fasting insulin concentrations and hyperinsulinemic responses to intravenous tolbutamide. These data suggested that idiopathic hypoglycemia was not a single entity and that a significant number of these patients had organic hyperinsulinism.

It is now recognized that organic hyperinsulinism can result from a variety of apparently different beta cell abnormalities: beta cell adenoma, diffuse beta cell hyperplasia, nesidioblastosis (ie, neoformation of beta cells from the ductal epithelium), and functional beta cell secretory disorders without detectable histologic abnormality. An islet cell adenoma of the pancreas is a rare finding in children; less than 50 cases have been reported in the literature. Many of these patients with beta cell tumors demonstrate marked hyperinsulinemic and hypoglycemic responses to leucine and intravenous tolbutamide. These responses are indistinguishable from those observed in children previously diagnosed as having idiopathic hypoglycemia. Ten of 13 children who had had partial pancreatectomy for idiopathic hypoglycemia showed increased numbers of beta cells in the exocrine portion of the pancreas. Nesidioblastosis cannot be diagnosed by routine staining methods; rather, insulin-specific staining techniques (eg, aldehyde-fuchsin and pinacynole metachromasia) are required to establish this diagnosis. This entity may account for many of the cases of idiopathic hypoglycemia that on routine histologic examination have normal-appearing islets of Langerhans. However, there may be instances of organic hyperinsulinemia in children in which a functional defect in insulin secretion exists that cannot be identified even by sophisticated histologic examination. At the present time one cannot utilize the plasma insulin response to fasting and provocative stimulatory agents to distinguish the entities of beta cell adenoma, beta cell hyperplasia, nesidioblastosis, and functional beta cell secretory disorders.

With currently available diagnostic procedures it would appear that the majority of patients who previously would have been diagnosed as cases of idiopathic hypoglycemia can now have the pathogenic basis of their disorder more clearly defined (Table 11). Since ketotic hypoglycemia is the most common form of childhood hypoglycemia, it seems reasonable to suggest that a large number of McQuarrie's original cases were ex-

amples of this disorder. His observations that a significant number of children with idiopathic hypoglycemia exhibited spontaneous remission of their disease with increasing age and had good responses to ACTH or cortisone therapy further support the suggestion that many of these patients had ketotic hypoglycemia. Although a few cases of symptomatic adults with leucine sensitivity have been reported, there is no documented instance in which a child with chronic hypoglycemia secondary to hyperinsulinemia exhibited spontaneous remission of the disease. Some think that the term idiopathic hypoglycemia should be discarded. With careful evaluation the majority of children with hypoglycemia will be found to have some form of ketotic hypoglycemia, a disorder easily distinguished from hyperinsulinemic states. Abnormalities of the beta cell will comprise the remainder of this group, and in only a rare child will no specific diagnosis be made.

The ultimate aim of therapy in childhood hypoglycemia is to prevent neurologic symptoms and sequelae, including mental retardation. Medical management of hyperinsulinemia has included the long-term use of glucocorticoids and dietary manipulation. In general the response to such treatment has been poor. The hyperglycemic effect of diazoxide is due, at least in part, to suppression of pancreatic insulin secretion, and this drug has been reported to be effective in treating many types of childhood hypoglycemia. Of 17 patients, 13 were reported to have a favorable response, 1 died 3 weeks after initiation of therapy in keto-acidosis, and 3 did not respond. The follow-up of these patients ranged from several weeks to 18 months. There have been several infants with proved pancreatic adenomas in which diazoxide was ineffective in controlling the hypo-

TABLE 11. Relative Incidence of Childhood Hypoglycemic Disorders*

Disorder	McQuarrie (1942–1954)	Kogut[†] (1964–1969)	SLCH (1969–1975)
Adrenal insufficiency	6	—	1
Hypopituitarism	1	—	7
Hypothyroidism	2	—	1
Hepatic enzyme defects	4	—	5
Maple syrup urine disease	—	—	2
Reye's syndrome	—	—	2
Ketotic hypoglycemia	—	13	40
Hyperinsulinism			
Pathologic diagnosis			
Beta cell adenoma	1	—	1
Beta cell hyperplasia	—	1[‡]	2[§]
Nesidioblastosis	—	—	2
Beta cell secretory abnormality	—	1[‡]	0
Nonoperative diagnosis			
Tolbutamide-sensitive	—	2"	0
Leucine- and tolbutamide-sensitive	—	3	0
Undiagnosed (idiopathic)	26	3	0
Total	40	23	63

* Transient symptomatic hypoglycemia of the neonate was not included.

† Patients with hepatic enzyme deficiencies and hypopituitarism were not included in this study.

‡ Patients demonstrated leucine sensitivity.

§ One patient was sensitive to both leucine and tolbutamide, whereas the second was sensitive only to tolbutamide.

" Patients previously classified as unknown were sensitive to tolbutamide but not to leucine.

glycemia. In a dosage range of 10 to 15 mg/kg body weight per day the side effects have consisted of hypertrichosis, advancement of bone age, mild hyperuricemia, and IgG deficiency.

There is no agreement on the therapeutic effectiveness of pancreatic surgery in children with hyperinsulinism. Obviously it is curative in beta call adenoma. The variable results reported with this procedure reflect, at least in part, the heterogeneity of the underlying pathology (ie, beta cell hyperplasia, nesidioblastosis, and functional beta cell secretory disorders) and the extent of the pancreatectomy. In 63 children reported by Hamilton in whom more than 50 percent of the pancreas was removed, 40 exhibited complete remission of symptoms, 7 were not benefited, 1 died as a result of surgery, and 15 were considered to have partial remission necessitating either reoperation or continued medical management to maintain euglycemia. Since subtotal pancreatectomy in a child performed by an experienced surgeon carries relatively little risk and the pathologic basis for hyperinsulinism cannot be defined by clinical testing, any child past the neonatal period with hypoglycemia and proved hyperinsulinemia is a candidate for pancreatic exploration. If an adenoma is not found after careful inspection and palpation, a subtotal pancreatectomy is indicated in which 75 to 85 percent of the pancreas is removed. Obviously long-term follow-up of these patients is required before definitive conclusions on the efficacy of surgical therapy can be made. However, current results would indicate that a significant number of children are benefited by this form of therapy.

Medical management continues to play an important role. In a small percentage of children no clue as to the etiology of hypoglycemia will be found, even following the most extensive diagnostic work-up presently available. In these children treatment with diet, diazoxide, and/or glucocorticoids should be considered in an attempt to prevent the consequences of chronic hypoglycemia. Medical management may also benefit children who continue to have hyperinsulinemia and hypoglycemia following subtotal pancreatectomy. However, if hypoglycemia cannot adequately be controlled medically in these patients, reoperation should be considered for removal of the remaining pancreas.

Substrate-limited Hypoglycemia

KETOTIC HYPOGLYCEMIA. Ketotic hypoglycemia is the most common form of childhood hypoglycemia. This disorder classically manifests itself between the ages of 18 months and 5 years and generally remits spontaneously before age 8 to 9 years. A presumptive diagnosis is made by documenting a low blood sugar in association with ketonuria, ketonemia, and typical symptoms of hypoglycemia. The definitive diagnosis is established by demonstrating an inability to tolerate a provocative ketogenic diet (ie, high fat, low carbohydrate, hypocaloric diet). Susceptible or affected

children develop severe hypoglycemia and ketosis on this diet within 24 hours.

Previous investigators have focused on hepatic gluconeogenic enzyme deficiencies and/or functional disturbances of insulin secretion as the causes of this syndrome. These studies have demonstrated several phenomena: glucagon evokes a normal glycemic response in these children in the fed state, indicating the presence of normal hepatic phosphorylase, amylo-1,6-glucosidase, and glucose-6-phosphatase activities; infusions of fructose and glycerol result in a prompt increase in blood glucose concentrations, thus indicating normal activities of fructose-1,6-diphosphatase and glucose-6-phosphatase; plasma glycerol levels in the fed and fasted states are no different from those of similarly treated control children, indicating that this substrate is not rate-limiting; responses to infusions of β-hydroxybutyrate do not differ from those of normal children; insulin levels are appropriately low.

Studies of children with ketotic hypoglycemia have shown that symptomatic hypoglycemia and ketonemia developed with 8 to 16 hours after the children are placed on a provocative ketogenic diet (1,200 kcal per 1.73 m^2 body surface area, 63 percent fat, 17 percent protein, 15 percent carbohydrate). Normal children exhibit similar findings after 32 to 36 hours on the same dietary regimen. Blood lactate and pyruvate concentrations are similar in both groups. Plasma alanine concentrations on either a normal or ketogenic diet are significantly lower in ketotic hypoglycemia children, as compared to normal children. In contrast to adults, even normal children develop hypoglycemia and ketonemia when calorically deprived for relatively short periods of time (32 to 36 hours). Plasma insulin concentrations during fasting progressively decrease to barely detectable levels. This fall in plasma insulin occurs despite more than a 100-fold increase in blood β-hydroxybutyrate. These findings support previous observations that hyperinsulinemia is not an etiologic factor in this disorder, and they demonstrate that ketone bodies are not significant insulinogenic secretogogues in children. Infusions of alanine (250 mg/kg body weight) produce a rapid rise in plasma glucose without significant changes in blood lactate or pyruvate concentrations. This response indicates that the entire gluconeogenic pathway from the level of pyruvate is intact, and hence a gluconeogenic enzyme defect can be excluded. Treatment with glucocorticoids prior to or during the provocative ketogenic diet prevents the development of hypoglycemia and ketosis. Within 4 to 6 hours following glucocorticoid administration, plasma levels of the gluconeogenic amino acids alanine and glutamine increase twofold to threefold. These results suggest that the protection from hypoglycemia afforded by glucocorticoid therapy is a result of its acute catabolic effect on muscle protein rather than induction of increased levels of hepatic gluconeogenic enzymes.

In other studies of patients with ketotic hypoglycemia comparable results were obtained with fasting alone, thus indicating that the usefulness of the ketogenic diet in provoking hypoglycemia and ketosis in these children is a consequence of its hypocaloric nature rather than its fat content. There may be no advantage in continuing the use of the ketogenic diet, since total caloric restriction can be used for diagnosis. The mechanisms responsible for the decreased supply of alanine in these patients remains unknown. Thus far, tests of adrenal and pituitary function have not shown any specific abnormalities in these children. Since the major source of endogenous gluconeogenic amino acids is skeletal muscle, a defect in any of the enzymes or hormone-sensitive sites involved in protein catabolism, oxidative deamination, transamination, or amino acid efflux in this tissue might represent a potential etiologic basis for this disorder. On the other hand, in the original clinical description of this syndrome it was pointed out that these children frequently are smaller than age-matched control subjects and present a history of transient neonatal hypoglycemia. Since the maintenance of a normal blood glucose level in the young child represents a more precarious balance between glucose demand and supply, any modest compromise of supply of endogenous gluconeogenic substrate such as is represented by a decreased muscle mass (independent of a specific enzyme or hormone defect) would predispose to the rapid development of hypoglycemia and ketosis. In this context, some of the children with ketotic hypoglycemia may constitute one end of a spectrum representing the normal distribution pattern of the organism's capacity to tolerate fasting. Other studies have implicated deficient adrenal medullary response in these children to insulin-induced hypoglycemia. Whatever the cause, it would seem reasonable to propose that the underlying deficit is present at birth but does not become manifest until the child is stressed with more prolonged periods of caloric restriction. Furthermore, as the supply of endogenous substrates increases relative to glucose demand (ie, with age), one would expect spontaneous remission to occur.

Ketotic hypoglycemia is a self-limited disorder that predictably remits by 8 to 9 years of age. Hypoglycemia usually occurs in association with intercurrent infections or during periods in which caloric restriction is sustained for 12 hours or more. Treatment consists of frequent feeding (four to five meals per day) of a high-protein high-carbohydrate diet. Parents should be instructed to test the child's urine for ketones during periods of illnesses, since ketonuria usually precedes hypoglycemia by several hours. Under these circumstances liquids with high carbohydrate content should be offered. If these cannot be consumed by the child, intravenous administration of glucose is required to prevent a hypoglycemic episode.

HYPOGLYCEMIA ASSOCIATED WITH ENDO-CRINE DEFICIENCIES. Hypoglycemia is a frequent occurrence in children with primary and secondary adrenal insufficienty (ie, Addison's disease, congenital adrenal hyperplasia, and isolated ACTH deficiency). A 20 percent incidence has been noted in panhypopituitarism, monotrophic growth hormone, or various combinations of trophic hormonal deficiencies including growth hormone and ACTH. The pathophysiology of the hypoglycemia in these endocrine disorders has generally been assumed to reflect decreased activity of gluconeogenic enzymes and accelerated rates of glucose utilization. Occasionally hypothyroidism has been implicated as a cause of hypoglycemia in children. The mechanism responsible for the hypoglycemia is unknown.

Hepatic Enzyme Deficiencies

GLYCOGEN STORAGE DISEASES. The glycogen storage diseases are inherited defects characterized by either a deficient or abnormally functioning enzyme involved in the degradation of glycogen. Although glycogen storage diseases type II (deficient lysosomal α-1,4-glucosidase) and type IV (amylo-1,4 $\rightarrow$ 1,6-trans-glucosidase, brancher enzyme), as well as those due to specific muscle enzyme defects, are not associated with hypoglycemia, the other forms are characterized by this abnormality (p. 729).

HEPATIC   FRUCTOSE-1,6-DIPHOSPHATASE DEFICIENCY. Hepatic fructose-1,6-diphosphatase deficiency is a newly described gluconeogenic enzyme defect. The presenting signs and symptoms are indistinguishable from those of glycogen storage disease type I. However, excessive glycogen storage does not occur, since the glycogenolytic pathway is intact. Hepatomegaly is secondary to lipid storage, but liver function studies are generally normal. Hypoglycemia, lactic-acidosis, keto-acidosis, hyperlipidemia, and hyperuricemia in this condition have the same pathogenesis as in glucose-6-phosphatase deficiency.

Five cases have been reported in children ranging in age from 5 months to 5.5 years at the time of diagnosis. One female infant died at 6 months, and the diagnosis was made by postmortem liver enzyme analysis; another died at 9 months with severe metabolic acidosis following extensive body burns. The other 2 females and 2 males were living at the time of the respective reports. In three of the five families there were 5 affected siblings who presented with hepatomegaly and died in the neonatal or early childhood period from unexplained metabolic acidosis. Postmortem histologic examination of the livers in 3 of the siblings revealed fatty infiltration similar to that found in the 5 index cases. Consanguinity was noted in two of the four families, and on the basis of available data this disorder appears to be inherited as an autosomal recessive trait.

Since the glycogenolytic system is intact, glucagon administration produces a hyperglycemic response in the immediate postprandial period, but not after a short fast. Glucose, galactose, maltose, and lactose are utilizable carbohydrates and can be stored as glycogen and metabolized. Since fructose, glycerol, and the gluconeogenic amino acids enter the gluconeogenic pathway at or below the level of fructose-1,6-diphosphatase, these substances cannot be converted to glucose. Infusions of these substances cause the accumulation of lactate and consequent lactic-acidosis and actually produce a rapid fall in the blood glucose level. The mechanism of this hypoglycemic effect has not been clarified, but one possibility is that the accumulation of triose phosphates below the level of fructose-1,6-diphosphatase may inhibit glycogenolysis in a manner similar to that resulting in the accumulation of fructose-1-phosphate in patients with hereditary fructose intolerance.

In 1 patient a diet containing 56 percent utilizable carbohydrate (glucose, maltose, and lactose), 12 percent protein, and 32 percent fat was effective in controlling the chronic lactic-acidosis and hypoglycemia. On this diet the patient has demonstrated normal growth and development; however, during infections associated with fever and vomiting, she develops lactic-acidosis, keto-acidosis, and plasma glucose concentrations of less than 3 mg/dl.

GLYCOGEN SYNTHETASE DEFICIENCY. Fasting hypoglycemia has been reported in identical twins and their younger siblings in whom liver biopsy studies in one twin have demonstrated fatty metamorphosis, absence of glycogen, and a lack of glycogen synthetase activity. Parr and associates observed a 4-month-old infant with hypoglycemia in whom no glycogen was demonstrable in muscle, liver, kidney, and adrenal glands. The liver showed fatty infiltration, absent hepatic glycogen synthetase and phosphorylase, and markedly diminished glucose-6-phosphatase. Similar histologic findings were also observed in 2 siblings who had clinical hypoglycemia. Since all of these studies were carried out on postmortem tissue, the significance of these findings is open to question.

GALACTOSE-1-PHOSPHATE URIDYL TRANSFERASE DEFICIENCY. Infants with galactose-1-phosphate uridyl transferase deficiency (galactosemia) (p. 713) are intolerant to products containing lactose and galactose; they present with hypoglycemia, diarrhea, and vomiting following meals, as well as failure to thrive. The occurrence of postprandial hypoglycemia in this disorder appears to be due to inhibition of phosphoglucomutase by galactose-1-phosphate, thereby resulting in acute inhibition of glycogenolysis.

FRUCTOSE-1-PHOSPHATE ALDOLASE DEFICIENCY. Fructose-1-phosphate aldolase deficiency (hereditary fructose intolerance) is dominated by symptoms of hypoglycemia and vomiting following ingestion of foods containing fructose. Fructosuria is present only after meals, and these patients frequently manifest hepatomegaly, jaundice, amino-aciduria, and failure to thrive. The hypoglycemia following fructose ingestion is a result of accumulation of fructose-1-phosphate, which inhibits the phosphorylase system and gluconeogenesis at the level of fructose-1, 6-diphosphate aldolase.

Maple Syrup Urine Disease

Maple syrup urine disease (MSUD) (p. 679) is an autosomal recessive disorder of oxidative decarboxylation of the α-keto acids of leucine, isoleucine, and valine. Hypoglycemia and profound hypoalaninemia are observed in patients with classical MSUD at times when their branched-chain amino acids and α-keto acids are markedly elevated. With correction of the plasma branched-chain amino acids, fasting alanine and glucose values have been observed to increase. Glycogen metabolism and gluconeogenesis from the level of the triose phosphates would appear to be intact, since glucagon and fructose elicit normal glycemic responses. Despite the lower plasma alanine concentrations, the etiology of the hypoglycemia in these children would not appear to be substrate-limited, since infusions of alanine prior to and following correction of the branched-chain hyperamino-acidemia do not result in a glycemic response. A defect in pyruvate carboxylase or phosphenol pyruvate carboxykinase also would seen unlikely, since an abnormal rise in blood lactate is not observed subsequent to alanine administration. However, a progressive and sustained rise in plasma glutamine occurs following alanine infusion. It would appear that an enzyme or enzymes regulating TCA cycle homeostasis are affected, perhaps by increasing intracellular branched-chain amino acids or their α-keto acid derivatives, which may divert substrates away from gluconeogenesis.

Reye's Syndrome

In 1963 Reye, Morgan, and Baral described 21 children who, following mild upper respiratory infections or varicella, developed protracted vomiting, hyperpnea, profound disturbances of consciousness (ranging from mild delirium to coma), and decorticate and decerebrate posturing that proceeded in many to apnea, flaccidity, and death (p. 713). Hypoglycemia is a prominent feature of children with Reye's syndrome who are less than 5 years of age. At the time these children are first seen they have a complex disorder of acid–base metabolism with a metabolic acidosis and respiratory alkalosis with a relatively normal arterial pH. Circulating concentrations of lactate, pyruvate, alanine, glutamine, and glutamate are twofold to tenfold elevated above normal values. These findings suggest that gluconeogenesis is compromised. This speculation is supported by in vitro studies that show no gluconeogenesis from pyruvate in hepatic biopsy tissue from 2 children with this syndrome. Plasma cortisol, glucagon, growth hormone, and probably epinephrine are elevated in response to the stress of this disease, resulting in increased mobilization of amino acids, fatty acids, and glycogen. Increased rates of amino acid mobilization superimposed on compromised hepatic and renal gluconeogenic mechanisms are most likely the etiology of these striking elevations of substrates. Whether the hypoglycemia observed in the younger patient is due to more severe hepatic involvement or other metabolic or toxic factors cannot be determined at this time.

The hypoglycemia must be treated with parenteral glucose, but whether glucose, peritoneal dialysis, exchange transfusion, or other therapeutic modalities have any specific effects in altering the course of this devastating illness remains to be determined. However, intensive supportive management is required if these acutely ill patients are to survive.

Drug-induced Hypoglycemia

ETHYL ALCOHOL. Ingestion of ethyl alcohol, particularly in young children, can lead to profound hypoglycemia, seizures, and in some cases death. Hypoglycemia has been observed in a number of adults following ethanol ingestion. Utilizing isotopic turnover techniques, hepatic gluconeogenesis has been documented to be decreased following the ingestion of ethanol in otherwise normal individuals. The metabolism of ethanol requires utilization of NAD with subsequent production of NADH. Accumulation of the reduced pyridine nucleotide prevents the conversion of substrate to glucose.

SALICYLATE AND RELATED COMPOUNDS. Salicylates and their ester derivatives, as well as acetometaphin, have been associated with hypoglycemia and ketosis. The pathophysiology of this disturbance in glucose homeostasis following salicylate ingestion is not well defined. The child with salicylism presents with signs and symptoms of vomiting, mental confusion or delirium, hyperventilation, and occasionally hypoglycemia. In the absence of a history of salicylate exposure or inappropriate salicylate administration, the diagnosis must still be suspected and plasma levels determined. However, clinically this entity may be confused with pneumonia, encephalitis, Reye's syndrome, or diabetic keto-acidosis.

ORAL HYPOGLYCEMIC AGENTS. Treatment of gestational diabetics with oral hypoglycemic agents (tolbutamide, chlorpropamide, or acetohexamide) near the time of parturition has been associated with profound life-threatening hypoglycemia in the infant within hours of delivery. The sulfonylurea compounds readily cross the placenta and stimulate insulin release from the fetal beta cells. Intravenous glucose must be provided for a number of days, and in some cases exchange transfusion is necessary to maintain the plasma glucose in a normal range. With the wide use of oral hypoglycemic agents the possibility of ingestion of these compounds must be considered in any hypoglycemic child, and the appropriate historical information must be sought.

DIAGNOSTIC EVALUATION

A detailed history is of utmost importance in evaluating a child with documented hypoglycemia or one suspected of having hypoglycemia. Historical factors helpful in defining the etiology of the hypoglycemia include the presence of absence of hypoglycemic symptoms at birth, age of onset, frequency of hypoglycemic episodes, specific food intolerance, temporal relationship to meals, family history compatible with hypoglycemia, and unexplained infant deaths. A large number of clinical diagnostic procedures are available that are helpful in defining the pathogenesis of the various hypoglycemic disorders, and a systematic approach

is necessary. The results obtained from history, physical examination, and initial fasting data should be a guide for further selective provocative stimulatory testing.

Hypoglycemia without hepatomegaly, ketonuria, or ketonemia should focus attention immediately on abnormalities of insulin secretion. Hyperinsulinism is best documented by fasting the patient and obtaining simultaneous plasma glucose and insulin levels. The normal 24-hour fasting plasma insulin level is rarely above 10 μunits/ml, except in marked obesity; levels less than 5 μunits/ml are generally noted. Plasma insulin levels greater than 10μunits/ml with a concomitant plasma glucose value less than 50 mg/dl, irrespective of whether the patient is fed or fasted, are distinctly abnormal and are an indication for further studies to document hyperinsulinism. Provocative testing of insulin secretion can be carried out with tolbutamide (20 mg/kg body weight, not to exceed 1 g, administered intravenously in 1 minute) and/or leucine (150 mg orally or 75 mg intravenously per kilogram of body weight). In normal children tolbutamide produces a transient decrease in plasma glucose (maximal fall does not exceed 50 percent of baseline), which returns to control levels within 60 to 90 minutes. Since the insulin secretory response to tolbutamide is rapid, it is imperative that blood samples be obtained at 2, 5, and 10 minutes after injection to ensure that the peak plasma insulin response will not be missed. Rarely do normal children exhibit peak plasma insulin levels in excess of 100 μunits/ml. Generally the hyperinsulinemic syndromes are associated with marked peak plasma insulin levels and clinically apparent hypoglycemic responses. Obviously a physician should be in attendance during the provocative testing, and the test should be terminated if the severity of the hypoglycemic symptoms so merit. Similar responses will be noted with leucine, except that after oral administration the peak insulin response will generally occur 15 to 30 minutes after ingestion. Obviously neither tolbutamide nor leucine should be administered to a hypoglycemic patient. At the present time there are clinical studies available to assess the frequency of positive and negative responses to these provocative agents in documented cases of organic hyperinsulinism in children. On the basis of reports of small series and individual case reports it would seem that the great majority of patients with this disorder will exhibit a positive response to one or both of these agents.

Symptomatic fasting hypoglycemia, having its onset after 18 months of age and being associated with ketonuria and ketonemia, without hepatomegaly, strongly suggests the diagnosis of ketotic hypoglycemia. The presence of marked ketonuria and ketonemia is strong presumptive evidence against a hyperinsulinemic state. This diagnosis can be confirmed by a carefully monitored 24-hour fast with frequent blood sampling for determination of insulin, ketones, lactate, and the gluconeogenic amino acid alanine. In this disorder the concentration of plasma insulin is very low (less than 5 μunits/ml), ketonemia is commensurate with the degree of hypoglycemia, and plasma lactate and pyruvate levels are normal, but plasma alanine is markedly decreased. Ketosis is also a common finding in gluconeogenic-enzyme-deficient states, but in contrast to the situation with children with hypoglycemia, blood lactate, pyruvate, and alanine values are markedly increased as a consequence of the block in gluconeogenesis. Since the gluconeogenic pathway is intact in patients with deficiencies in the glycogenolytic enzyme system, the main clinical feature differentiating this latter group from those with ketotic hypoglycemia is the marked hepatomegaly that is present from birth. Additional clinical tests that readily distinguish between ketotic hypoglycemia and the gluconeogenic and glycogenolytic enzyme disorders are the positive glycemic responses to glucagon and infusions of alanine that occur in the ketotic hypoglycemic child.

Several other disorders may be confused with ketotic hypoglycemia. Children with Addison's disease, primary ACTH deficiency, monotrophic growth hormone deficiency, or combined pituitary deficiencies may also present with a similar clinical picture. Severe growth retardation will be present with growth hormone deficiency and is an indication for further evaluation. Plasma cortisol levels at the beginning and termination of fasting may be informative in all patients presenting with ketosis and hypoglycemia. In addition, plasma growth hormone levels should be obtained under comparable conditions in children who are below the third percentile in height. If no increase in one or both of these hormones is noted during fasting, further provocative studies (eg, arginine infusion, oral L-dopa, metapyrone, etc) can be performed to evaluate the functional status of the pituitary and adrenal glands.

The diagnosis of galactosemia or hereditary fructose intolerance should be considered in infants presenting with hypoglycemia in the immediate postprandial period together with hepatomegaly and failure to thrive. In these disorders non-glucose-reducing substances (ie, galactose, fructose) will be present in the urine following meals. The definitive diagnosis of galactosemia is made by determining the galactose-1-phosphate uridyl transferase activity in red blood cells; a galactose infusion test is not required. Hereditary fructose intolerance is diagnosed by the hypoglycemic and hypophosphatemic responses produced by cautious intravenous infusion of fructose (0.25 g/kg body weight); the intravenous route of fructose administration obviates the distressful symptoms of nausea or vomiting associated with oral ingestion.

Fasting hypoglycemia, hepatomegaly, and signs and symptoms of severe metabolic acidosis (ie, episodic hyperventilation) are highly suggestive of either glucose-6-phosphatase or fructose-1,6-diphosphatase deficiency. Although each of these disorders has a similar clinical presentation, including hypoglycemia, hyperlactic-acidemia, ketosis, hyperlipidemia, and hyperuricemia, they may be readily distinguished by the responses to infusions of various gluconeogenic precursors. In both conditions alanine and fructose infusions do not produce a glycemic response but result in a rapid rise in blood lactate and pyruvate. Glycerol provides a similar response. However, caution must be used in administering this substrate intravenously, since acute hemolysis, hemoglobinuria, and renal failure have been associated with its use. Infusion of galactose provokes similar effects in patients with glucose-6-phosphatase deficiency, whereas in fructose-1,6-diphosphatase deficiency a normal glycemia response without demonstrable change in blood lactate is observed. Glucagon further differentiates between these two disorders in that the hormone will produce a prompt glycemic response in the fed state in fructose-1,6-diphosphatase deficiency but no significant response in glucose-6-phosphatase deficiency.

Hypoglycemia is rarely a problem in patients with a deficiency of amylo-1,6-glucosidase or in the phosphorylase enzyme system, but marked hepatomegaly and growth retardation are commonly present. These individuals exhibit normal blood glucose and lactate responses to infusions of alanine, galactose, and fructose, but the effects of glucagon are more variable; occasional positive responses have been found in patients with documented enzyme deficiencies. Hyperlactic-acidemia and hyperuricemia are not characteristic of these disorders, but ketosis may be present during episodes of hypoglycemia.

Definitive diagnosis of the various hepatic enzyme deficiencies is made by determining specific enzyme activities, glycogen content, and structure in liver biopsy specimens. Open liver biopsies are preferable to needle biopsies in order to obtain adequate tissue for the appropriate biochemical studies. Tissue specimens should be frozen immediately in liquid nitrogen and stored, preferably at −80 C, until assayed. In type I glycogen storage disease glucose-6-phosphatase is totally absent, and hepatic glycogen content is greater than 5 percent by weight. Occasionally a patient is seen with all the clinical stigmata of this disorder, including an elevated hepatic glycogen content, in whom the activities of glucose-6-phosphatase and other known glycogenolytic enzymes in the liver biopsy are normal. It has been suggested that in these rare patients there are factors as yet unidentified that are deficient but that are required for normal in vivo glucose-6-phosphatase activity. In fructose-1,6-diphosphatase deficiency the enzyme is totally absent, and hepatic glycogen content may be normal or low depending on the caloric intake immediately before the liver biopsy is obtained. Fructose-1,6-diphosphatase activity has been observed in white blood cells and may be a useful adjunct in the diagnosis of this enzyme deficiency disease.

Several subtypes of amylo-1,6-glucosidase deficiency have been described in which the enzyme deficiency is present in leukocytes and muscle as well as in liver. In these cases a definitive diagnosis can be established without a liver biopsy. The demonstration of normal enzyme activity in leukocytes does not exclude this diagnosis, and a large precentage of patients will remain undiagnosed unless determinations of hepatic enzyme levels and glycogen structure are undertaken.

The diagnosis of phosphorylase deficiency is complicated by the complex cascade of multiple enzyme systems involved in the final activation of this enzyme. Deficiency of phosphorylase *b* kinase can be established by demonstration of low or absent phosphorylase activity in leukocytes and its restoration to normal levels by the addition of phosphorylase *b* kinase. Normal phosphorylase activity in leukocytes, however, does not exclude a deficiency in the hepatic phosphorylase system, and therefore detailed enzyme analysis of liver is required.

With increasing knowledge of the subcellular, cellular, organ, and interorgan processes necessary for the maintenance of normal glucose homeostasis, our ability to define and categorize many of the hypoglycemic disorders of infancy and childhood on a pathophysiologic basis and to provide a rational approach to therapy has advanced, but many areas remain in which information is either rudimentary or nonexistent.

References

Colle E, Ulstrom RA: Ketotic hypoglycemia. J Pediatr 64:632, 1964

Cornblath M, Schwartz R: Carbohydrate Metabolism in the Neonate. Philadelphia, WB Saunders, 1966

Felig P, Marliss E, Pozefsky T, Cahill CR Jr: Amino acid metabolism in the regulation of gluconeogenesis in man. Am J Clin Nutr 23:986, 1970

Greenberg RE, Christiansen O: The critically ill child: hypoglycemia. Pediatrics 46:915, 1970

Illingworth B: Enzymatic defects as causes of hypoglycemia. Diabetes 14:333, 1965

Lubchenco LO, Bard H: Incidence of hypoglycemia in newborn infants classified by birth weight and gestational age. Pediatrics 47:831, 1971

Pagliara AS, Karl IE, DeVivo DC, Feigin RD, Kipnis DM: Hypoalaninemia: a concomitant of ketotic hypoglycemia. J Clin Invest 51:1440, 1972

GLYCOGENOSES

James B. Sidbury

The glycogen storage diseases are a group of heritable disorders associated with a quantitative or qualitative aberration of glycogen storage that cannot be accounted for by other physiologic mechanisms, as in the Mauriac syndrome, excessive insulin therapy in diabetes, or steroid therapy. Thirteen different enzymatically defined types of glycogen storage disease have been described. Types I through IV are those originally classifed by Cori; subsequent types have been added according to the chronology of their identification, except type O, which is so designated to reflect the associated deficiency of glycogen. Subtypes have been designated to reflect differences in clinical manifestations, differences in tissue distribution of the defective enzyme, or functional alteration of the enzyme in vivo without demonstrated in vitro deficiency (Table 12). All of the glycogenoses appear to be autosomal recessive conditions, except type IX, which is sex-linked. Clinically the glycogenoses can be divided into those primarily affecting liver (types O, I, III, IV, VI, IX, XI, XII) and the myopathic group (types II, V, VII, VIII, X).

Type O

Affected infants may have a seizure or apneic spell shortly after birth, or later when four hourly feedings are reduced to three feedings a day. The hypoglycemic seizures are indistinguishable from those of any other etiology. Mental retardation may become apparent as the infant grows older. Two families have been described, and in neither was there consanguinity. There was a sibship cluster of cases, and both males and females were affected. Biochemical evidence of heterozygosity has not been demonstrated, but the disease would appear to be autosomal recessive.

The primary clinical laboratory finding is fasting hypoglycemia. There is no rise of blood glucose in response to glucagon administration in the fasting state, but a rise is obtained 2 to 3 hours after a meal. Glycogen synthetase is markedly diminished in liver obtained at biopsy.

While fasting, the available glycogen becomes depleted because the rate of synthesis of glycogen is markedly decreased as a result of a deficiency of the

TABLE 12. Types of Glycogen Storage Disease

Type	Enzymatic Defect	Defect Demonstrated in:			
		Erythrocytes	Leukocytes	Liver	Muscle
O	UDPG–glycogen transferase	—	—	yes	yes
IG	Glucose-6-phosphatase	no	no	yes	yes
IIa	Lysosomal α-1,4-glucosidase	no	inconstant	yes	yes
IIb	Lysosomal α-1,4-glucosidase	no	inconstant	yes	yes
III	Amylo-1,6-glucosidase and/or oligo-1,4 → 1,4-glucantransferase	yes	yes	yes	yes
IV	Amylo-1,4 → 1,6-transglucosylase	yes	yes	yes	yes
V	Myophosphorylase	no	no	no	no
VI	Hepatic phosphorylase	no	yes	yes	no
VII	Phosphofructokinase	yes	yes	no	yes
VIII	Phosphohexosisomerase (inhibitor ?)	—	—	—	yes
IX	Phosphorylase kinase	no	yes	yes	no
X	Phosphorylase kinase	—	—	—	yes
XI	Phosphoglucomutase	—	—	yes	—
XII	Cyclic-AMP-dependent kinase	—	—	yes	—

enzyme primarily responsible for its synthesis. Thus an inadequate amount of glucose is produced by the liver to regulate blood glucose under fasting conditions. Transamination of amino acids and gluconeogenesis is not rapid enough or quantitatively sufficient to maintain the blood sugar alone in the infant, as judged by the findings in this condition and in types III, VI, and IX glycogenosis. The glucagon response in the fasting state reflects the lack of available glycogen, and the response following a meal demonstrates that the enzyme is not completely absent, for sufficient glycogen is synthesized to obtain a positive glucose response to glucagon.

Intravenous administration of glucose is indicated to correct severe hypoglycemia. Frequent feedings with relatively high sugar content are indicated for prevention. A high protein intake should also be helpful in maintaining gluconeogenesis maximally. ACTH was shown to be helpful in the initial study, and it may be of benefit in the induction of the enzymes involved in gluconeogenesis. The experience with type O glycogenosis to date has been poor. In the originally described family 1 child is mentally retarded, and in the second family the 4 affected children have died.

Type I

The infant with absent hepatic and renal glucose-6-phosphatase may be symptomatic in the neonatal period and may present with hepatomegaly and hypoglycemic convulsions. This is one of the few conditions associated with ketonuria in the neonatal period. The disease may be first noted in the later months of the first year on finding a very large liver during a routine examination. The infants are usually chubby but lag in linear growth. The skin is thin, the venules are prominent, and a prolonged bleeding time is demonstrable early. There is individual variability in the response to hypoglycemia. Some will have an almost undetectable blood glucose level after a 4- to 8-hour fast without symptoms of any kind; others will require frequent glucose feedings to prevent recurrent hypoglycemic convulsions after a similar fast.

From the end of the first year to about the fifth year of life is the most difficult period of management. The growth retardation, immense hepatomegaly, and characteristic general appearance (Fig. 12) persist. There is increased fatigability, and the activity of these children is subdued when compared with that of their peers. Infections, which these children do not handle well, may be associated with epistaxis, which can be severe. Mild upper respiratory infections are prolonged and often difficult to manage. Keto-acidosis, abetted by lactic-acidosis, may become rapidly profound with infections. Hypoglycemia is also a problem during these periods. Removal of the tonsils and adenoids and dental extractions are often associated with hemorrhage. From the fifth year until puberty, which is often delayed, management becomes easier. Some patients develop the capability to maintain the blood glucose in the non-hypoglycemia range with an overnight fast; others adapt

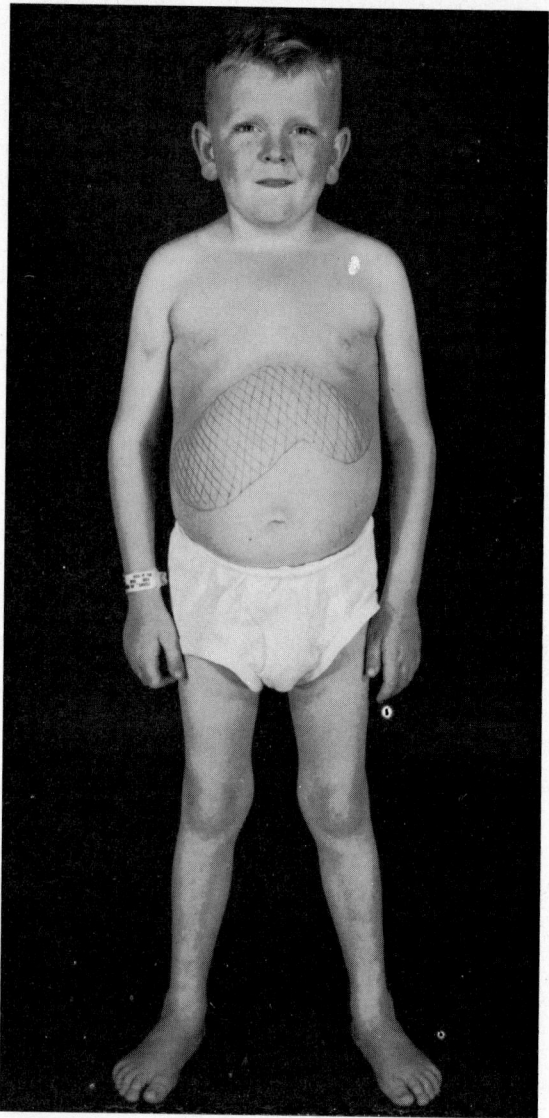

FIG. 12.   A 9-year-old boy with type I glycogen storage disease who shows the characteristic general appearance.

to the situation and arise at night to get carbohydrate-containing fluids or a snack. The enlarged liver, diminished stature, and variably increased adipose deposition persist after puberty. Stamina improves, but the patients are never hearty. Gout is a frequent problem in late adolescence, in the twenties, or later. Mental development is not affected.

The condition occurs in males and females equally and in siblings of unaffected parents. The frequency of consanguinity in the parents is not as high as might be anticipated. Detection of heterozygosity has been reported; the parents were found to have reduced glucose-6-phosphatase levels in ther intestinal mucosa. The evidence supports an autosomal recessive type of transmission. The incidence in Sweden is reported as 1 in 400,000 live births.

The clinical biochemical findings can be very helpful in differential diagnosis. These individuals show a fasting hypoglycemia, ketosis, hyperlactic-acidemia, elevated nonesterified fatty acids, and lipidemia. All of these abnormal values improve or return to normal with glucose administration. Hyperuricemia is also found. There may be a normal or a diabetic type of glucose tolerance curve, the latter being more frequent in older children and adults. There is no rise in blood glucose in response to administered epinephrine or glucagon in infants and young children, but there may be a delayed response in older children and adults. There is a rise in blood lactate in response to these agents.

Glucose-6-phosphatase is the final reaction product in the production of glucose in the liver and is common to glycogenolysis and gluconeogenesis. Thus a defect at this step mandates alimentary glucose for blood glucose maintenance. Since glucose cannot be released, stimulation of glycogenolysis results instead in a rise in lactate. Lowered blood glucose results in epinepherine release leading to mobilization of fatty acids and ketonemia. The increased ketones and particularly lactate competitively inhibit urate excretion by the renal tubules and result in hyperurincemia. There is some evidence for increased production, but this is of lesser consequence. There is increased glycerol phosphate as well as fatty acids, which accounts for the high lipid levels in the plasma. The high lipids are thought to be responsible for the platelet dysfunction that leads to the observed bleeding tendency.

The basic approach to management is administration of frequent high-carbohydrate feedings, because the individual is dependent on alimentary glucose to sustain the blood level. Portacaval shunt and tying off the portal vein have been used experimentally. Presumably this diverts more of the absorbed glucose to the systemic circulation rather than allowing it to be extracted by the liver. The basic defect remains, and the individual is still dependent on alimentary glucose for blood sugar regulation. Various modifications of hyperalimentation have been shown to return the aberrant blood chemical values to normal, and this improvement persists for some period after discontinuance of the infusion. Whether this approach will be of any practical value remains to be seen.

Infections need to be treated promptly, particularly in the first 2 years when there is more of a tendency to go rapidly into profound keto-acidosis. Sodium bicarbonate is recommended for the management of acidosis, since the blood lactate is characteristically high during these periods. Epistaxis is managed by conventional means. Hypoglycemia is readily corrected with oral glucose. In the adolescent period gout is increasingly likely; it is readily prevented and managed with allopurinol.

It is difficult to give a categoric prognosis. The severity of the condition is variable. In the first 2 years of life, death usually results from rapidly evolving profound acidosis triggered by infection. Hepatomas have been demonstrated at necropsy. Gout occurs some time after pubescence, and death has been reported at 40 years of age with gouty nephritis. Some of the older patients have shown signs of early angina and coronary symptoms. These observations represent very small numbers, and a true evaluation of prognosis must await further observations.

Type II

Type II glycogenosis is also known as generalized or cardiomegalic glycogenosis and as Pompe's disease (type IIa). The affected infant may be weak and have a poor sucking response from birth, or he may show no symptoms during the neonatal period and progress normally for 2 or 3 months. After this period there is steady retrogression, increasing irritability, feeding difficulty due to exertional dyspnea, cyanosis, increasing weakness or flaccidity, pooling of saliva in the pharynx, loss of reflexes, and progressive cardiomegaly. A progressively abnormal electrocardiographic pattern evolves characterized by a short P-R interval, very large QRS complexes, and deeply inverted T waves. Toward the end of the course of the disease the infant appears somewhat undernourished; spontaneous movements are weak and infrequent, and the tongue is often enlarged. The muscles are weak, although they are firm or even hard on palpation. The heart is very large, with weak heart sounds, and often a gallop rhythm is present. In type IIb the patient may present at 2 to 3 years of age in a state resembling pseudohypertrophic muscular dystrophy without cardiomegaly, and he may have a history of delayed motor development. Older patients have been described with a myopathic presentation. One individual has been described with late-onset myopathy.

The condition appears to be transmitted as an autosomal recessive disorder. There is a disproportionate number of affected males. Heterozygosity has been demonstrated in cultured fibroblasts. Type IIb also appears to be an autosomal recessive disorder, but its incidence is significantly lower than that of type IIa, which has been estimated to occur once in 400,000 live births.

The differential diagnosis includes congenital heart disease, primarily aberrant coronary vessels, truncus arteriosus, or endocardial fibroelastosis, as well as the floppy baby syndrome and cretinism. The firm and distinctly palpable muscles distinguish this condition from other floppy babies, and the protein-bound iodine concentration and a radiographic bone age survey assist in ruling out cretinism. Muscle biopsy permits a definitive diagnosis. Type IIb must be distinguished from other myopathies, primarily Duchenne's muscular dystrophy.

The usual clinical biochemical parameters of carbohydrate metabolism are normal. There is a marked increase in normal glycogen in the heart, skeletal muscle, liver, and neuronal cells. An absence of lysosomal α-glucosidase has been demonstrated in the tissues of these patients. With electron microscopy, engorgement of the lysosomes with glycogen can be demonstrated, whereas the amount of cytoplasmic glycogen appears normal. The relationship of the defect to the symptoms is not clear.

No effective treatment is known. Various dietary and hormonal modalities have been tried. Administrations of fungal α-glucosidase and human α-amylase have failed. Attempts to induce increased permeability of the lysosomes with large doses of vitamin A or hyperbarism have not been productive.

Type III

Clinical manifestations of type III may be very similar to those of type I. The liver may be equally large, but there is usually less growth retardation. Although clinical manifestations may be so mild that only the enlarged liver is present, all symptoms noted for type I glycogen storage disease, including hypoglycemia, may be found. As far as appearance, the boy in Figure 12 could very well have had type III glycogen storage disease. The clinical chemical findings in type III are distinguished from those of type I as follows: the fasting blood lactate values are normal; the lactate rise following glucagon or epinephrine is minimal; the lactate production from muscle with anoxic exercise is subnormal (see type V); the blood glucose response to glucagon or epinephrine 2 hours after a high-carbohydrate meal may be significantly improved over that in the fasting condition; the blood glucose rises following intravenous galactose administration; the serum uric acid concentration is normal or minimally elevated; the red cell glycogen concentration is often significantly elevated. The fasting blood sugar, blood ketone concentration, and serum nonesterified fatty acid values are of no assistance in distinguishing the two types.

The enzymes involved in debranching glycogen are amylo-1,6-glucosidase and oligo-1,4→1,4-glucantransferase. Either or both of these enzymes may be absent in either liver or muscle or both, on the basis of which four subtypes are defined. In each instance the glycogen in affected tissues is abnormal in structure, being short chain or limit dextrin in type. Thus far the data appear to be compatible with an autosomal recessive mechanism of transmission.

The treatment differs from that of type I glycogenosis in that a high-protein diet is helpful, utilizing gluconeogenesis to maintain the blood glucose. Many of these patients do not require any treatment. The prognosis for type III is considerably better than for type I in both morbidity and mortality. These children are sometimes management problems during the first 4 or 5 years of life, but they spontaneously improve thereafter. Around the time of puberty the hepatomegaly, lipemia, and fasting ketosis subside. The ultimate height is normal. Reproduction is normal. A myopathic syndrome has been observed in the third and fourth decades in 1 patient.

Type IV

There are now several patients reported with documented type IV glycogenosis. The patients presented at about 1 year of age with an enlarged nodular liver and splenomegaly. The clinical picture was no different from cirrhosis of any other origin. One patient had grossly abnormal liver function tests; in another they were only minimally deranged. Death usually results from portal hypertension, debilitation, and intercurrent infection. The glycogen isolated from a number of tissues of the body has been shown to be abnormal, having the characteristics of amylopectin; hence the designation of amylopectinosis, or long-chain glycogen storage disease. The glycogen formed has fewer than normal numbers of the 1,6-glucosidic branch points. This glycogen is also considerably less soluble than normal glycogen. The glycogen content of the tissues is not excessive. Hence an awareness of the possibility of the disorder and specific investigations of brancher enzyme activity or glycogen structure are required to detect further cases. Treatment is symptomatic. All patients have died by 5 years of age. The condition is transmitted as an autosomal recessive trait, and heterozygosity has been detected biochemically.

Type V

Type V glycogenosis, also known as McArdle's disease, results from complete absence or marked deficiency of phosphorylase in the striated muscles. The liver phosphorylase is normal, reflecting the separate genetic control of the two. Although generally regarded as becoming manifest in the middle to late teenage years, a careful history will reveal symptoms at a younger age. Three phases can be delineated: easy fatigability in childhood and lack of athletic prowess; severe cramps on exertion, sometimes associated with myoglobinuria, from 20 to 40 years of age; subsequent progressive atrophy and weakness of individual muscle groups. Several patients have been noted with tonic-clonic seizures who exhibited myoglobinuria after seizures. There are relatively few patients reported with this condition. The information available supports a recessive mode of transmission, although there is an unexplained preponderance of males. There are a few patients who show markedly reduced myophosphorylase activity. Usually the activity is absent, and no enzyme protein can be detected immunologically.

Diagnostically the muscle glycogenoses may be screened by performing blood lactate analyses following anoxic exercise. This is conveniently accomplished by inflating the blood pressure cuff above systolic pressure, having the subject exercise the hand vigorously for 1 minute, and collecting samples before the exercise and after release of the cuff at intervals of 1 minute for 5 minutes. The normal individual will show a twofold to threefold rise; the patient with muscle glycogenosis will show little or none. The definitive diagnosis is accomplished by assaying the glycogen content and activity of phosphorylase of a muscle biopsy. Treatment has not been effective. Strict control of seizures in those individuals at risk is clearly indicated. Vocational guidance is useful.

Type VI

Individuals with type VI clinically resemble those with types I and III. They have very large livers and may have hypoglycemia and ketonuria. Some have stunting of growth. The blood lactate is not elevated. The response of the blood glucose to glucagon may be normal or blunted. There is a normal rise of blood glucose with intravenous galactose. The liver phosphorylase activity is reduced, but the muscle phosphorylase is normal. Treatment is symptomatic. In the first 2 or 3 years of life supplementary dietary sugar may be needed for hypoglycemia. After that time a high-protein diet is effective. These patients improve with age.

Type VII

The original patients with type VII were Japanese siblings. One family with this type has been reported from the United States. The symptoms are very similar to those of individuals with type V glycogenosis. The studies of the original patients have shown that they lack the muscle isozyme of phosphofructokinase. The erythrocyte has a mixture of the liver and muscle isozymes; the red cells from these patients have reduced levels of phosphofructokinase, absence of the muscle isozyme, and mild hemolytic anemia.

Type VIII

A myopathy described in two Japanese brothers with symptoms and findings very similar to those found in McArdle's disease have been described. Administration of fructose before anoxic exercise results in a lactate response. Enzymatic assay of muscle homogenate produces results compatible with the presence of an inhibitor of phosphohexosisomerase.

Type IX

Clinically patients with type IX are difficult to distinguish from those with type I, III, or VI glycogenosis. The most prominent feature is hepatomegaly. The clinical chemical investigations may show fasting hypoglycemia, mild lactate and urate elevation, usually a normal glycemic response to glucagon, and a normal glucose rise with intravenous galactose. Males are primarily affected, but there is evidence that the female carrier may have an enlarged liver in the first 3 or 4 years of life without other symptoms. The condition is X-linked, in contrast to all of the other glycogenoses, which appear to be autosomal recessive. The affected males have resolution of all symptoms and signs around puberty. A high-protein diet can be prescribed if indicated.

Type X

The symptoms in type X muscle glycogenosis are similar to those in type V, and just as with type V they begin earlier in life than with types VII and VIII. The identification of the etiology of this type as a deficiency of phosphorylase kinase in muscle rests on histochemical methods. Standard biochemical methods have yet to be employed for demonstration of the enzyme deficiency.

Types XI and XII

Both types XI and XII present as a hepatomegalic form of glycogenosis. Type XI has been demonstrated to have deficient phosphoglucomutase. Type XII has been demonstrated to be deficient in the protein kinase necessary to activate phosphorylase kinase.

Undefined and Mixed Types

There is a small but significant number of patients in whom tissue enzyme analyses do not show an abnormality in the usual enzymes studies. There have also been patients who have had evidence of two distinct enzymatic defects related to glycogen metabolism, and there have been studies on siblings who have had different types of glycogen storage disease. Care must be taken in the handling of tissues in order to avoid factitious enzyme defects.

References

Cori GT: Glycogen structure and enzyme deficiencies in glycogen storage disease, Harvey Lect. 48:145, 1953

Moses, SW and Gutman A: Inborn errors of glycogen metabolism, In Schulman, I. (ed) Adv. Pediatrics 19:95, 1972.

Plasma Lipids and Lipoproteins

DISORDERS OF LIPIDS AND LIPOPROTEINS

PETER O. KWITEROVICH, JR.

Hyperlipidemia is usually accompanied by hyperlipoproteinemia, in which levels of one or more of the major plasma lipoprotein classes are also elevated. The familial hyperlipidemias and hyperlipoproteinemias are among the most common groups of inherited metabolic disorders in childhood. Premature ischemic heart disease (IHD) is often present in adult relatives of affected children. Early detection and treatment of children in these families consitute a challenge to the pediatrician and a model of great potential importance in the prevention of premature IHD. Normal absorption, transport, and metabolism of lipids and lipoproteins are discussed in Chapter 7.

THEORY

PLASMA LEVELS. Control of the plasma levels of cholesterol or any particular lipid or lipoprotein species is complex. The cellular synthesis of diverse lipids and

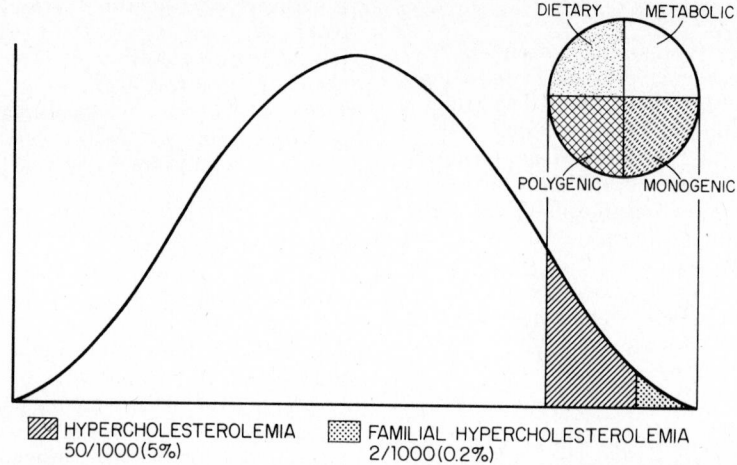

FIG. 13.   Diverse etiologies of hypercholesterolemia in childhood. An idealized distribution curve is drawn, in which hypercholesterolemia has been arbitrarily defined as the upper fifth percentile of the curve. Presumably only 1 in 25 of these children will carry the mutant gene for familial hypercholesterolemia, the most commonly recognized form of familial hyperlipidemia in childhood. Metabolic, dietary, polygenic, and other monogenic mechanisms of wide variety are contributing to an unknown degree to the hypercholesterolemia in the remaining children.

polypeptides and their intracellular packaging and secretion into the plasma compartment must be regulated. Many steps are involved in their intravascular metabolism, which is followed by cellular uptake and catabolism. The number of genetic loci and environmental perturbations (eg, diet) involved in any such series of processes is undoubtedly large. As a result the concentrations of plasma cholesterol and triglycerides and lipoproteins such as low-density lipoproteins (LDL) and very low density lipoproteins (VLDL) in a population of children are distributed over a wide range of values.

Irrespective of the environmental and genetic mechanisms responsible for the distribution of any atherogenic lipid or lipoprotein, one interested in the identification and treatment of individuals at risk for vascular disease logically focuses on the upper part of their distribution curves, as shown for plasma cholesterol in Figure 13. Workers interested in plasma lipids have arbitrarily chosen to label those children (or adults) with lipid values in the upper 5 percent of the curve as having hyperlipidemia. This selection is made with the understanding that the children in this part of the curve do *not* comprise all the children (or adults) at risk, but merely an enrichment of that subset.

CLASSIFICATION OF HYPERLIPIDEMIA AND HYPERLIPOPROTEINEMIA.   Hyperlipidemia (ie, hypercholesterolemia or hypertriglyceridemia or both) is defined in a given child when the concentrations of cholesterol or triglyceride or both exceed the arbitrary cutoff point at the upper 5 percent of the distribution curve for lipid values. Lipoproteins have also been used as the basis of classification of hyperlipidemia. Patients with hyperlipidemia have been classified into five major groups according to the plasma lipoprotein patterns on paper electrophoresis. Criteria for translation of hyperlipidemia into hyperlipoproteinemia have been defined by the World Health Organization. The classification of hyperlipidemia and hyperlipoproteinemia in childhood is summarized in Table 13, where the disorders are arranged numerically according to the Fredrickson classification scheme.

PRIMARY VERSUS SECONDARY HYPERLIPIDEMIA.   The finding of hyperlipidemia in a given child is not an etiologic diagnosis, and the first consideration is whether the hyperlipidemia or hyperlipoproteinemia is *primary* or *secondary* to one of a variety of metabolic diseases. A list of the secondary causes of hyperlipoproteinemia in children and young adults is found in Table 14. The most common causes in the first year of life are glycogen storage disease and congenital biliary atresia. Hypothyroidism, diabetes mellitus, and nephrotic syndrome are the most prevalent of the metabolic causes later in childhood. However, exogenous factors probably are the most prevalent causes of elevated lipids and lipoproteins in the first two decades of life. These include oral contraceptives, alcohol ingestion, and administration of steroids for such conditions as collagen vascular disease, rheumatic heart disease, asthma, and renal transplants. The possibility that hypertriglyceridemia is secondary to the nonfasting state, particularly in infants and very young children, must always be considered.

The diagnosis of primary hyperlipoproteinemia is one of exclusion, and its presence does not necessarily mean that it results from a single genetic mutation. For example, of the 50 children in 1,000 with a plasma cholesterol or LDL concentration above the upper 5 percent, presumably no more than 2 children represent a specific inherited form of hyperlipidemia under the

TABLE 13. Classification of Primary Hyperlipidemia and Hyperlipoproteinemia in Childhood

Fredrickson Type	Lipids	Lipoproteins	Prevalence in Childhood
Type I	Hypertriglyceridemia (severe) Hypercholesterolemia	Hyperchylomicronemia	Rare*
Type IIa	Hypercholesterolemia	Hyperbetalipoproteinemia	Common[†]
Type IIb	Hypercholesterolemia Hypertriglyceridemia	Hyperbetalipoproteinemia Hyperprebetalipoproteinemia	Uncommon[†]
Type III	Hypercholesterolemia Hypertriglyceridemia	Increased VLDL that have beta rather than prebeta mobility and an abnormal ratio of cholesterol to triglyceride	Very rare*
Type IV[‡]	Hypertriglyceridemia	Hyperprebetalipoproteinemia	Uncommon[†]
Type V	Hypertriglyceridemia (marked) Hypercholesterolemia	Hyperchylomicronemia Hyperprebetalipoproteinemia	Very rare*

The presence of these primary lipoprotein patterns in a child is usually indicative of familial hyperlipoproteinemia.

[†] *Since hypercholesterolemia and hypertriglyceridemia (as well as hyperbetalipoproteinemia and hyperprebetalipoproteinemia) are arbitrarily defined as the upper 5 percent of a population of children, the numbers with primary elevations of these lipids or lipoproteins are theoretically equal. In practice the children with primary hyperlipidemia who present to pediatricians or lipid clinics are enriched with the familial forms of these disorders.*

[‡] *In adult patients the hyperprebetalipoproteinemia may be severe enough to cause hypercholesterolemia in addition to marked hypertriglyceridemia. This very rarely occurs in children, who usually have a mild type IV pattern with normal levels of plasma cholesterol.*

TABLE 14. Etiologies of Secondary Hyperlipidemia and Hyperlipoproteinemia in Children and Young Adults

Exogenous
   Alcohol
   Contraceptives
   Steroid therapy
Endocrine and metabolic
   Acute intermittent porphyria
   Diabetes mellitus
   Hypopituitarism
   Hypothyroidism
   Lipodystrophy
   Pregnancy
Storage disease
   Cystine storage disease
   Gaucher's disease
   Glycogen storage disease
   Juvenile Tay-Sachs disease
   Niemann-Pick disease
   Tay-Sachs disease
Renal
   Chronic renal failure
   Hemolytic-uremic syndrome
   Nephrotic syndrome
Hepatic
   Benign recurrent intrahepatic cholestasis
   Congenital biliary atresia
Acute and transient
   Burns
   Hepatitis
Others
   Anorexia nervosa
   Idiopathic hypercalcemia
   Klinefelter's syndrome
   Progeria (Hutchinson-Gilford syndrome)
   Systemic lupus erythematosus
   Werner's syndrome

control of a single mutant gene (monogenic). The elevations in the other children are in all probability due to various dietary, polygenic, metabolic, and other unrecognized etiologies (Fig. 13).

LIPIDS AND LIPOPROTEINS AS DIAGNOSTIC TOOLS. Lipoprotein electrophoresis is not useful as a screening tool, since it is only semiquantitative. A complete quantitation of lipoproteins by ultracentrifugation is not usually accessible and is quite expensive. Extensive data indicate that a simple cholesterol determination is sufficient to identify about 90 percent of children at genetic risk for familial hypercholesterolemia (FH). Measuring LDL cholesterol is more diagnostic than measuring cholesterol alone, due in part to the lower high-density lipoprotein (HDL) concentrations in children with FH. The mean HDL cholesterol in children heterozygous for FH is 43 mg/dl, compared to a mean of 53 mg/dl in the unaffected offspring of parents heterozygous for FH.

The interrelationships between the total plasma cholesterol and the cholesterol carried by LDL, HDL, and VLDL may be summarized by the following formula: LDL cholesterol = total cholesterol − [HDL cholesterol + (total triglycerides/5)]. The concentration of cholesterol on VLDL in this formula is estimated by dividing the total plasma triglycerides by 5 (this is valid provided the patient is fasting, the triglycerides are below 300 mg/dl, and type III hyperlipoproteinemia is not present). This formula may be used to evaluate a child born to a parent with FH, using as a cutoff point an LDL cholesterol of 164 mg/dl. A child may be affected with FH with a cholesterol as low as 205 mg/dl, provided his HDL is only 30 mg/dl; conversely, a child with a cholesterol as high as 245 mg/dl ml may be normal if his HDL is 70 mg/dl or higher.

The same interrelationships are valid in the general population of children, except that those with hyperbetalipoproteinemia are a heterogeneous group. The routine quantitiative determination of HDL cholesterol is unfortunately not available in most laboratories; a pediatrician who wishes to estimate LDL might use an average mean value for HDL of 50 mg/dl. When this value is used, children with a total cholesterol of 225 mg/dl have hyperbetalipoproteinemia (type II hyperlipoproteinemia). A cholesterol over 210 mg/dl is suggestive and might be followed by repeated yearly analyses. The genetic interpretation of hyperbetalipoproteinemia in a given child requires information about the family. The presence of xanthomas, premature vascular disease, or severe hypercholesterolemia in a parent or grandparent strongly suggests that a familial problem is present. The absence of these findings in the family suggests that the hyperbetalipoproteinemia may be secondary to other dietary or metabolic factors or may be simply sporadic, with the etiology unknown.

A model similar to the one above is not available for comparison of the utility of measuring lipoproteins (VLDL) with that of measuring lipids (triglycerides) alone in the evaluation of a child with hypertriglyceridemia. Since the contributions of LDL and HDL to the total plasma triglyceride concentration are usually insignificant, there appears to be little theoretic basis for supposing that measurement of VLDL is any better than a fasting triglyceride determination.

NORMAL CONCENTRATIONS. The question of what constitutes a normal cholesterol or triglyceride value in a pediatric population appears to be a simple matter. Yet the answer is undoubtedly more complex early in life than in adulthood. The concentrations of plasma lipids and lipoproteins in any population are influenced by many factors, including age, sex, obesity, heredity, physical activity, social environment, seasonal variation, and diet. Most of the variables affect the levels of plasma lipids and lipoproteins in childhood, and at certain ages their effect is accentuated.

At Birth. From studies on the measurement of lipids and lipoproteins in umbilical cord blood, several common features may be derived: the concentrations of lipids and lipoproteins are significantly lower than later in life; the lipoproteins, and the lipids carried by them, do not cross the placental barrier; the distribution of values shows some positive skewness (as later in life);

the contributions to the plasma cholesterol concentration from the different lipoprotein fractions are proportionately different than in later life. A representative set of values is presented in Table 15. Of particular note is the distribution of plasma cholesterol in the different lipoprotein fractions in which HDL accounts for 50 percent of the total plasma cholesterol.

Birth to 1 Year. The low levels of plasma lipids and the distribution of the lipoproteins present at birth change drastically in the first few weeks of life and are characterized by a twofold to threefold increase in total cholesterol and LDL with a significantly smaller (30 percent) increase in HDL. The available triglyceride figures have been obtained only from nonfasting infants and are usually over 100 mg/dl. From age 1 week to 1 year there is a small (about 20 percent) increase in plasma cholesterol. Normal values for this period are not presented in Table 15 for several reasons. The available data are derived from studies in which different laboratory methods and sampling conditions were employed; second, diet has a dramatic effect on the concentrations of plasma cholesterol and triglycerides, particularly in the first 3 months of life. For example, infants fed breast milk or cow's milk have much higher plasma lipids than those fed a corn oil or soybean formula.

One Year to 20 Years. It has generally been accepted that the plasma lipid and lipoprotein levels remain relatively constant in the first two decades of life. Several recent studies have suggested that the cholesterol levels may be lower between 1 and 2 years of age than later in childhood, although conflicting results have been reported. Consequently a normal cholesterol value for the age of 1 year is presented in Table 15. Lipids and lipoproteins appear to remain relatively constant from the age of 2 years through young adulthood. However, several studies have suggested that the mean plasma cholesterol decreases 10 to 20 mg/dl during adolescence. Further studies are required, particularly large, well-planned longitudinal studies to investigate the effects of different variables including age, sex, and diet on the natural history of plasma lipids and lipoproteins in the first two decades of life. In the meantime, temporary guidelines for this age group are provided in Tables 15 and 16.

TABLE 15. Normal Plasma Lipid and Lipoprotein Concentrations* in First Two Decades of Life

Age	Total Cholesterol (mg/dl)	HDL Cholesterol (mg/dl)	LDL Cholesterol (mg/dl)	VLDL Cholesterol (mg/dl)	Total Triglycerides (mg/dl)
Birth	74 ± 11	37 ± 8	31 ± 6	6 ± 4	37 ± 15
Age 1 year	138 ± 29	†	†	†	†
Age 2–19 years					
Male	173 ± 34	49 ± 11	108 ± 33	9 ± 7	61 ± 34
Female	179 ± 33	53 ± 12	108 ± 10	11 ± 8	73 ± 34

Mean ± 1 standard deviation.
† *Not determined.*

TABLE 16. Suggested Guidelines for Abnormal Plasma Lipid and Lipoprotein Levels From Birth Through First Two Decades of Life*

Age	Cholesterol	LDL Cholesterol	Triglycerides
Birth	92	43	67[†]
1–2 years	198	140[‡]	140
2–19 years	225	164	140

Cutoff points are values that represent the limit for the upper 5th percentile; however, those for cholesterol and LDL cholesterol (ages 2–19 years) are values that mimimize misclassification (see text).

† *Triglyceride concentration at birth may be falsely high, secondary to a variety of perinatal events; the validity of plasma triglyceride in cord blood as a diagnostic criterion for hypertriglyceridemia has not been established.*

‡ *Not experimentally derived; estimated from the relationship between total and LDL cholesterol later in childhood.*

PRACTICE

SCREENING. Who to Screen. No unequivocal guidelines have yet been established for the screening of children for hyperlipidemia. One conservative but useful approach is to sample children who have a family history of hyperlipidemia or premature vascular disease in a parent or grandparent (ie, in males before age 50 years and females before age 60 years). Tamir and associates found that 30 of 85 children of men who had myocardial infarction before the age of 61 years had type II hyperlipoproteinemia regardless of the class of hyperlipoproteinemia found in the father. Glueck and associates found hyperlipidemia in 69 of 223 children screened because of premature myocardial infarction in one parent. Most of the children with hyperglyceridemia were older than 15 years. Chase and associates performed a similar study and found hyperlipidemia in 29 percent of children of victims of early heart attacks.

Screening limited to families such as those in the surveys mentioned above delays preventive treatment of affected offspring until the diagnosis is made in the parent. In many cases these children will already be in their late teenage years and early twenties. Conversely, routine screening of all children will miss about 60 percent of those patients who will develop familial hyperglyceridemia as adults. The issue is further confused by changes in plasma lipids with age, since they increase in the first year of life and apparently decrease during adolescence. The issue may be conceived in broader epidemiologic terms: that is, if all children with a cholesterol 1 standard deviation above the mean are potentially at risk, then screening of all children at entry into the first grade for cholesterol is not an unreasonable approach. In view of the present state of knowledge, it is recommended that as a *minimum* all children be screened for a fasting cholesterol and triglyceride if there is a family history of hyperlipidemia, premature vascular disease, sudden death, or xanthomas in a parent or grandparent or if the child has xanthomas or recurrent unexplained abdominal pain or is above the recommended weight for age. A routine determination of plasma cholesterol in all children and plasma triglycerides in adolescents and young adults is encouraged as part of the complete evaluation of these patients in the practice of pediatrics.

When to Sample. The suggestions for the age at which a blood specimen should be obtained range from birth (cord blood) to the late teenage years. The following guidelines are currently used in the Lipid Referral Clinic at the Johns Hopkins Hospital. When a parent is affected with hypercholesterolemia or xanthomas or both, all the children who are 1 year of age or older are screened. In the event of a pregnancy in such a family, an umbilical cord blood sample is obtained. If the parent has hypertriglyceridemia, all children 1 year of age or older are screened; should the results from the first test be normal, the sample is repeated in 1 year in obese children of a hypertriglyceridemic parent and every 2 to 3 years in their nonobese children. If a parent is referred because a close blood relative has premature ischemic heart disease, then the parent is first screened for hyperlipidemia. The children are screened subsequently if the parent has hyperlipidemia. Should a pediatrician in practice decide to screen *all* his patients, a single cholesterol determination after the age of 2 years and a cholesterol *and* triglyceride determination after the age of 12 years probably represent a simple and reasonably efficient screening approach. Those with a cholesterol above 200 mg/dl or triglyceride above 120 mg/dl should be resampled in 1 year.

How to Sample. For the most reliable results, the conditions for collection should be standardized, particularly if a child will require long-term follow-up. The sample should be obtained after a 12-hour overnight fast. If very young children cannot fast, limiting intake to clear juices on the morning the sample is drawn should minimize any possible dietary contribution to the plasma lipid levels. A venipuncture is usually necessary, since microtechniques for lipid determinations on capillary plasma from a finger stick are not ordinarily available or their standardization is not complete. Plasma is preferable to serum, since a clot can interfere with the evaluation of the presence of chylomicrons. A blood specimen drawn from a prone child should be obtained within 10 minutes, since a prolonged period of recumbency (20 minutes) will lower the plasma cholesterol level.

LABORATORY ANALYSES. Accurate and reproducible lipid data are essential for the physicians who plan to screen their patients for hyperlipidemia. In most areas a standardized research laboratory is not available. A good commercial or hospital laboratory should be chosen that measures cholesterol and triglycerides by methods solely set up for this purpose. For example, we have found that the mean cholesterol determined as part of a battery of tests (such as SMA-12) is 34 mg/dl higher than that measured by the Technicon AA-I method in our research laboratory. A good quality-control system assesses accuracy as well as precision of determinations. This is necessary to provide the pediatrician with reliable results, which are essential for both proper diagnosis and long-term follow-up of patients. The same principles are applicable to determinations of plasma cholesterol in the office with a commercially available kit. The relationship between the values the physician is obtaining in his office and those found in a reliable laboratory must be established. Duplicate samples can be analyzed blind by both methods in a pilot study. A system for continued monitoring of quality control can then be maintained.

INTERPRETATION OF RESULTS. The plasma may be analyzed qualitatively and quantitatively. The presence or absence of turbidity, lactescent, or milky plasma provides information about the presence and the nature of hyperglyceridemia. This is best assessed after the plasma has stood at 4 C overnight (Fig. 14). A cloudy plasma throughout the tube without a cream layer at the top is indicative of increased VLDL of endogenous origin; in that event the triglycerides are usually above 250 mg/dl. If a thick layer of chylomicrons is also present the patient has exogenous as well as endogenous hypertriglyceridemia; the triglycerides are ordinarily greater than 3,000 mg/dl. The finding of a clear plasma with a thin creamy layer of chylomicrons on the top of the tube usually indicates that the child

was not fasting for 12 hours; rarely the layer of chylomicrons will be so prominent as to suggest exogenous hyperglyceridemia. The triglycerides in a clear plasma are usually less than 150 mg/dl; however, the cholesterol and LDL may be significantly elevated.

Some temporary guidelines for the interpretation of quantitative lipid and lipoprotein data are provided in Table 16. The finding of elevated values in a child is an indication for further evaluation of the secondary etiologies of hyperlipidemia. Those children found to have primary hyperlipidemia should receive appropriate dietary therapy; some may also require treatment with a drug. The familial nature of the primary hyperlipidemia should be explored in the siblings and parents of such a child.

METABOLIC DISORDERS OF HYPERLIPOPROTEINEMIA

FAMILIAL HYPERCHOLESTEROLEMIA. Familial hypercholesterolemia (FH) or classic type II hyperlipoproteinemia is characterized by significant increases in the plasma concentrations of both total cholesterol and LDL cholesterol. Other aspects of the phenotypic presentation of this syndrome include tendon xanthomas, a striking predilection to premature ischemic heart disease, and development of arcus corneae early in life (Fig. 15). FH is transmitted as a mendelian dominant trait with complete expression of hypercholesterolemia and hyperbetalipoproteinemia in childhood. FH is the most commonly recognized form of familial hyperlipidemia in childhood. Estimates of 1 in 200 and 1 in 500 have been made for the incidence of affected

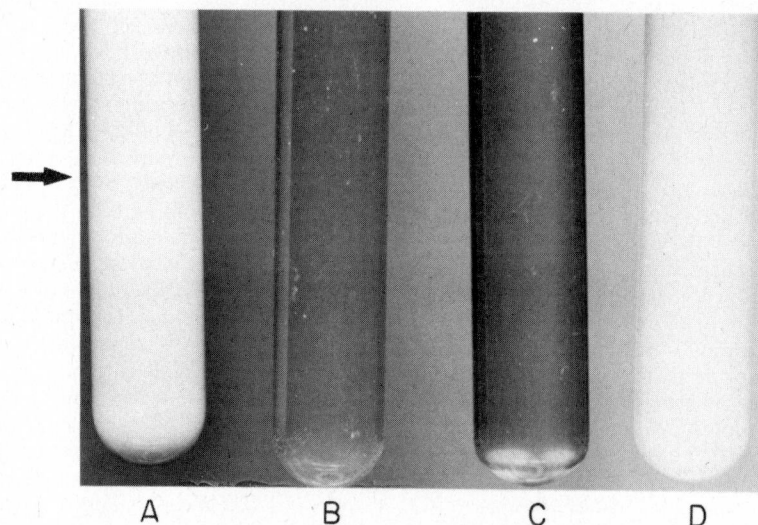

FIG. 14. Lipemic plasma. The presence of a thick chylomicron layer overlying a turbid layer of VLDL is seen in A. The point of demarcation between the two layers is indicated by an arrow. The plasma triglyceride concentration in this 9-year-old girl with type V hyperlipoproteinemia was over 6,000 mg/dl. Slight turbidity is present in B, the plasma from her 7-year-old sister with mild type IV hyperlipoproteinemia and a plasma triglyceride level of 160 mg/dl. The clear plasma seen in C is from the normal mother. The presence of a turbid plasma without chylomicrons is seen in the father (D), who had endogenous hypertriglyceridemia of 300 mg/dl.

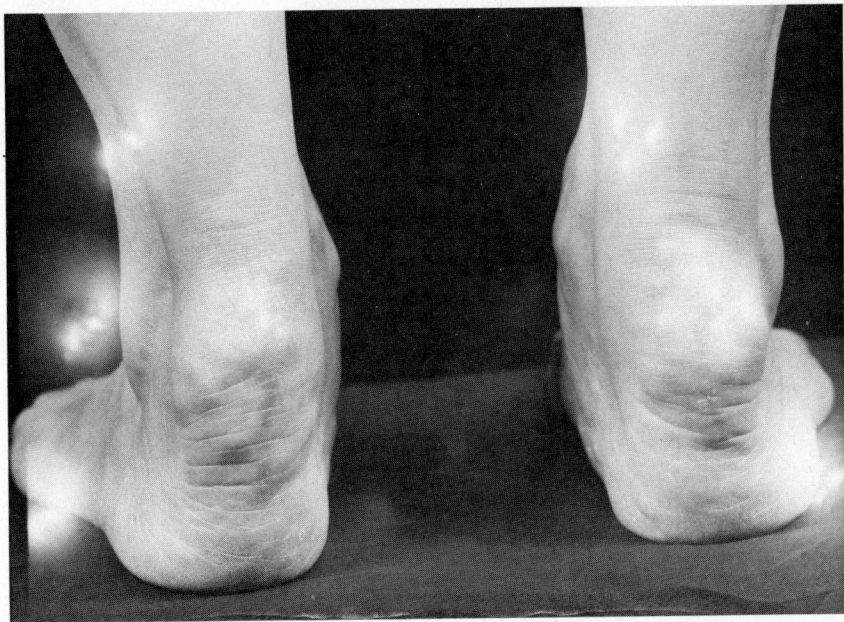

Fig. 15. Achilles tendon xanthomas (left). The tendons are markedly thickened in this 43-year-old woman with the clinical phenotype of heterozygous familial hypercholesterolemia and a type IIb lipoprotein pattern. Corneal arcus (right). A rather marked arcus in the same patient that involves both the superior and inferior aspects of the cornea.

heterozygotes. Glueck and associates have detected affected infants using mass screening of cord blood; however, follow-up at the age of 1 year, dietary evaluation, and detailed family studies were necessary to thoroughly document the familial nature of the disorder in each infant. The efficiency of detecting heterozygous children is considerably improved if the phenotype of the parent is known. Kwiterovich has shown that the heterozygous state of FH can reliably be detected at birth as elevated LDL cholesterol when the parent is known to have FH. A single dose of the mutant gene in the heterozygote child or young adult usually produces cholesterol and LDL cholesterol levels above 260 and 200 mg/dl, respectively.

The heterozygote child is clinically asymptomatic in the first decade; 10 to 15 percent of heterozygotes develop tendon xanthomas during the second decade, most commonly in the Achilles tendon and extensor tendons of the hands. Achilles tendinitis and tenosynovitis may be the initial clinical manifestation of FH in the teenage patient. The differential diagnosis of warm, erythematous, and painful Achilles tendons should include FH, along with juvenile rheumatoid arthritis, lupus erythematosus, acute rheumatic fever, and gonoccocal arthritis. Rarely, a young adult with FH will develop angina pectoris in the late teenage years.

The marriage of two heterozygote parents has occurred in approximately 100 kindreds. On the average, 1 of 4 children has been a homozygote. The cholesterol levels in these children are usually 600 to 1,000 mg/dl. The homozygous state of FH in many cases is first suggested in childhood by physical signs. Planar xan-

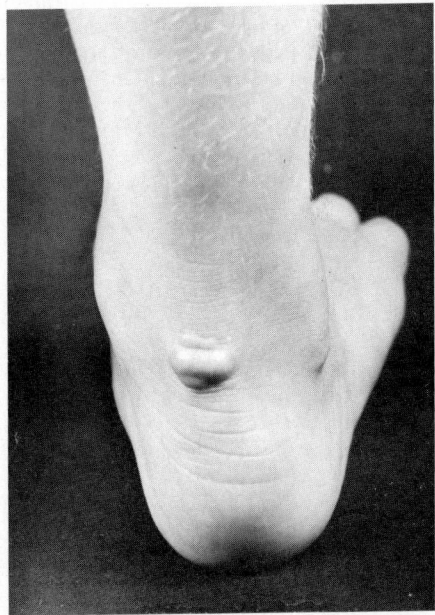

Fig. 16. Planar xanthoma. This somewhat raised lesion, orange in color and not involving the Achilles tendon, was found in a 6-year-old with the clinical and biochemical phenotype of homozygous familial hypercholesterolemia. Smaller planar xanthomas were found in more typical areas, such as the buttocks and in between the fingers. The plasma cholesterol was 800 mg/dl.

thomas, flat orange-colored lesions (Fig. 16), commonly occur by the age of 5 years, but they may be present at birth. They may be located on the buttocks and extensor surfaces, between the fingers, and in the popliteal fossae. Tendon and tuberous xanthomas usually develop between the ages of 5 and 15 years. Angina pectoris and myocardial infarction are ordinarily delayed to the second decade, but they have occurred as early as 6 years of age. The generalized atherosclerosis affects the aortic valve as well as the aorta and coronary vessels, usually resulting in aortic stenosis.

The probable biochemical defect underlying FH has been elucidated only recently. In heterozygotes for FH there is a decreased fractional catabolic rate of ^{125}I-LDL, which suggests a defect in the removal of LDL from the circulation. In homozygous children four interrelated defects in LDL and cholesterol metabolism have been described. Fibroblasts from skin biopsies of homozygotes grown in tissue culture have a marked inability to bind LDL, as compared to normal cells. This deficiency in functional cell membrane receptors for LDL is associated with faulty regulation of the rate-limiting enzyme of cholesterol biosynthesis, hydroxymethylglutaryl coenzyme A reductase (HMG CoA reductase), deficient proteolysis of LDL, and marked decrease in production of cellular cholesterol ester. Measurement of these four biochemical quantities in the heterozygote parents of these children has revealed that their functional capacity is approximately half that found in normal cells. Prenatal detection of the homozygote with FH appears technically feasible, since cultured fibroblasts derived from normal amniotic fluid have a level and a pattern of regulation of HMG CoA reductase activity similar to those of normal controls.

Recent studies in a larger number of homozygotes have shown significant heterogeneity in LDL binding and its associated cellular effects. Two kinds of genetic lesions appear to underly FH: receptor-negative and receptor-defective. Unlike the cells of the homozygotes, which were originally found to be receptor-negative, the receptor-defective cells have an LDL receptor capable of a low level of function.

PHENOCOPIES OF FAMILIAL HYPERCHOLESTEROLEMIA.   Because the measurement of cholesterol or LDL is a nonspecific biochemical test, many cases of primary (and usually mild) hypercholesterolemia will not be indicative of FH. Other clinical or family data are therefore necessary to confirm the diagnosis of heterozygosity in a given infant or child. Although the combination of xanthomas and hypercholesterolemia is clinically diagnostic of FH, normocholesterolemic xanthomatosis can occur in cerebrotendinous xanthomatosis, juvenile xanthogranuloma, xanthoma disseminatum, Schüller-Christian and Letterer-Siwe syndromes, and the recently described metabolic disorder β-sitosterolemia. In addition, xanthomas associated with secondary elevations of LDL can be found in congenital biliary atresia.

FAMILIAL DISORDERS OF TRIGLYCERIDE METABOLISM.   Metabolic disorders involving plasma triglycerides, VLDL, and chylomicrons are a heterogeneous group of diseases. The most common of these triglyceride disorders in childhood is probably endogenous hypertriglyceridemia (type IV hyperlipoproteinemia). The next most prevalent form of hyperglyceridemia in children is endogenous hypertriglyceridemia with increased LDL (type IIb hyperlipoproteinemia). It is presently not known what proportion of children with the latter lipoprotein pattern represent the genetic entity called familial combined hyperlipidemia, as opposed to FH. Approximately 10 percent of children with classic FH have endogenous hypertriglyceridemia. The rather severe hypertriglyceridemia associated with a combination of endogenous and exogenous hypertriglyceridemia (type V hyperlipoproteinemia) is usually expressed only in adulthood. However, there are a few examples of type V hyperlipoproteinemia in childhood. Finally, the most clearly distinct genetic disorder of glyceride metabolism is familial type I hyperlipoproteinemia, which invariably presents in the first decade of life; the disorder is rare, and only about 40 cases have been reported.

FAMILIAL   HYPERTRIGLYCERIDEMIA.   Hypertriglyceridemia (type IV hyperlipoproteinemia) appears to be inherited in some families as an autosomal dominant trait; it is characterized by significant increases in plasma concentrations of triglycerides and VLDL. One of 2 children born to an affected parent is therefore expected to have hypertriglyceridemia; however, only about 1 of 5 persons at risk who are less than 20 years of age have hypertriglyceridemia. The penetrance is therefore reduced to 0.40 (20 percent observed; 50 percent expected). The frequency of familial hypertriglyceridemia has been estimated to be 0.2 to 0.3 percent in the general adult population. If 2 children in 1,000 carry the mutant allele or alleles, only 1 per 1,250 will actually present with the monogenic form of hypertriglyceridemia (0.002×0.40). Therefore, presumably only 1 child of all the children ($N = 62.5$) in the upper 5th percentile of the triglyceride distribution of 1,250 children will have monogenic hypertriglyceridemia. Interpretation of the . meaning of the term hypertriglyceridemia in the other children is not possible at this time. The glucose intolerance, hyperuricemia, premature ischemic heart disease, and peripheral vascular disease seen in adults with endogenous hyperglyceridemia are not ordinarily seen in affected children. Court and associates found a significant number of obese children with endogenous hypertriglyceridemia; there was also a positive correlation between plasma triglyceride values and the degree and duration of obesity. Their plasma cholesterol concentrations were usually normal.

FAMILIAL COMBINED HYPERLIPIDEMIA.   Familial combined hyperlipidemia (FCH) is a syndrome in which three lipoprotein patterns (IIa, IIb, and IV) are expressed in approximately equal proportions among affected adult relatives. FCH is associated with a marked predilection to premature ischemic heart disease. Tendon xanthomas are reportedly not present. The working genetic hypothesis is that FCH is a major gene (dominant) disorder, but the degree of probable genetic heterogeneity is unknown. There is no strict counterpart to FCH in the Fredrickson classification scheme. The tendency to equate the type IIb lipoprotein pattern with FCH has led to some confusion. There appears to be delayed penetrance of FCH in patients less than 20 years of age. The finding of disparate lipoprotein patterns in a child and his parents is presumptive evidence of FCH. However, the presence of a type IIb lipoprotein pattern and tendon xanthomas should be considered the clinical phenotype of FH until proved otherwise.

ENDOGENOUS AND EXOGENOUS HYPERGLY-CERIDEMIA. Detection of endogenous and exogenous hyperglyceridemia (familial type V hyperlipoproteinemia) in a patient before the age of 20 years is rare. We have recently described the complete expression of type V hyperlipoproteinemia in a 9-year-old girl who had grossly cloudly blood during a routine evaluation. There was no history of abdominal pain, pancreatitis, or fat intolerance, although the hypertriglyceridemia was marked (> 6000 mg/dl). Abnormal physical findings were limited to lipemia retinalis. The child had both the fat and carbohydrate intolerance seen in adults with type V hyperlipoproteinemia. Low levels of lipoprotein lipase and mild hyperinsulinism were also present. We have recently found a second case of type V hyperlipoproteinemia in an 8-year-old boy with plasma triglycerides of 1000 mg/dl. He likewise had low levels of lipoprotein lipase. The sister of the first patient and all 4 siblings of the second patient had type IV hyperlipoproteinemia. The biochemical mechanisms underlying familial type V hyperlipoproteinemia are not clear, nor is its genetic relationship to simple endogenous hypertriglyceridemia well understood.

EXOGENOUS HYPERTRIGLYCERIDEMIA. Familial type I hyperlipoproteinemia is defined by a massive increase in the chylomicrons accompanied by marked hypertriglyceridemia (as high as 10,000 mg/dl) with a deficiency in lipoprotein lipase. The enzyme activity is measured in the plasma following an intravenous injection of heparin (postheparin lipolytic activity, PHLA). The enzyme activities of lipase that do not require apoC-II polypeptide as a cofactor are normal. The marked chylomicronemia, which is indicative of the inability to clear dietary fat, is manifested by a creamy layer found at the top of plasma left to stand at 4 C overnight. The marked hypertriglyceridemia of exogenous origin is accompanied by a somewhat elevated plasma cholesterol. The ratio of triglyceride to cholesterol is at least 5 and is usually 10. HDL and LDL are low.

Abdominal pain is the usual initial symptom, presenting as colic in the first year of life or as an acute abdomen later in childhood. Other clinical features may include eruptive xanthomas, hepatosplenomegaly, and lipemia retinalis. The PHLA deficiency and decreased chylomicron clearance are compatible with a catabolic defect. The disorder is rare and appears to be due to a homozygous state for a mutant allele. First-degree relatives may have endogenous hyperglyceridemia and low PHLA activity, but the heterozygote carriers cannot reliably be detected.

TYPE III HYPERLIPOPROTEINEMIA. Familial type III hyperlipoproteinemia is defined by the presence of a plasma VLDL that has an abnormal chemical composition and beta rather than prebeta electrophoretic mobility. Two lipoprotein species are present in the VLDL of these patients; one is similar in its composition and physical behavior to normal VLDL; the other contains more cholesterol and less triglyceride than normal VLDL (beta VLDL). The plasma cholesterol and triglyceride levels are both elevated, sometimes to a fairly equal degree, but concentrations can be extremely variable. This unusual lipoprotein pattern may be the phenotypic presentation of several different or closely related genetic abnormalities. Hypotheses concerning the mechanism of inheritance include that of an autosomal dominant trait or possibly a recessive trait. The biochemical defect that accounts for the increased amount of beta migrating VLDL is not known. Possibilities include a block in the normal metabolism of VLDL to LDL or a defective uptake of beta VLDL by the cell.

Premature vascular disease of both the coronary and peripheral vessels is common in this disorder. Tendon and tuberous xanthomas may occur; however, the clinical hallmark of the phenotype or phenotypes is the unusual yellow deposits in the creases of the palms (xanthoma striata palmaris). The palmar xanthomas and beta VLDL have been described in only 2 patients less than 20 years of age.

TREATMENT. HYPERCHOLESTEROLEMIA AND HYPERBETALIPOPROTEINEMIA. The object of therapy in primary type II hyperlipoproteinemia is to lower the cholesterol and LDL concentrations into the normal range. Dietary intervention is the first form of treatment; it will be most successful in those children with milder hypercholesterolemia (cholesterol levels of 225 to 250 mg/dl), a significant proportion of whom will not have FH. Most of the patients with a cholesterol level above 250 mg/dl will have FH; only a small proportion of these respond satisfactorily to diet alone. Most children with FH require the addition of a drug to lower the plasma cholesterol below 225 mg/dl.

Most of the published data on dietary therapy deal with children who are heterozygous or homozygous for FH. The first form of treatment is a diet in which the cholesterol is reduced to < 200 mg/day and the ratio of polyunsaturated to saturated fats (P/S ratio) is increased to 2.0. When this diet is given to school-age heterozygote children as outpatients, the total cholesterol and LDL cholesterol levels fall an average of 10 to 15 percent. Another 5 to 10 percent reduction is achieved on the metabolic unit, producing a maximum reduction of 20 to 25 percent. Only about 20 percent of children with FH achieve normal cholesterol levels on diet alone. Most children homozygous for FH have a similar mean percentage decrease, but homozygotes vary in their dietary responses and some of these children do not respond at all.

The types of foods offered to these children will depend on their ages. Infants can be placed on one of the commercially available formulas that are higher in polyunsaturated fat and lower in cholesterol than breast milk or cow's milk. This treatment lowers the cholesterol and LDL effectively into the normal range in infants with FH at 6 months of age. It is felt that this lowering of plasma cholesterol in the typical heterozygous infant will be the first step in the prevention of ischemic heart disease as an adult; however, this hypothesis is not proven. Other dietary modifications include selection of the appropriate commercial preparation of baby and junior foods and the kinds and amounts of solid foods.

The principles underlying the diet for children 1 through 12 years of age are similar; however, the sizes of the servings increase with age. For example, the daily quantity of lean meat, fish, or poultry prescribed is 2 to 3 ounces (up to 2 years); 3 to 4 ounces (2 to 5 years); 4 ounces (6 to 12 years). At age 2 years the amount of polyunsaturated oil added to the diet increases from 3 to 4 teaspoons. Children particularly like the foods that are to be avoided: hot dogs, regular hamburgers, luncheon meats, ice cream, and regular cheese. The diet can be made more palatable by substituting similar but acceptable foods: tuna sandwiches, homemade low-fat hamburgers, chicken, sherbet, and low-fat cheeses. Whenever possible, a knowledgeable dietitian should participate in planning treatment. This enables the family to follow the subtle nuances of the diet better (eg, adding 1 teaspoon of polyunsaturated oil for every 3 ounces of meat, and avoiding foods with hidden cholesterol, such as cakes and cookies).

No adverse effects have been reported in infants and children with FH treated with the above diet. However, potential problems should be considered, particularly in infants and young children who are undergoing rapid changes of growth and development. Impaired myelination of nerves in the first few years of life has been mentioned in this regard. The following facts make this highly unlikely: First, about 80 percent of the infants in this country already receive commercial formulas that are lower in cholesterol and higher in unsaturated fat than breast milk or cow's milk; their growth and development is normal, and the safety of these formulas is well established. Second, infants with FH who are treated develop a normal (not an abnormally low) plasma cholesterol concentration. Third, the brain and nervous tissue synthesize cholesterol from two-carbon precursors. Other possible side effects include the necessity of a dietary cholesterol challenge in infancy to induce cholesterol degrading enzymes, increased vitamin E requirements to prevent oxidation of polyunsaturated fats, and theoretic long-term psychologic effects. The long-term effect of a diet high in unsaturated fat, low in saturated fat and cholesterol, and high in plant sterol in children is not known. Domiciliary veterans who were treated with the above diet had a higher incidence (34 percent) of gallstones than the untreated group. The treated group had a higher mortality rate (1.7 percent) from malignant neoplasia than the controls (0.5 percent). The significance of these observations is obscure, particularly since the treated group had a prolonged life span and significantly fewer fatal atherosclerotic events. The plasma phytosterol levels in infants and children on this diet are significantly elevated, but the long-term effects of phytosterolemia are not yet known. In summary, dietary treatment appears to be relatively effective and safe.

Drug Therapy. Approximately 80 percent of heterozygous children and homozygotes will require drugs in addition to diet to lower cholesterol and LDL significantly. Cholestyramine (Questran) is presently the drug of choice. This anion-exchange resin binds bile acids and prevents their reabsorption. Cholesterol and LDL have been lowered to within the normal range in most heterozygous children treated with cholestyramine. The dosage of cholestyramine required to lower LDL into the normal range is directly proportional to the postdiet LDL levels and is not related to the body weight of the children. In some children an LDL level below 170 mg/dl can be achieved on as little as 4 g of cholestyramine per day, although the dosage usually required ranges from 8 to 16 g/day. The dose can be effectively and conveniently given twice daily. There are conflicting opinions as to whether the drug is more effective when combined with dietary treatment.

Agents other than cholestyramine have been used in these children. Colestipol (also a bile sequestrant) had achieved some success in lowering cholesterol and LDL. *p*-Aminosalicylic acid (PAS) has also been administered to a few children. PAS has significantly greater side effects than the bile sequestrants and does not appear to be as effective. Clofibrate has not been comparable to the bile sequestrants in its cholesterol- and LDL-lowering effects. D-thyroxine (Choloxin), the optical isomer of the naturally occurring hormone, has been used in hypercholesterolemic children at a dose of 0.05 mg/kg, up to a maximum dose of 4 mg. Although a substantial fall of LDL may occur with D-thyroxine, there has been considerably less experience with its use in children with FH than with the bile sequestrants. The use of nicotinic acid is usually reserved for the homozygotes.

The homozygote children may be divided into three groups: those who respond to cholestyramine alone (24 to 32 g/day), those who require nicotinic acid (up to 3 g/day) in addition to cholestyramine, and those who do not respond to any drug therapy. The response to therapy in these patients is highly correlated with differences in the biochemical characterization of their fibroblasts grown in tissue culture. Breslow and associates found that the homozygotes who responded to drug therapy had both a significantly higher binding affinity of LDL to cells and a greater suppression of HMG reductase activity by LDL.

The most common side effects of therapy with bile sequestrants are constipation, bloating, and nausea. The frequency and duration of these side effects in children are less than those in adults. Other side effects may include malabsorption of neutral fat and fat-soluble vitamins. Steatorrhea has occurred in adults receiving cholestyramine at dosages of 25 g/day or more. West and Lloyd found that 5 of 7 children who received comparable or greater dosage of cholestyramine per kilogram of body weight and who ate normal amounts of fat had some increase in stool fat, although this increase was marked in only 2 children. Steatorrhea can be minimized by using the lowest effective dosage of cholestyramine. The possible effects of steatorrhea and malabsorption of fat-soluble vitamins on growth and development must continually be considered when treating children. Therefore careful monitoring of growth and development and assessment of serum carotene, vitamin A, and prothrombin time are indicated. Glueck and associates found no systematic differences in serum vitamin A and E levels before and after therapy with cholestyramine. West and Lloyd found that serum folate levels were decreased in all of their series of 19 children with FH treated with cholestyramine; 6 of 12 children tested also had subnormal red blood cell folate. We have made a similar observation, but in only 5 of 20 treated children. Further investigation on possible folate deficiency is needed; one possibility is that some children with FH have an in situ deficiency in plasma or red cell folate. Homozygotes treated with nicotinic acid must be monitored for hepatic transaminase levels, hyperglycemia, hyperuricemia, and increased blood urea nitrogen.

Surgical Therapy. In addition to diet and drugs, surgery has been proposed as a therapeutic alternative to lower LDL in FH. *Partial ileal bypass* reduces hypercholesterolemia by decreasing cholesterol absorption and increasing fecal steroid excretion. The increase in cholesterol biosynthesis does not compensate for the above changes. The reduction in cholesterol levels appears constant and persistent (average 41.1 percent decrease over 9 years). However, the response to surgery is variable, and some patients, particular homozygote children, respond poorly. Patients with FH have an average increase in their triglyceride levels of 21.1 percent 1 year after surgery, an increase similar to that transiently present in patients treated with cholestyramine. This hypertriglyceridemia may be related to bile acid loss. Other side effects include an annoying diarrhea and the need for injections of vitamin B_{12}. Formal comparisons of this surgical procedure with drug therapy have not been made. For example, some patients may be very responsive to chemotherapeutic agents and resistant to surgery, and vice versa; some may respond to both modalities of treatment. Until this information is available, medical management of FH is recommended.

The *portacaval shunt* procedure was initially found to eliminate hyperlipidemia in patients with type I glycogen storage disease (hepatic glucose-6-phosphatase deficiency). A high complication rate, combined with the operative mortality (5 to 10 percent) and failure rate (10 percent), indicates that this procedure is not suitable for children and that it should be restricted to homozygous patients with severe arteriosclerotic vascular disease who are refractory to medical therapy.

HYPERTRIGLYCERIDEMIA. Treatment of hypertriglyceridemia in children rests on dietary therapy. The use of hypolipidemic agents is rarely, if ever, necessary. Dietary therapy is aimed at lowering the triglycerides of endogenous or dietary origin or both.

Endogenous Hypertriglyceridemia. In 33 children under 20 years of age with primary endogenous hypertriglyceridemia treated in the Johns Hopkins Lipid Research Clinic, mild hypertriglyceridemia (140 to 200 mg/dl) had disappeared in half the children at the time their second baseline sample was obtained. Since the glyceride elevations are usually mild and often transient, our initial dietary approach is a prudent type IV diet. In the child with normal weight for height, the restrictions include the following: concentrated sweets (eg, sodas, cookies, candies) are eliminated; other carbohydrate-containing foods (eg, breads, cereals, fruits, and milk) are allowed in restricted amounts. In most cases, if the child is also mildly overweight, elimination and restriction of these foods will correct the weight problem. The more stringent NIH type IV diet is prescribed in children when the prudent diet does not correct the hypertriglyceridemia, or when significant obesity is a problem and more stringent caloric limitation is needed, or when the triglycerides are above 200 mg/dl. Teenagers and young adults are also instructed to restrict the use of alcohol. The responses of the hypertriglyceridemic children to diet are quite rewarding.

Exogenous Hypertriglyceridemia. The massive chylomicronemia and hypertriglyceridemia seen in type I hyperlipoproteinemia respond quite well to a diet markedly reduced in fat content (10 to 15 g/day in a child), although this diet is difficult to maintain. Medium-chain triglycerides (MCT), which are absorbed directly through the portal vein, can be added to the diet as 15 percent of calories to increase compliance.

Exogenous and Endogenous Hypertriglyceridemia. Type V hyperlipoproteinemia is distinctly rare in children. In a 9-year-old patient an NIH type V diet, modified to contain 15 percent of the calories as MCT (40 percent carbohydrate, 20 percent protein, 25 percent fat as the other caloric sources), was successful for over a year in lowering the plasma triglycerides from 6,000 mg/dl to less than 150 mg/dl.

EARLY DETECTION. The preceding sections have provided guidelines for the early diagnosis and treatment of familial hyperlipoproteinemia. The ultimate goal in this approach is to prevent atherosclerosis through the treatment of hyperlipidemia. The reasoning that childhood is the appropriate age to begin is summarized below.

Premature Atherosclerosis. Convincing evidence of coronary atherosclerosis has been shown in many pathologic studies of the coronary vessels of young men in the military service, with 45 to 77.3 percent of the coronary vessels showing atherosclerosis varying in extent from gross to microscopic lesions. Aortic fatty streaks are present at all children over 3 years of age, and coronary fatty streaks are quite frequent in the second decade. The findings of Strong and McGill are consistent with the hypothesis that there is a gradual transition from fatty streaks to fibrous plaques and that advanced atherosclerotic lesions develop by progression and transformation of fatty streaks.

Hyperlipidemia and Premature Atherosclerosis. Fifty to 60 percent of survivors of premature ischemic heart disease have significant hyperlipidemia. Affected members in families with FH have a significantly greater incidence of premature vascular disease than nonaffected members. Many studies have shown familial aggregations of premature vascular disease and endogenous hypertriglyceridemia. The natural history of premature IHD in the affected parents of children with FH is so striking that even the most skeptical must consider the possibility that atherosclerosis starts in the first two decades of life in heterozygous children. This conclusion is strengthened by the fact that severe generalized atherosclerosis develops before 10 years of age in homozygous children.

Natural History of Premature Atherosclerosis. When the above evidence is considered together, it is reasonable to postulate that atherosclerosis has its genesis in childhood and is accelerated by the presence of hyperlipidemia. It has not yet been proved that treatment of susceptible patients at any given stage of atherosclerotic development will change or reverse the natural history of the disease process. Nevertheless, treatment of certain predisposed children and young adults appears judicious and prudent in view of information currently available.

METABOLIC DISORDERS OF HYPOLIPOPROTEINEMIA

ABETALIPOPROTEINEMIA. Abetalipoproteinemia (ABL) (Bassen-Kornzweig syndrome) (p. 1919) is a rare recessive genetic disease whose clinical expression in childhood includes fat malabsorption, severe hypolipidemia, retinitis pigmentosa, cerebellar ataxia, and acanthocytosis (Table 17). Three of the four major plasma lipoprotein classes (chylomicrons, VLDL, and LDL) are absent from the plasma. The concentrations of both plasma cholesterol and triglycerides are low (Table 18).

The disorder presents soon after an uncomplicated neonatal period with abdominal distension, steatorrhea, and decreased rate of growth. The misdiagnosis of celiac disease is often made. Neurologic signs such as clumsiness, ataxia, and decreased muscular strength usually begin before the age of 10 years. Muscular weakness may also be associated with ocular symptoms such as nystagmus and strabismus. Decreased visual acuity and scotomata accompany the development of atypical retinitis pigmentosa. The diagnosis is based on the demonstration of large intracellular fat particles in biopsy specimens of the jejunum, on the failure to form chylomicrons following a meal, and on the absence of beta apoprotein (apoB) in plasma as determined by immunochemical techniques.

The pathophysiology of ABL is not completely resolved. The digestion of dietary triglycerides and the uptake of free fatty acids and monoglycerides proceed normally. The mucosal cells fail to make chylomicrons, presumably because the apoB is not available. The jejunal cells become fat-laden, and most of the dietary fat is excreted in the stools. Some alternative pathway not requiring chylomicrons must become operative, because the essential fatty acid, linoleic acid, and fat-soluble vitamins such as A, D, E, and K are present in the plasma at low levels, and their concentrations are increased through dietary supplementation. Whether the relative deficiency of these dietary components due to malabsorption is responsible for the hematologic, retinal, and neurologic findings or whether these findings are related to the primary biologic lesion is not clear. A membrane defect of nutritional or genetic origin may be the common denominator underlying these pleiotropic effects.

The absence of chylomicrons, VLDL, and LDL indicates that apoB is necessary for their formation and secretion into the plasma. To link the absence of these lipoprotein classes to an intracellular deficiency of apoB requires several pieces of evidence. The first of these is that the apoA and apoC polypeptides are present in patients with ABL. HDL is also low in ABL, but the proportions of apoA-I and apoA-II are normal. The apoC polypeptides have an unusual distribution in the HDL of patients with ABL (Table 18). The lipid composition of HDL is also altered; the ratios of cholesterol ester to free cholesterol and lecithin to sphingomyelin are both decreased. The lack of three lipoprotein classes is not simply related to an absence of apoB in the plasma, since infusion of LDL into a patient with ABL was shown to be unable to raise plasma triglycerides. The removal rate of LDL in this same patient was normal, a finding incompatible with a marked increase in the catabolism of apoB. The possibility that a normal apoB is present intracellularly and that the defect is one of assembly or secretion has not been eliminated. The presence of abnormal Golgi zone as shown by electron microscopy of a hepatic biopsy, as well as the decrease in apoC-III$_2$ and the absence of apoC-III$_1$, suggests that there may be deficient glycosylation of these apoproteins. Finally, an incomplete or structurally altered apoB may be synthesized by the cell.

HYPOBETALIPOPROTEINEMIA. Hypobetalipoproteinemia (HBL) is characterized by low levels of LDL, usually defined as the lower 5th percentile of a normal distribution. This is reflected in diminished concentration of plasma cholesterol (Table 18). VLDL and plasma triglycerides are also frequently reduced. The same principles expounded for hyperbetalipoproteinemia are applicable to HBL. Within a group of subjects with arbitrarily defined HBL, the secondary causes are rare; they include anemia, dysproteinemias, hyperthyroidism, intestinal lymphangiectasia with malabsorption, myocardial infarction, severe infections, and trauma. Prior to 1972, four families with primary HBL had been desribed. The patients with HBL from these kindreds had few clinical symptoms (Table 17). The concentrations of fat-soluble vitamins in plasma were low to normal.

The degree of genetic heterogeneity underlying HBL

TABLE 17. Clinical Findings in Hypolipoproteinemia

Familial Disorder	Neurologic	Gastrointestinal	Hematologic	Ophthalmologic	Cardiologic	Biopsy Findings	Other Findings
Abetalipoproteinemia	Cerebellar ataxia	Severe fat malabsorption	Acanthocytes	Atypical retinitis pigmentosa	Arrhythmias	Gross intracellular fat in jejunal cells	—
Hypobetalipo-proteinemia	Usually absent*	Minimal fat malabsorption	Acanthocytes (occasionally)	Absent	None	None	—
Tangier disease	Relapsing peripheral neuropathy	Moderate splenomegaly, mild hepatomegaly	Absent	Corneal infiltration (adults)	Ischemic heart disease	Foam cells in bone marrow, skin, small nerves and rectum	Enlarged, orange tonsils
Lecithin-cholesteral acyltransferase deficiency	Absent	Absent	Normochromic anemia	Diffuse corneal opacities (childhood), corneal arcus	Accelerated atherosclerosis	Foam cells in bone marrow and renal glomeruli; sea blue histiocytes in spleen and bone marrow	Proteinuria with late renal insufficiency

*Spinocerebellar degeneration and peripheral neuropathy have been described in some patients.

TABLE 18. Laboratory Findings in Hypolipoproteinemia

Familial Disorder	Plasma Lipids			Plasma Lipoproteins			
	Cholesterol (mg/dl)	Triglycerides (mg/dl)	Phospholipid (mg/dl)	Chylomicrons	VLDL	LDL	HDL
Abetalipoproteinemia	Low (35–70)	Very low (1–10)	Low (76–83)	Absent	Absent	Absent	Low; apoC-III$_1$ absent; apoC-II high, apoC-III$_2$ low
Hypobetalipo-proteinemia	Low (55–146)	Low or normal (20–146)	Low or normal (110–170)	Low	Low	Low (10% of normal)	Normal
Tangier disease	Low (38–112)	Normal or high (116–332)	Low (70–144)	Low content of cholesterol	B mobility on electrophoresis, apoC polypeptides low	Low (10% of normal); cholesterol low; triglycerides high	Barely detectable amounts of mutant HDL†
Lecithin-cholesterol acyl transferase deficiency	Low, normal, or high (107–565)	Normal or high (105–900)	Normal or high (116–810)	*	B mobility on electrophoresis‡	Low amounts of abnormal LDL‡	Low amounts of abnormal HDL‡

*Chylomicrons appear to be abnormally catabolized in this order.
† Tangier HDL (HDL$_T$) contains unusual A-II lipoprotein particles and large disklike lipoproteins; the ratio of apoA-I to apoA-II is decreased (1:11, normal 3:1); the apoC polypeptides are decreased.
‡ VLDL, LDL, and HDL contain increased amounts of unesterified cholesterol and lecithin and decreased amounts of esterified cholesterol and lysolecithin; LDL contains a high-molecular-weight component (HM-LDL) and LP-X, the abnormal LDL usually found in obstructive jaundice.

is unresolved. Of interest in this regard is the recent description of two kindreds in which matings of HBL × HBL parents occurred. In one family there were 4 children: 1 normal, 1 with HBL, and 2 with clinical and biochemical features of ABL. Neither of the latter 2 children had any neurologic or ophthalmologic findings; however, each was below the age when these dysfunctions ordinarily appear. Further information on the natural history of homozygous HBL is provided in the second kindred. A 37-year-old woman presented with a hemorrhagic diathesis at parturition. The finding of acanthocytes suggested a disorder of apoB deficiency, and the patient was found to have a plasma cholesterol level of 31 mg/dl and a triglyceride level of 11 mg/dl. No chylomicrons, VLDL, or LDL were present. In contrast to the situation with ABL, there was minimal steatorrhea. The neurologic findings were mild, with "only minimal evidence of alteration of the sense of balance and decreased vibratory perception with reduction of deep tendon reflexes." Retinitis pigmentosa was present, but was of apparently minor clinical significance. Aggerbeck and associates have recently described a new kindred with HBL in which neurologic signs and symptoms of a spinocerebellar degeneration similar to those of Friedreich's ataxia are present in several affected members.

TANGIER DISEASE. Tangier disease is a rare metabolic disorder in which an abnormal plasma HDL is present in severely reduced concentrations. The compositions and amounts of the other lipoproteins are also abnormal (Table 18). The level of total plasma cholesterol is decreased, with normal or elevated concentrations of plasma triglycerides. The lipoprotein abnormalities are accompanied by a striking deposition of cholesteryl esters in different tissues. The major clinical manifestations reflect the lipid storage, and they include enlarged orange yellow tonsils, splenomegaly, and a relapsing peripheral neuropathy (Table 17). Mild hepatomegaly, lymphadenopathy, and corneal infiltration (in adulthood) may also occur. Foam cells can be demonstrated on biopsy of the skin, bone marrow, peripheral nerves, or rectum. The disorder can be detected in children, but the range at age of detection has varied from 3 to 48 years.

Tangier disease has been described in 17 patients from 3 kindreds. The pathophysiology of the pleiotropic effects of this disorder is not completely understood, but involves two apparently interrelated processes, ie, the presence of abnormal plasma lipoproteins and widespread lipid storage. The lipoprotein abnormalities are summarized in Table 18. The HDL in Tangier disease (termed HDL$_T$) is markedly abnormal; a chylomicronlike lipoprotein particle is present in the density range of HDL on a normal high-fat diet. These large, flattened lucent particles 1,000 Å in diameter disappear when a low-fat diet is fed. These observations suggest that HDL is necessary for the normal conversion of chylomicrons and VLDL to LDL. It has also been found that these abnormal lipoproteins are rich in cholesteryl esters, suggesting that these particles are the

ones sequestered by the reticuloendothelial cells in Tangier disease. The biochemical basis for intracellular deposition of cholesteryl esters is not known.

LECITHIN-CHOLESTEROL ACYLTRANSFERASE DEFICIENCY. The rare and unusual disorder familial lecithin-cholesterol acyltransferase (LCAT) deficiency is accompanied by quantitative and qualitative changes in the plasma lipoproteins (Table 18); these alterations result from the virtual absence of LCAT activity. The total concentration of plasma cholesterol may be low, normal, or elevated; however, the percentage of esterified cholesterol is only 10 to 15 percent (normally 60 to 70 percent exists as cholesteryl ester). The plasma triglycerides have been elevated in all but 2 patients, and the plasma is usually turbid. The major clinical findings include diffuse corneal opacities that can be detected in childhood, corneal arcus, proteinuria with late renal insufficiency, and normochromic anemia with decreased red cell life span. Foam cells are present in the bone marrow and renal glomeruli. In addition, sea blue histiocytes have been found in the bone marrow and spleen. Nine Scandinavian patients and 2 Sardinian brothers with LCAT deficiency have been studied. The abnormality in the lipid composition in all lipoprotein classes reflects the deficiency in LCAT, which ordinarily catalyzes the transfer of a fatty acid from lecithin to free cholesterol. The precise mechanism that accounts for the quantitative decrease in the plasma levels of apoB, apoA, and apoD is not completely understood.

TREATMENT. Patients with ABL, Tangier disease, and LCAT deficiency may all benefit from a low-fat diet. In ABL, steatorrhea can be controlled by reducing the intake of fat to 5 to 20 g/day. Lloyd has found that this measure alone can result in marked clinical improvement and growth acceleration. In addition, the diet should be supplemented with linoleic acid. It is unknown if the increase in the levels of this essential fatty acid in plasma has any beneficial clinical effect. Fat-soluble vitamins should be added to the diet. Rickets can be prevented by normal quantities of vitamin D, but up to 20,000 IU of vitamin A may be required to raise the level of vitamin A in plasma to normal. Enough vitamin K should be given to maintain a normal prothrombin time. The hemolysis of red blood cells by peroxide can usually be prevented by administration of vitamin E (100 mg/kg/day). In Tangier disease the feeding of a low-fat diet diminishes the presence of the abnormal lipoprotein species that are believed to be remnants of abnormal chylomicron metabolism (Table 18). The HM-LDL species found in LCAT deficiency is also thought to be a remnant of abnormal chylomicron metabolism. Its disappearance on a low-fat diet may have a beneficial effect, since HM-LDL may be involved in the pathogenesis of renal disease. Medium-chain triglycerides may be of some benefit in the administration of these low-fat diets, particularly in making them more palatable. Care must be exercised in ABL not to add too great a quantity of medium-chain triglycerides, since in large amounts they compete with the long-chain triglycerides for the binding sites in the portal blood-stream. Treatment of HBL is primarily symptomatic.

References

PLASMA LIPIDS AND LIPOPROTEINS

Fredrickson DS, Gotto AM Jr, Levy RI: Familial lipoprotein deficiency (abetalipoproteinemia, hypobetalipoproteinemia and Tangier disease). In Stanbury JB, Wyngaarden JB, Fredrickson DS (eds): The Metabolic Basis of Inherited Disease, 3rd ed. New York, McGraw-Hill, 1972, p 000

Nichols AV: Human serum lipoproteins and their interrelationships. Adv Biol Med Phys 11:109, 1967

CLASSIFICATION OF HYPERLIPIDEMIA AND HYPERLIPOPROTEINEMIA

Beaumont JL, Carlson LA, Copper GR, et al: Classification of hyperlipidemias and hyperlipoproteinemias, Bull WHO 43:891, 1970

Fredrickson DS, Levy RI, Lees RS: Fat transport in lipoproteins: an integrated approach to mechanisms and disorders. N Engl J Med 276:-32, 94, 148, 215, 273, 1967

NORMAL CONCENTRATIONS

Fredrickson DS, Breslow JL: Primary hyperlipoproteinemia in infants. Ann Rev Med 24:315, 1973

Friedewald WR, Levy RI, Fredrickson DS: Estimation of the concentration of low density lipoprotein cholesterol in plasma without use of the preparative ultracentrifuge. Clin Chem 18:499, 1972

Kwiterovich PO, Fredrickson DS, Levy RI: Familial hypercholesterolemia (one form of familial type II hyperlipoproteinemia). A study of its biochemical, genetic, and clinical presentation in childhood. J Clin Invest 53:1237, 1974

Tsang TC, Fallat RW, Glueck CJ: Cholesterol at birth and age 1: comparison of normal and hypercholesterolemic neonates. Pediatrics 53:458, 1974

SCREENING

Glueck CJ, Fallat RW, Tsang R, et al: Hyperlipemia in progeny of parents with myocardial infarction before age 50. Am J Dis Child 127:70, 1974

Tamir I, Bojamower Y, Leutow O, et al: Serum lipids and lipoproteins in children from families with early coronary disease. Arch Dis Child 47:808, 1972

METABOLIC DISORDERS OF HYPERLIPOPROTEINEMIA

Breslow JL, Spaulding DR, Lux SE, et al: Homozygous familial hypercholesterolemia. N Engl J Med 293:900, 1975

Brown MS, Goldstein JL: Familial hypercholesterolemia. Biochemical, genetic and pathophysiological considerations. Adv Intern Med 20:-273, 1975

Fredrickson DS, Levy RI: Familial hyperlipoproteinemia. In Stanbury JB, Wyngaarden JB, Fredrickson DS (eds): The Metabolic Basis of Inherited Disease, 3rd ed. New York, McGraw-Hill, 1972, p 545

——— Morganroth J, Levy RI: Type III hyperlipoproteinemia: an analysis of two contemporary definitions. Ann Intern Med 82:150,1975

Glueck CJ, Fallat R, Buncher CR, et al: Familial combined hyperlipoproteinemia: studies in 91 adults and 95 children from 33 kindreds. Metabolism 22:140, 1973

——— Heckman F, Schoenfield M, et al: Neonatal familial type II hyperlipoproteinemia: cord blood cholesterol in 1800 births. Metabolism 20:597, 1971

——— Tsang RC, Fallat RW, et al: Familial hypertriglyceridemia: studies in 130 children and 45 siblings of 36 index cases. Metabolism 22:1287, 1973

Goldstein JL, Dana SE, Brunschede GY, et al: Genetic heterogeneity in familial hypercholesterolemia: evidence for two different mutations affecting functions of low-density lipoprotein receptor. Proc Natl Acad Sci USA 72:1092, 1975

——— Hazzard WR, Schrott JG, et al: Hyperlipidemia in coronary heart disease. I. Lipid levels in 500 survivors of myocardial infarction. J Clin Invest 52:1533, 1973

——— Schrott HG, Hazzard WR, et al: Hyperlipidemia in coronary heart disease: genetic analysis of lipid levels in 176 families and delineation of a new inherited disorder, combined hyperlipidemia. J Clin Invest 52:1544, 1973

Kwiterovich PO: Neonatal screening for hyperlipidemia. Pediatrics 53:-455, 1974

Shapiro JR, Fallat RW, Tsang RC, et al: Achilles tendinitis and tenosynovitis. A diagnostic manifestation of familial type II hyperlipoproteinemia in children. Am J Dis Child 128:486, 1974

TREATMENT

Eder HA: Drugs used in the prevention and treatment of atherosclerosis. In Goodman LS, Gilman A (eds): The Pharmacological Basis of Therapeutics, 5th ed. New York, Macmillan, 1975, p 744

Farah JR, Kwiterovich PO, Neill CA: A study of the dose–effect relationship of cholestyramine in children with familial hypercholesterolemia. Pediatr Res 9:350, 1975

Fredrickson DS, Levy RI, Brunnell M, et al: The Dietary Management of Hyperlipoproteinemia: A Handbook for Physicians. US Department of Health, Education and Welfare, Public Health Service. Washington, DC, US Government Printing Office (No 75-110), 1974

Glueck CJ, Tsang RC: Pediatric familial type II hyperlipoproteinemia: effect of diet on plasma cholesterol in the first year of life. Am J Clin Nutr 25:224, 1972

Strong JP, McGill HC Jr: The pediatric aspects of atherosclerosis. J Atheroscler Res 9:251, 1969

West RJ, Lloyd JK: Use of cholestyramine in treatment of children with familial hypercholesterolemia. Arch Dis Child 48:370, 1973

HYPOLIPOPROTEINEMIA

Aggerbeck LP, McMahon JP, Scanu AM: Hypobetalipoproteinemia: clinical and biochemical description of a new kindred with "Friedreich's ataxia." Neurology 24:1051, 1974

Biemer JJ, McCammon RE: The genetic relationship of abetalipoproteinemia and hypobetalipoproteinemia: a report of the occurence of both diseases within the same family. J Lab Clin Med 85:556, 1975

TANGIER DISEASE

Alaupovic P, McConathy WJ, Curry MD, et al: Apolipoproteins and lipoprotein families in familial lecithin: cholesterol acyltransferase deficiency. Scand J Clin Lab Invest 33 [Suppl 137]:83, 1974

Ferrans VJ, Fredrickson DS: The pathology of Tangier disease. A light and electron microscopic study. Am J Pathol 78:101, 1975

LIPIDOSES

ROSCOE O. BRADY

Pediatricians are frequently confronted with infants whose primary difficulty is failure of development of motor and intellectual capabilities consistent with their age. The diagnosis of the disease process in these patients may be quite difficult. An attempt should be made to arrive at a correct solution, because prenatal diagnosis is presently available for many of these disorders, and effective treatment may be forthcoming for some of these diseases in the future. Remarkable progress has been achieved in the past few years toward elucidation of the biochemical abnormalities in heritable lipid storage diseases. Patients with these diseases present a wide variety of medical problems. Abnormalities of lipid metabolism should always be considered in infants whose mental development is slower than normal, especially if there is concomitant splenomegaly and hepatomegaly. The following section provides a brief review of the group of inherited disorders of lipid metabolism known as the sphingolipidoses.

Tay-Sachs Disease

Tay-Sachs disease (p. 1908) is the most common hereditable lipid disease. The gene frequency of this condition is 1 in 60 in persons of Ashkenazi Jewish ancestry, which means that 1 in 30 of these individuals is a heterozygous carrier of the trait. Somewhere around 100 infants with Tay-Sachs disease are born each year in the United States. The incidence is much less frequent in children of non-Jewish ancestry. The metabolic defect in Tay-Sachs disease has been identified as an absence of N-acetylgalactosaminidase in affected tissues.

CLINICAL MANIFESTATIONS. The hallmark of Tay-Sachs disease is severe and progressive mental retardation. Patients with this disease appear relatively normal until 5 to 7 months of age, when evidence of impairment of maturation of the central nervous system becomes manifested by inability to learn and by arrested motor development. These patients show progressive mental deterioration accompanied by amaurosis. Toward the end of the second year or early in the third year of life they become totally blind and die soon thereafter. There is usually a cherry-red spot in the macular region of the eyes of these patients. They have little or no organomegaly except for an increase of about 40 percent in head size compared with children of the same age.

PATHOPHYSIOLOGY. All of the lipids under consideration in this section have in common a portion of their molecule called ceramide, which consists of the amino alcohol sphingosine, to which a long-chain acid is linked through an amide bond to the nitrogen atom on carbon-2 of sphingosine (Fig. 42, p. 1907). In patients with Tay-Sachs disease an acidic glycolipid called GM_2 or Tay-Sachs ganglioside accumulates in neuronal cells in the form of concentrically layered membranous cytoplasmic bodies. These intracellular inclusions consist of cholesterol, phospholipid, and protein in addition to Tay-Sachs ganglioside. However, the only striking abnormality detected on chemical analysis of brain tissue from patients with Tay-Sachs disease is a marked increase in Tay-Sachs ganglioside, which normally constitutes about 5 percent of the total brain gangliosides. It has been shown that there is a complete absence of the N-acetylgalactosamine-cleaving enzyme in tissues of patients with Tay-Sachs disease.

These results complement the data obtained in other studies using artificial substrates, which revealed that there are two major isozymes in most human tissues that catalyze the hydrolysis of p-nitrophenyl-β-D-N-acetylgalactosaminide and 4-methylumbelliferyl-β-D-N-acetylgalactosaminide. These isozymes can be separated from each other by starch gel electrophoresis, and one of these enzymes, called Hex A, is completely absent in extracts of tissues from patients with Tay-Sachs disease. Together these studies provide good evidence that the metabolic defect in Tay-Sachs disease is the absence of an N-acetylgalactosamine-cleaving enzyme that participates in the catabolism of Tay-Sachs ganglioside.

DIAGNOSIS. Tay-Sachs disease can generally be diagnosed on the basis of the clinical findings. The diagnosis should be confirmed by laboratory tests. One procedure is based on the determination of hexosaminidase activity in tissue biopsy specimens using labeled Tay-Sachs ganglioside as substrate. Muscle tissue is a convenient source of enzyme for this assay. The disadvantage of this test lies in the difficulty and expense involved in the preparation of the substrate. For this reason methods have been devised to simplify the diagnosis using artificial substrates and more easily accessible enzyme sources, such as washed leukocyte preparations or serum samples. It has been shown that tests such as these permit the antenatal diagnosis of fetuses with Tay-Sachs disease by assay in amniotic cell cultures obtained following amniocentesis. The availability of tests for the identification of heterozygous carriers of Tay-Sachs disease is helpful for accurate genetic counseling.

TREATMENT. At the present time no therapy is available for this disorder. Therapeutic trials in the sphingolipidoses have been carried out using enzyme replacement. This procedure is fraught with a number if potential complications, primary among which is the danger of sensitization to a foreign protein, especially if other than human sources are used; there is also the problem that exogenously administered enzyme cannot pass through the blood-brain barrier.

Generalized Gangliosidosis

Generalized gangliosidosis is a very uncommon lipid storage disease characterized by psychomotor retardation, hepatomegaly, some degree of splenomegaly, and foam cells in the reticuloendothelial tissues. There is vacuolation of the lymphocytes, and skeletal abnormalities occur that involve the skull, trunk, vertebral bodies, and humerus. The neurons in the central nervous system are swollen and contain cytoplasmic inclusion bodies. The predominant material that accumulates in the brain and other tissues of these patients is monosialoganglioside. There is also some increase in keratosulfate in the tissues of these individuals.

The metabolic defect in patients with generalized gangliosidosis is a deficiency of a β-galactosidase, which catalyzes the hydrolysis of the terminal molecule of galactose of monosialoganglioside. There is only 7 percent of normal galactosidase activity in tissues from these patients judging by assays with p-nitrophenyl-β-galactopyranoside as substrate. This finding might suggest that other naturally occurring substances with a terminal galactose molecule such as galactocerebroside, ceramidelactoside, or ceramidetrihexoside might also accumulate. However, direct examination of the catabolism of these substrates using labeled glycolipids as substrates has revealed quite the opposite. The enzymatic hydrolysis of galactocerebroside was within normal limits in extracts of brain tissue from patients with generalized gangliosidosis, and the hydrolysis of ceramidelactoside and ceramidetrihexoside was actually increased 200 to 300 percent over that of age-matched controls. These findings amply demonstrate the pitfalls that must be scrupulously avoided when attempting to elucidate a metabolic abnormality based solely on data obtained with artificial substrates.

Gaucher's Disease

Patients with Gaucher's disease have been classified as having infantile, juvenile, and adult forms of the disorder on the basis of the rapidity of progression of hepatosplenomegaly, which exists in all of these patients, and the presence or absence of central nervous system difficulties. Patients with the infantile form of the disease show very rapid organ enlargement and impairment of neuronal function. The patients with the juvenile form are also characterized by rapidly progressive splenomegaly and hepatomegaly along with rarefaction of the long bones and pelvis; however, these children generally have no central nervous system derangement. Patients with the adult form of Gaucher's disease have slow enlargement of the spleen and liver and involvement of the long bones and pelvis, and they are frequently seen in hematology clinics because of a mild hypochromic anemia and prolonged clotting time due to thrombocytopenia. In all three forms of this disease large lipid-laden Gaucher cells that stain for both fat and carbohydrates are seen in bone marrow smears. There is usually an increase in serum acid phosphatase, which is not inhibited by tartrate.

PATHOPHYSIOLOGY. The enlarged systemic organs in patients with Gaucher's disease contain an increased amount of the sphingoglycolipid called glucocerebroside. The biochemical defect in this condition has been shown to be a deficiency of the β-glucosidase that catalyzes the hydrolysis of the glucose moiety of this compound. Tissues from patients with the infantile form of this disease are virtually devoid of glucocerebrosidase activity. Patients with the juvenile form have from 50 to 10 percent of normal glucocerebrosidase in their tissues. Patients with the adult form of Gaucher's disease have a rather wide range of activity of this enzyme in their tissues; it may be as much as 40 percent of the normal value. This scatter of cerebrosidase activity is clearly indicative of the genetic heterogeneity of Gaucher's disease. It is presumed that these differences are caused by alterations or deletions of the amino acid sequence in the enzyme, which of course is ultimately traceable to alterations of the DNA in the involved gene.

The major source of the glucocerebroside that accumulates in peripheral tissues of patients with Gaucher's disease is probably the glycolipids in senescent leukocytes, of which ceramidelactoside and hematoside are the chief components. Some glucocerebroside also arises from erythrocyte stroma that contains hematoside and globoside as major constituents. The glucocerebroside in neuronal cells in the brain probably arises in the course of turnover of gangliosides. It is currently assumed that patients with the juvenile and adult forms of Gaucher's disease have sufficient residual glucocerebrosidase activity in brain to prevent accumulation of this substance during the period of active ganglioside metabolism, and these patients are therefore spared difficulties of the nervous system.

DIAGNOSIS. The diagnosis of Gaucher's disease can usually be made on the basis of the organomegaly, the presence of Gaucher cells in marrow preparations, and the increase in serum acid phosphatase. A more specific test is now available for confirmation of the diagnosis that is based on measurement of glucocerebrosidase activity in washed leukocyte preparations. Sufficient cells can be obtained from a few milliliters of venous blood, and the assay is conveniently performed with ^{14}C-labeled glucocerebroside as substrate. Methods have been developed that permit accurate diagnosis using artificial substrates such as 4-methylumbelliferyl-β–D–glucopyranoside as substrate.

The enzymatic defect in Gaucher's disease can also be demonstrated by assaying glucocerebrosidase acting in extracts of skin fibroblasts grown in tissue culture. It is possible to identify heterozygous carriers of the Gaucher trait. In addition, it is now possible to diagnose Gaucher's disease in utero by assaying glucocerebrosidase activity in cultured fetal cells.

TREATMENT. Therapy for this disorder at the present time is symptomatic, and it is important to include genetic counseling. The concepts outlined for the treatment of Tay-Sachs disease can generally be applied to considerations of therapy of Gaucher's disease. Preliminary replacement trials have been carried out in patients with Gaucher's disease using glucocerebrosidase isolated from human placenta, and the results are encouraging.

Metachromatic Leukodystrophy

Patients with metachromatic leukodystrophy (MLD) present a number of signs of central nervous system derangement. The disease becomes evident in affected infants within the first 30 months of life and is manifested by weakness, speech and swallowing difficulties, ataxia, and paralysis. In addition, there is a decrease of the conduction velocity in peripheral nerves.

PATHOPHYSIOLOGY. An acidic glycolipid called sulfatide accumulates in brain, kidney, and bile ducts and stains metachromatically yellowish brown when tissue sections are treated with cresyl violet dye. The accumulated sulfatide may cause some renal and hepatic dysfunction. The metabolic defect in MLD has been shown to be a deficiency of an enzyme that catalyzes the cleavage of sulfuric acid from sulfatide. There are at least three sulfatases in human tissues whose activity may be assayed with the artificial substrate nitrocatechol sulfate. These enzymes are designated as arylsulfatases A, B, and C. In classic cases of MLD there is a consistent deficiency of arylsulfatase A. Sulfatide is considered to be the natural substrate of this enzyme. This information has provided the background for the development of a convenient diagnostic procedure based on the differential determination of arylsulfatase activity in leukocytes. The mean level of arylsulfatase A activity in leukocyte preparations from patients with MLD is only 10 percent of that found in control leukocyte preparations. Arylsulfatase B activity is within normal limits. The facility and reliability of this test make it the diagnostic procedure of choice at the present time. The diagnosis of MLD previously depended on measurement of the amount of sediment-bound urinary sulfatide or sulfatidase activity in urine; both of these determinations may vary with the volume, cellular composition, and degree of bacterial contamination of the urine.

TREATMENT.   There is no specific therapy. An unsuccessful attempt was made to treat MLD by intrathecal and intravenous administration of beef brain arylsulfatase A. The investigation was performed with care and included brain biopsy before and after administration of the enzyme; however, there was no histologic evidence of improvement. If urine does indeed contain significant sulfatidase activity, one might consider it as a potential alternative source for obtaining sphingolipid hydrolases.

Niemann-Pick Disease

Patients with Niemann-Pick disease are generally severely retarded and cachectic and have hepatosplenomegaly. There is some involvement of the long bones, although of a lesser degree than in patients with Gaucher's disease. Some patients with Niemann-Pick disease have an olive yellow coloration of the exposed areas of the skin, and about 30 percent of them have a cherry-red spot in the macula. A large waxy cell that stains for both lipid and phosphorus is seen in marrow preparations. Most of these patients seen in pediatric clinics are of the classic infantile type with rapidly progressive symptomatology. More recently, as our diagnostic acumen has increased, Niemann-Pick patients have been detected with less rapid progression of their disease.

PATHOPHYSIOLOGY.   The lipid that accumulates in various tissues of patients with Niemann-Pick disease is a phospholipid called sphingomyelin. The enzymatic defect in Niemann-Pick disease is now well established as a deficiency of the enzyme sphingomyelinase, which catalyzes the hydrolytic cleavage of the phosphorylcholine portion of this sphingolipid.

DIAGNOSIS.   A reproducible assay for sphingomyelinase activity has been developed using sonicated leukocyte preparations. The activity of this enzyme is markedly depressed in leukocytes obtained from patients with Niemann-Pick disease. This test provides both diagnostic and prognostic information, since the rapidity of progression of the disease is inversely related to the amount of residual sphingomyelinase activity. Similar findings have been obtained in sphingomyelinase assays in extracts of skin fibroblasts grown in tissue culture. Patients classified as Niemann-Pick type D (Nova Scotia variant) have normal sphingomyelinase activity in their cultured fibroblasts. It may be that this disease has been incorrectly classified and rightly belongs to the group of cholesterol storage diseases, although it is manifested by an ancillary and lesser accumulation of sphingomyelin.

Fabry's Disease

Fabry's disease was long considered to be a dermatologic disorder because of the occurrence of small, dark reddish purple macules and papules in the umbilical region, on the scrotum, and over the lateral iliac areas. The disease was called angiokeratoma corporis diffusum universale. It has subsequently been recognized that this condition is an X-linked inherited metabolic disorder in which hemizygous males manifest the disorder. The outstanding manifestation of the disease in these patients is a severe progressive impairment of kidney function that becomes increasingly difficult to manage in the third and fourth decades of life. Patients with Fabry's disease may also have electrocardiographic abnormalities and cardiac dysfunction. Ophthalmologic abnormalities, including cataracts, corneal opacities, and edema of the retina, are frequently present. There may also be bouts of fever, burning pains in the extremities, and disorders of the gastrointestinal system. Female carriers of the abnormal gene may be symptom-free or may have mild ocular and skin involvement.

BIOCHEMICAL LESION.   A glycolipid called ceramidetrihexoside accumulates in many tissues of patients with Fabry's disease. The high concentration of this material in kidney glomeruli is probably responsible for the impairment of function of this organ. The enzymatic defect in hemizygous males with Fabry's disease is a complete absence of the enzyme that catalyzes the hydrolysis of the terminal α-galactosyl moiety of ceramidetrihexoside. Heterozygous female carriers of this disease exhibit an intermediate level of activity of this enzyme in their tissues.

The most likely source of the accumulating ceramidetrihexoside seems to be globoside from senescent erythrocytes. Normally a small quantity of ceramidetrihexosidase is excreted in the urine. Increased levels of ceramidetrihexoside have been detected in the serum and urine of males with Fabry's disease. This compound is only very slightly soluble in water, and the increased quantities presented to the kidney in these patients may precipitate in the glomeruli.

DIAGNOSIS.   The diagnosis of Fabry's disease may be established by determining the level of α-galactosidase activity in biopsy specimens of tissue or leukocytes. The enzymatic assay is greatly facilitated by the use of appropriately labeled or fluorogenic substrates.

TREATMENT. A number of patients with Fabry's disease have been treated by renal transplantation to alleviate their renal insufficiency. The extensive current research directed toward the solution of difficulties related to organ transplantation should eventually permit the development of new and safer procedures. Enzyme replacement therapy has been attempted in patients with Fabry's disease, with a demonstrable but transient effect on ceramidetrihexoside excreted in urine.

Globoid Leukodystrophy

The etiology of globoid leukodystrophy (Krabbe's disease) (p. 1912) has been established following the demonstration of a deficiency of galactocerebroside β-galactosidase. Infants with this condition exhibit severe mental retardation, and "globoid bodies" are seen in histologic sections of brain tissue. These bodies are reported to contain cerebroside and sphingomyelin. Perhaps the most definitive chemical alteration in brain tissue of patients with Krabbe's disease is an increase in the ratio of cerebroside to sulfatide. Normally, there is about three times as much cerebroside as sulfatide in brain. In Krabbe's disease, this ratio may be as high as 12:1.

Investigations have shown a defect of sphingolipid catabolism in patients with Krabbe's disease involving a defect in breakdown of galactocerebroside.

References

Brady RO: Cerebral lipidosis. Ann Rev Med 21:317, 1970
——— Genetics and the sphingolipidoses. Med Clin North Am 53:-827, 1969
Greene HL, Hug G, Schubert WK: Metachromatic leukodystrophy. Treatment with arylsulfatase-A. Arch Neurol 20:147, 1969
Kampine JP, Brady RO, Kanfer JN, Feld M, Shapiro D: Diagnosis of Gaucher's disease and Niemann-Pick disease with small samples of venous blood. Science 155:86, 1967
Kolodney EH: Clinical and genetic aspects of the lipidoses. Semin Hematol 9:251, 1972
O'Brien JS: Tay-Sachs disease: from enzyme to prevention. Fed Proc 32:191, 1973

Okada S, O'Brien JS: Generalized gangliosidosis: beta-galactosidase deficiency. Science 160:1002, 1968
——— O'Brien JS: Tay-Sachs disease: generalized absence of a beta-D-N-acetylhexosaminidase component. Science 165:698, 1969
Percy AK, Brady RO: Metachromatic leukodystrophy: diagnosis with samples of venous blood. Science 161:594, 1968
Sandhof K, Andreae U, Jatkewitz H: Deficient hexosaminidase activity in an exceptional case of Tay-Sachs disease with additional storage of kidney globoside in visceral organs. Life Sci 7:283, 1968
Sloan MR, Uhlendorf BW, Kanfer JN, Brady RO, Fredrickson DS: Deficiency of sphingomyelin-cleaving enzyme activity in tissue cultures derived from patients with Niemann-Pick disease. Biochem Biophys Res Commun 34:582, 1969
Suzuki K, Suzuki K: Disorders of sphingolipid metabolism. In Gaul G (ed): Biology of Brain Dysfunction, Vol 2. New York, Plenum, 1973, p 1

MUCOPOLYSACCHARIDOSES
B. Shannon Danes

Acid mucopolysaccharides are among the primary constituents of the extracellular matrix synthesized by connective tissue cells. Disorders involving their synthesis or structure may lead to developmental changes that are recognized as abnormal clinical phenotypes known as genetic mucopolysaccharidoses.

CHEMISTRY. In 1884 Krukenberg isolated material from the extracellular matrix that he identified chemically as a polysaccharide and named chondroitic acid. Not until 1938 was the term mucopolysaccharide suggested by Meyer to describe "hexosamine-containing polysaccharides of animal origin occurring either in a pure state or conjugated with protein through a salt linkage." Several chemically different acid mucopolysaccharides are known to occur in specific connective tissues (Table 19). The exact macromolecular structure of the polysaccharide–protein complex is not known and probably shows considerable structural heterogeneity. The biosynthesis is thought to be a three-step process: synthesis of the protein core on the ribosome; a sequential addition of monosaccharide residues from appropriate sugar nucleotide precursors; and sulfation via phosphoadenosine-5'-phosphosufate. The second and third steps are presumed to occur in the membrane of the endoplasmic reticulum and Golgi apparatus.

Little is known about the catabolism of sulfated mucopolysaccharides, although it is evident that lyso-

TABLE 19. Mucopolysaccharides of Connective Tissue

Compound	Amino Sugar	Uronic Acid	Sulfate*	Tissue Occurrence
Hyaluronic acid	Glucosamine	Glucuronic acid	0	Vitreous humor, Wharton's jelly, synovial fluid
Chondroitin sulfate A	Galactosamine	Glucuronic acid	1	Cartilage
Chondroitin sulfate B (dermatan sulfate)	Galactosamine	Iduronic acid	1	Skin, blood vessels
Chondroitin sulfate C	Galactosamine	Glucuronic acid	1	Cartilage
Keratosulfate	Glucosamine	Galactose	1	Cartilage
Heparan sulfate	Glucosamine	Glucuronic acid, Iduronic acid	1	Aorta Liver

Moles per disaccharide repeating unit.

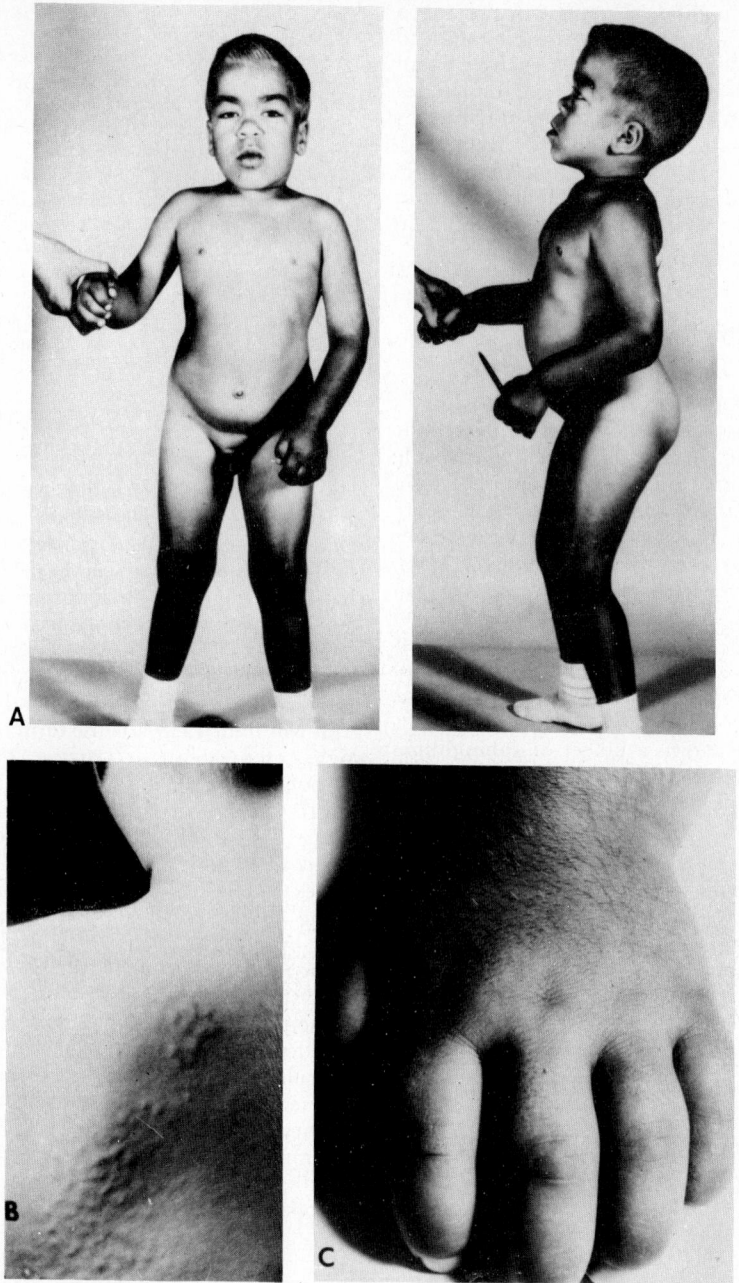

FIG. 17. Child with mucopolysaccharidosis type II (Hunter syndrome). *A.* General features. *B.* Nodular skin lesions on back thorax. *C.* Clawhands.

somes are involved. It appears from cell culture studies that two pools of mucopolysaccharides occur within a cell, a secretory pool that is small and turns over rapidly and a large separate storage pool that turns over slowly.

In 1952, from the livers of 2 patients with the Hurler syndrome, Brante isolated a substance with the properties of dermatan sulfate (chondroitin sulfate B); he suggested that the Hurler syndrome is an inborn error of mucopolysaccharide metabolism. In 1957 Dorfman and Lorincz demonstrated that two mucopolysaccharides, dermatan sulfate and heparan sulfate, were found in excess amounts in the urine of patients with the Hurler syndrome. Independently, Meyer and his colleagues found the same excessive mucopolysacchariduria. From cell culture studies it appears that these genetic disorders result from inability to degrade mucopolysaccharides.

CLINICAL FEATURES. Since the first definitive clinical description of this disorder by Hunter and Hurler, it has become apparent that several distinct disorders can be recognized, reflecting genetically transmitted disorders of acid mucopolysaccharide metabolism resulting in visceral storage of dermatan sulfate and heparan sulfate. In the brain there is also excessive cerebral storage of gangliosides GM_1, GM_2, and GM_3.

The general clinical features (Fig. 17) of this group of disorders are dwarfism, skeletal deformities, restriction of joint movements, deafness, abdominal hernias, hepatosplenomegaly, cardiac abnormalities, and usually mental retardation. The amount of mucopolysaccharides excreted in the urine may be increased or may be in the normal range (3 to 24 mg/24 hours), depending on the type (Table 20). Metachromatic inclusions are seen in the white blood cells in the peripheral blood and bone marrow. There is wide variation of these and other physical and laboratory findings reflecting storage of mucopolysaccharides in specific organs. Based on clinical, genetic, and biochemical studies, six distinct types have been delineated by McKusick:

TYPE I (HURLER SYNDROME). The Hurler syndrome is an autosomal recessive disorder associated with mental and physical deterioration in the newborn period. Diagnosis is usually made in the first year. Clinical features include gargoylelike facies with coarse features, lumbar gibbus, hydrocephalus, stiff joints, clawhands, excessive body hair, chest deformities, early and progressive clouding of cornea, and mental retardation. Dermatan sulfate and heparan sulfate are found in excessive amounts in the urine. Growth and development are markedly impaired, leading to death in childhood.

The lysosomal enzyme α-L-iduronidase is deficient in the Hurler syndrome. Dermatan sulfate and heparan sulfate appear in the urine, as both have iduronide as a component of their polysaccharide side chains, which are the sites of the degradative action of α-L-iduronidase.

TYPE IS (SCHEIE SYNDROME). Scheie syndrome is an autosomal recessive syndrome and has the least severe clinical manifestations. Stiff joints, coarse facies, cloudy cornea, and aortic regurgitation occur. The patients show the other general clinical stigmata to a minimal degree, with intelligence being usually normal. Increased amounts of dermatan sulfate and heparan sulfate are found in the urine. Decreased vision is the clinical problem in adults with this type.

Scheie first described this syndrome as a variant of the Hurler syndrome, which has been proved to be true. The same enzyme (α-L-iduronidase) is deficient in the Hurler and Scheie syndromes. The two syndromes are presumed to be allelic, like SS and CC hemoglobinopathies.

TYPE IH/S (HURLER-SCHEIE COMPOUND). On the basis of clinical phenotypes the Hurler and Scheie syndromes were considered to be separate disorders until in vitro complementation could not be demonstrated owing to a deficiency of α-L-iduronidase in both syndromes. McKusick hypothesized that the Hurler and Scheie syndromes were allelic and postulated the occurrence of genetic compounds (mixed heterozygotes) of the Hurler and Scheie genes; he described 4 clinical cases with intermediate clinical phenotypes laking enzyme activity. On the basis of enzyme deficiency it was not possible to determine which of the two mutated genes had been transmitted from each parent. From culture phenotypes Danes determined that the Hurler and Scheie genes could be distinguished in the heterozygote.

TYPE II (HUNTER SYNDROME). The Hunter syndrome is an X-linked recessive disorder usually less severe than type I. As in type I, the striking clinical features are stiff joints, dwarfing, hepatosplenomegaly, and gross facial appearance. Similarly, dermatan sulfate and heparan sulfate are increased in the urine. Features that distinguish type II from I are absence of gibbus and clear corneas. Deafness and mental retardation are not as profound as in type I, but they are progressive. Affected males usually live into adulthood, dying of cardiopulmonary impairment. There are severe and mild clinical forms of the Hunter syndrome.

The lysosomal enzyme deficient in both the mild and severe forms of the Hunter syndrome is sulfoiduronate sulfatase. As the same enzyme causes a sufficiently different clinical picture, the two forms of the Hunter syndrome are considered to be allelic. This sulfatase degrades sulfated iduronic acid residues. The clinical consequences of deficiency of this enzyme are similar to those of α-L-iduronidase deficiency. The degradation of mucopolysaccharides in the cornea does not appear to require sulfoiduronate sulfatase, thus indicating that the corneal tissue must be devoid of sulfoiduronate residues.

TYPE III (SANFILIPPO SYNDROME). The clinical features of the autosomal recessive Sanfilippo syndrome are central nervous system involvement, including mental retardation with only moderate somatic changes. Heparan sulfate is increased in the urine. Meyer and Hoffman found heparan sulfate normally in liver and not in bone and cartilage. This may explain the minimal skeletal abnormalities in this type, but it raises the question of the role of heparan sulfate in mental retardation. Because of minimal body impairment, patients live into adulthood. Severe mental retardation usually makes institutionalization necessary.

Although this disorder has a single distinct clinical phenotype, cultured fibroblasts from patients with the Sanfilippo syndrome fall into two subgroups (A and B), each manifesting a deficiency of a specific lysosomal enzyme required for the normal metabolism of sulfated mucopolysaccharides. The enzyme deficient in Sanfilippo A is heparan sulfate sulfatase; in Sanfilippo B it is *N*-acetyl-α-D-glucosaminidase.

TYPE IV (MORQUIO SYNDROME). The Morquio syndrome has been recognized as a distinct clinical chon-

TABLE 20. Characteristics of the Various Types of Mucopolysaccharidoses

Type (McKusick)	Eponym	Clinical Features Physical Involvement	Mental Retardation	Cloudy Cornea	Metachromasia in WBC	Mode of Inheritance	Urinary Mucopolysaccharides	Lysosomal Enzyme Deficiency
I	Hurler	+++	+++	+++	Present	Autosomal recessive	Dermatan sulfate Heparan sulfate	α-L-iduronidase
IS	Scheie	+	+/−	+++	Rare	Autosomal recessive	Dermatan sulfate Heparan sulfate	α-L-iduronidase
IH/S	Hurler-Scheie compound	+	+/−	+	Present	Autosomal recessive	Dermatan sulfate Heparan sulfate	α-L-iduronidase
II	Hunter (mild and severe)	++	+	−	Present	X-linked recessive	Dermatan sulfate Heparan sulfate	Sulfoiduronate sulfatase
III	Sanfilippo A	+	+++	−	Present	Autosomal recessive	Heparan sulfate	Heparan sulfate sulfatase
	Sanfilippo B	+	+++	−	Present	Autosomal recessive	Heparan sulfate	N-acetyl-α-D-glucosaminidase
IV	Morquio	+++	+/−	++	Rare	Autosomal recessive	Keratosulfate	N-acetylhexosamine sulfate sulfatase
V	(reclassified IS)							
VI	Maroteaux-Lamy	+++	−	+	Numerous	Autosomal recessive	Dermatan sulfate	N-acetylgalacto-samine-4-sulfatase
VII	β-glucuronidase deficiency	+,+++	+/−,+++	+/−,++	Present	Autosomal recessive	1 or more* AMPS	β-glucuronidase

*See text for mucopolysaccharides (AMPS) reported in urine of patients with β-glucuronidase deficiency.

Key to symbols: − absent; +/− mild or absent; + mild, ++ moderate, +++ severe.

754

drodystrophy since the descriptions in 1929 by Morquio and Brailsford. It was later considered to be a connective tissue disorder involving an inborn error of mucopolysaccharide metabolism, particularly kerato-sulfate. Since the first description of the Morquio syndrome many varieties of skeletal abnormalities have been included under this eponyn, but the term should be used only when generalized platyspondyly associated with corneal opacities, dental abnormalities, aortic regurgitation, and usually urinary excretion of keratosulfate are present. As some patients do not have keratosulfaturia, there are now considered to be two forms of the Morquio syndrome. These patients can be distinguished from those with the other mucopolysaccharidoses by the presence of distinct skeletal abnormalities and the absence of mental retardation, deafness, and gargoyle facies. Orthopedic and cardiopulmonary manifestations are the main clinical problems during adult life.

Matalon and Dorfman have suggested that the Morquio syndrome is due to a deficiency of a specific *N*-acetylhexosamine sulfate sulfatase. On the basis of the structure of the compounds excreted in the Morquio syndrome, the deficient enzyme may hydrolyze 6-O-sulfate linkages in mucopolysaccharides.

TYPE V. Type V has been reclassified IS.

TYPE VI (MAROTEAUX-LAMY SYNDROME). Growth retardation is the dominant feature of the autosomal recessive Maroteaux-Lamy syndrome. Dwarfism with stunting of both the trunk and limbs, genu valgum, lumbar kyphosis, anterior sternal protrusion, and corneal clouding are present. Although other general features occur, the distinctive characteristics are normal intelligence and severe osseous abnormalities. Increased amounts of dermatan sulfate are found in the urine. Metachromatic inclusions are found in all types of white blood cells of the peripheral blood. The life span is shortened in these patients due to progressive cardiovascular impairment. As there are mild and severe clinical forms of this syndrome, McKusick has postulated that the two forms are allelic.

The lysosomal enzyme deficient in this syndrome is *N*-acetylgalactosamine-4-sulfatase, which is required for the complete degradation of dermatan sulfate. Aryl-sulfatase B is also markedly diminished, but a role for this sulfatase in the degradation of dermatan sulfate has not been demonstrated.

TYPE VII (β-Glucuronidase Deficiency). With the assay of enzymatic activity of cultured fibroblasts, genetic disorders of aberrant degradation of mucopolysaccharides are being identified by specific enzymatic defects. Abnormal clinical phenotypes due to a deficiency of β-glucuronidase were first recognized by such in vitro studies. The clinical phenotypes have shown great variability with the same enzyme deficient in cultured cells. The following may be present: mental retardation, dysostosis, hepatomegaly, cloudy corneas, metachromatic inclusions in polymorphonuclear leukocytes, and mucopolysacchariduria (chondroitin sulfate, dermatan sulfate, or chondroitin sulfate and heparan sulfate have all been reported). Such heterogeneity of

clinical phenotype with the same enzyme deficiency suggests allelism (homozygosity for different alleles at the same locus). Mutations at the same or a different locus may be assumed to lead to different structural changes in the same enzyme, producing altered substrate recognition, which might explain the inability to degrade different mucopolysaccharides in the 4 patients so far reported.

MUCOLIPIDOSES. There are genetic disorders that have in common gargoylelike dysmorphism and dysostosis with visceral storage of mucopolysaccharides and lipids without mucopolysacchariduria. This heterogeneous group has now been identified as the mucolipidoses (p. 1904) and should be considered in the differential diagnosis of a patient with clinical features usually associated with the genetic mucopolysaccharidoses.

GENETICS. The mode of inheritance for all the types of mucopolysaccharidoses so far described is autosomal recessive, except for type II, which is inherited in an X-linked recessive fashion. The frequency for all types is very rare, less than 1 in 100,000 newborns. All types are widely distributed in all major ethnic groups.

Type II appears to be only one-fifth as frequent as type I. In the case of the X-linked recessive type II, one-third of the cases arise by new mutation in the X chromosome, which is transmitted to the affected son by his mother, and two-thirds arise from mutation of the X chromosome occurring in earlier generations.

Analyses of karyotypes have shown that number and morphology are normal. Heterozygote detection has been made possible through cell culture studies. Both cellular metachromasia and intracellular mucopolysaccharide content (measured as total uronic acid content and as synthesis by incorporation of ^{35}S-sulfate and ^{3}H-acetate) are increased in fibroblast and peripheral white blood cell cultures derived from heterozygotes. Degradation (measured as loss of ^{35}S-labeled mucopolysaccharides) is impaired. Lysosomal enzyme activity has been found to be intermediate in cultured cells from obligatory heterozygotes for the mucopolysaccharidoses for which an enzyme deficiency is known. McKusick's hypothesis that clinical variants represent genetic compounds (mixed heterozygotes) has broadened our concept of the genetic mucopolysaccharidoses.

PATHOGENESIS. Since the identification of the storage material as acid mucopolysaccharides, several explanations for the metabolic defect have been suggested but not experimentally proved. *A defect in binding protein:* Dorfman observed that mucopolysaccharides were more easily extracted from tissues of patients with the Hurler syndrome and that there was a deficiency in serine (important in the linkage of mucopolysaccharides to proteins) in such preparations, thus suggesting a defect in the binding protein. *A deficiency of degradative enzymes:* Van Hoof and Hers observed that the intracellular mucopolysaccharides stored in inclusion bodies, presumably derived from lysosomes, reflected a deficiency of a degradative enzyme in the tissue. Fibroblast culture studies have shown a storage of intracellular mucopolysaccharides with impairment in degradation of mucopolysaccharides. A deficiency of a specific lysosomal enzyme involved in the degradation of mucopolysaccharides has been identified for mucopolysaccharidoses I, IS, IH/S, II, II A and B, IV, VI, and VII in cultured fibroblasts and in tissues. The experimental evidence strongly supports the concept that the mucopolysaccharidoses are a group of phenotypically related but genetically distinct disorders with a specific lysosomal enzyme being the basic defect in each disorder. It may be proposed that a clinical phenotype will eventually be described for each lysosomal enzyme involved in the degradation of cellular mucopolysaccharides.

TREATMENT. Since the recognition that the genetic mucopolysaccharidoses are lysosomal diseases, attempts have been made to accelerate the degradation of intracellular mucopolysaccharides accumulating due to deficiencies of lysosomal hydrolases and to perform enzyme replacement. Vitamin A increased lysosomal instability in cell cultures, reducing intracellular mucopolysaccharide storage, but it had no influence on the progressive development of the clinical phenotype. Plasma infusions were tried as replacement enzyme therapy with definite progression of mucopolysaccharide storage in spite of infusions. Transplantation has been discussed as a possible means of enzyme replacement, but it has not been technically feasible.

References

Bach G, Friedman R, Weissmann B, Neufeld EF: The defect in the Hurler and Scheie syndromes: deficiency of α-L-iduronidase. Proc Natl Acad Sci USA 69:2048, 1972

——Eisenberg F, Cantz M, Neufeld EF: The defect in the Hunter syndrome: deficiency of sulfoidurinate sulfatase. Proc Natl Acad Sci USA 70:2134, 1973

Bergsma D: Skeletal dysplasias. Birth Defects p. 10, 1974

Danes BS, Bearn AG: Hurler's syndrome: a genetic study in cell culture. J Exp Med 123:1, 1966

Fluharty AL, Stevens RL, Sanders DL, Kihara H: Arylsulfatase B deficiency in Maroteaux-Lamy syndrome cultured fibroblasts. Biochem Biophys Res Commun 59:455, 1974

Kresse H, Neufeld EF: The Sanfilippo A corrective factor. J Biol Chem 247:2164, 1972

Matalon R, Dorfman A: Hurler's syndrome. An α-L-iduronidase deficiency. Biochem Biophys Res Commun 47:959, 1972

—— Arbogast B Dorfman A: Morquio's syndrome: a deficiency of chondroitin sulfate N-acetylhexosamine sulfate sulfatase. Pediatr Res 8:436, 1974

McKusick VA: Heritable Disorders of Connective Tissue, 4th ed. St Louis, CV Mosby, 1972, p 521

—— Hussels IE, Howell RR, Neufeld EF, Stevenson RE: Allelism, non-allelism, and genetic compounds among the mucopolysaccharidoses. Lancet 1:993, 1972

O'Brien JS: Sanfilippo syndrome : profound deficiency of alpha-acetylglucosaminidase activity in organs and skin fibroblasts from type B patients. Proc Natl Acad Sci USA 69:1720, 1972

O'Brien JF, Cantz M, Spranger J: Maroteaux-Lamy disease (mucopolysaccharidosis VI), subtype A: deficiency of a N-acetylgalactosamine-4-sulfatase. Biochem Biophys Res Commun 60:1170, 1974

PORPHYRIAS
BARRY H. KAPLAN

The porphyrias are a group of diseases in which there is a disruption in the pathway of the synthesis of heme, so that precursors of heme accumulate or are excreted in amounts far in excess of normal.

Biosynthesis of Heme

Proteins that utilize heme as a prosthetic group include not only hemoglobin but also the cytochromes, catalase, myoglobin, and others. Therefore heme is needed for many metabolic processes common to all cells, and it is synthesized by every cell in the body, except for the mature erythrocyte. Quantitatively, the most important sites of heme formation are the bone marrow, in which it is utilized for hemoglobin synthesis, and the liver, in which hemoproteins are needed for drug metabolism. The same pathway for biosynthesis of heme is used by all cells; it is shown in Figure 18.

The first step in the pathway, the combination of glycine and succinyl coenzyme A (CoA) to form δ-aminolevulinic acid (ALA), is catalyzed by the enzyme ALA synthetase and requires pyridoxal phosphate as a cofactor. α-Amino-β-ketoadipic acid may be an intermediate in the reaction. Heme exerts feedback inhibition on ALA synthetase, and this step is the major rate-controlling reaction in heme biosynthesis. In bacteria, ALA synthetase is subject to repression of synthesis of new enzyme molecules by heme, and it seems likely that repression by heme occurs in animal cells as well.

The second step in heme biosynthesis, the condensation of two moles of ALA to form porphobilinogen (PBG), is catalyzed by ALA dehydrase. The enzyme requires a sulfhydryl reductant for activity and is therefore exquisitely sensitive to sulfhydryl inhibitors such as lead ions. The formation of the tetrapyrrole uroporphyrinogen from four moles of PBG is a complex reaction in which the intermediates appear to be enzyme-bound. Isomers of porphyrinogens are classified according to the location of the groups in the β positions of the pyrrole rings. Of the four possible isomers of uroporphyrinogen and coproporphyrinogen, only types I and III are synthesized in nature.

Two important enzymes are needed to convert PBG to uroporphyrinogen III: uroporphyrinogen I synthetase, also called PBG deaminase, and uroporphyrinogen III cosynthetase, also referred to as uroporphyrinogen isomerase. In the absence of the cosynthetase, only uroporphyrinogen I is formed, and this isomer cannot be used for heme synthesis. Uroporphyrinogen III is converted to coproporphyrinogen III by successive decarboxylation of four acetate groups, a reaction catalyzed by a single enzyme, uroporphyrinogen decarboxylase. Protoporphyrin IX, the only naturally occurring protoporphyrin of 15 possible isomers, is formed from coproporphyrinogen III by a reaction

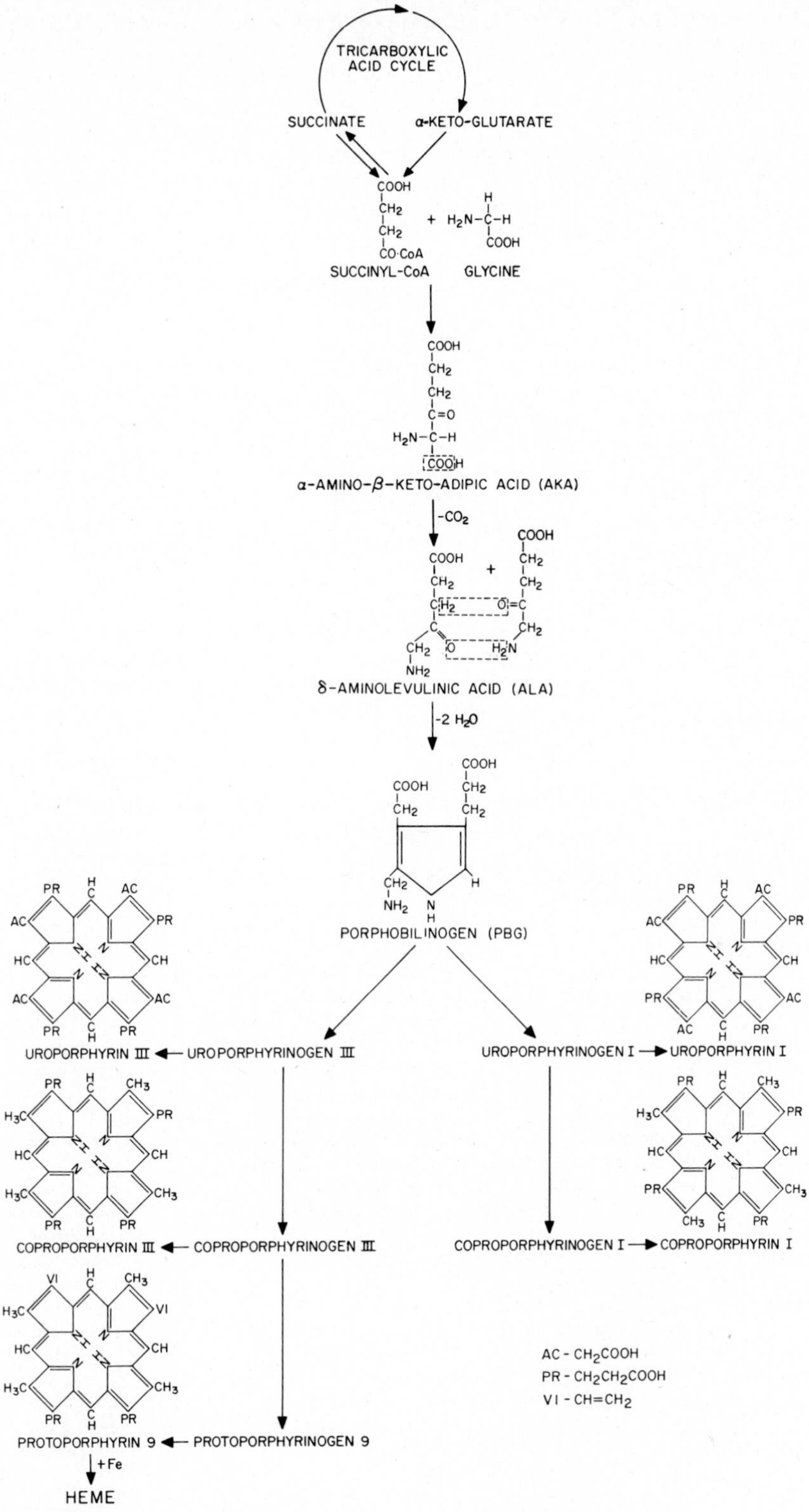

FIG. 18. Steps in biosynthesis of porphyrins.

requiring molecular oxygen. Finally, ferrochelatase (heme synthetase) catalyzes the synthesis of heme in the presence of ferrous iron and protoporphyrin IX.

The formation of ALA and the steps involving the conversion of coproporphyrinogen to heme occur within mitochondria; hence the enzymes involved in these reactions are particulate and have been very difficult to purify for study. Mature erythrocytes lack mitochondria and cannot synthesize heme, but enzymes for the steps from the formation of PBG to the synthesis of coproporphyrinogen are found in erythrocyte cytoplasm.

The tetrapyrrole precursors of protoporphyrin are in the form of porphyrinogens. The porphyrinogens contain methylene bridges between the pyrrole rings. These fully saturated bridges are readily oxidized in the tissues and excreta to methene bridges, a process that results in conversion of porphyrinogens to porphyrins. Porphyrinogens are colorless, but the methene bridges in porphyrins permit the formation of an extended conjugated ring system (ie, a sequence of alternating single and double bonds) that readily absorbs visible light. Porphyrins are therefore colored, and they typically have an intense absorption peak at about 400 nm called the Soret band. It is this property of porphyrins that results in the cutaneous manifestations of the porphyrias.

Normally, heme synthesis is so well regulated that only small amounts of the precursors are excreted. The early heme precursors, through uroporphyrinogen, are polar compounds excreted predominantly in the urine. Coproporphyrinogen is excreted both in the urine and through the bile into the feces; protoporphyrin, since it is largely nonpolar, is excreted almost entirely into the feces. Normal values for porphyrins and porphyrin precursors are given in Table 21.

Classification of Porphyrias

Historically, the porphyrias have been classified on the basis of the organ that seemed predominantly involved: hepatic or erythropoietic or both. However, genetic and biologic considerations make it clear that the enzymatic defects that result in these disorders are present in all tissues. Thus it seems more reasonable to classify the porphyrias in a manner that reflects the pathophysiology of the diseases. Those porphyrias associated with excretion of excessive amounts of porphyrin precursors (ie, ALA and PBG) are characterized by attacks of abdominal pain and neurologic disturbances. The disorders in which excessive amounts of porphyrins are present in the tissues or excreta typically have dermatologic manifestations. Therefore the porphyrias can be classified into a group that affects the early part

TABLE 21. Manifestations of Different Types of Porphyrias in Man

Form	Inheritance	Clinical Manifestations	Biochemical Findings
Acute intermittent porphyria (Swedish type)	Autosomal dominant with variable expression	Acute attacks of abdominal colic, hypertension, nervous system involvement, no photo sensitivity; usually after puberty	Increased urinary exretion of ALA and PBG during attacks and usually also during remission
Congenital erythropoietic porphyria	Autosomal recessive	Photosensitivity, severe dermatitis, hemolytic anemia, splenomegaly, erythrodontia; observed in early infancy and persistent through childhood and adult life	Increased amounts of uroporphyrin and coproporphyrin, mainly type I, in bone marrow, erythrocytes, plasma, urine and feces
Erythropoietic protoporphyria	Autosomal dominant with variable expression	Photosensitivity, mild dermatitis; usually first observed during childhood	Increased amounts of protoporphyrin in bone marrow, erythrocytes, plasma, and feces
Porphyria cutanea tarda		Photosensitivity and dermatitis; hepatic toxin required, especially alcohol	Increased excretion of urinary uroporphyrin; urinary coproporphyrin and protoporphyrin normal or slightly increased
Porphyria variegata (South African type)	Autosomal dominant with variable expression	Photosensitivity and dermatitis, acute attacks of abdominal and neurologic manifestations; usually after puberty	Increased amounts of coproporphyrin and protoporphyrin in feces during attacks and remission; and increased urinary excretion of ALA and PBG and porphyrins during acute attacks
Hepatic coproporphyria	Autosomal dominant with variable expression	Photosensitivity (rare), gastrointestinal, neurologic, and psychiatric manifestations similar to those in AIP; any age group	Increased amounts of coproporphyrin III in feces and urine; excessive urinary excretion of ALA and PBG during acute attacks

of the heme synthetic pathway, prior to the formation of uroporphyrinogen, a group that affects the later part of the pathway, and a group that affects both parts. The following is a list of the major kinds of porphyrias; the main clinical and biochemical features are summarized in Table 21.

Early pathway porphyria
    Acute intermittent porphyria

Late pathway porphyrias
    Congenital erythropoietic porphyria
    Erythropoietic protoporphyria
    Porphyria cutanea tarda

Mixed early and late pathway porphyrias
    Porphyria variegata
    Hepatic coproporphyria

Early Pathway Porphyria

ACUTE INTERMITTENT PORPHYRIA. Acute intermittent porphyria (AIP, Swedish type) is a not uncommon condition characterized chemically by the excretion of vastly increased amounts of PBG and ALA. Since only the early part of the heme synthetic pathway is affected, no dermatologic manifestations are present in these patients. The patients almost universally present with attacks of colicky abdominal pain, often associated with constipation, nausea, and vomiting. The pain in a typical attack persists for days to weeks and may result in surgical exploration, although leukocytosis and abdominal rigidity are usually absent. The majority of patients also have dark urine, particularly after the urine has been standing, and/or pain or paresthesias in the extremities. Tachycardia is a common sign, and many patients have hypertension during the acute attacks.

Neurologic findings include hallucinations, seizures, and cranial nerve weakness, but the hallmark of the disease is the development of flaccid paresis in one or more limbs. The paresis may progress to quadriplegia and respiratory paralysis in a small minority of patients, and death may result from pulmonary complications associated with ventilatory support. Hyponatremia (sometimes due to inappropriate release of antidiuretic hormone), hypercholesterolemia, and an elevated thyroid-binding globulin, are nonspecific laboratory abnormalities present in many of these patients.

During an acute attack the diagnosis of AIP can be established by performing a Watson-Schwartz test on the urine. This test, which is based on the reaction between PBG and *p*-dimethylaminobenzaldehyde (Ehrlich's reagent), can be made highly specific for PBG by appropriate extraction techniques. It is almost always positive during an acute attack and usually remains positive for months to years between attacks. When performed correctly, there are virtually no false positives.

Quantitative determination of urinary ALA and PBG reveals marked elevation up to 100 times the normal output. ALA and PBG levels tend to diminish between attacks, but they may remain elevated indefinitely. No other precursors of heme are found in significant excess. Some aspects of the pathogenesis of the disease have become clear. AIP is inherited as an autosomal dominant condition with variable penetrance. Patients with the mutant gene have about 50 percent of uroporphyrinogen I synthetase, as compared to their unaffected relatives. This deficit can be demonstrated in liver, circulating erythrocytes, cultured fibroblasts, and cells obtained by amniocentesis. The enzyme levels are low even in children or adults with no other biochemical or clinical manifestations of the disease. It has been estimated that more than 80 percent of the carriers of the mutant gene never manifest the disease.

As a compensatory mechanism for the partial block in heme synthesis, increased levels of ALA synthetase are present, so that adequate amounts of heme are made for hemoglobin and, under normal conditions, for hepatic drug-metabolizing enzymes. In situations in which the demand for heme exceeds the limited ability of these patients to supply heme, an acute attack may be precipitated.

The exact combination of factors resulting in an acute attack cannot always be identified. It is known that attacks are most common and most severe in women prior to menopause. Attacks are less common in men and are rare in children and postmenopausal women. There is a group of women whose attacks are related to events of their menstrual cycle. Furthermore, it has been shown that there is a marked reduction in steroid-5-α-reductase activity in patients with manifest AIP. It seems clear, therefore, that the hormonal milieu of the patient with the inherited enzymatic defect is important for expression of the disease.

There is a clear association between drug ingestion (particularly barbiturates, sulfonamides, and alcohol) and the acute attacks; decreased food intake is another factor that may induce attacks. The mechanism by which the abnormalities of heme synthesis produce the clinical syndrome of AIP remains to be elucidated. No specific morphologic changes have been identified, and it is not clear whether the symptoms are due to decreased production of heme or to a toxic effect of ALA and/or PBG.

Among the important aspects of the therapy of this disease is patient education in the avoidance of factors that precipitate attacks. Since the enzymatic defect can be detected even in childhood, close relatives of patients with AIP should be tested for the defect so that carriers can avoid these factors. Management of the acute attack includes supportive measures, especially treatment of hyponatremia; administration of large amounts of carbohydrates is also recommended. There is now strong evidence that heme, given intravenously as hematin, can reverse acute attacks; a prompt fall in ALA and PBG excretion associated with rapid clearing of symptoms has been noted in several patients treated with heme.

Late Pathway Porphyrias

CONGENITAL ERYTHROPOIETIC PORPHYRIA. The clinical manifestations of the rare congenital erythropoietic porphyria (CEP, Günther's disease), consisting of fewer than 100 reported patients, are the result of production of massive amounts of type I porphyrinogens. Dermatologic changes and hemolytic anemia are the cardinal features of this disorder. Typically, port-wine-colored urine appearing at birth or in early infancy is the first indication of disease. As the infant is exposed to light, a vesicular or bullous eruption develops in exposed areas. Secondary infection of these lesions results in scarring, mutilation, and loss of parts of digits. Red discolorations of the teeth resulting from deposition of porphyrins in bone and hypertrichosis are found in affected patients. Because of their grotesque appearance and avoidance of light, these patients may have been the basis of the werewolf legend. Most of the patients have a hemolytic anemia that occasionally can be severe and may require repeated transfusion. Splenomegaly is almost universal.

CEP is inherited as an autosomal recessive disorder. Biochemical studies indicate that the disease results from a marked decrease in uroporphyrinogen isomerase. Uroporphyrinogen I and coproporphyrinogen I are found in great excess in tissues and excreta. Fluorescence under ultraviolet light in the teeth, bones, bone marrow, urine, and fluid from bullae and vesicles is easily demonstrated. It seems likely that the absorption of light by porphyrins in the skin results in tissue damage by photochemical reactions. The hemolytic anemia is more difficult to explain because it cannot always be related to exposure to light. It is probable that shortened red cell survival results from damage directly inflicted on the erythrocyte by high levels of porphyrins.

Treatment for CEP includes protecting the patient as much as possible from light with wavelengths in the region of 400 nm by screening window light or using light bulbs that do not emit these wavelengths. The usual sunscreen creams for the skin are ineffective. There are a few reports of a favorable effect from administration of β-carotene in these patients. Splenectomy may be of some benefit in these patients. Transfusions of blood or even of hematin will depress the synthesis of porphyrins, but the long-term hazards of this kind of therapy must be kept in mind. It should be noted that hepatic dysfunction is not a feature of this disease, and there is no special drug sensitivity in these patients.

ERYTHROPOIETIC PROTOPORPHYRIA. Although erythropoietic protoporphyria (EPP) was recognized as a separate entity only in 1961, several hundred cases have been described since that time. Clinically it usually presents in infancy or childhood as one of the photosensitivity syndromes. The patients complain of intense pruritus, burning, or pain in exposed sites a few minutes to a few hours after exposure to light. Edema and erythema are typically present, but occasionally patients develop vesicles or a petechial rash. These symptoms and signs disappear within 12 to 48 hours after light exposure. Over a period of years the apparent severity of light sensitivity decreases. Chronic changes occur, including coarsening and lichenification of exposed areas of the skin.

Other manifestations of this disease include a very mild hypochromic anemia and a tendency to formation of gallstones containing large amounts of porphyrins. Recently it has become apparent that these patients have a high risk of developing cirrhosis; several have died from hepatic failure. Liver damage may be due to crystallized porphyrins, which have been demonstrated within the liver parenchyma, or to the effects of deranged heme biosynthesis.

The biochemical hallmark of this disease is a markedly elevated erythrocyte protoporphyrin content (5 to 100 times normal in symptomatic cases). Erythrocyte coproporphyrin III also may be mildly elevated. Plasma and fecal protoporphyrin levels are also variably elevated. The photosensitivity reaction results from light at 400-nm wavelength, and from pathologic studies it appears that the interaction of light and porphyrins occurs at or around the vasculature of the skin.

EPP is inherited as an autosomal dominant disorder with incomplete penetrance. Asymptomatic carriers of the mutant gene have abnormal protoporphyrin levels in erythrocytes and/or feces. Heme synthetase, the final enzyme of the heme synthetic pathway, is markedly depressed in liver, fibroblasts, bone marrow, and erythrocytes. No compensatory increase in ALA synthetase is found; presumably in these patients adequate amounts of heme can be made without detectable induction of this enzyme.

A new form of therapy has been developed for photosensitivity in these cases. When large amounts of β-carotene are given orally to these patients over a period of months, there usually is a striking improvement in tolerance to light. These changes have been confirmed by objective tests of the reaction of the skin to irradiation. β-carotene does not appear to act as a sunscreen; rather, it apparently quenches the photochemical reactions by interacting with energized protoporphyrin molecules. No side effects of this therapy have been observed. Hypervitaminosis A is not a problem. Attempts to use β-carotene in other dermatologic forms of porphyria have been unsuccessful, except for a few isolated reports in congenital erythropoietic porphyria.

PORPHYRIA CUTANEA TARDA. Porphyria cutanea tarda (PCT) encompasses a heterogeneous set of patients grouped together because of similar clinical features. They show a marked sensitivity of the exposed areas of the skin to minor trauma. Vesicles, ulcers, hyperpigmentation, and pseudosclerodermatous changes are frequently seen. Hypertrichosis, particularly over the forehead and preauricular areas, also is frequently noted. The patients excrete in the urine from 20 to 300 times the normal amount of uroporphyrin. Coproporphyrin excretion in the urine and feces may also be increased, but not by this order of magnitude. The characteristics of this disease differ from those in all of the other forms of porphyria. There is no obvious genetic basis for this disorder. Typically, it develops in middle-aged individuals. Only 6 cases have been described in children; liver disease and/or prolonged iron therapy were factors operative in these patients.

Most frequently the disease is found in male alcoholics, but its occurrence has been noted following administration of estrogens and birth control pills. Almost 25 percent of the patients have diabetes, and an association between systemic lupus erythematosus and PCT has been noted in a small group of patients. In 1 patient a hepatoma seemed to produce the uroporphyrin responsible for her disease; several other patients with liver metastases have developed the disorder. An epidemic of PCT developed in Turkey in 1956. It was eventually ascribed to the ingestion of hexachlorobenzene used as a fungicidal agent in wheat.

The mechanism by which these different etiologies result in PCT is assumed to be a toxic effect on liver metabolism. Deranged hepatic function in the form of BSP retention is almost universally present, and other liver function tests are also frequently abnormal. Striking red fluorescence and increased deposition of iron can be demonstrated in liver biopsy specimens. Although a hepatic toxin appears to be required and may be sufficient for development of the disease, a genetic predisposition may be present in many of these patients. Hepatic ALA synthetase has been shown to be normal, but recent data suggest these patients may have a deficiency in the conversion of uroporphyrinogen to coproporphyrinogen.

Treatment of these patients should be undertaken cautiously, since PCT is often an incidental finding and the disease itself is not life-threatening. When possible, ingestion of the toxic substance (ie, alcohol, estrogens, etc) should be discontinued. This action alone will eliminate the disease in a matter of months. Equally effective are repeated phlebotomies; this technique depletes the liver of the excessive iron stores that seem to be important in the development of PCT.

Other forms of therapy include alkalinization of the urine and administration of the ion-exchange resin cholestyramine. Both of these techniques increase porphyrin excretion. The antimalarial agent chloroquine forms a complex with uroporphyrin in the liver, and the complex is rapidly excreted. Enormous amounts of uroporphyrin are eliminated after a single treatment with chloroquine, and patients have a good remission of PCT; but the treatment is hazardous and therefore is not warranted in most of these cases.

Mixed Early and Late Porphyrias

PORPHYRIA VARIEGATA. In porphyria variegata (PV, South African type) abnormal excretion of both porphyrins and porphyrin precursors is observed; hence cutaneous lesions and abdominal and neurologic manifestations may be present. The cutaneous lesions closely resemble those described for PCT, and the abdominal and neurologic manifestations are indistinguishable from those of AIP, including the association of barbiturates and other drugs with acute attacks.

The disease is inherited as an autosomal dominant disorder with variable penetrance; it usually becomes manifest later in life than AIP. It is an uncommon disorder with worldwide distribution. The high incidence in South Africans can be traced to the descendants of an Afrikaner couple who were married at the Cape of Good Hope in 1688.

Patients who manifest PV have markedly increased fecal excretion of protoporphyrin, coproporphyrin, and porphyrin–peptide conjugates. The increase in fecal porphyrins is a constant feature and can be demonstrated even in children before the onset of dermatologic manifestations. About half the patients never experience attacks of abdominal or neurologic symptoms. In those who do, urinary excretions of ALA and PBG rise dramatically during the attacks and return toward normal between attacks.

The basic enzymatic defect remains to be elucidated. Hepatic ALA synthetase is markedly increased in these patients, but the other enzymes of heme biosynthesis, including heme synthetase, appear to be normal. It seems very likely that a deficiency in an enzyme closely related to protoporphyrin, possibly the one that converts protoporphyrinogen to protoporphyrin, causes this disorder. Therapy is limited to avoidance of factors known to induce acute attacks. Hematin may be tried in an effort to ameliorate severe symptoms.

HEPATIC COPROPORPHYRIA. Hepatic coproporphyria (HC) is a rare disease similar in most respects to AIP in its manifestations. Dermatologic symptoms have been reported, but they are uncommon. It is inherited as an autosomal dominant disorder and is characterized by excretion of a great excess of coproporphyrinogen III in the feces and sometimes in the urine. Protoporphyrin excretion may be mildly elevated. During acute attacks, urinary ALA and PBG levels approach those seen in AIP. The liver exhibits red fluorescence, and hepatic ALA synthetase levels are elevated. It is probable that the genetic lesion in HC is a deficiency of the enzyme that converts coproporphyrinogen to protoporphyrin. Treatment is similar to that used for AIP.

There are several known and suspected genetic defects in the porphyrias. None of the enzyme deficiencies is complete; a complete absence of one of these enzymes in such a vital pathway would probably be inconsistent with life. Several of the suspected defects remain to be verified, and many details of the enzymatic pathway and the interaction of genetic defects and environmental factors need to be clarified. Nevertheless, major advances in our understanding of the etiology and treatment of these disorders have taken place during the past few years, and they are reflected in more rational management of these patients.

References

Marver HS, Schmid R: The Porphyrias. In Stanbury JB, Wyngaarden JB, Fredrickson DS (eds): The Metabolic Basis of Inherited Disease, 3rd ed. New York, McGraw-Hill, 1972, 1087

Stein JA, Tschudy DP: Acute intermittent porphyria. Medicine 49:1, 1970

Schmidt H, Snitker G, Thomsen K, Lintrup J: Erythropoietic protoporphyria. Arch Dermatol 110:58, 1974

Ramsay CA, Magnus IA, Turnbull A, Baker H: The treatment of porphyria cutanea tarda by venesection. Q J Med 43:1, 1974

CHAPTER 15

Pediatric Ecology: Accidents, Poisonings, and other Environmental Hazards

Arnold H. Einhorn, *Associate Editor*

ENVIRONMENTAL HAZARDS

Arnold H. Einhorn

INTRODUCTION

Individual variations in the physical, physiologic, and behavioral characteristics of children are governed not only by genetic determinants but also by a myriad of environmental factors and influences. Environmental stimuli from surroundings that change more rapidly than ever constantly challenge the child's adjustment, both qualitatively and quantitatively, and exert major effects upon health status.

PEDIATRIC ECOLOGY

Ecology, which derives from the Greek *oikos,* meaning *home* or *house,* is defined as the relation of plants and animals to their environment and to one another. A dynamic concept of medical ecology has been formulated by May, who views disease not merely as the impairment of health but as the convergence within the host of environmental stimuli (organic, inorganic, or sociocultural). Bodily reactions actuated by these stimuli result either in ecologic *adaptation* (survival) or in *maladjustment* (illness and/or death). Disease becomes "that alteration of the living tissue that jeopardizes survival in the environment."

"Health," as defined by the World Health Organization, "is a state of complete physical, mental, and social well-being and not merely the absence of disease." In a broader ecologic context the health status of a child is a matter of individual physiologic and psychosocial adaptation or maladjustment to his environment. The achievement, maintenance, and restoration, if required, of optimal physical, intellectual, and emotional growth and development are the objectives laid down for the provision of child health care.

The pediatrician's role, as the child's primary physician, is to ensure for the child, on a continuing basis, the best possible adaptation, and to anticipate, prevent, and correct all factors apt to disrupt the complex interactions between the child's internal biologic systems and the total external environmental system. Rational pediatric practice requires thorough knowledge and judicious application of clinical ecology, thus identifying the "compleat pediatrician" of the present and of the future as the ecologist of the family unit.

THE CHILD'S ENVIRONMENT

The child's environment encompasses all substances, forms of life, forces, conditions, and influences under which he lives and to which he must adapt. Good health

TABLE 1. Environment

I. NATURAL ENVIRONMENT

A. Physical and Chemical Constituents

Air and other gases
Water and other liquids
Fire
Temperature, humidity, atmospheric pressure
Light, infra-red, UV, electromagnetic energies;
Vibration
Radiation
Solid elements and compounds: organic
                                                      inorganic

B. Living Organisms

Microorganisms
Macroorganisms, including man

C. Geography (direct relationship with A. and B.)

Climate, altitude
Temperature
Humidity
Luminosity
Flora and fauna

II. MAN-MADE ENVIRONMENT

A. "Altered" Natural Environment

e.g., buildings, transportation, food processing, etc.

B. "Situational" Environment

Family (or household unit)
Community, country, and/or ethnic group
Psychosocial environment
Socioeconomic environment
Nutritional environment
Educational environment
Recreational environment
Religion
Health care

ensues if the adaptation to the environment is satisfactory, and ill health when it is too stressful. The environment should not be considered in physical terms only; equally important for the child's individuality and his overall health are cultural, social, and psychologic factors.

Man's surroundings (Table 1) comprise a *natural environment* and a *man-made environment*. The latter includes finite products of varying size, consistency, and mobility; in addition, there are situations, circumstances, conditions, and resources that result from human groupings, associations, interactions, and activities, and which we have termed *situational environment*. (Table 1) Certain environmental conditions, such as air, water, food, and shelter, are essential requirements for survival. Others merely affect body functions, performance, and comfort without being fundamentally indispensable for the sustenance of life. Still others constitute, become, or are made into ecologic hazards.

ENVIRONMENTAL HAZARDS

Environmental hazards may be biologic (infections, parasitism, zoonoses); chemical (toxins, poisons, irritants, drugs, air and water pollutants); physical (ionizing radiations, vibrations, mechanical injury, noise, humidity, fire, heat); sociologic (poverty, overcrowding, social isolation, lawlessness); and psychologic (emotional stress, anxiety, insecurity, guilt, boredom, rebellion). The specific effects of the environment upon the individual child may depend entirely on the nature, size, or amount of environmental stimuli, as in poisoning. However, a quantitative assessment of the hazard is often difficult. The consequences of environmental influences upon each individual also depend on genetic factors and may vary considerably when genetic aberrations exist.

Effects of microorganisms in the environment are discussed in Chapter 12 and psychosocial factors are discussed in Chapter 3. Ecologic hazards of a physical, chemical, or unknown nature, as well as those associated with deliberate adult injury, are considered in this chapter.

Bibliography

ENVIRONMENTAL HAZARDS

Apley J: An ecology of childhood. Lancet 2:1, 1964

Carson R: Silent Spring. Houghton Mifflin Company, Boston 1962

Einhorn AH: The Child and His Environment, Pediatric Practice and Ecology. In Ecology and Pediatrics, Postgraduate Seminars, Vol 38. Karger-Verlag AG, Basel, London, New York, 1974, pp 1-5

Hanlon JJ: Principles of Public Health Administration, 5th edition. CV Mosby Co, St Louis, 1969

May JM: The Ecology of Human Disease. MD Publications Inc, New York, 1958

Purdon WP: Environmental Health. Academic Press, Inc, New York, 1971

ACCIDENTS IN CHILDHOOD
ARNOLD H. EINHORN

EPIDEMIOLOGY, INCIDENCE, ETIOLOGY

Advances in medicine and public health have resulted in a significant decline in childhood deaths in the past 40 years. However, deaths from accidents did not decrease to the same degree. Half of the deaths of children in the United States occur as a result of injuries, as compared with approximately 1 death in 10 in the general population. In 1974, in the United States, accidents disabled 11,000,000 persons and claimed approximately 105,000 lives. More than 14,000 accidental deaths occurred in children under 15 years of age, the total number exceeding that of the combined fatalities from five leading diseases: pneumonia, meningitides, congenital malformations, major cardiovascular disease, and cancer. Mortality statistics, however, only partly reflect the magnitude of the problem, for they do not take into account the heavy annual toll of over 100,000 permanently disfigured and crippled children. Although comparatively few case studies of accidental morbidity are recorded, it is estimated that nonfatal injuries outnumber lethal accidents by a ratio greater than 200 to 1. Accidents result in the loss of nearly 10 million school days in children between the ages of 6 through 16, or 23 days per 100 children per year.

The majority of injuries in children of all age groups are sustained in the home area. However, motor vehicle accidents rank first among those that are fatal, from birth to 14 years of age. Contrary to popular belief, more small children are killed and injured *inside* the vehicle than outside. Suffocation from accidental aspiration of objects or foods into the respiratory passages, smothering by bedclothes or plastic materials, and mechanical strangulation are the most frequent types of fatal home accidents in the first year of life. Deaths due to fire, burns, and explosion of combustibles range first among children 1 through 4 years old, and second among infants less than 1 year of age. The predominance of such causes relates to the fact that preschool children are apt to pull objects off stoves or play with matches if left unsupervised where dangerous heating or other hazardous equipment is accessible. Falls from heights (unprotected windows, fire escapes) constitute a major health hazard mainly for preschool boys in highly deteriorated slum dwellings, while older children tend to fall from dangerous play areas of lesser heights.

Accidents occur more frequently in boys than girls, and the injury rates are highest in the summer and lowest in the winter. Low-income groups appear to be at a higher risk. In children 1 through 4 years of age, causes of accidental deaths are the same for both boys and girls; beyond the age of 4 years, they are different in the two sexes. For children 5 through 14 years of age, drowning ranks first for boys and fourth for girls; motor vehicle traffic accidents to pedestrians is the leading cause of death in girls in this age group and the second ranking cause for boys. Four times as many accidental deaths occur among teen-age boys as among girls of the same age.

ECOLOGY OF ACCIDENTS

The variables elicited in the occurrence of most accidents are multiple and complex, involving an interplay of host, etiologic agent, and environment. The child's inexperience in the face of an unsafe environment probably constitutes the major determinant. The pattern of behavior of a particular child, his attitude, his personal traits, and his adjustment to noxious situations all play important roles.

Developmental sequences through which children progress from infancy to maturity determine in part the types of accidents that are more apt to occur at specific ages. A small infant may roll over, or propel himself enough to fall from an open crib, a bed, or any unprotected elevated surface. At the age when the infant crawls or toddles, he has a natural tendency to put objects in his mouth, and the ingestion of poisonous substances or other dangerous objects or foreign bodies becomes a hazard from 6 months through early childhood. With the acquisition of further mobility, the ability and urge to climb, the instinct to explore, to pull, and to grasp at objects, the accidents that take the most prominent place are falls, burns, scalds, electric shocks, and injuries from toppling furniture or colliding with heavy objects. Interest in moving and whirling objects is active long before caution has developed from painful experience. At a later age, the intense absorption of young children in play makes them reckless in street traffic, at water's edge, and in other dangerous settings. Throughout his growing years the child is in contact with an increasing variety of appliances, tools, or other objects that he may explore or use without proper supervision or guidance. This applies not merely to firearms, knives, and other sharp instruments, but also to matches, lamps, electrical equipment, kitchen utensils, tools, engines, and farm implements. As his social awareness grows, particularly in the school years, the child's temptation to accept a challenge becomes greater. He may try to demonstrate maturity by assuming prerogatives ordinarily reserved for adults.

Accident proneness or repeatism remains a subject of controversy. While virtually all accidents that occur in children could have been prevented, it is nonetheless reasonable to regard all children as inherently susceptible to accidents. Studies indicate that the child who frequently is involved in accidents is overactive, restless, and impulsive, and has less feeling of security at home. Children in the nonaccident group have been said to be quiet, more timid, submissive, studious, and to come from more closely united family groups. It has been stated also that parents of repeaters were frequently involved in accidents.

PREVENTION OF ACCIDENTS

Accidents are amenable to control, and the responsibilities of physicians and health agencies lie in the area of prevention. The same basic epidemiologic principles used to control communicable diseases can apply here and host, agent, and environment must be considered. It may not be possible to change the host readily, but the host can be safeguarded from hazards while both agent and environment are manipulated and made safer. Some examples are seat belts, safety glass for doors, noninflammable material, safe toys, safe play areas, and supervised recreation.

Accident prevention requires protection, education, and legislation. Children must be shielded from hazards when they are too young to be taught how to cope with them. Description or even enumeration of all possible measures of protection is beyond the scope of this book; however, a few important principles are worth mentioning. The infant must not be left where he can fall or roll over; he must not wear clothes that may choke him; he must have no access to places where he can drown, smother, scald, or burn himself; and he should not be given objects or toys with sharp edges or with detachable parts or tabs that could be pulled off and swallowed or aspirated. Even before the crawling stage, staircases should be guarded with proper gates and railings, low tables should be cleared of glass, pottery, and lamps, and the corners of tablecloths brought up out of reach. In the kitchen particular attention must be devoted to keeping the toddler at a safe distance from the stove and keeping handles of hot pots on the stove out of reach. Small children should not be permitted to touch matches or table lighters. Accessible electric outlets should be shielded by plastic plugs. Toys or household objects may be responsible for serious accidents when they happen to come under foot; the classic example is the roller skate left on a stair.

The exploring toddler, with his unsteady gait, must be protected from falling or from grasping dangerous objects. As the child gets older and begins to accept responsibility, dependence on protection is lessened while greater emphasis is placed on educational experience and graduated exposure. However, an irreducible segment of accident risk will remain. The development of legislation incorporating effective control measures and protection in the manufacturing of toys, clothing, furniture, paints, to name only a few, is an essential part of any accident prevention program.

The extent to which shielding and education are to be employed is a matter of judgment in which the characteristics of individual children and parents must be considered. Overprotection may be harmful; the child who is too rigidly kept off the street may, upon escaping excessive supervision, become more susceptible to unfamiliar traffic hazards. Fear of injury should not interfere with gradual exposure to the normal environment. The pediatric practitioner may have the opportunity to judge whether overexposure or overprotection from hazards exists. His advice may be helpful regarding the appropriate age to allow a child certain privileges or the use of potentially hazardous tools, instruments, or even toys, such as air rifles.

Parents can profit even more from education. While much can be accomplished through the media of communication, such as the press, radio, and television, direct parental instruction by the physician is of prime importance. This should begin at the earliest possible time and be reinforced with repetition and even demonstration at later stages.

Accident prevention should be an integral part of well-child supervision. Families could be *immunized* against accidents through safety education together with other well-baby procedures. The pediatrician's knowledge of the child's developmental level and of the household should enable him to provide anticipatory guidance with regard to the type of accidents most likely to occur at specific stages of the child's development and in a given family. During home visits, the physician should notice hazardous and unsafe conditions in the home and advise the family about corrective measures.

In addition every professional organization concerned with health and education, and every government agency involved in any aspect of public health and welfare, must be called upon to play a dominant role in safety education programs. Education of the public by professional educators, physicians, and individuals in allied health disciplines must be intensive and continuous and should permeate every phase and activity of daily living. Finally, medical organizations can be actively instrumental in introducing appropriate legislation.

Bibliography

ACCIDENTS

Committee on Accident Prevention, American Academy of Pediatrics. Accidents in Children, American Academy of Pediatrics, Chicago, 1969

Dickson DG, Schlesinger ER, Westaby Jr, et al : Medically attended injuries among young children. Am J Dis Child 107:618, 1964

Grosfeld JL (ed): Symposium on Childhood Trauma. Pediatr Clin North Am 22:2, 1975

Haddon W Jr, Suchman EA, Klein D: Accident Research Methods and Approaches. Harper and Row, New York, 1964

Haller JA Jr: Newer concepts in emergency care of children with major injuries. Pediatrics 52:485, 1973

Matheny AP Jr, et al: Assessment of children's behavioral characteristics. Clin Pediatr 11:437, 1972

Mathewson C Jr: Early management of trauma patient. Priority of care. Surg Clin North Am 52:531, 1972

Meyer RJ: Childhood injuries: approaches and perspectives. Pediatrics 44:865, 1969

National Center for Health Statistics, US Department of Health, Education, and Welfare. Final Statistics, 1974. US Public Health Service, Vol 24 (Suppl) February, 1976

National Safety Council, National Health Survey. Accidental Deaths and Injuries in 1974. In Accident Facts, National Safety Council. Chicago, 1975

Shelness A, Charles S: Children as passengers in automobiles: the neglected minority on the nation's highways. Pediatrics 56:271, 1975

Sieben RL, Leavitt RL, French JH: Falls as childhood accidents: an increasing urban risk. Pediatrics 47:886, 1971

Southard SC: The practicing pediatrician's role in accident prevention. Pediatr Ann 2:32, 1973

DROWNING
ARNOLD H. EINHORN

INCIDENCE, EPIDEMIOLOGY, ETIOLOGY

Drowning accidents constitute a major threat to young children. Excluding deaths in floods and cataclysms, mortality by submersion ranks third among the causes of accidental deaths in children 1 to 15 years of age. In 1973 and 1974, there were more than 8,000 annual fatal drownings in the United States, and 1,000 to 1,500 deaths each year from drowning in Great Britain; of these about one-third occurred in children under 15 years of age.

Boys are distinctly more prone to such accidents than girls. This preponderance in males is more evident in older children; from 5 to 14 years of age, 75 percent of the victims are boys; below the age of 5 years the ratio is 2 to 1. Both fatal drowning and near-drowning accidents have a year-round distribution. However, a seasonal peak is evident during the summer months, even in states where water activities responsible for the majority of drowning accidents, such as boating, fishing, swimming, water skiing, skin diving, and scuba diving, are possible throughout the year.

Younger children more commonly drown while left unattended in bathtubs or after a fall through the ice, than while swimming. They are also found submerged in unprotected backyard ponds or swimming pools; they may stray away unnoticed while adults are engrossed in lively conversations, or engaged in other activities. The vast majority of older children drown while swimming or while participating in other recreational water sports, especially boating, without having the proper experience and supervision; many drownings involve occupants of small boats. Contributory or precipitating causes include rough water conditions, cold exposure, overexertion, injuries, physical debility, heavy clothing, handicaps, intoxicants or drugs, and epilepsy. Among older children and adolescents who may be good swimmers deliberate hyperventilation before diving, for the purpose of lengthening the breathholding time underwater is a very dangerous practice. In such cases reduced arterial carbon dioxide tension produces peripheral and cerebral constriction and paresthesias, followed by a reduction of arterial oxygen tension, causing cerebral ischemia and hypoxemia and sudden loss of consciousness under water. Older children who drown in bathtubs usually have either epilepsy or other neurologic deficit or physical handicap. Drug abuse with mind-altering agents may be associated with home drownings in older children.

Private swimming pools rank high among the potential environmental hazards associated with an increasing number of childhood drownings. Community or quasipublic swimming pools, which are more likely to employ lifeguards and attendants and were once preponderant, are in the process of being outranked by the proliferation of private residential pools, often unsupervised and unprotected.

PATHOPHYSIOLOGY

In the vast majority of fatal drownings, death is caused by asphyxia with fluid aspiration (classic *wet drowning*). The succession of morbid events, which culminate in cardiorespiratory arrest and death, take place within a few minutes after immersion, and in general progress most rapidly in freshwater drowning. Schematically, the inhalation of even small amounts of fluid produces reflex closure of the glottis. If severe and prolonged, this laryngospasm is followed by movements of deglutition and frequently by vomiting. The ensuing asphyxia, if persistent and sufficiently pronounced, causes the glottis to relax, resulting in secondary flooding of the lungs with water and often also with gastric contents. Cardiac arrest may supervene very rapidly before, during, or after a terminal phase of apnea. However, in about 10 percent or less of immersion deaths, the glottis remains closed after the initial reflex laryngospasm, resulting in obstructive death, without aspiration, or *dry drowning.*

In animal models, depending upon whether the aspirated fluid is freshwater, or seawater, the consequent shifts in blood volume and the biochemical changes in extracellular fluid are quite different. In *experimental freshwater drowning* the aspirated hypotonic water rapidly moves from the lungs into the bloodstream and produces hemodilution, hypervolemia, hemolysis, hyponatremia, and ventricular fibrillation. In *experimental seawater drowning,* water drains from the plasma into the lungs filled with hypertonic seawater thereby considerably increasing the pulmonary edema and concomitantly causing hemo-concentration, hypervolemia, and a fall in blood pressure. Passage of seawater solute into the blood further increases hyperosmolarity and hypernatremia of serum.

In *human near-drowning victims* who survive either spontaneously or after resuscitation, the composition of the fluid in which the submersion occurred is far less important as regards effects and therapeutic implications than has been emphasized in the past. In human survivors, while certain differences exist between seawater and freshwater drowning, the main sequelae are virtually identical. Irrespective of whether the submersion occurred in fresh, in chlorinated, or in salt water, the central problem is acute asphyxia with hypoxemia and severe metabolic acidemia. The looming danger is *secondary drowning* or death from respiratory and circulatory failure, which may kill the victim as early as several minutes after resuscitation or as late as several days after the accident. In general death in freshwater is more rapid during the submersion before the victim can be rescued. In seawater victims on the other hand, secondary drowning is twice more lethal than with freshwater. Furthermore, pulmonary edema, which is a feature of both, tends to be intensified more dramatically after salt water aspiration, as intravascular water moves into the alveoli under the influence of the osmotic gradient. Consequently ventilation-perfusion disturbances may persist longer after seawater aspiration.

The major effects of any type of accidental drowning are on the lungs and circulation and relate to the arterial hypoxemia and metabolic acidemia. The aspirated fluid irritates the interalveolar septa and creates an inflammatory alveolitis and capillary congestion. The protein-rich exudate filling the alveoli interferes with oxygen diffusion, causes ventilation-perfusion disturbances, and is responsible for a considerable alveolar arterial oxygen gradient (Chap 28.). Lung compliance is greatly reduced not only by intraalveolar, frequently hemorrhagic, edema fluid, but also by significant interstitial pulmonary edema. Increasing hypoxemia leads to severe metabolic acidemia, which when severe reduces myocardial contractility and cardiac output. Bronchospasm and constriction of terminal airways secondary to irritation by the inhaled liquid and the presence of pink frothy sputum in the air passages may result in combined respiratory and metabolic acidemia and aggravate the asphyxia. In freshwater drowning, removal of pulmonary surfactant from the alveolar lining may increase alveolar surface tension and thus contribute to the stiffness of the lungs.

Electrolyte disturbances, hemolysis, and changes in blood volume and concentration, all related to the composition of aspirated fluid, are generally mild to moderate, if present at all; such disturbances rapidly improve after the respiratory and circulatory disturbances improve with ventilation, oxygenation, and correction of acidemia. In man ventricular fibrillation has not been demonstrated in freshwater victims but has rarely been reported in salt water immersions.

CLINICAL AND LABORATORY FEATURES

Symptoms and physical findings in survivors of near-drowning accidents vary. The victim may be in no difficulty whatsoever, have mild to severe respiratory distress, or be totally apneic.

Temperature elevations are frequent in symptomatic patients, sometimes reaching levels as high as 42 C and may be associated with significant polymorphonuclear leukocytosis. Neurologic symptoms are common, consisting of headaches, lethargy or agitation, disorientation, trismus, and sometimes convulsions or coma.

In patients with respiratory distress, symptoms may range from rapid shallow breathing to frank inadequacy of respiratory effort. The patient often is cyanotic, complains of chest pain, grunts, presents a hacking cough, and expectorates pink frothy sputum. Typical findings of pulmonary edema may be elicited, namely rales, rhonchi, and basal dullness. Cardiovascular manifestations include tachycardia, gallop rhythm or premature ventricular contractions, and hypo- or hypertension.

Measurements of arterial blood gases and pH are the most important laboratory determinations. Arterial Po_2 reduction and metabolic or combined metabolic and respiratory acidemia are the major disturbances. Hemoconcentration or hemodilution, hemolysis, and corresponding electrolyte changes usually subside with improvement of the blood gases and correction of pH. Drowning hemoglobinemia, hemoglobinuria and oliguria, transient azotemia, and proteinemia may develop after freshwater near-drownings. Return to normal renal function, following several days of hyposthenuric diuresis, is the usual course.

RADIOGRAPHY. Radiographic pulmonary findings may range from a few scattered patchy or fluffy parenchymal infiltrates to that of a picture indistinguishable from acute pulmonary edema. The most frequent radiographic appearance is that of diffuse and bilateral alveolar infiltrates usually concentrated in the perihilar and medial basal areas. In patients who are mildly to moderately ill, these perihilar infiltrates are partially confluent and may be symmetric or may change with the patient's position. In lungs *drowned by fluid* the opacity generally is homogeneous throughout both pulmonary fields, with few or no areas of relative sparing and with prominent air bronchograms. Such changes are considered radiographic expressions of hypoxic lung injury with possible contribution by gastric acid aspiration pneumonitis. In the least serious cases, on the other hand, there is a lack of any demonstrable radiographic abnormality, which does not necessarily exclude significant pulmonary pathology. However, as a rule if there are few radiographic abnormalities, there are also fewer clinical problems. Positive radiographic lung findings usually clear within 3 to 5 days. If infiltrates persist for one week or more, or increase, a superimposed bacterial pneumonia must be suspected. Once resolution of radiographic findings begins, it proceeds rapidly from the periphery toward the hilum, with complete disappearance in as little as 12 to 24 hours.

CLINICAL COURSE. The course of events after accidental submersion is highly variable. In general, both in seawater and freshwater drownings, the prognosis appears related to the degree and reversibility of pulmonary edema and cardiac failure and hypoxic central nervous system damage. Some factors may contribute to a poor prognosis, such as a large volume of aspirated fluid, a high degree of contamination of the water, and immersion in very cold water. The imminence of secondary drowning may be heralded by the recurrence of coma; the aggravation, despite ventilatory support and bicarbonate therapy, of pulmonary edema, hypoxemia, and acidemia; and the sudden collapse of central venous pressure. The development of hypercarbia is also an ominous indication of impending decompensation. Prompt and effective resuscitation may, however, dramatically reverse any unfavorable situation even in desperately ill patients. Sustained ventilatory and circulatory support are the two most important factors affecting the outcome in preventing the dreaded, often lethal, secondary drowning.

TREATMENT

Although the state of the victim may be unrelated to the apparent duration of submersion, speed is of the utmost importance in management. Central nervous system damage may become irreversible within three to seven minutes after the beginning of immersion and within less than one minute after cardiocirculatory arrest. Hypoxia, metabolic acidemia, and secondary circulatory failure are the immediate and major problems in near-drowning. The key to survival lies in the prompt establishment and maintenance of a reasonable arterial Po$_2$ and normal pH. The major difficulty in correcting hypoxemia consists in overcoming the reduced compliance of the stiffened water-laden lungs and the constriction of terminal airways.

Emergency Respiratory and Cardiocirculatory Resuscitation (Basic Life Support)

When reached, the drowning victim may be in no visible difficulty, in obvious respiratory distress, or totally apneic. If the patient is not breathing spontaneously, artificial inflation of the lungs should be started immediately, even while the victim is still in the water. After securing a reasonable airway by rapidly cleaning the oropharynx, the mouth to mouth technique should be used as soon as it is possible to stand in shallow water, in a boat, or on a surfboard, or the victim's head can be supported on some floating device. Time should not be wasted in fruitless attempts at external cardiac massage, impossible or ineffective, while the patient is in the water. Postural drainage is also of no value unless combined with adequate airway suction and assisted ventilation with positive end-expiratory pressure (PEEP).

After the victim is removed from the water and during transportation to the hospital, ventilatory assistance is continued, either by the mouth-to-mouth method or, if available, by manually operating a ventilating bag, preferably with oxygen supplementation.

Nasopharyngeal suction should be performed as soon as possible. If the carotid pulse cannot be felt, closed-chest cardiac massage must be performed concurrent with artificial ventilation as soon as the patient can be placed on a firm surface, in a horizontal position, and, if possible, with elevation of the lower extremities to increase venous return. External cardiac massage should be continued until a palpable spontaneous pulse returns and persists. Restoration of circulation may require concomitant intracardiac injection of epinephrine or isoprotenerol; cardiac or intravenous sodium bicarbonate administration; intravenous injection of calcium chloride and hypertonic glucose; rapid intravenous infusion of plasma expanders; and, if indicated and available, external electrical defibrillation (see p. 1499).

Advanced Cardiocirculatory Life Support

The drowning victim should be removed as promptly as possible to an intensive care facility, with advanced life support capabilities, staffed and equipped to provide the required respiratory mechanical assistance, cardiocirculatory support, clinical observation, and appropriate laboratory monitoring. Control or assistance of intermittent positive pressure ventilation (IPPV), preferably using a volume cycled device, is best combined with maintenance of positive end-expiratory pressure (PEEP) in order to prevent alveolar collapse during expiration. Frequent suctioning of the oropharynx is essential to maintain airway patency.

Orotracheal or nasotracheal intubation facilitates prolonged positive pressure breathing and removal of secretion. Placement of an endotracheal tube is mandatory not only in the comatose and apneic patient but also in the conscious patient if there is obvious respiratory distress and inadequate spontaneous ventilatory efforts and whenever positive pressure breathing by mask appears to be ineffective. Since drowning of severe degree is generally associated with vomiting, the tracheobronchial airway should be cleaned by suction under direct laryngoscopic visualization before the endotracheal tube is inserted. The stomach should be evacuated by nasogastric tube, and the tube left in place to prevent subsequent regurgitation of acid gastric contents into the airway and to alleviate acute gastric distension, which further reduces pulmonary volume. If artificial ventilation must be continued beyond 48 to 72 hours, a tracheostomy may be indicated.

Assisted ventilation, oxygenation, and circulatory support should not be restricted only to victims whose breathing is inadequate. In all patients who have been apneic, and in those who are or were cyanotic or unconscious, assisted intermittent positive pressure ventilation (IPPV) combined with positive end-expiratory pressure (PEEP) or continuous positive pressure ventilation (CPPV) should be continued, even after spontaneous breathing returns, as long as there is evidence of extensive pulmonary disease (edema and/or atelectasis); cardiac arrhythmia; blood volume disturbance; acid base and electrolyte imbalance; and hemolysis, hemoconcentration, or dilution.

The presence of breathing movements and coughing when the victim is removed from the water suggests that hypoxic damage and aspiration are probably slight. However, consciousness and absence of apnea are not synonymous with recovery in all patients. Lethal secondary drowning, especially after seawater drowning, threatens even those who were conscious and breathing after first being rescued. Hospitalization for close observation is therefore indicated in all instances of near-drowning until 24 hours after the submersion, preferably in an intensive care facility.

Monitoring

In addition to frequent assessment of vital signs, arterial blood pressure, central venous pressure, and respiratory, circulatory, and nervous system status, the following data should be monitored until normal: arterial pH and blood gases; hematocrit; red blood cell count and plasma hemoglobin level; blood clotting status; serum electrolytes and blood urea nitrogen; urinary volume; chemistry; cytology; concentration; and acidification. Follow-up chest radiography and repeat electrocardiography are also essential.

Fluids

Fluids must be quantitatively and qualitatively regulated to maintain circulatory integrity, correct acidemia and electrolyte disturbances, promote and maintain adequate urine output, and contribute to the relief of pulmonary and cerebral edema. As long as there is evidence of cerebral and/or pulmonary edema, intravenous fluids should be restricted to 1,000 ml/m^2/24 hours or less provided this amount of fluid adequately supports peripheral arterial and central venous pressures, and urinary flow. Fluctuations of blood pressure, central venous pressure, and urinary output and concentration should serve as criteria for flexible adjustments in the assessment of fluid volume requirements.

Initially salt-poor albumin or potassium-poor plasma analogue is best given at the rate of 10 ml/kg/hour for both freshwater and seawater drownings and continued until serum electrolytes stabilize. Except for the acidemia, electrolyte levels usually revert to normal quite rapidly after adequate assisted ventilation is instituted. The composition of subsequent solutions to be administered intravenously will vary in accordance with fluctuations of acid–base balance, individual electrolyte maintenance requirements, and urinary losses.

Correction of acidemia will require the administration of variable amounts of sodium bicarbonate adjusted to the degree of base deficit, until the arterial pH returns to at least 7.25 to 7.3.

Drug Therapy

If evidence of pneumonitis exists, or if there are indications that the fluid aspirated may be heavily contaminated, therapy with appropriate antibiotics is recommended. Evacuation of gastric contents, continuous gastric aspiration, and withholding oral intake appears desirable in all patients with respiratory distress. In case of severe hemolysis, partial exchange transfusion has been recommended but rarely seems indicated.

If aspiration into the lungs has been massive, systemic corticosteroids may be useful. They also may contribute to relief of cerebral edema, if present. Intravenous infusion of a hyperosmotic agent, such as mannitol, to reduce cerebral edema may be necessary. Diuretics, such as furosemide or ethacrynic acid, are advocated by some to alleviate pulmonary edema but strongly opposed by others because of their depleting effect on the vascular space.

CONCLUSION

While in victims of submersion no time should be wasted before instituting appropriate respiratory and circulatory resuscitation, it is equally important to support ventilation and circulation until all pulmonary, cardiocirculatory, metabolic, and neurologic disturbances are corrected. However, as is the case in accidental episodes of any type or nature, adequate prevention could forestall the need for such heroic therapy in almost every instance of drowning and preclude the tragedy of loss of life or irreversible and crippling handicaps.

Prevention

Most drownings result from lack of supervision, absence of adequate protection, inexperience, overconfidence, ignorance, and poor judgment. A prerequisite for the application of adequate preventive measures is awareness of and familiarity with circumstances conducive to such accidents (see p. 766).

Preventive measures consist mainly of education and training. Children must always be properly supervised by qualified adults in the vicinity of rivers, lakes, pools, ponds, and oceans; young children or children of any age with handicaps or epilepsy must never be left unattended in bathtubs; children should be taught as early as possible not only to swim or float, but also to maintain prudent swimming conduct. All family members, including the children, should be instructed in water safety and in first-aid resuscitation techniques. Communities must have active water safety and public education programs. Educational efforts directed toward parents should concentrate especially on families living in areas where subsidiary pools, including the portable above-ground type, are common.

Community action is even more important in protecting the child from all aquatic hazards. Appropriate regulations must be promulgated concerning construction, fencing, and supervision of all sites where perilous exposure may occur. Adequate enclosures must be provided for all pools and ponds.

The Committee on Accidents of the American Council of Pediatrics has made useful waterproofing recommendations that should be publicized by physicians and educators to help minimize the perils of water for children.

Bibliography

DROWNING

Committee on Accident Prevention, American Academy of Pediatrics. Perils of the Water: The Problems of Drowning and the Child. Committee Statement. Newsletter Supplement, 1968

Committee on Emergency Medical Services, National Academy of Sciences-National Research Council. Standards for cardiopulmonary resuscitation (CPPR) and emergency cardiac care (ECC). JAMA 227: Suppl 2, 1974

Dietz PE, Baker SP: Drowning. Epidemiology and prevention. Am J Public Health 64:303, 1974

Editorial. Drowning. Lancet 7770:691, 1972

Einhorn AH: Accidental Submersion in Children, in Edology and Pediatrics, Vol 38. Einhorn AH, Zurbrügg RP (eds), Karger-Verlag Ag, Basel, London, New York, 1974, pp 60-66

Giammona ST: Drowning. Pathophysiology and management. Curr Problems Pediatr 1:1, 1971

Geammona ST, Modell JH: Drowning by total immersion. Am J Dis Child 114:612, 1967

Hasan S, Avery WG, Fabian C, et al.: Near drowning in humans. A report of 36 patients. Chest (Suppl) 59:191, 1971

Hunter TB, Whitehouse WM: Fresh-water near-drowning. Radiological aspects. Radiology 112:51, 1974

Imburg J, Hartney T: Drowning and the treatment of non-fatal submersion. Pediatrics 37:684, 1966

Modell JH, Davis JH, Giammona ST: Blood gas and electrolyte changes in human near-drowning victims. JAMA 203:99, 1968

——— Calderwood HW, Ruiz BC: Effects of ventilatory patterns on arterial oxygenation after near-drowning in sea water. Anesthesiology 40:376, 1974

Moser RH: Drowning, a seasonal disease. JAMA 229:566, 1974

National Safety Council. In Accident Facts, Chicago 1974 and 1975

Redding JS: Resuscitation and treatment following submersion. Pediatrics 37:666, 1966

Rivers JF, Orr G, Lee HA: Drowning. Its clinical sequelae and management. Br Med J 2:157, 1970

Rosenbaum HT, Thompson WL, Fuller RH: Radiographic pulmonary changes in near-drowning. Radiology 83:306, 1964

BURNS IN CHILDHOOD
JOHN M. STEIN

INTRODUCTION

Burns, which are among the most common of severe childhood accidents, are almost always preventable. The depth to which the burn injury penetrates is a function of temperature, duration of exposure, and skin thickness. The very thin skin of the infant or young child may sustain a full-thickness (third-degree) injury, whereas identical exposure in an older child or adult may cause only partial-thickness (second-degree) burns.

ETIOLOGY

The most common etiology is scalding by spill or immersion. In *spill scalds,* a curious toddler usually pulls hot liquid onto himself, commonly burning the hand, arm, lateral side of the trunk, and lateral side of the face and neck. Such scald burns are generally, though not invariably, partial thickness (second-degree) in depth and are rarely fatal because of the limited extent of body surface involved. *Immersion scald* burns, which result when the child either climbs or is pushed into a tub of hot water, carry a higher mortality rate because larger portions of the body surface are involved. Although these also are generally partial thickness in depth, full-thickness (third-degree) injury may result with prolonged exposure to hot water, especially if the child cannot climb out of the tub himself.

Contact with hot utensils, flat irons, or stoves is also a common cause of injury. Such *contact burns* are often full thickness, occupy only a very small portion of the body surface, and are amenable to immediate excision and grafting.

Electrical burns are most often caused by relatively low-voltage household current. Typically, a child may bite an electric cord and sustain a small but disfiguring area of third-degree burn of the lips, or after introducing a hairpin or other metal object into an electric socket, suffer a limited burn of the fingers. These low-voltage injuries are not fatal unless the 60-cycle alternating current passes through the heart, causing ventricular fibrillation. High-voltage injuries (600 V or greater), generally seen in older children who play in electric transformer stations or on live railway lines, cause deep necrosis of muscle tissue and coagulation of blood vessels. The cutaneous injury is often minimal compared with the extensive volume of deep tissue damage. Loss of life is frequent, and loss of limb occurs in 30 percent of survivors. Special resuscitative techniques must be instituted immediately, including diuresis and alkalinization of urine to prevent hemoglobin precipitation in renal tubules, and early fasciotomy for limb decompression.

Flame burns generally cause full-thickness injury, especially when flammable clothing burns, and are often associated with pulmonary complications (see p. 777).

Chemical burns are usually caused by strong acid or alkaline agents such as those used as drain cleaners. Immediate treatment consists of washing off the offending agent with copious amounts of tapwater, preferably in a shower or bathtub. Burns of this nature are often the hallmark of the poorly supervised home environment or of deliberate child abuse. *Cigarette burns,* evident as single or multiple round lesions 0.5 cm in diameter, and usually differing in ages, are characteristic of child abuse.

INITIAL ASSESSMENT

If the burning process is still in progress, flames should be extinguished with cold water and cold water compresses applied to the burned area as quickly as possible. A chemical injury requires immediate and copious lavage with tapwater, which should be continued for one to two hours.

Initial attention is then directed, as with any severely traumatized patient, to the adequacy of airway and circulation. Early upper respiratory insufficiency is frequent in patients who have sustained their injuries in enclosed spaces. Direct laryngoscopic examination of the posterior pharynx and larynx must be performed immediately by an expert anesthesiologist. Adequacy of circulation is judged initially by the rate and quality of the pulse as well as the blood pressure and central venous pressure.

Associated injuries, such as bone fractures, central nervous system trauma, thoracic and abdominal injuries, are most frequently seen in automobile accident victims, in those who have jumped from a burning building, or in explosion victims and should take precedence over treatment of the burn itself. Associated intraabdominal, thoracic, and/or nervous system injuries should be treated without regard for the burn. Fluid resuscitation for the burn injury can be instituted along with treatment of the associated injury. The safest time for craniotomy, thoracotomy, and laparotomy is on the day of burn before the burn wound becomes infected. Fractures of long bones, which ordinarily would require internal fixation, are generally treated by traction or cast since the inserted foreign body may become infected.

As soon as possible sterile techniques should be instituted. The patient should be touched only with sterile gloves, and the entire team handling the patient should wear caps, gowns, and masks. Sterile bed linen is desirable, but if not immediately available, clean linen can be used. Early contamination of the burn wound with bacteria will lead to early septic complications.

If the child can talk, a detailed history of the circumstances of the burn should be obtained from him while initiating treatment. Patients with severe burns are often more lucid and cooperative in the first few hours after the injury than they are for a considerable time thereafter. It is particularly important to ascertain whether soot, smoke, or flames were inhaled. Inquiry about the child's feelings concerning those who were with him at the time of the accident may give considerable insight into the patient's emotional response to his burn.

In the case of major burns it is more efficient for one physician to take a history, examine, and treat the child while another obtains a detailed history from the parents. In order to avoid excessive contamination of the burns, traffic must be limited to a minimum within the burn treatment area, from which all nonessential personnel and curious onlookers must be barred.

Estimation of Burn Size

An approximate but clinically acceptable assessment of the body surface area involved can be obtained by using the Rule of Nines, which allots 9 percent of the total body surface to the head and neck, 9 percent to each upper extremity, and 18 percent to each of the following areas: anterior trunk, posterior trunk, and each lower extremity. A more exact estimate of burn surface can be obtained from a diagram such as Figure 1. The main difference between infancy and adulthood lies in the larger surface area for head and neck in the young. It is also convenient to remember that the palmar surface of the patient's hand at all ages represents 1 percent of the body surface area.

Burn Depth

The etiology of the thermal injury usually gives some indication of the depth of most of the burn. Very superficial or *first-degree burns* produce erythema without blistering, accompanied by pain and sensitivity to pin prick. Partial-thickness or *second-degree burns* are marked by blister formation or erythema with a wet exudative wound. Intact sensation to pin prick is variable, since in burns that extend deep *into* but not through the dermis, the cutaneous nerve endings may be damaged and insensitive. Areas of full-thickness or *third-degree burns* extend beyond the depths of the hair follicles and into the subcutaneous tissue. These areas are generally blanched and appear depressed; they swell less rapidly than the surrounding second-degree burn, and destruction of nerve endings renders them anesthetic.

Infants under two years of age have particularly thin

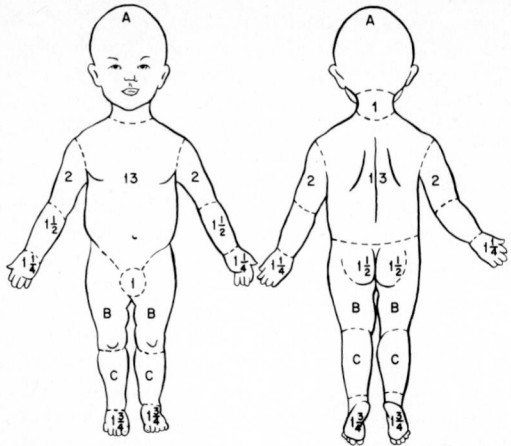

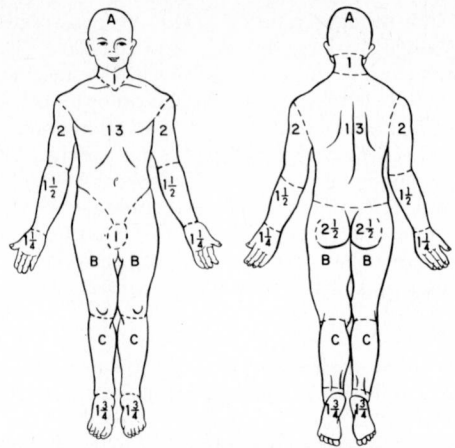

RELATIVE PERCENTAGES OF AREAS AFFECTED BY GROWTH

AREA	AGE 0	1	5
A = $\frac{1}{2}$ of Head	$9\frac{1}{2}$	$8\frac{1}{2}$	$6\frac{1}{2}$
B = $\frac{1}{2}$ of One Thigh	$2\frac{3}{4}$	$3\frac{1}{4}$	4
C = $\frac{1}{2}$ of One Leg	$2\frac{1}{2}$	$2\frac{1}{2}$	$2\frac{3}{4}$

% BURN BY AREAS

RELATIVE PERCENTAGES OF AREAS AFFECTED BY GROWTH

AREA	AGE 10	15	ADULT
A = $\frac{1}{2}$ of Head	$5\frac{1}{2}$	$4\frac{1}{2}$	$3\frac{1}{2}$
B = $\frac{1}{2}$ of One Thigh	$4\frac{1}{4}$	$4\frac{1}{2}$	$4\frac{3}{4}$
C = $\frac{1}{2}$ of One Leg	3	$3\frac{1}{4}$	$3\frac{1}{2}$

% BURNS BY AREA

FIG. 1. A. Relative percentage of areas affected by growth (infants and young children). (Lund and Bowden's modification of Berkow's table.)

FIG. 1. B. Relative percentage of areas affected by growth (older children and young adults). (Lund and Bowden's modification of Berkow's table.)

skin and are prone to full thickness burns, which by the usual criteria appear to be second-degree when first seen. There is a general tendency to underestimate depth and overestimate size of burns. Burns are not uniform over the entire injured surface. In any individual patient there are variations of depth due to differences in intensity of exposure to the thermal trauma, in body positions, and in skin thickness.

Admission Criteria

There are no strict criteria for the admission of burned children. For example, a child with cigarette burns or other suspicious burns suggesting child abuse may be admitted even if the area of involvement is small. In such cases notification of appropriate child protective authorities is mandatory and the physician is legally protected. A house fire destroying a family's living quarters may be sufficient reason for admitting burns of small surface areas. Maternal competence, the home situation, and other environmental circumstances must also be considered. A mother with a large number of children may be unable to devote the necessary attention to her burned child and may request admission of a child with moderate burns.

The conventional medical criteria for admission are:

Facial burns, especially those occurring in closed spaces where inhalation injury is considered.
Third-degree contact burns of 0.5 percent of the body surface or greater requiring immediate excision and primary autografting.

Partial- or full-thickness burns in older children of 20 percent or more of the body surface; in infants of 12 to 15 percent; and in neonates, 10 percent.
Partial- or full-thickness burns of the hands where functional impairment may result.
Burns of the perineum where ensuing difficulty in urination and/or fecal soilage may be anticipated.

AMBULATORY BURNS

The vast majority of burns are treated on an ambulatory basis, provided the child is closely followed and parents are given detailed written instructions. A short dissertation to the child and parents on burn prevention and emergency care (cold water, cleanliness, no application of butter or other ointment) is in order.

Most patients selected for ambulatory care will have suffered second-degree burns over a small portion of their body surface. The burned area should be gently cleansed with cold isotonic saline solution. Aqueous providone iodine solution may also be used, but the use of soaps and detergents is discouraged since they may injure cells further. The use of hexachlorophene is contraindicated since surface absorption may lead to neurotoxicity.

Controversy exists concerning the extent of initial debridement. It is the author's feeling that such initial debridement should be limited to the gentle removal of loose-hanging skin and that intact blisters and blebs should be left untouched. This therapy allows the second-degree burn to heal under the protective coating of the blister and leaves the burn relatively painless. Blisters are debrided once they rupture spontaneously or if the fluid they contain becomes cloudy due to infection. Others feel that all blisters and blebs should be debrided at the time of initial treatment in order to avoid infection. This therapy converts a relatively painless second-degree burn into a painful injury. In addition, there is some evidence that aggressive early debridement of second-degree burn delays subsequent wound epithelialization by a few days.

After the initial cleansing, the wound should be covered with a dressing, both to prevent bacterial contamination and for the patient's comfort. A single layer of gauze impregnated with a bland nonantibiotic ointment is applied directly to the burn, which is then covered with dry cotton gauze of sufficient thickness to protect the blisters and blebs. Paper tape may be used to hold the dressing in place but should be applied only to areas of unburned skin. More frequently circumferential dressings of roller-type gauze are employed. These should also be taped in place so that they do not ride up and down the extremities.

These superficial burns are not tetanus-prone and therefore do not require the administration of hyperimmune human antitetanus serum. Tetanus toxoid should be administered only if the child has not had previous adequate immunization.

Systemic antibiotics for ambulatory burns are not universally utilized, but the risk of early streptococcal cellulitis is sufficiently great that small doses of oral penicillin (or erythromycin in the allergic patient) for the first five days are generally recommended.

There is almost universal agreement that topical antimicrobial agents (see below) are not desirable in outpatient therapy; if the burn is severe enough to warrant topical antimicrobial therapy, the patient should be admitted.

A mild analgesic, such as aspirin or acetaminophen, should control pain in young children, and small doses of codeine may be prescribed for older ones. The injured part should be put at rest; this may require sedation in some children.

or the first week, dressings should be changed on alternate days to observe the healing process and the absence or presence of infection. At the time of dressing change, cloudy or ruptured blisters and blebs should be debrided. As healing proceeds dressing changes may be done less frequently and a competent parent may be able to change some of these dressings.

Even the most superficial second-degree burns will take at least two weeks to heal. Burns of greater depth may require as long as six to eight weeks to epithelialize spontaneously. A period of red discoloration follows epithelialization and may persist for nine months. Healed burned skin is shiny and atrophic. It is particularly susceptible to subsequent mechanical injuries and to sunburn, about which appropriate warning should be given to parents and children.

Pigmentation is a cosmetic problem for Black, Hispanic, and Indian patients. In the more superficial sec-

ond-degree burns pigment will grow darker than that in the surrounding normal skin. This dark pigmentation will persist for approximately 12 months. In deeper second-degree burns epithelialization occurs from the hair follicles and punctate return of pigmentation is frequently seen. These punctate areas generally coalesce to a relatively uniform pigmented area. However, normal pigmentation and normal skin texture rarely return into areas that have sustained deep second-degree injury.

IN-PATIENT MANAGEMENT

There is some tendency to overtreat patients with even minor burns when they are admitted to the hospital. Those who are hospitalized for social rather than medical indications should not be exposed to the inherent dangers of intravenous therapy, indwelling urinary catheters, frequent blood tests, and other measures appropriate for the more seriously burned. On the other hand, those whose burns involve 50 percent or more of the body surface of which a major portion is full-thickness burn are best treated at burn-care centers with facilities and staff for the care of large numbers of burns. Such centers, which have a specialized team for burn care, offer the child the greatest chance of survival with the least cosmetic and functional deformity.

Transfers

The transfer of very seriously burned patients to a burn treatment center should be arranged as early as possible. The referring physician must thoroughly examine the entire body surface and carefully note and diagram the extent of involvement. A secure intravenous line with a large-bore cannula should be established. All medications should be given intravenously. An indwelling urinary catheter should be inserted, attached to a closed collection system. The intravenous fluids (usually Ringers lactate) should be run at a rate to maintain urinary output at 0.25 ml/minute for infants under 1 year, 0.5 ml/minute for children 1 to 5 years, and 1 ml/minute for children over 5 years of age.

If respiratory difficulty is noted, laryngoscopy is recommended and, if necessary, endotracheal intubation performed. Paralytic ileus frequently accompanies major burns and nasogastric decompression should be instituted prior to transfer.

The referring physician should then contact the receiving burn treatment facility so that safe transfer can be accomplished. The receiving facility may have additional suggestions as to fluid therapy and topical burn care prior to transfer. The practice of first treating a major burn in an inadequate facility for a few days with the intention of calling upon a burn receiving hospital at the time of complications is unwise and harmful for the patient.

The details of therapy afforded by various burn facilities throughout the country are beyond the scope of this chapter. Most facilities of this type have developed an integrated team incorporating pediatricians or internists, surgeons, plastic surgeons, psychiatrists, orthopedists, and specialists in physical rehabilitation, along with a specially skilled nursing and ancillary staff.

Initial Therapy

The initial therapy given a child with extensive burns who is restless should not include intramuscular or subcutaneous administration of a narcotic, since the absorption of such a narcotic in hypovolemic shock is unreliable; the restlessness is often due to hypoxemia or hypovolemia and not to pain. Only after these conditions have been corrected should small incremental doses of narcotics be given intravenously.

Fluid Resuscitation

Many different formulas for resuscitation from burn shock have been devised. All formulas are merely estimates of the potential requirements of fluids and must be modified by adequate clinical and laboratory observations.

Because of the extreme permeability of capillaries in the burned area to molecules the size of albumin, an initial colloid-free fluid regimen has now been adopted generally. The classic fluids of the Brooke and Evans formulas have been displaced largely by the use of Ringers lactate during the first 24 hours post burn. Initial estimate of the volume of Ringers lactate required for resuscitation can be calculated as 4 ml of Ringers lactate/1percent burn/kilogram body weight. The actual volume administered should be modified to produce adequate urinary output (approximately 40 ml/m² body surface area/hour) and maintain pulse, blood pressure, serum osmolality, and serum electrolytes within normal limits.

Urinary output remains the single most effective parameter for ensuring adequate hydration. Low urine output should be treated with increased fluid administration rather than with diuretics. Mechanical causes, such as a nonpatent urinary catheter, should be investigated before a patient is declared oliguric. Factitiously elevated urinary output may be seen in patients who are undergoing osmotic diuresis, either due to endogenous or exogenous glucose or due to the administration of an osmotic diuretic, such as mannitol. The large urine volume is associated with high urinary specific gravity and/or glucosuria in such instances.

Systemic blood pressure should be measured frequently using a conventional but sterile blood pressure cuff, the doppler ultrasound oscillator technique, or direct arterial puncture.

If the patient receives adequate fluid resuscitation therapy, his urine output will be satisfactorily maintained. High serum osmolality, elevated serum sodium, and rising blood urea nitrogen and hematocrit all constitute evidence of dehydration. Arterial blood gases should be measured frequently. Acidemia indicates decreased tissue perfusion and should be treated with increased volumes of intravenous fluids and with additional sodium bicarbonate. Urine specimens should be measured for electrolyte content. Despite the initial release of potassium from injured cells, severe hyperkalemia is rarely a problem. On the other hand, with adequate urinary output potassium excretion increases and administration of additional potassium may be required within 8 to 12 hours after the burn. Determinations of serum and urinary potassium and electrocardiographic monitoring will be guides to potassium requirements.

Recent clinical and experimental work with hypertonic colloid-free resuscitative fluids has shown some promising results. These fluids contain 238 to 250 mEq of sodium with chloride, lactate, or bicarbonate anions. The hypertonic fluid regimen has the advantage of reducing the total volume of infused fluid since the hypertonic infusate draws extracellular and intracellular water into the intravascular space. Although hypertonic resuscitative fluids may become more commonly used in the future, they are not yet established in medical practice.

Rapid fluid shifts, which occur in burned patients, may produce cerebral edema and convulsions. Hypertension, often without bradycardia, is not uncommon in the burned child.

Within 24 to 36 hours postburn, the capillary permeability of the injured area returns to normal. At this time serum protein administration, preferably in the form of pooled, stored, hepatitis-free albumin solutions, should be administered to restore normal oncotic pressure to the serum.

Insensible water loss in burn patients is markedly increased because injury to the lipid-containing epidermis allows the evaporation of free water. Absolutely accurate intake and output measurements must be recorded and augmented by measurement of body weight on scales accurate to 10 g. In the properly resuscitated patient with burns exceeding 30 percent of the body surface a weight gain of approximately 10 percent of the preburn body weight will be noticed at the end of 24 to 36 hours. Thereafter, as capillary function returns to normal, diuresis should ensue and weight should return to preburn levels by the third or fourth postburn day. Diuretics, such as furosemide, may be required to hasten adequate diuresis. Careful monitoring of serum and urinary electrolytes is also required throughout this phase of diuresis.

Topical Burn Care

A variety of topical antibacterial agents is effective in reducing the numbers of bacteria present on the burn wound. None serves to render the burn wound sterile.

Silversulfadiazine (Silvadene) is a white aqueous cream, the application of which is relatively painless. Systemic absorption is small; argyria and sulfonamide precipitation in the kidneys are no problem and there are no resulting metabolic derangements. It is the most easily managed topical burn agent that can be employed either in open-wound care, applied every eight hours, or under dressings that are changed daily. It is the drug of choice for bacterial control in the severely burned patient.

Mafenide (Sulfamylon) is painful on administration, but because of its extreme solubility penetrates deeply into the burn wound to control bacterial growth. Although absorbed systemically, because of its solubility, it does not cause kidney stones. However, as a potent carbonic anhydrase inhibitor, it prevents the elimination of carbon dioxide, thus causing metabolic acidemia and hyperventilation. It does not, however, prevent secretion of gastric acid, which remains normal.

Aqueous silver nitrate in a concentration of 0.5 percent may be applied to the burn wound in thick gauze dressings saturated with this solution. The dressings must be changed frequently and soaked with the solution. The use of silver nitrate soaks on burns encompassing large portions of the body surface leaches out electrolytes, which must be replaced initially intravenously and later by mouth. In addition, the use of silver nitrate is messy since metallic silver stains on contact.

Povidine iodine (Betadine) ointment is a brown water-based cream that is moderately painful on application. It is an effective topical agent but generally reserved for those patients who demonstrate allergy to one of the sulfonamide preparations and in whom the use of silver nitrate is deemed impractical.

According to Feller of the National Burn Information Exchange, who has collected statistics from burn treatment facilities throughout the country, no difference in gross mortality rate can be attributed to any of the various topical agents. Timely debridement and early burn coverage with allograft or autograft are important factors.

Burns Wound Coverage

Partial-thickness burns will be covered by epithelium originating from hair follicles that have not been injured. As this type of healing occurs, small punctate islands of epithelium can be seen to migrate out from the hair follicles. They coalesce and wound closure is obtained.

Full-thickness burns contain no remnant epithelial elements and require skin grafting. The best currently available provisional skin coverage is fresh cadaver allograft. Such *allograft* is generally left in place for less than a week so that immune rejection is not a problem. The advantages of allograft covering are that it renders the burn pain-free, reduces the bacterial count on the burn surface, and acts as a test agent since the acceptance of allograft almost assures that a subsequently placed autograft will take.

Porcine *xenograft* is also frequently used as a provisional skin covering. Its commercial availability makes it more convenient to use, but it is generally felt to be inferior to cadaver allograft.

In addition to their use in areas of full-thickness burn, both allograft and xenograft may be applied to partial-thickness burns to reduce pain and hasten epithelial growth.

Final wound closure of full-thickness burns is accomplished by skin *autografting*. Split-thickness skin grafts are harvested from previously uninjured skin with the use of the dermatome, which cuts through the dermis removing the epidermis and a portion of the dermis. The donor site thus is analogous to a second-degree burn and will epithelialize spontaneously from the dermal elements and hair follicles left in place. The free skin graft thus obtained can then be placed on the granulating or excised full-thickness burn where it can be held in place with sutures, sterile tape, or a careful dressing technique.

Adequate pain medication and sedation should be provided for children as they emerge from anesthesia, since the donor sites are painful. Smooth emergence from anesthesia is essential to avoid dislodgment of the recently placed graft by the agitated child. Sedation and pain medication often must be continued for several days after grafting in order to allow the graft to adhere firmly, become vascularized, and take.

The most common causes of graft loss are mechanical displacement (hematoma under graft or squirming child) and bacterial infection. As soon as graft take is evident, active physical therapy to preserve function should be reinstituted.

Antibiotic Therapy

In the preantibiotic era, early and severe life-threatening burn infections with streptococci were frequent. It is therefore common practice to administer relatively low doses of prophylactic penicillin (300,000 units/24 hours) or erythromycin in the allergic child in the first five postburn days. Subsequent systemic antibiotics are determined by culture and sensitivities only. It is good practice to build a culture data bank on each burn patient by culturing several sites of the burn wound two or three times each week. After the first few days, all burn wounds will be colonized by some bacteria. The presence of such bacteria does not indicate that the wound has become infected. Cultures obtained by cotton swabs are the least informative since they give no quantitative information. Culture medium contact plates such as Rhodec plates give some information about the numbers of bacteria on the surface of the burn wound. It is best to obtain biopsy cultures, which give information as to the number of bacteria per gram of burn tissue. When the number of bacteria per gram of burn tissue exceeds 10^5, burn wound infection is very likely to be present. Invasive burn wound infection can also be diagnosed histologically by rapid section techniques wherein bacteria can be seen to invade unburned subcutaneous tissue.

It is most difficult to decide when and whether to treat a burned child with intensive antibiotic therapy. Many children who appear quite well, are alert, and eat well will have persistent fever and leukocytosis during much of their burn course. Intercurrent localized infections, such as pneumonias or urinary tract infections and infected intravenous sites, should, of course, be appropriately treated. However, to presume that there is burn-wound sepsis each time the patient becomes febrile and/or exhibits an elevated white count will lead to the substantial overuse of systemic antibiotics. On the other hand, the child who starts refusing food or exhibits irritability or irrationality should evoke suspicion of generalized sepsis. Although the usual objective findings of generalized sepsis are elevated body temperature and leukocytosis, in the burned child generalized sepsis may be associated with leukopenia and hypothermia. If such clinical manifestations develop and lead to the diagnosis of sepsis, intensive antibiotic therapy should be instituted *after* blood cultures, wound biopsies for culture and immediate pathologic section, urine cultures, and cultures at the site of the intravenous line are obtained. The antibiotics used will depend upon the data bank of culture material built up previously. Intense systemic antibiotic therapy, combined with appropriate surgical debridement, subeschar injection of antibiotics, and alteration of the topical agent, is appropriate therapy for invasive burn-wound sepsis. The margin for error is small, and the clinician is constantly treading the narrow path between overtreating minor infections and unduly delaying antimicrobial therapy of a true episode of burn-wound infection. The burned patient is often more susceptible to infection because his white cell function is depressed. On the other hand, antibiotics of the aminoglycoside group can cause deafness and renal failure as primary complications. In addition, prolonged intensive antimicrobial therapy allows the emergence of opportunistic organisms, including fungi, particularly candida and mucor, and systemic viral infections, such as Herpes simplex.

Nutrition

Adequate nutrition is extremely important. The large, metabolically active burn wound increases the metabolic rate two- to threefold. Excessive water evaporation through the injured skin costs the body 0.5 kcal/g of water evaporated. Fever, tachycardia, and hyperventilation, all frequent in the burned patient, further add to stress. Careful attention to both enteral and parenteral nutrition is required for a successful outcome.

Hyperglycemia secondary to gluconeogenesis stimulated by the stress of the burn is common during the early resuscitative phase. Therefore no attempt should be made during this period to provide high caloric intake, particularly in the form of glucose.

Soon after the resuscitative phase has passed, attention to nutrition must begin. The severely burned patient needs two to three times the normal caloric requirement. Large amounts of protein are lost through the burn wound in the form of exudate, and protein requirements for wound healing are great. Therefore a high protein intake should be provided, by mouth if possible, or alternatively by feeding tube or intravenously. It may even be necessary to resort to enteral and parenteral routes simultaneously. Intravenous hyperalimentation may be used, in which case the central

venous lines should be changed frequently to prevent sepsis.

Carbohydrate and fat intake must be adequate. The supplemental use of tasty milkshakes provides the necessary combination of the three food elements. These can often be given to children as a treat.

Vitamin supplementation is also important. Very large quantities of vitamin C are required to establish healthy granulation tissue; a minimum of 500 mg of vitamin C per day is recommended. Vitamin A is required for adequate wound epithelialization and should be supplemented in the diet. Many hospital diets are deficient in the water-soluble B vitamins, and these too should be added to the daily regimen.

PSYCHIATRIC CONSIDERATIONS

An important yet often neglected aspect in the care of the burned child concerns the psychologic interplay between the child and his parents and also the medical, nursing, and other ancillary staff caring for him. The average length of hospitalization of a child for burns is approximately 60 days; in very severe burns, an entire year may be spent in the hospital during the first admission. Subsequent readmissions for cosmetic or functional corrections may be required. The burn triggers a chain of short- and long-term interactions between the child, his family, and the hospital staff. A proportion of both the children and their parents have antecedent psychologic problems. Parental guilt feelings, invariably exceedingly strong, will often lead to unrealistic demands on the medical staff, including assurances that the burn will heal without scar or deformity. The parent may feel that the staff is providing inadequate attention to the child or that therapy causes excessive pain. Demands for parental visiting privileges may be excessive —or the opposite reaction may occur, when parents cannot bear to visit their child, who then feels completely rejected.

Another type of reaction is "It's your problem, doctor." With burns occurring through little or no fault on the part of the patient himself, and especially where litigation is possible, the philosophy that the patient and his parent have no role in the management of a burn occurs commonly. In this situation the child may be totally uncooperative during dressing changes and may refuse to participate properly in the activities of physical and occupational therapy undertaken to prevent deformity and contractures.

In general, behavior problems are minimized by treating children in areas where other children with burns are being treated. Dressing changes, physical therapy, and other treatments are then group norms, and the children can follow each other's progress.

Since the severe burn injury is a chronic disease, straightforwardness in physician-to-patient and family relationships is of utmost importance. Failure to maintain honest lines of communication invariably leads to distrust, often irreversible. An additional difficulty arises when a sibling, parent, or frient dies in the same accident. Protecting the child from such news may well cause an irretrievable break in communication. Soon after the acute resuscitative phase, if the child is communicative and inquires about it, he should be given the correct information.

During the hospitalization and especially prior to discharge of a particularly deformed and/or functionally limited child, psychiatric intervention is very important. In addition, the transition from hospital to home can be tempered by permitting first one-day then weekend passes before complete discharge.

COMPLICATIONS

Sepsis

Invasion of the burn wound with microorganisms is common. Even patients who do not appear septic may have daily temperature elevations generally associated with dressing changes or wound debridement. Such patients are treated with appropriate systemic antibiotics only if fever persists, blood cultures are positive, or disorientation, abdominal distension, leukopenia, or hypothermia occur. A markedly elevated white count per se, even to a level of leukemoid reaction, need not necessarily mandate antibiotic therapy.

Inspection of the wound may show pale granulation tissue, ulceration, or black necrotic areas, which confirm the diagnosis of invasive wound sepsis. After a biopsy is obtained for quantitative bacteriology and histology, aggressive systemic antimicrobial therapy should be instituted based on previous culture data, usually requiring a combination of gentamicin, carbenicillin, and one of the semisynthetic penicillins effective against staphylococci. Other measures for treatment of burn-wound sepsis are debridement, subeschar injection of antibiotics, and changing the topical agent being used on the burn wound.

Superinfection of the burn wound with Candida albicans or mucor yeasts is commonly associated with large dose and prolonged antibiotic therapy.

Septic foci in locations other than the burn wound include urinary tract infection, pneumonia, and suppurative phlebitis at the sites of intravenous lines and may cause the picture of generalized sepsis. Silent perforation of gastric or duodenal ulcers can mimic the septic picture.

Evaluation of a patient who appears septic is an emergency, and all possibilities must be urgently explored and thoroughly treated.

Pulmonary Complications

Pulmonary complications can affect the upper airway causing laryngeal edema and/or the lower airway where incomplete products of combustion (such as the aldehydes and ketones that result from burning wood and plastic) paralyze the ciliated respiratory epithelium.

Upper airway obstruction almost invariably accompanies severe burns around the face and neck. Edema of the epiglottis and laryngeal structures can occur in such patients, who should be examined by an experienced laryngoscopist at frequent intervals. The edematous upper airway should be bypassed by an endotracheal tube before obstruction occurs; tracheostomy is generally not required.

Lower airway injury is seen in patients who are burned while entrapped within a closed space. Very severe inhalation injury with paralysis of respiratory cilia and carbon monoxide poisoning can occur without any cutaneous burn whatsoever. Carbon monoxide poisoning (carboxyhemoglobin over 10 percent) should be reversed by intensive oxygen therapy. Considerable controversy exists concerning the desirability of long-term endotracheal intubation versus tracheostomy, the use of steroids, and prophylactic antibiotics.

Pulmonary infiltrates may have a number of additional causes. In the early resuscitative phase pulmonary edema may be produced by overhydration. Hypostatic pneumonias can occur if the patient is kept inactive. Blood-borne septic emboli can complicate burn wound sepsis.

Gastrointestinal Complications

The most common gastrointestinal complication consists of acute ulceration of the stomach and duodenum. *Curling's ulcers* are almost universally present in those patients who die of burns even if they do not contribute to the death. On the other hand, they occasionally bleed severely or perforate in those patients who survive. Perforation usually presents symptoms similar to sepsis, but can also occur with practically no symptoms. Upright chest films in a child who does not seem to be doing quite well may reveal free air as the only indication of this complication. Perforated ulcers should be repaired surgically. Surgical intervention for bleeding depends upon its rate but should be considered early since massive bleeding rarely subsides spontaneously and frequently recurs even if the initial hemorrhage ceases. Prophylaxis against ulceration with milk and antacids should be instituted as early as gastrointestinal function permits.

Intestinal obstruction at the level of the duodenum may be caused by superior mesenteric artery syndrome, especially in children who suffer considerable weight loss. Pancreatitis as a cause for intestinal dysfunction is relatively uncommon. Diarrhea can complicate antibiotic therapy and gavage feedings. Fecal impaction occurs in bedfast patients and should be anticipated by giving a stool softener.

Contractures

Many contractures can be prevented by aggressive physical and occupational, therapy which should start immediately upon hospitalization. Hand burns are particularly disabling and should be treated with decompressive escharotomies if indicated, elevation, active and passive exercises, and appropriate splinting techniques for the very start. Similarly contractures of the anterior neck and joints of the arms and legs can be prevented by early and constant positioning and exercise techniques, splints, and traction.

Despite attention to all details, some children, after recovering from thermal injury, exhibit severe hypertrophic scars and contractures. In many cases these can be treated without surgical release by early use of compression dressings combined with splints. Prolonged compression techniques extending over 6 to 12 months can reduce the irregularity of the hypertrophic scar and produce a more acceptable functional and cosmetic result. In addition, progressive application of splints to anterior cervical, elbow, axillary, and foot contractures can bring the extremities and neck more and more toward the proper position.

Surgical correction of contractures may be required if they are excessive or if the patient cannot tolerate the compression technique. Skeletal traction for stretching contracted limbs can also be successful.

Heterotopic bone formation may be visualized as periarticular calcification on radiographs of the elbows and hips. It is important to differentiate skin contracture from heterotopic bone before instituting aggressive therapy for contractures. Patients who have developed such heterotopic bone should not be forced to exercise the involved extremity. Spontaneous regression of heterotopic bone is the rule but occasionally surgical excision to restore adequate joint function is necessary.

Finally, some areas, particularly the face, the dorsum of the hand, and the lower portions of the calves and legs, may be so disfigured that the healed burn may have to be excised and replaced with new skin grafts. Such resurfacing, which is difficult, is best delayed until the healing burn scar has become quiescent, as evidenced by a change in color and consistency from inflamed red to relatively pliable white

SUMMARY

Successful management of the thermally injured patient requires attention to the smallest detail. Expertise in a variety of disciplines is required for total management of the patient. The team approach to the management of the burn patient is met with the highest success rate.

Bibliography

Baxter CR: Present concepts in the management of major electrical injury. Surg Clin North Am 50:1401, 1970

Bruck HM, Pruitt BA Jr: Curling's ulcer in children: a 12-year review of 63 cases. J Trauma 12:490, 1972

Bunchman HH II, Huang TT, Larson, DL et al: Prevention and management of contractures in patients with burns of the neck. Am J Surg 130:700, 1975

Burke JF, May JW Jr, Albright N, et al: Temporary skin transplantation and immunosuppression for extensive burns. N Engl J Med 290:269, 1974

Evans EB, Larson DL, Yates S: Preservation and restoration of joint function in patients with severe burns. JAMA 204:843, 1968

Hughes JR, Cayaffa JJ, Pruitt BA Jr, et al: Seizures following burns of the skin. Dis Nerv Syst 34:347, 1973

Janzekovic Z: A new concept in the early excision and immediate grafting of burns. J Trauma 10:1103, 1970

Joshi VV: Effect of burns on the heart: a clinicopathological study in children. JAMA 211:2130, 1970

Martin HL, Lawrie JH, Wilkinson AW: The family of the fatally burned child. The Lancet 21:628, 1968

Metcoff J, Buchman H, Jacobson M, et al: Losses and physiologic requirements for water and electrolytes after extensive burns in children. N Engl J Med 265:101, 1961

Moncrief JA: Burns. N Engl J Med 288:444, 1973

Nance FC, Lewis VL Jr, Hines JL, et al: Aggressive outpatient care of burns. J Trauma 12:144, 1972

Newsome TW, Eurenius K: Suppression of granulocyte and platelet production by Pseudomonas burn wound infection. Surg Gynecol Obstet 136:375, 1973

O'Neill JA Jr, Meacham WF, Griffin PP, et al: Patterns of injury in the battered child syndrome. J Trauma 13:322, 1973

Pruitt BA Jr, Erickson DR, Morris A: Progressive pulmonary insufficiency and other pulmonary complications of thermal injury. J Trauma 15:369, 1975

———— Foley FD: The use of biopsies in burn patient care. Surgery 73:887, 1973

Stein JM, Pruitt BA: Suppurative thrombophlebitis. N Engl J Med 282:1452, 1970

Zikria BA, Ferrer JM, Floch HF: The chemical factors contributing to pulmonary damage in smoke poisoning. Surgery 71:704, 1972

CHILDHOOD POISONINGS

ARNOLD H. EINHORN

An ever-increasing number of drugs and chemical household products abound in or around every home and represent potential sources of dangerous poisons for children. Adult negligence is largely responsible for accidental ingestion, primarily in very young children. There is a great need for adequate environmental protection, continuing public education, and appropriate legislation.

INCIDENCE, EPIDEMIOLOGY, AND ETIOLOGY

Accidental poisonings account for more than 3,600 deaths annually in the United States. While the total number of poisonings has continued to rise, since 1970 there has been a steady decline of deaths from poisonings in the 1 to 5 year age group, with a particularly significant drop in 1973. However, mortality is only part of the picture. The annual number of nonfatal poisonings is estimated to exceed 600,000 cases; many are left with permanent disabilities, some of which may be subtle. Thus intellectual impairment from chronic lead intoxication or from any toxic product that affects brain function may become apparent only when the child enters school.

The incidence of poisoning is highest in the 2-year and next highest in the one-year age group. Before the infant crawls he is less exposed to the danger of poisonings because of his relative immobility.

ECOLOGY OF POISONING

Host and Environmental Factors

The multiplicity of poisons and potential poisons (there are more than 250,000 manufactured chemical compounds in the United States) and the many routes of absorption are important ecologic factors in childhood poisoning. In addition the young child progressing through its normal development and exploratory curiosity is highly vulnerable. His vulnerability is compounded by the casual attitudes of the adults with whom he interacts and who contribute to make his environment unsafe and unprotected. Toxic episodes in children are almost always the product of adult negligence, ignorance, or poor judgment, and therefore preventable.

DEVELOPMENTAL MILESTONES. The normal toddler phase of oral exploration and insatiable curiosity and mobility and ever-growing urge to reach are major determinants in accidental poisonings. Toward the end of the first year infants who crawl and play on the floor are more likely to be poisoned by the contents of their mother's handbags or by household preparations that are generally stored on the floor, under the kitchen sink, or on low shelves. The 2- to 3-year-old child is likely to ingest products stored in cupboards, medicine chests, and bathroom cabinets including cosmetics, pharmaceutical products, and pesticides. After 4 years of age, the child becomes more cautious as he gains knowledge and experience, and the incidence of poisoning declines sharply, except in children with intellectual impairment. Accidental poisonings often occur in siblings; children of high-risk age groups who normally dislike sharing are paradoxically generous when it comes to toxic agents.

ACCESSIBILITY, CONFUSION, AND UNSAFE PRACTICES. Inadequate safety precautions in homes, particularly with regard to storage, facilitate the accessibility of toxic agents. One study showed that only in 6 percent of cases were toxic agents stored in locked medicine cabinets. In virtually all instances of poisoning, the substances involved are either improperly stored or carelessly placed within easy reach of children: on the floor, on low tables, in unlocked cabinets, or in women's handbags, a favorite and intriguing toy of children. In their own homes, physicians, dentists, pharmaceutic salesmen, and nurses are notoriously casual with potential poisons. Consequently, toxic episodes are more common in children of these professionals, due to the ready availability of samples.

Errors of mistaken identity are often made when medications of different nature, in bottles or jars similar in size, shape, or color, are placed side by side in medicine cabinets or other locations. The practice still prevails in the United States and Great Britain of dispensing medications without naming the drug on the label. It makes identification of potentially harmful agents difficult, predisposing to both accidental administrations by error and to delay in treatment when required.

Most containers in which drugs are distributed are readily opened by children. Efficiency of different types of safety devices on medication packages varies greatly and may give parents a false sense of security. Testing of package-opening abilities in children of *poison-prone* age by Jung and Done revealed that the snap-type *safety cap* is almost as easily removed as an ordinary screw cap. The palm-and-turn cap, although more difficult to manipulate, can still be opened by a significant percentage of children. However, the latter could be acceptable as child-resistant containers if, in addition, the maximum number of tablets and the potency of ingredients were strictly limited in each container. The safest method is unit packaging where tablets or capsules are sealed in individual compartments in foil or blister packs.

Removal of a toxic substance from its original container increases the risk of accidental poisoning. It is also not uncommon among certain cultural groups to buy large quantities of a product and redistribute it in unlabeled containers to friends and relatives. Dangerous preparations such as carbon tetrachloride, oil of wintergreen, kerosene, benzene, turpentine, ammonia, furniture polish, and pesticides involved in childhood poisoning are frequently found stored in drinking glasses, saucers, soda bottles, coffee cans, milk bottles, and fruit jars.

PARENTAL IGNORANCE. An important contributory factor is the lack of parental awareness of the potential toxicity both of many familiar household chemicals in daily use and of prescribed medications. Too often, parents fail to realize that the bad taste or the foul odor of a product is no protection against poisoning and that common household agents such as lye solution, gasoline, or kerosene may be ingested by a curious child who is looking for a drink or merely exploring. Physicians or pharmacists should accept the responsibility for warning parents explicitly of the inherent dangers of drugs to children.

CIRCUMSTANTIAL FACTORS. Accidental poisonings occur with greater frequency whenever there is a change, a disturbance, or deviation from the ordinary routine, such as during moving, preparation for vacation, painting the home, and during periods of stress, tension, illness, or death in the family. Visits to relatives or grandparents who are not used to the presence of children in their homes may provide access to potent medicines. Colors used to identify therapeutic agents can attract young children. There are indications that episodes of poisonings tend to recur in the same child or within the same family among siblings. Whether this repeatism is related to accident proneness of the child or the family or is the result of an accident-prone environment needs further study.

SOCIOECONOMIC FACTORS. A larger proportion of victims are children living in deprived social settings, with poor housing, overcrowding, and larger families. The higher incidence of childhood poisoning among the poor and disadvantaged is attributable to

TABLE 2. Ingredients Responsible for Toxicity in Common Household Products

Bleaches, Various Cleansing Agents, Detergents, Sanitizers, Disinfectants, Deodorants

Ammonia	Hydrochloric or Sulfuric Acid	Oxalic Acid
Benzine	Isopropanol	Phenol
Borates	Hypochlorites	Pine Oil
Carbon Tetrachloride	Kerosene	Quaternary Ammonium Compounds
Carbon Trichlorethane	Methanol	Surfactants
Cresol	Menthol	Turpentine
p-Dichlorobenzene	Na or K Hydroxide	Xylene
Formaldehyde	Naphthalene	

Cosmetics (Perfumes, After Shave Lotions, Nail Polish Removers, Hair Dyes)	Polishes, Solvents Paints, Waxes	Inks, Arts and Crafts Products
Acetone	Aromatic Hydrocarbons	Arsenic Oxide
Alcohols	Camphor	Cresols
Borax	Carbon Tetrachloride	Glycol
Essential Oils	Formaldehyde	Ketones
Lead Acetate	Methanol	Lead Oxide
Pyrogallol	Mineral Seal Oil	Oxalic Acid
Toluene	Mineral Spirits	Petroleum distillates
	Naphtha	Phenols
	Turpentine	Xylene

lack of supervision of children, poor storage facilities, and lack of information on the subject of poisons.

TOXIC AGENTS

Poisons can be ingested, inhaled, injected, or absorbed through the skin.

Ingestions

DRUGS AND HOUSEHOLD PRODUCTS. Drugs intended for internal medication cause 44 percent of all poisonings. Among these aspirin, hematinics, vitamins, antihistamines, tranquilizers, analgesics, and cough medicines are the chief offenders. Household chemicals rank next as leading poisons with soaps, cleaning agents, disinfectants, perfumes, and insecticides most frequently involved. Table 2 lists the ingredients responsible for toxicity in common household products

PLANTS. It is not uncommon for children to chew berries, leaves, or other plant constituents. More than 7,000 cases or 6 percent of all ingestions reported in 1974 to the National Clearinghouse for Poison Control Centers in the United States were plant ingestions. Ornamental plants, flowers, and shrubs (Table 3) found in the home, garden, and along suburban and rural roads may be responsible for atropinelike, digitalislike, cholinergic, or lysergic acid-type poisonings. The leaves of rhubarb contain oxalic acid; their ingestion may cause caustic burns of the esophagus and hypocalcemic convulsions.

FOODS. Even seemingly innocent edible foods may be a source of toxicity (Table 4). The exotoxin of *Clostridium botulinum* may contaminate the home-canned foodstuffs (see p.427). Contamination of wheat and rye

may cause ergotism and lathyrism. The former produces numbness of the extremities, striking circulatory changes that may lead to gangrene, skin changes, fixed miosis, and central nervous stimulation or depression; the latter causes degeneration of the posterior and lateral columns of the spine.

Poisoning by Inhalation

Inhalation of solvents, paints thinners, and the ingredients contained in insecticide sprays can be damaging to various organs, especially the nervous system, respiratory tract, and liver (Table 5). Camphor in some moth repellents and in camphorated oil may cause convulsions when inhaled. Methylbromide may be emanated from a leaky refrigerator and produce CNS toxicity. The inhalation of ethyl or isopropyl alcohol during spongebathing to reduce fever may result in alcohol intoxication and cause coma with or without hypoglycemia.

Glue and solvent sniffing continues to be a practice of school age children and preadolescents who deliberately inhale it to achieve a "high," using organic solvents contained in paint, thinners, nail polish removers, cleaning and lighter fluids, and aerosol propellants. These various substances possess certain narcotic effects and can induce states of inebriation and exhilaration. Ensuing EEG abnormalities, convulsions, and even fatalities have been documented.

Skin Absorption

The main poisons that may cause toxicity by absorption either through the broken or the intact skin are listed in Table 6. Severe poisoning may occur in infants

TABLE 3. Common Plants and Shrubs with Potential Toxicity

Plants	Plant Constituent	Poisonous Principle	Toxic Effect
Jimsonweed (Datura)	Seeds, roots, leaves	*Datura alkaloids*	Atropine-like effect
Nightshade (Solanaceae)	Berries, leaves	*Solanine, atropine*	
Lantana	Berries	*Lantanadene, lantanine*	
Morning glory (Heavenly blue)	Seeds	*Lysergic acid amide*	LDS-like effect
Larkspur (Delphinium)	Seeds	*Ajacine, delphinine*	CNS excitatory symptoms
Oleander	Leaves, flowers	*Nerioside, oleandroside*	CNS depression, paralysis miosis, bradyarrhythmia
Mountain laurel, (Yew, rhododendron, azalea)	All parts	*Taxine*	Cardiac, respiratory, and CNS depression (curare-like effect)
Foxglove	Leaves and seeds	*Digitoxin*	Digitalis-like effect
Lily of the Valley	All parts	*Convallatoxin*	
Green Hellebore	Roots and seeds	*Veratrum*	Circulatory and respiratory depressant
Monkshood (Aconite)	Roots, seeds, leaves	*Aconitine* (cholinergic)	Vagal stimulation bradycardia
Castor bean (Ricin)	Beans, seeds	*Ricin* *Ricinine*	Gastroenteritis, stupor, convulsions, circulatory collapse
Daphne	Bark, leaves, berries	*Daphnin*	Gastroenteritis, renal failure
Pokeweed (Black nightshade)	All parts (roots, shoots, unripe berries)	*Saponin*	Severe diarrhea, CNS depression coma
Poison Hemlock (Poison parsley)	Leaves and fruits during flowering	*Coniine*	Respiratory failure, convulsions
Christmas Plants			
Mistletoe	All parts	*b-Phenylethylamine and tyramine* (adrenergic)	Gastroenteritis, severe hypertension, tachy-dyspnea, CNS excitation mydriasis
Poinsettia	Sap, leaves	Unidentified	Skin and mucous membrane irritation gastroenteritis, severe
Holly (Ilex)	Red berries	*Ilicin*	Gastroenteritis severe dehydration
Vegetables			
Rhubarb	Leaves	*Oxalic acid*	Corrosive esophagitis, hypocalcemic convulsions (oxalic acid poisoning)
Potato	Leaves and sprouts	Unidentified	Depression with mental confusion
Mushrooms			
Amanita muscaria and Amanita phalloides	All parts	*Muscaria* *Phalloidine*	Parasympathomimetic effects Systemic poison

by misguided applications of boric acid, a worthless "antiseptic," to areas of denuded skin for treatment of eczema or diaper rash. *Boric acid toxicity* causes intense erythema, exfoliation of the skin, severe diarrhea and vomiting, and protracted convulsions. Neurologic symptoms may manifest themselves as late as one week after the poisoning. Boric acid poisoning is frequently fatal.

Aniline dyes freshly stamped on diapers have been responsible for nursery outbreaks of methemoglobinemia, causing severe cyanosis, coma, or convulsions in small infants. Sympathomimetic constituents of nose drops, such as tetrahydrozoline (Tyzine), dextroamphetamine (Benzedrine), or ephedrine, may be absorbed through the nasal mucosa and produce central nervous stimulation.

TABLE 4. Poisonings Associated with Ingestion of Edible Products

Agent Harmless to Adults in Moderate Amounts
Alcohol

Toxic Congeners of Edible Products
Lathyrism (Wheat)
Muscarinism (Mushroom)
Mussel Poisoning (Curare-Like-Effect)

Biologic Contamination
Botulism (Canned Food)
Ergotism (Wheat and Rye)

Chemical Contamination
"Ginger Jake" or *"Cooking Oil"* Paralysis
(Ortho-Tri-Cresyl-Phosphate)

TABLE 5. Substances Apt to Produce Toxicity by Inhalation

Acetone	Methyl bromide and/
Aniline	or chloride (refrigerant)
Chlorinated hydrocarbons	Nicotine
(DDT, dieldrin, chlordane,	Parathion
lindane)	Propyl alcohol
Camphor-naphthalene	Pyrethrum
Carbon monoxide	Turpentine
Carbon tetrachloride	
Cyanide	**Solvent sniffing**
p-Dichlorobenzene	**(glue sniffing)**
Fluoride	
Mercury vapors	Toluene
Methyl alcohol	Acetone
	Hexane

TABLE 6. Substances that May Produce Toxicity by Skin or Mucous Membrane Absorption

Skin	Phenol
Aniline	Thallium
Boric acid	Topical anesthetics
Chlorinated hydrocarbons (chlor-	Topical antihistamines
dane, toxaphene, etc.)	**Mucous Membrane**
Mercury	**(nose drops)**
Nicotine	
Organophosphates (parathion,	Dextroamphetamine (benzedrine)
malathion)	Ephedrine
	Tyzine (tetrahyrozoline HCl)

DIAGNOSIS

Unless the ingestion or the contact with poison has been witnessed or there is sufficient circumstantial evidence to suggest its occurrence, the diagnosis of poisoning may be exceedingly difficult. Presenting symptoms of intoxication, generally nonspecific, vary considerably and physical examination seldom offers a definite clue to the nature of the poison. Consequently, a high index of suspicion should be maintained, particularly in the high-risk age group. Poisoning should always be considered as a possible etiology in the presence of any sudden or progressive illness of unknown cause or in any situation where the differential diagnosis is an enigma.

Physical and/or Chemical Identification of Toxins

Some toxic agents may be identified by odor, rarely by their other physical attributes such as shape, size, or color. Thus the *odor* of vomitus, breath, or gastric aspirate may prove helpful in cases of poisoning with alcohol, benzene, kerosene, organophosphates, carbon tetrachloride, oil of wintergreen, phenol, ether, chloroform, or paraldehyde. The odor of violets in the vomitus or urine may suggest turpentine or eucalyptol poisoning; the odor of bitter almonds, cyanide poisoning; and a garliclike odor, phosphorus or arsenic. For some poisons, available rapid chemical tests are listed in Table 7.

Clinical Clues

It may require detailed and oriented questioning to obtain a positive history. A history of *pica*, if elicited, should call attention to the possibility of poisoning, particularly lead. The symptoms associated most frequently with acute poisonings are burning in mouth and throat, vomiting, nausea and respiratory difficulty, abdominal pain, diarrhea, circulatory collapse, altered consciousness, and/or seizures. These manifestations can, however, be produced by many other diseases. Some poisons produce characteristic clinical manifestations that may help to establish the diagnosis and to identify the agent, as summarized in Table 8.

TREATMENT

Every case of poisoning must be viewed and handled as an emergency. The primary objective of treatment is to rid the patient of the toxic substance and/or to prevent or counter the damaging effects that may already have occurred. Speed is critical for removal of ingested toxins, since they pass rapidly from the stomach into the intestinal tract, and from there into the circulatory system. Time should not be wasted searching for nonexistent antidotes. On the other hand, a therapeutic test in specific instances with antidotes such as narcan or atropine may help to establish a presumptive diagnosis. Overtreatment must be avoided, since it may at times be more harmful than the poison itself.

Telephone instructions to the parent to induce vomiting when the poisoning is first reported could be lifesaving. Vomiting may be induced by the parent by gagging the child with the blunt edge of a spoon or with the finger, which should be protected to prevent injury from biting. This procedure is more effective if preceded by a few small swallows of milk or warm water. It is essential to instruct the mother to hold the child on her lap in "spanking position"—head down and facing the floor—to prevent aspiration and to save the vomitus for later examination. In certain situations, such as ingestion of corrosive agents, vomiting is contraindicated (p. 1038).

Other first aid measures may be advised by the physi-

TABLE 7. Diagnostic Screening Tests

Poison	Test and/or reagent	Specimen	Ratio specimen/reagent	Result or reaction
Salicylates	Ferrichloride (10%) or phenistix	U,G	4:1	Purple color
Phenothiazines (except piperazine derivatives)	Ferrichloride (10%) gtt ii + H$_2$SO$_4$ (gtt vi), or phenistix	U,G	4:1 (gtt viii/2ml)	Pink — lilac color
Arsenic, mercury, antimony	Copper wire (Reisch test) (2 ml KCl+ Cu strip)	U,V	5:1 + Cu strip	Black deposit
Ferrous sulfate	1. K ferri-/ferro-cyanide test (10%)	V or GF	5:1	Prussian blue color
	2. Desferol infusion test	U	15 mg/kg	Brown color (wine)
Lead	Coproporphyrinuria ether+ glac. acetic acid (20 ml) + HCl(1.5n) (5 ml) + 0,1% alcoholated iodine (0,25 ml)	U	NA	Pink → red UV fluorescence (Wood's light)
Boric acid	Turmeric paper	U	NA	Brown color
Thallium	Platinum wire loop	U	NA	Green flame
Phosphorus	Luminescence	U,S,G,V	NA	Luminescence
Barbiturate	EEG			High frequency pattern

U = Urine, V = vomitus, G = gastric content, S = stools, F = filtrat, NA = not applicable.

cian before he arrives on the scene. If the poison was inhaled, as with carbon monoxide, the patient should be removed to another area that is well ventilated; artificial respiration may be required. If the toxic substance was spilled on the skin or eyes, washing the contaminated parts with copious quantities of water should be advised.

Poison Control Centers

Valuable information about poisons and assistance regarding specific treatment can be obtained from local poison control centers. The location of the nearest center should be known to every practicioner. In the United States, under the aegis of the Department of Health, Education, and Welfare, there are now more than 500 local poison control centers established in all states and territories. Some of these are staffed 24 hours a day by physicians. The National Clearinghouse for Poisons in Washington, DC, is also an invaluable resource for assistance to the pediatrician.

Treatment for poisoning is based on the following general principles of management (Table 9):

Rapid evacuation of the poison;
Administration of a specific antidote, if available, or of a chemical neutralizer;
Concurrent institution of supportive and symptomatic therapy.

Exclusive of poisons for which there are specific antidotes, speedy evacuation and supportive and symptomatic therapy are the mainstays of treatment and should be instituted immediately and concomitantly. While every attempt should be made to identify the toxic agent, gastric evacuation and institution of supportive therapy should not be delayed until the poison is identified.

Gastric Evacuation

The most effective initial approach is to remove from the stomach as much of the toxic agent as possible before it is absorbed. In many instances this can be accomplished either by inducing *emesis* mechanically or pharmacologically (syrup of ipecac) or by prompt *gastric lavage*. Contraindications to both gastric lavage and induced vomiting for fear of aspiration are poisoning with ammonia and other corrosive alkalis or acids, kerosene and other petroleum products, and in case of coma or convulsion, unless the patient has been intubated and the cuffed endotracheal tube is inflated. Gastric lavage is contraindicated after ingestion of corrosive alkali or acids because of the risk of perforation of the esophagus. In symptomatic patients with strychnine, glutethimide, barbiturate, or antihistamine poisoning prophylactic endotracheal intubation prior to gastric lavage is indicated because of the danger of laryngospasm.

Ipecac syrup USP,* an effective emetic, is the pharmacologic agent of choice to induce vomiting in cases

*Syrup of ipecac should never be confused with the highly toxic fluid extract of ipecac, which has caused serious illness and death; the fluid extract should never be available in the home or the hospital emergency room.

TABLE 8. Diagnosis of Poisoning Specific Manifestations

Central nervous system

Altered consciousness (somnolence, stupor, or coma)
Narcotics, hypnotics, sedatives, alcohols, tranquilizers, antihistaminics, psychoactive drugs, carbon monoxide

Convulsions
Amphetamine, strychnine, camphor, atropin, boric acid, ephedrin, oxalates and cholinesterase inhibitors, chlorinated hydrocarbons, fluoracetates, fluorides; also salicylates, dextropropoxyphene, gluthetimide, meperidine, alcohols, reserpin, diphenylhydantoin, carbon monoxide diphenhydramine

Hyperexcitability, agitation, confusion, garrulousness, and delirium
Belladonna alkaloids, cocaine, hallucinatory drugs, amphetamines, barbiturates, carbon monoxide

Extrapyramidal rigidity (drowsiness, lethargy; oculogyric crises)
Phenothiazine derivatives, reserpine

Muscle spasms
Strychnine, black widow spider and sting ray bites

Myoclonic movements
Piperazine derivatives, reserpine

Ataxia
Alcohol, diphenylhydantoin, dextropropoxyphene, dextromethorphan

Autonomous nervous system
Cholinergic syndrome (miosis, bradycardia, sweating, salivation, lacrimation)
Organophosphates, muscarin, reserpine

Specific ocular manifestations

Fixed mydriasis
Atropine, belladonna derivatives, gluthetimide, amphetamine, cocaine, ephedrine

Fixed miosis (pinpoint pupils)
Opiates, meperidine, dextropropoxyphene, pilocarpine, nicotine, muscarin, ergot, organic phosphoric esters

Ptosis
Botulism, thallium, dextropropoxyphene

Nystagmus
Diphenylhydantoin, dextropropoxyphene

Strabismus
Botulism

Specific skin manifestations

Cherry red color
Carbon monoxide

Pallor
Ergot, sympathomimetic derivatives

Cyanosis (methemoglobinemia)
Nitrates, nitrites, pyridium, potassium chlorate, aniline dyes, bismuth subnitrate, dinitrobenzene, phenacetin, sulfanilamide, toluidine, resercinol, xylidine

Flushing and dryness
Belladonna alkaloid, reserpine, alcohol, diphenhydramine (Benadryl)

Alternating flushing and pallor
Camphor

Sweating
Salicylates, quinine, organophosphates, pilocarpine, physostigmine

Exfoliative dermatitis
Boric acid

Cardiac rate and rhythm disturbances

Irregular
Digitalis, quinine, imioramine

Slow
Organophosphates, pilocarpin, physostigmine

Rapid
Amphetamines, aminophylline, belladonna alkaloids

Respiratory depression
Organophosphates, opiates and analgesics, cocaine, sedatives, tranquilizers

Oliguria/albuminuria
Mercury, lead

Gastrointestinal manifestations
Iron salts and other heavy metals, boric acid, cocaine, oxalates, fluorides, caustic agents, inorganic phosphorus, organic cholinesterase inhibitors

Specific systemic disturbances

Acidosis
Salicylates, methanol, quinine, formaldehyde, ethylene glycol, phenphormin

Hyperpyrexia
Salicylates, quinine, aminophylline, diphenhydramine (Benadryl), belladonna alkaloids, alcohol

---

of acute poisoning, except where vomiting is contraindicated. We do not use apomorphine, copper sulfate, or tartar emetic because of the toxicity of these agents. Syrup of ipecac is relatively safe in a dose of 15 ml after 1 year of age. Since most poisonous ingestions occur in the home, it is recommended that this effective emetic be stored and readily accessible in all homes with toddlers. Dangers inherent in the presence of ipecac in the home medicine chest has been eliminated by limiting the amount of syrup available for over the counter sale to 30 ml. However, if emesis fails to occur following ipecac administration, it will be absorbed and its own potential toxic effects will be added to those of the poison for which it was given. If a second dose proves ineffective, the stomach should be evacuated by other means. Although experimentally ipecac-induced vomit-

TABLE 9. General Principles in the Management of Poisoning

I Specific therapy

1. Gastric evacuation
2. Neutralizers
3. Antidotes

II General supportive

1. Restoration and/or maintenance of
   Circulation = i.v. fluids (and p.r.n. CCCM*/catecholamines/ defibrillation)
   Airway, ventilation, oxygenation = suction and p.r.n.: oral airway/endotracheal intubation/tracheostomy; assisted ventilation; O$_2$

2. Restoration and/or maintenance of
   Blood glucose
   Acid-base balance = (bicarbonate therapy)
   Fluid and electrolyte balance

3. Prevention and treatment of
   Cerebral edema: judicious fluid therapy and *p.r.n.:* mannitol, hypothermia, dexamethasone, hyperventilation
   Seizures: anticonvulsants

III Repeated assessments of patient's status

Consciousness and pupils
Cardiocirculatory status (BP; cardiac rate and rhythm; EKG)
Respiratory status (rate, pattern, pulmonary gas exchange)
Excretory status (urine output, concentration, pH, and chemistry)
Metabolic status (blood gases and pH, Ionogram, glucose)
Toxicology

CCCM = closed chest cardiac massage.

ing in dogs has been shown to be more effective in emptying contents of the stomach than gastric lavage, there is still considerable controversy regarding the relative merits of gastric lavage versus ipecac-induced emesis. The two modalities are probably not mutually exclusive and both can be used judiciously and advantageously. When emesis fails, gastric lavage may prove effective. However, since it may take 20 to 30 minutes for syrup of ipecac to induce emesis, the time element may preclude its use in severe poisonings, in which case gastric lavage would appear to be the method of choice. Pharmacologically induced emesis is not an effective procedure in phenothiazine poisoning, in patients who have taken an antiemetic or depressant drug, or when manifest toxic signs due to absorption of the poison have already appeared.

Antidotes, Chemical Neutralizers, Adsorbents, and Laxatives

Chemical neutralizing agents (milk, alkali, mild acids, nontoxic oxidizing or reducing substances), nonspecific adsorbents, and demulcents such as activated charcoal which decrease intestinal absorption of many poisons should be available in places where such emergencies are to be handled. Some chemical neutralizers (Table 10) modify the poison chemically into an inert or less toxic compound, decrease its systemic effects, and act as local antidotes.

Activated charcoal, to be kept in a "black bottle to catch the eye," is a very effective chemical adsorbent because of its broad spectrum of activity and its exceedingly rapid inactivation of the poison. Activated charcoal USP is treated to increase its adsorptive power. Other forms of charcoal are useless because they lack these properties. The value of activated charcoal as an emergency measure is confined to the first phase of therapy-inactivation of the poison before its absorption into the bloodstream. It is effective against most poisons, except cyanide, and more potent and safer than the so-called universal antidote, which contains tannic acid as well as charcoal. Burnt toast, which is frequently recommended as a substitute for activated charcoal, possesses no adsorptive capacity and is of no practical value in the treatment of poisoning. Ipecac and charcoal should not be given concomitantly since the former would be adsorbed, rendering both treatments ineffective.

Saline cathartics such as sodium or magnesium sulfate may be used to speed the elimination of poisons that have already left the stomach or cannot be recovered by gastric evacuation.

ANTIDOTES. Contrary to a widespread and erroneous belief there are, in fact, only very few effective specific antidotes (Table 11). The narcotic antagonist narcan, which is considerably safer than its predecessors nalorphin and levallorphan, promptly abolishes many of the effects of morphine, codeine, and mor-

TABLE 10. Chemical Neutralizers with Some Local Antidote Effect

Neutralizer	Poison
Activated charcoal	Alcohol, alkaloids, antibiotics, barbiturates, camphor, heavy metals, glutethimide, organophosphates, oxalic acid, phenol, *d*-propoxyphene, salicylates
Ammonium acetate	Formaldehyde
Bicarbonate, (Na)	Iron, methanol
Calcium gluconate or lactate	Fluorides, oxalic acid, and DDT
Formaldehyde sulfoxalate, Na	Mercury
Iodide, (Na or K)	Thallium
Starch	Iodide
Sulfate Salts (Na or Mg)	Barium Salts (acid soluble)

TABLE 11. Antidotes

Antidote	Poison
1. Atropine (antagonizes muscarinic effect/of acetylcholine) 0.2 mg/yr of age up to 2.0 mg	*Amanita muscaria* (1) (atropine)
2. 2-Pam (pralidoxime chloride), 25-50 mg/kg	Organic phosphate esters (1,2) (atropin and PAM)
Desferroxiamine (15 mg/kg/h x 6)	Iron
Ethyl alcohol (15-30 ml/q 4 h.)	Methyl alcohol
Methylene blue (1% sol.) 1 mg/kg	Nitrites, nitrate, aniline dyes
Naloxone H Cl (Narcan) inj, vial: 0.4 mg/ml - 0.01 mg/kg	Opiates, synthetic and 1/2 synthetic narcotics (heroin, meperidine, diphenoxylate, *d*-propoxyphene, methadone)
Nitrite amyl. Perles 0.3 ml (inhalation) Nitrite, sodium (3% sol. i.v.) 6-8 ml/m²at 3-5 ml/min Sodium thiosulfate (25% sol i.v.) 50 ml (12.5 g)	Cyanide

phinelike synthetic or semisynthetic compounds such as heroin, methadone, meperidine (Demerol), dextropropoxyphene (Darvon), and diphenoxylate (Lomotil). For the treatment of organic phosphate poisonings such as parathion, 2-PAM (2-pyridine aldoxime methiodide) has proved effective in conjunction with atropine. Amyl nitrite, by inhalation, and sodium nitrite and sodium thiosulfate, intravenously, may be lifesaving in cyanide poisoning, as may be methylene blue in methemoglobinemia.

Exchange Transfusion and Dialysis

In severe poisoning with dialyzable and nephrotoxic substances, exchange transfusions, extracorporeal hemodialysis, or peritoneal dialysis may be lifesaving procedures.

Exchange transfusion is practical only in very small children. In addition to the technical difficulties, it also carries the risk of serum hepatitis. This procedure may be helpful, however, for certain dangerous poisonings in which metabolites accumulate and have serious late effects such as methanol, ethylene glycol, and possible iron poisoning.

Dialysis effectively removes a variety of organic compounds from the blood such as barbiturates, salicylates, boric acid, carbon tetrachloride, anticonvulsants, and other materials. *Intermittent peritoneal dialysis* is safe and effective. It has a distinct advantage in that it can be instituted readily and requires a minimum of equipment. Improvements in equipment and technique have made this procedure increasingly useful; a plastic catheter is introduced through a hollow trocar used for ordinary abdominal paracentesis. The availability of commercially prepared dialyzing fluids greatly facilitates its use. The addition of 2 to 5 percent albumin to the dialyzing fluid increases the rate at which protein-bound poisons such as barbiturates and salicylates are removed.

Hemodialysis is less applicable to young children; it

should be performed only in specialized centers. The indications for its use have become progressively more limited in recent years.

PREVENTION OF CHILDHOOD POISONING

Pediatricians have a major responsibility in the field of poison prevention. Epidemiologic studies have shown that the vast majority of accidental poisonings in children is preventable by applying ordinary safety precautions in the packaging, use, handling, and storage of medicinal agents and household chemicals.

The pediatrician should inform and educate the general public about the danger and prevention of poisoning, guide and counsel individual families, and teach medical and paramedical hospital staff during training. It is also of major importance that he and his aides be familiar with the location and functioning of the nearest poison control center and that all instances of poisonings be reported, including untoward drug reactions.

In his community, on a regional and on a nationwide scale, the physician can motivate community groups and government agencies to inaugurate safety programs. Furthermore, every physician must feel a personal responsibility to see that on a nationwide scale the general public be adequately protected. The marketing of potentially toxic products must be subjected to stringent regulations. Distribution of dangerous preparations must be prohibited, unless sufficient protection is provided against the possible harmful effects by the use of safe packaging and danger warnings. The use of child-resistant containers to package solid prescription medications can reduce significantly the amount of accidental poisoning. In the United States, labeling of common household preparations is mandatory under the law, but labels are not always understood by all users. An important step toward the prevention of many iatrogenic poisonings is the obligatory inclusion of brochures and package circulars to physicians on new drugs specifying dosage, contraindications, side reactions and toxicity, and treatment of overdosage. Other nationwide safety measures that may contribute to reduce the danger of poisons are the voluntary or mandatory implementation of limits on the amount of tablets in a retail container to an amount quantitatively safe for children, a caution to be printed on each package to keep out of the reach of children, and the inclusion of a warning on the package, "In case of accidental overdose, contact a physician immediately."

Every physician must assume scrupulously safe personal habits and practices. All drugs should be ordered and dispensed at the lowest effective dosage; prescriptions should be limited to the smallest amounts of medicine sufficient to meet immediate needs. Specific and detailed recommendations, verbal and written, must be left with adult members of the family about the dosage, time interval, and internal or external use. Parents must be warned explicitly about the inherent danger for children for any drug that is prescribed or dispensed. It is good practice to instruct parents that whenever labels are lost from containers, their contents should be destroyed. Drugs must never be used if outdated, discolored, or in any way deteriorated. Explicit instructions must be given to destroy, and not merely to discard, all leftovers.

The pediatrician can and must contribute to rendering homes safer for children. His waiting room should contain educational material about the accidental poisoning problem and precautionary measures to be employed for its elimination. During home visits, he must observe possible existing poison hazards, prevail upon the families to eliminate them, provide education, and show the need for safe practices in the handling and safekeeping of drugs and other potentially dangerous substances. The importance of storing all hazardous preparations out of the reach of children must be repeatedly stressed. A safety list may profitably be distributed to parents.

In conclusion, in his role as the family ecologist, the pediatrician must constantly be guided by the principle that many more lives can be saved and an untold number of poisonings prevented if the available knowledge about household poison protection gained wider and more immediate application.

Bibliography

CHILDHOOD POISONINGS

Angle CR, McIntire MS, Meile RL: Neurologic sequelae in poisoning in children. J Pediatr 73:531, 1968

Arena JM: The general management of acute poisoning. Drug Therapy, May, 1973

——— Poisoning. CC Thomas, Springfield, Ill, 1975

Baltimore CL, Meyer RJ: A study of storage, child behavioral traits, and mother's knowledge of toxicology in 52 poisoned families and 52 comparison families. Pediatrics 42:312, 1968

Berenson MM, Temple AR: Detergent toxicity: effects on esophageal and gastric mucosa. Clin Toxicol 8:399, 1975

Bureau of Product Safety. US Department of Health, Education, and Welfare. Washington DC, Typical Poisonous Plants, US Government Printing Office, 0-49-626, 1973

Corby DG, Decker WJ: Management of acute poisoning with activated charcoal. Pediatrics 54:324, 1974

Cushman TM, Shirkey KC: Emergency management of poisoning. Pediatr Clin North Am 17:525, 1970

Deeths TM, Breeden GT: Poisonings in children—a statistical study of 1,057 cases. J Pediatr 78:299, 1971

Done AK: Poisoning from common household products. Pediatr Clin North Am 17:569, 1970

Einhorn AH: How Not to Poison Children. In Ecology and Pediatrics, Postgraduate Seminars, Vol 38. Einhorn AH, Zurbrügg R (eds), Karger Verlag, Basel, London, New York, 1974, pp 87–113

Gaultier M, Gervais P, Frejaville JP, Efthymiou M: Toxicologie, Vol 15. Flammarion Medicine Sciences, Paris, 1972

Gleason MN, Gosselin RD, Hodge HC: Clinical Toxicology of Commercial Products, 3rd ed. Williams and Wilkins, Baltimore, 1969

Hardin JW, Arena JM: Human Poisoning from Native and Cultivated Plants. Duke University Press, Durham, NC, 1974

Lampe KF: Systemic plant poisoning in children. Pediatrics 54:347, 1974

——— Fagerstrom R: Plant Toxicity. Williams and Wilkins, Baltimore, 1968

Lehr EL: Carbon monoxide poisoning. A preventable environmental hazard. J Public Health 60:289, 1970

McLean WC Jr: A comparison of ipecac syrup and apomorphine in the immediate treatment of ingestion of poisoning. J Pediatr 82:121, 1973

Mofenson HC, Greensher J: The unknown poison. Pediatrics 54:336, 1974

——— Greensher J: Peritoneal dialysis, an outline of the procedure. Clin Pediatr 11:534, 1972

Moss MH: Alcohol-induced hypoglycemia and coma caused by alcohol sponging. Pediatrics 46:445, 1970

National Clearinghouse for Poison Control Centers, US Department of Health, Education, and Welfare. Bureau of Drugs of the FDA, Bethesda (Maryland) Bulletins 1972 though 1975; Tabulations of 1973 reports May-June, 1974; Tabulations of Deaths from Accidental Poisoning 1971, 1972, and 1973, Sept-Oct. 1975.

Picchioni AL, Chin L, Laird HE: Activated charcoal preparations—relative antidote efficency. Clin Toxicol 7:97, 1974

Reid HSD: Treatment of the poisoned child. Arch Dis Child 45:428, 1970

Rosenbaum JL, Kramer MS, Raja R: Resin hemoperfusion. A new treatment for acute drug intoxication. N Engl J Med 284:874, 1971

Shirley HC: Ipecac syrup, its use as an emetic in poison control. J Pediatr 69:139, 1966

Sobel R, Margolis JA: Repetitive poisoning in children: a psychosocial study. Pediatrics 35:641, 1965

Wehrle PF, De Freest L, Penhollow J: Epidemiology of accidental poisoning in an urban population. The repeater problem. Pediatrics 27:614, 1961

Weissman N: Laboratory Aids in Toxicological Problems. Bio-Science Laboratories, Van Nuys, Calif, 1974

POISONING WITH SPECIFIC AGENTS

ARNOLD H. EINHORN

Harmful substances that can be ingested accidentally by a child are so numerous and so varied that it is impractical to include in this section a listing or description of all such substances and the specific therapy for each product. For such information reference should be made to textbooks of clinical toxicology, and valuable help can often be obtained from the nearest Poison Control or Information Center of which there are more than 500 in the United States.

The specific poisons discussed in detail in this section are especially frequent and important in children. The following have been selected for consideration in this section:

Therapeutic agents: salicylates and iron. Poisonings due to narcotics, sedatives, and stimulants are described in the section on Drug Abuse, (p. 809)

Household products: kerosene and organophosphate, insecticides. The effects and treatment of corrosive esophagitis secondary to the ingestion of caustic cleaning agents are discussed in the section on Gastrointestinal Diseases

Heavy metals: chronic lead poisoning

Venom: snake bites

SALICYLATE INTOXICATION

LAURENCE FINBERG

EPIDEMIOLOGY

Until 1973, salicylate poisoning, most often from aspirin, ranked as the most common reported poison ingested by young children in the United States. Aspirin is found in some form in virtually every household, primarily in two dosage forms: the "adult" tablet of 300 mg and the children's size of 75 mg. In addition, aspirin is an ingredient in many mixtures for analgesia and "cold" remedies and is frequently coupled with buffers and other adjuvants. The children's size may be flavored, making tablets more attractive; however, the risks of serious toxicity have generally been worse with adult tablet because of greater dosage and because the children's size is usually dispensed in small containers thus limiting total dosage.

During the past few years, improved safety packaging and a trend toward other antipyretics have reduced the overall incidence of salicylate poisoning in toddlers, and hospitalization figures have clearly fallen in many areas of the United States.

Acute single ingestions in toddlers, the most common type of salicylate poisoning, has a seasonal prevalance coinciding with the respiratory illness season probably because the drug is apt to be more readily accessible when the child or a family member has a mild febrile illness. The child suffering from an infection becomes more vulnerable to salicylate toxicity probably owing to depleted glycogen stores and increased oxygen demand.

CHEMISTRY AND PHARMACOLOGY

Salicylic acid is orthohydroxybenzoic acid. Aspirin is formed by acetylating the hydroxy group. Methyl salicylate or oil of wintergreen is another form of salicylate available in households because of its rubefacient quality in liniments. All of these compounds are absorbed from the duodenum, principally as salicylic acid following intestinal acetylase or demethylation activity; some aspirin (2 percent) is absorbed intact. Both salicylate salts and aspirin are absorbed very rapidly and com-

pletely, methyl salicylate more slowly, owing to its oily nature, which slows gastric emptying. Absorption is retarded by food in the stomach.

The toxic dosage on a single ingestion varies somewhat in individuals; 200 mg/kg of weight is virtually always toxic and symptomatic, but less than 100 mg/kg usually is without danger; in the intermediate ranges toxicity varies with individual vulnerability. Methyl salicylate probably has no greater toxicity than aspirin, but the liquid preparation is almost a pure compound with a density greater than 1. Thus, 5 ml of oil of wintergreen contains about 5,000 mg of methyl salicylate, an enormous dose for a toddler. The rate of absorption for aspirin on an empty stomach is very rapid with peak blood levels occurring in 90 to 120 minutes and complete absorption in a slightly longer time.

Once in the blood, salicylate (though not the small amount of intact aspirin absorbed) becomes bound to plasma albumin. The binding sites are quickly saturated even after a therapeutic dose. These bonds are not tight, permitting the salicylate to diffuse throughout body water. Since salicylic acid is a weak or poorly ionized acid, the ionized form will increase in the more alkaline regions wherever a pH gradient with an alkaline component exists.

Salicylate is slowly conjugated in the liver with glycine to salicyluric acid and with glucuronic acid to form acyl and phenolic glucuronides. These compounds are ultimately excreted in the urine together with some free salicylic acid; these three forms account for about 90 percent of the ingested dose.

Toxicity—Single Ingestion

The most striking and important toxic effects relate to a marked disturbance of acid-base physiology, which results from three independent types of toxicity.

An *encephalopathy* occurs with a particular predilection for the respiratory center of the medulla, which reacts with a primary hyperpnea. Whether the drug reaches the center's cells directly via the bloodstream or must first enter the cerebrospinal fluid through the choroid plexus has not been established; this effect occurs within a few minutes after a toxic level is reached in the plasma suggesting a direct route. In severe toxicity the central nervous system shows a diffuse encephalopathy with convulsions, but this occurs late in the course. A result of primary hyperventilation is a reduced P_{CO_2}, which causes a rise in plasma pH when no offsetting factors are present. Over the age of about 5 years, patients will usually show, for some time, a primary respiratory alkalemia.

Salicylate *uncouples oxidative phosphorylation* by an unexplained mechanism. This increases oxygen consumption and metabolism resulting in increased carbon dioxide and heat production tending to increase P_{CO_2}, but this effect is less than that of hyperpnea.

By *inhibiting dehydrogenase and aminotransferase enzymes,* salicylate blocks the Krebs cycle and profoundly alters carbohydrate metabolism. The net metabolic result of this toxic inhibition is the accumulation of the keto acids, acetoacetic and β-hydroxybutyric. These in turn reduce the HCO_3^- concentration of the extracellular fluid. This effect ultimately predominates over the first at any age; however, in the toddler and infant, the predominance is asserted very early because of the more rapid metabolism characteristic of this age.

The net result of these multiple toxicities on acid-base status may be quite confusing but in the toddler at least the picture is predictable. The PCO_2 will be very low, a metabolic acidosis will develop early, and within a few hours acidemia will occur. This in turn retards the excretion of salicylate because of the renal correction of acidemia through formation of an acid urine containing little or no free salicylate.

Toxic effects of salicylate usually only become manifest in the more chronic poisoning that accompanies overly vigorous therapy. The most important of these changes are *hematologic* and *renal.*

There are three known mechanisms by which salicylates promote hemorrhage. First, the acetyl radical of aspirin damages platelet ATP formation and thus makes them nonadherent. This takes place with therapeutic levels and permanently damages the affected platelets but not newly formed thrombocytes. The biologic consequence is reduced platelet function for about 48 hours after aspirin ingestion. A second effect is on prothrombin formation by the liver. While such an effect may be demonstrated in acute poisoning, it is not clinically significant except in chronic states. Also salicylic acid irritates gastric mucosa and may cause erosive bleeding. Again, except in chronic toxicity, the three effects rarely cause hemorrhage or require corrective therapy.

Renal epithelium is damaged by salicylate intoxication. In chronic poisoning or neglected acute poisoning, when coupled with secondary dehydration, oliguria or even anuria may occur.

Clinical Signs and Symptoms

As the discussion of the pathophysiology suggests, when the toddler has ingested a toxic dose of salicylates, the first visible sign will be hyperventilation. Anorexia, vomiting, dehydration, fever (paradoxically, but expectedly, from increased metabolism), coma, convulsions, and anuria may supervene. Hypernatremia from increased insensible water loss and diaphoresis may occur and, for poorly understood reasons, hypokalemia often occurs so long as urine formation continues.

In older children on continued therapy, tinnitus may be an early symptom of toxicity. In long-term toxicity, hemorrhage, liver damage, and albuminuria have all been observed.

DIAGNOSIS AND TREATMENT

Diagnosis is made primarily by history or by suspecting salicylate ingestion from symptoms and metabolic consequences. In the absence of a history, the diagnosis can be confused with acute lower respiratory infection, encephalitis, or diabetic acidosis. Confirmation of salicylate poisoning is obtained by measuring serum salicylate levels. In single-dose poisoning mild toxicity is generally associated with levels of 30 to 40 mg/100 ml; moderate toxicity with levels of 40 to 60 mg/100 ml; and severe toxicity with levels of over 60 mg/100 ml. Done has pointed out that because of the biphasic curve of salicylate levels caused by albumin binding followed by diffusion, a nomogram relating level to time after ingestion is a more reliable predictor of toxicity. Figure 2 shows this relationship.

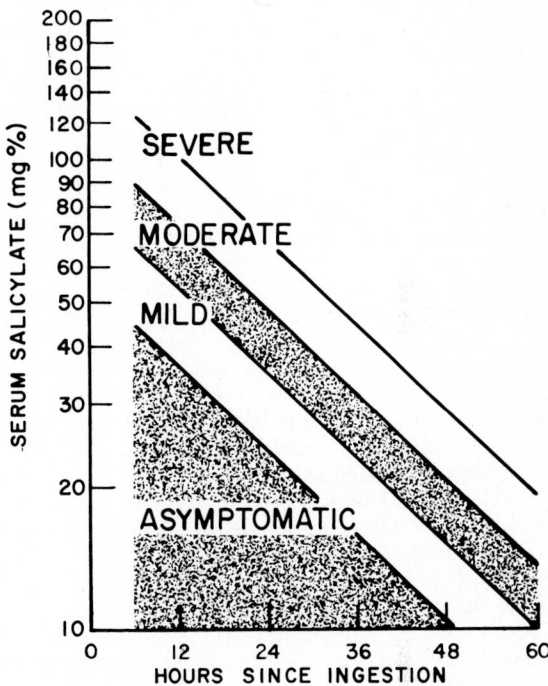

Fig. 2. Nomogram relating plasma salicylate concentration as a function of time following ingestion to severity of intoxication. (from Done AK, Pediatrics 26:800, 1960)

If the child is seen shortly after the ingestion, attempts should be made to remove the drug from the stomach. For this purpose, induction of emesis by ipecac or mechanically is more satisfactory than gastric lavage. Further treatment of single-toxic ingestion is aimed at prevention or correction of the pathophysiologic processes described above and removal of salicylate from the body. This requires appropriate fluid replacement and sufficient base to prevent or correct acidemia. Removal of the drug presents practical difficulties.

At present salicylate must be removed through the urine or by some exchange or dialysis procedure. No way is known to speed hepatic detoxification or to neutralize the molecule. If the patient is producing urine, theoretically the excretion of salicylate may be readily accomplished because an alkaline urine greatly enhances excretion owing to the diffusion of the anionic salicylate radical into an alkaline medium. Over the physiologic range of pH for urine, the excretion may be increased about 100-fold by securing a urine pH of 8 or greater. In practice, there are some difficulties. If the patient is severely acidemic, the amount of base necessary to infuse may be so enormous that the quantity of sodium salts needed (bicarbonate, lactate, or succinate) may produce hypernatremia and even pulmonary edema. Lesser amounts may fail to produce an alkaline urine.

Accordingly, the suggestion has been made that a carbonic anhydrase inhibitor, acetazolamide, be used to facilitate the administration of base. However, there is a theoretic risk if the acetazolamide were to be given without adequate base. Bicarbonate losses in the urine would produce further acidemia and thus facilitate entry of salicylate into the temporarily more alkaline cerebrospinal fluid and brain. This has been demonstrated in experimental animals. Therefore, use of acetazolamide must be preceded by an intravenous solution containing sodium bicarbonate or sodium lactate. When this is done the HCO_3^- concentration in serum rises throughout therapy. The concentration of base should be varied with the severity and duration of the acidosis or acidemia from as low as 1/18M (40 mEq/liter) to 1/6 M (167 mEq/liter). Once the urine has become alkaline—a catheter is warranted for collection—the lower concentration will suffice. Potassium salts should be added to therapy because of primary hypokalemia and because acetazolamide increases potassium loss. The infusion rate should be maintained at a high rate to maximize urine flow. The dose of acetazolamide is 5 mg/kg, intramuscularly, after the intravenous bicarbonate-containing solution is in place, repeated twice at 5-hour intervals.

We have treated over 1,000 hospitalized patients with this regimen, when the salicylate level was over 30 mg/100 ml. In several instances the level exceeded 150 mg/100 ml and in 2 cases it was over 200, a level at which a favorable outcome is not expected. Only one patient died during this time, not apparently related to adverse effect of therapy, and two others had a convulsion after being seen. One of these occurred prior to acetazolamide administration; the other occurred on the second day when the salicylate was largely excreted. With the exception of the above, all patients have done well, without sequelae. If acetazolamide is not used, similar fluid therapy is usually successful over a longer time, though one must guard against hypernatremic states.

When oliguria is present because of either preexisting or concomitant renal injury, either peritoneal or hemodialysis is in order for severe poisoning. Intermittent peritoneal dialysis, particularly incorporating a final concentration of 5 percent albumin, is a useful and relatively safe procedure for young infants and children. Exchange transfusion is very inefficient for this purpose and is not recommended. In chronic poisoning vitamin K administration is appropriate and so may be a platelet infusion if overt hemorrhage has occurred and the offending salicylate was aspirin.

Bibliography

Done AK: Salicylate intoxication. Pediatrics 26:800, 1960

Feuerstein RC, Finberg L, Fleishman E: The use of acetazolamide in the therapy of salicylate poisoning. Pediatrics 25:215, 1960

Hill JB: Experimental salicylate poisoning. Pediatrics 47:658, 1971

Levy G, Tsuchiya T: Salicylate accumulation kinetics in man. N Engl J Med 287:430, 1972

Reimold EW, Worthen HG, Reilly P: Salicylate poisoning. Am J Dis 125:668, 1973

Smith MJH, Smith PK: The Salicylates. Interscience, New York, 1966

Winters RW: In Winters RW (ed): The Body Fluids in Pediatrics, Chap 24. Little, Brown, Boston, 1973, p 483

IRON POISONING

Arnold H. Einhorn

The widespread usage of medicinal iron and iron-containing preparations has been paralleled by an increase in the incidence of acute iron poisoning in children. In 1973 iron-containing compounds ranked third in the United States among the drugs responsible for fatalities from poisoning in children under 5 years of age, and second in Great Britain and other Western European countries. The lay public is generally not aware of the inherent danger of iron. The product frequently is present in the victim's home as part of therapy prescribed either to the prenatal mother or to a member of the household. Unfortunately, specific warnings about the dangerous consequences of iron overdose to children are rarely conveyed to expectant mothers.

PRODUCTS

On the United States pharmaceutical market there are presently a large number and wide variety of iron-containing oral *hematinics*, differing in their iron composition. Some are dispensed as brightly and attractively colored pills or tablets, suggesting candies, or as pleasantly flavored and aromatized syrups. Ferrous sulphate is the product most widely prescribed and most often incriminated in toxic poisoning episodes; preparations with gluconate or fumarate salts are also used frequently.

Ferrous sulphate USP, the hydrated salt contains 20 percent elemental iron; the official tablets contain 300 mg of the salt (60 mg of iron); the syrup USP, 40 mg/ml of the salt (8 mg of iron); and the pediatric drops, 25 mg/ml of the salt (5 mg of iron). *Ferrous gluconate* contains only 12 percent and *ferrous fumarate*, 30 percent iron.

Iron also is incorporated in *vitamin tablets*, frequently without indication of the exact iron content. Some of these vitamin preparations are fruit-flavored, animal-shaped, and chewable. Marketed in bottles containing as many as 250 tablets, available without prescriptions, and without danger warning, they are usually considered safe by parents. In countries where chewable vitamin tablets are popular, as in Canada, there has been a corresponding increase in cases of iron poisoning.

Toxicity

Neither the true toxic dose nor the *minimal* lethal dose of iron for a child has been clearly established. The *mean* lethal dose has been estimated at 300 mg/kg elemental iron, but children can and have died after ingesting considerably lesser amounts. As little as 1,000 mg of ferrous sulphate (200 mg elemental iron) has caused death in toddlers; on the other hand, recoveries have also been reported from as much as 15 g. The Consumer Product Safety Commission in 1975 recommended that all drugs or food supplements providing the equivalent of 500 mg of elemental iron per total package come under the child resistant requirements of the Poison Packaging Act. This recommendation was based on definite evidence that 1,000 mg of elemental iron can be fatal in children younger than 5 years of age; the 500 mg was chosen in order to provide the necessary margin of safety to protect even the smallest toddlers from serious illness. In children the mortality rate after acute poisoning with large doses of iron has been reported to be as high as 50 percent.

Toxic Effects

Normally the gastrointestinal mucosa effectively controls the absorption as well as the elimination of normal dietary intake or of small excesses of ingested iron. Modest surpluses are eliminated in the stool as ferritin after conversion from ferrous (divalent) to ferric (trivalent) iron, which combines with apoferritin. This regulatory mechanism is inoperative when overwhelmed by excessive amounts of iron. Ingested in massive quantities the iron not only acts as a highly corrosive agent, ulcerating and necrotizing the gastric intestinal mucosa, but its direct absorption into the bloodstream may produce severe systemic toxicity from as early as 30 to 60 minutes to as late as several hours after ingestion.

Clinical Features

Manifestations of acute iron poisoning include:
Gastrointestinal symptoms: vomiting, and profuse diarrhea, both frequently bloody;
Metabolic disturbances: dehydration and severe metabolic acidemia;
Early and delayed *circulatory symptoms and signs:* pallor, hypotension, hypovolemic shock; and
Nervous system manifestations: convulsions and coma.
The clinical course, which may have a fatal outcome, characteristically progresses in three chronologic phases:

The *first phase* usually begins within 30 to 60 minutes after ingestion with vomiting and bloody diarrhea. Acidemia and circulatory collapse may develop concurrently or may follow within 4 to 6 hours. If no toxic symptoms appear within 6 to 12 hours after ingestion, or are limited to very mild gastrointestinal disturbances, it is unlikely that the disease will progress further. The untreated patient with severe clinical toxicity may die or improve either spontaneously or in response to supportive therapy.

The *second phase* is one of relative improvement, frequently misleading, lasting for 8 to 16 hours during which all symptoms will subside or are minimal.

A critical *third phase,* frequently fatal, may supervene about 24 to 48 hours after ingestion with progressive collapse, coma, and convulsions. This delayed third phase can be avoided or successfully treated.

Within 1 to 2 months after recovery, pyloric stenosis or obstruction secondary to gastric scarring may develop and may require surgery. Small bowel infarction, requiring small bowel resection, has also been reported as a complication of the acute toxicity.

Pathogenesis

The pathogenesis of shock has not been explained satisfactorily. It has been suggested that in addition to the corrosive gastritis, the ionic iron escaping into the circulation produces shock by its vasodepressant effect, by causing hemorrhagic necrosis of the liver, and by releasing vasodepressor material (VDM) identified as ferritin. Another mechanism has been postulated that attributes the shock to capillary congestion and increased permeability, resulting in a reduction of plasma volume and hemoconcentration. In a third hypothesis, the shock is ascribed to loss of plasma protein by destruction, renal excretion, and depression of protein synthesis due to liver damage. Which of these three mechanisms is singly or predominantly responsible is still obscure.

Diagnosis

In the absence of a history of ingestion the diagnosis should be considered in all children of 1 to 5 years of age in whom bloody diarrhea and/or vomiting is associated with hypotension or circulatory collapse, severe acidosis and dehydration, or convulsion and/or coma. The age of the patient, a recent pregnancy in any household member, and the admission of the presence of accessible therapeutic iron preparations in the home will enhance the suspicion. Supportive evidence of iron ingestion is provided by the recovery of particles in the lavage fluid or vomitus and radiographic visualization of radiopaque tablets. A serum iron level in excess of 350 µg/100 ml and/or a serum iron level exceeding the serum iron binding capacity by 50 µg/100 ml confirms the diagnosis of severe poisoning. If serum iron levels cannot be obtained the following semiquantitative tests provide evidence of elevated iron concentrations: dark red urine produced after 1 hour intravenous infusion of 15 mg/kg/hour of desferrioxamine in solution; a blue color reaction by ferrocyanide on gastric aspirate; and a red color elicited by bathophenantroline and hydroxylammonium on serum when the serum iron concentration exceeds 350 µg/100 ml (Fischer test).

TREATMENT

Treatment consists of:

Prompt evacuation and neutralization of gastric contents;

Supportive therapy instituted for the prevention and/or correction of shock, dehydration, and acidosis; the maintenance of airway, ventilation, and oxygenation; sustenance of renal function; and

Chelation with desferrioxamine, in severe intoxications.

Gastric Evacuation and Neutralization

Gastric lavage should be performed using a sodium bicarbonate or disodium phosphate duohydrate (Fleet phosphate R) containing solution that binds the iron into a noncorrosive and insoluble carbonate or phosphate precipitate. Part of the lavage solution should be left in the stomach in order to neutralize any residual iron. Intragastric administration of disodium phosphate, a saline cathartic, has the added advantage of accelerating the elimination of the iron from the gastrointestinal tract while further inactivating the ionic iron present in the bowel. Beyond the first 30 minutes after ingestion, induction of emesis by mechanical or pharmacologic means may be dangerous and should be avoided because of the corrosive effects of iron on the gastric mucosa. If there is profuse diarrhea or 3 hours or more have elapsed since the iron ingestion, rectal lavage with the same neutralizing solution may prevent damage to the rectosigmoid mucosa by iron fragments.

Supportive Therapy

In all instances of excessive iron ingestion, whether the patient is symptomatic or not, intravenous fluid should be started. Intravenous administration of blood and/or plasma analogues to combat peripheral vascular collapse and adequate fluids containing electrolytes to correct the acidosis and dehydration and maintain urinary function are essential in all severe cases. Excretion of chelated iron will not take place without adequate correction of the hypovolemia and maintenance of a satisfactory urinary output. All measures to ensure airway patency, maintenance of ventilation, and oxygenation must be instituted.

Chelation

The highly effective iron-binding compound, desferrioxamine, has been used since the early '60s with en-

couraging results in severe cases of iron intoxication. This chelating agent, specific for iron, is a siderochrome of microbial origin that had originally been successful in the treatment of hemosiderosis and hemochromatosis in man. In vitro its iron-binding capacity exceeds that of transferrin. Administered intravenously, desferrioxamine combines with iron to form ferrioxamine, which is excreted largely in the urine except for a small proportion that is metabolized in the body. The soluble hydrochloride or mesylate salt binds 9.3 mg of trivalent iron per 100 mg of chelate.

The recommended dose of desferrioxamine in children is 90 mg/kg to be given intravenously over a minimal period of 6 hours in 100 to 200 ml of 5 percent dextrose in water solution. The rate of infusion of the desferrioxamine should not exceed 15 mg/kg/hour. If the color of the urine continues to be orange or reddish brown, an indication of the presence of ferrioxamine, an additional course of 90 mg/kg of desferrioxamine is to be given over the next 12 hours. If needed, this dose may be repeated. The intramuscular route is also effective.

Parenteral desferrioxamine treatment should, however, be restricted to children with severe iron intoxication since excessive amounts of the iron complex ferrioxamine are potentially toxic. The iron toxicity should be regarded as severe if the amount of ingested iron is either known or proved to be large and/or the serum iron concentrations (normally 65 to 75 µg/100 ml) exceed, *within 4 to 6 hours of ingestion,* 350 µg/100 ml. Serum iron levels tend to decline 6 hours after ingestion regardless of the amount taken or the clinical condition.

Oral therapy with desferrioxamine is contraindicated. When given orally not only is iron absorption from the gastrointestinal tract not prevented, but it may result in toxicity secondary to passage into the circulation of large quantities of the iron chelate complex. Adverse reactions from the drug, such as hypotension, irritability, and convulsions, have been reported but may be minimized by precluding both the oral therapy and the rapid infusion of the chelating agent. Cataracts have been reported but only after chronic and prolonged usage.

If renal function is inadequate, peritoneal dialysis, hemodialysis, or exchange transfusion may be required as an additional means of removing chelated iron.

Bibliography

IRON POISONING

Aldrich RA: Acute iron toxicity. In Wallerstein RO, Mettier SR (eds): Iron in Clinical Medicine. University of California Press, Berkeley, 1958

Fischer DS, Parkman R, Finch SC: Acute iron poisoning in children. The problem of appropriate therapy. JAMA 218:1179, 1971

Gevirtz NR, Wasserman LR: The measurement of iron and iron-binding capacity in plasma containing desferrioxamine. J Pediatr 68:802, 1966

Herbert V: Drugs effective in iron-deficiency and other hypochromic anemias. Iron and iron salts. In Goodman LS, Gelman A (eds): The

Pharmacological Basis of Therapeutics, 5th ed. Macmillan, New York, 1975

Jacobs J, Greene H, Gendel BR: Acute iron intoxications. N Engl J Med 273:1124, 1965

Leikin S, Vossough P, Mochir-Fatemi M: Chelation therapy in acute iron poisoning. J Pediatr 71:425, 1967

McEnery JT, Greengaard J: Treatment of acute iron ingestion with desferrioxamine in 20 children. J Pediatr 68:773, 1966

Movassaghi N, Purugganan G, Leikin S: Comparison of exchange transfusion and desferrioxamine in the treatment of acute iron poisoning. J Pediatr 75:604, 1969

Viets C: Children's chewable vitamins with iron: their potential danger. Can Fam Physician, January 1974

Whitten CF, Gibson GW, Good MH, et al: Studies in acute iron poisoning. I Desferrioxamine in the treatment of acute iron poisoning: clinical observations, experimental studies, and theoretical considerations. Pediatrics 36:322, 1965

——— Studies in acute iron poisoning. II Further observations on desferrioxamine in the treatment of acute experimental iron poisoning. Pediatrics 38:102, 1966

POISONING BY NONMEDICINAL SUBSTANCES

Fatalities from pesticides in the United States account for less than 1 percent of total deaths from toxic substances, but in children less than 5 years of age they cause nearly one of every five deaths due to poisoning by nonmedicinal substances. The major ingredients responsible for toxicity in pesticides are listed in Table 12.

TABLE 12. Major Ingredients in Pesticides

I Organic

Chlorinated Hydrocarbons: (DDT, chlordane, toxaphene, d-d₁, dieldrin, aldrin)

Dinitrophenol/Cresol

Hydrocarbon Solvents: aliphatic (kerosene), aromatic (xylene, benzene)

Naphthalene, p-dichlorbenzene, Camphor

Nicotine

Phosphoric Esters: (malathion, parathion, tepp, ompa, carbamates)

Strychnine

Thiram

II Inorganic

antimony, arsenic, *barium Sulfate,* copper, *cyanide,* fluoracetates, *fluorides,* lead, mercury, *phosphorus* (inorganic), *thallium,* zinc phosphide

III Relatively Low Toxicity

Botanicals: pyrethrum, rotenone

Anticoagulant: warfarin, pival

ORGANOPHOSPHATE INSECTICIDE POISONING

Arnold H. Einhorn

DDT was banned from general use in the United States in 1973. Other chlorinated hydrocarbons such as aldrin, dieldrin, and chlordane were prohibited more recently. These agents have been replaced chiefly by organic ester compounds whose toxicity is in general much greater than DDT. As a result many of the insecticides available to the public and responsible for an increasing number of accidental poisonings are alkyl esters of phosphoric acid.

PRODUCTS

Included in this group are: compounds of *moderate or intermediary* toxicity such as abate, malathion, DDVP, EPN, dibrom, and diazinon; *highly dangerous* agents, such as ethion, methylparathion, demeton (systox), octomethyl pyrophosphoramide (OMPA), and parathion; and, *extremely toxic products,* such as tetraethyl pyrophosphate (TEPP), tetram, and paraoxon.

Parathion, the class compound of this group, has to be converted in the body to an active metabolite, paraoxon, before effects occur. The highly toxic parathion is considered of "intermediary" toxicity. The *mean* lethal dose of parathion, when taken orally, is estimated at 1.4 mg/kg. Yet, the ingestion of as little as 20 to 30 mg may be fatal in adults; children have died after swallowing only 2 mg or about 0.1 mg/kg; and death may result from a single drop of parathion in the eye.

TEPP (tetraethyl pyrophosphate) and *paraoxon* are direct-acting, considerably more potent than parathion, and their supremely toxic effects appear very shortly after exposure. The alkylphosphorylation of acetylcholinesterase by parathion, TEPP, and paraoxon is irreversible and the cholinergic effects may persist for several days.

Malathion, the first organic insecticide approved for household use, is comparatively less toxic. The *mean* lethal dose of malathion is approximately 800 mg/kg. Its anticholinesterase activity is relatively low, except on erythrocyte cholinesterase, which it depresses considerably. Although a safer product, about 100 times less toxic than parathion, malathion is by no means without danger. Several deaths from malathion have been reported. We have treated children in near-fatal condition following exposure to malathion.

The toxicity of the insecticides DDVP, EPN, diazinon, and dibrom is greater than that of malathion, but considerably less than that of parathion. Combined use of EPN or DDVP with malathion significantly potentiates the toxicity of the component ingredients.

TOXIC EFFECTS

The organophosphate compounds are inhibitors of carboxylic esterase enzymes, including *acetylcholinesterase* (erythrocyte and neural tissue) and *pseudocholinesterase* (liver, plasma) when ingested, inhaled, or absorbed through the skin or conjunctival mucosa. Toxicity of these insecticides in man is related primarily to the inactivation or inhibition of the acetylcholinesterase enzyme, which they affect by combining their phosphate radicals with the active site (esteratic site) of the enzyme. The enzyme inhibition results in excessive stimulation and overactivity of the parasympathetic nervous system and ultimately in its paralysis. The unopposed acetylcholine, which accumulates at the cholinergic synapses, produces muscarinic effects on the autonomic nervous system, nicotinic actions on the voluntary skeletal muscles, and central nervous system effects by accumulation in the brain and spinal cord.

CLINICAL COURSE

The time of onset, the nature of the initial symptoms, the intensity and sequence of clinical manifestations, and the rapidity of the course depend on both the portal of entry and the size of the dose. Clinical evidence of toxicity develops only after cholinesterase activity is reduced by more than 50 percent. In severe poisoning these values may fall below 10 percent of normal. Maximal enzyme inhibition usually occurs less than 6 hours after exposure.

In general, symptoms follow exposure without much delay; the time of death may range from less than 5 minutes to nearly 24 hours after a single, acute exposure. Toxic symptoms and signs are more severe and develop most rapidly after inhalation, often within a few minutes. The time interval is longer in gastrointestinal and cutaneous absorption, but shorter following ingestion than after skin absorption. After inhalation, ocular and respiratory effects generally appear first; gastrointestinal symptoms occur earliest after ingestion; and with dermal absorption, localized sweating and fasciculations of adjacent muscles are usually the initial manifestations.

Symptoms of organophosphate poisoning consist essentially of headaches; blurred vision; dizziness and mental confusion; weakness, convulsions, or coma; profuse sweating, lacrimation, and salivation; abdominal cramps and diarrhea; tightness of the chest, wheezing, and excessive bronchial secretions. Physical findings include miosis (sometimes terminal mydriasis); muscle incoordination and fasciculations; areflexia; comatose or convulsive state; wheezes, rhonchi, and diffuse crepitant rales of pulmonary edema; bradycardia; and mild to moderate hypertension.

If untreated, death occurs in the most severe cases. The cause of death is primarily respiratory failure associated with circulatory collapse. Respiratory failure is secondary to severe pulmonary edema and respiratory paralysis of both central and peripheral origin. Laryngospasm, bronchoconstriction, and excessive tracheobronchial secretions are important contributing factors.

Survivors generally recover without sequelae, even from severe poisoning. Liver functions may remain abnormal for weeks or even months in rare instances. Historically, adulteration of rum and cooking oil by triorthocresyl phosphate has left victims with persistent peripheral neuropathy, causing epidemics of paralysis (known as *Ginger Jake* paralysis) in the United States in the early '30s, and affecting thousands of consumers in Morocco and Tangiers in the '50s and '60s, respectively.

DIAGNOSIS

Recognition of organophosphate poisoning may be extremely difficult if exposure is not known. The pungently unpleasant and characteristic odor of the insecticide may be detected in the patient's breath, vomitus, or gastric aspirate. Suspicion should be aroused whenever sudden nervous system depression or excitation, rapidly progressing respiratory distress, excessive salivation, sweating, and diarrhea are associated with the evocative *triad of constricted pupils, bradycardia, and muscle fasciculations*. The differential diagnosis is mainly between pulmonary edema, all causes of either coma or convulsions, and narcotic or opioid overdose. However, in the latter instance miosis is associated neither with excessive respiratory secretions nor with diarrhea.

Whenever organophosphate poisoning is suspected in a patient whose condition is precarious, a therapeutic trial with atropine and pralidoxime is warranted. Evidence of increased tolerance to atropine should be regarded as diagnostic, especially if in response to atropine and/or pralidoxime signs and symptoms disappear early and dramatically; that is, miosis disappears, the frothy sialorrhea subsides, respiratory distress is relieved, and heart rate is accelerated.

If time permits, diagnosis can be facilitated by demonstrating p-nitrophenol by its yellow color reaction or by gas or thin-layer chromatography after the addition of sodium hydroxide to a steam distillate of stomach contents or urine. More specific is the estimation of inhibition of cholinesterase activity in blood. Normal values for both red blood cell and plasma or serum cholinesterase range from 0.6 to 1.3 ΔpH Michel units per hour. In organophosphate poisoning, levels of both erythrocyte acetylcholinesterase and serum "pseudocholinesterase" are reduced to below 50 percent of normal.

TREATMENT

Because the clinical course is so rapid, speed is of utmost importance. Treatment includes:

Gastric lavage with 5 percent sodium bicarbonate solution if the poison has been ingested. Because the solvent of the insecticide often is a petroleum product, mechanically or pharmacologically induced emesis is contraindicated.

Decontamination by washing the skin, hair, and fingernails with copious amounts of water and alcohol after all soiled clothing, including the shoes, are removed. Staff should wear gloves, mask, a rubber apron, and goggles, if necessary, to protect themselves from the poison.

Maintenance or restoration of an adequate airway; oxygen administration; and ventilatory assistance, if indicated.

Appropriate intravenous fluid and electrolyte therapy.

Concomitantly, *atropinization* of all symptomatic children, combined, in severe cases, with administration of a specific and highly effective systemic *cholinesterase reactivating oxime*.

Atropine effectively counteracts the muscarinic actions and some of the central nervous effects of acetylcholine. It does not affect the peripheral neuromuscular paralysis. It should be given intravenously in doses considerably larger (0.015 to 0.05 mg/kg) than those used ordinarily: for children under 2 years of age, 0.2 to 0.5 mg; from 2 to 10 years, 0.5 to 1.0 mg; and over 10 years of age, 1.0 to 2.0 mg. The initial dose should be repeated every 15 to 20 minutes until the acetylcholine effect subsides or signs of atropine toxicity appear— mydriasis, cutaneous flush, dryness of mucous membranes, and tachycardia. Tolerance of atropine is greatly increased in patients with organophosphate poisoning. Atropine therapy alone is sufficient in mild to moderate intoxication without central neurologic manifestations and/or without severe respiratory difficulty.

The *cholinesterase reactivating oximes* conteract both the muscarinic and nicotinic action of acetylcholine in all synapses and dramatically restore consciousness. These oximes reactivate the acetylcholinesterase by freeing the active unit of the alkylphospholylated enzyme. They have no effect on the accumulated acetylcholine in children with severe intoxication. While atropine therapy is continued, PAM (2-pyridine aldoxime methiodide, pralidoxime iodide) or the chloride salt Protopam chloride (pralidoxime chloride), in a dose of 25 to 50 mg/kg, should be administered intravenously in 5 to 10 minutes, as a 5 percent solution in 0.5 normal saline in 5 percent glucose, at a rate that should not exceed 200 mg/minute. If the muscle weakness persists or recurs, the dose may be repeated after 1 hour, and again, if needed, as soon as the effects of the cholinesterase reactivator seem to subside.

The different actions of atropine and of the oximes do not interfere with each other. The combination of an oxime with atropine is more effective than either drug alone. Both drugs should be used concomitantly in severe poisoning with significant muscle weakness, respiratory failure, severe bradycardia, coma, and/or convulsions. PAM and Protopam decrease the patient's tolerance to atropine, and great caution must be exercised in monitoring the effects of atropine when the two drugs are used concurrently.

In symptomatic organophosphate poisoning, the use of barbiturates as anticonvulsants, phenothiazines as antiemetics, theophylline derivatives as bronchodilators, and opioids as sedatives are all *contraindicated*.

Bibliography

ORGANOPHOSPHATE INSECTICIDE POISIONING

Bogusz MJ: Influence of insecticides on the activity of some enzyme contained in human serum. Clin Chim Acta 19:369, 1968

DuBois K: Basic Mechanisms Involved in Toxication by Organic Phosphate Pesticides. In Laboratory Diagnosis of Diseases Caused by Toxic Agents. Sunderman FW and Sunderman FW, Jr (eds) Warren Green, Inc, St. Louis, 1970, p 163

Eitzman D, Wolfson SL: Acute parathion poisoning in children. Am J Dis Child 114:397, 1967

Gleason MN, Gosselin RL, Hodge HC, Smith RP: In Gleason MN, Gosselin RL, Hodge HC, Smith RP (eds): Clinical Toxicology of Commercial Products, 3rd ed. Baltimore, Williams and Wilkins, 1969, p. 183-188

Goldin AR, et al: Malathion poisoning with special reference to the effect of cholinesterase inhibition on erythrocyte survival. N Engl J Med 25:1289, 1964

Hayes WJ Jr: Epidemiology and general management of poisoning by pesticides. Pediatr Clin North Am 17:629, 1970

Koelle GB: Anticholinesterase agents. In Goodman LS, Gilman A (eds): The Pharmacologic Basis of Therapeutics, 5th ed. Macmillan, New York, 1975

Kopel FG, et al: Acute parathion poisoning. J Pediatr 61:898, 1962

McQueen EG, Brosnan C, Ferry DG: Poisoning from a rose spray containing lindane and malathion. N Z Med J 67:533, 1968

Morse CS: Interconversion of cholinesterase measurements by the ΔpH method of Michel and the DTNB method of Garry and Routh. Clin Toxicol 7:389, 1974

Namba T, Nolte CT, Jacrel J, Grab D: Poisoning due to organophosphate insecticides. Acute and chronic manifestations. Am J Med 50:475, 1971

National Clearinghouse for Poison Control Centers Bulletin, Bureau of Drugs, Federal Drug Administration, US Department of Health, Education, and Welfare. Toxic Insecticides to replace DDT. Nov.-Dec. 1972 Tabulations of 1973 Report, May-June 1974

Quimby GE: Further therapeutic experience with pralidoximes in organic phosphorus poisoning. JAMA 187:203, 1964

Read WT, Combes MA: A new specific antidote for organic phosphate ester poisoning. Pediatrics 28:950, 1961

Sidell FR: Soman and Sarin: Clinical manifestations and treatment of accidental poisoning by organophosphates. Clin Toxical 7:1, 1974

Teitelman U, et al: Treatment of massive poisoning by the organophosphate pesticide methidathion. Clin Toxicol 8:277, 1975

Zavon MR: Poisoning from pesticides: diagnosis and treatment. Pediatrics 54:332, 1974

KEROSENE AND PETROLEUM PRODUCTS POISONING

Arnold H. Einhorn

In the United States during 1973, nearly 5,000 accidental ingestions of petroleum products by children under 5 years of age were reported to the National Clearinghouse for Poison Control Centers. From 1968 through 1973, 140 children of this age group lost their lives from poisoning by such compounds.

PRODUCTS

Kerosene and other petroleum distillates are derivatives of crude petroleum and mixtures of aliphatic and aromatic hydrocarbons. Liquid products most often accessible to young children and involved in toxic episodes in the home include cigarette and charcoal lighter fluids; kerosene, benzene, and naphtha; gasoline; solvents; mineral spirits, paint and lacquer thinners; mineral seal-oil containing furniture polishes; insecticide solvents; and oil paints, lacquers, and varnish. Among these substances furniture polish has become, in the United States, one of the most frequent types of petroleum products responsible for intoxications in toddlers.

TOXIC EFFECTS

The toxicity of petroleum distillates is related primarily to the danger of aspiration of the hydrocarbon into the respiratory tract, where it produces intense local irritation, pneumonitis, hemorrhagic bronchopneumonia, atelectasis, and/or pulmonary edema. Pneumatocele formation, pleural effusion, and pneumothorax may complicate the hydrocarbon pneumonitis. These pulmonary lesions may rapidly become extensive, and a fulminating course may lead to a fatal outcome in 2 to 24 hours after ingestion.

The aspirated compound damages the alveolar lining and the pulmonary capillaries and is primarily responsible for the pulmonary parenchymal injury. Alteration of intraalveolar surfactant has been demonstrated following experimental inhalation of petroleum hydrocarbons. However, some respiratory tissue damage possibly may result from indirect chemical injury secondary to excretion, through the lungs, of products absorbed from the gastrointestinal tract into the bloodstream.

The severity of respiratory difficulty usually parallels the extent of parenchymal disease. Fluid filled alveoli and altered interalveolar septa interfere with oxygen diffusion and interfere with ventilation-perfusion relationships. The resulting arterial-alveolar oxygen gradient may be considerable and severe hypoxia may produce or contribute to metabolic acidemia. Arterial hypoxemia and associated acidemia, if severe and prolonged, will, in turn, adversely affect myocardial contractility. Hypercarbia and respiratory acidemia occur only when airways are obstructed by excessive inflammatory secretions or by spasm of terminal bronchioles, and/or if the patient's nervous system is significantly depressed.

The ingestion of kerosene and other petroleum products, mainly benzene, gasoline, mineral seal oil, and lighter fluid, also can cause systemic and visceral toxic effects. These consist essentially of central nervous system depression, sometimes hypoplasia of the bone marrow, and rarely degenerative changes in the liver and kidneys.

Both pulmonary and central nervous system complications are more frequent as a result of vomiting, which is virtually unavoidable when more than 30 ml of petroleum distillates have been ingested. The respiratory complications are believed to be due primarily to aspiration of petroleum distillates into the lungs, rather than to absorption from the intestinal tract. However, patients have been known to develop pulmonary manifestations due to tracheal spillage in the absence of either vomiting or gastric lavage.

Aspiration hazards depend primarily on the viscosity and possibly on the surface tension of the hydrocarbon agent, while systemic toxicity is presumably related to its chemical composition and its volatility. Because of their low viscosity some compounds have low systemic toxicity but high aspiration hazards, even in small amounts. Thus, the incidence of pulmonary disease is higher after the ingestion of furniture polish than after any other petroleum product. Systemic toxicity is very serious with volatile products, especially benzene or petroleum ether, while the risk of aspiration is relatively minor. Others, such as lighter fluids, gasoline, kerosene, and mineral seal-oil containing furniture polishes, are not only very toxic systemically, but also readily aspirated because of their low viscosity. Viscous material, such as paint, glues, asphalt, and rubber cement, represent insignificant aspiration hazards; household fuel oil also produces little systemic or pulmonary effect.

CLINICAL FEATURES

The clinical picture of hydrocarbon poisoning is strikingly similar in most patients; only the severity of the manifestations varies. Early symptoms include a burning sensation in the mouth and throat, choking and gagging spells, cough, nausea, vomiting, and hemoptysis. Tachycardia, tachypnea, and auscultatory findings of pulmonary edema often appear shortly after the ingestion. In severe cases cyanosis, audible grunting, retractions and flaring, and signs of cardiac decompensation reflect the gravity of the pulmonary insult. Arterial hypoxemia and metabolic acidemia may be severe; arterial Pco_2 is usually normal or reduced but may be elevated if there is airway obstruction or if the patient is comatose. Typically, on chest radiography evidence of extensive pulmonary infiltration and emphysema may be demonstrated soon after the onset of symptoms, when physical signs are still minimal or even absent. In fact the time lag between the appearance of radiographic findings of pneumonitis and the appearance of clinical evidence of pulmonary disease may be considerable. Pneumothorax may occur secondary to kerosene ingestion.

Symptoms of central nervous system depression also may develop, usually manifested by generalized weakness, dizziness, mental confusion, lethargy or irritability, and convulsions or unconsciousness. Central nervous system involvement may either constitute the clinical expression of the systemic toxicity of the hydrocarbon compounds or result from hypoxic cerebral damage secondary to respiratory insufficiency.

TREATMENT

Gastric Evacuation

Extreme caution must be exercised in handling the patient so as not to provoke vomiting and aspiration. Mechanically or pharmacologically induced emesis is strictly contraindicated. Antiemetics are also dangerous. There is still considerable disagreement regarding the advisability of gastric lavage in the treatment of kerosene ingestion. Many experienced observers are opposed to gastric lavage on the grounds that it promotes vomiting, thereby increasing the risk of aspiration. Others feel that prompt and cautious removal of the poisonous substance by lavage, performed expertly, may be beneficial. We advise against this procedure except when the child is seen within 30 minutes after the ingestion of the hydrocarbon and when the quantity of the product ingested is known to be large (2 ml/kg or more); the risk of spontaneous vomiting is so great that it outweighs the potential danger of gastric lavage carried out with the utmost precautions to prevent aspiration. If more than 30 minutes have elapsed since ingestion, if the quantity swallowed is relatively small, and if the child already has vomited, lavage should not be performed. The careful administration of a saline cathartic may hasten elimination of the poison from the gastrointestinal tract.

Supportive Treatment

To be instituted concomitantly in an intensive or critical care setting in all patients with respiratory symptoms are:

Airway clearance and maintenance of airway patency;
Humidified oxygen administration adjusted to maintain adequate arterial oxygen tension;
Assisted or controlled intermittent positive pressure breathing if required, preferably by volume cycled ventilator, combined with positive end-expiratory pressure (PEEP);
Correction of metabolic acidemia with sodium bicarbonate therapy;
Maintenance of circulation, fluid and electrolyte equilibrium, and urinary output with appropriately balanced intravenous fluid.

Antimicrobial and Corticosteroid Therapy

Antibiotic should be used only if there is evidence or a strong possibility of superimposed bacterial infection of the respiratory tract. Corticosteroids may have a beneficial effect in the treatment and prevention of some of the more severe respiratory complications of chemical and aspiration pneumonitis. Their usefulness in poisoning due to hydrocarbon aspiration is, however, still the object of controversy.

Supervision of Therapy

In addition to intensive clinical observation of vital signs, color, respiratory, cardiac, and neurologic status, arterial pH and blood gases, fluid and electrolyte status, hematocrit, and urine output are monitored frequently. Whenever required, electrocardiography and repeat chest radiography are done. In patients who have ingested large amounts of highly volatile petroleum distillates, periodic assessments of the renal, neurologic, and hepatic status is particularly desirable.

Bibliography

KEROSENE POISONING

Ashkenazi AE: Experimental kerosene poisoning in rats. Use of C_{14}-labeled Hendecan as indicator of absorption. Pediatrics 28:642, 1961

Cooperative Kerosene Poisoning Study. Evaluation of gastric lavage and other factors in the treatment of accidental ingestion of petroleum distillate products. Pediatrics 29:648, 1962

Done AK: Poisoning from common household products. Pediatr Clin North Am 17:569, 1970

Eade N, Taussig LM, Marks MI: Hydrocarbon pneumonitis. Pediatrics 54:351, 1974

Giammona ST: Effects of furniture polish on pulmonary surfactant. Am J Dis Child 113:658, 1967

Gleason MN, Gosselin RL, Hodge HC, Smith RP (eds): Clinical Toxicology of Commercial Products, 3rd ed. Williams and Wilkins, Baltimore, 1969, pp 132-137

Marks MI, Chicoine L, Legere G, Hillman E: Adrenocorticosteroid treatment of hydrocarbon pneumonia in children—a cooperative study. J Pediatr 81:366, 1972

National Clearinghouse for Poison Control Centers. Tabulations of 1973 reports. Bulletin, May-June 1974, Tabulations of 1974 Deaths. Bulletin Sept-Oct. 1975

Steele RW, Conklin RH, Mark RH: Corticosteroids and antibiotics for the treatment of fulminant hydrocarbon aspiration. JAMA 219:1434, 1972

Wolfe BM, Brodeur AE, Shields JB: The role of gastrointestinal absorption of kerosene in producing pneumonitis in dogs. J Pediatr 76:867, 1970

Wolfsdorf J, Jundig H: Dexamethasone in the management of kerosene pneumonia. Pediatrics 53:86, 1974

LEAD POISONING

J. JULIAN CHISOLM, JR.

Lead intoxication (plumbism) is a chronic disorder. The chronic course may be punctuated by acute symptomatic episodes, the most serious of which is acute lead encephalopathy. Specific laboratory tests are needed to confirm the diagnosis because signs and symptoms are not specific and routine examination of blood and urine ordinarily does not reveal any abnormalities pointing to lead as the etiologic agent. Plumbism in preschool children is now recognized as a significant public health problem in the United States, where it is a reportable conditon in many communities.

Most cases are clearly related to *pica* for paint (and old putty) and are concentrated in areas of old dilapidated housing. About 85 percent of acute symptomatic episodes occur during the 6 warmer months of the year; there may be recurrences each summer. The reasons for the seasonal variation are poorly understood. Most cases of acute encephalopathy are reported in children 12 to 36 months of age. Valid incidence data are not available; however, current screening programs suggest that 5 to 15 percent of preschool children in the United States have increased lead absorption.

Plumbism should be considered in the differential diagnosis of mental retardation, seizure disorders, aggressive behavior disorders, or persistent pica in children of all ages. Although chelation therapy can apparently reduce mortality from acute encephalopathy to less then 5 percent, about 50 percent of the survivors sustain serious permanent brain damage. There is some evidence that mildly symptomatic or asymptomatic plumbism during the early preschool years may be associated with an increased frequency of behavioral problems, which become evident only after the child enters school.

ENVIRONMENTAL SOURCES

Lead is widely distributed in both natural and man-made substances. The concentration of lead in different items varies greatly, but is very low in most of the items to which children are exposed. The following concentrations are approximate: most public water supplies <0.015 μg Pb/ml; foods (fresh and in glass or plastic containers) <0.10 μg Pb/g; usual urban air <3 μg Pb/m^3; household dust and soil adjacent to homes, average values between 3,000 and 12,000 μg Pb/g; and paint containing 5 percent lead, 50,000 μg Pb/g.

Repetitive ingestion of a concentrated source such as lead-pigment paint accounts for most symptomatic cases, while exposure to a less concentrated source such as household dust in *old* houses may well account for minimally increased lead absorption in young children (blood lead concentration in the range of 30 to 50 μg/100 ml whole blood). Young children who live very close to lead smelters may also show mildly to moderately increased lead absorption. The following sources are responsible for sporadic cases of plumbism: retention of a metallic lead object (shot, fishing weight, bauble) in the stomach where lead is slowly dissolved; contamination of acidic foods and beverages (fruits, fruit juices, cola drinks, tomatoes, tomato juice, wine, cider) through storage in improperly lead-glazed ceramicware; chewing on old lead-painted toys and furniture; burning of battery casings or lead-painted wood in home fireplaces or stoves; sniffing leaded gasoline; use of lead nipple shields; and drinking rain or soft water stored in lead-lined cisterns or pipes.

Although modern interior paints do not contain lead pigments, the interior woodwork, painted plaster, and wallpaper of houses built prior to 1950 may contain layers of lead-pigment paints that have never been removed. *Several tiny flakes of such paint may contain 100 mg of lead or more.* Exterior paints may also contain lead pigments, so that flaking paint on porches, fences, and fire escapes must also be considered. Some old putty formulations contain lead. According to the United States Census Bureau, there were about 30 million residential dwelling units, including 7 to 8 million in a deteriorated state, which were built prior to 1950 but were still in use in 1970. Surveys indicate that 90 percent or more of such old housing stock contains significant amounts of lead on painted surfaces accessible to children. Recent experience shows that renovation of older homes must be undertaken with great care. The burning, scraping, and sanding of interior surfaces can result in the release of potentially hazardous amounts of lead into the rooms in fine particulate form. It is advisable for pregnant women, infants, and young children to avoid such exposure by seeking temporary residence elsewhere during the course of such work. Those doing the work must take precautions (ventilation, mask, protection of food, thorough damp cleanup, removal of debris, etc.). During the past decade, there has been a marked reduction in the use of lead in paint. A recent market survey indicates that the vast majority of residential paints do not now contain lead additives.

METABOLISM OF LEAD

The total body lead burden is divided into two main compartments. The compartment consisting of the soft tissues and an exchangeable fraction of bone lead is quite small, containing no more than 10 percent of the total in the adult. A much larger fraction is sequestered in bone, the other main component. The portion of lead in bone is greater in adults (over 90 percent) than it is in children (about 70 percent). Although the total body lead burden in normal persons may increase from 1 to more than 200 mg of lead during life, the increase is limited to increasing sequestration of lead in bone. The concentration of lead in the soft tissues remains low and relatively constant throughout life. The half-life of lead in the small mobile soft tissue compartment is estimated at 16 days, while the half-life of lead in bone is estimated at about 16 years. The toxic effects of lead are related to increases in the concentration of lead in the small soft tissue compartment, which occur when the rate of assimilation exceeds the rates of excretion and sequestration in bone. After excessive intake stops, soft tissue lead concentrations decrease very slowly over a period of months or years. A raised level of lead in shed deciduous teeth may provide evidence of increased lead absorption in the remote past, even though blood lead concentrations may have decreased to the normal range.

Absorption of lead from the intestine is related to age. In experimental animals, it is highest in the early suckling period (more than 70 percent) and lowest at maturity (about 1 percent). In young experimental animals, induced dietary deficiencies of calcium, copper, and iron, as well as administration of lead compounds in oils and as very fine particulates, increases absorption of lead from the intestine. When lead compounds used in paints are fed to animals before and after incorporation into a paint matrix, the paint matrix is found to reduce absorption by a factor of 3 to 4. In normal adult humans, about 5 to 10 percent of dietary lead is absorbed and most of the absorbed lead is excreted. Limited balance data in children indicate that about 50 percent of normal dietary lead is absorbed and about 20 percent is retained.

For children living in modern housing, as well as normal adults and newborns, blood lead concentration averages 15 to 20 μg/100 ml, range 10 to 35 μg/100 ml (Table 13). This reflects the assimilation of small

TABLE 13. Interpretation of Blood Lead (Pb-B) Data in Children

Group	μg Lead/100 ml in Whole Blood	
	Mean	Range
I. Epidemiologic Data		
Neonates	19	12–34[a]
Children less than 6-yr —modern housing	17	10–30[b]
Children less than 6-yr —old housing	28	15–60[b]
Children less than 6-yr —old housing	39	19–81[c]
II. Relation to Toxicity[d]		
No effect level		less than 30
Minimal inhibition of heme synthesis in some		30–49
Moderate inhibition of heme synthesis frequent; positive long bone x-rays in some; early symptoms in a few		50–79
Metabolic evidence of toxicity universal; clear-cut symptoms begin to appear		80–100
Metabolic evidence of toxicity universal; symptoms may be absent, but risk of acute encephalopathy great, immediate and unpredictable		more than 100

[a] *From Rosen, et al.: J Pediatr 84:45, 1974*
[b] *From Joselow, et al.: J Environ Health 37:10, 1974*
[c] *From Chisolm, et al.: J Pediatr 84:490, 1974*
[d] *Compiled from Chisolm et al.: Pediatrics 18:943, 1956; National Academy of Sciences: Lead, Airborne Lead in Perspective. Washington, DC, 1972; Zielhuis: Int Arch Occup Health 35:1-35, 1975*

amounts of lead from normal food, water, and air. Groups of young children in old poorly maintained housing show somewhat higher average values, reflecting additional assimilation of lead from household dusts and pica for paint and other nonfood items containing lead. In children with normal blood lead concentration (average = 20 μg/100 ml), daily fecal excretion averages 5 μg Pb/kg of body weight. In children with blood lead concentrations of at least 60 μg/100 ml, daily fecal collections have contained amounts ≧ 100 μg/kg body weight. In children with acute encephalopathy, amounts equivalent to 500 to 10,000 μg/kg body weight have been found. The occurrence and severity of plumbism depends largely upon how much leaded paint, dust, and dirt a child eats, how often he eats it, and how long his pica for lead-containing items persists.

ADVERSE EFFECTS OF LEAD

There is no known biologic requirement for lead. All recognized effects are adverse. The principal tissues affected are the erythroid cells of bone marrow, the central and peripheral nervous system, and the kidney. Acute lead poisoning is characterized histologically by eosinophilic intranuclear inclusion bodies in the kidney and liver and occasionally in bone and brain and by punctate basophilic stippling of normoblasts in bone marrow. Basophilic stippling of circulating red blood cells is inconstant. The inhibitory effects of lead on erythropoiesis are reversible; however, involvement of both the nervous system and the kidney may be followed by permanent irreversible injury. Clinical data and sensitive biochemical tests suggest that injury to the erythroid cells in the bone marrow probably precedes injury to the nervous system and kidney.

Lead interferes with the biosynthesis of heme at several steps (Fig. 3). This metabolic disturbance is characterized by the following combination, which is pathognomonic for plumbism: decreased activity of δ-aminolevulinic acid dehydratase (ALA-D) in erythrocytes, increased erythrocyte protoporphyrin (EP), increased excretion of δ-aminolevulinic acid (ALA-U) and coproporphyrin (CP-U) in urine, and normal excretion of porphobilinogen and uroporphyrin in urine. Excess lead impairs the uptake and utilization of iron, as well as the synthesis of globin in developing red cells. Red cell life span is decreased. A compensated hemolytic anemia results. Morphologically, the circulating erythrocytes are hyperchromic and microcytic. Except for occasional reticulocytosis, the morphology of the peripheral blood in children with plumbism closely resembles that of iron deficiency. In lead poisoning (and iron deficiency), the metalloporphyrin, zinc protoporphyrin, is the porphyrin found in circulating erythrocytes, while in erythrohepatic protoporphyria, a genetic disorder characterized by photosensitivity, free protoporphyrin IX is present in excess in red cells. The

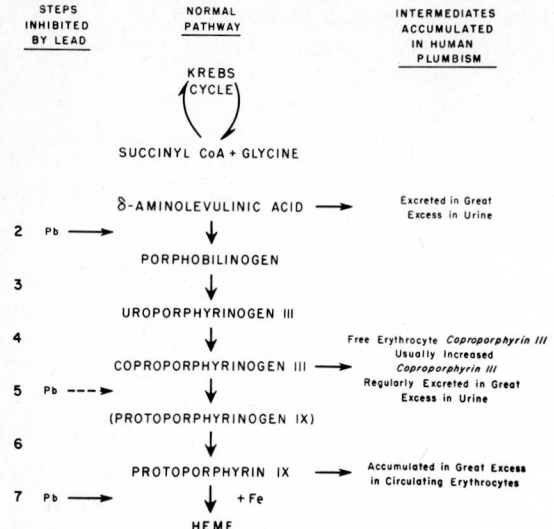

FIG. 3. Steps in biosynthesis of heme inhibited by lead. There is good evidence that lead partially inhibits the enzymes of steps 2 and 7. The origin of the coproporphyrinuria is not entirely clear.

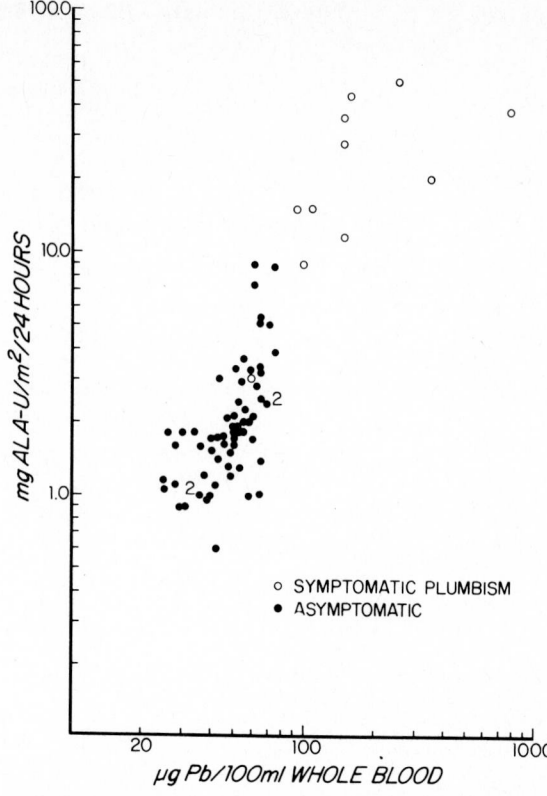

FIG. 4. Dose-effect relationship between blood lead concentration (Pb-B) and aminolevulinic acid excretion (ALA-U) in children. Most cases designated as "symptomatic plumbism" had acute encephalopathy. Note the general trend in ALA-U to increase sharply as Pb-B increases from 50 to 70 μg/100 ml; however, note the marked difference between individual patients. In some, ALA-U is within the normal range (less than 2 mg/M^2/24 hours). (From Chisolm, et al: J Pediatr 87:1152, 1975

concentration of zinc protoporphyrin is raised five- to tenfold in iron deficiency and to more than tenfold in plumbism (see p. 1122).

Most of the dose-response data in man are based on the relationship between blood lead (Pb-B) and various heme precursors. Toxicologic responses to lead appear to follow the law of random biologic variation. The relationship between Pb-B and ALA-U in children approximates the S-shaped curve predicted by this law (Fig. 4). ALA-U increases sharply as Pb-B rises above 50 μg/100 ml; however, the degree of increase varies widely among individuals. In the Pb-B ranges of 50 to 79 μg/100 ml, some individuals show normal or slightly increased ALA-U, while others show five- to tenfold increases. The relationship between Pb-B and erythrocyte protoporphyrin is similar (Fig. 5). In children with increased lead absorption, these measurements provide a means of identifying those who are experiencing the greater toxic effect. Prospective studies in adults show that hemoglobin begins to decrease as Pb-B rises above 50 to 60 μg/100 ml. Limited data suggest that there is an increased frequency of decreased hemoglobin (or hematocrit) in groups of children with Pb-B >40 μg/100 ml.

Acute encephalopathy is the result of massive cerebral edema and softening, which in turn stems from a diffuse vasculitis. Initially, there is an increase in capillary permeability with transudation of protein-containing fluid into the intervascular spaces of the brain. More severe lesions show necrosis of vessel walls with petechial hemorrhages. Neurons are irreversibly damaged.

Recently, clinical and experimental studies have focused on the central nervous system aspects of asymptomatic increased lead absorption. Experimen-

tally, slowed learning, hyperactivity, and aggressiveness have been produced in suckling animals by doses of lead insufficient to cause the histopathologic changes associated with severe encephalopathy. In these experiments, administration of excess lead is limited to the suckling period, but the behavioral effects do not become evident until later, usually at a time when blood lead concentration has returned to normal. Catecholamine metabolism is apparently altered. Juvenile and mature animals are less susceptible to these effects. Further work is needed to illuminate the relevance of these experimental observations for human lead exposure.

Studies in children with increased lead absorption have yielded conflicting results. Much of the controversy can be traced to their retrospective nature, inadequate control for confounding variables, and lack of a record of the degree of increase in lead absorption during infancy and early childhood. In the one long-term prospective study so far reported by de la Burde and Choate, cognitive function was only minimally affected; however, an increased frequency of poor performance

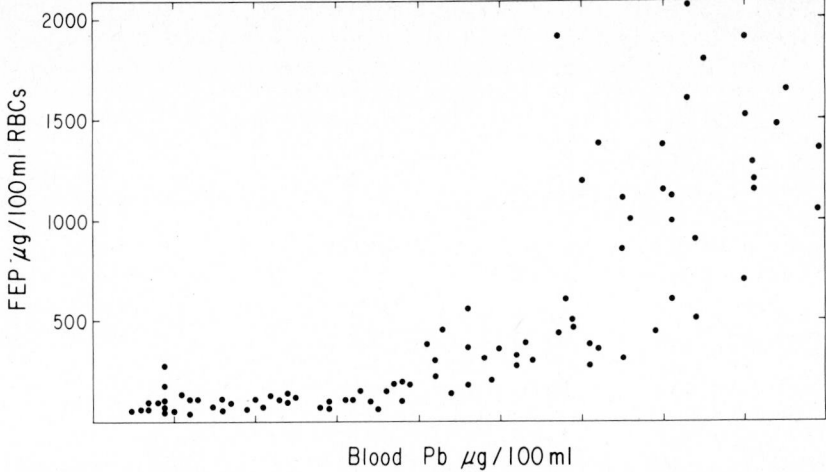

FIG. 5.   Dose-effect relationship between blood lead concentration and erythrocyte protoporphyrin. Again, note the variation in toxicologic response among individuals with Pb-B in the range of 50 to 79μg/100 ml of whole blood. Although erythrocyte protoporphyrin (EP) is also raised in iron deficiency, experimental data show that iron deficiency enhances the absorption, retention, and toxicity of lead. (From Piomelli, et al: J Lab Clin Med 81:932, 1973)

in school was observed. Behavioral aberrations, including short attention span, explosive behavior, and persistent temper tantrums, were considered the primary factors in impairing progress in school. These findings are similar to those reported by Byers and Lord in 1943, who noted that children with symptomatic plumbism, but without encephalopathy, later performed poorly in school despite relatively normal intelligence test results. Still at issue is the degree and duration of increase in lead absorption, the age at which it occurs, and the influence of other factors that play a role in the behavioral and learning problems found in school. In summary, the various clinical studies suggest that there is an increased frequency of neurologic deficits in groups of children who, during early childhood, eat leaded paint and sustain blood lead concentrations in excess of 50 to 60 μg/100 ml. Even so, it is likely that coexisting handicaps also play an important role in the final outcome.

Peripheral neuropathy is associated with chronic symptomatic plumbism. Motor weakness, with little or no sensory change, predominates. It is rarely, if ever, found in children < 3 to 4 years of age, and most of the reported cases have occurred in children with sickle cell disease. The Fanconi syndrome (hypophosphatemia with hyperphosphaturia, glycosuria, and generalized aminoaciduria) due to proximal renal tubular injury is a feature of severe acute poisoning. Albuminuria, and occasionally hematuria, have also been found in severe cases. Acute renal injury is reversible. Late lead nephropathy is characterized mainly by vascular injury, scarred contracted kidneys, and renal failure. The associated hyperuricemia and resultant gouty manifestations apparently reflect a selective decrease in the renal clearance of urate. It is a well recognized feature of chronic plumbism in adults, but it is rare in children.

PICA

The habit of pica—the repetitive search for and ingestion of nonfood items—is said to occur in about 50 percent of 1- to 3-year-old children. Frequency, intensity, and duration vary. Its physiologic and psychologic aspects are not well understood. Pica is variously attributed to inadequate mothering, emotional stress, and nutritional deficiencies. The preschool child with pica tends to be indiscriminate. He may eat paper, ashes, string, paint, putty, dirt, etc. Ordinarily, pica abates between 3 and 5 years of age, but under conditions of mental deficiency and severe psychosocial stress, it tends to become more selective and may persist throughout childhood.

Residence in old housing and blood lead values that remain which > 50 to 60 μg Pb/100 ml provide strong indirect evidence of pica for paint, despite a negative history of such ingestion. Although parents often report the eating of paper, they often deny seeing the child in the act of eating paint. Clinical experience further suggests that a child may indulge in pica when under the care of only one or two of the several adults (mother, father, grandparents, babysitters, etc.) who share responsibility for the child's care.

In the management of pica, the approach of Lourie and coworkers appears the most practical. Pica is viewed by this group as one of the responses to stress in a young child. Stress on the child may be potentiated by lack of mothering, marital conflict; other social, emotional, or financial difficulties; the arrival of a new infant; conflicts with grandparents and others; inability of the working mother to find an adequate substitute during her working hours; impulsive and immature parents —one or many of these factors may intensify pica in a particular child. The degree of success in ameliorating a child's pica often depends on the degree to which such family problems can be resolved. The medical social worker is generally the one best fitted to assist a mother in dealing with these problems. If, in a given case, the prospect of abating pica is remote (ie, mentally defective child, highly unfavorable family situation, very dilapidated home), transfer of the family into modern housing may be the only effective option. Placement in adequate day-care centers can be one of the most effective options, especially for the working mother.

CLINICAL FEATURES

Presenting complaints include the following: anorexia, vomiting, hyperirritability, slowing or regression in development, behavioral disorder characterized by irritability and aggression, seizures (responding to anticonvulsants), ataxia, and manifestations of increased intracranial pressure (persistent and forceful vomiting, coma, intractable seizures). Parents may also request tests for increased lead absorption because of pica or hyperactivity. Radiologic examinations for other conditions may inadvertently reveal radiopaque material in the bowel or evidence of lead deposition in the bone (Fig. 6). Clinical presentation tends to vary with age.

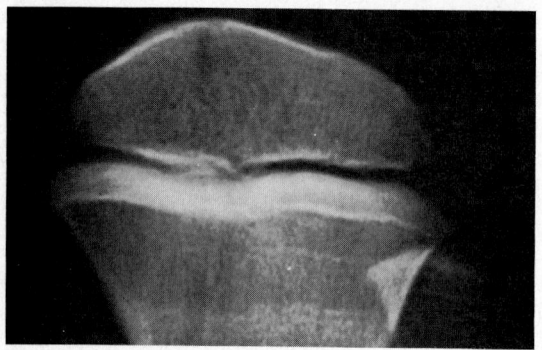

FIG. 6.   Radiogram of proximal end of tibia of child with lead intoxication. Continuous broad band of increased density at metaphysis is characteristic of plumbism and reflects the densely packed, irregular trabecular structure of bone being formed in presence of excess lead. This continuous broad band is to be distinguished from the multiple but discrete growth-arrest lines seen by x-ray in growing bones following a variety of illnesses.

Acute encephalopathy with cerebral edema is virtually always associated with blood lead levels of more than 120 µg/100 ml and is most prevalent during the summer in children under 3 years of age. Beyond this age, symptoms become chronic, but are usually less severe.

The following course is most common in children under 3 years of age who are actively ingesting excess lead. There is the insidious onset of anorexia, apathy, anemia, decreased play activity, hyperirritability, poor coordination and sporadic vomiting. Regression in newly acquired skill, particularly speech, is sometimes

reported. These complaints slowly intensify over a period of 3 to 6 weeks, after which acute encephalopathy may occur at any time. The onset of encephalopathy is heralded by the development over 2 to 5 days of gross ataxia, persistent, forceful vomiting, periods of lethargy or stupor, and finally, coma and intractable convulsions. Acute encephalopathy can also occur without these prodroma, but this is unusual. On the other hand, symptoms may regress at any point in the above sequence, if excess lead ingestion temporarily abates. Thus, a child may suffer recurrent symptomatic episodes without ever having obvious encephalopathy. Since there are no abnormal physical findings specific for plumbism in the young child, these nonspecific compaints may, at first, suggest an emotional disturbance or seem to be adequately explained either by some minor intercurrent infection, gastrointestinal disturbance, or by the associated iron-deficiency anemia, which is almost invariably present. Nor is the history uniformly reliable: pica may be denied even if the question is asked. For these reasons, the diagnosis of plumbism can be missed, if one relies entirely on history and physical examination.

Chronic plumbism may present as nonspecific mental retardation, behavior disturbance, convulsive disorder, or any combination thereof. Peripheral neuropathy, when seen in childhood, usually occurs during this chronic phase. Lead lines on the gingiva are occasionally seen in older children. In the older child, it is difficult without appropriate laboratory tests to distinguish between clinical manifestations due to continuing lead ingestion and those due to the residual cerebral injury of previous acute episodes.

LABORATORY DIAGNOSIS

Whole blood lead concentration is the most widely used index of current and recent lead absorption. At concentrations of lead up to at least 150 µg/100 ml whole blood, virtually all of the lead is bound to erythrocytes, and plasma lead is low and constant at about 3 µg/100 ml plasma. There is no clear evidence that red cell mass is a limiting factor in the capacity of blood to transport lead, except at very high concentrations. Correction of blood lead data on the basis of hematocrit is not warranted. While blood lead data are of great value in the study of groups, caution is needed in the interpretation of individual values. The precision of measurement is such that the 95 percent confidence limit for a single value is ± 5 µg /100 ml at best. Quantitative 24-hour collections of urine are needed for meaningful data. In asymptomatic children, the edathamil calcium disodium (CaEDTA) provocative test is sometimes helpful. In this test, 100 mg CaEDTA/M² is injected in divided dose at 12-hour intervals and urine lead output is measured in the 24-hour collection. (Alternatively, a single injection in a dose of 500 mg CaEDTA/M² followed by an 8-hour urine collection can suffice.) On the average, children with blood lead concentration more than 55 µg /100 ml will excrete more than 1.0 µg

Pb/mg CaEDTA given. For comparison, children with encephalopathy have been found to excrete 5.0 μg Pb/mg CaEDTA or more during the first day of treatment. This diagnostic test, while safe in asymptomatic cases, is hazardous in symptomatic cases in whom therapeutic amounts of chelating agents are needed. Collection of blood and urine requires special *lead-free* equipment to avoid contamination with exogenous lead.

The search for a simple screening test has led recently to a profusion of microfluorometric tests for erythrocyte protoporphyrin. Although they are not yet well standardized against each other, each method apparently measures a different but constant fraction of the zinc protoporphyrin present. For each method, values five to ten times greater than normal may signify iron deficiency, increased lead absorption, or both, while values more than ten times the normal value are indicative of significantly increased lead absorption, with or without iron deficiency. With ethyl acetate/acetic acid/hydrochloric acid extraction micromethods for free erythrocyte porphyrin, the average value in normals is 50 μg protoporphyrin per 100 ml of erythrocytes. Following treatment or termination of excessive lead intake, erythrocyte protoporphyrin may show little change for 1 to 3 months; thereafter, it decreases slowly but may not reach the normal range for 1 to 2 years or longer.

Reduction of ALA-D activity in erythrocytes to less than 15 to 20 percent of normal is indicative of incipient plumbism. Similarly, in symptomatic plumbism, plasma ALA exceeds 0.2 μg/ml and urinary ALA generally exceeds 6 mg/M^2/24 hours. Owing to the wide variation in concentration, measurements of ALA in random urine specimens from children may yield misleading information. The most useful emergency screening test in suspected symptomatic cases is the qualitative urine coproporphyrin test. The coproporphyrinuria of plumbism is much greater than that associated with acute infections and is exceeded only by the coproporphyrinuria of severe acute hepatic injury and some of the inborn errors of porphyrin metabolism. In moribund patients, this test is occasionally negative. The technique of Benson and Chisolm is designed to detect patients in whom blood lead exceeds 100 μg /100 ml.

Radiography of the abdomen may reveal radiopaque foreign material within the intestine. Such films are positive in about one-third of cases. Storage of excess lead in growing bone produces characteristic radiographic changes at the metaphyses of long bones (Fig. 6). The intensity and breadth of these *lead lines* are a function of the duration and degree of excessive lead absorption, but *are not related* to the severity of symptoms. Positive findings are generally associated with blood levels of lead sustained at more than 50 to 60 μg /100 ml. These levels are usually most prominent in children 2 to 5 years of age, although they have been found in older children. In children under 2 years of age, radiographs of long bones are often equivocal and may be negative, even in severely ill patients.

The diagnosis of acute encephalopathy usually can be made on the basis of the clinical picture and positive laboratory evidence of intoxication, but without resort to spinal fluid examination. Cerebral edema fluid can accumulate very rapidly in acute lead encephalopathy so that intracranial pressure is often dangerously high before obvious contraindications for lumbar puncture appear—that is, papilledema, retinal hemorrhages, bradycardia, bradypnea, and separation of sutures on skull radiographs. Lumbar puncture should be avoided in acutely symptomatic cases, unless other causes of increased intracranial pressure must be excluded. If lumbar puncture is attempted, cerebral spinal fluid should be collected *dropwise* and never allowed to spurt out. One milliliter is more than sufficient. In acute lead encephalopathy, the fluid shows normal sugar content, mild pleocytosis, and a moderate increase in protein content. Attempts to obtain fluid by ventricular tap are not warranted.

TREATMENT

Excessive lead intake must be stopped immediately! Therefore, environmental lead sources must be identified rapidly. Cases should be reported to the local health agency, which usually has the authority and responsibility for identifying and removing hazardous sources in the home. Because pica may be difficult to control, it is urgent that environmental hazards be removed. With each recurrence of acute symptomatic plumbism, prognosis worsens. If the source of lead is a painted toy, crib, or lead-glazed earthenware cup, the problem is simple. More often many interior and exterior areas of the home, accessible to children, contain flaking leaded paint. Proper abatement requires that all leaded paint be removed to the bare wood and that painted plaster be replaced or covered with wallboard. This is time consuming. Temporary residence should be found elsewhere for the child, while the repair work is in progress. Hospitalization should be coordinated with repairs in the home.

As the more serious cases generally come from multiproblem families, consultation with the medical-social service department is usually indicated. Children with pica who live in substandard housing require close follow-up until blood lead concentration declines and stabilizes near the normal range, in order to prevent recurrences. Therapy should also include correction of iron deficiency and other nutritional inadequacies and suppression of dust in the home. Intercurrent infections during the first 6 to 12 months after excessive intake of lead is terminated may be associated with exacerbations of plumbism. Effective management requires the sustained cooperative efforts of health department personnel, medical social worker, and pediatrician.

Chelation therapy is a valuable adjunct in the overall management of plumbism. In symptomatic cases, chelating agents can rapidly and safely lower the lead content of soft tissue, which is often followed by prompt clinical improvement. Although potentially lethal concentrations of lead in soft tissues may be reduced rapidly, the entire excess body burden of lead cannot be removed with available chelating agents. The oral use of chelating agents is hazardous if concurrent excessive lead ingestion occurs; under these conditions, absorption and retention of lead is increased. Once abnormal lead absorption is halted, they can be used effectively to reduce the lead content of tissue and to suppress metabolic toxicity more rapidly than can the body's normal physiologic mechanisms. Edathamil calcium disodium (CaEDTA), 2, 3-dimercapto-1-propanol (BAL), and d-penicillamine (PCA) are the three chelating agents used to treat plumbism. In the United States, d-penicillamine is classed by the FDA as an investigational drug when used for lead poisoning. It should not be used as initial therapy. Following initial 3 to 5 day courses of parenteral BAL-CaEDTA or CaEDTA alone, d-penicillamine given orally for 2 to 6 months can obviate the need for repeated parenteral courses of CaEDTA (Fig. 7). The sustaining oral dose of PCA should not exceed 750 mg/M^2/day. It must be given on an empty stomach at least 2 hours before meals. The contents of the capsule may be mixed with chilled fruit or fruit juice, but not with any other food.

In patients with acute symptoms, successful chelation therapy requires administration of a sufficient molar excess of chelating agent(s) over lead. If the dose is insufficient, heavy metal may redistribute within the body and toxicity may be enhanced. Once the mobilization and diuresis of lead into the urine are initiated, courses of BAL and CaEDTA should be completed *without interruption*. The highest dose consistent with safety is required for children with the highest soft tissue lead content, ie, those with acute encephalopathy. The rationale for the use of combined BAL-CaEDTA in the treatment of encephalopathy, as well as adverse side reactions, is described elsewhere.

For combined BAL-CaEDTA therapy, maximum safe dosage is as follows: BAL, 500 mg/M^2/24 hours; CaEDTA, 1,500 mg/M^2/24 hours. These drugs are injected deep, intramuscularly, at separate sites, simultaneously in divided dose every 4 hours for 5 days. This combination reduces blood lead concentration much more rapidly than does CaEDTA alone (Fig. 8), doubles urinary excretion of lead, suppresses toxic metabolic effects of lead on heme synthesis and renal tubular function (they are temporarily exacerbated if CaEDTA is used alone), and reduces mortality to less than 5 percent. Medicinal iron should not be given concurrently with BAL. For patients with less severe symptoms—metabolic evidence of toxicity and blood lead concentration in the 60 to 100 μg /100 ml range—dosage is reduced: BAL 333 μg/M^2/24 hours; CaEDTA, 1,000 mg/M^2/24 hours. Drugs are given intramuscularly in divided dose at 4- to 6-hour intervals for up to 5 days. BAL may be stopped after 3 days, if symptoms abate within 1 to 2 days.

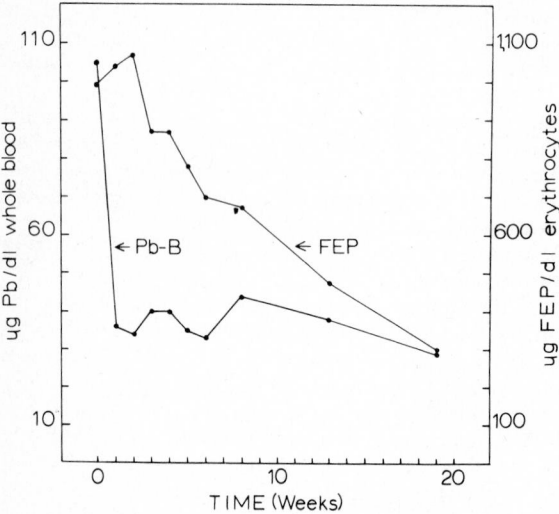

FIG. 7. Relationship between blood lead concentration (Pb-B) and erythrocyte protoporphyrin (EP) during chelation therapy. Patient received BAL-CaEDTA therapy for 5 days, followed by PCA for the next 19 weeks. Note that Pb-B decreases within 72 hours to less than 40 μg/100 ml whole blood and is maintained in this range thereafter; however, FEP changes little at first and then slowly declines, but after 19 weeks is not yet normal (less than 100 μg/100 ml erythrocytes). This illustrates discordance between Pb-B and FEP during PCA therapy; however, anticipated rebound in soft tissue lead levels, which follows brief courses of BAL-CaEDTA or CaEDTA alone, is minimized. (From Chisolm: unpublished data)

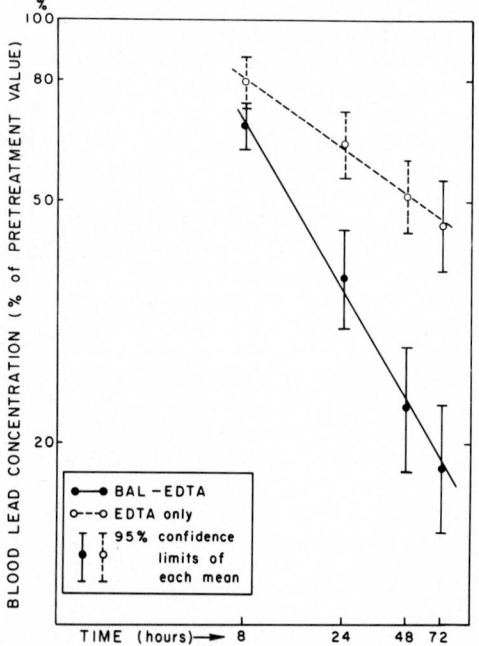

FIG. 8. Rate of decrease of blood lead concentration during first 72 hours of treatment with chelating agents: comparison between BAL-CaEDTA and CaEDTA only. Note that whole blood lead concentration is reduced to 50 percent of the pretreatment value in 15 hours in the BAL-CaEDTA group. Pretreatment values ranged between 100 and 798 μg Pb/100 g whole blood. (From Chisolm. J. Pediatr., 73:1, 1968)

In the treatment of *acute encephalopathy,* supportive therapy is just as vital to survival as chelation therapy. The critical determinants are *prompt* institution of BAL-CaEDTA administration, and restriction of parenteral fluids to basal requirements and a minimal estimate of deficit replacement. Oliguria, a difficult therapeutic problem, may result from dehydration secondary to protracted vomiting or from concurrent renal injury due to lead. Adequate, but not excessive, urine flow must be established before CaEDTA can be given. Ca-EDTA, which is not metabolized in the body, is removed exclusively by glomerular filtration. The following regimen is recommended: as soon as the patient is admitted, a continuous intravenous infusion of 10 percent glucose in water (10 to 20 ml/kg body weight) is given over a period of 1 to 2 hours. Should this fail to initiate urination, mannitol (1 to 2 g/kg body weight) is infused intravenously as a 20 percent solution at a rate of 1 ml/minute. As soon as urine flow is established, intravenous fluid therapy is restricted to basal water and electrolyte requirements and to a minimal estimate of the quantities required for replacement of deficits, convulsive activity, and fever. The intravenous infusion is adjusted hourly until the rate of urine flow is maintained within basal metabolic limits (0.35 to 0.50 ml urine secreted/calorie metabolized/24 hours). This is equivalent to a urinary output of 350 to 500 ml/ M^2/24 hours. This technique is used to avoid excessive fluid administration, which can further increase cerebral edema. Oral intake is prohibited until the patient is much improved. Convulsions are controlled with paraldehyde. (Diazepam will give quick but brief control.) Barbiturates are not given initially; instead, they are instituted on a long-term basis after several days. Body temperature is maintained at normal but not hypothermic levels. Oxygen is administered and cardiopulmonary function is artificially maintained, if necessary. No time is wasted in attempts to evacuate residual lead from the bowel by enema. After urine flow has been established, a matter of 2 to 3 hours at most, chelation therapy is started. A single injection of BAL is given first. Beginning 4 hours later and every 4 hours thereafter for the next 5 to 7 days, BAL and CaEDTA are injected simultaneously at separate intramuscular sites.

Surgical decompression and hypertonic solutions to relieve intracranial pressure and reduce the edema of acute encephalopathy are contraindicated. The use of steroids for this purpose is controversial. The judicious use of mannitol may, in selected cases, be helpful in ameliorating cerebral edema. Careful control of seizures is most important. Following the initial 5- to 7-day course of BAL-EDTA, transfer to a convalescent pediatric facility where PCA can be safely given is advisable. The onset of seizures following encephalopathy may be delayed for some months. Recurrence of seizures usually indicates insufficient dosage of anticonvulsants, lapse of medication, or recurrent lead ingestion. The degree of residual brain damage may not be fully evident for several years.

Screening programs are now causing many *asymp-tomatic children with increased lead absorption* to be referred to pediatric facilities for evaluation, treatment, and follow-up. In the management of these cases, quick identification and abatement of environmental hazards is the first priority. Attempts to abate pica, correction of nutritional deficiencies, and sustained follow-up are pediatric responsibilities. Only through sustained follow-up with repeated blood lead and erythrocyte protoporphyrin tests can the effectiveness of the environmental and pediatric management be judged. In these patients the selective use of CaEDTA (and PCA) is a valuable adjunct to reduce the lead content of soft tissue and minimize the risk of serious injury. Their use should be limited to children showing evidence of toxicity, as these are the ones likely to have the higher soft tissue lead content. Although there is no consensus on indications for CaEDTA (and PCA) therapy in asymptomatic cases, restriction of their use to patients who show one or more of the following is prudent: erythrocyte protoporphyrin greater than eight to ten times the average normal value (ie, FEP greater than 400 to 500 μg/100 ml erythrocytes); δ-aminolevulinic acid in urine greater than 3 mg/M^2/24 hours; plasma ALA greater than 0.2 μg/ml; ALA-D activity in blood less than 15 to 20 percent of normal; CaEDTA mobilization test, urinary lead output greater than 1 μg Pb/mg Ca-EDTA injected. Unless confirmed by at least one of the above tests or by a positive long-bone radiograph, levels of lead in blood in the range of 50 to 79 μg/100 ml are not sufficient indication for chelation therapy. The above tests may occasionally be positive in children with blood lead less than 50 μg/100 ml. Courses of parenteral CaEDTA (1,000 mg/M^2/24 hours, given in divided dose at 8- to 12-hour intervals) should be deferred for 1 to 2 days to allow evacuation of any lead in the bowel, and should be limited to 3 to 5 days.

PREVENTION

In the long run, reduction in mortality, morbidity, and residual nervous system injury associated with childhood plumbism will depend upon replacement or safe renovation of the substandard housing in which the disease is most prevalent. With the increasing use of residential paints that do not contain lead additives, childhood plumbism should eventually become a rarity. Meanwhile, systematic screening in high-risk areas with repeated micro tests for erythrocyte protoporphyrin, followed by confirmatory blood lead tests, provide the best practical means of detecting pediatric plumbism in the preclinical phase. This is especially important in 1- to 3-year olds in whom pica may be just beginning. For example, blood lead concentration in the range of 30 to 60 μg/100 ml may signify equilibration with a contaminated environment or, in a child with pica, it may signify an early increase in soft tissue lead; only through repeated testing can a decision be reached. The inadequacy of past case-finding techniques and brief courses of chelating therapy *after* the onset of intoxication is all too clear.

Bibliography

Barry PSI: A comparison of concentrations of lead in human tissues. Br J Industr Med 32:119, 1975

Beattie AD, Moore MR, Goldberg A: Tetraethyl-lead poisoning. Lancet 2:12, 1972

Benson PF, Chisolm JJ Jr: A reliable qualitative urine coproporphyrin test for lead intoxication in young children. J Pediatr 56:759, 1960

Betts PR, Astley R, Raine DN: Lead intoxication in children in Birmingham. Br Med J 1:402, 1973

Byers RK, Lord EE: Late effects of lead poisoning on mental development. Am J Dis Child 66:471, 1943

Carson TL, Van Gelder GA, Karas GG, Buck WB: Slowed learning in lambs prenatally exposed to lead. Arch Environ Health 29:154, 1974

Chisolm JJ Jr: Aminoaciduria as a manifestation of renal tubular injury in lead intoxication and a comparison with patterns of aminoaciduria seen in other diseases. J Pediatr 60:1, 1962

——————The use of chelating agents in the treatment of acute and chronic lead intoxication in childhood. J Pediatr 73:1, 1968

—————— Barrett MB, Mellits ED: Dose-effect and dose-response relationships for lead in children. J Pediatr 87:1152, 1975

De la Burde B, Choate MS: Early asymptomatic lead exposure and development at school age. J Pediatr 87:638, 1975

Emmerson BT: The clinical differentiation of lead gout from primary gout. Arthritis Rheum 11:623, 1968

Foreman H: Toxic side effects of ethylenediaminetetraacetic acid. J Chronic Dis 16:319, 1963

Lamola AA, Yamane T: Zinc protoporphyrin in the erythrocytes of patients with lead intoxication and iron deficiency anemia. Science 186:936, 1974

Landrigan PJ, Gehlbach SH, Rosenblum BF, et al: Epidemic lead absorption near an ore smelter: The role of particulate lead. N Engl J Med 292:123, 1975

Lead symposium. Postgrad Med J 51: 1975

Lin-Fu JS: Vulnerability of children to lead exposure and toxicity. N Engl J Med 289:1229, 1289, 1973

Millican FK, Layman EM, Lourie RS, Takahashi LY: Study of an oral fixation: pica. J Am Acad Child Psychiatr 7:79, 1968

National Academy of Sciences. Committee on Biologic Effects of Atmospheric Pollutants. Lead, Airborne Lead in Perspective., Washington DC, 1972

Park EA, Jackson D, Kajdi L: Shadow produced by lead in x-ray pictures of growing skeleton. Am J Dis Child 41:485, 1931

Perlstein MA, Attala R: Neurologic sequelae of plumbism in children. Clin Pediatr 5:292, 1966

Sayre JW, Charney E, Vostal J, Pless IB: House and hand dust as a potential source of childhood lead exposure. Am J Dis Child 127:167, 1974

Tola S, Hernberg S, Asp S, Nikkanen J: Parameters indicative of absorption and biological effect in new lead exposure: a prospective study. Br J Industr Med 30:134, 1973

SNAKEBITES

ARNOLD H. EINHORN

There are more than 2,700 species of snakes in the world. About 10 percent of these are poisonous. The worldwide incidence of poisonous snakebites is estimated to be approximately 300,000 annually, and the annual world mortality is believed to exceed 75,000. In the United States data collected primarily from 10 selected states with the highest snakebite rates indicate that each year approximately 7,000 individuals are bitten by poisonous snakes; of these 14 to 15 are fatal

bites. Children and adolescents are most frequently affected. One-fifth of all victims are less than 5 years of age, but by far the majority of all poisonous bites occur in boys 5 to 19 years old. Virtually all bites are inflicted on the extremities.

In the United States, the incidence of bites is highest in North Carolina but most fatalities have occurred in Arizona, Texas, Georgia, and Florida. Snakes, including venomous species, exist also in temperate zone states such as New York, Massachusetts, and Connecticut. In these locations, snakebites are restricted to the warmer months of the year, between April and October, when the snakes are not hibernating; exceptions are nearly always due to bites of captive reptiles. Bites of exotic poisonous snakes are increasing because of the greater availability of such animals and the growing popularity of reptile-keeping as a hobby.

All North American poisonous snakes, except the North American coral snake, are pit vipers (Crotalidae). These Crotalids include the *rattlesnake* (large rattler type Diamondback, pigmy rattler, massasauga, and sidewinder), the swampland infesting *cottonmouth* (or water mocassin), and the smaller *copperhead* (or highland mocassin).

Pit vipers have a characteristic heat-sensing pit midway between the eyes and nostrils on each side of the head. Their pupils are elliptical. Venom glands associated with fangs, which are enlarged grooved or tubular maxillary teeth, form the venom apparatus of the reptile. When the pit viper's mouth is open, well-developed hinged fangs, which ordinarily are folded against the roof of the mouth, protrude from the maxilla.

Coral snakes, which are Elapids, are smaller; they have smaller maxillae and deeply grooved and very anteriorly situated fangs, which have no pits. Their eyes are very small, with elliptical or semielliptical pupils. In the United States, most snakebites for which medical treatment is sought are inflicted by rattlesnakes and copperheads, and a smaller number by cottonmouth mocassins and coral snakes. In Europe and the Middle East the principal poisonous snakes are the Old World or True Vipers (comprising vipers, asps, and adders), which lack heat-sensing pits, but their pupils are elliptical and their fangs similar to those of the pit viper. The adder is the only poisonous snake in Great Britain.

TOXINS AND TOXIC EFFECTS

Snake venoms are toxins of unparalleled biochemical and pharmacologic complexity. Their constituents include at least 17 enzymes, primarily proteases, hyaluronidase, and phospholipases; several nonenzymatic polypeptides, glycoproteins; and several other compounds. The venom has direct myonecrotic effects, and the local neuro- and hemotoxicity that it exerts causes rapid and severe tissue destruction. The ensuing diffusion of substances contained in the venom produces systemic neurotoxic, cardiotoxic, hemotoxic, and nephrotoxic effects. Some factors in the poison elicit release of pharmacologically active compounds such as bradykinin and histamine from the tissues. Bradykinin causes vasodilatation and stimulates muscles of the mouth.

The systemic effects of venom include alteration of capillary permeability, with secondary loss of plasma into the extravascular space and considerable edema, hemolysis, thrombocytopenia, prolongation of prothrombin time, vasodilatation with pooling of blood in major vessels and hypovolemic shock, intravascular thrombosis, nervous system depression, impairment of myocardial contractility and conduction, and renal failure. In addition, snakebites occasionally may inflict rapid loss of digits, or even limbs, and necrosis of other body tissues. Permanent crippling and even loss of vision may occur.

The course of snakebite is unpredictable; the amount of venom available in the reptile's gland may differ in individual snakes and among different species; also the amount of poison injected in any given bite may vary. Poisonous snakes have the ability to withhold or control the volume of venom injected when striking. There also are individual variations in human response to the toxins of venom. As a rule, the toxic effects are quite rapid after a pit viper's bite. However, clinical evaluation of severity and prognosis may be difficult with the bite of a rattlesnake since the fangs are relatively long and venom may be injected subfascially. Systemic manifestations after envenomation by coral snakes and other Elapids, such as the cobra, may develop only after several hours.

DIAGNOSIS

Diagnosis is based on the history and the findings of fang or teeth marks, which are generally large and freely bleeding punctures. For identification it is preferable to examine the entire body of the offending snake rather than the head only. Pit vipers can be identified by turning the snake's belly upwards and noting a single row of subcaudal plates just below the anal plate. The differential diagnosis of snakebite involves primarily the distinction with other kinds of envenomations, such as arthropod stings and bites, which usually produce smaller punctures and do not bleed as readily. Immunologic studies on fluid collected around the puncture site may aid in the detection of snake venom.

SYMPTOMS AND SIGNS. The unpredictability of the clinical course after a poisonous bite has been stressed. When there is *no or minimal envenomation,* moderate or severe pain develops at the site of the wound where fang or tooth marks are visible. However, surrounding edema is less than 5 inches in the first 12 hours after the bite and there are few manifestations of systemic involvement.

In poisonous bites with *moderate to severe envenomation,* local excruciating pain occurs within minutes after the snakebite. At the site of injury a white wheal surrounds the site of puncture, soon followed by local redness and swelling which increases and extends rapidly (Fig. 9).

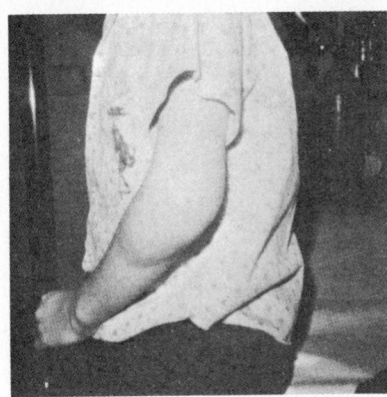

FIG. 9. Marked edema occurring within minutes after baby coral snakebite.

The skin becomes dark and purplish and sanguinous fluid oozes from the wound. In bites of the hand the entire area may become swollen in less than 1 hour.

Systemic ill-effects in severe cases include generalized weakness, giddiness and dizziness, profuse perspiration, nausea, and bloody vomiting. Subcutaneous and internal hemorrhage into the lungs and gastrointestinal and urinary tracts, will be manifest as epistaxis, hematemesis, melena, and hematuria. Severe loss of blood may cause hypovolemic shock and this may be aggravated by the effects of bradykinin release. Pupils may become dilated, the pulse weak, and respiration labored. Paralysis, loss of vision, convulsions, and coma may ensue and ultimately result in death.

After pit-viper and true-viper envenomation, hemorrhage, local swelling, and pain are the main symptoms. The swelling begins within minutes and lasts for days, but maximal swelling is reached during the first day. Massive hemorrhage, extensive diffusion, and a considerable degree of swelling are indicative of a bite in which a large amount of venom was injected.

The bite of a coral snake usually produces little or no swelling or edema at the site of the bite. The major clinical features of Elapid (coral snake, cobra) envenomation relate to the presence of neurotoxins, which accounts for the delayed clinical expression. Ptosis is very common and may be the earliest sign of systemic poisoning; it is often associated with strabismus and incoordination of speech. Generalized rhizomelic muscle weakness, without actual paralysis, is also quite typical. Other symptoms and signs include vertigo, convulsions, drowsiness, sometimes culminating in coma, and paralysis of respiration and deglutition.

TREATMENT

Severe or even moderately severe snakebite poisoning must be viewed as an emergency and treated vigorously. On the other hand, it is equally important to refrain from unnecessary use of heroic treatment if there is little or no evidence of envenomation and to avoid complications of the therapy itself. Before therapy is considered, it must be established that the offender is poisonous. If the bite is over one hour old and there is no local edema, pain, or tenderness and no evidence of fang puncture, the serpent was neither a viper nor an Elapid. If the snake is identified as nonpoisonous or the wound is not a serious one, incision is not warranted unless the bite of a coral snake is suspected. The wound is cleaned and the patient and parents are reassured.

Mild envenomation with only moderate pain at the site of the fang wounds, less than 5 inches of surrounding edema, and no systemic involvement can be adequately treated by cleansing the bitten area, making a linear incision through the skin from one fang mark to the other, gently expressing or suctioning the fluid from the local wound without maceration, and then injecting 10 ml of antivenin serum intramuscularly or intravenously.

Treatment of serious and critical bites is urgent and requires the combined use of bite excision, skin incision between the fang marks, early fasciotomy, and antivenom, steroid therapy, and antibiotics. Only immediately after the bite should a flat tourniquet be applied proximal to the wound, loose enough to permit easy introduction of one finger beneath it but tight enough to occlude superficial venous and lymphatic flow without interrupting arterial circulation. The tourniquet should be released for 1 to 2 minutes every 10 to 15 minutes for 1 to 2 hours. As edema progresses, the constricting band should be advanced centrally to keep just ahead of the swelling; it should be removed completely when antivenom is given and after incision and excision. Incision and gentle suction, or expression and excision, will eliminate appreciable quantities of venom only when performed during the first hour after the bite. The sooner these measures are instituted the larger the amount of venom that can be removed. Suction or expression of fluid must be very gentle and brief to avoid increasing local circulation and venous return. The bitten limb should be immobilized at heart level and should be neither elevated nor dependent. Similarly, muscular exercise, excitement, exertion, and excessive oral or intravenous fluid administration accelerate circulation time and propel the venom throughout the body; they should, therefore, be avoided.

The administration of specific *snake antivenin* is the mainstay of therapy and the treatment of choice. All victims of poisonous snakebites should be transported as rapidly as possible to a center where snake antivenin is available. The optimal dose of snake antivenin for children is not well established; it varies with the severity of the bite and accompanying symptoms. In severe bites with intense focal signs and moderate to severe systemic manifestations, the intravenous administration of 30 to 60 ml of snake antivenin diluted in 1,000 ml of saline is recommended. Studies with radioisotopes have shown that antivenin accumulates rapidly at the site of the bite when the intravenous route is used. Injection of antiserum into or near the area of the bite is of no particular value. In the United States the polyvalent pit viper antivenin is the only immunotherapeutic agent available and is effective against bites by all North American pit vipers. A major problem with bites by exotic poisonous snakes is the choice and availability of suitable antiserum. Pediatricians confronted with this situation may contact their local Poison Control Center or the Antivenin Index Center of the American Association of Zoological Parks and Aquariums in Oklahoma City (phone: 405-427-6232).

The administration of antivenin carries with it the risk of anaphylaxis to horse serum. A skin test should be performed before the antivenin is used and, if necessary, the patient must be gradually desensitized throughout the administration. Antihistaminics and epinephrine may also be necessary to control sensitivity reactions to horse serum antivenin.

Glucocorticosteroid therapy (intravenous hydrocortisone 5 mg/kg, first dose, then 10 mg/kg/24 hours in four divided doses) also may be a valuable adjunct to other measures in the treatment of snakebites. Glucocorticoids do not treat the snake envenomination per se. They are most likely of value for the prevention of shock and for the prevention or treatment of serum sickness secondary to the horse serum antivenin. If the patient is in hypovolemic shock, vasopressors alone cannot restore the lost blood volume. Whole blood or plasma analogues are necessary to maintain the blood pressure in such instances. Administration of fresh frozen plasma, specific antihemorrhagic blood factors, platelet transfusion, and vitamin K may be required to combat hemorrhage.

Tetanus antitoxin or toxoid and antibiotic therapy are indicated since all snakebites also introduce pyogenic microorganisms. In Elapid poisoning, respiratory failure may develop after a latent period. The patient may require appropriate measures to maintain or restore airway patency, and to provide oxygenation, ventilation, and respiratory support with intermittent positive pressure breathing if necessary.

Bibliography

SNAKEBITES

Boys F, Smith HM: Poisonous Amphibians and Reptiles. CC Thomas, Springfield, Ill, 1971

Brown JG: Toxicology and Pharmacology of Venoms from Poisonous Snakes. CC Thomas, Springfield, Ill, 1973

Henderson BM, Dujon EB: Snake bites in children. J Pediatr Surg 8:729, 1973

Minton SA Jr: Snakes and Snake Venoms in Venom Diseases. CC Thomas, Springfield, Ill, 1974

———— Snakebite: an unpredictable emergency. J Trauma 11: 1053, 1971

Mitrakul C, Impun C: The hemorrhagic phenomena associated with green pit viper bites in children. A report of studies to elucidate their pathogenesis. Clin Pediatr 12:215, 1973

Parrish HM: Analysis of 460 fatalities from venomous animals in the United States. Am J Med Sci 425: 129, 1963

———— Incidence of treated snakebites in the United States. Health Rep 81:269 1966

——— Nature of poisonous snakebites in New York. NY State J Med 1965

Russel FE: Treatment of rattlesnake bite. JAMA 207:159, 1969

Snyder R: Snake bites. Am J Dis Child 103:85 1962

Synder CC, Straight R, Glenn J: The snakebitten hand. Plastic Reconstr Surg 49:275, 1972

DRUG ABUSE

IRIS F. LITT
MICHAEL I. COHEN
S. KENNETH SCHONBERG

Drug abuse, an ancient and sporadic adult cultural phenomenon, has, in the past decade, become a diffuse and major psychosocial, legal, environmental, and health hazard for our youth. Drug use has broad implications for the young patient and the physician because of the potential for multisystem involvement at a time of accelerated physical and psychological maturation. The adverse effects of drugs upon mood, temperament, and behavior have become a problem of major import, with increasing medical and social significance. This section will be devoted to established patterns of abuse, newly emerging drug-usage trends, an analysis of the physiology, psychopharmacology, and organ system-related complications of drug abuse, and the health management issues of drug abuse in children and adolescents.

Our personal observations are based on a 7.5 year experience with approximately 14,000 drug-using adolescents between the ages of 10 and 21 years. These teenagers represent poverty level, and low- and middle-income families within New York City and the surrounding suburbs. There was one female for every five males in this group. Medical, social, and psychological appraisal of these teenagers was accomplished on an inpatient adolescent service and through several ambulatory care facilities for adolescents.

OPIATES

Opiates have been used for centuries for their ability to produce analgesia and euphoria. In the latter half of the 20th century these properties have been rediscovered and abused in epidemic proportions by adolescents, initially in the form of heroin and more recently as methadone.

Heroin

IDENTIFICATION, ADMINISTRATION, AND DOSAGE. Heroin is a semisynthetic derivative of the seed pods of Papaver somniferum, the opium poppy grown principally in Asia Minor. Acetylation of the parent morphine molecule to heroin renders it more potent as a respiratory depressant, analgesic, and euphoriant. In its pure form, heroin is a white, crystalline powder that is bitter to taste. When obtained by the youthful consumer, it is usually a mixture of heroin, lactose, and other adulterants. The lactose is added as a filler to dilute the opiate. A variety of other substances, such as quinine, procaine, or methylpyrilene, are used to disguise the sweet taste of lactose. The powdered mixture is commonly sold in small glassine envelopes, called *bags*, which, in 1975, ranged in price from $5 to $20. The content of individual envelopes varies widely and is limited only by the seller's resourcefulness and lack of scruples. The final concentration of heroin after adulteration may range from 1 to 20 percent, or 1 to 30 mg.

The adolescent's first introduction to heroin may be by the nasal route, called *snorting*. In most cases no more than one bag can be inhaled in a 6-hour interval, without producing irritation and erythema of the nasal mucosa. This discomfort, combined with a half-hour interval between administration and desired psychopharmacologic effect, frequently leads to the subcutaneous route of administration, called *skin-popping*. This has been a popular route for teenagers. The heroin is usually dissolved in heated water and then drawn up in a syringe or jagged-edged eyedropper, referred to as the *works*. We have found that the skin is rarely cleansed before it is punctured. Intravenous administration, or *mainlining*, results in almost immediate psychologic and physical gratification. Shooting up, or intravenous self-administration, is usually accomplished every 6 to 8 hours by the addict. Constant use of the same blood vessel will result in typical scars, termed *needle tracks*.

METABOLISM, PHYSIOLOGY, AND PSYCHOPHARMACOLOGY. Heroin is rapidly cleared from the blood, and 90 percent is excreted within 24 hours after administration. It is rapidly hydrolyzed to 6-monacetyl morphine and then to morphine. Detoxification proceeds by conjugation with glucuronic acid within the liver and then urinary excretion as free and conjugated morphine. Morphine can be detected in the urine, by thin-layer chromatography, up to 48 hours after administration. Quinine added to the heroin can be detected in urine up to 72 hours after the last dose.

Once heroin is converted to morphine, it may pass the placenta rapidly; maximal effects are observed in the fetus between 1 and 6 hours after the drug is administered to the mother. Controversy exists as to whether heroin is excreted in human breast milk.

In experiments at the cellular level, heroin as morphine, enhances glucose uptake and phospholipid production, inhibits hydrolysis and release of acetylcholine, and also increases production of 5-hydroxytryptamine by rat brain slices.

Heroin is desired because of its effectiveness in producing euphoria and relieving pain. The frequent occurrence of drowsiness, nausea, and vomiting following initial usage does not appear to be a sufficient deterrent to its abuse. Lowering of body temperature associated with heroin use appears to be a direct effect on the hypothalamus. Increased rate of release of antidiuretic hormone contributes to the relative oliguria of the heroin abuser. Heroin also increases the tone of the ureter and detrusor muscles. ACTH release is suppressed by chronic heroin use, and 17-hydroxy- and 17-ketosteroid levels are consequently lower. The electroencephalograph of the heroin user appears similar to that seen during normal sleep. Miosis caused by heroin appears to be a helpful clinical diagnostic sign of abuse, because it does not disappear as tolerance develops. Dilation of a miotic pupil following administration of an opiate antagonist such as naloxone is pathognomonic of opiate use. The test dose required to produce this effect is 0.4 mg of naloxone administered intravenously.

Heroin has four times the effect of morphine as a respiratory depressant, primarily by reducing the medullary response to carbon dioxide. The rate, minute volume, and tidal exchange are equally depressed. The medullary cough center is similarly depressed, and for this reason opiates have long been used as antitussives.

The physiologic effects of heroin on the gastrointestinal tract include increased tone of the antral portion of the stomach and first portion of the duodenum, which results in delayed gastric emptying time. Hydrochloric acid production and biliary and pancreatic secretions are all decreased by heroin. The constipating effect of opiates in the form of paregoric is well-known to pediatricians. Similarly, the action of heroin on the smooth muscle of the small and large intestine decreases propulsive contractions and augments anal sphincter tone, further contributing to the constipation that persists even as tolerance develops. Proliferation of hepatic smooth endoplasmic reticulum and focal areas of hepatocellular necrosis have been demonstrated in heroin users who have no evidence of clinical hepatitis, raising the possibility that the drug has a primary stimulatory and/or toxic effect on the liver. Studies in morphine- and methadone-addicted rodents have demonstrated that the activity of bilirubin glucuronyl transferase is enhanced.

The physiologic effects of heroin on the cardiovascular system are minimal. In normal subjects, morphine causes relaxation of the peripheral vascular bed without direct cardiac effects. In patients with aortic valvular disease, cardiac index, stroke index, and central venous pressure are increased after morphine administration.

MEDICAL COMPLICATIONS. Heroin became the leading cause of death among adolescents in New York City during 1969 and 1970. Because some sequelae of heroin abuse can be prevented and most others treated if diagnosed early, it is imperative that physicians be able to recognize these medical complications.

NEUROMUSCULAR. Among the heroin related neurologic diseases, disseminated *intracranial microabscesses*, secondary to septic emboli, are most common. These rarely produce symptoms and may only be appreciated at autopsy, unlike the less common solitary large abscess. *Staphylococcus aureus* is the usual etiologic agent. Noninfectious neurologic complications such as transverse *myelitis*, brachial and lumbosacral *plexitis*, and acute rhabdomyolysis are rare in the adolescent and develop primarily in patients reexposed to heroin after a period of abstinence. *Convulsive seizures* may occur as a complication of the cerebral edema of opiate overdose.

Neuropathy resulting from accidental injection into a peripheral nerve may cause ankle or wrist drop.

We have observed transient elevation of serum glutamic oxaloacetic transaminase activity associated with heroin withdrawal in the absence of other evidence of hepatic dysfunction. This effect may reflect mild striated muscle damage similar to that documented by electromyography and creatinine phosphokinase determinations in acute barbiturate withdrawal.

GASTROINTESTINAL. The gastrointestinal tract is the organ system having the greatest number of complications resulting from heroin abuse.

Approximately 10 percent of adult addicts described by Cherubin were found to have an active *duodenal ulcer*. One-third of the 18 deaths due to peritonitis at the Lexington Rehabilitation Center were secondary to an ulcer. This observation may appear inconsistent with the decreased production of hydrochloric acid that results from heroin use. However, the delayed gastric emptying time, coupled with the ability of heroin to mask pain, may contribute to this complication. Misinterpretation of peptic ulcer symptoms for those of acute withdrawal has been responsible for death from gastric perforation in several young addicts. Therapy in teenagers with ulcer diathesis, but without perforation, includes a relatively unrestricted diet with frequent antacid therapy. Sedatives are to be avoided because of their potential for abuse.

Chronic opiate abusers are constipated and frequently troubled by *hemorrhoids,* which are rare in nondrug abusing teenagers. With discontinuance of opiates, diarrhea associated with hyperactive bowel sounds occurs as a prominent component of the *abstinence syndrome,* usually within 48 to 72 hours of the last dose in the heroin user and after 6 days in the methadone addict.

A supply of heroin concealed in a condom and swallowed has led to *intestinal obstruction* in a small number of abusers. A still rarer cause of small bowel obstruction is the occasional practice of swallowing cotton pledgets through which heroin had previously been strained to remove particulate matter prior to injection. These pledgets contain powdered opiate and are a final reserve when all other supplies are gone.

Acute hepatitis is the single most common complication of heroin abuse in adolescents. Eighty percent of the teenage heroin users who required hospitalization in our program had this diagnosis. Of these, 11 patients developed hepatic encephalopathy, resulting in 6 deaths over a 7.5 year period.

Thirty-six percent of ambulatory, asymptomatic, heroin-using adolescents examined by our service had chemical evidence of hepatitis consisting of two or more abnormal liver function tests. Hepatitis is most often presumed to be viral in origin and related to the communal use of unsterilized needles. Observation of a few adolescents with hepatitis who had admitted only to having snorted heroin raises the possibility that heroin or one of its diluents may have a direct toxic effect on the liver. Support for this hypothesis is provided by the electron microscopic appearance of hypertrophied smooth endoplasmic reticulum and eosinophilic bodies in liver biopsies of some heroin addicts. Countervailing evidence of hepatic toxicity is found in human morphine addiction experiments. Our own experiments with liver explants grown in tissue culture with added opiate also failed to demonstrate liver function abnormalities. Approximately 500 heroin-using adolescents with hepatic dysfunction, followed by us, have had a prolonged clinical course marked by multiple exacerbations, quite different from the generally mild course seen with hepatitis in most children and adolescents who did not use drugs. The histologic appearance of liver biopsies in these patients is consistent with a diagnosis of chronic persistent hepatitis.

CARDIOPULMONARY. Any heroin user, whether addict or dabbler, who develops fever of unknown origin should be suspected of having *bacterial endocarditis.* This condition may occur in a patient with or without a history of a preexisting cardiac lesion. In Louria's series, only one-third of the patients had a history of or physical findings compatible with underlying cardiac pathology. Right-sided endocarditis is usually caused by *Staphylococcus aureus,* affecting a previously normal tricuspid valve, and may be associated with few, if any, clinical findings. Early diagnosis will be facilitated by examining the heroin addict in all positions, including squatting, in both phases of respiration, for auscultory evidence of acute tricuspid regurgitation. One of our 15-year-old addicts suffered two bouts of *Staphylococcus aureus* endocarditis affecting the triscupid valve and presented with findings of septic pulmonary emboli. Embolization to the brain, spleen, and kidney, as well as to the lungs, has been documented with tricuspid valve involvement. As in nondrug users, endocarditis affecting the left side of the heart is more often caused by streptococci or fungal agents, the latter particularly if previous valve damage exists. Septic emboli in the absence of pulmonary emboli is usually diagnostic of a left-sided lesion or a small intracardiac shunt. The initial diagnostic evaluation and therapeutic approach is similar to that of classic bacterial endocarditis as seen in children with rheumatic heart disease. Antimicrobial therapy will depend upon bacteriologic and fungal findings.

Angiothrombotic pulmonary hypertension is a rare complication of inadvertent intravenous injection of starch or other inert filler used to dilute heroin. Fibers of cotton used to strain heroin prior to injection may also play a role. Pulmonary granulomata may be caused in the same manner. While diagnosis must usually await postmortem examination of lung tissue with a polarizing microscope, it may be suspected in the heroin user with evidence of decreased lung volume and diffusion capacity. For unknown reasons, pneumonia is uncommon in the adolescent heroin user. However, radioisotopic studies have demonstrated abnormalities of regional lung perfusion in asymptomatic addicts. The combination of depressed cough reflex and delayed gastric emptying time described previously is the most plausible explanation for the high incidence of aspiration pneumonia in adult addicts.

Tuberculosis is found with greater frequency in adult heroin addicts than in the general population. However, in the heroin-using adolescent the incidence of tuberculosis, based on routine tuberculin skin testing, appears to be no higher than in his nonheroin-using peers. Similarly, the increased prevalence (5 to 9 percent) of asthma reported in adult heroin addicts has not been documented in adolescents who use heroin.

Pulmonary edema is prominent only in association with the heroin-overdose syndrome, which may be fatal. It is radiographically evident even in the absence of clinical signs. Follow-up evaluation of a small number of patients with pulmonary edema who have recovered suggests long-term sequelae, such as a reduced diffusing capacity. The pathogenesis of pulmonary edema in association with the heroin abuse is unknown.

GYNECOLOGIC. A variety of gynecologic disorders, including oligomenorrhea, amenorrhea, and menometrorrhagia, have been described in adult heroin addicts. *Amenorrhea* appears with striking frequency in adolescent heroin users. The rate at which menses returns after heroin use ceases varies inversely with the length of time the drug has been used. We have postulated that the production or release of gonadotrophin is inhibited by heroin, as has been demonstrated with ACTH release. The adolescent in whom a regular menstrual cycle has not yet been established appears more vulnerable to this effect that the adult heroin user.

Venereal diseases generally occur as a complication of heightened sexual promiscuity fostered by a frequent need to support heroin habituation through prostitution. Ironically, libido is actually decreased by heroin use. In addition, there is an increased prevalence of biologic false-positive serology studies (VDRL), the cause of which is not clear; the higher prevalence apparently does not correlate with the presence of active liver disease, which is also known to be associated with serologic false-positive VDRLs. A weakly reactive VDRL over a period of two weeks suggests a false-positive reaction. Confirmatory tests should be performed in such patients. However, it is prudent to commence treatment for syphilis on the basis of the screening test alone, since the patient may not return for follow-up.

In our experience the incidence of pregnancy in adolescent heroin users is no different from that in nonheroin using teenage girls. Assuming a greater risk of pregnancy associated with a high rate of prostitution in the former group, this observation may be additional evidence of anovulation in the heroin users and/or generally poorer health status.

The complications of pregnancy in the teenage heroin user, which are the same as those in the adult addict, include a higher rate of spontaneous abortion, stillbirths, and small-for-gestational-age infants. The combination of adolescence and heroin use results in a still higher-risk pregnancy, with danger extending into the newborn period because the abstinence syndrome frequently occurs in the neonate (p. 825). Although experimental administration of morphine sulfate to pregnant mice has resulted in exencephaly in offspring, we have not observed a higher incidence of congenital malformations in adolescent addict pregnancies.

DERMATOLOGIC.   *Skin abscesses* frequently complicate the use of an unsterilized needle for the subcutaneous or intravenous administration of heroin. Repeated use of the former route can also cause atrophy and *subcutaneous fat necrosis,* not unlike that found in patients with diabetes mellitus. The addition of sclerosing agents, such as mannite, used as adulterants in the heroin mixture to enhance its bitter quality, can result in necrotic *skin ulcers. Hyperpigmentation* of a vessel or lesions that resemble railroad tracts are indicative of intravenous use.

Cigarette burns around the upper chest may result from the user falling asleep with a lighted cigarette in his or her mouth after injection or from a street method of attempting resuscitation of an overdose victim by stimulation with a lighted cigarette. Bullae have been described on the skin of overdose victims, similar to those found in association with carbon monoxide or barbiturate intoxication, and analysis of the fluid from such bullae may be diagnostic, in that it may contain a high concentration of the responsible toxin.

Tattoos, either to disguise needle tracks or to facilitate identification among heroin users, are also common in adolescents. Superficial skin infections are easily managed with improved hygiene and appropriate antibiotic therapy. Plastic surgery for cosmetic repair of scars plays a specific and important role in the total rehabilitative effort of the teenage addict.

INFECTIOUS.   Bacteria within heroin injection paraphernalia, the lack of aseptic technique, and the possibility of altered immunologic status all contribute to the increased risk of infection in the drug user. Infectious complications of heroin abuse, such as *bacterial endocarditis, hepatitis,* and *cerebral abscesses,* have been previously mentioned. *Tetanus* is also observed with increased frequency in heroin users. Currently, the group with the highest incidence of tetanus is composed of older women addicts who have resorted to skin popping after their veins have sclerosed. The abscesses resulting from this method of administration provide excellent growth media for the clostridium organism. Among adolescents, in whom skin popping is often the preferred route of administration and in whom abscess formation is also common, tetanus is not as frequent a complication. The immunity acquired in childhood from tetanus immunizations probably accounts for this difference. A booster of tetanus toxoid would, nevertheless, seem indicated in all teenage drug users. Septic arthritis of the sternoclavicular and sternochondral articulations due to *Pseudomonas aeruginosa,* although rare, is more common in heroin users.

RENAL.   Seven of our heroin-abusing adolescent patients, all with elevated levels of SGPT and proteinuria, were found to have focal glomerulonephritis when evaluated by renal biopsy. Others have described immunocomplex deposits on the glomerular basement membranes of heroin addicts.

HEMATOLOGIC.   Significant peripheral eosinophilia has been observed in many of our adolescent users. Although we could find no explanation for this observation, the possibility exists that it expresses a state of hypersensitivity to heroin or one of its adulterants, which, in turn, could be related to the pathogenesis of the heroin overdose syndrome.

THE ABSTINENCE SYNDROME.   Heroin withdrawal is characterized by a syndrome progressing from yawning, to lacrimation, restlessness, dilated pupils, insomnia, goose flesh, muscle cramps, hyperactive bowel sounds, diarrhea, systolic hypertension, tachycardia, and, rarely, convulsions within 48 hours after the use of heroin has been discontinued. A seizure constitutes severe withdrawal even in the absence of other symptoms. Only 25 percent of the heroin-using teenagers we observed manifested some or all of these findings.

Evaluation of the withdrawal process was accomplished by use of an opiate withdrawal log (OWL) score (Table 14). This score was designed in an attempt to quantitate withdrawal. The OWL score also provides a means for following a patient systematically through a course of treatment.

Treatment of the abstinence syndrome or detoxification in adolescents is directed toward preventing the life-threatening complications of seizures and cardiovascular collapse. Chlorpromazine administration is undesirable in the case of the adolescent addict because of its potential for lowering the seizure threshold and for inducing hepatotoxicity and hypotension. Moreover, sudden death has been reported following its use in withdrawal. The inherent addictive potential of phenobarbital and its lack of superiority to other modalities makes it of little use in dealing with the adolescent. Methadone is effective in alleviating the symptoms of abstinence, but current treatment schedules require 7 to 10 days for this purpose. A treatment regimen for adolescent heroin users utilizing diazepam has been effective in our experience in eliminating signs of withdrawal within three days and in preventing seizures and cardiovascular collapse. Treatment is based on evaluation by the OWL score. Those who are scored as having *mild* withdrawal are treated with diazepam orally in a dose of 10 mg every 6 hours for 3 days. Patients in the *moderate* category are first given diazepam intramuscularly in two doses of 10 mg each, separated by an interval of 4 hours. This treatment is followed by the oral regimen described above. In *severe* withdrawal, diazepam is given intramuscularly in doses of 10 mg every 4 hours for the first 24 hours, the same intramuscular dose every 6 hours for the next 24 hours, and 10 mg orally every 6 hours for the third day. All medication should be discontinued when the OWL score falls below 2, usually within 3 days of onset of therapy. Occasionally, one 2.5-mg dose of diphenoxylate hydrochloride is necessary to control diarrhea. Insomnia will persist for as long as a month after onset of abstinence symptoms and is refractory to the usual sedatives. The patient should be made aware of this from the onset and warned of the danger of self-administration of other drugs in a search for sleep.

TABLE 14. Opiate Withdrawal Log (O.W.L.)

Symptoms	Items Receiving No Points	Items Receiving One Point Each	Items Receiving Two Points Each
1. Yawning	Absent		
2. Dilated pupils (> 8mm)	Absent	Present	—
3. Restlessnes	—	Moderate	Severe
4. Lacrimation	Absent	Present	—
5. "Goose flesh"	Absent	Present	—
6. Muscle cramps	Absent	Present	—
7. Insomnia	Slept for 7 hr or more/24 hr	Slept 4–7hr/ 24 hr	Slept less than 4 hr/24 hr
8. Hyperactive bowel sounds	Absent	Present after 48 hr from withdrawal of heroin	Present before 48 hr from withdrawal of heroin
9. Diarrhea	0–1 stools/12 hr	2–4 stools/12 hr	4 stools >/12 hr
10. Vital signs: Pulse Blood Pressure	<72 <108/70	72–100 or 110–140/70	> 100 or <140/70

The abstinence syndrome is clinically evaluated in each patient by scoring his symptom complex according to the above noted point system. An O.W.L. score of 1 to 5 points is considered "mild" withdrawal, 6 to 10 points is "moderate" withdrawal, and 11 to 15 points is "severe" withdrawal.
(From Litt, et al: J Pediatr 1971)

Many barbiturate-using adolescents started using the drug after they felt they have successfully kicked their heroin habit and merely desired something to induce sleep. Because we have had no experience treating the heroin addict with a history of a seizure disorder with diazepam, we would not suggest depending on this drug alone in detoxifying such a patient.

ACUTE HEROIN TOXICITY. DIAGNOSIS. The adolescent who presents with lethargy or coma, constricted pupils, respiratory depression, cyanosis, and/or rales should be considered *overdosed* until proved otherwise.

EMERGENCY TREATMENT. Treatment should be instituted immediately as follows:

Intubate the patient and administer oxygen by positive pressure.
Administer naloxone, 0.01 mg/kg intravenously. Dilation of previously constricted pupils after naloxone provides evidence of opiate toxicity.
Start intravenous fluid therapy.
Obtain serum samples for morphine, barbiturate, and glutethimide levels.
Perform blood gas and acid base studies.
Obtain urine for toxicologic analysis and carefully observe urinary output. A Foley catheter may be indicated.
Administer naloxone 0.01 mg/kg intravenously if the naloxone test (above) is positive. This may be repeated at 5-minute intervals until pulmonary ventilatory function improves.
A radiograph of the chest often reveals pulmonary edema. If present, the use of penicillin in therapeutic doses is recommended to prevent secondary infection.
Even if the patient becomes fully alert, hospitalization is warranted as a first step in the rehabilitation process.

It should be noted that the opiate overdose may be due to methadone, a situation seen with increasing frequency in children of adult addicts maintained on this drug who may keep it at home in orange juice. Treatment with naloxone should be continued at 4-hour intervals for 24 hours, as methadone is a longer-acting opiate than heroin.

Methadone

IDENTIFICATION, ADMINISTRATION, AND DOSAGE. Methadone is a synthetic narcotic that first came into clinical use in the early 1940s. At present federal restrictions limit its use to outpatient adjunctive therapy in the rehabilitation of narcotic addicts within licensed methadone maintenance programs. Paradoxically, it has become a major drug of abuse partly through illicit diversion from these programs.

Administered parenterally, methadone is almost identical to morphine in the dose required for analgesia, onset and duration of action, and its euphoric and sedative properties. It differs from both morphine and heroin in that it is effective when taken orally. Methadone is available in forms specifically designed to prevent intravenous abuse. The most widely dispensed preparation is a tablet or wafer containing 40 mg of methadone, plus both cellulose and corn starch. These two additives are insoluble and make intravenous abuse both difficult and foolhardy as they result in embolic sequelae. Another currently used preparation combines methadone and naloxone in a ratio of 20 to 1. The naloxone is inactive when taken by mouth but will prevent any opiate effect and precipitate withdrawal if this combined form is administered intravenously. The *street* methadone addict usually ingests a daily dose of between 40 and 100 mg, which at 1976 prices represents a $10 to $25/day habit.

METABOLISM, PHYSIOLOGY, AND PSYCHO-PHARMACOLOGY. By the oral route, methadone has an onset of action within 30 minutes and reaches peak plasma levels within 4 to 6 hours. It is excreted slowly, having a plasma half-life of approximately 22 hours. A major portion of ingested methadone appears in the urine and feces in the form of unknown biotransformation products, with less than 10 percent of the drug excreted unchanged. In addition, methadone metabolites are excreted into the intestinal tract via the bile. The principal pharmacologic actions of methadone are upon the central nervous system and smooth muscle. Its central nervous system effects include analgesia, release of antidiuretic hormone, depression of respiration and cough, sedation, and euphoria. Methadone increases intestinal smooth muscle tone, but diminishes the amplitude of its contractions and propulsive activity.

MEDICAL COMPLICATIONS. It is rare to find an opiate addict who is using either heroin or methadone exclusively. Far more commonly, the opiate of abuse is dependent upon availability rather than preference. Therefore the medical complications observed with methadone are a combination of those ascribed to either heroin or methadone.

The protean complications of heroin abuse have been previously detailed, and the consequence of illicit methadone abuse will only be described in those instances where significant differences exist. What is known regarding these consequences has been gained from the study of patients undergoing methadone maintenance treatment. The applicability of this information to the illegal methadone abuser is an assumption based on limited experience rather than controlled study.

With the exceptions of acute overdose and physiologic addiction, the medical complications of both illegal methadone abuse and medically sanctioned methadone maintenance are in the main benign. Those infectious complications so common among heroin addicts are generally not found in the teenager restricting his use to the oral ingestion of methadone. However, both the street methadone addict and the methadone maintained patient remain at high risk for other serious medical illnesses. These are usually secondary to prior somatic drug-related insult, current polydrug abuse including excessive alcoholic use, and continuance of a less than healthy and productive lifestyle.

Severe constipation is encountered in some 60 per-

cent of patients in the early months of methadone maintenance and laxative therapy may be required. This symptom tends to subside with time as the patient becomes tolerant of a constant dose. However, 20 percent of patients remain constipated for as long as methadone is administered. The high incidence of chronic persistent hepatitis found in adolescent heroin addicts is not significantly altered by prolonged methadone maintenance and the presumed abstinence from intravenous abuse.

A return to normal menstrual function is the rule in the adolescent girl placed on methadone as treatment for heroin addiction. Pregnancy may, therefore, be viewed as a consequence if not as a complication of maintenance therapy. Appropriate family planning information and services should be made available to all female drug users in the reproductive age who are being offered methadone therapy. Further gynecologic evaluation is indicated if amenorrhea persists after heroin is withdrawn or for more than the first 6 months of methadone maintenance. Pregnancy during methadone maintenance results in fewer small-for-dates infants than among heroin addicts but more than would be expected in a nondrug using population. Although differing criteria for the diagnosis of neonatal opiate withdrawal make comparisons difficult, methadone appears to cause more frequent, prolonged, and pronounced symptoms in the infant than does heroin. An increased incidence of sudden infant death syndrome within the first few months of life has been reported.

THE ABSTINENCE SYNDROME. The methadone withdrawal syndrome does not differ symptomatically from that of heroin. However, the onset is delayed and should not occur for at least 24 to 48 hours after the last dose. In addition, moderate symptomatology may persist for as long as one week. As with heroin abstinence, insomnia and anxiety may persist for a month after all other symptoms have subsided. The withdrawal syndrome may be treated with either diazepam, as outlined for heroin, or by the administration of methadone itself. An oral dose of 40 mg methadone once daily is sufficient to prevent withdrawal symptoms in all but the most excessive abuser. After one to two days at this dose, symptoms are usually controlled and the methadone can then be withdrawn slowly at roughly 5 mg/day, or alternatively the patient can be referred for continuing methadone maintenance. The patient on a methadone maintenance program who requires detoxification will similarly have his dose reduced slowly in a stepwise fashion and should experience few, if any, withdrawal symptoms.

ACUTE METHADONE TOXICITY. Clinical presentation of methadone overdose is identical to that of heroin (p. 810). Emergency treatment differs only from that of heroin overdose in that naloxone must be continued for a minimum of 24 hours. The overdosed patient will first respond dramatically to naloxone but, because of the increased length of action of methadone over heroin, may relapse into a fatal coma within 3 to 4 hours if the therapy is not continued.

The methadone maintained patient will often overdose with a drug other than an opiate, with tranquilizers, barbiturates, and alcohol being the predominant offenders. In these instances the administration of naloxone will not result in clinical improvement and may precipitate acute opiate withdrawal. In addition to being semicomatose, confused, and lethargic, the patient now becomes agitated and severely uncomfortable from opiate withdrawal. It is, therefore, best to reserve the use of naloxone to those instances in which coma or respiratory compromise mandate aggressive therapy.

METHADONE MAINTENANCE AS A THERAPEUTIC MODALITY. During the past decade, methadone maintenance has become the most prevalent form of therapy for adult heroin addicts in the United States. Initially, government regulations had restricted the use of methadone maintenance to individuals past their 18th birthday. More recently, the age limit has been reduced to 16 years. Furthermore, a handful of specially licensed programs has for a number of years been offering this form of therapy to adolescents of any age. In general the criteria for admission to a maintenance program include both a history of prolonged opiate addiction, usually at least 2 years, and proof of failure in a drug free treatment program. At present, most programs are funded by state or municipal agencies, although some privately sponsored programs do exist.

In both the adult and adolescent programs, methadone is administered daily as a substitute for heroin. In low doses of up to approximately 40 mg/day methadone will prevent physiologic opiate withdrawal. In larger doses of 80 to 100 mg/day tolerance to opiates is raised to a point where it becomes extremely difficult to achieve euphoria by the intravenous administration of heroin. Most adult patients are maintained in the higher dose range, while adolescents are offered the lower doses.

Negating the heroin *high* with methadone is referred to as *blockade.* In addition to the possible advantages of an orally administered, legal, and inexpensive drug that prevents withdrawal symptoms and interferes with heroin euphoria are the more subtle benefits derived from forcing the patient into daily contact with a medical and counseling staff. Once having obviated the need to procure illicit heroin, both patient and staff may now concentrate their energies on social, educational, and vocational rehabilitation. Using this combination of methadone maintenance and supportive services, these programs for adolescents have experienced moderate success in interrupting opiate abuse and returning young people to school and employment. When a stable, abuse-free lifestyle has been achieved, optimistically, within 1 to 2 years, an attempt can be made to proceed from methadone maintenance to complete opiate abstinence.

DEPRESSANTS

The recent increased use of depressants among teenagers appears to be related in part to the need for relief of insomnia associated with self-imposed heroin withdrawal, or the ability of barbiturates to potentiate a heroin high and modify an amphetamine binge. However, we suspect the major contributing factor to abuse is the depressant effect on mood and behavior in young people who are troubled, anxious, and unable to cope properly with adolescent life stresses.

IDENTIFICATION, ADMINISTRATION, AND DOSAGE. Synthetic central nervous system depressants (barbiturates and other sedative-hypnotic agents) are gaining in popularity among adolescents who abuse drugs. The more commonly used of this group are *Tuinal* (sodium amobarbitol and sodium secobarbital), *Doriden* (glutethimide or "Cibas"), and *Quaalude* (methaqualone or *soapers*). While these are prepared commercially for oral use, their abuse frequently involves intravenous administration following dissolution of pills or capsules in water. When barbiturates are appropriately prescribed for a seizure disorder, dosage falls in the range of 3 to 8 mg/kg/day. In the adolescent who has developed tolerance, self-administration may reach over 4,000 mg/day. However, tolerance to the lethal respiratory effect does not develop fully and many accidental deaths have occurred by inadvertent overdose. The usual therapeutic dose schedule for glutethimide is 0.125 to 0.5 g three times a day for sedation or hypnosis. In the nontolerant adolescent, 5 g will produce severe intoxication and 10 g may be fatal. Cross-tolerance develops within this category of drugs, a fact utilized in detoxification and treatment of the complications of depressant withdrawal.

Barbiturates and Glutethimide

METABOLISM, PHYSIOLOGY, AND PSYCHOPHARMACOLOGY. *Secobarbital* and *amobarbital,* the most commonly abused barbiturates, are short-acting. They are well absorbed from the stomach or subcutaneous tissue, detoxified in the liver, and excreted in urine. They pass the placental barrier and into breast milk. *Glutethimide,* on the other hand, is absorbed irregularly from the gastrointestinal tract. Because of its high lipid-to-water partition coefficient, it diffuses rapidly in vascular tissues. It is completely metabolized into the glucuronide and the glutaconimide, which are excreted into the intestine by way of the biliary tract. Urinary excretion of the metabolites is slow.

Barbiturates depress the central nervous system through their ability to raise the threshold of stimulation of neurons and prolong their time for recovery. For this reason they are used as anticonvulsants, hypnotics, anesthetics, and analgesics. *Respiratory depression* is a frequent complication of the effect of the drug on the medullary respiratory center. Barbiturates decrease the tone of the gastrointestinal tract and delay gastric emptying time. *Addiction* and *tolerance* develop within 1 or 2 months of the daily use of 500 mg or more of these sedatives.

The pharmacologic effects of *glutethimide* are very similar to those of secobarbital. However, glutethimide also acts as an anticholinergic to produce mydriasis, drying of the mouth, and decreased intestinal motility.

MEDICAL COMPLICATIONS. Complications of barbiturate or other sedative abuse result from the method of administration, idiosyncratic reactions, and accidental overdoses. An unsterile needle for the injection of sedatives is responsible for a high incidence of hepatitis and abscesses in this group of drug abusers, as in the heroin addict. The practice of crushing and dissolving tablets and capsules for intravenous use has been implicated in the production of talc and starch granulomata and emboli in the lung, with resultant pulmonary hypertension. A variety of skin lesions, including a measleslike exanthem, a scarlatiniform rash, and sweat-gland necrosis with bullae have been described in association with barbiturate use. The fact that the lethal dose does not change in the presence of tolerance to the other effects makes overdose common. Slurred speech, short attention span, emotional lability, nystagmus, and ataxia are characteristic of the sedative addict, who thus may be mistaken for an alcohol inebriate. Definitive diagnosis is made by analysis of serum or urine for barbiturates or other sedatives.

THE ABSTINENCE SYNDROME. Symptoms of withdrawal generally appear between 12 and 16 hours after the last dose of a short-acting barbiturate or glutethimide. Anxiety, restlessness, and tremors are the first symptoms to appear, followed in rapid succession by nausea, vomiting, and abdominal cramps. By 24 hours, the patient is weak with hyperactive reflexes and orthostatic hypotension and may experience a *major motor seizure* within 48 hours after his last dose if withdrawal is not appropriately treated. With the longer-acting barbiturates, seizures may not appear until 1 week after the last dose. Tachycardia and fever are also seen in glutethimide withdrawal.

The extremely high incidence of grand mal seizures following abrupt discontinuation of sedatives in an addict makes gradual withdrawal under close medical supervision imperative.

WHOM TO DETOXIFY:

Anyone using 500 mg/day or more of a barbiturate or any other sedatives for more than 1 month.

Anyone absuing sedatives regularly, regardless of amount, with a history of seizure disorder.

HOW TO DETOXIFY THE BARBITURATE OR GLUTETHIMIDE ADDICT:

Ascertain the usual total daily dose (termed X) and divide it into four equal doses. Therapeutically, use phenobarbital on a gram-for-gram substitution for the abused agent. If the patient's reliability is doubtful, assume that the true daily dose is half that stated and proceed as below.

If the last dose was taken more than 12 hours before the patient was seen, or if he manifests signs of tremor, restlessness, or hypotension, administer the first dose intramuscularly; otherwise administer this and all subsequent doses by the oral route.

If the history is accurate, the first dose should cause signs of mild toxicity, such as nystagmus, dysarthria, or ataxia. If these signs do not appear within 22 hours of the first dose, recalculate the total daily dose at X + 120 mg. The next dose, given 6 hours after the first, should therefore be 30 mg more than the first.

Continue to increase the dose until signs of mild toxicity appear.

Consider the total daily dose at which signs of mild toxicity appear as the maintenance dose.

On the second day of treatment give the initial day's maintenance dose divided in four equal parts.

On the third day reduce the total daily dose by 120 mg divided equally between the four doses.

Continue tapering at a rate of X-120 mg/day until half of the maintenance dose is attained.

Give half the maintenance dose for 2 days.

Continue tapering at a rate of X-120 mg/day. Stop tapering for a day or two if restlessness, tremor, anxiety, or drop in blood pressure develops and then continue as before to reduce at X-120 mg until no drug is being given.

Chlorpromazine is contraindicated in detoxification of the depressant addict.

Intravenous fluid administration and meticulous attention to intake and output will prevent iatrogenically induced barbiturate overdose in a patient who might otherwise become too lethargic to maintain adequate hydration.

ACUTE SEDATIVE DRUG TOXICITY. DIAGNOSIS. Toxicity from barbiturates resembles that from opiates in that the patient is comatose, in respiratory distress, often with constricted pupils unless hypoxic dilation has occurred, and manifests signs of shock. Bullae on the skin may be aspirated and their contents analyzed to determine the responsible drug. Tonic muscular spasms, convulsions, hypotension, and paralytic ileus are common in glutethimide overdose in which, in contrast to barbiturates, the pupils are usually dilated.

EMERGENCY TREATMENT:

A slurry of activated charcoal may be given if one sees the patient within 30 minutes of ingestion. This may still be effective after a longer period of time has elapsed because of the delayed gastric emptying caused by these drugs.

With a barbiturate, perform gastric lavage and/or induce vomiting. Never induce emesis if glutethimide is ingested; it may precipitate apnea. Save the first 10 ml of gastric aspirate for toxicologic analysis.

Maintain an adequate airway. Use oxygen if necessary but only by positive pressure. Keep the patient warm.

Start intravenous fluid therapy and monitor serum electrolytes, blood gases, and plasma barbiturate levels (3.5 mg/100 ml may be lethal with short-acting barbiturates, 8 mg/100 ml with the long-acting variety).

Urinary bladder catheterization is frequently helpful. Alkalinizing the urine has no effect on the excretion of short-acting barbiturates, but may be helpful with long-acting barbiturates. A high urine output will also be helpful.

Analeptics have no place in the treatment of barbiturate poisoning.

Hemodialysis may be effective in short- or long-acting barbiturate and glutethimide poisoning. However, dialysis is rarely indicated in a comatose patient solely because of coma, since supportive measures alone will suffice.

Methaqualone

In 1965 methaqualone (2-methyl-3-otolyl-4 (3H)-quinizaolinone), was marketed as a nonaddictive sedative-hypnotic agent. As has been the case with all other similarly touted drugs, methaqualone has subsequently been shown to be addictive and to produce severe toxicity when taken in excess. Its popularity as a drug of abuse relates to undocumented allegations of its aphrodisiac properties as well as early advertising in the medical literature claiming that this drug did not suppress REM sleep.

It appears to be the abused drug of choice by a widely diverse adolescent population, frequently used in conjunction with other drugs, alcohol, or marihuana. The drug is administered orally, frequently with wine or cider, in a dose of 250 to 500 mg. The euphoria, paresthesias, and a feeling of indestructability that follow even low-dose administration frequently result in automotive and other accidents.

Addiction may occur following ingestion of 2 g/day for as short a period as 30 days in adults. The *withdrawal syndrome* will appear within 3 to 5 days of abstinence in the addicted individual. Signs and symptoms consist of headache, anorexia, abdominal cramps, disturbed sleep patterns, and convulsions.

Detoxification, utilizing phenobarbital in a ratio of 1 mg of phenobarbital for each 10 mg of methaqualone, is appropriate. However, most patients may be detoxified with phenobarbital over 3 to 5 days rather than by the much slower process described for barbiturate and glutethimide withdrawal. The reasons for this remain unclear.

Absorption from the gastrointestinal tract is followed by glucuronidation within the liver. Methaqualone overdosage results from as little as 110 mg/kg body weight and is similar to the syndrome associated with overdose from any sedative, with the additional finding of muscular hypertonicity, increased deep tendon reflexes, and myoclonia in some patients.

Treatment of the intoxicated patient is mainly supportive, with peritoneal and hemodialysis offering little advantage. In contrast to treatment of phenobarbital overdose, forced diuresis is contraindicated in methaqualone overdosage because of the risk of precipitating congestive heart failure.

Methyprylon

A white, bitter powder, soluble in water and comparable in its hypnotic effect to secobarbital, methyprylon is utilized clinically as a sedative in a dose of 200 to 400 mg in adults. Its toxicity is similar to that of barbiturates, with hypotension and circulatory shock resulting from overdosage. Although the lethal dose is unknown, death has been reported following 6 g in an adult. A dose of approximately 1.5 g daily over a 60-day period has produced dependency in adults. The abstinence syndrome associated with abrupt discontinuance in the dependent patient consists of insomnia, hallucinations, and generalized convulsions. Detoxification in the addicted patient should proceed as with barbiturates, remembering that 10 mg of methyprylon is equivalent to 1 mg of phenobarbital.

STIMULANTS

Amphetamines

In the pursuit of a *high,* the drug-using adolescent may discover oral amphetamines. However, once the user has been introduced to an intravenous injection of a sympathomimetic amine, slow stimulation is incidental to achieving the main objective of immediate and complete excitation.

IDENTIFICATION, ADMINISTRATION, AND DOSAGE. Discovered in 1930s to have vasopressor action, by the 1940s amphetamines were abused by truck drivers and students alike for their ability to inhibit fatigue. In the 1950s they were abused by housewives and others for weight reduction and in the 1960s and 1970s by teen-agers for *kicks.* Amphetamines are sympathomimetic amines that act by inhibiting amine oxidase. A survey of medical students in a western university in 1965 revealed almost half to have used amphetamines at least once. In 1968, 22 percent of 11th and 12th graders in a California high school had experimented with them. The problem is not restricted to the United States; 7 percent of students in the 7th through 13th grades in Toronto had used stimulants, according to one report, and Sweden was heavily involved in an amphetamine crisis in the early 1970s.

The drug's effects can be appreciated within 30 minutes of oral administration, or within 5 minutes of subcutaneous injection. Intravenous injection is not recommended by pharmacologists, a fact ignored by teenagers, who prefer this route for the instantaneous effect.

Toxicologic analysis of a refrigerated casual specimen of urine or saliva will be diagnostic of amphetamine abuse.

METABOLISM, PHYSIOLOGY, AND PSYCHOPHARMACOLOGY. Amphetamines are well absorbed from the gastrointestinal tract. They are deaminated by the liver or excreted unchanged in the urine, where they may be detected from 3 hours to 3 days after ingestion.

Their peripheral manifestations result from a direct effect on adrenergic receptors of muscles and glands. Amphetamines stimulate the medullary respiratory center and the cerebrospinal axis and are utilized pharmacologically for their analeptic potential. In man, the psychic and psychomotor effects are dramatic. An initial oral dose of 10 mg results in mood elevation, wakefulness, self-confidence, greater concentration ability, increased strength, and appetite depression. Unfortunately, tolerance develops quickly to these effects, and depression, confusion, paranoia, and headache are common in the chronic user.

In higher doses, the usual physiologic effect is systolic and diastolic hypertension. A concomitant decrease in cerebral blood flow has been demonstrated. The effect on the gastrointestinal tract is variable, with gastric emptying time increased at first and later delayed. Hydrochloric acid production is unaffected. The ability of amphetamines to contract the trigone and relax the detrusor muscles of the urinary bladder is responsible for their use in enuresis. It is thought that the beneficial effect of amphetamines in the management of dysmenorrhea in the adolescent is related to their ability to diminish the amplitude of uterine contractions, although their effect on the central nervous system may also contribute to the beneficial results.

Speed, the term used for intravenously injected amphetamine, produces an immediate chill, racing pulse, blurred vision, dilation of the pupils, and elevated blood pressure. The user is consumed by a frenzy of activity directed at obtaining more drug to reproduce the alleged ecstasy effect, the so-called *speed binge.* If unobtainable, a profound fatigue and depression set in, called *crashing.* The victim sleeps for days and paranoia is marked.

MEDICAL COMPLICATIONS. The adolescent with dilated pupils, elevated blood pressure, rapid pulse, blanched mucous membranes, weight loss, and paranoia is possibly an amphetamine user. Hepatitis may result from the use of unsterilized needles. As with barbiturates, pulmonary granulomata and emboli may be the consequence of intravenous injection of capsules and tablets containing talc or starch. Intravenous use has also been implicated in cerebrovascular accidents, although this complication is rare. Angiitis has also been reported. Alterations in somatic growth have been documented in younger children receiving amphetamines for behavioral modification, and one wonders then about their affects on teenagers, who are in the midst of a major growth spurt.

ACUTE TOXICITY REACTIONS. DIAGNOSIS. Reactions consisting of vomiting, diarrhea, palpitation, arrhythmia, syncope, hyperpyrexia, and hyperreflexia, progressing to convulsion or coma, may result from as little as 30 mg, although there are reports of daily doses of 15,000 mg in chronic users.

TREATMENT OF ACUTE AMPHETAMINE POISONING.
Immediate hospitalization.
Gastric lavage.
Sedation with chlorpromazine.
Hypothermia mattress possibly indicated.

Based on experiments in monkeys, the lethal dose for children is thought to be 5 mg/kg, and for adults 20 to 25 mg/kg. The lethal dose in mice, however, is influenced by environmental conditions. While the LD_{50} for mice caged individually was 100 mg/kg, that for mice caged in groups was 25 mg/kg. Some investigators compare this rodent group–toxicity factor to the violence of speed users in a group setting. Tolerance definitely develops, as does psychic dependence.

TREATMENT OF AMPHETAMINE WITHDRAWAL. The treatment of the chronic user separated from his drug should consist of hospitalization with admission to a darkened and quiet room. A professional in attendance to reassure the patient is helpful, and observation should extend for approximately 48 to 72 hours. Suicide or homicide are possibilities after the patient awakens. Detoxification utilizing drug therapy is not necessary.

Cocaine

Cocaine is abused for the euphoric stimulation it produces as well as for its ability to cause pleasant hallucinations.

IDENTIFICATION, ADMINISTRATION, AND DOSAGE. Cocaine is derived from the leaves of Erythoxylon coca, indigenous to Peru, where the pre-Inca Indians discovered its stimulant properties. Cocaine (or benzolmethylecgonine) is structurally similar to many local anesthetics with which it shares the ability to block nerve conduction. It is well absorbed from mucous membranes and until recently its abuse involved chewing or nasal inhalation. However, subcutaneous and intravenous use are becoming increasingly more popular routes of administration.

METABOLISM, PHYSIOLOGY, AND PSYCHOPHARMACOLOGY. Most of that which is absorbed is detoxified by the liver and excreted in the urine as benzoylecgonine. Approximately 9 percent is excreted unchanged. Both forms can be detected by gas–liquid and thin-layer chromatography of the urine.

The systemic effects of cocaine include initial central nervous system stimulation, which manifests itself in restlessness, decreased fatigability, increased motor activity, increased respiratory rate, and emesis followed by eventual depression. The heart rate is increased as a result of central and peripheral sympathetic stimulation. This, in combination with centrally mediated vasoconstriction, produces hypertension initially. Vasoconstriction, a direct action on heat regulation centers, and increased muscular activity combine to make cocaine pyrogenic. The sympathomimetic actions of the drug are thought to result from its ability to prevent destruction of epinephrine or by increasing its cellular permeability.

Tolerance to these pharmacologic effects develops, and psychic dependence can be marked. The absence of characteristic withdrawal symptoms upon discontinuance of use in a chronic abuser suggests that physiologic addiction probably does not occur. Like the amphetamine abuser, the individual abusing cocaine is likely to develop paranoia. *Formication,* or the sensation of objects crawling on one's body, is another indication of mental deterioration.

MEDICAL COMPLICATIONS. Nausea, anorexia, emaciation, insomnia, tremors, and convulsions may occur in the chronic cocaine user. In addition, specific complications related to the route of administration occur. The most popular method of administration has been inhalation or sniffing. After prolonged use, this often results in perforation of the nasal septum. Subcutaneous injection causes ischemia secondary to the vasoconstrictive properties of the drug. This, in combination with the lack of sterile technique, is responsible for the frequent occurrence of abscesses at injection sites and the potential for bacterial endocarditis and tetanus, as described with heroin abuse. Intravenous injection of a large dose of cocaine may result in immediate death from cardiac failure due to a direct toxic action on the myocardium.

The current high cost of cocaine appears to be responsible for its use in combination with heroin, rather than alone. This combination is called a *speedball.*

Since physiologic addiction probably does not occur, we believe there is no clinical abstinence syndrome. Poisonings require the immediate intravenous administration of short-acting barbiturates in conjunction with support of respiratory efforts. A tourniquet about the extremity used for administration of the cocaine may prove helpful. Most of the drug is detoxified within 1 hour of administration so that prognosis is excellent if the patient can be adequately supported for a short period of time.

HALLUCINOGENS AND PSYCHEDELICS

Lysergic Acid Diethylamide (LSD)

This compound was first synthesized in 1938 from ergot and 5 years later was found to have profound hallucinogenic properties. Its structure is similar to ergonovine and both are oxytocics. LSD is thought to act on the central nervous system at the synaptic level, possibly by its effect on intracellular serotonin.

LSD is rapidly absorbed from the gastrointestinal tract and is widely distributed throughout the body, the greatest concentration being in the liver. There it is excreted as 2-oxy-LSD within 90 minutes of ingestion, although its central nervous system effects persist for days or longer. Radioactive LSD has been shown to pass the placenta in mice, but definitive evidence of its passage in humans is lacking. It is not yet known whether it can be transmitted to offspring through breast milk, but its wide diffusion throughout all body tissues makes this a likely possibility.

In man, LSD in doses of 20 mg have produced euphoria or dysphoria, visual or tactile distortions, or hallucinations and confusion. These effects may be relived without additional ingestion even months later in the so-called *flashback* phenomenon. Tolerance to these effects has been demonstrated and cross-tolerance exists to other hallucinogenic agents such as mescaline. Regular users may ingest 500 mg/dose.

Dilated pupils, hyperthermia, piloerection, hyperglycemia, and tachycardia are some of the sympathomimetic properties of the drug which may help in distinguishing an LSD abuser from a psychotic. In this regard it is helpful to recall that the latter frequently experiences auditory hallucinations, which are rare in the LSD patient, whose hallucinations are usually visual.

The use of LSD by college students and younger adolescents has reportedly declined in recent years as information concerning reputed associated chromoso-mal damage became widely known. The evidence of adverse effects of LSD on human pregnancy remains unclear.

Marihuana

IDENTIFICATION, ADMINISTRATION, AND DOSAGE. Marihuana is produced from the resin in the inflorescence, high leaves, fertilized ovary, and unripened fruit of *Canabis sativa.* This plant, also a source of hemp fiber and seed oil, grows in temperate and hot, dry areas, particularly near human habitation. Its hallucinogenic properties were reportedly known to man as early as 600 BC. Analysis of cannabis resin reveals cannabinol, cannabidial, cannabidiolic acid, tetrahydrocannabinol-carboxylic acid, cannabigerol, cannabichromic, and tetrahydrocannabinol. Cannabidiolic acid and cannabichromic possess sedative properties, while the hallucinogenic effects of marihuana appear to reside in the tetrahydrocannabinol (THC) fractions, especially $\Delta 9$, which have recently been synthesized. The pure synthetic form is a potent hallucinogen, even more so than LSD.

Marihuana is most commonly used in the form of *reefers* or *joints,* which are made by rolling the crushed leaves and flowers in paper. *Hashish,* the preferred form, has about eight times the potency of marihuana; it is smoked in a pipe. Because there is no accurate or simple method for toxicologic analysis of body fluids for marihuana, the exact extent of its use is difficult to ascertain. Based on various surveys, however, it can be concluded that at the present time, exclusive of alcohol, marihuana is the most extensively abused substance among adolescents in the United States.

$\Delta 9$ *THC,* 0.5 to 5.0 mg, or its equivalent of cannabis, is psychoactive by inhalation. Three times this amount is necessary to achieve the same effect by the oral route.

METABOLISM, PHYSIOLOGY, AND PSYCHOPHARMACOLOGY. Oral administration of tritium-labeled $\Delta 9$ THC to human volunteers results in absorption of 90 to 95 percent of the administered dose, while the biologic half-life is less than 72 hours. One to 2 hours after ingestion, at the time of peak psychologic effect, plasma levels of radioactivity are maximal and remain high for 6 hours, well after the subjective effects have passed. The level declines rapidly at 24 hours and more slowly thereafter. At the time of maximal radioactivity, $\Delta 9$ THC levels are low, while those of a metabolite 8, ii-di-OH-$\Delta 9$ THC are elevated. At 12 hours postingestion, plasma levels of $\Delta 9$ THC are increased more than twofold. By the inhalation route, 50 percent of THC is absorbed, resulting in a momentary increase in plasma radioactivity. The peak occurs 10 minutes later and most has disappeared by 60 minutes. There is extensive excretion of $\Delta 9$ THC and its metabolites in urine and feces, in a ratio of 1:3.

MEDICAL COMPLICATIONS. BEHAVIORAL. The sought-after effects of marihuana include elation and easy laughing. Other common effects include distortion in time perception, grandiosity, and loss of critical judgment. Since the late 1960s and the work of Weil and associates, a number of reports describing the pharmacologic effects of marihuana and its component fractions have appeared. Marihuana-induced impairment of immediate memory recall and performance of simple intellectual and psychomotor tests have been documented. In addition, it has also been demonstrated that doses of Δ9 THC comparable to those used socially caused decrement of performance of divided attention tasks, such as driving. Δ9 THC, in doses similar to those found to be hallucinogenic in humans, produces electroencephalographic and behavioral disruption in cats. Similar experiments in rats have suggested that tolerance develops to some of the EEG effects and that there is a rebound increase in integrated voltage following termination of chronic, daily administration.

Adverse reactions to marihuana do occur and appear to be correlated with personality structure rather than dose. Weil and coworkers described occasional depressive reactions, panic reactions, and toxic psychoses in the marihuana user without a history of other hallucinogen abuse or previous mental illness. Of these, the *panic reaction* is the most common and treatment should consist of gentle but authoritative reassurance that the patient is not psychotic and that the effects of the drug are only temporary. In those who have taken hallucinogens, marihuana use may cause flashbacks or the recurrence of hallucinations. Visual hallucinations or distortions in tactile and proprioceptive experience may occur at high doses of cannabis or THC. *Derealization* has been precipitated in schizophrenics who smoke marihuana. Adolescents are prone to develop a syndrome of passivity and lack of goal direction with chronic use.

Still unresolved are the questions of whether dependence and tolerance develop, and whether a true marihuana abstinence syndrome exists.

Marihuana has been condemned for its potential for causing later experimentation with heroin. While this may be true in some populations, we have found in a large inner-city ghetto adolescent population that for most heroin users the first contact was with glue sniffing rather than with marihuana.

CARDIOPULMONARY. Marihuana causes tachycardia in both novice and experienced subjects in 10 to 20 minutes after onset of smoking but prior to perception of the high. It has been suggested that marihuana affects heart rate through an alteration in autonomic tone. There exists, however, other evidence that this cardiovascular response is due to a direct action on myocardial contractility. Mild elevations in both systolic and diastolic blood pressure occur during the peak psychologic effect and disappear within 3 hours.

Respiratory rate is increased by marihuana smoking in the chronic, naive user but unchanged in the neophyte. Bronchoscopy and biopsy of the respiratory mucosa of hashish smokers who demonstrated signs of bronchitis showed atypical cells, loss of cilia, and epithelial cell hyperplasia.

ENDOCRINE. The clinical observation of gynecomastia associated with chronic high-dose marihuana

smoking prompted investigation of its effect on male reproductive physiology by Kolodny and associates. These studies failed to confirm the finding of gynecomastia or elevation of prolactin levels, but demonstrated dose-related suppression of plasma testosterone in otherwise normal young adult males who smoked marihuana for a minimum of 4 days a week for 6 months. The effect of marihuana in delaying development of a prepubertal male or one in early puberty has not yet been reported but is of obvious concern. Similarly, the possibility that Δ9 THC, which crosses the placenta, may depress fetal androgen levels has been raised but not confirmed. In female rodents, THC has been shown to accumulate in corpora lutea, to block the surge of LH secretion that normally occurs with proestrus, and to delay ovulation.

Although significantly higher glucose levels are found during a glucose tolerance test following the smoking of marihuana for 7 days than after an abstinence period, no impairment of insulin or growth hormone metabolism has been observed.

Δ8,–and Δ9 THC produce a marked decrease in body weight, which is maintained for the duration of the period of chronic administration in rats.

IMMUNOLOGIC. Chronic human marihuana smokers have been shown to have decreased cell-mediated immunity similar to that resulting from impaired T-cell immunity by in vitro testing. More recently, however, in vivo skin testing with 2.4 dinitrochlorbenzene has demonstrated no difference between chronic marihuana users and normal controls.

CARCINOGENIC POTENTIAL. Because both tobacco and *Cannabis sativa* are consumed by smoking, the possibility that the latter may be carcinogenic has been raised. Several reports, coupled with evidence of concentration of marihuana derivatives in the lung and placenta, serve to emphasize the importance of further study into the potential role of marihuana in carcinogenesis in humans.

TERATOGENIC POTENTIAL. Δ9 THC is embryocidal or fetocidal in early pregnancy in mice and is responsible for fetal growth retardation when administered at a later stage of pregnancy. Reports of teratogenesis in humans using marihuana have been difficult to substantiate because of associated polydrug abuse, including LSD, in these same mothers.

THERAPEUTIC POTENTIAL. Observations that THC can effect lowering of intraocular pressure and reduce edema, temperature, bronchospasm, pain, and bone marrow leukopoiesis have prompted speculation that this substance may have therapeutic potential in certain conditions. Further investigation and confirmation are necessary before these preliminary observations can have any clinical application.

Peyote (Mescaline)

Peyote is derived from the head or button of a cactus plant found in Texas and Mexico, which is dried and chewed or brewed into tea. First tried by the Aztecs, its hallucinogenic properties were realized by Indians who in 1885 banded together to form the Native American Church based on its use.

All the alkaloids thus far isolated from the peyote cactus are similar in structure to epinephrine; lophophorine, in the pure state, causes convulsion and death; pellotine causes drowsiness; anhalonidine stimulates the central nervous system; and mescaline induces hallucinations.

Less than half of the ingested mescaline is absorbed. Studies of radioactive mescaline indicate that it does not enter the neurons of the central nervous system. An indirect effect on serotonin has been postulated with blockade of epinephrine receptors a possible alternate mechanism of action.

Ingestion is followed by drying of lips, tongue, and skin, which is first flushed and then pale, dilated pupils, bradycardia, hypoglycemia, nausea and vomiting, and, in severe cases, by diarrhea and body odor. Insomnia, chest pain, uterine contractions, headache, and numbness may occur.

Hallucinations produced by peyote are visual, olfactory, or auditory. These are reportedly pleasant, although an occasional user experiences terror, tremor, or manic-depressive psychosis.

Mescaline, like LSD, has been shown to be teratogenic in early pregnancy in hamsters.

Nutmeg

The seed of the apricot like fruit of the tropical tree *Myristica fragrans* has long been known to have hallucinogenic properties. The physiologic effects of nutmeg are tachycardia, dryness of mucous membranes, and often headache, nausea, dizziness, and shortness of breath. These undesirable effects occur at the usual dose of one teaspoon.

STP (2,5-Dimethoxy-4-Methyl-Amphetamine or DOM)

STP causes visual hallucinations and psychoses similar to those produced by LSD, but more potent in that they may last up to a week after a single dose. The respiratory paralysis and death reported with its use are most likely the result of contamination with atropine, rather than from the drug itself.

GENERAL PRINCIPLES OF TREATMENT. Management of a *bad trip* or *bummer* whether from intoxication with a naturally occurring or synthetic hallucinogen requires a firm, authoritative, and reassuring approach. Repetitive defining of reality, eg, "This is a book—feel the book," is essential. Admission to a quiet, nonthreatening room with dim lighting is often helpful. If one finds difficulty establishing verbal contact, tranquilizers are indicated. Chlorpromazine is contraindicated for those hallucinogens with anticholinergic properties or additives. Since it is often difficult to know with certainty if such a substances has been taken, it may

be wise to *avoid the use of phenothiazine derivatives.* In such situations diazepam may be an effective alternative. The usual dose is 10 mg intramuscularly stat and then repeated in 2 and 4 hours if needed.

GLUE SNIFFING AND OTHER INHALANT ABUSE

Inhalants are used for their ability to produce exhilaration and euphoria. Solvent sniffing was first reported on the West Coast in the late 1950s and spread eastward a decade later as a phenomenon exclusively of children and adolescents. The plastic cement or glue used in making airplane models was the first agent so abused and popular in the young adolescent population of inner-city ghettos. Experimentation with other inhalants such as cleaning fluids, hair sprays, and various aerosols has recently characterized middle-income suburban teenagers.

The ritual of vapor inhalation takes many forms. It ranges from that of saturating a rag with the desired substance, pouring or squeezing it into a paper or plastic bag from which it is inhaled, placing it in a pan that is subsequently heated to promote rapid vaporization, or direct spraying of the posterior pharynx. Initial experimentation is usually a group phenomenon, while the habitué soon resorts to sniffing alone.

In the absence of routine toxicologic screening tests for the various substances abused by inhalation, the extent of such abuse is unknown. In the group of delinquent adolescents under our care, approximately 10 percent admitted to glue sniffing. The mean age of onset of this practice was 13 years. Inhalation of cleaning fluid, popular from 1967 for approximately 5 years, is now much less frequently observed. The mean age of this group was 15 years.

Plastic cement, or *airplane glue,* is a mixture of toluene and ethyl acetate. The popular *cleaning fluid* preparation most commonly used contains trichloroethylene and 1,1,1-trichloroethane.

Early uncontrolled studies have been cited to incriminate glue sniffing as a cause of brain damage, leukemia, and liver damage. None of these allegations has been substantiated. Indeed, we performed studies of liver function on over 750 glue sniffers and found no evidence of hepatic dysfunction.

On the other hand, *cleaning fluid inhalation* is, in our experience, a definite cause of hepatotoxicity and renal impairment. The sudden onset of vomiting, abdominal pain, and jaundice, in the absence of needle puncture marks, should alert the physician to the possibility of this form of abuse. Oliguria or anuria may be present. Bass described a syndrome of sudden sniffing death, consisting of sniffing followed in rapid sequence by exercise or a stressful situation and then death. Autopsies on these adolescent victims failed to elucidate the pathophysiology of the syndrome. He suggests that the myocardium may be sensitized by volatile hydrocarbons to the catecholamines released by the stress of the situation.

Death from suffocation resulting from the use of a

plastic bag as the vehicle for delivery of the volatile substance is reported with regularity. Particularly in the ghetto, glue sniffing is frequently performed on apartment house roofs. It is not uncommon under such circumstances for the intoxicated teenaager to misjudge distances or imagine he can fly and fall to his death.

Recently, a renal tubular acidification defect has been observed in toluene sniffers. Tolerance to the euphoric effects of glue develops, but there is no evidence of physiologic addiction. In the ghetto population, many heroin users report that glue sniffing provided their first contact with drugs. The vapor-inhaling teenager cannot be identified unless he is intoxicated at the time of examination and the odor detected, or if he suffers a complication of the inhalation. The toluene concentration can be determined in tissues at autopsy and the test should be performed in cases of suspicious deaths in teenagers.

ALCOHOL

The current epidemic of drug abuse notwithstanding, alcohol remains the most commonly abused pharmacologic agent in our society. Experimentation with alcohol still represents the first intoxicating experience for the majority of youth in this country, surpassing both tobacco and marihuana in frequency of use. Recent years have seen an ever increasing number of teenagers abusing alcohol. It is estimated that currently there are approximately 500,000 teenage alcoholics. Alcohol is unique among the major drugs of abuse in that it is legally obtainable without a prescription, the only restriction being one of age, which usually varies between 18 and 21 years among the states. This legality contributes to both easy availability and tacit societal approval of teenage usage.

IDENTIFICATION, ADMINISTRATION, AND DOSAGE. Alcohol, or ethanol, is a clear liquid with the chemical formula C_2H_5OH. The concentration of ethanol within beverages varies considerably, with whiskeys, wines, and beer containing approximately 40 to 50 percent, 8 to 12 percent, and 3 to 6 percent, respectively. The psychoactive effect of ethanol is dependent upon the plasma level achieved, which in turn is related to the type and quantity of beverage consumed and whether or not food was simultaneously ingested. A 4-ounce glass of whiskey consumed alone produces a plasma level of 65 to 90 mg/100 ml, whereas the same amount ingested with a meal results in a level of 30 to 50 mg/100 ml. The medicolegal definition of intoxication is a blood level of 200 mg/100 ml or more, and a level over 500 mg/100 ml may be incompatible with life.

METABOLISM, PHYSIOLOGY, AND PSYCHO-PHARMACOLOGY. Alcohol is absorbed throughout the length of the gastrointestinal tract, within 2 to 6 hours after ingestion. Diffusion is uniform among all tissues, including the placenta. Almost 98 percent of alcohol is metabolized by hepatic oxidation to acetalde-

hyde in the presence of alcohol dehydrogenase. The acetaldehyde is then converted to acetyl coenzyme A. The concentration of unmetabolized alcohol in urine equals that in alveolar air and rarely exceeds 0.05 percent of the blood level.

The psychoactive effect of ethanol is central nervous system depression mediated primarily by the reticular activating system. Disorganization of thought processes results from release of the cerebral cortex from this control system.

The analgesic effect of ethanol is appreciated by the laity and results from the ability of alcohol to raise the pain threshold by 30 to 40 percent, as well as its euphoriant potential. Vasodilation and hypothermia produced by ethanol are centrally mediated effects. The alcohol taboo in peptic ulcer disease has its basis in the fact that it stimulates gastric acid secretion and is irritating to the gastric mucosa. Oxidation of alcohol increases lipid production and accumulation of fat in liver and may be a factor in the production of fatty liver in the chronic alcoholic. Alcohol has an inhibitory effect on the release of antidiuretic hormone by the posterior pituitary.

MEDICAL COMPLICATIONS. The complications of chronic alcoholism seen in adults are cirrhosis, polyneuritis, Wernicke's ophthalmoplegia, and Korsakoff's psychosis. They are the results of presumed chronic nutritional deficiency attendant on the life of the alcoholic, as well as direct hepatotoxicity of ethanol. The usual brevity of the history of alcohol ingestion in the teenager is probably responsible for the absence of these complications in this age group. In our experience, the most frequent complications of alcohol abuse in the adolescent have been acute gastritis, acute pancreatitis, severe central nervous system depression, and secondary trauma. All of these usually result from a rather large and acute ingestion.

Gastrointestinal hemorrhage is the most serious clinical manifestation of acute erosive gastritis. Epigastric pain, anorexia, and vomiting are also usually present. These symptoms may subside without specific therapy other than antacids. However, persistent bleeding will frequently require gastric lavage with iced saline, vigorous antacid therapy, a bland diet, and further diagnostic studies.

Severe abdominal pain and profuse vomiting accompanied by elevations of serum amylase and lipase activity are indicative of *acute pancreatitis*. Treatment includes analgesia, gastric decompression, and maintenance of fluid, electrolyte, and colloid homeostasis. Chronic relapsing pancreatitis may result from this acute attack.

Management of the *central nervous system depression* accompanying alcoholic overdose is in the main supportive. Mixed ingestions, particularly with barbiturates, may cause sufficient respiratory depression to necessitate mechanical ventilatory assistance. The combination of vomiting and coma requires the insertion of a cuffed endotracheal tube to prevent the complication of aspiration pneumonia.

DRUG INTERACTIONS. Many medications utilized in the treatment of teenagers interact with alcohol. The anticonvulsant effects of diphenylhydantoin and sedative effects of barbiturates, diazepam, and meprobamate are all potentiated by acute alcoholic intoxication. Conversely, presumably due to enhanced microsomal enzyme activity, these same effects are diminished with chronic alcohol abuse. Also of import is the increased likelihood of gastrointestinal bleeding with aspirin, and the possibility of an antabuse-like syndrome when chloramphenicol, metronidazole, or quinacrine is administered at a time of alcohol ingestion.

THE ABSTINENCE SYNDROME. The teenage alcoholic should be defined on a psychosocial rather than a physiologic basis. We would classify as alcoholic any teenager drinking in excess as a response to behavioral or environmental problems or conversly the teenager in whom drinking was the cause of deterioration of either function or interpersonal relationships. It is not possible to denote clearly the length of time or the amount of alcohol ingestion that would place an adolescent at risk for withdrawal symptoms. At a minimum, daily use over a period of many weeks is necessary to produce addiction. Nevertheless, the withdrawal syndrome associated with alcohol addiction is a more common occurrence among teenagers in late adolescence than was previously appreciated. This phenomenon is particularly true among former opiate addicts. The clinical manifestations of abstinence generally include an early and minor withdrawal phase or less commonly a major withdrawal syndrome termed *delirium tremens*. The latter is rarely, if ever, seen in adolescents. The more benign withdrawal syndrome may have its onset as early as 8 hours after cessation of drinking and usually lasts no longer than 48 hours. Symptoms are essentially benign and include tremor, restlessness, mild diaphoresis, minimal disorientation, hallucinations, and rarely brief convulsions.

The treatment of the abstinence syndrome is aimed at minimizing the discomfort of the minor withdrawal phase and preventing death from circulatory collapse and hyperthermia. The latter are associated only with delirium tremens. General measures for the treatment of confusion, agitation, and anxiety include placing the patient in quiet surroundings and preventing self injury. Among the drugs commonly utilized for controlling the symptoms of minor withdrawal are paraldehyde, prochlorpromazine, chlorpromazine, promazine, promethazine, and chlordiazepoxide in addition to replacement of any fluid and electrolyte losses. We would suggest utilizing chlordiazepoxide in a dose of 25 mg every 6 hours for 3 days.

In contrast to the barbiturate withdrawal pattern, hyperthermia is more common and grand mal seizures are less frequent with alcohol withdrawal. While death may rarely eventuate, the teenager usually recovers within 1 week.

ANTABUSE THERAPY. Special mention must be made of the potential use of *disulfram* (antabuse) as an adjunct in the long-term rehabilitation of the teenage alcoholic. Disulfram prevents the metabolism of ethanol beyond the intermediate product acetaldehyde. In the patient maintained on antabuse the ingestion of even small amounts of alcohol will cause the accumulation of acetaldehyde and precipitate a syndrome marked by flushing, headache, tachycardia, hypotension, vertigo, nausea, and profuse vomiting.

When used daily, disulfram inhibits the impulse drinking done almost unconsciously by some alcoholics. It allows the patient to achieve abstinence and enter into a meaningful rehabilitative effort. The drug is administered orally once daily in an initial dose of 500 mg for 1 week followed by a maintenance dose of 250 mg. Medication may need to be continued indefinitely and should not be stopped before the patient has made sufficient rehabilitative progress to suggest that continued alcoholic abstinence is a reasonable expectation.

The drug is contraindicated in patients with cardiac decompensation, seldom a consideration in the adolescent, and in the face of an overt psychosis or serious brain damage. It should not be administered within 24 hours after the last ingestion of alcohol and patients must be cautioned to avoid alcohol in all forms including wine sauces, cough syrup, and other medications. The patient must be made aware that an antabuse–alcohol reaction may occur up to 5 days after the last dose of the drug.

GENERAL CONSIDERATIONS ABOUT THE ETIOLOGY AND MANAGEMENT OF TEENAGE DRUG ABUSE

During the past decade, drug abuse among teenagers has become a major national health problem that has left its mark on all sectors of our society. Postulations as to the etiology of this epidemic have been diverse and have often served to undermine rather than enhance the dialogue between adolescents and adults. The latter group attribute indiscriminate use of drugs variously to rebellion, accession to peer pressure, avoidance of the unpleasantness of life, and a manifestation of emotional or psychiatric illness. The adolescents themselves view substance abuse as a mystical and exciting experience, an opportunity for psychic self discovery, a way of coping in a nonrelevant adult-regulated society, and a natural phenomenon in our drug-oriented culture. The true causes are obviously as varied as the individuals who use drugs and so also must be the approaches to therapy.

Recommendations for long-term rehabilitation of the drug-using adolescent must and can be tailored to the needs of the particular teenager. Choosing between treatment resources requires the consideration of information on not only the history of drug involvement, but also the teenager's educational and vocational accomplishments and goals, family structure, current and past involvement with law enforcement and social agencies, evidence of prior psychiatric or emotional disturbances, and, of great importance, the patient's appraisal of his or her needs and tolerances for future care.

Although no specific criteria can be used to determine a proper referral, and all therapeutic resources may not be available within a particular community, certain general guidelines can be utilized to increase the possibility of long-term success. Counseling, that is discussion of problems with a professional other than a psychiatrist, is indicated for verbal teenagers from reasonable home settings without serious drug involvement or marked psychopathology. The decision between referral to individual or group counseling is best left to the patient's preference. Psychotherapy should be reserved for teenagers with a primary psychiatric problem and secondary drug abuse. A non-drug-oriented residence is a place to live and participate in group and individual therapy while continuing at school or work. Drug-oriented therapeutic communities offer similar counseling services but may initially forbid outside work or schooling. Either of these facilities may be appropriate for adolescents coming from disrupted, nonsupportive, or nonexistent homes. Although the therapeutic community may be a more appropriate setting for the deeply drug-involved teenager, we have encountered great reluctance on the part of adolescents to submit themselves to the incarceration and abrasive therapy attributed by them to those facilities. Methadone maintenance involves the daily administration of a synthetic narcotic to obviate opiate withdrawal and craving and block the euphoric effect of subsequently administered heroin. When offered in a program that concomitantly provides supportive and rehabilitative services, it may be indicated for the older adolescent with heavy opiate involvement and a history of failure in other therapeutic programs. Decisions regarding choice of referral for a particular patient must be made on the basis of location, availability of placement, financial considerations, the racial and ethnic make-up of the patient population at the referral resource, and past experience with the success rate of the specific therapeutic agency.

The role of physicians in this complex medical-social-psychologic problem is varied. They are often called upon to be a resource not only for the patient, but also for the family, the schools, and the community. One's ability to recognize and treat the stigmata and medical consequences of drug abuse has implications for both the physical and emotional health of the patients. The clinician's ability to detoxify a drug addict or adequately treat an overdose reaction may permit the additional role of initiating a suitable program of long-term rehabilitation. The physician should be prepared to take advantage of this opportunity.

Bibliography

GENERAL INFORMATION

Cohen MI, Litt IF: Accidental poisonings of drugs of abuse in children and adolescents. NIMH Monograph (National Clearinghouse for Drug Abuse Information). A Treatment Manual for Acute Drug Abuse Emergencies, Chap 3, pp 142–145, 1974

Goodman LS, Gilman A: The Pharmacological Basis of Therapeutics, 5th ed. Macmillan, New York, 1975
Litt IF, Cohen MI: The drug-using adolescent as a pediatric patient. J Pediatr 77:195, 1970
——— Schonberg SK: Drug abuse in adolescence. In Richter R (ed): The Medical Aspects of Drug Abuse. New York, Harper & Row, 1975

HEROIN

Banks T, Fletcher R, Ali N: Infective endocarditis in heroin addicts. Am J Med 55:444, 1973
Cherubin CE: A review of the medical complications of narcotic addiction. Int J Addictions 3:163, 1968
Harris WDM, Andrei J: Serologic tests for syphilis among narcotic addicts. NY J Med 67:2967, 1967
Karliner JS, Steinberg AD, Williams MH: Lung function after pulmonary edema associated with heroin overdose. Arch Intern Med 124:350, 1969
Litt IF, Cohen MI: End of an epidemic? J Pediatr 86: 293, 1975
——— Colli AS, Cohen MI: Diazepam in the management of heroin withdrawal in adolescence: preliminary report. J Pediatr 78:692, 1971
——— Cohen MI, Schonberg SK, et al: Liver disease in the drug-using adolescent. J Pediatr 81:238, 1972
Louria DB, Hensle T, Rose J: The major medical complications of heroin addiction. Ann Intern Med 67:1, 1967
Sapira JD: The narcotic addict as a medical patient. Am J Med 45:555, 1968

METHADONE

Jaffe GJ, Strelinger RW, Parwatikar S: Physical symptoms of patients on methadone maintenance. Proceedings Fifth National Conference on Methadone Treatment, Vol. 1. National Association for the Prevention of Addiction to Narcotics (NAPAN), New York, 1973
Kreek MJ: Physiologic implications of methadone treatment. Proceedings Fifth National Conference on Methadone Treatment, Vol. 2. National Association for the Prevention of Addiction to Narcotics (NAPAN), New York, 1973
Millman RB, Khuri ET, Nyswander MD: A model for the study and treatment of heroin addiction in an urban adolescent population. Proceedings Fourth National Conference on Methadone Treatment. National Association for the Prevention of Addiction to Narcotics (NAPAN), New York, 1972
Strauss ME, Andresko M, Stryker JC, et al: Methadone maintenance during pregnancy: pregnancy, birth and neonate characteristics. Am J Obstet Gynecol 120:895, 1974

DEPRESSANTS

Fiser RH, Maetz HM, Trenting JJ, et al: Activated charcoal in barbiturate and glutethimide poisoning of the dog. J Pediatr 78:1045, 1971
Smith DE, Wesson DR: Phenobarbital technique for treatment of barbiturate dependence. Arch Gen Psychiatr 24:56, 1971
Spear PW, Protass LM: Barbiturate poisoning—an epidemic disease. Med Clin North Am 57:1471, 1973

AMPHETAMINES

Csillag ER: Stimulant drugs—their use and abuse. Med J Austr 1:968, 1971
Grinspoon L, Hedblom P: Amphetamine abuse. Drug Therapy 83, 1972

MARIHUANA

Bech P, Rafaelsen L, Rafaelsen OJ: Cannabis: a psychopharmacological review. Danish Med Bull 21:106, 1974
Cottrell JC, Sohn SS, Vogel WH: Toxic effects of marihuana tar on mouse skin. Arch Environ Health 26:277, 1973

Kolodny RC, Masters WH, Kolodner RM, et al: Depression of plasma testosterone levels after chronic intensive marihuana use. N Engl J Med 290:872, 1974

Leuchtenberger C, Leuchtenberger R, Schneider A: Effects of marihuana and tobacco smoke on DNA and chromosomal complement in human lung explants. Nature 242:403, 1973

Weil AT, Zinbeig NE, Nelson JM: Clinical and psychological effects of marihuana in man. Science 162:1234, 1968

COCAINE

Fish F, Wilson WDC: Excretion of cocaine and its metabolites in man. J Pharm Pharmacol 21:1355, 1969

GLUE SNIFFING AND OTHER INHALANTS

Bass M: Sudden sniffing death. JAMA 212:2075, 1970

Litt IF, Cohen MI: Danger . . . vapor harmful: spot-remover sniffing. N Engl J Med 281:543, 1969

Taher SM, Anderson RJ, McCartney R, et al: Renal tubular acidosis associated with toluene "sniffing." N Engl J Med 290:765, 1974

HALLUCINOGENS AND PSYCHEDELICS

Taylor RL, Maurer JI, Tinklenberg JR: Management of "bad trips" in an evolving drug scene. JAMA 213:422, 1970

ALCOHOL

Bourne PG, Fox R: Alcoholism, Progress in Research and Treatment. Academic Press, New York, 1973

Kissin B, Gegleiter H: The Biology of Alcoholism, Vol. 3. Clinical Pathology. Plenum Press, New York, 1974

NEONATAL DRUG WITHDRAWAL

STEPHEN R. KANDALL

INTRODUCTION

The problem of drug addiction and abuse has become one of national significance, predominantly in but not restricted to, large urban areas. Many drug-using women are of childbearing age, and since these drugs cross into the fetal circulation via the placenta, it is not surprising that urban hospitals have had vast experience with passively addicted newborns. Many municipal hospitals in New York City are reporting neonatal drug dependency in 3 to 5 percent of the newborn infants.

During recent years a wide variety of drugs has been abused during pregnancy. Alcohol, amphetamines, barbiturates, codeine, ethchlorvynol (Placidyl), heroin (diacetyl morphine), meperidine (Demerol), methadone, methamphetamine, morphine, pentazocine (Talwin), and propoxyphene hydrochloride (Darvon) have all been incriminated in neonatal withdrawal. The changing distribution of abused drugs is illustrated by the analysis from the Bronx Municipal Hospital Center in New York City from 1971 to 1974, during which time the proportion of heroin abuse during pregnancy fell from 52.1 to 14.0 percent, while methadone, as the major drug used, rose from 12.5 to 42.0 percent.

FETAL EFFECTS

Effects of these drugs on the fetus have been recognized for many years. Heroin abuse is known to be associated with increased fetal wastage and neonatal death, both of which may be reduced with methadone maintenance under careful medical supervision. Fetal growth has been shown to be adversely affected by maternal heroin abuse. Infants born to heroin-abusing mothers have a mean birthweight of approximately 2,500 g, while those born to mothers using methadone have a mean birthweight of approximately 2,930 g, compared to a mean birthweight for nonaddicted infants of 3,200 g. One study suggests that larger doses of methadone early in pregnancy appear to be associated with higher birthweights in a dose-related fashion. It is also important to note that newborns of women who have abused heroin in the past have birthweights equivalent to those of infants born to mothers abusing heroin during the current pregnancy. Although gestational age is somewhat shortened in the drug-using groups, most pronounced with heroin, the lower weights are primarily due to intrauterine growth retardation rather than prematurity.

Meconium passage before birth is seen with increased frequency in infants of heroin-using mothers, but meconium aspiration occurs infrequently, suggesting that fetal meconium passage may be related to intrauterine withdrawal rather than acute or chronic hypoxic stresses. Transition from intrauterine to extrauterine life, as determined by the Apgar scores at one and five minutes, is accomplished without difficulty in the great majority of cases. The incidence of congenital anomalies is apparently not increased by maternal heroin and methadone use, but some other nonnarcotic drugs including LSD and alcohol have been implicated in an increased rate of malformations.

NEONATAL WITHDRAWAL SYNDROME

Symptoms of neonatal narcotic withdrawal can be divided into four main categories.

Central nervous system signs include tremulousness, irritability, excessive crying, reduced sleep periods, and a high-pitched cry. Skin abrasions may result from general hyperactivity. General neurologic dysfunction is often reflected in the incoordination of sucking and swallowing, leading to poor feeding despite a voracious appetite. Seizures, either generalized or myoclonic limb jerking, may occur either early in the course of withdrawal or after some delay. In some infants seizures may occur without progression through a period of marked tremulousness, especially in the methadone group. Treatment with anticonvulsants is indicated, but seizures may not respond well. Most of the infants studied have not shown seizure patterns by electroencephalographic study and the results of neurologic examinations were normal afterward despite the refractory nature of the convulsions.

Gastrointestinal signs, such as vomiting and diarrhea,

occur with the next highest frequency and are usually controlled with specific drug therapy. Dehydration may occur if treatment is not instituted.

Respiratory signs include tachypnea, with resulting respiratory alkalosis. The presence of respiratory distress (flaring, retractions, etc.) should not be attributed to withdrawal, however, and other causes of neonatal respiratory difficulty should be considered.

Autonomic nervous system signs of hyperpyrexia, yawning, sneezing, sweating, and lacrimation are of great help in diagnosing neonatal withdrawal because of their relative specificity. It is important to remember that all of the above signs may also be found in sepsis, metabolic disturbances (hypoglycemia, hypocalcemia, etc.), adrenal collapse, thyrotoxicosis, and central nervous system damage, such as meningitis, hemorrhage, etc. Before therapy is begun, a systematic search should be made for these other serious conditions.

More than 85 percent of infants born to methadone-maintained mothers will be symptomatic, while approximately 75 percent of the heroin group will show withdrawal symptoms. Babies should not show withdrawal if the mother becomes drug-free one month before delivery. It is not possible, however, to predict the severity of neonatal withdrawal from the amount of maternal drugs consumed. This may be due, as has been shown for methadone, to the poor correlation between maternal dosage and amounts of the drug detected in amniotic fluid, cord blood, urine, and breast milk. It seems clear that factors other than maternal dosage play a role in determining the severity of neonatal withdrawal. Treatment is needed more frequently in the methadone group than in the heroin group; higher doses of medication are needed for longer periods of time.

As soon as the umbilical cord has been cut, the passively addicted neonate is acutely deprived of its supply of maternal drug. Symptoms may appear at varying times after birth, related perhaps to the interval after the mother's last dose of narcotic. If a narcotic antagonist is given in the delivery room for presumed depression due to intrapartum sedative administration, symptoms may become apparent immediately.

In most infants addiction to heroin will usually be manifest within four days after birth, with an occasional infant presenting toward the end of the first week. Withdrawal from methadone will usually be obvious within the first few days after birth, but some infants may show initial or major symptoms only after a delay of 2 to 4 weeks. The accumulation of methadone in fetal tissue coupled with delayed metabolism and excretion of the drug may explain this phenomenon. When symptoms first appear in a delayed manner, consideration should also be given to neonatal phenobarbital withdrawal. Symptoms are quite similar to withdrawal from opiates; these include hyperactivity, excessive crying, tremulousness, sneezing, lacrimation, hyperphagia, vomiting, and diarrhea. Phenobarbital in doses of at least 90 mg/day for 12 weeks to the mother seem necessary to cause withdrawal symptoms in the newborn.

Although the syndrome of neonatal drug withdrawal is generally regarded as acute and confined to the first few weeks of life, it is now recognized that symptoms of hyperirritability, hyperreflexia, tremulousness, and poor socialization may last for 4 to 6 months. Although some preliminary studies have been reported, no longer-term neurobehavioral studies of large numbers of addicted babies have been published. Careful counseling should be provided in these cases to minimize disruption of the parent–child bond. Maternal use of drugs during pregnancy may also be associated with an increased incidence of sudden unexpected death in their offspring.

A history of drug abuse by the mother may not always be clear or may be denied. If heroin abuse is considered, the mother should be examined for needle marks, tatoos, and skin ulcerations. A history of maternal hepatitis, abscesses, cellulitis, thrombophlebitis, or bacterial endocarditis should also arouse suspicion. Concealment of an active drug history has proven to be less of a problem in recent years, since many women are registered in drug treatment programs, and punitive measures have been reduced in favor of therapeutic management of the mother. Those women not under treatment may find such help available to them during pregnancy or immediately following delivery. The peripartum period is generally regarded as an excellent time to offer help to the addicted patient since motivation may be high following the birth of a baby. Suspicion of drug usage can be confirmed by screening blood or urine for drug metabolites. Although thin-layer chromatography is used widely for mass screening, more accurate qualitative or quantitative determinations should be performed by gas–liquid chromatography or radioimmunoassay. Spectral analysis has also been employed by some laboratories. The use of highly specific and sensitive techniques may reveal unsuspected drug abuse.

Other physiologic effects, some of them possibly beneficial, have been reported in the newborn in association with maternal narcotic use during pregnancy. A lowered incidence of respiratory distress syndrome in prematurely born addicted infants has been noted and accelerated pulmonary maturation has been observed in experimental animals in which mothers were treated with narcotics. Increased concentrations of hemoglobin A and 2,3 diphosphoglycerate have been found in the cord blood of addicted newborns. Accelerated maturation of hepatic bilirubin conjugating systems and reduction of neonatal hyperbilirubinemia also have been suggested.

TREATMENT OF HEROIN AND METHADONE WITHDRAWAL

Principles of treatment include provision of general supportive care to make the infant more comfortable and treatment with specific drugs to control more severe withdrawal manifestations. Supportive measures, including swaddling and frequent feeding in a quiet, dimly lit room, may minimize the severity of withdrawal. Increased fluids and calories should be provided when increased needs are anticipated (diarrhea, vomiting, sweating, tachypnea, increased motor activity, etc.). Vital signs and intake and output should be closely monitored. If these supportive measures do not control the infant's discomfort, an opiate or nonspecific sedative may be employed.

Opiates: Paregoric USP (tincture of opium) can be administered orally and is generally quite safe. Treatment is begun with 0.2 ml every 3 hours; if symptoms are not controlled the dose is raised by 0.05 ml until a stabilizing dose is reached. In unusual cases in which more than 0.75 ml every 3 hours is needed, a tranquilizer may be added. The dose of paregoric must be tapered slowly, since symptoms may recur if the dose is lowered too rapidly. *Mild* symptomatology should be tolerated, however, as the dose is being reduced. Paregoric has been reported to restore the sucking reflex to normal more rapidly than nonspecific sedatives.

Nonspecific sedatives: Diazepam is administered every 8 hours intramuscularly in a dosage of 1 mg for mild, 1.5 mg for moderate, and 2 mg for severe withdrawal. Withdrawal of the medication can usually be accomplished within 2 weeks. Although this is often an advantage, the withdrawal syndrome has been known to recur after therapy has been terminated. Breakthrough symptoms, including seizures, have also been seen while diazepam was being administered. Theoretical objections to the use of diazepam because of its content of benzoate (part of the vehicle for solubilization of diazepam) have been raised. Benzoate may reduce the binding of bilirubin to albumin but this is probably of little clinical significance due to the rapid metabolism of benzoic acid to hippurate and its low concentration in the drug and in the blood. Chlorpromazine, administered at a dose of 2.2 to 3 mg/kg/day orally or intramuscularly in four divided doses, also has been used. It is usually possible to taper the dose over a 2 to 3 week period, but published experience with this agent has been limited primarily to its use in heroin withdrawal. Phenobarbital may also be administered in a total dose of 5 to 10 mg/kg/day for symptomatic relief. High doses may produce lethargy and poor feeding, preventing adequate intake of calories and fluids.

In general, the use of paregoric seems more physiologic in neonates exposed to narcotics in utero. In these infants sedatives may supress symptoms but do not provide proper relacement therapy. Diazepam, chlorpromazine, and phenobarbital, however, may be particularly effective in multiple drug withdrawal. The diagnosis should be made by appropriate urine testing. Phenobarbital withdrawal can best be controlled by the administration of phenobarbital in the above doses.

Recognition of the syndrome of neonatal drug withdrawal and treatment with any of the listed agents has dramatically reduced the mortality rate from rates of 34 to 93 percent in the early literature. Aside from one infant who died with delayed withdrawal outside of the hospital, we have had no deaths from acute withdrawal in our series of 280 babies.

MANAGEMENT DURING PREGNANCY

Although still very controversial, methadone maintenance programs appear to benefit the infant of the opiate-addicted mother despite somewhat more severe withdrawal symptoms than from heroin. Methadone maintenance appears to be more compatible with maternal and fetal well-being and affords the patient a better chance of proper prenatal care. Recommendations for drug management call for gradual detoxification to the drug-free state or to a maintenance dose compatible with the patient's physical and emotional well-being. Some mothers will not accept too severe a reduction in narcotic dose or the drug-free state and will leave a program entirely if reductions are too rapid. This often leads to poor medical care during pregnancy. All addicted and formerly addicted mothers should be designated as high-risk and followed in an appropriate clinical setting. A pediatrician with an interest in the problem should participate in the prenatal program to assist in drug control during pregnancy for optimal neonatal outcome and to prepare the mother for possible neonatal withdrawal. Social service personnel should also be actively involved to afford supportive intervention, psychosocial counseling, and compliance with local legal requirements.

Bibliography

Cobrinik RW, Hood RJ, Chusid E: The effect of maternal narcotic addiction on the newborn infant. Pediatrics 24:288, 1959

Goodfriend J, Shey IA, Klein MD: The effect of maternal narcotic addiction on the newborn. Am J Obstet Gynecol 71:29, 1956

Harper RG, Solish GI, Purow HM, et al: The effect of a methadone treatment program upon pregnant heroin addicts and their newborn infants. Pediatrics 54:300, 1974

Hill RM, Desmond MM: Management of the narcotic withdrawal syndrome in the neonate. Pediatr Clin North Am 10:67, 1963

Kandall SR, Gartner LM: Late presentation of drug withdrawal symptoms in newborns. Am J Dis Child 127:58, 1974

Naeye RL, Blanc W, Leblanc W, et al: Fetal complications of maternal heroin addiction: abnormal growth, infections, and episodes of stress. J Pediatr 83:1055, 1973

Neumann LL, Cohen SN: The neonatal narcotic withdrawal syndrome: a therapeutic challenge. Clin Perinatol 2:99, 1975

Rothstein P, Gould JB: Born with a habit: infants of drug-addicted mothers. Pediatr Clin North Am 21:307, 1974

Zelson C, Lee SJ, Casalino M: Neonatal narcotic addiction: comparative effects of maternal intake of heroin and methadone. N Engl J Med 289:1216, 1973

INTENTIONAL ACCIDENTS (MALTREATMENT OF CHILDREN, CHILD ABUSE, CHILD BATTERING, NONACCIDENTAL INJURIES)

ARNOLD H. EINHORN

INTRODUCTION

Willful physical abuse by adults is a significant cause of disability or death in young children. Pediatricians, as well as social workers, remained unaware of this danger for many years after the existence of nonaccidental injuries had been recognized and reported by radiologists and medical examiners. Caffey first emphasized the frequent association of chronic subdural hematoma in infants with multiple fractures of long bones. Silverman and subsequently Wooley and Evans stressed the probable relationship between unexplained skeletal lesions and intentionally inflicted injury. The term *battered child* was coined in 1962 by Kempe, who reported on several hundred victimized children hospitalized in a single year in various hospitals in the United States. It has been suggested that the emotional connotation of the name was deliberate and designed to attract the attention of medical and social professionals and to arouse public opinion. Currently the broader concept of maltreatment of children has evolved in relation to legal protective proceedings to include not only willfully inflicted serious physical injuries but also the physical and emotional harm or risk of injury attributable to passive parental negligence.

EPIDEMIOLOGY

It is difficult to assess the true incidence of the problem but it probably is underestimated. Medical and other health care personnel are reluctant to diagnose, record, and report child battering, which undoubtedly results in underreporting. The number of child-abuse cases reported annually in the United States has risen from 7,000 in 1967 to over 200,000 in 1974. Of 200,000 children in need of protective services, more than 30,000 were badly injured. The average age of the abused child is 4 years but most are under 2 years of age. The victimized children are equally divided as to sex. Mortality rates for children subjected to deliberate violence varies among different cities. The extrapolated overall death rate is estimated to be anywhere from 5 to 25 percent of abused children, with an average age at death of slightly under 3 years and a duration of exposure to battering of 1 to 3 years. It has been suggested that a significant proportion of *crib deaths* may actually be the result of parental assault. Sudden infant death should be suspicious whenever there is a long delay between the time the child was last seen alive and the discovery of death.

The majority of abusive parents are married, are in their mid-20s to early 30s; the father is slightly more often the abuser than the mother, but the most serious crimes are more frequently committed by the mother than by the father. In addition, the actual battering is not uncommonly done by a violent relative or a boyfriend of the mother who is living with the family. In many situations the abuse occurs in the presence of other family members. It is also felt that when one parent or friend of the parent victimizes the child, in some way the other permits the abuse to happen.

ETIOLOGY

The complex problem of child abuse, probably an index of social pathology, cannot be looked at as a homogeneous syndrome. The reasons and motivations that produce criminal actions against children are poorly understood. Parents of such children have been described as immature, antisocial, and unstable, often exhibiting uncontrollable violent impulses that readily explode. Some injuries are the result of crises, other are premeditated. Premeditation characterizes schizophrenia. Cigarette burns and poisoning, for example, are more likely to be premeditated than a physical attack that accompanies a family crisis. The availability of means of injury are important in crisis situations. Cultural differences probably also play an active etiologic role.

A high proportion of abusive parents have been abused as children themselves. A high prevalence of premarital conception, youthful marriages, unwanted pregnancies, coerced matrimony, social isolation, marital disharmony, financial difficulty, and poor work record are frequent circumstantial characteristics surrounding the family circle of the abused child. According to Helfer, the victim is often a different and very particular child who may be hyperactive, congenitally defective, or prematurely born. It is very unusual for *every* child in a given family to be abused.

Child battering is reported to be more frequent although by no means limited to socially deprived groups and ethnically disadvantaged minorities. Members of these groups are particularly susceptible because their life conditions are precarious, full of tensions and aggravations. A life of poverty and social rejection is inherently associated with psychologic stress, which in turn may be expressed in violence or neglect toward children. In many instances family ties are tenuous or nonexistent. Children may be unwanted and often considered a burdensome handicap against whom frustrations are readily aired. However, the association with poverty may be to a certain extent misrepresented. In affluent families most cases of abuse will come to the attention of private physicians who tend not to report the first injury as readily, while poor families seen in hospital settings and emergency departments are not thus shielded.

A crisis that leads to the acute episode of maltreatment does not constitute by itself an etiology but an important precipitating factor. Consequently, the solution of a crisis, while the underlying potentially dangerous situation remains, will lead to an almost unavoidable recurrence of the abuse.

CLINICAL MANIFESTATIONS

Many types of violence are used to abuse or even murder children, ranging from manual, pedal, or instrumental trauma to starvation, withholding of water, stabbing, shooting, drowning, strangulation, smothering, poisoning, and asphyxiation. Morbidity and mortality are also high among the siblings of abused children. Many cases probably go unrecognized, unreported, and untreated. Most likely, many *accidental deaths* or *sudden infant death syndromes* (SIDS) represent instances of deliberate injury inflicted on children by parents or caretakers and are made to simulate accidents. Caffey has postulated that frequent and forceful shaking of infants by the extremities may be responsible for intracranial and intraocular bleeding in the absence of external trauma to the head or fractures of the calvarium. Traction lesions of the periosteum of long bones also exist without associated fractures or traumatic changes of the overlying skin and without any history of trauma. This author links the existence of this *whiplash-shaken infant syndrome* with residual permanent brain damage and mental retardation. *Hypernatremic dehydration* following periodic water deprivation by psychotic mothers also has been reported as a form of child abuse.

A wide variety of findings can be documented in maltreated children ranging from the simple undernourished infant reported as a failure to thrive to the moribund and gasping victim. Nearly half of all battered children seen in emergency rooms have serious injury and 10 to 25 percent die. The more severely abused children usually are taken to hospitals with external evidence of body trauma. Others fail to thrive or have maternal deprivation syndrome, malnutrition, poor skin hygiene, irritability, repressed personality, rumination syndrome, and other circumstantial evidence of neglect. The overlap between physical abuse and both physical and affective neglect is considerable.

Common manifestations of child battering include a variety of skin lesions, burns, scars, abrasions, ecchymoses or lacerations, soft tissue swellings, craniocerebral injuries, intracranial bleeding, intraocular hemorrhage, intestinal perforations, pneumothorax, splenic, hepatic, and renal ruptures, pancreatic hematoma or pseudocyst, lesions of the genitalia, and rib or limb fractures in various stages of healing. Burns account for almost 50 percent of physical abuse cases. Many are intentionally injured more than once and lesions of varying ages can be seen. Radiographic bone changes may consist of metaphyseal fragmentation caused by twisting or pulling, periosteal hemorrhages followed by calcification, squaring of long bones secondary to new bone formation, or frank multiple fractures in various locations. Injury to the skeletal system even when recent may present without external evidence of trauma.

Severe physical abuse may leave serious difficulties in physical, emotional, and intelligence growth and development. Permanent neurologic sequelae are frequent. More durable damage may be produced by nonaccidental injury, neglect, and deprivation than by many organic diseases.

Diagnosis

Improved detection methods and earlier anticipatory case finding are vital. Outcome and long-term prognosis often are poor if one waits for overt and obvious signs of injury. Emergency room staffs should pay particular attention to all cases of injury to children under 3 years of age, especially if there is long delay after

injury in attending the hospital. It has been asserted, on the other hand, that in the prodromal stages of a precipitating crisis mothers may make several visits with their children for nonexistent complaints. Previous abuse of a sibling is very important in diagnosis.

In rare instances, there is no diagnostic difficulty when the character, circumstances, and nature of the trauma or other type of assault are so flagrantly extensive as to preclude anyone but an adult as the possible perpetrator. The abuse may occur in the presence of a witness, and even admission of direct or indirect guilt may be obtained.

More often, however, evidence of nonaccidental injury is lacking or concealed, and tracing the abuse by history may be exceedingly difficult. Parents who injure their children tend to seek medical attention for their mistreated child at different hospitals with each new episode of injury. A history difficult to relate to the injuries, evasions, contradictions, and conflicting statements about circumstances of neglect and battering should arouse suspicion, not only if marked discrepancies between clinical findings and historical data are elicited, but even if incongruities are slight. An inconsistent history that differs significantly from that reported by another observer or caretaker should also be an important warning.

Some phrases used by parents who mishandle their children have an ominously suggestive connotation. They often claim that the victim has bruising tendencies, falls easily, or has fallen off a table or a crib. The blame is commonly placed upon a sibling whose strength would be incompatible with injuries of such magnitude. A frequently telltale allegation is that the child was perfectly well the previous night when put to bed, but unable to move an extremity upon getting up in the morning.

There are physical clues that may help to identify victimized children or potential victims. Examinations of siblings for possible signs of abuse may also prove corroborative. A high index of suspicion should be maintained whenever children appear neglected, have poor hygiene, suffer from malnutrition, and present multiple soft tissue injuries, especially when there is clinical or radiographic evidence of trauma, even though a history of neglect and injury is denied. Facial bruises are valuable clinical findings. Patterns and distribution of facial bruising inflicted by slapping or by a fistblow are readily recognized and quite different from injuries sustained after accidents. The single bruise over the eye is very suggestive of battering. Bite marks leave unmistakable impressions, as do cigarette burns. The latter produce characteristic circular lesions, with old and fresh burns of various ages often coexisting anywhere on the body. Typical marks may also remain visible for days after a child has been struck on the back, trunk, or extremities by hand, with a belt, or any with other object.

Skeletal findings on radiography of the abused child must be differentiated from those of syphilis, scurvy, osteogenesis imperfecta, osteoid osteoma, coagulopathies, infantile cortical hyperostosis, hypervitaminosis A, severe rickets, hypophosphatasia, leukemia, and metatstatic neuroblastoma. (Chap. 32)

TREATMENT

Once suspicion of willful injury has been aroused or confirmed, methods for dealing with the abused child are, unfortunately, random and inadequate. Ideally the approach to child abuse is prediction and institution of preventive and rehabilitative measures. Increased experiences and familiarity with this problem hopefully will improve recognition of such cases at a stage when injuries are at a minimum. Whether children present with minor evidence of maltreatment or with the full maltreatment syndrome, they require identical and equally urgent investigation and management.

All abused or neglected children should be admitted to the hospital. Even if the condition warrants neither acute surgical intervention nor medical treatment, protective hospitalization is always mandatory in order to prevent possible repetition and to shield the victim from further harm. The assistance of social workers, psychiatrists, child protection agencies, and, if indicated, the law must be enlisted. Within hours of admission, all siblings should be examined for injuries or other evidence of neglect. Any adult who has inflicted multiple, life-threatening, and/or fatal injuries to a child may be psychotic or suicidal and will require emergency psychiatric evaluation.

For the continuing protection of the child a long-term therapeutic program must be planned that must be individualized to fit each particular situation. Episodic resolution of an acute crisis without helping the total situation will only lead to recurrent abuse. Depending on the circumstances one of the following courses of action may be envisioned: the child is completely and permanently removed from his home to a permanent surrogate family; removal is only temporary until the parents are considered sufficiently rehabilitated to make the home safe for the child; the child is returned to his home while his parents receive active rehabilitative treatment and adequate support; the child, together with his mother, remain institutionalized in a supervised environment (eg, halfway house) while the mother receives guidance and support.

In general, specialized hospital teams are suggested as a method of improving management, whatever the method of treatment selected. Physical mistreatment of a child is legally a form of neglect. Cases involving deprivation of food, clothing, education, medical care in various forms of parental guardianship are dealt with not as child abuse but under statutory definition of neglect. Since legal or other protection can be offered only if instances of abuse or neglect are known, it has become mandatory to report suspected or confirmed cases. The law requires physicians, nurses, social workers, and hospital administrators to report their suspicions to the police, law agencies, or special children's protective services operating in the community so that

cases can be investigated and appropriate measures taken for the safety of the child. State laws protect physicians against liability for reporting. Parents must be told if a report to protective agencies is contemplated or has been made. An aggressive and accusatory attitude toward such parents may isolate them completely and unnecessarily. A better understanding between physicians and parents is very important if it can be achieved.

The law merely provides a framework in which society can intervene to protect the child. Juvenile courts have power over neglected children but criminal sanctions do little to help the child or to prevent recurrences of similar events. In some states the law provides for protective services. In others, charters have been granted to voluntary agencies. The law is flexible and recognizes that rehabilitative treatment may produce improved circumstances. After rehearing, it may permit a change of disposition of the child and his return to his family. However, much of the legal protection is meaningless without community services and facilities to rehabilitate the families.

Finally, the danger of assuming too readily parental inadequacy or neglect should not be underestimated. A denial by parents or by caretakers may be truthful. There may in reality be no abuse whatever, or it may have been committed without any knowledge of the parents by a babysitter or even an older sibling. A child must never be separated unnecessarily from his family as a result of uninformed and precipitous protective action.

Bibliography

Adelson L: The slaughter of innocents. N Engl J Med 264:1345, 1962: 1880

Bleiberg N: Neglected child and child health conference. NY State J Med 65, 1880:1965

Bongiovi J, Locosso RD: Pancreatic pseudocyst occurring in the battered child syndrome. J Pediatr Surg 4:220, 1969

Buckler JM, Stool E: Failure to thrive. Am J Dis Child 114:652, 1967

Caffey J: Multiple fractures in the long bones of infants suffering from chronic subdural hematoma. Am J Roentgenol 56:163, 1946

———The whiplash shaken infant syndrome: manual shaking by the extremities with whiplash-induced intracranial and intraocular bleedings, linked with residual permanent brain damage and mental retardation. Pediatrics 54:396, 1974

Ebbin AJ, Gollub MH, Stein AM, Wilson MG: Battered child syndrome at the Los Angeles County General Hospital. Am J Dis Child 118:660, 1969

Elmer E, Gregg GS: Characteristics of abused children. Pediatrics 40:596, 1967

Fontana F: The Maltreated Child, 2nd ed. CC Thomas, Springfield, Ill, 1971

Green FC: Child abuse and neglect. A priority problem for the private physician. Pediatr Clin North Am 22:329, 1975

Gregg GS, Elmer E: Infant injuries: accident or abuse? Pediatrics 44:434, 1969

——— Physician child-abuse reporting laws and injured child. Psychosocial anatomy of childhood trauma. Pediatr Clin 6:720, 1968

Helfer RE, Kempe CH (eds): The Battered Child, 2nd ed. University of Chicago Press, Chicago, 1974

Holter JC, Friedman SB: Child abuse: early case finding in the emergency department. Pediatrics 42:128, 1968

Joyner N III: Symposium: Child Abuse (with participation of Solomon T, Helfer R, Fontana VJ, Isaacs JL, Lameron JS, Kelley FM, Kempe HC, Rausen AR). Pediatrics 51:799, 1973

Kempe CH, Silverman FN, Steele BF, et al: Battered child syndrome. JAMA 181:17, 1962

Krieger I: Food restriction as a form of child abuse in ten cases of psychosocial deprivation dwarfism. Clin Pediatr 13:127, 1974

Lipton GL, Roth EI: Rape: management problem in pediatric emergency room. J Pediatr 75:859, 1969

Newberger EH, Daniel JH: Knowledge and epidemiology of child abuse: a critical review of concepts. Pediatr Ann 5:140, 1976

Paulsen MG: Legal protection against child abuse. Children 13:43, 1966

Rowe DT, Leonard MF, Seashore MR: A hospital program for the detection and registration of abused and neglected children. N Engl J Med 282:950, 1970

Sanders RW: Resistance to dealing with parents of battered children. Pediatrics 50:853, 1972

Schmitte BD, Kempe CH: The pediatrician's role in child abuse and neglect. In Current Problems in Pediatrics. Gluck L Year Book Medical Chicago, Ill, 1975, pp 3–47

Silver B, Dublin CC, Lourie RS: Child abuse syndrome: the "gray areas" in establishing a diagnosis. Pediatrics 44:594, 1969

Silverman FN: Roentgen manifestations of unrecognized skeletal trauma in infants. Am J Roentgenol 69:413, 1963

Touloukian RJ: Abdominal visceral injuries in battered children. Pediatrics 42:642, 1968

Wooley PV, Evans WA: Significance of skeletal lesions in infants resembling those of traumatic origin. JAMA 158:539, 1955

THE SUDDEN INFANT DEATH SYNDROME

Eileen G. Hasselmeyer

The sudden infant death syndrome (SIDS) is defined as the sudden death of any infant or young child which is not expected by history and in which a thorough postmortem examination fails to demonstrate the cause of death. Other terms frequently used to describe the syndrome include crib death, cot death, sudden unexplained death, and sudden death in infancy. The definition of SIDS is one of exclusion. Nevertheless, in most cases, there are epidemiologic characteristics and clinical and postmortem clues that permit a diagnosis to be made with considerable certainty.

CLINICAL HISTORY

Infants who died of SIDS have usually been well cared for and considered to have been in good general health before death. However, in about one-half of the cases there is a history of a slight upper respiratory infection, but usually of such a minor degree that medical advice is not sought. A number of infants who have been reported were seen by a physician for a routine checkup within 24 to 48 hours before death, during which no major health problems were found.

It is generally believed that SIDS occurs almost in-variably during sleep, since the infant dies quietly without calling out. However, since the deaths are almost always unobserved, it is difficult to be certain about the state of the infant at the time of death. Findings of clenched fists, clutching of bedclothes, and the body wedged into the corner of the crib suggest some terminal struggle and vigorous motor activity at the end.

PATHOLOGY

Pathologists are in general agreement about the postmortem findings. The infants almost always appear clean, well nourished, and well developed. The skin surface and mucous membranes are not strikingly cyanotic in contrast to the cyanosis evident in the fingernails and around the lips. Frothy, frequently blood-stained, slightly mucoid fluid in the mouth and nostrils is observed in more than half the cases The diapers are usually soiled with urine and feces. The major internal findings are intrathoracic petechial hemorrhages, which are seen more consistently in cases of SIDS than in any other condition at this age. Histologically, mild to moderate inflammation of the upper respiratory tract is observed in about one-half of these infants. The lungs frequently exhibit some edema and congestion, but inflammatory infiltrates are seldom found. Lymphoid tissues (eg, lymph nodes, Peyer's patches) throughout the body are remarkably well preserved. The blood is characteristically in the fluid state and the right heart is mildly dilated. The adrenals are normal in weight for age. Agonal aspiration of vomitus is present in some but not in all cases.

DEMOGRAPHY

The sudden infant death syndrome is a worldwide major public health problem, with a striking consistency in its demographic characteristics. In the United States, an estimated 7,500 to 10,000 infants, predominantly between the ages of 1 and 5 months, die of SIDS. This syndrome is now recognized as the major cause of death in the country in infants between the first and twelfth months after birth.

Incidence

The average death rate from SIDS ranges between 2 and 3 per 1,000 live births, although the incidence is affected markedly by the distribution of a number of known variables described below, and perhaps by other unrecognized factors. A value as low as 0.31 per 1,000 live births has been reported from the Ashkelon District of Israel. Valdes-Dapena has reported that from 1961 through 1972 there was a dramatic decrease in the rate at which SIDS occurred among white infants and to a lesser extent among black infants in Philadelphia. The rate per 1,000 live births for white infants dropped from a mean value of 1.34 during 1961 to 1966 to 0.85 during 1967 to 1972; during these same periods the mean rate for black infants fell from 4.84 to 3.74. The reasons for these decreases are not apparent.

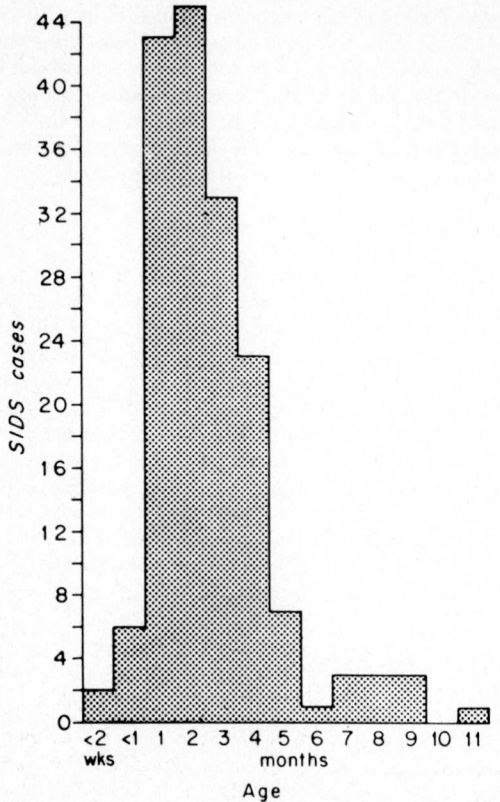

FIG. 10. The age distribution of 1970 cases of SIDS, January 1, 1965 to September 1, 1968 (From Bergman AB, Ray CG, Pomeroy MA, Wahl PW, and Beckwith JB: Studies of the sudden infant death syndrome in King County, Washington. III. Epidemiology, Pediatrics, 49:860, 1972. Reprinted with permission of the American Academy of Pediatrics)

Age

The age distribution of SIDS is considered to be the syndrome's single most characteristic demographic feature. The peak incidence is consistently found to be between the second and fourth months of life (Fig. 10). Comparatively few cases occur before 1 month of age, and there is a rapid decline in the incidence rate between 4 and 12 months. An occasional case is reported after 12 months of age.

Sex, Race, and Socioeconomic Level

The syndrome occurs more frequently in males than in females in a ratio of 3:2. The death rate is considerably higher in black than in white infants, in some series by factors as large as 3 or 4 to 1. While crib deaths occur in all socioeconomic levels, the frequency of cases is greater among the poor, which may account for the greater frequency among blacks.

Birth Weight, Gestational Age, and Multiple Births

Low birth-weight infants especially those born prematurely, and twins, appear to be at increased risk for SIDS (Fig. 11). Geertinger has reported tragic instances in which both twins succumbed to the syndrome simultaneously or within a very short period of each other.

Familial Occurrence

No definitive data exist that indicate a genetic basis for the syndrome, although there are families in which more than one infant died from SIDS. Frogatt has re-

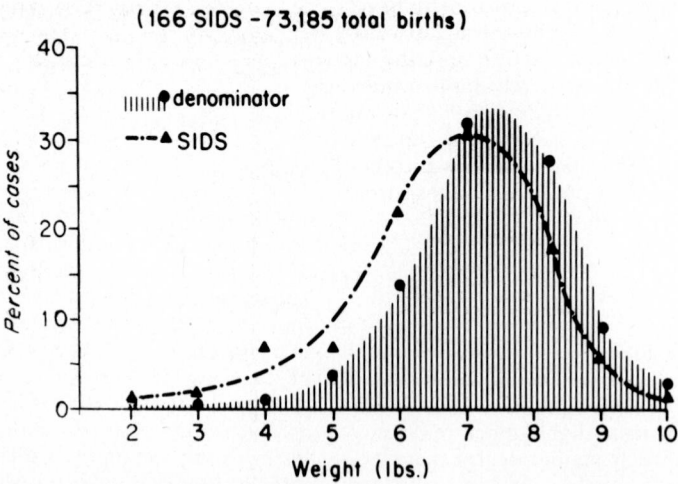

FIG. 11. The birth weight of 166 SIDS victims compared to other children born during the same time period, January 1, 1965 to September 1, 1968. (From Bergman AB, Ray CG, Pomeroy MA, Wahl PW, and Beckwith JB: Studies of the sudden death syndrome in King County, Washington. III. Epidemiology, Pediatrics, 49:860, 1972. Reprinted with permission of the American Academy of Pediatrics)

ported a recurrence rate in siblings of 11.1 to 22.1 per 1,000 siblings at risk. This is four to seven times the mean rate, representing a recurrence rate of about 2 percent.

Season, Geographic Area, and Time of Day

The occurrence of SIDS is higher between November and March, particularly in the United States and in urban areas, compared with rural areas. Geographic clustering of cases has been observed. Deaths due to SIDS occur more frequently between 12 midnight and 8:00 AM than during other periods of the 24 hours.

Perinatal and Postnatal Characteristics

With increasing maternal age, the risk of SIDS decreases, the rate per 1,000 live births being reported as 2.57 for mothers less than 20 years, 0.67 for those between 30 and 34 years, and 0.37 for mothers over 40 years. However, fewer cases of SIDS have been reported among first-born infants than among infants of subsequent birth order. After the first born, there is no evidence to suggest any difference in risk with increasing parity.

During pregnancy, mothers do not seem to differ from controls in the distribution of Rh factor, in prenatal exposure to x-ray, or in the incidence of toxemia, hydramnios, or vaginal bleeding. It has been reported, however, that mothers of SIDS cases made fewer prenatal clinic visits than other mothers, had more prior fetal losses, and were also more likely to have had "flu" during their pregnancy. Maternal anemia, proteinuria, vaginitis, and puerperal infections have been reported to be more common during the gestation. The prevalence of cigarette smoking during pregnancy has also been reported to be greater among mothers of subsequent SIDS cases.

Although no significant differences in the duration of the first state of labor has been found, a significantly shorter second stage of labor (14.1 minutes) has been reported for mothers of subsequent SIDS cases as compared with controls (23.7 minutes).

Postnatal growth of these infants has generally been considered to be normal. However, Peterson has recently reported impaired postnatal growth of these infants as measured by gain in weight, crown-to-head length, and head circumference from birth to demise. Naeye has studied 125 SIDS victims and matched controls followed prospectively from birth in the Collaborative Perinatal Project of the National Institutes of Health. He reports that postnatal growth was retarded in those SIDS infants who had appropriate birth weights for gestational age. The SIDS victims also differed from controls in the following factors: the prevalence of blood type B was higher; there were more with low Apgar scores; they required more neonatal resuscitation, positive respiratory pressure, and oxygen; they exhibited more temperature regulation problems; there was a greater frequency of respiratory distress syndrome; they received more antibiotics; feeding problems were more common; gavage feedings were required more often; and neurologic abnormalities were observed more frequently.

There is no difference in the distribution of SIDS among infants receiving cow's milk, breast milk alone, or a mixture of both. Some investigators have recently reported that the mean age of death is earlier in breastfed SIDS victims than in those who are not breastfed. SIDS infants are frequently described by their parents as being "good babies," "not demanding babies," "happy babies," "the best baby I ever had." In a study of the behavioral patterns before death of 46 SIDS victims, as reported by parents, in comparison with siblings, the SIDS babies were considered to be less responsive to environmental stimuli, less active physically, and generally more placid; they had a less vigorous suck and were more breathless and exhausted during feedings; they also had more abnormal cries.

ETIOLOGY AND PATHOGENESIS

Sudden, unexpected, and unexplained death in infancy has been recognized since biblical time. However, systematic study of these deaths began only in the 1940s with the publication of a series of papers by Werne and Garrow, between 1942 and 1953. They presented important evidence showing that in many sudden and unexpected deaths in infants, the cause of death was associated not with suffocation but with pathogenic mechanisms, probably inflammatory.

As a result of intensive investigations of SIDS between 1972 and 1975, it now appears that the pathogenesis of the syndrome is not through a single mechanism, as previously believed. Instead, a number of developmental, environmental, and pathophysiologic factors appear to be involved, which under a complex set of circumstances interact in such a way as to set up a sequence of events, which at some point becomes irreversible and leads to death.

Most of the hypotheses proposed over the years to explain SIDS have been refuted. The more popular of these included overlying and suffocation; status thymicolymphaticus; parathyroid insufficiency; upper respiratory tract inflammation; viremia and bacteremia; myocardial conduction system defects; hypersensitivity to cow's milk; and immunologic deficiencies. Intensive research during the 1970s has not only refuted and disproved most of these earlier suspicions concerning the cause and pathogenesis of SIDS but, more important has disclosed evidence suggesting a wholly different approach. Evidence is accumulating that, contrary to the widely accepted view that these infants were essentially healthy until their sudden unexpected death, they had abnormalities that may have been present since and even prior to birth. Evidence that these infants have preexisting difficulties includes anatomic pathologic findings suggestive of chronic stress and hypoxia; abnormalities in sleep state, cardiorespiratory function, and tissue oxygen utilization; postnatal growth retardation; and the infant's temperament and behavioral patterns between birth and death.

Etiologic mechanisms currently proposed to explain SIDS revolve around interrelated infectious disease processes and developmental, pathophysiologic, metabolic, and environmental phenomena. A number of them are closely tied to chronic stress and hypoxic states, while other mechanisms are concerned with cardiac, respiratory, and metabolic abnormalities. These include the following.

Chronic Oxygen Deficiency

The findings of Naeye, in SIDS victims, of hypertrophy and hyperplasia of the muscle mass surrounding the small pulmonary arteries, similar to those seen in normal infants and children living at high altitude, are regarded as suggestive that SIDS victims have had chronic hypoxia. These data provided the first presumptive evidence that SIDS victims may have been subjected to some type of chronic stress for varying periods of time before death. Naeye has also reported in some SIDS cases (a) deposits of brown fat around the adrenal glands at ages when such fat would be expected to be white, and (b) abnormal retention of hepatic extramedullary hematopoeisis. The latter observation, confirmed by Valdes-Dapena, is viewed as additional evidence of exposure of SIDS babies to prolonged periods of chronic stress and hypoxia.

Sleep Apnea

It has been proposed that prolonged sleep apnea, defined, in general, as the cessation of respiration for a period of 10 seconds or longer, may be involved in SIDS. Steinschneider reported that the incidence of sleep apnea in infants less than 2,500 g was significantly greater than in those with normal birth weights and that it occurs more frequently in conjunction with an upper respiratory tract infection. There appears to be an age-related effect. On the average spontaneous sleep apnea ceases to occur by 5 months of age, whereas sleep apnea associated with a nasopharyngitis continues until the sixth month of life.

Sleep Deprivation

The role of sleep deprivation in SIDS is being investigated in kittens. Kittens, like infants, exhibit sleep apnea and the frequency of apneic episodes is greatly increased following prolonged periods of lack of sleep. It has been observed that the ability of the kitten to awaken during a period of apnea is reduced in REM sleep state and following sleep deprivation. Spontaneous laryngeal spasms during REM sleep have also been observed, sometimes accompanied by arrhythmias. These arrhythmias may reflect respiratory insufficiency and hypoxemia during sleep.

These observations are important because a prolonged apneic period at a time when arousal mechanisms are suppressed could lead to an acute lack of oxygen in the tissues and associated central nervous system depression. Such depression could result in sudden death without pathologic findings. Moreover, a laryngeal spasm at a time when arousal mechanisms are depressed could precipitate irreversible respiratory failure.

Respiratory Control

Of particular importance to our understanding of SIDS are studies concerned with the young infant's ventilatory response to carbon dioxide and data showing an apparent increase in CO_2 responsiveness with gestational age. Furthermore, the load on the respiratory system is continually changing with alterations in posture, abdominal pressure, and nasal obstruction, which reduce the tidal volume. In adult man, load compensating mechanisms restore tidal volume to normal in about five breaths; in contrast, some infants show no evidence of progressive load compensation. The consequences in infants are more dangerous than in adults, since the intercostal muscles will be more affected than the diaphragm, and a tendency to collapse the rib cage may occur during REM sleep, coinciding with an increased airway resistance. Failure to compensate is particularly marked during REM sleep and in premature infants with histories of abnormal respiratory control, but it has been observed in some full-term infants as well. Infants in this age group spend a relatively greater time in REM sleep.

There are four infant reflex mechanisms that are of importance to SIDS because their disruption uniformly causes apnea and bradycardia. These include the peripheral chemoreceptor reflexes, the central chemoreceptor reflex, the Hering-Breuer reflex, and the reflex of the upper surface of the epiglottis. The role of these reflexes in the occurrence of SIDS is being intensely studied as it is becoming evident that they are closely related to respiratory control.

Laryngospasm

Because death is so sudden and quiet, it is thought to be caused by an instantaneous interruption of respiration, resulting from laryngospasm, and further that the threshold for development of the lethal event in susceptible babies is influenced by a balance of multiple factors (constitutional determinants, specific developmental stage, internal and external chemical milieu, irritation from a minor airway inflammation, and specific stage of sleep). In turn, an instantaneous catastrophic physiologic event, such as apnea with or without myotonic occlusion of the upper airway, occurs and this leads to sudden unexpected death.

Cardiac Abnormalities

Sudden death due to cardiac arrhythmias may be the cause of or contribute to the deaths in a manner not understood as yet. Bradycardia and sometimes arrhythmias have been reported with apneic episodes during sleep, especially those that occur during non-REM sleep. Such a mechanism might help explain the excess number of males in SIDS victims, since they generate a higher output of catecholamines during stress, which might predispose to fatal arrhythmias.

It has recently been hypothesized that a prolonged Q-T interval may contribute to or be the cause of some sudden and unexpected infant deaths. In a pilot study of 42 sets of parents of SIDS victims, prolongation of the Q-T interval was found in at least one member of 11 sets of parents, and in as many as 40 percent of the siblings, suggesting an autosomal dominant pattern of inheritance. In addition, an infant with a history of "near-miss" SIDS showed marked prolongation of the Q-T interval (see p. 1402).

A histologic analysis of myocardium in a group of 46 SIDS infants and 26 control infants revealed, in the ventricular septum of 22 percent of the infants with SIDS and 12 percent of the controls, small foci of normal-sized, disorganized cardiac muscle cells, resembling those in asymmetric septal hypertrophy (ASH). It is proposed that these may serve as a nidus for ventricular arrhythmias in some infants with SIDS and that the previous theory of myocardial conduction disturbances and arrhythmias in some infants with SIDS should be reevaluated.

Defective Gluconeogenesis

Hepatic phosphoenolpyruvate carboxykinase (PEPCK) activity has been reported to be decreased and defective in its response to divalent transition metals, such as Mn^{++} in victims of SIDS. Interestingly, the liver of one of the SIDS victims contained no detectable PEPCK. Another of the SIDS victims with low (0.09) PEPCK activity and no stimulation by Mn^+ had a sibling who earlier died of SIDS. The father of these two children was also the father of another SIDS victim, the latter by his first wife.

Based on these observations, Lardy has proposed that SIDS is caused by hypoglycemia, which results from impaired gluconeogenesis. Impaired gluconeogenesis would not be likely to be hazardous during the period of frequent feeding; however, with stressful bacterial or viral infection, a period of fasting, a cold environment, or a combination of any of these hazards, effective gluconeogenesis may be necessary for survival. A defect in the enzyme and hormone systems involved in regulating hepatic gluconeogenesis might be responsible for the reported deficiency in PEPCK; it is also possible that the enzyme deficiency is secondary to chronic hypoxemia.

Electrolyte Abnormalities

It has been hypothesized that SIDS results from a relative or absolute deficiency in magnesium (Mg) following rapid growth on cow's milk formula, the mineral composition of which is believed to be unbalanced for the human infant. It is proposed that mediators, including histamine, may be released during plasma Mg^{++} / Ca^{++} imbalance; in turn an exaggerated response, resulting in anaphylactic shock and death, might occur in a young infant with hypoglycemia or low adrenal corticoids and/or during cold stresses.

Investigators in the United Kingdom have found marked increases in sodium, chloride, and urea concentrations in the vitreous humor of some SIDS victims. These findings are suggestive of dehydration or of hyperosmolar seedings, but have not been reported in any SIDS cases in the United States.

Others

Additional hypotheses and explanations are being investigated either as the cause of the syndrome or as approaches to identifying infants at risk for SIDS. These include the role of anemia in potentiating apnea; CNS dysfunction above the brain stem; abnormalities of the carotid body; effects of acute metabolic conditions on central nervous system development, organization, and function; inability to metabolize free fatty acids; a lack of vitamin E or selenium; lack of secretory component of bronchopulmonary mucosa; nasal obstruction; cardio-vascular instability; biogenic amine metabolism; and tactile adaptive responses.

PSYCHOLOGIC CONSIDERATIONS

The sudden infant death syndrome is as much a human problem as it is a medical enigma. The psychologic impact upon the families of infants dying from SIDS is different from that which exists when an infant dies of other causes. SIDS is not generally recognized and understood as a specific cause of infant death, even by health and public safety officials who deal with the problem daily. As a consequence, the parents, particularly those in the lower socioeconomic bracket, may be accused of child abuse and neglect. In many instances parents are unable to explain the cause of death to a family and friends, which compounds the problem further. The sudden and unexpected death of an infant is frequently the beginning of a family crisis that affects the parents, siblings, relatives, and community. They all need emotional support, compassion, and reassurance that no one is to blame for the infant's death. Whenever possible, an autopsy should be performed. A definitive diagnosis of SIDS can provide some reassurance that the death was not due to an avoidable cause; the results of the necropsy can also help extend our knowledge of SIDS.

Professional counseling should be available immediately after the infant's death. The physician must anticipate a brief reaction of varying degree and assure the mother and father that this is normal. Families profit by being given adequate information about the syndrome. Well-informed health professionals can help ease the damaging repercussions of the tragedy by explaining that apparently healthy infants can die suddenly and unexpectedly from causes that are not known and that nothing the parents did or failed to do was responsible. Families should be told about the voluntary organizations of families that have lost babies to SIDS, which may be a source of comfort and support for more recent SIDS families. Follow-up of SIDS families is essential. Parents who appear to adjust well at first to the sudden and unexpected death of their infant may suddenly decompensate and be unable to relate to each other or their other children for months or even years after the experience.

When a baby dies from SIDS, siblings must be told what has happened. An older sibling cannot help feeling that something he did may have been responsible. His guilt feelings, like those of his parents, may persist and grow. A child too young to understand death nevertheless senses the parents' grief and guilt and may be frightened by it. A child old enough to understand about death should be told that the infant's death was due to a specific disorder limited to a few infants within a specific age range. Such information can help to reduce the child's anxiety about his own safety.

"Near-Miss" SIDS and Home Monitoring

There are a number of apparently healthy infants between the second and fourth month of life, the peak age incidence for SIDS, who are found to be cyanotic and apneic and recover after some form of resuscitory intervention. Since it cannot be known whether or not these infants would have died, the use of the term "near-miss" may be challenged. However, there have been several instances in which such infants have appeared to be quite well following the episodes and yet died subsequently of SIDS, sometimes within a week. It has been suggested, therefore, that infants having episodes of the type described are at high risk for dying of SIDS. They also represent one type of SIDS death for which means of prevention may be developed and applied.

The potential value and hazards in the use of monitoring systems is currently being investigated. Apnea and cardiac monitors are used extensively in pediatric intensive care units to give early warning of episodes requiring resuscitative intervention. Home monitoring is also being carefully investigated; Steinschneider, for example, is considering it for two types of patients: the otherwise healthy premature infant whose hospitalization is prolonged because of recurrent apneic and cyanotic episodes and the healthy infant who "develops" apneic and cyanotic episodes at home. Until the complex psychologic, physiologic, and technical aspects of this subject are better understood, the use of home monitoring equipment that is sold over the counter and advertised to prevent SIDS should be strongly discouraged, as recommended by the Committee on Infant and Preschool Child of the American Academy of Pediatrics. As stated in the Committee's report on home monitoring for SIDS: "In our present state of knowledge of SIDS, the most important functions of the pediatrician or family physician are to examine the patients he cares for and assure himself that they are in good health; to be well-informed about SIDS; and to give full emotional support to the family of a SIDS baby."

Bibliography

Beckwith JB: The sudden infant death syndrome. Curr Prob Pediatr 3:3, 1973

Bergman AB, Beckwith JB, Ray CG (eds): Sudden Infant Death Syndrome. University of Washington Press, Seattle, 1970

Committee on Infant and Preschool Child, American Academy of Pediatrics: Home monitoring for sudden infant death. Pediatrics 55:144, 1975

Friedman SB: Psychological aspects of sudden unexpected death in infants and children. Pediatr Clin North Am 21:103, 1974

Geertinger P: Sudden Death in Infancy. CC Thomas, Springfield, Ill, 1968

Hasselmeyer EG, Hunter JC: Sudden infant death syndrome. In Wynn RM (ed): Obstetrics and Gynecology Annual 1975. Appleton-Century Crofts, New York, 1975, pp 213–236

——— Research Perspectives in the Sudden Infant Death Syndrome 1975: A National Institute of Child Health and Human Development Research Reporting Workshop on the Sudden Infant Death Syndrome. US DHEW Public Health Service, National Institutes of Health, US DHEW Publication No. (NIH) 76

Marx JL: Crib death: some promising leads but no solution yet. Science, 189:367, 1975

Naeye RL: Pulmonary arterial abnormalities in the sudden infant death syndrome. N Engl J Med 289:1167, 1973

Peterson DR, Benson EA, Fisher LD, Chinn NM, Beckwith JB: Postnatal growth and the sudden infant death syndrome. Am J Epidemiol 99:389, 1974

Steinschneider A: Prolonged apnea and the sudden infant death syndrome: clinical and laboratory observations. Pediatrics 50:646, 1972

Sudden Infant Death Syndrome: Selected Annotated Bibliography, 1960–1971. US DHEW Public Health Service, National Institutes of Health. US DHEW Publication No. (NIH) 73-237, 1973

Sudden Infant Death Syndrome: Selected Annotated Bibliography, 1972–1974. US DHEW Public Health Service, National Institutes of Health. US DHEW Publication No. (NIH) 76-237, 1976

Valdes-Dapena MA: Sudden and unexpected death in infancy: a review of the world literature (1954–1966). Pediatrics 39:123, 1967

——— Sudden death in infancy: A report for pathologists. In Rosenberg HS, Bolande RP (eds): Perspectives Pediatr Pathol 2:1, 1975

Wedgewood RJ, Benditt EP: Sudden Death in Infants. US DHEW Public Health Service, National Institutes of Health. US DHEW Publication No. (NIH) 1412, 1966

Weitzman ED, Graziani L: Sleep and the sudden infant death syndrome: a new hypothesis. In Weitzman ED (ed): Adv Sleep Res 1:327, 1974

SUICIDE IN CHILDREN AND ADOLESCENTS

Joseph Richman

This discussion of suicide in children rests upon three basic foundations. The first is that such suicidal reactions represent a form of communication sounding a call for help. The plea, therefore, must always be listened to, even when the act is not a fatal one. The second is that suicide is to be understood developmentally, in terms of success or failure in meeting the tasks or roles typical of one's age, and the sequelae of task failure. The third is that the act of suicide in children is to a great extent socially determined and situationally based; it expresses a problem not only in the child but also in the family and society. These three aspects are intimately interrelated.

The implications of these principles are likewise threefold. First, the entire fate of the child may hinge upon the response of the important persons in his life to the appeal component of the suicide attempt. If the cry is answered early and constructively the suicide can be prevented, not only in the present but subsequently. Second, the most important life-saving agents are the family, the school, and the physician; the physician may play an especially important role by virtue of his position as a helping professional and the mediator between life and death. Third, suicide in children expresses problems in living rather than wishes for dying. Depending upon the fate of these components, the intrinsic drives for growth and fulfillment are either inhibited or given an opportunity to blossom. In our work with suicidal children, consequently, we treat the situation as the patient and aim primarily toward alleviating personal conflicts, family tensions, and school or peer conflicts, as well as carefully examining and evaluating the medical and organic components. In this approach the pediatrician or family doctor must become the doctor for the entire family.

DEMOGRAPHY

The suicide rate in children is relatively low compared with that of adults; nevertheless, there are compelling reasons to focus on the problems of the young. There are few happenings as poignant and sad as the self-inflicted death of a young person. Even if the rate is not as great as in the adult, suicide in the young is still a sizable problem. It is among the four major causes of death for individuals under 15 and second for young men at ages 15 to 24. There is evidence that the rate is increasing. Many of the underlying problems of suicide are common to all ages; anything that lowers the suicide rate at one age or among one group may reduce it for all. Suicide at all ages is probably the culmination of a disturbance that originated in childhood, and whatever can decrease the suicidal potential of children will have a favorable effect on the problem in adults.

In contrast to *completed* suicide, *attempted* suicide is more common in children than in adults. The rate is sufficiently high to indicate a problem of major proportions. Jacobziner estimated that there were 100 attempts for every completed suicide in children and adolescents. Lomanaco and Pfeffer have provided evidence that the amount of suicidal and self-destructive behavior in very young children, during latency and even earlier, is considerably greater than has been supposed.

Age and Sex

Suicide has been documented as early as the age of 2! Throughout the world the suicide rate increases with age. In males the increase is constant, while in females the suicide rate reaches a peak between the ages of 40 and 60 and then declines.

In both children and adolescents the male to female ratio of completed suicides is approximately 3:1. Among latency-age children, there are more recorded attempts at suicide by boys than by girls, but in adolescents the figures are reversed, there being from 3 to 10 female attempts for every male attempt.

Race

Among races in the United States, there are pronounced differences in the peak ages for suicide. For both white and nonwhite males, the completed suicide rate has been approximately the same up to age 35, after which it remains relatively constant and low for nonwhites, but rises steadily for whites. However, recent evidence indicates that the suicide rate in blacks is rising. For example, in 1969, Hendin reported that in New York City the suicide rate for black males under the age of 35 was twice that for whites. For nonwhite females, the suicide rate is uniformly low throughout all ages.

The figures for attempted suicides differ with ethnic groups, the rates being high in minority groups such as blacks and Puerto Ricans. However, a qualification should be noted. The statistics are derived largely from police files and from municipal and state hospital records, which include a higher proportion of poor people, especially Puerto Ricans and blacks. Suicide attempts of whites and of individuals belonging to the middle- and upper-class groups are less likely to be reported.

The emotional turmoil surrounding a suicide attempt is often particularly evident in the minority groups. Trautman described a characteristically intense episode of suicidal acting-out in Puerto Ricans, which he called *the suicidal fit,* while Gould observed a similar pattern, which he referred to as the *Puerto Rican syndrome.* The traits associated with these conditions tended to diminish with increasing acculturation.

It has been our observation, however, that impulsivity and dissociative trends are prominent in many individuals from all walks of life who attempt suicide. As our relationships with the people involved in a suicidal act became more intimate, ethnic and social differences tended to be minimized or disappeared. Among the families of higher socioeconomic classes, violence is more attenuated; also, less gross sexual deviation and less family disorganization were usually displayed. However, these apparently different characteristics now appear to us to be rather superficial. A greater acquaintance with the situation revealed, almost invariably, outbursts of uncontrolled aggression and either incestuous acting-out or other forms of sexual deviation. In contrast to Hendin, who considers the dynamics of suicide to vary in different countries and ethnic groups, it is our clinical impression that there are no major racial, ethnic, or socioeconomic differences in the dynamics of the suicidal individual and his family.

Religion

In general most studies of *completed* suicides report a lower rate among Catholics and Jews than among Protestants, while in most studies of *attempted* suicide there has been a tendency to disregard this variable. In our practice, however, there is a large percentage of Catholics and Jews among the young patients who attempt suicide. One can speculate that more distress would be required to drive a Catholic child to such an act, or that the completed act is more often concealed, or that the religious ban upon suicide does not apply with the same force to the more symbolic and less final behavior of the attempt. Further research into this area is needed to provide conclusive data.

Method

Boys use guns and hanging as the most frequent methods for completed suicide, while girls resort to pills. These sex differences remain constant throughout the life-span with, of course, many individual exceptions. The choice of less violent methods with their greater opportunities for rescue has been postulated as one basis for the lower suicide rate in females. In suicide attempts the most popular method in children and adolescents of both sexes is drugs. With increased age, however, the attempts tend to become more serious, the risk more lethal, and the intent to die closer to that of completed suicides.

Season

Jacobziner reported among adolescents more attempts in the spring, but in general no clear or consistent trends have been noted. Apart from any seasonal variations, weekends, holidays, and sometimes important anniversary dates are the most trying times for suicidally inclined youngsters.

DIAGNOSIS

In the literature a small tempest rages around the diagnostic characteristics of suicidal children and adolescents. Some report schizophrenia as the major diagnostic entity, others depression, and still others neuroses and character disorders.

The bulk of our youthful suicidal population was depressed and most were diagnosed as having character disorders. We tend to agree with Beck and his associates, however, that hopelessness is a more important variable than depression, even though the two are related. In general, however, the diagnosis of psychopathology in the adolescent or younger patient is of limited value. It usually tells little about the seriousness of the actual attempt or of the circumstances surrounding it. Furthermore, in focusing on the diagnostic characteristics, one tends to assign the reasons for the act to the personality disorder. As a result, the environmental and situational factors and the role of other significant persons are obscured or relatively disregarded. The diagnosis should not be ignored, but its meaning can be understood only in the total context.

MOTIVES AND PRECIPITATING EVENTS

A *precipitating event* refers to the existing situation or stresses instrumental in producing a suicidal act. A *motive* refers to the reason, purpose, or function of the act. The two are most often intertwined and inseparable, and are, therefore, best considered together.

Many difficulties lie in the path of examining and understanding these aspects. For example, not many children can say what event or motive precipitated their suicidal behavior. It is most valuable, therefore, to interview as many relatives and other significant persons as possible, both individually and as families. Such a procedure often reveals that the act serves a major function for the entire family.

The most helpful first step, in general, is to elicit the actual concrete circumstances surrounding the suicidal act. Typically, the motives and precipitants are more complex than suspected. Eleven major categories of individual motives for suicidal behavior in children and adolescents can be identified in addition to the social and family functions of the act. These include: (a) separation, object loss, and social disruption; (b) reunion wishes and fantasies; (c) aggression; (d) atonement; (e) precocious sexual disturbances; (f) manipulation and blackmail; (g) an attempt to escape from an unbearable situation; (h) school difficulties; (i) the expression of a disintegration of the personality; (j) a cry for help; and (k) a developmental crisis. In addition we have identified several social and family functions of the act.

Rather than attempting to discuss all of these, we shall focus upon the five individual motives and precipitants most important for the pediatrician to understand.

Separation, Loss, and Social Disruption

Suicide and the more serious suicidal attempts are often a reaction to the loss or threatened loss of a loved one, to which the person has been sensitized by losses in the past. Among the most consistent findings in the literature on suicide throughout the world is a history of parental loss, broken homes, and family disorganization. This motive, therefore, is intimately related to the family dynamics discussed in greater detail below. Rejection by friends, parents, and relatives and a greater sense of alienation from the other members of society appear relevant to this theme. It forms the most personal counterpart of the breakdown of integration between the individual and society, which Durkheim called *anomie*.

Aggression

Aggression in suicide appears in various forms. These include retaliation, thwarted or blocked hostility or anger, a need to punish the surroundings or others for perceived deprivation of love, and autoaggression. The most frequent precipitating event for a suicidal act in children and adolescents is a family quarrel. Aggression poses a suicidal threat when other forms of aggressive outlets are not available and when the person must endure not only his own aggression turned against himself, but the accumulated aggression of others. Under these conditions, suicide is simultaneously an act of aggression against the self *and* the significant other or others. Suicide really represents the last word in retaliation. The two-edged nature of aggression in suicide is often seen most clearly in cases where homicide or assault is followed by completed or attempted suicide. Such cases are more common than is generally known and the problem of suicide can be properly understood only when viewed as one aspect of the general problem of violence in individuals and society.

Manipulation and Blackmail

These include attention-getting, forcing reactions from the environment, attempts to control, and efforts to obtain more love. The interpersonal and family aspects of suicide are particularly evident in this category. We have been most impressed by the transactional, two-way nature of the interaction and the efforts to maintain a pathologic status quo involved in the manipulation.

School Difficulties

Assuming the role of a student and meeting the demands of school constitutes one of the primary tasks of growing up. For most children, school is the first major separation from home. Therefore, the child who cannot tolerate separation often is unable to make the required adjustment. School failure and tension about studies, together with parental demands and difficulties at home, are almost universal in suicidal children and adolescents. A pattern of strain and failure is found not only in children who still attend school, but in the past school history of the older suicidal person.

A Developmental Crisis

This broadly integrative concept covers the needs, role-related tasks, striving, and goals of the young person and the social and instinctual tensions characteristic of his age. During latency, when the first signs of suicidal behavior may become noticeable, the developmental task is that of establishing peer relationships and demonstrating adequacy in school. In the adolescent the developmental task is that of forming a clear identity rather than a diffusion of roles. The young suicidal person has invariably failed to meet expectations for his age-appropriate role at home, in school, and in his social life. His suicidal act expresses both an admission of a failure to meet the identity crisis and a regression to the infant–mother symbiosis.

We conclude that an understanding of the motives and precipitants of a suicidal act in childhood involves consideration of four aspects. First, the nature of the individual's personality, the stresses he is undergoing, and the resources he has available to him must be explored. Second, the role of the social and family network must be examined and understood. Most of the suicidal acts we studied became considerably more understandable in the light of the family patterns within which the behavior was embedded and in the light of the motives and stresses of the other significant persons. Third, the present here-and-now context must be explored, especially the current crises; and fourth, the historic background of the act must be studied. In all cases we found that the motives and precipitants of suicide were repetitive and cumulative. These unfortunate, unsuccessful, and repetitive experiences were designed to maintain regressive and infantile ties to the original family pattern.

THE FAMILY IN SUICIDAL CHILDREN AND ADOLESCENTS

In a recent study of the family relations of both aged and youthful subjects at the time of their suicide attempt, we found that the overt precipitants differed at different ages but that the underlying social and family functions were similar. The major covert family determinant was the effort to maintain a pathologic status quo. Other major features included an intolerance for mourning, depression, or the expression of neediness in the suicidal person, with a turning away by the family network; an intolerance for crises, with a similar turning away from the suicidal person; and a generation repetition compulsion. These family foundations of a suicidal act are more evident in younger than in older age groups, although present in both. As already noted, an impressive body of evidence has been accumulated documenting the prevalence of parental disturbances and family disorganization in the background of suicidal children and adolescents, stemming from the first years of life. Studies of these families reveal a high incidence of depriving and rejecting parents, destructive and grossly disturbed parent–child relationships, neglect, broken homes, and parental loss. It is not the parental loss in itself that is significant but the loss of parenting, which can occur also in ostensibly intact families.

The sheer bulk of the evidence of a disturbed and disorganized family background in suicidal children is incontestable. Although a disturbed family is characteristic of all children with emotional problems and is not the exclusive prerogative of suicidal children, its significance in suicidal behavior is not to be minimized. More studies are needed to understand the relationships between family structure and interactions and a suicidal resolution. Our studies form part of this endeavor. We have seen many features we consider characteristic of disturbed families in general, and some that are more specific to families in which suicidal actions occur. The latter include certain characteristic disturbances in the communication patterns of the family, in role distribution, and in the patterns of aggressive discharge or blocking of discharge.

Regarding the outcome of the aggressive impulses, the self-destructive activity was often a reaction to the destructive wishes of an important person. It was also a projection upon the suicidal child of the bad self of the parents and the entire family combined with a ubiquitous intolerance for separation. The relationship between the suicidal child and the family or other significant persons is a double-binding one in which they can neither separate nor remain together. The relatives communicate to the suicidal child that he is a burden. However, he is not only forbidden to leave the family, he is forbidden to establish relationships with others. The suicidal act occurs in a closed family system that excludes outsiders and within which the suicidal child is alienated and isolated, yet forbidden to move out.

Suicide is not necessarily the direct result of family and personal disturbances, be it a broken home, object loss, or occupational, social, or school failure. All of these are found in persons who are not suicidal. What is central is the way in which the disturbance is handled. In many of our cases of suicidal children we found a symbiosis with a mother who was rejecting and unable to empathize. No one was assigned age, sex, or socially appropriate roles in the family. Depression and low self-esteem were family characteristics. It was often a home in which the parents engaged in questionable behavior and the siblings were unreasonably aggressive, but only the patient was labeled as bad.

Our experiences indicate that the suicidal person was one who met with such difficulties in family relationships. Child, mother, and often the whole family, display intense infantile fixations. The implication is that how the developmental tasks at any age are met and mastered (or failed) depends upon how previous developmental crises were met and resolved. The time has come, therefore, for a developmental psychology of suicide. Lourie has pointed out that the developmental crises leading to early depressive and suicidal syndromes are based upon poor and distorted answers to the problems of earlier development. Suicidal behavior is then potentiated by events in the present.

The present, however, is much more than a mere trigger, since the suicidal act is not only based upon these early problems and fixations, but is a result of an entire network of present-day relationships in which each significant person plays his suicidogenic part. We hypothesize, therefore, that suicidal behavior in children is a pattern learned in the family, handed down from one generation to the next, and sustained by suicidogenic relationships in the present.

RECOMMENDATIONS AND CONCLUSIONS

An attempted suicidal act of a child is not wholly a tragedy. It is also a challenge and an opportunity that contains many positive potentials. Our data have led us to some recommendations regarding the role of the family, the school, and the doctor in the treatment and prevention of suicide.

First, early recognition of the potentially suicidal youngster is vital. An ounce of early intervention is far better than many pounds of later therapy. Special courses and training in the recognition of danger signs are desirable for physicians, teachers, guidance personnel, and all those who may be involved with the disturbed child. A program to detect the potentially suicidal child is needed. Pupils who tend to be loners or outcasts form the greatest suicidal risks. They need someone to talk to and someone to help them in becoming members of the social group.

Second, the school assumes a special role because it is the threshold of the larger society outside the home. For effective suicide prevention, the school and home should work closely together. Therapy and counseling services should be available in all schools at all levels. In addition to remedial and personal counseling for troubled pupils, we believe that every school, beginning with elementary school, should have a family counseling service available.

Third, sexual difficulties are as prevalent in the genesis of suicide as problems with aggression. Proper sex education, therefore, may help to prevent suicide.

Fourth, suicide is fostered by a violent and frustration-producing society. A social emphasis upon nonviolent means of solving national and international conflicts may prevent suicide.

Fifth, the teacher is a key figure. None of the psychiatric and social services in the schools can substitute for the sensitivity of the individual teacher, his awareness of the pupil who is in trouble and who may need him, and his availability when needed. The teacher's attitude can often make the difference between suicide or growth.

Sixth, the physician is a key figure, for reasons that have been discussed. The insensitivity of some doctors and teachers may have contributed to a suicidal act. There have also been many teachers and physicians whose influence has prevented suicides and preserved lives. However, there can be no statistics on persons who might have but did not commit suicide. Hence, their influence must go unnoticed, except in the lives and hearts of those they have met and touched. It is because of such individuals that there is hope that the cry for help will be answered.

Bibliography

Anonymous: Leading causes of death among insured lives. Statistical Bull 55:8, 1974

Dorpat TL, Jackson JK, Ripley HS: Broken homes and attempted and completed suicides. Arch Gen Psychiatry 12:213, 1965

Durkheim E: Suicide. Translated by Spaulding JA, Simpson G. The Free Press, New York, 1951

Gould RE: Suicide problems in children and adolescents. Am J Psychother 19:228, 1965

Hendin H: Black Suicide. Basic Books, New York, 1969

Jacobziner H: Attempted suicides in adolescence. JAMA 191:101, 1965

Lomonaco S, Pfeffer C: Suicidal and self-destructive behavior in latency age children. Presented at the Annual Convention of the American Academy of Child Psychiatry, San Francisco, Calif, Oct, 1974

Lourie RS: Suicide and attempted suicide in children and adolescents. In Yochelson L (ed): Symposium on Suicide. George Washington School of Medicine, Washington DC, 1967, pp 93–105

Richman J: Family determinants of attempted suicide. In Farberow NL (ed): Proceedings of the Fourth International Conference for Suicide Prevention, Los Angeles, Calif, 1968, pp 372–380

——— Age and the family determinants of attempted suicide. In Congress Abstracts, 10th International Congress of Gerontology, Jerusalem, Israel, 1975, p 162

——— Rosenbaum M: The family doctor and the suicidal family. Psychiatr Med 1:27, 1970

Rosenbaum M, Richman J: Suicide: the role of hostility and death wishes from the family and significant others. Am J Psychiatr 126:1652, 1970

Seiden RH: Suicide Among Youth. Bulletin of Suicidology Supplement, Washington DC, US Government Printing Office, Dec 1969

Shneidman ES, Farberow NL, Litman RE: The Psychology of Suicide. Science House, New York, 1970

Stengel E: Suicide and Attempted Suicide. Penguin Books, Baltimore, 1964

Trautman EC: The suicidal fit: a psychologic study in Puerto Rico immigrants. Arch Gen Psychiatr 5:76, 1961

Yacoubian JH, Lourie RS: Suicide and attempted suicide in children and adolescents. Clin Proc Child Hosp, 25:325, 1969

CHAPTER 16

Principles of Drug Disposition and Therapy in Infants and Children

Bernard L. Mirkin, *Associate Editor*

Biologic immaturity, its influence on mammalian response to drugs, and the ecology of therapeutics have become sources of increasing concern to the medical community and to society at large. Numerous investigations have shown that the reactivity of cells, tissues, and organ systems to pharmacologically active molecules is modulated by the maturational status of the affected structures. While the body of data available on the disposition, pharmacodynamics, and clinical effectiveness of drugs at different stages in mammalian development has greatly expanded in recent years, there still exists a compelling need to assess more accurately the benefits and potential hazards of contemporary therapeutic practices as applied to pediatric subjects.

The people involved in the disciplines of developmental pharmacology and pediatric clinical pharmacology have been engaged in defining the critical determinants that influence the disposition of drugs administered prenatally, at parturition, and during extrauterine life, so that a rational basis for therapeutic intervention in this population can be established. This chapter will consider these issues in detail.

PLACENTAL TRANSFER AND DRUG DISPOSITION IN THE MATERNAL-PLACENTAL-FETAL UNIT

The movement of pharmacologically active compounds across the placenta is affected by many factors, and the bidirectional transfer of molecules between the fetal and maternal circulations is dependent upon the smooth integration of these different processes. Due to the ethical and experimental difficulties such studies present, it has not been possible to achieve a detailed analysis of placental transfer in the human. Consequently most of the meaningful data relating to transplacental exchange of drugs has been obtained from a variety of animal models; the relevance of such studies for the human must be critically scrutinized. In general, the passage of pharmacologic agents across the placenta is determined by the physicochemical properties of the drug and the physiologic characteristics of the maternal-placental-fetal unit.

Physicochemical Properties of Drugs

LIPID SOLUBILITY AND DEGREE OF IONIZATION. Drug molecules that are lipophilic (ie, possess a high fat solubility) and that exist primarily in an unionized state at physiologic pH tend to diffuse more rapidly across the placenta and enter the fetal circulation in high concentrations. Compounds such as antipyrine and thiopental, each of which is poorly ionized at physiologic pH, traverse the placenta very rapidly, whereas bases with a high pKa and acids with a low pKa diffuse across biologic membranes quite slowly under similar conditions. Skeletal muscle relaxants such as succinylcholine and *d*-tubocurarine, which contain positively charged quaternary nitrogens, and the sulfated mucopolysaccharides such as heparin are highly ionized. As a consequence their transfer across the placenta is extremely slow, and only low concentrations are generally established within the fetal circulation. It should be noted, however, that apnea and flaccidity have been reported in some neonates whose mothers had been receiving these agents.

Some drugs, such as the salicylates, which are almost completely ionized at pH 7.4, appear to cross the placenta quite rapidly. The reason for this is that even though only small amounts of the molecule may exist in an un-ionized state at physiologic pH the quantity present readily traverses the placenta because of its high lipid solubility.

PROTEIN BINDING. The extent to which a drug is protein-bound may influence its placental passage. The pharmacologic importance of this dependence appears to vary markedly with whether the compound is lipophilic and nonpolar or lipophobic and highly polar. Compounds possessing a high degree of fat solubility are not significantly influenced by protein binding, since the transfer of these drugs seems to be proportional to placental blood flow. In contrast, those agents that diffuse across the placenta at slower rates, as a result of greater ionization and lesser lipid solubility, may be significantly affected by protein binding, since diffusion seems to be rate-limiting for such compounds.

Marked quantitative differences have been demonstrated in the extent to which drugs are bound to fetal, neonatal, and maternal sera. The binding of several different classes of drugs to maternal serum proteins seems to be substantially greater than that observed in fetal and neonatal sera. This has been shown, both in animal studies and in human studies, for sulfonamides, barbiturates, hydantoin anticonvulsants, and local anesthetic agents. Theoretically this could result in higher concentrations of free drug and a correspondingly greater pharmacologic response in the immature infant.

MOLECULAR WEIGHT.   Most therapeutic agents have molecular weights ranging from 250 to 500 daltons and cross the placenta quite readily, depending on their state of ionization and lipid solubility. Compounds with molecular weights between 500 and 1,000 daltons are generally considered to have slower transfer rates than those with lower molecular weights, although this has not been adequately studied. It has recently been demonstrated that digoxin (molecular weight 792 daltons) readily crosses the rodent placenta and human placenta but not the ovine placenta. While passage across the placenta of chemical compounds with molecular weights exceeding 1,000 daltons is severely impeded, certain proteins whose molecular weights are greater than 1,000 daltons can cross the placenta into the fetal circulation.

Characteristics of the Maternal-Placental-Fetal Unit

PLACENTAL BLOOD FLOW.   The movement of xenobiotics across the placenta is modified by hemodynamic changes in either the maternal or fetal placental blood flow. The extent to which highly lipid soluble drugs cross from the mother to the fetus appears to be directly proportional to maternal placental blood flow.

Alterations in placental blood flow may be caused by uterine contractions induced by spontaneous labor, removal of amniotic fluid, or administration of oxytocic drugs. Maternal uteroplacental perfusion can be reduced from 85 percent of total uterine flow to 75 percent by constriction of myometrial arterioles or by obstruction of the uterine venous outflow during contraction. Changes in fetal hemodynamics may also affect drug transfer to and from the fetus. The transplacental passage of local anesthetics from the mother to the fetus can significantly depress the fetal circulation, so that clearance of these compounds from the fetus is impaired.

The difference in pH of the maternal and fetal circulations may modify the maternal-fetal partitioning and the placental transfer of drugs, particularly any compound having a pKa similar to the pH of blood. The pH of umbilical vessel blood is normally 0.10 to 0.15 pH units lower than that of maternal systemic blood; consequently the concentration of un-ionized basic drug is higher in the maternal circulation than in the fetal circulation. The net effect of this pH difference is such that the overall transfer of drug from mother to fetus is enhanced, and fetal concentrations at equilibrium may exceed those of the mother.

PLACENTAL MATURATION.   The rate of drug diffusion across the placental membrane is proportional to the membrane cross-sectional area, the maternal-to-fetal concentration gradient, the physicochemical properties of the drug, and the thickness of the membrane. The thickness of the trophoblastic epithelium decreases in the last trimester, so that the thickness of the tissue layer or layers interposed between the fetal capillaries and maternal bloodstream decreases from 25 μ early in gestation to 2 μ at birth.

Most of the available information relating to drug transfer at different stages in gestation has come from studies in the pregnant rodent. These data suggest that drug transfer is slowest in midgestation and most rapid in the first and last trimesters. Similar studies with other types of placenta have not been performed, so that generalizations regarding the primate or human are not warranted at this time.

PLACENTAL METABOLISM OF DRUGS.   Several different types of aromatic oxidation reactions (eg, hydroxylation, N-dealkylation, and demethylation) have been shown to occur in placental tissue homogenates incubated in vitro with appropriate substrate. The drug-metabolizing activity of the placenta is significantly less than that of the maternal or fetal liver when compared on a unit weight basis. Consequently the physiologic significance of the placenta as a site for xenobiotic drug metabolism in the maternal-placental-fetal unit remains uncertain under in vivo conditions. However, the role of the placenta with respect to metabolic biotransformation of endogenous substrates such as the steroid hormones is of major biologic importance.

DISTRIBUTION OF DRUGS IN THE FETUS

Pharmacologically active molecules that have crossed the placenta are carried by the umbilical vein into the systemic fetal circulation. These compounds may undergo biotransformation in the fetal liver, they may bypass the fetal liver via the ductus venosus to enter specific fetal structures and/or body compartments, they may be excreted into the amniotic fluid by the fetal kidney and swallowed by the fetus to create an amniotic-enterohepatic recirculation, or they may be returned to the maternal circulation through the umbilical artery and placenta.

The fetal distribution of drugs is determined to a large extent by the relative permeability of the membranes surrounding specific organs and body compartments. Generally, the ease with which drugs diffuse across these delimiting structures is greater during fetal and neonatal existence than at later stages in maturation. While most drugs exhibit a rather widespread pattern of distribution in the fetus, unexpectedly high concentrations of drug may accumulate in tissues that are not normally considered to be primary target organs. This phenomenon has been observed with the anticonvulsant drug diphenylhydantoin. Following its administration to pregnant mice, the highest concentrations occur in maternal liver and maternal and fetal heart, with the brain (ostensibly the primary target organ) having the lowest concentration of any of the tissues studied. The blood-brain barrier is generally highly permeable to many drugs early in development, and it is somewhat surprising to find relatively low concentrations of diphenylhydantoin in fetal brain. The fetal brain possesses a low myelin and high water content, so that its affinity for lipophilic drugs is decreased, and this may counteract the increased membrane permeability present at this stage in ontogenesis.

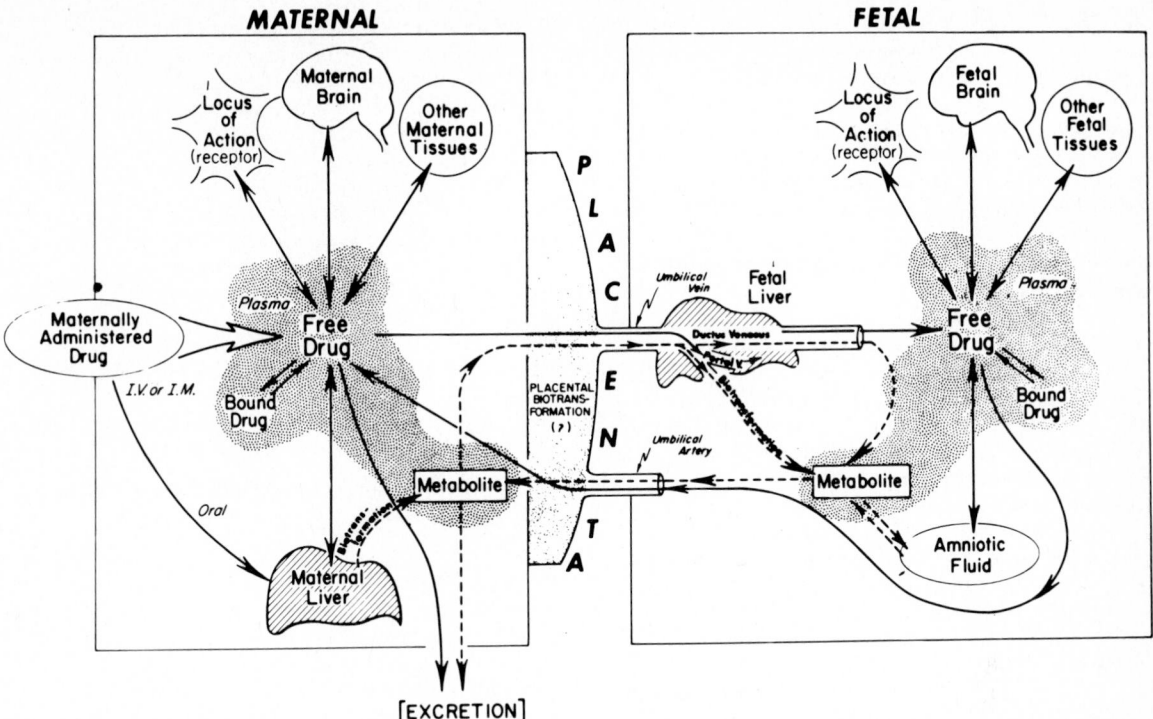

FIG. 1. Schematic representation of drug disposition in the maternal-placental-fetal unit. (Adapted from Mirkin: In Boreus (ed): Fetal Pharmacology, 1973. Courtesy of Raven Press.)

The overall distribution of drugs in fetal tissues is also considerably influenced by selective tissue uptake. Nonspecific lipid solubility appears to be a critical determinant in this regard, since many drugs are concentrated in organs with a high lipid content (eg, liver, ovary, and adrenal glands). Thus the unusually high levels of diphenylhydantoin that have been noted in the ovary, particularly the corpora lutea of this organ, may reflect the high affinity the drug has for lipids. Other types of highly specific binding sites have been identified, and it has been proposed that specialized cellular binding proteins may constitute another mechanism for selective drug distribution. An example of this can be found in the hepatic parenchymal cell, which contains a specific protein responsible for the binding of organic anions such as bilirubin. This protein appears to be absent or reduced at particular stages in development and in certain disease states, so that the binding of organic anions is impaired.

The fetal circulation and its distribution to specific organs have an extremely important role in determining the pattern of drug distribution in the fetus. The quantity of drug delivered to a given organ is directly proportional to the magnitude of its blood flow. All drugs reaching the fetal circulation via the umbilical vein enter the fetal liver, where blood flow may be diverted into the portal vein to perfuse the hepatic parenchyma or into the ductus venosus and thus bypassing the liver en route to the inferior vena cava. The extent

to which umbilical venous flow is shunted between these two circuits constitutes a major factor in determining the concentration of drug reaching the fetal right heart. These mechanisms are probably of greatest importance during the initial passage of a drug through the fetal circulation (eg, after a rapid maternal intravenous injection) and of lesser significance when steady-state conditions have been achieved.

Any increase in the quantity of blood flowing through the ductus venosus will decrease the proportion of drug carried to the fetal liver and probably diminish the amount of drug initially metabolized by this organ. The human fetal liver is able to oxidize numerous drug substrates with surprising effectiveness, in comparison to most subhuman species. While the true significance of hepatic drug metabolism in the fetus remains to be elucidated, it is highly probable that diversion of drug into the ductus venosus not only decreases the amount of drug metabolized per unit time but significantly elevates the concentration of pharmacologically active material presented to the fetal heart and central nervous system.

DISPOSITION OF DRUGS IN INFANTS AND CHILDREN

Fetal survival during transition from intrauterine to extrauterine environment is contingent on maturation of numerous physiologic processes required to establish self-sufficiency. Maternal systems for the elimination of drugs are no longer available, and the neonate must utilize its own, often poorly developed, physiologic and biochemical mechanisms. The well-known limitations of the neonate in this regard have led to the generalized and perhaps erroneous belief that most, if not all, therapeutic agents are more toxic to the newborn than to the adult.

Comparative toxicity of drugs in immature and adult mammals

The relative potencies of drugs administered during the newborn period can be readily established by comparing their respective toxicity ratios (adult LD_{50}/neonatal LD_{50}). The LD_{50} is calculated by administering increasing concentrations of drug to groups of animals and then determining the concentration that produces death in 50 percent of the treated animals. It should be recognized that such analyses are relatively nonspecific; they compare only acute toxicity and tend to demonstrate gross rather than subtle distinctions.

TABLE 1. Comparison of Acute Drug Toxicity in Newborn and Adult Rats[a]

Compound	Route of Administration	Toxicity Ratio (Adult LD_{50} /Neonate LD_{50})
Drugs of greater toxicity to the newborn		
Chloral hydrate	oral	1.8
Acetylsalicylic acid	oral	2.7
Desipramine	oral	2.5
Phenobarbital	oral	2.6
Chlorpromazine	IP[b]	4.2
Meprobamate	oral	4.3
Morphine	IP	6.4
Picrotoxin	IP	6.0
Dicumarol	oral	10.4
Drugs of equal or lesser toxicity to the newborn		
d-Amphetamine	oral	0.5
Strychnine	SC	0.4
Pentylenetetrazol	SC	0.6
Mercurial diuretics	SC	0.6
Isopropyl norepinephrine	oral	0.6
Codeine	SC	0.7
Menadione	IP	0.9
Meperidine	IP	1.0
Digitalis	IV	0.6–1.0

[a] *Adapted from Yeary: Applied Therap 9:918, 1967.*
[b] *SC = subcutaneous; IP = intraperitoneal; IV = intravenous.*

Central nervous system depressants such as chloral hydrate, phenobarbital, meprobamate, and chlorpromazine appear to be more toxic to the neonate than to the adult. Analgesics derived from the morphine al-

kaloids also follow this pattern, whereas the LD_{50} of meperidine is similar in both newborn and mature animals. In contrast, central nervous system stimulants such as strychnine, d-amphetamine, and pentylenetetrazol have a significantly lower LD_{50} in the neonatal rat than in the adult rat.

These toxicity data indicate that the neonatal animal is not categorically more sensitive to, or indeed more susceptible to, the toxic effects of a particular drug or group of drugs. In fact, the recommended dosage for some drugs such as digoxin and diphenylhydantoin is greater for children than adults in terms of body weight. It has become increasingly important, therefore, to identify those factors that modulate drug disposition in developing organisms so that more accurate predictions of pharmacologic reactivity can be achieved.

Determinants of Drug Disposition in Infants and Children

The processes that regulate drug disposition in man undergo significant changes during biologic maturation. These alterations in function may influence therapeutic strategies by modifying the manner in which specific physiologic processes affect drug disposition.

ABSORPTION. The movement of a drug from its site of administration into the systemic circulation is generally considered to constitute the process of absorption. It determines the quantity and rate at which drugs enter the bloodstream. Most drugs traverse biologic membranes exclusively by simple diffusion, and the transfer rates of such compounds are concentration-related. Specific physicochemical characteristics of the drug molecule and biologic properties of the organism exert a major regulatory influence on these kinetic events, as noted below.

PHYSICOCHEMICAL CHARACTERISTICS OF THE DRUG MOLECULE (pKA, LIPID SOLUBILITY). Compounds possessing a high lipid solubility or a pKa that allows a large percentage of the molecule to exist in the un-ionized state at the site of absorption will be readily absorbed. Thus an acidic or basic drug with a low pKa (eg, acetylsalicylic acid, pKa 3.5; caffeine, pKa 0.8) rapidly crosses the gastric mucosa to enter the systemic circulation of the stomach. Such drugs are more slowly, but not necessarily less completely, absorbed from the relatively alkaline milieu of the small intestine.

CHARACTERISTICS OF MEMBRANES TO BE CROSSED. Most membranes are lipoprotein in composition, so that compounds with high degrees of lipid solubility tend to pass through more readily. This appears to be of importance not only for absorption from the gastrointestinal tract but also for absorption from the renal tubule, the skin, and the lungs.

BLOOD FLOW AT SITE OF ADMINISTRATION. The rate of removal of a drug from an intramuscular or subcutaneous locus is largely limited by blood flow. Most molecules cross the capillary membranes by either diffusion or filtration; diffusion is the dominant mode of transfer for lipid-soluble drugs, whereas non-lipid-soluble compounds are primarily filtered across the capillary wall. Most drugs, regardless of their lipid solubility, traverse capillary walls at rates that far exceed the rates observed with other membranes. Consequently the uptake of drug from a parenteral site of administration is more likely blood-flow-limited than diffusion-regulated. Cardiovascular shock, local vasoconstriction (eg, following sympathomimetic agents), or impaired regional perfusion (eg, as occurs in diabetes or intrapulmonary shunting) are clinical situations in which drug uptake or absorption from a particular site may be diminished as a consequence of restricted blood flow.

Significant biochemical and physiologic changes occur in the human neonatal gastrointestinal tract shortly after parturition. There is a marked increase in gastric acidity, a prolongation of gastrointestinal transit time, and an increase in membrane permeability to specific substrates. Each modification in function exerts a marked effect upon the rate and magnitude of drug absorption, which ultimately influences the duration and intensity of drug action.

Compounds that are partially or totally inactivated by the low pH* of the gastric contents (eg, penicillin G, insulin) must not be administered via the oral route if a satisfactory therapeutic response is to be achieved. Any change in gastrointestinal transit time also exerts an important effect on the extent of drug absorption. Shortening of the gastric emptying time tends to substantially increase overall absorption, as it leads to a more rapid entry of drug into the lower gastrointestinal tract with its greater absorptive surface area. A compound with a low pKa (eg, salicylate), which would be expected to be better absorbed from the acidic environment of the stomach, also exhibits enhanced uptake if the gastric emptying time is decreased. An increase in lower gastrointestinal tract motility, such as may occur in diarrheal conditions, should tend to decrease overall absorption, since contact time with this large absorptive area is diminished. However, studies of antibiotic and digoxin absorption under such conditions have demonstrated excellent absorption. While the bioavailability of many pharmacologically active molecules may be substantially modified by developmental changes affecting gastrointestinal motility and physiology, each therapeutic agent must be considered individually.

The newborn is able to absorb a wide variety of chemical substances better than or as well as the adult. Some differences in absorption have been noted between premature and full-term infants following the administration of suspensions containing equivalent (per weight) doses of sulfonamide. The premature infant develops lower peak blood levels and appears to absorb the sulfonamide less efficiently than the full-term infant. Riboflavin is also absorbed to a much greater extent in older infants than in less mature newborns. This difference has been attributed to a deficiency in the active transport system required for movement of riboflavin across the intestinal membranes of the neonate.

Gastric pH ranges from 1 to 2.5 during the neonatal period.

Many varieties of antibiotic agents have been studied in sick infants and their respective absorption patterns characterized. Penicillin (procaine or phenoxypenicillin) is well absorbed from the gastrointestinal tract of the premature and the full-term neonate, and slightly higher blood concentrations have been reported to occur in the premature infant after administration of equivalent doses. Serum levels of nafcillin and ampicillin are much greater in the human neonate than in adults receiving comparable (per weight) doses. The percentage of ampicillin absorbed in the newborn also seems to be considerably greater, with about 66 percent of the dose absorbed as compared to 30 percent in the adult.

The penicillins, tetracyclines, cephalosporins, and their semisynthetic derivatives, as well as chloramphenicol, appear to be rapidly and efficiently absorbed in young infants. Therapeutically effective serum concentrations that persist for prolonged periods of time can be readily achieved by this route of administration. This pharmacokinetic pattern is attributable to the increased rate of absorption as well as to the decreased capacity for renal elimination and hepatic degradation present in the neonate.

Other classes of therapeutic agents, such as cardiac glycosides, are also satisfactorily absorbed in the newborn, and recent studies suggest an uptake pattern in infants resembling that of the adult. Peak serum levels of digoxin occur 1 hour after an oral dose, with excellent absorption observed even in the presence of severe congestive heart failure and diarrhea. In addition to data for the antimicrobial drugs, comprehensive data describing absorptive patterns in the newborn have been obtained for the following compounds: anticonvulsants (phenobarbital, diphenylhydantoin, diazepam), acetylsalicylic acid, aminophylline, and cardiovascular agents (propranolol). These examples differ significantly with respect to the kinds of drug molecules involved, and they clearly illustrate that the ability to absorb different types of substrates from the gastrointestinal lumen is well developed very early in neonatal life.

Drug absorption from other sites of administration must also be considered, particularly since they are frequently used in the treatment of sick infants and children. The mottling of skin commonly observed in the neonate is reflective of vasomotor instability and has prompted concern that the newborn infant may resemble the diabetic patient in manifesting a delayed uptake or absorption of drugs administered intramuscularly. Experiments utilizing neonatal and adult animals have shown the rates of disappearance of morphine from intramuscular sites of administration to be the same in both age groups. Comparable assessments in man have not been made, but certainly the clinical effectiveness of intramuscular injections in young infants and children has been extensively documented.

DISTRIBUTION. This process regulates the concentration of drug achieved in a specific body compartment or tissue and thereby influences the quantity of drug reaching a desired site of action. The distribution pattern of a pharmacologic agent is determined by many factors, among which tissue mass, blood flow, lipid content, and specific membrane permeability appear to be most important. Chemical compounds generally penetrate muscle, bone, and visceral structures more slowly than they permeate highly perfused organs such as the liver, kidney, and brain. Despite the limitations described, the relative masses of muscular and visceral structures are so great that any significant degree of uptake by these tissues can greatly modify the overall distribution of drugs in the body.

The composition of the tissues into which drugs distribute is very important in determining the volume of distribution of a drug. The human neonate has a much higher percentage of its body mass in the form of water than does the adult. Differences can also be observed between the full-term infant (70 percent of body weight as water) and the small premature infant (85 percent of body weight as water). Furthermore, the premature infant has much less total fat content; thus organs that generally accumulate high concentrations of lipophilic drugs in adults and older children may exhibit a lesser affinity for such compounds in less mature subjects.

While membrane permeability is frequently considered to be increased in immature mammals, comparative pharmacologic studies have revealed very significant differences between species. Consequently considerable attention should be given to the animal model utilized in a given study. The rat, rabbit, and chicken exhibit high degrees of permeability to drugs in terms of movement from the bloodstream into the central nervous system, whereas the guinea pig is much more resistant to such transfer at birth. Autoradiographic studies have demonstrated that a drug such as phenobarbital enters the white matter of the kitten's brain much more readily than in the adult cat. This has been attributed to the completion of myelinization during the later stages of ontogenesis, which causes a decrease in the ease of drug transfer across the blood-brain barrier.

Young rats (16 days postnatal) have a lower LD_{50} and are more sensitive to morphine than older rats (32 days postnatal). Brain concentrations of morphine determined at equivalent time intervals after injection are two to four times greater in the 16-day-old than in the 32-day-old animal. In sharp contrast, the LD_{50} of meperidine or heroin does not change with increasing age. This distinction may be due to the low lipid solubility of the latter compounds and their relatively poor affinity for the central nervous system, at least when compared with morphine. Morphine is at least 10 times more potent than equianalgesic doses of meperidine in depressing the respiratory response (minute volume) of infants to elevations in end-tidal P_{CO_2}.

It should be emphasized that the increased toxicity of certain analgesic agents in the young mammal may not be exclusively related to their accumulation in the brain. The concentrations of both morphine and meperidine in the neonatal rat brain are about two or three times

those observed in the adult; however, the neonatal LD_{50} for meperidine is similar to that of the adult. Therefore the greater toxicity of morphine in the less mature mammal may also reflect an enhanced sensitivity of specific receptors in the brain to this compound.

Another major factor influencing distribution is the extent to which the drug is protein-bound. The binding of drugs to plasma proteins in the fetus and neonate is less, strictly on a molar basis, than that observed in the adult. Consequently a greater percentage of the drug is potentially present in its unbound or free form and is available for diffusion in the immature individual. Albumin is the plasma protein with the greatest binding capacity, and interactions with both basic and acid compounds have been demonstrated. The general equilibrium equation for drug–protein interactions clearly illustrates that drugs with high affinity constants for the plasma proteins (ie, K_1 considerably greater than K_2) tend to have low volumes of distribution due to retention within the plasma compartment, whereas the volume of distribution will be greater if the affinity constant is low (Fig. 2).

PROTEIN BINDING OF DRUGS

$$[P] + [D] \underset{k_2}{\overset{k_1}{\rightleftarrows}} [PD]$$

$[P]$ = free protein concentration

$[D]$ = free drug concentration

$[PD]$ = drug–protein complex concentration

At equilibrium:

$$k_1 [P][D] = k_2 [PD]$$

$$\frac{[PD]}{[P][D]} = \frac{k_1}{k_2} = K = \text{association or affinity constant}$$

FIG. 2. Drug–protein interaction expressed in terms of mass-action law.

METABOLISM.   Drugs may act as substrates for a wide variety of mammalian enzyme systems, and the metabolism or biotransformation of pharmacologically active agents constitutes a major mechanism for the termination of drug action. Since most drugs exist mainly in a nonpolar state at physiologic pH, they are able to penetrate membranes that delimit body compartments, and they also tend to undergo reabsorption by the renal tubules. The biochemical reactions that xenobiotic compounds undergo convert them to more polar compounds, thereby decreasing lipid solubility and increasing water solubility so that clearance from the organism is enhanced.

The process of biotransformation occurs primarily in the liver and more specifically involves the drug-metabolizing system of the hepatic endoplasmic reticulum. Microsomal fractions isolated from liver homogenates contain most of the drug-metabolizing activity of this organ. The microsomal enzyme systems are able to catalyze an extraordinary number of metabolic reactions, which are mainly oxidative in nature but also include reductive and conjugating reactions. A drug commonly undergoes two or three such reactions before it is cleared from the body.

The versatility of the liver appears somewhat less remarkable if the drug-metabolizing reactions are visualized as simply representing different types of hydroxylation reactions. From this perspective the microsomal drug-metabolizing system can be considered to represent a mixed-function oxidase system in which the key components are NADP (nicotinamide-adenine dinucleotide phosphate), NADP-cytochrome C reductase (the flavin enzyme that oxidizes NADP), cytochrome P-450, and NADP-cytochrome P-450 reductase.

The ontogenesis of drug-metabolizing activity has been studied in many mammalian species utilizing both in vivo and in vitro techniques. As a rule, the capacity for drug metabolism in the early neonatal period is substantially less than that observed during later stages of postnatal development. The point in development at which enzymatic activity is maximal depends upon the specific enzymatic system under investigation. Certain reactions such as sulfuration achieve levels of activity during neonatal life that are much greater than those in the adult.

One of the earliest studies on the ontogenesis of mammalian drug metabolism used homogenates prepared from the livers of guinea pigs and rats at different ages. This investigation revealed that newborn guinea pigs had virtually no N-dealkylation, side-chain oxidation, or glucuronidation activity, nor did rats or rabbits. These observations are of great historical interest because parallel studies performed with specimens of human fetal and neonatal liver also confirmed the presence of low enzymatic activity and the absence of cytochrome P-450 in these tissues.

For over a decade it appeared that the human fetus and neonate, like the rodent, had an extremely impaired capacity for metabolizing drugs. Consequently data published between 1970 and 1972 demonstrating that extracts of human fetal liver contained quantities of cytochrome P-450 and NADP-cytochrome c reductase sufficient to catalyze drug-metabolizing reactions were extremely surprising. This was particularly so in view of the many investigations indicating that cytochrome P-450 and cytochrome-P-450-dependent reactions were not detectable.

Subsequent analyses explained how the discrepancy between the later investigations and earlier efforts had arisen. In essence, it was shown that the sedimentation characteristics of fetal liver homogenates differed markedly from those of adult livers. The fetal liver was more resistant to homogenization than the adult liver, and the highest fetal enzyme activity was obtained in the low-speed-contrifugation fractions, whereas in the adult the maximum activity was observed in the high-speed fraction. When the appropriate fractions were studied the enzyme levels in fetal and adult liver were found to be quite comparable when expressed either as activity or as amount per gram of liver tissue. In the fetus 8.6 + 1.7 nanomoles of cytochrome P-450 were present, as compared to 10.0 nanomoles in the adult. The activity of NADP-cytochrome C reductase was 1620 + 320 in the fetus and 2000 in the adult (expressed as nanomoles of cytochrome C reduced per minute). These similarities are even more striking when one considers that the human fetal liver constiues about 4 percent of total body weight, compared to 2 percent in the adult. Thus it is apparent that biologically immature humans can carry out drug-metabolizing reactions with a surprising degree of efficiency.

Another major aspect of drug metabolism in mammalian organisms is its relationship to the phenomenon of enzyme induction. In the present context enzyme induction will refer to any increase in drug-metabolizing activity that can be attributed to the prior administration of a specific drug molecule. It is not certain whether this is due to an enhancement of preexisting enzyme activity or to de novo synthesis of new enzyme provoked by administration of the xenobiotic agent.

The induction of hepatic microsomal systems has been extensively investigated, and as early as 1960 a significant increase in glucuronyl transferase activity was observed in the livers of newborn rats and guinea pigs given injections of benzpyrene. When the same experiment was performed with fetal livers obtained from pregnant rats receiving benzpyrene, no induction of enzyme activity was noted. Studies carried out in pregnant rabbits who were given phenobarbital also demonstrated the absence of enzyme induction in homogenates of fetal livers obtained more than 4 or 5 days prior to parturition. This species was similar to the rat in that induction was achieved only when the inducing agent was administered during the last few days of gestation, but not earlier.

The effects of drugs with known inducing action have been studied in pregnant women and children. It is quite clear that the elimination of bilirubin is facilitated and serum bilirubin levels are decreased in neonatal infants delivered from mothers receiving phenobarbital intrapartum. This has generally been assumed to reflect an increase in neonatal glucuronyl transferase activity. However, it is not certain whether the enzyme-inducing action of phenobarbital also enhances hepatic transport and clearance mechanisms of bilirubin, rather than only conjugation of this particular substrate. Enzyme-inducing agents have been used successfully to treat non-hemolytic hyperbilirubinemia as well as hyperbilirubinemia and hyperbiliacidemia associated with intrahepatic biliary atresia in older children.

EXCRETION. Several different routes of drug elimination exist in the body, such as the skin, the respiratory tract, and the biliary system, although the dominant mechanism is that of renal excretion. It should be noted that both nonmetabolized and metabolized drugs are removed from the body primarily via the kidney. Therefore renal insufficiency, whether it results from pathophysiologic causes or biologic immaturity, may produce a significant alteration in the rate of removal of a given drug from the body. Prolongation of drug action by extending its serum or tissue half-life may increase its overall toxicity. As a consequence it is often necessary to use lower maintenance doses in the presence of renal insufficiency in order to obtain a satisfactory therapeutic response.

Glomerular filtration in the human neonate is approximately 30 to 40 percent and tubular secretion 20 to 30 percent of that of the adult, when calculated on the basis of 1.73 m^2 of surface area. A substantial increase in function occurs during the initial five postpartum days in the human infant. On day five glomerular filtration rate and renal plasma flow have increased 50 percent from the initial postpartum period. On the seventh postpartum day glomerular filtration is approximately 50 percent of the adult value, and by 12 months it is equal to that of the adult.

The clearance rate of compounds that are primarily dependent upon the kidney for elimination tends to be significantly lower in the neonate. Penicillins, for example, are cleared from premature infants at a rate that is 17 percent of that of the adult, when compared on the basis of surface area, and 34 percent when adjusted to body weight. A decreased rate of renal elimination has also been observed with other semisynthetic penicillin derivatives (eg, ampicillin, methicillin, cephaloridine, and oxacillin) and aminoglycoside antibiotics (eg, kanamycin, neomycin, and streptomycin) in the neonate. Total body clearance of digoxin is directly dependent upon adequate renal function, and accumulation can occur in circumstances where glomerular filtration is decreased. Despite this, it is worth recalling that the dose of digoxin required for an adequate therapeutic response in the newborn is twice the dose that is administered to the adult on a per weight basis.

PHARMACOKINETICS AND DRUG DOSAGE IN PEDIATRICS

The time course of drug action, as well as the persistence of drug in the body, is determined by those factors that regulate drug disposition. Biologic responses to pharmacologic agents are generally considered as being elicited by the interaction of a receptor with an agonist (drug). Since the concentration of agonist tends to vary as a function of time, the intensity of effect produced is also altered proportionately. While the intensity and duration of effect may be enhanced by increasing the dosage and ultimately the concentration of drug (agonist) reaching the receptor site, this may also lead to the development of unanticipated adverse drug effects. Conversely, dosages that are too low may produce drug concentrations below the level of therapeutic

efficacy. Since a primary objective of clinical pharmacology is to optimize the risk–benefit relationship for the patient, it is crucial that dosage regimens, particularly in young children, be based upon rational guidelines.

It has long been recognized that the dosage of drug required to produce a therapeutic response in a child varies according to age and size, and numerous formulas for calculating drug dosage have been developed over the years in an effort to resolve this problem. Clinical rules based on age, weight, body surface area, and the relationships between an infant's age and weight and adult age and weight have been used, but none of these quasi-scientific mathematical expressions has proved satisfactory. Aside from their inability to adequately predict the appropriate dose for a given child, these formulations all possess a seminal flaw in that no consideration has been given to the importance of the dosing interval. In recent years the discipline of pharmacokinetics has attempted to define the time limits of pharmacologic action by analyzing the kinetics of drug disposition. Some of the basic concepts that may assist in the application of pharmacokinetic principles to the development of appropriate dosage regimens for children follow.

Volume of Distribution (V_D)

The parameter V_D is essentially a mathematical expression that represents the volume into which a drug appears to be distributed after administration of an intravenous dose: V_D = quantity of drug administered divided by plasma concentration of drug at zero time. The zero-time concentration is obtained by extrapolating a semilogarithmic plot of plasma concentration of drug versus time back to zero time (Fig. 3).

The volume of distribution for a given drug may suggest that it is distributed exclusively in body water, total blood volume, or plasma volume, but in point of fact this parameter may not have any physiologic significance. There are situations where the volume of distribution for a given drug is found to be measured in terms of thousands of liters, which indicates that the compound has distributed into some extravascular compartment and that very little of it can be found in the plasma compartment (which is 4 liters in the adult and less in the infant). The volume of distribution does not identify which tissue a drug has entered, and this can only be ascertained by analyzing specific tissues for the compound.

Subjects with nephrotic syndrome and low plasma albumin levels have been shown to have an increased volume of distribution, so that they tend to eliminate highly protein bound drugs more rapidly. The decreased protein binding also allows a greater percentage of drug to exist in the free form, so that the pharmacologic response to a given dose may be exaggerated under such conditions. Changes in distribution have been suggested as the basis for the difference in digoxin requirement observed in patients with thyroid disease. Hypothyroid subjects have consistently higher

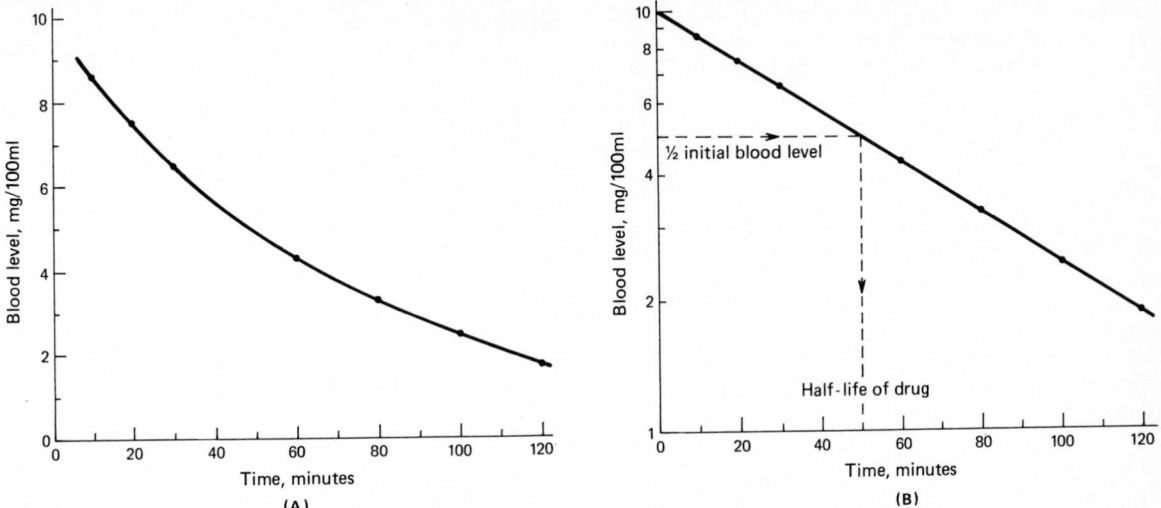

Drug X is injected intravenously into a subject and blood samples are taken at specific time intervals. Each sample is analyzed for its drug concentration, and the data obtained are as follows:

Time (in minutes) After IV Administration	Blood Level mg/100 ml
10	8.6
20	7.5
30	6.5
60	4.2
80	3.2
100	2.4
120	1.8

FIG. 3. Calculation of half-life. Tabulated data have been plotted on linear coordinates (A), producing an exponential function, and on semilogarithmic coordinates (B), producing a linear function. (Adapted from Cadwallader: Biopharmaceutics and Drug Interactions, Roche Scientific Monograph, 1971.)

and hyperthyroid subjects have consistently lower plasma digoxin concentrations than euthyroid individuals.

The volume of distribution is an important parameter primarily because it enables one to calculate the quantity of drug required to reach a specific blood level as well as the amount required to sustain that blood level over a given period of time.

Half-Life ($T_{1/2}$) and Elimination Constant (K_{el})

The biologic half-life of a drug is generally considered to be the time required for the drug concentration to reach one-half of the initial concentration observed at zero time (assuming that the drug has been completely absorbed at the time of observation). Viewed from another perspective it can also be defined as the time required for the body to eliminate 50 percent of the amount absorbed, whether by metabolic degradation or excretion, following establishment of equilibrium. It is important to emphasize that the biologic half-life of a drug is an integral characteristic of the drug itself and does not appear to be dependent on the route of administration. For most drugs the disappearance rate is proportional to the concentration of the drug at the time of determination, since the half-life is a first-order process under ideal clinical conditions. Once the biologic half-life has been estimated, the total drug requirements for a given time period can be determined and the dosage regimen adjusted to provide the optimum level required for treatment of the subject.

Mathematically the relationship between half-life and elimination constant is illustrated by the following equation: $T_{1/2} = 0.693/k_{el}$. This equation can be solved if only one of the unknowns has been estimated. In practical terms a half-life for a given drug is generally obtained by administering a dose of drug to the subject and then determining blood levels at different time intervals. A typical example is illustrated in Figure 3.

Following administration of a given drug dose to a patient, it requires four to five half-lives for that compound to achieve a steady state or a therapeutically effective drug level. Consequently, in clinical practice it is customary to use a loading oral dose or bolus injection of drug in conjunction with maintenance doses in order to decrease the time interval required for reaching optimum blood levels. Obviously compounds with very long half-lives (those greater than 24 hours) would require 4 to 5 days before approaching this level if only maintenance doses were used, and this is often clinically unacceptable.

The biologic half-life of a drug is markedly affected by postnatal age and a variety of pathophysiologic states. Compounds that are eliminated exclusively by the kidney, such as the penicillin and aminoglycoside antibiotics, have much longer half-lives in individuals with renal insufficiency. Drugs requiring hepatic biotransformation for termination of their action will also manifest a prolonged half-life wherever hepatic insufficiency due to maturational or pathologic causes occurs. Consequently, modifications must be made in the maintenance dose and the interval of administration for such compounds.

References

Ackerman E, Rane A, Ericsson J: The liver microsomal system in the human fetus—distribution in different centrifugal fractions. Clin Pharm Ther 13:652, 1972

Boreus L (ed?): Fetal Pharmacology. New York, Raven, 1973

Cadwallader DE: Biopharmaceutics and Drug Interactions. Roche Scientific Monograph, 1971

Heymann MA: Interrelations of fetal circulation and the placental transfer of drugs. Fed Proc 37:48, 1972

Jondorf W, Maikel R, Brodie B: Inability of newborn mice and guinea pigs to metabolize drugs. Biochem Pharm 1:352, 1958

Mirkin BL: Drug therapy and the developing human: who cares? Clin Res 23:106, 1975

Mirkin BL (ed): Perinatal Pharmacology. New York, Academic, 1976

Rane A, Sjoqvist F, Orrenius S: Drugs and fetal metabolism. Clin Pharmacol Ther 14:666, 1973

Yaffe S, Juchau M: Perinatal pharmacology. Ann Rev Pharmacol 14:219, 1974

Yeary RA: Drug toxicity in newborn animals. Applied Therap 9:918, 1967

CHAPTER 17

The Skin

Joseph McGuire, *Associate Editor*

INTRODUCTION

Man, with relatively sparse hair, exhibits a considerable expanse of skin. Because of its unique location as a limiting membrane, positioned between the individual and his environment, the skin is one of the best-described organs of the body.

In dermatology most diagnoses can be made from the morphology, configuration, and distribution of lesions. *Morphology* refers to the description of an individual lesion and is expressed by the following words: elevated, flat, pigmented, atrophic. *Configuration* refers to the patterning of the lesions; for example, annular, confluent, arcuate, linear. *Distribution* refers, of course, to the area of the body involved by the eruption.

These three types of descriptive analysis permit accurate pattern recognition of many skin diseases strictly from the clinical examination. In addition to careful inspection, histologic examination is often useful. A convenient aid to dermatologic diagnosis is the punch biopsy, which, when performed with local anesthesia, is no more effort for the physician or uncomfortable for the patient than a venipuncture. The biopsy tool, which resembles a cork borer, is the only special instrument required. The site can be closed with an adhesive dressing without suturing. A core of skin, 5 mm in diameter, is sufficient for adequate study of tissue by the pathologist.

The skin is a bilaminar organ (Fig. 1). The outer layer, the epidermis, is a relatively impermeable membrane, the chief function of which is to retard the exchange of liquids from either side. The effectiveness of this membrane is vividly demonstrated by the profuse fluid loss that follows damage to the epidermis by superficial thermal injury, pemphigus, or poison ivy dermatitis.

The epidermis consists of three functionally distinct compartments that correspond roughly to anatomic counterparts.

1. Stem cell population—these cells, which have the capacity to divide, correspond to the basal layer of the epidermis, which rests on a collagenous basal lamina. The entire dividing population includes some suprabasilar cells. In normal epidermis approximately 25 percent of the mitoses occur in suprabasilar cells.
2. Differentiating population—the Malpighian or prickle cells are a major component of the viable epidermis. These cells move outward into the stratum corneum. They are attached to each other by desmosomes. Movement from the basal layer to the stratum corneum requires about 2 weeks.
3. Fully (terminally) differentiated cells—the stratum cor-

neum is the outermost dead layer of the epidermis. These cells are thin squames, much larger in area than the viable cells of the epidermis. They are attached to each other by desmosomes, and the intercellular spaces also contain a lipid that arises intracellularly in membrane-coating granules. A transitional granular layer of cells, which contain granules of keratohyalin, usually is present beneath the stratum corneum. The granular layer and the stratum corneum form the impermeable barrier of the epidermis.

Supporting the epidermis is the dermis, which accounts for the main bulk of the skin. It is a relatively acellular fibrous tissue containing collagen and elastin

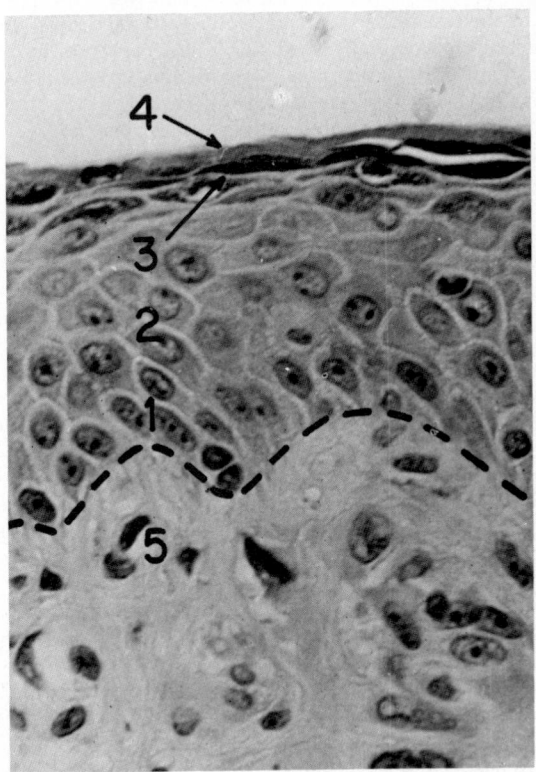

FIG. 1. Section of child's skin (×600). 1. Basal layer—location of cycling cells, the "stem cell" population of the epidermis. 2. Malpighian layer—differentiating epidermal cells. 3. Grandular layer—transitional zone between differentiating cells and stratum corneum. 4. Stratum corneum—compact layer composed of tightly adherent, dead, fully differentiated cells consisting predominantly of keratin and smaller amounts of cholesterol and phospholipid. 5. Dermis. The dermis is more cellular than normal because of the presence of a juvenile melanoma (benign).

fibers. In this chapter, diseases will be classified somewhat artificially into those affecting primarily the epidermis (keratinization), those affecting the dermis, blistering diseases, infectious disorders of pigmentation, and a miscellaneous group. These same descriptive terms will reappear in each section:

Macules—flat lesions
Papules—raised lesions
Vesicles—blisters less than 5 mm in diameter
Bullae—blisters greater than 5 mm in diameter

No attempt has been made to provide a complete catalog of skin diseases, and the reader is encouraged to consult references for more detailed and complete information.

DISEASES OF KERATINIZATION
ROBERT G. CROUNSE

Keratinization is the term applied to the differentiation of ectodermal tissues (hair, epidermis, and nails) into the final hardened end product. In each case, this product is eventually shed to the environment, either gradually, as is the case with human epidermis, or abruptly, as is the case with snake skin. It would be more appropriate to speak of disorders of the process of keratinization, the results of which will be, respectively, fragile (or absent) hair, scaling epidermis, and deformed nails. In these disorders other ectodermal systems may be affected, including the teeth and sweat glands. The observation of ectodermal disease in early life should also prompt a search for other systemic disorders, including aminoaciduria, deafness, immunologic defects, malnutrition, toxins, and others.

Epidermal keratinization. The paper-thin, cellular, outermost tissue of the skin, interposes a highly efficient barrier between man and his environment. Loss of sufficient amounts of this barrier, as in extensive burns, pemphigus, or toxic epidermal necrolysis, can be fatal. This layer is subject to continuous loss to the environment, and continuous regeneration from below. Imbalance in the rate of renewal, especially overproduction, results in a group of scaling or exfoliative disorders. The congenital forms are often termed *icthyosis;* the acquired forms include exfoliative dermatitis, psoriasis, and seborrheic dermatitis.

Although the precise role of lipids in orderly epidermal keratinization is not understood, their importance is emphasized by the examples of disordered keratinization associated with lipid imbalance, demonstrated by essential fatty acid deficiency in animals, in children, in Refsun's disease, and in Triparanol-induced icthyosis and hair loss.

Keratinization in the hair follicle is somewhat better defined biochemically. The fibrous, low-sulfur protein keratin is responsible for the highly ordered helical x-ray diffraction pattern of the hair shaft, and is, in turn, embedded in and stabilized by a group of amorphous, cementing proteins extensively cross-linked by disulfide bonds. It is the purposeful rupture and reformation of these disulfide bonds that result in the process known as permanent waving. Alterations in the synthesis of this group of high-sulfur proteins is apparently defective in certain cases of kwashiorkor (p. 214) and in trichoschisis, a congenital abnormality of the hair (p. 858).

Interpretation of hair follicle disorders requires an appreciation of two extraordinary features of the hair follicle. These are: (a) high rates of mitosis, metabolic activity, and protein synthesis, rendering the hair root extremely sensitive to mitotic or metabolic inhibitors, such as thallium or agents used in cancer chemotherapy; (b) the phenomenon of an inevitable and occasionally dramatic hair cycle or alternation of actively growing and totally resetting phases of hair growth. Approximately 90 percent of the hairs in the normal scalp are growing. Major changes in the normal growing/resting ratio, such as occur after birth, after pregnancy, and sometimes after high fever, result in unusual shedding of large number of resting hairs, so-called *telogen alopecia.*

Keratinization of the nail is poorly understood biochemically; kinetic events are similar to those of ectodermal tissues and subject to interruption by systemic events. Serious illness results in transverse lines, and local trauma to the proliferative matrix of the nail base causes nail dystrophy. The slow rate of growth of nails as compared to hair makes them less useful as a temporal guide to systemic events.

EPIDERMAL SCALING DISORDERS

The Ichthyoses

The precise classification of these congenital disorders of epidermal differentiation continues to be a vexing problem. Attempts to distinguish between forms of differences in epidermal cellular kinetics or inheritance patterns have been very helpful. For the moment, most cases of ichthyosiform dermatitis appearing during the first year of life can be classified as one of the following four types:

ICHTHYOSIS VULGARIS. Dryness and scaling on extensor surfaces characterize this genetically dominant form of ichthyosis (Fig. 2). Flexural sparing, onset after three months of age, and an atopic diathesis are supporting features. Histologically, the granular layer is reduced or absent. The horny layer is thickened (hyperkeratosis). Epidermal renewal rate is not accelerated, in contrast to other ichthyosiform dermatoses. Treatment is topical and symptomatic. The principle of restoration of relative flexibility to the thickened, dry stratum corneum is based upon the concept of hydration followed by the application of oil or grease to maintain hydration. The addition of an ounce or two of bath oil to the tub in theory leaves a protective coat on the hydrated skin during emergence. In practice a comparative trial of several ointments often provides the best individual compromise between cosmetic acceptability and therapeutic effect. The simple concept of hydration often results in dramatic improvement of a previously uninformed patient.

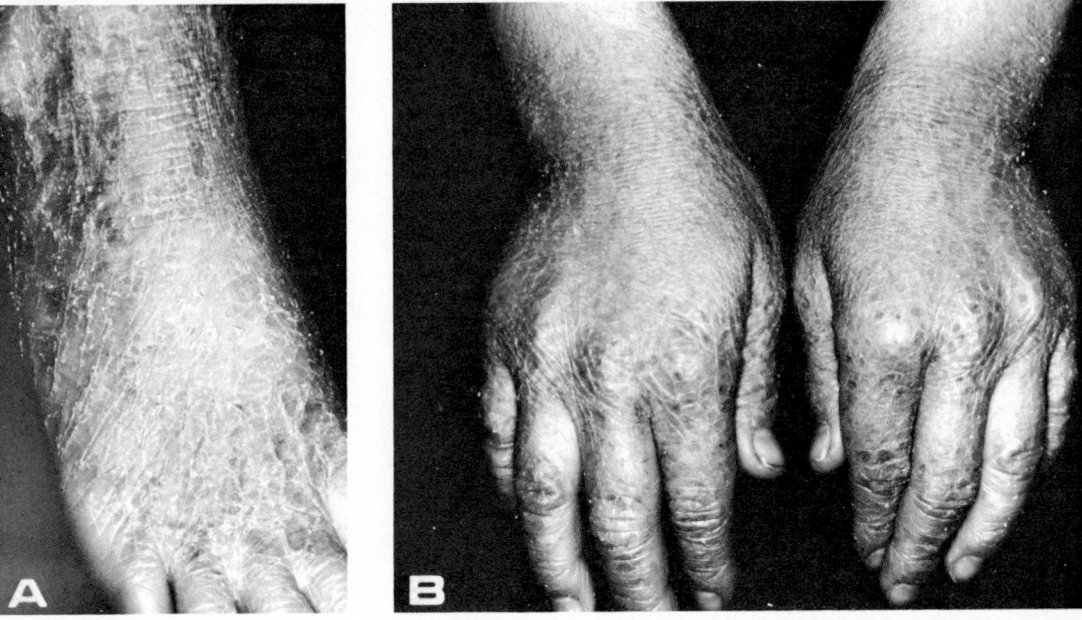

FIG. 2. Ichthyosis vulgaris in an 8-year-old girl. Ichthyosis vulgaris is a dominantly inherited disease characterized by retention of scale, especially in extensor areas. This disorder is often associated with atopy and is more troublesome when the humidity is low.

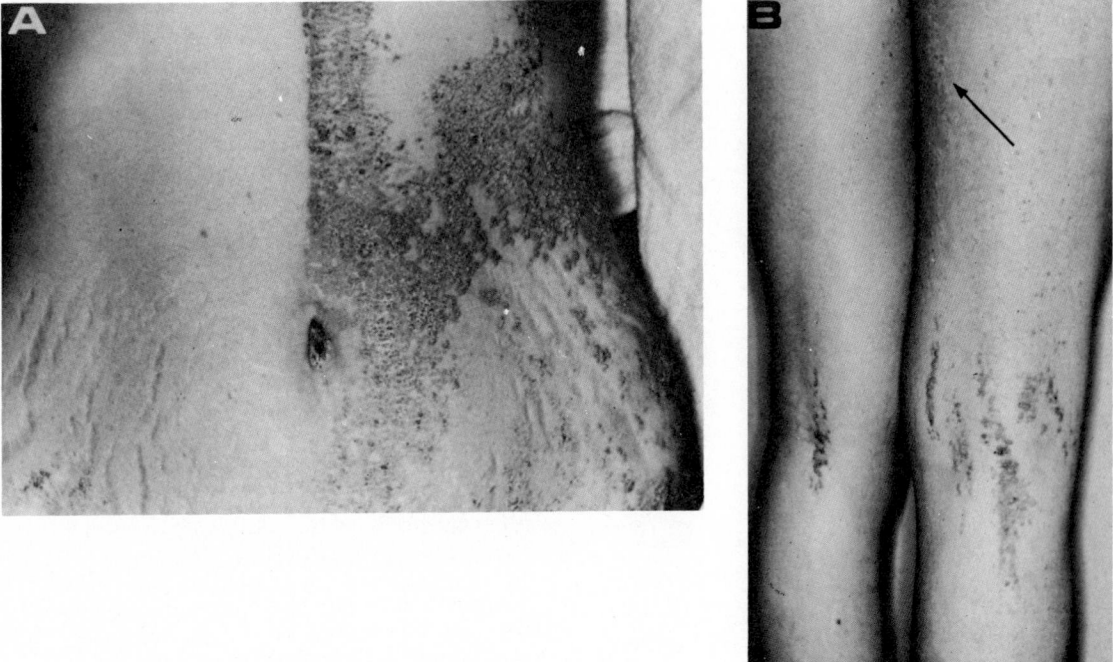

FIG. 5. Ichthyosis hystrix. **A.** Nevoid form of epidermolytic hyperkeratosis. Uncommon lesion in a young adult. Epidermal nevi may be linear or segmental and although they are usually present in early childhood, they may appear or become more extensive later in life. **B.** Bilateral distribution of epidermal nevus.

BULLOUS CONGENITAL ICHTHYOSIFORM ERYTHRODERMA (BULLOUS CIE).   This severe dominant disorder, also termed *epidermolytic hyperkeratosis,* by Frost and Van Scott, is characterized by blisters, background erythema, flexural involvement (Figs. 3 and 4, color plate 1), and rapid epidermal turnover. Lesions are frequently present at birth, but may abate spontaneously after puberty. Interestingly, some cases of severely localized forms of hyperkeratotic disorders previously termed icthyosis hysterix (Fig. 5), linear nevus, or palmar and plantar hyperkeratosis have been shown to exhibit histologic and cellular kinetic features of bullous CIE. Electron microscopic studies are consistent with faulty or incomplete keratinization but have not yielded etiologic clues. Secondary bacterial infection of bullae requires systemic antibiotics.

NONBULLOUS CONGENITAL ICHTHYOSIFORM ERYTHRODERMA (NONBULLOUS CIE). This disorder, also called lamellar ichthyosis (Fig. 6) is characterized by generalized scaling and redness; when it occurs with mental retardation and spastic paralysis, it is termed *Sjögren-Larsson* syndrome. Nonbullous CIE is a recessive disease ordinarily present at birth. In its most grave form it is apparently represented

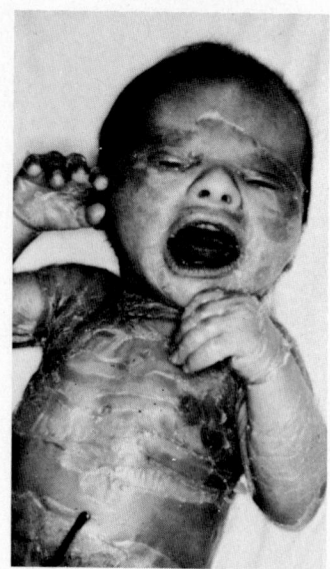

FIG. 7.   Collodion baby. This 4-day-old boy has the striking changes of lamellar exfoliation of the newborn: baked apple appearance with taut, split skin; ectropion, contraction bands around fingers and toes. The shiny tight membrane is shed within a few weeks and this child, now several years after the photograph, has normal-appearing skin with slight scaling on the neck. Other such infants have lamellar ichthyosis in later life.

by the bizarre *harlequin fetus.* Most infants with lamellar ichthyosis begin life as collodion babies with a cellophane-like covering present at birth (Fig. 7). Heavy scaling of scalp, palms, and soles is common in nonbullous CIE, as is ectropion; the latter may occur also secondary to other chronic scaling or bullous diseases. The histology is specific; there is increased thickness of the stratum corneum, granular layer, and overall epidermis; and some retention of nuclear remnants.

SEX-LINKED ICHTHYOSIS.   Careful clinical observation has separated this form of ichthyosis from those previously reported. Distinctive features include involvement of flexural areas and sides of the neck; occasionally delayed appearances (up to one year of age); and a classic, sex-linked pattern of inheritance with exclusive male involvement, sparing the palms and soles. Histologic sections may be helpful in confirming the diagnosis. Therapy is symptomatic and supportive; the diagnosis is benign but the course is prolonged.

Hyperkeratosis of the Palms and Soles (Keratoderma Palmaris et Plantaris)

Unusual thickening of the stratum corneum of the palms and soles without other skin abnormality can occur as diffuse scaling and fissuring or as discrete punctate lesions. Both forms may occur as an autosomal dominant trait, with expression during the first few years of life. Reports of successful treatment with topical vitamin A are encouraging. Systemic steroids may be

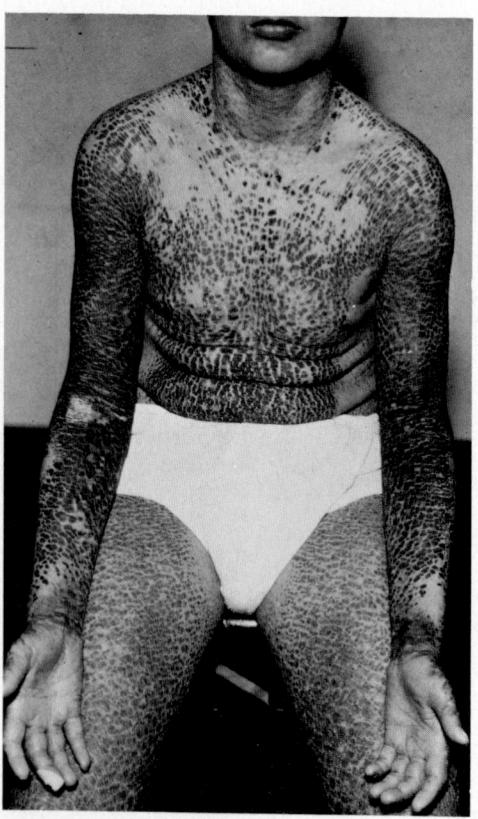

FIG. 6.   Lamellar ichthyosis. Angular, brownish scales involving most of the body, including flexural areas. The face is scaly, with ectropion formation. The clear areas on the flanks have been treated with retinoic acid.

effective but require prolonged administration with the attending hazards. Keratolytic ointments containing salicylic acid are still widely used.

The much quoted *mal de Meleda* refers to a recessive form of palmar and plantar hyperkeratosis traced to an inbred population on the Mediterranean island of Malta. Lesions on extensor surfaces and nail changes differentiate this syndrome clinically. Several other syndromes of combined defects, including palmar and plantar hyperkeratosis, occur, as described by Butterworth and Strean. Pathogenesis of these peculiar and localized disorders is not clear. Keratoderma following systemic administration of hypocholesterolemic agents reemphasizes the need to consider lipid involvement in the differentiation of tissues ordinarily associated primarily with protein synthesis.

Psoriasis

Psoriasis is a relatively common disease; its prevalence in the United States is probably about 2 percent. Onset is common before age ten and rare before age three, although it has been present at birth. The mode of inheritance of psoriasis is not clear; proposals range from simple dominant with incomplete penetrance to a system of three interdependent genetic loci, two recessive and one sex-linked. The possibility of genetic subpopulations within the diagnosis of psoriasis is quite real.

Typical lesions of psoriasis are red plaques surmounted by a silvery white scale, especially common about the elbows, knees, scalp, and penis (Fig. 8). In children an acute eruptive form, often poststreptococcal, has frequently been reported. Generalized and severe disease can occur. Major protein loss and negative nitrogen balance can result from the generalized exfoliation; enhanced transepidermal water loss and inadequate heat regulation can be significant.

The etiology of psoriasis is unknown; scaling is the result of markedly accelerated epidermal turnover. Histologic and electron microscopic changes reflect the apparently incomplete keratinization process.

Treatment of psoriasis is facilitated by some understanding of the pathophysiology of the process. The overproduction of keratinized stratum corneum and the necessity of regular scale removal can be understood by most without difficulty. When psoriasis is extensive it is often extremely valuable to parent, child, and physician to admit the child to the hospital for a combined treatment and education period. It is reassuring to the child to see that intensive topical therapy is effective when used properly. The separation of child and parent also helps identify the child's responsibility.

Topical therapy consists of application of coal tar products or anthralin on a regular daily basis. Topical steroids are also helpful in reducing scaling; however, the benefit of steroids is less sustained than that of tar. The systemic effects of steroids absorbed from the skin are negligible unless the site of application is large and

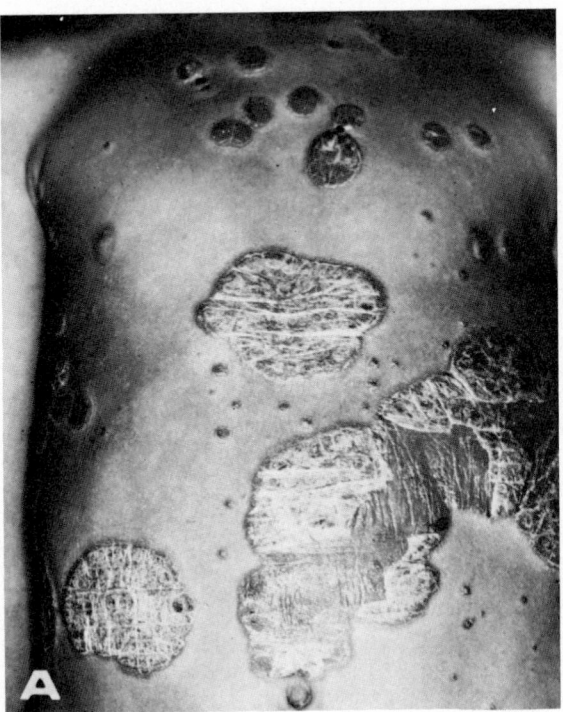 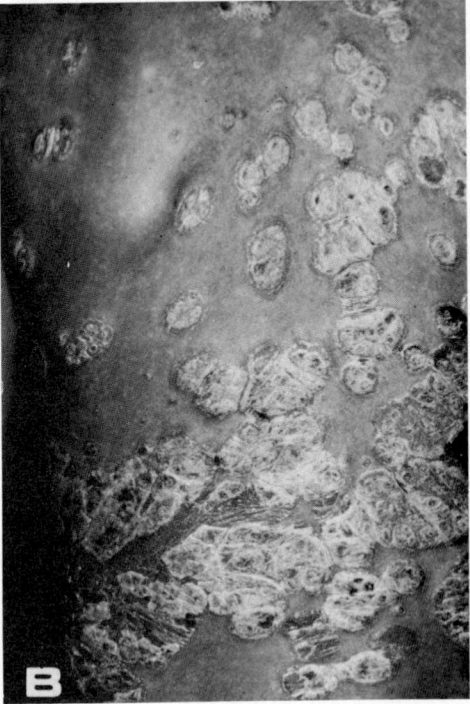

FIG. 8. Psoriasis. **A.** Extensive involvement in an 8-year-old boy with clinical evidence of disease since birth.
B. View of back of same patient.

occluded either naturally by body folds or by plastic wrap. A more substantial nuisance is the risk of local atrophy of the skin, which may occur with topical steroid therapy and occlusion and appears to be directly related to the potency of the steroid. Systemic therapy with steroids is almost never necessary in a child and only the most debilitating psoriasis would justify the use of oral methotrexate. Experience with orally administered methotrexate in children is small. In adults methotrexate, when administered in an interrupted oral schedule, is associated with very little toxicity.

The therapeutic effect of ultraviolet light on psoriasis must be balanced against its aging effect on skin. Long-wave ultraviolet light has been used to potentiate the effect of tar, and more recently there has been extensive trials of long-wave ultraviolet light (UVA) in conjunction with *psoralen*, which is photosensitizing. The long-term cutaneous damage produced by this approach is unknown.

Generalized Exfoliative Dermatitis

Causes of generalized exfoliative dermatitis include, besides psoriasis, such diseases as seborrheic dermatitis, which, when generalized in infancy, is termed *Leiner's disease;* and *pityriasis rubra pilaris*. Lymphoma and leukemia, as well as severe drug reactions, should be considered as possible causes. Pathophysiologic and therapeutic considerations described for generalized psoriasis apply to these as well. The generalized erythema and subsequent shedding of the horny layer following scarlet fever or severe measles is a benign self-limited process. An interesting observation in Leiner's disease is that the fifth component of complement is deficient, resulting in reduced serum opsonic function.

SEBORRHEIC DERMATITIS.   Erythema with yellowish, greasy appearing scales characteristically localized to the scalp, eyebrows, nasolabial folds, and presternal skin is typical of seborrheic dermatitis. Extensive scalp involvement with thick crusting is often called *cradle cap*. Facial involvement may suggest lupus erythematosus or photosenstivity. Heavy scaling with crusting and/or purpura should suggest Letterer-Siwe's disease. Major presternal involvement might indicate Darier's disease. However, seborrheic dermatitis is far more common than any of these. Treatment of seborrheic dermatitis is with topical medications, including corticosteroids and sulfur- or tar-containing preparations. The disorder recurs and requires continued therapy.

HAIR DEFECTS

Careful examination of hairs, collectively or individually, has become important in a variety of situations of particular interest to the pediatrician. Increasing reports of the strength of scanning electronmicroscopy, physical strength measurements, and biochemical evaluation of abnormal hair shafts or plucked roots emphasize awareness of the potential value of hair examination in the detection of inherited or acquired metabolic derangements.

ABNORMALITIES OF HAIR SHAFTS

Any child with complaints of slow hair growth or hair fragility should have a few hairs cut close to the scalp and examined microscopically with a 10 or 20 times objective. The structure of the shaft will be easier to examine if immersion oil or coverslip adhesive is dropped onto the hairs on the glass slide before the cover glass is applied. This examination may reveal factitial or inherited abnormalities of the hair shaft.

The abnormality called *trichorrhexis nodosa* (Fig. 9A), in which partial fracture sites of the hair shaft appear microscopically as interlocking paint brushes, has been noted in about one-half of the cases of argininosuccinicaciduria, an aminoaciduria with proved defect in the enzyme argininosuccinase. Trichorrhexis nodosa is most commonly produced by the trauma of grooming, especially in adults, but when present in a child should trigger a search for argininosuccinicaciduria or other congenital syndrome with which it has been associated.

Trichoschisis, a term recently applied to clean-faced fractures of the hair shaft, was observed in a child without abnormality other than aminoaciduria; examination of the hairs under polarized light revealed regular and alternating disappearance of the usual uniform birefringence. Amino acid analysis of this hair was compatible with a deficiency in a relatively specific group of high sulfur, amorphous hair proteins; similar proteins are known to be decreased in some cases of kwashiorkor.

Monilethrix (Fig. 9B), alternate fusiform constriction of the hair shaft, may be associated with other minor ectodermal abnormalities; association with argininosuccinicaciduria has not been confirmed. The period of alternation has not consistently varied with any known biologic period; however, lack of accurate measurements of growth rate in individual cases often has hampered clarification of such a relationship.

Pili annulati (ringed hair, Fig. 9C) is not associated with systemic disease. The defect is characterized quite literally by "holes" in the mass of the hair shaft, apparently representing absence of cortical cells rather than medullary abnormalities, as previously suggested.

Trichorrhexis invaginata (Fig. 9D) refers to an uncommon, ball-and-socket, bamboo joint defect of hair shafts, often occurring in conjunction with icthyosis linearis circumflexa; it is occasionally associated with nonspecific aminoaciduria and an autosomal recessive inheritance has been noted.

Pili torti refers to frequent and severe twisting of the hair shaft. It has been associated with a variety of ectodermal and neuroectodermal defects, the most recent of which is sensory neural hearing loss or Bjornstad's syndrome. Menkes' kinky hair syndrome is a serious X-linked recessive disorder in which there is progressive cerebral degeneration, growth retardation, and pili torti. Intestinal absorption of copper is reduced. Diffuse thinning of hair shaft may also be a sign of "cartilage hair hypoplasia"; focal thinning may be a sign of reversible toxicity from drugs or malnutrition.

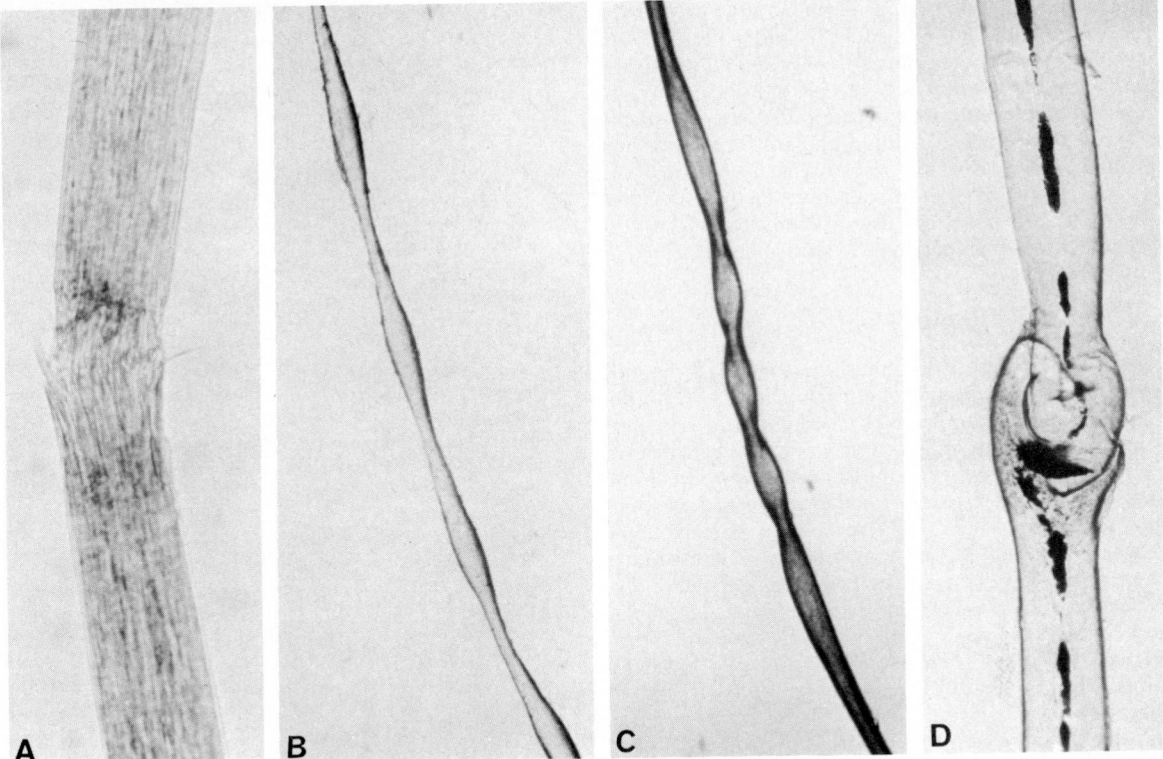

FIG. 9.   A.   Trichorrhexis nodosa. A common deformity of hair shaft that can be associated with aminoaciduria or produced by the trauma of grooming. **B.**   Monilethrix, which is often inherited as a dominant trait and in which there is regular periodic variation in the diameter of the hair shaft. **C.**   Pili torti. The hair is twisted on its long axis and is found in several rare syndromes, including Menkes. This hair is from a 1-year-old Black male with seizures and psychomotor retardation consistent with Menkes. Trichorrhexis nodosa was also present. **D.**   Trichorrhexis invaginata

LOSS OF SCALP HAIR

Diffuse thinning of scalp hair in children, especially if it occurs suddenly, should arouse suspicion of systemic toxicity, either iatrogenic or secondary to accidental ingestion of poison, such as thallium. Both of these circumstances result in damage to the growing, or "anagen," hair roots. Since about 90 percent of hair in the scalp normally is growing at any given time, and since they are distributed randomly, damage to all growing hairs will result in diffuse damage or loss. The injury may be quickly reversible, resulting in rapid recovery of the root and distal propagation of a constriction of the hair shaft often severe enough to cause easy breakage; if more severe, there may be atrophy and rapid loss of all anagen hairs. New hairs will replace them in a period of weeks, assuming the individual survives the *systemic toxic insult.*

Under some circumstances a large percentage of hairs are rapidly converted from a normal growing to a normal resting (telogen) stage; the microscopic appearance of these normal resting roots is readily differentiated from toxic atrophic roots, described above. This "telogen effluvium" occurs most often secondary to high fever (postfebrile alopecia); it also occurs postpar-

tum, postbirth, or following heparin therapy. *Anagen* and *telogen* alopecia can be readily distinguished by microscopic examination of the roots of hair being lost.

Focal or patterned hair loss in a child can usually be divided into scarring disorders, such as localized morphea and discoid lupus erythematosus, or sharply limited areas of hair loss without apparent scalp disease. In the latter instance two diagnostic possibilities predominate. *Trichotillomania* refers to self-induced breaking or pulling of the hairs from the scalp. Usually a stubble of shortened hairs remains, indicative of the difficulty of breaking hairs cleanly at the scalp surface by manual manipulation. Examination with ultraviolet lamp, a microscopic potassium hydroxide preparation, and culture will rule out infection with fungus. Trichotillomania may reflect severe psychopathology; fortunately it is more regularly associated with less severe behavior disturbances. In teenagers, a traction alopecia may result from grooming procedures, such as tight rollers and hot combs. Irregular spreading patches of balding, leaving absolutely bare and apparently normal scalp, are most likely lesions of *alopecia areata.* This peculiar idiopathic disorder is characterized histologically by incomplete formation of hair shaft by reasonably normal hair roots; hence it represents a true "disorder of keratinization." This disease may occur at any age. It may progress to complete loss of scalp and body hair. At least in the early stages, the process is reversible, either spontaneously or secondary to locally injected or systemically administered corticosteroids. Reports of increased coincidence of vitiligo and of "organ-specific autoimmune disease," especially hyperthyroidism, have not as yet yielded specific causative factors. Peculiar patterned alopecia is seen also with several of the syndromes of trisomy; its nature has not been clarified.

HIRSUTISM

Increased hairiness, or hirsutism, is clearly a diagnosis based in part upon semantics, in that it will be dependent upon culturally determined norms. In medical usage, it commonly refers to male-pattern hairiness in a female, or adult-type hairiness in a young child. Some instances dictate a search for endocrine disturbances due to tumors, glandular hyperplasia, or iatrogenic causes, which should not be overlooked. Hirsutism has been noted frequently in several types of mucopolysaccharidoses, in congenital erythropoietic porphyria, and in several other congenital syndromes. Focal thickening of the skin with sharply localized superimposed hirsutism, seen commonly on a wrist or forearm, is striking testimony to chronic trauma, often in a mentally defective child with a persistent habit of chewing or biting the involved area. In virtually all instances, the excess hair is simply a coarse terminal type of hair arising from the same follicle that previously produced the unnoticed or unobjectionable "vellus" or fine downy hair.

Removal of unwanted hair can be accomplished temporarily by a variety of commercially available depilatories, or permanently by electrolytic destruction of each individual hair root.

ABNORMALITIES OF THE NAIL

Nail deformations are common; however, both diagnosis and treatment are generally unsatisfactory. Thickened hypertrophic nails (*onychogryphosis*) may be regularly pared if desired. Spoon-shaped nails (*koilonychia*) are often congenital and idiopathic; occasionally they, together with distal loosening of the nail plate (*onycholysis*), draw attention to hypochromic anemia, polycythemia vera, or hyperthyroidism. Although *clubbing* (hippocratic nails) is most often congenital, it prompts consideration of systemic vascular or pulmonary disorder. Discolored or crumbly nails suggest bacterial or mycotic origin; ice-pick pits suggest psoriasis. Distortion of the nail with firm chronic inflammation surrounding the nail base is suggestive of *Candida albicans* infection. Any severe dermatitis involving the skin near the nail base and its underlying proliferative nail matrix can result in distortion of the nail. Brief systemic illnesses are frequently heralded as the cause of transverse lines or depressions propagated distally as the nail continues to grow.

Bibliography

DISEASES OF KERATINIZATION

Brown AC, Belser RB, Crounse RG, Wehr RF: A congenital hair defect: trichoschisis with alternating birefringence and low sulfur content. J Invest Dermatol 54:496, 1970

Brown AC, Crounse RG, Winkelmann RK: Generalized hair follicle hamartoma. Arch Dermatol 99:478, 1969

Crounse RG, Van Scott EJ: Changes in scalp hair roots as a measure of toxicity from cancer chemotherapeutic drugs. J Invest Dermatol 35:83, 1960

Gillespie JM: The Dietary Regulation of the Synthesis of Hair Keratin. In Symposium on Fibrous Proteins. Plenum Press, New York, 1967

Kligman AM: Pathologic dynamics of human hair loss: I. Telogen effluvium. Arch Dermatol 83:175, 1961

McCance RA, Widdowson EW: Calorie Deficiencies and Protein Deficiencies. Little, Brown and Co, Boston, 1968

Menkes JH, Alter M, Steigleder GK, Weakley DR, Sung JH: A sex-linked recessive disorder with retardation of growth, peculiar hair, and focal cerebral and cerebellar degeneration. Pediatrics 29:764, 1962

Menton DN: The effects of essential fatty acid deficiency on the skin of the mouse. Am J Anat 122:337, 1968

Mize CE, Herndon JH, Jr, Blass JP, et al: Localization of the oxidative defect in phytanic acid degradation in patients with Refsum's disease. J Clin Invest 48:1033, 1969

Winkelmann RK, Perry HO, Achor RWP, Kirby TJ: Cutaneous syndromes produced as side effects of triparanol therapy. Arch Dermatol 87:372, 1963

Zaias N: The embryology of the human nail. Arch Dermatol 87:37, 1963

THE ICHTHYOSES

Esterly N: The ichthyosiform dermatoses. Pediatrics 42:990, 1968

Esterly NB, Maxwell E: Nonbullous congenital ichthyosiform erythroderma. A case treated with methotrexate. Pediatrics 41:120, 1968

Feinstein A, Ackerman AB, Ziprkowski L: Histology of autosomal dominant ichthyosis vulgaris and X-linked ichthyosis. Arch Dermatol 101:524, 1970

Frost P, Van Scott EJ: Ichthyosiform dermatoses: Classification based on anatomic and biometric observation. Arch Dermatol 94:113, 1966

————— Weinstein GD: Vitamin A acid for ichthyosiform dermatoses and psoriasis. JAMA 207:1863, 1968

Hirone T: Electron microscopic studies of ichthyosis and congenital ichthyosiform erythroderma. J Electron Microsc 18:63, 1969

Wells RS, Kerr CB: Genetic classification of ichthyosis. Arch Dermatol 92:1, 1965

Wilgram GF, Caulfield JB: An electron microscopic study of epidermolytic hyperkeratosis. Arch Dermatol 94:127, 1966

HYPERKERATOSIS OF THE PALMS AND SOLES

Anderson PC, Martt JM: Myotonia and keratoderma induced by 20,25 diazocholestenol. Arch Dermatol 92:181, 1965

Butterworth T, Strean LP: Clinical Genodermatology. William and Wilkins Co, Baltimore, 1962

Heiss HB, Gross PR: Keratosis palmaris et plantaris treatment with topically applied vitamin A acid. Arch Dermatol 101:100, 1970

PSORIASIS

Brody I: The ultrastructure of the epidermis in psoriasis vulgaris as revealed by electron microscopy. J Ultrastructr Res 8:595, 1963

Freedberg IM, Baden HP: The metabolic response to exfoliation. J Invest Dermatol 38:277, 1962

Rothberg S, Crounse RG, Lee JG: Glycine-C[14] incorporation into the proteins of normal stratum corneum and the abnormal stratum corneum of psoriasis. J Invest Dermatol 37:497, 1961

Weinstein GD, Van Scott EJ: Autoradiographic analysis of turnover times of normal and psoriatic epidermis. J Invest Dermatol 45:257, 1965

HAIR DEFECTS

Altman J, Stroud J: Netherton's syndrome and psoriasiform ichthyosis. Arch Dermatol 100:550, 1969

Bradfield RB: Morphologic changes in human scalp hair roots during deprivation of protein. Science 157:438, 1967

Brown AC, Belser RB, Crounse RG, Wehr RF: A congenital hair defect: trichoschisis with alternating birefringence and low sulfur content. J Invest Dermatol 54:496, 1970

Caputo R, Ceccarelli B: Study of normal hair and of some malformations with a scanning electron microscope. Arch Klin Exp Dermatol 234:242, 1969

Chernowsky ME, Owens DW: Trichorrhexis nodosa; clinical and investigative studies. Arch Dermatol 94:576, 1966

Comaish S: Autoradiographic studies of hair growth and rhythm in monilethrix. Br J Dermatol 81:443, 1969

Crounse RG, Bollet AJ, Owens S: Tissue assay of human protein malnutrition using scalp hair roots. Trans Assoc Am Physicians 83:185, 1970

Cunliffe WJ, Hall R, Stevenson CJ, Weightman D: Alopecia areata, thyroid disease and autoimmunity. Br J Dermatol 81:877, 1969

Dawber R, Comaish S: Scanning electron microscopy of normal and abnormal hair shafts. Arch Dermatol 101:316, 1970

Efron ML: Diseases of the urea cycle. In Stanbury, Wyngaarden, and Fredrickson (eds): The Metabolic Basis of Inherited Disease. McGraw-Hill Book Co, New York, 1966

Gillespie JM: The Dietary Regulation of the Synthesis of Hair Keratin in Symposium of Fibrous Proteins. Plenum Press, New York, 1967

Menkes JH, Alter M, Steigleder GK, Weakley DR, Sung JH: A sex-linked recessive disorder with retardation of growth, peculiar hair, and focal cerebral and cerebellar degeneration. Pediatrics 29:764, 1962

O'Brien JS, Sampson EL: Kinky hair disease: II. Biochemical studies. J Neuropathol Exp Neurol 25:523, 1968

Pollitt RJ, Jenner FA, Davies M: Sibs with mental and physical retardation and trichorrhexis nodosa with abnormal amino acid composition of the hair. Arch Dis Child 43:211, 1968

Price VH, Thomas RS, Jones FT: Pili annulati, optical and electron microscopic studies. Arch Dermatol 98:640, 1968

Shih VE, Littlefield JW, Moser HW: Argininosuccinase deficiency in fibroblasts cultured from patients with argininosuccinic aciduria. Biochem Genet 3:81, 1969

Sims RT: "Beau's lines" in hair; reduction of hair shaft diameter associated with illness. Br J Dermatol 79:43, 1967

Slepyan AH: Traction alopecia. Arch Dermatol 78:395, 1958

Swanbeck G, Nyren J, Juhlin L: Mechanical properties of hairs from patients with different types of hair diseases. J Invest Dermatol 54:248, 1970

DISEASES OF THE DERMIS

J. Graham Smith, Jr.

Robert L. Anderton

The dermis consists of fibrous proteins, collagen, and elastin embedded in an aqueous matrix of ground substance.

Collagen, which is synthesized by fibroblasts, accounts for approximately 75 percent of the dry weight of the dermis. Hydroxyproline and hydroxylysine are the amino acids characteristically found in the collagen peptide chain. Light microscopy reveals coarse and wavy collagen fibers that are white and thin. In vivo, the fibers have a periodicity of 700 Å, possess high tensile strength, and have a high modulus of elasticity.

Certain disease states, such as acromegaly and hyperthyroidism, are associated with increased collagen synthesis and urinary hydroxyproline excretion; collagen synthesis and urinary hydroxyproline are decreased in dwarfs and cretins deficient in growth hormone. The only clearly identified human collagen diseases are scurvy, which is related to ascorbic-acid dependent hydroxylation of proline and lysine in collagen, and two recently described Ehlers-Danlos syndromes. Both of these Ehlers-Danlos variants are related to biochemical defects in collagen synthesis.

Elastic tissue, although invariably associated with collagen, differs from it morphologically, physically, and chemically. Elastin is synthesized by smooth muscle cells and fibroblasts. Microscopic examination reveals that the elastic fibers are delicate, straight, and freely branching. They form a lattice-like pattern and in general lie parallel to collagen fibers. The fibers are yellow, do not polarize light unless stretched, and have low tensile strength and a low modulus of elasticity. They fluoresce, and this fluorescence increases with aging. The mature elastic fiber has two morphologically different constituents, a microfibrillar component embedded in an amorphous matrix. The amorphous material has a predominance of nonpolar amino acids and has selective susceptibility to elastase digestion. The microfibrillar component has a predominance of polar amino acids and is susceptible to the action of a number of proteolytic enzymes. Embryologically the microfibrillar component forms as an aggregate structure well before any amorphous material is present. Thus these microfibrils may play an important role in the morphogenesis of the elastic fiber.

The ground substance is an amorphous, semifluid matrix comprised of various carbohydrate, lipid, and protein materials lying between fibers and cells. The major acid glycosaminoglycans found in the skin are hyaluronic acid and dermatan sulfate (chondroitin sulfate B). During the first year of life there is a marked decrease in acid glycosaminoglycans of the skin and a more gradual decrease from childhood through adulthood and older age. The decrease in hyaluronic acid is greater than that of chondroitin sulfate. Diseases such as myxedema and the various mucopolysaccharidoses (storage diseases associated with alterations in ground substance) are discussed elsewhere.

Nevus Sebaceous (Jadassohn)

This orange-yellow, hairless plaque is present at birth commonly on the scalp and face. During childhood the lesion is quiescent, but at puberty the lesion may become more verrucous and nodular (Fig. 10, color plate 1). Careful monitoring of the lesions is warranted as skin appendageal tumors may subsequently arise in the lesion. The lesion probably arises from matrix cells (primary epithelial germs) with a potential to differentiate toward hair, apocrine gland, and basal cell.

Histopathology reveals very small, underdeveloped

sebaceous glands and hair during the quiescent (child-hood) phase. At puberty the epidermis becomes papil-lomatous and many mature or nearly mature sebaceous glands are noted. Frequently, the hair follicles remain small, but cystic or hyperplastic apocrine glands may be noted. At a later stage, basal cell carcinoma may arise in 20 percent of lesions. Other tumors including syringo-cystadenoma papilliform; adenomatous tumors; hair follicle tumors; keratoacanthoma; sebaceous epitheli-oma; and, rarely, squamous cell carcinoma of the over-lying epidermis. The lesions should be excised electively.

APLASIA CUTIS CONGENITA

This condition is probably inherited as an autosomal dominant. Aplasia cutis congenita is frequently noted in the newborn infant as localized areas of scarring and erosion. The defect is primarily a solitary midline lesion (1 to 2 cm diameter) located on the vertex of the poste-rior scalp as a sharply marginated, raw, nonnecrotic, granulating, multishaped (circular, elongate, triangu-lar, or stellate), hairless defect (Fig. 11, color plate 2). The lesion, at times, is large, particularly when located on the extremities or trunk. Lesions may be multiple. The natural course is uneventful and most are healed at the time of birth. Healing results in scar formation.

The etiology and pathogenesis are unknown, but the two most likely explanations are: (a) The defect results from a local arrest of cutaneous development. Failure of the neural tube to close could represent a specific in-stance of such a developmental arrest. The location of the lesions, particularly midline of the scalp, suggests this origin. (b) Adhesions between amniotic membrane and fetal skin occur allegedly after enough amniotic fluid has accumulated to tear the fetal skin from the amniotic membrane. Some suggest that pressure necro-sis is responsible for the phenomenon while others ad-vocate drugs as possible causative agents. The former argument is very unlikely because pressure necrosis generally occurs two weeks after trauma and is clinically necrotic, whereas the aplasia lesions are noted immedi-ately after birth and are clean and nonnecrotic. The familial occurrence of the condition makes drug causa-tion alone unlikely.

The histopathology reveals, at times, an absence of epidermis, but when present, it is normal or atrophic. The dermis and subcutaneous tissues may also be in-volved as may muscle and bone. Elastic fibers may be normal, fragmented, or absent. All skin appendages are characteristically absent. Other associated abnormali-ties that have been described include focal dermal hypoplasia, constricting rings, hydrocephalus, cleft pal-ate, patent ductus arteriosus, and tracheoesophageal fistula.

FOCAL DERMAL HYPOPLASIA (GOLTZ SYNDROME)

Focal dermal hypoplasia (Goltz syndrome) is a rare mesoectodermal syndrome, generally noted in female infants at birth, and characterized by linear areas of thinned skin with herniation of the underlying fat. Ini-tially, the yellow areas are widely distributed and darker than the surrounding skin. Yellowish papillae represent underlying fat herniation. Associated ectomesodermal defects include optic atrophy, ocular defects, central nervous system abnormalities, nail dystrophy, dental hypoplasia, syndactyly, and polydactyly.

Histopathology reveals a greatly thinned dermis with subcutaneous fat noted just below the epidermis. The connective tissue remains in a thin band just below the epidermis and around the pilosebaceous structure. No effective therapy exists for this condition.

ALOPECIA MUCINOSA (FOLLICULAR MUCINOSIS)

This entity is characterized by hairless, well-demar-cated, slightly raised, erythematous indurated plaques with follicular keratotic prominence and fine scales most commonly located on the head and neck, but par-ticularly the face. Roughly one-half of the cases become more widespread. All races are involved, both sexes are approximately equally afflicted, and the highest inci-dence is in the middle-age group. The cause of the disease is unknown, but older individuals with evidence of multiple generalized lesions should be evaluated for underlying lymphoma.

Histopathology reveals mucinous alteration of the middle one-third of the external hair sheath and seba-ceous gland. The follicular bulb and papillae are charac-teristically spared; thus regrowth of hair may be anticipated following resolution of the disease. Therapy does not affect the course of this generally self-limited disease.

POROKERATOSIS (MIBELLI)

This condition is a genodermatosis with autosomal dominant inheritance. Clinically the lesions are asymp-tomatic, sharply demarcated keratotic anhidrotic plaques, with a raised, horny ridge (Fig. 12, color plate 2). The lesions occur most often in childhood and per-sist indefinitely. Porokeratoses occur worldwide and in all races. Males are afflicted two to three times as fre-quently as females.

The etiology of these lesions is unknown. The lesions begin as keratotic papules, generally follicular, located on the hands including the palms, but they have oc-curred on almost all areas of the body, including geni-talia and mucous membranes. The lesions may persist or gradually enlarge centrifugally in a circinate pattern. The peripheral lesion is an elevated ridge measuring 1 to 10 mm in height and is of variable color. The ridge may contain a shallow longitudinal furrow in numerous cylindrical keratotic plugs. Generally the resulting plaque is hairless and may cease to enlarge, but exten-sive lesions up to 29 cm have been described. Lesions are frequently single but may be multiple and coales-cent. Linear porokeratosis has been described.

Histopathology is diagnostic. The characteristic cor-noid lamellae exist in the raised border, which should be included in the specimen. The cornoid lamellae form a thickened column of keratin that is generally lighter in staining characteristics on hematoxylin and eosin stain. It extends outward from a notch in the malpighian layer and contains hematoxylinophilic particles. There is an absence of the granular layer, with a few dyskeratotic and vacuolated cells in the malpighian layer. The underlying dermis contains patches of lymphocytes and histiocytes.

Treatment is either by destruction (electrodesiccation or cryotherapy) or surgical excision if lesions are small, but recurrence may result. Although spontaneous disappearance may occur, the more common prognosis is that of a persistent, chronic, slowly extending plaque.

EHLERS-DANLOS SYNDROME

This multi-organ condition is characterized mainly by hyperextensibility of joints and skin that is fragile, bruises easily, and is excessively stretchable (Fig. 13). Within the last decade this syndrome has been subclassified into seven distinct forms. Table 1, adapted from McKusick, illustrates the variation in these clinical types.

Type 1 is the *classic gravis* Ehlers-Danlos syndrome, with its characteristic features, which include hyperextensible joints and multiple cutaneous defects. *Type 2* is the *benign (mitis)* type of Ehler-Danlos. Both the gravis and mitis types are autosomal dominant in inheritance. The biochemical defects responsible for types 1 and 2 are not known.

Type 3 has also been called the *benign hypermobility* type, as joint hyperextensibility is the predominant feature with minimal skin manifestations. Although marked joint laxity is present, the patients do not have profound scoliosis. Many of these patients do have the floppy mitral syndrome (Barlow's syndrome) as manifested by a midsystolic click and later systolic murmur.

Type 4, or arterial/ecchymotic (Sack-Barabas), is the most grave of the variants. Clinically, these patients have exceptionally stretchable and extraordinarily thin skin that is deficient in collagen. Subcutaneous veins are prominent and there is cutaneous ulceration. *Elastosis perforans serpiginosa,* which represents a transepidermal elimination of elastic fibers, is frequently present in these patients. Joint hypermobility is not excessive in this type of Ehlers-Danlos. Because of the very poor collagen that is synthesized in type 4, these patients develop their "malignant" problems as a consequence of rupture of large and intermediate size arteries. Spontaneous rupture of the bowel, as well as bowel diverticulae, are also quite common in this variety. The larger vessels, including the aorta, are not spared, and a tear may result; but general dissection is not expected. Although the precise biochemical defect is unknown, the defect may be in the synthesis of collagen.

Type 5 is not clinically distinct but is inherited as an X-linked recessive. *Type 6* syndrome described by Pinnell is the first of the Ehlers-Danlos syndromes to be characterized biochemically. A deficiency of procollagen lysyl hydroxylase results in hydroxylysine-deficient collagen, with inadequate cross links between collagen fibers. Clinically the patients have, in addition to those classic skin and joint changes noted in previous types, severe scoliosis and ocular fragility. The inheritance is autosomal recessive.

Type 7 Ehlers-Danlos clinically is characterized by loose-jointedness. The patients frequently are born with dislocated hips and have severe subluxations of the knees and other joints (arthrochalasis multiplex congenita). The skin is soft, velvety, and, at times, excessively stretchable. The patients are of short stature. The inheritance is as type 6, autosomal recessive. These patients have an enzymatic deficiency of procollagen protease or peptidase, which normally cleaves a terminal portion of the procollagen molecule after it has been excreted from the fibroblast.

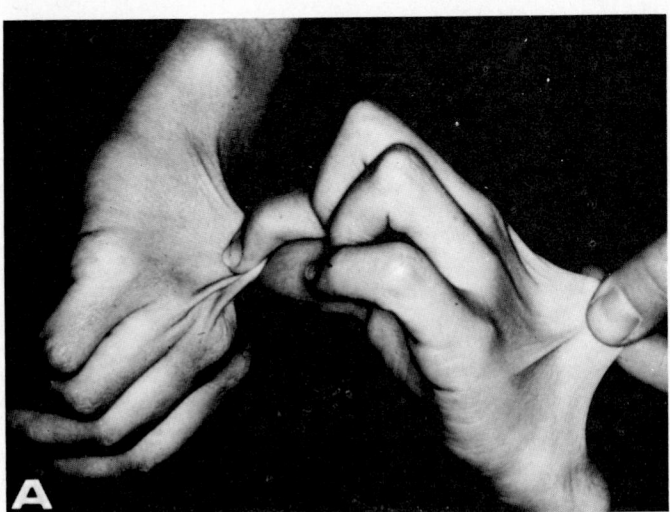
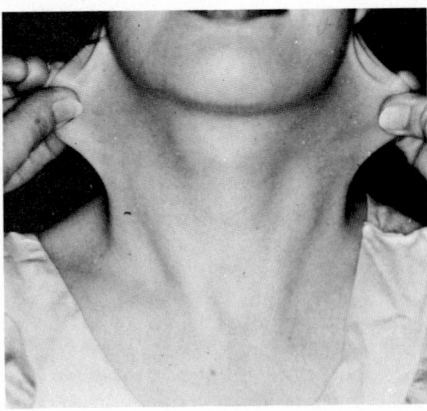

FIG. 13.   Ehlers-Danlos syndrome. Characteristic abnormal elasticity of skin.

TABLE 1. Forms of the Ehlers-Danlos (E-D) Syndrome

Number	Name	Clinical Features	Genetics	Biochemical Defect
E-D I	E-D, gravis type	Classic features, all severe	Autosomal dominant	Unknown
E-D II	E-D, mitis type	Classic features, all mild	Autosomal dominant	Unknown
E-D III	E-D, benign hypermobile type	Generalized marked joint hypermobility without skeletal deformity; skin features minimal	Autosomal dominant	Unknown
E-D IV	E-D, echymotic, arterial or Sack-Barabas type	Severe bruisability; very thin skin rupture of bowel rupture of large arteries; minimal joint laxity (eg limited to fingers)	?	In synthesis of type III collagen
E-D V	E-D, X-linked type	Stretchable skin striking; joint hypermobility minimal; skin fragility and bruisability variable	X-linked recessive	Unknown
E-D VI	E-D, ocular type; lysyl hydroxylase deficiency; hydroxylysine-deficient collagen disease	Scoliosis severe, skin features moderate; blindness from retinal detachment or ocular rupture	Autosomal recessive	Deficiency of procollagen-lysyl-hydroxylase
E-D VII	Arthrochalasis multiplex congenita; procollagen peptidase (or protease) deficiency	Short stature; severe joint laxity with congenital dislocations, moderate skin stretchability, and bruisability	Autosomal recessive	Deficiency of procollagen protease (or peptidase)

From McKusick VA: ED syndromes — an editorial. Ann Surg 109:475, 1974

KELOIDS AND HYPERTROPHIC SCARS

Both conditions represent abnormal responses to injury. Keloids may follow the most inconsequential injury and grow slowly in size, resulting in grotesque and disfiguring scars, particularly in Blacks and Orientals (Fig. 14). Keloids may occur anywhere; however, the central chest is a major site. Burns are said to incite this reaction more commonly than other types of injury.

Clinically, early keloids are pink and rubbery and later become firm and sometimes hyperpigmented. Pruritus and pain may be present. Clinically, keloids and hypertrophic scars differ: keloids generally extend well beyond the site of trauma, whereas hypertropic scars are limited primarily to the site of trauma. Keloids generally do not spontaneously regress, while hypertrophic scars commonly regress within 6 to 12 months.

Histologically, the mature keloid has conspicuous thick, glassy, pale-staining collagen with a few fibro-blasts and abundant mucinous ground substance, whereas hypertrophic scarring has a near absence of this collagen, scanty ground substance, and many fibroblasts. The cause of these reactions is unknown and response to treatment is unpredictable. Intralesional injections with steroids, and cryosurgery are often effective.

NECROBIOSIS LIPOIDICA

Necrobiosis lipoidica is a relatively uncommon disorder characterized clinically by the appearance of yellowish, atrophic plaquelike lesions often located on the shins (Fig. 15). Although it occurs in children, it is more common in the fourth decade and in females and is often associated with diabetes mellitus or abnormal glucose tolerance.

Histologically, the collagen in the lesions is swollen and homogenized and has an affinity for hematoxylin

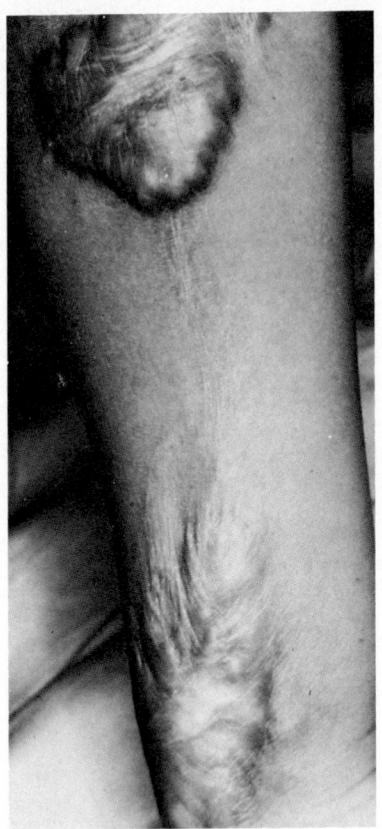

FIG. 14.   Keloid on arm of a child following burn.

stain (necrobiosis). The clinical course of necrobiosis lipoidica is one of chronicity and slow progression, and rarely of ulceration; in approximately 20 percent of cases, spontaneous remission occurs. Topical steroids with occlusion, intralesional corticosteroids, or excision followed by grafting may be of benefit, especially when there is ulceration.

GRANULOMA ANNULARE

Granuloma annulare is a fairly common childhood disorder characterized by annular lesions formed by the peripheral extensions of papules and nodules with central clearing (Fig. 16). The lesions are flesh-colored and characteristically involve the back of the hands and fingers and extensor aspects of the arms and legs but can involve any site. There may be scaling. In children granuloma annulare usually disappears spontaneously. The etiology is unknown, although generalized papular granuloma annulare is associated with diabetes mellitus.

Histologically, the lesions show the necrobiotic changes of collagen described in necrobiosis surrounded by palisading histiocytes. Multinucleated giant cells are found on occasion, and vascular changes are minimal except for perivascular lymphocytic cuffing. The lesions are asymptomatic and tend to involute spontaneously after a few months or years. Treatment is most difficult to evaluate because of the spontaneous involution of lesions, but intralesional corticosteroids and cryotherapy have been reported to pro-

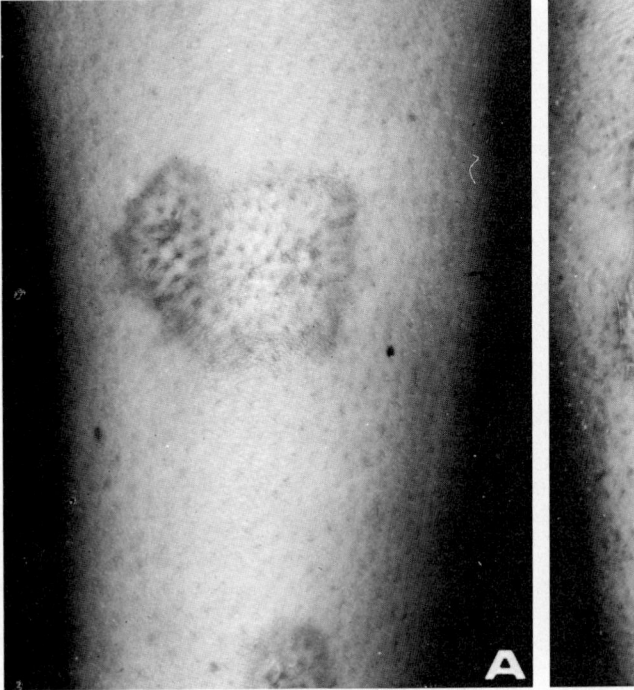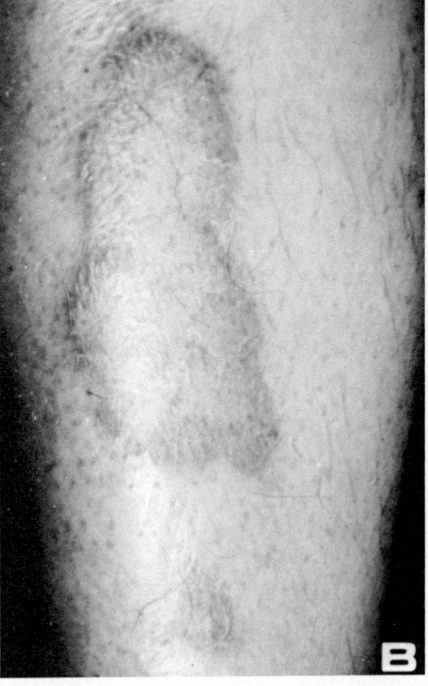

FIG. 15.   Necrobiosis lipoidica diabeticorum. **A.**   Early lesion, not yet atrophic, in a 13-year-old girl.
B. Yellowish elevated lesion on shin (a typical location). The lesion often is marked by telangiectasia and atrophy.

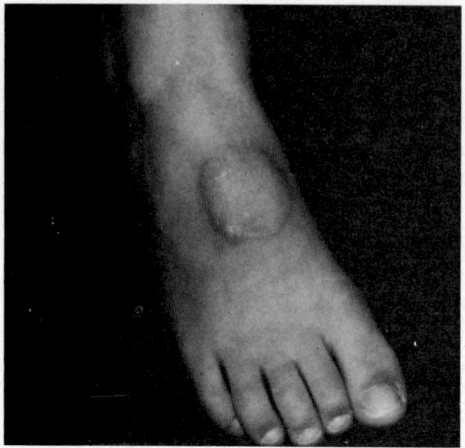

FIG. 16.   Granuloma annulare. Large annular lesion over the instep. Microscopically, there is necrobiosis and granuloma formation. The lesions heal without scarring.

duce regression of some lesions. The lesions must be distinguished from tinea circinata and alopecia mucinosa.

CUTIS LAXA

Cutis laxa (generalized elastolysis) is a very rare hereditary disorder characterized by loose, pendulous skin (Fig. 17). The disease appears to be inherited in an autosomal recessive fashion although a few cases of autosomal dominant inheritance have been noted. The

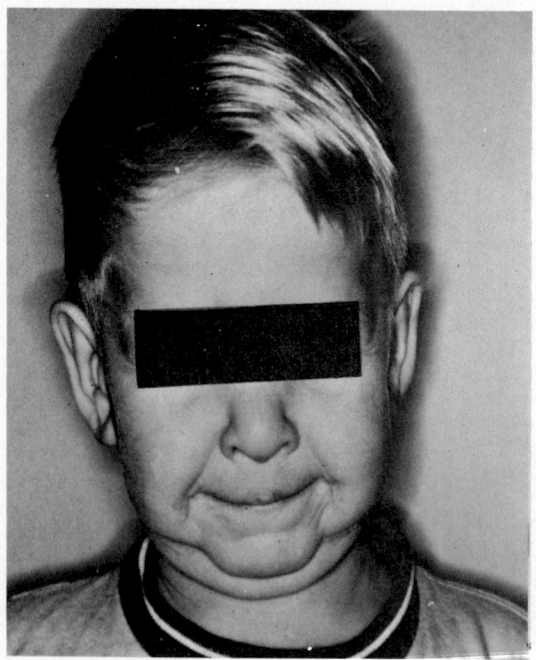

FIG. 17.   Epidermolysis bullosa simplex. Typical noninflammatory blisters at various stages of development and resolution.

basic defect appears to be related to an increased rate of degradation of elastic tissue, although abnormally synthesized elastic fibers could likewise be responsible for the peculiar features. The increased rate of degradation is supported by a report of a deficiency of elastase inhibiting substance in some affected individuals.

Both acquired and congenital forms of cutis laxa have been described. In the congenital form the skin changes are present at birth or shortly afterward, whereas in the acquired form the skin changes become manifest around puberty. On occasion they are not noted until middle or older age. The loose, pendulous skin of cutis laxa gives the afflicted child a prematurely aged appearance. Multiple organs may be affected because of the defect in supporting structure; notable abnormalities, including pulmonary emphysema, tracheobronchomegaly (Mounier-Kuhn Syndrome), gastrointestinal and urinary tract diverticulae, as well as rectal and vaginal prolapse, have been described.

Histologically, the elastic fibers appear to be reduced in size and number and show granular changes. Collagen fibers appear to be normal. In the absence of pulmonary emphysema, the prognosis in this disorder is reasonably good. Plastic surgery may improve the appearance of the face. Pulmonary function should be tested and pulmonary symptoms treated. There is no effective medical treatment for this disorder.

ELASTOSIS PERFORANS SERPIGINOSA

This elastic tissue disorder has frequently been associated with other conditions including Down's Syndrome, cutis hyperelastica, osteogenesis imperfecta, congenital heart disease, progeria, Rothmund-Thompson and Marfan's syndromes. Patients with Wilson's disease treated with penicillamine have developed an elastosis perforans serpiginosa-like condition.

Clinically the skin lesions are erythematous, skin-colored, keratotic papules with central scarring. These papules are annular (at times serpiginous) in configuration with a predilection for the nape of the neck, upper extremities, and face. The lesions are generally asymptomatic, but may be pruritic. Histologic changes reveal transepidermal elimination of elastic tissues. The base of the lesion underlying the perforation reveals a granulomatous infiltrate with both histiocytes and foreign body giant cells. The course of the condition varies, but spontaneous disappearance does occur. No effective treatment is known.

SUBCUTANEOUS FAT NECROSIS

This panniculitis afflicts healthy term infants, generally at the end of the first week or during the second week of life. Occasionally cases are described in three to four week-old infants. Although the cause is unknown, cases parallel the incidence of traumatic deliveries, and the location involved, ie, cheeks, neck, back, shoulders, buttocks, thighs, and deltoid areas, are more prone to obstetric trauma. The lesions vary from a few millimeters to 10 cm in diameter. They are generally very firm, freely movable but occasionally slightly elevated, and round to linear with a reddish to blue sharply demarcated border. At times the lesions become cystic and rarely ulcerate. The lesions generally run an uneventful course in several months without systemic symptoms, but subcutaneous calcification may occasionally occur.

Histopathology reveals a granulomatous infiltrate containing foreign body giant cells, some of which contain fat crystals on frozen section. The fat lobules appear enlarged. It is thought that the fat is altered secondary to ischemia during traumatic delivery and that the altered fat then incites the foreign body reaction in the subcutaneous tissue with production of the lesions. No definite therapy is known and, unlike sclerema neonatorum, with supportive therapy alone the prognosis is good.

SCLEREMA NEONATORUM

Sclerema neonatorum is an unusual condition characterized by progressive hardening of the subcutaneous tissue, often beginning in the first week of life. It primarily affects premature or full-term infants afflicted with intracranial hemorrhage or overwhelming pneumonitis. Clinically, these lesions begin on the buttocks, thighs, and hands; they rapidly progress to involve the entire subcutaneous tissue except that of the palms, soles, and genitalia. The skin is characteristically smooth, cool, tense, and mottled; it cannot be pitted, pinched into folds, or picked up easily. The infants are weak, cyanotic, and unable to regulate body temperature normally. They rapidly deteriorate, and death occurs in 75 percent of all cases.

Histologically, the fibrous trabeculae become thickened. There is absence of fat necrosis and inflammation is usual. Histochemical stains reveal an increase in saturated fats, primarily palmitic and stearic acid, with a decrease in oleic acid. Needle-shaped crystals may be seen within many fat cells. The crystals are doubly refractile and do not stain with fat stains.

The proposed etiology may be related to the poorly formed neonatal enzymes involved in the desaturation of palmitic and stearic acids to form oleic acids, eventuating in the abundant saturated fats as noted above. Because of the low unsaturated fat content, fat solidification occurs and might account for the clinical features.

Treatment should be supportive with particular attention directed toward temperature control. Although corticosteroids have been used, the results have not been encouraging.

CHRONIC ACIDEMIA

Metabolic and respiratory acidemia of greater than six to seven months duration result in an apparent systemic increase in elastic tissue with an apparent reduction of collagen. These alterations characteristically are associated with clinical changes, consisting of dry, scaly atrophic skin with generalized alopecia, poor wound healing, hemorrhagic tendencies, and wound dehiscence. The etiology of the connective tissue alterations is unknown.

CONNECTIVE TISSUE NEVI

These hamartomas commonly appear before age ten and may be present at birth. The morphology varies from flesh-colored papules and varied colored plaques to papillomatous or verrucous lesions. The plaques, also called *shagreen patch,* commonly occur in the lumbosacral area and frequently are associated with tuberous sclerosis. The histology varies; there may be increased collagen as in shagreen patch, increased elastic tissue as in juvenile elastoma, or decreased elastic tissue as in nevus anelasticus of Lewandowsky.

SCLEREDEMA OF BUSCHKE

Scleredema of Buschke, also called *scleredema adultorum,* is a rare disease of unknown cause. It begins suddenly as a diffuse, symmetric, nonpitting induration of the skin and generally subsides in 6 to 24 months, but relapses may occur. Females are afflicted more often than males. One-third of the cases occur before the age of 10, and one-half before the age of 20. Frequently ASO titers are elevated, which suggests a relationship to streptococcal hypersensitivity.

Clinically, the symmetric induration begins on the neck and gradually spreads to the face, shoulders, and chest. A febrile illness often precedes the skin changes by a few days to six weeks. The eruption is poorly marginated, infrequently involves the lower extremities, but may lead to joint difficulties related to the overlying edema. The tongue and oropharynx may be involved with resultant dysphagia; rarely pericardial, pleural, and joint effusions have been reported.

Histopathology reveals a normal-appearing epidermis. The dermal collagen is swollen and separated by clear spaces that stain for acid glycosaminoglycans and are thought to be hyaluronic acid. The appendageal structures and blood vessels appear normal. No effective treatment exists.

PSEUDOXANTHOMA ELASTICUM

Pseudoxanthoma elasticum is an uncommon genodermatosis (autosomal recessive) involving elastic tissue. The clinical features become more noticeable with aging. The *plucked chicken skin* appearance characteristically is noted in flexural areas, such as the axilla, neck, umbilicus, and groin. These white to yellowish papules increase in size and sometimes form reticulated patterns. Pseudoxanthoma elasticum is a systemic disease with involvement of the eye and arteries. Ocular findings are most notably, angioid streaks, sometimes frank hemorrhage, choroidal atrophy, and rarely blindness. Vessels throughout the body contain abnormal elastic tissue, which may result in hypertension, cerebrovascular accidents, pulseless extremities, and gastrointestinal hemorrhage. Pseudoxanthoma elasticum has occurred in conjunction with Paget's disease of the bone (osteitis deformans), sickle cell anemia, Marfan's Syndrome, and cutis hyperelastica.

Histologic abnormalities consist of an apparent increase in elastic tissue (primarily in the middle third of the dermis in contrast to solar elastosis where the clumped elastic tissue is in the upper one-third of the dermis). Additionally, calcium salts and acid glycosaminoglycans are found in the mid-dermis. Similar histopathologic abnormalities may also be found in the elastic membranes of vessels throughout the body. The condition is slowly progressive, eventuating in death. No therapy exists for this condition.

WEBER-CHRISTIAN

Weber-Christian disease (recurrent febrile nodular nonsuppurative panniculitis), more commonly found in adult females, rarely afflicts children. Multiple, tender, slightly nodular, dull-red swellings (1 to 2 cm in diameter) arise over the extremities. The lesions progresss with hyperpigmentation of the overlying skin and atrophy of the subcutaneous fat eventuating in a depressed hyperpigmented plaque. Rarely, liquefaction of the underlying fat results in the discharge of an oily yellowish-brown liquid. Characteristically the lesions appear in crops accompanied by fever, malaise, anorexia, and other symptoms related to panniculitis, in visceral organs and bone marrow.

Histopathologically the early lesions reveal fat necrosis, vasculitis, and acute inflammation. Older lesions reveal macrophage ingestion of fat (foam cells) with eventual fibrosis and deep dermal atrophy.

The etiology is unknown, but the process has been associated with recurrent infection, trauma, diabetes mellitus, systemic lupus erythematosus, and glomerulonephritis. Steroids have been used with equivocal results. Most cases resolve in two to five years.

ROTHMAN-MAKAI LIPOGRANULOMATOSIS SUBCUTANEA

In contrast to Weber-Christian disease, Rothman-Makai commonly afflicts children and is not associated with systemic disease. Characteristically subcutaneous nodules and plaques develop on the trunk and extremities. The nodules are firm and slightly tender with normal or slightly reddened areas overlying the skin. The lesions generally resolve without atrophy in 6 to 12 months. Rarely, they liquefy and drain an oily material.

Histopathologically the acute lesions reveal focal degeneration of fat cells, inflammatory cells, and vasodilation. Later, lipophagic histiocytes can be seen, and still later, fibrosis. The etiology is unknown and there is no effective treatment.

Bibliography

Blackburn WR, Cosman B: Keloids and hypertrophic scars. Arch Pathol 82:65, 1966

Curtis AC, Schulak BM: Scleredema adultorum. Arch Dermatol 92:526, 1965

Deeken JH, Caplan RM: Aplasia cutis congenita. Arch Dermatol 102:386, 1970

Finlayson GR, Smith JG, Moor MJ: Effects of chronic acidosis on connective tissue. JAMA 187:659, 1964

Goltz RW, Hult A-M, Goldfarb M, Gorlin RJ: Cutis laxa—a manifestation of generalized elastolysis. Arch Dermatol 92:373, 1965

——— Henderson RR, Hitch MM, OTT JE: Focal dermal hypoplasia syndrome. Arch Dermatol 101:1, 1970

Goodman RM, Smith EW, Paton D, et al: Pseudoxanthoma elasticum: a clinical and histopathologic study. Medicine 42:297, 1963

Gottlieb SK, Fisher BK, Violin GA: Focal dermal hypoplasia—a nine year follow-up of study. Arch Dermatol 108:551, 1973

Harper FB: The masquerade of Weber-Christian disease. Arch Surg 93:327, 1966

Hashimoto K, Kanzaki T: Cutis laxa. Arch Dermatol 111:861, 1975

Kellum RE, Ray TL, Brown GR: Sclerema neonatorum—report of a case and analysis of subcutaneous and epidermal-dermal lipids by chromatographic methods. Arch Dermatol 97:372, 1968

Laymon CW, Peterson WC: Lipogranulomatosis subcutanea (Rothman-Makai)—an appraisal. Arch Dermatol 90:288, 1964

MacDonald A, Feirvel M: A review of the concept of Weber-Christian panniculitis with a report of five cases. Br J Dermatol 80:355, 1968

Marks MB: Subcutaneous adipose derangements of the newborn. Am J Dis Child 104:122, 1962

Marshall J, Vogelpoel L, Weber HW: Primary elastolysis. S Afr Med J 34:721, 1960

McKusick VA: Multiple forms of the Ehlers-Danlos syndrome. Arch Surg 109:475, 1974

Mehregan AH: Elastosis perforans serpiginosa—a review of the literature and report of 11 cases. Arch Dermatol 97:381, 1968

Milunsky A, Levin SE: Sclerema neonatorum—clinical study of 79 cases. S Afr Med J 40:638, 1966

Muller SA, Winkelmann RK: Necrobiosis lipoidica diabeticorum—a clinical and pathological investigation of 171 cases. Arch Dermatol 93:272, 1966

Pass F, Goldfischer S, Sternlieb I, Scheinberg IH: Elastosis perforans serpiginosa during penicillamine therapy for Wilson disease. Arch Dermatol 108:713, 1973

Pope FM: Two types of autosomal recessive pseudoxanthoma elasticum. Arch Dermatol 110:209, 1974

Raque CJ, Wood MG: Connective tissue nevi. Arch Dermatol 102:390, 1970

Ross R, Bornstein P: The elastic fiber. I. The separation and partial characterization of its macromolecular components. J Cell Biol 40:366, 1969

Rudolph RI, Schwartz W, Leyden JJ: Bitemporal aplasia cutis congenita. Arch Dermatol. 110:615, 1974

Schorr WF, Optiz JM, Reyes CN: The connective tissue nevus—osteopoikilosis syndrome. Arch Dermatol 106:208, 1972

Smith JG Jr: The dermal elastoses. Arch Dermatol 88:382, 1963

Stankler L, Leslie G: Generalized granuloma annulare—a report of a case and review of the literature. Arch Dermatol 95:509, 1967

Wechsler HS, Fisher ER: Ehlers-Danlos syndrome. Arch Pathol 77:613, 1964.

BLISTERING DISEASES
ROGER W. PEARSON

A group of conditions in which blister formation is a prominent clinical feature is discussed here. In general, the etiology of these diseases is unknown or poorly understood. Diseases in which blistering is an occasional or regular clinical finding are discussed elsewhere. They include vesicular infectious diseases (such as certain viral infections, rickettsialpox, early congenital syphilis, bullous impetigo, and dermatophytosis), insect bite reactions, second-degree burns, incontinentia pigmenti, urticaria pigmentosa, lupus erythematosus, lichen planus, congenital ichthyosiform erythroderma, the various forms of cutaneous porphyria, drug eruptions, dyshidrotic eczema, and contact dermatitis.

The fact that children blister more easily than do adults is probably because the epidermis, particularly the horny layer, being thinner in children and the connective tissue being relatively immature, contains relatively more soluble collagen and water than adult skin. There may also be special biochemical properties of young skin that leave it more susceptible to attack by certain agents. (See Toxic Epidermal Necrolysis, p. 872).

EPIDERMOLYSIS BULLOSA (MECHANOBULLOUS DISEASES)

Epidermolysis bullosa is a term applied to a group of hereditary diseases in which noninflammatory blisters develop on the skin in response to mechanical trauma. Sometimes the tendency to form blisters is so great that the trauma may be inapparent. It is now possible to separate, on the basis of clinical, histologic, and genetic findings, six distinct diseases. There are some additional variant forms that defy classification because of the sparsity of cases and sketchy descriptions. Since only two of the major forms of the disease show lysis of the epidermis, it seems appropriate to reintroduce the term *mechanobullous diseases* for the group, since mechanical fragility is common to all members. The term *dystrophic* has resulted in frequent diagnostic errors because dystrophic nail and teeth changes also occur in junctional bullous epidermatosis (see below) and in the scarring diseases. New terms have therefore been introduced for some of the diseases (Table 2).

The erythropoietic forms of porphyria, porphyria cutanea tarda, and bullous congenital ichthyosiform erythroderma are also, technically, mechanobullous diseases, which may be confused with the above entities. They can usually be easily differentiated on the basis of clinical and laboratory data.

In all of the major mechanobullous diseases histologic examination of the skin gives useful information, and electron microscope examination is particularly valuable to establish the correct diagnosis early. Whenever possible, the lesions should be induced immediately before biopsy, by minimal mechanical trauma, since secondary alterations may destroy the diagnostic features if older lesions are taken. In instances where the skin is extremely fragile, biopsy of noninvolved skin may be adequate, the biopsy procedure itself providing sufficient trauma to produce the alterations.

Epidermolysis Bullosa Simplex (EBS)

This disease, inherited as an autosomal dominant, is characterized by the presence at birth, or development shortly thereafter, of vesicles and bullae at any site on the body following minor mechanical trauma (Fig. 18). Separation of skin layers occurs within a few minutes of injury, and frank blisters appear usually within 10 to 15 minutes. The palms and soles are usually relatively resistant to the process, especially as the child grows older. The lesions heal with remarkable rapidity and do not scar unless there has been considerable secondary infection. Heat decreases the blistering threshold, and cold raises the threshold to a near normal level. Mucous membranes are not frequently involved, and usually only during infancy or early childhood, the nails not at all, and general development is normal.

Although the disease may decrease in intensity at puberty, most if not all patients can expect lifelong activity of the disease; however, if reasonable care is taken in choice of occupation and recreational activities and the patient makes allowances for his disease, then it is a nuisance rather than a crippling illness.

Histologic examination of a freshly induced lesion reveals that the blisters are produced in the basal cell layer by disintegration of the cytoplasm of the cells. This process appears to be an exaggeration of the reaction pattern shown by normal basal cells in response to many types of injury. Probably the defect resides in the

TABLE 2. Epidermolysis bullosa

Type	Designation	Inheritance	Location of Pathology
Epidermolysis bullosa simplex	EBS	Dominant	Epidermal basal cells
Recurrent bullous eruption of hands and feet (Weber-Cockayne)	RBEHF	Probably dominant	Suprabasilar
Epidermolysis bullosa hereditaria "letalis"	EBHL	Recessive	Dermoepidermal junction
Dystrophic epidermolysis bullosa	DBD-R	Recessive	Papillary dermis
Dystrophic epidermolysis bullosa	DBD-D	Dominant	Superficial dermis
Dystrophic epidermolysis bullosa	DBD-A	Acquired	More superficial than DBD-R

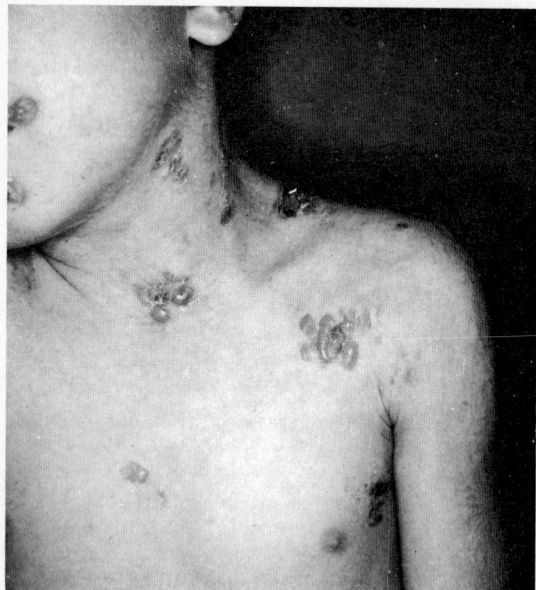

FIG. 18. Recurrent bullous eruption of the hands and feet (RBEHF). Blisters and thick calluses at sites of trauma.

cytolytic enzymes or the mechanism of their activation. An alternative possibility is that the cytoplasm itself is more susceptible than normal to cytolysis.

Treatment is prophylactic and consists primarily of avoidance of mechanical trauma. Most patients become expert early in life at setting their own limits of activity. Cooling of the skin immediately after injury is of great value, and air conditioning in warm climates is a wise investment. Antibiotic ointment and systemic antibiotics may be needed. Lubrication and powdering are useful in reducing friction; maceration, however, must be avoided.

Recurrent Bullous Eruption of Hands and Feet (Weber-Cockayne) (RBEHF)

This rather uncommon condition is characterized by recurrent blisters that develop after trauma on the palms and soles; they are generally mild. They appear less commonly on the dorsum of the hands and feet and rarely elsewhere. There is great variation in the intensity of trauma needed to induce the blisters. Usually the disease is first noted in early childhood, but occasionally it has a later onset. The lesions generally develop 30 minutes to 2 hours after trauma. They heal rapidly without scar formation.

The disease is usually inherited as an autosomal dominant trait, though there are some cases without an apparent hereditary basis. Relative amelioration of the process often occurs at puberty.

Although the blisters have been reported to occur at various levels within the epidermis, the histology of freshly induced lesions is characteristic. In contrast to EBS, there is lysis of cells *above* the basal layer, often

extending as high as the granular layer. There is also marked dyskeratosis. The pathology is identical to that found in "friction blisters" induced in normal individuals. Activation of cytolytic enzymes or increased substrate susceptibility, and decreased mechanical "strength" of cells are the most likely bases for the defect.

Treatment is similar to that of epidermolysis bullosa simplex (EBS). Although systemic steroid therapy has been advocated in rare severe cases, it is not advised in most instances.

Junctional Bullous Epidermatosis (JBE, Herlitz's Disease, or Epidermolysis Bullosa Hereditaria "Letalis", EBHL)

This autosomal recessive trait is apparent at birth and is characterized by vesicles, bullae, and erosions that occur following minimal trauma. Blisters or erosions usually can be induced easily in clear areas. The lesions heal very slowly without scar formation, unless there has been deep infection. The mucous membranes are usually affected, and the teeth are often dystrophic. The nails are frequently dystrophic or lost. Many patients die within a few weeks, some survive a few years, but few survive to adulthood. Some instances of alleged long survival were probably other mechanobullous diseases. With increasing use of steroid therapy and antibiotics it is reasonable to expect more long survivals.

General development is frequently impaired, although mental function is usually normal; severe anemia is often found. When death occurs the mechanism is frequently not apparent, though in some instances infection is the immediate cause. Histologically, blisters develop at the dermoepidermal junction. There is separation between the plasma membrane of the basal cells and the basement membrane.

Treatment consists of general supportive measures, air conditioning, gentleness in handling, protection from and treatment of local systemic infection, and judicious use of systemic anti-inflammatory steroids. Steroid therapy has been of value in some cases and apparently ineffective in others. Steroids are sometimes useful to help the patient through periods of increased activity of the disease. High dosage is usually required.

Dystrophic Epidermolysis Bullosa (Dermolytic Bullous Dermatosis) See Figures 19 and 20.

AUTOSOMAL RECESSIVE TYPE (DBD-R). This disease usually is present at birth and is characterized by blisters (often hemorrhagic) and erosions which tend to involve skin and mucous membranes at any location. The lesions heal slowly with scars and often with milia formation. After repeated episodes, especially on the hands and feet, there is gradual deepening of the scars. Contractures form, nails are lost, the skin of digits often fuses, and bone resorption may occur, so that marked limitation of motion results. Defects of the teeth are common. Eating may be difficult because of mucous

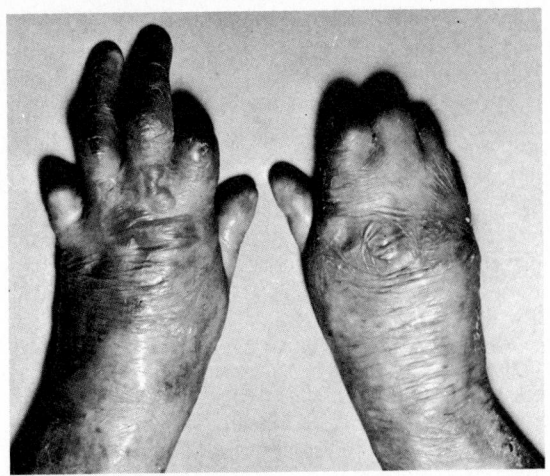

FIG. 19. Dystrophic epidermolysis bullosa. (Dermolytic bullous dermatosis). Recessive type. Moderately severe hand lesions, showing active blisters, scarring with contractures, and loss of nails.

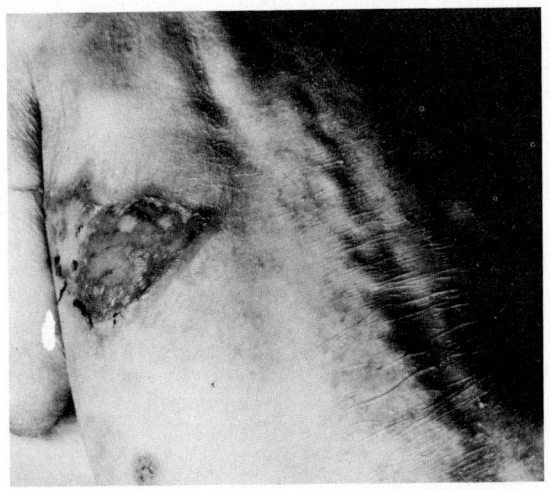

FIG. 20. Dermolytic bullous dermatosis. Recessive type. A large erosion, massive superficial scarring, atrophy, and milia formation.

membrane and teeth involvement. Secondary infection and anemia are common complications. General development is often slow and physical maturity may not be attained, but mental function is usually good. Some improvement often occurs at puberty and most patients reach adulthood. However, early death from infection or general debilitation or secondary amyloidosis may occur, especially in the more severely affected patients. Squamous cell carcinoma developing in scars is an occasional complication.

In warm weather the disease is aggravated, but local cooling of the skin does not prevent experimental blister induction as can be demonstrated in epidermolysis bullosa simplex.

Histologically, the blisters are clean dermoepidermal separations. Electron microscopic examination reveals

that the blisters form as a result of disintegration of the collagen of the papillary dermis. The defect in this disease is not known, but increased collagenase production in the skin of patients with DBD-R has been demonstrated. Whether the collagenase is responsible for the pathology is uncertain. An alternative possibility is that the collagen itself is defective.

Treatment consists of protection from trauma, control of infection, and general supportive measures. Surgeons generally do not attempt reconstruction of hands and feet in the presence of active disease, though recently more vigorous surgical attacks on the problem have been made. Excellent short-term improvement in mobility can be accomplished, but long-term prognosis must be guarded. Steroids have been of little or no value in small doses, but high doses are moderately effective, and useful if administered judiciously.

AUTOSOMAL DOMINANT TYPE (DBD-D). This disease presents at birth or in infancy. Vesicles and bullae occur chiefly on hands, feet, elbows, and knees. In childhood, any site on the skin may be involved. The lesions heal rather slowly with superficial scar formation and milia. Nail involvement is common, presenting typically as a clawlike dystrophy. Severe deformities of the hands and feet do not occur. Mucous membrane involvement is frequent but mild. At puberty moderate or sometimes substantial improvement occurs. General development is unaffected. The histology in this disease is similar to that of autosomal recessive dystrophic epidermolysis bullosa but with more superficial dermal alterations.

Treatment is aimed at reducing mechanical trauma to the skin. In most instances only moderate restriction of physical activities is required.

"ACQUIRED" TYPE (DBD-A). Mild dystrophic epidermolysis bullosa occurs occasionally without demonstrable hereditary background; it may develop during late childhood but more often in young adulthood. Some cases appear to have been induced by drugs (eg, arsenic, sulfonamides, and most recently penicillamine). Usually the manifestations are limited to the hands, feet, elbows, and knees, but more severe cases may occur. Blisters and erosions heal with superficial scar formation. Nail involvement is mild or absent. The pathology of the disease is similar to, but more superficial in depth than recessive dystrophic epidermolysis bullosa. Treatment is entirely symptomatic.

DERMATITIS HERPETIFORMIS (DH)

Although this disease is most frequent in adults, it also occurs in infants or children. Its chief features are grouped, tense vesicles or bullae that usually arise on erythematous or urticarial plaques; the disease is characterized by intense, often burning pruritus and a cyclic course. The lesions are symmetrical and frequently widespread, and the elbows, knees, groin, and buttocks are sites of predilection (Fig. 21). Papular, erythematous, or urticarial lesions may predominate, especially in mild cases, causing diagnostic confusion. Spontaneous exacerbations and remissions frequently occur, al-

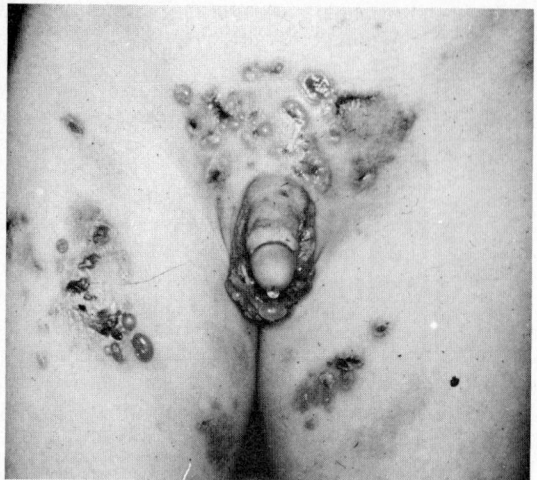

FIG. 21.   Dermatitis herpetiformis. Characteristic grouped vesicles and bullae, usually on an erythematous base.

though the disease tends to persist for several years. The morphology of the lesions may change from one episode to another. Sometimes figurate patterns develop as lesions spread. Individual lesions tend to heal after a relatively short course regardless of the general activity of the disease. The patient often excoriates the lesions. Healed lesions often become hyperpigmented. There is only rarely involvement of mucous membranes. General health is usually not affected, but blood eosinophilia is common. Small intestine abnormalities (frequently asymptomatic) are often found in patients with DH or in their relatives. The direct or indirect immunofluorescent basement membrane studies are negative. Histologically nonblistered areas show edema of individual dermal papillae with inflammatory cells including eosinophils. In well-developed blisters the base may be necrotic and the cavity filled with inflammatory cells, often predominantly eosinophils. The blister roof is usually not necrotic if the lesion is fresh.

Treatment consists of symptomatic management of the lesions with wet compresses and antibiotic or steroid ointments, and systemic administration of sulfones or sulfapyridine. Diaminodiphenyl sulfone is probably the drug of choice. Most children respond to relatively small doses of 25 to 100 mg daily. The chief side-reactions to the drug are mild hemolytic anemia and methemoglobinemia.

TOXIC EPIDERMAL NECROLYSIS (TEN) (SCALDED SKIN SYNDROME, LYELL'S DISEASE)

This recently characterized syndrome may occur at any age but is most common in infants and young children. Formerly, examples of the syndrome were likely to be diagnosed as acute "pemphigus," erythema multiforme, or unclassified toxic bullous eruptions. It is also now apparent that Ritter's disease is TEN in the newborn.

The onset of the disease may be explosive, or a single lesion may precede by a few hours or even days generalized involvement. In children purulent nasal discharge and perinasal and perioral impetigo are often the first lesions. In view of recent data clearly implicating a "toxin" of phage group 2 coagulase positive staphylococci in the pathogenesis of the disease in children, cases attributed to drugs in children are perhaps coincidental. In adults, however, drugs are clearly implicated in many, if not most, cases. Erythema is followed by loosening or loss of large sheets of epidermis, but occasionally the process occurs with minimal or no erythema. Slight frictional trauma to a noneroded area will loosen or erode the epidermis at that site (Nikolsky's sign). In eroded areas flaccid blisters often develop as fluid accumulates between the loosened layers. The entire skin including palms and soles may be involved and there may be erosive mucous membrane lesions. Children often spontaneously assume the knee-chest postion.

The skin is usually tender to light touch; fever and other signs of systemic toxicity usually are present. The active phase continues for about one week, and healing is usually complete by two weeks. Death is common in affected adults but uncommon in children (Figs. 22 and 23).

The disease is preceded in some instances by mild upper respiratory infections or a wide variety of other infectious and noninfectious diseases or by drug intake, but in other instances such factors have been absent.

Histology reveals separation at the dermoepidermal junction as a result of necrolysis and acantholysis of basal cells, or damage higher in the epidermis at the granular layer level. Most biopsy specimens from children have shown the granular layer pathology. At this higher level many cells have an acantholysis-like appearance. In contrast to pemphigus acantholysis, there may be actual splitting of desmosomes; in early lesions the alteration may be limited to a layer or two of cells. Later vacuolar degeneration at other levels may be

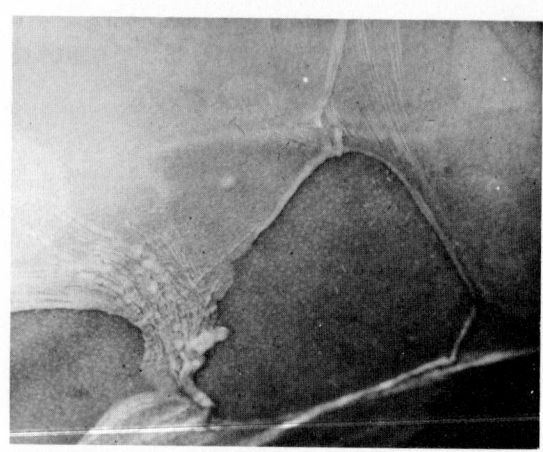

FIG. 22.   Toxic epidermolysis, childhood type. Characteristic loosening of large area of epidermis.

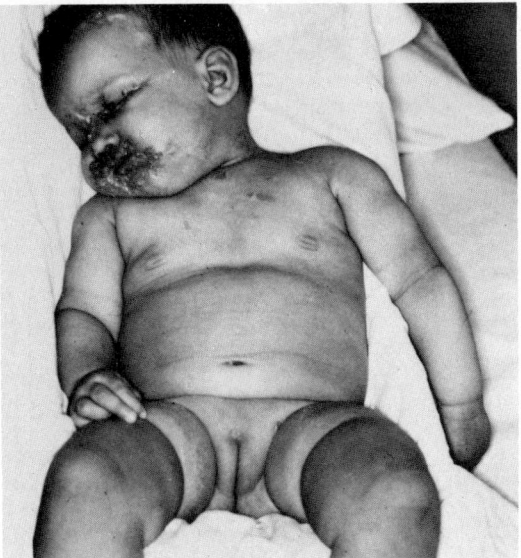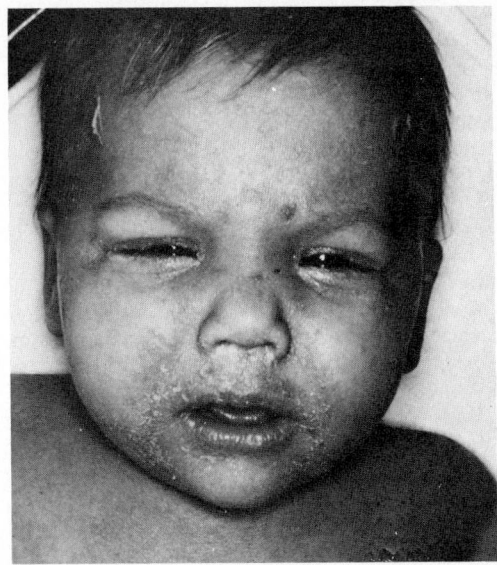

FIG. 23. Toxic epidermal necrolysis (Ritter-Lyell syndrome). Left. A 5½-month-old child with purulent conjunctivitis and nasal discharge for 4 days, impetigo about the mouth for 3 days, and blisters for 2 days. *Staphylococcus aureus.* Phage type II was cultured from her periorbital lesions. At the time of photograph the skin was generally erythematous and tender. There were blisters on the upper chest. She responded rapidly to antibiotic therapy. Right. A 6½-month-old girl with a 3-day history of eruption and nasal discharge. No bullae appeared spontaneously; however, Nikolsky's sign was positive. The child had the desquamative form of toxic epidermal necrolysis and responded rapidly to antibiotic therapy.

seen, and in basal layer (adult) cases the entire blister roof may be necrotic. In early lesions remarkably little inflammation is seen in the dermis, suggesting that the toxic process operative in this condition is relatively specific for the epithelium. Recently it has been demonstrated that a "toxin" from coagulase positive phage group 2 staphylococci can induce lesions in newborn mice similar clinically and histologically to childhood TEN. More mature animals are not susceptible. It is not known whether protection from the disease in more mature individuals results from substrate resistance or "inactivation" of the "toxin."

Treatment consists of reducing friction by removing clothes, gently applying lubrication, treatment of any local or systemic infections, administering prednisone in doses as high as 4 to 6 mg/kg/day, and general supportive care. In children the clinical course is characterized by spontaneous improvement; consequently, the improvement associated with the administration of steroids is difficult to evaluate. Observations on newborn mice suggest that steroids may have an adverse effect; however, steroids may be useful in selected infants and are indicated in adults whose disease is related to medications such as diphenylhydantoin.

Erythema Multiforme (EM)

This disease has an acute onset and can occur at any age. It is characterized by lesions that include erythematous macules, purpuric spots, papules, urticarial plaques, vesicles, and bullae. Individual lesions tend to develop central depressed brownish or violaceous areas that show epidermal necrosis histologically. When blisters develop, they occur on erythematous macular areas or urticarialike lesions. Concentric (iris-type) patterns of any type of lesion may develop, and may spread in striking polycyclic patterns (Fig. 24). Grouping may be present to some degree, causing confusion with dermatitis herpetiformis. Fortunately, the skin lesions are relatively asymptomatic. Distribution of the lesions favors the dorsum of the hands and neck, but lesions may be generalized. When mucous membranes are involved, there is usually an erosive stomatitis, often associated with fever, malaise, and other signs of systemic toxicity. When the conjunctiva and urethra are involved, the disease is sometimes called the *Stevens-Johnson syndrome.*

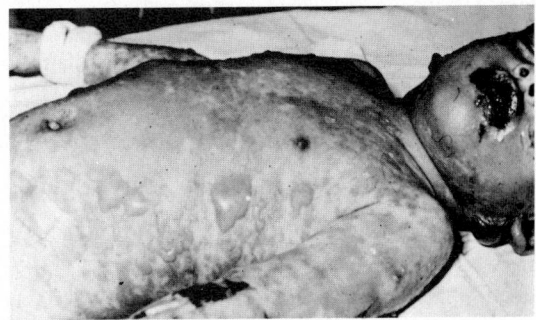

FIG. 24. Bullous erythema multiforme. Many vesicles and bullae on an erythematous base and erosive stomatitis.

However, it is difficult to separate this syndrome from other forms of bullous erythema multiforme.

Nevertheless, the concept of the Stevens-Johnson syndrome is important because of its severe clinical course, in contrast to the usual mild course of ordinary erythema multiforme. Typically, the onset is explosive, with fever, chills, malaise, and upper respiratory symptoms. Vesicles and pseudomembranous plaques that soon become hemorrhagic erosions usually develop first in the mouth, sometimes in the nasopharynx and on the lips. Most patients salivate profusely. Conjunctival involvement is generally erosive and may spread to the cornea. Severe corneal lesions may result in scar formation. When anal and urethral lesions occur, they are similar to oral lesions. Cutaneous involvement varies from none to generalized lesions of any morphologic erythema multiforme type. Maximal clinical activity occurs at seven to ten days; untreated, recovery occurs by four to six weeks. Milder forms of erythema multiforme usually have a somewhat shorter course. Mortality in severe erythema multiforme is usually "toxic" or due to intercurrent infection.

In some individuals erythema multiforme recurs regularly, particularly in spring and fall. Occasionally recurrences may be more frequent, and chronic forms have been described; the diagnosis is especially difficult in such cases.

Erythema multiforme has been associated with a great number of systemic conditions, including infections such as mycoplasma, streptococcus, herpes simplex, deep mycoses, and tuberculosis, connective tissue diseases, and sensitization to drugs; in most cases the cause is unknown. It is possible that many of these may be related to mild viral or mycoplasma infections.

Histologically, nonblistered lesions show edema of the upper dermis, angiitis of the small vessels, and often epidermal necrosis. Blisters are subepidermal. The blister roof is often necrotic, even in early lesions. Eosinophils may be present in the blister cavity, but lymphocytes usually predominate.

The treatment of erythema multiforme is dictated by the clinical state of the patient. Mild cases frequently respond to antihistamines. Anti-inflammatory steroids are indicated in cases with severe skin or mucous membrane involvement or when there is appreciable systemic toxicity. Prednisone, 2 to 6 mg/kg/day, or its equivalent, may be required to control the disease. The steroid should be reduced gradually to avoid relapse. Although response to systemic steroid administration may be dramatic, occasional patients do not respond at all. Kenalog in orabase adheres fairly well to mucosa and can be used on oral lesions. Mouthwashes with Dyclone solution reduce pain and facilitate eating.

Intravenous administration of nutrition and therapy is usually necessary in severe cases. Eye lesions are frequently responsive to local steroids, which should be used only after ophthalmologic consultation to rule out infection with herpes simplex. Skin lesions may be left alone if they are dry and asymptomatic; oozing lesions benefit from saline compresses, topical antibiotics, and/or steroids.

BULLOUS PEMPHIGOID (BP)

This disease is widely accepted as a distinct entity. It affects chiefly the elderly, but children may be affected. The onset is often insidious. Erythematous macules and plaques may precede blister development, but blisters frequently occur in nonerythematous areas. The erythematous lesions are sometimes arranged in patterns similar to those found in erythema multiforme. The blisters characteristically are tense bullae, but vesicles also occur. There is seldom any tendency to grouping of the lesions; the distribution is usually general, with some slight predilection for flexural surfaces. Rare cases of localized disease tend to involve the legs. There is sometimes involvement of the oral mucous membranes, consisting of erosions and an occasional intact blister. Most affected patients have mild to moderate pruritus or burning, though occasionally there is severe pruritus. Signs of systemic toxicity usually are absent. Individual lesions tend to heal quite rapidly, especially in children, but the natural course of the disease continues for months or years, with exacerbations and relative or complete remissions. In children the average total duration is usually about 4 years. Fatal cases have occurred only in adults, and then death is usually due to complications or concurrent disease.

Histologically, blisters develop at the dermoepidermal junction and are usually accompanied by mild inflammatory changes in the dermis. Early lesions may show tiny subepidermal vacuoles or, less commonly, edema and inflammation of papillae, thus resembling and causing confusion with dermatitis herpetiformis. The blister roof is sometimes necrotic, even in early lesions. Cells within the blister cavity may include many eosinophils, and there may be angiitis of the small vessels. The histology of bullous pemphigoid overlaps that of dermatitis herpetiformis and erythema multiforme, unless very early lesions are available for study so that, in a specific case, the histology may be helpful but not absolutely diagnostic. Only bullous pemphigoid shows positive immunofluorescent staining of the basement membrane area by direct or indirect techniques. These antibodies have not yet been shown to be involved in the pathogenic mechanism of the disease. In adults the disease is sometimes associated with malignancies or other severe systemic illness. In children it may be associated with other diseases, such as ulcerative colitis.

Treatment is with corticosteroids. Moderate doses are often sufficient, and it is frequently possible to reduce the dose to low maintenance levels or to discontinue the medication within a few weeks or months.

Bullous pemphigoid should not be confused with benign mucosal pemphigoid (ocular pemphigus, cicatricial pemphigoid), a disease that affects only adults and is characterized by erosions, especially of the oral, vaginal, and conjunctival mucous membranes, that frequently heal with scarring. On the skin, dermoepidermal blisters occasionally occur.

PEMPHIGUS (P)

Pemphigus (P) has been subclassified into four types —P. vulgaris, P. vegetans, P. foliaceus, and P. erythematosus (Senear-Usher syndrome)—but the current view is that there are only two basic types: P. vulgaris and P. foliaceus. P. vulgaris is extremely rare in children, and P. foliaceus is only slightly less rare. P. vulgaris and, to a lesser extent, P. foliaceus have an apparent predilection for Jewish people.

P. Vulgaris

This disease usually has an insidious onset. The initial lesions may occur anywhere on the skin as flaccid blisters of any size. On the oral mucosa, they usually appear as erosions. Blisters are easily eroded, and both erosions and intact blisters often enlarge, and heal slowly. Secondary infection is common. Usually, the blisters arise from normal-appearing skin, but the base is occasionally erythematous. Mild friction applied to uninvolved areas may result in loosening of the skin (Nikolsky's sign). Symptoms are more those of general discomfort than pruritus. The natural course of the disease is slow, with almost certain death following variable exacerbations and remissions. Treatment with high doses of anti-inflammatory steroids has greatly altered the formerly dismal picture.

P. vegetans is a variant of P. vulgaris in which there is apparent increased host resistance to the disease so that progression is retarded. The prognosis is considerably more favorable than that of classical P. vulgaris. This form is characterized by verrucous vegetations with a predilection for axillae and groin. Vesicles, bullae, and pustules may also be present.

P. Foliaceus

As with P. vulgaris, the onset of P. foliaceus is insidious. It most often presents early as very superficial erosions and flaccid bullae arising from erythematous patches. As partial healing and new blisters or erosions occur, the sloughed layers accumulate so that the lesions are crusted and scaly. Early lesions are frequently located with a butterfly distribution on the face, the scalp, upper chest, and back (Senear-Usher syndrome). Extension of the disease occurs by spread of old lesions or the development of new ones, sometimes producing figurate patterns. Uninvolved areas may show the Nikolsky sign. Gradually the entire skin surface may become involved, and at this stage blisters are uncommon. Mucous membrane lesions are rare. Pruritis and general discomfort are usually present. The prognosis in older patients is relatively favorable when judicious treatment is given, but spontaneous remissions also occur. Young patients remain in good health and are particularly likely to have a benign course with eventual remission.

Brazilian pemphigus (fogo selvagem) is clinically similar to P. foliaceus. Children and adolescents are frequently affected. The disease is localized to a relatively small area of the country, suggesting the possibility of an infectious etiologic determinant.

Histologically the hallmark of pemphigus is acantholysis, the loss of intercellular bridges with resultant separation of cells. In P. vulgaris the process occurs chiefly at the suprabasal level, whereas in P. foliaceus the process occurs at, or just beneath the granular layer. By direct or indirect immunofluorescent techniques antibodies localized between epidermal cells (or perhaps on cell membranes) may be demonstrated. The treatment of pemphigus is generally systemic administration of anti-inflammatory steroids in whatever dosage is necessary to achieve clinical control of the process. Use of an immunosuppressive is probably also effective but must be considered investigative. The long-term results in children are thought to be good.

BENIGN FAMILIAL PEMPHIGUS (HAILEY-HAILEY DISEASE)

This disease is characterized by vesicles, crusts, scales, vegetations, erythematous patches, and, rarely, bullae. The eruption is generally limited to a small area of the body, usually the neck, axillae, chest, or groin. Rarely plaques or erosions are present on the oral mucous membrane. The skin lesions are commonly secondarily infected. The disease is inherited as an autosomal dominant. Of particular interest is the fact that uninvolved skin responds to a variety of experimental insults with superficial acantholysis and dyskeratosis. These are also the chief histologic features of the natural disease. It appears that the defect involves increased susceptibility of the skin to the acantholytic type of response to injury, a response that all skin is capable of showing when appropriately injured.

Onset of the disease in childhood is rare. Adolescence and young adulthood are more common times for the initial lesions to appear. Repeated exacerbations and remissions throughout life are the usual course of the disease.

Therapy is largely directed against infection, which in the natural disease plays an important role. Local and systemic antibiotics and careful hygiene are of great value. Systemic anti-inflammatory steroids are also effective in high doses, but are usually not indicated because of the relative mildness of the disease. Topical steroids are often useful.

Hailey-Hailey disease is sometimes confused with Darier's disease, which may show blisters and crusts clinically and acantholysis histologically.

Bibliography

Bean SF, Good RA, Windhorst DB: Bullous pemphigoid in an 11-year-old boy. Arch Dermatol 102:205, 1970

Jordan RE, Bean SF, Triftshause CT, Winkelmann RK: Childhood bullous dermatitis herpetiformis. Negative immunofluorescent tests. Arch Dermatol 101:629, 1970

Lever W: Pemphigus and Pemphigoid. CC Thomas, Springfield, Ill, 1965

MacVicar DN, Graham JH, Burgoon CF: Dermatitis herpetiformis, erythema multiforme, and bullous pemphigoid: A comparative histopathological and histochemical study. J Invest Dermatol 41:289, 1963

Melish ME, Glasgow LA: The staphylococcal scalded-skin syndrome. Development of an experimental model. N Engl J Med 282:1114, 1970

Pearson RW: Studies on the pathogenesis of epidermolysis bullosa. J Invest Dermatol 39:551, 1962

Schroeter A, Sams WM Jr, Jordan RE: Immunofluorescent studies of pemphigus foliaceus in a child. Arch Dermatol 100:736, 1969

Silver HF: Epidermolysis bullosa hereditaria "letalis." Report of a case surviving for two and a half years. Arch Dis Child 32:216, 1957

INFECTIONS OF THE SKIN

JOSEPH W. BURNETT

BACTERIAL INFECTIONS (PYODERMA)

Streptococcal and Staphylococcal Infections

The pyodermas are cutaneous infections that occur at different levels of the skin and usually are caused by *Staphylococcus aureus* and/or Group A β-hemolytic streptococci. *Impetigo,* the superficial infection, involves primarily the upper epidermis. In *ecthyma,* the lower epidermis and dermis are the sites of infection. *Folliculitis* is a superficial infection of the hair follicle, whereas *furunculosis* is an infection of the deeper regions of the follicle. When organisms invade both the dermis and subcutaneous tissues the infection is termed a *cellulitis.*

ETIOLOGY AND EPIDEMIOLOGY. Pyodermas are a common group of diseases. Their epidemiology depends upon the nature of the bacterial pathogen, the level of the infection within the skin, and the presence or absence of bacterial infections in other regions of the body. These diseases may be spread by direct contact of susceptible individuals with contaminated crusts or debris.

It is futile to predict clinically whether an impetiginous lesion is caused by a streptococcus or a staphylococcus, since both microorganisms can often be recovered from the same lesion. Group A β-hemolytic streptococci are the most important biologic agents causing crusted impetigo. Bullous lesions may often be present in staphylococcal disease. Mixed infections of both microorganisms may cause pyodermas superimposed on other dermatologic diseases.

The epidemiology of these infections is complex. Concurrent cutaneous infections due to multiple strains of the same bacterial species may occur. The streptococci associated with pyoderma differ from those causing respiratory infections. Nonetheless, it appears that the streptococcus responsible for pyodermas may be transferred to the respiratory tract and the pathogenic staphylococcus appears to originate elsewhere on the skin.

Because the lesions of folliculitis and furunculosis appear as sharply circumscribed abscesses, they have been thought to be caused only by the staphylococcus. However, in a few instances, Group A β-hemolytic streptococci have been isolated from purulent material in these lesions.

The deepest cutaneous infection, cellulitis, involves the dermis and subcutaneous tissues. This disease usually is caused by either the streptococcus or the staphylococcus rather than by a combination of the two. In small children and in infants, *H. influenzae* may be the agent causing cellulitis.

PATHOLOGY. The pyodermas produce an acute inflammatory reaction in the skin. In impetigo this reaction occurs in the subcorneal epidermis where a vesicle containing bacteria, polymorphonuclear cells, and exudative fluid is formed. When the vesicle ruptures a crust containing fibrin and leukocytes lies directly on the prickle cell layer. A similar inflammatory infiltration appears in the lower epidermis and upper dermis in ecthyma, around the hair follicle in folliculitis and furunculosis, and in the dermis and subcutaneous tissues in cellulitis.

Because streptococci and staphylococci are ubiquitous, infection often occurs after trauma, which provides a foothold in the skin for the organism.

CLINICAL MANIFESTATIONS. Cutaneous infections may be localized at several different layers (Fig. 25). This location determines the severity and the communicability of the infection. The deeper the bacteria in the skin and the closer they reside in the dermal blood vessels, the more marked will be the constitutional symptoms and the greater the danger of septicemia. The more superficial bacterial infections have exudates on the skin surface and are therefore more communicable.

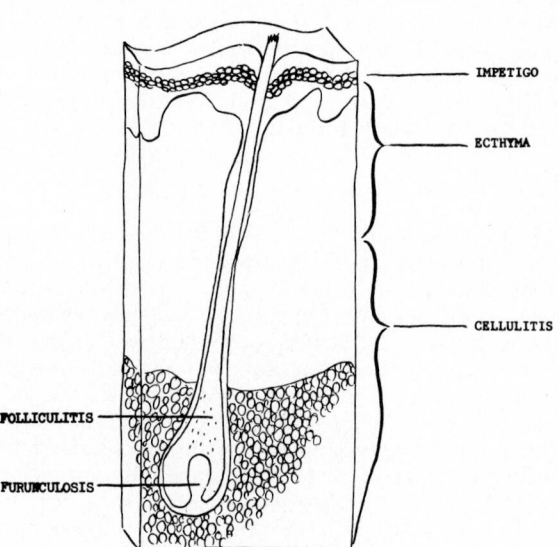

FIG. 25.   The location of various pyodermas within the skin.

The clinical appearance of pyodermas also varies according to the location of infection in the skin. The initial lesion of impetigo, a vesicle, is rarely seen; however, when vesicles do appear (bullous impetigo), they are multiple, whitish yellow, and may or may not have a thick wall (Fig. 26A and B). In streptococcal impetigo or in patients whose lesions are due to a mixed streptococcal and staphylococcal infection, the vesicles have usually ruptured, leaving a raw erythematous base covered with a yellow or honey-colored crust, the hallmark of the disease. Although fever and leukocytosis are not

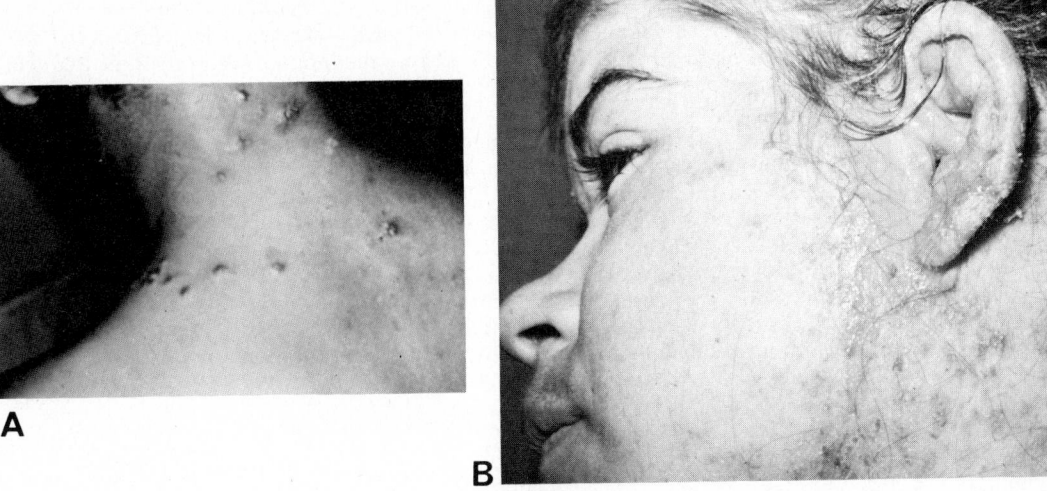

FIG. 26. **A.** Staphylococcal impetigo. **B.** Impetigo of the ear. Note the crusted exudative lesions and the edema of the ear.

usual, temperatures of 37.5 to 38 C may be recorded. Regional lymphadenopathy is present in most of the patients, especially those with streptococcal infections.

Ecthyma, an infection localized to the upper dermis and characterized by thick brown or black crusts covering raw, erythematous bases, is bacteriologically similar to impetigo and should be regarded as the same disease situated in a deeper plane of the skin.

One of the most common pyodermas occurs when preexisting dermatologic eruptions become secondarily infected. In these cases the underlying eruption becomes erythematous and is covered with a purulent exudate (Fig. 27).

Although yellow pustules surround hair follicles in both folliculitis and furunculosis, erythema, pain, and edema of the surrounding skin occur only in the lesions

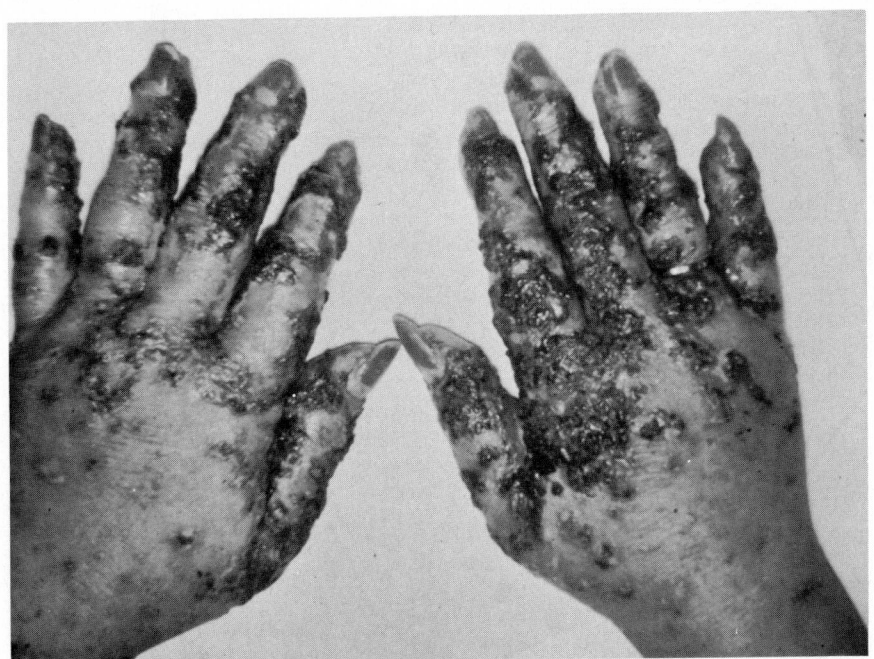

FIG. 27. Pyoderma. Superinfection of preexisting hand dermatitis.

of furunculosis, where the focus of infection is deeper. Chronic furunculosis may be an initial symptom of underlying diabetes, lymphoma, or agammaglobulinemia; however, the vast majority of cases occur in otherwise healthy individuals. Repeated phage typing of organisms from lesions of patients with furunculosis reveals that the same type of bacterium may be recovered from different furuncles in the same individual for prolonged periods of time.

Cellulitis may appear anywhere on the body, although the extremities, face, and regions around wounds are areas of predilection. Clinically, the affected skin is warm, erythematous, tender, edematous, and indurated. The patients usually have fever, malaise, and regional lymphadenopathy. The erythematous lesions of erysipelas are further characterized by rapidly advancing, well-demarcated borders. Occasionally vesicles or bullae may be present. Later, the lesions turn brown in color and finally desquamate.

Infections of the skin caused by certain strains of toxin-producing staphylococci may result in blistering and desquamation (scalded skin syndrome). This syndrome, seen mostly in children younger than six years, is a serious condition when it occurs in infancy (see p. 872).

Cellulitis due to *Haemophilus influenzae* should be considered in children of 6 to 24 months of age if the lesion appears on the face and the child has an elevated temperature. A characteristic purple color is seen in the affected skin in about half of the patients with *H. influenzae* cellulitis. A positive blood culture often confirms the diagnosis. Cellulitis due to pneumococci or haemophilus can occur in drug addicts who contaminate their injection equipment with saliva.

DIAGNOSIS. Gram-stained smears and cultures of purulent material or of the raw bases under the crusts will help confirm the diagnosis and determine the appropriate antibiotic by in vitro sensitivity tests. Culture inocula from cellulitis may be obtained by injecting and withdrawing sterile saline into the lesions. Serial serum antistreptolysin O titers are not as accurate as anti-DNase B and antihyaluronidase levels in cases of suspected streptococcal infections.

DIFFERENTIAL DIAGNOSIS. Facial impetigo may be differentiated from herpes simplex by smears or cultures. Cellulitis occurring on the malar region of the face may be confused with lupus erythematosus. Infected acne or inflamed sebaceous cysts may be misdiagnosed as furunculosis.

TREATMENT. Pyodermas should be considered as mixed infections caused by both Group A β-hemolytic streptococcus and *staphylococcus aureus*. Staphylococcal infections usually isolate themselves, their course may not be acute, and they may heal spontaneously. However, in some instances, especially in infants, septicemia may result, in which case prompt vigorous treatment is especially important. Streptococcal infections tend to progress more rapidly and early treatment is always important.

Topical antibiotics in the treatment of impetigo are inferior to systemic antibiotics. Because of the danger of inducing sensitivity by the topical application of an antibiotic agent, the antibiotic contained in such ointments should be one that is rarely used systemically.

Scrubbing the lesions, compresses, or frequent soap baths alone are insufficient therapy however; aseptic incision and drainage may be all that is necessary for some cases of furunculosis or folliculitis. Isolation procedures designed to prevent spread of the infection to other individuals should be enforced in cases where the lesions are either superficially located or draining purulent material. Therapy of chronic furunculosis is unsatisfactory. Staphylococcal vaccines have not been effective. An initial course of an antibiotic shown to be effective in vitro is the first step. Family members of patients with streptococcal lesions should be examined in order to detect carriers.

Erythrasma

Erythrasma is an asymptomatic cutaneous disease that appears in the toewebs, axilla, and inguinal regions.

ETIOLOGY. The etiologic agent of erythrasma (*Nocardia minutissima*), formerly regarded as a fungus, is now known to be a gram-positive bacillus (a Corynebacterium).

INCIDENCE AND EPIDEMIOLOGY. Erythrasma of the toewebs occurs in approximately 25 percent of the population. Axillary and pubic erythrasma is not uncommon. Generalized cutaneous erythrasma, however, is present mostly in tropical and subtropical areas. The mode of transmission is unknown.

PATHOLOGY. In erythrasma there is a mild inflammatory reaction involving only the superficial epidermis.

CLINICAL MANIFESTATIONS. The characteristic lesions of this disease include the following: scaling, fissuration, maceration of the toewebs, and dry, brown, slightly scaly, irregular, well-demarcated patches in the axillary, inguinal, submammary, and intergluteal areas. Coral red fluorescence, presumably due to porphyrins produced by these organisms, may be seen on Wood's light examination.

DIAGNOSIS. The diagnosis must be made clinically. Bacillary and coccoid forms are seen on microscopic examination of scrapings from the lesions. Tinea pedis and various pigmentary disorders are the most common diseases confused with erythrasma.

TREATMENT. Topical salicylic acid ointment is the therapy of choice. Although the erythrasma organism is sensitive to erythromycin as well as to other antibiotics, these drugs are usually not necessary to effect a cure. Some antibacterial bar soaps are effective in the prophylaxis and control of this disease.

VIRAL INFECTIONS

Herpes Zoster

Herpes zoster and chickenpox are infections caused by varicella-zoster (V-Z) virus, chickenpox being caused by an individual's initial exposure to this agent. The pathogenesis of herpes zoster is not known. The accepted theory is that zoster is caused by a reactivation of a latent varicella virus, although the possibility exists that zoster may occasionally be a result of exogenous reinfection.

ETIOLOGY. The viruses isolated from patients with zoster and varicella are regarded as the same agent because of similarities in ultramicroscopic morphology, tissue culture propagation, and antigenic cross-reactivity. The virus of varicella zoster is classified in the herpes virus group. It measures 200 μ in diameter, and DNA is its predominant nucleoprotein. The virus has been isolated from both vesicular and cerebrospinal fluid. Man is the only natural or experimental host. In vitro propagation of this agent can be readily performed in tissue culture systems prepared from a number of human tissues.

INCIDENCE AND EPIDEMIOLOGY. Zoster occurs sporadically at any time of year. The highest age incidence of the disease is between 40 and 70 years, although cases frequently appear at an earlier age. Approximately 50 percent of the population will suffer an attack of zoster before age 75. Zoster is unusual in infants, although it has been reported in a child 3.5 months of age.

Transmission of the disease is thought to occur by direct contact of susceptible individuals with infected crusts or vesicle fluids. Zoster patients are contagious for at least 5 to 7 days after the the vesicles appear, since virus can be isolated from the lesions during that period. Outbreaks of varicella have been initiated by exposing susceptible persons to zoster patients. The absence of virus from the nasopharynx might explain why zoster is not so contagious as varicella.

A history of recent exposure to either zoster or varicella is usually not obtained, a finding reinforcing the concept of latent virus reactivation. Mechanical and thermal trauma have been cited as factors capable of intitiating zoster attacks.

The appearance of zoster in the older age groups and in patients with leukemia or lymphoma may be explained by a decrease in antiviral immunity or T-cell incompetence.

PATHOLOGY AND PATHOGENESIS. The initial cytologic changes in zoster are margination of the nuclear chromatin and formation of an intranuclear inclusion body. An intraepidermal vesicle appears after the cells of the lower epidermal layers undergo balloon degeneration. A polymorphonuclear cell infiltration occurs in the corium, particularly around the blood vessels. Giant cells are seen in both the infected tisues and vesicular fluid. Similar cytologic changes may be visible in cells of the dorsal root ganglion, corresponding to the dermatome of zoster involvement. Likewise, involvement of anterior horn cells of the spinal cord and leptomeningitis can occur. The Landry-Guillain-Barré syndrome accompanying this disease may be a result of immunologic injury to the nervous system.

CLINICAL MANIFESTATIONS. Zoster produces a peripheral neuritis and a vesicular eruption. The latter is characterized by grouped vesicles on an erythema-

tous base located in the distribution of the infected spinal or cranial sensory nerves (Fig. 28). Some of the vesicles may be umbilicated. Within a few days the vesicles range from a clear to a white or yellow color as cells and detritus accumulate within the vesicular fluid. Hemorrhagic vesicles appear in rare instances and are not necessarily an ominous sign. When the vesicles rupture, a yellow crust or superficial ulcer remains. Some lesions later become gangrenous and necrotic, and assume a "punched-out" appearance. Regional lymphadenopathy, fever, and constitutional symptoms may accompany the eruption. Nerve root pain may precede, accompany, or follow the eruption; there is no correlation between the severity of the cutaneous lesion and the intensity of the pain. Cutaneous scarring can occur.

Zoster may affect any area of the body. The thoracic area is involved in more than 50 percent of cases, followed by the cervical, trigeminal, and lumbar areas in that order. Vesicular lesions on the mucous membrane of the mouth and eye appear in association with cutaneous lesions in that dermatome. Vesicles located on the face, between the tip of the nose and the inner canthus, signify involvement of the nasociliary nerve and possibly the cornea. Trigeminal zoster is not an uncommon complication of surgery performed on the gasserian

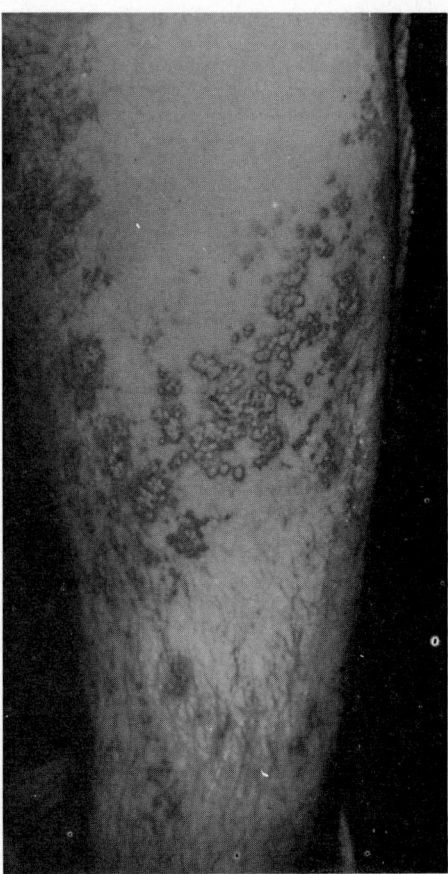

FIG. 28.   Herpes zoster. Grouped vesicle restricted in location.

ganglion. Zoster infection of the eye is accompanied by keratoconjunctivitis, scleritis, iridocyclitis, corneal ulceration, and scarring.

The neurologic symptoms include pain, loss of sensation, and motor weakness in the involved dermatome. Approximately 25 percent of the patients have a slightly elevated protein concentration or pleocytosis in cerebrospinal fluid. Autonomic motor symptoms, such as ileus or bladder paralysis, have been found in cases of zoster involving the lumbosacral dermatomes. Encephalitis has been reported, usually after cases of ophthalmic zoster. Persistent or severe pain during the active disease is unusual in children. Postherpetic neuralgia is rare in childhood.

One interesting type of herpes zoster is the generalized form. In these patients the eruption is initially restricted to a few dermatomes, but within a few days scattered single vesicles appear elsewhere on the body. Pulmonary infiltrates, presumably zoster pneumonitis, are present in some cases. Although a significant number of adult patients have an underlying lymphoma or other immunologic abnormality, this relationship has not been striking in children.

DIAGNOSIS. The diagnosis of zoster may be aided by examination of a smear of vesicle fluid for giant cells and intranuclear inclusion bodies (Fig. 29). Cultures of the vesicle fluid are the only conclusive diagnostic test. The demonstration of intranuclear inclusion bodies by biopsy is usually not necessary, but may be done to exclude smallpox infections, which are characterized by intracytoplasmic inclusions. Serologic tests for zoster include neutralization, complement fixation, and immunofluorescence assays. Antibody may be found in both "slow" and "fast" IgG components, whereas in varicella only the former fraction is positive. Diagnostic

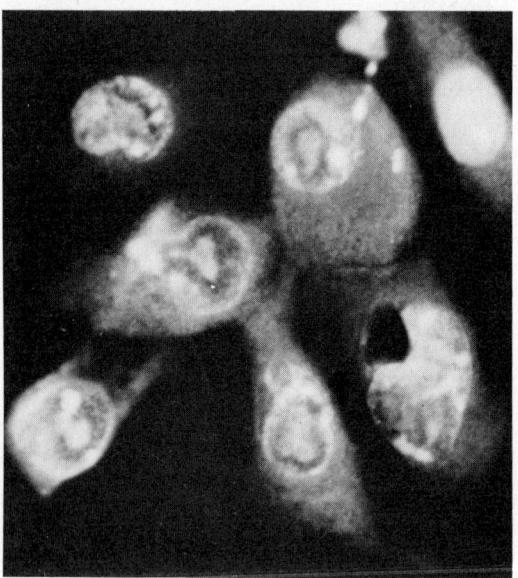

FIG. 29. Intranuclear inclusion bodies are visible within a primary culture of human cells infected with the V-Z virus.

gel diffusion studies can be performed with vesicular fluid and known specific antisera.

DIFFERENTIAL DIAGNOSIS. Smallpox may be differentiated from generalized zoster by physical examination, history, biopsy, and a smear of vesicular fluid. Eczema herpeticum and varicella may be confused with generalized zoster. Patients in whom neuralgia precedes the eruption may be thought to have pleurisy or peritonitis. Rickettsialpox may be differentiated from early zoster by the appearance of an initial bite, the presence of fever before the rash, the character of the eruption, and a complement fixation test.

Herpes simplex can be differentiated by culture and serologic tests from herpes zoster, which it sometimes mimics.

TREATMENT. No definitive therapy is available for this disease. Symptomatic relief may be obtained with analgesics and topical and open wet dressings. Corticosteroids, injected beneath the vesicles, may reduce the morbidity of the process. Because most zoster patients develop this disease despite the presence of antibodies, gamma globulin theoretically should be without benefit. Varicella can be prevented in susceptible individuals exposed to zoster patients by administering zoster-immune globulin promptly.

Molluscum Contagiosum

Molluscum contagiosum is a viral disease of the skin characterized by an umbilicated papule.

ETIOLOGY. Molluscum is classified as a pox virus because of its morphologic similarity with other viruses of that group. On ultramicroscopic examination molluscum particles have a dumbbell-shaped core with two surrounding envelopes. Its diameters have been estimated to be 300 by 200 mμ. Man is the only natural or experimental host. Lesions in the skin of human volunteers have been produced within two to seven weeks by subcutaneous inoculation of molluscum suspensions. Extracts of ground molluscum lesions inoculated into cell cultures prepared from various primate tissues produces a cytotoxic reaction within 48 hours. In vitro growth has been achieved in cell culture systems incubated at 30 C, but this procedure is tedious.

INCIDENCE AND EPIDEMIOLOGY. Molluscum lesions may appear at any age, but most occur in childhood. Epidemics have been reported from institutions caring for mentally retarded children and in the populations of various Pacific islands. It is reasonable to conclude that the virus spreads by direct contact, although the exact source in most cases ·is unknown. Autoinoculation is common.

PATHOLOGY AND PATHOGENESIS. The well-demarcated molluscum lesion is pear-shaped and has its base in the upper dermis. As the infected cells move upward toward the center of the lesion, they become more distorted. The first changes consist of an appearance of electron-dense intranuclear particles and later intracellular DNA bodies. The nucleus becomes compressed and marginated as the islands of DNA material, which contain virus, enlarge and coalesce to form inclusion bodies. The surrounding epidermis shows considerable acanthosis.

CLINICAL MANIFESTATIONS. The lesions are discrete, pearly gray, 1 to 5 mm, umbilicated papules, which appear anywhere on the skin (Fig. 30) or conjunctiva. A reactive keratitis or conjunctivitis may accompany lesions at the latter site. Usually there is no inflammation surrounding these lesions, unless they are traumatized or secondarily infected. Healing occurs without scarring in lesions free from bacterial superinfection.

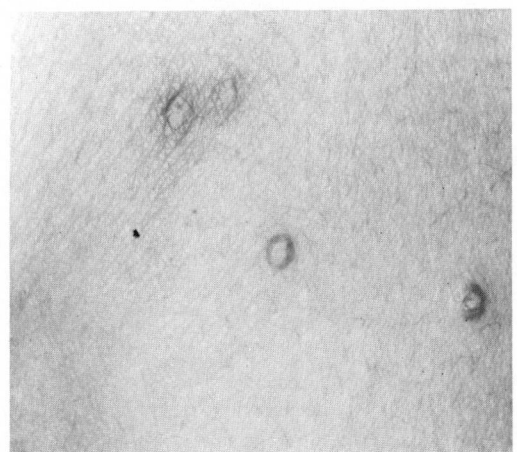

FIG. 30. Molluscum contagiosum. Typical lesions on the back of a 17-year-old boy. The umbilicated papule is produced by a virus resembling poxvirus.

DIAGNOSIS. The three best diagnostic procedures are staining smears of the expressed molluscum body (Fig. 31), examining a biopsy or inoculating a molluscum suspension into cell cultures in order to demonstrate the cytotoxic reaction.

The only other disease characterized by an umbilicated papule is lichen planus, which can be differentiated by its flexural distribution and purplish color. Molluscum has been confused with chickenpox, warts, papillomas, epitheliomas, furunculosis, and pyoderma.

TREATMENT. The easiest form of treatment is to remove the lesions with a sharp curette, under aseptic technique. Anesthesia is usually not necessary. Care must be taken to destroy all lesions to prevent autoinoculation.

Limited studies suggest that isatin, a thiosemicarbazine, may be effective in decreasing spread of the virus to susceptible persons during epidemics.

Warts (Verrucae)

Warts are a common viral disease characterized by flesh-colored, hyperplastic papules on the skin.

ETIOLOGY. Wart virus has been classified as a papova virus with a diameter calculated to be 38 mμ. This agent is a DNA virus. Filtered wart extracts in-

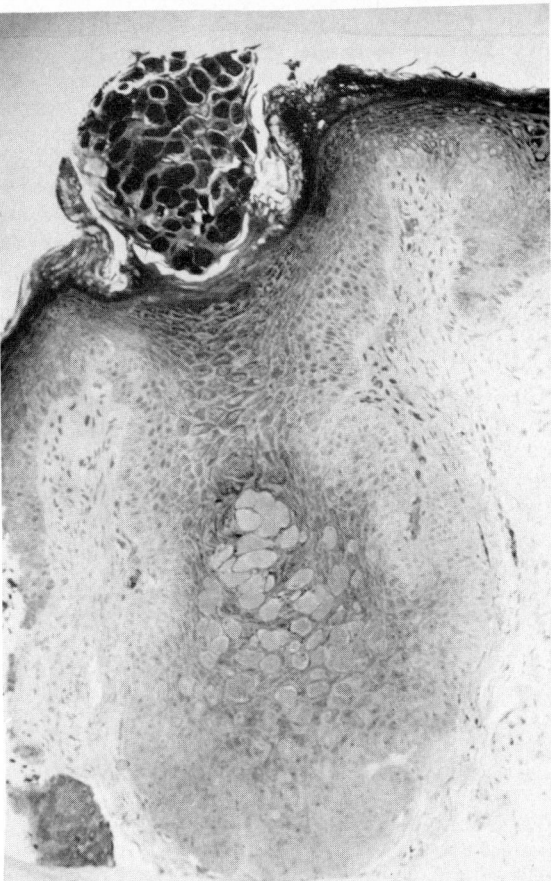

FIG. 31. Molluscum body. The well-demarcated epidermal lesion is shown with the large cytoplasmic inclusion seen in the cells of the granular and corneal layer.

jected into the skin of volunteers have produced lesions at the inoculation site after one to six months. In vitro propagation of wart virus has not yet been satisfactorily accomplished. No serologic procedures are available except as research tools.

INCIDENCE AND EPIDEMIOLOGY. Warts are one of the most common human dermatologic diseases; they are particularly prevalent in childhood but may occur at any age. The mode of transmission is unknown but thought to be due to direct contact. Autoinoculation can occur.

PATHOLOGY. The wart is a well-delineated hyperplastic papule extending in depth to the basal layer. There are acanthosis, parakeratosis, and hyperkeratosis within the lesion. The involved cells exhibit a progression of cellular alterations as they advance upward toward the surface. Viral packets have been discovered in both the cytoplasm and nucleus. The "dots" grossly visible on the top of warts represent thrombosed capillaries in the long thin dermal papillae, which extend high into the lesion.

CLINICAL MANIFESTATIONS. Warts are flesh-colored papules that may assume several morphologic types. *Plantar and palmar warts* are elevated or flat lesions that interrupt the natural skin lines and may, at times, be painful. Close examination may reveal punctate dots scattered over the surface. *Filiform warts*, commonly seen on the face and neck, are small fingerlike excrescences which protrude 1 to 10 mm above the skin surface. *Flat warts* are discrete, multiple, flesh-colored or slightly brown, stippled papules measuring 2 to 5 mm in diameter. These lesions appear commonly on the face or extensor arm surfaces (Fig. 32). Common warts, *verrucae vulgaris*, appear predominantly on the dorsal surface of the hands or periungual regions but may be seen anywhere. They measure 3 to 10 mm in diameter, are gray, brown, or flesh-colored, and are definitely elevated (Fig. 33). "Venereal" warts, *verrucae accuminata*,

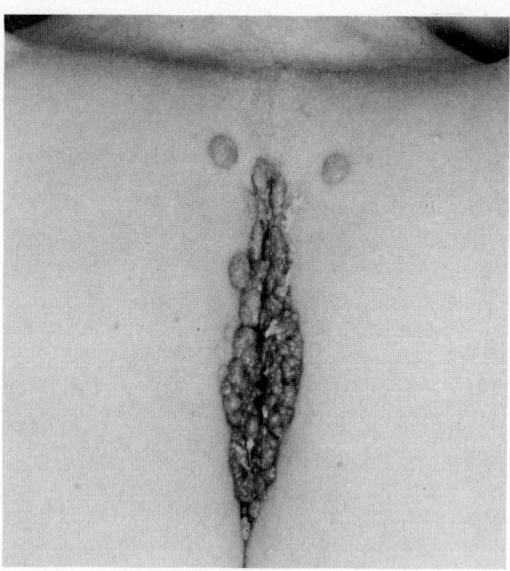

FIG. 34. Condyloma accuminatum. Perianal warts in 2-year-old boy. These genital or perianal warts are thought to be caused by the virus responsible for common warts.

occur on the genital regions; they are flesh-colored, wet, cauliflower papules that may be single or confluent (Fig. 34).

DIAGNOSIS.   The histologic picture of warts is pathognomonic (see under Pathology).

A plantar wart that obliterates the normal skin lines may be differentiated from a callus, which does not. Periungual fibromas in tuberous sclerosis may be misdiagnosed as warts. "Venereal" warts must be differentiated from the flat, raw condyloma lata by dark field examination and by the absence of a positive serology for syphilis. Flat warts may be misdiagnosed as acne, seborrheic keratoses, epidermal nevi, or freckles.

TREATMENT.   Warts are capricious in their behavior; some resolve spontaneously within a few months, but others will persist for prolonged periods of time. Cures by suggestion or hypnosis have been reported. In spite of such reports the only satisfactory treatment for warts are destructive measures. For verruca vulgaris the topical application of strong acids, such as 90 percent trichloroacetic acid, is used, although application of a plaster containing 40 percent salicylic acid is preferable in children because the procedure is relatively painless. Electrodesiccation, carbon dioxide snow, and liquid nitrogen are useful but painful. The treatment of choice for plantar warts is repeated applications of the salicylic acid plaster and for venereal warts topical podophyllin (25 percent solution in benzoin). Twelve percent salicylic acid in collodion, applied twice daily, may be effective against flat warts. The frequency of application for all keratolytic or acid treatments should be determined after the patient's reaction to one application has been observed. X-ray therapy or surgical excision should not be used. Recurrences are common regardless of the treatment.

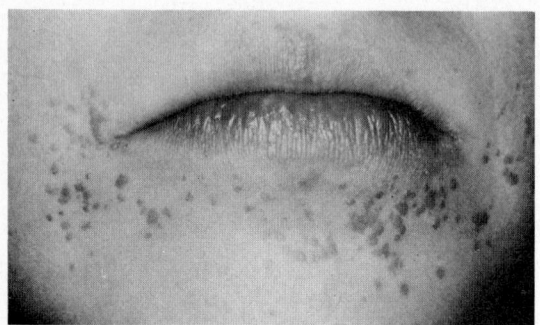

FIG. 32.   Flat warts (verruca plana). These warts often occur on the face and are thought to be caused by the same virus responsible for common warts (verruca vulgaris). Flat warts are usually skin-colored or slightly hyperpigmented.

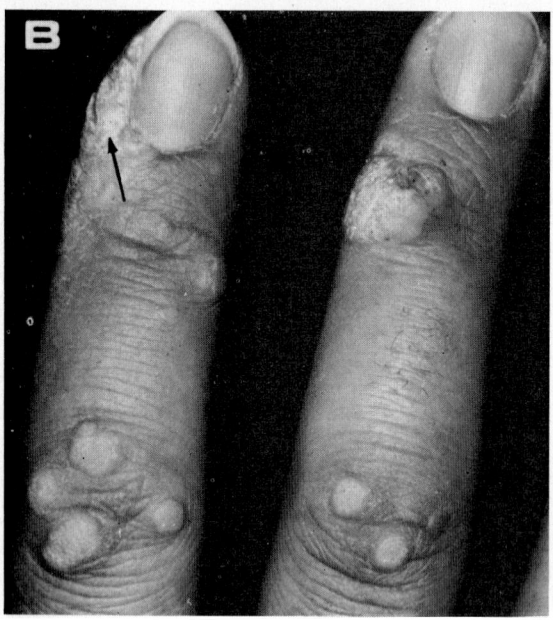

FIG. 33.   Verruca vulgaris. Warts in periungual location (arrow) sometimes produce deformity of the nail and are difficult to treat.

FUNGAL INFECTIONS

Many species of fungi are pathogenic to humans. The cutaneous infections caused by these organisms are commonly classified according to the depth of the pathologic process: ultrasuperficial, cutaneous, intermediate, and subcutaneous. Those fungi that cause primary subcutaneous lesions may produce a systemic infection, and conversely, systemic fungal infections may also cause cutaneous or subcutaneous lesions. Other classification schemes are based on the species of fungus, the anatomic sites of predilection, or the morphology of the lesion (Table 3). It is necessary to identify the species of invading organism as closely as possible in order to direct specific therapy and proper epidemiologic procedures.

Etiology and Clinical Manifestations

ULTRA SUPERFICIAL FUNGI. These organisms invade only the superficial skin, causing no symptoms or inflammatory reactions. *Tinea versicolor* is the cutaneous infection produced by *Malassezia furfur.* Asymptomatic, superficial, fawn or tan-colored, finely scaled lesions appear on the upper thorax, neck, axilla, and groin. In Blacks or suntanned Caucasians these lesions are hypopigmented and, except for scaling, might be misdiagnosed as vitiligo. There is no surrounding reactive erythema. The lesions are often confluent. Fungus structures consisting of round, thick-walled, refractile spherical spores and straight or curved, short or long, mycelial elements are seen microscopically.

CUTANEOUS FUNGAL INFECTIONS. Cutaneous fungal infections are caused by the "ringworm fungi" (dermatophytes). These organisms are divided into three common genera based on morphologic differences in their asexual spores (macroconidia) as seen on culture mounts. *Microsporum* species attack hair and skin. *Epidermophyton* invades nails and skin. *Trichophyton* may produce diseases in all three structures.

MICROSPORUM INFECTIONS. Microsporum species (*canis, audouini,* and *gypseum*) are the most common causes of *tinea capitis.* These fungi are characterized by single, spindle-shaped, thick-walled, rough macroconidia, and small microconidia. The latter are usually single, except in the case of *M. gypseum,* where grouping may be present. The microspora are naturally found in soil and on human or animal hosts. Although *M. canis* or *gypseum* may be transmitted to man from either young animals or other humans, *M. audouini* is probably transmitted only from human to human.

TABLE 3. Classification of Fungal Infections of the Skin

Dermatophyte	Clinical Appearance	Site of Predilection	Fluorescence Characteristic
Malassezia furfur	Tinea versicolor	Chest, back	
Microsporum			
canis	Less inflammatory scalp disease	Scalp (ectothrix)	Blue green
audouini	Scaly and inflamed scalp patches	Scalp (ectothrix)	Blue green
gypseum	Scaly and inflamed scalp patches	Scalp (ectothrix)	Some are blue green
Epidermophyton floccosum	Maceration	Toewebs	
	Starts on upper inner thigh	Tinea cruris onychomycosis not common	
Trichophyton			
mentographytes	Thickened white nails	Tinea pedis and onychomycosis	
verrucosum	Edematous, scaly may have pustules	Anywhere	
tonsurans	Black dot ringworm	Hair (endothrix)	
violaceum	Black dot ringworm	Hair	
schoenleine	Favus with scutula	Anywhere	
rubrum	Papulosquamous eruption granulomas	Hips, groin, palms, soles	

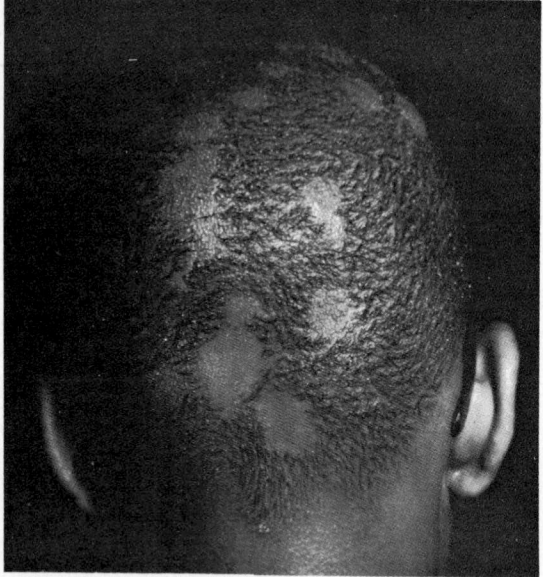

FIG. 35.   *Tinea capitis.*

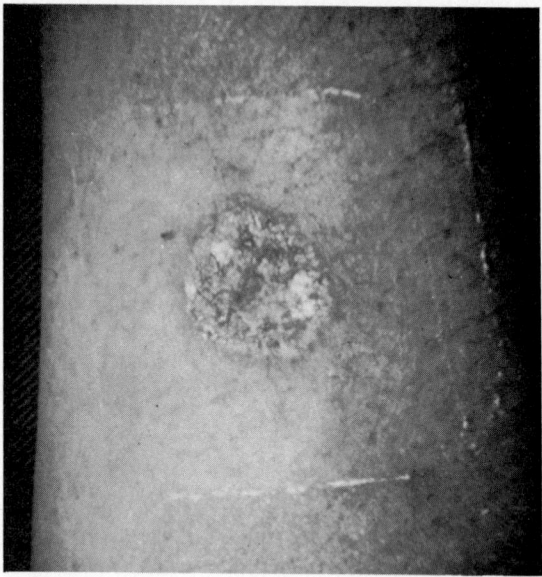

FIG. 36.   *Tinea circinata.* A clearing central scaly area surrounded by a peripheral ring of vesicles.

Hairs infected with microsporum species have mycelia within the hair shaft but spores on the hair surface (ectothrix). Microsporum infections produce well-demarcated, gray patches of partial alopecia and scaling (Fig. 35). A surrounding inflammatory reaction is more often seen in *M. gypseum* or *canis* infections than in those caused by *M. audouini.* One manifestation of the inflammatory reaction, *kerion celsi,* occurs after the infection has been present a few weeks. Kerions are large, localized, single or multiple, baggy, edematous lesions of the scalp containing considerable amounts of pus. The hair in this region is matted to the scalp by exudate. These purulent lesions are deeper than the ordinary scaly patches and are thought to represent an immune reaction of the host to the fungi. They are regarded as a favorable sign. Slow spontaneous resolution will follow unless secondary bacterial infections intervene. Microsporum infections of the glabrous skin are characterized by oval patches with central scaling and a peripheral ring or vesicles (Fig 36). The central scaly zone may heal as the peripheral area enlarges. These lesions are clinically indistinguishable from other causes of tinea corporis or tinea circinata. Adults are relatively resistant to these infections.

EPIDERMOPHYTON INFECTIONS.   The genus *Epidermophyton* contains only one species, *Epidermophyton floccosum.* This organism, which has club-shaped, thin-walled, two- to five-celled macroconidia, is found on humans and in the soil. Epidermophyton infects nails and skin. It is one of the common causes of *tinea pedis* (athlete's foot) or *tinea cruris.* The lesions in tinea pedis commonly begin in the fourth toeweb with maceration and fissuring. Other toewebs are soon involved as the eruption spreads over the foot. In the groin the disease starts as a scaly, elliptic patch on the inner thigh. The inguinal fold is spared initially, but within a few

weeks the eruption may spread, involving both the fold and pubic area. Epidermophyton lesions may or may not exhibit clearing in the center as the patch enlarges. Later, smaller, erythematous, satellite lesions appear around the larger, primary sites. Although not common, *onychomycosis* and tinea pedis can be produced by this organism.

TRICHOPHYTON INFECTIONS.   The genus Trichophyton contains six important species, which have smooth, thin-walled, two- to ten-celled, rounded macroconidia.

Trichophyton rubrum invades nails and epidermis, rarely hair. On the glabrous skin this organism causes dull, red, thick, scaly lesions without surrounding erythema or inflammation (Fig. 37). Complete or partial

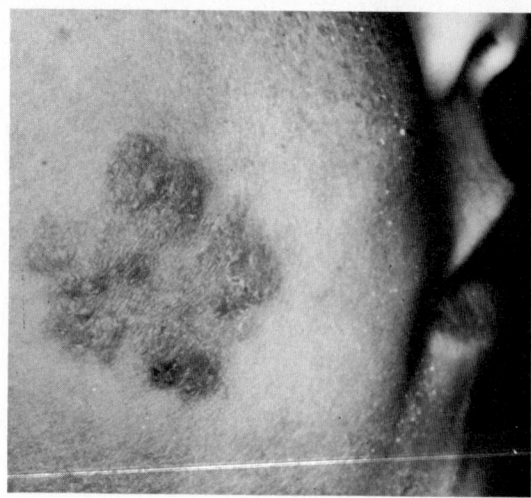

FIG. 37.   Trichophyton rubrum infection on the face of a healthy 5-year-old boy.

clearing of the center of the lesion is frequent except in lesions on the palm and sole. Unilateral involvement of a palm or sole is common. Unusual skin lesions produced by this organism include unilateral papulosquamous eruptions or granulomatous lesions of the lower leg (Majocchi-like granulomas). *T. rubrum* may produce generalized cutaneous eruptions, some with bizarre patterns, in chronically ill patients.

Trichophyton mentagrophytes is responsible for many cases of tinea pedis and onychomycosis of the toenails. Initially the nail becomes yellow or white at the distal margin as detritus and thickened white tissue accumulate underneath. Later the process advances proximally; grooves or ridges appear on the nail plate, and finally the nail may drop off. As long as the nailbed remains free of scar, regeneration will occur. *T. mentagrophytes* may produce tinea capitis and kerion celsi. Infections due to this organism are not common in prepubertal children.

Trichophyton verrucosum, which can be acquired from cattle, horses, mice, rabbits, or man, produces an inflammatory infection. The edematous, erythematous patches with elevated borders may contain vesicles or pustules. Kerion celsi is a common complication.

T. tonsurans is a cosmopolitan fungus, causing infections of the hair, skin, and nails. Because the spores of this organism are located inside the hair shaft (endothrix), the involved hairs fragment easily. These infections, known as *black dot ringworm,* appear as discrete, scattered, scaly patches containing dark stubs that remain after the hair fragments. *T. tonsurans* may produce circinate, gyrate, papulosquamous eruptions, mild seborrheic-like dermatitis, perifolliculitis, folliculitis, onychomycosis, and kerion.

In this country *T. violaceum* and *schoenleini* infections have been reported from areas of Kentucky and West Virginia and in immigrants. The former organism produces primarily a black dot ringworm. *T. schoenleini* infections (favus) involve the scalp and are characterized by crusted, yellow lesions with upward convexity (scutula). Underneath the scutula is an erythematous base that has a mousy odor. Because favus infections produce scarring, permanent alopecia is a common complication.

Dermatophytids are eruptions due to hypersensitivity of the host to invading fungi. These lesions appear at a site distant to the primary fungal infection. They must fulfill the following criteria: the absence of fungi in the suspected eruption, a proved fungal infection elsewhere on the skin, a positive intracutaneous tricophyton test, resolution of the suspected eruption after the distant fungal infection has been treated, and the history of appearance of the suspected "id" eruption only after irritation or inflammation of the primary fungal site. An id may be vesicular, lichenoid, exfoliative, erythematous, papular, or follicular. One common vesicular id, secondary to tinea pedis, appears on the sides of the fingers.

INTERMEDIATE FUNGI. *Candida albicans* causes infections of the skin and mucous membrane. It may also form granulomas and produce a disseminated disease.

This organism is the most common cause of an inflammatory paronychia and a white, macerated dermatitis in the fingerwebs (Fig. 38). A generalized, erythematous, papulosquamous eruption appears in rare instances, especially in patients with hypoparathyroidism or hypoadrenalism.

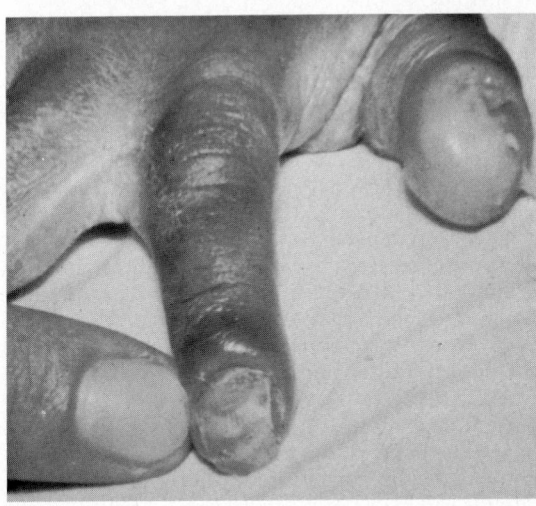

FIG. 38. Candidiasis. A macerating fissuring dermatitis of the fingerweb and paronychia, with fungal involvement of the nail plate.

Monilial infections occur in the mouth, rectum, vagina, and esophagus, where they may cause local pain. *Candida albicans* can cause infections of the canthi, the margins of the lips, and the skin folds of the body in the axillary, inguinal, and gluteal areas. Candida infections of the glabrous skin are characterized by sharp margins, bright erythematous color, and the appearance of satellite lesions. The satellite lesions differentiate candidiasis clinically from other forms of diaper rash. Candidiasis of the mucous membranes (thrush) is characterized by white patches surrounded by erythema. Thrush is a common disease in newborns. There is a direct correlation between maternal monilial vaginitis and thrush in the newborn. The disease is presumably acquired from the birth canal or from direct contact with children or contaminated articles in the newborn nursery.

SUBCUTANEOUS FUNGI. *Sporotrichum schenkii* is a pathogenic fungus found naturally on living or dead vegetation. The disease sporotrichosis is cosmopolitan, occurs at all ages, and is transmitted from soil or vegetation to man. No proven case of man-to-man transfer has been recorded. Cases have been seen after a thorn prick or in workers who have contact with hedges, barberry bushes, or peat moss. After an incubation period of approximately 3 to 12 weeks, the initial lesion appears. It is a freely movable, pink or purple, chancriform nodule that later ulcerates. Similar satellite lesions may appear along the path of lymphatic drainage. Painless movable lymphadenopathy is present. In a few cases the lesions may become furuncular or verrucous. Similarly a disseminated, nodular-ulcerative form of the disease has been reported.

DIAGNOSIS. All suspected fungal infections of the skin should be examined under ultraviolet light using the Wood's lamp. Blue-green fluorescence is present on eruptions due to *Microsporum audouini* and *canis* and in some lesions produced by *M. gypseum.*

Infected hairs or scrapings of the skin or nails in patients suspected of having fungal infections should be gently heated with 10 percent potassium hydroxide and examined microscopically. Specimens should be inoculated initially on Sabouraud's dextrose agar media at 25 C for four to six weeks. Once an agent has been isolated, subculturing on special media may be necessary for final identification.

In cases of suspected sporotrichosis, serologic tests and direct microscopic examination of human purulent material are not entirely dependable. The organism may be easily cultured at 25 C on blood agar or Sabouraud's dextrose agar media. Inoculation of infected material into rats or mice will produce peritonitis.

TREATMENT. The treatment of cutaneous fungal infection depends upon the species of invading organism and the depth of the pathology. All superficial and most cutaneous fungal infections can be treated primarily with keratolytic agents, 3 to 6 percent salicylic acid ointments, designed to "peel away" the infection. In special instances fungistatic preparations, such as diluted tincture of iodine, sulfur, short-chain fatty acids (undecylenic acid), tolnaftate, haloprogin, Castellani's paint, or Whitfield's ointment, may be used. These agents, with the exception of undecylenic acid, haloprogin, tolnaftate, and Whitfield's ointment have the disadvantage of coloring the skin. For this reason, salicylic acid is the main topical therapeutic preparation for these infections.

Tinea versicolor, one of the common ultrasuperficial fungal infections, responds well to tolnaftate or keratolytics, such as salicylic acid ointments. Solutions of 20 percent aqueous sodium thiosulfate are also effective topically. Acute or exudative lesions should be initially treated with soaks or water compresses before applying keratolytic agents. Lesions superinfected with bacteria should be treated with antibiotics before antifungal therapy is initiated.

The cutaneous fungal infections also respond to systemically administered griseofulvin, one micronized tablet (500 mg) daily for three to five weeks. The side effects of griseofulvin include headache, gastrointestinal upsets, fatigue, insomnia, reversible proteinuria, transient and reversible leukopenia, and photosensitivity. Patients given griseofulvin for prolonged periods have been shown to have increased urinary and fecal excretion of porphyrins and porphyrin precursors. This metabolic abnormality disappears after the drug is discontinued. Although there are no reports of patients receiving griseofulvin therapy developing photosensitivity characteristic of porphyria, it appears likely that such cases could occur. Since topical salicylic acid is inexpensive and free of side effect unless used in tremendous amounts, griseofulvin should be restricted to the following clinical situations: onychomycosis, *T. rubrum* infections of the palms or soles, fungal infections involving a large proportion of the body surface, tinea capitis, or dermatophytoses unresponsive to topical therapy.

The intermediate and subcutaneous fungal infections can be treated with nystatin or amphotericin B. Oral moniliasis is best treated with nystatin, which is available in a suspension containing 100,000 units/ml. One milliliter is given by dropper four times a day. An ointment containing 100,000 units of nystatin per milliliter is effective in treating cutaneous candidiasis. When treating monilial diaper rash, it is best to use the oral liquid as well as the local ointment, since oral lesions are often the initial source of infection. Generalized candidiasis is treated with systemic amphotericin B, since nystatin is not absorbed from the gastrointestinal tract and is not used in a parenteral form. *Nystatin* is effective only in candidiasis. *Amphotericin B* is used topically or parenterally for the other fungi discussed. If it is administered systemically, nephrotoxicity is a problem.

Topical haloprogin is effective and so is gentian violet solution, which, however, discolors the skin and clothes. There is suggestive evidence that hot soaks are a useful addition to the therapeutic program in sporotrichosis; however, oral potassium iodide is the therapy of choice. Treatment should be continued for several weeks after clinical resolution of the lesion.

PARASITIC DISEASES

Swimmers' Itch

Swimmers' itch is a pruritic dermatitis produced by an allergic reaction to nonhuman *Schistosoma cercariae* that have penetrated the skin.

ETIOLOGY AND EPIDEMIOLOGY. The cercariae of nonhuman schistosomes are widely found in both fresh and salt water. Although the disease is probably worldwide, most reported cases are from the Great Lakes region, New England, Hawaii, and Florida.

The cercariae penetrate the skin on exposed parts of the body during or immediately after bathing. Since man is an abnormal host, the parasite remains in the skin unable to complete its life cycle.

PATHOLOGY AND PATHOGENESIS. The cutaneous eruption is thought to be due to the reaction of the human host to schistosome antigens; thus, repeated contact with the cercariae is necessary before the patient is sensitized sufficiently to become symptomatic.

Pathologic examination of biopsies from lesions of swimmers' itch reveals nonspecific chronic inflammatory changes.

CLINICAL MANIFESTATIONS. Pruritus and transient urticarial lesions appear within minutes after penetration of the cercariae. A few hours later macules may be seen which are soon replaced by papules with erythematous halos. In some instances pustular and exudative lesions may be present. The pruritus returns and becomes intensive on the second or third day. Excoriation and secondary bacterial infection are common complications. Usually spontaneous resolution is complete within two weeks.

DIAGNOSIS. The diagnosis is usually made by history and examination.

Differential Diagnosis. The other three important eruptions affecting sea bathers are cymothoidism or related conditions, seaweed dermatitis, and seabathers' eruption. The first, cymothoidism, occurs after bathing in shallow salt water and is characterized by nonpruritic hemorrhagic puncta on exposed parts of the body. Seaweed dermatitis is an eruption caused by irritation of the skin by salt-water algae; it is localized to the skin under the loose parts of the bathing suit; to date cases have been reported only from northeastern Hawaii. Seabathers' eruption is thought to be a contact dermatitis from an unknown allergen in salt water; it appears in intertriginous areas as well as on the skin under the bathing suit.

Treatment. Careful drying immediately after bathing is a good prophylactic measure. Antihistamines are effective in reducing pruritus, and topical emollients may provide symptomatic relief.

Creeping Eruption (Larva Migrans)

Creeping eruption is a disease caused by the invasion of nonhuman hookworm larvae into the human skin.

ETIOLOGY AND EPIDEMIOLOGY. The larvae of *Ancylostoma braziliense* and *A. caninum* (cat and dog hookworms) enter human skin after direct contact. These organisms are found in excreta of dogs or cats infected with the adult worms. The highest incidence of the disease is in the southeastern United States where sandy soil and warm climate provide favorable conditions for the organism. Transmission is thought to occur by direct contact of the larva and the skin.

PATHOLOGY AND PATHOGENESIS. Most of the dermal tissue reaction present in a biopsy has been attributed to host hypersensitivity. However, in rare instances larvae may be found in the lower epidermis.

CLINICAL MANIFESTATIONS. The initial lesion, an erythematous papule, forms at the site of entry. Within two to three days the lesion becomes vesicular, and an erythematous, serpentine epidermal tunnel appears immediately behind the migrating larvae. As old tunnels heal, new ones are made. The eruption is present as long as the larvae remain viable, a period of days to several weeks. Approximately half of the patients have a peripheral eosinophilia. Loeffler's syndrome, presumably due to pulmonary migration of the larvae, is present in some cases.

DIAGNOSIS. The diagnosis is usually made by examination but may be proved by finding the larvae in a biopsy taken from the region of the skin immediately ahead of the advancing lesion.

The differential diagnosis includes other creeping eruptions such as myiasis or gnathostomiasis.

TREATMENT. This disease is self-limited. In cases in which only a few lesions are present, local freezing applied to the area ahead of the tunnel, where the larvae are presumed to be, may be effective. Variable results have been obtained with oral piperazine. *Thiabendazole,* 25 mg/kg twice daily, for 2 days, is effective.

In selected cases systemic corticosteroids or antihistamines may be required for relief since the pruritus can last long after the parasite has been killed.

INFESTATIONS OF THE SKIN

Insect Bite (See also pp. 361 and 668)

"Insect bite" is a term applied to a local cutaneous eruption caused by arthropods.

ETIOLOGY. A list of the habitats and characteristics of arthropods capable of inducing lesions in humans has been compiled in Table 4.

INCIDENCE AND EPIDEMIOLOGY. These eruptions are extremely common, especially in children. The epidemiology of any particular type of bite reflects the life cycle and ecology of the causative arthropod.

TABLE 4. Arthropods That Cause Cutaneous Lesions in Humans

	Common Name	Size (Approx)	Scientific Name	Habitat	Special Characteristics
	Scorpions	2-15 cm	Class—Arachnida Order— Scorpionidae	Southwestern USA Dry tropical areas Crevices	Painful
	Ticks	5 mm	Class—Arachnida Order—Acarina Family—Ixodidae Argasidae	Cosmopolitan Around grassy areas In nests or houses	Painless
	Mites Mouse mites	0.25-1.0 mm	Class—Arachnida Order—Acarina Family— Dermanyssidae	Cosmopolitan Nest parasite	Painless
	Spider mites	0.25-1.0 mm	Family— Tetranychidae	Around plants, in houses Cosmopolitan	Painless

TABLE 4. Arthropods That Cause Cutaneous Lesions in Humans (cont.)

	Common Name	Size (Approx)	Scientific Name	Habitat	Special Characteristics
	Chigger mites	0.25 mm	Family— Trombiculidae	Around grain, grasses, swamps, treeholes Cosmopolitan	Painless
	Follicle mites	0.25-1.0 mm	Family— Demodicidae	Cosmopolitan In man	Painless
	Grain mites	0.25-1.0 mm	Family— Pyentoidae	Cosmopolitan Around grass and straw	Painless
	Mange mites	0.25-1.0 mm	Family— Sarcoptidae	Cosmopolitan In man	Painless
	Brown spider	2.5 cm	Class—Arachnida Order—Araneidae Family— Loxoscelidae	Southern and central USA Central and So America Crevices, storage areas	May or may not be painful; necrotic bite
	Millipedes	5.0 cm	Class—Diplopoda	Cosmopolitan Around houses, stones, crevices	Painless
	Centipedes	5.0-7.0 cm	Class—Chilopoda	Cosmopolitan Around houses, stones, crevices	Painful nocturnal feeders, produce bite with two fang marks
	Buffalo gnats Blackflies	1-5 mm	Class—Insecta Order—Diptera	Widely distributed in USA, especially in hilly sections with swiftly moving water streams	Painful, daytime feeders; swarm in late spring and early summer
	Biting midge Punkies "NoSeeUms" Sandfly (misnomer)	0.5-5.0 mm	Class—Insecta Order—Diptera Family— Ceratopogonidae	Salt marches of Atlantic and Gulf coasts In decayed cactus, treeholes, seepage areas, ditches	Painful, bite at dawn and dusk; weak fliers; may occur in overwhelming numbers
	Horsefly Deerfly Greencads	7-30 mm	Class—Insecta Order—Diptera Family—Tabanidae	All over USA Breed in mud marshes	Very painful biters, daytime feeders
	Tsetse fly	6-15 mm	Class—Insecta Order—Diptera Family—Muscidae	Tropical Africa	Painful or painless; outdoor, daytime feeders
	Stable fly	6-15 mm	Class—Insecta Order—Diptera Family—Muscidae	Cosmopolitan Around large animals	Painless, daytime feeders
	Fleas	1-8 mm	Class—Insecta Order— Siphonoptera	Cosmopolitan Nest parasites	Painless, daytime or nocturnal feeders
		1 mm	Species—Tunga Penetrans	Pantropical	Female burrows in human skin to lay eggs, thereby producing blisters
	Blister beetle	1-3 cm	Class—Insecta Order—Coleoptera Family—Meloidae	Cosmopolitan	Painless; blisters form at site of bite; phototactic insects

TABLE 4. Arthropods That Cause Cutaneous Lesions in Humans (cont.)

Common Name	Size (Approx)	Scientific Name	Habitat	Special Characteristics
Caterpillar	2 cm	Class—Insecta Order— Lepidoptera	Cosmopolitan	Contact with caterpillar hairs produces urticaria
Ants Bees Wasps Hornets	1 cm 1-3 cm 1-3 cm 1-3 cm	Class—Insecta Order— Hymenoptera	Cosmopolitan	Stinging insects
Sandfleas	1-2 mm	Superclass— Crustacea Order—Amphipoda Isopoda	Cosmopolitan In shallow salt water	Produce hemorrhagic bites
Termites (Nasute)	3 mm	Class—Insecta Order—Isoptera	Pantropical In dead trees	Painful; ejectors of an irritant fluid
Lice	2 mm	Class—Insecta Order—Anopleura	Cosmopolitan In man and his clothes	Painless; produces little or no reaction to biting
Bedbugs	3-5 mm	Class—Insecta Order—Hemiptera Family—Cimicidae	Cosmopolitan Crevices, mattress seams, wallpaper	Nocturnal painless feeder
Kissing Bug	1-3 cm	Class—Insecta Order—Hemiptera Family— Reduviidae	Widely spread south of Pensylvania. In walls, floors, cracks, crevices, and rodent burrows	Nocturnal, may or may not be painful
Plant bug Leafhoppers	1-3 cm	Class—Insecta Order—Hemiptera Family— Ciccadellidae Aphidae Order— Thysanoptera	Cosmopolitan Plant feeders	Painful bite
Mosquito	2-8 mm	Class—Insecta Order—Diptera Family—Culicidae	Cosmopolitan	Painful bite
Sandfly	1-4 mm	Class—Insecta Order—Diptera Family— Psychodidae	Present but not common in USA, tropical areas, in treeholes, rodent burrows, and crevices	Nocturnal, weak fliers; may or may not be painful

PATHOLOGY AND PATHOGENESIS. The pathologic features of an insect bite initially include edema and a perivascular infiltration of both mononuclear and polymorphonuclear cells. Shortly afterward, many histiocytes, eosinophils, lymphocytes, and plasma cells appear. The infiltration may be granulomatous or may become so extensive that it is difficult to distinguish from lymphoma.

Arthropods may produce human cutaneous lesions by several mechanisms. Direct tissue injury may result from biting, stinging, or burrowing. Local urticarial reactions may be produced in two ways: by venoms introduced with a bite or sting, or by contact with various arthropod secretions or integumentary structures. Vesiculation may result from contact with the integumentary fluids of certain arthropods. Necrosis has been produced by the bite of certain spiders and, in some patients, by the bite or sting of arthropods. Finally, secondary abrasions, excoriations, and bacterial infections are often superimposed upon the original lesion.

CLINICAL MANIFESTATIONS. In general, arthropod infestations localize either on exposed areas of the skin or in regions of the body where clothing fits tightly. In these areas migratory movement of the insect is impeded, and feeding or defensive biting results.

The clinical picture of an arthropod bite consists of

two components: that produced by direct injury and that produced by species-specific hypersensitivity or toxicity. The latter is discussed in detail elsewhere (see p. 361). The mouth parts of an insect create a punctum which may be composed of single or multiple lacerations depending upon the structure of the weapon inflicting the wound. Patients who are either not sensitive or who have been "desensitized" by frequent bites will exhibit only a minimal reaction.

Papular urticaria is an eruption characterized by pruritic, papular lesions, with or without a surrounding wheal. This disease is thought to represent a papular response to an insect bite. However, in some cases the papular eruption may involve large areas of the body. Thus, it is not known whether each papule represents a bite or whether some of the lesions arise solely as a hypersensitive response.

DIAGNOSIS.   The diagnosis of an eruption caused by the bite of an arthropod is made by obtaining a history of possible exposure and recognizing the presence of lesions that have central puncta, necrosis, or a series of vesicles following the line of contact with the insect.

Because many arthropods produce identical cutaneous lesions, only a careful history and a subsequent search of the patient's environment will reveal the identity of the offending arthropod. In cases with urticarial lesions this history must include the activities of the patient during the entire 48-hour span prior to the bite.

TREATMENT.   Therapy of these lesions depends upon the extent of the allergic reaction, which is discussed elsewhere (p. 361).

Necrotic Arachnidism

Necrotic arachnidism is the term applied to necrotic cutaneous lesions produced by the bite of certain spiders.

ETIOLOGY.   The genus *Loxosceles* and *Latrodectus* includes medium-sized yellow or brown spiders, 10 to 15 mm in length, with six eyes arranged in an arc. "Wolf spiders" or lycosids have recently been found to cause significant cutaneous damage.

INCIDENCE AND EPIDEMIOLOGY.   There are two *Loxosceles* species of recognized medical importance: one indigenous to the United States, the other to South America. *Loxosceles reclusa* inhabits the south central portion of this country. It has been found in storage spaces, cellars, and closets. *Loxosceles laeta* is the South American species, which has been introduced into the United States.

PATHOLOGY.   Biopsies of spider bites show marked inflammation and necrosis of the epidermis, dermis, and underlying tissues. There is a similarity between these lesions and a localized Arthus reaction.

CLINICAL MANIFESTATIONS.   Almost identical clinical pictures are caused by both species. A wheal appears at the puncture site immediately after the bite. As necrosis evolves, this area becomes violaceous. Later an eschar forms. In some patients a systemic reaction with slight fever and a generalized scarlatiniform eruption occurs. Hemolysis, shock, and renal shutdown are occasionally present. There have been two fatal cases from bites of *Loxosceles* in the United States, one in a 4-year-old boy.

DIAGNOSIS.   The diagnosis can be made only by history and physical examination. Necrotic skin lesions can also occur in any disease characterized by multiple emboli or a vasculitis.

TREATMENT.   No specific treatment is currently available.

Pediculosis

Pediculosis is the disease produced from infestation of sucking lice.

ETIOLOGY.   Sucking lice (*Anoplura*) have flattened bodies, a protrusible proboscis at the tip of the head, and legs adapted for clinging to hairs.

The crab louse (*Phthirus pubis*) is light in color, measures approximately 1 mm in diameter, and has a crablike appearance. Its anterior legs are smaller than the posterior. This louse infests the pubic hairs especially, but in heavy infestations it may also be present in other hairy parts of the body, where it lays its eggs on the hair shaft.

The *head louse* (*Pediculus humanus capitis*) is also light in color and 2 to 3 mm long. It infests and lays its eggs in the scalp and other hairy areas of the body.

The *body louse* (*Pediculus humanus corporis*) spends most of its time in clothing, moving to the skin only to feed.

INCIDENCE AND EPIDEMIOLOGY.   Pediculosis is not rare. Transmission of the lice occurs by direct contact of susceptible people with infected hairs or clothing containing either eggs (nits) or adult lice.

PATHOLOGY.   The major lesions in pediculosis are inflicted by the host's scratching. Only inflammatory changes are found in biopsy specimens.

CLINICAL MANIFESTATIONS.   Lice produce pinpoint, flat, erythematous lesions at the feeding sites. Excoriations and bloody crusts are the most common lesions observed on infested patients. Secondary infections, exudation, and regional lymphadenopathy are a result of excoriation. In addition, postinflammatory hyperpigmentation may persist for several months.

Patients infested with scalp lice frequently consult physicians because of pyoderma and cervical lymphadenopathy.

DIAGNOSIS.   The diagnosis of pediculosis can be made by finding the lice or eggs. In pediculosis capitis and pubis, both ova and adults can be found attached to the hairs. In cases of pediculosis corporis the adult lice are located in greater numbers in clothing seams, but a few may be found feeding on the skin.

The differential diagnosis of pediculosis corporis includes other causes of generalized pruritus such as uremia, jaundice, malignancy, diabetes, and drug reactions. Frequently, pediculosis capitis is misdiagnosed as simple pyoderma.

TREATMENT.   *Benzene hexachloride* (Kwell) or any of several insecticide dusts may be applied to the body and clothes in the treatment of pediculosis corporis and to the infested areas of the body in cases of pediculosis capitis and pubis.

Scabies

Scabies is a disease resulting from an infestation of the skin by the mite *Sarcoptes scabiei*.

ETIOLOGY. The female measures 330 to 450μ in length and 250 to 350μ in width; the male is only about half as large.

INCIDENCE AND EPIDEMIOLOGY. Scabies is not an uncommon disease in this country. The peak seasonal incidence is during late summer and early autumn when campers and vacationers return from their trips. The mite migrates from one individual to another with facility.

PATHOLOGY AND PATHOGENESIS. Scabetic mites burrow in the skin, where the females deposit their eggs. After a few weeks the human host becomes sensitized to the antigens of the mite, and pruritus occurs. Biopsy specimens may include the mite, the ova and the epidermal tunnel. A chronic inflammatory infiltrate is present in both the epidermis and dermis.

CLINICAL MANIFESTATIONS. Because pruritus does not occur until the patient is sensitized, the infestation is usually well advanced before symptoms appear. Nocturnal pruritus is the most common chief complaint. Small, tortuous, burrow tracts with dark plugs at the entrance are found in the afflicted sites. The genital areas and the flexural creases, particularly between the fingers, are areas of predilection, although any region of the body may be attacked. Usually the scalp is spared. Asymptomatic or mildly pruritic hyperkeratotic lesions containing enormous numbers of acari are present in some neglected cases. In infants papulovesicular or vesiculobullous lesions are often seen, especially on the face and feet; atopic dermatitis may be mimicked. Secondary bacterial infection and excoriations are common.

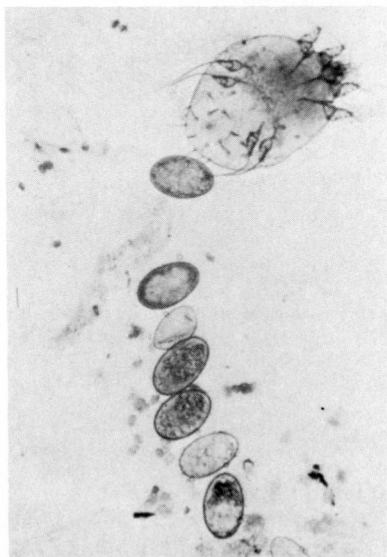

FIG. 39.   Female mite and eggs removed from the skin of a child by curettage.

DIAGNOSIS. The diagnosis of scabies may be confirmed by demonstrating the mite in the skin by probing the burrow with a needle or more easily by curetting a fresh lesion and examining the material on a glass slide (Fig. 39).

Scabies must be differentiated from other causes of pruritus such as pediculosis, uremia, jaundice, diabetes, malignancy, and drug eruptions. The lesions of factitial excoriations, although superficially resembling scabies, do not appear predominantly in flexural creases.

TREATMENT. *Crotamiton* cream (Eurax) or *benzene hexachloride* (Kwell) ointment are effective insecticide preparations, which should be applied twice daily for three to four days. Fifteen percent precipitated sulfur ointments and 25 percent benzyl benzoate emulsion are also effective drugs. All members of the family should be treated and the bedclothes sprayed with insecticides.

CUTANEOUS REACTION TO INFECTION

Erythema Nodosum

Erythema nodosum is a syndrome characterized by the appearance of painful, erythematous, subcutaneous nodules, usually on the extensor surfaces of the extremities.

ETIOLOGY. This syndrome is thought to be due to hypersensitivity to (a) drugs, such as iodides, bromides, penicillin, sulfonamides, and antipyrine; (b) infections, such as syphilis, lepromatous leprosy, tuberculosis, streptococcosis, meningococcal infections, lymphogranuloma venereum, cat scratch fever, coccidioidomycosis, and chancroid; and (c) miscellaneous diseases, such as sarcoidosis, ulcerative colitis, and regional enteritis. Streptococcal infections are the most common cause of this disease in American children. A great number of cases appear to occur de novo.

INCIDENCE AND EPIDEMIOLOGY. Erythema nodosum is a common syndrome in children over six years of age. A predominance of females has been observed in some series.

PATHOLOGY. The pathologic alterations in this syndrome are found in the dermis, where an infiltration of mononuclear cells is present. The capillaries are dilated, and areas of thrombosis and extravasation may occur.

CLINICAL MANIFESTATIONS. Erythematous, round or elliptical, tender nodules, ranging in size from 0.5 to 3 cm, appear in crops on the extremities. Although these nodules are firm, their border is not always well delineated. After a few days the lesions become purple, then brown, in color. Constitutional symptoms may accompany the eruption. Resolution usually takes place within three weeks without ulceration and without scarring. Recurrences are not uncommon.

DIFFERENTIAL DIAGNOSIS. Periarteritis nodosa and erythema indurata can be ruled out by biopsy. Erythema nodosum also may be confused with superficial, migratory thrombophlebitis and panniculitis.

TREATMENT. Treatment for this disorder depends upon the nature of the underlying disease. Analgesics are usually all that is necessary in most patients. Systemic corticosteroids and salicylates have been administered to those acutely ill patients having no conditions that would otherwise contraindicate such drugs.

Erythema multiforme is discussed elsewhere.

Bibliography

BACTERIAL INFECTIONS OF THE SKIN

Burnett JW: Management of pyogenic cutaneous infections. N Engl J Med 266:164, 1962

———— The route of antibiotic administration in superficial impetigo. N Engl J Med 268:72, 1963

Dajani AS, Ferrieri P, Wannamaker LW: Natural history of impetigo II etiologic agents and bacterial interactions. J Clin Invest 51:2863, 1972

Dillon HC Jr: Pyoderma and nephritis. Ann Rev Med 18:207, 1967

Dillon HC: The treatment of streptococcal skin infections. J Pediatr 76:676, 1970

Markowitz M, Bruton HD, Kultner AG: The bacteriologic findings, streptococcal immune responses and renal complications in children with impetigo. Pediatrics 35:393, 1965

ERYTHRASMA

Koostra JA: Prophylaxis and control of erythrasma of the toe webs. J Invest Dermatol 45:399, 1965

Sarkany I, Taplin D, Blank H: Incidence and bacteriology of erythrasma. Arch Dermatol 85:578, 1962

VIRAL INFECTIONS OF THE SKIN

HERPES ZOSTER

Brunnell PA, Miller LH, Lovejoy F: Zoster in children. Am J Dis Child 115:432, 1968

———— Ross A, Miller LH, Kuo B: Prevention of varicella by zoster immune globulin. N Engl J Med 280:1191, 1969

Gold E, Robbins FC: Isolation of cytopathogenic agents from cerebrospinal or vesicle fluid of patients with herpes zoster or varicella. Am J Dis Child 94:545, 1957

Luby JP: Varicella-zoster virus. J Invest Dermatol 61:212, 1973

Mersalis JG, Kaye D, Hook EW: Disseminated herpes zoster. Arch Intern Med 113:679, 1964

Muller SA: Association of zoster and malignant disorders in children. Arch Dermatol 96:657, 1967

Weller TH: Varicella: Herpes zoster. In Beeson PB, McDermott W (eds): Cecil-Loeb Textbook of Medicine, 11th ed. WB Saunders Co, Philadelphia, 1963, p 110

MOLLUSCUM CONTAGIOSUM

Burnett JW, Neva FN: Studies on the mechanism of molluscum contagiosum cytoxicity. J Invest Dermatol 46:76, 1966

Friedman-Kien AE, Vilcek J: Induction of interference and interferon synthesis by non-replicating molluscum contagiosum virus. J Immunol 99:1092, 1967

Prose PH, Friedman-Kien AE, Vilcek J: Molluscum contagiosum virus in adult human skin cultures; an electron microscopic study. Am J Pathol 55:349, 1969

Sutton JS, Burnett JW: Ultrastructural changes in dermal and epidermal cells of skin infected with molluscum contagiosum virus. J Ultrastruct Res 26:177, 1969

WARTS

Almeida JD, Howatson AF, Williams MG: Electron microscope study of human warts, sites of virus production and nature of the inclusion bodies. J Invest Dermatol 38:337, 1962

Blank H, Rake G: Viral and Rickettsial Diseases of the Skin, Eyes and Mucous Membranes of Man, Chap 9. Little, Brown & Co, Boston, Toronto, 1955, p. 156

Chapman GB, Drusin LM, Todd JE: Fine structure of the human wart. Am J Pathol 42:619, 1963

FUNGAL INFECTIONS OF THE SKIN

Conant NF: Manual of Clinical Mycology, 3rd ed. WB Saunders Co, Philadelphia, 1971

Lewis GM, Hopper ME: An Introduction to Medical Mycology, 4th ed. The Year Book Publishers, Chicago, 1958

Sulton RL Jr: Diseases of the Skin, 11th ed. CV Mosby Co, St Louis, 1956

Swartz JH: Current concepts in therapy: infections caused by dermatophytes. N Engl J Med 267:1246, 1962

PARASITIC DISEASES

SWIMMERS' ITCH

Cort WW: Studies on schistosome dermatitis. XI. Status of knowledge after more than twenty years. Am J Hyg 52:251, 1950

CREEPING ERUPTION

Lowenthal LJA: Evaluation of therapy in creeping eruption. Aust J Dermatol 2:171, 1954

Stauffer LW: Creeping eruption. Arch Dermatol 103:461, 1971

INFESTATIONS OF THE SKIN

INSECT BITES

Benjamini E, Feingold BF, Kartman L: Allergy to flea bites. III. The experimental induction of flea bite and by antigen prepared from whole flea extracts of Ctenocephilides felis. Exp Parasitol 10:214, 1960

Brook T: Résumé of insect allergy. Ann Allergy 19:288, 1961

Gordon RM, Lavopierre MMJ: Entomology for Students of Medicine. Blackwell Scientific Publications, Oxford, 1962

Herms WB, James MT: Medical Entomology, 6th ed. The Macmillan Co, New York, 1969

Ordman D: Desensitization to bee stings by intracutaneous injections of whole-bee extract. Br Med J 2:352, 1958

NECROTIC ARACHNIDISM

Atkins JA, Wingo CW, Sodeman WA: Necrotic arachnidism. Am J Trop Med 1:165, 1958

Pitts NC: Necrotic arachnidism. N Engl J Med 267:400, 1962

Redman JF: Human envenomation by a lycosid. Arch Dermatol 110:111, 1974

PEDICULOSIS

Sutton RL Jr: Diseases of the Skin, 11th ed. CV Mosby Co, St Louis, 1956, p 618

CUTANEOUS REACTION TO INFECTION

Doxiadis SA: Erythema nodosum in children. Medicine 30:283, 1951

Laurance B, Stone DGH, Philpott MG, et al: Aetiology of erythema nodosum, in children. Lancet 2:14, 1961

DISORDERS OF PIGMENTATION
JOSEPH McGUIRE

In addition to the basilar keratinocytes, which comprise the stem cell population of the epidermis, there is a second type of epidermal cell resting on the basal lamina—the melanocyte. These specialized secretory cells are derived from the neural crest, as are the sympathetic ganglia, adrenal medulla, Schwann cells *inter alia*.

These cells have elongated dendritic processes through which they transfer melanin granules to keratinocytes in the basal and malpighian layer. It is useful in considering the physiology and pathology of pigmentation to divide it into three separate processes:

1. Melanization
2. Intracellular pigment granule translocation
3. Pigment granule transfer and digestion

In step one, tyrosinase is synthesized on the rough endoplasmic reticulum and transferred to small vesicular structures in the Golgi region. These vesicular organelles are termed melanosomes and serve as the site for melanin synthesis. After the melanosome becomes completely melanized it is termed a stage IV melanosome or pigment granule. Tyrosinase catalyzes the oxidation of tyrosine to dopa (dihydroxyphenylalanine) and the subsequent oxidation of dopa to dopa quinone. Dopa quinone is further oxidized nonenzymically and its products form an insoluble polymer in association with the protein of the melanosome. These pigment granules are dispersed throughout the melanocyte and are then transferred to adjacent keratinocytes via the dendritic processes of the melanocyte.

Although intramelanocytic translocation of pigment granules has long been known to account for rapid color changes in frogs, fish, and reptiles, it has only recently been implicated in immediate pigment darkening, the transient darkening that occurs in the human after exposure to ultraviolet light. Delayed tanning, which persists for weeks following exposure to ultraviolet light, is associated with melanogenesis and increased transfer of pigment granules to keratinocytes. Abnormalities in these three steps are represented in various clinical disorders. In *vitiligo*, melanocytes are destroyed, in *piebaldism*, they were never present, in *albinism* melanocytes are present but tyrosinase is either abnormal or greatly reduced. In *pityriasis alba*, a form of hypopigmentation associated with mild atopic dermatitis, pigment granule transfer is abortive.

There is an inverse correlation between latitude and intensity of melanin pigmentation in the human. Tropical and subtropical populations tend to be more heavily melanized than temperate or more northerly located groups. It is therefore generally accepted that melanization is an important protective adaptive strategy against ultraviolet (UV) irradiation. Although the validity of this logic is unproved, melanin does protect the host from irradiation in two ways: absorption of light and absorption of radicals. The mechanism of UV-induced damage in biologic systems is thought to be through the generation of radicals, which produce thymine dimers in DNA. These dimers are excised in a repair process. Ultraviolet irradiation produces a greater concentration of free radicals in white skin than in nonwhite skin. Furthermore, melanin is a stable free radical and as such could function as a scavenger for the free radicals.

The destructive effects of ultraviolet light exposure are illustrated by the premature appearance of elastosis, actinic keratoses, and carcinomas in the exposed skin of albino Negroes in tropical climates. More pertinent and less generally appreciated, however, is the cumulative damage to the skin associated with chronic exposure to sunlight at temperate latitudes. Children, especially those of Celtic extraction and/or rufous complexions, can be permanently damaged by sunlight before they reach teenage. In general, the child who tans well and has brown eyes is relatively less damaged than the blue-eyed freckler. The cultural basis for sunbathing and acquisition of a suntan is obscure and is responsible not only for the actinic keratosis and many of the squamous cell carcinomas that appear later in life, but also for the prematurely aged appearance, loss of elasticity, and wrinkling in many people in the third and fourth decades of life.

Acute effects of ultraviolet irradiation are well known —erythema and blistering (Fig. 40). Chronic effects are atrophy, telangiectasia, and elastosis. In children these latter effects are definitely abnormal and are associated with xeroderma pigmentosum, the Rothmund-Thomson syndrome, and albinism. The best-known effect of ultraviolet light on skin apart from sunburn is tanning.

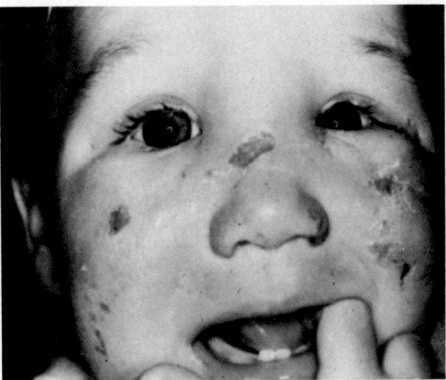

FIG. 40. Sunburn in a 1-year-old infant. There is periorbital edema, blistering, and erythema. Chronic damage from ultraviolet irradiation accounts for most of the changes associated with aging of the skin.

HORMONAL CONTROL OF PIGMENTATION

Although of considerable interest to physiologists, clinical abnormalities of pigmentation secondary to hormonal stimulation are uncommon in children. The pituitary secretes several peptides that have a direct darkening effect on the pigment cells of amphibia and, when administered systemically to man, produce darkening of the skin. α and β melanocyte-stimulating hormone (MSH) as well as ACTH in larger amounts, darken human skin. In Addison's disease, loss of feedback inhibition of the pituitary gland by steroidal products of the adrenal cortex results in increased secretion of both MSH and ACTH. In Addison's disease and the ectopic ACTH syndromes, β-MSH is responsible for the generalized darkening of the skin, nevi, palmar creases, and buccal mucosa in this disease; however, ACTH may also contribute to the melanocyte stimulation. The converse of this situation is seen in panhypopituitarism, where the skin is relatively hypo-. pigmented.

HYPOPIGMENTATION

Albinism (p. 678)

Albinism is a classic example of an inherited defect in enzyme synthesis. It is inherited as a recessive trait and is due to absent or defective tyrosinase synthesis in the melanocyte. The melanocyte is otherwise structurally normal.

Two forms of human albinism have been described: tyrosinase negative and tyrosinase positive. Individuals with the tyrosinase negative form are more lightly pigmented, and when their hair bulbs are incubated with tyrosine, no pigment is formed. In the tyrosine positive form of albinism, cutaneous and hair pigment is diluted, the irides are not so light as in the tyrosine negative form, and when hair bulbs are incubated with tyrosine, pigment is formed. Two families have been described in which there were normally pigmented offspring from tyrosinase positive and tyrosinase negative parents. These observations indicate that the genes for the two forms of albinism are not allelic.

Affected individuals have photophobia and often nystagmus. Hair color ranges from white to blond, iris color from light blue to hazel. The protective effect of melanin is demonstrated by the accelerated aging of albino skin with the appearance of keratosis, telangiectasia, and elastosis at an early age.

There is no treatment for albinism; prophylactic measures such as protective clothing and the use of chemical sun screens (Skolex, A-fil, Uval) should be employed when sunlight cannot be avoided.

Partial Albinism

Partial albinism, a dominant trait, is characterized by a white forelock and circumscribed areas of depigmentation on the skin. In the hypomelanotic skin from the white forelock area, no melanocytes are present. In other hypomelanotic areas in partial albinism, the melanocytes contain abnormal melanosomes.

Vitiligo

Vitiligo (Fig. 41) is a common but puzzling macular depigmentation of the skin affecting about 1 percent of people in the United States.

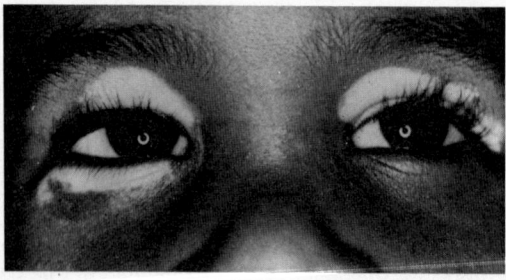

FIG. 41. Vitiligo in a Black boy with depigmentation around eyes. Loss of pigmentation commonly occurs around body orifices, eg, mouth, nose, nipples, eyes, navel, and on the dorsa of the hands.

One-half of these patients have relatives with vitiligo, and in half the onset is within the first two decades. Sites of trauma and pressure are often affected as well as areas around body orifices—eyes, mouth, nipples, umbilicus. The depigmented patches are usually noted during the summer, when tanning of the normal surrounding skin affords a striking contrast to the milky white area of pigment loss. Conversely, the vitiliginous patch may appear to improve in the wintertime as the surrounding suntan fades. As might be expected, the absence of melanin in vitiliginous areas results in enhanced sensitivity to sunlight. The border may be hyperpigmented. Occasionally, an intermediate degree of pigmentation may be seen between the central area of vitiligo and the normal skin. This represents partial pigment loss and heralds the progression of the depigmentation. The diagnosis can usually be made on clinical grounds; however, the use of a Wood's light facilitates identification of depigmentation in light-skinned individuals. Hair in areas of vitiligo may become depigmented or remain normal.

Basilar melanocytes are absent in well-established vitiligo; however, another type of epidermal dendritic cell, the Langerhans' cell, is present in normal or increased numbers. Ordinarily, Langerhans' cells, which can be demonstrated easily because of their ATPase activity, are present in the suprabasilar position. These dendritic cells have no desmosomes and contain racquet-shaped organelles which, unlike melanosomes, possess no tyrosinase activity. No role has yet been identified for the Langerhans' cell.

The course of vitiligo is capricious; it may progress to total depigmentation in less than a year, or it may remain relatively stable for decades. Spontaneous complete repigmentation is quite rare, although about half of the patients have some degree of repigmentation. Although vitiligo involves only the skin, it is associated with two systemic diseases—pernicious anemia and hyperthyroidism. Many patients relate their vitiligo to major trauma, either physical or emotional. The association of Addison's disease, pernicious anemia, and hyperthyroidism with vitiligo suggests that in vitiligo melanocytes may be destroyed through immunologic mechanisms.

The differential diagnosis of vitiligo includes partial albinism, which, however, is present at birth; depigmentation secondary to chemical exposure (monobenzyl ether of hydroquinone); and perihalo nevus (see below). The most common condition from which vitiligo must be differentiated in childhood is pityriasis alba.

Vitiligo may be treated with the topical or oral administration of 8-methoxypsoralen or trimethylpsoralen, which are photosensitizing agents. The medication is taken daily one to two hours before exposure to sunlight or applied to the skin. Ordinarily, treatment is carried out through the spring, summer, and early autumn when natural sunlight is available. Because of the photosensitizing property of psoralens, exposure to sunlight must be cautious, with a gradual increase in the length of exposure; otherwise a severe sunburn with blistering may result. Repigmentation occurs at the borders and within the patch of vitiligo in a perifollicular pattern. These spots coalesce to produce a fairly even pigmentation. Because of the demands made upon the patient by psoralen therapy, only highly motivated individuals should be treated. The simplest treatment is to darken the depigmented areas with dyes.

Halo Nevus

Halo nevus is a poorly understood condition in which a halo of depigmentation appears around a pigmented nevus, which itself eventually becomes depigmented and disappears (Fig. 42). The area then repigments spontaneously. Rarely, halo depigmentation may occur around a blue nevus or neurofibroma and even more rarely around a malignant melanoma.

There is a high incidence of halo nevi in vitiligo; however, they are not rare in otherwise normal children and may appear and resolve without coincident vitiligo.

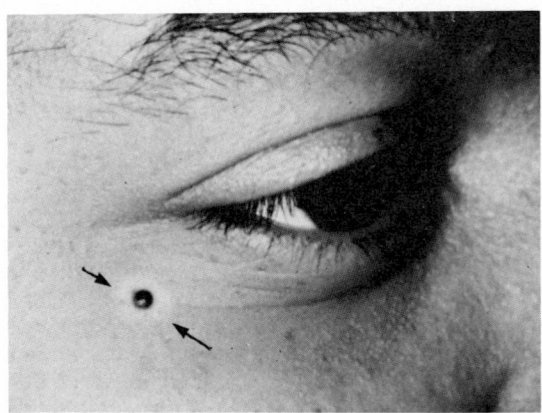

FIG. 42. Black girl with halo nevus on right cheek. Central pigmented nevus will probably become depigmented, then area will repigment.

Chediak-Higashi Syndrome

Chediak-Higashi syndrome is a rare lethal disorder associated with varying degrees of pigment dilution. In addition to apparent albinism, there are hepatosplenomegaly, recurrent infections, and severe infection or hemorrhage which usually are fatal before 10 years of age. The degree of pigment dilution in these patients is as in albinos is variable, and many of the children tan, especially those of dark-skinned parents; rarely, patients may even become hyperpigmented.

Anemia and leukopenia are common, and smears of peripheral blood reveal abnormally large granules in neutrophils and eosinophils. The dilution of skin color does not represent classical albinism but may be secondary to a structural abnormality of melanosomes which are several times larger than normal.

Waardenburg's Syndrome

An uncommon form of patterned leukoderma associated with congenital deafness occurs in Waarden-

burg's syndrome. Waardenburg defined the syndrome in 1951 with a clinical description of 161 affected individuals with the following findings:

Lateral displacement of the medial canthi and inferior lacrimal puncta	99%
Broad nasal root	78%
Eyebrows growing together	45%
Heterochromia iridum	25%
Deafness	20%
White forelock and occasional depigmentation of eyebrows	17%

Since then, it has been estimated that 2 percent of congenitally deaf children have this syndrome. It has been suggested that a developmental abnormality in the neural crest is responsible for the pigmentary changes and the absence of the organ of Corti. Heterochromia and the white forelock may disappear in childhood.

HYPERPIGMENTATION

Pigmented Nevus

The pigmented nevus (nevus cell nevus) or mole is the most common type of hyperpigmentation seen in childhood. It is usually absent at birth and appears in the first decade, often in crops. The nevus is composed of cells closely related to melanocytes. Nevus cells may contain melanosomes and melanin, and may be dopa oxidase and tyrosinase positive, depending on their location. The presence of nonspecific cholinesterase, an enzyme not found in melanocytes, in nevus cells of intradermal nevi may indicate that nevus cells are derived from a primitive cell of neural crest origin. Nonspecific cholinesterase is present in Schwann cells, which are also derived from neural crest.

Clinically, nevi may vary considerably in morphology. They may be flat, raised, or papillomatous and tan, brown, black, or blue in color.

The earliest form of nevus may be lentigo simplex, in which there is an increased number of melanocytes and sometimes elongation or budding of the rete ridges. Occasionally lentiges occur in a nevoid pattern (Fig. 43).

JUNCTIONAL NEVUS. Most nevi seen in children are of the junctional type; they consist of an accumulation of dopa positive, melanin-containing epithelioid cells which are arranged in nests in the lower epidermis and at the dermoepidermal junction. The cells are cuboidal and regular in shape. Junctional nevi are of interest because of their malignant potential, which fortunately is very small. The very large numbers of these lesions preclude their prophylactic removal.

Nevi are removed for two reasons: (a) cosmetic and (b) evidence of abnormal development. They should be excised if there is bleeding or crusting, color change or speckling of pigmentation, migration of pigment outside the margins of the nevus, or rapid growth. In the natural course of junctional nevi, nevus cells migrate toward the dermis and at the same time the lesions become more dome-shaped. When nests of nevus cells occur in the epidermis as well as freely in the dermis, they are termed *compound nevi.*

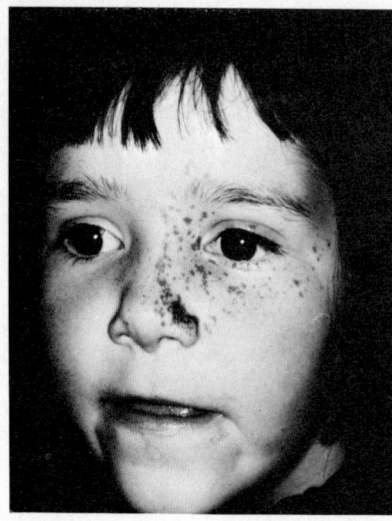

FIG. 43.   Nevoid lentigo. Patterned hyperpigmentation in "nevoid" distribution.

INTRADERMAL NEVUS.   This refers to a collection of nevus cells which are no longer associated with the dermoepidermal junction. The nevus is usually raised and may be a firm papule with varying degrees of pigmentation. The cells may contain melanin but are usually dopa negative. In the upper dermis they may be cuboidal, but in the lower dermis they are often spindle-shaped.

Although the classification of nevi into junctional, compound, and intradermal types is useful clinically, a thorough search for epidermal nests of nevus cells (evidence of junctional activity) will be productive in four of five clinically diagnosed intraepidermal nevi.

Several extensive surveys have confirmed the high incidence of junctional nevi in children, with a gradual decrease in number in older age groups. The converse relationship exists with intradermal nevi; they are rare in childhood and their incidence increases with age.

Removal of nevi for either cosmetic reasons or signs of abnormal development should be complete. Most small nevi can be removed with a punch biopsy. Larger lesions should be excised. Nevi on the palms, soles, genitalia, and sites of repeated trauma deserve special attention; however, their abundance makes wholesale removal impractical.

EXTENSIVE PIGMENTED NEVUS.   Extensive pigmented nevus (bathing trunk nevus) is a rare abnormality of pigment cell development which involves large areas of the body and is named according to its location—eg, bathing trunk, vest, cape, stocking, sleeve (Fig. 44). It is usually present at birth, unlike most other nevus cell nevi. Most are composed histologically of dopa oxidase and tyrosinase positive cells arranged as in a compound or intradermal nevus. The skin overlying the nevus is often hairy. In addition to their disturbing appearance, they are associated with a greatly increased incidence of melanoma, and despite their size, they can and should be surgically removed.

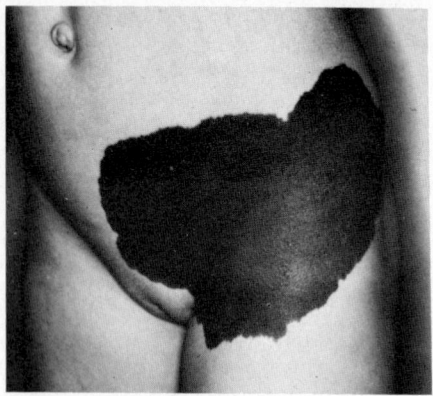

FIG. 44.   Nine-year-old girl with pigmented nevus present since birth. The nevus was excised and grafted. Histologic examination revealed compound nevus and at the time of surgery a black inguinal node contained melanophages.

Malignant Melanoma

Malignant melanoma (melanocarcinoma) is fortunately a rare diagnosis in children. It does, however, occur and shares the same dismal prognosis as melanoma in adults. A benign lesion, *juvenile melanoma,* which occurs in children and less commonly in adults, often causes considerable diagnostic difficulty, and must be differentiated from melanoma histologically. Clinically, juvenile melanoma may be located on any part of the body; however, there is a predilection for the face. It is smooth, elevated, usually hairless, and pink in color; however, it may be pigmented. It may resemble intradermal nevus or pyogenic granuloma. Ulceration is rare. Malignant melanoma in children is clinically similar to melanomas in adults. It is usually elevated and may vary from flesh color through deep red or black. Ulceration is frequent. Treatment is unsatisfactory; however, the best approach is wide primary excision with dissection of the draining lymphatic chain. The tumor is not sensitive to x-ray or chemotherapy.

Multiple Lentigines Syndrome

This syndrome is an example of associated neurologic and pigmentary abnormalities. First described in 1969, the mnemonic "leopard" designates the major findings: lentigines, ECG conduction defects, ocular hypertelorism, pulmonary stenosis, abnormalities of genitalia, retardation of growth, and deafness. The lentigines occur anywhere on the skin and often show mottled pigmentation. They vary in size from pinpoint to several centimeters (Fig. 45, color plate 2). Histologically they show the typical features of a lentigo: increased numbers of melanocytes and acanthosis.

Ephilis (Freckles)

Freckles are absent at birth and appear in early childhood. Freckling does not occur in areas unexposed to solar irradiation. Clinically freckles are flat and vary in color from tan to black. On histologic examination they contain fewer melanocytes than the normally pigmented surrounding skin; however, the melanocytes are larger and more active.

The pigmented macules, present around the mouth and across the bridge of the nose in Peutz-Jeghers syndrome, are histologically identical with freckles.

Mongolian Spot

In most Mongolian and in three-quarters of Black infants, there are present one or more bluish-gray areas of discoloration over the buttocks, sacrum, or back called Mongolian spots. These are collections of dopa-positive melanocytes in the dermis, which presumably have failed to migrate to the epidermis from the neural crest. They may occur on the face or trunk. Mongolian spots located on the buttocks and sacrum fade with age. They may be confused with extramedullary hematopoiesis in the newborn.

Xeroderma Pigmentosum

Xeroderma pigmentosum is a rare disorder inherited as an autosomal recessive. It is characterized by a profound sensitivity of the skin to the effects of sunlight. The disease is usually apparent in the first year of life and is heralded by a sunburn out of proportion to the amount of irradiation received. The course is relentless; first there is erythema, which may fade. Freckles appear, which enlarge, become more numerous, and are darkly pigmented. The eyes are usually involved, with corneal ulcerations, opacities, and pterygia. Telangiectasia next appears and the skin becomes dry and often atrophic. The changes resemble those of x-ray dermatitis. Tumors, benign and malignant, next appear, and the distressing appearance of these children reflects not only intrinsic changes in the skin but surgical attempts to remove ever-increasing numbers of basal cell tumors and epidermal carcinomas. Keratoses, papillomas, and angiomas also occur. Multiple basal cell tumors and epidermal carcinomas often are present by two or three years of age.

Although the skin exhibits a spectacular sensitivity to sunlight, no specific wavelength appears to be responsible for the damage. Areas that are shielded from sunlight do not deteriorate as rapidly as the skin of the face and hands.

The prognosis for patients with this disease is poor. Untreated patients usually do not survive beyond age 20, but with careful management some have lived more than 60 years. An interesting, as yet unexplained abnormality in many of these patients is aminoaciduria.

A variant of xeroderma pigmentosum is the *de Sanctis-Cacchione syndrome,* in which there are mental deficiency, microcephaly, gonadal underdevelopment, and dwarfism.

Fibroblasts cultured from normal human skin can repair DNA (unscheduled DNA synthesis) following ultraviolet irradiation. Fibroblasts from patients with xeroderma pigmentosum are unable to participate in this repair. Similarly, exposure of normal human skin to ultraviolet irradiation stimulates unscheduled (nonmitotic) DNA synthesis in the epidermis and upper dermal fibroblasts. Patients with xeroderma pigmentosum do not show this response. It is tempting to associate the high incidence of cutaneous malignancy in patients with xeroderma pigmentosum with their inability to repair damaged DNA.

Treatment of xeroderma pigmentosum, although discouraging, is effective in prolonging comfort, acceptable appearance, and life. The chief aim is to shield the patient from all solar radiation. Sunscreen ointments are obviously not as effective as simply staying indoors during the day. Careful periodic examination and removal of tumors while they are small are extremely important measures.

Incontinentia Pigmenti

Incontinentia pigmenti (*Bloch-Sulzberger syndrome*) is a rare abnormality, appearing almost exclusively in infant girls. It is characterized by three separate changes in the skin: (a) inflammatory vesicles located predominantly on the extremities; (b) linear verrucous and hyperkeratotic lesions on the extremities; and (c) irregular whorled patterns of pigmentation (Fig. 46). The pigmentation, which may have the pattern of veins in marble, often occurs in areas that are not involved by the vesicular, inflammatory, or verrucous changes.

The first signs of the disease are linear or grouped vesicles, usually located on the extremities. They may appear within the first two or three days after birth. New vesicles may appear and fade, to be replaced by inflammatory papules and hyperkeratotic warty lesions. The

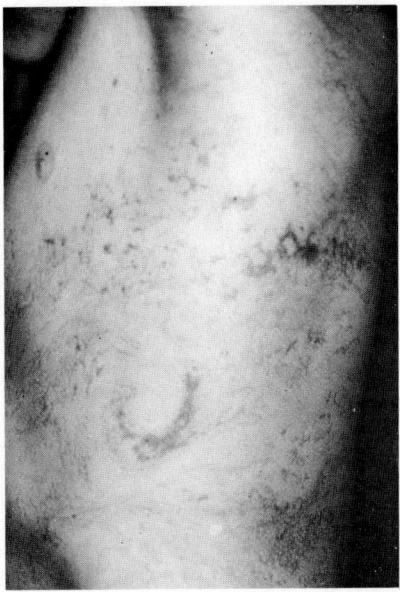

FIG. 46.   Seven-year-old girl with incontinentia pigmenti, showing whorls or irregularly scattered pigmentation.

pigmentation may be present at birth or appear within the first few years. It is brown to grayish-brown. The vesicular and verrucous lesions ordinarily resolve spontaneously within the first few years, and the pigmentation fades gradually, although usually some hyperpigmentation remains for life. In areas of pigmentation, there are extensive dermal deposits of melanin. It is because of this apparent inability of the epidermis to retain pigment that the syndrome was named incontinentia pigmenti.

In addition to the striking abnormalities of the skin, there are often defects of the central nervous system, teeth, or eyes. Eye changes, which occur in about one-third of the patients, include strabismus, optic atrophy, and cataract. At least one-third of the children with this disorder have central nervous system involvement, which may include mental retardation, microcephaly, hydrocephalus, or seizures. Dental abnormalities are common. There may be missing teeth, delayed dentition, or conical teeth (Fig. 47). Congenital heart disease has been found in some patients. Hair loss occurs in many of these children and resembles pseudodopelade.

The disorder is inherited either as an autosomal dominant, which is sex linked in its expression, or as a sex-linked gene on the X chromosome. In a few affected children karotypes have been examined and found to be normal.

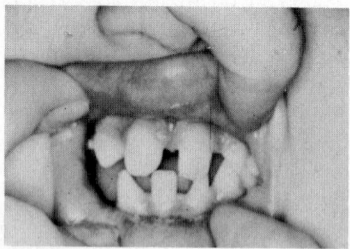

FIG. 47. Incontinentia pigmenti showing characteristic painted and absent teeth in a 7-year-old girl.

Acanthosis Nigricans

Acanthosis nigricans in children is a fairly uncommon condition in which skin markings are accentuated and the surface is velvety, rugose, and furrowed. The color may vary from tan to black. Sites of predilection are the neck, axilia, elbows (both flexor and extensor surfaces), groin, and occasionally the buccal mucosa. Involvement is usually bilateral, and when the lesion arises unilaterally, it may be impossible to differentiate from nevus unius lateralis.

The appearance of this disease is a serious omen in adults, many of whom develop internal malignancy. In children, the association has been made only once, in a teenage child, and no associated malignancy has been reported in younger children. Of greater significance in children is the frequent association of endocrine abnormalities of diverse types. Approximately one-third of

children with acanthosis nigricans have an endocrine abnormality—diabetes, Cushing's disease, adrenocortical hyperplasia, hypothyroidism or hyperthyroidism, or gigantism. Acanthosis nigricans is often present in children with lipodystrophic diabetes. Children with acanthosis nigricans in whom no endocrine abnormality can be demonstrated are regularly obese, and as techniques of endocrinologic investigation become more refined, perhaps more patients in this group will be found to have subtle endocrine abnormalities.

The sites of predilection of acanthosis nigricans are generally sites of friction and/or maceration. This suggests that a systemic predisposition can be evoked by local factors.

Familial occurrence of acanthosis, associated with obesity and malignancy, has been reported.

Acanthosis nigricans is chronic but often remits or improves when the obesity or underlying endocrinopathy is corrected. Local therapy has not been effective.

Café-au-lait Spot

Café-au-lait spots, which are a cardinal sign of neurofibromatosis (von Recklinghausen's disease), may also occur in epiloia and Gaucher's disease. These macular areas of hyperpigmentation are variable in size, light tan to brown in color, and usually have a regular border. They may be present at birth and are unrelated to exposure to sun. Histologically, there is an apparent increase in the number of melanocytes demonstrated by the dopa reaction. Café-au-lait spots may gradually increase in size and number throughout life and often precede the appearance of neurofibromas. In addition to discrete café-au-lait spots, patients with von Recklinghausen's disease often have diffuse freckling and hyperpigmentation. Solitary café-au-lait spots have no significance; six or more café-au-lait spots are practically always associated with neurofibromatosis.

In Albright's disease (polyostotic fibrous dysplasia) there are similar patches of hyperpigmentation, which, in contrast to café-au-lait spots in von Recklinghausen's disease, have irregular margins.

Bibliography

Abe K, Nicholson WE, Liddle GW, Island DP, Orth DN: Radioimmunoassay of β-MSH in human plasma and tissues. J Clin Invest 46:1609, 1967

Cleaver JE: Defective repair replication of DNA in xeroderma pigmentosum. Nature 318:652, 1968

Epstein J, Fukuyama K, Reed W, Epstein W: Defect in DNA synthesis in skin of patients with xeroderma pigmentosum demonstrated in vivo. Science 168:1477, 1970

Fitzpatrick TB, Szabo G, Hori Y, Sunone AA, Reed WB, et al: White leaf-shaped macules. Arch Dermatol 98:1, 1968

Kopf AW, Andrade R: A histologic study of the dermo-epidermal junction in clinically "intradermal" nevi employing serial sections. I. Junctional theques. Ann NY Acad Sci 100:200, 1963

——— Morrill SD, Silberberg I: Broad spectrum of leukoderma aquisitum centrifugum. Arch Dermatol 92:14, 1965

Lerner AB: Vitiligo. J Invest Dermatol 32:285, 1959

——— McGuire JS: Melanocyte-stimulating hormone and adrenocorticotrophic hormone, their relation to pigmentation. N Engl J Med 270:539, 1964

Reed WB, Dexter R, Corley C, Fish C: Congenital lipodystrophic diabetes with acanthosis nigricans. Arch Dermatol 91:326, 1965

——— May SB, Nickel WR: Xeroderma pigmentosum with neurological complications. Arch Dermatol 91:224, 1965

——— Becker SW Sr, Becker SW Jr, Nickel WR: Giant pigmented nevi, melanoma, and leptomeningeal melanocytosis. Arch Dermatol 91:100, 1965

Windhorst DB, Zelickson AS, Good RA: Chediak-Higashi syndrome: hereditary gigantism of cytoplasmic organelles. Science 151:81, 1966

ECZEMA (ATOPIC DERMATITIS)

Joseph McGuire

Eczema is a common chronic dermatitis characterized by exudation, lichenification, and pruritus. It occurs in a population defined as atopic by virtue of the presence of several related conditions including asthma, seasonal rhinitis, eczema, and recurrent urticaria. The prevalence rate of atopy in the general population is unknown, but a recent survey revealed that 19 percent of a large group of dermatologic patients, who did not have eczema, had a personal history of atopy; 23 percent had a positive family history of atopy and 34 percent had a positive personal or family history. See also Chap. 10.

Physiology

The skin of atopics responds abnormally to the intracutaneous injection of methacholine (mecholyl) by delayed blanching after initial erythema. In normal individuals an area of erythema appears around the site of injection and gradually fades. This paradoxical reaction is said to occur in 70 percent of patients with atopic dermatitis. Although the blanching suggests that vasoconstriction has occurred, direct examination of the capillaries does not support this assumption. The blanch produced by the injection of epinephrine into atopic skin is associated with decreased clearance and vasoconstriction. The pharmacology of the delayed blanch remains obscure.

Atopic reagin appears to be identical to immunoglobulin E, which is elevated in the sera of individuals with severe atopic dermatitis. Many individuals with moderate atopic dermatitis have normal levels of circulating IgE. Moreover, the amount of anti-IgE necessary to produce erythema and wheal reactions when injected into the skin is no different in patients with atopic dermatitis than in control groups.

The relationship of atopic dermatitis to other mediators of the immune reaction is not clear. Peterson and coworkers have reported that in a group of 23 patients with agammaglobulinemia and no detectable circulating globulin, 4 had atopic dermatitis.

The relationship of IgE and atopic dermatitis is puzzling, as is the role of IgE. Thymus-derived lymphocytes have the capacity to suppress IgE production. Thus diseases such as atopy may reflect depression of T lymphocyte function. Studies that require substantiation have shown that T-cell function is depressed in the atopic disease. It was also found that response to delayed skin tests SK-SD and candida were inverse to the degree of activity of eczema and that children with the most severe dermatitis showed marked delayed cutaneous anergy.

Pathology

Changes occur in both the dermis and epidermis, but the alterations are so variable that the clinical features of the disease tend to be more helpful for diagnosis than the histologic features. However, microscopic examination of the skin can sometimes be of great importance in differentiating atopic dermatitis from other diseases.

Histologic changes reflect the varying clinical picture. Early changes are acanthosis and parakeratosis. The inflammatory infiltrate varies in quantity with the clinical activity of the process and consists of lymphocytes and sometimes eosinophils. Spongiosis (intercellular edema), a prominent feature of contact dermatitis, is usually not a major feature of atopic dermatitis, except for the dyshidrotic form (pompholyx). Electron microscopy of exudative infantile eczema reveals lysosomes in the keratinocytes. The more chronic lichenified forms of eczema show hyperkeratosis, acanthosis, some degree of papillomatosis, and usually only scanty inflammatory infiltrate.

Clinical Forms

Long-term observations of individual patients, as well as statistical studies of large numbers of patients, both support the concept of including several clinically well-defined dermatoses within the general term atopic dermatitis. Although this "inclusive" approach to atopic dermatitis does not imply etiologic relationships, it is useful from a therapeutic standpoint and it tends to simplify an unnecessarily complicated area of dermatology. The basis for including the following clinical expressions in the category of atopic dermatitis is both the high incidence of history of atopic disease in these patients, and the changing pattern of dermatitis in a single patient (Table 5).

INFANTILE ECZEMA. In infancy, the creases of the neck may become exuded, moist, and sometimes secondarily infected with monilia. The cheeks have a healthy, rosy appearance, which, on close inspection, may be due to the presence of papules and crusting. Fissuring may occur behind the ears.

When the child becomes older, the pattern of involvement changes and becomes more scattered with extensor involvement. The lesions are usually dry and somewhat pruritic. Classic flexural involvement may occur at any age, but is most common after 4 years (Fig. 48, color plate 2).

DYSHIDROTIC ECZEMA. This is a well-established misnomer for a clinically well-defined dermatitis characterized by recurrent blistering eruptions on the palms and soles (Fig. 49). Although some of these children do have hyperhidrosis of the palms and soles, careful serial sections of the blisters establish their independence from the eccrine apparatus. This form of eczema is very pruritic and is sometimes misdiagnosed

TABLE 5. Changing Problems of Eczema at Various Ages

	Age	Site	Clinical Features
Infantile eczema	Infancy	Cheeks, neck creases ears, scalp	Exudative, moist, cheeks are rosy: papular
Flexural eczema	> 4 years	Antecubital popliteal areas, sides of neck, behind ears	Erythema, excoriation, skin becomes lichenified and taut
Dyshidrotic eczema (Pompholyx)	> 2 years	Palms, soles	Intensely pruritic, blisters occur on palms, soles and sides of fingers. Blisters may be minute or large. Frequently mistaken for dermatophytic infection
Nummular eczema	> 1 year	Extremities, trunk	Circular, papulovesicular patches, often extremely pruritic. Lesions may be sparse or numerous
Generalized atopic dermatitis	> 4-5 years	Generalized	Uncommon in young children, skin is generally lichenified with slight scaling. Hands and feet are cold, the eyelids are lichenified, infraorbital pigmentation and many excoriations. Involvement is worse in flexural areas

as contact dermatitis or dermatophytic infection. Opening the blisters on the hands and feet helps relieve the intense pruritus.

GENERALIZED ATOPIC DERMATITIS.   These unfortunate children itch in response to many stimuli such as heat, cold, wool, or anger. The skin becomes lichenified, taut, and scaly, and is often crossed with excoriations. Their eyelids and intraorbital folds are lichenified, which gives them an apprehensive, fatigued appearance.

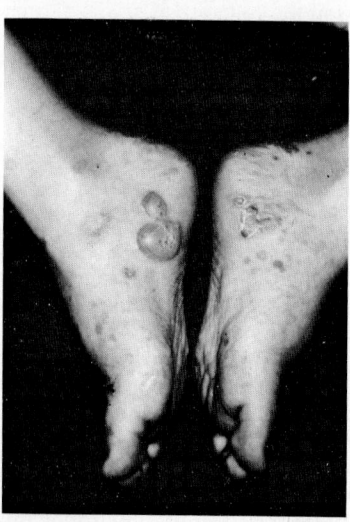

FIG. 49.   Dyshidrotic eczema (pompholyx). Recurrent blistering eruption on plams and soles. These lesions are not related to sweat retention as the name suggests. Pompholyx is probably one manifestation of atopic dermatitis. This child later had characteristic atopic dermatitis.

Ancillary Clinical Features

ICHTHYOSIS VULGARIS.   This is often associated with atopic dermatitis and, even in the absence of clinically distinctive ichthyosis vulgaris, keratosis pilaris may be present. These children often have dry, chapped skin in the wintertime. Prevention of scaling and chapping with local hydration and lubrication can sometimes preclude further development of eczema.

PITYRIASIS ALBA.   Pityriasis alba is a descriptive term for one or more oval or circular patches of depigmentation of varying degrees. There is often a fine scale and occasionally slight erythema. The lesions are located on the cheeks and trunk and often occur in children with evidence of atopy, especially eczema and hay fever. Pityriasis alba is thought by us to represent a form of atopic dermatitis; however, this is not a universally held concept. The lesions of pityriasis alba improve and repigment following the use of lubricants and topical steroids. In chronic eczema, there has been demonstrated a block in pigment transfer from the melanocyte to the keratinocyte. There may be a similar interference with this symbiotic relationship in pityriasis alba.

Complications

Atopic skin is especially susceptible to infections with microorganisms; among the more serious are herpes simplex (Fig. 50) and vaccinia. Impetigo is a common problem in these children. Because of the seriousness of Kaposi's varicelliform eruption (a vesicular eruption caused by herpes simplex or vaccinia) *these children should not be vaccinated or exposed to a freshly vaccinated individual* (p. 590).

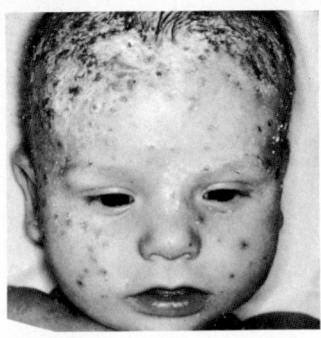

FIG. 50. Herpes simplex (eczema herpeticum). Infant with atopic dermatitis and multiple lesions of herpes simplex.

Associated Diseases

Allergic rhinitis, asthma, and vernal catarrh are frequent in children with atopic dermatitis. Cataracts occur frequently enough to be a recognized complication of the disease, although the relationship is obscure.

Ichthyosis vulgaris often coexists with atopic dermatitis. The Wiscott-Aldrich syndrome exhibits, in addition to atopic dermatitis, thrombocytopenia and cutaneous and pulmonary infection.

Other diseases occurring with increased frequency in children with atopic dermatitis are congenital agammaglobulinemia and phenylketonuria.

Prognosis

A 20-year follow-up of 492 patients with atopic dermatitis seen at the Mayo Clinic was conducted by a questionnaire to which 45 percent responded (Table 6). The median age of onset in the mild and severe groups was 4 months; the median age of complete clearing for the two groups was 21 years. The average duration of the disease was 27 years among the mild group and 32 years in the severe group. It is apparent from this study that the prognosis for complete clearing in childhood or early adulthood is not good, especially since any patient in the "cleared" group is subject to exacerbation.

Table 6. Twenty-Year Follow-up of Atopic Dermatitis

Present Condition (Percent)	Condition When First Seen	
	Mild	Severe
Completely Cleared	40	29
Better	48	55
Unchanged	1	13
Worse	11	3

Treatment

The form of treatment obviously is determined by the major clinical features. Therapy for acute weeping dermatitis differs from therapy for a chronic, lichenified dermatitis.

The use of antihistaminic drugs for pruritus, although widespread, is often disappointing. Sedation is often of the same magnitude as relief of itching. Hydroxyzine is the most useful drug currently used to control pruritus. The range of effective dosage is wide. Often the medication is required only in the evening or at bedtime when there is a marked exacerbation of pruritus. Hydroxyzine is not a very potent antihistaminic and it probably acts on the central perception of itch.

The value of open wet dressings cannot be overemphasized. The possiblity of infection must be constantly reviewed even in the absence of classic impetigo. If cultures show a pathogenic streptococcus or staphylococcus, the child should be treated with systemic antibiotics.

Lubricants are of great value in children with atopic dermatitis. In many children dry scaly pruritic skin appears to precede the more characteristic eczematous changes. The role of scratching and rubbing in the generation and perpetuation of eczematous changes is naturally suspect.

Topical steroid preparations can be extremely useful; however, they are often used ineffectively or to excess. Before application of topical steroids, the skin should be moistened with a damp cloth for a few minutes. After the steroid, a lubricant should be applied. The amount of the lubricant to be applied depends on the dryness of the skin and the relative humidity.

Continued application of topical steroids, especially the fluorinated compounds, to the skin can result in atrophy, particularly in areas where there is some degree of natural occlusion or where the skin is normally thin, such as the groin or medial thigh.

Systemic steroids are rarely required in children, and because of the prolonged adrenal suppression resulting from intramuscular administration, alternate day oral steroids are probably the safer choice. If atopic eczema is so severe that topical measures and oral antipruritics cannot control it, short-term hospitalization should be considered.

Bibliography

Lobitz WC, Campbell CJ: Physiologic studies in atopic dermatitis. Arch Dermatol 67:575, 1953

McGeady SJ, Buckley RH: Depression of cell-mediated immunity in atopic eczema. J Allergy Clin Immunol 56:393, 1975

Peterson RD, Page AR, Good RA: Wheal and erythema allergy in patients with agammaglobulinemia. J Allergy 33:406, 1962

OTHER DISEASES OF SKIN
Joseph McGuire

Miliaria (Poral Occlusion)

Miliaria is nearly universal in infancy. The lesions result from a combination of sweating and occlusion of the intraepidermal portion of the sweat duct. If the obstruction is very superficial, then only a fraction of the epidermis is lifted away from the skin by a drop of sweat, with the production of a minute transparent vesicle, miliaria crystallina, which often escapes notice. *Miliaria crystallina* is common in febrile illnesses and is not symptomatic. The lesions are so superficial that they may be removed by wiping the skin. This disease has no intrinsic importance and only reflects sweating and poral occlusion.

Miliaria rubra is produced by the same process, occurring deeper in the sweat duct. Sweat is retained behind the deeper occlusion and causes dilation and rupture of the epidermal portion of the sweat duct, with resulting swelling and inflammation. The lesions are symptomatic, often producing considerable itching and stinging—hence its familiar designation, prickly heat. The lesions appear in areas of maceration, under plastic pants, adhesive tape, and tight clothing, which occlude and cause the epidermal lining of the sweat duct to swell with obstruction of the lumen. Prickly heat is especially common in hot humid weather and in febrile illnesses with associated excessive sweating.

The lesions are small (2 to 5 mm) red papules, papulovesicles, and occasionally pustules that occur most often on the trunk. In severe cases the dermatitis may be generalized, with a resultant decrease in sweating and evaporative heat loss. Interference with heat loss may result in temperature elevation.

Effective therapeutic measures for miliaria rubra are based on the pathogenesis of the lesion. Reduction of environmental temperature and humidity is most important. Body temperature, when this is a contributing cause, is reduced by salicylates. Lightweight absorbent clothing should be worn.

Open wet dressings with *Burow's solution* promote drying and heat loss. Calamine lotion is an effective drying agent. When there is secondary bacterial or monilial infection, the specific antibiotic is added.

Pityriasis Rubra Pilaris

This rare chronic skin disease, which may begin in infancy or childhood, is characterized by red, horny papules that surround hair follicles. Large numbers of these papules cause the skin to appear erythematous. A characteristic clinical feature is occasional well-demarcated islands of normal skin surrounded by generalized involvement. The palms and soles are usually involved. They are red, thickened, and fissured. Papules are often present on the backs of the fingers. The scalp may be involved initially with severe seborrheic dermatitis, which may also affect the face. In children, facial involvement often produces a masklike appearance.

When there is extensive involvement, the diagnosis of generalized psoriasis is often difficult to rule out. Histologic diagnosis is usually possible.

The course of the disease is persistent and fortunately asymptomatic. In a few families it appears to be inherited as a dominant trait with incomplete penetrance. Treatment consists of lubrication and the use of keratolytics, such as salicylic acid. Oral vitamin A in large doses is definitely beneficial in occasional pa-

tients. Sunlight, which benefits psoriasis, has no effect on pityriasis rubra pilaris.

Pityriasis Rosea

Pityriasis rosea is a papulosquamous disease occurring primarily on the trunk. It is characterized by a herald patch—an erythematous annular lesion with a scaly border that precedes the generalized eruption by about a week. Infrequently, there may be a mild prodrome of fever and sore throat. The generalized eruption occurs mainly on the trunk, and the oval lesions lie with their axes along lines of cleavage. The lesions of the generalized eruption are usually smaller than the herald patch. They enlarge and are surrounded by a collarette of fine scales. In children the lesions may be urticarial or papulovesicular (Fig. 51).

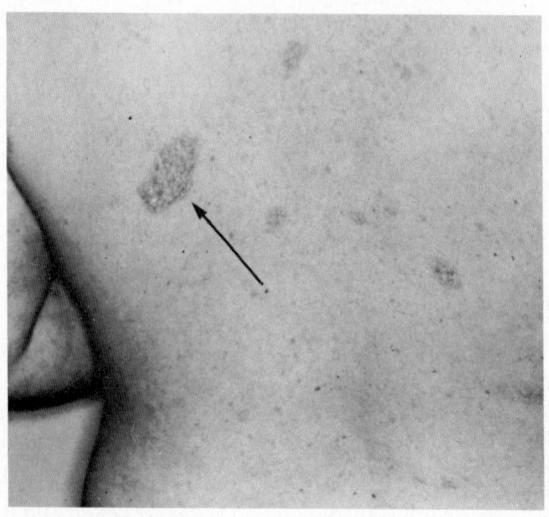

FIG. 51.   Pityriasis rosea. Herald patch (arrow) precedes the generalized eruption which can be papular, uricarial, or occasionally papulovesicular.

The occasional prodrome and the usual freedom from second attacks suggest a viral causation, although this has not been proved. The disease occurs frequently in children and young adults, rarely in infants. There is no evidence that it is contagious. The disease usually lasts for six to eight weeks, with or without treatment, but may persist longer.

The clinical features, the color, distribution, and morphology of the lesions are usually sufficient to establish a diagnosis. Although the disease itself is of trivial significance, it achieves distinction by being regularly misdiagnosed as tinea corporis. In older children, secondary syphilis must be ruled out.

If pruritus is troublesome, calamine lotion containing 0.5 percent phenol may be used topically. The oral administration of antihistamines is also effective for pruritus.

Lichen Planus

This member of the papulosquamous group of diseases is characterized by multiple polygonal, flat-topped papules with a predilection for the flexor aspects of the wrists and forearms and the lower legs; however, any part of the body may become involved. Involvement of the buccal mucosa is frequent, with a coalescence of minute white papules to form a linear or reticulated pattern. The typical lesion is usually only 1 to 2 mm in diameter; many of these may aggregate to form a plaque. Bullous forms of the disease also occur.

The disease is of unknown cause and mainly affects adults; it rarely affects children. A clinical feature shared with psoriasis is the Koebner phenomenon: new lesions appear on the skin at sites of trauma. The course of the disease is variable, often lasting a year. Lesions on the legs occasionally become hypertrophic and persist much longer.

In addition to the clinical features, which are fairly specific, there are characteristic histopathologic findings: a band of lymphocytic infiltrate immediately below the epidermis with destruction of the basement membrane of the epidermis. Differential diagnosis includes drug eruption and atopic dermatitis, in both of which there may be flat-topped papules. Oral lesions may be mistaken for thrush, and involvement of the genitalia may mimic seborrheic dermatitis or psoriasis.

Treatment is unsatisfactory and is directed toward the alleviation of pruritus, which may be severe. Topical steroids are often effective on the genitalia but usually have little effect elsewhere. The intralesional injection of triamcinolone acetonide into chronic plaques of hypertrophic lichen planus is often beneficial.

Lichen Nitidis

Lichen nitidis is a rare asymptomatic disease of unknown cause with no satisfactory treatment. Highly characteristic lesions permit easy diagnosis. The numerous, shiny, slightly elevated minute, flat-topped papules may occur anywhere, but the genitalia and abdomen are most often involved. Eczema is often characterized by similar small elevated flat-topped papules, especially in Blacks. These lesions, which are associated with pruritus and friction, are easily mistaken for the relatively uncommon lichen nitidis. The course of lichen nitidis is chronic, and the disease eventually resolves without residua.

Mucha-Habermann Disease

Mucha-Habermann disease (Pityriasis lichenoides et varioliformis acuta) is an uncommon disease characterized by recurrent crops of lesions that first appear as pink papules that form a central vesicle, then crust, and sometimes undergo an area of central hemorrhagic necrosis (Fig. 52). The lesions are usually asymptomatic; however, the onset is sometimes heralded by fever and malaise. The trunk and flexor aspects of the extremities are involved; the face is usually spared. The course is unpredictable. Many patients are clear within six to eight months; however, recurrent crops of lesions may appear for years (Fig. 53).

Although the etiology is unknown, the course of the illness suggests a viral etiology. The earliest histologic change is a lymphocytic infiltrate around dermal capillaries associated with epidermal edema.

There are febrile and scarring forms of the disease. Treatment is not satisfactory; systemic adrenocortical steroids or tetracycline may be tried.

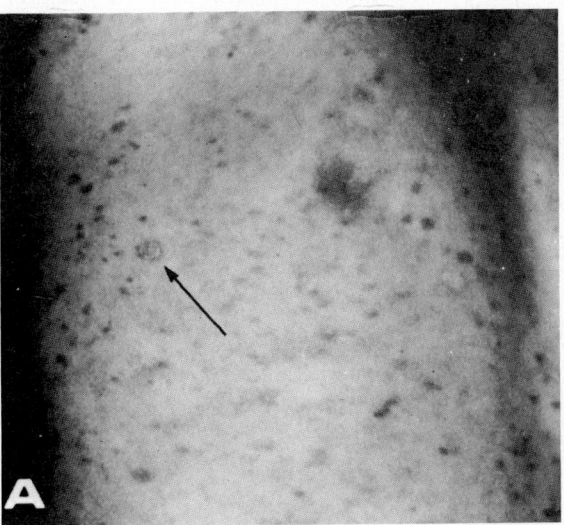
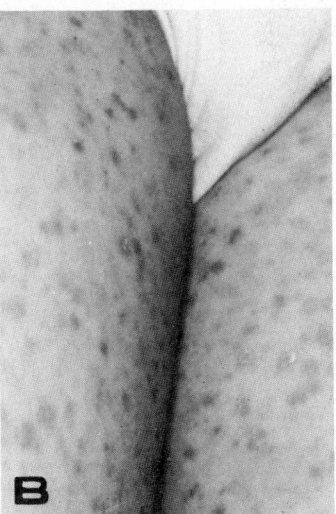

FIG. 52. Mucha-Habermann disease. **A.** Generalized distribution of lesions on trunk. This form of parapsoriasis is characterized by papulonecrotic lesions (arrow). **B.** Papular scaly lesions are distributed over extremities and trunk, usually sparing the face. The individual lesions are sometimes hemorrhagic.

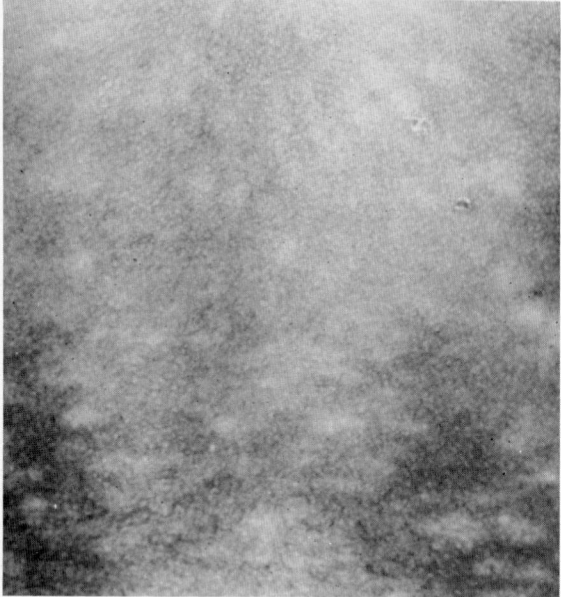

FIG. 53. Mucha-Habermann disease. The disease in this child is now quiescent and marked by postinflammatory hypopigmentation. Photograph is of back.

Gianotti-Crosti Syndrome

Gianotti-Crosti syndrome is a distinctive clinical syndrome charaterized by papules 0.5 to 1 cm in diameter located on the legs, thighs, and buttocks (Fig. 54). There is usually lymphadenopathy and sometimes mild

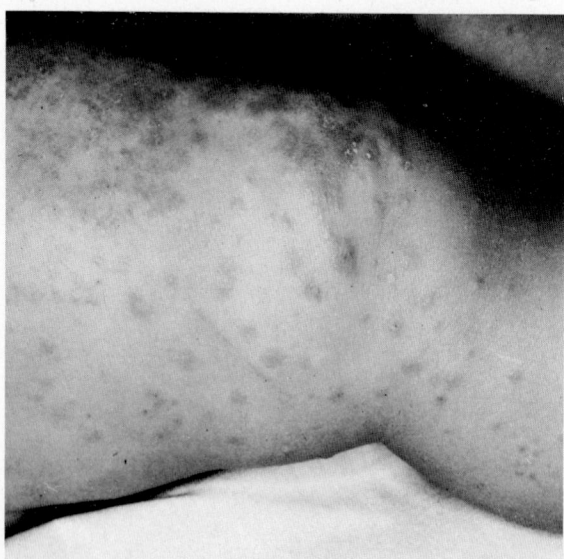

FIG. 54. Gianotti-Crosti syndrome. Red papules on legs of infant. The lesions may also occur on buttocks, extensor aspects of the arms, and on the face.

malaise. The lesions on the legs are occasionally purpuric. The disease may last up to 2 months. No therapy is indicated.

Urticaria Pigmentosa (Mastocytosis)

This disease has been classified into three groups, two of which have their onset in childhood. The lesions are characterized by collections in the dermis of tissue mast cells which stain metachromatically. Trauma or heat causes release of histamine from these cells, which leads to the formation of urticaria.

Distinguishing features of the three groups are:

I.   Solitary lesion with onset in childhood
II. Multiple lesions with onset in childhood
III. Multiple lesions with onset after childhood

GROUP I.   The lesions are often present at birth, but may appear during the first year. The lesions may be located anywhere on the trunk or extremities. Grossly, the lesions are yellow to tan in color and may range in size from a small papule to a large plaque. If a second lesion does not appear within 1 or 2 months, the patient can be placed in group I with fair assurance. Most of these solitary lesions are characterized by vesicle or bulla formation, and urticaria can be produced by rubbing (Darier's sign). These children improve spontaneously, and excision of the lesion is not indicated unless flushing or other symptoms necessitate it. Treatment is directed toward the pruritus.

GROUP II.   The lesions are macular or maculopapular and appear from birth to age 4 years. The site of involvement is usually the trunk. They vary in size and may be pink, yellow, or brown. Vesiculation is often present, and Darier's sign is almost always positive. Pruritus is the chief symptom and may be alleviated by the use of oral antihistamines. Rarely, blistering may precede the appearance of the typical maculopapular lesions of urticaria pigmentosa. Most of these children show either marked improvement or actual disappearance of the lesions by adolescence. Rarely, the disease persists unabated into adult life.

GROUP III.   In most of these patients, the lesions appear in adolescence or early adulthood. Located predominantly on the trunk, they are pink to brown in color and are usually macular or maculopapular. Darier's sign is usually postive and vesiculation is rare. These patients, in contrast to those in groups I and II, have a very chronic course.

In addition to involvement of the skin, there may be widespread and rarely fatal extracutaneous mast-cell infiltration of liver, spleen, and bone marrow. Systemic involvement is usually assocated with diffuse involvement of the skin.

The cause is unknown. Thirty-one patients have been described in 14 families with pedigrees suggesting autosomal dominant form of inheritance. All three types of mastocytosis were represented in these families. Most patients, however, do not have a positive family history. Treatment is directed toward reducing pruritus with antihistamines; air conditioning is an especially effective adjunct to therapy in warm weather. The pigmentation when present is due to melanin, the formation of which is stimulated by the mast cell or its products.

Nevoxanthoendothelioma (Juvenile Xanthogranuloma)

This benign tumor usually appears within the first few months of life. The individual lesions are elevated, dome-shaped, and smooth. Their color is sometimes yellow-orange but can also be tan. The lesions, which are characteristically located on the scalp, may also occur elsewhere, especially in extensor areas. The lesions are usually multiple and vary in size from a few millimeters to over a centimeter in diameter.

The disease is almost always uncomplicated and resolves spontaneously. Lesions involving the iris and ciliary body may result in glaucoma. The patients are normolipemic and the disease is not related to the more sinister histiocytosis. The earliest histologic event is the accumulation of histiocytes with secondary deposition of lipids.

The lesions must be distinguished from mastocytosis, which they may sometimes closely resemble.

Hemangioma

Hemangiomas and pigmented nevi are the most common developmental abnormalities of skin. They both produce considerably more apprehension than is warranted by their nature and prognosis. Hemangiomas, also termed vascular nevi, have practically no malignant potential and are of concern primarily because of their appearance, interference with function, ulceration, or hemorrhage after trauma. Most hemangiomas fall into one of the following three descriptive categories: port-wine stain, strawberry hemangioma, and cavernous hemangioma.

PORT-WINE STAIN.   The port-wine stain or *nevus flammeus* is pink to reddish purple and usually present at birth. The two most common sites are the nape of the neck and the center of the forehead, although the nevus may occur on any part of the body. The Sturge-Weber-Dimitri syndrome includes a port-wine vascular nevus, often in the distribution of the first division of the trigeminal nerve. The lesion is composed of mature capillaries, and although those located on the face and trunk tend to regress, most grow in relation to the affected part. Occasionally, the surface of the hemangiomas may become papular with age. In view of the persistent and benign course of the lesion, it is best left alone unless it is disfiguring. Small lesions may be excised, but dry ice and sclerosing agents are not effective. The nevi are not radiosensitive. The most acceptable treatment is a covering cosmetic. Attempts to tattoo pigment into these nevi to lighten the color have been only partially successful.

STRAWBERRY HEMANGIOMA.   The *nevus vasculosus* or strawberry mark usually appears a few days after birth as a tiny red spot. This is the only worthwhile time to interfere with its natural development; however, it is usually overlooked until after a few weeks of rapid growth. It then appears as a lobulated, elevated, bright red or red-purple, soft lesion. The lesion may persist, with slow growth for several years. The color then becomes mottled and the tumor begins to involute. The strawberry mark offers an almost irresistible temptation for the physician to interfere with its natural course.

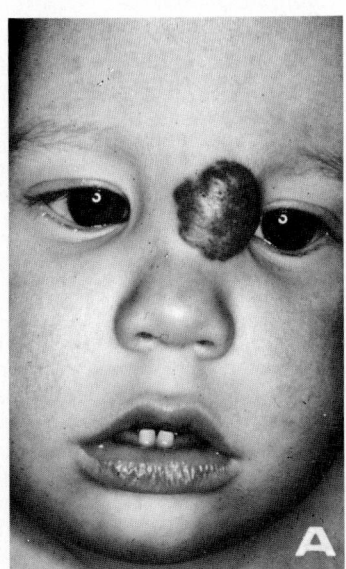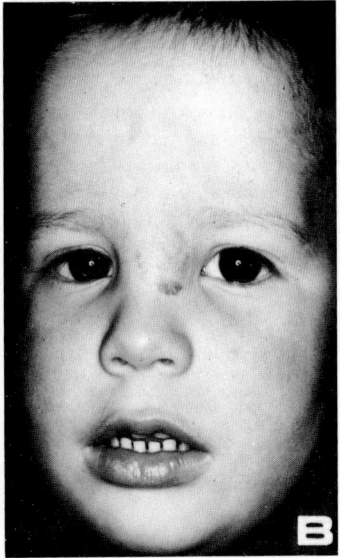

FIG. 55.   Strawberry hemangioma. **A.**   Lesion at its greatest size. **B.**   Same lesion as in A 26 months later, without treatment.

The ultimate cosmetic result is usually superior if impulses to treat the strawberry mark are resisted. Involution is usually nearly complete by age 6 or 7 and often occurs earlier. The dependability of this spontaneous resolution is confirmed by the absence of this lesion in adults, and there is little question that the cosmetic result is better if the lesion is not treated (Fig. 55).

In certain situations, treatment is required because the hemangioma interferes with feeding, respiration, or vision. Hemangiomas on the urethra or anus also require attention. Hemorrhage is rare and is usually the result of trauma or therapy. Ulceration is not so rare and may precede spontaneous resolution. Thrombocytopenic purpura has occurred in association with large hemangiomas, many of which are strawberry hemangiomas. The tumor apparently sequesters and destroys platelets.

The usual treatment by the application of carbon dioxide snow or dry ice is destructive and produces scarring. The strawberry hemangioma is radiosensitive, and x-ray is the preferred treatment for large lesions. Systemic steroids have been used successfully in the treatment of these nevi.

CAVERNOUS HEMANGIOMA. Cavernous hemangiomas are composed of mature blood vessels and do not involute, thus differing from strawberry hemangiomas. They are almost always present at birth and do not grow except in proportion to the area of body affected. The hemangioma may be raised or flat and may be predominantly subcutaneous in location. If intervention is necessary because of the position of the hemangioma, surgery is the only effective treatment. This can sometimes be carried out in stages, without the necessity of a graft. The mature blood vessels are not especially sensitive to x-ray. Several syndromes, eg, Parkes-Weber, are associated with cavernous hemangiomas.

OTHER VASCULAR ABNORMALITIES AND SYNDROMES. The spider nevus, or *nevus araneus,* is a common lesion of children, occurring in about one-fourth of children younger than 15 years. The dorsa of the hands, forearms, and face are most commonly involved. Unlike the nevus araneus in the adult, which is a fellow traveler with Laennec's cirrhosis, the appearance of this lesion has no medical significance in the child. There is a central vessel, which can often be seen to pulsate, with smaller radiating vessels. Although they are of little cosmetic consequence and often resolve spontaneously with age, electrocoagulation of the central vessel will usually cause the lesion to disappear.

There are many syndromes associated with hemangiomas:

In the *Sturge-Weber-Dimitri syndrome,* nevus flammeus in the trigeminal region of the face is associated with vascular abnormalities in the brain. Mental retardation, seizures, and contralateral hemiplegia are characteristic.

Parkes-Weber syndrome is a capillary or mature large vessel hemangioma on an extremity, with hypertrophy of that limb.

In the *von Hippel-Lindau syndrome* there are angiomas of the retina, brain, and skin.

In the *Maffucci syndrome,* there are enchondromas of the bone associated with multiple cavernous hemangiomas. The limbs may become seriously deformed, even to the point where amputation is necessary.

In *Louis-Bar (ataxia-telangiectasia) syndrome* there is progressive telangiectasia of the bulbar conjunctivae, ears, cheeks, and neck in association with cerebellar ataxia and retardation of growth. About half of these children have hypogammaglobulinemia; recurrent sinopulmonary infections are also characteristic of the syndrome.

The *Rendu-Osler-Weber syndrome* is characterized by multiple punctate small angiomas involving the tongue, nasal mucosa, lips, and fingertips. There are also telangiectases in the bowel and genitourinary tract, which occasionally bleed. The syndrome is inherited as a dominant and often presents in childhood as recurrent epistaxis.

Lymphedema

Lymphedema occasionally involves the lower extremities. It is usually apparent in infancy but may not present until puberty. It involves the distal or entire leg. The edema is solid and may be complicated by verrucous hypertrophy of the skin and recurrent infections. The disease may be unilateral. Lymphedema may have no apparent cause; it may be caused by postinflammatory fibrosis or may be a dominant trait labeled *Milroy's disease.* Treatment is unsatisfactory. Surgery has been carried out in many of these children with considerable resultant scarring. Elastic stockings are helpful. Histologically there are greatly dilated lymph vessels in the dermis and subcutaneous tissue.

Lymphangioma

There are several benign tumors of lymphatic channels in children. The most common is lymphangioma circumscriptum, which may be present at birth or appear during childhood. The lesions may occur in any location and consist of close-set, deep vesicles which may be clear or occasionally hemorrhagic. The lesion may resolve following treatment with liquid nitrogen.

THE NEWBORN SKIN

At birth, it is vital that the skin function as a relatively impermeable membrane to protect the organism from its new, dry environment. This transition from the warm, wet intrauterine existence is usually unmarked by notable disease except for two common findings: erythema toxicum and milia. The skin of the newborn is covered by vernix caseosa. The breasts are often hypertrophic, as are the scrotum and labia majora. A few infants exhibit pigmentation of the linea alba.

Although the role of the vernix caseosa is not established, its origin appears to be fetal rather than maternal, and no demonstrably good purpose is served by its removal.

Erythema Neonatorum (Toxic Erythema of the Newborn)

This eruption is ubiquitous in the newborn; its reported incidence is probably related to the frequency and care with which the infant is inspected. Early lesions are red macules that appear within the first few days of life. The macules, which may number in the hundreds, may fade or become papules, sometimes surmounted by a small pustule that contains a large number of eosinophils. No area of the body, including the palms and soles, is spared by this peculiar common eruption (Fig. 56, color plate 3).

Milia

Milia are tiny keratin inclusion cysts that occur on the nose and cheeks. Most milia disappear spontaneously; the few that persist can be easily removed by piercing the overlying skin and expressing them with a comedo extractor.

Diaper Rash

This diagnosis includes a number of separate entities that share one feature—the site of involvement, which is the area usually covered by the diaper.

The most common clinical picture is that of scaling, erythema, and maceration. Occasionally, lesions of miliaria rubra are present in the involved area. Nodular ulcerated lesions rarely occur and may resemble lesions of secondary syphilis. Pathogenesis is probably related to maceration, moisture, and sweat retention. The appearance of this type of lesion is promoted by occlusive rubber pants and prolonged intervals between diaper changes. Diarrhea, a frequent occurrence in infants, also contributes to the maceration of the skin.

Contact dermatitis is a rare event in infants but may occur following sensitization to a detergent or disinfectant used on the diapers. More often, in children the response to these agents is a primary irritant reaction.

Seborrheic and atopic dermatitis may also involve the diaper area and fall into the general designation of diaper dermatitis until involvement elsewhere helps establish the diagnosis.

A substantial number of eruptions in the diaper area are associated with or caused by monilia. Small, red, or eroded perianal satellite lesions, when present, strengthen the clinical impression. Positive diagnosis can be made by recovering candida from skin scrapings. Topical application of Mycostatin or Amphotericin B in combination with a topical steroid or Mycolog cream (Squibb) often dramatically improves the lesion.

Ammonia traditionally has been considered a major factor in the production of diaper rash. The evidence that ammonia generated by the bacterial decomposition of urea and other urinary substances is responsible for dermatitis is not conclusive. Other factors—maceration and irritation from feces and urine—are probably sufficient to account for most diaper rashes.

The treatment of diaper rash is directed toward cleansing and drying the involved area. The diaper should be changed as soon as possible after it is soiled. The diapers furnished by commerical diaper services, in addition to their convenience, are usually cleaner and freer of residual soap and detergent than diapers washed at home. Topical steroid lotions or creams promote clearing of seborrheic and atopic dermatitis and are often helpful in diaper rash of less clearly defined causation.

ADENOMA SEBACEUM

Adenoma sebaceum is the cutaneous manifestation of a widespread abnormality involving the brain (tuberous sclerosis), retina (glioma), heart (rhabdomyoma), and kidney (angiomyolipoma). Other cutaneous signs of the disease are periungual and subungual fibromas and a characteristic slightly raised plaque, the *Shagreen patch* (p 1929), which when present is usually located in the lumbosacral region. Café-au-lait spots and a variety of pigmented and vascular nevi may also be present.

An early aid to the diagnosis of adenoma sebaceum in a patient with seizures is the presence of macular leukoderma. The pigmentation in these oval areas is usually diminished but not absent (Fig. 57, color plate 3).

Epiloia refers to the triad of mental deficiency, epilepsy, and adenoma sebaceum (p 1930). Most patients with adenoma sebaceum are severely retarded; rarely there is little concomitant mental retardation. Epilepsy may be of any clinical type—grand mal, petit mal, or Jacksonian. (See also p 1842).

Adenoma sebaceum is usually not present at birth but appears in the first decade as small pink or flesh-colored, dome-shaped papules in the nasolabial fold. They also commonly occur on the cheeks and chin. They may be numerous and may become pedunculated and papillomatous. The disease is inherited as an incomplete dominant. Individual lesions of adenoma sebaceum may be removed by electrodesiccation or dermabrasion.

ACNE

Acne is a common problem, affecting to some degree practically every adolescent. It is characterized by comedones, papules, pustules, and cysts.

The pathogenesis of acne is closely linked to the response of the sebaceous gland to androgenic hormones, which cause hypertrophy and accompanying hypersecretion of the sebaceous glands. The role of androgens in acne is further emphasized by the observation that eunuchs do not develop acne and by the rarity of acne in children up to a few years preceding pubescence. There appear to be two further requirements for the appearance of acne: (a) the formation of a comedo or blackhead (a plug of sebum and keratin in the orifice of the follicle) and (b) tissue reaction to the comedo or to products that have accumulated behind the obstruction it creates. Large numbers of comedones may be present with very little accompanying inflammation or pustule formation. The other clinical extreme is also seen—ie, many inflammatory papules accompanied by few comedones. Usually, however, both are present.

The role of infection in the pathogenesis of acne, though unproved, appears likely. Two organisms, *Corynebacterium acnes* and *Staphylococcus albus,* are present in practically all acne lesions, whether they are open or closed comedones, papules, pustules, or cysts. Although their presence does not constitute proof of an etiologic relationship to acne, the concept is strengthened by the observation that injection of cultures of *C. acnes* into keratinous cysts causes inflammation and rupture of the cysts.

Free fatty acids are produced from sebum by the lipolytic action of *C. acnes.* Experimentally, inflammation resembling that seen in clinical acne can be produced by the intradermal injection of sebum or comedones. The free fatty acid component of sebum is especially irritating. These observations suggest that the leakage of sebum or fatty acids into the tissue is responsible, in some degree, for the inflammation of acne.

The significance of the lipolytic action of *C. acnes* is supported by the observation that killed *C. acnes* do not produce inflammation when injected into cysts of steatocystoma multiplex. Live cultures of *Staphylococcus albus* are similarly without effect when injected into cysts of steatocystoma multiplex.

Clinical Examination

The classification of clinical acne depends on the type and abundance of the several types of lesion: comedo, papule, pustule, cyst. The sites of predilection are the face, upper chest, back, and shoulders; however, the lesions may be restricted to a single area, such as the forehead or upper back.

The comedo or blackhead is probably the earliest clinical expression of acne and is often unaccompanied by inflammation. Various grades of activity of acne can be defined according to the number of lesions present. Although a combination of the various types of lesion is usually present, one type, eg, comedo, cyst, or pustule, may predominate. The comedo is easily recognized as a black dot in a patulous follicular orifice. The color is due to oxidation of lipid. A special form of excoriated acne (acne excoriée des jeunes filles) is rather common in adolescents who, acutely aware of their appearance, manipulate and excoriate otherwise imperceptible lesions, often producing a significant cosmetic problem.

Treatment

There is little evidence that therapy shortens the duration of the total course of acne. Judicious systemic and topical therapy does help control oiliness, follicular plugging, and cyst formation. The aim of therapy is to decrease in number and activity the lesions of acne and prevent scarring caused by cysts and large inflammatory pustules.

SYSTEMIC THERAPY. Administration of anovulatory agents often is associated with clinical improvement. Obviously this approach is limited to postmenarchal girls. Oral contraceptives containing large amounts of progestins may be associated with exacerbation of acne. The major systemic agent in acne is tetracycline. The most successful approach is to treat with 1 g daily until there is unequivocal clinical improvement. The dose is then gradually decreased, and eventually the antibiotic is discontinued after months to years of therapy, often with as little as 250 mg/day. Clindamycin, because of its association with pseudomembranous colitis, is no longer justified as a therapeutic alternative. Erythromycin, although more expensive than tetracycline, is useful in the therapy of acne. Systemic antibiotic therapy results in decreased numbers of corynebacteria and reduced hydrolysis of the sebum to short chain irritating fatty acids. Systemic antibiotics are used for pustular and cystic acne. Recurrent acne cysts, which often result in scarring, can be treated successfully with cryotherapy (liquid nitrogen) or intralesional injection of steroids.

TOPICAL THERAPY.

1. Drying agents—most of these preparations contain alcohol or acetone, salicylic acid, and/or sulfur. They are effective degreasers but have little effect on comedones or cysts.
2. Benzoyl peroxide—these compounds in concentrations of 5 or 10 percent effectively reduce the formation of superficial pustules and are important adjuncts to systemic antibiotics eventually replacing them after weeks to months of concurrent administration.
3. Retinoic acid—vitamin A acid has been a useful addition to acne therapy especially in the prevention of comedo formation. The inflammation and irritation that often occurs during the first few weeks of treatment with retinoic acid can be reduced by less frequent application or concommitant use of a topical steroid. For many children retinoic acid in combination with benzoyl peroxide is adequate therapy.
4. Erythromycin—topical antibiotics have been disappointing in the therapy of acne with the exception of erythromycin, which in a 2 percent concentration appears to be effective in reducing pustular, inflammatory lesions.

ULTRAVIOLET LIGHT. Sunlight benefits acne, although the high humidity and heat of summer may have the opposite effect. An ultraviolet lamp may be effectively used at home by the patient, who, in addition to shielding his eyes, must be careful to avoid burns. First exposure is usually limited to 15 seconds at a distance of 30 inches. The length of exposure is then increased by increments of 30 seconds until erythema is produced. Daily exposure is desirable; sporadic use of ultraviolet lamps often results in unexpected burning.

X-ray radiation is used infrequently by dermatologists and has no role in pediatric practice in the treatment of acne.

DIET. The efficacy of dietary restriction in acne, as in atopic dermatitis, is controversial. The simplest and least punitive method of determining the effect of diet on acne is to have each patient experimentally determine which foods, if any, make his acne worse. The foods most commonly implicated are those with high fat content: pork, french fried potatoes, potato chips, chocolate, nuts, milk. If the ingestion of these foods does not exacerbate a patient's acne, there is little reason to eliminate them from the diet. Unquestionably, there are patients in whom these foods do cause the acne to flare and who should avoid them; however, fatty foods should not be eliminated routinely.

SURGICAL. Comedones should be expressed after the face has been washed and then warmed with a hot towel. Pustules and inflamed cysts should be incised and aspirated when necessary. Cysts, especially those of a chronic nature, often resolve after the intralesional injection of triamcinolone acetonide.

OTHER. In some patients hygiene of the scalp and hair is related in an obscure way to the clinical activity of acne. Although it cannot be concluded that sebum from hair causes local inflammation where it touches the skin, acne of the forehead can often be improved by brushing the hair away from the forehead.

To a degree rarely seen in other diseases, encouragement, patience, and interest are effective therapeutic modalities in acne.

Bibliography

Caplan R: The natural course of urticaria pigmentosa. Arch Dermatol 87:146, 1963

Kirschbaum JO, Kligman AM: The pathogenic role of *Corynebacterium acnes* in acne vulgaris. Arch Dermatol 88:832, 1963

Miller R, Shapiro L: Bullous urticaria pigmentosa in infancy. Arch Dermatol 91:595, 1965

Nickel WR: Clinical spectrum of mastocytosis (urticaria pigmentosa) in man. Arch Dermatol 96:364, 1967

Shaw J: Genetic aspects of urticaria pigmentosa. Arch Dermatol 97:137, 1968

Shehadeh NH, Kligman AM: The bacteriology of acne. Arch Dermatol 88:829, 1963

Strauss JS, Pochi PE: Intracutaneous injection of sebum and comedones. Arch Dermatol 92:443, 1965

Szymanski FJ: Pityriasis lichenoides et varioliformis acuta. Arch Dermatol 79:7, 1959

Wenzl JE, Burgert EO: The spider nevus in infancy and childhood. Pediatrics 33:227, 1964

CHAPTER 18

The Mouth

Arnold H. Einhorn

ANATOMIC AND EMBRYOLOGIC CONSIDERATIONS

ANATOMY

The Oral Cavity

The mouth is the portal of entry and site of mastication of food, and contains the taste organs. The saliva which is secreted into the oral cavity not only serves to lubricate the aliments but also contains enzymes that initiate digestion. The oral cavity has two distinct regions: the *vestibule,* which is the portion bounded laterally by the lips and cheeks and medially by the teeth and the alveolar process; and the *oral cavity proper,* which lies within the dental arches and bones of the jaws and is limited posteriorly by the anterior pillars of the tonsilar fauces.

The Oral Mucosa

The thickness and structure of the mucosa lining the oral cavity varies with the specific functions of each region and depends upon the mechanical influences exerted upon them. The oral mucosa is composed of the *lamina propria,* a dense connective tissue with papillae which also carries blood vessels and nerves; and squamous *surface epithelium,* which is keratinized on the gingiva and hard palate.

Intraorally there are essentially three different types of mucosa: (a) the masticatory mucosa of the gingiva and the hard palate, which bear the major forces of mastication; (b) the lining mucosa of the lips, vestibule, upper and lower alveolar processes, floor of the mouth, inferior surface of the tongue, and the soft palate which are not exposed to major forces of chewing; and (c) the *specialized mucosa,* which lines the dorsum of the tongue and has a major role in taste perception. The epithelium of the masticatory mucosa is keratinized while that of the lining mucosa is not.

The Tongue

The surface of the tongue is rough and irregular. A V-shaped line separates its anterior portion or *body,* which is about two-thirds of its length, from its posterior part or *base.* The body is innervated by the lingual branch of the trigeminal nerve, the base by the glossopharyngeal nerve. The body is covered with keratinized epithelium and numerous fine-pointed, cone-shaped *filiform papillae* that produce a velvet-like appearance.

Interspersed between these are *fungiform papillae* (mushroom-shaped), which contain a few taste buds. In the front of the branches of the dividing V-shaped groove are the *vallate papillae* (walled-in), about eight to 10 in number. These contain von Ebner's glands, small serous glands, which serve to wash out soluble elements of food. At the angle of the V is located the *foramen cecum,* which represents the remnant of the thyroglossal duct. Posterior to the terminal sulcus, the surface of the tongue is irregularly studded with round or oval prominences, the lingual follicles containing lymph nodules, which together form the *lingual tonsil.* On the lateral border of the posterior parts of the tongue sharp parallel clefts of varying length, the *foliate papillae,* enclose taste buds.

TASTE. The primary taste sensations (sweet, salty, bitter, and sour) are perceived by different lingual areas. Sweet is tasted at the tip by the taste buds of the fungiform papillae; salt by those located at the lateral border of the body of the tongue. Bitter taste is perceived in the middle of the base by the vallate papillae, and sour by the foliate papillae in the lateral areas of the base. Sensory impulses from the receptors for bitter and sour tastes are carried by the glossopharyngeal nerve, and sweet and salty tastes are mediated by the intermediate facial nerve via the chorda tympani.

EMBRYOLOGY

The *primary oral pit,* or cavity, is first evident in the third-week human embryo, below the bulging forebrain, bounded caudally by the mandibular or first branchial arch and laterally by the maxillary processes. At the bottom of this pit is the *stomatodeum* or *primary oral plate* facing the blind end of the foregut. The primary oral cavity and the foregut communicate at 3 to 4 weeks, following rupture of the buccopharyngeal membrane. The *prolabium* or *anlage* of the upper lip structures forms at 5 to 6 weeks, conjointly with the premaxilla. The mandibular and maxillary processes originate from the first branchial arch. During early development, the mandible is small by comparison with the upper face. Its growth in width and length abruptly increases at the stages of palatal development, then arrests again, causing in the fetus a physiologic micrognathia that disappears at or soon after birth. In early embryonic life the oral orifice is very wide, but as the maxillary and mandibullary processes unite to form the cheeks its width is reduced.

In the fifth and sixth weeks of gestation a primary palate is formed; from it the upper lip and anterior portion of the maxillary alveolar process will develop.

While the primary palate is being formed the mandibular arch undergoes changes that lead to the appearance of a median furrow and two small pits on either side of the midline; these disappear by the union of the epithelial lining of their walls. The hard and soft palates develop from the secondary palate after the primary palate. Initially, the palatal shelves hang downward on each side of the tongue and later swing upward above the tongue. The premaxilla produces the aveolus with four central incisors. Primary and secondary palates join at the incisive foramen.

The tongue is derived from the first, second, and third branchial arches. In the midline of the base of the first arch and from the derivatives of the first and second branchial arches the thyroid gland develops by progressive downward growth and differentiation. A transitory duct, the thyroglossal duct, originates in this region, growing downward through the developing tongue to the future site of the gland. Its oral end is marked by the foramen cecum, and thyroglossal duct cysts may develop in this region from the foramen cecum to the isthmus of the thyroid gland. The palatine tonsil originates from the second pharyngeal pouch.

THE MOUTH OF THE NEWBORN

The oral cavity and perioral structures of the newborn infant normally exhibit several features present exclusively during the neonatal period.

Sucking pads develop soon after birth in most infants. *Sucking calluses* or corns appear frequently within days after birth on the central portion of the lips (Fig. 1). These consist of raised, cornified crusts or plaques protruding over the labial mucosa and persist only a few weeks. The alveolar ridges often are crowned tran-

sitorily by a thin, serrated, fringelike membrane. The frenulum of the upper lip is sometimes prominent, thick, and continuous with a deep notch in the alveolar ridge of the maxilla (Fig. 2).

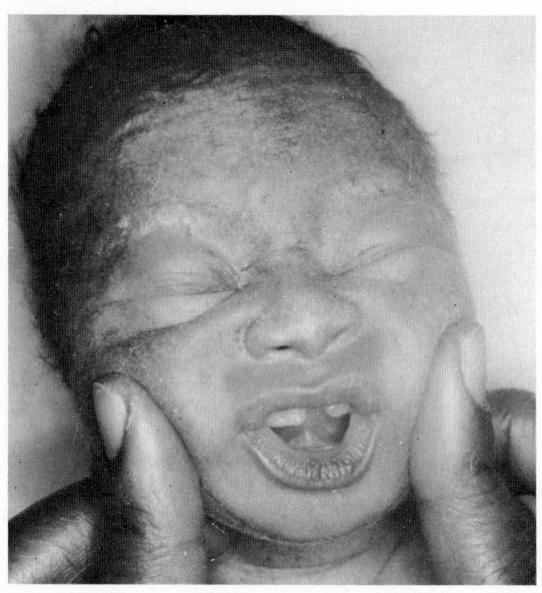

FIG. 2. Deep notched upper alveolar ridge continuing into a short labial frenulum.

On or near the gum margins newborns often have small, firm, white epithelial pearls or inclusion cysts which are shed after a few weeks or months. Bluish, translucent mucoceles (see below) are also occasionally present in the mouth of the newborn. Even more com-

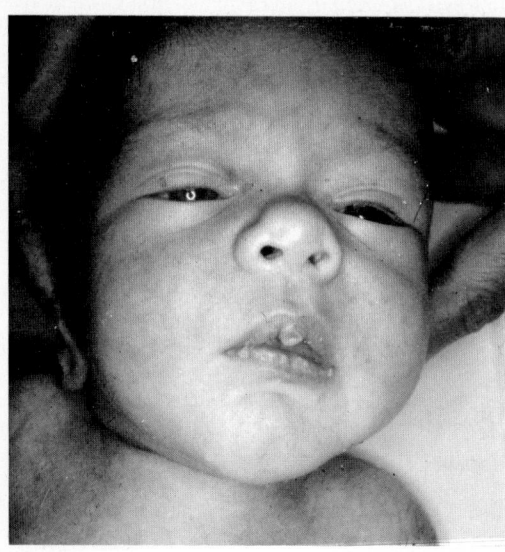

FIG. 1. Sucking calluses of the newborn.

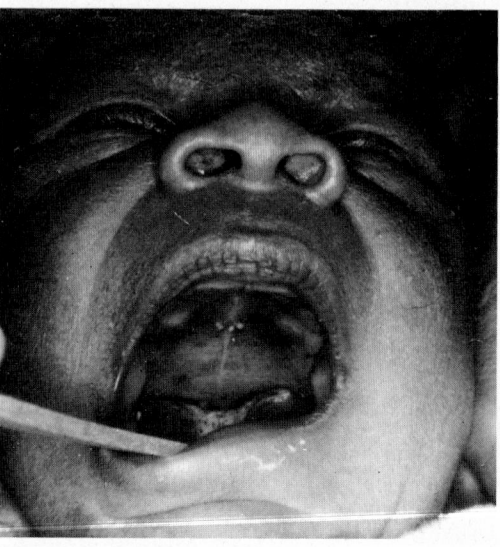

FIG. 3. Epstein's pearls.

monly, white or yellow-white bodies, pinhead sized or smaller, are found on the roof of the mouth, near the junction of the hard with the soft palate, just to either side of the median raphe (Fig. 3). They are known as *Epstein's or Bohn's pearls* and disappear quite rapidly.

Bednar's aphthae or pterygoid ulcers are superficial, elongated, oval-shaped ulcerations of the hard palate, about 1 cm or less in diameter, on either side of the midline above and somewhat medial to the tonsillar fossa. They are rare and generally believed to be traumatic abrasions resulting from attempts to clean the mouth at birth or from friction of the nipple. Less commonly there is a single ulcer, or a cluster of small ulcers, in the midline far back on the hard palate. As a rule these lesions are benign and disappear spontaneously within a few weeks. Petechial hemorrhages on the soft palate are seen sometimes after birth.

NATAL AND NEONATAL TEETH

Occasionally, one or more teeth (natal teeth) are present at birth; exceptionally, teeth may erupt in the first 30 days after birth (neonatal teeth). Usually, both natal and neonatal teeth are found in the position of the lower central incisors (Fig. 4). They are, as a rule, loosely attached to the gum margin and often shed spontaneously within a few days after birth. They may be either supernumerary or true deciduous teeth, and there is a familial incidence in about 15 percent of all reported cases; in several the inheritance pattern suggest an autosomal dominant trait. Natal teeth have been observed in association with cleft palate, cleft lip, and other median facial defects (p. 1752), chondroectodermal dysplasia (Ellis-van Creveld syndrome) (p. 2008),

oculomandibulodyscephaly with hypotrichosis (Hallermann-Streiff syndrome), and pachyonychia congenita (Jadassohn-Lewandowski syndrome).

Hallermann-Streiff syndrome (oculomandibulodyscephaly with hypotrichosis) comprises multiple craniofacial anomalies, mental retardation, short stature, and defects of hair, skin, and teeth. Dental abnormalities consist of natal teeth, subsequent dental hypoplasia, and partial anodontia. Micrognathia; microstomia; high and arched palate; hypoplasia of malar bones, mandibular rami and nasal cartilages; microphthalmia with cataracts; and brachycephaly with cranial bossing, form a complex of oculocranifacial malformations which produce a striking bird-headed appearance. The skin is atrophic; the hair is thin and rare with patchy or regional baldness and body hair, eyebrows, and eyelashes are sparse. Body growth is proportionately stunted; mental and motor retardation are marked.

Jadassohn-Lewandowski syndrome (*pachyonychia congenita*) is a hyperhydrotic form of ectodermal dysplasia. It is transmitted as an austosomal dominant trait and affects males more often than females. In addition to natal teeth and intraoral leukoplakia, it features congenital thickening of the anterior portion of the nails, plantar and palmar hyperkeratosis, plantar bullae, multiple verruca, and diffusely disseminated epidermal steatocystomas.

Bibliography

Bhaskar SN: Oral lesions in infants and newborn. Dent Clin North Am 10:421, 1966

Bodenhoff J, Gorlin RJ: Natal and neonatal teeth: folklore and fact. Pediatrics 32:1087, 1963

Hoefnagel D, Benirschke K: Dyscephalia mandibulo-oculo-facialis (Hallermann-Streiff syndrome). Arch Dis Child 40:47, 1965

Hooley JR: The infant's mouth. J Am Dent Assoc 75:95, 1967

Nichamin SJ, Kaufman M: Gingival microcysts in infancy. Pediatrics 31:412, 1963

Parmelle AH, Sr: The mouth of the newborn. Pediatr Clin North Am 3:847, 1956

Sicher H, Bhasker SN: Obran's Oral Histology and Embryology, 7th ed. St Louis, Mosby, 1972

Soderquist NA, Reed WB: Pachyonychia congenita with epidermal cysts and other congenital dyskeratoses. Arch Dermatol 97:31, 1968

Stark RB (ed): Congenital defects. In Cleft Palate, A Multidiscipline Approach. New York, Harper & Row, 1968

SOFT TISSUE LESIONS OF THE ALVEOLAR RIDGE AND FLOOR OF THE MOUTH

ERUPTION CYSTS

These benign, bluish, compressible, raised, and fluid-filled lesions occasionally arise from the alveolar ridge in association with erupting teeth. They are believed to

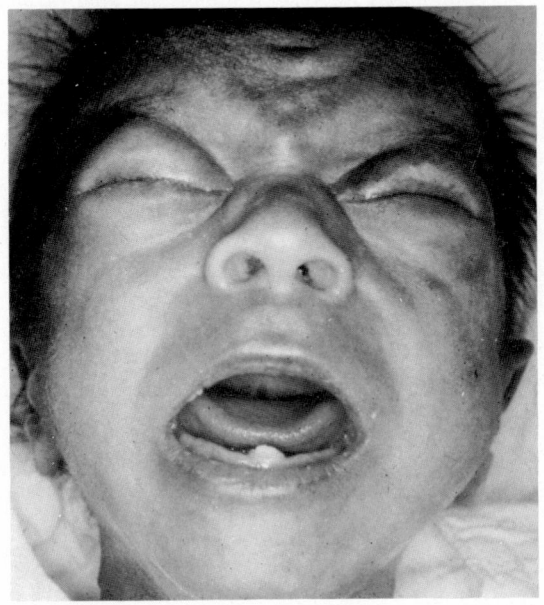

FIG. 4. Natal tooth.

be dentigerous cysts carried to the surface by the erupting tooth. They may rupture spontaneously and heal, but if they persist excision of the *roof* of the cyst may be necessary.

MUCOUS CYSTS (MUCOCELES)

Benign, circumscribed cysts, pea-sized or smaller, are seen occasionally in any area of the oral mucous membrane containing salivary glands (Fig. 5). They are thin-walled, translucent, glistening, bluish lesions, occurring most frequently on the labial or gingival mucosa, occasionally on the buccal region or on the lower aspect of the tongue. They are elevated, fluid filled, and compressible, and are due to the occlusion and/or traumatic rupture of minor salivary gland ducts, with secondary pooling of the saliva in the subepithelial tissue of the mucous membrane. Single or multiple, these cysts may either disappear spontaneously within a few months, or rupture, discharging a sticky mucoid material; they sometimes recur. Excision may be indicated if mucoceles recur or first appear at a later age and persist.

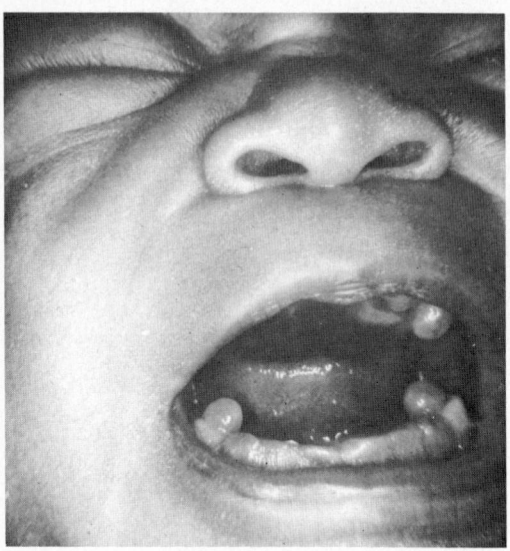

FIG. 5.   Multiple oral mucoceles in a newborn infant.

PERIPHERAL GIANT CELL REPARATIVE GRANULOMA

Painless, hemorrhagic, soft tissue growths can arise from the interdental papilla or from areas when deciduous teeth were recently shed. These are benign lesions, probably associated with trauma and exuberant repair rather than with neoplasia. Since their presence may lead to displacement of adjoining teeth, they are treated by local excision.

CONGENITAL EPULIS

This lesion (Fig. 6) is a benign, slow-growing, pedunculated, and usually asymptomatic soft tissue tumor present from birth. It arises from the anterior portion of the alveolar mucosa, more commonly from the maxillary than from the mandibular ridge, and occurs far more frequently in newborn girls than in boys. Surgical excision is indicated and is not usually followed by recurrence.

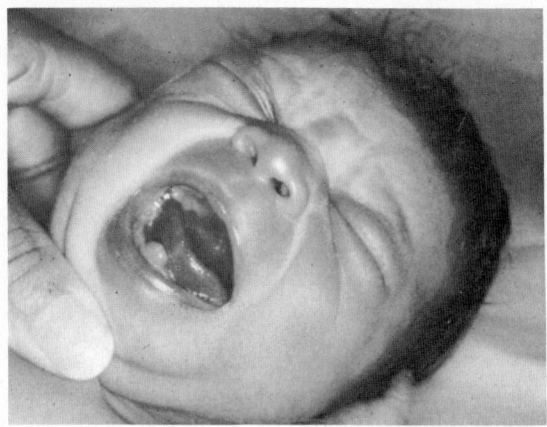

FIG. 6.   Congenital epulis.

HEMANGIOMAS

Hemangiomas, the most common tumors of childhood, can be seen in any of the oral soft tissue, including the tongue, the floor of the mouth, the gingiva, and the labial or buccal mucosa. These vascular anomalies may be of the cavernous or capillary type. Hemangiomas present usually as dark blue, diffuse, soft, partly raised, and compressible lesions that can be evacuated readily by stroking, remaining collapsed as long as pressure is applied, especially at the site of the feeding vessel. They bleed profusely when traumatized but may regress completely after trauma. They also vary considerably in size, ranging from small localized lesions of limited growth to extremely large tumors, which may grow rapidly and interfere with function and even be life-threatening (Fig. 7). Surgical excision is indicated for lesions that interfere with function. Small hemangiomas may be left alone, but adrenocortical steroids may be indicated if they are likely to be traumatized or to cause functional impairment. Many regress spontaneously.

RANULA

This condition (Fig. 8) is relatively rare in children but can be seen even in the newborn period. It is charac-

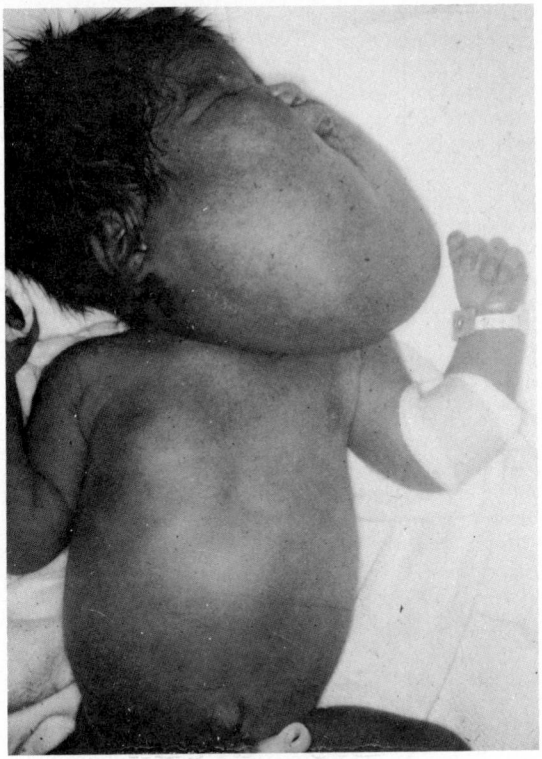

FIG. 7. Giant hemangioma.

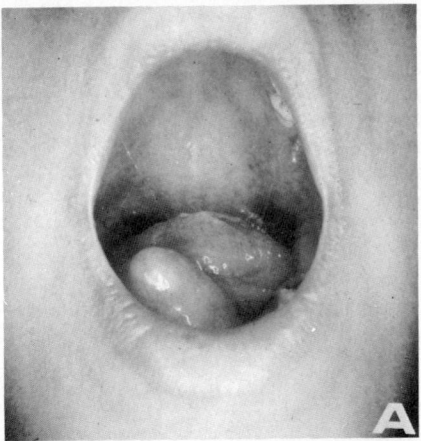

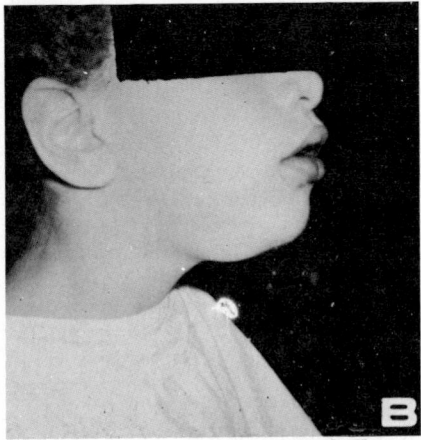

FIG. 8. Ranula. Protrusion of the mass with displacement of tongue.

terized by swelling of the tissues of the floor of the mouth, which displaces the tongue forward and laterally and may produce a visible bulge in the submandibular region. In most cases they represent sublingual salivary cysts but rarely may be lymphangiomatous. Treatment consists of surgical excision. However, when the size of the mass produces respiratory embarrassment, emergency aspiration or incision and drainage may be necessary as a temporary measure, followed at a later date by definitive excision.

Bibliography

Bhasker SN: Oral tumors in infancy and childhood. A survey of 239 cases. J Pediatr 63:195, 1963

Firfer HG, Stuteville OH: Congenital epulis. Oral Surg 15:781, 1962

Robinson HBG: Oral neoplasma of children. Pediatr Clin North Am 3:854, 1958

MALFORMATIONS OF THE LIPS, PALATE, AND JAW

OGIVAL PALATE

A high-arched palate without associated defects may be seen occasionally in the normal newborn but does not persist beyond early infancy in normal children.

However, this deformity is also one of the prominent craniofacial defects commonly present in a variety of skeletal abnormality syndromes. Thus, a high and narrow palate is a typical feature of those genetic affections of the skeleton, which are associated with the following.

Hypoplasia of the Lateral Facial Structures: mandibulofacial dysostosis of Treacher-Collins-Franceschetti (p. 1983).

Midfacial Hypoplasia without Associated Craniosynostosis: cleidocranial dysostosis (p. 2014), arachnodactyly or Marfan's disease (p. 2014), and Russel-Silver dwarfism (p. 1987).

Midfacial Hypoplasia Associated with Craniosynostosis: craniofacial dysostosis of Crouzon (p. 1980), acrocephalopolysyndactyly, or Carpenter's syndrome; and acrocephalosyndactyly, or Apert's syndrome.

In *Apert's syndrome* (acrocephalosyndactyly), a disorder of autosomal dominant inheritance, the combination of irregular craniosynostosis and considerable midfacial hypoplasia results in peculiarities of cranial shape and facial appearance, characterized by acrocephaly, high and prominent forehead with frontal bossing, flat facies, shallow orbits, supraorbital depressions, hypertelorism, downward slanting of the palpebral fissures, short and beaked nose, and high arched palate. The associated malformations of the extremities, consist primarily of syndactylism of digits and toes (p. 1988). The level of intelligence varies.

Carpenter's syndrome (acrocephalopolysyndactyly) is a clinical entity in which cranial and facial anomalies similar to those of Apert's syndrome are associated with mental retardation, obesity, and hypogenitalism. In addition to brachyturricephaly, hypertelorism, and high-arched palate, there is micrognathia. Associated malformations of fingers and toes consist of syndactyly, brachydactyly, polydactyly, and clinodactyly (p. 1988). The transmission of this disorder is probably autosomal recessive.

Midfacial Hypoplasia Associated with Microcrania

The *Rubinstein-Taybi syndrome* features short, broad, and angulated thumbs, abnormal dermatoglyphs, peculiarities of facial morphology, short stature, and mental retardation. The craniofacial defects are characterized by microcrania, midfacial hypoplasia, narrow and high-arched palate, narrow and prominent forehead, narrow and beaked nose with downward prolongation of the nasal septum, and antimongolian slanting of the palpebral fissures. There are also varied ocular defects, anomalies of the external ears, and cryptorchidism.

In *Long-Arm-Deletion syndrome,* mental deficiency, generalized hypotonia, physical growth retardation, and genital hypoplasia with cryptorchidism are associated with abnormalities of hands, feet, and dermatoglyphics, skin dimples, external ear defects and deafness, midfacial hypoplasia with high-arched palate and carp mouth, and microcephaly.

Diffuse Hypoplasia of the Face

Hallermann-Streiff syndrome (p. 913), progeria, and Seckel's bird-headed dwarfism.

Progeria is a disorder of unknown etiology and apparently sporadic occurrence. Affected individuals are short, thin, deformed and present a striking bird-headed facial appearance with pronounced senilelike features. Body configuration and facial morphology are the result of a combination of multiple congenital defects involving skeleton, skin, subcutaneous fat, hair, teeth, nails, and blood vessels. Premature aging and a short life span are related to the early onset in childhood of progressive arteriosclerosis, leading to anginal attacks and terminally to coronary occlusion.

Skeletal anomalies in this disorder consist of generalized dysplasias and hypoplasias and localized degenerative bone changes. Physical growth is markedly retarded. The calvarium is thin and poorly ossified; closure of the fontanel is delayed. Clavicles are characteristically short, limbs are thin, and joints are stiff and enlarged. The hips are deformed in coxa valga.

The face is hypoplastic, the chin small and receding, and the palate narrow and highly arched. The orbital cavities are relatively small and shallow, the eyes and nose are protuberant, and the scalp veins are prominent and dilated. An impression of hydrocephalus is produced by the contrast between the smallness of the face and the relative width of the forehead and cranium, further accentuated by progressive alopecia and the absence of eyebrows and eyelashes. The skin is thin and the nails are atrophic. The teeth are delayed in eruption, irregular, crowded, and partly missing. Subcutaneous fat gradually disappears over the entire body. Intelligence is normal. There is no effective treatment; death usually occurs in adolescence from coronary occlusion secondary to the generalized and progressive arterial atheromatosis.

Seckel's syndrome (bird-headed dwarfism) is a severe dysmorphic condition inherited as an autosomal recessive trait. Infants with this disorder are mentally retarded, have low birth weights, are small at birth, and remain short. A complex pattern of craniofacial anomalies creates a tragically grotesque, bird-headed, facial appearance. There is microcephaly with craniosynostosis. Facial hypoplasia involving mandible, palate, and malar bones is associated with large bulging eyes, prominent nose, receding chin, and low-set lobeless ears. The micrognathia, the beaklike protrusion of the nose, the protuberance of the eyes, the smallness of the face, and the virtual absence of forehead are all responsible for the birdlike look. There are multiple malformations of the bones and joints of the axial skeleton and of the extremities, including dislocation of the hips, hypoplasia or aplasia of one or several bones, and osseous deformities.

High arched palate also occurs in genetic syndromes in which the skeletal component of the facial abnormalities plays a less prominent role, as in variants of the pterygium syndrome, especially Turner's OX gonadal agenesis (p. 277), leprechaunism, Cockayne syndrome, Cornelia de Lange syndrome, and Marshall's type of ectodermal dysplasia.

Leprechaunism, a rare autosomal recessive disorder, is characterized by stunted physical growth, with mental and motor retardation and extreme emaciation; small hirsute, elfinlike, and prematurely senile facial appearance, with lack of facial subcutaneous fat; beaked nose; flaring nostrils; widely spaced prominent eyes; thick lips; narrow high-arched palate; large low-set ears; short neck; enlargement of breasts and external genitalia; and abnormalities of carbohydrate metabolism with hyperplasia of the islets of Langerhans.

Cockayne syndrome is an autosomal recessive disorder, comprising cachectic dwarfism with kyphosis, ankylosis, disproportionately long extremities, and large hands and feet; mental deficiency; microcranium with thick calvarium; lack of facial subcutaneous fat with prognathism, sunken eyes, and thin nose, producing a senile-like appearance; thin, pigmented, and photosensitive skin; retinal degeneration with pigmentation, optic atrophy, cataract, and pupillary sluggishness; prominent ears and partial deafness; cold, blue extremities; arteriosclerosis; ataxia and tremors; hepatosplenomegaly; and albuminuria (p. 1996).

Cornelia de Lange syndrome is a clinical entity which has occurred in siblings and is probably transmitted as an autosomal recessive trait. Children with this condition are short, mentally retarded; brachymicrocephalic, and hirsute. They have short extremities with tapering short fingers, oligodactyly, and proximally displaced thumbs; abnormal dermatoglyphics; defects of ribs and sternum; and hypoplastic nipples and umbilicus. Their facial appearance is striking and includes bushy eyebrows with synophris and long profuse eyelashes; flat nasal bridge with upturned tip and anteverted nostrils; increased distance from nasal base to vermilion of upper lip; midline notching of upper and lower lips; narrow high-arched palate with micrognathia; and low-set ears.

Marshall's type ectodermal dysplasia is a mildly hypohydrotic variant of ectodermal dysplasia. Additional features consist of midfacial hypoplasia with short depressed nose, low and flat nasal bridge, maxillary hypoplasia, and narrow high-arched palate; cataracts; and deafness.

MICROGNATHIA

Isolated hypoplasia of the mandible, of various degrees of severity, may occur without associated cleft palate or other congenital defect. The underdeveloped mandible is responsible for a characteristic birdlike facial appearance. When the micrognathia is relatively mild, there is no interference with breathing, but rarely the hypoplasia is severe and produces respiratory difficulty, requiring the same precautions as in the Pierre Robin syndrome in which the abnormality of the jaw is associated with cleft palate and glossoptosis (see below).

Micrognathia may be one of the congenital malformations induced by maternal use of aminopterin during pregnancy. The anomaly is also part of several chromosomal aberration syndromes, such as 18 trisomy, long-arm 21 deletion syndrome, 13-15 trisomy, and Cri du Chat syndrome (p. 282). In a number of genetic multidefect syndromes a hypoplastic mandible also constitutes one of the typical manifestations, as in Cornelia de Lange syndrome (see above), oculo-auriculo-vertebral syndrome of Goldenhar (p. 1952), progeria(see above),oculomandibulodyscephaly with hypotrichosis, or Hallermann-Streiff syndrome (p. 913) , Seckel's bird-headed dwarfism (see above), Russel-Silver dwarfism (p. 1987), mandibulofacial dyostosis of Treacher-Collins-Franceschetti (p. 1983) , and Smith-Lemli-Opitz syndrome.

Smith-Lemli-Opitz syndrome is a familial disorder, probably inherited as an autosomal recessive, characterized by mental retardation, short stature, skeletal defects, and urogenital abnormalities. In addition to micrognathia the major craniofacial anomalies consist of microcephaly; low-set slanted ears; epicanthus ptosis and strabismus; broad nasal tip and anteverted nostrils; and broad maxillary ridges. Hypospadias, cryptorchidism, syndactyly of the toes, and abnormal dermatoglyphics are also part of the syndrome.

PIERRE ROBIN SYNDROME

The clinical triad of micrognathia, cleft palate, and glossoptosis is known as the Pierre Robin syndrome (Fig. 9). Because of the underdeveloped mandible and the cleft palate, the tongue, too large for the space provided, drops backward into the pharynx, which it obstructs, thereby interfering with breathing. Episodes of cyanosis and respiratory distress associated with swallowing difficulty often occur soon after birth, particularly when the infant is in the supine position. Lateral radiographs of the neck may show the encroachment of the tongue upon the pharyngeal airway. Other nasopharyngeal anomalies, ocular defects (congenital glaucoma, congenital cataracts, progressive severe myopia, and retinal detachment), skeletal defects (spondyloepiphyseal dysplasia and rib dysplasia), and congenital cardiac defects often are associated with the orofacial anomalies. The Pierre Robin triad may be an isolated syndrome or may be part of a genetic dysmorphic syndrome in which the cleft palate and micrognathia are merely features of a constellation of anomalies (Micrognathia and Cleft Palate, p. 918).

In most cases the respiratory distress may be alleviated by placing the infant in prone position and maintaining this even during feedings. If the respiratory distress does not respond to positioning, it may be necessary to manage the infant for some time with endotracheal intubation. Newborn infants generally tolerate minimally reactive plastic tubes for comparatively prolonged periods. Insertion and maintenance of a plastic tube via the nasopharynx into the upper esophagus to slightly below the level of the larynx has been advocated as an effective method to hold the tongue forward and down, thereby ensuring an adequate open airway. In more extreme situations, which should occur rarely if the infant is carefully watched and appropriately managed, the tongue may have to be pulled forward by means of a traction suture inserted temporarily through the tip of the tongue. If either of these procedures has been necessary, a variety of methods have been advocated for the purpose of holding the tongue in a forward position during subsequent weeks or months. An artificial tongue-tie can be created, either by suturing the lingual undersurface to the mucosal aspect of the lower lip or by anchoring the tongue to the cartilaginous portion of the mandible. It has been reported that the desired effect can be achieved and maintained without operative glossopexy by means of a weight, exerting traction upon a suture passed through the midbody of the tongue.

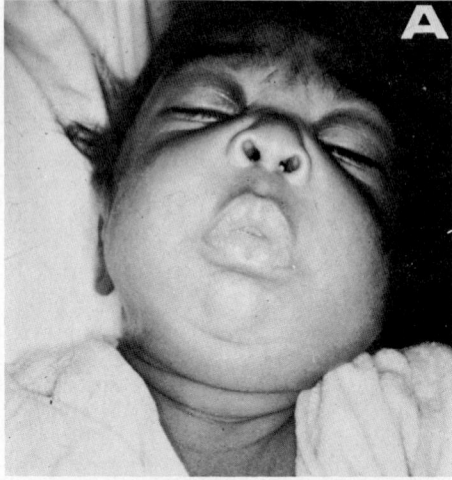

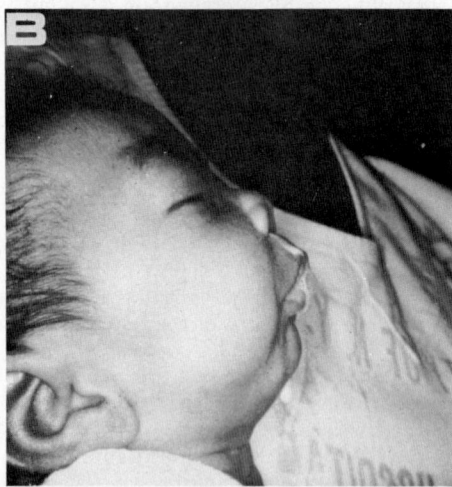

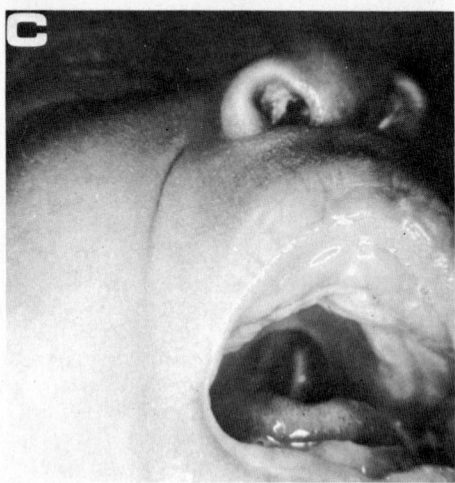

FIG. 9. Pierre Robin syndrome. A. On this anterior view, noticeable existence of respiratory distress (flaring of alae nasi and suprasternal retractions). B. Lateral view illustrating the micrognathia. C. Intraoral view shows wide posterior cleft palate.

Difficulty in feeding and provision of adequate nutrition may constitute a major cause for concern. Most infants survive and thrive with conservative management, namely careful positioning during feedings, either in upright or prone positon, combined with, very close supervision during the first few weeks or months after birth. Technical feeding problems generally can be overcome by using soft nipples or a lamb's nipple. Both winged cleft palate nipples and removable individually constructed acrylic palatine obturators are usually tolerated poorly. Prone feeding can be accomplished by using a lamb's nipple, either on a curved bottle (Takagi method) or on a curved J-shaped tube developed by the National Institutes of Health. A small number of infants who present major respiratory difficulty will require gavage feeding or even alimentation via gastrostomy.

CLEFT LIP AND CLEFT PALATE

Cleft lip (harelip) and cleft palate are developmental anomalies of the first branchial arch. The ensuing defects are of variable severity, some barely perceptible, others exceedingly handicapping functionally, cosmetically, and psychologically. However, even the most complex and disfiguring of these orofacial malformations is amenable to satisfactory correction, provided the numerous phases of treatment are competently planned and integrated. Successful management requires a comprehensive coordinated program involving multiple disciplines.

Cleft Lip

Cleft lip is a frequent congenital anomaly, occurring either alone or in conjunction with cleft palate. It is caused by incomplete fusion, during the second month of embryonic development, of the nasomedial or intermaxillary process with the more laterally placed maxillary process. Because the cleft deformity occurs during a period of intrauterine life when fetal growth is exceedingly rapid, structures of the face and mouth develop without the normal encircling restraints of muscles of the lips. A characteristic depression or flattening of the infant's midfacial contour may result from the disruption of normal antagonistic forces across the midline and the concomitant disturbance of growth of the facial segments involved. The facial cleft, even when not associated with cleft palate, may affect not only the lip but also the external nose, the nasal cartilages, the nasal septum, and the alveolar process.

The cleft is usually just beneath the center of one nostril; various degrees of completeness are recognized. There may be only a slight indentation of the lip, or the fissure may extend to the nostril, causing the latter to sag and to be flattened, with the tip of the nose deviated toward the noncleft side (Fig. 10). Although cleft palate may occur without cleft lip, the failure of lip fusion by 35 days of gestation may impair closure of the palatal shelves, which occurs later, and may be the cause for the cleft palate formation. The more complete the cleft in the lip the greater is the incidence of missing, malposed, supernumerary, or malformed teeth in the line of the cleft. The defect may occur bilaterally and may be symmetric or asymmetric. With double harelip, and particularly when cleft palate is also present, the unattached midline portion of the upper lip or *philtrum* may jut forward, out of line with the rest of the lip structures. Either single or double harelip may be accompanied by cleft palate.

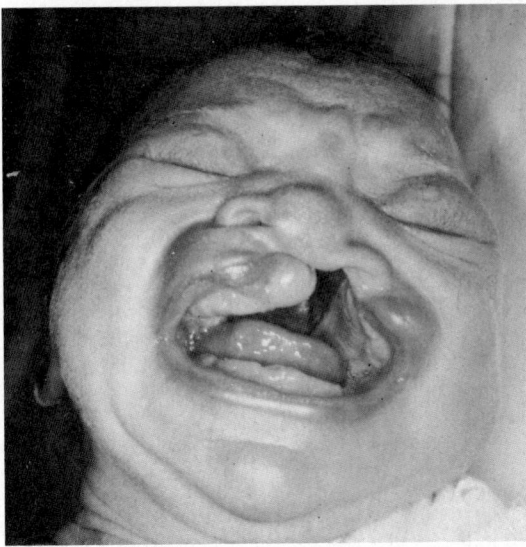

FIG. 11.   Cleft palate (type III). Complete cleft of soft and hard palates and alveolar ridge, unilateral.

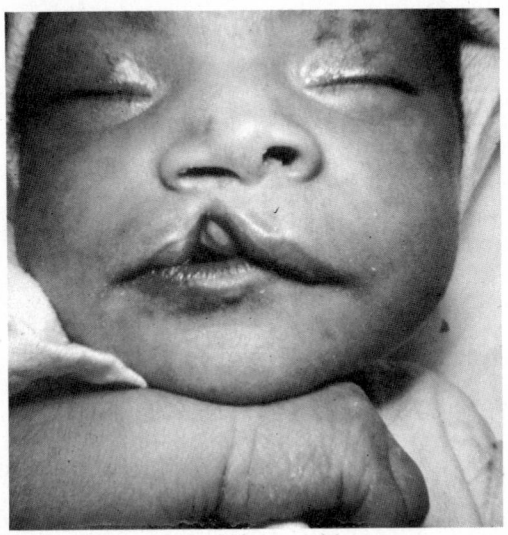

FIG. 10.   Cleft lip. Note sagging of the nostrils, unilateral nasal flattening, and deviation of tip to noncleft side.

Clefts of the palate have been classified into four types, depending on the anatomic extent of the defect: *type I*, cleft confined to the soft palate; *type II*, unilateral cleft of the entire soft and hard palate; *type III*, unilateral cleft of the entire soft and hard palate and the alveolar ridge (Fig. 11); and *type IV*, bilateral cleft of the entire palate and alveolar ridge (Fig. 12). There may also be partial or complete lack of development of the vomer

Feeding the infant generally presents no difficulty in cases of simple cleft lip with intact palate. Nursing at breast or bottle depends mainly on the suction developed by pressing the nipple with the tongue against the hard palate, rather than on closure of the lips. It is quite unnecessary to resort to large-holed nipples, droppers, or other devices in solitary cleft lip. Feeding is also not a consideration in the timing of primary surgical correction of the lip.

Cleft Palate

Cleft palate is often associated with harelip but may occur without it. All degrees are seen. The fissure may affect only the uvula and soft palate, or may extend forward to the nostril, involving the hard palate and the maxillary alveolar ridge. It may be unilateral or bilateral, the cleft occupying the midline posteriorly and as far forward as the alveolar process, where it deviates to the involved side, dividing the alveolar ridge usually between the tooth bud of the upper lateral incisor and that of the cuspid.

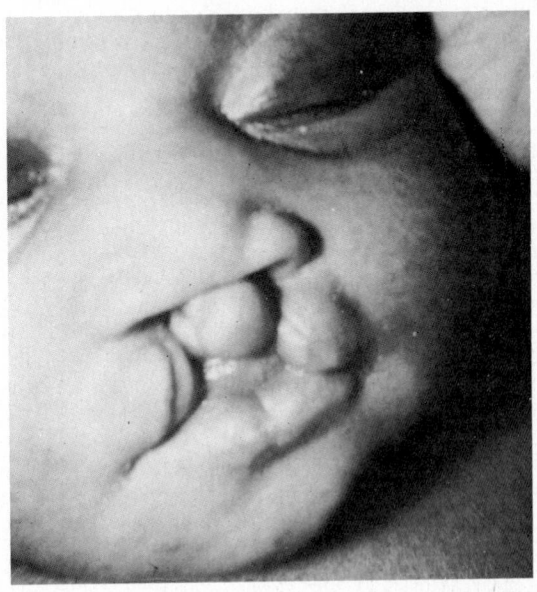

FIG. 12.   Cleft palate (type IV). Complete cleft of soft and hard palates and alveolar ridge, bilateral.

and nasal septum. In these cases the lateral palatal shelves may be quite rudimentary, leaving the nasal cavity in free communication with the oral cavity and permitting ready inspection of the turbinates, the fossa of Rosenmuller, and the adenoids. However, the philtrum, that portion of the lip just beneath the nasal septum, is almost always preserved even with extensive bilateral defects. Absence of the philtrum associated with hypertelorism, wide harelip, and cleft palate should suggest the diagnosis of arhinencephaly, a *median cerebrofacial agenesis* complex in which various segmental defects occur simultaneously in median structures of the face and brain (p. 1752).

Nutrition requires more careful consideration, and more patience is needed in feeding infants with cleft palate than with isolated cleft lip. Problems may arise from the presence of the deformity but are more often due to faulty technique or the existence of associated defects than to the cleft palate. Usually, the mechanical difficulties in sucking prevent the infant with cleft of the hard palate from establishing and maintaining an adequate supply of breast milk. However, most infants readily adjust to bottle feedings in spite of their deficiencies in sucking and swallowing. In most instances, despite leakage through the nose, little difficulty is encountered if the infant is fed unhurriedly, using either a soft nipple for premature infants or a lamb's nipple. Placing the infant in a sitting posture during nursing will minimize loss of fluids through the nose. We have found that "cleft palate nipples" with rubber palatal flaps are not only ineffective but often poorly tolerated, thereby enhancing the danger of aspiration of milk into the infant's lungs. In those rare instances in which the infant is debilitated and has poor suck, feeding with a medicine dropper or by gavage may be required. Semisolid and solid foods may be added to the nutritional regimen at the usual times; in fact, infants with cleft palate manage them somewhat more readily and efficiently than liquids.

GENETIC ASPECTS. In both cleft lip and cleft palate, a genetic pattern is suggested by the occurrence of comparable deformities among the forebears, but in some instances no such history can be obtained. Although both conditions show a familial tendency, fetal environmental factors also appear to play an important role. Breeding experiments with laboratory animals indicate that manipulations of the diet, administration of drugs, and a variety of other stresses applied to the pregnant female at the appropriate time in the gestation period will result in a relatively high incidence of analogous malformations. Comparable data regarding human experience are lacking.

Genetically, cleft lip (with or without cleft palate) and cleft palate (without cleft lip) behave as separate entities in regard to their familial distribution. Both categories appear to be etiologically heterogeneous, encompassing a variety of different types. The solitary form of cleft palate tends to be associated predominantly with other skeletal malformations, whereas harelip with or without cleft palate occurs more often in conjunction with anomalies of the central nervous system. The incidence of cleft palate is approximately two times as high in girls as in boys, whereas in most large series there is a higher incidence of harelip in males.

The incidence of cleft lip is about 1 in 1,000 births; isolated cleft palate has a frequency of about 1 per 2,500 births. Fraser estimates the recurrence risk of cleft lip in a sibship with one such child to be between 4 and 7 percent if neither parent is affected, and about 11 percent if one parent has the defect. With solitary cleft palate the recurrence risk for cases not associated with any other genetic malformation is about 3 percent, if both parents are normal and one child affected, and as high as 13 percent if one parent and one child are affected.

TREATMENT. The principle and details of surgical repair of both defects are beyond the scope of this discussion. The operative procedures employed are described in works on plastic surgery.

Many conflicting views in regard to the timing of the primary repair of the defects confront the pediatrician who assumes the responsibility of directing and coordinating the care of these children. There are obvious advantages to very early correction of the cleft lip, which generally may be done within the first 2 weeks after birth. However, operation on a debilitated or premature infant should be deferred somewhat longer, at least until a steady weight gain is assured and the initial hemoglobin fall has shown an upturn. Thrush, a common complication in newborns with cleft palate, constitutes a threat to the success of the operation, and if present, surgery should be delayed. In a vigorous infant it is safe and advantageous to operate within the first 48 hours. However, some surgeons prefer to wait until the infant is 1 or 2 months old.

Repair of bilateral cleft is technically more difficult, and the procedure is often performed in two steps. In experienced hands the results of surgery of cleft lip are usually quite satisfactory, although more than one operation may be required for cosmetic restitution. Excessively tight closure of the lip must be avoided. It may result in a significant lingual version of the upper incisor teeth, posterior displacement of the upper lip, and exaggerated fullness of the lower lip.

Operation on cleft palate is usually done at about 18 months of age. While early intervention enhances the risk of injury or dislocation of tooth buds, deferment adds to the technical difficulty of the procedure because of the greater ridigity of the parts. The aim of the surgery is to obtain an airtight closure of the palatal cleft and to preserve the mobility and length of the soft palate without disturbing the growing tooth buds. For cleft palate, multiple operations are required more often than in the case of simple cleft lip, and the cooperation of prosthodontist and orthodontist throughout the period of dental growth is essential for best cosmetic and functional results. Even with early closure the child may experience difficulty in sealing off the nasopharynx from the buccal cavity during deglutition and in the pronunciation of certain consonants. Speech training is almost always required.

Optimum care must also include specialized otologic

and audiologic surveillance. Both before and after operation, patients with cleft palate tend to suffer from repeated and often troublesome infections of the paranasal sinuses. Hypertrophy of tonsils and adenoids is an almost invariable accompaniment, and recurrent otitis media is common. With chronic nasopharyngitis, the risk of tubal deafness must always be borne in mind. All efforts should be made to keep such infections down to a minimum, and when indicated, they should be treated promptly with appropriate antibiotics. It also must be stressed that tonsils and adenoids may perform an essential function for intelligible speech in the child with a repaired palate. An ill-considered adenoidectomy may precipitate a severe and permanent speech deterioration.

In a therapeutic situation of this nature, in which the services of several different special disciplines must be brought into effective cooperation, the pediatrician almost inevitably serves as coordinator. On his shoulders rests the responsibility for ensuring that no single aspect of the problem is overlooked. He should provide guidance, counsel, and support to both the child and parent through the various traumatic exposures. He can be of great help in allaying the parents' anxiety and the child's fears of repeated anesthetics and operations, in building up the child's confidence and in dispelling the notion that the victim of cleft palate is inferior to other children.

FAMILIAL FIBROUS DYSPLASIA OF THE JAWS (CHERUBISM)

This familial and hereditary variant of osseous dysplasia of childhood and adolescence affects the jaws almost exclusively and generally occurs bilaterally. Painless and firm mandibular swelling constitutes the major and usually the only symptom. The enlargement of the jaw usually begins simultaneously in both rami and extends progressively; sometimes it may start on one side, subsequently growing forward to involve the other side. The resulting osseous deformity characteristically produces a rounded "cherubic" appearance of the face. In typical cases the mandibular swelling becomes apparent at about 2 to 5 years of age, increases either slowly or more rapidly between the ages of 4 to 8, and remains stationary until puberty, after which slow resolution takes place. Marked dental crowding and migration of the teeth may be associated with the gross orofacial distortion, but other symptoms are unusual. Cervical and submaxillary lymphadenopathy are common. Radiography reveals multiple and frequently multiloculated areas of radiolucency that enlarge progressively, with thinning and irregularity of the cortex.

The nature of this disease is still obscure. It has been suggested that cherubism represents a hereditary variant of polyostotic fibrous dysplasia. It affects boys more than girls and appears to be due to a dominant gene in which the penetrance is about 10 percent in males and 50 to 70 percent in females. The course is mostly benign and the disease self-limited. In general no treatment is necessary unless there is interference with speech and respiration. In rare instances, when growth of the bony lesion is rapid and produces severe, even life-threatening manifestations, surgical excision will be required.

Bibliography

OGIVAL PALATE

Coffin GS: Brachydactyly, peculiar facies and mental retardation. Am J Dis Child 108:351, 1964

Dekaban A: Metabolic and chromosomal studies in leprechaunism. Arch Dis Child 40:632, 1965

Goodman RM, Gorlin RJ: The Face in Genetic Disorders. St Louis, Mosby, 1970

Fujimoto WY, Greene ML, Seegmiller JE: Cockayne's syndrome: report of a case with hyperlipoproteinemia, hyperinsulinemia, renal disease, and normal growth hormone. J Pediatr 75:881, 1969

Harper RG, Orti E, Baker RK: Bird-headed dwarfs (Seckel's syndrome), a familial pattern of developmental, dental, skeletal, genital, and central nervous system anomalies. Pediatrics 70:799, 1967

Insley J: Syndrome associated with a deficiency of part of the long arm of chromosome no. 18. Arch Dis Child 42:140, 1967

Macdonald W B, Fitch KD, Lewis IC: Cockayne's syndrome, an heredofamilial disorder of growth and development. Pediatrics 25:997, 1960

McKusick VA, Mahloudji M, Abbott MH, et al: Seckel's bird-headed dwarfism. N Engl J Med 277:279, 1967

Pashayan H, Whelan D, Guttman S, et al: Variability of the de Lange syndrome: report of 3 cases and genetic analysis of 54 families. J Pediatr 75:853, 1969

Runbinstein JH, Taybi H: Broad thumbs and toes and facial abnormalities, a possible mental retardation syndrome. Am J Dis Child 105:588, 1963

Salmon MA, Webb J N: Dystrophic changes associated with leprechaunism in a male infant. Arch Dis Child 38:530, 1963

Smith DW: Recognizable Patterns of Human Malformations—Genetic, Embryologic, and Clinical Aspects. In Major Problems in Clinical Pediatrics. Philadelphia, Saunders, 1970

Summitt RL, Favara BE: Leprechaunism (Donohue's syndrome): a case report. J Pediatr 74:601, 1969

Temtamy SA: Carpenter's syndrome: Acrocephalopolysyndactyly. An autosomal recessive syndrome. J Pediatr 69:111, 1966

Thomson J, Forfar JO: Progeria (Hutchinson-Gilford syndrome), report of a case and review of the literature. Arch Dis Child 25:224, 1950

Villee DB, Nichols G, Jr, Talbot NB: Metabolic studies in two boys with classical progeria. Pediatrics 43:207, 1969

PIERRE ROBIN SYNDROME AND MICROGNATHIA

Berggren RB, Duran RJ: Pitfalls in the treatment of the Pierre Robin Syndrome. J Pediatr Surg 5:539, 1970

Crow ML, Holder TM, McCoy FJ, et al.: The use of temporary gastrostomy to prevent aspiration in Pierre Robin syndrome. Plast Reconstr Surg 35:494, 1965

Dennison WM: The Pierre Robin Syndrome. Pediatrics 36:336, 1965

Fine RN, Gwinn JL, Young EF: Smith-Lemli Opitz syndrome. Am J Dis Child 115:483, 1968

Goodman RM, Gorlin RJ: The Face in Genetic Disorders. St. Louis, Mosby, 1970

Goldberg MH, Eckblom RH: The treatment of the Pierre Robin syndrome. Pediatrics 30:450, 1962

Hoffman S, Kahn S, Seitchik M: Late problems in the management of Pierre Robin syndrome. Plast Reconstr Surg 35:504, 1965

Miller K, Allen RP, Davis WS: Rib gap defects with micrognathia: cerebrocostomandibular syndrome: Pierre Robin-like syndrome with rib dysplasia. Am J Roentgenol Radium Ther Nucl Med 114:253, 1972

Schreiner RL, McAlister WH, Marshall RE, et al.: Stickler syndrome in a pedigree of Pierre Robin syndrome. Am J Dis Child 126:86, 1973

Shah CV, Pruzansky S, Harris WS: Cardiac malformations with facial clefts. Am J Dis Child 119:238, 1970

Smith DW: Recognizable patterns of human malformation—genetic, embryologic, and clinical aspects. In Major Problems in Clinical Pediatrics. Philadelphia, Saunders, 1970

Smith JL, Stowe FR: The Pierre Robin syndrome. Glossoptosis, micrognathia, and cleft palate. A review of 39 cases with emphasis on associated ocular lesions. Pediatrics 27:128, 1961

Smith JL, Lemli L, Opitz JM: A newly recognized syndrome of multiple congenital anomalies. J Pediatr 64:210, 1964

Takagi Y, McCalla J, Bosma J: Prone feeding of infants with the Pierre Robin syndrome. Cleft Palate J 3:232, 1966

CLEFT LIP AND CLEFT PALATE

Bennett M, Ward RH, Tait CA: Otologic-audiologic study of cleft palate children. Laryngoscope 78:1011, 1968

Curtis EJ, Fraser FC, Warburton D: Cleft lip and cleft palate. Am J Dis Child 102:853, 1961

Fraser FC: The genetics of cleft lip and cleft palate. Am J Hum Genet 22:336, 1970

Goodman RM, Gorlin RJ: The Face in Genetic Disorders. St Louis, Mosby, 1970

Hagerty RF, Hill MJ: Midfacial contour in patient with cleft lip and cleft palate. Pediatrics 26:387, 1960

Landau W, Barry JM, Kock R: Arhinencephaly. J Pediatr 62:895, 1963

McKenzie J: The first arch syndrome. Arch Dis Child 33:377, 1958

McKusick VA: Genetics in medicine and medicine in genetics. Am J Med 34:594, 1963

Paradise JL, Bluestone CD: Early treatment of the universal otitis media of infants with cleft palate. Pediatrics 53:48 1974

Paradise JL, Bluestone CD, Felder H: The universality of otitis media in 50 infants with cleft palate. Pediatrics 44:35, 1969

Shah CV, Pruzansky S, Harris WS: Cardiac malformations with facial clefts. Am J Dis Child 119:238, 1970

Sicher H, Bhasker SN: Obran's Oral Histology and Embryology, 7th ed. St Louis, Mosby, 1972

Slaughter WB, Pruzansky S: Cleft lip and cleft palate. Pediatr Clin North Am 3:1029, 1956

Smith DW: Recognizable Patterns of Human Malformations. Genetic, Embryologic, and Clinical Aspects. In Major Problems in Clinical Pediatrics. Philadelphia, Saunders, 1970

Stark RB (ed): Cleft Palate. A Multidiscipline Approach. New York, Harper & Row, 1968

Thompson JS, Thompson MW: Genes in Differentiation and Development. In Genetics of Medicine. Philadelphia, Saunders, 1966

Yules RB: Hearing in cleft palate patients. Arch Otolaryngol 91:319, 1970

CHERUBISM

Anderson DE, McClendon JL: Cherubism: Hereditary fibrous dysplasia of the jaws, genetic considerations. Oral Surg 15: Suppl 2:5, 1962

Jones WA: Cherubism: A thumbnail sketch of its diagnosis and a conservative method of treatment. Oral Surg 20:648, 1965

Thompson N: Cherubism: Familial fibrous dysplasia of the jaws. Br J Plast Surg 12:89, 1959

THE TONGUE

MALFORMATIONS OF THE TONGUE

Macroglossia

Large, muscular tongues are occasionally familial; some orthodontists believe that these can cause malocclusion, particularly of the prognathous type. In many instances, enlargement of the tongue may be more apparent than real; a normal-sized tongue may seem larger when associated with underdevelopment of the jaws, especially in the absence of teeth.

True hypertrophy of the tongue is associated with mental retardation in cretinism, Down's syndrome, and Cornelia de Lange syndrome. In generalized gangliosidosis (p. 1908), and Hurler's disease (p. 1899) macroglossia is associated with mental deterioration, alveolar ridge hypertrophy, macrosomia, skeletal deformities, and stunted growth, and in Wiedemann-Beckwith syndrome with macrosomia, muscular hypertrophy, omphalocele, and abnormalities of carbohydrate metabolism.

Gross enlargement of the tongue of variable size, localized or diffuse, may be due to the presence of superficial or deep lymphangiomas or hemangiomas (Fig. 13). In the latter, treatment by surgery or with adrenocortical steroids may be indicated. In rare instances neurofibromatosis has been the cause of enlargement of the tongue.

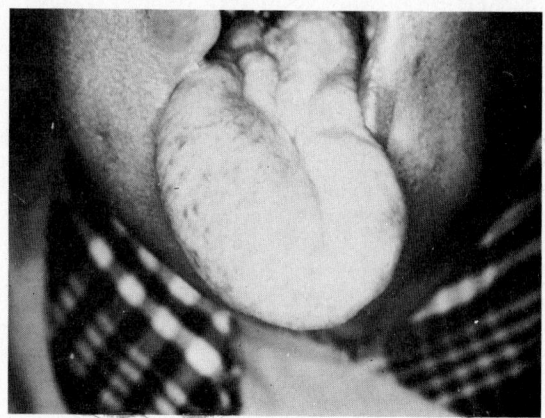

FIG. 13. Hemangioma of the tongue.

Microglossia (Tongue Hypoplasia)

Tongue hypoplasia is a much more rare anomaly than hypertrophy. It is usually accompanied by other congenital malformations.

Aglossia Congenita (Congenital Absence of the Tongue)

This condition is even more exceptional. It has been reported in conjunction with bony fusion of the jaws and other skeletal anomalies. In the *aglossia-adactylia syndrome,* absence of the tongue is associated with missing lower incisors, cleft or high arched palate, intraoral bands, hypertrophic submandibular and submaxillary salivary glands, and abnormalities of distal portions of the limbs, especially the digits.

Tongue-Tie

Congenital shortening of the frenulum interferes with protrusion of the tongue and causes a midline pucker when an effort is made to put out the tongue (Fig 14). In all probability it should be regarded as a normal variant (Fig. 14A). The assertion is sometimes made that tongue-tie impairs an infant's ability to nurse, and it is a common belief that persistent tongue-tie will eventually hamper speech, an hypothesis that has not been documented. If the tongue can be protruded

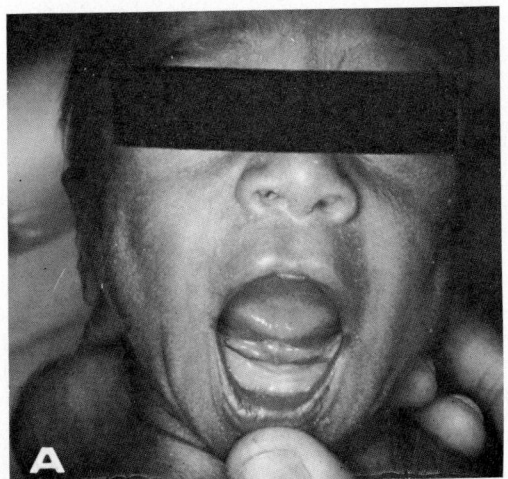

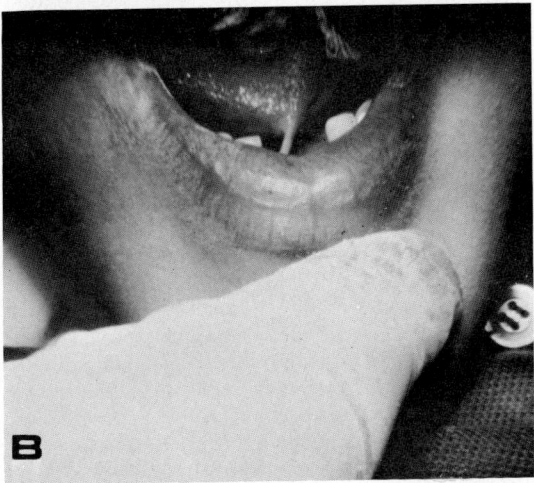

FIG. 14. Tongue-tie. A. "Normal" short frenulum of the newborn. B. True ankyloglossia.

beyond the lips, treatment is certainly not required. When an infant's tongue is found to be more closely bound, the parents are likely to persevere and persuade someone to release it. The operation, performed by cutting the frenulum close to the undersurface of the tongue, without anesthesia, probably does no harm; whether it does any good has not been evaluated. True *ankyloglossia* (Fig. 14B), where the frenulum is replaced by a short and thickened fibrous band that restricts the range of mobility of the tongue, is rare. This condition needs appropriate surgical repair.

Geographic Tongue

This condition is characterized by the appearance, upon the dorsum or margin of the tongue, of circular, elliptical, or crescentic red patches with gray margins. These gray margins, which are slightly elevated, are apparently due to thickening of the epithelial layer and the red areas to desquamation of the epithelium. It is a common condition, probably congenital. Usually, there are two to four red patches surrounded by a gray border, which is 1 to 2 mm wide and slightly elevated. From day to day, the configuration of the patches changes; the gray lines advance across the tongue from side to side or from base to tip, disappearing as they reach the border and run the same course (Fig. 15). Only the epithelium is involved, the deeper structures being unaffected. The duration of the disease is indefinite; it usually lasts for years but seems to clear up eventually. The cause is unknown. It is not accompanied by pain, salivation, or other symptoms of stomatitis and is of little practical importance. Treatment is unnecessary.

Fissured or Scrotal Tongue

This condition is characterized by deep, irregular fissures, often several millimeters deep, upon the dorsal surface. The condition generally occurs in families but is also found in Down's Syndrome. It is of no clinical significance. There is no convincing evidence that it is due to vitamin deficiency.

The Tongue in Familial Dysautonomia

Normally, the dorsal surface of the tongue is covered with conical, grayish white, filiform papillae. The larger and fewer red fungiform papillae are unevenly distributed near the margin and the tip. The vallate papillae are found posteriorly along the sulcus terminalis (p. 911). The tongue of the patient with dysautonomia is lacking in fungiform and vallate papillae and appears uniform and smooth. The absence of these papillae, in which the taste buds are normally concentrated, explains the taste deficit in these patients.

Choristomatic Cyst of The Tongue

Heterotopic islands of gastric mucosa have been found within the body of the tongue or in the floor of

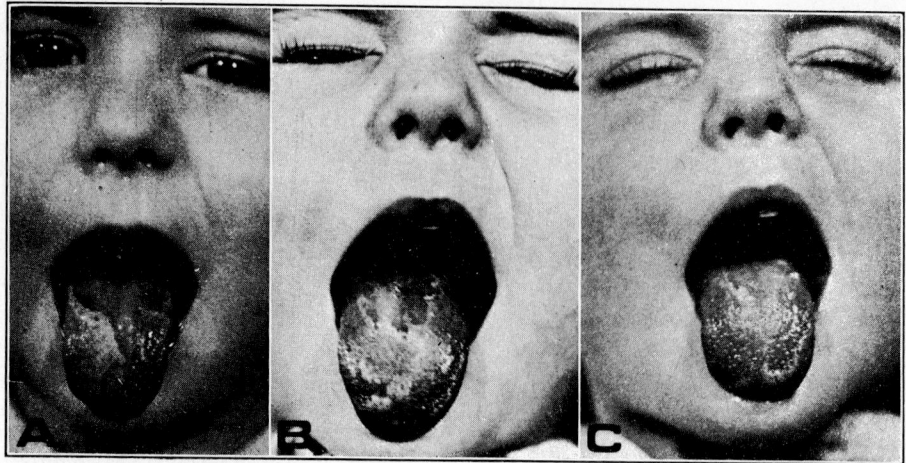

FIG. 15. Geographic tongue showing changing pattern of lesions. Patient 2.5 years of age. The interval between A and B is 14 days.

the mouth. The area anterior to the circumvallate papillae is the usual site of involvement. The lesions present as nonulcerated, elevated, or submerged masses, usually circumscribed and of slow growth. These choristomas may be asymptomatic or may interfere with feeding, deglutition, and speech. They are easily excised and usually do not recur.

Cleft Tongue

In the *orofacial digital syndrome,* an X-linked trait of dominant inheritance, limited to females and lethal to males, the tongue is characteristically cleft and lobulated. The tongue may be divided into two to four lobes, and hamartomas may exist between the lobes. Other oral anomalies of this syndrome include a pseudocleft in the middle of the upper lip, a transverse cleft of the hard palate, or asymmetric cleft of the soft palate; thick fibrous bands in the upper and lower mucobuccal folds; absence of lower lateral incisors; malposition of teeth; and supernumerary teeth.

In *Mohr syndrome,* an autosomal recessive trait, a midline cleft of the tongue is associated with a midline cleft of the lip, conductive deafness, and facial and digital anomalies.

Thyroglossal Cyst

In the course of embryonic development, anomalies of fusion of the pharyngeal arches may cause fistulae to persist, or strands of epithelium may survive resorption and lead to the formation of cysts. The number of possible varieties of these relatively common anomalies is great. Because of its attachment to the tongue, *thyroglossal cyst,* an embryonal rest of the oral cavity, will be discussed here, although its clinical manifestations occur, in most instances, in the region of the neck, the pharynx, or the larynx.

When remnants of the thyroglossal duct persist, they may give rise to the formation of cysts, and accumulation of secretions may produce a visible or palpable swelling. Such a cyst usually contains thick mucus and is lined by columnar, sometimes ciliated, epithelium; at time squamous epithelium is present and may even predominate. The mass is generally surrounded by a thick capsule of connective tissue, and a tube or cord of epithelium with a fibrous tissue envelope often penetrates the hyoid bone and extends upward to connect with the foramen cecum at the base of the tongue.

The common site of a thyroglossal cyst is at, or near, the midpoint of the hyoid bone, usually in the midline, sometimes a little to one side. It may, however, appear at any point between the thyroid gland and the foramen cecum. As a rule, pain and dysphagia are absent, except when the contents of the cyst become infected, in which case pain, tenderness, and rapid enlargement of the overlying skin will be present. In a small infant, a thyroglossal cyst at the base of the tongue rarely may cause breathing difficulty when the infant is in a supine position, which improves when the infant is placed on his abdomen. Not infrequently the lesion is discovered in childhood, sometimes by the parents, occasionally in the course of routine examination. It is usually quite firm, rises during swallowing, may be adherent to the overlying skin, and is almost always closely attached either to the hyoid bone or to the larynx. Transillumination often demonstrates the cystic structure but fails when the cyst contents have been rendered opaque by infection. In differential diagnosis, adenoma or abscess of the thyroid gland must be considered, although these are relatively rare. Since superficial cervical lymph nodes are generally situated toward the side of the neck, their enlargement is not apt to be mistaken for thyroglossal cyst. Lingual goiter or ectopic thyroid tissue situated high in the neck may be mistaken for thyroglossal duct cysts more readily. Such an error may lead to serious consequences, if the mass is removed and proves to be the only functional thyroid tissue present. Appropriate treatment in these instances is to give adequate thyroid hormone therapy to shrink the mass sufficiently to avoid surgery.

Treatment of thyroglossal duct cyst is surgical. Care must be taken to remove not only all of the cyst but also the entire epithelial tract. This excision usually sacrifices the central portion of the hyoid bone, with amputation of the superior projection of the epithelial remnant close to the foramen cecum.

Rupture of a thyroglossal cyst following infection, or drainage by a simple incision, leads to the formation of a cutaneous fistula. Cauterization is ineffective in preventing recurrence. The entire tract must be excised.

Acquired Lesions of the Tongue

Coated Tongue

The uniform white coating seen on the dorsal surface of the tongue in certain disease states is composed of dequamating epithelial cells, mucin, food debris, and various organisms. Under normal conditions, the saliva and the mechanical cleansing effect of mastication prevent such accumulation. In chronic mouth-breathing, and in febrile states accompanied by dehydration, especially with lack of food intake or diets limited to soft or liquid foods, such coating soon makes its appearance. No local treatment is necessary for ordinary white coating, which will disappear upon return to physiologic conditions.

In oral infections with *Candida albicans* (Oral thrush, (p. 927), the coating appears as discrete, flaky, white patches that bleed readily on removal. In *scarlet fever* (p. 499) the tongue, which is heavily coated at the onset of the pharyngitis, soon clears at the tip and along its margins. The swollen, hyperemic fungiform papillae that show through the coating give rise to the term *strawberry tongue.*

The Tongue in Deficiency Diseases

In *pellagra,* (p. 224) the tongue and oral mucous membranes are usually inflamed and swollen; the papillae are hypertrophied; the center of the tongue may be coated although the edges are clear. Glossitis may also accompany *riboflavin deficiency.* The "smooth tongue" resulting from atrophy of the filiform papillae and indicative of severe nutritional deficiency is rarely seen in children.

Ulcer of the Frenulum

Friction of the tongue against the sharp edges of the lower central incisors may cause ulceration of the frenulum in infants. It occurs typically in pertussis, but also in other conditions, especially in poorly nourished and

debilitated children. The ulcer may be confined to the frenum or may extend quite deeply into the tongue. It is usually 5 to 8 mm in diameter, and of a yellowish gray color. When associated with whooping cough it persists as long as severe spasms occur. The ulcer may be touched with alum or with gentian violet. If the lesion is extensive, it may require that the child be fed by dropper or by gavage for several days. Good oral hygiene must be maintained. Treatment of underlying chronic illness, and attempts at improving the child's nutrition are essential.

Bibliography

Adran GM, Beckett JM, Kemp FH: Aglossia congenita. Arch Dis Child 39:389, 1964

Bhaskar SN: Oral tumors of infancy and childhood: a survey of 239 cases. J Pediatr 63:195, 1963

Co-Te P, Dolman CL, Tischler B, et al: Oral-facial-digital syndrome. A case with necropsy findings. Am J Dis Child 119:280, 1970

Goodman RR, Gorlin RJ: The Face in Genetic Disorders. St Louis, Mosby, 1970

Gorlin RJ, Kalmins V, Izant RJ, Jr: Occurrence of heterotopic mucosa in the tongue. J Pediatr 64:604, 1964

Gorlin R: The oral-facial-digital syndrome. Cutis 4:1345, 1968

Guimaraes SB, et al: Thyroglossal duct remnants in infants and children. Mayo Clinic Proc 47:117, 1972

Keller EE, Bennett CG, Klingberg WG: Aglossia-adactylia syndrome. Am J Dis Child 116:549, 1968

Keynes G: Large thyroglossal cyst. Br J Surg 47:447, 1960

Kottmeier PK, Rosenthal S, Minkowitz S: Retropharyngeal abscess secondary to thyroglossal cyst. Am J Dis Child 109:160, 1965

Lewisohn MM, Lim DT: Apnea in the supine position as an alerting symptom at the base of the tongue in small infants. J Pediatr 66:1092, 1965

Lofgren RH: Respiratory distress from congenital lingual cysts. Am J Dis Child 106:610, 1963

Smith AA, Farbman A, Dancis J: Tongue in familial dysautonomia: A diagnostic sign. Am J Dis Child 110:152, 1965

Smith D: Recognizable patterns of human malformations—genetic, embryologic, and clinical aspects. In Major Problems in Clinical Pediatrics. Philadelphia, Saunders WB 1970

LESIONS OF THE GUMS AND ORAL MUCOSA

Gingival Hyperplasia

Enlargement of the gingivae is frequently observed in children and young adolescents as a consequence of unrelieved marginal gingivitis (see below). In hyperplasia of the gums associated with diphenylhydantoin therapy, the swollen gums are nodular, firm, and pink, presenting little or no evidence of inflammation; they almost cover the teeth. When the underlying neurologic disorders calls for continuing therapy, the development of gingival hyperplasia is not in itself adequate justification for discontinuing the drug. In the early stages of the condition, much can be done to check its progress by close attention to oral hygiene.

In diffuse, generalized *fibromatosis of the gingivae* (Fig. 16) the teeth may be completely covered by the exuber-

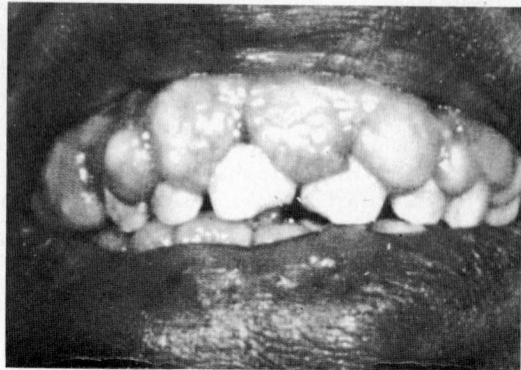

FIG. 16. Gingival fibromatosis.

ant soft tissues, producing the appearance of anodontia. Radiographic studies usually show that the developing teeth have left their bony crypts, the deciduous teeth presenting evidence of resorption in normal fashion for the patient's age. The teeth seem, however, unable to pierce the gums. Treatment consists of surgical removal, by stages, of the overlying gum.

INFLAMMATORY LESIONS OF THE ORAL MUCOSA

Inflammation of the oral mucous membranes may occur as a primary phenomenon or as a feature of systemic disease. When localized to the gums or tongue, it is designated as gingivitis or glossitis, the term stomatitis being reserved for more generalized lesions. In some instances the lesions are specific and their cause well identified, while in others they are less characteristic, the etiology being obscure or unknown. The clinical manifestations may vary from a mild generalized erythema to severe inflammation accompanied by vesiculation, ulceration, or even gangrene. Some degree of secondary infection follows any break in the surface membranes. Subjective symptoms range from mild soreness with increased salivation to pain sufficiently severe to result in dysphagia and dehydration.

Gingivitis, Stomatitis, and Gingivostomatitis

When inflammation involves only the gums, it is referred to as gingivitis; if intraoral mucosa other than the gum is affected it is termed stomatitis; and if all mucous membranes of the mouth are inflamed there is gingivostomatitis. The etiology of the inflammation may be local or systemic. A mild gingivitis or gingivostomatitis is quite common in children and requires no treatment.

ERUPTIVE GINGIVITIS. The localized reaction surrounding an erupting tooth, although usually mild and transient, occasionally may assume the characteristics of a hemorrhagic cyst when the tooth has difficulty in piercing the gum.

MARGINAL GINGIVITIS. Inflammation of the gingival margin and interdental papillae, associated with a variable degree of edema, exists commonly with poor oral hygiene. The tissues bleed easily upon slight trauma, as in brushing the teeth. There are no subjective symptoms in uncomplicated cases. Removal of sources of irritation combined with daily gingival massage usually eliminates this condition readily.

CATARRHAL GINGIVOSTOMATITIS. Any mild, generalized, nonspecific inflammation of the oral mucous membrane is commonly referred to as catarrhal stomatitis. Local—chemical, traumatic, or thermal—factors may produce such a generalized inflammation. In sensitive individuals certain antibiotic-containing mouthwashes or lozenges may produce severe local reactions far more disturbing than the condition they were intended to alleviate. Aspirin, when applied locally, may have a destructive effect upon the tissues, causing exfoliation of the mucosa and leaving a denuded surface. Habitual cheek-biting produces raw, ulcerative lesions that persist as long as the habit continues. Recovery of staphylococci, fusiform bacilli, or spirilla does not reflect the specific etiology, since these organisms frequently colonize any inflamed area of the mouth. Most cases of catarrhal stomatitis subside spontaneously within a few days after removal of the irritant, or after recovery from the underlying infection.

STOMATITIS ASSOCIATED WITH INFECTIOUS DISEASES. In *measles,* a characteristic enanthem (*Koplik's spots*) is pathognomonic of the disease. The lesions, which may be short-lived, appear approximately one day before the rash. The surrounding buccal mucosa is inflamed, edematous, and erythematous (p. 552). Severe and generalized stomatitis that may become ulcerative or gangrenous has been reported as a complication of *streptococcal infections.*

Diphtheria may extend onto the mucous membranes of the mouth, lips, and tongue (p. 433). Such wide distribution of the diphtheritic pseudomembrane is seen only in the severest cases, accompanied by extensive involvement of the pharynx and tonsils. The characteristic pseudomembrane in diphtheria is whiter, more opaque, and tougher than the exudate found in other infections. The subjacent tissues show less tendency to ulcerate.

In *varicella,* vesicles often develop on the oral mucous membranes especially on the soft palate, and posterior buccal mucosa, and also on the posterior pharynx. They may even appear 24 hours before the cutaneous eruption. The vesicles, which rupture readily, are surrounded by a red areola. They resemble nonspecific aphthae (p.927).

HERPANGINA. This term describes oral and pharyngeal manifestations of systemic infection associated with specific types of Group A Coxsackie viruses (types 2, 3, 4, 5, 6, 8, and 10). Shortly after onset of the infection the pharynx is diffusely congested, without focal lesions. Within 1 to 2 days, small vesicles appear on the faucial pillars, the tonsils, the edge of the soft palate, or on the posterior pharyngeal wall. In contrast to herpetic stomatitis (see below and p. 553), the anterior part of the mouth is usually spared. Systemic symptoms of fever, malaise, and anorexia are more prominent than local pain. The vesicles soon rupture, leaving shallow punched-out ulcers 2 to 5 mm in diameter which persist for several days usually outlasting the systemic symptoms. Regional adenopathy is minimal, and local complications are unknown.

HAND, FOOT, AND MOUTH DISEASE. This benign, self-limited, febrile illness caused by specific types of Coxsackie A virus (A5, A10, and A16) is characterized by a vesicular eruption affecting primarily the buccal mucosa and tongue and, less frequently, the gums and lips. A maculopapular eruption that secondarily becomes vesicular appears on the hands and feet, involving the palms, soles, and interdigital spaces of fingers and toes.

ACUTE LYMPHONODULAR PHARYNGITIS. Coxsackie virus A-10 may be responsible for a febrile illness, with headache and general malaise in which yellow or white nodular, nonvesicular lesions appear on the uvula, anterior pillars, and posterior pharynx.

HERPETIC GINGIVOSTOMATITIS (CHAP. 12, (p. 533). Primary infections with the virus of herpes simplex is a common cause of severe stomatitis in children. While the incidence of the disease is greatest between the first and sixth years of life, it may occur at any age. The onset is often insidious, with general malaise sometimes accompanied by mild upper respiratory symptoms. Food and even fluids are often refused. Children old enough to communicate verbally will complain of mouth soreness and pain on swallowing. The severity of systemic manifestations varies. Temperature elevations to 38.5 to 40.5 C frequently are observed. Dehydration of some degree may result from the dysphagia. Regional lymphadenopathy, which is present early in the disease, persists for some time after other symptoms have subsided.

Objective findings characteristically consist of a fiery red gingiva with swollen interdental papillae. Multiple small ulcers, which appear on the tongue, soft palate, and other parts of the buccal mucosa, have a yellowish white center with a hyperemic border. These aphthae represent ruptured vesicles, which may be noted fleetingly prior to their breakdown. Tags of gingival tissue adjacent to partially erupted teeth have a tendency to become ulcerated at their borders. The lips may develop painful fissures, extending outward toward the vermilion border. Occasionally, impetiginous vesicles appear upon the cutaneous portions of the lips. Pain, malaise, and fever subside after a few days. Healing of the gingivitis and aphthae is usually complete within 10 to 14 days, although lymphadenopathy may persist for 2 to 3 weeks.

Herpetic gingivostomatitis is self-limited, and its course is not greatly altered by local treatment. The use of irritating or caustic applications, such as silver nitrate, chromic acid, or sodium perborate, is contraindicated. The same is true for penicillin lozenges, which may produce glossitis. Systemic antibiotics have no beneficial effect and should not be given.

APHTHOUS STOMATITIS. Aphthae are small, circular or oval, painful ulcers involving the oral mucosa. The lesions are usually preceded by a small transient vesicle that soon loses its friable surface, leaving a shallow ulcer, 2 to 5 mm in diameter, surrounded by a red areola. Single ulcers of this type, occurring in the buccal sulcus, are commonly referred to as "canker sores." They may appear at any age, have a sudden onset, remain painful for 5 to 10 days, and heal without scarring. There is a slight induration, but usually no adenopathy. Food intake may be somewhat troublesome, but constitutional symptoms are absent. The origin of these single lesions is still debatable; in some instances herpes virus has been recovered, but its etiologic role has not been invariably borne out by subsequent rise in serum antibody level. Some cases have a traumatic origin. Mechanical irritation, as produced by the vigorous use of a stiff toothbrush, has often been implicated. Local applications of aqueous solution of gentian violet may prove helpful. Good oral hygiene must be maintained.

RECURRENT APHTHOSIS. Occasionally the aphthae are multiple; are distributed over the tongue, anterior pillars, buccal mucosa, and palate and tend to recur. New lesions develop while others are regressing. Clinically, these cases closely resemble herpetic gingivostomatitis, but the temperature is seldom elevated and there is little or no regional adenopathy. Pain may be severe enough to interfere with eating and talking. Complete healing occurs within 2 to 3 weeks, only to be followed by recurrence after a variable period of remission. This type of aphthosis was also once thought to be due to herpes simplex virus, but more recent work casts doubt on this etiologic hypothesis. While a specific allergen can seldom be incriminated, some cases reportedly have improved after antihistamine therapy.

DERMATOGINGIVOSTOMATITIS, EROSIVE. *Dermatogingivostomatitis* is a severe, diffuse, erosive, and painful stomatitis. It may result from rupture of intraoral vesicles or bullae, associated with typical erythematous, bullous, and iris skin lesions; exudative inflammation of conjunctival and anogenital mucosa; and marked systemic symptoms. It is a major feature of the *erythema multiforme exudativum* or ectodermosis erosiva pluriorificialis (Stevens-Johnson syndrome (p. 873). This syndrome may develop as a sensitivity reaction to drugs, or in association with a virus or mycoplasma infection.

Oral Thrush

Thrush is a mycotic stomatitis characterized by the appearance of small white flakes or patches on the oral mucous membranes usually on the tongue or the cheeks. It is common primarily in newborn infants but is seen sometimes in young infants and children with malnutrition or diabetes.

ETIOLOGY. The organism which produces thrush is *Candida albicans*. The structure of the fungus is readily visualized on a slide by adding one drop of a 10 percent potassium hydroxide solution to a small quantity of buccal exudate. The presence of *V. albicans* spores is very common in dust and in the atmosphere. Except in the newborn period, thrush is implanted with great difficulty on a healthy mucous membrane; its growth is favored by slight abrasions, lack of cleanliness, malnutrition, neoplasia, diabetes, antibiotic treatment, and hypoparathyroidism. Maternal vulvovaginal candidiasis appears to be the primary source of neonatal thrush. In utero infection of the fetus also has been reported. The infection also may be acquired from another patient, or from contaminated hands, bedding, or feeding equipment, but probably not from the air. It is relatively frequent in the first 2 to 3 months after birth and also in older infants suffering from harelip, cleft palate, or any other deformity of the mouth.

PATHOLOGY. The spores lodge between the epithelial cells and gradually separate the different layers. This implantation occurs before the formation of the white pellicle. Later the disease spreads on the surface of the mucous membrane and also penetrates the deeper structures. Invasion of the blood vessels is rare, but may cause thrombosis locally or dissemination to remote parts of the body. Growth of *Candida albicans* in the buccal cavity usually begins at several discrete points on the mucous membrane, with gradual spreading until some degree of coalescence takes place; a continuous membrane may thus be formed. The acid reaction of the mouth found in thrush is presumably a result of fermentation of sugar by the organisms.

SYMPTOMS. The essential feature of thrush is the development on the oral mucosa of small white flakes which resemble deposits of coagulated milk but which differ from milk curds in that they cannot be wiped off. If forcibly removed, they usually leave bleeding points. They usually appear first on the tongue or the inner surface of the cheeks. There may be only a few scattered patches, or the mouth and pharynx may be covered. Local pain and tenderness are conspicuously absent; the mouth is sometimes dry, and occasionally there is some difficulty in swallowing. Constitutional symptoms, if present, depend on some associated condition rather than on thrush.

DIAGNOSIS. The diagnosis is rarely difficult and in most cases is established by inspection. Manipulation with a tongue depressor readily permits differentiation between white deposits of thrush and milk curds. Coalescent thrush on the pharynx and fauces has been confused with diphtheria, although this mistake can hardly be made if all the facts are taken into consideration: age of the patient, involvement of the cheeks and tongue, absence of glandular enlargement or of constitutional symptoms. In case of doubt, microscopic examination of the deposit will establish the etiology. In cultures on Loffler's medium, the large, rounded or oval spores of the fungus are easily recognized.

PROGNOSIS. The cases involving only the mouth clear up readily, leaving no scar. Thrush is rarely a dangerous disease in itself. However, in the malnourished, or in the infant with harelip or cleft palate, it may prove tenacious and troublesome, at times even serious.

TREATMENT. Oral candidiasis may be prevented to a certain degree by attention to cleanliness of rubber nipples, bottles, and other objects which come into direct or indirect contact with the infant's mouth. Neonatal thrush is best prevented through mycologic screening and adequate therapy of all pregnant women who yield *Candida albicans* from the vagina. In infants with deformities of the mouth, and in institutional settings, the infection frequently develops despite all precautions. Local treatment is not essential, but recovery can probably be accelerated by the use of some mild antiseptic. A 1 percent aqueous solution of gentian violet on a swab may be applied several times a day. With such treatment the disease often improves; in the absence of treatment it may last several weeks. In obstinate cases, 1 to 2 ml of Nystatin U.S.P. may be applied locally four times a day, in the form of a freshly prepared solution containing from 100,000 to 200,000 units / ml. This drug can also be administered orally in the same dose three to four times a day with the formula.

Noma (Gangrenous Stomatitis, Cancrum Oris)

Noma is a slow-spreading gangrene involving the mucous membranes or mucocutaneous orifices. The mouth is the site most frequently involved, but the nose, external auditory canal, vulva, prepuce, or anus may also be affected. The disease, once invariably fatal, is now almost unknown in the United States. Usually, it develops following an infectious illness, most frequently measles, often on the site of previous local inflammation. It is a malignant infection primarily caused by *Borrelia* (Vincent's fusospirillar organisms) in a patient whose resistance to infection is greatly reduced.

The odor of the breath or a dusky spot on the cheek or lip may be the first symptom. In the mouth, a dark, greenish black, necrotic mass surrounded by edema is the usual finding. The cheek or lips may be two or three times their normal thickness. Externally the parts are tense and brawny from the swelling, the infiltration extending always beyond the gangrenous part. As the process extends, the teeth loosen and are extruded. Necrosis of the alveolar process of the jaw may occur, and perforation and extensive sloughing of one or both cheeks or of the lower lip may take place. The odor is very offensive; pain is rarely severe or may be absent; extensive hemorrhages are rare.

The prognosis, once extremely grave and inexorably fatal has been markedly altered since the advent of penicillin, which rapidly arrests the process. Intravenous penicillin therapy must be promptly instituted in large doses, 100,000/kg/day, obviating the need for surgical excision, once the treatment of choice. Plastic surgery may be needed after the process has been arrested.

Bibliography

Cherry JD, John CL: Herpangina: etiologic spectrum. Pediatrics 36:632, 1965

Cherry JD, John CL: Hand, foot, and mouth syndrome: report of six cases due to Coxsackie Virus, Group A, Type 16. Pediatrics 31:637, 1966

Dobias B: Moniliasis in pediatrics. Am J Dis Child 94:234, 1957

Dodd K Ruchman I: Herpes simplex virus not the etiologic agent of recurrent stomatitis. Pediatrics 5:883, 1950

Forman ML, Cherry JD: Enanthems associated with uncommon viral syndromes. Pediatrics 41:873, 1968

Hale BD, Rendtorff RC, Walker, LC: Epidemic herpetic stomatitis in an orphanage nursery. JAMA 183:1068, 1963

Higgins PG, Warin RP: Hand, foot, and mouth disease. A clinically recognizable virus infection seen mainly in children. Clin Pediatrics 6:373, 1967

Kozinn PJ, Taschadjian CL, Wiener H: Incidence and pathogenesis of neonatal candidiasis. Pediatrics 21:42, 1958

Lopez E, Aterman K: Intrauterine infection by *Candida*. Am J Dis Child 115:663, 1968

Nahmias AJ, Roizman B: Infection with Herpes-simplex viruses 1 and 2. N Engl J Med 289:781, 1973

Parrott RH, Wolf SI, Nudelman J, Naiden E, Huebner RJ, et al: Clinical laboratory differentiation between herpangina and infectious (herpetic) gingivostomatitis. Pediatrics 14:122, 1954

CHAPTER 19

The Teeth

SOLOMON N. ROSENSTEIN, D.D.S.

GROWTH AND DEVELOPMENT OF THE TEETH

EARLY DEVELOPMENT

The earliest sign of tooth development occurs during the sixth week of embryonic life and consists of unusually rapid proliferation of certain cells in the basal layer of the oral epithelium, along the free margins of the embryonic structures that are to become the upper and lower jaw arches. The thickened line in each arch, called the *dental lamina,* represents the anlage of that portion of the teeth derived from the ectoderm. Concomitantly, rounded swellings of additional cell proliferation arise at 10 different points in each arch; these are called *tooth buds* or tooth germs and are the primordia of the enamel organs of the 20 primary teeth at locations that correspond to their future positions in the primary dentition.

The *enamel organ* (Fig. 1), developing from the bud, is of ectodermal origin, determines the shape of the crown of the tooth, and gives rise to its enamel. With continued growth, as further cell proliferation occurs, the structural changes proceed inwardly from each arch margin and unequally at different parts. Layers of outer and inner enamel epithelium differentiate, with between them, the stellate reticulum consisting of branched reticular cells and a rich intercellular fluid. The inner enamel epithelium cells differentiate further to become *ameloblasts* or *enamel forming* cells.

As the tooth bud undergoes cell differentiation, invagination, and further growth through the various stages of enamel organ development, the cells in the mesenchymal structure of its inner aspect become the *dental papilla,* the formative organ of the dentine and pulp. The peripheral cells of the papilla, adjacent to the inner enamel epithelium, become the *odontoblasts,* which later form the dentine of the tooth. From the inner cells arise the structures that become the pulp.

While both the enamel organ and the dental papilla develop, the surrounding mesenchyme forms the dental sac from which cells later differentiate into cementoblasts and tissue cells that become the fibers of the periodontal membrane. The tissues associated with teeth and surrounding structures are listed in Table 1, and Figure 2.

LATER DEVELOPMENT

Primary Teeth

The inner aspect of the enamel organ becomes separated early from the adjacent dental papilla by a basement membrane; later this boundary becomes the dentino-enamel junction as the inner enamel epithelium begins to form the enamel. Inception of enamel formation, at any point, is immediately preceded by inception of dentine formation. Both develop in the enamel organ toward its periphery in a direction away from the dentino-enamel junction.

Enamel formation is considered to occur in two stages: (a) formation of organic enamel matrix in which some calcium salts are present; (b) maturation or calcification radiographically opaque. Once the inner enamel epithelial cells or ameloblasts reach the peripheral layer of outer enamel epithelial cells, the thickness of enamel is completely formed, the cells are reduced to a united enamel epithelium, and no more enamel can be formed

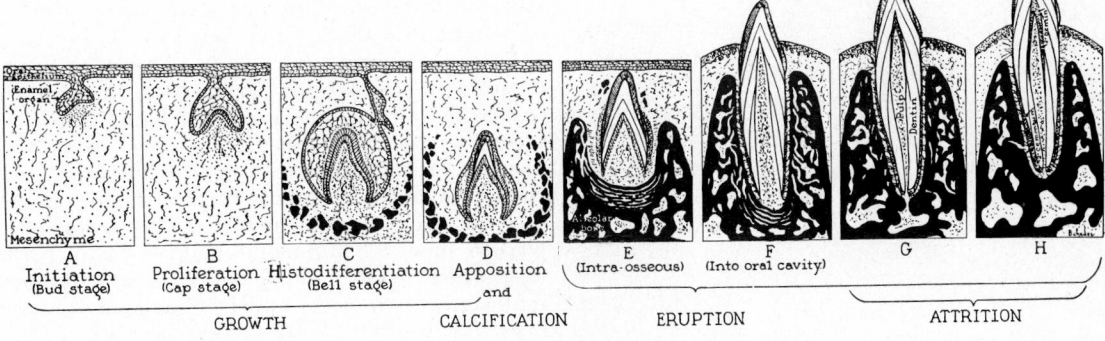

FIG. 1. Diagrammatic representation of life cycle of the tooth. (From Schour and Massler. *J Am Dent Assoc* 27:1785, 1940. Courtesy of the American Dental Association.)

TABLE 1. Classification of the Dental Tissues*

Tissue	Origin	Degree of Calcification	Function	Anatomic Classification	Regenerative Capacity	Disease	Special Fields of Dentistry
Enamel	Ectodermal	97%	Resistant to wear	Propriodontal	Nil	Enamel caries	Restorative dentistry
Dentin	Mesodermal	70%	Elastic strength	Propriodontal	Restricted	Dentin caries	Restorative dentistry
Pulp	Mesodermal	Uncalcified	Formation and vitality of dentin	Endodontal	Limited	Pulpitis	Endodontics
Cementum	Mesodermal	60%	Support	Periodontal	Good	Periodontitis Periodontosis	Periodontics
Periodontal Membrane	Mesodermal	Uncalcified	Support	Periodontal	Good	Periodontitis Periodontosis	Periodontics
Alveolar	Mesodermal	66%	Support	Periodontal	Good	Periodontitis Periodontosis	Periodontics
Gingiva	Ectodermal and mesodermal	Uncalcified	Investment and protection	Periodontal	Good	Gingivitis Gingivosis	Periodontics

*Adapted from: Schour, Noyes' Oral Histology and Embryology, 7th ed. Courtesy of Lea and Febiger.

at that area. When this occurs over the entire contour of the enamel organ, the contour of the tooth crown is completed and no further enamel formation can ever occur in that tooth.

In dentine formation odontoblasts migrate toward the middle area of the tooth; this process continues

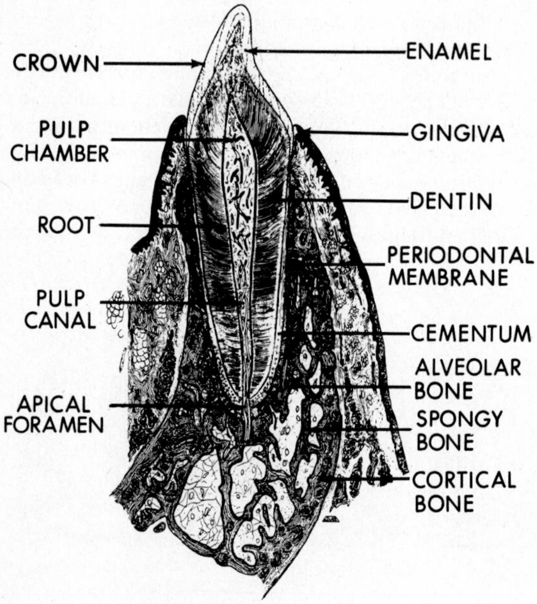

FIG. 2. Diagrammatic representation of the dental tissues. (From Schour. *Noyes' Oral Histology and Embryology*, 7th ed., 1953. Courtesy of Lea and Febiger.)

beyond the open end of the crown contributing to root formation and the lengthening of the tooth. The odontoblasts usually remain at the inner border of the dentine, lining the pulp, and dentinogenesis continues throughout the life of the tooth, with narrowing of the pulp area in the middle of the crown and root.

These structures become the 20 primary teeth, 10 in each arch, 5 in each quadrant: the central incisor next to the midline, then the lateral incisor, cuspid, first molar, and second molar. Although this represents the sequence of their positions in the completed dentition, their calcification and subsequent eruption occur in different order.

Permanent Teeth

The dental lamina also initiates development of the permanent teeth, which starts at about the fourth to fifth month in utero in two distinct steps for two groups of permanent teeth.

These permanent teeth, which are the successors of the primary teeth, are, in each quadrant, the permanent central incisor, lateral incisor, cuspid, first cuspid, and second cuspid. They arise from extensions from the lingual aspect of each enamel organ of the primary teeth and, continuing to grow lingually, become the anlage of each successor permanent tooth. This process takes place at about the fifth month in utero for the permanent central incisors and continues at particular times for the other permanent successor teeth until about ten months postnatally for the second bicuspid.

The permanent molars, which later are placed distally to the primary dentition, arise from the distal extension of the posterior part of the dental lamina in each quadrant, during the development of the second primary molars. The extension which gives rise to the anlage of the first permanent molar occurs at about 4 months in utero, at about 9 to 10 months postnatally for the second, and during the fourth to fifth year for the third permanent molar.

As each tooth bud is initiated, the cells of its dental lamina begin to disintegrate and disappear. Each tooth bud becomes an internal developing organ and goes through the stages of development and growth described above, to its eruption and continuing growth in root length.

CALCIFICATION

Primary Teeth

Calcification in the primary teeth is both prenatal and postnatal. It begins in all of the primary teeth before birth, usually during the fourth month, first in the central incisor crown, then in the other primary teeth in the following order: first molar, lateral incisor, cuspid, second molar. The crowns of all the primary teeth complete their calcification after birth, the central incisors within the first few months postnatally to the second molars at about 10 to 12 months.

Permanent Teeth

Calcification of the permanent teeth is a postnatal process, except for the first permanent molars, where it usually begins in the tips of the cusps before birth, during the eighth and ninth months.

All the anterior permanent teeth except the upper lateral incisors usually begin to calcify within the first 6 months of postnatal life; the upper central incisors, the lower central and lateral incisors, at about 3 to 4 months; the upper and lower cuspids at about 4 to 5 months. The upper lateral incisors begin to calcify later, at about the end of the first year and beginning of the second year. However, the crowns of all the incisor teeth usually complete calcification between 4 and 5 years, the cuspids at about 6 to 7 years. Disturbances in calcification in these teeth cannot be attributed to influences of diseases or disorders which occur later.

The bicuspids, or premolars, may begin to calcify between 1½ and 2½ years, although, in many instances the second bicuspids may not show evidence of calcification until appreciably later. As a rule, the upper bicuspids are ahead of the lowers, and the first is ahead of the second. Their crowns are usually completed by 6 to 7 years.

The first permanent molars, which usually have begun their calcification before birth will have crown calcification completed by about 3 years of age.

The second permanent molars usually begin calcification during the latter part of the third year and crown calcification is completed by about 7 years of age or shortly thereafter. By this time all the permanent teeth, except the third molars, if present, will have completed crown calcification.

The third molars may begin calcification after the seventh year.

ERUPTION

The eruption of a baby's first tooth is an important milestone for the baby and the parents; it marks the beginning of the period of the *primary dentition* which continues until the first permanent tooth makes its appearance. The period of the *mixed dentition* follows and extends to the time of exfoliation of the last of primary teeth. The period of the *permanent dentition* follows.

Mean Ages of Eruption of Primary Teeth

The onset of eruption of the primary dentition heralds an important change in oral habits and eating habits. From the earlier period of feeding through sucking, then eating only liquid and soft foods from a spoon, the child reaches the stage where he learns to incise foods with the front teeth and later to grind foods as the posterior teeth erupt. An increasing number of teeth prepares the child for eating the broad variety of regular foods.

The sequence of eruption of the teeth and the age at which these occur follow a certain pattern; the age at the first eruption is an important landmark of the child's development.

A handy guide for mean ages of eruption of the primary teeth in McBride's *Rule of 4*, starting with the first eruption at 6 to 7 months. Between eruption of different types of primary teeth, there is an approximate 4-month interval during which the other teeth of the same type are erupting, in each quadrant of the mouth. The first to erupt is usually a lower primary central incisor, followed shortly by its adjacent, homologous incisor; somewhat later an opposing upper central incisor erupts, followed by its homologous tooth. At about this time, or shortly thereafter, the first of the lateral incisors will erupt and, at short intervals, will be followed by the other lateral incisors. Rather infrequently the first tooth to erupt may be the upper central incisor; in these children the upper lateral incisor also may precede the eruption of the lower lateral incisor. This slight variation occurs very seldom and does not affect the rest of the pattern of dental development.

ERUPTION OF PRIMARY TEETH	
"Rule of 4"	
One Tooth	Age (mean)
1. Central Incisor	6-7 mos.
2. Lateral Incisor	11 mos.
3. First Molar	15 mos.
4. Cuspid	19 mos.
5. Second Molar	23-24 mos.

The first molar, the third type of primary tooth to

erupt, will appear in its normal posterior position, leaving a large space distal to the lateral incisor for the cuspid which has not yet erupted. Parents who express concern at the sight of this large posteriorly erupting tooth distal to a large space should be reassured that this sequence is normal.

The primary cuspids then erupt and are followed by the primary second molars, often called the 2-year molars.

Mean Ages of Eruption of Permanent Teeth

Later phases of development, such as exfoliation of the primary teeth and eruption of permanent teeth, will usually occur at average ages (see below) in children whose primary dentitions erupted at the normal time (Table 2). Exfoliation occurs as a result of progressive resorption of the roots of the primary teeth through osteoclastic action.

Toward the end of the sixth year the lower primary central incisors will begin to loosen as osteoclastic activity causes root resorption and the teeth approach exfoliation. At 6 to 6½ years one of the permanent successor incisors erupts, followed shortly by the adjacent central incisor. At about the same time or shortly thereafter one or more of the permanent first molars erupt distal to the primary molars. Parents are often unaware of this posterior extension of the dentition, since the first permanent molar usually erupts uneventfully, unless a gingival flap overlaying part of the new molar becomes irritated or mildly inflamed. These first permanent molars must be maintained in good position

and health, as they subsequently provide the major chewing surfaces and maintain the arch relationship when the primary molars are being exfoliated.

During the next half year the upper central incisor succession occurs, followed shortly by the loosening of the primary lower lateral incisors and eruption of their permanent successors at about 7 to 7½ years. Upper lateral incisor succession takes place at 8 to 8½ years.

There may appear to be a period of lessened activity at this time, during which the upper lateral incisors are continuing their eruption into normal positions in the dental arches. However, during this period intermittent resorption of the longer roots of the cuspids and the multiple roots of the primary molars is taking place. The remaining permanent successor teeth will usually erupt in the following order: first biscuspids at about 9½ years, and second bicuspids at about 10½ years. In most children cuspid succession follows the eruption of the first and second bicuspids at about 10½ years. Occasionally, cuspid succession in the lower jaw may precede the eruption of the second bicuspids.

The above changes will occur shortly before the permanent second molars begin to erupt just distal to the permanent first molars, the lower before the upper, at about 12 years.

The third molars, if present, begin to erupt after the seventeenth year. Their eruption is usually slow, with longer intervals during which the erupting tooth is partly covered by gum tissue while bone growth occurs to provide space for it. At such times the soft tissue may become inflamed; gentle cleansing will usually allay this troublesome condition. However, if bone growth is not

TABLE 2. Chronology of the Human Dentition.*

Tooth		Calcification Begins	Crown Completed	Eruption	Root Completed	Root Resorption Begins
Primary	I	14 wk†	4 mo	6-8 mo	1½-2 yr	5-6 yr
	II	16 sk†	5 mo	8-10 mo	1½-2 yr	5-6 yr
	III	17 wk†	9 mo	16-20 mo	2½-3 yr	6-7 yr
	IV	15½ wk†	6 mo	12-16 mo	2-2½ yr	4-5 yr
	V	18-19 wk†	10-12 mo	20-30 mo	3 yr	4-5 yr
Upper	1	3-4 mo	4-5 yr	7-8 yr	10 yr	
Permanent	2	1 yr	4-5 yr	8-9 yr	11 yr	
	3	4-5 mo	6-7 yr	11-12 yr	13-15 yr	
	4	1½-1¾ yr	5-6 yr	10-11 yr	12-13 yr	
	5	2-2½ yr	6-7 yr	10-12 yr	12-14 yr	
	6	8 mo†	2½-3 yr	6-7 yr	9-10 yr	
	7	2½-3 yr	7-8 yr	12-14 yr	14-16 yr	
	8	7-9 yr	12-16 yr	17-30 yr	18-25 yr	
Lower	1	3-4 mo	4-5 yr	6-7 yr	9 yr	
Permanent	2	3-4 mo	4-5 yr	7-8 yr	10 yr	
	3	4-5 mo	6-7 yr	10-11 yr	12-14 yr	
	4	1¾-2 yr	5-6 yr	10-12 yr	12-13 yr	
	5	2¼-2½ yr	6-7 yr	11-12 yr	13-14 yr	
	6	8 mo†	2½-3 yr	6-7 yr	9-10 yr	
	7	2½-3 yr	7-8 yr	12-13 yr	14-15 yr	
	8	8-10 yr	12-16 yr	17-30 yr	18-25 yr	

*Adapted from Logan and Kronfeld; Kraus and Jordan.
†In utero (average).

sufficient to permit the tooth to reach its normal, completely erupted state, more extensive dental procedures may be indicated.

Normal Range of Variation in Ages of Eruption

Knowledge of the mean ages at which dentitional changes occur is useful for guidance; however, developmental phenomena, such as calcification and eruption, occur according to individual patterns and show considerable variation.

For example, an infant who erupts his first tooth as early as 4 to 4½ months will probably erupt his first permanent molar at about 4½ years. This pattern will continue, with subsequent dental eruptions occurring at ages earlier than the average. On the other hand, the child who erupts his first tooth as late as 9 months of age will have subsequent eruptions at older ages, with the 6-year molar erupting, for example, at 7½ to 8 years. Occasionally the first tooth will not erupt until about 1 year of age, which although infrequent is still within the normal range, particularly when other developmental milestones are normal.

The multiple processes of dental development and growth are active over a long period of life, from the sixth week in utero to almost the end of childhood. In most individuals dental growth and development will occur normally. It is dentistry's purpose that a child should reach adulthood with a normal healthy dentition, essential for effective chewing, digestion, and the enjoyment of food. The social and cosmetic significance of healthy teeth and their role in optimal communication by speech are also major considerations.

BONE GROWTH

The entire process of tooth formation is accompanied by growth in both maxilla and mandible, which develop by intramembranous ossification.

Body of the Maxilla

The maxilla is formed from three bones: the maxilla proper, the premaxilla, and the prevomer. Ossification in the maxilla begins early in the seventh week of embryonic development. This bone will ultimately hold all the teeth of the upper jaw except the incisors. The premaxilla forms the anterior part of the mature maxilla and contains the structures which will become the incisors. Ossification of the premaxilla begins somewhat later than that of the maxilla proper. Fusion of these two bones to form the primary palate follows slightly thereafter, around the end of the eighth week. The primordia for the maxillary incisors appear in the premaxilla at about the middle of the eighth week. Fusion of the palatal processes of the maxillae to form the secondary palate usually starts during the ninth week.

The prevomer starts ossification at about the ninth week and is closely related to the premaxilla. It bears no teeth, but along with the premaxilla enters into formation of the primary palate.

Body of the Mandible

The mandibular arch appears during the sixth week of development as bilateral wings lateral to Meckel's cartilage. Their free ends continue to grow anteriorly toward each other to fuse, by the seventh week, at the future midline of the face. This fusion is usually completed during the eighth week. During the seventh week, the dental lamina has formed and will give rise to the structures that will become the lower primary teeth. Ossification of the bilateral plates of the developing mandibular arch also begins in the seventh week and continues in sequence, adding to the mandibular length and height, enclosing nerves and blood vessels, and the developing tooth structures.

Alveolar Processes

As tooth growth continues, bony septa appear between adjacent teeth. As the teeth proceed toward eruption locations, this bone, at the oral cavity end in the maxilla and mandible, extends from the body of the bone, enlarging the alveoli, which house and support the growing roots of the teeth. Growth of the alveolar processes continues with further eruption and root growth, and contributes to the increase in height or vertical dimension of each jawbone.

This type of bone growth occurs for the primary teeth, for the successor permanent teeth, and posteriorly for the roots of the permanent molars.

Other Bone Changes

Another type of bone growth occurs at ossification areas at the posterior portions of the bodies of the maxilla and the mandible, probably the result of functional activity. This growth provides the increase in the antero-posterior dimension, or length, of each arch, permitting growth and eruption of the permanent molars.

As these bone changes occur, the lower part of the face occupies a larger portion of the total head-face dimension and facial position moves in a downward and forward direction with further maturation.

POSTERUPTIVE CONDITIONS

Occlusion

Upon completion of each dentition following normal eruption of both the primary teeth and permanent teeth, the relation of lower and upper teeth should be that of normal occlusion. Normal occlusion essentially consists of: (a) even arch form in upper and lower jaws; (b) upper anterior teeth slightly overlapping the lower anterior teeth labially; (c) the posterior upper teeth slightly overlapping the lower posterior teeth bucally to part of the upper buccal cusps; (d) cusps interdigitating with the teeth in occlusion; and (e) the existence of a "normal" mesiodistal relation.

Marked aberrations from this pattern indicate malocclusions that should be investigated and corrected early, usually during the period of mixed dentition or early in the period of permanent dentition. Some early aberrant intermaxillary relationships can be corrected during the period of primary dentitions (Disorders of Occlusion, p. 942).

Maturational Changes

Posteruptively, the teeth continue to undergo changes. Some of these continue events of earlier growth stages, others are manifestations of maturation and aging. Attrition, or wear of biting surfaces secondary to function, promotes continuing dentinogenesis and other changes in the dentine and pulp. Dentinogenesis gradually narrows the coronal and root pulpal areas. Eruption does not subside even after the root of the tooth has attained its full length. To some extent it compensates some of the dimensional loss by attrition, and occurs as a result of continuing deposition of cementum at the root end and continued growth of the adjacent bone.

Bibliography

Kraus BS, Jordan RE: The Human Dentition Before Birth. Philadelphia, Lea and Febiger, 1965

McBride WC: Juvenile Dentistry, 5th ed. Philadelphia, Lea and Febiger, 1952

Provenza DV: Oral Histology. Philadelphia, JB Lippincott, 1964

Rosenstein SN: Dentistry for children. NY J Dent 22:327, 1952

Schour IN: Oral Histology and Embryology, 8th ed. Philadelphia, Lea and Febiger, 1960

Sicher H (ed): Orban's Oral Histology and Embryology, 5th ed. St Louis, cv Mosby, 1962

DEVELOPMENTAL DISORDERS OF TEETH

Dental development and growth occur from the sixth week of intrauterine life to the early part of the third decade of life. During this entire period, the multiple processes involved in tooth formation are all susceptible to various harmful influences.

Unlike bone, there is no ready metabolic inflow and outgo of calcium in any tooth structure already completed. During the period of tooth growth, any systemic disturbance or local trauma that affects tooth germ formation, enamel matrix formation, dentine formation, or calcification will leave its mark on the structure that is being formed at the time of the insult. Both the enamel and dentine may be affected, and the extent of the resulting defect will depend upon the severity and duration of the injury or disturbance.

The resulting malformation will usually appear as some form of hypoplasia or other malstructure of the part of the tooth, or teeth, in the process of being formed at the time of the insult or accident. When the disturbance is transitory, the resulting mark is fixed and normal growth will resume in the remainder of affected tooth or teeth (Figs. 3 and 4).

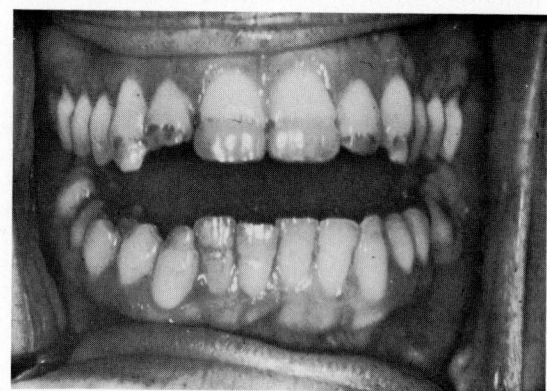

FIG. 3. Male, 31 years old. Patient had severe nephritis at 1½ years of age. Enamel hypoplasia, consisting of aplasia, pitting, and grooving present at all upper and lower incisors, cuspids, and first molars. (Courtesy of Dr. E. V. Zegarelli.)

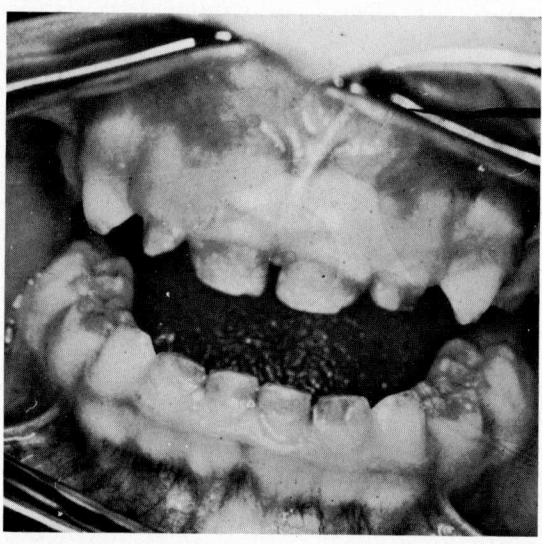

FIG 4. Female, 3 years old, premature birth. Hypoplasia of the enamel of the primary teeth involving large areas on the incisors and first molars, tips of the cuspids, and cusps and surface enamel at the mesio-occlusal portion of the second molars.

Examples of the effects of local factors may be observed following severe physical trauma to primary teeth. Young children frequently fall and strike, or are being struck by hard substances, which may cause shock to the teeth and adjacent structures, resulting in degeneration of the pulpal tissues. The blow to the teeth may be severe and the direction of force such, that comminuted fracture of the adjacent bone occurs or the primary teeth may be severely intruded. The developmental processes taking place in the successor teeth at that time can be disturbed and may delay their subsequent eruption. If the force of severe trauma is transmitted lingually during the period of enamel formation in the successor tooth, amelogenesis is disturbed and localized areas of variable size of enamel hypoplasia will be observed after its eruption.

Trauma and systemic disorders represent but two aspects of the total complex of developmental disorders of teeth. Genetic factors also influence tooth size and form. There are specific abnormalities involving entire dentitions, which can be traced back through generations, as in odontogenesis imperfecta. In other severe developmental disorders a genetic influence may be suspected, but has not yet been demonstrated. Dental anomalies may also occur in syndromes involving multiple developmental abnormalities; often such combinations of anomalies are associated with mental retardation and with chromosomal aberrations described in Chapter 8.

Disorders of development associated with facial anomalies will be accompanied by dental abnormalities if the disorders exist very early in life and/or involve disturbance of ectodermal or facial structures that contain developing teeth or their primordia.

The following conditions illustrate the effect on dental structures of systemic disturbances during dental development and the genetic influence on dental anomalies.

PREMATURITY: CEREBRAL PALSY

Enamel hypoplasia is highly prevalent among former premature infants (Fig. 4). In one recent study this dental abnormality was present in 45 percent of the children and was found to correlate significantly with neurologic, psychologic, and speech abnormalities. This finding suggests that the dental defects may be the result of the same damage. The time at which the insult occurred may be dated from the site of the hypoplastic lesion on the prenatally formed enamel of the primary teeth, particularly the incisors.

The prevalence of enamel hypoplasia is also higher in patients with cerebral palsy, especially among premature infants. In one study of children with cerebral palsy, 22 had been born prematurely and of these, 41 percent had enamel dysplasia. The enamel hypoplasia was found to be more pronounced in the athetoid and severely spastic children. Efforts to date the time at which enamel dysplasia occurred in these patients indicate that the largest number of dental abnormalities occur during the prenatal period, while a few occur in both the prenatal and early postnatal periods. Another significant relationship was also found between enamel dysplasia and blood incompatibilities.

TOOTH DISCOLORATION BY TETRACYCLINE

Administration of antibiotics of the tetracycline family may give rise to discoloration of children's teeth if the agent is taken during periods of tooth formation and growth. The darkened discoloration is the result of deposition of the medication in the dentine along the incremental lines of growth (lines of Owen). The primary or permanent dentition, or both, may be affected, depending upon the length and intensity of exposure to the drug, and the ages at which it occurred. Discoloration has also been observed in primary teeth of children who received no tetracycline-type medication, but whose mothers were treated with such therapy during pregnancy.

INHERITED DISORDERS

Dentinogenesis Imperfecta (Odontogenesis Imperfecta, Hereditary Opalescent Dentine)

Probably the most frequent of the inheritable disorders of abnormal dental structure formation, this condition is inherited as a non-sex-linked dominant characteristic. The dentine of both primary and permanent teeth is affected as a result of the failure of the odontoblasts to differentiate completely during the developmental stage of histodifferentiation. As a result dentine ground substance is formed, but the dentinal tubules may be irregularly arranged or absent. Formation of this type of dentine continues, with the further characteristic obliteration of pulp chambers and canals. The enamel is normal but root formation is usually abnormal.

Clinically, the crowns of the teeth have normal form and size. They are markedly translucent with abnormally dark color, usually grayish or bluish brown. Severe attrition occurs rapidly, with teeth frequently worn down to the gingival margins. Heroic restorative measures may be undertaken in efforts to prevent excessive attrition and early loss of teeth. In most instances full dentures are needed during the third or fourth decade.

Typical dentinogenesis imperfecta is frequently present in osteogenesis imperfecta.

Amelogenesis Imperfecta

Amelogenesis imperfecta is an inheritable anomalous condition involving the enamel. It is also a dominant and probably autosomal trait.

There are two types of amelogenesis imperfecta: one affects the matrix development and the other the maturation stage of enamel formation. Only the crowns of the teeth in both the primary and permanent dentitions are affected.

In teeth where matrix development is affected (*hereditary enamel hypoplasia*) all the enamel of all the teeth is involved, probably because of disturbance in activity of the ameloblasts. In severe cases the enamel may be very thin, and the teeth may have a conical appearance, as if the enamel caps were missing. The exposed surfaces may be hard where some enamel is present; decay may occur early.

Where the maturation stage of enamel formation is affected (*hereditary enamel hypocalcification*), the crowns of the teeth appear normal in size and shape, but the enamel is of poor quality, entirely opaque, and hypocalcified. The exposed structure may be soft, stain readily, and become abraded rapidly by mastication.

Missing Teeth

Anodontia, congenitally missing teeth, may be either partial or complete. One tooth or a bilateral pair of teeth may be missing in the permanent dentition. The maxillary lateral incisors are involved most frequently, the mandibular second bicuspid slightly less frequently, and the upper bicuspids occasionally. Missing teeth may be an isolated finding or may be part of a known syndrome. Where permanent lateral incisors or bicuspids

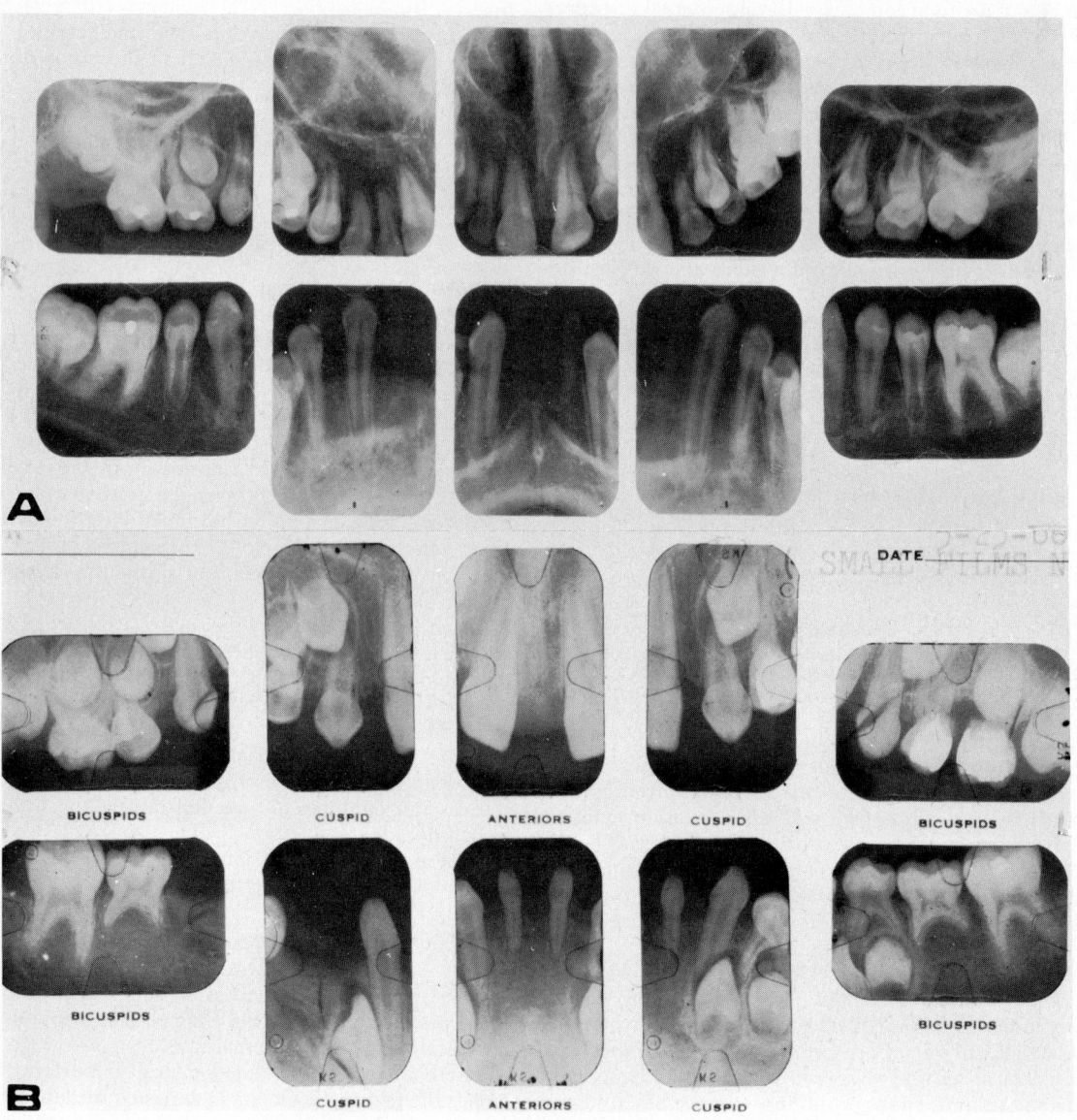

FIG 5.   Brother and sister with partial anodontia. Parents' dentitions are normal. Possible history of anodontia in a brother of paternal grandfather. A. Male, 11 years old. Missing lower permanent incisors and upper first bicuspids. Permanent teeth present are smaller than normal. B. Female, 7 years, 8 months. Missing upper right and left lateral incisors, left first bicuspid, right and left second and third molars, lower right and left incisors, right first bicuspid, right and left second bicuspids, second and third molars. Permanent teeth present are of normal size, but eruption is slow.

are congenitally missing, there will often be a family history of a similar occurrence.

Occasionally, anodontia may be more extensive, with absence of one or more primary teeth, but absence of any number of permanent teeth (Fig. 5). Dental management must be based on evaluation of the distribution of the existing teeth. Social considerations, important during adolescence, often dictate the need for dental restorative procedures. Planning for these children usually requires sequential treatment at different ages because of growth changes.

Hypophosphatasia

Hypophosphatasia (see also p. 246), a recessive, genetically transmitted condition, is characterized by low alkaline phosphatase in blood serum and other tissues and irregular and incomplete bone formation. The teeth are usually small and show early root resorption in the primary and permanent teeth (Fig. 6). In the latter this may occur within comparatively short periods after their eruption and be followed by early loss.

Dysautonomia

This congenital syndrome (see p. 1939) is manifested by disturbances of autonomic functions. Several of its features involve the oral cavity, such as abnormal chewing and swallowing, drooling, attacks of severe vomiting, insensitivity to pain, and tooth grinding. The latter is frequent in young patients of 2 to 3 years of age and may be so intense as to cause loosening and evulsion of primary teeth. Where the grinding pattern is severe, prevention of early loss of teeth may be attempted through use of a protective plastic bite plate.

Although the severity of periodontal involvement increases with age, the mean caries index is usually lower than in normal children. Smaller face size than in normal children has also been reported in dysautonomia. Orthodontic treatment can improve this problem of orofacial growth and appearance. The typically aberrant behavioral and speech patterns may require special efforts on the part of the dentist to establish rapport.

Osteopetrosis

Disorder of bone formation arises during fetal life and affects the entire skeletal structure. In the skull the basilar structures and orbits are usually involved and even the calvarium may be affected in severe cases. Facial appearance is peculiar in that the skull and upper face are large and the lower face is very small. The mandible is hypoplastic, with irregular sclerotic areas. Some teeth may be missing; those present have areas of hypocalcification. The first incisors may erupt within the average first eruption period, but subsequent eruptions are markedly delayed. Dental preventive measures should be instituted early to prevent caries at hypoplastic areas. Difficulty in dental management may be anticipated as a result of impaired vision and hearing, which are outstanding features of this condition.

Cleidocranial Dysostosis

The congenital absence of maxillary permanent lateral incisors, sometimes accompanied by other supernumerary teeth, may be found in cleidocranial dysostosis (p. 2014). This condition is inherited as a dominant factor. Other aberrant dental developmental phenomena may be unduly long retention of primary teeth and failure or long delay in the eruption of permanent teeth.

Ectodermal Dysplasia

Complete or almost complete anodontia is usually associated with the other systemic manifestations of ectodermal dysplasia (p. 2008), which affects all or most of the structures of ectodermal origin. Because of the absence of teeth, there is no development of alveolar processes. The body of the maxillar may be underdeveloped, but the body of the mandible is usually normal.

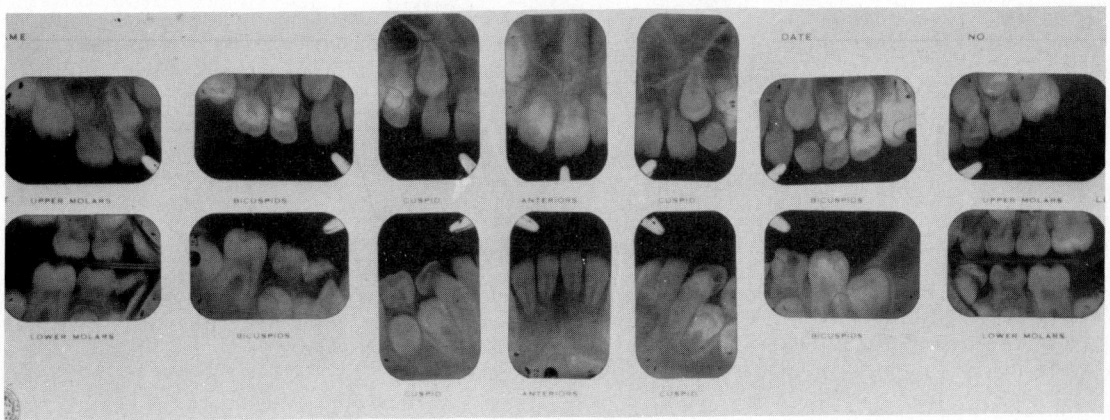

FIG 6.   Female, 11 years old, hypophosphatasia. Oral appearance negative for age; radiographs disclose incomplete and abnormal root formation.

Chondroectodermal Dysplasia

In this condition (p. 1593) the teeth that are present may be small and are often malformed. In the lower anterior region the teeth are frequently missing. There is also union of midportion of the upper lip to the anterior maxillary gingival tissue.

Oral Clefts

The genetic etiology of oral clefts is supported by a great deal of evidence, although experimental clefts have been produced using environmental influences.

The relationship between clefts and dental abnormalities varies because of differences in location and extent of the clefts. Clefts may involve the lip or the palate, or both (p. 918). In cleft palate the lack of fusion may extend anteriorly to include the premaxillary bone on one or both sides, thus affecting the future anterior alveolar process and the matrix areas that normally contain the primordia or future incisors. The resulting dental anomalies may involve lateral or central incisors or both, and may be manifested as malposed, malformed, missing, or supernumerary incisors. Restoration of missing teeth or removal of supernumerary teeth should be planned in accordance with stages of dentitional development. Regular dental care should be instituted early for these children to prevent premature loss of teeth and to maintain good oral health.

Chromosomal Aberrations

The number of recognized syndromes with orofacial anomalies related to chromosomal aberrations is increasing. In *Down's syndrome* (p. 1777) eruption of teeth may be delayed and one or more teeth may be missing or malformed. The cuspids are most frequently malformed; upper incisors may be malformed or missing; other teeth may also be abnormal in shape, and the entire dentition may be small. Periodontal disease is very common in trisomy 21, with severe bone loss often occurring early; necrotizing gingivitis may also be present. Malocclusion with mandibular prognathism and posterior cross-bite relationships are frequently found in these patients.

Cleft palate and lip are commonly observed in *trisomy 6, trisomy 13-15,* and *trisomy 18.* Other characteristic facial and cranial abnormalities also occur in these chromosomal aberration syndromes and in several sex-linked chromosomal syndromes.

Other Syndromes

Disturbances in dental morphologic development and eruption rates occur in other syndromes involving the head and neck. In Sturge-Weber's *encephalofacial angiomatosis* (p. 905), macrodontia has been observed, usually associated with delayed dental eruption on the affected side of the body, the result possibly of sclerosis of the bone in which the teeth are embedded.

The syndrome of *focal-dermal hypoplasia,* hypoplastic enamel, and microdontia has been reported to be common.

Bibliography

Cohen MM: Pediatric Dentistry, 2nd ed. Philadelphia, C V Mosby Co, 1961

Cuttita JA, Kutscher AH, Zegarelli EV, et al.: Discoloration of the teeth due to antibiotics of the tetracycline family. NY J Dent 35:89, 1965

Finn SB: Clinical Pedodontics, 2nd ed. Philadelphia, WB Saunders, 1962

Fraser FC: Experimental induction of cleft palate. In Congenital Anomalies of the Face and Associated Structures. Springfield, Ill, Thomas, 1961

Gordon EJ, Rosenstein SN: A study of the enamel of primary teeth in cerebral palsied children. NY Dent J 31:245, 1965

Hayward HL: The role of dentistry in the treatment of the cleft palate patient. NY J Dent 37:3, 1967

Kraus BS, Clark GR, Oka SW: Mental retardation and abnormalities of the dentition. Am J Ment Defic 72:905, 1968

Miller J: Dental enamel hypoplasia. Spastics' Q (London), 11:26, 1962

Public Health Service Publication No. 1487. Research Explores Cleft Palate. Washington, DC, Government Printing Office, 1966

Rathbun JC: Hypophosphatasia. Am J Dis Child 75:822, 1948

Reitman AA, Blacharsh C, Levy JM: Clinical evaluation of the dental aspects of familial dysautonomia: a preliminary report. J Am Dent Assoc 71:1436, 1965

Rosenstein SN: Dental findings in 2-year-old survivors of prematurity with 2 different neonatal antibacterial drugs. J Dent Child 31:342, 1964

Rosenstein SN: "Premature" infants: the relation of dental abnormalities to neurological and psychometric status at age two years. Dev Med Child Neurol 16:158, 1974

Sarnat BG, Schour I: Enamel hypoplasia (chronologic enamel aplasia) in relation to systemic disease: a chronologic, morphologic and etiologic classification. J Am Dent Assoc 28:1989, 1941, and 29:67, 1942

Watson AO, Massler M, Perlstein MA: Tooth ring analysis in cerebral palsy. Am J Dis Child 107:370, 1964

Zegarelli EV, Kutscher AH, Fahn B: Discoloration of teeth associated with intensive tetracycline therapy in infancy. NY J Med 63:2703, 1963

COMMON ACQUIRED DISORDERS OF THE TEETH AND SUPPORTING STRUCTURES

DENTAL DECAY

Dental decay is probably the most prevalent and almost entirely preventable disease of childhood. It has been reported that over 80 percent of preschool-age children and over 90 percent of the school children have some decay, with an appreciable incidence of teeth lost by extraction. The resulting loss of teeth by extraction in many children gives rise to severe malocclusion and such sequelae as facial disfigurement and loss of function.

Etiologic Considerations and Prevention

Susceptibility and immunity to decay involve constitutional systemic, local oral, genetic, and nutritional factors. Clinical studies of family groups have indicated *genetic factors* in tooth decay. In one study of a large population with comparable exposure to environmental factors in all families, mean decay experience (DMF, which is used as an index of tooth decay experience, represents the sum of decayed, missing, and filled teeth) of offspring was significantly correlated with the DMF of mothers.

Nutritional factors also play an important role. Fluoridation of the water supply to the extent of 1 to 1.5 parts of fluoride to 1 million parts of water in areas where fluoride is not naturally present in water is an important preventative measure. In children who have been born and raised in communities with fluoridation, there is over 60 percent reduction in decay, resulting in an increase in the number of adults with intact and complete dentitions.

A well-balanced diet of proteins, fats, carbohydrates, minerals, and vitamins is essential for good dental and oral health. Proteins enter into the formation of the protein matrix of dentin and enamel and is essential for tooth and bone formation. Vitamin A is essential for normal enamel formation, integrity of the oral soft tissues, and keratin formation; vitamin C is essential for normal dentine formation and for the integrity of the oral soft tissues and blood vessels. Vitamin D is indispensable for effective utilization of calcium and phosphorus during tooth formation and growth. Several vitamin B factors are involved in maintaining proper oral health, as exemplified by the relation of riboflavin to cheilosis, of niacin to glossitis and stomatitis of beriberi, and of pyridoxine to the oral microflora.

The beneficial effects of a well-rounded diet can be defeated by unfavorable oral environmental factors, primarily poor eating habits and poor choice of foods. Adherence to three regular daily meals and avoidance of carbohydrate snacks has been shown to result in a marked reduction in the incidence of dental decay. For growing children then, a snack in the middle of a long afternoon may be indicated, but should be limited to fruit, as an orange or a hard crisp apple, fruit juice, or a noncarbohydrate food, such as cheese. Fruit is superior to pastry as dessert because it is removed more readily from tooth surfaces. Toothbrushing following each meal eliminates food debris and microorganisms from the teeth.

Microorganisms and the acidic end products of enzymatic degradation of carbohydrates, which develop when carbohydrate foods remain on the teeth, two major oral factors related most closely to dental decay, are removed by thorough brushing immediately after meals.

Nighttime Bottle Caries Syndrome

Rampant decay in young children involving all or most of the teeth may be related to an early feeding habit, which consisted of giving a bottle of milk, juice, or syrup and water to an infant in the crib at naptime and at nighttime, while he is falling asleep (Fig. 7). Often, this practice continues until 3½ to 4 years of age, well past the age at which children normally discontinue using a bottle during mealtimes. A study disclosed that infants who took the feeding completely and discarded the bottle before falling asleep did not have a high incidence of decay; those who held the bottle in their mouths during sleep, with intermittent sucking, showed an interesting distribution of carious involvement. The lower incisors were usually entirely unaffected because the nipple was held in the tongue, which covered and protected the lower anterior teeth. All the upper teeth, especially the incisors and lower posterior teeth, became affected by decay, the severity depending upon the length of exposure to this habit.

The prolonged nighttime bottle habit may have another unfavorable aspect: these children, when too old to use the feeding bottle, tend to substitute other foods, usually of high carbohydrate content, and become almost constant between-meal nibblers. This continues their susceptibility to widespread decay.

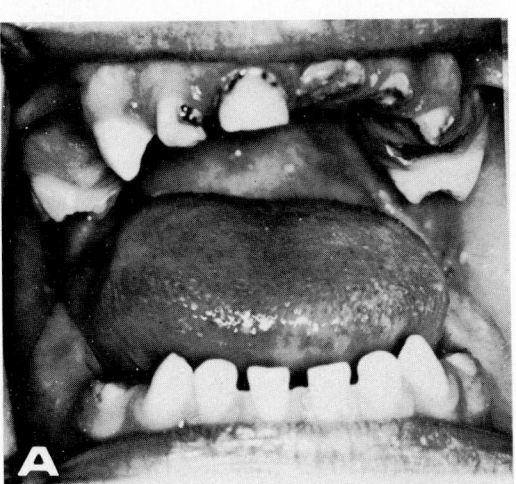
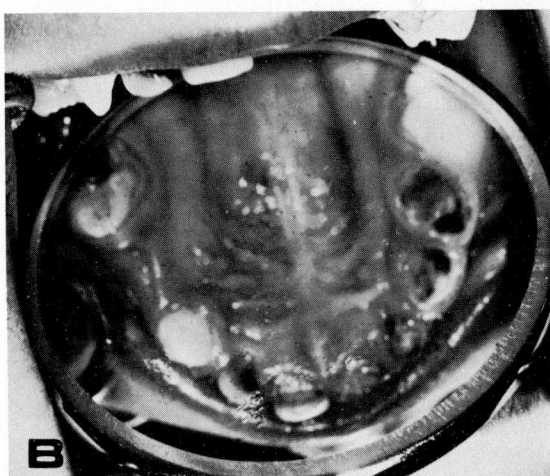

FIG 7. A. Labial view. B. Lingual view. Rampant decay in the primary dentition of a 4-year-old boy with history of bottle feeding during naptime and nighttime till 4 years of age. Lower anterior teeth are perfect and uninvolved because of protection from the tongue during sucking and swallowing. All upper teeth and lower posterior teeth are extensively decayed. Upper right second molar required early extraction.

Since the prolonged use of the bottle serves only to satisfy the need for sucking and relaxation, rather than a need for food, this habit should be discouraged and some other pacifier used, such as a large nipple or a bottle with water.

Prevention and Treatment

Regular visits to the dentist should be encouraged and should start shortly after the primary dentition is erupted. The dentist can detect early decay and, if present, institute corrective and preventive measures. Instruction should be given by the dentist to both the parent and the child in proper dental hygiene. Thus, the child becomes aware early of the need for good oral health and proper dental care.

Correct measures for home care include proper toothbrushing after meals and recommendations regarding eating habits. Through these measures, the dentist can also help prevent common disorders of the oral soft tissues and a large percentage of the disorders of occlusion.

COMMON SOFT TISSUE DISORDERS

These conditions include the simple forms of inflammation of marginal gingivae and interdental papillae, which result from lack of good oral hygiene. Proper toothbrushing and eating habits can prevent these mild conditions. However, in some instances this type of gingivitis secondary to lack of hygiene may give rise, at puberty, to hypertrophic and inflamed gingivae, which bleed easily.

Gingival hypertrophy occurs also in children on Dilantin therapy for seizures when adequate oral hygiene is not applied. This type of enlargement is mainly fibrous and appears firm; the presence of calcified masses, apparently heteroplastic bone, in gingival tissues has also been reported. It is almost axiomatic that regular dental prophylaxis and suitable home care procedures help greatly to prevent the occurrence of these gingival changes.

Both types of gingival hypertrophy will improve with appropriate dental treatment followed by a regimen of good home dental care. Where the Dilantin hypertrophy is excessive, gingival resection is usually indicated and should be followed by thorough instruction in suitable home care procedures. Other disorders of the gingivae are discussed in the section on diseases of the mouth (Chap. 18).

DISORDERS OF OCCLUSION

Malocclusion may become manifest in a variety of intermaxillary relationships. The child with a developing abnormality of occlusion can greatly benefit by early detection, evaluation, and correction if indicated. In certain forms of developing malocclusion, early intervention can prevent the need for extensive treatment later; in other forms it may be necessary to observe the subsequent course of development and defer the final decision on treatment.

A number of cases of malocclusion may be attributed to genetic factors that give rise to abnormal dimensional relationships between the jaw bones and the teeth they contain. These conditions require expert observation and evaluation to determine indications for treatment. However, a large proportion of malocclusions result from premature loss of primary teeth and early loss of first permanent molars. Loss of these teeth and ensuing development of malocclusion can be prevented by proper, early, and regular dental care. Tooth conservation procedures in children are very important preventive measures.

Other cases of malocclusion result from poor oral habits, such as thumb-sucking, lip-sucking, and tongue-thrusting. The effects of these oral habits on developing occlusions can be recognized early in the primary dentition; when intercepted early and properly managed, malocclusion in the permanent dentition may be prevented or attenuated.

Bibliography

Ast DB, Fitzgerald B: Effectiveness of water fluoridation. J Am Dent Assoc 65:581, 1962

Brash JC, McKeag HTA, Scott JH: The Etiology of Irregularity and Malocclusion of the Teeth, 2nd ed. London, Dental Board of the United Kingdom, 1965

Gustafson BE, Quensel CE, and Lande LS: The Vipeholm dental caries study; the effect of different levels of carbohydrate intake on caries activity in 436 individuals observed for 5 years. Acta Odontol Scand 2:232, 1964

Orland FJ, Blayney JR, Harrison RW, et al.: Experimental caries in germfree rats inoculated with enterococci. J Am Dent Assoc 50:259, 1955

DENTISTRY FOR HANDICAPPED CHILDREN

Dentistry is an important part of the total care and rehabilitation of handicapped children. This service is necessary to prevent adding dental disability to their other handicaps.

The teeth of children with conditions such as cerebral palsy are as susceptible to decay as those of other children. Without adequate dental care, decayed teeth will require extraction and thus many teeth may be lost unnecessarily. When they become young adults, the facial disfigurement and lack of oral function resulting from extensive edentulous areas may constitute obstacles to the vocational training and habilitation and to their prospects of becoming self-supporting. Furthermore, extensive restorative procedures required at that time may be doubly difficult and costly. These factors dictate the need for early care and preventive measures. These conditions apply equally to patients with cleft palate and lip, cardiovascular conditions, blood dyscrasias, neuromotor and physical disabilities, and metabolic disorders.

Visits for dental care must start at a young age for both institutionalized and noninstitutionalized handicapped children. They will permit the dentist to perform dental preventive procedures, provide instruction in oral home care, and create awareness of the need for good dental care early in life. Preventive dentistry measures can be made available readily for noninstitutionalized children through dental offices and treatment center clinics. For these children, it is necessary to obtain the aid of family members to implement oral hygiene home care procedures and recommended eating habits. Application of preventive dentistry and dietary control measures is usually easier for institutionalized children because of the availability of ancillary personnel.

Dentistry can be performed under the usual conditions, using local anesthesia in children with many types of handicaps, neuromuscular disabilities, mental retardation, metabolic and circulatory disorders, and others. The cooperation necessary to attain stability in the dental chair can be developed. These children may even benefit in general ways from their visits and look forward to the friendly reception of the dentist and his staff.

Where the patient's cooperation cannot be developed because of inability to comprehend its purpose, excessive dyskinetic movements, or extreme emotional disturbance, preoperative administration of combinations of sedatives and muscle relaxants has been found helpful. The agents used should be safe, effective in conservative dosages and proper combination, be eliminated rapidly, have no danger of addiction, and be discontinued after the first few visits when the patients have become oriented to the need for dental care.

Some very emotional and very handicapped patients may even require general anesthesia for their dentistry, particularly those with extensive decay. It provides the opportunity to complete all necessary treatment in one or two sessions, but it should be performed under optimal conditions, with adequate assisting personnel and all necessary safeguards. Subsequently, the children should visit their dentists for regular cleaning and orientation to dentistry under normal conditions.

Liaison should be established between the dentist who treats handicapped children and the pediatrician. An abstracted medical history should be available to the dentist, who should also be apprised of any special precautions that may be required for each individual handicapped child.

OTHER SPECIAL CONSIDERATIONS

Children with *diabetes* can usually be treated under normal conditions. Communication between the dentist and physician is important to inform the dentist of the extent of the child's condition and response to medication. Dental visits should be timed in relation to the schedule of insulin administration and meals; morning appointments are recommended to make dental treatment available after the medication has been taken and food has been eaten.

Children with *epilepsy,* who are treated with diphenylhydantoin sodium (Dilantin), must receive thorough instruction in intensive home-care oral hygiene procedures to prevent gingival hypertrophy. Mild hypertrophy may be controlled by thorough periodontal curettage and institution of intensive home care procedures. In the presence of extensive hypertrophy, practically covering tooth crowns, surgical removal of the hypertrophic tissue is usually indicated. Intensive home-care procedures and regular dental visits must be stressed in order to prevent recurrence.

In *cystic fibrosis of the pancreas* there may be discoloration of the teeth if the children have received tetracycline early. The extent of discoloration and its occurrence in the primary or permanent dentition will depend upon the length of administration and the age of the patient. Severe discoloration of anterior permanent teeth may give rise to social problems, as esthetics are important for adolescents and young adults, and corrective restorative procedures may be required. Rampant caries is also seen occasionally, related to unfavorable eating habits, prolonged use of the nursing bottle, and lack of good oral hygiene. With early and regular visits to the dentist, this condition can be prevented or corrected.

In *hemophilia* and other *blood disorders* dental and gingival disease may progress and become a severe hazard to the child's health.

Consultation with the child's hematologist should precede any dental treatment to determine the need for protective medication or hospitalization. All types of dental treatment must be done with extreme care to prevent injury to supporting tissues and dental pulps. Where bleeding can be expected, and with multiple dental procedures or extractions, hospitalization is indicated. Administration of fresh frozen plasma of the specific missing factor may be indicated. Treatments should be planned and coordinated in advance to make maximal use of the hospitalization period.

Children with cardiac lesions producing severe cyanosis often have poorly developed teeth and severe caries. Also it is important to use prophylactic antibiotic therapy before any dental work is done in children with cardiac lesions (p. 1471).

Children with *cyclic neutropenia* should receive regular conservative dental care to maintain good oral health. However, it is important to schedule restorative and periodontal treatment during the "well" periods when there are remissions in the neutropenic conditions.

In *scoliosis,* if the full body cast is the treatment, it should be designed to avoid reaching the lower jaw in order to prevent abnormal pressures, which can result in malocclusion. When the cast, or Milwaukee brace, remains in position for long periods of time and there is constant pressure on the mandible, it may cause abnormality in the shape of the bone, with a decrease in the vertical dimension of the intermaxillary relationship and abnormal positioning of the teeth. Whenever the Milwaukee brace or full body cast is used, an orthodontist should be consulted.

The benefits of early dental care, prevention of

premature tooth loss, indoctrination in home care procedures, and dental preventive measures should be made available to all handicapped children.

Bibliography

Adelson JJ: Some selective general anesthetic techniques for the problem patient. NY J Dent 34:332, 1964

Adelson JJ: The effect of dental treatment on behavior of handicapped patients. J Am Dent Assoc 71:1411, 1965

Green A: A preventive care guide for multihandicapped children: dental care begins at home. Rehab Lit 31:10, 1970

Rosenstein SN: On dentistry for the handicapped. Bull NJ Soc Dent Child 12:3, 1964

————— Dental management of the physically limited handicapped patient. Le Progres Odonto-Stomatologique, 4:57, 1971

————— Dental Care for the Handicapped. In Downey J, Low N (eds): The Child With Disabling Illness; Principles of Rehabilitation. Philadelphia, Saunders, 1974

————— Systemic and environmental factors in rampant caries in young children. NY Dent J 32:400, 1966

CHAPTER 20

Nose, Paranasal Sinuses, and Pharynx

ROBERT J. RUBEN

NOSE AND PARANASAL SINUSES

MORPHOLOGY

The significant development of the nose, and especially the paranasal sinuses, takes place after birth. The maxillary sinus is present at birth; located lateral to the nose and directly above the anterior portion of the palate, this sinus has a volume of approximately 0.5 ml. Occasionally there will be small ethmoid sinuses above and medial to the maxillary sinus. As the child grows the maxillary sinus increases in size. The ethmoid sinuses also increase in size and number. At about the age of 3 years there is present a rudimentary frontal sinus; at the age of 5 years the first signs of a developing sphenoid sinus are found. When the child reaches adolescence the paranasal sinuses reach their mature growth.

Diseases of the paranasal sinuses are dependent upon their anatomic location. The maxillary antrum and sphenoid sinuses are usually relatively constant, although the congenital absence of either has been known. The ethmoid sinuses are quite variable as to size, position, and symmetry. The following anatomic description is for the fully developed sinuses.

The *maxillary sinus* or *antrum* has as its medial border the lateral wall of the nose; anteriorly it runs from the inferior rim of the orbit to the superior portion of the palate, and the alveolar ridge, and forms the bony superstructure of the midface. It is encompassed within the malar bone. Inferiorly it forms the roof of the palate and anterolaterally the superior surface of the upper teeth. In early childhood the anterolateral part of its inferior portion contains the buds of all the deciduous and permanent teeth. The superior wall of the maxillary sinus is the orbital floor. The lateral portion forms the lateral extent of the malar bone and is part of the lateral bony support of the face. The posterior portion of the maxillary sinuses ends in the confluence of the superior, medial, inferior, and lateral walls. The general shape is similar to a pyramid with its anterior base supporting the face and the orbital rim supporting the orbital floor. Usually the maxillary sinus has one ostium, called the hiatus semilunaris, which opens from the superior one-third of the medial wall of the sinus into the nose under the posterior half of the middle meatus.

The *ethmoid sinus* cells are quite variable in number and are divided into three groups. The anterior ethmoid cells are found along the superior portion of the medial wall of the maxillary antrum and form a portion of the medial wall of the orbit in the anteroinferior floor of the frontal sinus. Anterior ethmoid cells are also found in the middle turbinate. The posterior ethmoid cells extend posteriorly to surround the sphenoid sinus and may run along the olfactory groove of the anterior cranial fossa. The third group includes those cells called the orbital ethmoid cells; these may be considered as an extension of the anterior ethmoids. They will form part of the floor of the frontal sinus laterally, along the superior orbital rim. Also, they can develop posteriorly to the orbital rim in the floor of the anterior cranial fossa. They will drain through variable ostia under the middle and superior turbinates.

The *sphenoid sinus* is usually made of two separate chambers. It is found posterosuperior to the posterior aspect of the bony nasal septum. Anteriorly it forms the posterior portion of the bony roof of the nasal cavity. Superiorly it is contiguous with the floor of the anterior cranial fossa. The posterior aspect forms the anterior wall of the sella turcica. Laterally it forms the wall of the anterior cranial fossa, and it is contiguous with the internal carotid artery, cavernous sinus, and the optic, trochlear, oculomotor, and abducens nerves. It drains usually through two ostia, one from each side of the anterosuperior wall under the posterior portion of the superior turbinate.

The *frontal sinus* has as its inferior border the anterior portion of the orbital roof. Anteriorly it forms the anterior surface of the frontal bone. Posteriorly it forms the anterior surface of the anterior cranial fossa. The frontal sinus is a midline structure that usually extends laterally about one-third of the superior orbital rim. Superiorly the anterior and posterior walls meet and create a more or less pyramidal sinus, with the base being the roof of the orbit. The frontal sinus is usually divided asymmetrically into two or more sinus spaces separated by the thin bony septum. There is usually, but not invariably, no connection between the right and left portions of the frontal sinus. Each half (right and left) of the frontal sinus drains through the nasofrontal duct that runs posteriorly to some of the anterior ethmoid cells and opens under the anterior third of the middle meatus.

The paranasal sinuses are contiguous with the orbit, anterior cranial fossa, pituitary, optic nerve, internal carotid artery, palate, and nose. Disease of the sinuses will have its most serious sequelae when the disease process leaves the sinus and involves these contiguous areas.

Anatomically the nose is divided into the external and internal nose. The external nose is what is most apparent. The external nose is covered by skin over a bony and cartilaginous framework. The rostral three-fifths of the nose is bony and consists of the nasal bones that join the malar bone laterally and the nasal process of the frontal bone superiorly. This forms a pyramid in which the base opens dorsally into the internal nose. Inferiorly the nasal bones are attached to a pair of cartilages called the upper lateral cartilages. The rostral two-fifths of the external nose (the nasal tip) is formed by two pairs of cartilages; the caudal pair are the upper laterals, and the rostral pair are the lower lateral cartilages. The lower lateral cartilages curve laterally to form the lateral border of the nostrils and medially to help form the ventromedial portion of the nostril, called the columella. During infancy and childhood the external nose grows in proportion to the face. The nasal bones and tip become more prominent. The normal growth pattern of the external nose can be altered by congenital or acquired disease. Any process that causes trauma to the nasal bones or external nasal cartilages may result in subsequent malformations of the matured external nose. Additionally, partial or total destruction or malformation of the nasal septum of the internal nose may result in extensive deformity.

The internal nose is divided into two passages by a midline structure called the nasal septum. Ventrally these passages open into the face through the nostrils, and dorsally they open into the nasopharynx through the choana. The nasal septum is covered by respiratory mucosa. The anterior one-third is cartilaginous, and the posterior two-thirds is bony, with the caudal portion being made up of the perpendicular plate of the ethmoid bone and the ventral portion by the vomer bone. The septum is attached rostrally to the floor of the nose of the maxillary crest and ends most ventrally at the maxillary spine. The floor of the internal nose is the roof of the palate. The lateral surface of the internal nose usually consists of three turbinates (Fig. 1). The inferior turbinate is placed most ventrally. Many times this is mistaken for a mass in the nose. The nasolacrimal duct drains from the medial portion of the orbit, under the ventral one-half of this turbinate. The middle turbinate is rostral and lightly dorsal to the inferior turbinate. The paranasal sinuses drain underneath this turbinate, usually the frontal sinus via the nasofrontal duct from the ventral one-third, the maxillary sinus via the hiatus semilunaris of the middle half, and the ethmoid sinuses from variable positions. The sphenoid sinus will drain dorsally and rostrally to the most distal portion of this turbinate. The superior turbinate is located rostrally and somewhat more dorsal to the most ventral portion of the middle turbinate. The turbinates are covered with respiratory mucosa that overlies an extremely vascular submucosa that can be considered as a type of erectile tissue. The roof of the internal nose is contiguous with the floor of the anterior cranial fossa. The mucosa covering the roof is olfactory mucosa and contains the olfactory receptor cells.

The blood supply to the nose is from both the external and internal carotid arteries. The external carotid artery supplies the posterior portion of the lateral nasal wall and the posterior and caudal portions of the septum via the internal maxillary artery. The external carotid arterial system also supplies the rostral ventral portion of the lateral nasal wall and the septum, through the greater palatine artery and the superficial labial artery. The internal carotid artery system, via the orbital artery, which divides into the anteroposterior

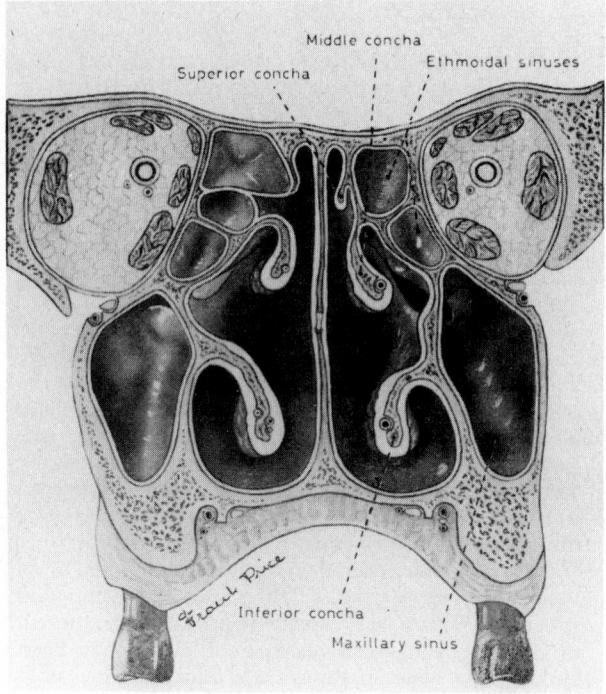

FIG. 1. Anatomy of coronal section of the internal nose and paranasal sinuses. (From Scott-Brown's *Diseases of the Ear, Nose and Throat*, vol. 1, ed. 3. John Ballantyne and John Groves (eds.). Philadelphia, J. B. Lippincott Co., 1971.

ethmoid artery, supplies the most rostral portions of the labionasal wall and nasal septum, both posteriorly and ventrally. There are numerous intranasal anastomoses.

PHYSIOLOGY

The nose has four main physiologic functions. The first of these is *olfaction*. The olfactory nerve enters the roof of the nasal cavity through the cribriform fossa of the ethmoid bone. The olfactory nerve or bulb is similar to the optic nerve in that it is part of the central nervous system. The dendrites enter the upper nose and terminate in the olfactory mucosa. The mechanism of olfaction is felt to be a recognition of different molecular shapes and sizes by olfactory mucosa. The sensitivity of the system is exquisite, eg, artificial musk can be detected at 4×10^{-5} mg/liter of air, and mercaptan is detected at 4×10^{-8} mg/liter of air.

The second and perhaps most important physiologic function of the nose is that of being an *air conditioner*. Almost all the air used for respiration enters the body through the nose. The nose sets the temperature of the air, regulates the humidity, and filters the air. The anatomic structure of the internal nose determines the efficiency with which these functions can be performed.

The nose is divided into two chambers by the nasal septum. Laterally there are the three turbinates, which serve to increase the surface area of the nose in a manner similar to the functioning of villi in the intestine. The nose is lined with respiratory mucosa consisting of cilia and mucus-secreting cells. The cilia and mucous blanket extract foreign materials and cause them to be propelled posteriorly, where they are swallowed with the mucus. The mucous cells give off water to the air. The turbinates are lined with respiratory mucosa. Submucosally the turbinates have an erectile tissue that has a very rich blood supply. This rich vascular bed serves to heat the air to an optimal temperature. Cold air entering the nose will be at body temperature after it goes through the nose and enters the nasopharynx.

The third physiologic function of the nose is in the area of *speech.* The nose, along with the nasopharynx, serves as a resonant cavity for speech. If the nose is obstructed, speech will sound hyponasal. If the nasopharynx and nose cannot be closed off, the speech will sound hypernasal; this is heard most commonly in children with uncorrected cleft palates.

The fourth function of the internal nose is to supply *optimal airway resistance.* When there is obstruction in the internal nose, the airway resistance will be increased; this is found to be associated with many forms of chronic lung disease. Whether the nasal condition is the causative agent is unclear, but it is certainly a contributing factor.

The paranasal sinuses are filled with air and lined with respiratory mucosa. These sinuses are also covered with a mucous blanket. The cilia are so arranged that they cause the mucus to be expelled from the natural orifices of the sinuses. The pathophysiology of the paranasal sinuses is relatively simple in concept. The main problem arises with infection of the sinuses. Infection increases the amount of mucus secreted and also causes edema of the mucosa. Edema can cause the natural orifices of the sinus to be occluded, but mucus is still secreted in the closed sinus. This mucus becomes infected and turns into pus. With further secretion the hydrostatic pressure is increased; this will cause venous compression, venous thrombosis, and death of bone, with resulting osteomyelitis. The pus will drain through the dead bone and into the surrounding tissue. Other causes of blockage of the sinus orifices are mucoceles, allergic polyps, neoplasms, osteomas, and trauma.

METHODS OF EXAMINATION

Physical Examination

The external nose may be examined by direct inspection and gentle palpation. Many times fractures of the nasal bone can be felt by gently palpating the contour of the nose. Occasionally crepitus is detected, indicating that the fracture has gone into the internal nose and air is communicating to the external nose. The internal nose may also be examined by means of direct inspection with a nasal speculum of appropriate size. This procedure is called anterior rhinoscopy. The presence and the nature of any discharge, the color of the mucous membrane, and the presence of any tumor or foreign body should be noted. Any tumor, after appropriate work-up, should be biopsied, usually under general anesthesia. The child with epistaxis should undergo anterior rhinoscopy to determine the site of bleeding. It is important to use a small suction catheter to evacuate the blood clots so that good visualization may be obtained.

Physical examination of the paranasal sinuses may also be made by direct observation and gentle palpation. When examining the paranasal sinuses, especially the maxillary antrum, attention should be given to the teeth of the superior alveolar ridge. The maxillary sinus may drain through the alveolar ridge, or a tooth abscess may be the cause of maxillary sinusitis. An infected tooth will be tender on palpation.

Any examination of the paranasal sinuses must include the orbit and the globes. Edema and erythema surrounding the orbit, or limitation of extraocular motion, are serious signs of orbital involvement secondary to sinus disease. Infections of the ethmoid, maxillary, and frontal sinuses can result in periorbital edema and infection. In more advanced cases the globe may be unable to move, which is a very grave sign indicating that the orbit has been invaded by either pus or tumor. Ophthalmoscopy should also be done to note the condition of the retina and its vessels. Neurologic examination is also indicated in infections and neoplastic disease of the paranasal sinuses, especially of the sphenoid and frontal sinuses.

Special Tests

RADIOGRAPHY. Radiography of the nose and paranasal sinuses is exceedingly useful in the diagnosis of nasal or facial bone fractures and in determining the presence of paranasal sinus pus or tumors. The use of radiographs in sinus infection is especially important in three types of sinusitis: acute sinusitis with possible spread to adjacent areas (eg, frontal lobe), any acute frontal sinusitis, and chronic sinusitis.

SINUS TRANSILLUMINATION. Sinus transillumination can be performed quite easily by placing a small incandescent lamp in the mouth of a child in a darkened room. The paranasal sinuses will show up as relatively symmetric reddish glowing masses. When the pupils are viewed in healthy sinuses a red color will be seen. In opaque diseased sinuses the transillumination will be asymmetric and the red reflex of the pupil will be absent.

DISEASES

Congenital

NOSE.   The most frequently encountered congenital malformations are those associated with *cleft palate*. The palatal abnormality involves the floor of the nose and in many instances the columella as well. The septal deformity, combined with the open palate, is associated with an almost universal incidence of chronic rhinitis and sinusitis. Even after the palatal defect is closed, many cleft-palate children still have severe chronic rhinitis and sinusitis.

Choanal atresia, is perhaps the most commonly encountered congenital malformation of the nose. The choanae are blocked due to a bony or membranous closure of the nasal air passage. The infant will present with severe respiratory distress, because newborns are obligatory nose breathers. If they cannot breathe through the nose, many newborn infants will not spontaneously breathe through the mouth. Great difficulty is encountered when the infant is feeding. Unilateral choanal atresia is also found. The diagnosis is usually not made until early childhood, when it presents as a unilateral chronic rhinitis with mucous discharge from just one nostril that is refractory to all treatment.

A number of newborns have very small choanae that are patent, as demonstrated by radiography and the passage of a small catheter. These children behave in a manner similar to those with bilateral choanal atresia. The first few months of life are marked by respiratory difficulty, especially when feeding or when the infant has an upper respiratory infection. These cases are best treated with gentle nasal suction. After the first 6 to 12 months they appear to do quite well, as the relative size of the choanae increases and they are no longer troubled.

There are a number of uncommon malformations of the external nose. *Dermoid cysts* usually arise in the ventral surface of the external nose at the junction of the nasal bone and the upper lateral cartilages. *Encephaloceles* can present as tumors either within the nose or externally or both. Any congenital mass, whether within the nose or on the surface of the nose, should be considered as a possible extension of the central nervous system. Radiographic examination should be undertaken first to determine the origin of the mass. They are all treated by planned surgical excision. Those cases in which the central nervous system is involved will in most instances need both rhinologic and neurosurgical care. *Clefts* and *fistulas* of the nose also occur. *Congenital syphilis* can result in a saddlelike deformity of the external nose. Additionally, it may be associated with nasoseptal perforations. *Congenital anosmia* has been reported as a genetically inherited disease associated with hypogonadism.

PARANASAL SINUSES.   There are very few congenital diseases of the paranasal sinuses. *Kartagener's syndrome* is one that consists of situs inversus, bronchiectasis, and chronic sinusitis. There may also be absence or diminution in size of any of the paranasal sinuses. This is most frequently seen in the frontal sinus, in which there may be aplasia of one or both sides.

Viral Disease

Viral infections of the nose are quite common. Viral upper respiratory infections are characterized by fever, irritability, malaise, and a clear discharge from the nose. Various viruses have been identified as causing acute viral rhinitis. These include rhinovirus, respiratory syncytial virus, influenza virus, and adenovirus. Viral infections cause edema, a large increase in nasal secretions, and destruction of the cells and the respiratory mucosa in the nose and paranasal sinuses. The damage from the viral infection will in many instances result in a secondary bacterial infection. The latter will be characterized by a change in nasal drainage from clear white to one that contains pus and is yellow to yellowish green in color. Epistaxis may also be a sequela of viral rhinitis due to destruction of the respiratory mucosa.

Bacterial Disease

ACUTE BACTERIAL INFECTIONS.   Acute bacterial rhinitis is most commonly associated with pneumococcus, β-hemolytic *Streptococcus,* or *Haemophilus influenzae.* The symptoms and signs consist of fever, irritability, leukocytosis and mucopurulent discharge, and not infrequently mild epistaxis. Similar bacterial agents will be found in acute sinusitis, which is almost invariably accompanied by acute rhinitis. Acute sinusitis, in addition to having the signs and symptoms of acute rhinitis, will be characterized by tenderness over the involved sinus and in some cases by edema over or adjacent to the sinus. Radiography will reveal fluid in the sinuses, which may appear opaque or have air–fluid levels. When taking radiographs for the possible diagnosis of acute sinusitis, the head should be in a vertical position so that the fluid levels can be seen.

There are five common complications of acute sinusitis. The first of these is spread from the ethmoid, maxillary, or frontal sinuses to the orbit. The infection enters the bone adjacent to the orbit and may allow free pus to drain into the orbit, which may result in blindness. Fortunately this condition is usually heralded by edema around the orbit and orbital cellulitis. The second complication usually occurs in frontal sinusitis, with bony erosion of the posterior bony plate of the frontal bone and extravasation of pus into the anterior cranial fossa. This may result in epidural abscess, subdural abscess, brain abscess, and/or meningitis. The third complication is when the acute sinusitis drains through the floor of the sinus, resulting in an oral-antral fistula. The fourth complication is found with acute maxillary sinusitis when the infection destroys the bony antrum and results in hyperplasia of the malar bone and facial asymmetry. The infection can also destroy the tooth buds of both deciduous and permanent teeth, which can produce subsequent orthodontic malformation. The fifth complication is thrombosis of the venous supply of the paranasal sinuses and extension of the infection through the infected veins into the cavernous sinus, with resultant cavernous sinus thrombosis.

Abscesses of the external nose are potentially serious problems. They can result in destruction of the cartilaginous framework of the nose, with consequent nasal deformity and increased air resistance due to the collapse of the nasal airway. They may also result in venous thrombosis, leading to cavernous sinus thrombosis. Abscesses of the internal nose are also liable to cause cavernous sinus thrombosis. A special problem is presented by an abscess in the nasal septum. This is commonly found secondary to a traumatic nasoseptal hematoma. The abscess, if untreated, can erode the nasal septum and leave a nasoseptal perforation. The perforation can cause external nasal deformity, chronic rhinitis, and severe epistaxis.

CHRONIC BACTERIAL INFECTION.   There are different bacteria associated with chronic rhinitis and sinusitis. These include β-hemolytic *Streptococcus*, anaerobic *Streptococcus*, pneumococcus, *Haemophilus influenzae, Staphylococcus aureus, Escherichia coli*, and *Pseudomonas aeruginosa*. The child with chronic rhinitis and/or sinusitis usually does not have fever, malaise, or leukocytosis. The primary symptom is a chronic mucopurulent, odoriferous discharge from the nose that can drain both anteriorly and posteriorly. The latter is often referred to as postnasal drip. Most children with chronic rhinitis and sinusitis have some form of primary disorder that results in the chronic infection. Some of these are nasal foreign bodies, nasal masses, nasoseptal deformities (eg, cleft palate), tumors of the nose and paranasal sinuses, allergy, and systemic reduction of immunity (eg, a decrease in humoral and cellular antibodies).

The complications of chronic rhinitis and sinusitis are the same as those of acute infection. Additionally, there is an increased association of chronic sinusitis with chronic chest disease. It is felt that the postnasal discharge of infected mucus contributes to the chronic pulmonary infection.

Fungal Infections

Fungal infections of the nose and paranasal sinuses are rare in children. They are usually associated with systemic abnormalities in the immune system. Their presentation is similar to that of chronic bacterial infections.

Neoplasms

Neoplasms in the nose and paranasal sinuses may present as chronic sinusitis and/or as a mass in the nose. Occasionally they can present as facial swelling or as an extension into the orbit, causing exophthalmos.

BENIGN TUMORS.   Most tumors of the nose and paranasal sinuses in children are benign. These include *congenital encephaloceles* and *gliomas* that are usually seen as masses in the internal nose. The most common benign tumor is the *allergic polyp*, which is found in the internal nose and paranasal sinuses. The polyp, or more frequently polyps, can fill the entire nasal space. They are soft masses of loose connective tissue and mucus, yellow to gray in color, and are usually associated with chronic rhinitis. There is also a high incidence of polyps in cystic fibrosis of the pancreas.

The paranasal sinuses are found to contain mucous cysts called *mucoceles;* when they are infected or filled with pus they are called pyoceles. These cysts can grow and erode the bony structures that encompass the sinuses and extend into adjacent structures or organs, eg, the orbit or anterior cranial fossa. *Osteomas* and *bone cysts* also occur. *Fibrous dysplasia* of the paranasal sinuses frequently appears at the end of the first decade of life and is characterized by obliteration of the sinus and a disfiguring overgrowth of bone. *Juvenile angiofibromas*, which probably start in the nasopharynx, are found in the nose, primarily in prepubescent boys (p. 956). This tumor can present as a reddish mass in the nasal cavity. Biopsy of such a tumor results in massive hemorrhage and should only be done under controlled conditions. After arteriography is completed the patient should be prepared for total removal of the tumor under general anesthesia.

MALIGNANT TUMORS.   Malignant tumors in the nose and paranasal sinuses are rare in children. The most common of these is the *rhabdomyosarcoma.* The outcome for these cases is poor. *Olfactory epitheliomas* (esthesioneuroblastomas) are occasionally found. *Metastatic tumors are seen in the paranasal sinuses, usually metastatic from the kidney. Lymphomas* are present, both in the internal nose and maxillary sinuses. They usually present as bluish red masses with occlusion of the nose. *Burkitt's lymphoma*, which is associated with the Epstein-Barr virus, has been reported as a sinus and nasal mass in North America.

Trauma

Blunt trauma to the nose and paranasal sinuses is a common injury resulting in fracture and/or dislocation of the bony and cartilaginous structures of the nose and paranasal sinuses. The etiology is varied. Nasal and facial trauma may be the result of almost all play activities and sports, especially contact sports and sports played with missiles, eg, baseball. Automobile accidents account for some of the more severe injuries. All facial fractures and nasal injuries associated with high impact velocity may be complicated by cerebral injury, eg, subdural hematoma or cerebral concussion and/or cervical spine injury. All these patients should be examined and observed for some period of time to ascertain the status of the central nervous system. Fractures of the nasal and facial bone (eg, paranasal sinuses) usually result in observable or palpable physical deformity. Radiography will demonstrate these fractures.

An especially important type of fracture is that of the malar bone, which encloses the maxillary sinus. Most commonly this bone will fracture at three places: the orbital rim, the zygomatic process of the maxillary bone, and the frontal process of the maxillary bone. This type of fracture can also involve the floor of the orbit and is often associated with limitation of the upward gaze of the eye due to edema and trauma to the inferior rectus muscle. There may be decreased sensation on the ipsilateral side of the face due to edema or disruption of the inferior branch of the trigeminal nerve as it passes through its foramen in the inferior orbital rim. These fractures can be associated with ecchymosis around the orbit, colloquially called a black eye. If not diagnosed and treated they can result in permanent disfigurement of the face, exophthalmos, and permanent diplopia due to the eye muscle defect.

Another serious fracture involves the orbital floor, with or without orbital fracture. This injury usually occurs due to blunt trauma to the globe, such as being hit by a fist or a ball, and it has several signs and symptoms similar to those in trimalar fractures of the malar bone. All patients with facial bone fractures should have an ophthalmologic examination to assess possible corneal laceration, extraocular muscle involvement, and intraocular hemorrhage or retinal displacement.

More complex fractures can involve all segments of the malar and nasal bones. Many of these can result in malocclusion of the teeth if the alveolar ridge and the malar bone are involved. Some of the more serious fractures may extend into the anterior cranial fossa and result in cerebrospinal fluid rhinorrhea. The cerebrospinal fluid can be detected as a crystal-clear fluid that drips either ventrally through the nostril or dorsally into the nasopharynx. The cerebrospinal fluid may be differentiated from normal mucous secretion because of its higher glucose content. The cerebrospinal fluid will usually cause a positive glucose reaction with the standard enzymatic test papers used for urinalysis, whereas normal nasal mucus will not.

Trauma to the external nose should present little difficulty in diagnosis. It is most often accompanied by epistaxis. Often there is an associated fracture or dislocation of the nasal septum. The nasoseptal injury can also occur without fracture of the nasal bone. The nasal septum will be displaced from its inferior attachment to the maxillary crest and occlude one or both nares. It will usually be accompanied by a nasoseptal hematoma visible as a bluish red swelling on either one or both sides of the septum. This type of injury can result in infection and/or septal perforation. The fractured dislocation of the nasal septum can result in an abnormal airway, the consequences of which can be chronic rhinitis, sinusitis, epistaxis, external nasal deformity, and possible chronic lung infection.

Foreign bodies impacted in the nose, especially in infants, are another form of trauma. The foreign body may be multiple, such as two or three plastic beads, or hydroscopic, such as a dried pea. When dry seeds are placed into the nose they can swell and occlude the nose, and they usually have to be removed under a general anesthetic. The complication of attempts at foreign body removal is often aspiration of the foreign body, when it is pushed through the choanae into the nasopharynx and is secondarily aspirated. Foreign bodies that are difficult to reach must be removed under general anesthesia with the child's head in a dependent position. As previously noted, long-standing nasal foreign bodies can present as chronic sinusitis or rhinitis.

Self-inflicted trauma caused by children cleaning the nose with their fingers is not uncommon, and it usually presents as episodic epistaxis. Examination usually reveals a small excoriated area on the anteroinferior portion of the nasal septum called Kiesselbach's triangle.

Allergy

Allergic rhinitis is a very common disease. It can present as nasal congestion, usually with a clear discharge and without fever. The most common allergies are to spores, pollens, dust, and animal dander. Food allergies play an important role in allergic rhinitis. The spore and pollen allergies are usually seasonal, as they occur only with exposure to the seasonal allergen. The mucous membrane of the nose in patients with allergic rhinitis will be pale, and the discharge can be quite copious. More serious nasal allergies result in the formation of nasal and sinus polyps and the eventual occurrence of chronic rhinitis and sinusitis.

Differential Diagnosis

Nasal Discharge

Nasal discharge is one of the more common signs of disease in childhood. Most often it is due to upper respiratory infection and resolves spontaneously. If the discharge does not clear, the cause must be determined. A clear white discharge is often associated with allergy; in rare instances it can be cerebrospinal fluid rhinorrhea. Those discharges that are yellow to yellowish green and are malodorous are usually associated with bacterial infections of the nose and paranasal sinuses. They may be due to any of the causes of acute bacterial rhinitis, sinusitis, or chronic rhinitis and sinusitis. In cases of purulent discharge, in addition to the physical examination of the nose and paranasal sinuses, radiographic examination may be necessary to differentiate between foreign bodies, congenital malformations, acquired malformations, allergic polyps, mucoceles, pyoceles, and other tumors. In all instances cultures of the discharge should be obtained in order to identify the bacteria and allow for appropriate antibiotic therapy, if indicated.

Facial Swelling

Facial swelling can result from different causes. The most common is trauma that results in ecchymosis and edema. All cases of facial swelling that are not due to renal, cardiac, nutritional, or allergic causes need radiography to determine if there are any associated fractures. Facial swelling may also be the result of spread of sinus infection to the face, forehead, and orbit. The latter is usually associated with fever and leukocytosis, and the patient may be quite toxic. They require radiographic examination and anterior rhinoscopy of the nose. A third and much rarer cause of facial swelling is extension of a benign or malignant tumor of the nose and paranasal sinuses. This can be found in rhabdomyosarcoma of the paranasal sinuses and in fibrous dysplasia. Occasionally a mucocele or pyocele will erode part of the frontal bone and extend into the upper orbital rim. A rare but distinct form of recurrent facial swelling is found in angioneurotic edema. This condition is characterized by episodes of facial swelling and is thought to be allergic.

Epistaxis

Nosebleeds are common in children and are usually caused by self-inflicted trauma to Kiesselbach's triangle. Recurrent episodes of epistaxis are associated with chronic rhinitis and sinusitis. The occurrence of severe epistaxis, other than that associated with nasal trauma, can represent major disease problems. These include structural alterations of the internal nose (eg, a septal perforation) and benign and malignant tumors of the nose and paranasal sinuses, especially juvenile angiofibromas and chronic rhinitis and sinusitis. Severe epistaxis is also associated with blood dyscrasias, especially leukemia. It appears to be somewhat more frequent in children with severe hypertension.

Hereditary hemorrhagic telangiectasia (Osler's disease) is a genetic disease, probably inherited as an autosomal dominant, that causes the growth of telangiectases throughout the body, including the surface of the internal nose. Epistaxis is also commonly seen in children with von Willebrand's disease.

Anosmia

Lack of the sense of smell is rare in children. It has been found on a genetic basis associated with hypogonadism. Occasionally it can represent impairment of the olfactory epithelium of the roof of the nose. This may be due to tumors of the olfactory groove (eg, olfactory neuroblastomas), tumors of the nose (eg, polyps), or chronic infection. Anosmia may also result from fractures through the anterior cranial fossae that go across the olfactory bulbs.

TREATMENT

Acute Rhinitis

The treatment of acute viral rhinitis consists of rest, antipyretics, and oral decongestants. Nose drops or topical applications to the internal nose should be used only in very young infants. Many times patients with underlying disease (eg, allergy) will become addicted to nose drops. The constant use of nose drops causes the mucosa to undergo metaplasia; the nose remains swollen with increased discharge, and the mucosa becomes refractory to any treatment with local medication. This condition is called *rhinitis medicamentosus*.

The treatment for acute bacterial rhinitis is the same as for viral rhinitis, with the addition of appropriate antibiotics. The latter should be instituted after culture has been taken. The usual course of acute rhinitis is about 1 week to 10 days.

Acute Bacterial Sinusitis

Acute bacterial sinusitis is similar to acute bacterial rhinitis. If there are any signs of extension of the disease to the orbit or central nervous system, parenteral antibiotics should be given and surgical drainage instituted. Extension of acute sinusitis is a life-threatening disease and must be treated promptly and adequately.

Chronic Rhinitis and Chronic Sinusitis

Chronic rhinitis and chronic sinusitis usually result from underlying disease. Many of these conditions (eg, benign tumors) can be treated surgically. Chronic sinusitis often develops secondary to acute infection, with closure of the small sinusoidal ostia. In these cases the sinus should be surgically drained and irrigated. In children this is usually done under general anesthesia. Antibiotics and oral decongestants play a small role in chronic rhinitis and sinusitis that come about from other anatomic and systemic diseases. Many times chronic rhinitis and sinusitis are associated with chronic or recurrent pulmonary disease. These cases must be treated with appropriate antibiotics, pulmonary drainage, and/or sinus and nasal surgery.

Allergic Rhinitis

Most often allergic rhinitis is of a seasonal nature and may be treated with oral antihistamines. When allergic rhinitis is chronic, it leads to infection or is associated with nasal polyps or asthma; then a more direct type of therapy is needed. The first step is to identify the causative allergen. The inhalant allergens appear to be best diagnosed with the use of skin testing, and the food allergens are most efficiently diagnosed with in vivo observation of the patient's leukocytes. When the allergens are identified, they should either be treated with desensitization or eliminated (the food allergens especially). Many cases will show a significant improvement with either part or all of this therapy. Patients in which there is no improvement may have to be treated with other antiallergic therapy. The use of systemic local steroids for the treatment of allergic rhinitis is not advocated because of the known complications and also because the patient may in time become refractory to the steroid therapy.

Epistaxis

The treatment of epistaxis consists of locating the source, determining the cause, and stopping the bleeding. The problem of finding the location and cause of the bleeding is discussed elsewhere . Most of the bleeds stop spontaneously. Those that persist can be stopped by gently aspirating the clot and lightly packing the nose with a small piece of Oxycel backed by some cotton next to the bleeding point. Small distinct arterial bleeders can be stopped with the use of very low voltage electrocautery. The cautery, if improperly used, can result in destruction of large areas of the septum, secondary infection, and more bleeding. Those bleeds that cannot be stopped with simple treatment will require anterior and posterior nasal packing. Occasionally it is necessary to ligate the internal maxillary artery and more rarely the external carotid artery.

Choanal Atresia

Bilateral choanal atresia is usually diagnosed at birth or a few hours later. Many infants rapidly learn how to breathe through the mouth. During the first few hours or days a small airway should be taped into the mouth. During feeding a nipple should be constructed that will allow both air and fluid to be taken. Any infant with bilateral choanal atresia should be considered to have a severe upper airway problem and should be kept in an intensive care unit with the same surveillance as for an infant with a tracheostomy. Many infants will be able to compensate for their lack of nasal breathing by the natural development of the pharyngeal airway. The eventual therapy is surgical. Adequate surgical therapy can be carried out at any time; however, it is technically more satisfactory if there is some palatal growth. If possible, the operation should be delayed until the age of 6 months or one year. Some infants cannot tolerate this delay and will experience continual respiratory problems. These infants should have at least one of the choanae opened during the first few days of life so that nasal breathing can be established.

Fracture

The treatment of fractures of the nose and paranasal sinuses is surgical. Most of these do not need to be corrected immediately. The child can usually be given thorough radiographic, ophthalmologic, and, neurologic examinations and prepared for general anesthesia. If possible, the delay should be no longer than 4 days, because at that time the bony fragments tend to become fibrous. The surgical correction of fractures should not be confined to just the external nose and face, but must be performed for fractures and dislocations of the nasal septum. Hematomas or abscesses of the septum should be divided as soon as possible.

PHARYNX

MORPHOLOGY

The pharynx is the main entrance for air into the larynx and lungs and for liquids and solids to the stomach via the esophagus. It is a muscular conduit that extends from the base of the skull and ends at the cricopharyngeal muscle sphincter, which is the entrance to the cervical esophagus. The pharynx is divided into three parts. The rostral portion, called the nasopharynx, is found in the rostral portion of the soft palate and extends to the base of the skull. The area from the caudal portion of the soft palate to the rostral portion of the upper glottis is called the oropharynx. The remaining portion, from the epiglottis to the cricopharyngeus, is called the hypopharynx.

The pharynx is derived essentially from the first two pharyngeal arches and pouches. At birth the pharynx is small in both its rostral-caudad and dorsoventral dimensions. During the first years of life it grows in both directions, but more so in the rostral-caudad dimension.

The eustachian tube is an outgrowth of the second pharyngeal pouch. At birth its course is relatively horizontal, and during the first decade of life the nasopharyngeal end of the eustachian tube assumes a position approximately 15 percent caudad to the middle ear portion.

The oropharynx and nasopharynx are encircled with a ring of lymphoid tissue called Waldeyer's ring. This includes the palatal tonsils on either side of the oropharynx, the lingual tonsils found on the rostral portion of the dorsal one-third of the tongue, the pharyngeal tonsil (the adenoids) on the rostral and dorsal wall of the nasopharynx, and small areas of lymphoid tissue on the lateral borders of the rostral portion of the hypopharynx. The precise embryologic derivation of these lymphoid structures is not known. It is thought that at least the palatine tonsils are derived from the ventral portion of the second pharyngeal pouch. The palatine tonsils are recognized as early as the fourteenth week of fetal life. At birth the lymphoid tissue of the pharynx is relatively small. Usually after the first 6 months of life this tissue begins to grow disproportionately to the size of the pharynx. The normal increase in size of the lymphoid tissue, especially the palatine tonsils and adenoids, is reached by the third to sixth years. Then the lymphoid tissue involutes; after puberty, if there has been no secondary disease, it becomes quite small. The normal adult palatine tonsil is a small mass that rarely exceeds 2 to 3 mm^3 in size. The adult adenoid can be less than 0.5 mm^3.

The pharynx is composed of three muscular sheaths that run rostral to caudad. These are the superior, middle, and inferior constrictor muscles which are innervated by the vagus nerve, and the stylopharyngeus which is innervated by the glossopharyngeal nerve. The muscles of mastication, the palate, and the tongue are coordinated with the pharyngeal musculature in swallowing, breathing, and speaking. The nasopharynx and hypopharynx are covered by mucosa. The oropharynx is covered with a noncornified squamous epithelium.

The eustachian tube runs from the rostral ventromedial wall of the middle ear cleft to the rostral dorsolateral wall of the nasopharynx. It is approximately 3.5 cm in length and has an hourglass shape. The middle ear portion is bony, and the nasopharyngeal portion is cartilaginous. The cartilage of the eustachian tube ends in a **C**-shaped cartilage opening medially. This cartilage is connected to two muscles, the levator veli palatini and the tensor veli palatini. The levator veli palatini is innervated by the glossopharyngeal nerve with contributions from the pharyngeal complex. The levator veli palatini is attached to the lateral caudal portion of the cartilage. The tensor veli palatini, innervated by the trigeminal nerve and possibly the glossopharyngeal nerve, is attached to the open rostral portion of the open side of the cartilage. Studies have shown that the levator veli palatini is relatively small in the first 6 years of life and may not play a major role in opening the eustachian tube until after the age of 6 years. The tensor tympani muscle, innervated by the trigeminal nerve, is found on the rostral medial portion of the eustachian tube. The bony portion of the eustachian tube is lined with a mucous membrane of low columnar ciliated epithelium. The cartilaginous portion is lined with pseudostratified columnar epithelium with both ciliated epithelium and mucus-secreting cells. Lymphoid cells are found frequently at the nasopharyngeal end of the eustachian tube and its submucosal lining. These lymphoid accumulations are called Gerlach's tonsil.

The histology of the palatine tonsils and the adenoids is somewhat different. The palatine tonsil is covered with a stratified squamous epithelium that invaginates to form 10 or 20 or more crypts in each tonsil. Arranged around the crypts are lymphoid follicles with secondary germinal centers. Lymphocytes, polymorphonuclear leukocytes, and plasma cells can be found in the palatine tonsil. The adenoid or pharyngeal tonsil is covered with a modified respiratory mucosa and does not form the crypts seen in the palatine tonsil. It also includes lymphoid germinal centers with lymphocytes, polymorphonuclear leukocytes, and plasma cells. As the tonsils and adenoids involute they are replaced by fibrous tissue.

PHYSIOLOGY

Airway and Deglutition

The pharynx must be patent so that air can enter the larynx. Most breathing is done through the nose. At birth the infant is primarily a nose breather. Respiratory distress is encountered in infants with blockage of the nose or nasopharynx (eg, choanal atresia or an encephalocele); these infants must learn to use their oropharynx for respiration. This appears to be dependent on the growth of the oropharynx. Some infants are able to do this quite readily; others cannot, and a nasal airway must be established.

Obstruction to the oropharynx also results in respiratory distress in the infant. This occurs in infants with small mandibles and glossoptosis, as in the Pierre Robin syndrome (p. 917). This condition is managed by maintaining the infant on its stomach so that the tongue will fall ventrally. A disproportionately large tongue and masses in the pharynx can also result in upper airway obstruction.

Deglutition is an important function of the pharynx.

Food, either liquid or solid, is formed into a bolus by the tongue. The bolus is propelled dorsally by the tongue and the palate and passes through the pharynx into the cricopharyngeus. Escape of the bolus through the nose or mouth or aspiration of food into the larynx, trachea, or bronchus is prevented by coordinated movements that close the nasopharynx, close the oropharynx, and elevate and close the larynx. The bolus of food is propelled on either side of the raised larynx rostrally and dorsally to the cricopharyngeus. The cricopharyngeus sphincter then opens, and the bolus passes into the cervical esophagus. Any disease process that interferes with either the structure or the function of the pharynx may result in aspiration and/or regurgitation of food through the nose and mouth. These types of dysphagia are seen in patients with cleft palate, in which there is nasal regurgitation, as well as in those with cranial nerve paralysis (eg, hydrocephalus accompanied by regurgitation and aspiration), neuromuscular disease (eg, Duchenne's muscular dystrophy, in which there may be both dysphagia and regurgitation), and masses that may obstruct the pharynx and result in either regurgitation and aspiration or dysphagia.

Speech

The pharynx participates in the speech mechanism. Air comes to the larynx after passing through the pharynx. Most sounds in the English language are dependent on the proper shape of the pharynx. Several sounds, such as *m* and *n*, require that air escape via the nose through the nasopharynx. When these sounds are abnormal, the condition is called hyponasality. Many sounds and combinations of sounds are dependent upon little or no nasal escape of air through a closed or partially closed nasopharynx. Most consonant sounds in the English language, especially *s* and *f*, require that the nasopharynx be closed. When these sounds are abnormal the condition is called hypernasality. This condition is seen in cleft-palate children and others with velopharyngeal insufficiency. This condition is observed in patients with a mass in the nasopharynx (eg, juvenile angiofibromas, adenoids, or other tumors) and also in patients with stenosis of the nasopharynx.

The air going through the nasopharynx and out of the nose is controlled by the velopharyngeal sphincter. The sphincter is formed ventrally by the dorsal rostral portion of the soft palate, laterally by the superior constrictors of the palate, and dorsally by the adenoids in children, and the formation of Passavant's ridge. The latter is formed from the muscles of the superior constrictors dorsally and is a ventral extension of the posterior wall of the pharynx, which meets the posterior portion of the soft palate.

Eustachian Tube

The eustachian tube serves to maintain in the middle ear an air pressure equal to that of the environment. This is achieved by frequent opening of the eustachian tube. The eustachian tube opens naturally with swallowing. Malfunction of the eustachian tube, with its subsequent sequela of otitis media, is divided into two types, anatomic and physiologic.

Anatomic blockage of the eustachian tube can result from any mass that occludes the tube. The most common of these in the nasopharynx are tumors, benign or malignant, such as hypertrophy of the adenoids or juvenile angiofibromas. Obstruction of the eustachian tube by an anatomic mass can also occur in the middle ear orifice from mucosal edema or a small polyp. Obstruction may also occur at any point in the tube due to edema or stricture.

Physiologic obstruction of the eustachian tube comes about from abnormalities in the tensor veli palatini or the levator veli palatini muscles, or their innervation. The tensor and levator palatini muscles are also the muscles that comprise the soft palate. This type of malfunction results in inability of the tube to open in response to negative pressure in the middle ear. There is also the possibility that negative pressure in the middle ear by itself may be another cause of tubal malfunction. The physiologic malfunction is seen in all those diseases that affect the palatal musculature and the shape of the nasopharynx, including cleft palates, submucosal clefts of the palate, and many of the cranial malformations associated with these diseases. There also seems to be an increase in tubal malfunction in children whose palates have extremely high arches.

Immunology

The lymphoid tissue of Waldeyer's ring has been shown to be capable of making certain antibodies. In vitro studies have demonstrated that the palatine tonsils are capable of making diphtheria antibodies, and clinical studies have shown that they are involved in the production of the polio antibody associated with secretory IgA. These immunologic observations agree with the clincial observations made before the development of poliomyelitis vaccine: children who had undergone tonsillectomies and adenoidectomies would have approximately the same attack rate of poliomyelitis, but the disease would be of much greater severity. This effect would be more pronounced if the tonsillectomy had been performed a short time before the polio infection.

It is suspected that the lymphoid tissues in Waldeyer's ring may have a role in the production of antibodies to antigens that pass through the pharynx. This tissue does not appear to be the sole source of these antibodies, and with the exception of the polio antibody, the contribution of the lymphoid tissue to overall antibody function is not known.

METHODS OF EXAMINATION

Physical Examination

Physical examination of the pharynx is carried out by having the child open his mouth and inspecting the soft and hard palate, the lateral palatal walls in which the palatine tonsils are found, and the lateral and posterior walls of the pharynx. Direct visual inspection will usually show the oropharynx and not the nasopharynx or the hypopharynx. A tongue depressor should not be used for the initial examination, as this can cause distortion of the pharynx and may cause gagging or vomiting. The oropharynx should be inpected for movement, for infection, and for abnormal masses. After this is completed the tongue depressor is gently inserted, and the posterior portion of the tongue is depressed. This will bring into view a portion of the rostral area of the hypopharynx and a lateral portion of the oropharynx, which lies directly dorsal to the palatine tonsils.

Digital palpation of the palate should be performed to reveal any submucosal clefts; these are commonly associated with a high arched palate and/or a bifid uvula. The usual finding is a depression in the middle of the soft palate and notching of the dorsal portion of the hard palate as it joins the soft palate.

Radiologic Examination

Radiography is one of the best methods for examination of the pharynx, both for masses and for function. Using soft tissue technique, lateral, anterior, and posterior views of the pharynx will reveal the contour of the pharynx and show whether any masses are present. Radiographs, either individual pictures or motion pictures taken during speech and swallowing, will show how the pharynx is functioning during these activities. The motion picture views can be taken with or without contrast media and are extremely useful in defining the competence of the velopharyngeal sphincter. Children with incompetent velopharyngeal sphincters are unable to close the nasopharynx and many times will demonstrate abnormal palatal motion.

Contrast radiography has also been used to demonstrate eustachian tube function. Eustachian tube blockage from adenoids can be demonstrated, as well as physiologic malfunction. Abnormal patency of the eustachian tube has also been identified with these techniques. In these instances the eustachian tube is abnormally open; it allows food and nasopharyngeal secretions to enter the middle ear and can serve as a cause of middle ear infection.

Endoscopy

Two types of endoscopes have been used to directly examine the nasopharynx: the nasopharyngoscope and the panendoscope. The nasopharyngoscope is inserted along the floor of the anterior nose. This allows for a direct view of the turbinates, nasopharynx, eustachian tube orifice, and adenoids. The panendoscope, a large instrument, is inserted through the mouth. When the viewing lens is turned rostrally, the entire nasopharynx is viewed. This instrument is used primarily in assessing velopharyngeal competence during speech. The use of both these instruments requires clinical skill and a cooperative patient.

DISEASES

Congenital Diseases

The most common congenital malformations of the pharynx are those associated with malformations of the soft and hard palates. These include all clefts of the palate. There are also submucosal clefts of the palate in children with bifid uvula. Congenital stenosis of the larynx has also been reported. At the dorsal junction of the oronasal pharynx, a congenital cyst called Thornwaldt's cyst may be found. This cyst can present as a small draining midline sinus. Encephaloceles may be found in the nasopharynx and may present as large smooth masses. Diverticula are found in the hypopharynx and may present as lateral neck masses or as smooth hypopharyngeal masses. Congenital nerve paralysis and paresis may be encountered, especially in children with hydrocephalus (eg, Arnold-Chiari syndrome) or other central nervous sytem malformation. These children may present with dysphagia and/or aspiration that may frequently be associated with laryngeal paresis and paralysis. Congenital absence of the palatine tonsils and/or pharyngeal tonsil has been seen in Di George's syndrome and X-linked agammaglobulinemia.

Infectious Diseases

VIRAL INFECTIONS. The same viruses associated with rhinitis and upper respiratory infection also infect the pharynx. Viruses account for approximately 15 percent of all acute pharyngitis. The signs and symptoms are similar to those of acute viral rhinitis. Infectious mononucleosis associated with the Epstein-Barr virus is one of the most severe viral infections of the pharynx. This infection is characterized by severe pharyngitis, fever, leukocytosis, atypical lymphocytes, a high heterophil antibody titer, lymphadenopathy, and splenomegaly. The appearance of the pharynx is quite striking in that it is erythematous and swollen. The pharynx may be coated with a white to yellowish gray exudate. Extreme hypertrophy of the palatine tonsils is also common. Some cases may result in upper airway obstruction and occasionally in spontaneous hemorrhage from the palatine tonsils.

BACTERIAL INFECTIONS. Bacterial infections of the pharynx are very common. They may present with fever, irritability, anorexia, sometimes vomiting and/or diarrhea, and occasionally a respiratory obstruction. Physical examination may reveal an erythematous pharynx, usually with hypertrophy of the tonsils, cervical adenopathy, and otitis media. Studies of the etiology of bacterial pharyngitis have shown *Haemophilus influenzae,* β-hemolytic *Streptococcus,* and pneumococcus to be the most common bacterial agents. *Haemophilus influenzae* appears to be more common than β-hemolytic *Streptococcus* in children less than 3 years of age. A pathogen may not be isolated in approximately 45 percent of cases. Diphtheria is a rare cause of pharyngitis and is characterized by a white to yellowish green membrane covering the entire pharynx. A diphtherial infection may result in upper airway obstruction necessitating tracheostomy or intubation, or in cardiac failure due to the diphtheria toxin.

Tonsillitis occurs in all cases of pharyngitis. The tonsillar crypts and stroma can become chronically infected and may contain abscesses. The tonsils may either hypertrophy or atrophy with chronic infection. The appearance of a chronically infected tonsil is quite variable. Sometimes large tonsils will be seen in which either pus or whitish caseous cellular debris may be expressed from the crypts. This is a common finding associated in many cases of chronic tonsillitis, but is not necessarily pathognomonic of chronic tonsillar infection.

The diagnosis of clinical tonsillitis is difficult. Many children have several episodes of bacterial pharyngitis each year with tonsillar involvement. This is sometimes called chronic tonsillitis. An important aspect of the diagnosis and treatment of these children is the relationship between their immune system and the recurrent infections. In a study of 30 children with chronic tonsillitis, the criteria for chronic tonsillitis was four or more episodes of pharyngitis and acute tonsillitis in 1 year. The children were divided into two groups on the basis of immunologic studies. One group had essentially normal immune systems, while the other showed a significant decrease in serum IgA. The children with low IgA also had *Haemophilus influenzae* infections. All the children underwent tonsillectomy, and those with low IgA appeared to have a higher incidence of pharyngitis postoperatively than those with normal IgA. Both groups of children appeared to have a decrease in tonsillitis postoperatively. These results suggest that the basis of repeated episodes of pharyngitis may be two general conditions, the first being clinically infected tonsils and the second a minor but significant deficiency in immunologic competence. The child with multiple episodes of pharyngitis should be suspected of having diminished immunologic competence, and appropriate diagnostic procedures should be carried out. If the immunologic mechanism appears to be well within the normal ranges, a diagnosis of primary tonsillitis can be made.

Bacterial infections of the pharynx and tonsils may result in abscesses in the surrounding tissues. The most common of these is the *peritonsillar abscess.* The abscess forms rostrally in the superior tonsillar space; it is evident on physical examination and produces trismus. There may be considerable swelling and erythema of the soft palate immediately rostral and medial to the abscessed tonsil. The uvula may be edematous and be deflected away from the infected node. *Parapharyngeal and posterior pharyngeal abscesses* also occur. They may present as a lateral neck mass and/or as a soft mass protruding into the oropharynx and/or hypopharynx.

All of these abscesses are potentially lethal, as they may spontaneously drain in several ways. The peritonsillar abscess can drain into the pharynx and cause aspiration of pus. It can also extend laterally and become a parapharyngeal abscess. The parapharyngeal and posterior pharyngeal abscesses may drain caudally by means of the fascial enclosures of the great vessels and reach the mediastinum. These will result in arterial rupture and/or mediastinitis. All of these abscesses are associated with edema and may result in upper airway obstruction and respiratory death.

Another bacterial infection, primarily of the oropharynx, is *Vincent's angina.* This infection usually presents in the second decade of life with ulcerations in the mouth, palate, tonsils, and pharynx; it may be associated with surgical lymphadenopathy and low-grade fever. It is caused by both the spirochete and fusiform *Fusobacterium.* Diagnosis can be made by staining some of the exudate and noting the two different bacteria. They are usually sensitive to penicillin.

Syphilis is also seen. Congenital syphilis can present as nasopharyngeal stenosis. Primary syphilis may be found in teenagers as a chancre on the soft palate or oropharyngeal wall.

Neoplastic Diseases

HYPERTROPHY. Marked hypertrophy of the palatine tonsils and adenoids in infants and younger children can result in chronic upper airway obstruction. Some children have been found to have marked hypertrophy of the palatine tonsils and adenoids, increased Pco_2, decreased Po_2, and right heart failure; they are symptomatic for some time before the right heart failure is evident. These infants and children may fall asleep while eating or playing; yet they sleep restlessly during the night. Their sleep is often accompanied by snoring. Their Pickwickian symptomatology is probably due to CO_2 narcosis. It is thought that the increase in CO_2 retention secondary to the chronic upper respiratory obstruction results in pulmonary hypertension and right heart failure. These children are dramatically relieved of their symptoms and signs by surgical removal of the tonsils and/or adenoids. This syndrome is also held to be responsible for sudden death in some young children. Marked hypertrophy of the adenoids may result in anatomic eustachian tube blockage. This blockage will result in repeated otitis media and possibly hyponasal speech. The diagnosis of an adenoidal mass can be made by either nasopharyngoscopy or radiology.

BENIGN TUMORS. *Juvenile angiofibroma* is the most common of the benign pharyngeal tumors of childhood. It usually occurs in boys and is first noted at the age of 5 or 6 years. It is a vascular tumor that grows from the nasopharynx into the choana, nose, and paranasal sinuses, and in some cases the orbit. The presenting signs and symptoms are nasal obstruction, rhinorrhea, epistaxis, otitis media, and occasionally hypernasal speech. It is seen as a bluish mass in the nose or nasopharynx. When this tumor is suspected, diagnostic studies should be carried out to show its extent and its vascular pattern. Most often a primary diagnosis is made with angiography (Fig. 2). Biopsies of this tumor are very dangerous; they can result in massive hemorrhage, and they should be done only under the

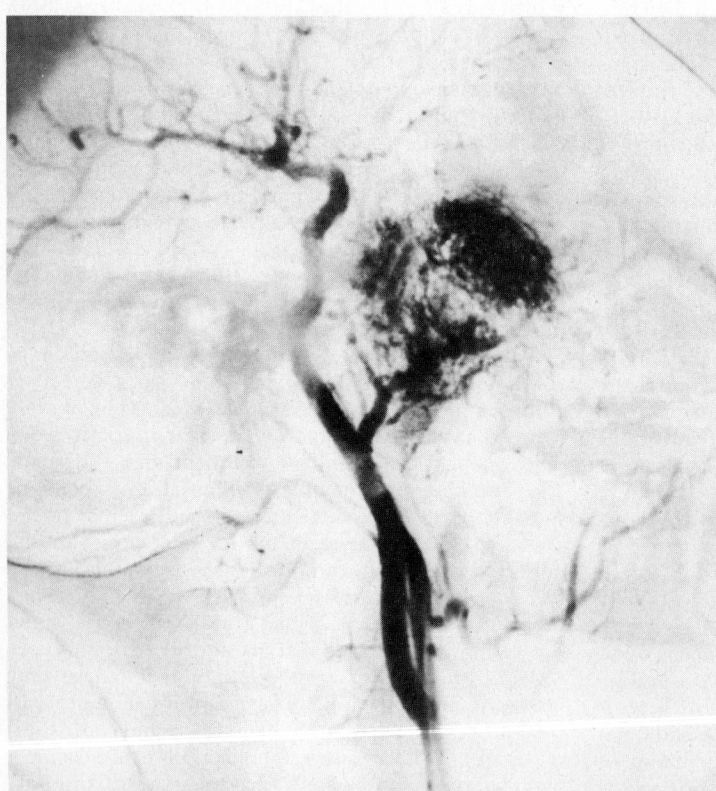

FIG. 2. Arteriogram showing the massive blood supply of Juvenile angiofibroma in nasopharynx of a child. (From the collection of the Department of Radiology, Albert Einstein College of Medicine. Acknowledgment to Drs. H. Goldman, L. Lutzker and B. Seife)

most controlled conditions, with intravenous fluids running and blood available for transfusion. Other benign tumors of the pharynx include hemangiomas, lymphangiomas, cysts, neurofibromas, cranial pharyngiomas, dermoids, and allergic nasal polyps.

MALIGNANT TUMORS.   Malignant tumors of the nasopharynx are rare in children. The most common of these are the rhabdomyosarcoma and teratoma. Carcinoma of the nasopharynx may be found in the first and second decades of life. All these tumors may result in blockage of the eustachian tube, with resulting otitis media. The more advanced tumors can invade the base of the skull and cause cranial nerve paralysis, most often of the vagal glossopharyngeus and hypoglossus.

TRAUMA.   Trauma of the pharynx is uncommon. Neck injuries may result in lacerations of the pharynx. These can lead to subcutaneous and mediastinal emphysema, with possible infection. Trauma to the nasopharynx may occur after operative procedures. Stenosis of the hypopharynx is associated with the ingestion of acids and caustics, especially in younger children.

DIAGNOSIS

Sore Throat

Sore throat is quite common in children, and it is usually associated with fever, lymphocytosis, and malaise. The cause can be either viral or bacterial infection. The viral infections usually, but not invariably, do not have exudate on the tonsils or pharynx, whereas the bacterial infections do. The major exception to this is infectious mononucleosis. Infectious mononucleosis may be associated with an increase in heterophil antibody, atypical lymphocytes, and other systemic signs. Many times infectious mononucleosis will be accompanied by an acute bacterial pharyngitis. The true nature of the infection often does not become apparent until after the usual therapy has been demonstrated to have little effect and the patient remains quite ill. Repeated episodes of pharyngitis may be associated with chronic tonsillitis and/or a decrease in immunologic competence. Sore throat associated with small ulcers will usually be Vincent's angina. Primary syphilitic chancre is uncommon and usually presents as a painless ulcer with very little general symptomatology.

Upper Respiratory Obstruction

The problem of upper respiratory obstruction may be related to the larynx or trachea, or to the pharynx. In the neonate and infant the problem of the nasal and pharyngeal airway must be considered in the differential diagnosis. If the breathing improves when the child is lying on his stomach, there is a strong possibility that the obstruction may be from the oropharynx or epiglottis. Radiography is very useful in the diagnosis of retropharyngeal masses that may be impinging on the posterior portion of the pharyngeal airway. Patients with retropharyngeal masses may breathe better when lying on their backs.

Nasal Regurgitation

Nasal regurgitation may be seen in any condition in which closure of the velopharyngeal sphincter is inadequate, which may result either from anatomic defects, such as cleft palate, or from any neurologic impairment of the velopalatal sphincter. Acquired neurologic diseases affecting the brainstem or cranial nerves that may present as nasal regurgitation include degenerative diseases, infectious diseases such as bulbar poliomyelitis, and any cause of increased cranial pressure.

Dysphagia and Aspiration

The inability to swallow may be caused by either an anatomic blockage of the esophagus or a neurologic defect. A significant cause of dysphagia in the neonate is esophageal atresia (p. 1015). Congenital diverticulum of the hypopharynx should also be considered in the differential diagnosis. Infants and children with progressive dysphagia, with or without aspiration, may have tumors of the hypopharynx or neurologic disease that causes interference with the swallowing mechanism. Aspiration may also be associated with laryngeal disease.

Hyponasal and Hypernasal Speech

Hyponasal speech occurs when the velopharyngeal sphincter is closed, which may be caused by masses in the nasopharynx (eg, massive adenoidal hypertrophy, juvenile angiofibromas) or stenosis of the nasopharynx from tumor or infection. Hypernasal speech may occur when the velopharyngeal sphincter cannot be totally closed. This occurs in children with cleft palates or submucosal clefts of the palate and in palatal paralysis or paresis. It is also found occasionally in children after adenoidectomy, most often in a child who has congenital shortening of the palate or a submucosal cleft of the palate.

Eustachian Tube Malformation: Recurrent Otitis Media

The cause of malfunction of the eustachian tube must be identified. The *anatomic* causes are due to tumor obstruction, usually at the nasopharyngeal end of the tube and most frequently adenoidal hypertrophy. Recurrent otitis media and chronic serous otitis media may be associated with any of the benign or malignant tumors in the nasopharynx. *Physiologic* obstruction may be associated with any abnormality of the soft palate and the base of the skull. These will be found in children with cleft palates, submucosal clefts, high arched palates, bifid uvulae, and other syndromes involving the palate and the base of the skull (eg, Apert's disease, Crouzon's disease, Klippel-Feil disease, and Turner's syndrome).

TREATMENT

Pharyngitis and Tonsillitis

Bacterial pharyngitis should be treated with antipyretics, oral decongestants, and antibiotics, if a bacterial etiology is proved. Those infections that recur more than three or four times a year should be considered to represent a possible deficiency in immunologic competence and/or chronic tonsillitis. Tonsillectomy should be reserved only for those children who have four or more repeated episodes of bacterial pharyngitis associated with tonsillitis and in whom the immunologic systems are felt to be adequate. Tonsillectomies are rarely indicated for children under 2 years of age. The efficacy of tonsillectomy in decreasing bacterial infections of the throat is dependent upon selection of cases in which tonsillitis is the major cause of the factor.

Tonsillectomy is a major procedure that has significant potential for the complications of hemorrhage and respiratory obstruction. A careful examination for any bleeding or dyscrasia should be part of the preoperative assessment of a child being considered for tonsillectomy or adenoidectomy. The operation should always be carried out under general anesthesia with an endotracheal tube in place. Rheumatic fever is not an indication for tonsillectomy. It has been shown that penicillin therapy will give better control of β-hemolytic *Streptococcus* than tonsillectomy alone.

Pharyngeal Abscesses

Peritonsillar, peripharyngeal, and retropharyngeal abscesses should be treated with high doses of parenteral antibiotics and surgical drainage. A child with a history of peritonsillar abscess should have a tonsillectomy performed after the infection has resolved.

Infectious Mononucleosis

Infectious mononucleosis is a potentially serious infection that can result in airway obstruction and spontaneous hemorrhage. In cases of severe tonsillar enlargement and inflammation, treatment with corticosteroids is quite effective. The response to systemic corticosteroids is usually dramatic, with swelling and inflammation resolving within 1 or 2 days after treatment. Corticosteroids should be used only after a definite diagnosis of infectious mononucleosis has been made, as demonstrated by the appearance of atypical lymphocytes and/or a high or increased heterophil antibody titer, since corticosteroids can lead to serious complications when used in bacterial infections.

Eustachian Tube Obstruction

If eustachian tube obstruction is anatomic, the occluding mass should be removed. This mass is most often the adenoid. Adenoidectomy is a simple procedure, as compared to tonsillectomy, and it has separate indications. The indications are proven eustachian tube obstruction or choanal obstruction with chronic rhinitis and sinusitis. Adenoidectomy is contraindicated in those cases in which there is physiologic malfunction of the eustachian tube resulting in otitis media. The removal of adenoids in such cases will not reduce the incidence of otitis media, but may make it worse and may also lead to increased velopharyngeal insufficiency with resultant hypernasal speech. Every child who is a candidate for an adenoidectomy should be examined to determine if there are any palatal malformations or nasopharyngeal malformations that would account for the otitis media. Children with recurrent otitis media due to physiologic eustachian tube obstruction are treated with ventilating tubes (p. 973).

References

Alpert JJ, Pickering MR, Warren RJ: Failure to isolate streptococci from children under the age of 3 with exudative tonsillitis. Pediatrics 38:663, 1966

Amjad H, Richburg FD, Adler E: Kartagener syndrome. JAMA 227:1420, 1974

Baer H: In vitro methods in allergy. Med Clin North Am 58:85, 1974

Bluestone C, Beery QC, Andrus WS: Mechanics of eustachian tube as it influences susceptibility to and persistence of middle ear effusions in children. Ann Otol Rhinol Laryngol 83:27, 1974

Brand KG: Bacteriology, basic and applied to otorhinolaryngology. In Paparella M, Shumrick D: Otorhinolaryngology, Vol 1. Philadelphia, WB Saunders, 1973, p 411

Bryan WTK, Bryan MP: Application of in vitro cytotoxic reactions to clinical diagnosis of food allergy. Laryngoscope 70:810, 1960

Donovan R, Soothill JF: Immunological studies in children undergoing tonsillectomy. Clin Exp Immunol 14:347, 1973

———— Clinical and immunologic studies on children undergoing tonsillectomy for repeated sore throat. Proc R Soc Med 66:413, 1973

Edison BD, Kerth JD: Tonsilloadenoid hypertrophy resulting in cor pulmonale. Arch Otolaryngol 98:205, 1973

Letson JA, Birck HG: Septal dermoplasty for von Willebrand's disease in children. Laryngoscope 83:1078, 1973

Mawson SR, Adlington P, Evans M: Controlled study evaluation of adenotonsillectomy in children. J Laryngol Otol 81:777, 1967

Morag A, Ogra PL: Immunologic aspect of tonsils. Ann Otol Rhinol Laryngol Suppl 19, 1975, p 37

Murakami Y, Kirchner JA: Mechanical and physiological properties of reflex laryngeal closure. Ann Otol Rhinol Laryngol 81:59, 1972

O'Connor JD: Phonetics. Middlesex, England. Penguin, 1973

Ogra PA: Effect of tonsillectomy and adenoidectomy on nasopharyngeal antibody response to poliovirus. N Engl J Med 284:59, 1971

Ogura JH, Suemitsu M, Nelson JR, et al: Relationship between pulmonary resistance and changes in arterial blood gas tension in dogs with nasal obstruction and partial laryngeal obstruction. Ann Otol Rhinol Laryngol 82:668, 1973

Petruson B: Epistaxis. A clinical study with special reference to fibrinolysis. Acta Otolaryngol [Suppl] (Stockh) Suppl 317, 1974

Ross RU, Christie SMK, Know JDE: Sore throat and cold, its causation and incidence. Br Med J 2:624, 1971

Ruben RJ, Weg N: Contraindications to adenoidectomy. Bull NY Acad Med 7:817, 1975

Schiff G: Viral diseases in otorhinolaryngology. In Paparella M, Shumrick D: Otorhinolaryngology, Vol 2. Philadelphia, WB Saunders, 1973, p 428

Weseman CM: Management of choanal atresia in the newborn. Laryngoscope 83:1160, 1973

CHAPTER 21

The Ear

ROBERT J. RUBEN

INTRODUCTION

The consideration of diseases of the ear in infants and children has several important facets, some of which are not immediately apparent. Usually attention is directed to the infectious problems. However, a diminution or total loss of hearing can profoundly influence the intellectual and behavioral development of a child; only recently have the more subtle effects of minimal hearing loss been documented. This chapter will stress both the physical and functional problems resulting from diseases of the ear.

MORPHOLOGY

Embryology

The ear can be divided into four portions (Fig. 1). These are: the outer ear, which includes the pinna, the external auditory meatus, and the external canal; the middle ear, which includes the eustachian tube, the middle ear cleft, and the mastoid; the inner ear or labyrinth, which includes the portion responsible for hearing, the cochlea, and the portion responsible for balance, the vestibular labyrinth; and the VIIIth cranial nerve with its cochlear and vestibular divisions. Also, any consideration of the development and morphology of the ear must include the facial nerve, which is intimately associated with the middle and the inner ear.

The external ear pinna and the external auditory meatus begin their development in the third month of fetal life and are formed by the sixth month. The middle ear cleft and eustachian tube also begin their development in the third fetal month. At birth, there is usually a single mastoid cell, called the *antrum*, and a middle ear cleft. The mastoid cells increase in number until pub-

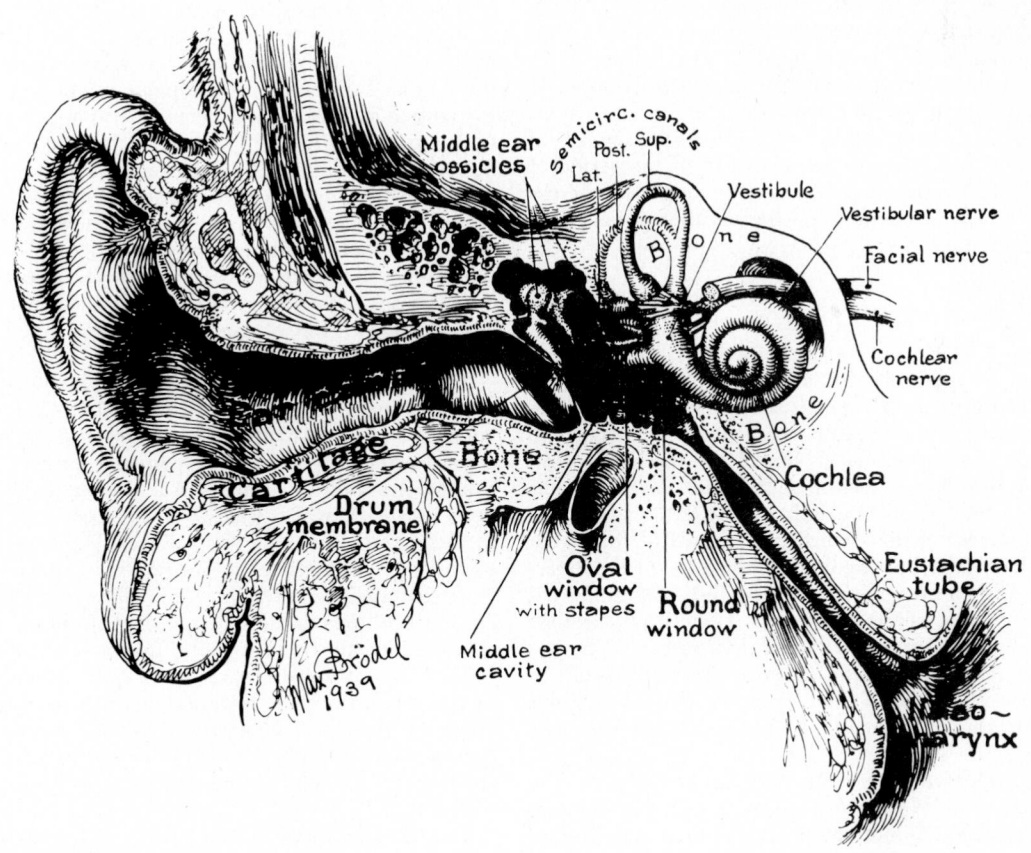

FIG. 1. Anatomic drawing of the ear. (Original illustration in the Brodel Collection of the Johns Hopkins Department of Art as Applied to Medicine)

erty, when they reach their adult configuration. Infectious diseases decrease the size and number of mastoid cells.

The ossicular chain, malleus, incus, and stapes, and the middle ear muscles develop from the first and second branchial arches. The tensor tympani muscle is derived from the first branchial arch and is innervated by a branch of the trigeminal nerve. The stapedius muscle is derived from the second branchial arch and is innervated by a motor branch of the facial nerve.

The position of the tympanic membrane changes with age. At birth it is more horizontal. At mature growth it is almost vertical in relation to the external canal. The eustachian tube is practically horizontal at birth; as the child grows, the pharyngeal end of the tube assumes a relatively lower position.

The inner ear is completely developed at birth. This includes the size of the bony capsule and the membranous portion of the labyrinth, which houses the cells that transduce sound. Since there are very few mastoid cells surrounding the bony labyrinth, it is quite easy to delineate the inner ear of an infant with simple mastoid radiography.

Normal central nervous system development is necessary if the bony labyrinth is to develop normally. If development of the central nervous system is abnormal, there may be abnormal development of the membranous labyrinth (its otic capsule). The mature inner ear is unable to replace any of its sensory cells. The sensory cells in the inner ear probably undergo their terminal mitosis during the second or third month of fetal life; any damage to these cells after this period of gestation will result in permanent hearing loss, the extent of which will depend on the number of cells that have been damaged.

Anatomy

The *auricle or pinna* consists of a cartilaginous frame covered by relatively thin skin. Any process that will cause swelling of the pinna, such as a hematoma or an abscess, will tend to cause necrosis of the cartilage. The external auditory canal is lined by squamous epithelium. The lateral portion of the canal is cartilaginous and one medial portion is bony. There is very little subcutaneous tissue, which accounts for the great amount of pain and swelling in infections of the external auditory meatus. Ceruminous glands of the external auditory canal secrete cerumen. Genetically, wet or sticky cerumen is dominant over dry cerumen. The wet type of cerumen is found in more than 90 percent of Caucasians and Blacks, whereas the dry cerumen is found in about 85 percent of Japanese and of American Indians.

The *tympanic membrane* (Fig. 2) at the medial end of the external auditory canal has an external layer of squamous epithelium, a middle layer of radial and circumferential connective tissue fibers, and an inner layer of modified respiratory mucosa. The lower four-fifths of the tympanic membrane, the *pars tensa*, is relatively

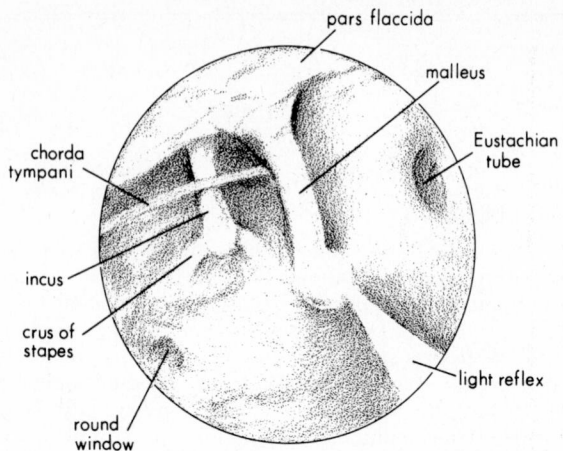

FIG. 2. Landmarks found in normal tympanic membrane. (From Ferguson and Kendig: Pediatric Otolaryngology, Vol. 2, 2nd ed. Philadelphia, WB Saunders Co, 1972)

rigid, whereas the upper portion, the *pars flaccida*, is looser. The handle of the malleus is attached vertically in the middle of the tympanic membrane and the chorda tympani runs horizontally on its upper third.

There are three *ossicles* in the middle-ear cleft. The most lateral of these is the *malleus*, which is attached to the medial surface of the tympanic membrane and is suspended by ligaments superiorly. It is attached to the tensor tympani by the ligament of the tensa tympani. Superiorly it is attached to the incus. The *incus* is suspended by ligaments and lies superior and posterior to the malleus. The incus has a process that extends posteriorly and then bends medially to articulate with the third bone, the *stapes*, which is shaped like a stirrup and articulates with the inner ear at a fossa, the oval window. The posterior crus of the stapes is connected to the stapedius muscle posteriorly.

The *middle ear cleft* (Fig. 1) is limited laterally by the tympanic membrane; inferiorly by the bulb of the jugular vein, anteriorly by the bony covering of the internal carotid artery and the eustachian tube orifice; superiorly by the middle cranial fossa; and medially by the bony labyrinth, which has two flexible portions related to the middle ear. The first of these is the *oval window* in which the footplate of the stapes is attached by a ligament; the second is the *round window*, which is covered by fibrinous tissue. Posteriorly the middle ear cleft is limited by the bone forming the mastoid or its air cells. It opens into the mastoid air cells superiorly and posteriorly through a small opening of less than 1 mm diameter, the aditus ad antrum. The middle ear cleft is covered with modified respiratory epithelium, which consists of epithelial cells, ciliated cells, and mucus-secreting cells.

The *facial nerve* runs through the middle ear cleft posteriorly, from superior to inferior and gives off the branch of the stapedius muscle and the chorda tympani. The latter travels through the middle ear, across the medial aspect of the superior portion of the tympanic membrane, exits anterosuperiorly, reaches the tongue, and is responsible for taste in the anterior two-thirds of the tongue.

The *eustachian tube*, which opens anterosuperiorly into the middle ear cleft, connects with the nasopharynx. The portion of the eustachian tube closer to the middle ear cleft is bony, whereas the nasopharyngeal end is cartilaginous. The tube is lined with respiratory mucosa. Areas of lymphoid tissue are also found, especially in children, underneath the lining of the eustachian tube and portions of the middle ear cleft. The tensor tympani muscle is adjacent to the eustachian tube, superiorly, and the internal carotid artery is medial to the bony portion of the eustachian tube. The cartilage of the nasopharyngeal end is attached to the tensor veli palatini and levator veli palatini muscles (Chap. 20).

The *mastoid cell system* is connected to the middle ear cleft through the aditus ad antrum. This leads posteriorly to the initial mastoid cell, the antrum. The mastoid cells increase in number during the growth of the child and may be found throughout the entire temporal bone, including the zygoma and the tip of the petrous portion of the temporal bone. The mastoid cell system superiorly borders the middle cranial fossa; posteriorly, the posterior cranial fossa and the sigmoid sinus; inferiorly, the mastoid tip; and medially mastoid cells can be found adjacent to the brain stem. Mastoid cells contain air and are lined with modified respiratory epithelium. These cells, which in the normal mastoid are flat epithelium, maintain their ability to dedifferentiate and redifferentiate, either into mucus-secreting cells or squamous epithelium.

The *inner ear or labyrinth* is enclosed in bone, the otic capsule or petrous portion of the temporal bone. The petrous bone may be connected to the subarachnoid space along the facial or auditory nerves, to the subdural space by the endolymphatic duct, to the middle ear via the round or oval window, and through vascular channels to the middle ear or dura.

The *cochlea* contains the receptor cells for hearing, is coiled, has from 2½ to 2¾ turns, and is divided into three compartments. The scala tympani and the scala vestibuli contain perilymph similar to cerebrospinal fluid; they interconnect at the most apical coil of the cochlea, called the helicotrema. The scala media, third compartment of the cochlea, is separated from the scala

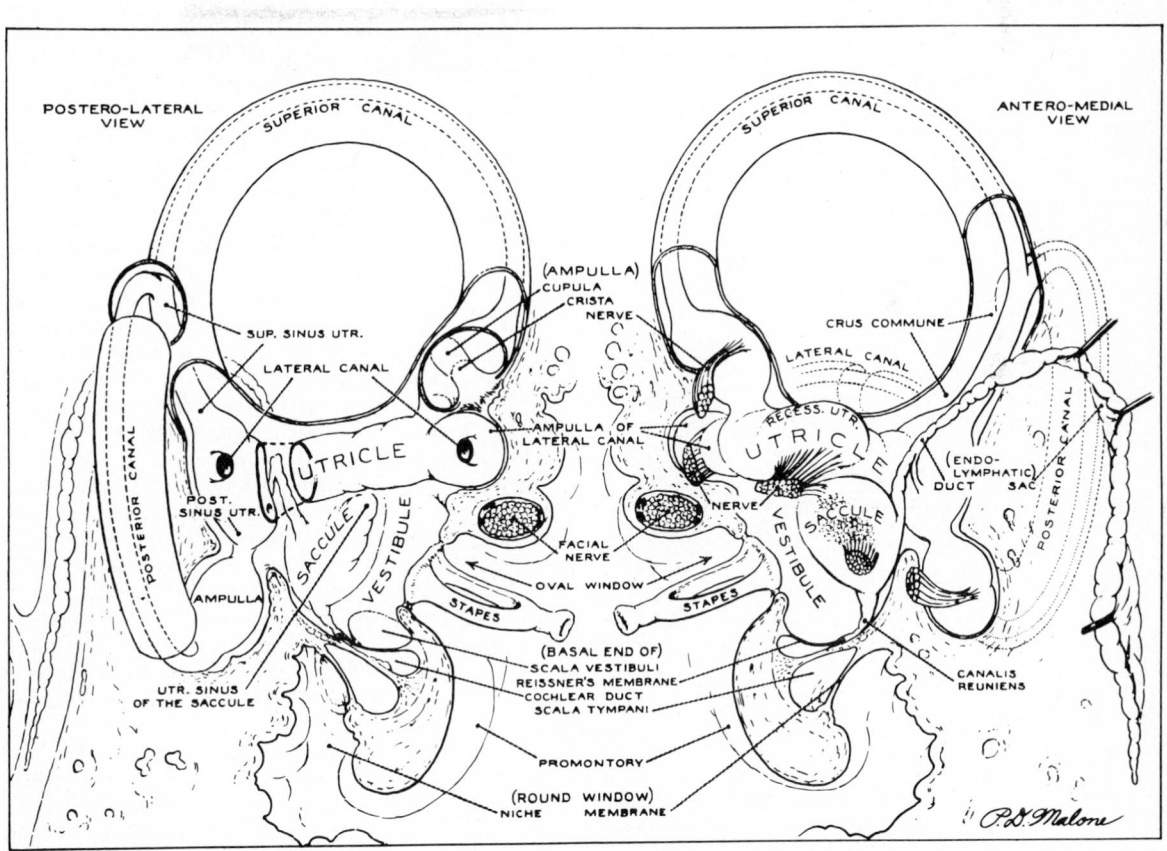

FIG. 3.   Anatomic drawing of sensory structures of the vestibular lab labyrinth. (Original illustration in the Brodel Collection of the Johns Hopkins Department of Art as Applied to Medicine)

vestibuli by Reissner's membrane, and from the scala tympani by the basilar membrane. It contains endolymph which is similar to intracellular fluid and has about 145 mEq/liter of potassium and 15 mEq/liter of sodium.

Within the scala media lies the *organ of Corti* with its receptor cells or hair cells, surrounded by supporting cells and covered by the tectorial membrane, which protrudes from the limbus. Efferent and afferent nerves pass from the center of the cochlea, the modiolus, and innervate the hair cells. The primary (spiral) ganglion cells of the afferent nerves are found in the modiolus. Efferent fibers are derived from cells in both olivary complexes in the brain stem. The vascular supply of the cochlea is derived from terminal branches of the internal auditory branch of the anteroinferior cerebellar artery.

The *vestibular labyrinth* is divided into two compartments, the outer filled with perilymph and the inner with endolymph. There are two types of end-organs in the vestibular labyrinth (Fig. 3). Static sense organs, the maculae of the utricle and saccule, consist of hair cells covered with a gelatinous material containing small calcium carbonate crystals called otoconia; they are thought to give information concerning static position sense. The other end-organs are the *cristae of the semicircular canals*, horizontal, superior, and posterior. They consist of ciliated receptor cells and are covered with a gelatinous material, the cupula. Any change in movement (eg, acceleration or deceleration) or position, will cause the endolymphatic fluid to move, displacing the cupula and stimulating the cilia. These receptor organs are all innervated by the vestibular division of the VIIIth nerve; the ganglion, Scarpa's ganglion, is located in the internal auditory meatus.

The *statoacoustic nerve or VIIIth nerve* has two divisions, cochlear and vestibular. The nerve runs through the internal auditory meatus to the midbrain. The fibers of the cochlear division synapse, for the most part, in the ipsilateral, dorsal, and cochlear nuclei, and some synapse in the contralateral cochlear nuclei. The fibers of the vestibular portion synapse in a similar manner with the vestibular nuclei of the brain stem.

The *facial nerve* is also found in the internal auditory meatus directly above the cochlear nerve. Several branches are given off beyond the internal auditory meatus. As mentioned above, the facial nerve is closely related to the inner and middle ears (Figs. 1 and 3).

PHYSIOLOGY

Hearing

The pinna has only a minor function of collecting sound, but the external auditory canal is an important conduit for sound to reach the tympanic membrane; if it is absent or closed, a severe conductive hearing loss results. The tympanic membrane and the middle ear ossicles serve as an acoustic transformer. The area of the tympanic membrane is approximately 18 times larger than that of the stapedial footplate. The middle ear apparatus functions in a manner similar to a hydraulic transformer in that the difference in the area between the tympanic membrane and the footplate enables sound energy to be concentrated by a factor of about 18. The middle ear muscles provide a governing mechanism, which is most apparent when very loud sounds are presented to the ear. The middle ear muscles will contract in such a manner as to reduce the amount of sound energy delivered to the oval window; thus, they serve as a protecting mechanism. The middle ear has an optimal condition for functioning as a transformer, a function that can be measured by its impedance. Any disease process that either increases or decreases impedance interferes with the efficiency with which sound can be transmitted through the middle ear and results in hearing loss. Impedance can be increased by increase in friction, mass, or stiffness of the system; this could be caused by fixation of one or more of the ossicles, or fluid in the middle ear cleft. Optimal impedance is decreased by conditions that result from ossicular disruption, either congenital or traumatic, or perforation of the tympanic membrane.

The inner ear converts acoustic energy into nerve impulses. This function is performed by the organ of Corti, most probably by the hair cells. The cochlea has a tonotopic organization. The high frequency sounds are best transmitted at the apical end of the cochlea. A loss of hair cells in the organ of Corti will raise the threshold of hearing. If the loss is greatest at the basal end, there will be a greater increase in the threshold for high frequency than for low frequency sounds. Any substantive loss of the organ of Corti will not only result in an increase in hearing threshold but also in a decrease in the ability to understand sounds. This is most apparent in hearing losses that affect the pure-tone range from 500 to 2000 Hz, an area of the auditory spectrum that conveys most of the sound energy in speech. Cochlear lesions also produce the phenomenon of recruitment, which is characterized by an abnormal increase in loudness function. The normal ear will have essentially lineal loudness function, ie, for each increment in acoustic energy there will be an equal increment in loudness perception. Ears in which there is hair-cell damage, especially outer hair-cell damage, will exhibit a disproportionately greater increase in perceived loudness for a given increment in acoustic energy.

Destruction of the cochlear nerve will result in a marked hearing loss; partial destruction, however, will result in only a moderate shift of threshold but in a great amount of distortion and large loss of intelligibility.

The inner ear can be stimulated in two ways. The normal mode of stimulation is via the transformer mechanism of the middle ear— *air conduction*. If the transformer mechanism malfunctions, the inner ear can still be stimulated by vibration of the bony capsule— *bone conduction*. This type of stimulation can serve to test whether a hearing loss is due to middle ear malfunction.

Vibration of the skull by a tuning fork or an oscillator will elicit in a normal ear air conduction thresholds approximately equal to those of bone conduction thresholds. Whenever bone conduction threshold is less than air conduction threshold there is a "bone air gap," which means there is some process interfering with the transformer mechanism of the middle ear. It also means that the function of the inner ear is better than would be assumed if only the threshold determined by air conduction is measured. Often bone conduction threshold will be normal and the air conduction threshold will indicate a moderate to severe hearing loss.

The ability of the cochlea to function probably begins during the last trimester of pregnancy. After birth, the infant less than 3 months responds to a loud sound with eye blink and a muscle jerk, but barely responds to soft sounds. After 3 months, there is less eye blink and muscle jerk, and after 8 months he will turn to localize the sound.

Concomitant with the development of hearing is the development of speech and language (p. 37).

Pressure Regulation in the Middle Ear

The middle ear cleft is connected to the nasopharynx by the eustachian tube and to the mastoid cell system by the aditus ad antrum. This connection to the nasopharynx and consequently to the atmosphere provides for drainage of the middle ear and regulates pressure in the air-filled middle ear and mastoid cavity. The eustachian tube, when not diseased, will open in about 50 percent of subjects when there is a pressure difference of about 5 cm H_2O between the nasopharynx and the middle ear. Conditions that cause interference with the connection between the middle ear and nasopharynx are discussed in Chapter 20 (p. 953). When the eustachian tube does not function properly, air becomes trapped in the middle ear and mastoid, the oxygen is absorbed, and air pressure in the middle ear cavity is lowered, creating a partial vacuum. Respiratory mucosa reacts to this negative air pressure by secreting either thin or thick fluid, which increases the middle ear mass and concomitantly its impedance, and causes conductive loss of hearing. The fluid in itself is also an excellent bacterial culture medium. The condition caused by this reaction to negative air pressure is called serous otitis media.

The respiratory lining of the middle ear cavity functions to remove foreign material, eg, bacteria, cellular debris, by the action of the mucus and the cilia. This material is thought to pass through the eustachian tube into the nasopharynx, where it is swallowed. The secretions in the middle ear are similar to plasma and have been found to contain IgG, IgM, and α_1 glycolipids. These secretions probably play an important role in the control of infections of the middle ear.

METHODS OF EXAMINATION

Physical Examination

The external ear should be inspected for malformations, especially abnormalities of the pinna or position, ectopic tags, and fistulas anterior to the tragus. The external auditory canal is examined to elicit patency, rule out infection, foreign body, and impaction of cerumen. Cerumen often obscures the view of the tympanic membrane, and if it must be removed this difficult procedure should be done without hurting the child. Occasionally the cerumen can be removed with a small blunt curette, but this instrument can produce a lacerated ear canal. The best method is to gently syringe the ear with 3 percent hydrogen peroxide solution in water at body temperature. A temperature much greater or much lower than body temperature will stimulate the semicircular canals and cause vertigo. If there is a known or suspected perforation of the tympanic membrane, the area should not be syringed, as it may spread infection into the middle and/or inner ear. Hard, dry cerumen may be softened by ear drops consisting of glycerine with hydrogen peroxide; 4 to 5 drops are instilled two to three times a day for 4 to 5 days.

The tympanic membrane is inspected by the use of an otoscope, which consists of a battery handle, a lens, and an ear speculum. There are two types of mountings for the lens and the speculum. The operating head consists of a small lens, with the ear speculum fitted-in at some distance, which allows the clinician to remove cerumen under direct magnified vision and to do other minor procedures. The diagnostic head consists of a large lens and a speculum in an airtight seal; a small rubber bulb can be attached and, by applying very gentle pressure, the tympanic membrane can be moved back and forth. The speculum should be inserted by gently lifting the pinna superiorly and laterally. This serves to straighten the external auditory canal and allow for a much better view of the tympanic membrane. The normal tympanic membrane (Fig. 2) is semitranslucent. Most of the following structures should be seen in the normal drum. The malleus runs vertically down the middle of the tympanic membrane in its upper two-thirds. Across the upper third, the chorda tympani is visible, running horizontally as a white line just below the pars flaccida. In the anterosuperior corner of the tympanic membrane is a dark shadow, the middle ear orifice of the eustachian tube. Directly posterior to the middle of the malleus and parallel to it, at one-third of its length, is the long process of the incus. In many instances, at the inferior margin of the incus, the crura of the stapes are seen, and on the posterior crus can be found another line running horizontally and posteriorly, which represents the tendon of the stapedius muscle. Immediately below the incus and posterior to the malleus is another dark shadow, which represents the round window. The "light reflex" can be seen anteriorly and inferiorly, but varies, depending on the source and intensity of the illumination and the angle from which the ear is viewed.

A tympanic membrane in which most of these structures cannot be seen, or which is not translucent or mobile, is abnormal. Most tympanic membranes are not normal. They are scarred, thickened, and have calcium deposits. A small sketch of each visualized tympanic membrane is quite valuable as part of the permanent record and as objective documentation of a developing or receding disease process.

SPECIAL TESTS

Radiography

Radiography of the mastoid and temporal bone is essential in serious ear diseases, such as chronic tympanomastoiditis, chronic otitis media, cholesteatoma, malformation, severe to profound hearing loss, etc. Mastoid films in infants will show not only the mastoid cells but also the inner ear structures. Tomography must be used in all patients with suspected middle ear malformation and in older children with suspected inner ear malfunction. In suspected disease of the internal auditory meatus and cerebropontine angle, systematic radiography with tomography of the internal auditory meatus is recommended at all ages.

Hearing Tests

These include behavioral testing and physiologic tests.

BEHAVIORAL TESTS. Behavioral testing is done differently for different age groups. Infants are usually tested by means of a free field examination during which both ears are tested simultaneously and the child's reactions to sounds are noted. Usually pure tones to which the infant does not respond optimally are not used. As the child matures, more sophisticated and accurate testing can be carried out using very simple conditioning techniques, eg, the child is conditioned to put a block in a basket each time a sound is heard. Behavioral and hearing tests in infants and young children are very difficult tasks. There are too few well-trained, clinical audiologists who can obtain precise, reliable, and repeatable results.

Most children about 3 years of age can be tested by conventional audiologic means. A set of earphones is placed on the child and his threshold for pure tones is

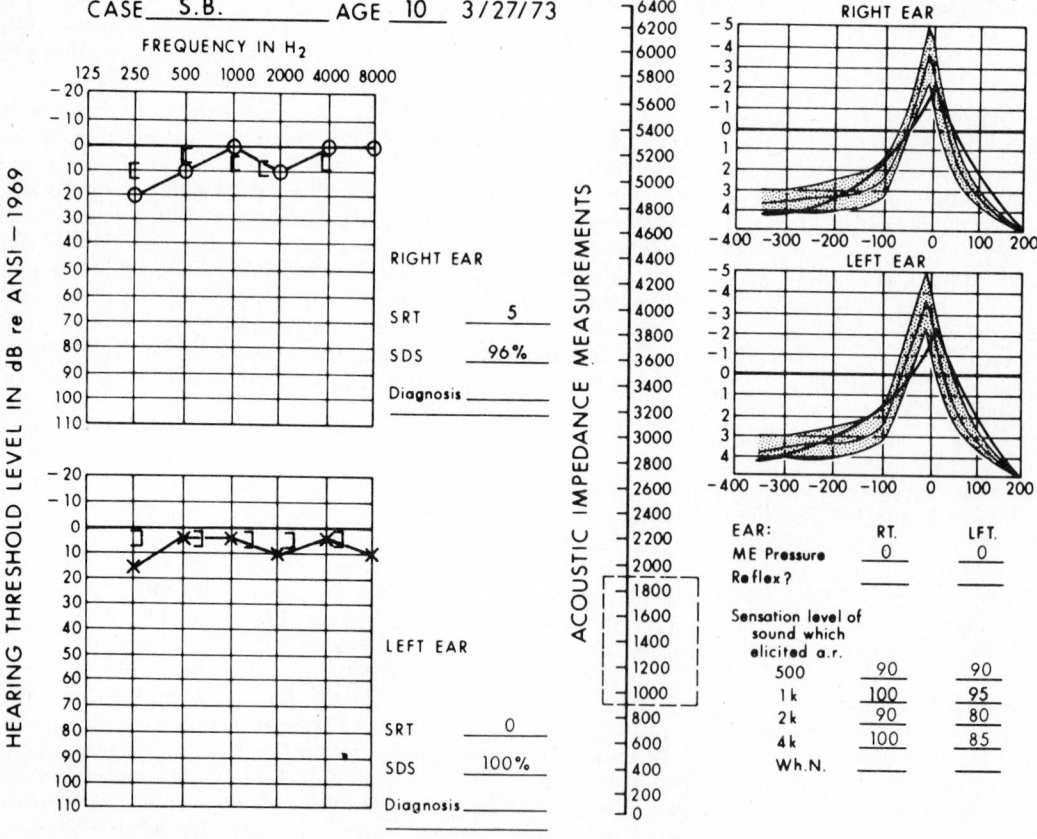

FIG. 4 Normal audiogram. On the left is the standard audiometric test. O = right ear conduction; [= right bone conduction; x = left ear air conduction;] = left bone conduction; SRT = speech reception threshold; SDS = speech discrimination score. On the right are the impedance function studies The tympanogram is in the upper right hand corner. ME = middle ear pressure; AR = acoustic reflex.

measured by air conduction and recorded on an audiologic form (Fig. 4). The hearing loss is given in decibels (dB). The greater the number of decibels, the greater the hearing loss. The one overall measure of the child's hearing is an average of the three speech frequencies: 500, 1000, and 2000 Hz.

There is much controversy as to what normal hearing should be. Normal hearing and average hearing range are not identical. Even with a mild loss of 10 to 20 dB, a child may have significant problems in learning and adaptive behavior; a loss greater than 30 dB will cause significant impairment. Losses greater than 20 dB should require some form of therapy—medical, surgical, or habilitative—to enable the child to acquire speech and language.

After the air conduction tests, a bone conduction test should be carried out. Again, the threshold value for the various frequencies is obtained. If both ears are similar in their air conduction threshold, or if one ear has a much lower threshold, the better ear should be masked by sound to prevent that ear from hearing the bone conduction sound. Masking is also performed in cases in which there appears to be a unilateral hearing loss, as the head will attenuate sound by only about 60 to 70 dB. A deaf ear may possibly appear to hear when it actually is receiving sound from the other side and gives a false audiogram called a shadow curve.

Tests are also made of the ability to discriminate sound by reading a list of phonetically balanced words (SDS) to the child at 30 to 40 dB above his speech reception threshold. The normal child should be able to distinguish more than 90 percent of such words. Difficulties in interpretation of the test arise when the language used is not the child's fundamental language. Special word lists have been prepared for Spanish-speaking children.

The loss of hearing is usually determined to be moderate, severe, or profound. The decibel notation is based on the pure tone average for the three speech frequencies and on the speech reception threshold (SRT). The SRT and pure tone average (PTA) should agree within plus or minus 5 dB.

PHYSIOLOGIC TESTS. IMPEDANCE TESTING. Measurement of acoustic impedance is very useful in the pediatric population. The impedance (p. 962) is measured by inserting a plug, which seals the ear, into the external auditory meatus. There are usually three connections leading into the external auditory meatus through the plug. One is connected to a pressure gauge, the second to a pure tone source, and the third to a calibrated microphone. The pressure in the external auditory meatus is equalized to that of the middle ear. Determination of the pressure in the middle ear is also useful in the diagnosis of eustachian tube dysfunction and serous otitis media. The intensity of the pure tone reflected from the tympanic membrane is then recorded by means of the tube connected to the microphone and is used to calculate the acoustic impedance. These determinations are carried out over a range of different pressures. The data are then plotted and the result is a quantitative measure of the physical properties of the tympanic membrane at different pressures. This graph is called a tympanogram (Fig. 4).

Impedance audiometry has been found useful in many screening activities. It is now used routinely for the assessment of hearing, especially in children with serous otitis media and in mentally retarded children in whom behavioral tests are difficult and unreliable. In a group of 50 mentally retarded children 60 percent were found to have a conductive loss.

ELECTROCOCHLEOGRAPHY. The electrical potentials generated from the hair cells of the inner ear, called the cochlear microphonics, and the VIIIth nerve action potentials can be recorded from either the external auditory meatus or the middle ear. This form of assessment requires specialized equipment and the use of averaging computers. Studies have shown that the risks in children are negligible. This mode of testing is primarily confined to those patients suspected of having a severe to profound hearing loss and/or for those in whom the behavioral test is either unreliable or its results ambiguous. The results of electrocochleography will give qualitative information concerning the severity of the hearing loss.

AUDITORY EVOKED RESPONSES. The recording of auditory evoked potentials from the central nervous system response to sound is another diagnostic tool used in children who are difficult to test. It also requires computer averaging and in some ways is similar to electrocochleography, although less reliable.

CONCLUSION. In testing a child's hearing, a combination of behavioral and impedance techniques will give precise and reliable information concerning the sound threshold, middle ear involvement, and types of disease that may be affecting the middle ear. In case of ambiguity, electrocochleography or auditory evoked response testing should be used if significant hearing loss is suspected. Every patient, regardless of age and psychologic or mental condition, can have a meaningful assessment of his hearing function with the use of current techniques. Any delay in diagnosis of hearing loss will result in a decreased ability to acquire speech and language, in intellectual retardation, and in severe psychologic disturbance.

Vestibular Testing

The vestibular portion of the inner ear can be easily assessed. In a study of the development of the vestibular response, infants with birth weights appropriate for gestational age elicited good vestibular responses, whereas in those who were small for gestational age the response was either very poor or absent.

Stimulation of the vestibular apparatus can be accomplished by rapidly rotating the child in order to produce nystagmus. The child is rapidly whirled around while held firmly in the arms, or in a more controlled fashion on a torsion swing or rotating chair. Most normal children, during the rotation, will have a short period of nystagmus, with the fast component moving in the direction of rotation. After the rotation has stopped, the fast component will reverse itself and move in the direction opposite to the rotation.

Irrigation of the external auditory canal with water at 35 to 44 C, ie, $\pm$ 4 C body temperature, is another means of inducing nystagmus. Normally, the fast component is directed away from the ear stimulated with cold water and toward the ear stimulated with warm water. If there is no reaction to this test, the external auditory canal should be irrigated with 3 ml of ice water. If nystagmus is not elicited, the ear may have hypofunction of the vestibular apparatus. The induced nystagmus can be recorded either visually or electronically. The visual observation of nystagmus is less satisfactory in young children in whom it may sometimes be difficult to assess cessation or direction of nystagmus. Electronystagmography, using the positive electrical potential between the cornea and the fundus, measures and records the voltage change produced by the movement of the globe in induced nystagmus. Duration, direction of fast and slow components, sensation, and other characteristics of nystagmus can be recorded easily.

Vestibular assessment is used primarily in children in whom the vestibular response is absent, as in some deaf children, especially those with deafness secondary to meningitis. A deaf child lacking a sense of balance may have a substantive delay in motor development which could be misinterpreted as mental retardation. The lack of an intact vestibular apparatus also can result in spatial disorientation in children who dive or swim underwater; drowning associated with such vestibular malfunction has been reported.

Facial Nerve Testing

The intimate relationship of the facial nerve to the temporal bone is very useful in diagnosing the source of pathology in both structures. The function of each of its branches can be tested. In a patient with peripheral facial paralysis the site of the facial nerve lesion can thus be determined. A deficit at a point in the internal auditory meatus where the facial nerve gives off a branch that provides fibers to the greater superficial petrosal nerve will cause diminution of tearing in the ipsilateral eye. Interruption of the facial nerve proximal to the origin of the stapedius will cause a diminution or absence of the middle ear muscle reflex, which is detectable by using impedance function equipment. A lesion proximal to the origin of the chorda tympani will result in a loss of taste in the anterior two-thirds of the tongue on the ipsilateral side.

DISEASES

Congenital

Severe to profound congenital deafness occurs in about 1:1000 live births. The congenitally deaf child may have the potential for normal intelligence, but may not be able to utilize his potential because of speech and language deficits. Congenital deafness is acquired in about 45 percent, genetic in 20 percent, and unknown in 35 percent of cases. The unknown category may include a large number of genetic cases, which are probably autosomal recessive, and new dominant mutations. Congenital deafness is a common symptom of many diseases. The following is a discussion of the more important and readily diagnosable diseases.

RUBELLA. The incidence of deafness associated with congenital rubella is 30 to 50 percent. Other associated defects, such as cataracts, retinopathy, congenital heart disease, prematurity, microcephaly, thrombocytopenia, etc., will be present in severely affected children (p. 583). The combination of hearing loss, decreased visual acuity, and central nervous system pathology makes habilitation difficult. The viral infection persists in these children, and in some instances persistent rubella infection may produce a progressive disease, so that some of the hearing loss in rubella children may occur after birth. All children with congenital rubella should be followed for several years to note changes in hearing acuity. Occasionally there is a conductive hearing loss in addition to the severe neurosensory loss, due to minor growth abnormalities of the middle ear. These children can be diagnosed using impedance assessment.

OTHER PRENATAL INFECTIONS. The *cytomegalic virus* is suspected of being one of the causes of congenital deafness, although there are few well-documented cases. The protozoa *Toxoplasma gondii* has been implicated, both clinically and pathologically, as a cause of congenital deafness, but is not common. Deafness resulting from *prenatal syphilis* is now also rare. It may be associated with other characteristics of congenital syphilis, including pear-shaped teeth and interstitial keratitis. The hearing loss is severe and of a neurosensory nature; it may present later in life, sometimes as a fluctuating hearing loss accompanied by dizziness.

KERNICTERUS. Children with severe kernicterus often have moderate to severe neurosensory hearing losses characterized by a greater loss in the high frequency tones. The lesion causing the hearing loss is thought to be gliosis of the secondary and tertiary acoustic nuclei. The hearing loss, which may not be detected for some years because of the residual hearing, can be alleviated by the use of a hearing aid. Moderate to severe hearing loss or high-tone loss will adversely affect speech and language development, as well as behavior. Since expectation for speech, language, and behavior would be based on the false premise that the hearing is normal, without a correct diagnosis the child will be inappropriately managed.

PREMATURITY. In a considerable number of children severe congenital deafness results from prematurity. The mechanisms responsible for hearing loss are not known, but it is thought that anoxia may be a contributing factor by causing nervous system damage.

OTOTOXICITY. Certain ototoxic medications traverse the placenta and result in neurosensory hearing loss. This has been most clearly documented for streptomycin and quinine. Consequently, any history of ototoxic therapy of the mother during gestation should prompt a detailed assessment of the child's hearing.

DEAFNESS WITHOUT ASSOCIATED ABNORMALITIES.   Pedigrees of inherited congenital deafness without associated anomalies have been well documented. These can be inherited as dominant, autosomal dominant, autosomal recessive, or sex-linked recessive traits. Neurosensory hearing loss of severe degree usually occurs, but it may be moderate or characterized by a high-tone loss. Unilateral deafness can also be inherited as an autosomal recessive or dominant. There are a number of kindred in whom congenital malformations of the middle ear, especially the footplate of the stapes, are inherited as autosomal dominant. Because these present with only moderate conductive hearing losses, diagnosis may be delayed.

CONGENITAL DEAFNESS ASSOCIATED WITH PIGMENTARY CHANGES.   Several deafness syndromes are associated with pigmentary changes. The most common is the *Waardenburg syndrome* (Fig. 5), which is inherited as an autosomal dominant. The syndrome (p. 895) consists of lateral displacement of the inner canthi of the eyes, prominent broad nasal root; a growing together of the eyebrows white forelock; heterochromia of the iris, and congenital deafness, either bilateral or unilateral. This syndrome is found in all racial groups throughout the world. The white forelock may disappear after the first year and, in some instances, there may be premature graying of the hair. The heterochromia of the iris will often not become apparent until after the first 6 months after birth. *Leopard syndrome*, in which the patient's skin is covered with multiple lentigines, is inherited as an autosomal dominant, with variable penetrance. The syndrome is also associated with ocular hypertelorism, pulmonary stenosis, abnormal genitalia, retardation of growth, and a profound to severe neurosensory hearing loss. *Albinism with congenital neurosensory hearing loss* is inherited as an autosomal dominant, autosomal recessive, or sex-linked.

CONGENITAL DEAFNESS ASSOCIATED WITH CARDIAC ABNORMALITIES.   Three well-recognized syndromes are associated with cardiac anomalies: the Leopard syndrome, Jervell-Lange-Nielsen syndrome, and pulmonary stenosis associated with conductive deafness.

The *Jervell-Lange-Nielsen syndrome* is inherited as an autosomal recessive trait and is found throughout the world. The affected children have severe to profound congenital neurosensory hearing loss and present with syncopal episodes. Sudden death has occurred in more than 50 percent of reported cases, probably due to ventricular fibrillation. Diagnosis is made on electrocardiography, which shows prolonged Q-T intervals and abnormal T waves.

Several cases have been reported of *pulmory stenosis with conductive hearing loss,* which appear to be transmitted as an autosomal dominant trait. The hearing loss is usually moderate to severe and can be alleviated by means of a hearing aid.

CONGENITAL DEAFNESS ASSOCIATED WITH THYROID ABNORMALITIES.   Abnormal thyroid function has been associated with several types of congenital deafness. Probably the most common of these syndromes is *Pendred's disease*, which is inherited as an autosomal recessive. The affected individuals usually have a severe congenital neurosensory hearing loss and many will develop a goiter during the first decade. The abnormality of the thyroid appears to be due to inability of the thyroid gland to change inorganic to organic iodine. The goiter is benign and is effectively treated with thyroid replacement (p. 1676). Deafness may also occur with endemic cretinism (p. 1671).

CONGENITAL DEAFNESS ASSOCIATED WITH EYE DISEASE.   *Retinitis pigmentosa* (Usher's syndrome), which is inherited as an autosomal recessive trait, is the most frequent form of congenital deafness associated with eye disease. The child is born with severe neurosensory hearing loss. There is also, in the first few months of life, a detectable pigmentary change in the retina, which continues to degenerate throughout

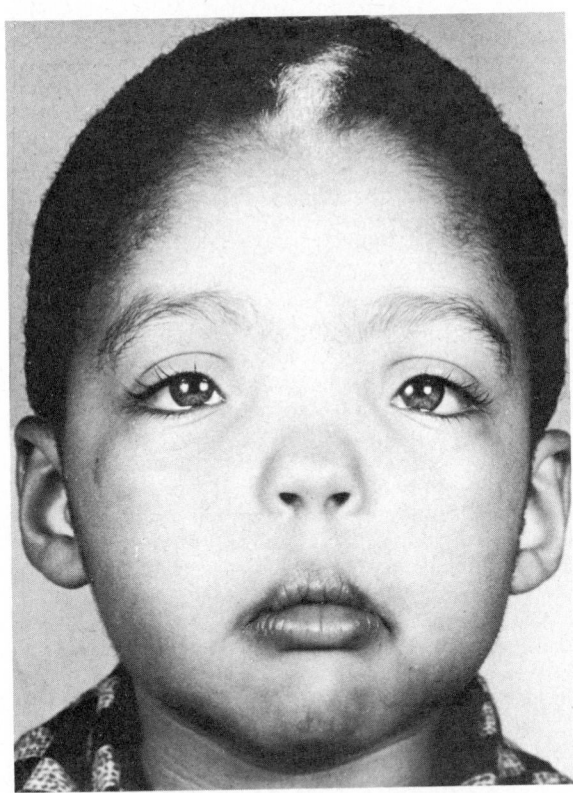

FIG. 5.   Patient with Waardenburg's syndrome. The patient has bilateral profound neurosensory hearing loss, a white forelock, increased intercanthal distance, abnormal medial canthi, blue eyes, and eyebrows which are beginning to join the midline. The nasal route is also somewhat broader than usual. (From Ruben RJ et al.: Otorhinolaryngology, Medcom Famous Teachings in Modern Medicine. New York, Medcom, 1971)

life. The first eye symptoms are a loss of night vision and a decrease in the visual fields, resulting in tunnel vision; in the second to third decade, many become functionally blind. The syndrome is often not diagnosed until after the eye signs become grossly apparent. Routine ophthalmoscopy is advisable in all congenitally deaf children, especially when there is a higher risk for autosomal recessive disease, as in consanguinity. Laurence-Moon-Biedl syndrome, which is characterized by obesity, hypogenitalism, polydactylia, and mental retardation, may be assoicated with retinitis pigmentosa and neurosensory hearing loss. About 10 percent of patients with the Laurence-Moon-Biedl syndrome have significant hearing loss.

CONGENITAL DEAFNESS ASSOCIATED WITH ABNORMAL FACIAL FEATURES.   *Mandibular facial dysostosis,* or Treacher-Collins syndrome, is inherited as an autosomal dominant with variable penetrance, a high mutation rate, and/or a large number of phenocopies. It consists of downward sloping of the palpebral fissure, causing antimongoloid slanting of the eye; coloboma, usually in the outer portion of the lid; hypoplasia of the facial bones—maldevelopment of the outer ear and/or middle ear; malocclusion; high-arched palate; macrostomia; blind fistulae between the corner of the mouth and ears; and atypical hair growth extending to the cheek. The hearing loss is usually conductive because of the malformation of the external auditory canal and middle ear.

In Goldenhar's *oculoauricular vertebral dysplasia* (p. 1996), the hearing loss is usually conductive and secondary to malformations of the external and middle ear. The *oto-palatal-digital syndrome* is inherited as a possible recessive and consists of conductive deafness, dwarfism, cleft palate, hypertelorism, broad nasal root, microsomia, and frontal occipital bossing. Congenital malformations of the external auditory canal and middle ear are also associated with Crouzon's craniofacial dysostosis (p. 1980) and Apert's acrocephalosyndactylia (p. 1987).

CONGENITAL   EAR   MALFORMATIONS. Atresia of the external auditory canal results in conductive hearing loss. Malformations may also affect the middle ear or both outer and middle ears. All ear malformations, even minimal deformities of the pinna, have a strong association with structural anomalies of the genitourinary tract, eg, horseshoe kidney, hydronephrosis, hypospadias, for which the patient should be investigated.

The bony labyrinth of the inner ear can also be affected by malformations. These cover a broad range from total aplasia of the inner ear to minor malformations of one of the semicircular canals. They can be diagnosed by radiography. Major malformations are frequently seen in anencephalics. Any infant with deafness due to a major malformation of the bony labyrinth should be suspected of associated central nervous system malformation.

Preauricular sinuses can be inherited or sporadic. Some patients with inherited preauricular sinuses also have conductive and/or neurosensory hearing losses.

These sinuses may become infected or drain and may require surgical removal.

Infections

VIRAL INFECTIONS.   The *herpes zoster virus* can infect the pinna, external auditory meatus, tympanic membrane, ear, and facial nerve. In this clinical complex, called the Ramsey-Hunt syndrome, small 1 to 2 mm blebs appear on the pinna and external auditory canal, associated with unilateral neurosensory hearing loss and facial nerve paralysis. The facial nerve paralysis usually resolves spontaneously, whereas the neurosensory hearing loss may be permanent.

In *bullous myringitis,* the tympanic membrane is covered with large, occasionally blood-filled blebs that cause pain but resolve spontaneously. Secondary bacterial infection may result in otitis externa and/or otitis media.

Mumps virus in infancy can infect the inner ear and cause profound neurosensory hearing loss, usually, but not always, unilateral. The inner ear infection is usually asymptomatic and without associated vestibular symptomatology. The hearing loss is, in general, discovered after the infection subsides. *Measles and smallpox* viruses, especially in the Orient, have been implicated as the cause of profound neurosensory hearing loss secondary to infections of the inner ear.

BACTERIAL INFECTIONS.   PINNA AND EXTERNAL AUDITORY CANAL.   The most common causative agent is *Pseudomonas aeruginosa,* and infection is not infrequent after swimming. The external auditory canal becomes very edematous. Since there is little subcutaneous tissue in the external auditory canal, swelling causes extreme pain, which is greatly exacerbated by even the slightest movement of the pinna. After the edema subsides, the external auditory canal is often filled with exudate and cellular debris, which may have to be cleared. Otitis externa can also follow acute or chronic otitis media due to contents of the middle ear draining into the external auditory canal.

Abscesses of the pinna and external auditory canal, usually due to *Staphylococcal aureus,* should be incised and drained. If there are any signs of systemic infection, appropriate antibiotics should be given. Infections of the preauricular sinus should first be treated with antibiotics and the sinus subsequently removed surgically.

ACUTE OTITIS MEDIA AND ACUTE MASTOIDITIS. Acute otitis media is among the most common problems in pediatric practice, and virtually every child has at least one infection. The most common etiologic agents are Pneumococcus and *H. influenzae,* but hemolytic streptococcus, *Neisseria,* and enteric bacteria may be responsible. Malformations of the palate and nasopharynx predispose to otitis media. Recurrent infections are common in children with cleft palate due to malfunction of the eustachian tube (p. 957), and in children with Apert's disease, Crouzon's disease, and Turner's syndrome. Frequent attacks of acute otitis occur in children with immune deficiency diseases and with hematologic disorders.

An upper respiratory infection often precedes the ear

infection. Otalgia, fever, and irritability are the main presenting features, but in infants, diarrhea and vomiting are common. In infants who are unable to express their complaint of ear pain, the diagnosis may not be made readily; it is important to consider this diagnosis in neonates, and particularly in premature infants, as it may present serious problems.

The diagnosis of otitis media is made by examining the tympanic membrane, which shows a loss of translucency and of landmarks. The drum may be red and inflamed, or covered with exudate; fluid levels often are seen behind it. Spontaneous rupture may create a small hole through which pus drains into the external canal; the fluid often is draining in a pulsatile manner. In otitis media, the pinna does not, as in external otitis, produce pain on movement. Most patients have a polymorphonuclear leukocytosis, but this may not occur in the neonate, particularly the preterm infant.

Tuberculous otitis media is rare and is usually not painful and not associated with fever. Often there are other evidences of tuberculosis, such as cervical adenopathy. The tympanic membrane often has several small perforations in tuberculous otitis.

With proper therapy and in the absence of predisposing factors, most instances of acute otitis media will resolve without sequelae, such as serous otitis media, chronic otitis media, labyrinthitis, meningitis, or facial nerve paralysis. Facial paralysis is related to the frequent presence of a congenital dehiscence in the bony covering of the facial canal in the middle ear. Appropriate antibiotic therapy and myringotomy usually result in complete recovery.

Occasionally acute otitis media will result in acute mastoiditis; this probably results from blockage of the aditus ad antrum by edema or an inflammatory polyp. Acute mastoiditis typically presents 1 to 2 weeks after the acute otitis media. Swelling behind the pinna, due to the collection of pus that has drained through necrotic bone from the mastoid to the space under the temporalis muscle, will displace the pinna anteriorly. Acute mastoiditis may also present as an abscess from the tip of the mastoid cell, draining into the sternocleidal mastoid muscle (Bezold's abscess) or draining extracranially through the zygomatic arch cell (zygomatic abscess). These three types of abscesses are often associated with collapse of the superior wall of the external auditory meatus, caused by free pus entering through the bony portion of the external auditory meatus and collecting under the skin of the external auditory canal. Radiographs of the mastoid in acute mastoiditis show a loss of the fine trabeculations of the mastoid cells, or a diminution of their clarity. These abscesses should be treated with both appropriate intravenous antibiotic therapy and surgical drainage.

CHRONIC OTITIS MEDIA AND TYMPANOMASTOIDITIS. Chronic otitis media and tympanomastoiditis are usually the result of acute otitis, especially in those children who are predisposed to recurrent acute otitis media. Both conditions manifest as chronically draining ears, usually accompanied by conductive hearing loss. Examination reveals a perforation of the tympanic membrane and occasionally a polyp in the external canal protruding from the tympanic membrane. The perforation may be large, involving almost the entire lower two-thirds of the drum, or it can be small in the pars flaccida. Chronic otitis media or tympanomastoiditis can produce serious sequelae. The chronic infection can cause destruction of the ossicular chain, leaving a permanent conductive hearing loss. Large tympanic membrane perforations usually do not heal spontaneously and also result in conductive hearing loss. Cholesteatoma and polyps are associated with chronic otitis media. A polyp is usually pathognomonic of an underlying cholesteatoma.

Cholesteatoma is a benign tumor of a thin layer of squamous epithelium that sheds its epithelial debris into a sac and usually rests on a layer of granulation tissue. It is felt to be due to either invagination of squamous epithelium from the lateral surface of the tympanic membrane, or metaplasia of the respiratory mucosa lining the middle ear cavity. Some cholesteatomas are congenital in origin (p. 969). Cholesteatomas are usually found in the posterosuperior portion and middle ear and present with small perforations in the posterior portion of the pars flaccida. There often is little or no discharge from the ear. As they grow they erode bone and also serve as the cause for continuing infection of the ear. Their growth destroys the ossicular chain and may erode the bony capsule of the facial nerve, with resulting paralysis. They also erode the superior and posterior walls of the mastoid cavity, impinging upon the dura of the middle and posterior cranial fossae and allowing for the formation of epidural and subdural brain abscesses and/or meningitis. Rarely, they may be found in the apex of the petrous portion of the temporal bone, where they can affect the trigeminal, oculomotor, facial, and statoacoustic nerves, causing decreased facial sensation and facial pain, lateral rectus palsy, deafness, vestibular impairment, and facial nerve paralysis (Gradenigo's syndrome).

Chronic otitis media may also result in a change in the lining of the middle ear and tympanic membrane, known as tympanosclerosis, which on otoscopy appears as white depostis of calcium in the middle layer of the tympanic membrane. Tympanosclerosis of the middle ear can immobilize the ossicular chain with significant conductive hearing loss.

Labyrinthitis is another complication of chronic otitis media, which can be either bacterial, causing irreversible deafness, or irritative and present as vertigo and hearing loss, which may be reversible.

Chronic otitis media is most frequently due to *Pseudomonas aeruginosa;* Staphylococcus, and Streptococcus are also common. Occasionally, acute necrotizing otitis media secondary to streptococcus may occur without antecedent chronic otitis media.

SEROUS OTITIS MEDIA.   Serous otitis media is a very common and frequently undiagnosed middle ear disease. It is due to a collection of sterile thin or viscid fluid in the middle ear. The condition has been called "glue ear." The symptoms in young children are subtle, usually consisting of irritability and mild or moderate conductive hearing loss. Occasionally the child may pull or rub the ear, but severe pain or fever are not associated with this condition. The tympanic membrane is thickened and pale or opaque, and normal landmarks are lost, but there is no inflammation. Air fluid levels often can be seen behind the tympanic membrane, which moves sluggishly or not at all on pneumo-otoscopy; sometimes the drum is markedly retracted medially, apparently because the eustachian tube is not able to open properly to equalize air pressure. Middle ear mucosa subjected to repeated episodes of either acute or serous otitis media undergoes metaplasia, with an increase in the number of secretory cells and in the amount of secretion into the middle ear cleft.

Serous otitis media occurs in virtually every patient with a cleft palate or other nasopharyngeal malformation. It also is common with pharyngeal obstruction of the eustachian tube, due to adenoidal hypertrophy and nasopharyngeal tumors. Children with serous otitis media are more prone to acute otitis media. In addition, psychologic and behavioral problems may result from hearing loss. Children with intermittent or chronic mild to moderate hearing losses during the language formative years, from birth to 5 to 6 years, often have a significant decrease in their verbal and language abilities. It is thought that alleviation of the hearing impairment can prevent the psychologic and intellectual consequence.

Diagnosis of the disease is based primarily on a high index of suspicion and is made by otologic examination but primarily by impedance assessment. Serous otitis media characteristically increases the impedance and produces a large negative pressure in the middle ear.

INNER EAR.   Bacterial infections of the inner ear are usually associated with infections of the middle ear or with bacterial meningitis, and generally result in a permanent, profound neurosensory deafness. The infection proceeds through the round or oval windows, or is secondary to cholesteatoma, which has eroded part of the bony capsule of the inner ear. They are serious and may spread to the meninges. Bilateral labyrinthitis following bacterial meningitis is a relatively common cause of profound neurosensory deafness in children. All children with meningitis should have their hearing tested after recovery. Occasionally bacterial labyrinthitis may follow temporal bone fractures.

FUNGAL INFECTIONS.   Fungal infections of the middle ear are uncommon and usually occur in the external auditory meatus as a complication of external otitis. Candida infections of the middle ear may occur in children with other debilitating diseases.

Neoplasms

Tumors of the ear are rare in childhood, the most common being acquired cholesteatoma and polyps. Congenital cholesteatomas usually are found in the petrous portion of the temporal bone. Rare cases of glomus tumor (paragangliomas), benign chondromas, and osteomas have been reported in the middle ear cleft. Monostotic fibrous dysplasia of the temporal bone has been observed in which the bone overgrowth re-

sults in stenosis of the external auditory canal, blockage of the eustachian tube, chronic otitis media, and conductive hearing loss.

Acoustic neuromas of the statoacoustic nerve, benign tumors of the temporal bone, have been reported in the first and second decades, presenting as unilateral deafness. They initially affect the superior vestibular portion of the statoacoustic nerve and then the cochlear division. The tumors have been found bilaterally and are transmitted as an autosomal dominant trait.

Eosinophilic granulomas are diagnosed by biopsy and respond well to treatment (p.1228). Rhabdomyosarcomas grow very rapidly. They usually present as a tumor of the pinna or external auditory canal. The treatment is a combination of radiotherapy, chemotherapy, and surgery, but the prognosis is poor.

Degenerative Diseases

The inner ear may be involved by genetic degenerative diseases which may, or may not, be associated with other anomalies. The hearing loss may affect all frequencies or only high or low frequencies. The age of onset and rate of progression are variable.

The most common degenerative condition of the inner ear is associated with *Alport's syndrome.* This syndrome is probably transmitted as an autosomal dominant, with variable penetrance and greatest effect in males. A progressive high-tone hearing loss, usually the first symptom to appear, is associated with glomerulonephritis. The renal disease, which often leads to renal failure and death, especially in males, should be recognized early if treatment is to succeed. All children with high-tone hearing loss, especially if their hearing loss is progressive, should have a thorough renal workup.

Congenital deafness is also associated with *renal tubular acidosis,* inherited as a possible autosomal recessive. Two rare autosomal recessive diseases, associated with neurosensory hearing loss, are *Refsum's disease,* an abnormality of phytic acid metabolism, and *Norrie's disease,* in which the child is born blind and then develops progressive neurosensory hearing loss.

Genetically determined bony diseases may result in mixed conductive and neurosensory hearing loss. *Osteopetrosis* (p. 2016). when inherited as an autosomal recessive, appears in early infancy. Hypertrophy of the bone, which narrows the foramina of the nerves, may cause blindness as well as deafness. Radiographic findings are quite pathognomonic. *Osteogenesis imperfecta* (p. 2011), inherited as an autosomal dominant with variable penetrance, is almost always associated with mixed hearing loss due to the abnormal development of the ossicles and otic capsule. *Otosclerosis,* an autosomally dominant inherited disease, is confined to the ear and usually manifests itself as a progressive conductive hearing loss in the third decade. However, in a significant number of patients hearing loss begins in the second decade. Otosclerosis must be differentiated from congenital malformations of the footplate of the middle ear in which results of surgery are considerably less favorable.

Acquired degenerative disease in the inner ear can result from the use of ototoxic drugs, most commonly kanamycin, neomycin, dihydrostreptomycin, streptomycin, gentamycin, aspirin, and quinine. Whenever these drugs are used for prolonged periods or if there is any suspicion of renal failure, the patient should be monitored with serial audiography and, in some instances, with serial electronystagmography. If labyrinthine involvement can be detected early and the drug discontinued, total loss of labyrinthine function can sometimes be prevented. Occasionally degeneration of the inner ear cannot be arrested.

Meniere's syndrome is rare in children. It is characterized by episodic vertigo, neurosensory hearing loss, nausea, and vomiting (p. 972). Idiopathic facial palsy, or *Bell's palsy*, occurs in children, often in association with pain in the mastoid region. The paralysis is usually total but most cases resolve spontaneously.

Trauma

Injuries to the pinna may result in hematoma, which can become infected. The hematoma and/or the abscess may cause destruction of the cartilaginous framework of the pinna, causing a deformed or cauliflower ear.

Foreign bodies in the external auditory canal can damage the canal and rupture the tympanic membrane. This may also result from an improper attempt to remove the foreign body. A foreign body in the ear of a child should be removed under general anesthesia with the aid of an operating microscope and proper instruments. Removal of foreign bodies from the ear of an awake child is quite painful and very difficult. It may cause the foreign body to be impacted further into the external auditory canal and possibly rupture the tympanic membrane. Improper removal of a foreign body may even result in fracture of the ossicular chain, with permanent conductive hearing loss or even a neurosensory hearing loss.

Temporal bone fractures occur with severe head injuries and may affect the middle ear, the inner ear, or both. They can result in conductive, neurosensory, or mixed hearing loss, and/or facial nerve paralysis, depending on the structures involved. Unless there are indications for immediate surgery, as in sudden facial nerve paralysis, they should be observed. About 60 percent of cases with conductive hearing loss will resolve spontaneously in 3 to 6 weeks, while those with neurosensory hearing loss show little or no improvement. Patients with conductive hearing loss who do not improve may need some form of surgical therapy.

Cerebrospinal fluid otorrhea is a serious complication of temporal bone fractures. It develops when the fracture involves either the posterior or middle cranial fossa. The cerebrospinal fluid may drain through the ruptured tympanic membrane or down the eustachian tube into the nasopharynx. Cerebrospinal fluid otorrhea will usually subside spontaneously. The use of "prophylac-

tic" antibiotics in noninfected cases is controversial. Infected cases should be treated with appropriate antibiotics. Any temporal bone fracture increases the risk for later development of meningitis, as the temporal bone heals by fibrous and not bony union. The fibrous healing creates a potential pathway to the meninges for the flora of the upper respiratory system, via the middle ear and mastoid.

Sound trauma is occasionally seen in children and more often in adolescents. Loud blasts, such as from a firecracker held next to the ear, can cause a permanent loss of hair cells in the inner ear, with resulting neurosensory hearing loss. Constant exposure to loud noise, such as guns and high-intensity amplified sound, may produce a partial hearing loss. Significant individual susceptibility exists to sound trauma. Hearing loss from sound trauma usually affects only the higher frequencies.

Allergy

A number of cases of external otitis media develop on an allergic basis. A special instance is represented by children who become allergic to their hearing aid inserts. The use of a nonallergic type of hearing aid bulb may solve this problem. Occasionally, allergic otitis externa, usually in association with allergic serous otitis media, occurs in children with severe asthma or general allergy. The middle ear mucosa is similar to other respiratory mucosa in that it reacts to allergens. Many cases of serous otitis media are thought to be related to allergy.

DIAGNOSIS

Hearing Loss

The type, extent, and etiology of any hearing loss must be determined. Hearing loss may be conductive, neurosensory, or mixed. The extent can be either mild, moderate, severe, or profound, or only a portion of the frequency spectrum may be abnormal. This can be measured with the use of the various audiometric tests described above (p. 964).

Determining the etiology of hearing loss in order to provide proper therapy, habilitation, and/or genetic guidance is most difficult in the congenitally deaf child. Not all studies should be performed in every child. The possibility of genetic deafness should be assessed by family history and by ascertaining whether or not there is consanguinity. Audiometric studies of parents and siblings can uncover unsuspected hearing losses and help to confirm the diagnosis of genetic disease. Children with malformations of the external or middle ear should be investigated for possible genitourinary malformations. Whenever deafness is suspected of being congenital, rubella antibody titers should be obtained in serum samples from the patient and the mother. Ophthalmologic and neurologic examinations are important. One study has shown that 23 percent of the genetically deaf have major neurologic, and 26 percent significant ophthalmologic abnormalities. Deafness is rarely an isolated manifestation of a disease process. The objective of assessing the child with a hearing loss is to uncover not only the etiology but associated lesions.

The earlier the diagnosis of hearing loss is made, the better the results for the child. Neonatal screening tests have been moderately successful in defining congenitally deaf infants. Maintenance of a high-risk registry is helpful in pointing out which infants may be at risk. A combined high-risk registry and neonatal screening program should reveal most deaf infants. The consequences of delay in diagnosis of a hearing loss are very serious. The child may be considered retarded and/or psychotic and receive incorrect therapy for these conditions. Delaying appropriate treatment may lead to retardation and behavioral disturbances.

Mentally retarded children appear more sensitive to a hearing loss than children with normal intelligence. Even a moderate hearing loss in the mentally retarded child may aggravate intellectual and behavioral retardation. It is important to assess the hearing ability of all these children.

Vestibular impairment often results in delayed motor development. If it is associated with congenital deafness, the likelihood is great that the child will be diagnosed as mentally retarded.

Otitis

External otitis should be differentiated from secondary external otitis associated with acute or chronic otitis media. A foreign body in the external canal may cause infection, with edema and exudate, and an incorrect diagnosis of external otitis media may be made.

The differential diagnosis of acute otitis media includes the Ramsey-Hunt syndrome (herpes zoster of the external auditory canal, neurosensory deafness, and facial paralysis), otitis externa, bullous myringitis, tympanosclerosis, and hemotympanum, a rare condition that presents with decreased hearing, conductive hearing loss, and a blue appearance of the tympanic membrane. *Hemotympanum* is due to a collection of blood in the tympanic membrane; it is not associated with great pain and usually resolves spontaneously, although a myringotomy may be necessary. The myringotomy must be done with great caution, since occasionally the bulb of the jugular vein, unprotected by its bony cover, protrudes as a blue mass behind the inferior portion of the tympanic membrane.

The diagnosis of acute otitis media in young infants and neonates is sometimes difficult. A surprisingly high incidence of acute and chronic otitis media has been found at autopsy of newborn, particularly premature, infants. Acute otitis media should be considered in the differential diagnosis of irritability and diarrhea in young infants.

Chronic otitis media or tympanomastoiditis is diagnosed by history and examination. Intermittent discharge from the ear is common and is often exacerbated by upper respiratory infections. Cholesteatoma, or tumors of the ear, should be considered in all cases. In some cases of chronic otitis media with cholesteatoma, normal hearing may be present as the cholesteatoma can complete the ossicular chain. The diagnosis of chronic otitis media should be based on a combination of intermittent drainage from the ear, abnormal tympanic membrane, perforation, positive radiographs, and usually, but not invariably, a conductive hearing loss.

In serous otitis, the initial presenting symptoms may seem unrelated to the ear. The patient may be seen because of an apparent behavioral problem, poor school work, or inattentiveness secondary to the intermittent hearing loss. Serous otitis media is a disease with exacerbations and remissions, and several examinations may be necessary to make the diagnosis.

Dizziness, Vertigo, and Nystagmus

Dizziness, vertigo, and nystagmus in any child should be correlated with the anatomic location and, if possible, to the specific disease. The following investigations should be carried out to differentiate between inner ear, VIIIth nerve, eye, and/or central nervous system disease: physical examination of the ear, the eye, and the central nervous system; audiologic impedance evaluation; electronystagmographic analysis of vestibular function; and radiographs of the skull and temporal bones.

Congenital nystagmus is not to be confused with spasmus nutans in which nystagmus is associated with voluntary head nodding and torticollis (p.1939). Spasmus nutans usually begins 1 to 2 months after birth, whereas congenital nystagmus is present within the first few weeks. Spasmus nutans usually resolves, whereas congenital nystagmus may persist beyond the fifth year.

Acquired nystagmus may be due to blindness, central nervous system disease, or labyrinthine dysfunction (p. 1748). Nystagmus from inner ear disease is usually horizontal, whereas nystagmus from central nervous system disease may be vertical, rotary, pendular, or horizontal. Electronystagmographic analysis usually shows a decrease in vestibular function in cases of labyrinthine disease; they also often have dizziness and vertigo.

Primary labyrinthitis presents with sudden vertigo, and the patient has residual unsteadiness to which he adjusts within a few months. In secondary labyrinthitis due to chronic otitis media or cholesteatoma, vertigo is usually episodic and not severe; the examination will reveal the chronic otitis. Occasionally both vertigo and nystagmus may be elicited by changing the pressure in the middle ear by pneumo-otoscopy. A tumor of the VIIIth nerve will present as intermittent episodes of unsteadiness; the patient usually does not have true vertigo, ie, the sensation of rotary movement; and the hearing tests will point to an VIIIth nerve lesion. Meniere's syndrome is associated with repeated episodes of severe vertigo, which may last for hours or days, often accompanied by nausea and vomiting. The associated hearing loss will have the audiometric characteristics of cochlear involvement.

Facial Nerve Paralysis

Testing of the facial nerve may localize the lesion. In facial nerve paralysis due to central lesions, the muscles of the forehead are not involved because they have a bilateral supply from upper motor neurones. Congenital peripheral facial palsy, Mobius syndrome, is often associated with middle and inner ear malformations and is inherited as an autosomal dominant. Facial nerve paralysis may be associated with trauma during delivery and is thought to be secondary to compression of the fallopian canal in the middle ear. Temporal bone fractures may cause peripheral facial nerve paralysis at any point along its course. Tumors of the internal auditory meatus often cause peripheral facial paralysis. All cases of facial nerve paralysis need an otologic examination, radiography of the temporal bone, audiometric and impedance assessment, and vestibular testing.

TREATMENT

External Otitis

The initial treatment, after collecting culture material from the external ear, aims at reducing the edema and relieving the pain. Burow's solution (2 percent acetic acid in aluminum acetate) on a cotton wick kept damp with the solution is maintained in place for 1 day. Then, eardrops combining corticosteroids and appropriate antibiotics are used; about 5 drops are instilled four times a day for one week. In case of fever or other systemic signs, appropriate antibiotics may be indicated. Exudate and cellular debris should be removed gently once or twice a week until the infection subsides.

Acute Otitis Media and Acute Mastoiditis

After cultures are taken from the nasopharynx and if the tympanic membrane is perforated from the external auditory canal, initial treatment includes ampicillin orally, 100 to 150 mg/kg/24 hours for a minimum of 7 days, and an oral decongestant for 3 to 5 days. The antimicrobial agent may be continued or modified in accordance with culture results or clinical response. Patients with acute mastoiditis, or with facial nerve paralysis, labyrinthitis, or meningitis should be hospitalized and treated with immediate myringotomy and appropriate intravenous antibiotics in high doses. Pus should be examined by direct smear and culture.

Chronic Otitis Media and Tympanomastoiditis

The treatment is primarily surgical; it is elective and designed to alleviate disease, create a safe ear, and whenever possible to restore hearing. If there is only tympanic membrane perforation, reconstruction of the tympanic membrane should be performed after con-

trolling infection. Cases of suspected or confirmed cholesteatoma should have immediate surgery to remove the mass, in view of the risk of serious complications. Immediate surgery is also indicated in cases of labyrinthine, facial nerve, or central nervous system involvement.

Serous Otitis Media

Nasal decongestants may be tried for a 5-day period; this is not usually successful as most cases are secondary to anatomic or functional disturbances in the eustachian tube. If the otitis is not relieved within 2 to 3 weeks, or if it recurs repeatedly, surgery may be indicated. In some children, adenoidectomy alone is adequate, while in others myringotomy is also indicated. An allergic evaluation is most important, as treatment of allergies may relieve the condition (p. 345). If these procedures are not successful, insertion of ventilating tubes into the tympanic membrane is recommended; this is done under general anesthesia but can be performed as ambulatory pediatric surgery. The tubes permit middle ear pressure to be equal to atmospheric pressure and, it is felt, may permit the mucosa to revert to normal. Replacement is necessary if the tube becomes clogged or is displaced. The duration for maintaining tubes in place is variable, but in some cases, as in children with cleft palate, they have been kept in place for 3 to 6 months. In about 10 percent of cases, acute otitis media develops, requiring local, or if indicated, systemic antibiotic therapy. Indications for the use of ventilating tubes is a subject of some controversy at this time.

Congenital Malformations

Minor malformations of the pinna can be successfully treated by reconstructive surgery; the results are less satisfactory with major anomalies. Since pinna malformations do not interfere with hearing, the effects are largely psychologic. Since surgical reconstruction may require numerous procedures, it should be delayed until adolescence. At that age the patient can cooperate and can participate in the decision as to whether the procedure should be done. Many may elect to hide the malformed ear with their hair.

In malformations of the external auditory canal and middle ear, hearing can be restored by use of a hearing aid. Minor anomalies can usually be treated surgically with success. With major malformations, the chances for establishing normal hearing are not very good, and there is the risk of producing facial nerve paralysis or total deafness. Unilateral anomalies do not impair hearing and do not require treatment in early childhood.

Deafness

Severe and profound deafness detected in early infancy can be treated by use of hearing aids and intensive auditory training. There are special infant auditory training centers in many areas. The parents will carry out most of the early habilitative therapy but constant medical supervision of the deaf child is needed to detect progressive hearing loss or other diseases. Whether or not a child should be instructed only in oral communication, sign language, or in both, is still very controversial. It is felt that it is most important that the child acquire language of any sort; once a language basis is established, more sophisticated oral communication can be developed.

In older children and adolescents who have moderate to severe neurosensory hearing losses, the only therapy available is the use of a hearing aid, combined with proper aural habilitation. Many of these children will not accept the hearing aid. Ideally, the patient should achieve acceptance of the aid by himself, a process that takes considerable patience and support from parents and physician. Hearing aids also are useful in children with moderate or significant hearing loss in which surgical therapy cannot restore normal hearing, as in refractory serous otitis media and bilateral tympanomastoiditis. Although the patient appears to hear, the hearing is greatly diminished and there may be substantive difficulty in school. These patients should be encouraged to wear their hearing aids continually.

In children with profound unilateral hearing loss it is important to arrange for proper seating in the school room. Some older children may avail themselves of a special hearing aid, called a Cros aid, which has a microphone on the deaf side and a speaker on the hearing side. Thus, the child will be able to hear with the good ear the sound transmitted from the deaf side.

Children with vestibular dysfunction should be discouraged from participating in activities that require vestibular orientation, particularly diving and underwater swimming.

Most communities have some structure for supplying either diagnostic and/or habilitative resources for the hearing-impaired child. Information about community resources can usually be obtained from otorhinolaryngologic clinics, hearing and speech centers, and handicapped children's programs, which exist in each state. Any child with a hearing loss should be considered as a child with a treatable disease. The problems in securing the most efficacious treatment are not only medical but are tied to the social, economic, political, and philosophic attitudes in each community.

Bibliography

Bland RD: Otitis media in the first six weeks of life. Pediatrics 49:187, 1972

Bonding P, Lorenzen E: Chronic secretory otitis media: Long term results after treatment with grommet tubes. Oto-Rhino-Laryngology 36:227, 1974

Brookhauser PE, Bordley JE: Congenital rubella deafness. Arch Otolaryngol 98:252, 1973

Brun RA: Deafness in Laurence-Moon-Biedl syndrome. Br J Ophthalmol 34:65, 1950

Crowley DE, Davis H, Beagley HA: Survey of the clinical use of electrocochleography. Ann Otolaryngol 84:297, 1975

Dudding BA, Gorlin RJ, Langer LO: The oto-palatal-digital syndrome. A new symptom complex consisting of deafness, dwarfism, cleft palate, characteristic facies and generalized bone dysplasia. Am J Dis Child 113:214, 1967

Eviatar L, Eviatar A, Naray I: Maturation of neurovestibular responses in infants. Dev Med Child Neurol 16:435, 1974

————Eviatar A: Vertigo in childhood. Clin Pediatr 13:940, 1974

Fine PJ: Deafness in infancy and early childhood. New York, Medcom Press, 1974

Fraser GR, Froggatt P, James TN: Congenital deafness associated with electrocardiographic abnormalities, fainting attacks and sudden death. Q J Med 33:361, 1964

————Association of congenital deafness with goiter—Pendred's syndrome. Ann Hum Genet 28:201, 1965

————Causes of profound deafness in childhood. In Wolstenholm GEW, Knight J (eds): Sensorineural Hearing Loss. London, Churchill, 1970, p 5

Friedmann I, Fraser GR, Froggatt P: Pathology of the ear in the cardioauditory syndrome of Jervell and Lange-Nielsen and recessive deafness with electrocardiographic abnormalities. J Laryngol Otolaryngol 80:451, 1966

Glorig A, Gerwin K: Otitis Media. Springfield, Ill. Thomas, 1972

Gorlin RJ, Anderson RC, Blaw M: Multiple lentigines syndrome complex consisting of multiple lentigines, electrocardiographic conduction abnormalities, ocular hypertelorism, pulmonary stenosis, abnormalities of genitalia, retardation of growth, sensory neural hearing loss and autosomal hereditary pattern. Am J Dis Child 117:652, 1969

Hall J: Cochlea and the cochlear nuclei in asphyxia. Acta Otolaryngol Suppl 194:1, 1964

Holm VA, Kunze LH: Effect of chronic otitis media on language and speech development. Pediatrics 43:833, 1969

Howie VM, Ploussard JH: Otitis media: a clinical and bacteriological correlation. Pediatrics 45:29, 1975

Iversen UM: Hereditary nephropathy with hearing loss: Alport's syndrome, Acta Pediatr Scand Suppl 245, 1974

Johnson WW: Survey of middle ears: 101 autopsies of infants. Ann Otolaryngol 70:377, 1961

Konigsmark BW: Hereditary deafness in man. N Engl J Med 281:713;774;827, 1969

Melish ME, Hanshaw JB: Congenital cytomegalovirus infection. Am J Dis Child 126:190, 1973

Nance WE, Unger EJ, Sweeney A: Evidence for autosomal recessive inheritance of the syndrome of renal tubular acidosis with deafness. Birth Defects 7:70, 1970

Nutilla A: Dystrophia retinae pigmentosa—Dysacousis syndrome, A study of Usher's or Halgren's syndrome. Am J Hum Genet 18:57, 1970

Peckham CS, Sheridan M, Butler NR: School attainment of seventeen-year old children with hearing difficulties. Dev Med Child Neurol 14:592, 1972

Rapin I: Hypoactive labyrinth and motor development. Clin Pediatr 13:922, 1974

————, Ruben RJ, Lyttle M: Diagnosis of hearing loss in infants using auditory evoked responses. Laryngoscope 80:712, 1970

Rees DO, Collum M, Bowen DI: Radiographic aspects of oculo-auricular vertebral dysplasia. Br J Radiol 45:15, 1972

Refsum S: Heredopathia atactica polyneuritiformis. J Nerv Ment Dis 116:1046, 1952

Ruben RJ: Development of the inner ear of the mouse: a radioautographic study of terminal mitoses. Acta Otolaryngol Suppl 220:1967

————, Rozycki D: Diagnostic screening for the deaf child. Arch Otolaryngol 91:429, 1970

————Rozycki DL: Clinical aspects of genetic deafness. Ann Otolaryngol 80:255, 1971

Stool SE, Randall P: Unexpected ear disease in infants with cleft palate. Cleft Palate J 4:99, 1967

————, Anticaglia J: Electric otoscopy, a basic pediatric skill. Clin Pediatr 12:420, 1973

Van de Calseyde P, Blaton V, Peeters H: Protein pattern of middle ear effusion in serous otitis media behind an intact drum. Acta Otolaryngol 71:153, 1971

Waardenburg PJ: A new syndrome combining developmental anomalies of the eyelid, eyebrows and nose root with pigmentary defects of the iris and head hair, with congenital deafness. Am J Hum Genet 3:195, 1951

Warburg M: Norrie's disease. Acta Ophthalmol Suppl 89, 1966

Wilber LA: Significance and detection of conductive lesions in children with multiple handicaps. J Commun Disord 7:31, 1974

Worthington EL: Index: Handbook of Ototoxic Agents, 1966-1971. Baltimore, Johns Hopkins University Press, 1973, pp 439

Young DF, Eldredge R, Nager R, et al.: Hereditary bilateral acoustic neuroma. Birth Defects 7:73, 1971

CHAPTER 22

Gastrointestinal Tract

MURRAY DAVIDSON, *Associate Editor*

NORMAL GASTROINTESTINAL TRACT

DIGESTION AND ASSIMILATION

Digestion, absorption, and assimilation of foodstuffs in infants and children are similar to those in adults. However, in infancy gastrointestinal capacity and digestive ability are limited and the gastrointestinal tract is more easily upset. During periods of stress, particularly those imposed by infection, the infant's intestinal tolerance may be impaired to such an extent that nutrition cannot be maintained through the usual pathways for digestion and assimilation. By 2 years of age most of these limitations are no longer operative.

GASTROINTESTINAL MOTILITY

Sucking and Swallowing

Opening and closing movements of the mouth have been demonstrated prenatally in human fetuses as young as 8.5 weeks. Newborn infants weighing more than 1,500 g usually have little difficulty coordinating sucking and swallowing. Consecutive sucks occur in small bursts of 3 to 4 in the neonate and in more efficient groupings of 10 to 30 after several days of life. The mechanism has been studied by recording pressures in the oral cavity and by cineradiographic techniques with both artifical and natural nipples coated with radiopaque materials. The infant grasps the nipple between tongue and hard palate, and alternate suction and compression help pass the milk to the pharynx. Suction is created by withdrawing the tongue from the hard palate, and compression is created by its reapposition to that surface. It has been documented that the volumes obtained from artifical nipples under normal conditions are the same as those provided from the mother's breast. The infant can breathe during this process because continuity of the respiratory tract is not interrupted. With onset of swallowing there is sudden elevation of the posterior part of the tongue, which forces the contents of the posterior pharynx into the esophagus, while the epiglottis simultaneously closes the entry to the larynx and the muscles of the soft palate close the entry to the nose. When the act of swallowing is initiated, a variable amount of air is present in the posterior pharynx. A portion of this air is swallowed and propelled by the bolus of food acting as a piston. By the age of 6 months the average child is no longer able to coordinate sucking and swallowing with breathing. The pattern at this age becomes more like that of the adult, in whom breathing and swallowing occur at different times. Attempts to do both simultaneously may result in aspiration.

Attempts of a young infant to move semisolid food to the back of his mouth with his tongue are clumsy during the early weeks of life; by the age of 3 months he is usually able to do this easily. Thus efforts to administer such foods prior to this age sometimes meet with failure. Newborn infants generally exhibit no difficulty in passing swallowed material to the stomach, despite the fact that records made in the first days of life demonstrate incoordinated esophageal peristaltic activity. In most infants the pattern rapidly becomes normal, although in mental retardates uncoordinated and delayed swallowing patterns may persist for several weeks.

Gastric Motility

Interpretation of the data on the emptying of the infant's stomach is difficult because of variations in techniques of study by different authors. Influences such as the state of health of the infant, his degree of hunger at the time of study, the type of meal fed, the times and volume of feeding, the possible psychic stresses induced during radiographic studies, and the positions in which studies are performed are variables that have been largely uncontrolled. Air has been demonstrated to traverse the pylorus within minutes after birth. The pylorus will open almost immediately as feedings reach it. In one study the average time for opening of the pylorus after a barium meal reached the cardia was 90 sec. Infants fed in the upright position or on their right sides displayed the shortest interval between the time the barium meal entered and left the stomach. However, in other positions emptying was only slightly longer. Air was also less likely to pass into the duodenum when the infants were fed upright than when fed in other positions.

The motility of the stomach is markedly affected by the addition of fat to a meal. When fat first enters the duodenum and absorption begins, it evokes the elaboration of enterogastrone, a hormone that inhibits gastric motility and secretion. As a result, a fatty meal stays in the stomach much longer than a fat-free meal. Saturated fatty acids are particularly effective in delaying stomach emptying. Among other ingested materials, large milk curds or chunks of solid food also delay opening of the pylorus.

Emptying is retarded if the stomach contains increased amounts of mucus or if the muscular tone of the organ is lax—conditions normally present in low-birthweight infants and induced in larger infants and children by fever, infection, and states of malnutrition.

Factors contributing to earlier emptying are feedings of larger volume and of increased carbohydrate content, greater degrees of denaturation or fragmentation of protein particles, and low temperature of foods. Osmolality of ingested food also plays an important role. Relatively isosmotic material passes through the pylorus more readily than extremely hypotonic or hypertonic foods. Studies of emptying time of the stomach in low-birth-weight infants by use of aqueous or milk mixtures with barium have demonstrated significant emptying in 3 to 4 hours on all feedings; complete emptying occurs by 5 hours with aqueous mixtures and by 7 to 8 hours with milk. Variations ranging from 1.5 to 25 hours for complete emptying have been reported in full-term infants.

Intestinal Motility

Transit time through the intestines has been measured in only a limited number of children using relatively crude techniques such as feeding of colored markers, manometry, and radiography. Wide variations are reported in all age ranges. Lönnerblad found that the small-intestine transport time of a barium meal varied from 0.5 to 6 hours in patients less than 1 year old. Radiographs of the small intestine in infants differ from those seen in older children and adults in that the contrast medium progresses more slowly, appears in clumps, and usually does not have the feathery appearance caused by the intestinal mucosa. The explanation of this difference is a matter of dispute, attributed by some to an increased secretion of mucus in early life, by others to difficulty in fat assimilation. Development of the normal adult pattern commonly takes place by the end of the first year, but it is delayed in the presence of the malabsorption syndrome.

Two types of motility occur in the large intestine. Closely approximated segments may simultaneously be engaged in different types of resting activity involving mixing of contents or exchanges of fluid, electrolytes, and nutriments. In other periods these local patterns are diminished, and coordinated propulsive motility supervenes to push the colonic contents analward. Such coordinated mass movements occurring during feeding produce the gastrocolic reflex. Fluid introduced into the sigmoid or descending colon induces a propulsive state toward the terminal rectum, while fluid introduced into the rectum produces immediate relaxation and accommodation by this intestinal segment, slowly followed by patterns associated with fluid absorption.

DEFECATION

Although passage of material through the gastrointestinal tract from the upper esophagus to lower colon is under autonomic control, defecation is entirely a voluntary act. Although it has not been confirmed by sufficient study, it may be possible that peristalsis in the colon induced by feedings results in bowel movements in infants. However, normal individuals do not usually defecate involuntarily beyond the initial months of life, regardless of the vigor of colonic peristalsis. Instead, material projected into the rectum distends that organ. If the volume is appreciable or if the process occurs when there is a particularly resistant state of rectal muscular tone, receptors in the lower rectal mucosa are activated to set up the reflex urge to defecate. Voluntary expulsion occurs following increase in intraabdominal pressure by the Valsalva maneuver, during which there is descent of the diaphragm and contraction of the rectus muscles. It is necessary that this increased force against the pelvic contents be coordinated with simultaneous squatting and application of leverage via the feet to pinch off the upper rectum from the rest of the colon by action of the pelvic sling muscles. If such leverage is not applied, squeezing of the rectal contents may aid in retention, with gradual subsidence of the urge to defecate and additional drying of the mass.

DIGESTIVE SECRETIONS AND ABSORPTION

Mouth and Pharynx

The normal adult secretes from 1 to 2 liters of saliva daily; accurate measurements of daily volume of saliva are not available in infants and children. The parotid component is relatively watery, whereas the submaxillary gland produces both aqueous and mucinous fractions. Electrolyte levels are always hypotonic relative to serum, but they have been shown to rise with increased secretory rates and to be somewhat higher in the neonatal period. The protein content is mainly from amylase and mucopolysaccharides, including the blood group fractions and immunoglobulins, especially IgA. The quantities of saliva and salivary amylase are reported to be small for several weeks after birth, but they are apparently adequate for the needs of the infant's digestion. Beyond 3 months of age amylase is found in increasing amounts, particularly if starch is fed.

Stomach

Coagulation of casein is an important gastric function usually attributed to rennin. However, this enzyme, which is present in the gastric juice of the newborn calf, has not been demonstrated in the human infant. Gastric acidity aids in milk curdling, the solubility of casein being minimal at the isoelectric point (pH 4.7). Gastric pepsin also has milk-clotting properties. The curd of breast milk, which is low in casein, is soft and friable, in contrast to that of raw cow's milk, which is tough and less easily broken up and digested. Measures to influence the character of the curd have played a large part in the history of artifical feeding.

The volume of gastric secretion and its acidity have been measured early in life and are at adult levels in a considerable proportion of both low-birth-weight and full-term newborn infants. However, beyond the first days of life the ability to secrete acid is impaired for a number of weeks, especially among infants of low birth weights or in malnourished children of higher weights. The increase in volume and acidity of gastric secretion in response to histamine stimulation in older children has been found similar to that of adults, using weight or surface area as a standard of reference.

It is thought that proteolytic digestion does not occur to any appreciable degree in the infant's stomach, since pH levels beyond the immediate newborn period are commonly above 4.0 in the breast-fed infant and over 5.0 among those who are bottle-fed. At these levels of acidity conversion of pepsinogen to pepsin is impeded, since peptic digestion is effective only at a pH below 3.0. Nevertheless, some gastic proteolysis does occur at the higher pH that prevails in early life. This activity may be attributed either to the higher plasma pepsinogen levels of the first weeks of life, resulting apparently from supplemental maternal cortiocosteroids, or to the presence of the enzyme cathepsin, which is effective over a wider range of pH that extends from 2.0 to 5.0. Pure cathepsin has not been isolated, but its activity has been demonstrated to be distinct by heating and inactivating pepsin at 70 C.

Small Intestine

Most protein hydrolysis is accomplished by the peptidases of pancreatic juice that are secreted in inactive zymogen forms and are activated by a variety of agents, including enterokinase, from the duodenal mucosa. The active peptidases of the pancreas include trypsin, chymotrypsin, and the carboxypeptidases. At least four other enzymes that have effects on digestion of protein or nucleic acids have been isolated from pancreatic secretions: pancreatic elastase, pankrin, ribonuclease, and deoxyribonuclease. Although the precise kinetics of the individual enzymes have not been studied in infants, proteolytic activity has been demonstrated even in young low-birth-weight infants. Failure of protein hydrolysis is virtually confined to situations in which insufficient pancreatic secretions enter the intestine. The most frequent cause in children is cystic fibrosis of the pancreas (p. 993). It may also occur in rare cases of congenital atresia of the common bile duct in which the pancreatic duct empties into the atretic bile duct. Failure to activate the precursor forms of the peptidases because of a congenital enterokinase deficiency may infrequently simulate conditions in which pancreatic secretions are excluded. Unsplit protein may also appear in the stools because of tough curd formation in the stomach, inadequate mastication of solid foods, or states of hyperperistalsis.

There is some controversy as to whether proteins are completely broken down to amino acids before absorption or whether in the course of digestion certain polypeptide complexes are absorbed intact. Although it has been shown that biologic traces of unsplit protein are absorbed and it may be presumed that the same is true of peptides, their importance as nutrients has not been demonstrated. Peptide levels in portal blood are negligible. However, high titers of enzymes capable of protein hydrolysis are found in mucosal cells, and polypeptides can be shown to disappear from the intestinal lumen before digestion. Thus, although the hydrolysis of proteins to amino acids in the digestive tract is believed to be virtually complete under normal conditions, there is limited evidence suggesting auxiliary avenues of digestion. Absorption of amino acids occurs in the upper small intestine. The L forms in low concentration may be absorbed against a concentration gradient, suggesting specific active transport mechanisms. In high concentrations absorption may occur principally by simple diffusion.

Salivary and pancreatic amylase digestion of starch and glycogen results in splitting of more than 90 percent of these substrates into maltose and the remainder (which come from the branching points of chains in the polysaccharide structures) into isomaltose. Pancreatic amylase is delayed in development; it reaches full activity at 4 to 6 months of age. Maltose, isomaltose, and two disaccharides that occur naturally (sucrose and lactose), together with other rare disaccharides, are hydrolyzed by specific disaccharidases into their component monosaccharides. The disaccharidases are located in the outer cell layer of epithelium of the intestinal villi, mainly (although not entirely) concentrated in the brush border. Complete hydrolysis probably takes place at this membrane, although some may occur within the mucosal cell after absorption of the disaccharide.

At least four and perhaps five individual disaccharidases are present that are capable of digesting maltose. Two of these are also able to split sucrose, and one can hydrolyze isomaltose. Two β-glycosidases capable of hydrolyzing lactose have been described, one concentrated in the brush border and the other in the cytoplasm of the mucosal cells. Significant sucrase and isomaltase activities are demonstrable in the 12-week fetus. Maltase activity develops more slowly, but all of the α-glycosidase activites are comparable to those of adults by 6 to 7 months of fetal life. The β-glycosidases develop more slowly and reach normal levels of activity only at the end of gestation. Babies born prematurely usually display decreased lactase activity during the first 3 days of life. On a comparative basis, maltase activity is about three times as great as that for sucrase-isomaltase and six to eight times greater than that for lactase in the normal child. Lactase activity usually decreases gradually after the first year of life, and only rarely is the level of activity of this early period maintained into adult life. The enzymes are distributed relatively evenly over the entire small intestine, but activities are somewhat lower in the duodenum and terminal ileum.

Glucose and galactose are absorbed against a concentration gradient by an active transport mechanism that is energy- and sodium-dependent. It is generally believed that fructose is absorbed by passive diffusion; however, some authors believe that it, too, is absorbed by an active process of a very low order of magnitude. The absorption of monosaccharides facilitates absorption of water and sodium (solvent drag).

Faulty splitting of disaccharides, followed by their unmodified appearance in stools, is rare and is confined to disaccharidase deficiency states. Starch may escape digestion to a variable extent under normal circumstances. Intracellular starch, which is present in vegetable cells unruptured by processing, is often demonstrable in normal stools. Starch that is extracellular (ie, from ruptured vegetable cells) often appears in stools of young infants. Unfortunately such starch is often regarded as indicative of incomplete digestion due to inadequate amylase activity; however, it has been shown that it results from release of starch from the cellulose coating in which it was encased when it passed to the lower colon following bacterial digestion of the cellulose.

Balance studies of carbohydrate digestion and absorption do not provide valid information, since the unabsorbed carbohydrate is fermented in the intestine. Holt and Somersalo overcame this difficulty by feeding ^{14}C-tagged carbohydrate; they found more than 98 percent absorption of ingested starch, even by low-birth-weight infants.

A negligible amount of fat splitting occurs in the stomach, although some emulsification results from mechanical activity there. Triglyceride is insoluble in the luminal water. Secreted pancreatic lipase functions at the oil water interface and splits off the two α fatty acids leaving a β monoglyceride. The secreted bile salts are amphiphilic, i.e., one end of the molecule is water soluble (polar) and the other is lipid soluble (nonpolar). They orient so that their nonpolar ends surround the lipid soluble fatty acids and monoglycerides and produce a physiochemical complex called a micelle. Since all of the polar portions of this complex face outward to the water interface, the micelle is rendered soluble. The micelle disaggregates at the intestinal mucosa and the fatty acids and monoglycerides are absorbed through the trilaminar lipoprotein membrane of the intestinal cell. The bile salts remain in the lumen and pass to the ileum, where they are reabsorbed to enter the bloodstream and be reexcreted in the bile. This recirculation of conjugated bile salts is referred to as the enterohepatic circulation.

Absorbed fatty acids and monoglycerides are reesterified in the upper intestinal mucosa to triglycerides; they become encased by lipoproteins, cholesterol, and phospholipids to form chylomicrons and pass through the mucosal cells to the lacteals and the lymphatic system in this form. It is believed that triglycerides of fatty acids below 10 carbons (short- and medium-chain) are able to be absorbed intact and to pass directly into the portal circulation.

Overall fat digestion and absorption are readily measured by means of fat balance. After the neonatal period, 95 percent of the intake of most fats is absorbed. Slightly lower figures are often obtained during the early weeks of life, and markedly reduced figures are encountered in premature infants. The chemical constitution of the fat affects the ease of absorption, short-chain fats and those containing unsaturated linkages being more readily assimilated. The premature infant commonly absorbs from 40 to 85 percent of the intake of butterfat. In the belief that the difficulty of fat absorp-

tion in premature infants might be limited to absorption through the lacteals, Snyderman and her associates fed fats with extremely short chains (tributyrin and triaxetin) and found that these materials were absorbed almost completely. We have demonstrated a deficiency of bile salt secretion in small prematurely born infants that correlates with their degree of steatorrhea. As the babies grow the elaboration of bile salt improves, and fat absorption proportionately increases.

The assimilation of fat in conditions of malabsorption is favored by finer mechanical subdivision or by surface-active agents such as bile salts; however, the effect is very small. Treatment with surface agents seems indicated only in patients in whom bile salts are deficient, such as those with biliary atresia or with surgical removal of the ileum, which is the site of bile salt reabsorption. In patients with other forms of malabsorption, the use of fats with higher proportions of short-chain fatty acids or unsaturated fatty acids may improve absorption. According to Holt, an even more effective method of increasing fat absorption is to give more fat, since the percentage of ingested fat that is absorbed is appreciably influenced by the intake. Hence, even though the stool loss is increased by increasing the intake, the absolute quantity of fat absorbed is also increased correspondingly.

FLUID EXCHANGE AND COLONIC FUNCTION

There is no portion of the gastrointestinal tract of man in which the mucosa may be regarded as impermeable to movement of water in either direction. Net changes in amounts of water at any point are dependent on many factors: the state of hydration of the individual, the quantities of water available in the intestinal tract, the effects of feeding, the osmolality of gastrointestinal contents, the nature of the luminal solutes and their normal mechanisms of digestion and absorption, the site within the intestinal tract, and the tonus of the intestinal musculature. Techniques devised to assess these factors often lack specificity and precision. Balance studies are relatively crude and unphysiologic. Investigations using isolation of segments between balloons are subject to undetected errors such as leaks. Many calculations are based on assumptions of unidirectional flux in a system that almost constantly undergoes multidirectional flux, ie, into and out of the mucosal cells. Finally, it is not possible to assess the constant influences on luminal contents of additions from and losses to the adjacent segments of the intestinal tract.

The handling of water appears to be passively linked to that of solutes in terms of both quantity and rate of movement. Expressed in terms of unit serosal surface area, the rates of influx of water from isotonic solutions are approximately equal in the jejunum and ileum; both appear to be more rapid than that in the colon. However, limited measurements have indicated that the mucosal surface area, per unit length or per unit serosal surface, is greater in the jejunum than in the ileum. This ratio is also considerably higher in all areas of the small intestine than in the colon. This implies that the unidirectional flow rates per unit mucosal surface are faster in the colon than in the small bowel and faster in the ileum than in the upper small intestine. However, the osmotic permeability of all areas of the small and large intestine is sufficiently high that solute transport from isotonic solutions is quickly followed by flow of enough water to maintain isotonic conditions in the gut lumen.

Although the underlying mechanism for absorption of isotonic solutions is not entirely defined, most workers infer from available data that it is based on active sodium transport. Various studies indicate that sodium and water absorption are facilitated by the solvent drag effect of active glucose absorption in the upper small intestine. These effects seem less influential in the lower ileum or colon. Differences in patterns of sodium and water movements are also apparent from studies with adrenal hormones. Levitan and associates were unable to show any effect of aldosterone on ileal water and electrolyte composition, but they found significant increases in colonic sodium absorption. In our own studies of colonic absorption of sodium we have observed that the absence of intraluminal potassium produces a movement of potassium out of the mucosa while sodium from isotonic fluids moves in the opposite direction, although the exchange is not stoichiometric. The mechanism is probably responsible for the fact that the ratio of sodium to potassium in ileal water is reported to range from 12 to 1 up to 20 to 1, whereas in the stool the ratio is less than 1 to 3. Chloride absorption and bicarbonate secretion in the small and large intestine have a similar relationship, but are influenced considerably by intraluminal pH and by serum potassium levels. With hypokalemia and tissue potassium depletion the permeability of gut mucosa to chloride is adversely affected.

The colon of the normal adult normally absorbs about 400 ml of water per day; the figure for infants is probably proportionately higher. Various calculations have shown that this colonic activity represents less the 20 percent of the total fluid and electrolyte absorbing capacity and suggest why resection of extensive portions of the colon is usually followed rapidly by readjustment and fairly normal stool formation.

Material arriving in the rectum is usually semiliquid. This is the final area for water absorption, and the consistency of the stool passed is determined largely by the activity of the segment. The young infant has a smaller capacity for retention of material in the rectum than the older child and the adult; this results in stools that have a smaller volume and an increased water content and are passed more frequently.

INTESTINAL BACTERIA AND STOOL

Bacteria are usually absent from the gastrointestinal tract at birth, but they invade it quickly via both mouth and anus within the first hours of life. By the end of 24 hours an intestinal flora is firmly established. The duodenum, particularly the first portion, is usually sterile, a phenomenon attributed to the discharge of acid chyme from the stomach. Farther down the intestinal tract, organisms are found in increasing numbers, being most abundant in the colon. Aerobic cultures reveal the ever-present coliform organisms and many varieties of lactobacilli, streptococci, and staphylococci. Yeasts are often found when special efforts are made to cultivate them. By far the most frequent organisms, in infants as well as adults, are various species of *Bacteroides*; these are pleomorphic, gram-negative, non-spore-bearing organisms that, being anaerobic, are not usually reported in stool cultures. The bacterial flora is influenced to a considerable extent by the diet. In the breast-fed infant lactobacilli are always conspicuous, and a gram-positive flora predominates; in artifically fed infants the proportions of protein and sugar in the formula affect the bacterial flora, a relatively high protein intake favoring the growth of the coliform organisms. Fatty acids tend to check the growth of a number of organisms, notably staphylococci. When fat is completely removed from the infant's diet, the stools tend to become loose and mushy for a variable length of time. What part the bacterial flora plays in this change is not clear.

The role of the intestinal bacteria in the maintenance of health would seem to be important, as has been demonstrated by studies of germ-free animals. Bacteria appear to be important for the synthesis of essential nutrients and also as natural sources of antibiotics that protect against pathogenic microorganisms. The known B vitamins are all synthesized by the intestinal bacteria, particularly by coliform organisms. It is not clear whether these are essential for human nutrition. However, useful synthesis occurs for folic acid and biotin, and there is evidence that synthesis in the intestine may be an important source of vitamin K in the early days of life.

In ruminant animals and in certain other herbivora the bacteria of the gut perform functions they do not perform in man: they are a major nutritional protein source, and enzymes they produce are capable of hydrolyzing cellulose and synthesizing ascorbic acid as well as certain essential amino acids.

Many intestinal microorganisms elaborate substances that inhibit the growth of other organisms. The colon bacilli are particularly noteworthy in this respect; they elaborate a variety of so-called colicins, the most powerful of which is colicin K. Demonstration that *Lactobacillus bifidus* is conspicuous in the flora of the breast-fed infant and that in circumstances of poor hygiene the breast-fed infant tends to suffer less from infection has led to the view that this organism possesses specific virtue in combating infections. A number of attempts have been made to encourage an abundant *L. bifidus* flora in infants. However, evidence is still awaited that a predominant growth of these organisms has virtue.

The intestinal bacteria may under certain circumstances exert untoward effects. They may compete with the body for available nutrients, and some of them, particularly certain strains of *Escherichia coli*, are potential pathogens to debilitated and small infants. Several strains with specific antigenic structure have been incriminated as etiologic agents in epidemics of infantile diarrhea. The presence of such strains in the stools of infants is not necessarily associated with disease, for they are at times found in healthy carriers. Enteropathogenic strains of E. coli are generally noninvasive and produce an enterotoxin which adheres to jejunal microvilli, is probably absorbed into the mucosal cell, and stimulates production of cyclic AMP. This leads to secretory diarrhea. Strains of E. coli not typable as enteropathogenic are reported to cause the "Traveler's Diarrhea" experienced by older children and adults by a similar mechanism. Certain strains of enteropathogenic E. coli have also been described that do not produce enterotoxin but cause a severe shigella-like diarrhea by invasion of the colonic mucosa. Whether enteropathogenic strains arise from mutations of nonpathogenic colon bacilli, whether they become pathogenic from transfer of R factors by known pathogens, or whether they are invariably acquired by contact is not clear.

The increased use of antibiotics and the popularity of high-protein diets have tended to destroy the balance of the intestinal flora, suppressing some organisms and permitting others that are potential pathogens to flourish. The emergence of resistant staphylococci and pathogenic strains of coliform organisms may well be related to these practices.

Although the importance of the stool as a guide to the feeding of infants was overemphasized in the past, there is no doubt that valuable information concerning the infant's digestion can be obtained from this source.

The first rectal discharges after birth consist of meconium. It is composed of bile and intestinal secretions high in nitrogenous and mucopolysaccharide content, with squamous epithelial cells and hair that have been swallowed in utero. The absence of epithelial cells in meconium may be of diagnostic aid in intestinal obstruction in the newborn. Normal meconium contains representative amounts of the amylolytic, tryptic, and lipolytic activities secreted by the pancreas. Bacteria are absent from meconium in the first hours of life. A dark brownish green semisolid, it is usually passed four to six times a day for the first 2 or 3 days. When the milk supply becomes well established, the appearance changes to that of normal milk feces.

The stools of a healthy breast-fed infant may have the color of egg yolk, but are usually paler and often green. The quantity passed in 1 day usually ranges from 30 to 45 g. They are seldom entirely smooth and homogeneous, but contain, in general, a large number of small light yellow particles. Their consistency is sometimes pasty, often rather loose, although never watery under normal conditions. They have a slighty sour but not unpleasant odor. The reaction is acid, usually between pH 4.5 and 5.1. This acidity is due largely to the presence of organic acids but partly also to carbon dioxide, the loss of which accounts for the reaction becoming less acid on standing. The number of stools passed by most breast-fed infants in the early weeks of life is from two to four daily. After the first month the usual number is two or three per day, although many infants have only one and others have four or more. The average child passes approximately 100 to 150 g of stool per day during the first 5 years of life. Stool water content may be up to 80 percent of a formed stool and is rarely less

than 70 percent. Total osmolality of a normal stool ranges from 200 to 250 mOsm/liter, the values increasing as stools become softer. Values for sodium and chloride are variable, but except in severe and prolonged diarrhea they are always considerably lower than simultaneous concentrations of these electrolytes in serum.

The stools of an infant fed on cow's milk are usually firmer, more homogeneous, and less frequent than those of a breast-fed infant. However, the stools of infants on low-protein formulas may more closely resemble the stools of breast-fed babies. In infants fed cow's milk the color of the stool is likely to be paler and the odor more unpleasant. The reaction is less constant and tends to be more alkaline, the pH ranging between 4.6 and 8.3. The undigested masses appearing in the stools of infants taking milk are usually spoken of as curds. In infants given raw cow's milk these may take the form of bean-sized lumps composed of coagulated casein with an envelope of soap. They are of no pathologic importance. A different type of curd that is small and white or yellowish white and consists almost entirely of fat is seen in conditions where fat is not being digested completely.

In the past, alterations in the gross characteristics of the stool were interpreted as indications of impairments in the digestion of protein, fat, or carbohydrate—a foul odor pointing to indigestion of protein with overgrowth of putrefactive bacteria, the presence of gross fat indicating fat indigestion, the presence of vegetable material or a frothy stool suggesting carbohydrate indigestion. Although these changes in the gross appearance of the stool do suggest incomplete digestion of specific foodstuffs, they give only qualitative information, not information concerning the quantity that is being digested. They should not be used as indications for withdrawing specific foods from the diet, as was done formerly.

The pigment of the infant's stool shows variations that are not seen in later childhood. Partly because of swallowed air and party because of the peculiarities of the intestinal flora on a milk diet, the reducing power of the infant's intestinal contents is distinctly less than in later life and is subject to greater variations. As a consequence the bilirubin of the bile is incompletely reduced to stercobilin; a variable amount of bilirubin is excreted unchanged, and bilirubin crystals can sometimes be identified in the stools microscopically. Bilirubin is readily oxidized by the oxygen of the air to green biliverdin. Because of such oxidation one frequently sees a yellow stool become green on standing.

Absence or diminution of biliary secretion results in pale stools. However, a pale stool in an infant does not necessarily mean that bile pigment is absent; it may be due to the fact that nearly all of the pigment exists as the colorless stercobilin. Such stools will darken on standing and are thus easily distinguished from acholic stools. The normal fecal color in older children is due mainly to dipyrrole pigments and to pigments formed in the intestine by bacterial action.

Abnormal pigments may be found in the stool after ingestion of various vegetables. Black stools may result from bleeding in the upper intestine, or they may occur with the administration of any heavy metal that forms a black sulfide, iron being the most common of these. Bacteria may contribute to stool color (eg, red staining of stools and diapers in the presence of *B. serratio*). Streaks of blood due to small anal fissures may be associated with constipated stools. In dysentery, flecks of blood and mucus are found. Larger hemorrhages may occur with any type of ulcerative lesion of the intestine. In intussusception the stools contain blood and mucus without appreciable quantities of fecal matter.

Microscopic examination of the stools gives little information that cannot be obtained on inspection. However, chemical examination has yielded information of fundamental importance in regard to the absorption of both organic and inorganic foodstuffs. The chief clinical value of stool analysis is in the disorders of fat assimilation. An excess of fat in the stools may be evident as gross steatorrhea, but the appearance is often deceptive, since chemical studies may reveal a marked loss of fat that has not been suspected. Impairment of fat assimilation cannot be accurately assessed by measuring the percentage of fat in individual stools, since this is subject to considerable variation. It may be recognized by balance studies or by measuring the total fat excreted over a minimum period of 3 or 4 days. Normally from 2 to 3 g of lipids are excreted per day by infants and young children; a daily excretion in excess of 5 g is evidence of poor absorption. When there is marked interference with absorption, the feces may contain more than 10 g per day. Defective fat absorption is seen in diarrheal states, in many acute and chronic infections, in prematurity, in celiac disease, in disorders of pancreatic secretion, and in bile salt deficiency syndromes.

Absence of significant quanitities of proteolytic enzymes in the stool occurs in cystic fibrosis of the pancreas and at times in other pancreatic disorders.

References

Ames MD: Gastric acidity in the first ten days of life of the prematurely born baby. Am J Dis Child 100:252, 1960

Ardran GM: A cineradiographic study of breast feeding. Br J Radiol 31:156, 1958

———— Kemp FH: A correlation between sucking pressures and movements of the tongue. Acta Paediatr Scand 48:261, 1959

———— Lind J: A cineradiographic study of bottle feeding. Br J Radiol 31:11, 1958

Borgstrom B, Lindquist B, Lundh G: Digestive studies in children. Am J Dis Child 101:454, 1961

Ebers DW, Smith DI, Gibbs GE: Gastric acidity on the first day of life. Pediatrics 18:800, 1956

Grayzel HG, Elkan B, Moghazeh M, Schneck L, Garza S: Plasma pepsinogen levels in the newborn. Am J Dis Child 103:759, 1962

Gryboski JD: The swallowing mechanism of the neonate. I. Esophageal and gastric motility. Pediatrics 35:445, 1965

Hirsch J, Ahrens EH, Blankenhorn DH: Measurements of the human intestinal length in vivo and some causes of variation. Gastroenterology 31:274, 1956

Holt LE Jr: Role of Carbohydrates in Infant Feeding. Advances in Chemistry, Series XII. New York, Interscience, 1955, p 104

Hood JH: Effect of position on amount and distribution of gas in the intestinal tract of infants and young children. Lancet 2:107, 1964

Hunt JN: The osmotic control of gastric emptying. Gastroenterology 41:59, 1961

Kron REJ, Ipsen J, Goddard KE: Consistent individual differences in the nutritive sucking behavior of the human newborn. Psychosom Med 30:151, 1968

Lönnerblad L: Transit time through the small intestine; a roentgenologic study of normal variability. Acta Radiol[Suppl] (Stockh) 10:88, 1951

Olsen E: Studies on Intestinal Flora of Infants. Copenhagen, Munksgaard, 1949

Salisbury DM: Bottle-feeding: influence of teat-hold size on suck volume. Lancet 1:655, 1975

Silverio J: Gastric emptying time in the newborn and the nursling. Am J Med Sci 247:732, 1964

Snyderman SE, Morales S, Holt LE Jr: The absorption of short chain fats by premature infants. Arch Dis Child 30:83, 1955

Strawczynski H, Beck IT, McKenna RD, Nickerson GH: The behavior of the lower esophageal sphincter in infants and its relationship to gastroesophageal regurgitation. J Pediatr 64:17, 1964

Symposium on physiology and pathology of digestion in infancy. Bibliotheca Paediatrica. Ann Paediatr [Suppl 64] Basel, Karger, 1957

Tantibhedhyangkul P, Hashim SA: Medium-chain triglyceride feeding in premature infants: effects on fat and nitrogen absorption. Pediatrics 55:359, 1975

Törnwall L, Lind J, Peltonen T, Wegelius C: The gastrointestinal tract of the newborn. I. Cineradiographic findings. Ann Paediatr Fenn 4:209, 1958

Symptomatic Conditions

VOMITING

Murray Davidson

In infants and young children, vomiting may occur from a great variety of causes; although some of these are trivial, vomiting may also indicate serious disease. A distinction is sometimes made between regurgitation (in which one or two mouthfuls of food are brought up at one time with little effort or distress) and true vomiting (in which the stomach virtually empties itself). As a rule regurgitation results from minor feeding disorders. Vomiting of larger volumes need not necessarily indicate serious disease, but if it is persistent and recurrent the symptom requires investigation.

The pathophysiologic mechanism of vomiting is often misunderstood and therefore symptomatically mistreated. In virtually all instances the stomach is atonic and distended, and the force for vomiting is supplied by strong contractions of the abdominal musculature. The column of food is usually not held up at the pylorus, but in the duodenum, which is in spastic contraction during nausea and vomiting; the afferent stimuli to the vomiting center in the central nervous system arise from the duodenum.

Only in those rare instances in which there is obstruction at the pylorus does vomiting occur from a stomach in which vigorous contractions are taking place. Thus hypertrophic pyloric stenosis is one of the few conditions in infants in which the stomach empties by reverse peristalsis, a condition that usually induces projectile vomiting.

NEONATAL VOMITING. In the newborn, vomiting may be benign and self-limited, probably caused by irritating material swallowed during the birth process. The presence of blood requires determination of the type of hemoglobin by alkaline denaturation (Apt test) to indicate its probable origin (maternal or infant). Intracranial pathology, septicemia, and certain metabolic abnormalities, particularly those associated with chronic acidosis, may result in persistent and projectile vomiting by a newborn. With congenital anomalies of the gastrointestinal tract, vomiting is common. Specific obstructive lesions are discussed later in this chapter. A history of polyhydramnios in the mother or the finding of a single umbilical artery at delivery should alert the physician to an increased likelihood of one of the congenital gastrointestinal anomalies. Bile-stained or fecal vomiting virtually always indicates gastrointestinal obstruction. Generally speaking, the higher the level of obstruction the earlier the symptoms appear. In malformations of the ileum, colon, or rectum, vomiting is less constant and appears later.

STOMACH OVERDISTENSION. Gastric overdistension is especially common in infants; it may result from swallowing air and/or from ingestion of too large a volume of food. The vomiting is not accompanied by other evidence of disease. It occurs effortlessly within a few minutes after nursing; it may be produced by moving the infant or by undue pressure on the stomach. Air swallowing, as previously explained, is normal. Excessive gastric air is one of the most common causes of overdistension and vomiting in the first 6 months of life. Breast-fed infants may swallow excessive air when the supply of milk is small or when the nipples are retracted. In bottle-fed infants it may result from feeding with a nipple with inadequate aperture. With both breast- and bottle-fed infants prolonged feeding time causes excessive air ingestion.

Some infants swallow air between feedings; this may be caused by sucking on pacifiers or by sucking the thumb or fingers. Hunger may at times lead to vomiting, because the infant is apt to suck other objects that are within reach and thereby swallow considerable air between feedings. However, in general the mother is more likely to believe that the infant's cry of discomfort is due to hunger and not to distension with air; this may lead to frequent feedings of excessive quantities of milk. Infants may not always indicate that they are satiated, and they will often respond to stimulation by the breast or bottle by sucking, even if this ultimately aggravates their discomfort.

In artificially fed infants the bottle should be held in a position that will keep the neck of the bottle always filled with liquid. Regurgitation due to air swallowing can be prevented by feeding the infant in the semierect position to maintain the air bubble at the cardiac end of the stomach, by limiting sucking periods to approximately 20 minutes, by encouraging intervals of about 4 hours between feedings, and by patiently holding the infant upright over the shoulder for a few minutes after feeding and patting him gently on the back until belching occurs. In general, it is wise to interrupt a feeding at least once for this purpose.

Persistent cases of such functional vomiting may require thickening of liquid feedings by adding 2 tablespoonfuls of infant cereal to an 8 ounce bottle of milk, and in some instances it may be necessary to switch to formulas containing a vegetable oil. The addition of the latter offers two advantages; vegetable oil may pass from stomach to small intestine more easily and may result in less malodorous vomitus, in the event that the child continues to regurgitate despite all efforts. Sedation and antispasmodics are unphysiologic because of the atonic stomach, and they are usually ineffective.

INFECTION. Vomiting is seen in association with many infections, both enteric and parenteral. It may occur at the onset of any acute febrile disease. The vomiting may or may not persist; it may also outlast the underlying disease. Infants and young children may develop vomiting even with a common cold or an attack of otitis media. Severe vomiting accompanied by such vigorous (anterograde) gastric peristalsis as to suggest pyloric stenosis may be observed in neonates with infection of the urinary tract. Vomiting due to infection often bears no definite relationship to the intake of food; it may be delayed for some hours after a meal. In general, when vomiting results from parenteral infection or other systemic disease the desire for food may be impaired. The ingestion of toxic substances or of food contaminated by bacterial toxins may also lead to vomiting. Treatment in cases associated with infections is usually not specific and is directed to parenteral rehydration, whenever the patient's condition requires it.

As children grow older, vomiting due to improper feeding technique or parenteral infections becomes less frequent. Dietary indiscretions and acute febrile illness may lead to short-term bouts of emesis that are usually self-limited.

Epidemics of nausea and vomiting, thought to be due to a viral infection, affect adults as well as children. The specific diagnosis and its infectious etiology are usually not established; the latter is merely postulated from the presence of many cases of vomiting in the community at the same time. Many affected individuals suffer the complete picture of nausea, vomiting, diarrhea, abdominal pain, slight elevation of temperature, and often moderate pharyngeal hyperemia. The condition is more severe in children, who may have an explosive onset and more persistent periods of vomiting. Frequently they suffer intense thirst, but vomit as soon as they drink any amount of liquid. In this condition the stomach is atonic, and gastric secretions are diminished. The latter slows the rate at which the water achieves isotonicity, which is required for its passage to the duodenum. Proper management is based on severe restriction of intake, which should be limited to very small amounts (1 ounce per hour) of carbonated sodas, fruit punch, or sweetened weak tea until at least 8 to 10 hours have passed without nausea and vomiting. The symptoms usually subside completely after 24 to 72 hours.

CENTRAL NERVOUS SYSTEM DISEASES. Vomiting is a feature of organic nervous system disease with increased intracranial pressure or hemorrhage. Cerebral vomiting is usually forcible or projectile and may bear no relationship to meals. In meningitis the effects of parenteral infection and disease of the central nervous system are combined, and vomiting is rarely absent. Vomiting among children may also be reflex from irritation of the pharynx. It may be excited by paroxysms of coughing, particularly in pertussis.

Acute attacks of abdominal epilepsy (p. 1860) as a cause of vomiting are probably diagnosed more frequently than is warranted. The diagnosis should require that the child have an abnormal electroencephalographic tracing and other features of epilepsy and that the attacks may be aborted by administration of parenteral barbiturates. Dilantin is very effective prophylactically as long-term therapy. Abdominal migraine is equally difficult to diagnose with accuracy. In older children progression of a beginning attack may be interrupted by oral administration of 1 to 2 mg of ergotamine tartrate combined with 50 mg of caffeine. These medications are usually ineffective once the attack is established, but their efficacy in preventing progression of early symptoms is a valuable diagnostic test.

METABOLIC CAUSES. Vomiting is common in advanced renal insufficiency, adrenocortical insufficiency associated with congenital adrenal hyperplasia, diabetic acidosis, renal tubular acidosis, lactic acidosis, isovaleric acidosis, and congenital galactosemia.

DRUGS. Vomiting may be caused by many drugs, including digitalis, sulfonamides, broad-spectrum antibiotics, acetylsalicylic acid, various anesthetic agents, and a variety of poisons.

HABIT VOMITING. Habit is a potent factor in causing vomiting to continue when it has occurred frequently from another cause. There is no question that some infants and children vomit far more readily than do others. Habitual vomiting may be encouraged by injudicious attitudes on the part of the parents in regard to the child's meals, especially when food is forced because of the mistaken notion that a child must be fed a certain quantity of food at a certain time, disregarding his own inclinations. This form of habitual vomiting commonly makes its appearance early in the second year of life. Prompt diagnosis of the causes and adequate explanation and orientation to proper parental attitudes are necessary. If habitual vomiting goes untreated and symptoms become pernicious, it may be difficult to distinguish the condition from cyclic vomiting.

CYCLIC VOMITING. Cyclic vomiting, also known as recurrent, periodic, or acetonemic vomiting, is characterized by attacks of vomiting that recur at irregular intervals without apparent cause. The attacks usually begin between the ages of 2 and 4 years, but they may date from infancy. Almost invariably the condition sub-

sides before puberty. The attacks are of variable length, some lasting only a few days and others more than a week. They usually occur several times a year and are separated by intervals during which the child is entirely normal. Children with the fixed-habit type of vomiting are less likely to have such long symptom-free periods. Children with either habit or cyclic vomiting do not have any demonstrable underlying pathology.

Severe bouts of cyclic vomiting are often associated with ketosis, dehydration, and fever. In some instances headache, general malaise, and anorexia may occur as prodromal symptoms. The vomiting may be so persistent and severe that it leads rapidly to prostration. Parenteral treatment with appropriate electrolyte solutions is sometimes necessary.

Cyclic vomiting probably should not be regarded as a disease entity. In some instances it appears to be precipitated by nonspecific stimuli (such as infection, emotional upset, or fasting) in susceptible individuals who also may possess an unusual tendency to develop ketosis and hypoglycemia. For many of these children small frequent feedings and a late evening snack are suggested to forestall early morning exacerbations. In other instances the mechanism appears to be quite different; such diverse causes as food allergy and partial intestinal obstruction have been implicated. Millichap and associates have described a group of patients in whom they attributed cyclic vomiting to an episodic disorder arising in the brain; they believe that it should be classified as an autonomic epilepsy. Vomiting in patients with familial dysautonomia may be of this type.

The cycle may be broken with one of the phenothiazine derivatives given rectally or by injection. These agents are especially useful in this type of vomiting, but they must be prescribed with caution because of their serious side effects. Unfortunately they are too frequently prescribed in less severe vomiting of infants and children, in which case their potential toxicity outweighs any possible benefits. Perphenazine (Trilafon), chlorpromazine (Thorazine), or prochlorperazine (Compazine) may be given as rectal suppositories in doses of 0.2 mg/kg body weight. Medication may be repeated at 8-hour intervals in lower dosages, with a maximum daily dose of 0.4 mg/kg for children up to 40 kg and 16 mg/day for those over that weight. These agents tend to induce drowsiness which may initially be useful in overcoming the vomiting. They may also cause undesirable extrapyramidal manifestations, although rarely with the dosages recommended.

CHALASIA OF ESOPHAGUS. Vomiting and regurgitation may arise from disturbances in the esophagus. Congenital surgical problems leading to obstructive vomiting are described elsewhere in this section (p.1014). A rare congenital problem is chalasia, or an abnormally relaxed cardiac orifice. In this condition ingested material is refluxed effortlessly into the esophagus after its passage to the stomach. The functional abnormality is readily demonstrated by fluoroscopic examination with barium. Unless there is marked pyloric obstruction, hiatal hernia, or severe peptic esophagitis from acid reflux, the condition is self-limited and disappears after the first few months of life. The only treatment usually required is to maintain the infant almost constantly in a vertical position. If hiatus hernia or severe pyloric obstruction accompanies chalasia, surgical repair may be necessary before the symptoms subside.

ACHALASIA (CARDIOSPASM). While it is slightly more frequent than chalasia, this lesion is still extremely rare in children; it is more common in adults. In children the symptoms usually first appear some time after 5 years of age. In this condition there is gradual distintegration of the myenteric ganglia of the lower end of the esophagus. The nervous elements that remain provide disorganized peristalsis; with parasympathomimetic stimulation they respond maximally, as per Cannon's law, and spasm of the entire esophagus results. This pathophysiologic mechanism explains the symptomatology. Swallowing difficulties and vomiting occur intermittently, and during the early period of slow insidious onset there may be no difficulties for days at a time. Occasionally the primary difficulty is caused mainly by the spasm and functional narrowing at the lower end of the esophagus, where a chunk of swallowed food, usually meat, may lodge and produce substernal fullness. Such obstructions are usually relieved by washing down the impacted food with fluids. In other patients disordered motility and spasm produce the sensation of substernal pain and difficulty even when they swallow water or their own saliva. Vomiting is never forceful, but consists of drooling and regurgitation after a variable length of time. With passage of time a megaesophagus develops, with a typical funnel-shaped narrowing at the cardiac end of the esophagus (Fig. 1). In advanced cases esophagitis with pressure necrosis and ulceration of the esophageal mucosa are seen. Some patients suffer repeated bouts of pneumonia from aspiration and may develop bronchiectasis or lung abscesses.

Anticholinergic and antispasmodic drug therapy is usually ineffective. Medical management includes maintaining nutrition with high-calorie liquid diets when necessary. Most patients ultimately require dilation with bougies. Pneumatically controlled application of pressure from a rubber balloon to "fracture" the stenosing lower esophageal fibers, or a pyloromyotomy of the lower esophagus (Heller procedure), is sometimes necessary. In all patients who have had surgical splitting of muscle fibers at the cardioesophageal junction or pyloromyotomy, interruption of vagal fibers and postprandial vertical positioning of the patient are advised to minimize the undersirable effects of the incompetent lower esophagus with its tendency to reflux.

SURGICAL CONDITIONS INVOLVING ABDOMINAL ORGANS. Vomiting is a prominent symptom in surgical conditions such as hiatus hernias, appendicitis, peritonitis, intussusception, volvulus, abdominal trauma, internal herniations, incarcerated hernias, and twisted ovarian cysts. These conditions are discussed under their appropriate headings elsewhere in this chapter.

References

Adams HD: Esophageal amyenteric achalasia. Surg Gynecol Obstet 119:251, 1964

Benedict EB: Bougienage, forceful dilatation, and surgery in treatment of achalasia; a comparison of results. JAMA 188:355, 1964

Berenberg W, Neuhauser EBD: Cardio-esophageal relaxation (chalasia) as a cause of vomiting in infants. Pediatrics 5:414, 1950

Cassella RB, Brown AL, Sayre GP, Ellis FH Jr: Achalasia of the esophagus: pathologic and etiologic considerations. Ann Surg 160:474, 1964

Craig WS: Vomiting in the early days of life. Arch Dis Child 36:451, 1961

Douglas EF, White PT: Abdominal epilepsy—a reappraisal. J Pediatr 78:59, 1971

Forshall I: The cardio-oesophageal syndrome in childhood. Arch Dis Child 30:46, 1955

Hoyt CC, Stickler GB: A study of 44 children with the syndrome of recurrent (cyclic) vomiting. Pediatrics 25:775, 1960

Hughes JG: The etiology of vomiting in infancy and childhood. Pediatr Clin North Am 2:483, 1955

Millichap JG, Lombroso CT, Lennox WG: Cyclic vomiting as a form of epilepsy in children. Pediatrics 15:705, 1955

Polonsky L, Guth PH: Familial achalasia. Am J Dig Dis 15:291, 1970

Redo SF, Bauer CH: Management of achalasia in infancy and childhood. Surgery 53:263, 1963

Shaw EB, Dermott RV, Lee R, Burnbridge TN: Phenothiazine tranquilizers as a cause of severe seizures. Pediatrics 23:485, 1959

Sorsdahl OA, Gay BB Jr: Esophageal achalasia in childhood. Am J Dis Child 109:141, 1965

Swenson OS, Oeconomopoulos CT: Achalasia of the esophagus in children. J Thorac Cardiovasc Surg 41:49, 1961

Thomson J: Neuro-muscular incoordination of the cardia in the newborn. Arch Dis Child 25:52, 1950

Vantrappon G, et al: Treatment of achalasia with pneumatic dilatations. Gut 12:268, 1971

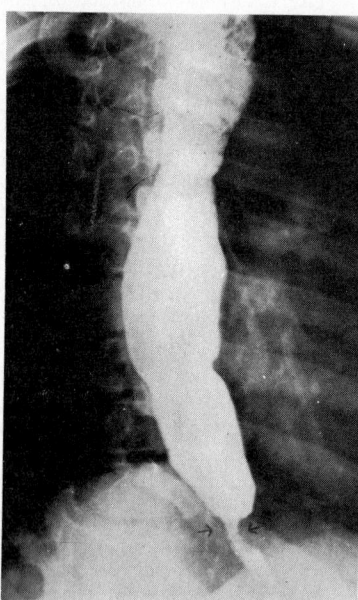

FIG. 1. Achalasia of the esophagus. Right anterior view after barium swallow.

RUMINATION SYNDROME

ARNOLD H. EINHORN

Some young infants acquire the ability to induce at will the regurgitation of previously ingested food, much in the manner of ruminant animals. This singular habit is seen primarily in infants from extremely underprivileged homes. When it develops into a regular pattern it leads to weight loss, growth failure, severe malnutrition, dehydration, and electrolyte imbalance. If the process is not recognized and arrested, it may even progress to death from starvation.

The habit of rumination (merycism) usually commences between the ages of 3 and 6 months and may persist for many months. The onset has been reported to occur exceptionally as early as 5 weeks and as late as 1 year after birth. Among 43 of our own patients with infantile rumination, this syndrome started before 3 months of age in two infants only. Both infants had undergone surgery at birth for upper airway obstruction; they were breathing via tracheostomy tubes and were being fed exclusively through gastrostomy. At the ages of 8 and 11 weeks these two infants began voluntarily bringing up part of their stomach contents and mouthing the material vigorously before reswallowing it, seemingly seeking to recapture the oral gratification of feeding, of which they were being deprived.

In the early decades of the twentieth century this syndrome was quite common; reports in the literature were numerous, and mortality rates were estimated to be in the vicinity of 20 percent. Although today its incidence has considerably declined, it still occurs, probably more frequently than the scarcity of reports in the current literature would indicate. The prevalence of this syndrome in the past was apparently related to the general social and economic deprivation of the time. Richmond suggests that overall improvement of infant care may account for its decreased incidence.

Numerous speculations have been made concerning the nature and etiology of merycism. The illness is generally regarded as psychosomatic in nature, an emotional derangement secondary to a distressful environment. It does not appear to be the result of any organic abnormality, anatomic or physiologic. Lack of stimulation and disruption or deprivation of a close mother–infant relationship are the major etiologic factors of the rumination syndrome. Such conditions are fostered especially by adverse environmental circumstances that are found primarily in homes with precarious social and economic conditions. Surroundings equally unsuitable for appropriate parent–infant interaction may prevail in instances of profound and chronic familial disharmony, maternal psychopathology, and prolonged institutionalization.

The following observations were made by us on 43 infant ruminators hospitalized in our service and followed until well after recovery from their aberrant behavior. The ratio of males to females was approximately 2 to 1. All were offspring of parents living in slums. However, 9 infants, including the 2 patients previously mentioned who had undergone neonatal surgery, had never left the hospital before the onset of their rumination. Seven of these infants, who were abandoned by their parents, remained in the hospital after birth pending foster home placement. Custodial care of these social boarders was good, but was given in a depersonalized hospital setting by varied staff members without any attempt to create surrogate mother figures. In this group of patients total lack of parent–infant interaction was coupled with incomplete deprivation. The remaining 35 infants were all hospitalized after failing to thrive in a home environment of extreme poverty. All but 1 of the 43 infants were born out of wedlock. Even where both parents were living together this arrangement was at best temporary, and the emotional climate pervading each home was extremely insecure. Drug addiction, admitted to by seven mothers, probably existed in several others, and also in some of the fathers. The only married parents were both narcotics users. Some of the mothers of our ruminators appeared either very dull, apathetic, or immature; in some, frank psychopathology was documented. Evidences of child battering in other siblings, alcoholism, and prostitution were apparent or were admitted to by several mothers.

The episodes of rumination in the affected infant may take place at any time between feedings, provided the infant is alone and not in the proximity of objects likely to attract or occupy his attention. Since the infants do not usually ruminate when distracted, it is often difficult to observe them performing their deliberate regurgitation. Even the parents of these infants seldom witness it. Typically, the following events occur in rapid succession during the act. Motionless at first, as if plunged in deep meditation, the infant frowns and grimaces, curls his lower lip, protrudes his tongue, and projects his mandible forward. His head slightly extended, he arches his back and stiffens his abdominal muscles, making at the same time rhythmic chewing movements until food is brought up with evident ease, a mouthful at a time. A portion of the regurgitated stomach contents is rechewed and partially reswallowed. Variable quantities of this material ejected to the outside without force run along the corner of the mouth onto the infant's shirt, which remains constantly wet and sour smelling, usually around one side of the neck. The losses of fluids, electrolytes, and nutrients may be considerable. Some infants introduce one or several fingers or objects into their mouths to help them accomplish the rumination. The infants often show obvious signs of satisfaction, as if the rumination procedure produced a sense of accomplishment. We have occasionally observed fleeting but frank smiles on the faces of these habitually unsmiling youngsters on successful completion of their regurgitation.

The disorder may go unrecognized for long periods of time if the diagnosis is not systematically considered in evaluating infants with failure to thrive. Physicians who are unfamiliar with the relatively rare rumination syndrome tend to mistake it for habitual vomiting. Rumination should be strongly suspected in any emaciated young infant from an economically disadvantaged home who has vomitus constantly plastered over his chin, neck, and upper shirt, but who is never actually seen vomiting. Once the suspicion is aroused the diagnosis can readily be confirmed by furtive observation. In rumination the regurgitation is self-induced and is followed by rechewing and reswallowing of the expelled material. Vomiting is distressing and involuntary; rumination is effortless and accomplished with evident control. Furthermore, the infantile ruminator, far from suffering the discomforts related to the act of vomiting, evidently derives sensory pleasure from sucking and mouthing the regurgitated matter. In addition to the state of malnutrition of variable severity, the outward appearance of the infantile ruminator is striking. These infants are quiet, sad, and singularly wide-eyed. When alone and not engaged in their odd practice they seem lost in inner contemplation. They may continue to produce sucking movements even though their mouths are empty. While they may lie immobile for hours with a vacant gaze and seem detached from their surroundings, any external stimulation evokes a rapid change in comportment and draws their immediate and clinging attention. Intensely, searchingly, untiringly, and often without turning their heads, they follow every gesture or movement of any bystander or any unaccustomed moving object. The melancholy of their facial expressions and the alertness, inquisitiveness, and intensity of their foraging gazes, paired with the gauntness and ascetic quality of their features, produce in these infants the appearance of wise old men. Associated neurotic traits such as autistic posturing, excessive genital and fecal play, body rocking, and rolling and banging of the head have been reported by Richmond to be more frequent in ruminating infants.

The rumination syndrome may be exceedingly difficult to control. Mechanical devices such as chin straps and a variety of physical treatments including aversive conditioning by electric shock have been recommended as means of preventing or inhibiting rumination. Such methods have proved worthless; those of a punitive nature are at best undesirable. The use of thickened feedings or solid food is sometimes effective in milder cases. In instances where infants are able to ruminate only when they use a finger, toy, or some other object, elbow restraints can be of value. The most successful results are obtained by distracting the patient after feedings, holding him, and providing him with attention during and after nursing. When the continued presence, comfort, and physical contact of the mother or any other adult cannot be constantly assured, distraction with multicolored or moving objects and the company of other children can greatly contribute to the infant's improvement. Permanent control of the habit may be anticipated only by furthering or reestablishing a close, warm, and comfortable mother–child relationship or its closest equivalent. Major emphasis must be placed on correction of the social, emotional, or educational deficiencies in the human environment of the infant that carry the responsibility for the deprivation and the disruption in mother–infant relationship.

References

Fullerton DT: Infantile rumination. Arch Gen Psychiatry 9:593, 1963

Gaddini RDB, Gaddini E: Rumination in infancy. In Jessner L, Pavenstedt E (eds): Dynamic Psychopathology in Childhood. New York, Grune & Stratton, 1959, p 166

Hollowell JG, Gardner LI: Rumination and growth failure in male fraternal twins, associated with disturbed family environment. Pediatrics 36:565, 1965

Luckey RE, Watson CM, Musick JK: Aversive conditioning as a means of inhibiting vomiting and rumination. Am J Ment Defic 73:139, 1968

Menking M, Wagnitz JG, Burton JJ, Coddington RD, Sotos JF: Rumination—a near fatal psychiatric disease of infancy. N Engl J Med 280:802, 1969

Patton RJ, Gardner LI: Influence of family and environment: "the syndrome of maternal deprivation." Pediatrics 30:957, 1967

Richmond JB, Eddy E, Green M: Rumination: a psychosomatic syndrome of infancy. Pediatrics 22:49, 1958

Rothney WB: Rumination and spasmus nutans. Hosp Practice 4:102, Sept 1969

Stein ML, Rausen AR, Blau A: Psychotherapy of an infant with rumination. JAMA 171:2309, 1959

GASTROINTESTINAL BLEEDING

MURRAY DAVIDSON

HEMATEMESIS. Vomited blood is not uncommon in the newborn period. True gastric hemorrhage may occur from ulcers in states of anoxemia, in septicemia, in hemorrhagic disease of the newborn, and in hiatus hernia of the stomach from erosion of the esophageal muscosa by regurgitated gastric juice.

Vomited blood in newborns is not necessarily from the infant's stomach. Vomiting of blood swallowed during the birth process may be delayed up to 2 or 3 days. The most reliable means for distinguishing maternal blood from infant's blood is the semiquantitative test for fetal hemoglobin by alkali denaturation (Apt test). Trauma to the nasopharynx caused by a suction tube is another source of vomited blood in newborn infants. Infants at the breast may draw blood from a fissure or ulcer in the mother's nipple. Alarmingly large amounts of blood may be vomited in these circumstances; yet the child's condition remains good. Examination of the mother will generally reveal the source of the trouble. It may sometimes be noted that vomiting of blood follows nursing from one breast and not from the other.

In older infants and children vomited blood may also come from a source other than the gastrointestinal tract. The nose and pharynx are the most common sources, especially with nosebleeds and after tonsillectomy. Although peptic ulceration is the most common cause of true upper gastrointestinal bleeding in all age groups, a very important cause of hematemesis in children is rupture of esophageal varices. These varices develop as a collateral venous network in portal hypertension due to cirrhosis of the liver or obstruction of the extrahepatic portal vein system. These lesions may be congenital or acquired. The acquired form rarely may be due cavernomatous transformation of the portal vein or frequently may be due to pylethrombophlebitis. The latter may be secondary to infection of the umbilical cord or may follow catheterization of the vessel. Hematemesis is usually the first sign of the condition; the varices may rupture without warning, and bleeding may be massive. Episodes of hemorrhage recur unless the portal hypertension is corrected surgically by some type of portacaval shunt. Other less common causes of bleeding from the esophagus in children are erosions of the mucosa associated with hiatus hernia, regurgitation of gastric juice as in chalasia (p.1018), and thoracic gastrointestinal duplications that open into the esophagus and are lined by secreting gastric mucosa. As in adults, children who bleed from peptic ulcers may have displayed no previous signs of ulcer, and bleeding may continue to the point of exsanguination. Abscesses and neoplasms of the stomach may cause hemorrhages.

Hemorrhage is seen with various systemic conditions such as thrombocytopenia, leukemia, scurvy, hemophilia, and purpura and rarely in infections such as malaria and hemorrhagic measles. Liver poisons, such as phosphorus, may lead to hypoprothrombinemia and bleeding. Fatal hemorrhage has been reported after the swallowing of a foreign body.

If the hemorrhage is rapid and vomiting is prompt, the blood may be bright red; if blood has been in the stomach for a period of time it is dark brown and black, resembling coffee grounds. The stools, which invariably contain blood if there is bleeding from the stomach, are black and tarry in appearance if considerable blood is present; otherwise the presence of blood may be detected only be chemical tests. Whether symptoms of shock are present will depend on the amount and rapidity of blood loss.

A vital part of management of gastrointestinal hemorrhage is to keep the patient quiet and immobilized; sedation appropriate for the clinical condition may be necessary. If a good deal of blood has been lost, supportive transfusions with whole blood to replace cells and blood volume are required. Hematocrits must be followed frequently and regularly to evaluate continuing losses of blood. The pulse should be carefully watched; if there are signs of vascular collapse, transfusion is urgently indicated. Whether food or water should be given by mouth during the period of hemorrhage and observation depends on the diagnosis; if the diagnosis is in doubt, no feedings should be given. With known peptic ulcerations, frequent small amounts of antacids or milk are useful. If bleeding is due to esophageal varices, food should be withheld for at least 24 hours after the hemorrhage has been controlled. Fluids should be given parenterally as indicated. Gastric cooling and/or passage of an occluding Sengstaken-Blakemore catheter have been employed for control of upper gastrointestinal hemorrhage. Specific treatment should be directed toward the primary condition causing the hematemesis.

HEMATOCHEZIA AND MELENA. Hematochezia, the appearance of gross blood in the stool, is usually associated with bleeding from the lower intestines. Melena, or tarry stool, indicates the presence of blood from the upper gastrointestinal tract that has been altered by secretions during its passage to the rectum. However, massive gastric bleeding may be followed by recognizable unaltered blood in the stool, while slow oozing of blood from the lower ileum may occasionally result only in tarry stools. Blood losses up to about 15 ml/day may occur from any point in the intestinal tract without a gross change in appearance of the stools of children, although tests for occult blood will be strongly positive.

Conditions associated with hematemesis usually lead to melena or occult blood in the stool. Intussusception and, more rarely, midgut volvulus are associated with bloody stools, the blood being characteristically mixed with mucus to give the classic currant jelly stool. In acute dysentery, diarrhea and gross bleeding are common.

The presence of blood in the stools in children is a prime example of the principle that the diagnostic implications of symptoms and findings in children may be quite different from in adults. The possibility that such bleeding in an adult is from a malignancy dictates an

TABLE 1. Rectal Bleeding in Children

Causes	Newborn	1 wk–2 yr	2–13 yr
		Age Groups	
1. Swallowed blood	+++*	−	−
2. Trauma to rectum	+*	±	−
3. Milk allergy	+	+*	−
4. Bleeding diathesis	++*	+*	+*
5. Peptic ulceration	++*	++*	+*
6. Developmental anomalies	±	++*	+*
7. Meckel's diverticulum	−	++*	+*
8. Intussusception	−	++*	+*
9. Fissure in ano	−	++++	++++
10. Polyps	−	++*	+++*
11. Portal hypertension	−	+*	++*
12. Ulcerative colitis	−	±*	+++*
13. Cancer	−	−	−

Bleeding may be massive.

attitude of immediacy in approach. The probability of a malignancy in a child with this finding is so remote that the same attitude should not prevail. A number of reported series of children admitted to hospitals for investigation of rectal bleeding indicate that in a considerable percentage no etiologic diagnosis is established despite repeated sigmoidoscopic, radiographic, and other examinations. Since fissure in ano often accounts for more than 50 percent of children with rectal bleeding in whom a diagnosis is established, one may safely postpone more extensive investigations while a course of mineral oil therapy is prescribed. This therapeutic approach to rectal bleeding is probably more important for evaluation than are repeated instrumentations and barium enemas. If bleeding persists after a few weeks of treatment with oral doses of liquid petrolatum, investigation is warranted.

The data in Table 1 have been compiled from a number of sources. The 13 causes of rectal bleeding in children are listed in the order of ages at which they are initially encountered. The frequency of occurrence is indicated semiquantitatively by the number of plus signs; a minus sign indicates negligible incidence. Thus, although swallowed blood may be a source of rectal bleeding at other ages than in the newborn period, its occurrence is so rare at these times as to deserve a minus sign. On the other hand, fissure in ano is so much more common a cause of rectal bleeding than all others that it is rated four plus signs in the 1-week to 2-year age group. The chart makes clear that cancer is not a serious problem, and repeated definitive studies are therefore not indicated for this possibility. Most of the conditions in this table are discussed individually elsewhere in this chapter.

References

Abrams B, Lynn HB: Rectal bleeding in children. Am J Surg 104:831, 1962

Brayton D: Gastrointestinal bleeding of "unknown origin"; a study of cases in infancy and childhood. Am J Dis Child 107:288, 1964

Gans SL, Ament M, Christie DL, Liebman, WM: Pediatric endoscopy with flexible fibrescopes. J Pediatr Surg 10:375, 1975

Malt R: Control of massive upper gastrointestinal hemorrhage. N Engl J Med 286:1043, 1972

Spencer R: Gastrointestinal hemorrhage in infancy and childhood: 476 cases. Surgery 55:718, 1964

DIARRHEA

MURRAY DAVIDSON

ACUTE DIARRHEA

The subject of acute diarrhea and its causes and management are discussed elsewhere in detail (p. 264). Certain supplemental general features of the subject, especially those related to gastrointestinal function, are discussed in this section. They are also related to the problem of chronic diarrhea, which is discussed principally in this chapter.

PATHOLOGIC CHEMISTRY AND PHYSIOLOGY. The mechanism responsible for the hyperperistalsis of acute diarrhea is not accurately known. Pathogenic organisms, endotoxins, and directly irritating materials may play a role. The loss of nutrients in diarrhea is due only in part to hyperperistalsis, which prevents adequate time for absorption; there may be disturbances in enzyme functions, impairment of the inherent assimilatory mechanisms, and also disturbances in fluid and electrolyte movements. These factors do not necessarily operate simultaneously. In some severe cases fluid absorption may be impaired to such an extent that symptoms of shock appear some hours before diarrhea is evident. Likewise, with recovery, balance studies have shown that it is not uncommon for poor assimilation of fat to persist for days or even weeks after hyperperistalsis has subsided. The extent to which assimilation of individual nutrients is impaired varies widely in individual cases. Of the calorigenic foodstuffs, protein assimilation is relatively little affected; even moribund infants with severe diarrhea may continue to absorb and retain nitrogen. Assimilation of fat is usually affected and may be markedly impaired in severe cases. It is readily measured by balance studies; in cases of moderate severity only 50 to 70 percent of the intake may be absorbed, whereas in the most severe cases absorption may fall to 20 percent of the intake or even less. A flat postabsorptive blood sugar curve and the passage of considerable flatus are commonly regarded as evidence of impaired carbohydrate absorption. These findings, however, do not necessarily indicate a serious defect of absorption; disturbed motility or delayed gastric emptying may be responsible. The postabsorptive sugar curve is related to rate rather than to completeness of absorption. The only accurate method of measuring carbohydrate absorption involves balance studies with labeled carbohydrate in which the intake and stool output of tagged carbon are measured. This method has not been applied to infants with diarrhea. In exceptional infants failure of carbohydrate assimilation may be based on temporary deficiencies of the appropriate disaccharidases, especially of lactase, or of the ability to absorb monosaccharides (p. 1002).

Most serious for the welfare of the infant are the disturbances in water and electrolyte balance in diarrhea. The loss of water and electrolyte in the stools is promptly reflected by a reduction of blood volume and interstitial fluid volume. The loss of extracellular fluids is responsible for a series of pathologic processes that are discussed elsewhere (p. 262). Stool losses of water in severe cases of diarrhea may range from 250 to 500 ml or more per day, amounting to 10 to 15 times the normal, and electrolyte losses may also approach a 10-fold increase over normal. In some instances a relative deficit of water predominates and hyperelectrolytemia develops. This condition and the opposite disturbance, hypoelectrolytemia, are discussed in detail elsewhere (p. 266).

PATHOLOGY. Except in *Shigella* infections, in which ileocolitis is often found, and in patients with staphylococcal enterocolitis, in whom ulcerations may occur (p. 497), nothing striking is usually seen grossly in the gastrointestinal tract of children with acute diarrhea. The intestines are likely to be distended but otherwise normal. Parenteral infection may be present but frequently is absent. Although melena or hematemesis may have occurred, the site of bleeding is seldom demonstrated. Anatomic changes from dehydration, loss of fluid from the subcutaneous tissues, and reduction of muscle volume are less conspicuous at autopsy than during life. In long-standing cases evidences of malnutrition are prominent. Fatty liver is a fairly frequent finding. Thrombosis of the cerebral venous sinuses is found in some fatal cases, and subdural effusions and hemorrhages have been described. A rare lesion is calcification of the renal epithelium.

NUTRITIONAL TREATMENT. Parenteral fluid and electrolyte therapy of hospitalized patients with diarrhea is discussed elsewhere (p. 264). The home treatment of infants with mild diarrhea should be expectant; patients should be observed especially closely for the development of constitutional symptoms. Special attention should be paid to the intake of fluids, which in young infants should not be allowed to fall below 150 ml/kg (day). However, feeding should be infrequent and of relatively large amounts each time, rather than the small frequent feedings that are often ordered; the latter tend to induce frequent bowel movements. Lowering the fat content of the milk presumably serves to shorten the course of mild diarrhea and to lessen the chance of a mild attack increasing in severity. This concept has not been studied adequately and has been challenged by some who recommend that an infant with mild diarrhea be offered usual amounts of normal diet. If diarrhea remains mild or if moderate diarrhea subsides rapidly, parenteral therapy may not be required. Charcoal, kaolin, pectin, apple pulp, carrot soup, carob flour, and synthetic resins have been suggested in an effort to diminish the number of stools. In our experience these remedies are of limited value. In the hope of arresting the diarrhea, oral solutions of glucose and electrolytes are often substituted for the milk feeding. There is no objection to this procedure if properly used, and isotonic solutions of glucose should be encouraged, but excessive or improper use of electrolyte mixtures has been held responsible for the apparent increase in the incidence of hypernatremia (hyperelectrolytemia) in dehydrated infants. This applies especially if these solutions are used in addition to milk.

Controversy prevails as to the desirability of restricting oral food in infants with acute diarrhea who require hospitalization for parenteral fluid and electrolyte management. In cases with vomiting it must obviously be withheld. The debatable question arises when vomiting is not a problem. There is no question that the administration of feedings to a patient with an intolerant intestine increases the volume of diarrheal stools and that the reduction of oral intake decreases them. This finding has been generally interpreted as indicating that the administration of oral food decreases the tolerance of the intestine and that resting the intestine promotes recovery. The procedure followed by those who interpret the evidence in this way is to omit all oral food for a period of 24 hours or perhaps longer, postponing its resumption until dehydration has been brought under control and the stools have become less voluminous and watery. It is then cautiously introduced in a stepwise manner. Should the stools again become increasingly loose and frequent, the conclusion is drawn that the introduction of oral food was premature, and a second period of oral starvation is instituted. Various modifications of this general plan are used. In the belief that only caloric food is harmful, some physicians give water and electrolytes by mouth from the start; others give glucose, water, and electrolytes, withholding only protein and fat. The belief prevails that the attack of diarrhea is shortened by such dietary management.

A different point of view was expressed by Park in 1924; he advocated disregarding the stools and thinking rather of the assimilation of the food by the child. His view, however, did not gain wide acceptance in the absence of physiologic data on different regimens. Chung undertook such studies in 1948, obtaining results that supported Park's views. He and his associates were able to show that although administration of oral food increased stool losses in patients with infantile diarrhea, as well as in those with other forms of intestinal intolerance, it also increased the quantities of nitrogen, fat, and electrolytes absorbed. They further made a comparison of the duration of diarrhea in a group of infants with summer diarrhea in which half the patients were subjected to early fasting while the other half were allowed an adequate oral intake from the start. Their findings suggested that oral feedings merely demonstrated intolerance, rather than adding to it, and did not delay recovery. These investigators were inclined to view instances in which patients had deteriorated under oral feeding, as compared with parenteral fluid therapy, as being due not to any noxious effect of the oral food but rather to the fact that oral food was substituted for parenteral therapy instead of being used as a supplement to needed parenteral fluid.

Oral feedings are less controversial if they are relied on simply as a source of calories and nutriment and are *expected to induce additional losses of fluid and electrolyte* in the recovery phases of acute diarrhea. Adoption of such an attitude permits earlier institution of oral feedings with simultaneous prolonged administration of intravenous fluids properly designed for daily maintenance needs as well as for replacement of losses induced by the feedings. Use of combined oral feeding and parenteral fluid and electrolyte regimens has been successful in a number of instances of protracted diarrhea with resistant infections. Parenteral therapy can be relaxed in the combined oral–intravenous treatment only when it is clear that sufficient fluids are being *absorbed* from the oral intake.

PARENTERAL NUTRITION.   The majority of fatalities in diarrhea occur in long-standing cases in which profound inanition develops. Combined oral nutrition with prolonged parenteral fluid therapy is usually successful in forestalling this dire result. Some investigators have tried to sustain both nutrition and fluid-electrolyte metabolism by the parenteral route alone. Emulsified fat suitable for intravenous use has been made available from time to time. Although it is the most potent source of calories and it has been shown that it is rapidly burned, the difficulty has been the occurrence of reactions usually attributable to the emulsifying agent. Intralipid®, the newest such agent, appears to be safe in this respect. Commercial protein hydrolysates and amino acid mixtures are nonantigenic and can be given safely intravenously. Although these preparations are effective sources of nitrogen, positive nitrogen balance cannot be achieved unless sufficient calories are simultaneously supplied from other sources to prevent their conversion by gluconeogenesis to sources of energy. Amino acid mixtures are excellent culture media, and care must be used to avoid contamination. Cloudy solutions should never be used.

In total parenteral nutrition the deep veins are cannulated so that hypertonic glucose solutions may be successfuly administered without fear of venous thrombosis. This calorie source, together with amino acid mixtures and adequate fluid and electrolyte, offers both parenteral feeding and fluid-electrolyte replacement. It is indicated much more frequently following surgery for congenital lesions of the gastrointestinal tract than in persistent diarrhea, since in our experience the latter patients do just as well with combined nutritional feedings orally and fluid-electrolyte administration parenterally. Morbidity is lower with this combined treatment than with deep venous alimentation, which is associated with the dangers of septicemia, hyperammonemia, hyperglycemia, hyperosmolality, increased mucosal drainage, and hepatic enlargement.

Neonatal Necrotizing Enterocolitis

Necrotizing enterocolitis is a virulent form of diarrhea among neonates and is particularly prevalent among low-birth-weight infants. The etiology is unknown, but mesenteric vascular ischemia with resultant hypoxia of the intestinal mucosa has been suggested as the probable pathogenetic mechanism. Initially the condition is not remarkably different from other types of diarrhea in the neonate. The lethargy, irritability, distension, anorexia, vomiting, and poor body temperature regulation are not unusual among low-birth-weight infants with diarrhea from any cause. However, the history of respiratory difficulty at birth, increased apneic episodes, and blood in the stools should alert the physician to the possibility of this serious condition. A persistent patent ductus arteriosus is commonly associated with necrotizing enterocolitis in the premature infant. Pneumatosis intestinalis, the presence of air in the submucosa and/or subserosal surfaces of the colon, which

is virtually always present, is pathognomonic. Increased air in the bowel lumen or in the peritoneum (indicating perforation of gangrenous bowel) may be seen, but this is not a specific sign. Barium examination, which is unnecessary for demonstration of condition, is contraindicated because it may lead to perforation.

Once the condition is suspected, oral feedings should be discontinued and parenteral fluid therapy instituted, with intermittent or continuous gastric suction. Antibiotic therapy should be given using combinations of ampicillin and kanamycin. Plain and upright radiography of the abdomen should be performed every 6 to 12 hours to follow the progress of the infant. In some cases the symptoms will regress after 48 to 72 hours. However, the mortality exceeds 50 percent in most series, and there is an increasing tendency to approach the situation aggressively. If deterioration occurs with medical management, surgery may be indicated, even in the absence of signs of perforation. Resection and primary anastomosis should be carried out for localized lesions; in more extensive cases resection and exteriorization with ileostomy or colostomy are recommended. The extensive nature of the surgical procedure often dictates a prolonged period of parenteral alimentation, which may be life-saving.

Chronic Diarrhea

Persistence of acute diarrhea may presage a chronic problem in any individual case. More frequently chronic diarrhea tends to develop insidiously. Rational therapy of chronic diarrhea depends to a large extent on precise knowledge of its etiology and pathophysiology. The underlying process in a patient with acute diarrhea is much more likely to be self-limited than in one with chronic symptoms.

Although, as in acute diarrhea, loose or watery stools may result from a disorder of the normal fluid and electrolyte balance in the distal colon, involvement of this area by the disease occurs in only a limited number of types of chronic diarrhea. In many instances the disturbance of colonic function is secondary to small-bowel malfunction; for example, inflammatory exudates may be passed from the small intestine into the colon and have a deleterious effect on colonic salt and water absorption, patients with disturbed enterohepatic circulation of bile salts in the small bowel pass the unabsorbed salts to the colon where they interfere with normal salt and water absorption, or in patients with disaccharidase deficiencies excess disaccharides may exert an osmotic effect and withdraw colonic fluid. In each of these instances there may be little or no objective evidence to suggest disease of the colon; yet the small-intestine disease may produce chronic watery diarrhea of the type usually associated with large-bowel diseases. In other forms of chronic diarrhea the stools, instead of being watery or loose, are more likely to be large, bulky, and somewhat softer than normal stools. In these patients the only defect in intestinal function may be a profound disturbance in fat digestion or absorption, with little or no alteration in the handling of other nutriments or of water and electrolytes.

The inflammatory diseases that are associated with chronic diarrhea may involve either small or large intestine or both; they include regional enteritis, ulcerative colitis, and pseudomembranous enterocolitis of congenital megacolon. Other forms of chronic diarrhea include the various malabsorption syndromes and functional chronic diarrhea.

MALABSORPTION SYNDROMES

In 1888 Gee described a chronic nutritional disorder of children characterized by abdominal distension and persistent diarrhea with large, greasy, foul-smelling stools that he referred to as the celiac affection and that subsequently was called celiac disease. Unfortunately, a wide variety of entities differing from each other in causation and in course but presenting in common the symptom of persistent or recurrent diarrhea were ultimately ascribed to this group and gathered under the title of the celiac syndrome, synonymous with malabsorption syndrome. Clinical entities that have been distinguished in the malabsorption syndrome are usually classified into groups based either on the mechanism of the defect (such as digestive, absorptive, or exudative) or on the specific types of foodstuffs (fat, protein, carbohydrate) primarily involved in the absorption defect. In the following presentation both patterns are fused. The initial description is of a digestive defect, cystic fibrosis of the pancreas.

Cystic Fibrosis

In 1938 Anderson defined the clinical entity cystic fibrosis of the pancreas and suggested that demonstration of pancreatic exocrine insufficiency in duodenal fluid collected from these children could be used for establishing the diagnosis during life. The next 10 to 15 years witnessed remarkable advances in the descriptive aspects of this disease. It was recognized to be generalized, to involve all exocrine glands, to be a genetic disease inherited as an autosomal recessive, to have an incidence variously estimated at 1 per 1,000 or 1 per 4,000 fetuses in the Caucasian population, and to occur in all other races at lesser frequencies. Secretions from the mucus-producing glands are thickened, which once led to the now abandoned name of mucoviscidosis. Electrolytes (sodium, chloride, and potassium) are elaborated in increased concentrations from the sweat glands.

Symptoms of the disease are clearly not restricted to the gastrointestinal tract. However, primarily the gastrointestinal manifestations are discussed in this section. Serious pulmonary involvement often represents the overwhelming difficulty for a particular patient (p. 1563). Liver involvement (p. 1100), genetic patterns (p. 1563), abnormalities of male genitalia (p. 1565), secondary effects on the heart and circulation (p. 1565),

and signs of allergy and nasal polyposis (p. 343). are all described elsewhere.

PATHOGENESIS. The precise pathogenesis remains unknown. Pancreatic exocrine glands and the goblet cells of the intestinal epithelium, as well as other mucus-producing glands in the body, secrete viscid mucus that inspissates the glands and ducts, causing obstruction. The factors contributing to the tenacity and increased viscosity of the mucus are not clearly defined; Dische suggested an abnormal ratio between fucose and sialic acid concentrations in the mucoprotein fractions of duodenal juice, obtained from patients with cystic fibrosis. It is not clear precisely what relationship exists between the widespread mucus abnormality and the elevated concentrations of sodium, potassium, and chloride that are secreted in sweat. Concentrations of these electrolytes and of bicarbonate are also abnormal in the watery portions of various exocrine glandular secretions, including those from the salivary glands and pancreas. Agents, possibly humoral, that inhibit ciliary activity of various invertebrates have been detected in the saliva and in other secretions from patients. An abnormal lipoprotein has been isolated from stools and from rectal tissue of patients.

The predominant gross and microscopic pathology is related to obstruction of lumina by the tenacious secretions. Accumulations are observed in the acini or ducts or within individual goblet cells. The sublingual salivary glands, which normally secrete considerable mucus, are hypertrophied and severely affected. On the other hand, the parotid glands contain considerably fewer mucus-secreting elements and display only minimal changes. The lumina of goblet cells throughout the stomach, small intestine, and colon are usually distended with retained secretions. The mucosa of the entire gastrointestinal tract as well as the area over the salivary glands of the buccal mucosa is usually coated with a layer of tenacious thickened mucus. In most of these areas fibrosis secondary to ductal obstruction is uncommon. However, in the pancreas, distension of the lumina of the acini and ductules by eosinophilic-staining inspissated material is followed by gradual flattening of the epithelium, atrophy of the secretory cells, and replacement of the atrophied tissue by fibrotic changes. The islands of Langerhans are not intrinsically affected, and the total number of beta cells appears normal early in life. Only among patients who have survived into the late second and third decades of life have there been reports of gradual replacement of the islets by fibrous tissue with subsequent development of diabetes mellitus. The pancreatic lesion is progressive and may be very minimal at birth. At the end stage the pancreas is virtually entirely replaced by fat and fibrous tissue with clusters of islet cells. It is usually smaller than normal and is firm and irregular with a gritty feel.

The lesion extends to the liver by a similar process. The biliary ductules suffer obstruction, and ultimately fibrous tissue replaces them. Cirrhosis of the liver is present at autopsy in approximately 25 percent of the patients. The lesions in the pancreas and the liver need not be uniform in all areas.

CLINICAL PICTURE. Many children with cystic fibrosis exhibit abnormal stool and feeding patterns from birth and experience difficulty gaining weight, despite voracious appetites. Although frequent diarrhea is not common, the stools are bulkier and much larger than in normal children of the same age. Incomplete digestion of fat and protein tends to promote growth of bacterial flora in the lower portions of the gastrointestinal tract. The bacterial mass and excess undigested food result in the characteristic increased bulk and greasy appearance of the poorly formed stools. Their odor is usually extremely foul and pungent.

The increased appetite in these patients is probably related to absence of the pyloric reflex. Enterogastrone is released in normal subjects by the duodenal mucosa as soon as free fatty acids are elaborated in the duodenum. The hormone enters the circulation and closes the pylorus via neuronal mediation. The sequence of events does not occur in patients with cystic fibrosis, since in the absence of pancreatic lipase free fatty acids do not appear. Under these circumstances, regardless of their content of lipid, meals tend to move continuously through the pylorus. The satiety that normally follows eating rapidly disappears, and these patients are prepared to eat again much sooner than normal subjects. The increased appetite in these children disappears when proper therapy with substitution by pancreatic enzymes is provided.

Pulmonary manifestations may dominate in the early months of life (p.1565). The child with severe pulmonary infection may, as a result of overwhelming illness, demonstrate poor appetite because of debility and weakness. However, the history of ravenous appetite with poor weight gain prior to the onset of the respiratory symptoms may usually be elicited on careful questioning.

The major foodstuffs that patients with cystic fibrosis fail to digest properly are fat and protein. Because of deficiency or total absence of pancreatic lipase, these children suffer from steatorrhea. Different types of lipids are usually absorbed with considerable variation in all forms of steatorrhea. The absence of lipase in cystic fibrosis is partial in some individuals and complete in others, and there are variations in the interactions between pancreatic lipase and bile salts that are not yet clear. An intestinal lipase may be active in some individuals. These factors, and possibly others that remain unknown, cause marked variations in balance studies performed among patients with cystic fibrosis; they vary from time to time, not only between patients but even in individuals. Because the defect is maldigestive, this is one of the few malabsorptive conditions of childhood in which triglycerides instead of individual fatty acids are found in the stool. Stools will therefore be grossly oily. Since these patients waste fat, their absorption of vitamins A, D, E, and K is impaired, and they should receive supplemental amounts of these essential nutrients in water-miscible preparations. The initial manifestation of vitamin K deficiency may be hemorrhage into the skin.

Patients with cystic fibrosis have azotorrhea and ex-crete increased amounts of nitrogen in their stools as a consequence of the absence of proteolytic activity. Normal individuals usually absorb 97 to 98 percent of dietary protein, while some patients with cystic fibrosis may absorb as little as 40 percent. In infants hypoproteinemic edema may develop if the early onset of diarrhea is incorrectly diagnosed as milk allergy and is improperly treated with substitution of soybean preparations. In the absence of proteolytic enzymes the soy protein is even less well digested than that from cow's-milk formulas, thus leading to protein starvation. Ultimately the severe depletion of proteins, primarily albumin, leads to anasarca.

Prior to the development of clinical tests for sweat electrolyte concentrations in 1950, determinations of activity of amylase, among other enzymes in the pancreatic juice, were utilized for diagnosis. There was significant clinical reduction in this parameter among most patients. Multiple abnormalities of secretory activity by the salivary glands include changes in electrolyte concentrations, increases in calcium output leading to turbidity, changes in protein content, and increased mucus from those glands that secrete mucus. However, the depression of amylase output from both the salivary glands and pancreas is rarely sufficient with usual diets to produce disturbances of starch digestion that are of clinical significance. Untreated patients may often develop the protuberant abdomen generally characteristic of children with malabsorptive conditions. In addition, children with cystic fibrosis are especially prone to recurrent episodes of rectal prolapse (p. 1059).

MECONIUM ILEUS. The earliest manifestation of cystic fibrosis occurs at birth as meconium ileus. The clinical picture is similar to that of certain other forms of intestinal obstruction during the neonatal period; it is discussed elsewhere, together with its surgical therapy (p. 1026). The problem arises from prenatal complete obstruction of a portion of the small intestine, usually the terminal ileum, by tenacious inspissated meconium. The intestine is narrowed distal to the obstructed area, whereas the proximal segment is markedly distended. Perforation and peritonitis of the dilated intestine may occur in utero or within a few hours after birth, as a result of ischemia of the bowel wall. If the perforation is intrauterine, meconium peritonitis with calcification follows and may be demonstrated radiographically. Healing of the prenatal tear may lead to development of atresia or stenosis of the affected bowel segment. Approximately 30 percent of infants with meconium ileus have associated volvulus. It is not clear why only a small proportion of patients with cystic fibrosis suffer from meconium ileus. Although normal meconium consists primarily of carbohydrates, meconium in these patients shows increased protein content. Presumably the altered meconium composition reflects congenital absence of tryptic digestion, and the variations in the degree of pancreatic achylia at birth among patients would explain differences in incidence. However, the initial meconium may vary in different individuals. Intestinal activity forces air bubbles into this sticky material and leads to a characteristic spongy radiographic picture.

Meconium Ileus Equivalent. Older children, teenagers, and young adults are increasingly susceptible to intestinal obstruction from material impacted into lumina already narrowed by hyperplastic mucus-secreting glands. The combined effects of pancreatic insufficiency and the abnormal mucopolysaccharide secretion by intestinal goblet cells lead to formation of solid tenacious fecal material. Under normal circumstances the fecal stream is liquid. The precise locus of such an obstruction is usually in the lower small intestine and/or colon. A mass is frequently palpable in the right lower quadrant and is often demonstrable as an obstructing mass on plain film radiography or by contrast studies.

DIFFERENTIAL DIAGNOSIS. A very important aspect of the differential diagnosis of this condition is for the physician to appreciate that the disease represents the most common lethal gene inherited among Caucasians and that it outweighs—by far—the combined incidence of all other causes of malabsorption in children. Therefore a high index of suspicion must exist for this disease. If the diagnosis so much as crosses the physician's mind, the relatively simple diagnostic sweat test should be performed. Cystic fibrosis of the pancreas should be considered in virtually all children who fail to thrive and in whom a clear-cut alternative diagnosis is not established. At specific ages more specific presenting patterns should suggest the diagnosis.

In newborn infants with intestinal obstruction, meconium ileus must be differentiated from atresia or stenosis of the gastrointestinal tract unrelated to this diagnosis. Additionally, newborn infants with Hirschsprung's disease may demonstrate delay in the initial passage of meconium; in lieu of this, or in addition to it, their symptomatology of vomiting and distension may appear to be related to lower small-bowel obstruction and may represent an important differential from meconium ileus.

In addition to those who fail to thrive, children who present with repeated lower respiratory tract infections or recurrent bronchiolitis must also be suspected of having cystic fibrosis of the pancreas. Alternatively, such infants might have congenital defects of the respiratory tract leading to repeated infection or might be prone to such infections because of immune deficiency syndromes. Infants with failure to thrive may suffer from absence of some or all specific pancreatic enzymes without having cystic fibrosis of the pancreas. These children may have one of the pancreatic lesions, as discussed below, or they may be failing to pass pancreatic juice into the duodenum as in certain rare instances of annular pancreas. Other malabsorptive diseases, as described below, must be considered. Among the additional reasons that infants fail to gain weight and thrive are congenital cardiac defects, congenital renal anomalies with renal insufficiency, and severe parental deprivation. Most of these various problems are associated with poor appetites, in contrast with cystic fibrosis, in which children display voracious appetites except in the presence of infections.

Cystic fibrosis should be suspected among older children (in some instances as late as the second decade of life) in whom chronic respiratory problems have been thought of as atypical cases of asthma or allergy without specific proof of diagnosis. In other patients in whom bronchiectasis is diagnosed without a clear cause, cystic fibrosis must be ruled out.

DIAGNOSIS. The most frequently performed test for diagnosis of cystic fibrosis of the pancreas is the quantitative analysis of chloride and sodium concentration in the sweat. Although occasionally there are reports that patients with this disease have normal concentration of sweat electrolytes, the test is positive in over 99 percent of cases. The laboratory in which the test is performed must be experienced in the procedure, with its own well-established techniques and range of values. The collections should be performed only by technicians trained to perform this procedure regularly and with uniformity.

Sweat is collected after a current of 3 to 4 mamp is applied for 60 sec over an area of the arm on which a piece of gauze saturated with a 0.2 percent solution of pilocarpine nitrate has previously been placed. The current ensures that the pilocarpine will be iontophoresed under the skin and will induce sweating. A preweighed small pad of gauze is then applied over this surface, covered with a small patch of plastic sealed on all sides, and kept in place for 1 hour. The gauze pad with its sweat is placed in a small Erlenmeyer flask that has also been preweighed. The difference in weight before and after collections is measured; an aliquot of distilled water is added to the flask, and it is shaken mechanically for 1 to 2 hours so that there will be complete mixing. A number of potential sources of error must be avoided in the determination. These include failure to utilize flasks, gauze, plastic, and other equipment that are salt-free, introduction of salt from one's own fingers because of poor technique in collection, and collection of so little sweat that dilution factors become overwhelmingly important in calculation errors. In our laboratory no determinations are made if less than 100 mg of sweat are collected; both chloride and sodium are measured. Other laboratories collect sweat from two sites simultaneously to ensure reliability. Appropriate safeguards are essential in this most important test.

Normal sodium and chloride levels range between 5 and 50 mEq/liter. This range covers the normal variations in different age groups. Patients with the disease tend to have values that range from 70 to 180 mEq/liter. There is thus a very clear separation between the patient and the normal control. Siblings of affected individuals sometimes show modest elevations, as do the parents, but these are usually in the intermediate range, (between 40 and 70 mEq/liter). Suspects who register in this intermediate range should have the test repeated once or several times to establish a clear-cut diagnosis. In addition, among normal individuals the sweat sodium exceeds chloride, as it does in extracellular fluids in the body, while in patients the two tend to be equal or slightly reversed (ie, chloride higher than sodium). We have no explanation for this observation;

although it is not absolutely reliable in all cases, it has been helpful in certain doubtful cases.

Prior to 1950, tests for pancreatic function were important because the sweat abnormalities were not appreciated. They are now rarely carried out for clinical purposes. However, where necessary, duodenal fluid may be collected and the volume, pH, and electrolyte and bicarbonate concentrations and enzyme activities determined. Although the deficiency is not universal, at least 80 percent of patients demonstrate some abnormalities. The fasting specimen usually shows reduced volume, increased viscosity, lower pH (from poor bicarbonate output and failure to neutralize acid from the stomach), and reduced activities of the pancreatic enzymes, lipase, amylase, trypsin, chymotrypsin, and carboxypeptidase. Stimulation with secretin-pancreozymin, as is performed in pancreatic function tests for other conditions, fails to improve the lower baseline values in patients with cystic fibrosis. Specific substrates for trypsin (TAME, toluenesulfonyl L-arginine methyl ester) and chymotrypsin (BTEE, *N-benzoyl* L-tyrosine ethyl ester) are currently available and may be incubated with a small specimen of stool to assay these enzymes without need for duodenal intubation. A specimen from a control of similar age should always be assayed simultaneously to ensure the reliability of the results obtained. A simpler test exists that does not distinguish specific enzymes but merely evaluates proteolytic activity by study of the dissolution of gelatin on unexposed x-ray film. This test is more reliable in infants than in older children, in whom proteolytic enzymes from bacteria may dissolve the gelatin. Variations in the digestibility of the film gelatin from different firms (whether or not patients have been receiving antibiotics or other drugs) introduce other unpredictable factors in this test. As with the synthetic substrates, it is imperative that control specimens be incubated at the same time as the patient's specimen, because time of exposure, temperature, and other factors affect the results.

TREATMENT. The treatments of pulmonary lesions and of other complications of patients with cystic fibrosis are discussed elsewhere (p. 1568). The management of the pancreatic insufficiency is relatively simple, but must be individualized. In general, fats are less well tolerated than are proteins or carbohydrates. A high-protein high-carbohydrate diet is usually suggested, since most children who have poor lipase activity may continue not to tolerate a diet with normal fat content despite pancreatic replacement therapy. This fat intolerance is related to the difficulty with which lipase is preserved in the various pancreatic extracts.

A number of commercial pancreatic preparations are available for enzyme replacement therapy. Among the most popular is Viokase, a defatted pancreatic preparation that is not an extract. Cotazym has become popular in recent years because of the unsubstantiated belief that lipase is best preserved in this preparation. Powdered preparations of pancreatin USP and Panteric granules (enteric-coated bits of pancreatin powder) are also used in infants when it is difficult to administer tablets and capsules. The powders and granules are usually diluted in small amounts of applesauce or some other fruit and are given with meals. Complete correction is rarely achieved. The preparations are biologic materials and are not of uniform potency. The shelf life and deterioration with exposure to light and moisture render their potency variable. The physician must constantly be alert to individual needs of patients and adjust diets and drug doses accordingly. It is our own practice to pay particular attention to appetite for dosage determination. The voracious appetite of an inadequately treated patient usually is reduced to more normal levels once the pancreatic extract dose is optimal and absorption is more adequate.

Medium-chain triglycerides (8 to 12 carbons) may be digested by the intracellular lipase in the mucosa of the intestine and do not depend on pancreatic lipase. Feeding of medium-chain triglyceride formulas to infants usually leads to stools that are less frequent, bulky, oily, and offensive. In some patients a significant weight gain occurs; however, this improvement is not universal.

The fat-soluable vitamins A, D, and E should be administered in accordance with current recommended daily allowances in a water-miscible form to all patients with pancreatic insufficiency. There is no evidence that the increased bulk or fat content of the stools is inherently deleterious. The calcium loss in the stools is reduced by adequate vitamin D therapy.

The treatment for meconium ileus in the newborn is surgical (p.1026). Older children with the equivalent condition may be treated conservatively with medical therapy, which consists of irrigation of the site twice daily with 100 to 200 ml of a 10 percent solution of *N*-acetylcysteine. If the lesion is in the colon the material is usually given by rectal enema or directly to the site of the obstruction by a catheter passed retrograde to this point. For lesions of the lower ileum a decompressing Miller-Abbott tube is passed to the site of obstruction for the purpose of irrigations. In some instances detergents (eg, 1 percent solution of Tween 80) are administered in similar amounts to the obstructed site in alternation with the *N*-acetylcysteine. The addition of oral mineral oil to the regimen after the initial mass has begun to disintegrate tends to prevent reaggregation. The first episode of difficulty with the meconium ileus equivalent should lead to upward adjustment in dose and in frequency of administration of pancreatic supplementation, which will often prevent recurrences. In some patients it has been necessary to continue the Tween 80 or *N*-acetylcysteine alone or in combination with mineral oil orally on a daily basis as a supplement to pancreatic enzymes.

Some patients with fecal impaction develop intussusception and/or volvulus. A majority of the intussusceptions are ileocolic, with the lead point frequently being a dense accumulation of thick inspissated material in the terminal ileum. Such patients may require surgery, but reduction by cautiously performed barium enema may be successful in uncomplicated cases (p. 1057). Volvulus around the site of impaction may occur at any time and is always a surgical emergency.

PROGNOSIS. The outlook for patients with cystic fibrosis has been improving. In the early years following definition of this disease, more than 80 percent of the diagnosed patients died within the first 2 years. Since 1945 there has been stress on earlier detection and early institution of antibiotic therapy, as well as improvement in evaluation and management of pulmonary disease and complications and improved nutrition with pancreatic replacement therapy and use of medium-chain triglycerides; thus today the prognosis is significantly better. While children still die in depressing numbers, most deaths are now in the latter part of the first decade and in the second decade of life. While it is still a difficult problem to treat and there is still the certainty of premature death, there is considerable gratification in following patients who survive and function more normally for ever-increasing lifespans. Data now appear regularly regarding sterility in adult males and the status of the offspring of females with the disease.

Lipid Malabsorption

The major defect in the patients described by Gee in 1888 was probably defective absorption of lipids. The disease entities that involve defective fat absorption tend to remain constant throughout the life span, and mechanisms of studying the disorders are equally applicable to children and adults. The ability to digest fat may be evaluated by both direct and indirect means. Measured meals have been fed and digestive and assimilative activities permitted to occur, following which the residue has been measured in material aspirated from tubes terminating at specific locations in the gastrointestinal tract or from stools collected for varying periods. The usual balance study technique involves collection of stools for 72 to 96 hours from a subject on a measured fat intake. Some authors utilize 5-day collections and discard those of alternate days, pooling the samples of days 1, 3, and 5 for the determination of average fat losses in the stool. Fat absorption is also assessed after feeding measured amounts of radioiodine that has been incorporated into specific saturated and unsaturated long- and short- chain fatty acids, into triglycerides of known fatty acid composition, or into fatty mixtures (Lipiodol). Although a disadvantage of such procedures is that radioisotopes must be used in young children, differential studies with a group of such agents make it possible in some instances of doubt to pinpoint whether a defect exists primarily in digestive or absorptive activity. The measurement of split and unsplit fat in the stool and the ratio of saturated to unsaturated fatty acid patterns have been utilized as indications of fat digestion and of the amount of exogenous versus endogenous fat in the specimen. These techniques are useful in a semiquantitative sense, but they cannot be interpreted with certainty when the results are not clear-cut. Perhaps amplification with more precise methods such as gas–liquid chromatography will make this type of study even more valuable in the future.

A variety of tolerance curves is employed in study of fat digestion and absorption. A chylomicron count is a crude measurement by microscope of the number of fat particles in the bloodstream after ingestion of a fatty meal. It was formerly popular to test for the differential effects of both water-miscible and fat-soluble preparations of vitamin A. Vitamin A levels in blood are measured at 1 and 5 hours after feeding either water-miscible or oily preparations of the vitamin. In the normal individual a significant rise over the baseline is expected from both. In those individuals in whom there is a defect in the digestion of vitamin A but not in absorption, as with pancreatic insufficiency, the fat-soluble preparation is not absorbed, but the tolerance curve for the water-soluble form is normal. In individuals with absorptive defects, feeding either form of vitamin A yields a low tolerance curve. Some authors do not carry out a tolerance test, but simply interpret a low fasting carotene level as indicating malabsorption. However, this interpretation is less reliable in children than in adults, since supplementation of the diet with water-miscible preparations may maintain a normal fasting carotene level even in patients with malabsorption.

Disorders of lipid absorption may be due to abnormalities of lipolysis, mucosal cell transport, or lymphatic transport of fat. However, it is difficult to pinpoint the precise mechanism causing steatorrhea in premature infants or in patients with conditions such as neurogenic tumors with increased catecholamine secretion or dysgammaglobulinemia.

ABNORMALITIES OF LIPOLYSIS. Abnormalities of lipolysis are due principally to pancreatic insufficiency, which in children is virtually restricted to cystic fibrosis of the pancreas. However, on rare occasions isolated deficiencies of specific pancreatic enzymes have been described. Pancreatic lipase may also be destroyed by the acid pH of the upper small intestine in patients with hypersecretion of gastric acid.

CONGENITAL PANCREATIC HYPOPLASIA. Congenital hypoplasia of the exocrine pancreas with neutropenia, hypoplastic anemia, thrombocytopenia, or pancytopenia is probably, after cystic fibrosis, the next most common cause of pancreatic insufficiency in childhood. Steatorrhea and retarded growth are the main clinical problems; metaphyseal dysostosis and dwarfism occur regularly. Treatment of the digestive disturbances in these patients is the same as for cystic fibrosis, but the growth retardation and hematologic abnormalities appear to be irreversible. Metaphyseal dysostosis requires orthopedic corrective measures. The frequency is estimated as approximately 1 in 20,000 live births, and an autosomal recessive pattern of inheritance is suggested. Immunoglobulin deficiency may possibly play a role. Those patients with neutropenia and possible immune deficiencies require aggressive antimicrobial treatment to prevent deterioration from frequent infections, primarily of the skin and respiratory tract. Pulmonary involvement may lead to confusion with cystic fibrosis. However, the diseases are easily differentiated by sweat electrolyte determinations, which are normal in this syndrome.

ISOLATED LIPASE DEFICIENCY.   This extremely rare disease is characterized by severe steatorrhea beginning shortly after birth. The duodenal juice contains normal amounts of amalyse and proteolytic activity, whereas lipase is low. Prognosis is favorable. The patients are fed low-fat diets. Supplementation of normal-fat-containing diets with pancreatic extracts is not effective because of the poor preservation of lipase in the commercial preparations. Although there have been no reports on the effects of medium-chain triglyceride formulas in the diets of such patients, one would expect that they might be useful.

CONJUGATED BILE SALT DEFICIENCY.   In those conditions in which normal hepatic function is impaired or in which there is obstruction to flow of bile into the duodenum, the critical levels of conjugated bile salts essential to the formation of micelles may not be reached, and solubilization will be impaired. In addition to liver diseases, this problem may occur in those instances in which chronic stasis of the small bowel results in bacterial overgrowth of this region with resultant deconjugation of the bile salts by the organisms. Such bacterial overgrowth is encountered in a variety of conditions, including decreased acidity (as with achlorhydria following resections of the stomach), malrotations, multiple small-intestine strictures, and jejunal diverticula and duplications. Another factor that interferes with the effectiveness of conjugated bile salts in micellar formation is disturbance in the enterohepatic circulation resulting from extensive disease of the distal small bowel or absence of this segment after surgery for a congenital obstruction or an acquired inflammatory disease.

ABNORMALITIES OF MUCOSAL CELL TRANSPORT OF LIPIDS.   IDIOPATHIC CELIAC DISEASE.   Idiopathic celiac disease (gluten-induced enteropathy), which is relatively rare in the United States, is characterized by malabsorption of fat. In this disease, in contrast to cystic fibrosis of the pancreas, there does not appear to be any deficiency in lipolysis. The major clinical manifestations as well as the physiologic and biochemical abnormalities observed in patients with idiopathic celiac disease can be attributed to the malabsorption of fat and the resulting malnutrition. In virtually all respects idiopathic celiac disease in children is identical with nontropical sprue as seen in adults, and the latter term has now generally been abandoned in favor of celiac disease in all age groups.

Etiology.   The exact cause and pathogenesis of celiac disease are still unknown. There is some evidence that a genetic constitutional factor may play a role; in some families it has occurred in more than one child. Symptoms suggesting celiac disease during early childhood have been reported in the medical history of a number of adults. In addition, there is evidence that intolerance to certain proteins plays a par_ in most instances of the disease. A close correlation is observed between the ingestion of wheat flour and exacerbations. The disturbing factor in wheat lies in a protein moiety, gluten, particularly its gliadin component. Oral administration of glutamine, the amino acid that comprises 43 percent of the nitrogen of gliadin, has no demonstrable effect on a patient with celiac disease, but the feeding of various peptide fractions of gliadin is deleterious to these patients. Patients with celiac disease have been described who show no sensitivity to gluten but who demonstrate steatorrhea following ingestion of small amounts of cow's-milk β-lactoglobulin or soy protein. In other instances it has been demonstrated that steatorrhea following ingestion of cow's milk precedes the frank onset of gluten sensitivity. These observations suggest the possibility that a variety of proteins may play specific roles in individual patients.

A variety of nonspecific stresses may initiate or aggravate symptoms. Chief among these are parenteral infections; they appear to have effects no different from those seen in many normal infants. What differentiates the patient with celiac disease is the prolonged duration of his response, as well as the often minor nature of the infections and the persistence of the pattern beyond infancy. In this sense the difference between the normal and the celiac subject is one of degree. One child passes through acute infections, even in infancy, without any disturbance of digestion; another develops diarrhea that may outlast evidence of infection for 1 or 2 weeks; in a third, whom we label a celiac, the disturbance of assimilation persists for months, and the tendency to it extends beyond the age of infancy. Most pediatricians agree that emotional stress may initiate or aggravate the symptoms in the absence of infections. Opinions are more disparate concerning the effect of the fat content of the diet.

Pathology.   A major advance in the diagnosis of celiac disease has been the introduction of the peroral biopsy technique. Many kinds of tubes and capsules may be employed, but the principle common to all involves the sucking in of a small knuckle of upper intestinal mucosa, which is amputated relatively atraumatically and is withdrawn for examination. Although rare instances of protracted bleeding or perforation have been encountered, thousands of biopsies have been performed without incident. The tissue recovered may be examined by light and electron microscopy, studied chemically for enzymes and other constituents, or assayed for immune substances. Microscopic examination is of particular value for the diagnosis and follow-up of patients with celiac disease.

Mucosal lesions of the small intestine are apparent on gross and microscopic examination. Loss of villi with obliteration of intervillous spaces can be demonstrated by light microscopy. The mucosal cells tend to become more cuboid than columnar, and there is disturbance in the normal basal position of their nuclei. The crypts are deeper, and increased mitoses can be observed in the cells that line them. The monocellular population of the lamina propria is also increased. Electron micrographs reveal decreases and shortening of microvilli. The changes can be shown to be reversible in patients treated by exclusion of gluten from the diet. The specificity of the lesion for celiac disease is sometimes questioned, since similar changes in villi may occur in some inflammatory conditions and in other instances of malnutrition. However, among such patients the findings are usually not as generalized and are less intense than those observed so uniformly in all patients with untreated celiac disease.

Other anatomic changes observed in a limited number of autopsies are those of inanition. There is conspicuous atrophy of fat, lymphoid tissue, and muscle; a small heart is not an uncommon finding. Evidence of infection or of specific deficiencies may be encountered. There may be a fatty liver.

Pathologic Physiology.   The view that starch ingestion has an adverse effect on celiac disease is no longer widely held. It is the specific protein of flour rather than the starch that is responsible. Starch itself is reasonably well absorbed, and the presence of extracellular starch granules in the stools carries no sinister significance. A flat or nearly flat blood sugar curve following oral ingestion of glucose or the pentose sugar xylose is commonly found in idiopathic celiac disease. It is by no means specific for this condition, since it is also encountered in severe malnutrition of any cause and in some chronic disorders affecting hepatic function. Using isotope-labeled glucose in tolerance tests on patients with celiac disease, Somersalo was able to demonstrate that the absorption of glucose was minimally affected; the flat tolerance curve was attributed to delay in the rate of absorption.

The assimilation of protein is affected relatively little in the celiac patient. Except during episodes of diarrhea, from 80 to 90 percent of the nitrogen intake is absorbed, and blood amino acid curves after a test dose of casein or gelatin follow a normal pattern. However, hypoproteinemia and nutritional edema are sometimes encountered. In some of these cases they result from diversion of essential amino acids to abnormal metabolic pathways by intestinal flora. In other cases it has been possible to demonstrate that the hypoproteinemia results from excessive losses of serum proteins into the gastrointestinal lumen, while in still other cases the hypoproteinemia may reflect overall malnutrition. It has been our impression that the hydrolability often seen in these patients is related to hypoproteinemia. Such patients, when affected by an intercurrent acute digestive upset, may lose weight so precipitously and develop alarming symptoms of dehydration so rapidly as to justify the term celiac crisis.

The fundamental defect in celiac disease is malabsorption of fat, the unabsorbed fat of the feces being virtually completely split. As in the normal subject, the unsaturated and short-chain fats are more readily absorbed; the unabsorbed fecal fats are therefore the longer chain saturated fatty acids. To what extent and in what manner the atrophic changes described in the intestinal villi are responsible for the deficit in absorption are not known. The earlier view that the fat intolerance was induced by fat and could be ameliorated by limiting the fat intake has little support.

Symptoms.   In most patients with celiac disease the symptoms begin during infancy, although rarely before 6 months of age. Only exceptionally does the process begin later than 3 years of age. Although breast feeding will not prevent the development of celiac disease, it has a tendency to postpone the time of appearance of symptoms, probably because many breast-fed infants are introduced to solid foods, including wheat cereal, at a later time. The development of the frank clinical picture is inevitably insidious, but it often follows one or more acute episodes. A common story is that the infant suffered from one or more attacks of acute diarrhea, perhaps associated with respiratory infections and accompanied by vomiting. Recovery from these symptoms seems to be incomplete. The appetite is not restored, and normal weight gain is not resumed. The stools, although numbering only one to three a day, tend to be mushy and unusually bulky; they are foul and often frothy.

If the condition persists the picture of chronic malnutrition becomes established. There is loss of subcutaneous fat that is particularly conspicuous in the buttocks. Muscular activity is diminished, and the muscles lose their tone; the abdomen becomes distended. There is a change in disposition, with the child becoming fretful. Sleep is often disturbed.

Exacerbations of the acute digestive disturbances occur at irregular intervals. Often they are precipitated by obvious infections; at other times these may not be as apparent, and other causes may be implicated. In those patients in whom sensitivity to protein has been demonstrated, relatively minor dietary indiscretions may produce exacerbations of the disease. During these episodes acute diarrhea may develop, sometimes of alarming severity; vomiting may also occur, and loss of weight may be precipitous, obliterating several months' gains. The hydrolability and marked anorexia of these patients are often very striking.

With persistence of the celiac state evidence of malnutrition becomes more conspicuous, and specific deficiencies may make their appearance. Anemia is one of the most common; usually it is microcytic, but occasionally the macrocytic type more characteristic of adults is encountered. There may be hypoproteinemia and nutritional edema. Symptoms due to deficiency of fat-soluble vitamins may develop in severe and long-standing cases. Tetany and rickets as complications of celiac disease, which are apparently more common in Europe, are seen rarely in this country. Osteoporosis may be the only expression of vitamin D deficiency. The osteoporotic bones are fragile, and fractures of the long bones may occur. Hypoprothrombinemia due to deficient absorption of vitamin K is occasionally seen, but hemorrhage is rare. Frank vitamin A deficiency is virtually unknown in celiac patients in the United States, despite the fact that it is a common complication in other parts of the world. Clinical deficiencies of the B group are rare, although thiamine deficiency has been reported. Delay in growth and in skeletal maturation is commonly found, and if the condition persists for years there may be some permanent impairment of growth.

The prognosis in the individual case must be based

largely on prolonged observation of the patient. There is generally a period of quiescence in late childhood and adolescence, even without treatment, that is referred to as the latent period. However, evidence is accumulating that mucosal lesions, mild degrees of steatorrhea, and less than optimal growth may result from failure to adhere to a strict diet during this age period. Intellectual development is not permanently impaired by the nutritional disturbance. Although celiac patients frequently appear dull, they progress normally with convalescence. Alarming numbers of cases are now beginning to appear in which long-standing disease has ended in lymphomas and reticulum cell sarcomas of the small intestine. It is too early to make further comment on this subject.

Diagnosis. In the presence of chronic malnutrition and typical stools, steatorrhea must be established before the diagnosis of celiac disease can be made. Steatorrhea is most accurately measured by a complete fecal collection for a period of several days. Children with celiac disease absorb less than 90 percent of ingested fat and show fecal loss of fat greater than 3 to 5 g/day. There has been an unfortunate tendency to make the diagnosis in many children who suffer one or more acute digestive upsets from which they may recover entirely, as well as a tendency to make the diagnosis in many children with the "irritable colon syndrome". To label such children as celiac often results in their being placed on sharply restricted diets and becoming the objects of undue concern. Once steatorrhea has been demonstrated in the individual patient, other causes of this condition must be ruled out before the diagnosis of idiopathic celiac disease is tenable.

Of special importance to the differential diagnosis is the demonstration that apathy, negativism, anorexia, and evidences of abnormal absorption may be reversed after a short period of intake of a gluten-free diet. The abnormalities observed on peroral biopsy specimens of the upper intestinal mucosa are also reversible, but only after a number of months on a gluten-free diet.

Radiography of the small intestine in celiac disease usually reveals a clumping segmentation pattern similar to that seen in the normal young infant. However, such a pattern is abnormal when seen after the first year; its presence is not confined to celiac disease, but its absence would make one question that diagnosis. Radiography is also employed to rule out the possibility of a short-circuiting congenital anomaly that might result in steatorrhea.

Treatment. Successful therapy in celiac disease depends on maintaining the patient's nutrition from the point of view of calories and specific nutrients and on treating intercurrent complications, especially infections. Attempts should be made to avoid excessive psychologic stress.

In those patients sensitive to gluten, complete elimination of this protein from the diet and substitution of corn, rice, soybean, or buckwheat flour for wheat, rye, barley, and oats often have a striking effect. It has been our experience with such children that strict adherence to such an elimination regimen permits complete freedom from symptoms. The efficacy of an elimination diet has also been well demonstrated in instances of sensitivity to the β-lactoglobulin of cow's milk. Patients should otherwise receive a nutritious diet that is rich in other proteins.

The view that carbohydrates are not well tolerated by patients with celiac disease can probably be attributed to the occasional instance in which extreme mucosal changes result in temporary acquired disaccharidase deficiency or glucose-galactose intolerance. In these instances, until successful regeneration of villi has occurred in response to a gluten-free diet, it may be necessary to avoid lactose or sucrose.

Restriction of fat has been widely advocated with a view to decreasing fecal losses and with the hope that partial rest of the disordered function of fat assimilation will promote recovery. On the other hand, those who have employed generous fat intakes, even prior to the introduction of the gluten-free diet, have not been impressed with unfavorable effects on tolerance. Balance studies have shown that even high levels of fat do not affect the percentage absorbed; they increase the fecal loss of fat but also increase the absolute amount absorbed by the patient, and they produce no consistent effect on the assimilation of other foodstuffs. When fats are to be given there is some advantage in replacing butter in part by vegetable oil, which contains a higher proportion of the more readily assimilable unsaturated fatty acids. Feeding of medium-chain triglycerides, which contain fatty acids ranging from 8 to 12 carbons, yields virtually quantitative absorption, presumably directly into the portal circulation.

Fat-soluble vitamins should be provided in increased quantities to compensate for impaired absorption. Anemia should be watched for and treated appropriately with iron if it is of the usual microcytic variety, or with folic acid when it is macrocytic. Other drugs play little part in therapy.

Some patients, especially those with hypoproteinemia, seem to be unusually hydrolabile and may develop alarming symptoms of fluid loss and shock with great rapidity. The management of these acute episodes differs in no way from that of hypovolemic shock in general.

The psychologic disturbances of the celiac patient should not be overlooked. Patients who are markedly undernourished are often petulant and difficult to manage, requiring a combination of patience and firmness that is not always available. Emotional tensions in the family may compromise the environment needed for convalescence and recovery and may exercise an unfavorable influence on the child's digestion. Mothers of these patients are often tense, apprehensive, and overprotective. The aura of mystery conveyed to the lay mind by the term celiac and the rigid systems of control often employed may perpetuate an attitude of invalidism, which must be guarded against.

NONSPECIFIC DISORDERS OF MUCOSAL CELL TRANSPORT. In addition to the villous atrophy and mucosal cell disorganization associated with ingestion of specific proteins, such as gluten in celiac disease, many other noxious agents are associated with a similar effect on the mucosa of the small intestine. In most instances the clinical manifestations and the laboratory tests for steatorrhea are similar to those in celiac disease. However, the condition is not improved by feeding a gluten-free diet, although in some instances authors report some crossover between onset from another cause and worsening of the disease with gluten ingestion.

Tropical sprue. Is a condition similar to celiac disease that is encountered in patients from warm countries. In tropical sprue there is a greater monocellular and eosinophilic infiltration of the lamina propria of the blunted villi. Reported improvement with long-term antimicrobial therapy has suggested an infectious etiology. Additional beneficial effects from withdrawal of gluten from the diet have also been observed in certain instances. In addition, megaloblastosis is the rule in tropical sprue, and folic acid therapy is beneficial. This is in contrast to celiac disease, in which there is depression of serum folate levels, but rarely a macrocytic anemia.

Malabsorption of lipids occurs in certain skin diseases, particularly *dermatitis herpetiformis* (p. 871) and *acrodermatitis enteropathica,* and in a limited number of these instances abnormal upper intestinal mucosal biopsies are reported. These diseases are not related to gluten ingestion. Acrodermatitis enteropathica, which is related to an abnormality of zinc metabolism, is also probably associated with immunoglobulin insufficiency. It is improved by feeding unpasteurized human milk, a source of secretory IgA and by administration of supplemental zinc sulfate. Additional causes of upper intestinal mucosal abnormalities are infiltration with parasites, particularly *Giardia lamblia,* prolonged or intensive irradiation or treatment with drugs of the antifolic-acid group, and infiltration of the bowel wall by tumors or by inflammatory diseases. Circulatory disturbances, chiefly vascular occlusions or chronic heart failure, have also been observed to lead to villous atrophy and impaired lipid absorption.

ABETALIPOPROTEINEMIA. Abetalipoproteinemia (acanthocytosis) is a rare hereditary disorder of mucosal cell transport in which there is a congenital deficiency in the ability to synthesize β-lipoprotein. These patients demonstrate abnormalities of the central nervous system, ocular defects, and red blood cell membrane deficiencies (p. 1919). It is from the last abnormality that the secondary name of acanthocytosis is derived.

The gastrointestinal manifestations in this disease are associated with the inability to transport absorbed fat from the intestinal mucosa. Since the intestinal mucosal cells cannot synthesize β-lipoprotein, they are unable to invest the triglycerides reconstituted after fatty acid absorption with a protein envelope containing this substance. This limits chylomicron formation, and lipid cannot be transported into the lymphatic system. However, carbohydrate tolerance tests are normal, in contradistinction to most other diseases with fat malabsorption. Peroral intestinal biopsy specimens have a characteristic frosted appearance imparted by heavy fat

accumulations. The site of pileup in the mucosal cell is easily demonstrated on light microscopic examination of specimens stained for fat.

Treatment consists of a low-fat diet. Feeding of medium-chain triglycerides results in a decrease in steatorrhea and improved general nutrition. However, this treatment does not improve the basic defect and has no influence on the ocular, red blood cell, or central nervous system lesions.

ABNORMALITIES OF INTESTINAL LYMPHATIC TRANSPORT. Mechanical blockage of the lymphatics is encountered in a number of conditions and is associated with steatorrhea. Increased pressure on the intestinal lymphatics results in dilation of the lacteals in the villi. In many of these diseases fat losses are of less importance than the exudation of protein.

Among the many acquired diseases in which this abnormality may occur are lymphomas, leukemia, infectious lymphadenopathy (as in tuberculosis or parasitic infestations), and scarring of the submucosa after irradiation. Widespread congenital obstructive abnormalities of the lymphatic system (Milroy's disease) may be associated with dilation of intestinal lacteals; the disease may also be confined to lymphatics of the mucosa. The latter condition is known as congenital lymphangiectasia and may be widespread over the intestine or confined to a localized segment of small bowel. The peroral biopsy is characteristic.

Administration of a low-fat diet or of medium-chain triglycerides in the diet reduces protein loss and steatorrhea in these patients. If the condition is secondary to a primary disease that can be ameliorated with reduction of the pressure in the intestinal lymphatics, the symptoms improve or subside. Occasionally it can be demonstrated radiographically that the lymphangiectasia is confined to a limited area of the intestine in which the mucosal patterns are strikingly disordered; in such instances surgical excision of the affected region affords complete cure.

Carbohydrate Malabsorption

POLYSACCHARIDES AND STARCH INTOLERANCE. The concept of starch intolerance is not useful. In his initial report of celiac disease in the United States in 1908, Herter reported that the children were made worse by ingestion of certain starchy foods. However, he clearly did not believe that this was intolerance to starch, since on the basis of his empiric observations he did not advise withholding starch but rather recommended substitution of certain starchy foods for others. With the demonstration of the pathogenetic role of the protein complex gluten from wheat and rye, the lack of any effect of starch in this disease is established. Nevertheless, in the 40 years between Herter's report and the elucidation of the role of gluten, pediatricians focused their attentions on starch and made the diagnosis of starch intolerance in many children, who were then treated with rigid starch-poor diets. The routine microscopic examination of stools for starch became the standard test to establish the diagnosis. It has been established that this test is not reliable and that many normal children pass undigested starch in their stools. The diagnosis of starch intolerance is not tenable by the criteria currently in use and should not be made. Virtually all children diagnosed as having starch intolerance have the condition termed *irritable colon of childhood.* Occasionally children with sucrase-isomaltase deficiency might be expected to be intolerant to starches. However, isomaltose makes up only a small fraction of most starches, and the rare clinical problems are relatively minor when they do occur and are limited to the early months of life.

DISACCHARIDE AND OLIGOSACCHARIDE MALABSORPTION
PHILIP SUNSHINE
AND
NORMAN KRETCHMER

Abnormalities of sugar digestion and absorption have been recognized for many years, but it was not until 1958 that Durand described an infant who suffered from vomiting, diarrhea, and failure to thrive and who had both lactosuria and amino-aciduria. The following year Holzel and associates described siblings who were unable to hydrolyze lactose and who had fermentative diarrhea. These observations led to recognition of lactose malabsorption and subsequently sucrose-isomaltose malabsorption as distinct entities in infants and children that could cause failure of growth and develop-

TABLE 2. Classification of Sugar Malabsorption

Congenital abnormalities
   Glucose-galactose malabsorption
   Sucrose-isomaltose malabsorption
   Lactose malabsorption
Acquired or secondary disaccharide malabsorption
   associated with:
      Infectious diarrhea in infancy and childhood
      Kwashiorkor or severe malnutrition
      Gluten-induced enteropathy
      Cystic fibrosis
      Ulcerative colitis or granulomatous enterocolitis
      Blind-loop syndrome
      Severe *Giardia* infestation
      β-lipoprotein deficiency
      Extensive resection of the small intestine
      Immunologic deficiency syndromes
      Necrotizing enterocolitis
      Drug ingestion (colchicine, neomycin, birth control medication)

ment. Initially all of these defects were thought to be related to a congenital deficiency of the disaccharidases. It soon became apparent that carbohydrate malabsorption could be an acquired abnormality associated with other defects that could damage or alter the normal intestinal epithelia. Sugar malabsorption syndromes may be classified as either congenital or acquired defects (Table 2).

CONGENITAL ABNORMALITIES. Glucose-Galactose Malabsorption. Although these patients may have normal activities of intestinal disaccharidases, they have a congenital inability to absorb actively either glucose or galactose. The defect is inherited as an autosomal recessive disease and affects both the intestine and the kidney. Ingestion of either glucose or galactose by these patients will produce severe watery diarrhea, but intravenous infusions of either glucose or galactose are metabolized normally. The patients also have decreased urinary clearance of these monosaccharides, and glycosuria is a common finding. The mucosal morphology is normal, but the accumulation of either glucose or galactose by the intestinal cells is defective. Sodium absorption, sodium activation of invertase, Na^+-K^+-dependent ATPase activity, and absorption of L-amino acids are all normal. The basic defect appears to be either absence or alteration of a binding protein that is located in the brush border membrane of the microvilli and that facilitates the binding and movement of glucose and galactose into the epithelial cell. Fructose, which is absorbed normally, may be used as the source of carbohydrate in the diet of these infants.

Transient malabsorption of monosaccharides has been described in patients who have had resection of portions of the small intestine, in certain infants who have had acute episodes of gastroenteritis, and in some newborns following perinatal hypoxia or asphyxia. These infants develop watery diarrhea, metabolic acidosis, and often severe hypoglycemia. The mechanism responsible for the defect is not clearly understood, but it may be due to the presence of increased concentrations of deconjugated bile acids secondary to bacterial overgrowth. Another mechanism that has been postulated is the presence of increased intestinal contents that overlie the surface membrane of the intestine and prevent the sugars from making contact with the brush border itself. Often the infants will not tolerate any feeding that contains more than 1 to 2 percent carbohydrate. If the basic pathophysiology can be corrected, these patients will begin to tolerate normal carbohydrate intake after several weeks or months.

Sucrose-Isomaltose Malabsorption. The sucrose-isomal-tose malabsorption defect is due to congenital deficiencies of both intestinal sucrase and isomaltase. It is inherited as an autosomal recessive disorder. The defect is much more common than congenital lactose malabsorption. In many patients the clinical manifestations of the disorder are not severe. Most infants ingest either breast milk or formulas that contain lactose and will not have any clinical manifestations until sucrose or starch-containing foods are added to their diets. If the infant is fed a proprietary formula containing sucrose, the clinical signs may be manifested in the early neonatal period. Cereals, especially those with added sucrose, are poorly tolerated. Although isomaltose constitutes only 4 or 5 percent of dietary starch, the presence of this sugar in starch-containing foods is thought to be responsible for producing diarrhea in these patients. These patients do not hydrolyze oligosaccharides such as maltotriose or even maltotetrose readily, and the presence of these sugars in the intestinal lumen will accentuate the diarrhea.

As these children mature they are able to tolerate increasing amounts of sucrose and starch, despite the fact that the specific activities of both sucrase and isomaltase remain decreased. The morphology of the small intestine is normal as shown by light microscopy, and the activities of trehelase, β-galactosidases, and various other digestive enzymes are within normal ranges.

Sucrose-isomaltose malabsorption is one of the rare genetic disorders in which two enzymatic activities are affected. There are many investigators who believe that only one enzyme is involved and that the enzyme has two active sites for hydrolysis of both disaccharides. Attempts to identify two separate enzymes by ion exchange, gel filtration, or trypsin inhibition techniques have not been successful, and heat inactivation offers the only tenuous data indicating that there are two separate enzymes.

Congenital Lactose Malabsorption. The defect of congenital lactose malabsorption is rare, and few cases have been documented in the neonatal period that persist into late infancy and childhood. Many patients appear to have either a delay in development or maturation of intestinal lactase or an acquired defect secondary to mucosal damage. Because of the difficulty in diagnosing the entity precisely, the exact incidence of the defect and the mode of inheritance have not been elucidated. Although the incidence of congenital lactose malabsorption is low, the prevalence of lactose malabsorption in adults is quite high. About 10 percent of Caucasians, 70 to 80 percent of American blacks, and an even greater percentage of Orientals will manifest lactose malabsorption as adults even though they were able to digest lactose as infants. Many Greek Cypriots, southern Italians, Arabs, Jews, Eskimos, and North and South American Indians also have a very high incidence of lactose maldigestors in their adult populations.

Why some people lose their ability to digest lactose as adults while others retain this ability has not been elucidated. A cultural historical hypothesis has been advanced to explain this phenomenon. Supposedly, during the early stages of human evolution man had a developmental pattern of intestinal lactase similar to that of other land mammals, wherein the activity is very high during the nursing period and decreases to low levels after weaning and remains low in the adult; however, during evolution a mutation occurred that allowed certain groups to retain their ability to digest lactose into adult life.

Investigators have postulated that such genetic selection occurred initially among pastoralists and then among others who had the opportunity to consume large quantities of milk. Those adult humans who can digest lactose, including many Scandinavians, French, Germans, Dutch, Poles, Czechs, and northern Italians, as well as particular African tribes such as the Fulani and Tussi, transmit this ability as a dominant characteristic. Those who are unable to digest lactose lose their ability to do so at varying times during development. The Yoruba tribe in Nigeria become lactose maldigestors by the age of 2 to 3 years, the Bagandas by the age of 3 to 4 years, the Pima and Papago American Indians of the southwestern United States and most American blacks by 4 to 5 years of age.

The problem of lactose malabsorption is universal, and before any large-scale milk supplementation program is begun for any group of people, the ability of that population to digest lactose should be evaluated carefully in order to prevent the consequences that may occur following ingestion of milk.

ACQUIRED ABNORMALITIES. The acquired defects of carbohydrate absorption are responsible for the presenting of problems in the greatest number of patients. It appears that any disorder that can damage the intestinal cell can produce disaccharide malabsorption. This is especially true in patients with gluten-induced enteropathy or infections that damage the small intestine. Lactase appears to be the digestive enzyme most readily affected and is usually the last to reappear after the small intestine has returned to normal function. The enzyme is usually low in activity as compared to sucrase and maltase, and any disorder that affects the small intestine usually will affect lactase primarily. In adults the intestine has a rapid turnover rate that in normal patients may be between 48 and 72 hours. If the intestine is damaged, the turnover rate may be prolonged. Although conclusive data in humans are lacking, there are indications in laboratory animals that the turnover rate in suckling animals is markedly prolonged and may approach 6 to 7 days. Thus any damage to the mucosa in suckling animals would require almost twice as long to repair as would the adult mucosa, and the activities of intestinal disaccharidases, especially lactase, might be depressed for a greater period of time.

Cystic Fibrosis. Approximately 15 percent of patients with cystic fibrosis have lactose malabsorption. The mechanism by which this takes place has not been determined. This disaccharidase deficiency occurs even when the intestinal morphology appears to be grossly normal.

Necrotizing Enterocolitis. Many infants with necrotizing enterocolitis will demonstrate decreasing ability to digest carbohydrates as an initial manifestation of their disease. Also, many infants will be unable to digest carbohydrates adequately during the recovery period of their illness.

Drugs. Certain drugs such as colchicine and neomycin have a unique capability of depressing the activity of various disaccharidases, especially lactase, even though the gross morphology of the intestine may not be affected. In laboratory animals small amounts of colchicine appear to exert their effect directly on the differentiated cell of the villus without affecting cellular renewal or proliferation.

PATHOPHYSIOLOGY. When patients with carbohydrate malabsorption ingest the sugar to which they are intolerant, a watery fermentative diarrhea ensues. The sugar that is not hydrolyzed remains in the lumen of the intestine; and although small amounts may passively diffuse across the cell membrane, most of the unhydrolyzed sugar will pass through the small intestine unchanged. The sugar will act as an osmotic hydrogogue and cause an increased amount of fluid to accumulate in the intestinal lumen. In the distal ileum and colon, bacteria ferment the sugar to lactic and acetic acids, and these molecules can act so as to increase the water content within the lumen of the bowel. Lactic and acetic acid may be irritating to the colon as well and may perpetuate the water loss. The stool is watery, with low pH (4.0 to 5.0), and is irritating to the rectoanal area.

The unhydrolyzed sugar that passively diffuses into the intestinal cell is usually excreted unchanged in the urine. Although it has not been proved, it appears that the disaccharide or oligosaccharide is toxic to both the intestinal cell and the renal tubular cell. Other sugars as well as various amino acids are in turn poorly reabsorbed from the renal tubule, and significant mellituria and amino-aciduria may result.

CLINICAL MANIFESTATIONS.   The clinical manifestations of carbohydrate malabsorption are fairly characteristic and do not depend on the specific disaccharide or oligosaccharide involved. However, the earlier in infancy the disorder becomes manifest, the more serious are the complications. Infants with lactose malabsorption are the most severely affected because of marked fluid and electrolyte imbalance and also because it takes longer for the intestine to recover normal function. Severe fermentative diarrhea associated with abdominal cramping, dehydration, and acidosis are common findings in these patients. Although it is not mentioned widely in the literature, another common finding in infancy is vomiting, which occasionally may be present in the absence of diarrhea. Initially the infants may demonstrate a voracious appetite in order to compensate for intestinal losses, but after a period of time they become lethargic, irritable, and anorectic. Steatorrhea is encountered in some patients with carbohydrate intolerance and is usually a sign that the small intestine has suffered significant damage. It is usually not encountered in patients with congenital defects early in the course of their disease.

If the disorder is unrecognized in infancy, dehydration, acidosis, and mucosal damage will result and irreversible damage to the small intestine will ensue. The infant can develop protein-losing enteropathy and intractable and unrelenting diarrhea and may succumb in a severely malnourished state. Older infants and children do not seem to have a protracted course, and many patients with sucrose-isomaltose malabsorption appear to tolerate these sugars more readily as they mature.

The patients who have acquired carbohydrate malabsorption usually regain their ability to hydrolyze the carbohydrate to which they are intolerant when the basic pathophysiology has returned to normal. Some children with lactose malabsorption have recurrent abdominal pain and similar complaints, as do adults with the irritable colon syndrome.

Adults usually have minimal signs and symptoms of carbohydrate malabsorption that include bloating, abdominal cramps, and loose stools. In fact, some adults who recognize their intolerance will use milk or lactose as a cathartic.

DIAGNOSIS.   If a patient is suspected of having carbohydrate malabsorption, diagnostic procedures should be performed without delay. Screening procedures such as examining fresh stools or rectal swabs for acidity and reducing substances have been advocated, but they are not helpful and are often misleading in very young patients. If the patient has not ingested the carbohydrate to which he is intolerant, the changes in the stool may not be detected.

Disaccharide and monosaccharide tolerance tests are useful as screening procedures, although there is a great deal of debate as to their validity. If the emptying time of the stomach is delayed, a very slow rise in blood glucose may be noted. Also, measurements of glucose concentration in capillary blood tend to be greater than those of venous blood and may therefore alter the interpretation of results.

In most instances an increase in the concentration of glucose in blood greater than 25 mg/100 ml within 1 hour after ingestion of 2.0 to 2.5 g disaccharide per kilogram of body weight indicates that significant hydrolysis of sugar has occurred. Some investigators have indicated that a rise of 20 mg/100 ml or greater is normal after the ingestion of lactose, but that a much greater increase is usually found after the ingestion of sucrose. The patient should be carefully observed for development of abdominal cramps or watery diarrhea within 2 to 6 hours following ingestion of the test substance. If a patient has normal elevation in concentration of glucose in blood and no symptoms following ingestion of the sugar, the diagnosis of carbohydrate malabsorption cannot be made. However, if the rise in concentration of glucose in blood is less than 25 mg/100 ml, a diagnosis may be suspected.

Radiographic techniques utilizing lactose in a barium mixture have been utilized to demonstrate marked outpouring of fluid into the lumen of the colon in patients with lactose malabsorption. This increased fluid loss occurs in the area of the splenic flexure. Analysis of hydrogen in breath after ingestion of lactose has been used to identify lactose malabsorbers. As fermentable substances reach the colon, increased colonic luminal hydrogen will be absorbed and excreted via the respiratory tract. Although this technique is noninvasive, it requires the use of elaborate and expensive equipment.

Several authors have attempted to identify patients with *congenital* lactose malabsorption and distinguish them from those with *acquired* lactose malabsorption by the presence of lactosuria; if lactosuria were present, the patient would be diagnosed as having the acquired form of the disease. Data from laboratory animals as well as affected adults raise doubts about the diagnostic significance of this finding. The presence of lactosuria depends not only on the mucosal structure and function and the activity of the disaccharidase but also on the amount of substrate presented to the mucosa.

Biopsies of the mucosa of the small bowel and direct assay of the disaccharidases are the best methods of correctly diagnosing the disorder. Initially research tools, the biopsies and assays have now been adapted for clinical diagnosis. If biopsies are taken from the duodenum or jejunum that has been damaged, the activities of the enzymes are decreased. If activity ratios such as sucrase to lactase or isomaltase to lactase are used, the interpretations may be made with greater validity. Although the techniques for biopsy and assay are the most reliable diagnostic tools available, there are rare occasions when the results may be misleading. Therefore one must use the clinical features, laboratory diagnosis, and mucosal assays to arrive at a correct diagnosis.

TREATMENT. Treatment is almost always dietary in nature and consists of removing the offending sugar or sugars from the diet. Patients who have glucose-galactose malabsorption are the most difficult patients to treat, and fructose must be the only sugar in their diet. Patients with lactose malabsorption will thrive on a diet in which milk intake is reduced. They usually do not have to be placed on a diet completely free of milk and milk products; they will thrive if they do not drink milk with meals. Newborns and small infants must be fed formulas that do not contain lactose; they will grow and develop if they are fed soybean, meat-base, or other formulas in which sucrose, glucose, or maltose has been substituted for lactose (Table 3). On occasion, an infant will tolerate little or no carbohydrate, and a carbohydrate-free formula will have to be given. Infrequently a patient will have such extensive mucosal damage that an intractable diarrhea will result. These patients have to be maintained on hypercaloric intravenous feedings that contain 15 to 25 percent glucose, 2 to 3 percent hydrolyzed protein or amino acids, vitamins, and electrolytes. They can then be fed very small amounts of oral nutriments until they regain their ability to digest and absorb food normally. Sometimes this treatment

may require several months before any oral feedings are tolerated.

Patients with sucrose-isomaltose malabsorption can be managed quite well simply by omitting sucrose-containing foods from their diets. A starch-free diet is usually not necessary, as the infants and children may tolerate a small to moderate amount of starch without difficulty. The parents can usually determine the amount of starch their child can tolerate by observing the effect of diet on the frequency and amount of stool excreted by the patient. As these children mature the amount of starch they can tolerate increases, so that they can usually ingest a fairly normal diet.

Protein Malabsorption

Gastric achylia is uncommon in children, but in rare instances in which partial or total gastrectomy is performed for tumors or congenital defects, achlorhydria may result. Although gastric achlorhydria primarily induces disordered protein digestion, secondary problems of malabsorption often complicate the deficiency. The lack of hydrochloric acid may lead to decreased pancreatic secretion or to excessive multiplication of flora of the upper small intestine. These effects result in further decrease of proteolysis and disturbed lipid digestion and absorption.

Deficiency of exocrine secretion of the pancreas results in an assimilatory defect caused by incomplete splitting of protein. In the United States pancreatic insufficiency of this type in children occurs almost exclusively in cystic fibrosis of the pancreas, a congenital condition in which deficiency of the exocrine secretion of the pancreas is only one part of a more generalized

TABLE 3. Composition of Carbohydrates in Various Milks

Milk	Lactose	Sucrose	Glucose	Maltose	Dextrin or Starch
Human milk	X				
Cow's milk	X				
Goat's milk	X				
Evaporated milk	X				
Alacta	X				
Olac	X			X	X
Similac	X				
Enfamil	X				
Nutramigen		X			X
Probana	X		X		X
Soyalac		X	X	X	X
ProSobee		X	X	X	X
Mull-soy		X			X
Baker's	X		X	X	X
Isomel		X	X	X	X
Meat-base		X			X
Portagen	X	X			X
Pregestimil			X		X
CHo-Free (dextrose, sucrose, or lactose may be added)					

disorder (p. 993). The pancreatic insufficiency of this disease is by far the most common cause of malabsorption among children. Patients have been described with isolated pancreatic deficiencies associated with bone marrow insufficiencies that result in neutropenia, anemia, and thrombocytopenia. Some of these patients display marked growth retardation and show evidence of metaphyseal dysostosis on radiography. Among children with this syndrome who have died, post-mortem examinations have showed extensive replacement of pancreatic tissue with fat; hence the alternative name *congenital lipomatosis* of the pancreas.

Isolated Trypsinogen and Intestinal Enterokinase Deficiencies. A congenital isolated absence of trypsinoge results in a deficiency of all proteolytic enzymes, since chymotrypsinogen and procarboxypeptidase are not activated in the absence of tryptic activity. It is unclear whether this disease is different from the entity described by Haddorn in which the complete absence of pancreatic proteolytic activity in the duodenal fluid was based on a congenital absence of enterokinase. The latter enzyme is secreted by the duodenal mucosa and activates the zymogens. Although patients with this deficiency behave from birth as if their pancreatic secretory function were impaired and respond favorably to feedings of pancreatic extracts, it can be shown that the salutary effect of such extracts is in the activation of the patient's own trypsinogen. This can be demonstrated in vitro by addition of either trypsin or enterokinase to the duodenal fluid from an affected child. Duodenal secretions of such patients are otherwise normal in volume, electrolyte and bicarbonate content, and lypolytic and amylolytic activities. They can be stimulated with secretin and pancreozymin. Intestinal morphology on examination of peroral biopsy is normal. Symptoms that are most frequent are those of hypoproteinemia, anemia, and failure to thrive because of decreased protein digestion. Patients respond to feedings of hydrolyzed proteins, which are especially useful in neonates, or to small supplements of pancreatic extracts with meals.

EXUDATIVE ENTEROPATHY. PROTEIN-LOSING GASTROENTEROPATHY. Excessive leakage of plasma proteins into the gastrointestinal tract has been demonstrated as a cause of hypercatabolic hypoproteinemia. The condition has been described in association with a variety of anatomic abnormalities: giant hypertrophy of the gastric mucosa, obstruction and dilation of the lymphatic drainage of the intestinal mucosa (lymphangiectasia), granulomatous diseases of the intestine, and ulcerative colitis. Exudative enteropathy has been attributed to ingestion of cow's milk protein; it has been demonstrated in gluten-induced enteropathy and has been observed by us in a patient with a secreting neuroblastoma.

Children with this condition suffer from edema. Where generalized lymphatic abnormalities play a role, edema may be unequally distributed. Disturbances of growth are frequent and gastrointestinal complaints inconstant. The disease is usually suspected when hypoproteinemia is found without proteinuria. Definitive diagnosis rests on demonstration that the protein losses are into the intestine. Intravenous injection of ^{131}I-labeled albumin has limitations, since intestinal enzymatic activity splits the exuded albumin, with variable reabsorption of the resultant amino acids and radioactive iodine. In one technique that overcomes this difficulty, resins such as Amberlite IRA-400 or Deacidite FF (Permutit) are fed orally to bind the exuded radioiodine. Another technique substitutes a synthetic ^{131}I-labeled polyvinylpyrrolidone, but variations in molecular size and properties not entirely similar to those of serum albumin limit the effectiveness of the test. We prefer injection of 20 to 30 μCi of ^{51}Cr-labeled albumin. The radioactive chromium is poorly absorbed after digestion and is readily assayed in 4-day stool collections. Patients with the disease demonstrate excretion well in excess of the normal daily rate of 0.01 to 0.1 percent of the injected dose. However, because of greater stability of the iodinated albumin, chromated albumin should be used only for quantitating albumin leaks; ^{131}I-albumin is a better measure of total albumin turnover.

The picture varies with the specific cause, but patients generally display greater depression of serum albumin than of the globulins, except for gamma globulin, which may be specifically depressed. Diarrhea and steatorrhea are inconstant findings. In cases where the primary condition can be alleviated, as in localized intestinal mucosal abnormalities, in gluten-induced enteropathy, or in inflammatory diseases such as regional enteritis and ulcerative colitis, the hypoproteinemia improves. For the majority of patients therapeutic efforts are generally not rewarding. Diuretics, salt restriction, and periodic injections of albumin are employed for symptomatic relief. In patients with lymphangiectasia and steatorrhea, low-fat diets or diets in which medium-chain triglycerides have been substituted for long-chain saturated fatty acids are of considerable value, not only in improving steatorrhea but also in reducing protein losses.

MILK-ASSOCIATED GASTROENTEROPATHY. Wilson and associates have reported children with increased protein loss associated with red cell transudation and iron-deficiency anemia that responded to withdrawal of cow's milk protein from the diet. As these children matured they regained their tolerance for whole milk. Waldmann and associates described additional findings in children who probably suffer from the identical problem and labeled the condition allergic gastroenteropathy. Their patients had diarrhea, steatorrhea, growth retardation, anemia, hypoproteinemia and edema, respiratory and/or skin allergies, and peripheral eosinophilia. Studies of the gastrointestinal tract revealed it to be the site of red cell and protein losses. Microscopic examination of peroral biopsies revealed normal villous architecture with increased amounts of eosinophils and plasma cells in the lamina propria. We have confirmed their finding that not all children improve simply by withdrawal of milk and milk products from their diets. In certain instances beef also must be scrupulously avoided in all its forms, since other bovine proteins may be secreted in milk. Corticosteroids may be helpful but usually are unnecessary if proper dietary eliminations have been carried out.

Cow's milk may also be involved in other gastrointestinal disorders. Infants occasionally display a marked intolerance during the first weeks of life that expresses itself in vomiting or in rectal bleeding that may be profound and may be associated with severe diarrhea, simulating ulcerative colitis. Tolerance for cow's milk is usually normal by the end of the first year of life in these patients. In a patient in whom we observed steatorrhea related to the ingestion of cow's-milk β-lactoglobulin, there was ultimate spontaneous improvement. On the other hand, Kuitunen and associates observed patients who had malabsorption induced by ingestion of cow's milk and whose intestinal mucosa had blunted villi. Others have suggested that gluten intolerance, presumably a permanent defect, may develop secondarily in similar children.

Amino Acid Malabsorption

The various hereditary amino-acidopathies are presented in detail elsewhere (p. 673). A number of these involve disturbances of specific digestive and absorptive functions in the small intestine. If patients with phenylketonuria and maple syrup urine disease are fed a diet rich in tryptophan, they do not achieve anticipated serum levels, and they pass excessive amounts in the stool and excrete elevated amounts of indoles in the urine. The latter quite certainly arise from bacterial breakdown of the unabsorbed tryptophan by intestinal bacteria, since their appearance in urine can be suppressed with oral feeding of neomycin. In cystinuria the renal tubular defect in transportation of cystine, cysteine, hemocysteine, ornithine, lysine, and arginine is also shared by the intestinal villi and has been confirmed by in vitro studies. The defect in absorption is especially important for lysine. It has been reported that the combination of excessive urinary losses and poor absorption of this essential amino acid may be an important factor in the subnormal growth exhibited by patients with cystinuria.

Hartnup disease is a recessive condition in which the transport mechanism for the monoamino–monocarboxylic amino acids is deficient. These include alanine, serine, threonine, phenylalanine, lysine, tryptophan, histidine, and citrulline. Findings with tryptophan are the same as in phenylketonuria, (eg, poor absorption, excessive indole formation). In addition, it is postulated that the neurologic signs these patients demonstrate may be due to colonic absorption of decarboxylated products of some of these amino acids: histamine, phenylalanine, tryptamine, and tyramine. In oasthouse syndrome malabsorption of amino acids may be less important than excessive losses of methionine and branched-chain amino acids into the stool. Diarrhea results from irritation caused by products of bacterial degradation of the excessive intraluminal methionine, and the symptoms improve with antibiotics or with a low-methionine diet.

IRRITABLE COLON SYNDROME

The irritable colon syndrome (chronic nonspecific diarrhea), which is by no means uncommon in pediatric practice, is characterized by recurrent episodes of loose stools that occur for the most part in children from 6 months to 3 years of age. Steatorrhea and malabsorption of protein do not occur, and although accurate studies of carbohydrate absorption are wanting, the normal growth of these children belies any significant loss of this foodstuff either. The fundamental difficulty appears to be irritability of the colon.

The cause of the condition is unknown. There is a strong familial tendency, often with a similar history in siblings; not infrequently adults in the family suffer from an irritable colon. Various stresses may initiate diarrheal episodes; mild infections, usually of the respiratory tract, allergic reactions, and emotional stresses can often be identified as precipitating factors. In other instances such factors are not apparent. The possibility that unrecognized viral infections are involved remains to be investigated. Pathogenic bacteria have not been identified in the stools.

The episodes of diarrhea are commonly observed toward the end of the first year, before which there may have been a history of constipation. The onset is often insidious but may be dramatic. A diarrheal attack may last a few days or may continue for weeks, the intervals between attacks showing great variability. Constitutional symptoms such as fever and leukocytosis are absent, and the appetite remains unaffected. In fact, except for the looseness of the bowels, the child seems altogether well, and unless his diet is restricted he continues to gain weight normally. The number of stools varies from 3 to 10 per day. Frequently all or a majority of them will be passed within the space of a few hours in the early part of the day, and during the remainder of the day the child will be free of symptoms. Apart from the fact that they tend to be loose, the stools are not abnormal. Mucus is often present, and in the more severe cases there may be excoriation of the buttocks. In the few instances in which balance studies have been carried out, the only defect of absorption has been that of water. The presence of extracellular starch granules in the stools carries no untoward significance, nor does stainable fat in the feces imply that fat absorption is defective.

Diarrheal episodes usually cease between 3 and 4 years of age; only in rare instances do they occur after the age of 5 years. During interludes between diarrheal exacerbations, and especially following their complete cessation, the child frequently has chronic constipation.

The chief importance of this condition lies in its differentiation from the various causes of the malabsorption syndrome. Unless the diet has been unduly restricted, evidence of malnutrition is not present, nor can steatorrhea be demonstrated by chemical means. Pathogenic bacteria are not recovered from the stools, which contain neither pus nor blood. The characteristic features of cystic fibrosis of the pancreas are wanting. In our experience gastrointestinal allergy has played little part; we have not encountered instances in which the stools contained abundant eosinophils. The diagnosis is rarely difficult. We have, however, encountered occasional instances of low-grade *Salmonella* infection that have simulated it closely.

The treatment is largely expectant. Reassurance that the condition does not involve loss of nutrients, is not caused by the food, and requires no special diet will do much to allay needless parental concern and to avoid invalidism on the part of the child. It can confidently be predicted that the condition will improve with time, although it may not disappear altogether, even in adult life. The avoidance of stress situations, if this can be accomplished, may be expected to lessen the activity of the colon. Little can be accomplished by diet. We have observed during motility studies that ingestion of ice water induces propulsive activity in the colon (although it does not normally do so) in individuals suffering from diarrheal diseases and specifically in children with this syndrome. We therefore advocate avoidance of iced foods for these children. Cohlan and associates showed that diiodohydroxyquin (Diodoquin) decreased the number of stools in a considerable number of patients, as contrasted with a placebo. The mechanism of action of this agent in ameliorating the condition is unknown. It should not be prescribed in clinical practice; development of subacute myelo-optic neuritis and total blindness has been reported following prolonged administration.

References

NEONATAL NECROTIZING ENTEROCOLITIS

Frantz ID III, L'Heureux P, Engel RR, Hunt CE: Necrotizing enterocolitis. J Pediatr 86:259, 1975

Santulli TV, Schullinger JN, Heird WC: Acute necrotizing enterocolitis in infancy. Pediatrics 55:376, 1975

CYSTIC FIBROSIS

Andersen DH: Cystic fibrosis of the pancreas and its relation to celiac disease; clinical and pathologic study. Am J Dis Child 56:344, 1938

Bodian M (ed): Fibrocystic Disease of the Pancreas: A Congenital Disorder of Mucus Production—Mucosis. New York, Grune & Stratton, 1953

Darling RC, di Sant'Agnese PA, Perera GA, Andersen DH: Electrolyte abnormalities of the sweat in fibrocystic disease of the pancreas. Am J Med Sci 225:67, 1953

di Sant'Agnese PA, Talamo RC: Pathogenesis and physio-pathology of cystic fibrosis of the pancreas. Fibrocystic disease of the pancreas (mucoviscidosis). N Engl J Med 277:1287, 1343, 1399, 1967

Dische Z, di Sant'Agnese P, Pallavicini C, Youlos J: Composition of mucoprotein fractions from duodenal fluid of patients with cystic fibrosis of the pancreas and from controls. Pediatrics 24:74, 1959

Fleischer DS, DiGeorge AM, Auerbach VH, Huang NN, Barness LA: Protein metabolism in cystic fibrosis of the pancreas. J Pediatr 64:349, 1964

Gibson LE, Cooke RE: A test for the concentration of electrolytes in sweat in cystic fibrosis of the pancreas utilizing pilocarpine by iontophoresis. Pediatrics 23:545, 1959

Handweger S, Roth J, Gorden P, et al: Glucose intolerance in cystic fibrosis. N Engl J Med 281:451, 1969

Johansen PG, Anderson CM, Hadorn B: Cystic fibrosis of the pancreas.

A generalized disturbance of water and electrolyte movement in exocrine tissues. Lancet 1:455, 1968

Lowe CU, May CD, Stauffer HM, Neuhauser EDB: Fibrosis of the pancreas: enterogastrone and the "duodenal mechanism" in relation to increased appetite. Am J Dis Child 79:91, 1950

Sarsfield JK, Davies JM: Negative sweat tests and cystic fibrosis. Arch Dis Child 50:463, 1975

Shwachman H, Redmond A, Khaw KT: Studies in cystic fibrosis: report of 130 patients diagnosed under 3 months of age and over a 20-year period. Pediatrics 46:335, 1970

MALABSORPTION SYNDROME

Anderson CM: Histologic changes in duodenal mucosa in coeliac disease: reversibility during treatment with wheat gluten-free diet. Arch Dis Child 35:419, 1960

——— Intestinal malabsorption in childhood. Arch Dis Child 41:571, 1966

——— Townley RR, Freeman M, Johansen P: Unusual causes of steatorrhea in infancy and childhood. Med J Aust 2:617, 1961

Asquith P: Celiac disease. Immunology. Clin Gastroenterol 3:213, 1974

Barry RE, Read AE: Celiac disease and malignancy. Q J Med 42:665, 1973

Chung AW, Morales S, Snyderman SE, Lewis JM, Holt LE, Jr: Studies in steatorrhea: effect of the level of dietary fat upon the absorption of fat and other foodstuffs in idiopathic celiac disease and cystic fibrosis of the pancreas. Pediatrics 7:491, 1951

Clark PA: The use of *d*-xylose excretion test in children. Gut 3:333, 1962

Collins JR: Small intestinal mucosal damage with villous atrophy—a review of the literature. Am J Clin Pathol 44:36, 1965

Cortner JA: Giardiasis, cause of celiac syndrome. Am J Dis Child 98:311, 1959

Davidson M: Clinical conference: the celiac syndrome. Pediatrics 21:508, 1958

——— Bauer CH: The value of microscopic examination of the stool for extracellular starch in the diagnosis of starch intolerance. Pediatrics 21:565, 1958

——— Burnstine RC, Kugler MM, Bauer CH: Malabsorption defect induced by ingestion of beta lactoglobulin. J Pediatr 66:545, 1965

Gee S: On the coeliac affection. St Bartholomew's Hosp Rep 24:17, 1888

Herbst JJ, Sunshine P, Kretchmer N: Intestinal malabsorption in infancy and childhood. Adv Pediatr 16:11, 1969

Herskovic T, Sinawer SJ, Goldsmith R, Klein R, Zamcheck N: Intestinal lymphangiectasia. Pediatrics 40:345, 1967

Hooft C, Kriekemans J, VanAcker K, Devos E, Traen S, Verdonk G: Sjögren-Larsson syndrome with exudative enteropathy. Helv Paediatr Acta 22:447, 1967

Isselbacher KJ, Scheig R, Plotkin GR, Caulfield JB: Congenital betalipoprotein deficiency: an hereditary disorder involving a defect in the absorption and transport of lipids. Medicine 43:347, 1964

Lamy M, Frezal J, Polonovski J, Druez G, Rey J: Congenital absence of beta-lipoproteins. Pediatrics 31:277, 1963

MacDonald WC, Dobbins WO, Rubin CE: Studies of the familial nature of celiac sprue using biopsy of the small intestine. N Engl J Med 272:448, 1965

MacMahon RA: Massive resection of intestine in infancy. Aust NZ J Surg 35:202, 1966

McNeish AS, Anderson CM: Celiac disease. The disorder in childhood. Clin Gastroenterol 3:127, 1974

Margileth AM: Acrodermatitis enteropathica. Am J Dis Child 105:285, 1963

Mistilis SP, Skyring AP: Intestinal lymphangiectasia. Am J Med 40:634, 1966

Robertson AF, Putz J: Serum and erythrocyte fatty acids in case of acrodermatitis enteropathica. J Pediatr 70:279, 1967

Rubin CE, Dobbins WO III: Peroral biopsy of the small intestine. A review of its diagnostic usefulness. Gastroenterology 49:676, 1965

Salt HB, Wolf OH, Lloyd JK, et al: On having no beta-lipoprotein. A syndrome comprising a-beta-lipoproteinemia, acanthocytosis, and steatorrhoea. Lancet 2:325, 1960

Sheldon W, Tempany E: Small intestine peroral biopsy in coeliac children. Gut 7:481, 1966

Stickler GB, Hallenbeck GA, Flock EV, Rosevear JW: Catecholamines and diarrhea in ganglioneuroblastoma. Am J Dis Child 104:598, 1962

Visakorpi JK, Immonen P, Kuitunen P: Malabsorption syndrome in childhood. The occurrence of absorption defects and their clinical significance. Acta Paediatr Scand 56:1, 1967

Weijers HA, van de Kamer JH: Celiac disease and wheat sensitivity. Pediatrics 25:127, 1960

——— van de Kamer JH, Dicke WK: Celiac disease. In Advances in Pediatrics, Vol 9. Levine SZ, Chicago, Year Book, 1957, p 277

Weir DG, Hourihane DO: Celiac disease during the teenage period. The value of serial serum folate estimations. Gut 15:450, 1974

Winawer SJ, Broitman SA, Wolochow DA, Osborne MP, Zamcheck N: Successful management of massive small bowel resection based on assessment of absorption defects and nutritional needs. N Eng J Med 274:72, 1966

CARBOHYDRATE MALABSORPTION

Ament ME, Ochs HD, Davis SD: The structure and function of the gastrointestinal tract in 39 cases of primary immunodeficiency syndromes. Medicine 52:227, 1973

Auricchio S, Rubino A, Mürset G: Intestinal glycosidase activities in the human embryo, fetus and newborn. Pediatrics 35:944, 1965

Bayless TM, Rosensweig NS: A racial difference in incidence of lactase deficiency. JAMA 197:968, 1966

Crane RK: A perspective of digestive-absorptive function. Am J Clin Nutr 22:242, 1969

Dahlqvist A, Lindberg T: Development of the intestinal disaccharidase and alkaline phosphatase activities in the human foetus. Clin Sci 30:517, 1966

Davidson M: Disaccharide intolerance. Pediatr Clin North Am 14:93, 1967

Deren JJ, Broitman SA, Zamcheck N: Effect of diet upon intestinal disaccharidases and disaccharide absorption. J Clin Invest 46:186, 1967

Doell RG, Kretchmer N: Studies of small intestine during development. I. Distribution and activity of β-galactosidase. Biochim Biophys Acta 62:353, 1962

Durand P: Lattosuria idiopathica in una paziente con diarrea cronica ed acidosi. Minerva Pediatr 10:706, 1958

Eggermont E, Loeb N: Glucose-galactose intolerance. Lancet 11:343, 1966

Gracey M, Burke V: Sugar-induced diarrhoea in children. Arch Dis Child 48:331, 1973

Gray GM: Intestinal digestion and maldigestion of dietary carbohydrates. Ann Rev Med 22:391, 1971

——— Carbohydrate digestion and absorption: role of the small intestine. N Engl. J Med 292:1225, 1975

Hamilton JD, McMichael HB: Role of the microvillus in the absorption of disaccharides. Lancet 11:154, 1968

Herbst JJ, Hurwitz R, Sunshine P, Kretchmer N: Effect of colchicine on intestinal disaccharidases: correlation with biochemical aspects of cellular renewal. J Clin Invest 49:530, 1970

———Sunshine P, Kretchmer N: Intestinal malabsorption in infancy and childhood. Adv Pediatr 16:11, 1969

Holzel A, Schwarz V, Sutcliffe IW: Defective lactose absorption causing malnutrition in infancy. Lancet 1:1126, 1959

Huang SS, Bayless TM: Milk and lactose intolerance in healthy Orientals. Science 160:83, 1968

Johnson JD, Kretchmer N, Simoons FJ: Lactose malabsorption: its biology and history. Adv Pediatr 21:197, 1974

Koldovsky O: Development of the Functions of the Small Intestine in Mammals and Man. Basel, Karger, 1969

——— Sunshine P, Kretchmer N: The digestion of carbohydrates during postnatal development. Gastroenterology, 50:596, 1966

Leavitt MD, Donaldson RM: Use of respiratory hydrogen (H_2) excretion to detect carbohydrate malabsorption. J Lab Clin Med 75:937, 1970

Meeuwisse GW, Dahlquist A: Glucose-galactose malabsorption: a study with biopsy of the small intestinal mucosa. Acta Paediatr Scand 57:273, 1968

Paes IG, Searl P, Rubert MW, Faloon WW: Intestinal lactase deficiency and saccharide malabsorption during oral neomycin administration. Gastroenterology 53:49, 1967

Sunshine P, Kretchmer N: Studies of small intestine during development. III. Infantile diarrhea associated with intolerance to disaccharides. Pediatrics 34:38, 1964

Townley RRW, Khaw KT, Shwachman H: Quantitative assay of disaccharidase activities of small intestinal mucosal biopsy specimens in infancy and childhood. Pediatrics 36:911, 1965

Wilson FA, Dietschy JM: The intestinal unstirred layer: its surface area and effect on active transport kinetics. Biochim Biophys Acta 363:112, 1974

PROTEIN MALABSORPTION

Bookstein JJ, French AB, Pollard HM: Protein-losing gastroenteropathy: concepts derived from lymphangiography. Am J Dig Dis 10:573, 1965

Burch GE, Phillips JH Jr: Protein-losing gastroenteropathy. Am J Med Sci 245:109, 1963

Burns B, Gay B Jr: Menétrier's disease of the stomach in children. Am J Roentgenol Radium Ther Nucl Med 103:300, 1968

Holt PR: Dietary treatment of protein loss in intestinal lymphangiectasia: the effect of eliminating dietary long chain triglyceride on albumin metabolism in this condition. Pediatrics 34:629, 1964

Jeffries GH, Chapman A, Sleisenger MH: Low-fat diet in intestinal lymphangiectasia: its effect on albumin metabolism. N Engl J Med 270:761, 1964

Parfitt AM: Familial neonatal hypoproteinemia with exudative enteropathy and intestinal lymphangiectasia. Arch Dis Child 41:54, 1966

Tift WL, Lloyd JK: Intestinal lymphangiectasia. Long-term results with MCT diet. Arch Dis Child 50:269, 1975

Waldmann TA, Steinfeld JL, Dutcher TF, Davidson JD, Gordon RS: The role of the gastrointestinal system in "idiopathic hypoproteinemia." Gastroenterology 41:197, 1961

Yssing M, Jensen J, Jarnum S: Dietary treatment of protein-losing enteropathy. Acta Paediatr Scand 56:173, 1967

MILK-ASSOCIATED GASTROENTEROPATHY

Davidson M, Burnstine RC, Kugler MM, Bauer CH: Malabsorption defect induced by ingestion of beta lactoglobulin. J Pediatr 66:545, 1965

Fallström SP, Winberg J, Andersen HP: Cows' milk induced malabsorption as a precursor of gluten intolerance. Acta Paediatr Scand 54:101, 1965

Kuitunen P, Visakorpi JK, Hallman N: Histopathology of duodenal mucosa in malabsorption syndrome induced by cow's milk. Ann Paediatr Fenn 205:54, 1965

Shiner M, Ballard J, Smith ME: The small intestinal mucosa in cow's milk allergy. Lancet 1:136, 1975

Waldmann TA, Wochner DR, Laster L, Gordon S Jr: Allergic gastroenteropathy—a cause of excessive gastrointestinal protein loss. N Engl J Med 276:761, 1967

Wilson JF, Heiner DC, Lahey ME: Milk-induced gastrointestinal bleeding in infants with hypochromic microcytic anemia. JAMA 189:568, 1964

AMINO ACID MALABSORPTION

Hooft C, Carton D, Snoeck J, et al: Further investigations in the methionine malabsorption syndrome. Helv Paediatr Acta 23:334, 1968

Rosenberg LE, Crawhall JC, Segal S: Absorption—intestinal transport of cystine and cysteine in man: evidence for separate mechanisms. J Clin Invest 46:30, 1967

IRRITABLE COLON SYNDROME

Cohlan SQ: Chronic nonspecific diarrhea in infants and children treated with diiodohydroxyquinoline. Pediatrics 18:424, 1956

Davidson M, Sleisenger MH, Almy TP, Levine SZ: Studies of distal colonic motility in children. I. Non-propulsive patterns in normal children. II. Propulsive activity in diarrheal states. Pediatrics 17:807, 1956

——— Bauer CH: The value of microscopic examination of the stool for extracellular starch in the diagnosis of starch intolerance. Pediatrics 21:565, 1958

——— Wasserman R: The irritable colon of childhood (chronic non-specific diarrhea syndrome). J Pediatr 69:1927, 1966

Fleisher DI, Hepler RS, Landaw JW: Blindness during diiodohydroxyguin (Diodoquin®) Therapy: A case report. Ped 54: 106, 1974

Pittman FE, Westphal M: SMON and inflammation of the colon. Lancet 2:566, 1973

Prugh DG, Schwachman H: Observations in "unexplained" chronic diarrhea in early childhood. Am J Dis Child 90:496, 1955

ABDOMINAL PAIN

MURRAY DAVIDSON

Recurrent abdominal pain is a common complaint in pediatric practice; it has been estimated that approximately 1 in 10 school-age children suffers with the problem. An organic cause for the condition is found in less than 10 percent of these children. Although repeated and potentially harmful investigations are to be avoided, the diagnosis of serious or treatable conditions causing recurrent abdominal pain must be made without delay. Certain guidelines are useful for suggesting how diligent the diagnostic work-up should be.

Organic causes are more likely if the pain is sharply localized and constant, especially if it occurs during the night and awakens the child from sleep. Severity of pain is not a good guide, since more emotional children and parents may subjectively exaggerate a symptom, while more phlegmatic patients may minimize a complaint. Pains that are generalized over the periumbilical area or in the middle of the lower abdomen are less likely to be organic than those that are lateralized. The presence of anemia, persistent or recurrent fevers, elevation of erythrocyte sedimentation rates, marked loss of appetite, vomiting, or weight loss may point to an organic cause of abdominal pain, and such findings should be explained adequately. It is sometimes pointed out that patients with pain in more than one part of the body (such as limb pain or headaches in addition to abdominal pains) are less likely to have an organic disease. This is generally true, but regional enteritis and other inflammatory or immunologic disorders may present with such multiple and not easily definable symptoms. Similarly, obviously disturbed interpersonal relationships between parents and children often suggest a primary emotional cause for the complaint; however, when it is severe the child's disability may be the cause of great frustration, especially where there have been recurrent ineffective reassurances by physicians that the problem is not organic.

The major organic cause for recurrent abdominal pain is disease of the urinary tract, and every patient with the complaint deserves urinalysis. Within the gastrointestinal tract a number of conditions, such as peptic ulcer, regional enteritis, Meckel's diverticulum, gastrointestinal tumors, and ulcerative colitis, may present with chronic abdominal pain as the major symptom. We have observed abdominal pain as a severe and unexplained prodromal complaint in a number of patients who subsequently developed unequivocal diabetes mellitus.

Psychogenic causes vary, and careful interview is necessary. Among the predominant causes are guilt and anxiety in the child with respect to parental discord, physical or emotional illness of a parent, or overwhelming family financial problems that have been allowed to worry the child. School or learning difficulties, inability to handle hostile feelings toward parents or siblings, and age-related problems such as sexual feelings in early adolescence may all be transposed into abdominal pain. The major avenues for treatment lie in patient counseling by the interested pediatrician after he has become thoroughly acquainted with the basis of the symptoms. In some instances psychiatric referral is indicated.

An important type of recurrent abdominal pain, which we believe is often present and tends to bridge the gap between psychologic and organic causes, is related to the tendency to constipation. Colicky or paroxysmal abdominal pain results from distension of the intestine when exaggerated peristalsis occurs in the presence of some degree of obstruction. Among individuals genetically predisposed to constipation there is increased tone in the distal colon, which may progress in some to unremitting spasm when they are under physical or emotional stress. If such individuals simultaneously are troubled by flatulence and trapping of gas that they are unable to pass, severe pain may result. Some individuals with lactose insufficiency may, as a result of the balance between doses of lactose ingested and the degree of such insufficiency, suffer more from flatulence and abdominal pain than from diarrhea. In some instances certain foods to which patients are allergic or otherwise intolerant may increase intestinal gas production. A number of patients who have been severely troubled over long periods with such symptoms have been relieved when managed by the type of regimen described below for patients with constipation.

Acute abdominal pain is associated with such surgical problems as appendicitis, volvulus, or intussusception. In acute mesenteric adenitis pain is usually present. However, it is doubtful that diagnoses such as chronic appendicitis and chronic mesenteric adenitis, which were formerly frequently applied, are at all tenable in modern pediatrics. Intermittent porphyria may in rare cases be a cause of abdominal pain.

Paroxysmal Fussing

Paroxysmal fussing (infantile colic) is defined as a symptom complex of early infancy characterized by evidence of intermittent abdominal pain of varying degrees of severity for which no organic or obvious physiologic cause can be demonstrated. It is an ill-defined condition that seems to consist primarily of pain associated with symptoms ranging in degree from general fussiness to paroxysms of agonized crying. The symptoms usually start after feeding and become worse late in the day. Besides the typical unhappiness, as exemplified by clenching the fists and flexing the legs, the infant often makes sucking movements and appears to be searching for food. Usually these infants have a great deal of gas, manifested by excessive belching, flatus, and rumbling. The passage of gas occasionally is followed by temporary relief, thus supporting the theory that loops of intestine distended from collected air cause colic. It is most common in the firstborn, usually starting at 2 to 4 weeks of age and lasting through the third or fourth month. It is difficult to state what percentage of infants have colic, since a certain amount of fussiness is natural, and crying that may be considered normal in one household or in one infant may be regarded as intolerable in another.

There is little agreement as to the cause of infantile colic. Physiologic immaturity of the intestinal tract, a constitutional predisposition to hypertonicity, hunger, improper feeding, allergy, or a reaction to tenseness in the home have all been described as etiologic factors. A careful history is important, not only for obvious medical reasons but also to provide an opportunity for the mother to discuss her attitudes and feelings. A thorough physical examination must exclude such conditions as disease of the central nervous system, detectable congenital defects of the gastrointestinal or genitourinary tracts, and other organic causes. This investigation should include a rectal examination, since gentle dilation of a tight rectal sphincter frequently will give rather spectacular and sometimes permanent relief. The finding of such spasm on rectal examination suggests that this type of colic may be related to a predisposition to later constipation and to functional gastrointestinal problems and that the difficulty may have a pathogenesis not unlike the colic described in the preceding section. Except for a very questionable psychologic advantage to the parents, changing the formula is useless except in the rare instances of milk allergy or flatulence from lactose intolerance.

Treatment of infantile colic is often not very satisfactory. Stress should be placed on feeding in the upright (sitting) position and on careful burping to prevent as much swallowed air as possible from entering the intestines. Most physicians restrict the use of drugs to severely disturbed patients. Among the drugs that have been recommended are paregoric, phenobarbital, and various anticholinergic agents. In a number of instances we have been impressed that administration of 10 to 15 drops of an alcoholic beverage, given in 2 ounces of warm, slightly sweetened water, has been associated with passage of flatus and temporary relief of symptoms. Applications of heat to the abdomen and stimulation of the rectum with a Vaseline-covered thermometer tip or glycerine suppository appear to have the same effect. Until an exact cause can be found, drug therapy should be secondary, and sympathetic support for family is of utmost importance. The pediatrician must give parents adequate time and display a patient and interested attitude. Despite the fact that treatment often does not meet with success, the doctor's interest will serve to help the parents and the infant through a trying but self-limited experience.

References

Aldrich CA, Sung C, Knop C: The crying of newly born babies. III. The early period at home. J Pediatr 27:428, 1945

Apley J: The Child with Abdominal Pains, 2nd ed. Oxford, Blackwell, 1975

———— The child with recurrent abdominal pain. Pediatr Clin North Am 14:63, 1967

Bayless TM, Huang SS: Recurrent abdominal pain due to milk and lactose intolerance in school-aged children. Pediatrics 47:1029, 1971

Christensen MF, Mortensen O: Long term prognosis in children with recurrent abdominal pain. Arch Dis Child 50:110, 1975

Green M: Diagnosis and treatment: psychogenic, recurrent, abdominal pain. Pediatrics 40:84, 1967

Jorup S: Colonic hyperperistalsis in neurolabile infants; studies in so-called dyspepsia in breast-fed infants. Acta Pediatr [Suppl] 41:85, 1952.

Marshall DG: Diagnosis and treatment: recurrent abdominal pain in children—a surgeon's viewpoint. Pediatrics 40:84, 1967

Rambar AC: Colic in infants—general considerations. Pediatrics 18:829, 1956

Wessel MA, Cobb JC, Jackson EB, Harris GS Jr, Detwiler AC: Paroxysmal fussing in infancy, sometimes called colic. Pediatrics 14:421, 1954

———— Use of methyl scopolamine nitrate in the treatment of paroxysmal fussing (colic) in infancy. N Engl J Med 257:14, 1957

Winsey HS, Jones PF: Acute abdominal pain in childhood: analysis of a year's admissions. Br Med J 1:653, 1967

CONSTIPATION

Murray Davidson

Constipation is defined as a state in which bowel movements are hard, infrequent, and difficult to pass. These attributes are commonly related, since colonic stasis causes infrequent stools and, by allowing more time for water absorption, predisposes to hard stools, which are difficult to pass. However, infrequent defecation and difficult defecation may occur independently. A marked reduction in food intake may result in infrequent but easy passage of feces; on the other hand, anal stenosis or fissure may cause a soft stool to be passed with difficulty. Such conditions should not be regarded as constipation.

Constipation in children may in rare cases result from disturbances in propulsion of material into the lower colon due to hypothyroidism, diabetes, neuromuscular disorders, prolonged bed rest, or obstruction by space-occupying lesions. An infrequent but important anatomic anomaly that causes constipation by interfering with peristalsis in the colon is Hirschsprung's disease or congenital aganglionosis.

In the most common form of constipation, so-called functional constipation, there is excessive drying of rectal contents associated with difficulty in evacuation. The tendency to this problem is probably constitutional and hereditary, as evidenced by frequent strong family histories, by greater concordance among monozygous than among dizygous twins, and by the fact that some infants experience constipation from the first days of life even though they are ingesting the same formula that does not evoke constipation in the vast majority. Motility studies of the distal colon have demonstrated that certain children with constipation have increased frequencies of pressure wave patterns that are presumed to be associated with altered fluid absorption; they also display the ability to resist development of propulsive activity following parasympathomimetic drug stimulation. Ziskind and Gellis have shown that constipated children absorb increased amounts of water from their rectums.

Infants fed on cow's milk, with its higher content of casein and calcium salts, tend to have bowel movements that are harder and less frequent than those of breast-fed infants. When higher protein feedings are used, such as unmodified cow's milk, protein milk, or formulas fortified with calcium caseinate, the constipating effect is more striking. In older children, overemphasis on milk may result in diminished intake of residue foods; conversely, children who tend to be constipated may have diminished appetites and may prefer milk to other foods. Thus two factors tend to aggravate the symptoms of constipation: first, smaller boli reach the rectum as a result of low intake of roughage; second, individuals who are disposed to constipation reduce the quantity of rectal contents by excessive water resorption. Both mechanisms result in a lessened urge and further drying of the mass into small, pelletlike formations.

SYMPTOMS. Passage of constipated stools may be accompanied by rectal pain, and if anal fissures result, the stool surface may be streaked with blood. Infrequently, excessive straining with constipated stools may be associated with rectal prolapse; in adults it is believed to lead more commonly to hemorrhoids. With developing awareness that evacuation is under voluntary control, children may deliberately begin to withhold the stool in the latter part of the first year after birth. Such children, by grunting, turning red, and squeezing, appear to make attempts to defecate, but actually they are able to accomplish withholding by diminishing the effectiveness of the feet as a fulcrum; they develop a personal pattern whereby they avoid squatting or they do not rest both feet squarely on the ground when the intraabdominal pressure is raised. Both of these activities are necessary for normal defecation (p. 978). Gradual distension of the rectum by the retained stool results in increased ability to withhold larger quantities before urgency is experienced. This leads to abdominal distension, decreased frequency of

stool passage, increased pain, and difficulty in passing the larger and firmer stool masses. The decreased appetite frequently observed in constipated individuals is exaggerated at this stage. Parents complain that the stool is often large and firm enough to interfere with the toilet plumbing. Frequent involuntary passage of the relatively liquid material that slithers around the large bolus of hard material may result in paradoxical diarrhea, or encopresis, after a number of days without bowel movement. Children rarely exhibit symptoms such as headache and general malaise that are often reported by adults with fecal impactions.

DIFFERENTIAL DIAGNOSIS. Infants who strain and pass small stools must have digital examinations of their rectums. Rarely, a firm constriction will be encountered at the anus, dilation of which by the examining finger may be followed by copious passage of stool. If the rectal examination permits ready entry of the finger, this usually implies that the tightness is due to muscle spasm rather than to the extremely rare instance of a sphincteric anomaly. In addition, if the examining finger palpates stool in the rectum, organic and neurogenic obstructions above this level are virtually ruled out.

In the older child in whom chronic constipation has led to the development of large infrequent stools, the question of Hirschsprung's disease may be raised. The mistaken impression has arisen that either early onset of symptoms or marked infrequency of bowel movements favors the diagnosis of Hirschsprung's disease and does not occur in chronic constipation. We believe that the presence or absence of the urge to defecate is a more reliable differential diagnostic criterion. Since the proprioceptors that initiate this reflex urge are located just proximal to the internal sphincter, failure of patients with congenital aganglionic megacolon to propel material to this site results in rare activation of this reflex. Also, the presence or absence of stool on rectal examination will suggest the proper diagnosis. In doubtful cases a trial period of therapy with large doses of mineral oil, as outlined later, may be of diagnostic benefit since patients with Hirschsprung's disease will not respond. The barium enema, biopsy findings, and motility abnormalities diagnostic of Hirschsprung's disease will be described later.

TREATMENT. In the infant the objective should be to alter the consistency of the feces in such a way that they can readily be passed. In most instances this objective may be accomplished by increasing the concentration or changing the type of carbohydrate in the formula. Lactose appears to be slightly more laxative than cane sugar; malt-dextrin preparations per se exert no laxative effect. Substitution of certain carbohydrate preparations such as honey, molasses (dark cane syrup is preferable to light), brown sugar, and malt soup extract is effective. The addition of solid foods to the infant diet, especially prunes, apricots, and fibrous vegetables, may be of some benefit.

Although it is often recommended, additional water probably has the effect merely of increasing urinary rather than stool water. However, nonabsorbable hygroscopic substances, which to some extent retain water in the gut, may be given to soften the stool. One teaspoonful of agar sprinkled in the food once or twice daily may be used for this purpose; the surface-active agent dioctyl sodium sulfosuccinate (Colace) at a dosage of 5 mg/kg/24 hours divided into three or four doses is widely used.

The question of the desirability of regular bowel habits is often argued. It has been clearly demonstrated that retention of fecal material for more than 24 hours (and indeed for considerably longer) produces no untoward results. For the majority of children who are not constipated, daily movements are not necessary, and parents should be reassured in this regard. However, the inherent tendency to be constipated beyond infancy is best combated by development of regular bowel habits; this is possible only in children above 3 years of age who may be motivated and trained in this direction. Attempts at toilet training at too early an age (before 2.5 to 3 years) may result in voluntary withholding; such attempts should be discouraged. During training the use of a "potty" chair that sits on the floor is preferable to the seat that is attached to the adult toilet because the former provides better leverage for evacuating hard stools. Even those attachable seats that provide a footrest are not suitable because they do not permit the small child to bend the knees properly and squat.

Older children who exhibit symptoms of chronic constipation, with or without significant resistance to bowel movement and development of fecal impactions, require a more thorough regimen that involves three phases:

In the first phase hypertonic phosphate enemas (1 ounce for every 20 pounds of body weight to a maximum of 4 ounces) are given morning and evening in pairs, 1 hour apart. When the second enema of a pair yields clear returns, evacuation of preexistent impactions is assumed to be complete. Saline enemas may be substituted, but tap water enemas must be avoided because of the hazard of water intoxication.

Light-grade mineral oil given orally is prescribed on an individual basis. Children receiving sufficient amounts of mineral oil should pass three to five large, loose, unformed bowel movements daily, but they should not have leakage of oil between times. In fact, overflow soiling of oil due to retention of solid fecal masses is an indication of inadequate doses of oil; paradoxically, such soiling subsides when the dose is increased. It is our general practice to start with approximately 1 to 2 ounces daily for every 10 pounds of body weight and to increase the dose by 0.5 to 1 ounce daily until the desired response is achieved. The mineral oil is preferably chilled and taken directly from a glass. Half the total dose is given in the morning and the other half at bedtime, in order to interfere as little as possible with the absorption of fat-soluble vitamins and lipids from meals taken during the day. Children are permitted to drink sweetened fluids or juice immediately after taking the medication to eliminate the oily sensation from their mouths.

Youngsters who develop three to five soft bowel movements daily during the first phase of management are continued on the same doses of oil for a second period of approximately 3 months duration while they develop a regular daily pattern. Following this phase the oil is withdrawn gradually; to ensure lasting success the physician must continue to offer interest, encouragement, and patient handling of overanxious parents for considerable periods. In a few instances continuance of symptoms beyond the second phase of management may indicate a deep-seated emotional problem for which psychiatric help is necessary. In the majority of cases, however, the development of regularity is the end of the problem for the remainder of childhood and adult life.

The continuing use of laxatives, suppositories, and enemas should be discouraged, and children should not be made dependent on them. Little may be expected from involved and restrictive dietary management of chronic constipation. Nevertheless, in the continuing management of constipation, a daily intake of prunes and bran flakes, with reduction in milk intake to 1 pint daily to reduce casein and calcium intake and substitution of adequate fruit juices and water, may be of some value.

References

Brazelton TB: Child-oriented approach to toilet training. Pediatrics 29: 121, 1962

Carlson SS, Asnes RS: Expectations and attitudes toward toilet training compared between clinic and private practice mothers. J Pediatr 84:148, 1974

Davidson M, Kugler MM, Bauer CH: Diagnosis and management in children with severe and protracted constipation and obstipation. J Pediatr 62:261, 1963

Mercer RD: Constipation. Pediatr Clin North Am 14:175, 1967

Ziskind A, Gellis SS: Water intoxication following tap-water enemas. Am J Dis Child 96:699, 1958

RECTAL INCONTINENCE AND PRURITUS ANI

THOMAS V. SANTULLI AND MURRAY DAVIDSON

The most important cause of inability to control fecal evacuations (encopresis) by children is the overflow soiling that follows overdistension of the rectum from prolonged chronic constipation and fecal impactions. Not infrequently the condition appears rather suddenly among children over 5 years of age in whom the underlying constipation and gradually increasing periods between bowel movements have previously gone unnoticed. If such patients are not adequately examined to establish the true nature of the condition, the focus of diagnosis and management may be misdirected toward improving the children's attitudes and motivating them to exert better control with reprimands, bribery, or vain attempts at psychotherapy. Unable to satisfy such wishes because of the involuntary nature of the symptom, such youngsters may take to hiding their soiled undergarments; when this act is discovered it is often regarded as further proof of the psychogenic origin of the soiling and of the contrariness of the patients. Appropriate treatment that may be curative consists of the management of extreme constipation discussed previously.

Other less common causes of rectal incontinence are paraplegia due to myelitis following injury to or disease of the spinal cord, spina bifida, and comatose states. The condition may also occur from chronic stretching of the sphincter by rectal prolapse of long standing, or it may be the result of scarring at the sphincter following surgery in the area for imperforate anus or congenital megacolon. Treatment of this assorted group of conditions is often unsatisfactory. For incontinence of neurogenic origin the best chance for improvement lies in surgical correction of the underlying lesion, if this is possible. For local problems at the anus or sphincter it is important to determine whether incontinence is due to poor control or to too tight an outlet with resultant retention and overflow. In the latter states sphincterotomy may be helpful. Many operative procedures involving muscle and tendon transplants have been tried for loose sphincters, but none has been completely satisfactory. It is seldom necessary to treat this group of conditions by the establishment of a permanent colostomy. Most of these patients for whom no definitive

procedure is available can best be managed by symptomatic treatment consisting of local cleanliness, constipating foods, avoidance of fecal impactions, use of bulk-type laxatives such as psyllium seed, agar, or methyl cellulose, and periodic enemas as needed to maintain an empty rectum and lower colon.

Anal itching may result from moist underclothing and overflow soiling. Pruritus ani is also associated with hemorrhoids, fissures, and oxyuriasis. It results in scratching, restlessness, and irritability. Anal pruritus of nocturnal periodicity is almost always due to pinworm infestation. Treatment consists of local cleanliness and removal of the underlying cause. The anal area should be cleansed by washing or wiping with soft cotton rather than with toilet tissue. Drying powders or hydrocortisone ointment are beneficial.

References

Ellison FS: Anal fissure occurring in infants and children. Dis Colon Rectum 3:61, 1960

Mentzer CG: Anorectal disease. Pediatr Clin North Am 3:113, 1956

Santulli TV: Miscellaneous anal diseases. In Benson CD, et al (eds): Pediatric Surgery. Chicago, Year Book, 1962, p 854

Turell R, Pomeranz AA, Denmark SM: The colon and anorectum in pediatric practice. Int Abstr Surg 103:209, 1956.

Malformations of the Gastrointestinal Tract

ABNORMALITIES OF DEVELOPMENT CAUSING OBSTRUCTION
MURRAY DAVIDSON

Gastrointestinal symptoms based on congenital malformations may initially appear at any age. Most lesions of major significance are associated with symptoms occurring early in life, often in the newborn period. Manifestations of gastrointestinal tract obstruction are the most common complaints. Atresias and severe degrees of stenosis of the lumen cause intrinsic obstructions, while the accessory lumina produce extrinsic pressure; ie, cysts, diverticula, or duplications are obstructing when they become distended with secretions or trapped intestinal contents and impinge on the main tract. The higher the lesion and the more complete the obstruction, the earlier the obstructive symptoms appear in an infant. Interpretation of objective signs is the same as for older individuals; eg, whether vomitus contains bile depends on whether the obstruction lies above or below the biliary tract outflow into the duodenum.

Radiographic findings of intestinal obstruction in infants are similar to those in older children, and contrast medium is sometimes helpful for delineating the level of obstruction. In the newborn, normal passage of air through the gastrointestinal tract is an ideal contrast medium. It is almost always unnecessary in newborns to

introduce barium or a similar material. Another important difference between the neonate and older individuals is that at least 50 percent of newborns with atresias as low as the terminal ileum may pass meconium, and the presence or absence of stools becomes a reliable guide to diagnosis only after the initial meconium stools have been passed.

Atresia of the gastrointestinal tract was formerly presumed to occur in utero as a malfunction of a normal ontogenetic mechanism, namely failure to complete the normal recanalization process. This mechanism probably still accounts for some of the foregut and hindgut abnormalities. However, the midgut has not been shown to develop a solid stage. There is a strong body of evidence that most lesions of the small and large intestines arise from compromise of the fetal circulation to part of the developing gut, eg, from an intrauterine volvulus. The resulting gangrenous loop of intestine is ultimately resorbed and may leave an atretic segment connecting two patent areas. In some cases evidence of intrauterine peritonitis may be seen.

References

Dykstra G, Sieber WK, Kiesewetter WB: Intestinal atresia. Arch Surg 97:175, 1968

Louw JH: Jejunoileal atresia and stenosis. J Pediatr Surg 1:8, 1966

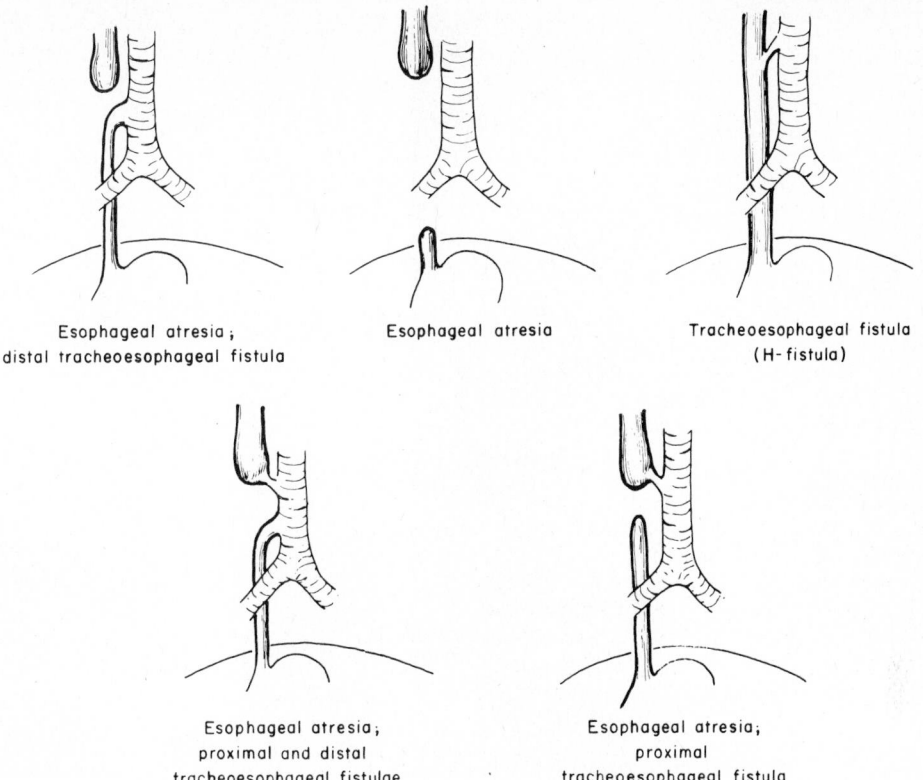

Esophageal atresia;
distal tracheoesophageal fistula

Esophageal atresia

Tracheoesophageal fistula
(H- fistula)

Esophageal atresia;
proximal and distal
tracheoesophageal fistulae

Esophageal atresia;
proximal
tracheoesophageal fistula

FIG. 2. Esophageal atresia and distal tracheoesophageal fistula. The air bubble in the neck and upper thorax outlines the dilated, blind-ending upper esophageal pouch. The finding of air in the stomach confirms the presence of a distal tracheoesophageal fistula.

ESOPHAGEAL MALFORMATIONS

JOHN H. SEASHORE

ESOPHAGEAL ATRESIA AND TRACHEOESO-PHAGEAL FISTULA. Congenital malformations of the esophagus have an incidence of about 1 in 4,000 live births. A number of classifications have been proposed, but it is most helpful to define these malformations in terms of descriptive anatomy, as shown in Fig. 2. Esophageal atresia with distal tracheoesophageal fistula is the most common type; esophageal atresia without tracheoesophageal fistula occurs much less frequently. Esophageal atresia with proximal tracheoesophageal fistula, atresia with both proximal and distal fistulae, and tracheoesophageal fistula without atresia (H-type fistula) are rare. The incidences of these types in a national survey conducted by the Surgical Section of the American Academy of Pediatrics are shown in Table 4.

The blind-ended proximal esophagus has a capacity of only a few milliliters; it rapidly fills with swallowed oral secretions that overflow into the pharynx, resulting in drooling and occasionally in aspiration. Esophageal atresia should be suspected in any newborn infant who has excessive oral secretions and drooling with or without mild respiratory distress. When feedings are offered

the baby promptly and often forcefully regurgitates and usually aspirates, producing the characteristic triad of coughing, choking, and cyanosis. Esophageal obstruction must be ruled out before a second feeding is offered. Atelectasis and pneumonia occur early and progress rapidly. In the usual case with distal tracheoesophageal fistula, pulmonary complications are com-

TABLE 4. Incidence of Types of Tracheoesophageal Anomalies

Esophageal atresia, distal tracheoesophageal fistula	916 (86.6%)
Esophageal atresia, no fistula	82 (7.7%)
Tracheoesophageal fistula, no atresia	44 (4.2%)
Esophageal atresia, proximal tracheoesophageal fistula	9 (0.8%)
Esophageal atresia, proximal and distal tracheoesophageal fistulae	7 (0.7%)
Total	1058 (100%)

Courtesy of the Surgical Section, American Academy of Pediatrics, 1964. (Source: Holdez TM, Cloud DT, Lewis EL, Pilling GP: Esophageal atresia and tracheoesophageal fistula: A survey of its members by the Surgical Section of the American Academy of Pediatrics. Ped 34:542, 1964)

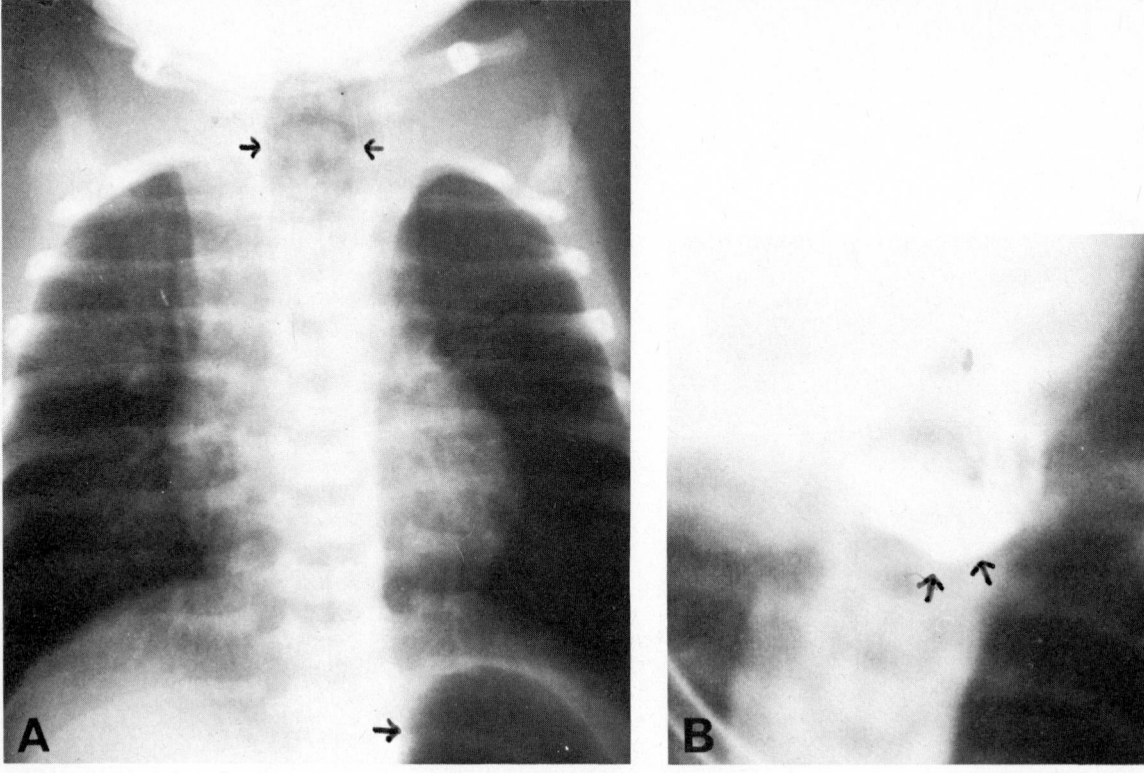

FIG. 3. Esophageal atresia. Contrast material introduced through the esophageal tube demonstrates the obstucted proximal esophagus.

pounded by reflux of air and gastric secretions into the tracheobronchial tree through the fistula, causing severe chemical irritation. The right upper lobe is most commonly involved, probably because of its proximity to the tracheoesophageal fistula.

Once the diagnosis of esophageal atresia is suspected, a plastic radiopaque catheter should be passed through the nose into the esophagus. Inability to advance the catheter beyond the upper esophagus confirms the diagnosis. Even if the catheter appears to advance, it is essential to obtain anteroposterior and lateral radiographs, since the soft catheter occasionally may become coiled in the blind upper esophageal pouch. A simple air esophagram may sometimes outline the obstructed esophagus (Fig. 3). The diagnosis should be clear at this point, but if there is doubt it is permissible to introduce a small amount (0.5 to 1 ml) of non-water-soluble radiopaque material into the catheter under fluoroscopic observation. The small amount of contrast material outlines the blind pouch without overfilling it and causing aspiration (Fig. 3). The plain radiograph should include the abdomen, since air in the stomach confirms the presence of a distal tracheoesophageal fistula. Associated intestinal obstruction may also be apparent on the film.

Repeated aspiration and gastroesophagotracheal reflux cause rapidly progressive respiratory distress,

and these infants invariably die if they are left untreated. As soon as the diagnosis is established, a sump catheter should be passed into the upper esophageal pouch for constant aspiration of secretions. The infant should be elevated at an angle of 45 degrees to minimize reflux of gastric contents through the fistula. Immediate gastrostomy under local anesthesia provides decompression of the gastrointestinal tract and further reduces the risk of reflux. Hydration, acid–base balance, and pulmonary toilet must be attended to constantly. Supplementary oxygen may be necessary. Antibiotic therapy should be instituted if pneumonia is present. These initial measures permit a period of observation during which the infant is examined for the presence of other anomalies, which occur in almost half of these patients. Congenital heart disease and intestinal obstruction may require prompt attention.

One-stage primary repair is preferred in the full-term infant who does not have other life-threatening anomalies. Right thoracotomy and extrapleural dissection provide adequate exposure. The tracheoesophageal fistula is divided, and esophageal continuity is restored by end-to-end anastomosis. Alternatively, the fistula may be ligated and an end-to-side anastomosis performed, avoiding dissection of the poorly vascularized distal esophagus. The latter method entails less risk of stricture, but there is perhaps slightly greater risk of recurrence of the fistula. Vigorous measures to prevent or treat pneumonia and atelectasis must be continued in the postoperative period. Gastrostomy feedings should be started as soon as gastrointestinal function resumes. Oral feedings should be cautiously begun 7 to 10 days after operation in uncomplicated cases. Over 90 percent of this group of infants should survive.

Premature infants and babies with severe pneumonia or other serious malformations have a much poorer prognosis. A staged approach is preferable for these patients. In the first stage the fistula should be divided, using local anesthesia if necessary. Constant sump drainage of the upper esophagus and intensive nursing care should be continued. Primary esophageal anastomosis should be performed when the infant is larger and is free of pneumonia and when associated anomalies are either resolved or stable.

Postoperative *complications* are not uncommon. *Anastomotic leak* occurs in about 17 percent of patients. Mortality is high, but the leak frequently closes spontaneously if oral feedings are withheld. Empyema resulting from a leak is less common if an extrapleural approach has been used. *Stricture* of the anastomosis develops in 40 percent of patients following end-to-end anastomosis and may require frequent dilation. Resection of the stricture and reanastomosis are occasionally required. Stricture is rarely seen after end-to-side anastomosis. *Recurrent tracheoesophageal fistula* occurs in about 5 percent of patients. All patients with esophageal atresia have *abnormal motility of the distal esophagus* characterized by failure of propagation of peristaltic waves, reverse peristalsis, and occasionally pooling of swallowed material in the esophagus. In some patients these abnormalities may contribute to feeding difficulties or to recurrent aspiration.

A few patients continue to have pulmonary infections for months or years following repair of esophageal atresia as a result of recurrent aspiration. Persistent stricture is a major factor in some patients. Hiatal hernia and gastroesophageal reflux occur with increased frequency in these patients and may cause aspiration directly or by contributing to persistent anastomotic stricture. The abnormal distal esophageal motility is responsible for aspiration in some patients.

Infants with esophageal atresia without tracheoesophageal fistula characteristically have such a long atretic segment of esophagus that primary anastomosis is not feasible. Occasionally a patient with the common form of atresia and distal tracheoesophageal fistula will also have an unusually large gap. In these patients the fistula, if present, is divided, gastrostomy is performed for feeding, and a cervical esophagostomy is created to drain oropharyngeal secretions. The esophagus is reconstructed by interposition of a segment of colon when the infant weighs at least 10 kg.

Infants who have tracheoesophageal fistula without atresia are able to swallow, but they have frequent attacks of coughing, choking, and cyanosis with feedings. The diagnosis may be difficult to establish and may not be made until the baby is a few weeks or months of age. Repeated esophagograms performed by an ex-

perienced radiologist may be necessary to demonstrate the fistula. The fistula is most commonly in the cervical region and is best approached through a supraclavicular incision.

CONGENITAL ESOPHAGEAL STENOSIS. Congenital stenosis of the esophagus is much less common than acquired stricture. Differentiation of these lesions may be difficult. Congenital stenosis usually produces dysphagia in the first week of life. Dilatation with graded bougies is usually effective. Reestablishment of the stenosis is rare in this congenital form of the disease, in contrast to the experience with acquired strictures.

CONGENITAL ESOPHAGEAL DUPLICATIONS. Duplications of the esophagus are rare cystic lesions of foregut origin commonly located in the posterior mediastinum in close proximity to the esophagus, but usually not in communication with it. Duplications are occasionally tubular and may extend through the diaphragm to communicate with the proximal gastrointestinal tract. The intestinal epithelium secretes fluid and mucus into the closed cyst, which enlarges progressively. The lesion may become apparent on routine chest radiography or may cause symptoms by compression of neighboring intrathoracic structures. Hemorrhage and perforation may occur if the cyst is lined with gastric epithelium. Complete excision is indicated and is usually curative.

ESOPHAGEAL DIVERTICULA. Congenital esophageal diverticula are uncommon, but they may arise at any level of the esophagus, notably in the posterior midline of the hypopharynx at the level of the cricopharyngeus muscle or just above the diaphragm. Diverticula in the upper third of the esophagus may be related embryologically to tracheoesophageal fistula. Careful radiographic identification of the origin and extent of the diverticulum should precede surgical excision.

Traumatic pseudodiverticulum of the pharynx, while rare, is important because it may mimic esophageal atresia. Perforation of the hypopharynx may result from passage of a variety of tubes or even a finger into the mouth of the newborn baby. Associated spasm of the cricopharyngeus muscle may prevent passage of a tube or of radiopaque contrast material into the normal esophagus; radiographs show only the false passage posterior to the esophagus that may be mistaken for the blind proximal pouch of esophageal atresia. If the lesion is recognized, it may be possible to pass a feeding tube into the stomach under fluoroscopic observation. At times, a gastrostomy may be required for feeding. The injury usually heals without cervical drainage or other surgical intervention. Thoracotomy for an erroneous diagnosis of esophageal atresia is obviously contraindicated.

ESOPHAGEAL HIATAL HERNIA. *Sliding hiatal hernia* is an abnormal anatomic condition in which a portion of the stomach herniates intermittently or constantly through the esophageal hiatus of the diaphragm and the esophagus is relatively shortened. *Gastroesophageal reflux* is the regurgitation of gastric contents into the esophagus or even into the pharynx. Hiatal hernia by itself rarely causes symptoms. Gastroesophageal reflux, while usually associated with hiatal hernia, may occur in the absence of demonstrable anatomic abnormality. Reflux may be asymptomatic; it may cause varying degrees of vomiting or may lead to progressive peptic esophagitis and eventual stricture formation.

Gastroesophageal reflux is caused primarily by incompetence of the lower esophageal sphincter, which normally acts as a high-pressure barrier between the stomach (slightly positive pressure) and esophagus (slightly negative pressure). The presence of an intra-abdominal segment of esophagus and the acute angle of entry of the esophagus into the stomach presumably contribute to prevention of reflux in the normal patient. The obliteration of these two factors by hiatal hernia may partially explain the frequent association of reflux and hiatal hernia.

Nonbilious postprandial vomiting occurs to varying degrees in most newborn babies; manometric studies demonstrate very low resting pressure of the lower esophageal sphincter in normal neonates. Sphincter pressure reaches normal adult levels by 4 to 6 weeks of age. *Chalasia* or persistent gastroesophageal reflux and vomiting beyond this age may or may not be associated with hiatal hernia. Gastroesophageal reflux or hiatal hernia or both may be demonstrated by careful contrast radiographs of the upper gastrointestinal tract (Fig. 4). Cineradiography may be especially useful. Esophagoscopy is indicated if there is suggestion of the presence of severe esophagitis or stricture.

Severe or prolonged reflux and vomiting may lead to a number of secondary life-threatening complications. Growth failure is not uncommon. Chronic occult aspiration of gastric contents, particularly at night, produces recurrent pneumonia or chronic pulmonary disease in a significant number of patients. Pneumonia is the most common cause of death in children with hiatal hernia. Peptic esophagitis from constant reflux of gastric acid may cause gastrointestinal bleeding or anemia. Continued esophagitis eventually leads to transmural *esophageal stricture* and progressive dysphagia, which compound the problems of growth failure and aspiration pneumonia.

These serious complications notwithstanding, the natural history of symptomatic gastroesophageal reflux and hiatal hernia in most infants is gradual spontaneous improvement over a period of months, probably related to maturation of the lower esophageal sphincter. About 80 percent of infants are asymptomatic by the age of 2 years, even if untreated. Postural treatment is the cornerstone of medical therapy. The infant should be maintained at an angle of 45 degrees in an infant seat, 24 hours per day if necessary. Improvement is more rapid and the percentage of patients ultimately cured is slightly greater if postural treatment is rigorously followed. Thickening of the formula may be helpful. Antacids and parasympatholytic drugs are of no value in infants, but they may be useful in the older child. Postural therapy in the child with persistent symptoms

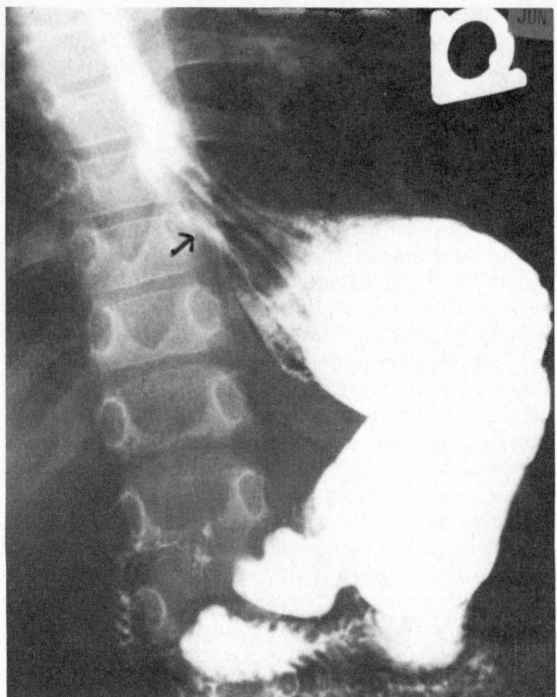

FIG. 4. Sliding esophageal hiatal hernia demonstrated by barium study. Gastric rugae are clearly seen extending into the mediastinum. The gastroesophageal junction is at the level of the 8th thoracic vertebra.

beyond the age of 2 years and in the occasional patient who first becomes symptomatic in later childhood consists primarily of elevation of the head of the bed to minimize nocturnal reflux.

Surgical intervention is necessary in about 10 percent of patients with symptomatic gastroesophageal reflux. Failure of vigorous medical management for a period of at least 2 months is the usual indication for operation, which should not be delayed longer if the life-threatening symptoms discussed above are still present. A number of surgical procedures are available that effectively prevent gastroesophageal reflux. Anatomic repair of the hernia, which is incorporated in most operations, is of secondary importance. The choice of operation depends on the specific pathology and the surgeon's preference. Excellent or good results should be achieved in about 90 percent of patients. Significant esophageal stricture is treated by dilation and an antireflux operation to prevent continuing esophagitis. Dilation alone provides only temporary relief. Esophagoplasty or partial esophageal replacement is necessary if the stricture cannot be dilated. Complications are frequent, and more than one operation may be necessary. Ultimately, about 75 percent of patients with stricture achieve a satisfactory outcome.

Paraesophageal hernia is a herniation of the stomach through a separate defect in the diaphragm adjacent to the esophageal hiatus. The gastroesophageal junction usually remains below the diaphragm, and reflux is not common. Paraesophageal hernias frequently become incarcerated and strangulated, and they may also cause gastric ulceration with bleeding or perforation. Prompt surgical repair of the hernia is always advisable.

References

Bettex M, Kuffer F: Long-term results of fundoplication in hiatus hernia and cardioesophageal chalasia in infants and children. J Pediatr Surg 4:526, 1969

Borrie J: Duplication of the esophagus. Br J Surg 48:611, 1961

Carcassonne M, Bensoussan A, Aubert J: The management of gastroesophageal reflux in infants. J Pediatr Surg 8:575, 1973

Carre IJ: The natural history of the partial thoracic stomach (hiatus hernia) in children. Arch Dis Child 34:344, 1959

———— Postural treatment of children with a partial thoracic stomach ("hiatus hernia"). Arch Dis Child 35:569, 1960

Darling DB, Fisher JH, Gellis SS: Hiatal hernia and gastroesophageal reflux in infants and children: analysis of the incidence in North American children. Pediatrics 54:450, 1974

Filler RM, Randolph JG, Gross RE: Esophageal hiatus hernia in infants and children. J Thorac Cardiovasc Surg 47:551, 1964

Forshall I: The cardioesophageal syndrome in childhood. Arch Dis Child 30:46, 1955

Girdany BR, Sieber WK, Osman MZ: Traumatic pseudodiverticulums of the pharynx in newborn infants. N Engl J Med 280:237, 1969

Gryboski JD, Thayer WR, Spiro HM: Esophageal motility in infants and children. Pediatrics 31:382, 1963

Haight C: Congenital esophageal atresia and tracheoesophageal fistula. In Mustard WT, Ravitch MM, Snyder, Jr. WH (eds): Pediatric Surgery. Chicago, Year Book, 1969, p 357

Holder TM, Cloud DT, Lewis JE, Pilling GP: Esophageal atresia and tracheoesophageal fistula: a survey of its members of the Surgical Section of the American Academy of Pediatrics. Pediatrics 34:542, 1964

Kehrer B, Oesch A, Bettex M: Manometric studies of esophageal motility in infants with hiatus hernia. J Pediatr Surg 7:499, 1972

Kirkpatrick JA, Cresson SL, Pilling GV: The motor activity of the esophagus in association with esophageal atresia and tracheoesophageal fistula. Am J Roentagenol Radium Ther Nucl Med 86:884, 1961

Koop CE, Hamilton JP: Atresia of the esophagus: increased survival with staged procedures in the poor-risk infant. Ann Surg 162:389, 1965

Lind JF, Blanchard RJ, Guyda H: Esophageal motility in tracheoesophageal fistula and esophageal atresia. Surg Gynecol Obstet 123:557, 1966

Moncrief JA, Randolph JG: Congenital tracheoesophageal fistula without atresia of the esophagus. J Thorac Cardiovasc Surg 51:434, 1966

Pieretti R, Shandling B, Stephens CA: Resistant esophageal stenosis associated with reflux after repair of esophageal atresia: a therapeutic approach. J Pediatr Surg 9:355, 1974

Seashore JH, Woodward ER: Transthoracic fundoplication for short esophagus in children. Arch Surg 109:374, 1974

Touloukian RJ, Pickett LK, Spackman T, Biancani P: Repair of esophageal atresia by end-to-side anastomosis and ligation of the tracheoesophageal fistula. J Pediatr Surg 9:305, 1974

GASTRIC MALFORMATIONS
Thomas V. Santulli

Portions of the stomach sometimes lie in the thoracic cavity in patients with *diaphragmatic hernia* or *eventration*

of the diaphragm. In such instances the cardia is usually in its normal position, while the greater curvature protrudes through the diaphragmatic defect or occupies the dome of the eventration. In *esophageal hiatal hernia* (p. 1017) the upper part of the stomach, which has not completed its descent in embryonic development, protrudes into the thoracic cavity through a congenitally enlarged diaphragmatic hiatus; the esophagus itself is of normal length. Varying degrees of this abnormality are seen. In the rare *congenitally short esophagus* the stomach tends to occupy a vertical position, with its upper portion fixed at a supradiaphragmatic level. In *situs inversus* the stomach may be situated on the right side of the abdomen.

Malformations of the stomach are much less frequent than those of other parts of the alimentary tract. *Duplication of the stomach* may cause hematemesis or may produce a cystic mass that is palpable in the epigastrium or that is seen by fluoroscopy to impinge on the gastric lumen, causing partial obstruction. *Diverticula* rarely are seen, usually associated with a defect in the muscular coat, so that the wall locally consists only of mucosa and serosa. Rarely, there may be *congenital atresia* or *stenosis of the pylorus* in the form of a complete or incomplete web. This may cause vomiting leading to dehydration and starvation. *Ectopic gastric mucosa* may be found in a Meckel's diverticulum or elsewhere in the intestine and may cause peptic ulceration and hemorrhage.

Congenital Hypertrophic Pyloric Stenosis

Congenital hypertrophic pyloric stenosis is a relatively common condition characterized by persistent vomiting, constipation, failure to gain weight (or actual loss of weight), marked visible gastric peristalsis, and usually a palpable pyloric mass. Unless it is recognized early and treated properly it may result in prolonged morbidity. It is seen in early infancy, usually in the first 2 months of life, but seldom in the first 2 weeks; only in exceptional instances do symptoms appear in the first few days after birth. Four-fifths of the cases occur in male infants, and firstborn children are more commonly affected. There is some evidence for a genetic factor; with identical twins both are usually affected, while the same is not true of nonidentical twins. Multiple cases may occur in one family or in successive generations in the same family. The incidence of pyloric stenosis apparently varies in different parts of the world. According to Wallgren, the incidence in Sweden in live births is 1 in 150 boys and 1 in 775 girls. Comparatively large numbers of cases are reported in North America, England, and northern Europe, while reports are scanty from Latin America, and the condition is said to be rare in Africans.

PATHOGENESIS AND PATHOLOGY. The pathogenesis of the stenosis is obscure. Markedly hypertrophied pyloric muscle has in rare instances been found in stillborn infants, indicating an inception of the process before birth. On the other hand, Wallgren, who gave barium feedings to 1,000 unselected newborn infants for fluoroscopic examination of the stomach and the duodenum, was unable to find any sign of obstruction or pyloric hypertrophy at that age. Five of these infants subsequently developed pyloric stenosis. Such evidence suggests a postnatal onset. Earlier writers usually argued that hypertrophy of the muscle appeared first and spasm later. In favor of this view is the marked variation in the intensity of spasm encountered from one case to another. On the other hand, the development of hypertrophy of smooth muscle secondary to spasm is a more familiar sequence, and the primary role of spasm is further supported by the favorable response to antispasmodic drugs. Several investigators have found in infants with pyloric stenosis certain degenerative changes in the nerve cells of the myenteric plexus of the pylorus that have been interpreted as a response to excessive vagal stimulation. The nature of the stimulus is not known.

The appearance of the pylorus is remarkably uniform. It constitutes a hard whitish mass about 2 cm long and 1.5 cm in diameter. Its lumen may be so narrow as barely to admit a fine probe, while the normal pylorus will usually admit a No. 21 sound, French scale. Frequently water cannot be forced through the stenosed pylorus, probably because the mucous membrane is thrown into folds. The walls of the stomach are hypertrophied, especially toward the pyloric end. The stomach is dilated; its lower border may extend well below the level of the umbilicus. On section the pylorus is much thickened and considerably elongated; the lower end may project into the duodenal lumen somewhat as the uterine cervix projects into the vagina. On microscopic examination the thickening is seen to affect chiefly the muscle of the circular layer, which is increased to two or three times its normal width. The other coats are thickened, but to a much lesser degree. The hypertrophied smooth muscle cells contain a large amount of glycogen. The uniformity with which the pylorus is found to be enlarged at operation argues against the existence of pure pylorospasm. Failure to palpate the pylorus in atypical cases does not justify the conclusion that hypertrophy is absent.

CLINICAL FEATURES. In the majority of instances the clinical picture evolves in a typical sequence. Symptoms usually appear between the second and third weeks of life, rarely in the first few days, and they may appear up to 12 weeks after birth. A delay in onset is more commonly seen in premature infants. The typical history is that of an infant who, having taken feedings and gained weight regularly in the first week or two, begins to vomit without evident cause.

VOMITING. Initially vomiting occurs occasionally, then repeatedly; in a short time it becomes more forceful and then projectile. It is more forceful than that seen in any nonobstructive condition. An infant will often fairly shoot out the contents of the stomach, sometimes to a distance of 3 or 4 feet; food is also often regurgitated through the nose. Vomiting usually occurs directly after feeding, and characteristically nursing is resumed with avidity.

The vomitus usually consists only of food; it rarely contains bile. The absence of bile is a critical point in establishing the level of the obstruction above the ampulla of Vater. In some patients coffee-ground vomitus appears as a consequence of gastritis. In these instances the partially digested blood should not be confused with the green staining of gastric secretions that occurs with reflux of bile into the stomach. Vomiting does not usually occur at night unless the infant is nursed at that time. In general, the bulk of a feeding is expelled at one time, and the amount vomited may be greater than the feeding just taken, indicating considerable retention. In spite of marked retention, frequent regurgitation of small amounts of feeding is unusual, in contrast to vomiting from several other causes. Some of these patients vomit regularly after every feeding, while others retain two or three feedings in succession. The frequency of vomiting varies from once or twice to six or eight times a day.

Owing to loss of fluid, the infant may become markedly dehydrated; the skin becomes dry and inelastic, and the urine is scanty. Excessive loss of acid in the gastric secretions may lead to alkalosis, hypokalemia, and occasionally tetany. The typical electrolyte picture includes marked reduction of plasma chloride and elevation of bicarbonate (p. 262); however, metabolic acidosis is not uncommon.

STOOLS. Constipation is the rule, and it follows a reduction in the volume of food reaching the intestine because of the excessive vomiting. Occasionally, even when vomiting is severe, there may be frequent small stools consisting mostly of bile-stained mucus.

WEIGHT. Progressive deterioration in nutritional status is one of the most striking features, and close observation of weight is one of the best guides to the progress of the baby. The subcutaneous fat is depleted more than is muscle, so that the patient, in spite of his small size, may present a muscular appearance. If the loss amounts to as much as one-fourth of the maximum body weight previously attained, the condition should be considered critical. In such instances the body temperature may be subnormal.

PERISTALSIS. On examination of the abdomen the epigastrium is usually prominent, in contrast to the lower half of the abdomen, which may be sunken. The characteristic gastric peristaltic waves are best seen immediately after taking a feeding, with the patient observed in a strong light directed tangentially to the contour of the anterior abdominal wall. If the waves do not appear spontaneously, they can often be stimulated by gentle friction or tapping on the epigastrium. The wave begins in the left upper quadrant as a ball-like prominence and slowly moves toward the right, proceeded by a depression or trough. The wave may progress past the midline and fade as it approaches the obstructed pylorus. Sometimes one wave is quickly followed by another. Typical gastric contractions are rarely mistaken for anything else and are virtually pathognomonic of pyloric or duodenal obstruction.

PYLORIC MASS. Palpation of the infant's abdomen for the pyloric hypertrophy or tumor requires both patience and experience. The examination is facilitated if the stomach is empty and a pacifier is used to relax the abdominal muscles, as well as by taking care that the palpating fingers are warm. Compressing the stomach with the opposite hand may help displace the pylorus under the examining finger. The hardened pylorus can be felt in most instances about 3 to 5 cm below the right costal margin and just lateral to the right rectus muscle, sometimes quite superficially. The mass feels about as large as a medium-size olive. It may be obscured by distension of the stomach or by enlargement of the liver. The pylorus may be displaced on its duodenal attachment by the gastric enlargement that occurs in cases of long standing. In spite of its excursion, the direction and course of the peristaltic waves aid the examiner in finding it. The mass may be felt only during active gastric peristalsis, and when it contracts actively under the examining finger its identity is unmistakable. The character of the tumor is thus more important than its position. It is best felt after vomiting or after emptying the dilated stomach. If the tumor cannot be felt from the right side, the examiner should attempt palpation from the baby's left side. Palpation of the tumor has been reported in 68 to 100 percent of patients with pyloric stenosis, depending on the thoroughness, patience, and experience of the examiner.

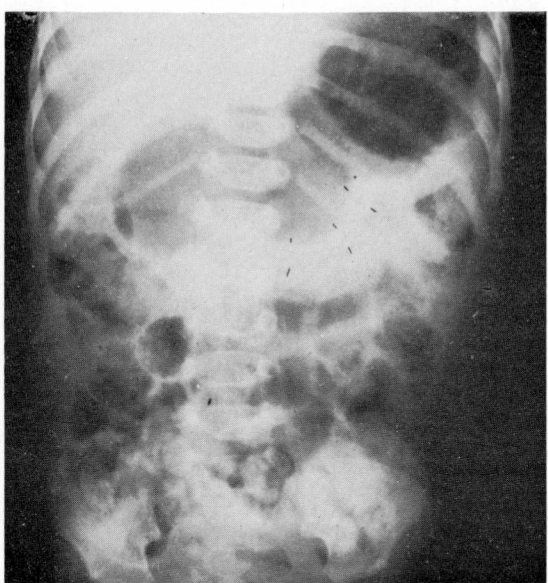

FIG. 5. Plain roentgenogram in hypertrophic pyloric stenosis illustrating the dilation of the gas-filled stomach. Note also the static wave, best seen along the greater curvature.

GASTRIC RETENTION. Prolonged retention of food in the stomach is one of the characteristic features of pyloric stenosis. In healthy infants the stomach is found virtually empty 3 hours after feeding, and it is often empty at the end of 2 hours. If pyloric stenosis is present, food in considerable quantity is invariably found after 3 hours and, unless vomiting has occurred, usually after 4 hours. A large gastric residue, which consists of both food and gastric secretions, may persist even after vomiting or fasting for many hours. Gastric retention may be estimated by aspiration of the stomach contents.

DIAGNOSIS. The history of posnatal onset, with almost uninterrupted progression of symptoms and absence of bile in the vomitus, is characteristic. The presence of visible gastric peristaltic waves and a palpable pyloric mass establishes the diagnosis and allows initiation of treatment early in the course of the disease.

In atypical cases and in those infants where the tumor cannot be palpated with certainty, radiographic examination may be necessary. A plain film of the abdomen often shows a large gas-filled stomach (Fig. 5). Contrast material will show elongation and narrowing of the pyloric channel with delayed opening. The gastric emptying time is usually but not always prolonged, and gastric peristaltic waves are easily visualized. The base of the duodenal bulb is frequently indented and tipped superiorly (Fig. 6).

Pyloric stenosis may be mistaken for cerebral disease because of the projectile nature of the vomiting. In general, the major difficulty is to distinguish it from vomiting associated with improper feeding, chalasia of the esophagus (p. 985), or parenteral infection. In these conditions projectile expulsion of the food usually does not occur, and the other essential features of pyloric stenosis are lacking; with infections, anorexia and other manifestations are often present.

Congenital obstruction of the duodenum or other part of the small intestine may lead to persistent, forcible vomiting; if the obstruction is high up it may even lead to visible gastric peristalsis. In these cases, whether due to stenosis or duodenal compression from congenital bands, the symptoms appear soon after birth, and the vomitus contains bile, except in the very rare instance of supraampullar obstruction.

COURSE. In severe cases peristalsis and vomiting are little influenced by changes in feeding. Unless proper treatment is instituted, the loss of weight is continuous, amounting to 50 to 100 g/day, and could be fatal in 4 to 6 weeks.

In mild cases the symptoms, although characteristic, are much less marked. Gastric peristalsis and the palpable pyloric mass are present, but the vomiting may be only occasional, and the loss of weight is not so relentless. There may even be periods of improvement in which the infant gains weight. In this group some of the patients do well with medical treatment; the symptoms gradually abate, and by the age of 6 to 8 months all evidence of obstruction has disappeared. The muscular hypertrophy recedes less rapidly. Pyloric muscle enlargement has been found at autopsy in children dying of intercurrent disease as long as 6 months after the disappearance of all symptoms. A chronic form of infantile stenosis that persists into later childhood has been reported but is extremely rare.

TREATMENT. In most American clinics operative correction for all patients with hypertrophic pyloric stenosis is regarded as the treatment of choice. Uniform

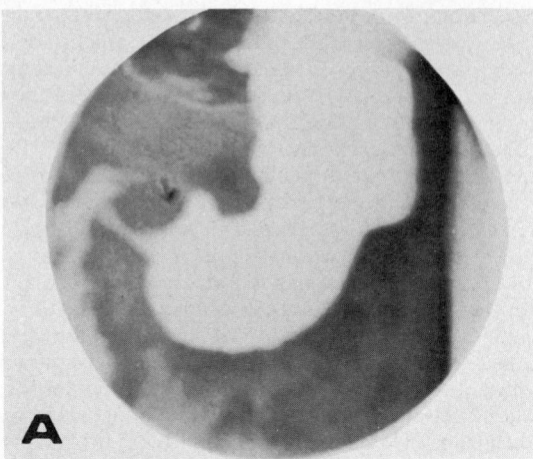

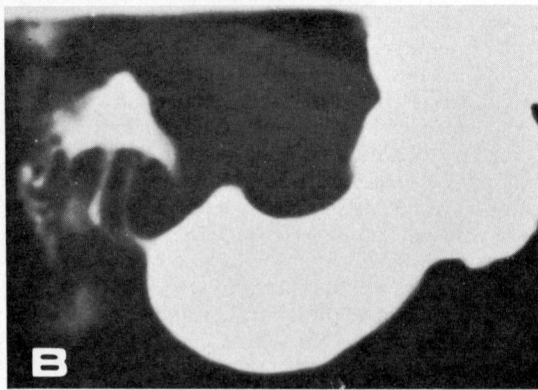

FIG. 6. Barium contrast study in hypertrophic pyloric stenosis. A. Peristaltic contraction is seen ending abruptly in the antrum near its junction with the pyloric canal. The narrowing and elongation of the pyloric channel are illustrated by the stringlike appearance of the barium. B. The double tracks of barium in the pyloric channel noted in this case are related to asymmetric narrowing of the lumen of the canal. (The single track of barium usually seen, as in A, results from more concentric narrowing of the pyloric lumen.) The barium also outlines the duodenal bulb, which is indented and tilted superiorly. The duodenal lumen forms a circumferential cuff or fornix around the projecting pyloric muscle tumor, resulting in the umbrellalike appearance of the bulb.

success is expected, with almost immediate relief of symptoms, a gain in weight beginning within a week, and a short hospital stay. Experience in many of the larger pediatric centers now indicates a mortality of less than 1 percent. It should be emphasized, however, that successful treatment requires facilities that are especially adapted for the preoperative and postoperative care of these infants.

Medical treatment in some of the milder cases has been reported to yield a degree of success comparable to that of early surgery. Considerable skill and effort are needed to bring this about, and the hospital stay is greatly prolonged in comparison to that with surgical treatment. The choice of procedure is therefore influenced to a considerable extent by experience with the method employed and by the medical and surgical talent available. In a controlled study Mellin and associates compared the results of medical and surgical therapy and concluded that operative treatment was preferable in experienced hands.

SURGICAL TREATMENT.   The current low operative risk has been achieved by proper preparation of the patient, especially by the correction of dehydration and metabolic derangements. The Fredet-Ramstedt operation is the accepted procedure: The pyloric mass is incised along its longitudinal axis, and the hypertrophied muscle layers are split along the entire length of the tumor. The divulsion is extended into the contiguous antrum for a short distance, and the muscle fibers are separated down to the submucosa without opening the lumen of the stomach. The intact mucosal and submucosal layers pout between the disrupted smooth muscle, thereby maintaining the opening in the pyloric channel.

Postoperative treatment is important. Parenteral fluids are given until oral intake is adequate. The following scheme of feedings is recommended: Nothing is given orally for the first day. Thereafter, 30 ml of 5 percent glucose and water are given; this is repeated in 3 hours. Milk is then started, consisting of 30 ml of half-strength formula that is progressively increased. Larger quantities of a formula providing 0.6 calorie/ml are given according to the following schedule: 40 ml every 3 hours for 4 feedings, 50 ml every 3 hours for 4 feedings, 60 ml every 3 hours for 8 feedings, 75 ml every 3 hours for 8 feedings, 90 ml every 4 hours for 6 feedings, 105 ml every 4 hours for 6 feedings, and 120 ml every 4 hours for 6 feedings. Subsequent increases or other modifications are made according to individual requirements. The customary vitamin supplements are withheld during the immediate postoperative period and are resumed usually on the fifth day after operation.

Any vomiting during the first few days after operation almost always stops and the infant does well after the stomach has been evacuated by tube. Complications are rare, but they include perforation of the duodenum at the time of operation, persistent obstruction due to incomplete separation of the circular muscle, intestinal obstruction due to postoperative adhesions, and dehiscence of the abdominal wound. Most patients resume daily weight gain early in the postoperative period and are ready for discharge from the hospital 3 to 7 days after surgery.

MEDICAL TREATMENT.   Based on the theory that the pylorus will in time open up spontaneously if nutrition can be maintained, medical treatment includes drug therapy and refeeding. When a feeding has been vomited, food may be retained if the infant is immediately refed, which can be done two or three times. Feedings should be small; they should be perhaps slightly more concentrated than breast milk and not too frequent. Stomach washing has little effect.

Treatment with antispasmodics to relax the pylorospasm is recommended by some authorities as the medical alternative to operation. Atropine methyl nitrate (Eumydrin) has been used, with claims of great success. It is said to be much less toxic than atropine. Eumydrin is used in aqueous (1:10,000) or alcoholic (0.6 percent) solution. The alcoholic solution is preferable in that it can be applied by dropper to the base of the infant's tongue, where it is absorbed locally, and the amount used can be accurately determined. The aqueous solution, given by mouth, deteriorates rapidly and must be freshly prepared each week. The infant should first be treated with appropriate fluids and electrolytes, parenterally if necessary. The drug is then given 15 to 20 minutes before each feeding, starting with doses of about 0.05 mg and working up quickly to amounts of about 0.3 mg. Immediate effects on the vomiting are infrequent, but usually there is some improvement by the fourth day. Some weight gain should appear in the first week. The dosage of Eumydrin should be adjusted to the individual patient and may be increased when the response is not adequate. Parenteral fluids may be continued if necessary. Expert nursing care is essential; the situation is not necessarily beyond the scope of a cooperative mother, but she should receive careful instructions and constant support.

It is by no means clear that the pharmacologic effect of Eumydrin must be continuously maintained for medical treatment to be effective. For unknown reasons good results have been obtained in typical cases when the drug has been given only once a day or when it has been discontinued after only 1 to 2 weeks of therapy. It is possible that a vicious circle is interrupted by Eumydrin treatment. Thus the optimal length of time that treatment should be continued varies. Comparable success has been reported with the use of methscopolamine nitrate (Skopyl), a pharmacologically related drug that exerts its principal effect by decreasing gastric tone. Its toxic action is somewhat less conspicuous than that of atropine derivatives. Toxic effects of Eumydrin include mydriasis, flushing, dry mouth, and fever; these are easily handled by omitting the next dose. A more serious symptom is abdominal distension due to gastric atony or paralytic ileus, which may supervene in spite of improvement in the vomiting. Fatalities have occurred when the drug was continued in the presence of distension.

The consensus on medical treatment is that a small proportion of patients respond rapidly and can be discharged from the hospital as quickly as operated patients. For the majority, however, the situation is only slowly brought under control, and 4 or 5 weeks of close observation in a hospital are needed to achieve success. A few respond poorly, and it is only by the most skillful efforts that they can be carried through with this regimen. The treatment adopted in the individual case will depend in large part on the experience of the medical and surgical personnel at hand. When skilled pediatric surgical talent is available, it is questionable whether medical treatment should be given even a brief trial in mild cases; certainly it should be abandoned if weight cannot be maintained.

References

Becker JM, Schneider KM, Fischer AE: Pyloric atresia. Arch Surg 87:413, 1963

Donovan EJ, Santulli TV: Duplication of the alimentary tract. Ann Surg 126:289, 1947

Gross RE, Holcomb GW Jr, Farber S: Duplications of the alimentary tract. Pediatrics 9:449, 1952

Woolley MM, Gwinn JL, Mares A: Congenital partial gastric antral obstruction. Ann Surg 180:265, 1974

CONGENITAL HYPERTROPHIC PYLORIC STENOSIS

Alarotu H: The histopathologic changes in the myenteric plexus of the pylorus in hypertrophic pyloric stenosis of infants (pylorospasm). Acta Paediatr 45:579, 1956

Benson CD, Lloyd JR: Infantile pyloric stenosis. Am J Surg 107:429, 1964

Clark MB, Norman JN: Alkalosis in pyloric stenosis. Lancet 1:1244, 1964

Day LR: Medical management of pyloric stenosis. JAMA 207:948, 1969

Donovan EJ: Congenital hypertrophic pyloric stenosis. Ann Surg 124:703, 1946

Freisen SR, Boley JO, Miller DR: The myenteric plexus of the pylorus: its early normal development and its changes in hypertrophic pyloric stenosis. Surgery 39:21, 1956

Lynn HB: The mechanism of pyloric stenosis and its relationship to preoperative preparation. Arch Surg 81:453, 1960

Mellin GW, Santulli TV, Altman HS: Congenital pyloric stenosis. J Pediatr 66:649, 1965

Nielsen OS: Histological changes of the pyloric myenteric plexus in infantile pyloric stenosis: studies on surgical biopsy specimens. Acta Paediatr 45:636, 1956

Scharli A, Seiber WK, Kiesewetter WB: Hypertrophic pyloric stenosis at the Children's Hospital of Pittsburgh from 1912 to 1967. J Pediatr Surg 4:108, 1969

Wallgren A: Preclinical stage of infantile hypertrophic pyloric stenosis. Am J Dis Child 72:371, 1946

Woolley MM, Felshen BF, Asch MJ, Carpio N, Isaacs H: Jaundice, hypertrophic stenosis, and glucuronyl transferase. J Pediatr Surg 9:59, 1974

SMALL INTESTINE MALFORMATIONS
Mark M. Ravitch

A wide variety of congenital malformations may lead to neonatal intestinal obstruction. Their presenting signs and symptoms are frequently similar. Physical examination, observation of the vomitus, and radiographic studies will generally provide the diagnosis of intestinal obstruction and frequently the specific kind and location. In general it is immaterial whether the obstruction is complete or incomplete, since even incomplete obstruction will require early operative relief. Hydramnios is often associated with any congenital anomaly of the alimentary tract.

Normal newborn babies regurgitate readily, but seldom vomit, and almost never do they vomit bile. Although distension is usual in neonatal intestinal obstruction, it may not occur with high obstructions, since vomiting appears early and may evacuate the obstructed proximal bowel. Vomiting in the newborn, whether or not bile is present and whether or not the baby is distended, should prompt appropriate radiographic studies.

Radiography usually establishes the diagnosis of obstruction and frequently indicates its nature. With complete obstruction the proximal loops are usually dilated, and there is absence of air in the colon. Barium swallow is rarely necessary and may actually give less information than a plain film. An enema of thin barium or of a water-miscible contrast solution will tell whether the colon is distal to the obstruction and will also indicate the presence of incomplete rotation of the intestine. In any instance in which there is a high probability of intestinal obstruction, a gastric tube should be placed for constant suction, intravenous fluids should be started, and operation should be undertaken.

ATRESIA AND STENOSIS

ETIOLOGY. Intrinsic obstructions of the intestine may range from narrowing of the lumen of variable length or partial occlusion by a crescentic diaphragm to complete occlusion by a diaphragm or actual solid replacement of a segment or several segments of the bowel, or even to a total deficiency of a segment or several interrupted segments of bowel and their mesentery. There is abundant evidence that atresia, at least beyond the ligament of Treitz, derives from an intrauterine pathologic process that results in destruction of a portion of the bowel. The causative lesions have been demonstrated by fetal experimental surgery to be occlusions of mesenteric vessels, intussusceptions, volvulus, herniation, and strangulation in abdominal wall defects (gastrochisis). In children with one or several complete interruptions of the bowel, bile, squames of vernix caseosa, and/or lanugal hairs have been demonstrated in segments between or distal to interruptions and in the meconium of children with intestinal atresias. All these findings are considered evidence that the bowel was patent from end to end and functioning before the development of the atresia. In the duodenum, actual absence of a segment is much rarer, and a complete membrane is the most common form of obstruction. Here it is still conceivable that the old theory of a failure of canalization of the once completely obstructing epithelial plug is the mechanism involved. Neonatal intestinal obstruction, as a result of a lesion extrinsic to the bowel, is seen in annular pancreas, in malrotation or nonrotation, and in herniation, particularly diaphragmatic hernia.

Neonatal Duodenal Obstruction

The classic sign of duodenal atresia (Fig. 7) is the radiographic double bubble showing one fluid level on the left, in the stomach, and another on the right, in the hugely dilated duodenum, with absence of air distally. In the vast majority of cases the obstruction is beyond the ampulla of Vater, and the vomitus contains bile. The common mechanism is a diaphragm of mucosa that may have a tiny central perforation or may be incomplete and crescentic. A substantial proportion of patients, in some series up to 35 percent, are children with Down's syndrome. Vomiting begins within a few hours of birth, except in children with incomplete obstructions. Annu-

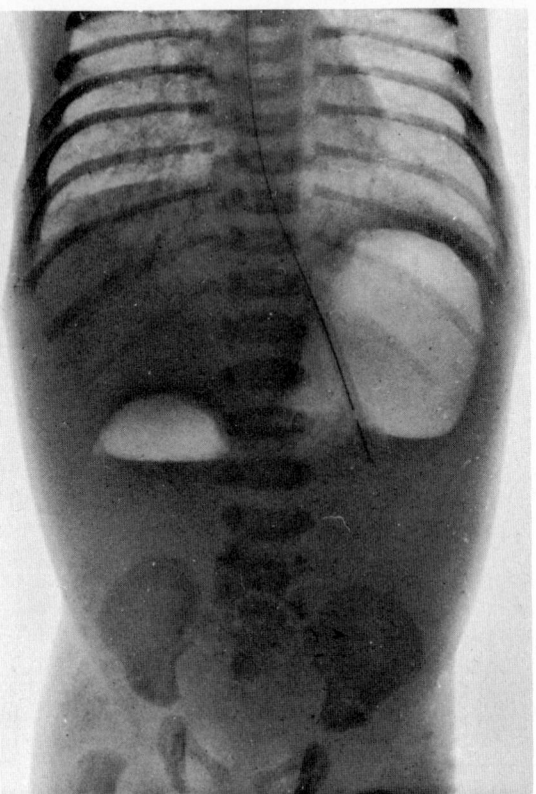

FIG. 7. Duodenal atresia. Note the double-bubble sign, the huge dilation of the duodenum, and the absence of air in the rest of the intestinal tract. This child, like 25 to 30 percent of patients in most series, had Down's syndrome.

lar pancreas (Fig. 8) causes duodenal obstruction by encircling the duodenum with a ringlike constricting mass of pancreatic tissue that results from fusion of the dorsal and ventral pancreatic anlagen. Curiously, the condition may cause no disturbance until adult life. In a substantial proportion of cases that are symptomatic in the neonatal period, an associated intrinsic obstruction of the duodenum exists. The radiographic picture is similar to that of duodenal atresia, but the site of obstruction is usually in the third portion of the duodenum; the obstruction may be complete or incomplete.

Duodenal atresia is best treated by either duodenojejunostomy or duodenoduodenostomy, making sure in either instance, by passing a catheter in both directions, that one is not dealing with two mucosal diaphragms, a not uncommon situation. Gastrojejunostomy, which leads to anastomotic ulcers, is contraindicated.

Annular pancreas is treated similarly by duodenoduodenostomy or duodenojejunostomy. There is frequently an intrinsic obstruction, and operative division of the pancreatic ring has proved to be unsatisfactory because the pancreas may be closely adherent to the duodenum or even intramural. Pancreatitis or pancreatic fistula may result, or inflammation following

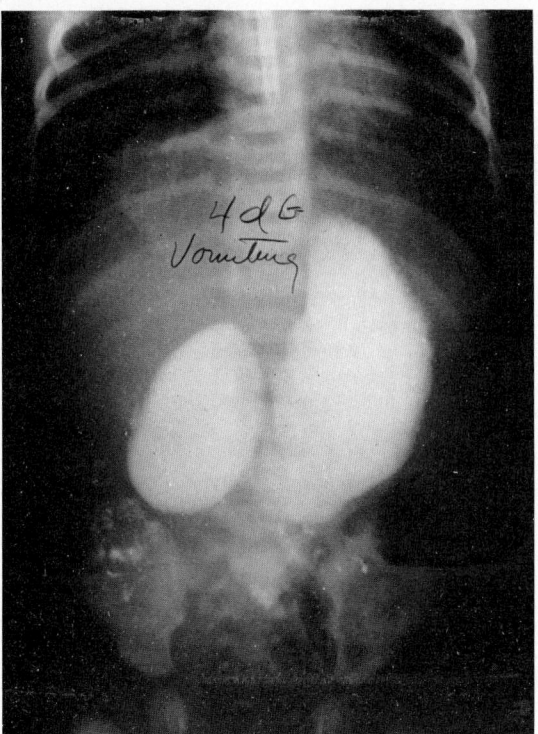

FIG. 8. Annular pancreas. Ordinarily a contrast meal is not required for diagnosis. Note the hugely dilated duodenum and the incomplete obstruction demonstrated by the passage of barium and air into the distal bowel.

division of the pancreas may cause a secondary inflammatory obstruction.

Duodenal Obstruction by Ladd's Bands. Peritoneal bands from the nonrotated or incompletely rotated cecum in the left upper quadrant to the peritoneum in the right upper quadrant, traversing and obstructing the duodenum, may produce a picture of incomplete duodenal obstruction. The contrast enema will show the incomplete rotation of the colon and alert the physician to the possibility of this type of obstruction.

Anomalies of Rotation

ETIOLOGY. The portion of the intestine extending from the duodenum to the middle of the transverse colon is formed from the embryonic midgut loop. In early fetal life this loop projects into the exocoelom in the umbilical cord, receding in about the ninth or tenth week into the endocoelom, the true abdominal cavity. As is shown in Figure 9, the reentering gut normally rotates in a counterclockwise direction about its nutrient vessel, the superior mesenteric artery; on completion of the rotation it will lie anterior to the duodenum and behind the transverse colon. The mesentery of the midgut subsequently fuses with the peritoneum of the posterior abdominal wall, forming a diagonal line of attachment extending from the duodenojejunal fossa in the left upper quadrant downward and to the right. This complicated process may in a number of ways fail to be completed properly. The midgut, or a portion of it, may remain inside the umbilical cord, producing an omphalocele with a small or large separation of the recti, the herniated viscera being covered only by translucent amniotic membrane. In such instances atresias of the intestine are common and anomalies of rotation invariable.

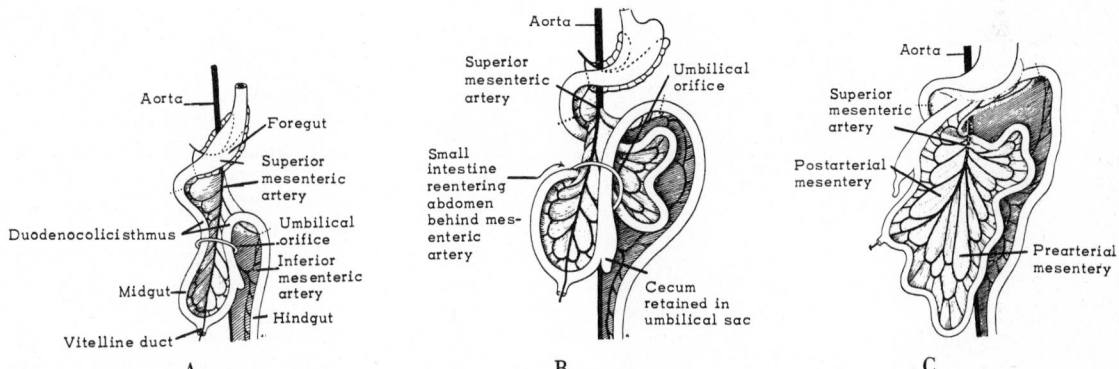

FIG. 9. Developmental rotation of the intestinal tract in embryonic life. A. At about the eighth week of intrauterine life most of the small intestine and part of the large intestine occupy the cavity of the umbilical cord, lying outside the abdominal cavity. Turning on the axis of the superior mesenteric vessels, the midgut loop has rotated about 90 degrees, so that the proximal portion lies to the right, the distal portion to the left of the midsagittal plane (first stage of rotation). B. At about the tenth week, as this extruded portion of the gut is returned to the abdominal cavity, the proximal coils pass from behind the superior mesenteric vessels; distal portions of the intestine leave the umbilical cord last, coming to lie in the right half of the abdominal cavity (second stage of rotation). C. At the completion of the second stage of rotation the transverse colon lies anterior to the superior mesenteric vessels, which in turn lie anterior to the duodenum; the duodenojejunal junction is at the left of the midsagittal plane. (Adapted from Gardner and Hart: Arch Surg 29:942, 1934.)

Anomalies of rotation, which may occur independently of omphalocele, may consist of incomplete rotation, nonrotation, or reverse rotation. Intestinal obstruction occurring as a result of incomplete rotation may be caused by the peritoneal bands passing from the cecum in the left upper quadrant to the posterior parietal peritoneum on the right across the duodenum, which is not rotated and which passes straight down on the right. Alternatively, and much more ominously, the obstruction may be due to a volvulus of the entire small bowel, whose mesentery has no fixation, so that the bowel hangs free on the mesenteric stalk. Since the volvulus involves the entire small bowel, the obstruction is high. In this case distended small-bowel loops do not appear, for when the baby vomits the proximal intestine empties. Thus distension may not occur until the circulation of the twisted bowel has been compromised and a mass of engorged and necrotic bowel becomes visible and palpable as the baby goes into shock. Delaying surgery for only a few hours in a vomiting baby who has volvulus of the midgut may mean the difference between reduction of viable bowel and the near-hopeless problem of resecting the entire small intestine, and perhaps right colon, for gangrene.

Some duodenal bands that are associated with incomplete rotation do not obstruct the duodenum sufficiently to bring the patient to operation in infancy; in other instances the volvulus of the entire small bowel on its mesentery fails to produce complete intestinal obstruction or complete vascular occlusion. Such children may suffer for months or even years with malnutrition before the diagnosis is made and relief is given by operation. The condition has often been mistaken for cyclic vomiting of metabolic origin, malabsorption syndrome, and even psychoneurosis. The barium swallow in these chronic cases will usually show the duodenum descending directly from the pylorus without the usual C loop and sometimes an oblique irregularity of the bowel that is the effect of the twist of the volvulus. Barium enema will confirm the abnormal position of the colon.

In the neonate, intestinal obstruction due to an anomaly of rotation demands urgent operation. Rapid evisceration permits appraisal of the situation, derotation of an existing volvulus, and division of abnormal bands constricting the duodenum.

Atresia of Jejunum and Ileum

Atresia of the jejunum and ileum (Fig. 10) produces the nonspecific picture of neonatal intestinal obstruction, bilious vomiting, distension, and absence of stools. The higher the obstruction the earlier the onset of vomiting; the lower the obstruction the greater the distension and the more numerous the loops of dilated bowel. Hydramnios is common. While in some infants the obstruction is incomplete and is due to a local stenosis, in other patients portions of the bowel may be missing or occluded in one or several segments. Immediate operation is the treatment; it may be made difficult by the enormous disproportion between the dilated proximal bowel and the tiny unused distal bowel. Survival of 70 to 90 percent of patients can be expected, depending on the size of the infant, the association of other anomalies, and delay in operation.

Meconium Ileus

The clinical picture in the infant with meconium ileus is essentially that of neonatal intestinal obstruction. Radiographically the granular appearance of viscid meconium in the right side of the abdomen speckled with tiny air bubbles and the "rabbit pellets" of inspissated meconium in the colon are characteristic. The knowledge that previous siblings have had this condition is particularly helpful in making the diagnosis. A variety of operative treatments—enterotomy and evacuation, enterotomy and irrigation with acetylcysteine, resection of the terminal ileum containing the obstructing mass of meconium, and either anastomosis or double-barreled enterostomy— have all yielded substantial salvage. The irrigation of the colon in the unoperated baby with 15 to 20 ml of a dilute 4 percent acetylcysteine solution or the radiocontrast material Gastrografin, which contains a small amount of the detergent Tween 80, may liberate the adherent meconium in the terminal ileum and allow the baby to be relieved without operation. This procedure is not to be recommended when there is radiographic evidence of massive distension, since in these babies there probably is some additional complicating factor resulting from the in-

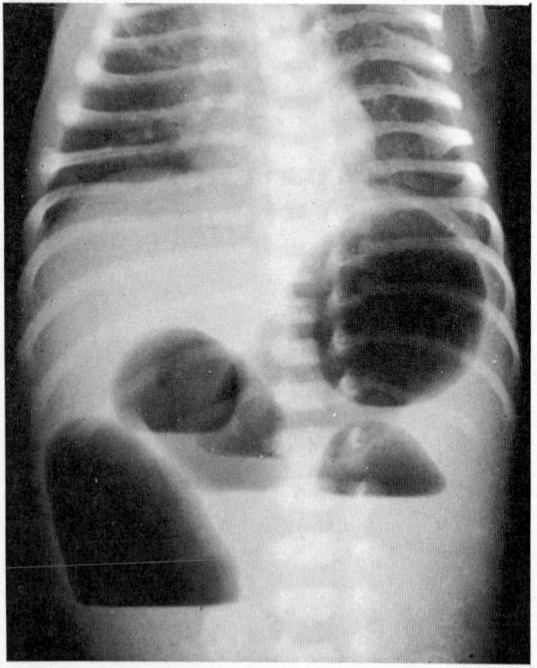

FIG. 10. Jejunal atresia is diagnosed by the dilation of a modest number of loops of small bowel. The enormous discrepancy in size between this dilated bowel and the contracted, unused neonatal distal bowel presents a technical problem in the restoration of continuity.

trauterine obstruction (meconium peritonitis, volvulus, or atresia). The ultimate prognosis is that for any child with cystic fibrosis (p. 993), which is apparently no different from the prognosis in children with cystic fibrosis who do not present with meconium ileus.

Meconium Peritonitis

Meconium peritonitis is the result of an intrauterine rupture of the intestine, with escape of the contents into the peritoneal cavity. The initiating obstruction may be atresia or meconium ileus in association with cystic fibrosis. Often by the time of birth the perforation has resealed, and in rare cases no cause for the initiating obstruction is found. In an infant with neonatal intestinal obstruction in which radiography shows obvious calcification varying from speckles to sheets in an area where there are no gas-filled loops, one may confidently make the diagnosis of meconium peritonitis.With a widespread inflammatory reaction, operation may be extremely difficult. In what has been termed the cystic form of meconium peritonitis the extruded meconium becomes encapsulated in the neighborhood of the perforation, and it is possible to resect en masse the sac of meconium and the malformed bowel that has perforated.

Hirschsprung's Disease

Hirschsprung's disease is characterized by intestinal aganglionosis. It may manifest itself in the newborn as an incomplete or a total intestinal obstruction, occasionally with perforation of the distended proximal bowel. Radiographic films show numerous dilated loops of small bowel; in the infant it may be difficult to be certain whether a distended loop is colon or small intestine. Contrast enema carefully performed may be diagnostic, showing a narrow rectum and sigmoid and dilated proximal colon. The enema in any case may lead to the discharge of inspissated meconium and yield temporary relief.

Meconium Plug

In some infants with neonatal intestinal obstruction a diagnostic contrast enema results in extrusion of a large formed meconium cast of the distal bowel, following which all symptoms are relieved. Occasionally the obstructing meconium plug is in the transverse colon or the splenic flexure. If it is not dislodged following Gastrografin irrigations, operation is required. These children prove not to have cystic fibrosis or any other underlying disease and remain perfectly well after the plug has been eliminated.

Neonatal Intestinal Perforation

The possibility of neonatal intestinal perforation should be suspected whenever an infant who seems not to be doing well, who rejects feedings, or who may have vomited only once or twice suddenly becomes massively distended. A plain film may show an extraordinary degree of pneumoperitoneum (Fig. 11) or only a small amount of air below the diaphragms. Operation obviously is to be undertaken at once. The etiologic possibilities are the following: spontaneous rupture of the stomach, usually proximally on the greater curvature (it may represent either actual rupture from emetic force or perforation by a gavage tube, but is probably not indicative of a congenital anatomic weakness); perforation of a gastric or duodenal ulcer; a postnatal blowout

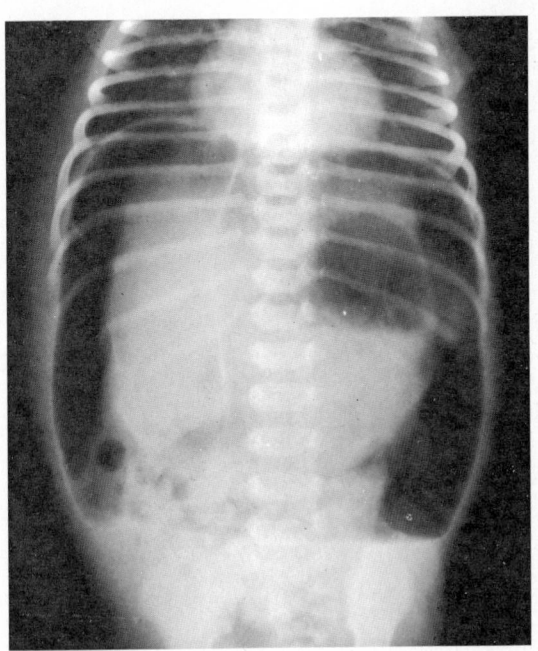

FIG. 11. Neonatal perforation in a 7-day-old infant who refused feedings and suddenly became distended because of perforated gastric ulcer. Perforated duodenal ulcer or neonatal gastric rupture, without ulceration, could also have been the cause.

proximal to an atresia or stenosis; a perforation of the cecum or appendix in a child with Hirschsprung's disease; perforation of the rectum by thermometer or rectal tube; or perforation of the small or large bowel on an unexplained basis.

Duplications of Intestinal Tract

Duplications of the intestinal tract (enteric cysts) are spherical or tubular structures with serosal covering, mucosal lining, and usually a muscular wall in common with the segment of bowel to which they are attached. The duplications are usually separated from the lumen of the bowel by a heavy muscular wall and occasionally are entirely detached. The smallest ones may be submucosal, protruding into the lumen, and may cause intussusception. Symptoms otherwise are produced by the distension, size, and displacement of a large blind cyst, by obstruction from compression of the attached bowel, or from bleeding when a cyst lined by gastric mucosa communicates with the neighboring bowel and produces a peptic ulcer.

Treatment is by resection of the cyst with the attached bowel, although in certain locations, particularly if a tubular cyst is very long and would require resection of a long segment of bowel, it may be preferable to peel the mucosa from the cyst. Cysts behind the duodenum, which are not susceptible of extirpation, may be treated by anastomosis to the duodenum. None of the embryologic theories thus far offered to explain the formation of enteric cysts appears to be valid.

In the mediastinum so-called duplications of the esophagus occur. Although they are closely attached to the

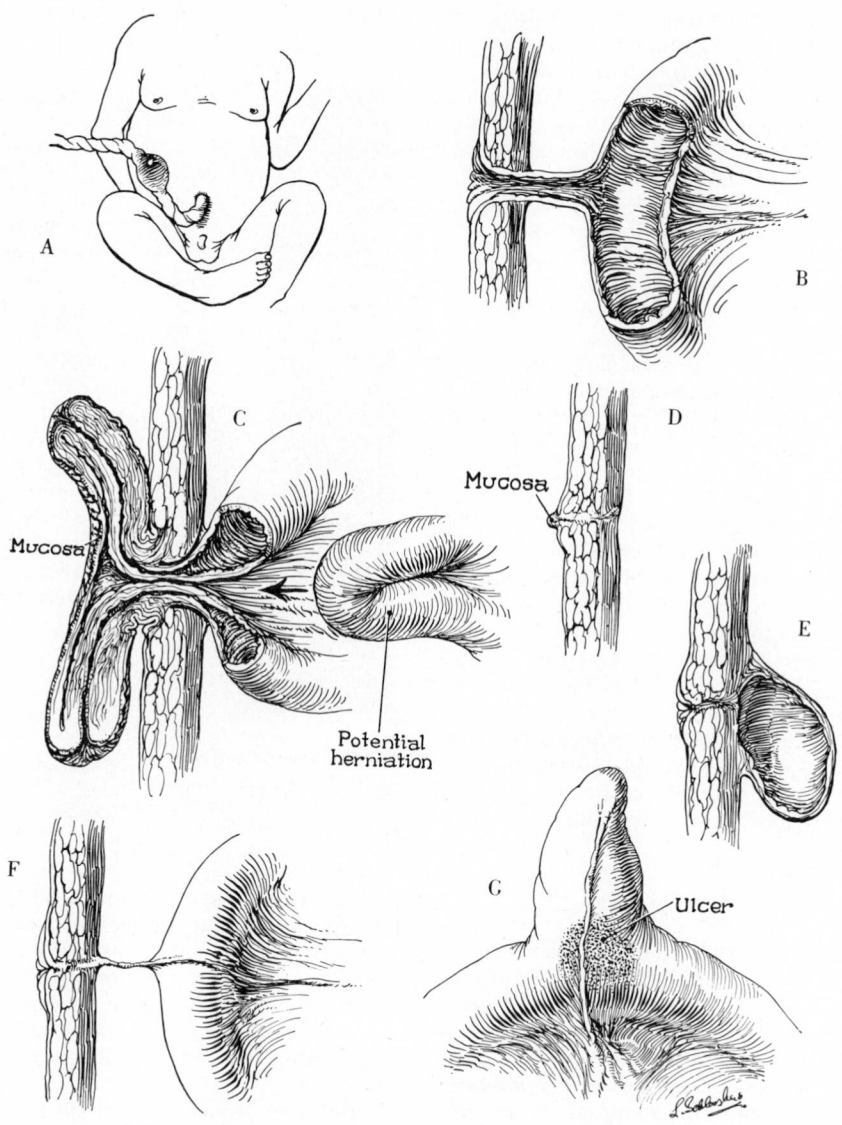

FIG. 12. Some of the possible types of vitelline duct (omphalomesenteric duct) remnants. A. Epithelial cyst in the cord, rare type. Cysts in this position may also be due to collections of Wharton's jelly. B. Patent omphalomesenteric duct connecting ileum with umbilicus and constituting a fecal fistula. C. Prolapse of proximal and distal loops of ileum through the orifice shown in B. This may be complicated by a hernia between the prolapsed loops. D. Mucosal polyp or pouch in external surface of umbilicus, often confused with an umbilical granuloma. E. Extraperitoneal mucosal cyst that may communicate with the surface, in which case there is a continuous discharge of mucus. F. Persistence of the vitelline artery, which may act as a band to obstruct another loop of bowel or may serve as the focal point for a volvulus. At times an epithelium-lined cyst occurs in the middle of such a band. G. Meckel's diverticulum showing the characteristic vascular supply and a peptic ulcer.

esophagus, they are in fact lined by gastric mucosa and occasionally have prolongations passing down through the diaphragm that communicate with the lumen of the small intestine. These cysts are almost invariably associated with thoracic vertebral malformations, not uncommonly in the same patients with intraabdominal intestinal duplications of the ordinary variety.

Complete duplication of the colon is also usually associated with vertebral malformations as well as with duplications of the bladder and urethra and external anal orifices and/or fistulas. The multiple duplications and associated vertebral anomalies that are encountered with esophageal and colonic duplications suggest a more complicated origin for these lesions than for the more common isolated enteric cysts. Incomplete caudal twinning has been suggested to be the genesis of such complex duplications of the colon.

Meckel's Diverticulum and Persistent Vitelline Duct

The omphalomesenteric duct, or vitelline duct, connects the midgut of the embryo to the yolk sac. From the seventh to the twelfth week of fetal life the duct gradually becomes obliterated, leaving ordinarily no connection with the bowel. However, any or all portions of the omphalomesenteric duct may persist. Figure 12 shows some of the possible types of vitelline duct remnants.

Symptoms are related to the nature of the persistence. No more than a fibrous cord representing the omphalomesenteric vessels may exist connecting the small intestine to the umbilicus. and this may serve as the focal point for a volvulus or as a band under which another loop of bowel may be caught. At times a cyst of intestinal structure occurs in the umbilical cord at some distance from the umbilicus; it is treatable by mere ligation and division of the cord. At the other extreme, the ileum may connect widely with the umbilicus by a side arm of bowel, forming a fecal fistula. In some instances a portion of the mucosa may persist at the umbilicus, presenting either as a cherry-red mass that simulates a peculiarly stubborn granuloma or as a mucosal cyst under the umbilicus, with or without an external communication. At times the cordlike remnant of the vitelline vessels between the intestine and the umbilicus may contain, in its midportion, a cyst lined by intestinal mucosa.

Most important is the true *Meckel's diverticulum,* an outpouching of the ileum that may occur anywhere from the ileocecal valve to a point 3 feet or more proximal to the valve in the adult (Fig. 12). The incidence of Meckel's diverticulum is variously given as 1 to 2 percent. It may be a slender process, like a vermiform appendix, or a bell-shaped outpouching several inches wide at the base and several inches long. Symptoms arise from two circumstances: slender diverticula resemble vermiform appendices, and diverticulitis in them produces a disease that is indistinguishable from appendicitis and is treated in the same way; many of the diverticula contain ectopic gastric mucosa, and peptic ulcers develop in the neighboring ileal mucosa. Such ulcers occasionally perforate, but more commonly bleed.

In infants and children painless intestinal bleeding (passage of large quantities of fresh blood in the stool in the absence of hematemesis) is strongly suggestive of a peptic ulcer associated with a Meckel's diverticulum. The hemorrhage is rarely exsanguinating but may be extremely severe. Fresh blood may alternate with changed blood. A massive hemorrhage leads to rapid evacuation of bright red blood, followed, as bleeding subsides, by slow evacuation of changed blood. Repeated hemorrhage is common, and operation should be performed in chronic cases on suspicion, after the stomach and colon have been studied and found normal. Meckel's diverticula are rarely found by contrast radiography. A technetium scan may show an area of radioactivity in the abdomen suggesting that gastric mucosa in a Meckel's diverticulum has picked up the isotope. In acute cases, operation for massive hemorrhage may have to be performed without these studies. Resection of the diverticulum is curative, but at times a broad attachment of the diverticulum to the intestine may require resection of a segment of bowel. Occasionally Meckel's diverticula do not bleed until later in life. Hemangiomas of the bowel, isolated or diffuse, or duplications of the gut may give rise to intestinal hemorrhage similar to that from a Meckel's diverticulum. Meckel's diverticulum is one of the more common mechanical lesions that lead to intussusception.

Ordinarily, if a Meckel's diverticulum is encountered in the course of abdominal surgery for another condition, it is resected.

Mesenteric Cysts

Cysts of the mesentery produce symptoms of mechanical bowel obstruction either by direct infringement on and compression of the lumen or by initiating volvulus. They may be chylous, filled with opaque creamy material, or lymphatic. Lymphatic cysts are usually unilocular and thin-walled, but they occasionally appear as diffuse lymphangiomas of omentum or mesentery. Diagnosis is seldom made before operation because the cysts are usually so soft and flabby as not to be palpable. Symptoms arise either from compression or twisting of the bowel, causing obstruction, or from inflammation in the cyst, clinically simulating appendicitis. The attachment to the bowel is frequently so intimate as to require resection of the bowel with the mesenteric cyst.

References

Abrami G, Dennison WM: Duplications of the stomach. Surgery 49:794, 1961

Amadeo JH, Ashmore HW, Oponte GE: Neonatal gastric perforation caused by congenital defects of the gastric musculature. Surgery 47:1010, 1960

Basu R, Forshall I, Rickham PP: Duplications of the alimentary tract. Br J Surg 47:477, 1960

Beardmore HE, Wiglesworth FW: Vertebral anomalies and alimentary duplications. Pediatr Clin North Am 96:457, 1958

Benson CD, Linkner LM: The surgical complications of Meckel's diverticulum in infants and children. Arch Surg 73:393, 1956

———— Lloyd JR: Atresia and stenosis of the jejunum and ileum. In Mustard WT, Ravitch MM, Synder Jr. WH (eds): Pediatric Surgery, 2nd ed. Chicago, Year Book, 1969

deLorimier AA, Fonkalsrud EW, Hays DM: Congenital atresia and stenosis of the jejunum and ileum. Surgery 65:819, 1969

Dykstra G, Sieber WK, Kiesewetter WB: Intestinal atresia and stenosis of the jejunum and ileum. Surgery 64:661, 1968

Feggetter S: A review of the long-term results of operations for duodenal atresia. Br J Surg 56:68, 1969

Holsclaw DA, Eckstein HB, Nixon HH: Meconium ileus—a 20 year review of 109 cases. Am J Dis Child 109:101, 1965

Jackson JM: Annular pancreas and duodenal obstruction in the neonate. Arch Surg 87:379, 1963

Jewett TC, Duszguski DO, Allen JE: The visualization of Meckel's diverticulum Te 99m pertechnetate. Surgery 68:567, 1970

Kiesewetter WB: Meckel's diverticulum in children. Arch Surg 75:914, 1957

Kittle CF, Jenkins HP, Dragstedt LR: Patent omphalomesenteric duct and its relation to the diverticulum of Meckel. Arch Surg 54:10, 1947

Louw JH, Barnard CN: Congenital intestinal atresia, observations on its origin. Lancet 2:1065, 1955

Martin LW: Meconium ileus. Am J Dis Child 109:99, 1965

Mellish RW, Koop CE: Clinical manifestations of duplication of the bowel. Pediatrics 27:397, 1961

Moore TC, Battersby JS: Congenital cysts of the mesentery. Ann Surg 145:428, 1957

Parrish RA, et al: Spontaneous rupture of the gastrointestinal tract in the newborn. Ann Surg 159:244, 1961

Pollock WF: Intestinal obstruction in the newborn. Surg Gynecol Obstet 119:104, 1964

Ravitch MM: Hindgut duplications, doubling of colon and genitourinary tracts. Ann Surg 137:588, 1953

————In Mustard WT, Ravitch MM, Synder Jr. WH (eds): Pediatric Surgery, 2nd ed. Chicago, Year Book, 1969

Rogers CSR: Pneumoperitoneum in the newborn. Surgery 56:842, 1964

Santulli TV: Meconium ileus. In Mustard WT et al (eds): Pediatric Surgery, 2nd ed. Chicago, Year Book, 1969.

———— Blanc WA: Congenital atresia of the intestine; pathogenesis and treatment. Ann Surg 154:939, 1961

Snyder WH Jr, Chaffin L: Embryology and pathology of the intestinal front-presentation of 48 cases of malrotation. Ann Surg 140:368, 1954

———— Malrotation of the intestine. In Mustard WT et al (eds): Pediatric Surgery, 2nd ed. Chicago, Year Book, 1969

Spencer R: The various patterns of intestinal atresia. Surgery 64:661, 1968

Wang CA, et al: Anomalies of intestinal rotations in adolescents and adults. Surgery 54:839, 1963

Wilmore DW, Groff DB, Bishop HC, Dudrick SJ: Total parenteral nutrition in infants with catastrophic gastrointestinal anomalies. J Pediatr Surg 4:181, 1969

CONGENITAL AGANGLIONIC MEGACOLON

MURRAY DAVIDSON AND MERVIN SILVERBERG

Congenital aganglionic megacolon (Hirschsprung's disease) is a malformation of the parasympathetic system characterized by absence of the intramural ganglion cells of the submucosal (Meissner's) and myenteric (Auerbach's) plexuses that produces a disorder of stool propulsion. As a result of obstruction by the abnormally innervated distal colon, the proximal normal bowel becomes distended; ie, megacolon develops and the distal segment is narrowed.

The pathophysiology of the narrowed bowel is not entirely clear. Some authors believe that it is not spastic, but simply fails to participate in normal peristalsis. Others suggest that the obstruction associated with this narrowed segment may be due in part to tonic contraction of its smooth muscle, since adrenergic innervations appear to be disturbed. The entire rectum is usually involved, but the proximal extent of the defect above the rectum is variable. In more than half the patients aganglionosis extends to the midsigmoid colon. In others, varying lengths of the colon are abnormal. Ten to 15 percent of all cases extend beyond the left side of the colon, and in rare instances part or all of the small bowel may be aganglionic. Segmental involvement has been reported on one occasion. In other instances very short segments of aganglionosis, not even reaching the rectosigmoid, have been associated with the picture of megarectum, colonic dilation extending virtually to the anal canal.

The incidence in the general population is reported to be higher than 1 in 5,000. Support for the role of genetic factors in the pathogenesis of this condition is derived from evidence that there is a familial incidence of 2 to 4 percent, a preponderance of affected males, and an association with Down's syndrome. Additionally, a hereditary disease that has been related to specific gene defects and that is analogous to that of man occurs in the mouse. Hair changes result from reduced numbers of pigment cells in the mouse's coat, and the bowel changes are initially identical and are associated with absence of colonic ganglion cells.

The most common early clinical presentation is that of delay in passage of meconium, in association with abdominal distension, in the first days of life. This apparent intestinal obstruction may be complicated by perforation of the proximal colon, cecum, or appendix, if these structures are distended and have thinned-out walls. Digital examination of the small-caliber rectum often results in a copious gush of meconium or fecal material, with apparent relief of the obstructive features. These cases may be confused with the so-called self-limited meconium plug syndrome. They should be followed closely for signs of continuing fecal retention as a clue to the possible presence of congenital aganglionic megacolon.

A second common presenting syndrome in the first weeks of life is severe persistent or recurrent diarrhea due to secondary enterocolitis. The condition arises more commonly among infants with long segments of aganglionic bowel. Peritonitis, mucosal ulceration, and septicemia develop frequently in this condition, and the mortality rate is about 75 percent. In older children enterocolitis is rare, and they display the more characteristic symptoms of Hirschsprung's disease, ie, persistent abdominal distension and stool retention. Malnutrition, anemia, rectal bleeding due to ulcers from colonic stasis, protein-losing enteropathy, and recurrent systemic infections have all been reported as complicating features of the disease.

Physicians frequently are assured that the symptoms of this disease may readily be distinguished from those of chronic voluntary stool withholding because the patients with congenital megacolon have a history of difficulty going back to the neonatal period. It is apparent from the foregoing that some children may present no such history, others may have had diarrhea, and only some will have been constipated. Conversely, children with voluntary withholding may have had a prior history of colic and bowel difficulty that goes back to birth. The most important distinguishing features in differential diagnosis were pointed out above in the discussion of constipation and are reiterated here. The stool, which is retained in patients with Hirschsprung's disease, generally does not reach the distal area of the rectum. This produces two major differential findings. Since the proprioceptors that initiate the urge to defecate are located just proximal to the internal sphincter, this reflex is

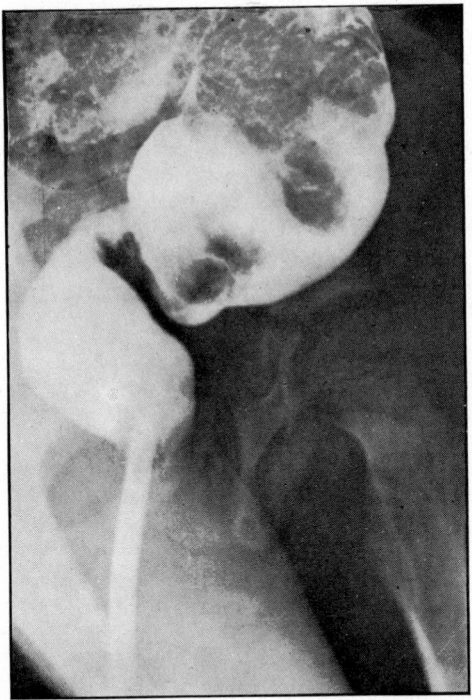

FIG. 13. Congenital megacolon in an 8-year-old boy. Transition segment at rectosigmoid junction.

rarely activated in children with congenital aganglionic megacolon. Second, on repeated digital examinations of the rectum this segment is virtually always found to be empty, despite large amounts of retained material.

The mainstays of diagnosis are the barium enema and rectal biopsy. Radiocontrast studies before the age of 6 weeks often will not show a transition zone. In the young child, especially if frequent enemas have been given to decompress the colon, sufficient time may not have elapsed to permit the segment proximal to the aganglionic area to become dilated. Failure to evacuate barium adequately after examination should alert the radiologist to the correct diagnosis even in the absence of the typical transition zone (Fig. 13). Excessive amounts of administered barium may obscure the typical appearance in the older infant and child. Total colonic aganglionosis is often associated with an apparently normal barium enema (ie, no transition zones or dilated areas are visualized), although narrowing and shortening of the normal-caliber colon with rounding of the flexures should be apparent in such a colon, and these signs may be considered presumptive evidence of the disease. If there is any reasonable doubt and the infant's clinical condition permits temporizing, a rectal biopsy should be done. Wedge biopsies taken deep enough to contain elements of the intramuscular plexus are preferred, since these ganglion cells are more easily identifiable. To obviate administration of general anesthesia and any of the rarely encountered postoperative complications such as stricture, bleeding, or sepsis in very ill infants, simple rectal suction biopsy has become popular. In experienced hands, demonstration of submucosal ganglia (Meissner's plexus) is adequate to exclude the diagnosis in many cases. However, absence of ganglia from tissue secured by this technique should not be considered diagnostic of Hirschsprung's disease, since such biopsy specimens may be too small or too superficial or may be taken from areas too close to the internal sphincter, wherein there is usually a paucity of ganglia. Manometric diagnostic studies show dissociation of stimulated motility between the normally innervated and aganglionic segments and abnormal contractile responses of the internal sphincter to rectal distension. Distension of the rectum is normally followed by prompt relaxation of the internal sphincter. This response is not obtained in children with Hirschsprung's disease. The recording from this site in affected children either shows an increase of pressure or no change from the baseline value.

Treatment of aganglionic megacolon may be either symptomatic or definitive. In the acutely ill and distended child, emergency correction of fluid and electrolyte imbalance and hypoproteinemia, with appropriate treatment of sepsis, is mandatory. Following restoration of reasonable homeostatic balance, the patient should be provided with an emergency colostomy in a segment in which normal ganglia have been identified on pathologic review of frozen sections. In less urgent situations stool evacuation may be achieved by enemas. Only small isotonic enemas should be used, since serious complications have followed the use of tap water, hypertonic phosphate solutions, or large saline enemas. With severe impaction, frequent mineral oil or warm saline instillations, retrograde or through a colostomy, are useful.

Definitive surgical procedures are designed to establish regular and spontaneous defecation, maintain complete continence, and avoid ultimate sexual impotence. Several different surgical techniques are offered, each intended to best serve the operative objectives of its originator. All the methods now include some form of sphincterotomy or sphincter dilation to correct the sphincteric achalasia that is demonstrable on motility study. The individual procedures contribute very little to overall mortality. A majority of deaths are due to irremediable imbalances in the nutritional or fluid-electrolyte conditions of patients preoperatively, the most important factor in death being development of pseudomembranous enterocolitis. The latter condition is not an infrequent complication in the postoperative period, and its precise cause and treatment are unknown.

A number of disorders simulate aganglionic megacolon clinically and have often been considered collectively as pseudo-Hirschsprung's diseases. Abnormal, decreased, or absent intramural ganglion cells are noted in Chagas' disease, immaturity of ganglion cells, and a number of unnamed conditions. Segmental dilation of the colon, achalasia of the distal colon with normal ganglia, and colonic disorders associated with congenital colonic anomalies, vascular insufficiency of the colon, hypothyroidism, and central nervous system diseases usually simulate aganglionosis, but normal ganglion cells may be demonstrated. Ehrenpreis has postulated that one mechanism for postnatal degeneration of ganglion cells in the myenteric plexuses and a possible cause of congenital aganglionosis is a vascular accident that results in poor oxygenation of the affected segment.

References

Aldridge RT, Campbell PE: Ganglion cell distribution in the normal rectum and anal canal. A basis for the diagnosis of Hirschsprung's disease by anorectal biopsy. J Pediatr Surg 3:475, 1968

Bill AH Jr, Chapman ND: The enterocolitis of Hirschsprung's disease. Its natural history and treatment. Am J Surg 103:70, 1962

Bodian M, Carter CO: A family study of Hirschsprung's disease. Ann Hum Genet 26:261, 1963

——— Carter CO, Ward BCH: Hirschsprung's disease. Lancet 1:302, 1951

Bowden DH, Goodfellow AM, Munn ND: Hirschsprung's disease in the neonatal period; a report of five cases, four of which involved the small intestine. J Pediatr 50:321, 1957.

Davidson M: Congenital aganglionosis. In Code CF (ed): Handbook of Physiology—Alimentary Canal. Washington, DC, American Physiological Society, 1968, p 2783

——— Bauer CH: Studies of distal colonic motility in children. IV. Achalasia of the distal rectal segment despite presence of ganglia in the myenteric plexuses of this area. Pediatrics 21:746, 1958

——— Sleisenger MH, Steinberg H, Almy TP: Studies of distal colonic motility in children. III. The pathologic physiology of congenital megacolon (Hirschsprung's disease). Gastroenterology 29:803, 1955

Dobbins WO, Bill AH Jr: Diagnosis of Hirschsprung's disease excluded by rectal suction biopsy. N Engl J Med 272:990, 1965

Ehrenpreis T: Long-term results of rectosigmoidectomy for Hirschsprung's disease, with a note on Duhamel's operation. Surgery 49:701, 1961

——— Pseudo-Hirschsprung's disease. Arch Dis Child 40:177, 1965

——— Some newer aspects on Hirschsprung's disease and allied disorders. J Pediatr Surg 1:329, 1966

Emanuel B, Padorr MP, Swenson O: Familial absence of myenteric plexus (congenital megacolon). A study of six families. J Pediatr 67:381, 1965

Fraser GC, Berry C: Mortality in neonatal Hirschsprung's disease: with particular reference to enterocolitis. J Pediatr Surg 2:205, 1967

Koop CE: The choice of surgical procedures in Hirschsprung's disease. J Pediatr Surg 1:523, 1966

Lawson JON, Nixon HH: Anal canal pressures in the diagnosis of Hirschsprung's disease. J Pediatr Surg 2:544, 1968

Moseley PK, Segar WE: Fluid and serum electrolyte disturbances as a complication of enemas in Hirchsprung's disease. Am J Dis Child 115:714, 1968

Passarge E: The genetics of Hirschsprung's disease. Evidence for heterogeneous etiology and a study of 63 families. N Engl J Med 276:138, 1967

Swenson O: A new surgical treatment for Hirschsprung's disease. Surgery 28:371, 1950

——— Follow-up on 200 patients treated for Hirschsprung's disease during a ten year period. Ann Surg 146:706, 1957

——— Neuhauser EBD, Picket LK: New concepts of the etiology, diagnosis and treatment of congenital megacolon (Hirschsprung's disease). Pediatrics 4:201, 1949

Tobin F, Reid NCRW, Talbert JL, Schuster MM: Non-surgical test for the diagnosis of Hirschsprung's disease. N Engl J Med 278:188, 1968

ANORECTAL MALFORMATIONS

THOMAS V. SANTULLI

Malformations of the anus and rectum, frequently referred to as imperforate anus, are among the most common congenital anomalies, occurring about once in every 5,000 births. They consist of a variety of lesions ranging from a mild congenital stenosis of the anus that requires only simple dilation to complex deformities that present some of the most vexing and discouraging problems in management.

In recent years the original classification of Ladd and Gross has been changed in order to relate the clinical appearance more directly to embryologic derivation and certain anatomic features of these anomalies. Chief among these features is the relationship of the termination of the bowel, even as a fistula, to the puborectalis sling of the levator ani musculature, the principal muscle of continence. Accordingly the current classification divides the anomalies into three main groups (Table 5): the low or translevator group, in which the bowel is through the sling; the intermediate, in which the bowel is at the sling; and the high or supralevator, in which there is arrested development above the sling. This grouping is important because the high anomalies carry a far greater mortality and morbidity and have a much higher incidence of associated malformations, especially urologic and vertebral, than the low or intermediate anomalies. Also, correction of the low anomaly is generally associated with a far better functional result, since the termination of the bowel has passed through the puborectalis sling. High anomalies are found in 50 percent of the males and in only 20 percent of the females. The various types of anomalies and their associated fistulae are illustrated in Figure 14.

TABLE 5. Anorectal Anomalies

Male	Female
Low (translevator)	**Low (translevator)**
At normal anal site	Same
Anal stenosis	Same
Covered anus, complete	Same
At perineal site	Same
Anocutaneous fistula	Same
(covered anus, incomplete)	
Anterior perineal anus	Same
	At vulvar site
	Anovulvar fistula
	Anovestibular fistula
	Vestibular anus
Intermediate	**Intermediate**
Anal agenesis	Same
Without fistula	Without fistula
With fistula	With fistula
Rectobulbar	Rectovestibular
	Rectovaginal, low
Anorectal stenosis	Same
High (supralevator)	**High (supralevator)**
Anorectal agenesis	Same
Without fistula	Without fistula
With fistula	With fistula
Rectourethral	Rectovaginal, high
Rectovesical	Rectocloacal
	Rectovesical
Rectal atresia	Same
Miscellaneous	
Imperforate anal membrane	
Cloacal exstrophy	
Others	

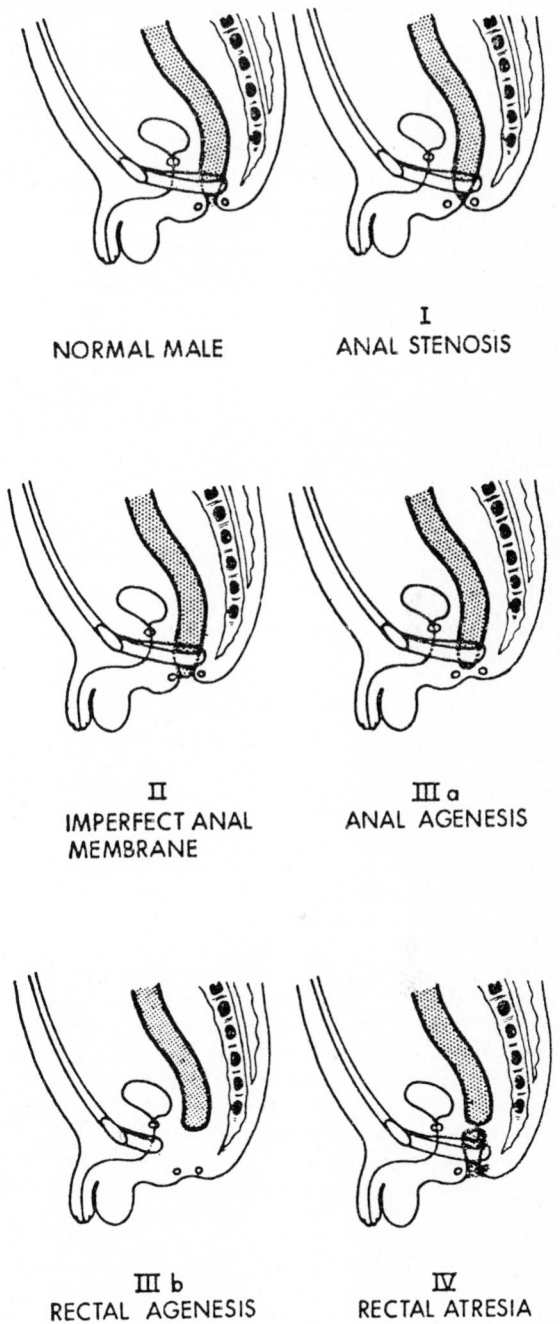

NORMAL MALE

I
ANAL STENOSIS

II
IMPERFECT ANAL
MEMBRANE

III a
ANAL AGENESIS

III b
RECTAL AGENESIS

IV
RECTAL ATRESIA

The low and intermediate groups represent abnormalities in the embryologic formation of the anus and/or perineum. The high anomalies represent embryologic malformations of the rectum and anus. Anorectal stenosis and rectal atresia are probably not embryologic defects. They should be considered as acquired malformations best explained as secondary stenosis or atresia in the fetus resulting from a vascular accident to an already normally formed bowel.

The diagnosis can usually be made soon after birth by careful examination of the perineum or vagina. When the normal anal site is imperforate, there is usually a depression (anal dimple) where one would expect to find the anus. In most cases the anal dimple is sharply defined; in others it may be less evident. The skin is more deeply pigmented than the surrounding skin, and the lines seem to converge to a central point within the external anal sphincter muscle that surrounds the dimple. Puckering can be seen at this point when the muscle contracts.

A careful search should be made for a fistula. A fistula to the perineum or the urinary tract (usually urethral, rarely vesical) will be found in about 70 percent of the males. About 90 percent of the females have a fistula communicating with the perineum or the vagina. Rectourinary fistulae in the female are extremely rare. A fistula to more than one site does not occur.

FIG. 14. Types of malformations of the anus and rectum schematically represented and compared with the normal male. Possible fistulous connections are omitted. Note the relationship of the termination of the bowel to the puborectalis sling of the levator ani muscle. (From Santulli TV et al: Surg Clin North Am 45:1253, 1965.)

Outlining the rectal pouch by radiographs taken with the baby held in the upside-down position may be helpful in determining the level of the termination of the bowel; together with the clinical findings they are of some value in planning the surgical approach. They are of little or no value in patients who present a visible fistula on the perineum or vagina.

The most important contribution of radiography to the evaluation of patients with imperforate anus lies in the detection of accompanying vertebral and urologic abnormalities. Some abnormality of the sacral spine may be found in over 50 percent of the high-anomaly group, and the accompanying neurologic defects may significantly affect the functional results in these patients. When the sacrum is grossly abnormal the incidence of urologic abnormalities is also high and may exceed 70 percent. Hence voiding cystourethrograms and intravenous pyelograms should be done early in all patients with imperforate anus. About 40 percent of the patients have other developmental anomalies, and half of these may be serious. The most commonly associated major anomalies are congenital heart disease, atresia of the esophagus, hydronephrosis, ureterovesical reflux, and malformation of the spine.

Treatment is determined by the specific type of anomaly present. Careful and thorough assessment of the anomaly is done before any surgical correction is carried out. In general, most of the low anomalies are corrected by the perineal approach (anoplasty or cutback procedure). Since the bowel has already traversed the puborectalis sling in these anomalies, the surgical principle is to create the minimal disturbance of this bowel-to-sling relationship in creating an adequate anal opening.

The baby with a high anomaly should have a preliminary divided sigmoid colostomy performed in the newborn period, followed by definitive abdominoperineal or sacroabdominoperineal procedure between 9 and 12 months of age, with the bowel carefully brought through the puborectalis sling of the levator ani muscle. The colostomy is then closed at a later date.

Regardless of the form of treatment utilized, it is essential that these children be followed closely for many years; great care must be taken to guard against stricture, impaction, and rectal inertia from long-standing constipation. Dilations, cathartics, stool softeners, and cleansing enemas are all adjuncts that may be used advisedly and under medical supervision to ensure good bowel function.

The overall mortality is about 10 percent; surgical procedures to correct the malformations account for 1 percent of the deaths, prematurity and associated anomalies for the remainder.

Almost all patients with low anomalies should be continent. The functional results in the high anomaly depend on the type of anomaly, the surgical corrective procedures, and the associated neurologic deficits, if any. Long-term follow-up is essential in assessing the results in high anomalies. Overall, in our group 60 percent are considered to have normal anal function, 20 percent satisfactory, and 20 percent unsatisfactory (total or near-total incontinence, frequent fecal impactions, or permanent colostomy).

References

Berdon WE, Baker DH, Santulli TV: The radiologic evaluation of imperforate anus. An approach correlated with current surgical concepts. Radiology 90:466, 1968

Hiatt RB, Santulli TV: Important factors influencing the treatment of imperforate anus. Dis Colon Rectum 5:110, 1962

Kiesewetter WB: Imperforate anus: the role and results of the sacro-abdomino-perineal operation. Ann Surg 164:655, 1966

Louw JH: Congenital abnormalities of the rectum and anus. Curr Probl Surg, May 1965

Nixon HH: Imperforate anus. In British Surgical Practice and Surgical Progress. London, Butterworth, 1961

Palken M, Johnson RJ, Derrick W, Bill AH: Clinical aspects of female patients with high anorectal agenesis. Surg Gynecol Obstet 135:411, 1972

Santulli TV, Schullinger JN, Amoury RA, Berdon WE: Malformations of the anus and rectum. Surg Clin North Am 45:1253, 1965

——— Imperforate anus. In Mustard WT et al (eds): Pediatric Surgery, 2nd ed. Chicago, Year Book, 1969, p 983

——— Kiesewetter WB, Bill AH Jr: Anorectal anomalies: a suggested international classification. J Pediatr Surg 5:281, 1970

——— Schullinger JN, Kiesewetter WB, Bill AH Jr: Imperforate anus: a survey from the members of the Surgical Section of the American Academy of Pediatrics. J Pediatr Surg 6:484, 1971

Stephens FD, Smith ED: Ano-rectal Malformations in Children. Chicago, Year Book, 1971

Wiener ES, Kiesewetter WB: Urologic abnormalities associated with imperforate anus. J Pediatr Surg 8:151, 1973

MALFORMATIONS OF THE ABDOMINAL PARIETES

Thomas V. Santulli

Umbilical Hernia

Umbilical hernia is a common lesion in infants and children; while it is often annoying, it is rarely serious. It results from a muscular and fascial defect of the abdominal wall where the wall was pierced by the blood vessels of the umbilical cord. The peritoneum that protrudes through this defect is completely covered by skin. Although separation of the rectus muscles, if present, is usually confined to this region, the separation may extend upward and downward in the midline (diastasis recti). The hernia is seen especially in infants born prematurely and in those who are poorly nourished or who suffer from rickets or cretinism. It is more frequent in blacks than in other races and is about twice as common in girls as in boys.

The protruding mass is usually from 1 to 2 cm in diameter. It can be easily reduced; the edge of the hernial ring and fascial defect may be felt. With larger masses and a larger ring there may be local tympany, and a gurgling sound is heard on reduction. Incarceration of the contents (omentum or intestine) is extremely rare, but it does occur.

In a great majority of patients the fascial ring gradually becomes smaller, and the hernia disappears spontaneously; even fairly large hernias will close. The value of adhesive strapping, which was once widely practiced, is open to question. If the hernia has not disappeared by the end of the fourth year, operation may be necessary.

Inguinal Hernia and Hydrocele

Inguinal hernia is common and is seen much more frequently in boys than in girls. The great majority are of the indirect variety; direct inguinal hernia is uncommon in infancy and childhood. About 60 percent are found on the right side and 20 percent left, and 20 percent are bilateral.

Embryologically, as the testis descends through the inguinal canal a projection of peritoneum (processus vaginalis) is carried downward into the scrotum. Normally the lowermost part of this process, which lies in the scrotum alongside the testis, is pinched off to form the tunica vaginalis, while the remainder closes off up to the internal ring and atrophies. Any portion of the processus vaginalis may remain patent. If all of it stays open a complete congenital hernia results; when only the upper part is patent the hernia is said to be incomplete, as the sac is not in continuity with the tunica vaginalis. Central portions of the processus vaginalis may persist and give rise to hydrocele of the spermatic cord (or canal of Nuck in the female). Combinations of hernia and hydrocele are common.

Most hernias in the pediatric age group contain small bowel; female infants may have an ovary or fallopian tube in the sac. A sliding type of hernia in the female infant involving ovary or fallopian tube is relatively common.

Inguinal hernias may appear at any age, frequently soon after birth or during the first few months of life. There is a history of recurrent swelling in the inguinal area or scrotum that is usually easily reduced. If the mass is not present during physical examination the diagnosis can be made from the characteristic history and from palpable thickening of the spermatic cord. In infants and young children the diagnosis cannot be made by palpation of an enlarged internal ring through the invaginated scrotum, as in the adult, since the ring is too small to admit the tip of the finger. Gentle palpation of the lower part of the inguinal area near the pubis will frequently give the sensation of rubbing silky surfaces together if a hernial sac is present (silky sign).

A history of incarceration can be obtained in about 20 percent of children with inguinal hernia up to 1 year of age. It may occur anytime, but it is most common in the first 3 months. When this complication develops, the inguinal mass is usually painful and the child is fretful. Vomiting occurs and there may be abdominal distension. Although it is uncommon, strangulation does occur, and infarction of the small bowel, ovary, or testis (most common) may result.

All inguinal hernias are potentially dangerous and should be surgically corrected early in life. Operation is deferred only in the infant with a serious associated illness that would contraindicate surgery, in which case the hernia may be temporarily treated by some form of truss (yarn truss or elastic belt with a rubber pad over the inguinal region). For incarceration, reasonable attempts should be made to reduce the hernia. This is best accomplished by adequate sedation, Trendelenburg position, and gentle taxis. If these measures are unsuccessful or if there are signs of strangulation, immediate operation is indicated.

The results of surgical treatment are excellent; recurrence is rare, and morbidity and mortality are extremely low.

Femoral hernia is rare in the pediatric age group. The hernia protrudes through the femoral canal below the inguinal ring. Surgical repair is necessary.

Hydroceles, being fluid filled sacs, are diagnosed by transillumination. The lesions are benign and self-limited. Surgery is not necessary; the fluid absorbs spontaneously and the hydrocele disappears, almost always before the first birthday.

Epigastric Hernia

Epigastric hernia is an unusual hernia of the linea alba that is due to a midline fascial defect above the umbilicus. It varies from a few millimeters to several centimeters in diameter and may occur anywhere between the xiphoid and the umbilicus. The lesion may be painful; it is frequently tender. A small subcutaneous mass can be felt that usually represents properitoneal fat herniated through a defect in the line alba. Surgical repair is usually indicated.

Diaphragmatic Hernia

Diaphragmatic hernia (p. 1542) is a protrusion of abdominal organs into the chest through a defect in the diaphragm. It occurs in two forms, the congenital and the post-traumatic; the latter is rare in early life. In the congenital type, which occurs more frequently on the left side, the defect is caused by a failure of fusion of the various parts of the embryonic diaphragm and may appear in one of several areas of the diaphragm. Most commonly it occurs in the posterolateral portion along the pleuroperitoneal canal or the foramen of Bochdalek; less frequently it occurs at the esophageal hiatus or in the retrosternal areas (the foramen of Morgagni). In most instances of hernia through the posterolateral defect there is free communication between the thoracic and abdominal cavities; rarely there may be a thin peritoneal sac covering the abdominal viscera in the chest. The small intestine, the right side of the colon, the stomach, and the spleen may be found in the thoracic cavity. There is usually an associated malrotation with nonfixation of the intestine. With right-sided hernias a part of the liver may be in the thorax. The homolateral lung is usually collapsed and may be hypoplastic, the mediastinal structures are shifted to the opposite side of the chest, and the contralateral lung is often partially compressed and may also be hypoplastic. Hernias at the esophageal hiatus usually have a peritoneal sac that limits the upward progress of abdominal viscera; the sac rarely contains more than the stomach. Retrosternal hernias (through the foramen of Morgagni) have a sac in about half of the cases; only a part of the transverse colon, stomach, or liver may be herniated.

Usually symptoms are present at birth; in rare instances the patient may be several weeks or months old before any significant abnormality is suspected. There may be respiratory, circulatory, or digestive disturbances (p. 1542). In severe cases cyanosis is evident immediately after birth. There is rapid respiration, dyspnea, overdistension of the involved chest, and a sunken abdomen. Other symptoms may at times suggest intestinal obstruction; occasionally acute, but more often chronic or intermittent, vomiting is prominent. Pain is seldom present, but there may be unexplained episodes of anorexia and dyspnea. The physical signs are variable, and in some cases no abnormality may be detected, even when the condition is known to be present. Sometimes the findings suggest pneumothorax; at other times there is so much dullness and suppression of breath sounds as to suggest pleural fluid. The heart may be displaced to the opposite side. In infants, intestinal peristaltic sounds are not usually heard over the involved side, as they commonly are in older patients.

The diagnosis can be made by plain radiography of the chest, which demonstrates a shift of the heart to the opposite side, the characteristic mottled appearance of air-filled loops of intestine in the involved hemithorax, and the relative absence of intestinal shadows in the abdomen (see Fig. 36, p. 1543). Ingestion of barium or other radiopaque medium is usually not necessary to establish the diagnosis; indeed, this should be avoided if possible. When the diagnosis is not clear on plain radiographs, barium may be required to differentiate congenital lung cyst or postpneumonic pneumatoceles. In the less frequent esophageal hiatal hernia and retrosternal hernia, which show little if any respiratory symptoms, radiographic studies of the gastrointestinal tract with contrast media are necessary.

The need for surgical repair is urgent; with conservative therapy 75 percent of these patients die before the end of the first month, with most deaths occurring within the first few days. Expectant treatment is dangerous because of the threat of sudden distension of the intrathoracic intestine, which may lead to acute respiratory distress and death. Except for small esophageal hiatal defects that are asymptomatic at the time, all congenital diaphragmatic hernias require immediate surgery as soon as the condition is recognized, regardless of the extent of the herniation and the condition of the child. Even in asymptomatic cases operation should be done early in order to avoid the serious complications of intestinal obstruction or incarceration.

Diaphragmatic Eventration

Less common than diaphragmatic hernia, diaphragmatic eventration is due to an abnormal thinness of the diaphragmatic muscle; in some instances there is complete absence of the muscle layer in a part of the diaphragm. This defect results in stretching of the diaphragm, allowing abdominal viscera to ascend into the hemithorax. Two forms are generally recognized. In true congenital eventration the phrenic nerve is normal; however, faradic stimulation does not cause contraction of the muscular elements of the diaphragm. Acquired eventration is due to unilateral phrenic nerve palsy resulting from birth injury to the brachial plexus; faradic stimulation in acquired cases causes contraction of the diaphragm.

If the diaphragm is markedly elevated and compresses the ipsilateral lung, there is acute respiratory embarrassment in the newborn period, with dyspnea, cyanosis, and shift of the mediastinal structures to the opposite side; the symptoms and radiographic findings may be indistinguishable from those of true diaphragmatic hernia. In less severe cases there may be a combination of respiratory and gastrointestinal symptoms in later life.

Treatment is usually not necessary in the mild case. When symptoms are present, surgical intervention is indicated. Plication operations are usually successful in repairing localized defects; in rare instances of extensive muscle deficiency the use of mersilene or other synthetic prosthesis has been successful.

Omphalocele and Gastroschisis

Omphalocele (hernia into the umbilical cord, exomphalos) is a rare and serious anomaly that consists of a herniation of abdominal viscera into the base of the umbilical cord. The covering of the protruding mass is thin and translucent, consisting of a fusion of the peritoneum and the amniotic membrane; it is not covered by skin as is the umbilical hernia (Fig. 15). The mass varies in size from a small protrusion to complete eventration in which nearly all the abdominal organs are outside the body. The defect in the abdominal wall may be quite small, measuring up to 2 cm in diameter, or it may be enormous, extending to the flanks. Malrotation of the portion of the alimentary tract supplied by the superior mesenteric artery is commonly associated.

The condition must be recognized at the time of delivery in order to avoid injury to the contained viscera when ligating the umbilical cord. Treatment consists of immediate coverage of the mass by sterile gauze moistened with warm saline, since the thin sac will soon dry and rupture, which may lead to infection and death. Operation is urgently required. Small omphaloceles are simple to repair; the sac is excised, its contents placed in the abdomen, and the defect in the abdominal wall closed. Large omphaloceles, especially those containing the liver, may be extremely difficult to treat. Furthermore, there is a relatively high incidence of associated anomalies, such as intestinal atresia, that may affect the prognosis. However, some of these large lesions may be successfully repaired by multiple operations. The first procedure consists of extensive mobilization of the skin of the abdominal wall in order to cover the mass and its sac, which must be kept intact. Silastic, mersilene, or a similar type of synthetic material should be used to cover the viscera if the sac has been ruptured. Later, when the peritoneal cavity has sufficiently enlarged to contain the viscera, the large defect of the abdominal wall (ventral hernia) should be corrected by a second operation.

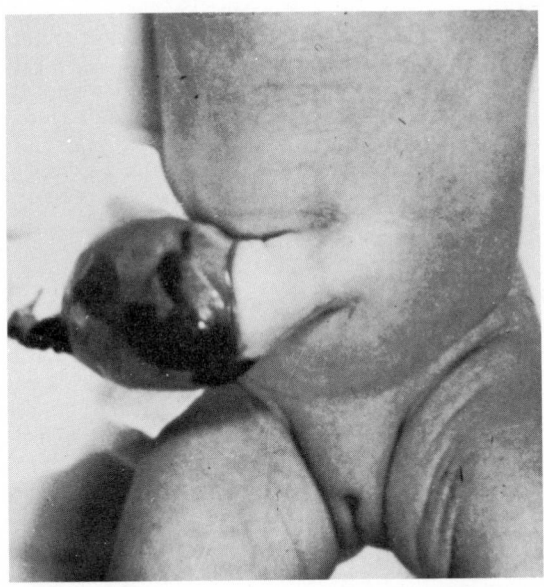

FIG. 15. Omphalocele or hernia into the base of the umbilical cord. The thin sac covering the viscera consists of a fusion of the peritoneum and amniotic membrane.

In giant omphaloceles, nonoperative treatment occasionally may be successful. Care must be taken to keep the sac intact. The application of 2 percent aqueous solution of Merthiolate to the sac several times a day may be beneficial. In time the herniated mass diminishes in size as the viscera gradually recede into the enlarging abdominal cavity, and epithelization of the sac occurs.

Gastroschisis is a defect in the abdominal wall similar to omphalocele, but occurring at a point other than the umbilicus. The umbilicus is normally inserted, the viscera protruding through an extraumbilical defect. There is no membranous covering of the exteriorized intestine, which is thickened, embedded in a mass of adhesions, and covered with a gelatinous exudate. The lesion may be successfully treated by covering the viscera with silastic or similar type of synthetic material that is sutured to the edges of the peritoneal and fascial

defect in the abdominal wall, creating a silo. Gradual and progressive manual compression of the protruding mass of viscera is accomplished over a period of days or weeks, and final closure of the abdominal wall defect is achieved when all the viscera have been reduced into the enlarging peritoneal cavity.

References

UMBILICAL HERNIA

Benson CD: Umbilical hernia. In Mustard WT, Ravitch MM, Synder Jr. WH (eds): Pediatric Surgery, 2nd ed. Chicago, Year Book, 1969, p 689

Halpern LJ: Spontaneous healing of umbilical hernia. JAMA 182:851, 1962

Sibley WL III, Lynn HB, Harris LE: Infantile umbilical hernia. Minn Surg 55:462, 1964

INGUINAL HERNIA AND HYDROCELE

Clatworthy HW Jr, Thompson AG: Incarcerated and strangulated inguinal hernia in infants: a preventable risk. JAMA 154:123, 1954

Fonkalsrud EW, deLorimier AA, Clatworthy HW Jr: Femoral and direct inguinal hernias in infants and children. JAMA 192:597, 1965

Kiesewetter WB, Parenzan L: When should hernia in the infant be treated bilaterally? JAMA 171:127, 1959

Potts WJ, Riker WL, Lewis JE: The treatment of inguinal hernia in infants and children. Ann Surg 132:566, 1950

Santulli TV, Shaw A: Inguinal hernia: infancy and childhood. JAMA 176:110, 1961

Snyder WH Jr, Greaney EM Jr: Inguinal hernias. In Mustard WT, Ravitch MM, Synder Jr. WH (eds): Pediatric Surgery, 2nd ed. Chicago, Year Book, 1969, p 692

Swenson O: Diagnosis and treatment of inguinal hernia. Pediatrics 34: 412, 1964

DIAPHRAGMATIC HERNIA

Allen MS, Thomson SA: Congenital diaphragmatic hernia in children under one year of age: a 24 year review. J Pediatr Surg 1:157, 1966

Baffes TF: Diaphragmatic hernia. In Mustard WT, Ravitch MM, Synder Jr. WH (eds): Pediatric Surgery, 2nd ed. Chicago, Year Book, 1969, p 342

Berdon WE, Baker DH, Amoury R: The role of pulmonary hypoplasia in the prognosis of newborn infants with diaphragmatic hernia and eventration. Am J Roentgenol Radium Ther Nucl Med 103:413, 1968

Boles ET, Schiller M, Weinberger M: An improved management of neonates with congenital diaphragmatic hernia. Arch Surg 103:344, 1971

Dibbins AW, Wiener ES: Mortality from neonatal diaphragmatic hernia. J Pediatr Surg 9:653, 1974

Jackson TM: Congenital diaphragmatic hernia. Arch Surg 95:102, 1967

Johnson DG, Deaner RM, Koop CE: Diaphragmatic hernia in infancy: factors affecting the mortality rate. Surgery 62:1082, 1967

Ravitch MM, Handleman JC: Lesions of the thoracic parieties in infants and children. Surg Clin North Am 32:1397, 1952

Snyder WH Jr, Greaney EM Jr: Congenital diaphragmatic hernia: 77 consecutive cases. Surgery 57:576, 1965

Thompson SA: Diaphragmatic hernia in infancy and childhood. Surg Clin North Am 34:997, 1954

DIAPHRAGMATIC EVENTRATION

Bisgard JD: Congenital eventration of the diaphragm. J Thorac Surg 16:484, 1947

Stauffer VG, Rickhaus PP: Acquired eventration of the diaphragm in the newborn. J Pediatr Surg 7:635, 1972

OMPHALOCELE AND GASTROSCHISIS

Lewis JE Jr, Kraeger RR, Davis RK: Gastroschisis: ten year review. Arch Surg 107:218, 1973

Mahour GH, Weitzman JJ, Rosencrantz JG: Omphaloceles and gastroschisis. Ann Surg 177:478, 1973

Moore TC, Stokes GE: Gastroschisis. Surgery 33:112, 1953

Rickham P: Rupture of exomphalos and gastroschisis. Arch Dis Child 38:138, 1963

Schuster SR: A new method for the staged repair of large omphaloceles. Surg Gynecol Obstet 125:837, 1967

Inflammatory Diseases

ESOPHAGUS

JOHN H. SEASHORE

Acute Esophagitis

Acute pharyngeal infections, which are so common in childhood, rarely involve the esophagus. Thrush occasionally extends into the esophagus, but the pharyngeal component produces more symptoms. Peptic esophagitis resulting from gastroesophageal reflux has been discussed under hiatal hernia (p. 1017). Acid-peptic damage to the esophageal mucosa may permit bacterial invasion of the esophageal wall, which contributes to the inflammatory response and eventual scarring.

Corrosive Esophagitis

Ingestion of poisonous substances is a major cause of morbidity and mortality in children, especially among toddlers, who are mobile, curious, and unable to read labels. Lye (sodium hydroxide) is the main constituent of most household drain cleaners, which are all too frequently used and stored without appreciation of their devastating potential. The liquefaction necrosis caused by lye and other strongly basic caustic agents produces deep and penetrating chemical burns following even brief contact. Full-thickness burns of the face, lips, and oral cavity are not uncommon. The esophagus is particularly susceptible to lye injury. Full-thickness burns may lead to esophageal perforation in the early postburn period. Circumferential burns involving the muscle layers frequently result in stricture as the injured tissue is replaced by scar tissue. Swallowed lye is rapidly neutralized in the stomach, but gastric necrosis and perforation may occur following ingestion of large quantities. Solid crystals of lye produce the most severe injury if they reach the esophagus. Liquid lye causes more diffuse and superficial injury, but is more likely to reach the esophagus and is quite capable of causing stricture or perforation. Liquid lye is more likely to be aspirated, thus leading to rapidly progressive laryngotracheal edema and respiratory distress.

All children who are known to have ingested lye or who are suspected of having ingested lye should be hospitalized. Induction of emesis and passage of a nasogastric tube are contraindicated, since the risk of aspiration or perforation is much greater than the chance of recovering unneutralized lye from the stomach. Burns of the face and lips should be cleansed and treated with topical antibiotic ointment. The child should be given nothing by mouth until the extent of injury has been determined; pain and spasm from oropharyngeal burns often cause the child to refuse oral fluids. Careful observation for respiratory distress is mandatory. Tracheostomy is occasionally necessary.

About one-third of children who ingest lye sustain some esophageal damage that can be identified only by direct visualization. Significant esophageal injury can occur even if oropharyngeal burns are not visible. Esophagoscopy should be performed within 24 hours of ingestion. If the esophagus is normal, the child may be discharged as soon as he is able to eat and drink adequately. If any esophageal burn is visualized, the esophagoscope should be immediately withdrawn to avoid perforating the friable esophageal wall. Corticosteroid treatment, instituted within 24 hours of injury and continued for 2 weeks, is considered effective in preventing esophageal stricture. Antibiotic therapy with ampicillin is recommended to prevent invasive bacterial infection if the esophagus appears damaged. Oral feedings should be started as soon as the patient can swallow. Esophageal perforation, manifested by sudden fever and chest pain, is a serious complication in the early postburn period. Early recognition and prompt closure of the perforation, in conjunction with mediastinal drainage, is essential. Even with vigorous treatment the mortality of esophageal perforation is significant.

A barium swallow should be obtained after 2 weeks of steroid therapy, or sooner if dysphagia develops. Treatment should be discontinued if the esophagus appears normal, but monthly follow-up is essential because strictures may develop late even after adequate steroid therapy. The appearance of esophageal stricture (Fig. 16) at this time or later is an indication for esophageal dilation. One or two dilations occasionally suffice, but generally a series of regular graded dilations is necessary to relieve the obstruction. Bypass of the esophagus with a segment of interposed colon may be required if the stricture persists despite adequate dilations.

Burns of the oral cavity usually heal without significant sequelae, but scarring from deep and extensive burns may necessitate complex reconstruction. Full-thickness facial burns may require grafting or late scar revision. Caustic agents other than lye are occasionally ingested. Esophageal injury from houshold bleach (sodium hypochlorite) is usually confined to the mucosa and rarely causes stricture. Concentrated acids produce coagulation necrosis, which limits the depth of esophageal burn. Gastric injury is much more common after ingestion of acids.

Paraesophageal Mediastinal Abscess

Mediastinal abscess is uncommon in childhood. Suppurative mediastinal lymphadenitis, extension of a retropharyngeal abscess, and tuberculosis of the thoracic vertebrae are occasionally causative factors. The most

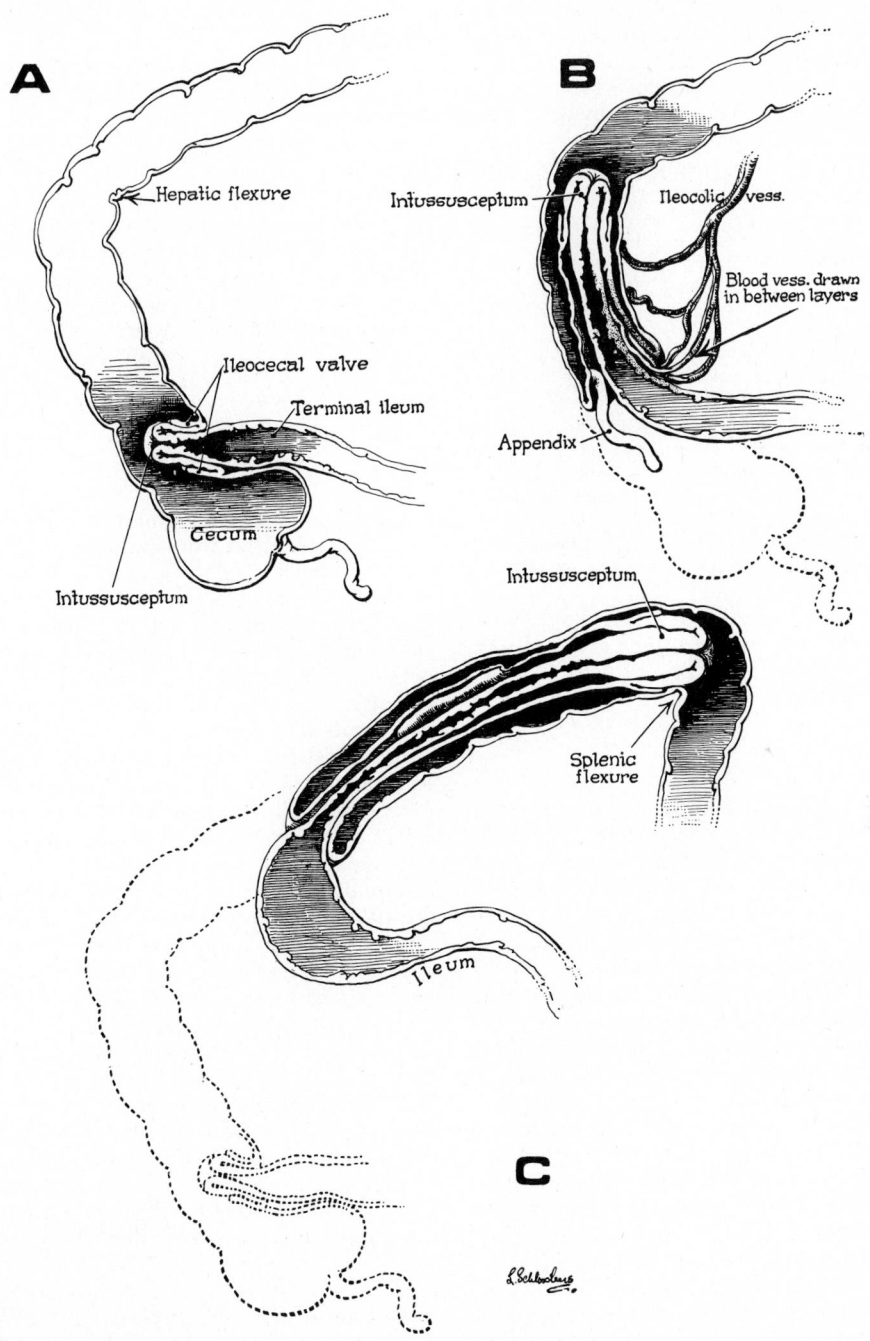

FIG. 16. Progress of intussusception. As the intussusception is passed along by peristaltic action, the appendix is drawn in between its layers (B), and the telescoping of the bowel pulls it away from its normal position (C).

common etiology of mediastinal abscess is esophageal perforation by a foreign body or by instrumentation. Spiking fever, chest pain, respiratory distress, and occasionally dysphagia are the predominant symptoms. Subcutaneous crepitus may be felt in the neck as air dissects upward from the mediastinum. The child is gravely ill. Radiography of the chest may demonstrate widening of the mediastinum or air in the mediastinum. Contrast radiography of the esophagus may demonstrate a site of perforation. Broad-spectrum intravenous antibiotic therapy and prompt surgical drainage of the mediastinum are essential if the patient is to survive. An upper mediastinal abscess can occasionally be drained through a low cervical incision. In most cases thoracotomy is necessary for adequate drainage, especially if the abscess has ruptured into the pleural cavity. Feeding gastrostomy is indicated if an esophagopleural fistula develops.

References

Haller JA, Andrews HG, White JJ, Tamer MA, Cleveland WW: Pathophysiology and management of acute corrosive burns of the esophagus. J Pediatr Surg 6:578, 1971

Knox WG, Scott JR, Zintel HA, Guthrie R, McCabe RE: Bouginage and steroids used singly or in combination in experimental corrosive esophagitis. Ann Surg 166:930, 1967

Leape LL, Ashcraft KW, Scarpelli DG, Holder TM: Hazard to health—liquid lye. N Engl J Med 284:578, 1971

Middelkamp JN, Ferguson TB, Roper CL, Hoffman FD: The management and problems of caustic burns in children. J Thorac Cardiovasc Surg 57:341, 1969

STOMACH
THOMAS V. SANTULLI

Acute Gastritis

Inflammatory lesions of the stomach are comparatively uncommon in early life. They may occur in severe gastroenteritis, in parenteral infections, or from the introduction of irritant drugs or poisons. In contrast to the situation in adults, hyperacidity is rarely the cause.

Corrosive gastritis usually results from ingestion of caustic acids. Less frequently, lye, ammonia, carbolic acid, hypochlorite solutions (Clorox), and other basic corrosives are responsible. Some cases have been caused by an excessively strong solution of calcium chloride. The lesions in the stomach are much influenced by the quantity and concentration of the irritant and by the quantity of food in the stomach. Strong acids usually act more intensely in the pharynx and esophagus, since spasms of the muscles of these parts often prevent the agent from reaching the stomach. The gastric lesions may affect the mucous membrane diffusely or may produce irregular ulcerations, especially along the greater curvature. Perforation may occur. In severe cases death takes place within a few hours; dark ragged ulcers are found, with the surrounding mucosa being intensely congested and with extravasations in places. If death is delayed there is intense

inflammation, often with the production of a pseudomembrane. Recovery may result in a cicatricial contraction of the stomach with partial obstruction.

The immediate symptoms are intense pain, a sense of constriction in the throat, and vomiting, sometimes of blood. The effects of the caustic may be seen in the mouth. Collapse follows rapidly. If the patient survives, acute gastritis persists for some time, often associated with esophagitis and enteritis. Dehydration may be a serious problem.

Treatment consists of early gastric lavage. However, if 1 hour or more has elapsed, lavage is quite useless, and therapy should be confined to the treatment of pain and shock and the prevention of esophageal stricture, especially after the swallowing of lye (p. 1038).

Membranous gastritis is occasionally found in association with diphtheria, bacillary dysentery, or streptococcal infections of the pharynx. *Candida* infection of the mouth may extend down the esophagus and involve the gastric muscosa. These lesions are usually first detected at post-mortem examination.

PEPTIC ULCER
MERVIN SILVERBERG

Peptic ulcers in infants and children are reported with variable frequencies from different parts of the United States. In most large pediatric centers the condition is viewed as relatively uncommon. It has been argued that many cases are missed because of justifiable reluctance to subject children to radiographic studies. About 2 percent of adults with peptic ulcer are reported to have had symptoms since childhood. Pain attributed to peptic ulceration is usually in the epigastrium, but it is often indistinguishable from functional abdominal pain, which is ubiquitous in children. The main diagnostic aid is a careful radiographic study to demonstrate an ulcer crater or deformity due to scarring. Gastric ulcers are best seen with small amounts of barium and proper positioning of the patient, so that all stomach regions are visualized in profile and en face. Distension of the duodenal bulb is essential to obtaining information on duodenal ulcers. Hypotonic radiographic studies may be necessary using intramuscular propantheline (15 to 30 mg). Where there is a high index of suspicion but a single negative study, radiographic examination should be repeated. It is debated whether presumptive or secondary radiographic features such as spasm and thickened folds of the duodenum are of value, particularly in the apprehensive child. Gastric acid studies in children, including the augmented histamine stimulation test, show an unusually broad range of normal values without consistently significant differences from ulcer patients.

CLASSIFICATION. Three varieties of peptic ulcer disease are recognized: *Acute infantile* and *secondary ulcers* are most common in the preschool child. Hemorrhage and perforation with peritonitis may be presenting manifestations. Lesions occur with equal frequency in the stomach and duodenum. The newborn infant is particularly vulnerable in the first 48 hours of life. This may be the result of a combination of stress and hypoxia. The increased gastric acidity and parietal cell mass normally observed during this early period probably play a contributing role. Secondary ulcers occur with greater frequency in children than in adults. Ulcers of the stomach or duodenum occur in association with severe infections, malignant disease, burns (Curling's ulcer), neurologic disorders (Rokitansky-Cushing ulcer), and ulcerogenic drugs such as corticosteroids. Other disorders associated with peptic ulcers in greater numbers than would be expected by chance are cirrhosis of the liver, chronic pulmonary disease, hypoglycemia, and congenital pyloric stenosis. These children frequently present with severe gastrointestinal bleeding or perforation, and the morbidity is compounded by the underlying illness.

Adult type or *chronic ulcers* may occur at any age between infancy and late adolescence. The major presenting manifestions vary with the age of the child. Many younger children complain more of periumbilical than of epigastric pain, and the relationship of symptoms to the ingestion of food is variable. Pain is often aggravated by food intake and is frequently accompanied by vomiting, in contrast to the characteristic relief of pain reported by adults with ulcer when they eat. Pyloric canal ulcers are rare, but when they occur vomiting may be particularly severe and prolonged due to pylorospasm. Adolescents more often report symptoms like those of adults; their pain is localized to the epigastrium and is usually relieved with food intake. There is a high incidence of peptic ulcers among teenage heroin users (p. 810).

The ulcer is located in the duodenum in 90 percent of these cases, the posterior wall of the bulb being a particular site of predilection. The male-to-female ratio for incidence is approximately 1.5:1. About 20 to 30 percent of children experience painless and occult bleeding leading to iron-deficiency anemia; melena and hematemesis are occasionally encountered. Significant or characteristic emotional problems are reported in 25 to 50 percent of these children, who are often described as anxious, intense, and introverted. School phobias are among the most common of the psychosocial problems in these patients. A family history of ulcer diathesis is found in at least 25 percent of cases.

Most children respond well to an antiulcer regimen and are free of complaints within 3 months. However, when followed for periods exceeding 1 year, as many as 50 percent are reported to show persistent complaints or to develop recurrences during later childhood or adolescence, with a typical chronic history of episodic or intractable discomfort, bleeding, or obstruction. Although the incidence of complications in children appears to be high, it is more likely due to delayed diagnosis.

Zollinger-Ellison syndrome and related disorders: Severe peptic ulcer disease often is associated with non-beta-cell islet adenomas secreting a gastrinlike material measured in serum or plasma by radioimmunoassay. Blood gastrin levels usually exceed 300 pg/ml, whereas in other varieties of peptic ulcer disease values are below 200 pg/ml. In patients with equivocal serum gastrin elevation, a calcium challenge or infusion test will usually produce diagnostic levels of serum gastrin and increased acid secretion. Patients with this type of peptic ulcer do not have hyperinsulinemia. Most of them demonstrate gastric hypersecretion of such magnitude that histamine augmentation does not significantly increase the basal acid output. In patients with other varieties of peptic ulcer disease, basal gastric acid per hour is usually less than 60 percent of the amount secreted after a maximal dose of histamine or histalog.

The ulcers in this syndrome are usually single and large; they are located in the duodenum and are associated with intractable and persistent symptoms usually resistant to amelioration by medical therapy. They form a high proportion of multiple and postbulbar ulcers. Severe watery diarrhea and malabsorption of fat and vitamin B_{12} due to excessive gastric secretions may complicate the already difficult course for these patients.

A number of related syndromes have been described. Multiple endocrine adenomas involving the parathyroid, pancreatic islets and pituitary glands may be associated with multifocal peptic ulcers resistant to medical therapy (Wermer's syndrome). These adenomas may be hormonally active in various combinations. Peptic ulcer disease has also been associated with syndromes involving a severe choleralike illness and profound hypokalemia, islet cell tumors of the pancreas that secrete multiple unrelated hormones, islet cell hyperplasia, or hyperparathyroidism.

PATHOGENESIS. The pathogenesis of peptic ulcer involving either stomach or duodenum is controversial. It is believed that abnormal levels of gastric acid and pepsin in various combinations, in addition to locally impaired tissue resistance, may explain the development of a focal lesion rather than diffuse ulceration. Hereditary factors play a role, and there is considerable evidence to suggest that patients with both gastric and duodenal ulcers have higher levels of anxiety and greater sensitivity to stress than control subjects. Increased acid-pepsin appears to be related in part to hypergastrinemia, increased acid secretion, and defective acid disposal by the duodenum. It is generally believed that mucosal resistance deficiency is more important in gastric ulcers and acid-pepsin excess is more important in duodenal lesions. Decreased mucosal resistance is associated with one or more of the following: local defects of the mucosa and muscular anatomy of the stomach and duodenum, derangements in mucosal blood flow, defects in mucus production, abnormalities in rate of cell renewal, and preexisting inflammatory disease of the stomach and duodenal mucosa.

Acute infantile and secondary ulcers seem to be related to mucosal ischemia, the presence of acid-pepsin, and disruption of the gastric mucosal barrier, which leads to increased retrodiffusion of hydrogen ion. Bile reflux into the stomach may further aggravate the retrodiffusion of hydrogen ion and possibly produce mucosal ischemia itself. Additionally, some of these patients have been shown to have high circulating serum gastrin levels.

THERAPY. Therapeutic measures vary according to the type of ulcer. Acute ulcer manifestations in older children respond best to regular frequent neutralization of gastric acidity by foods and antacids. Initially, dietary and antacid regimens should be introduced on an hourly basis using 10–20 ml of antacid (such as Maalox®) alternating with 1 to 3 ounces of a milk–cream mixture. The intervals should be increased as the symptoms improve, and a normal unrestricted diet, except for caffeine, may be introduced once the patient becomes asymptomatic. The use of frequent snacks is controversial. However, bedtime snacks are best avoided, since they may delay return to the basal secretory state and are associated with high nocturnal acidity. Moderately large amounts of antacid (5–20 ml) should be given prophylactically during the subsequent 2 to 3 months. They are used most effectively 1 hour after a meal, when there is maximal acid production and when they will be retained the longest in the stomach. A second dose 3 hours after the meal may be of some value. A large bedtime dose is important to reduce acidity overnight. Liquid antacids are usually more effective neutralizers, although there is a wide range of effectiveness. Postcibal anticholinergic agents such as propantheline (1.5 mg/kg/24 hours) may be prescribed three times a day and at bedtime during the symptomatic period of therapy. The optimal effective dose appears to be near the level at which side effects such as dryness of the mouth and photophobia are produced. These should be continued at bedtime for at least 1 year, and 5–20 ml of antacids should be prescribed whenever the ulcer complaints recur. Severe bleeding should be treated with blood volume replacement, cold saline gastric lavages, and nasogastric suction. In 20 percent of cases with hematemesis the gastric aspirate will be negative for blood. In these cases flexible fiberoptic endoscopy has been very useful in demonstrating the ulcer and source of bleeding before any radiographic studies are necessary. Endoscopy has also been useful in confirming the diagnosis of peptic ulcer when all other studies have been negative or equivocal.

Surgical procedures have been restricted to the emergency complications of perforation, severe hemorrhage, and obstruction. That the child with chronic complaints would benefit from earlier surgical intervention has been suggested by some authors, but this remains to be proved. Vagotomy and pyloroplasty or antrectomy give best results in both emergency and elective surgery. Patients with ulcerogenic tumor syndromes must be explored and the tumor or tumors removed. Preoperative arteriography occasionally may help to identify the tumor site. Even when this is practical, but especially if such a tumor is difficult to locate or has metastasized, or in cases where islet tissue is diffusely involved, total gastrectomy has been recommended as the operation of choice for definitive treatment of the ulcer. Infants and children with resected stomachs have been shown to thrive under careful dietary management.

References

Baida M, McIntyre JA, Dietel M: Peptic ulcer in children and adolescents. Arch Surg 99:15, 1966

Classen M: Endoscopy in benign peptic ulcer. Clin Gastroenterol 2:315, 1973

Collins DL, Black JH, Mullinger MM: Gastrectomy in early childhood. Am J Dis Child 109:149, 1965

Habbick BF, Melrose AG, Grant JC: Duodenal ulcer in childhood: a study of predisposing factors. Arch Dis Child 43:23, 1968

Jackson RH, Blair EL, Dawson PJ, Reed JD, Watts WPT: Gastrin activity of tumour tissue in a child with the Zollinger-Ellison syndrome. Lancet 2:908, 1963

Lucas C, Benson CD: Chronic bleeding duodenal ulcer in childhood managed by hemigastrectomy and vagotomy. Surgery 61:478, 1967

Michener WM, Kennedy RLJ, DuShane JW: Duodenal ulcer in childhood. Am J Dis Child 99:135, 1960

Muggia A, Spiro HM: Childhood peptic ulcer. Gastroenterology 37:715, 1959

Nuss D, Lynn HB: Peptic ulceration in childhood. Surg Clin North Am 51:945, 1971

Raffensperger JG, Condon JB, Greengard J: Complications of gastric and duodenal ulcers in infancy and childhood. Surg Gynecol Obstet 123:1269, 1966

Ravitch MM, Duremdes GD: Operative treatment of chronic duodenal ulcer in childhood. Ann Surg 171:641, 1970

Robb JDA, Thomas PS, Orszulok J, Odling-Smee GW: Duodenal ulcer in children. Arch Dis Child 47:688, 1972

Rosenlund ML: The Zollinger-Ellison syndrome in children. A review. Am J Med Sci 254:884, 1967

Schwartz DL, White JJ, Saulsbury F, Heller JA Jr: Gastrin response to calcium infusion: an aid to the improved diagnosis of Zollinger-Ellison syndrome in children. Pediatrics 54:599, 1974

Singleton EB, Faykus MH: Incidence of peptic ulcer as determined by radiological examinations in the pediatric age group. J Pediatr 65:858, 1964

Tudor RB: Peptic ulceration in childhood. Pediatr Clin North Am 14:109, 1967

Wilson SD, Ellison EH: Total gastric resection in children with the Zollinger-Ellison syndrome. Arch Surg 91:165, 1965

PANCREATITIS

MURRAY DAVIDSON

Probably the most common form of acute pancreatitis in children is associated with mumps. Severe epigastric pain, vomiting, and diarrhea develop several days after the parotid swellings and may persist for about a week. Trauma to the abdomen is the next most common cause, accounting for about 30 percent of the cases. Sadly, the increasing incidence of child battering is making this a more prominent antecendent to the development of pancreatitis in small children. Blunt trauma that is often forgotten by the time the symptoms of pancreatitis appear is thought to cause injury as a result of a shock wave traveling through the abdomen and compressing the fixed retroperitoneal gland. Small hemorrhages and destruction of acinar tissue lead to release and activation of proteolytic enzymes that extend the destructive phenomenon.

Acute pancreatitis and chronic relapsing pancreatitis

in childhood may be associated with autosomal dominant patterns of transmission. Recurrent pancreatitis has been observed in association with familial hyperlipemia and with hyperparathyroidism. Rarely, the disease may be associated with a familial pattern of amino-aciduria, specifically lysinuria and cystinuria.

Acute hemorrhagic pancreatitis also occurs, often without clear antecedent causes. It may be a complication of glucocorticoid therapy, and children on such therapy may suddenly develop severe abdominal pain, nausea, vomiting, abdominal distension, possibly complicated by signs of shock. Hypocalcemia, hyperglycemia, and elevation of serum amylase with leukocytosis usually are evident after a number of days. The prognosis is grave. Ascites, acute vascular collapse, and renal failure are the complications that precede death.

Because the pain of pancreatitis may vary from mild to very severe and because abdominal pain is so common in children, the diagnosis is often overlooked if it is not incapacitating. Characteristically the pain is located near the midepigastrium, and because of the retroperitoneal location of the pancreas it tends to bore directly through to the back. As the disease progresses the pain may become generalized and involve the entire abdomen. Nausea and repeated vomiting are the next most common symptoms. Ileus and abdominal distension frequently accompany pancreatitis, probably as a reaction to the swelling of the pancreas and irritation of the adjacent peritoneum. However, fluid and electrolyte shifts associated with the hypovolemia of the disease may also play a role. Fever, which is present in 60 percent of patients with acute pancreatitis, is rare in the chronic form. Children with acute pancreatitis may develop hypovolemia, resulting in shock.

Pseudocyst formation secondary to a leak of pancreatic fluid into the lesser sac of the omentum is a frequent complication of pancreatitis. These non-epithelial-lined cavities contain plasma, blood, pancreatic products, and inflammatory exudate. They vary in size from very small to huge. They are presumably due to obstruction of outflow from the acini, which are secreting excessive quantities of pancreatic fluid during the disease. The abdomen becomes painfully distended, and a tumor may be palpable in the left upper quadrant.

A small amount of ascites is common in pancreatitis; it results from exudation and transudation of fluid from the pancreas and serous surface. However, pleural effusions are also common, especially in the left thorax. These effusion tend to have high concentrations of amylase and lipase. Mild jaundice may occur due to compression of the common duct as a result of edema and inflammation of the head of the pancreas, which it closely approximates or through which it passes.

DIAGNOSIS.   The patient with acute pancreatitis often appears acutely ill, restless, and uncomfortable. The discomfort is usually aggravated in the recumbent position and somewhat relieved in the sitting position, with trunk flexed and arms pressed against the abdomen. The pain is continuous and is not colicky and rarely changes in pattern. Mild icterus may be present.

If shock is a factor the patient may be cold, clammy, and possibly confused. Because of ileus the abdomen is often distended and bowel sounds are decreased. Patients with pulmonary complications may have restricted thoracic expansion. Severe hypocalcemia may be manifested by a positive Chvostek sign that may progress to frank convulsions.

Laboratory confirmation of pancreatitis rests primarily on determination of serum amylase, which is not universally reliable. Amylase levels may return to normal 5 to 7 days following the initial rise, despite continuing disease. The diagnosis of acute pancreatitis complicating mumps is especially difficult, since serum amylase levels are elevated from parotitis alone. Serum lipase determinations should also be obtained.

A diagnostic paracentesis or thoracentesis is useful in the presence of suspected pancreatitis associated with ascites and/or pleural effusion. The fluid may or may not be hemorrhagic, but in the presence of pancreatitis it usually contains high concentrations of amylase and lipase, even with normal serum levels of these enzymes. Hypocalcemia is common in acute pancreatitis; in severe cases the values may be below 7.0 mg/100 ml.

The differential diagnosis is much easier in children than in adults because disorders such as gall bladder disease, penetrating or perforated peptic ulcers, carcinoma of the pancreas, and angina pectoris are not included for consideration. However, a high index of suspicion is important, since abdominal pain in children is common and generally is not suspected of being associated with pancreatitis. In the presence of pleural effusion, other causes of pneumonia must be differentiated.

TREATMENT.   The medical therapy of acute pancreatitis is largely empiric and is based on the theoretical objective of putting the gland to rest. Gastric suction limits entry of acid gastric contents into the small intestine, decreases release of secretin and cholecystokinin, and reduces air passage into the intestine, thus preventing aggravation of the existing ileus. The efficacy of anticholinergic drugs such as atropine and propantheline bromide, which normally reduce basal pancreatic secretion, has not been proved in pancreatitis. Although they lower gastric acidity, they also increase ileus and may predispose to tachycardia and arrhythmias, which should be avoided among patients with signs of shock. If narcotics are necessary to relieve pain, these agents should be very cautiously prescribed. Since narcotics tend to elevate serum amylase, blood volume must be maintained to combat hypovolemia and shock. Fever is frequent, but proved bacterial infections are uncommon. A combination of ampicillin and kanamycin is generally recommended despite the lack of controlled evidence of efficacy.

If a large pseudocyst is discovered, surgical intervention is not necessarily indicated, since many either spontaneously reabsorb with time or spontaneously rupture into the intestinal tract. A delay of approximately 4 weeks is recommended after discovery of the pseudocyst to allow for spontaneous resolution or for the wall of the cyst to ripen and provide a tissue that will retain sutures and reduce fistula formation if operation is required. The preferred surgical technique consists of mobilization of the pseudocyst followed by marsupialization into the stomach or upper small intestine. The latter will depend on size, location, and the surgeon's judgment with respect to the best placement of the fistula to maintain adequate drainage and to prevent reaccumulation.

References

Collet RW, Kennedy RLJ: Chronic relapsing pancreatitis associated with hyperlipemia in an eight-year-old boy. Proc Mayo Clin 23:158, 1948

Davidson P, Costanza D, Swieconek JA, Harris JB: Hereditary pancreatitis: a kindred without gross aminoaciduria. Ann Intern Med 68:88, 1968

McElroy R, Christiansen PA: Hereditary pancreatitis in a kinship associated with portal vein thrombosis. Am J Med 52:228, 1972

Sarsfield JK, Davies JM: Negative sweat tests and cystic fibrosis. Arch Dis Child 6:463, 1975

Sibert JR: Pancreatitis in children: a study in the north of England. Arch Dis Child 6:443, 1975

INTESTINES
MARK M. RAVITCH

Appendicitis

Acute appendicitis is the most common lesion requiring laparotomy in children. It occurs in all age groups. It is rare in young infants, although it has been reported in the first few days of life. Males are more frequently affected than females in a ratio of more than 2 to 1.

ETIOLOGY AND PATHOLOGY. The underlying cause of acute appendicitis is usually obscure. In occasional instances acute enteritis seems to merge into appendicitis. This sequence is particularly dangerous in mass outbreaks in schools and summer camps, where an enteritis that does not clear up may go on to perforation before the appendicitis is recognized. An acute upper respiratory infection may precede an attack of appendicitis. In a number of cases a fecalith or a worm plays an obvious role by obstructing the lumen of the appendix, distending the appendix and impairing its blood supply. The anatomic structure of the appendix (a long narrow intestinal diverticulum supplied by a single artery) explains its predisposition to disease. Mucosal inflammation produces edema and resultant obstruction of the lumen. Distension follows, the intraluminal tension increases, and there is interference with the blood supply. Ulceration, infection, and gangrene result. At times the lumen may remain free of obstruction, and instances of spontaneous recovery from appendicitis believed to be frequent are probably attributable to the absence of obstruction in those cases. In infants, necrosis and perforation are more common than in older children. This difference is probably accounted for by the more delicate structure of the appendiceal wall in younger children, as well as by infants' lower resistance to infection in general. The relatively smaller omentum of the infant increases the seriousness of perforation.

SYMPTOMS. Typically, the succession and array of symptoms of appendicitis include anorexia, cramplike abdominal pain beginning in the epigastrium and migrating to the right lower quadrant, vomiting, localized pain and tenderness, and muscular rigidity. However, in a great many instances, particularly in children under 5 years of age, the symptoms are atypical or difficult to elicit. Abdominal pain is probably the most invariable symptom. The early generalized cramplike pain is frequently dismissed in children as mere colic. Vomiting is a very common early sign. Either constipation or diarrhea may be present. If the appendix is long enough to dip down into the pelvis, there may be pain on urination, usually at the end of micturition when the bladder has contracted, pulling away from the inflamed tissues.

Abdominal palpation in an infant or child with an acute abdominal disorder calls for the exercise of the greatest gentleness and patience. The response of a child to a single abdominal palpation is not to be trusted; often repeated and very gentle examination is required until the child is quiet. Muscle spasm is frequently absent or undetectable in infants. Rebound tenderness is an important sign particularly useful in infants. Evidences of rebound tenderness in an infant are the sudden cry or grimace when the hand is released and an involuntary flexion of the right thigh. Rectal examination is of the greatest importance. After the finger has been fully introduced, the child should be allowed to settle down before manipulation is begun. There may be merely tenderness localized in the right side or a bogginess in the cul-de-sac, suggesting a diffuse peritonitis with exudation of a considerable quantity of pus; palpation of a mass may reveal the presence of an appendiceal abscess. Abdominal distension is a late sign and indicates peritonitis rather than appendicitis. Fever is more likely to be present and to be higher than in adults, but its presence is chiefly a nonspecific indication of an acute infectious process. The leukocyte count tends to be elevated, but it is neither reliable nor consistent. The finding of leukocytosis merely indicates that some acute inflammatory process must be present and that the child should not be dismissed until its source is discovered. It is not at all rare for an infant or child with an illness allegedly of 1 or 2 days' duration to be first seen with a well-walled-off appendiceal abscess obviously of greater duration.

Appendicitis may be confounded with colic or indigestion, and, in infants, with intussusception. Differentiation from an acute gastrointestinal upset is always difficult and may even be impossible. In gastrointestinal upsets the pain is likely to be less severe, while repeated vomiting and diarrhea are likely to be prominent. The possibility of a strangulated inguinal hernia should always be considered in infants with abdominal pain and vomiting. In older children an iliac adenitis that drains a trivial infection of the foot may very closely mimic appendicitis. In infants with abdominal pain and tenderness, radiologic examination of the chest is a wise diagnostic measure. Pneumonia may be difficult to differentiate from appendicitis, and the abdominal signs may closely resemble those of appendicitis at a time when the pulmonary physical signs are still obscure. Fever, leukocytosis, and prostration all tend to be more marked with pneumonia than with appendicitis, and manifestations of pulmonary disease such as dyspnea and dilation of the alae nasi are helpful. However, we have seen an instance in which a child in the hospital with veritable right-sided lobar pneumonia developed appendicitis that was permitted to go on to abscess formation before this diagnosis was made. The abdominal pain that accompanies acute rheumatic fever may frequently precede the appearance of joint pains and carditis and is readily confused with appendicitis. The crises of sickle cell anemia may simulate appendicitis. The condition called mesenteric adenitis (p. 1045- 6) closely resembles appendicitis clinically. The so-called Brenneman syndrome is a frequent source of diagnostic difficulty. In this condition patients with acute upper respiratory infections, particularly tonsillitis, develop abdominal pain, tenderness, muscular rigidity, and even rebound tenderness of such a degree as to overshadow the primary pharyngeal infection, which may not be discovered until after a negative abdominal exploration. Primary bacterial peritonitis (p. 1052) may be confused with appendicitis. In these conditions high fever and prostration are likely to be present, and diarrhea is common. If there is any likelihood that one of these conditions is present, as in a child with nephrosis or with vaginal discharge, an attempt should be made to establish the diagnosis by aspiration of pus from the peritoneal cavity with a short-beveled needle. If the diagnosis of a primary peritonitis can thus be established by a smear showing only pneumococci or only gonococci, operation is unnecessary, and the treatment may be left to antibiotics. If mixed or gram-negative organisms are found, it is good evidence of peritonitis of perforative origin, requiring operation. A large number of other abdominal conditions, such as torsion of an ovarian or mesenteric cyst, pyelitis, and the onset of acute nephritis, may be confused with appendicitis. The acute exanthematic diseases are occasionally ushered in by abdominal pain indistinguishable from that of appendicitis, and at times appendicitis occurs in association with such diseases. Abdominal allergy and abdominal epilepsy are occasionally responsible for acute attacks of pain.

The fundamental point in the differential diagnosis is as follows: while every attempt should be made to arrive at an accurate diagnosis, the clinical picture of appendicitis is so varied and uncertain that more harm will result from too rigid adherence to fixed diagnostic criteria than from ready resort to operation. The safest approach is to operate at once whenever there is a reasonable possibility that a child may have appendicitis. *If a child has abdominal tenderness and if his history and physical examination do not disclose features incompatible with appendicitis, operation should be performed.* The mortality from appendectomy, if the appendix is normal, or inflamed but unruptured, is almost nil. Furthermore, since appendicitis does not spare children with known rheumatic fever, sickle cell anemia, or other acute or chronic

diseases, the removal of a normal appendix in general will do little harm to such a patient. If two of every three unruptured appendices removed are acutely inflamed, one may probably be satisfied. Hypercritical attempts at diagnostic accuracy before resort to operation invite perforation of the appendix and grave complications or death.

As long as the patient remains a diagnostic problem opiates are to be avoided for fear of obscuring surgical signs. Cathartics should never be given to patients with abdominal pain. A gentle enema will frequently relieve colonic distension, which may mimic appendicitis. In remote areas where operation is impossible, penicillin in large doses, as shown by war experience, may tide the patient over. Apart from such instances, one should operate whenever the diagnosis of appendicitis is made. If children are brought in late in the disease suffering from dehydration and loss of fluids, 2 or 3 hours before operation may profitably be spent alleviating the intestinal distension, restoring fluid balance parenterally, and administering antibiotics if perforation is suspected.

In the postoperative treatment of patients with perforated appendices, the mortality, morbidity, and length of hospitalization have been greatly lowered by the use of antibiotics, indwelling intestinal tubes, and large transfusions of blood plasma to replace the protein-rich fluids that are lost into the lumen of the intestine, the wall of the intestine, and the peritoneal cavity. These measures should be employed prophylactically in such patients without waiting for paralytic ileus, hemoconcentration, and electrolyte imbalance.

After a simple appendectomy through a McBurney incision, the patient may be permitted unrestricted activity as soon as he wishes after recovering from anesthesia. The child may eat a normal diet as soon as peristalsis reappears. Prophylactic appendectomy is not advised as a routine measure, but it has been recommended for children who are about to be taken to remote areas for a protracted stay.

Although untreated appendicitis characteristically is a recurrent disease, we do not recognize a condition in which the appendix is chronically mildly inflamed and produces vague symptoms and "a run-down condition." When a child has appendicitis he either recovers spontaneously or gets worse. If he recovers spontaneously the appendix causes no symptoms until the next acute attack.

Mesenteric Adenitis

The name mesenteric adenitis is given to a condition that produces an acute illness characterized by abdominal pain, nausea, and vomiting, often in association with an upper respiratory infection. The pain may be severe, but the patient is generally not particularly ill. Pain and tenderness are usually more diffuse than in appendicitis, while rebound tenderness and muscle spasm are likely to be absent. Fever and leukocytosis are common. At operation the appendix is found to be normal; the mesenteric lymph nodes at the ileocecal junction and along the terminal ileum are enlarged and often appear succulent, with occasional edema of the mesentery and a little clear, free fluid. On section the nodes show a nonspecific hyperplasia. Cultures for viruses and pathogenic bacteria have been reported to be negative or have yielded so wide a variety of organisms as to lose significance. Mesenteric adenitis is not a well-defined entity; no specific etiology or pathognomonic lesion has been demonstrated, and the symptoms are nonspecific. Moreover, autopsies on children dying of any cause, including violent trauma, frequently show large mesenteric lymph nodes.

References

Aird I: Acute non-specific mesenteric lymphadenitis. Br Med J 2:680, 1945

Benson CD, Coury JJ Jr, Hagge DR: Acute appendicitis in infants; a 15-year study. Arch Surg 64:561, 1952

Brenneman J: The abdominal pain of throat infections. Am J Dis Child 22:493, 1921

———— Abdominal pain in children. JAMA 127:691, 1945

Firor HV, et al: Perforating appendicitis in infants. Surgery 56:581, 1964

Hoefer PFA, Cohen SM, Greeley DM: Paroxysmal abdominal pain, an epileptic equivalent. Trans Am Neurol Assoc 75:183, 1950

Hurwitt ES: Acute appendicitis occurring during the course of other diseases. N Engl J Med 236:20, 1947

Longino LA, Holder TM, Gross RE: Appendicitis in childhood; a study of 1,358 cases. Pediatrics 22:238, 1958

Minervini F, Santulli TV: Acute appendicitis in early childhood. J Pediatr 52:324, 1958

Postlethwait RW, Campbell FH: Acute mesenteric lymphadenitis. Arch Surg 59:92, 1949

Shaw EB: Appendicitis in childhood. Pediatrics 22:235, 1958

Stanley-Brown EG: Acute appendicitis during the first five years of life. Am J Dis Child 108:1348, 1964

REGIONAL ENTERITIS

MERVIN SILVERBERG AND MURRAY DAVIDSON

Regional enteritis is a chronic nonspecific enteritis characterized by one or more combinations of noncaseating granulomata, necrotizing or cicatrizing inflammation, and external or internal strictures and fistulas. The inflammatory process usually involves all layers of the gut wall, often including the subtending mesentery and regional lymph nodes. Although there are many earlier references in the literature, the full importance of the disease was not recognized until Crohn, Ginzburg, and Oppenheimer in 1932 described 14 pateints in whom the lesion was limited to the ileum; hence their term terminal ileitis, referring to its principal location in over 80 percent of cases. Since that time the disease process has been shown to involve all areas of the gastrointestinal tract, continuously or serially, from esophagus to anus. When confined to the colon alone the condition may be difficult to distinguish from chronic ulcerative colitis, and it is estimated that 20 to 30 percent of all patients with chronic inflammatory disease of the colon suffer from regional enteritis. From 10 to 15 percent of patients in all large adult series are reported to have onset of disease below the age of 15 years, and about half experience onset before 21 years

of age. At the other extremes, some cases are reported to start in the neonatal period.

PATHOGENESIS. Regional enteritis is at present understood only by its clinical and pathologic features. No known pathogenesis has been defined, and no experimental animal model has been found. Indeed, there is no proof that regional enteritis may not have multiple etiologies. There is evidence that it may be a disease of altered immunologic reactivity, occurring at least in part on a hereditary polygenic basis. A transmissible agent may be involved, but it is none of the known bacterial, viral, or mycotic organisms. In 5 to 10 percent of cases a family history of chronic inflammatory disease of the bowel is reported. A slight predominance in males has been noted among children, and in the United States it is more common in Jews and less common blacks and Hispanics than in the general white population. It also occurs with greater frequency than expected in association with ulcerative colitis, ankylosing spondylitis, and atopic disorders, both in the individual and in the family. Despite many reports to the contrary, it is unlikely that it is closely related to sarcoidosis.

The onset is abrupt in less than 10 percent of children, in whom the pathology is restricted to the terminal ileum, and it simulates acute appendicits or intestinal obstruction. These patients are usually diagnosed at laparotomy, half of them undergoing an uneventful and apparently permanent recovery. The remainder develop the clinical picture of chronic regional enteritis, frequently involving other areas of the intestine, within weeks to months of the surgery. Although certain of the clinical manifestations vary with the anatomic site and extent of involvement, abdominal pain is the rule. Children most commonly also present with chronic constitutional complaints, ie, failure to thrive, persistent or recurrent fevers, weight loss, and anorexia. The type of anemia encountered with chronic inflammations, in which both serum iron concentration and total iron binding capacity are low, is found in most cases and occasionally may be the presenting problem. Diarrhea, although not infrequent, is usually intermittent and is rarely explosive, bloody, or accompanied by steatorrhea. Patients often are troubled by borborygmi, bloating, and flatulence.

Perianal or perirectal abscesses and fistulae are somewhat less frequent than in adults, but when they occur these lesions may antedate any other systemic or abdominal complaints. Digital clubbing, aphthous stomatitis, iritis, erythema nodosum, arthritis, and pyoderma gangrenosum are associated abnormal findings and in some cases may precede the gastrointestinal manifestations. Growth failure and sexual infantilism are major concerns in the adolescent, and an otherwise asymptomatic patient may seek help primarily for these complaints.

Growth hormone studies usually reveal normal or increased circulating levels following appropriate challenge. With extensive ileal disease or the presence of areas of stasis anywhere in the small bowel, steatorrhea may contribute to excess loss of nutriments due to bile salt deficiency. Occasionally delayed growth may be noted for 1 to 2 years before any other clinical manifestations surface. Fistulous connections often develop between adjacent involved loops of intestine and occasionally between a diseased area and normal colon, the bladder, or the abdominal wall. Free perforations with diffuse peritonitis, amyloidosis, and protein-losing enteropathy are less frequent complications. Liver disease is uncommon, although abnormalities of liver function tests occur in one-third of patients. Urinary tract disorders, especially ureteral obstruction and urolithiasis due to uric acid and oxalic acid stones, are increasingly being recognized.

Radiographic changes in the prestenotic phase of the disease are often subtle and difficult to recognize. Radiograms may be completely normal for 1 to 2 years. Early abnormalities affect the ileocecal valve area, resulting in thickened mucosal folds, with some rigidity and separation of the bowel loops. Eventually a cobblestone pattern is noted. The progressive constriction of affected segments results in the final picture of rigid pipe stems or string signs, with skip areas of apparently normal intestine intervening.

DIFFERENTIAL DIAGNOSIS. Many disorders of the small bowel are difficult to differentiate from regional enteritis. Abdominal pain, fever, laboratory evidence of inflammation, and diarrhea of some degree are common to all. Patients with appendicitis are less likely to have a chronic course and diarrhea. Nongranulomatous ulcerative jejunoileitis is usually associated with malabsorption, severe weight loss, and hypoproteinemia. Lymphoma is commonly associated with intestinal obstruction and intussusception. Signs of extraintestinal involvement are helpful. Tuberculosis is almost never seen in the absence of pulmonary disease, although the latter may be subclinical with minimal radiographic findings. Fungal infections such as actinomycosis or histoplasmosis are extremely rare, but special cultures and skin tests are useful. Terminal ileitis due to a gram-negative polymorphic coccoid or ovoid *Yersinia* should be excluded by appropriate cultures or serologic studies.

THERAPY. Therapeutic regimens utilized over three decades suggest that medical management should be the major form of treatment, with surgical intervention restricted to specific complications. This approach is mainly due to the high incidence of recurrence of disease and complications that ranges between 50 to 85 percent. Surgical intervention is indicated for complications such as intestinal obstruction or fistulization. The adolescent with short stature and delayed sexual development usually will benefit from resection if the disease is localized. Growth spurts and catch-up growth have occurred together with accelerated sexual maturation.

Supportive measures are important to maintain nutrition, hydration, and comfort. Except during exacerbations, when it may be prudent to reduce the intake of raw fruits and vegetables or highly seasoned foods, an ad lib diet is best ordered to avoid compounding the severe anorexia. Supplements of 5,000 IU vitamin A, 400 IU of vitamin D, and 50 to 200 mg of ascorbic acid should be prescribed daily. Additional vitamin D may be indicated when there is need to improve calcium absorption. Among chronic patients with subtotal obstruction or fistulization, high caloric central venous alimentation or the use of oral commercial elemental low-residue diets have been helpful in reversing the debilitating malnutrition in preparing patients for surgery. In some cases the improvement has been sufficient to avoid surgery.

Electrolyte and mineral losses, mainly of potassium and calcium, may be excessive with severe diarrhea and/or with adrenocorticosteroid therapy, and supplementation is often necessary. Extensive ileal involvement may result in bile salt deficiencies due to interruption of the enterohepatic circulation, with resultant steatorrhea. Occasionally the excess unconjugated bile salts in the colon may cause a negative balance for water and electrolytes. The resultant diarrhea will respond to 3 to 16 g of cholestyramine in divided doses, if the degree of steatorrhea is not marked. Prescription of a diet in which half of the ingested fat has been replaced by a source of medium-chain triglycerides may not only lessen steatorrhea but also may result in significant weight gains among such patients. Anticholinergic drugs such as propantheline bromide (Pro-Banthine), 2 to 3 mg/kg/day administered every 4 hours and at bedtime, are often helpful for relief of abdominal discomfort. Selected patients experience improvement of most of their complaints after administration of nonabsorbable sulfonamide such as salicylazosulfapyridine (Azulfidine) in divided doses totaling 2 to 8 g/day.

Many patients respond only transitorily to these measures and some not at all. Corticosteroids are eventually required for most. Initially, prednisone should be administered at a dosage of 2 mg/kg/day for 10 to 14 days and then withdrawn very slowly over a period of 6 to 8 weeks. Occasionally the child may exacerbate repeatedly during attempts to taper doses of prednisone, and 10 to 40 U daily of intramuscular ACTH may be introduced to facilitate steroid withdrawal. Short 14- to 21-day courses of prednisone may be useful for subsequent relapses; although Azulfidine may not be dramatic in its salutary effects on a severe bout of the disease, once a child has improved with steroids this sulfonamide may be helpful in maintaining a better state of health and may permit more prolonged intervals between steriod therapy.

Other immunosuppressive agents such as 6-mercaptopurine and azathioprine have been reported to be beneficial in a limited number of complicated cases, but these drugs cannot as yet be recommended for general use in the majority of patients. Generally, initial therapeutic dosages are recommended well below that required for total immunosuppression, ie, 1.25 mg/kg body weight of 6-mercaptopurine and 2 mg/kg body weight of azathioprine. Maintenance dosages are usually about half the initial levels and should be introduced 2 to 3 months after starting the medications. These drugs may be used combined with corticosteroids, and they have been helpful in weaning patients off the latter. In the absence of bone marrow depression or vomiting, long-term use for 4 to 6 years has not been associated with any adverse effects. Diarrhea, if prominent, usually subsides, with general improvement of the patient.

As a rule, 75 percent of these patients suffer chronic indolent courses with variable degrees of debilitation and incapacitation. The requirements for and hazards of long-term steroid therapy, together with the high risk of postoperative recurrence, emphasize the therapeutic dilemma in treating many patients with this disease.

References

Barber KW, Waugh JM, Beahrs OH, Saner IWG: Indications for and the results of the surgical treatment of regional enteritis. Trans Am Surg Assoc 80:146, 1962

Chrispin AR, Tempeny E: Crohn's disease of the jejunum in children. Arch Dis Child 42:631, 1967

Crohn BB, Yarnis H: Regional Ileitis, 2nd ed. New York, Grune & Stratton, 1958

Davidson M: Ulcerative colitis and regional enteritis. In Green MG and Haggerty RJ (eds): Ambulatory Pediatrics. Philadelphia, WB Saunders, 1968, p 696

————— Chronic ulcerative colitis and Crohn's colitis in the pediatric patient. In Kirsner and Shorter (eds): Inflammatory Bowel Disease. Philadelphia, Lea & Febiger, 1975, p 154

————— Medical therapy and prognosis of chronic ulcerative colitis and Crohn's in children. In Kirsner and Shorter (eds): Inflammatory Bowel Disease. Philadelphia, Lea & Febiger, 1975, p 300

Gotlin RW, Dubois RS: Nyctohemeral growth hormone levels in children with growth retardation and inflammatory bowel disease. Gut 14:191, 1973

Harris BH, Hollabaugh RS, Clatworthy HW: Surgery for developmental and growth failure in childhood granulomatous enteritis. J Pediatr Surg 9:301, 1974

Miller RC, Larsen E: Regional enteritis in early infancy. Am J Dis Child 122: 301, 1971

Soper RT, Silber DL, Holcomb GW Jr: Gastrointestinal histoplasmosis in children. J Pediatr Surg 5:32, 1970

VanHeerden JA, Sigler RM, Lynn HB: Regional enteritis in children: surgical aspects. Mayo Clin Proc 42:100, 1967

Weber J, Finlayson NB, Mark JBD: Mesenteric lymphadenitis and terminal ileitis due to Yersinia pseudotuberculosis. N Engl J Med 283:172, 1970

Winkleman E: Regional enteritis in adolescence. Pediatr Clin North Am 14:141, 1967

ULCERATIVE COLITIS

MURRAY DAVIDSON AND MERVIN SILVERBERG

Ulcerative colitis is the most common chronic inflammatory disease of the bowel. The mucosa of the colon is friable and often frankly ulcerated and covered with exudate. The primary complaints are abdominal pain and diarrhea, frequently associated with rectal bleeding. The disease may involve either the entire large intestine or portions of it, and the clinical course is variable. *Proctitis* is a form of the disease limited to the segment distal to the rectosigmoid junction. This clinical variety is different at different ages. It is not very common in children, but when present it usually heralds spread to full-blown disease in more proximal areas of the colon. In adults this limited form of disease is a frequent finding and is generally regarded as having a good prognosis.

ETIOLOGY.   The exact pathogenesis of the disease remains obscure. Elevated white blood count and sedimentation rate, fever, and pus cells in the stool, all common findings, suggest that the disease may be an infectious process. In some patients the initial presentation has been associated with a well-documented bacterial or amebic dysentery that has persisted after the specific infection has cleared. However, despite frequent and diligent attempts to prove a relationship with bacteria or viruses, no specific pathogenic organism has been demonstrated.

Focus on the gastrointestinal tract as a major central and peripheral lymphoid organ has been accompanied by a great deal of work attempting to relate ulcerative colitis to some immunologic or hypersensitivity disorder. Sera of these patients contain circulating antibodies to many different antigens, but they do not appear to be related to the severity, duration, or extent of the disease. Furthermore, these antibodies are neither tissue- nor species-specific; they are often found in normal individuals, and they persist after colectomy, suggesting that their presence is a secondary event with only a questionable relationship to pathogenesis. The possible cytotoxic effects of lymphocytes and bacterial antigens in patients with ulcerative colitis have been investigated with inconclusive results. Milk allergy has been suggested as an important pathogenic factor, but results of clinical studies are contradictory. Circulating immunoglobulins IgA, IgM, and IgG do not consistently differ from those of control subjects, and studies of tissue-fixed immunoglobulins have not been revealing.

Although there is general agreement that psychologic factors are important in children with ulcerative colitis, there are differences of opinion concerning their etiologic role. Many of the patients are dependent, passive, rigid, and oversensitive, with an excessive need for love, and with mothers who are domineering, punitive, and lack warmth. Failure of all patients and all mothers to show these characteristics has led to the impression that these features may not be of primary importance. It is likely that there are multiple determinants that play an etiologic role, including personality patterns of both mother and child, as well as environmental influences such as separation phenomena. Whichever emotional factors are important, there is little question that once the disease is established exacerbations and remissions are often associated with changes in emotional state.

SYMPTOMS.   *Diarrhea* and *abdominal pain* are the most common presenting features, often with rectal bleeding and occasionally with tenesmus. In rare cases the rectal bleeding precedes any changes in fecal consistency. Characteristically the stools are loose to watery and contain small amounts of feces mixed with variable quantities of pus and mucus. The bowel movements occur mainly during the night and early morning hours, but in severe attacks they are continuous throughout the day.

Clinically apparent *dehydration* and depletion of electrolytes occurs only in severe attacks. However, patients with milder but persistent diarrhea may display marginal insufficiencies that are easily thrown into severe depletion states during brief exacerbations.

Anemia is common in ulcerative colitis, although there is disagreement as to its etiology and relationship to rectal bleeding. Many patients suffer from iron-deficiency anemia, while others with persistent bleeding have little or no red cell deficit. In some children, particularly in those with a chronic continuous course of illness, anemia is related to defects in hematopoiesis and iron transport, often in the face of minimal blood loss per rectum. This type of anemia may be further compromised by excessive protein exudation into the gastrointestinal tract; as a rule it responds poorly to oral or parenteral iron administration. In a small number of cases excessive hemolysis has been demonstrated, presumably due to absorbed bacterial toxins, medications such as sulfonamides, or autoimmune processes such as microangiopathic hemolytic anemia.

Liver disease is an uncommon complication in children, although mild abnormalities of liver function tests are frequently reported. Fatty metamorphosis is the most common histologic finding; it has been attributed to nutritional deficiencies or absorption of toxic materials. Hepatitis acquired by parenteral therapeutic measures, or due to an immunologic disturbance, is the second most common lesion. Pericholangitis and biliary or postnecrotic cirrhosis have been noted in long-standing cases, but they are unusual in children.

Erythema nodosum occurs in about 1 to 2 percent of cases, usually during an attack, occasionally preceding all gastrointestinal manifestations. *Pyoderma gangrenosum, erythema multiforme, papulonecrotic lesions,* and *erythematous plaques* are encountered in an appreciable number of children. *Uveitis* and *arthritis,* which often coexist with *aphthous ulcerations* and skin lesions during exacerbations of the disease, may be more troublesome to the patient than the colonic symptoms.

DIAGNOSIS. Before making the diagnosis of idiopathic nonspecific ulcerative colitis, other identifiable causes of colonic inflammation and diarrhea must be ruled out. Repeated stool examinations for amebic and bacterial infections must be performed. On the other hand, the diagnosis of ulcerative colitis should be considered in patients with early onset of painless rectal bleeding without diarrhea.

The two most important tools for diagnosis of ulcerative colitis are sigmoidoscopy and barium enema. With sigmoidoscopy a friable, easily bruised mucosa is seen more commonly than are frank ulcers or exudates. In many instances no abnormalities are observed until the epithelial surface is gently swabbed with a cotton pledget, following which a shower of petechiae and small bleeding points develops. This finding is associated with microscopic evidence of mucosal inflammation and cellular infiltration of the small vessels of the bowel wall. Among patients with long-standing disease, muscular spasm, as well as shortening and narrowing of the colonic lumen, may make sigmoidoscopy

difficult. A rectal biopsy adds little to the diagnosis, although in rare cases histologic study of grossly normal appearing mucosa may demonstrate pathology, eg, increased cellularity of the lamina propria, microscopic abscesses, or granulomas.

As greater experience is accumulated with flexible fiberoptic colonoscopy, reports are beginning to appear of the value of the procedure in children. Questions that remain unresolved from limited rigid-tube sigmoidoscopy (which permits examination of only the distal 22 cm) and that may remain unclear from radiographic studies are amenable to answer by this technique.

Barium enema may appear entirely normal for periods as long as 2 to 3 years after onset of the disease. Conversely, the first examination, within days or weeks of onset, may show evidence of advanced disease. Minimal lesions are represented simply by loss of mucosal integrity, progressing to the pseudopolypoid appearance. Decrease of colonic haustrations with marked shortening and narrowing to a pipe-stem lumen are later findings. However, in some patients the colon has a remarkable potential for returning toward a normal appearance when the clinical picture improves.

Patients with this illness generally should have sigmoidoscopy performed annually and barium enema every 1 to 2 years before adolescence, with semiannual examinations after this age because of the dangers of complications. The clinical picture in individual patients may require deviation from this schedule, making it desirable to examine some children more frequently or to postpone studies in others because of illness.

Ulcerative colitis must be distinguished from regional enteritis restricted only to the colon (Crohn's disease of the colon, granulomatous colitis). In nonspecific ulcerative colitis the disease is essentially mucosal, with almost invariable involvement of the rectum, while granulomatous disease is usually transmural and discontinuous and may spare the rectum. Radiographic differences are useful in selected cases, although interpretation is often based on a great deal of personal bias. A normal rectum, cecal deformity, strictures, fistulae, cobblestone appearance of the mucosa, and longitudinal ulcerations that are presumably submucosal in location are all suggestive of granulomatous disease. The differential diagnosis is greatly facilitated in the 10 percent of patients with granulomatous disease in whom small-bowel disease is simultaneously demonstrable.

CLINICAL COURSE. Two clinical patterns are observed in children. *Remitting colitis* is the more common type and is associated with recurrent relapses that are often stormy and are interspersed between symptom-free periods. Patients with this pattern of disease usually present with bloody diarrhea and may experience considerable rectal bleeding even during diarrhea-free periods. In *chronic continuous colitis* there are no complete remissions at any time. The diarrhea may be deceptively mild and more tolerable than the complications that develop in patients with this type of disease. Despite frequent absence of rectal bleeding, intractable anemia and other signs of poor nutrition such as hypoproteinemia and failure to gain weight are problems.

These patients are more prone to bouts of fever and development of arthritis, fistulas, and abscesses than are those with the remitting pattern.

Children with the remitting pattern of the disease usually either appear to be entirely well after 2 or 3 years or develop the chronic continuous type. Although many of the clinical features of the chronic continuous pattern of disease are common to those attributed to granulomatous colitis, histopathologic examination of surgical specimens does not always reveal granulomas. Conversely, some patients whose biopsies or surgical specimens do not support the diagnosis of granulomatous disease subsequently develop clear-cut ileocolitis. Both granulomatous and nonspecific ulcerative colitis have been reported to occur in the same family, and they have similar epidemiologic and genetic characteristics. Colitis is a familial disease, and together with regional enteritis most large series report that approximately 10 percent of patients have affected relatives. The disease occurs in Jews about 10 times as often as in all other groups combined, and it is encountered with lowest frequency among nonwhites.

Some patients, though not all by far, suffer one or the other of the various colonic complications. Enterocolic fistulas or abnormal communications between bowel and skin, usually anorectal fistulas, occur. Some patients develop the ominous complication referred to as toxic megacolon, with acute dilation and stasis. The exact cause of this complication is unknown, but it is likely that electrolyte imbalance is an important contributing factor.

These is no increased tendency to develop adenomatous polyps in these patients. Heaped-up remnants of colonic mucosa that remain between the ulcers of this disease lead to a pseudopolypoid appearance on radiographic examination. These lesions are inflammatory and are not premalignant. Cancer of the colon occurs in an appreciable percentage of children with ulcerative colitis. Although the factors that predispose to development of carcinoma are unknown, its occurrence appears to be particularly related to duration of disease for more than 5 to 10 years and to onset in early childhood. Actuarial calculations indicate that the likelihood of developing colonic cancer is 20 percent per decade after the disease has been present for ten years.

THERAPY. *Dietary restrictions* are often imposed, but their value is questionable. Patients are frequently treated with diets free of highly seasoned foods and roughage. There are few clinical or experimental data to indicate that these foods make the disease worse. Studies of concurrent lactase deficiency in the small intestine have been conflicting. Tolerance tests can be used to determine the presence of specific sugar intolerance in individual patients. More frequently, an initial short-term trial of milk and milk product withdrawal is arbitrarily attempted during the acute phase of illness to observe for a possible relationship between either lactose intolerance or "allergy" to cow proteins and the pathogenesis of symptoms. Such a relationship has not been observed by us very often, and milk is usually reintroduced after 1 to 2 months. Children are otherwise permitted a free intake, keeping in mind that unnecessary dietary manipulations compromise the already capricious intake of these ill children. The ideal self-chosen diet is rich in calories, high in protein, and supplemented with 5,000 IU vitamin A, 400 IU vitamin D, and 50 to 200 mg vitamin C each day.

As in many other chronic diseases in children, excessive restriction of physical activity is unnecessary and frustrating to both physician and patient. While hospitalization is useful for the initial evaluation, and a brief period of increased rest may he helpful in aborting attacks in patients who have been in remission, children generally do better if allowed free choice of activity.

Psychotherapy is an important consideration in ulcerative colitis, but there is need for individualization. Most patients can be managed by the personal physician alone if he is sensitive to the damaging effects of diagnostic procedures, the fears of the chronically ill child, and the anxieties and helpless feelings of parents. He must be a good listener and must spend time in gaining the confidence of the child and family. As a rule, the constant availability of one sympathetic physician who explains, is honestly optimistic, is reassuringly frank, and is attuned to problems of individual families will maintain an ideal doctor–patient relationship and will be sufficient for chronic care of the child. For the very immature, labile child whose parents may be unable to cope with his needs, a team approach with psychiatric help is sometimes desirable.

Antispasmodic agents are used to control abdominal pain. Propantheline bromide (Pro-Banthine), 2 to 3 mg/kg/day, should be prescribed before meals and at bedtime, with optimal results obtained when atropine side effects are noted. *Antidiarrheal drugs* are frequently prescribed, but they do not produce much effect as long as the inflammatory process remains active. Diphenoxylate hydrochloride (Lomotil), 2.5 to 5 mg three or four times daily, or preparations containing opiates (eg, Donnagel-PG, tincture of paregoric) are the preparations most often utilized. One must be aware of the danger of possible intestinal atony from overdosage with these agents.

The anemic child requires *iron supplements* or even blood replacement . Oral ferrous sulfate should be used in appropriate doses, except when gastrointestinal intolerance necessitates the intramuscular or intravenous administration of the iron-dextran complex Imferon. Patients with the granulomatous and chronic continuous forms of colitis are often unable to utilize exogenous iron. They are best treated with small transfusions of packed red blood cells if anemia becomes severe.

Salicylazosulfapyridine (Azulfidine), 2 to 8 g/day, is useful and constitutes the initial therapy in most patients. Its mode of action is not clear, but it has been shown to suppress symptoms for prolonged periods in individual patients. Although not dramatic in aborting severe attacks, such agents may be used for maintenance therapy to reduce the frequency of relapses. Soluble, absorbable sulfonamides, penicillin, streptomycin, or broad-spectrum antibiotics may be prescribed in usual therapeutic doses for periods of 1 to 2 weeks during acute febrile periods, especially if steroids are being given.

Antiinflammatory and *immunosuppressive drugs* provide the most certain control of acute and deteriorating symptomatology. Prednisone administered over a period of 6 to 8 weeks is used most frequently by us. Dosage is 2.0 mg/kg/day in divided doses for 10 to 14 days, followed by a slow withdrawal for the duration of treatment. In up to 30 percent of patients other authors report more prolonged periods of therapy. Complications of steroid administration, such as osteoporosis, hypertension, excessive weight gain, and hypokalemia, must be anticipated in such patients, and they should be treated prophylactically or at the time they arise. Attempts to avoid steroid side effects by alternate-day administration have not been universally successful in this disease. Rectal instillations of corticosteroids at bedtime may be an adjunct in patients with severe urgency and frequency of defecation. It is preferable that enemas generally not be prescribed for chronic home use, since this may develop into an important point of contention between mother and child. It is much more useful in the hospitalized child and for *self-administered* home use by the late adolescent and young adult.

Corticotropin (ACTH, 20 to 80 U) is usually restricted to specific hospitalized cases or to patients in whom steroid withdrawal repeatedly results in exacerbation of the disease. Unfortunately, children often find frequent regular injections of the aqueous or gel preparations objectionable, and prolonged use is therefore undesirable.

Conclusions vary from unbridled enthusiasm to pessimistic caution with regard to the use of 6-mercaptopurine or azothioprine. Our own experience is as variable as are the reports in the literature. However, among patients who do not respond well and who require virtually continuous courses of steroids, the immunosuppressive agents in dosages of 1.25 mg/kg 6-mercaptopurine and 2 mg/kg azothiaprine have sometimes proved valuable for maintenance of a state relatively more free of symptoms. The hazards of bone marrow depression, malignancy, and a high rate of relapse are very real, and regular physical examination and close supervision of the peripheral blood picture are mandatory.

In both acute and chronic disease there is wide divergence of opinion as to the indications for surgical intervention and the nature of the operation to be employed. Fulminant ulcerative colitis requiring early surgical management is fortunately rare in childhood. Perforation, impending perforation, and the presence of cancer are undisputed indications. Severe hemorrhage is uncommon, and surgery is rarely if ever indicated. Criteria for elective surgery are usually based on degree of clinical disability, failure of growth and development, and in those patients with disease exceeding 10 years' duration, the fear of cancer. The criterion of surgery for a prolonged duration of clinical symptomatology varies with different authors from 1 to 9 years. We believe that patients with chronic continuous disease in whom there is no concomitant small-intestine involvement may benefit from early surgery, especially preadolescent children with growth retardation, who tend to grow normally after total colectomy and ileostomy. When considering surgery in long-standing cases, it is necessary to take into account the high risk of carcinoma, which outweighs the small mortality from elective colectomy.

Total colectomy with permanent ileostomy is the operation most likely to produce a cure. Most appliances that can be utilized with an abdominal ileostomy now make it possible for such a patient to lead a normal life. Introduction of the continent ileostomy operation by Kock is of particular benefit to growing children and adolescents. With proper preparation, patients with the disease make an excellent emotional adjustment to surgery. There is usually marked physical improvement, disappearance of complications, and a complete change for the better in the emotional status of all members of the family.

References

Ament ME: Inflammatory disease of the colon: ulcerative colitis and Crohn's colitis. J Pediatr 86:322, 1975

Berger M, Gribetz D, Korelitz BI: Growth retardation in children with ulcerative colitis: the effect of medical and surgical therapy. Pediatrics 55:459, 1975

Broberger O, Lagercrantz R: Ulcerative colitis in childhood and adolescence. Ad Pediatr 14:9, 1966

Davidson M: Management of ulcerative colitis in children. Am J Surg 107:3, 1964

——— Current concepts: juvenile ulcerative colitis. N Engl J Med 277:1408, 1967

——— Ulcerative colitis and regional enteritis. In Green MG, and Haggerty RJ (eds): Ambulatory Pediatrics. Philadelphia, WB Saunders, 1968, p 696

——— Bloom A, Kugler M: Chronic ulcerative colitis of childhood: an evaluative review. J Pediatr 67:3, 471, 1965

——— Chronic ulcerative colitis and Crohn's colitis in the pediatric partient. In Kirsner and Shorter (eds): Inflammatory Bowel Disease. Philadelphia, Lea & Febiger, 1975, p 154

——— Medical therapy and prognosis of chronic ulcerative colitis and Crohn's colitis in children. In Kirsner and Shorter (eds): Inflammatory Bowel Disease. Philadelphia, Lea & Febiger, 1975, p 309

Ehrenpreis T: Surgical treatment of ulcerative colitis in childhood. Arch Dis Child 41:137, 1966

Engel GL: Studies of ulcerative colitis. II. The nature of the somatic processes and the adequacy of psychosomatic hypothesis. Am J Med 16:416, 1954

——— Studies of ulcerative colitis. III. The nature of the psychologic process. Am J Med 19:231, 1955

Goldberg HI, Carbone JV, Margulis AR: Roentgenographic reversibility of ulcerative colitis in children treated with steroid enemas. Am J Roentgenol Radium Ther Nucl Med 103:365, 1968

Jackson DD, Yalom I: Family research on the problem of ulcerative colitis. Arch Gen Psychiatry 15:410, 1966

Korelitz BI, Gribetz D, Danziger I: The prognosis of ulcerative colitis with onset in childhood. I. The presteroid era. Ann Intern Med 57:582, 1962

——— Gribetz D, Danziger I: The prognosis of ulcerative colitis with onset in childhood. II. The steroid era. Ann Intern Med 57:592, 1962

——— Gribetz D, Kopel FB: Granulomatous colitis in children: a study of 25 cases and comparison with ulcerative colitis. Pediatrics 42:446, 1968

Lagercrantz R, Hammerstrom S, Perlmann P: Autoimmunity in ulcerative colitis. Acta Paediatr Scand [Suppl] 14:111, 1967

McDermott JF Jr: Children with ulcerative colitis. Their own perception of the disease. Psychosomatics 7:163, 1966

Michener WM: Ulcerative colitis in children. Problems in management. Pediatr Clin North Am 14:159, 1967

Schneider KM, Becker JM, Korelitz BI, Krasna IH, Kark AE: The surgical treatment of ulcerative colitis in childhood—a study of 38 cases. J Pediatr Surg 3:12, 1968

Tumen HJ, Valdes-Dapena A, Haddad H: Indications for surgical intervention in ulcerative colitis in children. Am J Dis Child 116:641, 1968

ANORECTAL CONDITIONS
THOMAS V. SANTULLI

Anorectal Abscesses

Perianal abscesses are relatively common in infancy. Deeper ischiorectal abscesses may also occur, usually from infection of any anal crypt. Primary infection of these crypts of Morgagni may cause perianal suppuration, with subsequent formation of anal fistulas. There is a painful swelling overlying the perianal area or ischiorectal fossa with redness, heat, and induration. Fluctuation occurs late. Treatment consists of early incision and drainage followed by warm baths and local cleanliness. In about one-half of the cases of surgical or spontaneous drainage of these abscesses a fistula in ano will result.

Fistula in Ano

Fistula in ano is the end result of progression of an abscess that originates in an anal crypt of Morgagni. The diagnosis is based on the presence of an opening in the perianal area that usually can be probed upward into the involved anal crypt within the anus. A history of one or more episodes of perianal drainage, spontaneous or surgical, with intermittent purulent discharge is common. In some cases recurrent fistulas may communicate with an abscess in the lower pelvic or perirectal area. Such abscesses originally arise from internal fistulous tracts from the appendix, small intestine, cecum, or sigmoid and may indicate a chronic inflammatory disease, eg, regional enteritis. Treatment consists of fistulotomy with wide exposure of the entire tract, including the internal opening.

PERITONITIS
THOMAS V. SANTULLI

Inflammation of the peritoneum may be classified as acute or chronic, primary or secondary, localized or diffuse, bacterial or nonbacterial. Acute peritonitis may occur at any time in infancy and childhood. In the newborn period it is usually but one manifestation of sepsis. It may also occur from perforation of the intestine, with spilling of meconium into the peritoneal cavity.

Acute Primary Peritonitis

Acute primary or idiopathic peritonitis has almost disappeared since effective antibacterial agents have been available. The oganisms responsible for most of these infections (pneumococci or hemolytic streptococci) are effectively controlled by early antibacterial treatment. Both sexes are about equally affected with acute primary peritonitis; most of the cases occur in children from 1 to 6 years of age. The peritonitis is diffuse, involving the general peritoneal cavity; localized abscesses are not as common as in secondary peritonitis. The fluid is generally thin and contains large amounts of fibrin, which eventually causes many adhesions between loops of intestine.

The onset is usually sudden, the child becoming acutely ill with fever as high as 40.5 C and prostration. Sometimes there has been a preceding upper respiratory infection. An older child experiences diffuse abdominal pain and tenderness with boardlike rigidity; in younger patients the abdomen may be soft and doughy. Anorexia and vomiting are rarely absent. Leukocytosis is marked (sometimes as high as 50,000 cells/mm^3), with 80 to 90 percent polymorphonuclear leukocytes.

When there are no localizing signs to indicate a secondary type of peritonitis, some have advocated needle aspiration of the peritoneal fluid to establish the diagnosis. If streptococci or pneumococci are seen on direct smear, in the absence of *Escherichia coli*, the diagnosis of primary idiopathic peritonitis may be made and appropriate chemotherapy instituted. Blind needle aspiration always carries the risk of perforating a loop of intestine that may be adherent to the abdominal wall. It may be safer to take the child to the operating room, where a very small incision can be made in the right lower quadrant of the abdomen, preferably under local anesthesia, in order to obtain some fluid for smear that can be examined immediately. If the character of the fluid and morphology of the organisms establish the presence of primary peritonitis, the procedure is terminated. If secondary peritonitis is found, as indicated by the character of the fluid and the presence of *E. coli* in the smear, the incision is enlarged and appropriate surgical treatment is carried out as described below. The mortality from primary peritonitis should be very low if antibiotic treatment is instituted early in the disease.

Patients with nephrotic syndrome have an unusual susceptibility to primary peritonitis during the active stages of renal disease. Although the same organisms described above were isolated in these patients before 1960, it now appears that the epidemiology has changed since the use of steroids in these patients. Gram-negative organisms, as well as the pneumococcal and streptococcal organisms, are now found. These patients should be treated with parenteral broad-spectrum antimicrobial therapy. We use ampicillin and kanamycin initially.

Acute Secondary Peritonitis

Acute secondary peritonitis is much more common than primary peritonitis. The most frequent cause is appendicitis with perforation, which should always be suspected when peritonitis appears without obvious explanation. Other important causes are primary inflammations of other abdominal viscera, from which extension to the peritoneum may occur, as in volvulus, intussusception, Meckel's diverticulum, perforating ulcers, and rupture of a viscus. The infection is caused by a variety of organisms; the most common, in order of frequency, are some type of *E. coli*, other gram-negative enterobacteriaceae, nonhemolytic streptococci, staphylococci, and *Clostridium perfringens* (welchii).

The fluid is usually purulent, and in rapidly progressing cases there is an extensive exudation of fibrin, with formation of pockets containing pus among the coils of intestine. The process may become localized and result in a peritoneal abscess, which may be found in the pelvis, the subhepatic area, or the subphrenic space or among loops of small intestine. In children pelvic abscesses frequently rupture spontaneously into the rectum.

As in adults, the symptoms in older children are usually well marked and are sufficiently characteristic, but in infants the symptoms are often obscure. In some cases the acute toxemia and hypovolemia resulting from peritoneal exudation cause rapid prostration and death, and the disease may be found at autopsy when not suspected during life.

As a rule the signs of the preceding abdominal illness, usually appendicitis, increase in severity, the temperature rises, usually between 38.5 C and 41 C, and ileus and dehydration are invariably present; vomiting and intestinal obstruction ensue. Older children complain of pain that may be localized or general; in younger children pain is indicated by crying and fretfulness. The abdomen becomes distended and tympanitic. There is marked tenderness on pressure and rebound tenderness, as well as rigidity of the abdominal wall that may be both localized and diffuse.

The systemic symptoms are those of a serious disease; the pulse is weak, rapid, and compressible. In severe cases there may be hiccough, cold extremities, and collapse. In infants convulsions may occur. A polymorphonuclear leukocytosis of 10,000 to 25,000 cells/mm^3 is almost invariable present, but it may be absent in some cases of the gravest type.

In the most severe forms of diffuse peritonitis the course is short; without treatment these patients may succumb within days or even hours. In other cases the course is slower and the process is more apt to be localized. Development of a peritoneal abscess is indicated by continued fever, often spiking in nature, with chills and sweating. The inflammatory mass may be palpable externally or by rectum.

Residual adhesions persisting after the infection has been overcome sometimes give rise to obstructive symptoms later, and operation may be necessary to relieve intestinal obstruction.

Treatment consists of correction of hypovolemia and electrolyte imbalance with blood, fluids, and electrolytes, early operation, and antibiotics; aspiration of intestinal contents through a Miller-Abbott intestinal tube is indicated for paralytic ileus. A period of preoperative preparation is important but should not be prolonged.

Localized Peritonitis

Local collections of exudate or abscesses may form in the pelvis, subhepatic area, or subphrenic space or among loops of intestine and delay recovery; some eventually resorb or rupture into the bowel, usually the rectum; others need to be drained. Subphrenic abscess, usually on the right side, is uncommon in children. Although the most frequent cause is a focus of suppuration in the abdomen, such as perforated appendicitis with peritonitis, it may represent metastasis for a more remote infection by way of the bloodstream or in rare instances direct extension of pneumonia or empyema downward through the diaphragm. The symptoms and physical signs may resemble those of empyema, but more often the symptoms appear as a gradual exacerbation of the primary intraperitoneal disease. There may be higher elevation of the temperature, increasing malaise, anorexia, and upper abdominal pain. Hiccough may occur. Tenderness and spasm are found over the upper abdomen or costal margin on the right or left side, and a mass or local bulging with edema may be present. Radiography in the upright position may show haziness in the lower lung field, with an indistinct diaphragmatic shadow and a collection of pleural exudate or, less frequently, a fluid level with gas just beneath the diaphragm. Diagnostic aspiration of the abscess is often unreliable and may be dangerous; contamination of the pleura is to be avoided. Incision and drainage, usually employing the posterior or extraperitoneal approach, as well as appropriate intravenous antibiotic treatment, are necessary.

Chronic Peritonitis

The most common form of chronic peritonitis is tuberculous (p. 473). Other less common types include the widespread adhesive peritonitis that sometimes follows acute diffuse peritonitis, calcified meconium peritonitis (p. 1027). with extensive adhesions resulting from perforation of the intestine in the prenatal period, and nonspecific inflammatory peritonitis accompanying chylous ascites (p. 1060) or ascites due to portal hypertension.

References

Golden GT, Shaw A: Primary peritonitis. Surg Gynecol Obstet 135:513, 1972

Gross RE (ed): Primary peritonitis. In The Surgery of Infancy and Childhood. Philadelphia, WB Saunders, 1953, p 384

Harken AH, Schochat SJ: Gram positive peritonitis in children. Am J Surg 125:769, 1973

Ladd WE, Swan H: Subdiaphragmatic abscess in children. N Engl J Med 229:1, 1943

Speck WT, Dresdale SA, MacMillan RW: Primary peritonitis and the nephrotic syndrome. Am J Surg 127:267, 1974

Miscellaneous Surgical Topics

FOREIGN BODIES

THOMAS V. SANTULLI AND RAYMOND A. AMOURY

Between the ages of 1 and 4 years the habit of swallowing foreign substances is very common. The most common are detached parts of toys, marbles, pebbles, buttons, and coins. Not only are smooth articles swallowed, but also, with equal readiness, sharp ones such as pins of every variety, bits of glass, fragments of bone, nails, and small toy knives and forks; extraordinary objects are sometimes swallowed. At the time of swallowing, choking or coughing attacks, severe pharyngeal pain, and sometimes slight hemorrhage may occur.

Foreign bodies in the esophagus are, in general, the most difficult to manage. Only large objects and those with sharp edges and angles are apt to become impacted; others pass into the stomach and rarely give trouble. A foreign body may become impacted at any point in the esophagus, most commonly in its upper portion, about the level of the fourth cervical vertebra. If allowed to remain it may lead to ulceration or perforation. The ulceration may occur into the trachea or into the posterior mediastinum, producing retroesophageal or mediastinal abscess. A tracheoesophageal communication leads to aspiration pneumonia and sometimes to lung abscess.

If the foreign body lodges in the throat it may give rise to gagging. In the esophagus itself it may cause dysphagia, vague sensations of discomfort, or no symptoms at all. In many cases respiratory symptoms predominate, such as dry cough and tracheal gurgling, and little or no obstruction to swallowing is observed. Some patients will tolerate liquid foods perfectly well, while attempts to take solid or semisolid foods precipitate attacks of choking or vomiting. When there is laceration of the esophagus, ulceration and inflammation are likely to follow. In such instances there is pain and soreness on swallowing. It is well to remember that foreign bodies (or, indeed, a food bolus) are much more likely to become impacted in the esophagus if a preexisting stricture is present.

Opaque foreign bodies can be localized accurately by radiography. A flat object, like a coin, will usually lie in the frontal plane if it is in the esophagus and in the sagittal plane if in the larynx. All foreign bodies that lodge in the esophagus should be removed. Sounding is valueless and may cause further impaction of the object; the removal should be left to an expert esophagoscopist. Clumsy attempts to remove an object impacted in the entrance of the esophagus not infrequently result in its aspiration into the larnyx, with resulting asphyxiation. Most foreign bodies can be withdrawn with the esophagoscope, although sometimes it is more convenient to push them down into the stomach.

Once foreign bodies have entered the stomach, 90 to 95 percent of them will pass uneventfully through the gastrointestinal tract. During passage of the object through the intestine there may be complaints of pain, but in the great majority of instances there are no symptoms whatever, even with sharp or angular bodies. Impaction and perforation, while possible, are rare. Progress may be impeded at the pylorus, the horizontal part of the duodenum, the duodenojejunal junction, and the ileocecal area. The usual time required for a foreign body to traverse the intestinal tract is 2 to 12 days, but it may be considerably longer. We have known a safety pin to be retained in the intestinal tract for 8 months without producing any symptoms and then to be passed spontaneously; its presence in the stomach was demonstrated radiographically 2 hours after it was swallowed. If the body swallowed is smooth it passes through the anus without difficulty; sharp bodies may produce severe anal pain and sometimes rectal bleeding.

Diagnosis is often a matter of much difficulty, and without radiography positive verification is impossible. Often when the physician is called because this condition is suspected by parents the alarm turns out to be false; the object thought to have been swallowed is discovered in the child's crib.

Although most foreign bodies, including open safety pins, pass through the intestinal tract without causing any symptoms whatever, certain objects are potentially dangerous enough to justify interference. The relationship between the size of the foreign body and the size of the child is important. Objects over 5 or 6 cm in length may be expected to cause trouble in the younger child, and their progress should be observed carefully; these may include some bobby pins, hairpins, and long needles. If such a foreign body has already passed the pylorus, radiographic observations of its progress should be made periodically; if it remains stationary for a week or 10 days, there is cause for some concern. Operation is indicated at the first sign of perforation—tenderness, rigidity, fever, nausea, and vomiting. With the more innocuous foreign bodies, especially those that are disk-shaped, expectant treatment is almost always successful. The diet need not be changed. No emetics or cathartics should be administered.

Quite distinct from accidental swallowing of foreign bodies is the practice of pulling off and swallowing hair, fur from rugs, wool from toys or blankets, shreds from clothing, and a great variety of other substances. In infants the quantity of the substance is generally small, and usually it provokes vomiting, or the material is speedily passed by rectum. Occasionally the substance does not pass in the stools and accumulates to form an intestinal mass that may be associated with obscure and sometimes severe symptoms of long duration. More often the mass forms in the stomach. These gastric tumors, or *bezoars,* are usually composed of hair from the patient's own head, although hair from toys, brushes, and other sources is occasionally found in them. They are more frequently seen in older children than in infants, and usually in those with long hair. The habit of trichophagy may continue for years, until a mass of considerable size has formed, sometimes attaining a weight of 1 to 1.5 kg.

The symptoms of such a hair ball in the stomach (*trichobezoar*) are usually indefinite. Epigastric pain or vague gastric distress is common, but vomiting is not especially marked. The general health may suffer but little for a long time. Foul breath is not infrequent. On palpation the abdominal mass is readily felt. The tumor may be mistaken for malignancy, a displaced spleen or kidney, fecal impaction, or a mesenteric cyst. Radiographic examination may show an extensive filling defect. A correct diagnosis may not be made until operation is performed. In a few instances the tumor has disappeared after catharsis, but the risk involved is obvious. With surgical removal the outcome is almost always favorable.

In sharp contrast to the hair balls are the food balls (*phytobezoars*) sometimes found in the stomach. These form quite suddenly as a result of the ingestion of some mucilaginous material that adheres to whatever food happens to be present in the stomach, producing a heterogeneous solid mass. Such tumors have followed the ingestion of varnish, shellac, tar, or powdered agar. A more frequent cause in this country is the persimmon; this fruit, particularly if not quite ripe, forms a mucilaginous product on reaching the stomach. Instances are recorded in which a persimmon debauch has been followed within a few hours by symptoms of gastric distress as the result of a large persimmon bezoar occupying the entire stomach. The drug salol, once popular as an intestinal antiseptic, also has a tendency to produce these bezoars.

Mineral concretions (*gastroliths*) occasionally occupy the stomach of young subjects. They have been observed after the administration of magnesium, bismuth, or iron salts. We have recently seen one that consisted largely of barium sulfate employed for a contrast meal some weeks before. The conditions responsible for their formation are obscure.

References

Benson CD, Lloyd JR: Foreign bodies in the gastrointestinal tract. In Mustard WT, Ravitch MM, Synder Jr. WH (eds): Pediatric Surgery, 2nd ed. Chicago, Year Book, 1969, p 825

Friedlander FC, Kushlick P: Trichobezoar. Arch Dis Child 29:556, 1954

Holinger PH, Johnston KC: Foreign bodies in the air and food passages. Pediatr Clin North Am 1:827, 1954

Laff HS, Allen RP: Management of foreign bodies in the alimentary tract. J Pediatr 48:563, 1956

ESOPHAGEAL VARICES
John H. Seashore

Extrahepatic or intrahepatic portal vein obstruction causes portal hypertension and increased flow of blood through collateral venous channels, including the submucosal veins of the esophagus. These dilated and tortuous esophageal varices are easily ruptured and may bleed massively. Respiratory infection, esophagitis, and aspirin ingestion have all been incriminated as causes of bleeding from esophageal varices.

Varices are an important part of the differential diagnosis of upper gastrointestinal hemorrhage in children. Sudden massive hematemesis is frequently the first manifestation of portal hypertension. The diagnosis is confirmed by barium esophagram, esophagoscopy, or arteriography. Hemorrhage from esophageal varices is usually tolerated better by children than by adults, especially if the portal hypertension is due to extrahepatic portal vein obstruction. Bed rest, sedation, transfusion, and nasogastric suction, to keep the stomach free of blood and clots, may be sufficient treatment for the acute episode. Gastric lavage with iced saline reduces blood flow through major collateral veins and may be helpful in controlling hemorrhage.

Definitive treatment of esophageal varices requires some type of portal-systemic venous shunt to control portal hypertension. Since the long-term patency of shunts is directly proportional to the size of the veins used, it is advisable to defer the shunting operation until the major splanchnic veins of the child are at least 1 cm in diameter, usually at about 10 years of age. Repeated episodes of hemorrhage are remarkably well tolerated by most children, and many temporizing procedures are available to support the child through these early years. Esophagoscopy and injection of sclerosing agents directly into the varices is a useful procedure. Constant infusion of Pitressin through an indwelling catheter in the superior mesenteric artery may dramatically reduce collateral venous flow and bleeding from varices. Transthoracic ligation of the varices and gastric division are effective operations, but they do not permanently prevent recurrent hemorrhage. The Sengstaken-Blakemore tube is a dangerous instrument in children and should only be used to control exsanguinating hemorrhage while the child is prepared for emergency operation.

Prognosis of children with bleeding esophageal varices is generally good if the portal hypertension is due to extrahepatic portal vein obstruction. The prognosis with intrahepatic obstruction is largely determined by the primary hepatic pathology.

STOMACH DILATION AND GASTRIC PERFORATIONS
Thomas V. Santulli

Acute Dilation

Acute dilation (gastric paralysis) is a rare condition in childhood; although it may occur in infancy, most of the cases we have seen have been in older children. It is encountered in association with dilation of the intestine in severe infections, such as pneumonia or typhoid fever, in states of extreme inanition, in hypokalemia, and also postoperatively. The disturbance is probably neurogenic in origin, with normal peristalsis being inhibited; however, secretion continues actively. The condition is characterized by progressive prostration and collapse, by upper abdominal distension and by the vomiting of large amounts of fluid, which is usually colorless, although sometimes it is bile-stained or darkened by the presence of changed blood. Acute dilation of the stomach is a serious, often fatal complication. Treatment consists in keeping the stomach empty by continuous gastric suction and in maintaining fluid balance. Transfusion may be required to combat shock. We have seen the condition subside and recur again within a few days. Great caution must be used in resuming oral feeding after such an episode.

Chronic Dilation

Chronic dilation may be obstructive or atonic in origin, or it may result from overfeeding. Pyloric stenosis and congenital malformations of the duodenum are the most common causes of obstruction. Atonic dilation may be encountered in severe rickets as a manifestation of general muscular atony; it is also seen in older subjects with visceroptosis. Some degree of dilation is not uncommon in the digestive disorders of infancy.

Symptoms depend on the cause of the dilation. When the stomach does not empty in the normal time and when the amount vomited exceeds the quantity of food taken at the last meal, one may assume that dilation is present. The stomach can usually be outlined by percussion; if its lower border is below the umbilicus, dilation may be assumed. Occasionally a dilated colon is mistaken for stomach dilation. More accurate information is obtained by radiographic study.

The ultimate prognosis in chronic dilation is good, provided the underlying factors can be dealt with, although the dilation may persist for months.

Gastric Perforations

Spontaneous perforation or rupture of the stomach, although not a common lesion, must be suspected in any infant, premature or full-term, who in the first few days of life exhibits respiratory distress and rapidly increasing abdominal distension. An *upright* radiograph of the abdomen will usually show considerable quantities of free air in the peritoneal cavity and will establish the diagnosis of perforated viscus. If the pneumoperitoneum is massive, the stomach is the most likely source (see Fig. 11).

Abdominal exploration with closure of the perforation should be carried out as soon as possible after the diagnosis is made. Preoperatively, nasogastric suction, vitamin K by intravenous administration, oxygen, and systemic antibiotic treatment should be promptly instituted. If respiratory embarrassment secondary to sudden abdominal distension is severe, a 19 or 20 gauge needle inserted through the upper abdominal wall will allow for escape of air from the peritoneal cavity and may dramatically improve the infant's condition while preparations are being made for emergency operation. It should be emphasized that multiple perforations may occur and that several deaths have been caused by failure to recognize all sites at the time of exploration.

In extremely rare instances perforation of the stomach may be associated with total distal obstruction, as in pyloric or upper duodenal atresia. However, the exact cause of so-called spontaneous perforation or rupture is unknown. It is probably related in some way to sudden increases in intragastric pressure. The amount of pressure required to rupture the stomach is variable and is dependent on the degree of prematurity of the infant and factors that may weaken the gastric wall, such as intubation, sepsis, and peptic ulceration. Recent evidence casts some doubt on the widely accepted theory that a congenital deficiency of muscle fibers in the stomach wall is the underlying cause of spontaneous gastric rupture.

References

Inouye WY, Evans G: Neonatal gastric perforation: a report of six cases and a review of 143 cases. Arch Surg 88:471, 1964

MacGillivray PC, Stewart AM, MacFarlane A: Rupture of the stomach in newborn infants due to congenital defects in gastric musculature. Arch Dis Child 31:56, 1956

Rees JR, Redo FS: Neonatal gastric necrosis and perforation treated by gastrectomy and esophagogastric anastomosis. Surgery 64:472, 1968

Shaw A, Blanc WA, Santulli TV, Kaiser G: Spontaneous rupture of the stomach in the newborn: a clinical and experimental study. Surgery 58:561, 1965

——— Perforations of the GI tract in newborn infants. Hosp Practice 6:131, 1971

INTESTINAL OBSTRUCTION BEYOND THE NEONATAL PERIOD

MARK M. RAVITCH

The term ileus denotes any type of intestinal obstruction. *Mechanical ileus* may be due to a variety of causes: compression by a neoplastic or inflammatory mass, constriction in a herniation through a natural orifice or beneath adhesive bands, twists or angulations due to adhesions, volvulus due to abnormal fixation of the bowel at one point or to complete lack of fixation, intussusception, tumors involving the bowel, ingested foreign bodies, fecal concretions, masses of ascarids, congenital atresias and stenoses, meconium ileus, or aganglionosis. The order of probability in the differential diagnosis of intestinal obstruction varies with the age of the patient. In the newborn, atresia, malrotation, aganglionosis, meconium ileus, and meconium plug are the chief possibilities. In the first 2 years after the neonatal period, incarcerated hernia and intussusception are the most common causes of mechanical ileus; thereafter the field broadens.

The onset of mechanical ileus is characterized by intestinal pain that is severe, griping, and periodic. Borborygmi offer corollary evidence of increased peristalsis. In an uncommunicative child, periodic restlessness associated with simultaneous increase in intestinal sounds is diagnostic. In general, in low obstruction distension appears early and the onset of vomiting may be delayed; in high obstruction vomiting is an early symptom and death may occur without distension. The rapid loss of great quantities of fluid and electrolytes in high obstruction is one of its principal dangers. However, the fluid that backs up in the bowel in low obstruction is just as effectively lost to the body as if it had been vomited.

Mechanical intestinal obstruction is an acute surgical emergency. The diagnosis should be made and treatment instituted on the basis of cramps and vomiting in a child in whom another cause is not established for these symptoms. Distension, obstipation, persistent failure to pass either feces or flatus, absence of peristaltic sounds, the presence of intestinal patterns, dehydration, electrolyte disequilibrium and tachycardia, and radiographic evidence of dilated loops and fluid levels are late results of obstruction seen only in neglected patients. A mass is felt only when ileus is caused by a palpable tumor or when strangulated bowel, as in volvulus, becomes sufficiently engorged and distended to be palpable. Tenderness appears when the bowel is becoming gangrenous or is perforating. Plain radiographs of the abdomen with the patient erect and recumbent reveal distended loops long before they are discovered by physical examination. The presence of fluid levels and distended loops is corroborative evidence of intestinal obstruction, but it is not required. The barium swallow has no place in the study of this condition.

Treatment is operative and immediate. It is impossible to determine clinically whether one is dealing with a mechanical obstruction that will produce gangrene (volvulus, adhesive bands) or one that may not (intrinsic tumors, kinks due to adhesions), and the surgeon is rarely justified in temporizing. If obstruction is incomplete there may be some justification for delay and study in spite of the ever-present risk that the obstruction will become complete. The stomach must be emptied before induction of anesthesia, and a Cantor or Miller-Abbott indwelling intestinal tube is best inserted at once. Before operation, rehydration should be started with electrolyte solution; blood and plasma may be needed. Large doses of any of several antibiotics have been found to ameliorate the effects of experimental strangulating obstruction. Administration of antibiotics is therefore begun as soon as the diagnosis has been made and while preparations for operation are under way. Dependence on indwelling tubes for relief of mechanical intestinal obstruction is dangerous and rarely defensible.

After operation, no food or water should be given by mouth until passage of feces and flatus demonstrates the patency and muscular sufficiency of the alimentary canal. The period of intravenous alimentation may last a week or more. Fluid removed by intestinal intubation must be replaced parenterally in addition to the calculated daily requirements, and allowance must be made for the loss of protein-containing fluid into edematous bowel wall and into the peritoneal cavity. In infants, parenteral nutrition may be required through centrally placed silastic catheter.

Paralytic ileus may occur in massive peritonitis, after extensive operative procedures, following release of a low mechanical obstruction late in the disease, or in severe bodily injuries or overwhelming infections. The abdomen is greatly distended. There is absence of peristaltic waves, cramps, and borborygmi, and the pain is only a constant dull ache from distension. Intestinal tonus has been destroyed and the alimentary stream is stagnant. Treatment is directed at relief of the primary condition, at decompression of the intestine with indwelling tubes, and at maintenance of fluid balance. If the bowel is not completely paralyzed, pharmacologic stimulation may be attempted with Pitressin, Prostigmin, or Mecholyl. Pharmacotherapy is most likely to be effective early, before extreme distension has destroyed the tonus of the bowel. These drugs all have potent side effects and must be administered with caution. Operative intervention is not employed, and resort to ileostomy and similar measures has been abandoned. As in mechanical ileus, nothing is given by mouth until intestinal function has been restored.

Intussusception

Intussusception is produced by the invagination of one portion of the intestine into another. Characteristically it affects infants in the first 2 years of life, although in some parts of the world, as in Nigeria, a later onset is common. In 152 cases seen at the Johns Hopkins Hospital from 1893 to 1948, 61 percent occurred in children from the fourth through the tenth month of life, and the peak incidence was in the seventh, eighth, and ninth months. It affects males more frequently than females in the ratio of 3 to 2 and white children more often than black children. Most of the victims are well nourished and in good health up to the time of onset. A large number of the patients seem to occupy late positions in their mothers' obstetric careers.

The cause is rarely clear. An area of thickening in the intestinal wall, or a mass incorporated in it, could conceivably act like a foreign body and be propelled by the normal peristaltic activity of the gut. However, in only less than 10 percent of the cases, and in only 2.5 percent of those under the age of 2 years, does a polyp, Meckel's diverticulum, nodule of ectopic pancreatic tissue, or other local lesion serve as the exciting cause. The marked development of the lymphoid nodules of the intestine, coinciding as it does with the age incidence of intussusception, has been thought by some to be a contributing factor. Peyer's patches enlarged to tumorlike proportions have been found in some instances. In infancy the disproportion between the calibers of cecum and ileum is greater than in later life and may be facilitating the occurrence of intussusception. Attempts have been made to correlate the incidence of adenovirus in the stools and the occurrence of intussusception, with results that are equivocal.

Of 123 cases in which data were available, in 103 the intussusception began at or near the ileocecal valve, in 14 well up in the small bowel, and in 6 in the colon. Attempts at greater precision in localization are apt to be inaccurate, and the use of compound anatomic designations tends to obfuscation.

PATHOLOGY.   Once an intussusception forms it is clear that the leading point or intussusceptum is constant (Fig. 16), while any increase in length occurs at the expense of the sheathing or receiving loop, the intussuscipiens. Compression of the mesenteric vessels between the two inner layers and the presence of the **U**-shaped angulation of the mesenteric vessels at either end of the intussuceptum lead to venous stasis, engorgement, edema, exudation, further vascular compression, and ultimately gangrene, Discharge of blood is one of the first results, and the early evacuation of quantities of mucus is correlated with the appearance of great numbers of goblet cells in the mucosa of the intussusceptum. The tension of the mesentery on the intussusceptum tends to arch the bowel in a curve with its center at the mesenteric root. Edema and compression obstruct the intestine, although most patients should be relieved of their intussusception before they have come to suffer from ileus. The rapidity of appearance of gangrene is highly variable. At times the bowel is viable and reducible after a week; at other times an intussusception may become irreducible within 24 hours. Spontaneous sphacelation of the intussusception and passage of the slough through the rectum is a rarity chiefly of historic interest.

SYMPTOMS.   The clinical picture of acute intussusception is so striking and so characteristic that once it is seen it should be easily recognized thereafter. A well-nourished infant between 4 and 11 months of age suddenly cries out with obvious abdominal colic and vomits. The attacks of colic recur regularly, in the intervals leaving a flaccid or prostrated infant, but rarely one who appears normal. There is usually one normal stool, evacuating the colonic contents. Thereafter, only blood or blood and mucus are passed. Lassitude or collapse increases. The abdomen is relaxed, soft, and nontender, except at times directly over the palpable intussusception. Signs of ileus (distension, vomiting, and tachycardia) gradually supervene.

The initial symptom in almost half of the cases is *abdominal pain* and in the other half *vomiting.* In a few cases bloody rectal discharge is the first recognized symptom, but this occurs chiefly in infants in the first year of life who have failed to attract attention with their less dramatic earlier symptoms. The pain is characteristically episodic and cramplike and at first very severe. Pain may appear to decrease in intensity late in the course of intussusception, when intestinal dilation produces atony.

Vomiting appears initially as a reflex symptom, but if the patient has been neglected it takes on the character of the vomiting in intestinal obstruction. In one study, 141 of 152 patients (93 percent) vomited before treatment was begun, and 75 percent of infants under 1 year of age began to vomit in the first 3 hours of disease. It is of interest that in 8 percent of the cases studied the patients took and retained food after the onset of symptoms, and in 42 percent they accepted food but were unable to retain it.

Bloody stools are the telltale sign of intussusception. In all, blood was seen in 138 of 152 cases (91 percent). In 95 percent of patients under 2 years of age blood was observed in the stool or in the rectum, but only in 65 percent of these older than 2 years. Frequently one normal stool is passed, after which obstruction becomes complete and no feces or flatus appear. Characteristically blood is passed admixed with mucus in the classic currant-jelly stool, but at times only a thin bloody fluid (prune-juice stool) appears. Feces continue to be mixed with the blood in enough instances to warrant caution in making the diagnosis of dysentery solely on the basis of bloody diarrhea, particularly since in a small number of cases of intussusception the obstruction is incomplete and there is continuing diarrhea. In many cases blood is first observed on the examining finger, emphasizing the importance of rectal examination.

PHYSICAL EXAMINATION.   The child is characteristically listless and apathetic or even prostrate. The abdomen is flaccid and flat until signs of obstruction supervene and distension appears. More than a third of the patients present with a temperature of 38.5 C or higher. Fever is more common and higher in the younger infants. Pulse and respiratory rates tend to be elevated. In three-fifths of the cases there is a leukocyte count of over 12,000 cells/mm^3.

Prostration is present in over half the cases. Great torpor and severe depression are indicative of grave progression of the disease. Dehydration is dependent on the extent of the vomiting and the intestinal obstruction. Surprisingly early in the disease the infant may be severely dehydrated, with lax skin and deeply sunken eyes.

The abdomen is at first flat or scaphoid, and in this condition the mass formed by the intussusception may be visible. The abdomen is soft and nontender, although palpation of the mass itself may elicit slight tenderness and muscular resistance. Early in the progress of intussusception the mass passes into the hepatic flexure, behind the liver and right costal margin, and may be difficult or impossible to feel for a time. The mass is most readily felt when thrown into prominence by vigorous peristalsis during a cramp and is usually described as tubular or sausage-shaped. In almost 90 percent of the cases the mass is felt abdominally or rectally. In 6 of a group of 152 patients, a mass was felt rectally when none was palpable on abdominal examination. In 11 patients (7.2 percent) the intussusception presented through the anus.

PROGNOSIS.   The duration of the pathologic process is an obvious determining factor in the production of necrosis of the bowel. Death is rare in cases treated within 24 hours. The mortality rises with the duration of symptoms until 96 hours, at which point there emerge a number of cases of nonstrangulating chronic intussusception that lower the mortality figures. In some instances intussusception may reduce itself spontaneously. High fever is of grave prognostic significance, although in a third of our fatal cases the temperature was below 38.5 C on admission. Dehydration likewise indicates dangerous progression of the disease. Until World War II mortality reports of 20 to 30 percent were common. In most large clinics there has been a steady downward progression in mortality rates from intussusception, and one should now expect no deaths except in patients moribund when first seen.

TREATMENT. Definitive treatment should be instituted at once, subject only to the necessity for administration of appropriate preoperative fluid or blood to combat dehydration or shock. If treatment is by hydrostatic pressure reduction, fluid or blood administration may be started simultaneously.

Hydrostatic pressure reduction is the method of choice in the treatment of intussusception. The discomfort of hydrostatic pressure reduction is much less than that of operative reduction; the complications, in the absence of anesthesia or incision, are fewer, and the period of hospitalization is much shorter. Reduction of an intussusception by hydrostatic pressure is a surgical procedure to be instituted under the direction of the surgeon while the operating room is held in readiness. We do not agree with those who refuse barium enemas to distended babies or to children who have had symptoms longer than some arbitrarily established duration.

As in any intestinal obstruction, a tube is passed into the stomach for constant suction. Blood or electrolytes are started. A Foley bag catheter with a 45-ml balloon is inserted into the rectum just beyond the sphincters, and the balloon is distended. The catheter is left ungreased so that it can be expelled only with difficulty, and the buttocks are tightly strapped with adhesive. A barium suspension, from a maximum height of 3 feet above the table, is permitted to run into the bowel under fluoroscopic observation. The barium will usually be seen to run rapidly into the rectum and colon until the head of the barium column meets the point of the intussusceptum. At this point the rounded head of the advancing barium column suddenly becomes concave, forming a meniscus around the point of the intussusceptum much as a column of barium in the vagina would outline the cervix. As pressure increases the meniscus lengthens, the horns extending until suddenly the intussusceptum is pushed back and the meniscus flattens out again. This process is continued until the entire colon fills readily and until barium can be seen to flow freely into the ileum. So long as reduction continues, however slowly, the flow of barium should be uninterrupted and the reduction continued. Successful reduction is denoted by the following criteria: (1) free flow of barium well into the small bowel; (2) disappearance of the mass; (3) passage of feces or flatus; (4) clinical relief of the patient; and (5) recovery in the stool of charcoal given by mouth. The intussusception can almost invariably be reduced at least to the cecum; if there is doubt about complete reduction, it is necessary only to make a small McBurney incision either to confirm the reduction or to complete it by pushing the last small tip of ileum through the ileocecal valve.

At the completion of successful reduction of the intussusception charcoal instilled in the stomach through a tube should be recovered by enema in 6 hours, further to confirm reduction. Recurrence (2 to 6 percent) is apparently no more likely after hydrostatic pressure reduction than after manual operative reduction; although the adhesions after operation might make recurrence less likely, they are responsible for a significant number of cases of subsequent intestinal obstruction. Resection is more common in patients treated primarily by operation. Clinical and experimental evidence indicates that with 3 feet of pressure, rupture of the bowel does not occur and gangrenous bowel will not be reduced. The incidence of specific pathologic lesions causing intussusception is so low, and the lesions in themselves usually benign, that no concern need be felt over the possibility that such a lesion might be missed unless a second intussusception occurs.

References

Benson CD, Lloyd JR, Fischer H: Intussusception in infants and children. Arch Surg 86:745, 1963

Gross RE, Ware PE: Intussusception in childhood: experiences from 61 cases. N Engl J Med 239:645, 1948

Ravitch MM: Intussusception in Infants and Children. Springfield, Ill, Charles C Thomas, 1959

RECTUM AND ANUS
Thomas V. Santulli

Prolapse of Rectum

Prolapse is the abnormal descent or protrusion through the anus of one or more coats of the rectum. When mucous membrane alone descends, the prolapse is said to be partial or incomplete; if all coats of the bowel are involved, it is complete (procidentia). In the latter the mucosal folds of the protruding mass are concentric; in partial prolapse they are arranged radially. In infancy the rectal mucosa, which is loosely attached to the underlying muscularis, may be normally redundant. Mucosal prolapse is frequently seen under the age of 3 years, with most of the cases occurring in the first year. Certain anatomic features in the young age group predispose to prolapse: the nearly vertical course of the rectum, which has little of the lateral and anteroposterior curves of the adult organ, the flat surfaces of the infantile sacrum and coccyx, the relatively low position of the rectum in relation to other pelvic organs, and the lack of support furnished by the levator ani muscles. Spontaneous cure usually results with increasing age and normal growth; as the pelvis loses its vertical plane the sacrum becomes hollowed out, the muscular layers of the rectum and its supports are better developed, and the mucosal redundancy disappears.

Any condition that increases the intraabdominal pressure and is responsible for frequent and sudden straining efforts at stool may precipitate prolapse, as in constipation, diarrhea, polyps, worms, phimosis, whooping cough, and excessive vomiting. Malnutrition with consequent disappearance of the ischiorectal fat may be a contributing factor.

Repeated episodes of prolapse of the rectum occur frequently in infants and young children with cystic fibrosis which is probably related to the frequent stools and malnutrition, since prolapse usually disappears with improved dietary control. It has been stated that cystic fibrosis is the most common cause of prolapse of the rectum in the pediatric age group. Its repeated occurrence in a patient known to have a ravenous appetite is suggestive of the disease.

Complete prolapse sometimes occurs in debilitated or malnourished patients. It may also be seen in children with meningomyeloceles as a result of partial or complete sphincter paralysis and in patients with exstrophy of the urinary bladder.

The protrusion usually comes on gradually at stool and recedes spontaneously. When recurrent, it often remains permanently extruded and rarely may become strangulated or gangrenous. Blood and mucus may be passed by rectum due to the engorgement. Secondary inflammatory changes occur in the mucosa, resulting in ulceration.

Although most prolapses reduce spontaneously, some may require manual replacement. The lesions usually regress with growth of the child. They can frequently be managed by simple measures or by correcting the cause. Constipation should be controlled by stool softeners; paregoric may be helpful in checking tenesmus in diarrhea; polyps should be removed. In severe and chronic cases operative intervention may be necessary, consisting of excision of the prolapsed mucosa or temporary packing of the presacral space with gauze through a posterior approach in order to produce adherence of the rectum to the sacrum. Rarely are more radical procedures necessary in children.

Fissure in Ano

Anal fissure or anal ulcer is a superficial tear in the anal canal at the mucocutaneous junction. It occurs commonly in infancy as the result of trauma from the passage of a hard bulky stool or explosive diarrhea. In infancy the lesions are usually multiple and may occur in any part of the anus; in older children and adults they are usually located posteriorly, sometimes anteriorly, but rarely in the lateral quadrants. In the acute fissure the base is shallow and the edges are clean, soft, and usually sharply defined. In the more chronic form, as the edges become thickened and undermined, there will frequently be found a tag of edematous skin at the peripheral or distal end of the fissure, the sentinel pile. Severe pain on defecation and bleeding are the cardinal symptoms. The blood is characteristically bright red, streaking the surface of the stool. Constipation may be the cause or the result of a fissure in ano.

Almost all of the fissures in this age group will heal with conservative measures consisting of warm baths, drying and anesthetic ointments, and treatment of constipation with stool softeners. The instillation of warm olive or mineral oil before defecation and gentle dilation of the external and sphincter are helpful. Treatment should be continued for several weeks after the apparent healing and disappearance of symptoms. If these simple measures fail and the fissure assumes a chronic appearance with fibrosis and undermined skin edges, surgical excision is necessary.

Hemorrhoids

Hemorrhoids are not often seen in children, but they may be found in patients with chronic constipation. True internal hemorrhoids are rare; external hemorrhoids and tags are more common. Pain, protrusion, and bleeding are the usual symptoms. Treatment of the underlying constipation will usually correct the condition. Operation is rarely necessary, but it may be needed for acute external thrombosed hemorrhoids.

References

di Sant'Agnese PA, Vidaurreta AM: Cystic fibrosis of the pancreas. JAMA 172:2065, 1960

Fowler R: Anatomy and treatment of rectal prolapse in childhood. Aust Paediatr J 3:90, 1967

Kulczycki LL, Schwachman H: Studies in cystic fibrosis of the pancreas: occurrence of rectal prolapse. N Engl J Med 259:409, 1958

Santulli TV: Prolapse of the rectum. In Mustard WT, Ravitch MM, Synder Jr WH (eds): Pediatric Surgery, 2nd ed. Chicago, Year Book, 1969, p 1007

ASCITES

THOMAS V. SANTULLI

The term ascites, which denotes an excessive collection of fluid in the general peritoneal cavity, is usually confined to noninflammatory extravasations. Ascites fluid is of low specific gravity, contains few cellular elements, and is amber and usually clear. It is seen in nephrosis, heart failure, constrictive pericarditis, portal hypertension due to liver cirrhosis or thrombosis of the portal or hepatic veins, and nutritional edema. It may accompany any condition causing pressure on the inferior vena cava above the entrance of the hepatic veins. Fluid accumulation within the peritoneal cavity is also encountered in some cases of tuberculous peritonitis and advanced abdominal malignancy. Ascites in the newborn may be associated with urinary tract obstruction, usually posterior urethral valves. It is presumed to be due to extravasation of urine from the renal pelvis.

The symptoms consist of abdominal distension, fullness, and discomfort due to the fluid accumulation. Small amounts of fluid in the peritoneal cavity are difficult to detect. Large amounts are, as a rule, easy to identify. The abdomen is moderately or greatly distended, with the skin of the abdominal wall tense or shiny and the umbilicus often pouting. The superficial veins are dilated, especially about the umbilicus, and with significant accumulations a fluid wave can be elicited. In infants and children, shifting dullness alone is not pathognomonic of ascites, since it may be caused by a change in position of the intestinal contents.

Cysts of the omentum or mesentery, celiac syndrome with conspicuous abdominal distension, and occasionally severe megacolon are to be differentiated from ascites. Rarely, hydronephrosis may be difficult to distinguish. The prognosis and treatment depend on the cause.

Chylous Ascites

Chylous ascites is a rare form of ascites in which the abdominal fluid contains fat. The color may be bluish white, milky, or creamy, and the fluid after standing will have at its surface a lipid layer, the thickness of which serves as a rough measure of total fat content; after a diet rich in fat the content has been as high as 5 percent in some cases.

Cases that appear in the first year of life are usually due to *congenital* malformation of the central or peripheral lymph channels. *Acquired* cases are due to obstruction of the thoracic duct, which may result from neoplasm, inflammation, or obstruction to the intestine, as in malrotation or incarcerated inguinal hernia. Other causes are filariasis with obstruction of the thoracic duct by the parent worm, trauma to the thorax or abdomen, or surgical injury of the duct.

The diagnosis of chylous ascites, or chyloperitoneum, is made by aspiration and inspection of the fluid. The fat content of the fluid varies directly with the quantity of fat in the diet; its protein content usually remains more or less constant at 2 or 3 g/100 ml.

The treatment is directed at the cause of the condition if this is known. In the absence of obvious cause, conservative management consisting of a low-fat, high-protein, high-vitamin diet and aspiration of the fluid is indicated. In most cases the fluid reaccumulates rapidly, and repeated paracenteses may be necessary. In some instances the patient may recover after several aspirations without the cause ever being known. When many aspirations are necessary the loss of fat may be minimized by a low-fat diet or medium-chain triglycerides; but loss of protein, which is considerable, is less easily controlled, and hypoproteinemia may result. In most cases surgical exploration is indicated to search for the cause.

References

Gribetz D, Kanof A: Chylous ascites in infancy. Pediatrics 7:632, 1951

Nix JT, Albert M, Dugas JE, Wendt DL: Chylothorax and chylous ascites; a study of 302 selected cases. Am J Gastroenterol 28:40, 1957

Vasko JS, Tapper RI: The surgical significance of chylous ascites. Arch Surg 95:355, 1967

Warwick WJ, Holman RT, Quie PG, Good RA: Chylous ascites and lymphedema. Am J Dis Child 98:317, 1959

Wegner ES: Congenital chylous ascites, apparently cured by Routte's operation (venous peritoneal anastomosis). Am J Dis Child 47:586, 1934

Whittlesey RH, Ingram RP, Riker WL: Chylous ascites in childhood, report of five cases. Ann Surg 142:1013, 1955

ALIMENTARY TRACT NEOPLASMS

Mark M. Ravitch and Thomas V. Santulli

Benign polyps are the most common intestinal tumors. They usually are confined to the colon, and the most frequent symptom is bleeding. The blood is generally bright red and may be present on the surface of the stool or mixed with the stool; occasionally it is passed free into the toilet bowl. The character of bleeding is determined to some degree by the distance of the lesion from the anus. Rarely is the bleeding in large amounts. Diagnosis is made by digital examination of the rectum or by proctosigmoidoscopy; occasionally the lesion may protrude from the anus.

Juvenile polyps are usually single, occasionally mutliple, and only rarely are they numerous. They may be sessile or pedunculated and may reach a size of 2 or 3 cm; they are most commonly found in the rectum. Grossly they are smooth and spherical, and histologically the surface is covered by only a single layer of flattened cells, which have frequently been entirely abraded. The stroma of the polyp is composed of a loose myxomatous tissue in which there are numerous large mucus lakes, lined by tall columnar cells. Serial section of such a polyp shows that these mucus lakes communicate with the surface, and the histologic appearance is entirely different from the arborization, with numerous irregular clefts, of a true adenomatous polyp.

Juvenile polyps are self-limited and possibly inflammatory in origin. They do not lead to the development of malignancy, and they frequently become infarcted and are expelled. The differential diagnosis between a juvenile and an adenomatous polyp cannot be made radiographically. If one is within reach of the sigmoidoscope and is removed in this manner and found to be a juvenile polyp, there is no need for operation to identify the nature of other more proximal polyps in the same child.

Adenomatous polyps in the rectum are of interest primarily because of bleeding and occasional prolapse. In the small bowel they are of interest chiefly because of their propensity for causing intussusception, the usual cause of their discovery. They may cause painless bleeding and diarrhea. Polyps are occasionally multiple, and they may be responsible for repeated episodes of intussusception. There are a number of syndromes of familial involvement with intestinal polyps. In the *Peutz-Jeghers syndrome* scattered polyps of colon, small intestine, and stomach occur in association with the characteristic melanin pigmentation of the lips, buccal mucosa, tongue, palms, and soles. The Peutz-Jeghers polyps are hamartomatous and have almost never been known to lead to malignant degeneration. On the other hand, *polypoid adenomatosis of the colon,* one of several familial syndromes associated with colonic polyps, invariably leads to the development of cancer if the colon or entire colonic mucosa is not removed by one or another operation. Bloody diarrhea is the usual presentation. Symptoms of familial polyposis rarely become apparent until after the first decade. Carcinomatous degeneration in childhood has been reported.

Lipomas, myomas, angiomas, and other tumors of the small bowel occur infrequently. The first two manifest themselves chiefly by obstructive symptoms, and the angiomas by bleeding. Occasionally the angiomatous process may be so diffuse as to involve the entire small intestine and make resection impossible. At operation the angiomas may appear remarkably innocuous, showing only unimpressive telangiectatic vessels on the serosal surface and a questionable thickening and darkening of the mucosa here and there.

Carcinoids, or tumors of the argentaffine cells of Kulchitsky in the mucosa of the small intestine, are of low-grade malignancy and are late to metastasize; they are often cured simply by resection. In children they are most likely to be discovered accidentally in a resected appendix, the most common sites for such tumors being the appendix and the terminal ileum. The carcinoid generally is not recognized at the time of the appendectomy and is discovered by the pathologist. Under these circumstances no further operation need be undertaken, for carcinoids of the appendix are rarely malignant.

Lymphosarcoma is the most common malignant tumor of the bowel in childhood. It is an insidious tumor, usually extending to the point of total infiltration of the intestine and becoming incurable before causing any symptoms, which are chiefly those of intestinal obstruction. Bleeding is a rare symptom. In the terminal ileum, the site of predilection for this lesion, lymphosarcoma tends to produce chronic intussusception into the cecum. The occurrence of intussusception after infancy should lead to suspicion of this diagnosis. Resection of the primary mass, subsequent radiotherapy, and the addition of the currently available chemotherapeutic agents are followed by only occasional cures.

Ectopic pancreatic tissue occurs in the stomach, duodenum, or ileum. The ectopic pancreatic tissue is often found in a Meckel's diverticulum. Submucosal nodules of ectopic pancreatic tissue are an occasional cause of intussusception, but they rarely cause any other problem.

Any resectable tumor of the bowel should be removed, since even benign tumors may have serious consequences by serving as the focal point of intussusception.

References

Knox WG, Miller RE, Begg CF, Zintel HA: Juvenile polyps of the colon, a clinico-pathologic analysis of 75 polyps in 43 patients. Surgery 48:201, 1960

Mestel AL: Lymphosarcoma of the small intestine in infancy and childhood. Ann Surg 149:87, 1959

Middelkamp JN Haffner H: Carcinoma of the colon in children. Pediatrics 32:558, 1963

Pickett LK, Briggs HC: Cancer of the gastrointestinal tract in childhood. Pediatr Clin North Am 14:223, 1967

Ravitch MM: Polypoid adenomatosis of the entire gastrointestinal tract. Ann Surg 128:283, 1948

Riner L, Silverstein J, Tope JW: Benign neoplasms of small intestine—collective review. Int Abstr Surg 102:1, 1956

Santulli TV: Intestinal polyposis associated with muco-cutaneous pigmentation (Peutz-Jeghers syndrome). In Mustard WT, Ravitch MM, Snyder Jr WH (eds): Pediatric Surgery, 2nd ed., Chicago, Year Book, 1969, p 891

Troll MM: Aberrant pancreatic and gastric tissue in the intestinal tract. Arch Pathol 38:375, 1944

Wenzl JE, Bartholomew LG, Hollenback GA, Stickler GB: Gastrointestinal polyposis with mucocutaneous pigmentation in children (Peutz-Jeghers syndrome). Pediatrics 28:655, 1961

CHAPTER 23

The Liver

Lawrence M. Gartner and Irwin M. Arias, *Associate Editors*

In recent years advances in biochemical, morphologic, and immunologic techniques and concepts have contributed greatly to an understanding of the pathogenesis, diagnosis, and treatment of liver disease in infants and children. This chapter will review these liver diseases, emphasizing their pathophysiology.

ANATOMY OF THE LIVER

GENERAL ANATOMY

RACHEL MORECKI

Normal liver function depends on the structural and functional integrity of the liver and the individual hepatic cell to assure normal blood supply and excretion of metabolites and bile.

Architectural Design

The mature human liver is a spongelike organ with spaces (lacunae) separated by one-cell-thick plates or laminae. In the neonate and throughout the first year of life these plates are two cells thick. The lacunar surfaces are lined by the liver parenchymal cells (hepatocytes), which project into the lacunae as active microvilli. Centrally located in the lacunar space is the sinusoid (hepatic capillary) surrounded by the pericapillary space of Disse. The walls of the sinusoids are made up of large, flat reticuloendothelial Kupffer cells. These cells are not adherent to each other, but overlap like roof shingles, leaving interstices between them. The perisinusoidal space contains supporting structures made up of reticular fiber bundles, connective tissue cells, and fat storage cells. A functional unit of approximately 1 mm^3, the lobule, can be defined in the liver surrounding a central vein and limited by the adjacent portal tracts. The liver is contained within a fibrous capsule. The outermost layer of liver parenchymal cells (subcapsular cells) is called the limiting plate.

Liver Vasculature

The liver vasculature is composed of the portal venous system, the hepatic venous sytem, the hepatic arterial system, and the sinusoids. Major branches of the portal vein penetrate the liver at the porta hepatis; they are coated by connective tissue derived from the liver capsule, which also incorporates branches of the hepatic artery, bile duct, and lymph vessels. This tubular package of conduits and connective tissue, known as the portal canal or portal tract, arborizes throughout the liver. Through inlet venules portal blood reaches the sinusoids by penetrating the limiting plate. From the sinusoids blood flows into the central veins (the smallest branches of the hepatic vein) via outlet venules. Central veins drain into sublobular veins and then into larger branches, which eventually emerge from the porta hepatis as the main hepatic vein. Each portal tract contains one large and two small branches of the hepatic artery. From these arterioles arise tiny branches (arterial capillaries) that pierce the limiting plate and open into the sinusoids.

Parenchymal Cell (Hepatocyte)

The parenchymal cells (hepatocyte) vary in size from 10,000 n^3 to 60,000 n^3, depending on their locations within the plates, and are variably polygonal in shape (octahedral, pentahedral, decahedral, and dodecahedral). Each hepatocyte faces the pericapillary space (vascular pole), has grooves that delimit bile canaliculi to form the biliary pole, and makes contact with adjacent liver cells.

Bile Ducts

The smallest receptacle for excreted bile is the bile canaliculus, a structure formed by grooves adjoining hepatocytes. The adjoining liver cells are bound by continuous bands (terminal bars) that seal off the canaliculus from the space of Disse and therefore from the sinusoids. Bile in canaliculi drains into bile ductules. Small ductules are bound by simple squamous cells, while those of larger diameter are lined by cuboidal or columnar epithelium. The periportal ductules (canals of Herring) empty into the portal bile ducts and from there into larger ducts, ultimately reaching the right and left hepatic ducts, which unite outside the liver to form the main hepatic duct. The hepatic duct unites with the cystic duct from the gallbladder to form the common bile duct, which enters the descending limb of the duodenum at the muscular sphincter called the ampulla of Vater.

References

Elias H, Sherick JC: Morphology of the Liver. New York, Academic, 1969

Biava CG: Studies on Cholestasis: an evaluation of the fine structure of normal human bile canaliculi. Lab Invest 13:840, 1964

Bouiller CH: The Liver: Morphology, Biochemistry, Physiology, Vol I. New York, Academic, 1963

SUBCELLULAR ANATOMY OF LIVER PARENCHYMAL CELL

SIDNEY GOLDFISCHER

The introduction of electron microscopy to the study of the liver has resulted in identification of subcellular anatomic structures (organelles). This section will summarize current knowledge of the ultrastructure of the hepatic parenchymal cell, which is represented schematically in Figure 1. Much of this knowledge has been derived from studies combining the use of electron microscopic, histochemical, biochemical, and cell fractionation techniques. Although the detail seen in electron micrographs is impressive, caution must be used in interpretation because of artifacts and inadequate sampling. Interpretation of static images must also be tempered by the consideration that the liver cell is synthesizing, conjugating, hydrolyzing, storing, excreting, secreting, and absorbing a variety of materials including proteins, lipids, carbohydrates, and heavy metals, and probably doing all of these at the same time.

Plasma Membrane

The plasma membrane of the hepatocyte is an active participant in the functioning of the cell. The sinusoidal, lateral, and bile canalicular portions of the plasma membrane differ in appearance and enzymatic activity. The surface area of the membranes forming the sinusoidal surface and the bile canaliculi is greatly increased by fingerlike microvilli that project into the lumen of the sinusoid and canaliculus. Tight junctions formed by fusion of the external layers of the opposing plasma membranes on each side of the bile canaliculus probably serve to limit direct exchange of material between blood and bile. The canalicular membrane has high levels of hydrolase activity toward all nucleoside phosphates, including adenosine triphosphate (ATP). Such ATPase activity suggests that active transport may occur in canalicular membranes. In bile secretory failure of intrahepatic or extrahepatic origin, canalicular microvilli are distorted and lose their nucleoside phosphatase activity. The lateral and sinusoidal surfaces show greatly increased ATPase activity, which may represent a change in polarity of hepatocellular excretory processes during bile secretory failure.

The sinusoidal surface is a two-way passage. Lipids, glucose, amino acids, and other materials enter the liver across this membrane; cholesterol, albumin, and fibrinogen and the other proteins involved in coagulation are secreted into the circulation across this membrane. Small, coated vesicles, together with tubular and vacuolar invaginations formed from the plasma membrane, probably function in transporting proteins and lipids across the sinusoidal membrane into the cytoplasm.

Nucleus

The nucleus functions as the principal site for the regulation of hereditary characteristics. The deoxyribonucleic acid (DNA) of the nucleus is localized in the chromatin, which represents the chromosomes of interphase nuclei. Heterochromatin is that portion of the chromosome that has remained condensed during interphase; it is considered relatively inactive. It appears as densely stained clumps of fine fibrous material largely around the nuclear periphery and adjacent to the nucleolus. The metabolically active euchromatin, however, is poorly stained and difficult to identify in routine ultrathin sections.

Ribonucleic acid (RNA) is present in the nucleolus. The nucleolus consists of a granular and a fibrous component. Available evidence indicates that the fibrous component contains protein and DNA and the granular component contains RNA molecules that are precursors to the RNA of the large ribosomal subunit.

The nucleus is surrounded by a pair of membranes that enclose a space called the perinuclear cisterna. The outer membrane is studded with ribosomes, and the

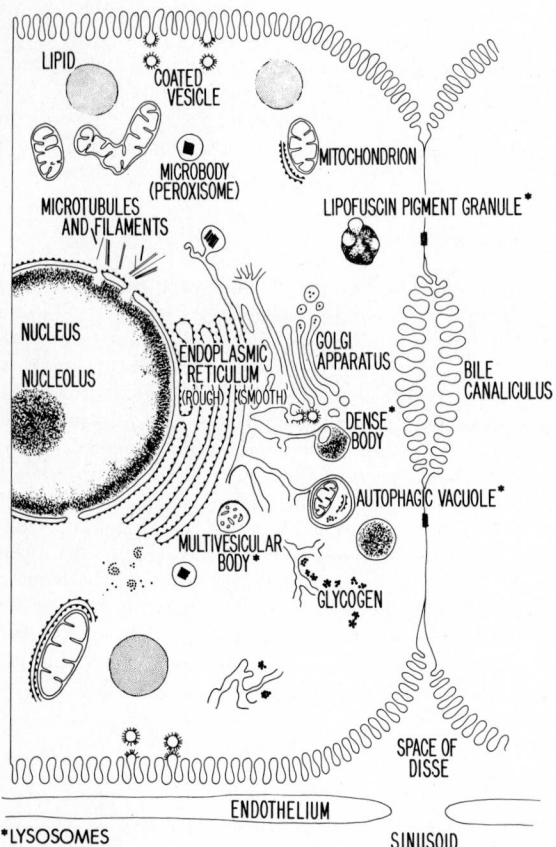

FIG. 1. Rat liver cell. The fine structure of this cell, which has been studied most extensively by electron microscopy, is similar to that of human hepatocytes. In man the smooth endoplasmic reticulum often appears as irregularly shaped vesicles, and the peroxisomes normally do not have cores.

nuclear cisterna is continuous with and enzymatically similar to endoplasmic reticulum. The paired nuclear membranes often fuse and show discontinuities called nuclear pores. It is not known whether the pore represents a true hole or whether it is sealed by a diaphragm derived from the fused membranes.

Endoplasmic Reticulum

The endoplasmic reticulum is a continuous system of rough-surfaced (granular) and smooth-surfaced (agranular) cisternae and tubules. Continuities are often found between the nuclear envelope and the rough-surfaced endoplasmic reticulum, and available evidence strongly suggests that the smooth endoplasmic reticulum is formed from the rough endoplasmic reticulum . The membranes of the rough endoplasmic reticulum are studded with ribosomes, which consist of RNA and protein and are the sites at which amino acids are incorporated into protein. Free ribosomes are also seen in the cytoplasm in ordered arrays. Studies of fetal liver suggest that the rough endoplasmic reticulum evolves from an early stage in which ribosomes are scattered freely in the cytoplasm and subsequently form polysomes, from which membranes of the rough endoplasmic reticulum are derived.

Protein, after synthesis by ribosomes on the rough endoplasmic reticulum, is believed to be transported in the cisternae of the endoplasmic reticulum. This has been demonstrated in guinea-pig pancreas by Palade and associates. Triglycerides are apparently synthesized in the endoplasmic reticulum of liver from fatty acids absorbed at the cell surface. In rats fed orotic acid, β-lipoprotein synthesis is deficient. Consequently lipid accumulates within the cisternae of the endoplasmic reticulum. This is similar to what occurs in the intestinal epithelium of children with absence of β-lipoproteins (acanthocytosis), where massive amounts of triglycerides accumulate and conversion to chylomicra does not take place. It is believed that protein and lipids move from the endoplasmic reticulum to the Golgi apparatus. The smooth endoplasmic reticulum is the main site of drug-metabolizing enzymes. Many compounds such as phenobarbital appear to induce proliferation of the smooth endoplasmic reticulum. Glucuronyl transferase, which catalyzes the formation of glucuronides of bilirubin, various drugs, and endogenous steroids, is found in the smooth endoplasmic reticulum. Newborn infants metabolize various drugs poorly and have reduced enzyme activity associated with the smooth endoplasmic reticulum. Morphologic studies in newborn and fetal rats reveal comparatively little smooth endoplasmic reticulum until approximately the end of the first day after birth. The smooth endoplasmic reticulum also appears to be the site at which peroxisomes (microbodies), some dense bodies, and autophagic vacuoles are formed.

The microsomal fraction of liver which is obtained by ultracentrifugation, is composed mainly of endoplasmic reticulum. In addition to various drug-metabolizing enzymes and glucuronyl transferase, the microsomal fraction also contains many other enzymes, including those concerned with the intermediary metabolism of proteins, lipids, and carbohydrates, and enzymes of heme biosynthesis and of an electron transport chain. It is possible to separate the microsomes into smooth and rough endoplasmic reticulum subfractions. Thus most drug-metabolizing enzymes are localized in the smooth endoplasmic reticulum, but the precise localizations of the other enzymes mentioned have not been fully elucidated. Several microsomal enzymes, including glucose-6-phosphatase, which is absent in type I (von Gierke's) glycogen storage disease, can be demonstrated in the endoplasmic reticulum of normal liver by cytochemical staining methods.

Golgi Apparatus

Although it is unimpressive in size, the fine structure of the hepatocyte Golgi apparatus is typical and consists of three or four parallel saccules that are dilated at the edges and associated with vacuoles and small vesicles that are probably derived from the saccules. Much remains to be learned concerning the role of the Golgi apparatus, particularly in the liver cell, but the available evidence points to an important role in secretion. The predominantly pericanalicular location of the Golgi apparatus suggests that it plays a role in the elaboration and transport of bile. In bile secretory failure in the rat, the Golgi apparatus is greatly enlarged. The Golgi apparatus appears to be the site at which sugars are incorporated into glycoproteins. Reasonably pure Golgi apparatus fractions have recently been isolated from rat and bovine liver and other tissues. UDP galactose, N-acetylglucosamine galactosyl transferase, and other sugar transferases are concentrated in these fractions.

Peroxisomes (Microbodies)

Highly purified preparations of intact rat liver microbodies are greatly enriched in four oxidases; three of these, uricase (urate oxidase), L-D-hydroxy acid oxidase, and D-amino acid oxidase, form hydrogen peroxide, which is in turn destroyed by the fourth oxidase, catalase. Peroxisomes are round organelles that are slightly smaller than mitochondria and are delimited by a single membrane. In many species they contain a core or nucleoid that may be crystallike. In general, a correlation exists between the presence of microbody cores and uricase activity found in normal human livers. Peroxisomes are absent from hepatocytes and renal tubular cells in Zellweger's cerebrohepatorenal syndrome.

Microtubules and Filaments

Thin filaments that are 40 to 50 Å wide and microtubules that are 250 to 300 Å wide are concentrated around the nucleus and bile canaliculi of the human hepatocyte. Although little is known of the functions of these intracellular elements, it has been suggested that they may be contractile and responsible for either intracellular movements or maintenance of cellular form.

Lysosomes

Lysosomes contain more than three dozen acid hydrolases that are capable of degrading virtually all components of the cell and are therefore well equipped to serve as an intracellular digestion system. Material that is taken into the cell by pinocytosis and phagocytosis (endocytosis) and cytoplasmic constituents such as mitochondria, glycogen, and fragments of endoplasmic reticulum may be incorporated into lysosomes. The latter phenomenon, known as autophagia, is prominent in stress situations such as starvation and after partial hepatectomy, but also occurs in normal cells. It is believed that autophagia provides the cell with a means of metabolizing its own structures under stress as well as removing organelles following damage by toxins or disease.

Lysosomes are not usually seen in light microscopic study of hematoxylin-eosin preparations. However, following staining for acid phosphatase, lysosomes can be identified by electron microscopy as well as light microscopy. In the liver the lysosomes are localized along bile canaliculi. Electron-dense granular and membranous materials, called dense bodies or residual bodies, are found within lysosomes. They are believed to be the undigested residue of hydrolysis. Electron micrographs demonstrate that human liver lysosomes often contain an insoluble, lipid, dense melaninlike pigment. Such lysosomes, called lipofuscin pigment granules, are considered to be residual bodies and appear to increase in number with aging. Lipofuscin pigment granules are yellow brown and may be seen in routine histologic preparations. In hemosiderosis and hemochromatosis iron is deposited in lysosomes. In Wilson's disease lysosomes contain high concentrations of copper. In bile secretory failure of intrahepatic or extrahepatic causes lysosomes contain dense material thought to be bile.

Another type of lysosome whose precise function is not known is the multivesicular body. Multivesicular bodies are membrane-delimited structures containing varying numbers of small smooth vesicles that may originate from endoplasmic reticulum or the Golgi apparatus.

A large number of hereditary storage diseases, including type II glycogenosis (Pompe's disease), Gaucher's disease, Hurler's disease, and metachromatic leukodystrophy, that had previously been believed to be unrelated now appear to be lysosomal diseases. Patients suffering from these disorders are deficient in various lysosomal hydrolases, which leads to an unceasing accumulation of the appropriate substrate within lysosomes. Eventually the affected cells, filled with huge lysosomes that are distended by accumulated substrate (eg, glycogen in Pompe's disease, kerasin in Gaucher's disease), can no longer function. Prolonged intravenous administration of the deficient hydrolase to a 3-

month-old child with type II glycogenosis has resulted in marked histologic improvement of the child's liver, with disappearance of the enormous glycogen-packed lysosomes. This type of therapy may eventually prove to be of great value.

Glycogen

Glycogen occurs in two forms within liver cells. The less common type is composed of single, roughly spherical, beta particles. These particles are often found within liver cell nuclei in adult patients undergoing metabolic stress; in children glycogen nuclei are often found in normal specimens of liver. Cytoplasmic glycogen appears as tightly packed accumulations of particles that resemble the beta particles and are referred to as glycogen rosettes or alpha particles. Alpha particles are present in almost all liver cells in close association with the smooth endoplasmic reticulum. There is disagreement as to whether this association reflects a role of the endoplasmic reticulum in the synthesis or phosphorolytic breakdown of glycogen.

Small amounts of glycogen are found in autophagic vacuoles, which are a type of lysosome. This glycogen is normally degraded by a lysosomal enzyme (acid maltase) that hydrolyzes linear oligosaccharides and the outer chains of glycogen to glucose. In children suffering from one of the rarer hereditary glycogen storage diseases, type II glycogenosis (Pompe's disease), the phosphorlylase enzymes are normal; however, acid maltase is absent. Consequently in the liver glycogen accumulates within lysosomes, which become greatly distended.

Mitochondria

The mitochondrial fine structure is characteristic. Mitochondria are delimited by an outer smooth membrane that is separated by a short distance from an inner membrane, which is folded into numerous cristae that project like baffles into the inner compartment (matrix). A few smaller dense granules that appear to be sites at which cations like calcium accumulate are scattered within the mitochondrila matrix. DNA fibrils and granules resembling ribosomes have been found in mitochondria.

It has been estimated that there are more than a thousand mitochondria in a single parenchymal liver cell. In mitochondria oxidation of a variety of substrates is coupled with esterification of inorganic phosphate to produce adenosine triphosphate (ATP). Energy is stored in the high-energy phosphate bonds of ATP and is available for essential cell functions.

The mitochondria also have several important secondary functions. For example, they are vital in gluconeogenesis from pyruvate, they are able to oxidize fatty acids, and they contain the enzyme Δ-aminolevulinic acid synthetase, which catalyses the rate-controlling step in porphyrin synthesis.

Mitochondria are sensitive indicators of cell damage. Mitochondrial swelling, gigantic and bizarre-shaped mitochondria, and the formation within mitochondria of unknown crystallike materials composed of filaments and rods have been described in various hepatic disorders. These changes are not specific and may, in fact, be seen in normal liver. The metabolic defects associated with these altered forms are generally not known. In Zellweger's cerebrohepatorenal syndrome structural changes are associated with a defect in electron transport.

References

de Duve C: Tissue fractionation: past and present. J Cell Biol 50:20D, 1971

———— Baudhuin P: Peroxisomes (microbodies) and related particles. Physiol Rev 46:323, 1966

Dingle IT, Fell HB (eds): Lysosomes in Biology and Pathology. New York, Wiley, 1969

Goldfischer S, Moore CL, Johnson AB, et al: Peroxisomal and mitochondrial defects in the cerebro-hepato-renal syndrome. Science 182:62, 1973

———— Novikoff AS, Albala A, Biempica L: Hemoglobin uptake by rat hepatocytes and its breakdown within hepatocytes. J Cell Biol 44: 513, 1970

Hug G, Schubert WK: Lysosomes in type II glycogenosis. J Cell Biol 35:C1, 1967

Loewy AG, Siekevitz P: Cell Structure and Function. New York, Holt, Rinehart & Winston, 1969

Ma MH, Biempica L: The normal liver cell. Cytochemical and ultrastructural studies. Am J Pathol 62:353, 1971

———— Goldfischer S, Biepica L: Morphology of the normal liver cell. In Popper H, Schaffner F (eds): Progress in Liver Diseases, Vol IV, New York, Grune & Stratton, 1972, p 1

Mahley RW, Hamilton RL, Lequire VS: Characterization of Lipoprotein particles isolated from the Golgi apparatus of rat liver. J Lipid Res 10:433, 1969

Novikoff AB: Mitochondria (chondriosomes). In Brachet J, Mirsky AE (eds): The Cell, Vol 2. New York, Academic, p 299

———— Essner E: The liver cell. Some new approaches to its study. Am J Med 29:102, 1960 Palade GE: Structure and function at the cellular level. JAMA 198:143, 1966

Steiner JW, Phillips MJ, Miyai K: Ultrastructural and subcellular pathology of the liver. Int Rev Exp Pathol 3:65, 1964

Tolbert NE: Compartmentation and control in microbodies. In Symposium of the Society for Experimental Biology, No. XXVII, Cambridge, 1973, p 215

BILIRUBIN METABOLISM
Lawrence M. Gartner

Jaundice, a yellow discoloration of skin, sclerae, and other body tissues due to accumulation of bilirubin, is a sign of major importance in many pathologic and functional disorders involving the hepatic, biliary, and hematologic systems. Yellow skin may also occur in individuals ingesting excessive amounts of β-carotene-containing foods such as carrots or sweet potato, but the sclerae do not become pigmented and the serum van den Bergh reaction remains normal.

In neonates icterus of sclerae or skin is not apparent until the serum bilirubin exceeds approximately 5.0 mg/dl, whereas in older children and adults icterus will be clinically apparent at serum bilirubin concentrations above 2.0 mg/dl. Clinical evaluation of the intensity of icerus is inaccurate, and the serum bilirubin concentration should be measured, particularly in the neonate. The normal total bilirubin concentration in serum after the neonatal period is less than 1.0 mg/dl. The normal direct-reacting bilirubin concentration in serum is less than 0.5 mg/dl.

BILIRUBIN PRODUCTION

Bilirubin is derived from multiple sources. Approximately 80 percent of the bilirubin excreted results from breakdown of the hemoglobin of mature, circulating erythrocytes. The circulating red blood cell has an aver-

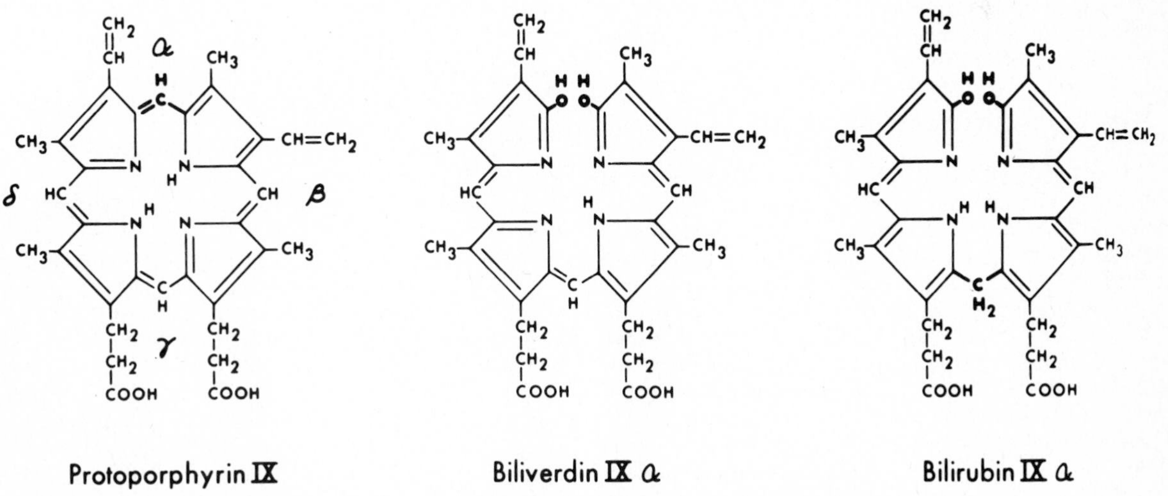

Protoporphyrin IX   Biliverdin IX α   Bilirubin IX α

FIG. 2.   The molecular structure of protoporphyrin IX, biliverdin IXα, and bilirubin IXα, the naturally occurring isomers of the bile pigments. Protoporphyrin is the pigment moiety to which iron and globin are attached to form hemoglobin. (From Troxler RF: Gastroenterology 56:143, 1969.)

age life span of 120 days, at which time mechanical fragility increases and the cell is lysed in the reticuloendothelial system. Hemoglobin consists of heme, an iron-porphyrin complex, combined with globin (Fig. 2). The pathway by which hemoglobin is converted to bilirubin is not known with certainty. Recent studies indicate that all reticuloendothelial cells contain a microsomal heme oxygenase capable of oxidizing the porphyrin ring of heme at the α-methene bridge to form the tetrapyrrole biliverdin (Fig. 2). The carbon atom of the α-methene bridge is oxidized quantitatively to carbon monoxide, on an equimolar basis. Since heme degradation is the only endogenous source of carbon monoxide, measurement of carbon monoxide production rates either by timed collection of expired air or by estimation of blood carboxyhemoglobin concentrations affords a reasonably accurate measure of heme degradation and therefore of bilirubin production. All heme proteins, including cytochromes, contribute to carbon monoxide and bilirubin production.

Iron released during hemoglobin catabolism is stored as ferritin. Globin is degraded to its component amino acids for reutilization in the synthesis of proteins. Biliverdin is reduced to bilirubin in the reticuloendothelial system by bilirubin reductase as well as nonenzymatically by various reducing substances. One gram of hemoglobin will theoretically produce 34 mg of bilirubin.

Approximately 20 percent of the bile pigment excreted into the intestine is derived from sources other than the destruction of mature, circulating erythrocytes. This may be further subdivided into bilirubin production resulting from pathways related to erythrocyte formation and pathways independent of erythrocyte formation. The relative contributions from each of these sources in the human are not known with certainty, but they may be approximately equal. In the former pathway, heme not entering the circulation as erythrocytes contributes to bilirubin synthesis. In the latter pathway, bilirubin may be derived from nonerythrocyte heme proteins such as myoglobin, catalase, peroxidase or cytochromes.

SERUM TRANSPORT OF BILIRUBIN

Unconjugated bilirubin is nearly insoluble in serum water at physiologic pH and is transported in plasma primarily bound to albumin, with small amounts associated with other plasma proteins only at high serum bilirubin concentrations. One mole of albumin is capable of binding at least 2 moles of bilirubin in vivo and 3 moles or more in vitro. Thus at a molar ratio of two, 1 g of albumin can bind approximately 16 mg of bilirubin, permitting a serum unconjugated bilirubin concentration of between 50 and 75 mg/dl. The first binding site is believed to afford a tighter bond than the second binding site. The affinity of subsequent sites is considerably weaker. In clinical experience high concentrations of unconjugated bilirubin are rarely attained. Certain organic anions, especially sulfonamide drugs and certain free fatty acids, alter bilirubin transport by albumin

and enhance the movement of bilirubin into tissues, particularly brain. The precise mechanism of this effect has not been fully elaborated. As will be discussed subsequently, the albumin–bilirubin bond in neonates is a critical factor in the production of kernicterus.

UPTAKE OF BILIRUBIN BY LIVER CELLS

The mechanism and regulation of hepatic uptake of bilirubin are not well understood. Animal studies suggest that the process involves carrier-mediated diffusion of pigment from plasma across the hepatic cell–plasma membrane into the cytoplasm. Bilirubin enters the liver cell free of albumin to which it was previously bound. Two hepatic cytoplasmic proteins, ligandin (Y protein) and Z protein, function as intracellular acceptors of bilirubin, sulfobromophthalein (BSP), and other anions, including corticosteroids. Ligandin is the primary receptor protein for bilirubin and accounts for 5 percent of the total cytoplasmic protein of the liver cell. Reduction in these proteins may result in diminished entry of bilirubin. The plasma bilirubin concentration is largely determined by the rate of bilirubin uptake by the liver cell and the rate of bilirubin production.

BILIRUBIN CONJUGATION

Bilirubin must be made water-soluble in order to be excreted into bile. This is accomplished by conjugation of bilirubin primarily with glucuronic acid. One mole of bilirubin acquires 2 moles of glucuronic acid on the carboxyl groups of the propionic side chains (Fig. 2), forming an ester-linked bilirubin diglucuronide (pigment II of Cole and Lathe). Glucuronic acid used in this process is derived from uridine diphosphoglucuronic acid (UDPGA), and the transfer is catalyzed by glucuronyl transferase, an enzyme associated with the endoplasmic reticulum of the hepatocyte. Glucuronic acid is derived from glucose by the following enzymatic steps in the liver cell:

$$\text{glucose-1-PO}_4 + \text{uridine-5-(PO}_4)_3 \xrightarrow{\text{uridyl transferase}}$$
$$\text{uridine diphosphoglucose (UDPG)} + \text{pyrophosphate}$$

$$\text{UDPG} + \text{DPN} \xrightarrow{\text{UDPG dehydrogenase}} \text{UDPGA} + \text{DPNH}$$

Free glucuronic acid is not a precursor of UDPGA in man.

Chromatographic examination of icteric serum and bile reveals a component identified as pigment I that contains equimolar amounts of bilirubin and glucuronic acid, thus suggesting that it may be bilirubin monoglucuronide. Pigment II contains 2 moles of glucuronic acid per mole of bilirubin and is therefore bilirubin diglucuronide. The biologic existence of pigment I is uncertain. It may represent a complex of free bilirubin and bilirubin diglucuronide. The clinical importance of pigment I in icteric serum is uncertain, and for the present its measurement should not influence treatment. When it is present, conjugated bilirubin in serum is also bound to albumin.

Bilirubin also forms water-soluble conjugates with other carbohydrates, including xylose and glucose. In the human these conjugates account for a small portion of the total conjugates formed. Other conjugates of bilirubin, such as sulfate and taurine, have been prepared synthetically; however, their biologic importance is uncertain.

Naturally occurring metabolites such as thyroxine, and drugs such as morphine, may also be conjugated with glucuronic acid, resulting in biologic inactivation and enhanced solubility in water. The latter facilitates their excretion by the liver or kidney. Whereas bilirubin is conjugated with glucuronic acid by an ester linkage, most drugs and other naturally occurring substances form ethereal glucuronide conjugates. Hepatic bilirubin conjugation normally has a potential capacity approximately 100 times greater than required.

Hepatic Cell Bilirubin Excretion

The excretion of conjugated bilirubin from the liver cell into bile is probably energy-dependent, and when stressed to capacity by increased bilirubin load presented to the liver, it limits overall transfer of bilirubin from plasma to bile. Other organic anions, such as sulfobromophthalein and cholecystographic dyes, which are rapidly transferred from the liver cell into bile, share this excretory pathway with conjugated bilirubin. In the normal rhesus monkey hepatic excretory capacity exceeds the required activity by approximately 50-fold. Severe reduction of hepatic excretory function or marked increase in bilirubin entering the hepatocyte results in accumulation of conjugated bilirubin in the liver cell and plasma.

Transport of Bilirubin in Bile Ducts and Intestines

Conjugated bilirubin in bile is conducted via the intrahepatic and extrahepatic bile ducts into the gallbladder and ultimately into the duodenum. In the gallbladder and intestinal tract conjugated bilirubin may be partially hydrolyzed to unconjugated bilirubin by β-glucuronidase or the alkaline intestinal pH. Unconjugated bilirubin (but not conjugated bilirubin) can be partially reabsorbed by intestinal tract epithelium, particularly in neonates.

The bacteria of the small and large intestine reduce conjugated and/or unconjugated bilirubin to a group of colorless compounds that react with Ehrlich's aldehyde reagent and are called urobilinogens. These compounds are subsequently oxidized to stercobilins, which give the brown color to normal feces. Following administration of broad-spectrum antibiotics and sulfonamides, which substantially decrease intestinal bacterial counts, urobilinogens are not formed, and unchanged bilirubin may be excreted in the feces. Normally about 70 percent of the urobilinogen formed each day is reabsorbed in the ileum and ultimately excreted by the liver, and to a small extent by kidney. Fecal and urinary excretions of urobilinogen are increased in hemolytic disease. Urinary urobilinogen excretion is also increased in parenchymal liver disease, but may be absent with complete biliary obstruction.

Van den Bergh Reaction

The functional classification of jaundice largely depends upon the biochemical nature of the serum bilirubin (ie, whether the serum bilirubin is unconjugated or conjugated). Serum unconjugated and conjugated bilirubin concentrations are reasonably approximated as indirect- and direct-reacting bilirubin respectively, by the van den Bergh reaction. The reaction of bilirubin as direct or indirect is independent of protein binding. In the reaction bilirubin is coupled with diazotized sulfanilic acid to produce a red dipyrrolazo derivative that is estimated colorimetrically. Methodologically the direct reaction is performed first, and the intensity of color is measured 1 minute after addition of the reagents. An accelerator (methanol or caffeine) is added, and color is measured 10 to 30 minutes later. The difference between the total and the direct-reacting portion is the indirect-reacting portion. Falsely high concentrations of direct-reacting pigment may be obtained in the van den Bergh reaction if the serum contains excessive bile acids, urea, and other substances.

References

Arias IM: Formation of bile pigment. In Handbook of Physiology, Alimentary Canal V. 1967, p 2347

——Transfer of bilirubin from blood to bile. Semin Hematol 9:55, 1972

Billing BH, Cole PG, Lathe GH: The excretion of bilirubin as a diglucuronide giving the direct van den Bergh reaction. Biochem J 65:774, 1957

Gartner LM, Arias IM: Formation, transport, metabolism and excretion of bilirubin. N Engl J Med 280:1339, 1969

——Hollander M: Disorders of bilirubin metabolism. In: Assoli N, Pathophysiology of Gestation, Vol III. New York, Academic, 1972, p 455

Goresky CA, Fisher MM (eds): Jaundice. Hepatology Research and Clinical Issues, Vol 2. New York, Plenum, 1975

Gray CH: Bile Pigments in Health and Disease. Springfield, Ill, Charles C Thomas, 1961

Heirwegh KPM, Van Hees GP, Leroy R, et al: Heterogeneity of bile pigment conjugates as revealed by chromatography of their ethyl anthronilate azopigments. Biochem J 120:877, 1970

Israels LG: The bilirubin shunt and shunt hyperbilirubinemia. In Popper H, Schaffner F (eds): Progress in Liver Diseases, Vol III. New York, Grune & Stratton, 1970, Chap 1

Lathe GH: The degradation of haem by mammals and its excretion as conjugated bilirubin. Essays Biochem 8:107, 1972

Lemberg R: The chemical mechanism of bile pigment formation. Rev Pure Appl Chem 6:1, 1956

Lester R, Schmid R: Intestinal absorption of bile pigments. II. Bilirubin absorption in man. N Engl J Med 269:178, 1963

Levi AJ, Gatmaitan Z, Arias IM: Two hepatic cytoplasmic protein fractions, Y and Z, and their possible role in the hepatic uptake of bilirubin, sulfobromophthalein, and other anions. J Clin Invest 48:2156, 1969

London IM, West R, Shemin D, Rittenberg D: On the origin of bile pigment in normal man. J Biol Chem 184:351, 1950

Maisels MJ: Bilirubin: on understanding and influencing its metabolism in the newborn infant. Pediatr Clin North Am 19:447, 1972

Odell GB: The dissociation of bilirubin from albumin and its clinical implications. J Pediatr 55:268, 1959

Robinson SH: Formation of bilirubin from erythroid and non-erythroid sources. Semin Hematol 9:43, 1972

Schmid R: Hyperbilirubinemia. In Stanbury JB, Wyngaarden JB, Fredrickson DS (eds): The Metabolic Basis of Inherited Disease. New York, McGraw-Hill,

Tenhunen R, Marver HS, Schmid R: Microsomal heme oxygenase. Characterization of the enzyme. J Biol Chem 244:6388, 1969

With TK: Bile Pigments: Chemical, Biological and Clinical Aspects. New York, Academic, 1968

BILE ACID METABOLISM

NORMAN B. JAVITT

Bile acids or their salts comprise the major organic components and functional agents in bile because of their important role in intestinal fat absorbtion. The role of bile acids in hepatic physiology and pathophysiology is only partially understood.

TYPES OF BILE ACIDS

Bile acids are categorized as primary or secondary. Primary bile acids are synthesized de novo from cholesterol in vivo. Secondary bile acids are formed by further alteration of primary bile acids by intestinal bacteria. Altered bile acids may be further modified by the liver before being excreted in bile. In the neonate secondary bile acids are occasionally found in meconium and are probably derived via the placenta from the mother, since the fetal gastrointestinal tract is sterile.

All bile acids are conjugated in the liver before being excreted in bile. In fetus and neonate virtually all bile acids are conjugated with taurine. In postnatal life bile acid conjugation with glycine increases, perhaps as a result of expansion of the glycine pool by a milk diet.

PRIMARY BILE ACID SYNTHESIS.   The hepatocyte is the only cell having all the enzymes necessary for conversion of cholesterol to bile acids. Three classes of primary bile acids are formed by the hepatocyte: monohydroxy, dihydroxy, and trihydroxy (Fig. 3).

MONOHYDROXY BILE ACIDS.   The cholesterol molecule (Fig. 3) has a saturated hydrocarbon side chain that must be oxidized to form a carboxylic acid. Normally this occurs with simultaneous shortening of the side chain by 3 carbons to reduce the molecule from 27 carbons to 24 carbons. This derivative, known as 3β-hydroxy-5-cholenoic acid (Fig. 3), is normally present in meconium. There is preliminary evidence that this bile acid, which has a steroid ring configuration identical to that of cholesterol, may not be derived from the same cholesterol pool as dihydroxy and trihydroxy bile acids. Since meconium also contains 26-hydroxycholesterol, one possible pathway for cholenoic acid synthesis is from cholesterol to 26-hydroxycholesterol to 3β-hydroxy-5-cholenoate, a sequence present in the rat and hamster. In these species, 3β-hydroxy-5-choleno-

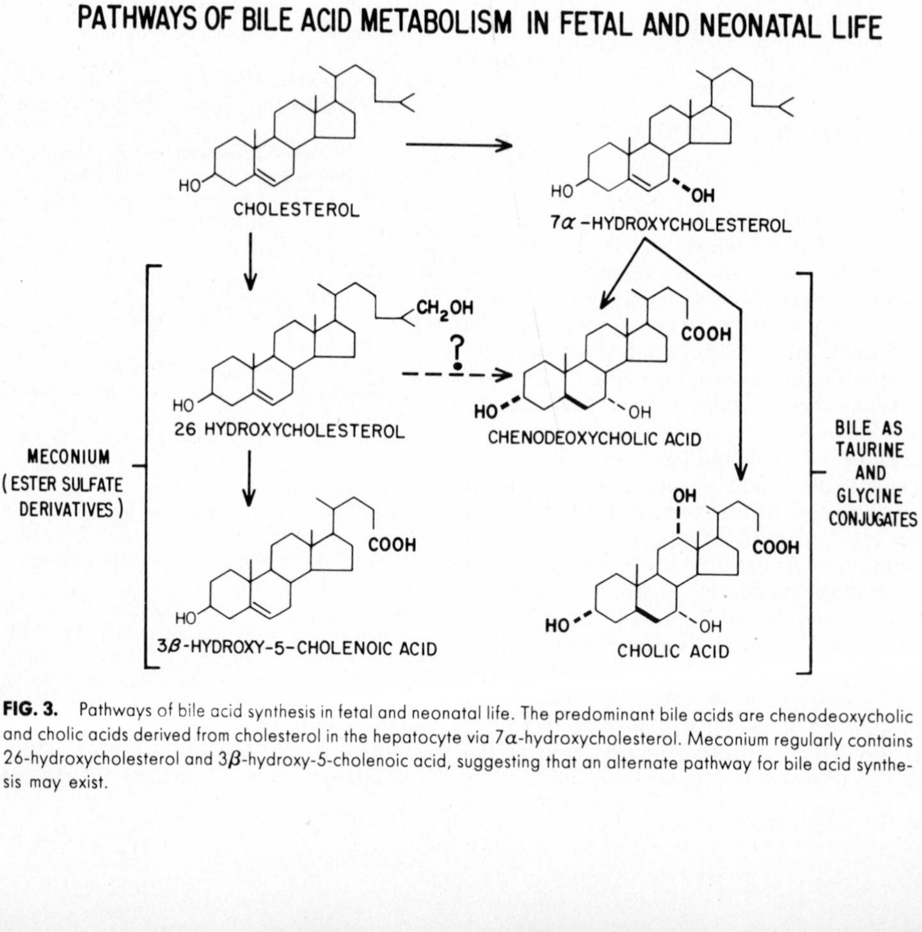

PATHWAYS OF BILE ACID METABOLISM IN FETAL AND NEONATAL LIFE

FIG. 3.   Pathways of bile acid synthesis in fetal and neonatal life. The predominant bile acids are chenodeoxycholic and cholic acids derived from cholesterol in the hepatocyte via 7α-hydroxycholesterol. Meconium regularly contains 26-hydroxycholesterol and 3β-hydroxy-5-cholenoic acid, suggesting that an alternate pathway for bile acid synthesis may exist.

ate is metabolized to another monohydroxy bile acid, 3 α-hydroxy-5β-cholanoate or lithocholic acid. Although lithocholic acid can be classified as a primary bile acid according to this scheme and has been reported to occur in newborn meconium, most lithocholic acid found in adult bile is derived from chenodeoxycholic acid as a consequence of intestinal bacterial activity. Therefore lithocholic acid is usually classified as a secondary bile acid.

The formation of ester sulfate conjugates is a well-recognized pathway for metabolism of steroid hormones and is actively utilized in fetal and neonatal life. Less polar bile acids (ie, cholenoic) and their intermediates (26-hydroxycholesterol) are also found in meconium as ester sulfates. It is uncertain whether the enzyme system for sulfation of hormones is the same as that for 26-hydroxycholesterol and monohydroxy bile acids.

DIHYDROXY BILE ACIDS. Chenodeoxycholic acid (3α, 8α, 5β-cholanoic acid) is the only primary dihydroxy bile acid synthesized in the liver of man. The major pathway for synthesis is via either 7α-hydroxycholesterol or theoretically, 26-hydroxycholesterol. The initial and rate-limiting step in bile acid synthesis from cholesterol is believed to be 7α-hydroxylation.

Chenodeoxycholic acid is normally found in bile as glycine and taurine conjugates. The normal liver extracts more than 90 percent of bile acids returning from the intestine; therefore the concentration in the systemic circulation is low (< 1 μg/ml), and there is very little excretion in urine. Increase in serum levels as a result of hepatobiliary disease results in increased urinary excretion, and approximately 80 percent of chenodeoxycholic acid conjugates occur as monoester and diester sulfates. It is not known where sulfation occurs or how essential esterification is for renal excretion.

TRIHYDROXY BILE ACIDS. Cholic acid (3α, 7α, 12α, 5β-cholanoate) is the only primary trihydroxy bile acid synthesized in human liver and is found in bile as glycine and taurine conjugates. In common with chenodeoxycholate, it is only found in appreciable amounts in urine in the presence of hepatic or biliary tract disease. In contrast to chenodeoxycholate, about 30 percent of cholate conjugates present in urine are ester sulfates.

SECONDARY BILE ACID SYNTHESIS. DIHYDROXY BILE ACID. Deoxycholic acid (3α, 12α-dihydroxy-5β-cholanoate) is synthesized from cholic acid by bacteria, primarily in the large intestine, and is a major component of fecal bile acids. A small fraction of deoxycholic acid is reabsorbed and returns to the liver where it is conjugated, excreted in bile, and reabsorbed by active transport in the ileum to return once again to the liver. Once bacterial flora have colonized the intestine of the neonate, a pool of deoxycholate begins to accumulate and ultimately accounts for 25 percent of the total bile acid pool. The rate at which bacterial colonization occurs in early life is variable, and it is not possible to predict when deoxycholate should be detectable in infancy.

MONOHYDROXY BILE ACID. Lithocholic acid (3α-hydroxy-5β-cholanoate) may be formed de novo from cholesterol in the liver as primary bile acid, but virtually all lithocholic acid found in feces is a secondary bile acid derived from chenodeoxycholic acid as a result of bacterial dehydroxylation of the 7α position of the steroid ring. A very small fraction of lithocholic acid produced in the large intestine is reabsorbed and returns to the liver where it is conjugated and excreted in bile. In addition, some lithocholic acid undergoes ester conjugation with sulfate.

Lithocholic acid conjugates have no greater aqueous solubility than the nonconjugated (free) bile acid, both of which can precipitate in the canaliculi of the biliary tree. Sulfation greatly increases water solubility and reduces the possibility of precipitation.

HEPATIC TRANSPORT OF BILE ACIDS

The term organic anion transport is generally used to describe the ability of the liver to secrete into bile a variety of compounds that are organic carboxylic or sulfonic acids. The concentration of these compounds in bile can be several hundredfold greater than in simultaneously obtained plasma, and one can compute transport kinetics that resemble enzyme kinetics. An active or membrane-mediated transport system for these compounds is believed to exist. Certain of these organic anions, such as conjugated bilirubin and DBSP (phenoldibromophthalein disulfonate), compete with each other for secretion into bile, suggesting that they share a common transport system.

The bile acids can also be classified chemically as organic carboxylic (nonconjugated and glycine conjugates) and sulfonic acids (taurine conjugates); they appear to have a transport system that can be distinguished from that involving other organic anions. The molecular basis for this specificity is not known, but under physiologic conditions bile acid excretion augments rather than inhibits the capacity of the liver to secrete bilirubin and other organic anions. The daily hepatic excretory load of bile acids is approximately 10-fold greater than for bilirubin, and in most species that have been studied the maximum capacity to excrete bile acids is roughly 10 times greater than for bilirubin or DBSP. There is no evidence that conjugated bilirubin competes with bile acids or that bile acids compete with bilirubin for the same excretory pathway.

BILE FLOW AND BILE ACID EXCRETION

Hepatic bile is more than 95 percent water. Water flow into the biliary tree is believed to occur at two anatomic sites: bile canaliculi that are formed by specialization of the cell membranes of hepatocytes and ductules that are lined with columnar epithelium.

Ductular water flow occurs in response to hormones such as secretin or in response to vagal stimulation. A clear solution of inorganic salts, chiefly sodium chloride and bicarbonate, is produced; the mechanism is thought to be similar to transport across other epithelial surfaces.

Canalicular bile flow is augmented by excretion of bile acids. At high rates of bile acid excretion, a linear relationship exists between canalicular bile flow and bile acid excretion. Other organic anions such as bilirubin conjugates or DBSP do not show this relationship, perhaps because of the relatively small amounts that are excreted in bile. Bile acids, perhaps because of their effect on bile flow, increase the maximum capacity to excrete other organic anions.

Canalicular bile flow does not decrease in proportion to the decrease in bile acid excretion that occurs when bile drainage is diverted externally to reduce the bile acid pool. At low rates of bile acid excretion there is no apparent relationship between canalicular bile flow and the rate of bile acid excretion. Certain drugs such as phenobarbital increase canalicular bile flow without enhancing bile acid excretion. It seems, therefore, that other molecular mechanisms may generate canalicular water flow, which has been designated as bile-salt-independent canalicular bile flow.

GALLBLADDER BILE

Hepatic bile flows into the gallbladder between meals, and the solute concentration of organic components increases as water and inorganic salts are transported out of the gallbladder by the epithelial-lined surface. Cholesterol and bilirubin conjugates can, under certain conditions, precipitate in the gallbladder and provide a nidus for gallstone formation.

Cholesterol is maintained in solution as a macromolecular complex containing lecithin and bile acid, which is termed a mixed micelle. Cholesterol can be secreted by liver in man in a supersaturated state, and when stored in the gallbladder it may crystallize as the solvent volume contracts. The rate at which this phenomenon occurs is dependent on the degree of supersaturation, which is determined by the proportions of lecithin, bile salt, and possibly other components such as proteins and minerals. When sufficient bile acid is secreted by the liver, the bile is undersaturated with respect to cholesterol, and crystallization does not occur.

The conjugates of bilirubin have not been prepared in pure form; thus little is known of their physical properties. Although they are more water-soluble than unconjugated bilirubin, they migrate with the macromolecular complex during ultracentrifugation of bile and are probably included within the micelle structure. Precipitates of bilirubin in bile occasionally occur, but the mechanisms are not understood.

BILE ACID POOL SIZE AND ENTEROHEPATIC CIRCULATION OF BILE ACIDS

The normal neonate has a bile salt pool of 290 mg/m^2, which is approximately one-half that of the adult. The rate of synthesis of primary bile acids in the neonate is also approximately one-half of that in the adult when expressed on a surface-area basis. There is no apparent physiologic relationship between bile salt pool size and surface area or body weight.

The availability of bile salt to augment lipolysis of fat and micellar solubilization of fatty acids in the intestine is a function of bile salt pool size, efficiency of gallbladder contraction, and return of bile acids from the ileum to the liver and gallbladder. Intestinal absorbtion of fat in some neonates and in most premature infants is less efficient than in adults and may be related to a constricted bile acid pool. Since fecal bile acid excretion is not excessive compared to pool size, ileal absorbtion of bile acids is normal. Factors regulating bile salt pool size in the neonate have not been identified, and considerable variation may exist.

METHODS OF MEASUREMENT

Serum and urine bile acid concentrations can be determined by enzymatic, gas chromatographic, or mass spectrometric techniques. Enzymatic methods measure total bile acids, while the latter two methods permit quantitation of specific bile acids and differentiation between conjugated and unconjugated bile acids. None of these methods is available as a routine clinical chemical determination.

References

Anderson KE, Javitt NB: Bile formation. In Becker FF (ed): The Liver, Normal and Abnormal Function, Part A. New York, Marcel Dekker, 1974, Chap 12

——— Kok E, Javitt NB: Bile acid synthesis in man: metabolism of 7 α-hydroxycholesterol-^{14}C and 26-hydroxycholesterol-[3]H. J Clin Invest 51:112, 1972

Back P, Ross K: Identification of 3β-hydroxy-5-cholenoic acid in human meconium. Hoppe Seylers Z Physiol Chem 354:83, 1973

Javitt NB: Bile salts and hepatobiliary disease. In Schiff L (ed): Diseases of the Liver, 4th ed. Philadelphia, Lippincott, 1975, Chap 4

Watkins JB, Ingall D, Szczepanik P, Klein P, Lester R: Bile salt metabolism in the newborn. N Engl J Med 288:431, 1973

METHODS OF EXAMINATION IN LIVER DISEASE

FREDRIC DAUM AND MICHAEL I. COHEN

Although they are never a substitute for a thorough history and physical examination, a wide variety of chemical, enzymatic, isotopic, radiographic, and morphologic studies play a critical role in the management of patients with liver disease by helping to elucidate the etiology, severity, and chronicity of the problem. Some of these studies indicate the extent of hepatic cellular damage, while others test the capacity of the liver either to synthesize a substance or to clear it from the blood. Normal values for many of these tests are age-dependent.

Serum and Urine Chemical Determinations

BILIRUBIN. Jaundice signifies an elevated serum bilirubin concentration, which indicates an imbalance between the rate of bilirubin production or intestinal reabsorption and the rate of bilirubin disposal by the liver. Hyperbilirubinemia is a critical measure of hepatic function and of hepatobiliary and/or hematologic dysfunction. A detailed discussion of bilirubin metabolism and measurement will be found on p. 1067.

ALBUMIN. Determination of total serum albumin provides information regarding the duration and severity of hepatocellular pathology. Albumin is synthesized in the liver by ribosomes in the endoplasmic reticulum. The liver produces 120 to 200 mg of albumin per kilogram of body weight daily in the adult. Because serum albumin has a half-life of 17 to 20 days, several weeks elapse before hepatic injury results in significant reduction in the serum albumin concentration.

The normal serum albumin concentration varies with age, and the lowest values occur during the neonatal period, when the mean serum albumin is 2.5 g/dl. In older children 3.0 to 3.5 g/dl is considered the lower limit of normal. Albumin concentrations in serum may be determined by one of several electrophoretic techniques with quantitative scanning, dye binding, or immunodiffusion. In the presence of hyperbilirubinemia dye-binding methods for determination of albumin often yield falsely low values due to displacement of the dye bilirubin. Newer techniques utilize dyes such as bromcresol green that are free of bilirubin competition and yield accurate results.

Pronounced hypoalbuminemia resulting from decreased hepatic synthesis occurs in children with fulminating hepatitis, chronic active hepatitis, or decompensated cirrhosis. Persistent hypoalbuminemia suggests hepatocyte destruction and a poor prognosis. Several conditions unrelated to disease of the liver may also deplete the serum albumin. These include protein-losing enteropathies, renal disease, severe malnutrition and malabsorption, thermal burns, and dilutional problems related to plasma volume.

Severe hypoalbuminemia (less than 2.0 g/dl) may result in ascites even in the absence of liver disease. In the presence of liver disease and/or portal venous hypertension, hypoalbuminemia of less severe degree contributes to development of ascites.

GLOBULINS. Serum globulin abnormalities occur in a variety of illnesses, including acute and chronic liver diseases. Utilizing electrophoretic, immunoelectrophoretic, and radioimmunoassay techniques, a large number of plasma proteins may be quantitated. Although an abnormality in the serum globulin fraction is not diagnostic of a specific liver disease, such information is helpful when used in conjunction with history, physical examination, and other available laboratory data.

With standard electrophoretic techniques, gamma globulins are often shown to be elevated in many different liver diseases, particularly chronic active hepatitis. Elevations of IgG, and to a lesser degree IgA, suggest chronic active hepatitis and/or cirrhosis. Normalization of the serum concentration of these globulins is one measure of therapeutic effectiveness in chronic active hepatitis. Increased titers of smooth muscle antibodies and antimitochondrial, antiglomerular, antinuclear, and antierythrocyte antibodies (positive Coombs test) have also been described in patients with chronic active hepatitis.

Specific serum globulin abnormalities may be associated with specific hepatic lesions. Elevation of α-fetoprotein, an α_1-globulin, suggests the presence of a teratoma or hepatoma, although similar abnormalities occur in children with biliary atresia and hepatitis. In children with α_1-antitrypsin deficiency, the α_1-globulin band on electrophoresis is low or almost absent. Ceruloplasmin, an α_2-globulin, is deficient in the sera of almost all patients with Wilson's disease. Detection of hepatitis B_s antigen and/or antibody is the most specific means of differentiating hepatitis B from other varieties of viral hepatitis.

Serum albumin and globulin concentrations should be viewed as individual determinations. A reversal of the albumin–globulin ratio has little meaning in itself, as it may reflect either depressed albumin synthesis or increased globulin production, or a combination of the two. The administration of blood products may artificially alter albumin and globulin levels for 2 to 4 weeks.

UROBILINOGEN. Urobilinogen is the metabolic product of bacterial conversion of bilirubin in the lumen of the distal small intestine. A portion of the urobilinogen is absorbed across the intestinal mucosa to return via the portal circulation to the liver, where it is then excreted into bile. The fraction of intraluminal urobilinogen not reabsorbed is further converted to urobilin and stercobilin, the normal brown pigment in stool.

The appearance of urobilinogen in urine indicates either compromised hepatic uptake and excretion of urobilinogen, as in severe hepatitis or cirrhosis, or an increased load of bile pigment, as in hemolytic disorders. In contrast, in disorders with obstruction to flow of bile into the intestinal tract, urobilinogen formation may be minimal or absent, and urine urobilinogen may be negative.

Sequential testing for urinary urobilinogen may assist in evaluating the progress of hepatic excretory function. During recovery from extrahepatic biliary obstruction or severe cholestasis, urine urobilinogen, which was previously absent, may increase to high levels and then return to normal levels. Low concentrations of urinary or fecal urobilinogen do not exclude total biliary obstruction. Loss of conjugated bilirubin from intestinal epithelial cells into the lumen with subsequent formation of urobilinogen permits accumulation of urobilins in low concentration in stool and urine in spite of complete biliary obstruction.

Because urobilinogen is a weak organic anion it is found mainly in the afternoon or evening urine; testing of morning specimens should be avoided. Despite hepatobiliary pathology, antibiotics may alter intraluminal bacterial flora and limit conversion of bilirubin to urobilinogen. The healthy person excretes less than 3 mg of urinary urobilinogen and 40 to 280 mg of fecal urobilinogen every 24 hours.

LIPOPROTEIN X. An abnormal low-density serum lipoprotein (LP-X) occurs in patients with obstructive liver disease. Infants with neonatal hepatitis may show a decrease in serum concentration of LP-X after cholestyramine therapy, while those with extrahepatic biliary atresia have persistent elevations of this lipoprotein. The diagnostic usefulness of LP-X in differentiating extrahepatic biliary obstruction from intrahepatic disorders remains to be established.

AMMONIA AND UREA NITROGEN. Dietary protein is digested to peptides and amino acids. Deamination by bacterial ureases in the distal small intestine and colon leads to production of ammonia, which enters the portal vein and is subsequently converted in the normal liver to urea. Kidney and muscle also produce small amounts of ammonia.

As a test of liver function, determination of serum ammonia nitrogen concentration has been helpful in differentiating hepatic from other types of encephalopathy. The relationship of hyperammonemia to the severity and pathogenesis of hepatic encephalopathy is uncertain. Hyperammonemia has also been associated with excessive parenteral amino acid infusions, inherited deficiency of ornithine transcarbamylase, portal hypertension with shunting between the portal vein and systemic venous channels, Reye's syndrome, and liver failure. Quantitation of serum ammonia nitrogen concentrations is complex, and the means are not available to all clinicians. Although there are slight variations in the venous and arterial ammonia levels, the normal blood ammonia nitrogen does not exceed 75 to 100 μg/100 ml. The failing liver is often unable to convert ammonia to urea. Extremely low blood urea nitrogen concentrations signal severe hepatic dysfunction.

GLUCOSE. Hypoglycemia develops in association with various forms of liver disease. Glycogen storage diseases (especially types I, III, IV, and VI) and galactosemia are manifested by hypoglycemia early in the disease. In other acquired and inherited diseases of the liver hypoglycemia may occur at a later stage when cirrhosis has developed. In children below the age of 5 years with Reye's syndrome, low blood glucose values are common. Serial determinations of serum glucose may be useful in following acute severe hepatopathies as well as chronic, smoldering forms of liver disease.

CHOLESTEROL. Total serum cholesterol is a determination usually given little attention in pediatric patients. Its concentration may be modestly elevated following acute extrahepatic biliary obstruction and may be reduced in acute hepatitis. The most dramatic elevations of serum cholesterol are seen in infants with paucity of intrahepatic bile ducts (intrahepatic biliary hypoplasia), where concentrations in excess of 1,500 mg/dl may occur, usually in association with cutaneous xanthomata.

SERUM ENZYME DETERMINATIONS

TRANSAMINASES. A sensitive indicator of hepatocellular damage is elevation of serum glutamic pyruvic transaminase (SGPT) and serum glutamic oxaloacetic transaminase (SGOT). SGPT is specific for liver, whereas SGOT may also derive from myocardial, renal, cerebral, or skeletal muscle tissue. Transaminases normally are present within the intact hepatocyte, and injury to the cell membrane, with or without cell death, results in leakage of these enzymes into plasma. In healthy infants under the age of 2 months, the concentrations of SGPT and SGOT are generally less than 125 to 150 Karmen units, while a level of 40 to 50 Karmen units is the upper limit of normal in older infants, children, and adolescents. The highest concentrations of SGPT and SGOT are most frequently associated with acute hepatocellular injury due to viral or toxic hepatitis and Reye's syndrome. In Reye's syndrome there is seldom histologic evidence of hepatic necrosis or inflammation, but there is extensive, diffuse fatty infiltration.

Although they are associated with hepatocellular injury, the levels of SGOT and SGPT do not correlate with the amount of cellular necrosis, and fulminant hepatic necrosis may result in only moderate increases in the activities of these enzymes. Nonetheless, a serum concentration in excess of 500 Karmen units usually denotes primary hepatocellular necrosis, while less marked transaminase abnormalities are noted in cirrhosis, infiltrative diseases of the liver, and intrahepatic and extrahepatic biliary obstruction.

The patient's serum should be separated from the red cell component and frozen or analyzed immediately. If serum is allowed to remain at room temperature there will be a loss of transaminase activity. Even under ideal conditions SGOT and SGPT activities may normally fluctuate by as much as 30 Karmen units in paired specimens.

ALKALINE PHOSPHATASE. Alkaline phosphatase represents a group of isoenzymes originating in bone, liver, intestine, placenta, kidney, and white blood cells. In healthy persons serum alkaline phosphatase activity is primarily derived from bone and liver. Although intestinal alkaline phosphatase is affected by food intake and increases noticeably after a fatty meal, it accounts for less than 20 percent of the total serum alkaline phosphatase activity. There is a narrow range of normal serum alkaline phosphatase activity in adults, whereas in children and teenagers the normal values are increased approximately twofold during periods of rapid osseous growth.

Elevations of serum alkaline phosphatase activity occur in a wide variety of hepatic and skeletal disorders. Specific alkaline phosphatase isoenzyme determinations may be useful in distinguishing hepatic disease from disorders of other tissues. Increased serum alkaline phosphatase activity in liver disease results from accelerated enzyme synthesis within the liver and its subsequent regurgitation into the circulation. A marked increase in serum alkaline phosphatase activity in children with liver disease suggests mechanical bile duct obstruction or cholestasis. Less profound elevations occur with focal hepatic lesions such as granuloma, metastatic lesions to the liver, or abscesses.

5'-NUCLEOTIDASE (AMPase). Serum 5' nucleotidase activity using AMPase substrate is highly specific for liver dysfunction. Increased serum 5'-nucleotidase activity suggests bile stasis from either intrahepatic or extrahepatic biliary obstruction. It may be useful in determining whether an elevation of alkaline phosphatase activity is the result of hepatic disease.

Γ-GLUTAMYL TRANSPEPTIDASE (GGTP). γ-Glutamyl transpeptidase also has origins in multiple organ systems and is elevated in most liver diseases.

OTHER ENZYMES. Lactic dehydrogenase (LDH) activity in serum has generally not been considered useful in evaluation of hepatic disorders because of its widespread tissue distribution. The use of specific isoenzyme measurements may render it more useful. Creatine phosphokinase (CPK) is not derived from liver, but its elevation in serum indicates muscle or brain damage and is useful in discriminating origins of elevated SGOT activity.

COAGULATION STUDIES. The integrity of the normal coagulation process is dependent on adequate nutritional input, absorption of precursors, and hepatic protein synthesis. Severe liver disease is manifested by deficiencies in factor V and in the vitamin-K-dependent factors II, VII, IX, and X. An abnormal prothrombin time most often indicates a decreased level of one or more of these vitamin-K-dependent factors. If the abnormal prothrombin time is due to poor nutritional intake or intestinal malabsorption of vitamin K, 1 to 5 mg of parenteral vitamin K will correct the defect in 8 to 12 hours. Generally an abnormality in serum prothrombin time correlates well with the severity of hepatocellular disease, and when markedly prolonged it may be the first clue to impending hepatic coma.

DYE CLEARANCE STUDIES

Bromosulfophthalein (BSP) is a phenolphthalein derivative that when injected intravenously is taken up by hepatocytes. Hepatic excretion into bile is the rate-limiting step and is partially dependent on prior conjugation with glutathione in the liver. Plasma clearance depends primarily on hepatic excretion of the dye into bile, but is also related to hepatic uptake, storage capacity, and conjugating capacity.

The test is performed in the fasting state. Immediately after an initial blood specimen is obtained, BSP (5 mg/kg body weight) is injected intravenously. No dye must be allowed to escape subcutaneously, as this may result in tissue necrosis. Precisely 45 minutes later a second blood sample is obtained from a venous site different from that of the initial injection. The concentration of dye is determined spectrophotometrically and compared with a standard of 10 mg/dl. At the time of injection of BSP the initial serum concentration should be 10 mg/dl, assuming a plasma volume of 50 ml/kg body weight. The result is expressed as percent-

age retention of dye at 45 minutes. In healthy infants less than 1 month of age, up to 15 percent of the administered dose may be present in the serum at 45 minutes. In older children and adolescents a level of retention greater than 5 percent of the administered dose is considered abnormal.

The BSP clearance study is a nonspecific test of liver disease, since it measures such diverse functions as hepatic uptake, glutathione conjugation, and excretion. However, in patients with previously documented liver disease, serial BSP studies may provide information regarding improvement or deterioration of hepatic function. Parenchymal liver disease, cholestasis, and extrahepatic bile duct obstruction will usually lead to excessive BSP retention.

Abnormal BSP retention occurs despite a normal hepatobiliary system (1) when an excessive dose is administered or the study is performed within 1 week of cholecystography, (2) during febrile episodes, shock, heart failure, or anemia, or (3) after recent synthetic androgen therapy.

ISOTOPIC TECHNIQUES AND LIVER SCANNING

Radioactive substances are useful in determining size, shape, and position of the liver as well as the presence of intrahepatic space-occupying lesions. Because of its superior physical properties, technetium (^{99m}Tc-sulfur colloid) has replaced iodine-labeled rose bengal (^{131}I-RB), and gold colloid (^{198}Au colloid) as the most commonly used agent for routine liver scans. More recently, gallium citrate (^{67}Ga-citrate) has been noted to exhibit increased uptake in pyogenic liver abscesses, primary liver carcinoma, Hodgkin's disease involving the liver, and liver metastases.

Focal intrahepatic space-occupying lesions such as tumors, abscesses, cysts, hemangiomata, and vascular malformations may be identified if they are larger than 2 cm in diameter. These lesions will be appreciated as areas of either increased uptake (hot) or decreased uptake (cold), depending on the isotope used. Sequential liver scanning of neoplasms or abscesses after appropriate therapy is of value to gauge the effectiveness of treatment. Suspected intrahepatic lesions prior to liver biopsy or surgery, or liver injury after abdominal trauma, may be localized with scanning techniques. Cirrhosis of the liver may be manifested by patchy uptake of radioisotope, probably secondary to diminished hepatic blood flow, and if the preparation used is incorporated by reticuloendothelial cells, the spleen may exhibit increased uptake.

Radioiodinated rose bengal may also be used to test hepatic excretory function. Unlike ^{99m}Tc-sulfur colloid and ^{198}Au colloid, which are taken up from the circulation by the Kupffer cells (macrophages) of the liver, ^{131}I-RB is taken up by the hepatocytes and excreted into bile in a manner similar to that of bilirubin, but without prior conjugation. Measurement of ^{131}I-RB in stool is a useful index of the severity of bile secretory failure or of the completeness of obstruction of extrahepatic biliary drainage, and therefore it is helpful in differentiating severe neonatal hepatitis from extrahepatic biliary atresia. Excretion of more than 10 percent of the administered dose in stool in the 72 hours following intravenous administration of the contrast material suggests that the excretory defect or obstruction is incomplete and is compatible with neonatal hepatitis, whereas excretion of less than 5 percent of the administered dose suggests complete extrahepatic biliary obstruction or atresia. Excretions between 5 and 10 percent are less conclusive. Completeness of collections must be assured, and stool must be carefully separated from urine during the entire period of collection.

An alternative procedure to discriminate between these two conditions has been suggested to eliminate the need for 72 hours of stool collection. Scanning of the abdomen for significant accumulation of radioactivity in the intestinal tract has been shown to correlate significantly with excretion of more than 10 percent of the rose bengal administered. The technique, although simpler, lacks the accuracy and certainty of the stool collection technique and requires administration of approximately 10 times as much ^{131}I. Prior administration of cholestyramine to concentrate the dye in the intestine is said to improve the sensitivity of this test.

Although the relatively small dose of ^{131}I is not likely to damage the thyroid gland, it is advisable to block thyroid gland uptake of radioactive iodine by prior administration of one drop of Lugol's solution, followed by one drop per day for each of the 3 days following ^{131}I-RB administration.

RADIOGRAPHIC TECHNIQUES

Plain radiographs of the abdomen may demonstrate calcifications within the liver or biliary system. Opacities within the liver parenchyma may represent primary or metastatic neoplasms, vascular lesions, cysts, or specific infectious processes, while those in the biliary system usually reflect calculi. On occasion unsuspected air in the biliary tree or portal venous system may also be noted. Fluoroscopy to evaluate movement of the right hemidiaphragm with respiration may be useful in diagnosing a perihepatic abscess or fluid collection.

Radiographic examinations using opaque contrast material are available for study of the biliary tract. Oral cholecystography is used to visualize the gallbladder and cystic duct; intravenous cholangiography is used for the biliary duct system. Nonopaque calculi, appearing as filling defects, are easily identified. However, in the presence of active hepatocellular disease or conjugated hyperbilirubinemia exceeding 3 to 5 mg/dl, neither examination will visualize the biliary structure. Sensitivity to iodides is a contraindication to cholecystography.

Operative cholangiography appears to be safer and more informative than percutaneous transhepatic cholangiography for evaluation of suspected extrahepatic biliary obstruction. However, the future availability of fine and highly flexible needles may make percutaneous cholangiography feasible and useful, even in the newborn. Similarly, choledocho-pancreatico-duodeno-graphy via a fiberoptic gastroscope may prove to be an additional aid in the near future in selected children and adolescents in defining obstructions of the biliary tree without surgical intervention.

Esophagography, splenoportography, and selective angiography and venography are helpful in the diagnosis of portal hypertension in children with or without liver disease. Esophagography with barium sulfate is a moderately accurate technique for the demonstration of esophagogastric varices in children, but is virtually without hazard. Splenoportography with manometry and selective angiography permits evaluation of the patency of the portal system, the caliber of the splenic vein, and the presence of other significant anastomotic channels. However, neither technique is without hazard, especially in the young child; they require highly skilled personnel and specialized equipment.

LIVER BIOPSY

Percutaneous liver biopsy in children by the Menghini method has become a mainstay in the evaluation of serious, protracted, or clinically confusing hepatic dysfunction. The procedure serves as an important diagnostic aid as well as a means of following the course of a variety of liver diseases.

Contraindications to percutaneous hepatic biopsy are severe abnormalities in coagulation, the presumed presence of intrahepatic vascular lesions, cysts, or pyogenic abscesses, and massive ascites. Severe cholestasis from obstructive liver disease is not a contraindication to liver biopsy in pediatrics. Bile peritonitis and bile pleuritis, which are occasionally reported in adult patients after biopsy, are seldom if ever noted in children.

Prior to performance of percutaneous liver biopsy, hematocrit, platelet count, and prothrombin time must be obtained. Blood should be typed and cross-matched, and a surgeon should be available for at least 24 hours after biopsy in the relatively rare event of significant or intractable postbiopsy hemorrhage. A platelet count of less than 75,000/mm^3 or a prolonged prothrombin time increases the risk of intra-abdominal bleeding after biopsy. In such patients if biopsy is still considered essential, fresh frozen plasma and/or platelets may be administered prior to biopsy and again 8 to 12 hours later. Alternatively, an open surgical biopsy may be preferred, but bleeding may remain a problem.

Potentially hepatotoxic medications must be avoided for sedation. Demerol (2 mg/kg) and Phenergan (1 mg/kg) administered intramuscularly about 1 hour before the biopsy are usually adequate. With suspected severe hepatitis, cirrhosis, or hepatic failure premedication should be avoided if possible. If sedation is necessary to achieve the biopsy doses should be reduced by one-half. Using sterile technique the Menghini needle is inserted transthoracically in the anterior axillary line through the diaphragm and into the liver for less than 0.1 sec, while suction is applied with the attached syringe, and a core of liver tissue, approximately 1 cm in length is withdrawn. A compression bandage is applied over the puncture site for the next 24 hours, during which careful observation of the patient's vital signs and hematocrit is essential.

The liver tissue obtained by biopsy is generally processed for light microscopic evaluation using various staining techniques. In selected clinical situations, electron microscopy, histochemical staining, enzymatic determinations, and culture for possible infectious agents are invaluable complementary studies to light microscopic appraisal.

Performance of biopsy in infants and children is safe in experienced hands. The risk of serious complications is probably less than 1 percent. Hemorrhage into the peritoneum, penumothorax, intrahepatic hematoma, arteriovenous fistula, portal vein biliary fistula, bile peritonitis, laceration of the liver or biliary tree, and hemobilia are complications that have been reported. In children the transcostal-transdiaphragmatic route minimizes the risk of laceration of the liver, even if the child takes a breath while the needle is in the liver, and the diaphragm helps to tamponade any bleeding from the liver surface.

ENDOSCOPY

Examination of the upper gastrointestinal tract through a pediatric fiberoptic endoscope is a useful technique that is not yet applicable to the smaller child and infant. In older children and adolescents esophagogastric varices from portal hypertension are easily visualized, and direct catheterization of the common duct through the ampulla of Vater in the duodenum using the fiberoptic endoscope permits direct bile sampling and radiographic examination of the biliary tree.

References

Braunstein P, Song CS: The uses and limitations of radioisotopes in the investigation of gastrointestinal diseases. Am J Dig Dis 20:53, 1975

Cohen MI, Gartner LM, Blumenfeld O, Arias IM: Gamma glutamyl transpeptidase: measurement and development in guinea pig small intestine. Pediatr Res 3:5, 1969

Davidsohn I, Henry JB (eds): Todd-Sanford Clinical Diagnosis by Laboratory Methods, 14th ed. Philadelphia, WB Saunders, 1969

Henley KS, Schmidt E, Schmidt FW: Enzymes in Serum: Their Use in Diagnosis. Springfield, Ill, Charles C Thomas, 1966

Hill PG, Sammons HG: An assessment of 5'-nucleotidase as a liver function test. Q J Med 36:457, 1967

Kaplan MM: Alkaline phosphatase. N Engl J Med 286:200, 1972

Mendeloff AI, Kramer P, Ingelfinger FJ, Bradley SE: Studies with bromsulfalein. II. Factors altering its disappearance from the blood after a single intravenous injection. Gastroenterology 13:222, 1949

Menghini G: One-second biopsy of the liver—problems of its clinical application. N Engl J Med 283:582, 1970

O'Brien D, Rodgerson DO: Interpretation of biochemical values. In Kempe CE, Silver HK, O'Brien D (eds): Current Pediatric Diagnosis and Treatment. Los Altos, 1970, Lange Medical, 1970, p 854

Obrinsky W, Denley ML, Brauer RW: Sulfobromophthalein sodium excretion test as a measure of liver function in premature infants. Pediatrics 9:421, 1952

Osserman EF, Takatsuki K: The plasma proteins in liver disease. Med Clin North Am 47:679, 1963

Porter M, Riley HD Jr, Graham H: Needle biopsy of the liver in infants and children. J Pediatr 65:176, 1964

Salz JL, Daum F, Cohen MI: Serum alkaline phosphatase activity during adolescence. J Pediatr 82:536, 1973

Switzer S: Plasma lipoproteins in the differential diagnosis of liver disease. Gastroenterology 53:790, 1967

Wroblewski F: Serum enzyme alterations in diseases of the liver and biliary tract. Med Clin North Am 44:699, 1960

Yudkin S, Gellis SS, Lappen F: Liver function in newborn infants, with special reference to excretion of bromsulphalein. Arch Dis Child 24:12, 1949

Zein M, Discombe G: Serum gammaglutamyl transpeptidase as a diagnostic acid. Lancet 2:748, 1970

HYPERBILIRUBINEMIA

Unconjugated hyperbilirubinemia can theoretically result either from increased production or from reduced hepatic uptake or conjugation of bilirubin. The functional defect in *conjugated hyperbilirubinemia* is either decreased excretion of conjugated bilirubin by the parenchymal liver cell or damage to the intrahepatic or extrahepatic biliary system. Whenever conjugated bilirubin is increased in serum, the concentration of unconjugated bilirubin is also increased.

UNCONJUGATED NEONATAL HYPERBILIRUBINEMIA
LAWRENCE M. GARTNER

Icterus neonatorum or jaundice of the newborn is a descriptive term encompassing a large variety of diseases and physiologic variations. Moderately elevated serum unconjugated bilirubin concentrations in normal newborn infants are so common that the term physiologic jaundice is often used. Severe unconjugated hyperbilirubinemia results from superimposition of additional factors on the physiologic limitations present in the normal neonate. Conjugated hyperbilirubinemia in the newborn is infrequent and results from hepatic biliary tract, or rarely hematologic, pathology (p. 1085).

Physiologic Jaundice of the Newborn

Serum unconjugated bilirubin concentrations transiently exceed 2.0 mg/dl during the first week of life in approximately 90 percent of all newborn infants. Clinical icterus is not usually detectable during the first 24 hours of life unless there is hemolytic disease or some other superimposed disorder. The average maximum serum bilirubin concentration in normal full-term infants is approximately 6 mg/dl and will occur during the second to fourth days of life. In premature infants the rate of increase in serum bilirubin concentration is similar to that in full-term infants, but the higher mean maximal levels of 10 to 12 mg/dl are not reached until the fifth to seventh days of life. Serum unconjugated bilirubin concentrations attained in physiologic jaundice are not associated with kernicterus in full-term infants, but they may be in preterm infants under certain circumstances (see below and also p. 1138). Concentrations of serum bilirubin exceeding 10 mg/dl in full-term infants and 14 mg/dl in premature infants suggest that additional factors are superimposed on the normally occurring physiologic jaundice. In full-term infants serum bilirubin concentrations may remain elevated above the normal adult level of 1.0 mg/dl for up to 12 days, while in premature infants normal bilirubin concentrations may not be achieved until the second month of life. The diagnosis of physiologic jaundice may be considered in any newborn with mild unconjugated hyperbilirubinemia, but it is only established by excluding known causes of neonatal jaundice. For this reason all jaundiced newborn infants should have the following laboratory tests performed: (1) maternal blood group and Rh types; (2) infant blood group, Rh type, and Coombs' test; (3) total and and direct-reacting serum bilirubin concentrations; (4) hemoglobin or hematocrit determination; (5) examination of erythrocyte morphology; (6) reticulocyte count; (7) white blood cell count and urinalysis. In infants with severe hyperbilirubinemia more extensive studies are indicated to rule out the disorders enumerated in the following section.

The etiology of physiologic jaundice is not fully understood, although mechanisms to explain its development have been suggested. Since the bilirubin in these infants is unconjugated, four possible mechanisms can be considered: (1) increased production of bilirubin either from destruction of mature, circulating erythrocytes or from other sources; (2) impairment of uptake of bilirubin from plasma by the liver cell; (3) defective hepatic conjugation of bilirubin with glucuronic acid; (4) increased enterohepatic circulation of bilirubin:

1. Survival times of circulating erythrocytes in full-term and premature infants are significantly reduced, to approximately 70 to 90 days as compared to 120 days in the normal adult or older child. This could double the rate of bilirubin synthesis, but it would not alone account for the concentrations of bilirubin observed in newborns. Excessive synthesis of bilirubin from sources other than circulating erythrocytes must also be considered, since the newborn has a vast amount of erythropoietic tissue at the time of birth. Within the first 2 days of life erythropoiesis virtually ceases. It is likely that much of the residual heme in this inactive erythropoietic tissue is degraded in the same manner as that of the circulating erythrocytes, contributing significantly to an increased rate of bilirubin synthesis. In the newborn rhesus monkey bilirubin production and/or enteric reabsorption of bilirubin are increased sevenfold over those observed in the adult monkey.

2. Transport of bilirubin from serum into the liver cell has not been investigated in newborn human infants because of the unavailability of suitable techniques. It has been demonstrated, however, that newborn guinea pigs and monkeys have markedly defective hepatic uptake of bilirubin. Furthermore, ligandin (Y protein), the major hepatic cytoplasmic organic anion-binding protein, is relatively deficient in the newborn guinea pig, monkey, and man, thus suggesting that this deficiency may limit hepatic uptake of bilirubin. Reduced hepatic blood flow in neonates may also retard transport of unconjugated bilirubin from plasma into

the liver. Studies in newborn monkeys suggest that the slow return of the serum bilirubin to normal in the healthy neonate may result from combined relative deficiency in hepatic uptake of bilirubin and from the increased load of bilirubin presented to the liver.

3. Deficiencies in hepatic glucuronide-conjugating pathways have been demonstrated in newborn infants and animals. In newborn guinea pigs, uridine diphosphoglucose dehydrogenase activity is reduced, thus decreasing production of uridine diphosphoglucuronic acid (UDPGA). It is not known, however, whether the availability of UDPGA is a limiting factor in bilirubin glucuronide formation during the newborn period. Deficiency of glucuronyl transferase activity has generally been considered to be responsible for physiologic jaundice, but definitive studies to establish the rate-limiting step in overall transfer of bilirubin from plasma to bile in newborns with physiologic jaundice have not been performed until recently. Studies in the newborn rhesus monkey reveal that the early phase of physiologic jaundice results from deficiency of glucuronyl transferase activity combined with an excessive load of bilirubin presented to the liver. In this early phase (usually up to days 3 to 5 in the human) conjugation is the rate-limiting step. If conjugation were normal, increased bilirubin load alone should be insufficient to produce bilirubin retention. The degree of conjugating deficiency, although severe, should be insufficient to produce physiologic jaundice in the absence of an increased bilirubin load. Glucuronyl transferase activity probably reaches normal adult levels by the end of the second week of life, as judged from studies in both newborn guinea pigs and monkeys. The relative inability of the liver of the newborn infant to form glucuronides also accounts for impaired drug metabolism and for consequent toxicity, such as the peripheral vascular collapse (gray baby syndrome) observed following administration of relatively large doses of chloramphenicol to neonates (p. 406). In the premature exaggerated pattern of physiologic jaundice (with occasional pathologic sequelae) appears to result primarily from a marked delay in the rate of maturation of glucuronyl transferase.

Although factors regulating maturation of glucuronyl transferase activity are unknown, inhibition of the enzyme may be biologically important. Urine and serum obtained from normal women during the second and third trimesters of pregnancy inhibit hepatic glucuronyl transferase activity in vitro. Several progestational steroids isolated from pregnancy sera competitively inhibit glucuronyl transferase activity in vitro. Attempts to correlate inhibition of glucuronyl transferase activity by normal maternal sera with the occurrence and severity of physiologic jaundice have been unsuccessful. Markedly increased serum levels of inhibition are also observed, however, in the syndrome of transient familial neonatal hyperbilirubinemia (p. 1079). Pregnane-3α, 20β-diol, an inhibitory steroid, has been isolated from the milk of certain mothers and is associated with prolonged unconjugated hyperbilirubinemia in their breast-fed infants.

4. In newborn infants, unlike older children, bilirubin is probably not chemically reduced to urobilinogens in the intestine because of the limited number of enteric bacteria. Therefore excess unconjugated bilirubin in the intestinal tract may theoretically result in increased absorption by the intestinal mucosa, thus presenting an exaggerated load of bilirubin to the liver. Meconium also may contribute to increased enteric reabsorbtion of bilirubin in the neonate, since it contains a large quantity of bilirubin. Oral administration of substances such as agar, which bind bilirubin and prevent its intestinal reabsorption, reduce the severity of physiologic jaundice.

SEVERE OR PROLONGED UNCONJUGATED HYPERBILIRUBINEMIA OF THE NEWBORN
LAWRENCE M. GARTNER

Many factors or diseases may be superimposed on the normally occurring physiologic jaundice of the newborn, which results in severe or prolonged unconjugated hyperbilirubinemia, sometimes with increased risk of kernicterus. Among these are (1) exaggerated erythrocyte destruction, (2) inherited deficiency of glucuronyl transferase (types I and II), (3) breast-feeding jaundice, (4) transient familial neonatal hyperbilirubinemia, (5) drug-related jaundice, (6) maternal diabetes and jaundice, (7) pyloric stenosis and jaundice, (8) miscellaneous (hypothyroidism, hypoxia, mongolism, starvation).

Exaggerated Erythrocyte Destruction

The classic situation in which severe hyperbilirubinemia of the newborn results from exaggerated erythrocyte destruction is erythroblastosis fetalis secondary to Rh or major blood group incompatibility between infant and mother. The pathogenesis of this syndrome is discussed elsewhere (p. 1134). Although the excessive destruction of erythrocytes and production of bilirubin in this disease usually begin in utero, the serum bilirubin concentration in cord blood is either normal or only modestly increased. The placenta is capable of transporting unconjugated bilirubin from fetal to maternal plasma for excretion by maternal liver. In cases of severe erythroblastosis, particularly following successful intrauterine transfusion, cord-blood direct-reacting bilirubin concentrations up to 40 mg/dl have been observed. Markedly elevated direct-reacting bilirubin concentrations may persist for 1 to 2 weeks in these cases. These and other observations suggest that the human placenta cannot efficiently transfer conjugated bilirubin and that severe hemolytic disease with marked increase in bilirubin production either stimulates hepatic uptake and conjugation of bilirubin or reduces the already limited hepatic excretory capacity for bilirubin in utero.

Infants with severe hemolytic disease become clinically icteric as early as 30 minutes after delivery. With less severe hemolysis, icterus may not be observed until after the second day of life. In some infants with significant hemolysis, jaundice does not become severe, which suggests that in these infants hepatic uptake, conjugation, and excretion are adequate to handle the increased load.

During the neonatal period hemolysis may also occur as a result of congenital spherocytosis, pyknocytosis, minor blood group incompatibilities, sepsis, and resorption of blood from hematomas or ecchymoses. Deficiency of erythrocyte glucose-6-phosphate dehydrogenase (G-6-PD) activity (p. 1169). may result in episodic hemolysis during the neonatal period, which may occur without a known inciting agent, after exposure to certain drugs such as phenacetin or chemicals such as naphthalene, or with infection. Hemolysis may follow administration of large doses of vitamin K$_3$ to either mother or newborn, ingestion of mothballs containing naphthalene prior to parturition, or inhalation of naphthalene vapors by neonates.

Hemolysis in G-6-PD-deficient individuals may occur at any time in life. In older individuals hemolysis more commonly results in anemia without icterus, whereas during the neonatal period, when hepatic mechanisms are relatively deficient, icterus almost always develops. In general, hemolysis occurring during the first week of life produces predominantly unconjugated hyperbilirubinemia. After the second week of life, hemolysis may be associated with significantly increased serum concentrations of both conjugated and unconjugated bilirubin, particularly if there is coexistent hepatic damage. The use of vitamin K$_3$ has been discontinued; it has been replaced by vitamin K$_1$. Administration of 1.0 mg of vitamin K$_1$ oxide to newborns with or without G-6-PD deficiency does not produce hemolytic disease and yet is more than adequate to prevent hemorrhagic disease of the newborn.

Large numbers of infants with G-6-PD deficiency and severe neonatal hyperbilirubinemia have been described in many areas of the world, particularly in Greece. In Israel, however, where there is a high incidence of G-6-PD deficiency in certain portions of the population, the incidence of associated neonatal jaundice is low. This difference suggests that an additional factor may be operative in those infants who develop marked hyperbilirubinemia. Infants with severe hyperbilirubinemia and G-6-PD deficiency may require exchange transfusion if kernicterus is to be prevented. The diagnosis of G-6-PD deficiency requires demonstration of increased hemolysis and reduced erythrocyte G-6-PD activity.

Inherited Deficiency of Glucuronyl Transferase Activity

Two forms of lifelong glucuronyl transferase deficiency may be clearly distinguished on the basis of clinical, chemical, and genetic findings. The type I abnormality has previously been called the Crigler-Najjar syndrome. The type II syndrome was described more recently and is often not recognized until adolescence or later, although it may present as exaggerated neonatal jaundice.

Type I glucuronyl transferase deficiency is a rare syndrome inherited as an autosomal recessive and characterized by the onset of severe jaundice within the first 3 days of life. Unconjugated hyperbilirubinemia persists throughout life at serum concentrations ranging from 20 to 32 mg/dl as a result of an almost total inability of the liver to conjugate bilirubin with glucuronic acid. In the absence of repeated exchange transfusions, many infants develop kernicterus resulting in death during the first week of life. Patients with the type I syndrome who survive the first weeks of life often have severe neurologic impairment. Occasional individuals reach childhood without neurologic signs, even without exchange transfusions. These survivors occasionally develop signs of kernicterus later in life. Hepatic glucuronyl transferase activity measured in vitro is virtually absent in these individuals when bilirubin is used as the glucuronide receptor. With other substrates used either in vitro (O-aminophenol) or in vivo (menthol or salicylamide), hepatic conjugating activity is reduced or absent. Gallbladder is very light in color and contains little bilirubin and no bilirubin glucuronide. Both parents have a partial deficiency (approximately 50 percent of normal) in the ability to form glucuronides of bilirubin and other substrates both in vivo and in vitro, although they do not have hyperbilirubinemia. A similar enzymatic defect has been found in a mutant strain of Wistar rats (Gunn) that also have lifelong unconjugated hyperbilirubinemia and develop kernicterus during the neonatal period. The Gunn rat has a normal capacity for the excretion of administered conjugated bilirubin.

The second type of glucuronyl transferase deficiency (type II) is similar to the first but is characterized by greater variation in the serum bilirubin concentration from one affected individual to another. The range of unconjugated serum bilirubin concentrations observed is from normal to 22 mg/dl. The mode of inheritance appears to be that of an autosomal dominant with marked variability in penetrance, which accounts for those individuals with detectable defects in glucuronyl transferase activity but normal or only mild elevations of serum bilirubin concentration. Abnormalities of conjugation and a history of chronic jaundice are found only in one parent and in members of one parental lineage. Gallbladder bile is pigmented and contains traces of bilirubin glucuronide. In this syndrome, as in the type I, glucuronyl transferase activity is markedly deficient. Although some patients may not be noted to be icteric until adolescence, chronic hyperbilirubinemia may begin during the first days of life, and kernicterus, although very rare in the type II syndrome, has been reported in two cases. The type I and type II syndromes are not known to have occurred in the same families.

Administration of phenobarbital in doses of 5 mg/kg/day to children and 30 to 90 mg/day to adults with the type II disorder of glucuronyl transferase results in dramatic decreases of the serum bilirubin concentration within 1 to 2 weeks. Similar administration to patients with the type I disorder does not change the serum bilirubin concentration. The mechanism of the response to phenobarbital is uncertain. The observed differences between types I and II probably reflect differences in the structure of a single glucuronyl transferase or in the control of protein synthesis. The administration of phenobarbital offers a relatively simple means for differentiation of the two syndromes and reduction of hyperbilirubinemia in patients with type II glucuronyl transferase deficiency.

Either of these two syndromes may be suspected in a newborn whose serum bilirubin concentration either continues to rise into the second week of life or does not decline at that time. In the absence of hemolytic disease, hypothyroidism, intestinal obstruction, or breast feeding, the diagnosis is more strongly suspected, but efforts to rule out other causes of prolonged or persisting unconjugated hyperbilirubinemia must be undertaken. Chronic unconjugated hyerbilirubinemia in one parent strengthens the likelihood of the infant having the type II syndrome.

A definitive diagnosis requires persistence of hyperbilirubinemia beyond the fourth week of life, demonstration of deficient hepatic conjugation either in vivo or in liver in vitro, and appropriate deficiencies in one or both parents. Recovery of bile by duodenal intubation and demonstration of concentrations of bilirubin in bile below 5 mg/dl support the diagnosis of type I syndrome.

The management of the newborn with either of these two syndromes requires maintenance of serum bilirubin concentrations below 20 mg/dl for the first 3 to 4 weeks of age. In the type I syndrome repeated exchange transfusions are not feasible for this period of time, and most clinicians have utilized phototherapy to reduce the serum bilirubin concentrations. It is not known whether this method of treatment reliably prevents brain damage from bilirubin encephalopathy, but there is no other suitable therapy for long-term management. Prevention of hypoxia, acidosis, infection, hypothermia, and hypoglycemia may reduce the risk of kernicterus.

If there is marked reduction in serum bilirubin concentration following phenobarbital administration, thus leading to the presumptive diagnosis of type II syndrome, the drug should be stopped for a brief period of time to demonstrate a rise in bilirubin and a second decline when phenobarbital treatment is reinstituted.

BREAST-FEEDING JAUNDICE. Approximately 1 in every 200 breast-fed infants develops severe and prolonged unconjugated hyperbilirubinemia that cannot be explained by any other mechanism than breast feeding. Unlike infants with erythroblastosis fetalis, transient familial neonatal hyperbilirubinemia, or inherited glucuronyl transferase deficiency, severe jaundice is not present in these breast-fed infants during the early days of life. Significant elevations develop on the fourth to seventh days of life. Maximum concentrations of serum unconjugated bilirubin, in some cases as high as 15 to 25 mg/dl, occur during the second and third weeks. Following this period, hyperbilirubinemia gradually decreases and may either disappear by the end of the third week or persist for as long as 10 weeks.

Interruption of nursing for 2 to 4 days results in rapid decline in hyperbilirubinemia, while interruption of nursing for 6 to 9 days usually returns the serum bilirubin concentration to normal. Except for jaundice, these infants appear entirely well and are thriving. Approximately 75 percent of infants nursed by these mothers develop the syndrome. Kernicterus has not been observed, presumably because the peak concentrations of unconjugated bilirubin occur after the end of the first week of life. Kernicterus can occur during this time of life in full-term otherwise healthy infants, but only with serum bilirubin concentrations higher than those that *usually* occur in this syndrome. Breast milk obtained from the mothers of infants with this syndrome contains pregnane-3α,20β-diol, which competitively inhibits glucuronyl transferase in vitro. Administration of this same compound to newborn infants at the end of the first week of life produces significant reversible unconjugated hyperbilirubinemia. The isomer found normally in urine and serum, but not in milk, of both pregnant and nonpregnant women, is pregnane-3α,-20α-diol, an equally inhibitory steroid. During lactation, and only during lactation, these women excrete increased amounts of the abnormal isomer in urine as well as in milk, which suggests that the actively secreting mammary tissue is the source of the abnormal steroid. Several recent studies have demonstrated that certain free fatty acids (especially linoleic acid) are potent inhibitors of glucuronyl transferase in vitro and that milk from the mothers of infants with the breast-feeding jaundice syndrome contains increased concentrations of the inhibitory free fatty acids. The relationship between pregnanediol and free fatty acids in milk has not yet been studied. The ability of linoleic acid to produce jaundice in infants has not been determined. In contrast to the syndrome of transient familial neonatal hyperbilirubinemia (see below), sera from these nursing mothers does not significantly inhibit glucuronyl transferase activity.

Despite continuation of breast feeding, hyperbilirubinemia gradually disappears in all of these infants, accompanied in some cases by a spontaneous and concurrent disappearance of inhibitor from the milk. In other cases the inhibitor remains in the milk over a prolonged period, and disappearance of jaundice must be attributed to maturation of the infant's hepatic glucuronyl transferase activity.

Although this syndrome may be suspected on the basis of the family history and the temporal relationship of jaundice to breast feeding, a definite diagnosis requires demonstration of inhibition of glucuronyl transferase by milk in vitro. All other causes of unconjugated hyperbilirubinemia must be excluded, since they may present in a similar manner. The occurrence of this syndrome in breast-fed infants should not lead to the interdiction of breast feeding of infants with this syndrome or of infants in general. Despite their jaundice, infants with the breast-feeding jaundice syndrome are vigorous and do not suffer any sequelae from it. In those rare cases when hyperbilirubinemia exceeds 20 mg/dl during the first 3 weeks of life, interruption of

nursing for 2 to 4 days will usually result in significant reduction of hyperbilirubinemia. Resumption of nursing will produce only a small increase of 1 to 3 mg/dl of sera, followed by a progressive slow decline. If the serum bilirubin concentration is less than 20 mg/dl and is either stable or falling slowly, and the child is clinically well and has been in the past, nursing should not be interrupted.

TRANSIENT FAMILIAL NEONATAL HYPERBILIRUBINEMIA. In this rare syndrome all infants born to the mother develop severe unconjugated hyperbilirubinemia within the first 4 days of life. Jaundice spontaneously subsides during the second to third weeks of life. These infants frequently develop kernicterus unless an exchange transfusion is performed. Known causes of severe hyperbilirubinemia have been excluded in these infants. Sera obtained from normal women during the second and third trimesters of pregnancy and immediately following delivery inhibit glucuronyl transferase activity to a small degree in vitro. Sera from mothers of infants with transient familial neonatal hyperbilirubinemia, and sera from the infants themselves, are 4 to 10 times more inhibitory. The inhibitory effect of maternal sera gradually decreases, becoming normal by about the fourteenth postpartum day. Inhibition by infant sera is slightly less than that observed with maternal sera, but it follows a similar course. The inhibitor has not been identified; the association with pregnancy suggests that it is a progestational steroid. Although the syndrome is familial, inheritance of the disorder has not been demonstrated. Diagnosis requires demonstration of increased inhibition of glucuronyl transferase activity by sera from mother and infant in vitro.

DRUG-RELATED JAUNDICE. The administration of several drugs to neonates is associated with exaggerated unconjugated hyperbilirubinemia, either as a result of hemolysis or interference with hepatic conjugation of bilirubin. Vitamin K_3 given in large doses to newborns or to pregnant women at term may cause hemolysis in the newborn, especially in the presence of G-6-PD deficiency. In recent years this problem has been avoided by use of vitamin K_1 oxide instead of vitamin K_3.

In years past, administration of the antibiotic novobiocin to newborn infants increased the incidence of severe unconjugated hyperbilirubinemia approximately threefold. Novobiocin is a noncompetitive inhibitor of glucuronyl transferase in vitro. The increased frequency with which inhibitors of glucuronyl transferase produce unconjugated hyperbilirubinemia in neonates may result from the relatively low endogenous activity of the enzyme in neonatal liver. Although streptomycin and chloramphenicol also inhibit glucuronyl transferase activity in vitro, neither of these antibiotics has ever been noted to increase the severity or frequency of jaundice in neonates, nor do any other antibiotics currently in use.

MATERNAL DIABETES AND JAUNDICE. Compared with normal infants of the same gestational age, infants of women with either frank or gestational diabetes have an increased incidence and prolongation of neonatal unconjugated hyperbilirubinemia. These infants also have higher hemoglobin concentrations than normal, which could result in increased bilirubin formation. It is not known whether this factor or possible derangements in endocrine factors that alter hepatic bilirubin metabolism result in exaggerated hyperbilirubinemia. Early feeding (prior to 12 hours of age) reduces the intensity of hyperbilirubinemia in these infants.

PYLORIC STENOSIS AND JAUNDICE. Infants with pyloric stenosis (p.1019) occasionally develop unconjugated hyperbilirubinemia coincident with the onset of vomiting, or more rarely they have persistent unremitting jaundice from birth. Serum bilirubin concentrations may be as high as 5 to 20 mg/dl. Although two infants with this syndrome have been reported to have direct-reacting hyperbilirubinemia and mechanical obstruction of the common bile duct, this has not been found in any other case. With careful search for elevated serum bilirubin concentrations in infants with pyloric stenosis, it may be found that hyperbilirubinemia is more common than was realized merely from the appearance of clinical jaundice in infants with pyloric stenosis. Chemical studies of hepatic function, radiographic studies of the bile ducts, and histologic examination of liver biopsy specimens are normal. Neither the severity of pyloric obstruction nor the degree of dehydration and electrolyte imbalance correlates with the occurrence of jaundice. Pyloromyotomy is usually followed by rapid disappearance of hyperbilirubinemia. Congenital obstruction of either the duodenum or jejunum is also associated with an increased incidence of severe unconjugated hyperbilirubinemia, as is Hirschsprung's disease or any other cause of obstipation. The mechanism by which intestinal obstruction causes jaundice is unknown, but it may relate to enhancement of intestinal bilirubin reabsorption and/or reduction in glucuronyl transferase activity.

MISCELLANEOUS CONDITIONS ASSOCIATED WITH NEONATAL UNCONJUGATED HYPERBILIRUBINEMIA. Anoxia and respiratory distress during the first few days of life may increase the incidence and severity of unconjugated hyperbilirubinemia, particularly in premature infants. Experimental birth asphyxia in monkeys increases the severity of the normally occurring neonatal unconjugated hyperbilirubinemia.

The interval between birth and the onset of feeding may be related to the severity of unconjugated hyperbilirubinemia in premature infants. Studies on this question in premature infants are not in agreement, although early feeding of infants of diabetic mothers does reduce the severity of the unconjugated hyperbilirubinemia.

Prolonged and sometimes severe unconjugated hyperbilirubinemia is seen in approximately 10 percent of infants with congenital hypothyroidism. The mechanism is unknown. Congenital hypothyroidism should always be considered in an infant with prolonged neonatal jaundice.

KERNICTERUS

LAWRENCE M. GARTNER

Kernicterus or bilirubin encephalopathy is characterized pathologically by bilirubin staining and necrosis of neurons in the basal ganglia, hippocampal cortex, and subthalamic nuclei of the brain. Other areas of the central nervous system are less commonly affected. The clinical syndrome and pathologic lesions result from entry of unconjugated bilirubin into neurons, which causes a toxic encephalopathy. Conjugated hyperbilirubinemia does not cause kernicterus.

Kernicterus may present clinically as lethargy, rigidity, opisthotonus, high-pitched cry, fever, and convulsions; it may result in death. Survivors often have cerebral palsy, frequently of the choreoathetoid type, deafness, mental retardation, and other neurologic defects in infancy or early childhood. These late manifestations of kernicterus may also occur in some infants without clinical signs of bilirubin encephalopathy in the newborn period. Subtle forms of brain damage, such as diminished cognitive function, may be late sequelae of bilirubin encephalopathy in the absence of any other neurologic impairments. Premature infants are particularly susceptible to this type of insult.

Bilirubin encephalopathy is most likely to occur during the third to seventh days of life, but it may develop at older ages, including adolescence in those children with persisting severe unconjugated hyperbilirubinemia. From a small number of neonatal cases, statistical evidence supporting the concept of a critical serum concentration of unconjugated bilirubin above which a significant number of infants will develop kernicterus has been accumulated only for full-term infants with erythroblastosis. An unconjugated serum bilirubin concentration of 20 mg/dl or greater occurring during the first week of life is accepted as an indication for exchange transfusion in such infants. Critical serum bilirubin concentrations have not been established for full-term infants without hemolytic disease or for premature infants with or without hemolytic disease. It is extremely unlikely that a single serum bilirubin concentration, even when adjusted for gestational age, birth weight, or prior clinical condition, could predict the development of bilirubin-related brain damage. In premature infants kernicterus can occur at serum bilirubin concentrations as low as 9.0 mg/dl, especially when associated with hemolytic disease, asphyxia, respiratory distress syndrome, hypoglycemia, acidosis, sepsis, meningitis, and hypothermia. In low-birth-weight infants with these complications, serum bilirubin concentrations lower than those in infants without such complications should be taken as an indication for exchange transfusion. Table 1 lists the serum bilirubin concentrations recommended as levels that should not be exceeded during the first 14 days of life, adjusted by birth weight and clinical status. Sudden deterioration or change in clinical status may be an early and unexpected sign of bilirubin encephalopathy that indicates the need for immediate exchange transfusion. It is not known to what degree bilirubin-dependent brain damage is reversible.

Of great importance in the development of kernicterus is the capacity of serum albumin to bind unconjugated bilirubin, thus enabling bilirubin to remain in solution in plasma. Reduction in total albumin concentration, displacement of bilirubin from albumin, or reduction in albumin binding capacity or affinity of bilirubin will increase the amount of unbound or potentially unbound bilirubin in the circulation. This may increase deposition of unconjugated bilirubin in many tissues, including the brain, and may result in reduction of serum bilirubin concentrations. Physiologic derangements such as acidosis or marked increase in unesterified fatty acids due to either starvation or hypothermia may also alter albumin binding of bilirubin. Certain drugs, particularly sulfonamides, markedly increase the risk of developing kernicterus, presumably by altering the binding of bilirubin to albumin. Recent studies using newer techniques for estimation of plasma protein binding capacity suggest that minimal brain damage in some older children correlates with poor albumin binding reserve, despite only moderate elevations of unconjugated bilirubin during the newborn period. The use of some of these newer dye-binding and chromatographic techniques would be expected to indicate more precisely which infants require treatment and which do not, independently of serum bilirubin concentrations. The actual benefits from the use of these techniques require further evaluation, however.

In severe erythroblastosis the aim of therapy is to alleviate the anemia, prevent further hemolysis, restore the blood volume to normal, and prevent kernicterus by removal of unconjugated bilirubin. In the forms of hyperbilirubinemia not associated with hemolysis, the major object of therapy should be to prevent brain damage. Exchange transfusion has for many years been the standard mode of therapy in both hemolytic and nonhemolytic hyperbilirubinemia. The risk of the procedure and the length of time required for its performance have led to development of other means of removal of bilirubin. The administration of phenobarbital to patients with type II glucuronyl transferase deficiency results in a marked decrease in serum bilirubin concentrations, presumably due to stimulation of the deficient conjugating enzyme. Similar treatment of pregnant women during the last trimester of pregnancy and of the infants immediately following delivery has been shown to reduce the peak concentration of bilirubin in infants with physiologic jaundice. A dose of approximately 5 mg/kg/day has been used for newborns and 60 mg/day for mothers. Treatment of the newborn infant alone, without prior treatment of the mother during pregnancy, is also effective, but to a lesser degree. At least 2 or 3 days of treatment of the infant are required before any effect is observed. Therefore this is not suitable therapy for an infant who develops hyperbilirubinemia during the second or third day of life. Phenobarbital probably increases hepatic bilirubin excretion, both by stimulation of glucuronyl transferase activity and by enhancement of hepatic uptake of bilirubin resulting from increased synthesis of the hepatic cytoplasmic bilirubin-binding protein Y. Since phenobarbital has respiratory depressant effects and may adversely alter other enzyme systems and result in maternal and neonatal addiction, its use is not without potential danger, and it requires careful observation of the infant. At the present time phenobarbital is recommended only for those mothers with documented high risk for a severely affected infant with erythroblastosis or some other cause of severe neonatal jaundice. For this type of infant, prior treatment with phenobarbital will reduce the number of exchange transfusions required.

Phototherapy

Exposure of infants to increased intensities of light in the visible range, particularly blue light (wavelengths between 420 and 470 nm), results in increased oxidation of bilirubin or conversion by other mechanisms to products that are not yet fully identified. Studies in animals and more limited studies in infants have demonstrated that the photo-oxidation products of bilirubin are excreted in urine and bile as water-soluble materials. Increased excretion of unconjugated bilirubin in bile has also been demonstrated in rats and humans following phototherapy. Normal full-term and premature infants exposed to fluorescent light for periods of 1 to 3 days demonstrate peak serum bilirubin concentrations approximately one-half those of infants not exposed to increased light intensities. The effectiveness of phototherapy in infants with hemolytic disease is less predictable. Although the use of phototherapy has become widespread throughout the United States, there are still many unanswered questions regarding its

TABLE 1. Recommended Maximal Total Serum Bilirubin Concentrations (mg/dl)[a]

	Birth Weight (g)				
	less than 1250	1250–1499	1500–1999	2000–2499	2500
Uncomplicated course	13	15	17	18	20
Complicated course[b]	10	13	15	17	18

[a] *Direct-reacting bilirubin concentrations are not subtracted unless they amount to more than 50 percent of the total serum bilirubin concentration.*
[b] *Complications include perinatal asphyxia and acidosis, postnatal hypoxia and acidosis, significant and persistent hypothermia, hypoalbuminemia, meningitis and other significant infection, hemolysis and hypoglycemia.*

safety and effectiveness. The major question is whether phototherapy is effective in preventing the development of either frank kernicterus during the newborn period or milder forms of brain damage thought to be associated with bilirubin toxicity. Phototherapy may or may not have direct effects on plasma protein binding of bilirubin, circadian rhythms, physical growth, or neurologic development. Whether light exposure should be continuous or intermittent, and which intensities and wavelengths should be used, also require further evaluation. It has been generally agreed, however, that the infant's eyes must be covered during the period of light exposure to prevent possible retinal damage.

If phototherapy is to be used, it is essential that therapy be initiated at serum bilirubin concentrations well below those considered to place the baby at risk of kernicterus, since it may require 12 to 24 hours before a reduction in serum concentration is effected. Should phototherapy be ineffective, exchange transfusion should be undertaken when the critical level is reached (Table 1).

References

Arias IM, Gartner LM, Cohen M, et al: Chronic non-hemolytic unconjugated hyperbilirubinemia with glucuronyl transferase deficiency: clinical, biochemical, pharmacologic and genetic evidence for heterogeneity. Am J Med 47:395, 1969

———— Gartner LM, Seifter S, Furman M: Prolonged neonatal unconjugated hyperbilirubinemia associated with breast feeding and a steroid, pregnane-3-(α), 20(β)-diol, in maternal milk that inhibits glucuronide formation in vitro. J Clin Invest 43:2037, 1964

———— Wolfson S, Lucey JF, et al: Transient familial neonatal hyperbilirubinemia. J Clin Invest 44:1442, 1965

Behrman RE, Hsia DYY: Summary of a symposium on phototherapy for hyperbilirubinemia. J Pediatr 75:718, 1969

Blanc WA, Johnson L: Studies on Kernicterus. J Neuropathol Exp Neurol 18:165, 1959

Boggs TR Jr, Bishop H: Neonatal hyperbilirubinemia associated with high obstruction of the small bowel. J Pediatr 66:349, 1965

———— Hardy JB, Frazier TM: Correlation of neonatal serum total bilirubin concentrations and developmental status at age eight months. J Pediatr 71:533, 1967

Brown AK, Zuelzer WW: Studies on the neonatal development of the glucuronide conjugating system. J Clin Invest 37:332, 1958

Crigler JF, Najjar VA: Congenital familial nonhemolytic jaundice with kernicterus. Pediatrics 10:169, 1952

Doxiadis SA, Valaes T: The clinical picture of glucose-6-phosphate dehydrogenase deficiency in early infancy. Arch Dis Child 39:545, 1964

Gartner LM, Arias IM: Studies of prolonged neonatal jaundice in the breast-fed infant. J Pediatr 68:54, 1966

———— The transfer of bilirubin from blood to bile in the neonatal guinea pig. Pediatr Res 3:171, 1969

———— Bernstein J: Kernicterus and prematurity: the development of nuclear jaundice at relatively low serum concentrations of bilirubin. Jewish Memorial Hosp Bull 10:125, 1965

———— Snyder R, Chabon RS, Bernstein J: Kernicterus: high incidence in premature infants with low serum bilirubin concentrations. Pediatrics 45:906, 1970

———— Hollander M: Disorders of bilirubin metabolism. In Assali N (ed): Pathophysiology of Gestation, Vol III. New York, Academic, 1972 p 455

———— Lee KS: Bilirubin binding, free fatty acids and a new concept for the pathogenesis of kernicterus. In Blondheim SH (ed): Proceedings of the International Symposium on Bilirubin Metabolism in the Newborn. New York, National Foundation, 1975

———— The functional basis of physiologic jaundice of the newborn. In Goresky CA, Fisher MM, (eds): Jaundice, Vol 2. New York, Plenum, 1975, p 257

Hsia DYY, Allen FH Jr, Gellis SS, Diamond LK: Erythroblastosis fetalis. VIII. Studies of serum bilirubin in relation to kernicterus. N Engl J Med 247:668, 1952

———— Dowben RM, Shaw R, Grossman A: Inhibition of glucuronyl transferase by progestational agents from serum of pregnant women. Nature 187:693, 1960

Johnson JD: Current Concepts: neonatal nonhemolytic jaundice. N Engl J Med 292:194, 1975

Kandall S, Saldana LR, Gartner LM: Hemolytic disease of the newborn (erythroblastosis fetalis). In Conn HF (ed): Current Therapy, 1975. Philadelphia, WB Saunders, 1975, p 246

Lathe GH, Walker M: The synthesis of bilirubin glucuronide in animal and human liver. Biochem J 70:705, 1958

Lee KS, Gartner LM, Zarafu I: Fluorescent dye method for determination of the bilirubin-binding capacity of serum albumin. J Pediatr 86:280, 1975

Lischner HW: Genesis of neonatal jaundice. Biochem Clin 3:57, 1964

Maisels MJ: Bilirubin: on understanding and influencing its metabolism in the newborn infant. Pediatr Clin North Am 19:447, 1972

McKay RJ Jr, Lucey JF: Bilirubin metabolism and "physiologic" jaundice. N Engl J Med 270:1292, 1964

Phototherapy in the Newborn. Final Report of the Committee on Phototherapy in the Newborn. Washington, DC, National Research Council. National Academy of Sciences, 1974

Taylor PM, Wolfson JH, Bright NH, et al: Hyperbilirubinemia in infants of diabetic mothers. Biol Neonate 5:289, 1963

Thaler MM: Neonatal hyperbilirubinemia. Semin Hematol 9:107, 1972

Vaisman S; Gartner LM: Pharmacologic treatment of neonatal hyperbilirubinemia. Clinics in Perinatology 2:37, 1975

Wolfson S, Arias IM, Lucey JF, McKay RJ Jr: Transient familial neonatal hyperbilirubinemia. J Clin Invest 44:1442, 1965

UNCONJUGATED HYPERBILIRUBINEMIA IN THE OLDER CHILD

IRWIN M. ARIAS

Whereas developmental aspects of bilirubin metabolism influence the pathogenesis of congenital as well as acquired jaundice in neonates, jaundice in older children usually results from diseases and mechanisms similar to those found in adults. Some of the acquired or inherited syndromes seen in adults may have their onset in childhood or during adolescence. In older children and adults the first clinical manifestation of hyperbilirubinemia is jaundice of the sclerae, which is observed when the serum bilirubin concentration exceeds approximately 2 mg/dl.

Unconjugated Hyperbilirubinemia With Hemolysis

Hemolytic disease or ineffective erythropoiesis occurring in the older child with a normal liver is rarely associated with unconjugated hyperbilirubinemia in excess of 3 to 4 mg/dl. Hemolysis in association with liver disease such as cirrhosis or hepatitis results in predominantly conjugated hyperbilirubinemia because of further restriction of hepatic excretory capacity resulting from cell loss or injury. The conjugated fraction may also be increased to a modest degree in more chronic forms of hemolysis, since the ability of the normal liver cell to excrete conjugated bilirubin into bile is rate-limiting in the overall transfer of bilirubin from blood to bile.

Unconjugated Hyperbilirubinemia Without Overt Hemolysis

The term *Gilbert's syndrome* has been used to describe any older child or adult with chronic unconjugated hyperbilirubinemia not attributed to overt hemolysis. All signs and laboratory tests of hepatic function are normal. The serum bilirubin fluctuates from normal to 5 or 6 mg/dl and is entirely unconjugated. There is no bilirubinuria. This syndrome is associated with a variety of acquired diseases and may follow viral hepatitis. The disorder is benign, and liver biopsy and repeated liver function tests are not indicated. The mechanism of this syndrome and its pathogenesis remain controversial. Impaired transfer of bilirubin from plasma into the liver (uptake) and reduced hepatic glucuronyl transferase activity have been claimed.

Gilbert's syndrome results from many etiologic factors and may be classified as follows: (1) In compensated hemolytic disease the hemoglobin concentration and reticulocyte count may be normal, but ^{51}Cr-labeled erythrocyte life span is shortened, resulting in increased bilirubin formation. (2) Rarely, patients have Gilbert's syndrome in association with increased production of bile pigment from sources other than mature circulating erythrocytes. ^{51}Cr-labeled erythrocyte life span is normal, but there is a substantial increase in fecal urobilinogen excretion. (3) Drugs such as novobiocin and flavaspidic acid occasionally produce unconjugated hyperbilirubinemia in older children and adults as well as in neonates. The mechanism is uncertain; however, inhibition of glucuronyl transferase activity in vitro and competition with bilirubin for binding to Z protein have been observed. (4) Mild unconjugated hyperbilirubinemia occurs in older children and adults with thyrotoxicosis. Jaundice disappears following successful treatment of hyperthyroidism. This contrasts with the situation in newborns, in which thyroid deficiency is associated with unconjugated hyperbilirubinemia. The mechanism is unknown. (5) Following portacaval shunt surgery in patients with cirrhosis, chronic unconjugated hyperbilirubinemia occasionally develops and disappears following splenectomy. (6) Gilbert's syndrome also occurs as an inheritable disorder that appears to be transmitted as an autosomal dominant characteristic. (7) In other patients the disorder is associated either with a wide variety of acquired diseases or with no disease and with no evidence for inheritance.

Etiologic diagnosis of chronic unconjugated hyperbilirubinemia in older children and adults requires extensive and frequently highly specialized techniques. On the other hand, with the exception of compensated hemolytic disease, Gilbert's syndrome is a cosmetic disorder that probably most often results from different genetically determined alterations in the formation, transport, and disposition of bilirubin. It is the responsibility of physicians to recognize this commonly occurring benign disorder and to avoid overdiagnosis and overenergetic treatment. This syndrome of mild unconjugated hyperbilirubinemia is not a manifestation of chronic active liver disease or cirrhosis, and it rarely, if ever, requires treatment other than reassurance. Unconjugated hyperbilirubinemia, regardless of etiology, is accentuated by fasting, exercise, sepsis, alcohol, pregnancy, and rarely menstruation. Recognition of these associations will help to alleviate anxiety when worsening of jaundice is observed.

References

Arias IM: Inheritable and congenital hyperbilirubinemia. Models for the study of drug metabolism. N Engl J Med 285:1416, 1971

Fleischner G, Arias IM: Recent advances in bilirubin formation, transport, metabolism and excretion. Am J Med 49:576, 1970

Foulk WT, Butt HR, Owen CA, Whitcomb FF, Mason HL: Constitutional hepatic dysfunction (Gilbert's disease): its natural history and related syndromes. Medicine 38:25, 1959

CONJUGATED HYPERBILIRUBINEMIA OF THE NEWBORN

JAY BERNSTEIN

Conjugated hyperbilirubinemia occurring shortly after birth accompanies a large number of acquired and inherited disorders. Conjugated bilirubin is the major bile pigment found in extrahepatic biliary atresia, neonatal giant cell hepatitis, and hepatitis due to known infectious agents and metabolic disorders. Although it is not necessarily the predominant serum pigment in severe erythroblastosis fetalis, significant elevations of conjugated bilirubin may be present in serum. Cholestasis and predominantly conjugated hyperbilirubinemia can occur without morphologically apparent hepatocellular injury, although the latter is usually present. Histologic evidence of cellular injury may vary considerably, and neither inflammatory cell infiltration nor cholestasis is a constant finding in jaundiced neonates.

The single most common cause of conjugated hyperbilirubinemia in early infancy, which accounts for approximately 50 percent of cases, is extrahepatic biliary atresia; the second most common is neonatal giant cell hepatitis. The differential diagnosis of these two conditions is a major clinical problem with important therapeutic implications.

Biliary Atresia and Neonatal Hepatitis

Biliary obstruction and neonatal hepatitis share many clinical features and may have a common etiology or inciting agent. Extrahepatic biliary atresia may be an acquired lesion rather than a congenital malformation.

TABLE 2. Differential Diagnosis of Neonatal and Early Infantile Conjugated Hyperbilirubinemia

A. Hepatitis of infectious origin
  1. Viral
      Giant cell hepatitis of presumed viral origin
      Hepatitis B
      Congenital rubella infection
      Congenital cytomegalovirus infection
      Congenital or neonatal coxsackie, echo, herpes, or vari-
        cella infection
  2. Bacterial
      Syphilis
      Tuberculosis
      Listeriosis
  3. Parasitic
      Toxoplasmosis
B. Biliary tract obstruction
    Extrahepatic biliary atresia
    Extrahepatic biliary stenosis and choledochal cyst
    Spontaneous choledochal perforation
    Bile plug syndrome
    Tumors (hepatoma, bile duct sarcoma, hemangiomatosis)
    Fibrocystic disease and meconium ileus
    Calculi
    Paucity of intrahepatic bile ductules
C. Toxic hepatitis
    Bacterial sepsis and pyelonephritis
    Diarrhea
    Intestinal obstruction (ileum)
    Intravenous alimentation
    Infantile histiocytosis
D. Hemolytic disease
    Severe erythroblastosis fetalis
E. Heredofamilial and metabolic disease
    Familial giant cell hepatitis and biliary atresia
    Trisomy E with giant cell hepatitis and biliary atresia
    Polysplenia syndrome with biliary atresia
    Ductular hypoplasia with skeletal and cardiac malforma-
      tion and retarded development (Alagille syndrome)
    Down's syndrome, leprechaunism
    Cerebrohepatorenal syndrome (Zellweger's syndrome)
    Dubin-Johnson and Rotor syndromes
    Wilson's disease
    α_1-Antitrypsin deficiency
    Idiopathic neonatal hemochromatosis
    Fibrocystic disease
    Galactosemia and fructosemia
    Tyrosinemia
    Niemann-Pick disease, Gaucher's disease
    Wolman's disease
    Glycogenoses III and IV
    Indian childhood cirrhosis
    Familial hepatosteatosis
    Cholestatic syndromes
      Paucity of intrahepatic biliary ductules
      Paucity of intrahepatic biliary ductules with lym-
        phedema
      Benign recurrent cholestasis
      Byler's disease
      Fatal familial cholestasis

The pathogenetic concept in which a single etiologic agent injures liver cells or biliary epithelium or both is based on clinical and morphologic observations. It is generally assumed that the primary etiologic agent is viral. Epidemiologic data have been used to support a possible role for hepatitis B virus and also for rubella virus. The latter has been demonstrated to cause both hepatitis and intrahepatic ductal injury. Hepatic cell necrosis, giant cell transformation, and inflammatory cell infiltration may occur alone or in association with biliary atresia. Atresia of the biliary tract resulting from ductal epithelial damage may be extrahepatic or intrahepatic or both. Despite the frequent concurrence of biliary and hepatocellular lesions, one or the other pattern is usually dominant.

Extrahepatic biliary atresia accounts for 90 percent of cases presenting with extrahepatic mechanical obstruction of the biliary tree. A small number of these are accounted for by choledochal cyst, biliary stenosis, and mucobiliary plugs. The etiology and pathogenesis of choledochal cyst are probably the same as for biliary atresia; however, the obstruction is incomplete and of limited length and leads to proximal dilatation or cyst formation. The lesion is usually accompanied by hepatic giant cell transformation. Mucobiliary plugs and stenosis, and hypoplasia constitute a group of uncertain etiology in which biliary epithelial injury may be the primary event. Sludging of bile in the extrahepatic bile ducts may accompany classic neonatal hepatitis.

The lesion in biliary atresia may be diffuse or segmental; it may involve all or several of the extrahepatic ducts and may be accompanied by occlusion of intrahepatic ducts and cholestasis in dilated canaliculi and hepatocytes. Secondary changes in the liver are severe, progressing from bile duct proliferation and portal fibrosis to biliary cirrhosis. Progressive obliteration of intrahepatic bile ducts may occur in later stages. Giant cell transformation of liver cells is seen in about one-third of cases.

Neonatal hepatitis simulates biliary atresia by producing an obstructive type (bile secretory failure) of jaundice. In the majority of cases an etiology cannot be established, although a virus seems to be the likely agent. In the minority of cases an infectious agent can be identified. These include *Toxoplasma*, syphilis, *Listeria*, cytomegalovirus, rubella virus, herpesvirus, varicella virus, and coxsackie virus. Direct liver involvement occurs in these diseases, varying from mild giant cell transformation and cholangiolitis in rubella to severe zonal necrosis in herpes simplex infection. Specific diagnosis requires elaborate procedures such as viral isolation or fluorescence antibody tests, as in toxoplasmosis. Elevated serum immunoglobulin (IgM) levels in cord blood are presumptive evidence of antenatal infection. The presence in cord blood of IgM-specific antibody to an infectious agent more firmly establishes congenital infection. This is particularly useful for rubella, cytomegalovirus, toxoplasosis, and syphilis. Hepatitis B virus causes hepatitis in infants, usually as a result of transmission of virus from the mother at the time of delivery. Despite development of hepatitis B_s antigenemia and chemical and histologic changes of hepatitis at 2 to 4 months of age, it has not been demonstrated to cause neonatal *giant cell hepatitis.*

Histologically, neonatal hepatitis liver cells are changed into large, multinucleate, syncytial giant cells.

Giant cell transformation is not a specific lesion; it is a response to hepatocellular damage that is also seen in toxic injury and bacterial sepsis. Degenerative or toxic hepatocellular changes in hepatitis also include cytoplasmic swelling, bile stasis, pigment retention, and glycogen accumulation. Alterations in liver cells may be inconspicuous; the histopathologic diagnosis of neonatal hepatitis requires demonstration of an inflammatory reaction. Inflammatory cells infiltrate the lobules and portal areas and must be differentiated from hematopoietic cells that occupy the same areas and may have a similar appearance.

Males with neonatal hepatitis outnumber females by 2 to 1, whereas in biliary atresia there is no gender predominance. Biliary atresia and hepatitis occur most often as isolated lesions, but they are occasionally seen in association with other conditions. Both have been observed with increased frequency in trisomy E. A possible relationship between the chromosomal abnormality and viral infection remains conjectural. Biliary atresia occurs with unexpectedly high frequency (up to 50 percent of cases) in a syndrome characterized by polysplenia, partial or complete abdominal heterotaxia, symmetrically placed liver, situs inversus of the abdominal organs, intestinal malrotation, and respiratory-tract, vascular, and cardiac malformations.

CLINICAL PRESENTATION. In both extrahepatic biliary atresia and hepatitis, jaundice is usually first observed at 1 to 6 weeks of age. Approximately 50 percent of infants with atresia are anicteric until the second or third week of life and only very rarely develop conjugated hyperbilirubinemia during the first 48 hours. Infants with extrahepatic biliary atresia have never been noted to be icteric at birth. In contrast, approximately 20 percent of infants with hepatitis have elevated direct-reacting bilirubin concentrations in cord blood and are icteric at birth or shortly thereafter. Infants with atresia characteristically have complete biliary obstruction with gray or white stools, although there may be an earlier period of several days when jaundice is apparent but stool color is normal. Babies with hepatitis also may have acholic stools, but bile secretory failure is partial, as demonstrated by the presence in the stool of intravenously administered radioiodinated rose bengal, a dye that is excreted in bile by hepatocytes (p. 1075). In both conditions the urine contains bilirubin. Although urobilinogen is generally absent from stools and urine in biliary atresia and hepatitis with severe cholestasis, trace amounts are occasionally found. Both conjugated and unconjugated fractions of serum bilirubin are increased. Despite complete biliary obstruction the serum bilirubin concentration in atresia is usually less than 12 mg/dl during the first few months of life and often rises later. The serum bilirubin concentration may be higher in hepatitis, but is not a reliable point of differentiation.

LABORATORY DIAGNOSIS. Serum glutamic oxaloacetic transaminase (SGOT) and serum glutamic pyruvic transaminase (SGPT) levels are usually higher in hepatitis than in biliary atresia, but use of these tests to differentiate the two conditions is unreliable. Serum alkaline phosphatase activity is also elevated in both conditions. A mild hemolytic anemia with reticulocytosis is present in most cases of hepatitis and occasionally in biliary atresia. Liver function tests cannot be expected always to differentiate these two conditions because of the simultaneous occurrence of atresia and hepatitis. With the use of suitable laboratory studies, however, diagnostic accuracy approaches 95 percent. The major objective of diagnosis is to identify infants with complete or nearly complete mechanical obstruction of any portion of the extrahepatic biliary duct system with or without associated intrahepatic atresia or hepatitis. Measurements of ^{131}I in stools after intravenous administration of rose bengal (see p. 1075) may be helpful in identifying jaundiced infants with acholic stools who have extrahepatic bilary atresia. It has also been suggested that serum levels of α-fetoprotein are elevated in hepatitis but not in biliary atresia. The erythrocyte peroxide hemolysis test is said to be positive only in biliary atresia. Serum lipoprotein X (LP$_X$) concentrations may also help to differentiate the two conditions. Each of these techniques needs careful evaluation as a potentially reliable index of diagnostic differentiation.

HISTOPATHOLOGIC EXAMINATION. Hepatic biopsy will often confirm the diagnosis. Percutaneous needle biopsy usually suffices and avoids anesthetic and surgical risks. The characteristic histologic abnormality of extrahepatic biliary obstruction is prolifera-

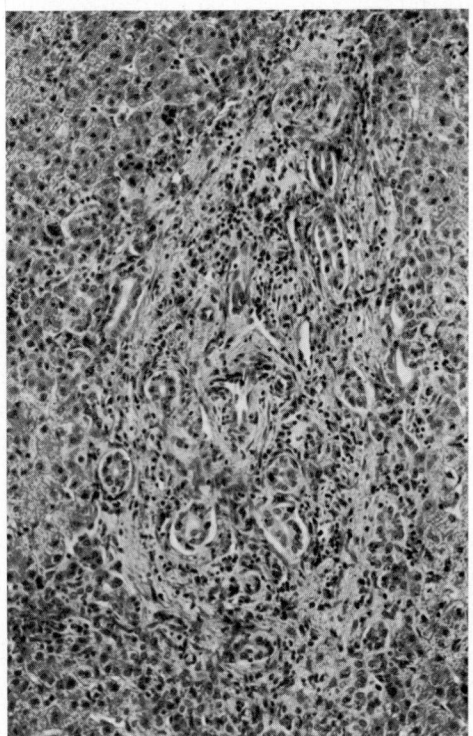

FIG. 4. Typical changes in the portal area of a young infant with extrahepatic biliary atresia: bile duct proliferation, fibrosis, medial hypertrophy of hepatic artery (H&E, $\times$ 75).

tion of intrahepatic bile ducts in the portal areas of the liver lobule, a lesion common to all forms of extrahepatic obstruction (Fig. 4). The single most common cause of incorrect diagnosis is over interpretation of bile duct proliferation, small degrees of which may occur in hepatitis and α_1-antitrypsin deficiency in association with partial or transient obstruction of large bile ducts.

Another source of confusion in the interpretation of liver biopsies can result from the rare situation in which extrahepatic biliary atresia and a paucity of intrahepatic ducts co-exist. A paucity of intrahepatic ducts occurs either as an isolated finding or in association with giant cell hepatitis. If the paucity of intrahepatic ducts is a primary phenomenon it prevents developmental proliferation; if it evolves slowly as a destructive process after the development of complete extrahepatic obstruction, proliferation decreases or disappears. A paucity of intrahepatic ducts, regardless of time of development, is associated with a clinical syndrome characterized by conjugated hyperbilirubinemia, hypercholesterolemia, xanthomatosis, and, rarely, lymphedema of the lower extremities. Due to its slow progression to cirrhosis, a paucity of intrahepatic ducts is compatible with a life span of 10 to 15 years and possibly longer; when associated with extrahepatic biliary atresia, it delays hepatic decompensation and prolongs life. The explanation for this protective effect is unknown.

MANAGEMENT. When diagnostic studies are inconclusive or when they indicate extrahepatic biliary obstruction, surgical exploration is indicated to establish the presence of extraphepatic obstruction and its cause. At the time of surgical exploration cholangiography should also be performed, when feasible, either through the gallbladder or directly into a portion of the duct system. A wedge biopsy of the liver should be obtained. In the past, biliary anastomosis to the intestinal tract was attempted only when a dilated portion of the extrahepatic duct system proximal to the obstruction was found.

Biliary anastomosis to the intestinal tract was then attempted. Recent developments, based upon the techniques of Kasai, have encouraged more aggressive approaches in all cases with occluded bile ducts. Thus if a large channel for classic anastomosis is not available, the fascial layer in which the hepatic duct normally resides is isolated and transected, and a small segment is taken for histologic examination. A jejunal segment is anastomosed to the porta hepatis, inserting the tongue of tissue into the lumen of the jejunum. The jejunal segment is then brought to the skin surface for external drainage. A second cutaneous jejunostomy connects to the remainder of the bowel. This jejunal loop is used to return bile from the proximal loop into the intestine. At a later time, perhaps at 6 months, the integrity of the bowel is reestablished. The purpose of separation of the bowel lumen from the hepatoptosis-enterostomy is to prevent development of ascending cholangitis. Ascending bacterial infection is the major complication of this procedure. The optimal time for surgery is uncertain, but it is probably best not to delay beyond 3 to 4

months. The effectiveness of this procedure in establishing drainage is variable, but it is initially effective in more than one-half of the cases. Even when good drainage of bilelike material is established, cirrhosis and portal hypertension may develop in a high proportion of cases. The complications of cirrhosis are discussed in another section (p. 1101).

Some obstructive lesions may be transient, and it may be appropriate to delay surgery until approximately 3 months of age, since later reexplorations and postmortem dissections have disclosed patent ducts that have escaped earlier surgical detection. Occasional reports of spontaneous recovery in infants diagnosed at surgery and by biopsy as having atresia may mean that partial and transient obstruction occurs and potentially patent ducts may persist. Further experience with the Kasai procedure should establish the optimal time for surgery. Prior to the introduction of the newer surgical procedures, the majority of infants with this disease died, usually by 2 years of age, a pattern that may possibly be changing. Survivors into late adolescence have occasionally been reported.

Failure of surgical intervention for biliary atresia to prevent cirrhosis or progression of neonatal hepatitis to cirrhosis may lead to consideration of hepatic transplantation. Although this is still a difficult and highly experimental procedure carrying a lifelong obligation for medical management to prevent rejection, it has been successful in prolonging life in some infants. Infants with the polysplenia syndrome are not candidates for transplantation because of the vascular anomalies.

Most infants with neonatal hepatitis recover with only supportive management; there is no specific therapy. Treatment with phenobarbital in sporadic neonatal hepatitis does not seem justified. A small number of infants with hepatitis progress to cirrhosis and portal hypertension. These complications occur more frequently in cases of familial hepatitis, which may have a different etiology than sporadic disease (see below).

Familial and Hereditary Conjugated Hyperbilirubinemia of the Newborn

Classic biliary atresia and giant cell hepatitis occur together in families, thus raising questions about genetic contributions to their etiology. Nothing in the histologic or clinical appearance of the familial disorders distinguishes them from sporadic cases. In some familial cases there has been an intrahepatic accumulation of iron, suggesting that they represent primary perinatal hemochromatosis.

Giant cell hepatitis, hepatitis with obliterative cholangitis, hepatitis with biliary atresia, and biliary stenosis are encountered in the trisomy E syndrome, in which hepatobiliary abnormalities have a high prevalence. Since the hepatic lesions are partly inflammatory and are presumed to be of viral etiology, these associations have led to speculation that the chromosomal abnormality predisposes of viral infection. A familial, inherited disorder characterized by benign recurrent cholestasis has been described in which giant cells are the major histologic characteristic in the newborn period. Despite continued episodic cholestasis, giant cells disappear later in childhood.

Familial giant cell hepatitis must be differentiated from a group of heterogeneous familial cholestatic syndromes that are usually not accompanied by giant cell transformation and other pathologic features of hepatitis. The nosology of these abnormalities is far from satisfactory. Some children have benign recurrent or chronic cholestasis, whereas others have progressive fatal liver disease. A histopathologic feature common to many of these conditions is a paucity, or "atresia," of intrahepatic bile ducts. The clinical syndrome has recently been designated by that histopathologic feature as the "paucity of intrahepatic bile ducts" syndrome. It may also occur without evidence of a familial occurrence. Some of the familial cases and rare sporadic cases of bilary hypoplasia have severe lymphedema and apparent absence of the lymphatic system in the lower extremities. Paucity of intrahepatic ducts may also occur in association with extrahepatic biliary hypoplasia or atresia; it also occurs in association with unusual facies, vertebral malformations, cardiac murmur, and retarded mental, physical, and sexual development. The condition is compatible with relatively prolonged survival; jaundice frequently diminishes after infancy.

Laboratory findings in infants with paucity of intrahepatic bile ducts are essentially identical with those in neonatal hepatitis and biliary atresia, except for elevated serum cholesterol levels, which sometimes exceed 1,500 mg/100 ml in patients with a paucity of intrahepatic ducts. Xanthomatosis over the knees, elbows, neck, hands, and eyelids is common and often leads to the correct diagnosis. Hypercholesterolemia of this magnitude is never seen in giant cell hepatitis or extrahepatic atresia alone. Steatorrhea, fat-soluble vitamin malabsorption, and growth retardation are common. Phenobarbital and cholestyramine are reported to enhance bile salt excretion and decrease pruritus in these disorders, as well as to reduce hypercholesterolemia.

The prognosis in paucity of intrahepatic ducts is better than in extrahepatic biliary atresia. Cirrhosis may develop, but it is usually delayed until 5 to 15 years of age.

The pathogenesis of these cholestatic syndromes is unknown. In certain subgroups of these infants, cholestasis may result from primary abnormalities of bile salt metabolism. Among these is *Byler's disease,* a disorder described in a large Amish kindred with recurrent episodes of severe cholestasis with progressive hepatic necrosis and cirrhosis. There is neither giant cell transformation nor paucity of intrahepatic ducts. Hypercholesterolemia is absent.

Other Causes of Conjugated Hyperbilirubinemia

Sepsis is seldom a cause of increased unconjugated bilirubin, but in recent years it has become a frequent cause of conjugated hyperbilirubinemia of the newborn. Jaundice is particularly common in association with coliform infection and pyelonephritis in infant boys.

Pneumococcal infections may also be associated with conjugated hyperbilirubinemia. Older children with chronic debilitating diseases may also be affected. In the newborn, jaundice characteristically begins de novo after the period of physiologic hyperbilirubinemia. Infants present with poor feeding, lethargy, and irritability. Laboratory studies show moderate azotemia, acidosis, hyperbilirubinemia, normal or only mildly elevated serum transaminase activities, and slight hemolysis. Antibiotic therapy of the underlying infection results in prompt abatement of jaundice. Histopathologic studies reveal bile stasis and, occasionally, evidence of hepatocellular damage. There is no evidence of bacterial involvement of the liver. Jaundice and cholestasis occur occasionally in association with enteritis and diarrhea as remote effects of intestinal disease rather than as the result of ascending cholangitis.

Conjugated hyperbilirubinemia occurs and may persist for weeks in severe erythroblastosis fetalis, after an initial period of severe unconjugated hyperbilirubinemia. Conjugated hyperbilirubinemia is also seen occasionally at birth in severely anemic and hydropic babies with Rh erythroblastosis, especially in those surviving intrauterine transfusions. Histologic studies reveal hepatocellular necrosis and giant cell transformation. The cause of cellular injury has not been determined, but anemia and hypoxia may play a role.

Conjugated hyperbilirubinemia may develop in both newborns and older children receiving parenteral alimentation with amino acid mixtures and hypertonic glucose. Since all infants treated in this fashion suffer from other serious diseases, several factors may be responsible for cholestasis. Toxic effects of one or more of the amino acids in the mixture, deficiency of essential fatty acids, deficiency of trace metals, and osmotic diuresis with dehydration have been suggested to explain bile secretory failure. Reduction in amino acid concentration usually ameliorates jaundice and elevated serum transaminase activities. The liver is infiltrated with fat, and a ceroidlike pigment accumulates within liver cells in addition to bile pigment. Giant cell transformation and hepatocellular necrosis are present occasionally, and there is usually severe cholestasis.

References

Aagenaes O: Hereditary recurrent cholestasis with lymphoedema—two families. Acta Paediatr Scand 63:465, 1974

———— Matlary A, Elgjo K, Munthe E, Fagerhol M: Neonatal cholestasis in alpha-l-antitrypsin deficient children. Acta Paediatr Scand 61: 632, 1972

———— van der Hagen CB, Refsum S: Hereditary recurrent intrahepatic cholestasis from birth. Arch Dis Child 43:646, 1968

Alagille D: Clinical aspects of neonatal hepatitis. Am J Dis Child 123: 287, 1972

———— Odièvre M, Gautier M, Dommergues JP: Hepatic ductular hypoplasia associated with characteristic facies, vertebral malformations, retarded physical, mental and sexual development, and cardiac murmur. J Pediatr 86:63, 1975

Alpert LI, Strauss L, Hirschhorn K: Neonatal hepatitis and biliary atresia associated with trisomy 17-18 syndrome. N Engl J Med 280:16, 1969

Ballow M, Margolis CZ, Schachtel B, Hsia YE: Progressive familial intrahepatic cholestasis. Pediatrics 51:998, 1973

Bernstein J, Brown AK: Sepsis and jaundice in early infancy. Pediatrics 29:873, 1962

Brent RL, et al: Persistent jaundice in infancy. J Pediatr 61:111, 1962

Brough AJ, Bernstein J: Conjugated hyperbilirubinemia in early infancy. A reassessment of liver biopsy. Hum Pathol 5:507, 1974

——— Chang CH, Bernstein J: Conjugated hyperbilirubinemia in infancy associated with parenteral hyperalimentation. J Hematol (in press)

Chandra RS: Biliary atresia and other structural anomalies in the congenital polysplenia syndrome. J Pediatr 85:649, 1974

Craig JM, Landing BH: Form of hepatitis in neonatal period simulating biliary atresia. Arch Pathol 54:321, 1952

Danks DM, Campbell PE, Clarke AM, Jones PG, Solomon JR: Extrahepatic biliary atresia. The frequency of potentially operable cases. Am J Dis Child 128:684, 1974

Dunn PM: Obstructive jaundice and haemolytic disease of the newborn. Arch Dis Child 38:54, 1963

Dupuy JM, Frommel D, Alagille D: Severe viral hepatitis type B in infancy. Lancet 1:191, 1975

Finegold MJ: Cholestatic syndromes in infancy. In Bolande RP, Rosenberg HR (eds): Perspectives in Pediatric Pathology, Vol 3. Chicago, Year Book (in press)

Greco MA, Finegold MJ: Familial giant cell hepatitis. Report of two cases and review of the literature. Arch Pathol 95:240, 1973

Haas L: Intrahepatic cholestasis in the newborn. Arch Dis Child 43:438, 1968

Hamilton JR, Sass-Kortsak A: Jaundice associated with severe bacterial infection in young infants. J Pediatr 63:121, 1963

Hays DM: Biliary atresia: the current state of confusion. Surg Clin North Am 53:1257, 1973

Javitt NB, Morrissey KP, Siegel E, et al: Cholestatic syndromes in infancy: Diagnostic value of serum bile acid pattern and cholestyramine administration. Pediatr Res 7:119, 1973

Kasai M, Kimura S, Asakura Y et al: Surgical treatment of biliary atresia. J Pediatr Surg 3:665, 1968

Kattamis CA, Demetrios D, Matsaniotis NS: Australia antigen and neonatal hepatitis syndrome. Pediatrics 54:1257, 1974

Landing BH: Considerations of the pathogenesis of neonatal hepatitis, biliary atresia and choledochal cyst—the concept of infantile obstructive cholangiopathy. Prog Pediatr Surg 6:113, 1974

Lawson EE, Boggs JD: Long-term follow-up of neonatal hepatitis: safety and value of surgical exploration. Pediatrics 53:650, 1974

Lilly JR: The Japanese operation for biliary atresia: remedy or mischief? Pediatrics 55:12, 1975

Porter CA, Mowat AP, Cook PJL, et al: α-1-antitrypsin deficiency and neonatal hepatitis. Br Med J 3:435, 1972

Rager R, Finegold M: Cholestasis in immature newborn infants: Is parenteral alimentation responsible? J Pediatr 86:264, 1975

Sass-Kortsak A, Bowden DH, Brown RJK: Congenital intrahepatic biliary atresia. Pediatrics 17:383, 1956

Schweitzer IL, Wing A, McPeak C, Spears RL: Hepatitis and hepatitis-associated antigen in 56 mother-infant pairs. JAMA 220:1092, 1972

Sharp HL, Carey JB Jr, White JG, Krivit W: Cholestyramine therapy in patients with a paucity of intrahepatic bile ducts. J Pediatr 71:723, 1967

———Krivit W: Hereditary lymphedema and obstructive jaundice. J Pediatr 78:491, 1971

Stiehl A, Thaler M, Admirand WH: Effects of phenobarbital on bile salt metabolism in cholestasis due to intrahepatic bile duct hypoplasia. Pediatrics 51:992, 1971

Strauss L, Bernstein J: Neonatal hepatitis in congenital rubella. Arch Pathol 86:317, 1968

———Valderrama E, Alpert LI: Biliary tract anomalies: the relationship of biliary atresia to neonatal hepatitis. Birth Defects 82:135, 1972

Thaler MM, Gellis SS: Studies in neonatal hepatitis and biliary atresia. I–IV. Am J Dis Child 116:257, 262, 271, 280, 1968

Valman HB, France NE, Wallis PG: Prolonged neonatal jaundice in cystic fibrosis. Arch Dis Child 46:805, 1971

Zeltzer PM, Neerhout RC, Fonkalsrud EW, Stiehm ER: Differentiation between neonatal hepatitis and biliary atresia by measuring serum-alpha-fetoprotein. Lancet 1:373, 1974

CONJUGATED HYPERBILIRUBINEMIA IN THE OLDER CHILD

IRWIN M. ARIAS

Conjugated bilirubin, as well as other organic anions such as porphyrins, various drugs, sulfobromophthalein, indocyanine green, steroids, and other metabolites are excreted into the bile, presumably by an active transport system. With the exception of bile acids, these substances are excreted by a common mechanism. Impaired biliary excretion of bile acids occurs in obstructive jaundice and bile secretory failure (cholestasis). The result is conjugated hyperbilirubinemia, bilirubinuria, increased concentrations of cholesterol and bile salts in serum, and enhanced serum alkaline phosphatase activity. Morphologically the liver shows signs of cholestasis.

Acute viral hepatitis accounts for most cases of conjugated hyperbilirubinemia in children. This disease is discussed in another section (p. 525 and p. 1092). Mechanical obstruction due to calculi, abdominal tumors, enlarged lymph nodes, or primary carcinoma results in either acute or chronic conjugated hyperbilirubinemia; if it is not relieved biliary cirrhosis can develop. These entities are rare in childhood. Calculi in the bile ducts or gallbladder may occur in association with chronic hemolytic disease.

Drugs and Conjugated Hyperbilirubinemia

A large number of chemical substances and drugs are associated with the development of hepatic necrosis, bile stasis, and fatty degeneration. Jaundice may or may not occur, depending upon the severity of the hepatic damage. Jaundice due to bile secretory failure (cholestasis), rather than to parenchymal liver cell damage, may also occur following administration of drugs. Approximately 2 percent of individuals receiving chlorpromazine, independent of the dose administered, develop conjugated hyperbilirubinemia and elevation of serum alkaline phosphatase activity. Many of these patients also show eosinophilia. Abnormal retention of sulfobromophthalein is regularly found. Within 2 weeks after withdrawal of the drug, jaundice and hepatic function usually return to normal. Hypersensitivity may be the mechanism by which chlorpromazine and several other drugs produce jaundice with cholestasis. Several synthetic steroids, including C-17 alkylated anabolic steroids and naturally occurring and synthetic estrogens, may produce conjugated hyperbilirubinemia when administered in high dose. Although jaundice occurs only rarely with these drugs, sulfobromophthalein excretion by liver is frequently abnormal. Histologic changes demonstrating bile stasis and canalicular dilatation are variable. Complete recovery occurs following withdrawal of the drug.

Recurrent Familial Cholestasis

This rare disorder of unknown etiology is characterized by multiple episodes of conjugated hyperbilirubinemia. Pruritus also occurs and is probably secondary to retention of bile acids. Pathologically there is intense cholestasis. Remissions and exacerbations are spontaneous, and there is complete functional and morphologic return to normal during remission. A congenital origin has been postulated, based on the early age of onset and familial occurrence. Total serum bile acids are elevated during clinical exacerbations, and in some cases elevations of circulating monohydroxy bile acids, such as the hepatotoxic lithocholic acid, have been recorded. Cholestasis, pruritus, steatorrhea, and failure to thrive are frequently encountered. Cholestyramine, a bile acid sequestring agent, is effective in controlling the clinical manifestations in the benign forms, but it is only of transitory value in the more severe varieties. A benign recurrent form may follow what appears to have been neonatal hepatitis, but this type usually has an onset after the first year of life.

Another variant has been found in a geographically isolated population in southern Norway and their descendents in the United States. Lymphatic abnormalities, especially lymphedema of the lower extremities, may develop early in infancy or more commonly may surface during adolescence. Intrahepatic bile ducts are deficient in number, as in the syndrome of paucity of intrahepatic ducts. More virulent variants have been described, with death occurring before the child is 10 years of age. Some of these patients are mentally and physically retarded; others have lymphedema or hemangiomata.

Byler's disease, a disorder in the Amish, is characterized by diarrhea and recurrent episodes of severe cholestasis with progressively worsening liver function and cirrhosis, leading to death in the first decade of life. Excessive visceral deposition of ceroid is also reported to produce hepatomegaly and occasionally cholestasis and cirrhosis; the basic defect in these patients is unknown, and it is likely that it is a secondary disorder. Bile secretory failure (cholestasis) may also be associated with Hodgkin's disease, cirrhosis due to any cause, and sickle cell disease.

Dubin-Johnson and Rotor Syndromes

Two inherited disorders with mild conjugated hyperbilirubinemia are the Rotor syndrome and the Dubin-Johnson syndrome. In both syndromes the transfer of various organic anions (including bilirubin) from liver to bile is defective. Bile acid excretion is normal, and plasma bile acid concentrations are normal. Chronic conjugated hyperbilirubinemia resulting from these disorders is usually detected during adolescence or early adulthood but it may be noted as early as the second year of life. Sulfobromophthalein retention is abnormal in both syndromes, particularly in the Rotor syndrome. Radiologic visualization of the gallbladder with iodopanoic acid is usually abnormal in the Dubin-Johnson syndrome and normal in the Rotor syndrome. Other conventional tests of hepatic function are normal in both. The Dubin-Johnson syndrome is characterized by a diagnostic abnormality in urinary coproporphyrin analysis. Total urinary coproporphyrin excretion is normal; however, more than 90 percent is in the form of the coproporphyrin I isomer, which suggests a defect in porphyrin metabolism or excretion. Obligate heterozygotes have an intermediate defect, and the disorder is transferred with the characteristics of an autosomal recessive trait. Patients with the Rotor syndrome have an elevated total urinary coproporphyrin excretion with a relatively increased amount of coproporphyrin I isomer. This abnormality is also transmitted with the characteristics of an autosomal recessive trait. In Israel the Dubin-Johnson syndrome occurs largely in Persian Jews, in whom it occurs with a gene frequency of approximately 1 per 1,400. Pathologically, cholestasis is absent in both syndromes; however, in the Dubin-Johnson syndrome the liver cells contain a black pigment that has physical and chemical properties of melanin. The pigment probably results from accumulation, oxidation, and polymerization of metabolites that are normally excreted in bile. The life expectancy of patients with both the Dubin-Johnson syndrome and the Rotor syndrome is normal. In each of these disorders hyperbilirubinemia is usually mild, but it may be converted into overt jaundice by infection, pregnancy, oral contraceptives, alcohol, and surgery. These factors are responsible for the high frequency with which these patients are incorrectly diagnosed and subjected to inappropriate treatment.

References

Arias IM: Inheritable and congenital hyperbilirubinemia. Models for the study of drug metabolism. N Engl J Med 285:1416, 1971

Dubin IN: Chronic idiopathic jaundice: a review of 50 cases. Am J Med 24:268, 1958

————Johnson FB: Chronic idiopathic jaundice with unidentified pigment in liver cells (a new clinicopathologic entity with a report of 12 cases). Medicine 33:155, 1954

Fleischner G, Arias IM: Recent advances in bilirubin formation transport, metabolism and excretion. Am J Med 49:576, 1970

Rotor AB, Manahan L, Florentin A: Familial non-hemolytic jaundice with direct van den Bergh reaction. Acta Med Philippines 5:37, 1948

Williams R, Cartter MA, Sherlock S, Scheuer PJ, Hill KR: Idiopathic recurrent cholestasis: a study of the functional and pathological lesions in 4 cases. Q J Med 33:387, 1964

Wolkoff A, Cohen L, Arias IM: The inheritance of the Dubin-Johnson syndrome. N Engl J Med 288:113, 1973

————Wolpert E, Pascasio F, Arias IM: Rotor's syndrome: a distinct inheritable pathophysiologic entity. Am J Med (in press)

HEPATITIS

FREDRIC DAUM
AND
MICHAEL I. COHEN

ACUTE VIRAL HEPATITIS (SEE P. 525)

For many years two types of viral hepatitis have been defined on the basis of the probable route of inoculation. Serum hepatitis virus was thought to be transmitted only by inadequately sterilized syringes or contaminated blood products, while infectious hepatitis virus was believed to be transmitted only by the fecal-oral route. However, it has been demonstrated that "serum" hepatitis can develop after ingestion of infectious material, and the two varieties of acute viral hepatitis are now identified as types A and B.

The duration of the incubation period is the only distinguishing feature between these two forms of acute viral hepatitis. The initial symptoms and signs of serum hepatitis (hepatitis B) usually occur 45 to 180 days after contact, while acute infectious hepatitis (hepatitis A) generally becomes clinically apparent 15 to 30 days after exposure. However, children and drug abusing teenagers are frequently unable to identify the time of contact with an infected individual.

In recent years our knowledge of the epidemiology, immunology, and clinical manifestations of hepatitis B has been enormously advanced by identification of Australia antigen, a particle in the circulation and liver that either contains the virus or is associated with the virus of hepatitis B. The newest designation for the antigen is hepatitis B surface antigen (HB_sAg). An antibody (HB_sAb) to the agent has also been identified in patients who have had type B hepatitis. The virology and communicability aspects of hepatitis are discussed in Chapter 12.

CLINICAL MANIFESTATIONS. The signs and symptoms of both hepatitis A and B are similar, and it is virtually impossible to distinguish clinically between them. The prodromal phases of both are of variable duration, and common symptoms include fatigue, anorexia, nausea, and vomiting. Fever, chills, headache, arthralgia, and right upper quadrant pain often characterize the preicteric phase. Diarrhea and pruritus, which are frequently noted in adult patients, are uncommon in children. On occasion the chief complaint may be an urticarial eruption or other rash similar to that seen in Schönlein-Henoch purpura, which usually disappears prior to onset of jaundice. Transient arthralgia and arthritis may precede jaundice in both types of hepatitis, with involvement especially of proximal interphalangeal joints in hepatitis B, although all joints may be affected.

In contrast to adults, children with hepatitis frequently remain anicteric, although severe and prolonged jaundice may also occur. When jaundice is absent the diagnosis is made on the basis of history, a tender liver on physical examination, and appropriate laboratory tests. Prior to the onset of scleral icterus, there is often a history of dark urine and light stools. Splenomegaly is present in approximately 10 to 15 percent of patients. Jaundice, when it develops, may persist for 7 to 14 days, or for as long as 10 to 12 weeks, while other symptoms and signs usually abate within the first month. Continued anorexia, vomiting, and lethargy usually indicate more severe hepatic destruction.

The infant born to a mother with HB_sAg-positive hepatitis during pregnancy or to a mother who is an asymptomatic carrier of HB_sAg may become positive for the same antigen immediately after delivery or up to 2 to 3 months of age. Only rarely do clinical signs of hepatitis develop in these HB_sAg-positive infants, but serum transaminase elevations often occur transiently at from 1 to 4 months of age. Such children may become chronic carriers of hepatitis B_s antigen. Persistent inflammatory changes in the liver have also been observed, but the ultimate outcome in these infants is not yet known.

There are no substantive data to suggest that acute viral hepatitis during any stage of pregnancy is teratogenic, mutagenic, or oncogenic.

LABORATORY STUDIES. Elevations in serum glutamic pyruvic transaminase (SGPT) and serum glutamic oxaloacetic transaminase (SGOT) activities are sensitive indicators of hepatocellular destruction. The intrahepatic obstructive phase of hepatitis is clinically manifested by jaundice with a moderate rise in the total serum bilirubin to 5 to 15 mg/dl and occasionally higher. More than half of the total serum bilirubin is in the conjugated or direct-reacting fraction. Increases in serum alkaline phosphatase activity and cholesterol concentration also indicate bile secretory failure. In acute viral hepatitis the serum albumin concentration is normal, while mild elevations in the gamma globulin fraction may be observed. Markedly prolonged prothrombin time frequently provides the earliest chemical clue to incipient hepatic failure. The diagnosis of hepatitis B may be confirmed if the patient's serum is positive for either HB_sAg or HB_sAb.

MANAGEMENT. Although bed rest is generally recommended for patients with acute hepatitis during the active phase of the disease, there continues to be uncertainty about the need for such restricted activity in children. Similarly, reduction of fat intake has been recommended to alleviate gastrointestinal discomfort. Moderate restrictions of activity and dietary fat may be indicated, but further study of the effect of this type of management on the course of hepatitis is needed. In the face of impending hepatic coma, bed rest is recommended. Hospitalization usually becomes necessary if the child is dehydrated or is unable to retain fluids, or whenever there is a serious threat of spread of infection to others. A prothrombin time more than 5 sec longer than control and/or changes in the patient's behavior are signs of impending hepatic coma and also warrant hospitalization. Parenteral vitamin K (5 mg) should be given in an attempt to correct this clotting abnormality. Abnormalities of other laboratory tests, including the serum bilirubin concentration and alkaline phosphatase activities, are no reasons for hospitalization.

Stool and needle precautions are advised for about 2 to 4 weeks after the onset of symptoms. If the patient's serum is negative for hepatitis B$_s$ antigen and antibody, and infectious hepatitis (hepatitis A) is considered the likely diagnosis, close playmates of younger patients, household contracts, and dating partners of teenagers should be given gamma globulin intramuscularly (0.02 to 0.04 ml/kg body weight) if exposure has occurred within the previous 4 to 6 weeks. Classmates with whom there has been only casual contact need not be immunized. All medications that are potentially hepatotoxic should be avoided. The teenager should be advised to abstain from all alcoholic beverages until liver function tests have returned to normal. Steroids and other immunosuppressive agents have no documented role in the management of acute viral hepatitis.

PROGNOSIS. One cannot clinically predict which child with acute viral hepatitis will develop severe hepatic necrosis. Even anicteric, mildly symptomatic patients may develop acute liver failure. Rapid deterioration usually occurs within 10 days of the onset of clinically evident hepatic disease. During childhood and adolescence approximately 1 percent of all patients with clinically apparent acute viral hepatitis develop acute hepatic failure with encephalopathy, and despite therapy, 70 percent of these patients may succumb.

Medical follow-up of children with acute viral hepatitis should include frequent monitoring of chemical tests of liver function. Continued abnormalities for more than 12 to 20 weeks after the onset of symptoms, signs, or chemical derangement require further evaluation because of the possibility of development of chronic liver disease. A few children with acute viral hepatitis continue to have hepatocellular destruction, leading to chronic liver disease, portal hypertension, functional hypersplenism, and ascites. In all cases progressing to chronic or persisting hepatic derangements, consideration should be given to other diagnoses For example, initial presentation of α_1-antitrypsin-deficiency hepatopathy may be confused with classic acute viral hepatitis, but this inherited metabolic disorder unfailingly proceeds to chronic liver disease.

OTHER HEPATIC INFECTIONS

INFECTIOUS MONONUCLEOSIS. Infectious mononucleosis (see also p. 1094), which is caused by the Epstein-Barr (EB) virus, is a common cause of acute hepatitis among older children and teenagers. These patients usually have fever, exudative pharyngitis, lymphadenopathy, and occasionally splenomegaly. Clinical jaundice is usually absent. Even without tender hepatomegaly, chemical evidence of hepatitis is often present in later stages. Although liver dysfunction associated with infectious mononucleosis is usually mild and complete recovery is expected, hepatic coma has been described. The diagnosis of hepatitis associated with the Epstein-Barr virus rests partially on the presence of a positive heterophil antibody in the patient's serum, atypical monocytes seen on peripheral blood smear, and a rise in the EB virus titer.

CYTOMEGALOVIRUS. Cytomegalovirus (CMV) (see also p. 520) produces a syndrome often indistinguishable from that of infectious mononucleosis. The patient's history includes malaise, fever, myalgia, and possibly a sore throat. Physical examination reveals lymphadenopathy, occasionally splenomegaly, and pharyngitis without tonsillar exudate. The liver is rarely tender or enlarged. Serum transaminase activities may be slightly elevated, while the majority of chemical tests are normal. SGPT and SGOT activities usually return to normal 2 to 6 weeks after the onset of symptoms. There is a prominent atypical lymphocytosis, but the heterophil anitbody test is persistently negative. A rise in antibody titer of CMV can be determined by the complement-fixation method or by indirect hemagglutination studies. Cytomegalovirus may also be cultured from the urine and nasopharyngeal secretions of infected individuals. Liver biopsy may be useful in making the diagnosis, since characteristic cytoplasmic inclusion bodies may be seen in infected cells. This same infection during pregnancy may produce widespread hepatic and central nervous system damage in the fetus (p. 520).

OTHER VIRAL AGENTS. Herpes simplex virus type I, adenovirus, echovirus, coxsackievirus, influenza virus (Hong Kong variety), and mumps virus may also produce acute hepatitis, although rarely. Treatment includes general supportive measures and close observation.

TOXOPLASMOSIS. *Toxoplasma gondii,* (see also p. 520) a protozoan, may cause an acute hepatitis clinically indistinguishable from infectious mononucleosis or cytomegalovirus infection. A Sabin-Feldman dye test or an indirect fluorescence antibody test should be performed on any child with hepatitis in the presence of lymphadenopathy with or without splenomegaly where there is no hematologic or serologic evidence of infectious mononucleosis.

VENERAL DISEASES. Gonorrhea and syphilis, which are currently found in epidemic proportions among teenagers, may also involve the liver. In gonococcal perihepatitis (Fitz-Hugh-Curtis syndrome) there is seeding of the liver capsule with gonococcal organisms that have exited from the fimbriated openings of the fallopian tubes in the adolescent female with gonococcal salpingitis. The patient is symptomatic with right upper quadrant pain and tenderness, and serum transaminase activities may be minimally elevated. Other liver function tests are normal. After 48 hours of penicillin therapy, right upper quadrant discomfort generally subsides, and enzyme levels return to normal. Secondary syphilis may also produce hepatitis. Congenital syphilis, if untreated, often progresses to severe hepatic inflammation and necrosis during the first few months of life.

CHRONIC HEPATITIS

Chronic hepatitis is defined as protracted inflammatory reaction in the liver as demonstrated by chemical hepatic dysfunction, abnormal histopathology, and a clinical course continuing without improvement for at least 6 months. The following two relatively distinct forms of chronic hepatitis have been appreciated.

Chronic Persistent Hepatitis

Chronic persistent hepatitis is characterized by the conspicuous absence of symptoms or signs of hepatitis, by mildly elevated SGOT and SGPT activities, and by a nonspecific histologic pattern on liver biopsy. It is the most common form of chronic hepatitis among adolescents, perhaps relating to the high incidence of drug abuse in this age group. Antecedent infections with hepatitis A or B, infectious mononucleosis, and exposure to hepatotoxins have all been associated with chronic persistent hepatitis. Older children and teenagers with inflammatory bowel disease and normal serum chemistries may also have histologic changes on biopsy consistent with this condition.

The patient may present after an acute attack of hepatitis, and liver function tests may remain abnormal for more than 6 months. Usually there are few symptoms except for occasional lethargy and anorexia. More commonly, abnormal serum liver enzyme activities are discovered incidentally, and physical examination is normal. Serum transaminase activities are mildly abnormal, in the range of 50 to 350 Karmen units. The serum bilirubin, cholesterol, alkaline phosphatase, total protein, albumin, and globulin fractions are usually within normal limits. Liver biopsy reveals a mononuclear cell infiltrate in the portal triads. There may be mild necrosis of adjacent periportal hepatocytes and minimal fibrosis, but lobular architecture is preserved.

Although there have been no prospective follow-up studies regarding the prognosis of children with chronic persistent hepatitis, evidence has accumulated to show that adults usually recover from the illness without specific therapy. A normal diet without modification of physical activities is recommended. There appears to be no indication for the use of steroids or other antiinflammatory agents. To minimize the potential for further hepatic injury, teenagers with chronic persistent hepatitis should avoid alcoholic beverages or the use of any potentially hepatotoxic medication until there is no longer chemical evidence of disease.

Chronic Active Hepatitis

Chronic active hepatitis (chronic aggressive hepatitis, lupoid hepatitis, plasma cell hepatitis), which was initially reported in teenage and young adult females with multiple manifestations of autoimmune disease and markedly elevated gamma globulin levels, has also been recognized in younger children. In most cases the initiating disease, toxin, or infectious agent is unknown, although it may develop after what is thought to be viral hepatitis or drug-induced toxic hepatitis. A multifactorial origin is likely, although the possibility of a single autoimmune mechanism cannot be excluded.

In approximately 50 percent of patients the onset of illness occurs during adolescence or early adulthood. Females comprise 70 to 80 percent of the patients. The initial clinical and laboratory features are commonly indistinguishable from those of acute viral hepatitis. The onset may be acute, with a prodrome of anorexia, nausea, arthralgia, and fever, or more insidious, with vague nonspecific complaints including an anicteric phase in approximately 20 percent of cases. It is in this latter group that clinical evaluation of manifestations such as epistaxis and amenorrhea may lead to discovery of the chronic active hepatitis. Hepatomegaly, with or without tenderness, and splenomegaly are variable in the pediatric patient. Spider nevi may be present. Endocrine disturbances including gynecomastia, acne, hirsutism, striae, obesity, and cushingoid facies are frequent in adolescents. Ascites, edema, and hepatic encephalopathy are late features consistent with cirrhosis of the liver and portal hypertension. Extrahepatic involvement includes arthritis, hemolytic anemia, ulcerative colitis, thyroiditis, pleuritis, glomerulonephritis, and dermatologic manifestations such as erythema nodosum.

In children hyperbilirubinemia is an inconsistent finding, with the total serum bilirubin rarely exceeding 10 mg/dl. Serum transaminase activities are variable, but may exceed 1,500 Karmen units. Hypoalbuminemia corresponds to the severity and chronicity of hepatocellular damage. The prothrombin time is usually abnormal, and defects in fibrinogen and thrombin time are common. There is a marked increase in the globulin component, particularly the IgG portion of the gamma fraction. Elevations in serum IgM and IgA have also been described. Thrombocytopenia, neutropenia, and a normochromic, normocytic anemia (which is expected in the later stages of the disease when portal hypertension and hypersplenism are established) can also be seen earlier in the precirrhotic stages. Coombs-positive hemolytic anemia has been reported, as has peripheral eosinophilia. Occasionally the sera of such patients are positive for lupus erythematosus (LE) cells, antinuclear antibodies, smooth muscle antibodies, antiglomerular antibodies, and antimitochondrial antibodies; however, there are no characteristic immunologic patterns by which the diagnosis can be made.

When hepatic biopsy can safely be performed it is a valuable diagnostic tool, if one accepts the limitations of sampling error. Microscopic examination reveals an inflammatory infiltrate involving the portal tracts and extending into the parenchyma, with extension of fibrous tissue around small collections of hepatocytes that then become necrotic (piecemeal necrosis), thus leading to formation of intralobular septa. The infiltrate consists of lymphocytes and plasma cells. The lobular architecture is disturbed and patchy fibrosis is common. Bone marrow examination usually reveals large numbers of plasma cells.

Discussion of therapy for children with chronic active hepatitis must take into account the fact that all major clinical drug trials have either excluded children or included only very few children. Improvement in survival rate has been described among adult patients receiving prolonged courses of corticosteroid therapy. Corticosteroids increase appetite, reduce lethargy, fatigability, and fever, relieve arthralgia, and improve the general sense of well-being in these patients, while serum transaminase activities and bilirubin concentrations return to normal. It remains unclear, however, whether the progression to cirrhosis is impeded by steroid treatment, or even if histologic improvement occurs.

Some clinicians prefer to initiate therapy with 6-mercaptopurine (6-MP), an antimetabolite. In some cases 6-MP has been as effective as steroids, while avoiding the growth-arresting effect and other serious complications of corticosteroids. Azathioprine, an analogue of 6-MP, is contraindicated for use in patients with liver disease, since it must be metabolized by the liver to the active form, 6-MP. Irregular conversion of azathioprine to 6-MP may result from serious hepatic damage. Failure to respond to steroids may indicate the need to start 6-MP therapy. Conversely, failure to respond to 6-MP may dictate the addition of corticosteroids.

Two modes of corticosteroid therapy may be used. In the first, an initial dose of 1 to 2 mg/kg/day oral prednisone is reduced gradually after 2 to 4 weeks of therapy to a dose at which the SGPT activity is generally less than 100 Karmen units and the patient is asymptomatic. After 4 to 6 months of this lower dosage regimen, if hepatic biopsy reveals no further evidence of active hepatocellular disease, steroids may be discontinued. If exacerbation occurs, a similar brief therapeutic plan might be reinstituted. Under the second plan, long-term maintenance of these patients on continuous low-dose, alternate-day prednisone therapy is continued for years without interruption even if there is no evidence of active disease. Most reports indicate that short-term therapy fails to sustain a remission and that therapy must be maintained for many years or even indefinitely.

In the child who develops severe side effects from steroids, lower doses of prednisone in conjunction with 6-MP may produce or sustain the desired remission. With 6-MP therapy alone or in combination with steroids, a dose of 1.5 mg/kg/day is usually satisfactory and safe, but requires frequent determinations of hemoglobin, white blood cell count and differential, and platelet count. Daily doses should never exceed 2.0 mg/kg/day.

The overall goal of therapy is induction of a clinical remission, the prevention of further intrahepatic destruction, and avoidance of cirrhosis and hepatic failure. Currently there are few data on children to suggest the optimal approach to achieve these results with a minimum of untoward side effects.

Toxic Hepatitis

Hepatotoxic reactions are of two clearly discernible types; non-dose-related hypersensitivity and dose-related direct toxin types. In some situations the clinical course and liver histology suggest toxic hepatitis, but the agent cannot be identified.

Liver disease associated with a variety of pharmacologic agents is in most instances probably the result of acquired hypersensitivity to the offending agent and is often associated with fever, rash, arthralgia, and eosinophilia. Some drugs, such as halothane, primarily cause hepatic cell necrosis, as evidenced by serum transaminase activities. Other agents, such as estrogen-containing oral contraceptives, methyltestosterone derivatives, and phenothiazines, predominantly produce cholestasis with conjugated hyperbilirubinemia and little or no increase in serum transaminase activities. Symptoms usually subside within a few days after withdrawal of the drug, while blood chemical abnormalities require several weeks to return to normal.

Phosphorus, arsenic compounds, carbon tetrachloride, tetrachloroethylene, and trichloroethane produce hepatocellular necrosis, steatosis, and mild to moderate cholestasis. The length of exposure to these toxins and the dosage received usually determine the extent of tissue damage. If recovery ensues, there is often resolution of all liver pathology.

After discontinuation of the offending agent, management of toxic hepatitis with or without hepatic encephalopathy is identical to that of acute viral hepatitis. The efficacy of steroids in toxic liver states remains similarly controversial and uncertain.

References

Anand OP, Tamburro CH, Leevy CM: Detrimental effect of exercise in hepatitis. Gastroenterology 60:739, 1971

Becker MD, Scheuer PJ, Baptista A et al: Prognosis of chronic persistent hepatitis. Lancet 1:53, 1970

Blumberg GS, Gerstley BJS, Hungerford DA, et al: A serum antigen (Australia antigen) in Down's syndrome, leukemia and hepatitis. Ann Intern Med 66:924, 1967

DeGroote J, Desmet VJ, Gedegk P, et al: A classification of chronic hepatitis. Lancet 2:626, 1968

Dubois R, Silverman A, Slovis TL: Chronic active hepatitis in children. Am J Dig Dis 17:575, 1972

Fernandez R, McCarty DJ: The arthritis of viral hepatitis. Ann Intern Med 74:207, 1971

Goldstein GB, Lam KC, Mistilis SP: Drug-induced active chronic hepatitis. Am J Dig Dis 18:177, 1973

Klatskin G: Toxic and drug-induced hepatitis. In Schiff L (ed): Diseases of the Liver. Philadelphia, Lippincott, 1963, p 453

Kouba K, Jira J, Zitova D: Hepatic involvement in the course of acquired toxoplasmosis. Acta Paediatr Scand 60:482, 1971

Krugman S, Giles JP, Hammond J: Infectious hepatitis: evidence for two distinctive clinical, epidemiological and immunological types of infection. JAMA 200:365, 1967

Litt IF, Cohen MI, Schonberg SK, Spigland I: Liver disease in the drug-using adolescent. J Pediatr 81:238, 1972

Mackay IR, Wood IJ: Lupoid hepatitis: a comparison of 22 cases with other types of liver disease. QJ Med 31:485, 1962

McMahon J, Ellicott C, Green R: Infectious mononucleosis complicated by hepatic coma. Am J Gastroenterol 51:200, 1969

Mistilis SP, Blackburn CRB: Active chronic hepatitis. Am J Med 48:484, 1970

————Lam KC: Treatment of chronic hepatitis. In Progress in Liver Diseases, Vol IV. New York, Grune & Stratton, 1972, p 419

————Skyring AP, Blackburn CRB: The natural history of active chronic hepatitis. I. Clinical features, course, diagnostic criteria, morbidity, mortality and survival. Aust Ann Med 17:214, 1968

Panush RS, Wilkinson LS, Fagin RR: Chronic active hepatitis associated with eosinophilia and Coombs'-positive hemolytic anemia. Gastroenterology 64:1015, 1973

Repsher LH, Freebern RK: Effects of exercise on recovery from infectious hepatitis. N Engl J Med 281:1393, 1969

Rosenblate HJ, Eisenstein R, Baldwin D, et al: Nonviral hepatitis in drug addicts. Arch Pathol 95:18, 1973

Schweitzer IL, Wing A, McPeak C, et al: Hepatitis and hepatitis-associated antigen in 56 mother-infant pairs. JAMA 220:1092, 1972

Soloway RD, Summerskill WHJ, Baggenstoss AH, et al: Clinical, biochemical and histological remission of severe chronic active liver disease: a controlled study of treatments and early prognosis. Gastroenterology 63:820, 1972

DISORDERS OF BILE ACID METABOLISM

NORMAN JAVITT

BILE ACID EXCRETORY FAILURE

The normal liver transports bile acids at a mean rate of 1.2 g/kg of liver per 24 hours. However, since transport is not constant over a 24-hour period, but increases during the few hours following meals, the hourly excretory capacity for bile acids is considerably higher than is suggested by the 24-hour average. When the hepatocyte is damaged it cannot maintain this high transport rate, and serum bile acid concentrations increase. With mild hepatic dysfunction, bile acid retention in serum may be the only detectable biochemical abnormality. Since bile acids must traverse the entire length of the biliary tree, partial or complete mechanical obstruction to flow can also elevate the serum bile acid concentration, which is a sensitive indicator of an abnormal hepatobiliary system, but does not specify the nature or site of the disease process. In addition to disturbances in bile acid transport resulting from hepatobiliary disease, primary disturbances in bile acid metabolism and transport may also occur; however, these are conjectural at this time.

Elevated Serum Bile Acid Concentrations

The concentration of total conjugated bile acid in serum obtained from healthy humans (adult and newborn) 3 hours or more after the last meal ranges from 1 to 2 μg/ml. A slight rise in serum bile acid concentration occurs following eating and usually reaches a peak at 2 hours. A normal range for the 2-hour postprandial serum bile acid has not been established, but a rise greater than twice the fasting value is probably abnormal. Given a normal bile acid pool, decreased hepatic extraction of bile acids from plasma occurs early in hepatocellular disease and is one of the last specific functions to return to normal.

Elevation of serum bile acid concentration following an overnight fast indicates that the liver lacks the capacity to remove bile acids from serum even when an interval as long as 12 hours has elapsed since bile acids entered the intestine. Under these circumstances, following breakfast and gallbladder contraction a marked elevation in serum bile acid concentration can be expected. In neonates receiving frequent feedings it is particulary treacherous to relate changes at any one time in serum bile acid concentrations to a particular therapy. A minimum of at least two specimens should be studied, one prior to the first feeding of the day and the other 1 or 2 hours following an evening feeding.

In the adult, elevated plasma cholic acid concentration indicates either intrahepatic or extrahepatic cholestasis, while an increase in the plasma chenodeoxycholate concentration is suggestive of either cirrhosis or hepatitis. The usefulness of this differentiation in children is uncertain.

NEONATAL CHOLESTATIC SYNDROMES In both neonatal giant cell hepatitis of unknown etiology (p. 1088) and extrahepatic biliary atresia (p. 1085) serum bile acids are elevated, and the predominant bile acid is chenodeoxycholate. In infants who die within a year, plasma chenodeoxycholate may be 80 to 90 times greater than plasma cholate. Monohydroxy bile acids such as lithocholate or 3β-hydroxy-5-cholenoate are found in serum only in trace amounts. Urine of infants with extrahepatic biliary atresia contains monohydroxy bile acids derived from an undefined metabolic pathway. The use of agents such as cholestyramine to bind bile acids in the intestinal tract and prevent their enterohepatic circulation appears to have long-term beneficial effects in children with a paucity of intrahepatic bile ducts; but until it can be shown that such therapy prevents cirrhosis, one must be cautious in predicting effectiveness.

BILE ACIDEMIA IN OTHER LIVER DISEASES In order to classify a disease with hyperbilirubinemia as resulting primarily from defective bilirubin transport or metabolism, serum bile acid concentrations should be normal. In both Gilbert's syndrome (unconjugated hyperbilirubinemia, p. 1085) and Dubin-Johnson syndrome (conjugated hyperbilirubinemia, p. 1091) serum bile acids are normal in both quantity and quality. Similarly, in Reye's syndrome (fatty viscera with encephalopathy, p. 1099) neither hyperbilirubinemia nor bile acidemia is seen; there is no evidence for a defect in hepatic excretory function. In contrast, however, in the bronze baby syndrome associated with phototherapy, conjugated hyperbilirubinemia and accumulation of the bronze pigment may be associated with bile acidemia, as noted in two reported cases, thus suggesting the presence of cholestasis.

References

Back P: Identification and quantitative determination of urinary bile acids excreted in cholestasis. Clin Chem Acta 44:199, 1973

Javitt N, Morrissey K, Siegel E, et al: Cholestatic syndromes in infancy: diagnostic value of serum bile acid pattern and cholestyramine administration. Pediatr Res 7:119, 1973

Kaplowitz N, Kok E, Javitt N: Postprandial serum bile acid for the detection of hepatobiliary diseases. JAMA 225:292, 1973

Sharp HL, Mirkin BL: Effect of phenobarbital on hyperbilirubinemia, bile acid metabolism and microsomal enzyme activity in chronic intrahepatic cholestasis of childhood. J Pediatr 81:116, 1972

METABOLIC DISORDERS OF THE LIVER

MERVIN SILVERBERG

The liver is affected by numerous metabolic disorders, but in only a few do biochemical derangements result in significant liver disease (Table 3). These may be grouped into four general areas of disordered metabolism: carbohydrate, protein, lipid, and miscellaneous diseases in which the exact etiology has not been determined.

DISORDERS OF CARBOHYDRATE METABOLISM

GALACTOSEMIA AND FRUCTOSEMIA. Galactosemia (p. 713) and hereditary fructose intolerance or fructosemia (p. 715) show several similarities: (1) ingestion of the offending nutrient results in vomiting, hypoglycemia, and failure to thrive; (2) hepatocellular disease and renal tubular dysfunction develop as a result of accumulation of toxic subtrates, ie, galactose-1-phosphate and fructose-1-phosphate, respectively.

In galactosemia, deficiency of the enzyme galactose-1-uridyl transferase is responsible for the failure to metabolize galactose-1-phosphate, which may cause severe and often irreversible damage to the cornea and the central nervous system. Hepatomegaly and both conjugated and unconjugated hyperbilirubinemia occur early in infancy, within a few days after starting milk feedings. Occasionally hyperbilirubinemia may be primarily of the unconjugated variety at the onset. Development of ascites early in the course of the disease should alert one to the possibility of galactosemia. In the untreated child cirrhosis, portal hypertension, and occasionally hepatic failure become evident before the first year of life. Hepatic manifestations are usually reversible with rigid adherence to a galactose-free diet from before the age of 3 months and for an indefinite period of time.

Vomiting and/or voluntary avoidance of fruits and other fructose-containing foods are protective mechanisms that are most effective in the case of fructose intolerance. The liver disease is usually milder than that seen with galactosemia, and older undiagnosed children with self-imposed restrictions usually have virtually normal liver function.

GLYCOGEN STORAGE DISEASES. Ten enzymatically defined glycogenoses have been described (p. 729), with various qualitative and quantitative abnormalities of glycogen deposition in various tissues. Liver glycogen may account for more than 5 percent of the wet weight in some types; however, excessive fat accumulation in the liver is the major cause of hepatomegaly. Elevated serum transaminase activities frequently occur; with the exception of types V, VII, VIII, and X, which primarily involve skeletal muscle; hepatomegaly is common to all. Types III and IV are associated with hepatocellular dysfunction and fibrosis.

In the branching enzyme defect (type IV), deficiency of amylo-1,4→1,6-transglucosylase results in hepatic cirrhosis, splenomegaly, and portal hypertension during early infancy. None of the 10 reported patients, 9 of whom were males, has survived beyond the fourth year of life. Progressive liver failure is attributed to amylopectin, which is a relatively insoluble plantlike polysaccharide having long outer chains and consisting of heterogeneous fractions. In none of these cases has the concentration of the abnormal glycogen exceeded 4 percent of the wet liver weight. Patients with deficiencies of debrancher enzymes (type III), amylo-1,6-glucosylase, or oligo-1,4→1,4-glucotransferase occasionally develop extensive hepatic fibrosis without cirrhosis. Portal transposition or shunt, and central venous alimentation, have been successful in severely affected cases with types I or III.

DISORDERS OF PROTEIN METABOLISM

α_1-**ANTITRYPSIN DEFICIENCY.** Numerous hepatic disorders have been described that are as-

TABLE 3. Hepatic Manifestations of Metabolic Disorders

Metabolic Disorders	Neonatal Hepatitis	Clinical Phenotypes Infantile Cirrhosis	Juvenile Cirrhosis and/or Hepatomegaly
Galactosemia	+[a]	++	+
Hereditary fructose intolerance	+	++	+
α_1-antitrypsin	++	++	+
Hereditary tyrosinemia	++	++	+
Bile acid secretory disorders	++	++	+
Cerebrohepatorenal syndrome of Zellweger	+	++	−
Brancher type IV glycogenosis	+	++	−
Cystic fibrosis	+	−	++
Niemann-Pick disease	+	−	−
Wolman's disease	+	−	−
Gaucher's disease	+	−	+
Wilson's disease	−	−	++
Familial hepatic cholesterol ester storage disease	−	−	++
Glycogenosis types I–III, VI, IX	−	+	+

[a] + = less common; ++ = very common; − = rare or never.

sociated with reduced serum levels of the glycoprotein protease inhibitor (PI) α_1-antitrypsin. The latter accounts for approximately 90 percent of the serum protease inhibitory activity and is the major fraction of serum α_1-globulins. It is also an acute-phase reactant and may be increased in the circulation in response to acute and chronic physiologic stresses, eg, infection. The inheritance of serum α_1-antitrypsin is determined by a series of more than 11 codominant PI alleles that are completely expressed. M is the most common allele and is present in the normal phenotype. The Z allele in the homozygous state is associated with the most severe quantitative deficiency and the clinical syndromes.

Hereditary deficiencies of this glycoprotein inhibitor were initially found in adults suffering from chronic obstructive lung disease that resulted in emphysema. The first reports in the pediatric age group involved an unrelenting infantile cirrhosis with no apparent pulmonary involvement. More recently, some of the affected infants have shown clinical improvement without any specific therapy. Lung disease in association with α_1-antitrypsin deficiency is rare in children, but has been reported in a few cases of infantile cirrhosis as early as 2 years of age.

Liver disease in infants often begins with acute cholestasis indistinguishable from that of idiopathic neonatal hepatitis. Some cases revert clinically, with loss of jaundice and improving liver function tests. Usually there is little or no improvement in liver histopathology, and infants in remission develop progressive hepatomegaly and deteriorating liver chemistries. Antitrypsin inhibitor deficiency may account for 10 to 20 percent of all cases of neonatal cholestasis.

Another phenotype of the PIZZ variety is seen in the child who presents beyond the first year of life with cirrhosis and portal hypertension, with or without hepatomegaly. Some children have a remote history of neonatal cholestasis; most do not. Histologic studies reveal cirrhosis that may be quiescent or in various degrees of active fibrosis and cellular infiltration. In this disorder a very diffuse type of fibrosis is noted, rather than the predominantly portal fibrosis associated with hepatitis.

In all affected patients with liver involvement, distinctive intracytoplasmic eosinophilic hyaline globules are seen in periportal hepatocytes. These globules stain with periodic acid Schiff (PAS); they are resistant to diastase digestion and are immunologically similar to α_1-antitrypsin. Similar accumulation is seen in adults with lung disease and α_1-antitrypsin deficiency, even in the absence of clinical and histologic liver disease. This suggests that the antitrypsin deposits may not be responsible for hepatic damage.

HEREDITARY TYROSINEMIA. A number of phenotypes of hereditary tyrosinemia have been described that vary with the age of the patient and have a worldwide distribution. The earliest manifestations occur in the first 6 months of life, with signs and symptoms attributed to acute hepatic necrosis. Hepatomegaly, failure to thrive, and jaundice occur in over half the cases. Hypoglycemia, hypoproteinemia, and a hemorrhagic diathesis are common presenting features; death occurs in 90 percent of untreated cases. A more slowly progressive chronic phenotype includes survivors of the infantile hepatic necrosis stage who present with nodular cirrhosis, portal hypertension, and renal tubular insufficiency. In the older child a complete Fanconi syndrome may predominate, with the liver disease occasionally assuming subclinical proportions. It is probable that acute and chronic forms are clinical phenotypes of the same mutual autosomal recessive allele. Many children surviving to an older age succumb to a virulent multifocal primary hepatic malignancy.

The basic defect is still controversial, with the most favored theory supporting a deficiency of liver p-hydroxyphenylpyruvic acid (pHPPA) oxidase. It has also been postulated that pHPPA oxidase inhibition may be due to another unidentified enzyme defect. The deficiency state results in elevation of serum and urine tyrosine and its keto-acid derivatives. Hypermethioninemia is frequently noted, and results in a characteristic odor when it is excreted in urine and sweat, probably because of the concurrent deficiency of methionine-activating enzymes and cystathionine synthetase.

Carefully monitored dietary restriction of phenylalanine and tyrosine will reverse many of the renal tubular abnormalities and will usually improve hepatic function. Progressive hepatic failure has occurred, however, in the face of apparently adequate treatment. Dietary management has also been valuable in the prophylaxis of asymptomatic siblings that are homozygous for the disease. Transitory formes frustes have been noted in selected cases of neonatal hepatitis, infantile galactosemia, and hereditary fructosemia.

DISORDERS OF LIPID METABOLISM

The liver has a very rapid turnover of lipid and is therefore one of the major sites for storage of excess or abnormal lipids, particularly in liposomes. Hepatosplenomegaly is found in most varieties of lipid storage disease.

NIEMANN-PICK DISEASE. Niemann-Pick disease (p. 750) may be associated with early cholestasis, which is indistinguishable from idiopathic neonatal hepatitis.

GAUCHER'S DISEASE. Occasionally patients with Gaucher's disease (p. 749) develop portal hypertension, cholestasis, cirrhosis, cholelithiasis, and cholangitis, in decreasing order of frequency. In the infantile form of Gaucher's disease, opisthotonic posturing of the head is often seen, leading to the mistaken diagnosis of kernicterus due to conjugated hyperbilirubinemia and neonatal hepatitis. In infants with Gaucher's disease, identification of the characteristic storage cells in liver may be very difficult because of their rarity.

CHOLESTEROL STORAGE DISEASES. Excessive storage of cholesterol esters in liver, adrenal, and intestinal mucosa has been noted in Wolman's disease or familial visceral xanthomatosis (p. 738). All patients that have been reported have died in early infancy. Familial hepatic cholesterol ester storage disease that occurs in older children has a more benign course; septate cirrhosis of the liver develops in all patients.

LIPOATROPHIC DIABETES MELLITUS. Hyperlipemia followed by hepatomegaly with fatty metamorphosis and sometimes cirrhosis occurs in lipoatrophic diabetes mellitus. This condition is usually associated with *acanthosis nigricans,* generalized absence of subcutaneous fat, and insulin-resistant diabetes mellitus without ketosis and is frequently noted around puberty. Patients are hirsute, and affected females appear rather masculine. There is an increased prepubertal growth rate, but mature height is either normal or reduced.

Miscellaneous Metabolic Disorders

REYE'S SYNDROME. Reye's syndrome is a distinct clinicopathologic entity characterized by fatty infiltration of the liver, kidney, pancreas, brain, and heart, associated with various stages of altered consciousness and hepatic dysfunction. The disease occurs in children from the newborn period through 15 years of age all over the world. It is endemic in Thailand and often epidemic in the United States. The patients usually develop acute encephalopathy after a mild upper respiratory illness, often associated with vomiting (especially blood-tinged or having the appearance of coffee grounds). Blood studies at the time of onset of coma reveal moderately to markedly elevated transaminase activities, as well as ammonia and creatine phosphokinase in the majority of cases. Less than half of the patients are hypoglycemic (usually those less than 5 years of age), and serum bilirubin concentration is normal or only minimally elevated. The liver may be of normal size, or there may be mild to moderate hepatic enlargement due to uniform fatty swelling of hepatocytes, associated with mild peripheral lobular necrosis. In rare cases no evidence of fatty metamorphosis can be detected by light microscopy, thus suggesting that the hepatic dysfunction is not secondary to the fatty changes. Between 25 and 100 percent of untreated patients succumb within a few days, with increased intracranial pressure secondary to cerebral swelling as a major contributing factor. Survivors show dramatic improvement, but often have neurologic sequelae; hepatic abnormalities always return to normal either within a few days or up to 1 month after onset of coma.

The exact etiology remains obscure, despite numerous hypotheses that have been proposed and investigated. Common viral infections have been circumstantially implicated. These include, in order of frequency, influenza B, varicella, echovirus, coxsackievirus, adenovirus, rhinovirus, influenza A, herpes simplex, and rubeola. Some studies have suggested that an interaction between a potential toxin (such as an insecticide) and the virus renders the host vulnerable. Ingested toxins such as aflatoxin and hypoglycin have been implicated in related disorders in Thailand and Jamaica, respectively. Circulating potential endogenous toxins such as ammonia, certain amino acids (glutamine, glutamic acid, alanine, lysine, and ornithine), and certain medium-chain free fatty acids (C-8 caprylic) have been found to be markedly elevated in the serum of patients with Reye's syndrome. These abnormalities of protein, urea, and fatty acid metabolism are probably secondary to a more basic disturbance within the hepatocyte, muscle cell, or any other cell affected in the disease. It is not clear whether the neurologic disturbance is primary and independent of hepatic dysfunction or secondary to the accumulation of these toxins or others that are as yet undefined. Understanding this relationship would aid enormously in designing appropriate therapy. The suggestion has also been made that Reye's syndrome may result from the impact of a viral or toxic agent on an inherited metabolic defect that would otherwise not be clinically manifest. Thus elevated serum ammonia nitrogen concentrations have been postulated to result from exacerbation of a partial defect in hepatic ornithine transcarbamylase activity.

The major thrust of the various therapeutic regimens has been directed toward clearing of theoretical endogenous and exogenous toxins. The techniques utilized include exchange transfusions, peritoneal dialysis, saline washout, administration of glucose and insulin, and administration of *l*-citrulline to reduce hyperammonemia due to a possible defect in orithine transcarbamylase, a urea-cycle enzyme. Supportive therapy may be equally effective. At present no distinct superiority has been noted for any of these measures, and in larger studies survival rates for each usually hover around 50 percent. Since survival rates are higher for older children, it is essential that comparisons of therapies utilize age-matched populations; or better yet they should be based upon well-controlled clinical trials performed simultaneously.

It has also been recognized that in some patients hepatic abnormalities (transaminase elevations, hepatomegaly, delayed prothrombin time) may not be apparent at the time of onset of neurologic disturbance. The changes may appear 24 to 72 hours later and persist thereafter for many weeks. It is essential to observe all patients with idiopathic seizures, coma, and even psychoses for hepatic abnormalities if this diagnosis is to be made.

WILSON'S DISEASE. Hepatic or abdominal manifestations of Wilson's disease (p. 1921) predominate in 80 percent of all patients presenting under the age of 15; they include atypical hepatitis, hypersplenism, portal hypertension, and cirrhosis. In rare cases a fulminant course is observed with rapid onset of hepatic failure. Histologically the disease progresses from mild fibrosis with excessive copper deposition in asymptomatic preschool patients through subacute necrosis to nodular cirrhosis in older children. Liver function may improve with treatment, which consists of a low-copper diet and a copper-chelating agent (penicillamine). Removal of copper from the liver in advanced cases may improve liver function.

CEREBROHEPATORENAL SYNDROME. The cerebrohepatorenal syndrome (Zellweger's syndrome) is associated with hepatic fibrosis and cirrhosis in all cases surviving beyond 2 to 3 months of life. The syndrome is characterized by seizures, severe retardation of development, profound hypotonia, glaucoma, congenital stippled epiphyses, and cysts of the renal cortex. The typical facies is characterized by hypertelorism, a high forehead, and pursed lips. Infants fail to thrive and usually die before 6 months of age. Hyperbilirubinemia, elevated transaminases, and hypoprothrombinemia develop at around 2 to 3 months of life, along with hepatomegaly and splenomegaly. Excessive lipid and iron stores are found in brain, liver, and kidneys. Electron microscopy of the liver, brain, and muscle has revealed small, dense, grossly abnormal mitochondria and absent peroxisomes. Histochemical and biochemical analysis has demonstrated functional absence of the nonheme iron protein of the electron transport chain prior to the cytochromes. It has been assumed that all of the previously described abnormalities are secondary to this defect in electron transport. The syndrome occurs with a frequency of 1 in 100,000 live births. Autosomal recessive inheritance has been established. A defect in the heterozygote has not yet been described.

HEPATIC STEATOSIS. A damaged liver from any cause is prone to accumulate all lipid fractions, which results in a nonspecific fatty liver. Cirrhosis rarely results from a fatty liver in children, but transitory hepatomegaly and abnormal liver function tests are commonly encountered. Various disorders involving excessive mobilization of lipids may also lead to accumulation of fat in the liver (eg, diabetes, hyperphagia, corticosteroids, and protein-calorie deficiency). The administration of steroids in high doses to a child with a normal liver and free access to food may result occasionally in massive caloric intake and equally massive hepatomegaly with accompanying fat storage in hepatocytes. Restriction of caloric intake will result in complete amelioration of this disorder. Drugs such as tetracycline, hydrocarbons, and heavy metals may also interfere with hepatic lipid metabolism and produce the same pathology.

CYSTIC FIBROSIS. Asymptomatic focal hepatic fibrosis may be found in virtually all older children with cystic fibrosis (p. 993), regardless of the clinical status of the child. In poorly controlled cases hepatomegaly and steatosis often occur. Rarely, young infants may present with prolonged neonatal cholestasis attributed to inspissated bile secretions, which may be evident as eosinophilic concretions on light microscopy. These cases may be indistinguishable from the neonatal hepatitis syndrome. Biliary cirrhosis resulting in portal hypertension is found in some older children and adolescent patients and rarely may be the initial manifestation of cystic fibrosis.

References

Cottrall K, Cook PJL, Mowat AP: Neonatal hepatitis syndrome and alpha-l-antitrypsin deficiency: an epidemiological study in southeast England. Postgrad Med J 50:376, 1974

Donnell GN, Bergren WR, Ng WG: Galactosemia. Biochem Med 1:29, 1967

Eriksson S, Larsson C: Purification and partial characterization of PAS-positive inclusion bodies from the liver in alpha-1-antitrypsin deficiency. N Engl J Med 292:176, 1975

Glasgow JFT, Lynch MJ, Hercz A, Sass-Kortsak A: Alpha-l-antitrypsin deficiency in association with both cirrhosis and chronic obstructive lung disease in two sibs. J Med 54:181, 1973

Glick TH, Lilosky WH, Levitt LP, Mellin H, Reynolds DW: Reye's syndrome: an epidemiologic approach. Pediatrics 46:371, 1970

Goldfischer S, Moore CL, Johnson AB, et al: Peroximal and mitochondrial defects in the cerebro-hepato-renal syndrome. Science 10:62, 1973

Hermann RE, Mercer RD: Portacaval shunt in the treatment of glycogen storage disease. Surgery 65:499, 1969

Huttenlocher PR: Reye's syndrome: relation of outcome to therapy. J Pediatr 80:845, 1972

Kahane D, Berant M, Wolman M: Primary familial xanthomatosis with adrenal involvement (Wolman's disease). Pediatrics 42:70, 1968

Levin B, Oberholzer VG, Snodgrass GJAI, Stimmler L, Wilmers MM: Fructosemia. An inborn error of fructose metabolism. Arch Dis Child 38:220, 1963

Mowat A: Encephalopathy and fatty degeneration of viscera—Reye's syndrome. Arch Dis Child 48:411, 1973

Partington M, Scriver CR, Sass-Kortsak A: A conference on hereditary tyrosinemia. Can Med Assoc J 97:1045, 1967

Reye RDK, Morgan G, Baral J: Encephalopathy and fatty degeneration of the viscera. A disease entity in childhood. Lancet 2:749, 1963

Scriver CR, Larochell J, Silverberg M: Hereditary tyrosinemia and tyrosyluria in a French Canadian geographic isolate. Am J Dis Child 113:41, 1967

Sharp HL, Bridges RA, Krivit W, Freier EF: Cirrhosis associated with alpha-l-antitrypsin deficiency. A previously unrecognized inherited disorder. J Lab Clin Med 73:934, 1969

Smetana HF, Hadley GG, Sirsat SM: Infantile cirrhosis. An analytic review of the literature and a report of 50 cases. Pediatrics 28:107, 1961

Stanbury JB, Wyngaarden JB, Fredrickson DS (eds): The Metabolic Basis of Inherited Diseases, 3rd ed. New York, McGraw-Hill, 1972

Talamo RC: The alpha-l-antitrypsin in man. J Allergy Clin Immunol 48:240, 1971

Tysob KRT, Schuster SR, Schwachman H: Portal hypertension in cystic fibrosis. J Pediatr Surg 3:271, 1968

CIRRHOSIS

FREDERIC DAUM AND MICHAEL I. COHEN

Cirrhosis in childhood is relatively uncommon. It is histologically characterized by extensive bands of fibrous tissue linking one portal area with another. Based on clinical and histopathologic features, cirrhosis may be classified as either biliary or postnecrotic cirrhosis. Common etiologic factors include infectious and toxic agents, anatomic abnormalities, metabolic disturbances, and autoimmune phenomena. Regardless of etiology, the eventual result is restricted blood flow to the liver cell, with progressive necrosis, loss of liver cell function, and portal hypertension.

Clinical Presentation

BILIARY CIRRHOSIS. The most common cause of biliary cirrhosis in young children is extraheptic biliary atresia. Jaundice is usually present from the outset, and cirrhosis rapidly occurs when the lesion is not surgically corrected by approximately 4 months of age. The initial presentation and pathology in extraphepatic biliary atresia are discussed elsewhere (p. 1085). Growth, which is normal early in the disease, slows after 6 months of age. The abdomen is protuberant, initially because of hepatomegaly and later because of splenomegaly and ascites. By 6 months of age the liver often shrinks considerably. Distended superficial abdominal veins are notable. Liver and spleen are firm and nontender. Ascites may become severe and ultimately restrict diaphragmatic excursion, resulting in respiratory distress. Clubbing and cyanosis of the nailbeds, angiomatous spider nevi, hypertrophic osteoarthropathy of small and large joints, and cardiac enlargement are manifestations of arteriovenous shunting that appear toward the end of the first year of life. The etiology of these circulatory changes is poorly understood. Pruritus becomes noticeable at about 1 year of age and rarely prior to 1 year. Most patients die before the age of 3 years, often by 18 months. Death is due to rupture of esophageal varices, peritonitis, or hepatic failure with coma.

The effect of the recently developed hepatoporticoenterostomy (Kasai procedure) in preventing biliary cirrhosis in children with biliary atresia is controversial. In some patients establishment of bile drainage prior to 4 months of age results in apparent cure; however, in other patients, despite bile drainage, cirrhosis progresses.

In the older child and teenager, cystic fibrosis is the most common cause of biliary cirrhosis. The process is often clinically and chemically silent. Jaundice and ascites are absent until late in the illness, while portal hypertension, splenomegaly, and upper gastrointestinal bleeding from esophageal varices are common.

POSTNECROTIC CIRRHOSIS. In the young child postnecrotic cirrhosis is rare. There is usually a history suggesting preceding neonatal hepatitis or metabolic disturbance. Jaundice is variable, while signs of portal hypertension frequently occur. Postnecrotic cirrhosis in the older pediatric population usually results from previous acute viral hepatitis or chronic active hepatitis. Wilson's disease (p. 1921) must be considered in any child over the age of 18 months with postnecrotic cirrhosis. α_1-antitrypsin deficiency should be considered at any age.

The clinical findings in postnecrotic cirrhosis are variable. Some patients have no complaints and appear healthy. Many are fatigued, irritable, and depressed, and adolescents may complain of decreased libido. Failure to thrive and delay in pubertal maturation are not clearly related to the degree of hepatic dysfunction or histologic destruction. Postnecrotic cirrhosis is often manifested solely by primary or secondary amenorrhea or epistaxis. Pruritus is infrequent, and jaundice appears late. The liver may be small or large, depending on the extent of scarring, while splenomegaly and ascites relate to the severity and duration of portal hypertension. Hemorrhoids seldom develop in children even when portal hypertension is significant. Signs of hypertrophic osteoarthropathy are usually present with advanced cirrhosis. In adolescents with jaundice and ascites, body image is often distorted, but this problem is seldom expressed. Amenorrhea and gynecomastia often evoke crises in sexual identity for adolescent patients.

Laboratory Appraisal

Chemical studies of hepatic dysfunction may suggest cirrhosis, but they are not pathognomonic. SGPT and SGOT activities are usually elevated to 50 and 400 Karmen units, but decline in the terminal stages. The serum bilirubin concentration may be normal in postnecrotic cirrhosis, but it is always elevated and predominantly conjugated in biliary cirrhosis. Serum alkaline phosphatase, gamma glutamyl transpeptidase, and 5′-nucleotidase activities vary with the degree of bile secretory failure. Serum cholesterol concentrations are variable. The BSP test is abnormal. A decrease in serum albumin concentration depends on the amount of functional liver tissue, dietary protein intake, and fluid and electrolyte dynamics. Hypergammaglobulinemia is common in patients with postnecrotic cirrhosis and chronic active hepatitis. Coagulation is often impaired because of depressed synthesis of vitamin-K-dependent factors II, VII, IX and X and fibrinogen. Functional hypersplenism results in thrombocytopenia, leukopenia, and normochromic and normocytic anemia. The serum concentrations of calcium and magnesium are often low, and diuretic therapy may complicate the already existent hyponatremia and hypokalemia.

Definitive diagnosis of cirrhosis requires histologic confirmation. Adequate specimens of liver may be obtained by either percutaneous needle biopsy or open surgical biopsy. Histologic diagnosis of cirrhosis should not be confused with congenital hepatic fibrosis, in which the lobular architecture is normal.

Hepatic scans with technetium pertechnetate reveal mottled or uneven uptake in cirrhosis. Increased uptake of radioisotope by the spleen suggests portal hypertension. Esophageal and gastric varices are visualized by barium sulfate esophagraphy in less than half of affected children. Fiberoptic esophagogastroscopy improves the frequency of visualization. Various radiographic techniques are used to determine whether portal hypertension is intrahepatic or extrahepatic. These include splenoportography, angiography, and measurements of wedged hepatic and umbilical vein pressures.

Complications

A major complication of biliary and postnecrotic cirrhosis is portal hypertension with hypersplenism, bleeding from esophageal varices, and ascites. The signs of portal hypertension are evident early in extrahepatic biliary atresia and are usually late manifestations of biliary cirrhosis secondary to cystic fibrosis. In older children with postnecrotic cirrhosis, splenomegaly, hypersplenism, and/or upper gastrointestinal bleeding are often the first manifestations of liver disease. Ascites and peripheral edema usually appear later. Bacterial contamination of ascitic fluid, particularly by pneumococcal, streptococcal, or coliform organisms, may cause peritonitis.

Nutritional defects in children with cirrhosis pose significant problems requiring constant attention. Although a moderate degree of steatorrhea, presumably due to abnormalities in bile acid metabolism, is common in children with cirrhosis, fat and caloric losses in the stool are probably insufficient to account for severe growth retardation, especially in children with extrahepatic biliary atresia. Steatorrhea appears to be an important factor in the development of rickets in growing children with cirrhosis: bone fractures suggest abnormalities in vitamin D and calcium metabolism. Infants and children with normal skeletal radiography and normal to borderline calcium and phosphorus concentrations in serum, may have diminished levels of 25-hydroxycholecalciferol. Factors in the development of rickets are malabsorption of fat-soluble vitamins (including vitamin D), formation of soaps by intraluminal precipitation of fat and calcium, and the inability of damaged liver to hydroxylate cholecalciferol.

In children with end-stage cirrhosis, hepatic failure slowly results in coma and death. The precipitating events leading to coma include gastrointestinal hemorrhage, sepsis, electrolyte imbalance, sedatives, and hepatotoxic medications.

Management

Some diseases that result in cirrhosis can be prevented or their complications can be ameliorated by nutritional modification, pharmacotherapy, or surgery. Medium-chain triglycerides that are absorbed directly into the portal circulation promote better growth and reduce the formation of calcium soaps and secondary rickets. Parenteral preparations of vitamin D and K are available, as are water-soluble vitamins A, E, and K. Oral 25-hydroxy vitamin D_3 has been successfully used in young children with cirrhosis.

When treating patients with increasing accumulations of ascitic fluid, it is essential to restrict dietary intake of sodium. Attempts to impose dietary restrictions are often met with resistance because foods low in salt are often not palatable. Therefore a very low salt diet should be maintained only until the desired therapeutic effect has been achieved. Moderate water restriction will minimize hyponatremia, but no amount of water and electrolyte therapy will completely correct the low serum sodium concentration of the severe cirrhotic. Administration of sodium does not correct the serum sodium concentration, but it increases the severity of ascites.

When respiratory distress results from abdominal

distension secondary to ascites, diuretic therapy is useful. Spironolactone and chlorothiazide often result in modest diuresis without major serum electrolyte abnormalities. Furosemide and other more potent (and dangerous) diuretics should be reserved for patients who are in severe distress or who are unresponsive to milder diuretic management. Hypokalemia and hyponatremia may result from therapy with furosemide or ethacrynic acid and may precipitate hepatic failure and coma. The realistic goal of diuretic therapy for ascites is to relieve respiratory distress and not to remove all ascitic fluid. Selected patients with cirrhosis and severe hypoalbuminemia may benefit from intravenous infusion of salt-poor albumin prior to diuresis.

Diagnostic paracentesis should be performed in patients with peritonitis or rapidly accumulating ascites without discernible cause. Paracentesis for relief of discomfort should be performed only when adequate diuresis cannot be achieved by diuretic agents and salt and water restriction.

The use of prophylactic antibiotics to prevent bacterial contamination of ascitic fluid and peritonitis is controversial; however, any child with fever and ascites should be suspected of having peritonitis, usually caused by pneumococci.

Cholestyramine, a bile-acid-binding anion-exchange resin, may provide relief from pruritus. The usual dose is 9 to 12 g/day. However, it may cause severe constipation leading to symptoms and signs of acute intestinal obstruction.

Oral iron supplementation is recommended for children with cirrhosis and iron-deficiency anemia. The most common cause of iron deficiency in these patients is frequent, intermittent, or mild gastrointestinal bleeding.

In patients with upper gastrointestinal bleeding, localization of the specific site should be attempted by barium esophagram, esophagoscopy, and/or angiography. Catheterization of the superior mesenteric artery and infusion of posterior pituitary extract to cause vasoconstriction and decrease mesenteric and retrograde variceal blood flow may be effective in controlling variceal hemorrhage.

For infants with uncorrectable biliary atresia or other types of cirrhosis, only supportive measures are available. Liver transplantation is an experimental treatment undergoing evaluation. Obtaining suitable donor liver plus the ongoing struggle to control the rejection process continue to be problems, but transplantation remains a possibility.

The overall prognosis in infants, children, and adolescents with cirrhosis and portal hypertension is poor. Each of the above therapeutic modalities has only a temporizing effect and improves longevity without altering overall mortality.

References

Cohen MI, Gartner LM: The use of medium-chain triglycerides in the management of biliary atresia. J Pediatr 79:379, 1971

Craig JM, Gellis SS, Hsia DYY: Cirrhosis of the liver in infants and children. Am J Dis Child 90:299, 1955

di Sant'Agnese PA, Blanc WA: A distinctive type of biliary cirrhosis of the liver associated with cystic fibrosis of the pancreas; recognition through signs of portal hypertension. Pediatrics 18:387, 1956

Klatskin G: Newer concepts of cirrhosis. Arch Intern Med 104:899, 1959

Kopel FB: Gastrointestinal manifestations of cystic fibrosis. Gastroenterology 62:483, 1972

Nusbaum M, Baum S, Kuroda K, et al: Control of portal hypertension by selective mesenteric arterial drug infusion. Arch Surg 97:1005, 1968

Sharp HL, Carey JB Jr, White JG, Krivit W: Cholestyramine therapy in patients with a paucity of intrahepatic bile ducts. J Pediatr 71:723, 1967

Smetana HF, Hadley GG, Sirsak SM, Infantile cirrhosis; analytical review of literature and report of 50 cases. Pediatrics 28:107, 1961

Indian Childhood Cirrhosis

R. K. Chandra

An enlarged, readily palpable liver is a common physical sign in children living in tropical countries. Fatty infiltration, nonspecific reactive hepatitis, tuberculosis, parasitic infestation, and cirrhosis are the common underlying pathologic states. In India cirrhosis of the liver occurs frequently and is a major cause of mortality in children 1 to 4 years of age. The well-recognized types of cirrhosis discussed above account for only one-third of such cases. In the others a characteristic syndrome has been observed that has unique clinical features, histopathology, biochemical epiphenomena, and immunologic abberrations. The geographic localization of this syndrome principally to the Indian subcontinent has led to the designation Indian childhood cirrhosis.

The clinical course follows one of two patterns. In the majority of patients the onset at the age of 6 to 24 months is gradual, with vague symptoms such as distension of the abdomen, mild pyrexia, frequent pale pasty stools, and either anorexia or a voracious appetite. In some cases mild transient jaundice may be seen. Within a few weeks the liver becomes palpable and has a sharp firm edge; the surface is either smooth or granular and nontender. Subsequently there is progressive hepatomegaly, ascites, splenomegaly, and edema. Death is due to hepatic coma and accompanies deepening jaundice and bleeding, especially into the gastrointestinal tract. In very young infants 3 to 9 months old, the onset may be acute, with hepatitislike features including jaundice, hyperpyrexia, and poor appetite and with a rapid progression within weeks to fatal hepatic coma.

The syndrome is familial; several siblings may be affected in succession. Both sexes are involved, but there is a significant male preponderance of about 4 to 1. The closely inbred Brahmin and Banya communities are especially at risk. Genealogic analyses suggest that the genetic predisposition is inherited on an autosomal recessive basis. Dermatoglyphics of cirrhotic children differ from those of healthy controls, although no pattern is diagnostic. Chromosomes are normal in number and morphology.

Histomorphology is characteristic. The liver may be enlarged or normal, or rarely even small; it is bile-stained and finely granular. Biliary passages are patent. Microscopy shows widespread degeneration of liver cells with little attempt at regeneration; there is creeping fibrosis encircling single or clustered ballooned necrotic hepatocytes with pale vesicular nuclei and an intracytoplasmic eosinophilic material that is indistinguishable from Mallory's acholic hyaline. Ultrastructurally this material is made up of a tangled mass of fibrils and electron-dense particles possibly derived from the endoplasmic reticulum. In the early stages there are no significant changes in the bile ducts or hepatic veins. There is a mild inflammatory exudate; fatty infiltration is conspicuously absent.

Biochemical tests show varying degrees of hepatic cell dysfunction. In the majority of cases serum α-fetoprotein is raised. The continued or renewed synthesis of this protein through depression of the embryonic gene has been suggested to indicate a peculiar hepatocytic immaturity that makes it more vulnerable to injury. In addition, gastric acid output in response to maximal augmented histamine stimulation is severely reduced; this could be due to the release of histaminase from degenerating liver cells. Serum copper and ceruloplasmin are raised. Plasma zinc is low, due to increased excretion in the urine. There is generalized aminoaciduria and mellituria, possibly a result of renal tubular reabsorptive defect, although no specific pattern is detected on urinary chromatography. Serum α_1-antitrypsin is normal or elevated, although PI typing has not been done. Serum immunoglobulins are markedly elevated. Serum hemolytic complement and C3 levels are often low. Many patients show complement activation in vivo, and a few may have circulating immune complexes. Hepatitis B surface antigen (HB_sAg) has been detected in the serum and other body fluids in 5 to 20 percent of patients in different series. There is a higher incidence of HB_sAg in family members as well. Cell-mediated immunity is slightly depressed, which is commensurate with inanition associated with the disease. Recently a lack of cell-mediated immune reactivity specifically to HB_sAg has been demonstrated in these patients; it may have etiopathogenetic significance.

No definite cause has been found that would explain all the known features of Indian childhood cirrhosis. It is possible that more than one pathway may lead to the same clinicopathologic syndrome. Malnutrition and established metabolic causes of cirrhosis have been ruled out as primary etiologic factors. Genetic predisposition probably plays a contributory role. No local toxin has been detected consistently, but a description of hepatic lesions histologically similar to Indian childhood cirrhosis resulting from ingestion of aflatoxin-contaminated food by a group of malnourished children supports a toxic etiology. Clinical and epidemiologic data and the demonstration of HB_sAg suggests that viral infection may play a causative role. Hepatitis virus or viruses may initiate hepatocytic injury, which is then perpetuated by secondary immunologic mechanisms. The failure to mount an adequate specific cell-mediated immune response can result in persistent antigenemia and formation of immune complexes and progressive liver damage ending in death.

Management is supportive. No form of therapy has been successful in halting the progression of the established disease process. There is controversy about the definition of the early hepatic lesion, and thus claims of survival and cure of early cirrhosis are questionable.

References

Achar ST, Raju VB, Sriramachari S: Indian childhood cirrhosis. J Pediatr 57:744, 1960

Chandra RK: Immunological picture in Indian childhood cirrhosis. Lancet 1:537, 1970

——Indian childhood cirrhosis. Clinical, biochemical, genealogical, histomorphological and immunological observations. Med Chir Dig 3:63, 1974

—— The liver and biliary system. In Anderson CM (ed): Pediatric Gastroenterology. Oxford, Blackwell, 1975

Liver Diseases Subcommittee, Indian Council of Medical Research: Infantile cirrhosis of the liver in India. Indian J Med Res 43:369, 1955

Nayak NC, Sagareyia K, Ramalingaswami V: Indian childhood cirrhosis: the nature and significance of cytoplasmic hyaline of hepatocytes. Arch Pathol 88:631, 1969

PORTAL HYPERTENSION

LAWRENCE M. GARTNER

Portal venous hypertension results when the flow of portal blood to the liver is obstructed either within the liver or along the extrahepatic portal vein. A major cause of portal hypertension in children is thrombosis (cavernous transformation) of the portal vein, the etiology of which is usually unknown. Omphalitis, umbilical vein catheterization, and intra-abdominal infection in infancy may be associated with portal vein thrombosis. Hepatic function and histology are normal. Although thrombosis of the portal vein probably occurs in the neonatal period, the onset of bleeding from esophageal varices, which is almost always the presenting symptom in this disorder, does not occur until 6 months to 15 years later. Variceal hemorrhage is manifested by hematemesis, melena, sudden onset of anemia, or shock. Hemorrhage is usually not fatal when hepatic function and morphology are normal. Other signs of extrahepatic portal obstruction are splenomegaly, distended abdominal veins, thrombocytopenia, leukopenia, and anemia. Following the sudden loss of a large volume of blood, the spleen may not be palpable; however, after blood transfusion or spontaneous restoration of blood volume, splenomegaly may reappear.

The second major cause of portal hypertension in children is cirrhosis, which may be postnecrotic or biliary. In biliary cirrhosis, portal hypertension follows months or years of jaundice, pruritus, and progressive deterioration of hepatic function. In postnecrotic cirrhosis of any cause, progressive deterioration of hepatic function may be insidious, but clinical and laboratory signs of hepatic damage are usually evident prior to clinical recognition of portal hypertension.

In schistosomiasis of the liver, hepatic function remains normal until very late in the disease, and portal hypertension and massive splenomegaly occur as initial manifestations. This sequence results from intrahepatic portal venous obstruction by schistosome eggs and the associated inflammation. Markedly elevated serum alkaline phosphatase activity is usually observed in schistosomiasis of the liver, but its cause is obscure. In endemic areas, such as northeastern Brazil, China, and Africa, schistosomiasis is the predominant cause of portal hypertension in children and may be associated with infantilism.

A relatively rare cause of portal hypertension is congenital hepatic fibrosis with polycystic disease of the liver, kidneys, and/or spleen. Hepatic fibrosis may exist with or without hepatic cysts. Approximately one-half of children with polycystic disease of the liver have renal polycystic disease. The hepatic cysts are variable in size, occasionally large enough to be identified by hepatic scanning or angiography. The initial symptom is usually hematemesis secondary to esophageal varices. Jaundice and laboratory evidence of liver disease are usually absent. Portal hypertension is thought to result from a paucity of hepatic portal venules rather than fibrosis or the cysts. Massive hepatomegaly is common, and an enlarged abdomen may be the first indication of hepatic disease.

Although it is extremely rare in infants and children, obstruction of hepatic vein blood flow due to thrombosis or tumor (Budd-Chiari syndrome) may result in catastrophic illness with sudden hepatic enlargement, vascular collapse, portal hypertension, or secondary splenic enlargement.

Ascites is generally absent in diseases such as congenital hepatic fibrosis and extrahepatic portal vein thrombosis and portal hypertension with normal hepatocellular function. Ascites is common in disorders that cause reduced hepatic cell function, such as cirrhosis.

The diagnosis of portal hypertension requires demonstration of esophageal and/or gastric varices by barium swallow or endoscopy, or elevated portal venous pressure by splenic pulp manometry or umbilical venous catheterization. Percutaneous splenic venography usually reveals the site and extent of portal venous obstruction and frequently reveals portal systemic venous anastomoses. The latter information is critical in determining the type of surgery to be performed. When portal hypertension is secondary to cirrhosis or congenital hepatic fibrosis, percutaneous splenic venography or umbilical venography reveal dilated collateral venous channels, normal portal vein, and intrahepatic circulatory changes. Percutaneous aspiration needle biopsy is often helpful in differentiating intrahepatic from extrahepatic causes of portal hypertension. Oral aspirin use is contraindicated in all patients with portal hypertension, as it is a frequent cause of esophageal variceal hemorrhage.

Surgical relief of portal hypertension offers the only means by which subsequent hemorrhagic episodes may be prevented. The decision to perform surgery and the choice of technique depend on the location of the obstruction, frequency and severity of previous bleeding, degree of hypersplenism, and availability of vessels of sufficient size to permit successful anastomosis. Occasionally operative risks are so great that surgery should not be undertaken. Portal venous surgery in patients with normal hepatic histology and function should cure the disease without risk of hepatic damage from diversion of portal blood. In patients with cirrhosis, although successful surgery for portal hypertension may prevent subsequent bleeding from esophageal varices, hepatic function often deteriorates, resulting in death from hepatic insufficiency.

Hypersplenism secondary to splenomegaly suggests the need for splenectomy. Removal of the spleen without simultaneous vascular shunt anastomosis to relieve portal hypertension may lead to esophageal hemorrhage. Anastomosis of the inferior vena cava to the superior mesenteric vein (mesocaval shunt) offers the best surgical approach for relief of portal hypertension in small children. Portacaval anastomosis is not applicable for the child with portal vein thrombosis. Splenorenal anastomosis in smaller children often results in poor shunt flow and thrombosis.

References

Hsia DYY, Gellis SS: Portal hypertension in infants and children. Am J Dis Child 90:290, 1955

Oski FA, Allen DH, Diamond LK: Portal hypertension—a complication of umbilical vein catheterization. Pediatrics 31:297, 1963

Sherlock S: Diseases of the Liver and Biliary System, 3rd ed. Philadelphia, FA Davis, 1963

Vorhees AB Jr, Harris RC, Britton RC, Price JB, Santulli TV: Portal hypertension in children: 98 cases. Surgery 58:540, 1965

HEPATIC FAILURE

Michael I. Cohen and Fredric Daum

Hepatic failure is a pathologic state of diverse etiology and manifestations that occurs when liver cell function cannot sustain minimal metabolic needs of the patient. It is characterized by an altered state of consciousness, chemical evidence of hepatocellular dysfunction, abnormal electroencephalogram, and usually increased blood concentrations of ammonia. Hepatic failure may be acute or chronic and may develop during the course of any type of acute or chronic liver injury.

One cannot predict which individual with acute viral or toxic hepatitis will develop severe hepatic necrosis and clinical encephalopathy. Even anicteric, mildly symptomatic patients may suddenly develop liver failure and die within days. Early clinical manifestations of hepatic coma (stage I) are alternating lethargy and excitation, changes in personality, inappropriate response to simple commands, slurred speech and poor handwriting, and inability to perform elementary calculations and recall commonly known names, places, and dates. Hyperreflexia and a shrinking liver may be associated with these manifestations. This stage may be followed by drowsiness and bizarre behavior, with trem-

ors and asterixis (ie, flapping of the hands when held elevated) (stage II). Stage III is characterized by marked sleepiness, incoherent speech, mental confusion, and severe asterixis. As the state of consciousness worsens, unresponsiveness and loss of pain occur, and asterixis and deep tendon reflexes disappear (stage IV). Deepening coma eventually requires ventilatory assistance. The EEG is abnormal during stages II, III, and IV and is characterized by slow triphasic waves.

Liver function tests, including serum ammonia levels, bilirubin concentrations, and transaminase activities, are abnormal and of little prognostic significance. Only a progressive increase in prothrombin time over a period of hours to days is predictive of hepatic encephalopathy. A child with hepatitis and a prothrombin time 5 sec greater than control should be hospitalized. Falling plasma glucose and urea concentrations may also indicate progressive inability of the liver to maintain glycogenolysis and ammonia metabolism, respectively.

Hepatic histology, when a biopsy is technically feasible, may suggest the etiology and specific therapy; however, in most instances the cause of hepatic coma is unknown, and therapy is supportive. This includes correction of hypoglycemia, hyperammonemia, hemorrhage, fluid, electrolyte, and mineral imbalances, infection, seizures, and respiratory depression. Although the pathophysiologic relationship between an elevated serum ammonia concentration and hepatic encephalopathy remains obscure, efforts are aimed at reducing hyperammonemia by withdrawing dietary protein, reducing conversion of urea to ammonia by urease-producing intestinal bacteria through the use of oral antibiotics, using enemas to remove residual protein and blood, and decreasing intestinal absorption of ammonia by reducing the pH of colonic fluid.

To sterilize the distal small intestine and colon, 250 to 1,000 mg of neomycin or kanamycin are administered by nasogastric tube every 6 hours, while 250 to 500 mg of the same antibiotics in about 250 to 500 ml of warm saline solution may be infused by a high colonic enema. As an alternative or adjunct to these antibiotics, lactulose can be administered by mouth and/or rectum. This synthetic carbohydrate is not metabolized by the human intestinal mucosa, but is degraded by colonic bacteria, thus releasing lactic acid that decreases the pH of the colonic luminal contents and converts freely diffusible NH_3 to nondiffusible NH_4^+. The latter is excreted in feces and lowers the plasma ammonia concentration. Vitamin K (5 mg) should be injected intramuscularly or intravenously in an attempt to correct the prothrombin deficiency noted in almost all patients with hepatic coma.

The usefulness of corticosteroids in management of hepatic coma remains questionable. Mortality appears unaffected and may be worsened. Other immunosuppressive or anti-inflammatory agents offer no benefit in management of hepatic coma. Sedatives, hypnotics, analgesics, and psychoactive agents are contraindicated. In therapy for the child with hepatic coma and concomitant seizure activity, caution in drug dosage is critical. Before any central nervous system depressants are used, staff and equipment for support of ventilation must be available.

Despite exchange transfusion, plasmapheresis, cross-circulation, peritoneal dialysis, plasma-rich hepatitis B_s antibody infusions, and asanguineous hypothermic total body perfusion, the high mortality in pediatric patients with acute hepatic encephalopathy remains unchanged. Since the specific etiologic factors in hepatic coma are not discernible, supportive therapy with intensive nursing care and close clinical and laboratory observation still provides the best hope for survival.

The pediatric patient who recovers from an episode of hepatic coma may be at risk for development of cirrhosis, portal hypertension, and esophageal varices. Long-term evaluation is essential in the management of these children.

References

Berger RL, Liversage RM Jr, Calmers TC, et al: Exchange transfusion in the treatment of fulminating hepatitis. N Engl J Med 274:497, 1966

Chalmers TC: Pathogenesis and treatment of hepatic failure. N Engl J Med 263:23, 77, 1960

Cohen MI, Schonberg SK, Witover S: The use of plasmapheresis during exchange transfusion for hepatic encephalopathy. J Pediatr 75:431, 1969

Gazzard BG, Weston MJ, Murray-Lyon IM, et al: Charcoal haemoperfusion in the treatment of fulminant hepatic failure. Lancet 1:1301, 1974

Kersh ES, Rifkin HR: Lactulose enemas. Ann Intern Med 78:81, 1973

Redeker AG, Yamahiro HS: Controlled trial of exchange transfusion therapy in fulminant hepatitis. Lancet 1:3, 1973

Schenker S, Breen MD, Horjumpa AM: Hepatic encephalopathy; current status. Gastroenterology 66:121, 1974

Trey C, Burns DG, Saunders SF: Treatment of hepatic coma by exchange transfusions. N Engl J Med 274:473, 1966

Zieve L: Pathogenesis of hepatic coma. Arch Intern Med 118:211, 1966

TUMORS OF THE LIVER

JAY BERNSTEIN AND A. JOSEPH BROUGH

Primary tumors of the liver are relatively uncommon in children, accounting for only 1.5 percent of all tumors. They comprise perhaps 10 percent of abdominal neoplasms. Approximately two-thirds of such tumors are discovered in the first 3 years of life; the peak incidence is at 1 year of age. Some hepatic tumors are present at birth.

The most common clinical abnormality is painless abdominal enlargement. Jaundice rarely occurs, and abnormalities of liver function tests are uncommon. Excretory urography is often helpful in differentiating between hepatic abdominal tumors and extrahepatic tumors such as neuroblastoma or Wilms' tumor. Hepatic calcification, sometimes due to bone formation, as in teratomas or hamartomas, can be seen radiographically, simulating metastatic neuroblastoma. Scintillation radionuclide imaging, ultrasound echography, celiac axis angiography, splenoportography, cholecystography, and cholangiography are valuable in localizing areas of involvement and demonstrating important anatomic relationships that must be known if surgical therapy is

considered. The specific diagnosis of a hepatic tumor can be determined only by pathologic examination of tissue obtained by needle or open biopsy. Although radiologic studies may suggest operability or inoperability, a laparotomy is necessary for determining the extent and resectability of a tumor.

HEPATOCELLULAR CARCINOMAS AND HEPATOBLASTOMAS. Hepatocellular neoplasms constitute approximately one-half of primary hepatic tumors in childhood. Carcinomas are usually primary in the sense that they are not associated with preexisting cirrhosis. Hepatocellular tumors include both hepatoblastoma and hepatocellular carcinoma, the former a less differentiated tumor that often contains mesenchymal elements. The mesenchymal components include variable amounts of hematopoietic tissue, osteoid, bone, cartilage, and muscle. Both types of tumors are often associated with an increase in the serum globulin α_2-fetoprotein, but it is not specific for hepatic tumors, since elevations occur in association with benign hepatic diseases as well. Epithelial differentiation in hepatoblastoma can occasionally lead to squamous metaplasia, melanin production, and gonadotropin production with precocious puberty. The incidence of congenital malformations in patients with hepatoblastoma is unexpectedly high. Both types of hepatocellular tumors are associated relatively frequently with osteoporosis and with the combination of hyperlipemia, hypercholesterolemia, and lipid histiocytosis. The prognosis in hepatoblastoma has been reported to be relatively good in comparison with the outcome in hepatic carcinoma, but other reports and our own updated series lead to less sanguine conclusions (Table 4).

TABLE 4. Hepatic Tumors in Childhood: Children's Hospital of Michigan 1950–1975

Type	Total
Hepatoblastoma	16
Hepatocellular carcinoma	8
Hepatic sarcoma	2
Lymphangioma (benign)	3
Hemangioma (benign)	6
Mesenchymoma (benign)	1
"Hepatic neuroblastoma"	6[a]

[a] Two deaths not related to tumor.

Hepatocellular carcinomas generally have had a poor prognosis, despite a frequently benign histologic appearance. The well-differentiated hepatocarcinoma cannot always be differentiated from the rare hepatic adenoma, and the usual criteria of malignancy, such as cellular atypia and vascular invasion, are often lacking. Malignant hepatomas invade local vessels and metastasize to other portions of the liver, to the lungs, to the peritoneum, and to lymph nodes. Direct extension through the vena cava also occurs.

MESENCHYMAL TUMORS. Malignant mesenchymal tumors are rare. One in particular, an embryonal sarcoma or rhabdomyosarcoma, has been discussed extensively in the literature. It may arise in the liver or more commonly in the extrahepatic biliary tree. Growth into and along the common duct causes intermittent mild jaundice. The tumors are similar histologically to embryonal rhabdomyosarcomas seen elsewhere. The prognosis is exceedingly poor. Chemotherapy and irradiation are only palliative.

BENIGN TUMORS. Benign tumors of the liver include hepatocellular adenomas, hemangiomas, lymphangiomas, mesenchymomas, and so-called hamartomas. Adenomas have been reported as complications of the use of contraceptives in young women. Hemangiomas may grow to considerable size and produce symptoms by pressure. They may be solitary or part of a generalized visceral hemangiomatosis. They have been observed to opacify during excretory urography. Both cavernous and endotheliomatous tumors occur. Such tumors occasionally behave as arteriovenous fistulas, with an audible bruit and cardiomegaly. Thrombosis of the vascular channels can lead to consumption of clotting factors and secondary thrombocytopenia. Traumatic rupture of a vascular tumor can lead to exsanguinating hemorrhage. Lymphangiomas can become enormous, and the loculi contain fluid indistinguishable from hepatic lymph. They may be superficial or pedunculated, and they are rarely associated with visceral lymphangiomatosis. Hamartomas contain epithelial and mesenchymal elements arranged in disorderly fashion, and they are sometimes regarded as tumorous malformations.

HEPATIC CYSTS. Hepatic cysts of biliary origin can arise as part of polycystic disease or as isolated lesions. The latter are usually unilocular and lined by biliary epithelium. They may develop as the result of localized ductal obstruction and distension. They contain mucus and bile in varying amounts and at times are surrounded by dense fibrous capsules.

METASTATIC TUMORS. Metastatic tumors of the liver are far more common than primary tumors. Of particular interest is so-called hepatic neuroblastoma, ie, marked hepatomegaly due to extensive infiltration by neuroblastoma in very young infants. The tumor is presumed to arise in the adrenal, although demonstration of an adrenal mass is frequently lacking. The babies present with abdominal distension, and mild anemia, and the diagnosis is usually established by liver biopsy and histopathologic examination. The prognosis in our experience has been extremely good. Most cases have been treated with irradiation, resulting in complete resolution of the tumor and long-term survival. Spontaneous resolution has also been known to occur without specific therapy, but it must be recalled that fatalities in the period prior to radiation therapy were not uncommon.

TREATMENT. Surgical extirpation of primary tumors is the accepted form of therapy at present. Resection of very large tumors involving the right or left hepatic lobes is practicable by modern surgical techniques. Benign tumors should be excised preferably in toto; partial resection may be necessary if complications due to enlargement or rupture occur. Hamartomas that are pedunculated can easily be excised; however, those deep within the parenchyma, producing no symptoms, may be left in situ after a definitive diagnosis has been made.

References

Davis GL, Kissane JM, Ishak KG: Embryonal rhabdomyosarcoma (sarcoma botrioides) of the biliary tree. Report of five cases and a review of the literature. Cancer 24:333, 1969

Howat JM: Major hepatic resections in infancy and childhood. Gut 12:212, 1971

Ishak KG, Glunz PR: Hepatoblastoma and hepatocarcinoma in infancy and childhood. Report of 47 cases. Cancer 20:396, 1967

Kasai M, Watanabe I: Histologic classification of liver-cell carcinoma in infancy and childhood and its clinical evaluation. A study of 70 cases collected in Japan. Cancer 25:551, 1970

Keeling JW: Liver tumours in infancy and childhood. J Pathol 103:69, 1971

McArthur JW, Toll GD, Russfield AB, et al: Sexual precocity attributable to ectopic gonadotropin secretion by hepatoblastoma. Am J Med 54:390, 1973

Schiodt T: Hepatoblastoma and hepatocarcinoma in infancy and childhood. Report on the pathology of eight cases from the University Hospital, Copenhagen. Acta Pathol Microbiol Scand [Suppl 212] 1970

Yang S-S, Brough AJ, Bernstein J: Tumors of the liver in early infancy: hepatoblastoma. Michigan Med 71:539, 1972

CHAPTER 24

Blood and Blood-forming Tissues

PETER R. DALLMAN, *Associate Editor*

THE RED CELL

PETER R. DALLMAN

DEVELOPMENTAL CHANGES IN RED CELL PRODUCTION AND FUNCTION

Sites of Production

During development, the size of the developing embryo rapidly becomes too large to allow for oxygenation of tissues by simple diffusion. By 2 weeks of gestation, the production of red blood cells starts within the newly developing vessels of the yolk sac; shortly thereafter, circulating red cells play the major role in the delivery of oxygen to the tissues. At 8 weeks of gestation the site of red cell maturation shifts primarily to the liver sinusoids, and the production of white cells and platelets begins. The production of these cellular elements in the liver, and in lesser amounts in the spleen and lymph nodes, reaches a peak at about 5 months. Thereafter, hepatic blood formation declines, but it does not disappear entirely during the remainder of gestation. Hematopoiesis in the bone marrow begins near the fifth month of gestation and increases rapidly, soon filling the entire marrow space.

BONE MARROW. During the last third of gestation, the marrow is the main organ for maturation of the cellular elements of the blood. In the newborn and during early infancy, hematopoietic marrow fills the bony cavities of the entire axial skeleton, the long bones, and many membranous bones. For this reason, during the first year, the tibia is often chosen as a convenient site for bone marrow aspiration. With advancing age, hematopoietic tissue gradually retreats centrally to the vertebrae, sternum, pelvis, scapulae, skull, and proximal ends of the femora and humeri. Of these sites, the iliac crest or posterior superior iliac spine is used most commonly for bone marrow aspiration in children beyond the age of infancy. The vertebral posterior spinous process provides an alternative.

EXTRAMEDULLARY HEMATOPOIESIS. In diseases characterized by hemolysis, the normal rate of red cell production can increase up to eightfold, causing a concomitant increase in the volume of hematopoietic tissue. Blood production first expands from the ends of the long bones toward the middle of the shafts to replace the fatty marrow. Next, the production of blood cells extends to extramedullary sites, particularly in the liver and spleen. In infants and children, hemolytic disease results in a relatively greater enlargement of the liver and spleen than in adults because most of the bony sites are already filled with red marrow (Fig. 1). In chronic hemolytic disease the expanded volume of red marrow within the bones results in loss of trabeculae and in outward displacement and thinning of the cortex, which are detectable radiographically.

Rate of Production, Normal Values

THE FETUS. The concentration of hemoglobin and the hematocrit both increase gradually and at similar rates, almost doubling during gestation. The mean concentration of hemoglobin increases from 10 g/dl at 12 weeks to 14 g/dl at 24 weeks; near the end of gestation, values increase more slowly, reaching 16.5 g/dl in the cord blood of the term infant. Corresponding values for hematocrit increase in proportion from 33 to 40 to 51 percent, respectively. In contrast, the red blood cell count more than triples during fetal life, from about 1.5 million/mm^3 at 12 weeks of gestation to 4.7 million at term. This disproportionate increase in number is explained by the marked reduction in red cell volume

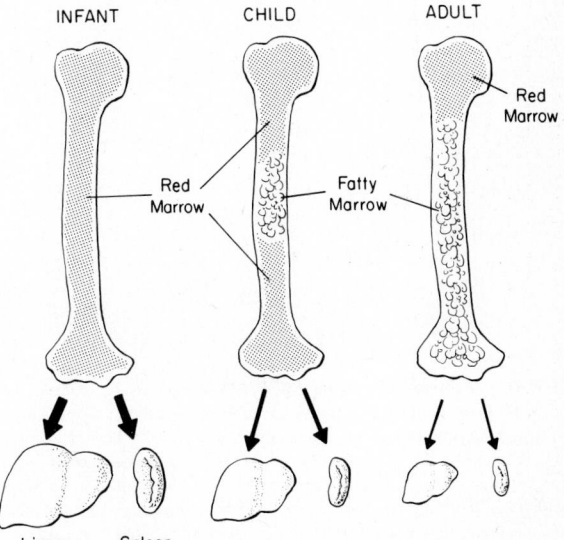

FIG. 1. Sites of hematopoiesis. With maturation, red marrow is partly replaced by fatty marrow in the shafts of the long bones. In the adult, in addition to the vertebrae and the pelvic bones, hematopoietic tissue is largely restricted to the proximal ends of the femur and humerus. In response to hemolysis, there is extension of marrow in the long bones. In the infant whose skeletal hematopoiesis has little room for expansion, the extent of extramedullary hematopoiesis in the liver and spleen is more marked than in the adult.

from a mean of 180 femtoliters (fl) at 12 weeks to 108 fl at term. The difference in red cell size in the fetus compared with the adult (mean 90 fl) is so great that it has been applied to the intrauterine diagnosis of red cell disorders. Thus, a sample of blood obtained from the placenta can be identified as fetal, maternal, or a mixture of the two from the size distribution of the cells as determined by an electronic counter (Fig. 2).

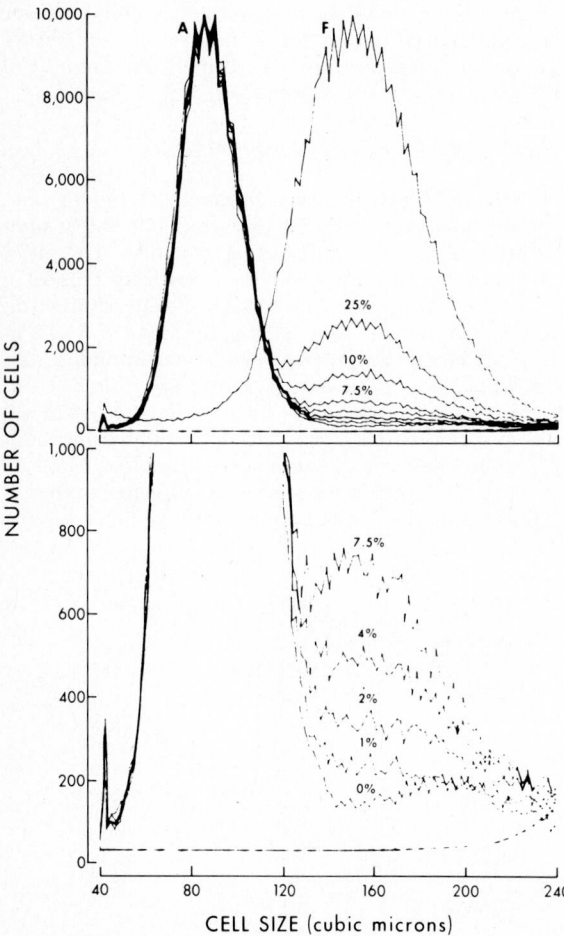

FIG. 2. Mean red cell volume (MCV) in the fetus and the mother. The quantitative contribution of fetal and maternal blood can be estimated in a sample of blood from the placenta by determining the size distribution of the red cells on an electronic counter; a larger peak at an MCV of 160 fl indicates a predominance of fetal cells whereas a major peak at an MCV of 90 shows that primarily maternal blood is being sampled. A cubic micron is equivalent to an fl. (From Kan; unpublished data)

THE NEWBORN. The umbilical cord is the most convenient site for sampling blood at birth. Normal values for cord blood are shown in Table 1. During the first few days after birth, there is a discrepancy between venous and capillary values. The concentration of capillary hemoglobin is consistently about 2 g/dl higher than in venous blood, and the hematocrit is approximately 6 percent higher. This discrepancy reflects an increase in concentration of blood cells as they traverse the capillaries, due to the transient seepage of plasma out of the capillary bed. The apparent rise in hemoglobin, hematocrit, and red cell counts between birth and 1 to 3 days of age (Table 1) may be attributable to the sites of sampling: cord blood and capillary blood, respectively. After 1 to 2 weeks of age, the difference between venous and capillary values is too small to be of clinical significance.

POSTNATAL ERYTHROPOIESIS. The rate of division and differentiation of nucleated red blood cells in bone marrow is controlled by a humoral substance, termed erythropoietin, which is produced primarily in the kidney. Its rate of production is increased in response to tissue hypoxia, and it in turn stimulates production of red cells. The resulting increase in concentration of hemoglobin restores tissue oxygenation to normal. The relative polycythemia of the newborn is attributable to the hypoxic intrauterine environment, which stimulates erythropoietin production in the fetus and results in a high rate of erythropoiesis. After birth, as oxygen from the lungs begins to saturate the arterial blood, the amount of oxygen delivered to the tissues increases. In response to the change from a placental to a pulmonary oxygen supply during the first few days of life, levels of erythropoietin and rate of erythropoiesis decrease. This is reflected in a decline in the percentage of erythroid precursor cells in the bone marrow from an average of 35 percent at birth to 15 percent after 1 week (Table 1) and in the concurrent obliteration of the remaining sites of extramedullary hematopoiesis. In the peripheral blood the decreased production of red cells is reflected in the disappearance of nucleated red blood cells and a precipitous fall in the reticulocyte count. A marked depression in the rate of red blood cell production continues for 6 to 8 weeks following birth. During this period of rapid growth, the rate of red cell destruction is also greater than in later life, with a lifespan of about 90 days compared with 120 days. As a consequence of decreased production and increased destruction, the hemoglobin and hematocrit values drop to their lowest mean values of 11.5 g/dl and 35 percent, respectively, between 8 and 12 weeks. After 6 to 8 weeks of age, red cell production increases, and the rate of production is sufficient to maintain a stable hemoglobin concentration, despite the tripling of blood volume and weight that occurs during the first year of life.

In the premature infant the postnatal fall in hemoglobin and hematocrit is more marked than in the term infant, even with what is considered optimal nutrition (see sections on iron, p. 1119, and vitamin E, p. 1166). Between 2 and 3 months of age, values fall to a mean of about 9.5 g/dl and 28 percent, respectively, in infants with a mean birth weight of 1,800 g.

In the preschool and preadolescent child, erythropoiesis more than keeps pace with growth, and there is a gradual rise in hemoglobin, hematocrit, and red cell count. Values in male and female first begin to diverge

TABLE 1. Red Blood Cell Values at Various Ages: Mean and Lower Limit of Normal (−2 SD)*

Age	Hemoglobin (g/dl)		Hematocrit (%)		Red Cell Count (10¹²/liter)		MCV (fl)		MCH (pg)		MCHC (g/dl)	
	Mean	−2 SD	Mean	−2 SD	Mean	−2 SD	Mean	−2 SD	Mean	−2 SD	Mean	−2 SD
Birth (cord blood)	16.5	13.5	51	42	4.7	3.9	108	98	34	31	33	30
1 to 3 days (capillary)	18.5	14.5	56	45	5.3	4.0	108	95	34	31	33	29
1 week	17.5	13.5	54	42	5.1	3.9	107	88	34	28	33	28
2 weeks	16.5	12.5	51	39	4.9	3.6	105	86	34	28	33	28
1 month	14.0	10.0	43	31	4.2	3.0	104	85	34	28	33	29
2 months	11.5	9.0	35	28	3.8	2.7	96	77	30	26	33	29
3 to 6 months	11.5	9.5	35	29	3.8	3.1	91	74	30	25	33	30
0.5 to 2 years	12.0	10.5	36	33	4.5	3.7	78	70	27	23	33	30
2 to 6 years	12.5	11.5	37	34	4.6	3.9	81	75	27	24	34	31
6 to 12 years	13.5	11.5	40	35	4.6	4.0	86	77	29	25	34	31
12 to 18 years—female	14.0	12.0	41	36	4.6	4.1	90	78	30	25	34	31
male	14.5	13.0	43	37	4.9	4.5	88	78	30	25	34	31
18 to 49 years—female	14.0	12.0	41	36	4.6	4.0	90	80	30	26	34	31
male	15.5	13.5	47	41	5.2	4.5	90	80	30	26	34	31

* Compiled from the following sources: Dutcher: Lab Med 2:32, 1971; Koerper et al: J Pediatr 89:580 1976; Marner: Acta Paediatr Scand 58:363, 1969; Matoth, et al: Acta Paediatr Scand 60:317, 1971; Moe: Acta Paediatr Scand 54:69, 1965; Okuno: J Clin Pathol 25:599, 1972; Oski and Naiman: Hematological Problems in the Newborn. Saunders, 1972, p 11; Penttilä et al: Suomen Lääkärilehti 26:2173, 1973; and Viteri et al: Br J Haematol 23:189, 1972. Emphasis is given to recent studies employing electronic counters and to the selection of populations that are likely to exclude individuals with iron deficiency. The mean ± 2 SD can be expected to include 95 percent of the observations in a normal population.

1111

in adolescence. In the female, the gradual preadolescent increase in concentration of hemoglobin continues into early puberty, then levels off. In the male, hemoglobin production not only keeps pace with the accelerated growth that accompanies sexual maturation, but is sufficient to elevate its concentration to the substantially higher values characteristic of the adult. This higher value in the mature male, as compared with the female, is attributable to androgen secretion. Blood values at any single age during adolescence fall into a broad range, particularly in boys; values in sexually mature boys will approach those of an adult, whereas sexually immature boys will have values similar to those of children 6 to 12 years of age.

RETICULOCYTES AND NUCLEATED RED CELLS.   Both of these immature red cell elements are found in large numbers in the peripheral blood of the fetus, reflecting a very active rate of erythropoiesis. In the term newborn infant the reticulocyte count averages about 300,000/mm³ or 5 percent of total red cells. The reticulocyte count remains high during the first 3 days, then drops rapidly to values below 2 percent by 7 days after birth. Persistence of a high reticulocyte count between 1 and 6 weeks of age is abnormal and suggests a hemolytic process or blood loss; after 6 weeks an increase in reticulocyte count coincides with increased erythropoietic activity. Reticulocytes are more abundant in premature infants, with values as high as 10 percent at birth; subsequently the changes are similar to those in term infants. There is a rapid fall to values below 2 percent between 1 and 6 weeks of age; between 4 and 6 weeks, an increase of reticulocytes to 2 to 8 percent heralds the resumption of more active erythropoiesis; after 5 months of age, the reticulocyte count remains below 2 percent.

Nucleated red blood cells are almost invariably present at birth, an average of about 500/mm³ in the term infant and 1,000 to 1,500/mm³ in the preterm infant; the smaller the infant, the higher the average number. Equivalent values, expressed as percentage of white cell count, are 3 percent in term and 6 to 9 percent in premature infants. After birth, the number of nucleated red cells decreases about 50 percent every 12 hours, so that it is unusual to observe any nucleated red cells in the term infant or more than an occasional one in small premature infants after the first week.

BLOOD VOLUME.   The interpretation of hemoglobin values in terms of oxygen delivery to the tissues depends to some degree on variations in blood volume. Fortunately, the normal blood volume is relatively stable throughout most of life; the major developmental changes and individual variations in blood volume occur during the perinatal period. In the term newborn infant, the average blood volume is 85 ml/kg, with a range of 50 to 100 ml/kg body weight. The method of umbilical cord clamping is the most important variable. When the cord is clamped early, the mean blood volume 30 minutes after delivery is 78 ml/kg, in contrast to 99 ml/kg when cord clamping is delayed; the difference between the two groups is due to a difference in red cell rather than plasma volume. After a few

months of age, no difference in blood volume can be detected as a function of early or late cord clamping. It can be assumed, however, that late cord clamping eventually results in a more generous and long-lasting supply of storage iron derived from degradation of the additional red blood cells. Premature infants have an average blood volume of 90 ml/kg body weight, which is somewhat larger than in the term infant. The volume increases to a mean of 105 ml/kg during the first few days after birth. In both premature and term infants the blood volume decreases during the first few months. Thereafter, the average blood volume is 75 to 77 ml/kg, which is similar to that in older children and adults.

Fetal and Adult Hemoglobin

The red cell is more specialized in composition than most other cells in the body. Its major compound, hemoglobin, accounts for more than 95 percent of the total protein and for about 90 percent of the dry weight of the cell. Hemoglobin has a molecular weight of 68,000 daltons; it has four subunits, each containing one iron atom linked to a porphyrin ring to form the heme moiety, which in turn is attached to a globin chain. Each molecule of hemoglobin contains two pairs of identical globin chains. The type of globin chain is designated by a Greek letter and a subscript to indicate the number of that type of chain per molecule.

The rate of alpha (α) chain synthesis is high throughout life, beginning early in fetal development, but there is an orderly sequence of changes in the synthesis of the other predominant globin chains. The production of the embryonic epsilon (ϵ) chain is restricted to early fetal life and is soon supplanted by the gamma (γ) chain synthesis. Clinically, the most significant change is from γ to beta (β) synthesis during the perinatal period (Fig. 3).

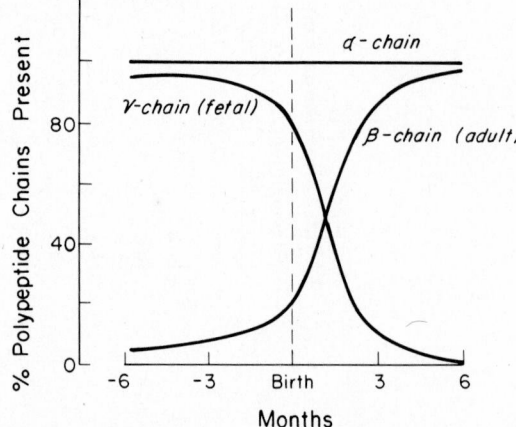

FIG. 3.   Globin chain synthesis in the fetus and during the neonatal period. The amount of α-chain synthesis is expressed as 100 percent. With maturation the corresponding percentage of γ chain synthesis decreases as production of β-chain increases, accounting for the shift from fetal to adult hemoglobin.

The types of hemoglobin that are produced change in a corresponding manner. Between 8 and 12 weeks of gestation, there is a brief period during which small amounts of hemoglobin containing the embryonic ϵ chain are produced; hemoglobin Gower 1 contains four ϵ chains (ϵ_4) and Gower 2 is made up of two α and two ϵ chains ($\alpha_2 \epsilon_2$). From 12 to 34 weeks of gestation, hemoglobin F ($\alpha_2 \gamma_2$) accounts for 90 to 95 percent of the total hemoglobin. It then declines at a rate of 3 to 4 percent per week until term. Some hemoglobin A ($\alpha_2 \beta_2$) is produced throughout fetal life and accounts for at least 5 to 10 percent of the total; this early production of a small percentage of β chains is of importance in the prenatal diagnosis of hemoglobinopathies since the most common abnormalities of hemoglobin structure (S and C) and of hemoglobin production (thalassemia) involve this chain (see p. 1148).

At birth, hemoglobin F (fetal hemoglobin) averages about 75 percent and hemoglobin A accounts for most of the remainder. However, measurement of hemoglobin synthesis in cord blood reticulocytes by isotopic techniques indicates that rates of production of hemoglobin A and F are roughly equal. The apparent discrepancy between rate of synthesis and the total amount present is explained by the fact that most of the hemoglobin present in the newborn was synthesized weeks to months earlier, during the period when production of hemoglobin F predominated. In newborns with hemolytic anemia the percentage of hemoglobin A is higher than normal due to the increased rate of destruction of old hemoglobin F-rich red cells and the increased production of new cells containing more hemoglobin A.

The rate of decline of fetal hemoglobin after birth is shown in Figure 4. The production of hemoglobin F

ties of the β chain, such as sickle cell anemia and thalassemia, the rate of decline in fetal hemoglobin is much slower than average, and values continue to be elevated throughout life.

Hemoglobin A_2 ($\alpha_2 \delta_2$) makes up a small fraction of the total hemoglobin. Its production begins late in gestation, and normally it accounts for 2 to 3 percent of total hemoglobin after the first few months postnatally. Developmental changes in red cell enzymes are discussed on p. 1169.

Oxygen Delivery

CHARACTERISTICS OF OXYGEN DELIVERY DURING DEVELOPMENT. The function of hemoglobin is to combine reversibly with oxygen, allowing red blood cells to pick up oxygen from the lungs and deliver it to the tissues. This function can be depicted in quantitative terms by the *oxygen dissociation curve* (Fig. 5). The oxygen saturation of a red cell suspension is plotted against the oxygen tension or partial pressure (Po_2); the oxygen tension at which hemoglobin

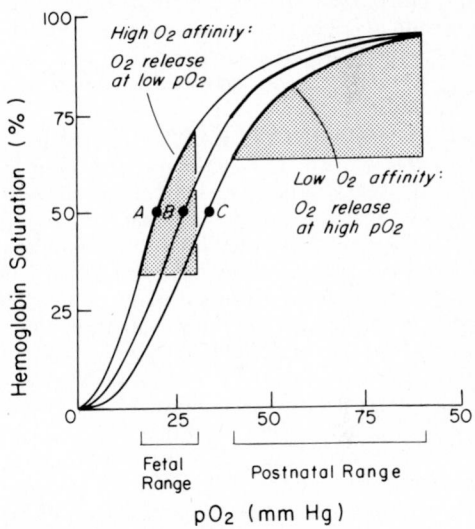

FIG. 5. Oxygen dissociation curve in the newborn (curve A), the normal adult (curve B), and the adult exposed to hypoxia (curve C). See text for explanation.

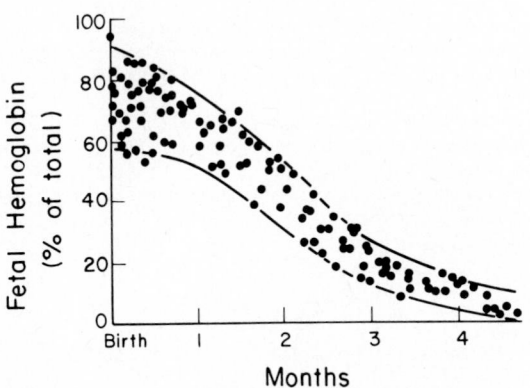

FIG. 4. Decline in percentage of fetal hemoglobin after birth in 17 normal infants (120 observations). The lines enclose the estimated range of normal. (Adapted from Garby: Acta Paediat 51:245, 1962.)

after birth does not stop entirely but proceeds at a markedly reduced rate. By 4 months of age, hemoglobin F has decreased to less than 20 percent; at 1 year, values average less than 2 percent but may occasionally be as high as 5 to 10 percent. In individuals with abnormali-

becomes 50 percent saturated is designated as P_{50}. In the adult the P_{50} averages 27 torr (mm Hg). The curve of the fetus or newborn is shifted to the left, denoting a higher oxygen affinity. On this curve, the P_{50} is 20 torr; thus an oxygen saturation of 50 percent can be attained at a Po_2 that is 7 torr lower than that required in the adult. This higher oxygen affinity of fetal blood favors the extraction of oxygen from the maternal circulation; thus an oxygen saturation of 70 percent can be attained in the fetal placental veins despite the relatively low Po_2 of 30 torr. In the peripheral vessels of the fetus, a decrease in Po_2 to 15 torr results in the release of about half of that oxygen. Although the high oxygen affinity of fetal blood suits the conditions of the intrauterine environment it does not allow the release of as large a proportion of oxygen to tissues after birth. Although blood Po_2 increases within minutes of delivery, the shift to the right to an oxygen dissociation curve that is more favorable for extrauterine conditions is not reached for several weeks. By 3 months of age, the curve reaches a position where it remains throughout the remainder of life. The experimental use of adult blood for replacement transfusion of asphyxiated newborn infants is an attempt to facilitate the release of oxygen to the tissues by substituting blood with a lower oxygen affinity.

In response to the hypoxic stimuli of high altitude, cyanosis, and anemia, there is a compensatory shift of the oxygen dissociation curve to the right from the normal childhood and adult position, resulting in an increased P_{50} within 6 to 24 hours. This indicates that the red blood cell has developed a decreased affinity for oxygen, allowing more oxygen to be released to the tissues. In anemia the facilitation of oxygen delivery partly compensates for the lower oxygen-carrying capacity of the blood. Similarly, in the adaptation to high altitude or cyanosis, a shift of the oxygen dissociation curve to the right allows improved oxygen delivery to tissues within a day, long before the oxygen-carrying capacity of blood can be increased by stimulation of erythropoiesis.

2,3-DIPHOSPHOGLYCERATE (2,3-DPG). The basis for the gradual shift of the oxygen dissociation curve to the right after birth was obscure until about 10 years ago. At that time it was found that certain organic phosphates can decrease the affinity of hemoglobin A for oxygen by competing for binding sites. Of these organic phosphates, 2,3-DPG is the most important in modulating the interaction between hemoglobin and oxygen. Because hemoglobin F has a lower affinity for 2,3-DPG than does hemoglobin A, it is able to bind oxygen more tenaciously, accounting for an oxygen dissociation curve that is shifted to the left. The postnatal shift of the oxygen dissociation curve to the right is therefore indirectly attributable to the decreasing production of hemoglobin F and its replacement by hemoglobin A. The shift of the oxygen dissociation curve to the right in response to high altitude, cyanosis, and anemia results from an increase in the red cell concentration of 2,3-DPG. This increases the competition with oxygen for binding sites and decreases the affinity of the red blood cell for oxygen.

Postnatal changes in oxygen delivery to the tissues are a function not only of the percentage of fetal hemoglobin and the concentration of 2,3-DPG, but also of the concentration of hemoglobin. The result of the interaction of these three factors is depicted in Figure 6, where the oxygen-carrying capacity of the blood is plotted against oxygen tension. At any oxygen saturation, the oxygen content of a given sample of blood is a function of hemoglobin concentration. The volume of oxygen unloaded to the tissues between the arterial and venous Po_2 can be estimated from each of the two curves. At birth, the ability of the blood to unload oxygen is relatively low because of its high oxygen affinity.

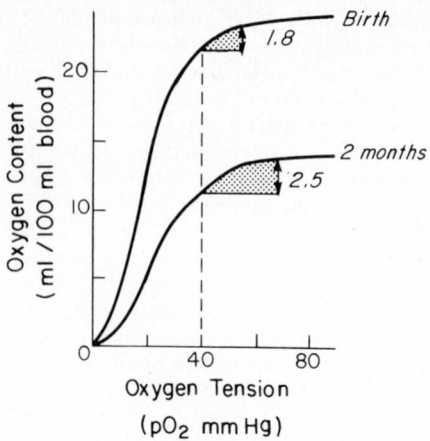

FIG. 6. Oxygen equilibrium curves of blood from term infants at birth and 2 months of age. Double arrows represent the oxygen-unloading capacity between a given "arterial" and "venous" Po_2. (Adapted from a figure in Delivoria-Papadopoulos et al Pediatr Res 5:235, 1971.)

By 2 months of age, the total oxygen-carrying capacity of blood decreases, in parallel with the fall in hemoglobin concentration. Despite this apparent handicap, the capacity to unload oxygen actually increases. This can be attributed to the postnatal rise in hemoglobin A, which binds 2,3-DPG and lowers the oxygen affinity of blood.

Blood stored for more than a week loses a large portion of its 2,3-DPG and may not function optimally in delivering oxygen to tissues until 6 to 24 hours after transfusion. This is a consideration that affects the selection of red cell preparations for transfusion (p.1216).

References

Delivoria-Papadopoulos M, Roncevic N, Oski FA: Postnatal changes in oxygen transport of term, premature and sick infants: the role of red cell 2,3-diphosphoglycerate and adult hemoglobin. Pediatr Res 5:235, 1971

Guest GM, Brown EW: Erythrocytes and hemoglobin of the blood in infancy and childhood. III. Factors in variability, statistical studies. Am J Dis Child 93:486, 1957

Oski F, Naiman JL: Hematologic Problems in the Newborn. Philadelphia, WB Saunders, 1972

Stockman JA, III: Anemia of Prematurity. Semin Hematol 12:163, 1975

ANEMIA

Peter R. Dallman and William C. Mentzer

Anemia can be defined as a lower than normal value for hemoglobin, or hematocrit, or number of red cells per cubic millimeter. The lower limit of the normal range is set two standard deviations below the mean at any given age (Table 1). By this arbitrary but clinically convenient definition, 2.5 percent of normal individuals will be mistakenly classified as anemic. Conversely, some individuals may have values in the low part of the normal range that are subnormal for them and that may be recognized only if the values are increased in response to treatment with iron or after the resolution of an infection, or other illness.

ETIOLOGIC CLASSIFICATION OF ANEMIAS

I. Impaired Production of Red Cells and Hemoglobin

    A. Nutritional anemias
       1. iron deficiency
       2. megaloblastic anemia

    B. Anemia of infection and chronic disease

    C. Aplastic and hypoplastic anemia

II. Accelerated Destruction of Red Cells

    A. Extracorpuscular defects
       1. erythroblastosis fetalis
       2. autoimmune and drug induced hemolytic anemia
       3. abnormalities of the vasculature or plasma
       4. splenic enlargement

    B. Intracorpuscular defects
       1. abnormalities of hemoglobin structure and synthesis
       2. abnormalities of the red cell membrane
       3. abnormalities of red cell metabolism

III. Blood Loss

APPROACH TO DIAGNOSIS

The diagnosis of anemia in children is facilitated by bearing in mind the *relative frequency* of its various causes. Iron deficiency is by far the most common, and the anemia of infection and chronic disease is second in frequency. Next are conditions such as the hemoglobinopathies and hemolytic disease of the newborn, but their incidence depends on the racial makeup of the population. Other causes of anemia, such as malignancy, aplastic anemia, inherited disease of the red cell membrane or red cell metabolism, are relatively rare, except where such patients become concentrated in referral hospitals.

Aspects of the *patient's history* that should be emphasized include diet, evidence of recent infection or chronic disease, ethnic background, and exposure to drugs or toxins. Age at onset of symptoms is important because disorders of the red cell membrane and enzymes are often evident at birth, whereas more commonly encountered hemoglobinopathies, such as sickle cell disease or β-thalassemia, are usually not clinically apparent before 3 months of age. A family history indicating dominant inheritance suggests a defect of the erythrocyte membrane or of hemoglobin, whereas recessive or sex-linked inheritance is characteristic of most enzymopathies. The diagnosis of an inherited anemia such as spherocytosis is often suggested by a family history of anemia, jaundice, splenomegaly, splenectomy, or the early appearance of gallstones.

Several aspects of the physical examination deserve special attention. Tachycardia and pallor are present only if the anemia is relatively severe. The presence of bruising may suggest blood loss due to a deficiency of clotting factors. Petechiae are present with thrombocytopenia and indicate a disease that affects not only the red blood cell but other elements of the blood. Jaundice, with or without splenomegaly, is recognized as evidence of a hemolytic process. Enlargement of the lymph nodes or liver or other signs of systemic disease also may indicate the source of anemia.

Laboratory Diagnosis

The most useful laboratory tests for the diagnosis of anemia include the *red cell indices,* the *blood smear,* and the *reticulocyte count* (Table 2). With the red cell indices and the blood smear, anemias can be classified primarily by *red cell size and morphology,* and with the reticulocyte count they can be distinguished *in kinetic terms.*

RED CELL INDICES. The mean corpuscular volume (MCV) has become an accurate and routine determination with the increased use of electronic particle counters. However, evaluation of the MCV must take into account the normal developmental changes in red cell size, particularly in infancy and early childhood (Table 1). The most prevalent anemias in childhood are those associated with a *low MCV.* One simple scheme for *screening based on the MCV* done by electronic counter can be depicted as follows:

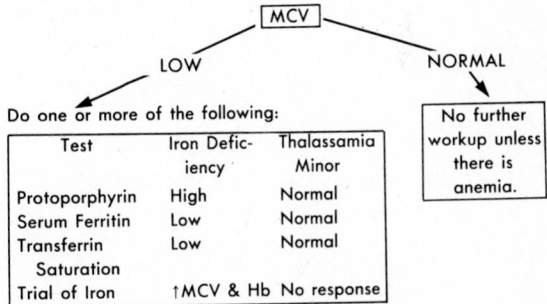

Test	Iron Deficiency	Thalassamia Minor
Protoporphyrin	High	Normal
Serum Ferritin	Low	Normal
Transferrin Saturation	Low	Normal
Trial of Iron	↑MCV & Hb	No response

If the MCV is low the differential diagnosis is primarily between iron deficiency and thalassemia minor. The distinction can be made in several ways depending on the clinical setting and on the laboratory tests that are available (p. 1122 and 1155). This scheme allows the detection of most cases of iron deficiency and reserves the use of more expensive tests such as hemoglobin electrophoresis only for those patients suspected of having thalassemia trait. A hemoglobin value of less than 9 g/dl with a low MCV is almost always associated with iron deficiency. A normal MCV is often found in the anemia of chronic disease and in acute bone marrow failure. A high MCV is usually associated with reticulocytosis, vitamin B_{12} or folate deficiency, liver disease, or chronic hypoplastic anemia.

PERIPHERAL BLOOD SMEAR. The peripheral blood smear provides the easiest and most readily available means of identifying abnormalities in the shape of the red cells. It is first examined under low power to identify the portion of the smear in which the red cells are well separated from one another and are primarily biconcave in appearance. This part of the smear is then used to systematically examine red cells, white cells, and platelets under the oil immersion lens. Distinctive abnormalities of red cell shape are nearly always evident

TABLE 2. Approach to Laboratory Diagnosis of Anemia

	Blood Smear	Reticulocyte Index*
Low MCV		
Iron deficiency	Hypochromia in severe cases	Low
Chronic disease	No characteristic changes	Low
Lead intoxication	Hypochromia and occasional stippling in severe cases	Low
Thalassemia trait	Aniso and poikilocytosis, target cells	Normal
Thalassemia	Aniso and poikilocytosis, target cells, nucleated RBC	High
Hemoglobin CC or C thalassemia	Target cells, spherocytes	High
Spherocytosis (also high MCHC)	Spherocytes	High
Normal MCV		
Chronic disease	No characteristic changes	Low
Malignancy		
with marrow involvement	WBC and platelets decreased, leukoerythroblastic (teardrop and nucleated RBC, leukocytosis immature forms)	Low
without marrow involvement	Variable	Low, normal
Acute aplastic or hypoplastic anemia	WBC and platelets decreased in aplastic anemia	Low
Acute blood loss, early	Usually none	Normal
late	Polychromatophilia	High
High MCV		
Folate and vitamin B₁₂ deficiency	Hypersegmentation of polys, macro-ovalocytosis	Low
Chronic aplastic or hypoplastic anemia	WBC and platelets decreased in aplastic anemia	Low
Active hemolysis—any cause	Polychromatophilia and morphologic changes characteristic of particular type of anemia, eg, RBC fragmentation in hemolytic uremic syndrome	High

High: > 3, low: < 2

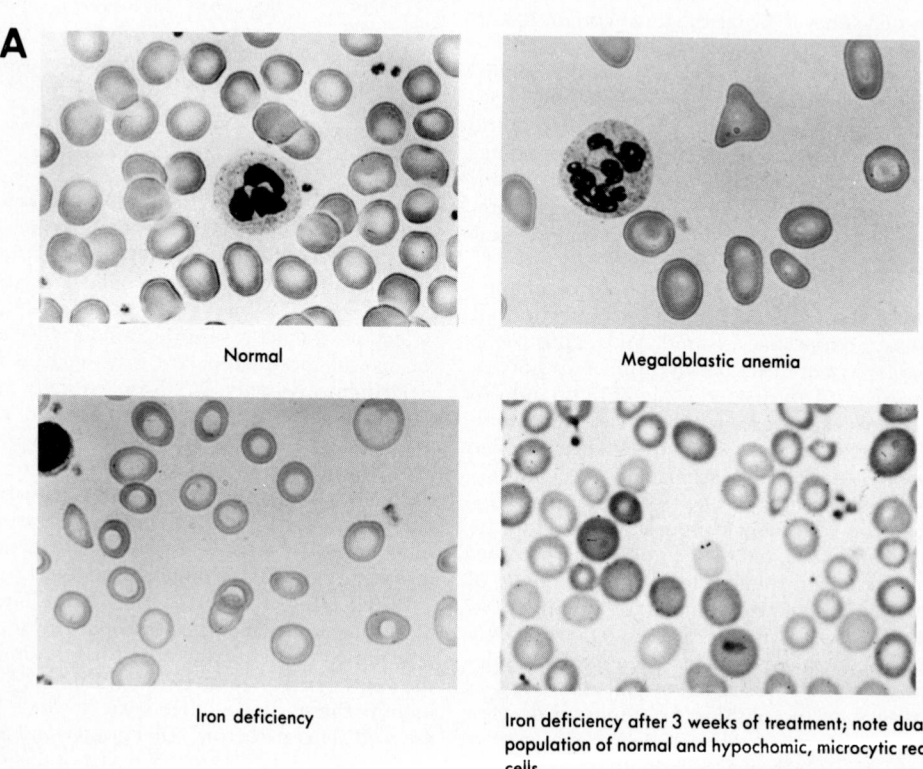

Normal

Megaloblastic anemia

Iron deficiency

Iron deficiency after 3 weeks of treatment; note dual population of normal and hypochomic, microcytic red cells.

FIG. 7.   Red cell appearance in various diseases. **A.** Peripheral blood morphology: nutritional anemias. (Continued)

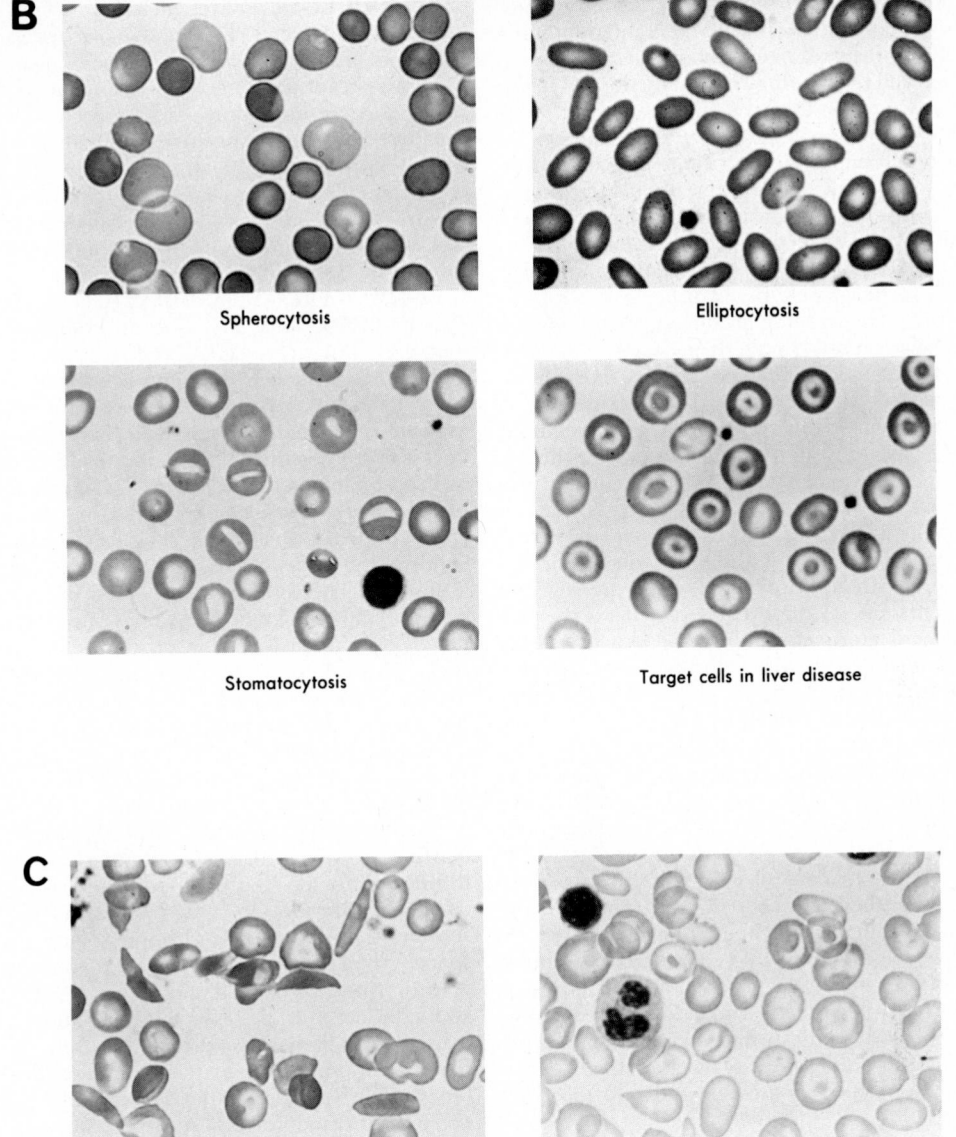

B

Spherocytosis

Elliptocytosis

Stomatocytosis

Target cells in liver disease

C

Sickle cell anemia

Hemoglobin H disease

Thalassemia trait

Microangiopathic hemolytic anemia

FIG. 7. (cont.). **B.** Membrane abnormalities. **C.** Hemoglobinopathies and other conditions.

in red cell membrane disorders (spherocytosis, stomatocytosis) and in the common hemoglobinopathies (sickle cell disease, hemoglobin C, thalassemia). However, red cell morphology is usually normal in enzymopathies. Common abnormalities of red cell morphology are shown in Figure 7. Abnormalities in number, size, and morphology of white cells and platelets must also be evaluated as they often indicate the presence of a disease that affects the production or destruction of all cellular elements of the blood.

RETICULOCYTE COUNT. Since the number of reticulocytes in peripheral blood reflects the rate at which new red cells are being produced, anemia can be assessed in kinetic terms. In the steady state, when production and destruction are balanced, the reticulocyte count also reflects the rate of destruction. However, it should be appreciated that 3 to 5 days are required before a reticulocyte response is manifest after the beginning of an acute hemolytic episode. A high reticulocyte count can be anticipated when there is marked polychromatophilia on the blood smear and an otherwise unexplained elevation in the MCV, since reticulocytes are larger than mature red cells. In severely anemic patients, the reticulocyte count reflects the rate of erythropoiesis more accurately if the *reticulocyte index* is estimated. This index corrects for the longer persistence of the reticulocyte in the circulation that is seen in anemic patients due to premature release of reticulocytes from the bone marrow. It also allows for the conversion of reticulocyte percentage to a figure that reflects their absolute number. A rough approximation of the reticulocyte index is adequate for differential diagnosis and can be based on the following figures: if the hemoglobin or hematocrit is 25 percent below the normal mean for the age, divide the reticulocyte count by 2; if either is 50 percent below the normal mean, divide the reticulocte count by 4. A reticulocyte index above 3 indicates increased production and an index below 2 suggests decreased production of red blood cells. The reticulocyte index will be inappropriately low when hemolysis is predominantly intramedullary, since relatively few reticulocytes are released into the peripheral blood.

MEASURES OF HEMOLYSIS. Abnormalities associated with *intravascular* hemolysis include an increase in plasma hemoglobin, a decrease in serum haptoglobin, and an increase in urinary hemosiderin. Serum unconjugated bilirubin may be elevated when *extravascular* hemolysis is present. The degree of hyperbilirubinemia is a function of both the extent of hemolysis and the rate of hepatic conjugation and clearance. *Carbon monoxide production,* measured in a closed rebreathing system, allows an accurate assessment of total heme catabolism, since endogenous CO is derived solely from cleavage of the tetrapyrrole ring of heme. In certain cases it may be useful to measure the survival of circulating red cells labeled with ^{51}Cr and to determine the extent to which such cells are sequestered within the spleen. A more comprehensive evaluation of red cell kinetics requires the use of ^{59}Fe.

BLOOD LOSS. Assessment of occult intestinal blood loss is difficult. The stool guaiac measurement is relatively insensitive to the presence of small but clinically significant amounts of blood, whereas the benzidine and orthotolidine reactions are excessively sensitive and may be positive in the absence of blood loss. If more accurate measurement of occult blood loss is warranted, it may be achieved by determining the rate of appearance of ^{51}Cr- or ^{59}Fe-labeled red cells or ^{131}I-labeled serum albumin in the stool or by measuring the loss of ^{59}Fe from the body in a whole-body counter.

BONE MARROW ASPIRATION AND INTERPRETATION. It is necessary to evaluate both bone marrow cellularity and morphology, particularly when malignancy, bone marrow failure, or certain storage diseases are suspected. On most occasions a bone marrow aspirate is adequate for diagnosis, but on occasion it is necessary to perform a needle bone marrow biopsy as well. In infants under 1 year of age, adequate samples of bone marrow may be obtained from the tibia or iliac crests or from a vertebral spinous process. In older children the posterior iliac crest is the preferred site of aspiration. The child is placed either in a supine position or lying on his side with knees drawn up. Approximately 1 hour prior to the procedure, premedication such as a combination of meperidine (Demerol) 2 mg/kg, promethazine (Phenergan) 1 mg/kg, and chlorpromazine (Thorazine) 1 mg/kg may be given intramuscularly. Following antiseptic preparation of the skin, a local anesthetic is injected first as an intradermal bleb, then into subcutaneous tissue, and finally into periosteum at the projected site of aspiration. The bone marrow needle, with trocar in place, is introduced through the infiltrated skin and firmly seated in bone, using a rotary motion. Often there will be a distinct sensation of the needle dropping into the marrow space. When the needle is firmly in place, a large 10- or 20-ml syringe is attached and strong negative pressure applied. Care must be taken not to withdraw more than 0.2 to 0.5 ml of marrow, as further withdrawal will only lead to dilution of the marrow sample with peripheral blood. The syringe may be wetted with a 10 percent solution of disodium EDTA, or alternatively, the marrow specimen without anticoagulant may be expelled onto a watchglass placed on ice to retard coagulation. Using a small micropipet or a microhematocrit tube, an attempt is made to obtain bone marrow spicules from which smears are prepared. Coverslips are preferred for preparation of smears, since the morphology is more uniform and less distorted by this method. A portion of the marrow specimen may be allowed to clot and may be fixed, sectioned, and stained in order to evaluate marrow cellularity. If a bone marrow biopsy is indicated in addition to an aspirate, a small core of bone marrow and an aspirated sample for coverslip smears may be obtained using a pediatric bone marrow biopsy needle such as the Jamshidi needle. The bone marrow must be evaluated in relation to normal developmental changes in the proportion of erythroid, myeloid, and lymphoid elements (Table 3).

TABLE 3. Differential Counts of Bone Marrow in Infants and Children

	Birth	1 wk	3-11 mo	1-12 yr	Adults*
Neutrophilic Series	53	66	43	50	54 (34-74)
Eosinophilic Series	3	3	3	5	3 (1-5)
Erythrocytic Series	35	15	12	21	26 (15-36)
Lymphocytes and Others	9	16	14	24	17 (10-24)
M : E Ratio	1.6	4.6	3.8	2.6	2.3

* Mean values and 95% confidence limits for normal adults are from Wintrobe: Clinical Hematology. Philadelphia, Lea & Febiger, 1974, p 62. Mean values in infants and children are derived from: Divany: Arch Dis Child 15:159, 1940; Gairdner et al: Arch Dis Child 27:214, 1952; Lundmark: Acta Paediatr Scand Suppl 162, 1966; Shapiro and Bassen: Am J Med Scl 202:341, 1941; and Sturgeon: Pediatrics 7:642, 1951. There are insufficient data for children to provide accurate confidence limits.

NUTRITIONAL ANEMIAS

PETER R. DALLMAN

Iron, folate, and vitamin B_{12} are required for the proliferation and maturation of red blood cells. Iron is a constituent of all body cells, but only in the red blood cell is it present in high concentration; the synthesis of hemoglobin consumes about 70 percent of the iron assimilated from the diet each day. Folate and vitamin B_{12} are required for the synthesis of DNA in all proliferating cells, and a deficiency of either results in a delay of cell division that is apparent not only in blood but also in other tissues with a rapid rate of cell renewal. The main cause of anemia in all three deficiencies is decreased red cell production. In addition, there is also some degree of increased destruction of immature red cells in the bone marrow, termed ineffective erythropoiesis, and of mature cells in the peripheral blood. Vitamin E deficiency is different from the other forms of nutritional anemia in that it is characterized primarily by red cell destruction in the peripheral blood (p. 1166). Hemolysis occurs when there is insufficient vitamin E to protect the red cell membrane from oxidative injury.

Iron Deficiency

Iron deficiency can be defined as a diminution in body iron of sufficient degree to restrict the production of hemoglobin and other iron compounds that serve a metabolic or enzymatic function.

IRON METABOLISM. Dietary iron is needed primarily for the production of heme proteins, which function in the transport, storage, and utilization of oxygen. These metabolically functional iron compounds account for about 70 percent of the total of 35 to 70 mg/kg of iron in the body. Most of the remaining 30 percent is present in the iron storage compounds, ferritin and hemosiderin, which are located primarily in the liver, spleen, bone marrow, and skeletal muscle. Almost all iron compounds in the body are continuously broken down and replaced; the iron that is released by the degradation of hemoglobin and other iron proteins is efficiently reutilized for replacement of these compounds by new synthesis. Very little iron is lost from the body, normally less than 15 μg/kg/day in the child. In the adult, the assimilation of iron need only be equivalent to iron losses for the prevention of iron deficiency; in the child, additional iron is required for growth.

Iron balance is normally maintained within narrow limits at each stage of growth and development through regulation of intake by the placenta in the fetus and by the intestinal mucosa after birth. Although the quantity of iron absorbed from the diet is regulated by the intestinal mucosa, it is also a function of the quantity and form of iron present in the food and of the interaction of iron in the food with other dietary components and with intestinal secretions.

The iron content of a mixed diet is very close to 6 mg/1,000 calories. Breast milk and cow's milk are unusually poor in iron and contain less than 1.5 mg/1,000 calories (0.5 to 1.0 mg/liter). Iron in food is primarily in the form of ferric complexes; a smaller amount is in the heme proteins, hemoglobin, and myoglobin, which are present in meat. In the process of digestion, the ferric iron complexes are partly broken down, and the iron is reduced to the ferrous form, which is more readily absorbed. This is facilitated by hydrochloric acid in the gastric juice. Absorption takes place in the small intestine. Assimilation of ionic iron is enhanced by the formation of readily absorbed complexes with other components of the diet, such as fructose, ascorbic acid, and probably most important, amino acids, including histidine and lysine. Iron absorption is decreased by the formation of insoluble phosphates and oxalates, which is favored by the alkaline environment of the small intestine.

Dietary iron in the form of heme protein is handled differently from iron salts; heme is split from the globin portion of the molecule in the intestinal lumen and is assimilated intact. A heme-splitting enzyme within the mucosal cell then releases ionic iron.

The dietary source of iron strongly influences assimilation. The range of iron absorption from a variety of biosynthetically labeled foods averages from less than 1

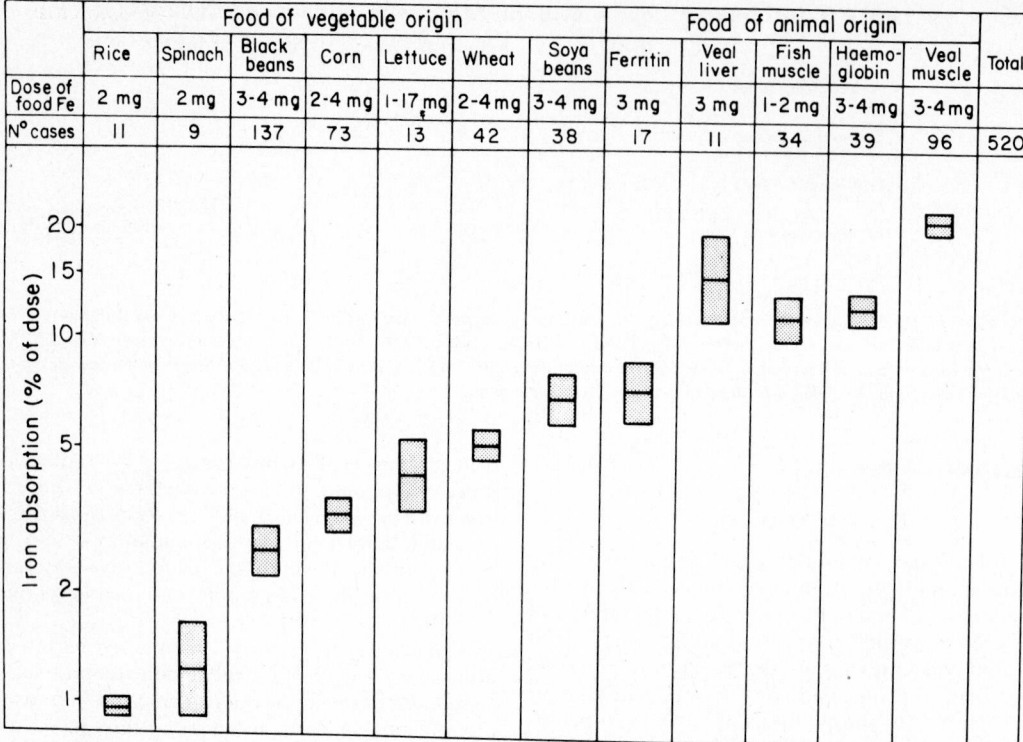

	Food of vegetable origin							Food of animal origin					
	Rice	Spinach	Black beans	Corn	Lettuce	Wheat	Soya beans	Ferritin	Veal liver	Fish muscle	Haemo-globin	Veal muscle	Total
Dose of food Fe	2 mg	2 mg	3-4 mg	2-4 mg	1-17 mg	2-4 mg	3-4 mg	3 mg	3 mg	1-2 mg	3-4 mg	3-4 mg	
N° cases	11	9	137	73	13	42	38	17	11	34	39	96	520

FIG. 8. Iron absorption from biosynthetically labeled food. Collaborative study of the Departments of Botany and Medicine, University of Washington at Seattle, USA, and the Department of Pathophysiology, Instituto Venezolano de Investigaciones Científicas, Caracas, Venezuela. The horizontal line represents the geometric mean, and the shaded area shows the limits of one standard error. (From WHO Tech Rep Ser, 503 1972.)

to over 20 percent (Fig. 8). Food of vegetable origin is at the lower end of this range, whereas meat and animal products are at the upper end. About 5 percent of the iron present in fortified milk formulas is absorbed, and absorption of iron from fortified infant cereals is probably similar.

The regulation of iron entry into the body takes place in the mucosal cell of the intestine (Fig. 9). This cell, by virtue of its 2- to 3-day life span, constitutes a temporary holding zone for iron between the intestinal lumen and the blood. In the iron-loaded individual, iron is taken up and largely retained by the mucosal cell, to be returned to the luminal contents by desquamation. In contrast, in iron deficiency, iron crosses through the mucosa into the circulation, and very little is retained within the cell to be lost by desquamation. The mechanism by which this mucosal regulation takes place is not understood. It is known that absorption depends on both the amount of available iron in the diet and body iron stores. The more iron ingested, the lower the percentage absorbed, and the lower the body iron stores, the larger the percentage of iron retained. Normally the diet contains 5 to 20 times the amount absorbed. In response to increased hematopoiesis, iron absorption is enhanced. This normally has the beneficial effect of facilitating recovery from blood loss. However, in

chronic hemolytic states, such as thalassemia, it may lead to iron overload, even with ingestion of a normal diet. In individuals with normal rates of erythropoiesis, body iron is maintained at a relatively constant level over a wide range of iron intake.

PATHOGENESIS. Etiologic factors in the development of iron deficiency include insufficient dietary intake of iron, dilution of body iron by rapid growth, and blood loss; many cases result from a combination of all three. In individuals with an adequate dietary intake of iron, hemoglobin iron normally increases roughly in proportion to body weight. However, during the periods of most rapid weight gain in infancy and adolescence, the diet is often iron-poor. Intestinal blood loss can be a contributing factor to the development of anemia in infants, but it is rarely associated with gross anatomic lesions, such as ulcer or carcinoma, which are common in adults.

DEVELOPMENTAL FACTORS IN SUSCEPTIBILITY. In the full-term infant, iron deficiency is uncommon before 6 months of age because of the abundance of iron stores present at birth and the normal postnatal decrease in concentration of hemoglobin. After these stores have been virtually consumed, dietary iron must be adequate to provide for rapidly rising total body hemoglobin. During the first year after birth,

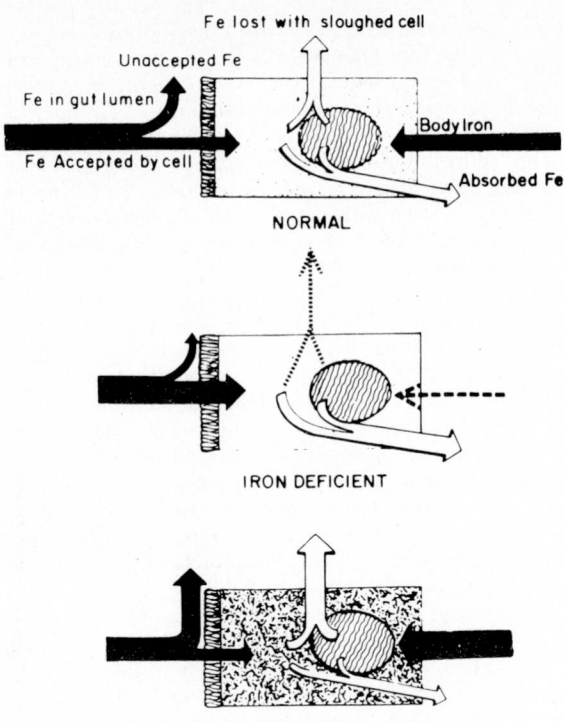

Fe lost with sloughed cell

Unaccepted Fe

Fe in gut lumen

Fe Accepted by cell

Body Iron

Absorbed Fe

NORMAL

IRON DEFICIENT

IRON LOADED

FIG. 9. Regulation of iron absorption at the intestinal mucosa. The mucosal cell normally accumulates iron from the intestinal lumen as well as from systemic sources. A portion of the iron enters the body, whereas the remainder is lost when the cell is sloughed into the intestinal lumen at the end of its 2- to 3-day lifespan. In the iron-deficient patient, more iron, primarily from the lumen, enters the cells to be transferred to the body, and little iron is retained in the cell to be lost by desquamation. In iron-loaded individuals, increased iron from systemic sources is incorporated into the developing mucosal cell, and absorption of dietary iron is decreased (except in hemolytic anemia). The iron in the cell is then lost with cell death. (From Conrad: Blood 22:406, 1963.)

about 135 mg of iron is required for the doubling of the red blood cell mass that occurs during this period. Lesser amounts are needed for the production of other iron compounds, such as myoglobin and the cytochromes. Since neonatal iron stores average less than 15 mg/kg out of a total body iron of 75 mg/kg, most of the increment in iron must come from exogenous sources. Infants of low birth weight (premature infants and twins) have lower iron stores at birth, in proportion to their smaller size; yet their rate of growth is more rapid than that of the term infant. Consequently, they may deplete their iron stores as early as 2 months of age. Severe cases of iron deficiency are most common between 6 months and 3 years, when the rate of growth is still rapid and when milk, a uniquely iron-poor food, usually accounts for a major portion of the diet.

Iron loss often contributes to the development of iron deficiency in infants. Among severely iron-deficient infants (Hb < 8 g/dl), about half are found to have occult intestinal blood loss. The blood loss is often related to the consumption of large amounts of fresh unprocessed cow's milk and contributes significantly to the development of iron deficiency. In some of these patients, blood loss is reversed by substituting heat-processed cow's milk formula or soy-based formula for fresh cow's milk, whether or not iron is administered. This suggests an intestinal sensitivity to a protein component of milk, such as lactalbumin, which is usually denatured or modified by heat processing.

In the preschool and preadolescent child, iron nutrition is generally improved since there is greater opportunity to obtain iron from a mixed diet. However, in parts of the world where hookworm infestation is a significant cause of intestinal blood loss, severe iron-deficiency anemia remains common throughout childhood. In adolescence, the incidence of mild iron-deficiency anemia increases again, as there is an acceleration in rate of growth. Additional factors are the onset of menstrual losses in girls and the androgen-related rise in hemoglobin concentration in boys. Iron lack continues to be prevalent in both sexes until the early twenties; subsequently it is common only in women.

Blood loss due to anatomic lesions is easy to overlook in children because of its rarity. It should be suspected when anemia persists or recurs after iron treatment, when intestinal blood loss persists despite substitution of processed formula for fresh cow's milk, or when severe anemia occurs after infancy. In the perinatal period, causes of bleeding include fetal–maternal hemorrhage, placental injury at the time of delivery, and twin-to-twin transfusion through placental communications. Beyond infancy, recurrent iron deficiency, particularly in the absence of abdominal pain, should suggest *Meckel's diverticulum*, often a cause of intermittent bleeding and the most common lesion associated with painless intestinal blood loss in children. Other congenital anomalies, such as intestinal duplications and hemorrhagic telangiectasia, are less common but may also result in iron-deficiency anemia. Bleeding peptic ulcer is rare in children, but as in the adult, it is usually accompanied by abdominal pain.

Primary *pulmonary hemosiderosis*, another unusual condition involving iron loss, should be considered when chronic pulmonary disease and hypochromic anemia coexist. In this disorder, although the chronic loss of blood is into the lung parenchyma rather than through removal from the body, the iron is not available for reutilization. This is also the case in Goodpasture's syndrome (progressive glomerulonephritis with intrapulmonary hemorrhage).

Rare disorders of iron metabolism may result in a hypochromic microcytic anemia, even though there is no blood loss or lack of dietary iron. Such defects include abnormalities of iron mobilization from storage sites and a congenital lack of transferrin.

Mild iron deficiency due to any cause tends to be self-correcting because iron absorption from food is increased as iron stores in the body diminish. In severe iron deficiency, and in some cases of apparent milk intolerance or more generalized malabsorption, the absorption of iron be decreased. This can contribute to the persistence of iron deficiency despite adequate dietary intake, and in occasional cases it may account for initial failure to respond to oral iron treatment.

CLINICAL MANIFESTATIONS. The symptomatology of iron deficiency is nonspecific. Mild iron deficiency is usually diagnosed on the basis of laboratory screening or, fortuitously, when a child is seen for an intercurrent infection. The findings in severe iron-deficiency anemia are likely to be similar to those of other anemias. Fatigue, decreased exercise tolerance, irritability, loss of appetite, and pallor may be noted, but the gradual onset of the anemia, which is characteristic of nutritional iron lack, may escape notice even when the hemoglobin is below 6 g/100 ml. Tachycardia and cardiomegaly are found when anemia is severe, but they are rarely the initial clues to the diagnosis.

In addition to the anemia, iron deficiency may also cause abnormalities in epithelial tissues, but these are rarely apparent, even in children with severe anemia. Epithelial abnormalities include thin and brittle fingernails that assume a concave shape (koilonychia or spoonnail) and atrophy of the papillae of the tongue. Inflammation of the mucous membranes of the mouth, vagina, and anus are described in the older literature but are now rare, perhaps because of a decreased severity of other coexistent deficiency states. Abnormalities of intestinal function occur in some cases and include decreased absorption of fat, vitamin A, and xylose, occasionally associated with an atrophic appearance of the villi in the small intestine. It is uncertain how frequently these intestinal changes result from iron deficiency or, alternatively, in which cases the iron deficiency is merely one facet of a more generalized, primary malabsorptive disease. An example of the latter is the iron deficiency associated with depletion of serum protein and copper on the basis of exudative loss through the intestinal mucosa. In general, intestinal abnormalities resolve with iron treatment. However, a concurrent change in the diet that has previously consisted of excessive quantities of fresh cow's milk may account for improvement of intestinal pathology in most of these cases.

LABORATORY DIAGNOSIS. The development of iron deficiency proceeds in a well-defined sequence that facilitates its diagnosis and staging. *Depletion of iron stores* is followed by a *fall in serum transferrin saturation,* which ultimately results in the decreased production of hemoglobin that is clinically recognized as *anemia.* When the transferrin saturation becomes depressed below 10 to 15 percent, the rate of production of hemoglobin decreases, and newly produced red blood cells gradually become smaller and less well filled with hemoglobin. However, anemia is a delayed manifestation of iron deficiency, clinically evident only after months of suboptimal hemoglobin production, since red cells that were produced under conditions of iron adequacy live out their normal 120-day life span.

The laboratory diagnosis of iron deficiency, is based primarily on the detection of anemia and microcytosis.

Most cases are discovered by routine laboratory screening with the microhematocrit, the spectrophotometric assay of hemoglobin as cyanmethemoglobin, and/or electronic red cell sizing and counting.

Most patients with dietary iron deficiency, who are detected by laboratory screening, have a relatively mild anemia, with a hemoglobin concentration of 9 to 11 g/dl. In children with more severe anemia there is an increased likelihood of discovering substantial intestinal blood loss. A low MCV is of diagnostic value, but as in the case of anemia, it is important to bear in mind developmental differences (Table 1). Around 1 year of age, when infants are most commonly screened for anemia, an MCV below 70, the lower limit of normal for this age, should suggest iron deficiency. The lower limit of normal for the preschool child is 75. The blood smear may be unrevealing in mild iron-deficiency anemia, in contrast to the morphologic abnormalities that characterize thalassemia minor (p. 1156); in more severe cases of iron-deficiency anemia, the blood smear shows microcytic hypochromic cells with moderate poikilocytosis.

The serum iron is decreased, whereas the iron binding capacity is increased, in iron-deficiency anemia. These changes result in a decreasing saturation of transferrin, which is of greater clinical usefulness than either value taken alone. There is a marked day-to-day variability in the concentration of serum iron in addition to a substantial diurnal variation, with high values in the morning and low values in the evening. Serum iron levels in infancy have a mean value of about 70 μg/dl at 1 year, which is somewhat lower than the 110 μg/dl in adults; lower limits of normal are about 30 μg/dl in infancy and 65 μg/dl in the adult. The normal iron binding capacity remains stable at 200 to 400 μg/dl after the first few months. A transferrin saturation below 16 percent is believed to restrict the rate of hemoglobin production in the adult; the corresponding figure for infants is probably lower, below 10 or 12 percent.

The erythrocyte protoporphyrin level is elevated when iron lack restricts hemoglobin production. Protoporphyrin is the compound that combines with iron to produce heme. Measurement of blood levels is used to screen for both iron deficiency and lead intoxication, which also results in elevated values. Abnormally high values may also be present in patients with infection or chronic disease. Despite its lack of specificity, the erythrocyte protoporphyrin has the important advantage of remaining elevated until iron-deficiency anemia has been reversed by treatment; consequently, its diagnostic value is not affected by a recent iron-rich meal or initiation of iron treatment.

Storage iron can be evaluated by Prussian blue staining of *iron in bone marrow* aspirate or biopsy, quantitated on a 0 to 4+ scale. This primarily reticuloendothelial iron represents the reserve available for the synthesis of hemoglobin, and its abundance usually parallels the reserve of iron stores as a whole. Determination of bone marrow iron stores is less useful in infants and adolescents than in adults, since storage iron is normally marginal during rapid growth and there is little difference between normal and deficient individuals.

Analysis of *serum ferritin* should provide a simple and practical measurement of iron stores as the assay becomes generally available. Ferritin is normally present in serum, but in such small quantities (7 to 140 ng/ml) that it remained undetected until recently. The size of iron stores and the serum ferritin concentration are closely correlated under most conditions. Thus, iron stores within the normal range and in conditions of deficiency and overload can be estimated in a small sample of serum. A low concentration has been found only in association with iron deficiency, but inappropriately elevated values may be present in infection, chronic disease, and malignancy.

Other laboratory findings may include evidence of occult intestinal blood loss, particularly in infants. Mild thrombocytosis is common with intestinal blood loss, whereas other cases of severe iron deficiency may be accompanied by mild thrombocytopenia.

DIFFERENTIAL DIAGNOSIS. This includes other causes of microcytic hypochromic anemia such as thalassemia minor (p. 1156) and lead poisoning (p. 797). In both conditions, serum iron levels are usually normal or elevated. In lead poisoning erythrocyte protoporphyrin is usually far more elevated than in iron deficiency; basophilic stippling of red cells is detectable in only some cases. It can be particularly difficult to distinguish iron-deficiency anemia from the anemia of chronic disease or infection, especially when the two coexist. Both conditions can be characterized by mild anemia, an elevated erythrocyte protoporphyrin, and a low serum iron. In simple iron deficiency, MCV is decreased and total iron binding capacity (TIBC) is normal or elevated; in chronic disease MCV is either normal or low and TIBC is normal or depressed. A depressed serum ferritin (below 7 ng/ml) is diagnostic of iron deficiency, whereas infection and chronic disease are associated with normal or elevated values. A serum ferritin of less than 25 ng/ml in anemic patients with rheumatoid arthritis, chronic renal disease, or other chronic disorder suggests coexisting iron deficiency. A therapeutic trial of iron (p. 1119) will effectively decrease the degree of anemia in such cases.

TREATMENT. The treatment of choice for most cases of iron deficiency is oral administration of ferrous sulfate. This iron salt remains the standard against which the efficacy of a multitude of other compounds is measured. It is low in cost, and it is as well tolerated as a comparable amount of iron in other therapeutically effective preparations. Gastrointestinal symptoms following oral ferrous sulfate treatment are not as common in children as in adults; if they occur, a reduction of the dose or administration with meals will generally solve the problem. The teeth may become stained by iron, but this is not permanent and can be minimized by administering liquid medication toward the back of the tongue.

An oral dose of iron at 3 mg/kg/day is sufficient in most cases and should theoretically be adequate for a maximal hematologic response. No more than 6 mg/kg/day need be given under any circumstances. Administration of this amount in divided doses, two or three times a day, results in better absorption and reduces the likelihood of gastrointestinal intolerance. Reticulocytosis occurs after 3 to 7 days of treatment. Recovery from anemia then takes place at a maximum rate of 0.25 to 0.4 g/dl/day of hemoglobin or about a 1 percent per day rise in hematocrit. If iron deficiency is discovered as an incidental finding in a patient with an infection, the response to iron is often delayed until the infection is resolved.

THERAPEUTIC TRIAL. Dietary iron deficiency accounts for the vast majority of anemias in otherwise healthy infants and children. This makes an elaborate diagnostic evaluation unnecessary in the typical case of mild anemia; a trial of iron medication is often justified on the basis of anemia and microcytosis alone. If the child seems otherwise well, this is an economical, practical, and safe course, with the stipulation that the results of the therapeutic trial be monitored. The reticulocyte response is usually of small magnitude and is not practical to monitor in cases of mild anemia. The response in hemoglobin, hematocrit, and MCV is slow but easier to establish. Normal values should be reached after 3 to 4 months of therapy, by which time microcytic cells will have been completely replaced. If the values are still abnormal, a more extensive diagnostic evaluation is indicated. In order to avoid iron overloading, the duration of therapy should only extend 2 to 3 months after the anemia has been corrected; this is sufficient time to allow for the restitution of depleted iron stores, provided that the cause of the deficiency has been corrected.

Intramuscular or intravenous iron in the form of iron-dextran (Imferon) is rarely warranted, except when administration of oral iron has been unsuccessful or when oral iron might aggravate an underlying intestinal disease. The therapeutic response is not significantly more rapid than with oral medication, the injections are often painful, and skin discoloration may occur even if care is taken to avoid backflow into subcutaneous tissue. Severe anaphylactic reactions are rare but have resulted in death. Therefore, parenteral iron should be used only when there is a compelling reason to substitute it for oral medication, as for example after there has been an apparent lack of response to oral therapy. The incidence of malabsorption of oral iron has recently been reported to be more common than previously thought. However, failure to administer medication as directed is still the most frequent cause for unexplained persistent iron-deficiency anemia.

If *intramuscular* or *intravenous* iron is used, the total dose of Imferon (50 mg elemental iron/ml) can be calculated by estimating the iron deficit as follows: about 2.5 mg of elemental iron per kilogram body weight is required to raise the hemoglobin concentration 1 g/dl, and an additional 10 mg/kg should be added to the total dose to allow for iron stores to be replenished and to make up for incomplete absorption from the site of injection. Tolerance to parenteral iron should be checked by administering a small test dose. Intramuscular injections distributed over several days are less painful than a single large injection.

Blood transfusion is indicated rarely as an adjunct in the treatment of iron deficiency to partially correct very severe anemia more rapidly than is possible with iron medication. The infant with a hemoglobin below 4 to 5 g/dl has very little margin for safety between precarious cardiovascular compensation and heart failure. If the risk of blood transfusion is warranted to bring the hemoglobin to a less precarious level, packed red cells should be given either at a very slow rate or, alternatively, at the same rate at which the patient's anemic blood is withdrawn (p. 1218).

Nutritional counseling to prevent recurrence of a dietary deficiency is important, but it should be realized that culturally-based eating patterns may not be modified easily. However, in infants who have been milk-fed, an improved appetite and weaning from the bottle, as the child gets older, may automatically provide a more iron-rich diet. When iron deficiency has been related to excessive ingestion of cow's milk, which can be associated with intestinal blood loss, substitution of processed milk formula is warranted, as well as encouragement to use a more varied diet.

PREVENTION.   Iron lack is unique among the classic deficiency syndromes in that its overall prevalence is stable or may actually be increasing, whereas scurvy, rickets, and pellagra have become rarities. The focus of interest is therefore shifting from treatment to prevention. Table 4 lists the recommended daily dietary allowances for iron according to age and sex. In the growing child and in the female between adolescence and menopause, iron intakes far below these amounts are common. In the United States the incidence of iron deficiency is high throughout late infancy, childhood, and adolescence. The peak incidence is between 6 months and 3 years of age, and at all ages the incidence of iron deficiency is highest in children from low-income families.

In the United States iron is used to fortify infant cereals, proprietary milk formulas, and enriched flour and other cereal products. For many years infant cereals were fortified with reduced iron of relatively large particle size or with sodium ferric pyrophosphate or similar products, which recent studies indicate are poorly absorbed. In the past few years the use of reduced iron of small particle size has been adopted for supplementation of most infant cereals. This form of iron appears to be almost as well absorbed as ferrous sulfate. Milk-based infant formulas are supplemented with 12 mg of iron as ferrous sulfate per reconstituted quart, which is effective in preventing iron deficiency.

RECOMMENDATIONS FOR INFANTS.   Iron supplements in some form should start no later than 6 months after birth in term infants and within 3 months in preterm infants. In formula-fed infants the most convenient and best sources of supplemental iron are iron-fortified formula and iron-fortified cereal. Formula is the more reliable vehicle for those infants who, for a variety of reasons, are fed solid foods only sporadically. When formula is used, it is the major source of calories

and is therefore a good vehicle for a relatively constant and predictable amount of iron supplement. In breast-fed infants one or two portions of iron-fortified cereal per day is the best source; iron drops are an alternative. The dose of iron drops should not exceed 1 mg/kg/day for term infants and 2 mg/kg/day for preterm infants up to a maximum of 15 mg/day. No more than a 1-month supply should be kept in the home to reduce the risk of accidental poisoning. Infant formula is preferable to pasteurized milk as a substitute for breast feeding during the first 6 to 12 months, since cow's milk may contribute to iron deficiency by increasing gastrointestinal blood loss. Breast milk or infant formula should be the main source of calories for infants for at least the first 6 months. After 6 months of age, formula intake should not exceed 1 liter or quart, and unmodified milk should not exceed 0.75 liter or quart per day, or it will displace supplemental foods from the diet, particularly iron-fortified cereals.

CHILDREN AND ADULTS.   The greatest impact on iron nutrition during the next decade is likely to result from current proposals to increase iron supplementation of a broad range of flour products from the present level of 13.0 and 16.5 mg/pound to 40 mg/pound. This increase should assure an adequate iron supply for children beyond infancy. Plans for a continuous system of nutritional surveillance of the general population under the auspices of governmental agencies should help in evaluating the efficacy of this form of fortification (Table 4).

TABLE 4. Recommended Daily Dietary Allowances (RDA) for Iron (1974)

Group	Age Range (yr)	RDA for Iron (mg)
Infants	0–0.5	10
	0.5–1	15
Children	1–3	15
	4–10	10
Males	11–18	18
	18+	10
Females	10–50	18
	51+	10
Pregnant		18
Lactating		18

Prevention of iron deficiency is a more complex and urgent problem in the underdeveloped countries where the prevalence of hookworm infestation and the predominance of cereals and starches in the diet are responsible for a high incidence of iron deficiency. Vehicles for supplementation are limited, since most food products do not go through commercial processing. Cereal staples, such as rice and wheat, and such products as sugar have been used as vehicles when they form a relatively constant and predictable fraction of the diet. However, the absorption of such supplemental iron often remains low because the diet is poor in foods of animal origin that facilitate iron assimilation. The forms and amounts of iron best suited for supplementing staple foods are being actively investigated.

MEGALOBLASTIC ANEMIA

Megaloblastic anemia is uncommon in children; its causes in order of frequency include folate deficiency, vitamin B_{12} deficiency, and hereditary orotic aciduria. Megaloblastic anemia is usually first suspected on the basis of an increased mean red cell volume. However, it should be borne in mind that an MCV in excess of 100 fl is normal in the newborn and that reticulocytosis of any cause can also result in an increased MCV. In neither case are megaloblastic abnormalities of cell maturation evident in the bone marrow, nor are hypersegmented neutrophils present in the peripheral blood.

Folate Deficiency

The metabolic role of folates is to serve as cofactors in reactions that involve the transfer of single carbon units. An example is the conversion of deoxyuridylate to thymidylate, the nucleotide that is unique to DNA. The role of folate in DNA synthesis probably accounts for the megaloblastic cell morphology that characterizes folate deficiency. Cells in rapidly proliferating tissues such as bone marrow grow to an abnormally large size and accumulate RNA but require longer than normal to synthesize sufficient DNA to enter mitosis.

During development the supply of folate to the fetus is adequate even in the presence of mild folate deficiency in the mother. Folate levels in cord blood are normally more than twice those in maternal blood. During the first few weeks after birth mean levels of blood and serum folate drop rapidly to values slightly below those of the normal adult; levels remain relatively stable throughout the remainder of the first year, and then rise to adult values. In the premature infant, blood and serum folate are commonly depressed between 1 and 3 months of age, especially if evaporated milk formula is fed (see below). Folate fortification can be given in the form of processed formula or vitamin drops.

Folate deficiency may be due to deficient dietary intake, malabsorption, or drug interactions. A *dietary lack of folate* is most common under circumstances that increase the requirement, such as rapid body or cell growth. This is most evident in the premature infant, during pregnancy, and in severe chronic hemolytic states, such as sickle cell anemia (p. 1149). Infants require about ten times as much folate on the basis of body weight as do adults. The recommended intake of folates for infants is 50 μg per day. Although folate is widely distributed in most foods, milk is a relatively poor source of this vitamin. Breast milk and pasteurized cow's milk contain about 35 μg/liter (3.5 μg/dl); this is less than the amount present in most foods and close to that required to sustain rapid growth in infancy—about 50 μg/day. Heat treatment lowers the folate content of milk further. Thus sterilizing the formula in a boiling water bath decreases the folate content by half. Evaporated milk has less than 20 μg of folate per reconstituted liter. Goat's milk is an even poorer source of folate, and severe megaloblastic anemia may result if it is the main source of calories. The heat lability of folate is not as marked in commercial formulas in which the vitamin is stabilized by the addition of ascorbic acid.

Intestinal bacteria may supplement the dietary folate supply, but the quantitative importance of this source is not known. Folate-containing bacteria reside mainly in the colon, a site from which the vitamin is poorly absorbed; nevertheless, the partial elimination of intestinal bacteria by prolonged use of broad-spectrum antibiotics is associated with folate deficiency.

Folate deficiency due to *malabsorption* is common, particularly in infancy, in such chronic diarrheal states as tropical sprue, gluten intolerance, and idiopathic steatorrhea. At least two mechanisms are likely to be responsible. First, diarrhea may result in a deficiency in intestinal conjugase. Consequently, the conjugated polyglutamate forms of folate that predominate in the diet may not be broken down to the monoglutamate form that can be absorbed. Thus, a small dose of monoglutamic folate can produce a prompt therapeutic response, whereas a large dose of polyglutamic folate has no effect. Second, diarrhea may interfere with the normal enterohepatic circulation of folate by excessive losses due to rapid intestinal passage.

DRUG INTERACTIONS. Folate analogues such as methotrexate react with dihydrofolate reductase and interfere with the conversion of normal dihydrofolate substrates to the active tetrahydro forms. Consequently, hypersegmentation of neutrophils and megaloblastic changes in bone marrow and peripheral blood are common concomitants of this form of antimetabolite therapy. A different mechanism is responsible for the folate deficiency associated with the use of oral contraceptives, diphenylhydantoin, and other anticonvulsants. These drugs interact with polyglutamates in the intestinal lumen and interfere with their digestion to the absorbable monoglutamate form. Administration of pteroylglutamic acid (PGA), which is unconjugated, reverses the folate deficiency, whereas an increase in polyglutamic folate is ineffective unless the drug is also stopped.

DIAGNOSIS. As a deficiency of folate progresses, abnormalities develop in the following sequence: low serum folate, hypersegmentation of neutrophil nuclei, low red cell folate, megaloblastic bone marrow, and macrocytic anemia. Most cases are mild and do not progress through this entire sequence. Hypersegmentation of neutrophil nuclei is the single most useful laboratory aid to early diagnosis, since it is easy to detect on a smear of peripheral blood. Even when deficiencies of both iron and folate coexist, hypersegmentation is usually present, whereas red cell indices and serum folate levels become less reliable. Hypersegmentation is suspected when there are numerous neutrophils with nuclei having four or more lobes; in quantitative terms, an average of more than 3.4 nuclear lobes per cell in 100 neutrophils is abnormal. Confirmation of the diagnosis is then obtained by a determination of serum, whole blood, and/or red cell folate, by bone marrow aspiration or by a therapeutic trial of folate (see below). Although serum folate reflects recent dietary changes, it may be too sensitive to normal dietary fluctuations to be an ideal test of chronic folate status. Nevertheless, it remains the best way of confirming the existence of folate deficiency of recent onset. Red cell and whole blood folate levels are better indices of chronic folate status. The folate content of newly produced red cells appears to reflect current folate availability. As with hemoglobin, the folate complement of the red cell is established during its early development in the marrow. Therefore, a deficiency does not become evident until new folate-deficient cells replace most older cells that live out their normal lifespan. A serum folate below 3 ng/ml is subnormal; the lower limit for whole blood folate is 50 ng/ml. When the value falls below 20 ng/ml whole blood in infants, the marrow will be megaloblastic in more than half the cases.

The development of macrocytic indices occurs later, usually concurrently with anemia and with other noticeable abnormalities in red cell morphology. Variations in cell size are marked in megaloblastic anemia; most cells are larger than normal, but many are small and distorted in shape. Megaloblastic changes in the bone marrow affect all cell lines and are similar in both folate and vitamin B_{12} deficiency. Many large erythroid precursors contain nuclei with a finely granular chromatin pattern and prominent nucleoli. The cytoplasm usually appears too mature for the nucleus and has the eosinophilic staining characteristic of abundant hemoglobin. Cells of the myelocytic series are also enlarged and have nuclei that appear immature.

TREATMENT. A therapeutic dose of folate, 0.5 mg/day of pteroylglutamic acid (ten times the daily requirement), may be given only when the diagnosis of deficiency is firmly established. A suitable maintenance dose to prevent deficiency is 0.1 mg/day, an amount that is present in some multivitamin preparations. Folic acid is available in 0.25- and 1-mg scored tablets. Folate in liquid for oral use is not commercially available at present, but can be prepared by diluting the injectable form from 5 mg/ml to a convenient potency, such as 0.1 mg/ml. As in iron deficiency, marrow morphology shows a return toward normal within 1 or 2 days. The appearance of the reticulocytosis by 7 to 10 days and the rate of rise in hemoglobin and hematocrit are also comparable to the response to treatment of iron deficiency.

A therapeutic trial may be indicated, where specific diagnostic studies cannot be done, to distinguish between folate and vitamin B_{12} deficiency. A dose of 50 to 100 µg of folate per day orally or parenterally, or 0.3 to 1.0 µg per day of vitamin B_{12} parenterally, is adequate to produce a prompt reticulocyte response specific to each of the deficiencies. A larger dose of folate can correct anemia due to vitamin B_{12} deficiency, but it may aggravate the neurologic manifestations.

A deficiency of folate often calls attention to a diet inadequate in many other aspects. A multiple vitamin and mineral supplement, which includes no more than 0.1 mg folate per day, may be indicated.

Vitamin B_{12} Deficiency

Vitamin B_{12} deficiency in children assumes importance because of the danger of irreversible neurologic damage, unless it is diagnosed and treated early, and because most causes of the deficiency require continuing therapy throughout life. Most cases of vitamin B_{12} deficiency involve a defect in absorption. Deficient dietary intake of the vitamin is very unusual.

REQUIREMENTS AND SOURCES. The normal human diet contains a considerable excess of vitamin B_{12} over the normal requirements of less than 1 µg/day in the adult and 0.1 µg/day in the infant, necessary for normal erythropoiesis. Deficiency is rare except in strict vegetarians (vegans) who avoid all animal products, including milk and eggs. Among such groups, megaloblastic anemia with neurologic changes may occur even in breast-fed babies because of a subnormal concentration of vitamin B_{12} in maternal milk. Animal products are the sole source of vitamin B_{12}, but the vitamin is not synthesized in the tissues of animals. It is unique among nutrients in that it enters the food chain entirely through synthesis by bacteria, particularly those in the intestine of ruminants.

The absorption of physiologic amounts of vitamin B_{12} is dependent upon the vitamin forming a complex with a specific mucoprotein (intrinsic factor) produced by parietal cells of the stomach. The complex is taken up specifically by the distal ileum. Vitamin B_{12} is then freed from the complex and released into the circulation. In the plasma, vitamin B_{12} is bound to a β-globulin transport protein (transcobalamin II). The vitamin is stored primarily in the liver. In the newborn liver these stores are large, averaging about 25 µg, and are rarely depleted before 1 year of age.

PATHOGENESIS. Causes of vitamin B_{12} deficiency are summarized in Table 5. With the exception of the rare dietary deficiency, most cases of vitamin B_{12} deficiency result from an absence or abnormality of intrinsic factor from the gastric mucosa or from interference with absorption of the vitamin–intrinsic factor complex.

The term *pernicious anemia* is generally reserved for those cases in which there is a deficiency of intrinsic factor. Two types of pernicious anemia are distinguished in children; in both, absorption of vitamin B_{12} becomes adequate if intrinsic factor is supplied.

The so-called *juvenile pernicious anemia* occurs in older children and is the same in most respects as pernicious anemia in the adult. Gastric atrophy and decreased secretion of acid and pepsin are commonly associated with antibodies to intrinsic factor or to parietal cells. Concurrent endocrinopathies may also be present. Often there are associated manifestations of immune deficiency, such as selective IgA deficiency, chronic candidiasis, or abnormal cellular immunity as manifested by a lack of in vitro responsiveness of lymphocytes to phytohemagglutinin. It has been postulated that the immune deficiency may be the primary defect leading to parietal cell damage or endocrine and tissue damage or

TABLE 5. Vitamin B$_{12}$ Deficiency in Children

	Earliest Age at Onset	Familial Incidence	Abnormal Schilling Test
I. Diet			
A. Related to maternal deficiency	Less than 4 mo		
B. Related to child's diet	Over 6 mo		
II. Inadequate Absorption			
A. Lack of intrinsic factor			
1. Congenital	Over 6 mo	X	X
2. Addisonian type (juvenile)	Over 10 yr	*	X
B. Competition for vitamin B$_{12}$ in intestinal lumen—fish tapeworm or bacteria in blind loops	Over 6 mo		
C. Abnormality of absorptive site—ileal resection of regional ileitis	Over 6 mo		X
D. Abnormality of transcotbalamin II, the serum vitamin B$_{12}$ transport protein	Less than 1 mo	X	X
E. Unknown mechanism			
1. Syndrome of vitamin B$_{12}$ malabsorption and proteinuria	Over 6 mo	X	X
2. Associated with pancreatic insufficiency, celiac disease, and other forms of less specific malabsorption	Over 6 mo	X	X

* *Endocrinopathy in siblings.*

both. Although there is no clear inheritance pattern, endocrinopathies or immune deficiencies may be present in siblings.

In contrast, in *congenital pernicious anemia* the disease is usually evident before 3 years of age. Although secretion of normally active intrinsic factor is lacking, gastric mucosa is normal with respect to morphology and secretory function. There are no demonstrable antibodies or associated endocrinopathies, and long-term follow-up does not show progression to the typical adult form of pernicious anemia. An autosomal recessive inheritance pattern is suggested by a high incidence of consanguinity and the occurrence in siblings.

Other causes of deficiency are not properly called pernicious anemia since there is no lack of intrinsic factor. These include removal of the vitamin from the intestinal lumen by parasites or bacteria. This is a cause of megaloblastic anemia in individuals with heavy infestations of fish tapeworm (*Diphyllobothrium latum*). It is restricted to areas in which raw or smoked fresh-water fish form an important part of the diet, as in parts of Scandinavia. Bacterial consumption of vitamin B$_{12}$ in intestinal diverticuli or blind loops also can result in removal of the vitamin before it is absorbed.

Vitamin B$_{12}$ is unusual among dietary constituents in having an absorptive site restricted to a small segment of the intestine, the distal half of the ileum. Surgical removal of this area of bowel for treatment of intussusception, regional enteritis, or congenital malformation results in a severe and lifelong deficiency. Chronic disease of this tissue, most commonly due to regional en-

teritis, can also produce a deficiency of vitamin B$_{12}$, but usually one that is mild and manifested primarily by a low serum concentration of the vitamin. Vitamin B$_{12}$ absorption and transport are also decreased in a rare inherited deficiency or abnormality of transcobalamin II. Presumably the transport protein is necessary as an acceptor to assure normal transport of the vitamin across the ileal mucosa. An additional cause of vitamin B$_{12}$ deficiency in children is an apparently specific absorptive defect usually associated with proteinuria. It is postulated that these may be only two manifestations of a more widespread defect in membrane transport. Consanguinity is associated, and an autosomal recessive pattern of inheritance is suspected.

Progression of vitamin B$_{12}$ deficiency in infancy is very slow, since neonatal liver stores normally are ample. Exceptions are the development of megaloblastic anemia in the infant of a mother with pernicious anemia and the inherited deficiency of transcobalamin II. If intrinsic factor is present, as in dietary vitamin B$_{12}$ deficiency, the onset of deficiency is even more delayed because vitamin B$_{12}$ lost in bile and pancreatic juice is normally reabsorbed.

DIAGNOSIS. Depression of serum vitamin B$_{12}$ and the appearance of hypersegmented neutrophils are the earliest clinical manifestations. Late findings of vitamin B$_{12}$ deficiency include megaloblastic changes in the bone marrow followed by megaloblastic anemia, leukopenia, thrombocytopenia, and mild jaundice; they are similar to those of folate deficiency. However, neurologic manifestations are generally quite distinct from those of folate lack. They include posterior and lateral column demyelinization in the spinal cord and associated paresthesias, sensory deficits, loss of deep tendon reflexes, slowing of mental processes, confusion, and memory defects. Neurologic changes may precede anemia. The biochemical basis for the neuropathy is uncertain. Inappropriate administration of moderate or large doses of folate (well in excess of 0.1 mg/day in an adult) to vitamin-B_{12}-deficient individuals can aggravate neurologic disease.

Diagnosis of vitamin B_{12} deficiency can be suspected when serum B_{12} is less than 100 pg/ml. The serum folate is usually normal or elevated. If the dietary history indicates a normal vitamin B_{12} intake, then absorption of ^{57}Co-vitamin B_{12} may be determined by the Schilling test. A standard dose (0.5 μg) of the labeled vitamin is given orally after an overnight fast; 2 hours later a flushing dose of 1,000 μg of vitamin B_{12} is given parenterally. This allows the excretion of labeled vitamin B_{12} into the urine in readily detectable amounts. Less than 7 percent of the administered label is recovered in the urine in 24 hours if there is a lack of intrinsic factor or a defective absorption of vitamin B_{12} for other reasons. If absorption is impaired, the Schilling test is repeated with oral intrinsic factor. Enhancement of urinary excretion of the label with intrinsic factor confirms the diagnosis of intrinsic factor deficiency. The availability of assays for intrinsic factor in gastric juice provides an additional diagnostic tool. Absence of acid in gastric secretions after histamine stimulation may be helpful in distinguishing between the two forms of pernicious anemia in children, although a gastric biopsy provides a more definitive answer. The urinary excretion of methylmalonic acid is increased in vitamin B_{12} deficiency and is another means of detecting the deficiency state.

TREATMENT. Most cases of vitamin B_{12} deficiency require treatment throughout life. Optimal doses for children are not as well defined as those for adults. For a therapeutic trial, parenteral administration of 0.3 to 0.1 μg of vitamin B_{12} (cyanocobalamin or hydroxycobalamin) per day may be employed, allowing 7 to 10 days for the appearance of polychromatophilia and reticulocytosis. If the diagnosis is firmly established, several daily doses of 25 to 100 μg may be used to initiate therapy. Alternatively, in view of the ability of the body to store vitamin B_{12} for long periods, maintenance therapy can be started with the first of a series of monthly intramuscular injections. Doses ranging between 50 μg and 1,000 μg once a month have been used successfully.

Hereditary Orotic Aciduria

Megaloblastic anemias produced by deficiencies of folic acid or vitamin B_{12} should be distinguished from the rare disorder of pyrimidine biosynthesis, hereditary orotic aciduria. This defect may manifest with megaloblastic anemia, leukopenia, retarded growth and development, and excessive urinary excretion of orotic acid. It appears to be inherited as an autosomal recessive trait. The heterozygotes are detectable by enzyme assays but are hematologically normal and are asymptomatic. Patients with the disorder are unresponsive to therapy with folic acid or vitamin B_{12} but may improve when fed yeast extracts containing uridylic and cytidylic acid.

References

IRON DEFICIENCY

American Academy of Pediatrics, Committee Statement: The ten-state nutrition survey: a pediatric perspective. Pediatrics 51:1095, 1973

Committee on Nutrition, American Academy of Pediatrics; Iron balance and requirements in infancy. Pediatrics 43:134, 1969

Council on Foods and Nutrition: Iron in enriched wheat flour, farina, bread, buns, and rolls. JAMA 220:855, 1972

Dallman PR: Tissue effects of iron deficiency. In Jacobs A (ed): Iron in Biochemistry and Medicine. London, Academic, 1974

——— Nutritional anemia. In Nathan DG, Oski FA (eds): Hematology of Infancy and Childhood. Philadelphia, WB Saunders, 1974, p 103

Finch CA, Monsen ER: Iron nutrition and the fortification of food with iron. JAMA 219:1462, 1972

Gorten MK, Cross ER: Iron metabolism in premature infants. II. Prevention of iron deficiency. J Pediatr 64:509, 1964

Herbert V: Drugs effective in iron-deficiency and other hypochromic anemias. In Goodman LS, Gilman A (eds): The Pharmacologic Basis of Therapeutics, 5th ed. New York, Macmillan, 1975, p 1309

Hoag MS, Wallerstein RO, Pollycove M: Occult blood loss in iron deficiency anemia of infancy. Pediatrics 27:199,1961

Piomelli S, Davidow B, Guinee VF, Young P, Gay G: The FEP (free erythrocyte porphyrins) test: a screening micromethod for lead poisoning. Pediatrics 51:254, 1973

Schulman I, Smith CH: Studies on the anemia of prematurity. III. The mechanism of anemia. Am J Dis Child 88:582, 1954

Siimes MA, Addiego JE, Dallman PR; Ferritin in serum: The diagnosis of iron deficiency and iron overload in infants and children. Blood 43:581, 1974

Wilson JF, Lahey ME, Heiner DC: Studies on iron metabolism: further observations on cow's milk-induced gastrointestinal bleeding in infants with iron deficiency anemia. J Pediatr 84:335, 1974

Woodruff CW, Wright SW, Wright PR: The role of fresh cow's milk in iron deficiency. II. Comparison of fresh cow's milk with a prepared formula. Am J Dis Child 124:26, 1972

FOLATE DEFICIENCY

Burland WL, Simpson K, Lord J: Response of low birthweight infants to treatment with folic acid. Arch Dis Child 46:189, 1971

Drugs and folic acid utilization. Nutr Rev 29:34, 1971

Erbe RW: Inborn errors of folate metabolism. N Engl J Med 293:753, 807, 1975

Herbert V: Experimental nutritional folate deficiency in man. Trans Assoc Am Physicians 75:307, 1962

Herbert V: Drugs effective in megaloblastic anemias. In Goodman LS, Gilman A (eds): The Pharmacologic Basis of Medical Practice, 5th ed. New York, Macmillan, 1975, p 1324

Matoth Y, Pinkas A, Zamir R, Mooallem F, Grossowicz N: Studies on folic acid in infancy. I. Blood levels of folic and folinic acid in healthy infants. Pediatrics 33:507, 1964

VITAMIN B_{12} DEFICIENCY

Gräsbeck R, Gordin R, Kantero I, Kuhlbäck B: Selective vitamin B_{12} malabsorption and proteinuria in young people. A Syndrome. Acta Med Scand 167:289, 1960

Hakami N, Neiman PE, Canellos GP, Lazerson J: Neonatal megaloblastic anemia due to inherited transcobalamin II deficiency in two siblings. N Engl J Med 285:1163, 1971

Katz M, Lee SK, Cooper BA: Vitamin B$_{12}$ malabsorption due to a biologically inert intrinsic factor. N Engl J Med 287:425, 1972

McIntyre OR, Sullivan LW, Jeffries GH, Silver RH: Pernicious anemia in childhood. N Engl J Med 272:981, 1965

Pearson HA, Vinson R, Smith RT: Pernicious anemia with neurologic involvement in childhood. J Pediatr 65:334, 1964

Valman HB, Roberts PD: Vitamin B$_{12}$ absorption after resection of ileum in childhood. Arch Dis Child 49:932, 1974

COPPER DEFICIENCY

The chief metabolic role of copper is as an essential component of cytochrome oxidase, the terminal oxidase of the electron transport chain required for the oxidative production of cellular energy in the form of ATP. The enzyme tyrosinase is also a copper-containing protein and is required for melanin synthesis. Thus, copper deficiency in animals decreases the activity of cytochrome oxidase in many tissues and results in loss of hair pigment. The anemia that accompanies copper deficiency is attributed to the role that copper plays in iron transport (see below).

During development, the fetus accumulates large stores of copper, particularly in the liver. After birth, an adequate copper intake of 0.04 to 0.15 mg/kg/day in the growing child and 2 to 5 mg/day in the adult is provided by most diets. Dietary copper deficiency in man has been recognized primarily under unusual or iatrogenic dietary circumstances, such as when copper is inadvertently omitted from a chronic intravenous alimentation regimen or when only milk is used to treat cases of severe combined nutritional deficiency states. Milk is unusually poor in copper, containing only about 0.12 mg/liter.

Copper balance, in contrast to iron balance, is regulated by excretion as well as absorption. Much of the copper absorbed from the diet is promptly excreted in the bile, with a lesser amount lost through the intestinal mucosa. Some of the excreted copper can be reabsorbed, but with chronic diarrhea copper deficiency can be aggravated through interference with this enterohepatic circulation. The hypocupremia of exudative enteropathy is thought to be due to the intestinal loss of ceruloplasmin, along with other serum proteins, such as albumin.

Copper deficiency can be the consequence of an inherited defect in copper absorption as in Menkes's syndrome (kinky hair syndrome, p. 1923). This potentially treatable disorder is characterized by a low serum copper, slow growth, kinky hair, cerebral degeneration, and X-linked pattern of inheritance. Death before age 3 years is usual. There is a striking similarity between the clinical features of this syndrome and severe nutritional copper deficiency in infants.

Plasma copper exists in two forms; a small amount is loosely bound to albumin and is probably involved in transport, while the larger fraction is tightly bound to an α_2-globulin, known as ceruloplasmin or ferroxidase. This blue green protein catalyzes the oxidation of ferrous iron to the ferric form in which it is bound to plasma transferrin. This may explain why copper deficiency, which results in a depression of serum ceruloplasmin, mimics certain of the findings of iron deficiency, such as low serum iron and hypochromic anemia.

DIAGNOSIS. A low concentration of serum copper is an early manifestation of copper deficiency. The lower limit of normal is 70 μg/dl except in the newborn, where it is 45 μg/dl . Anemia is not found consistently, but when present it is generally mild and hypochromic. Leukopenia and marked neutropenia are characteristic and can provide the first clues to the diagnosis.

Treatment of the deficiency with 0.2 mg/kg/day (two to three times the estimated daily requirement) in the form of 0.5 percent copper sulfate (about 2 mg of copper per milliliter) given orally results in prompt reticulocytosis and correction of the anemia and neutropenia. The medication should be kept out of reach of children, as it can cause fatal poisoning. Menkes' syndrome requires parenteral treatment; optimal regimens have not been established. Dietary circumstances that lead to the deficiency can be corrected once copper lack is recognized.

References

Cordano A, Baertl JM, Graham GG: Copper deficiency in infancy. Pediatrics 34:324, 1964

Danks DM, Campbell PE, Stevens BJ, Mayne V, Cartwright E: Menkes's kinky hair syndrome, an inherited defect in copper absorption with widespread effects. Pediatrics 50:188, 1972

Frieden E: Ceruloplasmin, a link between copper and iron metabolism. Nutr Rev 28:87, 1970

Gubler CJ: Copper metabolism in man. JAMA 161:530, 1956

Karpel JT, Peden VH: Copper deficiency in long-term parenteral nutrition. J Pediatr 80:32, 1972

ANEMIA OF INFECTION AND CHRONIC DISEASE

PETER R. DALLMAN

Next to iron deficiency, this is the most common type of anemia. It is frequently associated with chronic infection, rheumatoid arthritis, systemic lupus erythematosus, cystic fibrosis, immune deficiency disorders, malignancy, and renal failure. The laboratory findings and pathogenesis vary to some extent, depending on the primary disease, but the following features are common to most cases:

Shortened red cell survival. This is due to extracorpuscular factors that affect both patient's cells and transfused cells; probably increased phagocytic removal of red cells by a stimulated reticuloendothelial (RE) system is an important mechanism.

Impaired erythropoietin and marrow response. The hypoxic stimulus of anemia in many patients with chronic disease fails to trigger as much erythropoietin response as would be expected in the normal individual. Normally, the bone marrow can compensate for mild hemolysis by an increased rate of red cell production. In chronic disease this marrow response is impaired.

Impaired utilization of iron. Most of the iron needed for production of hemoglobin is normally salvaged from the breakdown of senescent red cells in the RE system; this is supplemented by a smaller supply from the absorption of dietary iron. In chronic disease there is interference with both routes. Even if RE iron stores are ample, as shown by a marrow aspirate, the release of iron to serum is diminished. In an analogous fashion, iron absorption is decreased despite ample dietary iron.

Diagnosis

Elaborate diagnostic studies of the anemia are usually discouraged because of the multiple etiologic factors and because other aspects of the disease demand more attention. The anemia is usually mild, with normocytic or microcytic red cells. In patients with renal disease, anemia tends to be more severe. The serum iron, iron binding capacity, and transferrin saturation may be normal or decreased. The bone marrow, stained for iron, shows reduced or absent iron in erythroid precursors despite the presence of RE iron. When iron deficiency coexists with the anemia of chronic disease, stainable iron is absent from both normoblasts and RE cells. This association often occurs when chronic intestinal blood loss results from prolonged aspirin or corticosteroid therapy.

When coexisting iron deficiency is suspected, a 2- to 4-month therapeutic trial of iron (3 to 6 mg elemental iron/kg/day) is warranted. Alternatively, intramuscular iron may be used (p. 1123). In either case, it is futile to administer iron on a long-term basis unless there is some evidence of a therapeutic response, such as increased hemoglobin concentration and increased mean corpuscular volume. Transfusion of packed red cells may be necessary in the most severe cases, usually patients with renal disease. Unfortunately, the effect is transient because of shortened survival of transfused cells and probably also due to further suppression of hematopoiesis. In chronic renal disease blood may have to be transfused very slowly or given as a partial exchange transfusion in order to reduce the risk of producing cardiac failure.

References

Cartwright GE, Lee GR: Annotation. The anaemia of chronic disorders. Br J Haematol 21:147, 1971

Douglas SW, Adamson JW: The anemia of chronic disorders: studies of marrow regulation and iron metabolism. Blood 45:55, 1975

Hypoplastic and Aplastic Anemia

William C. Mentzer

Either a deficiency in bone marrow erythrocyte precursors or an arrest in their maturation may result in inadequate production of erythrocytes. Anemia associated with suppression of erythropoiesis only is generally referred to as *hypoplastic anemia*. *Aplastic anemia* is the term used when the production of platelets and granulocytes is also impaired. Hypoplastic or aplastic anemia may occur without identifiable cause or as a result of bone marrow injury by infections, radiation, or chemicals. Inherited failure of erythrogenesis, occurring alone, is known as the *Diamond-Blackfan syndrome* or *congenital hypoplastic anemia*. When all three major cell lines in the bone marrow are involved, the resulting syndrome is termed *Fanconi's aplastic anemia*. These defects will be discussed below, while isolated inherited defects in granulopoiesis (congenital neutropenia, p. 1180, or thrombopoiesis, p. 1208) are described elsewhere.

Acquired Aplastic Anemia

Bone marrow hypoplasia or aplasia is common in children exposed to ionizing radiation or treated with cytotoxic chemotherapeutic agents. In sufficient doses, these agents will produce marrow aplasia in all exposed individuals. A variety of other agents may induce marrow aplasia only in certain susceptible individuals, while the majority remain unaffected. Insecticides such as chlordane, DDT, or lindane, solvents (particularly those containing benzene, such as model airplane glue), and drugs such as chloramphenicol, tridione, mesantoin, and sulfonamides have been associated with acquired aplastic anemia in children. The disorder may also follow infectious hepatitis. Even after the most meticulous evaluation, no specific etiology is discovered in 20 to 50 percent of cases.

In most patients the onset is insidious and is characterized by the gradual appearance of symptoms related to anemia or bleeding. Infection at the onset is uncommon. Occasionally, aplastic anemia will be discovered on routine examination in the absence of clinically significant symptoms. The most common findings on examination are those related to anemia (pallor, tachycardia) or to bleeding (petechiae, purpura, epistaxis). The spleen may be palpable in about 10 percent of cases, but is never markedly enlarged. Hepatomegaly is rare, and adenopathy is absent. The hematocrit and platelet count are subnormal; the absolute granulocyte count is usually decreased but may occasionally be normal. The absolute lymphocyte count is depressed in fewer than 50 percent of patients. There are no characteristic morphologic abnormalities evident on the peripheral blood smear. The erythrocytes are usually normocytic or macrocytic. Failure of erythropoiesis is reflected by a subnormal reticulocyte count and by an increase in the iron saturation of serum transferrin, due to diminished utilization of iron for erythropoiesis. Evaluation of marrow cellularity is difficult with an aspiration alone and usually requires bone marrow biopsy. Myeloid elements are usually absent or greatly diminished, although small islands of normal myeloid activity may be preserved. Nonmyeloid cells, such as plasma cells, lymphocytes, and histiocytes, may suffer little reduction in numbers, but there may be an increase in marrow fat.

Other causes of pancytopenia should be considered in evaluating such patients. Infiltration of the marrow by leukemia or by solid tumor can be excluded by careful evaluation of the bone marrow biopsy specimen. A cellular megaloblastic marrow with peripheral pancytopenia suggests the diagnosis of folate or B_{12} deficiency. Congenital aplastic anemia may be suspected when skeletal abnormalities of upper extremities, microphthalmia, and abnormal skin pigmentation are present. Paroxysmal nocturnal hemoglobinuria (p.1148) may present as pancytopenia and marrow aplasia. The correct diagnosis can be established by the acid hemolysis or sucrose lysis test.

The mortality rate in acquired aplastic anemia is about 70 percent, and in some referral centers that see only the more severe cases, the rate may be even higher. In 35 to 50 percent of patients, the disease is fatal within 4 to 6 months, while in the remainder it runs a more protracted course. In general, those patients destined for short survival may be identified at the onset of the disease by their more severe peripheral pancytopenia and reticulocytopenia, and by evidence of more extreme bone marrow aplasia on biopsy, as evidenced by a higher percentage of nonmyeloid elements on differential counting of bone marrow cells. Severely affected patients tend to have a more abrupt onset, to be male, and to have early clinical evidence of hemorrhage.

Identification and elimination of any agent suspected of initiating bone marrow failure are essential preliminaries in the treatment of aplastic anemia. Complete lists of such agents are available in references cited at the end of this section. Support with blood component transfusions to provide adequate levels of red cells and platelets is usually required. If bone marrow transplantation is a possibility, random donors rather than family members should be used to provide blood components for transfusion so as not to sensitize the patient to a prospective marrow donor's cells. In neutropenic patients, potentially lethal infections may produce few or no symptoms. A high index of suspicion of infection, thorough and frequent cultures, and vigorous use of antibiotics may be necessary. Intravenous carbenicillin and gentamicin is one regimen that has proved effective in the treatment of suspected sepsis in the febrile neutropenic patient when no specific organism has been identified. The prophylactic use of antibiotics in such patients, however, cannot be justified. Administration of androgens may stimulate partial or complete bone marrow recovery in some patients. The most commonly used androgens are oxymetholone (1 to 6 mg/kg/day, orally), testosterone enanthate (10 to 20 mg/kg/week, intramuscularly), or methyltestosterone (1 to 2 mg/kg/day, orally). The erythropoietic marrow is most sensitive to androgen therapy, while thrombopoiesis and granulocytopoiesis are less regularly influenced. The response to androgens is slow. An appreciable effect may not be seen until treatment has continued for 3 to 6 months. Since patients that survive for this length of time already have a much more favorable prognosis, the proposed beneficial effect of androgens has been somewhat difficult to evaluate. However, it is clear that certain patients do benefit from prolonged androgen therapy. The side effects of androgens include virilization, fluid retention, hepatotoxicity, and an increase in the rate of skeletal maturation. The latter may be minimized by addition of prednisone (0.5 mg/kg/day, maximum 20 mg/day) to the therapeutic regimen. There also appears to be an increased incidence of malignant hepatoma in patients on prolonged androgen therapy.

The short survival and poor response to androgen therapy of certain patients with severe aplastic anemia have provided impetus for evaluation of early bone marrow transplantation in such disorders. Since exposure to repeated transfusions and infections diminishes the likelihood of successful marrow engraftment, early marrow transplantation has been advocated for patients with severe aplastic anemia (such as that which follows infectious hepatitis) for whom a compatible HL-A-matched sibling donor has been identified. Preliminary results indicate that survival following early marrow engraftment can exceed 50 percent. Bone marrow transplantation is expensive and not widely available; it involves a major commitment of a family's financial and emotional reserves. Furthermore, the long-term consequences of marrow transplantation have not yet been fully evaluated. Nevertheless, considering the high mortality of acquired aplastic anemia and the promising results of early marrow transplantation, it seems warranted to evaluate the prospects for a marrow transplant at the onset of aplastic anemia. Androgen therapy may be instituted while HL-A typing of patient and family is under way. If there is no improvement within 3 to 4 weeks and a suitable donor is available, bone marrow transplantation should be seriously considered.

Congenital Aplastic Anemia

The onset of inherited aplastic anemia is usually delayed until well after birth. The initial hematologic manifestations of the disorder, which usually appear between the ages of 5 and 10 years, resemble those seen in acquired aplastic anemia. Anemia, either with or without hemorrhage, is the usual presenting feature. Examination of the peripheral blood reveals a macrocytic and normochromic anemia, often accompanied by granulocytopenia and thrombocytopenia. As the disorder slowly progresses, bone marrow becomes increasingly devoid of normal hematopoietic elements and closely resembles the bone marrow seen in severe acquired aplastic anemia. At the onset, however, the typical findings of bone marrow failure may be absent, and erythroid hyperplasia, often with megaloblastic features, may be noted. A variety of chromosomal abnormalities, not characteristic of acquired aplastic anemia, are frequently present in congenital aplastic anemia. Chromatid exchanges and chromatid and isochromatid breaks are the usual abnormalities encountered. In the majority of patients with constitutional aplastic anemia, other congenital anomalies are present and are of great aid in diagnosis. The most common anomaly is skin hyperpigmentation due to increased deposition of melanin, particularly on the trunk, neck, and skin folds.

Skeletal malformations of the upper extremities are also prevalent; aplasia or hypoplasia of thumb or radius or both structures is most common. Occasionally, a reduction in the normal number of carpal bones, syndactyly, or supernumerary thumbs may be present. About 25 percent of patients exhibit renal malformations, such as horseshoe kidney, ectopy, or absence of one kidney. Decreased birth weight, short stature, microcephaly, microphthalmia, strabismus, and, in males, hypogenitalism are commonly encountered. Less common are mental retardation, cryptorchidism, and deafness. About 1 in 10 patients will develop acute leukemia, usually monomyelogenous; this rate is considerably greater than the 1 in 2,500 characteristic of the general population in the United States. Patients with the hereditary skin condition dyskeratosis congenita may exhibit hematologic findings of constitutional aplastic anemia, but usually lack renal and skeletal anomalies; such patients commonly develop squamous epithelioma of the throat and other malignancies.

The inheritance pattern has not yet been fully defined. Although occasional examples of vertical transmission have been recorded, both parents are usually clinically normal. The incidence of consanguinity is increased, suggesting a recessive mode of inheritance. The clinical expression of the disorder varies considerably, with some patients exhibiting skeletal anomalies, but no hematologic manifestations, while others develop aplastic anemia despite the absence of other congenital anomalies. Although family members are usually clinically normal, in some instances chromosomal abnormalities similar to those that occur in anemic patients have been discovered, and the incidence of leukemia appears to be slightly higher in relatives of patients with constitutional aplastic anemia than in non-relatives. The peripheral blood lymphocytes of relatives are abnormally susceptible to malignant transformation in vitro by the oncogenic virus SV 40. An undue susceptibility to cancer is thus suggested by both clinical and experimental evidence.

The treatment of constitutional aplastic anemia is similar to that outlined for acquired aplastic anemia. The response to combined treatment with androgens and corticosteroids is more rapid, often occurring within several weeks. Patients who respond usually remain hormone-dependent and require continuing maintenance therapy, although it is often possible to lower dosage. A beneficial effect of androgen therapy is most likely to be seen on erythropoiesis, while it is uncommon for thrombopoiesis to be favorably influenced. The 5-year survival of about 50 percent is better than that obtained in acquired aplastic anemia, and many patients with constitutional aplastic anemia survive for more than 10 years following the onset of hematologic manifestations.

CONGENITAL HYPOPLASTIC ANEMIA

Inherited failure of erythropoiesis without accompanying abnormalities in the production of white cells or platelets is termed congenital hypoplastic anemia (Diamond-Blackfan syndrome). Anemia, usually present at birth, increases gradually, eventually resulting in pallor and weakness. The disorder is clinically apparent by 6 months of age in 90 percent of patients, but occasionally the onset may be delayed for several years. Congenital hypoplastic anemia is rare, and affected infants are usually Caucasian. There is no sex predilection. Characteristic congenital anomalies are present in 33 percent of the patients; those encountered most often are the phenotype of Turner's syndrome and bifid, double, or triphalangeal thumbs. Renal, cardiac, palatal, and other skeletal anomalies are seen occasionally. Hepatosplenomegaly and lymphadenopathy are not features of congenital hypoplastic anemia. The anemia is macrocytic and unaccompanied by abnormalities in white cell count or platelet count; red cell morphology is usually normal. In older patients, fetal hemoglobin concentration is usually elevated, occasionally to levels of 15 to 20 percent. Other elements of fetal erythropoiesis, such as an increase in red cell membrane i antigen concentration and increased activity of certain erythrocyte enzymes, are also often present. The reticulocyte count is low, and few or no erythroid precursors are present in the marrow.

The diagnosis of congenital hypoplastic anemia is usually made without difficulty. Lack of reticulocytosis and bone marrow erythroid hyperplasia readily distinguishes the disorder from blood loss anemia. Between 1 and 2 months of age, it may be difficult to distinguish congenital hypoplastic anemia from the late anemia of erythroblastosis, unless the previous history is known. Erythroid hypoplasia is a normal developmental feature during this period, and there may be little or no reticulocytosis in response to mild hemolytic anemia. However, in cases of isoimmunization, the concentration of hemoglobin seldom falls below 5 to 6 g/dl, without stimulating erythropoiesis in the bone marrow and producing a reticulocyte response. The increase in bone marrow lymphoid elements often encountered in congenital hypoplastic anemia may result in confusion with acute lymphocytic leukemia. White cell and platelet abnormalities, which are not a feature of congenital hypoplastic anemia, should suggest a diagnosis of aplastic anemia.

The pathogenesis of congenital hypoplastic anemia is not well understood. The rapid appearance of normal erythropoiesis following successful corticosteroid therapy indicates that erythroid precursor cells are present, but that an unknown maturational factor is lacking. This factor is probably not erythropoietin, since serum erythropoietin levels are unusually high in congenital hypoplastic anemia and the hormone has normal biologic activity in vivo. In vitro bone marrow cultures from patients with congenital hypoplastic anemia form erythroid colonies, unless the bone marrow is completely devoid of erythroid precursors. Such cultures, however, must be provided with large amounts of erythropoietin in order to exhibit erythroid colony formation.

Although the disorder is undoubtedly congenital, only sporadic instances of vertical transmission have been noted. Occasionally, more than one sibling in a family is affected. It is possible that full expression of the disease requires that both an inherited predisposition and an as yet unrecognized environmental factor be present. Increased concentrations of tryptophan metabolites have been detected in the urine of many patients with congenital hypoplastic anemia, suggesting an abnormality of riboflavin metabolism. Because experimental riboflavin deficiency will induce hypoplastic anemia, it has been suggested that an abnormality of riboflavin metabolism may play a pathogenetic role in the development of congenital hypoplastic anemia. Riboflavin intake and gastrointestinal absorption appear to be normal in congenital hypoplastic anemia, but the transport of riboflavin across the erythrocyte membrane is subnormal. The relationship of such abnormalities to hypoplastic anemia is conjectural, since prolonged treatment with high doses of oral riboflavin has no favorable influence upon the disease. The successful engraftment of bone marrow from a normal sibling donor in 1 patient with congenital hypoplastic anemia indicates that the underlying defect is likely to reside in the erythroid stem cell, rather than in those environmental factors necessary for erythropoiesis.

Treatment with oral corticosteroid therapy will produce reticulocytosis within 5 to 7 days, followed by a rise in hemoglobin concentration to normal or near-normal levels in approximately two-thirds of all patients. Some erythropoietic response is noted in 80 percent of patients. The customary initial therapeutic dose is 20 to 30 mg/day of prednisone by mouth. Larger amounts may be required in an occasional patient. Once an adequate erythropoietic response is obtained, the corticosteroid dosage is gradually lowered, until the least amount of medication required to maintain adequate erythropoiesis is discovered; in some patients, as little as 5 mg of prednisone several times weekly may be adequate. In order to minimize long-term effects of corticosteroids upon growth, maintenance corticosteroids should be given on an intermittent basis, such as every other day, three times weekly, or one week out of three. Once the diagnosis of congenital hypoplastic anemia has been established, steroid therapy should not be delayed unduly, since there is a lower response rate in patients treated initially at an older age. About 25 percent of patients will undergo spontaneous remission eventually and thereafter require no further steroid therapy; such a remission is unpredictable and can occur at any age. A few patients not responsive to steroid therapy may benefit from androgen therapy. The only other effective therapy is by repeated transfusions of red blood cells, but with this form of treatment, eventual death from transfusion hemosiderosis may be anticipated (see thalassemia, p. 1115). Bone marrow transplantation has been attempted only once. Donor marrow was successfully engrafted and evidence of erythropoiesis obtained, but the patient died of infection.

Acquired Hypoplastic Anemia (Transient Erythroblastopenia)

Brief episodes of erythroid hypoplasia may follow viral infections. These usually go undetected in individuals whose red cell life span is normal. In chronic hemolytic anemia, where the red cell life span may be greatly shortened, a brief episode of erythroid hypoplasia may lead to severe anemia rapidly (see sickle cell disease, p. 1149). The specific virus responsible for such marrow aplastic crises usually remains unidentified. Red cell hypoplasia may also follow the use of certain drugs, notably Dilantin, and is sometimes seen in malnutrition and in association with thymic tumors.

Occasionally, suppression of erythropoiesis may be of longer duration and occur without recognizable antecedent cause. This disorder, termed *transient erythroblastopenia of childhood*, may occur throughout infancy and childhood, but seems to be most common between the ages of 6 months and 4 years. Its onset closely resembles that of congenital hypoplastic anemia, but within a period of weeks to several months, spontaneous marrow recovery is noted. Anemia may be severe, with the hemoglobin value dropping to a level of 3 to 4 g/dl. Differentiation of transient erythroblastopenia from congenital hypoplastic anemia is important in order to avoid chronic steroid therapy, which is unnecessary in transient erythroblastopenia. The older age of onset and the absence of associated congenital anomalies help distinguish transient erythroblastopenia from congenital hypoplastic anemia. In addition, the red cells in transient erythroblastopenia are not macrocytic and do not contain an increased percentage of fetal hemoglobin or membrane i antigen. Erythrocyte glycolytic enzyme activity is low or normal in transient erythroblastopenia, consistent with the presence of an older population of erythrocytes, whereas the activity of certain enzymes (glyceraldehyde 3-phosphate dehydrogenase, enolase, aldolase, glutathione peroxidase) is often greatly increased in congenital hypoplastic anemia. It is unusual for an individual to experience more than a single episode of transient erythroblastopenia.

Myelophthisic Anemia

Invasion of the bone marrow by granulomatous infection, tumor, or myelofibrosis may result in an anemia characterized hematologically by reticulocytosis and the appearance of teardrop and nucleated red cells in peripheral blood, increased numbers of leukocytes, including many immature forms, and giant platelets. Such changes in the blood, termed leukoerythroblastic anemia, are evidence of extramedullary hematopoiesis and are often accompanied by hepatosplenomegaly. Malignant disorders (p. 2025) and granulomatous infections (p. 324) are dealt with elsewhere, while two other unusual causes of leukoerythroblastic anemia, myelofibrosis and osteopetrosis, will now be briefly discussed.

Idiopathic myelofibrosis is rare in children and usually fatal within 1 year, although 1 exceptional patient survived more than 5 years. The disorder occurs in females more often than in males by a factor of 2:1. Leukoerythroblastic anemia is present at onset, and hepatosplenomegaly, fever, weight loss, fatigue, and weakness are noted often. Bone marrow biopsy reveals fibrosis, and ferrokinetic studies usually demonstrate that hematopoiesis is predominantly extramedullary. As in adults with myelofibrosis, there may be premature destruction of the patient's own red cells due to hypersplenism. However, since the spleen may also be the predominant site of erythropoiesis, splenectomy should be considered only in occasional cases in which hemolysis is severe and there is ferrokinetic evidence of substantial erythropoietic activity outside the spleen. Therapy with androgens or corticosteroids appears to have little favorable effect.

Osteopetrosis (p. 2016) has no hematologic manifestations in the benign dominant form, but in the lethal recessive form, leukoerythroblastic anemia, often with thrombocytopenia, is noted soon after birth. Both spleen and liver are usually enlarged and are sites of extramedullary hematopoiesis. Hypersplenism may be a significant cause of hemolytic anemia and thrombocytopenia. Splenectomy is often of benefit but, as in myelofibrosis, should only be considered if the spleen is not the major site of blood cell production. Oral prednisone therapy may considerably alleviate the hematologic abnormalities in some cases and allow splenectomy to be postponed or avoided. The cause of osteopetrosis is unknown. A congenital form of the disorder that exists in mice can be corrected by bone marrow transplantation, but there is as yet no experience with marrow transplantation in humans with osteopetrosis.

References

Boxer LA, Camitta BM, Berenberg W, Fanning JP: Myelofibrosis—myeloid metaplasia in childhood. Pediatrics 55:861, 1975

Camitta BM, Nathan DG, Forman EN, Parkman R, Rappaport JM, Orellana TD: Posthepatitic severe aplastic anemia—an indication for early bone marrow transplantation. Blood 43:473, 1974

Camitta BM, Rappeport JM, Parkman R, Nathan DG: Selection of patients for bone marrow transplantation in severe aplastic anemia. Blood 45:355, 1975

Camitta BM, Thomas ED, Nathan DG, Santos G, Gordon-Smith EC, Gail RP, Rappeport JM, Storb R: Severe aplastic anemia: a prospective study of the effect of early marrow transplantation on acute mortality. Blood 48:63, 1976

Diamond LK, Shahidi NT: Treatment of aplastic anemia in children. Semin Hematol 4:278, 1967

Diamond LK, Wang WC, Alter BP: Congenital hypoplastic anemia. Adv Pediatr, in press, 1976

Dosik H, Hsu LY, Todaro GJ, Lee SL, Hirschhorn K, Selirio ES, et al: Leukemia in Fanconi's Anemia: cytogenetic and tumor virus suscepti-bility studies. Blood 36:341, 1970

Fanconi G: Familial constitutional panmyelopathy, Fanconi's anemia. I. Clinical aspects. Semin Hematol 4:233, 1967

Li FP, Alter BP, Nathan DG: The mortality of acquired aplastic anemia in children. Blood 40:153, 1972

Lynch RE, Williams DM, Reading JC, Cartwright GE: The prognosis in aplastic anemia. Blood 45:517, 1975

Schwartz E: Aplastic and hypoplastic anemias. In Nathan DG, Oski FA (eds): Hematology of Infancy and Childhood. Philadelphia, WB Saunders, 1974, p 151

Sjölin S: Studies on osteopetrosis. II. Investigations concerning the nature of the anaemia. Acta Paediatr 48:529, 1959

Steier W, Van Voolen GA, Selmanowitz VJ: Dyskeratosis congenita: relationship to Fanconi's anemia. Blood 39:510, 1972

Storb R, Thomas ED, Buckner CD, et al: Allogenic marrow grafting for treatment of aplastic anemia. Blood 43:157, 1974

Wang WC, Mentzer WC: Differentiation of transient erythroblastopenia of childhood from congenital hypoplastic anemia. J Pediatr, in press, 1976

Williams DM, Lynch RE, Cartwright GE: Drug-induced aplastic anemia. Semin Hematol 10:195, 1973

Yu JS, Oates RK, Walsh KH, Stuckey SJ: Osteopetrosis. Arch Dis Child 46:257, 1971

HEMOLYTIC DISEASE OF THE NEWBORN (ERYTHROBLASTOSIS FETALIS)

RODERIC H. PHIBBS

In 1932 Diamond and associates suggested that three clinical syndromes, anemia of the newborn, icterus gravis neonatorum, and universal edema of the fetus or hydrops fetalis, were all part of the spectrum of a single disease they named erythroblastosis fetalis. A decade later Levine found that the basis for the disease was an isoimmune hemolytic anemia in the fetus caused by transplacental passage of anti-Rh antibody from the maternal circulation. Usually the Rh-negative mother has been sensitized by a transplacental transfusion of Rh-positive cells during an earlier pregnancy with an Rh-positive fetus.

Following these discoveries there were major improvements in therapy, including exchange transfusion to prevent brain damage (kernicterus) from high levels of unconjugated (indirect) bilirubin and premature delivery to prevent stillbirth of severely affected fetuses. Amniocentesis and analysis of bilirubin pigment in amniotic fluid provided a much more accurate assessment of the severity of disease in the fetus, and in 1963 Liley introduced intrauterine transfusion of the most severely affected fetuses to prevent stillbirth and prolong intrauterine life until the fetus was mature enough to be delivered. At the same time improved methods of neonatal intensive care lowered the gestational age at which an affected fetus could be delivered with a good chance of survival.

The most recent advance is the prevention of sensitization of Rh-negative mothers by an injection of anti-Rh antibody (RhoGAM) after each delivery of an Rh-positive infant. This prophylaxis, which has been available for less than a decade, is rapidly altering both the frequency and severity of erythroblastosis. But, because prophylaxis only prevents sensitization, and does not help once sensitization has occurred, severely affected infants are still being born to mothers sensitized prior to the use of prophylaxis. In addition, prophylaxis only prevents Rh isoimmune disease, and there will still be cases of erythroblastosis due to antibodies against other blood group antigens and other forms of hemolytic anemia in the fetus, for example, due to G6PD deficiency or α-chain hemoglobinopathies.

The discussion of hemolytic disease due to Rh incompatibility that follows is also largely applicable to erythroblastosis due to other causes.

MATERNAL SENSITIZATION

Rh Blood Groups and Sensitization

The inheritance of Rh type is best understood in terms of the CDE nomenclature of Fischer and Race. The Rh blood group system is composed of three sets of allelic antigens, C and c, D and d, E and e; a person can be homozygous or heterozygous for each (eg, CC, Cc, or cc). Only 5 of the 6 antigens that should theoretically be present have been identified (C, c, D, E, and e). No d antigen has yet been found. The D antigen is most often the cause of disease. By convention, presence of the D antigen makes a person Rh-positive, and its absence makes one Rh-negative, regardless of the state of the other antigen sites.

The frequency of the D antigen varies among different races. In the average mixed white population about 15 percent are Rh-negative and 85 percent Rh-positive (35 percent homozygous or DD and 50 percent heterozygous or Dd). Among North American blacks only 5 percent are Rh-negative , and almost no Orientals are Rh-negative. The incidence of erythroblastosis due to Rh incompatibility is correspondingly reduced in these races.

When a woman who lacks one of the Rh antigens receives blood that contains that antigen, it is possible she will become sensitized and produce antibodies against the antigen. This can occur with a blood transfusion or with leakage of fetal blood into the maternal circulation during pregnancy or delivery, or following an abortion. Sensitization is most likely if the blood (fetal or donor) has the D antigen (Rh-positive) and the mother lacks it (Rh-negative), because D is by far the most antigenic of the Rh antigens.

In the typical case of Rh disease the mother is Rh-negative(dd) and the father is Rh-positive (DD or Dd). If the father is homozygous (DD), all fetuses will be Rh-positive (Dd); if he is heterozygous (Dd), half may be Rh-positive (Dd) and half Rh-negative (dd). Small numbers of fetal erythrocytes cross the placenta and enter the maternal circulation during the second and third trimesters of pregnancy. Rarely, this is sufficient to produce detectable sensitization and mild hemolytic disease in the fetus during the first pregnancy, but usually there are no detectable maternal antibodies and no fetal disease during the first pregnancy. At delivery, there is often a larger fetomaternal transfusion, but the volume rarely exceeds 10 to 15 ml, and sensitization of the mother most commonly occurs at this time. Some mothers will have detectable anti-D antibodies within the next 6 months; others may not but may still develop antibodies early in their next pregnancy if that fetus is also Rh-positive. Since these are IgG antibodies, they will cross the placenta into the fetal circulation and cause hemolysis.

Sensitization with other Rh antigens can also occur, and a mother who is Rh-positive can have a baby with erythroblastosis. For example, if she is homozygous CDe/CDe (16 percent of the population) and her husband is Rh-negative cde/cde, the fetus will be Rh-positive (Cc Dd ee). The mother can be sensitized by the c antigen on fetal red cells, and maternal anti-c can then cross the placenta and cause destruction of the fetal red cells, which have the c antigen. This type of sensitization of the Rh-positive mothers is uncommon, but does occur with anti-c, anti-E, and anti-C, in descending order of frequency.

An Rh-negative person who receives Rh-positive blood does not invariably become sensitized. Two factors known to influence sensitization are ABO type and dose of antigen. Incompatibility in the ABO blood group system will often protect the fetus from Rh disease. If the mother lacks the A or B antigen she will have naturally occurring anti-A or anti-B antibodies (or both if she is group O) of the IgM class, which do not cross the placenta. These will attack the donor cells, causing their rapid removal from the circulation and often preventing the D antigen on the cells from sensitizing the mother.

The dose of antigen is also important and will depend both on the volume of donor blood and on the number of D antigen sites on each erythrocyte. Heterozygous cells (Dd) have roughly half as many antigen sites as homozygous cells (DD). This is unimportant in erythroblastosis, since the mother is usually sensitized by cells from her own fetus, and since she is Rh-negative (dd) her fetus cannot be homozygous Rh-positive (DD). However, the number of antigen sites is also affected by other Rh antigens present. For example, CDe/cde cells have one-third more D antigen sites than do cDE/cde cells, even though both are heterozygous for D. Such factors help to explain why only about 10 percent of Rh-negative mothers with Rh-positive fetuses become sensitized.

Management

DETECTION OF SENSITIZATION.   When naturally occurring IgM antibodies attach to corresponding antigens on the red cell membrane, they will cause the cells to agglutinate when they are suspended in saline; this is the standard method of detecting such antibodies. IgG antibodies, which can cross the placenta and cause erythroblastosis, will not do this, and a special method, the Coombs' test, is required to detect such antibodies in the serum of a pregnant mother or on the cells of a newborn infant. Coombs' reagent is an antibody against human IgG. When IgG is bound to antigens on red cells and Coombs' reagent is added, it binds to the IgG molecules and agglutinates the cells.

The *indirect Coombs' test* is used to detect antibodies in the mother's serum by mixing her serum with cells of known antigenic type. They will coat the cells, and when the cells are then mixed with Coombs' reagent they will agglutinate. If the mother's serum has IgG antibodies against an antigen on the test cells, the antibody can be identified by testing her serum against various test cells of known antigenicity. The concentration of antibody in the mother's serum is usually estimated by titration. A test that is still positive at a 1:8 dilution usually is considered significant.

The *direct Coombs' test* simply mixes Coombs' reagent with cells from a patient with suspected erythroblastosis; if the cells agglutinate, they are coated with IgG. The more antibody on the red cells the stronger the agglutination, as estimated on a scale of 1 to 4+. In the case of erythroblastosis fetalis a positive direct Coombs' test on the infant's blood indicates maternal IgG has crossed the placenta and attached to the antigens on the infant's red cells.

All pregnant mothers should have their serum tested for antibodies early in pregnancy and, if the initial test is negative, again later in pregnancy. The test is performed against a panel of test red cells, which allows detection of antibodies against most red cell antigens, not only the D antigen. If a mother has an antibody, it must be identified and the father's red cells tested for the matching antigen. If he has the antigen, it can be on the fetal red cells, and erythroblastosis may develop. One must then evaluate the severity of disease in the fetus throughout pregnancy.

PREVENTION OF SENSITIZATION. If the mother is Rh-negative and has not been sensitized by a previous pregnancy or abortion, she is a candidate for treatment with anti-D antibody (RhoGAM) after delivery of her infant. The infant should have a blood type and direct Coombs' test immediately after birth (usually done on cord blood), and if the infant is found to be Rh-positive and direct-Coombs'-negative, RhoGAM should be administered to the mother within 72 hours of delivery to prevent sensitization. If pregnancy in an Rh-negative mother is terminated by an abortion or the infant is delivered stillborn, so that no blood typing can be done, RhoGAM still should be administered.

Some individuals who are thought to be Rh-negatove by routine testing may in fact be Rh-positive because their red cells contain the D^u allele, which is a weaker form of the D antigen and does not react with routine testing sera. Before deciding whether to give RhoGAM, Rh-negative women should be tested for the D^u antigen, since if they have it, they are in fact Rh-positive and do not need RhoGAM. An Rh-negative infant should also be tested for the D^u antigen, because if he has it, he is actually Rh-positive, and his mother should be given RhoGAM to prevent sensitization if she is Rh-negative and unsensitized.

The dose of RhoGAM given is 300 μg, which is sufficient to prevent sensitization by the usual transfusion of fetal blood at delivery. It will not be effective in the occasional case of a larger fetomaternal transfusion. When a newborn infant of an Rh-negative mother shows evidence of an extensive intrauterine hemorrhage, the physician caring for the mother must be advised of this situation. The infant's blood must be typed, and if it is Rh-positive, the mother's blood should be examined for evidence of fetal blood cells to estimate the volume of the hemorrhage. If it is judged to be large (p. 125) the dose of RhoGAM must be increased proportionately (10 μg/ml fetal blood) to prevent sensitiza-

tion. Once a mother has been sensitized, it is impossible to desensitize her later with hyperimmune globulin.

DISEASE IN THE FETUS

Hemolysis in Utero

Maternal anti-D antibodies cross the placenta into the fetus slowly, with an equilibration half-time of about 3 weeks. Therefore there will be a considerable delay between a rise in maternal antibody concentration and its effect on the fetus; this explains, in part, why maternal antibody titer is not a better predictor of severity of disease.

Once in the fetal circulation, the antibodies attach to the corresponding antigen sites on the fetal erythrocytes and cause hemolysis. The sensitivity of red cells to destruction is directly proportional to the number of antibody molecules on each cell. This, in turn, is determined by both the number of antigen sites (see above) and the concentration of maternal antibody in fetal plasma. The antibody-coated cells are removed by phagocytosis, primarily in the spleen but also to some degree in the liver and other parts of the reticuloendothelial system (extravascular hemolysis). This contributes to hyperplasia of the reticuloendothelial system and splenic enlargement. However, the capacity of the spleen to trap and lyse such cells is limited, and when the red cells are coated with very large amounts of antibody, there will also be hemolysis in the bloodstream (intravascular hemolysis), causing hemoglobinemia. With rare exception, anti-Rh IgG antibodies do not cause a complement-fixing reaction, which is associated with intravascular hemolysis and may cause disseminated intravascular coagulation.

BILIRUBIN. The hemoglobin released by extravascular hemolysis is converted into unconjugated (indirect) bilirubin, which rapidly crosses the placenta into the mother's circulation where it is taken up by her liver and conjugated. As a result there is never a high concentration of bilirubin in the fetus, and at birth the concentration in umbilical cord blood rarely exceeds 7 mg/dl, even with very severe disease. Some bilirubin also enters the amniotic fluid, probably as a component of the fluid that leaves the pulmonary capillaries to form the fetal lung fluid, which then passes up the bronchial tree to contribute to the formation of amniotic fluid (p. 1504). The fluid suctioned from the trachea of a severely erythroblastotic infant during the first hour after birth is often visibly stained with bilirubin. The presence of higher than normal concentrations of unconjugated bilirubin in fetal plasma may also cause premature induction of the liver's conjugating system, resulting in slightly higher levels of direct bilirubin in erythroblastotic fetuses (p. 125).

Hematopoiesis

The fetus responds to anemia with an increased release of erythropoietin and increased rate of hematopoiesis. Normally, fetal erythropoiesis occurs in the liver and spleen, resulting in hepatosplenomegaly and, toward the end of gestation, in bone marrow. In severe cases the liver and spleen become massively enlarged and are vulnerable to trauma during labor and delivery; most cases of intrapartum rupture of the spleen occur in infants with erythroblastosis.

LIVER. In severe erythroblastosis there is hepatic cellular necrosis, that differs in histologic appearance from other forms of liver disease. The liver is filled with erythroid precursors, which, it is speculated, could cause hepatic damage by compressing blood vessels and bile canaliculi. Evidence of liver damage includes high concentrations of conjugated bilirubin (4 to 10 mg/dl at birth) in umbilical cord blood, low serum albumin concentrations and occasional ascites in the absence of peripheral edema or pleural effusions, suggesting the presence of portal hypertension.

PANCREAS. There is islet cell hyperplasia and hyperinsulinism in erythroblastotic infants. It has been suggested that free hemoglobin in the plasma binds to and inactivates insulin; the compensatory increase in insulin production causes islet cell hyperplasia.

GROWTH. Despite all of these problems, fetal growth usually is normal, but maturation of certain organ systems may be impaired. Appearance of pulmonary surfactant is delayed, and this increases the risk of subsequent hyaline membrane disease (p. 1519).

Hydrops Fetalis

Hydrops fetalis refers to an excessive accumulation of fluid by the fetus, ranging from mild peripheral edema to massive anasarca, which fixes the limbs in extension and almost obliterates facial features. The placenta is correspondingly large, edematous, and pale. The capillaries of the placental villi appear immature and incompletely developed, and there is polyhydramnios. Some authors reserve the term hydrops for the more severe forms and use *prehydrops* to indicate the milder. Hydrops usually develops in utero, but occasionally an infant born without edema will develop it during the first few hours. Generally, hydrops occurs when there is severe hemolysis and moderate or severe anemia, but some fetuses with profound anemia are not hydropic, whereas some with only moderate anemia are.

The cause of hydrops is uncertain, and three mechanisms have been suggested: (1) decreased synthesis of albumin secondary to severe liver damage, with hypoalbuminemia and a low plasma colloid osmotic pressure, which allow fluid to leave the intravascular compartment and accumulate in tissues; (2) fluid accumulation because of increased capillary permeability secondary to chronic anemia and tissue hypoxia; and (3) chronic high-output heart failure secondary to anemia causing fluid retention, hypervolemia, and increased filtration of fluid through capillaries into tissue. The first two mechanisms are probably more important. Hydropic infants do not have larger blood volumes than do nonhydropic erythroblastotic infants but they do have lower concentrations of serum albumin and lower plasma colloid osmotic pressure, and they usually have evidence of tissue asphyxia at birth.

DIFFERENTIAL DIAGNOSIS OF HYDROPS. Hydrops is not unique to Rh hemolytic disease. It can occur with other forms of hemolytic anemia in the fetus, such as G6PD deficiency, α-thalassemia, and rarely, ABO incompatibility. It can occur also in some diseases in the absence of anemia. The differential diagnosis includes intrauterine viral and protozoan infections, congenital neuroblastoma, cardiac arrhythmias, cardiac malformations such as severe tricuspid insufficiency, premature closure of the foramen ovale in utero, adenomatoid malformation of the lung, renal vein thrombosis, congenital nephrosis, multiple congenital anomalies such as trisomy E, twins (usually in the recipient of a twin-to-twin transfusion), chorioangioma of the placenta, chorionic vein thrombosis, and umbilical vein thrombosis. In some cases no cause is found; many of these infants are not anemic but often have very low concentrations of serum albumin.

Stillbirth

In the more severe cases there is a substantial risk of intrauterine death that increases progressively toward the end of pregnancy. Stillbirth occurs in about 15 percent of all affected fetuses. It is rare before 28 weeks of gestation; about half the cases occur between 28 and 37 weeks and the other half thereafter, if there is no medical intervention.

Severity of Disease

Usually the second affected fetus has more severe disease than the first; there is then no increase in severity. This does not mean that the first affected fetus will have mild disease; many require premature delivery or intrauterine transfusion, and about 3 percent of all first affected pregnancies will end in stillbirth, if there is no early medical intervention. Disease tends to be more severe in twin pregnancies, but both twins are not always affected. Mothers carrying severely affected fetuses may develop a syndrome indistinguishable from toxemia of pregnancy and will show signs of polyhydramnios if the fetus develops hydrops.

The titer of anti-Rh antibody in maternal blood is not a very good indicator of the severity of disease in the fetus. In general, the antibody titer is higher in more severe disease, but occasionally it is low in the presence of severe disease or high in the presence of an Rh-negative fetus with no disease. Radiographic and ultrasonic examination of the fetus is discussed in Chapter 5, but these techniques are useful only in detecting the presence of severe disease. The concentration of bilirubin pigment in amniotic fluid increases in proportion to the severity of hemolysis and is the most accurate indicator; it can be followed with repeated amniocentesis. This method of analysis and the interpretation of the results are discussed elsewhere (p. 125).

Management

Prenatal screening should detect sensitized mothers, and the severity of fetal disease should be evaluated in affected pregnancies. The choices in management consist of permitting the pregnancy to go to term, delivering prematurely, or giving intrauterine transfusions followed by premature delivery at a later date. The decision is based primarily on the results of amniotic fluid analysis (see Fig. 1, p. 126).

Premature delivery is performed when the risks of continued intrauterine life are estimated to be greater than those of premature birth. In a recently published series of severe cases the average gestational age ranged from 34 to 36 weeks, and many were delivered much earlier, superimposing many of the problems of prematurity, such as asphyxia, hyaline membrane disease, decreased bilirubin conjugation, and hypoglycemia, on those of erythroblastosis. Intrauterine transfusions are generally reserved for those so severely affected that they are unlikely to survive long enough in utero to reach an age when they can be delivered with a reasonable chance of surviving. It is essential to perform amniocentesis early enough to detect severe disease before hydrops develops because, once a fetus is hydropic, intrauterine transfusion is rarely successful. The first transfusion can be performed as early as 25 weeks gestation, if necessary.

An intrauterine transfusion is done by injecting packed red blood cells that are compatible with the mother's serum (usually group O, Rh-negative, low titer anti-A and anti-B) into the fetal peritoneal cavity. The red cells are slowly absorbed into the lymphatics of the mesentery and on the abdominal side of the diaphragm; they pass to the thoracic lymph duct and thence into the left subclavian vein. Most of the transfused blood reaches the circulation within 3 days of transfusion. The timing and risks of intrauterine transfusions are discussed on p. 126.

DISEASE IN THE NEWBORN

Pathophysiology after Birth

ANEMIA. The degree of anemia at birth varies widely, depending on severity of disease; the hematocrit may be normal or as low as 10 percent. The peripheral blood may contain large numbers of reticulocytes and earlier red blood cell precursors, including erythroblasts, the characteristic from which erythroblastosis fetalis takes its name. Nucleated red blood cells often reach 10,000 to 100,000/mm^3 in the severely affected newborn. The number of nucleated red blood cells is not a particularly reliable indicator of severity of disease; the number in peripheral blood fluctuates widely over short periods of time, and acute stress even without hemolysis can mobilize these cells from the bone marrow for brief intervals. The increase in reticulocytes is a more reliable indicator of severity of hemolysis; this ranges from 15 to 20 percent of the red cell count in moderate disease to 80 percent in very severe cases.

Hemolysis will continue after birth as long as there are Rh-positive cells and antibodies, which have a half-life of about 3 weeks. Patients with very mild disease will not be anemic or sufficiently jaundiced to require exchange transfusion in the first days after birth but may become anemic over the next few weeks. More severely affected infants will require at least one exchange transfusion, which will replace about 85 percent of Rh-positive with Rh-negative cells (see below) but will only remove a small portion of the maternal anti-D antibody, which is widely distributed in tissues and can reenter the circulation. During the first few days after birth new Rh-positive cells continue to be produced at an increased rate in response to the stimulus of hemolysis, and these, with Rh-positive cells not removed by exchange transfusion, are available for continued hemolysis. Severely affected infants who have had one or more exchange transfusions may become anemic again at a few months of age if they had very high concentrations of maternal antibody at birth. As the Rh-negative cells from donor blood die off, they are replaced by new Rh-positive cells, which can be attacked by any remaining antibody. In the most severe cases the direct Coombs' test will become weakly positive again at several months of age.

BILIRUBIN. After birth, unconjugated (indirect) bilirubin can no longer be cleared by the placenta, and its concentration rises in proportion to the rate of hemolysis. The concentration usually reaches a peak during the first week after birth and then declines as the liver's ability to conjugate and excrete bilirubin increases. Figure 10 shows the course of an infant with moderately severe disease. Commonly there is a transient rise of conjugated (direct) bilirubin to 2 to 4 mg/dl as the concentration of unconjugated (indirect) bilirubin falls. This is due to a transient accumulation of conjugated bilirubin, presumably because the rate of conjugation temporarily exceeds the excretory capacity. Rarely, with severe disease and liver damage, the direct bilirubin may rise to very high levels, 20 to 40 mg/dl, for a week or more, but as hepatic function improves this falls to normal.

Unconjugated bilirubin is cytotoxic if it enters cells, and it has a predilection for the basal ganglia of the brain, producing a particular type of encephalopathy known as *kernicterus*. Normally, unconjugated bilirubin is bound to albumin in the plasma and will not enter cells in significant amounts unless it reaches a concentration that exceeds the capacity of albumin to bind it or the cell's permeability and susceptibility to bilirubin are altered. A variety of processes interact in erythroblastotic infants to increase the risk of kernicterus in the first few days after birth. Many infants have lower plasma concentrations of albumin either from liver injury (see above) or prematurity and hence have a lower capacity to bind bilirubin. They are often acidemic, and a lower pH decreases the binding affinity of albumin for bilirubin. Very high levels of free fatty acids, as may occur with hypoglycemia and drugs such as salicylates and sulfonamides, compete with binding sites on albumin and thus increase free bilirubin levels. Processes

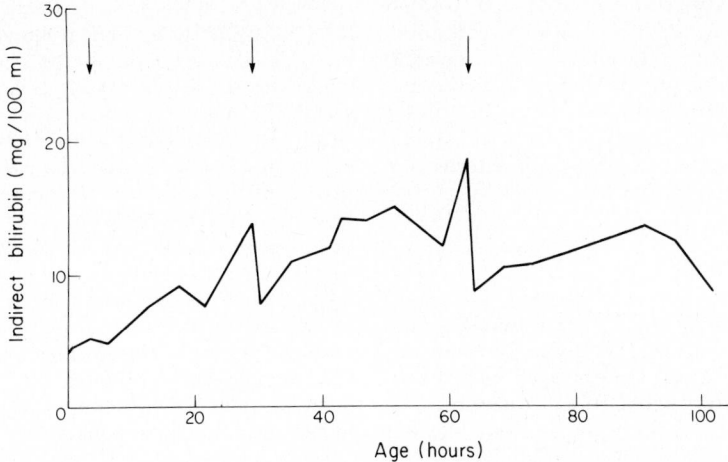

Fig. 10.   Course of bilirubinemia in a 36-week gestation, 2400-g infant with moderately severe erythroblastosis. Arrows indicate exchange transfusions. The first was a one-volume exchange (180 ml) and the others were 2-volume exchanges (400 ml each).

such as hypoxia and acidemia may increase cellular permeability and susceptibility to bilirubin toxicity in addition to their effects on albumin binding. Neonatal bilirubin metabolism, toxicity, and the findings in kernicterus are discussed in detail elsewhere.

GLUCOSE.   After birth, the infant no longer has a steady supply of glucose from its mother across the placenta, and pancreatic islet cell hyperplasia can cause hypoglycemia. This may occur at any time in infants with either mild or severe disease and is particularly likely if an infant is not fed or is given an intravenous infusion of glucose that is then discontined abruptly. In addition to interfering indirectly with the binding of bilirubin by albumin, hypoglycemia can be a direct cause of brain damage.

COAGULATION.   Coagulation abnormalities occur in many of the more severely affected infants. Purpura may be present at birth or may develop in the first few days, and infants with severe coagulation disorders may suffer pulmonary, intracranial, or generalized hemorrhages that are often lethal. The disorder is probably due to a combination of factors, including accelerated intravascular coagulation, deficient production of clotting factors secondary to liver damage, and splenic sequestration of platelets in cases with splenomegaly. Thrombocytopenia is the most common abnormality; it may be present at birth but often develops during the first hours or days after birth.

HYDROPS FETALIS.   Hydrops may interfere with the normal onset of ventilation after birth. Pleural effusions or elevation of the diaphragm by ascites will restrict lung expansion, and pulmonary edema will interfere with exchange of respiratory gases. The low serum albumin and colloid osmotic pressure present an additional problem; therapy that raises colloid osmotic pressure will draw a large volume of extravascular fluid into the circulation and produce congestive heart fail-

ure. Typically, this occurs on the second or third day associated with the increase in albumin concentration during or following a full exchange transfusion. The hypoalbuminemia of hydropic infants also increases the risk of kernicterus (see above).

CARDIORESPIRATORY   DISTRESS.   Infants with severe erythroblastosis, with or without hydrops, usually are delivered prematurely and commonly become asphyxiated during delivery. They may have hypoxemia, metabolic acidemia, and, if not vigorously ventilated after birth, respiratory acidemia. The asphyxia and cardiopulmonary insufficiency are not only a consequence of premature birth. Asphyxia of some degree occurs during the birth process; in the fetus with anemia it is likely to be more severe because the blood oxygen-carrying capacity is decreased. The more anemic an erythroblastotic fetus, the greater is the fall in pH of scalp blood in the latter part of labor.

Asphyxia causes pulmonary and systemic vasoconstriction, which raises aortic and central venous pressures; with relief of asphyxia this is reversed and intravascular pressures fall. If pressures are normal at birth, often they will fall to hypotensive levels as arterial pH and PO₂ rise; if pressures are increased at birth, they will usually fall to normal or, less often, to hypotensive levels. The hypotension responds to blood volume expansion, suggesting that circulating blood volume was inadequate in these infants at birth. Uncommonly, some of these infants have high central venous pressure and normal or high aortic pressure, even after relief of asphyxia; these respond to a reduction of blood volume, suggesting that they were in congestive failure.

The course of the asphyxiated erythroblastotic infant during the hours after birth usually follows one of three patterns: many respond rapidly to resuscitation and signs of respiratory difficulties disappear in a few minutes; some have transient respiratory distress requiring increased inspired oxygen and occasionally assisted ventilation, but they begin to improve within 12 hours and are usually well within 48 hours; others develop typical severe hyaline membrane disease, which is the most common cause of death. Many of the consequences of hyaline membrane disease, such as hypoxia and acidosis, also increase the risks of kernicterus (see above).

Management

Some aspects of management, such as initial evaluation, prevention of kernicterus and hypoglycemia, and late care, apply to all cases. Others, such as management of cardiorespiratory sequelae, coagulation problems, and hydrops only apply to the severely affected case, which should be identified before delivery.

PREPARATION. Proper care demands close coordination between obstetrician and pediatrician. Those who will care for the infant must attend the delivery and be prepared to initiate diagnostic studies to evaluate the infant and to begin immediate therapy if required. Preparations must include the immediate availability of appropriately crossmatched blood (see below). In the case of a severely affected prematurely born infant there are so many components of care, each urgent, that there should be a team of experienced personnel at the delivery, each with assigned responsibilities.

EVALUATION AT BIRTH. Evaluation of severity of disease in the infant includes looking for evidence of anemia, development of jaundice, edema, and hepatosplenomegaly. At birth the umbilical cord should be doubly clamped with two pairs of hemostats, 20 cm or more apart. The cord is then cut between each pair to give an isolated length of cord 20 cm long and clamped at each end, trapping the blood in the vessels. A blood specimen is aspirated from one of the vessels, with a needle and syringe. If blood cannot be collected in this way, it should be obtained by venipuncture or aspiration from an indwelling umbilical artery or venous catheter. Blood collected from the draining end of a cut umbilical cord will be contaminated with amniotic fluid and almost worthless. If capillary blood is used it should be appreciated that it has a higher hematocrit than venous or arterial blood (p.1110). Appropriate blood studies include hematocrit or hemoglobin concentration, reticulocyte count, leukocyte count, examination of the blood smear, platelet count, blood grouping and typing, direct Coombs' test, albumin concentration, and both conjugated and unconjugated bilirubin levels. Total bilirubin alone is unacceptable because it may be high from an elevated conjugated bilirubin, and it is only the level of unconjugated bilirubin that determines the need for exchange transfusion to prevent kernicterus. All these measurements should be done on all patients as emergencies, so that the results will be available quickly. A positive Coombs' test even in an Rh-negative infant should be considered presumptive evidence of hemolytic disease of the newborn.

PREVENTION OF KERNICTERUS. MEASUREMENTS OF BILIRUBIN. The frequency with which bilirubin is determined depends upon the severity of disease. There are no absolute rules, but, in general, bilirubin should be measured about every 2 to 4 hours if it is rising rapidly (0.5 mg/dl/hour or faster) or is within 5 mg/dl of the level considered dangerous for that particular infant (see below). It can be measured less often when it is rising more slowly, is at a lower absolute level, or has begun to fall (Fig. 10, during the first 20 hr). In the first hours after birth, it is important to define the initial rate of rise of bilirubin by frequent measurements in all cases. If the rise in bilirubin is extremely rapid, multiple exchange transfusions may be needed to control the hyperbilirubinemia (Fig. 11). This situation must be detected as soon as possible to control the hyperbilirubinemia adequately.

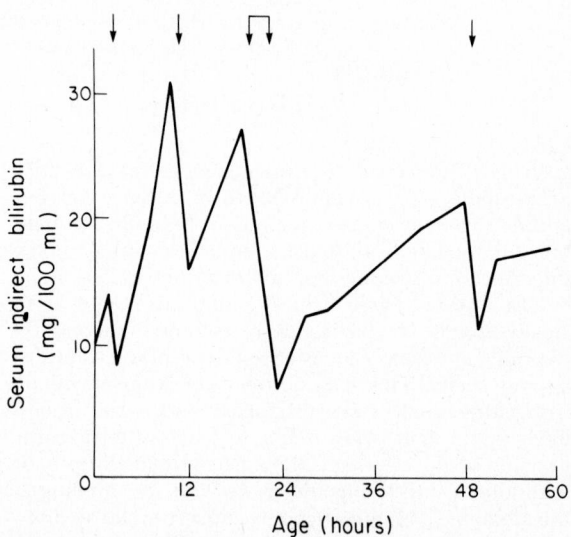

FIG. 11. Course of bilirubinemia in a 36-week gestation infant with severe erythroblastosis. Each single arrow indicates a standard 2-volume exchange transfusion, the double arrow, a 4-volume exchange transfusion. The rapidly rising bilirubin after the first exchange was a clue that a 4-volume exchange might be needed. The second 2-volume exchange halved the bilirubin concentration but, since it was 17mg/100 ml at the end, continuing the exchange would have removed much more bilirubin. The 4-volume exchange reduced bilirubin to one-fourth the pre-exchange level, and the postexchange rise was much slower. Note delay in repeat exchanges due to failure to anticipate the need for several units of donor blood.

ALTERATION OF BILIRUBIN BINDING. Factors capable of reducing the capacity of plasma albumin to bind bilirubin should be avoided if possible, or otherwise should be detected and corrected. Hypoalbuminemia may be corrected with infusions of 1 g/kg salt-poor albumin to raise the serum albumin concentration to about 3 g/dl. Venous pressure should be maintaned to avoid development of congestive failure. Blood gas measurements will detect acidemia and hypoxia in infants with severe cardiopulmonary disease, but in those with mild respiratory distress, significant acidemia is likely to be overlooked. Unless an erythroblastotic infant appears entirely well, one should measure at least the pH of peripheral capillary blood to rule out serious acidosis. Treatment of acidemia and hypoxia is discussed elsewhere (p.1507). Marked increases in free fatty acids usually can be avoided by providing an adequate caloric intake and preventing hypoglycemia. Similarly it is usually possible to avoid using drugs that interfere with bilirubin binding.

CONTROL OF BILIRUBIN LEVEL.   Once the various factors that influence bilirubin toxicity have been evaluated, one can decide on a safe upper limit of unconjugated bilirubin for the individual infant (p. 1082). Frequently the bilirubin level can be maintained below this level by phototherapy but if it approaches the dangerous level, exchange transfusion is indicated. The factors influencing bilirubin toxicity should be continually reevaluated; if they change for the worse, the level at which exchange is indicated may have to be revised downward.

PHOTOTHERAPY.   This is a proven method of reducing the concentration of unconjugated bilirubin in hemolytic disease, and it substantially reduces the need for exchange transfusions to control the hyperbilirubinemia after the first day. Phototherapy is based on the fact that visible light degrades fat-soluble unconjugated bilirubin that deposits in the skin to water-soluble monopyrroles and dipyrrholes that are not neurotoxic and can be eliminated by the kidney. The mechanism of action is discussed on page 1083. The effect of phototherapy is slower than that of exchange transfusion, but it is greater in the long run; it cannot replace exchange transfusion in the first hours after birth in infants with moderate or severe disease when anemia or a rapidly rising bilirubin level is present. In practice, phototherapy and exchange transfusion are often used in combination in the moderate or severely affected infant.

EXCHANGE TRANSFUSION.   Exchange transfusion can control the level of unconjugated bilirubin both by removing bilirubin and by removing Rh-positive antibody-coated cells before they are hemolyzed. An exchange is indicated if the concentration of indirect bilirubin is approaching the safe limit or if it is rising at such a rapid rate that it may approach that limit within a few hours (Fig. 11). A rate greater than 1 mg/100 ml/hour generally indicates a dangerously rapid rise that warrants early exchange.

Indications for exchange to prevent jaundice by removing antibody-coated cells are no longer clear-cut. Allen and Diamond devised graphs for predicting which infants would ultimately reach the dangerous level and need exchange transfusion and so could be exchanged earlier to reduce hemolysis. In the more severe cases early exchange transfusion can reduce the need for second or third exchanges. However, as phototherapy has reduced the number of repeat exchanges, it is no longer clear when early exchange is warranted. Usually full

exchange transfusion can be delayed until 3 to 4 hours after birth when the infant is in a more stable condition and can better tolerate the stress of the procedure.

Selection of donor blood.   Once an exchange transfusion is decided upon, appropriate donor blood should be available immediately. This requires advance preparation, particularly in infants with severe disease in whom a second exchange may be needed shortly after completion of the first. Figure 11 illustrates the risks of underestimating the need. Donor blood must be crossmatched against maternal serum to ensure that it is compatible; crossmatching against only the infant's serum is less accurate. Generally group O Rh-negative blood with a low titer of anti-A and anti-B antibodies is used. When an infant is group A or B, it is possible to use donor blood of the same group, if the mother's group is also the same. Blood crossmatched before delivery for use at delivery must be group O, since the infant's ABO group is not known; in actual practice it is usually easiest to use group O Rh-negative blood for all cases. After the first transfusion, donor blood for succeeding transfusions must be crossmatched against both mother and infant because of antibodies in the earlier donor's blood that may now be in the infant's circulation.

Technique of Exchange.   Traditionally exchange transfusions have been done by a catheter passed through the umbilical vein without much concern for the location of the catheter tip. Improper location and management of the catheter can cause complications such as acute necrotizing enterocolitis, air embolus, and portal vein thrombosis, and also may give misleading information regarding venous pressure. The techniques of umbilical vessel catheterization and methods for proper placement of the umbilical venous catheter tip are described elsewhere (p. 168). If an umbilical venous catheter is used for exchange transfusion, the catheter tip should be in the inferior vena cava or right atrium, where blood flow is large and the blood withdrawn and injected during transfusion is only a small proportion of total flow. Pressure measured in this site provides central venous pressure. Many erythroblastotic infants require insertion of an umbilical artery catheter for cardiopulmonary care, and this catheter can also be used for transfusions. If both artery and vein are catheterized, the exchange transfusion can be done by infusion through one catheter while simultaneously withdrawing through the other.

If only one catheter is in place, one must repeatedly withdraw an aliquot of infant blood and replace it with an equal volume of donor blood. Theoretically, the washout would be more effective if one used large aliquots, but within the range of practicality, aliquot size has little effect. Thus an exchange of 500 ml, using 30-ml increments, is no more efficient than one using 5- or 10-ml increments, and the latter is safer.

Effects of Exchange Transfusion.   The procedure is simply a flushing out of the intravascular space. Generally a volume equal to twice the infant's estimated blood volume (body weight in kg $\times$ 85 $\times$ 2), is exchanged. An exchange of this volume should take at least 30 minutes, but averages 60 to 90 minutes. As it proceeds, proportionately more of the blood removed is donor blood that was infused earlier. Thus the amount of infant's blood removed per volume of blood transfused gradually diminishes as shown:

Vol. transfused/infant's blood vol.	% infant's blood vol. replaced
0.5	40
1.0	65
2.0	85
3.0	95

These figures on the efficiency of an exchange only indicate the washout of the vascular compartment, and do not reflect the removal of bilirubin. Unlike red cells, bilirubin is distributed in a much larger space than the intravascular compartment, and as soon as plasma concentration falls, bilirubin moves from the extravascular space into the plasma. Although proportionately more bilirubin is removed than red cells, bilirubin concentration drops less than would be anticipated on the basis of the volume exchanged (Fig. 12). The standard two-volume exchange removes an amount of bilirubin equal to twice what was in the circulation at the start of the exchange and reduces bilirubin concentration by 50

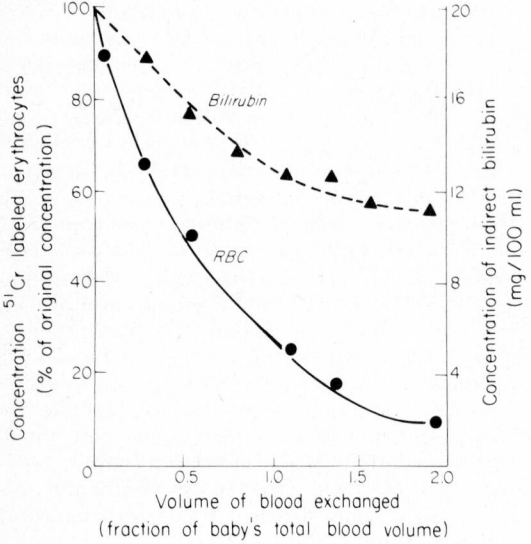

FIG. 12. The efficiency of an exchange transfusion in a 2,865 g newborn. Chromium-labeled red cells had previously been infused into the infant's circulation; the fall in their concentration (solid line) during the exchange transfusion is a measure of the efficiency with which the vascular compartment is washed out. Note that the fall in indirect bilirubin concentration (dotted line) is not as great. The difference between the two lines is due to the indirect bilirubin that moved from extravascular areas into the vascular compartment during the procedure. The baby had a total of 33.2 mg of indirect bilirubin in his intravascular compartment at the start of the exchange. A total of 43.9 mg of indirect bilirubin was removed by the procedure, yet the serum concentration was only halved, and 18.9 mg remained in his vascular space at the end, so that 29.6mg moved into the vascular space during the exchange. (Graph derived from the data of Sproul and Smith.)

percent. After such an exchange, reequilibration of bilirubin between extravascular and intravascular spaces continues for 30 minutes, causing a rapid rise or rebound of bilirubin to 60 to 75 percent of the preexchange level. Thereafter it rises more slowly due to continued hemolysis (Fig. 10). Thus bilirubin should be measured at the beginning and end of the exchange, 30 to 60 minutes later, and then after 2 to 3 hours to establish the new rate of rise. The amount of bilirubin removed by a two-volume exchange can be increased by as much as 50 percent by infusing 1 g/kg body weight of salt-poor albumin shortly before the start of an exchange. This increases plasma binding capacity for bilirubin and draws more bilirubin into the circulation from the extravascular compartment. Increasing the duration of the exchange does not increase bilirubin removal significantly, unless the procedure is prolonged to 4 to 6 hours.

Certain precautions are necessary to obtain the most benefit from an exchange transfusion and to avoid serious problems. The donor blood must be agitated repeatedly or it will settle, and the infant will receive very dilute blood at the end of the exchange, leaving him anemic. The donor blood should be warmed to at least room temperature before starting the exchange or it will produce severe hypothermia in the infant; blood should be warmed slowly since temperatures above 37 C will cause hemolysis. Unless donor blood is very fresh it will have a low concentration of platelets and will leave the infant thrombocytopenic; however, except in infants who were severely thrombocytopenic before, the platelet count after exchange is rarely low enough to cause bleeding. It should be checked after exchange transfusion in these infants. Citrate phosphate dextrose (CPD) anticoagulant will cause a mild metabolic acidosis because of its acidic pH. However, it is preferable to acid citrate dextrose (ACD) anticoagulant which has an even lower pH. Healthy infants can usually compensate for the acidemia, but those with respiratory disease, or premature infants, cannot. Developing metabolic acidema should be corrected by infusion of alkali. In critically ill infants it is better to avoid acidemia by measuring pH of donor blood and adding enough THAM buffer to raise the pH to 7.15 to 7.20. Both CPD and ACD anticoagulants act by binding calcium and are present in excess in the donor blood. Infusions of 1 ml of 10 percent calcium gluconate diluted in 4 ml of 5 percent glucose in water usually are given after every 100 ml exchanged to prevent hypocalcemia; it should be given slowly over 1 to 2 minutes while monitoring the electrocardiogram to detect arrhythmias. Both ACD and CPD-anticoagulant blood contains so much glucose that marked hyperglycemia occurs. This stimulates the hyperplastic pancreas to release insulin; the excessive supply of glucose ends abruptly when the exchange is completed, and profound hypoglycemia can occur within 20 minutes. This must be prevented by starting a parenteral infusion of 10 percent glucose immediately after the end of the exchange, measuring the blood glucose repeatedly, and gradually reducing the glucose infusion, as tolerated. If the donor blood is more than a week old, it may be hyperkalemic due to release of intracellular potassium from hemolyzed red cells, causing hyperkalemia in the infant.

Many of these problems can be resolved by use of fresh blood. CPD blood less than 4 days old is not very acidic and has a nearly normal potassium. If less than 1 to 2 days old, some viable platelets are preserved and clotting factor activity is close to normal. An alternative is to use fresh heparinized blood, which has a disadvantage in that it leaves the infant temporarily heparinized (heparin half-life is about 4 hours). Heparin may be permitted to degrade, or heparinization can be reversed with protamine (p. 1218); however, protamine may cause cardiac arrhythmias and itself may act as an anticoagulant.

HYPOGLYCEMIA. All erythroblastotic infants should be tested frequently for hypoglycemia until they have a stable intake of carbohydrate that proves adequate to prevent hypoglycemia. Testing with Dextrostix can be done at the bedside on capillary blood specimens. The same principles of management of hypoglycemia in infants of diabetic mothers apply to erythroblastotic infants (p. 177).

BLEEDING PROBLEMS. Severely affected infants who are thrombocytopenic at birth require repeated platelet counts to evaluate the state of their coagulation system. In the presence of severe thrombocytopenia, investigation for the possibility of disseminated intravascular coagulation (DIC) should be carried out (p. 1214). Infants with clinical bleeding must be treated. Those with thrombocytopenia without bleeding usually do not require treatment unless the platelet count is below $50,000/mm^3$ and they otherwise have an increased risk of serious bleeding, eg, if they are premature and weigh less than 1,750 g or if they have cardiorespiratory distress. Severe thrombocytopenia can be corrected with transfusions of concentrated platelets, which can also supply a significant amount of all essential clotting factors. If an exchange transfusion is needed for other purposes, use of fresh blood that is less than 1 day old has the advantage over platelet transfusions of not increasing blood volume and reducing the hematocrit.

MANAGEMENT OF SEVERELY AFFECTED INFANT WITH OR WITHOUT HYDROPS. The treatment of asphyxia (p. 1507), must be combined with correction of the more urgent hematologic disorders. Therapy cannot follow a routine program but must be guided by repeated measurements of PaO_2, $PaCO_2$, pH, hematocrit, and aortic and central venous pressures. The aorta and inferior vena cava should be catheterized immediately after birth to make these measurements and also provide a route for exchange transfusion. It is particularly important that central venous pressure be measured properly (p. 168); if it is not done carefully, misleading information may be obtained. Pleural effusions or ascites sufficient to distend the abdomen should be relieved to allow adequate ventilation. Caution should be exercised during paracentesis to avoid puncturing the enlarged liver and spleen, which may extend into the lower quadrants of the abdomen. Significant anemia requires rapid correction by a small exchange transfusion with packed red blood cells crossmatched against the mother's serum before delivery, and ready for use at birth. Raising blood oxygen-carrying capacity is helpful in the management of asphyxia. Generally, an exchange of 20 to 40 ml/kg body weight will raise the hematocrit to 35 to 45 percent, but this should be checked by repeated measurements.

Manipulations of blood volume should be based on measurements of aortic and central venous pressures, which should be recorded as soon as the catheters are in place. In the presence of asphyxia, abnormal pressures could be due to the asphyxia, to an abnormal blood volume, or to both; it may be impossible to separate the causes. Asphyxia should be treated promptly, the anemia corrected, and the changes in pressures following treatment observed closely. Pressures persistently subnormal after initial treatment suggest an inadequate blood volume, requiring expansion; a persistently high central venous pressure with normal or high aortic pressure suggests hypervolemia, requiring phlebotomy. In practice, the former is relatively common and the latter uncommon in the first hours of life. When indicated, blood volume should be changed by repeated small increments or decrements, using changes in intravascular pressures, changes in blood gas tensions, and the general condition as a guide to further changes in volume. Figure 13 shows findings during the first hour after birth in a typical case.

Moderate or severe hydrops may require additional treatment. Initiation of a diuresis is usually followed by a general improvement in the cardiorespiratory condition. Sometimes diuresis begins during resuscitation; it may be induced by raising the low concentration of albumin in the plasma with infusion of salt-poor albumin in an initial dose of 1 g/kg body weight. If serum albumin concentration is raised by this method or by exchange transfusion, central venous pressure should be monitored in case excessive fluid is drawn into the circulation and produces congestive heart failure. Albumin should not be given unless central venous pressure is low or normal; if it rises above normal afterward phlebotomy is indicated. As an alternative to albumin one may use a potent fast-acting diuretic, such as ethacrynic acid (1 mg/kg, intravenously) or furosemide (1 mg/kg intramuscularly or intravenously), to induce a diuresis. These should not be given if central venous pressure is already low.

LATE CARE. Erythroblastotic infants should be followed with repeated measurements of hematocrit and reticulocyte counts and should be examined in the first months after birth for physical signs of development of late anemia. There is no absolute level of hematocrit that always requires transfusion, and moderate anemia with hematocrit levels greater than 25 percent is often well tolerated. The first evidences of difficulty usually are poor feeding, decreased activity, and, later, resting tachycardia. Treatment consists of transfusions of packed cells to raise the hematocrit to 30 to 35 percent. Usually by 6 to 8 weeks, reticulocytes will appear in the blood, and thereafter the infant will main-

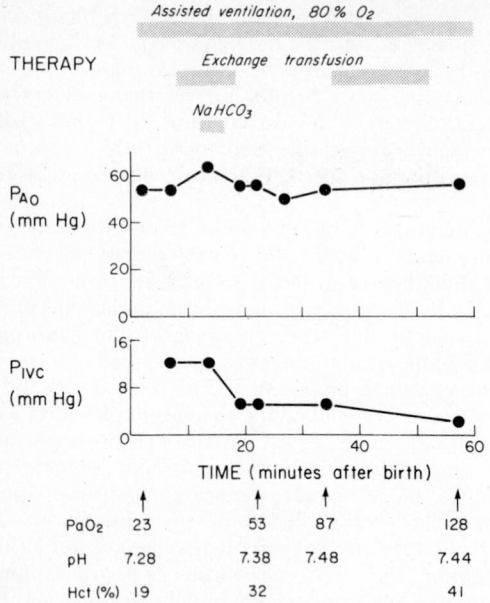

FIG. 13. First hour of life of an infant with severe erythroblastosis fetalis, born at 34.5 weeks gestation, weighing 2400 g. The 1-minute Apgar score was 1. Blood from the artery of the umbilical cord had a hematocrit of 19 percent, a reticulocyte count of 78 percent, an indirect bilirubin of 5.6 mg/100 ml, direct bilirubin of 1.7 mg/100 ml, and albumin of 2.2 mg/100 ml and a platelet count of 60,000/cm. The infant had moderately severe generalized edema but no ascites or pleural effusion. Aorta and inferior vena cava were catheterized via the umbilical artery and vein respectively. Exchange transfusions were with packed red blood cells, infused into the inferior vena cava while equivalent volumes were simultaneously removed via the arterial catheter. Blood volume was not reduced. Note the high central venous pressure which rapidly falls to normal as hypoxia is relieved. The infant had transient respiratory distress that cleared completely before 24 hours of age.

tain adequate hematocrit levels. A disadvantage of transfusions between 1 and 6 weeks is that the hematocrit is maintained at a high level only temporarily because erythropoiesis is suppressed.

INFANTS WHO RECEIVED INTRAUTERINE TRANSFUSIONS. All of these infants are delivered prematurely, and many still have severe disease, including hydrops. In most cases about half the red cells in circulation are donor cells; the remainder are infant cells. These infants usually develop severe hyperbilirubinemia and require exchange transfusion. About 33 percent will have virtually 100 percent donor blood in their circulation and hematocrits of 35 to 45 percent. In these infants the transfusions have suppressed their erythropoiesis so completely that they have almost no reticulocytes, even if mildly anemic. The blood is Rh-negative by direct Coombs' test and positive by indirect Coombs' test. The infants often have little or no hyperbilirubinemia because they have so few Rh-positive cells to be hemolyzed, and they may require only small transfusions to correct anemia. They tend to become very

anemic during the first few months, require close attention to hematocrit and reticulocyte count, and may need several transfusions.

There have been a few documented cases of graft-versus-host reactions in infants transfused in utero who also required exchange transfusions after birth (p. 322). It is postulated that the intrauterine transfusions created a state of immune tolerance that allowed the lymphocytes from the exchange transfusion to survive and cause the disease. It is not certain whether this can be prevented by irradiating the donor blood used for the intrauterine transfusion and for the postnatal exchange transfusions to kill donor lymphocytes. Many infants who receive intrauterine transfusion followed by postnatal exchange transfusions develop an intense maculopapular rash that tends to become confluent, and they have thrombocytopenia and eosinophilia in the first week, similar to the early manifestations of graft-versus-host reaction. However, the abnormal findings disappear and there is no further evidence of immunologic disorder; this phenomenon is unexplained.

Many infants have physical evidence of trauma secondary to intrauterine transfusions, including hematomas in the flank, rare renal injury and, commonly, scars from the needle punctures over the trunk. Many of these infants develop unexplained abdominal distension during the first week and often have very large umbilical hernias for 1 to 2 years after birth and weak anterior abdominal musculature that gives them a pot-belly appearance for a few years. These findings presumably are related to distension of the abdomen with donor blood in utero. Several studies have now shown that infants transfused in utero tend to have few serious physical or neurologic handicaps when they reach later childhood.

ABO HEMOLYTIC DISEASE

A mother who is group O has naturally occurring anti-A and anti-B antibodies in her circulation. If her fetus is group A or group B, erythroblastosis may occur. Most naturally occurring anti-A and anti-B are IgM antibodies, which do not cross the placenta. Some mothers have relatively high levels of IgG anti-A or anti-B, which have the potential for causing erythroblastosis, since IgG does cross the placenta. Group O mothers have higher levels of IgG anti-A than do group B mothers and higher levels of IgG anti-B than group A mothers. Thus, disease almost always occurs when the mother is group O. Disease rarely occurs when the mother is group A and the infant group B. At present, no practical system of screening can detect those mothers who are likely to have affected fetuses, but this is not a serious problem because the disease is usually mild.

Even though anti-A and anti-B IgG are more potent hemolysins than anti-D IgG, ABO disease tends to be mild. In a group A or B individual the antigens are not limited to the red blood cell membrane but occur in many tissues. As a result much of the antibody that does cross the placenta to the fetus attaches to these other antigens rather than to those on the red cells. Infants with ABO disease tend to have very little antibody on their red cells and only a weakly reactive direct Coombs' test.

First pregnancies may be affected because sensitization occurs early in life through contact with A and B antigen. The disease does not worsen with succeeding affected pregnancies; if anything, it tends to become milder. Because hemolysis is mild, the infants are similar to those with very mild cases of Rh hemolytic disease. The typical patient has little or no anemia at birth, a +1 or +2 positive direct Coombs' test, and microspherocytes in peripheral blood. Hyperbilirubinemia is milder and usually requires no exchange transfusion if phototherapy is used. Hydrops due to ABO disease is rare. The principles of management are the same as for Rh hemolytic disease.

References

Allen FH Jr, Diamond LK: Erythroblastosis fetalis including exchange transfusion technique. N Engl J Med 257:659, 705, 1957

Baum JD, Harris D: Colloid osmotic pressure in erythroblastosis fetalis. Br Med J 1:601, 1972

Bowman JM, Friesen RF, Bowman WD, McInnis AC, Barnes PH, Grewar D: Fetal transfusion in severe Rh isoimmunization. JAMA 207:1101, 1969

Cashore WJ, Karotkin EH, Stern L, Oh W: The lack of effect of phototherapy on serum bilirubin-binding capacity in newborn infants. J Pediatr 87:977, 1975

Chassels JM, Wigglesworth JS: Hemostatic failure in babies with rhesus isoimmunization. Arch Dis Child 46:38, 1971

Diamond LK, Blackfan KD, Baty JM: Erythroblastosis and its association with universal edema of the fetus, icterus gravis neonatorum and anemia of the newborn. J Pediatr 1:269, 1932

Driscoll SC, Steinke J: Pancreatic insulin content in severe erythroblastosis fetalis. Pediatrics 39:448, 1967

Dunn PM: Obstructive jaundice and hemolytic disease of the newborn. Arch Dis Child 38:54, 1963

Graham HM, Morrison M, Casey E: Severe ABO haemolytic disease due to high titre IgG anti-B in an A$_2$ mother. Vox Sang 27:363, 1974

Hathaway WE, Mahasandana C, Makowski EL: Cord blood coagulation studies of infants of high risk pregnant women. Am J Obstet Gynecol 121:51, 1975

Hobel CJ: The influence of anemia on the acid-base state of the fetus and newborn. Am J Obstet Gynecol 106:303, 1970

Kitchen WH, Krieger VI, Smith MA: Human albumin in exchange transfusion. J Pediatr 57:876, 1960

Liley AW: The use of amniocentesis and intrauterine transfusions in erythroblastosis fetalis. Pediatrics 35:836, 1965

Lind T, Anderton K, Tacchi D: Early induction of labour in cases of rhesus isoimmunization. Lancet 1:585, 1969

Lund HT, Jacobsen J: Influence of phototherapy on the biliary bilirubin excretion pattern in newborn infants with hyperbilirubinemia. J Pediatr 85:262, 1974

Maisels MJ, Pathak A Nelson NM: The effect of exchange transfusion on endogenous carbon monoxide production in erythroblastotic infants. J Pediatr 81:705, 1972

Moller J, Ebbeson F: Phototherapy in newborn infants with severe rhesus hemolytic disease. J Pediatr 86:135, 1975

Odell GB, Cohen S: Albumin priming in the management of hyperbilirubinemia by exchange transfusion. Am J Dis Child 102:699, 1961

Parkman R: Graft-versus-host disease after intrauterine and exchange transfusion for hemolytic disease of the newborn. N Engl J Med 290:359, 1974

Phibbs RH, Harvin D, Jones G, Talbot C, Cohen M, Crowther D, Tooley WH: Development of children who had received intrauterine transfusion. Pediatrics 47:689, 1971

———Johnson P, Kitterman J, Gregory GA, Tooley WH: Cardiorespiratory status of erythroblastotic infants: relationship of gestational age, severity of hemolytic disease and birth asphyxia to idiopathic respiratory distress syndrome and survival. Pediatrics 49:5, 1972

———Johnson P, Tooley WH: Cardiorespiratory status of erythroblastotic newborn infants: II. Blood volume, hematocrit and serum albumin concentration in relation to hydrops fetalis. Pediatrics 53:13, 1974

Richings J: Later progress of infants who received transfusions in utero for severe rhesus haemolytic disease. Lancet 1:1220, 1973

Schiff D, Aranda JV Colle E, Stern L: Metabolic effects of exchange transfusion II. Delayed hypoglycemia following exchange transfusion with citrated blood. J Pediatr 79:589, 1971

Sisson TR, Kendall N, Glauser SC, Knutson S, Bunyaviroch E: Phototherapy of jaundice in newborn infants. I. ABO blood group incompatibility. J Pediatr 79:904, 1971

Sproul A, Smith L: Bilirubin equilibration during exchange transfusion in hemolytic disease of the newborn. J Pediatr 65:12, 1964

Townsend L, Kitchen WH: Perinatal mortality associated with mode of induction of labour in Rh immunized patients. Aust NZ J Obstet Gynaecol 9:183, 1969

Van Praagh R: Causes of death in infants with hemolytic disease of the newborn (erythroblastosis fetalis). Pediatrics 28:223, 1961

Zipursky A: The universal prevention of Rh immunization. Clin Obstet Gynecol 14:869, 1971

AUTOIMMUNE AND DRUG-INDUCED HEMOLYTIC ANEMIA

BERTRAM H. LUBIN

In immune hemolytic anemia, an antibody becomes bound to the surface of the red cell and shortens its survival. Fixed macrophages within the reticuloendothelial system remove both antibody and portions of the red cell membrane, producing spherocytes that have limited deformability and become trapped, particularly in the spleen. Some antibodies may also fix complement, which binds to the membrane and results in intravascular lysis of the red cell.

The diagnosis of immune hemolytic anemia is based on the Coombs' test, which is used to detect antibody or complement on the surface of the erythrocyte. In the direct Coombs' test, antiserum against human globulin is incubated at 37 C with the patient's washed erythrocytes (p. 1136). If the cells agglutinate, the test is positive. The Coombs' antiserum can be made specific for complement or immunoglobulin, but most commercial antiserum will not detect complement alone. When the amount of antibody on the surface of the cell is small, the direct Coombs' test may be negative. Such small quantities of antibody may be eluted from the cell, concentrated, and tested against normal cells. The patient's serum may also contain antibody against red cells. This antibody can be measured by incubating the serum with normal cells and enzyme-treated cells. After the cells are washed, they are reincubated with Coombs' antiserum and observed for agglutination. This test is called the indirect Coombs' test. Positive reactions with maximal activity at 37 C are called warm antibodies, and those that react maximally at 4 C are called cold antibodies. In situations where both the direct and indirect Coombs' tests are negative, specific complement fixation techniques may be used to detect small numbers of IgG molecules on the surface of the red cell.

ACQUIRED IMMUNE HEMOLYTIC ANEMIA

The acquired immune hemolytic anemias have at least two distinct types of clinical course that may be predicted on the basis of the mode of onset and the specificity of the Coombs' test.

The acute transient form of this disease usually has its onset in the first 4 years of life. Typically, a previously well child presents with the fulminant onset of pallor, fever, and anorexia following a viral illness. Scleral icterus, splenomegaly, hemoglobinemia, and hemoglobinuria may be observed. The patient frequently has tachycardia, and when the hemoglobin is markedly decreased he may be in shock. The hemoglobin may be as low as 2 g/dl but usually is 4 to 6 g/dl. The reticulocyte count is usually elevated, although reticulocytopenia may be observed during the initial stages of the disease. The platelets may be decreased, and the total leukocyte counts may be either increased or decreased. The indirect bilirubin is elevated and the haptoglobin is decreased. Examination of the peripheral blood smear reveals rouleaux formation, microspherocytes, polychromasia, basophilic stippling, nucleated red cells, and fragmented erythrocytes.

Immunohematologic studies in most patients with acute transient disease reveal a warm antibody. Complement is frequently found on the surface of the red cell. Less often, specific Coombs' reagents reveal IgG or a mixed reaction involving both complement and IgG. When IgG is present, the antibody is usually against all Rh antigens. An unusual autoantibody, sometimes associated with the acute transient form of autoimmune hemolytic anemia, is the Donath-Landsteiner antibody. This antibody is peculiar in that it is an IgG antibody that binds to the surface of the red cell at 4 C and fixes complement on the cell. When the incubation temperature is raised to 37 C, the cell hemolyzes. In adults the Donath-Landsteiner antibody is found in association with syphilis, but in children there is no association with a specific infection.

The prognosis in patients with the acute idiopathic transient form of autoimmune hemolytic anemia is good. Treatment with prednisone, 2 to 6 mg/kg/day, is usually successful in diminishing the rate of hemolysis. The mechanisms of action are believed to be decreased removal of red cells by the reticuloendothelial system and diminished antibody production. The dose of corticosteroids should not be tapered until hemolysis has subsided. It is important to lower the dose very slowly, because abrupt discontinuation of steroids often results in a recurrence of disease manifestations. Under unusual circumstances, when the degree of anemia is severe and the patient is in cardiorespiratory distress, a transfusion or partial exchange transfusion with packed cells should be considered. It is often impossible to crossmatch the patient due to the positive direct and indirect Coombs' reactions. Therefore, group O, Rh-negative cells with the most compatible crossmatch should be used. Due to the persistence of antibody in the patient, transfusions frequently do not result in an increase in hemoglobin. A one- or two-volume exchange transfusion may be required in extreme situations as a temporary measure while steroids are taking effect. Under these circumstances, the higher dose of corticosteroids should be used immediately.

After the initial period, the hemoglobin, reticulocyte count, and Coombs' test should be followed frequently. Decreased rate of hemolysis is evidenced by an increase in the hemoglobin concentration and a decrease in the reticulocyte count. Improvement may occur despite persistence of the red cell antibody. The Coombs' test may remain positive for as little as 2 weeks or as long as 1 year after the onset of the clinical disease. Thus, the administration of steroids should not be based upon the Coombs' reaction but on the degree of hemolysis.

In patients with *Mycoplasma* pneumonia and mononucleosis, there may be a positive Coombs' test and an acute transient form of hemolytic anemia. In these disorders the antibody has its maximal activity at 4 C and has minimal activity at 37 C. Although the Coombs' test may be positive, hemolytic anemia only occurs when the antibody titer is very high (ie, 1:1024). The antibody is often directed against the I antigen on the surface of the red cell in *Mycoplasma* infections and the I antigen in mononucleosis. Patients with hemolytic anemias associated with these infectious diseases have mild courses that rarely require treatment and improve as the basic disease improves.

The chronic idiopathic form of autoimmune hemolytic anemia usually has an insidious onset but also may present in an acute fashion. Chronic autoimmune hemolytic anemia may be present in patients with chronic hepatitis, cytomegalic inclusion disease, chronic thrombocytopenic purpura, and autoimmune disorders, such as systemic lupus erythematosus. Sometimes the hemolytic anemia is recognized before the primary disease becomes apparent. The common feature of many of these disorders is their association with a defect in the immune response. The prognosis is worse than in the acute transient form where there is a primary disease; prognosis depends on how successfully it can be managed. The patient is noted to be jaundiced and may have intermittent episodes of hemoglobinuria and hemoglobinemia. The chronic anemia is less severe than in the acute form of the disease. Reticulocytosis is usually present, and thrombocytopenia and neutropenia are observed occasionally. The spleen is often enlarged and hepatomegaly also may be found. The peripheral blood smear is similar to that in the acute form. Patients with the chronic form of autoimmune hemolytic anemia have a warm antibody. However, in contrast to the acute form, there is usually IgG or IgG plus complement on the surface of the red cells, or rarely complement alone. The response to corticosteroids is generally poor. Relapses are common and may, in the more severe cases, warrant a trial of immunosuppressive agents, such as Imuran or Cytoxan. When none of these is successful and hemolysis is significant, splenectomy should be considered. The degree of splenic sequestration and destruction of red cells is estimated by monitoring over the spleen after injection of normal cells labeled with ^{51}Cr. Marked splenic sequestration is of some help in predicting the effectiveness of splenectomy. The decision to remove the spleen should be based on the patient's clinical condition rather than any specific value of hemoglobin or reticulocyte count. The clinical course of autoimmune hemolytic anemia in children is different from that in adults. Adults most commonly have chronic disease with a poor response to therapy and a high rate of mortality. Postinfectious immune hemolytic anemia is very rare in adults but common in children.

DRUG-INDUCED HEMOLYTIC ANEMIA

Drug-induced hemolytic anemia accounts for 16 percent of the acquired immune hemolytic anemia in adults, but drugs are rarely a cause of hemolysis in children. The three drugs most commonly implicated in adults are penicillin, α-methyldopa, and Keflin.

Penicillin, when given in high doses (20 million IU/day intravenously) can bind to the red cell membrane and act as a haptene; an antibody is then formed against the combination of red cell membrane and penicillin. This antibody is IgG and can be detected on the patient's red cells with the direct Coombs' test. The indirect Coombs' test is normal unless the red cells are first incubated with penicillin. Three percent of adult patients receiving massive doses of intravenous penicillin will develop a positive direct antiglobulin test, and a small percentage of these will develop hemolytic anemia. Hemolysis may occur within 1 week after initiation of therapy and promptly subsides following the discontinuation of penicillin.

α-Methyldopa (Aldomet) is the most common cause of drug-induced hemolytic anemia. Approximately 15 percent of patients receiving α-methyldopa will develop a positive Coombs' test. This will occur within 3 to 6 months after treatment has been initiated and is dose-dependent. Hemolytic anemia occurs in less than 1 percent of these patients. The mechanism of the Aldomet-induced autoantibody is not known. The Coombs' test may remain positive for a period of several weeks to 2 years after discontinuation of the drug, but clinical improvement in those cases with hemolytic anemia occurs rapidly. When Aldomet is used in the management of pediatric patients with renal disease and hypertension, autoimmune hemolytic anemia should be considered as a possible contributing factor to the anemia associated with renal disease.

Therapy with Keflin can result in a positive Coombs' test by the nonimmunologic adsorption of proteins on the surface of the red cell. This reaction is not associated with hemolysis. In rare situations, Keflin may be a haptene, similar to penicillin, in which case a hemolytic anemia may develop. The nonspecific adsorption of protein to the surface of the membrane results in a false-positive Coombs' test in 3 percent of adult patients taking Keflin. This reaction is dependent upon the dose and duration of therapy. Similar data have not been collected in children. When patients receiving Keflin require blood transfusions, crossmatching may be complicated by this nonimmunologic reaction. By notifying the blood bank that Keflin is being used, these difficulties can be resolved.

References

Dacie JV, Worlledge SM: Autoimmune hemolytic anemias. Prog Hematol 6:82, 1969

Garratty G, Petz LD: Drug-induced immune hemolytic anemia. Am J Med 58:398, 1975

Gilliland BC, Baxter E, Evans RS: Red-cell antibodies in acquired hemolytic anemia with negative antiglobulin serum tests. N Engl J Med 285:252, 1971

Habibi B, Homberg J, Schaison G, Salmon C: Autoimmune hemolytic anemia in children—a review of 80 cases. Am J Med 56:61, 1974

Petz LD, Garratty G: Laboratory correlations in immune hemolytic anemias. In Vyas GN, Stites DP, Brecher G (eds): Laboratory Diagnosis of Immunologic Disorders. Philadelphia, Grune & Stratton, 1975

Zuelzer WW, Mastrangelo R, Stulberg C, Poulik MD, Page R, Thompson R: Autoimmune hemolytic anemia. Natural history and viral immunologic interactions in childhood. Am J Med 49:80, 1970

DESTRUCTION OF RED BLOOD CELLS DUE TO ABNORMALITIES IN VASCULATURE OR PLASMA

WILLIAM C. MENTZER

MECHANICAL INTRAVASCULAR HEMOLYSIS. Destruction of red blood cells may result from impact with abnormal surfaces, turbulent blood flow, and shearing by fibrin strands or platelet–fibrin aggregates. Mechanical fragmentation of red blood cells leads to the formation of spherocytes, microcytes, and schistocytes (cells with an irregular shape that have one or more pointed protrusions). Reticulocytosis is indicative of the degree of hemolysis. Serum haptoglobin is low or absent, serum hemoglobin may be elevated, and hemosiderin is often present in the urine. When hemolysis is of long standing, loss of iron as urinary hemosiderin may be sufficient to superimpose iron-deficiency anemia on the chronic hemolytic process. Thrombocytopenia may be present in certain settings (hemangioma, intravascular coagulation) either as an isolated finding or associated with a deficiency of clotting factors.

Mechanical intravascular hemolysis within large vessels, or *macroangiopathic hemolytic anemia*, is most commonly associated with abnormal turbulent blood flow over the surface of a diseased heart valve or a heart valve prosthesis. With mild degrees of hemolysis, a compensated hemolytic state can often be maintained, particularly if iron is given to replace what is lost in the urine as hemosiderin. The hemolysis associated with a valve prosthesis may intensify during recovery from cardiac surgery as increased physical activity results in increased cardiac output. Where hemolysis is severe, requiring frequent blood transfusions, surgical revision of the valve prosthesis may be necessary, but often the degree of hemolysis does not justify the risk of a second operation.

Microangiopathic hemolytic anemia, or mechanical intravascular hemolysis within small blood vessels, may occur in disseminated intravascular coagulation (p. 1214), localized intravascular coagulation (hemolytic-uremic syndrome, thrombotic thrombocytopenic purpura, (p. 1207), cavernous hemangioma (Kasabach-Merritt syndrome), or malignant hypertension. Damage to the endothelial lining of small vessels, sometimes accompanied by the deposition of fibrin strands or fibrin–platelet aggregates, is the component responsible for mechanical destruction of red cells in these diseases. Studies in vitro have demonstrated that forced passage of red blood cells through a fibrin meshwork will produce morphologic changes of mechanical fragmentation identical to those changes observed in vivo. Thrombocytopenia and clotting factor deficiencies are characteristic of disseminated intravascular coagulation and may be found in some cases of localized intravascular coagulation, such as cavernous hemangioma. In hemolytic uremic syndrome, thrombocytopenia is usually an isolated finding and may be largely due to mechanical destruction, as is the case with red blood cells, rather than to consumption within clots (p. 1207). Therapy in these conditions is directed at the underlying cause of the abnormality in the microcirculation.

HYPERSPLENISM Hemolysis associated with splenic enlargement is discussed on p. 1197.

LIVER DISEASE The lipid composition of the red blood cell membrane may be altered by changes in plasma lipids induced by either hepatocellular disease or biliary obstruction. Target cells are frequently observed in liver disease, but have no adverse effect on red blood cell survival. They are the morphologic consequence of excess membrane lipid, which results in a buckled, redundant red blood cell membrane. Rarely, severe hepatocellular disease is associated with hemolytic anemia. Spur cells, which resemble the acanthocytes characteristic of abetalipoproteinemia, are seen in the blood, and their appearance often indicates a fatal prognosis, with death due not to hemolytic anemia but to liver disease. Treatment is directed at the underlying liver disease.

PAROXYSMAL NOCTURNAL HEMOGLOBINURIA (PNH). Red blood cells in this acquired disorder are abnormally susceptible to complement-mediated lysis, even in the absence of antibody directed against erythrocytes. Hemolysis is intravascular, resulting in hemoglobinemia, hemoglobinuria, and hemosiderinuria. The lower plasma pH associated with sleep may accentuate nocturnal hemolysis, as implied by the name of the disorder. Exposure of PNH red blood cells to acid plasma at 37 C in vitro also causes their lysis and is the basis of the best-known diagnostic test for PNH, the Ham or acid lysis test. The sucrose hemolysis test, in which cells and serum containing complement are incubated in a low-ionic-strength isotonic sucrose medium, also demonstrates any susceptibility to complement-mediated lysis of red blood cells. Leukopenia and thrombocytopenia are commonly encountered in PNH; the disorder often resembles aplastic anemia. Major thrombotic episodes occasionally occur. The disease may terminate in leukemia.

Therapy consists of treatment of iron deficiency resulting from urinary iron loss and transfusion of blood components as necessary. Androgens and corticosteroids may be beneficial in selected cases in which marrow failure rather than hemolysis predominates (p. 1132).

INFANTILE PYKNOCYTOSIS   is a poorly defined syndrome characterized by a hemolytic anemia during the neonatal period, which resolves spontaneously after several months. Jaundice may be severe enough to require exchange transfusion. Dense, contracted, spiculated erythrocytes, or pyknocytes, appear in the blood, sometimes in great numbers. It is of interest that such cells may also be seen in smaller numbers in normal infants. Presumably an extracorpuscular factor, transiently present during early infancy, is responsible for hemolysis in the most severely affected patients. The Coombs' test is negative, and there is no blood group incompatibility.

References

Brain MC: Destruction of red cells by the vasculature and the reticuloendothelial system. In Nathan DG, Oski FA eds): Hematology of Infancy and Childhood. Philadelphia, WB Saunders, 1974, p 241

———— Microangiopathic hemolytic anemia. Br J Haematol (Suppl) 23:45, 1972

Bull BS, Kuhn IN: The production of schistocytes by fibrin strands (a scanning electron microscope study). Blood 35:104, 1970

Inceman S, Tangün Y: Chronic defibrination syndrome due to giant hemangioma associated with microangiopathic hemolytic anemia. Am J Med 46:997, 1969

Lieberman E: Hemolytic-uremic syndrome. J Pediatr 80:1, 1972

MacWhinney JB Jr, Packer JT, Miller G, Greendyke RM: Thrombotic thrombocytopenic purpura in childhood. Blood 19:181, 1962

Marsh GW, Lewis SM: Cardiac haemolytic anaemia. Semin Hematol 6:133, 1969

Miller DR, Baehner RL, Diamond LK: Paroxysmal nocturnal hemoglobinuria in childhood and adolescence. Pediatrics 39:675, 1967

Tuffy P, Brown AK, Zuelzer WW: Infantile pyknocytosis: common erythrocyte abnormality of the first trimester. Am J Dis Child 98:227, 1959

Abnormalities of Hemoglobin Structure and Function

Clinical abnormalities may result from structural abnormalities of globin due to substitution of one or more amino acids, from reduced synthesis of normal globin chains, from accumulation of various intermediates of heme synthesis, from changes in concentration of substances that regulate hemoglobin oxygen affinity, and from abnormalities in glutathione metabolism or methemoglobin reduction. The first two possibilities will be considered further now, while the other three abnormalities will be discussed later (see Erythrocte Metabolism, p. 1167).

SICKLE CELL DISEASE

BERTRAM H. LUBIN AND WILLIAM C. MENTZER

Although sickle cell disease was recognized in Africa more than 100 years ago, it was not until 1910 that the first case was reported in the United States. The disease is due to a structurally abnormal hemoglobin; the difference between sickle and normal adult hemoglobin is the substitution of the neutral amino acid valine for the positively charged glutamic acid in the sixth position of the β-globin chain. The difference in electrical charge allows for the electrophoretic separation of sickle from normal adult hemoglobin.

Sickle cell disease can be defined as a condition in which sickling of the red cells results in a significant and chronic clinical disorder. Sickle cell anemia, sickle β-thalassemia, and sickle-hemoglobin C disease are the commonest forms of sickle cell disease. The estimated frequency of sickle cell anemia in newborn blacks in the United States is 1:600, whereas sickle-hemoglobin C disease (1:800) and sickle β-thalassemia (1:1,700) are less common. In each condition, at least one β-globin gene directs the synthesis of sickle β chains; the other, allelic β-globin gene may also direct the production of sickle chains (sickle cell anemia), may be thalassemic (sickle β-thalassemia), or may code for another structural mutation (eg, sickle-hemoglobin C disease).

PATHOPHYSIOLOGY

The rigid, deformed sickle cell is easily damaged by mechanical stress associated with its passage through the vasculature. The result is a chronic hemolytic anemia with a rate of red cell destruction two to eight times normal. The degree of anemia is relatively constant in any individual patient unless red cell production is suppressed, for example by infection, or alternatively if hemolysis is accelerated by the concomitant presence of another hemolytic process such as G6PD deficiency. Because of its decreased deformability, the sickled erythrocyte is susceptible to entanglement and sequestration wherever blood flow is sluggish. Such rigid, misshapen cells also increase whole blood viscosity, thus compromising blood flow, often to the extent of producing clinically apparent local ischemia, thrombosis, and/or infarction, resulting in a vaso-occlusive crisis.

The conversion of the red blood cell from normal biconcave disks to sickle forms requires first the deoxygenation of hemoglobin and then the transformation of deoxyhemoglobin S from a sol to a gel phase. In the gel phase sickle hemoglobin has been polymerized, forming parallel fiber bundles that distort the cell into a sickle form. This polymerized sickle hemoglobin can revert to the soluble form upon reoxygenation, allowing the cell to return to its original, unsickled shape. However, approximately 10 percent of the circulating erythrocytes remain irreversibly sickled despite reoxygenation. The defect appears to reside in the cell membrane, since hemoglobin S within these oxygenated irreversibly sickled cells may not be polymerized.

The total number of reversibly and irreversibly sickled cells in the blood is inversely related to the oxygen saturation of hemoglobin. Hypoxia and acidemia, by decreasing the oxygen saturation of hemoglobin, promote sickling. In the arterial circulation the PO_2 is about 95 torr; hemoglobin is fully saturated with oxygen and only irreversibly sickled cells are seen. In the venous circulation the PO_2 is about 40 torr; hemoglobin is approximately 60 percent saturated with oxygen, and as many as 70 percent of the cells may be sickled. The tendency to sickle is also related to the concentration of hemoglobin, particularly hemoglobin S, within the cell. Since hypertonicity of the blood plasma increases the intracellular concentration of hemoglobin S, hypertonic dehydration also promotes sickling.

CLINICAL MANIFESTATIONS

There are two major *types of crisis* in sickle cell disease, anemic and vaso-occlusive; each can have multiple clinical manifestations (Table 6). *Anemic crises* most commonly result from a transient decrease in the rate of red cell production in the bone marrow. Such decreased production, also termed an aplastic crisis, is often associated with a bacterial or viral infection and is heralded by a fall in the reticulocyte count. (*aplastic crisis*) Due to the short life span of the circulating sickle erythrocyte, a transient decrease in red cell production

TABLE 6. Clinical Manifestations of Sickle Cell Disease

Ocular-tortuous conjunctival vessels
    proliferative retinopathy.
Cardiac-high-output failure
Pulmonary-infarction
    infection (pneumococcal, *Mycoplasma*)
    actelectasis (infection, obstruction, infarction)
Gastrointestinal and hepatic
    gallbladder (bilirubin stones)
    splenic (sequestration, infarction, functional
    asplenia
Musculoskeletal-infarction (aseptic necrosis, pain, hand-foot syndrome)
    infection (*Salmonella* osteomyelitis).
Genitourinary and renal-concentrating defects, hematuria, nephrosis
    priapism
Endocrine-delayed secondary sex characteristics
Immune system-susceptibility to infections
    defect in the alternate pathway of complement
    asplenism
    phagocytic defects
    lymphoid hyperplasia (enlarged tonsils and
    adenoids)
Skin-ulceration
Hematopoietic–anemia (aplasia, hemolytic, megaloblastic)
    phagocytic defects
    hyperuricemea
Neurologic-stroke, convulsions, visual disturbance
Psychiatric-dependence, addiction, separation, maturation

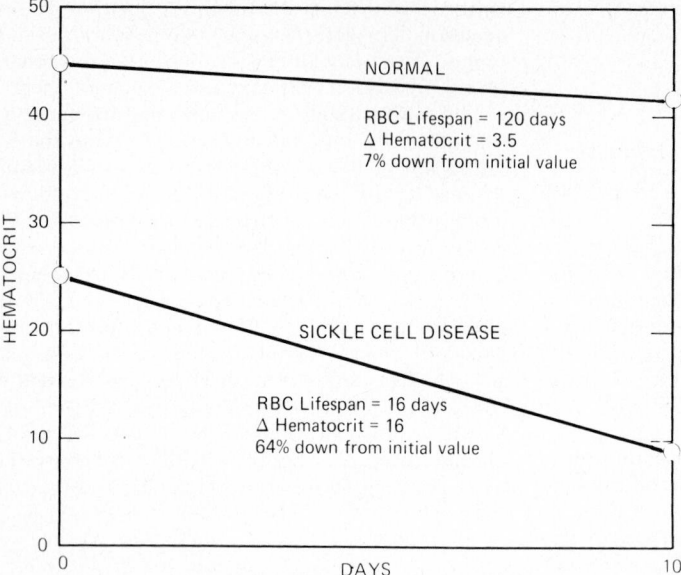

Fig. 14. Aplastic Crisis: The short life span of the sickle erythrocyte results in a rapid drop in hematocrit when red cell production is curtailed.

that would go unrecognized in the normal individual may rapidly result in profound anemia (Fig. 14). Two other types of anemic crisis are caused by an increased rate of sequestration or destruction of red cells. A *splenic sequestration crisis* is characterized by a rapidly enlarging spleen, which, in the most severe cases, sequesters a large proportion of the red cell mass, resulting in profound anemia and cardiovascular collapse. Severe anemia may develop within hours, as illustrated in Figure 15. Such crises, which may occur spontaneously or following a viral infection, are a major cause of death during the first 5 years of life. A *hyperhemolytic crisis* or a condition in which there is an even greater rate of hemolysis than usual, is characterized by anemia, reticulocytosis, and increasing jaundice. It is often associated with red cell glucose-6-phosphate dehydrogenase deficiency, which is also common among blacks (p. 1169). *Vaso-occlusive crises* are the most common type of crisis in sickle cell disease. A vaso-occlusive episode can involve any organ system and lead to permanent ischemic damage. Vaso-occlusive crises in young children are frequently associated with painful swelling over the hands and feet. This so-called *hand-foot syndrome* may be the initial manifestation of sickle cell disease. The swelling usually resolves within 2 weeks and often within a few days. Radiographic changes characteristic of aseptic necrosis of bone often appear about 10 days after the onset of the clinical manifestations and also resolve spontaneously. Painful crises often involve the abdomen in infants and young children and can be readily misinterpreted as representing gastrointestinal spasm (colic). Painful crises occur in the low back, abdomen, and long bones in older children and young adults; they often develop without warning and may last from a few hours to several weeks; exceptionally they persist for several months. The emotional impact of such un-

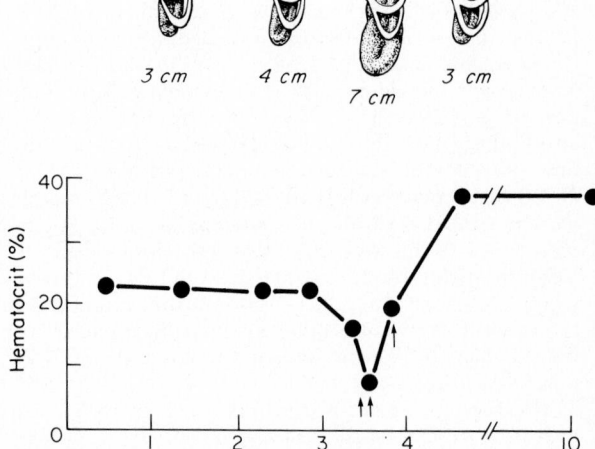

FIG. 15. Splenic Sequstration Crisis. During a viral infection, a 16-month old infant developed splenomegaly and life-threatening anemia. An identical twin had died of a similar complication 1 week earlier. Management included exchange transfusion (indicated by arrows) and eventually splenectomy.

predictable crises and their disruptive effect on schooling and later work is a significant handicap to these patients. Vaso-occlusive crisis occur at all ages and eventually lead to the prevalence in adults of permanent organ damage affecting the kidney, liver, lung, and central nervous system.

Infections

Patients with sickle cell disease are extremely susceptible to infections. Defects in the functional capacity of the spleen (p.1169), the alternate pathway of complement activation, and the phagocytic and killing capacity of granulocytes may explain this undue susceptibility, but the defect in splenic function appears to be the main factor. As in patients who lack a spleen, infections in patients with sickle cell disease may progress rapidly from mild manifestations to sepsis, shock, and death. The spleen not only fails to filter bacteria, but also does not normally promote the production of opsonizing antibodies. From about 5 months to 5 years of age, the spleen may be enlarged but incapable of normal reticuloendothelial function, as can be demonstrated by its failure to take up ^{99}technetium-sulfur colloid. In early childhood, this functional asplenia can sometimes be reversed by partial exchange transfusion with normal red cells. Later in life, the spleen becomes small and fibrotic due to repeated infarctions. However, in the older child and young adult, bacterial septicemia is less frequent, as there has been an opportunity to develop humoral immunity to many strains of bacteria and consequently there is less dependence on splenic filtration of bacteria. Bacterial septicemia is most commonly secondary to pneumococci, but *Haemophilus influenzae, Staphylococcus aureus,* or *Mycoplasma pneumoniae* may also be found. *Salmonella* osteomyelitis is also associated with sickle cell disease, but rarely progresses to generalized sepsis.

Pneumonia is a frequent complication in sickle cell disease. It may be accompanied by infarction and atelectasis. Such pulmonary problems often begin with chest or abdominal pain. Although the chest roentgenogram may be normal at first, within 24 hours segmental changes may be found, and bilateral pulmonary consolidation may ensue rapidly.

Natural History

The earliest clinical manifestations of sickle cell disease rarely begin before 4 months of age. In younger infants, sickling is uncommon because the fetal hemoglobin concentration is greater than 20 percent and the hemoglobin S concentration is less than 80 percent. Thereafter, the clinical manifestations of sickle cell disease tend to increase as the patient gets older; the highest mortality is in the first decade of life. Death in this period is mainly due to bacterial septicemia and the splenic sequestration syndrome. Sudden death may occur in either. During and after the second decade of life, there is an increasing incidence of gallstones attribut-

able to chronic hemolysis and increased production of bile pigment. Other clinical problems include leg ulcers and failure of organs, such as the heart, kidney, or liver. Cardiac problems are attributed to the stress of chronic anemia. High-output failure may occur, particularly in the patient with severe anemia. Renal complications include an inability to produce concentrated urine, pyelonephritis, hematuria, nephrosis, and nephritis. Liver enlargement and failure may occur due to infarction, bile stasis, or infection. Infarction of retinal vessels may lead to proliferative retinopathy, retinal detachment, and loss of vision.

Alterations in growth and development occur in patients with sickle cell disease. Both the bone age and height age are decreased, frequently resulting in growth retardation prior to puberty. The onset of puberty and development of secondary sex characteristics may be delayed by several years, but normal adult height is almost always eventually achieved.

Severe neurologic manifestations can occur in both young children and older patients with sickle cell anemia. Hemiplegia, convulsions, coma, and visual disturbances are the most frequent clinical findings. Such complications, which may develop acutely and progress rapidly, require prompt treatment. Hemiplegia and other cerebral vaso-occlusive phenomena are rarely reversible if they have persisted for more than a week.

The frequency and severity of clinical manifestations vary markedly in patients with sickle cell disease. In some, painful crises occur monthly or even more often, whereas others remain symptom-free for periods of several years. The percentage of hemoglobin S is an important determinant of clinical severity. Patients with sickle-hemoglobin C disease and most with sickle-thalassemia have fewer complications than do those with homozygous sickle cell anemia. Additional undefined factors must account for variability in clinical course when no differences in hemoglobin composition exist.

LABORATORY EVALUATION

The laboratory evaluation of a patient with suspected of having sickle cell disease should include an examination of the peripheral blood smear, a complete blood count with red cell indices, reticulocyte count, hemoglobin electrophoresis on cellulose acetate (pH 8.8) and citrate agar (pH 6.4) quantitative determinations of hemoglobins A, S, A_2, and F or other variant hemoglobins, and family studies. The peripheral blood smear in sickle cell anemia will show sickle cells, polychromatophilic macrocytes, and occasional spherocytes. The presence of nuclear remnants (Howell-Jolly bodies) in the red cells indicates functional asplenia. In sickle-β-thalassemia, hypochromic microcytic cells, target cells, and occasional sickle cells are noted. In sickle-hemoglobin C, target cells and rare sickle forms will be seen. It should be noted that a low mean corpuscular volume will help to distinguish patients with sickle-β^0-thalassemia (see p. 1161 for classification of the thalassemias) from those with sickle cell anemia. Thalassemia trait is associated with microcytic red cells, while in sickle cell anemia the predominance of young red cells results in macrocytosis.

Typical hemoglobin electrophoretic patterns on cellulose acetate and citrate agar are shown in Figure 16.

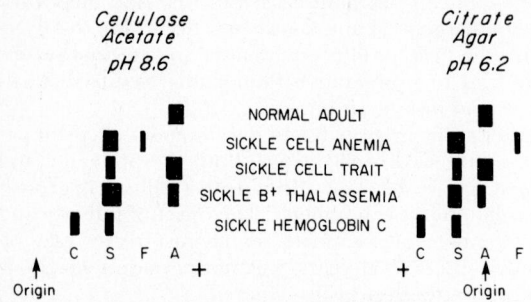

FIG. 16. Comparison of electrophoretic pattern on cellulose acetate (pH 8.6) and citrate agar (ph 6.2). Citrate agar separates hemoglobin F from S and is therefore very useful in the newborn period.

Not all hemoglobins migrating in the S position on cellulose acetate are sickle hemoglobin. For example, hemoglobin D (not shown in the figure) migrates in the S position on cellulose acetate (pH 8.8) but migrates differently from S on citrate agar (pH 6.2). Important ancillary laboratory findings in patients with sickle hemoglobin on cellulose acetate hemoglobin electrophoresis are listed in Table 7. The quantitative measurement of hemoglobins S and A is important. Individuals with sickle cell trait (AS) have more hemoglobin A than S. Due to the thalassemia gene, patients with sickle-β^+-thalassemia (p. 1161) have more hemoglobin S than A.

Typical hematologic data obtained in patients with sickle cell anemia are listed in Table 8. Results vary between patients but usually tend to remain constant in the same individual; baseline information for each patient is therefore of prognostic value. The reticulocyte count is particularly important, as a fall in value may predict an aplastic crisis. Leukocytosis is normally found in patients with sickle cell disease. The specific gravity of the urine is usually less than 1.010.

TREATMENT

Despite our knowledge regarding the molecular de-

fect in sickle cell anemia and the nature of the sickling process in vitro, little progress has been made in the treatment of this disorder.

GENERAL MANAGEMENT.   There is an unfortunate tendency to emphasize episodic treatment of crises in sickle cell disease to the neglect of general care. The social and emotional problems encountered in a chronic, severe disease such as sickle cell anemia require sympathetic attention at a time when the patient is free of pain and able to devote his energies toward developing a positive, productive approach to life. Continuing care provided at regular intervals, including immunization and a complete evaluation at least once a year, is important in management. Clinical examination should focus on growth, sexual development, evaluation of cardiopulmonary, endocrine, hepatic, renal, and neurologic function, and an inspection of the optic fundi. At these times, studies may include a complete blood count and tests of kidney function (BUN, serum creatinine, urine specific gravity) and liver function (serum enzymes, bilirubin, and alkaline phosphatase). Chest and abdominal roentgenograms, electrocardiograms, examination for gallstones, ophthalmologic consultation, pulmonary function tests, and other more expensive and time-consuming studies are necessary in some individuals. In some older patients, progressive damage to specific organ systems is the inexorable consequence of repeated occlusive crises. Such organ damage can best be detected by systematic and regular evaluation as outlined above. Treatment of the consequences of organ damage may require an increasing commitment of time and resources as the patient grows older. Other adults have a benign course that is virtually subclinical.

INFECTIONS.   Because of the relatively high frequency, sudden onset, and serious consequences of septicemia, usually due to pneumococci, in children with sickle cell disease, the sudden appearance of an unexplained fever should be viewed as a medical emergency. When the temperature is higher than 38 C, it is appropriate to obtain at least one blood culture and promptly institute therapy with intravenous penicillin, 50,000 IU /kg stat and at 6-hour intervals subsequently. The need for prompt therapy should be emphasized, since death from overwhelming sepsis may occur within a few hours of presentation. Where fever is of several days duration or is accompanied by physical signs, such as a rash, that indicate the infection is not of pneumococcal origin, immediate intravenous antibiotic therapy may not be appropriate. In such circumstances, antibiotics can be given orally if indicated clinically. Pro-

TABLE 7. Differential Diagnosis of Patients With Sickle Hemoglobin

Percent Hemoglobin				MCV	H (g/dl)	Reticulocytes
	S	A	F			
Sickle cell anemia	90–95	0	5–10	↑	5–8	Markedly increased
Sickle β^0-thalassemia	90	0	10	↓	8–11	Slightly increased
Sickle β^+-thalassemia	50	40	10	↓	8–11	Slightly increased
Sickle cell trait	40	60	Normal	Normal	Normal	Normal

TABLE 8. Hematologic Data in Sickle Cell Disease

	Normal Average	Sickle Cell Average	Range
Hemoglobin	12	7.5	5.5–9.5
Hematocrit	36	22	17–29
Reticulocytes	1.5	12	5–30
Nucleated RBC	0	3	1–20
WBC	7,500	20,000	12–35,000

phylaxis by immunization with polyvalent purified pneumococcal polysaccharide antigen or by daily oral administration of penicillin has been suggested and is currently being evaluated. *Salmonella* osteomyelitis should be treated with appropriate doses of ampicillin or chloramphenicol.

ANEMIC CRISES. The treatment of anemic crises includes reversing the primary cause, such as infection, if possible. If the anemia is symptomatic or rapidly progressive, prompt administration of blood is required, ideally in the form of packed red blood cells. The volume administered should not exceed 15 ml/kg body weight. If cardiac failure is suspected, partial exchange transfusion is safer than simple transfusion, since rapid changes in blood volume are avoided. In children with severe *splenic sequestration crisis,* partial exchange transfusion should be carried out immediately. Exchange transfusion with a total of 35 ml packed red blood cells/kg body weight (hematocrit 70 to 75 percent) will replace about 60 percent of the patient's sickle cells with normal erythrocytes; this should be adequate to reverse splenic sequestration. It is important to ensure that the donor blood does not contain sickle hemoglobin, since donors are not usually screened for sickle trait. A needle or intravenous catheter, preferably 19 gauge or larger, is placed in each antecubital fossa; from 25 to 100 ml of blood are removed initially. Packed cells are then administered into one antecubital vein, either by drip or by syringe, depending upon the necessity for speed. After the desired aliquot has been infused (usually 25 to 100 ml), an equivalent amount of mixed venous blood is withdrawn from the other antecubital vein. The process is repeated until the total calculated amount of packed cells has been administered. A quantitative hemoglobin electrophoresis or sickle prep may be carried out at the conclusion of the procedure to verify the extent to which normal cells have replaced sickle cells. The percentage of cells that fail to sickle after a 1-hour incubation in 2 percent sodium metabisulfite reflects the proportion of normal cells.

Recurrent splenic sequestration crises warrant consideration of splenectomy. The knowledge that autosplenectomy by repeated infarction will eventually occur without surgical intervention should be balanced against the risk of recurrent sequestration crises. In young children the risk of recurrence is substantial, but in children over 5 years the risk is slight, and splenectomy is not necessary. Increased postoperative susceptibility to infection is a less important consideration in weighing the risk of splenectomy in sickle cell anemia, since functional asplenia customarily develops in infancy and the risk of infection is increased even in the presence of an enlarged, though poorly functioning, spleen.

Megaloblastic anemia may occur in sickle cell disease, particularly where the dietary intake of folate is marginal, since there is an increased requirement for folate as the result of the increased rate of erythropoiesis. Many hematologists suggest that all patients with sickle cell disease take supplementary folate, 1 mg daily by mouth; others limit supplementary folate therapy to those occasions when the patient's dietary intake is restricted by acute illness.

Hemolytic crises are uncommon in sickle cell disease and should suggest the possibility of a complicating disorder, such as autoimmune hemolytic anemia or G6PD deficiency. It is well to evaluate all patients with sickle cell disease for the presence of G6PD deficiency, since the African variant of G6PD is present in at least 10 percent of black patients, and potentially serious hemolytic reactions can be prevented by prior counseling in the avoidance of hemolytic drugs.

VASO-OCCLUSIVE CRISES. The vaso-occlusive crises are usually painful but may be difficult to diagnose, particularly in the small infant who cannot localize pain well and in the older child with abdominal pain in whom a variety of other diagnoses, including appendicitis, may be suggested by the physical findings. Once surgical causes of abnormal pain have been excluded as far as possible, appropriate analgesia should be provided. Codeine 0.5 mg/kg/4 hours or meperidine (Demerol) 1 mg/kg/4 hours is usually effective in controlling pain. Such analgesics are rarely required for more than 7 to 10 days, and the risk of addiction appears to be small. Therapy should be directed to elimination of factors such as hypertonicity, acidosis, or hypoxia, which may foster further sickling of red cells. Correction of even mild dehydration is essential, since sickling is facilitated by hyperosmolarity of the plasma environment. In planning appropriate maintenance *fluid therapy,* it should be recalled that older patients with sickle cell disease are incapable of concentrating urine, thus increasing their maintenance fluid requirements to 1.5 to 2 times the usual volume. Due to the impaired concentrating ability of the kidney, urine specific gravity measurements are an unreliable guide to the adequacy of hydration, and reliance must be placed on hematocrit, body weight, and clinical criteria, such as skin turgor and moistness of mucous membranes. Acidemia, when present, should be corrected by the administration of intravenous bicarbonate because an acid environment favors sickling. The dose may be calculated from the serum bicarbonate, or 3 mEq/kg/12 hours may be given as an approximation of average need. The use of alkali therapy in patients without acidemia is probably of no value. Administration of oxygen by mask or tent is of benefit only in the rare patient who is hypoxemic, since delivery of oxygen to the site of vascular occlusion is limited by local circulatory stasis rather than by oxygenation of arterial blood. Prolonged use of oxygen therapy for many days is hazardous, since it may suppress erythropoietin production and produce transient erythroid hypoplasia.

The only reliable means of terminating or preventing a vaso-occlusive episode that is available currently is replacement transfusion, carried out as outlined above. Such treatment generally should be limited to life-threatening crises involving vital organs such as the brain, heart, or lungs. Prophylactic partial exchange transfusion also should be considered prior to surgical procedures requiring general anesthesia. Reduction of hemoglobin S concentration to less than 30 percent provides protection from vaso-occlusive crises during and after anesthesia. Blood replacement therapy is probably not necessary prior to spinal or local anesthesia, unless regional hypoxemia or hypoperfusion is anticipated. The use of chronic blood replacement therapy to provide an interval of weeks or months free from the possibility of sickling is a standard practice in the management of the last trimester of pregnancy in patients with sickle cell disease and has been used in other patients to provide time for organ recovery following prolonged or particularly severe episodes of vaso-occlusive crises. It also may be necessary to allow chronic ulcers, which often develop in the lower extremities of older patients, to heal. As a general rule, however, the hazards customarily associated with transfusion, notably hepatitis, antigenicity, and iron overload, limit the use of chronic transfusion programs to the indications listed.

ANTISICKLING AGENTS.   No antisickling agent has been found clinically valuable despite intensive research. Double-blind evaluations of intravenous urea and of oral sodium cyanate have failed to demonstrate a beneficial effect in preventing vaso-occlusive crises. Oral sodium cyanate will increase the lifespan of sickle erythrocytes in vivo and ameliorate anemia. Toxic manifestations, including weight loss, anorexia, somnolence, peripheral neuropathy, and cataracts, have occurred in patients receiving prolonged treatment with oral sodium cyanate and have limited its usefulness. Extracorporeal therapy in which erythrocytes are removed from the patient, treated with cyanate, washed, and returned to the patient may eventually prove to be safe and effective, but this requires further evaluation. Other antisickling agents, such as nitrogen mustard and dimethyl adipimidate, are effective in vitro, but have not as yet undergone clinical trial.

PREVENTION.   The inadequacies of currently available therapy for sickle cell disease and the availability of simple and accurate methods for the identification of sickle cell trait justify efforts to prevent sickle cell disease by appropriate genetic counseling of parents at risk. Where the hemoglobin types of both the prospective mother and the father are known, the odds of sickle cell disease appearing in their children should be carefully explained. Methods currently being developed for antenatal detection of sickle cell disease in the offspring of affected parents should prove to be valuable for the prevention of sickle cell disease. The sickle cell gene can be detected in midtrimester fetuses, providing that an effective and safe means for obtaining fetal blood becomes available. Preliminary studies indicate that localization of the placenta by ultrasound, followed by aspiration of a placental blood sample with an amniotomy needle, usually yields an adequate sample of fetal blood. Direct venipuncture of fetal blood vessels after their localization by amnioscope offers an alternative approach currently under investigation. At present, intrauterine diagnosis is available only on a limited basis.

SICKLE CELL TRAIT

Sickle cell trait refers to the heterozygous inheritance of the hemoglobin S β-globin gene. In sickle cell trait, the red cell concentration of hemoglobin S is approximately 40 percent and that of hemoglobin A, 60 percent. The high concentration of hemoglobin A prevents the cell from sickling under normal oxygen tensions. In vitro, hemoglobin must be less than 5 percent saturated with oxygen to induce sickling of 15 percent of sickle trait erythrocytes. Such extremely hypoxic conditions may occur in vivo in the spleen. Splenic infarcts have been documented in individuals with sickle cell trait who were flying in unpressurized aircraft at an altitude over 7,000 feet. Hypoxia accompanying anesthesia may also induce sickling if oxygen tension is sufficiently low. Except for rare circumstances, the relationship between vaso-occlusive episodes and sickle cell trait is not sufficiently well established to warrant specific precautions or alterations in life style. Furthermore, there is no evidence to implicate sickle cell trait as a cause of early death, since in American blacks, at least, there is no reduction in the frequency of sickle cell trait with increasing age.

The peripheral blood smear, hemoglobin, hematocrit, red cell indices, and reticulocyte count are normal in sickle cell trait. In some individuals, hyposthenuria and hematuria may result from sickling in the renal medullary capillaries. The extreme hypertonicity of the renal medulla fosters sickling, probably by increasing the concentration of hemoglobin S within the red cell.

Screening for sickle cell disease has detected many individuals with sickle cell trait. As the incidence of sickle cell trait in American blacks is 1 in 12 and of sickle cell disease is 1 in 600, fifty individuals with sickle cell trait will be detected for each patient with sickle cell disease. The advantages of identifying individuals with sickle cell trait are related primarily to family planning. Thus, it is important that screening is available to adolescents and young adults and that it is voluntary and includes adequate counseling and education. The benign nature of the trait must be stressed. When both prospective parents have sickle cell trait, the options for the family include: risking pregnancy knowing there is a 1 in 4 chance of having a child with sickle cell disease, intrauterine diagnosis and abortion of fetuses with sickle cell disease, adoption, and birth control. Most screening efforts have failed to evaluate the personal and community impact of sickle cell screening. The disadvantages of identifying an individual with sickle cell trait include anxiety regarding the diagnosis, the common confusion between the diagnosis of sickle cell trait and sickle cell disease, and unfavorable treatment at work or school or in applying for insurance as a result of misinformation regarding sickle trait on the part of teachers, supervisors, and other personnel. These disadvantages can be eliminated almost completely by appropriate education and counseling.

References

Abramson H, Bertles JF, Wethers DL (eds): Sickle Cell Disease: Diagnosis, Management, Education and Research. St Louis, Mosby, 1973

Austrian R, Lukens J, Seeler RA: Pneumococcal infections in sickle cell anemia. Am J Dis Child 123:614, 1972

Diggs LW: The crisis in sickle cell anemia: hematologic studies. Am J Clin Pathol 26:1109, 1956

———— Sickle cell crises. Am J Clin Pathol 44:1, 1965

Motulsky AG: Frequency of sickling disorders in U.S. blacks. N Engl J Med 228:31, 1973

Nathan DG, Pearson HA: Sickle cell syndromes and hemoglobin C disease. In Nathan DG, Oski FA (eds): Hematology of Infancy and Childhood. Philadelphia, WB Saunders, 1974, p 419

Pearson HA, Diamond LK: Sickle cell disease. Pediatrics 48:629, 1971

———— O'Brien RT: Sickle cell testing programs. J Pediatr 81:6, 1972

———— O'Brien RT, McIntosh S, Aspnes GT, Yang M: Routine screening of umbilical cord blood for sickle cell diseases. JAMA 227:420, 1974

———— Spencer RP, Cornelius E: Functional asplenia in sickle cell anemia. N Engl J Med 281:923, 1969

———— Hemoglobin S-thalassemia syndrome in Negro children. Ann NY Acad Sci 165:83, 1969

Portnoy BA, Herion JC: Neurological manifestations in sickle cell disease with a review of the literature and emphasis on hemoplegia. Ann Intern Med 76:643, 1972

Powars DR: Natural history of sickle cell disease – the first ten years. Semin Hematol 12:267, 1975

Serjeant GR: The Clinical Features of Sickle Cell Disease. Amsterdam, North Holland, 1974

Smits HL, Oski FA, Brody JI: The hemolytic crisis of sickle cell disease: the role of glucose-6-phosphate dehydrogenase deficiency. J Pediatr 74:544, 1969

Watson RJ, Burko H, Megas A, Robinson M: The hand-foot syndrome in sickle cell disease in young children. Pediatrics 31:975, 1963

THALASSEMIA

William C. Mentzer

The thalassemia syndromes result from the diminished synthesis of one or more of the globin polypeptide chains which combine to form hemoglobin (Fig. 17). Reduced synthesis of α, β, γ, or δ chains, either singly or in combination, may be present. Several different abnormalities in the biochemical pathways that lead to globin chain synthesis may give rise to the clinical and hematologic picture of thalassemia. Thus, Oriental forms of the α-thalassemia syndrome appear to be due to deletion of one or more α globin genes. In β-thalassemia, diminished amounts of functional messenger RNA, due either to RNA instability, reduced RNA synthesis, or synthesis of nonfunctional RNA, may result in reduced globin chain synthesis. Although only normal globin chains are produced in these disorders, there are also unusual forms of thalassemia in which abnormal globin chains are synthesized. For example, unequal crossing over at the $\delta\beta$-gene loci may result in the synthesis of a $\delta\beta$-fusion product, which can combine with α chains to form hemoglobin Lepore. Hemoglobin Constant Spring, a tetramer formed of two normal β chains and two abnormally elongated α chains, is the result of a mutation at the normal site of termination of α-globin chain synthesis. Because both hemoglobin Lepore and hemoglobin Constant Spring are synthesized quite slowly, the overall effect on hemoglobin production resembles that of other forms of thalassemia. Certain other structural gene mutations, such as hemoglobin E or Q, are also associated with reduced synthesis of the abnormal globin chain.

The *incidence* of thalassemia varies markedly according to ethnic group. α-thalassemia trait is most prevalent in southeastern Asia, is found in 2 to 7 percent of American black newborns, and is less common in the Mediterranean regions. The incidence of the β-thalassemia gene exceeds 5 percent in certain areas of Italy, Greece, Sardinia, Sicily, India, and southeastern Asia and is about 0.8 percent in American blacks. Because those areas of the world in which thalassemia is prevalent coincide with former endemic regions of malaria, the persistence of the thalassemia gene in such populations may reflect a protective effect of the gene against malaria.

Hematologic abnormalities resulting from the mild reduction in globin chain synthesis seen in thalassemia heterozygotes (trait) are usually limited to hypochromia, microcytosis, and mild anemia. More profound reduction of globin synthesis, usually found only in homozygotes, is accompanied by hemolysis and by severe anemia. Hemolysis is a consequence of imbalance in the synthesis of the two major types of globin

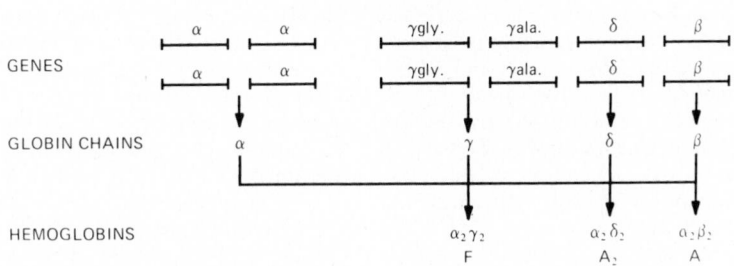

FIG. 17. Biochemical pathways leading to globin chain synthesis in Thalassemia.

chains (α and β). Impaired synthesis of one type of globin chain limits the formation of hemoglobin tetramers that require that chain. Continued production of the other type of globin chain at a normal rate results in accumulation of excess globin chains that are unable to participate in normal tetramer formation for lack of suitable partners. Such uncombined globin chains are readily precipitated within the erythrocyte, forming insoluble inclusion bodies. In β-thalassemia, inclusions of excess α chains form so rapidly during erythroid maturation that rapid hemolysis occurs within the bone marrow prior to the release of such cells as reticulocytes. In α-thalassemia, β-chain tetramers (β_4 or hemoglobin H) precipitate more slowly, after red cells have left the marrow. Once formed, hemoglobin H inclusion bodies are rapidly removed from the red cell by reticuloendothelial cells of the spleen, resulting in membrane damage, fragmentation, and eventual hemolysis.

HETEROZYGOUS β-THALASSEMIA (β-THALASSEMIA MINOR OR TRAIT). A number of genetically distinct abnormalities of β-globin chain synthesis may produce the clinical picture of thalassemia minor (Table 9). The degree to which the synthesis of normal β-globin chains is suppressed and the amount of residual γ-chain synthesis appear to be important determinants of the severity of the heterozygous state. This varies from the silent carrier who is clinically completely normal to the severely affected carrier with significant lifelong hemolytic anemia. In most heterozygotes, anemia and clinical symptoms are absent, but on occasion mild anemia and pallor may be evident. Rarely, more severe manifestations, including jaundice, gallstones, reticulocytosis, and anemia (hemoglobin 7 to 9 g/100 ml), may occur. Anemia may be accentuated by pregnancy but otherwise usually fluctuates little in severity. Life expectancy in β-thalassemia minor is normal.

Table 9 lists nine genetically distinct β-chain abnormalities, which usually can be distinguished in heterozygotes by quantitative determination of A_2 and F hemoglobin, complete blood count with red cell indices, and staining for red cell inclusion bodies. Measurement of globin chain synthesis by peripheral blood reticulocytes in vitro has demonstrated only a rough correlation between the degree of reduction in β-chain synthesis and the clinical severity of the thalassemia gene. In part, this is due to the fact that studies in reticulocytes reflect only the final stages of hemoglobin synthesis; most hemoglobin is produced at an earlier stage in erythroid development. In Caucasian and Oriental heterozygotes, it has not been possible by in vitro synthesis studies to separate β^0-thalassemia trait, where no β chain is synthesized by the thalassemic globin gene, from β^+-thalassemia trait, where some β chain is synthesized. However, it may be inferred that both parents have the β^0 form of thalassemia trait if a homozygous offspring is totally incapable of β-chain synthesis. On the other hand, if a β-thalassemia gene is inherited along with a β-chain structural abnormality, such as sickle hemoglobin, any hemoglobin A present must be derived from the thalassemic β-globin gene locus and indicates the presence of β^+-thalassemia. The absence of hemoglobin A in this setting is consistent with β^0-thalassemia. Identification of the severity of the thalassemia gene in prospective parents may be of value in predicting the severity of the disease in their homozygous offspring.

In thalassemia minor, examination of the blood reveals microcytosis, target cells, a variable degree of hypochromia, and often some degree of basophilic stippling. The red blood cells are resistant to osmotic lysis. The mean corpuscular volume and mean corpuscular hemoglobin are subnormal, but the red blood cell count is often elevated. Microcytosis, an increased red count, and the presence of target cells in a patient of the appropriate ethnic background should suggest thalassemia trait. These findings, however, often are confused with those of iron deficiency and may result in unnecessary and often prolonged iron therapy. Confirmation of the diagnosis requires hemoglobin electrophoresis. Variants of β-thalassemia minor are best distinguished by quantitation of A_2 and F hemoglobins (Table 9). When β-thalassemia trait is complicated by coexisting iron deficiency, the A_2 hemoglobin level may fall to the normal range, masking the presence of thalassemia trait. In such a setting, electrophoresis should be repeated after iron deficiency is corrected.

HOMOZYGOUS β-THALASSEMIA (β-THALASSEMIA MAJOR)

CLINICAL MANIFESTATIONS. The clinical onset of β-thalassemia major occurs gradually after birth as the normal postnatal decline in γ-chain synthesis (Hb F) reveals the defect in production of β chains. The rapidity with which symptoms develop depends on the rate of decline in γ-chain synthesis and the degree of impairment of β-chain synthesis. The fetus and the newborn infant are clinically and hematologically normal, even though in vitro measurements already demonstrate reduced or absent β-chain synthesis. Such measurements allow the diagnosis of β-thalassemia major to be made in the fetus or newborn infant before clinical manifestations of the disease appear. At the age of 6 to 12 months, the infant begins to demonstrate pallor, irritability, anorexia, fever, and often an enlarging abdomen.

Examination of the blood reveals a hypochromic and usually microcytic anemia (Fig. 7). Distorted microcytes, target cells, basophilic stippling, and an occasional macrocyte are evident. The reticulocyte count, although elevated, rarely exceeds 5 percent. Nucleated red cells are present, often in very large numbers. Fetal hemoglobin concentration is always elevated beyond the normal for age but varies considerably. For example, in older children and adults, the percentage of hemoglobin F may range from 13 to 95 percent. Hemoglobin A is absent in β^0-thalassemia but may be present, although in reduced concentration, in β^+-

TABLE 9. β-Thalassemia Minor Variants

Disorder	Genotype*	% A$_2$	% F	Globin Chain Synthesis Ratios[†] Mean (Range)	Other
Normal controls	δβ δβ	3.7	2	1.0 (0.90–1.10)	——
δβ-Thalassemia trait (silent carrier)	δβ (δβ)$^{thal?}$	2.3–2.9	0.8–1.6	0.63 (0.60–0.69)	Clinically and hematologically normal
δβ-Thalassemia trait	δβ (δβ)^{thal}	3.7	5–20	0.72 (0.71–0.74)	——
β⁺-Thalassemia trait (blacks)	δβ δ(β)^{thal}	3.0–7.5	0.0–5.5	0.84 (0.52–1.38)	——
β-Thalassemia trait (with increased Hb F)	δβ δ(β)$^{thal,?}$	4.0–7.0	5.0–15.0	——	May represent combined inheritance of β-thalassemia trait + a form of hereditary persistence of fetal hemoglobin
α,β-Thalassemia trait	δβ δ(β)^{thal} and α$_1^{thal}$	3.2–3.4	1.2	1.04 (1.03–1.05)	——
Hemoglobin Lepore trait	δβ (δβ)^{lepore}	1.2–2.6	1.3–14.0	0.52 (——)	Electrophoresis shows 6-15% Lepore hemoglobin. β⁰ + β⁺-thalassemia genes can be separately identified only in families where homozygous β-thalassemia or a β structural abnormality is also present (see text)
β⁺-Thalassemia trait (Caucasians, Orientals)	δβ δ(β)^{thal}	4.0–6.0	1.0–5.0	0.56 (0.43–0.71)	
β⁰-Thalassemia trait (Caucasians, Orientals, blacks)	δβ δ(β)$^{thal 0}$	4.0–6.0	1.0–5.0	0.53 (0.46–0.65)	
Inclusion body β-thalassemia trait	δβ δ(β)^{thal}	3.1–5.3	1.5–12.2	0.72 (0.60–0.80)	Severe — α-chain inclusions in bone marrow

* The δ- and β-globin gene loci are designated for each of two paired chromosomes. Parentheses enclose genes thought to be thalassemic.

[†] Measured in peripheral blood reticulocytes in vitro. reticulocytes are incubated for several hours with radioactive amino acids. The globin chains are then isolated by chromatography and the amount of radioactivity incorporated into α and β chains is taken to reflect the relative synthesis of these two chains. Ratio shown is β/α, (β+α)/α, or (β+ Lepore)/α.

1157

thalassemia. The relative percentage of A_2 hemoglobin may be reduced, normal, or elevated; thus, in contrast to β-thalassemia trait, the determination of A_2 hemoglobin is of little diagnostic value.

Periodic *transfusions* are usually required by 1 to 2 years of age in order to maintain life. Later, clinical manifestations are determined in large measure by the transfusion policy adopted. In children receiving transfusions only for severe, symptomatic anemia, the hemoglobin level usually ranges between 4 and 10 g/dl . At the lower hemoglobin concentrations, irritability, fatigability, listlessness, and anorexia may occur; the parent, and often the child, can usually determine when transfusions are required. Cardiac dilatation and hemic murmurs are customary findings. Frank cardiac failure may accompany exacerbations of anemia that occur during acute infections because of transient erythroid hypoplasia. Scleral icterus is usually present, and bilirubin gallstones may form in adolescence as a consequence of chronic hemolysis and hyperbilirubinemia. However, there is rarely any evidence of crises due to sudden acceleration of hemolysis. Red blood cell destruction is predominantly intramedullary. Compensatory hypertrophy of the erythroid marrow at the expense of bone may produce disfiguring cosmetic changes. Involvement of the cranial bones leads to enlargement of the head due to frontal and parietal bossing; enlargement of the maxilla causes protrusion of the upper frontal teeth, with forward and upward displacement of the upper lip. Marked malocclusion is common. The malar eminences are prominent; the bridge of the nose is broadened, deepened, and depressed; the eyes have a mongoloid slant; and an epicanthal fold is frequently present. Expansion of the marrow space also may result in bone pain and susceptibility to pathologic fractures of the long bones or vertebrae. Compensatory extramedullary hematopoiesis in the liver and spleen causes abdominal enlargement. With continued hemolysis and extramedullary hematopoiesis the spleen may become enormous, producing lumbar lordosis and abdominal discomfort, anorexia, and occasionally vomiting due to pressure. Hepatomegaly develops somewhat more slowly, but the liver also reaches a very large size.

Children who are transfused to maintain a hemoglobin above 10 g/dl have few or none of the clinical manifestations just described (see Treatment). The use of blood transfusions and antibiotics has reduced the mortality formerly associated with infections in early childhood, but infections still are common. Fairly normal growth in height and weight is usual during the first 4 to 5 years in children transfused regularly. Thereafter, retardation of growth is increasingly evident, and the final height achieved is usually strikingly subnormal. Slow growth results primarily from failure of skeletal maturation, particularly through the adolescent years. Sexual maturation is also delayed or absent, and hypogonadism is common in both boys and girls. Intellectual development is normal.

The cause of death in many patients is attributed to iron excess. Gastrointestinal absorption of iron is increased as a consequence of the chronic hemolytic anemia. In addition, there is a progressive increase in the body iron burden of approximately 250 mg with each unit of blood transfused (the total body iron is 3.5 g in a normal adult male). Such relentless iron accumulation leads to darkening of the skin due to deposition of both melanin and iron in the dermis. Iron accumulation in other tissues, notably the liver, pancreas, endocrine glands, and heart, may result in fibrosis and permanent organ damage. Diabetes mellitus, hepatic insufficiency, and endocrine gland disturbances may occur. The most serious complication is the often fatal cardiac failure that follows bizarre atrial and ventricular arrhythmias in some adolescents and young adults.

Treatment

Regular transfusions are essential for survival in most cases of homozygous β-thalassemia. Where the supply of blood is limited, the goal of transfusion therapy is modest—to maintain hemoglobin levels above 5 or 6 g/dl so as to preserve life and allow the patient some measure of activity. More generous transfusion programs, termed hypertransfusion, which maintain a minimum hemoglobin level of 10 g/dl by regular transfusions every 3 to 4 weeks, offer significant advantages over a limited transfusion regimen. Exercise tolerance and sense of well-being are enhanced, and signs and symptoms of chronic cardiac failure are eliminated. The bony deformities and tendency to pathologic fractures are decreased, and massive hepatosplenomegaly is also usually eliminated or ameliorated. If hypertransfusion is started in early infancy, preliminary evidence suggests that physical growth is also enhanced. The major disadvantage is the increased accumulation of excess iron that accompanies the administration of extra units of blood. This disadvantage is partially offset by a reduction in the increased iron absorption that accompanies chronic anemia, since anemia is largely prevented by transfusion. Furthermore, there is evidence in mice that iron overload is less damaging to the myocardium when severe anemia is prevented. Hyper-transfusion does not appear to increase the duration of life in thalassemia major, but a considerable improvement in the quality of life usually is achieved.

The use of iron chelators to minimize the problems of iron toxicity in thalassemia is still under investigation. The efficacy of the best iron chelator currently available, desferrioxamine, can be enhanced by the daily administration of oral ascorbic acid. Heavily iron-overloaded thalassemic patients given daily oral ascorbic acid and intramuscular desferrioxamine, as well as large doses of intravenous desferrioxamine with each transfusion, can be placed in negative iron balance. Unfortunately, current chelating regimens become increasingly less effective as the concentration of tissue iron falls, and it has not yet proved possible to prevent iron accumulation in the young child or to reduce tissue iron concentration to subtoxic levels in the older individual. The high cost, discomfort, and possibility of unfavorable reactions are disadvantages of chronic chelation regimens.

Splenectomy is considered in patients whose transfusion requirement increases out of proportion to growth. Splenectomy also may be helpful in alleviating pressure symptoms due to the massive splenic hypertrophy often noted in patients maintained on a low transfusion regimen. In this situation, a more generous transfusion regimen can sometimes decrease the size of the spleen and remove the need for splenectomy. The increased risk of bacterial septicemia that follows splenectomy in younger children(p.1196) appears to be accentuated in thalassemia. If splenectomy is undertaken, appropriate precautions, such as immunization with polyvalent pneumococcal polysaccharide vaccine or prophylactic antibiotic therapy for a period of 1 to 2 years postsplenectomy, should be considered (p. 1196).

As in most patients with severe chronic hemolytic anemia, the folic acid requirements of thalassemic children are increased. Supplementation of the daily diet with 1 mg of folic acid is warranted, especially if red blood cell folate levels are low or neutrophils are hypersegmented.

In the absence of definitive treatment for β-thalassemia major, emphasis has been placed upon screening populations at risk for the thalassemia trait, followed by genetic counseling. Prenatal diagnosis of β-thalassemia, using samples of fetal blood obtained by placental aspiration, is being undertaken currently in a few centers.

With the best therapy currently available, most patients die during childhood, although an increasing number are surviving beyond the age of 20 years. Future prospects for more effective therapy in β-thalassemia include the refinement of methods for bone marrow transplantation, the development of techniques for gene replacement, and exploration of the possibility that the gene controlling the synthesis of γ chains can be reactivated. That an increase in γ chains (and in hemoglobin F concentration) will prevent clinical manifestations of β-thalassemia is clearly indicated by the absence of clinical abnormalities in the fetus and newborn with homozygous β-thalassemia. The milder clinical course in β-thalassemia homozygotes who also have an α-thalassemia gene suggests that agents capable of reducing α-chain synthesis might also be of potential therapeutic value in β-thalassemia major.

β-Thalassemia Intermedia

Occasionally, the clinical course may be milder than that just described, despite genetic evidence that the patient has homozygous thalassemia. The hemoglobin level may remain between 6 and 9 g/dl even in the absence of transfusion therapy. Both parents are usually found to have microcytosis and evidence of β-thalassemia trait on hemoglobin electrophoresis. The milder clinical course in such patients is usually due to the homozygous inheritance of a milder thalassemia gene, such as δβ-thalassemia (Table 9), or to the doubly heterozygous inheritance of one severe and one mild thalassemia gene, as for example with the simultaneous inheritance of β-thalassemia and the silent carrier state for β-thalassemia. The homozygous inheritance of two severe β-thalassemia genes may be mitigated by the concurrent inheritance of an additional gene for α-thalassemia. Even though total globin chain synthesis is lower in such patients than in patients with homozygous β-thalassemia, there is less imbalance between α- and β-globin chain production and therefore less inclusion-body formation and diminished hemolysis.

α-Thalassemia

α-Thalassemia is common in southeastern Asia. In this population, it has been shown to be due to deletion of one or more of the four α-globin genes normally present (Table 10). The severity of the disorder depends primarily on the number of α-globin genes deleted. Heterozygotes in whom a single α-globin gene is deleted are known as *silent carriers of α-thalassemia* and are clinically and hematologically normal. They may be identified at birth by the presence of small amounts of Barts hemoglobin (γ_4) on electrophoresis. Since trace amounts of Barts hemoglobin may also be seen at birth in nonthalassemic individuals, the tentative diagnosis of the silent carrier state for α-thalassemia can only be confirmed by the detection of hemoglobin H disease in a parent or offspring of the propositus (see below). One type of silent carrier state that can be identified easily is that resulting from inheritance of a gene coding for the abnormally elongated α-chain mutant, hemoglobin Constant Spring. A reduction in α-globin chain synthesis equivalent to the silent carrier state results from inheritance of this mutant, because the mutant chain is synthesized at a very slow rate. Since the small amount (1 to 2 percent) of hemoglobin Constant Spring synthesized can be detected on hemoglobin electrophoresis, this type of mild α-thalassemia can be identified without the need for extensive family studies. *Heterozygotes* in whom two of four α-globin genes are deleted exhibit microcytosis, are occasionally mildly anemic, and, in

TABLE 10. α-Thalassemia Syndromes

	Number of Globin Genes Deleted	Barts (γ_4) Hemoglobin (% at birth)	Clinical Manifestations
α-Thalassemia trait	1	1–2	None
α-Thalassemia trait	2	5–6	Microcytosis, occasional mild anemia
Hemoglobin H disease	3	20–40	Chronic hemolytic anemia
Homozygous α-Thalassemia	4	> 50	Hydrops fetalis

general, resemble subjects with β-thalassemia trait. At birth, microcytosis and the presence of a modest amount of Barts hemoglobin on hemoglobin electrophoresis are noted. Barts hemoglobin disappears by 3 to 6 months of age, and the hemoglobin electrophoresis thereafter is completely normal. Microcytosis, however, persists throughout life. The disorder is readily confused with iron deficiency and should be suspected when ever a patient with microcytosis and mild anemia fails to respond to an adequate course of iron therapy (p. 1123). Definitive diagnosis may not always be possible or practical in this mild disorder since it may require complete family studies as well as in vitro studies of globin-chain synthesis.

When a patient has inherited both forms of heterozygous α-thalassemia described above (silent carrier and deletion of two α-globin loci), the disorder that results is known as *hemoglobin H disease.* Because three of four α-globin genes are deleted, there is a marked imbalance between α- and βchain synthesis. The accumulation of excess β chains results in the formation of hemoglobin H (β_4) inclusions and leads to chronic hemolytic anemia due to trapping of the inclusion-containing cells in the reticuloendothelial system. Laboratory findings

include microcytosis, hypochromia, spherocytosis, and reticulocytosis. The concentration of hemoglobin usually ranges between 7 and 10 g/dl, but the anemia may be more severe in some patients. The diagnosis may be confirmed by finding hemoglobin H on electrophoresis and by the discovery of erythrocyte inclusion bodies when the blood smear is stained with brilliant cresyl blue. Hemoglobin H is readily precipitated by oxidants, and the administration of many of the same agents that cause hemolysis in G6PD deficiency (see Table 11) may lead to exacerbation of hemolysis in hemoglobin H disease. Patients with hemoglobin H are also susceptible to anemic crises due to transient suppression of erythropoiesis following infections.

If all four α-globin genes are deleted, severe erythroblastosis fetalis, with stillbirth or immediate postnatal death, occurs as a consequence of *hydrops fetalis.* In the absence of α-chain synthesis, such fetuses are incapable of synthesizing any of the normal human hemoglobins, apart from embryonic hemoglobins. At birth, hemoglobin electrophoresis reveals predominantly Barts hemoglobin (γ_4) with some hemoglobin H (β_4) and embryonic hemoglobins. The high oxygen affinity of Barts hemoglobin and hemoglobin H renders them

TABLE 11. Some Agents Reported to Produce Hemolysis in Patients with G6PD Deficiency*

Antimalarials
    Primaquine
    Pamaquine
    Pentaquine
    Plasmoquine
    Quinocide
    Quinacrine (Atabrine)
    Quinine (*C*)

Sulfonamides
    Sulfanilamide
    N^2-Acetylsulfanilamide
    Sulfacetamide (Sulamyd)
    Sulfamethoxypyridazine (Kynex, Midicel)
    Salicylazosulfapyridine (Azulfidine)
    Sulfisoxazole (Gantrisin)
    Sulfapyridine

Nitrofurans
    Nitrofurantoin (Furadantin)
    Furazolidone (Furoxone)
    Furaltadone (Altafur)
    Nitrofurazone (Furacin)

Antipyretics and Analgesics
    Acetylsalicylic acid (in large doses)
    Acetanilide
    Acetophenetidin (Phenacetin)
    Antipyrine (*C*)
    Aminopyrine (*C*)
    p-Aminosalicylic acid

Sulfones

Others
    Dimercaprol (BAL)
    Methylene blue
    Naphthalene
    Phenylhydrazine
    Acetylphenylhydrazine
    Probenecid
    Vitamin K (large doses of water-soluble analogues)
    Chloramphenicol (*C*)
    Quinidine (*C*)
    Fava beans (*C*)
    Chloroquine
    Nalidixic acid (Negram)
    Orinase

Infections
    Respiratory viruses
    Infectious hepatitis
    Infectious mononucleosis
    Bacterial pneumonias

Diabetic Acidosis

(*C*), to date, only Caucasians
* From Oski FA, Naiman JA: Hematologic Disorders in the Newborn 1972, p 8. Courtesy of W.B. Saunders.

relatively ineffective as respiratory pigments, thus leading to the intrauterine manifestations of severe hypoxia, even though the actual hemoglobin level in fetal blood may be as high as 9 to 10 g/dl.

In some populations, such as black Americans, α-thalassemia may be the consequence of a gene that causes reduced synthesis of α chains rather than the complete absence of α-chain synthesis seen with gene deletion. This form of α-thalassemia is milder than in Orientals and has not been reported to result in hydrops fetalis in the homozygote.

γ-THALASSEMIA

An infant has been described with fairly severe hypochromic, microcytic anemia in the newborn period, which gradually improved during the first year of life. Studies of globin chain synthesis suggested that this infant had inherited a mild β-thalassemia gene from one parent and a gene for partial suppression of γ-chain synthesis from the other parent. The severe hemolytic anemia during the newborn period was the result of depressed γ- and β-globin chain synthesis at a time when both γ- and β-chain synthesis is normally relatively active.

HEREDITARY PERSISTENCE OF FETAL HEMOGLOBIN (HPFH)

Deletion of the β-globin (and probably δ-globin) gene locus is of little consequence if there is also a failure of the normal developmental switch from γ- to β-chain synthesis. This circumstance results in the preservation of fetal hemoglobin synthesis throughout adult life. In heterozygotes, hemoglobin F levels of about 30 percent are usual, while in homozygotes, hemoglobin F is the only hemoglobin present. Despite complete absence of one or both β-globin genes, neither heterozygote nor hemozygote exhibits any of the clinical manifestations of thalassemia. Heterozygotes are completely normal, while homozygotes may be mildly polycythemic, probably due to the increased oxygen affinity of hemoglobin F. Appropriate stains (see Betke-Kleihauer stain) show that all the red cells contain increased amounts of fetal hemoglobin.

HPFH also may occur without reduction in β- or δ-globin chain synthesis. In such cases, fetal hemoglobin levels are lower than 30 percent, although still above the normal level of 1 to 2 percent. In a few instances, fetal hemoglobin distribution in red cells has been clonal (restricted only to some cells) rather than homogeneous.

When HPFH and sickle trait coexist, clinical symptoms are few or nonexistent, even though the percentage of sickle hemoglobin may be as high as 70 to 80 percent. The high concentration of fetal hemoglobin (20 percent or more) within each cell renders sickling difficult under physiologic conditions.

SICKLE β-THALASSEMIA

Inheritance of sickle trait and $β^0$-thalassemia trait can produce a disease indistinguishable from sickle cell anemia. Since only sickle β chains are synthesized, the concentration of hemoglobin S may approach 100 percent. Variable persistence of γ-chain synthesis results in fetal hemoglobin levels of 0 to 20 percent. Unlike HPFH, fetal hemoglobin in sickle β-thalassemia is heterogeneously distributed, creating subpopulations of red cells with variable susceptibility to sickling.

In sickle $β^+$-thalassemia, some hemoglobin A is made (occasionally as much as 30 percent), decreasing the relative concentration of hemoglobin S. Increased amounts of hemoglobin F and A, as well as a decrease in the total red cell hemoglobin concentration due to the thalassemic reduction of globin chain synthesis, reduces the tendency to sickle. For this reason, sickle β-thalassemia is usually a milder disease than sickle cell anemia.

References

Barry M, Flynn DM, Letsky EA, Risdon RA: Long-term chelation therapy in thalassemia major: effect on liver iron concentration, liver histology and clinical progress. Br Med J 2:16, 1974

Braverman AS, McCurdy PR, Manos O, Sherman A: Homozygous beta thalassemia in American blacks: the problem of mild thalassemia. J Lab Clin Med 81:857, 1973

Engelhard D, Cividalli G, Rachmilewitz EA: Splenectomy in homozygous beta thalassemia: a retrospective study of 30 patients. Br J Haematol 31:391, 1975

Forget BG, Kan YW: Thalassemia and the genetics of hemoglobin. In Nathan DG, Oski Fa (eds): Hematology of Infancy and Childhood. Philadelphia, WB Saunders, 1974, p 450

—— Nathan DG: Thalassemia. Ann Rev Med 26:345, 1975

Kan YW, Holland JP, Dozy AM, Charache S, Kazazian HH: Deletion of the β-globin structure game in hereditary peristence of foetal hoemoglobin. Nature 258:162, 1975

—— Golbus MS, Trecartin R: Prenatal diagnosis of homozygous β-thalassemia. Lancet 2:790, 1975

Knox-Macaulay HHM, Weatherall DJ, Clegg JB, Bradley J, Brown MJ: The clinical and biosynthetic characterization of αβ-thalassemia. Br J Haematol 22:497,

Lie-Injo LE: Alpha-chain thalassemia and hydrops fetalis in Malaya: report of five cases. Blood 20:581, 1962

—— Ganesan J, Clegg JB, Weatherall DJ: Homozygous state for HB Constant Spring. Blood 43:251, 1974

Nathan DG, Gunn RB: Thalassemia: the consequences of unbalanced hemoglobin synthesis. AM J Med 41:815, 1966

Pearson HA, O'Brien RT, McIntosh S: Screening for thalassemia trait by electronic measurement of mean corpuscular volume. N Engl J Med 288:351, 1973

Schwartz E: The silent carrier of beta thalassemia. N Engl J Med 281:-1327, 1969

—— Atwater J: α-Thalassemia in the American Negro. J Clin Invest 51:412, 1972

Stamatoyannopoulos G, Fessas P, Papayannopoulou T: F-thalassemia: a study of thirty-one families with simple heterozygotes and combinations of F-thalassemia with A$_2$-thalassemia. Am J Med 47:194, 1969

—— Woodson R, Papayannopoulou T, Heywood D, Kurachi, S: Inclusion-body β-thalassemia trait. A form of β-thalassemia producing clinical manifestations in simple heterozygotes. N Engl J Med 290:939, 1974

Third Conference on Cooley's anemia. Ann NY Acad Sci 232:1, 1974

Weatherall DJ, Clegg JB: The Thalassemia Syndromes, 2nd ed. Oxford, Blackwell, 1972

Weatherall DJ: Biochemical phenotypes of thalassemia in the American Negro population. Ann NY Acad Sci 119:450, 1964

UNSTABLE HEMOGLOBINS

BERTRAM H. LUBIN

The unstable hemoglobins usually have an amino acid substitution in the central hydrophobic core of the hemoglobin molecule where heme is bound to globin. Such substitutions weaken the internal structure of the molecule and facilitate the oxidation of heme iron. This results in an increased production of methemoglobin and may also affect the oxygen affinity of the hemoglobin. The substitutions may occur either in the α- or in the β-globin chain. Unstable hemoglobins are susceptible to spontaneous loss of heme, leading to the appearance of pigmented heme degradation products, dipyrroles, in the urine. The loss of heme greatly reduces the stability of the hemoglobin tetramer, and the globin chains dissociate to form insoluble precipitates, either spontaneously or on exposure to oxidants. Such precipitates, called Heinz bodies, bind to erythrocyte membrane, induce a defect in cation permeability, and increase cell rigidity. The Heinz bodies are removed from the red cells by the spleen, resulting in cell damage and reduced cell life span.

The inheritance pattern is autosomal dominant, as in the case of other abnormal hemoglobins; only heterozygotes have been detected. The isolated appearance of an unstable hemoglobinopathy in a family where both parents are hematologically normal is usually attributed to spontaneous mutation.Anemia, jaundice, splenomegaly, reticulocytosis, and dark urine are variable in severity. Discoloration of the urine is primarily due to dipyrroles rather than bilirubin. The peripheral blood smear may reveal polychromatophilia, spherocytes, schistocytes, and basophilic stippling; the clinical consequences of having an unstable hemoglobin depend upon the instability and oxygen affinity of the molecule. In patients with hemoglobin Zurich, clinical symptoms only occur following infection or ingestion of the same group of oxidant drugs that affect individuals with glucose-6-phosphate dehydrogenase deficiency. In hemoglobin Köln, the most common of the unstable hemoglobins, an increase in oxygen affinity results in mild tissue hypoxia. This stimulates erythropoietin production and increases the hemoglobin level; anemia, if present, is usually very mild. In contrast, patients with hemoglobin Hammersmith exhibit spontaneous denaturation of the hemoglobin molecule. This hemoglobin variant is associated with a decreased oxygen affinity. Patients with hemoglobin Hammersmith have severe hemolytic anemia, with reticulocyte counts of 20 to 50 percent.

The diagnosis of an unstable hemoglobin should include demonstration of Heinz bodies following incubation of whole blood with 1 percent methyl violet. In patients who have intact spleens, incubation for 24 to 48 hours may be required before the Heinz bodies are noticed. In those who have been splenectomized, Heinz bodies will be seen following a short incubation period. The two most convenient screening tests for unstable hemoglobins are the isopropanol precipitation test and the heat instability test. In the isopropanol test, incubation of buffered solutions of unstable hemoglobin with 70 percent isopropanol, pH 7.4, 37 C for 1 hour, results in denaturation of the molecule and spontaneous precipitation. Isopropanol breaks the weakened hydrophobic bonds in the abnormal hemoglobin molecule, and the dissociated globin chains then precipitate. In the heat instability test, hemolysates are prepared in 0.1 M phosphate buffer, pH 7.4, and incubated for 1 hour at 50 C. Precipitation will be observed in many of the unstable hemoglobins. The oxyhemoglobin dissociation curve in cases with unstable hemoglobins may show either an increase or a decrease in oxygen affinity. Hemoglobin electrophoresis is abnormal in most of the unstable hemoglobins. Although most common amino acid substitutions that result in instability of hemoglobin involve the exchange of one neutral amino acid for another with no net change in charge, the spontaneous loss of the heme group from the globin chain results in abnormal electrophoretic mobility. The abnormal band will disappear if heme is first added to the hemolysate. In some cases, more sensitive techniques, such as isoelectric focusing, may be required to identify the abnormal hemoglobin. When the amino acid substitution involves the β chain, free α chains may also be present. If a patient has Heinz bodies and no hemoglobin abnormalities are detected, a glycolytic enzyme defect should be considered.

The treatment of patients with unstable hemoglobins is supportive. Supplemental folic acid, 1 mg/day, may be beneficial to patients with significant chronic hemolysis. Splenectomy, which may reduce but does not eliminate hemolysis, is customarily reserved for more severe cases of hemolytic anemia. Many of the oxidant drugs that accelerate hemolysis in G6PD deficiency (see Table 11) also precipitate unstable hemoglobins in vivo and may produce a hemolytic crisis. Such drugs should be avoided, when possible, in patients with unstable hemoglobins. As in other hemolytic anemias, patients with unstable hemoglobins may have aplastic marrow crises following infections and may, on rare occasions, require transfusion.

References

Bellingham AJ, Huehns ER: Compensation in haemolytic anaemias caused by abnormal haemoglobins. Nature (Lond) 218:924, 1968

Bunn HF: The unstable hemoglobins (congenital Heinz body hemolytic anemia). In Nathan DG, Oski FA (eds): Hematology of Infancy and Childhood. Philadelphia, WB Sanders, 1974, p 406

Jandl JH, Simmons RL, Castle WB: Red cell filtration and the pathogenesis of certain hemolytic anemias. Blood 18:133, 1961

Rifkind RA: Heinz body anemia: an ultrastructural study. II. Red cell sequestration and destruction. Blood 26:433, 1965

White JM, Dacie JV: The unstable hemoglobins-molecular and clinical features. Prog Hematol 7:69, 1971

INBORN ABNORMALITIES OF THE RED CELL MEMBRANE

WILLIAM C. MENTZER

The red cell membrane consists of two layers of lipid, each formed of phospholipids and unesterified cholesterol. The lipid bilayer is in a state of dynamic equilibrium with plasma lipids, so that membrane lipid composition reflects changes in plasma lipids. Phospholipids cannot be synthesized de novo by erythrocytes, but an ATP-requiring acylation reaction allows their synthesis from plasma lysophospholipids and free fatty acids. Thus, to a limited extent, the red cell membrane is capable of self-renewal and self-modification in lipid composition.

A variety of glycoproteins and proteins are also found on the inner and outer membrane surface. Red cell blood group antigens, present on the external membrane surface, are glycoproteins. A filamentous, contractile membrane protein, spectrin, located primarily on the inner membrane surface, is thought to play an important role in the regulation of cell shape. Active transport of Na^+ and K^+, essential for the maintenance of osmotic equilibrium, is carried out by Na^+-K^+ ATPase, a protein molecule penetrating the entire thickness of the lipid bilayer from the external to the internal membrane surface. The passive entry of anions and water into the cell is thought to be by way of charged pore like channels through the interior of individual proteins which span the membrane.

The state of the red blood cell membrane is an important determinant of cell volume, shape, and plasticity. Inherited abnormalities in the plasma lipid environment, in the structure or function of membrane protein, or in the pathways of membrane lipid renewal may lead to abnormalities in erythrocyte shape, which are usually readily detected on the peripheral blood smear and which are often accompanied by hemolysis. Inheritance of the membrane disorders is almost always autosomal dominant. Since usually there are associated abnormalities of cation transport, cell cation content, and cell water content, the red cell size (MCV) and hemoglobin concentration (MCHC) are often abnormal. Derangements in the osmotic equilibrium of the cell are also reflected in vitro by abnormalities in the osmotic fragility test. In certain cases, abnormalities of plasma lipids, membrane phospholipids, or membrane cholesterol content are also present.

HEREDITARY SPHEROCYTOSIS

Hereditary spherocytosis is the commonest congenital hemolytic anemia in populations of northern European origin. It also occurs in other ethnic groups, but less frequently. The incidence of hereditary spherocytosis in the United States is approximately 1 in 4,500.

Pathophysiology

Many abnormalities of red cell metabolism have been described in hereditary spherocytosis, but their underlying cause is still undefined. The permeability of spherocytic red cells to sodium is two to three times greater than normal. This abnormality, once thought to be the primary defect, is now considered to be secondary to a more fundamental membrane abnormality. Recent evidence suggests that spherocytosis is a consequence of structural alterations in the contractile membrane protein, spectrin. The structural configuration of spectrin appears to be regulated by the extent to which it is phosphorylated, a process mediated by one or more ATP-dependent protein kinases present in the erythrocyte membrane. Abnormally low protein kinase-mediated phosphorylation of spectrin has been reported in hereditary spherocytes and may be responsible for the unusual shape and other abnormalities of the red cell.

The spleen plays an important role in the evolution of spherocytes. Reticulocytes in patients with hereditary spherocytosis are not spherocytic. Transformation to the spherocytic shape normally takes place by gradual splenic conditioning of the abnormal erythrocytes. The erythrocytes traversing splenic pulp must be sufficiently deformable to pass through pores in the splenic sinusoids whose diameters are 2μ or less. Because spherocytes are more rigid than normal cells, they are less able to traverse such pores and, consequently, may be detained within the spleen.

The abnormal Na^+ permeability of spherocytes must be offset by an increase in active transport of Na^+ out of the cell if cation balance is to be maintained. Active transport requires energy in the form of ATP, which in the mature erythrocyte can only be generated through glycolysis. Because the acidic, hypoglycemic environment of the spleen inhibits glycolysis, the increased ATP requirements of spherocytes go unmet.

Continued consumption of energy to support active cation transport when unaccompanied by regeneration of ATP leads to metabolic depletion, which, in the spherocyte, results in susceptibility to loss of membrane lipid and thus membrane surface area. Since the loss of red cell membrane occurs without a reduction in cell volume, the cell becomes increasingly spherical in order to accommodate its contents. With assumption of the spherical shape, the cell becomes even less deformable and is subject to further metabolic depletion and lipid loss, since lack of deformability favors further retention by the spleen. Eventually, lysis of spherocytes occurs within the spleen. The importance of the spleen in the pathogenesis of hemolysis in hereditary spherocytosis is clearly demonstrated by the virtual abolition of hemolysis that follows splenectomy. However, following splenectomy spherocytes do not disappear from the blood smear, indicating that, although erythrocyte survival is enhanced, the underlying membrane defect is not altered.

Genetics

Autosomal dominant inheritance is usually apparent. In 10 to 25 percent of cases, however, the family history is negative. In some instances, this reflects the presence, in one parent, of mild subclinical spherocytosis. For this reason, other family members should be studied when an index case of spherocytosis is discovered. Such studies should not be limited to blood counts, but should include a careful examination of the peripheral blood smear and an osmotic fragility test. In occasional families, the only abnormality evident in relatives may be an increase in erythrocyte sodium permeability. Where no parental abnormality is found, the appearance of spherocytosis in an offspring has been attributed to spontaneous mutation. Analysis of a large family in which both spherocytosis and a crossover between the eighth and twelfth chromosome occurred has suggested that the gene for spherocytosis is localized either to the short arm of chromosome 12 or close to the centromere of chromosome 8.

Clinical Manifestations

The usual features of chronic hemolytic anemia (jaundice, reticulocytosis, and splenomegaly) are present to varying degrees in spherocytosis. Significant hemolytic anemia and hyperbilirubinemia may become evident soon after birth. Conversely, the disease may be so mild as to evade detection until the sixth or seventh decade. The clinical severity of spherocytosis tends to be relatively consistent within families, although it varies widely from family to family. Hemolysis may be fully compensated, without anemia or jaundice, and reticulocytosis can be the only manifestation of increased red cell production and destruction. Anemia, when present, is usually of moderate degree; hemoglobin levels below 8 g/100 ml are rare. Commonly, acute exacerbations of anemia are the result of transient suppression of erythropoiesis by acute viral infections. Occasionally, a hemolytic crisis, resulting in a precipitous fall in hemoblobin levels, may follow an acute viral or bacterial infection. Bilirubin gallstones are a common occurrence in adults, but may also be encountered during childhood, particularly after the first decade. Leg ulcers are an occasional feature of spherocytosis in adults, but are rare in children.

An essential component of the *laboratory diagnosis* of spherocytosis is the appearance on the peripheral blood smear of small, dense, spherical cells that show little or no evidence of the normal biconcavity. Spherocytes may be abundant or may comprise only 1 to 2 percent of the total cell population. Red cells that are not spherocytic are usually normal in appearance. Different areas of the blood smear should be carefully examined because loss of red cell biconcavity is a common artifact on the thin part of the smear. Increased polychromasia, reflecting reticulocytosis, is evident in most cases. The MCV is at or below the lower limit of normal for age, despite reticulocytosis which tends to raise the MCV. The MCHC is usually greater than normal and often as high as 37 to 38 percent. The spherical shape of the spherocyte allows little room for expansion when the cell is subjected to osmotic swelling; therefore, spherocytes are more likely to rupture than normal cells when

they are suspended in hypotonic solutions in vitro. Increased fragility of spherocytes in the osmotic fragility test reflects this difference. When spherocytes are rare, there may be insufficient cells to produce an abnormality in osmotic fragility, or the abnormality may be manifested only in a small subpopulation of osmotically fragile cells that will be missed unless a complete fragility curve is obtained. The incubated osmotic fragility study, in which red cells are studied after 24 hours of incubation at 37 C, is more sensitive and is often diagnostic when studies conducted with fresh blood are equivocal or negative. In other conditions, such as red cell enzyme abnormalities, there may also be a fragile subpopulation evident on the incubated osmotic fragility pattern, but a marked shift of the entire curve towards greater fragility is characteristic only of spherocytosis.

The diagnosis of spherocytosis may be obscured by coexisting obstructive hepatobiliary disease. Alterations in plasma lipids, especially cholesterol, which result from biliary obstruction, lead to the accumulation of excess red cell membrane lipid and an increase in membrane surface area. Under these conditions, the loss of membrane required to form spherocytes is balanced by rapid reaccumulation of membrane lipid due to the abnormal plasma lipid environment. A previously abnormal osmotic fragility may be converted to normal, since normal cell shape and cell volume-to-surface-area relationships have been reestablished.

Differential diagnosis

The presence of spherocytes on the peripheral blood smear is by no means diagnostic only of hereditary spherocytosis. Spherocytes may be seen following thermal injuries and in association with mechanical or antibody-mediated hemolysis. In the newborn, ABO incompatibility commonly results in spherocytosis. Determination of parental blood groups may confirm the possibility of ABO incompatibility, but as the Coombs' test is often very weakly positive, or negative, the diagnosis is sometimes uncertain until 2 to 3 months have elapsed. Since ABO incompatibility is a self-limited disease, hemolytic anemia and spherocytes will disappear within this interval, whereas the abnormalities will persist in hereditary spherocytosis. Spherocytes are commonly seen in autoimmune hemolytic anemia, which should be ruled out by a Coombs' test and other appropriate studies. Occasional spherocytes are often noted in sickle cell disease, but the appearance of characteristic sickle cells usually makes the diagnosis apparent. In homozygous hemoglobin C disease, spherocytes coexist with target cells on the blood smear. Hemoglobin electrophoresis will serve to identify such hemoglobinopathies. Intravascular hemolysis, due to such conditions as hemangioma, disseminated intravascular coagulation, or the hemolytic uremic syndrome, may result in the appearance of appreciable numbers of spherocytes. Such conditions may be suspected when the blood smear reveals not only spherocytes but also schistocytes and other evidence of red cell fragmentation. Although there is no laboratory test whose results are uniquely abnormal in hereditary spherocytosis, the diagnosis usually can be made by a careful analysis of the clinical status of the patient, the family history, the peripheral blood smear, the red cell indices, and the osmotic fragility test. The presence of similar laboratory abnormalities in one parent is often of greatest diagnostic help.

Treatment

The hemolytic anemia in hereditary spherocytosis is virtually abolished by splenectomy. The operation is customarily deferred until at least the age of 3 to 4 years in order to minimize the risk of infection following splenectomy. Measures to reduce the risk of infection after splenectomy are discussed on page 1196. If significant hemolysis persists after splenectomy, the diagnosis of spherocytosis is probably incorrect, and other erythrocyte abnormalities should be suspected (see below). Occasionally, an accessory spleen, overlooked at splenectomy, may enlarge sufficiently to produce a recurrence of hemolysis. The presence of an accessory spleen should be suspected if Howell-Jolly bodies are not present on the blood smear, as would be anticipated after splenectomy. Confirmation requires a spleen scan. Patients with spherocytosis may have an increased requirement for folic acid due to their accelerated rate of erythropoiesis, and it is advisable to provide 1 mg of supplemental folic acid daily until the spleen has been removed and hemolytic anemia abolished.

ELLIPTOCYTOSIS

The incidence of elliptocytosis is approximately 1 per 2,500 in the United States. Like spherocytosis, the disorder is inherited as an autosomal dominant. In 85 to 90 percent of cases, elliptocytes are merely a morphologic curiosity unaccompanied by any shortening of red cell life span. The remaining 10 to 15 percent of individuals with elliptocytosis exhibit evidence of chronic hemolytic anemia. In most cases, hemolysis is well compensated and is characterized by reticulocytosis without significant anemia. The osmotic fragility of fresh erythrocytes is normal, but following 24 hours in incubation at 37 C, an increased fragility usually is seen. Rarely, a patient has more severe hemolysis, accompanied by anemia. In such patients, the osmotic fragility of fresh blood, as well as incubated blood, is abnormal. In this *severe variant* of elliptocytosis, the peripheral blood smear contains not only elliptocytes, but also microspherocytes, fragmented microcytes, and erythrocytes that appear to be undergoing a process of budding or fission. Such morphologic changes resemble those seen in patients with thermal injury. In some of the patients with elliptocytosis and uncompensated hemolysis, budding and fragmentation of erythrocytes can be produced in vitro by exposure to an elevated temperature (45 C) for 15 to 60 minutes. Similar changes in normal erythrocytes or in hereditary spherocytes are not seen below 49 C. Although such studies

suggest the presence of a structurally unstable red cell membrane, the basis for the defect is unknown, as in spherocytosis. During the neonatal period, erythrocyte morphology may be unusually bizarre in cases with severe hemolysis. Large numbers of pyknocytes and fragment forms may be more evident than elliptocytes on the blood smear. Characteristic elliptocytes may appear only gradually within a few months after birth. Neonatal hemolysis and hyperbilirubinemia may be sufficiently severe to require exchange transfusion. The role of the spleen in the pathogenesis of hemolysis resembles that described in hereditary spherocytosis, and splenectomy also eliminates hemolysis in most patients with the hemolytic forms of elliptocytosis. In some patients with severe hemolysis, splenectomy may reduce, but not completely eliminate, the hemolytic process. No therapy is required for patients without hemolysis.

STOMATOCYTOSIS AND RELATED ABNORMALITIES OF CATION PERMEABILITY

Stomatocytes are red cells with a slit like area of central pallor when examined on the peripheral blood smear and with a cup or bowl shape in wet preparations. Such cells are often encountered as an artifact, unassociated with any clinical abnormality. Occasionally, however, stomatocytes may be the predominant morphologic abnormality in patients with hereditary hemolytic anemia. Where inheritance has been clearly established, an autosomal dominant mode of transmission has been found. In some families, hemolysis is mild and characterized only by reticulocytosis. In a small number of patients anemia is much more severe, with jaundice, splenomegaly, reticulocyte counts occasionally as high as 40 percent, and an irregular requirement for blood transfusion. Sodium and potassium permeability is increased, sometimes to a marked degree, in red cells from such patients, leading to alterations in cation content. When the red cell cation content is increased, swelling occurs due to the concurrent obligate osmotic movement of water. When net cation content is decreased, there is loss of cell water and the creation of a shrunken, dehydrated, rigid red cell. Either water excess or deficiency may predominate in the red cells of hereditary stomatocytosis syndromes. The abnormalities in cell cations and water content are reflected in the red cell indices and osmotic fragility. Swelling due to water excess, termed hydrocytosis, is associated with an increase in the MCV, a decrease in the MCHC, and an increase in osmotic fragility. Conversely, shrinkage due to water loss, called desiccytosis, results in a normal or low MCV, an increase in MCHC, and a decrease in osmotic fragility. In both types of stomatocytes, erythrocyte glycolysis may be markedly accelerated to supply energy for the increased active transport of cations that is required to maintain osmotic equilibrium. As is the case in hereditary spherocytosis, such metabolically hyperactive cells are unable to maintain an adequate supply of ATP in the acidic, hypoglycemic splenic environment. Thus, the spleen contributes to hemolysis in such disorders. The underlying membrane defect responsible for the changes in permeability is unknown. A decrease in the phosphorylation of spectrin, similar to that noted in spherocytosis, has been described in 1 patient with stomatocytosis. Splenectomy usually decreases, but does not eliminate the hemolysis in stomatocytosis. Complete in vitro correction of the cation permeability defects in one case of severe stomatocytosis has been achieved experimentally with dimethyl adipimidate, a bifunctional cross-linking imidoester. Treated cells regain many of the properties of normal red cells, including size, cation content, water content, and deformability. The toxicity of these compounds is unknown, and therapeutic use in human subjects is only a theoretic possibility.

Atypical Cases

Disturbances in cation permeability associated with additional morphologic abnormalities have also been described. In one kindred, a marked defect of K^+ permeability was coupled with a lesser defect in Na^+ permeability. The result was net cation loss, desiccytosis, and the appearance of target cells, fragmented cells, acanthocytes, and peculiar cells with hemoglobin "puddled" at either pole. In several patients with high-sodium low-potassium red cells and hemolytic anemia, the predominant morphologic abnormality on the peripheral blood smear was the presence of target cells rather than stomatocytes. However, typical bowl- or cup-shaped red cells were seen on wet preparations in several of these patients, and incubation of the abnormal red cells in hypertonic saline resulted in the replacement of target cells by large numbers of stomatocytes on the blood smear. An excessive amount of phosphotidylcholine was found in membranes of these red cells. These cases differ from typical stomatocytosis where the lipid composition of the membrane is normal. In one family with hemolytic anemia and target cells, accumulation of phosphotidylcholine was due to a block in the normal conversion of phosphotidylcholine to phosphotidylethanolamine.

Hemolytic anemia and stomatocytosis may also occur without abnormalities in erythrocyte cation permeability. A characteristic finding in many such patients, who are usually of Mediterranean origin, has been the presence of chronic abdominal pain.

Inheritance of the Rh null gene type may be associated with stomatocytosis and hemolytic anemia.

References

Cooper RA, Jandl JH: The role of membrane lipids in the survival of red cells in hereditary spherocytosis. J Clin Invest 48:736, 1969

Cutting HO, McHugh WJ, Conrad FG, Marlow AA: Autosomal dominant hemolytic anemia characterized by ovalocytosis; a family study of seven involved members. Am J Med 39:21, 1965

Dacie JV: Hereditary elliptocytosis. In The Hemolytic Anemias, Congenital and Acquired. Part 1. The Congenital Anemias. New York, Grune & Stratton, 1960, p 151

——— Hereditary spherocytosis. In The Hemolytic Anemias, Congeni-

tal and Acquired. Part I. The Congenital Anemias. New York, Grune & Stratton, 1960, p 82

de Gruchy GC, Loder PB, Hennessy IV: Haemolysis and glycolytic metabolism in hereditary elliptocytosis. Br J Haematol 8:168, 1962

Ducrou W, Kimber RJ: Stomatocytes, haemolytic anemia and abdominal pain in Mediterranean migrants. Med J Aust 2:1087, 1969

Geerdink RA, Helleman PW, Verloop MC: Hereditary elliptocytosis and hyperhaemolysis. A comparative study of 6 families with 145 patients. Acta Med Scand 179:715, 1966

Glader BE, Fortier N, Albala MM, Nathan DG: Congenital hemolytic anemia associated with dehydrated erythrocytes and increased potassium loss. N Engl J Med 291:491, 1974

Greenquist AC, Shohet SB: Phosphorylation and dephosphorylation in the erythrocyte membrane. In Brewer GJ (ed): Erythrocyte Structure and Function. New York, Alan R Liss, 1975, p 515

Jacob HS Yawata Y, Matsumoto N, Abman S, White J: Cyclic nucleotide- membrane protein interaction in the regulation of erythrocyte shape and survival: defect in hereditary spherocytosis. In Brewer GJ (ed): Erythrocyte Structure and Function. New York, Alan R Liss, 1975, p 235

Jandl JH, and Cooper RA: Hereditary spherocytosis. In Stanbury JB, Wyngaarden JB, Fredrickson DS eds): The Metabolic Basis of Inherited Disease. New York, McGraw-Hill, 1972, p 1323

Mentzer WC, Smith WB, Goldstone J, Shohet SB: Hereditary stomatocytosis: membrane and metabolism studies. Blood 46:659, 1975

——— Lubin BH, Emmons S: Correction of the permeability defect in hereditary stomatocytosis by dimethyl adipimidate. N Engl J Med 294:1200, 1976

Nathan DG, Shohet SB: Erythrocyte ion transport defects and hemolytic anemia: "Hydrocytosis and desiccytosis." Semin Hematol 7:381, 1970

Oski FA, Naiman JL: Defects characterized by abnormalities of red cell morphology. In Hematologic Problems in the Newborn, 2nd ed. Philadelphia, WB Saunders, 1972, p 120

Shohet SB, Lux SE: The red blood cell membrane and mechanisms of hemolysis. In Nathan DG, Oski FA (eds): Hematology of Infancy and Childhood. Philadelphia, WB Saunders. 1974, p 190

——— Nathan DG, Livermore BM, Feig SA, Jaffe ER: Hereditary hemolytic anemia associated with abnormal membrane lipid. II Ion permeability and transport abnormalities. Blood 42:1, 1973

Wiley JS, Ellory JC, Shumann MA, Shaller CC, Cooper RA: Characterisitics of the membrane defect in the hereditary stomatocytosis syndrome. Blood 46: 337, 1975

Zarkowsky HS, Mohandas N, Speaker CB, Shohet SB: A congenital haemolytic anaemia with thermal sensitivity of the erythrocyte membrane. Br J Haematol 29:537, 1975

VITAMIN E DEFICIENCY
Peter R. Dallman

Vitamin E deficiency manifests itself as a mild hemolytic anemia and is most prevalent in small premature infants 1 to 3 months after birth and in children with malabsorption of fat. The vitamin E compounds are antioxidant and protect the lipid of cell membranes against oxidative damage. The most biologically active compound is α-tocopherol, which also is the most abundant of these compounds in food (1 IU of vitamin E is equivalent to 1 mg α-tocopherol).

Factors that favor the development of vitamin E deficiency include decreased vitamin E in the diet, malabsorption of the vitamin, a diet rich in polyunsaturated fatty acids, and administration of supplemental iron. In the premature infant who develops mild hemolysis all of the last three factors usually are present. In terms of diet, the vitamin E content of cow's milk or breast milk is adequate to meet body needs if it is well absorbed. However, small premature infants have poor intestinal absorption of naturally occurring tocopherols and alpha-tocopherol acetate (a medicinal form of the vitamin Aquasol E USP Pharmaceutical) until they reach the age of about 12 weeks or a body weight of about 2,000 g. A water-soluble form of the vitamin, alpha-tocopherol polyethylene glycol-1000 succinate (TPGS), is better absorbed by premature infants during this period and is already being used in some commercial vitamin preparations (Poly-vi-sol). The dependence of the premature infant on vitamin E is particularly great because body stores of the vitamin are disproportionately low at birth—3 mg of α-tocopherol in a 1,000 g premature infant, compared with 20 mg in a 3,500 g infant. In all age groups, absorption of vitamin E from food requires fat in the diet and the presence of bile; the latter is the basis for vitamin E deficiency in biliary atresia.

The requirement for vitamin E depends on the degree of saturation of fats in the diet. Diets particularly rich in unsaturated fats produce a corresponding change in the composition of fatty acids in cell membranes. The membranes are then more susceptible to damage resulting from lipid peroxidation, and the requirement for the antioxidant effect of vitamin E is increased. Consequently, 5 IU/day of vitamin E is the estimated requirement for adults whose diet contains little unsaturated fatty acid, but 30 IU/day is needed if the diet is rich in polyunsaturated fats. The daily requirement for vitamin E during the first year has been tentatively estimated to be 0.4 IU/day, if, as in breast milk, butterfat is the major source of dietary lipid, and 1.5 IU/day if polyunsaturated fats predominate, as in most artificial formulas. Breast milk contains a low proportion of polyunsaturated fats, including only 8 percent linoleate. In contrast, in some artificial formulas in which milk fat is replaced by vegetable oil, linoleate may account for over 50 percent of the fatty acids. Vitamin E levels in breast milk and cow's milk are similar. In order to take into account the higher content of unsaturated fatty acids in proprietary formulas, they are routinely fortified to contain at least 5 IU/liter.

Diagnosis

Hematologic manifestations include a normochromic, normocytic anemia and an elevation of the reticulocyte count, though rarely above 10 percent. Red cell morphology is characterized by the presence of acanthocytes, cells with up to eight irregular, pointed, thorny projections from an irregular central mass. However, acanthocytes are also a relatively common and reversible finding in infants with an adequate supply of vitamin E and are therefore of limited help in establishing a diagnosis. Thrombocytosis also may be present.

A serum concentration of α-tocopherol below 0.5 mg/dl is considered evidence for vitamin E lack. The concentration of vitamin seems to be partly a function of the serum lipids to which it is bound. This is a potential source of error when the concentration of serum lipids is markedly abnormal. The lipid composition of the red cell membrane is as important as the vitamin E intake in determining the cell's resistance to oxidative damage. The red cell peroxide hemolysis test provides a crude estimate of this by measuring the resistance of the red cell membrane to incubation in hydrogen peroxide. Although the peroxide hemolysis test is often closely correlated with serum α-tocopherol, it seems to reflect the fatty acid composition of the diet rather than vitamin E status. The only physical manifestation characteristic of vitamin E deficiency is edema of the legs, labia, and eyelids in infants.

The role of vitamin E deficiency in anemia of premature infants between 1 and 3 months of age is often difficult to establish. Normally, the postnatal low point in hemoglobin concentration and hematocrit is reached during this period, and is followed by an increase in erythrocyte production, which is heralded by a rise in the reticulocyte count. Against this normal background of profound changes in hematopoiesis, the diagnosis is difficult to make on the basis of anemia and an elevated reticulocyte count, and the therapeutic response to vitamin E is hard to evaluate.

Therapy

In preterm infants TPGS is the preferred form of vitamin E because it is best absorbed. At present it is available only as a component of the multivitamin preparation, Poly-Vi-Sol, and can be given at a dose of 5 IU/day. Vitamin E alone is available only as α-tocopherol acetate (Aquasol E, USP Pharm) which is not absorbed as well. Use of a formula with a low percentage of polyunsaturated fatty acids and avoidance of excessive iron supplementation reduce the vitamin E requirement and make it unlikely that a premature infant will develop a deficiency.

References

Gross S, Melhorn DK: Vitamin E-dependent anemia in the premature infant. III. Comparative hemoglobin, vitamin E, and erythrocyte phospholipid responses following absorption of either water-soluble or fat-soluble d-alpha tocopheryl. J Pediatr 85:753, 1974

Melhorn DK, Gross S, Childers G: Vitamin E-dependent anemia in the premature infant. I. Effects of large doses of medicinal iron. II. Relationships between gestational age and absorption of vitamin E. J Pediatr 79:569, 581, 1971

Oski FA, Barness LA: Hemolytic anemia in vitamin E deficiency. Am J Clin Nutr 21:45, 1968

Ritchie JH, Fish MB, McMasters V, Grossman M: Edema and hemolytic anemia in premature infants. N Engl J Med 279:1185, 1968

Williams ML, Shott RJ, O'Neal PL, Oski FA: Role of dietary iron and fat on vitamin E deficiency anemia of infancy. N Engl J Med 292:887, 1975

ABNORMALITIES OF ERYTHROCYTE METABOLISM

William C. Mentzer

The mature erythrocyte is a simple cell, highly specialized to handle its major function—gas transport. Because it lacks a nucleus and organelles such as ribosomes or mitochondria, it cannot replicate, synthesize proteins, or generate ATP via oxidative pathways.

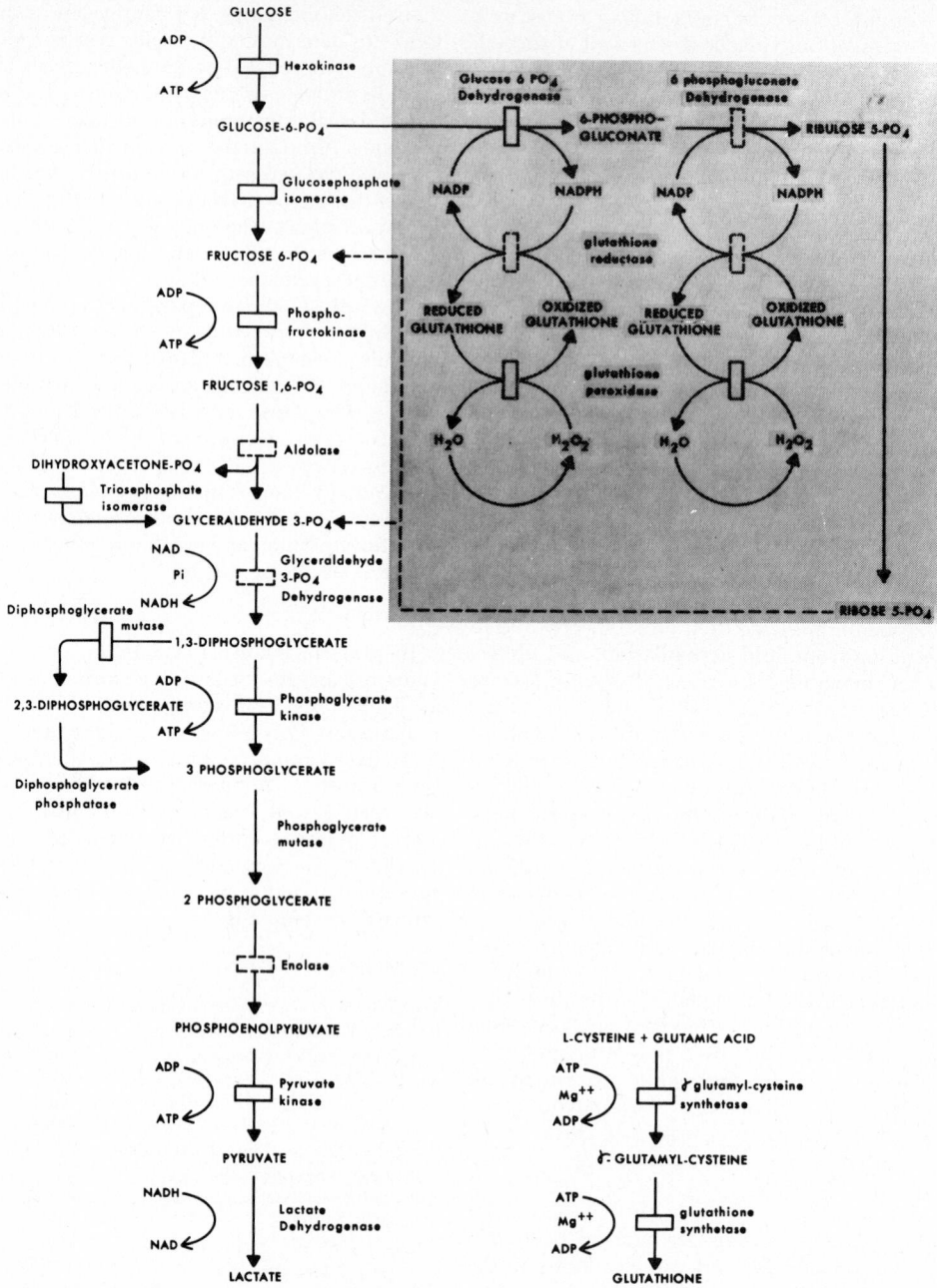

FIG. 18. Glucose metabolism in mature erythrocytes. The hexose monophosphate shunt and glutathione metabolism are shown within the shaded area. Reactions involved in the synthesis of glutathione are indicated in the lower right. Solid bars indicate enzymatic deficiencies whose association with hereditary hemolytic disorders is well established, while open bars signify enzymatic deficiencies, whose relationship to hemolytic disorders requires further verification.

Despite these handicaps, the red cell survives in the circulation for a period of about 120 days. This requires a continuing source of energy for the synthesis of ATP and the maintenance of hemoglobin in a functional state. Lacking mitochondria, the mature erythrocyte must meet its limited requirements for ATP entirely from glycolysis (Fig. 18). ATP is needed in order to initiate the first several reactions in the glycolytic sequence, to maintain cell shape and flexibility, for renewal of membrane phospholipids, for active transport of cations, and for the synthesis of pyridine nucleotides, glutathione, and flavin adenine dinucleotide. Glycolysis also recycles NAD to NADH, an essential cofactor in the enzymatic reduction of methemoglobin.

Approximately 95 percent of the glucose metabolized by the red cell passes directly through the Embden-Meyerhof pathway. The remaining 5 percent is diverted through the hexose monophosphate shunt, the sole source of NADPH in the mature erythrocyte. The reduction of oxidized glutathione, catalyzed by the enzyme glutathione reductase, requires NADPH. This reaction provides a continuing source of reduced glutathione, essential for the protection of cell constituents, such as hemoglobin, enzymes, and membrane, from oxidative damage. The shunt is also a source of ribose pyrophosphate, utilized in the synthesis of ATP.

Oxidative threats to red cell integrity are countered by three different mechanisms, each involving glutathione. Reduced glutathione may reduce an exogenous oxidant directly or may return an oxidized cellular component such as hemoglobin to its functional, reduced state. Reduced glutathione also participates in the glutathione peroxidase-mediated conversion of hydrogen peroxide to water. In each reaction, glutathione is oxidized. Subsequent recycling of oxidized glutathione to the reduced state requires a normally functioning hexose monophosphate shunt.

Enzyme proteins of the Embden-Meyerhof and hexose monophosphate shunt pathways are degraded as erythrocytes age. Since the red cell cannot synthesize new enzyme protein, a gradual loss of enzyme activity is a normal feature of erythrocyte aging. Death of the cell after an average life span of 120 days may in part be determined by deterioration of enzymatic machinery to a level inconsistent with further survival. Because of the limited number of alternative metabolic pathways in the red cell, an enzymatic defect in any of the pathways of glucose metabolism can result in serious metabolic deficiencies, leading to impairment of cellular function and shortening of the cell lifespan.

DISORDERS OF THE HEXOSE MONOPHOSPHATE SHUNT AND METABOLISM OF GLUTATHIONE

Enzyme deficiencies of the hexose monophosphate shunt or of the pathway leading to the production of reduced glutathione can cause premature destruction of erythrocytes, presumably from oxidative damage. When the enzymatic deficiency is mild, there may be little or no hemolysis under normal conditions. However, when there is a demand for increased activity of these reaction sequences, as for example when the action of oxidant drugs or chemicals leads to the formation of hydrogen peroxide, a severe hemolytic episode may occur.

Glucose-6-Phosphate Dehydrogenase (G6PD) Deficiency

More than 100 million people throughout the world are G6PD-deficient. The deficiency can occur in any ethnic group, although it is uncommon in Caucasians from non-Mediterranean regions. The incidence of G6PD deficiency exceeds 1 percent of the male population in Greece and is even higher in other Mediterranean and Middle Eastern countries. Approximately 5 percent of Chinese and 10 percent of American black males are G6PD-deficient.

G6PD is located on the X chromosome and has a sex-linked recessive pattern of inheritance. Clinical manifestations of the deficiency are ordinarily encountered in male hemizygotes or female homozygotes. Female heterozygotes are usually clinically normal. In female heterozygotes both enzyme-replete and enzyme-deficient red cells are present, since either the normal or mutant X chromosome may be active. The percentage of G6PD-deficient cells characteristic of each heterozygote is determined by random inactivation of the X chromosome during embryogenesis and remains fairly constant thereafter. Some heterozygotes may have sufficient numbers of enzyme-deficient red cells so as to resemble deficient male hemizygotes, while others may have almost no enzyme-deficient cells and be indistinguishable from normal. Because cells with normal enzyme activity as well as enzyme-deficient cells are present, it is often impossible to distinguish heterozygotes from normal by the use of screening tests or quantitative assays that measure enzyme activity in cell mixtures. There are methods for identification of heterozygotes, based on the analysis of G6PD activity in single cells on a blood smear, but they are time-consuming and not available routinely.

The most common clinical manifestation of G6PD deficiency is episodic acute hemolysis, usually following infections or the ingestion of certain drugs or other hemolytic agents (see Table 11). Rarely, a patient with G6PD deficiency will exhibit chronic, lifelong hemolytic anemia, jaundice, and splenomegaly, with a susceptibility to more severe anemic crises when erythropoiesis is suppressed during infections. Administration of hemolytic agents to such individuals will further accelerate the rate of hemolysis and may be lethal.

Hemolytic episodes are characterized by increasing pallor, jaundice, dark urine, back pain, and, in the most severe cases, shock, cardiovascular collapse, and death. Between hemolytic episodes, anemia is absent and erythrocyte survival may be normal. In blacks, G6PD activity is near normal in reticulocytes and young erythrocytes; it declines rapidly as cells age, resulting in a population of older, enzyme-deficient cells that are susceptible to hemolysis. Following administration of a hemolytic agent, older erythrocytes are hemolyzed, but younger, enzyme-replete cells remain intact. In blacks, an abrupt fall in hematocrit, associated with hemolysis of older, enzyme-deficient red cells, is followed by reticulocytosis and a gradual return of the hematocrit to normal levels, even with continued administration of the hemolytic agent. A period of equilibrium is reached subsequently, in which anemia is absent and there may be only minimal evidence of continued hemolysis. During this period, G6PD activity is sufficient to avoid hemolysis in all but a small proportion of cells each day. It may be difficult to diagnose G6PD deficiency during the recovery and equilibrium periods since only young, enzyme-replete red cells remain in the circulation. In the more severe Mediterranean G6PD deficiency, both young and old erythrocytes are enzyme-deficient and are thus equally susceptible to hemolysis. Since all red cells are enzyme-deficient, the diagnosis usually can be made even during a hemolytic episode.

G6PD deficiency is most likely to be associated with neonatal jaundice in Oriental and Mediterranean infants, even in the absence of exposure to a recognized hemolytic agent. In blacks, an increased incidence of jaundice is seen in premature but not in mature G6PD-deficient infants. In the Mediterranean and the Orient, red cells from certain G6PD-deficient individuals are susceptible to hemolysis when fresh, dried, or even cooked fava beans are ingested. The hemolytic principle contained in the fava bean has not yet been identified, but can be transmitted through breast milk and possibly through the placenta to the unborn fetus.

The variable clinical manifestations of G6PD deficiency are, in greatest measure, due to differences among the numerous mutant forms of the enzyme. Some variants are not associated with episodic or chronic hemolysis. Approximately 100 variant forms of G6PD have been distinguished on the basis of their differing enzyme kinetics, pH of optimal enzyme activity, electrophoretic mobility, and stability in vitro. The relatively few variant enzymes that have been purified and subjected to amino acid analysis have all differed from normal only by the substitution of a single amino acid. Reduced synthesis of structurally normal enzyme protein has not been demonstrated unequivocally, but remains a theoretical possibility.

The normal enzyme in nonblacks is known as the B enzyme. The A-plus variant enzyme, present in about 30 percent of American blacks, migrates more rapidly than the B enzyme on electrophoresis. This variant has normal activity and is not associated with hemolysis. The enzyme usually associated with hemolysis in blacks is another variant whose electrophoretic migration is identical to that of the A-plus variant enzyme. Because enzyme activity is abnormally low, this enzyme is known as the A-minus variant. Other G6PD variants are named after the city or region in which they were first discovered (G6PD Canton, G6PD Mediterranean, and so on).

Hemolysis in G6PD deficiency results from a failure to generate sufficient NADPH to recycle the reduced glutathione that is essential for the protection of cellular components from oxidation. In the presence of an oxidant, hemoglobin is oxidized progressively to met-

hemoglobin, sulfhemoglobin, and denatured globin-glutathione complexes, which eventually precipitate as insoluble inclusions called Heinz bodies. The presence of such red cell inclusions, as well as oxidative damage to the membrane and possibly to enzymes, leads to irreversible cell damage and hemolysis. Heinz bodies, which can be detected by staining a blood smear with crystal violet, may be present only early in an episode of hemolysis because red cells that contain inclusion bodies are rapidly destroyed.

The diagnosis of G6PD deficiency is made by quantitative assay of enzyme activity in red cell lysates. Various screening tests, which in essence measure the ability of the erythrocyte to generate NADPH in vitro, are also available. In the fluorescent spot test, a buffered red cell lysate is incubated briefly with substrates of the G6PD reaction, glucose-6-phosphate and NADP. Fluorescence of the reaction mixture following incubation indicates that NADPH, a fluorescent compound, has been generated and that red cell G6PD activity is adequate. To assess fluorescence, a few drops of reaction mixture are placed on filter paper and inspected with a UV lamp. Another screening test that is more sensitive in the detection of female carriers is the ascorbate-cyanide test. Addition of ascorbic acid to a sample of whole blood results in the generation of small amounts of hydrogen peroxide within the red cell. If glutathione metabolism and the hexose monophosphate shunt are intact, hydrogen peroxide is rapidly converted to water; if not, hydrogen peroxide accumulates and forms methemoglobin, which imparts a characteristic chocolate brown color to the blood. If no abnormality is present, the blood remains red. Cyanide is added at the outset to block catalase, which otherwise would provide an alternate pathway for removal of hydrogen peroxide. This screening test has the virtue of simplicity and can detect a relatively small population of G6PD-deficient cells. However, it is not specific for G6PD deficiency and will detect other abnormalities of the hexose monophosphate shunt or of glutathione metabolism.

Screening tests for G6PD may be used to confirm the cause of a hemolytic episode. They are also useful in identifying susceptible individuals in order to avoid agents known to produce hemolysis (see Table 11). There is controversy regarding the value of mass screening for G6PD deficiency, since with certain common variants, (such as the A-minus variant in blacks) hemomon variants hemolytic episodes have been infrequent and usually mild. Screening, particularly of males from susceptible ethnic groups, seems reasonable prior to administration of potentially hemolytic agents, such as antimalarials, sulfonamides, or nitrofurans. G6PD-deficient individuals should be provided with a list of such agents and counseled regarding the risk associated with their use. In counseling, it should be recalled that Caucasian G6PD-deficient subjects are susceptible to certain hemolytic agents that do not cause hemolysis in blacks (see Table 11). In the event of a hemolytic episode, discontinuance of the suspected drug is usually prudent in black G6PD-deficient patients and is mandatory in patients with G6PD Mediterranean or other more severe variants in which all erythrocytes are enzyme-deficient and susceptible to hemolysis. In black patients, continued administration of an oxidant drug may be better tolerated than an initial dose, since most enzyme-deficient cells will already have been destroyed.

Other Abnormalities of the Hexose Monophosphate Shunt

Inherited deficiencies of glutathione reductase, 6-phosphogluconate dehydrogenase, glutathione peroxidase, and the two enzymes involved in the synthesis of glutathione, glutamyl cysteine synthetase and glutathione synthetase, have been described and may result in either episodic or chronic hemolysis. Unlike G6PD deficiency, these disorders have an autosomal recessive pattern of inheritance or, in the case of glutathione reductase, an autosomal dominant one. Their diagnosis requires quantitative assay of red cell enzyme activity in vitro or the detection of reduced levels of erythrocyte glutathione. The ascorbate-cyanide test is abnormal in all hexose monophosphate shunt disorders and is the most useful preliminary screening test for such disorders.

Flavin adenine dinucleotide (FAD) is a required cofactor for activation of erythrocyte glutathione reductase. Dietary riboflavin deficiency, which can produce FAD deficiency, may result in diminished glutathione reductase activity. Measurement of erythrocyte glutathione reductase activity is thus a convenient assay for dietary riboflavin deficiency. By the same token, the attribution of a hematologic disturbance to glutathione reductase deficiency should be made only after ensuring the adequacy of dietary riboflavin intake.

DISORDERS OF GLYCOLYSIS (EMBDEN-MEYERHOF PATHWAY)

Inherited deficiencies of Embden-Meyerhof glycolytic pathway enzymes may result in chronic hemolytic anemia. Inadequate glycolytic synthesis of ATP appears to be the common denominator responsible for shortened red cell survival in these disorders. Unique features that are associated with particular glycolytic enzymopathies are highlighted in Table 12. With the exception of such features, the clinical manifestations, genetics, and treatment of these enzymopathies are so similar that it is convenient to describe them as a group rather than individually.

Clinical Manifestations

Jaundice, reticulocytosis, and splenomegaly are found in most anemic patients. The severity of hemolysis varies depending on the degree to which erythrocyte glycolysis is impaired. In an individual patient, however, the degree of hemolysis fluctuates little in intensity. Gallstones and anemic crises due to transient erythroid hypoplasia may occur in the more severely anemic patients.

Erythrocyte morphology is usually normal, aside from the macrocytosis and polychromatophilia that customarily accompany reticulocytosis. However, after splenectomy, a variable number of contracted, spiculated cells may appear. The unincubated osmotic fragility curve is normal. After incubation, a fragile tail of hemolysis may be evident. The spontaneous hemolysis of erythrocytes incubated under sterile conditions in saline for 48 hours is increased. The abnormalities in autohemolysis are usually substantially improved by the addition of glucose to the incubation medium, although in some cases of pyruvate kinase deficiency autohemolysis is paradoxically accentuated by the addition of glucose. Because the autohemolysis test is abnormal in spherocytosis, paroxysmal nocturnal hemoglobinuria, and certain other hemolytic anemias, it is not a specific screening test for erythrocyte enzymopathies. Diagnosis of these conditions requires quantitative enzyme assay. The availability of such assays is limited, but screening tests are available widely for the more common enzymopathies, notably pyruvate kinase deficiency, glucose phosphate isomerase deficiency, and triose phosphate isomerase deficiency.

As in G6PD deficiency, clinical variability is the consequence of numerous biochemically distinct variant forms of the defective enzyme. This is particularly true of pyruvate kinase deficiency, where more than 20 variants have been associated with hemolytic anemia. Several of these variants have near normal activity at the artificially high substrate concentrations employed in the usual in vitro assay, but are inactive at the lower substrate concentrations actually found within erythrocytes. Modification of the usual assay to include measurement of enzyme activity at low substrate concentrations will identify such variants.

Incidence and Genetics

Glycolytic enzymopathies are rare in all populations but are most frequently encountered in individuals from northern Europe. Inheritance is autosomal recessive except for phosphoglycerate kinase deficiency, which is sex-linked. Anemic individuals are either homozygotes or double heterozygotes. In the latter situation, family studies may be useful in determining the biochemical nature of the two enzyme variants, which, inherited together, have caused anemia.

Pathophysiology

Mechanisms of hemolysis have been evaluated more extensively in pyruvate kinase deficiency than in other glycolytic enzymopathies. Hemolysis in pyruvate kinase deficiency appears to result from the inadequate synthesis of ATP. ATP depletion causes a defect in membrane cation permeability. Potassium is lost from the cell faster than sodium is gained. Since ATP is unavailable for the active transport of cations to restore normal cation gradients, progressive potassium loss occurs, producing a reduction in cell cation content accompanied by an obligate osmotic loss of cell water. The

TABLE 12. Enzyme Deficiencies of Embden–Meyerhof Pathway

Enzyme		Tissues Involved	Clinical Features	Red Cell & Metabolites		Other Remarks
				ATP	2,3-DPG	
Hexokinase	AR*	RBC	CNSHA	↓	↓	Increased hemoglobin O_2 affinity, decreased exercise tolerance for degree of anemia
Glucosephosphate isomerase	AR	RBC, WBC, skin fibroblasts, plasma	CNSHA	↓, N	N	Spiculated microspherocytes sometimes observed
Phosphofructokinase	AR	RBC, muscle	CNSHA myopathy (muscle glycogen storage disease)	↓	—	
Aldolase	AR (?)	RBC	CNSHA, mild mental retardation	—	—	Only one case thus far described
Triose phosphate insomerase	AR	RBC, WBC, muscle, serum, CSF	CNSHA, severe progressive neurologic disorder	↓	—	Dihydroxyacetone phosphate accumulates in RBC, increased susceptibility to infection
Glyceraldehyde 3-phosphate dehydrogenase	AR (?)	RBC, ?WBC	CNSHA (?)	—	—	Hemolysis accentuated by dapsone in one patient, enzyme deficiency may occur without hemolytic anemia
Phosphoglycerate kinase	Sex-linked, R	RBC, WBC	CNSHA, mental retardation	N	N,↑	Dihydrooxyacetone phosphate accumulates in RBC
2,3-DPG mutase	AR, AD	RBC	CNSHA (hemolysis may be severe)	N,↑	↓	Increased hemoglobin O_2 affinity
Enolase	?	RBC	Chronic anemia	—	—	Acute hemolytic anemia produced by nitrofurantoin, spherocytes
Pyruvate kinase	AR	RBC, liver	CNSHA	—	—	Decreased hemoglobin O_2 affinity, increased exercise tolerance for degree of anemia

*AR = autosomal recessive, AD = autosomal dominant; CNSHA = congenital nonspherocytic hemolytic anemia; N = normal.

ATP-depleted erythrocyte is a rigid cell that assumes the shape of a crenated sphere. Dehydrated, stiff, ATP-depleted red cells are susceptible to sequestration by the spleen. The acidic, hypoglycemic, hypoxic environment of the spleen may then produce further metabolic depletion. The immediate cause of hemolysis in such cells is not understood, but is presumed to be a consequence of ATP depletion. In general, reticulocytes are immune to the sequence of events just outlined, as long as an alternate source of ATP synthesis, such as oxidation phosphorylation, is available. However, reticulocytes, which have greater metabolic requirements for ATP than do mature erythrocytes, may be particularly vulnerable to metabolic depletion, if ATP synthesis is compromised. Inhibition of oxidative phosphorylation by hypoxia may compromise ATP synthesis severely in reticulocytes with defective glycolysis, since no alternate energy source is then available. Sequestration of reticulocytes within the spleen, which is hypoxic as well as acidic and hypoglycemic, represents an unusually severe metabolic stress for such cells and may lead to their immediate destruction. In fact, in pyruvate kinase deficiency and possibly in certain other glycolytic enzymopathies, hemolysis of reticulocytes plays a major role in the pathogenesis of anemia. In such conditions, there is a paradoxical rise in reticulocyte count following splenectomy, sometimes to levels as high as 60 to 90 percent, reflecting the enhanced survival of reticulocytes previously destroyed by the spleen.

Deficient enzyme activity along the Embden-Meyerhof pathway usually results in altered concentration of glycolytic intermediates above and below the site of deficient enzymatic function. In particular, the concentration of 2,3-DPG may be greatly altered. Because 2,3-DPG is an important regulator of hemoglobin oxygen affinity, changes in its concentration may have important implications for oxygen transport. Indeed, the clinical effects of anemia are modified to a significant degree by the intracellular concentration of 2,3-DPG characteristic of each glycolytic enzymopathy. Anemia may result in few or no symptoms in pyruvate kinase deficiency, where 2,3-DPG levels are high, enhancing oxygen transport. In hexokinase deficiency, the same degree of anemia may be severely symptomatic because 2,3-DPG levels are subnormal.

Treatment

Splenectomy, although not curative, has usually lessened the intensity of hemolysis in severely anemic patients. In patients with mild anemia, splenectomy seldom results in significant improvement. Daily supplemental folic acid should be given to patients with severe hemolysis, and blood transfusion may occasionally be required, particularly following transient bone marrow aplasia.

OTHER DISORDERS OF ERYTHROCYTE METABOLISM

Enzyme abnormalities associated with hemolytic anemia

Red cell adenylate kinase deficiency has been associated with chronic hemolytic anemia. Deficiency of erythrocyte pyrimidine 5'-nucleotidase produces moderately severe hemolytic anemia with pronounced basophilic stippling of the erythrocytes. Stippling is thought to result from retarded ribosomal RNA degradation. Pyrimidine 5'-nucleotides accumulate to an extraordinary degree within the erythrocyte and can be detected by simple ultraviolet spectral analysis, useful in screening for the disorder. Both adenylate kinase deficiency and pyrimidine 5'-nucleotidase deficiency appear to follow an autosomal recessive mode of transmission.

Enzyme abnormalities thought to be secondary to other hematologic disorders

The activity of numerous erythrocyte enzymes may be abnormal in a miscellaneous group of conditions that include acute and chronic leukemias, dyserythropoietic anemias, Fanconi's aplastic anemia, and Diamond-Blackfan syndrome. Although various of patterns have been seen, the most commonly reported has been a relative reduction in erythrocyte pyruvate kinase and glutathione reductase activity and an unusual increase in the activities of enolase, hexokinase, aldolase, and glyceraldehyde-3-phosphate dehydrogenase. It is speculated that such abnormalities may result from chromosomal alterations, from stress or dyserythropoiesis, or from the reappearance of fetal erythropoiesis. The enzyme abnormalities have not been implicated in the pathogenesis of anemia but have proved useful in the differential diagnosis of certain of these conditions, notably Diamond-Blackfan syndromes (see p. 1132).

EFFECT OF ABNORMAL SERUM PHOSPHATE ON 2,3-DPG AND ERYTHROPOIESIS. In uremia, where serum phosphate concentration may rise, an organic phosphate-mediated decrease in hemoglobin oxygen affinity may occur. Conversely, in hypophosphatemia, such as that sometimes seen during hyperalimentation, an increase in oxygen affinity may result from the fall in red cell organic phosphate levels. When the serum phosphate drops below 0.5 mg/100 ml, ATP depletion may be so extreme as to result in hemolytic anemia, which can be subsequently corrected by the administration of phosphate.

References

Baugham MA, Valentine WN, Paglia DE, Ways PO, Simons ER, DeMarsh QB: Hereditary hemolytic anemia associated with glucose-phosphate isomerase (GPI) deficiency—a new enzyme defect of human erythrocytes. Blood 32:236, 1968

Beutler E: Abnormalities of the hexose monophosphate shunt. Semin Hematol 8:311, 1971

———— Scott S, Bishop A, Margolis N: Red cell aldolase deficiency and hemolytic anemia: a new syndrome. Clin Res 21:727, 1972

Beutler E: Effect of flavin compounds on glutathione reductase activity: in vivo and in vitro studies. J Clin Invest 48:1957, 1969

Bowin P, Galand C, Hakim J, Kahn A: Acquired erythroenzymopathies in blood disorders: study of 200 cases. Br J Haematol 31:531, 1975

Gilman PA: Hemolysis in the newborn infant resulting from deficiencies of red blood cell enzymes: diagnosis and management. J Pediatr 84:625, 1974

Jacob HS, Amsden T: Acute hemolytic anemia with rigid red cells in hypophosphatemia. N Engl J Med 285:1446, 1971

Konrad PN, Richards F, Valentine WN, Paglia DE: γ glutamyl-cysteine synthetase deficiency. N Engl J Med 286:557, 1972

———— McCarthy DJ, Mauer AM, Valentine WN, Paglia DE: Erythrocyte and leukocyte phosphoglycerate kinase deficiency with neurologic disease. J Pediat 82:456, 1973

McCann SR, Finkel B, Cadman S, Allen DW: Study of a kindred with hereditary spherocytosis and glyceraldehyde-3-phosphate dehydrogenase deficiency. Blood 47:171, 1976

Mentzer WC Jr: Pyruvate kinase deficiency and disorders of glycolysis. In Nathan DG, Oski FA (eds): Hematology of Infancy and Childhood. Philadelphia, WB Saunders, 1974, p 346

Mohler DN, Majerus PW, Minnich V, Hess CE, Garrick MD: Glutathione synthetase defiency as a hereditary hemolytic disease. N Engl J Med 283: 1253, 1975

Necheles TF, Maldonado N, Barquet-Chediak A, Allen DM: Homozygous erythrocyte glutathione-peroxidase deficiency: clinical and biochemical studies. Blood 33:164, 1969

Piomelli S: G6PD deficiency and related disorders of the pentose pathway. In Nathan DG, Oski FA (eds): Hematology of Infancy and Childhood. Philadelphia, WB Saunders, 1974, p 346

Schneider AS, Valentine WN, Baughan MA, Paglia DE, Shore NA, Heins HL Jr: Triosephosphate isomerase deficiency. In Beutler E (ed): Hereditary Disorders of Erythrocyte Metabolism. New York, Grune & Stratton, 1968, p 265

Stefanini M: Chronic hemolytic anemia associated with erythrocyte enolase deficiency exacerbated by ingestion of nitrofurantoin. Am J Clin Pathol 58:408, 1972

Szeinberg A, Kahana D, Gavendo S, Zaidman J, Ben-Ezzer J: Hereditary deficiency of adenylate kinase in red blood cells. Acta Haematol 42:111, 1969

Valentine WN, Oski FA, Paglia DE, Baughan MD, Schneider AS, Naiman JL, Hereditary hemolytic anemia with hexokinase deficiency. N Engl J Med 276:1, 1967

———— Konrad PN, Paglia DE: Dyserythropoiesis, refractory anemia, and "preleukemia": metabolic features of the erythrocytes. Blood 41:857, 1973

———— Fink K, Paglia DE, Harris SR, Adams WS: Hereditary hemolytic anemia with human erythrocyte pyrimidine 5' - nucleosidase deficiency. J Clin Invest 54:866, 1974

Waterbury L, Frenkel EP: Hereditary nonspherocytic hemolysis with erythrocyte phosphofructokinase deficiency. Blood 39:415, 1972

METHEMOGLOBINEMIA

WILLIAM C. MENTZER

Methemoglobin is a form of hemoglobin in which heme iron has been oxidized to the ferric state. As a result, it can no longer reversibly bind oxygen and is therefore useless as a respiratory pigment. Normally, about 1 to 3 percent of all hemoglobin is oxidized to methemoglobin each day. However, there are several mechanisms for the enzymatic reduction of methemoglobin that prevent the accumulation of levels greater than 1 to 2 percent of total hemoglobin. Under normal circumstances, NADH-dependent methemoglobin reductase accounts for nearly all methemoglobin reduction. NADPH methemoglobin reductase can be utilized as an alternate pathway when NADH methemoglobin reductase is deficient, but it normally contributes little to the reduction of methemoglobin. Methemoglobin reductase activity in cord blood is only about 70 percent of that normally found in adults, and the level of activity in fetal blood is even lower. Normal adult values appear to be reached between 7 weeks and 6 months after birth.

An increase in the concentration of methemoglobin in the blood, termed *methemoglobinemia*, occurs whenever there is a disturbance in the usual balance between oxidation and reduction of heme iron. This can result from inherited abnormalities of red cell enzymes or of hemoglobin, or from exposure to drugs or toxins. Accumulation of methemoglobin to concentrations above 1.5 g/dl imparts a chocolate brown appearance to the blood and a slate gray cyanotic hue to the skin and mucous membranes. As the percentage of methemoglobin increases, progressively more symptoms of hypoxia may be encountered.

Methemoglobin reductase deficiency

An inherited deficiency of NADH-methemoglobin reductase may result in either intermittent or chronic methemoglobinemia. The disorder is rare and appears with greatest frequency in inbred populations, such as Eskimos or American Indians. The pattern of inheritance is autosomal recessive. Homozygotes generally exhibit lifelong cyanosis. The methemoglobin level is customarily 10 to 25 percent of total hemoglobin, but this level may be increased by exposure to certain oxidant drugs. Despite the presence of methemoglobinemia, these patients appear to have a normal life span and usually have few symptoms. About 12 percent of homozygotes are mentally retarded, for reasons that are not well understood. Heterozygotes do not normally have methemoglobinemia but may develop it upon exposure to certain oxidant drugs (see Table 13). They may also exhibit spontaneous methemoglobinemia during the newborn period, perhaps because their heterozygous deficiency state accentuates the normally low levels of methemoglobin reductase during this period of life.

A number of electrophoretic variants of methemoglobin reductase have been discovered. Not all variants have been associated with reduced enzyme activity and susceptibility to methemoglobin formation. NADPH-methemoglobin reductase deficiency has also been described. Because the major burden of methemoglobin reduction is borne by NADH-methemoglobin reductase, methemoglobinemia is not a feature of NADPH-methemoglobin reductase deficiency.

M Hemoglobins

Certain alterations in hemoglobin structure, involving substitution of amino acids in the region of the

TABLE 13. Oxidants Reported to Cause Methemoglobinemia

1. Analgesics
    Acetophenetidin
2. Anesthetics
    Benzocaine (topical , rectal)
    Prilocaine (obstetrical)
3. Aniline derivatives
    Marking dyes (topical)
    Disinfectants (topical)
    Crayons
4. Antimalarials
5. Nitrites
    Nitrate contamination of well water
    Bismuth subnitrate
    Nitroglycerin
    Nitrate food additives
6. Pyridium
7. Sulfonamides
8. Vitamin K analogues

heme pocket, lead to a marked increase in the rate of spontaneous oxidation of hemoglobin to methemoglobin. These hemoglobinopathies, known collectively as the *hemoglobin M disorders,* exhibit an autosomal dominant pattern of inheritance. Three substitutions involving the α-globin chain and two involving the β-globin chain have been described. Infants with the α-chain mutant are cyanotic from birth, while those inheriting the β-chain abnormality do not exhibit cyanosis until later in infancy, when the normal increase in β-chain synthesis results in the accumulation of sufficient hemoglobin M. The M hemoglobinopathies are benign disorders, not associated with any reduction in life span. Their clinical significance lies in the need to distinguish them from other more serious causes of cyanosis, such as congenital heart disease or pulmonary disease.

Toxic methemoglobinemia

A variety of drugs and chemicals may increase the rate of oxidation of hemoglobin and produce methemoglobinemia (Table 13). Newborns are particularly susceptible to such agents because hemoglobin F is more readily oxidized to methemoglobin than is hemoglobin A and because levels of NADH-methemoglobin reductase are lower in the erythrocytes of newborns than in those of adults.

Diagnosis

The discovery of clinical cyanosis usually first suggests the possibility of methemoglobinemia. If a freshly obtained blood specimen is chocolate brown in color and does not become red when aerated by mixing, a presumptive diagnosis of methemoglobinemia can be made. Spectrophotometric analysis of the concentration of methemoglobin is required to confirm the diag-

nosis. When methemoglobinemia is acute in onset, exposure to chemicals or drugs should be suspected. When methemoglobinemia has been chronic, the family history may be helpful in distinguishing between NADH-methemoglobin reductase deficiency, which has an autosomal recessive mode of inheritance, and hemoglobin M, which is transmitted as a dominant trait. The M hemoglobinopathies can also be identified by hemoglobin electrophoresis at pH 7, by their distinctive absorption spectrum, which differs from that in other forms of methemoglobinemia, and by the failure of methylene blue to reduce methemoglobin in vitro. Methylene blue does reduce methemoglobin in the blood of patients with a deficiency of erythrocyte methemoglobin reductase or toxic methemoglobinemia. The diagnosis of NADH-methemoglobin reductase deficiency can be confirmed by measuring activity of the enzyme in the patient's red cells, but the assay is not widely available.

Treatment

The first step in treatment is to remove any oxidant drugs or chemicals suspected of initiating methemoglobinemia. Rapid conversion of methemoglobin to hemoglobin can be achieved by the intravenous infusion of a 1 percent solution of methylene blue in saline at a dose of 1 to 2 mg/kg body weight except in patients with hemoglobin M. In patients with a deficiency of NADH-methemoglobin reductase, oral methylene blue, 1.5 to 5 mg/kg/day in divided doses, may be required chronically. The reduction of methemoglobin by methylene blue is mediated by NADPH-methemoglobin reductase and requires an intact hexose monophosphate shunt as a source of NADPH. For this reason, it is advisable to screen methemoglobinemic individuals for G6PD deficiency prior to the use of methylene blue, since the drug will not only be ineffective for the treatment of methemoglobinemia in such patients, but may actually cause hemolytic anemia. Ascorbic acid (5 to 8 mg/kg/day orally in divided doses) is commonly used for chronic methemoglobinemia due to NADH-methemoglobin reductase activity, but it is slower and less effective than methylene blue in treating acute episodes of methemoglobinemia. Where methemoglobin exceeds 50 percent of total hemoglobin, the potential for serious complications or death may justify the use of exchange transfusion in addition to or as a substitute for intravenous methylene blue.

References

Comings DE: Hemoglobinopathies producing cyanosis. In Williams WJ, Beutler E, Erslev AJ, Rundles RW (eds): Hematology. New York, McGraw-hill, 1972, p 434

Feig SA: Methemoglobinemia. In Nathan DG, Oski FA (eds): Hematology of Infancy and Childhood. Philadelphia, WB Saunders, 1974, p 378

Jaffé ER, Hsieh HS:DPNH-methemoglobin reductase deficiency and hereditary methemoglobinemia. Semin Hematol 8:417, 1971

Oski FA, Naiman JL: Methemoglobinemia. In Hematologic Problems in the Newborn. Philadelphia, WB Saunders, 1972, p 169

WHITE BLOOD CELLS

PETER R. DALLMAN

All white cells are specialized in some aspect of defending the body against foreign cells, microorganisms, and protein. The different types of white cells fall into two major functional categories: those that are primarily phagocytic and those involved in the immune response. *Phagocytic* cells include neutrophils, monocytes, eosinophils, and basophils. Cells that participate in an *immune response* are lymphocytes and plasma cells; they are discussed further in Chapter 9. Monocytes engage in both functions; they are phagocytic cells, but they also appear to process antigen as an initiating event in the production of antibody. Each type of white cell serves a specialized function and is under independent synthetic control.

Neutrophils

MATURATION.   In contrast to the red blood cell, most of the life cycle of the neutrophil takes place in the bone marrow. In the marrow, neutrophil maturation takes 10 to 14 days, and neutrophil precursors outnumber red cell precursors (Table 3, p. 1119). Mature neutrophils are released into the circulation where they remain briefly, with a disappearance half-time of about 6 hours. They then move rapidly into the tissues and remain there for about 1 day.

GRANULES.   Mature neutrophils contain two kinds of granules. The primary or azurophilic granules are produced first, during the proliferative stages of promyelocyte and myelocyte maturation. They contain hydrolytic enzymes, cationic proteins and myeloperoxide. Secondary or specific granules are produced mainly during the postmitotic stages of metamyelocyte maturation and eventually outnumber primary granules in the mature cells. Secondary granules contain lactoferrin (an antibacterial protein) and acid phosphatase.

NUMBER.   The neutrophil count in blood depends on the rate of entry of cells from the marrow, the rate of migration to tissues, and the proportion of cells that are marginated. Normally the rates of entry and departure are equal, and about half of the neutrophils are circulating, whereas the other half are marginated or transiently adherent to the capillary wall. Some marginating cells are mobilized with exercise or administration of epinephrine, causing a transient neutrophilia. With bacterial infection, there is an increased rate of mobilization of neutrophils to sites of inflammation. Usually, this is more than compensated for by a prompt release of mature and near mature (band) neutrophils from the storage pool of the marrow, which results in neutrophilia. The storage pool contains 10 to 20 times as many cells as are in the circulation and serves as a temporary supply for the several days that are required before an increased number of mature cells can be derived from more rapid division of myeloid precursors. Neutrophilia associated with glucocorticoid therapy is due to a different mechanism. Glucocorticoids tighten the junctions between endothelial cells so that neutrophils are less able to migrate to inflammatory sites and therefore accumulate in the circulation. The increased susceptibility to localized infection in patients receiving steroid therapy is partly attributable to fewer neutrophils at the site of inflammation.

Neutropenia most commonly results from decreased production of myeloid cells in the bone marrow and/or an absent or decreased marrow storage pool. Another cause of neutropenia is an increased rate of destruction of cells, sometimes attributable to white cell antibodies or splenic sequestration. Decreased survival of neutrophils in the circulation can be documented by kinetic studies with neutrophils incubated with radioactive diisopropylfluorophosphate ($DF^{32}P$), but this procedure is not routinely performed in most medical centers. More generally available is the urine or serum muramidase (lysozyme), a neutrophil breakdown product that is elevated when there is an increased rate of neutrophil destruction.

FUNCTION.   The *phagocytic function* of the neutrophil takes place primarily in the tissues and involves the following steps:

Chemotaxis, which refers to the movement of the neutrophil to the site of inflammation. This takes place within a period of several hours. Bacteria attract neutrophils primarily through activation of the complement system. Chemotaxis is also dependent on the mobility of the neutrophil and its ability to traverse the capillary wall.

Recognition or *opsonization*. The neutrophil recognizes what is to be phagocytosed at an inflamed site after specific serum proteins called opsonins have coated the invading particles. The most important of these opsonins are the C3 component of complement and antibodies of the IgG class.

Ingestion takes place next, when the neutrophil's pseudopods surround the particle and fuse to form a membrane-bound, intracellular vesicle or phagosome.

Degranulation is the process by which neutrophil granules fuse with the phagosome. This allows the discharge of these previously packaged hydrolytic enzymes into the phagosome where the particle can be digested without damage to the cell itself.

Killing of bacteria takes place through hydrolytic digestion and is facilitated by the generation of hydrogen peroxide, the acidity of the phagosome contents (pH 3.5 to 4), and the action of antibacterial proteins (lactoferrin and cationic proteins). Some bacteria (streptococci and pneumococci) contribute to their own death because they generate peroxide but lack the enzyme catalase, which breaks it down. Other bacteria (*Staphylococcus aureus*) contain catalase and are more resistant to both self-generated and neutrophil-generated peroxide. Such bacteria are the source of the most serious infections when the neutrophil lacks the capacity to generate hydrogen peroxide on either an acquired or congenital basis (see chronic granulomatous disease, p. 326). Ingestion, degranulation, and killing take place with surprising speed over a period of a few minutes.

Monocytes

These cells mature in the bone marrow over a period of 1 to 3 days; their life span in the circulation is about 1 day. Subsequently they may either participate in the inflammatory reaction or differentiate into tissue macrophages. The monocytic phagocytes that enter sites of inflammation do so more slowly than neutrophils, reaching a peak number after about 1 day rather than by 6 hours. Those monocytes that become tissue macrophages or RE cells are long-lived. They undergo changes in morphology and function that are characteristic of their final location in the sinusoids of the spleen, in the liver, as Kupffer cells, or in the bone marrow, lymph nodes, lung, etc. Although monocytic cells have fewer lysosomal granules than neutrophils, they are efficient in phagocytosis, digestion, and killing. Monocytes also are involved in delayed hypersensitivity and play a role in the processing of antigen. They are increased in number in chronic infection, in granulomas, and in certain viral infections.

Eosinophils and Basophils

These cells resemble neutrophils in their marrow production, brief life span in the circulation, and ultimate appearance at sites of inflammation. The eosinophil is believed to serve the specialized function of ingesting antigen-antibody complexes. Eosinophilia usually appears to reflect some type of hypersensitivity reaction. Persistent eosinophilia is most commonly associated with allergic conditions (asthma, hay fever, eczema, and chronic rhinitis) and with parasitic infestations (trichinosis, toxicara canis, filariasis, ascariasis, and taenia). Less frequent causes of eosinophilia are drug reactions (penicillin and iodides), rheumatoid disease (periasteritis nodosa), malignancy (Hodgkin's disease), and skin disorders (dermatitis herpetiformis).Basophil granules are rich in histamine and heparin, but the function of this distinctive but rare cell is not known.

Lymphocytes

These cells in the peripheral blood represent a small fraction of the total, most of which are located in the thymus, lymph nodes, and spleen. Normal morphologic differences among lymphocytes primarily represent different stages in the cell's life cycle. Most lymphocytes are slightly larger than red blood cells and contain a narrow ring of cytoplasm around a nucleus that virtually fills the cell. Other lymphocytes are larger and have a more generous amount of cytoplasm that is more irregularly shaped. In infants, large lymphocytes sometimes contain nucleoli; these are probably proliferating cells. Lymphocytes are classified on the basis of their function as T (thymus-dependent) lymphocytes or B (bone-marrow-derived) lymphocytes (see p. 301), but these cannot be distinguished morphologically. T cells participate in the cell-mediated immune response,

whereas B cells differentiate into plasma cells which synthesize immune globulins. In the peripheral blood about 70 percent of lymphocytes are T cells, and most of the remainder are B cells.

Lymphocyte kinetics differ from neutrophil and erythrocyte kinetics; there is a continuous recirculation of lymphocytes to and from solid tissues that makes use of a separate circulatory system, the lymphatics. Another distinctive characteristic is that some B and T lymphocytes have a life span of at least several years, in contrast to the much shorter life span of all other circulating cells. Both types of lymphocytes originate in the bone marrow, but T cells require the thymus for their differentiation. B cells also proliferate in the germinal centers of the lymph nodes and spleen at a rate that is increased after stimulation by an antigen.

DEVELOPMENTAL CHANGES IN NUMBER

The number of white cells and the proportion of each cell type in the circulating blood are helpful in the diagnosis and management of many illnesses. There are marked developmental changes in normal values that must be taken into consideration in the interpretation of results (Table 14). The mean *white cell count* at birth is high, and there is a broad range of normal. There is a further brief rise in the mean value at 12 hours after birth, followed by a rapid fall until the end of the first week. Thereafter values are stable until 1 year of age. Subsequently, there is a slow, steady fall in white cell count throughout childhood, until the values characteristic of adult life are reached at 21 years of age.

Differential cell counts indicate the relative proportions of different kinds of white cells in the blood, but they have less physiologic meaning than absolute counts of each type of cell. In the differential count, *neutrophils* account for about half the white cells at birth. There is a transient rise within 12 hours due to mobilization of marginated cells; this is followed by a decrease to a mean of about 32 percent between 1 month and 1 year. Neutrophil counts as low as 20 percent are relatively common in normal infants; after infancy, there is a slow increase in neutrophils throughout childhood to the mean adult value of 59 percent. If a differential cell count suggests neutropenia, it is important to determine whether the feather edge of the blood smear (the last part of the slide to be smeared out) includes a disproportionate number of neutrophils. Neutrophils are sticky cells and may be pushed to the edge of the blood smear unintentionally, leaving behind mostly mononuclear cells on the part of the slide that is used for the differential count.

Lymphocytes account for about 30 percent of the white cells in the newborn. The proportion of lymphocytes then increases rapidly within the first month to remain near an average of 60 percent until 2 years of age; a count of 75 percent lymphocytes is not unusual in this age range. During infancy, lymphocytes often are large and may contain nucleoli. Their immature appearance and increased number, particularly during mild,

TABLE 14. Normal Leukocyte Counts*

Age	Total Leukocytes		Neutrophils†			Lymphocytes			Monocytes		Eosinophils	
	Mean	(Range)	Mean	(Range)	%	Mean	(Range)	%	Mean	%	Mean	%
Birth	18.1	(9.0–30.0)	11.0	(6.0–26.0)	61	5.5	(2.0–11.0)	31	1.1	6	0.4	2
12 hr	22.8	(13.0 38.0)	15.5	(6.0–28.0)	68	5.5	(2.0–11.0)	24	1.2	5	0.5	2
24 hr	18.9	(9.4–34.0)	11.5	(5.0–21.0)	61	5.8	(2.0–11.5)	31	1.1	6	0.5	2
1 wk	12.2	(5.0–21.0)	5.5	(1.5–10.0)	45	5.0	(2.0–17.0)	41	1.1	9	0.5	4
2 wk	11.4	(5.0–20.0)	4.5	(1.0– 9.5)	40	5.5	(2.0–17.0)	48	1.0	9	0.4	3
1 mo	10.8	(5.0–19.5)	3.8	(1.0– 9.0)	35	6.0	(2.5–16.5)	56	0.7	7	0.3	3
6 mo	11.9	(6.0–17.5)	3.8	(1.0– 8.5)	32	7.3	(4.0–13.5)	61	0.6	5	0.3	3
1 yr	11.4	(6.0–17.5)	3.5	(1.5– 8.5)	31	7.0	(4.0–10.5)	61	0.6	5	0.3	3
2 yr	10.6	(6.0–17.0)	3.5	(1.5– 8.5)	33	6.3	(3.0– 9.5)	59	0.5	5	0.3	3
4 yr	9.1	(5.5–15.5)	3.8	(1.5– 8.5)	42	4.5	(2.0– 8.0)	50	0.5	5	0.3	3
6 yr	8.5	(5.0–14.5)	4.3	(1.5– 8.0)	51	3.5	(1.5– 7.0)	42	0.4	5	0.2	3
8 yr	8.3	(4.5–13.5)	4.4	(1.5– 8.0)	53	3.3	(1.5– 6.8)	39	0.4	4	0.2	2
10 yr	8.1	(4.5–13.5)	4.4	(1.8– 8.0)	54	3.1	(1.5– 6.5)	38	0.4	4	0.2	2
16 yr	7.8	(4.5–13.0)	4.4	(1.8– 8.0)	57	2.8	(1.2– 5.2)	35	0.4	5	0.2	3
21 yr	7.4	(4.5–11.0)	4.4	(1.8– 7.7)	59	2.5	(1.0– 4.8)	34	0.3	4	0.2	3

Numbers of leukocytes are in thousands per cubic millimeter; ranges are estimates of 95% confidence limits, and percentages refer to differential counts.
* From Albritton EC (ed): Standard Value in Blood, 1952. Courtesy of W.B. Saunders.
† Neutrophils include band cells at all ages and a small number of metamyelocytes and myelocytes in the first few days of life.

nonbacterial infections, may give the false impression of malignancy.

The *absolute count* per cubic millimeter of each cell type can be obtained by multiplying the total leukocyte count by the percentage of that cell type in the differential count. Absolute values for neutrophils and lymphocytes have more clinical relevance than relative values, because each type of cell has a distinct function and the proliferation of each s under separate control in health and disease. Absolute counts also show relatively smooth and gradual developmental trends. The aforementioned exception is the rise in neutrophils during the first 12 hours after birth. The average number of *neutrophils* per cubic millimeter decreases rapidly from a mean above 10,000 during the first day of life and then maintains a value near 3,500/mm^3 for 2 years. The neutrophil count rises to the adult mean of 4,400/mm^3 at about 3 years of age. A neutrophil count below about 1,000/mm^3 is associated with an increased risk of infection. *Immature neutrophils* are common in the peripheral blood of the newborn. Metamyelocytes and myelocytes may be as high as 2,000 and 750 cells/mm^3, respectively, during the first 3 days. In the premature infant, the upper limits of normal are even higher, 3,000 and 1,000/mm^3, respectively, during the first 3 days, and an occasional myelocyte may be found up to 2 weeks after birth. Rarely, even promyelocytes and blast cells are seen in healthy newborn infants.

The absolute *lymphocyte* count in early infancy starts at a value that is more than twice that found in the adult, 5,500 compared to 2,500/mm^3. The number of lymphocytes then increases further to reach a peak of about 7,000/mm^3 between 6 months and 1 year of age. This is followed by a gradual decrease during early childhood to a value of 3,500/mm^3 at 6 years of age and a slower subsequent decline to the adult value of 2,500/mm^3. A lymphocyte count below 1,500/mm^3 in infants and children suggests the possibility of defective cellular immunity and the risk of graft-versus-host disease from blood transfusion.

Monocytes are most abundant in the first weeks of life and then gradually decline to a much lower adult value. *Basophils* follow a similar pattern, which is less evident because their average number remains below 1 percent of a differential count throughout development. Developmental changes in circulating *eosinophils* are not great. Eosinophils are most abundant in infancy and decline during childhood. The upper limit of normal is regarded as 5 percent, but higher values are common in individuals with mild allergies.

References

Cline MJ: The White Cell. Cambridge, Harvard Univ Press, 1975
Stossel TP: Phagocytosis. N Engl J Med 290:717, 774, 833, 1974

Neutropenia

William C. Mentzer

The normal number of neutrophils in the peripheral blood is a function of age. Neutropenia, or a deficiency in circulating granulocytes, is present in adults and older children if the absolute granulocyte count is less than 1,800/mm^3. In infants between 2 weeks and 1 year of age the lower limit of normal is 1,000/mm^3. The incidence of infections, particularly those associated with bacteria, increases in direct proportion to the severity of neutropenia. If the immune system is otherwise normal, an absolute granulocyte count of 500/mm^3 or even less may be tolerated for years without a substantial increase in infections. If the immune defenses are compromised, as during the administration of chemotherapy for leukemia, a significant rise in the frequency of severe infections is seen at absolute granulocyte levels below 1,500/mm^3.

Neutropenia reflects an alteration in the normal balance between production and destruction of white cells. Decreased delivery of granulocytes to the peripheral blood may result from diminished differentiation of stem cells into committed granulocyte precursors, an arrest in the normal sequence of granulocyte maturation, or impaired release of mature granulocytes from the bone marrow. Increased removal of granulocytes may result from sequestration of cells within an enlarged spleen, from destruction by antibody-mediated processes, or from compromised survival due to intrinsic defects of the granulocyte. Occasionally, as in some cases of cirrhosis, both increased destruction and decreased production may coexist and together result in neutropenia.

Normally, about half of the neutrophils within the bloodstream are circulating freely, whereas the other half are adherent to the walls of capillaries. A shift of more granulocytes into the marginating pool at the expense of the circulating pool may result in apparent neutropenia (pseudoneutropenia), even though the total number of granulocytes in the blood remains normal.

Diminished production of granulocytes underlies the neutropenia regularly observed after sufficient exposure to ionizing radiation or to certain drugs used in the chemotherapy of cancer. As these agents also suppress erythropoiesis and thrombopoiesis, they are discussed further elsewhere (see aplastic and hypoplastic anemia, p. 1130) Other drugs produce neutropenia in only an occasional recipient who is presumed to have an inherent sensitivity to the drug. For example, a single dose of aminopyrine or its derivatives may lead to a profound fall in the blood neutrophil count within hours. The mechanism of this neutropenia appears to be immunologically mediated destruction of neutrophils. Other drugs, such as chloramphenicol, phenothiazides, propylthiouracil, sulfonamides, diphenylhydantoin, and trimethyl oxazolidine, act to suppress granulopoiesis. The resultant neutropenia appears only gradually days or weeks after the institution of drug therapy.

The distinction between drugs that cause neutropenia by an immunologic mechanism and those that do not is of more than academic interest. In the former group agranulocytosis occurs as a sudden, rapidly progressive event that is not dose- or time-related.

Therefore, even frequent blood counts during treatment will not serve to identify the patient in danger. With the more slowly acting agents, progressive neutropenia may be detected in time to stop the offending agents before symptoms appear.

Infiltration of the marrow by tumor cells or deficiencies of folate or B_{12} also may diminish the production of granulocytes. The *Schwachman-Diamond syndrome* of hereditary pancreatic insufficiency and bone marrow hypoplasia customarily results in neutropenia, anemia, and thrombocytopenia. Other features of the syndrome are steatorrhea and growth retardation without the pulmonary infections or abnormal sweat test characteristic of cystic fibrosis. The cause of diminished granulocyte production is unknown but may relate to malabsorption of nutrients essential for granulopoiesis.

Congenital Neutropenias

Suppression of granulopoiesis may be periodic and result in *cyclic neutropenia.* The cycle length is usually about 3 weeks (range 14 to 30 days), and during the neutropenic phase recurrent episodes of stomatitis, fever, or skin infections may be noted. There is evidence of some rhythmic variation of the granulocyte count in normal individuals, and cyclic neutropenia may be the result of a pathologic exaggeration of this normal oscillation.

Suppression of granulopoiesis is more constant in other forms of congenital neutropenia. *Infantile genetic agranulocytosis* is a rare form of neutropenia in which severe, recurrent episodes of bacterial sepsis begin shortly after birth. The pattern of inheritance appears to be autosomal recessive. The phagocytic and bactericidal capabilities of blood monocytes and eosinophils, whose numbers may exceed 50 percent of all circulating leukocytes, offer some degree of compensation for the absence of neutrophils. Nevertheless, death from infection occurs prior to 3 years of age in 80 percent of such children. Granulopoiesis in the bone marrow is arrested, usually at the myeloid stage of development, and it is uncommon to find more than a rare polymorphonuclear leukocyte in either bone marrow or peripheral blood. Under in vitro culture conditions, bone marrow from some patients may exhibit normal granulocyte maturation despite evidence of myelocyte arrest in vivo. However, in 2 brothers granulopoiesis became normal only when bone marrow was incubated with normal plasma, implying the lack of a plasma factor. Infusion of normal plasma subsequently led to an increase in blood neutrophil count in 1 brother, but this has not been successful in other patients with this condition. Occasionally, there may be a transient rise in the blood neutrophil count during episodes of infection. This suggests that the potential for normal granulopoiesis exists, but that there is a deficiency of a maturational factor.

Neutropenia associated with defects of cellular or humoral immunity is usually characterized by reduced or absent production of granulocytes. The most severe of these defects is *reticular dysgenesis* in which there is thymic aplasia or hypoplasia with reduced or absent circulating lymphocytes and impairment of cellular immunity. There is either no evidence of granulopoiesis or an arrest of granulocyte maturation at the myeloid stage. Death from overwhelming bacterial or viral infection usually occurs in early infancy. Cellular immunity is also impaired in the syndrome of *cartilage-hair hypoplasia and leukopenia.* The main features of this syndrome are autosomal recessive inheritance, short-limbed dwarfism, fine sparse hair, normal humoral immunity, neutropenia, lymphopenia, and abnormal lymphocyte function as evidenced by impaired delayed hypersensitivity and reduced lymphocyte transformation in vitro. Affected individuals are unusually susceptible to fatal varicella infections, which is probably as a result of the abnormalities in cellular immunity rather than as a consequence of neutropenia.

Neutropenia may be encountered in *agammaglobulinemia* and in the *hypogammaglobulinemias,* particularly those associated with an increase in IgM. The marrow may be cellular or hypocellular, often with a maturation arrest. Neutropenia, which may be transient, chronic, or cyclic, is usually attributed to decreased production, but in some patients there is also evidence of increased utilization or destruction of granulocytes.

Ineffective myelopoiesis or *myelokathexis* is a condition in which neutropenia is the consequence of impaired granulocyte release from the marrow. An excess of mature granulocytes accumulates within the marrow; many of these have a hypersegmented and abnormally lobulated nucleus and vacuolated cytoplasm. Such cells can be released under the stress of severe infection or following the administration of pyrogen, but their subsequent survival in the peripheral blood is less than normal.

Antibody-mediated destruction of granulocytes may occur in a variety of clinical settings. *Drug-associated neutropenias* have already been mentioned. *Autoimmune neutropenia* may also follow certain viral infections and may be associated with systemic lupus erythematosus, rheumatoid arthritis, or Hashimoto's thyroiditis, or no cause may be found. *Neonatal isoimmune neutropenia* is due to the transplacental passage of a maternal leukoagglutinin to fetal neutrophils. The disorder is analogous to erythroblastosis fetalis, except that granulocytes rather than red cells participate in the reaction with antibody. However it should be emphasized that leukoagglutinins present in the mother's circulation do not invariably cause granulocytopenia in the infant. The infants of certain granulocytopenic mothers, particularly those with systemic lupus erythematosus, also may have neutropenia due to transplacental passage of maternal antibodies. In this case, the same antibody is responsible for neutropenia in both mother and child. The neutropenia resolves as the maternal antibody disappears from the infant's circulation within the first several months of life. Severe, sometimes fatal infections may occur during the neutropenic phase.

Splenic neutropenia refers to the abnormal sequestration and destruction of granulocytes by an enlarged spleen. Splenomegaly due to portal hypertension, storage diseases, or chronic hemolytic anemia, or without recognized cause, may be associated with neutropenia and also, in many instances, with anemia and thrombocytopenia (p. 1197).

Chronic granulocytopenia in childhood is a relatively benign condition, beginning in infancy and lasting for several years. Infections, although frequent, are usually not life-threatening and can be controlled by antibiotic therapy and suitable local measures. The bone marrow is cellular and exhibits normal granulocyte maturation up to the band stage. Mature polymorphonuclear leukocytes are lacking, but when bone marrow is cultured in vitro, mature granulocytes rapidly appear. This has been interpreted as indirect evidence of increased granulocyte destruction in vivo, leading to rapid removal of mature granulocytes. Direct measurements of a shortened granulocyte survival time in this condition are not available.

In *Chediak-Higashi syndrome,* a disorder characterized by albinism, photophobia, nystagmus, excessive sweating, decreased production of tears, and an autosomal recessive mode of inheritance, striking giant lysosomal granules are present in the neutrophils and lymphocytes. There is an increased susceptibility to viral and bacterial infection. Despite their morphologic abnormalities, neutrophils, in this condition, retain their ability to phagocytose and kill bacteria; susceptibility to infection may relate, at least in part, to neutropenia, which usually appears as the disease progresses. Available evidence indicates that neutropenia in Chediak-Higashi syndrome is a consequence of increased destruction of granulocytes within the bone marrow.

Diagnosis

A thorough search for recent exposure to radiation, drugs, or chemicals capable of inducing neutropenia should be the initial step in evaluation. Serial white blood counts obtained weekly for at least 1 month will establish whether neutropenia is transient, cyclic, or chronic. A search should be made for the giant granules of Chediak-Higashi disease, the peculiar nuclear lobulation and cytoplasmic vacuolization characteristic of myelokathexis, and other abnormalities of granulocyte morphology. White blood counts should be obtained in other family members if hereditary neutropenia is suspected. In some cases, it is important to measure the functional competence of granulocytes as well as to quantitate their numbers (p. 325). In addition, since neutropenia may be a component of more general disorders of the immune system, evaluation of humoral and cellular immunity should be carried out in patients with chronic neutropenia. Various infiltrative diseases of the bone marrow that cause neutropenia, such as leukemia, storage diseases, or granulomatous infections, can best be discovered by evaluation of a bone marrow aspirate or biopsy. Evaluation of myelopoiesis in the marrow also aids in distinguishing diminished production of granulocytes from increased destruction.

In the former situation, diminished numbers of myeloid elements or an arrest in myeloid maturation will be found, while in the latter setting evidence of abundant granulopoiesis will be obtained. If destruction of granulocytes is suspected, serologic evidence of leukocyte antibodies should be sought. Muramidase, an enzyme contained within granulocytes and monocytes, is released into the serum when these cells are destroyed. Thus, an increase in the level of muramidase in serum or urine may reflect increased destruction of granulocytes, while low muramidase levels are more compatible with diminished granulocyte production. Other, more precise measures of neutrophil kinetics, such as determination of the survival of $DF^{32}P$-labeled neutrophils, are technically complex and not widely available.

Treatment

An essential component of treatment is removal of any physical or chemical agents implicated in the pathogenesis of neutropenia. Patients with autoimmune neutropenia may benefit from alternate-day prednisone therapy, whereas other forms of neutropenia are generally not responsive to corticosteroids. Some cases may be improved by splenectomy, if splenomegaly is present. However, in other cases splenectomy may merely add the susceptibility to infection associated with asplenia to that which accompanies neutropenia. Infusions of fresh normal plasma have resulted in a rise in the blood neutrophil count in a very few patients with infantile genetic agranulocytosis and cyclic neutropenia, but plasma infusions have been without effect in other patients. In hypogammaglobulinemia associated with an increased serum level of IgM, treatment with intramuscular gamma globulin has been associated with an increase to normal in the blood neutrophil count.

In most patients with neutropenia there exist no known means of favorably influencing the neutrophil count, and treatment is aimed at minimizing the consequences of repeated infections. Vigorous antibiotic therapy of established infections is imperative, but prophylactic use of antibiotics is not beneficial and may be harmful. Evidence is accumulating that granulocyte transfusions are beneficial in the infected neutropenic patient. There are insufficient data to evaluate the potentially favorable influence of bone marrow transplantation in patients with severe neutropenia.

References

Boxer LA, Greenberg MS, Boxer GJ, Stossel TP: Autoimmune neutropenia. N Engl J Med 293:748,1975

Broun GO, Herbig FK, Hamilton JR: Leukopenia in Negroes. N Engl J Med 275:1410, 1966

Cline MJ: The White Cell. Cambridge, Harvard Univ Press, 1975

Gitlin D, Vawter G, Craig JM: Thymic alymphoplasia and congenital aleukocytosis, Pediatrics 33:184, 1964

Higby DJ, Yates JW, Henderson ES, Holland JF: Filtration leukapheresis for granulocyte transfusion therapy. N Engl J Med 292:761, 1975

Hugeley CM Jr: Drug-induced dyscrasias. II Agranulocytosis, JAMA 188:817, 1964

Kauder E, Mauer AM: Neutropenias of childhood, J Pediatr 69:147, 1966

Lux SE, Johnston RB Jr, August CS, Say B, Penchaszadeh VB, Rosen FS, McKusick VA: Chronic neutropenia and abnormal cellular immunity in cartilage-hair hypoplasia. N Engl J Med 282:231, 1970

Morley AA, Carew JP, Baikie Ag: Familial cyclic neutropenia. Br J Haematol 13:719, 1967

Schwachman H, Diamond LK, Oski FA, Khaw KT: The syndrome of pancreatic insufficiency and bone marrow dysfunction. J Pediatr 65:645, 1964

Wreidt K, Kauder E, Mauer AM: Defective myelopoiesis in congenital neutropenia. N Engl J Med 283:1072, 1970

Zuelzer W: "Myelokathexis"—a new form of chronic granulocytopenia. N Engl J Med 270:699, 1964

——— Bajoghli M: Chronic granulocytopenia in childhood. Blood 23:359, 1964

LYMPHOCYTES

PETER R. DALLMAN

Atypical Lymphocytes.   In infants and young children, and less frequently in older individuals, febrile illnesses presumably of viral origin are often associated with atypical lymphocytes or so-called *activated lymphocytes*. Atypical lymphocytes are most common in infectious mononucleosis and cytomegalic inclusion disease. They are also seen after blood transfusions and are believed to represent a cellular immune reaction to a foreign antigen. Atypical or activated lymphocytes are larger than the typical lymphocyte; the cytoplasm is abundant and often irregular in shape; in some cases, cells are characteristically indented and deformed by surrounding red cells. The cytoplasm may be pale blue, or may stain the deep intense blue characteristic of plasma cells; it reflects the presence of abundant ribosomes. The nucleus is also often irregular in shape and may contain nucleoli.

Lymphopenia is discussed in Chapter 9, page 314 (see also normal values, Table 14, p.1178).

Lymphocytosis (see normal values, p.1178, Table 14). Elevated lymphocyte counts commonly accompany febrile illnesses, with respiratory and/or gastrointestinal manifestations. Markedly elevated counts above 50,000/mm^3 are occasionally seen and are commonly associated with pertussis. Although such elevated counts may suggest leukemia initially, the differential diagnosis is rarely difficult. The morphology of the lymphocytes is rarely similar to that of the lymphoblast; splenomegaly, neutropenia, and thrombocytopenia are rarely present, and the bone marrow shows all normal cellular elements and only sometimes a modest increase in the percentage of lymphocytes.

LYMPH NODES

PETER R. DALLMAN

It is characteristic of infancy and childhood that the lymphoid tissues respond to infection with marked swelling and hyperplasia. Moreover, the enlargement may persist for a long time after the primary exciting cause has subsided. This tendency is noted in all parts of the body. In the upper respiratory tract it manifests itself by the hypertrophy of the tonsils and adenoids, but it occurs in any of the external or internal lymph nodes. With advancing age, lymphoid structures become relatively smaller, and the response of regional nodes to acute infections tends to diminish. The tonsils, adenoids, and cervical nodes tend to diminish in size around the seventh or eighth year and may shrink markedly at the time of puberty.

The prominent lymphoid response in early life has been attributed to the fact that the child has not acquired resistance to many infectious agents. It is characteristic not only of tuberculosis but of many pyogenic infections that a first infection meets with little resistance at the portal of entry; it travels rapidly to the regional lymph nodes, where it may cause considerable reaction. A subsequent infection with the same organism finds the body with a certain degree of acquired resistance; the infectious agent encounters difficulty in getting beyond the portal of entry and may never reach the regional lymph nodes.

Acute Adenitis

In young patients swelling and inflammation of regional lymph nodes frequently outlast the original infection or greatly overshadow it in clinical importance. In infants acute adenitis often comes close to being a disease in itself. Cervical adenitis most commonly follows infections of the upper respiratory tract. The occipital, preauricular, and postauricular nodes are affected in scalp infection. Adenitis may also occur in the nodes of the submental region, the axilla, and the groin, or even in internal nodes like the mesenteric and retroperitoneal groups. Suppuration of internal nodes is fortunately exceedingly rare.

In the majority of cases of acute suppurative adenitis, β-hemolytic streptococci are found, but pneumococci, staphylococci, and other organisms occur, depending on the location and specific nature of the primary process. In acute cervical adenitis the responsible organism may or may not be isolated from pharyngeal cultures. Unless an abscess forms, one does not learn with certainty what organism is responsible or whether viable organisms are present at all. Some of the respiratory viruses cause enlargement and tenderness of regional lymph nodes; in these infections suppuration rarely occurs unless there is secondary bacterial involvement.

Some swelling of the node occurs at the height of the primary infection, but the size of the node may increase to 5 cm or more in diameter, even after the primary infection has resolved. Size alone does not indicate whether an abscess will form or the node will shrink rapidly. There is a great deal of variation in clinical course, but the total duration of the process is rarely less than a week, and often the gland remains enlarged for months.

In primary infections of the throat the ensuing adenitis is often bilateral, particularly in young patients, and more than one gland may be involved on each side. Cervical adenitis often causes stiffness of the neck as a protective reaction, which may be as definite as in meningitis. With great swelling, the soft tissues of the lateral pharyngeal wall may be displaced medially, simulating peritonsillar or retropharyngeal abscess, and the voice may be affected. In the most severe examples of adenitis there is marked inflammation of the periglandular tissues, with pain, tenderness, and local heat. In many cases the node remains firm throughout this period; in others it becomes so soft at the height of the swelling as to suggest fluctuation; in still others it becomes frankly fluctuant and may point, requiring drainage. Prompt treatment of adenitis with systemic antibiotics will usually prevent suppuration and as a rule will control constitutional symptoms within 48 hours. Penicillin will cope successfully with most infections caused by hemolytic streptococci or pneumococci. For staphylococcal infections other agents often are required. Local application of cold may give some relief from pain until defervescence commences. Surgical drainage is not indicated unless the node is large and frankly fluctuant. Spreading of the infection to adjacent nodes or development of diffuse cellulitis is often the result of premature surgical intervention, and extensive scarring can occasionally result.

Chronic Adenitis

The most common cause of chronic lymphadenitis is persistent pyogenic infection within the area drained; familiar examples are cervical adenopathy secondary to repeated upper respiratory infections; enlargement of the preauricular, occipital, and cervical nodes in eczema of the face and scalp; and palpable epitrochlear nodes in many nail-biters who develop digital infections. Unexplained generalized enlargement of the lymph nodes should suggest infectious mononucleosis, leukemia, lymphosarcoma, acute reticuloendotheliosis, or syphilis. Tuberculous adenitis of superficial nodes is usually confined to the neck. The possibility of Hodgkin's disease, lymphogranuloma venereum, tularemia, or cat-scratch disease should not be overlooked. Patients with a history of recurrent fever, eczema, staphylococcal infection, and repeated pneumonia should be suspected of having an underlying immune deficiency. In some instances all of the causes mentioned can be excluded, and the diagnosis remains obscure even after biopsy.

LEUKEMIA
Joseph Simone

Cancer kills more children in the United States than any other disease. Leukemia, the most common form of cancer in childhood, is characterized by the abnormal accumulation of immature leukocytes which, at diagnosis, are proliferating more slowly than normal marrow cells. The disease appears to originate in the bone marrow and causes signs and symptoms mainly by impeding production of normal blood cells. Leukemia differs from other forms of cancer in that it is always dis-

seminated at the time of diagnosis and may involve any organ. Except for the apparent site of origin, leukemias and malignant lymphomas have much in common and may behave like different facets of the same basic disease.

TYPES OF LEUKEMIA. Nearly all children with leukemia have the acute variety in which the malignant cells remain primitive and do not mature normally. There are two types of acute leukemia in children, distinguished by the cytologic features of the predominant malignant cell. Acute lymphoblastic (lymphocytic) leukemia (ALL), the more common variety, accounts for about 80 percent of cases; most of the remainder are acute myelogenous leukemias (AML), a cytologically heterogeneous group with cells having granulocytic or monocytic features. AML may be subdivided further by cytomorphology into myeloblastic, myelomonocytic, promyelocytic, monocytic, histiocytic, or erythroleukemic, but there are no major differences in therapy or prognosis. The clinical manifestations of ALL and AML are similar, but it is important to distinguish the two because of the major therapeutic and prognostic differences.

Chronic leukemias are rare in children, accounting for only 2 percent of cases. Chronic myelocytic leukemia may be of the juvenile or adult variety. Some features distinguishing the juvenile type include absence of the Philadelphia chromosome, thrombocytopenia rather than thrombocytosis, less marked leukocytosis, a high percentage of monocytes with monocytic rather than granulocytic colony formation in vitro, and a relative unresponsiveness to chemotherapy. The median survival of children with the juvenile type is about 1 year compared to 3 years for those with the adult type. Chronic lymphocytic leukemia probably does not occur in children.

Neonatal or congenital leukemia may be apparent at birth or may develop several weeks later. While the clinical features and therapy are generally the same as in older children, in neonates the prognosis is much worse, and the proportion with AML is greater. The differential diagnosis includes sepsis, hemolytic disease of the newborn, congenital thrombocytopenia, toxoplasmosis, syphilis, rubella, cytomegalovirus infection, and other malignant tumors. An important consideration in infants with Down's syndrome is a leukemoid picture that may be indistinguishable from AML, except that it may regress spontaneously without specific therapy. In view of this possibility and the relative ineffectiveness of therapy for both AML and neonatal leukemia, chemotherapy is probably not indicated for the infant with Down's syndrome and features of AML.

Etiology

The cause of human leukemia (and lymphoma) is unknown. Because viruses cause leukemia in certain species of mice, birds, and cats, many believe the same is true for man. Thus far, however, efforts to identify a human leukemia virus have failed. Occasional reports of an increased frequency of leukemia in small geographic areas (clusters), the association of Epstein-Barr virus with Burkitt's lymphoma, and the granulomatous features of Hodgkin's disease have spurred the search for an infectious agent. However, neither vertical nor horizontal transmission of these diseases has been demonstrated. Leukemia has been associated with high doses of ionizing radiation, chronic exposure to hydrocarbons such as benzene, and certain drugs such as chloramphenicol. In the pediatric age group, the association of genetic disorders and leukemia is of greatest interest. Children with Down's syndrome, Bloom's syndrome, congenital immunodeficiency syndromes, and Fanconi's anemia are at greater risk of developing leukemia than the population at large. If leukemia develops in one of monozygous twins, there is a 25 percent chance of leukemia in the second twin. Although these associations are of considerable interest, they account for only a small fraction of cases.

Incidence

Acute leukemia occurs at any age, including the newborn period. There is an incidence peak of acute leukemia in the pediatric age group between 2 and 6 years of age. The annual incidence in the United States is about 4 cases per 100,000 children under 15 years of age, resulting in about 4,000 new cases. The incidence is greater among boys than girls (1.3 to 1) and among whites than nonwhites (2 to 1). The higher incidence among white children and in the 2-to 6-year age group is due mainly to the greater incidence of ALL. In AML, there is no peak age incidence in childhood, and the incidence in whites and nonwhites is approximately the same.

PATHOGENESIS

In normal bone marrow, complex control mechanisms regulate the number of stem cells that divide and differentiate as distinguished from those cells that remain to maintain the stem cell pool. In contrast, the leukemic blast cells divide without apparent control, fail to mature, and therefore accumulate. In the marrow, leukemic proliferation inhibits the production of normal erythrocytes, granulocytes, and platelets, which results in anemia, infection, and hemorrhage. Leukemia cells may infiltrate any organ and cause enlargement and dysfunction. The liver, spleen, and lymph nodes are nearly always involved, the kidneys, gonads, meninges, and gut commonly, and the eyes, endocrine glands, heart, and lungs occasionally.

Clinical Manifestations

The symptoms of acute leukemia range from explosive to insidious in onset and days to months in duration. The number and severity of symptoms differ widely from patient to patient. Some asymptomatic patients are diagnosed as having leukemia during routine examination, while others have died within hours of diagnosis from sepsis or hemorrhage. Manifestations

due to the decrease in normal blood cells include fatigue, lassitude and pallor, fever and infection, petechiae, ecchymosis, and mucosal or visceral hemorrhage. Bone and joint pain, sometimes migratory, is a common manifestation of acute leukemia in children and frequently is mistaken for rheumatoid arthritis or rheumatic fever. Hepatosplenomegaly may result in abdominal enlargement and discomfort. Lymph nodes may be moderately enlarged, but massive enlargement is unusual. Less common presenting manifestations due to leukemic infiltration include enlargement of the salivary and lacrimal glands (Mikulicz syndrome), subcutaneous nodules (leukemia cutis), and testicular enlargement. Central nervous system involvement may cause cranial nerve palsy, increased intracranial pressure, or papilledema. Eye findings also include retinal hemorrhage and infiltration of the retina or anterior chamber of the eye. Gingival infiltration with hypertrophy occurs in a small percentage of children and is almost always associated with AML, particularly the monocytic forms. Infiltration of the tonsils, adenoids, or appendix may lead to surgical intervention before the diagnosis of leukemia is suspected.

Laboratory Findings

Initial blood cell counts in children with acute leukemia are not uniform. Although the blood cell count may be completely normal, one usually finds some or all aspects abnormal. The total leukocyte count ranges from less than 1,000 to over 1 million/mm^3, with a median of 13,000/mm^3. Absolute granulocytopenia is common, the majority of the cells being lymphocytes or blasts. The platelet count is usually below normal, often below 50,000/mm^3. The hemoglobin level ranges from 2 to 15 g/dl with an average of 7 g/dl.

Although the diagnosis of leukemia may be made by history, physical examination, and the blood counts, examination of bone marrow is mandatory for confirmation. A bone marrow aspiration is a relatively simple procedure that may be performed in children with an 18-gauge bone marrow needle (see p. 118). The site of aspiration is usually the posterior iliac spine, elsewhere on the iliac crest, or the vertebral spinous process. Sternal aspirations are traumatic and dangerous in small children and are rarely necessary. Bone marrow aspiration generally reveals almost complete replacement with blast forms, with a concomitant reduction of normal cells. Because the marrow is so packed with leukemic cells, aspiration of a satisfactory sample may be difficult or impossible. A bone marrow biopsy may be necessary to establish the diagnosis and to distinguish the condition from aplastic anemia. The infant or pediatric size Jamshidi needle has been most satisfactory for this purpose.

Radiographic abnormalities include transverse radiolucent bands in metaphyses of long bones, periosteal elevation, generalized rarefaction, and, rarely, osteolytic lesions. Enlargement of the kidneys, presumably due to leukemic infiltration, is a common finding; the BUN and serum uric acid may be elevated even before therapy is instituted. Although central nervous system manifestations or cerebrospinal fluid pleocytosis are seen in less than 1 percent of patients, leukemia cells are found at the time of diagnosis in cerebrospinal fluid examined by cytocentrifuge in 2 to 3 percent of patients with ALL and 10 percent of patients with AML. This important finding may have dire prognostic significance. A chest radiograph may reveal an enlarged mediastinal shadow due to infiltration and enlargement of the thymus or perihilar lymph nodes. The leukemia cells of patients with mediastinal involvement often have a surface characteristic in common with thymus-derived lymphocytes, demonstrated by the formation of spontaneous rosettes with sheep erythrocytes (E+ cells). Such patients do not respond to therapy as well as patients without these features.

Differential Diagnosis

A wide variety of disorders may be confused with leukemia. Petechiae, ecchymoses, and unusual bleeding may be observed in idiopathic thrombocytopenic purpura (ITP), hemophilia, and connective tissue disorders, such as the Ehlers-Danlos syndrome. Pancytopenia is a manifestation of aplastic anemia and may be associated with severe infections. Leukocytosis is observed in a wide variety of infections. Children with pertussis may have a marked lymphocytosis for weeks afterward. Infectious mononucleosis can be most difficult to distinguish from leukemia, especially when there is fever, infection, anemia, thrombocytopenia, enlargement of liver, spleen, or lymph nodes, and atypical cells in the blood. Fever with bone and joint pain should also raise the possibility of rheumatic fever, rheumatoid arthritis, and osteomyelitis. Leukemia may be confused with other malignancies, primarily Hodgkin's disease, non-Hodgkin's lymphoma, and neuroblastoma. Neuroblastoma may invade the bone marrow with cells that are difficult to distinguish from lymphoblasts and cause pancytopenia and osteolytic lesions. Other tumors that may invade the marrow, although much less commonly, include rhabdomyosarcoma, Ewing's sarcoma, Wilms' tumor, osteogenic sarcoma, and carcinomas. The reticuloendothelioses also may involve the bone marrow. These conditions often are distinguished from leukemia by other means, but the ultimate test is examination of the bone marrow. A bone marrow biopsy may be necessary since aspiration does not always provide a sufficient sample for interpretation, especially to distinguish leukemia from aplastic anemia. The distinction of acute leukemia from non-Hodgkin's lymphoma with involvement of the bone marrow is difficult, if not impossible, unless the bone marrow was initially free of tumor. Many believe these diseases to be fundamentally the same and to differ only by apparent site of origin.

Therapy

GENERAL. The objective of the initial management of the child with acute leukemia is to relieve symptoms, combat and prevent complications, and begin specific chemotherapy. Prompt and thorough assessment with considered and orderly action will include the following major points: (1) Establish the diagnosis and cytologic type of leukemia. A Wright-stained aspirate of bone marrow usually is sufficient. If the aspirate is inadequate, a bone marrow biopsy may be necessary. Special cytochemical stains may be helpful for distinguishing ALL from AML. Lymphoblastic cells often contain large cytoplasmic granules or "blocks" that stain pink with periodic acid-Schiff. Myeloblasts often contain cytoplasmic granules stained by peroxidase, Sudan black and naphthol AS-D chloroacetate esterase stains: monoblasts may stain like myeloblasts except for a positive reaction to α-naphthol acetate esterase. When the distinction remains unclear despite an adequate marrow sample and special stains, it is preferable to make a presumptive diagnosis of ALL and treat accordingly. This is done for two reasons: ALL is the more common type, and, with its far better prognosis, there is a great deal more to lose from inappropriate therapy. (2) Inform the family of the diagnosis, prognosis, and plan of therapy as soon as possible. (3) Determine the extent of leukemic involvement by measurement of organ enlargement and by radiographs, especially of the chest. The cerebrospinal fluid should be examined for leukemic cells, but the lumbar puncture must be atraumatic in order to avoid contamination with cells from the blood. If this occurs, the lumbar puncture is repeated after several days. (4) Assess liver, kidney, and cardiopulmonary function as well as the fluid and electrolyte status. Manage any disorders and assure adequate hydration to avoid accumulation of catabolic products (especially uric acid) and delayed detoxification and excretion of drugs. The danger of crystalluria and renal shutdown is greatest during the first few days of treatment when leukemic cells are destroyed rapidly. Allopurinol, 100 to 150 mg/m^2/12 hours, given for the first few days will usually prevent accumulation of uric acid, and sodium bicarbonate, 1 g/m^2/6 to 8 hours, may be added to alkalinize the urine because uric acid is highly soluble at alkaline pH. Sufficient fluids are given to assure an adequate urine flow to prevent deposition of purine catabolites, such as xanthine, hypoxanthine, or uric acid. (5) Correct anemia with packed red cell transfusions and treat thrombocytopenic bleeding with platelet transfusions. However, platelets should not be given only because the platelet count is low. Many patients will never have more serious bleeding than petechiae. Persistent mucosal bleeding, a progressive increase in hemorrhage, and suspected hemorrhage in a vital organ, such as the brain, are indications for platelet transfusion. One should be alert to other factors predisposing to hemorrhage, such as tissue infiltration, liver dysfunction, and disseminated intravascular coagulation. (6) Treat infections or suspected infections. Fever may be due to the leukemic process itself, but more often it is due to infection, especially when temperatures exceed 38 C. Infections often are overlooked because normal leukocytes may be insufficient to cause a characteristic inflammatory tissue reaction or because the site is obscure (perineum, paranasal sinuses, gingiva). Thus, the lack of inflammatory leukocytes in urine or cerebrospinal fluid does not rule out infection. The usual search for an organism or site of infection should be instituted and broad-spectrum antibiotic therapy started promptly. Until an organism is isolated, oxacillin and gentamicin may be given by vein every 6 hours, and if *Pseudomonas* infection is suspected, carbenicillin, every 6 hours, is added. Prolonged use of antibiotics should be avoided. If there is no response after 4 to 5 days, antibiotics should be stopped and all cultures repeated. If there is a response, antibiotics may be stopped after the patient has been afebrile for 2 to 3 days. Although most infections respond to antibiotics, the use of granulocyte transfusions may be warranted if fever and sepsis persist, when a suitable donor and appropriate facilities are available. One should avoid deep venipunctures, intramuscular injections, and bladder catheterization, which may cause bleeding and provide foci for infection. (7) Begin specific chemotherapy. The more useful chemotherapeutic agents for acute leukemia are listed in Table 15. The effectiveness of these agents depends on the type of leukemia, the phase of treatment (induction of remission or maintenance of remission), and the biologic variation of the tumor and host. All chemotherapeutic agents may have toxic side effects. To a large extent, toxicity is a function of pharmacokinetics and of factors that may modify the toxic threshold, such as infection and irradiation.

RATIONALE OF SPECIFIC THERAPY.   Ever since Jacob Furth and colleagues demonstrated, 40 years ago, that a single leukemia cell transplanted into a histocompatible normal mouse could proliferate and kill the animal, the ultimate goal of therapy has been the destruction of every last leukemia cell. It is debatable whether this is feasible, or even necessary. Possibly, host defenses are capable of controlling the growth of small numbers of leukemia cells. It has been estimated that patients with acute leukemia have 10^{12} leukemia cells, weighing 1 kg, at diagnosis and that reducing that number to 10^9 (1 g) or less induces remission. The ideal therapeutic agent would rapidly destroy all leukemia cells, with no toxic effects on normal cells. Also, a method for detecting and quantitating residual leukemia cells during remission would provide a precise guide for therapy. Since no such agent or method currently exists, therapy must depend on giving agents in dosages and schedules that are more toxic for leukemia than for normal cells. The leukemocidal effectiveness of therapy given during remission can be judged only by the duration of remission and whether remission continues after therapy is stopped.

SPECIFIC THERAPY OF ACUTE LYMPHOBLASTIC LEUKEMIA (ALL).   The drugs of choice for remission induction of ALL are prednisone, 40 mg/m^2/day in divided doses, and vincristine, 1.5 mg/m^2/week. These agents destroy leukemia cells rapidly, with minimal toxicity and little impairment of normal hematopoiesis, and are effective in almost all children with ALL. Although the addition of other effective agents, such as asparaginase or daunorubicin, may not significantly influence the attainment of remission, the destruction of an additional fraction of leukemia cells may favorably influence the duration of remission. Pyogenic infection may be rapidly fatal during this period and should be treated vigorously and promptly. Leukopenia is not a valid reason for withholding vincristine and prednisone.

About 90 percent of children with ALL will achieve complete *remission* after 4 weeks of therapy. Complete remission means that there is no detectable leukemia in the blood, bone marrow, and cerebrospinal fluid; the hematopoietic activity of the bone marrow has returned; and there is no evidence of serious infection or complications. If no further therapy is given after this point, the patient will relapse within a few months, because viable leukemia cells persist, even though they are undetectable by current methods. The remainder of therapy, therefore, is aimed at continuing the destruction of the invisible leukemia cells and maintaining a state of remission for as long as possible. As soon as the patient attains remission, some modern regimens employ a 1- to 12-week intensive course of chemotherapy, which may consist of the same agents used for remission induction or continuation therapy. This is an attempt to achieve a rapid additional reduction of the leukemia cell population while the patient is better able to tolerate chemotherapy and before resistant clones emerge. Whether or not this intensive course is given, all programs require administration of continuation or *maintenance chemotherapy*. The most effective agents for this phase of therapy are methotrexate and mercaptopurine, although some regimens include other agents such as cyclophosphamide, cytosine arabinoside, or periodic "pulses" of vincristine and prednisone.

An important innovation of therapy during remission is the use of *preventive central nervous system therapy*. As the duration of remission and survival has lengthened, the frequency of central nervous system involvement has increased, often occurring while the bone marrow has remained in remission. In recent years the central nervous system has become the initial site of relapse in approximately one-half of children. The apparent reason for this complication is the failure of antileukemic drugs to penetrate the meninges and cerebrospinal fluid in effective concentrations. On the theory that leukemia cells are in the meninges at the time of diagnosis, "preventive" central nervous system therapy attempts to eradicate these cells while they are few in number and undetectable by clinical manifestations. Early studies have shown that administration of 500 or 1,200 rads of craniospinal irradiation or a single dose of intrathecal methotrexate is ineffective for preventing this complication. However, 2,400 rads craniospinal irradiation or 2,400 rads cranial irradiation with simultaneous intrathecal methotrexate reduce the frequency of initial relapse in the central nervous system to less than 10 percent. A common schedule of central nervous system therapy begins a few days after remission is achieved

TABLE 15. Chemotherapeutic Agents Commonly Used for Acute Leukemia

Agent Common Dose	Type	Most Effective Use	Marrow Toxicity	Immuno-Suppression	Other Toxic Effects
Prednisone 40 mg/m²/day	Corticosteroid ? Membrane effect	Remission induction-ALL	No	Yes	Salt and water retention, increased appetite, hypertension, hyperglycemia, protein catabolism, osteoporosis
Vincristine 1.5 mg/m²/wk	Periwinkle alkaloid Inhibits mitosis by preventing spindle formation	Remission induction-ALL	Little	Yes	Peripheral neuropathy, constipation, jaw pain, hair loss
Methotrexate 20-40 mg/m²/wk	Folate antagonist Blocks folic acid reductase, inhibits purine synthesis	Remission maintenance-ALL Intrathecal therapy	Yes	Yes	Mucosal ulceration, hepatic cirrhosis, encephalopathy, megaloblastosis
Mercaptopurine and thioguanine 50-100 mg/m²/day	Purine analogues Block purine synthesis	Remission maintenance-ALL Remission induction and maintenance-AML	Yes	Yes	Mucosal ulceration, hepatic dysfunction
Cyclophosphamide 200-300 mg/m²/wk	Alkylating agent Cross-links DNA, inhibits replication	Remission maintenance-ALL Remission induction and maintenance-AML Limited efficacy in both	Yes	Yes	Nausea, vomiting, hair loss, hemorrhagic cystitis
Cytosine arabinoside 50-300 mg/m²/wk	Pyrimidine analogues Inhibits DNA polymerase	Remission induction and maintenance-AML Less effective for ALL	Yes	Yes	Nausea, vomiting, mucosal ulceration, hepatic dysfunction
Asparaginase 10,000-50,000 units/m²/wk	Enzyme Deprives cell of asparagine	Remission induction-ALL	Little	Yes	Allergic reactions, anaphylaxis, hepatitis, pancreatitis, hypofibrinogenemia
Daunorubicin and adriamycin 20-50 mg/m²/wk	Anthracycline antibiotics Bind DNA, prevent transcription	Remission induction-AML and ALL	Yes	Yes	Mucosal ulceration, hair loss, myocardial damage

and employs a 2.5 -week course of cranial radiation (the ports must include *all* meninges) and simultaneous intrathecal methotrexate, 12 mg/m^2 twice weekly for five doses (maximum single dose, 15 mg). Another method being tested for prevention of central nervous system leukemia is the use of intrathecal methotrexate monthly with aggressive, multiple-agent systemic chemotherapy. Preventive central nervous system therapy is associated with side effects such as temporary hair loss, meningismus, back pain, nausea, and headache. Several weeks after completion of irradiation to the brain, a self-limited syndrome of somnolence and lassitude may appear, which lasts several days to weeks. Rare but serious side effects associated with intrathecal methotrexate administration include leukoencephalopathy and transverse myelitis with paraplegia. Brain irradiation followed by intravenous methotrexate in doses exceeding 50 mg/m^2/week has also been associated with leukoencephalopathy.

Chemotherapy during remission must be given in maximum-tolerated dosages to achieve the best possible result. A useful guide for dosage adjustment is to keep the patient free of serious side effects, with the total leukocyte count between 2,000 and 3,500/mm^3 and the total granulocyte count above 500/mm^3. Individual tolerance varies considerably from patient to patient and time to time.

Relapse is the reappearance of leukemia at any site in the body. With modern combination chemotherapy and adequate preventive central nervous system therapy, relapse occurs most often in the bone marrow. Hematologic relapse may be heralded by the reappearance of anemia, granulocytopenia, thrombocytopenia, enlargement of the liver or spleen, bone pain, fever, or a sudden decrease in chemotherapy tolerance. Since relapse results from the growth of a leukemia cell population that has become resistant to chemotherapy, therapy must be changed and an attempt made to reinduce remission.

Second remissions are achieved in most patients with ALL, but since the most effective agents for maintaining remission will have been used and the cells will have become resistant, there is no very effective regimen to maintain the second remission. Consequently, the second remission usually is shorter than the first, and eventually there will be resistance to all chemotherapeutic agents.

Central nervous system relapse may occur despite the use of preventive therapy. With routine lumbar punctures every 3 months, the diagnosis usually is made by finding leukemia cells in the cerebrospinal fluid before symptoms of increased intracranial pressure develop. Administration of intrathecal methotrexate, 12 mg/m^2/week, will usually clear leukemia cells from the cerebrospinal fluid within a few weeks. In addition to intrathecal methotrexate, intrathecal cytosine arabinoside, 30 to 60 mg/m^2, and craniospinal irradiation in palliative doses of 500 to 1,500 rads also have been used. Central nervous system leukemia seldom is eradicated with these measures, and recurrence is common. With higher doses of irradiation (2,500 to 3,500 rads),

it may be possible to eradicate this disease. Once the cerebrospinal fluid has cleared, one may give intrathecal chemotherapy monthly in an attempt to prevent or delay exacerbation.

Patients may have repeated episodes of central nervous system leukemia while bone marrow remains in initial remission. There is no need for major changes in the systemic chemotherapy in this circumstance. However, dosage adjustment may be necessary with the added toxicity to the bone marrow of intrathecally administered drugs that diffuse into the peripheral blood.

Testicular leukemia is another common form of recurrence and is found in 5 to 10 percent of boys with ALL. It should be suspected whenever there is painless swelling or hardness of the testis. The diagnosis is confirmed by needle biopsy, which in some centers is done routinely in both testes because of the significant chance of bilateral disease. Radiotherapy is the treatment of choice. As with central nervous system involvement, testicular relapse may occur independent of relapse elsewhere. However, simultaneous relapse at more than one site is common. Therefore bone marrow, cerebrospinal fluid, and testes should be examined carefully when relapse is found at any one site.

SPECIFIC THERAPY OF ACUTE MYCLOGENOUS LEUKEMIA (AML). Unfortunately, therapy for AML has been far less successful than that for ALL. Remission is successfully achieved in 30 to 70 percent of patients; it lasts an average 6 to 9 months, and the average survival is about 1 year. The most effective chemotherapeutic agents for AML are cytosine arabinoside, daunorubicin, thioguanine, mercaptopurine, and vincristine. For AML, however, there is no therapeutic parallel to the rapid effectiveness and low toxicity of vincristine and prednisone for ALL. Because therapy is less effective and the therapeutic index narrower, complications are more frequent, and supportive measures assume even greater importance. Several chemotherapeutic regimens have been moderately successful, but none is sufficiently superior to warrant specific recommendation.

Complications

INFECTION. Children with leukemia are more susceptible to infections due to the myelosuppressive and immunosuppressive effects of the disease and of the therapy. During periods of granulocytopenia, the child is more likely to develop sepsis, pneumonia, and cellulitis. Gram-negative sepsis is especially devastating. Organisms such as *Pseudomonas, Klebsiella,* and *E. coli* may enter the blood-stream through small intestinal ulcerations, infected gingiva, perineal lesions, or paronychia. Although once thought to be characteristic of *Pseudomonas* sepsis, cutaneous septic emboli and septic shock can occur with a wide variety of organisms. Disseminated fungal infections are more likely to occur in patients with prolonged exposure to broad-spectrum antibiotics or corticosteroids.

Although any infection may occur at any time in the

course of the illness, or during remission, life-threatening infection is more likely to be caused by nonbacterial organisms. *Pneumocystis carinii* pneumonia has become increasingly frequent. Predisposing factors include malnutrition, thoracic irradiation, and aggressive combination chemotherapy. The cardinal features are fever, tachypnea, cyanosis, and cough, with a paucity of auscultatory findings. The chest roentgenogram most often reveals diffuse alveolar infiltration, but the initial film may show lobar, perihilar, or no apparent infiltration hours before the diffuse pattern emerges. All patients have some degree of arterial hypoxia. The organism is identified by special stains of material obtained by needle aspiration or open biopsy of the lung; if it is untreated, the mortality approaches 100 percent. Even with administration of pentamidine isethionate or trimethoprim and sulfamethoxazole and optimal supportive care, the mortality is 25 percent.

Varicella should be avoided diligently and significant exposures reported immediately so that chemotherapy may be stopped. Zoster immune globulin (0.3 mg/kg) or plasma (10 ml/kg) may modify the disease when given within 48 hours of exposure. Although this infection has a benign course in most leukemic children, about one-third develop visceral dissemination with pneumonia, hepatitis, or meningoencephalitis, which are fatal in about one-fourth. Thus, varicella has a fatal outcome in about 1 of 12 children with leukemia.

A wide variety of organisms may cause *meningoencephalitis,* an especially important infection because it is easily confused with central nervous system leukemia or the transient effects of central nervous system therapy. Headache, meningismus, fever, and cerebrospinal fluid pleocytosis and protein elevation may occur with all three conditions. Examination of cerebrospinal fluid cells with Wright's stain usually distinguishes normal from leukemic cells, especially with cytocentrifuge preparations, but additional samples may be required.

TOXIC EFFECTS OF THERAPY. In addition to marrow and immune suppression, chemotherapy and radiotherapy may cause a wide range of immediate and late side effects. The more common toxic manifestations are shown in Table 15. Both the toxic and the therapeutic effects of giving two or more agents may be additive or synergistic, especially with the potent suppressors of marrow and immune function, such as thioguanine, mercaptopurine, cytosine arabinoside, and cyclophosphamide. The combination of corticosteroids and asparaginase may cause nonketotic hyperglycemia of sufficient severity to require insulin therapy. Vomiting tends to be more severe when cyclophosphamide and cytosine arabinoside are given together. Encephalopathy is more likely to occur with high-dose intravenous methotrexate following brain irradiation. Cyclophosphamide-induced hemorrhagic cystitis is more frequent following pelvic irradiation.

With the increasing duration of remission and survival, the possible late effects of therapy have become more important. In addition to the potential carcinogenic and mutagenic effects of therapy, functional impairment of the gonads, liver, brain, heart, or any organ

may emerge years later. Thus, new methods of therapy will be judged not only by efficacy, but also by the price paid in short- and long-term toxicity.

EXPERIMENTAL THERAPY. New chemotherapeutic agents are developed continually, but few remain sufficiently promising after in vitro and animal testing to warrant trials in humans, and a mere handful prove to be of significant clinical value. Two other forms of therapy under study in humans are noteworthy. The goal of immunotherapy is to stimulate or direct the patient's own immune system to destroy residual malignant cells. Immunization during remission with live BCG organisms is a form of nonspecific or adjuvant therapy aimed at boosting the immune system. Despite initial claims of efficacy, there is no convincing evidence that BCG is effective for ALL. BCG has apparently prolonged survival in patients with AML but has not significantly improved the duration of remission. Some explain this observation as evidence that BCG stimulates hematopoietic stem cells and, consequently, increases tolerance to chemotherapy rather than directly causing leukemia cell destruction. BCG and other bacteria have been injected along with leukemia cells in an attempt to stimulate a tumor-specific immune reaction, but results have not been impressive thus far.

Another form of therapy under study is *bone marrow transplantation,* which has a twofold rationale. First, since marrow toxicity limits dosage in therapy, marrow transplantation would permit administration of therapy that destroys both the leukemia and the normal marrow. Second, if the patient's immunity is completely suppressed so that the marrow graft is not rejected, the graft may take and produce immunocompetent cells that destroy any remaining leukemia cells in the recipient because the leukemic cells are recognized as foreign. Unfortunately, the leukemia often recurs, opportunistic infections are frequent, and the grafted cells may attack normal tissues, causing graft-versus-host disease, any of which may be fatal. An intriguing and disturbing observation is the development, in several successfully grafted patients, of leukemia in the *donor* cells. One likely explanation is that a leukemogenic agent remains active in the recipient. Although some promising results have been achieved in marrow transplantation, it is a costly and difficult procedure that requires considerably more development in specialized centers.

Prognosis

The prognosis for children with ALL has changed considerably in the past 10 years. With the most effective regimens reported to date, over 90 percent of children will attain remission and 50 percent will survive 5 years or more free of any evidence of leukemia. In fact, therapy has been stopped in some long-term survivors, and most have continued to enjoy remission for months or years. Although there is no way to predict accurately which child will have such a gratifying response, a number of prognostic factors have been identified. Features present at diagnosis that are associated with a poor prognosis include a very high leukocyte count (greater than 100,000/mm^3), central nervous system involvement, mediastinal enlargement, age less than 2 or over 10 years, and massive hepatosplenomegaly. For children with AML, the response to therapy is so poor that individual features have little prognostic significance. However, marked thrombocytopenia and leukocytosis are associated with a poorer prognosis.

PATIENT FAMILY PHYSICIAN RELATIONSHIP. A child with leukemia and his family face an extremely difficult time. They need a physician who is hopeful, truthful, compassionate, understanding, accessible, informative, and knowledgeable. While they understand that several physicians may be involved in the care, they prefer and need one physician who can assume ultimate responsibility and give direction and is willing to give continuous comprehensive care. Whether that physician is a hospital-based specialist, pediatrician, internist, or generalist is less important than his ability and willingness to take consistent responsibility for the myriad needs of the patient.

The child should be told of plans and procedures in language that is understandable and appropriate for him or her. Withholding the diagnosis from children, especially those of school age, is a self-defeating and fruitless exercise, since children today often guess or are told the truth by a playmate. To provide some idea of the nature of leukemia, it is useful to describe it by analogy. One may compare the disease to the overgrowth of a farmer's field by weeds (leukemia cells), preventing the growth and export of crops (normal blood cells). Since the weeds cannot be removed manually, it is necessary to give chemicals that destroy the weeds and allow the normal crops to grow. Physicians and family often mistakenly believe that the child is as concerned with the possibility of death as they are. In fact, children are most concerned with the immediate implications of leukemia, for example, whether there will be separation from family, pain, disfigurement, lengthy hospitalization, or missed time at school. It is important for the child to learn to trust the physician and other medical personnel. He should never be told that a procedure will be painless when it is not. Some patients and parents become very knowledgeable about the disease and may know as much as or more than the physician about certain details; instead of creating resentment, this should be viewed as an asset that provides another observer on the scene to aid the physician in management. Physicians may become emotionally attached to a patient or his family. This need not be avoided, so long as the physician sustains the necessary patient–physician relationship and sound medical judgment. The physician must realize that, above all, the patient and family want in him an expert physician, not a pal or buddy.

When the leukemia becomes resistant to therapy and death is imminent, the patient and his family need a physician more than ever to help the child to die. The family must be made to understand that there is no known effective therapy remaining, and that the goal of management must change from destroying leukemia cells to providing comfort. Once this decision is made, chemotherapy, transfusions, antibiotics, blood counts, and other laboratory tests are no longer necessary. The child need be hospitalized only if proper supportive care or pain medication cannot be given at home. For pain that cannot be controlled by oral analgesics, morphine is the drug of choice and is most effective when given by continuous intravenous infusion. Children themselves seldom ask the physician at this time whether they are going to die, probably because they already know or suspect the truth and do not want to confront the physician with an uncomfortable question. Should the child ask, however, he probably knows already, and to deny this is worse than useless. Although guidelines can be provided for management of children during this difficult period, the medical staff must adopt an approach suitable to the particular patient and circumstances. Most of all, the patient needs palpable demonstration that that the medical staff is readily available and willing to listen, to comfort, to provide any possible service, and simply to be there. Even patients who are at home should not be abandoned; telephone communication can provide welcome support to the family.

Plans should be made to maintain communication with the family after the child dies. A discussion of autopsy findings is a useful vehicle, but one should take the opportunity to determine whether any family member, especially a sibling, is having problems eating or sleeping (nightmares) or difficulty in functioning at work or at school; sometimes professional help is indicated.

References

Aur RJA, Simone JV, Hustu HO, Verzosa MS: A comparative study of central nervous system irradiation and intensive chemotherapy early in remission of childhood acute lymphocytic leukemia. Cancer 29:381, 1972

———Simone JV, Hustu O, Verzosa MS, Pinkel D: Cessation of therapy during complete remission of childhood acute lymphocytic leukemia. N Engl J Med 291:1230,1974

———Simone J, Hustu HO, Walters T, Borella L, Pratt C, Pinkel D: Central nervous system therapy and combination chemotherapy of childhood lymphocytic leukemia. Blood 37:272, 1971

Feldman S, Hughes WT, Daniel CB: Varicella in children with cancer: seventy-seven cases. Pediatrics 56:388, 1975

Goldin A, Sandberg JS, Henderson ES, Newman JW, Frei E III, Holland JF: The chemotherapy of human and animal acute leukemia. Cancer Chemother Rep 55:309, 1971

Hagbin M, Tan CC, Clarkson BD, Mike V, Burchenal JH, Murphy ML: Intensive chemotherapy in children with acute lymphoblastic leukemia (L-2 protocol). Cancer 33:1491, 1974

Holland JF, Frei E III (eds): Cancer Medicine. Philadelphia, Lea & Febiger, 1973

———Glidewell O: Chemotherapy of acute lymphocytic leukemia of childhood. Cancer 30:1480, 1972

Hughes WT, Feldman S, Cox F: Infectious diseases in children with cancer. Pediatr Clin North Am 21:583, 1974

Hustu HO, Aur RJA, Verzosa MS, Simone JV, Pinkel D: Prevention of central nervous system leukemia by irradiation. Cancer 32:585, 1973

Lascari AD: Leukemia in childhood. Springfield, Ill, Charles C Thomas, 1973

Price RA, Jameson PA: The central nervous system in childhood leukemia. II. Subacute leukoencephalopathy. Cancer 35:306, 1975

———Johnson WW: The central nervous system in childhood lymphocytic leukemia—I. The arachnoid. Cancer 31:520, 1973

Simone J: Acute lymphocytic leukemia in childhood. Semin Hematol 11:25, 1974

———Holland E, Johnson W: Fatalities during remission of childhood leukemia. Blood 39:759, 1972

Smith KL, Johnson WW: Classification of chronic myelocytic leukemia in children. Cancer 34:670, 1974

MALIGNANT LYMPHOMAS

Joseph Simone

Malignant lymphomas are a form of cancer arising in lymph nodes or other lymphoid tissue such as the tonsils, thymus, or Peyer's patches. In comparison to leukemia, they are relatively rare in children, constituting about 10 percent of all childhood neoplasms. The lymphomas customarily are divided into Hodgkin's and non-Hodgkin's types with further subdivision by histopathology and extent of disease.

HODGKIN'S DISEASE

Hodgkin's disease is characterized by a progressive, painless enlargement of regional lymph nodes. It is considered to be unicentric in origin, arising in a single node or anatomic group of nodes. The usual mode of progression is a predictable pattern of extension to contiguous nodes. Subsequent involvement of other tissues, including the spleen, liver, bone marrow, lung, and other organs, may occur and thereby account for many of the protean manifestations.

Etiology and Epidemiology

Although an infectious agent has been suspected because of the granulomatous appearance of the involved lymphoid structures, the etiology is unknown. Despite certain clinical manifestations and laboratory abnormalities, that suggest an inflammatory process, Hodgkin's disease is regarded as a neoplastic process. Its association with such disorders as lupus erythematosus, rheumatoid arthritis, infectious mononucleosis, and impaired immune responsiveness has led to an intense search for common or related predisposing factors. Additionally, an infrequent but apparently causal relationship has been noted between the administration of hydantoin derivatives and the development of pseudolymphoma. Although this type of lymphoid hyperplasia has certain histologic features common to Hodgkin's disease and other lymphomas, the absolute criteria for malignancy have been lacking, and regression of the lymphadenopathy has occurred following withdrawal of the offending agent. More recently, however, in a group of patients receiving anticonvulsant therapy the criteria of malignant lymphoma were definitely met, with persistence and progression of lymphoid pathology following cessation of antiseizure therapy. Whether the atypical hyperplasia observed during anticonvulsant therapy is precancerous or whether the agents are truly carcinogenic in certain sensitive individuals requires further clarification.

Hodgkin's disease is rare before the age of 5 years, with a gradual rise in incidence until adolescence, after which there is a striking increase that persists through age 30. Its incidence is greater among males throughout the pediatric age group, with a male-to-female ratio of 3 to 1 for children 5 to 11 years old, and 1.5 to 1 for patients 11 to 19 years old. The reported incidence of Hodgkin's disease in the 0 to 39-year age group in the United States and Western Europe is twice that observed in Australia and five times that in Japan. The incidence of Hodgkin's disease is somewhat lower among blacks than Caucasians.

Several studies have shown that close relatives of a patient with Hodgkin's disease have a slightly but significantly increased risk of developing the disease compared with the population at large. Cases have been reported in parent and child, siblings, husband and wife, and unrelated neighbors, often within months or a few years of one another. Although these reports tempt one to invoke a causative environmental agent, convincing evidence is lacking.

Pathology

Although any organ may be involved, Hodgkin's disease characteristically is a disease of lymph nodes. A *sine qua non* of histologic diagnosis is the presence of neoplastic reticulum cells (Hodgkin's cells), the most easily recognized form of which is the multinucleated Reed-Sternberg cell. The histologic features may include sparse to abundant concentrations of neoplastic, inflammatory, reactive, and stromal cells, lymphocytes, collagen, and fibrous tissue. The distinctive combination of features provides a means for histologic classification that has prognostic and therapeutic relevance. The Rye classification, currently used most often, includes four major categories: (1) lymphocytic predominance, (2) nodular sclerosis, (3) mixed cellularity, and (4) lymphocytic depletion. They are listed in relative prognostic order from best to worst. To some degree, the anatomic distribution, clinical extent (stage) of disease, pattern of spread, and age-related frequency differ by histologic type.

Clinical Manifestations

The signs and symptoms depend upon the site and the extent of involvement. Most commonly the first manifestation is a painless, progressive enlargement of a superficial lymph node or group of nodes, especially in the neck, where 60 percent of cases occur initially. Axillary and inguinal adenopathies are less frequent. Mediastinal adenopathy may be suggested by a persistent nonproductive cough, although this site of involvement may be initially asymptomatic. Unexplained abdominal pain may be due to enlargement of retroperitoneal nodes. Systemic symptoms of low-grade fever or intermittent fever lasting several days with afebrile periods of days or weeks (Pel-Ebstein fever), anorexia, nausea, and weight loss are usually absent when the disease is localized; pruritus, a relatively common symptom in adults, is an infrequent complaint in children, even with extensive involvement.

Differential diagnosis of the adenopathy includes chronic pyogenic and tuberculous adenitis, cat-scratch disease, infectious mononucleosis, and hydantoin hypersensitivity, as well as other malignant lymphomas, reticuloendothelioses, or metastatic tumors, especially those arising in the nasopharynx or neck. It is essential to obtain an adequate amount of tissue by biopsy for histologic examination. One must be wary of the sometimes malignant appearance of "reactive hyperplasia," especially in lymph nodes that drain areas of chronic infection such as those in the inguinal area.

Hematologic Findings

There is no characteristic abnormality of the blood in Hodgkin's disease. In localized disease, the complete blood count is usually normal. With more extensive disease, patients may have anemia or polymorphonuclear leukocytosis; in advanced disease leukopenia and lymphopenia often occur and Reed-Sternberg cells may occasionally be seen in the peripheral blood. Because these cells are rare in bone marrow aspirates, bone marrow biopsy is usually necessary to document the presence or absence of involvement; bone marrow biopsy is recommended for children with clinical stage III or IV disease, radiographic bone lesions, hematologic abnormalities, or elevation of serum alkaline phosphatase. Although not specific, elevations of the erythrocyte sedimentation rate and serum copper can be useful indicators of disease activity when done serially during remission.

Clinical Staging

A careful clinical, laboratory, and radiographic evaluation is mandatory for accurate staging. In addition to a detailed history and thorough physical examination, a complete blood cell count, urinalysis, posteroanterior and lateral chest films, skeletal survey, excretory urogram, bipedal lymphangiogram, and liver function tests, including BSP dye excretion, should be obtained. In the presence of hilar adenopathy, whole lung tomograms should be performed.

The staging of Hodgkin's disease by extent of disease provides a rational basis for determining therapy and defining prognosis. The following staging definitions are based on the original classification by Peters as modified at a 1971 workshop at Ann Arbor, Michigan.

Stage I. Involvement of a single lymph node area (I), or a single extralymphatic site (I_E).

Stage II. Involvement of two or more lymph node areas on the same side of the diaphragm (II), or localized involvement of one extralymphatic organ or site and one or more lymph node regions on the same side of the diaphragm (II_E).

Stage III. Involvement of lymph node regions on both sides of the diaphragm (III), which may also include localized extralymphatic involvement (III_E), splenic involvement (III_S), or both (III_{ES}).

Stage IV. Diffuse or disseminated involvement of one or more extralymphatic sites with or without lymph node involvement. To include all patients with liver or bone marrow involvement. All stages are subclassified A or B to indicate absence or presence of unexplained fever, night sweats, or unexplained loss of 10 percent or more of body weight in the preceding 6 months.

There has been considerable debate over the advisability and value of staging laparotomy, which usually includes biopsies of periaortic nodes, mesenteric nodes, and liver, as well as a splenectomy. Staging laparotomy is the only reliable technique for determining the extent of abdominal disease. With this procedure, as many as one-half of patients thought to have stage I or II disease will be found to have stage III or IV disease. The risk of inaccurate staging and inadequate or excessive therapy must be weighed against the trauma, surgical risk, and the risk of fulminating sepsis after splenectomy. In many centers, this procedure is performed in all patients except those in whom therapy would not be changed regardless of the findings. Others would exclude children with stage I disease only if an exhaustive and completely satisfactory diagnostic workup proved negative and if the localized primary involvement was in a particularly favorable location, for example, high in the right neck.

Therapy

As new data accumulate, treatment for Hodgkin's disease continues to be modified. Specific therapy depends on the anatomic location, the clinical stage, and the histologic type, and requires the coordinated efforts of radiotherapist, chemotherapist, pathologist, and surgeon, as well as megavoltage radiation equipment. *Radiotherapy* is the cornerstone of treatment for clinical stages I, II, and IIIA; 3,500 to 4,500 rads in 3 to 4 weeks is considered the usual tumoricidal dose. Radiotherapy is given to involved areas and often is extended to adjacent lymphoid tissues or to most lymphoid tissues (total nodal radiotherapy), depending on the sites of known tumor, the clinical stage, and histologic type. Regardless of clinical staging, radiotherapy may be indicated for potentially dangerous local disease, such as airway obstruction, spinal cord compression, or vertebral disease that may lead to spinal cord compression.

The primary form of therapy for clinical stages IIIB and IV is multiple-agent chemotherapy, although radiotherapy may also have a role. The major types of chemotherapeutic agents employed for Hodgkin's disease include the alkylating agents (nitrogen mustard, cyclophosphamide, chlorambucil, procarbazine, nitrosoureas [BCNU, CCNU]), vinca alkaloids (vincristine, vinblastine), antibiotics (adriamycin, bleomycin), corticosteroids (prednisone), and dimethyltriazenoimidazole carboxamide (DTIC). These agents may be used singly only for palliation of advanced relapsing Hodgkin's disease. In all other instances multiple agents are given. The more widely used combinations are MOPP (nitrogen mustard, vincristine [Oncovin], procarbazine and prednisone) and MVPP (in which vinblastine is substituted for vincristine). The drugs are given in 14-day courses followed by 14-day rest periods for at least 6 cycles. Other effective combinations include adriamycin, bleomycin, vinblastine, and DTIC; or CCNU, adriamycin, and vinblastine, which are especially useful for patients with disease refractory to MOPP.

Radiotherapy alone is sufficient for clinical stage I and some forms of stage II disease; the best results for stage IIIA have been achieved with combined chemotherapy and radiotherapy, and chemotherapy alone is suitable for most patients with stage IV disease. However, a number of therapeutic questions have not been resolved: Should chemotherapy be given for stage IIB in addition to extended-field radiotherapy? For patients with stage IIIA disease receiving chemotherapy, should radiotherapy be limited to involved fields or extended? Does limited or delayed radiotherapy have a role in stage IIIB and IV disease?

The risk of immediate and late toxic effects of radiotherapy or combination chemotherapy is considerable and is compounded when both are used. Many of the complications of leukemia and its therapy also occur in patients with Hodgkin's disease. Even before therapy is given, patients with Hodgkin's disease often have defects in delayed hypersensitivity, and during immunosuppressive therapy, patients experience an increased frequency of viral, fungal, and protozoal infections. Varicella zoster and *Pneumocystis carinii* infections may be fatal. The initial therapeutic effort offers the best chance for cure of Hodgkin's disease, and it is imperative that treatment be delivered by those best able to provide all necessary facets of specific and supportive therapy. For the management of Hodgkin's disease, the reader is referred to the excellent paper by Kaplan and Rosenberg and the classic and comprehensive monograph by Kaplan.

Prognosis

Hodgkin's disease can no longer be considered an invariably fatal disease. If one considers all clinical stages and histologic types, about 80 percent of patients survive 5 years or more, 60 percent survive relapse-free for 5 years or more, and 50 percent survive relapse-free for 10 years or more. This is probably true for children as well as adults. In recent years the prognosis for patients with clinical stage IIIA disease has approached that of stages I and II. However, 5-year relapse-free survival is achieved in only 25 percent of patients with stage IV disease.

References

Kaplan HS: Hodgkin's Disease. Cambridge, Harvard Univ Press, 1972
————Rosenberg SA: Management of Hodgkin's disease. Cancer 36:796, 1975

Smith KL, Johnson D, Hustu O, Pratt C, Fleming I, Holton C: Concurrent chemotherapy and radiotherapy in the treatment of childhood and adolescent Hodgkin's disease. Cancer 33:38, 1974

NON-HODGKIN'S LYMPHOMA (NHL)

These lymphomas are heterogeneous by histopathology, site of origin, and clinical manifestations. Formerly termed lymphosarcoma, reticulum cell sarcoma, or giant follicular lymphoma, classification (see below) according to predominant cell type and architectural pattern has been adopted widely. NHL in childhood differs significantly from Hodgkin's disease and from NHL in adults with regard to clinical behavior, pathology, mode of spread, and response to treatment. In childhood NHL, the malignant cells appear undifferentiated or poorly differentiated, and the pattern of infiltration is diffuse; therapy is less effective and control of the primary tumor is more difficult; dissemination occurs earlier and more often, and consequently the overall mortality rate is higher. However, intensive combined-modality treatment with radiation and combination chemotherapy has improved results in recent years. In children, NHL is 3 to 4 times more common than Hodgkin's disease. The prototype patient is a boy aged 9 to 11, reflecting the male-to-female ratio of 3:1 and the older average age than in acute leukemia.

Pathology

The histologic classification of NHL continues to be the subject of considerable interest and investigation. The Rappaport classification subdivides NHL into (1) undifferentiated, Burkitt and non-Burkitt, (2) lymphocytic, well or poorly differentiated, (3) mixed, histiocytic and lymphocytic, and (4) histiocytic. Each is classified as nodular (follicular pattern) or diffuse. This classification has little prognostic significance in childhood NHL because the mixed and nodular types, which have a more favorable prognosis, are extremely rare in children. New approaches to classification which may be more important are based on in vitro characteristics of the tumor cells, such as the capacity for blastic transformation in response to mitogens, the ability to synthesize immunoglobulin, and surface features in common with thymus-derived lymphocytes. Thus, mediastinal NHL may arise from thymic or T cells and abdominal NHL from bone marrow or B cells. The prognostic significance of these types in childhood NHL has not been defined.

Clinical Manifestations

The clinical presentation of NHL depends on the anatomic site(s) and extent of involvement. NHL may appear to arise in the abdomen, mediastinum, head-neck region (tonsils, adenoids, sinuses), peripheral lymph nodes, or central nervous system, and involvement of the orbit, breast, skin, bone, or reproductive organs is not rare. Primary disease in the abdomen often presents as intussusception. Mediastinal involvement may obstruct major blood vessels or the airway with a risk of sudden death due to respiratory arrest. Systemic symptoms not attributable to local infiltration are rare and may include low-grade fever, malaise, and anorexia. The interval from onset of any symptoms to diagnosis averages 2 to 6 weeks, even in children presenting with widespread disease, malignant ascites, or pleural effusion.

A multifocal presentation involving the jaw and abdomen is characteristic of a variant of NHL known as the *Burkitt type.* It is rare in America but endemic in tropical Central Africa and New Guinea. The diagnosis of Burkitt's lymphoma requires a combination of features, since no one symptom or sign is pathognomonic. The child with Burkitt's lymphoma often presents with jaw tumor, abdominal swelling, paraplegia, or an extranodal tumor in an unusual location. Involvement of spleen, mediastinum, or peripheral lymph nodes and the development of a frankly leukemic picture are most unusual in the African Burkitt type in contrast to other types of childhood NHL. The histologic pattern features uniform dark-stained primitive cells interspersed with an abundance of pale-stained macrophages (starry-sky pattern). Tumors from African patients with Burkitt's lymphoma contain the Epstein-Barr virus genome, whereas this is not demonstrated consistently in American cases.

Development of diffuse bone marrow involvement is common in children with NHL, but central nervous system involvement is relatively rare. Diffuse marrow infiltration develops in about one-third of children and is especially common in those who initially have primary tumors in the mediastinum. No objective method exists for distinguishing acute leukemia from NHL with diffuse bone marrow involvement at initial presentation. For practical purposes, one may diagnose NHL in patients who have less than 25 percent tumor cells in the presence of normal hematopoietic elements in the bone marrow and an otherwise compatible clinical presentation; a diagnosis of acute leukemia is made in patients with a lymphoreticular malignancy who have over 25 percent tumor cells in the bone marrow at initial presentation. The features of central nervous system involvement in NHL are similar to those observed in ALL, but focal neurologic findings, such as paraplegia and cranial nerve palsy, are more common in NHL. The presence of either a leukemia-like picture or central nervous system disease generally precludes long term survival.

Like Hodgkin's disease, the diagnosis of NHL requires a good biopsy of the primary tumor mass or regional nodes. Although the diagnosis may be suspected on the basis of cytologic examination of malignant ascites, pleural effusion, or bone marrow, diagnosis by these methods is less secure and informative. Rarely, mediastinal tumors threaten respiratory obstruction, and initiation of life-saving radiotherapy or chemotherapy may be necessary prior to lengthy diagnostic studies or biopsy. Differential diagnosis includes rhabdomyosarcoma, Ewing's tumor, neuroblastoma, histiocytosis, Hodgkin's disease, and other benign and malignant causes of adenopathy.

Other abnormalities depend on the site and extent of disease. Roentgenograms may show a mediastinal mass and pleural effusion, ascites, displacement of retroperitoneal structures, renal enlargement, or intestinal filling defects, often in the ileocecal region. The blood count is usually normal in the absence of marrow involvement. Elevations of serum uric acid and lactic dehydrogenase is common with massive disease. Because involvement of the bone marrow and central nervous system is so common, a bone marrow aspirate and lumbar puncture should be done as soon as the diagnosis of NHL is suspected. Liver and spleen scan, brain scan, bone scan, and whole-body ^{67}Ga scans may reveal clinically unsuspected sites of involvement.

Staging

The lymphangiogram is a useful means of assessing disease below the diaphragm in NHL as in Hodgkin's disease. Exploratory laparotomy may be necessary for diagnosis but is of little value for staging purposes because of the high frequency of disseminated disease, the noncontiguous patterns of involvement, and the scant likelihood that the results of such a procedure will alter treatment. However, as in Hodgkin's disease, the clinical stage or extent of NHL at diagnosis has prognostic significance. About one-half of patients have tumor limited to a single lymph node group or anatomic site, and these have a far better prognosis than those with more extensive involvement. Application of the Ann Arbor system developed for Hodgkin's disease is awkward in NHL because of the virtual absence of a true stage III NHL in children and the poor prognosis with the disease when it is confined to the mediastinum (stage I). Children with tumor involving an entire body cavity, such as an abdominal primary with omental metastases and ascites, and those with central nervous system or bone marrow involvement also have a very poor prognosis. Until a better method of clinical staging is developed for childhood NHL, the Ann Arbor system is of some use if the above qualifications are kept in mind.

Treatment

The treatment of NHL consists of megavoltage irradiation of the tumor plus combination chemotherapy. Extensive experience with radiotherapy alone as primary management for NHL has demonstrated convincingly that there is an unacceptably high rate of relapse outside the irradiated field, usually at extranodal sites, such as pleura or bone marrow. Unlike Hodgkin's disease, therefore, even children with stage I or II NHL should receive combination chemotherapy because of the great likelihood of occult disease. Nonetheless, radiotherapy is an important therapeutic modality for NHL and should be used with curative intent (3,500 to 4,000 rads) for all patients with stage I and II disease. For patients with evidence of generalized disease, radiotherapy may be directed to areas of bulky tumor to effect rapid regression with portals limited to the involved field. Extended-field irradiation as the primary mode of therapy, as used in Hodgkin's disease, is unsuitable for NHL. Patients with primary tumor of the abdomen require whole-abdominal irradiation, usually to a dose of 2,400 rads, with additional radiation to the area of demonstrable tumor. Radiotherapy may be given for palliation of advanced disease or for the immediate relief of distressing or life-threatening local symptoms, such as respiratory obstruction, paraplegia, cranial nerve palsies, or intestinal obstruction.

Combination chemotherapy should be instituted with agents of established efficacy such as vincristine, cyclophosphamide, prednisone, and adriamycin in maximally tolerated doses. Complete remission is the immediate goal and usually requires 6 to 9 weeks of chemotherapy. Therapy must be started cautiously in those patients because massive tumor lysis may be expected to produce hyperuricemia, hyperkalemia, and possible renal shutdown. Adequate hydration and allopurinol should be employed prophylactically.

Although infections at initial presentation are less common than in acute leukemia, they can be just as serious and should be treated promptly and vigorously.

After complete remission has been achieved, it is necessary to continue therapy. While the value of preventive central nervous system therapy has not been established, in some centers a regimen of intrathecal chemotherapy is given. However, the risk of initial relapse in the central nervous system is small for patients with stage I disease and does not appear to justify preventive therapy. The chemotherapy given during remission is similar to that used for acute leukemia. Most regimens employ some combination of mercaptopurine, methotrexate, and cyclophosphamide, or repeated courses of the same agents used for induction of remission.

Relapse in NHL often occurs within 6 months. Relapse after 12 months of complete remission is uncommon when chemotherapy is continued for the usual total of 18 to 24 months. Lymphomatous relapse, leukemic conversion, or central nervous system invasion often signal a short duration of subsequent survival. When leukemic transformation occurs, the chemotherapeutic approach is the same as one would use for hematologic relapse of acute leukemia.

Prognosis

The duration of survival for children with NHL is improving. An initial therapeutic approach based on palliation with single-agent chemotherapy or low-dosage radiation is no longer justifiable. About 75 percent of children with localized (stage I) NHL survive the disease, excluding patients with mediastinal primary disease who have a high rate of relapse despite intensive combination therapy. Approximately 40 to 50 percent of patients with regional disease (stage II) may be cured. The outlook for patients with more extensive disease is poor, with only a 10 to 20 percent survival.

Cyclic multiple-agent regimens, which are inherently very toxic and require highly skilled supervision, have had promising results in recent years and deserve further investigation.

References

Aur RJA, Hustu HO, Simone JV, Pratt CB, Pinkel D: Therapy of localized and regional lymphosarcoma of childhood. Cancer 27:1328, 1971

Glatstein E, Kim H, Donaldson SS, Dorfman RF, Gribble JT, Wilbur JR, Rosenberg SA, Kaplan HS: Non-Hodgkin's lymphomas. VI. Results of treatment in childhood. Cancer 34:204, 1974

Lemerle M, Gerard-Merchant R, Sarrazin D, Sancho H, Tehernia G, Flamant F, Lemerle J, Schweisguth O: Lymphosarcoma and reticulum cell sarcoma in children. A retrospective study of 172 cases. Cancer 32:1499, 1973

Murphy SB, Davis LW: Hodgkin's disease and the non-Hodgkin's lymphomas in childhood. Semin Oncol 1:17, 1974

——— Frizzera G, Evans AE: A study of childhood non-Hodgkin's lymphoma. Cancer, 36:2121, 1975

Wollner N, Leiberman P, Exelby P, D'Angio G, Burchenal J, Fang S, Murphy ML: Non-Hodgkin's lymphoma in children: results of treatment with LSA$_2$-L$_2$ protocol. Br J Cancer 31 (Suppl 2):337, 1975

SPLEEN

PETER R. DALLMAN

The thin abdominal wall in young children makes it easier to palpate the spleen than in adults. In addition, the spleen is proportionally larger in the neonatal period and is palpable in about 30 percent of normal newborns and 15 percent of infants below 6 months of age. Subsequently, the normal incidence of a palpable spleen diminishes gradually.

CIRCULATION. Blood enters the spleen through the splenic artery, which branches promptly into trabecular arteries. Each trabecular artery branches into central arteries which are surrounded by a collar of white pulp. The white pulp is made up of masses of T and B lymphocytes, which are segregated into separate zones. The main branch of the central artery continues through the white pulp into the red pulp where it branches into an open circulation, without well-defined capillary walls. This open circulation consists of a spongelike reticular network within which lie numerous elongated venous sinuses separated by cylindrical cellular cords (splenic cords). The venous sinuses drain into the trabecular veins, which return the blood to the portal circulation. This drainage system usually contains no valves, so that the pressure in the red pulp is the same as in the portal vein.

Most blood cells traverse this splenic labyrinth rapidly by percolating through the reticular network directly to the venous sinus. Smaller numbers of cells are diverted for sorting in either the white or red pulp. Lymphocytes are delivered to the outer marginal zone of the white pulp, and over a period of hours they either migrate slowly back to the para-arterial lymphatics or they are sorted into respective T cell and B cell zones. The T cells form the matrix of the white pulp in which globular masses of B cells are embedded. The diverted red cells are forced through such small slits between the splenic cords in the red pulp that particulate matter, such as nuclear remnants, is retained and plucked out of the cell. The red cells are also screened by fixed macrophages which remove old, abnormal, and antibody-coated cells (see below). When the spleen is enlarged and functioning abnormally, the proportion of red cells that is forced to traverse the slits between the cords increases, and the amount of time that the average blood cell remains within the spleen is lengthened substantially. The resulting hypoxic and acidotic cellular environment may lead to premature cell destruction (see below).

FUNCTION. The functions of the spleen include (1) removal or sequestration of red cells, platelets, and lymphocytes; (2) removal of particulate elements from the cytoplasm of young red blood cells; and (3) resistance to infection by filtration of bacteria from the blood and by the production of opsonizing antibody. *Red cell removal* is through the action of phagocytic tissue macrophages, which line the splenic cords and venous sinuses of the red pulp. These are considered part of the reticuloendothelial (RE) system. The splenic portion of the RE system is more sensitive to antibody-coated or metabolically abnormal cells than is any other part of the body.

A related function of the spleen is culling or *removal of particulate elements,* especially from young red cells. The red cell has an average diameter of 7.5 μm, but is extraordinarily flexible. This property is put to its greatest test in the spleen when the red cell traverses the slits between the splenic cords, which may spread apart no more than 1 μm. Large or rigid cytoplasmic particles, such as nuclear remnants (Howell-Jolly bodies), precipitated globin (Heinz bodies), ferritin-containing vesicles, and mitochondria, are pinched off and left behind to be eliminated by phagocytosis. Usually, the red cell membrane seals over after the particulate elements have been plucked out without any damage other than the loss of a minute amount of membrane. When there are many abnormal cells in slow transit across the splenic cords, the circulation through the spleen as a whole is slowed, and macrophages increase in number. These events lead to splenic enlargement and increased splenic sequestration of cells.

When the spleen is removed, other reticuloendothelial organs, particularly the liver, gradually take over the normal function of removing senescent red cells and platelets so that their life span is not prolonged. When a splenectomy is performed for idiopathic thrombocytopenic purpura, the liver may continue to remove antibody-coated platelets from the circulation and account for the persistence of thrombocytopenia. After splenectomy, nucleated red cells may appear in the circulation, and there is often a thrombocytosis and a moderate lymphocytosis that is sometimes transient but occcasionally long lasting.

RESISTANCE TO INFECTION. The spleen plays two roles in the resistance to infection. It first filters out certain encapsulated pneumococci and other organisms. Subsequently it produces a specific antibody that serves as an opsonin and promotes clearance of the remaining organisms from the blood. The filter function of the spleen assumes critical importance when the body has not been previously challenged to develop opsonizing antibody, as for example against a new infecting strain of pneumococci.

INFECTION AFTER SPLENECTOMY AND IN CONGENITAL AND FUNCTIONAL ASPLENIA. Individuals without a functioning spleen are subject to a form of sepsis that is rapid in onset and unusually severe and that can lead to sudden death if not recognized and treated promptly. Pneumococci are responsible in more than half of such cases, *Haemophilus influenzae* in about a quarter, and *Staphylococcus aureus,* group A streptococci, coliforms, and meningococci in most of the remaining cases.

Asplenia

The diagnosis of anatomic or functional asplenia may be first suspected from the presence of red cell inclusions, particularly Howell-Jolly bodies, on a peripheral blood smear. Confirmation of the diagnosis is obtained when no splenic shadow is noted on scanning over the abdomen after the infusion of [99]technetium- sulfur colloid, which is normally taken up by the entire RE system. Functional asplenia occurs in children with sickle cell anemia, initially due to stasis of sickled cells in the splenic circulation and later to malfunction of the splenic reticuloendothelial cells (p. 1153).

Congenital absence of the spleen may occur alone or, more commonly, in association with partial situs inversus or anomalies of the heart and great vessels. The most frequent lesions of the heart are endocardial cushion defects, pulmonary artery stenosis or atresia, and large atrial septal defects (p. 1359).

The risk of fulminant infection postsplenectomy or in functional asplenia depends on the child's age and the nature of his basic disease. The risk is greatest in the first few years; it diminishes gradually but never quite disappears. Older children and adults are thought to be safer because they are more likely to have developed opsonizing antibodies through previous exposure to a larger number of bacterial strains. In children with post-traumatic splenectomy, idiopathic thrombocytopenic purpura, and spherocytosis, the risk of infection is relatively low. In contrast, life-threatening infections are more common in sickle cell anemia and thalassemia, probably because other parts of the RE system are involved by the disease and can compensate less well for loss of the spleen. The risk is even greater in diseases which affect other aspects of immune defenses, eg, Wiskott-Aldrich syndrome.

MANAGEMENT. The management of functional or anatomic asplenia lies mainly in prevention. First, elective splenectomy for hemolytic disease due to conditions such as spherocytosis can usually be postponed beyond the age of 3 to 5, except in the severest cases. When the splenectomy becomes necessary, immunization of patients with polyvalent pneumococcal vaccine shows promise of offering partial protection, especially to young children who have not previously had the opportunity to be exposed to many of the potentially pathogenic strains.

Prophylactic penicillin may be given continuously as a single daily dose for 1 to 2 years after splenectomy in children who are not old enough to voice complaint of mild symptoms; with older children, parents are advised to administer penicillin at the first suspicious sign of a febrile and/or respiratory illness. Close medical supervision is essential.

Hypersplenism

Blood formation in the spleen is normally restricted to the last two-thirds of gestation, but the hematopoietic potential of the organ is preserved when the need arises. Severe anemia or hypoxemia may lead to extramedullary blood formation with splenic enlargement; this is more marked in infants and children than in adults (Fig. 1, p. 1109). In some instances the benefits of increased blood production are partly or completely offset by a concomitant increase in sequestration and elimination of cells. This has been termed hypersplenism.

Hypersplenism is characterized by splenomegaly accompanied by anemia, thrombocytopenia, and neutropenia, either singly or in combination. The bone marrow shows normal or increased cellularity with increased numbers of immature forms in one or more of the three cell lines. The pathogenesis can be described as an exaggeration of the trapping and/or phagocytic function of the spleen directed at one or more of the particulate elements of the blood. It can occur with splenomegaly due to a wide variety of causes.

Hypersplenism in respect to red cells may be suspected by demonstrating the rapid destruction of normal transfused erythrocytes and documented by the accumulation of excess radioactivity in the spleen after transfusion of the patient's own red cells tagged with ^{51}Cr or in the course of a ferrokinetic study with ^{59}Fe. Hypersplenism in respect to platelets is suspected when infusion of radioactively labeled platelets (the patient's own, if a count of over 50,000 permits) is followed by detection of increased radioactivity over the spleen and recovery of less than 50 percent in the circulation. Normally only about 30 percent of the infused platelets marginate in the spleen and other sites.

In conditions where the cells that cause splenic enlargement also accumulate in the marrow, eg, Gaucher's disease, kinetic studies are necessary to determine to what extent marrow invasion or splenic destruction is responsible for a decreased number of circulating red cells, white cells, or platelets.

Splenomegaly may be a helpful clue in arriving at a diagnosis. Causes of splenic enlargement can be categorized under the headings of infection, hemolytic disease, extramedullary hematopoiesis due to bone marrow suppression, portal and splenic hypertension, malignancy, and storage disease. Splenic enlargement is often associated with evidence of hypersplenism, but this is rarely the patient's most serious clinical problem.

Acute and chronic *infection* and *inflammatory disease* commonly cause splenomegaly as part of a more generalized hyperplasia of lymphatic and reticuloendothelial tissues. In the newborn, splenomegaly as part of the *torch syndrome* (p. 149) may characterize intrauterine infections with toxoplasmosis, rubella, cytomegalovirus, and herpes simplex. At other ages, splenomegaly is a common feature of infectious mononucleosis, malaria, subacute bacterial endocarditis, tuberculosis, and many other infections. Chronic inflammatory diseases such as systemic lupus erythematosus and rheumatoid arthritis often are associated with splenomegaly.

In some *hemolytic diseases*, such as hereditary spherocytosis, the spleen may be enlarged through engorgement of the phagocytic reticuloendothelial cells by senescent red cells and their breakdown products. In more severe hemolytic anemias, such as thalassemia and hemolytic anemia of the newborn, extramedullary hematopoiesis in the spleen is often an additional cause of massive enlargement. Extramedullary hematopoiesis is also marked in conditions of *bone marrow suppression or obliteration* , such as osteopetrosis.

In *portal hypertension* the spleen becomes enlarged in response to an elevated blood pressure in the portal system, and hypersplenism may develop. An additional consequence of increased portal pressure is the development of collateral circulation that includes esophageal and gastric varices. The most serious clinical problems related to splenic enlargement are those associated with thrombocytopenia due to splenic trapping. Since most cases of severe portal hypertension are associated with advanced liver cirrhosis, a depression of coagulation factors is usually combined with the thrombocytopenia. This makes it all the more difficult to arrest the esophageal bleeding initiated by the mechanical factors of elevated blood pressure in fragile varices.

In the early stages of portal hypertension the spleen may be soft in consistency and may shrink temporarily after an acute bleed from esophageal varices. Later there is fixed enlargement due to fibrosis and proliferation of reticular tissue (see diagnosis and treatment of portal hypertension, p. 1104, and bleeding manifestations of liver disease, p. 1213).

The forms of *malignancy* most commonly associated with splenomegaly are leukemia, lymphoma, and Hodgkin's disease. In all cases the cause of the splenic enlargement is infiltration with tumor rather than extramedullary hematopoiesis in response to invasion of the bone marrow. Benign cysts of the spleen may also result in a palpable spleen or splenic mass.

The *storage diseases* associated with splenomegaly include Gaucher's disease and Niemann-Pick disease. In Gaucher's disease (p. 749) the basis of the splenomegaly is believed to be the failure of the phagocytic reticuloendothelial cells to rid themselves of the sphingolipid, glucosyl ceramide. The glucosyl ceramide accumulates in the RE cells, primarily from the membranes of phagocytosed red blood cells, but it cannot be broken down due to the congenital lack of the catabolic enzyme, glucocerebrosidase. The characteristic Gaucher cells present in bone marrow, liver, and spleen are simply the glucosyl-ceramide-laden tissue macrophages. The appearance of these cells is characteristic, but in thalassemia major and in chronic myelogenous leukemia there may be a small number of enlarged macrophages with a similar appearance. In an analogous manner, in Niemann Pick disease, macrophages with foamy cytoplasm are laden with sphingomyelin due to lack of the catabolic enzyme, sphingomyelinase.

Malformations

Accessory spleens are found so frequently in the region of the splenic hilus as to justify their being regarded as a normal variant rather than a true malformation. Following surgical removal of the spleen, any remaining splenic tissue is prone to undergo compensatory hypertrophy and to take over the spleen's functions. When splenectomy is undertaken as a therapeutic measure, as in some of the blood dyscrasias, removal of accessory spleens is recommended for lasting success. Accessory spleens can often be detected by scanning after an injection of [99]technetium-sulfur colloid.

INJURY

Rupture of the spleen may follow major trauma to the abdomen. Splenic injury may also follow relatively minor trauma in instances where the spleen is enlarged in the course of some illness, such as infectious mononucleosis. Immediately after injury the patient may faint, but he usually revives within a short time and often appears to suffer from nothing more than superficial contusions. Within the next few hours there may be evidence of shock and internal hemorrhage and sometimes fever and vomiting. Although the physical findings vary greatly according to the nature and severity of the injury, persistent or increasing abdominal pain and tenderness are characteristic. In most instances this is especially marked in the left upper quadrant, but it usually extends in some degree to the entire abdomen. Rebound tenderness and muscle spasm are usually noted. Pain in the left shoulder may be constant or may be elicited only on abdominal palpation. Shifting dullness or other signs of free fluid are rare, even when the amount of blood recovered at operation is as great as 500 ml. A leukocytosis of about 20,000/mm^3 is commonly found.

In some instances, an initial trauma lacerates the spleen or causes subcapsular bleeding without complete rupture. The patient may complain of symptoms of moderate severity at the time of injury. A few days to months later, a second, sometimes very mild injury results in rupture with all the symptoms of the acute abdominal catastrophe.

Rupture of the spleen occasionally is observed in the newborn from trauma suffered either during a difficult delivery (breech) or in the course of resuscitation. It is most likely to occur in infants with severe erythroblastosis fetalis. The objective symptoms are similar to those described. Abdominal hemorrhage may be suspected when there is evidence of shock and a distended, rigid abdomen.

Either at the time of the original injury or in the course of surgery, splenic tissue may be seeded through the peritoneal cavity, forming implants which thrive under the stimulus of splenectomy. This condition, commonly called *splenosis*, has no serious clinical consequences but may produce a bizarre picture at subsequent laparotomy.

Splenic rupture or subcapsular hemorrhage can be diagnosed by scanning over the spleen after an injection of [99]technetium-sulfur colloid. Splenectomy is the only treatment for rupture of the spleen, since the risk of death from shock and hemorrhage is great in unoperated patients.

References

Chen LT, Weiss L: The role of the sinus wall in the passage of erythrocytes through the spleen. Blood 41:529, 1973

Crosby WH: Splenectomy in hematologic disorders. N Engl J Med 286:1252, 1972

Eraklis AJ, Kevy SV, Diamond LK, Gross RE: Hazard of overwhelming infection after splenectomy in childhood. N Engl J Med 276:1225, 1967

Jacob HS: Hypersplenism: mechanisms and management. Br J Haematol 27:1, 1974

Kabins SA, Lerner C: Fulminant pneumococcemia and sickle cell anemia. JAMA 211:467, 1970

Pearson HA, Cornelius EA, Schwartz AD, Zelson JH, Wolfson SL, Spencer RP: Transfusion-reversible functional asplenia in young children with sickle-cell anemia. N Engl J Med 283:334, 1970

Robinson MG, Watson RJ: Pneumococcal meningitis in sickle cell anemia. N Engl J Med 274:1006, 1966

Weiss L, Tavassoli M: Anatomical hazards to the passage of erythrocytes through the spleen. Semin Hematol 7:372, 1970

HEMOSTASIS
WILLIAM E. HATHAWAY

Hemostasis depends upon an interaction between blood vessel structure, platelets, and the coagulation system. Even though these are difficult to separate physiologically, hemostasis will be discussed from two aspects: the vessel–platelet interaction and the coagulation system.

VESSEL–PLATELET INTERACTION. The series of reactions involved in the formation of a hemostatic plug is the primary means by which bleeding is arrested at the capillary and small vessel level (Fig. 19). It can be summarized as follows: *vascular injury* exposes the endothelial collagen fibers and provides a site for the *adhesion* of platelets. Adhesion also requires the presence of plasma coagulation factors, including the von Willebrand factor. As the platelets adhere to the vessel wall, their granular contents are discharged into the adjacent plasma. *Aggregation* of additional platelets is facilitated by the substances that are released, including ADP, that causes nearby platelets to aggregate, and serotonin, that increases the contractility of the vessel. *Plug formation:* Concurrently in the coagulation system, the thromboplastic material (tissue factor) released as a result of vascular injury initiates extrinsic clotting, which results in the formation of thrombin. This process is facilitated by the release of phospholipid (platelet factor 3) and a heparin-neutralizing factor (platelet fac-

THE HEMOSTATIC PLUG

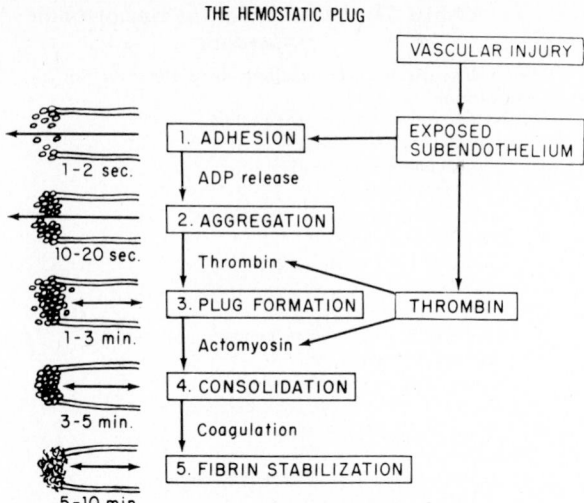

FIG. 19. The hemostatic plug. Platelet adhesion to subendothelial tissue structures, especially collagen, basement membrane and microfibrils, follows within a second or two of any break in the endothelium. (From Harker: Hemostatis Manual, 1974, p 5. Courtesy of FA Davis.)

TABLE 16. Nomenclature of Blood Coagulation Factors

I	Fibrinogen
II	Prothrombin
III	Thromboplastin, tissue factor
IV	Calcium
V	Proaccelerin, accelerator globulin
VI	Number not now used
VII	Proconvertin
VIII	Antihemophilic factor (AHF); antihemophilic globulin (AHG)
IX	Plasma thromboplastin component (PTC); Christmas factor
X	Stuart-Prower factor
XI	Plasma thromboplastin antecedent (PTA)
XII	Hageman factor
XIII	Fibrin-stabilizing factor

Platelet factors
Platelet factor 3 (PF-3) —phospholipoprotein
Platelet factor 4 (PF-4) – antiheparin

tor 4) from the platelets. *Consolidation and Fibrin stabilization:* Fibrin is formed, and the mass of platelets and fibrin is pulled together into a tight hemostatic plug by a contractile protein within the platelet, thrombosthenin, and by the stabilization of polymerized fibrin (see below). This mechanism for arrest of bleeding at the small vessel level can be independent, to a large extent, of the coagulation system; hence the observation that the bleeding time, which measures platelet plug formation, is usually normal in hemophilia.

COAGULATION. The coagulation system, consists of a sequence of reactions by serine proteases on their specific substrates, and is shown in simplified form

in Figure 20. The accepted nomenclature for the coagulation factors is listed in Table 16. Coagulation may be initiated by either of two pathways. *Intrinsic coagulation* is initiated by the surface activation of factor XII, accelerated by the presence of prekallikrein (Fletcher factor), which links the coagulation system to the kinin system, and progresses through the stepwise activation of factors XI and IX. Activated factor IX forms a complex with VIII, phospholipid, and calcium to activate factor X. The reactions in this pathway are time-consuming and account for most of the delay in in vitro clotting tests. *Extrinsic coagulation* is initiated by the release of tissue factor (a complex lipoprotein) from parenchymal and vascular tissues, which leads to the formation of a complex of factor VII, tissue factor, and calcium, which activates factor X. This pathway is extremely rapid in its action. The last steps in coagulation are shared in common by the two pathways. The formation of thrombin is mediated by the action of activated factor X, factor V, and phospholipid. Thrombin then

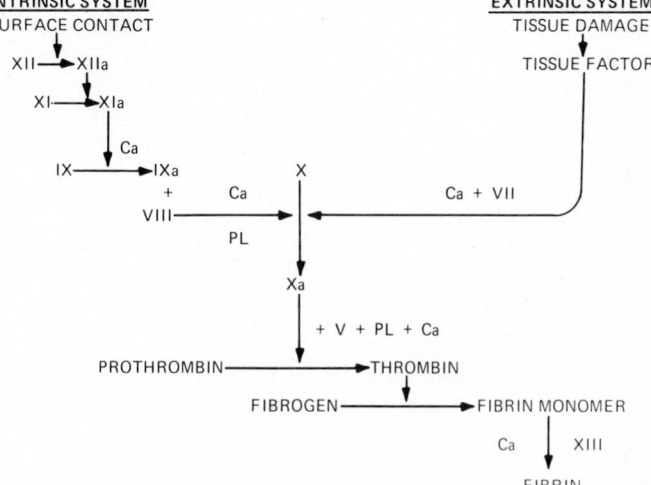

FIG. 20. Scheme of blood coagulation, see Table 1 for coagulation factor designations. The suffix a denotes the activated factor with enzyme activity. Ca = calcium ions; PL = phospholipid.

accelerates the polymerization of fibrinogen to fibrin. The fibrin clot that finally results is stabilized by a cross-linking enzyme, factor XIII.

FIBRINOLYSIS. The fibrinolytic system helps to limit formation of excessive clot at the site of injury. The system is activated by a number of substances that convert inert precursor, plasminogen, to the fibrinolytic enzyme plasmin. When fibrin is degraded by plasmin, the resulting "fibrin degradation products" (FDP) then inhibit further conversion of fibrinogen to fibrin. FDP are removed from the blood over a period of hours by the liver.

INHIBITORS. Protease-inhibitors work to keep the activated clotting process in control. Among the most important is an α_2-globulin designated antithrombin III (AT-III), which is also the heparin cofactor. AT-III, antiplasmin, and other antiproteases bind the activated serine proteases irreversibly and thereby neutralize their procoagulant and fibrinolytic effect.

BLEEDING TENDENCY

Initial Diagnostic Approach: Use of Screening Tests

The history and physical findings are important in the classification of a patient with a bleeding tendency. A carefully constructed family pedigree may indicate the hereditary nature of the bleeding manifestations (sex-linked in VIII and IX deficiency; autosomal dominant in von Willebrand's disease; recessive in factor V and VII deficiency). Characteristic of the hemophilias are bleeding at circumcision (although not invariably), deep hematomata, and hemarthroses if the disorder is severe. In contrast, thrombocytopenia and abnormalities of platelet function frequently are manifested by epistaxis, bruising, and petechiae. Patients with factor XIII deficiency characteristically have umbilical cord bleeding in the neonatal period. Prolonged hemorrhage following tooth extractions or after nasopharyngeal surgery, such as tonsillectomy or adenoidectomy, is a reliable symptom of an abnormal bleeding tendency. Negative personal history and family history are rare in a child with hereditary hemorrhagic disease, unless the child is very young or the disease is quite mild. Nevertheless, one should be aware of the possibility that mild hemophilia may result in bleeding only with severe trauma or major surgery.

Children with positive family history of bleeding or significant hemorrhagic episodes in the past, or those who are scheduled for major surgery (including tonsillectomy and adenoidectomy), should have certain laboratory tests performed to determine and classify a potential bleeding diathesis. These screening tests should also be done in any patient who shows active bleeding without known cause. Experience has indicated that a carefully performed battery of tests will aid in diagnosis of the hemostatic disorders shown in Table 17. A study of Table 18 indicates that all of the tests should be done so as not to miss a specific disor-

TABLE 17. Classification of Hemorrhagic Disorders

Disorders due to abnormalities of platelet–vessel interaction
  Hereditary hemorrhagic telangiectasia
  Connective tissue diseases
    Osteogenesis imperfecta
    Marfan's syndrome
    Ehlers-Danlos syndrome (cutis hyperelastica)
  Secondary vasculitis
    Systemic lupus erythematosus
    Sepsis
  Scurvy
  Schönlein-Henoch syndrome (anaphylactoid purpura)
Thrombocytopenias
  Increased destruction or trapping
    Idiopathic thrombocytopenic purpura
    Immunologic drug purpura
    Splenomegaly
    Acute infection and inflammatory disorders
    Hemolytic uremic syndrome
    Thrombotic thrombocytopenic purpura
    Giant hemangioma
    Cyanotic congenital heart disease
    Intravascular coagulation
    Isoimmune thrombocytopenias
    Wiskott-Aldrich syndrome
  Decreased production
    Leukemia and other malignancies
    Aplastic anemias
    Drugs and toxins
    Hereditary thrombocytopenias
    Thrombopoietin deficiency
Disorders of platelet function
  Thrombasthenia or Glanzmann's disease
  Bernard-Soulier giant platelet syndrome
  Platelet release abnormality
    Storage pool disease
    Abnormal release mechanism
  von Willebrand's disease
  Acquired disorders
Disorders of coagulation system
  Congenital deficiencies
    Factor VIII (classic hemophilia A, AHF deficiency) and von Willebrand's syndrome
    Factor IX (PTC deficiency, Christmas disease)
    Factor XI (PTA deficiency)
    Factor XIII (fibrin-stabilizing factor deficiency)
    Factor XII (Hageman trait)
    Fletcher factor (prekallikrein deficiency)
    Factor I (afibrinogenemia, dysfibrinogenemia)
    Factor II (hypoprothrombinemia, dysprothrombinemias)
    Factor V (parahemophilia)
    Factor VII (hypoproconvertinemia)
    Factor X (Stuart deficiency)
    Combined factor deficiencies
  Acquired deficiencies due to decreased production
    Vitamin-K-dependent coagulation factors
      Liver disease
      Altered bowel flora
      Malabsorption
      Coumadin treatment
    Hypothyroidism
  Acquired deficiencies due to increased destruction
    Disseminated intravascular coagulation
    Purpura fulminans
    Necrotizing enterocolitis
    Localized venous and arterial thrombosis
  Pathologic anticoagulants

TABLE 18. Use of Screening Tests for Classification of Hemorrhagic Disorders

Condition	Platelet Count	BT*	PTT	PT	TT
Afibrinogenemia	N	Mild Abn	No clot	No clot	No clot
Dysfibrinogenemia	N	N	N	Mild Abn	Abn
II, V, X deficiencies	N	N	Abn	Abn	N
VII deficiency	N	N	N	Abn	N
VIII, IX, XI, XII deficiencies / Fletcher factor deficiency	N	N	Abn	N	N
XIII deficiency	N	N	N	N	N
von Willebrand's disease	N	Abn	Abn	N	N
Platelet function defects	N or low	Abn	N	N	N
DIC	Low	Abn	Abn	Abn	Abn
Severe liver disease	N or low	N or Abn	Abn	Abn	N or Abn
Uremia	N or low	Abn	N or mild Abn	Abn	Abn

* BT = bleeding time; PTT = partial thromboplastin time; PT = prothrombin time; TT = thrombin time; N = normal for age; Abn = abnormal prolongation of clotting test time.

der. The screening tests include: (1) the *platelet count* and/or estimation of platelet number on the blood smear; (2) the *bleeding time* by the Ivy or template method, using a blood pressure cuff at 40 mm Hg, which is a measure of the platelet–vessel interaction; (3) the *partial thromboplastin time* (PTT), which measures thrombin generation in the intrinsic pathway and is a function of all the coagulation factors except factor VII; the PTT is commonly done by use of an activating agent (celite or kaolin), which may shorten the clotting time excessively and mask a mild defect if not carefully controlled; (4) the *prothrombin time* (PT or Quick test), which measures thrombin generation in the extrinsic pathway and is a function of factor II, V, VII, and X activity, in addition to estimating the fibrinogen level; the PT is normal in mild deficiencies of fibrinogen (100 to 200 mg/dl); and (5) the *thrombin time* (TT), which estimates the amount and function of fibrinogen and is particularly sensitive to the presence of fibrin degradation products or heparin. The latter tests (PTT, PT, and TT) are performed on citrated plasma, usually collected by venipuncture using careful two-syringe technique to avoid contamination by tissue juice (tissue factor), and put into a tube that contains the appropriate amount of citrate for the volume of plasma. The usual proportion of citrate to total volume of sample of whole blood is 1 to 10 and is appropriate for a hematocrit of 40 + 10 percent. (0.5 ml citrate solution and 4.5 ml of blood are usually added to make a final volume of 5.0 ml.) With low or high hematocrits, the ratio of citrate solution to plasma should be maintained by modifying the volume of blood added to 0.5 ml of citrate as follows: 20% hematocrit, 3.5 ml; 30%, 4.0 ml; 60%, 7.0 ml; and 70%, 10.0 ml. In infants smaller volumes of blood can be used with tubes containing smaller volumes of citrate (such as 0.1 or 0.25 ml), but the ratio of citrate to blood must be maintained.

Depending upon the history, clinical situation, and results of the screening tests, additional laboratory determinations, such as fibrinogen level, clot retraction, specific factor assays (activity and antigenic measurement), platelet function tests, prothrombin consumption, factor XIII, and heparin assay, may be indicated to establish a diagnosis. These tests are discussed below.

Developmental Aspects

Coagulation factors, clotting tests, and platelet–vascular interaction in the perinatal period are compared to normal values for older children and adults in Table 19. Term infants and most preterm infants show a normal *platelet–vessel interaction,* as evidenced by normal bleeding times. Only in very small preterm infants does capillary fragility appear to be increased. Platelet number in normal term and premature infants is within the normal adult range. Platelet retention in glass bead filters (platelet adhesiveness) is also similar to normal adult values. However, platelet factor 3 release and in vitro platelet aggregation to ADP, epinephrine, collagen, and thrombin are impaired in most premature and many term infants. This mild platelet function defect occurs only transiently in the neonatal period. The few biochemical studies available (low phosphofructokinase, increased phosphoglycerate kinase, and decreased stainable glycogen) also suggest metabolic differences in fetal platelets.

Many *coagulation factors* are decreased in activity in the fetus and newborn. Of greatest clinical significance are the *vitamin-K-dependent factors* (II, VII, IX, X), which are low at birth and often fall to even lower levels during the first week, unless vitamin K is given soon after deliv-

TABLE 19. Hemostatic and Coagulation Data for Normal Subjects in Perinatal Period*

Subject	Activated PTT (sec)	Prothrombin Time (sec)	Thrombin Time (sec)	Platelet Count (per cu mm)	Bleeding Time (min)	Capillary Fragility	Platelet Adhesiveness	Platelet Aggregation
		Screening Tests				Vascular–Platelet Interaction		
Normal adult or child	44	13	10	300,000 ± 50,000	4 ± 1.5	N	N	N
Fetus, early 10–15 wk	—	—	—	Platelets present	—	Inc	—	Abn to collagen, epi
Preterm 27–31 wk	—	23	—	275,000 ± 60,000	—	Inc	N	Abn to ADP, collagen
Preterm 32–36 wk	70	17 (12–21)	14 (11–17)	290,000 ± 70,000	4 ± 1.5	N	N	Abn to ADP, collagen
Term, AGA	55 ± 10	16 (13–20)	12 (10–16)	310,000 ± 68,000	4 ± 1.5	N	N	Abn to ADP, collagen, epi

Subject	I mg/dl	II	V	VII + X	VIII	IX	XI	XII	XIII	Plasminogen (%)	Euglobulin lysis time (min)	Antithrombin III (%)	Fibrin split products (μg/ml)
	Coagulation Factors Percent of Adult Value									Fibrinolytic-Anticoagulant System			
Normal adult or child	315 ± 60	100	100	100	100	100	100	100	100	100	140	100	0–7
Fetus, early 10–15 wk	< 120	—	81	18	—	—	—	—	—	0 to trace	Inc	—	—
Preterm, 27–31 wk	270 ± 140	30 ± 10	72 ± 25	32 ± 15	70 ± 30	27 ± 10	—	—	100	25	95	—	0–10
Preterm, 32–36 wk	226 ± 70	35 ± 12	91 ± 23	39 ± 14	98 ± 40	—	—	30	100	40	95	48	0–7
Term, AGA	246 ± 55	98 ± 15	56 ± 40	105 ± 16	28 ± 35	30 ± 8	51	100	43	84	55	55	0–7

* From Hathaway WE: Semin Hematol 12:175 1975.

The values represent smoothed means, ± 1 SD or ranges from cord blood samples or venous samples in first 24 hr of life.

AGA, average for gestational age; N, normal value for older child or adult; Inc, increased; Dec, decreased; Abn, abnormal; epi, epinephrine; PTT, partial thromboplastin time.

ery. Factors XI and XII are also moderately reduced; whether this represents a true deficiency or is related to a deficiency of prekallikrein (Fletcher factor) remains to be seen. In contrast, fibrinogen and factors V and VIII are within normal adult range, except for slightly low values in very small premature infants. The fibrin stabilizing factor (XIII) exists at adult levels after later fetal life. All factors that are physiologically low in the term infant (II, VII, IX, X, XI, XII) reach normal adult levels in a few weeks, except factors IX and XI and Fletcher factor, which may require months to reach adult levels.

Knowledge of the decreased levels of coagulation factors allows one to understand the neonatal alterations in commonly used *screening tests* of blood clotting. The partial thrombin time (PTT), a measure of thrombin generation in the intrinsic pathway, is prolonged mostly because of low factors XII, XI, and IX and Fletcher factor. The prothrombin time (PT), an estimate of thrombin generation in the extrinsic pathway, is increased due to deficiencies of factors II, VII, and X. The prolonged thrombin time in newborns is more difficult to understand in view of normal fibrinogen levels. Inhibitors of the fibrinogen–fibrin conversion (such as heparin or fibrin degradation products) or the existence of a fetal fibrinogen molecule could explain this observation.

Falsely abnormal coagulation studies can result from *heparin contamination,* particularly in sick newborn infants if blood is drawn through an indwelling catheter after infusion of dilute heparin to keep the line open. Small amounts of heparin have a profound effect on the thrombin time, a lesser effect on the partial thrombin time (PTT), and least influence on prothrombin time (PT). It may be possible to distinguish the effect of heparin with a reptilase time. Reptilase is a potent snake thrombin that is not inhibited by heparin. If a prolonged thrombin time (TT) is due to heparin, the reptilase time will remain normal.

Despite prolongation of the PTT, PT, and TT and the above noted deficiencies of clotting factors, the whole blood of the preterm or term infant clots more quickly than the whole blood of children and adults. This hypercoagulability can be demonstrated by the whole blood clotting time, the thrombelastogram (a clotting instrument showing the dynamics of clot formation), and the thrombin generation test. This paradoxic hypercoagulability has been attributed to a deficiency of naturally occurring anticoagulants or protease inhibitors, the most potent of which is antithrombin III (AT-III).

Fibrinolytic activity is increased in the newborn infant, but it decreases to adult levels in a few days. Since plasminogen is decreased at birth, the increased fibrinolytic activity may be related to high activator levels. Despite elevated fibrinolytic activity, fibrin degradation products are not significantly elevated in normal infants.

Abnormalities of Blood Vessel–Platelet Interaction

Many hemorrhagic disorders are characterized by defective hemostasis at the site of a small vessel injury but no abnormality of the coagulation system. Some of these disorders appear to be due to a defect of blood vessels, some due to abnormal numbers or function of platelets, and some due to a defect in the interaction between the platelet and the blood vessel (Table 7). The following disorders are characterized by vascular abnormalities with or without concurrent platelet disorders.

HEREDITARY HEMORRHAGIC TELANGIECTASIA. (Rendu-Osler-Weber disease) is characterized by multiple small angiomas involving the skin and mucous membranes that tend to bleed either spontaneously or as a result of trauma. It is transmitted by a simple dominant pattern of inheritance and affects both sexes equally. The individual lesions consist of multiple dilations of capillaries and venules 1 to 4 mm in size, that are slightly raised, are bright red, and fade partially on firm pressure. The telangiectases are present in childhood and tend to increase in number and distribution with age. Bleeding may occur from any involved site and is frequently manifested as recurrent epistaxis in childhood. Gastrointestinal, pulmonary, and urinary bleeding also occur. Results of screening tests for hemostasis are usually normal; however, decreased platelet aggregation has been noted. Treatment of bleeding is by topical hemostatic agents (thrombin, Oxycel, Surgicel) when the site is accessible. Chronic and acute blood loss may be great enough to require treatment of the resultant anemia with iron and occasionally with transfusions.

CONNECTIVE TISSUE DISORDERS. A bleeding tendency manifested by easy bruising and hemorrhage after trauma or surgical procedures is seen with connective tissue disorders, such as osteogenesis imperfecta, Marfan's syndrome, and Ehlers-Danlos syndrome (cutis hyperelastica). Prolonged bleeding times and defects of platelet aggregation are sometimes observed in these patients. The most significant bleeding tendency occurs in cutis hyperelastica, where there is marked hyperelasticity of the skin and hyperextensibility of the joints. The skin is fragile and splits on slight trauma. Prolonged bleeding may occur as a result of gaping wounds and inadequate tissue support for small blood vessels. Wound healing is slow, and the scars are thin and weak. No effective therapy is known, but attempts should be made to provide protection from trauma.

SECONDARY VASCULITIS. Systemic lupus erythematosus and related diseases, as well as severe viral and bacterial infections, may produce vasculitis and associated bleeding. Inflammation of the small blood vessels may cause increased permeability and hemorrhage into the surrounding tissues. Vasculitis-related bleeding may present with petechiae, purpura, or hemorrhage into such organs as lung, kidney, brain, or gut. Meningococcemia without either intravascular coagulation or severe thrombocytopenia can produce widespread cutaneous hemorrhages due to direct infection and inflammation of blood vessels. Subacute bacterial endocarditis also may be associated with petechiae or purpuric eruptions resulting from bacterial embolization.

SCURVY. In scurvy (ascorbic acid deficiency), bleeding occurs in the skin, mucous membranes, and soft tissues and as painful subperiosteal hemorrhages. The small vessel bleeding may be due to a defect in formation of intact endothelium or abnormal platelet metabolism or both (p. 228).

ANAPHYLACTOID PURPURA. Anaphylactoid purpura (Schönlein-Henoch syndrome, allergic purpura, p. 382) usually occurs as a hemorrhagic rash in association with gastrointestinal symptoms (Henoch's purpura), joint manifestations (Schönlein's purpura), and renal involvement. It is a generalized vascular disorder resulting from acute aseptic vasculitis involving arterioles and capillaries. The inflammatory lesions in and around the vessel walls are similar to those found in periarteritis nodosa and other conditions seemingly related to hypersensitivity. The disorder is most common in children 4 to 15 years of age.

ETIOLOGY AND PATHOGENESIS. Although anaphylactoid purpura is generally considered to be related to hypersensitivity, a definite allergen is rarely identified. A few patients have a history of antecedent infection with a β-hemolytic streptococcus, and in several cases recurrences of this syndrome have been associated with streptococcal infection. Exposure to viruses (smallpox vaccination, hepatitis-associated antigen) may precede the onset. Occasionally a specific food or drug idiosyncrasy has been implicated, but rarely conclusively.

CLINICAL MANIFESTATIONS. These depend upon the sites involved by the widespread vasculitis. The most frequent areas of involvement are skin, joints, gastrointestinal tract, and kidneys. Rash, abdominal pain, and joint pain are the most common presenting manifestations. The rash is variable, but usually progresses from recurrent crops of urticarial lesions to a pink or red maculopapular eruption, which becomes hemorrhagic and then fades, leaving a brownish discoloration of the skin that may persist for several weeks. The distribution of the rash is quite characteristic, usually involving the buttocks, posterior thighs, and extensor surfaces of the arms and legs, while sparing the face, trunk, palms, and soles. Marked, painful edema of the scalp may occur, especially in younger patients. Single or multiple joints may be puffy, warm, painful, and tender; the swelling is due to periarticular involvement rather than intra-articular bleeding. Abdominal mani-

festations are frequently responsible for bringing the patient to medical attention and are also the source of most serious acute complications. Recurrent colicky abdominal pain, vomiting, and melena are common and result from edema and hemorrhage from and into the intestinal wall. Perforation may occur, and there is a predilection to intussusception. Occasionally the abdominal symptoms may precede development of the typical rash. Renal involvement occurs frequently and may be manifested as gross or microscopic hematuria.

LABORATORY FINDINGS. Anemia and leukocytosis may occur as a result of blood loss. Eosinophilia is noted only in some patients. Tests of hemostatic function are normal. Urinary abnormalities include hematuria, proteinuria, and increased casts. Since the renal involvement may not be manifested until late in the disease, urinalysis should be repeated frequently.

DIAGNOSIS. The characteristic maculopapular rash with its peculiar distribution usually can be distinguished from the flat purpuric rash of thrombo cytopenia, and frequently the diagnosis can be made on inspection. The normal platelet count differentiates the Schönlein-Henoch syndrome from thrombocytopenic purpura. Likewise, the entirely normal coagulation studies distinguish this disorder from primary hemorrhagic disorders. In some instances, however, the rash may be atypical, or the visceral and joint manifestations may precede the appearance of the rash. In such situations an acute surgical abdomen may be the first impression in patients with abdominal pain, or acute rheumatic fever may be suspected in patients with prominent articular manifestations. In patients with high fever and a more petechial type of eruption, meningococcemia may be suspected.

COURSE AND PROGNOSIS. In most instances the disease is limited to a single episode that subsides in 6 weeks. The course is variable, however, and some children have repeated episodes with remissions and exacerbations recurring for months or years. Renal involvement is the most serious chronic consequence of the disorder. While the majority of children make a complete recovery, some develop chronic nephritis and eventual renal failure.

Treatment is primarily symptomatic and supportive. If throat culture reveals group A β-hemolytic streptococci, appropriate antibacterial therapy should be initiated. Short-term steroid therapy (prednisone, 1 to 2 mg/kg/day) may be useful in the presence of marked scalp edema, persistent joint pain, or severe abdominal colic. In the latter, steroids may help prevent the development of intussusception by decreasing the amount of edema and hemorrhage in the bowel. Steroid therapy does not influence the course of the skin rash, nor does it alter the incidence of renal involvement. Skin testing and elimination diets, often employed to detect specific allergens, are rarely rewarding.

THROMBOCYTOPENIAS

It is useful to distinguish the thrombocytopenic disorders due to increased destruction of platelets from those associated with decreased production. Most thrombocytopenias are due to increased platelet destruction, usually accompanied by a compensatory increase in the rate of production. Consequently, the megakaryocytes in bone marrow may be either normal or increased in number, and there may be a shift to an increased number of immature megakaryocytes, with eight or fewer lobulations of the nuclei. Large young platelets, which are functionally very active, predominate on the peripheral blood smear, and hemostasis is often better than one would predict from the platelet count. In the disorders of production, the few platelets that remain in the peripheral blood tend to be small when examined on a smear or when a size distribution curve is obtained on an electronic counter. Megakaryocytes are absent or decreased in number in the bone marrow aspirate.

In the diagnostic evaluation of thrombocytopenias it is important to determine whether other elements of the blood are involved. Coexisting abnormalities of the white cells and/or red cells may indicate disease involving the bone marrow or spleen. When thrombocytopenia is associated with abnormalities in coagulation, the probability of consumption of platelets and clotting factors in disseminated intravascular coagulation (p. 1214) should be considered.

Thrombocytopenia Associated with Increased Destruction

IDIOPATHIC THROMBOCYTOPENIC PUR-PURA (IMMUNE THROMBOCYTOPENIC PUR-PURA, ITP). ETIOLOGY AND PATHOGENESIS. Although it has been clearly demonstrated that an antiplatelet factor with characteristics of an antibody is present in the plasma of many patients with ITP (particularly adults), attempts to identify such a factor regularly by in vitro tests have led to variable results, especially in children. Despite the failure of present methods to demonstrate antiplatelet antibody consistently in ITP, most investigators believe that the basic mechanism involves an immunologic response. The mechanism probably varies depending upon the triggering agent (virus, drug, unknown factors) but results in sensitization or alteration of the platelets in such a manner that they are prematurely destroyed or removed from the circulation.

The spleen is implicated in ITP as a site for removal of sensitized platelets from the circulation and as a source of antibody production. In the presence of severe platelet sensitization, the liver also functions as a major organ of platelet sequestration. The bone marrow aspirate shows evidence for a compensatory increase in platelet production, ie, increased numbers of younger megakaryocytes.

While ITP occurs in both children and adults, there are significant differences in the manifestations of the disease in the two age groups. The incidence is much greater in children, and there is no sex difference, compared with a 3:1 predominance of females over males in adults. ITP in children is found to follow viral infections (rubella, rubeola, varicella, miscellaneous respiratory infections) in up to 80 percent of the cases; this association is not as common in adults. Prompt spontaneous remission occurs in 80 to 90 percent of children in contrast to a high incidence of a more chronic course in adults.

CLINICAL MANIFESTATIONS. Bleeding into the skin, either spontaneously or following minor trauma, is the most common feature of ITP. The onset is often abrupt. The lesions may be widespread and may range from pinpoint petechiae to large ecchymoses. Nosebleeds and bleeding from mucous membranes frequently accompany the purpura and may lead to significant blood loss. Central nervous system bleeding, the most serious complication, may occur early in the course of the disease but is quite uncommon. Joint hemorrhage is rare.

Physical examination, apart from evidence of hemorrhage, is generally unrevealing. Enlargement of the spleen and lymph nodes is rare; its presence requires a careful search for other causes of thrombocytopenia such as leukemia, Gaucher's disease, or systemic lupus erythematosus.

LABORATORY FINDINGS. Thrombocytopenia, with platelet counts usually below $50,000/mm^3$, is the most significant finding. The reduction in platelet number may be confirmed by the sparsity of platelets on the stained blood smear, where the few platelets are often of the relatively large size that characterizes young platelets. The rest of the blood count is normal unless anemia and leukocytosis are seen in response to hemorrhage. Clot retraction is poor to absent. Prothrombin time, partial thromboplastin time, and thrombin time are normal. Bone marrow examination is essential for accurate diagnosis and usually reveals an increased number of megakaryocytes, with a predominance of immature forms. Erythroid hyperplasia may be noted in response to significant blood loss.

COURSE AND PROGNOSIS. ITP is a self-limited disease in most children; 80 to 90 percent make a spontaneous recovery, usually within 3 months from the onset of illness. Relapses are uncommon but may occur up to several years following the initial episode, especially in association with an intercurrent infection. In about 10 percent of cases, thrombocytopenia persists longer than a year. During the period of thrombocytopenia the severity of bleeding manifestations is variable and often is not correlated directly with the platelet count. Petechiae are often absent despite platelet counts below $25,000/mm^3$, probably because these few remaining platelets are primarily young and functionally more competent than the older platelets that predominate in thrombocytopenia due to decreased production.

TREATMENT. Significant blood loss should be replaced with packed red cells or whole blood. Active bleeding may be arrested with platelet transfusions, but the survival of transfused platelets is brief, and only a temporary improvement in hemostasis is achieved. Restriction of activity during the acute phase is advisable.

Because of the high incidence of spontaneous recovery from ITP in children, conservative management is generally recommended. Treatment with corticosteroids is used widely, but there is no evidence that the incidence of eventual recovery is influenced by such therapy. Low doses of prednisone (about 0.5 mg/kg/day in divided doses) appear to decrease the bleeding tendency before the platelet count has returned to normal. This effect is thought to result from alteration of vascular permeability. A higher dose of prednisone, 1 to 2 mg/kg/day in divided doses, may be associated with a rise in the platelet count in some patients. However, this effect may be transient and limited to the duration of a 2- to 3-week course of treatment. Prolonged use of prednisone can suppress platelet response and actually prolong the duration of thrombocytopenia.

The role of steroid therapy in ITP still remains unsettled, and its routine use is not advised. A reasonable approach is to individualize, limiting the use of prednisone to children presenting with extensive active bleeding manifestations, particularly mucous membrane, subconjunctival, or retinal hemorrhages. Patients with only easy bruising and scattered petechiae or with minimal epistaxis should be followed conservatively, regardless of the platelet count. When prednisone is used, it should be given in divided doses of 1 to 2 mg/kg/day for 2 weeks to try to achieve both a capillary and a platelet effect. Prednisone is then tapered and stopped during the third week regardless of the platelet-count response, thus avoiding the possibility of marrow suppression. The use of prednisone during the initial phase of ITP in children, with the aim of preventing serious bleeding manifestations, has become widespread. But it should be kept in mind that serious bleeding manifestations tend to occur early in the course of illness, often before the patient is seen; the incidence of symptomatic central nervous system bleeding is very low (probably about 1 percent), and in some cases may be related to other thrombocytopenic states (such as thrombotic thrombocytopenic purpura). Functional impairment of platelets with drugs like aspirin should be avoided (p. 1209).

CHRONIC ITP. When severe thrombocytopenia persists beyond 6 to 12 months it is appropriate to weigh the possible benefits of *splenectomy* against the risk of postsplenectomy sepsis. Measures for reducing the incidence of postsplenectomy infection are discussed elsewhere. Splenectomy results in recovery in about two-thirds of children who develop chronic ITP. History of an earlier platelet response to prednisone and demonstration of splenic sequestration of labeled platelets are factors that favor recovery after splenectomy. Since spontaneous remission may occur 2 years or longer from the onset of the illness, it may be justified to delay splenectomy in any child tolerating the thrombocytopenic state without serious clinical bleeding problems or undue restrictions of physical activity. While immunosuppressive agents have been used in the treatment of ITP in adults, there is little experience with their use in children.

IMMUNOLOGIC DRUG PURPURA. A variety of drugs are capable of sensitizing certain individuals so that subsequent exposure to the drug leads to acute thrombocytopenia. The antibody formed may react with the specific drug, and subsequent absorption of this antigen (drug)–antibody complex onto the platelet surface may lead to destruction of the latter. Lysis of platelets may be demonstrated in vitro and requires the specific drug, serum from the drug-sensitive patient, platelets from any donor, and complement. Several tests are available to detect drug sensitization. Drugs that may induce such a response in susceptible individuals include quinidine, quinine, digitoxin, chlorothiazide derivatives, chlorpropamide, meprobamate, phenylbutazone, sulfonamides, and antihistamines. The thrombocytopenia resulting from this process usually resolves spontaneously on elimination of the offending drug.

SPLENOMEGALY. Splenomegaly (p.1206; see hypersplenism, p.1197) resulting from a variety of conditions associated with thrombocytopenia may be due to sequestration and/or destruction of platelets by the enlarged spleen. Megakaryocytes are plentiful in the marrow in most of these disorders, which include congestive splenomegaly with portal hypertension (Banti's syndrome), thalassemia major, Gaucher's disease, reticuloendotheliosis, Hodgkin's disease, and others. Splenectomy may attenuate the thrombocytopenia in many instances, even though the underlying disease is not affected. Platelet kinetic studies, with monitoring over the spleen, help to distinguish those cases in which the spleen is removing platelets; these have the best chance of benefiting from splenectomy.

ACUTE INFECTIONS AND OTHER DISORDERS. Thrombocytopenia has been associated with tuberculosis, typhoid fever, measles, rubella, varicella, scarlet fever, endocarditis, infectious mononucleosis, and other infectious diseases. Thrombocytopenia is also a common manifestation of lupus erythematosus. When it accompanies acquired autoimmune hemolytic anemia, it is referred to as Evan's syndrome.

THROMBOCYTOPENIA ASSOCIATED WITH THROMBUS FORMATION. Increased destruction of platelets with thrombosis and damage to organs may occur in a virtually isolated manner or in combination with consumption of coagulation factors (see arterial thrombosis, p. 1214). Conditions associated primarily with platelet destruction include *hemolytic uremic syndrome, thrombotic thrombocytopenic purpura, giant hemangioma, cyanotic congenital heart disease,* and *small vessel arterial thrombosis.* In all of these conditions antiplatelet agents (aspirin and dipyridamole, see below) show more therapeutic promise than anticoagulation therapy with heparin.

HEMOLYTIC UREMIC SYNDROME AND THROMBOTIC THROMBOCYTOPENIC PURPURA. These closely related and overlapping conditions are characterized by hemolytic anemia and thrombocytopenia but rarely show evidence of disseminated intravascular coagulation (DIC). In both conditions platelet survival is markedly diminished whereas the rate of fibrinogen degradation usually is normal. Red cell morphology is characterized by distorted, fragmented shapes and microspherocytes.

The term hemolytic uremic syndrome is generally applied to the condition in infants and young children that typically follows an episode of bloody diarrhea and in which renal manifestations of hematuria, oliguria or renal shutdown, and uremia predominate. Neurologic manifestations are common but do not appear to be thrombotic in origin. Most patients recover completely if they can be tided over the period of renal shutdown with careful fluid and electrolyte management. Long-term sequelae are restricted to chronic renal disease. Rarely, there are recurrent episodes. Heparin therapy has not proved to be effective in most cases. Agents that inhibit platelet aggregation, such as the combination of aspirin and dipyridamole, are being tested, but their effectiveness is still uncertain.

Thrombotic thrombocytopenic purpura is the term applied to a similar but usually fatal condition, primarily in adults, in which neurologic manifestations predominate over the renal ones. Paresthesia, personality disorders, convulsions, and coma may occur, but hematuria, proteinuria, and uremia are also common. Although early reports indicated moderate success with heparin, aspirin-dipyridamole therapy may prove more effective (aspirin 10 mg/kg/day and dipyridamole 3 to 5 mg/kg/day).

GIANT HEMANGIOMA. Sequestration of platelets, leading to severe thrombocytopenia and bleeding, may occur secondary to giant hemangioma in infants. Increased consumption of coagulation factors occurs in some cases. Recovery follows surgical removal, prednisone therapy, or spontaneous regression of the hemangioma.

CYANOTIC CONGENITAL HEART DISEASE. Thrombocytopenia may occur in children with severe polycythemia associated with cyanotic cardiac lesions. The degree of platelet deficiency is proportional to the severity of the hypoxia and is frequently seen when the hematocrit is 70 percent or higher. Results of platelet survival studies are abnormal in these patients and indicate a peripheral destruction of platelets. Cyanotic patients with significant thrombocytopenia should be prepared for surgery by a partial exchange transfusion with plasma and platelet concentrates to lower the hematocrit and raise the platelet count.

INTRAVASCULAR CLOTTING. Thrombocytopenia in the syndromes associated with intravascular clotting will be discussed in the section on acquired coagulation defects (p. 1213).

NEONATAL THROMBOCYTOPENIC PURPURA. Thrombocytopenia occurs in about half of newborn infants of women who have or have had ITP,

including those who have normal platelet counts after splenectomy. The disease in the infant apparently results from *transplacental transmission of an antiplatelet antibody* from mother to infant. A similarly acquired thrombocytopenia may occur in infants of mothers with systemic lupus erythematosus. In *isoimmune thrombocytopenic purpura,* there is evidence that the mother is sensitized to the infant's platelets, which are of a different immunologic type. Maternal antibodies directed against the infant's platelets are produced during pregnancy and cross the placenta, causing thrombocytopenia in the newborn infant (a mechanism analogous to isoimmunization of red blood cells in erythroblastosis fetalis). It may be difficult to make a specific diagnosis, since serologic tests for platelet antibodies are not generally available and, where available, are not always diagnostically reliable. In both types of neonatal thrombocytopenia the firstborn infant may be affected, and disease tends to occur in subsequent infants. Hemorrhagic manifestations appear within minutes to hours after birth and include skin, mucous membrane, vaginal, and central nervous system bleeding.

TREATMENT. Recommendations vary according to the severity of the clinical manifestations. Mild cases can be managed with simple observation, since the major risk of trauma has passed when the baby has been delivered. Prompt transfusion with platelet concentrates is useful when bleeding manifestations are prominent at birth, even though survival of transfused platelets may be brief. Transfusion of a platelet concentrate obtained from the mother is most effective if the disorder is on an isoimmune basis. The routine use of corticosteroids in neonatal thrombocytopenia remains a debated issue, as in ITP, but they may be of benefit to tide the severely affected infant over the dangerous neonatal period by a brief course of prednisone, 1 to 2 mg/kg/day in divided doses. In severely bleeding infants, exchange transfusion is recommended to remove antibody. The disease is self-limited when antibody has been passively transmitted from the mother. Serious perinatal complications may occur in up to one-third of the cases, but the subsequent prognosis is excellent. Most infants achieve a normal platelet count within 6 to 8 weeks.

Thrombocytopenia in the neonatal period may also be *secondary to a variety of systemic diseases,* including severe erythroblastosis fetalis, sepsis, cytomegalic inclusion disease, toxoplasmosis, rubella, leukemia, and congenital anemia.

A rare type of congenital thrombocytopenia is associated with bilateral absence of the radius (TAR syndrome). Megakaryocytes are decreased in the marrow, and a transient leukemoid blood picture may suggest congenital leukemia. Despite persistence of thrombocytopenia, these infants tend to do well if they escape fatal bleeding during the neonatal period.

BONE MARROW DISEASE. Replacement of the marrow by leukemia, metastatic neuroblastoma, lymphosarcoma, or other malignancies may result in severe thrombocytopenia due to decreased megakaryocytes. Aplastic and hypoplastic anemias, whether congenital, idiopathic, or secondary to drugs, chemical toxins, or irradiation, are also commonly associated with amegakaryocytic thrombocytopenia. Agents known to cause thrombocytopenia by damaging the bone marrow include benzol, chloramphenicol, DDT, gold salts, neomycin, nitrogen mustards, organic arsenicals, organic hair dyes, phenobarbital, streptomycin, tridione, and others. Treatment of these bone marrow disorders is discussed on page 1130.

HEREDITARY THROMBOCYTOPENIAS. Consideration of this heterogeneous group of disorders becomes important in the differential diagnosis of ITP in the young child or in the child with chronic thrombocytopenia. One disorder, characterized by a decreased number of normal and large-size platelets, is rarely associated with renal disease and deafness and has an autosomal recessive inheritance. The May-Hegglin anomaly (giant platelets, Döhle inclusion bodies in the granulocytes) and other large platelet syndromes, with both normal and shortened platelet survival and a rare association with nephritis, are transmitted by a dominant pattern. Most of the reported cases of familial thrombocytopenia are sex-linked and represent either the typical Wiskott-Aldrich syndrome (p. 316) or variants thereof.

Treatment of thrombocytopenic manifestations is mainly symptomatic. Splenectomy is contraindicated in any of the Wiskott-Aldrich syndromes, since overwhelming sepsis has been observed frequently after splenectomy. Similarly, corsticosteroid treatment has little or no effect on the platelet count and predisposes to serious infection.

THROMBOPOIETIN DEFICIENCY. A chronic congenital thrombocytopenic purpura refractory to corticosteroids and splenectomy, but regularly responding to infusions of fresh or fresh-frozen plasma, has been reported in a child and is thought to be due to a congenital deficiency of a platelet-stimulating factor (thrombopoietin).

Thrombocytosis

Thrombocytosis is relatively common in infants and children as an incidental finding in the evaluation of some other clinical disorder. An elevated platelet count is usually first suspected on the basis of numerous platelets on a peripheral blood smear and is then confirmed with a platelet count. Most cases of thrombocytosis probably result from an increased rate of platelet production, possibly mediated by thrombopoietin. Platelet survival is usually normal, and a prolonged platelet lifespan has not been documented. The abnormality is usually of brief duration. Conditions most commonly associated with thrombocytosis are asplenia, iron deficiency, vitamin E deficiency, and use of vinka alkaloids. Thrombocytosis may also be seen in the myeloproliferative disorder of Down's syndrome, megaloblastic anemia, hyperadrenalism, graft-versus-host reaction, nephrotic syndrome, infections, and treatment with citrovorum factor or corticosteroid.

Adults with severe thrombocytosis (greater than 1 million/mm^3) have a substantially increased risk of developing thrombosis and hemorrhage. In children, however, symptomatic cases are rare but have included hemiplegia and electrocardiographic evidence of myocardial infarction. Because of the rarity of such cases in children, the substantial risk of complications of anticoagulant or antimetabolite therapy seems to outweigh the possible benefits in what is usually a self-limited condition. On the other hand, inhibition of platelet aggregation by the less toxic combination of acetylsalicylic acid and dipyridamole may prove advisable in selected cases.

Disorders of Platelet Function

Abnormalities of platelet function should be suspected in patients with a bleeding time inappropriately prolonged for the platelet count. Normally, the bleeding time does not become prolonged until the platelet count falls below 100,000/mm^3. In general, there is a history of petechiae, ecchymoses, and/or epistaxis of mild to moderate severity. The hemostatic screening tests, except for bleeding time, are normal. Clot retraction may be poor. In some cases, withdrawal of a drug, such as aspirin, may correct the abnormality. However, in many instances, tests of platelet aggregation must be performed in order to make a specific diagnosis. These tests are based on the transmission of light through a platelet-rich suspension. An increased amount of light is transmitted when the platelets clump in response to the addition of collagen, ADP, epinephrine, or ristocetin. Most of the disorders described in this heading can be grouped into one of the following categories.

THROMBASTHENIA (GLANZMANN'S DISEASE) an autosomal recessive disorder, is characterized by absent platelet aggregation with ADP, decreased clot retraction, and abnormal membrane proteins. Platelet survival and morphology are normal. Treatment of this condition consists of platelet transfusions when warranted by clinical manifestations. Steroids are not beneficial.

BERNARD-SOULIER GIANT PLATELET SYNDROME is an autosomal recessive disorder characterized by large and bizarre-shaped platelets. Most aggregation studies (including ADP) are normal; abnormal aggregation in response to ristocetin has been reported. Thrombocytopenia and shortened platelet survival are observed. Increased numbers of large platelets may be seen in the asymptomatic heterozygous carriers.

PLATELET RELEASE DEFECT DUE TO ABSENT STORAGE POOL (OR STORAGE POOL DISEASE) is a disorder of platelet function wherein a deficiency of the storage pool of ADP can be demonstrated. The platelets are morphologically normal except for decreased numbers of electron-dense bodies on electron microscopy. There is decreased aggregation with epinephrine and collagen in the face of normal aggregation to ADP. Inheritance is either autosomal recessive or dominant. The patients with Hermansky-Pudlak syndrome (albinism with ceroid deposits in bone marrow macrophages) have a platelet function defect of the same type. The tiny platelets of the *Wiskott-Aldrich syndrome* also show similar morphologic and aggregation defects.

PLATELET RELEASE DEFECT WITH NORMAL STORAGE POOL is a heterogenous group of disorders wherein the basic defect is the failure of the platelet to release ADP despite a normal storage pool of adenine nucleotides. Inheritance is variable but frequently dominant. Aggregation with epinephrine and collagen is decreased, whereas aggregation with ADP is normal. The defects of platelet function seen in type I glycogen storage disease and in subjects who have taken aspirin fall into this category.

VON WILLEBRAND'S DISEASE (PSEUDO-HEMOPHILIA). von Willebrand's disease is a relatively common hereditary bleeding disorder occurring in both sexes and inherited as an autosomal dominant trait. It is characterized by a prolonged bleeding time and a variable deficiency of factor VIII (antihemophilic factor). Unlike hemophilia, the clinical manifestations of von Willebrand's disease are characterized by skin and mucous membrane bleeding. Nosebleeds and easy bruising are the most common manifestations, whereas hemarthroses are rare. Menorrhagia may be a serious problem. Bleeding following dental extraction and operative procedures is extremely variable but may be serious, particularly in patients with the lowest factor VIII activity. The severity of the disorder in terms of laboratory findings and clinical manifestations varies considerably among families, among different affected members of the same family, and, at times, in the same individual on different occasions. The hemostatic defect in von Willebrand's disease is characterized by a reduction in the plasma factor VIII (both factor VIII activity and antigenically determined factor VIII concentration). The prolonged bleeding time appears to be due to a deficiency of a plasma factor, factor VIII antigen, which is normally present on the platelet and the blood vessel endothelial cells. This factor is necessary for platelet adhesion to glass beads (platelet adhesiveness) and platelet aggregation by the antibiotic ristocetin. Platelet aggregation in vitro by ADP, collagen, and epinephrine is normal in this disorder.

A patient with the severe form will display a prolonged bleeding time, a prolonged PTT due to deficient factor VIII activity, decreased amounts of factor VIII antigen, deficient platelet adhesion to glass beads, and decreased aggregation of platelets to ristocetin. Also, after transfusion of factor VIII antigen (from normal or classic hemophilic plasma), the patient will show a temporary increase in factor VIII activity, which is greater and more prolonged than can be accounted for by the factor VIII activity in the transfused plasma. Diagnosis in mild cases may be extremely difficult. In addition, variants are described in which only some of the abnormalities are noted.

Local hemostatic measures are usually effective in stopping nosebleeds. However, nasal packing and replacement of blood loss may be necessary occasionally. Serious bleeding is best treated by transfusion of cryoprecipitated factor VIII concentrate, as used for treatment of classic hemophilia. Fresh frozen plasma is also effective. The dose is usually based on the factor VIII content, and enough material is given to correct the PTT or to raise the factor VIII level to at least 40 percent (p. 1211). Although this treatment may correct the bleeding time only transiently, it is usually effective in arresting hemorrhage. Factor VIII concentrate, given daily or every other day, is also valuable as prophylactic treatment when elective surgery or major dental surgery procedures are undertaken. The use of ε-aminocaproic acid (an inhibitor of fibrinolysis) may be of help in the treatment of nasal bleeding in von Willebrand's disease (p. 1211).

Familial disorders similar to von Willebrand's disease have been described in which laboratory abnormalities consist of a prolonged bleeding time associated with mild to moderate deficiency of factor IX or factor XI. The relationship of these cases to classic von Willebrand's disease is not known.

ACQUIRED DISORDERS OF PLATELET FUNCTION. Platelet function is frequently influenced by the plasma environment in which platelets reside. Abnormal plasma components are probably the basis for the decreased function of platelets, as follows: in uremia, guanidosuccinic acid, urea, phenolic compounds; in cirrhosis, fibrin degradation products and phospholipids; in disseminated intravascular coagulation, fibrin degradation products; in Waldenström's macroglobulinemia, abnormal globulins; in systemic lupus erythematosus, antibodies; and in infections, antigen–antibody complexes or viruses. Deficiency of vitamin C or B_{12} can also decrease platelet function. Decreased platelet function has been documented in many myeloproliferative disorders, such as polycythemia vera, myelofibrosis, primary thrombocythemia, Down's syndrome, and the myeloproliferative disorder associated with a missing C chromosome. In thrombocytosis, platelet function is normal. Many pharmacologic agents decrease platelet function. Clinically, the most important of these include aspirin, dipyridamole, antihistamines, glyceryl guaiacolate, carbenicillin, and phenylbutazone. Usual doses of aspirin (10 mg/kg) double the bleeding time in the average normal individual.

DISORDERS OF COAGULATION

Congenital Deficiencies

HEMOPHILIAS. Prior to 1952, the term hemophilia was reserved for a severe hemorrhagic disorder of males caused by a congenital deficiency of factor VIII activity (antihemophilic factor). Since that time, it has been recognized that specific hereditary deficiencies of factors IX and XI are also associated with similar hemorrhagic manifestations, so that the term *hemophilia* is now used to describe all of these disorders.

FACTOR VIII DEFICIENCY (CLASSIC HEMOPHILIA, AHF DEFICIENCY). Classic hemophilia is the most common hereditary deficiency of a coagulation factor that has severe clinical manifestations. The estimated incidence is 1 per 10,000 white male births in the United States and is probably similar in other races. The disease is due to a functionally abnormal factor VIII molecule present in normal amounts, as has been demonstrated by normal factor VIII antigen levels. Hemophilia is transmitted by the female as a sex-linked recessive trait. Thus, a positive family history may include brothers, sons of sisters, maternal uncles and grandfather, and maternal aunts' sons. The female carrier is usually asymptomatic, but in many instances can be shown to have a subnormal level of factor VIII activity (30 to 50 percent). About 40 percent of known carrier females have normal levels of factor VIII (50 to 200 percent). New techniques allow the detection of carriers with normal factor VIII activity by comparison with measurements of factor VIII antigen. A significant excess of antigen compared to activity indicates the carrier state with approximately 95 percent accuracy. In the affected male, deficiency of factor VIII may be severe with levels of less than 1 percent to mild levels of 5 to 25 percent. The severity of clinical manifestations is directly related to circulating factor VIII activity, which remains fairly constant in the individual patient and among affected males in the same family.

CLINICAL MANIFESTATIONS. Severe factor VIII deficiency is demonstrable at birth and may be recognized by serious hemorrhage following circumcision. However, failure to bleed excessively after circumcision does not rule out the diagnosis, since this procedure is tolerated without bleeding in many hemophilic infants. In the absence of trauma, significant hemorrhagic symptoms may not occur until the infant begins to walk, when excessive bruising is usually noted. Thereafter, recurrent bleeding, both spontaneous and following minor trauma, is a life long problem. Hemorrhage may occur in any area but most often leads to soft tissue bleeding and painful hemarthroses, particularly involving the knees, ankles, and elbows. Acute bleeding into a joint space or bursa produces severe pain, swelling, heat, tenderness, and limitation of motion. Repeated joint hemorrhages may result in extensive damage to synovial membranes, articular surfaces, epiphyseal plates, and metaphyses with ultimate contracture, ankylosis, and severe crippling if proper therapy is neglected. Bleeding may also occur into the skin, muscles, abdominal organs, gastrointestinal tract, peritoneal cavity, retroperitoneal area, and central nervous system. Hematuria is a frequent manifestation. Nosebleeds occur but are rarely troublesome, in contrast to disorders involving platelets. Severe trauma and surgical procedures may lead to extensive bleeding. It is not uncommon for phases or cycles of increased incidence of apparently spontaneous bleeding episodes to occur in individual patients. Although widely recognized, this phenomenon is not explained. Physical examination is unrevealing in the absence of hemorrhagic manifestations, unless chronic deformities have resulted from previous bleeding episodes.

DIAGNOSIS. The simplest and most sensitive of the screening tests is PTT, which is elevated when levels of factor VIII activity are below about 40 percent of normal. The whole blood clotting time is markedly prolonged only in severe hemophilia; only 1 to 2 percent of normal factor VIII level will produce a normal clotting time. Tests measuring platelet number and function are all normal (platelet count, bleeding time, platelet adhesiveness, clot retraction) as are the prothrombin time and fibrinogen concentration.

Confirmation of the diagnosis requires either a specific assay for factor VIII activity or the correction of a prolonged PTT by administration of factor VIII concentrate. The latter may be appropriate when the specific assay is not available and when therapy is needed for a bleeding complication. Assays for factor VIII activity are usually done by methods based on the PTT or thromboplastin generation test. The factor VIII activity is expressed as percent of a normal standard. The level of factor VIII antigen is normal in classic hemophilia, in contrast to von Willebrand's disease. It can be measured by immunologic methods, using a crossreacting animal antibody.

TREATMENT. The treatment of classic hemophilia is based primarily on the administration of factor VIII in the form of plasma or a concentrate of factor VIII derived from plasma. Local measures may be beneficial but constitute an addition to, rather than a substitute for treatment with factor VIII concentrates. Local pressure and/or topical application of hemostatic agents (thrombin, Oxycel, Surgicel) may be useful in treating superficial abrasions or very minor lacerations. When suturing is indicated, it should be done under coverage of factor VIII concentrate. Cauterization is contraindicated because it may lead to intractable bleeding. Immobilization of an affected limb and application of cold may add to the comfort of the patient. However, prolonged immobilization should be avoided as it results in muscle wasting and increases the risk of rebleeding when normal activity is resumed. Aspirin and aspirin-containing medications should never be used because they predispose to bleeding by inhibiting platelet function. Acetaminophen (Tylenol) can be substituted as an analgesic or antipyretic.

SOURCES OF FACTOR VIII. One of the most useful factor VIII concentrates is the cold-precipitable fraction of plasma described by Pool, which can be prepared in any blood bank. It is obtained by first quick-freezing plasma, and then thawing at 4 C; the precipitate that is formed is then separated. It can be stored frozen and later redissolved in about 10 ml of the original plasma or saline at room temperature. Depending on the efficiency of the blood fractionation center, the average bag of cryoprecipitate contains 75 to 150 units of factor VIII. One unit is defined as the factor VIII activity in 1 ml of average fresh normal plasma, eg, plasma with 100 percent factor VIII activity contains 1 unit/ml. Many commercial concentrates of factor VIII are available with a known amount of activity per vial. These lyophilized materials are made from pooled plasma, thus increasing the hepatitis risk over single-donor cryoprecipitate. However, they can be stored without refrigeration and, therefore, are convenient for self-administration by patients who are traveling. They are also useful when large doses are needed in management of serious bleeding, in surgery, and in patients with low titer factor VIII inhibitor. Replacement of factor VIII also can be achieved by transfusion of fresh, fresh-frozen, or lyophilized plasma. However, these unconcentrated sources are suitable primarily for treatment of mild bleeding episodes. One rarely achieves a peak factor VIII activity of greater than 20 percent with a dose of 10 ml/kg of fresh frozen plasma, and with larger doses there is a risk of hypervolemia. Regardless of the source of factor VIII, its rate of disappearance in the hemophilic patient is the same, with a half-life averaging 12 hours. The presence of active bleeding, fever, infection, or a circulating inhibitor of factor VIII increases the rate of disappearance.

DOSE. Specific treatment of acute bleeding depends on providing the patient with an amount of factor VIII that will achieve and maintain hemostasis until the particular hemorrhagic manifestation has subsided. As a general rule, transfusion of 0.5 units factor VIII/kg body weight should result in a 1 percent rise of factor VIII activity in the recipient. This is a useful guide, regardless of the source of factor VIII.

General therapeutic guidelines are as follows: severe and life-threatening hemorrhage requires initial levels between 50 and 100 percent and maintenance levels above 25 percent. More common periarticular or soft tissue bleeding of intermediate severity requires initial levels of about 40 percent and may respond to a single dose if treated early. Mild bleeding episodes can be arrested with initial levels of about 20 percent; 5 to 10 percent is effective in preventing spontaneous bleeding during normal activity. Specific problems will be discussed in more detail below.

Maintenance therapy requires administration of half the initial dose every 12 hours, this being the average interval during which half the activity in the originally infused material has disappeared. A treatment interval of 24 hours is more convenient and often adequate, even though it results in greater fluctuation of factor VIII activity; an average of 75 percent of the original activity is lost before the next infusion.

Management of Specific Bleeding Problems. *Joint, periarticular, and large soft tissue bleeds* are effectively treated by transfusion to a 40 percent factor VIII level, using the appropriate dose of cryoprecipitate or commercial concentrate. A brief period of traction or splinting may be indicated to prevent contractures. Cold compresses and analgesics (not aspirin) can be used to reduce pressure from swelling and to relieve pain. Aspiration of the acute hemarthrosis may be helpful after severe hemorrhage, but is rarely necessary if prompt and adequate replacement therapy is given. Rapid relief of joint pain usually follows adequate therapy long before objective improvement in the joint is detectable. Rehabilitative measures should be planned to prevent muscular atrophy and to maintain functional position of the affected extremity. However, extreme caution must be taken to avoid stretching beyond the comfortable range of motion without adequate factor VIII coverage, as this increases the risk of rebleeding. Gradual return to normal

activities is usually possible as pain and swelling subside. The orthopedist and the physical therapist may provide valuable guidance in rehabilitation.

In treating *severe and life-threatening bleeding* manifestations, such as hemorrhage into the pharynx or neck leading to dyspnea or dysphagia, central nervous system bleeding, suspected retroperitoneal bleeding, or bleeding from deep lacerations, or in preparing a patient for required surgical procedures, initial levels of 50 to 100 percent are required. Maintenance above about 25 percent for as long as 2 weeks may be needed to maintain hemostasis, particularly after surgery. It is therefore apparent that the availability of a large supply of factor VIII concentrate must be assured before elective procedures are undertaken. A tentative dosage schedule can be estimated, based on an average 12-hour biologic half-life of factor VIII. It is useful to monitor levels of factor VIII in the patient by factor VIII assay or by the degree of correction of the patient's PTT, since there are marked individual differences in the rate of factor VIII disappearance. Elective surgery should not be undertaken until the patient has been checked for the presence of an inhibitor (see below).

Hematuria may be unresponsive to treatment with factor VIII but frequently can be treated successfully without transfusion. Spontaneous hematuria, unassociated with known severe trauma, will usually subside on treatment with prednisone, 2 mg/kg, for 5 days. Gross hematuria often disappears within 48 hours after initiation of steroid therapy. Prednisone also has been recommended for the rehabilitation period following acute hemarthrosis or for chronic "effusions" in joints, but its effect in these situations has not been evaluated objectively.

ε-Aminocaproic acid (EACA) in mouth bleeding promotes hemostasis when used in conjunction with factor VIII concentrates. EACA is an inhibitor of the fibrinolytic enzyme system, which is particularly active in mucosal tissue. Indications for its use are bleeding of the oral mucosa, gums, tongue, or frenulum and bleeding from a tooth extraction. It is given in a dose of 200 mg/kg in conjunction with an initial administration of factor VIII (to a 40 to 50 percent level). A maintenance dose of 100 mg/kg/6 hours is continued for 2 to 5 days until complete healing occurs. EACA is contraindicated in suspected renal bleeding and has not proven helpful in soft tissue or joint hemorrhages.

FACTOR VIII INHIBITORS IN HEMOPHILIA. A specific circulating inhibitor of factor VIII, an antibody of the IgG type, develops in about 10 percent of hemophilic patients at some time in life. The presence of inhibitor may be first suspected when the patient fails to have the expected symptomatic response or correction of a prolonged PTT after treatment with factor VIII. Laboratory confirmation of the presence of an inhibitor is based on incubation of the patient's plasma with normal plasma, followed by determination of factor VIII activity or PTT. An inhibitor in the patient's plasma results in the inactivation of factor VIII in normal plasma. There is no evidence that the development of an inhibitor is related to the number of transfusions a patient receives. Therefore, replacement therapy in acute bleeding episodes should not be withheld for fear of inducing an inhibitor. In the presence of an inhibitor, transfused factor VIII is rapidly destroyed, and transfusions of factor VIII should be avoided if possible, as they predispose to development of a higher titer of inhibitor. The use of immunosuppressive drugs does not appear to be successful in preventing a rise in antibody titer after transfusion. In dire circumstances, exchange transfusion followed by large doses of concentrated factor VIII may be life-saving. Transfusions of prothrombin complex or factor IX concentrates, which contain activated coagulation factors, may be effective in controlling hemorrhage in patients whose inhibitor titer is too high to use factor VIII. The inhibitor usually subsides with time.

GENERAL CARE.   In addition to specific treatment for bleeding episodes, complete care of the hemophilic child should include prophylactic dental measures and routine immunizations given orally, intradermally, or slowly through a small needle if intramuscularly. Careful counseling of parents and the child regarding the limitations and requirements of hemophilia is most important in attempting to prevent the emotional invalidism and disturbed parent–child relationships that may arise.

The institution of *home treatment,* in areas where it can be medically supervised, allows the child and his family to become virtually self-sufficient in management of his disease. The rate of hospitalizations is decreased dramatically because bleeding manifestations are treated promptly with factor VIII concentrate kept at home. Most patients and their families first rely heavily on outpatient medical advice and telephone consultations but quickly become expert in recognizing those bleeding manifestations that they can treat with factor VIII and those that require prompt medical attention in addition.

FACTOR IX DEFICIENCY (PTC DEFICIENCY, CHRISTMAS DISEASE). Factor IX deficiency is transmitted as a sex-linked trait and accounts for about 15 percent of all patients with hemophilia. The clinical manifestations are indistinguishable from classic hemophilia, and this disorder also occurs in mild to severe forms. Factor IX assays indicate levels as low as 20 to 40 percent in some of the carriers, although a normal level does not eliminate the possibility of the carrier state. Diagnosis is suspected in the laboratory by a prolonged PTT and is confirmed by specific assays.

The principles of therapy are essentially the same as for factor VIII deficiency, except for the sources of factor IX. Since factor IX is stable in refrigerated plasma or blood, it is not necessary to use freshly drawn blood or plasma for transfusions; plasma stored as long as 21 days will provide adequate factor IX. Fresh frozen or lyophilized plasma may also be used, but there is some loss of factor IX in their preparation. Commercially prepared concentrates of factor IX are available and presently are the mainstay of transfusion therapy. The biologic half-life of factor IX is about 22 hours, but the initial rate of disappearance is more rapid, since approximately half of the transfused factor IX activity passes rapidly into the extravascular space. Consequently, a larger dose is given initially: 1 unit of factor IX activity/kg body weight. The need for repeated doses of plasma or concentrate to treat severe bleeding episodes is similar to that described for factor VIII deficiency.

FACTOR XI DEFICIENCY (PTA DEFICIENCY). This is the least common form of hemophilia and differs from factor VIII and IX deficiency in several respects. Deficiency of factor XI is transmitted as an autosomal recessive trait and occurs in both sexes, primarily in patients of Jewish ancestry. The homozygote manifests severe factor XI deficiency that is associated with hemorrhagic problems similar to those present in severe factor VIII or IX deficiencies, but the symptoms are usually considerably milder. The carrier rarely develops clinical bleeding. Treatment of bleeding episodes is with 10 ml/kg of fresh frozen plasma.

FACTOR XIII DEFICIENCY (FIBRIN-STABILIZING FACTOR DEFICIENCY). Congenital deficiency of factor XIII is a rare familial hemorrhagic disorder and is probably transmitted as an autosomal recessive trait. Prolonged umbilical bleeding, bruising, hematoma formation, and central nervous system hemorrhage are the most frequent manifestations. All of the usual tests of hemostatic function are normal. The defect is detected by testing for solubility of the patient's fibrin clot in 5-M urea, normal clots being insoluble, whereas factor-XIII-deficient clots are readily dissolved. Hemorrhagic symptoms respond readily to transfusion with plasma.

FACTOR XII DEFICIENCY (HAGEMAN TRAIT). Deficiency of factor XII is not a hemorrhagic disorder but is mentioned here to call attention to the marked laboratory abnormalities associated with this hereditary trait. The homozygous state is associated with severe lack of factor XII, which results in marked abnormalities of several coagulation tests, including the clotting time, prothrombin consumption test, and PTT. Since these patients are not subject to abnormal bleeding, specific identification of their deficiency, which is usually found as an abnormal result in a screening test, is important. This may be accomplished by specific assay or correction studies. Factor XII is required for contact activation of the coagulation process in vitro; however, the in vivo contribution of factor XII to the hemostatic process is not known.

FLETCHER FACTOR (PREKALLIKREIN) DEFICIENCY. This rare coagulation factor deficiency (Fletcher factor) produces an extremely prolonged PTT in the absence of any bleeding tendency. The activated PTT tends to correct during prolonged (9- to 12-minute) incubation of the clotting mixture. Fletcher factor is probably plasma prekallikrein, which is the precursor of the kinin system. Subjects with this deficiency have no known associated clinical abnormalities of hemostasis or inflammation.

Another intrinsic coagulation factor necessary for optimal contact activation (prolonged PTT without bleeding manifestations) has been noted to be deficient on a hereditary basis. This factor has been termed contact activation cofactor or Fitzgerald factor.

HEREDITARY AFIBRINOGENEMIA AND DYS-FIBRINOGENEMIA. Congenital afibrinogenemia and dysfibrinogenemia are rare disorders that are due to absent or functionally defective fibrinogen. They occur in both sexes and are transmitted as an autosomal recessive trait. The dysfibrinogenemias are named for the cities in which they were first described, ie, fibrinogen Zurich, Baltimore, Paris, and so forth, and are characterized by prolonged thrombin and prothrombin times with a normal level of fibrinogen by turbimetric and immunologic methods. Clinical manifestations include bruising, epistaxis, and bleeding following trauma but may be quite mild. Congenital hypofibrinogenemias also occur in which clotting is delayed, but a very small clot is eventually formed.

Treatment of acute bleeding episodes or preparation for surgery may be accomplished by transfusions of plasma, fibrinogen concentrates, or cryoprecipitate. The minimal hemostatic level is 80 to 100 mg/dl. The rate of disappearance of transfused fibrinogen is biphasic; 50 percent disappears within 48 hours, and thereafter the biologic half-life is 4 to 5 days.

PROTHROMBIN, FACTOR V, FACTOR VII, AND FACTOR X DEFICIENCIES. Isolated deficiencies of prothrombin (hypoprothrombinemia), factor V (parahemophilia), factor VII, or factor X (Stuart-Prower factor deficiency) are rare hemorrhagic disorders. Combined congenital deficiencies of some of these factors have also been reported. An abnormal prothrombin time is found in each disorder, but specific assays are required to establish the diagnosis. Treatment of bleeding episodes is by use of fresh plasma or plasma concentrate. Vitamin K is of no value in treatment of the congenital deficiencies of vitamin-K-dependent factors.

Combined coagulation factor deficiencies have been reported in rare cases. These include factors V and VIII, VIII and IX, and VIII and abnormal fibrinogen.

Acquired Deficiencies: Decreased Production

VITAMIN-K-DEPENDENT COAGULATION FACTORS. Combined deficiencies of the vitamin-K-dependent factors (factors II, VII, IX, and X) frequently result from interference with intake, absorption, or utilization of vitamin K, as in liver disease, malabsorption, altered bowel flora, coumadin treatment, or a combination of several of these factors as occurs in the newborn. Such deficiencies are most readily detected by a prolonged prothrombin time, and the degree of individual factor depression may be measured by specific assays. Treatment with vitamin K may reverse such deficiencies unless parenchymal liver disease is severe. Blood or plasma may be required to manage hemorrhagic symptoms.

The vitamin-K-dependent factors are often depressed in the newborn infant. Rarely, the deficiency is severe enough to result in spontaneous bleeding manifestations, or hemorrhagic disease of the newborn. Older infants with chronic diarrhea are also susceptible to vitamin K deficiency.

Administration of vitamin K in a single small dose (1 mg), either intramuscularly or orally at the time of birth will prevent the fall of prothrombin and factors VII, IX, and X in full-term infants. This measure is recommended as prophylaxis for hemorrhagic disease of the newborn in all newborn infants. The natural oil-soluble preparations of vitamin K are preferred for this purpose, since large doses of the synthetic water-soluble preparations have been associated with hyperbilirubinemia and kernicterus. Hemorrhagic disease of the newborn or vitamin K deficiency in the older infant may be treated effectively with 1 to 2 mg vitamin K_1 intravenously. Serious bleeding may require transfusion of fresh whole blood or frozen plasma, since several hours may be required for vitamin K to be effective.

FACTORS VIII AND IX DEFICIENCIES ASSOCIATED WITH CONGENITAL HYPOTHYROIDISM. Moderate deficiencies of factors VIII and IX have been observed in congenital hypothyroid patients and have been associated with bleeding following operative procedures or dental extractions. Treatment of the hypothyroid state has corrected the coagulation factor deficits.

LIVER DISEASE. The hemorrhagic complications seen in severe liver disease may be due to decreased production of coagulation factors or to disseminated intravascular coagulation (DIC) or both. All of the clotting factors are produced in the liver (factor VIII is made elsewhere as well); therefore their circulating levels reflect the protein synthetic capacity of the liver parenchymal cells. Deficiency of factor VII (biologic half-life of 4 hours) is the first coagulation factor abnormality seen in liver damage and may manifest itself as a prolonged prothrombin time. Significant depressions of fibrinogen (half-life of several days) are seen much later. In severe liver disease, such as overwhelming hepatic necrosis or far-advanced cirrhosis, all coagulation screening tests are markedly prolonged; in mild disease only the prothrombin time may be affected. Thrombocytopenia is seen occasionally in severe liver disease, although the mechanism usually is not clear. Increased fibrinolysis, with or without DIC, may be manifested by the detection of increased fibrin degradation products and shortened euglobulin lysis times. Therefore, the diagnosis of DIC in patients with liver disease should be made with great caution. A decreasing or low level of factor VIII is the most useful laboratory sign of DIC in these instances, since factor VIII activity and antigen often are greatly elevated in uncomplicated hepatitis and cirrhosis.

Treatment of the bleeding episodes consists of replacement of decreased platelets and clotting factors as needed with platelet concentrates and fresh frozen plasma. In the infant, exchange transfusion may be helpful temporarily, especially in severe fetal hydrops with secondary liver necrosis. Heparinization is rarely warranted, even when DIC is suspected. Patients with severe liver disease tolerate heparin very poorly.

Acquired Deficiencies: Increased Destruction

INTRAVASCULAR COAGULATION SYNDROMES   Pathologic intravascular coagulation may be seen in two groups of disorders: (1) disseminated intravascular coagulation (DIC) throughout the body, with widespread microthrombi and frequently a diffuse bleeding diathesis due to consumption of platelets and coagulation factors; and (2) localized venous or arterial thrombosis often restricted to a single vessel or organ. Although these groups may overlap, it is useful to discuss them separately.

DISSEMINATED INTRAVASCULAR COAGULATION (DIC, defibrination syndrome, consumption coagulopathy) is a complication of many diseases and is triggered by many events, including sepsis, hypoxia, acidosis, and tissue damage. The condition may be acute, as in septic or hemorrhagic shock or asphyxia, or chronic, as in sickle cell anemia, polycythemic states, or diffuse malignancies. Depending upon the severity of the process, a variable decrease in circulating clotting factors (fibrinogen, II, V, and VIII) and varying elevation of fibrin degradation products (FDP) may be observed. In the severe episodes, all screening tests (Table 3) are abnormal; in the mild episodes, only transient thrombocytopenia and increased FDP may be seen.

Treatment consists of removing the triggering event if possible and, if the patient is at risk of serious hemorrhage, correcting of the deficit in platelets and clotting factors by transfusion of platelet concentrates (1 platelet pack per 7 kg is estimated to raise the platelet count by 50,000) and/or fresh frozen plasma (10 ml/kg). If the triggering event cannot be removed and/or serious damage is likely due to microthrombi, *heparinization* (100 units/kg as a loading dose and 100 units every 4 to 6 hours) may be necessary in addition to replacement therapy with platelets and clotting factors. The dose of heparin can be intermittent, but a more even therapeutic effect is obtained by continuous infusion. Heparin therapy may be monitored by the activated PTT, which should be kept at 1.5 to 2 times the normal or baseline level.

PURPURA FULMINANS is an acute, frequently fatal disorder characterized by sudden appearance of large ecchymotic areas, which are commonly located on the lower extremities and are often symmetric. The syndrome is usually preceded for several days to a month by an infectious disease, scarlet fever or varicella being the most frequent. The lesions rapidly enlarge and may lead to gangrene of an entire extremity. The edges of the lesions are usually sharply demarcated, and central bullae may develop. Fever, vomiting, and oliguria are usually present, and the patient may develop shock. Laboratory evidence of DIC may be detected. Widespread microthrombi involving many organs, including the kidney, have been demonstrated. The mortality rate is high, and amputation and plastic repair often have been required in survivors. Prompt heparinization can be life-saving.

NECROTIZING ENTEROCOLITIS (p. 992), which occurs primarily in sick newborn infants, usually presents with significant thrombocytopenia; DIC may also be seen in the more severely affected infants. If severe DIC is present, exchange transfusion is helpful in preparing the infant for surgery; otherwise, platelet transfusions are indicated for therapy of associated bleeding manifestations.

Antifibrinolytic agents such as ϵ-aminocaproic acid have no role in the intravascular coagulation syndromes, even though increased fibrinolysis frequently is present as well.

LOCALIZED VENOUS AND ARTERIAL THROMBOSES (with or without thromboemboli) are occasionally seen with vascular stasis, malignancies, renal disease, severe inflammatory disease such as ulcerative colitis or regional enteritis, and infection. The diagnosis is usually made by history and physical findings substantiated by venogram, arteriogram, or lung scans. The different patterns of platelet and coagulation factor consumption, characteristically associated with venous and arterial thrombi, have been elucidated by studying the turnover of labeled platelets and fibrinogen. For example, in *venous thrombosis* (eg, with immobilization following trauma) the "red thrombus" that forms resembles clotted blood, and there is increased consumption of both platelets and fibrinogen. Laboratory findings may include either depressed or normal platelet count and fibrinogen concentration because normal values can be maintained by a compensatory increase in production with rates of destruction that are about 2 to 3 times normal. Results of the TT, PTT, PT, and FDP are variable. In general, *large vessel thrombosis*, whether venous or arterial, is treated by heparinization. In *small vessel arterial thrombosis*, which is usually associated with the formation of small white platelet thrombi on foreign surfaces (prosthetic devices, denuded epithelium, and areas of vasculitis) in the arterial circulation, there is increased consumption of platelets, but the rate of fibrinogen disappearance may be normal. The only laboratory abnormalities may be a depression in the platelet count and/or a slight increase in FDP. In arterial thrombi associated with abnormal surfaces (vasculitis, heart valve prosthesis, hemolytic uremic syndrome) the use of agents that inhibit platelet aggregation (aspirin 10 mg/kg/day and dipyridamole 3 to 5 mg/kg/day) may return platelet survival to normal and arrest progression of the thrombi.

Pathologic Anticoagulants

Imbalance of hemostasis leading to hemorrhagic manifestations may result from pathologic anticoagulants arising spontaneously or in association with a variety of disease states. Anticoagulants against specific clotting factors (factors VIII, IX, and XI) occur in the hemophilias, and an anticoagulant against factor VIII may develop in otherwise normal individuals, particularly postpartum women and older adults. The latter circumstance results in an acquired hemophilia-like state, with a marked decrease in factor VIII secondary to the specific anticoagulant.

Circulating anticoagulants occur in a small percentage of patients with lupus erythematosus. These anticoagulants tend to act as antithromboplastins and antithrombins and may be detected by prolongation of the PTT, PT, and PTT performed with mixtures of the patient's plasma with normal blood or plasma. Significant hemorrhage is uncommon despite these abnormalities, and the anticoagulants frequently subside following steroid treatment of the lupus. Heparin-like anticoagulants have been reported with urticaria pigmentosa and mast cell leukemia.

References

Abildgaard CF: Current concepts in the management of hemophilia. Sem in Hematol 12:223, 1975

Addiego JE, Mentzer WC, Dallman PR: Thrombocytosis in infants and children. J Pediatr 85:805, 1974

Allen DM, Diamond LK, Howell DA: Anaphylactoid purpura in children (Schönlein-Henoch syndrome); review with a follow-up of the renal complications. Am J Dis Child 99:833, 1960

Arenson EB, August CS: Preliminary report: treatment of the hemolytic-uremic syndrome with aspirin and dipyridamole. J Pediatr 86:957, 1975

Bennett B, Forman WB, Ratnoff OD: Studies on the nature of antihemophilic factor (factor VIII). J Clin Invest 52:2191, 1973

Biggs R (ed): Human Blood Coagulation Haemostasis and Thrombosis Oxford, Blackwell, 1972

Bloom AL: Intravascular coagulation and the liver. Br J Haematol 30:1, 1975

Corrigan JJ: Oral bleeding in hemophilia: treatment with epsilon aminocaproic acid and replacement therapy. J Pediatr 80:124, 1972

Czapek EE, Deykin D, Salzman EW: Platelet dysfunction in glycogen storage disease type 1. Blood 41:235, 1973

Duthie RB, Matthews JM, Rizza CR, Steel WM: The Management of Musculo-Skeletal Problems in the Haemophilias. Oxford, Blackwell, 1972

Ekert H, Firkin BG: Recent advances in haemophilia and von Willebrand's disease. Vox Sang 28:409, 1975

Goldschmidt B, Sarkadi B, Gardos G, Matlary A: Platelet production and survival in cyanotic congenital heart disease. Scand J Haematol 13:110, 1974

Harker LA, Slichter SJ: The bleeding time as a screening test for evaluation of platelet function. N Engl J Med 287:155, 1972

———— Slichter SJ: Platelet and fibrinogen consumption in man. N Engl J Med 287:999, 1972

Hathaway WE: Care of the critically ill child: the problem of disseminated intravascular coagulation. Pediatrics 46:767, 1970

———— Bleeding disorders due to platelet dysfunction. Am J Dis Child 121:127, 1971

———— Heparin therapy in acute meningococcemia. Editorial comment. J Pediatr 82:900, 1973

———— The bleeding newborn. Semin Hematol 12:175, 1975

———— Alsever J: The relation of "Fletcher factor" to factors XI and XII. Br J Haematol 18:161, 1970

Hilgartner MW: Hemophilic arthropathy. Adv Pediatr 21:139, 1974

Lammi AT, Lovric VA: Idiopathic thrombocytopenic purpura: an epidemiologic study. J Pediatr 83:31, 1973

Murphy S, Oski FA, Gardner FH: Hereditary thrombocytopenia with an intrinsic platelet defect. N Engl J Med 281:857, 1969

Pechet L, Chesney C, Colman RW: Variants of von Willebrand's disease. N Engl J Med 288:1129, 1973

Pool JG, Shannon AE: Production of high potency concentrates of anti-hemophilic globulin in a closed-bag system. N Engl J Med 273:1443, 1965

Quick AJ: Telangiectasia: its relationship to the Minot von Willebrand syndrome. Am J Med Sci 254:585, 1967

Regan DH, Lackner H: Defibrination syndrome: changing concepts and recognition of the low grade form. Am J Med Sci 266:84, 1973

Riedler GF, Straub PW, Frick PG: Thrombocytopenia in septicemia. A clinical study for the evaluation of its incidence and diagnostic value. Helv Med Acta 36:23, 1969

Rosenberg RD: Actions and interactions of antithrombin and heparin. N Engl J Med 292:146, 1975

Saito H, Ratnoff OD, Waldmann NR, Abraham JP: Fitzgerald trait. Deficiency of a hitherto unrecognized agent, Fitzgerald factor, participating in surface-mediated reactions of clotting, fibrinolysis, generation of kinins, and the property of diluted plasma enhancing vascular permeability (PF/dil). J Clin Invest 55:1082, 1975

Schulman I, Pierce M, Lukens A, Currimbhoy Z: Studies on thrombopoiesis. I. A factor in normal human plasma required for platelet production; chronic thrombocytopenia due to its deficiency. Blood 16:943, 1960

Shapiro SS, Hultin M: Acquired inhibitors to the blood coagulation factors. Semin Thrombosis Hemostasis 1:336, 1975

Simone JV, Abildgaard CF, Schulman I: Blood coagulation in thyroid dysfunction. N Engl J Med 273:1057, 1965

Simons SM, Main CA, Yaish HM, Rutzky J: Idiopathic thrombocytopenic purpura in children. J Pediatr 87:16, 1975

Stuart MJ: Inherited defects of platelet function. Semin Hematol 12:233, 1975

Wedemeyer AL, Lewis JH: Improvement in hemostasis following phlebotomy in cyanotic patients with heart disease. J Pediatr 83:46, 1973

Weiss HJ: Platelets: physiology and abnormalities of platelet function. N Engl J Med 293:531, 580, 1975

William WJ: Thrombocytosis. In Williams WJ, Beutler E, Erslev AJ, Rundles RW: (eds): Hematology. New York, McGraw-Hill, 1972, p 1162

Zimmerman TS, Ratnoff OD, Littell AS: Detection of carriers of classic hemophilia using an immunologic assay for antihemophilic factor (factor VIII). J Clin Invest 50:255, 1971

USE OF BLOOD AND BLOOD PRODUCTS
Peter R. Dallman

Blood and blood products usually are used as replacement therapy when there is decreased production or excessive loss of one or more blood components. Their use can be life-saving. However, because of the high risk of complications (p. 1219), it is important to weigh the anticipated benefits against the known risks and to be guided by clinical considerations rather than the desire to correct abnormal laboratory values.

All blood products are expensive, and many are in very short supply; it is rare that all components present in whole blood are needed in any single clinical situation. Selection of the appropriate blood fraction will permit more efficient use of a scarce commodity and is better for the patient. Fractions of blood in common use are listed in Table 20. The uses of albumin, fibrinogen, immune serum globulin, and Rho (D) immune globulin are discussed in other chapters. The uses of fresh frozen plasma and of concentrates of coagulation factors are described on pages 1210 and 1212 and in Table 20.

TABLE 20. Blood Components in Common Use

Blood Component:* Volume and Activity	Indication for Use	Dose	Duration of Effectiveness	Effectiveness After Repeated Use	Complications
1. *Whole blood* 450–500 ml/unit	Restoration of blood volume after acute blood loss; exchange transfusion[†]	2 ml/kg raises Hct 1%	Red cell loss of about 1%/day	Red cell survival may remain normal after many transfusions but there is an increasing risk of developing antibodies to minor RBC blood groups WBC,[‡] and platelets[‡]	Acute intravascular hemolysis with ABO incompatibility
2. *Packed red cells:* 250–350 ml/unit	To increase oxygen delivery to tissues; severe anemia	1 ml/kg raises Hct 1%; Max amount: 15 ml/kg at one time; Max rate: 5-6 ml/kg/hr			Slower extravascular hemolysis with Rh and minor blood group incompatability
3. *Leukocyte-poor red cells:* buffy coat removed 200–250 ml/unit	Same as 2 and to prevent febrile reactions due to WBC antibodies				Febrile reactions due to WBC antibodies[‡]
4. *Frozen red cells:*[§] 200 ml/unit	Same as 2 and to prevent febrile and anaphylactic IgA reactions				Urticaria, anaphylactic Ig A reactions
5. *Platelet concentrate:* 30–50 ml/unit	Severe thrombocytopenia	1 unit of platelets/7 kg raises platelet count about 50,000	Loss of about 50%/day	Rapid decrease in life-span due to development of antibodies	Risk of infection with 2–3 days storage at room temperature, febrile reactions (WBC antibodies), urticarial reactions (anti-IgA)
6. *Fresh frozen plasma:* 200–250 ml/unit	Replacement of clotting factor or immune globulin, burns, expansion blood volume	1 ml/kg raises clotting factor activity about 2%	Half-life of clotting factor ranges from 6 hr to 5 days	Continued effectiveness, but danger of hypervolemia restricts the volume used.	Urticarial reactions (anti-IgA)
7. *Cryoprecipitate:* Average of 100 units of factor VIII activity per 10–25-ml bag	Hemophilia	1 unit of activity/kg raises factor VII activity in plasma by 2%	Half-life averages 12 hr	Continued effectiveness except in rare patient who develops antibodies against factor VIII	Rare anti-IgA urticarial reaction
8. *Pooled factor VIII concentrate:* 250–1000 units of factor VIII activity per 10 to 30 ml					Increased risk of hepatitis
9. *Pooled concentrate of II, VII, IX, X:* Proplex 500 units of factor IX activity per vial	Factor IX deficiency	1 unit of factor IX raises factor IX activity in plasma by 2%	Half-life averages 24 hr	Usually continues to be effective	Intravascular thrombosis when used in liver disease or DIC, increased risk of hepatitis

Albumin, fibrinogen, immune globin, Rho immune globulin and leukocytes are not included.

* *Each unit or bag of No. 2 to No. 7 is prepared from a single unit of blood; No. 8 and No. 9 are purified from large pools of plasma and are associated with an increased risk of hepatitis.*

† *Blood less than 1 week old.*

‡ *Less common with leukocyte-poor blood.*

§ *Washed cells can also be used in patients who are deficient in IgA.*

WHOLE BLOOD

Whole blood rarely is required when the purpose is to improve oxygen delivery, since packed red cells provide the same oxygen-carrying capacity in a smaller volume. The most important indication for the use of whole blood is the rapid restoration of normal blood volume and red cell mass after acute hemorrhage. Restoration of the blood volume is generally the more vital of the two. Clinical evidence of acute blood loss includes an elevated pulse rate and a fall in systolic blood pressure; other findings are pallor, vasoconstriction, sweating, and oliguria. These manifestations indicate that the extent of blood loss is in excess of 20 to 30 percent of the total. Replacement of blood with a volume equivalent to the estimated loss should be prompt. After massive blood transfusion, laboratory studies may also indicate a need for clotting factors and/or platelets. Labile clotting factors (such as factors V and VIII) and viable platelets are not adequately replaced by stored whole blood. Consequently fresh-frozen plasma and platelet concentrates may be given in addition to whole blood, or packed red blood cells. Estimates of the degree of blood loss by hemoglobin or hematocrit within a few hours of an acute hemorrhage are likely to be misleading. Both values may remain normal and fail to indicate blood loss until the plasma volume has been expanded with fluid from extravascular sources. Such equilibration may not be complete until 2 to 3 days later.

Indications for Fresh Whole Blood (Stored Less Than 1 Week)

In contrast to most situations, in which stored blood can be used, fresh whole blood (often collected on the previous day) is commonly used to prime the equipment used for extracorporeal circulation, as in hemodialysis units and in heart-lung machines. In some centers fresh platelet-poor blood is used to prime the equipment, and the platelets from the same units of blood are administered after the procedure. This avoids damage to transfused platelets in the equipment. Fresh whole blood also may be used to assure a high red cell 2,3-DPG content after exchange transfusions for hemolytic disease of the newborn and idiopathic hyperbilirubinemia. Fresh blood also supplies clotting factors in these situations, since even the labile factors V and VIII usually retain more than 50 percent of their original activity if the blood is used within 1 week. (The choice of anticoagulant and effects of blood storage are discussed on page 1218).

Walking Donors

It has become a common and probably overutilized practice to give small replacement transfusions to sick newborn infants, especially preterm babies with respiratory distress, when large amounts of blood have been withdrawn for the determination of blood gases and other laboratory tests. Ideally, the transfused blood should have a near-neutral pH to avoid aggravating acidemia, and it should retain the original levels of 2,3-DPG to assure optimal oxygen delivery. The need for an efficient system for providing a series of small transfusions is met in some large hospitals by a walking donor program. In such programs, hospital personnel serve repeatedly as donors for the relatively small individual amounts of blood needed to transfuse infants. Such donors should meet the standards of the American Association of Blood Banks and be tested periodically for hepatitis-associated antigen. When needed, blood is drawn from the donor into a syringe containing 2 units of heparin per milliliter of blood to be drawn. An aliquot is appropriately crossmatched, and the remainder is then administered to the patient through a filter as soon as possible. The procedure avoids wasting larger amounts of blood when only 10 to 30 ml are needed, but it also requires strict attention to aseptic technique and the proper use of anticoagulants. There is a great deal of concern among blood banking experts about the safety of such transfusions, since it is difficult to maintain the careful quality control that blood bank personnel have developed. Under present conditions, there is a need for reconciling convenience with safety, but even more important is the development of better criteria for such transfusions and methods for monitoring sick infants with less blood sampling.

RED CELL PREPARATIONS

Packed Red Blood Cells

Since the purpose of most transfusions is to improve the oxygen-carrying capacity of the blood, packed red blood cells are usually the preparation of choice. This is the component of blood remaining when most of the plasma has been removed. Transfusions of packed red cells are used in such conditions as hypoplastic anemia, hemolytic anemia, leukemia in relapse, or chronic renal failure. They may also be used in sickle cell anemia as a source of red cells resistant to sickling, thus reducing the chance of thrombotic crisis in high-risk situations, such as late pregnancy or major surgery. In thalassemia, transfusions not only improve oxygen delivery but also suppress the excessive and harmful endogenous production of nonviable cells.

White-cell-poor Preparations

In individuals who require repeated transfusions, it may be preferable to use blood preparations from which most of the white cells have been removed, especially if the patient has developed febrile reactions thought to be due to white cell antibodies. Leukocyte-poor blood is also used in potential transplant recipients to reduce the risk of sensitization to tissue antigens. White-cell-poor preparations include red cells from which most leukocytes have been removed by centrifugation or from which neutrophils have been removed by passing blood through a fiber filter and frozen red cells in which washing has removed most of the white cells and freezing has ruptured most of the remaining ones. Frozen red cells are also useful for stockpiling rare red cell types.

Dose and Rate of Administration of Whole Blood and Red Cells

About 2 ml/kg of whole blood (PVC ~ 35 percent) are required to raise the patient's hematocrit by 1 percent. Using packed cells, leukocyte-poor cells, or washed cells that are prepared to a hematocrit of about 75 percent, about 1 ml/kg is required to raise the hematocrit by 1 percent.

The greatest volume of blood that can be administered safely at one time depends on the clinical situation. With acute hemorrhage, large amounts of blood (estimated to be equivalent to the amount that has been lost) can be administered rapidly and safely. At the other extreme, the patient with severe anemia or chronic renal disease may already be on the verge of cardiac failure and cannot tolerate more than 2 to 3 ml/kg given at a slow rate. In such patients a safe way of administering blood is to infuse high-hematocrit blood in increments of 10 to 20 ml, alternating with the removal of the same volume of the patient's low-hematocrit blood. Even under these circumstances, vital signs should be monitored carefully in order to detect impending heart failure.

Under ordinary conditions, when cardiovascular reserve is adequate, it is safe to administer a maximum of 15 ml/kg packed red cells at a rate not to exceed 5 ml/kg/hour (a minimum of 3 hours for a transfusion of 15 ml/kg). Some patients with a chronic transfusion requirement may tolerate a maximum of 20 ml/kg of packed red cells, with careful monitoring of blood pressure and pulse rate. Blood should be given more slowly for the first 15 to 30 minutes, since this will allow for the detection of unexpected transfusion reactions before the patient has received a large volume.

Anticoagulants in Common Use

Most donor blood is collected into a container in which there is an anticoagulant mixture of either citrate, phosphate buffer, and dextrose (CPD) or a more acid mixture of citrate and dextrose (ACD). In both mixtures, citrate acts as an anticoagulant by chelating ionic calcium. Ordinarily, this removal of calcium is of no clinical consequence. However, during exchange transfusions or with the transfusion of massive amounts of blood, there may be transient hypocalcemia, rarely leading to tetany or cardiac arrest. In these situations, it is advisable to administer ionic calcium intravenously in a dose of 0.5 to 1.0 ml of 10 percent calcium gluconate solution after each 100 ml of blood infused (p.1142).

With storage, ACD and CPD blood becomes increasingly acid, and there is gradual loss of 2,3-DPG in the red cells. Blood freshly drawn into ACD has a pH of 6.9. After a week, pH drops to 6.8. CPD blood is less acid, with an initial pH of 7.1 and a pH of 7.0 after 1 week. Blood stored more than 7 days in ACD or more than 10 days in CPD has lost sufficient 2,3-DPG to have a left-shifted oxygen dissociation curve, similar to that of fetal blood. Such blood has a high oxygen affinity and releases less oxygen to the tissues than does fresh blood (p.1114). When stored blood is transfused into the patient, the 2,3-DPG level within the transfused red cells is gradually restored to normal, but this requires 8 to 24 hours following transfusion and consequently delays the full therapeutic effect. The use of CPD blood is advantageous in clinical situations that are characterized by acidosis and hypoxia because it has a more neutral pH and retains a normal 2,3-DPG for a longer period of storage than ACD blood.

Heparin is a useful anticoagulant for blood used in exchange transfusion and open heart surgery. It has a slightly alkaline pH, and there are no problems related to hypocalcemia. The major disadvantage of heparin is that blood must be used within 24 to 48 hours of collection because there is no glucose in the medium to maintain red cell metabolism and because the anticoagulant effect of heparin is gradually lost. Therefore heparinized blood is often wasted if it is ordered but not used. Heparin is normally cleared from the blood at the rate of 50 percent every 4 hours. After an exchange transfusion, the residual heparin in the circulation is sufficient to slow blood clotting for a few hours. Some physicians administer 1.5 units of protamine for every unit of heparin calculated to be remaining after an exchange transfusion in order to further reduce the small risk of spontaneous hemorrhage.

PLATELET TRANSFUSION

Platelet concentrates have become available widely in recent years and are used increasingly to arrest bleeding due to thrombocytopenia or abnormalities of platelet function. One unit of platelet concentrate contains about 50 percent of the platelets present in a unit of blood. One unit per 7 kg body weight will raise the platelet count by about $50,000/mm^3$. Administering platelets sufficient to raise the count above $50,000/mm^3$ is adequate to arrest most types of bleeding due to thrombocytopenia, and a count above $25,000/mm^3$ may be adequate to stop bleeding that is not life-threatening. Concentrates can be stored at room temperature (22 C) up to 72 hours. Such unrefrigerated platelets have a biologic half-life of about 1 to 2 days, a marked improvement over the shorter survival formerly obtained with refrigerated platelet concentrates. The short survival of platelets requires administration of platelets daily or every other day when maintenance of the platelet count is justified on clinical grounds.

Platelet concentrates are contaminated to some extent with red cells, which can sensitize the Rh-negative individual. Rh-negative girls who require platelet transfusions and who have a disease with a good prognosis should receive platelets from Rh-negative donors when possible. A simple means of assessing the usefulness of a platelet transfusion in terms of platelet survival is by two or more determinations of the platelet count after infusion. Unfortunately, an increase in platelet number is not necessarily correlated with improved platelet function, as judged by reversal of a prolonged bleeding time or correction of hemorrhagic manifestations. In fact, there is evidence that storage of platelets at room temperature results in some loss of platelet function, which is only regained gradually after transfusion.

The best use of platelet concentrates is in the treatment of hemorrhagic manifestations in acute and self-limited thrombocytopenic conditions, especially those in which the mechanism for thrombocytopenia is decreased production. However, even when thrombocytopenia is due to an increased rate of destruction, a platelet transfusion is often effective in stopping hemorrhage, even though only a very brief rise in platelet count is achieved. Platelet transfusions may be life-saving in neonatal thrombocytopenias, which usually run a brief but sometimes fatal course.

Prophylactic use of platelet transfusions in chronically thrombocytopenic patients is rarely practical because of the short survival of platelets and the likelihood that platelet antibodies will develop. Demonstrable isoimmunization is rare with 10 or fewer units of platelets but becomes increasingly frequent with continued infusion. The development of platelet antibodies is associated with shortened platelet survival. For this reason, it is usually better to treat patients with aplastic anemia, malignancies (leukemia), and thrombocytopenias of unknown etiology only for specific hemorrhagic complications.

When a patient has become refractory to platelets from random donors, there may still be a response to platelets from a histocompatible donor (usually a sibling) or from a partly compatible donor (usually a parent). Indeed, some patients with aplastic anemia have been effectively treated for long periods solely with platelets from one histocompatible sibling. Another situation in which the selection of the donor can be critical is isoimmune thrombocytopenia of the newborn (p. 1207). This disorder is due to maternal antibodies against the platelets of the newborn. Since maternal platelets are not affected, platelets obtained from the mother have a good survival in the infant. The mother's red cells can be reinfused into her circulation after the platelets have been separated.

Platelet Concentrates as Sources of Clotting Factors

Units of platelet concentrate are usually suspended in 20 to 40 ml of plasma. In the newborn this volume of plasma often exceeds 10 ml/kg and can be sufficient to improve hemostasis in conditions characterized by a deficiency of both platelets and clotting factors (see disseminated intravascular coagulation, p. 1214).

Fresh blood is a poor source of platelets, since an excessive volume must be given in order to produce a substantial rise in the platelet count. The platelet count can be raised by no more than 15,000/mm^3 after 10 ml of fresh whole blood per kilogram of body weight are administered, and even to achieve this effect the blood must be given within 24 hours of the blood donation. Platelet-rich plasma is a slightly more concentrated source of platelets and also contains other coagulation factors, but a relatively large volume is required for the administration of few platelets. Ten milliliters per kilogram can raise the platelet count no more than 30,000/mm^3.

LEUKOCYTE TRANSFUSION

Granulocyte transfusions are used experimentally in a few specialized centers to treat granulocytopenic patients with life-threatening infection. It remains difficult to isolate sufficient functioning granulocytes from a single individual, and current procedures involve some risk to the donor. The short half-life of neutrophils in the circulation is an additional handicap. Recent studies indicate that clinical benefit is most likely when the donor is HL-A matched and more than one leukocyte transfusion is administered.

TRANSFUSION REACTIONS

It is estimated that over 0.5 percent of blood transfusions are followed by a transfusion reaction. Certain precautions can be taken to minimize this risk. A history of the patient's responses to previous transfusions should be obtained, particularly in respect to febrile and allergic reactions which are most common. This allows for premedication with antipyretic agents or antihistamines, which reduce the severity of these manifestations. Next, one must make sure that the patient's blood sample is clearly and accurately labeled and that the identity of the unit of blood is carefully checked before administration. Serious hemolytic transfusion reactions are most frequently due to administration of blood to the wrong recipient. Emergency use of universal donor blood (type O, Rh-negative, low titer anti-A and anti-B) that has not been crossmatched should be avoided as much as possible since the use of such blood substantially increases the risk of transfusion reactions. The rate of administration of the blood should be slow at the beginning of the transfusion—about 0.5 ml/kg/hour for the first 15 to 30 minutes. Close observation during this period allows for prompt cessation of the transfusion, if necessary.

Classification of Transfusion Reactions

Most transfusion reactions fall into one of four categories: febrile, allergic, bacterial, or hemolytic. *Febrile reactions* are the most common and are generally due to the presence of incompatible leukocytes or platelets in the blood. The reaction usually starts about 1 hour after the beginning of the transfusion but may be delayed for as long as 24 hours. Some reactions are characterized initially by a chilly sensation followed by frank chills and then fever, which may be accompanied by headache, nausea, and vomiting. A mild febrile reaction, with an elevation in temperature of only about 1 C, does not necessarily require stopping the transfusion, particularly in patients who have a history of this type of reaction. Rarely, patients with leukoagglutinins have a more severe febrile reaction lasting from a few hours to 2 days and associated with transient pulmonary infiltrates. Such patients are likely to have cough and dyspnea as prominent clinical manifestations. Leukoagglutinins are often demonstrable, but even if they are not, patients may be helped in the future by the use of blood from which most of the white cells have been removed. Leukocyte-poor red cell preparations are described on page 1217. When possible, the transfusion of such preparations of red cells must be scheduled in advance with the blood bank to allow for preparation of these less commonly used forms of blood.

Allergic reactions start shortly after the beginning of a transfusion and are usually characterized by itching and urticaria. More severe manifestations may include abdominal pain, bronchospasm, and an anaphylactic reaction. Eosinophilia is noted in some cases. In some instances this type of reaction can be attributed to the passive transfer of food reagins from the donor to a sensitive recipient. This type of reaction, generally in a severe form, is also present in patients with IgA deficiency who have antibodies against the IgA present in donor blood. Approximately 1 out of 400 individuals is estimated to be IgA-deficient. With a severe allergic reaction, the blood should be discontinued and the patient's pretransfusion blood sample should be checked for the presence of IgA-and antibodies to IgA. If the patient has antibodies to IgA, frozen red cells may be used or, if available, blood from IgA-deficient donors. In mild allergic reactions with only a few hives, an antihistamine may be given and administration of blood continued more slowly and with close observation. Epinephrine is effective in more severe cases. In patients with a history of previous allergic transfusion reactions, administration of antihistamine 0.5 to 1 hour prior to the start of the transfusion may be effective.

Reactions due to *bacterial contamination* are fortunately rare. They are characterized by severe chills, fever, and confusion. In the most severe cases, hypotensive shock may be accompanied by disseminated intravascular coagulation and can rapidly lead to renal shutdown and death. In blood stored under the usual conditions of refrigeration, gram-negative bacteria are responsible for most severe reactions. *Pseudomonas* and coliform organisms can multiply in stored blood despite refrigeration. Septic reactions are readily confused with hemolytic transfusion reactions (see below) because of the similarity in severity of the manifestations. The diagnosis can be established by demonstrating bacteria in a Gram stain of the donor blood.

The transfusion must be stopped promptly and appropriate intravenous antibiotic therapy begun. If there is evidence of disseminated intravascular clotting, treatment with heparin, fresh-frozen plasma, platelets, and/or fresh blood must be begun promptly (p. 1214) In

recent years the use of platelet concentrates has also been associated with bacterial transfusion reactions, since the storage of platelets at room temperature for 2 to 3 days increases the risk of bacterial growth. The risk of such bacterial contamination is minimized by careful aseptic technique in the blood bank and by prompt administration of platelets after they are obtained from the blood bank.

Hemolytic transfusion reactions are also characterized by a rapid onset of symptoms. Patients may experience restlessness, anxiety, flushing of the face, precordial discomfort or pain, an increase in pulse and respiratory rate, generalized tingling sensations, and pain in the back and thighs. There may be nausea and vomiting as well as chills and fever. If the transfusion is stopped rapidly, there may be no serious complications. However, some patients progress to shock, renal shutdown, and disseminated intravascular coagulation. Such patients may exhibit hemorrhagic tendencies, such as oozing from the mucous membranes and the venipuncture site. Hemoglobinemia and hemoglobinuria are usually present but may be transient. The renal involvement appears to be due to a combination of hemoglobinemia, disseminated intravascular coagulation, and decreased renal perfusion, resulting in a precipitation of hemoglobin and deposition of fibrin in the glomeruli.

Severe hemolytic transfusion reactions are due to *intravascular* breakdown of transfused cells due to ABO incompatibility. Naturally occurring anti-A and anti-B are mostly in the IgM category and bind complement. This results in rapid intravascular destruction of the red cells. Other hemolytic transfusion reactions are much milder, and many are not clinically apparent. Mild transfusion reactions are usually due to IgG antibodies not in the ABO system, which bind to the red cell membrane and result in the *extravascular* removal of the red cell by the reticuloendothelial system, primarily the spleen. In such cases chills and fever may be delayed as much as an hour, and acute renal failure is not characteristic. Most extravascular hemolysis is attributable to the Rh system, usually in an Rh-negative individual (dd) who has developed anti-D after exposure to Rh-positive blood. However, reactions may occur in Rh-positive individuals. As in hemolytic disease of the newborn, such cases are most commonly due to anti-c and E antibodies.

In some cases, a hemolytic transfusion reaction may be delayed 1 to 2 weeks. This is due to the triggering of a booster reaction to an antigen in the donor blood and results in the development of a positive Coombs' test. Such a reaction may be suspected when there is a more rapid decrease in the concentration of hemoglobin than anticipated. Such cases may at first be wrongly identified as Coombs'-positive hemolytic anemia if the history of transfusion is overlooked.

General Aspects of Management

When anything more severe than a mild febrile or allergic reaction is suspected, the transfusion should be stopped but the vein kept open with intravenous fluids.

Blood pressure and urine output should be monitored. A fresh sample of patient's blood without anticoagulants is sent to the blood bank with the unadministered remaining donor blood and a brief description of the reaction. The first post-transfusion urine is analyzed for free hemoglobin. The workup of suspected transfusion reactions is summarized in Table 21. Therapy of hemolytic transfusion reactions is focused on the prevention of renal complications, as these are most serious. The maintenance of renal blood flow and urinary output are fostered as follows: an osmotic diuresis is attempted with a trial of mannitol; shock is treated with compatible transfusions of blood; disseminated intravascular clotting, when present, is treated with heparin, platelets, and clotting factors, and maintenance of blood pressure and renal perfusion by α-adrenergic blocking agents (the latter is advisable only for physicians experienced in the use of these medications).

TABLE 21. Workup of Suspected Transfusion Reactions

A. Hemolytic
  1. Tests of red cell destruction: plasma hemoglobin, urine hemoglobin, haptoglobin, methemoglobin, and bilirubin
  2. Tests for disseminated intravascular clotting —— PT, PTT, TT, fibrinogen, protamine test, fibrin degradation products
  3. Serologic tests:
     a. Retype patient and donor blood to rule out error in identifying the unit of blood or error in the crossmatch
     b. Direct Coombs' test of patient's cells to detect surface immunoglobin
     c. Indirect Coombs' test of donor's cells and patient's serum to detect presence of antibody in patient's serum against donor's cells
     d. Indirect Coombs' test of patient's cells and donor's serum to detect antibody in donor's serum against patient's cells
  4. Renal function: urine output
B. Other transfusion reactions
  1. Leukocyte agglutinins
  2. IgA and anti-IgA in patient's pretransfusion sample
  3. Anaerobic and aerobic cultures of donor blood

TRANSMISSION OF INFECTIOUS DISEASE BY BLOOD

Hepatitis, malaria, syphilis, and brucellosis have long been recognized to be transmissible by blood transfusion. In recent years, cytomegalic inclusion virus and EB virus have been identified as additional infectious diseases that can follow a transfusion.

The risk of viral hepatitis can be minimized by using blood obtained from volunteer donors rather than from commercial sources and, when possible, avoiding blood preparations that are prepared from pooled plasma. Both viral hepatitis type A (infectious hepatitis or short-incubation hepatitis) and viral hepatitis B (serum hepatitis or long-incubation hepatitis) may be transmitted by transfused blood. The risk of hepatitis B is sub-

stantially decreased by checking the donor blood for hepatitis-B-associated antigen (Australia antigen). At present, the most reliable means of detecting the antigen is by radioimmunoassay. Even the careful screening of blood for hepatitis B antigen is unlikely to detect more than one-half of hepatitis carriers. The administration of hepatitis-B-antigen negative blood can still result in an incidence of post-transfusion icterus of about 1 percent and a 3 percent incidence of elevated liver enzyme levels. Hepatitis can be transmitted by all commonly used blood fractions, except for gamma globulin, albumin, and plasma protein USP. The latter two are heat-treated preparations.

COMPATIBILITY TESTING

Whenever possible, blood that is ABO- and Rh-compatible and has been typed and crossmatched should be used. The term *universal donor* for type O, Rh-negative blood approaches validity only when most of the plasma has been removed from the preparation of red cells or when units of blood with low anti-A and anti-B titers are selected. When blood with a high titer of anti-A or anti-B is transfused into recipients who are type A, B, or AB, transfusion reactions due to destruction of the recipient's cells can occur. It is impractical to routinely administer blood compatible for rarer red cell antigens, as Kell, Duffy, and so forth. An exception is made in those patients, usually recipients of many transfusions, who have developed antibodies to one of these weaker antigens. Such antibodies are usually detected in the Coombs' crossmatch. The risk of developing alloantigenic antibodies as a result of a transfusion is estimated to be about 1 percent. In order to avoid the future risk of erythroblastosis in offspring, it is particularly important to avoid administering Rh-positive cells to Rh-negative female recipients. It should be noted that platelet concentrates may contain sufficient red cell contamination to be antigenic (p. 1218).

For the use of blood products to treat deficiencies of coagulation factors see pages 1209 - 1213, especially in reference to factor VIII deficiency, page 1210, and factor IX deficiency, page 1212.

References

Adner MM, Fisch GR, Starobin SG, Aster RH: Use of "compatible" platelet transfusions in treatment of congenital isoimmune neonatal thrombocytopenic purpura. N Engl J Med 280:244, 1969

Bailey DN, Bove JR: Chemical and hematological changes in stored CPD blood. Transfusion 15:244, 1975

Blankenship WJ, Goetzman BW, Gross S, Hattersley PG: A walking donor program for an intensive care nursery. J Pediatr 86:583, 1975

Buchholz DH, Young VM, Friedman NR, Reilly JA, Mardiney MR Jr. Bacterial proliferation in platelet products stored at room temperature transfusion-induced Enterobacter sepsis. N Engl J Med 285:429, 1971

———— Blood transfusion: merits of component therapy. J Pediatr 84:1, 165, 1974

Chaplin H Jr, Beutler E, Collins VA, Giblett ER, Polesky HF: Current status of red-cell preservation and availability in relation to the developing national blood policy. N Engl J Med 291:68, 1974

Goldfinger D, McGinniss, MH Chaplin H Jr, et al: Rh-incompatible platelet transfusion—risk and consequences of sensitizing immunos-uppressed patients. N Engl J Med 284:942, 1971

Huestis DW, Bove JR, Busch S: Practical blood transfusion. Boston, Little, Brown, 1969

Krugman S: Viral hepatitis and Australia antigen. J Pediatr 78:887, 1971

Lostumbo MM, Holland PV, Schmidt PJ: Isoimmunization after multiple transfusions. N Engl J Med 275:141, 1966

Mollison PL: Blood Transfusion in Clinical Medicine, 5th ed. Philadelphia, FA Davis, 1972

Myhre BA (ed): Blood Component Therapy, 2nd ed. Washington, DC, American Association of Blood Banks, 1975.

Oberman HA: Replacement transfusion in the newborn infant: a commentary. J Pediatr 86:586, 1975

Prince AM, Szmuness W, Millian SJ, David DS: A serologic study of cytomegalovirus infections associated with blood transfusions. N Engl J Med 284:1125, 1971

Schwartz AD, Pearson HA: Aspirin, platelets, and bleeding. J Pediatr 78:558, 1971

Stuart MJ, Murphy S, Oski FA, Evans AE, Donaldson MH, Gardner FH: Platelet function in recipients of platelets from donors ingesting aspirin. N Engl J Med 287:1105, 1972

Turner AR, MacDonald RN, Cooper BA: Transmission of infectious mononucleosis by transfusion of pre-illness plasma. Ann Intern Med 77:751, 1972

Vyas GN, Perkins HA, Fudenberg HH: Anaphylactoid transfusion reactions associated with anti-IgA. Lancet 2:312, 1968

——— Perkins HA, Schmid R (eds): Hepatitis and Blood Transfusion; Proceedings. New York, Grune & Stratton, 1972

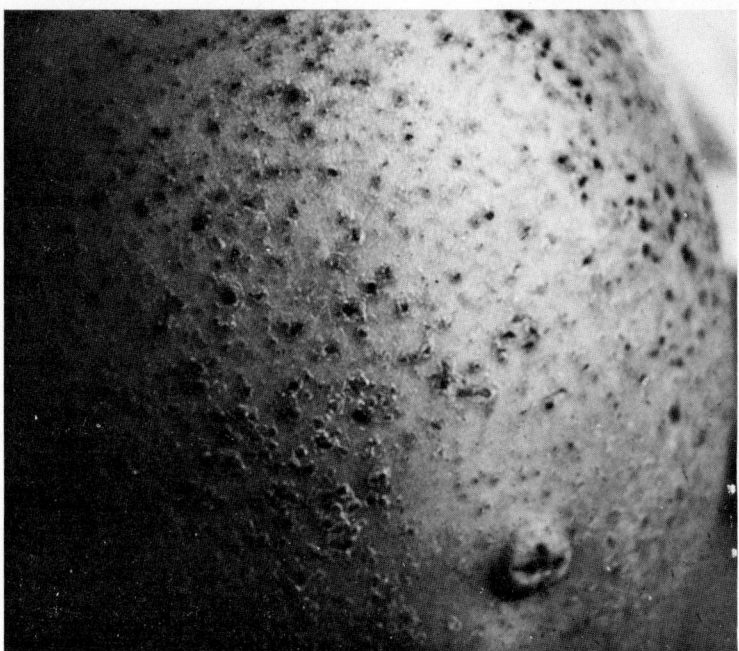

Fig. 1. Scaly and crusted cutaneous lesions on abdomen of 8-month-old infant with Letterer-Siwe disease.

child with that ailment was estimated to be about 1,400 times normal. These findings are regarded as an indication of neonatal origin of Letterer-Siwe's disease.

Clinical Manifestations

Characteristically, widespread involvement of viscera, skin, and gingival mucosa is present at the onset, often but not always without demonstrable skeletal lesions initially.

Typical cases feature a characteristic cutaneous eruption; gum lesions; enlargement of spleen, liver, and lymph nodes; a febrile systemic illness; and hypoplastic anemia, leukopenia, thrombocytopenia, and hemorrhagic phenomena. Skeletal changes may occur if the course of the disease is less acute. Widespread visceral histiocytic infiltration not suspected during the child's life may be found at autopsy.

The *skin eruption* is often the first symptom to attract attention. Cutaneous involvement rarely is the only manifestation. The rash (Fig. 1) typically starts at the hairline and then tends to become generalized, usually remaining most marked over the trunk, on the scalp, behind the ears and in the auditory canal, in the groin and axillae, and in all skin folds. The individual lesions are greasy, scaly, crusted maculopapules, sometimes considerably elevated. Although they blanch under pressure, their color often appears dark red or purplish, simulating hemorrhagic vesicles. Palms and soles may be the site of a desquamative erythrodermia. Later in

the disease, with the development of thrombocytopenia, localized or generalized *petechiae* may be observed. The infiltrative exanthema also may become the site of hemorrhages and even ulcerate. Hemorrhagic skin lesions and thrombocytopenia are indicative of a grave prognosis and may occur in conjunction with disseminated intravascular coagulation (DIC). A nonhemorrhagic rash does not, however, preclude the existence of diminished platelets. The skin eruption may be very pruriginous and its appearance may suggest eczema or seborrheic dermatitis. However, the presence of petechiae, the distribution of the lesions, and a tenacious eruption persisting despite adequate therapy for seborrheic dermatitis or eczema, distinguishes the infiltrative histiocytosis from atopic dermatitis.

Intraoral lesions, if present, consist of gingival swelling frequently combined with ulceration, bleeding, infection, and drooling and there is often a fetid odor. Histologically these oral lesions reflect histiocytic infiltration. If teeth have erupted, there is dental malposition, crowding, and loosening. *Dental extrusion* is a typical feature of histiocytosis X and may be the reason for seeking medical advice.

Generalized *lymphadenopathy,* moderate to marked *splenomegaly,* and *hepatomegaly* are almost always present. *Obstructive jaundice* produced by a portal lesion may be the first sign. *Hepatic dysfunction* with hypoproteinemia, edema, and ascitis may be present with or without associated hyperbilirubinemia. Evidence of hepatic dysfunction is regarded as an ominous factor.

Hemolytic uremic syndrome and *disseminated intravascular coagulation* (DIC) have been reported in association with Letterer-Siwe disease.

Pulmonary involvement is frequently demonstrable. Respiratory difficulties may actually herald the onset of the disease. Small infiltrative nodules, interstitial pneumonitis, and lung cysts are not uncommon. Radiography of the chest may reveal bilateral diffuse reticulonodular densities. When cysts are present, the typical roentgenologic appearance of *honeycomb lungs* is produced. Pneumothorax following the rupture of subpleural lung cysts represents a typical complication in the course of Letterer-Siwe disease; in 2 of our patients, death was directly attributable to this complication. The combination of honeycomb lung and recurrent episodes of pneumothorax should suggest the possibility of reticuloendotheliosis. In patients who succumb, extensive histiocyocitic infiltration of the pulmonary parenchyma can be demonstrated.

If the disease runs a subacute course, localized *osseous defects* may be found in the skull and other bones. Two of our own patients with neonatal malignant histiocytosis X had extensive bone defects. Characteristic areas of rarefaction, seen on radiography, are comparable to those of Hand-Schuller-Christian disease.

Anorexia, failure to thrive, daily temperature elevations, pallor, or hemorrhagic manifestations commonly are prominent features and, at times, the presenting complaints.

Course

In most instances, regardless of the mode of onset, the disease tends to run a downhill course. Without therapy, progression and dissemination of the morbid process generally are rapid, even fulminating, and early fatal termination is the rule rather than the exception.

Histologic Diagnosis

When the disease is suspected on the basis of a typical skin rash or other findings, the diagnosis is most readily confirmed by biopsy and histologic examination of involved tissue, in particular skin lesions, gingival lesions, and/or lymph nodes. Whenever possible it is desirable to obtain a biopsy from a site, in addition to the skin, in order to increase the probability of establishing the diagnosis. Early in the disease the histology consists of proliferation of mononuclear histiocytes without vacuolization and with minimal surrounding reaction. When survival has lasted several months, the lesions tend to become granulomatous, with *foam cells,* eosinophils, and multinucleated giant cells. *A touch preparation* of serous material exuding from a skin lesion after scraping the overlying epidermis with a scalpel (a simple and rapid procedure described by Moore), may facilitate the diagnosis when skin lesions are present.

CHRONIC DISSEMINATED HISTIORETICULOENDOTHELIOSES

Histiocytosis X, Chronic Disseminated, Histologically Benign Type or Hand-Schüller-Christian Syndrome

Originally this syndrome described a classic triad: *exophthalmos, membranous bone defects,* and *diabetes insipidus;* it was seen in older children or young adults and often followed a comparatively benign course. It is now appreciated that in this particular entity, typical lesions may be found in virtually every organ of the body. The concept of this syndrome has been broadened to include all instances of the disease complex in which skeleton, viscera, and soft tissues are affected at the onset, regardless of the patient's age.

Pathology

While skin, middle ear, and bones are most conspicuously affected, most other soft tissues and organ systems are also commonly involved. Granulomatous lesions, originating in the base of the skull, especially in the sphenoidal sella turcica, and exerting pressure on the pituitary and the *tuber cinereum,* are responsible for the diabetes insipidus. Lesions in the orbit produce the exophthalmos. Involvement of the mastoid or petrous portion of the temporal bone causes the chronic otitis media, while displacement or extrusion of teeth results from granulomata of the mandible or maxilla.

Histologically, the lesions, when fully developed, are xanthomas. In their early stage the infiltrating histiocytes contain no visible lipids, and some eosinophils can be observed. The typical xanthomatous granuloma is yellowish, of miliary size, contains lipid-filled foam cells, and is surrounded by a zone of fibrosis of variable width. As the lesion ages, some lipid-containing cells disintegrate, and free cholesterol crystals and giant cells may be seen in the center. Eventually, only a fibrous scar remains if healing takes place.

Clinical Manifestations

Clinical manifestations of the Hand-Schüller-Christian syndrome are most varied. The disease begins most commonly during early or late childhood; the time of onset is rarely in infancy. Any or all of the three original manifestations of the classic triad may be absent; in fact, the combination of all three is rare. A cutaneous eruption sometimes in crops, a chronic ear discharge, and diabetes insipidus are the most common reasons for seeking medical advice. Dental loosening, loss of teeth, or ulcerative lesions of the gum may be the first symptoms to attract attention. Fever may be present but is inconstant. Neurologic manifestations associated with increased intracranial pressure are rare. When they occur, they may indicate central nervous infiltration and

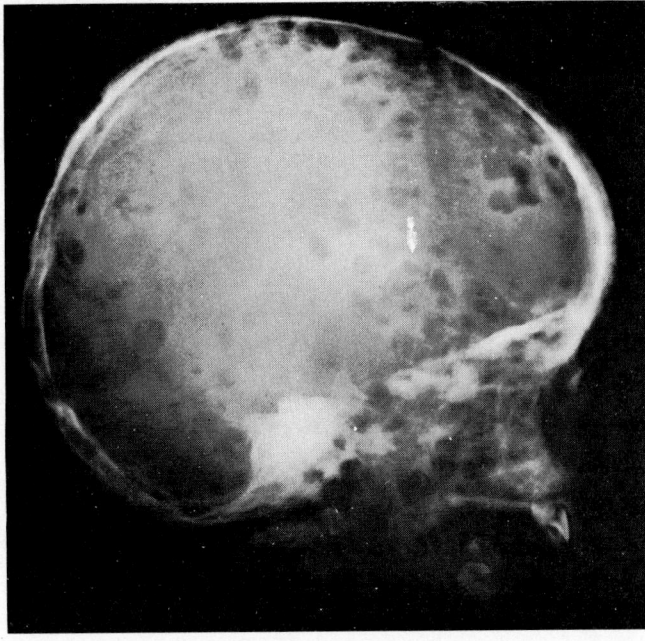

Fig. 2. Radiogram of skull in reticuloendotheliosis, showing multiple defects. Patient 3½ years of age.

carry a poor prognosis. However, the raised intracranial pressure may be secondary to an osteolytic lesion strictly confined to one cranial bone and readily amenable to therapy (excision or radiotherapy).

Stunting of growth with delayed skeletal maturation, a very prominent feature in one of our patients, may be considerable. Growth retardation may be secondary to diabetes insipidus or may result from lesions directly affecting the pituitary, either by infiltration or compression. *Exophthalmos* is the feature of the triad most rarely encountered. Single or multiple granulomatous lesions may be present in the orbit without producing proptosis.

Skin lesions are variable. In their early state they are often similar to seborrheic dermatitis or may present the greasy, scaly, crusted, and reddish maculopapular appearance identical with that of acute reticuloendotheliosis. In the course of months, however, the reddish-brown lesions turn yellow and, microscopically, cholesterol droplets appear in the cells. Ecchymoses, xanthomas, granulomas, ulcerations, and bronze discolorations of the skin are sometimes observed.

Visceral manifestations are likely to become more striking in very young children. Enlargement of the spleen, liver, and lymph nodes may be considerable; jaundice may occur. In some instances lymph nodes are sufficiently prominent to suggest lymphoma. At times splenomegaly, hepatomegaly, or adenopathy is moderate or may not be observed at all. There may be a miliary, mottled, or patchy infiltration of the lung fields, often relatively asymptomatic. Thyroid lesions have been found at autopsy or in biopsy material even without clinical evidence of enlargement of the gland. In fatal cases miliary xanthomatous lesions are found in nearly every organ of the body, including the brain.

Skeletal lesions are most striking. Flat as well as long bones are affected. The calvarium of the skull is the most common site of involvement. Defects of the skull can be discovered clinically or can be palpated as soft tissue nodules overlying lytic lesions demonstrable radiographically (Fig. 2). In long bones, pathologic fractures may lead to the discovery of destructive foci (Fig. 3). The osteolytic lesions are responsible for the exophthalmos, the diabetes insipidus, the chronic otitis media, and the dental problems (see above, under Pathology). They may also produce neurologic manifestations, labyrinthine dysfunction, and even benign intracranial hypertension or pseudotumor cerebri. In flat bones the osseous lesions present a typical radiologic appearance, featuring sharply defined punched-out areas, round or ovoid, with no reaction in the surrounding bone. In long bones, however, involvement of the cortex results in a destructive lesion with periosteal new bone formation, which may suggest a neoplasm, tuberculosis, or late syphilis. The bone defects may heal spontaneously or persist for many years.

Laboratory Findings

Radiography of the skeleton and histologic examinations of biopsies of skin and bone lesions or lymph nodes constitute the major laboratory diagnostic aids. Blood lipids are characteristically not elevated. Eosinophilia has been reported but is inconstant. Anemia,

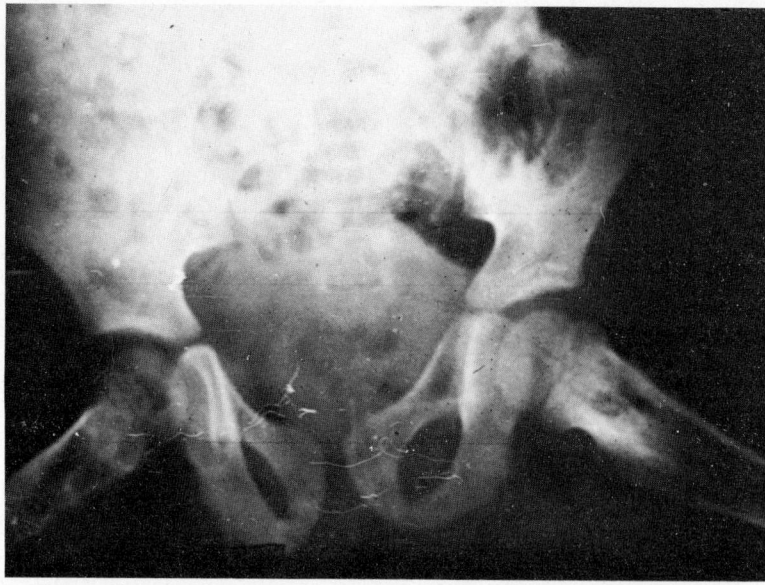

Fig. 3.   Radiography of 7½-year-old boy with Hand-Schüller-Christian syndrome. Destructive lesions are discernible in upper end of both femurs; note healed fractures on the right.

leukopenia, and thrombocytopenia may be present but are observed less commonly than in acute reticuloendotheliosis.

Course

The course is extremely variable. Some children recover completely from the disease even after lesions have continued to occur in new sites for several years. In others diabetes insipidus may persist after cranial bone lesions disappear. The polydipsia and polyuria usually respond to variable doses of vasopressin. Those in whom the disease is fatal may survive anywhere from several months to several years. The course is often shorter and more progressive in younger children. In patients older than 10 years of age the prognosis for arrest of bone lesions is excellent.

EOSINOPHILIC GRANULOMA

Histiocytosis X, Solitary Form, Benign Type

This condition was originally described as a circumscribed bone lesion, usually solitary, primarily seen in older children and running essentially a benign course. Microscopically it was characterized by infiltration of round cells with no vacuoles and no fibrosis. In some instances eosinophilia was present.

Lichenstein described the relationship between this solitary type and other forms of reticuloendotheliosis. Green and Farber described the subsequent evolution of the lesions, vacuolization of histiocytes, disappearance of eosinophils, and appearance of fibrosis. Eosinophilic granuloma is now generally regarded as one mode of onset of granulomatous reticuloendotheliosis rather than as a separate disease.

Clinically, the bone lesion may be tender; in some instances local pain or swelling may attract attention. A fracture may be the presenting complaint. The radiographic findings are identical with those described in Schuller-Christian disease. Fortunately, in most instances this particular clinical variant does not progress beyond the stage of the solitary, circumscribed bone lesion.

Treatment of the Histioreticuloendothelioses

DISSEMINATED HISTIOCYTOSES. Efforts to arrest the disease have not been entirely successful, especially when the clinical disease starts before 6 months of age. However, improved survival has been achieved, presumably from the effects of better supportive therapy, antimicrobial agents, corticosteroids, and chemotherapy. The great majority of favorable responses are believed to be the result of chemotherapy.

A wide variety of antiproliferative chemotherapeutic agents are being used, either alone or in combination, to induce remission and for maintenance. These include antimetabolites (6-mercaptopurine [6-MP] and methotrexate), alkylating and immunosuppressive agents (cyclophosphamide, chlorambucil), vinca alkaloids (vincristine VCR, Vinblastin VBL), and antibiotics (daunomycin).

No single drug or combination has emerged as the therapy of choice. Several children's cancer study groups are performing prospective studies to establish the superiority of any single, or combinations of therapeutic regimens. With existing treatment methods, the results are variable and unfortunately often transient. Moreover, effectiveness of therapy is difficult to evaluate since remissions do occur either spontaneously or after antimicrobial therapy. The question usually remains open as to whether these patients are saved by treatment or whether their illness abated spontaneously.

Comparative therapeutic trials, using various regimens, have shown that single drugs, such as VCR, VBL, or cyclophosphamide, and combinations, such as prednisone (PDN)+VBL, PDN+methotrexate, or PDN+6-MP, are about equally efficacious in achieving complete or good remissions in about 45 to 65 percent of patients with disseminated histiocytosis X.

Dosage and duration of treatment presently recommended by Lahey, when using the following chemotherapeutic agents, are:

Prednisone (PDN)—daily and orally in three divided doses of 2mg/kg/day for 6 weeks, then 1 mg/kg/day for 4 weeks, and then tapered for 2 weeks and discontinued.

Vinblastine (VBL)—intravenously, once weekly, in an initial dose of 0.15mg/kg, increased weekly by 0.05 mg/kg until the white blood cell count is less then 3,000/mm^3 and continued weekly thereafter at the largest dose tolerated without resulting in a leukopenia of less than 3,000/mm^3.

6-Mercaptopurine (6-MP)—daily, oral doses of 2.5 mg/kg/day for 6 to 10 weeks.

On the basis of available data gained from the study previously mentioned under Prognostic Factors (p. 1224) Lahey recommends that at the present time it seems appropriate to employ relatively simple therapy for patients without organ dysfunction and with *benign* histology. More aggressive therapy is indicated in patients with organ dysfunction, whose histology is of the *malignant* variety and in whom the onset of the disease occurs in infancy.

Supportive therapy is important in patients with disseminated histiocytosis X and includes early recognition of infections and their treatment with appropriate antimicrobial agents, administration of red blood cells and platelets, and correction of any acid base or respiratory disturbance. Splenectomy has been recommended if hypersplenism appears responsible for persistent cytopenia.

Before therapy is instituted with agents that have immunosuppressive properties, the patient's immunologic status should be evaluated thoroughly, including skin testing for delayed hypersensitivity and serum immunoglobulin determinations. If immunizations are required, killed antigen must be used. Patients with Lettere-Siwe should not be given live attenuated vaccines, and/or unirradiated blood or blood products. If both humoral and cellular immunocompetence are severely and persistently depressed, the feasibility of a bone marrow transplantation should be considered as a possible form of therapy.

In *Hand-Schüller-Christian* disease, radiotherapy and adrenal corticosteroids, either singly or in combination, may cause rapid retrogression of osteolytic bone lesions. The response to chemotherapy of the effects of histiocytic infiltration on other organ and systems is, in general, less spectacular, inconsistent, and often only temporary. Surgical excision is recommended for lesions easily accessible. Vasopressin tannate (Pitressin) may help alleviate the discomfort caused by diabetes insipidus.

EOSINOPHILIC GRANULOMA. In *eosinophilic granuloma* curettage is the treatment of choice because it constitutes definitive therapy, provides a specimen for pathologic examination, and avoids the hazards of irradiation. Complete healing occurs often after local curettage; and relapses after surgery are exceedingly rare. Only if the size, the location, or the number of lesions make surgery impractical, or if the operative procedure entails a risk of considerable disability, is radiotherapy required. The lesion is relatively radiosensitive. The total tumor dose of radiation, although not definitely established in children, varies in most instances from 500 to 1,500 rads. Chemotherapy is not indicated.

Bibliography

Ahnquist G, Holyoke JB: Congenital Letterer-Siwe disease (reticuloendotheliosis) in a term stillborn infant. J Pediatr 57:905, 1960

Avery ME, McAfee JG, Holyoke JB: Course and treatment of reticuloendotheliosis (eosinophilic granuloma, Schüller-Christian disease and Letterer-Siwe disease). Am J Med 22:636, 1957

Batson R, Shapiro M, Christie A: Acute nonlipid disseminated reticuloendotheliosis. Am J Dis Child 90:323, 1955

Beier FR, Thatcher LG, Lahey ME: Treatment of reticuloendotheliosis with vinblastine sulfate. J Pediatr 63:1087, 1963

Braunstein GD, Whitaker JN, Kohler PO: Cerebellar dysfunction in Hand-Schuller-Christian disease. Arch Intern Med 132:387, 1973

Cederbaum SD, Niwayama G, Stiehm ER, et al.: Combined immunodeficiency presenting as the Letterer-Siwe Syndrome. J Pediatr 85:466, 1974

Esterly NB, Swick HM: Cutaneous Letterer-Siwe disease. Am J Dis Child 117:236, 1969

Freundlich E, Amit S, Montag Y, Suprun H, Nevo S: Familial occurrence of Letterer-Siwe disease. Arch Dis Child 47:122, 1972

Glass AG, Miller RW: U.S. mortality from Letterer-Siwe disease, 1960-1964. Pediatrics 42:364, 1968

Green WT, Farber S: "Eosinophilic or solitary granuloma" of bone. J Bone Joint Surg 24:499, 1942

Hertz CG, Hambrick GW: Congenital Letterer-Siwe disease. Am J Dis Child 116:553, 1968

Jackson AH, Griffith JF: Histiocytosis X with benign intracranial hypertension. Dev. Med Child Neurol 17:783, 1975

Kepes JJ, Kepes M: Predominantly cerebral forms of histiocytosis X. Acta Neuropathol 14:77, 1969

Lahey ME: Prognosis in reticuloendotheliosis in children. J Pediatr 60:664, 1962

———Histiocytosis X—an analysis of prognostic factors. J Pediatr 87:184, 1975

———Histiocytosis X—comparison of three treatment regimens. J Pediatr 87:179, 1975

Latorre H, Kenney FM, Lahey ME, Drash A: Short stature and growth hormone deficiency in histiocytosis X. J Pediatr 85:813, 1974

Leiken S: The histiocytoses. Pediatr Ann 85:35, 1975

Lichtenstein L: Histiocytosis X: Integration of eosinophilic granuloma of bone, "Letterer-Siwe disease," and "Schüller-Christian disease" as related manifestations of a single nosologic entity. Arch Pathol 56:84, 1953

Lucaya J: Histiocytosis-X. Am J Dis Child 121:289, 1971

Mauger DC: Letterer-Siwe's disease: a case complicated by disseminated intravascular coagulation and responding to heparin therapy. Pediatrics 47:435, 1971

Moore TD: A single technique for the diagnosis of nonlipid histiocytosis. Pediatrics 19:438, 1957

Nelson P, Santamaria A, Olson RL, Nayak NC: Generalized lymphohistiocytic infiltration. Pediatrics 27:931, 1961

Oberman HA: Idiopathic histiocytosis. A clinical study of 40 cases and review of the literature on eosinophilic granuloma of the bone, Hand-Schüller-Christian disease and Letterer-Siwe disease. Pediatrics 28:307, 1961

Roland AS, Merdinger WF, Froeb HF. Recurrent spontaneous pneumothorax: A clue to the diagnosis of histiocytosis. N Engl J Med 270:73, 1964

Rogers DL, Benson TE: Familial Letterer-Siwe disease. J Pediatr 60:550, 1962

Rube J, delaPava S, Picken JW: Histiocytosis X with involvement of brain. Cancer 20:486, 1967

Schoeck VW, Peterson RDA, Good RA: Familial Letterer-Siwe disease. Pediatrics 32:1033, 1963

Siegel JS, Coltman CA: Histiocytosis X: Response to vinblastine sulfate. JAMA 197:403, 1966

FAMILIAL FORMS OF RETICULOENDOTHELIOSIS

Several varieties of reticuloendotheliosis have been reported, which actually constitute atypical variants of, or diseases related to, histiocytosis. In spite of some differences in clinical expression and histologic findings, there appears to be no valid reason to separate these entities from the nonlipid acute reticuloendothelioses.

Nelson and his group reported a disease fatal in three siblings, termed *generalized lymphohistiocytosis* and characterized by fever, anemia, leukopenia, thrombocytopenia, lymphadenopathy, hepatosplenomegaly, pneumonia, and meningitis. Histologically, there was extensive visceral infiltration of many organs and tissues by large lymphocytes and histiocytes. The leptomeninges, the central nervous system, and neurohypophysis were involved. The bones and skin were not affected. Involvement of the central nervous system was given as one of the grounds for separating this condition from Letterer-Siwe disease.

Almost identical clinical features were reported by Farquhar in *familial erythrophagocytic lymphohistiocytosis* (*familial hemophagocytic reticulocytosis*), also a multisystem and familial disease. Clinical and pathologic findings include splenomegaly and hepatomegaly; pancytopenia and atypical lymphocytes in the peripheral blood; and associated infiltration of the bone marrow, spleen, liver, and lymph nodes by histiocytes showing active phagocytosis of erythrocytes and leukocytes. Frequently a severe bleeding disorder is present in which thrombocytopenia is associated with afibrinogenemia. Other plasma clotting factors remain normal and there is evidence of fibrinolysis. The existence of this particular combination of coagulation anomalies, without disseminated intravascular coagulation, may help to establish the diagnosis of familial hemophagocytic reteculocytosis.

Subsequently cases were reported of Farquhar's disease with central nervous system involvement. Lesions of the central nervous system have also been found in Letterer-Siwe disease. Consequently, the diffuse infiltrative characteristics of both Nelson's and Farquhar's reticulosis remain the only features that still distinguish them from the granulomatous lesions of Letterer-Siwe disease.

Another multisystem familial syndrome, *familial reticuloendotheliosis with eosinophilia*, has been described by Omenn. This clinical and histologic entity characteristically includes: onset in early infancy, failure to thrive, generalized erythematous scaly skin eruption, alopecia, lymphadenopathy, hepatosplenomegaly, eosinophilia, and widespread histiocytic infiltration. Severe, bizarre, and chronic bacterial and fungal infections occur repeatedly. Typically both humoral and cellular immune systems are severely impaired. The mode of inheritance appears to be autosomal recessive. Despite therapy, the outcome in this syndrome, which is also very similar to Letterer-Siwe disease, has been uniformly fatal.

Bibliography

FAMILIAL RETICULOENDOTHELIOSES

Farquhar JW, Claireaux AE: Familial haemophagocytic reticulosis. Arch Dis Child 27:519, 1952

McClure PD, Strachan P, Saunders EF: Hypofibrinogenemia and thrombocytopenia in familial hemophagocytic reticulosis. J. Pediatr 85:67, 1974

Miller DR: Familial reticuloendotheliosis: concurrence of disease in five siblings. Pediatrics 38:986, 1966

Nelson P, Santamaria A, Olson RL, et al.: Generalized lymphohistiocytic infiltration. Pediatrics 27:931, 1961

Omenn GS: Familial reticuloendotheliosis with eosinophilia. N Engl J Med 273:427, 1965

SARCOIDOSIS
ARNOLD H. EINHORN

Sarcoidosis, often referred to as Boeck's sarcoid, is a chronic granulomatous process of unknown cause that may affect any one or any number of organs and systems. It produces in general only mild symptoms despite extensive tissue involvement. Characteristically, the disease tends to progress slowly, with relapses and remissions, ultimately burning itself out in the course of years. The clinical manifestations are due mainly to pressure phenomena exerted by enlarged structures.

Epidemiology, Incidence, and Etiology

The disease is rarely observed in children. In 1956 in McGovern and Merritt's first comprehensive review of childhood sarcoidosis compiled from the world literature through 1953, only 113 cases were reported in children less than 15 years of age; 135 additional cases have been subsequently documented in children, 59 of these from the United States. However, there is growing evidence that clinically silent forms of this disease occur more frequently in children than is generally suspected. In these asymptomatic forms bilateral hilar adenopathy, often combined with pulmonary parenchymal lesions, can be demonstrated radiographically. An increasing number of such cases have been detected primarily in countries (Hungary and Japan) where mass chest radiographic surveys are performed on children. In the United States the diagnosis of sarcoidosis usually is made in children at a considerably later stage than it is in adults.

Epidemiologic studies have provided no clues concerning etiology or pathogenesis of this disorder. There appears to be no clear-cut difference in sex distribution. Cases affecting siblings have been reported but have occurred so rarely that, although not excluded, a genetic factor is unlikely. The distribution of the disease is universal; the highest known prevalence rate is in Sweden. In the United States there are areas with high attack rates of sarcoidosis in the South Atlantic and the Gulf States, and endemic areas in New England and the Midwest. The unusually high incidence of the disease in one rural county in Virginia among workers handling peanuts and peanut products is striking but unexplained. Such an association suggests the possible role of environmental factors. Ethnic factors also appear to influence not only the prevalence but also the clinical patterns of the disease. In the United States sarcoidosis is much more common in Blacks and in Puerto Ricans. Ocular, skin, and peripheral lymph node involvement is significantly more frequent in Blacks and Puerto Ricans, but chronic pulmonary insufficiency, sometimes fatal, is more common in Caucasians.

The possibility of an infectious etiology has been raised because of the occasionally febrile course, because of the resemblance of the histologic lesions to tubercles, and because in some families more than one member has been affected, sometimes simultaneously. However, efforts to recover an infectious agent have been unsuccessful. The belief, once prevalent, that the disease is a form of tuberculosis in an anergic subject now has few adherents. A distinct feature is the patient's inability to react to tuberculin and to other delayed hypersensitivity skin tests in the presence of normal circulating antigen-antibody production. Patients who were positive reactors to tuberculin before the onset of sarcoidosis often do not react during the course of the illness and regain tuberculin sensitivity after recovery. This observation led to the suggestion that the depressed skin reactivity possibly results from impaired immunologic mechanisms caused by the disease. Persistence of insensitivity to tuberculin after recovery has also been reported. The latter observation may lend support to an alternative hypothesis that the inability to develop and maintain delayed hypersensitivity is a constitutional immunologic defect that precedes the disease and may be a prerequisite to its development.

Pathology

The fundamental pathologic lesion, which may be found in virtually any organ or tissue, consists of granulomata of tubercle like structure composed principally of epithelioid cells, together with varying number of Langhans-type giant cells, and surrounded by lymphocytes. Central necrosis is inconspicuous or absent. Giant cells often contain refractile, stellate, basophilic inclusions. Tubercle bacilli cannot be found, either by acid-fast staining of tissue sections or by culture. In the course of time the lesion may be replaced by fibrosis, hyalinization, or both. The tissues most frequently involved are lymph nodes, lungs, skin, eye, and bones, especially of the hands and feet.

Clinical Manifestations

The clinical picture is extremely variable. The most striking feature of sarcoidosis is the *multisystem involvement.* Signs and symptoms depend on the organs and tissues affected, hence the great diversity of clinical manifestations. As a rule the onset of symptomatic sarcoidosis is insidious. In the child as well as in the adult, cough, chest pain, and weight loss are symptoms that occur most frequently. Constitutional symptoms, such as fever, anorexia, fatigability, and malaise, are usually absent, although they may have been observed. The enlargement of one or more peripheral lymph nodes, the presence of skin lesions, parotid swelling, pain in the extremities, or a disturbance of vision, may be the presenting complaint, but may also indicate that the disease process is well advanced.

Peripheral lymphadenopathy, second in frequency only to mediastinal adenopathy, may be generalized. The involved nodes usually are discrete and nontender. The *spleen and liver* may be enlarged. Swelling of the *parotid glands* may be conspicuous.

Specific *skin lesions* are found in more than a third of patients with systemic sarcoidosis and usually are associated with severe disease. They represent dermal sarcoid granulomata and vary widely in their clinical morphology. Cutaneous lesions occur most often on the face, and in children carry a bad prognosis. They may appear as yellowish waxy miliary papules or larger, somewhat lichenoid, conglomerates, or as flat, smooth, purplish, or deep pigmented papules or plaques 1 cm or more in diameter. Typical erythema nodosa lesions are not uncommon, especially in girls of dark-skinned ethnic groups.

Ocular manifestations may result in severe impairment of vision. The eye involvement may take the form of keratitis, iritis, iridocyclitis, uveitis, glaucoma, or rarely retinitis. Flame-shaped hemorrhages in the retina have also been observed. Excessive lacrimation, with involvement of the eyelids and lacrimal glands, may be present. The formation of synechiae sometimes interferes with normal contraction of the pupils. When the lesions affect the eye, fibrotic uveitis may produce partial or total blindness, which makes the involvement of this organ one of the most dreaded complications of this disease.

A characteristic syndrome of sarcoidosis is the so-called *uveoparotid fever* in which tender swelling of the parotid or other salivary glands is associated with uveitis and sometimes with fever or peripheral facial paralysis.

Pulmonary and osseous lesions most frequently cause no symptoms and are discovered only through careful radiologic studies. The classic skeletal lesions are sharply defined punched-out areas of bone rarefaction in the phalanges or other small bones. The radiographic findings observed in the lung vary considerably. Hilar lymphadenopathy is considered the hallmark of sarcoidosis and is recognized on radiography in virtually every child with sarcoidosis. The bilateral hilar adenopathy may exist alone or in combination with parenchymal mottling. The pulmonary densities, if present, may consist of flocculent infiltrations, miliary nodules, focal streaking, or pulmonary reticulations. The most common manifestations of sarcoidosis in the lungs closely simulate the radiographic picture of miliary tuberculosis. With massive enlargement of hilar nodes, the patient may have shortness of breath on exertion. Extensive pulmonary disease can be associated with pneumothorax.

Respiratory function studies in sarcoidosis have shown little correlation between functional abnormalities and radiographic changes. Impaired diffusion, reduced lung compliance, and lowered vital capacity were the most common findings and correlated closely with severity of clinical symptoms and duration of illness. The dyspnea, if present, appeared to be secondary to diminished vital capacity.

Joint involvement clinically resembling rheumatoid arthritis has been described. Joint manifestations quite distinct from those of rheumatoid arthritis have also been reported. In such instances the distinguishing features of the sarcoid arthritis consist of the large "boggy" effusion, with thickening of joint membranes, involvement of tendon sheaths, minimal pain and limitation of motion, and the absence of osteoporosis, which is unusual in rheumatoid arthritis. Rheumatoid factor has been found in the sera of a number of patients with sarcoidosis. The presence of this factor appears unrelated to the presence or absence of joint symptoms and to be of little prognostic significance.

OTHER SYSTEMS. Sarcoid granulomas can involve the myocardium and exceptionally the pericardium. The most frequent manifestations of sarcoid heart disease, excluding cor pulmonale, are conduction defects ranging from complete heart block to supraventricular and ventricular arrhythmias.

Symptoms of diabetes insipidus and amenorrhea due to pituitary lesions have been reported, but are rare. Sarcoid infiltration of the thyroid and/or of the adrenal gland may lead to fibrosis and failure of either or both glands and cause hyperthyroidism, Hashimoto's thyroiditis, and/or Addison's disease. A sarcoidal mass infiltrating the testis of a young boy has been reported. The central nervous system is rarely affected. In a small number of children paralysis of the facial nerve has been associated with uveoparotid fever. Striated muscle sarcoidosis can produce muscle weakness or pseudohypertrophy. Deafness can be a presenting symptom. In one child hoarseness was associated with the presence of a sarcoid nodule on the vocal cords; in another patient extensive laryngeal infiltration caused almost complete airway obstruction at a time when the pulmonary parenchymal disease had improved.

The kidneys are among the less frequently affected organs in childhood sarcoidosis. However, several instances of kidney involvement with various degrees of renal failure have been recorded, some in association with polyarthritis. The most common findings are proteinuria, pyuria, hematuria, intermittent glycosuria, and granular casts. Clinical symptoms are usually mild and do not correlate with the severity of histologic lesions observed on biopsy or autopsy. Persitent hypertension is exceptional. Since parenchymal renal granulomas are often microscopic, they are not thought to be the cause of the impairment of renal function. The hypercalcemia of sarcoidosis with or without nephrocalcinosis or nephrolithiasis is believed to be primarily responsible for the renal complication of this disease. A fairly good correlation appears to exist between the severity of renal symptoms and the duration and degree of hypercalcemia. Renal insufficiency is usually associated with hypercalcemia.

Course and Complications

Sarcoidosis runs a chronic course characterized by remissions and exacerbations with a tendency to ultimate healing in the child. Fatalities are infrequent. Childhood sarcoidosis could be considered essentially a benign disease but for three troublesome complications: pulmonary fibrosis, fibrotic uveitis, and nephrocalcinosis. However, even very severe impairment of pulmonary function does not necessarily indicate grave prognosis. Skin lesions in children carry an ominous connotation, chiefly because of the greater association with either blindness or severe restrictive lung disease. Unsuspected tuberculosis has complicated the course of some patients and has caused their death. *Cryptococcus neoformans meningitis* has been responsible for the fatal outcome in one child with diffuse systemic Boeck's sarcoid.

Laboratory Findings and Diagnosis

The diagnosis can be established by an assessment of the clinical manifestations, the radiographic findings in lungs and bones, in combination with certain laboratory abnormalities, and the histologic features of a biopsy. Most patients have an elevated serum protein due to an absolute increase of serum globulins, with elevation of α_2 and γ globulins and reversal of the albumin/globulin ratio. Serum complement activity may be increased. Activation of the complement system (primarily of C_3) is particularly marked in the early stages of the disease and often returns to normal as symptoms subside. Hypercalcemia occurs quite commonly and is an important complicating factor in sarcoidosis. The hypercalcemia is believed to be due to hypersensitivity to vitamin D. Eosinophilia is found more frequently in children than in adults. There are no other characteristic changes in blood count, blood chemistries, or sedimentation rate.

The tuberculin test is negative, except in some, but not all patients who have both sarcoidosis and tuberculosis. Depression of delayed-type hypersensitivity is also demonstrable with other antigens including pertussis and mumps. Dissociation between defective cellular antibodies and the normal circulating antibody response may be used as a diagnostic aid in sarcoidosis. A negative mumps skin test with a positive mumps complement-fixation test, although not specific for sarcoidosis, can nonetheless be considered significant in support of this diagnosis.

The diagnosis is most readily confirmed by biopsy and histologic examination of a lesion. An enlarged, peripheral lymph node, the scalene fat pad, a skin lesion, or muscle are tissues most suitable and most accessible for biopsy.

The *Nickerson-Kveim* or *Kveim-Siltzbach skin test* is helpful in differentiating sarcoidosis from other granulomatous diseases, provided the test is carried out under rigid control, with confirmation by biopsy. The test is based on the reaction that follows the intracutaneous injection of 0.2 ml of antigen prepared from sarcoid tissue. Material used for the test must be adequately tested on known cases of sarcoid before it can be used for diagnosis. The test is positive when a sarcoid lesion forms at the injection site in the course of a few weeks. It must be interpreted by histologic examination of the papule, removed by punch biopsy 6 or 8 weeks after the injection. Although a positive Kveim test offers strong confirmation of the diagnosis, a negative result does not exclude sarcoidosis. Irregularities in response to the test depend in large part on differences in the properties of the antigenic material used.

Treatment

There is no specific therapy for sarcoidosis. The indications for treatment with adrenal corticosteroids and the magnitude of the benefits derived from such therapy are still the subject of controversy. The true value of any treatment in a disease with such a high spontaneous remission rate is difficult to assess. However, there is general agreement that the adrenal corticosteroids alleviate symptoms and decrease the extent of organ involvement, at least temporarily. Therapy with adrenal corticosteroids is recommended for patients with active ocular disease, persistent hypercalcemia, central nervous system or myocardial involvement, disfiguring skin lesions, hypersplenism and progressive pulmonary disease. Both symptoms and lesions may improve or disappear completely under the influence of steroid therapy, but often recur when such treatment is terminated. However, relapses after withdrawal of therapy are often only temporary and may be followed by lasting improvement, without reinstitution of adrenal corticosteroids. A low-calcium diet may lower hypercalcemia, but in the majority of cases diet, alone, or in combination with sodium sulfate, is not effective. Corticosteroids have been successful in resolving the hypercalcemia, followed by a striking and permanent return to normal renal function. Longitudinal studies of serial pulmonary functions were carried out over several years on sarcoid patients. These have shown steroid therapy to be beneficial for patients with restrictive pulmonary disease, particularly if the pretreatment impairment was great and therapy was given early in the course of the disease.

Bibliography

Bautista A: Childhood sarcoidosis involving joints and kidneys. Am J Dis Child 119:259, 1970

Beier FR, Lahey ME: Sarcoidosis among children in Utah and Idaho. J Pediat 65:350, 1964

Emirgil C, Sobol BJ, Williams Jr MH: Long term study of pulmonary sarcoidosis, the effect of steroid therapy as evaluated by pulmonary function studies. J Chron Dis 22:69, 1969

Israel HL, Jones M: Immunologic defect in patients recovered from sarcoidosis. N Engl J Med 273:1003, 1965

James DG: Immunology of sarcoidosis. Lancet 7515:526, 1967

————Treatment of sarcoidosis. Lancet 7464:633, 1966

Jasper PL, Denny FW: Sarcoidosis in children. J Pediatr 73:499, 1968

Holden KR, Heller RM: Childhood sarcoidosis. Am J Dis Child 129:103, 1975

Karlish AJ, McGregor GA: Sarocidosis, thyroiditis, and Addison's disease. Lancet 2:330, 1970

Kendig EL: Sarcoidosis among children, a review. J Pediatr 61:269, 1962

————The clinical picture of sarcoidosis in children. Pediatrics 54:289, 1974

Kirschner BS, Holinger PH: Laryngeal obstruction in childhood sarcoidosis. J Pediatr 88:263, 1976

Kogut MD, Newman LL: Renal involvement in Boeck's sarcoidosis. Pediatrics 28:40 1961

Lofgren S: Concepts of sarcoidosis. In 3rd International Conference on Sarcoidosis. Acta Med Scand 425:1, 1964

McGovern JP, Merritt DH: Sarcoidosis in childhood. Adv Pediatr 8:97, 1956

Oreskes I, Silzbach LE: Changes in rheumatoid factor activity during the course of sarcoidosis. Am J Med 44:60, 1968

Scholz DA : Effect of steroid therapy on hypercalcemic and renal insufficiency in sarcoidosis. JAMA 169:682, 1959

Shiff AD, Blatt CJ, Colp CC: Recurrent pericardial effusion secondary to sarcoidosis of the pericardium. N Engl J Med 281:141, 1969

Siltzbach LE, Greenberg GM: Childhood sarcoidosis—a study of 18 patients. N Engl J Med 279:1239, 1968

Ting EY, Williams MH: Mechanics of breathing in sarcoidosis of lung. JAMA 192:123, 1965

CHAPTER 26

The Kidneys and Urinary Tract

CHESTER M. EDELMANN, JR., *Associate Editor*

MORPHOLOGIC DEVELOPMENT

JAY BERNSTEIN

The development of the metanephros or definitive kidney begins in the fifth week of embryonic life when a diverticulum of the wolffian or mesonephric duct establishes contact with the caudal mesenchyme of the nephrogenic cord. This diverticulum, the ureteric bud, develops into the renal collecting system, which includes the ureter, pelvis, calyces, and collecting ducts. The mesenchyme or metanephric blastema forms the renal secretory system, including glomeruli, convoluted tubules, and loops of Henle.

The ureteric bud divides into the first generation of branches, the primary cranial and caudal pole tubules, which eventually give rise to the major calyces. Subsequent branching gives rise to the minor calyces and collecting ducts of the renal pyramids. Secretory activity of the first nephrons causes dilatation and consequent remodeling of the metanephric duct and its branches to form the pelvis and calyces, the outflow of urine possibly being temporarily impeded by epithelial septa at the caudal end of the ureter. The relationship of continuing formation and accumulation of urine to subsequent organogenesis is not clear; that the former may have a profound effect on development is suggested by the frequent association of congenital urinary tract obstruction and parenchymal maldevelopment of the kidney.

Proliferation of and differentiation within the metanephrogenic mesenchyme lead to the development of glomeruli and tubules in juxtaposition to the growing collecting ducts. A condensation of mesenchyme appears near the growing end, at the ampulla of the collecting tubule, and this cellular mass is transformed into a nephric vesicle by the development of a lumen. The cells forming the vesicle undergo alignment into a simple columnar epithelium. As it grows the vesicle becomes kinked into an **S**-shaped structure in which a glomerulus is formed at the blind, free end and continuity with the collecting system is established at the other. Capillaries grow into the cleft at the free end of the kinked vesicle to form the glomerular vessels, establishing circulation through blood vessels in the adjacent mesenchyme. Basement membrane material appears between juxtaposed endothelial and epithelial cells and becomes progressively thicker with advancing age, from approximately 100 nm to slightly more than 300 nm at full maturity. It may be more permeable in the fetal and neonatal periods than in later life, but its capacity to form an ultrafiltrate seems to be unaffected, since the urine is free of proteins even in prematurely born infants. In its definitive form the glomerulus is composed of a rete or network of freely anastomosing capillaries. With age these assume a lobulated appearance, although numerous intercapillary connections persist. The solid central portion of the glomerulus is referred to as the stalk. It contains cells morphologically different from capillary endothelium; they are believed to function in phagocytosis by clearing the glomerulus of unfilterable macromolecules and in secretion by responding to mineralocorticoid deficiency by developing granules similar to those in cells of the juxtaglomerular apparatus.

Continued growth of the vesicle leads to further elongation and coiling, with development of the proximal and distal convoluted tubules and the intervening loop of Henle. The first portion of the distal convolution remains in close proximity to the hilar arterioles of the glomerulus, and together they undergo specialization to form the complex known as the juxtaglomerular apparatus. The epithelial cells in that part of the distal convolution differentiate into the macula densa, and specialized cells develop between and in the walls of the afferent and efferent arterioles. Secretion of renin has been attributed to granular epithelioid cells in the walls of the hilar arterioles. Agranular "lacis" cells form the juxtaglomerular cell mass and are continuous with and morphologically similar to the mesangial cells of the glomerular stalk. In early infancy this complex is poorly developed; it usually does not appear as a well-defined structure before the age of 2 years.

Nephrogenesis proceeds at the periphery, and the growth of the kidney is thus centrifugal. The central portion of the cortex near the corticomedullary junction contains the developmentally older glomeruli, whose loops of Henle dip into the medulla and whose efferent arterioles form the arteriolae rectae of the medulla. The peripheral cortex contains the more recently formed glomeruli and tubules. These are the cortical nephrons, whose loops of Henle do not reach into the medulla. The deeper glomeruli are also larger than those developing more peripherally, and a number of them, particularly those around the arcuate vessels, normally undergo involution and resorption in the early neonatal period.

During development of the inner cortex new nephrons are formed at the growing ampullary end of the collecting duct in more or less successive fashion. The collecting ducts branch as they grow and induce the formation of new nephrons, but by differential growth the terminal portions of all nephrons maintain their points of attachment on the ampullae. The nephrons are therefore carried forward into the cortex, leaving approximately six divisions of the ducts free of attached nephrons and, as a result, the medullary pyramids free of glomeruli. Since the older nephrons remain attached at the ampullae of the collecting ducts as new nephrons are developing, they form arcades that drain peripherally, generally in groups of four to seven, with the last segments of the collecting tubules finally entering the collecting ducts. The last portions of the collecting ducts grow peripherally, commonly without branching, and beyond the arcades subsequent nephrons are attached individually and directly to the collecting ducts in the peripheral cortex. Approximately 20 percent of nephrons are formed by 3 months of gestation and about 30 percent by 5 months. At the end of a full-term gestation each kidney contains between 850,000 and 1,000,000 nephrons.

Knowledge of the postnatal growth and maturation of the kidney is fragmentary. Physical growth during organogenesis depends upon the formation of new units and enlargement of existing units. Formation of new nephrons ordinarily ceases before full fetal maturity (approximately 36 weeks gestation), and an infant of low birth weight exhibits a degree of nephrogenesis more commensurate with gestational age than with size. Nephrogenesis continues for a variable period of time postnatally in premature infants, but it may possibly end earlier than it would have had the fetus remained in utero. Nephrogenesis may also occasionally cease prematurely in a normally developing fetus. It is not known whether these factors affect subsequent renal development. Renal growth during infancy and childhood ordinarily follows a predictable allometric curve, and kidney size correlates to a strikingly high degree with both age and the usual parameters of somatic growth. However, in patients with intrinsic renal disease, cerebral abnormalities, and some form of congenital heart disease, renal size may be considerably less than expected.

Maturation of the kidney has been assessed both by the histologic appearance of glomeruli and by the size and disposition of the tubules. The rate of glomerular maturation is variable, and immature forms are present normally for months after birth. Superimposed diseases, such as inflammation and urinary tract obstruction, may lead to a persistence of abnormally immature forms and even to regressive changes in normally formed glomeruli. The differences among glomeruli disappear as rapid growth in the outer cortex leads toward greater homogeneity. Glomerular size (average diameter 100 μ at birth, increasing to approximately 300 μ) also follows a regular growth curve in childhood and may be either retarded or accelerated by certain diseases. Cyanotic congenital heart disease, for example, is often associated with striking glomerular enlargement. Glomerular function increases during early infancy, but it is quite clear that even immature glomeruli can function once capillary circulation has been established. Increasing glomerular blood flow and filtration rate in childhood are reflected in increasing glomerular size and surface area of the capillary bed.

Measurements of microdissected specimens have confirmed the expected postnatal increase in tubular length and volume; tubular length, like glomerular size, becomes more homogeneous. However, tubular growth is relatively greater than glomerular enlargement, and this is undoubtedly a factor in maintaining glomerulotubular balance as the glomerular filtration rate increases postnatally. Differential tubular growth results in a spreading out of glomeruli and their redistribution in the cortex; it is responsible also for a diminution in the number of cortical nephrons as additional loops of Henle become included within the enlarging medulla. Thus tubular growth with increasing tubular mass leads to increasing cortical capacity for transport and metabolic functions and to increasing medullary capacity for concentrating urine.

Cytostructural changes play a much smaller role in the phenomenon of tubular maturation. Although histochemical studies have in general shown increasing enzymatic activity postnatally, electron microscopy has demonstrated few ultrastructural differences between immature fetal and mature adult tubular epithelial cells. Characteristic ultrastructural features in cells of the newly formed proximal convoluted tubule can be shown in fetal kidneys at the same time that glomerular vascularization can be demonstrated, ie, when glomerular structure is capable of maintaining ultrafiltration and when the tubular lumen presumably contains filtered glomerular fluid. The ultrastructural features are not appreciably changed under experimental conditions, such as, for example, increasing the transport capacity of the tubular epithelial cells. This apparent discrepancy between structural and functional differentiation can be interpreted to mean that tubular maturation, in the sense of postnatal induction of enzymatic activity or transport capacity, may be related to quantitative enhancement of existing cellular systems. Thus renal maturation is only slightly related to the continuing differentiation of individual cells, perhaps more so to physical growth with changing and more efficient anatomic interrelationships among nephrons, ducts, and blood vessels, and perhaps most to increasing blood flow with increasing substrate-specific workload and hormonal stimulation.

References

Bernstein J, Meyer R: Some speculations on the nature and significance of developmentally small kidneys (renal hypoplasia). Nephron 1:137, 1964

DuBois AM: The embryonic kidney. In Rouiller C, Muller AF (eds): The Kidney, Vol 1. New York, Academic, 1969, p. 1.

Fetterman GH, Shuplock NA, Philipp FJ, Gregg HS: The growth and maturation of human glomeruli and proximal convolutions from term to adulthood; studies of microdissection. Pediatrics 35:601, 1965

Fujikura T, Froehlich LA: Birth weight, gestational age, and renal glomerular development as indices of fetal maturity. Am J Obstet Gynecol 113:627, 1972

McCrory WW: Developmental Nephrology. Cambridge, Harvard Univ Press, 1972

Oliver J, Rubenstein M, Meyer R, Bernstein J: Congenital abnormalities of the urinary system. III. Growth of the kidney in childhood—determination of normal weight. J Pediatr 61:256, 1972

——— Nephrons and Kidneys. A Quantitative Study of Developmental and Evolutionary Mammalian Architectonics. New York, Hoeber, Harper & Row, 1968

Potter EL: Normal and Abnormal Development of the Kidney. Chicago, Year Book, 1972

Vernier RL, Birch-Andersen A: Studies of the human fetal kidney. I. Development of the glomerulus. J Pediatr 60:754, 1962

———Studies of the human fetal kidney. II. Permeability characteristics of the developing glomerulus. J Ultrastruct Res 8:66, 1963

Zamboni L, De Martino C: Embryogenesis of the human renal glomerulus. I. A histologic study. Arch Pathol 86:279, 1968

PHYSIOLOGY AND FUNCTIONAL DEVELOPMENT OF THE KIDNEY

Adrian Spitzer

The limited variability of the internal environment that is necessary for the development and subsequent maintenance of the organism is in large part the result of the activity of the kidneys. As stated by Homer Smith, father of modern renal physiology: "In the last analysis, composition of the plasma is determined not by what the body ingests but by what the kidneys retain and what they excrete." Hence it is probably correct to say that the excretory function of the kidney is only incidental to its regulatory function. Conceptually, however, the regulatory and excretory functions of the kidney should not be considered identical. The kidney of the newborn, for instance, has an excretory capacity that is entirely adequate under usual circumstances, but its ability to respond to changes is slow and quantitatively limited. At any age excretory rates of the diseased kidney may be normal at a time when regulatory function is significantly deficient, as is evidenced by distortions in the composition of the body fluids.

A thorough understanding of the mechanisms underlying the excretory and regulatory functions of the kidney, as well as knowledge concerning the capacity of the organ to fulfill its role at different ages and in various states of disease, are of paramount importance in providing optimal medical care of the child.

FETAL KIDNEY

During intrauterine life the kidney is able to perform most of the functions that characterize the adult organ. The development of the human fetus, however, does not seem to depend on the capacity of the kidneys to retain or excrete substances, these regulatory and excretory functions being assumed by the placenta. This conclusion is supported by the fact that children with bilateral renal agenesis may be born without other abnormalities.

Renal plasma flow, as determined in experimental animals, is low during intrauterine life, and renal vascular resistance is high. This might contribute to the low tubular secretory rates observed during this period, although immaturity of the secretory mechanisms per se is of major importance.

Formation of urine by the human fetal kidney begins toward the end of the first trimester. This coincides with the differentiation of the brush border in the proximal

tubules and the onset of transport by the renal tubular epithelium, as has been evidenced by accumulation of dyes in tubular segments isolated from human fetuses. No information is available regarding glomerular filtration rate (GFR) or rate of urine flow in the human fetus. In the sheep, however, in which formation of urine starts at about 2 months of gestation, there is a progressive increase in the rates of both glomerular filtration and urine flow up to about 4 months of intrauterine life. During the remaining month of gestation, despite a continuing increase in GFR, a decrease in urine flow occurs. This is likely to be the result of the onset of function of the newly formed loops of Henle, which have a high capacity to reabsorb salt and water.

Fetal urine is hypotonic to plasma, as a result of low concentrations of electrolytes and urea. The fetal kidney is able to excrete an acid urine with a pH of about 6, but the capacity to increase the excretion of H^+ following administration of an acid load is limited.

Neonatal Kidney

Following placental separation there is a prompt increase in renal blood flow due to a decrease in renal vascular resistance. The nature of the mechanism that underlies the decrease in resistance is still controversial. Morphologic studies suggest a role for epithelioid cells that are present in the precapillary branches of the so-called dormant organs (lungs, gut, kidney). These cells have been found to shrink immediately after birth, but the stimulus for this change is unknown. Accompanying the increase in renal blood flow there is a marked increase in functional capacity. However, definite limitations in many renal functions persist during the newborn period and to a lesser degree during most of the remainder of infancy.

Glomerular Function

The first step in the formation of urine is ultrafiltration of plasma across the semipermeable membranes of the glomerular capillaries. Micropuncture studies in single nephrons of experimenatal animals have shown that at arterial pressures comparable to those found in adult man glomerular capillary pressure is around 50 mm Hg. Opposing filtration is the pressure in the proximal tubule, about 10 mm Hg, and the colloid osmotic pressure of the plasma proteins, approximately 25 mm Hg. Thus the effective hydrostatic pressure for filtration is about 15 mm Hg. These forces, together with the surface of the glomerular capillary available for filtration and the permeability characteristics of the capillary membrane, determine the rate of glomerular filtration.

In young infants glomerular filtration rates have been found to be low in comparison to those in adults, even when corrected for kidney weight or body surface area. Moreover, it has been suggested that in the immature kidney not all the glomeruli participate equally in the process of filtration. The more recently formed glomeruli, which are located in the superficial cortex, have a lower filtration rate than the deeper and more mature ones. During the first week of life the value for total total kidney GFR is about 35 ml/minute/1.73 m². A steady progression occurs, so that at the end of the first year the corrected values for GFR are close to those found in adults. Because of the wide range of normal variation, however, individual measurements of GFR during infancy may be difficult to interpret. The search for an explanation for the low rates of glomerular filtration during infancy currently points toward a multicausal phenomenon.

One of the factors found to play a role in experimental animals is a relatively high resistance in the afferent and efferent glomerular arterioles. For example, an 88 percent decrease in intrinsic renal vascular resistance was found to occur in the piglet during the first 6 weeks of extrauterine life.

Low capillary permeability is another contributing factor. The clearance of dextran with a molecular weight of 15,000 daltons is close to zero in the newborn infant, whereas the adult is able to filter dextran molecules up to a weight of about 50,000 daltons. The calculated effective pore radius is 20 Å in the newborn, compared to 40 Å in the adult. The net result is a low hydrostatic pressure available to move fluid through the glomerular capillary membrane (effective filtration pressure). An increase in filtration pressure and an increase in the surface area of the filtering membrane have been shown to be the main contributors to the increase in GFR observed during development.

The role that the tubule may play in controlling glomerular filtration is not yet defined. Experimental evidence points toward the existence of a regulatory mechanism whereby a low tubular reabsorptive capacity results in a low rate of filtration. Since, during most of infancy, striking limitations exist in the reabsorptive capacity of the tubules, such a mechanism might have a significant influence on the rate of glomerular filtration.

Tubular Function

REABSORPTIVE MECHANISMS. The urinary output represents only a small fraction of the glomerular ultrafiltrate. In adult man about 175 liters of filtrate containing some 25,000 mEq of sodium chloride are reabsorbed daily, compared with about 9 liters of fluid and 1,300 mEq of sodium chloride reabsorbed by the kidney of the newborn. However, relative to body weight or the size of the extracellular compartment the rates in the newborn and the adult are similar, representing a turnover of about four times the total body content of sodium and water.

In the mammalian nephron about 70 to 75 percent of the filtered sodium chloride and fluid is reabsorbed in the proximal convolution. Simultaneous measurements of electrochemical potential gradients and the direction and magnitude of net ion movement permit characterization of the nature of these reabsorptive mechanisms (Fig. 1). When net transport takes place against an electrochemical gradient, and thus requires energy, it is called active. Therefore active transport excludes pas-

sive diffusion or bulk movement of fluid. It includes, on the other hand, carrier-mediated transport along an electrochemical gradient, provided the process is energy-consuming and the rate of transport exceeds that expected to occur as a result of the electrochemical forces operating at the level of the respective membrane. Substances actively reabsorbed by the proximal tubule include sodium, amino acids, calcium, phosphate, potassium, organic anions, and vitamin D.

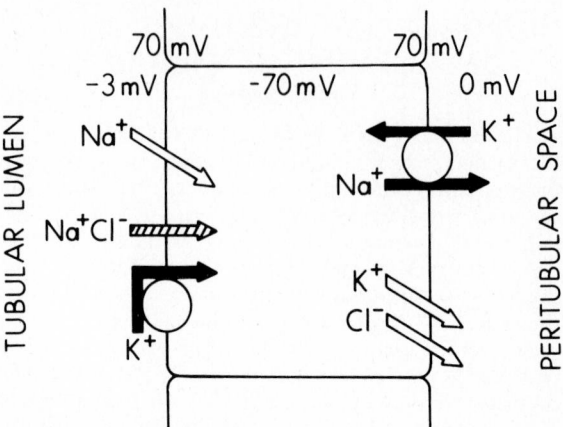

FIG. 1. Ion transport by a cell of the proximal tubule. Open arrows represent passive diffusion, cross-hatched arrows carrier-mediated passive transfer, and solid arrows active transport. The figures represent electrical potential differences.

Sodium diffuses from the proximal tubule into the cell along an electrochemical gradient, but its extrusion from the cell takes place against such a gradient. Potassium is transported actively into the cells, while outward movement occurs by diffusion. Chloride ions are reabsorbed passively in proximal tubules, but the exact nature of the process at the luminal membrane is not known (it may be ionic diffusion or carrier-mediated transport). Transport of chloride out of the cells occurs along an electrochemical gradient.

In the loop of Henle about 15 percent of the filtered sodium is reabsorbed, primarily in conjunction with the concentrating and diluting mechanism (see below); the remaining 10 to 15 percent is reabsorbed in the distal tubule. Virtually all filtered potassium is reabsorbed in the proximal tubule, the excreted moiety being added to the distal tubular fluid by active secretion. The nature of chloride transport in the distal nephron is still controversial, although there is considerable evidence for its active transport in the thick ascending limb of the loop of Henle and perhaps the early portion of the distal tubule. Whereas the proximal tubule reabsorbs most of the substances present in the glomerular filtrate, either in an indiscriminate fashion or with only gross regulation, the distal nephron (distal convoluted tubule and collecting duct) performs the "fine tuning" that allows the kidney to fulfill its regulatory function (Fig. 2).

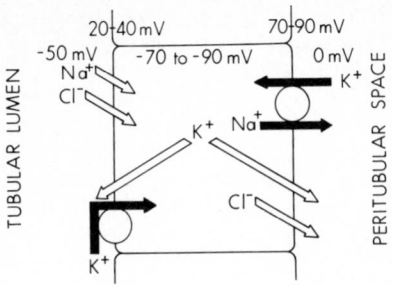

FIG. 2. Ion transport by a distal tubular cell (see legend for Figure 1).

SECRETORY MECHANISMS.

SECRETORY MECHANISMS. Two mechanisms for active tubular secretion of organic substances, both of which operate in the proximal tubule, have been characterized. One serves as a transport pathway for a variety of organic acids, including creatinine, p-aminohippurate (PAH), and penicillin; the other transports organic bases such as guanidine, choline and histamine.

Knowledge concerning the capacity for tubular transport in the developing kidney is limited. One micropuncture study showed that the capacity for sodium reabsorption by the proximal tubule of young rats was low in comparison to adult animals. The renal clearance of certain amino acids is higher in infants than in children older than 3 years. The Tm* for glucose has been found to be 313 ± 71 mg/minute/1.73 m² in infants, 362 ± 96 mg/minute/1.73 m² in children 18 months of age and older, and 364 ± 35 and 303 ± 29 mg/minute/1.73 m² in adult men and women, respectively. The Tm for PAH has been found to be 20 ± 6 mg/minute/1.73 m² in full-term infants; the mean increases to 40 at 3 months of age and to 50 at 6 months. In the adult it is 80 ± 16 mg/minute/1.73 m².

GLOMERULOTUBULAR INTERRELATIONSHIPS

It is well established that under varying experimental conditions proportionality exists between the amount of a substance filtered and the amount that is reabsorbed. This relationship can be demonstrated for the function of the whole kidney as well as for the function of individual nephrons; for example, the fraction of sodium reabsorbed in the proximal tubule is constant over a wide range of filtration rates. This phenomenon has been named glomerulotubular balance.

Studies performed almost half a century ago showed a strong morphologic predominance of glomerular tissue over tubular tissue in newborn animals; more recently this finding has been confirmed in humans. In one study in a full-term infant the diameter of the

* The Tm, or tubular transport maximum, of a substance is the highest rate at which it can be reabsorbed or secreted by the tubule. It is a measurement used to evaluate renal functional capacity.

glomeruli averaged 116 μ and the length of the proximal tubule 1.79 mm. This compares to a glomerular diameter of about 200 μ and a proximal tubular length of about 20 mm in the adult. Thus whereas the increase in glomerular size is less than twofold the increase in proximal tubular length exceeds tenfold. The mean ratio of glomerular surface to proximal tubular volume has been found to be 27.8 in a full-term infant, 13.4 in a 3-month-old infant, and 3.1 in an adult. These ratios indicate that in the infant the glomeruli are disproportionately large relative to the proximal tubules. Nephron heterogeneity also characterizes the developing kidney, with tubules varying in length over a tenfold range, but with a rather small variation in glomerular size. The fact that these morphologic features are more prominent in the renal cortex (which is ontogenetically and phylogenetically newer than the medullary area) and that they disappear with age demonstrates their relationship to development.

Functional characteristics of the kidney during early life are considered to be the consequence of morphologic glomerulotubular imbalance. The concentrations of glucose and bicarbonate in the serum, at which they appear in the urine, are lower in infancy than later in life. The net percentage of filtered amino acids and phosphate reabsorbed by the tubules is low. The average penicillin-to-inulin clearance ratios in the urine have been found to be 2.0 in premature infants and 4.4 in older children. Since penicillin is actively secreted by the tubule and inulin concentration is a measure of GFR, this finding is considered to support the hypothesis of greater immaturity of tubular function than glomerular function in early life.

However, micropuncture experiments performed in puppies and guinea pigs have shown that fractional reabsorption of fluid in the proximal convoluted tubule remains relatively constant during development. This finding indicates that proportionality between filtration and reabsorption is maintained despite morphologic imbalance between glomerulus and tubule. Further support for this concept is derived from new studies of renal glucose transport in puppies and in infants in which the ratio of Tm glucose to GFR was found to be equal to or greater than that in the adult.

Simultaneous measurements of GFR and effective renal plasma flow (ERPF) in early infancy have revealed values of filtration fraction (GFR/ERPF) ranging from 0.32 to 0.34, as compared to a range of values of 0.19 to 0.20 in adult man. Initially these data were interpreted as providing additional evidence for glomerular preponderance. Subsequently the extraction ratio of PAH was found to range between 0.50 and 0.80 during the first 3 months of life, representing, on the average, 30 percent less than the adult value of 0.95. Correction for this extraction ratio yields a mean filtration fraction of 0.23, a value that is only slightly higher than that observed in the adult.

More recent studies on the intrarenal distribution of blood flow suggest that a significant part of the blood going to the cortex at this age may represent nutrient flow that is not filtered. In addition, a higher proportion of the total renal blood flow is distributed to the juxtamedullary nephrons. The fraction of postglomerular flow that passes through the vasa recta thus bypasses the secretory sites of the proximal tubules. Under these circumstances the ratio of GFR to ERPF does not represent an index of the balance between glomerular and tubular function, and the filtration fraction does not have the generally accepted physiologic meaning.

Progress in histochemistry has made possible the mapping of enzymatic activity in the developing kidney of experimental animals. In agreement with the finding of structural immaturity of the outer cortex, little enzymatic activity has been found in this area. Even in tubules that have reached morphologic maturity the activities of mitochondrial ATPase and of succinic dehydrogenase are less than in the adult. In contrast, the activity of enzymes of mitochondrial origin in the medulla is greater than in the adult kidney.

The mechanism or mechanisms responsible for enzymatic maturation have not been determined. One possible contributing factor is substrate-induced stimulation. Several studies have shown that the capacity to secrete PAH increases significantly following ingestion of a high-protein diet. The capacity of the tubules to transport organic acids can be enhanced by administration of penicillin, which is excreted by active secretion.

In summary, during intrauterine life glomerular development prevails over tubular development, and medullary development precedes and exceeds cortical development. In early postnatal life glomerular filtration rates are low as a result of relatively impermeable basement membranes, small surface areas for filtration, and low net driving force for filtration. Despite on apparent morphologic glomerular preponderance, functional glomerulotubular balance is maintained during development. However, because of the low levels of GFR and because the rate of reabsorption of most substances is close to the maximum transport capacity of the tubules, the kidney is limited in its ability to adapt under conditions of stress.

Renal Control Mechanisms

The complex systems that control homeostasis are of two principal types: steady state and negative feedback. In a steady-state system a change in one variable is minimized by a change in one or more covariables. Only the variable and the effector organ are involved in such a mechanism and the degree of control achieved is not very high. The concentrations in plasma of urea and creatinine seem to be under the control of a simple steady-state mechanism in which the glomeruli represent the end organs.

The negative-feedback systems are much more complex and are able to provide a much finer degree of control. They can either be located within the effector organ itself or be remote from it. In a negative-feedback system the change in the controlled variable determines a change in a servomechanism that causes a change in the opposite direction in the effector organ. Such systems control the metabolism of salt and water and probably control, in part, acid excretion.

In general the steady-state systems are better developed in infancy than the more complex negative-feedback systems. In the following section the mechanisms controlling three essential body constituents (water, sodium, and hydrogen ion) will be considered.

CONTROL OF WATER EXCRETION. Under usual circumstances about 99 percent of the water filtered by the glomeruli is reabsorbed passively by the tubules as a result of the active transport of solute. In order to maintain the osmolality of the body fluids in the face of wide variations in intake and extrarenal loss, the amount of water excreted per unit of urinary solute can be varied over a tremendous range. The mature kidney is able to produce a urine as dilute as 50 mOsm/liter under conditions of water diuresis and as concentrated as 1,300 mOsm/liter during antidiuresis.

There are three distinct areas for water movement along the nephron: (1) the proximal tubule, where the amount of water reabsorbed is totally dependent on the reabsorption of solute and where both the reabsorbate and the fluid delivered into more distal parts of the nephron are always isosmotic; (2) the distal tubule, including the loop of Henle, where the amount of water that is reabsorbed varies but is always somewhat less than the rate of reabsorption of solute, with the tubular fluid ultimately becoming hypotonic; and (3) the collecting duct, where the amount of water reabsorbed is determined not only by the rate of solute reabsorption and the permeability characteristics of the membrane but also by the capacity of the medulla to concentrate solute. The last two segments, namely the distal nephron (including the loop of Henle) and the collecting duct, are involved in the process of urinary concentration and dilution and need to be considered in more detail.

In order to understand this process some knowledge about countercurrent multipliers is necessary (Fig. 3). The descending and ascending limbs of the loops of Henle are arranged as two parallel tubes connected in a hairpin manner, in which flow takes place in opposite directions. This structure, which is able to transport sodium actively, has therefore the characteristics of a countercurrent multiplier. In such a system small differences in gradients can be multiplied as a function of length. In the particular instance of the kidney, the active transport of chloride out of the thick ascending limbs of the loop of Henle coupled with the relative impermeability to water of this site produces hypertonicity of the interstitium, causing passive movement of water out of and net movement of sodium chloride and urea into the descending limb. The ascending limb of the loop of Henle, the distal tubule, and the cortical collecting duct are relatively impermeable to urea. Therefore, urea becomes concentrated in those segments as water is reabsorbed. Under the influence of antidiuretic hormone (ADH) the medullary collecting duct is highly permeable to urea. This solute diffuses passively into the medullary interstitium, thus enhancing the hyperosmolality of this area. The high concentration of urea in the interstitium results in passive diffusion into the descending limb. Current evidence suggests that active transport of chloride is confined to the thick ascending limb, the thin limb of the loop of Henle playing a passive role in movement of water and recycling of urea from the collecting duct. Ultimately a steady state is reached in which the interstitium and the fluid in the descending limb become more and more concentrated from the cortex to the medullary tip, and fluid in the ascending limb becomes more and more dilute on its way up toward the cortex.

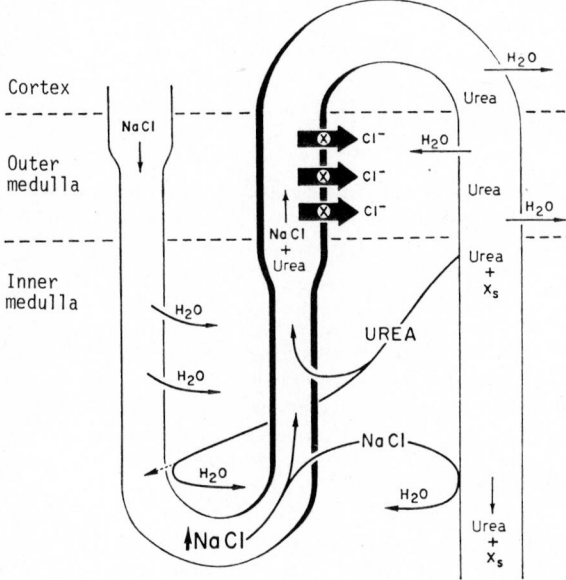

FIG. 3. Countercurrent mechanism in the formation of hypertonic urine. Shown is the model of Kokko and Rector in which all inner medullary structures function as purely passive equilibrative segments without active transport processes. The heavy black arrows indicate active chloride reabsorption from the thick ascending limb. X_s = non-reabsorbable solute. (From Kokko JP et al: In Villarreal H (ed). Proc 5th Int Cong Nephrol (Mexico 1972) Vol. 2, 1974, by permission).

This system allows for urinary dilution as well as concentration. In the absence of antidiuretic hormone (ADH) the distal and collecting ducts are impermeable to water, and the dilute fluid that leaves the ascending limbs of the loops of Henle becomes progressively more dilute as additional solute is removed in these structures. Maximal water diuresis, therefore, represents maximal trapping of water within the nephron, coupled with maximal outward transport of sodium chloride.

Increase in the tonicity of blood is a stimulus for secretion of ADH, which acts to render the collecting duct permeable to water. Hypotonic fluid leaving the loops of Henle and the distal convolution becomes isotonic as it equilibrates with the interstitium of the cor-

tex. Concentration of the urine occurs during its passage through the collecting duct as it traverses the medulla, with passive outward movement of water being induced by the progressively increased hypertonicity of the interstitium. Urinary concentration and dilution obviously are not all-or-none phenomena, because the rate of urine flow (ie, the rate of excretion of water) varies inversely with the amount of ADH present as a continuous function.

During the first few days of life the newborn does not respond to a water load. By the end of the first week the response to a decrease in plasma osmolality is prompt, and the degree of urinary dilution achieved is comparable to that observed in the adult. However, the rate of urinary flow is lower, and the infant excretes water at a decelerating rate and stops completely before the entire load has been eliminated. This suggests an immaturity of the underlying control mechanism and renders the infant more vulnerable to excess administration of water.

The capacity of the infant to concentrate urine in response to water deprivation matures more slowly than does the diluting capacity. Following maximal stimulation, young infants usually are unable to concentrate their urine to more than 700 mOsm/liter, as compared to 1,300 mOsm/liter in the older child or adult. Among contributing factors in this limitation are the shortness of the loops of Henle and probably a low capacity of the tubules to reabsorb sodium chloride. Of even greater importance, however, may be the infant's low rate of excretion of urea, which results from the strongly anabolic state that characterizes this period of life. When an infant is fed urea or a high-protein diet his ability to concentrate urine approaches that found in adults.

Information concerning the rate of release of ADH and the sensitivity of the end organ to ADH is incomplete, and the mechanisms involved are the subject of controversy. During osmotic diuresis, urines hypotonic to plasma have been observed in infants, possibly indicating incomplete equilibration between tubular and interstitial fluid. This could be due to relative impermeability of the tubules or to unavailability of or impaired responsiveness to ADH, or a combination of both.

It should be emphasized that the limitation in concentrating capacity observed during the first few weeks of life does not signficantly jeopardize the well-being of the infant; because of a relatively large surface area the infant loses large amounts of water via nonrenal routes (skin and lungs). In view of this, an increase in concentrating capacity to mature levels would save only trivial amounts of water.

CONTROL OF SODIUM EXCRETION. Sodium is the major cation of the extracellular fluid and therefore is directly linked to variation in extracellular volume. Its reabsorption and excretion are tightly controlled by a complex mechanism that is only partially defined. No secretory mechanism for sodium exists; sodium is excreted only to the degree that the amount reabsorbed is smaller than the amount filtered. The latter is directly proportional to the rate of glomerular filtration, which is controlled through the sympathetic nervous system and unidentified intrarenal and extrarenal mechanisms. Tubular reabsorption is controlled by the adrenal cortex, by peritubular physical factors, and by other mechanisms related to variations in intravascular volume or filling.

The lack of a secretory mechanism for sodium has been explained on the basis of the phylogenetic need of terrestrial vertebrates to conserve, rather than to excrete, sodium. Since ontogenesis repeats phylogenesis, one would expect to find the newborn better equipped to withstand the stress of sodium deficiency than that of sodium excess. The response of infants to sodium restriction has not been tested adequately. Considerable data are available, however, suggesting significant limitations in response to sodium loading.

When a sodium solution is administered intravenously to an adult there is an almost immediate increase in urine volume, the excess fluid being excreted within 2 or 3 hours. A proportionately similar volume of saline infused into an infant elicits after a much longer delay only a small increase in the rate of urine flow; the excretion of the excess load takes three to four times longer.

Infants fed diets with high sodium content develop a measurable expansion of their extracellular compartments, and when switched abruptly to such a regimen they may become edematous. No careful study has been done in order to test the capacity of the infant to adjust to relatively small changes in sodium intake. The tolerance to variation in sodium intake arising from the differences in sodium content of proprietary formulas suggests that the newborn is able to handle an intake of sodium varying between 5 and 20 mEq/day. For an older infant receiving a diversified diet the amount can increase to 50 mEq/day. However, recent evidence indicates that when an infant between 5 and 7 months of age is given a diet with a sodium content in excess of 50 mEq/day he starts retaining sodium. It is not known to what degree sodium is retained before a new steady state is reached. It is likely that a relatively high degree of expansion is needed in order to elicit a response of the control mechanism.

ACID–BASE REGULATION. The important role played by the bicarbonate–carbonic acid buffer system in acid–base homeostasis derives not from its high buffering capacity (this is restricted by its pK, which is remote from the normal pH of the blood) but from the fact that its two components are regulated by very effective physiologic systems: the concentration of carbonic acid is controlled by the respiratory system, and the concentration of bicarbonate is controlled by the kidney.

The net effect of intermediary metabolism is the production of a hydrogen ion load that must be neutralized by an equivalent amount of buffer, approximately 50 to 100 mEq/1.73 m^2/24 hours. This is accomplished by the active secretion of hydrogen ion by the renal tubular cells (Fig. 4), which results in reabsorption of filtered bicarbonate and thus its conservation, as well as formation of new bicarbonate by net excretion of hydrogen into the urine in combination with a number of buffers.

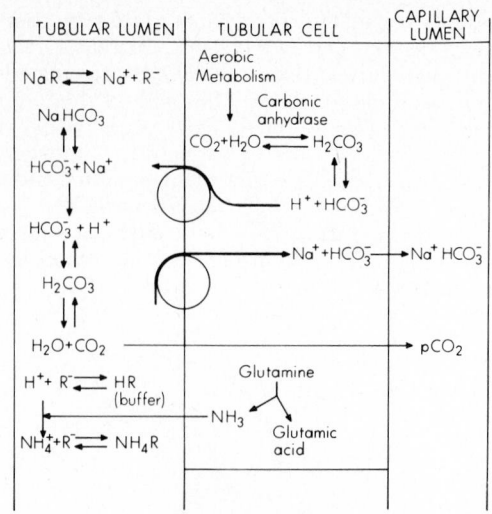

FIG. 4. Mechanisms involved in reabsoprtion of filtered bicarbonate and excretion of hydrogen ion in urine.

Hydrogen ion that is excreted following titration within the tubule of filtered substances such as phosphate and creatinine is referred to as titratable acid. Additional hydrogen ion is excreted as ammonium ($NH_4{}^+$) following titration of ammonia (NH_3), which is synthesized by the tubule from glutamine and other amino acids and secreted into the distal nephron.

Although immediately following birth the newborn seems to be in a state of relative acidemia when compared to his mother, blood samples collected at 1 day of age from the left atria of full-term infants have been found to have a mean pH of 7.40. This does not hold true for premature infants, whose blood pH can remain acid for several weeks. The main feature of this acidotic state is a relatively low concentration of bicarbonate in plasma, secondary to the inability of the immature kidney to conserve this ion. In the adult the threshold for bicarbonate (ie, the plasma concentration below which urine is bicarbonate-free) ranges between 25 and 27 mmole/liter; during the first year of life, in contrast, it is in the range of 21.5 to 22.5. Furthermore, depending on dietary intake, young infants may excrete little phosphate in their urine and as a consequence be limited in their capacity to excrete titratable acid. Production of ammonia by the kidney in response to administration of acidifying salts also is low by adult standards. After 1 month of age, however, infants fed cow's-milk formulas excrete hydrogen ion at rates comparable to those observed in older children. They are unable, however, to increase these rates substantially in response to acid loading, which suggests again that the kidney is working close to its maximum capacity. This fact, when considered with the low threshold for bicarbonate, explains why the ability of the infant to maintain the pH of body fluids within the normal range is so often overtaxed during states of disease.

References

Barnett HL: Kidney function in young infants. Pediatrics 5:171, 1950

Edelmann CM Jr: Developmental renal physiology. In Becker EL (ed): Cornell Seminars in Nephrology. New York, Wiley, 1973, p 95

————Spitzer A: The maturing kidney. J Pediatr 75:171, 1950

McCance RA: Age and renal function. In Black DAK (ed): Renal Disease. Philadelphia, FA Davis, 1962, p 157

Nash MA, Edelmann CM Jr: The developing kidney: immature function or inappropriate standard. Nephron 11:91, 1974

Pitts RF: Physiology of the Kidney and Body Fluids, 2nd ed. Chicago, Year Book, 1968

Smith HW: Renal function in infancy and childhood. In: The Kidney. New York, Oxford Univ Press, 1951, p 492

Vernier RL, Smith FG Jr: Fetal and neonatal kidney. In Assali NS (ed): Biology of Gestation, Vol 11. New York, Academic, p 225

Vogh B, Cassin S: Correlations of renal function and morphogenesis in the embryo and neonate. In Sunderman FW, Sunderman FW Jr (eds): Laboratory Diagnosis of Kidney Disease. St Louis, Warren H Green, 1970, p 21

CLINICAL EVALUATION OF RENAL FUNCTION

Adrian Spitzer

No single test is able to provide comprehensive information about the status of the kidney. The tests available measure specific aspects of regulation and of urine production; several may be necessary in order to define adequately the clinical condition of the patient.

Urine Analysis

Prompt examination of a freshly voided random urine specimen is of great value in the examination for renal disease. If urine is not examined soon after voiding, formed elements may have disappeared. Thus, although the first urine specimen in the morning has the advantage of being concentrated, it may not be possible in the nonhospitalized patient to perform the appropriate examinations without undue delay.

Urine should be free of protein when tested with 10 percent sulfosalicylic acid or with paper strips impregnated with bromphenol blue (Albustix). Both these methods detect as little as 5 to 10 mg of protein per dl of urine. It should be recognized that if the urine is very dilute significant degrees of proteinuria can escape detection. Not infrequently proteinuria is found on a single examination in an apparently healthy child. Repeat examination usually is negative. Persistently positive results, even if proteinuria is minimal, necessitate further investigation.

Examination of the urinary sediment following centrifugation of 10 ml of urine for 5 minutes should reveal no more than two to four white blood cells per high-power field, usually no red cells, and rarely any casts. Casts are cylindrical masses of agglutinated material formed in the distal parts of the nephron from protein or from protein and cells. The presence of more than a few cellular casts in the sediment is indicative of renal disease. Red cell casts are pathognomonic of glomerulonephritis but are not specific for any type.

Bacteriuria is evaluated by direct examination of the urinary sediment for the presence of organisms, as well as by cultural methods. These are discussed on page 1324.

The Addis count was devised in order to examine urine quantitatively, making it possible to express results as rates of excretion of cells and casts rather than concentrations. In addition, the Addis count specimen may be used conveniently to determine rates of excretion of protein and as a test of concentrating performance. The child should be instructed to have a normal noon meal and then, except for a dry supper, to thirst and fast totally until the following morning. Starting in the evening, just prior to going to bed, the bladder is emptied and the time of this "discard" specimen is noted. A timed collection of urine is then begun, which includes all urine passed during the night (if any) as well as the first urine voided the next morning. Under these conditions urinary osmolarity in healthy children age 2 to 16 years averages 1,090 mOsm/liter, with a range of 870 to 1,310 (mean $\pm$ 2 SD). Data in children below 2 years of age are limited, but a concentration of at least 800 mOsm/liter should be achieved by subjects between 3 months and 2 years of age. During the period 1 week to 3 months an osmolarity varying between 400 and 800 is expected. Winberg provides the following equation for estimating the maximum concentrating capacity of children under 3 years of age: $y = (415.5x) - 62.9$, where y is milliosmols per kilogram of H_2O and x is the logarithm of age in days. The standard deviation around the regression line described by this equation was 145 mOsm/kg H_2O.

Good correlation is found under most circumstances between concentrating performance and GFR. Significant impairment in concentrating ability in association with normal GFR may be indicative of an acquired disorder, such as pyelonephritis (p. 1322), potassium deficiency (p. 1312), or hypercalciuria (p. 1311). It may also be found in specific diseases such as sickle cell anemia (p. 1149), diabetes insipidus (p. 1615), or nephrophthisis.

The great majority of Addis count specimens reveal no protein when tested by conventional chemical methods. Up to 50 mg of protein per 12 hours is usually considered normal in the adult, although data from our laboratory suggest that 10 to 20 mg may be the upper limit of normal in children.

The numbers of cells and casts in a measured aliquot of urine are estimated quantitatively in a counting chamber. An amount of urine equivalent to that passed in a period of 20 minutes is centrifuged for 5 minutes at 3,500 rpm and the sediment is resuspended in a volume of 1 ml. All nine large squares on one side of a standard counting chamber (0.9 mm^3) are examined. The sum of each element times 40,000 represents the rate of excretion of that element per 12 hours.* Up to 1 million white blood cells and 250,000 red blood cells per 12 hours is considered normal in children; values of

500,000 to 750,000 red blood cells may be normal in adults. Since no more than 5,000 casts per 12 hours are excreted by normal subjects, under the conditions outlined for the Addis count casts usually are not found in the absence of disease.

Tests of Renal Function

PLASMA UREA AND CREATININE. The elimination of most waste products from plasma depends on the adequacy of the filtering process. In dehydration, circulatory failure, and intrinsic renal disease the rate of glomerular filtration drops and the concentrations of the excretory products in the blood rise. This inverse relationship permits the use of the concentrations of urea and creatinine in plasma or serum to assess renal function. When the production rate is constant (which is not the case in the growing individual) the relationship between levels in plasma and GFR is hyperbolic, as seen in Figure 5. It should be appreciated that filtration

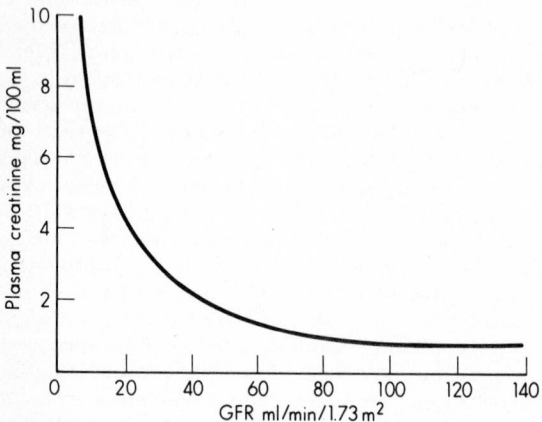

FIG. 5. Relationship between concentration of creatinine in the serum and rate of glomerular filtration. A similar correlation applies to urea.

rate can be less than 50 percent of normal with the urea or creatinine level still within what is loosely considered normal limits. For urea this is explained by the relatively wide range of values in the normal population that is due in part to differences in levels of protein intake. Plasma creatinine levels are less influenced by protein intake, but they are affected more than urea by technical difficulties in measuring plasma creatinine accurately. The issue is further complicated by changes in plasma

---

* The volume of the aliquot is calculated as follows: aliquot volume = (20 × total volume)/(length of collection (minutes)). This fraction represents one thirty-sixth of a 12-hour period. The volume in which the cells are counted is 0.9 mm³. The number of cells per 1.0 ml is calculated by multiplying the actual count by 1,000/0.9. Therefore actual cell count × 36 × 1,000/0.9 = cell count per 12 hours.

---

concentrations that occur with age. It is frequently overlooked that the creatinine concentration in the plasma of an infant is usually not higher than 0.4 mg/dl, whereas it can be as high as 0.9 mg/dl in a 15-year-old child. Thus levels of creatinine well within the accepted normal range for older children and adults might in infants signify a substantial impairment in glomerular filtration. The regression statistics for the relationship between age and plasma creatinine (Pcr) are as follows: Males: Pcr (mg/dl) = 0.35 ± 0.03 age. Females: Pcr (mg/dl) = 0.37 ± 0.02 age. The regression lines for the two sexes diverge progressively above the age of 4 years, reaching a difference of about 0.1 mg/dl in young adults.

CLEARANCE METHODS. The rate of excretion of a substance by the kidney is not a measure of intrinsic excretory capacity, since the rate of excretion depends also on the intake or rate of production. A better estimate of renal capacity is gained from the amount of blood (or plasma) that would have to have been cleared completely of the substance per unit time to provide for the rate of excretion observed in the urine. This value, referred to as the renal clearance, is given by the formula:

$$\frac{U \times V}{P} = C$$

in which U and P are, respectively, concentrations in urine and plasma (or serum) of the substance under consideration, V is the rate of urine flow, and C is the renal clearance of that substance. Conventionally clearances are expressed in milliliters per minute related to some unit of body size, usually 1 or 1.73 m² of body surface area.

GLOMERULAR FILTRATION RATE. Estimates of GFR probably provide a better assessment of the progression of renal disease than any other test of renal function. A substance used to measure the rate of glomerular filtration should not be bound by plasma proteins, should be freely filtered at the glomerular level, must be neither secreted nor reabsored by the tubule, and must be physiologically inert. Inulin, a polymer of fructose, has been found to fulfill all these requirements, and consequently its clearance is used as the reference for measurement of GFR. The drawbacks in its use are the necessity for continuous intravenous infusion and the rather elaborate chemical analysis required. Clearances of inulin in the adult male and female are, respectively, 127 (21.5)* and 117 (16.4) ml/minute/1.73 m². In the first few days of life GFR in full-term infants may be as low as 25 to 30 ml/minute/1.73 m². It reaches 50 to 60 ml/ minute/1.73 m² by several weeks, from which point it gradually increases, reaching adult levels by 12 to 18 months of age.

Although each has its limitations, both urea and creatinine clearances provide reasonable estimates of

---

* Here and in the following text the values are given as the mean followed in parentheses by the value of one standard deviation.

GFR. At rates of urine flow above 2 ml/minute approximately 60 percent of filtered urea is excreted. Since the portion excreted falls unpredictably when the rate of urine flow is below 2 ml/minute, it is essential to maintain rates above this level throughout the collection periods. To this end the subject is given water to drink at a rate of 20 ml/kg of body weight over a period of 60 to 90 minutes. The bladder is emptied and three 20-minute collection periods are carried out. Following voiding of the third specimen a single blood sample is obtained. Since serum urea changes very little in the postabsorptive state and GFR in man is not influenced by diet, breakfast need not be withheld. It is important, however, that the child remain supine at quiet bed rest throughout the test.

Assuming that under these conditions 60 percent of filtered urea is excreted, the normal rate of urea clearance is 0.6 times 127 ml/minute/1.73 m^2, or 75 ml/minute/1.73 m^2. The lower limit of normal is 60 ml/minute/1.73 m^2.

Creatinine clearance has the advantage of being much less dependent on rate of urine flow. The clearance can be performed as described above for urea, or it can be performed on 12- or 24-hour urine specimens, thus minimizing collection and timing errors. Since creatinine is filtered as well as secreted into the urine its clearance is greater than the true GFR. However, because of the presence of interfering chromogens in the plasma the level of creatinine in plasma is usually overestimated, and hence the clearance comes close to the true GFR.

In chronic renal disease, when GFR has fallen to 25 ml/minute or below, urea and creatinine clearances provide a very accurate estimate of GFR. At this stage of disease, as discussed in the next chapter, there is marked hyperperfusion of the residual nephrons resulting in excretion of close to 100 percent of filtered urea. At the same time, filtered creatinine provides most of the creatinine excreted, with relatively little coming from tubular secretion. Thus urea clearance is just below the true GFR, creatinine clearance is just above it, and the mean is equal to GFR.

Recent progress has made possible the use of mathematical analysis of plasma disappearance curves for measurements of GFR. This method obviates the need for urine collections. Several isotopes have been used for this method, substituting isotope counting for tedious and often inaccurate chemical determinations. Because of their short half-lives and the fact that they, too, are excreted solely by glomerular filtration, ^{125}I-iothalamate and ^{51}Cr-EDTA are suitable isotopes. The amount of radiation from one procedure is about 40 μr, which is only one-fifth the amount of daily background radiation in New York City.

When accurate chemical measurements can be performed, GFR can be estimated from the disappearance curve of nonradioactive inulin injected as a bolus. Finally, a rough estimate of GFR can be obtained from measuring serum creatinine and using the formula GFR (ml/minute/1.73 m^2) = 0.55 L(cm)/Pcr (mg/dl), where L is length and Pcr is plasma creatinine.

RENAL BLOOD FLOW. Since almost all the postglomerular blood perfuses the renal tubules before entering the venous drainage, certain substances that are actively secreted by the tubules, such as p-aminohippurate (PAH), are removed almost completely from the blood on one passage through the kidney. At plasma levels of PAH below 4 to 5 mg/dl an average of only 10 percent of the renal arterial concentration is found in renal venous blood. Arterial minus venous concentration divided by arterial concentration (termed the extraction ratio) ranges from 0.85 to 1.0. Measurement of the clearance of PAH therefore provides a close estimate of renal plasma flow (RPF). Renal blood flow (RBF) can be calculated with knowledge of the hematocrit (Hct):

$$RBF = \frac{RPF}{1 - Hct}$$

Values of PAH clearance in adult males and females are, respectively, 643 (140) and 585 (128) ml/minute/1.73 m^2. The average value for children age 2 to 12 years has been found to be 654 (120). In patients with renal disease PAH extraction varies widely and unpredictably, and thus its clearance is an unreliable measure of renal plasma flow. Although PAH clearance has been of great value in physiologic investigation, it has limited use in clinical assessment.

A single-injection method based on the analysis of the plasma disappearance curve of ^{131}I-orthoiodohippurate can be used for measurement of RPF. It has the advantages previously mentioned with regard to isotope techniques. The procedure results in about 14 μr of total body radiation.

The fraction of renal plasma flow filtered is referred to as the filtration fraction (FF); it is calculated from the ratio of C_{In} to C_{PAH}. Values of 0.20 (0.03), 0.21 (0.04), and 0.20 (0.04) have been found in adult males, adult females, and children age 2 years and over, respectively. Since values for PAH clearance in young infants range from 20 to 50 percent of adult values, FF at this age has been calculated to be as high as 0.5. However, even at low concentrations of PAH in plasma the extraction ratio in young infants may be considerably below 0.9, resulting in falsely low values of RPF and proportionately high values of FF.

EXCRETION OF HYDROGEN ION. Tests of renal acidifying mechanisms are useful in evaluating patients with either specific tubular abnormalities or generalized disturbances in tubular functions.

Total CO_2 and pH are measured in blood and in one or two 1-hour collections of urine. A dose of ammonium chloride calculated to reduce blood total CO_2 by 4 to 6 mmole/liter is administered orally over the next hour. This dose is calculated on the assumption that total body water is 60 to 70 percent of body weight. For example, a patient weighing 10 kg is to be tested. His blood CO_2 is 23 mmole/liter, and it is planned to lower this to 18. The dose of ammonium chloride required is $0.7 \times 10 \times (23 - 18) = 35$ mEq or 1.8 g of ammonium chloride (1.0 mEq of ammonium chloride = 53 mg). Urine is collected at hourly intervals for the following

4 to 5 hours. Maximal values in normal infants and children are shown in Table 1.

TABLE 1. Excretion of Hydrogen Ion

	Infants During First Year of Life	Children 3 to 15 Years
Urine pH	$\leqq$5.0	$\leqq$5.5
Titratable acid μEq/min/1.73 m^2	62 (43–111)	52 (33–71)
Ammonium μEq/min/1.73 m^2	57 (42–79)	73 (46–100)

Total acid excretion is impaired in chronic renal failure, hypercalcemia, potassium deficiency, and tubular disorders (notably distal tubular acidosis), although ammonium excretion is normal in potassium deficiency and most tubular disorders. In early chronic renal failure, on the other hand, ammonium excretion may be impaired at a time when total acid excretion is normal.

Radiography, Sonography, and Imaging Techniques

The normal kidney has a smooth outline. An irregular edge may be indicative of scarring following infection or of vascular obstruction. It should be differentiated from lobulation, which is characteristic of the fetal kidney but can persist into extrauterine life. The size of the kidney varies with age (Table 2). A large

TABLE 2. Kidney Size[a]

Surface Area (m^2)	Right Kidney (cm)	Left Kidney (cm)
0.2	6.2	6.0
0.3	6.6	6.6
0.5	7.6	7.6
0.7	8.5	8.6
1.0	9.9	10.2
1.2	10.8	11.3
1.5	12.2	12.8

[a] *The length of the kidneys as a function of body surface area. The range around each mean is approximately $\pm$ 1 cm. (From Olbing: Harnwegsentzündungen bei Kindern und Jugendichen, 1971. Courtesy of Thieme, Stuttgart.)*

kidney may be the result of hypertrophy or hydronephrosis. A small kidney, in the pediatric age group, is in most instances a congenitally dysplastic or hypoplastic organ. Since 90 percent of renal calculi are radiopaque, radiographic examination should be done in all patients with renal colic. Occasionally nephrocalcinosis will be seen, the most common cause in children being distal renal tubular acidosis.

Until recently the study of the gross morphology of the kidney and urinary tract could be performed only by radiologic techniques. During the last few years methods such as sonography and radioisotopic scanning have been added as diagnostic modalities. Their main advantage consists in the elimination or significant diminution of the hazards related to radiation and instrumentation.

Sonography is based on the ability of ultrasound waves (2 to 5 MHz) to travel through body tissues and be reflected back from tissue interfaces. The patterns obtained permit differentiation between structures of varying density and between solid and hollow formations. The method has proved useful in localizing and outlining the kidneys, in identifying intraabdominal and retroperitoneal tumors, in establishing the diagnosis of cystic disease, and in detecting the presence of urine in the bladder prior to needle aspiration.

Imaging techniques are based on the detection of radiolabeled substances with very short half-lives. They have been used successfully in the evaluation of a variety of kidney conditions, such as congenital malformations, obstructive uropathy, renovascular disorders, and evaluation of kidney transplant. The type of examination depends upon the nature of the clinical problem. Static studies with ^{197}Hg-chlormerodrin or ^{99m}Tc-iron ascorbate can be used to determine kidney localization and size; dynamic studies with technetium-99m compounds and ^{131}I-orthoiodohippurate can be used for assessing the adequacy of renal blood flow and tubular secretion. Quantitation of renal scans provides information regarding renal function.

Although the impact of these new techniques on the practice of nephrology is increasing steadily, they do not match standard radiographic methods in the quality of detail they provide. Radiography remains for the time being the method of choice for visualization of the fine structural abnormalities of the urinary tract. Its usefulness is enhanced by such versatile procedures as rapid-sequence photography for the diagnosis of renal vascular hypertension, tomography for the diagnosis of renal tumors, and angiography for the diagnosis of renal vascular anomalies.

Intravenous and retrograde pyelography, cystography, renal angiography, and renography are discussed further in the sections on urogenital disorders (p.1327) and hypertension (p. 1484).

Percutaneous Renal Biopsy

Percutaneous needle biopsy has been applied extensively in the past decade to the diagnosis and study of renal disease. Its safety and its value for both clinical and research purposes are now firmly established. Examination of renal tissue is of special value to the clinician in the resolution of diagnostic problems (as in children discovered fortuitously to have proteinuria and microscopic hematuria), as a guide to therapy (as in patients with the nephrotic syndrome unresponsive to adrenocortical steroid therapy), as a means of determining progression of disease, and in determining prognosis.

To ensure minimal risk to the patient and maximal likelihood of obtaining tissue adequate for study, percutaneous renal biopsy should be done only by those thoroughly trained in the procedure. Contraindications to percutaneous biopsy include the presence of only one functioning kidney, pyelonephritis, dysplastic-hypoplastic and cystic disorders, and obstructive urologic conditions; in these instances an open surgical biopsy is indicated. Also, hypertension must be controlled with appropriate therapy before a renal biopsy is attempted. Adequate studies must be done to ensure absence of any type of bleeding disorder. Following the procedure the patient should be kept in bed under close observation for 24 hours or as long as significant hematuria persists. Transient microscopic hematuria occurs in most patients; gross hematuria is observed rarely.

In exposing the patient to the risk and discomfort attendant to such a procedure, the physicians carrying out the renal biopsy assume the responsibility for proper and complete evaluation of the tissue: specimens must be placed in appropriate fixatives and solutions, and the material must be delivered to the laboratory promptly together with the pertinent and necessary clinical information. The laboratory must accept as part of this commitment the responsibility for doing the procedures necessary to obtain the maximal information: light microscopy, immunofluorescence, and electron microscopy. The local laboratory not capable of performing those procedures is obligated to seek assistance from a regional or central laboratory that does have the necessary facilities. Such reference laboratories exist in all parts of the country, and there is no excuse for incomplete workup of biopsy specimens.

References

Barnett HL, Sereny F: Kidney function tests in infants and children. Pediatr Clin North Am 2:191, 1955

Ben-Bassat M, Stark H, Robson M, Rosenfeld J: Value of routine electron microscopy in the differential diagnosis of the nephrotic syndrome. Pathol Microbiol (Basel) 41:26, 1974

Lippman RW: Urine and Urinary Sediment, 2nd ed. Springfield, Ill, Charles C Thomas, 1957

Reubi FC: Clearance Tests in Clinical Medicine. Springfield, Ill, Charles C Thomas, 1963

Silkalns GI, Jeck D, Earon J, et al: Simultaneous measurement of glomerular filtration rate and renal plasma flow using plasma disappearance curves. J Pediatr 83:749, 1973

Schwartz GJ, Haycock GB, Edelmann CM Jr, Spitzer A: A simple estimate of glomerular filtration rate in children derived from body length and plasma creatinine. Pediatrics (in press)

———Haycock GB, Spitzer A: Plasma creatinine and urea concentrations in children: normal values for age and sex. J Pediatr 88:828, 1976.

Sunderman FW, Sunderman FW Jr: Laboratory Diagnosis of Kidney Diseases. St Louis, Warren H Green, 1970

Winberg J: Determination of renal concentration capacity in infants and children without renal disease. Acta Pediatr Scand 48:318, 1959

UREMIA: PATHOPHYSIOLOGY AND TREATMENT

CHESTER M. EDELMANN, JR.

Uremia is conveniently discussed under the headings acute renal failure and chronic renal failure. This section will deal with the pathophysiology and treatment of each, without regard to specific diagnostic entities.

ACUTE RENAL FAILURE

The term acute renal failure is applied to the clinical syndrome of oliguria and sudden loss of renal homeostasis. Oliver's pathologic studies following traumatic and toxic injury revealed the presence of cellular necrosis in the proximal tubules when the syndrome followed exposure to certain toxins (mercuric ion, arsenic, carbon tetrachloride, diethylene glycol, and sulfonamides), in addition to the more characteristic widespread but patchy disruption of the basement membrane throughout the nephron. The latter lesion may be the only change observed when this syndrome follows a number of heterogeneous incidents, such as thermal burns, crush injury, incompatible blood transfusion, prolonged anesthesia, surgical shock, utilization of the pump oxygenator, and possibly severe diarrheal dehydration. No correlation can be shown between the clinical features and the histologic abnormalities. Moreover, in children with acute renal failure postmortem examination of the kidneys frequently reveals no significant morphologic abnormality. Despite the suggestion from the earlier studies that tubular obstruction and disruption were the causes of acute renal failure, more recent observations indicate that the common denominator is prolonged renal ischemia, and the former abnormalities are not found in most cases.

In the absence of significant morphologic changes in the glomeruli the reduced inulin clearance and the oliguria of acute renal failure have been attributed to fairly complete reabsorption of glomerular filtrate; however, it now seems more likely that they are due to glomeruli that are perfused with blood but do not filter.

Acute renal failure may also be caused by extensive glomerular damage, as in acute glomerulonephritis, rapidly progressive glomerulonephritis, Goodpasture's syndrome, and the hemolytic-uremic syndrome; it is also seen in association with bilateral occlusion of the renal arteries, sickle cell crisis, myoglobinuria, and a number of other diseases.

Acute cortical and tubular necrosis is not commonly observed in the pediatric age group. Most cases have been reported in the newborn and have been attributed to obstetric complications, asphyxia, erythroblastosis, sepsis, dehydration, and hemorrhage. Acute papillary necrosis following administration of radiographic material is an infrequent but important complication of angiographic procedures. Scattered reports of renal cortical and medullary necrosis in older infants and children have been attributed to the usual factors, including circulatory collapse, infection, nephrotoxins, vascular disease, burns, and transfusion reactions.

DIAGNOSIS. The diagnosis of acute renal failure may at times be extremely difficult. It is important early to rule out two conditions that may mimic true renal failure and that frequently are amenable to specific therapy. The first of these, termed prerenal failure, refers to decreased renal blood flow and glomerular filtration rate and oliguria secondary to cardiovascular insufficiency. Initially the process is rapidly reversible, and there may be no renal parenchymal lesions, although if renal ischema persist renal damage may be severe. Prerenal failure is seen in association with vascular collapse, blood loss, hypotension, and severe dehydration. Postrenal failure refers to absence of urine secondary to urinary tract obstruction. Radiographic studies and ureteral catheterization may be necessary to make the diagnosis.

The alert physician, aware of situations in which renal failure may develop, should watch the urinary output in order to detect significant oliguria that is not a response to dehydration. In general a urine output of less than 400 ml/m^2/day (approximately 15 ml/kg) in a well-hydrated child indicates some degree of renal failure. The excretion of small quantities of isotonic or hypotonic urine is highly suggestive of acute renal failure. However, a moderately concentrated urine may be elaborated during the early stages, in which case fluids should be administered cautiously until better hydration is established. Urine should be collected hourly, through an indwelling catheter if necessary. If urine flow and clinical status are evaluated at hourly intervals the situation is usually more clearly defined within 2 to 3 hours, provided arterial hypotension is not present. Potassium salts should not be administered in rehydration therapy until the possiblity of acute renal failure has been excluded.

TREATMENT. No effective measure for reversing the acute pathologic process is available. Attempts at flushing out the kidney may result in congestive heart failure and death. The therapeutic goal is to maintain normal body composition while awaiting spontaneous recovery. Efforts should be directed toward restoration of blood and extracellular volumes if they are deficient. Administration of fluids to differentiate between oliguria due to dehydration and true renal failure has been discussed above. Infusion of intravenous fluid, 20 ml/kg of body weight over a 30-minute period, usually will suffice. This may need to be repeated.

The use of intravenous mannitol in the prevention of acute renal failure has been proposed. Current evidence indicates that when given early in the course of prerenal failure it may prevent development of renal lesions and progression to true renal failure. The dose is 0.5 g/kg of body weight given as 2.5 ml/kg of a 20 percent solution.

WATER BALANCE. During renal failure the water requirement is limited to that needed to replace urinary output plus insensible loss. From this must be subtracted metabolic water available from the high rate of tissue catabolism that is usually present. Water intake thus should be limited to 200 to 300 ml/m^2/day, plus urinary output. The most accurate gauge of adequacy of water balance is careful daily measurement of body weight. A weight loss of about 0.5 percent per day indicates an appropriate water intake.

ELECTROLYTE BALANCE. Urine output and sodium concentration should be measured daily. Provided that overhydration has not occurred, sodium losses should be replaced, preferably with sodium lactate or bicarbonate, to correct or prevent acidosis. Replacement of other electrolyte losses need not occasion concern; the problem is to prevent their accumulation in excess. Hyponatremia is unlikely to be a sign of sodium deficiency, but rather an indication of excess water. Furosemide and ethacrynic acid are useful agents in patients with acute renal failure. The enhanced excretion of sodium and water that may result from vigorous diuretic therapy may greatly increase the ease of maintaining fluid and electrolyte balance.

Serious acute hyperkalemia usually can be avoided by adherence to the principles described for the management of acute renal failure. Serum potassium level should be followed closely in conjunction with frequent use of the electrocardiogram. If serum potassium rises above 6 mEq/dl, or if sequential changes of potassium intoxication are seen in the electrocardiogram, therapy with a cation-exchange resin should be instituted (see below). The emergency treatment of advanced potassium intoxication consists of administration of intravenous sodium bicarbonate (2.5 mEq/kg of body weight) or hypertonic glucose (1 ml/kg of body weight of 50 percent solution). These measures are only temporary and should be followed promptly by dialytic management.

CALORIC REQUIREMENTS. Tissue catabolism, with release of intracellular potassium and of phosphate and other acid products, may be prevented in large part by maintaining good nutrition. This is done with the use of nonprotein electrolyte-free foods, although attainment of full caloric intake is almost an impossible task in the face of severe renal failure. At least one-fourth and preferably one-half of the calories should be provided as carbohydrate. Fat may be given in moderate amounts to the oliguric patient, but protein is best avoided. Ethyl alcohol, given orally or intravenously, can be used to supplement caloric intake. There is evidence to suggest that the use of anabolic agents such as norethandrolone may aid in minimizing protein catabolism.

INFECTION. The most common cause of death in patients with acute renal failure is infection, particularly of the respiratory or urinary tract. So-called prophylactic antibiotics should not be used, but rather patients should be observed closely for development of infection and treated vigorously if it occurs.

DIALYSIS. Dialytic therapy can be used, when indicated, even in the smallest infant. Further details concerning performance of peritoneal and extracorporeal dialysis are given below. Indications for this procedure include renal failure extending beyond 7 to 10 days or severe volume overload, acidosis, or hyperkalemia. Blood urea nitrogen in excess of 100 to 150 mg/100 ml usually indicates a degree of uremia that warrants dialysis.

RECOVERY PHASE. Recovery from acute renal failure is frequently accompanied by a period of obligatory diuresis during which modification of the glomerular filtrate appears to be impaired. Adequate and appropriate fluids must be provided to prevent sodium depletion, hypovolemia, and acidosis. Following cessation of the diuretic phase, evidence of renal tubular defects (eg, isosthenuria, renal tubular acidosis) may persist for many months.

Chronic Renal Failure

PATHOPHYSIOLOGY. During the past two decades the pathophysiology of renal insufficiency has been elucidated in considerable detail by many investigators, particularly through the work of Bricker and his associates. Prior to their work the diseased kidney was considered a disorganized and distorted structure, exhibiting a variety and heterogeneity of functional disturbances that varied from one kidney to another, from one disease to another, and from one patient to another. It is now apparent that despite the variety of pathologic lesions encountered in the various forms of renal disease the functional pattern that emerges during progression of renal insufficiency and the adaptation of functional impairment that takes place are remarkably uniform.

The major factor leading to disturbances in uremia is the reduction in total functional renal mass that occurs during the course of progressive disease. As the number of remaining nephrons decreases the task of maintaining homeostasis imposes increasingly greater demands on each residual nephron. In order to maintain balance with regard to substances that are excreted into the urine primarily by tubular secretion, enhanced capacity for secretion by each nephron must develop. The capacity for such increase obviously is limited, and at some point in the continuing loss of nephrons the demand for secretion must exceed the functional capacity. For substances that are excreted into the urine primarily by glomerular filtration, balance is maintained by decreasing tubular reabsorption. In this regard, also, the capacity to maintain balance ultimately is exceeded as the rate of glomerular filtration falls to such levels that complete compensation is no longer possible.

Moreover, the adaptive mechanisms by which the organism is able to reject a larger and larger portion of the filtered load may themselves lead to disturbances in homeostasis. For example, phosphate balance is maintained in renal insufficiency by the excretion of a larger and larger percentage of filtered phosphate through the development of increasing degrees of secondary hyperparathyroidism. Although this serves a useful purpose with regard to maintaining phosphate balance, secondary hyperparathyroidism leads to all the osseous complications observed in primary hyperparathyroidism. The ability to maintain homeostasis by stressing certain control systems at the expense of causing disturbances in other areas has been described by Bricker as the trade-off hypothesis, and the reader is directed elsewhere for further discussion of this important concept.

In addition to impairment of the ability to maintain a balance of water and electrolytes as uremia progresses, various end products of metabolism tend to accumulate due to decreased rate of glomerular filtration and tubular secretion. Although the precise substances leading to specific disturbances have not been identified, it appears likely that they are related, at least to a major extent, to products of nitrogen metabolism and that they cause many of the nonspecific disturbances of uremia such as hematologic and neurologic abnormalities.

Treatment directed toward the biochemical and metabolic disturbances of renal insufficiency—as opposed to treatment directed toward the disease process per se—thus consists of supporting the kidney in its attempts to maintain homeostasis. This is accomplished by reducing the work load imposed upon the kidney, by appropriately modifying the diet, and by administering various pharmacologic agents.

TREATMENT. Treatment of patients with chronic renal insufficiency is nonspecific unless there is a recognizable and treatable underlying condition. Therefore, it is extremely important, whenever possible, to make a precise diagnosis of the cause of chronic renal insufficiency. Successful treatment of infants and children with impairment of renal function due to pyelonephritis, particularly when associated with correctable forms of obstructive uropathy, provides a striking example of the importance of this principle.

DIET. Regulation of the diet is a primary means of treating disturbances, such as chronic uremia, in which there is a decreased ability to handle some of the end products of the metabolism of food. Unfortunately such regulation usually involves reduction of the intake or the intestinal absorption of certain foods that in the infant or child are important for growth. Therefore arbitrary unneccessary restrictions should be avoided. Although these patients frequently grow very slowly, a palatable well-balanced diet adequate to meet caloric and other nutritional needs should be provided.

In the asymptomatic infant or child with chronic renal insufficiency, no change should be made in the usual well-balanced diet. Patients with more severe degrees of renal insufficiency do require dietary regulation, involving particularly intake of protein, osmotically active solutes, and certain electrolytes and minerals such as sodium, calcium, and phosphate.

Each 100 g of dietary protein, which is essential in the maintenance of a positive nitrogen balance, requires renal excretion of approximately 70 mEq of acid. In order to provide essential protein and yet not induce metabolic acidosis in patients with severe renal insufficiency, dietary protein should be limited initially to 0.3 to 0.5 g/kg of body weight per day. This amount can be increased empirically as tolerated. Protein-containing foods should be limited to those of high biologic value that provide a rich mixture of essential amino acids; these include meat, fish, eggs, cheese, and milk. The intake of high-protein vegetables, particularly those of the bean family, should be markedly curtailed. Cow's milk is an excellent source of protein of high biologic value, but because of its high sodium, potassium, and phospate content it may need to be restricted or completely removed from the diet.

Remarkable clinical improvement has been reported in patients with advanced chronic uremia given a diet designed to provide a minimal intake of protein in the form of essential amino acids. Although further clinical trials with this type of low-protein diet are needed, the experience reported has been successful enough to warrant clinical application. It should be noted that several authors have emphasized the failure of adults to adhere to strict, unpalatable dietary regimens. We have applied the principle underlying this type of therapy with success to infants and small children, using naturally available foods and less vigorous attempts at dietary control. Low-protein, low-electrolyte products such as Controlyte and Resource Baking Mix are of considerable value in providing caloric intake in the form of bread, cookies, milk shakes, etc. Infants with severe renal insufficiency often do very well on formulas with low concentrations of both electrolytes and protein.*

Abitrary restriction of dietary sodium is one of the most common errors in treatment of patients with renal disease. The child with hypertension, edema, or obvious salt intolerance needs restriction of dietary sodium to as little as 0.2 mEq/kg/day, whereas certain patients with chronic renal disease tend to be salt-losers and require sodium supplementation. In the absence of these complications, a normal sodium intake should be allowed. Certain milks with low sodium content (for example Lonalac) that are excellent for infants and children with cardiac impairment may be dangerous in children with renal disease owing to their high potassium content.

Most patients with renal insufficiency can be allowed to ingest water ad libitum, their water intake being regulated by their own thirst mechanisms. However, there may be a decrease in renal ability to conserve water, requiring the provision of adequate water to prevent dehydration and hemoconcentration, particularly in hot weather and during febrile illnesses. Children allowed free access to water usually present no problem, but disturbances in water balance may occur in the infant or the sick child whose water intake is regulated by the parent or the physician.

Anorexia, nausea, and vomiting are frequent disturbances in chronic uremia. Early in the course of renal insufficiency gastrointestinal symptoms usually respond well to simple restriction of dietary protein; in the more advanced stages they may be exceedingly resistant to treatment. Phenothiazines, such as prochlorperazine (0.4 mg/kg/24 hours) or chlorpromazine (2 mg/kg/24 hours) given in three or four oral doses may be very effective.

ACIDOSIS.   Patients with mild degrees of acidosis are usually asymptomatic and require no therapy other than modification of diet. The child who remains acidotic despite restriction in dietary protein may require more specific therapy.

Correction of acidosis requires administration of alkali, given usually in a dosage of 1 to 3 mEq/kg/day. After prolonged ingestion of diets low in protein and high in carbohydrate, patients with chronic acidosis may develop potassium depletion and therefore may require a mixture of sodium and potassium salts, as in the following formula, which provides 25 mEq of each cation per 15 ml: sodium citrate ($Na_3C_6H_5O_7 \cdot 5H_2O$) 97 g, potassium citrate ($K_3C_6H_5O_7 \cdot H_2O$) 90 g, and water, quantum sufficit, 500 ml. If there is severe reduction in GFR, potassium depletion is less likely, and the potassium load of this solution may be excessive. In these instances a solution of sodium citrate alone can be given.* Aluminum hydroxide, used primarily to correct hyperphosphatemia, may also serve to correct acidosis. A dosage of 50 to 150 mg/kg/day may be given.

Respiratory compensation of metabolic acidosis, resulting in low Pco_2 in blood, may be of extreme importance in preventing severe acidosis in the patient with impaired renal mechanisms for hydrogen-ion excretion. Interference with alveolar ventilation secondary to pneumonia, sedatives, or thoracic surgery may result in profound acidosis and sudden death.

DISTURBANCES IN HANDLING OF WATER AND SOLUTES.   The rare patient requiring sodium supplementation to combat excessive salt losses has been mentioned. Much more common, however, is the child whose ability to excrete sodium is reduced to the level where ingestion of normal amounts of dietary sodium is excessive and results in edema. Frequently correction is achieved by restriction of sodium intake to 0.2 to 1 mEq/kg/day. When this measure is not successful diuretic therapy may be given. Hydrochlorothiazide appares to be the drug of choice and is given in a dosage of 2 to 4 mg/kg/day. Recent experience with furosemide in children suggests that it is a most useful diuretic. We have used it in a dosage of 1 to 2 mg/kg given orally once or twice a day.

HYPERKALEMIA AND HYPOKALEMIA.   Significant elevation of extracellular potassium concentration is not a common finding in patients with chronic renal insufficiency unless there is a marked reduction in GFR, oliguria, or acidosis. In these instances exogenous sources of potassium such as drugs and antibiotics, candy, and fruits must be carefully controlled. Diuretics may be useful in promoting urinary losses of potassium. Sodium polystyrene sulfonate (Kayexalate), a sodium–potassium-exchange resin, is especially effective. It can be given orally or rectally in a starting dosage of 0.5 to 1.5 g/kg/day, with subsequent adjustment of the dosage according to need. One gram will exchange approximately 1 mEq of potassium.

---

* *Two such preparations, Similac PM 60/40 and SMA New Formula S-26, are commercially available.*

* *Although it is not tolerated by all patients, some find sodium bicarbonate (baking soda) to be a convenient form of therapy. One gram contains 11.9 mEq of sodium. One measuring teaspoon is approximately 3.7 g and thus provides about 44 mEq.*

Hypokalemia due to anorexia, diarrhea, vomiting, or the injudicious use of diuretic drugs may also occur in patients with chronic uremia. An increase in potassium intake is a simple corrective measure; it may be given in a dosage calculated to provide a daily supplement of 3 to 5 mEq/kg.*

HYPOCALCEMIA AND BONE DISEASE. Hypocalcemia is commonly seen in patients with chronic renal disease. Although it usually causes no symptoms, muscle cramps, weakness, tetany, and convulsions may be seen occasionally. Therapy is aimed at symptomatic control and consists of a diet low in phosphate and oral administration of aluminum hydroxide and calcium. The calcium is usually given in the form of calcium lactate,† calculated to provide 10 to 20 mg of calcium per kilogram of body weight per day. Without supplemental vitamin D, patients with chronic renal insufficiency usually remain in negative calcium balance despite oral calcium supplementation; however, recent evidence suggests that the use of calcium carbonate may reduce the dosage of vitamin D required.

The hypocalcemia of chronic renal disease and renal osteodystrophy can be attributed in major part to a disturbance in vitamin D metabolism, notably impaired ability of the kidney to convert 25- hydroxy cholecalciferol to the 1,25-dihydroxy form, which is the active metabolite of vitamin D. Therefore, the use of pharmacologic doses of vitamin D to overcome so-called vitamin D resistance has been advocated. However, vitamin D may induce hypercalcemia and metastatic calcification and therefore should be used with caution. Widespread arterial calcification in the absence of hypercalcemia has been reported. We recommend its use only in patients in whom other measures have not been successful, and then with careful monitoring of concentrations of calcium and phosphate in serum. The product serum calcium times phosphorus should not be allowed to exceed 70. A dosage of 25,000 to 50,000 units of vitamin D daily may be given initially, but dosage levels as high as 400,000 units per day may be necessary. Recent experience with the use of various metabolites and analogues of vitamin D in uremic patients suggests that one or more of these may be useful in the prevention or treatment of uremic osteodystrophy. At present, however, their use remains experimental.

The quantitative importance of acidosis in the pathogenesis of uremic osteodystrophy is unclear, but it seems to play some role. Correction of acidosis, therefore, is an integral part of therapy.

The bone disease that follows chronic renal insufficiency generally falls into one of two catergories: rickets (or osteomalacia) or osteitis fibrosa. Vitamin D is the treatment of choice for the former. In osteitis fibrosa serum calcium levels may be normal or slightly reduced,

suggesting that an unusually severe degree of secondary hyperparathyroidism may play a major role. Doses of vitamin D adequate to cause healing may result in dangerous degrees of hypercalcemia. On occasion partial parathyroidectomy in such patients may be indicated (see also p. 252).

HYPERTENSION. Control of hypertension can be a large factor in prolonging survival in patients with chronic renal disease. Therapy is empirical, the particular drug and effective dose being determined by trial in each patient.

Hydrochlorothiazide, which was discussed previously, may be successful in controlling mild elevations of blood pressure, especially in patients with a tendency toward sodium retention.

Reserpine is perhaps the safest and simplest antihypertensive agent available. A dosage of 0.01 to 0.02 mg/kg/day in one or two divided doses is often effective and usually completely without side effects, although somnolence, headaches, nasal stuffiness, and diarrhea may be seen at higher levels. When reserpine alone does not bring about normotension, hydralazine is given in addition. The effective dosage of this drug varies enormously. Therapy should be initiated at low dosage levels and adjusted over a period of days to weeks until the desired response or side effects are noted. An initial dosage of 1 or 2 mg/kg/day in four divided doses can be tried with careful monitoring of the blood pressure. Doses as high as 20 mg/kg may be required. Side effects include nausea, hypotension, headaches, and tachycardia. If blood pressure has not returned to normal levels with those agents, guanethidine or α-methyldopa can be given, in starting dosages of 0.2 to 0.3 mg/kg/day and 10 mg/kg/day, respectively. Guanethidine is given as a single daily dose; α-methyldopa is divided into two or three doses daily.

ANEMIA. The anemia of chronic renal disease is rarely symptomatic, although it may be persistent and severe. There is no specific therapy, assuming that iron deficiency and other nutritional deficiencies such as vitamin D, folic acid, and vitamin B_{12} have been ruled out. Blood transfusions are of only temporary value; they depress the bone marrow and are not without hazards. Sudden, unexpected, and unexplained deaths have followed transfusions of whole blood in patients with chronic renal insufficiency. Sensitization of patients from administration of blood may be of importance if renal transplantation is subsequently considered. If anemia is severe and symptomatic the infusion of washed red blood cells may be recommended; they appear to cause fewer reactions than whole blood and are relatively free of leukocytes.

The transfusion must be given slowly and with extreme caution, since patients with renal insufficiency may be very sensitive to small changes in vascular volume; severe hypertension may be noted after administration of blood. Concomitant administration of a potent diuretic such as furosemide has been advocated.

GROWTH FAILURE. The cause of growth failure in chronic renal disease is uncertain, although poor nutrition, chronic acidosis, negative calcium balance, and

---

* One gram of potassium chloride contains 13.4 mEq of potassium. Potassium Triplex is a palatable liquid preparation that contains 15 mEq/5ml.

† One gram of calcium lactate, $Ca(C_3H_5O_3)_2 \cdot 5H_2O$, contains 130 mg of calcium. Several propiertary preparations are available.

chronic infection may play important roles. Therapy is directed toward each separate problem or complication in an attempt to provide as healthy a milieu as possible for growth. The possible beneficial effect of anabolic steroids has not been established.

NEUROMUSCULAR AND PSYCHOLOGIC DISTURBANCES. It is important to realize that the irritative neuromuscular phenomena commonly seen in patients with chronic uremia, including muscle twitching and convulsions, are rarely due to hypocalcemia and thus respond poorly to calcium therapy. This is probably due to the protective effect of the associated acidosis and elevated level of serum magnesium. Other than the rare instance in which hypocalcemia can be implicated, therapy is nonspecific and unsatisfactory, consisting merely of sedation.

Other types of neuromuscular disturbances include a variety of mental symptoms, ranging from depression to psychosis, and peripheral neuropathy. Treatment other than dialysis is not available.

Management of a child with chronic renal insufficiency must include psychologic support not only of the child but also of his family. Considerable understanding of child development and of the defenses used by children of different ages is required for this aspect of treatment. As in other serious diseases in which the cause is not know, the parents and older patients need to be reassured repeatedly that they are not responsible for the disease. In an illness such as chronic uremia in which medical treatment is usually so inadequate it is also important for the physician to examine repeatedly how his own feelings may be affecting his relationship with the patient and his family.

EFFECT ON UNRELATED INTERCURRENT DISTURBANCES. The presence of chronic renal insufficiency in an infant or child must be taken into account in the treatment of unrelated intercurrent disturbances. For example, toxic amounts of potassium may inadvertently be given in the form of potassium penicillin, and the concentrations of other drugs excreted by the kidneys may reach abnormally high levels if they are given in the usual dosage. Kunin has provided excellent data concerning appropriate dosages of antibiotics in patients with renal failure. A guide to the use of other drugs has been prepared by Bennett, Singer, and Coggins. Finally, there is the recurrent and difficult problem of assessing to what extent chronic renal insufficiency may be contributing to such common events as recurrent respiratory infections and particularly psychologic disturbances.

IMMUNOSUPPRESSANT DRUGS. At present there are only limited data concerning the value of these drugs in the treatment of patients with chronic renal insufficiency. Earlier experience indicated that adrenocorticosteroids were of little if any value, and there was even some suspicion that in addition to their known undesirable side effects they accelerated loss of kidney function in some patients. There is suggestive evidence that treatment with other immunosuppressant drugs, such as azathioprine or cyclophosphamide, may arrest or retard progression of chronic renal impairment in patients with certain types of chronic glomerulonephritis. The data are preliminary, and general recommendations regarding use of these drugs cannot be given. Children considered candidates for such therapy should be evaluated by investigators actively engaged in studying the effects of these drugs in patients with chronic renal disease.

DIALYSIS. Peritoneal dialysis has been used frequently in the treatment of infants and children with acute renal failure, and to a much lesser degree in patients with chronic renal failure. The procedure, which is technically simpler than hemodialysis, is tolerated even by small infants. The 2-liter exchanges commonly employed in adults are too large for children. In older children a 1-liter exchange is used. In younger children and infants 50 to 100 ml/kg per exchange has been recommended. Commercially available catheters are suitable for use in children and are inserted after distending the abdomen by installation through a No. 18 needle of a volume of fluid equal to one exchange. This permits positioning the catheter within the peritoneal cavity so that free return of fluid is obtained. Commercial dialysis fluid with or without added potassium is used, with 5 mg of heparin per liter. Usually 1.5 percent glucose dialysis fluid is employed. If it is desired to remove additional fluid from the patient, a mixture of equal parts of 1.5 percent and 7 percent glucose may be employed. The use of 7 percent glucose dialysis fluid alone should be avoided in order to prevent excessively rapid transfer of fluid.

Peritoneal urea clearances relatively greater than those obtained in adults have been reported in children. It has been suggested that this is due to greater permeability of the peritoneal membrane or to the fact that the peritoneal surface area is greater relative to body size than in adults. Dialysis can be maintained continuously for period of 48 to 72 hours or longer, as needed clinically, with the risk of peritonitis increasing as the duration of dialysis is prolonged.

A major disadvantage of peritoneal dialysis is the large loss of protein and amino acids in the peritoneal fluid. This may be particularly troublesome in patients being maintained chronically.

Children with terminal renal failure have been maintained with chronic hemodialysis for periods of several years. The technical problems are greater than in adults, particularly with regard to maintenance of cannulas. Recent experience with surgically created internal arteriovenous fistulas (which obviate the need for cannulization) is encouraging. In children special attention must be paid to nutritional requirements, and in many instances nutritional supplements may be necessary. Despite the improved success with chronic hemodialysis in children, its major role, apart from the treatment of acute renal failure, remains the maintenance and preparation of children for renal allotransplantation. The techniques of hemodialysis in children are essentially the same as in adults, but they are beyond the scope of this text.

TRANSPLANTATION. As survival figures following renal homotransplantation steadily improve this proce-

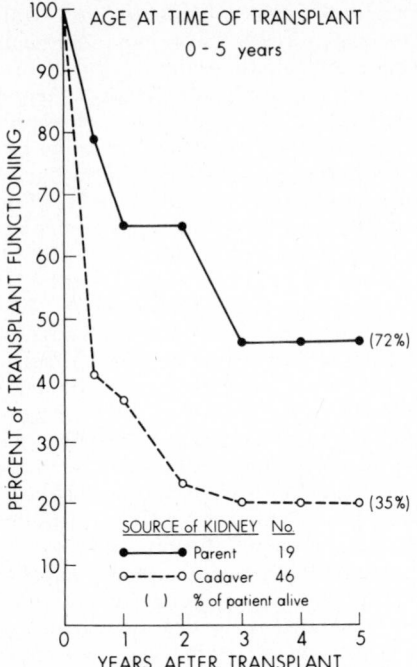

FIG. 6. Patient and kidney survivals following transplantation in children up to 5 years of age. (From Greifer and Barnett: Ped Ann 3:82, 1974.)

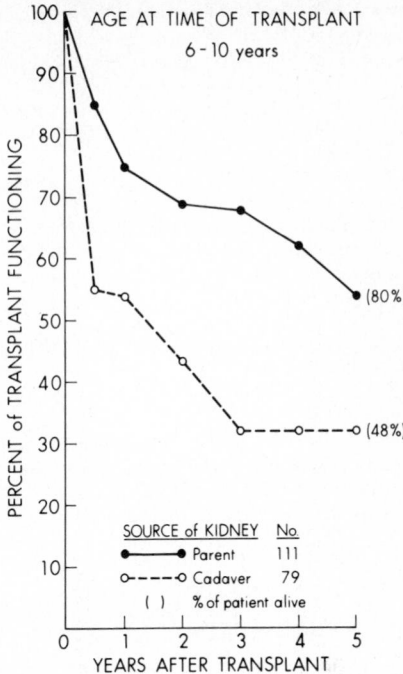

FIG. 7. Patient and kidney survivals following transplantation in children 6 to 10 years of age. (From Greifer and Barnett: Ped Ann 3:82, 1974.)

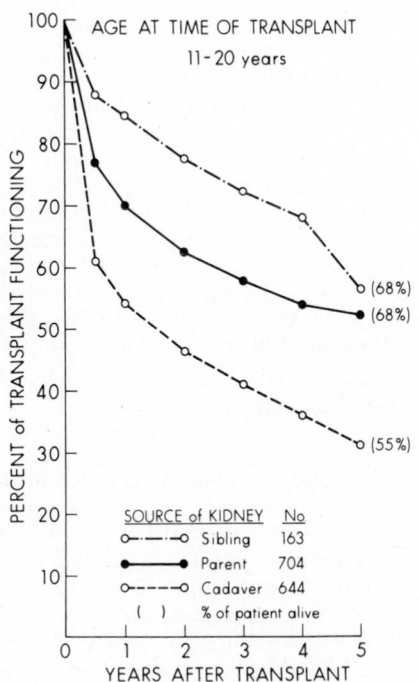

FIG. 8. Patient and kidney survivals following transplantation in children 11 to 20 years of age. (From Greifer and Barnett: Ped Ann 3:82, 1974.)

dure becomes more and more the one of choice in the management of terminal renal failure. This is particularly true for children, in whom chronic dialysis as definitive therapy generally has not been successful. Experience with transplantation in children is summarized in Figure 6, 7, and 8, which are constructed from data in the National Transplant Registry. It can be seen that patient and kidney survivals are comparable to the experience in adult patients.

The decision regarding renal transplantation cannot be undertaken lightly; not all children with chronic uremia can be considered suitable candidates. Nevertheless, after careful evaluation of all the medical, social, and psychologic aspects, with regard to both the patient and his family, the procedure should be considered for most children, in whom it can be a most profitable undertaking.

References

Barratt TM: Renal failure in the first year of life. Br Med Bull 27:115, 1971

Bennett WM, Singer I, Coggins CH: Guide to drug dosage in adult patients with impaired renal function. JAMA 223:991, 1973

Bernstein J, Ruben M: Congenital abnormalities of urinary system: II. Renal cortical and medullary necrosis. J Pediatr 59:657, 1961

Bricker NS: On the pathogenesis of the uremic state. An exposition of the "trade-off hypothesis." N Engl J Med 282:953, 1970

———Klahr S, Lubowitz H, Riesselbach RE: Renal function in chronic renal disease. Medicine 44:263, 1965

———Wessler S, Avioli LV: Renal osteodystrophy. Therapy based on mechanism. JAMA 211:97, 1970

Cameron JS: The treatment of chronic renal failure in children by regular dialysis and by transplantation. Nephron 11:221, 1973

DeLuca HF: The kidney as an endocrine organ for the production of 1,25-dihydroxy-vitamin D_3, a calcium-mobilizing hormone. N Engl J Med 289:359, 1973

de St Jeor ST, Carlston BJ, Tyler FH: Planning low-protein diets for use in chronic renal failure. J Am Diet Assoc 54:34, 1969

Dobrin RS, Larsen CD, Holliday MA: The critically ill child: acute renal failure. Pediatrics 48:286, 1971

Eastwood JB, Bordier PJ, DeWardener HE: Some biochemical, histological, radiological and clinical features of renal osteodystrophy. Kidney Int 4:128, 1973

Editor: Pathogenesis of oliguric acute renal failure. N Engl J Med 282:1370, 1970

Fine RN, Korsch BM, Grushkin CM, Lieberman E: Hemodialysis in children Am J Dis Child 119:498, 1970

———Rosoff L, Grushkin CM, Donnell GN, Lieberman E: Total parathyroidectomy in the treatment of renal osteodystrophy. J Pediatr 76:32, 1970

Korsch BM, Stiles Q, et al: Renal homotransplantation in children. J Pediatr 76:347, 1970

Grushkin CM, Fine RN: Growth in children following renal transplantation. Am J Dis Child 125:514, 1973

Jones-Boulton JM, Cameron JS, Bewick M, et al: Treatment of terminal renal failure in children by home dialysis and transplantation. Arch Dis Child 46:457, 1971

Korsch BM, Negrete VF, Gardner JE, et al: Kidney transplantation in children: psychosocial follow-up study on child and family. J Pediatr 83:399, 1973

Kunin CM: A guide to use of antibiotics in patients with renal disease. A table of recommended doses and factors governing serum levels. Ann Intern Med 67:151, 1967

LaPlante MP, Kaufman JJ Goldman R et al: Kidney transplantation in children. Pediatrics 46:665, 1970

Lilly JR, Giles G, Hurwitz et al: Renal homotransplantation in pediatric patients. Pediatrics 47:548, 1971

McEnery PT, Gonzalez LL, Martin LW, West CD: Growth and development of children with renal transplants. Use of alternate-day steroid therapy. J Pediatr 83:806, 1973

Massry SG, Coburn JW: Renal osteodystrophy. Pathogenesis, clinical features, and treatment. Kidney 5:1, 1972

Oliver J, MacDowell M, Tracey A: The pathogenesis of acute renal failure associated with traumatic and toxic injury; renal ischemia, nephrotoxic damage and the ischemuric episode. J Clin Invest 30:1307, 1951

Potter D, Belzer FO, Rames L, et al: The treatment of chronic uremia in childhood. I. Transplantation. Pediatrics 45:432, 1970

——— Potter D, Larsen D, Levman E, et al: Treatment of chronic uremia in childhood. II. Hemodialysis. Pediatrics 46:678, 1970

RENAL ABNORMALITIES IN THE NEWBORN

JAY BERNSTEIN

Renal disease in the newborn may present as an obvious congenital malformation, as an abdominal mass with hematuria or evidence of infection, or nonspecifically as failure to thrive. The majority of infants with renal disease have a congenital malformation or some form of gross obstructive uropathy. Some renal abnormalities in the newborn are congenital but are acquired late in gestation; others are postnatal in origin. Renal tumors in newborns are uncommon, although metanephric neoplasms do occur in the form of a relatively benign variant, the so-called mesoblastic nephroma.

The presence of oligohydramnios observed at the time of delivery is often the first indication of a renal abnormality in the newborn. The clinical clues to renal disease may not be obvious during the first 2 to 3 days of life, but evidence of disordered renal function usually is apparent by the end of the first week. More than 90 percent of normal newborns urinate within 24 hours, and more than 99 percent within 48 hours. The urinary output of 30 to 60 ml/day in the first 2 days increases to 100 to 300 ml/day at the end of the first week. A failure to pass urine suggests severe renal maldevelopment or urinary tract obstruction. A diminished urinary output (less than 15 to 20 ml/kg/24 hours) may be secondary to obstructive malformations, to renal parenchymal disease, or to prerenal abnormalities. Causes of hypovolemia and prerenal oliguria include hemorrhage, fetal–maternal transfusion, diarrhea, and maternal diabetes. The kidneys are normally palpable in the newborn, and their enlargement, diminution, or absence can be important clues to the presence of renal disease. Ascites and edema may also be signs of renal disease. Palpable abdominal flank masses reflect cystic disease, tumors, obstruction, or circulatory disturbances of the kidney. Hematuria is a very important sign of renal disease; it is found particularly with acquired vascular or circulatory disorders, but also with cystic disease and urinary tract obstruction. The criteria for assessing hematuria, pyuria, and cylindruria are similar to those used in older patients. The concentration of urinary protein is ordinarily below the level of detection of the usual screening procedures, and detectable proteinuria in the newborn should be regarded as abnormal. The concentration of urea in the serum is ordinarily low in the first weeks, and elevations commonly reflect dehydratation; after the first few days of life a urea nitrogen value greater than 10 mg/dl in the presence of normal hydration requires investigation. Finally, it is a truism of medical practice that multiple malformations are clues to other malformations; renal and urinary tract abnormalities are often associated with anogenital anomalies.

Congenital Abnormalities

The most readily recognized renal malformation clinically is *bilateral agenesis*, ie, complete absence of the kidneys. This anomaly is associated with oligohydramnios and amnion nodosum, a peculiar facies, and misshapen and low-set ears; this collection of malformations has come to be known as Potter's syndrome which has been obscured also after prolonged leakage of amniotic fluid in the absence of renal disease. Oligohydramnios and abnormal ears are seen with other forms of renal maldevelopment. The former results from decreased urination during intrauterine life, and the latter

have been recognized in individuals of all ages with relatively minor renal anomalies. Most cases of bilateral agenesis are sporadic; such infants are commonly born prematurely and are also often small for their ages. The major clinical problem in babies surviving delivery and the first few hours of life is respiratory distress secondary to pulmonary hypoplasia. Vigorous resuscitative measures often result in interstitial emphysema and pneumothorax. Esophageal and duodenal atresia, imperforate anus, and colonic agenesis may be associated anomalies. Caudal malformations occur with some frequency; sirenomelic monsters frequently have no kidneys.

Infantile polycystic disease is a developmental abnormality that involves both the kidney and liver. The kidneys are enlarged and diffusely spongy, with more or less uniform dilatation of collecting ducts and somewhat less regular dilatation of convoluted tubules and glomeruli. The hepatic portal areas are enlarged, and in section they appear to contain dilated anastomosing bile ducts, which in all likelihood are interconnecting flattened cisternae that surround the portal blood vessels. Cystic pancreatic and pulmonary changes have occasionally been described, but their presence may signify other forms of cystic disease, reflecting the extreme heterogeneity of what is customarily called polycystic disease. Severe diffuse polycystic disease is a cause of renal nonfunction, but newborns often die because of respiratory impairment due to coexistent pulmonary hypoplasia. The abdomen is frequently greatly distended by huge kidneys that may have been present in intrauterine life and may cause fetal dystocia. Oligohydramnios and Potter's facies are common complications. Less severe degrees of cystic involvement are compatible with renal function and survival beyond the newborn period. The condition is familial and is transmitted as an autosomal recessive inheritance. It is different from the classic adult type of polycystic disease, which is an autosomal dominant condition; it is also to be differentiated from other forms of generalized cystic renal disease, including Meckel's syndrome (encephalocele, microcephaly or hydrocephalus, ocular abnormalities, polydactyly, cleft palate and lip, genital abnormalities, polycystic liver), Jeune's asphyxiating thoracic dystrophy (chondrodystrophy, dwarfism, neonatal respiratory impairment, pancreatic cysts, hepatic dysgenesis), Zellweger's syndrome (abnormal facies, hypotonia, cerebral maldevelopment, ocular abnormalities, stippled epiphyses, hepatic dysgenesis), bilateral multicystic dysplasia, and generalized cystic renal dysplasia.

Renal dysplasia results from altered development and differentiation of both the collecting system and nephrons. Among the important types or patterns of dysplasia in the newborn period is the condition of severe dysplastic hypoplasia, often referred to as aplasia, in which only a small nubbin of renal tissue is identifiable grossly. Multicystic dysplasia is closely related, being distinguished grossly by numerous, often large, renal cysts; it is almost always associated with ureteropelvic

occlusion. This is, incidentally, the most common form of cystic disorder in newborns. Renal dysplasia is commonly associated with malformations of other systems, particularly cardiovascular and alimentary. Bilateral involvement in either condition is, of course, a cause of renal nonfunction; it may be accompanied by stigmata of Potter's syndrome and is lethal within the first few days of life. The enlarged multicystic kidneys usually are palpable on abdominal examination; the bladder is hypoplastic and the infant does not pass urine. Unilateral multicystic kidney, either in newborns or in older children, is discovered most often as an abdominal or flank mass, and excretory urography fails to demonstrate renal function on the affected side. However, total body opacification with high-dose urography does demonstrate accumulation of contrast medium within the septa of the cystic kidney. The unilateral cystic kidney is usually treated by nephrectomy; careful urographic evaluation of the opposite kidney is necessary because of the frequency of associated and sometimes correctable abnormalities.

Posterior urethral valves in newborns often are accompanied by renal dysplasia, the severity of which appears to be related to the degree of urinary obstruction. Severe valvar obstruction can be the cause of bladder dilatation and hydroureter (Fig. 9) very early in life and may be a cause of anuria in the newborn. In this regard, the presence of bilateral renal masses and a midline suprapubic mass in a newborn male should be taken as prima facie evidence of urethral or bladder neck obstruction until appropriate diagnostic measures can be undertaken.

Acquired Abnormalities

Glomerulonephritis in the newborn is uncommon, and the few reports of chronic glomerulonephritis remain medical curiosities. The congenital nephrotic syndrome (p. 1288) may be regarded as a form of primary glomerular disease. The nephrotic syndrome also occurs in immune-deposit disease secondary to congenital syphilis and toxoplasmosis.

Acute pyelonephritis in the newborn can be a severe infection. It occurs most often in males and results from coliform septicemia. Clinical or anatomic evidence of an underlying anomaly of the urinary tract is usually not present. The initial sign is often jaundice due to conjugated hyperbilirubinemia, presumably resulting from toxic injury to the liver. Mild hemolysis may also be present early in the course and may contribute to the accumulation of unconjugated bilirubin. The usual clinical findings are nonspecific, and irritability and anorexia are common. Recognition may be delayed because of little or no clinical evidence to implicate the urinary tract. The infection responds to prompt and vigorous antibiotic therapy, but in severe cases the course is rapid and the child may be moribund before the gravity of his illness is appreciated. Acute infections can and do occur in infants who have anatomic urologic abnormalities. In such cases the outcome may hinge on the prevention of recurrent or chronic pyelonephritis; surgical relief of the underlying lesion is mandatory. Milder renal infections are also difficult to diagnose because they are too often asymptomatic. Pyuria may be lacking, and the diagnosis rests on the demonstration of bacteriuria. Because of the difficulty in collecting noncontaminated urine from newborns, suprapubic aspiration is frequently employed. Radiographic studies have shown normal kidneys and normal urinary tracts in most cases; some have enlarged kidneys with poor function. Successful treatment usually leaves no residual renal abnormality. Renal parenchymal damage and scarring may be related to urinary tract abnormalities and to persistent reflux.

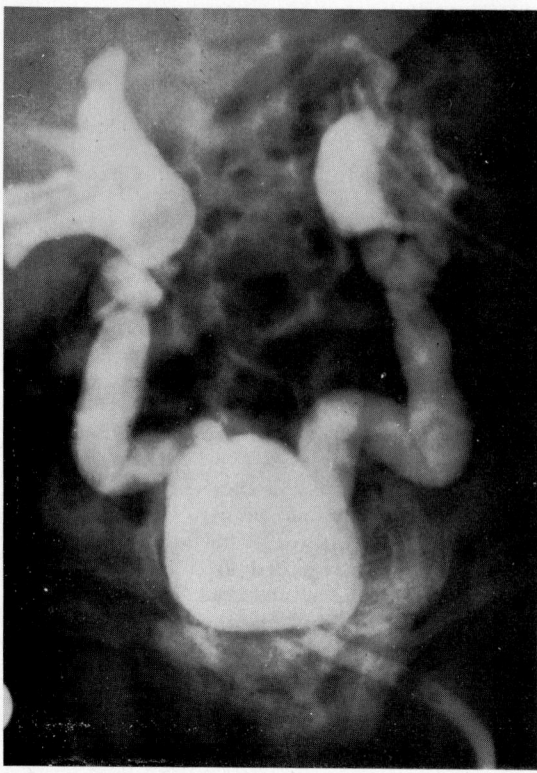

FIG. 9.   Bilateral hydroureter and hydronephrosis secondary to a posterior urethral valve in a newborn. The greatly enlarged kidneys and bladder were easily palpable on physical examination.

The most common forms of acquired renal disease in the newborn fall into the general category of *circulatory disturbances*. Some are clearly the result of ischemia and anoxia, such as infarction of the kidney following vascular occlusion. Others, such as cortical necrosis, presumably result from transient or functional alterations in renal blood flow. A transitory syndrome of renal enlarg-

ment and hematuria in newborns indicates that some circulatory disturbances are reversible. This group of renal abnormalities presents an ill-defined clinical problem in which recognition of the anatomic lesion is not often possible. Any of these lesions may be present in an infant with enlarged kidneys, azotemia, and hematuria, although the same findings are also equally compatible with the diagnosis of a congenital malformation of the urinary tract.

Vascular occlusion may result from either arterial or venous thrombosis. The former (p. 1317) is often embolic, from a primary thrombus lying within the ductus arteriosus, and it has also been reported to follow catheterization of the umbilical artery. Renal infarction may be unilateral, but aortic occlusion or multiple emboli can cause bilateral necrosis. Flank masses and hematuria are the clinical evidences of renal involvement; infants develop severe, acute hypertension and may present with congestive heart failure without obvious cause. Embolic lesions also appear in the extremities, gastrointestinal tract, and head, and portions of the thrombus that extend into the pulmonary artery can embolize to the lungs.

Renal venous thrombosis (p.1318) involves the major vessels or their tributaries or both. Renal infarction often ensues, resulting in renal enlargement and oliguria with hematuria. Renal involvement is often asymmetric. At times the lesion can be shown to have developed before birth. Clinical findings are commonly nonspecific, including vomiting, anorexia, fever, lethargy, and shock. Excretory urography in the acute stages shows delayed or poor function. The diagnosis may be confirmed by a venogram of the inferior vena cava. Arteriography shows stasis and narrowing of intrarenal branches and lack of venous filling.

Renal venous thrombosis in newborns, as in older children, occurs as a complication of diarrhea and dehydration. It has in the recent past also been relatively frequent in babies born to diabetic mothers, presumably because of the infants' hypovolemia and dehydration. In the last few years, however, this lesion has been found to be far less common than earlier, probably because of better fluid management and rehydration of distressed infants. It also occurs in newborns who have polyuria and dehydration from other causes, such as anencephaly. Another factor of possible pathogenetic importance is disseminated intravascular coagulation, for which the frequent occurrence of thrombocytopenia and depletion of certain clotting factors have been cited as evidence; however, it is not clear that these findings are anything more than the effects of extensive local thrombosis. Therapeutic measures include rehydration; the effectivenesses of anticoagulation remains undemonstrated. Prompt surgical extirpation has been advocated in the treatment of unilateral infarction, but in recent years several observers have favored more conservative therapy. There are several reports of recovery after caval embolectomy and some reports of recovery after nonsurgical management of bilateral infarction. Late complications of conservative therapy include renal atrophy with nonfunction, occasional renal hypertension, and possible tubular dysfunction.

Anoxic lesions of the kidney in which vascular occlusion cannot be demonstrated include cortical and medullary (Fig. 10) necrosis. These conditions, which

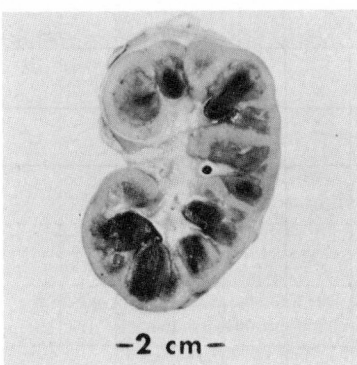

FIG. 10. Renal medullary necrosis in a newborn. The medullary pyramids are partially hemorrhagic; the cortex is not involved.

may be separate or combined, have been reported infrequently in the past, but the descriptions of "hemorrhagic nephritis" and "hemorrhagic infarction" of the kidneys in newborns probably include many examples of cortical and medullary necrosis. Cortical necrosis also has been confounded with infarction due to renal vein thrombosis on the grounds that they are different stages of the same process, but there is no evidence that the two are related. In recent experience cortical and medullary necroses have become the most common forms of renal necrosis in the newborn. Both are associated with anemic or asphyxial shock. Blood loss may have resulted from uteroplacental hemorrhage, twin–twin transfusion, fetal–maternal transfusion, or severe hemolytic disease. Maternal toxemia has been relatively frequent among babies suffering from fetal asphyxia. Cortical necrosis has been observed in stillborn infants, and a variable degree of cortical involvement accompanies medullary necrosis. Both cortical and medullary necroses are accompanied by focal necrosis in other organs. Both conditions are usually bilateral, and both can be responsible for renal enlargement and hematuria. Cortical necrosis is sometimes accompanied by an unexplained thrombocytopenia, and clinical or histopathologic evidence of intravascular coagulation has been found on occasion, although very few cases of documented disseminated intravascular coagulation have also shown renal cortical necrosis. Medullary necrosis in infants with congenital heart disease has recently been related to the toxicity of large doses of angiographic contrast medium, and medullary necrosis in infants with severe hyperbilirubinemia and kernicterus seems to be secondary to the direct toxic effects of unconjugated bilirubin concentrated in the renal medulla.

Prognosis of cortical and medullary necrosis is related to the nature and severity of the associated and underlying conditions, as well as to the severity of the renal lesion. Treatment is supportive, except that renal failure may be ameliorated by peritoneal dialysis. The effectiveness of anticoagulant therapy, which is used on the assumption that intravascular coagulation plays a role, remains to be demonstrated. In surviving infants the kidney undergoes fibrosis and scarring, producing within weeks a radiographically characteristic pattern of cortical calcification. Medullary pyramids are deformed, leading to pyelocalyceal distortion and papillary cavitation. Prolonged survival may be attended by impaired function, and glomerular insufficiency has been observed in cases with relatively good preservation of tubular function. Selective tubular dysfunction might also result from disproportionate tubular atrophy around areas of cortical necrosis, as suggested in some survivors of venous thrombosis.

Transient renal impairment has been observed in newborns suffering from asphyxia and from the respiratory distress syndrome. Urinary output may be diminished, and functional studies have shown depressed GFR and diminished urea and creatinine clearances. These abnormalities may be regarded as a form of prerenal failure, perhaps related to reduced renal cortical blood flow. Renal concentrating capacity is also impaired in asphyxiated newborns, and studies of tubular function have shown impaired dilution and acidification. Older studies had shown increased numbers of cells and casts in the urinary sediment of asphyxiated babies, suggesting tubular epithelial injury. Frank tubular necrosis is, however, an uncommon lesion, and the poor correlation between these functional observations and the histopathologic findings indicates that renal impairment most likely results from reduced cortical perfusion rather than from an anatomic tubular necrosis.

References

Arneil GC, MacDonald AM, Murphy AV, Sweet EM: Renal venous thrombosis. Clin Nephrol 1:119, 1973

Belman AB, King LR: The pathology and treatment of renal vein thrombosis in the newborn. J Urol 107:852, 1972

Bernstein J: Heritable cystic disorders of the kidney: the mythology of polycystic disease. Pediatr Clin North Am 18:435, 1971

——— Brough AJ, McAdams AJ: The renal lesion in syndromes of multiple congenital malformations. Cerebrohepatorenal syndrome; Jeune asphyxiating thoracic dystrophy; tuberous sclerosis; Meckel syndrome. Birth Defects 10:35, 1974

Brough AJ, Zuelzer WW: Renal vascular disease. Pediatr Clin North Am 11:533, 1964

Dimmick JE, Hardwick DF, Ho-Yuen B: A case of renal necrosis and fibrosis in the immediate newborn period: association with the twin-to-twin transfusion syndrome. Am J Dis Child 122:345, 1971

Dunbar JS, Nogrady B: Excretory urography in the first year of life. Radiol Clin North Am 10:367, 1972

Emanuel B, Aronson N: Neonatal hematuria. Am J Dis Child 128:204, 1974

Ford KT, Teplick SK, Clark RE: Renal artery embolism causing neonatal hypertension: a complication of unbilical artery catheterization. Radiology 113:169, 1974

Groshong TD, Taylor AA, Nolph KD, Esterly J, Maher JF: Renal function following cortical necrosis in childhood. J Pediatr 79:267, 1971

Gruskin AB, Oetliker OH, Wolfish NE, et al: Effects of angiography on renal function and histology in infants and piglets. J Pediatr 76:42, 1970

Leonidas JC, Berdon WE, Gribetz D: Bilateral renal cortical necrosis in the newborn infant: roentgenographic diagnosis. J Pediatr 79:623, 1971

Littlewood JM: 66 Infants with urinary tract infection in first year of life. Arch Dis Child 47:218, 1972

McDonald P, Tarar R, Gilday D, Reilly BJ: Some radiologic observations in renal vein thrombosis. Am J Roentgenol Radium Ther Nucl Med 120:368, 1974

Moore ES, Galvez MB: Delayed micturition in the newborn period. J Pediatr 80:867, 1972

——— Perlman M, Williams J, Hirsch M: Neonatal pulmonary hypoplasia after prolonged leakage at amniotic fluid. Arch Dis child 51 349, 1976

Sherry SN, Kramer I: The time of passage of the first stool and first urine by the newborn infant. J Pediatr 46:158, 1955

Siegel SR, Fisher DA, Oh W: Renal function and serum aldosterone levels in infants with respiratory distress syndrome. J Pediatr 83:854, 1973

Stark H: Renal vein thrombosis in infancy. Recovery without nephrectomy. Am J Dis Child 108:430, 1964

——— Geiger R: Renal tubular dysfunction following vascular accidents of the kidneys in the newborn period. J Pediatr 83:933, 1973

Svenningsen NW, Aronson AS: Postnatal development of renal concentration capacity as estimated by DDAVP-test in normal and asphyxiated neonates. Biol Neonate 25:230, 1974

Torrado A, Guignard LS, Prod'hom LS, Gautier E: Hypoxaemia and renal function in newborns with respiratory distress syndrome (RDS). Helv Paediat Acta 29:399, 1974

Wigger HJ, Bransilver BR, Blanc WA: Thromboses due to catheterization in infants and children. J Pediatr 76:1, 1970

ABNORMALITIES OF RENAL DEVELOPMENT

JAY BERNSTEIN

HYPOPLASIA AND DYSPLASIA; CYSTIC DISORDERS AND POLYCYSTIC DISEASE

Developmental disturbances of the kidneys include various forms of hypoplasia (reduction of mass), dysplasia (abnormal differentiation), and cystic disease. The genetic basis of some conditions, such as bilateral polycystic disease, is widely accepted, but heritable conditions account for a minority of these structural abnormalities (Table 3). Most human malformations occur without overt evidence of either abnormal inheritance or exogenous injury to the fetus. Renal dysplasia, however, may be related to obstructive anomalies of the urinary tract, and in this sense the renal maldevelopment is conditioned by environmental factors. Also, renal growth and development continue after birth, and postnatal injury can result in growth retardation and developmental arrest of the kidneys.

Many developmental abnormalities are cystic, but the practice of regarding all kidneys that contain cysts as polycystic is neither justified nor appropriate. Cysts of the renal parenchyma are encountered in both dysplastic and polycystic kidneys. Cysts may also be encountered in conditions that clearly are acquired rather than

TABLE 3 Inherited Structural Abnormalities of the Kidney

I. Polycystic disease[a]
    A. Infantile polycystic disease
    B. Adult polycystic disease
II. Cortical cysts in malformation syndromes[a]
III. Medullary sponge kidney[a]
IV. Hereditary and familial dysplasia
    A. Generalized cystic dysplasia with cerebral maldevelopment (Meckel's syndrome)
    B. Cerebrohepatorenal and Jeune's syndromes
    C. Beckwith-Wiedemann syndrome
    D. Lenz's microphthalmia syndrome
V.   Hereditary unilateral agenesis and agenesis-aplasia syndrome
VI. Hereditary hydronephrosis

[a] See Table 4.

developmental (eg, cystic arteriolar nephrosclerosis in the adult) and in conditions in which they seem to be secondary to another renal abnormality (eg, tubular cysts in the congenital nephrotic syndrome). Cysts do not appear to be of specific pathogenetic significance, and they may develop in normally formed, dysplastic, atrophic, or scarred nephrons (Table 4).

Renal Hypoplasia

Renal hypoplasia may take several forms. Small kidneys with normal parenchyma (so-called dwarf kidneys) are usually unilateral and are frequently found in association with other congenital abnormalities. Although the abnormality is usually asymptomatic during infancy, it has been regarded as a predisposing factor in the development of hypertension and chronic pyelonephritis. Consequently the presence of inflammation and scarring in small kidneys makes it very difficult to differentiate hypoplasia from the shrunken kidney with secondary atrophy. Bilateral hypoplasia, while occasionally associated with histologically normal development, is more often associated with marked hypertrophy of individual nephrons. In this form of maldevelopment, known as oligonephronic hypoplasia or oligomeganephronia, the kidneys are extremely small and contain a reduced number of lobes; there may be only one or two medullary pyramids. The nephrons are also markedly reduced in number, but the glomeruli are enlarged. Measurements of microdissected specimens have shown tubules to be increased approximately 4 times in length and 17 times in volume.

The clinical manifestations of oligonephronic hypoplasia include impaired concentrating ability, with po-

TABLE 4. Classification of Renal Cysts

I. Renal dysplasia
  A. Multicystic dysplasia
    1. Unilateral multicystic kidney
    2. Bilateral multicystic dysplasia
  B. Focal and segmental cystic dysplasia
  C. Cystic dysplasia associated with lower urinary tract obstruction
  D. Familial cystic dysplasia
II. Polycystic disease
  A. Infantile polycystic disease
    1. Polycystic disease of early infancy
    2. Polycystic disease of childhood
    3. Congenital hepatic fibrosis
  B. Adult polycystic disease
III. Renal cysts in hereditary syndromes
  A. Meckel's syndrome
  B. Zellweger's cerebrohepatorenal syndrome
  C. Jeune's asphyxiating thoracic dystrophy
  D. Tuberous sclerosis complex and Lindau's disease
  E. Cortical cysts in syndromes of multiple malformations
IV. Renal cortical cysts
  A. Diffuse glomerular cystic disese
  B. Peripheral cortical microcysts
  C. Juxtamedullary cortical microcysts
  D. Simple cysts, solitary and multiple
V. Renal medullary cystic disorders
  A. Medullary sponge kidney
  B. Medullary cystic disease complex
    1. Familial juvenile nephronophthisis
    2. Medullary cystic disease
    3. Renal-retinal dysplasia
VI. Miscellaneous parenchymal renal cysts
  A. Inflammation and necrosis
    1. Medullary necrosis
    2. Lithiasis
    3. Tuberculosis
    4. Echinococcosis
  B. Neoplasia
    1. Cystic degeneration of carcinoma
    2. Multilocular cystadenoma (benign cystic nephroma)
    3. Dermoid cyst
  C. Endometriosis
  D. Traumatic intrarenal hemotoma
VII. Extraparenchymal renal cysts
  A. Pyelogenic cyst (pelvic diverticulum)
  B. Parapelvic cyst (lymphangiectasia)
  C. Perinephric cyst

lyuria, polydipsia, and bouts of dehydration beginning in the first weeks or months of life. Growth retardation is a prominent feature, and anemia is frequent. Proteinuria is generally moderate. Salt-wasting may be present. Renal function may be diminished early, but GFR, renal plasma flow, and tubular functions often remain stable for years. Progressive glomerular insufficiency does appear, however, and is associated with glomerular obsolescence, tubular atrophy, and cortical fibrosis. Renal failure, commonly beginning in the second decade, terminates in uremia. A familial incidence has been observed only rarely. The differential diagnosis includes principally medullary cystic disease and familial juvenile nephronophthisis, with which oligomeganephronia shares a number of clinical features, particularly concentrating defect and growth retardation. It is distinguished, however, by its usual lack of familial occurrence, the early onset of proteinuria, and its distinctive histologic features. Treatment early in the course is to prevent and combat dehydration; later treatment of renal insufficiency includes chronic dialysis and allotransplantation.

A segmental form of hypoplasia, sometimes referred to as Ask-Upmark kidney, is associated with hypertension in children and young adults. This abnormality, which is to be differentiated from chronic pyelonephritis and from the segmental lesions of reflux nephropathy, consists of one or more hypoplastic and atrophic lobes that appear as depressions or transverse grooves on the capsular surface. The abnormal segments overlie elongated calyces or pelvic recesses that extend under the narrow parenchyma almost to the indented capsular surfaces. The cortical portions of the involved areas are extremely thin and the medullary pyramids extremely small. The abnormal portions of cortex may contain a few hyalinized glomeruli or sometimes may seem to be aglomerular, and the tubules are severely atrophic. Some authors have regarded the lesion as a true congenital malformation; however, it could well be an acquired lesion that originated during later gestation or in childhood and resulted in renal growth arrest and localized atrophy. Urinary tract abnormalities are found in a minority of cases, but the frequency of coincidental reflux and obstruction is too low for them to be of pathogenetic significance.

Hypertension may be very severe; resection of the kidney or involved segment is sometimes curative. The pathogenesis of the hypertension is not clear, since the involved segments contain neither normal glomeruli nor juxtaglomerular apparatus. Plasma renin concentrations have been inconsistent, as has hyperplasia of juxtaglomerular apparatus in the adjacent normal kidney. Therapeutic failures after uninephrectomy may be due to a high prevalence of bilaterality. Medical antihypertensive treatment can be effective in patients with bilateral involvement, but malignant hypertension and renal failure are potentially lethal complications.

Renal Dysplasia

Renal dysplasia is defined as abnormal development of nephronic and ductal structures resulting in total or partial renal malformation. The abnormalities under consideration must be differentiated from cystic disease on the one hand and hypoplasia with structurally normal parenchyma on the other. Histologic examination of a typical dysplastic kidney discloses conglomerates of seemingly disorganized tubules and glomeruli, and dysplastic kidneys contain abnormally differentiated structures that have a fetal or primitive appearance. Structures that can be regarded as resulting from embryonic maldevelopment are (1) primitive ducts that are lined by relatively tall columnar epithelium, often ciliated, and are surrounded by fibromuscular collars and (2) nests of metaplastic cartilage. The former, located frequently in the medulla, appear to be altered derivatives of the metanephric duct; the latter, principally cortical, derive from metanephric blastema. Primitive nephronic elements (glomeruli and tubules) are generally present, and cysts, which may or may not be present, are regarded as coincidental findings.

The association of renal dysplasia with other anomalies of the urinary tract is of the order of 90 percent. It is believed that the significance of this association lies in the obstructive nature of most ureteral and lower urinary tract anomalies. Patterns of malformations correlate to some degree with the nature and severity of the obstructive lesion. Unilateral ureteral anomalies are associated with ipsilateral and lower urinary tract anomalies with bilateral dysplasia. Segmental anomalies, as in the syndrome of ectopic ureterocele, are associated with segmental dysplasia. Severe degrees of urinary tract obstruction, as in posterior urethral valves, are associated with dysplasia; mild obstruction rarely is. Cortical dysplasia is generally most marked and is sometimes present only in the outer portion (that is, in the part of the cortex formed late in development after urinary excretion has already begun in the inner portion). The association of dysplasia and urinary tract obstruction may be coincidental, but the patterns that have been observed do support the hypothesis that a causal relationship exists.

CLINICAL FORMS OF DYSPLASIA.   The majority of dysplastic kidneys are sporadic malformations without evidence of heritable causation; a few are familial or occur in syndromes of multiple malformation. Several types of dysplasia can be recognized as clinicopathologic entities, although a sizable group remains unclassified.

Multicystic kidneys and *aplastic kidneys* differ only by the occurrence in the former of gross cysts. The degree of cyst formation varies, and therefore the two abnormalities are not clearly separable. They are similar malformations, both commonly unilateral and both occurring bilaterally in newborns as lethal malformations. Both are also associated with malformations of other systems, particularly alimentary and circulatory. Microscopic examination shows structural disorganization and the histologic features of dysplasia. The multicystic kidney is invariably associated with ureteropelvic occlusion; the aplastic kidney also seems to be, but the point has not been critically evaluated. Bilateral multicystic dysplasia is the single most common cystic disorder of the newborn. Unilateral abnormalities are often asymptomatic and are therefore found in patients of all ages. Unilateral aplasia may be associated with a variety of vague signs and symptoms, some of which possibly are related to recurrent infection. Hypertension is an important late complication. Of particular interest in children is the unilateral multicystic kidney, which presents as an abdominal mass and which may be associated with nonspecific complaints. Abnormalities of the other kidney do occur and may impair the prognosis, but multicystic dysplasia is not a progressive disease that will eventually involve the opposite side. It is rarely associated with hypertension, at least in pediatric practice. Males

predominate, and the lesion is somewhat more common on the left. The kidney does not function, although excretory urography with high doses of contrast medium (total body opacification) results in opacification of the cystic mass, perhaps because the solid portions and septa of the cystic kidneys contain rudimentary metanephric lobules. Endoscopic examination often shows absence of the ureteral orifice or ureteral nonpatency. Surgical extirpation has been the preferred treatment, despite the infrequency of complications, possibly because of the difficulty in differentiating it from Wilms' tumor.

General dysplasia is the term used to describe small, malformed kidneys that retain a semblance of normal architecture and a limited ability to function. Most clinical studies of "renal hypoplasia" have dealt with this type of malformation. There are fewer lobes than normal, a feature that is apparent grossly and radiographically, and radiographic studies often delineate pyelocalyceal deformities. Symptoms, in addition to those deriving from renal insufficiency, are related to infection that occurs in two-thirds of cases and to lithiasis that occurs in one-third of cases. Hypertension develops in 20 to 25 percent, although not always as the result of pyelonephritis. Infants with bilateral dysplasia of this type often have multiple congenital malformations.

Cortical dysplasia is seen in association with lower urinary tract obstruction, its incidence being in general related to the severity of obstruction. Extensive cortical dysplasia may nullify surgical relief of posterior urethral valves. Medullary dysplasia, another associated abnormality, may be partly responsible for a diminished ability to concentrate urine after surgical reconstruction.

The *hereditary dysplasias* comprise a heterogeneous group of genetically unrelated conditions. A severe form of cystic dysplasia with marked nephronic hypoplasia is seen in Meckel's syndrome (microcephaly or posterior encephalocele, polydactyly, cleft palate and lip, genital anomalies, and hepatic ductular dysgenesis with cysts). Renal dysplasia is also encountered in newborns with Zellweger's cerebrohepatorenal syndrome (p. 1100) and in Jeune's syndrome of asphyxiating thoracic dystrophy (p.1593). Infants surviving the first few days of life have shown evidence of renal insufficiency. Dysplasia, predominantly medullary, has also been seen in older children with cerebral maldevelopment and renal failure. A form of medullary dysplasia characterized by widely separated, immature ducts and an increase in stroma frequently accompanies the Beckwith-Wiedemann syndrome of macroglossia, omphalocele, and visceromegaly (p. 922). The kidneys are considerably enlarged, but the functional significance of the abnormality has not as yet been established.

Cystic Disorders of the Kidney

Cystic conditions of the kidney comprise a heterogeneous group of both heritable and acquired conditions that have been classified on the basis of clinical–pathologic correlation (Table 4). The important cystic conditions in childhood include renal dysplasia (discussed in the preceding section), polycystic disease, and several lesions encountered in association with certain constellations of congenital malformations. The majority of cystic abnormalities fall into the first group and are not heritable; most heritable abnormalities, on the other hand, are cystic and fall into the second and third groups.

POLYCYSTIC DISEASE. Most studies have supported the division of polycystic disease into infantile (autosomal recessive) and adult (autosomal dominant) forms. The morphologic and clinical features of typical recessive disease in newborns and typical dominant disease in adults are reasonably distinctive. However, only recently have studies of cystic disease in older children been undertaken to clarify the natural history of the condition and to delineate clinical–pathologic patterns. The concepts that have emerged are based on clinical, genetic, radiographic, and morphologic observations.

Infantile polycystic disease encompasses at least two major subgroups. It is possible, despite morphologic and clinical overalp, to differentiate (1) the large, spongy kidneys that are encountered in newborns and are accompanied by hepatic abnormalities and (2) the predominantly medullary disease in older children that is often asymptomatic but is accompanied by hepatic changes that lead to portal hypertension. However, this separation may be artificial if these differences reflect first the severity of cyst formation at birth and second the evolution of the renal and hepatic lesions with age. The separation of infantile polycystic disease into a fewer or greater number of subtypes will depend ultimately upon extended clinical and genetic studies.

The first subgroup includes those kidneys designated elsewhere as "hamartomatous," "rein en éponge," and "Potter type i." The kidneys are greatly enlarged and diffusely spongy. The usual lobar configuration is preserved, a point of differentiation from cystic forms of renal dysplasia. Slightly increased connective tissue may be present among the tubular elements, but significant fibrosis ordinarily is not present. Microdissection studies have shown that the most consistent and prominent site of dilation is in the collecting tubules, and histologic examination may also show dilation of glomerular spaces and convoluted tubules. The medullary ducts characteristically are dilated, and ectasia of the collecting ducts may be seen grossly. The condition is usually associated with cystic changes in the liver, in which the biliary passages appear to be mildly dilated, tortuous, and anastomosing ducts or cisterns that surround the portal vein. Massive enlargement of the kidneys can produce sufficient abdominal distention in the fetus to result in dystocia. The majority of infants born live die within the first few days of life, although survival into infancy has been described. Newborns suffer from respiratory distress and may develop congestive heart failure. Excretory urography may show poor excretion of contrast medium, and delayed excretion results in a mottled nephrogram with retention of contrast medium in small cysts. The condition may appear either sporadically or in more than one sibling of a single generation. It has not been reported in the offspring of unaffected siblings, nor has consanguinity been noted in the parents. The sibling involvement and horizontal familial transmission are nonetheless consistent with an autosomal recessive abnormality.

The second subgroup seems to lack clinical or pathologic homogeneity. Renal cortical involvement is irregular, and medullary tubular ectasia predominates, often to the point of being readily detectable by excretory urography. The medullary cysts may be radiographically indistinguishable from those of medullary sponge kidney, a disease that is exceedingly uncommon in childhood. Some infants surviving the newborn period suffer from progressive renal insufficiency, and the degree of renal failure has been correlated in a general way with the extent of cyst formation. Older children have progressively more hepatic fibrosis than those with early infantile renal failure. These cases have been designated as congenital hepatic fibrosis, although the hepatic lesion is variable enough to include severe fibrosis in some cases and nonobstructive biliary dilatation in others. Patients with the latter often develop recurrent cholangitis, which may be responsible for the presenting symptoms. Portal hypertension is more often the principal clinical problem, and renal involvement is an incidental radiographic finding. Whether the early infantile and later types of polycystic disease are distinct entities or stages in the evolution of one entity is still a matter of debate.

The adult type (autosomal dominant) of polycystic disease does on occasion occur in childhood. These patients may have large flank masses, proteinuria, and various formed elements in the urine. Hypertension and the classic evidence of progressive renal failure sometimes occur. Adult polycystic disease can be differentiated pathologically from the infantile type. The familial character of the disorder is quite typical, with repetition in several generations demonstrating an autosomal dominant mode of inheritance.

RENAL CORTICAL CYSTS. Multiple cortical microcysts are encountered in several malformation syndromes. They cannot in most instances be regarded as either polycystic disease or renal dysplasia, and they appear to be of no functional or clinical significance. Such lesions have been seen in the autosomal trisomy syndromes D and E, the lissencephaly syndrome, the oral-facial-digital syndrome, the Marden-Walker syndrome, the Ehlers-Danlos syndrome, congenital cutis laxa, and several other syndromes of multiple malformation. The cerebrohepatorenal syndrome and Jeune's syndrome have, as noted elsewhere (p. 1260), been associated in some cases with cortical microcysts and in others with more severe degrees of cyst formation and cystic dysplasia. Tuberous sclerosis may be singled out as distinctive. Renal cysts are variably present. They are generally of tubular origin and are lined by hyperplastic cells; they are often of sufficient size to produce radiographic distortion and to be associated with renal functional impairment. Several patients with renal cysts in early childhood have been reported to have had hypertension and variable renal insufficiency before other manifestations of the syndrome became evident. The practice of applying the term polycystic indiscriminately to this miscellany has little more than descriptive value.

References

RENAL HYPOPLASIA

Batzenschlager A, Weill-Bousson M, Guerbaoui M: L'hypoplasie segmentaire aglomérulaire du rein. I. Lésions rénales associées. Sem Hop Paris 50:601, 1974

Bernstein J: Developmental abnormalities of the renal parenchyma—renal hypoplasia and dysplasia. In Sommers SC (ed): Pathology Annual 1968. New York, Appleton, 1968, pp 213–247

——— Meyer R: Some speculations on the nature and significance of developmentally small kidneys (renal hypoplasia). Nephron 1:137, 1964

Carter JE, Lirenman DS: Bilateral renal hypoplasia with oligomeganephronia. Oligomeganephronic renal hypoplasia. Am J Dis Child 120:537, 1970

Dein RW, Walker D, Hackett RL: The Ask-Upmark kidney. A case report. Arch Pathol 96:10, 1973

Elfenbein IB, Baluarte HJ, Gruskin AB: Renal hypoplasia with oligomeganephronia. Light, electron, fluorescent microscopic and quantative studies. Arch Pathol 97:143, 1974

Fetterman GH, Habib R: Congenital bilateral oligonephronic renal hypoplasia with hypertrophy of nephrons (oligoméganéphronie). Studies by microdissection. Am J Clin Pathol 52:199, 1969

Godard G, Vallotton MB, Broyer M: Plasma renin activity in segmental hypoplasia of the kidneys with hypertension. Nephron 11:308, 1973

Rosenfeld JB, Cohen L, Garty I, Ben-Bassat M: Unilateral renal hypoplasia with hypertension (Ask-Upmark kidney). Br Med J 2:217, 1973

Royer P, Habib R, Broyer M, Nouaille Y: Segmental hypoplasia of the kidney in children. Adv Nephrol 1:145, 1971 (Chicago, Year Book)

Van Acker KJ, Vincke H, Quatacker J, Senesael L, Van Den Brande J: Congenital oligonephronic renal hypoplasia with hypertrophy of nephrons (oligonephronia). Arch Dis Child 46:321, 1971

RENAL DYSPLASIA

Beckwith JB: Macroglossia, omphalocele, adrenal cytomegaly, gigantism, and hyperplastic visceromegaly. Birth Defects 5:188, 1969

Bernstein J: The morphogenesis of renal parenchymal maldevelopment (renal dysplasia). Pediatr Clin North Am 18:395, 1971

——— Brough AJ, McAdams AJ: The renal lesion in syndromes of multiple congenital malformations. Cerebrohepatorenal syndrome; Jeune asphyxiating thoracic dystrophy; tuberous sclerosis; Meckel syndrome. Birth Defects 10:35, 1973

Buchta RM, Viseskul C, Gilbert EF, Sarto GE, Optiz JM: Familial bilateral renal agenesis and hereditatry renal adysplasia. Z Kinderheilkd 115:111, 1973

Cain DR, Griggs D, Lackey DA, Kagan BM: Familial renal agenesis and total dysplasia. AM J Dis Child 128:377, 1974

Johannessen JV, Haneberg B, Moe PJ: Bilateral multicystic dysplasia of the kidneys. Beitr Pathol 148:290, 1973

Kyaw MM: Roentgenologic triad of congenital multicystic kidney. Am J Roentgenol Radium Ther Nucl Med 119:710, 1973

Leonidas JC, Strauss L, Krasna IH: Roentgen diagnosis of multicystic renal dysplasia in infancy by high dose urography. J Urol 108:963, 1972

Newman L, Simms K, Kissane J, McAlister WH: Unilateral total renal dysplasia in children. Am J Roentgenol Radium Ther Nucl Med 116:778, 1972

Risdon RA: Renal dysplasia. I. A clinico-pathological study of 76 cases. II. A necropsy study of 41 cases. J Clin Pathol 24:57, 65, 1971

Young LW, Wood BP, Spohr CH, Panner B: Delayed excretory uro-

graphic opacification, a puddling effect, in multicystic renal dysplasia. Ann Radiol (Paris) 17:391, 1973

POLYCYSTIC RENAL DISEASE

Bernstein J: Hereditary disorders of the kidney. I. Parenchymal defects and malformations. In Bolande RP, Rosenberg H (eds): Perspectives in Pediatric Pathology, Vol 1. Chicago, Year Book, 1973

———Heritable cystic disorders of the kidney: the mythology of polycystic disease. Pediatr Clin North Am 18:435, 1971

———The classification of renal cysts. Nephron 11:91, 1973

Blyth H, Ockenden BG: Polycystic disease of kidneys and liver presenting in childhood. J Med Genet 8:257, 1971

Carter CO: Polycystic disease presenting in childhood. Birth Defects 10:16, 1974

Elkin M, Bernstein J: Cystic disease of the kidney—radiological and pathological considerations. Clin Radiol 20:65, 1969

Jørgensen M: A stereological study of intrahepatic bile ducts. 3. Infantile polycystic disease. Acta Path Microbiol Scand [A] 81:670, 1973

———A stereological study of intrahepatic bile ducts. 4. Congenital hepatic fibrosis. Acta Path Microbiol Scand [A] 82:21, 1974

Kaye C, Lewy PR: Congenital appearance of adult-type (autosomal dominant) polycystic kidney disease. Report of a case. J Pediatr 85:807, 1974

Landing BH, Wells TR, Reed GB, Narayan MS: Diseases of the bile ducts in children. In Gall EA, Mostofi F, (eds): The Liver. Baltimore, Williams & Wilkins, 1973, Chap 22

Lieberman E, Salinas-Madrigal L, Gwinn JL, et al: Infantile polycystic disease of the kidneys and liver: clinical, pathological and radiological correlations and comparison with congenital hepatic fibrosis. Medicine 50:277, 1971

Murray-Lyon IM, Shilkin KB, Laws JW, Illing RC, Williams R: Nonobstructive dilatation of the intrahepatic biliary tree with cholangitis. Q J Med 164:477, 1972

Potter EL: Normal and Abnormal Development of the Kidney. Chicago, Year Book, 1972

Weiss L, Reynolds WA, Saeed SM, Cabal L: Congenital hepatic fibrosis and polycystic disease of kidneys with the roentgen appearance of medullary sponge kidney. Birth Defects 10:22, 1974

POSTURAL PROTEINURIA
CHESTER M. EDELMANN, JR.

Postural, or orthostatic, proteinuria is a condition in which significant protein excretion occurs in the upright position, particularly in hyperlordosis, but disappears or is reduced to normal levels (less than 25 mg/24 hours) during recumbency. The incidence of orthostatic proteinuria is not known, but the condition is said to be common, occurring in as many as 2 to 5 percent of adolescents. In the survey by Randolph and Greenfield of almost 4,000 children ranging in age from 3 weeks to 16 years who were screened for urinary tract disease, proteinuria was observed on at least one occasion in more than one-third. However, reexamination of the children with one positive test revealed no persistent, intermittent, or postural proteinuria in the entire group. Wagner and associates detected proteinuria on initial testing in 5.4 percent of 4,807 children aged 5 to 18 years. Only 1.1 percent had a positive second test. A number of these were thought to have orthostatic proteinuria.

The pathophysiology is not fully understood. Increased glomerular filtration of protein has been suggested, although diminished tubular reabsorption cannot be excluded. Elevated inferior vena caval pressure has been observed concomitantly with orthostatic protein excretion, but artificial elevation of the pressure in recumbency fails to reproduce this effect. Proteinuria has been induced in susceptible individuals by the application of tourniquets to the legs and by norepinephrine administration. Alternatively, it has been suggested that the protein may be derived from renal papillary lymph, although other studies strongly suggest a vascular orgin.

Orthostatic proteinuria has been shown to be nonselective and similar to the slight proteinuria present in normal subjects, suggesting that orthostatic proteinuria may simply reflect an exaggeration of the normal state. However, the technical difficulties in determining selectivity in normal subjects in the presence of very minimal proteinuria and the possibility of nonrenal sources of protein make this interpretation uncertain.

Erect posture and ambulation usually increase the rate of protein excretion in patients with renal disease. If renal abnormalities are mild protenuria may be demonstrable only in the erect or lordotic position. Therefore proteinuria cannot be classified as benign simply because it can be made to disappear during recumbency. King reported that one-third of 191 apparently healthy young males with postural proteinuria had developed constant proteinuria when examined 5 to 8 years later. Robinson and associates in a study of army recruits with a condition they termed fixed and reproducible orthostatic proteinuria, demonstrated significant abnormalities on renal biopsy in one-half. A 10-year follow-up evaluation was performed in 43 of the 64 young men initially studied. Although half continued to have proteinuria, clinical or laboratory evidence of progressive renal disease was not found in a single patient.

Light microscopy generally has revealed either no abnormalities or minimal alterations in glomerular structure; focal abnormalities in the glomeruli have been seen with electron microscopy. Lange and associates have reported the finding of gamma globulin and complement, suggesting the presence of immune complexes. Thus considerably more attention must be directed toward this condition than has been recommended in recent years, and all such patients should be investigated thoroughly. Long-term follow-ups of many patients are needed before the true significance of postural proteinuria can be determined.

Herdman and associates reported cessation or diminution of proteinuria in four of five patients with orthostatic proteinuria in response to adrenocortical steroid therapy and suggested that a diagnostic trial of steroid therapy in this condition might separate out patients with benign disease from those with a poorer prognosis.

The diagnosis of postural proteinuria is easily established by comparison between rates of excretion of protein in a timed overnight specimen (eg, an Addis count) and in a specimen obtained in the erect, and preferably lordotic, position. If postural proteinuria is found patients should have appropriate investigation to discover specific etiology and pathology. In the absence of demonstrable abnormality patients should be followed for possible subsequent development of overt renal disease.

References

Glover SN, Phillippi PJ, Lecocq FR, Longelier PR: Fixed and reproducible orthostatic proteinuria. I. Light microscopic studies of the kidney. Am J Pathol 39:291, 1961

Herdman RC, Michael AF, Good RA: Postural proteinuria. Response to corticosteroid therapy. Ann Intern Med 65:286, 1966

Lecocq FR, McPhaul JJ, Robinson RR: Fixed and reproducible orthostatic proteinuria. V. Results of a 5 year follow-up evaluation. Ann Intern Med 64:557, 1966

Lowgreen E: Studies on benign proteinuria with special reference to the renal lymphatic system. Acta Med Scand [Suppl] 5:300, 1966

Randolph MF, Greenfield M: Proteinuria. A six-year study of normal infants, preschool and school-age populations previously screened for urinary tract disease. Am J Dis Child 114:631, 1967

Robinson RR, Glenn WG: Fixed and reproducible orthostatic proteinuria. IV. Urinary albumin excretion by healthy human subjects in the recumbent and upright postures. J Lab Clin Med 64:717, 1964

Ruckley VA, MacDonald MK, MacLean PR, Robson JS: Glomerular ultrasructure and function in postural proteinuria. Nephron 3:153, 1966

Thompson AL, Durrett RR, Robinson RR: Fixed and reproducible orthostatic proteinuria. VI. Results of a 10-year follow-up evaluation. Ann Intern Med 73:235, 1970

Wagner MG, Smith FG Jr, Tinglof BO, Cornberg E: Epidemiology of proteinuria. A study of 4,807 school children. J Pediatr 73:825, 1968

GLOMERULONEPHRITIS

CHESTER M. EDELMANN, JR.

Glomerulonephritis is a term used to include a number of diseases of the kidney that affect primarily the glomeruli. These diseases are distinguished from primary vascular disorders, nephropathies associated with systemic diseases, toxic and infectious disorders of the kidneys, congenital parenchymal malformations, and so forth. Although they are considered collectively, since they exhibit many similarities in clinical courses and histologic abnormalities, it should be emphasized that these diseases undoubtedly have diverse causes, and their nosologic relationships are unclear.

Addis considered that all forms of glomerulonephritis began with an acute stage, even though the disease at that stage might not be clinically apparent. Longcope and Ellis subsequently divided glomerulonephritis into two groups, depending on whether the onset was acute or insidious. They recognized that recovery was the common course following acute glomerulonephritis, whereas failure to recover was most common when the onset was insidious.

In addition to these clinical classifications, attempts have been made to classify glomerulonephritis on the basis of the histologic changes within the kidney. More recently, classifications based on underlying immunologic mechanisms have been proposed. It is apparent, however, that no classification, clinical, pathologic, or immunologic, is completely satisfactory. The same disease may present clinically with an abrupt explosive onset and be labeled acute glomerulonephritis or may be detected fortuitously and ultimately be labeled chronic progressive glomerulonephritis. Conversely, patients presenting with any given clinical picture may have a wide variety of underlying histologic lesions.

Unfortunately, too little is known of the cause of most forms of glomerulonephritis to make possible a classification based on etiology. The classification used here, therefore, is based mainly on the various clinical syndromes that have been identified. This of necessity must result in some degree of confusion and redundancy. For example, lupus erythematosus, hereditary nephritis, and membranoproliferative glomerulonephritis all may present with a clinical picture indistinguishable at onset from acute postinfectious glomerulonephritis. As described here, however, acute glomerulonephritis refers to the last condition. The various diseases that may present clinically with the nephrotic syndrome are mentioned in the discussion of that condition. Nevertheless, the bulk of the section on the nephrotic syndrome deals with the idiopathic form commonly observed in children. Without this somewhat arbitrary restriction, many forms of progressive glomerulonephritis would need to be discussed under each of the headings acute glomerulonephritis, the nephrotic syndrome, and chronic progressive glomerulonephritis.

Attempts have been made to point out the interrelationships between the various clinical and pathologic syndromes, but the reader should be aware that distinctions often are arbitrary and a certain degree of compromise cannot be avoided.

References

Heptinstall RH: Glomerulonephritis: historical outline and classification. In Pathology of the Kidney. Boston, Little, Brown, 1966, p 235
White RHR: Glomerulonephritis in children. Br J Hosp Med May 1970, p 746

ETIOLOGY AND PATHOGENESIS

CLARK D. WEST

Currently most forms of acquired glomerulonephritis are considered to have their origin in an immune reaction. In the vast majority of the cases in children the sequence of the reaction is thought to be formation of antibody by the host, combination of antigen with antibody in the circulation, and deposition of a portion of the immune complexes thus formed in the glomerulus. The immune complexes almost immediately activate the complement system so that complement components deposited in the glomerulus may be found by immunofluorescence studies, and in some types of nephritis serum complement levels are low. The contribution of the complement reaction to the glomerular inflammation has not been established.

In rare instances in children nephritis can result from the formation of antibody to fixed antigen of the glomerular basement membrane (GBM). In this form, known as anti-GBM disease, the antibody reacts directly with basement membrane in situ and complexes do not circulate.

For a better understanding of the genesis of the types of glomerulonephritis produced by circulating immune complexes, the constituents of the immune reaction can be considered separately. The antigen that reacts with antibody in the circulation has not been identified with absolute certainty in any form of the disease. In acute poststreptococcal glomerulonephritis there is evidence that the antigen is a constituent of the plasma membrane of the streptococcus. In lupus nephritis the antigen is thought to be desoxyribonucleic acid. In the nephritis of chronic bacteremia, which occurs with subacute bacterial endocarditis and in patients with chronically infected ventriculoatrial shunts for relief of hydrocephalus, the antigen most likely derives from the invading organism. There is some evidence suggesting that in some cases of membranous glomerulopathy the glomerular deposits contain an antigen derived from the renal tubular epithelium. However, in other forms of chronic glomerulonephritis the nature of the antigen is not known. In animals it has been noted that certain chronic viral infections are often accompanied by glomerulonephritis. In these experimental diseases there is evidence that the antigen of the complex is derived from the virus, but similar evidence for this origin of antigen in the chronic nephritides in man has not been found.

A second requirement for the genesis of glomerulonephritis is the production of antibody, which in all types of glomerulonephritis is made by the host. In a few forms of glomerulonephritis free antibody of the type thought to be a constituent of the complex has been detected in the circulation. Thus in lupus nephritis an antibody reacting with nuclear material is readily demonstrated in serum, and in the nephritis of chronic bacteremia abundant antibody to the invader is found. In acute poststreptococcal nephritis antibody reactive with material deposited in the glomerulus has been detected by indirect means. However, in membranous glomerulopathy, membranoproliferative glomerulonephritis, the nephritis of anaphylactoid purpura, and other chronic nephritides, a circulating antibody that might possibly be responsible for the disease has so far escaped detection.

From studies in animals it seems likely that a variable fraction of the complexes formed in human glomerulonephritis may be removed from the circulation by the reticuloendothelial system. The fraction removed by this system probably depends on the size of the complexes and on their other characteristics. The hepatosplenomegaly often observed in such conditions as the nephritis of chronic baceremia and lupus nephritis probably reflects reticuloendothelial system hyperactivity produced by the circulating complexes. Complexes not removed by the reticuloendothelial system appear to deposit preferentially in the glomerular capillaries. The vulnerability of this site appears to be the result of the large volume of plasma being filtered in this bed. In animals the deposition of circulating complexes has been shown to be favored by histamine. In the presence of this agent endothelial cells of small vessels contract, allowing the complexes to deposit against the endothelial side of the capillary basement membrane. In serum sickness nephritis in the rabbit the release of histamine from platelets, apparently occurring as a result of an immune reaction, favors glomerular deposition of circulating complexes, and in the presence of an antihistamine the nephritis is less severe. The contribution of histamine release to glomerular complex deposition in nephritis in man has not been established, and the value of antihistamines in therapy has yet to be demonstrated.

With glomerular deposition of complexes identified as the nephritogenic event in most forms of glomerulonephritis, the question arises why glomerular morphology differs markedly in the various forms. Observations in animals have to a large extent answered this question. The glomerular morphology produced would appear to be dependent on the ability of the complexes to penetrate the glomerular basement membrane. For instance, following injection of ferritin, a macromolecule that cannot penetrate the basement membrane, it has been found by study of glomerular ultrastructure that the molecule initially penetrates the capillary endothelium and accumulates against the basement membrane in the subendothelial space. Moving in the subendothelial space the ferritin reaches the capillary waist and enters the mesangium, where under the influence of macrophagelike action of the mesangial cells the macromolecules coalesce into deposits that are often intracellular. Eventually the macromolecules disappear from the mesangium, probably via the lymphatics. Impenetrable immune complexes would appear to take the same route and by their pholgogenic properties produce mesangial hyperplasia. According to this concept membranoproliferative glomerulonephritis of the type characterized by subendothelial deposits is a prime example of a type produced by impenetrable complexes. Here complexes are abundant in the subendothelial space and in the mesangium, and there is marked mesangial proliferation; subepithelial deposits are rarely observed. Membranous glomerulopathy appears to be an example of a disease produced by penetrable complexes. After passage through the basement membrane the complexes responsible for this disease presumably are collected into deposits by the epithelial cells and reside in a subepithelial location. In this disease it is rare to see subendothelial or mesangial deposits, and the mesangium is usually not hypercellular. In a number of nephritides the complexes appear to be heterogeneous as to penetrability, and deposits are found in all three locations: subendothelially, subepithelially, and in the mesangium. Examples are acute poststreptococcal nephritis and certain stages in the development of lupus nephritis. Variability in the penetrability of the complexes in these diseases could be the result of differing ratios of antibody to antigen at the time the complexes form, differences in the valence of antibody, and perhaps differences in antigenic structure. The mechanism by which focal glomerulonephritis is produced in diseases such as the nephritis of anaphylactoid purpura is not fully understood.

In Goodpasture's syndrome and in certain rare cases of rapidly progressive glomerulonephritis the target of the antibody is an antigen present in the glomerular basement membrane. This antibody also reacts with antigen in the basement membrane of the lungs, and it is thought that the lung antigen stimulates antibody production. Thus in Goodpasture's syndrome the renal involvement usually follows the pulmonary manifestations. In this disease fluorescein-labeled antibody to IgG is seen deposited in a linear fashion along the basement membrane, whereas in forms of nephritis produced by circulating complexes fluorescence with labeled antibody to IgG or complement components is confined to discrete deposits located in the capillary wall or in the mesangium.

The concept that complement is involved in the production of glomerular inflammation in this disease has arisen from two sources: (1) the observation that complement components are usually found by immunofluorescence studies to be deposited in the glomeruli and (2) the fact that several forms of glomerulonephritis are accompanied by hypocomplementemia. The hypocomplementemia now appears to be the result of the presence of complement-reactive material in the circulation; reaction of plasma complement components with immune complexes deposited in the glomeruli probably contributes little to the hypocomplementemia. Understanding the significance and nature of the hypocomplementemia requires some familiarity with the complement system.

It now appears that the pivotal component of the complement system is C3, or β_1C-globulin, which is present in serum in a concentration of 90 to 200 mg/100 ml. Two and perhaps three pathways lead to activation of this component. One is the classic pathway in which immune complexes or aggregated gamma globulin activate C1, which in turn activates C4 and C2 to form the complex C$\overline{42}$. The C$\overline{42}$ complex is highly reactive with C3. Another pathway is the alternate pathway activated by complex polysaccharides that bypasses C1, C4, and C2 and involves properdin, properdin factor D, properdin factor B, and perhaps other serum proteins. In this pathway the activation of C3 occurs by cleavage of properdin factor B, with one of the cleavage products activating C3 in much the same way as it is activated by C$\overline{42}$. The third pathway, as yet not fully defined, is apparently activated only when immune complexes are abundant; it is designated the C1 bypass. This pathway involves, in order, C1, properdin, perhaps other proteins, and finally properdin factor B; properdin factor B presumably activates C3 as in the alternate pathway. Complexes that activate this bypass mechanism would also activate the classic pathway.

The activation of C3 via these three pathways has two effects. First, the activated C3 sets in motion a positive-feedback machanism, which results in further C3 activation. Thus C3b, the activated form of C3, sets in motion the reaction by which properdin factor D activates properdin factor B. This results in formation of more C3b. This feedback would continue to cycle if it were not for an inhibitor known as the C3b inactivator. This enzyme cleaves C3b into two relatively nonreactive breakdown products, C3c and C3d, also known as $\beta_1 A$ and $\alpha_2 d$. Second, the activated C3 in turn activates the terminal components of the complement pathway (C5 through C9).

In the course of the complement reaction various biologically active breakdown products of complement are generated that are phlogogenic and have other effects. These include chemotactic factors and anaphylatoxins, and if the reaction takes place on a cell wall the end result may be lysis of the cell.

The hypocomplementemia frequently observed in lupus nephritis and in the nephritis of chronic bacteremia has a complement profile characteristic of classic pathway activation, with low levels of C1, C4, and C2. Such a profile would be expected with an immune complex in the circulation. It is possible that in these diseases the C1 bypass mechanism is also activated. In acute poststreptococcal glomerulonephritis the complement profile is not so typical of classic pathway activation as in the two previously mentioned diseases, in that C1 is often in normal concentration but serum properdin levels are significantly reduced. The exact mechanism of activation in this disease is not known. In membranoproliferative glomerulonephritis C1 and C4 may be in somewhat reduced concentration, but the levels of C3 are most markedly affected. The mechanism of the C3 reduction is thought to be via a complement reactive factor known as the nephritic factor that activates the alternate pathway. In this disease the levels of the circulating nephritic factor and of C3 do not correlate well with the clinical course of the disease, and the mechanism by which this alternate pathway activator participates, if at all, in producing the glomerulonephritis is obscure. In all these nephritides studies of the metabolism of C3 have shown that C3 synthesis may be reduced, presumably by a negative feedback imposed on the synthetic mechanism by the presence of circulating C3 breakdown products.

From the above observations it could be inferred that in lupus nephritis and in the nephritis of chronic bacteremia the serum levels of the complement components reflect the presence of complement-reactive circulating complexes, and therefore the severity of the hypocomplementemia may in a general way parallel the severity of the nephritis. In acute poststreptococcal and membranoproliferative glomerulonephritis, on the other hand, the levels are of value as a diagnostic aid but do not reliably reflect events in the kidney. Thus in approximately 10 percent of the patients with acute poststreptococcal glomerulonephritis and 20 percent of those with membranoproliferative glomerulonephritis reduced serum complement levels may never be observed, and yet the nephritis may be severe.

The nephritides in which serum complement levels are normal, such as rapidly progressive nephritis and the nephritis of anaphylactoid purpura, often give evidence of a glomerular complement reaction, as attested by the fact that complement components may be found deposited in the glomeruli. Presumably, a complement-reactive factor does not circulate in these diseases.

The contribution of the complement reaction in the glomerulus to the glomerular inflammation has not been determined. The phlogogenic by-products of the reaction, anaphylatoxins and chemotactic factors, may be swept away from the site of the reaction too rapidly to be effective. The property of immune adherence, which is bestowed on a surface when C3b is deposited, may, if conferred on the capillary walls by a complement reaction, cause passing polymorphonuclear leukocytes to adhere, thus contributing to acute inflammation. It is possible that a complement reaction in the mesangium would be more phlogogenic than one in the capillary walls. It is known that complement components (at least C3) rather rapidly diffuse into the mesangium, and a reaction there may contribute to the mesangial hyperplasia frequently observed when there are mesangial deposits. Studies in experimental animals have indicated that experimental nephritis can occur under conditions in which the complement system is blocked, although in the presence of an intact complement system the disease is often more severe and the proteinuria less selective.

References

Cochrane CG: Mediation of immunologic glomerular injury. Transplant Proc 1:949, 1969

Farquhar MG, Palade GE: Functional evidence for the existence of a third cell type in the glomerulus. J Cell Biol 13:55, 1962

Germuth FG Jr, Rodriquez E: Immunopathology of the Renal Glomerulus: Immune Complex Deposit and Anti-basement Membrane Disease. Boston, Little, Brown, 1973

Kniker WT, Cochrane CG: The localization of circulating immune complexes in experimental serum sickness. The role of vasoactive amines and hydrodynamic forces. J Exp Med 127:119, 1968

Merrill JP: Glomerulonephritis. N Engl J Med 290:257, 1974

Müller-Eberhard HJ: Complement. Ann Rev Biochem 38:389, 1969

Nicol PAE, Lachmann PJ: The alternate pathway of complement activation. The role of C3 and its inactivator (KAF). Immunology 24:259, 1973

Treser G, Semer M, Ty A, et al: Partial characterization of antigenic streptococcal plasma membrane components in acute glomerulonephritis. J Clin Invest 49:762, 1970

West CD, Ruley EJ, Forristal J, Davis NC: Mechanisms of hypocomplementemia in glomerulonephritis. Kidney Int 3:116, 1973

ACUTE GLOMERULONEPHRITIS

CHESTER M. EDELMANN, JR.

Acute glomerulonephritis is characterized by the sudden onset of proteinuria and hematuria 1 or 2 weeks following a respiratory infection, in association with a variable degree of edema, hypertension, and oliguria. Performance of percutaneous renal biopsies soon after the onset of what appears clinically to be acute glomerulonephritis has led to the recognition that many of the chronic progressive glomerulopathies may be initiated or exacerbated by a syndrome that is indistinguishable clinically from acute postinfectious glomerulonephritis. It is the latter disease that will be discussed in this section.

ETIOLOGY. Experimental work and clincial observations both suggest that acute nephritis most commonly represents an altered tissue reaction following infection with group A β-hemolytic streptococci. Other infectious agents, including other bacteria and viruses, have been implicated, and it is likely that there are diverse etiologies. Differences in clinical course and renal histology dependent upon etiology have not been established, and only acute poststreptococcal nephritis will be described here in detail.

Although infection with group A streptococci precedes the acute episode in most instances, the rate of attack varies widely. It has been possible to demonstrate a rise of antistreptolysin O titer in 70 to 90 percent of afflicted children. It has been shown that most of the infections that precede acute nephritis are caused by type 12 or 4 hemolytic streptococci; less frequently other types (types 1, Red Lake, and 25) are implicated. The infection is usually·followed by a latent period before the nephritis becomes evident.

It is now generaly accepted that acute glomerulonephritis is a form of immune-complex disease, the antigenic component of the immune complex being related somehow to the streptococcus. However, most attempts at demonstrating streptococcal components or products in the deposits in the kidney have been unsuccessful. Lange and associates demonstrated in the serum of patients with acute glomerulonephritis antibody that reacted with the glomerular capillary wall of patients with early acute glomerulonephritis. The antibody appeared to be specific for streptococcal plasma membrane and presumably was reacting in the glomerulus with streptococcal material.

INCIDENCE. The incidence of acute nephritis in children is difficult to asssess. Systematic examination of the urine in children recovering from streptococcal infections has provided clinical evidence that many patients with acute glomerulonephritis are not diagnosed because they are either asymptomatic or have such mild sysmptoms that the disease is not suspected and the urine is not examined. The performance by Dodge and associates of percutaneous renal biopsies in family contacts of patients with acute glomerulonephritis has now confirmed the diagnosis in such children not suspected of having the disease. Although the proportion of patient who may be undiagnosed cannot be estimated with any assurance, the figure is probably high enough that any epidemiologic studies must be interpreted on the basis that the population being described is the empirical one composed of recognized or manifest cases. Reports of patients with poststreptococcal glomerulonephritis with minimal or no urinary findings, which may be more frequent in children than in adults, complicate epidemiologic analyses even further.

An analysis of the age of onset of clinically recognizable acute glomerulonephritis in 214 children during their first 12 years of life showed a peak incidence between 6 and 7 years, with about 60 percent of cases between ages 5 and 10 and 90 percent between 2 and 12 years of age (Fig. 11). Although it is not unknown, the disease is rare in patients under 1 year of age, probably because of the low incidence of streptococcal infections during that period. The high incidence during early school years may be related to the correspondingly high prevalence of streptococcal infections during that time.

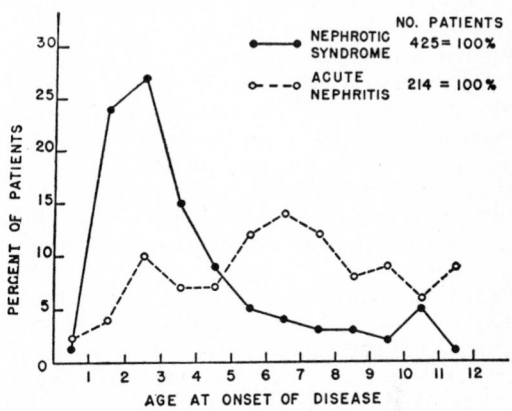

FIG. 11. Age of onset of acute nephritis in 214 patients and age of onset of the nephrotic syndrome in 425 patients. (From Barnett, Forman, and Lauson: Adv Pediatr 5:53, 1952.)

In acute nephritis associated with pharyngitis there is a distinct predominance of males over females, in some series as high as two to one, in contrast to nephritis assocated with pyoderma, in which the sex distribution is equal. Familial incidence is directly related to familial occurrence of respiratory and skin infections.

CLINICAL FEATURES. Clinical manifestations of acute glomerulonephritis usually occur after an asymptomatic period following infection, rarely while the acute infection is still present. The preceding infection is usually one involving deep tissues of the upper respiratory tract, such as tonsillitis, otitis media, or cervical adenitis, and is followed by a latent period of about 10 days. Not infrequently, particularly in warm climates, infections of the skin, (notably impetigo) precede glomerulonephritis, in which case the latent period averages 3 weeks. In some instances there is no knowledge of a preceding infection. Coexistence of active rheumatic fever and acute glomerulonephritis is rare, although it does occur; it was observed twice in one series of 140 patients with rheumatic fever.

There is marked variation in the intensity and distribution of symptoms and signs at the onset and during the early stage of acute nephritis. In many instances the symptoms and the urinary findings are so mild that unless they are specifically looked for, the disease goes unrecognized. It is probable that the number of such unrecognized cases greatly exceeds those recognized.

The usual clinical manifestations of acute nephritis are a mild degree of edema, urinary abnormalities (hematuria, proteinuria, and cylindruria), and varying degrees of hypertension. The possiblity of a child presenting with minimal or even no urinary abnormalities must not be overlooked. In one group of 144 hospitalized patients 77 percent had urinary abnormalities, edema, and, hypertension; 9 percent had urinary abnormalities and edema; 6 percent had urinary abnormalities and hypertension; and only 8 percent had urinary abnormalities alone. Abdominal pain is present in more than half of all patients. Other less frequent symptoms are low-grade fever, anorexia, vomiting, and headache. Evidences of the preceding infection may persist in the respiratory tract or skin.

The early phase of acute nephritis in children is made perilous by three possible complications: hypertensive encephalopathy, cardiac failure, and acute renal failure. Early recognition and prompt treatment of these complications are of greatest importance. Although usually present soon after the onset of disease, they may develop several days later, a fact that necessitates close observation.

Edema is present in most patients, although fluid retention may not be apparent until the patient has lost several pounds of weight in association with a diuresis. Edema is almost certainly due to primary renal retention of salt and water; the theory attributing it to generalized increased vascular permeability has been discarded.

Symptoms and signs referable to the heart occur in many patients with acute nephritis, and heart failure dominates the clinical picture in some. Paroxysmal or persistent dyspnea, orthopnea, apical gallop rhythm, cardiac enlargement, venous engorgement, enlarged liver,and pulmonary edema may appear suddenly during the course of the disease or may be the first manifestation of the disease. Radiographic evidence of pulmonary edema is seen in as many as 60 percent of cases. The cause of heart failure in acute nephritis is not certain, but it is probably attributable to an increase in blood volume secondary to retention of sodium and water. Although cardiac work may be aggravated by accompanying hypertension, it seems clear that failure is not due to hypertension per se. Evidence for myocarditis is lacking.

Hypertensive encephalopathy is characterized by headache, vomiting, irritability or apathy, convulsions, transitory paralyses, and coma. Temporary complete blindness occurs occasionally. The cause of the elevated blood pressure is unknown. The hypertension of acute nephritis is attributed to expanded vascular volume or to vasospasm, the cerbral symptoms being caused by cerebral ischemia and anoxia. Papilledema may or may not be present. Blood pressure may be as high as 160 to 200 mm Hg systolic and 100 to 140 mm Hg diastolic. Severe renal failure (p. 1147) is a less common complication of acute nephritis in children. It is characterized by marked oliguria or anuria.

LABORATORY FINDINGS. Although urinary abnormalities may be minimal, proteinuria is almost always present, ranging from 1+ to 4+. Quantitatively there is usually not more than 1 g of protein in a 12-hour overnight collection, and there may be as little as 25 or 50 mg. Gross or microscopic hematuria is almost always present, the urine usually being reddish brown or smoky in appearance. The supernatant usually is brownish, indicting hemolysis and release of hemoglobin that has been converted to acid hematin. The urinary sediment also contains many white blood cells and epithelial cells and hyaline, granular, and red blood cell casts. Early in the disease white blood cells in the urine may predominate, thus suggesting a urinary tract infection. These urinary abnormalities may vary independently in severity and duration.

In nephritis associated with pharyngitis the antistreptolysin O titer is usually elevated, the degree and duration of the elevation being related to hemolytic streptococcal infection rather than to the severity or duration of glomerulonephritis. Antistreptolysin O response following streptococcal impetigo is uncommon. Hypocomplementemia is demonstrable in 90 percent or more of cases and is very useful in differential diagnosis. With the exception of lupus erythematosus, the finding of a transiently low complement level in a patient presenting clinically with acute nephritis almost assures the diagnosis of postinfectious glomerulonephritis.

Mild hypoalbuminemia is commonly found and is usually dilutional in origin. Occasionally it is caused, at least in part, by severe proteinuria. Almost one-half of children have moderate degrees of hypercholesterolemia as part of a generalized hyperlipidemia. The cause of these elevations is unknown. Hypoalbuminemia and hyperlipidemia in association with proteinuria and edema may lead initally to the diagnosis of the idopathic nephrotic syndrome.

Moderate elevation of body temperature and leukocytosis may be present during the first few days. Mild anemia is usually present, being attributable to expansion of the vascular volume. Hemolysis and bone marrow depression are either absent or play only minor roles. Unexplained thrombocytopenia has been reported and may be related to the preceding infection, although this finding should alert the physician to the possiblity of a hemolytic-uremic syndrome. Elevation of the erythrocyte sedimentation rate develops during the course of acute glomerulonephritis. Transient electrocardiographic changes consisting of premature beats, T-wave inversion, and prolongation of the P-R interval may occur.

Renal functional impairment is usually present from the onset. The most characteristic alteration is reduction in GFR. Urea and creatinine clearances are usually depressed, with the blood urea and creatinine concentrations correspondingly increased. Renal plasma flow is usually normal or slightly increased, rarely decreased. The filtration fraction characteristically is low. This low filtration fraction indicates that the functional alteration, like the morphologic one, is predominantly glomerular. Ability to excrete water may be maintained but is frequently impaired. Maximal concentrating capacity is retained throughout in about 40 percent of patients with acute glomerulonephritis; in the remainder it may be impaired either early or late. The few observations on other tubular functions, such as extraction ratio of *p*-aminohippurate and maximal rates of tubular transport of PAH and glucose, indicate that these functions frequently are impaired to some degree. Return of the various renal functions to normal generally lags behind clinical improvement; decreased glomerular filtration and impaired concentrating capacity may persist after blood pressure has returned to normal and edema has disappeared.

PATHOLOGY. Renal biopsies in cases diagnosed clinically as acute postinfectious glomerulonephritis show a variety of histologic lesions, not all of which are properly regarded as acute glomerulonephritis. It seems apparent that long-standing renal disease, such as Alport's syndrome and familial hematuria, may undergo exacerbation and that other renal diseases, such as membranoproliferative glomerulonephritis, can have their clinical onset following an actue infection. Without regard to the etiologic implications of these observations, the histologic differentiation of these types from typical acute glomerulonephritis is of the utmost importance in determining prognosis. Acute proliferative glomerulonephritis is a nonsuppurative inflammatory disease that characteristically involves virtually all glomeruli. The most striking abnormality is hypercellularity, compounded of swelling and proliferation of the capillary endothelial cells and proliferation of the mesangial or intercapillary cells, the combination sometimes being referred to as endocapillary proliferation. The glomeruli are usually enlarged, sometimes considerably, and they are ischemic, despite the presence of leukocytes within the capillary lumens. Immunofluorescence studies have demonstrated in typical cases granular deposits of immunoglobulin (IgG), complement, and properdin around the capillary walls. Electron microscopic studies have shown subepithelial deposits of electron-dense material, forming localized bumps or humps that contain immune complexes. Occasional electron-dense deposits may be seen within or beneath the basement membrane. Deposits of material similar to basement membrane are also found among the mesangial cells in the glomerular stalks, and the mesangial cells are enlarged and increased in number. The epithelial cells are variably swollen, with focal fusion of the foot processes. In what is ordinarily regarded as more severe involvement, glomerular capillaries may be thrombosed, with focal necrosis of the capillary tufts. Leakage of fibrin into Bowman's space elicits proliferation of the glomerular epithelium (extracapillary proliferation) to form crescents. Tubular necrosis and disruption are occasionally seen with severe glomerular inflammation.

Some cases are predominantly exudative and others proliferative, apparently without reflecting significant clinical differences. The histologic severity of the glomerular lesion seems to be correlated in a general way with the severity of the clinical course, and cases of permanent renal impairment are found among those children who had acute glomerulonephritis as their initial disease. Histologic resolution of the inflammatory process is protracted beyond the duration of the clinical disease. Most cases in childhood go on to complete recovery, with perhaps only focal glomerular scarring. It may be anticipated that focally necrotic or damaged glomeruli will heal with scarring and that extensive damage and glomerular sclerosis will lead to a glomerular deficit with functional impairment. It should be noted in this regard that 50 to 75 percent of children with extracapillary and endocapillary proliferative glomerulonephritis (that is, with severe crescent formation) experience resolution of their disease and that they appear not to be left with renal insufficiency. The question of whether continuing glomerular sclerosis and obsolescence following acute glomerulonephritis is a residuum of the initial lesion or a reflection of chronic disease remains unresolved. There is no evidence at all that mild or unrecognized or clinically silent lesions of this type progress to chronic glomerulonephritis. The differentiation of other, potentially chronic, lesions therefore becomes all the more important.

DIFFERENTIAL DIAGNOSIS. The onset of the classic manifestations of acute glomerulonephritis (urinary abnormalities, edema, and hypertension) following infection in a child usually establishes the diagnosis without difficulty. When there are only urinary abnormalities the diagnosis is more difficult. Transient urinary abnormalities may occur in the course of dehydration, heart failure, infections, and drug intoxications. Their persistence for a week without other explanation suggests the diagnosis of primary glomerular disease. Differentiation from postural proteinuria may require careful observation.

Urinary tract infection should be considered in the differential diagnosis even in the absence of specific sysmptoms. Urine cultures, with quantitation of bacteriuria, serve to establish the daignosis. Benign recurrent hematuria may mimic acute nephritis in almost every respect, and it is differentiated on the basis of the absence of hypocomplementemia and the clinical course (p. 1323).

Not infrequently the onset of some type of progressive glomerulonephritis, particularly membranoproliferative disease, mimics acute glomerulonephritis. Exacerbation of preexisting chronic nephritis also may easily be mistaken for acute disease. The history and prior urinalyses, in addition to renal biopsy close to the onset of recognized disease, are of value in the differential diagnosis. Additional conditions that have to be considered are renal disease associated with Schönlein-Henoch syndrome, systemic lupus erythematosus, and periarteritis nodosa.

It should be emphasized that despite typical clinical and laboratory findings the diagnosis of acute poststreptococcal glomerulonephritis cannot be established with certainty without histologic examination of the kidney. Therefore a renal biopsy should be performed in all atypical cases, in all cases that are unusually severe, and in patients who are not following the expected course of recovery.

TREATMENT. The preventive treatment of acute nephritis consists in the prevention of streptococcal infections. An epidemic of acute nephritis at Red Lake,

Minnesota, was prompty terminated by mass prophylaxis with benzathine penicillin. However, once the infection is clinically evident the incidence of nephritis can be decreased only slightly, if at all, with early and adequate treatment with antibiotics. After the nephritis itself has developed antibiotics fail to affect its course. They are indicated only when there is evidence of persistent streptococcal infection.

No therapeutic measure has been demonstrated that can favorably influence the course of acute glomerulonephritis. Prompt recognition and treatment of the early complications, based on sound understanding of the disturbed physiology, constitute the most urgent aspects of treatment.

EDEMA AND CONGESTIVE FAILURE.   Salt restriction is the most important and frequently the only measure required in the therapy of edema. Patients demonstrating severe degrees of edema and oliguria may require management, including dialysis, as described under *acute renal failure* (p. 1247). Diuretics are usually ineffective, although a trial of furosemide or ethacrynic acid may be warranted. Patients with evidence of circulatory congestion and pulmonary edema may respond well to elevation of the head of the bed, phlebotomy, rotating tourniquets, positive-pressure oxygen, and morphine. The value of digitalis is still debated, but it probably should be given in the desperately ill patient.

HYPERTENSION.   When there is evidence of rising blood pressure, or when the diastolic value exceeds 90 mm Hg, antihypertensive therapy should be given. Magnesium sulfate has been used widely for the treatment of hypertension, but with development of more effective and less toxic agents it is no longer indicated. A combination of reserpine (80 to 150 μg/kg) and hydralazine (250 to 500 μg/kg) given intramuscularly constitutes the treatment of choice. Often only a single dose is necessary, but the drugs should be given repeatedly as needed, with appropriate modification of dosage (see p. 1489).

In situations with marked rises in blood pressure requiring more urgent control, diazoxide appears to be the drug of choice; it will produce a drop in blood pressure within a few minutes.

BED REST.   Although traditional therapy of acute glomerulonephritis has included prolonged bed rest, a much less restrictive policy is now generally recommended. Bed rest is indicated as long as there are clinical manifestations of active disease, such as edema, hypertension, or gross hematuria. These usually subside within 2 or 3 weeks, after which the patient feels quite well. At this state the patient may be allowed out of bed, with activity gradually being resumed. Within a few weeks most children are back in school, but exhausting and competitive acivities are prohibited until the Addis count returns to normal. This policy of early ambulation is well supported by many observations, especially the controlled studies of Akerrén and Lindgren in Sweden.

DIET.   Although protein restriction has been advocated in the past, present evidence indicates that it is without value. Illingworth and associates treated 42 cases by allocating them randomly to two dietary regimens: severe protein restriction and ordinary ward diet. Each patient was observed for a minimum period of 1 year, and strict criteria of cure were applied. Their investigation failed to reveal any advantage in restricting protein. Similarly, Mortensen placed 44 patient alternately on low- and high-protein diets. Evaluation of these patients 2 years after discharge revealed that those on the high-protein diet recovered more rapidly than those on the restricted diet. It appears, then, that the only time that protein need be restricted is if acute renal failure occurs during the initial stage of acute nephritis. The same principle applies to the salt content of the diet, which should be that of a normal diet except during the period of hypertension, edema, and oliguria.

ANTIBIOTICS.   Recommendations vary concerning the prevention and treatment of infections in children recovering from acute nephritis. Although continuous prophylactic adminstration of antibiotics has been recommended, we do not believe this is justified. As has been pointed out, second attacks are rare. The situation differs from that in rheumatic fever in that the number of nephritogenic types of streptococci is limited; the great majority of attacks are caused by type 12, and a permanent immunity to this type results from an attack.

COURSE AND PROGNOSIS.   In the great majority of instances the course of acute glomerulonephritis in children is benign. In the past the majority of deaths have been due to extension of the preceding streptococcal infection, congestive heart failure, or hypertension with central nervous system complications. Deaths from these causes are now rare; in a prospective study of 362 children with acute glomerulonephritis there were no deaths attributable to them. Early deaths from acute renal failure, which appears to be more frequent and more severe in adults than in children, have been almost totally eliminated with the use of peritoneal dialysis or hemodialysis.

In the course of 1 to 3 weeks edema, gross hematuria, and hypertension, if they have been present, ordinarily have disappeared, and the patient usually feels quite well. Abnormal laboratory findings usually last somewhat longer. Functional impairment, as shown by azotemia or impaired clearances of urea, creatinine, or inulin, may persist for 1 or 2 months, occasionally as long as 6 months. Addis counts remain abnormal somewhat longer, usually not more than 6 months but sometimes for more than a year. If renal function has returned to normal one can confidently predict that the urinary abnormalities will do so, although somewhat later, and permanent recovery is practically assured (Fig. 12). The probability of a second attack is less than the probability of a first attack in the population at large, because permanent immunity develops against the particular nephritogenic strain of streptococcus that has caused the attack.

The proportion of patients who fail to heal following what appears clinically to be acute glomerulonephritis is generally estimated to range from 15 to 30 percent in adults and from zero to 10 percent in children. These estimates, previously based on clinical data alone, must be reexamined to include the relationship between the clinical and pathologic features of the disease. Understanding the nature and course of the disease or diseases in these patients requires additional information on several important questions. The one that has been argued most extensively is whether acute glomerulone-

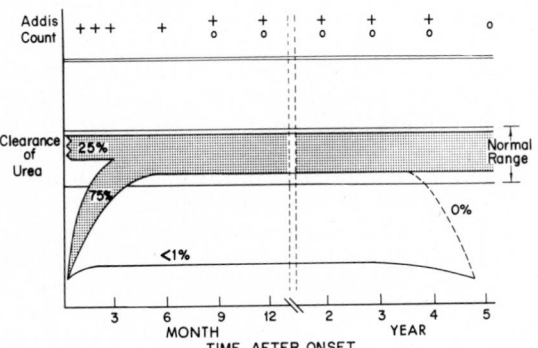

FIG. 12. Schematic representation of the course of acute glomerulonephritis in children.

phritis in children is an antecedent of chronic nephritis in adults. Prospective studies have revealed complete healing in such a high proportion of children that a relationship with chronic nephritis in adults seems very unlikely. However, at least two possible situations could negate this suggestion. Acute glomerulonephritis in children whose clinical features are so mild that the disease is not recognized could, unlike the recognized form, lead to latent disease first manifested as chronic nephritis of unknown cause in adults. However, the experience of most, though not all, pediatric nephrologists suggests that the severity of the clinical manifestions correlates with the severity of the pathologic change in the glomerulus and with the patient's prognosis. It seems unlikely, therefore, that complete healing would occur less frequently in children with the mildest clinical disease.

The preceding discussion does not exclude completely the second possibility—that what appears clinically to be complete healing may be associated histologically with pathologic processes that might lead to future disease after a long latent period. Persistent histologic alterations observed in renal biopsy of children who clinically have recovered completely provide tentative support for this concept. However, until much more evidence is at hand it does not seem reasonable to assume that there is a relationship between acute glomerulonephritis in children and chronic nephritis of unknown cause in adults.

Another important unanswered question concerns the nature of the disease or diseases in children with apparent acute glomerulonephritis that fails to heal. Percutaneous renal biopsy has shown that some patients in these groups have had preexisting glomerular

disease, the proportion being lower in children than in adults. Such exacerbations of preexisting renal disease may follow streptococcal as well as other infections, which in itself does not establish the diagnosis of acute poststreptococcal glomerulonephritis. In other patients what appears to be acute glomerulonephritis is in fact the onset of one of the many types of progressive glomerulonephritis.

Excluding these patients there remains a very small number of patients with typical acute poststreptococcal glomerulonephritis who do develop chronic renal disease. These children usually have severe symptoms initially, with depressed renal function that may improve but does not return to normal. Thus their progression is from what appears to be acute glomerulonephritis directly to chronic renal insufficiency over a period of months or years. Renal biopsies suggest that in these children so many glomeruli were destroyed in the initial episode that chronic renal insufficiency developed even though there was no continuing activity of the initial disease process.

Children apparently do not develop chronic nephritis after a latent stage of several years during which renal function is normal and Addis count abnormal. If children go through such a course it must be extremely rare, and no justification exists for trying to explain from such a sequence the large number of cases of chronic nephritis seen in adults.

References

Addis T: Glomerular Nephritis; Diagnosis and Treatment. New York, Macmillan, 1948

Akerrén Y, Lindgren M: Investigation concerning early rising in acute haemorrhagic nephritis. Acta Med Scand 151:419, 1955

Baldwin DS, Gluck MD, Schacht RG, Gallo G: The long-term course of poststreptococcal glomerulonephritis. Ann Intern Med 80:342, 1974

Bernsteen J,: ...

Dodge WF, Spargo BH, Travis LB, et al: Poststreptococcal glomerulonephritis. A prospective study in children. N Engl J Med 286: 273, 1972

————Spargo BH, Bass JA, Travis LB: The relationship between the clinical and pathologic features of poststreptococcal glomerulonephritis. A study of the early natural history. Medicine 47:227, 1968

Edelmann CM, Jr, Greifer I, Barnett HL: The nature of kidney disease in children who fail to recover from acute glomerulonephritis. J Pediatr 64:879, 1964

Fish AJ, Herdman RC, Michael AF, Pickering RJ, Good RA: Epidemic acute glomerulonephritis associated with type 49 streptococcal pyoderma. II. Correlative study of light, immunofluorescent and electron microscopic findings. Am J Med 48:28, 1970

Greifer I: Clinicopathology and natural history of acute glomerulonephritis. In Metcoff J (ed): Acute Glomerulonephritis, 17th Annual Conference on the Kidney. Boston, Little, Brown, 1967, p 165

Hall WD, Blumberg RW, Moody MD: Studies in children with impetigo. Bacteriology, serology, and incidence of glomerulonephritis. Am J Dis Child 125:800, 1973

Hoyer JR, Michael, AF, Fish AJ, Good RA: Acute poststreptococcal glomerulonephritis presenting as hypertensive encephalopathy with minimal urinary abnormalities. Pediatrics 39:412, 1967

Illingworth RS, Philpott MG, Rendle-Short J: A controlled investigation of the effect of diet on acute nephritis. Arch Dis Child 29:551, 1954

Jennings RB, Earle DP: Poststreptococcal glomerulonephritis: histopathologic and clinical studies of the acute, subsiding acute, and early chronic latent phases. J Clin Invest 40:1525, 1961

Joseph MC, Polani PE: The effect of bed rest on acute hemorrhagic nephritis in children. Guys Hosp Rep 107:500, 1958

Kandall S, Edelmann CM Jr, Bernstein J: Acute poststreptococcal glomerulonephritis. A case with minimal urinary abnormalities. Am J Dis Child 118:426, 1969

Kaplan EL, Anthony BF, Chapman SS, Wannamaker LW: Epidemic acute glomerulonephritis associated with type 49 streptococcal pyoderma. I. Clinical and laboratory findings. Am J Med 48:9, 1970

Lewy JE, Salinas-Madrigal L, Herdson PB, Pirani CL, Metcoff J: Clinicopathologic correlations in acute poststreptococcal glomerulonephritis. Medicine 50:453, 1971

Strife CF, McAdams AJ, McEnery PT, Bove KE, West CD: Hypocomplementemic and normocomplementemic acute nephritis in children: a comparison with respect to etiology, clinical manifestations and glomerular morphology. J Pediatr 84:29, 1974

Travis LB, Dodge WF, Beathard GA, et al: Acute glomerulonephritis in children. A review of the natural history with emphasis on prognosis. Clin Nephrol 1:169, 1973

Treser G, Ehrenreich T, Ores R, et al: Natural history of "apparently healed" acute poststreptococcal glomerulonephritis in children. Pediatrics 43:1005, 1969

Van Ackar KJ,...

Wannamaker, LW: Differences between streptococcal infections of the throat and of the skin. N Engl J Med 282:23, 1970

RAPIDLY PROGRESSIVE GLOMERULONEPHRITIS

CHESTER M. EDELMANN, JR.

The term rapidly progressive glomerulonephritis refers to a severe form of glomerulonephritis that follows a very rapid course varying from a few weeks to a few months; it commonly ends in uremia that requires maintenance hemodialysis or renal transplantation. The cause and pathogenesis are unknown; some cases may represent a severe form of acute poststreptococcal glomerulonephritis, but more often the disease appears to be a separate entity.

Most reported cases have been in young adults, but a number of children have been described as well. The clinical onset may be acute or insidious. Proteinuria and hematuria are present, and azotemia progresses rapidly. Histologic examination of the kidneys customarily shows marked glomerular epithelial proliferation that forms crescents, a finding that has come to be regarded as characteristic of the condition and has given rise to the name crescentic glomerulonephritis. Mesangial proliferation, on the other hand, has been quite variable —severe in some instances and negligible in others. Immunofluorescence studies have most often shown only fibrin in the crescents and a lack of immunoglobulin. A few cases have had linear deposition of IgG, as in Goodpasture's syndrome, but the significance of the observation is controversial. Subepithelial localization of IgE has been described in a few cases.

Differential diagnosis must take into consideration acute poststreptococcal glomerulonephritis, hypersensitivity angiitis, lupus erythematosus, hemolytic-uremic syndrome, Schönlein-Henoch nephritis, and in adults Wegener's granulomatosis, all of which can have prolonged oliguric nephritis with the histologic picture of severe extracapillary proliferative glomerulonephritis.

No treatment has been demonstrated to be effective, although claims have been made for the beneficial effects of both heparin and immunosuppressive agents.

CHRONIC PROGRESSIVE GLOMERULONEPHRITIS OF NONSPECIFIC ETIOLOGY

CHESTER M. EDELMANN, JR.

Chronic nephritis encompasses a group of many diseases rather than a single entity. It is characterized by bilateral, nonsuppurative disease of the kidneys, with continued loss of nephrons, progressive reduction in renal function, and ultimate renal insufficiency. Considered here are those conditions associated with primary glomerular diseases. Progressive glomerular diseases associated with systemic diseases such as anaphylactoid purpura, metabolic diseases such as diabetes mellitus, and collagen diseases such as lupus erythematosus are discussed elsewhere. It is difficult to estimate the frequency with which chronic nephritis in children is associated with these various conditions. It would appear, however, that in most instances it arises de novo. The end stage comprises the pathologic features of glomerular obsolescence, tubular atrophy, and cortical fibrosis. Secondary vascular changes and chronic inflammation complicate the histologic picture. Occasionally remnants of the active process provide a clue to the initial lesion. Much more information can be obtained by studying renal biopsies during the course of disease.

ETIOLOGY AND MORPHOLOGIC CLASSIFICATION. In children, as in adults, chronic nephritis may develop insidiously in the absence of any evidence of previous kidney disease, it may manifest with a nephrotic syndrome, or it may begin with what appears to be acute nephritis. It has been suggested that a common cause of chronic nephritis in adolescents and adults is acute poststreptococcal glomerulonephritis in childhood that has usually gone unrecognized. However, there is no convincing evidence for the progression, following a prolonged latent phase, of acute to chronic glomerulonephritis in either children or adults (see p.1269). The cause and pathogenesis of most forms of chronic glomerulonephritis are unknown, although recent evidence suggests that immune mechanisms and disorders of coagulation may play a major role (see p.1264). Renal biopsy has served to group the various nephritides into a number of histologic patterns, even though it is most likely that each morphologic type includes a number of different entities.

One histologic pattern found in children is *diffuse proliferative glomerulonephritis,* with crescent formation and hyalinization and sclerosis of glomeruli. The clinical features in such patients are extremely variable. They usually progress insidiously and may be detected fortuitously. The patient may present initially with what appears clinically to be acute glomerulonephritis, despite evidence of chronic disease by renal biopsy; uncommonly in children the first manifestation is the nephrotic syndrome; other children present for the first time in terminal renal failure. The pathogenesis of disease is entirely unknown, and there is no specific laboratory test. The course of the disease in these patients may be slow or rapid. They do not appear to be affected by any form of therapy. It must be remembered that some of these cases will eventually be found to have Alport's syndrome.

Focal glomerulonephritis refers to a histologic pattern in which only some of the glomeruli reveal abnormalities, in contrast to the diffuse involvement seen in most types of nephritis. This form of glomerular disease has been found in association with collagen disease; it may occur as a complication of bacteremia, particularly bacterial endocarditis, and it apparently may occur without known cause. Focal glomerulonephritis has been observed in some cases with IgA-IgG nephritis (Berger's disease)(p.1263),which can progress to glomerular scarring and obsolescence. The early impression of Berger's disease as a relatively benign condition with only rare examples of serious disease has given way to the realization, as the result of long-term studies, that a large number of such patients eventually develop renal insufficency. The renal lesion may be focal in systemic disease like Schönlein-Henoch purpura and systemic lupus erythematosus, both of which are associated with mesangial deposition of IgA. Therefore the histologic finding of focal glomerulonephritis is not to be regarded as indicative of a single disease—a view also supported by the extreme variability in clinical expression.

There are no distinctive clinical or laboratory features. Urinary findings vary from minimal abnormalities to massive proteinuria and gross hematuria. Reduction in renal function is usually only moderate and may be entirely absent. Evidence of preceding streptococcal or other infection is lacking. Differential diagnosis consists simply of ruling out known specific renal disease. In the absence of identifiable etiology, and with the histologic demonstration of focal renal involvement, the diagnosis of focal glomerulonephritis is made. Some cases appear to be self-limiting, although since focal glomerulonephritis is a pathologic diagnosis associated with a variety of diseases its course is extremely variable. Renal failure has been reported, although the disease may continue for many years. Treatment is entirely symptomatic unless a specific etiology is determined.

Membranoproliferative glomerulonephritis is a specific type of glomerular disease in children that often is associated with persistent or recurrent hypocomplementemia, although not all patients with hypocomplementemia have this histologic lesion. It appears to be the same disease as described under the term lobular glomerulonephritis. It commonly presents with the nephrotic syndrome, but it may develop insidiously or have an abrupt onset similar to that of acute poststreptococcal glomerulonephritis, with which it may be confused.

Membranoproliferative glomerulonephritis occurs in two principal morphologic forms: (a) subendothelial deposits with mesangial interposition and double-contour basement membranes and (2) intramembranous dense deposits. Either pattern may be associated with epithelial crescents, mesangial sclerosis and hyperlobulation (lobular glomerulonephritis), or extramembranous deposits separated by argyrophilic spikes. In the first type deposits of immunoglobulin (predominantly IgG) and complement are found along the peripheral capillary walls between the basement membrane and endothelium, and granular deposits of complement are also present in the mesangium. In the second type the lamina densa of the capillary wall is thickened by intramembranous electron-dense deposits of complement, which are present also as granular deposits in the mesangium. Properdin may also be localized to the peripheral capillary wall. The second type (dense-deposit disease) is associated with persistent hypocomplementemia, and because of its highly distinctive morphologic appearance, it has been recognized to recur in renal allografts. The clinical differences between the two types are otherwise minor. However, dense-deposit disease with crescents does have a relatively rapid progressive course and an extremely poor prognosis. Membranoproliferative glomerulonephritis with subendothelial deposits containing tubular epithelial antigen has been identified as a form of immune-complex nephropathy in patients with sickle cell disease, and some patients with viral hepatitis develop nephritis with the histologic appearance of membranoproliferative disease. Membranoproliferative glomerulonephritis with dense deposits is seen in association with hereditary lipodystrophy, usually the syndrome of partial lipodystrophy.

The course of membranoproliferative glomerulonephritis may be rapidly progressive, but it usually extends over a period of many years and involves progressive uremia and ultimate loss of renal functioning requiring maintenance hemodialysis and renal transplantation. It has been pointed out that patients may have normal function and be totally asymptomatic over a period of years, a circumstance not to be misinterpreted as indicating a good prognosis. At times the serum complement level may return to normal, despite clinical and histologic evidence of continued active disease.

Pure membranous nephropathy is usually detected during the investigation of a child with the nephrotic syndrome; however, it may be found in patients with minimal, asymptomatic proteinuria. The course of this disease is usually quite protracted, and patients characteristically are well for many years prior to developing renal failure. It should be noted that some children with membranous nephropathy develop spontaneous remissions and occasionally complete resolution.

In patients with the nephrotic syndrome complete clinical and biochemical remission may occur, and patients with proteinuria as the only manifestation may have a return to an entirely normal urine; nevertheless, renal biopsy demonstrates steady progression of disease, and recovery is not to be anticipated. Recent evidence suggests that this may be another example of immune-complex disease, although the nature of the antigen is not known (see p.1281).

CLINICAL FEATURES. As noted above, patients with chronic nephritis may have few if any symptoms for long periods of time. Indeed, the condition may be detected by the chance finding of asymptomatic proteinuria or hematuria. If it has been preceded by the nephrotic syndrome there is often a period of months or even years during which the tendency toward edema subsides and the proteinuria decreases.

Hypertension, with significant elevation of diastolic pressure, is often present. Ophthalmoscopic examination in patients with hypertension shows constricted retinal vessels, edema, exudates, or hemorrhages. Even with persistent reduction of kidney function children may continue to grow through mid-childhood and begin to have symptoms only during adolescence. When symptoms do develop lassitude and fatigability are common, and anemia is almost invariably present. There may be headache, restlessness, and insomnia. Muscular pains and twitchings are frequent, and there may be convulsions associated with hypertension. Rickets may become clinically manifest, and tetany may be present. Pericarditis is unusual in children.

As the condition advances the patient tends to become drowsy; he may develop Cheyne-Stokes respiration; death follows, usually preceded by coma. The nature of the factors responsible for these manifestations remains obscure. Acidosis and dehydration play a limited part in the symptomatology. Nitrogen retention may be marked, but the symptoms cannot be attributed to or correlated with the level of any known nitrogenous constituent of the blood. Despite this uncertainly it seems likely that retention of some end product of metabolism is responsible.

LABORATORY FEATURES. The most consistent laboratory finding in chronic glomerulonephritis is proteinuria. The degree of proteinuria is extremely variable, and particularly in the late stages of the disease it may be minimal. The urinary sediment contains abnormal numbers of red blood cells and leukocytes, and as the disease progresses large, broad renal-failure casts appear. Renal functional impairment may be minimal early, but it becomes marked as the disease progresses. Gradually all the clinical and laboratory features of uremia develop (p. 1247).

PATHOPHYSIOLOGY. The disturbed physiology of chronic glomerulonephritis can be related directly to the process of progressive nephron destruction and production of renal insufficiency. The consequences of the resulting uremia have been discussed in an earlier section (p.1247).

DIFFERENTIAL DIAGNOSIS. The findings of persistent proteinuria and hematuria in association with reduced renal function are suggestive of chronic glomerulonephritis, but they are not sufficient to rule out other conditions. A search must be made for specific diseases, such as hereditary nephritis, lupus erythematosus, and renovascular hypertension. Urine cultures are essential in excluding pyelonephritis, while radiographic examination of the urinary tract may be necessary to rule out obstructive uropathy and congenital malformations, and renal biopsy may be extremely helpful in diagnosing other conditions.

COURSE AND PROGNOSIS. Recovery does not occur once a child has passed into the hypertensive, uremic phase of the disease. However, occasionally a patient who has had proteinuria for years has apparently healed completely. Without histopathologic examination the nature of the disease in such patients remains uncertain. Chronic glomerulonephritis has an extremely variable course, making estimates of its duration very uncertain. The onset of azotemia usually indicates that end-stage renal disease will be reached within a few years, but survival for many years is encountered. Some estimate of the course of the disease may be obtained from serial determinations of serum levels of urea or creatinine, or from estimates of GFR. When function falls below 10 to 15 percent of normal the patient is usually near the terminal phase of the disease.

TREATMENT. There is still no form of therapy that appears to reverse the course of chronic nephritis; however, during much of the course, and often over a period of many months or years, symptomatic treatment can be of great importance to the patient. Details of medical treatment and of dialysis and transplantation are given in the discussion of uremia (p.1247). Prolonged restriction of activity is not recommended unless it is demanded by the symptomatic state of the patient. The child should be encouraged to attend school and to participate in other activities within his limitations. No special changes in diet are needed early in the course of chronic nephritis, and needless restrictions should be avoided. Thus far the evidence of favorable effects from treatment with adrenocorticosteroids, other immunosuppressant drugs, or anticoagulants is not conclusive. Individual case reports suggest that in some patients the process of progressive nephron destruction may be slowed or even halted by such therapy.

References

RAPIDLY PROGRESSIVE GLOMERULONEPHRITIS

Anand, JK, Trygstad CW, Sharma HM, Northway JD: Extracapillary proliferative glomerulonephritis in children. Pediatrics 56:434, 1975

Lewis EJ: Rapidly progressive glomerulonephritis. Kidney 6:1, 1973

McPhaul JJ Jr, Newcomb RW, Mullins JD, et al: Participation of immunoglobulin E (IgE) in immune-mediated glomerulonephritis. Kidney 5: 292, 1974

Kincaid-Smith P, Saker BM, Fairley KF: Anticoagulants in "irreversible" acute renal failure. Lancet 2:1360, 1968

Lowgren E:...

Urizar RE, Tinglof B, McIntosh R, et al: Immunosuppressive therapy of proliferative glomerulonephritis in children. Am J. Dis Child 118:411, 1969

CHRONIC PROGRESSIVE GLOMERULONEPHRITIS

Edelmann CM Jr, Greifer I, Barnett HL: The nature of kidney disease in children who fail to recover from apparent acute glomerulonephritis. J Pediatr 64:879, 1964

Habib R, Kleinknecht C, Gubler MC: Extramembranous glomerulonephritis in children: report of 50 cases. J Pediatr 82:754, 1973

———— Kleinknecht C, Gubler MC, Levy M: Idopathic membranoproliferative glomerulonephritis in children: report of 105 cases. Clin Nephrol 1:194, 1973

——— Loirat C, Gubler MC, Levy M: Morphology and serum complement levels in membranoproliferative glomerulonephritis. Adv Nephrol 4:109, 1974

Heptinstall RH, Joekes AM: Focal glomerulonephritis. A study based on renal biopsies. Q J Med 28:329, 1959

Herdman RC, Edson JR, Pickering RJ, et al: Anticoagulants in renal disease in children. Am J Dis Child 119:27, 1970

Hyman LR, Burkholder PM: Focal sclerosing glomerulonephropathy with hyalinosis. J Pediatr 84:217, 1974

Jenis EH, Sandler P, Hill GS, et al: Glomerulonephritis with basement membrane dense deposits. Arch Pathol 97:84, 1974

McAdams AJ, McEnery PT, West CD: Mesangiocapillary glomerulonephritis: changes in glomerular morphology with long-term alternate-day prednisone therapy. J Pediatr 86:23, 1975

Myers BD, Griffel B, Naveh D, Jankielowitz T, Klajman A: Membranoproliferative glomerulonephritis associated with persistent viral hepatitis. Am J Clin Pathol 60:222, 1973

Olbing H, Greifer I, Bennett BP, Bernstein J, Spitzer A: Idiopathic membranous nephropathy in children. Kidney Int 3:381, 1973

Peters DK, Charlesworth JA, Sissons JGP, et al: Mesangiocapillary nephritis, partial lipodystrophy, and hypocomplementaemia. Lancet 2:535, 1973

Vallota EH, Forristal J, Davis MC, West CD: The C3 nephritic factor and membranoproliferative nephritis. J Pediatr 80:947, 1972

West CD: Hypocomplementemic glomerulonephritis. Kidney 6:1, 1973

——— McAdams AJ: Serum β_1C globulin levels in persistent glomerulonephritis with low serum complement: variability unrelated to clinical course. Nephron 7:193, 1970

Westberg NG, Naff GB, Boyer JT, Michael AF: Glomerular deposition of properdin in acute and chronic glomerulonephritis with hypocomplementemia. J Clin Invest 50:642, 1971

GLOMERULONEPHRITIS IN SYSTEMIC DISEASE

CHESTER M. EDELMANN, JR.

Schönlein-Henoch Syndrome

The Schönlein-Henoch syndrome is discussed in detail elsewhere (p. 382); this section will treat only the renal manifestations. Anaphylactoid purpura appears to be more common in children than in adults, with a peak incidence in childhood at the age of 3 to 5 years, although cases in infants as young as 6 months have been reported. Most series report more males than females, but a higher incidence in females has also been reported. Most cases occur during the winter and spring months. A history of preceding respiratory infection is common, but there is no convincing evidence that the condition is related to antecedent streptococcal infection. Reports in the literature vary considerably with regard to the frequency of renal involvement in this disease, but probably one-fourth to one-half of children have obvious renal disease. In our own experience only 6 of 24 children with Schönlein-Henoch syndrome had abnormal urines, as judged by repeated Addis counts, whereas 21 demonstrated histologic abnormalities on biopsy. The pathogenesis of the syndrome is unknown. The multiorgan involvement and diffuse vasculitis suggest the possibility of a hypersensitivity reaction to drugs, foods, or infectious agents.

Renal involvement usually becomes apparent within a few days to a few weeks after the onset of the skin, joint, and gastrointestinal manifestations. The clinical features vary from minimal urinary abnormalities to severe, rapidly progressive nephritis and often are indistinguishable from the features of acute glomerulonephritis, the diagnosis of Schönlein-Henoch nephritis being suggested by the accompanying joint, skin, or gastrointestinal involvement. Serum concentration of complement (C3) is consistently normal. Infrequently a nephrotic syndrome is seen. Renal biopsy early in the course of the disease reveals most commonly a focal proliferative glomerulonephritis. The renal lesion may vary in severity from minimal change to diffuse, severe proliferative and necrotizing glomerulonephritis. Prognosis and the development of complications such as the nephrotic syndrome may be correlated with the severity of the lesions and the number of crescents, the latter presumably reflecting the degree of glomerular disruption. On occasion a membranoproliferative lesion with endothelial deposits may be present. Immunofluorescence studies have prominent mesangial localization of IgA, C3, and properdin, usually in a diffuse distribution even when the glomerulonephritis seems histologically to be focal; IgG is also present.

Most studies suggest that more than 90 to 95 percent of children with Schönlein-Henoch nephritis recover completely. Reports indicating a poorer prognosis are probably due to selection of patients with the most severe degree of renal involvement. Even in severe cases the course is usually a self-limiting one, with return of urine to normal over a period of a few weeks to a few months; however, some children are seen with a chronic course, with repeated remissions and exacerbations. Renal damage may be extensive enough to cause permanent reduction in renal function and renal insufficiency.

Although adrenocorticosteroids cause prompt remission of most manifestations of the disease, they have not been shown to have a beneficial effect on the renal disease in the child with severe nephritis or the nephrotic syndrome. A few patients appear to have benefited from azathioprine or cyclophosphamide, but an adequate evaluation has not been done.

Systemic Lupus Erythematosus

Infection and renal failure continue to be the major causes of death in children with systemic lupus erythematosus (SLE). General aspects of the disease are discussed in detail elsewhere (p. 375); the discussion here will focus on the renal involvement.

ETIOLOGY AND PATHOGENESIS. Twenty years after the discovery of the LE cell by Hargraves it was shown that the LE cell phenomenon was the result of alteration of cellular nuclei by a humoral factor (antinuclear antibody) and subsequent phagocytosis of the altered nuclear material. Lupus erythematosus glomerulonephritis is now recognized as an example of immune-complex disease (p. 1264); a variety of nucleoproteins serve as the antigens and can be found in the circulation associated with antinuclear antibody in the form of soluble immune complexes. These complexes, together with complement, have been demonstrated in the kidneys of patients with glomerulonephritis and presumably are causative of the disease in that organ.

It would appear that lupus arises from a combination of genetic and environmental factors. A major environmental factor is sunlight. A number of drugs including hydralazine, isoniazid, several anticonvulsants, and several antibiotics also may be included as environmental factors, although there is some question whether spontaneous and drug-induced lupus are identical. The origin of the nucleoprotein and the relationship to environmental factors are not known. The sera of patients with SLE contain a variety of antibodies implicating a number of different antigens.

INCIDENCE.   SLE occurs in all races and in children of all ages, with a peak in adolescence. The ratio of girls to boys is about 4 to 1. Only 42 patients age 15 years or under who had SLE were encountered at the hospitals of New York University over an 18-year period. Hagge and associates reported on 41 children seen at the Mayo Clinic from 1945 to 1967. Although no precise data are available concerning the incidence of SLE in the pediatric age group, these data provide some idea of the rarity of the disease. Nevertheless, SLE maintains an important place among the various nephritides that may progress to renal failure.

CLINICAL FEATURES.   Meislin and Rothfield reported a mean time between onset of disease and diagnosis of 3.3 years, thus demonstrating the insidious manner in which SLE may present. Often an erroneous initial diagnosis, such as rheumatic fever or rheumatoid arthritis, is made.

Half of children with SLE present with joint involvement, and many have either skin manifestations or neurologic symptoms. At times asymptomatic proteinuria and/or hematuria may be the presenting complaint, but usually by the time renal involvement is apparent the diagnosis of SLE is readily established. Renal disease occurs in two-thirds or more of children with lupus. A clinical picture of acute or progressive glomerulonephritis may be present, and rapidly progressing uremia is encountered occasionally. Most patients with renal involvement have the nephrotic syndrome at some point in the course of their disease. A constitutional deficiency of the C2 component of complement has been reported to be associated with the clinical pattern of lupus.

In the absence of therapy lupus nephritis is an ultimately fatal process, terminal uremia occurring after a period of months to many years. Meislin and Rothfield reported 70 percent survival 5 years after diagnosis in children without renal disease at onset and 45 percent in children with renal disease. At 10 years these figures fell to 55 and 20 percent, respectively, and by 20 years to 30 and 5 percent.

PATHOLOGY.   Histologic examination in cases with renal involvement shows several different patterns: focal and diffuse proliferative glomerulonephritis and membranous nephropathy. Focal lesions have been associated generally with a milder clinical course, but focal nephritis might on occasion progress to more diffuse involvement. Severe glomerular lesions may be associated with fibrinoid degeneration and focal necrosis. Crescents are common. Subendothelial deposits in the capillary wall lead to focal segments of marked thickening known as wire loops. Immune complexes are readily identified within the glomeruli by specific immunofluorescence; immune complexes may be mesangial and subepithelial, in addition to the characteristic subendothelial deposits. Antibodies against DNA can be identified in the deposits. The presence of renal involvement correlates in general with other clinical evidence of activity. Renal lesions may be progressive, although minimal lesions respond to therapy and often show little progression over periods of several years.

THERAPY.   There is accumulating evidence that patients with lupus nephritis benefit from administration of adrenocorticosteroids or other cytotoxic immunosuppressant drugs. Treatment may not only suppress clinical and laboratory manifestations of disease but also produce both functional and histologic improvement. Currently we recommend that patients be treated initially with steroids alone. If nontoxic doses are not successful in producing complete control of the disease, as judged by examination of the urine and of serum factors, other drugs such as azathioprine or cyclophosphamide may be added to the regimen.

Shur and Sandson have reported on the usefulness of immunologic factors in judging activity of disease in patients with SLE. They found that very low complement levels and high titers of complement-fixing antibodies to DNA were always associated with active disease, whereas the absence of these abnormalities usually indicated inactive renal disease. A 50 percent fall in serum complement level usually accompanied or preceded the onset of active nephritis. Thus serial immunochemical observations may be of value as guides to therapy.

Polyarteritis Nodosa

This disease is rare in children, although it occurs at all ages, including infancy. The male-to-female ratio is approximately 2 to 1. The kidneys are involved in 75 to 85 percent of cases. Lesions within the kidney include the typical vasculitis that is also found in other organs, as well as a type of glomerulitis with capillary microthrombi, focal fibrinoid necrosis, and crescent formation.

Etiology and pathogenesis are not known, but the disease is thought to be one of hypersensitivity. In the so-called chronic (or macroscopic) form medium-size vessels are involved, and often several organ systems are affected. Renal involvement may manifest as flank pain and gross hematuria or as subacute glomerulonephritis. Hypertension is frequent. The course varies from months to years.

At times polyarteritis follows an acute fulminating course, beginning with a clinical syndrome resembling severe acute glomerulonephritis. Progression to terminal uremia may occur within a few weeks. Involvement of small-caliber arteries has led to its designation as the *microscopic form* of polyarteritis. In infants, polyarteritis presents with fever, rash, conjunctivitis, and rhinitis. Although the kidneys are involved in most cases, death usually occurs from lesions of the coronary arteries. There is evidence that corticosteroid therapy is of benefit in adult subjects, but the experience in children has been too limited to evaluate its usefulness.

Goodpasture's Syndrome

The form of glomerulonephritis associated with diffuse pulmonary hemorrhage, which was reported by Goodpasture in 1919, usually involves young adults, with only rare reports in children; males predominate 5 or 6 to 1. There is no evidence for streptococcal etiology. Patients present with cough, dyspnea, and hemoptysis followed in days, weeks, or months by the clinical and laboratory features of severe acute glomerulonephritis. Blood pressure initially is usually normal, and edema is uncommon. Rales, rhonchi, and wheezes usually are present, and anemia is evidenced by pallor.

Pulmonary infiltrates are seen radiographically, and at autopsy the alveoli are distended with red blood cells and hemosiderin-laden macrophages. Histologic examination of the kidneys reveals severe extracapillary proliferation forming glomerular crescents. The capillary tuft is most often collapsed and shows little mesangial proliferation. The lesion initially may be focal and associated with capillary thrombosis and deposition of fibrin in the glomerular tuft. Progression of the lesion leads to more diffuse involvement, and glomerular fibrosis and sclerosis may ensue. Immunofluorescence examination has shown linear deposits of IgG and β_1 C-globulin on the basement membranes of the alveoli, alveolar capillaries, and glomerular capillaries. Lerner and associates have eluted the immunoglobulins from the kidneys of patients and by injection into monkeys have induced nephritis with a similar pattern of linear deposition, thus confirming the hypothesis that this syndrome is caused by autoantibodies to glomerular and alveolar basement membranes. Although anti-GBM antibodies are present in all cases, the mechanism of immunization and the source of the immunizing antigen are unknown. Patients with this syndrome have had an unusually high frequency of exposure to industrial solvents.

Diffential diagnosis must consider acute glomerulonephritis with pulmonary congestion, uremic pneumonitis, pneumonia complicated with nephritis, polyarteritis nodosa, and idiopathic pulmonary hemosiderosis. There is a difference of opinion whether the last entity is in fact different from Goodpasture's syndrome.

In the review by Benoit the mean survival time in those who died was 15 weeks; in the series reported by Proskey and associates it was 41 weeks, and only 13 of 56 patients survived. Treatment with adrenocorticosteroids and various immunosuppressant agents and anticoagulants has been tried, but there is no firm evidence that any of these treatments is successful. Many of the severe cases progress to death in uremia, unless the course is interrupted with dialysis and transplantation.

Hemolytic-Uremic Syndrome

This condition has been described for several decades under a variety of names, but the term hemolytic-uremic syndrome was first used by Gasser and associates, who reported five children with sudden onset of intravascular hemolysis and acute renal failure. Four of the five were infants, and it has been recognized subsequently that the disease is seen predominantly in young infants and only rarely after the age of 2 years. There is no sex predilection. The hemolytic-uremic syndrome is an uncommon condition, but occasional outbreaks and a number of instances of close association with various infectious agents have suggested that infectious disease may be a common precedent. The wide geographic variation in incidence is unexplained. Many features of the disease have suggested an immune process, but the Coombs' test usually is negative; serum complement levels are not depressed, and only rarely have immunoglobulins been demonstrated in the kidney.

Many aspects of the hemolytic-uremic syndrome are similar to those of the Shwartzman reaction: the occurrence in young subjects, the onset following infection, the finding of fibrin in glomerular capillaries and arterioles, and the selective involvement of the kidneys. These observations have led to the hypothesis that intravascular coagulation is the initial event in the disease, although primary damage to blood cells or blood vessels cannot be ruled out. The following sequence of events has been proposed: following the onset of diffuse intravascular clotting, fibrin is deposited in the glomerular capillaries and arterioles, resulting in patchy fibrinoid necrosis. Red blood cells and platelets passing through these damaged vessels are injured, resulting in hemolytic anemia, platelet destruction, and thrombocytopenia. If the process is not too severe gradual recovery may take place, otherwise death in renal failure will ensue.

The course of the disease is quite characteristic. Following several days of acute gastroenteritis an infant or young child, previously well, develops the clinical features of acute glomerulonephritis. In addition a severe hemolytic anemia is present from the onset or develops within a few days. Thrombocytopenia and its complications also are usually present. The course is one of prolonged renal failure with repeated hemolytic episodes.

Mild to severe neurologic signs, including irritability, ataxia, convulsions, and coma, commonly are seen. The disease may either progress rapidly to death (in 5 to 10 percent) or gradually abate over a period of several weeks. Both neurologic and renal sequelae are seen, the incidence relating apparently to the severity of the initial process.

In the reports of Gianantonio and associates complete recovery was observed in 60 percent of those cases considered initially to be mild, in contrast to fewer than 15 percent of those considered severe. In 76 patients followed for 1 to 8 years healing was observed in only 33; another 20 appeared to be in the process of stabilization or recovery; 7 had died or were uremic, and there were signs of progressive renal disease in the remainder.

Renal lesions in this syndrome fall into two overlapping general categories. The patients described originally by Gasser and associates had cortical necrosis; those reported by Royer and associates had a form of severe glomerulitis, termed thrombotic microangiopathy. Fibrinoid necrosis and thrombosis of arterioles and glomeruli are seen in both. Electron microscopy discloses subendothelial deposits of fibrillary and granular material believed to be, at least in part, fibrin. The glomeruli in thrombotic microangiopathy are the site of striking endothelial and mesangial swelling. Focal or partial glomerular necrosis is often observed, suggesting a transition stage to cortical necrosis. Renal biopsies in survivors may show patchy glomerular scarring and residual vascular lesions, and the possibility of subsequent chronic progressive glomerulonephritis cannot be excluded.

Therapy remains unsatisfactory. The management of acute renal failure, which may require dialysis, is discussed on p. 1248. Severe hemolysis may necessitate blood transfusions. Corticosteroids, although not adequately evaluated, do not appear to be of value. Therapy with heparin has been proposed, but there is little evidence that it is of value. In the only controlled trial of heparin the results were negative. Dipyridamole and aspirin have been proposed as antiplatelet factors, but these drugs remain untested. There has been considerable experience with streptokinase therapy, with the conclusion by some authors that its early use may diminish morbidity and mortality, but controlled trials have not been conducted.

Thrombotic Thrombocytopenic Purpura

Thrombotic thrombocytopenic purpura (TTP) is a generalized vascular or hematologic disease characterized by fever, purpura, and neurologic manifestations. It is described fully in the section on hemorrhagic disorders (p. 1207), and therefore only those aspects relating to the kidney will be discussed here. The kidneys are often involved in TTP, and examination of the urine reveals proteinuria, gross or microscopic hematuria, white blood cells, and casts. Renal function varies from normal to severely depressed, but some degree of azotemia is usually present. Pathologic examination reveals large, bland, thrombotic masses in intralobular arterioles and glomeruli. A focal proliferative glomerulitis is occasionally present in addition to the vascular lesion, but the striking endothelial alterations of the hemolytic-uremic syndrome are not seen. Differential diagnosis must consider the hemolytic-uremic syndrome and SLE. The cause of TTP is unknown. It runs a chronic or fulminating course. Therapy is not available, and the outcome is invariably fatal.

Septicemia

With the arrival of the antibiotic era pyelonephritis and renal abscess formation, which may occur as suppurative complications in patients with sepsis, have become uncommon. This type of disease will not be considered further in this section, which focuses on the nonsuppurative involvement of the kidney during bloodstream infection.

Chronic bacteremia has been implicated as the precursor of severe renal disease in a variety of clinical situations, including bacterial endocarditis, infection from prosthetic devices placed in the circulation (such as ventriculoatrial shunts), malaria, and syphilis. In addition, transient urinary abnormalities and acute glomerulonephritis have been reported in association with a large number of viral diseases, although a clearcut causal relationship has not been established for most. Nevertheless, it is of interest that severe progressive renal disease in many species is a common consequence of viral infection.

There is considerable evidence that the renal disease that may occur during the course of chronic bacteremia (which may present as acute glomerulonephritis, progressive nephritis, or the nephrotic syndrome) is immunologically determined and not the consequence of septic emboli. The mechanism appears to be the formation in the circulation of soluble antigen–antibody complexes that deposit in the glomerular capillary walls, the so-called immune-complex renal disease (see p. 1264). In patients with the nephrotic syndrome secondary to *Plasmodium malariae* infection, specific antigen and IgG, IgM, and β_1C-globulins have been demonstrated in the glomeruli. Bacterial endocarditis is associated with a focal, proliferative glomerulonephritis that may go on to glomerular sclerosis. Immunofluorescence studies have demonstrated the presence of immune complexes. Shunt nephritis is characterized by subendothelial deposits and the histologic pattern of membranoproliferative disease. In a patient with an infected ventriculoatrial shunt *Micrococcus* antigen was present along with immunoglobulin and complement. In many of these patients serum complement is reduced. Treatment consists of eradication of the infection, which does not preclude the possibility of progressive renal disease. Immunosuppressive therapy has been without effect.

References

Ayoub EM, Hoyer J: Anaphylactoid purpura: streptococcal antibody titers and β_1C-globulin levels. J Pediatr 75:193, 1969

Evans DJ, Williams DG, Peters DK, et al: Glomerular deposition of properdin in Henoch-Schönlein syndrome and idiopathic focal nephritis. Br Med J 3:326, 1973

Hurley RM, Drummond KN: Anaphylactoid purpura nephritis: clinicopathological correlations. J Pediatr 81:904, 1972

Koskimies O, Rapola J, Savilahti E, Vilska J: Renal involvement in Schönlein-Henoch purpura. Acta Paediatr Scand 63:357, 1974

Meadow SR, Glasgow EF, White RHR, et al: Schönlein-Henoch nephritis. Q J Med 41:241, 1972

Urizar RE, Michael A, Sisson S, Vernier RL: Anaphylactoid purpura. II.

Immunofluorescent and electron microscopic studies of the glomerular lesions. Lab Invest 19:437, 1968

SYSTEMIC LUPUS ERYTHEMATOSUS

Agnello V, Koffler D, Kunkel HG: Immune complex systems in the nephritis of systemic lupus erythematosus. Kidney Int 3:90, 1973

Alarcón-Segovia D, Ibáñez G, Velázquez-Forero F, Hernández-Ortíz J, González-Jiménez Y: Sjögren's syndrome in systemic lupus erythematosus. Ann Intern Med 81:577, 1975

Baldwin DS, Lowenstein J, Rothfield NF, Gallo G, McCluskey RT: The clinical course of the proliferative and membranous forms of lupus nephritis. Ann Intern Med 73:929, 1970

Bergstein JM, Wiens C, Fish AJ, Vernier RL, Michael A: Avascular necrosis of bone in systemic lupus erythematosus. J Pediatr 85:31, 1974

Cade R, Spooner G, Schlein E, et al: Comparison of azathioprine, prednisone, and heparin alone or combined in treating lupus nephritis. Nephron 10:37, 1973

Cameron JS, Boulton-Jones M, Robinson R, Ogg C: Treatment of lupus nephritis with cyclophosphamide. Lancet 1:846, 1970

Comerford FR, Cohen AS: The nephropathy of systemic lupus erythematosus. An assessment of clinical, light, and electron microscopic criteria. Medicine 46: 425, 1967

Dillard MG, Dujovne I, Pollak VE, Pirani CL: The effect of treatment with prednisone and nitrogen mustard on the renal lesions and life span of patients with lupus glomerulonephritis. Nephron 10:273, 1973

Donadio JV Jr, Holley KE, Wagoner RD, Ferguson RH, McDuffie FC: Treatment of lupus nephritis with prednisone and combined prednisone and azathioprine. Ann Intern Med 77:829, 1972

Dujovne I, Pollak VE, Pirani CL, Dillard MG: The distribution and character of glomerular deposits in systemic lupus erythematosus. Kidney Int 2:33, 1972

Gabrielsen AE: Lupus erythematosus: A disease of D.N.A. discard? Lancet 2:1116, 1974

Gibson TP, Dibona GF: Use of the American Rheumatism Association's preliminary criteria for the classification of systemic lupus erythematosus. Ann Intern Med 77:754, 1972

Ginzler EM, Nicastri AD, Chen C-K, et al: Progression of mesangial and focal to diffuse lupus nephritis. N Engl J Med 291:693, 1974

Grishman E, Porush JG, Lee SL, Churg J: Renal biopsies in lupus nephritis. Nephron 10:25, 1973

Grossman J, Schwartz RH, Callerame ML, Condemi JJ: Systemic lupus erythematosus in a l-year-old child. Am J Dis Child 129:123, 1975

Hagge WW, Burke EC, Stickler GB: Treatment of systemic lupus erythematosus complicated by nephritis in children. Pediatrics 40:822, 1967

Hayslett JP, Kashgarian M, Cook CD, Spargo BH: The effect of azathioprine on lupus glomerulonephritis. Medicine 51:393, 1972

Hoffer D, Agnello V, Carr RI, Kunkel HG: Variable patterns of immunoglobulin and complement deposition in the kidneys of patients with systemic lupus erythematosus. AM J Pathol 52:305, 1969

Jacobs JC: Systemic lupus erythematosus in childhood: report of 35 cases. Pediatrics 32:257, 1963

Keeffe EB, Bardana EJ Jr, Harbeck RJ, Pirofsky B, Carr RI: Lupus meningitis. Antibody to deoxyribonucleic acid (DNA) and DNA:anti-DNA complexes in cerebrospinal fluid. Ann Intern Med 80:58, 1974

Koffler D, Agnello V, Kunkel HG: Polynucleotide immune complexes in serum and glomeruli of patients with systemic lupus erythematosus. Am J Patho 74:109, 1974

Meislin AG, Rothfield N: Systemic lupus erythematosus in childhood. Analysis of 42 cases, with comparative data on 200 adult cases followed concurrently. Pediatrics 42:37, 1968

Pollak, VE, Pirani CL: Renal histologic findings in systemic lupus erythematosus. Mayo Clin Proc 44:630, 1969

Ritchie RF: Antinuclear antibodies: their frequency and diagnostic association. N Engl J Med 282:1174, 1970

Rothfield NF: Diagnosis of lupus erythematosus and rheumatoid arthritis in children. Pediatr Clin North Am 18:39, 1974

Sharon E, Kaplan D, Diamond HS: Exacerbation of systemic lupus erythematosus after withdrawal of azathioprine therapy. N Engl J Med 288:122, 1973

Steinberg AD, Kaltreider HB, Staples PJ et al: Cyclophosphamide in lupus nephritis: a controlled trial. Ann Intern Med 75:165, 1971

POLYARTERITIS NODOSA

Arroyave HC, Quiroga ZG, Gordillo PG, Bessodo MYL: Polyarteritis nodosa. Bol Med Hosp. Infant Mex 24:549, 1967

Frohnert PP, Sheps SG: Long-term follow-up study of periarteritis nodosa. Am J Med 43:8, 1967

Harrison CV, Loughridge LW, Milne MD: Acute oliguric renal failure in acute glomerulonephritis and polyarteritis nodosa. Q J Med 33:39, 1964

Krous HF, Clausen CR, Ray CG: Elevated immunoglobulin E in infantile polyarteritis nodosa. J Pediatr 84:841, 1974

Leff R, Harrer WV, Baylis JC, Jackson L, Faber K: Polyarteritis nodosa in two siblings. Am J Dis Child 121:67, 1971

Roberts FB, Fetterman GH: Polyarteritis nodosa in infancy. J Pediatr 63:519, 1963

GOODPASTURE'S SYNDROME

Dixon FJ: The pathogenesis of glomerulonephritis (editorial). Am J Med 44:493, 1968

Goodpasture, EW: The significance of certain pulmonary lesions in relation to the etiology of influenza. Am J Med Sci 158:863, 1919

Halgrimson CG, Wilson CB, Dixon SJ, et al: Goodpasture's syndrome. Treatment with nephrectomy and renal transplantation. Arch Surg 103:283, 1971

Lerner FA, Glassock RJ, Dixon FJ: The role of antiglomerular basement membrane antibody in the pathogenesis of human glomerulonephritis. J Exp Med 126:989, 1967

Lewis EJ, Schur PH, Busch GJ, Galvanek E, Merrill JP: Immunopathologic features of a patient with glomerulonephritis and pulmonary hemorrhage. Am J Med 54:507, 1973

Proskey AJ, Weatherbee L, Easterling RE, Greene JA Jr, Weller JM: Goodpasture's syndrome. A report of five cases and review of the literature. Am J Med 48:162, 1970

Siegal RR: The basis of pulmonary disease resolution after nephrectomy in Goodpasture's syndrome. Am J Med Sci 259:201, 1970

HEMOLYTIC-UREMIC SYNDROME

Abildgaard CF: Recognition and treatment of intravascular coagulation. J Pediatr 74:163, 1969

Avalos JS, Vitacco M, Molinas F, Penalver J, Gianantonio C: Coagulation studies in the hemolytic-uremic syndrome. J Pediatr 76:538, 1970

Chan JCM, Eleff MG, Campbell RA: The hemolytic-uremic syndrome in nonrelated adopted siblings. J Pediatr 75:1050, 1969

Gasser C, Gautier E, Steck A, Siebenmann RE, Oechslin R: Hämolytisch-urämische Syndrome. Schweiz Med Wochenschr 85:905, 1955

Gervais M, Richardson JB, Chiu J, Drummond KN: Immunofluorescent and histologic findings in the hemolytic uremic syndrome. Pediatrics 47:352, 1971

Gianantonio CA, Vitacco M, Mendilaharzu F, Gallo GE, Sojo ET: The hemolytic-uremic syndrome. Nephron 11:174, 1973

Herdman RC, Edson R, Pickering RJ, et al: Anticoagulants in renal disease in children. Am J Dis Child 119:27, 1970

Katz J, Krawitz S, Sacks PV, et al: Platelet, erythrocyte, and fibrinogen kinetics in the hemolytic-uremic syndrome of infancy. J Pediatr 83:739, 1973

McCoy RC, Abramowsky CR, Krueger R: The hemolytic uremic syndrome, with positive immunofluorescence studies. J Pediatr 85:170, 1974

Mettler NE: Isolation of a microtatobiote from patients with hemolytic-uremic syndrome and thrombotic thrombocytopenic purpura and from mites in the United States. N Engl J Med 281:1023, 1969

Monnens L, Kleynen P, Van Munster P, Schretlen E, Bonnerman A: Coagulation studies and streptokinase therapy in the haemolytic-uraemic syndrome. Helv Paediatr Acta 27:45, 1972

Powell HR, Ekert H: Streptokinase and anti-thrombotic therapy in the hemolytic-uremic syndrome. J Pediatr 84:345, 1974

Proesmans W, Eeckels R: Has heparin changed the prognosis of the hemolytic-uremic syndrome. Clin Nephrol 2:169, 1974

Stuart J, Winterborn MH, White RHR, Flinn RM: Thrombolytic therapy in haemolytic-uraemic syndrome. Br Med J 3:217, 1974

Tune BM, Groshong T, Plumer LB, Mendoza SA: The hemolytic-uremic syndrome in siblings: a prospective survey. J Pediatr 85:682, 1974

———— Leavitt TJ, Gribble TJ: The hemolytic-uremic syndrome in California: A review of 28 non-heparinized cases with long-term follow-up. J Pediatr 82:304, 1973

Van Wieringen PMV, Monnens LAH, Schretlen EDAM: Haemolytic-uraemic syndrome. Epidemiological and clinical study. Arch Dis Child 49:432, 1974

Vitacco M, Avalos JS, Gianantonio CA: Heparin therapy in the hemolytic-uremic syndrome. J Pediatr 83:271, 1973

Vitsky BH, Suzulei Y, Strauss L, Churg J: The hemolytic-uremic syndrome. Am J Pathol 57:627, 1969

Willoughby MLN, Murphy AV, McMorris S, Jewell FG: Coagulation studies in haemolytic uraemic syndrome. Arch Dis Child 47:766, 1972

THROMBOTIC THROMBOCYTOPENIC PURPURA

Amorosi EL, Ultmann JE: Thrombotic thrombocytopenic purpura. Report of 16 cases and review of the literature. Medicine 45:139, 1966

Berberich FR, Cuene SA, Chard RL Jr, Hartmann JR: Thrombotic thrombocytopenic purpura. Three cases with platelet and fibrinogen survival studies. J Pediatr 84:503, 1974

SEPTICEMIA

Adeniyi A, Henrickse RG, Houba V: Selectivity of proteinuria and response to prednisolone or immunosuppressive drugs in children with malarial nephrosis. Lancet 1:644, 1970

Allison AC, Houba V, Hendrickse RG, et al: Immune complexes in the nephrotic syndrome of African children. Lancet 1:1232, 1969

Bhorade MS, Carag HB, Lee HJ, Potter EV, Dunea G: Nephropathy of secondary syphilis. A clinical and pathological spectrum. JAMA 216:1159, 1971

Braunstein GD, Lewis EJ, Galvanek EG, Hamilton A, Bell WR: The nephrotic syndrome associated with secondary syphilis. Am J Med 48:643, 1970

Burch GE, Chu KC, Colcolough HL, Sohal RS: Immunofluorescent localization of coxsackievirus B antigen in the kidney observed at routine autopsy. Am J Med 47:36, 1969

Editor: Viruses and renal disease. JAMA 204:219, 1968

Gutman RA, Striker GE, Gilliland BC, Cutler RE: The immune complex glomerulonephritis of bacterial endocarditis. Medicine 51:1, 1972

Hendrickse RG, Glasgow EF, Adeniyi A, et al: Quartan malarial nephrotic syndrome. Lancet 1:1143, 1972

Kaufman DB, Logan L, McIntosh RM: The nature of the antibody in a patient with immune complex renal disease. Pediatr Res 3:363, 1969

———— McIntosh R: The pathogenesis of the renal lesion in a patient with streptococcal disease, infected ventriculoatrial shunt, cryoglobulinemia and nephritis. Am J Med 50:262, 1971

Keslin MH, Messner RP, Williams RC Jr: Glomerulonephritis with subacute bacterial endocarditis. Arch Intern Med 132:578, 1973

Levy RL, Hong R: The immune nature of subacute bacterial endocarditis (SBE) nephritis. Am J Med 54:645, 1973

Moncrieff MW, Glasgow EF, Arthur LJH, Hargreaves HM: Glomerulonephritis associated with staphylococcus albus in a Spitz Holter valve. Br Med Bull 48:69, 1973

Morel-Maroger L, Sraer J-D, Herreman G, Godeau P: Kidney with subacute endocarditis. Arch Pathol 94:205, 1972

Rames L, Wise B, Goodman JR, Piel CF: Renal disease with staphylococcus albus bacteremia. A complication in ventriculoatrial shunt. JAMA 212:1671, 1970

Stickler GB, Shin MH, Burke EC, et al: Diffuse glomerulonephritis associated with infected ventriculoatrial shunt. N Engl J Med 279:1077, 1968

Wegmann W, Leumann EP: Glomerulonephritis associated with (infected) ventriculo-atrial shunt. Clinical and morphological findings. Virchows Arch [Pathol Anat] 359:185, 1973

Wiggelinkhuizen J, Kaschula ROC, Uys CJ, Kuijten RH, Dale J: Congenital syphilis and glomerulonephritis with evidence for immune pathogenesis. Arch Dis Child 48:375, 1973

IDIOPATHIC NEPHROTIC SYNDROME OF CHILDHOOD

CHESTER M. EDELMANN, JR.

The nephrotic syndrome is characterized by proteinuria, hypoproteinemia, hyperlipemia, and edema. The great majority of children who develop the nephrotic syndrome have neither recognizable systemic disease (as judged by any clinical or laboratory examination) nor evidence of exposure to toxic agents. In these children, whose disorders appear to represent a variety of primary glomerular disease, the condition is referred to as the idiopathic nephrotic syndrome of childhood (INS). The nephrotic syndrome may occur infrequently in children, although commonly in adults, during the course of various systemic disorders (Schönlein-Henoch syndrome, lupus erythematosus, sickle cell anemia, cyanotic congenital heart disease, malaria, syphilis, tuberculosis, diabetes mellitus, amyloidosis, multiple myeloma), following renal vein thrombosis, or as a result of drug toxicity (Tridione, mercurials, penicillamine, tolbutamide, bismuth and gold salts). Whether the nephrotic syndrome that follows a bee sting or exposure to poison oak or poison ivy is different from the idiopathic disease in unknown.

Approximately 80 percent of children with INS have the so-called minimal-change disease, which is designated as such because light microscopy of renal tissue reveals few or no abnormalities. These patients generally respond well to treatment and have a good prognosis. The other 20 percent of children with INS demonstrate a variety of histologic lesions, including almost all forms of glomerulonephritis. These patients usually fail to respond to therapy and have a grave prognosis.

INCIDENCE. The incidence of INS in children in the United States has been estimated variously to be 1.9, 2.3, and 2.8 cases per 100,000 white children below 10 years of age. Schlesinger et al. reported an incidence of 1.9 cases per 100,000 white children and 2.8 cases per 100,000 nonwhite children under 16 years of age; they found the number of active cases to be 15.7 per 100,000 children below the age of 16. The age of onset peaks at 2 to 3 years, with more than half the patients between 1 and 4 years and three-quarters under 7 years of age. Our recent experience with more than 500 patients confirms previous impressions that 60 to 65 percent of the patients are male.

ETIOLOGY. The cause of the nephrotic syndrome is unknown. Even when it occurs in association with some systemic disorder or following toxic exposure, the pathogenic relationship is not clear, and the association is not a consistent one. Many nephrologists consider minimal-change disease to be related to hypersensitivity, with a poorly understood antigen–antibody reaction involving the kidneys. Evidence in favor of this formulation includes the apparently increased incidence of allergic disease in patients and their families, the production of a similar disease in experimental animals using a variety of immunologic techniques, and the favorable effects of adrenocorticosteroids and other immunosuppressant drugs. It must be recognized that none of these constitutes a firm basis for including this condition among the diseases of immune origin. Furthermore, serum complement activity in these patients is normal, and neither gamma globulin nor components of the complement system are found deposited in renal tissue. Finally, the mechanisms of action are not understood for any of the drugs found useful in these patients.

Another type of immunologic abnormality in the minimal-change nephrotic syndrome has recently been reported. Patients with minimal-change disease were found to have elevated levels of serum IgM as compared with normals or with patients with the nephrotic syndrome associated with the various forms of glomerulonephritis. All patients with the nephrotic syndrome had reduced levels of IgG and IgA. Although these levels increased during remissions, the levels of IgM remained elevated. From these data it has been suggested that the primary defect in minimal-change disease may be immunologic, consisting of deficiencies in the T-cell function that mediates conversion of IgM synthesis to IgG synthesis.

FAMILIAL FORMS. The occurrence of the nephrotic syndrome in siblings or in consecutive generations of the same family is infrequent. Two forms of heritable nephrosis can be identified. One form, congenital or infantile nephrosis (p. 1288), differs from idiopathic childhood nephrosis by its appearance before 3 months of age (often at or shortly after birth) and by its lack of responsiveness to steroid therapy, its poor prognosis, and its distinctive morphologic appearance. The other form, familial childhood nephrosis, simulates sporadic childhood nephrosis in clinical picture and pathologic findings. The possibility that it is a heritable disorder arises only when the syndrome occurs in more than one member of the same family and follows the same clinical course.

CLINICAL FEATURES. The most important clinical feature is proteinuria, although edema is the symptom commonly calling attention to the disease. The onset of edema is usually insidious, but it may be abrupt. It is usually noted first about the eyes and often is more apparent to the parents than to the physician. The edema may progress slowly or rapidly; not uncommonly, however, it tends to subside and reappear over a period of weeks. The first evidence of periorbital edema is often attributed to a cold, although frank respiratory symptoms are usually wanting. It may be misinterpreted as allergic in origin. Sooner or later the edema becomes generalized, with ascites and occasionally pleural effusion, and the true nature of the disease becomes apparent.

The presence of clinical edema is not necessary for the diagnosis of the nephrotic syndrome, and it should be considered as a secondary manifestation of the disease. The degree and duration of edema are very variable. Some children remain edematous, if they are left untreated, whereas others have repeated remissions and exacerbations.

Significant findings on physical examination generally are limited to those associated with edema. Marked skin pallor may be present. The large abdomen produced by ascites is common, and labial or scrotal swelling is often seen. More severe degrees of edema may be associated with dilated veins of the anterior abdominal wall, umbilical hernia, and rectal prolapse. The liver is enlarged in many children during the active stage; it decreases in size with recovery. Treatment with adrenocorticosteroids has dramatically altered the clinical course of nephrosis in the majority of children, particularly in those with minimal-change disease. If initiated early it may prevent the appearance of massive edema and in many cases will prevent its recurrence after a remission.

Susceptibility to infection is increased during periods of edema. Peritonitis, which may be accompanied by bacteremia and cellulitis, is the most common of these. In the past, pneumococcal infection was common, but infections with other organisms are now more frequent. The presence of ascites may mask the classic signs of peritonitis, which therefore must be suspected whenever an edematous child develops fever and looks sick.

Minor skin irritations and infections are commonly seen during periods of massive edema. These occur around the genitalia, the eyes, and other areas where swelling causes pressure on opposing skin surfaces. A curious erysipeloid infection of the skin is occasionally encountered. It differs from erysipelas in having less induration and no very sharp edge; the infectious agent in such cases is not known.

Malnutrition is common in children in whom the active stage of the disease is prolonged. Poor appetite and loss of protein in the urine are responsible. Malnutrition and consequent reduction in muscle mass tend to be obscured by the edema, although changes in the quality of the hair may reveal it. Striking changes also may be observed in the cartilage of the ear. Despite the poor nutrition, which in only rare instances may persist for many months, there is apparently no residual growth impairment if recovery from the disease occurs and prolonged high-dosage steroid therapy has not been required.

Gastrointestinal disturbances not associated with infections are frequently observed. Diarrhea is especially common during periods of massive edema and has been attributed to edema of the intestinal mucosa. Respiratory difficulty resulting from abdominal distention, with or without pleural effusion, may be disturbing and occasionally alarming. The fact that children in the active stage of the nephrotic syndrome are sometimes irritable and depressed is less surprising than that they are ever otherwise. Even in the presence of massive edema, which appears so uncomfortable to others, many children remain in remarkably good spirits.

LABORATORY FEATURES. In addition to edema, the nephrotic syndrome is characterized by altered laboratory examinations, and these play a major role in establishing the diagnosis and evaluating prognosis and act as guides to treatment.

Proteinuria is consistently present during the active stage, the daily protein excretion varying from as little as a few hundred milligrams in the small child to 15 g or more per day. This protein is predominantly albumin, reflecting its low molecular weight. Nevertheless, tests of urinary protein selectivity, which reflect clearance ratios of proteins of various molecular weights, have yielded variable results. Most children with minimal-change disease have highly selective proteinuria, ie, almost exclusively albuminuria, in contrast to those with various forms of glomerulonephritis who more often have nonselective proteinuria, ie, excretion of low- and high-molecular-weight proteins. Thus there is a rough correlation between the selectivity index on the one hand and either the likelihood of steroid response or the histologic classification on the other. However, exceptions to the rule that highly selective proteinuria indicates a steroid-responsive, minimal-change patient and poorly selective proteinuria a steroid-unresponsive patient with glomerulonephritis are too numerous to make this test very helpful clinically.

Fifty percent of children have hematuria at the onset, but in most this is minimal. Only 20 percent of children with minimal-change disease exhibit hematuria in excess of 100,000 RBC/hour m^2 BSA, in contrast to 60 percent of children with other lesions. Thus the presence of this degree of hematuria at onset makes the likelihood of something other than minimal-change disease almost 50 percent.

Hypoproteinemia, hypoalbuminemia, and hyperlipemia are characteristic, cholesterol being the only lipid that is commonly measured. Total serum protein averages 4.0 g/dl with most values falling between 3 and 5; albumin averages 1.5 g/dl, with a range of 0.5 to 2.5. Characteristically α_2-and β-globulins are markedly elevated and γ-globulin is depressed. Cholesterol, which in one series averaged 730 ± 81 mg/dl, may vary from normal to as high as 1,500.

Serum calcium concentration is uniformly reduced, often to as low as 6 mg/100 ml, but the deficit is largely in the protein-bound fraction, so that tetany almost never occurs. The sedimentation rate is usually markedly elevated. The third component of complement (C3) usually is normal in children with INS. When found to be depressed it usually reflects the presence of membranoproliferative glomerulonephritis and almost always augurs a poor prognosis.

Tests of renal function yield variable results. Maximum concentrating ability and acidification of the urine usually are retained, and as a rule frank azotemia is absent. Glomerular filtration rate ranges from normal to considerably depressed, as many as one-fifth of children with minimal-change disease having values below 35 ml/minute/m^2. The occasional observation of urea and inulin clearances significantly above normal remains unexplained.

RENAL PATHOLOGY. Studies of renal biopsies during the last two decades have led to a classification of glomerular lesions in INS unassociated with systemic disease, and this classification forms the basis of several important clinicopathologic correlations (Table 5).

TABLE 5. Classification of Histologic Lesions Encountered in Idiopathic Nephrotic Syndrome of Childhood

Minimal change disease	80%
Focal glomerular lesions	9%
Pure mesangial hypercellularity	2%
Diffuse proliferative glomerulonephritis:	
Membranoproliferative	5%
Other	2%
Membranous nephropathy	1%
Other	1%
	100%

The most common histologic finding in children with INS is minimal-change disease, a histologic pattern with only minor differences from normal glomerular structure. This designation allows for mild degrees of stalk hypercellularity, slight leukocytosis, and focal mesangial thickening. Tubular abnormalities, including focal calcification and disruption by extruded casts, may also be seen. The presence of an occasional, totally obsolete, hyalinized glomerulus does not alter the diagnosis. Electron microscopy of biopsies with minimal-change disease has consistently shown, as in all types of the nephrotic syndrome, fusion of the foot processes of glomerular epithelial cells. Evidence has been presented to show that fusion is secondary to excessive glomerular filtration of protein, but it has also been suggested that the fusion reflects a primary abnormality in which the ability of epithelial cells to maintain the basement membrane is impaired. Electron microscopic studies have failed to demonstrate abnormalities in the glomerular basement membranes, except for occasional thickening in cases with long-standing disease. In such cases there may also be mild mesangial thickening associated with wrinkling of the basement membranes. Immunofluorescence studies for glomerular deposition of immune complexes and complement have generally been negative. This pattern of minimal change, including the variations noted above, has usually (90 to 95 percent) but not invariably been associated with a good initial response to steroid therapy and with a good prognosis. Some of the patients do, however, develop sclerosing glomerular changes later in their courses and may develop late steroid resistance.

Another type of glomerular lesion, when seen early in the course of disease, has altogether different therapeutic implications. Sclerosis and hyalinosis involving a portion of the glomerular tuft (Fig. 13), even if found in only one of numerous glomeruli, signal a relatively poor response to steroid therapy and an ultimately poor prognosis. Affected glomeruli are always most numerous at the corticomedullary junctions. The glomerular lesions are usually accompanied by patchy tubular atro-

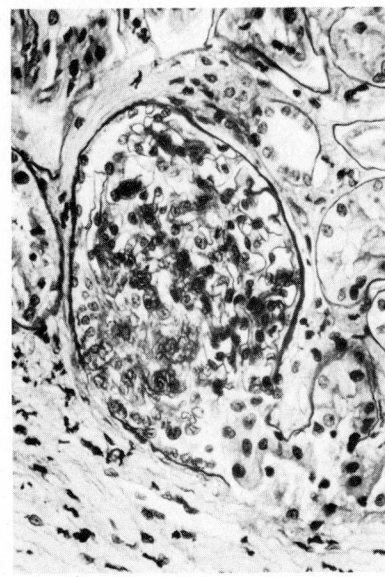

FIG. 13.   A juxtamedullary glomerulus contains a localized area of sclerosis associated with focal proliferation of epithelial cells. It is associated with mild, diffuse mesangial hypercellularity and appears to be an early stage in the development of segmental sclerosis (PAS stain, ×300).

phy. Immunofluorescence often shows IgM and C3 within sclerotic areas; this finding may reflect entrapment of serum protein and is not generally regarded as convincing evidence of immune injury and pathogenesis. These cases have significantly more hypertension and hematuria at the onset, and they commonly develop a course of progressive functional deterioration that terminates in renal failure. The recognition of this lesion (despite its extremely focal distribution) and its differentiation from minimal-change disease are clearly of great importance in avoiding steroid toxicity from a futile course of prolonged medication.

A third pattern of glomerular disease in children with the idiopathic nephrotic syndrome is membranous or so-called epimembranous nephropathy. This lesion is distinctly less common in children than in adults. It is characterized by marked thickening of the capillary walls, as seen by light microscopy, and by selective staining of the basement membrane, with a pattern of spikes or protrusions on the epithelial sides of the basement membranes (Fig. 14). Immunofluorescence discloses finely granular deposits of IgG and C3 around the capillary walls. Electron microscopy shows that these deposits are initially separated by spiked projec-

tions of material similar to basement membrane and are later covered over the incorporated into greatly thickened membranes. There is no evidence that the membranous lesion is a stage in the progression of minimal-change disease, although the former has on very rare occasions been observed to follow proliferative glomerulonephritis. In the usual case, the membranous lesion is present from the onset; it may increase in thickness with duration of the disease and progress to glomerular involution. This lesion is commonly associated with hematuria at the onset of the disease, and

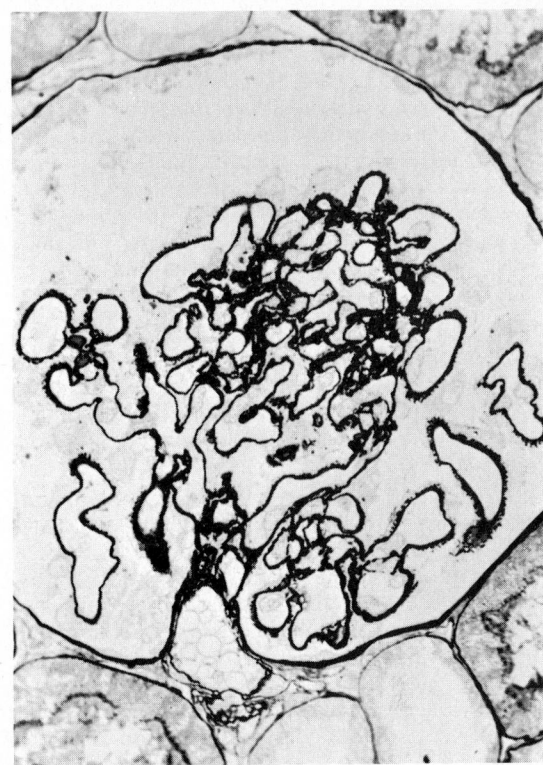

FIG. 14.   Membranous nephropathy in INS; note thickening of basement membrane, with subepithelial spikes (Jones' periodic acid-silver methenamine stain, ×350).

it appears not to be affected by steroid therapy. However, clinical improvement has been observed in as many as one-fourth of cases, presumably unrelated to therapeutic intervention; in some cases histologic resolution has also been demonstrated.

A relatively small number of children have nephrotic syndrome secondary to glomerulonephritis. The most frequent form in childhood is membranoproliferative glomerulonephritis (p. 1273), which has been associated with a very poor response to therapy and usually with progression to renal failure. Proliferative and exudative glomerulonephritis is in some instances post-streptococcal, and in these patients the prognosis has been relatively good, with a tendency to rapid, often spontaneous, cure. Proliferative glomerulonephritis may be accompanied by sclerosis and diffuse crescent formation, which are regarded as indicators of poor prognosis.

The nephrotic syndrome may appear during the course of glomerulonephritis associated with systemic disease: Schönlein-Henoch purpura (p. 1275), systemic lupus erythematosus (p. 1275), and hemolytic-uremic syndrome (p. 1277). The nephrotic syndrome develops occasionally in the course of Alport's syndrome (p. 1295), and it has been described as a complication of numerous other diseases. Of particular importance in pediatric patients is congenital syphilis (p. 505), in which the lesion, an immune-complex nephritis, may be proliferative or epimembranous or both. Renal vein thrombosis as a cause of INS in childhood appears to be extremely uncommon. It has in most instances been regarded as a secondary phenomenon, since nephrotic children are frequently dehydrated and develop venous thromboses; however, a recent study suggests the possibility that renal vein thrombosis damages tubules, leading to the release of tubular antigens and to the development of nephrotoxic antigen–antibody complexes.

PATHOPHYSIOLOGY.   There are striking changes in nephrosis in the metabolism of protein, lipids, electrolytes, and water. However, a great deal of evidence points to increased glomerular membrane permeability to protein as the basic disturbance in this condition.

MEMBRANE PERMEABILITY.   It is generally accepted that abnormal permeability of the glomerular basement membrane to normal plasma protein accounts for the proteinuria of the nephrotic syndrome. Decreased tubular reabsorption of filtered protein may play a secondary role, but cannot adequately explain the amounts of protein encountered clinically. Although increased passage of protein through a defective basement membrane is associated morphologically with obliteration of the foot processes and formation of vacuoles and hyaline droplets, the nature of the glomerular lesion is entirely unknown.

PROTEIN METABOLISM.   Although it is generally agreed that proteinuria is the major cause of hypoproteinemia, increased rates of catabolism of protein also occur and apparently explain some of the discrepancies between intensity of proteinuria and degree of hypoalbuminemia. Protein loss through the gastrointestinal tract, as in protein-losing enteropathy, has been reported in a few patients.

The usual pattern of hypoproteinemia is low albumin, normal or low α_1-globulin, elevated α_2-globulin and β-globulin, and low γ-globulin. Occasional patients show increase in the γ-globulin fraction, particularly those with SLE.

LIPID METABOLISM.   Patients with the nephrotic syndrome exhibit marked hyperlipemia. In addition to the elevation in serum cholesterol there are proportional increases in the concentrations of phospholipids and even more marked increases in the concentrations of triglycerides, which is the primary cause of the latescent appearance of serum. All of the serum lipids exist in association with proteins as lipoproteins.

The cause of hyperlipemia remains obscure. Markedly elevated cholesterol is rarely seen in the presence of normal serum albumin. However, normal or only moderately elevated levels of cholesterol are commonly observed in association with hypoalbuminemia.

ELECTROLYTE AND WATER BALANCE.   The mechanism of edema formation in patients with the nephrotic syndrome is complex. As described above, loss of protein in the urine at a rate that exceeds the synthetic capacity of the liver results in hypoproteinemia. Decrease in the concentration of albumin in blood reduces the oncotic pressure of plasma, shifting Starling's force to favor movement of fluid from the vascular compartment into the interstitium. When this is of sufficient magnitude to be detected clinically, it is recognized as edema. Another consequence of this fluid shift is contraction of the vascular volume, which acts as a stimulus to the kidney to increase the reabsorption of filtered sodium and water; this action of the kidney is mediated by hyperaldosteronism, increased release of antidiuretic hormone, and other mechanisms which influence renal hemodynamics and alter glomerulotubular balance. A reduction in renal plasma flow and GFR, which occurs in some patients, may also contribute to decreased urinary excretion of sodium and water. Net retention of salt and water by the kidney does serve to preserve the vascular volume; however, the hypoalbuminemia allows a considerable portion of this additional fluid to enter the interstitial space, furthering formation of edema. Ultimately the patient comes into a steady state in which Starling's forces are balanced and intake of sodium and water is equal to renal excretion. This edematous state persists until there is a reduction in the rate of proteinuria, resulting in a shift of Starling forces back to normal, expansion of the vascular volume, and a diuresis of sodium and water. It must be recognized that the logical synthesis of the mechanism of edema formation in the nephrotic subject must be considered incomplete since the orderly progression described here does not seem to apply to all patients, who at times increase or decrease their edema without detectable changes in the forces cited.

RENAL TUBULAR FUNCTION.   Defects in tubular function, including amino-aciduria, phosphaturia, glycosuria, polyuria, renal tubular acidosis, and concentrating defects, have been described. Since these are absent in the majority of patients with the nephrotic syndrome, it is uncertain whether they represent abnormalities that develop during the course of prolonged proteinuria or whether they are instances of primary damage to both glomeruli and tubules.

DIFFERENTIAL DIAGNOSIS.   The combination of edema, proteinuria, hypoproteinemia, and hyperlipemia defines the nephrotic syndrome; differential diagnosis concerns the underlying diseases with which it may be associated. All the conditions mentioned above, including the various types of glomerulonephritis, must be considered. In the clinically typical patient with normocomplementemia and no evidence of either systemic disease or glomerulonephritis the diagnosis of minimal-change disease can be established with reasonable certainty by demonstrating a complete clinical and laboratory response to adrenocorticosteroid therapy. When there is evidence of systemic disease or glomerulonephritis, and in all steroid-nonresponsive patients, diagnostic investigation should include histologic examination of tissue obtained by percutaneous renal biopsy to permit morphologic as well as clinical classification.

TREATMENT. Nephrosis is a trying disease for the physician, the family, and the patient himself. Treatment must include measures directed toward control of the outstanding clinical feature (edema) and, more important, measures directed toward favorable modification of the course of the disease and its ultimate prognosis. In addition, because of the chronicity of the disease and the uncertainty of the outcome, the child with nephrosis and his parents need more than the usual amount of psychologic support from the physician.

In recent years there have been several major advances in the treatment of children with the nephrotic syndrome. First was the development of antibacterial agents, which have almost eliminated the severe infection that was the principal cause of death in these children. Another advance was the development of the therapeutic use of adrenocorticosteroids, which in most instances permits complete control of the edema and appears to favorably modify the underlying disease and the ultimate outcome. The availability of potent diuretic agents constitutes another advance that permits control of severe edema in patients prior to their response to adrenocorticosteroid therapy or in those who are refractory to such therapy. Finally, it now appears that other immunosuppressant or cytoxic drugs may be effective in the management of steroid-responsive, but steroid-toxic, children.

GENERAL MEASURES. The diet of the nephrotic child is that suitable for the normal child. Salt needs to be restricted only during periods of edema, at which time foods are not salted during cooking, a shaker is not provided, and excessively salty foods are avoided. The protein content of the diet is not altered. No restrictions are placed on the activity of the child beyond those he himself may impose during periods of edema. It is important to maintain associations with other children, but because exacerbations of proteinuria and edema may follow common upper respiratory tract infections, some limitations are advisable. For example, when contacts with other children during visits or playtimes are planned, more than the usual amount of attention is paid to the possibility of infection in the other children. Although exposure to large groups is best avoided, patients are encouraged to attend kindergarten and regular school classes.

Serious intercurrent infections are a real hazard for the nephrotic child. Although continuous prophylaxis with antibiotics is not recommended, it is advisable to administer antibiotics after definite exposure to bacterial infection and to use these agents promptly and more liberally for therapy of possible bacterial infection, particularly during periods of edema. In the past most serious infections were due to pneumococci, but at present they are caused more frequently by other organisms, particularly gram-negative bacilli and staphylococci. Until the infecting organisms can be identified, a broad-spectrum antibiotic is indicated.

ADRENOCORTICOSTEROIDS. Although recommendations for specific adrenocorticosteroids and dosage schedules vary considerably, the basic aim of all regimens is to maintain the patient free from proteinuria* with the minimal dosage of adrenocorticosteroids. We are not convinced that any one of the suggested therapeutic regimens for adrenocorticosteroids has any clear advantage over the others, including the following plan that we currently use. This plan is relatively easy to follow, it utilizes one of the less expensive drugs, and it involves oral medication exclusively.

INITIAL TREATMENT. Adrenocorticosteroid therapy is started as soon as the diagnosis is established, prednisone being given orally for 28 days in a dosage of approximately 60 mg/m²/day in three divided doses up to a maximum of 80 mg/day. With this regimen diuresis will occur in the majority of patients within 7 to 21 days, and the urine will become free from protein (less than 50 mg/m² BSA per 12-hour night specimen). Following completion of this 28-day course of therapy, daily dosage is reduced to 40 mg/m² and is given three consecutive days out of each week for an additional 4 weeks. Patients receive no additional prednisone unless there is a return of proteinuria.

TREATMENT OF REFRACTORY PATIENTS. Our experience has been that patients with minimal-change disease who do not respond to an initial treatment of 4 weeks of daily therapy and 4 weeks of intermittent therapy often do respond to continuing steroid therapy given in an intermittent dosage. Patients with minimal-change disease who do poorly clinically and remain severely nephrotic, and children with other forms of INS unresponsive to steroid therapy, should be considered for treatment with other drugs.

TREATMENT OF RECURRENCES. Patients showing recurrences of proteinuria lasting more than 2 or 3 days are begun again on their initial dosage or prednisone, which is continued until the urine is free from protein for 3 days. Therapy is then changed to the lower dosage, given on an intermittent basis for an additional 4

*Daily determination of urinary protein concentration is performed at home by the parents on the first urine specimen in the morning using 10 percent sulfosalicylic acid or Albustix. This test constitutes the simplest and yet the most important means of assessment of disease activity. It has been extremely valuable in judging adequacy of treatment.

weeks, as during the initial course of therapy. If there are frequent recurrences with this regimen, patients are considered for combined therapy with an immunosuppressant agent.

Alternate-day steroid therapy in which a single dose, equivalent to twice the usual daily dose, is given once every 48 hours has not been successful in our experience, although good results have been claimed by others. Properly designed controlled clinical trials have not been done. Until the therapeutic efficacy and the supposed freedom from steroid toxicity of this dosage schedule has been tested against other dosage schedules, recommendations regarding its use remain uncertain.

In addition to hypothalamic-pituitary-adrenocortical suppression, other side effects of steroid therapy are frequently seen in children with the nephrotic syndrome who are treated with relatively high dosages over prolonged periods of time. However, extensive experience indicates that with proper precautions serious side effects such as vertebral compression fractures, arrested growth, and severe Cushing's syndrome are not seen more frequently in children with the nephrotic syndrome than in children receiving steroids for other reasons.

Occasionally a child is encountered in whom tapering of steroids after many months of therapy at high dosage is associated with symptoms of headache, lethargy, weakness, anorexia, and vomiting. Treatment is accomplished by providing the minimal dosage of steroid that is adequate to alleviate the symptoms. After a period of 2 to 3 months therapy is stopped. If symptoms reappear treatment is given for another period of 2 to 3 months. In rare instances supportive therapy may be required for as long as 1 year before treatment can be discontinued completely.

The nephrotic syndrome that is related etiologically to certain drugs such as Tridione usually resolves after discontinuation of the offending agent. If not, it is questionable whether adrenocorticosteroids should be used. At present we would tend not to give them until several weeks or even months after the drug has been stopped. Drugs implicated in producing the nephrotic syndrome should be withheld permanently, since their repeated administration may subsequently result in irreversible disease.

DIURETICS.   Sodium restriction, although capable of slowing accumulation of edema during an exacerbation of the nephrotic syndrome, is usually not successful in eliminating edema. In recent years numerous diuretic agents have become available that in combination with moderate sodium restriction contribute significantly to control of edema.

Since the majority of patients exhibit satisfactory diuresis within 2 to 3 weeks after beginning adrenocorticosteroid therapy, diuretic agents are not given initially. But in refractory patients, or before diuresis has occurred in very edematous patients who become more edematous during treatment, diuretics may provide important symptomatic relief.

Hydrochlorothiazide, in a dosage of 2 to 4 mg/kg/day, is the agent used initially in patients whose edema is not severe. The thiazide drugs are relatively nontoxic. Hypokalemia is usually not seen if a child is eating a normal diet, but it may be avoided by giving potassium supplements. Elevated concentration in serum of uric acid is frequently found. The other side effects, including thrombocytopenia, skin rashes, jaundice, pancreatitis, and hyperglycemia, are either extremely rare or have not been reported in children.

In patients with severe degrees of edema we have developed the following schedule of diuretic therapy, which has proved extremely successful. In hypoalbuminemic patients, salt-poor human albumin is given first, in a dosage of 0.5 g/kg for patients whose serum albumin is between 1.5 and 2.0 g/dl, and 1 g/kg if the serum albumin is lower. The albumin is infused slowly over the course of 1 hour. Furosemide is given by intravenous injection after an additional 30 to 60 minutes of equilibration, in a dose of 1 mg/kg. This entire course may be repeated every 4 to 6 hours as needed.

IMMUNOSUPPRESSANT AND CYTOTOXIC DRUGS. The use of drugs such as nitrogen mustard, cyclophosphamide, chlorambucil, methotrexate, 6-thioguanine, and azathioprine has been advocated in the treatment of patients refractory to other forms of therapy, but the value of these agents in such patients has not been established. The limited data available from controlled studies have been negative, and it is difficult to make recommendations regarding their use.

There has been considerable recent experience with steroid-responsive, frequently relapsing children in whom prednisone therapy has resulted in serious complications, including vertebral compression fractures, arrested growth, and severe Cushing's syndrome. Treatment with cyclophosphamide, either alone or in combination with low-dosage prednisone, has been successful in inducing and maintaining remissions, thus permitting gradual resolution of steroidal side effects. The use of this drug in appropriately selected patients may prove to be a major advance in the management of these steroid-dependent children. The decision to use cyclophosphamide, however, must involve consideration of the potentially serious gonadal toxicity of this agent.

Since the use of immunosuppressant and cytotoxic drugs must still be considered experimental, patients considered candidates for such treatment should be managed by, or in consultation with, investigators actively engaged in studying the effect of these drugs in patients with the nephrotic syndrome.

COURSE AND PROGNOSIS.   There are indications that steroid therapy has modified the outcome of the nephrotic syndrome quite apart from its diuretic effect. In the antibiotic era, before the introduction of steroids, a group of 60 children showed the following figures: 33 (55 percent) were recovered or recovering, 18 (30 percent) had died during the active stage, and 9 (15 percent) had developed renal insufficiency (3 of the 9 had died). Riley and associates have since collected data on 779 nephrotic children from 18 clinics. They were followed for a 5-year period in an effort to evaluate the effect of prolonged and intensive steroid therapy. The survival rate in the control group was 60 percent, as compared with 75 percent in the group under intensive steroid therapy. A longer period of observation is needed before a final evaluation can be made, since patients who appear to be doing well at the end of 5 years of steroid therapy may subsequently do less well and may ultimately develop renal insufficiency. The situation is further obscured by the fact that in neither of these series is it possible to separate patients with minimal-change disease from those with other forms of INS.

Ninety-five percent or more of children with minimal-change disease have a total response to initial adrenocorticosteroid therapy, with loss of all clinical and laboratory evidences of disease. The subsequent course in these children tends to follow one of three general patterns: (1) 20 percent do not again develop evidence of disease and therefore appear to have recovered; (2) 50 percent or more relapse from time to time, but infrequently; (3) the remainder have frequent relapses and are referred to by some authors as being steroid-dependent. Relapses in the last two categories may occur over a period of many years, but the patients continue to respond to repeated courses of treatment and presumably go on to ultimate recovery. Patients who relapse infrequently require relatively little steroid therapy and generally do not experience difficulty with steroid toxicity. In contrast, patients who relapse often may require such frequent treatment that severe steroid toxicity becomes the major problem.

Fortunately only a small percentage of children with minimal-change disease fail to attain complete remission in response to initial steroid therapy. In most of these remission is ultimately to be expected following prolonged therapy with steroids or a course of cyclophosphamide. The prognosis in totally unresponsive patients may be grave, with renal insufficiency ensuing over a period of years. Much less often a patient previously steroid-responsive becomes nonresponsive after one or more successfully treated relapses. Recent evidence suggests that at least some of these patients may respond to cyclophasphamide and subsequently be amenable once more to steroid treatment.

Patients with INS unrelated to minimal-change disease commonly are resistant to all forms of therapy, as shown in Table 6. Except for the relatively small number who go into spontaneous or drug-induced remission, the prognosis is guarded. It is not possible early in the course of disease to predict with certainty which course a given child will follow. It is now recognized that the various laboratory tests, which are abnormal more often in patients who are steroid-resistant and who do poorly, serve to identify patients with glomerulonephritis rather than to determine prognosis in patients with minimal-change disease. In the latter group we have found no correlation between the subsequent course and age, sex, or the presence or absence of hematuria or poorly selective proteinuria.

The best prognostic feature at the onset of disease, other than findings on renal biopsy, is initial response to adrenocorticosteroid therapy. Complete cessation of proteinuria following treatment with steroids indicates a favorable prognosis; in complete or absent response often is associated with a grave outcome, fewer than one-third of such children having minimal-change disease.

Finally, criteria of recovery must be considered in formulating therapy and must be included as an important aspect of discussions with the family. Recovery from the nephrotic syndrome must be defined as permanent subsidence of all the manifestations of the disease. Although one can never be absolutely certain that proteinuria may not recur at some future date, if 2 or 3 years have elapsed on a steroid-free regimen without recurrence of proteinuria permanent recovery is virtually assured.

References

Prospective, controlled trial of cyclophosphamide therapy in children with the nephrotic syndrome. Lancet 2:423, 1974

Abramowicz M, Arneil GC, Barnett HL, et al: Controlled clinical trial of azathioprine in children with nephrotic syndrome. Lancet 1:959, 1970

Ackerman GL, Nolan CM: Adrenocortical responsiveness after alternate-day corticosteroid therapy. N Engl J Med 278:405, 1968

Arneil GC: Management of the nephrotic syndrome. Arch Dis Child 43:257, 1968

———Lam NC: Long-term assessment of steroid therapy in childhood nephrosis. Lancet 2:819, 1966

Barnett HL, Forman CW, Lauson HD: The nephrotic syndrom in children. Adv Pediatr 5:53 1953

Browth RB, Burke EC, Stickler GB: Studies in nephrotic syndrome. I. Survival of 135 children with nephrotic syndrome treated with adrenal steroids. Mayo Clin Proc 40:384, 1965

Cameron JS: Nephrotic syndrome. Br Med J 4:350, 1970

———Blanford G: The simple assessment of selectivity in heavy proteinuria. Lancet 2:242, 1966

——— White RHR: Selectivity of proteinuria in children with the nephrotic syndrome. Lancet 1:463, 1965

Churg J, Habib R, White RHR: Pathology of the nephrotic syndrome in children. Lancet 1:1299, 1970

Cornfield D, Schwartz MW; nephrosis: a long-term study of children treated with corticosteroids. J Pediatr 68:507, 1966

Drummond KN, Michael AF, Good RA, Vernier RL: Nephrotic syndrome of childhood. Immunologic, clinical and pathologic correlations. J Clin Invest 45:620, 1966

TABLE 6. Clinical Status Following 8 Weeks of Treatment with Prednisone

Lesion	Number	Percentage in Remission
Minimal-change disease	300	92
Segmental glomerular sclerosis	28	14
Membranoproliferative	20	0
Other	21	38

Duffy JL, Cinque T, Grishman E, Churg J: Intraglomerular fibrin, platelet aggregation, and subendothelial deposits in lipoid nephrosis. J Clin Invest 49:251, 1970

Giangiacomo J, Cleary TG, Cole BR, Hoffsten P, Robson AM: Serum immunoglobulins in the nephrotic syndrome. N Engl J Med 293:8, 1975

Groshong T, Mendelson L, Mendoza S, Bazaral M, Hamburger R: Serum IGE in patients with minimal-change nephrotic syndrome. J Pediatr 83:767, 1973

Habib R: Focal glomerular sclerosis. Kidney Int 4:355, 1973

——— Gubler MC: Les lésions glomérulaires focales des syndromes néphrotiques idiopathiques de l'enfant: A propos de 49 observations. Nephron 8:382, 1971

——— Kleinknecht C: The primary nephrotic syndrome of childhood: classification and clinicopathologic study of 406 cases. Pathol Annu 6:417, 1971

Hayslet JP, Kashgarian M, Bensch KG, et al: Clinico-pathological correlations in the nephrotic syndrome due to primary renal disease. Medicine 52:93, 1973

——— Krassner LS, Bensch KG, Kashgarian M, Epstein FH: Progression of "lipoid nephrosis" to renal insufficiency. N Engl J Med 281:181, 1969

Hyman R, Burkholder PM: Focal sclerosing glomerulonephropathy with hyalinosis. J Pediatr 84:217, 1974

Jenis EH, Teichman S, Briggs WA, et al: Focal segmental glomerulosclerosis. Am J Med 57:695, 1974

Lieberman E, Heuser E, Gilchrist GS, Donnell GN, Landing BH: Thrombosis, nephrosis, and corticosteroid therapy. J Pediatr 73:320, 1968

Moore HL, Katz R, McIntosh R, et al: Unilateral renal vein thrombosis and the nephrotic syndrome. Pediatrics 50:598, 1972

Riley CM, Davis RA, Fertig JW, Barger AP: Nephrosis of childhood: statistical evaluation of the effect of adrenocortical-active therapy. J Chronic Dis 3:640, 1956

Rothenberg MB, Heymann W: The incidence of the nephrotic syndrome in children. Pediatrics 19:446 1957

Saxena KM, Crawford JD: The treatment of nephrosis. N Engl J Med 272:522, 1965

Schlesinger ER, Sultz HA, Mosher WE, Feldman JG: The nephrotic syndrome. Its incidence and implications for the community. Am J Dis Child 116:623, 1968

Siegel NJ, Kashgarian M, Spargo BH, Hayslett JP: Minimal change and focal sclerotic lesions in lipoid nephrosis. Nephron 13:125, 1974

Soyka LF: The nephrotic syndrome. Current concepts in diagnosis and therapy; advantages of alternate day steroid regimen. Clin Pediatr (Phila) 6:77, 1967

West CD, Hong R, Holland NH: Effect of cyclophosphamide on lipoid nephrosis in the human and on aminonucleoside nephrosis in the rat. J Pediatr 68:516, 1966

——— McAdams AJ, McConville JM, Davis NC, Holland NH: Hypocomplementemic and normocomplementemic persistent (chronic) glomerulonephritis; clinical and pathological characteristics. J Pediatr 67:1089, 1965

White RHR: The familial nephrotic syndrome. I. A European survey. Clin Nephrol 1:215, 1973.

——— Cameron JS, Trounce JR: Immunosuppressive therapy in steroid-resistant proliferative glomerulonephritis accompanied by the nephrotic syndrome. Br Med J 2:853, 1966

——— Glasgow EF, Mills RJ: Clinico-pathologic study of nephrotic syndrome in childhood. Lancet 1:1353, 1970

Wittig HJ, Goldman AS: Nephrotic syndrome associated with inhaled allergens. Lancet 1:542, 1970

MISCELLANEOUS NEPHROPATHIES

CHESTER M. EDELMANN, JR.

Infantile Nephrosis (Congenital Nephrosis)

The nephrotic syndrome occurs infrequently during the first year and particularly during the first three months of life; when it does it presents certain characteristic features: a high familial incidence, almost complete resistance to therapy, and a fatal outcome. Many of these cases have occurred in newborn and premature infants. Most instances of the nephrotic syndrome in infancy are of the so-called Finnish type. Rarely the nephrotic syndrome in infants is associated with congenital syphilis, toxoplasmosis, and renal vein thrombosis. In addition some forms of the nephrotic syndrome encountered in older children, including minimal-change disease, focal segmental glomerular sclerosis, and membranous nephropathy, have been reported in infants, although very rarely before the age of 6 months.

At least 112 families with congenital nephrosis have been described, with the great majority being from Finland or of Finnish origin. From a genetic study of 57 Finnish families Norio concluded that the disease is transmitted as an autosomal recessive. Hallman, Norio, and Kouvalainen pointed out features of the disease that indicate an onset during intrauterine life: almost without exception the placenta is very large; the birth weight is low, at least partly because of prematurity; proteinuria and characteristic changes in serum proteins are seen immediately after birth in a great majority of cases; wide cranial sutures at birth indicate that the ossification process is already delayed in utero; polycythemia and especially the advanced erythroblastosis occasionally seen in newborns with congenital nephrosis probably derive from impaired function of the large edematous placenta.

Studies of renal biopsies from patients with infantile nephrosis have shown several different lesions, some of them apparently unique to early infancy and some similar to the glomerular lesions in older childhood. The following descriptions are based on Habib's classification. Approximately one-third to one-fourth of infants have had so-called microcystic kidneys, or the Finnish type of infantile nephrotic syndrome. The cysts, seen histologically near the corticomedullary junctions, are dilated tubules, predominantly proximal in location. There is no evidence that they are the primary abnormality or that they constitute a developmental error. The glomeruli may initially be normal, with electron microscopy showing only fusion of foot processes, but they do undergo progressive sclerosis. Although early death is common, children are said to die of complications (eg, infection) rather than of renal failure. Immunologic studies have been negative, and despite some earlier reports to the contrary, there is no convincing evidence that the disease is immunologically mediated. The renal cortical arterioles are often remarkably hyperplastic. Successful renal transplantation has been reported. Another lesion that is apparently unique to early infancy is diffuse mesangial sclerosis that leads to small, dense, retracted glomeruli and to progressive renal insufficiency. The cases are familial and have an early onset; the prognosis is poor and is unaltered by therapy. This lesion accounts for one-fifth of all cases. Approximately one-fourth of all patients will have minimal glomerular change. The clinical onset is slightly later, and the condition appears to be steroid-sensitive, as in later childhood. It is occasionally familial.

Segmental glomerular sclerosis also occurs in early infancy, perhaps in one-fifth of all cases. The lesion is similar to that seen in older cases of the nephrotic syndrome and is steroid-resistant. It also has a poor prognosis. A small number of cases will have membranous nephropathy, which seems to be nonfamilial. Its histologic appearance and clinical manifestations are similar to those seen in older children. Finally, the nephrotic syndrome in early infancy has occurred with increasing frequency in association with congenital syphilis. Histologic studies have shown an immune-complex nephritis with variable mesangial proliferation. A similar lesion has been described in a case of early infantile nephrotic syndrome associated with congenital toxoplasmosis. The relationship of the nephrotic syndrome to renal vein thrombosis in early infancy remains debatable, but most workers feel that the vascular lesion is almost always secondary.

The clinical picture and laboratory findings in congenital nephrosis do not differ from those of the nephrotic syndrome in older children, except for the age of the patients. Most of them have developed edema during the first month of life; exceptionally it has been present at birth. Although the serum cholesterol is usually elevated in these infants, as in children and adults with the nephrotic syndrome, the distribution of values is shifted to the left due presumably to the developmentally lower values in young infants.

Susceptibility to infection and to water and electrolyte imbalance is exaggerated because of the young ages of these patients. Steroid therapy fails to induce a remission and may complicate the management of the disease. Most patients survive but a few months, succumbing as a rule to fluid and electrolyte disorders, inanition, and intercurrent infection usually before the development of renal failure. Exceptionally an infant who develops the disease toward the latter part of the first year will show the favorable response that is seen in the older child, most likely representing an instance of minimal-change nephrotic syndrome, which does occasionally occur in the young infant even within the first few months of life. Successful therapy with a combination of immunosuppressive drugs has not been reported, but additional experience with this form of treatment is needed. Most attempts at renal transplantation have been unsuccessful.

Recurrent Hematuria

This designation probably represents a number of disorders characterized by multiple episodes of gross hematuria that occur over a period of months or years. The term benign recurrent hematuria is also used, thus implying an invariably good prognosis. It would appear, however, that recovery does not take place in many cases; and since those with a poor prognosis cannot be differentiated at onset from those with a truly benign course, the term benign probably should be abandoned.

The onset commonly mimics acute poststreptococcal glomerulonephritis, although hypertension, reduced renal function, and edema usually are absent. However, instead of following the expected course for acute nephritis, recurrent bouts of gross hematuria ensue, often with considerable proteinuria. The acute episodes are usually preceded by a viral respiratory infection, and abdominal symptoms may be striking. Between episodes the patient is asymptomatic, the only abnormality being residual microscopic hematuria with or without minimal or moderate proteinuria. In some patients urinalyses have been reported to have returned to normal during asymptomatic periods.

Histologic findings in the kidney are heterogeneous, including IgA-IgG mesangial nephritis (Berger's disease), focal glomerulonephritis, focal glomerulosclerosis, and minimal-change disease with ultrastructural alteration of the basement membrane. IgA-IgG nephritis may run a protracted course, with recurrence but with little or no change in renal function; but glomerular sclerosis does occur and can be responsible for progressive renal insufficiency. In some instances the deposits of IgA are present around the peripheral capillary wall (even in an epimembranous location) and have been associated with progressive glomerular sclerosis; other cases with similar distributions of deposits have shown clinical resolution. The differentiation of severe glomerular lesions with extensive immune deposits from Schönlein-Henoch purpura may be exceedingly difficult on morphologic grounds.

Recurrent hematuria has been reported as a familial disease, although in such instances great caution must be exercised in making this diagnosis because familial nephritis of the form that progresses to uremia may be present for many years without evidence of renal damage. Since even minimal urinary abnormalities may be evidence of severe progressive renal disease, the diagnosis of recurrent hematuria should not be made in familial or nonfamilial cases without thorough examination, including renal biopsy.

The clinical course may be as long as 10 years. During this time there is often progressive loss of renal function and scarring and glomerular obsolescence on renal biopsy. It appears that in many instances complete recovery ultimately ensues, although longer follow-ups of many patients are needed to determine this with certainty.

Balkan Nephropathy

A peculiar form of renal disease has been reported in certain rural areas of Bulgaria, Romania, and Yugoslavia. Several members of one family may be affected, and the disease is often seen in children. Urinary findings are minimal, hypertension is unusual, and there is a striking loss of concentrating capacity. Patients progress slowly but relentlessly to chronic uremia without passing through a nephrotic stage. Pathologically the tubules seem to be primarily involved, exhibiting degenerative changes with severe interstitial fibrosis. Ultimately the kidneys are extremely contracted with extensive fibrosis and almost total absence of recognizable nephric elements in the outer part of the cortex. No clue to etiology has been found. Although therapy is not available, those moving out of an endemic area appear to escape the disease.

Hyperuricemia and Gout

It is estimated that as many as two-thirds of patients with gout have renal involvement, but this disease has been reported only rarely in childhood, and few of these patients have had overt renal manifestations. Rosenthal and associates described an infant from a gouty family with elevated levels of uric acid in the blood and symptoms of uremia at age 2 months. Several adolescents are included in the report by Duncan and Dixon of familial gout and renal disease with hypertension. Hyperuricemia with uric acid nephropathy is also observed in patients with Lesch-Nyhan syndrome, in patients with glycogen storage disease, in patients who have had prolonged diuretic therapy, and in patients having acute cytolytic therapy for malignant disease such as leukemia.

Renal damage occurs primarily from parenchymal deposition of urates, particularly in the renal pyramids, and precipitation within the tubules, with subsequent nephron loss. In addition, stones are present in approximately one-fifth of patients. Finally, patients with gout seem to be unusually prone to develop pyelonephritis.

Hypercalcemia and Hypercalciuria

Hypercalcemia and/or hypercalciuria are seen in a variety of clinical situations, including immobilization, vitamin D intoxication, idiopathic hypercalcemia of infancy, hyperparathyroidism, hyperthyroidism, sarcoidosis, multiple myeloma, and malignancy. Nephrocalcinosis with severe generalized renal damage and ultimate renal insufficiency may result.

In the absence of demonstrable nephrocalcinosis and prior to depression of glomerular filtration rate, characteristic changes in renal function may be noted. The most prominent of these is a rapidly developing and equally rapidly reversible concentrating defect, produced apparently by impairment of production of the usual medullary gradient of hyperosmolality. Another finding in patients with hypercalcemia, with the notable exception of hyperparathyroidism, is metabolic alkalosis. Parathormone release appears to lower the renal threshold for bicarbonate; thus parathormone inhibition due to hypercalcemia might be the cause of the alkalosis. Other patients with calcium nephropathy, particularly those with idiopathic hypercalcemia and vita-

min D intoxication, develop the features of renal tubular acidosis.

Treatment consists of determining and correcting the underlying causes of hypercalcemia or hypercalciuria. Early changes of calcium nephropathy, including degenerative and necrotic changes in the tubular epithelium of Henle's loop, distal convoluted tubule, and collecting duct, are reversible. As the process advances calcium is deposited interstitially, and changes of chronic inflamation may be noted. Ultimately glomeruli may be sclerosed, apparently because of tubular obstruction and nephrocalcinosis.

Potassium Depletion

Potassium depletion severe enough to cause renal impairment is not often encountered in infants and children, but it does occur, particularly under two circumstances: in chronic gastrointestinal loss and secondary to hyperadrenalism.

It appears that potassium depletion must be of fairly long duration and of considerable magnitude before the kidney is affected, although there are instances in which abnormalities have occurred apparently after only a few days of potassium loss. Potassium depletion in man is associated with characteristic histologic changes in the kidney, namely swelling and degeneration of tubular epithelial cells, particularly in the proximal convolution. This differs from the situation in the rat, in which the predominant lesion is in the collecting ducts. Although the renal lesions appear to be reversible, there are a few reports of anatomic changes of pyelonephritis and interstitial nephritis.

The physiologic consequences of potassium nephropathy include (1) a concentrating defect, (2) limitation in production of a hydrogen-ion gradient, and (3) increase in the renal bicarbonate threshold. However, it has recently been suggested that the elevation in renal bicarbonate threshold and resulting metabolic alkalosis seen in patients with potassium depletion are due in most instances to an accompanying deficiency of sodium chloride. An additional consequence of potassium depletion that has been demonstrated primarily in rats is a marked increase in susceptibility to pyelonephritis. The role of potassium depletion as a predisposing factor for pyelonephritis in man requires further study.

Treatment generally consists of administration of potassium, which must be given cautiously, particularly in patients with impaired renal function. Conditions such as primary hyperaldosteronism must receive specific therapy before potassium repletion can be accomplished.

Drugs, Metals, and Other Nephrotoxins

Renal damage may occur from a variety of pharmacologic and toxic agents. Damage may be either mild and reversible or so severe that acute or chronic renal failure occurs. A number of agents have been shown to have their effect on the proximal tubule and to produce features of the Fanconi syndrome. These include tetracycline, oxalic acid, and lead and other heavy metals (including mercury, cadmium, uranium, copper, and bismuth). In addition, heavy metals may cause either acute tubular necrosis or chronic nephropathy. Many organic solvents are capable of producing severe renal damage by a number of different mechanisms. The most common of these is carbon tetrachloride, which causes acute proximal tubular necrosis and oliguric renal failure. Recovery in children usually is complete. Ethylene glycol is metabolized partially to oxalate; deposition of calcium oxalate crystals causes proximal tubular obstruction and dilatation. Propylene glycol causes acute intravascular hemolysis and consequent renal damage. Diethylene glycol causes severe renal cortical necrosis.

Certain antimicrobials are nephrotoxic. Sulfonamides cause obstructive uropathy by crystallization within the tubules or ureters. Streptomycin, Vancomycin, kanamycin, neomycin, polymyxin, colistin, bacitracin, amphotericin B, and dimethoxyphenylpenicillin are all toxic to the renal tubular epithelium. Hematuria or proteinuria or both give the first indication of renal toxicity, generally preceding development of azotemia. Discontinuation of treatment usually leads to a fairly prompt return of urine to normal, but the nephrotoxicity of neomycin, amphotericin B, and bacitracin may be permanent. Methicillin therapy has been associated with an interstitial nephritis in which immunologic studies have shown antibodies to tubular basement membrane. The nephrotic syndrome has been attributed to ingestion of a variety of drugs and metals, including trimethadione, tolbutamide, penicillamine, gold, bismuth, mercury, and thallium.

A great deal of attention has been directed in recent years to analgesic nephropathy. Severe interstitial nephritis with extensive renal damage apparently does occur, although the dosage must be tremendous and must be given over very long periods. Earlier reports focused on phenacetin as the major toxic agent, but it is possible that other analgesics may be implicated as well. Chronic glomerular disease with the nephrotic syndrome has been observed in a number of heroin addicts. Some have progressive glomerular sclerosis and others an immune-complex nephritis. Rapid deterioration of renal function is common. Most such patients have been black males, a factor that may or may not be of significance in the development of the renal complication, the pathogenesis of which is uncertain. Finally, there have been a number of reports of acute oliguric renal failure secondary to the intravascular administration of various media in the course of radiographic studies. Infants appear to be particularly susceptible

Diabetes Mellitus

Prior to the discovery of insulin, no renal deaths in patients with diabetes mellitus were reported. Renal failure now accounts for more than half the deaths in such patients. However, in the pediatric age group significant clinical signs of renal involvement in patients with diabetes mellitus are extremely rare, since the so-called diabetic nephropathy usually takes 10 years or more to develop, despite notable exceptions. Nevertheless, even young patients with diabetes mellitus may be found to have minimal proteinuria if carefully tested, and renal abnormalities have been demonstrated histologically early in the course of the disease, as well as in patients with so-called prediabetes. The nephrotic syndrome has occasionally developed in diabetic children —possibly a chance occurrence. In a study of 123 children with diabetes mellitus Moss reported a tendency for blood pressure to increase significantly at about 13 years of age, as compared to normal controls; he postulated that this reflected a prehypertensive state due to subclinical renal vascular disease.

There is still controversy as to the possible correlation between the degree of clinical and biochemical control and diabetes and the likelihood of emergence of renal and other complications. There is no question, however, that diabetic nephropathy may develop even in the patient with the best control of disease.

The renal lesions of diabetes mellitus are numerous, comprising a severe nephropathy that affects glomeruli, tubules, vessels, and interstitium; however, renal lesions in childhood diabetes are relatively mild. Biopsy studies disclose focal thickening of the glomerular basement membranes and mesangium, and hyaline deposits appear at the vascular poles. Electron microscopy in the earliest stages shows minimal thickening of basement membranes and accumulation of hyaline material or material like basement membrane beneath endothelium and among mesangial cells—changes that appear to be progressive. Similar abnormalities have been detected in renal biopsies of diabetic children with the nephrotic syndrome.

The high prevalence of pyelonephritis in patients with diabetes mellitus was originally interpreted as reflecting an unusual susceptibility of these patients to bacterial infection of the urinary tract. It is now recognized that the frequency of infection is probably due to the frequency of urethral catheterization rather than the diabetic process per se. However, an unusually severe complication of pyelonephritis, necrotizing renal papillitis, is much more common in the diabetic than in the nondiabetic population. This condition, which represents ischemic necrosis of the papilla, develops during an episode of acute infection. Papillary tissue that is sloughed may be recovered in the urine. Characteristic filling defects can be observed radiographically.

The only treatment of diabetic nephropathy, apart from optimal clinical management of the diabetes per se, is treatment of urinary tract infection. Established diabetic nephropathy is treated as is any type of chronic renal insufficiency (p. 1249).

Sickle Cell Disease

Patients with sickle cell disease have functional and morphologic abnormalities involving many organ systems. Renal manifestations include a concentrating defect, hematuria, the nephrotic syndrome, and a peculiar type of progressive nephropathy that may lead to renal insufficiency. Priapism, a common urologic complication in adults, is rare in children.

The incidence of sickle hemoglobin in American blacks has been estimated to be 8 percent, and 2 to 3 percent of these have sickle cell disease. The proportion demonstrating renal involvement is unknown, but the concentrating defect and hematuria are seen in patients with SA and SC hemoglobin as well as patients with sickle disease. Progressive nephropathy apparently is limited to the latter group.

CLINICAL AND LABORATORY FEATURES.

During the first few years of life GFR and RBF in patients with sickle cell disease tend to be normal or elevated for age, similar to the findings in patients with other types of chronic anemia. These functions subsequently decrease, however, so that characteristically they are reduced to below normal by early adult life.

Studies in adults have suggested that as many as one-third of affected patients may have hematuria; although this abnormality is not uncommon in children, precise figures are not available. Hematuria may be unilateral or bilateral in origin. The left kidney is involved four times as often as the right, and a similar male-to-female ratio of 4:1 has been described. Passage of clots may lead to renal colic.

The concentrating defect is not present early in life but is almost constant after 2 or 3 years of age. Initially this abnormality may be reversible, but by adolescence it appears to be a permanent defect.

Published reports of the nephrotic syndrome associated with sickle cell disease are rare, but it is probably not such an uncommon disorder, since we have seen several instances in the past few years. This form of the nephrotic syndrome is totally resistant to steroid therapy, and we have had one patient in whom severe sickle crisis was produced by administration of prednisone.

Chronic renal insufficiency and uremia secondary to sickle cell disease, with all clinical and laboratory manifestations of chronic glomerulonephritis, also have been reported, although rarely. We have treated four children with this condition and have found evidence of early renal insufficiency in a number of other children. This suggests that generalized renal damage secondary to sickle cell disease may be more common than realized.

PATHOLOGY.

Pathologic studies of young patients show certain abnormalities that can be correlated with the known alterations of renal function. Scarring and tubular obliteration in the inner medulla, presumably the result of anoxic injury, may be responsible for the irreversible concentrating defect that appears in late childhood. A more severe, acute lesion is papillary necrosis, which occurs in both the homozygous and heterozygous forms of the disease. Pelvic and medullary hemorrhages are particularly common and often are the only pathologic findings in kidneys removed for gross

unilateral hematuria. These lesions presumably result from vascular stasis, a state that would be enhanced by the tendency of erythrocytes to undergo sickling in the hypoxic and hypertonic environment of the medulla.

Changes are also present in the cortex, where the glomeruli are markedly congested. During childhood the glomeruli, particularly in the inner cortex, appear to undergo striking progressive enlargement, considerably in excess of normal growth. This finding is undoubtedly related to the increased glomerular filtration rate seen in the same age group. However, increased vascularity gives way to progressive ischemia and sclerosis, apparently leading in some individuals to glomerular obliteration and chronic renal insufficiency. Less severe changes may underlie the decline of glomerular filtration in older patients. Other abnormalities include focal tubular necrosis and scarring, tubular hemosiderosis, and cortical infarcts. The nephrotic syndrome occurs with somewhat greater frequency than might be anticipated were it a chance association. In most of these instances renal biopsy has, in our experience, shown minimal glomerular change. Some patients, however, seem to have a membranoproliferative lesion with subendothelial deposits of immune complexes in which antibody is directed against a tubular epithelial antigen. It has been suggested that ischemic tubular damage is the initial event and leads to the release of and sensitization against tubular protein. The occasional occurrence of renal vein thrombosis might also initiate tubular damage leading to a similar sequence of events.

PATHOPHYSIOLOGY.

The cause of hematuria in patients without generalized renal damage or chronic renal insufficiency is probably related to papillary congestion and necrosis secondary to red cell sickling, stasis, and hypoxia. Similarly, the concentrating defect appears to be best explained by sickling of erythrocytes in the vasa recta during descent into the hypertonic, relatively hypoxic, renal medulla. Vascular stasis may exaggerate the normal degree of hypoxia and thus interfere with medullary sodium transport in the loop of Henle or impair countercurrent exchange mechanisms of the vasa recta. Osmotic diuresis with its associated increase in medullary blood flow might be expected to reverse intravascular sickling in the kidney by lessening medullary hypoxia and decreasing medullary hypertonicity. Thus it is of interest that the maximal rate of reabsorption of free water during osmotic diuresis in patients with sickle cell anemia is normal or close to normal, which supports the hypothesis that the concentrating defect is caused by intravascular sickling. Further evidence relating disturbed function specifically to the sickling phenomenon is the ability to correct the concentrating defect in young subjects by administration of multiple blood transfusions.

The pathogenesis of the nephrotic syndrome and renal insufficiency in patients with sickle cell disease is unknown, but the latter may result from the occurrence of multiple small infarctions over the course of many years. The tendency for renal insufficiency to occur with advancing age lends support to this suggestion.

Radiation Nephritis

Radiation nephritis usually results from inclusion of the kidneys in the field of x-ray therapy. The most frequent circumstance in children is following abdominal irradiation for Wilms' tumor. Luxton has established the following classification of the various patterns of disease: acute radiation nephritis, chronic radiation nephritis, benign hypertension, late malignant hypertension. Although other authors have not found it possible to fit all patients into this scheme, and there does appear to be a considerable degree of overlap, the classification has clinical usefulness.

Acute radiation nephritis occurs within a few months to a year following x-ray exposure; it may be manifested by abnormal urine, symptoms of uremia, or hypertension. Death may occur from malignant hypertension or uremia. If recovery is to take place, improvement is usually noted within several months of onset. Even with recovery there is usually residual renal damage. Chronic radiation nephritis may occur as a sequel to acute radiation nephritis or evolve asymptomatically following irradiation of both kidneys. Benign essential hypertension with minimal renal abnormalities may occur within a year following x-ray therapy. Late malignant hypertension has been seen up to several years following irradiation in patients with chronic radiation nephritis and in patients with exposure of just one kidney. The prognosis is ominous.

In a long-term follow-up of children who had undergone nephrectomy and radiation for malignant disease, Mitus and associates concluded that normal renal function can be preserved if x-ray exposure is kept below 1,200 r. This figure agrees well with the finding of Luxton that adults are able to tolerate 1,700 r to both kidneys. Avioli and associates found that RPF and GFR decreased progressively as radiation dosage exceeded 400 r. At dosages of 2,000 to 2,400 r a progressive decrease in GFR was observed that persisted up to 12 months after radiation.

The renal lesion progresses from the acute stage of cortical edema and glomerular ischemia to the chronic lesion of glomerular sclerosis, tubular atrophy, and cortical fibrosis. The kidney becomes small and atrophic. Vascular changes are usually prominent. The small vessels undergo fibrinoid necrosis, medial fibrosis, and hyalinization. However, hypertension is common, and secondary vascular changes may be superimposed on the primary lesions. Tubular atrophy generally parallels the degree of glomerular sclerosis, although on occasion the former is present to an excessive degree.

Hepatorenal Syndrome

Renal failure in patients with terminal liver disease is encountered frequently in adults, but rarely if ever in young children. Morphologic lesions in the kidneys are variable and involve both glomeruli and tubules. However, the low GFR and RBF appear to be due to altered hemodynamics rather than to a specific anatomic or biochemical defect. This view is supported by the fact that kidneys from patients with the hepatorenal syndrome function promptly when transplanted into recipients without hepatic disease.

The functional pattern of oliguria, azotemia, low concentration of sodium in serum and urine, and high urinary specific gravity is similar to that observed experimentally during decreased renal perfusion. In most patients with cirrhosis, cardiac output is adequate and plasma volume is normal or increased. Despite this there appears to be a general hypoperfusion of all vital organs, including the kidneys, as is seen in congestive heart failure or hypovolemia. The cause of renal hypoperfusion is unknown, and Papper has suggested that other mechanisms, such as abnormalities in the intrarenal circulation, should be considered in the pathogenesis of renal failure.

No specific treatment is available. Transient improvement has been noted in response to volume expansion, and reversal of renal failure has been reported following portacaval shunting.

References

INFANTILE NEPHROSIS

Bouton JM, Coulter BS: The nephrotic syndrome of infancy. Acta Paediatr Scand 63:769, 1974

Fetterman GH, Feldman JD: Congenital anomalies of renal tubules in a case of "infantile nephrosis." Am J Dis Child 100:319, 1960

Habib R, Bois E: Hétérogénéité des syndromes néphrotiques à début précoce du nourrisson (syndrome néphrotique [infantile]). Etude anatomo-clinique et génétique de 37 observations. Helv Paediatr Acta 28:91, 1973

Hallman N, Norio R, Kouvalainen K: Main features of the congenital nephrotic syndrome. Acta Paediatr Scand [Suppl] 172:75, 1967

——— Norio R, Rapola J: Congenital nephrotic syndrome. Nephron 11:101, 1973

Hoyer JR, Kjellstrant CM, Simmons RL, Najarian JF, Mauer SM: Successful renal transplantation in 3 children with congenital nephrotic syndrome. Lancet 1:1410, 1973

Kaplan BS, Bureau MA, Drummond KN: The nephrotic syndrome in the first year of life: is a pathologic classification possible? J Pediatr 85:615, 1974

——— Wiglesworth FW, Marks MI, Drummond KN: The glomerulopathy of congenital syphilis—an immune deposit disease. J Pediatr 81:1154, 1972

Norio R: Heredity in the congenital nephrotic syndrome. A genetic study of 57 Finnish families with a review of reported cases. Ann Paediatr [Suppl] 12:27, 1966

Oliver J: Microcystic renal disease and its relation to "infantile nephrosis." Am J Dis Child 100:312, 1960

Rapola J, Savilahti E: Immunofluorescent and morphological studies in congenital nephrotic syndrome. Acta Paediatr Scand 60:253, 1971

Shahin B, Papadopoulou ZL, Jenis EH: Congenital nephrotic syndrome associated with congenital toxoplasmosis. J Pediatr 85:366, 1974

Wiggelinkhuizen J, Kaschula ROC, Uys CJ, Kuijten RH, Dale J: Congenital syphilis and glomerulonephritis with evidence for immune pathogenesis. Arch Dis Child 48:375, 1973

Yuceoglu AM, Sagel I, Tresser G, Wasserman E, Lange K: The glomerulopathy of congenital syphilis. A curable immune-deposit disease. JAMA 229:1085, 1974

RECURRENT HEMATURIA

Davies DR, Tighe JR, Jones NF, Brown GW: Recurrent haematuria and mesangial IgA deposition. J Clin Pathol 26:672, 1973

Finlayson G, Alexander R, Juncos L, et al: Immunoglobulin A glomerulonephritis. A clinicopathologic study. Lab Invest 32:140, 1975

Glasgow E, Moncrieff M, White R: Symptomless haematuria in childhood. Br Med J 11:687, 1970

Hendler E, Kashgarian M, Hayslett J: Clinicopathological correlation of primary haematuria. Lancet 1:458, 1972

Johnston C, Shuler S: Recurrent haematuria in childhood. A five-year follow-up. Arch Dis Child 44:483, 1969

Lannigan R, Insley J: Light and electron microscope appearances in renal biopsy material from cases of recurrent haematuria in children. J Clin Pathol 18:178, 1965

Levy M, Beaufils H, Gubler MC, Habib R: Idiopathic recurrent microscopic hematuria and mesangial IgA-IgG deposits in children (Berger's disease). Clin Nephrol 1:63, 1973

Lowance DC, Mullins JD, McPhaul JJ Jr: Immunoglobulin A (IgA) associated glomerulonephritis. Kidney Int 3:167, 1973

Rogers PW, Kurtzman NA, Bunn SM Jr, White MG: Familial benign essential hematuria. Arch Intern Med 131:257, 1973

Roy LP, Fish AJ, Vernier RL, Michael AF: Recurrent macroscopic hematuria, focal nephritis, and mesangial deposition of immunoglobulin and complement. J Pediatr 82:767, 1973

Singer DB, Hill LL, Rosenberg HS, Marshall J, Swenson R: Recurrent hematuria in childhood. N Engl J Med 279:7, 1968

van de Putte LBA, de la Riviere GB, van Breda Vriesman PJC: Recurrent or persistent hematuria. Sign of mesangial immune-complex deposition. N Engl J Med 290:1165, 1974

Zollinger HU, Gaboardi F: Verzögerte Heilung einer diffusen intra- und extracapillären Glomerulonephritis mit IgA-Depots. Virchows Arch [Pathol Anat] 354:349, 1971

BALKAN NEPHROPATHY

Editor: The Balkan nephropathy. Lancet 1:304, 1966

Hall PW III, Dammin GJ, Griggs RC, et al: Investigation of chronic endemic nephropathy in Yugoslavia. II. Renal pathology. Am J Med 39:210, 1965

Wolstenholme GEW, Knight J: The Balkan Nephropathy. Boston, Little, Brown, 1967

HYPERURICEMIA AND GOUT

Editor: Gout and the kidney. Lancet 1:961, 1968

Gutman AB, Yü TF: Uric acid nephrolithiasis. J Med 45:756, 1968

Nyhan WL, Oliver WJ, Lesch M: A familial disorder of uric acid metabolism and central nervous system function. II. J Pediatr 67:257, 1965

Rosenthal IM, Gaballah S, Rafelson ME Jr: Gout in infancy manifested by renal failure. Pediatrics 33:251, 1964

HYPERCALCEMIA AND HYPERCALCIURIA

Heinemann HO: Metabolic alkalosis in paitents with hypercalcemia. Metabolism 14:1137, 1965

Manitius A, Levitin H, Beck D, Epstein FH: The mechanism of impairment of renal concentrating ability in hypercalcemia. J Clin Invest 39:693, 1960

Richet G, Ardaillou R, Amiel C: Alcalose métabolique rénale de l'hypercalcémie. In Hamburger J (ed): Actualités Néphrologiques de l'hôpital Necker, 1963. Paris, Editions Médicales Flammarion, 1963, p 145

Stark H, Barnett HL, Edelmann CM Jr: Renal effects of hypercalciuria in immobilized children. Proc Soc Exp Biol Med 118:870, 1965

POTASSIUM DEPLETION

Holliday MA, Segar WC, Bright NH, Egan T: The effect of potassium deficiency on the kidney. Pediatrics 26:950, 1960

Kassirer JP, Schwartz WB: Correction of metabolic alkalosis in man without repair of potassium deficiency. Am J Med 40:19, 1966

DRUGS, METALS, AND OTHER NEPHROTOXINS

Abramowicz M, Edelmann CM Jr: Nephrotoxicity of anti-infective drugs. Clin Pediatr (Phila) 7:389, 1968

Balslov JT, Jorgensen HE: A survey of 499 patients with acute anuric renal insufficiency. Am J Med 34:753, 1963

Eknoyan G, Györkey F, Dichoso C, Györkey P: Nephropathy in patients with drug addiction. Evolution of pathological and clinical features. Virchows Arch [Pathol Anat] 365:1, 1975

———— Györkey F, Dichoso C, et al: Renal involvement in drug abuse. Arch Intern Med 132:801, 1973

Emmerson BT: Metals and the kidney. In Black DAK (ed): Renal Disease. Philadelphia, FA Davis, 1967, p 561

Friedman EA, Sreepada Rao TK, Nicastri AD: Heroin-associated nephropathy (editorial). Nephron 13:421, 1974

Gilberg EE, Khoury GH, Hogan GR, Jones B: Hemorrhagic renal necrosis in infancy: relationship to radiopaque compounds. J Pediatr 76:49, 1970

Gilman A: Analgesic nephrotoxicity. A pharmacologic analysis. Am J Med 36:167, 1964

Gruskin AB, Oetliker OH, Wolfish NM, et al: Effects of angiography on renal function and histology in infants and piglets. J Pediatr 76:41, 1970

Hollenberg NK, Adams DF, Oken DE, Abrams HL, Merrill JP: Acute renal failure due to nephrotoxins. Renal hemodynamic and angiographic studies in man. N Engl J Med 282:1329, 1970

Kilcoyne MM, Daly JJ, Gocke DJ, et al: Nephrotic syndrome in heroin addicts. Lancet 1:17, 1972

Kunin CM: Nephrotoxicity of antibiotics. JAMA 202:204, 1967

Sreepada Rao TK, Nicastri AD, Friedman EA: Natural history of heroin-associated nephropathy. N Engl J Med 290:19, 1974

DIABETES MELLITUS

Balodimos MC, Legg MA, Bradley RF: Diabetic glomerulosclerosis in children. Diabetes 20:622, 1971

Beisswenger PJ, Spiro RG: Studies on the human glomerular basement membrane. Composition, nature of the carbohydrate units and chemical changes in diabetes mellitus. Diabetes 22:180, 1973

Fisher ER, Perez-Stable E, Amidi M, Saruer ME, Danowski TS: Ultrastructural renal changes in juvenile diabetics. JAMA 202:291, 1967

Kefalides NA: Biochemical properties of human glomerular basement membrane in normal and diabetic kidneys. J Clin Invest 53:403, 1974

Osterby R: Morphometric studies of the peripheral glomerular basement membrane in early juvenile diabetes. I. Development of initial basement membrane thickening. Diabetologia 8:84, 1972

———— The number of glomerular cells and substructures in early juvenile diabetes. A quantitative electron microscopic study. Acta Pathol Microbiol Scand 80:785, 1972

Urizar RE, Schwartz A, Top F Jr, Vernier RL: The nephrotic syndrome in children with diabetes mellitus of recent onset. Report of five cases. N Engl J Med 281:173, 1969

Westberg NG, Michael AF: Immunohistopathology of diabetic glomerulosclerosis. Diabetes 21:163, 1972

SICKLE CELL DISEASE

Bernstein J, Whitten CF: A histologic appraisal of the kidney in sickle-cell anemia. Arch Pathol 70:407, 1960

Elfenbein B, Patchefsky A, Schwartz W, Weinstein AG: Pathology of the glomerulus in sickle cell anemia with and without nephrotic syndrome. Am J Pathol 77:357, 1974

Levitt MF, Hauser AD, Levy MS, Polimeros D: The renal concentrating defect in sickle-cell disease. Am J Med 29:611, 1960

McCoy RC: Ultrastructural alterations in the kidney of patients with sickle-cell disease and the nephrotic syndrome. Lab Invest 21:85, 1969

Strauss J, Pardo V, Koss MN, Griswold W, McIntosh RM: Nephropathy associated with sickle-cel anemia: an autologous immune complex nephritis. I. Studies on nature of glomerular-bound antibody and antigen identification in a patient with sickle cell disease and immune deposit glomerulonephritis. Am J Med 58:382, 1975

Strom T, Muehrcke RC, Smith RD: Sickle cell anemia with the nephrotic syndrome and renal vein obstruction. Arch Intern Med 129:104, 1972

Van Eps LWS, Pinedo-Vells C, de Vries GH, de Koning J: Nature of concentrating defect in sickle-cell nephropathy. Microangiographic studies. Lancet 1:450, 1970

Walker BR, Alexander F, Birdsall TR, Warren RL: Glomerular lesions in sickle cell nephropathy. JAMA 215:437, 1971

RADIATION NEPHRITIS

Arneil GC, Emmanuel IG, Flatman GE, et al: Nephritis in two children after irradiation and chemotherapy for nephroblastoma. Lancet 1:960, 1974

Luxton RW: Radiation nephritis. A long-term study of 54 patients. Lancet 2:1221, 1961

——— Kunkler PB: Radiation nephritis. Acta Radiol 2:169, 1964

Madrazo A, Suzuki Y, Churg J: Radiation nephritis. Acute changes following high dose of radiation. Am J Pathol 54:507, 1969

Mitus A, Tefft M, Fellers FX: Long-term follow-up of renal functions of 108 childen who underwent nephrectomy for malignant disease. Pediatrics 44:912, 1969

O'Malley B, D'Angio GJ, Vawter GF: Late effects of roentgen therapy given in infancy. Am J Roentgenol Radium Ther Nucl Med 89:1067, 1963

Phillips TL, Ross G: A quantitative technique for measuring renal damage after irradiation. Radiology 109:457, 1973

HEPATORENAL SYNDROME

Editor: Renal resurrection. N Engl J Med 280:1414, 1969

Epstein M, Berk DP, Hollenberg NK, et al: Renal failure in the patient with cirrhosis. The role of active vasoconstriction. Am J Med 49:175, 1970

Koppel MH, Coburn JW, Mims MM, et al: Transplantation of cadaveric kidneys from patients with hepatorenal syndrome. Evidence for the functional nature of renal failure in advanced liver disease. N Engl J Med 280:1367, 1969

Papper S, Vaamonde CA: Renal failure in cirrhosis—role of plasma volume. Ann Intern Med 68:958, 1968

Reynolds TB, Lieberman FL, Redeker AG: Functional renal failure with cirrhosis. The effect of plasma volume expansion. Medicine 46:191, 1967

Shear L, Kleinerman J, Gabuzda GJ: Renal failure in patients with cirrhosis of the liver. I. Clinical and pathologic chracteristics. Am J Med 39:184, 1965

HEREDITARY NEPHROPATHIES
Jay Bernstein

The hereditary nephropathies encompass a number of unrelated inherited disorders. Our awareness and knowledge of them have increased greatly in the last 15 years, and the lists of variants, subgroups, and eponyms have grown accordingly. At least part of this rapid development can be attributed to a greater awareness of hereditary renal disease and to increasing accuracy in differentiating hereditary nephritis from acquired glomerulonephritis. The frequent use of renal biopsy has led to more reliable clinicopathologic correlation and enabled us to establish certain categories of nephropathy, but the need for defining hereditary nephropathy and for classifying its individual components has become increasingly more urgent.

The hereditary nephropathies include several primary renal diseases and certain clearly systemic diseases; in neither group is the basic structural or metabolic defect known (Table 7). The group does not

TABLE 7. Hereditary Nephritis

Hereditary progressive nephritis with and without neurosensory deafness (Alport's syndrome)
Familial bening hematuria
Hereditary onycho-osteodysplasia (nail-patella syndrome)
Hereditary acro-osteolysis
Juvenile megaloblastic anemia (Imerlund's syndrome)
Asphyxiating thoracic dystrophy (Jeune's syndrome)
Medullary cystic diseases

include other heritable systemic disorders, such as cystinosis, diabetes mellitus, and sickle cell anemia, in which the renal component, although major, is obviously secondary. It also does not include heritable disorders of tubular transport and function, which are considered elsewhere (p. 1300). It does include hereditary and familial nephritis, a heterogeneous group with primary glomerular involvement, and the medullary cystic disorders, a heterogeneous group with primary tubular involvement. The distinction between glomerular and tubular disease may not be sharp (as in the nephropathy of Jeune's syndrome), and the differentiation of hereditary nephropathy from developmental abnormality may be unclear and even arbitrary. Nevertheless we assume, for the conditions under discussion, initially normal renal morphogenesis with subsequent structural and functional deterioration. Finally, for convenience, several conditions are discussed elsewhere in this volume: familial and congenital nephrotic syndrome (p. 1288) and glomerulonephritis associated with the syndrome of partial lipodystrophy (p. 746).

Hereditary Nephritis

The recognition of hereditary hematuria dates back to Guthrie's studies at the turn of the century. The relationship between nephritis and deafness was observed by Alport in his study of the same kindred 25 years later, and his name is often used to designate that syndrome. A significant incidence of ocular abnormalities, among them lens deformities and cataracts, is also seen. From investigations of large families it appears that individuals may be affected by some or all manifestations, but it is not certain whether hereditary nephritis in families without deafness is a separate genetic disease or a variant of the more complete syndrome.

Alport's syndrome of *hereditary progressive nephritis* (HPN) with neurosensory deafness characteristically begins in childhood with episodic hematuria. Attacks of gross hematuria are often precipitated by streptococcal or upper respiratory tract infections, and clinical manifestations may closely resemble typical postinfectious actue glomerulonephritis with edema, mild oliguria, and azotemia. Hypertension is said to be relatively uncommon. Hematuria persists or recurs after the other signs subside, and the patient may suffer recurrent attacks of pyuria, cylindruria, and dysuria. Proteinuria is variable and occasionally is severe enough to result in the nephrotic syndrome. Attacks are characteristically not associated with reduction of serum complement.

The diagnosis of HPN in the absence of a family history or of auditory and ocular findings is difficult, both in patients with recurrent attacks of nephritis and in those with insidious onset of renal failure. Renal biopsies have shown minimal changes early in the course of disease, with later progression to glomerular sclerosis and cortical atrophy. Mesangial thickening and sclerosis and segmental sclerosis are seen in some cases, but mesangial and epithelial proliferation and crescent formation predominate in others. Capsular thickening and periglomerular fibrosis progress to cortical fibrosis and tubular atropy. Interstitial accumulations of mononuclear cells are partly inflammatory infiltrates and partly tubular epithelial remnants. A characteristic, but by no means specific, finding is the presence of numerous interstitial lipid-containing foam cells, particularly along the medullary rays in the inner cortex. Their presence, even in the absence of other findings, is suggestive of hereditary nephritis, but interstitial foam cells are also common in the idiopathic nephrotic syndrome.

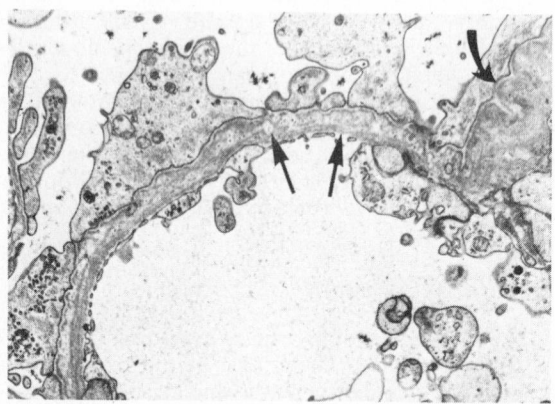

FIG. 15.   Electron microscopy of the glomerular capillary wall in the hereditary progressive glomerulonephritis of Alport demonstrates splitting and lamellation of the basement membrane (straight arrows). The lamina densa is thickened and multilayered, enclosing numerous small electron-dense granularities. There is also some thickening of the basement membrane at its mesangial reflection (curved arrow). The epithelial foot processes are irregularly swollen (×46,000).

A distinctive abnormality in the glomerular capillary basement membrane has been observed by electron microscopy. The basement membrane, which consists normally of a single electron-dense lamina, is split into multiple strands or lamellae (Fig. 15). The lesion may not be specific, in that somewhat similar changes with perhaps a focal distribution can be seen in the idiopathic nephrotic syndrome with focal segmental glomerular sclerosis and in several other forms of nephritis. However, the typical lesion, with a lamellated basement membrane containing numerous electron-dense granularities, seems to be characteristic of HPN. It may not be found in all cases of HPN (again raising the question of genetic heterogeneity), but when it is present it is found in all affected members of the family. A similar and sometimes more striking lesion is found in tubular basement membranes; they have a markedly thickened, laminated, and garlanded appearance. The festoons of basement membrane contain numerous lipid droplets, and foamy macrophages are seen in the adjacent interstitial tissue. The proximity of the foam cells to the lipid-laden basement membranes suggests that the former arise from imbibition of that lipid. The ultrastructural abnormality may identify the primary lesion in HPN—perhaps, as has been suggested by Spear, an abnormality in the structure of collagen within the basement membrane, an abnormality that could account for the otic and ocular manifestations of the syndrome.

Although HPN is distributed equally between males and females, males are affected earlier and more severely than females, often dying of renal failure by the third or fourth decade. Thus clinical studies of large kindreds will frequently uncover a greater number of affected females, many with mild or subclinical disease. The clinical pattern among members of a single kindred is usually consistent. Females often remain asymptomatic, their disease being discovered only on screening by urinalysis or audiometric testing. There are many exceptions to this rule, however, and girls have been observed to develop renal failure in childhood. Neurosensory deafness occurs in approximately 40 percent of affected individuals and can be used as a clinical marker in family studies; lenticular abnormalities are seen in approximately 15 percent, mostly males. These and other observations on the sex ratios of affected sibships have complicated the genetic analysis of HPN, but the disease is probably transmitted as an autosomal dominant. The observation that minimally affected, asymptomatic females have the same ultrastructural changes in their glomerular basement membranes as the more severely affected males suggests that the differences between the males and females may be determined by hormonal or other sex-related factors, rather than by sex-related transmission of the abnormal gene.

Both the renal disease and deafness are progressive, so that the two may seem to be more commonly associated in older patients; deafness has been estimated to be present in one-half of patients with HPN and renal failure. The hearing loss seems to result from an abnormality in the organ of Corti, or perhaps in the eighth nerve, although the pathologic lesion has not been precisely located. The hearing defect is not helped much by prosthetic devices.

Several nonrenal inherited abnormalities have been described in association with HPN, thus leading to the identification of a number of "variants." The most frequent has been *hyperprolinemia,* which in some reports has been present in only the index case and siblings, whereas renal disease and deafness had been found in previous generations. Pathologic studies have been inconclusive in establishing identity with HPN, but it appears on clincial grounds that the hyperprolinemia and nephritis are genetically separate, coincidental diseases. Other coincidental diseases have included familial neurologic abnormalities, familial myopathy, familial platelet abnormalities, and familial ichthyosis. In each of these the renal disease has been indistinguishable from HPN, apparently being transmitted by autosomal dominant inheritance.

Not all patients with familial hematuria develop renal insufficiency, and HPN should be differentiated from benign hematuria, which occurs both sporadically and in families. Cases of *familial benign hematuria* tend to have persistent hematuria, perhaps with periodic exacerbation. In many instances there has been no deterioration of renal function over long periods of observation, and a few cases have had only minimal functional abnormality. The condition is not associated with hearing loss. The clinical disease is probably genetically heterogeneous, since it has in most instances been transmitted as an autosomal dominant and in others possibly as a recessive. Recognition and differentiation from HPN, which is of considerable importance in determining prognosis, can be difficult both clinically and pathologically. Renal biopsies have shown proliferative glomerulonephritis in some instances and minimal glomerular changes in others. Ultrastructural studies might differentiate HPN and benign hematuria on the basis of the ultrastructural lesion described above. Some ultrastructural studies in benign hematuria have shown marked attenuation of the glomerular basement membrane, with gaps in the lamina densa, but it must be remembered that similar abnormalities are seen focally in HPN and perhaps in other diseases.

HPN should also be differentiated from several other types of hereditary nephritis that are unrelated to Alport's syndrome. A diffuse nephritis develops in 30 to 40 percent of patients with the *nail-patella syndrome* or hereditary onycho-osteodysplasia (HOOD). The characteristic clinical features include hypoplastic and dystrophic nails, hypoplastic or absent patellae, abnormally developed radial heads, and posterior iliac horns. An occasional finding is abnormal pigmentation of the iris. HOOD is transmitted as an autosomal dominant condition, and the abnormality is linked to the gene locus for ABO blood groups. Renal involvement is typically indicated by the presence of proteinuria, at times sufficiently severe to result in the nephrotic syndrome. Patients also suffer from hypertension. Approximately 25 percent of patients with renal disease develop renal failure. Renal biopsies early in the disease may show only thickening of glomerular basement membranes. Progressive glomerular sclerosis with tubular atrophy and cortical fibrosis lead to typical features of chronic nephritis. Electron microscopy has demonstrated thickening of the glomerular basement membrane with areas

of lucency that contain collagen fibers, which are not normally found in the basement membrane. The lesion in HOOD, like that in HPN, appears to reside in the collagen of the glomerular basement membrane, but the lesions are morphologically dissimilar, and there is no genetic relationship between the two.

The syndrome of *hereditary acro-osteolysis* is associated with severe hypertension and renal abnormalities. The disease is transmitted by autosomal dominant inheritance. It is not to be confused with disappearing-bone disease (Gorham's disease). The syndrome of osteolysis begins clinically as childhood arthritis, progressing to destruction of bones at the wrists and ankles. Fragments of bone are often extruded through the skin, and severe deformities result. Hypertension and abnormal urinary sediment have been reported in high percentages of involved families, but the overall frequency of these complications is not clear. Early findings include minimal proteinuria, increased urinary white cells, and microscopic hematuria. The lesion progresses to renal failure with severe tubular atrophy, cortical fibrosis, severe vascular sclerosis, and glomerular involution. It has been characterized as a glomerulonephritis, but much of the abnormality appears to be ischemic, perhaps as the result of hypertensive vascular disease. Whether a glomerular lesion exists independently of vascular disease is not certain, but clinical study has served to dissociate renal involvement and hypertension. The pathogenesis of the nephropathy is unknown.

Juvenile megaloblastic anemia (Imerlund's syndrome) with selective malabsorption of vitamin B_{12}, despite the adequate secretion of intrinsic factors, is regularly associated with proteinuria. The proteinuria, which often is found coincidentally with the onset of anemia, usually persists after correction of the anemia by treatment with vitamin B_{12}. Studies of renal function occasionally show nonspecific amino-aciduria, but are negative for evidence of progressive renal disease. Gross abnormalities of the urinary tract have been demonstrated by excretory urography. No significant glomerular abnormalities were described in the single reported case with adequate renal biopsy. The customary clinical manifestations of weakness, lethargy, glossitis, and neurologic abnormalities are related to the anemia and vitamin B_{12} deficiency.

Renal disease accompanies the syndrome of *asphyxiating thoracic dystrophy* (ATD), known also as Jeune's syndrome. These children, who have a form of chondrodystrophy, suffer from severe respiratory distress at birth because of thoracic deformity. Survivors often subsequently develop renal failure, the frequency of which has not been determined. The renal abnormality is characterized early by impaired concentrating ability and impaired proximal resorption of bicarbonate, urate, phosphate, amino acids, and glucose. Thus the initial lesion appears to be a form of tubular injury; this interpretation has been supported by morphologic studies, that show frequent tubular dilatation. Moreover, pathologic studies have shown a complex pattern of tubular injury with considerable variability among cases: (1) diffuse nephritis with patchy tubular atrophy, irregular tubular dilatation, glomerular obsolescence, and cortical fibrosis; (2) peripheral cortical microcysts; (3) diffuse cystic degeneration of normally developed tubules; and (4) generalized cystic dysplasia with abnormal ductal differentiation and metaplastic cartilage. Thus the renal lesion in ATD appears to encompass intrauterine maldevelopment, early postnatal tubular damage, and late nephropathy. The different patterns suggest that the primary abnormality, presumably a heritable metabolic defect, may in some cases interfere with renal organogenesis and in others interfere with tubular function and structure, causing secondary glomerular obsolescence. The condition is transmitted by autosomal recessive inheritance, and microscopic asymptomatic hepatic and pancreatic lesions are present in addition to the renal and osseous abnormalities.

Therapy is limited to supportive measures, except that intercurrent infections are treated specifically. Steroids and immunosuppressive agents have not been helpful. Renal allotransplanatation has been performed with some success.

Medullary Cystic Disorders

The uremic medullary cystic diseases are a group of genetically separate, predominantly tubular disorders with cysts located in the renal medulla. Despite their heterogeneity, they have in common several clinical and morphologic features, and they often cannot be easily differentiated in the evaluation of a given case. Therefore it has been proposed that they constitute a single clinical entity, a view that currently seems untenable. We follow the concepts of Schimke and Gardner in recognizing (1) *familial juvenile nephronophthisis* (FJN), a condition of autosomal recessive inheritance with onset predominantly in childhood; (2) *medullary cystic disease* (MCD), a condition of autosomal dominant inheritance or sporadic occurrence with predominantly adult onset; and (3) *renal-retinal dysplasia,* a group of conditions probably heterogeneous, of autosomal recessive inheritance with onset predominantly in childhood and with progressive retinal degeneration. On the basis of the information currently available the renal lesions of the Laurence-Moon-Bardet-Biedl syndrome and of Alström's syndrome are included in the last group. The medullary cystic diseases with progressive renal deterioration must be differentiated from (1) medullary sponge kidney (Cacchi-Ricci), a disease of adults, rarely of children, that is commonly associated with nephrolithiasis and its complications; (2) medullary tubular ectasia, which is the characteristic abnormality of infantile (autosomal recessive) polycystic disease and of congenital hepatic fibrosis; and (3) medullary cavitation secondary to medullary necrosis, renal tuberculosis, and nephrolithiasis (Table 8).

The two conditions FJN and MCD were originally described independently, the former in siblings who had frequent parental consanguinity and who showed urinary concentrating defects, severe growth retardation, and severe renal atrophy and the latter as sporadic cases of progressive renal failure, severe anemia, excessive renal salt loss, and medullary cysts. However, the two were quickly found to be virtually indistinguishable clinically and pathologically and were thought to be identical; certainly the terms as used in the literature are not a reliable basis for differentiation. The distinction between FJN and MCD indicated above depends on genetic evaluation and on family history, and individual sporadic cases without a characteristic onset may well remain in an indeterminate group.

TABLE 8. Renal Medullary Cysts: Differential Diagnosis

A. Uremic medullary cystic disorders
  1. Medullary cystic disease (MCD)
  2. Familial juvenile nephronophthisis (FJN)
  3. Renal-retinal dysplasia
    a. Retinitis pigmentosa
    b. Congenital optic atrophy of Leber
    c. Laurence-Moon-Bardet-Biedl syndrome
    d. Alström syndrome
B. Medullary sponge kidney
C. Infantile polycystic disease
  1. Medullary tubular ectasia
  2. Congenital hepatic fibrosis
D. Medullary and papillary necrosis

Clinical studies in both conditions are characterized by the early findings of polyuria, growth retardation, and normochromic anemia. Proteinuria and formed elements in the urine are uncommon, and other clinical signs and symptoms are often minor prior to the stage of renal failure. Hypertension is rare, except as a terminal complication of renal failure. Anemia, however, is often severe and out of proportion to the degree of renal failure. Functional studies show impaired concentrating ability; renal failure develops insidiously and inexorably. Evidence of tubular dysfunction, although inconstant, includes glycosuria, amino-aciduria, and impaired acidification, and evidence of proximal tubular damage may be among the earliest manifestations. An inability to conserve sodium ion may lead to severe hyponatremia that resembles Addison's disease except that hyperkalemia is absent and the abnormality is unresponsive to mineralocorticoid therapy. The histories of familial involvement and of polyuria are strong clues to the diagnosis in patients with renal failure.

Pathologic studies have shown extensive interstitial and tubular changes, although an early biopsy may show negligible abnormality. Tubular atrophy becomes marked and out of proportion to glomerular involvement, and there is cystic dilatation of Henle's loops and of collecting ducts. Microdissection reveals numerous diverticula of the distal convoluted tubule, descending limbs, and collecting ducts. Localized ductal dilatation, particularly in the medullary portions of collecting ducts, reaches gross proportions. The cysts in cases recognized through family studies have varied, and at times they have been inconspicuous or absent; therefore it must be assumed that cysts are necessary neither to the clinical state nor to pathologic progression of the disease. It may also be assumed that sporadic cases without cysts might go unrecognized morphologically. The pathogenesis of the cysts and the cause of the nephropathy in both FJN and MCD are unknown. There is no evidence, despite the cysts, of a developmental abnormality, and both conditions may be due to nephrotoxic metabolites or other heritable metabolic defects. Glomeruli are at first normal, but periglomerular fibrosis progresses to glomerular sclerosis. Interstitial fibrosis and inflammatory cell infiltrates are prominent, causing confusion with chronic interstitial nephritis.

In the condition designated as renal-retinal dysplasia renal involvement is functionally and morphologically similar to the renal abnormality in FJN and MCD. The characteristic ocular abnormality has been progressive retinal degeneration in cases of retinitis pigmentosa and cases of congenital blindness due to retinal atrophy and aplasia (Leber's optic atrophy). The Laurence-Moon-Bardet-Biedl syndrome (mental retardation, hypogonadism, obesity, and retinitis pigmentosa) has included in some cases a renal lesion compatible clinically and morphologically with medullary cystic disease, and Alström's syndrome (deafness, diabetes mellitus, obesity, and retinitis pigmentosa) has included a renal lesion with concentrating defect and severe tubular atrophy. These conditions are all transmitted by autosomal recessive inheritance.

Treatment is supportive, including provision of adequate amounts of fluid and electrolyte. Renal transplantation has been employed with some success.

References

HEREDITARY PROGRESSIVE NEPHRITIS

Chazan JA, Ambler M, Kalderon A, Cohen JJ, Zacks J: Vascular deposits causing ischemic myopathy in uremia: two brothers with hereditary nephritis. Ann Intern Med 73:73, 1970

Churg J, Sherman RL: Pathologic characteristics of hereditary nephritis. Arch Pathol 95:374, 1973

Epstein CJ, Sahud MA, Piel CF, et al: Hereditary macrothrombocytopathia, nephritis and deafness. Am J Med 52:299, 1972

Gaboardi F, Edefonti A, Imbasciati E, et al: Alport's syndrome (progressive hereditary nephritis). Clin Nephrol 2:143, 1974

Grünfeld JP, Bois EP, Hinglais N: Progressive and nonprogressive hereditary chronic nephritis. Kidney Int 4:216, 1973

Hill GS, Jenis EH, Goodloe S Jr: The nonspecificity of the ultrastructural alterations in hereditary nephritis: with additional observations on benign familial hematuria. Lab Invest 31:516, 1974

Hinglais N, Grünfeld JP, Bois E: Characteristic ultrastructural lesion of the glomerular basement membrane in progressive hereditary nephritis (Alport's syndrome). Lab Invest 27:473, 1972

Kaufman DB, McIntosh RM, Smith FG Jr, Vernier RL: Diffuse familial nephropathy: a clinicopathological study. J Pediatr 77:37, 1970

Kissane J: Hereditary disorders of the kidney. Part II. Hereditary nephropathies. In Rosenberg HS, Bolande RP (eds): Perspectives in Pediatric Pathology, Vol 1. Chicago, Year Book, 1973, p 147

Knepshield JR, Roberts PL, Davis CJ, Moser RH: Hereditary chronic nephritis complicated by nephrotic syndrome. Arch Intern Med 122:156, 1968

Kopelman H, Sastoor AM, Milne MD: Hyperprolinemia and hereditary nephritis. Lancet 2:1075, 1964

Preus M, Fraser FC: Genetics of hereditary nephropathy with deafness (Alport's disease). Clin Genet 2:331, 1971

Sherman RL, Churg J. Yudis M: Hereditary nephritis with a characteristic renal lesion. Am J Med 56:44, 1974

Spear GS: Alport's syndrome: a consideration of pathogenesis. Clin Nephrol 1:336, 1973

Spear GS: Pathology of the kidney in Alport's syndrome. Pathol Annu 9:93, 1974

Spear GS, Slusser RJ: Alport's syndrome: emphasizing electron microscopic studies of the glomerulus. Am J Pathol 69:213, 1972

FAMILIAL BENIGN HEMATURIA

Hill GS, Jenis EH, Goodloe S Jr: The nonspecificity of the ultrastructural alterations in hereditary nephritis: with additional observations on benign familial hematuria. Lab Invest 31:516, 1974

Marks MI, Drummond KN: Benign familial hematuria. Pediatrics 44:590, 1969

Rogers PW, Kurtzman NA, Bunn SM Jr, White MG: Familial benign essential hematuria. Arch Intern Med 131:257, 1973

HEREDITARY ONYCHO-OSTEODYSPLASIA

Bennett WM, Musgrave JE, Campbell RA, et al: The nephropathy of the nail-patella syndrome: clinicopathologic analysis of 11 kindred. Am J Med 54:304, 1973

Hoyer JR, Michael AF, Vernier RL: Renal disease in nail-patella syndrome: clinical and morphologic studies. Kidney Int 2:231, 1972

Morita T, Laughlin LO, Kawano K, et al: Nail-patella syndrome: light and electron microscopic studies of the kidney. Arch Intern Med 131:271, 1973

HEREDITARY ACRO-OSTEOLYSIS

Marie J, Lévêque B, Lyon G, Bêbe M, Watchi J-M: Acro-ostéolyse essentielle compliquée d'insuffisance rénale d'évolution fatale. Presse Med 71:249, 1963

JUVENILE MEGALOBLASTIC ANEMIA

Imerslund O: Idiopathic chronic megaloblastic anemia in children. Acta Paediatr Scand [Suppl 119] 49:1–115, 1960

Mohamed SD, McKay E, Galloway WH: Juvenile familial megaloblastic anaemia due to selective malabsorption of vitamin B_{12}: a family study and a review of the literature. Q J Med 139:433, 1966

ASPHYXIATING THORACIC DYSTROPHY

Bernstein J, Brough AJ, McAdams AJ: The renal lesion in syndromes of multiple congenital malformations: cerebrohepatorenal syndrome; Jeune asphyxiating thoracic dystrophy; tuberous sclerosis; Meckel syndrome. Birth Defects 10:35, 1974

Edelson PJ, Spackman TJ, Belliveau RE, Mahoney MJ: A renal lesion in asphyxiating thoracic dysplasia. Birth Defects 10:51, 1974

Gallet J-P, Olivier C, Sarrut S: Dystrophie thoracique, malformation oculaire et néphropathie tubulo-interstitiele chez deux fréres. Ann Pédiatr 20:813, 1973

Gruskin AB, Baluarte HJ, Cote ML, Elfenbein IB: The renal disease of thoracic asphyxiant dystrophy. Birth Defects 10:44, 1974

Shokeir MHK, Houston CS, Awen CF: Asphyxiating thoracic chondrodystrophy: association with renal disease and evidence for possible heterozygous expression. J Med Genet 8:107, 1971

MEDULLARY CYSTIC DISEASE AND JUVENILE NEPHROPHTHISIS

Alexander F, Campbell S: Familial uremic medullary cystic disease. Pediatrics 45:1024, 1970

Gardner KD: Evolution of clinical signs in adult-onset cystic disease of the renal medulla. Ann Intern Med 74:47, 1971

Giselson N, Heinegard D, Holmberg C-G, et al: Renal medullary cystic disease or familial juvenile nephronophthisis: a renal tubular disease. Am J Med 48:174, 1970

Ivemark BI, Ljungqvist A, Barry A: Juvenile nephronophthisis: a histologic and microangiographic study. Acta Paediatr 49:480, 1960

Makker SP, Grupe WE, Perrin E, Heymann W: Identical progression of juvenile hereditary nephronophthisis in monozygotic twins. J Pediatr 82:773, 1973

Mongeau JG, Worthen HG: Nephronophthisis and medullary cystic disease. Am J Med 43:345, 1967

Strauss MB, Sommers SC: Medullary cystic disease and familial juvenile nephronophthisis: clinical and pathological identity. N Engl J Med 277:863, 1967

RENAL-RETINAL DYSPLASIA

Alton DJ, McDonald P: Urographic findings in the Bardet-Biedl syndrome. Radiology 109:659, 1973

Goldstein JL, Fialkow PJ: The Alström syndrome: report of three cases with further delineation of the clinical, pathophysiological, and genetic aspects of the disorder. Medicine 52:53, 1973

Senior B: Familial renal-retinal dystrophy. Am J Dis Child 125:442, 1973

DISORDERS OF RENAL TUBULAR FUNCTION

JUAN RODRIGUEZ SORIANO

Renal tubular disorders may be defined as conditions in which specific tubular dysfunctions exist in association with little or no impairment of glomerular function. This definition applies only to the early stages of disease, since secondary glomerular damage may appear later, as in the Fanconi syndrome with cystinosis, or in renal tubular acidosis with nephrocalcinosis and secondary pyelonephritis. In addition, decreased glomerular function and elevation of blood urea may be seen as prerenal phenomena early in the disease if a tubular defect in the conservation of water or solute is present (p. 1239).

Defects of tubular function may be single or multiple. Analysis of the disorder may be complicated by the fact that a defect may not represent a primary specific abnormality, but rather a secondary functional one. For example, a concentrating defect may be due to potassium deficiency; hyperkaliuria may be caused by secondary hyperaldosteronism; hypercalciuria may result from acidosis; an increased phosphate clearance may be due to acidosis itself or may result from secondary hyperparathyroidism. The reversibility of the abnormality when the primary cause is corrected establishes the defect as functional, but such a clear distinction between functional and specific defects is not always possible.

The cause of many renal tubular disorders is unknown, but in most either a hereditary or an acquired cause may be traced. Genetic disorders may modify renal function in two ways: through a primary abnormality in a specific tubular function (eg, primary renal glycosuria) or secondarily by the toxic effect on the renal tubule of accumulated metabolites consequent to an extrarenal metabolic block (eg, galactosemia). Both primary and secondary causes may present with identical symptomatology, and they may be indistinguishable on the basis of functional and urinary findings. For this reason a descriptive rather than an etiologic classification is followed in this section.

RENAL GLYCOSURIA

Primary renal glycosuria results from a defect in proximal tubular reabsorption of glucose. Glomerular filtration rate and other tubular functions are normal. Most cases are believed to be inherited as autosomal dominant characteristics but in some cases both parents have been normal, suggesting an autosomal recessive trait.

This condition undoubtedly is present at birth, but its detection may be delayed until adult life. It is a benign condition, and patients generally are asymptomatic, except for the rare occurrence of hypoglycemia. The presence of glucose in the urine concurrent with normal blood levels establishes the diagnosis. In the obvious case glycosuria is constant, even during fasting, but in some cases it can be detected only postprandially.

Two types of renal glycosuria have been recognized. In so-called type A or "renal diabetes" both the renal plasma threshold and the maximal rate of glucose reabsorption (glucose Tm) are low (see p. 1239). This is believed to represent a true tubular defect, although the abnormality in the transport mechanism is completely unknown. This type of renal glycosuria may occur as an isolated defect but more often is associated with other tubular abnormalities as part of the Fanconi syndrome.

In type B or "pseudorenal diabetes" the Tm of reabsorption is normal, but there is a low renal plasma threshold, with a resultant marked splay of the titration curve of glucose reabsorption. This type may represent an exaggerated heterogeneity of the nephron population, either functional or anatomic or both. The overall rate of glucose reabsorption is normal at high plasma levels, but at lower levels a disparity exists in the saturation of glucose transport in individual nephrons.

Type B glycosuria is usually considered to be present only as an isolated abnormality without other tubular defects. However, in glucoglycinuria (p. 1302) this type of glycosuria is seen, and we have studied one child with this defect who had a similar abnormality in bicarbonate reabsorption.

The separation of types A and B as two different entities is still a matter of speculation. It is now known that, at least in the rat, the splay of the titration curve of glucose reabsorption increases when the extracellular volume is expanded, a factor not controlled in most studies. Moreover, in one kindred studied by Elsas and Rosenberg both types A and B coexisted in the same family, suggesting the possibility of different degrees of the same inherited defect rather than two distinct types of disease.

It is known that some amino acids share the same transport processes in the renal tubule and the intestinal mucosa. In renal glycosuria the curve of the glucose tolerance test is frequently flattened, suggesting a defect in the transport of glucose through the intestine. However, studies in one family, utilizing the in vitro incubation of jejunal mucosa with radioactive glucose, failed to show an abnormality in cellular uptake. In contrast, in glucose-galactose malabsorption, a familial disease with defective intestinal absorption of both of these sugars (p. 1002), an abnormality in the renal tubular transport of glucose has been demonstrated. These studies suggest that at least two mechanisms are responsible for glucose transport and that only one is shared by both the gut and the kidney.

In the few cases of renal glycosuria studied the kidney was histologically normal. However, Monasterio and associates have reported alterations in the ultrastructure of proximal tubular cells.

The differentiation of renal glycosuria from diabetes mellitus is essential in order to avoid dangerous therapeutic errors. The glucose oxidase test will differentiate other types of mellituria.

No therapy is indicated. The amount of glucose in the urine is independent of the carbohydrate intake, and no dietary restrictions are needed.

AMINO-ACIDURIAS

The amino acids present in the glomerular filtrate normally are reabsorbed almost completely in the proximal tubule. Urine of the normal adult contains less than 1 percent of the filtered amino nitrogen, mainly in the form of glycine, taurine, histidine, and glutamine, which are the only amino acids detected when urine is analyzed by paper chromatography. However, it can be demonstrated by ion-exchange chromatography that most of the plasma amino acids are present in urine, although in very small amounts. The rate of excretion of amino acids in infants and children is comparatively greater than that in adults. Healthy children excrete α-amino nitrogen at a rate of about 2.5 mg/kg body weight per day, and infants as much as 8.5 mg/kg. The pattern of urinary excretion of amino acids in children is similar to that in adults, but it may differ markedly in small infants, especially prematures, who excrete predominantly threonine, serine, proline, glycine, and alanine. The percentage tubular reabsorption of all amino acids is lower in infancy, reflecting a state of glomerulotubular imbalance (see p. 1239).

Tubular reabsorption of amino acids is accomplished by a number of specific energy-dependent active transport processes. The efficiency of tubular reabsorption of an individual amino acid is related to its chemical structure, steric configuration, and concentration in plasma. It appears that there are several distinct transport sites for individual amino acids or groups of amino acids and the competitive and noncompetitive mechanisms of inhibition of uptake occur at the various sites.

Transport sites common to more than one amino acid have been identified on the basis of physiologic studies or characteristic findings in patients with specific diseases. The first site involves the dibasic amino acids (lysine, arginine, and ornithine). This transport system is defective in cystinuria, an inherited disorder leading to impaired intestinal absorption and marked urinary hyperexcretion of cystine as well as the dibasic amino acids (p. 689). In a condition called hyper-

dibasic amino-aciduria, the defect is limited to the dibasic amino acids, without involvement of cystine (p. 1302). This suggests that there are two renal mechanisms for dibasic amino acid transport, only one of which includes cystine. This amino acid seems to be transported also in a specific site, since in so-called hypercystinuria only the excretion of cystine is elevated in the urine.

A second transport mechanism involves the acidic amino acids (glutamic and aspartic acids). This transport site has been identified only in the dog. Imino acids (proline and hydroxyproline) and glycine are involved in a transport system that is defective in familial iminoglycinuria. Affected individuals excrete excessive amounts of all three compounds (p. 1302). Neutral amino acids, other than glycine and the imino acids, share a common transport mechanism, since they are all characteristically increased in Hartnup disease (p. 689). The β-amino compounds (β-alanine, β-aminoisobutyric acid, and taurine) share a transport system distinct from that transporting α-amino acids, as has been shown in patients with β-alaninemia.

In many instances the absorption of amino acids at the level of the jejunal mucosa appears to involve mechanisms similar to those in the renal tubule, since identical defects in transport have been identified. For example, in cystinuria and in Hartnup disease intestinal and tubular absorption of the same group of amino acids is defective. However, in familial iminoglycinuria in vitro studies using intestinal biopsy specimens revealed no defect in mucosal uptake. It is possible, as in cystinuria, that further study of this disorder will reveal the presence of more than one genetic type.

Increased urinary excretion of amino acids is due to one of the following mechanisms: (1) *saturation* of tubular transport due to an increased filtered load, the level of the amino acid or acids in plasma being elevated (overflow amino-aciduria); (2) *competition* between the reabsorption of amino acids sharing a common transport site, when the concentration in plasma of one of them is increased (combined amino-aciduria); (3) *selective abnormality* leading to a specific defect in the reabsorption of an individual amino acid or a group of amino acids (specific renal amino-aciduria); (4) *generalized abnormality* involving a large and heterogeneous group of amino acids due to nonspecific dysfunction of the proximal tubule (nonspecific renal amino-aciduria). In the renal amino-acidurias, specific or nonspecific, the plasma amino acid levels characteristically are normal. Only these types will be considered in this section.

CYSTINURIA. The importance of this defect is that patients are prone to urolithiasis. Tubular reabsorption of cystine, lysine, arginine, and ornithine is abnormal (see also p. 690). This disorder is discussed in detail on page 689 .

HARTNUP DISEASE. This is a disorder in which there is abnormal tubular transport of the neutral amino acids, with the exception of the imino acids and glycine. A peculiar rash is present, and there are central nervous system manifestations. The disease is described in detail on page 689 .

HYPERCYSTINURIA. In this disorder there is a defect of a specific site that handles only the transport of cystine. This mutation, transmitted as an autosomal dominant, seems to be limited to the kidney. Clinically, as in "classic" cystinuria, there is a tendency to the formation of urinary calculi.

DIBASIC AMINO-ACIDURIAS. Increased urinary excretion rates of dibasic amino acids have been observed by several investigators in apparently different inborn errors of metabolism.

In "familial protein intolerance with deficient transport of basic amino acids" described by Finnish authors the children have recurrent vomiting, diarrhea, failure to thrive, hepatomegaly, and diffuse hepatic cirrhosis. They have low blood urea concentration, hyperammonemia, and leukopenia. The symptoms are exacerbated by high-protein diets. Urinary excretion of basic amino acids (lysine, ornithine, and arginine) is elevated, but no defect is evident in intestinal transport. No amino-aciduria has been detected in the parents.

The condition "hyperdibasicamino-aciduria" was described by Whelan and Scriver in 13 of 33 members of a French Canadian family. The proband was an 18-month-old girl studied because of small stature and a mild malabsorption syndrome. Neither defect could definitely be linked to the amino-aciduria, which appeared to be inherited as an autosomal dominant. Affected individuals, who are mostly asymptomatic, excrete excessive amounts of lysine, ornithine, and arginine. Cystine is excreted in normal amounts; concentrations in plasma are normal after oral administration of cystine but are lower than in control subjects after administration of lysine, indicating a concomitant defect in the intestinal absorption of the dibasic amino acids.

Oyanagi and associates described a condition they called congenital lysinuria. The children affected have recurrent diarrhea and vomiting, which become milder with increasing age. The urinary excretion of basic amino acids is markedly elevated in the patients, but is normal in the parents. Intestinal transport of basic amino acids is also impaired.

The conditions described might represent allelic mutations of the gene locus for transport of basic amino acids, and the differences found between different families probably are due to genetic heterogeneity.

FAMILIAL IMINOGLYCINURIA. This entity results from the defective tubular reabsorption of proline, hydroxyproline, and glycine. Only a few families, mostly of Jewish origin, have been described. The disease is inherited as an autosomal recessive. Patients are generally asymptomatic, but a few subjects have been mentally retarded. The original case presented with convulsions and high spinal fluid protein.

In the homozygotes the urinary excretion of proline, hydroxyproline, and glycine is increased. Heterozygotes for the defect have hyperglycinuria only, without concomitant hyperimino-aciduria. This finding suggests that there is more than one renal transport system for glycine and the amino acids: one common for all three compounds and a second (or possibly more) responsible for a selective absorption of glycine or the imino acids. In the homozygotes the common system is severely affected, with the selective system permitting partial reabsorption of glycine and the imino acids; in the heterozygotes the activity of the common system appears to be less affected, permitting reabsorption of virtually all the filtered proline and hydroxyproline but only part of the glycine. The intestinal transport of glycine and imino acids in this condition has been found to be normal by most authors, but it was impaired in two patients, most likely indicating the presence of more than one genetic type.

HEREDITARY GLYCINURIA. This condition was described by DeVries and associates in a single family; it was transmitted as an autosomal dominant and was present in three consecutive generations. The only clinical manifestations were those associated with recurrent nephrolithiasis. Urinary excretion of glycine was markedly elevated; concentrations in plasma were normal. Chemical analysis of one calculus revealed primarily calcium oxalate, but 0.5 percent of free glycine also was found. Jejunal transport of glycine was not investigated.

GLUCOGLYCINURIA. This condition was described by Käser and associates in 14 members of a single family. Type B renal glycosuria was present in association with a marked excretion of glycine. The patients were asymptomatic except for the propositus, who had cystic fibrosis.

LATE VITAMIN-D-RESISTANT RICKETS WITH HYPERGLYCINURIA. This entity is similar to the more common *familial hypophosphatemia* (p. 243) except for the presence of excessive urinary excretion of glycine and its late onset in adolescence and early adulthood. Scriver and associates reported a case in which glycinuria and hyperphosphaturia were associated with renal glycosuria and abnormal excretion of glycylproline.

The relationships, if any, among the various entities of abnormal excretion of glycine are unknown. Differentiation from *idiopathic hyperglycinemia* (p. 682), in which the hyperglycinuria depends on an overflow mechanism, is important.

β-AMINOISOBUTYRIC-ACIDURIA. This finding has no clinical significance. The urinary excretion of metabolite is of interest as a genetic marker.

NONSPECIFIC RENAL AMINO-ACIDURIAS. The presence of a generalized amino-aciduria is indicative of nonspecific tubular damage and generally is associated with other tubular abnormalities. This type of amino-aciduria usually is not characteristic, most of the plasma amino acids being present in the urine in excessive amounts. However, some differences in the pattern of amino-aciduria may be found, depending on the etiology of the tubular dysfunction. Thus cystine is characteristically increased in Wilson's disease, proline in cystinosis, and lysine and tyrosine in Lowe's syndrome.

Generalized amino-aciduria is characteristically present in vitamin-D-deficiency rickets and may be found as an isolated tubular abnormality in cases of congenital lactose intolerance, hereditary intolerance to fructose, galactosemia. Wilson's disease, heavy-metal poisoning, and malnutrition.

DISORDERS OF PHOSPHATE TRANSPORT

Between 85 and 95 percent of filtered phosphate normally is reabsorbed in the proximal tubule. The rate of reabsorption is controlled by parathyroid hormone, which acts to inhibit reabsorption and thus to enhance urinary excretion. Calcitonin, a recently discovered hormone that has an effect on serum calcium opposite to that of parathyroid hormone, also increases the urinary excretion of phosphate (see also p. 235).

Variation in phosphate reabsorption is poorly reflected by urinary excretion of phosphate, which is dependent mainly on oral intake and concentrations in plasma. Determination of phosphate clearance, or better, the coefficient of tubular reabsorption of phosphate (TRP), is necessary.* Since TRP varies with the concentration of phosphate in plasma, the latter value must be taken into consideration when the TRP is interpreted. This is the basis of the *phosphate excretion index* (PEI), which is calculated from the regression between the percentage of filtered phosphate that is excreted and the concentration of phosphate in serum. Children 2 to 15 years of age have lower values of PEI than adults, reflecting a higher reabsorption of phosphate at the same concentration in plasma (see Nordin and Fraser in References).

Although these calculations are useful in clinical medicine, the range of values obtained in normal subjects is very large, overlapping that of patients with proved hypoparathyroidism and hyperparathyroidism. The maximum rate of tubular reabsorption of phosphate ($Tm_{phosphate}$) would seem to be a more precise means of assessment, but its calculation requires a phosphate infusion and determination of glomerular filtration rate. The same disadvantage applies to determination of the "theoretical renal phosphate threshold." In this test a progressive increase in serum phosphate is produced by infusing buffered sodium

phosphate in increasing amounts over a period of 3 hours. The regression of urinary phosphate on serum phosphate is calculated, and the point at which the regression line cuts the abscissa is defined as the theoretical renal phosphate threshold. This technique seems especially useful in patients with osteomalacia in order to test the sensitivity of the renal tubule to a physiologic dose of vitamin D.

Decreased tubular reabsorption of phosphate is found in both hyperparathyroidism and specific tubular dysfunctions involving phosphate transport. The distinction between these two conditions may be difficult, since secondary hyperparathyroidism often accompanies renal tubular abnormalities. An increase in phosphate reabsorption during induced hypercalcemia or during low phosphate intake favors the primacy of the hormonal mechanism, although this response does not exclude a primary tubular defect. Determination of concentration of immunoreactive parathyroid hormone in serum constitutes the best method of distinguishing between the possibilities.

An isolated defect in renal tubular transport of phosphate is now believed to be the primary abnormality in hereditary hypophosphatemia (familial vitamin-D-resistant rickets) (see p. 243). This defect seems to depend on the loss of a parathyroid-hormone-sensitive component of phosphate transport. Until recently the most widely accepted theory was a primary abnormality in intestinal absorption of calcium and phosphorus, with secondary hyperparathyroidism. This explanation is no longer tenable following the demonstration of normal serum levels of parathyroid hormone in this disease.

In another type of vitamin-D-resistant rickets (so called pseudo-vitamin-D-deficient rickets or vitamin D dependency) the defect lies in impaired synthesis of the most active metabolite of vitamin D, 1,25-dihydroxycholecalciferol, probably due to an inherited deficiency of 25-hydroxyvitamin-D_1-hydroxylase in the kidney. In this condition, as in vitamin-D-deficiency rickets, the low tubular reabsorption of phosphate is directly related to secondary hyperparathyroidism. Serum levels of immunoreactive parathyroid hormone are significantly increased, and a strong correlation is present between the degree of secondary hyperparathyroidism and the severity of the tubular dysfunction of both phosphate and amino acid transport.

Decreased phosphate clearance or increased TRP is present in primary hypoparathyroidism and in pseudohypoparathyroidism, a disorder characterized by congenital unresponsiveness of the proximal tubule to parathyroid hormone (p. 250). The clinical syndrome includes short stature, brachydactylia and other skeletal malformations, and often mental retardation. Two types of the disease have been identified. In type I the administration of parathyroid hormone does not increase urinary cyclic AMP, but upon administration of dibutyryl cyclic adenosine 3',5'-monophosphate a phosphaturic response is observed. In type II the administration of parathyroid hormone results in a marked increase in urinary cyclic AMP, with no phosphaturic

---

The formula for calculation of TRP is derived as follows:

$$(1) \quad TRP = \frac{reabsorbed\ phosphate}{filtered\ phosphate} \times 100$$

$$(2) \quad TRP = \frac{filtered\ phosphate\ -\ excreted\ phosphate}{filtered\ phosphate} \times 100$$

$$(3) \quad TRP = [1 - \frac{excreted\ phosphate}{filtered\ phosphate}] \times 100$$

Filtered phosphate is calculated as the product of glomerular filtration rate (GFR) and plasma phosphate concentration, and GFR usually is estimated from creatinine clearance. Therefore, substituting in (3):

$$(4) \quad TRP = [1 - (U_p V \div \frac{U_{cr} V}{P_{cr}} P_p)] \times 100$$

$$(5) \quad TRP = [1 - \frac{U_p P_{cr}}{U_{cr} P_p}] \times 100$$

where U_p, P_p, U_{cr}, P_{cr} are, respectively, urine and plasma concentrations of phosphate and creatinine, and V is rate of urine flow. It can be seen that the value for V cancels out in the final equation, signifying that TRP can be calculated without knowing rate of urine flow, and therefore an untimed urine specimen can be used.

response, thus suggesting a more distal metabolic block.

Multiple Dysfunction of Proximal Renal Tubule

The name Fanconi syndrome or de Toni-Debre-Fanconi syndrome is given to a group of disorders involving multiple functional disturbances of the proximal tubule, including defects in the reabsorption of glucose, amino acids, and phosphate. Tubular proteinuria, acidosis, inadequate renal conservation of sodium and potassium, and a defect in maximum renal concentrating ability may all be present. However, cystinosis was soon found to be the most common etiology of the primary form in children, and many other causes or entities with an associated Fanconi syndrome have been disclosed. In current terminology the designation Fanconi syndrome is given to any nonspecific, complex, proximal tubular dysfunction, complete or partial, regardless of etiology (Table 9).

PATHOPHYSIOLOGY AND CLINICAL AND LABORATORY FEATURES. The Fanconi syndrome is probably caused by nonspecific enzymatic damage to the proximal tubule. The multiple endogenous and exogenous toxins producing this syndrome, the finding of multiple renal tubular dysfunctions following vascular accidents of the kidney in the newborn period, and the experimental production by maleic acid, which impairs ATP synthesis and inhibits the enzyme Na-K-ATPase, sustain the above hypothesis. Details concerning specific etiologies are discussed below.

The histology of the kidney may be normal or may show nonspecific lesions of tubular damage. In cases of cystinosis all gradations from normal structure to chronic renal disease can be found. Clay and associates found by microdissection a straight, short proximal tubule (swan neck) in both childhood cases of cystinosis and adult cases of the idiopathic type. They believed it represented a congenital malformation directly responsible for the tubular dysfunction. This interpretation is questionable because recent evidence indicates that the anomaly represents an atrophic, secondary change. Vacuolization of distal tubular cells can be found in cases with potassium deficiency.

The clinical picture varies depending on both the degree of tubular dysfunction and the etiology. However, characteristic symptomatology is common to all forms with complete dysfunction of long-standing duration. Failure to thrive and growth retardation are constant. Bone lesions of rickets or osteoporosis or both are frequent, despite adequate intake of vitamin D, and may dominate the clinical picture. Polyuria is found occasionally and in the early months of life may cause unexplained fever, dehydration, and constipation. Muscular weakness and paralysis caused by potassium deficiency may also be present.

Serum analysis reveals hypophosphatemia and normal levels of calcium. Alkaline phosphatase is increased if there is active osteomalacia. Hyperchloremic acidosis and hypokalemia are frequently present. Rarely a patient may present with metabolic alkalosis due to chronic renal loss of sodium and potassium. Serum amino acid levels are normal.

The urine contains glucose, and there is a generalized amino-aciduria of nonspecific renal type. The rate of excretion of phosphate in urine may be normal, but an increased phosphate clearance or decreased coefficient

TABLE 9. Fanconi Syndromes

Primary	Glyco-suria	Amino-aciduria	Hyper-phos-phaturia	Rickets, Osteo-porosis	Tubular Acidosis	Hypo-kalemia	Hypo-calcemia	Concen-tration Defect
Primary								
Cystinosis	++	++	++	++	+	+	−	+
Idiopathic	++	++	++	++	+	+	−	+
Luder-Sheldon syndrome	++	++	+	+	+	−	−	−
Lowe's syndrome	±	++	++	++	+	−	−	±
Secondary								
Tyrosinemia	++	++	++	++	+	+	−	+
Galactosemia	±	++	−	−	±	−	−	−
Glycogen storage disease	±	±	±	±	−	−	−	−
Wilson's disease	±	++	±	±	±	−	−	−
Fructose intolerance	−	+	−	−	+	−	−	−
Nephrotic syndrome with tubular dysfunction	++	++	+	+	++	++	++	+
Heavy metals	++	++	±	±	−	−	−	−

++ *almost always present.*
+ *often present.*
± *rarely present.*
− *absent.*

of phosphate reabsorption (TRP) is found. Tubular proteinuria frequently is present.

The urine pH is 6.0 or higher, and rates of excretion of titratable acid and ammonium are low. However, most patients are able to elaborate an acid urine and to excrete adequate hydrogen ion when appropriately stimulated, indicating that the acidosis is of the proximal type caused by a defect in bicarbonate reabsorption (p. 1308). Both the plasma threshold and maximal rate of reabsorption of bicarbonate have been found low in cases of Fanconi syndrome of varied types.

Hypercalciuria is not constant, and when it is present it probably depends more on the rate of sodium excretion than on the existence of a metabolic acidosis. Even when hypercalciuria is present, nephrocalcinosis and lithiasis are exceptional, in contrast to the situation with distal renal tubular acidosis. A defect in maximum concentrating ability may be present; it probably results from the potassium deficiency and hypercalciuria rather than from a specific tubular defect.

TREATMENT. The course, prognosis, and specific treatment of the Fanconi syndrome depend on etiology. Secondary dysfunctions will in general disappear after withdrawal of the offending cause or treatment of the primary disease. Some general therapeutic measures applicable to all types of the disease will be considered here.

The bone lesions of rickets and osteomalacia are resistant to vitamin D and require doses in excess of 25,000 IU per day. Some children require as much as 400,000 IU per day, and often remineralization cannot be achieved even with these large doses. Careful monitoring of concentration of calcium in blood and rate of excretion in urine is necessary to avoid vitamin D toxicity. Correction of the acidosis is an important measure, but in contrast with distal renal tubular acidosis, rachitic lesions will not heal until vitamin D is given. The amount of sodium and potassium citrate or bicarbonate necessary to control the acidosis is generally much greater than that required in distal renal tubular acidosis. It should be given every 2 to 4 hours, day and night, in a dose sufficient to keep the blood pH and total CO_2 within the normal range. As much as 10 mEq/kg/day of citrate or bicarbonate may be required. Rampini and associates have shown that the correction of the acidosis is greatly facilitated by the administration of hydrochlorothiazide, which probably acts by causing sodium loss with a consequent decrease in extracellular volume, resulting in increased proximal tubular reabsorption of sodium and, concurrently, bicarbonate. Unpublished observations have demonstrated the same effect with other potent diuretics. Surprisingly the bone lesions also may heal rapidly during diuretic therapy, even in the absence of vitamin D administration, perhaps reflecting increased reabsorption of both phosphate and calcium. The administration of potassium is mandatory if hypokalemia is present. In these cases the administration of diuretics may be dangerous. When polyuria is present water requirements should be evaluated carefully, especially during infancy. Finally, it must be realized that in spite of all these measures growth and development often remain poor.

PRIMARY FANCONI SYNDROMES. The *idiopathic Fanconi syndrome* is most often seen in adults, but it occasionally occurs in children. About 50 cases have been reported. In a few cases there has been a suggestion of autosomal recessive inheritance, but in one family the complete syndrome was observed in two generations, indicating transmission as an autosomal dominant. The onset is often during the second year of life, and the clinical picture is that of the complete Fanconi syndrome. In contrast with cystinosis, glomerular function may not be affected during its evolution, and patients may attain adult life, although severely retarded in growth. Renal insufficiency may occur, however, and a renal transplant may be required. In one 14-year-old patient with idiopathic Fanconi syndrome homotransplantation was followed by the appearance of glycosuria, amino-aciduria, and proximal renal tubular acidosis in the transplanted kidney. In many cases clinical onset is delayed until adulthood. Exclusion of cystinosis is obligatory in any isolated Fanconi syndrome appearing in childhood, since the diagnosis of cystinosis implies a fatal prognosis. Only after a repeatedly negative search for cystine, including examination of leukocytes, can a Fanconi syndrome be labeled idiopathic.

Luder-Sheldon syndrome was described in a family with glucoamino-aciduria in three generations. Over the course of many years the three affected members of the last generation developed vitamin-D-resistant rickets and tubular acidosis.

Oculocerebrorenal dystrophy (Lowe's syndrome) was described in 1952 by Lowe, Terrey, and MacLachlan. It associates the Fanconi syndrome with mental retardation and severe congenital ocular abnormalities. It is a hereditary condition transmitted by a sex-linked recessive gene, all the affected members being males. A few cases of Lowe's syndrome in females have been reported; they probably represent a metabolically similar but genetically different entity. The inital demonstration of development of cataracts in female carriers has not been confirmed. Chromosomal analyses have been normal, and no specific metabolic block has been detected. Abnormalities of amino acid excretion during ornithine administration have been reported, but their significance is unknown.

The age of onset is variable, ranging from the early months of life to late childhood. The presence of cataracts is almost constant, and they frequently coexist with congenital glaucoma (hydrophthalmos). Nystagmus is common and is probably secondary to blindness. The involvement of the nervous system is very characteristic and combines severe mental retardation with marked muscular hypotonia and tendinous areflexia. Paralyses are never found. Patients may emit a continuous distressing cry. Cryptorchidism is reported in one-fourth of the cases.

A peculiar type of Fanconi syndrome is also seen: tubular proteinuria is always present, glycosuria is rare, amino-aciduria is only moderate, a concentrating defect is exceptional, and hypokalemia has never been found. Lowe and associates reported a characteristic organic aciduria; however, this finding has not been confirmed. Osteoporosis is the most frequent bone lesion, but rickets may also be present. Retardation in growth and development becomes evident during the evolution of the disease. Development of glomerular insufficiency does not generally occur, but the prognosis nevertheless remains poor due to severe mental retardation and poor vision. Histologically the kidney shows severe tubular involvement with epithelial atrophy, enormous dilatation of tubules, and interstitial fibrosis. Glomerular changes are minimal, although progressive glomerular obsolescence has occasionally been described.

The differential diagnosis includes other conditions in which there is an association of cerebral, ocular, and renal abnormalities. A frequent error is the indiscriminate diagnosis of Lowe's syndrome in a severely retarded child with rickets, amino-aciduria, and ocular anomalies. In many such cases rickets is due to deficiency of vitamin D from inadequate nutrition and lack of sunlight.

There is no specific therapy, but adequate measures to control bone lesions and acidosis should be undertaken.

SECONDARY FANCONI SYNDROMES. CYSTINOSIS.

This disease is an inborn error of metabolism first recognized at autopsy by Abdehalden in 1903 and established as a clinical entity by Lignac in 1924. It is also known under the names of Lignac-Fanconi syndrome or cystine storage disease. The disorder is characterized by the existence of the Fanconi syndrome in association with deposits of cystine crystals in many tissues of the body. Tubular dysfunction represents a secondary abnormality, but often appears to be a primary condition, the cystine storage being undetected. The incidence is estimated to be between 1 and 2 in 40,000 of the general population. In one-third

of reported cases there has been a familial distribution, the disorder being inherited as an autosomal recessive.

Recent studies have shown that the defect in cystinosis is the excessive storage and subcellular compartmentalization of cystine in the lysosomes, and not a defect in the normal degradation of cystine, as was formerly believed. Plasma cystine levels are normal, but the cellular content of cystine is markedly elevated, as much as 100 times normal in peripheral leukocytes or fibroblasts cultured from cystinotic patients. Leukocytes and fibroblasts obtained from parents of these children average five or six times the normal content of free cystine, thus permitting the first biochemical identification of the heterozygote. The tubular dysfunction is believed to represent a toxic effect of the stored cystine on sulfhydryl-containing enzymes, since the clinical prognosis seems to be related to the degree of cystine storage. The intralysosomal compartmentalization of cystine may be the result of an impaired mechanism of degradation of the amino acid within the cellular organelle or of a defective membrane system associated with the egress of cystine from the lysosome.

The clinical symptomatology arises form involvement of kidney, intestine, eyes, liver, spleen, thyroid, and lymph nodes. Three phenotypes are recognized: a fatal infantile form, a benign adult form, and an adolescent form of intermediate clinical severity. The main differences are outlined in Table 10. Children with the infantile form present a clinical picture dominated by the tubular symptomatology, with progressive glomerular insufficiency and death in uremia. The clinical onset occurs in the first months of life, but in rare cases it may be delayed until late childhood (adolescent form). The earliest abnormality, detected in the apparently normal siblings of affected children, is the appearance of amino-aciduria. Soon thirst, vomiting, constipation, chronic dehydration, unexplained fever, and failure to thrive become evident. Growth retardation becomes

TABLE 10. Phenotypic Features of Three Different Types of Cystinosis[a]

Feature	Infantile Form	Adolescent Form	Adult Form
General			
Onset of symptoms	infancy	2nd decade	(incidental)
Life expectancy	late childhood	unknown	probably normal
Somatic growth	impaired	normal	normal
Rickets	present	appear in 2nd decade	normal
Hypopigmentation	present	absent	absent
Ocular			
Retinopathy	present	absent	absent
Cystine in cornea	present	present	present
Photophobia	present	absent	occasional
Renal abnormalities			
Glomerular failure	present 1st decade	present 2nd decade	absent
Tubular failure	generalized (Fanconi syndrome)	generalized (Fanconi syndrome)	absent
Morphology of nephron	swan-neck lesion	swan-neck lesion	unknown
Cystine level			
Plasma	normal	normal	normal
Granulocyte	increased (4–14 μmole/g	increased (3–6 μmole/	increased (1–4
Skin fibroblast	protein)	g protein)	μmole/g protein)
Inheritance	autosomal recessive	probably autosomal recessive	unknown

[a] From Goldman et al: Pediatrics 47:979, 1971.

more and more severe, and signs of rickets may become predominant. When renal function is studied during the early stage, glomerular filtration rate is normal, but multiple tubular dysfunctions usually are found. Sometimes only isolated abnormalities are present: glycosuria, amino-aciduria, or hyperchloremic acidosis. Death may occur during this stage from acute hypokalemia, acidosis, or overwhelming infection. Hepatomegaly, lymphadenopathy, and rarely, splenomegaly may appear. Photophobia, if noted, should suggest strongly the diagnosis of cystinosis. This has been attributed to the presence of refractile bodies in the cornea and conjunctiva, but probably is due to a peripheral pigmentary retinopathy, which is almost always present in the severe form. In the benign adult form corneal deposits are present but photophobia is rare.

After a variable period glomerular insufficiency becomes evident and tubular symptomatology improves or disappears. This amelioration is only apparent and is due to the progressive destruction of nephrons. After a number of years the glomerular insufficiency becomes so severe that the symptomatology is dominated by the uremic syndrome. Maintenance dialysis and transplantation are usually required before puberty.

The adolescent form, which is probably also inherited as an autosomal recessive, is characterized by delayed age of onset (generally in the second decade of life), mild nephropathy, and absence of retinopathy and pigmentary changes. The intracellular concentration of free cystine in the cultured fibroblast is lower than in fatal infantile cystinosis and slightly higher than in the benign adult form. Prognosis is apparently influenced by the severity of cystine retention, and glomerular insufficiency may develop in the second decade of life. The adult form, or benign cystinosis, is characterized by the presence of cystine crystals in the eye and the bone marrow. There are none of the associated renal or peripheral retinal abnormalities that are typical of nephropathic cystinosis. Patients with the benign disorder are asymptomatic and presumably have a normal life expectancy.

Cystine crystals are rectangular or hexagonal, and they are easily seen under polarized light in peripheral leukocytes, bone marrow aspirates, rectal mucosa, liver, spleen, or lymph nodes. In about 80 percent of cases they can be seen by slit-lamp examination of the cornea and conjunctiva. Cystine is soluble in aqueous solution and in formalin, and therefore an alcoholic fixative should be chosen for pathologic studies. The absence of cystine crystals in a single bone marrow aspiration does not exclude the condition, and repeated trials may be necessary. The best way to diagnose this entity is by a determination of the cystine content of peripheral leukocytes; an increase is pathognomonic of cystinosis.

Treatment in infantile and adolescent forms is symptomatic. The use of diuretics greatly facilitates the correction of the acidosis and the healing of bone lesions, but careful attention must be paid to the development of severe hypokalemia. The initial impression of the usefulness of penicillamine has not been confirmed, and the beneficial effect of a diet poor in cystine and methionine also remains controversial. The demonstration that dithiothreitol removes cystine from cultured cystinotic fibroblasts has not led to therapeutic application, since its toxicity precludes its use in patients. A number of patients with cystinosis have received homotransplants. There is evidence that the grafted kidneys accumulate cystine in the interstitial tissue but not intracellularly, and no tubular dysfunction dependent on cystine storage has appeared.

CONGENITAL CIRRHOSIS WITH FANCONI SYNDROME AND TYROSINURIA. This entity, first reported by Baber in 1956, consists of congenital cirrhosis of the liver and multiple tubular dysfunctions. Tyrosine is present in abnormal amounts in blood and urine, and the term tyrosinemia has been suggested. A high degree of consanguinity has been reported. The disease appears to be inherited as an autosomal recessive. Gentz and associates have suggested that the condition is an inborn error of tyrosine metabolism associated with lack of *p*-hydroxyphenylpyruvic acid oxidase; *p*-hydroxyphenylpyruvic acid is increased in the urine, suggesting an identity with the condition described by Medes as tyrosinosis (p. 677). However, the conditions appear to be different on both clinical and biochemical grounds.

In cases with very early onset the clinical picture is dominated by liver involvement and is similar to that of galactosemia and hereditary fructose intolerance. It especially can be confused with the latter disease, in which blood tyrosine levels frequently are elevated. In less severe cases the Fanconi syndrome is the predominant feature. Hepatomegaly is constant. Death may occur during the early months of life from hepatic insufficiency or may be delayed several years, in which case the development of malignant hepatoma has been reported. Differential diagnosis also must include Wilson's disease in addition to other tubular disorders. The finding of tyrosinemia and tyrosinuria is not adequate to establish the diagnosis, which should be made, if possible, by demonstration of the enzymatic deficiency.

The outcome of the disease invariably is fatal. The effects of a diet low in phenylalanine and tyrosine are very promising, with excellent results reported on tubular dysfunction and rate of growth. The effect on hepatic function, however, is very poor, and the early forms continue to have a very severe prognosis.

GALACTOSEMIA. Galactosemia (see also p. 713) is an inborn error of galactose metabolism caused by an absence of galactose-1-phosphate uridyl transferase. The accumulation of galactose-1-phosphate has toxic effects in many body tissues, especially liver, brain, lens, and kidney. The renal toxic effect is primarily an isolated amino-aciduria, but tubular proteinuria, true glycosuria, and tubular acidosis also may appear. The tubular abnormalities disappear quickly when a diet without lactose and galactose is instituted.

GLYCOGEN STORAGE DISEASE. Occasionally a patient with the hepatorenal form of glycogen storage disease may demonstrate tubular dysfunction, as in the original case of Fanconi and Bickel in which the patient presented with glucoaminophosphaturia. Tubular dysfunction is probably dependent on accumulation of glycogen in the renal proximal tubular cells (p. 729).

WILSON'S DISEASE.   The most frequent renal abnormality in Wilson's disease (see also p. 1921) is aminoaciduria. Glycosuria, increased phosphate and urate clearances, and hyperchloremic acidosis may also be found. Hypercalciuria is very frequent, and urinary lithiasis has been reported in adult cases. The tubular abnormalities probably depend on toxic accumulation of copper. Treatment of the disease by D-penicillamine improves the hepatic and neurologic symptoms, but the effect on tubular dysfunction is less evident.

HEREDITARY INTOLERANCE TO FRUCTOSE.   Aminoaciduria and hyperchloremic acidosis may be present in this disease (see also p. 715). A defect in bicarbonate reabsorption has been documented by Morris. The toxic substance is probably fructose-1-phosphate.

NEPHROTIC SYNDROME.   The presence of tubular abnormalities during the evolution of the idiopathic nephrotic syndrome is exceptional. Only 19 cases of a complete Fanconi syndrome have been described in children. It is not known if these patients have a specific entity or a particular evolution of a noncharacteristic idiopathic nephrotic syndrome.

The clinical picture is rather uniform. During the initial period the nephrotic syndrome is uncomplicated, and normal renal histology and funtion are present. Later, tubular function becomes progressively affected with marked hypokalemia and tetany. Nephrocalcinosis has been noted in four children from two unrelated families. In a later stage glomerular insufficiency is severe, and the patients in all reported cases have died

in uremia. The administration of steroids has been ineffective.

EXOGENOUS TOXINS.   Proximal tubular damage may follow exposure to many toxic substances. Heavy metals, including lead, cadmium, uranium, and mercury, are notorious. Chisolm and Leahy found that amino-aciduria and glycosuria were almost constant in lead poisoning in children and reported a case with associated increased phosphate clearance and rickets. Other potentially toxic substances include Lysol, 3-methylchromone, and some antibiotics, including outdated tetracycline and amphotericin B. The tubular abnormality disappears after removal of the toxic substance.

Renal Tubular Acidosis

Although renal acidosis is always tubular in origin, it can conveniently be classified into glomerular or tubular on the basis of the underlying pathophysiology. Glomerular acidosis is present in patients with chronic renal insufficiency and is part of the uremic syndrome. Tubular acidosis is a condition in which glomerular function is either normal or relatively less impaired than tubular function. Used in this general sense, renal tubular acidosis (RTA) represents a syndrome and includes varied forms.

Two mechanisms are involved in renal excretion of acid (p.1242): reabsorption of filtered bicarbonate, which is primarily a proximal function, and excretion of hydrogen ion in the form of titratable acid and ammonium, which is primarily a distal function. Abnor-

TABLE 11. Renal Tubular Acidosis

	Proximal	Distal
Etiology		
Primary	Infantile (transient)	Infantile isolated associated with congenital nerve deafness
Secondary	Adult (vitamin D deficiency?) Fanconi syndrome Cystinosis Lowe's syndrome Primary and secondary hyperparathyroidism Vitamin D deficiency Medullary cystic disease Renal transplantation Osteopetrosis Cyanotic congenital heart disease Leigh's syndrome	Adult Primary hyperparathyroidism with nephrocalcinosis Primary hyperthyroidism with nephrocalcinosis Idiopathic hypercalciuria with nephrocalcinosis Vitamin D intoxication Hypergammaglobulinemic states Medullary sponge kidney Hepatic cirrhosis Amphotericin B nephropathy Renal transplantation
Diagnosis		
Urine pH	4.5–7.8 depending on level of plasma bicarbonate	Always above 6.0 regardless of level of plasma bicarbonate
Bicarbonate threshold	Decreased	Normal
Hydrogen-ion excretion	Normal, below bicarbonate threshold	Impaired, below bicarbonate threshold
Therapy	Resistant to alkali therapy Effect of diuretics	Sensitive to alkali therapy No effect of diuretics

malities of these mechanisms will therefore be associated, with (1) loss of bicarbonate into urine due to a defect in bicarbonate reabsorption, termed proximal RTA, (2) impaired excretion of hydrogen ion as titratable acid or ammonium or both, termed distal RTA, or (3) a combination of 1 and 2 (Table 11).

PROXIMAL RTA. In this condition hyperchloremic acidosis results from a depression in the renal threshold of excretion of bicarbonate caused by a defect in reabsorption of bicarbonate in the proximal tubule. Under ordinary circumstances virtually all filtered bicarbonate is reabsorbed. If the concentration of bicarbonate in plasma exceeds the level of the renal threshold, bicarbonate reabsorption is incomplete, and urinary excretion gradually lowers the concentration to a level below the threshold. At this point the excretion of bicarbonate ceases and a new steady state is reached. The level of the bicarbonate threshold changes with age: in adults bicarbonate begins to be excreted in urine when the concentration in plasma exceeds 25 to 26 mmole/liter, whereas in infants bicarbonate is present in urine when the plasma level exceeds 22 mmole/liter. Patients with proximal RTA have bicarbonate thresholds below normal for their ages. Therefore bicarbonate is present in the urine when the concentration in plasma is below that found in normal individuals; a steady state is maintained with the plasma bicarbonate in the acidemic range. This can be increased into the normal range only by giving large amounts of bicarbonate orally or intravenously, although this is associated with large losses of bicarbonate in the urine. When therapy is stopped the acidemia quickly reappears, due not only to continued loss of bicarbonate into the urine but also to inhibition of the distal mechanisms of hydrogen-ion secretion, as the distal tubule is flooded with bicarbonate-rich fluid. Only by giving large amounts of bicarbonate on a continuous basis can levels of bicarbonate in plasma be elevated to and maintained within the normal range.

An important feature in these patients is their unimpaired ability to lower urinary pH and to excrete adequate amounts of titratable acid and ammonium when their bicarbonate concentration in plasma is below their threshold. As a consequence they may easily be overlooked when using the usual methods for detecting RTA.

The exact nature of the defect is unknown. A deficiency of carbonic anhydrase appears to be excluded, as is evidenced by a normal response to the administration of the enzyme inhibitor acetazolamide, although a deficiency in that enzyme was suspected by Donckerwolcke and associates in a girl with this syndrome. There may be a primary defect in bicarbonate reabsorption or an abnormality in sodium reabsorption in the proximal tubule leading secondarily to impaired bicarbonate reabsorption. The recent finding in a patient with primary proximal RTA of a marked excess of duodenal secretion of bicarbonate associated with decreased secretion of chloride would suggest a defective exchange mechanism of chloride and bicarbonate in both the kidney and the intestine.

Primary proximal RTA refers to the occurrence of hyperchloremic acidosis due to an isolated defect in bicarbonate reabsorption, in the absence of any other abnormality in glomerular or tubular function. The only clinical manifestation is retarded growth; the complications observed in patients with distal RTA, such as interstitial nephritis, bone lesions, nephrocalcinosis, nephrolithiasis, polyuria, and hypokalemia, are absent. Most patients with this condition have been males. Functional evaluation of these patients reveals the presence of a low bicarbonate threshold. When distal acidifying capacity is examined as levels of serum bicarbonate below the renal threshold, all subjects excrete a urine of strongly acid pH, with rates of excretion of titratable acid and ammonium within the normal range. Treatment consists of administration of sodium bicarbonate or citrate in amounts adequate to maintain the plasma concentration within the normal range. The starting dosage is 5 to 10 mEq/kg/24 hours given in fractional doses spread over as much of the 24-hour period as is practical. The prognosis of these patients seems to be good; all the patients we have studied have been taken off therapy after several years of treatment without reappearance of the acidosis. During administration of adequate alkali therapy there is usually slow but progressive catch-up growth.

Secondary proximal RTA has been demonstrated in association with other tubular dysfunctions in patients with idiopathic or secondary Fanconi syndrome (cystinosis, Lowe's syndrome, tyrosinemia, glycogen storage disease, Wilson's disease, hereditary fructose intolerance, nephrotic syndrome, multiple myeloma, renal amyloidosis, and toxicity to outdated tetracycline, 3-methylchromone, and heavy metals), in patients with vitamin-D-deficiency rickets, medullary cystic disease, osteopetrosis, cyanotic congenital heart disease, and subacute necrotizing encephalomyelopathy (Leigh's syndrome), or following renal transplantation.

In 1953 Lightwood and associates described a transient form of renal tubular acidosis in infants with anorexia, vomiting, constipation, and failure to thrive. Rickets and nephrocalcinosis usually were absent radiologically. Most of the infants were male. The response to alkali therapy was dramatic, and the patients were said to recover by 2 years of age. The pathophysiology of the acidosis in these infants was unclear, since few precise studies of hydrogen-ion excretion were performed. Latner and Burnard presented considerable evidence for a defect in bicarbonate reabsorption in six patients, but on the basis of other evidence the defect was generally accepted as an inability to acidify the urine. Lightwood's syndrome thus became recognized as a transient, self-limited form of distal RTA in infants. It is of interest that these patients were mainly males, nephrocalcinosis and rickets were strikingly absent, and very high dosage therapy was required to maintain their blood bicarbonate within the normal range. These features can now be recognized as characteristic of proximal rather than distal RTA. In addition, although a large number of these infants were diagnosed in various parts of Great Britain in the late 1940s and early 1950s, the disease subsequently all but disappeared, suggesting that its frequency at that time was the result of some unrecognized environmental factor. There is evidence that the condition may have been due to vitamin D intoxication or to toxicity to sulfonamides or mercury. Therefore it seems reasonable to conclude that in most instances Lightwood's syndrome represented a secondary form of proximal RTA. This is of considerable importance, since it implies that the diagnosis of primary distal RTA in an infant most likely establishes the existence of a permanent defect.

DISTAL RTA. In distal RTA the primary defect is an inability to establish adequate gradients of hydrogen ion between blood and tubular fluid, despite low levels of serum bicarbonate. The inability to lower urinary pH to less than 6.0 or 6.5 is the most distinctive feature. The exact nature of the acidification defect is unknown. The hypotheses suggested implicate either the energetic mechanism necessary to pump hydrogen ion (or to reabsorb sodium) across the tubular membrane or, more likely, an increased rate of passive diffusion of hydrogen ion from the tubular lumen back into the cell. Defects in the carbonic anhydrase system are unlikely, since enzyme activity in the renal tissue has been found normal in most patients. However, an inactive mutant form of red cell carbonic anhydrase B has been described in a family whose affected individuals presented with infantile RTA and nerve deafness. Failure of patients with distal RTA to increase urinary Pco_2 to the same extent as normals during bicarbonate loading has suggested that a limitation in the rate of secretion of hydrogen ion in the distal nephron is the basic defect. The frequent association between hypergammaglobulinemic states and distal RTA is rather striking; this observation, together with the presence of antibodies to cells of the loop of Henle and the deposit of immunoglobulin in tubular cells in some patients, supports the suggestion of an autoimmune pathogenesis in some cases of this syndrome.

Primary distal RTA (Butler-Albright syndrome) is a disorder that occurs predominately in females (about 70 percent) and usually is not diagnosed until after 2 years of age, frequently not until adult life. However, several cases unquestionably have begun in infancy, presenting with vomiting, constipation, anorexia, polyuria, dehydration, and failure to thrive. The majority of cases are sporadic, but at least 18 families with RTA have been reported. Inheritance appears to be of the autosomal dominant type, with a variable degree of expression.

Growth retardation is most evident beyond early infancy and may represent the only clinical abnormality. Bone lesions are frequent, although they usually are absent early in life. Rickets and osteomalacia often are present during childhood and adolescence, accompanied by generalized bone demineralization. Nephrocalcinosis is an almost constant finding and may be demonstrated radiographically. Calcium deposits preferentially in the renal medulla, which can become completely petrified. Urolithiasis also is common, but occurs less frequently in children than in adults. The

intravenous pyelogram is otherwise normal if obstructive uropathy caused by the lithiasis is not present.

Analysis of blood reveals a low pH and low concentration of bicarbonate, with elevation of the chloride. Moderate hyponatremia and hypokalemia may be present, although the serum potassium is not a good index of the degree of potassium deficiency because of the associated acidemia. Periodic paralysis caused by severe potassium deficiency is not exceptional. The concentration of phosphate in blood is low, with normal or even high levels of calcium. The alkaline phosphatase level may be elevated if active osteomalacic lesions are present. Glomerular filtration rate is normal in the young child, but a progressive decrease may occur over the years as a consequence of progressive parenchymal damage. It should be noted that evaluation of glomerular function is best performed after prolonged administration of alkali therapy and correction of the contracted extracellular space.

Urinary pH is usually above 6.0 or 6.5, with low rates of excretion of titratable acid and ammonium. A low degree of proteinuria may be found. Leukocyturia is frequent and may accompany sterile urines or be secondary to urinary tract infection. Polyuria due to a concentrating defect is marked. In the early stages the hyposthenuria may be corrected by adequate control of the acidosis and potassium deficiency, but subsequent to nephrocalcinosis and tubular damage it becomes fixed.

The phosphate clearance is increased either as a direct consequence of the acidemia or as a manifestation of secondary hyperparathyroidism. Hypercalciuria is a constant feature when acidosis is present and reverts completely to normal after adequate alkali therapy. Hyperkaliuria results mainly from secondary hyperaldosteronism triggered by sodium depletion. A low excretion of citrate is characteristic and is probably secondary to intratubular acidosis and potassium deficiency. Normal urinary levels of citrate can be obtained only after persistent administration of alkali and potassium. Hypercalciuria, hypocitraturia, and alkaline urine are important factors in the development of nephrocalcinosis. The pathophysiologic interrelationships in this disease are presented schematically in Figure 16. Other tubular functions usually are normal. Amino-aciduria is usually not present, although two reports have noted it, with disappearance following correction of the acidosis and hypokalemia. The histology of the kidney is normal in the early stages, but later variable degrees of calcium deposition and interstitial nephritis are observed.

The prognosis of primary distal RTA is good if the diagnosis is established early enough to prevent the development of nephrocalcinosis, secondary pyelonephritis, and tubular damage.

Treatment consists of correction of the acidemia, following which the bone lesions heal without need for large doses of vitamin D and growth rate accelerates, with patients often regaining their earlier normal growth pattern or even evidencing catch-up growth. Calcium excretion reverts to normal, and further calcium deposits may be prevented. Potassium should be

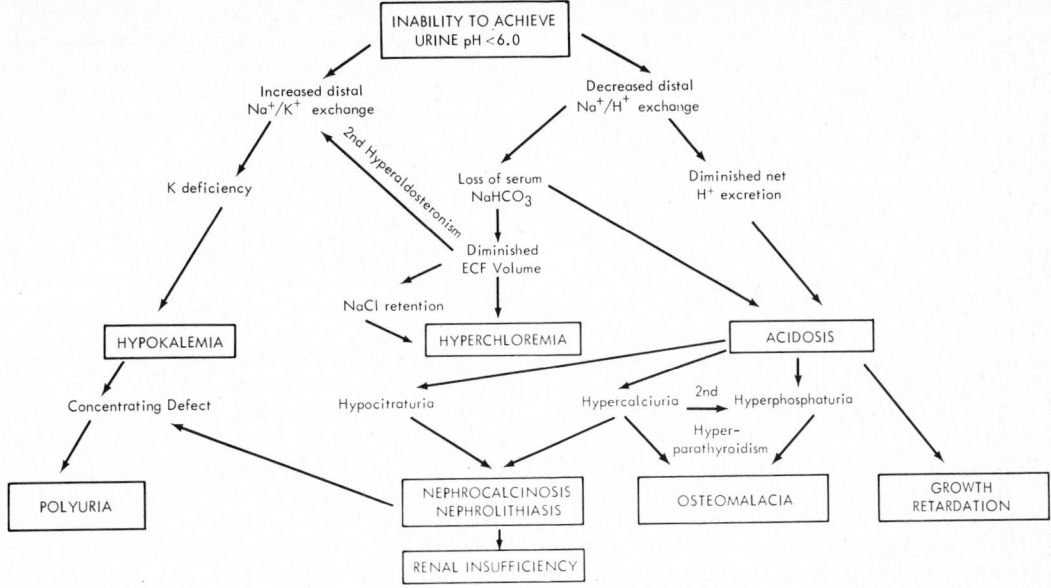

FIG. 16. Interrelationships of the metabolic complications of distal RTA. (From Rodriquez-Soriano and Edelmann: Ann Rev Med 20:363, 1969.)

given regardless of the level of serum potassium; in instances of severe hypokalemia potassium should be given prior to the correction of acidemia. A useful mixture is a solution of sodium and potassium citrate: 100 g of each salt diluted in 1 liter of water provides approximately 2 mEq/ml. A dose of 2 to 5 mEq/kg is adequate, but it must be adjusted in each case according to changes in blood pH and bicarbonate and changes in rate of excretion of calcium in urine. In some cases correction of the acidemia may permit continued excessive excretion of calcium, resulting in further calcium deposition. Calcium excretion falls to normal following increased intake of citrate. When distal RTA appears in infancy significant bicarbonate wasting frequently is present, requiring the administration of doses of alkali almost as large as those necessary in proximal RTA. The bicarbonate wasting appears to depend on an associated and transitory defect of proximal reabsorption of bicarbonate that diminishes progressively with age.

Secondary distal RTA may be associated with a number of systemic or renal conditions including starvation, malnutrition, hyperparathyroidism, hyperthyroidism, vitamin D intoxication, amphotericin B nephropathy, hypergammaglobulinemic states (idiopathic hypergammaglobulinemia, hyperglobulinemic purpura, Sjögren's syndrome, cryoglobulinemia, active chronic hepatitis, sarcoidosis), hepatic cirrhosis, medullary sponge kidney, and a variety of genetically transmitted disorders (hereditary fructose intolerance with nephrocalcinosis, Ehlers-Danlos syndrome, Fabry's disease, hereditary elliptocytosis); it probably also may be found following renal tubular necrosis and renal homotransplantation. The occurrence in a single family of individuals with nephrocalcinosis and distal RTA and individuals with hypercalciuria but without either nephrocalcinosis or RTA suggests that a picture identical to that of primary distal RTA may develop secondarily to long-standing hypercalciuria.

Idiopathic Hypercalciuria

Idiopathic hypercalciuria is a frequent cause of recurrent lithiasis in adults. It occurs less frequently in children, however, and few cases have been described. The most frequent presenting symptom is growth retardation in association with renal abnormalities such as proteinuria and decreased concentrating capacity. Clinical manifestations also include urolithiasis, nephrocalcinosis, distal RTA, and vitamin-D-resistant rickets. Some children present a more benign type resembling that usually seen in the adult; the symptomatology depends upon the formation of urinary calculi. Calcium excretion exceeds 5 mg/kg/day. Acidemia is not present, and hypercalciuria does not decrease after administration of sodium bicarbonate. Serum calcium is normal and serum phosphorus may be normal or low. Renal histology is normal or shows variable degrees of interstitial nephritis. In the cases studied intestinal absorption of calcium has been normal, thus pointing to a renal tubular abnormality as the cause of the hypercalciuria. However, kidney transplantation from a hypercalciuric father to a normocalciuric son has not been followed by any abnormality.

There is no specific therapy. Thiazide diuretics, which are known to decrease calcium excretion, are being evaluated. Decreased calcium excretion has been noted following restriction of dietary sodium, which at present constitutes the most effective method of treatment. In adult patients with this disorder the highest success rate in lowering urinary calcium has been achieved by the association of thiazides and cellulose phosphate, although the effect of this therapy still waits confirmation in idiopathic hypercalciuria of childhood.

Sodium-losing Disorders

PSEUDOHYPOALDOSTERONISM. This entity, first described by Cheek and Perry in 1958, is believed to represent a failure of the renal tubule to respond to aldosterone, with secondary excessive loss of sodium in the urine, as well as hyponatremia and hyperkalemia. About 11 cases have been reported to date, with marked predominance of males over females. Several cases have been observed in the same kindred. Affected infants are normal at birth, but after 1 or 2 weeks they exhibit vomiting, anorexia, failure to thrive, and if treatment is delayed, severe marasmus, with delayed skeletal and psychomotor development. During episodes of dehydration, often triggered by intercurrent infection, patients may have marked collapse or even coma.

The concentration of sodium in plasma is low, and moderate hyperkalemia is present. Despite dehydration and hyponatremia, a high rate of excretion of urinary sodium continues. The excretion of 17-ketosteroids and 17-hydroxysteroids is normal, but the excretion of aldosterone is abnormally high, up to 900 μg/24 hours. Aldosterone secretion rates are also very elevated during the active phase of the disease and remain so even after the serum electrolytes and the growth rate have been normalized under the influence of salt supplementation. Plasma renin values are also increased, indicating that the hyperaldosteronism is due to hyperactivity of the renin-angiotensin system secondary to salt depletion. The administration of DOCA or aldosterone fails to modify the urinary excretion of sodium. The accepted pathogenesis, an unresponsiveness of the distal tubule to aldosterone, has recently been challenged, since the administration of spironolactone provoked in one patient a tremendous aggravation of the salt loss. Morever, in six patients in whom aldosterone secretion was measured there was an inverse correlation between sodium intake and aldosterone production. An alternative hypothesis would be a disturbance of sodium reabsorption in the proximal tubule or in the ascending loop of Henle, with secondary hyperaldosteronism. This hyperaldosteronism may be unable to fully compensate for the excessive amounts of sodium reaching the distal tubule. This hypothesis would be in accordance with the finding of normal aldosterone receptor mechanisms in the intestine.

Seven Jewish children from five families have been described with a similar syndrome of salt wastage, very high plasma renin activity, and normal or high plasma aldosterone levels; however, they differ from patients with classic pseudohypoaldosteronism by having a positive response to exogenous salt-retaining steroids and a normal or only slightly raised level of plasma aldoster-

one. This syndrome probably depends on either a partial block of aldosterone synthesis with formation of salt-losing metabolites or a partial defect in the enzymatic conversion of angiotensin I to angiotensin II. In neither case do renal tubular abnormatites seem to be present.

Differentiation from the salt-losing forms of congenital adrenal hyperplasia and adrenal insufficiency is clinically difficult and depends upon appropriate investigation of steroid metabolism. Hypertrophic pyloric stenosis, cystic fibrosis, inappropriate ADH secretion, and other salt-losing nephropathies (see below) also should be considered.

The administration of supplementary sodium chloride is the treatment of choice. A dose of about 5 g/day is required, following which there is usually a dramatic decrease in vomiting as well as a weight gain and enhanced skeletal and psychomotor development. There is some evidence that after some months or years the need for supplementary sodium chloride decreases, but sufficient data from long-term follow-ups are not yet available.

SALT-LOSING NEPHROPATHIES. Excessive urinary loss of sodium occurs together with other tubular abnormalities in the Fanconi syndrome, in distal renal tubular acidosis, and in other tubulopathies; it is also found in association with generalized renal disease. Limitation of renal capacity to conserve sodium is common in most cases of uremia, but usually a balance between input and output is maintained, with urinary wastage becoming evident only under conditions of salt deprivation. However, in exceptional cases (termed salt-losing nephritis) the urinary loss of sodium is so marked during periods of normal intake that patients may appear to have Addison's disease. This syndrome has usually been associated with chronic pyelonephritis, medullary cystic disease, or hereditary polycystic disease. The condition apparently is rare in children, the youngest patient reported being an adolescent. However, urinary sodium loss of lesser degree is seen in children with bilateral renal hypoplasia or dysplasia, obstructive uropathy, juvenile nephrophthisis, and interstitial nephritis.

It is important to realize that the salt-losing defect associated with tubular or generalized renal disease is often unrecognized. Dehydration may be minimal and the serum sodium may be normal due to compensatory contraction of the extracellular space. However, even in these patients administration of extra sodium is followed by improved well-being, weight gain, and increases in rates of glomerular filtration and renal plasma flow.

Potassium-losing Disorders

PSEUDOHYPERALDOSTERONISM. This hereditary condition (Liddle's syndrome), which is probably transmitted as an autosomal dominant, was described in 1964 by Liddle, Bledsoe, and Coppage in six siblings with hypertension, hypokalemic alkalosis, and negligible aldosterone secretion. The disorder seems to be caused by an unusual tendency of the kidney to reabsorb sodium and excrete potassium even when mineralocorticoids are almost completely absent. This syndrome probably reflects a generalized, inherited abnormality of sodium transport, since the defect is also present in erythrocytes. These patients differ from normal subjects and from patients with primary aldosteronism in that their electrolyte excretion is unaffected by the administration of either an inhibitor of aldosterone synthesis or an aldosterone antagonist. Giving both an inhibitor of tubular sodium transport (triamterene) and supplementary potassium chloride serves to normalize the blood pressure and correct the hypokalemia.

HYPERPLASIA OF JUXTAGLOMERULAR APPARATUS WITH HYPERALDOSTERONISM AND HYPOKALEMIC ALKALOSIS.

In 1962 Bartter and associates reported a new syndrome characterized by hypokalemic alkalosis, hyperaldosteronism with normal blood pressure, and hyperplasia of the juxtaglomerular apparatus (Bartter's syndrome). About 25 cases have been reported in the literature under such varied names as renal tubular alkalosis, congenital hyperaldosteronism, chronic idiopathic hypokalemia, and congenital hypokalemia. Several familial cases have been described; it is probably inherited as an autosomal recessive.

Symptoms first occur during infancy, but the diagnosis may be delayed for many years. The earliest symptoms are polyuria, polydipsia, a tendency toward dehydration, salt craving, constipation, vomiting, and anorexia. Growth retardation is constant, becoming more marked as the child gets older. These patients do continue to grow throughout childhood, and with a delayed adolescent growth spurt they may attain normal adult height, even in the absence of any treatment. Muscular weakness is frequent, and very often recurrent tetany is present. A dilated viscus (megacolon, dilated ureter) is often found. A few patients have presented with nephrocalcinosis. The blood pressure characteristically is normal. The outstanding biochemical feature is the marked hypokalemia, often accompanied by hyponatremia, hypochloremia, and metabolic alkalosis. Erythrocytosis, hypomagnesemia, hypercalcemia, and hyperlipemia may also be found. Aldosterone secretion and excretion rates are markedly elevated if potassium deficiency has been corrected previously. Cortisol and corticosterone production are normal. Plasma renin activity and angiotensin level are characteristically elevated. The response to expansion of intravascular volume by means of albumin infusion or high sodium load, which inhibits the angiotensin-aldosterone system, is paradoxic in some cases; neither secretion of aldosterone nor plasma renin activity is changed by these measures. However, in other cases a normal, although somewhat blunted, response has been reported. Methyldopa and propranolol will also suppress the hyperreninemia, but this effect is lost with continous administration of methyldopa. The long-term effectiveness of propranolol is unknown. Angiotensinase levels are significantly reduced.

Renal pathology is characteristic. The glomeruli reveal marked hypertrophy of the juxtaglomerular apparatus and a variable degree of hyalinization. The tubular lesions of potassium deficiency may be present. The zona glomerulosa of the adrenal gland is hypertrophic, with marked lipid infiltration.

The pathogenesis of this syndrome remains obscure. Bartter and associates believed that the primary defect was in inability of the vascular wall to respond to angiotensin and that the subsequent increase in angiotensin led to increased aldosterone secretion and potassium loss. A central point in this hypothesis was the normotension and the decreased response to administration of angiotensin. However, this resistance to the pressor effect of angiotensin may be secondary to the hyperreninemia (tachyphylaxis), since it has been found in many other patients with conditions producing chronically elevated renin levels (malignant or renovascular hypertension, liver cirrhosis with ascites, and sodium depletion).

An alternative explanation more recently proposed suggests that the primary cause is a renal tubular defect in proximal reabsorption of sodium with increased delivery of sodium into the distal nephron and enhanced exchange with potassium, even after correction of secondary hyperaldosteronism. An abnormality of sodium reabsorption in the loop of Henle has been reported in one patient. The capacity of these patients to conserve sodium normally is explained by a compensatory increase in distal sodium reabsorption. This theory explains the absence of hypertension on the basis of chronically decreased intravascular volume despite increased aldosterone secretion rate and plasma renin activity and the persistence of hypokalemia despite correction of the hyperaldosteronism. The finding of an increased permeability to sodium in the red cell membrane suggests that the abnormality of sodium transport is present in cellular membranes other than in the renal tubule.

A third hypothesis explains the findings on the basis of a primary, but not autonomous, hyperreninemia. The previously mentioned defect in sodium transport across epithelial membranes could conceivably affect the juxtaglomerular cells as well and lead to excessive renin production. The diminution of effective blood volume could be mediated by the natriuresis and increased urinary volume caused by the direct effect of angiotensin II on the kidney.

Finally, a fourth hypothesis attributes the condition to renal overproduction of prostaglandins, with consequent loss of sodium, secondary hyperreninemia and hyperaldosteronism, potassium loss, and peripheral vasodilatation preventing hypertension. Support for this hypothesis has been obtained from measurement of urinary excretion of prostaglandins and a favorable effect from chronic administration of inhibitors of prostaglandin synthesis.

Differential diagnosis must consider primary aldosteronism; the very high levels of renin and angiotensin in Bartter's syndrome differentiate the two conditions. The more rare tumor in the juxtaglomerular apparatus causes autonomous oversecretion of renin, but hypertension is constantly observed. Patients with secondary hyperaldosteronism due to renovascular or malignant hypertension or associated with edematous states should be differentiated easily. Other potassium-losing disorders such as the Fanconi syndrome, distal RTA, Liddle's syndrome, and some types of pyelonephritis must also be considered.

The prognosis is poor, and death may occur suddenly due to acute electrolyte imbalance or intercurrent infection. There is some evidence that progressive glomerular insufficiency may appear over a period of years.

Therapeutic administration of potassium is mandatory, but if given alone it is quickly lost in the urine without correction of the hypokalemia. The best results are obtained by simultaneous administration of spironolactone (Aldactone) with sodium and potassium supplements. Dosage must be adjusted to obtain an equilibrium between intake and excretion. Magnesium supplements may be necessary. In one patient the simultaneous administration of spironolactone and propranolol has resulted in a prolonged period of normalization of serum potassium, but this therapy remains experimental. The usefulness of prostaglandin inhibitors awaits further clinical testing.

Potassium-retaining Disorders

SHORT STATURE, HYPERKALEMIA, AND ACIDOSIS. This condition (Spitzer's syndrome) was first described in an 11-year-old boy by Spitzer and associates in 1973. A second case, in a 9-year-old boy, was reported by Weinstein and associates in 1974. Previous reports of hyperkalemia and metabolic acidosis without renal failure may represent the same entity. Both patients presented with short stature, metabolic acidosis, and persistent hyperkalemia. Glomerular filtration rate and endocrine function were normal. Although the acidosis was explained by a low renal bicarbonate threshold, correction of the acidosis by sodium bicarbonate therapy did not influence the hyperkalemia. During treatment with thiazide diuretics both serum potassium and bicarbonate concentrations became normal. This entity may represent a primary abnormality in renal excretion of potassium. The resulting hyperkalemia would induce the urinary loss of bicarbonate and the systemic acidosis. Correction of acidosis and hyperkalemia by the continuous administration of thiazides and sodium bicarbonate has resulted in resumption of normal growth in Spitzer's patient, but it did not improve growth in Weinstein's patient.

Magnesium-losing disorders

Chronic hypomagnesemia is rare in childhood, and when it occurs it is usually associated with defective intestinal absorption of magnesium or, more rarely, with hyperaldosteronism or hyperparathyroidism. A probable tubular defect of magnesium reabsorption was described in 1974 by Booth and Johanson in a 5-year-old girl who presented with carpopedal spasm and failure to thrive. Evalution showed normocalcemia and normokalemia associated with hypomagnesemia, hyperamino-aciduria, and intermittent glycosuria. Studies with ^{28}Mg showed no defect in intestinal absorption. Treatment with supplemental oral magnesium did not result in an immediate effect on growth but did significantly raise the serum magnesium level. Amino-aciduria and glycosuria persisted despite treatment.

Nephrogenic Diabetes Insipidus

Nephrogenic diabetes insipidus (NDI) (see also p. 1616) is a hereditary disorder characterized by insensitivity of the renal tubule to antidiuretic hormone (ADH). Most of the affected patients are male, suggesting a sex-linked transmission. Heterozygous females may exhibit some degree of polyuria with limitation of concentrating ability. This type of inheritance contrasts with ADH-deficient diabetes insipidus, which when genetically determined is transmitted as an autosomal dominant.

NDI appears shortly after birth. Polyuria and polydipsia generally are not appreciated, and the infant presents with a nonspecific picture of vomiting, anorexia, constipation, unexplained fever, recurrent dehydration, and failure to thrive. In some of these infants thirst is virtually absent (occult diabetes insipidus). A marked retardation in psychomotor development is often present; it has been attributed both to the chronic hyperelectrolytemia and to the lack of environmental stimulation, most of the infant's time being spent in drinking and sleeping.

In older children beyond 3 or 4 years of age polyuria, polydipsia, and retarded growth persist, but a more normal balance between intake and output is possible, and secondary complications generally are absent.

Examination of the serum, especially in infants, reveals increased concentrations of sodium, chloride, and urea secondary to the negative water balance. Despite dehydration and hemoconcentration, urine is dilute, with a specific gravity between 1.001 and 1.005 (40 to 200 mOsm/kg). During severe dehydration, with very decreased glomerular filtration rate, urinary osmolality may increase, but rarely to hypertonic levels. Administration of vasopressin changes neither the volume nor concentration of the urine. A water-deprivation test to assess maximum urinary concentrating ability is not necessary for the diagnosis; it is hazardous and should be avoided.

Insensitivity to ADH is the only primary tubular abnormality in NDI, but during dehydration proteinuria and amino-aciduria may be present. Glomerular filtration rate is normal if hydration is adequate.

In most cases the intravenous pyelogram is normal. Although marked bladder distension and hydronephrosis have been attributed to the high rate of urine flow, such findings should suggest the diagnosis of obstructive uropathy with secondary diabetes insipidus, and adequate urologic studies should be done.

Histologically the kidney is normal, although a shortened proximal segment has been demonstrated by microdissection by Darmady and associates; this finding needs confirmation. In one case studied by electron microscopy, glomerular immaturity and mitochondrial changes in the tubules were noted, suggesting an abnormality in mitochondrial membrane lipids.

The complete pathogenesis of NDI is unknown. ADH is present in blood and urine, and neurohypophyseal lesions are not found. It is believed at present that the intracellular intermediate in the action of vasopressin is cyclic 3′,5′-AMP, the formation of which is stimulated by the action of vasopressin on the adenylcyclase system. An abnormality in the cellular production of cyclic AMP could account for the tubular insensitivity to the hormone, in a manner similar to the mechanism that has been described in patients with tubular insensitivity to parathyroid hormone. This hypothesis has received support from the observation that intravenous administration of vasopressin does not result in a significant increase of cyclic AMP in the urine, in contrast to normal individuals or patients with vasopressin deficiency. Studies in mice with inherited vasopressin-resistant diabetes insipidus suggest that the defects may lie in the cellular action of vasopressin and not in a deficient activity of adenylcyclase.

Differential diagnosis must consider the hereditary form of ADH-deficiency diabetes insipidus, which also may start very early in life; the response to vasopressin serves to separate these conditions. Several renal disorders may present with a syndrome of vasopressin-resistant diabetes insipidus: obstructive uropathies, hypercalcemia, hypercalciuria with or without RTA, potassium-losing disorders, and a special group of chronic renal diseases that includes bilateral renal hypoplasia, medullary cystic disease, and familial nephrophthisis. It also may be present in renal periarteritis nodosa, renal amyloidosis, and Sjögren's syndrome. Some adults with malignant hypertension present with nocturnal diabetes insipidus only; during the day the urine is hypertonic to plasma and the patient is oliguric. A polyuric syndrome similar to NDI has been described after administration of various drugs such as lithium, demethylchlortetracycline, vincristine, and methoxyflurane.

The prognosis is favorable if the diagnosis is made early in life and adequate therapy is instituted; however, between 5 and 10 percent of patients die in infancy, and in some cases both mental growth and physical growth are irreversibly retarded.

Therapy consists in giving water in the amount and frequency necessary to compensate for the obligatory urinary loss. In older children this aim is easily attained, but great difficulties may be encountered in infancy, especially when thirst is absent. Administration of solute-poor milk reduces urinary water requirements and helps to maintain an adequate water balance.

The discovery that thiazide diuretics decrease urinary output has enormously facilitated the management of these patients, especially during infancy. The decrease of urinary volume observed following administration of the diuretic is accompanied by an increased concentration of urinary solute and decreased clearance of free water. It has been shown that the effect is mediated through sodium depletion, with increased proximal reabsorption of sodium and water and decreased delivery of fluid to the distal tubule. Giving sodium chloride interferes with the antidiuretic effect, which is maximal on a low-sodium intake. Furthermore, the effect can be produced by other diuretics and is not an exclusive property of the thiazides. Different drugs such as chlorpropamide, clofibrate, and carbamazepine have an antidiuretic effect in ADH-deficiency diabetes insipidus, but they are without effect in the nephrogenic form.

References

RENAL GLYCOSURIA

Brodehl J, Franken A, Gelissen K: Maximal tubular reabsorption of glucose in infants and children. Acta Paediatr Scand 61: 413, 1972

Elsas LJ, Rosenberg LE: Familial renal glycosuria: a genetic reappraisal of hexose transport by kidney and intestine. J Clin Invest 48:1845, 1969

——— Hillman RE, Patterson JH, Rosenberg LE: Renal and intestinal hexose transport in familial glucose-galactose malabsorption. J Clin Invest 49: 576, 1970

AMINO-ACIDURIAS

Brodehl J, Gellissen K: Endogenous renal transport of free amino acids in infancy and childhood. Pediatrics 42:395, 1968

Greene ML, Lietman PS, Rosenberg LE, Seegmiller JE: Familial hyperglycinuria. Am J Med 54:265, 1973

Oyanagi K, Miura R, Yamanouchi T: Congenital lysinuria: a new inherited transport disorder of dibasic amino acids. J Pediatr 77: 259, 1970

Rosenberg LE, Durant JL, Elsas LJ: Familial iminoglycinuria. An inborn error of renal tubular transport. N Engl J Med 278: 1407, 1968

Scriver CR: Hartnup disease. A genetic modification of intestinal and renal transport of certain neutral alpha-amino acids. N Engl J Med 273: 530, 1965

——— Use of human genetic variation to study membrane transport of amino acids in kidney. Am J Dis Child 117:4, 1969

Tancredi F, Guazzi G, Auricchio S: Renal iminoglycinuria without intestinal malabsorption of glycine and imino acids. J Pediatr 76:386, 1970

DISORDERS OF PHOSPHATE TRANSPORT

Albright F, Burnett CH, Parson W, Reifenstein EC Jr, Roos A: Osteomalacia and late rickets: the various etiologies met in the United States with emphasis on that resulting from a special form of renal acidosis; the therapeutic indications for each etiological sub-group and the relationship between osteomalacia and milkman's syndrome. Medicine 25:399, 1946

Bell NH, Avery S, Sinha T, et al: Effects of dibutyryl cyclic adenosine 3′,5′-monophosphate and parathyroid extract in calcium and phosphorus metabolism in hypoparathyroidism and pseudohypoparathyroidism. J Clin Invest 51:816, 1972

Fanconi A, Fischer JA, Prader A: Serum parathyroid hormone concentrations in hypophosphataemic vitamin D resistant rickets. Helv Paediatr Acta 29:187, 1974

Glorieux F, Scriver CR: Loss of parathyroid hormone-sensitive component of phosphate transport in X-linked hypophosphatemia. Science 175:997, 1972

Rodriguez HJ, Villarreal H Jr, Klahr S, Slatopolsky E: Pseudohypoparathyroidism type II. Restoration of normal renal responsiveness to parathyroid hormone by calcium administration. J Clin Endocrinol Metab 39:693, 1974

Scriver CR: Rickets and the pathogenesis of impaired tubular transport of phosphate and other solutes. Am J Med 57:43, 1974

Thalassinos NC, Leese B, Latham SC, Joplin GF: Urinary excretion of phosphate in normal children. Arch Dis Child 45:269, 1970

FANCONI SYNDROME

Abbassi V, Lowe CU, Calcagno PL: Oculo-cerebro-renal syndrome. A review. Am J Dis Child 115:145, 1968

Brubacker RF, Wong VG, Schulman JD, Seegmiller JE, Kuwabara T: Benign cystinosis. Am J Med 49:546, 1970

Burgess JL, Birchall R: Nephrotoxicity of amphotericin B, with emphasis on changes in tubular function. Am J Med 53:77, 1972

Burke EC, Holley KE, Stickler GB: Familial nephrotic syndrome with nephrocalcinosis and tubular dysfunction. J Pediatr 82:202, 1973

Elsas LJ, Hayslett JP, Spargo BH, Durant JL, Rosenberg LE: Wilson's disease with reversible tubular dysfunction. Ann Intern Med 75:427, 1971

Fanconi G: Der Frühinfantile nephrotisch-glykosurische Zwergwuchs mit hypophosphatamischer Rachitis. Z Kinderheilkd 147:299, 1936

Goldman H, Scriver CR, Aaron K, Delvin E, Canlas Z: Adolescent cystinosis: comparisons with infantile and adult forms. Pediatrics 47:979, 1971

—— Scriver CR, Aaron K, Pinsky L: Use of dithiothreitol to correct cystine storage in cultured cystinotic fibroblasts. Lancet 1:811, 1970

Holmes LB, McGowan BL, Efron ML: Lowe's syndrome: a search for the carrier state. Pediatrics 44:358, 1969

Houston IB, Boichis H, Edelmann CM Jr: Fanconi syndrome with renal sodium wasting and metabolic alkalosis. Am J Med 44:638, 1968

Hunt D, Stearns G, McKinley JB, et al: Long-term study of family with Fanconi syndrome without cystinosis (DeToni-Debré-Fanconi syndrome). Am J Med 40:492, 1966

Kramer HJ, Gonick HC: Effect of maleic acid on sodium-linked tubular transport in experimental Fanconi syndrome. Nephron 10:306, 1973

Lowe CU, Terrey M, MacLachlan EA: Organic-aciduria, decreased renal ammonia production, hydrophthalmos, and mental retardation. Am J Dis Child 83:164, 1952

Luder J, Sheldon W: A familial tubular absorption defect of glucose and amino acids. Arch Dis Child 30:160, 1955

Morris RC Jr: An experimental renal acidification defect in patients with hereditary fructose intolerance. I. Its resemblance to renal tubular acidosis. J Clin Invest 47:1389, 1968

Pallisgaard G, Goldschmidt E: The oculo-cerebro renal syndrome of Lowe in four generations of one family. Acta Paediatr Scand 60:146, 1971

Rodriguez-Soriano J, Houston IB, Boichis H, Edelmann CM Jr: Calcium and phosphorus metabolism in the Fanconi syndrome. J Clin Endocrinol 28:1555, 1968

Schneider JA, Wong V, Bradley K, Seegmiller JE: Biochemical comparisons of the adult and childhood forms of cystinosis. N Engl J Med 279:1253, 1968

Schulman JD, Wong VG, Kuwabara T, Bradley KH, Seegmiller JE: Intracellular cystine content of leukocyte populations in cystinosis. Arch Intern Med 125:660, 1970

Uzman LL, Denny-Brown D: Amino-aciduria in hepatolenticular degeneration (Wilson's disease). Am J Med Sci 215:599, 1948

RENAL TUBULAR ACIDOSIS

Albright F, Burnett CH, Parsons W, Reifenstein EC Jr, Roos A: Osteomalacia and rickets: the various etiologies met in United States with emphasis on that resulting from a special form of renal acidosis; the therapeutic implications for each etiological sub-group and the relationship between osteomalacia and milkman's syndrome. Medicine 25:399, 1946

Buckalew VM Jr, Purvis ML, Shulman MG, Herndon CN, Rudman D: Hereditary renal tubular acidosis. Medicine 53:229, 1974

Chanarin I, Loewi G, Tavill AS, Swain CP, Tidmarsh E: Defect of renal tubular acidification with antibody to loop of Henle. Lancet 2:317, 1974

Donckerwolcke RA, Van Stekelenburg GJ, Tiddens HA: A case of bicar-bonate-losing renal tubular acidosis with defective carboanhydrase activity. Arch Dis Child 45:769, 1970

—— Van Stekelenburg GJ, Tiddens HA: Therapy of bicarbonate-losing renal tubular acidosis. Arch Dis Child 45:774, 1970

Györy AZ, Edwards KDG: Renal tubular acidosis. A family with an autosomal dominant genetic defect in renal hydrogen ion transport, with proximal tubular and collecting duct dysfunction and increased metabolism of citrate and ammonia. Am J Med 45:43, 1968

Huth EJ, Webster CD, Elkinton JR: The renal excretion of hydrogen ion in renal tubular acidosis. III. An attempt to detect latent cases in a family; comments on nosology, genetics, and etiology of the primary disease. Am J Med 29:586, 1960

Latner AL, Bunard ED: Idiopathic hyperchloremic renal acidosis of infants: observations on the site and nature of the lesion. Q J Med 19:285, 1950

Lightwood R, Butler N: Decline in primary infantile renal acidosis: aetiological implications. Br Med J 1:855, 1963

McSherry E, Sebastian M, Morris RC Jr: Renal tubular acidosis in infants: the several kinds, including bicarbonate-wasting, classic renal tubular acidosis. J Clin Invest 51:499, 1972

Morris RC Jr: Renal tubular acidosis. Mechanisms, classification and implications. N Engl J Med 281:1405, 1969

—— Fudenberg HH: Impaired renal acidification in patients with hypergammaglobulinemia. Medicine 46:57, 1967

—— Sebastian A, McSherry E: Renal acidosis. Kidney Int 1:332, 1972

Nash MA, Torrado A, Greifer I, Spitzer A, Edelmann CM Jr: Renal tubular acidosis in infants and children. Clinical course, response to treatment and prognosis. J Pediatr 80:738, 1972

Rodriguez-Soriano J: The renal regulation of acid-base balance and the disturbances noted in renal tubular acidosis. Pediatr Clin North Am 18:529, 1971

—— Boichis H, Stark H, Edelman CM Jr: Proximal renal tubular acidosis: a defect in bicarbonate reabsorption with normal urinary acidification. Pediatr Res 1:81, 1967

—— Edelmann CM Jr: Renal tubular acidosis. Ann Rev Med 20:363, 1969

—— Vallo A, Garcia-Fuentes M: Distal renal tubular acidosis in infancy: a bicarbonate wasting state. J Pediatr (in press)

—— Vallo A, Chouza M, Castillo G: Proximal renal tubular acidosis in tetralogy of Fallot. Acta Paediat Scand 64:671, 1975

Schoeneman M, Lifshitz F, Diaz-Benssusen S: The transport of bicarbonate by the small intestine of a patient with proximal renal tubular acidosis. Pediatr Res 8:735, 1974

Shapira E, Ben-Yoseph Y, Eyal FG, Russell A: Enzymatically inactive red-cell carbonic anhydrase B in a family with renal tubular acidosis. J Clin Invest 53:59, 1974

Vladutin AO: Renal tubular acidosis: an autoimmune disease? Lancet 1:265, 1973

Wrong O, Davies HE: The excretion of acid in renal disease. Q J Med 28:259, 1959

IDIOPATHIC HYPERCALCIURIA

Finn WF, Cerilli GJ, Ferris TF: Transplantation of a kidney from a patient with idiopathic hypercalciuria. N Engl J Med 283:1450, 1971

Rose GA, Harrison AR: The incidence, investigation and treatment of idiopathic hypercalciuria. Br J Urol 46:261, 1974

Royer P, Balsan S: Effet d'un regime pauvre en chlorure de sodium dans le "syndrome d'hypercalciurie idiopathique avec nanisme et troubles rénaux" de l'enfant. Schweiz Med Wochenschr 96:412, 1966

SODIUM-LOSING DISORDERS

Postel-Vinay MC: Sodium balance, aldosterone excretion and secretion rates, study of colon receptors to aldosterone in a 9-year-old boy known as a case of pseudohypoadrenocorticism. Acta Paediatr Scand 61:261, 1971

Proesmans, W, Geussens H, Corbeel L, Eckels R: Pseudohypoaldosteronism. Am J Dis Child 126:510, 1973

Rösler A, Theodor R, Gazit E, Boichis H, Rabinowitz D: Salt wastage, raised plasma renin activity, and normal or high plasma-aldosterone: a form of pseudohypoaldosteronism. Lancet 1:959, 1973

POTASSIUM-LOSING DISORDERS

Bartter FC, Pronove P, Gill JR Jr, MacCardle RC: Hyperplasia of the juxtaglomerular complex, with hyperaldosteronism and hypokalemic alkalosis. Am J Med 33:811, 1962

Cannon PJ, Leeming JM, Sommers SC, Winters RW, Laragh JH: Juxtaglomerular cell hyperplasia and secondary hyperaldosteronism (Bartter's syndrome); a re-evaluation of the pathophysiology. Medicine 47:107, 1968

Chaimovitz C, Levi J, Better OS, Oslander L, Benderli A: Studies on the site of renal salt loss in a patient with Bartter's syndrome. Pediatr Res 7:89, 1973

Fanconi A, Schachenmann G, Nüssli R, Prader A: Chronic hypokalemia with growth retardation, normotensive hyperrenin-hyperaldosteronism (Bartter's syndrome), and hypercalciuria. Helv Paediatr Acta 26: 144, 1971

Gardner JD, Lapey A, Simopoulos AP, Bravo EL: Abnormal membrane sodium transport in Liddle's syndrome. J Clin Invest 50: 2253, 1971

——— Simopoulos AP, Shibolet S: Altered membrane sodium transport in Bartter's syndrome. J Clin Invest 51:1565, 1972

Godard C, Valloton MB, Broyer M, Royer P: A study of the inhibition of the renin-angiotensin system in renal potassium wasting syndromes, including Bartter's syndrome. Helv Paediatr Acta 27:495, 1972

Liddle GW, Bledsoe T, Coppage WS Jr: A familial renal disorder simulating primary aldosterone secretion. In Baulieu EE, Robel P (ed): Aldosterone. Oxford, Blackwell, 1963, p 353

Modlinger RS, Nicolis GL, Krakoff LR, Gabrilove JL: Some observations on the pathogenesis of Bartter's syndrome. N Engl J Med 289: 1022, 1973

Simopoulos AP, Bartter FC: Growth characteristics and factors influencing growth in Bartter's syndrome. J Pediatr 81:56, 1972

White MG: Bartter's syndrome. Arch Intern Med 129:41, 1972

POTASSIUM-RETAINING DISORDERS

Spitzer A, Edelmann CM Jr, Goldberg LD, Henneman PH: Short stature, hyperkalemia and acidosis: a defect in renal transport of potassium. Kidney Int 3:251, 1973

Weinstein SF, Allan DME, Mendoza SA: Hyperkalemia, acidosis, and short stature associated with a defect in renal potassium excretion. J Pediatr 85:355, 1974

MAGNESIUM-LOSING DISORDERS

Booth BE, Johanson A: Hypomagnesemia due to renal tubular defect in reabsorption of magnesium. J Pediatr 85:350, 1974

NEPHROGENIC DIABETES INSIPIDUS

Abelson H: Nephrogenic diabetes insipidus. A study of the fine structure of the kidney in a seven-month-old male. Pediatr Res 2:271, 1968

Bell NH, Clark CM Jr, Avery S, et al: Demonstration of a defect in the formation of adenosine 3', 5'-monophosphate in vasopressin-resistant diabetes insipidus. Pediatr Res 8:223, 1974

Crawford JD, Kennedy GC: Chlorothiazide in diabetes insipidus. Nature 183:891, 1959

Dousa TP, Valtin H: Cellular action of antidiuretic hormone in mice with inherited vasopressin-resistant urinary concentrating defects. J Clin Invest 54:753, 1974

DeSousa RC: Diabète insipide. Quelques aspects récents. Schweiz Med Wochenschr 104:1045, 1974

Earley LE, Orloff J: The mechanism of antidiuresis with the administration of hydrochlorothiazide to patients with vasopressin-resistant diabetes insipidus. J Clin Invest 41:1988, 1962

CIRCULATORY DISTURBANCES

CHESTER M. EDELMANN, JR.

RENAL CORTICAL NECROSIS

In childhood renal cortical necrosis is seen most frequently in association with dehydration, infection, and shock. The clinical picture is that of acute renal failure. Initially patients are usually described as feeling well and there are no physical findings. Blood pressure usually remains normal. Total anuria is not uncommon, as distinguished from acute tubular necrosis. The urine is grossly abnormal, with protein, red blood cells, white blood cells, and less commonly casts. The course and treatment are those of the uremic syndrome. Most reported cases have ended fatally, although it is very likely that the survival rate is appreciable among less severely affected patients.

Pathologic examination shows patchy or diffuse ischemic necrosis of the cortex, occasionally accompanied by medullary necrosis. The necrosis is often hemorrhagic and is usually bland. Vascular occlusion of arterioles and glomeruli by fibrinous masses is sometimes seen, but thrombi cannot be demonstrated in all cases.

The pathogenesis of renal cortical necrosis, with its severe cortical destruction and almost total sparing of the medulla, is unknown. The initiating factor, toxic or other, may cause vasospasm of the small renal vessels, but there is considerable evidence that intravascular coagulation, as part of a spontaneous Shwartzman reaction, is responsible.

RENAL ARTERY OCCLUSION

Renal artery occlusion has been reported rarely in infants and children. The usual etiology is either infection or trauma, and one or both renal arteries may be involved. Other causes include neurofibromatosis, compression by neoplasm, the vasculitis of lupus erythematosus and polyarteritis nodosa, aneurysm, and embolic occlusions. Clinical manifestations vary with the etiology and specific circumstances. Pain, fever, nausea, and vomiting are frequently seen. The kidney is often palpably enlarged. Hypertension may or may not be present. Woodard and associates have called attention to the occurrence in infants of hypertension and congestive heart failure, in the absence of renal enlargement. The urine usually contains red blood cells and protein, but may be normal. Gross hematuria is rare. Function of the involved kidney usually is severely impaired. London and associates have reported elevations in serum and urinary lactic dehydrogenase in adults with renal artery occlusion, and this may be a worthwhile examination in infants and children. Definitive diagnosis, of course, is established by renal arteriography.

In the absence of early diagnosis, cortical necrosis or

renal infarction with irreversible damage may ensue. Treatment is surgical: thrombectomy, arterial reconstruction, or nephrectomy.

RENAL VENOUS OBSTRUCTION

Renal venous obstruction with hemorrhagic infarction of the kidney, which is almost always due to venous thrombosis, was first described by Rayer in 1837. In many instances the diagnosis has been made postmortem, but increasing awareness of the condition permits clinical diagnosis in many instances.

Thrombosis of the renal vein leading to hemorrhagic infarction is seen most frequently in newborn infants, in association with diarrhea, vomiting, and dehydration. Suggested explanations for the higher incidence in infants have included a greater tendency toward dehydration, the low blood pressure characteristic of the newborn infant, a low rate of renal blood flow, the frequency of septicemia, birth trauma, and anomalous venous circulation. However, the condition may occur under a variety of situations in every age group; when there is no apparent predisposing cause it has been referred to as primary renal vein thrombosis. A number of reports suggest an increased incidence for infants of toxemic and diabetic or prediabetic mothers. In adult subjects renal vein thrombosis occurs as a complication of renal amyloidosis and diabetes mellitus, an association not seen in children.

In somewhat less than one-half of the cases in infants and young children the thrombosis is demonstrated to be bilateral, although involvement of both kidneys may be a much more frequent occurrence. In unilateral cases in girls (although apparently not in boys) it occurs more frequently on the left than on the right side. Combined thrombosis of renal veins and inferior vena cava has been reported, but is far less frequent than renal vein thrombosis alone.

The clinical diagnosis of renal vein thrombosis depends on the sudden appearance of a mass in the flank, accompanied by gross hematuria. However, hematuria and albuminuria are not essential to the diagnosis, since the urinary findings may be quite trivial and even absent. Fever, leukocytosis, vomiting, diarrhea, and dehydration may precede or follow the appearance of the mass, or they may be absent. Significant anemia is found in one-third of young infants and two-thirds of older children. Thrombocytopenia is found in 90 percent of cases and may be associated with evidence of intravascular coagulation and a hemolytic-uremic syndrome. Hypertension commonly is recorded in older subjects. In the cases reported in infants blood pressure has usually not been recorded, although there are instances of hypertension. Isolated proteinuria and the combination of massive edema and the nephrotic syndrome, which are common forms of presentation in adults, appear to be the result of gradual thrombosis of the renal veins. These forms of presentation are extremely rare in the pediatric age-group. The major laboratory aids to diagnosis are an excretory urogram and radioisotopic scan, which reveal nonfunctioning of the kidney, and an in-ferior vena cavagram. Renal arteriography, with particular attention to the venous phase, has been advocated.

Differential diagnosis must consider Wilms' tumor, hydronephrosis, multicystic kidney, and retroperitoneal hemorrhage.

Renal thrombosis is a serious condition; if it is not promptly treated the mortality may be as high as 95 percent. Nephrectomy was once considered to be the best form of treatment in unilateral cases, although it is now well established that recovery may take place (even full return of renal function) with intensive medical therapy alone. Extension of the thrombus to involve the contralateral kidney is often given as a reason for nephrectomy, but this sequence is not well documented. Medical therapy is the only course in instances of bilateral involvement, and a number of patients in this category have recovered. If renal vein thrombosis is diagnosed early in its development in older children and adults, thrombectomy may be of value, although the thrombus frequently extends far intrarenally. Indeed, many authors feel that in infants the thrombus begins in the arcuate and interlobular vessels and then extends to involve both smaller and larger veins. Anticoagulant therapy to prevent dissemination of the clot and fibrinolytic therapy to promote dissolution may be of value, but they have not been adequately evaluated.

RENAL ARTERIOVENOUS FISTULA

This rare abnormality occurs as a congenital defect and also secondary to trauma. In a review in 1967 Malloy and associates found 24 cases of congenital fistula in the literature and added three more. There have now been several instances of fistula secondary to the trauma of needle biopsy. The clinical picture includes hypertension, congestive heart failure, local thrill and bruit, and hematuria. The diagnosis is established by angiography, and the treatment is surgical, nephrectomy being required in most instances.

References

RENAL CORTICAL NECROSIS

Bernstein J, Meyer R: Congenital abnormalities of the urinary system. II. Renal cortical and medullary necrosis. J Pediatr 59:657, 1961

Mauer SM, Nogrady MB: Renal papillary and cortical necrosis in a newborn infant: report of a survivor with roentgenologic documentation. J Pediatr 74:750, 1969

Rieselbach RE, Klahr S, Bricker NS: Diffuse bilateral cortical necrosis. A longitudinal study of the functional residual nephrons. Am J Med 42:457, 1967

RENAL ARTERY OCCLUSION, RENAL VENOUS OBSTRUCTION, AND RENAL ARTERIOVENOUS FISTULA

Arneil GC, MacDonald AM, Murphy AV, Sweet EM: Renal venous thrombosis. Clin Nephrol 1:119, 1973

Belman AB, Susmano DF, Burden JJ, Kaplan GW: Nonoperative treatment of unilateral renal vein thrombosis in the newborn. JAMA 211: 1165, 1970

Lowry MF, Mann JR, Abrams LD, Chance GW: Thrombectomy for renal venous thrombosis in infant of diabetic mother. Br Med J 3:687, 1970

McFarland JB: Renal venous thrombosis in children. Q J Med 34:269, 1965

Smith GH, Remmers AR, Dickey BM, Sarles HE: Intrarenal arteriovenous fistula and systemic hypertension following percutaneous renal biopsy. Report of a case. Nephron 5:24, 1968

Stark H: Renal vein thrombosis in infancy. Recovery without nephrectomy. Am J Dis Child 108:430, 1964

Verhagen AD, Hamilton JP, Genel M: Renal vein thrombosis in infants. Arch Dis Child 40:214, 1965

Woodard JR, Patterson JH, Brinsfield D: Renal artery thrombosis in newborn infants. Am J Dis Child 114:191, 1967

UROLITHIASIS

Martin A. Nash

The precipitation and growth of crystalline material in the genitourinary tract has fascinated and puzzled medical scientists since antiquity. While they are fairly common in adults, urinary stones in the pediatric population are relatively rare, at least in the United States. In some areas of the world urinary lithiasis in children is endemic and presents a major health problem. For example, a recent survey from two hospitals in New Delhi disclosed stones in 600 children occurring over a 2-year period. Sixty percent were bladder calculi. The etiology of these is elusive, but their occurrence appears to be more frequent in the lower socioeconomic classes, suggesting an environmental or dietary factor related to poverty. In the United States bladder stones are exceedingly rare in the absence of a neurogenic bladder or foreign body.

Urinary stone disease occurs more frequently in males, although this sex preponderance is not borne out in all surveys. From wide experience Williams suggests that the majority occur in children under 4 years of age, with a peak in the second and third years.

Calculi are composed of a crystalline fraction embedded in an organic matrix that comprises 2.5 to 10 percent of the stone by weight and consists of various proteins. The crystalline fraction is composed of one or more of the following: calcium phosphate, calcium oxalate, or magnesium ammonium phosphate; less commonly uric acid and cystine; and rarely xanthine. The analysis of calculi traditionally has been performed by chemical means that serve to identify chemical radicals but not crystalline structure. The recent application to stone analysis of the tools of minerology and crystallography has demonstrated the large number and great complexity of crystals that precipitate as calcium salts in human stone disease.

PATHOGENESIS AND PROPHYLAXIS. Theories of the pathogenesis of stone formation have revolved around the two components: matrix and crystal. At the present time it appears that while the protein matrix acting as an adhesive is important in the growth of stones, disturbances in these urinary proteins are not inciting events in their formation.

Consideration of the cause of precipitation of crystals in urine can be approached usefully through an examination of the behavior of urine as an aqueous solvent. It is clear that far greater amounts of calcium, phosphate, oxalate, uric acid, and cystine can be held in solution in urine than in distilled water. This superiority of urine to water as a solvent can be explained to a great extent by an examination of the factors that determine the capacity of an aqueous solvent.

QUANTITY OF SOLVENT. Obviously the greater the quantity of solvent for a fixed amount of solute the more dilute the solution and the lesser the probability of precipitation. The quantity of solvent, ie, the rate of urine flow, has been implicated in some cases of endemic stone formation in dry climates where water drinking is minimal and in areas where chronic gastroenteritis with subsequent dehydration and oliguria is prevalent. The virtues of increasing fluid intake in stone-formers is apparent.

CONCENTRATION OF IONS. For a fixed quantity of solvent the greater the amount of a specific solute the greater the likelihood that the solubility constant will be exceeded and precipitation will occur. However, it is not the ionic concentration per se that is important but the ionic activity, since the chance of two molecules interacting is decreased by the presence of other particles. Many substances in urine (Na^+, Cl^-, SO_4^{--}, Mg^{++}, urea) contribute to the total ionic strength and thus enhance solubility. An increased quantity of solute in the urine is of prime importance in many diseases. For example in hyperparathyroidism, vitamin D intoxication, distal renal tubular acidosis, immobilization, thyrotoxicosis, and sarcoidosis the rate of calcium excretion may be increased above normal. The quantity of uric acid for excretion is augmented in gout, the Lesch-Nyhan syndrome, and the leukemias, especially while under treatment with cytotoxic drugs. Oxalate excretion is increased in hyperoxaluria of both types. There is a marked elevation of cystine excretion in cystinuria. There are a few reports of xanthine stones associated with the metabolic disorder xanthinuria. Theoretically there may be an increase in the occurrence of xanthine stones with the wide use of the xanthine oxidase inhibitor allopurinol, although stones have been seen only rarely as a complication of therapy. Although 50 percent of children and adults with urinary stones do not have an associated identifiable disease, approximately one-half of these patients are hypercalciuric, either constantly or intermittently.

Treatment directed toward decreasing the amount of solute excreted includes limiting the intake of foods containing high amounts of calcium, purine (uric acid), or sulfoproteins (cystine). However, since 60 percent or more of oxalic acid is produced endogenously, decreasing oxalate intake is of little benefit. Other approaches include decreasing the formation of uric acid by inhibiting the enzyme xanthine oxidase with the drug allopurinol and converting cystine into a more soluble disulfide by the administration of penicillamine. Recent evidence suggests that some patients with a familial occurrence of calcium stones demonstrate an augmented excretion of calcium after a glucose load. This work must be confirmed, however, before carbohydrate limitation can be recommended as therapy. It should be noted that decreasing the calcium intake in patients without hypercalciuria may increase oxalate excretion and actually enhance the possibility of stone formation. Such dietary manipulations must be monitored closely to avoid this consequence. Thiazides may be used to increase renal calcium reabsorption and thereby decrease its excretion.

pH. Solubility varies markedly with changes in pH. Calcium phosphate and magnesium ammonium phosphate are more soluble at a pH less than 6 and uric acid at a pH greater than 6. Cystine demonstrates little increase in solubility up to pH 7, but further increases in pH greatly augment its solubility.

The importance of pH as a pathogenetic factor is suggested in several clinical situations. The majority of uric acid stone-formers show neither hyperuricemia nor increased uric acid excretion, but as a group these patients have a lower mean urine pH than controls and thus a favorable environment for uric acid precipitation. Therapy is directed at alkalinization of the urine by administration of sodium bicarbonate or citrate. The vast majority of patients with magnesium ammonium phosphate stones have urinary tract infection with a urea-splitting organism (such as *Proteus*), which releases ammonia and renders the urine alkaline, thus favoring magnesium ammonium phosphate precipitation. Treatment is directed toward eradication of infection and acidification of the urine by administration of ammonium chloride, ascorbic acid, or methionine. The frequent occurrence of urolithiasis in distal renal tubular acidosis may be related partially to persistent urine alkalinity. Although there is no way to acidify the urine, because of the nature of the intrinsic defect treatment of systemic acidosis decreases the rate of excretion of calcium. In urine, as opposed to water, the solubility of oxalate is increased with alkalinization, which is most likely related to a consequent absolute decrease in calcium excretion and an increase in both the rate of excretion and the degree of ionization of citrate. Urinary alkalinization in this instance has not been evaluated as a therapeutic measure.

SUBSTANCES WITH A PARTICULAR SOLUBILIZING ACTION. Magnesium ions have been shown to exert a greater influence on solubility than can be explained by their contribution to the total ionic strength. This action is presumably due to the formation of complex ions that further reduce the activities of precipitable ions. Citrate has been found to have a similar virtue to an even greater degree, probably due to the same mechanism. Pyrophosphate can be shown to increase the solubility of calcium oxalate and calcium phosphate; two small peptides have been identified that increase calcium phosphate solubility, presumably by inhibiting the aggregation of tiny clusters of ions.

Some patients with idiopathic calcium phosphate stones have been shown to have a decreased ratio of urinary Mg^{++} to Ca^{++}. Rats on Mg^{++}-deficient diets show an increased incidence of calcium deposition in the proximal tubules. There are several reports of patients with recurrent calcium lithiasis who have remained stone-free on oral magnesium therapy. This treatment may be useful for those patients with a decreased ratio of urinary Mg^{++} to Ca^{++}, but controlled studies are needed before a recommendation can be made. The concentration of citrate in urine is decreased in patients with distal renal tubular acidosis, but there is no practical way to increase it since oral citrate is quickly metabolized to bicarbonate. Oral phosphate will increase urinary pyrophosphate, but favorable results from this therapy are not universal, and recent evidence suggests that in some patients it may be deleterious.

TIME. Time has an adverse effect on solubility. For example, precipitates often are seen in urine specimens that have been allowed to stagnate in their collection bottles. The factor of time is important when urinary stasis is present, such as in ureteropelvic obstruction, megaureter, and neurogenic bladder. Treatment consists of relief of obstruction and establishment of adequate drainage.

PRESENCE OF A NIDUS. A precipitate may be induced in a saturated solution by addition of a crystal of the solute or, under some circumstances, by addition of a nonspecific particle. An important factor in stone formation is the presence of a nidus on which crystallization may take place, such as an indwelling catheter, a postoperative or self-introduced foreign body, or debris from infection. Two-thirds of patients with stones are infected either primarily or secondarily, *Proteus* and *Escherichia coli* being the predominant organisms. Treatment of a nidus obviously involves removal with either surgery or antibiotics.

The relative frequency with which the factors discussed above are important etiologically in children with stones is uncertain. Approximately 30 percent of stones are associated with significant anomalies of the genitourinary tract, and 10 percent are related to metabolic disorders, leaving 50 to 60 percent idiopathic. This percentage will decrease as more knowledge is gained concerning the factors affecting urine as a solvent.

CLINICAL PICTURE. Two-thirds of children with stones are discovered incidentally or during a work-up for urinary tract infection. Presenting symptoms are hematuria, fever, flank pain, recurrent urinary tract infection, or persistent pyuria. It should be noted that the symptoms attributed to trigonitis (frequency, dysuria, terminal hematuria) are the same symptoms presented by patients with bladder calculi, in both cases symptoms being produced by irritation of the trigonal area.

DIAGNOSIS. The diagnosis of urinary tract stones should be considered in any child with the above symptomatology or urinary findings. The approach to etiology in a child with a stone will more profitably be based on a consideration of abnormalities in the nature of urine as a solvent rather than on the perfunctory elimination of named diseases. These factors, as discussed above, are summarized in Table 12, along with some of the underlying diseases. The evaluation should include a search for a family history of stones or metabolic diseases, urine culture, radiographic examination of the urinary tract (uric acid and xanthine stones are the only radiolucent ones), determination of the capacity for urinary acidification (administering ammonium chloride if necessary), and multiple analyses of

24-hour rates of excretion of calcium (normal ≤ 2 to 4 mg/kg on a usual diet, 300 mg in adults), oxalate (50 mg/24 hours/1.73 m^2), and cystine* (normal < 70 mg/g creatinine). Analysis of urine for citrate and magnesium is interesting but not essential for treatment. The serum should be analyzed for urea nitrogen and creatinine as indices of renal function, as well as for calcium, phosphorus, alkaline phosphatase, uric acid, and electrolytes (with special attention to bicarbonate as an indication of acidosis). A urea or creatinine clearance is helpful as an estimate of renal damage and as a basis for later evaluation of renal function. Of primary importance is a chemical analysis of stone composition. It should be noted that a small uric acid stone may lead to obstruction, infection, and subsequent stone growth by deposition of magnesium ammonium phosphate. In fact, patients who form calcium stones have a higher incidence of hyperuricemia and hyperuricuria than do controls, thus suggesting that the primary abnormality may be the formation of a uric acid nucleus followed by calcium deposition. Failure to recognize the composition of this nucleus would lead to misdirected and deleterious pH therapy.

TREATMENT. Urinary stones too large to pass spontaneously must be removed surgically. Prophylaxis to prevent recurrence involves appropriate alteration of urine composition by the methods discussed above. Stones secondary to a metabolic disorder can be expected to recur unless the underlying abnormality is corrected. In contrast to the situation in adults, recurrence of stones of the idiopathic variety in children appears to be infrequent. Severe and irreversible renal damage unfortunately results occasionally in silent urinary stone disease; however, it should be preventable by early detection and treatment.

TABLE 12. Factors Contributing to Stone Formation

Composition of Stone	Contributory Factors
Calcium phosphate	Hypercalciuria
	Hyperparathyroidism
	Vitamin D intoxication
	Distal RTA
	Immobilization
	Thyrotoxicosis
	Sarcoidosis
	Idiopathic
	High-calcium diet (in susceptible individuals?)
	Alkaline urinary pH
	Decreased urinary citrate
	Decreased urinary pyrophosphate (?)
	Decreased urinary Mg^{++}/Ca^{++} ratio (?)
	Foreign body
	Urinary stasis
Calcium oxalate	All of above except pH
	Hyperoxaluria
	Types I & II hyperoxaluria
	Ethylene glycol poisoning
	Pyridoxin deficiency
	Methoxyflurane anesthesia
	Ileal disease
	Massive doses ascorbic acid
	Hyperglycinuria
Magnesium ammonium phosphate	Infection with urea-splitting organism
	Alklaine urine
	Foreign body
	Urinary stasis
Uric acid	Hyperuricosuria
	Gout
	Lesch-Nyhan syndrome
	Hematologic malignancies
	High-purine diet
	Acid urine
Xanthine	Xanthinuria
	Acid urine
	Allopurinol therapy
Cystine	Cystinuria
	Acid urine

References

Daeschner CW, Singleton EB, Curtus JC: Urinary tract calculi and nephrocalcinosis in infants and children. J Pediatr 57:721, 1960

Gershoff SN: The formation of urinary stones. Metabolism 13:875, 1964

Halzbach RT, Pak CYC: Metastable supersaturation: physicochemical studies provide new insights into formation of renal and kidney tract stones. Am J Med 56:141, 1974

Hodgkinson A, Nordin BEC (eds): Renal Stone Research Symposium. London, J&A Churchill, 1969

Myers NAA: Urolithiasis in childhood. Arch Dis Child 32:48, 1957

Prien EL, Prien EL Jr: Composition and structure of urinary stone. Am J Med 45:654, 1968

Williams DI, Eckstein HB: Urinary lithiasis. In Williams DI (ed): Pediatric Urology. London, Butterworth, 1968, p 323

Williams HE: Nephrolithiasis. N Engl J Med 290:33, 1974

---

* *The nitroprusside test on a random urine specimen will give an adequate indication of markedly increased cystine concentration. To 5 ml of urine are added a few drops of ammonium hydroxide and 2 ml of fresh 5 percent NaCN. After 10 minutes for equilibration a few drops of 5 percent sodium nitroprusside are added. A deep purple color indicates a positive reaction. False-positives occur from ketonuria.*

INFECTIONS OF THE URINARY AND GENITAL TRACTS

MARK ABRAMOWICZ

CYSTITIS AND PYELONEPHRITIS. The urinary tract is one of the most common sites of infection. Although there is considerable variability in clinical presentation, site of infection, and extent of involvement, the feature common to all urinary tract infections is the presence in the urine of significant numbers of bacteria. Bacteriuria per se may not always indicate active infection of the urinary tract, but it defines the population at risk and therefore for practical purposes should be considered synonymous with urinary tract infection. Clinically it is usually not possible to localize infection specifically to the bladder or to the kidney. Therefore the term urinary tract infection (UTI) will be used to refer to either or both conditions.

INCIDENCE AND PREVALENCE. Less than 1 percent of apparently healthy newborns have UTI. Underlying congenital malformations are rare in these infants. Although sex distribution varies, there appears to be a slight preponderance of males. As many as 1 or 2 percent of females and 0.5 percent of males beyond the neonatal period but below 2 years of age have UTI. In contrast to newborns, as many as 80 percent of these patients have associated congenital malformations or malfunctions of the urinary tract.

In a survey of school-age children by Kunin and associates bacteriuria was found in 1.2 percent of girls and 0.03 percent of boys. Most of these children were asymptomatic, but 40 percent had positive radiographic findings, most commonly caliectasis. This abnormality in 13 percent of those with asymptomatic bacteriuria suggests that this condition sometimes is associated with pyelonephritis. In girls the cumulative rate of bacteriuria over the first 7 years of school was 2.9 percent, with an annual mean conversion rate of 0.3 percent. If further study finds no change in the conversion rate in adolescence, it can be projected that 5 percent of girls will have bacteriuria by the time of graduation from high school.

ETIOLOGY. The bacteria responsible for most UTI are enteric organisms, including *E. coli, Aerobacter aerogenes, Proteus, Pseudomonas aeruginosa,* and enterococci; less than 10 percent of infections are caused by staphylococci. *E. coli* accounts for approximately one-half to three-fourths of initial infections and a lower proportion of recurrent infections. Certain *E. coli* serotypes, namely, 04, 06, 02, 01, and 75, commonly cause UTI; however, this relationship probably reflects their ubiquity rather than a particular pyelopathogenicity. Enteropathogenic *E. coli* serotypes are rare in urinary tract infection.

Pure cultures are the rule; it is even uncommon to find more than one serotype of *E. coli* infecting urine at one time, although several strains are usually present in feces. A mixed flora in urine is most often the result of contamination, but truly mixed infections may be seen in patients with chronic or complicated infections, especially after instrumentation. In the majority of patients the organism cultured from the urine can also be isolated from the stool.

Most recurrences of UTI are associated with a new serologic type of *E. coli* or another species altogether. This makes it unlikely that protoplasts of *E. coli* play an important role in recurrent infection, despite the fact that these L forms have been cultured from infected renal tissue.

Circulating antibodies often can be demonstrated in patients who have evidence of pyelonephritis. Usually no antibody response is seen when infection is limited to the lower urinary tract. Antibody-coated bacteria (detectable by immunofluorescence) can usually be observed in urine specimens from patients with pyelonephritis, but usually not in urine from patients with infection limited to the lower urinary tract.

The role of viruses in the pathogenesis of UTI has not been convincingly demonstrated. Type II adenovirus has been implicated as an etiologic agent in acute hemorrhagic cystitis in children.

PATHOGENESIS. Bacteria usually invade the urinary tract by an ascending route. Hematogenous spread is probably a rare event, since (1) most urinary tract infections are with gram-negative organisms, all of which are potent pyrogens, and (2) most cases of bacteriuria, symptomatic or not, do not follow an obvious bacteremia. Gram-positive infections with staphylococci and enterococci are more likely to be blood-borne. Lymphatic spread from the gastrointestinal tract or from the bladder upward has never been proved.

The normal bladder rids itself in some way of invading bacteria. Voiding and dilution probably play important roles in this, although there is always a small amount of urine left in the bladder, and bacteria multiply there very easily. In patients with obstruction or bladder dysfunction this bladder clearance mechanism fails. Vesicoureteral reflux may occur, and ureteral peristalsis may be disturbed.

Other factors besides obstruction that are associated with frequent and persistent UTI include stasis, abnormal renal vasculature, calculi, or the presence of islets of dysplastic tissue. All of these possess a potential for causing obstruction of some degree, but a purely mechanistic view of the pathogenesis of UTI is not adequate to explain all the observations. In experimental animals partial obstruction of a ureter does not necessarily produce infection localized to the obstructed side; complete obstruction does tend to localize infection, but bacteria injected into a completely obstructed kidney usually disappear.

The reported incidence of underlying uropathy in patients with bacteriuria varies widely, depending on the criteria for selection of patients, the choice of diagnostic tests, and their interpretation. However, some of the more reassuring reports with regard to absence of uropathy come from studies in which contamination was not convincingly ruled out.

Certain systemic disorders, as well as pregnancy, are associated with an increased incidence of UTI, although in most the cause is not apparent; these include cirrhosis of the liver, hypertension, hypokalemia, and perhaps diabetes mellitus.

Chronic pyelonephritis may follow either single or multiple acute infections. In the absence of urologic abnormality it is not known why the infection resolves rapidly in some patients, whereas in others it persists. The possible roles of immune mechanisms in the host and transformation of L forms of bacteria have aroused speculation from observations in experimental pyelonephritis, but there are few data relevant to human disease. The role of bacterial infection in the pathogenesis of chronic pyelonephritis has been questioned because of the frequent failure to elicit a history of infection or to demonstrate bacteriuria in such patients. Using immunofluorescence techniques Aoki and associates have been able to identify bacterial antigen in the kidneys of patients with so-called abacterial pyelonephritis, which suggests that renal infection did in fact play a role in the pathogenesis of their disease.

CLINICAL AND LABORATORY FEATURES. Infants with *acute pyelonephritis* usually present with nonspecific symptoms, including fever, anorexia, vomiting, diarrhea or constipation, jaundice, and anemia. In newborn infants acidosis and abnormal weight loss during the first days of life are prominent features. The classic description of acute pyelonephritis in older children includes rigors, chills, and high fever; suprapubic, abdominal, and flank pain; vomiting and malaise; and occasionally central nervous system signs such as meningism, stupor, delirium, or convulsions. However, this clinical picture is rarely seen, and in most instances the symptoms of pyelonephritis are less severe. Urinalysis usually reveals proteinuria, leukocyturia, microscopic hematuria, and almost invariably bacteriuria.

Chronic pyelonephritis combines the features of chronic infection with those of progressive renal insufficiency; in addition, symptoms of acute pyelonephritis may occur during exacerbations. In many instances chronic pyelonephritis is limited to one kidney or to one renal pole, and the symptomatology is that of acute and chronic infection without evidence of renal insufficiency. Leukocyturia may be continuous, intermittent, or absent. Significant bacteriuria is not always present. In cases with reduced renal function it can be inferred that the disease process is bilateral and diffuse, and renal biopsy may contribute to the diagnosis. An intravenous urogram (IVU) may reveal impaired function and general or local contraction and narrowing, the kidney appearing compressed medially against the vertebral column, with calyces, pelvis, and ureter lying in one straight vertical line. The calyces may appear either blunted and clubbed or narrowed and elongated. There is an irregular diminution of parenchyma. When the disease process is unilateral there usually is hypertrophy of the contralateral kidney.

Infections of the lower urinary tract cause few systemic signs other than fever; local symptoms include painful urination, burning, frequency, urgency, low abdominal or suprapubic pain, and retention that may be secondary to pain. Enuresis, hematuria, and foul-smelling urines may also be present.

Many cases of UTI evolve insidiously with almost total absence of symptoms. In retrospect one may uncover suggestive signs, such as unexplained bouts of fever, malaise, or low-grade abdominal pain.

PATHOPHYSIOLOGY. In acute pyelonephritis glomerular filtration rate usually remains normal. A decreased capacity to concentrate urine has been described that persists for 4 to 6 weeks after subsidence of clinical symptoms. Extremely severe metabolic acidosis has been observed in infants with acute pyelonephritis that suggests the possibility of a defect in urinary acidification. At any given level of glomerular filtration rate, however, concentrating capacity and ability to excrete hydrogen ion in pyelonephritis usually are lower than in other forms of chronic renal disease.

In chronic pyelonephritis, as the disease progresses, diminution in total renal function ensues, and the complete picture of chronic renal insufficiency may evolve.

PATHOLOGY. Except in young infants the kidney in acute infections is usually enlarged, with a smooth capsular surface that only rarely is marred by superficial abscesses. The pelvic mucosa may be involved, and wide yellow streaks may radiate from pelvis to capsule. Microscopically there is edema, congestion, polymorphonuclear infiltration of the interstitium, abscess formation, and distended tubules filled with exudate consisting of leukocytes, bacteria, and debris. Excessive tubular dilatation may result in necrosis. The brunt of the inflammation is borne by the medulla. However, glomeruli may be involved either in the exudative process or in periglomerular fibrosis.

At a later phase plasma cells and lymphocytes replace the polymorphonuclear leukocytes, and when healing occurs an interstitial scar is formed. In fatal cases the inflammation extends and produces a swollen kidney studded in its entirety with abscesses and disrupted tubules.

In chronic pyelonephritis the kidney is usually contracted and has an irregularly scarred surface and an adherent thickened capsule. The calyces and pelvis are fibrosed and distorted by wedge-shaped parenchymal scars. The thickness of the parenchyma is diminished, often unevenly. Glomeruli show proliferation, crescents, and hyalinization and are surrounded by intense pericapsular fibrosis. They are clustered together in wedges by the interstitial scarring. Bands of fibrosis and nests of lymphocytes, eosinophils, and plasma cells disrupt the renal architecture. Tubules are atrophied and dilated and may contain colloid casts. Productive endarteritis, hyperplastic arteriosclerosis, or fibrinoid arteriolar necrosis may be present, as well as foci of calcification.

DIAGNOSIS. Regardless of which collection technique is employed, a negative culture usually can be considered a valid result, since under ordinary conditions, in a patient who is not under treatment, a false-negative urine culture is rare. When the culture reveals bacteria the number of organisms in the urine specimen must be quantitated in order to distinguish contaminated from truly infected urine. In toilet-trained children infected urines contain more than 10^5 organisms per milliliter, in contrast to contaminated urines, which contain fewer than 10^3 organisms per milliliter. Counts between 10^3 and 10^5 are of equivocal significance. In younger children and infants the possibility that urine does not remain in the bladder long enough to allow bacteria to enter a logarithmic growth phase cannot be excluded, so that lower counts of plausible organisms may represent true infection and should be repeated. However, in younger children and infants who have other convincing evidences of infection, bacterial counts are seldom less than 10^5.

Urine obtained by suprapubic puncture or from the upper urinary tract by retrograde catheterization should not contain any bacteria if sterile technique is employed. Therefore any growth from these sources may be important, but it should be noted that low counts in bladder aspirates are rare in patients with other evidence of true infection.

Low bacterial counts or sterile urine in the presence of true infection may be seen with rapid urine flow, urine pH of less than 5.0 or more than 8.5, the presence of an antibiotic or chemotherapeutic agent in the urine, or complete ureteral obstruction.

Of the many ways proposed for circumventing the tedious performance of quantitative bacterial cultures, examination of the gram-stained urinary sediment has proved of value; it also provides immediately available information. Bacteria seen in the smear of an uncentrifuged urine specimen indicate more than 10^5 organisms per milliliter, while few or no organisms indicate less than 10^5. Following centrifugation, many bacteria on smear reflect counts over 10^5; few or no organisms represent less than 10^3. A simple and inexpensive culture technique that uses agar-coated microscope slides for quantitative culture is available and has been found to be highly reliable. A number of other tests have been proposed based on color alteration of an indicator in the presence of products derived from bacterial metabolism. Correlation between the results of these tests and bacterial counts, however, has shown them to be inadequate, even for screening, since they yield an unacceptable number of false negative results. In any case, standard bacteriologic methods are needed to identify the organisms and determine their antibiotic sensitivity.

Since an increased rate of excretion of white blood cells is present in many cases of UTI, leukocyturia should suggest this diagnosis. However, pus cells may be absent in as many as 20 percent of cases of true infection, and their presence may be related to other causes, such as vaginal contamination, glomerulonephritis, nephrocalcinosis, or urolithiasis; they may also result from a functional renal disturbance secondary to dehydration or hypotension. White blood cell casts suggest renal involvement, and when these are accompanied by significant bacteriuria the combination favors a diagnosis of pyelonephritis.

Red blood cells may appear in urine in infection of either the lower or the upper tract. Microscopic hematuria is found in urethritis and hemorrhagic cystitis, or it may be due to an underlying urologic abnormality such as hydronephrosis, duplication, ureterocele, or lithiasis.

Proteinuria in UTI is usually of small magnitude, ranging from trace to $2+$. It is interesting that regardless of its magnitude the electrophoretic pattern is typical: globulins predominate and are equally distributed among alpha, beta, and gamma.

TREATMENT. Oral sulfonamides are most often used for initial treatment of acute infection with sensitive organisms or before sensitivities are known. Ampicillin and tetracyclines are alternative choices for oral treatment of acute infections, but there is no evidence that these agents are more effective than sulfonamides in patients with fever or other toxic signs. Tetracyclines should not be given to children less than 9 years old when an alternative is available, since mottling of permanent teeth has been reported after the use of tetracyclines in this age group.

Subsequent treatment is guided by response to therapy and the results of the culture and antibiotic sensitivity test · Should the patient responds to initial therapy a sensitivity report of resistance to the drug can be ignored, since some disks that evaluate sensitivity simulate antibiotic concentrations in blood, and urine concentrations are much higher when the antibiotic is excreted by the kidney. Infections can be cured by sterilizing the urine alone, so that agents with little or no tissue activity such as acidifying drugs or nitrofurantoin can eradicate bacteriuria, even when there is evidence of renal parenchymal involvement. Although some laboratories report sensitivities for neomycin, this drug should never be given parenterally because of its severe ototoxicity.

In chronic or complicated infections sensitivity tests should be used to guide therapy. The usual organisms in such difficult cases are *Klebsiella, Aerobacter, Proteus, Pseudomonas,* and resistant strains of *E. coli*. Oral drugs that may be useful in these infections, in addition to sulfonamides and ampicillin, include carbenicillin indanyl sodium, cephalexin, methenamine hippurate, methenamine mandelate, nitrofurantoin, or sulfamethoxazole-trimethoprim. Parenteral carbenicillin and gentamicin should be reserved for severe infections resistant to other drugs.

In patients with diminished renal function the dosage schedules must be altered if the drug to be used is excreted by the kidneys. Specific recommendations for these alterations have been published by Bennett and others.

In acute uncomplicated infections controlled studies have demonstrated that 10 days of treatment are as effective as 2 months of treatment in eradicating bacteriuria and preventing recurrences. Most initial infections will show clinical improvement within 24 hours and sterile urine within a few days. A "cure" is determined by several negative cultures following discontinuation of therapy.

The patient should be followed with repeated urinalysis and cultures for at least 2 years, since symptomatic or asymptomatic recurrences of bacteriuria are common. Some experts recommend long-term antimicrobial prophylaxis for patients with recurrent or chronic infections. If long-term prophylaxis is to be used drugs such as methenamine mandelate or methenamine hippurate, which are used with an acidifying agent, have the advantage that they do not promote emergence of resistant strains.

Recognition and treatment of an associated urologic abnormality are mandatory; *complete radiologic and urologic evaluation should be undertaken in every patient shown to have significant bacteriuria.* IVU may be performed within a week of diagnosis. A voiding cystourethrogram should not be done until the urine is sterile in order to avoid obtaining positive results that may be due to the infection rather than to an intrinsic abnormality. In patients with obstructive or other urologic anomalies there may be no response to therapy until the underlying lesion has been corrected. *It should be emphasized that restricting the radiographic investigation to patients who have a past history of pyuria or symptoms of infection will result in overlooking children with important and correctable urologic abnormalities.*

There is no unanimity as to what should be done when certain urologic or radiographic abnormalities are found. Perhaps the most controversial of these is the presence of ureteral reflux, which can be transient or medically reversible and which is not invariably corrected by surgical intervention. The best indications for surgery in a patient with reflux would seem to be loss of renal parenchyma, progressive ureteral dilatation, or infection that does not respond to adequate medical therapy. Certainly it has become clear that the surgical correction of apparent bladder neck obstruction often is of no benefit to the patient, and major surgery of uncertain value should be reserved for the most difficult cases or those in whom anatomic obstruction is unquestionable. In the case of distal urethral obstruction a controlled trial of meatotomy in girls with meatal stenosis demonstrated no effect of the procedure in lowering the recurrence rate of UTI.

COURSE AND PROGNOSIS. UTI may represent (1) an isolated single episode of infection of the upper or lower urinary tract, (2) one of many recurrent acute infections, or (3) an acute episode in the course of chronic infection. Symptomatic uncomplicated UTI responds quickly to therapy or may improve spontaneously. Nevertheless, one-third or more of these patients may relapse within 1 year. Although UTI associated with uropathy may not be curable until there is correction of the underlying abnormality, subjective symptoms and urinary findings may disappear with treatment only to return when therapy is discontinued.

Although some studies have indicated that the severity rather than the rate of recurrence is related to the presence or absence of underlying uropathy, a much higher rate of recurrence has been observed in most studies of patients with urologic abnormality. In the great majority of recurrences the infective organism differs from the initial one. Thus recurrence usually represents new infection rather than relapse of latent infection.

Although the urine will be rendered sterile by treatment in 75 to 80 percent of patients with chronic pyelonephritis, the infection almost always recurs, and patients with bilateral disease may progress ultimately to renal failure. In cases of unilateral chronic pyelonephritis with either hypertension or severe recurrent disease, nephrectomy may be curative.

Xanthogranulomatous Pyelonephritis

In this disease the renal parenchyma is wholly or regionally replaced by inflammatory tissue consisting of masses of lipid-laden histiocytes surrounded by mononuclear infiltrates and fibrosis. Several cases have been reported in childhood. Etiology is unknown. The disease usually is preceded by long-term, low-grade urinary infection, often with *Proteus* bacilli, with local suppuration, microobstruction, and lithiasis. The clinical signs are those of UTI and of an increasing renal mass. Radiographically an enlarged nonfunctioning kidney is found, usually with calyceal deformity. Treatment consists of nephrectomy.

Renal Tuberculosis

Tuberculosis is now a rare form of pyelonephritis in childhood. It occurs by hematogenous spread from primary lesions in the lungs or infected cervical nodes; however, the primary lesion may heal before renal involvement is evident.

Initially tubercles form in the glomeruli of both kidneys. Most of these heal spontaneously. Only 4 to 5 percent of lesions progress to the point of slough, with shedding of organisms and white blood cells in the urine. With progression the medulla is colonized; this secondary lesion is usually unilateral. Tubercles coalesce and caseate, and as their contents slough a paracalyceal cavity becomes evident on IVU and there is a marked increase in the excretion of white cells, red cells, and organisms in the urine. The time lag from initial seeding to demonstrable calyceal deformity may range from months to years. Gradually an entire pyramid may become caseated; if the caseum is retained it creates a roundish, solidified, sometimes calcified bulge; if the caseum is evacuated, a jagged cavity appears. With time the cavity may contract, and a capsular indentation will mark its emplacement.

The infection may spread across the pelvic cavity to other calyces or down to the ureter and bladder. Involvement of the ureter may cause stricture, rigidity, and proximal dilatation. Tuberculous cystitis occurs in most patients with moderately advanced renal tuberculosis, producing typical trigonitis and disseminated ulceration. If the inflammation penetrates through the mucosa into the muscle, fibrosis will result in a rigid, contracted malfunctioning bladder. In male children with advanced renal tuberculosis the prostate, vas, and epididymis may be infected. Presenting symptoms may be dysuria, loin pain, or painless hematuria. Tuberculosis of the urinary tract often evolves insidiously; over one-fourth of pediatric cases are asymptomatic and are discovered by the incidental finding of leukocyturia; in others it is discovered by doing routine urine cultures following pulmonary or miliary tuberculosis.

Treatment is usually medical. Even nonfunctioning kidneys are now left in situ and observed, provided the urine can be sterilized. Hypertension, secondary infection of advanced tubercular lesions, or intractable pain are indications for surgery.

During therapy the tests of erythrocyte sedimentation rate, urinalysis, cultures, and IVU should be repeated every 4 to 6 months; similar tests are done at yearly intervals following cessation of therapy. Improved general state, return of urine to normal, and repeated negative cultures indicate success of treatment. Following a 2-year course of therapy over 85 percent of cases remain negative for 5 to 10 years.

Perinephritis and Perinephric Abscess

Perinephritis is an infection of the tissue surrounding the kidney; it is usually unilateral and may occur at any age. There is a slight preponderance of females.

ETIOLOGY. Perinephritis is probably the result of hematogenous spread. However, it may occur after blunt local trauma or by extension from a renal abscess, pyelonephritis, or an adjacent osteomyelitic focus.

CLINICAL MANIFESTATIONS. Onset may be abrupt, with chills, high fever, and prostration, or insidious, with a variable period of flank tenderness, pain, low-grade fever, and the gradual development of psoas spasm. At the height of disease there is marked lumbar pain, spasm, lameness, persistent flexion of the thigh, indefinite local swelling, and a fluctuating temperature. If it is untreated the symptoms may persist for many weeks, followed by spontaneous resolution. In two-thirds of cases suppuration occurs, with formation of an abscess, which may rupture into the peritoneal cavity, viscera, thorax, urinary tract, iliocostal space, or groin.

DIAGNOSIS. Urinary abnormalities are present mainly in cases that occur as a complication of pyelonephritis. Radiography may show edema around the kidney, an obliterated psoas shadow, scoliosis with concavity facing the affected side, and sometimes atelectasis and pleural fluid in the corresponding hemithorax. The kidney usually is displaced anteriorly, caudally, and laterally. On fluoroscopy there may be a decreased diaphragmatic excursion on the affected side, and IVU reveals markedly decreased renal excursion and sometimes pelvic deformation. Diagnosis may be confirmed by needle aspiration.

TREATMENT. Treatment consists of analgesics and appropriate chemotherapy. If the responsible organism has not been identified by culture of blood or urine, antibiotics covering a broad range of organisms including staphylococci should be administered. Surgical drainage may be required. Prognosis usually is excellent.

Balanoposthitis

Balanoposthitis is an inflammation of the glans and the prepuce that may occur at any age. It originates from poor local hygiene, infected regional dermatitis, or urethritis; it may also follow a combination of mechanical and infectious factors, such as phimosis, forceful manipulation of the foreskin, and masturbation. The inflamed glans and prepuce are red, painful, edematous, and purulent. The meatus may be narrowed or encrusted, with resultant dysuria. The infection usually does not extend into the urinary tract.

Treatment consists of sitz baths, irrigations, and local applications of antibiotics in solution or ointment. Systemic therapy rarely is necessary. A dorsal slit of the foreskin may be required when the edema is such that the preputial cavity cannot be exposed. Circumcision may be advisable, but only after recovery from the acute episode.

Urethritis

Urethritis usually presents as an inflammation of the distal two-thirds of the urethra, with dysuria, frequency, leukocyturia, and urethral discharge. Urine voided initially is positive, while midstream specimens may be negative. Similarly, a comparison of spontaneously voided urine with that obtained by chatheterization may confirm the diagnosis.

Most instances of urethritis are nonspecific or nonbacterial, but gonococcal urethritis is not uncommon. It may be seen in infants, although most cases occur in patients over 7 years of age. Infection in older patients in nearly all cases is the result of direct sexual encounter or handling of the genitalia by an infected person. The symptoms of gonococcal urethritis are more severe than those of nonbacterial urethritis. Extension up the urethra may produce cystitis, prostatitis, or epididymitis. Reiter's triad (conjunctivitis, arthritis, and urethritis) is very rare in children. Gonococcal vaginitis is also seen.

Diagnosis is made by stained smear and culture of urethral discharge, and occasionally urine culture and stain may also be positive. Treatment consists of appropriate antibiotic therapy.

Prostatitis and Prostatic Abscess

Prostatitis is a rare entity in childhood. It may occur as an extension of tuberculosis or gonococcal urethritis or be of nonspecific bacterial origin. Presenting symptoms are frequency, dysuria, leukocyturia, terminal hematuria, perineal pain, and fever. Diffuse edema and tenderness are evident on rectal examination. Cultures of the uretheral discharge should be obtained, preferably following prostatic massage.

Prostatic abscess occurs mainly in infancy and is believed to originate by hematogenous spread. The causative organisms are usually staphylococci or coliform bacilli. Treatment consists of incision and drainage combined with chemotherapy.

Nonspecific Vulvovaginitis

The term vulvovaginitis is applied to a group of infections affecting the vulva, the vagina, and often the urethra. Nonspecific vaginitis may be seen at any age, even in infancy, but is most frequent after the second year of life. A local cause is usually responsible, such as pinworms, scabies, a local lesion of varicella, or, most commonly, poor hygiene. It may follow local trauma, especially from the introduction of foreign bodies. Masturbation may be a contributing cause. Unexplained, self-limited attacks frequently occur in otherwise healthy girls.

Urinary frequency or enuresis is sometimes seen and may be the presenting symptom. The disease generally begins as a subacute catarrhal inflammation, the discharge being the first and often the only symptom. It is white or yellowish and rarely profuse; in some cases a foul odor is present. Blood-stained discharge often results from a foreign body. When the discharge is abundant there may be excoriations of the labia and the skin of the thighs. The mucous membranes are swollen and red. Microscopic examination of the discharge usually shows fewer pus cells and more epithelial cells than are seen in gonorrhea. Organisms may be numerous or comparatively infrequent, and it is common to observe several types in a single preparation, ie, both cocci and bacilli, gram-positive as well as gram-negative. Diphtheroids and *E. coli* are found in the great majority of cases, with a doubtful pathogenic role. Among the organisms of etiologic significance occasionally encountered are β-hemolytic and other forms of streptococci, *Staphylococcus aureus*, and *Trichomonas*. With hemolytic streptococcal infections the same strain is at times recovered from the nose and throat in association with a respiratory infection.

Simple cleansing measures consisting of sitz baths and local irrigations with warm saline solution should be prescribed. In some cases the condition will disappear within a few days with these measures alone. Antibacterial agents given by mouth may be dramatically effective in cases that accompany a respiratory infection; they should also be used in cases with associated lymph node enlargement and those resistant to local therapy. Specific local therapy includes instillation of acidifying solutions, such as dilute acetic acid (vinegar), and introduction into the vagina of urethral suppositories of 0.2 percent nitrofurazone or aminoacridine. The latter treatment is especially effective against *Trichomonas*. Mycotic infections may be treated with topical administration of 0.5 percent gentian violet or nystatin. In refractory or recurrent cases the possibility of a foreign body must be investigated thoroughly.

References

Aoki S, Imamura S, Aoki M, McCabe WR: "Abacterial" and bacterial pyelonephritis. Immunofluorescent localization of bacterial antigen. N Engl J Med 281:1375, 1969

Aronson AS, Gustafson B, Svenningsen NW: Combined suprapubic and clean-voided urine examination in infants and children. Acta Paediatr Scand 62:396, 1973

Bennett WM, Singer I, Coggins CH: Guide to drug usage in adult patients with impaired renal function. JAMA 223:991, 1973

Bergström T, Larson H, Lincoln K, Winberg J: Studies of urinary tract infections in infancy and childhood. XII. Eighty consecutive patients with neonatal infection. J Pediatr 80:858, 1972

Edelmann CM Jr, Ogwo JE, Fine BP, Martinez AB: The prevalence of bacteriuria in full-term and premature newborn infants. J Pediatr 82:125, 1973

Freeman RB: Does bacteriuria lead to renal failure? Clin Nephrol 1:61, 1973

Hatch CS, Cockett ATK: Xanthogranulomatous pyelonephritis. J Urol 92:585, 1964

Hodson CJ: Radiologic diagnosis of renal involvement. In O'Grady F, Brumfitt W (eds): Urinary Tract Infection. London, Oxford Univ Press, 1968, Chap 13

Houston IB: Urinary white cell excretion in childhood. Arch Dis Child 40:313, 1965

Jones SR, Smith JW, Sanford JP: Localization of urinary-tract infections by detection of antibody-coated bacteria in urine sediment. N Engl J Med 290:591, 1974

Kunin CM: Emergence of bacteriuria, proteinuria, and asymptomatic urinary tract infections among a population of school girls followed for 7 years. Pediatrics 41:968, 1968

——— The natural history of recurrent bacteriuria in school girls. N Engl J Med 282:26, 1970

Lattimer JK: Current concepts—renal tuberculosis. N Engl J Med 273:208, 1965

Norden CW, Kass EH: Bacteriuria of pregnancy—a critical appraisal. Ann Rev Med 10:431, 1968

O'Grady F, Brumfitt W (eds): Urinary Tract Infection. London, Oxford Univ Press, 1968

Rollestan GL, Shannon FT, Utley WLF: Relationship of infantile vesicoureteric reflux to renal damage. Br Med J 1:460, 1970

Savage DCL, Wilson MI, McHardy M, Dewar DAE, Fee WM: Covert bacteriuria of childhood. A. Clinical and epidemiological study. Arch Dis Child 48:8, 1973

Thomas V, Shelokov A, Forland M: Antibody-coated bacteria in the urine and the site of urinary tract infection. N Engl J Med 290:588, 1974

UROLOGY

Selwyn B. Levitt

Congenital Urogenital Disorders

GENERAL CONSIDERATIONS

CLINICAL PRESENTATION. The nature of the anomaly and the age of the child are the most important factors determining the mode of presentation of congenital urogenital disorders. Anomalies of the external genitalia, such as hypospadias, epispadias (Fig. 17), exstrophy (Fig. 18), and ambiguous genitalia (Fig. 19), are strikingly obvious at birth. Internal anomalies, however, are much less simple to diagnose, and the physician must be aware of the associated conditions that should arouse suspicion of the presence of internal anomalies.

The genitourinary tract is involved in as many as 30 to 40 percent of children with congenital anomalies of other systems. Oligohydramnios should suggest the possibility of renal agenesis, severe hypoplasia, or complete bladder outflow obstruction, since fetal urine contributes significantly to the formation of amniotic fluid. The classic Potter facies, characterized by low-set ears, hypertelorism, pronounced epicanthal folds, flattened

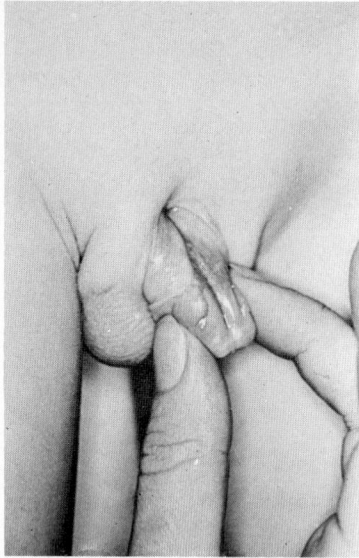

FIG. 17. Penopubic variety of epispadias in a patient with urinary incontinence.

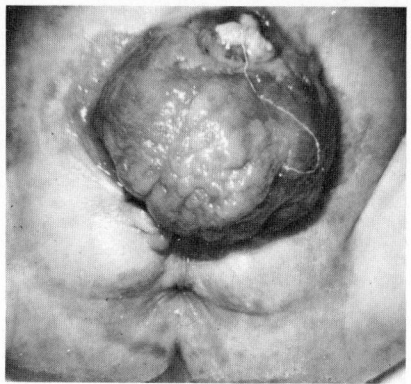

FIG. 18. Exstrophy. Epispadias in a female.

nose, and micrognathia, may also be present in these patients. Small deformed ears are a common concomitant of renal anomalies, often on the ipsilateral side if the renal lesion is unilateral. A single umbilical artery, which is estimated to occur in approximately 0.7 to 1.1 percent of newborns, indicates an increased general incidence of anomalies of organ systems, including the genitourinary tract. However, the majority of genitourinary anomalies, as well as other anomalies, occur in those newborns who do not survive the perinatal period. Those children with single umbilical vessels who survive (86 percent in the collaborative study conducted by the National Institutes of Health) do not seem to manifest a higher incidence of clinically signifi-

cant genitourinary disease up to the age of 4 years. However, the children in the NIH study did not have routine screening intravenous pyelograms. Feingold and associates found urinary tract anomalies in 33 percent of the infants they studied with intravenous urography. None of these babies had symptoms or abnormal renal findings on physical examination.

Absent abdominal musculature together with undescended testes is associated consistently with marked dilation of the urinary tract; these constitute the triad of the prune-belly syndrome. An infant with a major anomaly, such as an anorectal malformation, abnormality of the cloaca, or tracheoesophageal fistula, should be investigated for associated urologic anomalies. Myelomeningoceles and sacral deformities are often accompanied by neurogenic vesical dysfunction; if three or more segments of the sacrum are absent the association is invariable. A lax anus with absent anocutaneous reflex confirms this suspicion. Kidneys in the normal neonate are palpable, owing to their low lumbar position and to the minimal resistance of the abdominal

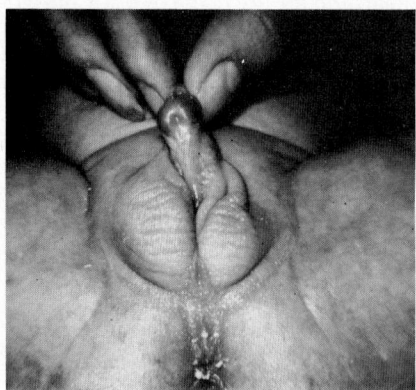

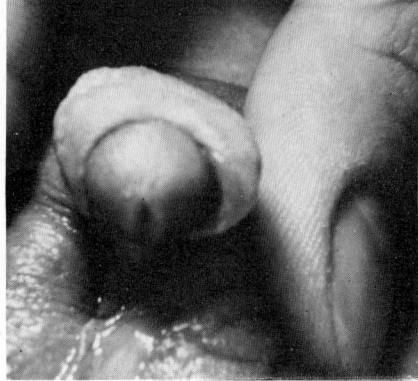

FIG. 19. Ambiguous genitalia showing bifid scrotum or rugated labia majora, penis with chordee, and scrotal hypospadias or hypertrophied clitoris with urogenital sinus.

wall. Large kidneys suggest either cystic disease of the kidneys or, less frequently, hydronephrosis; neoplasms occur but are much less common.

The most common presentation of an obstructive anomaly in the neonate or older infant is unexplained fever, often associated with vomiting and diarrhea. Symptoms and signs of obstruction per se are rare modes of presentation before toilet training has been achieved. The child's stream is rarely observed by the parent, and diapers conceal the normal intermittent pattern of micturition because they are usually wet. Thus the opportunity to observe a poor urinary stream or dribbling may be missed. Even in the older child or teenager congenital obstructions frequently are not recognized, since the individual has never micturated with a normal uninterrupted stream and thus may not recognize his abnormal pattern of voiding.

Obstructive anomalies not detected at birth often present later with signs and symptoms of urinary tract infection. Initial treatment of these infections may procure a good symptomatic response, satisfying both patient and physician. Unsuspected underlying pathology may then continue to progress silently until either frequent reinfection or evidence of renal failure leads to further investigation. If the lesion in such patients had been detected at the time of the original infection it might have been corrected by surgery, with a good anatomic and functional result. Thus, despite opinions to the contrary, it is our strong belief that *intravenous urography and voiding cystourethrography are mandatory studies in any neonate, infant, or toddler, male or female, who has had a documented urinary tract infection.*

DIAGNOSTIC PROCEDURES. Intravenous urography is used routinely for evaluation of the urinary tract and is a safe procedure at all ages. Mortality is extremely rare; for example, at the Hospital for Sick Children in London only one death has occurred in the past 30 years.

In performing urography the intravenous route of injection is preferable; subcutaneous injection, usually in the subscapular region, may occasionally be necessary, but it should be appreciated that high quality of visualization may be lost with this technique. Positioning is important in order to move gas-filled bowel away from the renal areas. Prone films and filling of the stomach with a feed or carbonated drink often are helpful. When there is poor visualization with a standard dose, urography should be repeated with a larger dose. Films taken immediately after injection, during the vascular phase of the study, show a total bodygram effect from opacification of vascular tissue. Masses that are highly vascular opacify, whereas cystic lesions are outlined by a negative shadow. This technique is also useful in demonstrating parenchymal thickness in hydronephrosis.

Formerly the finding on conventional urography of one nonfunctioning and one normal kidney led to ablative surgery rather than plastic reconstruction. Better visualization with demonstration of adequate parenchymal thickness has led to more conservative reconstructive procedures, with very encouraging results. The author has performed 38 consecutive pyeloplasties in the past 6 years for hydronephrosis secondary to ureteropelvic junction obstruction. The patients were not nephrectomized at the initial operation, and no subsequent nephrectomies have been required for pain, secondary calculus formation, hypertension, or pyonephrosis. No kidneys in the postoperative follow-up period have been shown radiographically to have deteriorated, and function studies performed at the time of the pyeloplasties revealed that even the most damaged kidneys contributed at least 10 percent of overall renal function. Therefore any hydronephrotic kidney secondary to ureteropelvic junction obstruction that visualizes on high-dose intravenous urography is potentially salvageable. When using a high dose it must be recognized that the rapid injection of a large amount of contrast material, with its large osmotic load, may be hazardous in patients with cardiac impairment, due to volume overload, and also in dehydrated infants, in whom vascular collapse may occur during the diuretic phase of the study.

Voiding cystourethrography should be regarded as an obligatory part of the radiologic work-up of any child suspected of having vesicoureteral reflux or obstructive uropathy. It is preferable, although not always possible, to do the study in the unanesthetized child. In the acutely ill or uremic child suspected of having obstructive uropathy, antibiotics should be administered 24 to 48 hours before the cystourethrogram in an attempt to prevent exacerbations of pyelonephritis and gram-negative septicemia. A No. 5 or No. 8 pediatric feeding tube makes an ideal catheter for infants or toddlers of either sex; it is simple to pass and is atraumatic. In older children a Foley catheter may be more appropriate. Lubasporin is a satisfactory antibiotic-impregnated lubricant. A 12 to 15 percent solution of a water-miscible contrast medium such as diatrizoate is used. Fluoroscopy provides maximun information regarding vesicoureteral reflux and bladder configuration and function, as well as urethral anatomy; when properly done it also involves the least amount of radiation. The initial specimen of urine obtained by catheterization during this procedure should be cultured.

Voiding cystourethrography has emerged as the best and most accurate indicator of urethral pathology in the male. In the female, however, the urethral configuration as seen on a single voiding film may be too readily interpreted as indicative of obstructive disease. Urethral patterns in the female previously regarded as obstructive have been found to correlate poorly with other indications of obstruction, such as residual urine, bladder trabeculation, bougie à boule urethral calibration, and pressure–flow studies. Sequential voiding with spot films, which show dynamic changes in the urethra, has provided an explanation for many of the urethrographic variations described as pathologic when recorded on a single film. Ascendant Lipiodol, a low-density contrast material in oily solution, can be injected together with the water-miscible contrast material when performing the cystogram. Since it floats on top of the urine rather than mixing with it, any residual noted on a film taken the following day suggests incomplete bladder emptying.

Aortography and selective renal angiography may be helpful in the differential diagnosis of abdominal masses. Inferior vena cavography has little value in pediatric urology; it may be useful in the diagnosis of renal vein thrombosis or aid in determining the extent of an abdominal mass.

Cystoscopy and retrograde urography in children must always be done under general anesthesia. It should be noted that high-dose urography may obviate the need for retrograde studies. The smallest possible instruments should be used in the male to prevent postendoscopy edema and difficulty with micturition. With the miniature instruments now available no child should be denied a full urologic evaluation when it is indicated.

BLADDER AND URACHUS

EMBRYOLOGY. The urorectal septum divides the cloaca into a ventral vesicourethral segment and a dorsal rectal moiety. The upper half of the vesicourethral canal, which is continuous with the allantois, forms the definitive bladder. Normally the allantois undergoes retrogressive changes, with complete obliteration of its lumen, and the residual fibrous cord or urachus passes from the apex of the bladder to the umbilicus. Anomalous closure of the allantois most often results in a patent urachus, which appears clinically as a urinary fistula opening at the umbilicus. A small uncomplicated patent urachus may close spontaneously, but if it persists extraperitoneal excision and bladder closure are required. Other abnormalities include urachal cysts (if the lumen is obliterated at both ends), blind-ending urachal sinuses, and urachal diverticuli.

ANATOMY AND PHYSIOLOGY. The bladder detrusor is composed of interlacing bundles of smooth muscle fibers and elastic tissue that extend down into the posterior urethra. The muscular arrangement at the vesicourethral junction constitutes the bladder neck, which is no longer considered to be a true sphincter but rather an integral portion of the detrusor mechanism, the only true sphincter being the skeletal muscle of the urogenital diaphragm or external urinary sphincter.

Both the autonomic pelvic nerves and the somatic internal pudendal nerves emanate from the conus medullaris, which lies at the level of the first lumbar vertebra in the adult and slightly lower in the child. The conus contains the sacral segments of the spinal cord and is the integrating center for the spinal reflex for micturition (Fig. 20). This simple segmental reflex is modified by voluntary and involuntary impulses descending from the suprasegmental level; these may be facilitory or inhibitory.

Motor innervation to the detrusor is autonomic, predominantly parasympathetic, and is derived from sacral spinal segments S-2, S-3, and S-4, which reach the bladder as the pelvic nerve or nervi erigentes. The sympathetic system from the lower thoracic and upper lumbar cord plays only a minor role. Proprioceptive (appreciation of bladder fullness) and exteroceptive (hot and cold sensation) impulses are carried by afferent fibers that return to the cord in the pelvic nerve. The somatic internal pudendal nerve (S-3 and S-4) contains the afferent and efferent supply to the striated external sphincter and posterior urethra. The external sphincter

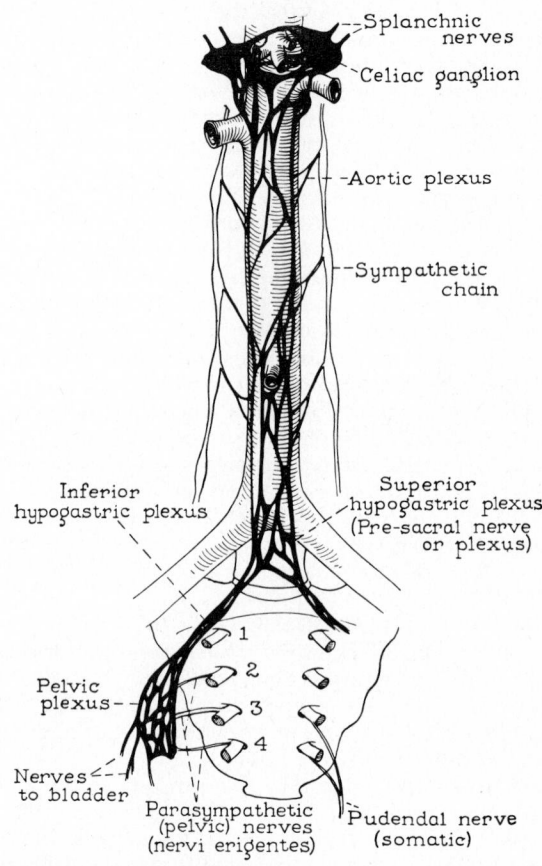

FIG. 20. Nerve supply of the bladder. (From Campbell and Harrison: Urology, 3rd ed, Vol 1, p 112. Courtesy of WB Saunders Company.)

was formerly thought to be supplied solely by the somatic pudendal nerve. Modern histochemical techniques have shown that it is also influenced by autonomic fibers.

Normal bladder function, in which the bladder is emptied completely and voluntarily at intervals, depends upon an intact nerve supply as well as the inherent properties of the bladder muscle and elastic tissue. Reflex activity and sensation are under nervous control, whereas tone and rhythmic contractility do not require participation of the central nervous system. During the first years of life the child's bladder empties reflexly at intervals varying from 30 minutes to 3 hours. Bowel actions and penile erections occur similarly. The infant who is always wet, whose diapers are damp within a few minutes of changing, and who is never seen to project his urine with force may have an abnormality in bladder function. Micturition following instillation of cold water into the bladder (ice-water test of Bors) indicates an intact autonomic reflex arc. An intact somatic arc is confirmed by a normal anocutaneous and bulbocavernosus reflex. Cystometry provides information concerning residual urine, bladder capacity, accomodation, and the threshold and force of the detrusor contraction.

URINARY RETENTION. In the newborn urinary retention must be differentiated from true anuria. The neonate may not pass urine for 24 to 48 hours, the exact cause of which is undetermined; it may be related to deposition of urates or Tamm-Horsfall proteins in the renal tubules. The bladder does not become distended and no treatment is required. True retention in the male infant is most often due to temporary obliteration of the urethral meatus with epithelial debris, particularly when there is a coronal hypospadias associated with meatal stenosis. Probing of the meatus on the glans dorsal to the hypospadiac opening may reveal a blind sinus extending for a variable distance. Membranous or posterior urethral atresia as a cause of urinary retention should be suspected from the inability to pass a catheter. Posterior urethral valves, although only an occasional cause of acute retention in the newborn, often will allow easy retrograde passage of a catheter. Voiding cystourethrography is the most accurate means of demonstrating the nature and site of these obstructions. In the female, hydrocolpos secondary to obstructing vaginal septae or an imperforate hymen occasionally may produce acute urinary retention.

In the older infant or toddler acute retention is due to a variety of causes, including painful meatal ulcers in boys, fecal impaction with rectal distension, urethral strictures, vesical or urethral diverticuli, impacted urethral calculi, or urethral prolapse of lobules of a bladder tumor. Acute inflammatory lesions of the prostate or a prostatic abscess occasionally may be responsible. Chronic retention of urine usually presents as overflow incontinence with a painless, overdistended, easily palpable suprapubic mass. Often renal failure or complicating infection is the factor that draws attention to the condition.

ENURESIS. All children lack voluntary bladder control during the first year or two of life. Physiologic urinary continence is already present in the newborn baby, although voiding occurs at frequent intervals. The act of micturition is a simple reflex phenomenon, but the baby is perfectly dry between each act of micturition. Physiologic continence gives way to social continence in most children somewhere between 1 year and 4 years of age. Daytime control is usually attained before nighttime continence.

Enuresis is the inappropriate voiding of a normal stream of urine beyond the age at which one would expect normal voluntary urinary control. Enuresis can be nocturnal only or nocturnal and diurnal. Many children with purely nocturnal enuresis have in addition daytime frequency and urgency. Enuresis can be primary (that is, there never having been a period of dryness) or secondary. Secondary enuresis implies a recurrence of the symptom following a short or long period of continence.

Nocturnal enuresis is an extremely common disorder, with an estimated prevalence in the United States of 5 million children. Bloomfield and Douglas followed 5,386 children from birth and found that at age 6 years 1.8 percent of boys and 4.1 percent of girls were still wet by day; 11.9 percent of boys and 8.4 percent of girls were bedwetters. Two years later nocturnal enuresis persisted in 8 percent of boys and 6.4 percent of girls. It is of interest that Levine reported that 1.2 percent of navy recruits were enuretic. At all age levels nocturnal enuresis is more common in boys. A familial factor is common. Gregor found one parent to have been enuretic in 47 percent of his cases; in 35 percent a sibling had enuresis. Socioeconomic factors also may play a role.

The etiology of enuresis remains conjectural. A great number of theories have been advanced, ranging along a spectrum beginning with subtle organic GU pathology as the causal agent in virtually every case, through theories that consider enuresis to be a neurologic or endocrine diathesis, to hypotheses that maintain that the symptom is related exclusively to psychiatric or sociologic factors (see Chap. 3). Minor degrees of urethral and bladder neck obstruction have been described by some urologists. However, improper development of bladder capacity and uninhibited detrusor contractions, as determined by cystometry, are the urologic lesions most frequently cited. Abnormal detrusor function has been ascribed to delayed development of inhibitory control of the bladder reflex arc consequent to delayed myelinization of the central or peripheral nerves. Arnold believes that certain children have an "inborn familial diathesis toward uninhibited bladder contractions which expresses itself in the absence of tranquility of cerebral process."

Immature electroencephalographic patterns have been found in enuretic children. Some with electroencephalographic evidence of seizure activity were reported to have the most severe degrees of enuresis, and thus it has been suggested that enuresis in some cases may be an epileptic equivalent. Inadequate nocturnal increase in ADH has also been postulated as a cause of enuresis. Breneman believes that food allergy is an important factor. The behaviorists state that enuresis is a symptom of deficit and is due to a failure of conditioning. On the other hand, many psychiatrists consider enuresis a manifestation of antisocial aggressive behavior. Despite the many theories (and each form of investigation seems to come up with a new answer), it is generally recognized that there is no one factor responsible for all cases. Enuresis is probably an example of a delay in the development of a physiologic function provoked at times by local disorders or psychologic problems, but often neither of these factors is clinically obvious.

From the clinician's point of view one of the major difficulties when confronted with a child apparently suffering from enuresis is weighing the possibilities of an organic urinary tract abnormality being present and deciding whether to subject the child to the full range of urinary tract investigation. The implications of the term enuresis, then, are (1) that it constitutes a functional abnormality rather than an organic one, (2) that the prevalence of organic abnormalities in the urinary tract is no greater in children with true enuresis than in the general population, and (3) that if such a combination of organic abnormalities and true enuresis occurs it is coincidental. That the basis of enuresis in most cases is functional would appear to be validated by the appreciable spontaneous remission rate and by the excellent cure rate with enthusiastic management. In fact, most patients are cured within 6 months of consulting the physician. Forsythe and Redmond have shown that even without treatment the spontaneous cure rate in the 5- to 9-year-old age group is 14 percent per year, and in the 10- to 19-year-old age group it is 16 percent per year. These rates mean that one of seven patients is spontaneously cured each year. It is most important to recognize that not all wetting is enuresis, either before of after the age of 4 years. A detailed history allows simple enuresis to be differentiated from wetting, which is part of a general urologic problem. The child who is still in diapers may be hard to evaluate, since the parents will often report that he is always wet. However, more careful questioning will usually reveal the true state of affairs. There are two key questions that allow classification of the various forms of incontinence (see Table 13): When does the wetting occur? How or under what circumstances does it occur? Simple bedwetting or nocturnal enuresis is almost exclusively a functional disorder.

Many enuretics, although wet only at night, have daytime urgency and frequency. Infection and bladder calculi must be considered, the latter being suggested by painful micturition. Other causes of frequency include chronic renal failure and diabetes mellitus and insipidus. Dribbling incontinence due to retention with overflow is excluded by abdominal palpation. Neurogenic bladders that never fill because of poor resistance at the bladder outlet are almost always associated with other somatic neurologic signs, such as perineal anesthesia and absent or poor rectal tone, impaired bowel control, and footdrop and disturbances in gait. An absent sacrum is readily apparent, and other forms of spinal dysraphia such as diastometamyelia may be revealed by a pit or hairy mole on the back. An ectopic ureter produces dribbling incontinence despite normal micturition at regular intervals. Incontinence associated with coughing or straining (stress variety) is uncommon in children, but may occur with some forms of neurogenic bladder or epispadias or following operations to relieve bladder neck or urethral obstruction.

The numerous theories concerning the etiology of functional enuresis are matched by the diversity of treatments that have been proposed. These include bladder training with fluid restriction at night, drug therapy (including Dilantin, dextroamphetamine, propantheline, and imipramine), psychotherapy, and urologic manipulation. The most uniformly successful treatments appear to be timed training for diurnal enuresis and alarm-bell conditioning for nocturnal wet-

TABLE 13. Classification of Incontinence in Children Based Upon Two Key Questions

When does it occur?	Nighttime only
	Nighttime as well as daytime
How does it occur?	Under what circumstances?

Types of Urinary Incontinence

1. Pure nocturnal enuresis	Functional or psychogenic abnormality (if there have been dry intervals, "leaks" in the "plumbing" are excluded for all practical purposes)
2. Giggle incontinence	A functional self-limiting abnormality
3. Urge incontinence	Functional
	Organic causes
	Urinary tract infection
	Bladder outlet or urethral obstruction
	Neuropathic bladder dysfunction secondary to:
	Myelodysplasia and spinal dysarhaphia
	Occult bladder neuropathy
	Spinal cord tumors and abscesses
	Measles and other forms of viral encephalitis
	Renal failure with polyuria
4. Dribbling incontinence (always organic)	With normal-interval micturition = ectopic ureter with or without duplication of the collecting system
	Without normal-interval micturition:
	Neurogenic bladder
	Epispadias
	Status after YV-plasty
	Persistent urogenital sinus (female hypospadias)
	Obstructive uropathy with overflow incontinence
5. Stress incontinence (always organic)	Neurogenic bladder
	After YV-plasty

ting. Tofranil (imipramine) is the most successful drug for the functional enuretic. It is given 1 hour before bedtime in a dose of 25 to 50 mg. After 1 to 2 months the dosage is gradually reduced.

When a child presents with pure nocturnal enuresis associated with a perfectly normal daytime voiding pattern, no further work-up, apart from a urine analysis and culture, is indicated. A reassuring, confident explanation by the physician and a positive attitude regarding cure will go a long way toward defusing what may be a disturbingly tense home situation. The doctor needs to show concern and involvement, and the child must be included directly in the therapy so that he cures himself. Charts and stars allow for a detailed record and also involve the child in his treatment. Operant conditioning and a reward for dry nights are frequently helpful. Tofranil or the alarm bell may be required in addition if simple operant conditioning is not successful. Fluid restriction does not appear helpful in most studies unless excessive intake is truly documented. Lifting the child before the parents go to bed may be helpful, and if it results in a dry bed we see no reason to discourage the procedure; it should be discontinued at intervals in order to determine whether the methods suggested above are effective. The alarm bell is effective in most children and seems to have a lower rate of recurrence after discontinuation than does Tofranil. It is well to remember that the alarm-bell system may take up to 4 months to effect a cure, whereas benefit from Tofranil usually occurs within the first week or two. Successful results using the alarm bell require that the system be tested to be sure that it works, that it be continued for a sufficient period of time, and that the switch turning off the alarm be out of reach from the bed, thus requiring the child to get up. In addition the system must be thoroughly and carefully demonstrated before beginning its use.

Radiographs of the spine are not indicated unless there are neurologic symptoms or signs. Ten percent or more of radiographs of the spine in children will reveal some degree of spina bifida occulta. Furthermore, intravenous urography and cystography are not indicated unless there is a strong suggestion of a major anatomic fault or there is a proven urinary tract infection. The policy of requesting intravenous urography on every bedwetting child over the age of 5 years is not justified.

Those children who exhibit diurnal urgency and frequency as well as nocturnal symptoms, but who have none of the stigmata associated with true organic wetting (as gauged by a thorough history, physical examination, normal observed voiding stream, and negative urine analysis and culture), may be managed similarly without radiologic or urologic evaluation at the outset. Bladder training, increasing the intervals between voiding, and Tofranil by day are useful additions to the regimen used for those children with nocturnal wetting alone. Radiologic evaluation including intravenous urography and voiding cystourethrography are reserved for those children with documented urinary tract infections and for those with organic incontinence.

An association of urinary tract infection and enuresis might well be expected, since both are common disorders. Stansfeld reported a 5 percent incidence of urinary tract infection in girls with occasional bedwetting and a 10 percent incidence in those who wet their beds practically every night. Conversely, 16 percent of children with urinary tract infections present with pure enuretic symptoms; however, successful treatment of these infections will leave 70 percent with persistent enuresis.

Children who fail to respond to therapy despite conscientious treatment may be candidates for radiologic and urologic studies. Geist and Antolak report that sterile vesicoureteral reflux may be responsible for enuretic symptoms. However, they noted that the majority with only nocturnal enuresis continued to be enuretic despite successful treatment of their reflux. Moreover, daytime enuresis persisted in a proportion of children with successfully treated reflux, whereas some with persistent reflux were cured spontaneously of their diurnal wetting. Mahoney found obvious or potentially obstructive lesions in 96.5 percent of his patients. He stated that "simple bedwetting is, with rare exceptions, organic in nature and fundamentally obstructive in etiology." He failed to mention cure rates following correction of the lesions, but noted that voiding dynamics were generally improved. Posterior urethral valves have been reported by some authors to be common in enuretic boys. However, it is generally recognized that urethral valves are comparatively rare and are almost always accompanied by difficulty with voiding, in addition to wetting. Williams reported a few cases of idiopathic dilation of the bladder neck, but Scott and associates and Clayton and associates have shown these to be variations of normal urethrographic appearances during different phases of micturition.

In summary, the prevalence of organic abnormalities in the urinary tract appears to be no greater in children with simple enuresis than in the general population. There are data suggesting the contrary, but they are probably inaccurate because the cases investigated radiologically or urologically have in general not been carefully defined and diagnosed. Many have not been true enuretics, but rather children with incontinence or symptomatic wetting, and clear-cut objective criteria of abnormality have been lacking. There does appear to be a higher incidence of vesiocoureteral reflex in enuretic children, but seccessful treatment of their reflux often leaves them with persistent enuresis. Enuretic children without documented urinary tract infections should be given an adequate trial of bladder training, drugs, operant conditioning, and the alarm bell before considering radiologic or urologic evaluation.

Endoscopic and surgical methods of treatment are reserved for cases in which unquestionable pathology has been demonstrated. Thus such treatment is directed specifically at elimination of obstruction and only incidentally at the eradication of enuresis. Psychiatric treatment should be reserved for those children exhibiting other manifestations of behavior disorders and evident emotional disturbance.

It is wise to maintain a certain skepticism with regard to all methods of treatment. Barbour and colleagues found the 75 percent of children were cured over a period of 5 years but that the cure was not related to any particular type of treatment.

NEUROGENIC BLADDER. The most common cause of neuropathic bladder dysfunction in children is myelomeningocele, or spina bifida cystica, the incidence of which in the United States has been reported to vary from 1.1 to 2.5 per 1,000 births; approximately 25 percent of these are stillborn. If immediate closure of the myelomeningocele is accomplished more than 70 percent will survive 1 year and most will live into the second decade.

Although myelodysplasia is the most common type of neuropathic bladder dysfunction occurring in children, other causes must not be overlooked. Agenesis of three or more sacral segments is associated invariably with severe loss of pelvic nerve supply. Operative trauma from excision of a sacrococcygeal tumor or from an abdominal-perineal pull-through procedure for Hirschsprung's disease or anorectal anomaly is not an uncommon cause of neurogenic bladder. Spinal dysraphia, traumatic paraplegia, extradural spinal cord metastases, and abcesses are rare causes. Neurogenic bladders occasionally develop after measles or other forms of viral encephalitis, as well as following tuberculous meningitis.

More than 90 percent of myelomeningoceles involve the lumbosacral spine. Extensive myelodysplasia affects the whole sacral outflow, thus destroying the bladder reflex arc and rendering it an autonomous or lower motor type of neurogenic bladder. In the complete form of this lesion there is no vesical sensation, no voluntary micturition, and no reflex bladder emptying. Detrusor contractions are initiated by bladder distension; they are myogenic in nature and poorly coordinated and result in inadequate bladder emptying. However, the extent of neural involvement in myelomeninigocele is variable, seldom resulting in as complete a lesion as in traumatic paraplegia, so that some afferents and efferents usually are intact. When the sensory elements are more severely affected than the motor, there may be features of the atonic bladder. If the long tracts of the spinal cord are dyplastic above the level of the overt lesions, features of the uninhibited or upper motor neuron bladder may be present as well.

Various classifications of the neurogenic bladder resulting from myelodysplasia have been offered. Two main types are recognized. In the first the bladder is flaccid, thin-walled, and free of trabeculation; urethral resistance is low and does not allow the bladder to distend. Manual expression permits easy bladder expressibility; the upper tract usually is not dilated, and infection is easily controlled. In the second type the bladder is grossly hypertrophied and trabeculated, and urethral resistance is high, so that manual expression is difficult and incomplete. The upper tract commonly is dilated, and reflux frequently is present. Infection may be difficult to control. Many cases fall between these extremes, and the features in a given patient may change over a period of time, in some instances as a result of secondary infection.

Examination should attempt to elicit a sensory level, but in the newborn this is often difficult. Absence of perineal sensation and the anocutaneous reflex, with poor rectal tone, indicates efferent or motor denervation. However, preservation of perineal sensation does not necessarily mean that the efferents are intact.

Since renal failure is an important cause of death in these patients, treatment is directed toward preventing obstruction and infection. An intravenous urogram is done as soon as the back wound is healed. This examination identifies associated upper tract anomalies, which have been reported to be present in 20 percent of cases; in addition it establishes a baseline for subsequent studies, that are done yearly until the child is stabilized, and then biennially. Urine cultures are performed every 3 months. Suprapubic aspiration is the most reliable method of obtaining urine. This procedure is particularly applicable because most of these children have anesthesia of the suprapubic area.

Voiding cystourethrograms are not done routinely, since instrumentation of the bladder in these children is accompanied by a significant incidence of infection. Furthermore, vesicoureteral reflux in newborns with myelomeningocele is unusual. Congenital anomalies of the vesicoureteral junction do not appear to be an associated abnormality in children with myelodysplasia, as suggested by some authors. Rather, the later high incidence of reflux seen in older children with myelodysplasia seems to be related to recurrent infections and to progressive neuropathic bladder dysfunction. We reserve voiding or expression cystourethrograms for those children who present with or who develop upper urinary tract changes or who become infected de novo.

Infections are treated with appropriate short courses of antibiotics. Long-term therapy is reserved for infections that recur frequently. The usual cause in such cases is inadequate bladder emptying due to relatively high outlet resistance. This can be managed in a variety of ways. Pharmacologic manipulation of the bladder outlet using drugs such as phenoxybenzamine, an α-adrenergic blocking agent, has been shown to be effective in lowering bladder outlet and urethral resistance, thus accomplishing more complete bladder evacuation. This treatment may be combined with Urecholine if the detrusor is hypotonic. Endoscopic resection of the bladder neck or YV-plasty may be used in conjunction with pharmacologic drugs if the latter prove insufficient alone. Johnston and Kathel have reported effective bladder drainage and upper urinary tract decompression in neonates with overdistended bladders by simply overdilating the posterior urethra and bladder neck, which can be performed easily in girls through the urethral meatus. In boys it must be done through a perineal urethrotomy because of the narrow penile urethra. Some 20 percent of babies were found to have distended incompletely expressible bladders shortly after neurosurgical closure of their myelomeningoceles, and a high proportion of them showed upper tract dilatation on intravenous urography.

The exact site of obstruction in these children remains a topic of debate. Johnston and Farkas, on the basis of urethral pressure profile measurements, believe that the dilated posterior urethra that is often seen in such cases results from paresis of the musculature of the proximal urethra above the relatively undistensible membranous urethra within the rigid perineal membrane rather than from external sphincter spasm. They contend that urethral resistance does not have to be greater than normal to be obstructive when there is a defective detrusor muscle. Others, notably Stark, as well as Zachary and Lister, have implicated the external urethral sphincter as the obstructive site and have reported good results with pudendal neurectomy and with external sphincterotomy. More recently a great deal of enthusiasm has been voiced for intermittent urethral catheterization in those cases where simple manual expression or Urecholine fails to empty the bladder adequately. Rabinovitch and Lyon and associates have reported good results with intermittent catheterization in the hands of trained and responsible parents. Electrical stimulation of the detrusor muscle itself or of its nerve supply has been employed, but the method has practical and technical difficulties and for the present must be regarded as experimental.

Ileal or sigmoid conduits or external urinary diversion were until recently considered by many authors to be the treatments of choice in children with myelodysplasia, since the child was kept dry and this was thought to be the best method of preserving the upper urinary tract. However, it is now clear that diversion does not alway preserve renal parenchyma, and the longer one follows these patients the more deterioration is seen. Most recent work suggests that permanent external urinary diversion should be reserved as the procedure of last resort. Conservative treatment as outlined above to gain better bladder emptying, combined with antireflux operations where indicated, as well as effective treatment of infection, should be tried for initial treatment.

Treatment is aimed not only at prolonging life but also at improving the quality of life. This involves producing a bladder that will provide adequate dry periods between voidings. Constant wetting with its attendant malodor, excoriation, and bedsores will reduce patients to miserable social outcasts. If adequate dry periods cannot be attained with bladder training, including voiding on schedule, credé, drugs, and the surgical procedures listed above, males are fitted with a penile collecting device or alternatively are given a trial of intermittent catheterization. There is, of course, no adequate collecting device for females. Thus if intermittent catheterization is not feasible or is unsuccessful a procedure to divert the urine must be performed. The site of the stoma must be carefully chosen so as not to interfere with orthopedic appliances. The isolated ileal or sigmoid conduit is the best form of diversion, but cutaneous ureterostomies may be preferable when the ureters are grossly dilated. Hip surgery, if indicated, should precede diversion, since management of the stoma in a child with a double hip spica can present a formidable problem.

PENIS

PREPUCE. The preputial skin normally is redundant. In newborns the visceral surface frequently is adherent to the glans penis; these adhesions usually resolve spontaneously during infancy. Accumulation of smegma from the preputial glands admixed with retained urine may produce chemical irritation or permit secondary infection, resulting in balanitis or balanoposthitis. In such cases the adhesions are lysed, allowing retraction of the prepuce; release of the retained infected smegma and resolution of the inflammation with local treatment is then readily accomplished. Recurrent episodes of balanoposthitis or balanitis associated with inability to retract the prepuce because of a narrow preputial opening (*phimosis*) is best treated by elective circumcision after the acute inflammation has subsided. *Paraphimosis* results in a patient with mild phimosis when the prepuce is retracted behind the glans, becomes edematous, and then cannot be reduced. If it is left untreated vascular obstruction results and gangrene of the glans can occur. Older children must be sedated in order to reduce the paraphimosis. Occasionally a dorsal slit through the constricted preputial ring is necessary. Circumcision is indicated, but should be delayed until the edema has resolved.

Circumcision is the most common urologic operation performed in infancy and childhood. Extreme phimosis with ballooning of the prepuce on micturition, phimosis with complicating balanoposthitis, and an espisode of paraphimosis are indications for circumcision. Campbell reported five fatalities in children with severe phimosis and secondary obstructive uremia. Ritualistic circumcision of the neonate is practiced by Jews, among whom, it is interesting to note, carcinoma of the penis is virtually nonexistent. The prevalence of carcinoma of the cervix in the female partners of circumcised men also seems to be lower, but this claim has not been confirmed. Circumcision is not altogether a benign procedure. Complications include postoperative hemorrhage, which is not uncommon and may be alarming. Medical and religious authorities consider a recongnized familial bleeding tendency as a definite contraindication. Partial or even complete amputation of the glans is not unknown, and extensive burning and subsequent sloughing of part of the penis may follow the use of diathermy. Excessive removal of penile skin can lead to scarring and contractures. Insufficient removal of mucosa can result in recurrent phimosis. Deeply placed sutures have produced urethral fistulae. Meatal ulcers due to ammoniacal dermatitis and diaper rash are much more common in circumcised boys and may lead to meatal stenosis. Circumcision is contraindicated in boys with hypospadias or genital anomalies that might require preputial skin for later surgical reconstructions. The anesthetic risk for the older infant is low but cannot be disregarded. In a series of 90,000 circumcisions Gardner found a mortality rate of 0.018 percent.

HYPOSPADIAS. Hypospadias is a common urogenital anomaly in which the external urethral meatus lies on the ventral aspect of the penis proximal to the normal site (Fig. 21); it occurs in approximately 1 in 160 male children. The urethral groove normally closes ventrally by progressive fusion of the urogenital folds from behind forward. In patients with hypospadias it fails to complete its development. Because the posterior urethra develops from a separate embryologic anlage (the urogenital sinus), continence is never deficient. More than 50 percent of cases are of the minor glandular and subcoronal types. Penile, penoscrotal, and scrotal hypospadias account for 30 to 40 percent, and the remaining small number are of the perineal type. The minor forms frequently are associated with meatal stenosis. Other features include chordee and lack of normal ventral preputial skin, or the presence of fibrous bands that produce ventral curvature of the glans and penile shaft. Together these features give the penis a hooded or cobra-head appearance. When the urethral meatus opens proximal to the penoscrotal junction the scrotum remains incompletely fused; in the perineal type it is completely bifid.

There is a tendency for hypospadias to be familial. Recent data suggest a low prevalence of associated anomalies of the upper urinary tract. This is in sharp contrast to previously published data, where anomalies were reported to range from 11 to 25 percent. The author, in collaboration with Lutzker, reviewed 80 urograms performed in 120 children with uncomplicated hypospadias. Eight children had anomalies that we would regard as variations of normal. These included six partial uncomplicated duplications, one malrotated kidney, and one lobulated kidney. Two children had mildly dilated ureters, one with and one without reflux; neither required treatment. Treatment was required in only one patient, a boy with a ureteropelvic junction obstruction. Thus the incidence of anomalies requiring treatment was less than 1 percent. The findings in this small unpublished series were recently corroborated by a much larger series by McArdle and Lebowitz, who reviewed 200 urograms in uncomplicated hypospadiacs. Six children (3 percent) had anomalies, which included two horseshoe kidneys, one pelvic kidney with reflux, two duplicated collecting systems, and one absent kidney. Only one required treatment. Previous studies attempting to define the incidence of upper tract anomalies in uncomplicated hypospadias have been inaccurate and misleading. Minor variants such as duplications and malrotation, nonexistent entities such as bladder neck obstruction, reflux without infection or upper tract changes, and enlarged utricles have been included. The prevalence of significant upper tract anomalies appears to be no greater than in the general population if the criteria of Donahue and associates are used.

Cryptorchidism occurs in about 15 percent of cases of hypospadias and is often bilateral. The severe forms of hypospadias, especially with incomplete scrotal fusion and undescended testes, should be evaluated carefully to exclude problems of intersex (see p. 1695).

Initial treatment of glandular hypospadias is aimed at alleviating meatal stenosis, if it is present. A dorsal meatotomy should be done as soon as the condition is diagnosed. In the neonate no anesthesia is required, and the procedure can be done in the nursery simply by dividing the septum between the dorsal blind pit and the urethra itself. If there is no chordee nothing further need be done. However, excision of the redundant dorsal hood (a modified circumcision) will improve the cosmetic appearance of the penis considerably.

Patients with chordee require straightening of the penis. Formerly this was accomplished by one of several surgical techniques, all of which resulted in the urethral meatus retracting to a more proximal position after excision of the chordee or fibrous bands. This so-called first stage was generally performed between 12 and 18 months of age. The second stage, urethroplasty to advance the meatus, was generally deferred until age 3½ to 4½ years. Moreover, the parents were cautioned that often more than two stages would be required, since fistulae were not at all uncommon with standard urethroplasties. In 1968 Allen and Spence described a new technique for correction of glandular and coronal hypospadias with chordee, which involved straightening of the penis without the need to free the urethra. This innovative operation left the urethral meatus at its preoperative location and thus eliminated the need for a urethroplasty. The operation is based upon the observation made earlier by Smith and later Nesbit that all chordee were not due to fibrous bands distal to the meatus. Cutaneous tethering proximal to the meatus often causes ventral bowing of the glans and the shaft, and thus extensive freeing of these skin bands can accomplish the straightening just as effectively. Soon thereafter King described a further modification of the Spence-Allen operation that allowed straightening of the penis as well as a distal urethroplasty in the distal penile types of hypospadias with mild to moderate chordee. Fistulae occur rarely with this technique, and thus for the first time the surgeon was armed with a reliable, effective, and relatively simple single-stage operation for correcting the majority of hypospadias. Hodson has described an excellent, although technically more difficult, single-stage operation for penile hypospadias with even marked chordee. His operation utilizes the prepuce for creating the new urethra as well as for covering the resulting skin defect secondary to the straightening. In effect, the experienced urologist can now accomplish successful repairs in a single stage in most children with hypospadias. The repair is generally performed when the patient is between 1 and 4 years of age. Staged procedures are presently reserved by this author for a small group of severe hypospadiacs (10 to 15 percent of the total) where the meatus opens at or proximal to the proximal third of the penile urethra. The ultimate goal is a straight penis with a urethral meatus placed sufficiently distal to allow the child to stand when urinating and to direct his stream without difficulty. Such a result will permit normal coitus, and the cosmetic appearance of the penis should be satisfactory.

EPISPADIAS-EXSTROPHY COMPLEX. Classic exstrophy of the bladder with epispadias is the most common manifestation of a series of anomalies ranging from simple mild epispadias to complete cloacal exstrophy. It occurs once in every 30,000 to 50,000 births, and thus about 100 children with exstrophy are born each year in the United States. The ratio of males to females is 2 to 1. There is no prominent familial predisposition, although isolated cases of exstrophies occurring in the same family, in siblings, and in twins have been reported.

The anomaly results from a failure of midline fusion of the mesodermal structures in the infraumbilical abdominal wall. Muecke has reproduced the anomaly in chicks by placing a minute plastic disk over the cloacal membrane, thus obstructing mesodermal migration. Multiple organ systems in the lower abdomen are involved, including the genitourinary tract, the musculoskeletal tract, and in the severest forms the intestinal tract. There is shortening in the sagittal plane as well as midline failure, so that the umbilicus is displaced downward and the anus forward, and the scrotum is somewhat anteriorly situated and typically flat. The bladder is completely everted, and the ureteral orifices can be seen to efflux urine, constantly bathing the abdominal wall and perineum. The penis is short and flat, and the urethra appears as a short mucosal strip on the dorsum of the penis. There is wide diastasis of the symphysis pubis and the rectus muscles. There is almost always an umbilical hernia, and inguinal hernias are common. The weak pelvic floor commonly allows rectal prolapse, which may be severe. Upper urinary tract anomalies are unusual.

Treatment is aimed at preserving renal function, preventing the complications of continued incontinence (which no appliance can control), construction of a penis in the male, and improving the appearance of the abdominal wall and genitalia. The continual incontinence and the ulcerated, inflamed, exposed bladder render most children with untreated exstrophy very irritable and bad-tempered, which serves to accentuate hernias and aggravate rectal prolapse.

Pyelonephritis usually does not occur in early infancy, but over a period of time infection and obstruction take their toll in untreated patients; about two-thirds die before age 21. Those who survive have an increased liability to neoplastic change in the exposed bladder epithelium.

Early treatment consists of measures to protect the skin of the perineum and abdominal wall from excoriation. Vaseline gauze and various barrier creams, in addition to frequent diaper changes, are important. Definitive treatment involves primary closure of the bladder (with or without iliac osteotomies) or urinary diversion. Those children with very small bladders are best diverted, since they have the smallest chance of attaining continence with reconstructive surgery. Moreover, they appear more prone to develop upper tract damage if continence is achieved. Ureterosigmoidostomy is probably the diversion of choice, providing the anus is continent, since it avoids an external appliance.

If possible it should be deferred until the child is old enough to cooperate in timed evacuations. Primary reconstruction in the suitable case with a large pliable bladder seems worthwhile, since it offers the patient the possibility of normalcy or near normalcy that cannot be claimed for any other form of therapy. The reported results suggest that the two-stage approach, involving bladder closure followed by later combined anti-incontinence and antireflux surgery, offers the best chance of attaining continence with the least risk to the upper urinary tract. Such a program of staged reconstruction in selected cases results in good urinary control in about 20 to 40 percent of children. However, a proportion of these subsequently require diversion for deterioration of their upper tracts secondary to obstruction, persistent infection, and bladder calculi.

Incontinent boys can occasionally be controlled with an external penile collecting device, so that closure may represent a reasonable compromise for those whose upper tracts remain stable and free of major infection. For boys who cannot be fitted with an incontinence device, and for incontinent girls, urinary diversion is the treatment of choice. Ureterosigmoidostomy is preferred when the ureters are undilated, since this allows for an adequate antireflux ureterocolonic anastomosis. Where the ureters are significantly dilated or where anal continence is inadequate, urinary diversion is best made into an isolated ileal or sigmoid loop. Since the epispadias-exstrophy complex involves multiple organs, reconstructive surgery in most cases involves not merely closure or diversion of the urinary tract but also cosmetic surgery of the genital and abdominal wall as well as hernia repair.

Various schedules are used by different surgeons to rehabilitate these children. In boys, genital reconstruction, particularly dorsal chordee release, is generally carried out early in the reconstructive program, since it is more difficult to accomplish once the penile urethra has been closed. More recently, surgical techniques for penile lengthening have been developed. These are generally performed in adolescence or early adulthood (see Fig. 21 for summary of different plans of reconstruction). In girls, genital reconstruction and cosmetic surgery to create mons veneris and normal female-appearing escutcheon is generally deferred until after puberty.

Children with epispadias usually are incontinent. Reconstructive bladder neck surgery together with closure of the urethra should be attempted. Williams reported on 27 such children in 1965; he achieved successful control in 70 percent of the girls and 47 percent of the boys. For those few children with epispadias but no incontinence, simple closure of the urethra suffices, and a good cosmetic and functional result can be obtained.

TESTIS

CRYPTORCHIDISM. The testes develop from the medial aspects of the urogenital ridges, which extend from the thorax to the sacrum. By differential growth, with cranial degeneration and caudal differentiation, the testes come to lie opposite the internal inguinal rings by the sixth month of gestation. In the last trimester they traverse the inguinal canals and reach the scrotum. Scorer, on the basis of 1,700 examinations,

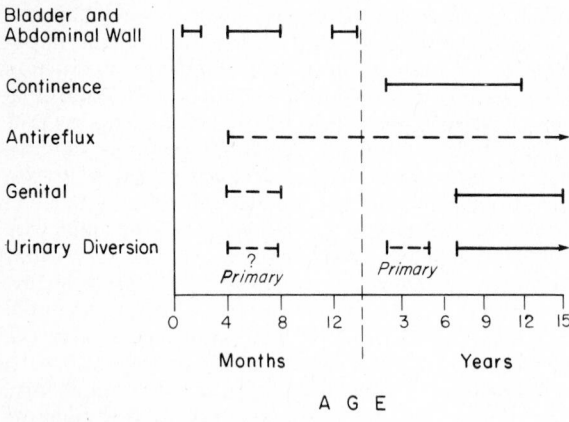

FIG. 21. Surgical reconstruction of the child with complete exstrophy-epispadias. A summary of timetables used in various centers for the rehabilitation of these children. (Courtesy of Dr. S. J. Kogan.)

defined a descended testis in the full-term neonate as one that with gentle traction can be coaxed 4 cm below the pubic arch, with 2.5 cm as the minimum distance in prematures. Most testes descend fully within 6 weeks after birth in full-term infants and within 3 months in prematures. With this definition, Scorer found the prevalence of cryptorchidism to be 30 percent in prematures, 4 percent in full-term infants, and 0.66 percent at 1 year of age. Since the prevalence of cryptorchidism in adults is between 0.28 and 0.8 percent, the belief that formerly was widely held, that undescended testes frequently descend spontaneously and completely at puberty, is untenable. Spontaneous complete descent after infancy is uncommon, and even if it does occur the testis may have suffered degenerative changes proportionate to its delay in reaching the scrotum. Late spontaneous descent, therefore, is to be neither expected nor desired.

Cryptorchidism is more common on the right side and is bilateral in approximately 20 percent of cases. There are two main types. In the incompletely descended variety the testis stops somewhere along its normal path of descent and may be found anywhere between the abdomen and upper part of the scrotum. Most of these testes are located at the superficial inguinal ring or within the inguinal canal. The second variety is the ectopic testis, which is located most commonly in the superficial inguinal pouch between Scarpa's fascia and the external oblique aponeurosis. However, it may also be found in pubic, femoral, or perineal locations.

It is important to differentiate undescended testes from retractile testes, since no treatment is required for the latter condition. In childhood an active cremasteric reflex elevates the testis in response to cold, stress, or merely palpation; however, careful examination reveals that it can be manipulated into the bottom of the scrotum. Failure to differentiate retractile from undescended testes has invalidated many statistical analyses of the prevalence of cryptorchidism, its spontaneous resolution, and its response to gonadotropins.

Embryologic studies suggest that descent is controlled by production of testosterone by the testis under the influence of chorionic or possibly fetal pituitary gonadotropic hormone. The pathogenesis of nondescent is obscure. The occurrence of undescended testes in siblings as well as in fathers and sons suggests a genetic etiology. Hormonal deficiencies have been postulated, but they seem unlikely in view of the absence of other endocrinopathy and the poor response of the unilateral undescended testis to exogenous gonadotropin. In the majority of instances hormonal stimulation appears to be adequate, and the testis either fails to respond because of an intrinsic deficiency or is prevented from descending by an anatomic hindrance. Fibrous bands, a narrow inguinal canal, and inadequate length of spermatic vessels frequently are noted at surgery, but they are just as likely to be the result as the cause of the condition.

Histologic examination of the undescended testis after the age of 5 years reveals a lag in development as compared with the normally descended contralateral organ. At and after puberty the undescended testis degenerates rapidly. Fertility is unusual in untreated bilateral cryptorchid men, and many reports show a fertility rate of less than 30 percent in untreated patients with the unilateral variety. In contrast, Gross reported a rate of fertility exceeding 80 percent in his treated bilateral cryptorchids and even more encouraging figures for fertility in patients treated for unilateral nondescent.

Torsion, trauma, and malignancy are more common in undescended testes than in normal testes. The increased risk for malignancy overall is about 20-fold, and abdominal varieties are probably even more prone to develop neoplastic change. However, perspective must be maintained despite these alarming statistics, since testicular tumors are rare. Although the cryptorchid has about a 1.5 percent chance of developing a tumor, the majority of these are seminomas, with an excellent prognosis. Orchiopexy, although it does not change the malignant potential, does allow easy examination and prompt recognition should a tumor develop. Where malignancy has developed the average delay before presentation has been 15 years. The bilateral cryptorchid is particularly at risk, a tumor in one testis indicating a chance of malignancy in the other of 1 in 4.

The prevalence of urinary tract anomalies in cryptorchid boys has been reported to be as high as 20 percent in some series. An attempt was recently made by Watson and associates to reconcile the high incidence of silent upper tract disease reported in the literature with the widely held clinical conviction that significant findings are rare. Four hundred cases, including 84 of their own asymptomatic cryptorchid boys, were critically analyzed (Table 14.) Significant anomalies were found in 3 percent. They concluded that "since the cryptorchid patient carries an above average risk of silent upper tract disease careful clinical attention must be given to this possibility in every case. Clearly any additional evidence of upper tract disease or the presence of other congenital anomalies makes IVU mandatory. However, routine urography in the otherwise asymptomatic patient should only be undertaken with the realization that, contrary to previous reports in the literature, this test will result in a low yield of truly significant upper tract disease." Infants with bilateral impalpable undescended testes should have buccal smears to exclude cases of female pseudohermaphroditism, such as congenital adrenal hyperplasia with complete fusion of the urogenital folds and a normally appearing penile urethra.

TABLE 14. Upper Urinary Tract Anomalies in 400 Asymptomatic Cryptorchid Boys: Composite Analysis[a]

	No. Cases	Percent
Duplicated collecting system	11	2.75
Ureteral dilatation (without demonstrated reflux)	10	2.50
Renal malrotation (without obstruction)	6	1.50
Ureteropelvic junction obstruction (2 cases with significant secondary hydronephrosis[b])	5	1.25
Hydronephrosis, bilateral[b]	4	1.00
Ectopia of kidney or ureter (without obstruction)	4	1.00
Renal hypoplasia[b]	3	0.75
Horseshoe kidney	3	0.75
Calyceal diverticulum (1 with calculus within)	3	0.75
Ureteral reflux with secondary renal parenchymal loss[b]	2	0.50
Nonvisualization of ipsilateral kidney with contralateral megaloureter[b]	1	0.25

[a] *From Watson et al: J Urol 8:789, 1974.*
[b] *These cases constitute clinically significant upper tract pathology by Donohue's criteria.*

Treatment of the true undescended and ectopic unilateral testis is surgical; the optimum age is 5 years. The writer does not recommend a trial of hormonal treatment in boys with a unilateral undescended testis, as has been advocated by some. However, patients with bilateral undescended testes may benefit from a course of gonadotropin. Dougherty reported success in bringing about descent in one-third of such patients using Follutein (chorionic gonadotropin) in three doses of 3,300 units each over a 10-day period. Patients who do not respond should have surgical exploration, except in the situations qualified below. Failure to locate a testis in the groin should direct the surgeon to a thorough exploration of the pelvis and abdomen on that side, since agenesis accounts for only 2 percent of impalpable un-

descended testes. An intraabdominal testis may on occasion require a two-stage orchiopexy to bring it into good position within the scrotum. The author prefers high ligation of the testicular vessels, provided that good collateral circulation through vasal, cremasteric, and gubernacular vessels has been demonstrated prior to transection. This allows the testes to be brought well down into the scrotum in a single operation.

Bilateral impalpable undescended testes in an otherwise normal phenotypic male should be differentiated from congenital bilateral anorchia. The presence of functioning testicular tissue can be reliably identified by a human chorionic gonadotropin (HCG) test, in which serum testosterone levels are measured by radioimmunoassay before and after the intramuscular administration of 1,500 units of A.P.L. on alternate days for three doses. A negative HCG response with no rise in serum testosterone in the child with raised levels of serum gonadotropins obviates the need for extensive surgical exploration.

TORSION.   In the absence of trauma the sudden or gradual onset of groin pain associated with testicular swelling and scrotal edema must be considered to be testicular torsion until proved otherwise. Mumps orchitis and epididymo-orchitis must be differentiated, but they are rare conditions in the prepubertal child. Torsion of müllerian and wolffian duct vestiges may mimic testicular torsion. However, excision of these gangrenous twisted appendages results in less morbidity than if they are treated conservatively. Idiopathic testicular infarction is a rare condition that may simulate torsion. Its etiology is obscure, and it may involve only a portion of the testis.

Torsion of the spermatic cord may be supravaginal, with only a loose attachment of the tunica vaginalis to the scrotal wall; this variety predominates in infancy. The intravaginal type occurs where the tunica covers the whole epididymis and extends unusually far up the spermatic cord. The testis and epididymis are suspended from the tunica by a narrow vascular pedicle that can readily twist. This is the more common variety in older children. Torsion of a redundant mesorchium where wide separation of the testis and epididymis occurs is a rarer abnormality that results in testicular strangulation without epididymal involvement.

Treatment consists of prompt exploration, detorsion, and fixation of the testis to the scrotum. Since the predisposing anomaly is bilateral in at least 50 percent of cases, fixation of the opposite side should be accomplished during the same operation.

HYDROCELE.   Primary vaginal hydrocele in children is the result of incomplete obliteration of the processus vaginalis. It is always communicating, even though the very small connection with the peritoneal cavity may be difficult to demonstrate. Spontaneous cure is likely and usually occurs within the first few months of life. However, some may take as long as a year to close, and unless the hydrocele is associated clinically with a hernia or is very large when first seen or continues to enlarge, no treatment is required in the first year.

Encysted hydroceles of the cord have the same pathogenesis. They can be differentiated from vaginal hydroceles by the fact that the testis is palpable distally. They are distinguished from tumors of the cord by transillumination and by their fluctuant cystic feel. Treatment is the same as for vaginal hydroceles.

FEMALE GENITALIA

Examination of the female genitalia may reveal significant abnormalities. *Vaginal aplasia* may be recognized by an absent vaginal opening or a shallow depression. Associated serious upper urinary tract anomalies have been reported in 30 to 50 percent of cases. *Epispadias,* although extremely rare without associated exstrophy, can occur as an isolated anomaly. *Vaginal cysts,* which derive from the epoophoron or Gartner's duct, may present at the level of the hymen. Differential diagnosis must consider a paraurethral cyst, a urethral diverticulum, an ectopic ureterocele, or hydrocolpos associated with a bulging obstructing hymen. Suprapubic and rectal examinations are done to exclude the pelvic mass of hydrocolpos, and probing of the vagina assures its patency. Ureteroceles are usually associated with duplications of the upper tract, and thus intravenous urography and voiding cystourethrography are helpful. *Hydrocolpos* most often results from vaginal obstruction above the hymen, and no bulging or cystic mass is visible. Septa most commonly occur at the junction of the upper and middle thirds of the vagina and result from failure of fusion between the sinovaginal bulbs of the urogenital sinus and the fused müllerian ducts. *Adherent labia minora* is not a congenital condition but results from mild trauma in the presence of the hypoestrogenic state of childhood. Vulvovaginitis may be the precipitating factor. The adhesions are readily lysed mechanically, and recurrence is prevented by the application of dienestrol cream. *Urethral prolapse* is occasionally seen in girls following a period of coughing or straining. Resection or ligation of the prolapsed mucosa may be required. There is little or no tendency for urethral meatal stenosis to occur. *Hymenal polyps* occur not infrequently. Very rarely mesonephric carcinoma or sarcoma botryoides will be detected by the discovery of a vaginal mass that appears similar.

Girls with anorectal anomalies may have rectovaginal or rectovesical fistulas. Low anorectal anomalies in the female are associated only occasionally with urinary tract abnormalities, whereas these are present in two-thirds of patients with high anomalies.

OBSTRUCTIVE UROPATHY AND ANOMALIES OF KIDNEYS AND URETERS

Obstructive uropathy refers to an impedance to normal urinary flow that may be located anywhere along the course of the urinary drainage system. It may be organic or functional; in neonates, infants, and children it is usually congenital.

Ureteropelvic Obstruction

Hydronephrosis due to obstruction at the ureteropelvic junction is the most common upper tract obstruction encountered in children. It is slightly more common in boys than in girls. When it is unilateral the left side is more commonly involved than the right. Bilateral involvement has been reported in 11 to 25 percent and is more common in infants than in older children. In some patients the pathology in the opposite kidney becomes overt only after ablative surgery on the first side. Hydronephrosis is encountered at all ages, but most often during the first 6 months of life, when it is discovered most frequently as an abdominal mass. In later childhood abdominal or flank pain or hematuria following minor trauma is the more common mode of presentation. In infants transillumination in a darkened room using a fiberoptic light source may reveal the cystic nature of the mass. The diagnosis may be made with high-dose intravenous urography, with early films to outline the parenchymal thickness and later films to delineate the site of obstruction and extent of pyelocaliectasis. Ultrasonography will identify the cystic nature of the mass and will exclude a Wilms' tumor or mesonephric blastoma, although occasionally differentiation from multicystic kidney and from tumor with extensive necrosis and hemorrhage is difficult.

The basic cause of the obstruction is still in dispute. Compression of the ureter by aberrant vessels has been implicated frequently. Fibrous bands, a high insertion of the ureter into the pelvis, and organic stenosis account for some cases. The most widely favored explanation, however, suggests a functional obstruction, with peristaltic waves from the renal pelvis failing to be transmitted to the ureter across the ureteropelvic junction. Murnaghan explains this dysfunction on the basis of an interruption of the circular element of the musculature. Vesicoureteral reflux must be excluded as a cause of ureteropelvic obstruction, particularly in patients with infection, since secondary acquired obstructions may result.

The treatment is surgical and involves plastic repair of the ureteropelvic junction. Nephrectomy may be required, but conservative procedures generally should be tried first, since most kidneys are salvageable and contralateral kidney disease is not uncommon. Often the radiographic appearance of the grossly dilated pelvis and calyces changes little postoperatively, but progression of disease is prevented. Excellent clinical response, including absence of pain, infection, and complicating calculi, can be expected.

Horseshoe Kidney

Horseshoe kidney occurs in about 1 of every 600 individuals. It results from incomplete ascent, failure of rotation, and fusion of the two metanephric blastemal masses. The isthmus is at the lower pole in more than 90 percent of cases, and ureteral duplication as well as obstruction, particularly at the ureteropelvic junction, is fairly common. Many children experience vague abdominal pain that is difficult to explain in the absence of complicating infection, hydronephrosis, or calculi. Surgical division of the isthmus for relief of pain has been advocated, but its efficacy is dubious. Many horseshoe kidneys function normally and require no treatment at all. Those with obstruction should have appropriate corrective surgery. Horseshoe kidneys have been reported with increased frequency in Turner's syndrome.

Ectopic Kidney

An ectopic kidney is usually associated with a normally placed contralateral kidney. It derives its importance from the frequent association with ureteropelvic or ureteral obstruction as well as vesicoureteral reflux. The usual site is pelvic or sacroiliac, but rare cases of thoracic kidney have been reported. The lower abdominal location renders the organ easily palpable on abdominal or bimanual examination. It can be differentiated from a ptotic kidney, which is rare in children, by its anomalous short vessels and short ureter. Should the ectopic organ cross the midline during embryologic development, fusion usually results and is termed crossed fused ectopia. The crossed organ in such situations lies below and medial to the normally placed one. Pelvic ectopia is not uncommonly associated with anorectal abnormalities and may be found incidentally at the time of an abdominal-perineal pull-through procedure for anorectal agenesis.

Obstruction of Ureter and Ureterovesical Junction

Megaureter or megaloureter is literally a large, dilated ureter. However, in urologic parlance the term generally implies chronic ureteral dilatation without overt organic obstruction. Hydroureter, in contrast, is a dilated ureter consequent to organic obstruction, either of the ureter itself or of the bladder or urethra. Megaureters may be divided into those with free vesicoureteral reflux and those without reflux, in which there is an impediment to emptying of the lower ureter of a functional nature. In the latter, referred to as primary obstructive megaureter, the basic pathology is unexplained, and the ureter is dilated in all but its terminal segment. Cases with other congenital anomalies, such as ureteral duplication, ectopia, and ureterocele, are not included in this definition, although the obstructive element may be very similar.

Primary obstructive megaureter is mainly a disease of early life. Males predominate; the left side is much more frequently involved than the right, and bilateral disease is common, particularly during infancy. Infection is the most common complication. However, pain, hematuria, or uremia may be the presenting features.

Management is conservative in those with mild disease. Failure to clear infection or radiographic demonstration of progression of the dilatation necessitates excision of the obstructing segment and ureteral reim-

plantation. If the disease is unilateral and the kidney has been destroyed by hydronephrotic atrophy, nephroureterectomy is the preferred treatment.

Vesicoureteral reflux is occasionally associated with massive ureteral dilatation, which is referred to as the refluxing megaureter. The distinction between simple and massive dilatation is somewhat arbitrary, but suggests certain characteristics. These ureters show marked permanent dilatation on intravenous urography, as well as on retrograde cystography, that is distinct from the distensibility of ureters that is often seen during reflux, in which the dilatation is transitory and disappears rapidly with ureteral emptying. Cinegraphic studies reveal ineffective peristalsis, and the ureter is slow to empty. Severe hydronephrosis and marked parenchymal atrophy are the rule. Refluxing megaureters are usually encountered in early infancy, and the kidneys, in addition to hydronephrotic atrophy, may show dysplastic areas containing primitive tubules and glomeruli.

The capacity of the bladder, particularly when both ureters are involved, may be quite large, leading to the designation megaureter-megacystis syndrome. The walls of the bladder are smooth, and there is no trabeculation. The trigone may be large and the ureteral orifices spread widely apart. Despite the large capacity of the bladder, it is able to empty completely, although it may refill rapidly by return of refluxed urine from the megaureters. The large bladder capacity in megaureter-megacystis syndrome is thought to develop as a result of the unusually large volumes of urine that the viscus is required to accommodate. Swenson and Brenner have suggested that megaureter-megacystis syndrome is analagous to Hirschsprung's disease, but exhaustive histologic studies by Liebowitz and Bodian have shown that the ganglion cells in the bladder wall are normal in number and distribution.

Treatment is dependent upon the amount of remaining renal function and the capacity of the ureters to regain their tone. Preliminary temporary diversions may be required to assess these factors before embarking on reconstructive surgery or deciding upon permanent urinary diversion. However, most recent reports suggest a preference for primary reconstruction and ureteral tapering without preliminary upper tract diversions.

Ureteral Anomalies: Duplication, Ectopia, Ureterocele

The ureter develops embryologically as an outgrowth or bud from the wolffian duct. It then grows toward the caudal end of the nephrogenic cord, divides successively to form the pelvocalyceal system and collecting tubules, and in the process induces differentiation of the metanephric blastema to form the definitive kidney. Early division of the ureteric bud results in incomplete ureteral duplication, whereas an accessory bud arising directly from the wolffian duct produces complete duplication, with each ureter opening separately into the bladder or onto an ectopic site. Both buds grow into the undivided metanephrogenic mass, so that the resulting duplicated kidney is one continuous parenchymal structure with two collecting systems. The incidence of complete duplication is 1 per 150 births. The process frequently is bilateral. The sex incidence is equal, but females are recognized more frequently owing to complicating urinary tract infections. Ureteral duplication must be distinguished from a bifid renal pelvis, which is a normal variant occurring in 10 percent of the population.

Many duplicated ureters function normally. However, complications are not uncommon. The bifid ureters in the incomplete variety may show dilatation above their points of juncture as a result of abnormal peristalsis. In complete duplications where both ureters open into the trigone, the ureter opening cephalad and lateral, which serves the lower moiety of the duplicated kidney, has a shorter submucosal tunnel than its fellow and is thus more prone to reflux. Thus chronic pyelonephritis in the lower element is not uncommon. In such cases ureteral reimplantation or heminephroureterectomy may be necessary.

The complications and modes of presentation of ectopic ureters vary with the sex of the child and the position of the ectopic opening. In females, where the orifice usually is at the bladder neck, infection is often the first evidence of abnormality. When the orifice opens into the distal urethra, vagina, or vestibule, persistent wetting associated with normal micturition is the rule and is quite diagnostic. In the male the ectopic ureter enters the posterior urethra, ejaculatory duct, or vas. Epididymitis or urinary tract infection is the first evidence of abnormality. Intravenous urography, voiding cystourethrography, and endoscopy confirm the diagnosis. The ectopic ureter and renal segment that it subserves are usually markedly dilated and dysplastic; treatment is usually excision.

The ectopic ureter may be complicated by a ureterocele, which refers to ballooning of the submucosal portion of the ureter within the bladder. Females are affected seven times more frequently than males. Both sides are equally affected, and bilateral disease occurs in about 10 percent. The renal element involved characteristically is small and dysplastic, while the ureter is grossly dilated. The ureterocele may be so large as to obstruct both ureters as well as the bladder neck. Prolapse may occur in girls and appear as a pink swelling at the urethral meatus. Complicating infection is generally the mode of presentation. Standard treatment includes uncapping of the ureterocele and heminephroureterectomy. The ipsilateral ureter is reimplanted into the bladder employing an antirefluxing technique.

The simple ureterocele, involving the termination of a single normally situated ureter, results from stenosis of the ureteric orifice. It produces flank pain and may become infected. Diagnosis is established by intravenous urography, which demonstrates a typical cobra-head appearance at the ureteral termination. Cystoscopy confirms the diagnosis. Treatment requires uncapping of the ureterocele. Ureteral reimplantation by an antireflux technique is necessary in some cases.

Obstruction of Bladder Neck and Urethra

Minor degrees of obstruction to bladder outflow in the female are difficult to diagnose. Indeed, most authors now question whether obstruction is ever a factor in children with recurrent urinary tract infection, enuresis, or difficulty with urination. Voiding cystourethrograms in girls are difficult to interpret even when multiple films are taken during the act of micturition. Bougie à boule calibration of the urethra is often not diagnostic, since the range of normal is so large; furthermore, correlation with the findings on voiding cystourethrography is inconstant. Urethral calibration as a method of diagnosing obstruction has been criticized by those who regard the obstructive element as functional rather than organic. Endoscopic methods are notoriously inaccurate in demonstrating minor degrees of obstruction. Physiologic methods of testing, including measurement of detrusor pressures and flow rates and calculations of urethral outflow resistances, have such wide variations even in normal subjects that they are of limited value. Obstructions due to meatal stenosis, distal urethral stenosis, and bladder neck contraction do exist, but their prevalence rate remains in great dispute.

Urethral meatal stenosis is probably the most common outlet obstruction in the male child, particularly in circumcised infants. Most cases are acquired secondarily to meatitis and meatal ulcers. Diagnosis is made by observation of the voided stream, which is narrowed and forceful. Calibration confirms the stenosis. Ventral meatotomy may be required. The congenital variety is usually associated with glandular and subcoronal hypospadias. Dorsal meatotomy will relieve the obstruction in these cases.

Meatal stenosis only rarely results in serious outlet obstruction; the most severe examples of this in early infancy are caused by *posterior urethral valves,* which are saillike mucosal folds arising from the lower aspect of the verumontanum. Their cusps extend laterally and downward to become attached to the walls of the urethra. The resulting obstruction is severe, with elongation and dilatation of the posterior urethra and gross trabeculation of the bladder with cellules and saccules. Marked ureteral dilation, elongation, and tortuosity are the rule. Hydronephrotic renal atrophy is often severe, and various degrees of cystic dysgenesis complete the picture. The majority of cases present within the first year of life, with more than half of these in the first 3 months. Infants presenting in the neonatal period usually represent the most severe cases and have a high mortality rate if they are not treated promptly. Presentation within the first week is usually due to signs of renal failure or secondary infection. The bladder is distended and typically is very firm owing to gross hypertrophy of the detrusor muscle. Hydronephrotic kidneys may be palpable.

The status of the upper tracts is demonstrated with

high-dose intravenous urography and with tomography if necessary. A voiding cystourethrogram will demonstrate the classic picture of valves. Other less common causes of obstruction to be ruled out include urethral diverticulae, anterior urethral valves, posterior urethral polyps, trigonal cysts, Marion's disease (bladder neck obstruction), and urethral fibroelastosis.

Transurethral fulguration of the valves is performed after preparation for surgery, which involves rehydration and correction of electrolyte imbalance and may require 24 hours or more; a period of peritoneal dialysis may be needed. Perineal ureterostomy can often be avoided by using the newer, smaller Storz operating endoscope. When severe infection is present, or in patients with serious renal functional impairment or massive hydronephrosis, it is safer simply to divert the urine by high-loop ureterostomy, with definitive surgery being performed at a later date.

PRUNE-BELLY SYNDROME

Absence or deficiency of the abdominal wall musculature is one of a series of congenital defects of the anterior abdominal wall. These can involve the umbilicus alone (umbilical hernia, hernia into the cord, omphalocele), the paraumbilical abdominal wall (gastroschisis), the infraumbilical wall (ranging from simple epispadias to a cloacal anomaly), or the whole abdominal wall, as in the triad of prune-belly syndrome. Frölich reported the first case of absent abdominal wall musculature in 1839, but Parker in 1895 recognized the urologic implications and described the classic triad of absent abdominal wall musculature, bilateral undescended testes, and urinary tract anomalies. This syndrome was once considered rare, but to date 245 cases have been reported, most of them in the past 20 years. Almost all of the reported cases have involved males. The literature now covers nine females with deficiency of the abdominal wall musculature, but in six there were no associated urinary tract anomalies. Several of these had other multiple congenital anomalies.

Abnormalities of the urinary tract can range from mild to severe, with gross dysplasia involving the entire urinary tract, including kidneys, ureter, bladder, and urethra. The associated uropathy is in general so severe that 20 percent of reported infants are stillborn or die within the first month, and 50 percent are dead within 2 years. However, long-term survival has been recorded in two patients who survived to 60 and 70 years. The etiology remains obscure. Since the disease is almost entirely confined to males, a cytogenetic sex-linked abnormality has been suspected. However, for this to be so, an affected female could derive only from the mating of an affected male subject with a heterozygous female. Since no fertile males have been recorded, this cannot be the explanation. Moreover, a sex-linked recessive gene should result in examples of two or more affected brothers. However, apart from the report of Harley and associates concerning two siblings with missing number 16 chromosomes, and the report of Petersen and associates concerning affected twin boys with no chromosomal anomalies, no familial incidence has been recorded. Furthermore, seven sets of monozygotic twins discordant for the syndrome as well as one affected male of homozygous triplets have been reported, which further suggests that a nongenetic developmental disorder is move likely. Chromosomal studies, apart from those reported by Harley and associates, have been normal.

Urethral obstruction was thought at one time to be an essential part of the syndrome, and in fact it was postulated that severe obstruction resulted in a massively dilated urinary tract with secondary pressure atrophy of the abdominal wall musculature. However, in the many cases with similar obstructive distension due to posterior urethral valves the abdominal wall has been normal. Moreover, recent electron microscopic studies of the abdominal muscle demonstrating loss of coherence and orderly arrangement in the two bands, agglomeration of glycogen granules, and disruption of mitochondria (changes consistent with hypoplasia) support the theory of developmental arrest rather than secondary atrophy. Most recent authors have not been able to demonstrate definite organic obstructions in more than 10 to 20 percent of their cases. Williams and Burkholder measured detrusor pressures, maximum flow rate, and urethral resistance in five older children with the syndrome and found all parameters to be normal. Nunn and Stephens were not able to demonstrate abnormal pressure gradients between the bladder neck and urethral bulb in three of their patients. When it is present the obstruction is usually secondary to atresia or marked stenosis of the membranous portion of the urethra, although posterior urethral valves also occur. Roger and associates suggested that organic urethral obstruction without a patent urachus defines a lethal variant of this syndrome. Laxity of the abdominal wall and lack of counterpressure has been proposed as the cause of the urinary tract dilation. However, the absence of urinary anomalies in omphaloceles or large hernias makes this theory untenable. Audren and associates suggested that estrogen might cause dilation of the bladder and ureters and also cause failure of testicular descent. The facts that the external genitalia of these boys are unquestionably male and that seven sets of twins discordant for the syndrome have occurred contradict this theory. Ganglion cells are normal at the trigone and the bladder neck and within the ureters. The pelvic parasympathetic nerves and anterior spinal nerves are intact. The syndrome seems to suggest a dysplasia of the urinary tract and anterior abdominal wall secondary to some general disturbance in embryogenesis between 6 and 10 weeks of gestation.

The diagnosis of this syndrome is simple. The abdominal wall is lax and the skin wrinkled, giving the appearance of a wizened prune. Later, as the subcutaneous tissue increases, the skin smooths out and the abdomen is then more appropriately described as pot belly. The muscular weakness varies in degree and location, but is most common in the lower abdomen. The umbilicus is displaced upward. In infancy the weak belly leads to a flaring out of the lower chest with a wide subcostal margin. The diaphragm tends to be flattened, and because of a weakened cough mechanism, such a child is subject to respiratory complications. If anesthesia is required it must be carefully planned, and careful attention in the postoperative period is mandatory to avoid retention of secretions and postoperative atelectasis. These children need their accessory muscles for adequate ventilation, and a posture favoring efficient action of these muscles is helpful. Constipation may be a problem. An abdominal binder is all that is required to support the abdominal wall; surgical plication of the abdominal wall is unnecessary. The weakness becomes less significant as the patient grows older, and healing of abdominal wounds is uneventful.

The scrotum is hypoplastic. All but four of the reported patients have had bilateral undescended testes, usually in an intraabdominal position overlying the ureters. Orchiopexies are difficult and usually require two stages or high transection of the spermatic vessels, relying on the vasal arteries for adequate blood supply. Anomalies of the gastrointestinal tract are common, particularly malrotation. There is no record of any patient being fertile. Other features include talipes equinovarus, which is commonly present.

Urinary tract anomalies, though almost always present, can only be clearly defined radiographically. The anomalies may include a very large capacity bladder with its apex attached to the abdominal wall. A urachal diverticulum or patent urachus may be present; the bladder neck and posterior urethra are widely dilated and taper down to a membranous urethra of normal caliber. In most cases, as mentioned earlier, no organic obstruction is evident, although some have atresia or stenosis of the membranous or whole anterior urethra. A tubular utricular diverticulum may be present, arising from the urethra at the level of the verumontanum. Reflux is usually present, with the ureters showing massive irregular dilatation, usually most pronounced in the middle and lower thirds. Renal dysplasia is frequently present. Histologically the bladder and ureters are thickened. Patchy absence of muscle fibers with fibrous tissue replacement is the rule.

Treatment is difficult and must be individualized. The prognosis is largely dependent on the degree of renal dysplasia. Those with organic urethral obstruction require immediate high tubeless urinary diversion. Loop cutaneous ureterostomy is probably the procedure of choice, although in general these children have the greatest degree of renal dysplasia. When the urethra is patent, as in the majority, aggressive medical management of the frequent urinary tract infections is necessary, with careful monitoring of renal function. Staged reconstruction, including ureteral tailoring and reimplantations, reduction cystoplasty, and tailoring pyeloplasties, are feasible in some children. Urinary diversion by ureterostomies or ileal conduits may become necessary for those with uncontrolled infection, progressive dilatation, or decreasing renal function. Successful reconstruction is possible in selected cases even many years after urinary diversion provided that renal function is stable.

Vesicoureteral Reflux

The normal urinary tract has a delicately balanced ureterovesical valve mechanism that permits orderly flow of urine from the renal pelvis into the bladder and prevents its regurgitation back into the kidney. The anatomic and functional features that characterize the normal flap-valve mechanism include (1) an oblique entry of the intramural ureter into the bladder, (2) adequate length of the intramural ureter and especially the submucosal segment (the ratio of submucosal tunnel length to ureteral diameter has been shown to average 2.4:1 in newborns), (3) good support from the bladder musculature, (4) adequate distal fixation to a normal trigone by the ureterotrigonal ligaments, and (5) normal ureteral flexibility and peristalsis.

Several well-conducted studies in normal premature and full-term neonates, in children of different ages, and in adults have demonstrated that reflux at any age is an abnormal phenomenon. Moreover, Booth and associates, in a series of intrauterine fetal cystograms obtained at the time of fetal peritoneal blood transfusion for erythroblastosis fetalis, observed reflux in only 1 of 28 studies. When restudied at age 1 year this baby continued to exhibit bilateral reflux despite the absence of urinary tract infection, which suggests that the reflux was due to a congenital ureterovesical junction abnormality and that even in the fetus reflux should be considered abnormal.

Vesicoureteral reflux is due to a congenital deficiency of the longitudinal muscle of the submucosal ureter. The deficiency may be mild or severe, resulting in a spectrum of abnormalities that can be determined by measuring submucosal ureteral tunnel length and observing the appearance of the ureteral orifice. Mild abnormalities may allow the ureterovesical junction to remain competent under normal circumstances. However, when stressed by a minor bladder outlet obstruction, or by bladder dysfunction with increased intravesical pressure, or by a superimposed bladder infection, reflux will ensue. Amelioration of these stress factors allows the ureterovesical junction to return to its former competent state. The neonate and infant seem particularly prone to develop reflux in the presence of secondary stress situations, as seen with irritative contrast materials, high-pressure nonphysiologic instillation of dye into the bladder, and bladder infections. With growth the submucosal ureter elongates and the delicate ratio between submucosal tunnel length and ureteral diameter increases, making compromise of the antireflux mechanism less likely. Complete duplication of the collecting system, with implantation of the lower pole ureter more lateral and cephalad in the bladder, allows for a shorter submucosal tunnel and is classically associated with reflux into that ureter and therefore into the lower pole of the duplication. The well-known familial incidence of reflux, which may be genetically influenced, is further evidence in support of a congenital anomaly. Several authors have reported more than one member of a family affected with reflux where asymptomatic siblings of symptomatic patients have been studied.

Vesicoureteral reflux has been detected in 20 to 70 percent of children undergoing radiologic evaluation for recurrent urinary tract infections. Very young children with urinary tract infections have a particularly high prevalence of demonstrable reflux, especially boys. A systematic evaluation of the child with urinary tract infection is therefore essential for accurate diagnosis and prognosis and in planning appropriate therapy. Reflux may also result from iatrogenic causes, as seen following decompression of a ureterocele or implantation of a ureter into the bladder by a faulty technique.

Reflux can be suspected from intravenous urography but is best demonstrated in the conscious child during voiding cystourethrography, using image intensification and fluoroscopy. Expression cystography under anesthesia has been shown to be misleading and will fail to demonstrate reflux in as many as 50 percent of cases. Minor reflux occurs only on voiding (ie, high-pressure reflux) and may be present at one examination and absent at the next. More severe reflux occurs during filling of the bladder, as well as during voiding (low-pressure type), and is less likely to disappear spontaneously, especially if associated with ureteral dilatation and grossly abnormal ureteral orifices detected cystoscopically.

The clinical significance of reflux lies in the fact that it provides a ready pathway for bacteria to ascend from the bladder to the kidney, and therefore it can permit a lower urinary tract infection to develop into pyelonephritis. Reflux over long periods of time may also damage the ureteral and pelvic musculature, causing dilatation, loss of elasticity, and impaired peristalsis.

Vesicoureteral reflux appears to play a major role in focal pyelonephritic scarring in children. "Infected" reflux seems to carry the greatest risk of scarring, particularly in the very young when the reflux is severe and is associated with intrarenal extravasation. Sterile reflux unless severe or associated with lower urinary tract obstruction or a neurogenic bladder, does not seem to result in pelvocalyceal or parenchymal scarring, at least in the short term. Hodson recently showed that "sterile" high-pressure intrarenal reflux in pigs caused parenchymal scarring. Whether sterile intrarenal reflux due to pyelotubular backflow can result in scarring in humans is as yet not clear and must await further clarification.

Focal chronic pyelonephritis is a frequent complication that occurs in as many as 30 percent of children with major reflux. Reflux itself may predispose the child to recurrent infection by virtue of the refluxed urine returning to the bladder and acting as a residual after voiding. However, there is evidence to suggest that recurrent urinary tract infection is no more common in children with reflux than in those without reflux.

Younger children tend to have a relatively low incidence of pyelonephritis, as detected radiographically. However, with time an increasing number develop scarring that reflects continued exposure to infection, which may occur with mild as well as with severe degrees of reflux. Alternatively, scarring that is not obvious on initial radiography but that appears later or seems worse might represent failure of the parenchyma (damaged early by infection) to grow in proportion to the normal adjacent kidney tissue. The latter evolution would suggest that the scars seen on sequential urograms actually result from a single pyelonephritic episode early in infancy. Resolution of this question has important clinical implications.

Treatment is directed toward keeping the urine sterile and eliminating reflux. Antibacterial agents, adequate fluid intake, attention to proper perineal hygiene, and regular double voiding will accomplish this goal in about 50 percent of patients with mild reflux. Smellie has presented strong arguments for long-term chemotherapy for as long as reflux is observed. She has been able to maintain 76 percent of 84 children with reflux completely free from infection. Even more important, follow-up examinations in 24 of 26 refluxing children who initially had normal urograms showed normal renal growth and no fresh scars.

The indications for abandoning conservative therapy in favor of surgery would appear to be failure to attain the therapeutic goals of elimination of infection, protection of the kidneys from scarring, and spontaneous cessation of reflux within a reasonable period of time. More severe degrees of reflux, with moderate to marked ureterectasis on intravenous and voiding cystourethrography and grossly patulous displaced ureteral orifices as seen cystoscopically, will seldom experience spontaneous cure; these are best managed by early surgical correction. Fresh scarring, an inability to render the urine sterile with antibacterials, and follow-up radiologic studies showing marked ballooning of the ureter and pelvis indicate the need for antireflux surgery. It is also important that treatment be individualized, based upon the likelihood of parental and child compliance, when recommending a conservative program. The child from a family in difficult economic circumstances runs excessive risks and may be less likely to adhere to a long-term medical regimen with frequent follow-up visits. Parents must be brought into the decision-making process, especially in the gray areas of persistent, moderately severe, sterile reflux. Some parents, on learning the success rate of the reimplantation procedure, the chances of the problem not resolving spontaneously, and the possible risks of long-term reflux, will elect for an early surgical solution. They prefer to avoid the longer course of antibiotics and radiologic follow-up studies and the attendant apprehension during the child's formative years. Others will put off the decision for as long as the issue is in doubt.

In experienced hands the rate of success of antireflux surgery for relatively normal or moderately dilated ureters varies from 90 to 98 percent. In advanced, severely dilated ureters the success rate drops precipitously. Success implies absence of reflux with no further dilatation of the collecting system. Sterile urine is achieved without antibiotics in more than two-thirds of these children within a year of surgery. In children who continue to have recurrent bacteriuria the infection seems to be localized to the lower tract, since follow-up urography usually shows no evidence of progressive pyelonephritic scarring.

It is well to remember that the ultimate prognosis with regard to the serious implications of focal pyelonephritic scarring in children is unclear. Autopsy studies in children suggest that chronic pyelonephritis is an unusual cause of childhood death, except in the first year of life when associated with gross urologic anomalies. Adult autopsy studies begin to show significant numbers of deaths from chronic pyelonephritis only in women after age 45. However, it is difficult to conclude from these figures that chronic pyelonephritis is secondary to reflux, urinary tract infection, and scarring incurred during childhood. The reason for this dilemma is the pathologist's difficulty in separating chronic bacterial pyelonephritis from other forms of interstitial nephritis. This dilemma notwithstanding, there are patients who come to dialysis and transplantation centers with end-stage renal failure in early adulthood. These patients have classic histologic criteria of chronic pyelonephritis with vesicoureteral reflux, with or without a childhood history of recurrent urinary tract infections; they have no history of phenacetin abuse, do not have segmental hypoplasia, and are not arteriosclerotic or diabetic.

The problem with respect to urinary tract infections and vesicoureteral reflux seems to be our inability to predict which children will ultimately progress to end-stage renal failure. A rational approach in our present stage of ignorance would therefore appear to be identification of those children with urinary tract infections who have reflux, with the aim of eliminating the potentially damaging effects of this combination by treatment that involves the least morbidity.

NEOPLASMS OF GENITOURINARY TRACT

The genitourinary tract is the primary site in 6 to 10 percent of all malignant tumors in children. The prognosis for tumors treated before they have spread beyond the confines of the involved organ is encouraging. Malignant tumors of the genitourinary tract in infants and children can be classified into three groups: the one encountered most frequently is the nephroblastoma or Wilms' tumor; sarcoma botryoides or rhabdomyosarcoma arising from the urogenital sinus is less common and more lethal; the third group comprises the gonadal tumors, which are usually benign teratomas but can behave malignantly.

Nephroblastoma

Wilms' tumor is the most common malignant tumor of the genitourinary tract. It occurs in about 1 in 10,000 live births, and approximately 500 patients with Wilms' tumor are seen each year in the United States. If two siblings are affected the likelihood of a third child developing Wilms' tumor is 20 percent. The majority present between 6 months and 3 years of age. Sex incidence is equal. The tumor is bilateral in 5 to 10 percent of cases. Associated anomalies include aniridia, congenital hemihypertrophy, and genitourinary malformations.

A firm abdominal mass is the presenting sign in most children. Pain related to rapid growth and hemorrhage into the tumor are not infrequent. Hematuria occurs in about 30 percent. Fever is often seen, and hypertension has been reported in up to 60 percent. Spontaneous rupture with presenting signs of an acute abdomen may occur. Clinical evidence of spread is present in approximately 20 percent of cases when first seen, the usual site of metastasis being the lung. Other relatively common sites include lymph nodes and liver. The intravenous urogram demonstrates a renal mass lesion, usually with calyceal distortion. Nonfunction is unusual, and calcification is present in about 10 percent. Differential diagnosis must consider hydronephrosis, cystic kidney disease, other renal tumors, and neuroblastoma. Ultrasonography is a new technique that can assist in clarification of the location and density of intraabdominal masses. Arteriography may be useful in the differential diagnosis where reasonable doubt still exists after intravenous urography and ultrasonography. Delineation of the vascular supply may help to establish the origin of the tumor in large masses. Inferior vena cavagrams can be very helpful in establishing extension of tumor into the renal vein and vena cava, particularly when the IVU shows nonvisualization. Diagnostic studies to determine the presence or absence of metastatic disease should include a chest radiograph with whole lung tomograms and liver scan.

The vast majority of children with Wilms' tumors can now be treated successfully. The best long-term results are achieved when an interdisciplinary team works in close cooperation throughout the patient's course. A tentative management plan regarding surgery, radiotherapy, and chemotherapy should be made prior to the initiation of any treatment, although the findings at surgery may require modification of this plan. Surgical exploration should be performed as soon as the work-up is completed. However, where the tumor is very large, making operative risk and likelihood of tumor spillage great, surgery is best deferred. Vincristine has been shown to produce dramatic shrinkage of large inoperable Wilms' tumors with as little as two weekly doses of 1.5 mg/m^2 given intravenously; it is now generally advocated to shrink tumors in preference to pre-operative radiotherapy. Surgery includes (1) a transabdominal or thoracoabdominal approach, (2) thorough inspection of the liver, nodes, and contralateral kidney for evidence of tumor, with biopsy of suspicious areas, (3) removal of the tumor in toto without rupture or spillage if at all possible, and (4) paraaortic lymph node dissection. The extent of the tumor bed and any residual tumor are marked with clips for subsequent radiation therapy. A more complete staging of the tumor can be made postoperatively and treatment plans with respect to radiation and chemotherapy tailored accordingly. Radiotherapy to the tumor bed is usually recommended beginning within 10 days of surgery, except in children under 1 year of age. The details of radiotherapy are dependent upon the age of the child and upon the extent of the tumor. For patients with stage I disease (tumor confined to kidney and completely resected) there soon may be sufficient evidence from the National Wilms' Tumor Study to indicate that radiation is unnecessary in localized lesion of this type. As long-term survival rates with Wilms' tumors improve there is increasing concern to minimize radiation therapy whenever possible in order to avoid the long-term toxic effects that have been observed on liver, bone, and kidney. Actinomycin D in a daily dosage of 15 μg/kg for 5 days is given once the diagnosis of Wilms' tumor is confirmed on frozen section, except in children under 1 year old. The use of actinomycin D to both potentiate local radiation effect and eradicate distant micrometastases has resulted in an improvement in long-term survival. Repeated courses of actinomycin D 6 weeks after surgery and then every 3 months for 18 months does significantly decrease the relapse rate and the associated morbidity. However, there does not appear to be a significant difference in long-term survival for those children receiving multiple-course chemotherapy as opposed to single-course therapy. Combination chemotherapy using vincristine and actinomycin D has achieved statistically significant increased disease-free rates in group II (tumor extending beyond the kidney but completely resected) and group III patients (residual nonhematogenous tumor confined to the abdomen) in the National Wilms' Tumor Study. Even stage IV tumors with hematogenous spread to the lung are potentially curable with aggressive therapy. Surgical extirpation of a solitary lung metastasis, when not adjacent to the mediastinum or involving the pleura, is recommended. When multiple lung metastases are present, or when the tumor is adjacent to the mediastinum or involves the pleura, radiotherapy and chemotherapy are preferred. Surgery for multiple lung metastases is reserved for those cases where the lesions initially shrank and then became fixed in size and where no new lesion developed after waiting several weeks. Bilateral Wilms' tumors or Wilms' tumor in a solitary kidney can be removed by partial nephrectomy. Where tumor spillage appears likely, excision of the kidney and tumor with subsequent "bench" surgery excision of tumor and autotransplantation of the remaining kidney is feasible. Where one kidney is almost totally replaced by tumor and the other is partially involved it may be preferable to nephrectomize the most involved kidney and at the same time or later (after chemotherapy or radiation therapy) do a partial nephrectomy on the less-involved side. Gross hematogenous liver metastases carry the gravest prognosis, and almost all such children will succumb to their disease within a relatively short period of time.

The overall rate of recovery from Wilms' tumor is about 60 percent. Most patients can be regarded as cured if there has been no recurrence 2 years after chemotheraphy has been discontinued. Neonatal tumors are rarely true Wilms' tumors, but rather are fibromatous variants with an excellent prognosis following nephrectomy alone.

Tumors of Urogenital Sinus

Rhabdomyosarcoma arises in the base of the bladder, posterior urethra, or vagina. Presenting symptoms and signs include strangury, urinary retention, and the passage of grapelike masses. Hematuria is uncommon, but vaginal bleeding sometimes occurs. Local extension or distant spread to lungs, lymph nodes, liver, bone, and bone marrow is common at the time of diagnosis. Most children present before the age of 4 years. Radical surgical extirpation has resulted in an overall cure rate of 53 percent for tumors in the vagina and base of the bladder, although those in the prostate carry a very poor prognosis and only isolated cases of long-term survival have been reported. Prior to 1966 no patient with inoperable or metastatic rhabdomyosarcoma had been treated successfully and experienced long-term survival. However, more recently several long-term survivors with incompletely removed tumors have been reported following the use of supervoltage radiotherapy (doses from 5,000 to 6,000 rads delivered over 5 to 6 weeks) in conjunction with intensive combination chemotherapy (actinomycin D, vincristine, and Cytoxan, as recommended by Sutow and Sullivan). In contrast to the situation with other embryonic malignant tumors such as nephroblastoma and neuroblastoma, cure rates in the younger age groups have been much lower than those in children over 1 year old. Combined therapy, including radical anterior pelvic exenteration, postoperative regional radiation, and simultaneous prolonged courses of actinomycin D, vincristine, and Cytoxan, offers the best chance for cure.

Testicular Tumors

Primary testicular tumors constitute about 3 percent of urologic neoplasms in children. They present as painless scrotal swellings that must be differentiated from hydroceles, hernias, torsion, and hemorrhagic infarctions. The pediatrician must be wary of unusual scrotal masses and, in particular, enlarging hydroceles. Of note is the presence of a hydrocele in as many as 46 percent of children with testicular neoplasms.

Testicular neoplasms can be divided into those of germ cell origin and those of other origin, the former accounting for 60 percent of the total. Teratomas are the most common variety; they are slow growing and benign, but can become malignant in later life. Embryonal cell carcinoma is the most common malignant germ cell tumor in childhood. Orchioblastoma (yolk sac tumor or endodermal sinus tumor) has a distinct histologic picture and tends to occur in infants. Debate continues as to whether it is a distinct entity or merely a form of embryonal cell carcinoma. Teratocarcinomas account for the remaining malignant germ cell tumors. Seminomas as well as choriocarcinomas have not been reported in infants or prepubertal adolescents. Those tumors not of germ cell origin, although rare, occur more often in children than in adults. Sarcoma is most frequently encountered, followed by interstitial cell tumor, malignant lymphoma, and Sertoli cell tumors. Paratesticular tumors are embryonic sarcomas.

Leukemic infiltration of the testes is usually present in children dying of leukemia. However, clinical testicular enlargement during or apart from bone marrow relapses can occur. Gonadoblastomas arise from the dysgenetic gonads of patients with intersexuality. Treatment of testicular tumors involves radical orchiectomy. Incisional biopsy is mentioned only to be condemned; the only place for it, or for needle biopsy, is in known leukemia. Benign tumors of germ cell origin and other origin require no further therapy. Orchioblastomas (yolk sac tumors) do not require retroperitoneal lymph node dissection for cure in children under 1 year of age. After that age many authors recommend lymph node dissection for orchioblastoma as well as for embryonal cell carcinoma, teratocarcimona, and rhabdomyosarcoma. Radiotherapy and chemotherapy are generally reserved for those children with paraaortic lymph node metastases and for those with general dissemination. It is important to remember that no single treatment regimen has been conclusively demonstrated to be of advantage, since combined prospective treatment trials have never been carried out in these relatively rare tumors.

Ovarian Tumors

Ovarian tumors are often difficult to diagnose. Vague abdominal pains are usual, but on occasion torsion is encountered. Teratomas are the most common types, and most are benign. Granulosa cell tumors may present with isosexual precocity. Dysgerminomas occur in later childhood; treatment of these tumors is salpingo-oophorectomy. Invasive lesions require wider excision, including the uterus and both appendages, followed by radiation.

TRAUMA

Serious trauma has reached epidemic proportions in our complex, urban, mechanized society. Accidents are the leading cause of childhood mortality and account for 40 percent of childhood deaths in the United States. Abdominal injuries presently rank third among accidental causes of death in children, following burns and head injuries. The alarming rise in automobile accidents, which increases steadily each year, has resulted in greater numbers of children with blunt abdominal trauma and urologic injury.

Recent reports suggest that renal injuries account for as many as 1 in 1,000 pediatric hospital admissions. In some series the kidney is the most frequently involved intraabdominal organ following blunt trauma. This particular predisposition to renal injury can be explained by certain features peculiar to children: kidneys (1) are relatively larger in children than in adults, (2) are surrounded by less perinephric fat, (3) have a lower situation that allows less protection from the rib cage, (4) maintain their lobulations that represent areas of weakness, and (5) have a higher incidence of anomalies.

Preexisting renal disease is found in 13 to 23 percent of children evaluated for renal trauma. Hydronephrosis is the incidental lesion discovered most often, but Wilms' tumor and cystic kidneys are also encountered. Other viscera are frequently injured in conjunction with the renal injury, particularly in vehicular accidents. In general, the more severe the kidney injury the greater the likelihood of multiorgan involvement.

Most childhood renal injuries result from direct blunt trauma secondary to falls, vehicular accidents, and blows to the abdomen. The peak incidence occurs in the group 10 to 14 years of age. Males predominate in all reports, with an average ratio of 3:1, probably reflecting the more rugged types of play that older boys indulge in. Right and left kidneys are involved equally. Bilateral injuries occur in 2 to 3 percent of cases. Left-sided injury is more common in the United States when the child is the victim of a pedestrian-automobile collision.

The kidney may be contused or lacerated. Lacerations may be incomplete, involving the parenchyma and capsule only, or complete, with involvement of the pelvocalyceal system resulting in urinary extravasation. The most serious injury is the shattered fragmented kidney. Deceleration injuries, such as those that occur with falls from a height, can result in avulsion of the vascular pedicle; these children often present in shock.

Diagnosis is based on history of abdominal trauma and the presence of hermaturia, loin pain, bruising, and tenderness. Significant bleeding and urinary extravasation result in a flank mass. Intravenous urography shows decreased concentration in contused kidneys or frank extravasation from complete lacerations. Vascular injuries produce spasm and thrombosis, resulting in nonvisualization on the intravenous urogram. In such cases angiography and selective renal arteriography are of great value and help to differentiate vascular spasm from thrombosis. Demonstration of a thrombotic renal artery occlusion should be followed by prompt transabdominal exploration, thrombectomy, and repair of the vessel, if possible. However, even with expeditious surgery the vast majority of these kidneys are lost.

Adequate visualization of the kidney is the key to classification of extent and type of injury and to planning management and anticipating sequelae. High-dose infusion intravenous urography is recommended by most authors as the first and most useful radiologic investigation in children suspected of having renal injuries. The technique is safe and simple and in most instances produces nephrograms and pyelograms superior to those obtained by standard intravenous urography. Urograms are mandatory even in suspected renal trauma or when the injury appears slight, in order to exclude underlying pathology. Early study within a few hours of injury allows optimal visualization before parenchymal swelling becomes a major factor. Most children will void upon request, thus permitting excellent voiding cystourethrograms without the need for catheterization. Arteriography is reserved for those cases where infusion urography is not diagnostic or where nonvisualization of one or both kidneys occurs. It is also of immense value to the surgeon in those cases where exploration appears indicated, since excellent delineation of the extent of injury, including arterial supply, is obtained. This valuable information allows maximal salvage of renal tissue by conservative surgery. Cystoscopy and retrograde pyelography are recommended only when infusion urography and arterography do not adequately visualize the collecting system or when ureteral injury is suspected. The renal scan with ^{197}Hg-chlormerodrin is a simple study that is highly accurate and rapidly performed; it is totally free of the allergic problems that may on occasion complicate iodide studies. Its prime indication is as a screening procedure for those children who are allergic to Hypaque and are suspected of having sustained renal injury. Because of its ease of performance and low radiation dose it is probably the ideal study for long-term serial follow-up of patients with renal injuries. It should, if possible, be performed as part of the primary work-up of the patient in whom further follow-up studies are anticipated.

Most renal injuries are contusions that respond to conservative therapy, including strict bed rest and careful monitoring of vital signs. An expanding flank mass, severe continuous or persistent hematuria, ureteral avulsion, and shattered kidneys are indications for prompt surgical intervention. Complete lacerations with mild urinary extravasation can frequently be managed conservatively. However, in the author's opinion wide parenchymal separation with gross urinary extravasation is best managed by surgery at a propitious time, usually 2 to 7 days after injury when ischemic segments of kidney have become clearly demarcated, when hemorrhage is relatively easy to control, and when perirenal infection usually has not supervened. Morse has reported a very high kidney salvage rate by partial nephrectomy using this approach. Although salvage of functioning renal tissue is desirable and would seem particularly important to children who still face the hazards of military service, athletics, or child-bearing, nephrectomy is not a disaster if a normal contralateral kidney is present; and this procedure does in general lead to a brief uneventful recovery. Nevertheless, the extra convalescent period that conservative operations may entail seems justified. If nephrectomy must be done, children are advised to avoid unnecessary exposure to potential sources of abdominal trauma such as contact sports.

The true incidence of the late complications of renal trauma is probably not reflected in the literature because of inadequate follow-up of asymptomatic patients. Contusions without urographic abnormalities do not appear to be followed by late sequelae. However, severe contusions with urographic changes require careful clinical and radiologic follow-up. Scarring is common, and growth of recognizably damaged kidneys is abnormal. Scarring may produce obstructive uropathy or a parapelvic pseudocyst (urinoma). Calcification of the cyst wall may occur. Ischemia may result in later hypertension. These complications, aside from hypertension, almost invariably become apparent within the first year following injury. Although its true incidence is unknown, from the available information it would ap-

pear that hypertension secondary to renal trauma rarely develops during childhood.

Acute complications of renal trauma include mortality, which is most unusual when the kidney is the sole organ involved; most of the reported deaths in children with renal trauma occur secondary to other injuries. Perinephric hematomas may become secondarily infected, resulting in a perinephric abscess. Delayed hemorrhage may occur with conservative treatment or following reparative surgery; it usually occurs between 10 days and 4 weeks following the injury.

Penetrating injuries are unusual in children, but they occasionally occur. The ureter is more likely to be involved in this type of injury. Exploration may be required to control hemorrhage or to exclude lacerations of other intraabdominal viscera. Bladder injuries may result in intraperitoneal or extraperitoneal rupture. The former is more common and usually occurs as a result of blunt trauma applied to a full bladder, with rupture occurring at the bladder dome. Extraperitoneal extravasation is usually associated with pelvic fracture. Children with hematuria resulting from indirect trauma, especially when the trauma is poorly localized, as in automobile accidents, must have a retrograde cystogram in addition to intravenous urography. Ruptures of the bladder are easily overlooked on the latter examination. It should be remembered that the bladder may also be perforated from within by careless passage of an endoscope or metal bougie. "Spontaneous" intraperitoneal perforations have also been reported in neonates and young children with underlying bladder pathology.

Mortality rates of unsuspected or untreated bladder injuries are very high. Electrolyte disturbances secondary to peritoneal autodialysis, later peritonitis and perivesical necrosis, and infection from concentrated urine with superimposed infection almost always prove fatal unless adequate drainage is established. With prompt recognition of bladder injuries and early adequate bladder drainage by suprapubic cystostomy and suture of the lacerations the outlook for complete recovery is excellent.

Urethral injuries usually result from instrumentation or pelvic fractures. Most cases involve males. Rupture of the urethra above the urogenital diaphragm results from serious crush injuries with pelvic fracture dislocations. The puboprostatic ligaments are ruptured and the posterior urethra becomes avulsed at the prostatic apex. Complete separation of bladder and urethra can occur. These children are usually severely shocked and have marked bruising, swelling, and lower abdominal tenderness. Large pelvic hematomas are the rule. There is inability to void, and catherization of the bladder is not possible. Cystostomy drainage without any attempt at reapproximation of the severed, avulsed urethral segments appears to be the treatment of choice. Posterior urethral strictures commonly follow and are treated by one of the established urethroplasty techniques.

Attempts to reestablish continuity of the urethra immediately following injury by "railroading" techniques, traction sutures, or balloon catheters generally result in strictures that are subsequently more difficult to handle. Moreover, impotence, incontinence, and difficulty with ejaculation occur much more frequently with this form of therapy.

Anterior urethral lacerations result from instrumentation or occasionally from straddle injuries. Treatment involves catheter drainage for partial lacerations, and complete lacerations require diversion by cystostomy and subsequent urethral repair.

Penile injuries with pants zippers are fairly common. Local anesthesia generally is sufficient to allow removal of the clothing, but on occasion surgical removal under general anesthesia is required. Iatrogenic injuries from circumcision are discussed on page 1335.

Contused testes may occur from direct blows. Minor blows are often mistakenly held responsible for testicular symptoms caused by torsion. Trauma is treated with scrotal elevation, immobilization, and application of ice packs. Exploration is required in cases of rupture.

References

Backhouse KM: The gubernaculum testis hunteri: testicular descent and maldescent. Ann R Coll Surg Engl 35:15, 1964

Barnhouse D: Prune belly syndrome. Br J Urol 44:356, 1972

Booth EJ, Bell TE, McLaine C, Evans APT: Fetal vesicoureteral reflux. J Urol 113:258, 1975

Boyarsky S: The Neurogenic Bladder. Baltimore, Williams & Wilkins, 1967

Campbell EB, Young JD Jr: Enuresis and its relationship to electroencephalographic disturbances. J Urol 96:947, 1966

Caucci M: Clinical and statistical appraisal of seven hundred orchidopexies, operative technique and follow-up. Int Surg 45:218, 1966

Elbadawi A, Schenk EA: A new theory of the innervation of bladder musculature, part 4. Innervation of the vesicourethral junction and external urethral sphincter. J Urol 111:613, 1974

Forsythe WI, Redmond A: Enuresis and the electric alarm. Study of 200 cases. Arch Dis Child 49:259, 1974

Froelich LA, Fujikura T: Follow up of infants with single umbilical artery. Pediatrics 52:1 1973

Geist AJ: Clinical problems of children with sterile reflux. J Urol 108:343, 1972

Giebink GS, Ruymann FB: Testicular tumors in childhood. Am J Dis Child 127:433, 1974

Grosfeld JL, Smith JP, Clatworthy HW Jr: Pelvic rhabdomyosarcoma in infants and children. J Urol 107:673, 1972

Halligren B: Enuresis, a clinical and genetic study. Acta Psychiatr Scand [Suppl] 114:32, 1957

Harley LM, You Chen Rattner WH: Prune belly syndrome. J Urol 108:174, 1972

Hendren WH: Posterior urethral valves in boys: a broad clinical spectrum. J Urol 106:298, 1971

Hilson D: Malformation of ears as sign of malformation of genitourinary tract. Br Med J 2:785, 1957

Hodgson NB: A one stage hypospadias repair. J Urol 114:118, 1975

Hutchison RJ, Nogrady MD: Late sequelae of renal trauma in the pediatric age group. J Can Assoc Radio 24:3, 1973

Johnson N: Torsion of the testis—a plea for bilateral exploration. Med J Aust 1:653, 1960

Johnston JH, Farkas A: Congenital neuropathic bladder. Practicalities and possibilities of conservational management. Urology 56:719, 1975

——— Kathel OL: The obstructed neurogenic bladder in the newborn. Br J Urol 43:206, 1971

Levitt SB: Urologic trauma in childhood. In Edelmann CM Jr (ed): Pediatric Nephrology. Boston, Little, Brown, 1975

Lowell W, Rogers Ostrow, T: The prune belly syndrome. J Pediatr 83:786, 1973

Lyon RP, Scott MP, Marshall S: Intermittant catheterization rather than urinary diversion in children with myelomeningocele. Trans Am Assoc Genitourin Surg 66:78, 1974

McArdle R, Lebowitz R: Uncomplicated hypospadias and anomalies of upper urinary tract. Urology 5:712, 1975

McDonald P, Hiller HG: Angiography in abdominal tumors of childhood. Clin Radiol 19:1, 1968

MacGregor M: Pyelonephritis lenta. Arch Dis Child 45:240, 1970

Mahony DT: Studies of enuresis. I. Incidence of obstructive lesions and pathophysiology of enuresis. J Urol 106:951, 1971

Martin LW, Pedro MR: An evaluation of 10 years' experience with retroperitoneal node dissection for Wilms' tumor. J Pediatr Surg 4:6, 1969

Meadow R: Practical aspects of the management of nocturnal enuresis. In Kolvin I, MacKeith RC, Meadow SR (eds): Bladder Control and Enuresis. Philadelphia, JB Lippincott, 1973, Chap 21

Mininberg DT, Montoya F, Okada K, Galioto F, Presutti R: Subcellular muscle studies in the prune belly syndrome. J Urol 109:524, 1973

Morse TS, Smith JP, Howard WHR, Howe MI: Kidney injuries in children. J Urol 98:693, 1967

Murphy S, Jackson N, Hammar S: Neurological evaluation of adolescent enuretics. J Pediatr 45:2, 1970

Nash DFE: Urinary problems of spina bifida. Dev Med Child Neurol 11:106, 1969

Nashold B, Friedman H, Glenn JF, Grimes HJ: Electromicturition in paraplegia, implantation of a spinal neuroprosthesis. Arch Surg 104:195, 1972

Rabinovitch HH: Bladder evacuation in child with myelomeningocele. J Urol 3:425, 1974

Retik AB: Urinary reflux in children: an approach to management. Hospital Practice: 125, 1974

Rogers LW, Ostrow PT: The prune belly syndrome. J Pediatr 83:786, 1973

Rolleston TMJ, Maling TMJ, Hodson CJ: Intrarenal reflux and the scarred kidney. Arch Dis Child 49:531, 1974

Rose JS, Glassberg KI, Waterhouse K: Intrarenal reflux and its relationship to renal scarring. J Urol 113:400, 1975

Scott JES: Urinary diversion in children. Arch Dis Child 48:199, 1973

Shopfner CE: Modern concepts of lower urinary tract obstruction in pediatric patients. Pediatrics 45:194, 1970

Smelle JM, Normand ICS: Urinary Tract Infection. Symposium. London, Oxford Univ Press, 1968

Stansfeld JM: Enuresis and urinary tract infection. In Kolvin I, MacKeith RC, Meadow SR (eds): Bladder Control and Enuresis. Philadelphia, JB Lippincott, 1973, p 102

Stanton L, Williams DI: The wide bladder neck in children. Br J Urol 45:60, 1973

Stark G: Pudendal neurectomy in management of neurogenic bladder in myelomeningocele. Arch Dis Child 44:238, 698, 1969

Watson RA, Lennox KW, Gangai MP: Simple cryptorchidism; the value of the excretory urogram as a screening method. J Urol 113:789, 1974

Welch KJ, Kearney GP: Abdominal musculature deficiency syndrome: prune belly. J Urol 113:693, 1974

Wilbur JR, Etcubanas E: Advances in diagnosis and treatment of solid tumors in children. In Schulman I (ed): Advances in Pediatrics, Vol 21. Chicago, Year Book, 1974 p 281

Williams DI:. Pediatric Urology. London, Butterworth,1968

——— Hulme-Moir I: Primary obstructive megaureter. Br J Urol 42:140, 1970

CHAPTER 27

Circulatory System

Julien I. E. Hoffman, *Associate Editor*

FETAL CIRCULATION AND CARDIOVASCULAR ADJUSTMENTS AFTER BIRTH

Abraham M. Rudolph

Although dramatic changes in the circulation occur after birth, when the function of gas exchange is transferred from the placenta to the lungs, there is continuous development of cardiovascular function both before and after birth. Knowledge of the developmental changes in the circulation is important to our understanding of variations in postnatal adaptation and the effects of cardiac lesions on the circulation. Little information is available regarding physiology of the circulation in the human fetus, and most of our knowledge is derived from studies in fetal lambs; in general, the course of this circulation and its responses to stress are probably similar to those in the human, but there may be species differences.

COURSE AND DISTRIBUTION OF FETAL CIRCULATION. In adult animals blood circulates serially through the right side of the heart to the lungs and then through the left side of the heart to the systemic circulation to return to the right heart (Figs. 1 and 2). Cardiac output is the volume of blood circulating per minute. In the fetus the series circulation does not occur, as blood from both ventricles is distributed to the lower body. It is convenient to consider cardiac output in terms of the total output of the two ventricles; this is expressed as combined ventricular output (CVO).

Blood oxygenated in the placenta returns to the fetal body through the umbilical veins, which enter the portal venous system. A variable proportion (20 to 80 percent) of umbilical and portal venous blood passes through the hepatic microcirculation to the hepatic veins, which drain into the inferior vena cava; the remainder bypasses the liver through the ductus venosus,

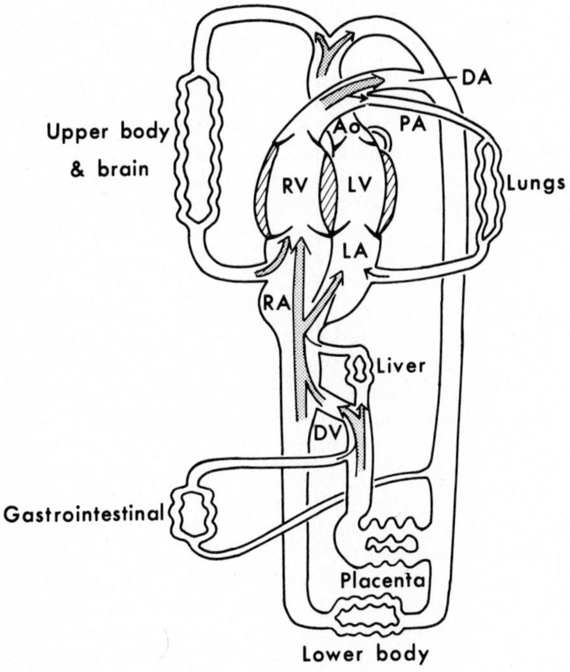

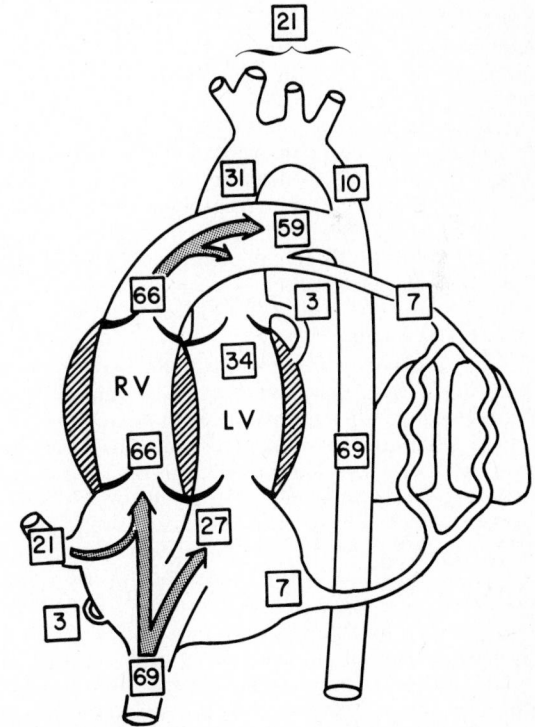

FETAL CIRCULATION

FIG. 1. Course of fetal circulation; for description see text. DA, ductus arteriosus; Ao, aorta; PA, pulmonary artery; RV, right ventricle; LV, left ventricle; LA, left atrium; RA, right atrium; DV, ductus venosus.

FETAL CIRCULATION-DISTRIBUTION OF C. V. O.

FIG. 2. Percentages of combined ventricular output ejected by the left (LV) and right (RV) ventricles and passing through the major vascular channels are shown (numbers in squares). For description see text.

a channel connecting the portal sinus with the inferior vena cava. It is not known what regulates the proportions of blood passing through the ductus venosus and the liver; the ductus venosus is not very reactive to changes in blood gases and pH, nor to vasoactive agents. In the proximal inferior vena cava, the venous blood draining the lower body mixes with that from the ductus venosus and the hepatic veins. This represents about 70 percent of the total volume of blood returning to the heart. About one-third of the inferior vena caval blood passes directly through the foramen ovale into the left atrium, while the remaining two-thirds enter the right atrium and right ventricle. Superior vena caval blood is directed toward the tricuspid valve, and in normal fetuses an insignificant volume of superior vena caval blood passes through the foramen ovale. About 20 percent of the CVO returns to the heart through the superior vena cava, and thus the right ventricle receives and ejects about 66 percent of the combined ventricular output. The major portion of blood ejected into the pulmonary trunk passes through the ductus arteriosus to the descending aorta (58 percent of CVO); only 7 to 8 percent of the CVO (or only 10 to 15 percent of the blood ejected by the right ventricle) is distributed to the pulmonary circulation. The left atrium receives the blood returning to the heart from the lungs (7 to 8 percent of CVO) and the inferior vena caval blood that crosses the foramen ovale (25 percent of CVO). The left ventricle thus receives and ejects about 33 percent of the CVO. About 3 percent of the CVO enters the coronary arteries, and 20 percent of the CVO supplies the head, brain and neck, upper body, and arms. The remaining 10 percent of CVO that is ejected by the left ventricle passes across the aortic isthmus to the descending aorta. The proportions of CVO distributed to various fetal organs, as determined in near-term lambs, are: myocardium 3 to 4 percent, lungs 7 to 8 percent, gastrointestinal tract 5 to 6 percent, brain 3 to 4 percent, kidneys 2 to 3 percent, placenta 40 percent. Combined ventricular output is about 500 ml/kg fetal weight/minute, and umbilical-placental flow is about 200 ml/kg/minute.

The oxygen tension of fetal arterial blood is considerably lower than that in the adult. Umbilical venous blood has an oxygen tension of about 30 to 35 torr. This mixes with portal venous and inferior vena caval blood, and the oxygen tension of inferior vena caval blood entering the heart is about 26 to 28 torr. In the left atrium a small volume of blood with a low oxygen tension returning through the pulmonary veins reduces the oxygen tension of the blood passing from the inferior vena cava through the foramen ovale. Venous blood returning through the superior vena cava has an oxygen tension of about 12 to 14 torr, and this combines with the inferior vena caval stream passing through the tricuspid valve to give a resultant oxygen tension of right ventricular and pulmonary arterial blood of about 18 to 19 torr. The oxygen tension of blood entering the left ventricle and the ascending aorta and its branches is about 23 to 25 torr, but descending aortic blood, which is a mixture of bloods

passing through the ductus arteriosus and the aortic isthmus, has a lower tension of 20 to 22 torr.

Since the fetus is surrounded by amniotic fluid in the uterus, all fetal vascular pressures are recorded in relation to amniotic cavity pressure. Vena caval pressures are 3 to 5 mm Hg above, and left atrial pressure is 2 to 4 mm Hg above, amniotic cavity pressure. Right and left ventricular systolic pressures are usually equal, with a systolic level of 65 to 70 mm Hg in the latter part of gestation. Pulmonary arterial and aortic systolic and diastolic pressures are also usually equal, with systolic levels of 65 to 70 mm Hg and diastolic levels of 30 to 35 mm Hg. In late gestation right ventricular and pulmonary arterial systolic pressures are often 5 to 8 mm Hg higher than those in the left ventricle and aorta; this is probably related to mild constriction of the ductus arteriosus.

FETAL MYOCARDIAL PERFORMANCE. Cardiac output is more sensitive to changes in resting heart rate in the fetus than in the adult. In the fetus an increase from resting heart rate of about 160 beats per minute to about 240 beats per minute results in a 15 percent increase in cardiac output, but a fall in heart rate to 120 beats per minute causes a 20 to 25 percent drop in cardiac output. The marked reduction of cardiac output with a decreased heart rate is related to the limited ability of the fetal heart to increase stroke volume. Friedman has shown that isolated strips of myocardium from fetal lamb hearts develop less tension per unit mass of muscle than tissue obtained from adult sheep hearts. In fetal lambs in utero the heart is not able to maintain its stroke volume as well as in the adult animal when outflow resistance to the ventricles is increased. Also, when an increase in volume load is placed on the fetal ventricles by a rapid intravenous infusion, the fetal heart does not increase its output as much as the adult heart subjected to a similar volume load. There is considerable evidence indicating that there is better performance of the heart with advancing gestation. It is not known whether myocardial function continues to improve after birth, nor is it known when the heart develops adult characteristics.

The improvement of myocardial performance during gestational development is in part related to morphologic changes in heart muscle. Fetal muscle has a higher water content and fewer contractile elements than adult muscle; however, there may also be differences in metabolism of the muscle. Another factor that may account for the lesser function of fetal myocardium is the lack of sympathetic innervation. In adults, local release of norepinephrine from sympathetic nerve endings is an important inotropic mechanism that may be absent in the fetus, since sympathetic innervation of the myocardium proceeds at varying rates in different species. In the rat and rabbit no sympathetic nerve endings are demonstrable in the myocardium at birth, and innervation develops after 2 to 3 weeks; but in the guinea pig, innervation starts about the middle of gestation and is complete at the time of birth. Although the pattern of innervation of the human heart is not known, it is probably not fully developed at birth. The lesser performance of the myocardium of the fetus may be important in determining the ability of the premature infant to respond to increased volume and pressure loads.

CIRCULATORY CHANGES AFTER BIRTH. Two dramatic events that occur immediately after birth are cessation of the umbilical-placental circulation and establishment of an adequate pulmonary circulation. The umbilical vessels are very reactive to mechanical stimulation, particularly stretch; in natural birth in animals the umbilical vessels constrict after being torn or bitten. The vessels also constrict when exposed to an increase in oxygen tension, and the rise in systemic arterial oxygen tension after birth is probably responsible for maintaining constriction; severe hypoxia could result in relaxation of the vessels and cause hemorrhage. Removal of the placental circulation markedly reduces venous return through the inferior vena cava. The cessation of umbilical venous return also reduces flow through the ductus venosus, which closes within 3 to 7 days after birth, probably passively as a result of the reduced flow and pressure. It is possible that constriction of its wall by changing oxygen tension or by vasoactive agents also contributes to ductus venosus closure.

CHANGES IN PULMONARY CIRCULATION. The low pulmonary blood flow in the fetus is related to the high pulmonary vascular resistance. The small precapillary arteries in the fetal lungs have a thick medial smooth muscle layer, and maintained constriction of these vessels is responsible for the high pulmonary vascular resistance. The pulmonary vessels are very reactive to several physiologic and pharmacologic influences. A decrease in oxygen tension or in the pH of the blood perfusing the pulmonary vessels results in

their constriction. The pattern of response of pulmonary vascular resistance in fetal and newborn animals is shown in Figure 3; it is apparent that the vasoconstrictor responses to hypoxemia and acidemia are additive. Acetylchloline, histamine, tolazoline, and β-adrenergic catecholamines are potent vasodilators of the fetal pulmonary vessels, and recently it has been shown that bradykinin and prostaglandin E_1 are pulmonary vasodilators in the fetus. Ventilation of the lungs with air results in a 4-fold to 10-fold increase in pulmonary blood flow associated with a marked fall in pulmonary vascular resistance. This decrease in vascular resistance can be explained partly by the physical expansion of the alveoli with gas, but the main factor is the increase in oxygen tension to which the vessels are exposed. Before birth the precapillary vessels are exposed to pulmonary arterial blood with an oxygen tension of approximately 18 torr. Expansion of the alveoli with air subjects the vessels to a higher oxygen tension, since oxygen diffuses into vessels proximal to the capillaries. The effects of oxygen are exerted largely locally, although it is possible that a minor effect may be produced through chemoreflex mechanisms; the pulmonary vasodilator effects of oxygen may result from a direct local effect on the smooth muscle or from a chemical mediator. It has been suggested that an increase in oxygen tension results in release of bradykinin, which is responsible for pulmonary vasodilatation after birth; but this does not completely explain the effects of oxygen, since bradykinin levels are elevated for only a short period.

While the ductus arteriosus is still widely patent, the pulmonary arterial pressure remains at systemic arterial levels; but constriction of the ductus separates the aorta and pulmonary artery, so that pulmonary arterial and right ventricular pressure fall when there is the normal fall in pulmonary vascular resistance.

The initial decrease in pulmonary vascular resistance results from release of hypoxemia-induced vasoconstriction. In the 6 to 8 weeks following birth there is a further progressive fall associated with thinning of the smooth muscle layer in the media. The patterns of change of pulmonary vascular resistance, pulmonary arterial pressure, and blood flow are shown in Figure 4. The postnatal maturation of the pulmonary vessels is disturbed by conditions that interfere with normal oxygenation after birth, such as lung disease or exposure to high altitude, and also by congenital cardiac lesions, particularly those associated with pulmonary hypertension.

CLOSURE OF FORAMEN OVALE. In the fetus more than half of inferior vena caval blood is derived from umbilical venous return. Removal of the placental circulation results in a marked fall in the amount of inferior vena caval blood returning to the heart and a small drop in right atrial pressure, while the increase in pulmonary blood flow results in a rise in pulmonary venous return and elevation of left atrial pressure. This small increase in left atrial pressure and decrease in right atrial pressure closes the valvelike flap of the foramen ovale. In many infants the foramen ovale is incompletely closed, and a small opening with a small

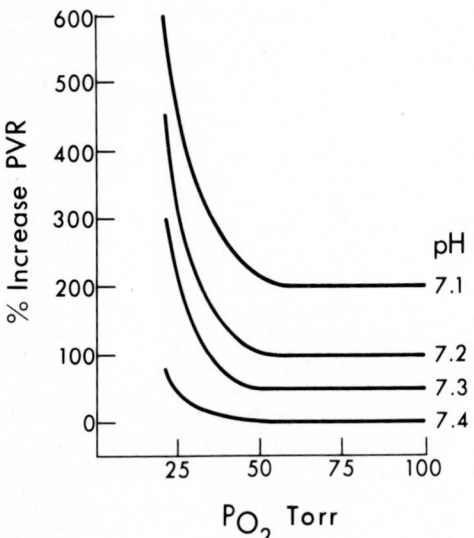

FIG. 3. Responses of pulmonary circulation to hypoxia and acidemia. At PO_2 levels of 50 to 100 torr, metabolic acidemia results in a moderate increase in pulmonary vascular resistance (PVR). Hypoxia alone causes a modest rise of PVR, but a combination of acidemia and hypoxia produces severe pulmonary vasoconstriction.

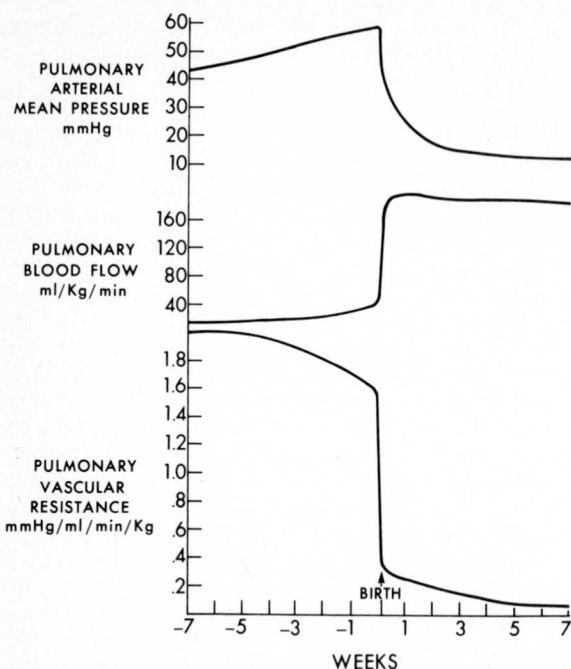

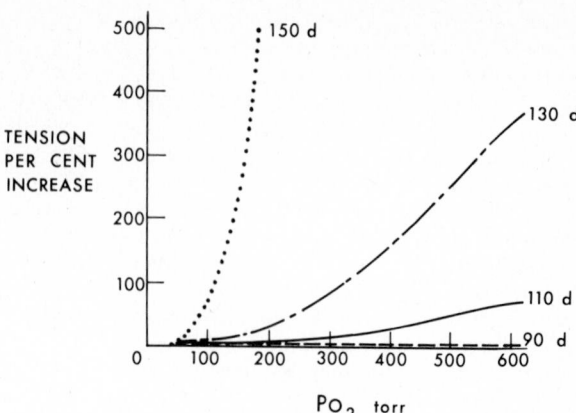

FIG. 5. Responses to oxygen of the ductus arteriosus in fetal lambs of varying gestational ages are shown. Term gestation is 150 days. Little constrictor response is noted at 90 days gestation. The initial level of PO_2 at which constriction occurs decreases, and the magnitude of response increases, with advancing gestation.

FIG. 4. Changes in fetal pulmonary arterial pressure, pulmonary blood flow, and pulmonary vascular resistance in the perinatal period. Pulmonary vascular resistance decreases during the latter part of gestation, mainly because of an increase in the number of pulmonary vessels associated with growth; it falls dramatically at birth, due to the vasodilator effect of ventilation of the lungs with air; a further gradual decrease occurs as pulmonary vascular smooth muscle regresses. Pulmonary blood flow increases slightly during fetal growth, then increases dramatically after birth. Pulmonary arterial pressure falls rapidly immediately after birth, and then more gradually, to reach adult levels after 6 to 8 weeks.

left-to-right shunt is present for several months. A small opening without left-to-right shunting may persist throughout life in about 15 to 20 percent of people. In early infancy and sometimes in later life, if right atrial pressure is raised above that in the left atrium, the foramen ovale may open and right-to-left shunting of blood may occur.

CLOSURE OF DUCTUS ARTERIOSUS. During fetal life the ductus arteriosus is a large channel with a diameter similar to that of the descending aorta. The ductus has a large amount of smooth muscle in the media, in contrast with the contiguous aorta and pulmonary artery, which have largely elastic tissue. It was once thought that the ductus is passively kept open by the pressure within it; however, recently it has been suggested that prostaglandin E_1 or E_2, which dilate the ductus, may be released locally in the wall and maintain its patency. The ductus arteriosus constricts rapidly after birth and in most mature infants is functionally closed within 10 to 15 hours. Permanent closure by thrombosis, intimal proliferation, and fibrosis is complete within 3 weeks. Constriction of the ductus after birth is related to the increase in systemic arterial oxygen tension; the pattern of response of the ductus to

oxygen tension in a full-term lamb is shown in Figure 5. It is not known whether oxygen affects the ductus smooth muscle directly or whether it acts through a chemical mediator; the ductus is constricted by acetylcholine and bradykinin, so that the effect of oxygen could result from local release of one or the other of these vasoactive substances.

The ductus arteriosus in very young fetuses does not respond to an increase of oxygen tension to levels as high as 600 torr. With advancing gestation there is a decrease in the level of oxygen tension that initiates constriction and a decrease in the level at which the peak effects are observed. The lesser responsiveness of the ductus to oxygen in the immature fetus is not due to lack of muscular development, as constriction can be induced by acetylcholine. The high incidence of persistent patency of the ductus arteriosus in premature infants is probably due to lack of maturity of the mechanism for oxygen-induced constriction. In most of these infants spontaneous closure of the ductus occurs within 2 to 3 months after birth.

While the ductus arteriosus is still patent after birth, the reduction in pulmonary vascular resistance will result in a left-to-right shunt through the ductus. If pulmonary vascular resistance is increased by hypoxia, right-to-left shunting of blood will occur through the ductus. If systemic arterial oxygen tension does not increase normally after birth, the ductus may remain patent; there is thus a high incidence of patent ductus arteriosus in people who are born and who continue to live at high altitudes (above about 3,000 m).

CHANGES IN CARDIAC OUTPUT AND DISTRIBUTION. The combined ventricular output in the fetus is about 500 ml/kg fetal body weight/minute, with about 330 ml/kg/minute being ejected by the right ventricle and 170 ml/kg/minute by the left ventricle. After birth there is an increase in total output of the heart during the first few days, with each ventricle ejecting about 400 ml/kg/minute. There is thus little change in right ventricular output, but a marked increase in left ventricular output. The cardiac output per kilogram of body weight falls rapidly during the first 3 months and then gradually falls to about 100 ml/kg in the adult. The increase in cardiac output after birth is probably due mainly to the increase in oxygen consumption per kilogram of body weight. Other factors may also contribute, such as a high percentage of fetal hemoglobin. Reduced adult hemoglobin binds very rapidly with 2,3-diphosphoglycerate, and at the tissue site release of oxygen from hemoglobin is potentiated. There is reduced binding of fetal hemoglobin to 2,3-diphosphoglycerate that will not permit this potentiation of oxygen release so that a larger blood flow may be required to deliver oxygen to the tissues.

CHANGES IN HEART RATE AND BLOOD PRESSURE. Resting fetal heart rate averages 160 to 180 beats per minute. During the newborn period the heart rate averages about 120 beats per minute during sleep and increases to 140 to 160 beats per minute while the infant is awake. In premature infants the resting heart rate is higher, averaging 120 to 140 beats per minute. Heart rate gradually decreases with advancing age. Systemic arterial blood pressure in the fetus at term is about 60/35 mm Hg, as referred to amniotic cavity pressure. Arterial pressure in the mature infant averages 70/50 mm Hg, but it is lower in the premature infant. Arterial pressure gradually increases with advancing age.

References

Dawes GS: Foetal and Neonatal Physiology. Chicago, Year Book, 1968

Friedman WF, Lesch M, Sonnenblick EH (eds): Neonatal Heart Disease. New York, Grune & Stratton, 1973

Rudolph AM: Congenital Diseases of the Heart. Chicago, Year Book, 1974

EMBRYOLOGY
PAUL STANGER

CARDIAC CHAMBERS AND GREAT ARTERIES. During the first month of gestation the primitive cardiac tube forms; it is made up of four segments in series—three chambers (the sinuatrium, the primitive ventricle, and the bulbus cordis) and a single main artery (the truncus) (Fig. 6). Blood enters the caudal end via the sinuatrium and leaves via the truncus. During the second month of gestation there is a transition from this simple tubular arrangement to a heart with two pumping systems in parallel, each system having two chambers and a great artery. The increase in the number of components is accomplished by division of the proximal and distal segments into paired structures, ie, the sinuatrium into the right and left atria and the truncus into the aorta and pulmonary artery. While the two atria form, the atrioventricular canal is divided by the endocardial cushions into a tricuspid and mitral inlet, both of which connect to the primitive ventricle. In contrast

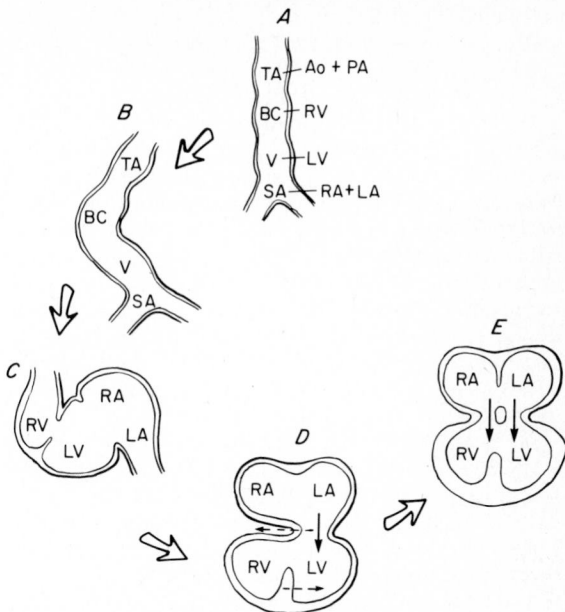

FIG. 6. Transition from straight cardiac tube to four-chambered heart. A. Straight cardiac tube stage with four segments in series. The sinuatrium (SA) is destined to become the right and left atria (RA, LA); the primitive ventricle (V) is precursor to the left ventricle (LV); the bulbus cordis (BC) becomes the right ventricle (RV); the truncus arteriosus (TA) subsequently divides into the aorta (Ao) and main pulmonary artery (PA). The proximal and distal ends of the tube are fixed. B. Differential growth results in the tube bending toward the right. C. The bulboventricular portion of the tube doubles over on itself, so that the right and left ventricles lie side by side. D. The right and left atria still connect to the left ventricle by the atrioventricular (AV) canal. The AV canal migrates toward the right, so that it lies over both ventricles. E. The anterior and posterior endocardial cushions meet and divide the AV canal into tricuspid and mitral orifices.

to the formation of paired atria and two great arteries by division, the left and right ventricles form from the primitive ventricle and bulbus cordis, which are initially in series but with the forming of a loop come to lie side by side (Fig. 6). The transition to a double pumping system involves alignment of each ventricle with its respective atrioventricular valve proximally and the great arteries distally. The proximal alignment is achieved by rightward migration of the atrioventricular canal and leftward migration of the ventricular septum, so that the right ventricle connects to the right atrium. At the distal end of the cardiac tube the transition is more complex. The distal end of the bulbus cordis divides into two muscular portions: the subaortic conus and the subpulmonic conus. The subpulmonic conus increases in length; however, the subaortic conus resorbs as the aorta migrates posteriorly to connect with the left ventricle.

Clearly, there are many possible places for error in such a complex developmental process. Failure of the ventricles to realign with the tricuspid valve over the right ventricle results in double-inlet left ventricle (single ventricle); both atrioventricular valves or a common atrioventricular valve connect to a large left ventricle, and in addition there is a rudimentary right ventricular outflow chamber. At the other end of the cardiac tube, failure of the truncus to divide into aorta and main pulmonary artery results in the various types of truncus arteriosus. Abnormalities of conal resorption are considered the cause for many congenital cardiac lesions in which there is abnormality of great artery connections to the ventricles. For example, failure of resorption of either subaortic conus or subpulmonary conus results in persistence of connection of both great arteries to the right ventricle (double-outlet right ventricle); or resorption of the subpulmonary conus instead of the subaortic conus results in the pulmonary artery arising from the left ventricle and the aorta from the right ventricle (transposition of great arteries).

ATRIAL SEPTUM. The primitive common atrium is divided into two chambers by a septum that forms from three structures: septum I, septum II, and a small portion of endocardial cushion tissue (Fig. 7). Septum I arises as a crescent-shaped structure from the atrial roof and grows toward the atrioventricular (AV) canal to leave an interatrial opening (ostium primum) of decreasing size. Before the ostium primum closes, multiple perforations develop in the cephalad portion of septum I; they coalesce to form the ostium secundum

and permit continued right-to-left flow when the ostium primum is obliterated. Septum II begins to form at the roof of the atrium just to the right of septum I. This septum grows along the atrial wall, but its free concave margin remains open centrally as the fossa ovalis. The thin tissue of septum I serves as a one-way valve, the valve of the foramen ovale, and permits passage of blood from right to left.

Defects of the atrial septum may be of three types: foramen ovale or secundum defects, primum defects, sinus venosus defects. Secundum defects occur when there is insufficient foramen ovale valve tissue to permit closure of the foramen; they may also be the result of a short valve or fenestrations of the valve.

STRUCTURES DERIVED FROM ENDOCARDIAL CUSHIONS. The AV canal initially connects to the primitive ventricle, but it subsequently overlies both ventricles, probably due to shifting of the AV canal toward the right and shifting of the lower ventricular septum toward the left (Fig. 6). The projection and fusion of the dorsal and ventral endocardial cushions divide the canal into tricuspid and mitral channels. The endocardial cushions also form the lowermost portion of the atrial septum, the uppermost portion of the ventricular septum, and portions of the septal leaflets of the tricuspid and mitral valves. Deficiency of development in

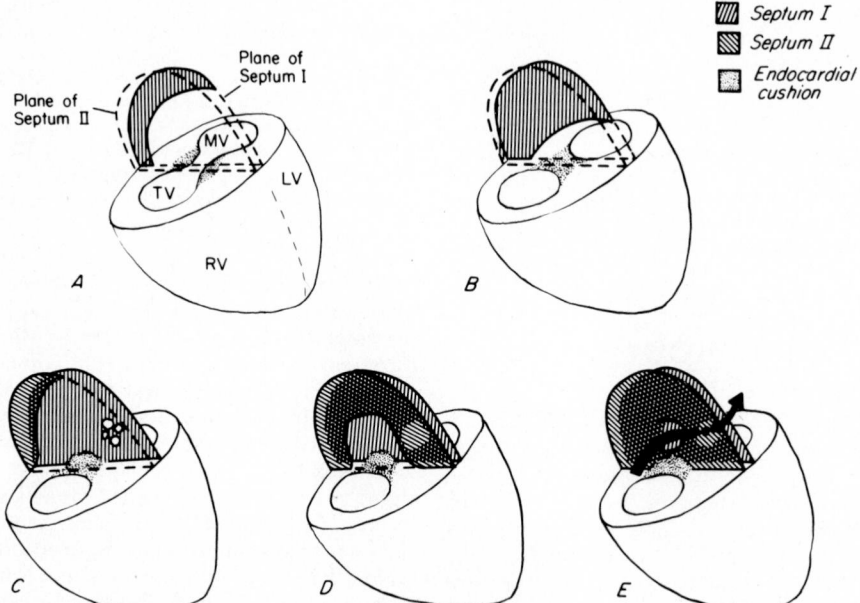

FIG. 7. Formation of the atrial septum and foramen ovale. A and B. Septum I begins to form at the superior-posterior aspect of the sinuatrium and separates the chamber into right and left atria. C. Perforations form in the anterosuperior portion of septum I. At the same time septum II begins to form to the right of septum I. D. The perforations in septum I coalesce to form a discrete opening. E. Septum II forms a complete septum, with the exception of a central opening with a prominent muscular rim at its superior margin. This opening, the fossa ovalis, is covered by the tissue of septum I (the valve of the foramen ovale). Note that there is a small portion of atrial septum just above the AV valves that is formed by endocardial cushion tissue. The latter also forms the uppermost portion of the ventricular septum, as well as portions of the tricuspid and mitral valves. RV and LV, right and left ventricles; TV and MV, tricuspid and mitral valves.

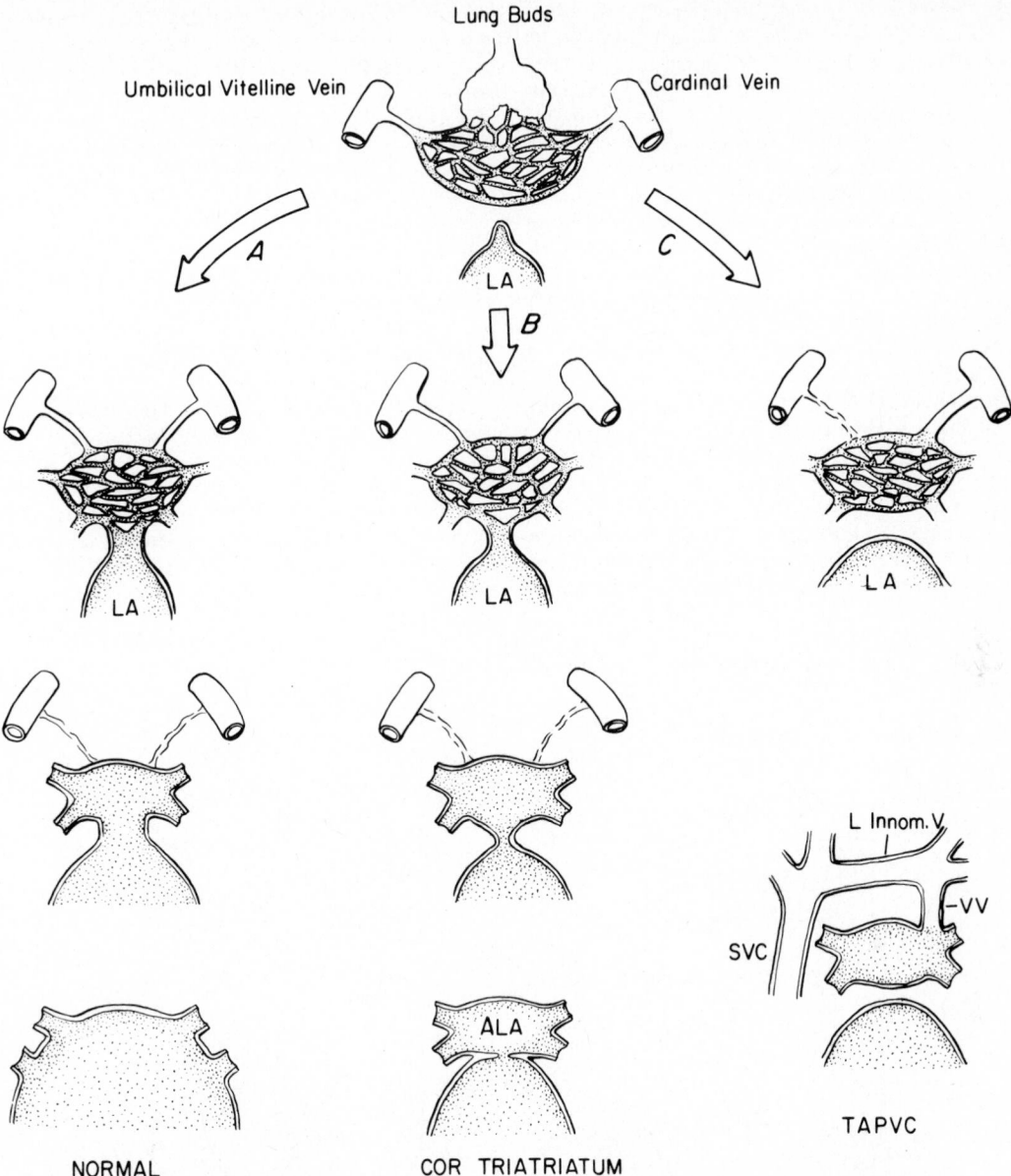

FIG. 8. Embryology of normal pulmonary veins, cor triatriatum, and total anomalous pulmonary venous connection. The lungs are formed from the lung bud, an outgrowth of the primitive foregut. The blood supply of the lungs is initially from the splanchnic plexus, and venous drainage is initially via the umbilico-vitelline or anterior cardinal veins. The left atrium is close to the splanchnic plexus. The common pulmonary vein begins as a diverticulum at the posterior portion of the left atrium just to the left of the atrial septum. A. Normal pulmonary venous development. The common pulmonary vein connects to the splanchnic plexus and establishes drainage to the left atrium. Once this drainage is established, the communications to the umbilico-vitelline and anterior cardinal veins atrophy. The common pulmonary vein becomes incorporated into the left atrium. B. Cor triatriatum. Narrowing of the common pulmonary vein—left atrial junction results in formation of a stenotic membrane that separates the left atrium from a chamber receiving the pulmonary veins, ie, the accessory left atrium (ALA). C. Total anomalous pulmonary venous connection (TAPVC). Failure of the common pulmonary vein to establish connection with the splanchnic plexus results in persistence of drainage to either the umbilico-vitelline vein or anterior cardinal vein. VV, vertical vein; L innom V, left innominate vein; SVC, superior vena cava.

this region may result in varying degrees of endocardial cushion defects. The least severe is the atrial septal defect of the ostium primum type, which usually has a large defect in the lowermost portion of the atrial septum and is associated with an anterior (septal) mitral leaflet cleft and a displaced mitral valve as well as a hemodynamically insignificant ventricular septal defect below the AV valves. The most severe type of endocardial cushion defect is the primitive AV canal with large contiguous atrial and ventricular defects, a common AV valve straddling the ventricular septum, and deficiency of AV valve tissue. Other less common types of endocardial cushion defects include isolated mitral clefts or isolated ventricular septal defects in the region closed by the endocardial cushions.

PULMONARY VEINS. The lung buds are an outgrowth of the primitive foregut, and early in fetal life venous drainage is by the splanchnic plexus to the cardinal and umbilico-vitelline veins (Fig. 8). The common pulmonary vein arises from the posterior left atrium as a small outpouching that enlarges and communicates with the splanchnic plexus. As pulmonary venous drainage via the common pulmonary vein increases, the anas-

tomoses to the cardinal and umbilico-vitelline venous systems disappear. The common pulmonary vein becomes incorporated into the posterior left atrial wall, and the pulmonary veins then connect directly to the left atrium. Should the common pulmonary vein fail to develop or fail to establish communications to the splanchnic plexus, the primitive venous connections persist and result in anomalous pulmonary venous connection to derivatives of the cardinal system (superior venae cavae) or umbilico-vitelline (portal) venous system. A closely related anomaly is cor triatriatum, in which the common pulmonary vein is poorly incorporated into the left atrium, so that there is a stenotic membrane between the common pulmonary vein and the left atrium.

AORTIC ARCH SYSTEM. The ventral and dorsal aortas, as well as their cervical extensions, the ventral and dorsal aortic roots, are connected by six pairs of aortic arches (Fig. 9). The aortic arches make their appearance sequentially, and three of these paired arches (arches I, II, and V) disappear without leaving permanent remnants, while another (arch III) forms the connection between the internal and external carotid

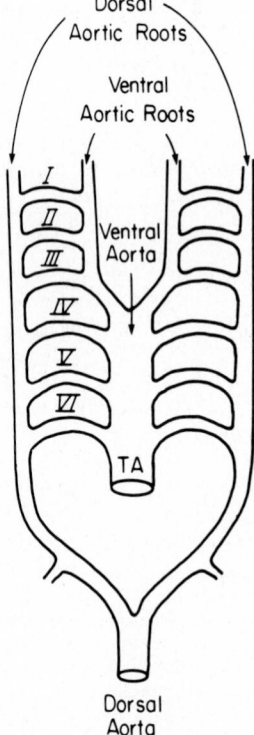

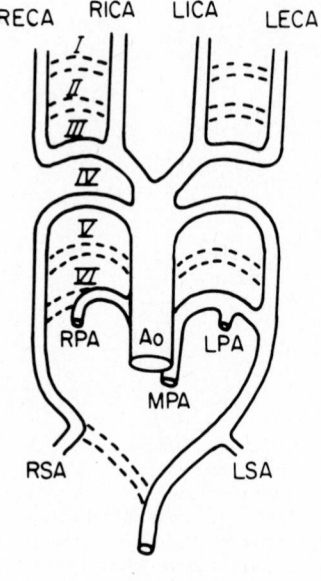

FIG. 9. Schematic diagram of the embryonic aortic arch system. On the left is a schematic of the truncus arteriosus (TA) and the six arches that connect it to the dorsal aorta. The six arches appear sequentially, and those that regress do so at different times. Involution of the various aortic arches and portions of the dorsal aortic roots, as well as persistence of other segments, results in formation of the normal arterial pattern shown on the right. The structures are drawn to show their aortic arch derivations rather than their final anatomic positions. TA, truncus arteriosus; Ao, aorta; MPA, main pulmonary artery; RPA, right pulmonary artery; LPA, left pulmonary artery; RECA and RICA, right external and internal carotid arteries; LECA and LICA, left external and internal carotid arteries; RSA and LSA; right and left subclavian arteries.

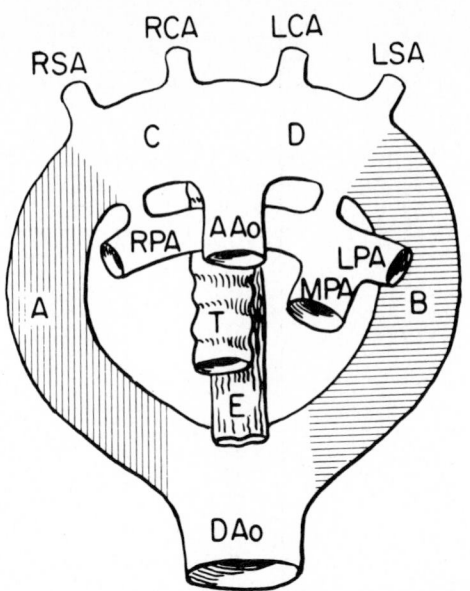

FIG. 10. Schematic diagram of Edwards' hypothetic double aortic arch and bilateral ductus arteriosi. Regression in shaded area A results in the normal left aortic arch; regression in shaded area B results in right aortic arch. Regression at location C results in left aortic arch and anomalous right subclavian artery, while regression at D results in right aortic arch and anomalous left subclavian artery. T, trachea; E, esophagus; MPA, main pulmonary artery; RPA and LPA, right and left pulmonary arteries; RSA and LSA, right and left subclavian arteries; RCA and LCA, right and left carotid arteries. These are the four most common types of arch anomalies; however, the number of possible arch anomalies is large, since regression can occur at almost any location. Lack of regression results in a double aortic arch.

arteries. The proximal portions of the sixth arches become the right and left pulmonary arteries, and the distal left sixth arch becomes the ductus arteriosus; rarely the distal right sixth arch persists as a right ductus arteriosus. The fourth aortic arches persist bilaterally; however, they form different structures on each side. The left fourth arch becomes the segment of aortic arch between the left carotid and subclavian arteries, and the right fourth arch becomes the proximal portion of the right subclavian artery. The aortic arch system and the arterial structures that it subsequently forms are diagrammed in Fig. 9. Edwards has devised a hypothetic double aortic arch system that greatly simplifies the understanding of aortic arch anomalies (Fig. 10). The embryology of any aortic arch anomaly is readily apparent if one postulates regression of an aortic arch at an appropriate location; if there is no arch regression, then there will be a double aortic arch.

References

Langman J, Van Mierop LHS: Development of the cardiovascular system. In Moss AJ, Adams FH (eds): Heart Disease in Infants, Children and Adolescents. Baltimore, Williams & Wilkins, 1968

Netter FH, Van Mierop LHS: Embryology. In Netter FH (ed): The Ciba Collection of Medical Illustrations, Vol 5, Heart. Summit, N.J., Ciba Pharmaceutical Co., 1969, p 112

Stewart JR, Kincaid OW, Edwards JE: An Atlas of Vascular Rings and Related Malformations of the Aortic Arch System. Springfield, Ill, Charles C Thomas, 1964

CARDIAC MALPOSITIONS

PAUL STANGER

A heart that is abnormally placed in the thorax is said to show malposition. Such hearts commonly show abnormalities of chamber localization and great artery attachments as well as associated septal defects, valve anomalies, and outflow obstructions. Describing the basic structure of such a complex heart requires description of three cardiac segments (the atria, the ventricles, and the great arteries), and these descriptions should include not only positional interrelationships but also connections of ventricles to atria and great arteries.

SITUS AND ATRIA. The right and left atria may be regarded as extensions of the systemic and pulmonary veins, respectively, so that the body situs indicates the position of atria. Body situs is determined by certain organs that are normally asymmetric. The normal body configuration, *situs solitus* (Fig. 11), is characterized by a right lung with three lobes, a left lung with two lobes, correspondingly asymmetric tracheobronchial branching, a liver with a major lobe on the right, a left-sided stomach and spleen, right-sided venae cavae, morphologically distinct atria, and a specific orderly arrangement of the gastrointestinal tract. *Situs inversus* is characterized by a mirror-image configuration of the asymmetric organs, including the gastrointestinal tract. In addition to the above two asymmetric forms of situs, two roughly symmetric body configurations have been found with *asplenia* and *polysplenia*. Asplenia is characterized by bilateral right-sidedness, with bilateral three-lobed lungs, each with a typical right bronchial branching pattern, a horizontal liver with equal-size lobes, and bilateral morphologic right atria, each with a sinoatrial node. The absent spleen may also be regarded as a feature of bilateral right-sidedness. In contrast, polysplenia is characterized by bilateral left-sidedness involving lungs, bronchi, and the atria. There are multiple (2 to 30) roughly equal-size spleens with a total mass equal to that of a normal spleen; this is in contrast to accessory spleens, which are small splenic masses in addition to the normal spleen. The spleens are clustered together on both sides of the dorsal mesogastrium. Malrotations of the bowel are common in both asplenia and polysplenia.

VENTRICLES. The primitive cardiac tube normally bends to the right and forms a d-loop (p. 1355). As a result, the anatomic right ventricle lies to the right of the anatomic left ventricle. Such a loop is appropriate or *concordant* for a situs solitus individual; that is, the right atrium connects to the right ventricle and the left atrium to the left ventricle. Conversely, an l-loop is concordant for a situs inversus individual (Fig. 6). Occa-

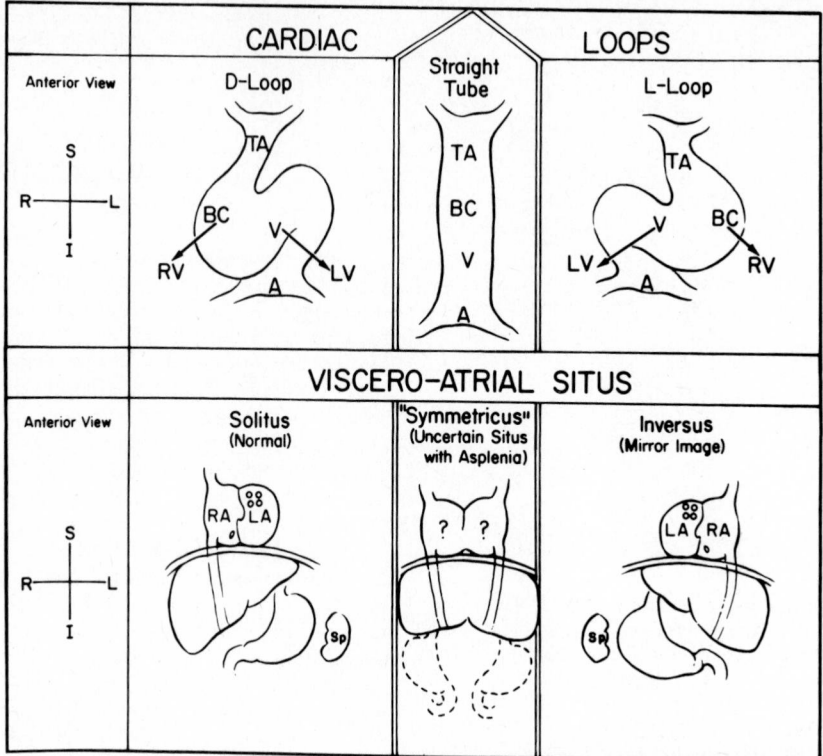

FIG. 11. Abnormalities of chamber and great vessel localization. S, superior; I, inferior; R, right; L, left; TA, truncus arteriosus; BC, bulbus cordis; V, primitive ventricle; A, atrium; RV, right ventricle; LV, left ventricle; RA, right atrium; LA, left atrium; Sp, spleen.

sionally a discordant loop forms (l-loop in situs solitus or d-loop in situs inversus), and the anatomic right atrium connects to the anatomic left ventricle and anatomic left atrium to anatomic right ventricle.

GREAT ARTERIES. Great arteries may be described in terms of their ventricular connections and their positional interrelationships. Ventricular attachments may be normal (pulmonary artery from right ventricle, aorta from left ventricle), double-outlet right or left ventricle (DORV and DOLV), or transposition (aorta from right ventricle, pulmonary artery from left ventricle). The positional interrelationships may be described as *d* (dextro), in which the aortic valve is to the right of the pulmonary artery, *l* (levo), in which the aortic valve is to the left, or *o* (ortho), where the aorta is directly in front of the pulmonary artery; these terms are not to be confused with d-loops and l-loops. In most cases the great artery interrelationships reflect the ventricular interrelationships; however, there are enough exceptions that description of both segments is preferable.

As a general rule the right ventricular infundibulum (or conus) is the most anterior cardiac structure and connects with the anterior great artery. Accordingly, normally related great arteries usually have an anterior pulmonary artery, transpositions have an anterior aorta, and double-outlets tend to have side-by-side vessels. Vessels arising from the left ventricle almost always lack a conus, and consequently their valves are more caudad than those arising from the right ventricle.

Discordant loops (solitus/l-loop or inversus/d-loop) are almost always associated with transposition of the great arteries. The sequential arrangement of chambers and great arteries in these patients is such that the flow is potentially normal, and for this reason these lesions have been called (physiologically) corrected transposition of the great arteries. Any abnormal circulation in these hearts is the result of associated abnormalities such as septal defects, AV valve stenoses, or regurgitation, which occur in nearly all cases. The conduction pathways are also abnormal, and they may cause varying degrees of AV block.

Van Praagh has devised two nomenclatures for describing complex hearts. A modification of his second nomenclature, which is somewhat simpler and has fewer abbreviations, is given below:

Situs
   solitus
   inversus
   asplenia
   polysplenia
Ventricles
   d-loop: morphologic RV to right of morphologic LV
   l-loop: morphologic LV to right of morphologic RV

d- or l- single ventricle: outlets of both atria to a large primitive ventricle with small outlet chamber that has no AV valve; as the outflow chamber is the RV outflow, its position determines *d* or *l* designation

Great arteries
  d-: aortic valve to right of pulmonic
  l-: aortic valve to left of pulmonic
  o-: aortic valve directly anterior
    -normal: PA from RV, Ao from LV

-DORV: PA and Ao from RV
-DOLV: PA and Ao from LV
-trans: Ao from RV, PA from LV
-malposition: unusual arrangement of vessels not conforming to above

Hence segmental sets may be described as follows: Solitus/d-loop/*d*-trans is the usual case of transposition of the great arteries in situs solitus; inversus/d-loop/

Table 1. Most Common Cardiac Anomalies Found in Each Type of Body Configuration

Segmental Set	Common Name	Associated Cardiac Anomalies	Miscellaneous
Solitus/d-loop/*d*-normal	Normal heart of situs solitus; may have abnormal cardiac position due to dextroposition (cardiac displacement due to extracardiac forces) or dextrorotation (rightward pivoting of the ventricular portion of the heart)	Variable, but usually atrial septal defects, ventricular septal defects, or patent ductus arteriosus.	
Solitus-/l-loop/*l*-trans	Corrected transposition of situs solitus	High incidence of ventricular septal defect and/or pulmonic stenosis, Ebstein's malformation of the systemic ventricle, and AV block	
Inversus/l-loop/*l*-normal	Normal heart of situs inversus	Usually normal, but sporadic cases with associated lesions including transposition	
Inversus/d-loop/*d*-trans	Corrected transposition of situs inversus	High incidence of ventricular septal defect and/or pulmonic stenosis, Ebstein's malformation of systemic ventricle, and AV block	
Asplenia/d- or l-loop		Almost all have transposition of the great arteries, severe pulmonic stenosis or atresia, and AV canal with large ventricular septal defect or single ventricle; two-thirds have anomalous pulmonary venous connection to venae cava or portal system	Severe cyanosis from birth on; symmetric liver and bronchi; malrotation of bowel common; Heinz or Howell-Jolly bodies on peripheral blood smear
Polysplenia/d-/or l-loop		Most commonly have left-to-right shunts through atrial septal defects, ventricular septal defects, endocardial cushion defects, and double-outlet right ventricle; transposition and pulmonic stenosis are unusual. Pulmonary veins may connect to either or both atria; two-thirds have interruption of the inferior vena cava	Cyanosis usually mild or absent; congestive heart failure common; malrotation of bowel common; symmetric liver, but less so than in asplenia; superior P axis in ECG common; occasional biliary atresia

d-trans is corrected transposition of the great arteries in situs inversus; asplenia/d-single/*d*-trans is single ventricle with aorta from small outlet chamber and pulmonary artery from large single ventricle in asplenia. Additional defects (eg, septal defects, stenoses, anomalous veins) must be described separately. Some of the common associated anomalies are listed in Table 1.

Cardiac position within the thorax may be influenced by external forces, eg, a hypoplastic right lung or left eventration may cause displacement toward the right. A heart that is predominantly in the left hemithorax is termed levocardia and is normal for situs solitus. If the heart is mainly in the right hemithorax it is referred to as dextrocardia, dextroposition, or dextroversion. Since each of these terms is used in different ways by different people, some of whom use them to indicate ventricular position, it is better to describe the heart as being in the right or left hemithorax and then go on to add descriptions of the cardiac chambers and great vessels. In the absence of such external factors, cardiac position is most closely related to concordance or discordance of the bulboventricular loop. Concordant loops nearly always have normal ventricular postion for that situs, ie, left-sided heart for situs solitus and right-sided for inversus. Exceptions are few and tend to be accompanied by less severe, if any, cardiac abnormalities. Discordant loops in situs solitus or inversus and all loops in asplenia and polysplenia have variable cardiac position, eg, an l-loop in situs solitus (or asplenia or polysplenia) can have a right-sided, left-sided, or midline heart. Similarly, a d-loop in situs inversus, asplenia, and polysplenia can have any position.

References

Stanger P, Benassi RC, Korns ME, Jue KL, Edwards JE: Diagrammatic portrayal of variations in cardiac structure. Circulation 37 [Suppl IV]:, 1968

Van Mierop LHS, Gessner IH, Schiebler GL: Asplenia and polysplenia syndrome. Birth Defects 8:74, 1972

Van Praagh R, Van Praagh S, Vlad P, Keith JD: Anatomic types of congenital dextrocardia. Am J Cardiol 13:510, 1964

AUSCULTATION
JULIEN I.E. HOFFMAN

This section will not deal with the principles of auscultation nor the mechanisms of sounds and murmurs; they are adequately dealt with in many texts. It will describe those aspects of auscultation that are specific to children with congenital heart disease.

The first heart sound and its alterations do not differ in children and adults, and its abnormalities will be discussed later in individual sections. It is important to distinguish the first heart sound, especially if it is split, from systolic clicks. Systolic clicks fall into two main groups, the ejection and the nonejection clicks. Systolic ejection clicks arise early in systole, at the base of the heart, so that although they may be early enough to be confused with a first heart sound, the fact that they are better heard at the base than at the apex serves to distin-

guish them. In addition, the clicks are, as their name implies, high-pitched and clicking, rather than having the dull, lower pitched quality of the first heart sound. Systolic ejection clicks occur frequently whenever there is an enlarged great vessel at the base of the heart. Thus they may occur with an enlarged aorta in valvar aortic stenosis, bicuspid aortic valve, or tetralogy of Fallot, with the large single vessel of a truncus arteriosus, and with a large pulmonary artery due to valvar pulmonic stenosis, idiopathic dilatation of the pulmonary artery, or pulmonary hypertension, although they are relatively uncommon when there is a large pulmonary artery due to a large left-to-right shunt. These clicks are due either to the opening snap of a semilunar valve or to sudden distension of the arterial wall in systole. Nonejection clicks are usually later in systole and are heard at the lower left sternal border or at the apex. When a ventricular septal defect is closing spontaneously, there is often an aneurysm of the membranous ventricular septum, which is pushed into the right ventricle with each systole; the snap as it reaches its limit is often audible in early or midsystole at the lower left sternal border. At the apex there may be an early or midsystolic click, often followed by a midsystolic or late systolic murmur of mitral incompetence, and these are the hallmarks of mitral valve prolapse (billowing mitral valve syndrome).

The second heart sound and its changes are similar in children and adults, but for a few important differences. In the newborn infant with moderately elevated pulmonary arterial pressure and thin chest wall, pulmonic closure is often as loud as aortic closure and is heard at the lower as well as the upper left sternal border. Even in the first few years of life a normal pulmonary closure may be almost as loud at the upper left sternal border as is the aortic closure at the upper right sternal border. However, if the second heart sound is heard loudest at the upper left sternal border, then one must think seriously of the possibility of malposition of the aorta. Thus in *l*-transposition of the great arteries (corrected transposition) the aorta is anterior and to the left, so that the aortic closure is unusually loud and is heard best at the upper left sternal border. This sign may also be present in a *d*-transposition of the great arteries (classic transposition of the great arteries), even though the aortic valve is not on the left side of the sternum. In the tetralogy of Fallot the aorta is wide and dextroposed, and the pulmonary artery that is anterior to it is smaller than usual. The second heart sound is usually single and is loudest at the lower left sternal border.

Absence of splitting of the second heart sound is important because a single second sound may indicate atresia or severe stenosis of a semilunar valve. However, certain sources of confusion should be appreciated. In newborn infants with rapid heart and respiratory rates, the splitting may be too narrow to appreciate, even though it may be present on a phonocardiogram. In *d*-transposition of the great arteries the pulmonary artery is posterior, so that pulmonic closure may be too soft to be heard, even though it is present.

Very wide splitting of the second heart sound suggests right bundle branch block, pulmonic stenosis, or atrial septal defect, as in adults. Occasionally it occurs in normal children examined when supine; on sitting them up, the width of the splitting decreases markedly, and the respiratory variation becomes more prominent, thus separating this from pathologic splitting of the second sound. It should be noted, too, that infants and very young children with large atrial septal defects may have normal splitting and respiratory variation of the second heart sound for reasons that are not understood.

INNOCENT MURMURS. Murmurs that are due to normal turbulence and vibration and that do not indicate present or future heart disease may be termed innocent or benign murmurs. They are also often called functional murmurs, but this term is confusing because in a sense all murmurs are related to cardiac function. Furthermore, the murmur of mitral incompetence due to left ventricular dilatation in anemia is functional and will disappear when the hemoglobin rises, but it is by no neans benign. One or more of these innocent murmurs can be heard in almost every child provided that the child cooperates and the room is quiet. With age and increasing thickness of the chest wall, the murmurs become harder to hear and may be detected easily in only about 15 or 20 percent of adolescents and adults. Some people retain these murmurs throughout life. There are six distinct types of innocent murmurs, all of which can and should be diagnosed by their specific features, rather than by failing to identify the murmur as being due to a known organic lesion.

SYSTOLIC MURMURS. Still's murmur, also termed vibratory or musical murmur, is heard best at the apex and lower left sternal border. The murmur is midsystolic and lasts about half of systole or less; it is diamond-shaped (crescendo–decrescendo) and is seldom more than grade 2/6 in intensity. Its characteristic feature is its musical quality, much like that of a plucked string instrument. It is usually low-pitched, with regular frequencies commonly between 90 and 120 Hz, that is, about one and one-half octaves below middle C. The mechanism of production is uncertain, but vibrations of the semilunar valve cusps or chordae tendineae have been suggested. The musical quality, timing, and shape easily distinguish this murmur from other murmurs in the lower precordium. Mitral incompetence murmurs are usually apical, with radiation to the axilla and back; they are high-pitched and blowing and either pansystolic or late systolic in timing. Ventricular septal defects have murmurs that are harsh, loud, and pansystolic, or if the defect is very small the murmurs may be very early in systole and have a high-pitched whistling quality.

The basal ejection systolic murmur is heard best at the upper right or left sternal border; it is also midsystolic, relatively short, diamond-shaped, and usually not over grade 2/6 in intensity. Unlike Still's murmur, however, it is not only in a different site but is high-pitched and blowing, with no musical component. The murmur is due to the fact that at the beginning of systole blood just above the aortic and pulmonic valves is not moving and is sheared away from the wall when blood is ejected

from the ventricles. The most likely difficulty in diagnosis is in separating these murmurs from those due to pulmonic or aortic stenosis or a bicuspid aortic valve. The distinction may not be easy, since the innocent and the pathologic murmurs have similar mechanisms of origin. If there is mild stenosis (for severe stenosis can be diagnosed from other features) the murmur is usually harsher, and there may be a systolic ejection click. If the murmur is soft and blowing and there is no other evidence of heart disease, it is probably wisest to regard it as innocent in order to avoid producing a cardiac neurosis.

The carotid bruit is heard in the supraclavicular regions along the carotid arteries. Like the basal ejection murmur, it is diamond-shaped, high-pitched, and blowing; it is usually grade 2/6 in intensity. However, it is heard best above the clavicles and is very short and early, being over within the first quarter or third of systole. It is probably due to turbulence in the carotid arteries as the blood is accelerated early in systole. Its extreme shortness and predominant supraclavicular site make it easy to diagnose. The murmurs of aortic or pulmonic stenosis may transmit to the neck, but they will then be heard best below the clavicles and will be longer. Internal carotid arterial obstructive lesions are rare in children, and the bruits of thyrotoxicosis are accompanied by typical signs of that lesion.

The physiologic peripheral pulmonic stenosis murmur is heard best in the axillae and back, although it may also be heard at the upper sternal border. The murmur is again diamond-shaped, usually not more than grade 2/6 in intensity, midsystolic, and relatively short. It is blowing and rather high-pitched. It is due to the fact that at birth and for some weeks after birth the right and left pulmonary arteries are much smaller than, and come off at a sharp angle from, the large main pulmonary artery. As a result there is turbulence and an actual loss of pressure head as blood passes from main to branch pulmonary arteries, and with this there is a soft stenotic murmur. As the child grows, the vessels alter until the branch pulmonary arteries are similar in diameter to the main pulmonary artery and come off from it at a more gentle curve. There is no turbulence at that time, and the murmurs disappear, usually by about 3 months of age.

All of these systolic murmurs, then, are relatively short, soft, and diamond-shaped. They are all louder in the supine than in the erect position because stroke volume is greater when supine. For the same reason (greater cardiac output) these murmurs all get louder with exercise, anxiety, or fever, and this phenomenon does not help to differentiate them from pathologic murmurs.

CONTINUOUS MURMURS. The venous hum is heard under the clavicles and in the neck; it is more often heard on the right side than on the left side, but it can be present on both. The murmur is very low-pitched; it can be grade 3–4/6 in intensity and is usually continuous, but with no clear relationship to the cardiac cycle. It may vary with respiration. The murmur is due to blood draining down the jugular veins. As blood flows from the collapsed cervical veins to the dilated intrathoracic veins, the vein walls flutter and cause the low-pitched murmur. This explains the continuous nature of the murmur, its lack of relation to the cardiac cycle, and the effect of respiration. It also explains why the murmur is often absent in the supine position, since the neck veins are distended and there is no point of transition between collapsed and distended veins. For the same reason the murmur can often be abolished by altering the position of the head (tilting, rotating), since this alters flow in the neck veins; it can also be abolished by occluding the veins in the neck with the thumb or by having the subject do a Valsalva maneuver. The murmur may be mistaken for a patent ductus arteriosus, if it is on the left side, or for other arteriovenous fistulae. Its characteristics and changeability make it easily diagnosed.

A continuous murmur (the mammary souffle) may be heard over the breasts in pregnant or lactating women. It is usually not loud. The setting makes the diagnosis easy, and it is important not to diagnose underlying heart disease.

SIGNIFICANCE.   These murmurs are of great importance because of the marked cardiac anxiety that people have. Murmurs are equated with heart disease and sudden death in many people's minds, and if the doctor transmits uncertainty to the patient there can be great harm done. In some studies it has been found that there has been more anxiety in parents and children and more restriction of the children with innocent murmurs than of those with moderate congenital or rheumatic heart disease. Therefore the approach should be to assess the child's health and cardiac status by a thorough history and physical examination, with particular attention to the characteristics of the murmurs. It is important to emphasize that since it is possible to have an innocent murmur with a cardiac abnormality, for example a cardiomyopathy, the assessment of cardiac normality must be made from all aspects of the cardiovascular examination, not only from the murmur.

Once an innocent murmur *and* a normal heart have been diagnosed, the parents should usually be given a full explanation to the effect that the heart is normal and the murmur is a normal phenomenon. It may help to explain that normal turbulence causes murmurs, much as flowing water in a hose or pipe has a swishing sound or a river flowing around a bend ripples and splashes. For many parents it is essential to make sure that they realize that the murmur is not an indication of slight heart disease and that it is of no importance whether it goes away or stays. It is, of course, not always possible to be sure that a murmur is innocent, particularly in infants who are difficult to examine. In that instance it is reasonable to explain to the parents that the murmur is either normal or may be indicative of mild heart disease and that further following of the child or cardiac consultation will probably help to make the definitive diagnosis.

PATHOLOGIC MURMURS.   Murmurs that are due to organic heart disease differ from innocent murmurs in quality, intensity, position, and radiation, and they may often be associated with other abnormal features of the cardiac examination. They will be discussed in detail in sections dealing with specific cardiac lesions.

References

Caceres CA, Perry LW: The Innocent Murmur. Boston, Little, Brown, 1967
Castle RF, Craige E: Auscultation of the heart in infants and children. Pediatrics 26:511, 1960
McKusick VA: Cardiovascular Sound in Health and Disease. Baltimore, Williams & Wilkins, 1972
Nadas AS, Fyler DC: Pediatric Cardiology. Philadelphia, WB Saunders, 1972

CARDIAC CATHETERIZATION
PAUL STANGER

As techniques for cardiac surgery became available, the need for accurate anatomic and physiologic diagnosis of cardiac disease increased, and this encouraged the development of cardiac catheterization and angiography. Not only did catheterization serve as a diagnostic tool, it brought about a clearer understanding of abnormal hemodyamics and provided sound physiologic explanations for clinical findings.

TECHNIQUE.   Catheters are placed in peripheral vessels either percutaneously or by cutdown and isolation of the vessels. Percutaneous techniques have several advantages: local infections and arterial complications are less frequent, the same vessels may be used repeatedly, and in older children the relatively deep femoral vessels are more accessible. In patients with congenital heart disease the use of the femoral approach often permits passage of a venous catheter into the left side of the heart through a patent foramen ovale, an atrial septal defect, or a ventricular septal defect, thus avoiding retrograde arterial catheterization.

Catheter manipulation is performed under fluoroscopy with image intensification to reduce radiation exposure. Most catheters are semirigid, and the position of the catheter tip is controlled by twisting the catheter. Flow-directed ballon-tipped catheters are particularly useful for difficult manipulations. Special catheters are used for intracardiac phonocardiography and His bundle electrocardiography.

OXYGEN SATURATIONS.   Small blood samples are obtained in each of the major vessels and cardiac chambers, and the presence or absence of shunts is determined by measuring oxygen saturations rapidly by reflectance oximetry. This information must be interpreted with caution, as streaming from different veins may influence saturations, especially in the venae cavae and right atrium. Superior vena caval blood contains streams with much variability of saturation. Similarly, hepatic venous blood with medium saturation mixes with highly saturated renal streams and less saturated femoral venous streams in the inferior vena cava. The lowest oxygen concentrations are found in coronary sinus blood, and since the coronary sinus enters just above the tricuspid valve, a sample in the right ventricle may be a little less saturated than one in the right atrium. Because of streaming, an increase in oxygen saturation of 10 percent at the right atrial level, 3 percent at the ventricular level, or 2 percent at the pulmonary arterial level is required to indicate a left-to-right shunt and must be verified by another technique, usually angiocardiography. Furthermore, an increase in oxygen saturation at a given level does not necessarily indicate a left-to-right shunt at that level. For example, an increase in oxygen saturation at the right atrial level may indicate streaming alone, or it may indicate shunting of oxygenated blood coming from any left-sided structure (Table 2). Similarly, an increase in oxygen saturation at the right ventricular level may be the result of one of several factors: streaming alone, anomalous pulmonary venous connection to the coronary sinus with streaming, atrial septal defect with streaming (usually a small to moderate shunt), ventricular septal defect, ruptured sinus of Valsalva, coronary arteriovenous fistula with streaming, or aorticopulmonary shunt with pulmonary insufficiency. In general, an increase in oxygen saturation at a given level may be the result of a shunt at that level, at a more proximal level with streaming, or at a more distal level with regurgitation.

Oxygen saturation data are of limited use in identifying the second of two large shunts. A patient with a large left-to-right atrial shunt will have blood with a very high oxygen saturation entering the right ventricle. A second shunt of equal magnitude at the ventricular level will produce a relatively small, if any, further increase in oxygen saturation. Similarly, oxygen saturations may not indicate a large left-to-right shunt through a patent ductus arteriosus if there is a large left-to-right ventricular shunt. In view of all these limitations, the sites of communication are best delineated by selective angiocardiography. Indicator dilution curves may be used for localizing shunts; however, they are also influenced by streaming and regurgitation. Although they can be used to detect much smaller shunts than can be detected with saturation data, their importance has decreased as the detail provided by angiograms has improved.

Normal right-sided oxygen saturations vary between 65 and 80 percent, depending on cardiac output and hemoglobin concentration. In patients breathing room air, left-sided saturations are invariably less than 100 percent (usually 94 to 98 percent). The P_{O_2} in room air is about 150 torr, and about 110 torr in the alveolus. Because of a small alveolar–arterial gradient, pulmonary venous P_{O_2} is 85 to 100 torr—values that correspond to 95 to 98 percent saturation on the oxyhemoglobin dissociation curve (p. 1113).

FLOW, SHUNT, AND RESISTANCE. Flows and shunts may be calculated by the Fick method, by angiographic volumes, or by indicator dilution techniques using cold saline and thermistor catheters or indocyanine green dye and photometric methods. As the Fick technique is by far the most widely used, it will be described in detail (Fig. 12).

Flow through an organ may be estimated if one measures the amount of substance (indicator) added to or removed from blood as it passes through that organ, the concentration of the substance in arterial blood flowing to that organ, and the concentration of the substance in venous blood leaving that organ:

$$F = \frac{i}{c_V - c_A}$$

where F is flow per minute, i is indicator added per minute, c_V is venous concentration of indicator, and c_A is arterial concentration of indicator. To calculate flow through the lungs:

$$Q_P = \frac{V_{O_2}}{C_{PV} - C_{PA}}$$

where Q_P is pulmonary flow (liters/minute), V_{O_2} is oxygen consumption (ml/min), C_{PV} is pulmonary venous oxygen content (ml/liter blood), and C_{PA} is pulmonary arterial oxygen content (ml/liter blood).

Note that the calculation requires oxygen content rather than oxygen saturation. Oxygen *saturation* refers to the proportion of hemoglobin in blood that is combined with oxygen. It is expressed as a percentage and is independent of hemoglobin concentration. In contrast, oxygen *content* refers to the total amount of oxygen in a volume of blood and includes physically dissolved oxygen. It is expressed as milliliters of oxygen per 100 ml blood, or volume percent, or it may be expressed as milliliters of oxygen per liter of blood. Clearly, the oxygen content of blood with a 50 percent oxygen saturation and a hemoglobin concentration of 20 g/100 ml will be nearly twice that of blood with a 50 percent oxygen saturation and a hemoglobin concentration of 10 g/100 ml. Oxygen *capacity* refers to the total content of oxygen that hemoglobin contains when it is 100 percent saturated.

In patients breathing room air the physically dissolved oxygen is negligible in comparison with the oxygen bound to hemoglobin. A close approximation of the arteriovenous oxygen content difference may be obtained by multiplying the arteriovenous oxygen saturation difference by the oxygen capacity:

$$Q_P = \frac{V_{O_2}}{(sat_{PV} - sat_{PA})(O_2 \text{ capacity})}$$

TABLE 2. Causes of Increased Right Atrial Oxygen Saturation

From	Via
Pulmonary vein	Anomalous pulmonary venous connection
Left atrium	Atrial septal defect
Left ventricle	LV-to-RV communication Ventricular septal defect and tricuspid regurgitation Endocardial cushion defect with LV-to-RA shunt
Aorta	Ruptured sinus of Valsalva Coronary arteriovenous fistula

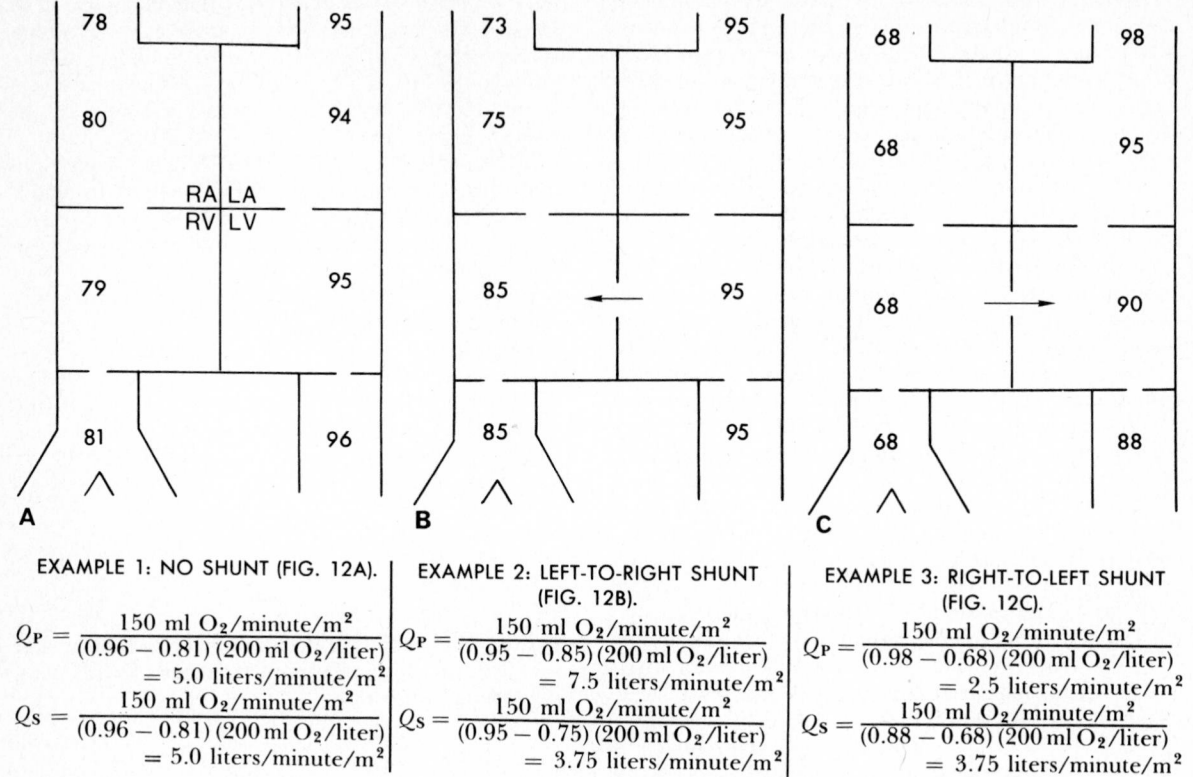

EXAMPLE 1: NO SHUNT (FIG. 12A).

$$Q_P = \frac{150 \text{ ml O}_2/\text{minute/m}^2}{(0.96 - 0.81)(200 \text{ ml O}_2/\text{liter})}$$
$$= 5.0 \text{ liters/minute/m}^2$$
$$Q_S = \frac{150 \text{ ml O}_2/\text{minute/m}^2}{(0.96 - 0.81)(200 \text{ ml O}_2/\text{liter})}$$
$$= 5.0 \text{ liters/minute/m}^2$$

EXAMPLE 2: LEFT-TO-RIGHT SHUNT (FIG. 12B).

$$Q_P = \frac{150 \text{ ml O}_2/\text{minute/m}^2}{(0.95 - 0.85)(200 \text{ ml O}_2/\text{liter})}$$
$$= 7.5 \text{ liters/minute/m}^2$$
$$Q_S = \frac{150 \text{ ml O}_2/\text{minute/m}^2}{(0.95 - 0.75)(200 \text{ ml O}_2/\text{liter})}$$
$$= 3.75 \text{ liters/minute/m}^2$$

EXAMPLE 3: RIGHT-TO-LEFT SHUNT (FIG. 12C).

$$Q_P = \frac{150 \text{ ml O}_2/\text{minute/m}^2}{(0.98 - 0.68)(200 \text{ ml O}_2/\text{liter})}$$
$$= 2.5 \text{ liters/minute/m}^2$$
$$Q_S = \frac{150 \text{ ml O}_2/\text{minute/m}^2}{(0.88 - 0.68)(200 \text{ ml O}_2/\text{liter})}$$
$$= 3.75 \text{ liters/minute/m}^2$$

FIG. 12.

where sat$_{PV}$ is pulmonary venous oxygen saturation and sat$_{PA}$ is pulmonary arterial oxygen saturation.

In the absence of right-to-left shunting, an aortic sample is preferable to a pulmonary venous sample, since it is a mixture of blood from all four pulmonary veins. Similarly, a pulmonary arterial sample is a representative mixture of systemic venous blood.

In a steady state the amount of oxygen utilized in the tissues is equal to the amount taken into the lungs, and systemic flow is calculated with the same equation and oxygen consumption. In the absence of any shunts the systemic arteriovenous oxygen difference is the same as the pulmonary arteriovenous oxygen difference, and the calculated flows are equal. If there are shunts, then pulmonary and systemic flows must be calculated separately, the former from oxygen contents in pulmonary veins and pulmonary artery, the latter from aorta and mixed venous blood.

The following are examples of flow and shunt calculations. In each the oxygen consumption (V_{O_2}) is assumed to be 150 ml/minute/m^2, and the hemoglobin (Hb) concentration is assumed to be 14.7 g/100 ml blood or 147 g/liter blood. Since 1 g Hb combines with 1.356 ml O$_2$, then

$$O_2 \text{ capacity} = \left(\frac{147 \text{ g Hb}}{\text{liter blood}}\right)\left(\frac{1.356 \text{ ml O}_2}{\text{g Hb}}\right) = \frac{200 \text{ ml O}_2}{\text{liter blood}}$$

The aortic saturation of 0.96 was used instead of the pulmonary venous saturation in the calculation of Q_P because it is mixed pulmonary venous saturation.

The most distal saturation that is proximal to the left-to-right shunt is used in the calculation, as it is usually the best mixed venous sample available. Left-to-right shunt $= Q_P - Q_S = 3.75$ liters/minute/m^2.

Right-to-left shunt $= Q_S - Q_P = 1.25$ liters/minute/m^2.

The calculation of bidirectional shunts requires an additional concept, that of effective pulmonary flow (Q_{EP}), which may be defined as the volume of systemic venous blood per minute that flows through the lungs. This volume does not include blood that is shunted in either direction. In a patient with only a left-to-right shunt, it is equal to systemic flow ($Q_P - Q_{EP}$ is the left-to-right shunt), while in a patient with only a right-to-left shunt it is equal to pulmonary flow ($Q_S - Q_{EP}$ is the right-to-left shunt). In patients with bidirectional shunting the arteriovenous difference used in the calculation of effective pulmonary flow employs the mixed systemic venous and mixed pulmonary venous oxygen contents.

Left-to-right shunt $= Q_P - Q_{EP} = 0.75$ liters/minute/m^2; right-to-left shunt $= Q_S - Q_{EP} = 2.0$ liters/minute/m^2.

There are two types of shunts: physiologic and ana-

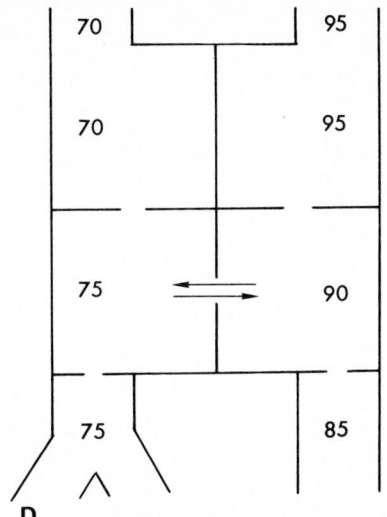

D   **E**

EXAMPLE 4: BIDIRECTIONAL SHUNTING
(FIG. 12D).

$$Q_P = \frac{150 \text{ ml } O_2/\text{minute/m}^2}{(0.95 - 0.75)\,(200 \text{ ml } O_2/\text{liter})}$$
$$= 3.75 \text{ liters/minute/m}^2$$

$$Q_S = \frac{150 \text{ ml } O_2/\text{minute/m}^2}{(0.85 - 0.70)\,(200 \text{ ml } O_2/\text{liter})}$$
$$= 5.0 \text{ liters/minute/m}^2$$

$$Q_{EP} = \frac{150 \text{ ml } O_2/\text{minute/m}^2}{(0.95 - 0.70)\,(200 \text{ ml } O_2/\text{liter})}$$
$$= 3.0 \text{ liters/minute/m}^2$$

$$Q_P = \frac{150 \text{ ml } O_2/\text{minute/m}^2}{(0.95 - 0.75)\,(200 \text{ ml } O_2/\text{liter})}$$
$$= 3.75 \text{ liters/minute/m}^2$$

$$Q_S = \frac{150 \text{ ml } O_2/\text{minute/m}^2}{(0.75 - 0.50)\,(200 \text{ ml } O_2/\text{liter})}$$
$$= 3.0 \text{ liters/minute/m}^2$$

$$Q_{EP} = \frac{150 \text{ ml } O_2/\text{minute/m}^2}{(0.95 - 0.50)\,(200 \text{ ml } O_2/\text{liter})}$$
$$= 1.67 \text{ liters/minute/m}^2$$

FIG. 12.

tomic. A physiologic left-to-right shunt is pulmonary venous blood that is recirculated through the lung; a physiologic right-to-left shunt is systemic venous blood that passes directly into the systemic arteries. In contrast, an anatomic shunt is one that passes through a defect at a given level within the heart. The following example of tricuspid atresia illustrates both types of shunts (Fig. 12E).
Physiologic left-to-right shunt = $Q_P - Q_{EP}$ = 2.08 liters/minute/m²; physiologic right-to-left shunt = $Q_S - Q_{EP}$ = 1.33 liters/minute/m². Anatomic left-to-right shunt = the shunt through the ventricular septal defect, which is the total pulmonary flow (3.75 liters/minute/m²); anatomic right-to-left shunt = the shunt through the atrial septal defect, which is the total systemic flow (3.0 liters/minute/m²).

In the above example the anatomic right-to-left and the anatomic left-to-right shunts include some systemic venous blood that crosses through the atrial septal defect and returns to the right side via the ventricular septal defect; this systemic venous blood ultimately enters the pulmonary circulation and thus is not shunted in the physiologic sense.

In patients with transposition of the great arteries, the pulmonary and systemic circulations are in parallel. The effective pulmonary flow indicates the degree of mixing of the two circulations. By definition, the effective pulmonary flow is the volume of systemic venous blood that passes directly into the lungs, and in transposition the only systemic venous blood to follow that pathway is the anatomic shunt from the systemic to the pulmonary circulation. Furthermore, in transposition the anatomic right-to-left and left-to-right shunts must be equal over a period of time, or one of the two parallel circulations will empty into the other.

PRESSURES. Pressures are monitored continuously during catheter manipulation to assist in determining catheter position, and they are recorded in each chamber and vessel entered. Differences in pressure from site to site help to localize obstructions and are essential to assessing their severity (Table 3).

VASCULAR RESISTANCE. The resistance to blood flow in the pulmonary and systemic circulations is calculated from the equations

$$R_P = \frac{\text{mean PA pressure} - \text{mean PV or LA pressure}}{Q_P}$$

$$R_S = \frac{\text{mean aortic pressure} - \text{mean RA pressure}}{Q_S}$$

Table 3. Average Normal Ranges of Intracardiac and Intravascular Pressures

	Infants and Children	Newborn period
Right atrium	a = 5–8; v = 2–6; M = 2–6	M = 0–4
Right ventricle	15–25/2–5	35–80/1–5
Pulmonary artery	15–25/8–12 (M = 10–16)	35–80/20–50 (M = 25–60)
Pulmonary wedge	a = 6–12; v = 8–15; M = 5–12	
Left atrium	a = 6–12; v = 8–15; M = 5–10	M = 3–6
Left ventricle	80–130/5–10	
Systemic artery	90–130/60–80 (M = 70–95)	65–80/45–60 (M = 60–65)

Adapted from Rudolph AM: Congenital Diseases of the Heart, 1974. Courtesy of Year Book Medical Publishers.

where R_P is pulmonary vascular resistance (resistance units/m^2), Q_P is pulmonary flow (liters/minute/m^2), R_S is systemic vascular resistance (resistance units/m^2), and Q_S is systemic flow (liters/minute/m^2). When pressures are measured in millimeters of mercury, resistance units are equivalent to millimeters of mercury per liter per minute. Most of the resistance to flow is at the arteriolar level, and the calculated resistance is inversely related to the cross-sectional area of the arteriolar lumina. In the systemic circulation the calculated resistance is a mean value for several different vascular beds. The normal systemic vascular resistance varies between 15 and 30 units/m^2. Although it is quite high at birth, the pulmonary vascular resistance reaches values near adult values after 6 to 8 weeks. In order to compare these values at different ages, they are usually related to surface area. Normal values in children and adults are 1 to 3 units/m^2. Evaluation of pulmonary vascular resistance and its responsiveness to pulmonary vasodilators is discussed elsewhere (p. 1438).

SELECTIVE ANGIOCARDIOGRAPHY. Positioning a catheter in a particular chamber and rapidly injecting iodinated contrast medium permits delineation of most cardiovascular structures radiographically. The concentration of contrast medium is greatest in the injected chamber, and consequently its anatomy and motion are most clearly defined. As the contrast material passes into more distal chambers or vessels, dispersion and dilution cause a loss of definition. Multiple injection sites are often necessary to obtain a complete anatomic diagnosis.

Angiograms may be recorded on cine film at 30 to 60 frames per second or on large films that are rapidly changed at 6 to 8 frames per second. Although large films show anatomic details better, small shunts and ventricular movement are better seen on cine film. Biplane angiograms yield more information than single-plane angiograms with the same volume of contrast material, which is an important consideration in patients with complicated abnormalities who require multiple angiograms and in newborns who may have a low tolerance to contrast medium. A video replay system permits immediate examination of angiograms. This not only ensures that the desired information has been recorded but also minimizes delays in treating critically ill newborns.

ADDITIONAL TESTING. A variety of additional tests may be done during the procedure. The effect of exercise on patients with moderately severe obstructive lesions may be assessed with ergometer or handgrip exercise. An isoproterenol infusion simulates exercise conditions; however, this is less satisfactory. Bundle of His electrograms may be recorded by positioning a bipolar electrode catheter near the bundle of His; the technique is of particular value in determining the site of atrioventricular block. Pacing may be used at catheterization in order to assess the effect of increased heart rate on patients with pulmonic stenosis, aortic stenosis, or aortic insufficiency. Rapid atrial pacing may bring out atrioventricular block that is not apparent at slower rates.

RISKS. Cardiac catheterization can lead to serious complications, including serious arrhythmias, arterial obstruction, reactions to contrast medium, hemorrhage, cardiac perforation, hypoxemic episodes, infections, and death. Pericatheterization deaths are rare except in neonates. In most instances the neonates are critically ill, often with uncorrectable lesions, and catheterization is but one event in a relentless downhill course. Older children at particular risk of death are those with a very high pulmonary vascular resistance and no means of shunting. In these children vagal episodes leading to decreased systemic output and death may occur during the catheterization or during the following day. The actual risk varies with the age and illness of the child, the type of lesion, and the experience of those doing the catheterization. In laboratories with extensive experience of catheterizing sick children, about 1 child per 1,000 will die because of the catheterization. Almost always this will be due to a complication such as an arrhythmia occurring in an already ill child. If the infants are desperately ill and have emergency studies, some will die during or just after the study, but not because of it. About 3 percent of the children may have significant but nonfatal complications.

INDICATIONS. Not only do the indications for cardiac catheterization vary from institution to institution, they may also vary among cardiologists in the same center. There is some agreement that neonates with cyanotic congenital cardiac disease require immediate cardiac catheterization, as they are at great risk of deteriorating rapidly, usually when the ductus arteriosus closes. Many of these infants require prompt anatomic diagnosis in order to facilitate emergency surgery, and in some a balloon atrial septostomy performed at cardiac catheterization may be life-saving.

Similarly, if a newborn has congestive cardiac failure in the first days after birth and the cause is an anatomic cardiac abnormality (in contrast to an arrhythmia or metabolic abnormality alone), it is unlikely that the infant will respond to medical management alone. Any infant with congestive heart failure requires catheterization; however, infants beyond the first days of life can usually have their congestive heart failure stabilized with medication before proceeding to the catheterization.

In older infants and children, cardiac catheterization is usually indicated whenever a condition is severe enough to require surgical intervention. In some conditions such as pulmonic stenosis, severity can be assessed reasonably accurately on clinical grounds. In others, most notably aortic stenosis, clinical assessment may be considerably in error. In some centers patients with patent ductus arteriosus, coarctation of the aorta, or atrial septal defect do not undergo cardiac catheterization prior to surgery. Clearly, in such cases one must weigh the relative risks of incomplete or erroneous diagnosis and the risks of cardiac catheterization.

References

Braunwald E, Swan HJC: Cooperative study on cardiac catheterization. Circulation 37 [Suppl 3]:, 1968

Rudolph AM: Congenital Diseases of the Heart. Chicago, Year Book, 1974

Zimmerman H: Intravascular Catheterization. Springfield, Ill, Charles C Thomas, 1974

ECHOCARDIOGRAPHY
Norman H. Silverman

This section is an introduction to understanding how echocardiographic signals are interpreted; a formal review of the subject matter may be found in the References. It is important to note that the echocardiogram forms a part of the investigation of patients with cardiac disease, and information gained from the history, physical examination, electrocardiogram, and chest roentgenogram is helpful in facilitating echocardiographic diagnosis.

Ultrasound is that frequency of sound above the audible range of 20,000 Hz. In general, the sound frequency used in medical work ranges from 2 to 5 MHz. The ultrasound is transmitted from a piezoelectric crystal similar to those found in record players. When an electrical field is applied to this crystal, electrical energy is converted into mechanical energy, so that the crystal vibrates (piezoelectric phenomenon) and sets up sound waves in the particular frequency of the crystal. An important property of ultrasound is that its course is unidirectional, like that of a light beam. When an ultrasonic transducer is applied to the surface of a particular part of the body and a short burst of electrical energy excites the crystal, a pulse of ultrasound waves is beamed through the tissue. This beam of sound has approximately the same diameter as the crystal (0.5 to 1.25 cm). As the sound waves pass through the body they encoun-

ter tissues of different densities, and they travel through different tissues with different velocities; the density times the velocity is called the impedance of a tissue. At the interface between two tissues of different impedances, a number of changes in the sound beam occur, just as a beam of light striking a glass is reflected or refracted. Some of the sound waves pass through the tissue in the direction of the beam, some are refracted and pass off in directions different from that of the original beam, and some are reflected, giving rise to the echo signal. If the interface is nearly perpendicular to the sonic beam, the reflected sound travels back at the same speed at which it entered and returns to the chest wall–transducer interface. The sonic energy excites the piezoelectric crystal of the transducer, which now acts as a receiver, and the mechanical energy is converted into electrical energy, just as vibrations from a phonograph record are converted into electrical energy. The electrical energy passes up the transducer cable to an amplifier. Most commercially available instruments transmit a pulse for 1 μsec and for 999 μsec act as receivers. This cycle is repeated so that 1,000 depth samplings are obtained each second.

The velocity of sound transmission in soft tissue and blood is approximately 1,500 m/sec. The time delay between sound transmission and reception of each sound reflection allows the electronic timing circuitry in the ultrasonic scope equipment to calculate the distance between the transducer and the interface producing each echo pulse. One thousand depth samplings per second allow virtually continuous plotting of the distances between the echo signals recorded from multiple depths and the transducer. The signals, after suitable amplification, can be displayed as spikes, with their amplitudes corresponding to the strength of the echo and their position marking the depth of each interface. This is called amplitude modulation (A mode), and it has been used in neurology and ophthalmology. However, the echocardiographic instrument can also display motion of structures with respect to depth. By converting the spike into a dot, with brightness proportional to the amplitude of the echo spike, dots of varying brightness can be displayed on the echoscope with respect to depth from the transducer. This is called brightness modulation or B mode. The repetitive pulse–reception cycle allows continuous plotting of the distances between the transducer and the reflected surfaces as they move in time (M mode).

The amplified output is usually displayed on an oscilloscope. Although direct Polaroid photographs can be made of the signal, continuous recording from a stripchart recorder is more satisfactory. The phonocardiogram, carotid pulse, jugular venous pulse, or apex cardiogram tracings may also be used in order to relate cardiac motion to left- and right-sided cardiac physiology.

EXAMINATION TECHNIQUE. The infant or child may be examined in the supine position; slight rotation so that the left side is more dependent than the right sometimes facilitates examination. Sedation is not usually required, but patience and reassurance are, since cooperation of the young child with the examiner is extremely helpful. The transducer is usually applied directly to the chest wall at the left sternal edge at the third and fourth intercostal spaces, and a water-soluble jelly is used to make airless contact between the transducer and skin, since air is a poor transmitter of ultrasound. The so-called echocardiographic window corresponds to the lingular reflection where no lung tissue is interposed between the heart and the chest wall. In the infant and young child, in whom the sternum and ribs are unossified, the window is much larger because cartilage does not interfere with the conduction of echoes. On the other hand, with mechanical ventilation, hyperinflation of the lung may considerably diminish the size of the window. It is also possible to obtain echo signals from the aorta, pulmonary arteries, and left atrium from the suprasternal notch by angling the transducer downward toward the heart. A 5-mm-diameter transducer is preferable for examining smaller patients than the standard 1.25-cm size used for adults.

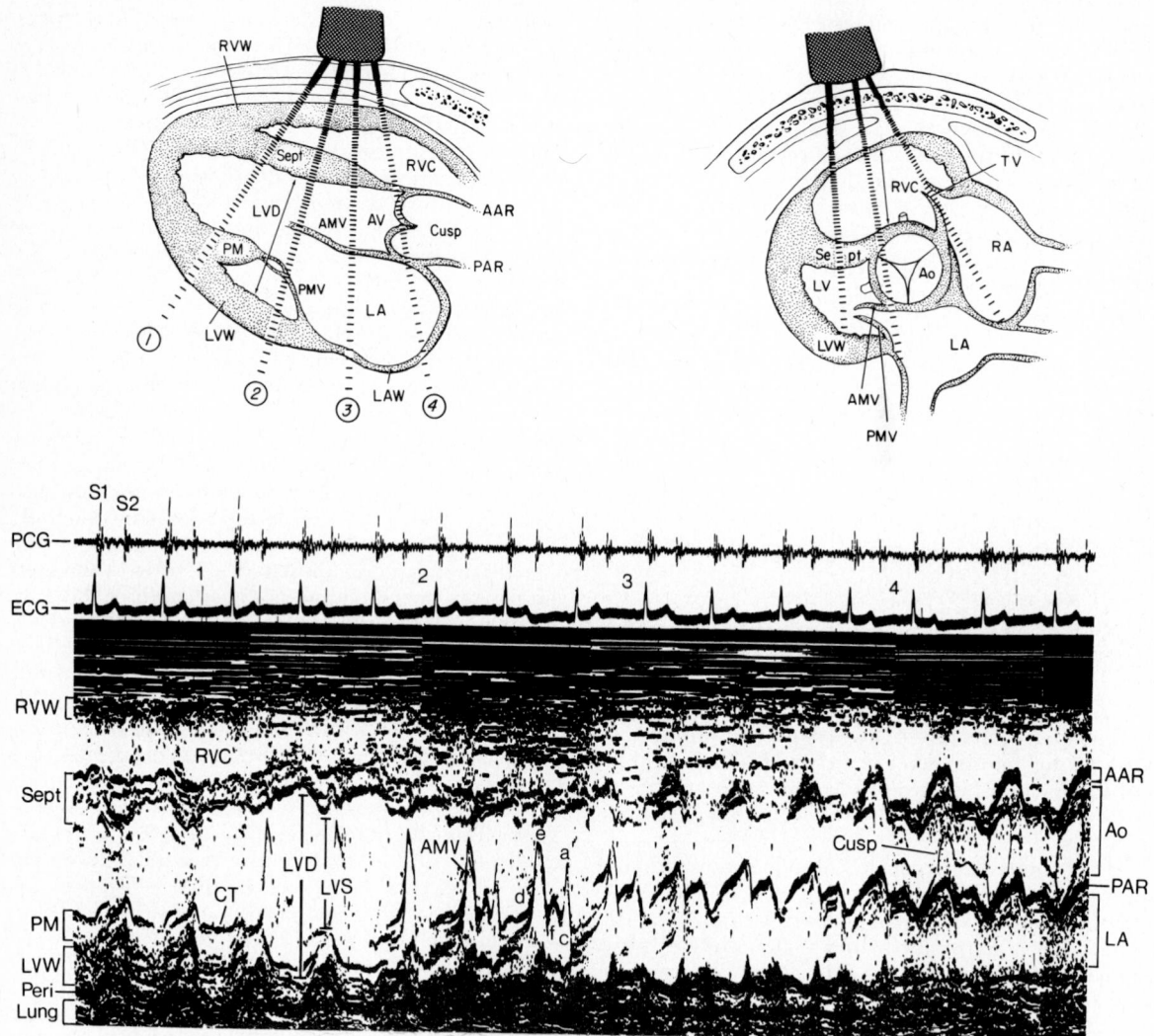

FIG. 13. Sagittal section (top left) and horizontal section (top right) through the heart to demonstrate transducer position and angulations. The bottom echogram is a composite sweep of the echocardiogram recorded as the transducer is swept from a caudal to cranial direction with the transducer pivoting on the chest wall. The positions of the transducer are recorded from 1 through 4. RVW, right ventricular wall; RVC, right ventricular cavity; Sept, interventricular septum; PM, posterior papillary muscle; CT, chordae tendineae; LVW, left ventricular wall; peri, pericardium; AMV and PMV, anterior and posterior mitral leaflets. The various points used to define mitral motion (d, e, f, a, and c) are shown. LA, left atrium; AV, aortic valve; AAR and PAR, anterior and posterior aortic roots. The aortic cusps are shown in position 4. The left atrium is recorded posterior to the aortic root echoes. ECG, electrocardiogram; LVS, left ventricular dimension in systole; LVD, left ventricular dimension in diastole; LAW, left atrial wall; PCG, phonocardiogram. See text for details.

Frequencies of 5MHz are preferable for premature infants and newborn infants, but for older children the standard adult transducer with a frequency of 2.25 MHz is satisfactory.

The echocardiograms obtained from a standard position are displayed in Figure 13. It is possible to sweep the echo beam from the apex of the heart along the axis of the left ventricle and into the aorta by pivoting the transducer on the chest wall. In position 1, or slightly above this area, the beam passes progressively through the chest wall, right ventricular free wall, right ventricular cavity, interventricular septum, left ventricular cavity, mitral chordae tendineae, left ventricular posterior wall, and lung. Note that contraction of the muscle causes thickening in systole and thinning in diastole. The right ventricular cavity appears smaller than that of the left ventricle because the sonic beam is not directed through the major axis of the cavity and because the right ventricle has a crescentic rather than a spherical cross section. The ventricular septum moves posteriorly during systole, and the left ventricular posterior wall moves anteriorly, thus diminishing the minor axis of the left ventricular cavity. It is believed that the left ventricular cavity has its major cross-sectional diameter in this plane or in plane 2 (described below) in infants and younger children. As the echocardiographic beam is gradually rotated from position 1 to position 2 (Fig. 13), both leaflets of the mitral valve are traversed by the sonic beam, giving rise to the most characteristic echo. With the onset of diastole the mitral valve opens and the ventricle undergoes rapid filling. The anterior mitral leaflet shows a rapid high-amplitude motion toward the transducer, while the posterior leaflet throughout diastole moves as a mirror image of the anterior leaflet and has a smaller amplitude posterior motion. The end-systolic point is termed the *d* point, and the maximal opening is termed the *e* point. At the end of rapid filling the anterior mitral leaflet moves posteriorly to the *f* point. If diastole is long enough, low-frequency oscillations of the mitral leaflets are seen, due to continued forward flow of blood between the left atrium and left ventricle. With atrial contraction (which follows the P wave on the electrocardiogram) the anterior leaflet again moves toward, and the posterior leaflet away from, the transducer. Following atrial relaxation the valve begins to close prior to ventricular systole, which begins at point *b* (not always clearly defined). The valve closes completely at point *c*. With the onset of ventricular systole the echo signals from the apposed anterior and posterior mitral valve leaflets move gradually toward the transducer while ventricular blood is ejected into the aorta. The diastolic pattern of anterior mitral leaflet inscribes an **M**-shaped pattern, while that of the posterior leaflet has a smaller **W**-shaped motion that is not always well recorded.

As the echo beam is swept farther cranially and medially to position 3, the posterior mitral valve leaflet echo gives way to the echo from the posterior left atrial wall. The anterior mitral leaflet still can be recorded, and ventricular septal echoes and right ventricular structures are seen anterior to it. With continuing sweep cranially and medially the mitral valve echoes become attenuated. The echo beam then passes through the right ventricle anteriorly, the left ventricular outflow area and the left atrium posteriorly. At position 4 more cranially and medially the echo beam passes through the right ventricular wall and cavity and then into the parallel echo signals obtained from the aortic root; the left atrium is seen posteriorly. The aortic valve leaflets within the aortic root move toward and away from the transducer after inscription of the QRS complex. These leaflets stay open for the duration of systole and then move into the middle position between the parallel aortic root echoes during diastole; this boxlike configuration of systolic motion is not always completely shown, and neither is the diastolic echo. The anterior portion of the box is believed to arise from echo signals obtained from the right coronary cusp leaflet of the aortic valve. Behind the aortic root the left atrium is seen. Note from Figure 13 that the diameters of the left atrium and aorta are roughly similar.

Right ventricular structures are easily recordable in most children. By rotating the transducer medially and inferiorly from the aortic region, the tricuspid valve echocardiogram can be recorded (Fig. 14). Its configuration is similar to that seen with the mitral valve, but it is located more anteriorly. Usually only the anterior leaflet can be recorded, but the posterior leaflet often may be seen in children. Anteriorly the right ventricular free wall is seen. Behind the tricuspid valve a variety of structures can be shown, depending on the direction of the echo beam (Figs. 13 and 14): either the right atrium and the aorta or the ventricular septum, the mitral valve, and the left ventricle.

By pointing the beam superiorly and laterally off the aortic root echo recorded in the third or second left interspace, the pulmonary valve echoes can usually be identified in most children. Because of angulation of this valve, only the posterior valve leaflet usually can be seen. The systolic portion is therefore recorded only as half a box, although especially with younger patients a more complete signal can be obtained. An *a* wave corresponding to the right atrial contraction can usually be identified in the pulmonary valve echo.

The echocardiogram thus has the potential of identifying cardiac structure and position. Using the information from a plain posteroanterior roentgenogram and the echocardiogram, important information can be obtained in cardiac malpositions (p. 1359) and complicated forms of intracardiac congenital defects. Thus the echocardiogram can determine whether there are two great arteries at the base of the heart, whether they are normally placed, and whether one of them is hypoplastic. Normally the aortic valve echo is posterior, inferior, and to the right of the pulmonary valve echo; this relationship is termed the *d* position of the great arteries. In complete situs inversus the aortic valve echo is still posterior and inferior, but to the left of the pulmonary valve echo; this is the *l* position of the arteries. In *d*- and *l*-transpositions the aortic valve echo is anterior, superior, and respectively to the right or left of the pulmonary valve echo. Identification of each great ar-

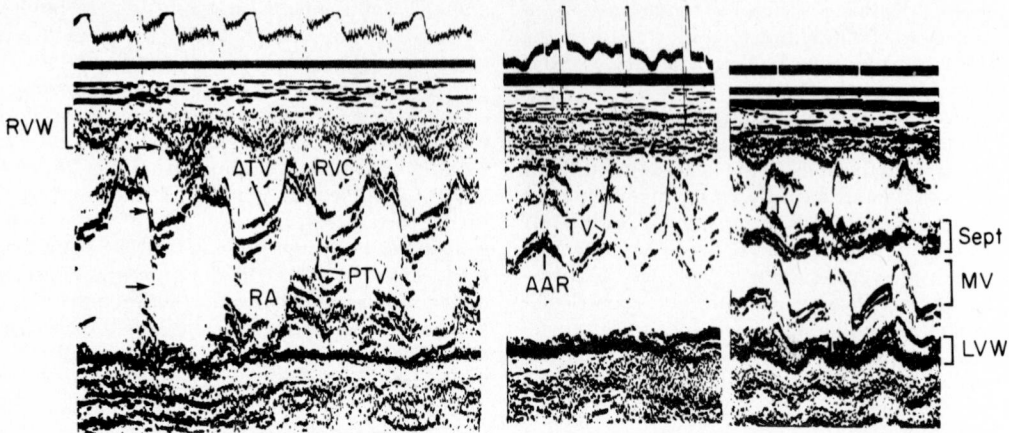

FIG. 14. Different views of the tricuspid valve obtained with different transducer angulation. TV, tricuspid valve; ATV, anterior tricuspid valve leaflet; PTV, posterior tricuspid valve leaflet; RA, right atrium. The other abbreviations are the same as for Figure 13. See text for details.

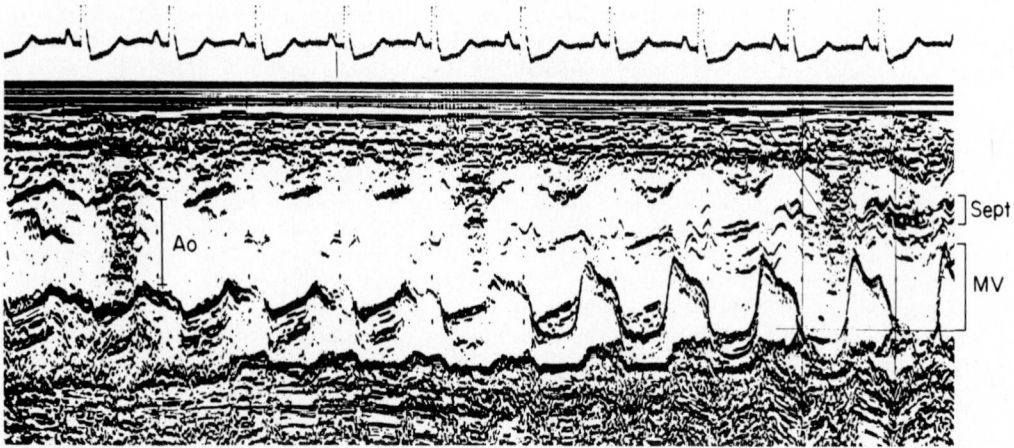

FIG. 15. Echocardiographic sweep from the aorta to the left ventricle and mitral apparatus in tetralogy of Fallot. Note that the anterior aortic root echo is anterior to echoes from the ventricular septum and that there is discontinuity between these structures, suggesting the presence of a ventricular septal defect. The posterior aortic root appears to be continuous with the anterior mitral leaflet.

tery is best made from the fact that in the absence of paradoxic splitting of the second heart sound the aortic valve echo shows valve closure before that in the pulmonary valve echo.

The echocardiogram can also be used to demonstrate relationships of the great arteries to the ventricular septum and mitral valve. Thus in the *tetralogy of Fallot* and *truncus arteriosus* the echoes of the anterior root of the aorta or truncus override those of the ventricular septum (Fig. 15); the posterior part of the great artery and the mitral valve are in continuity, as shown by the posterior great artery echo being at the same level as the mitral valve echo during systole. If the posterior great artery echo is anterior to the systolic mitral valve echo, then the aortic and mitral valves may not be contiguous and a *double-outlet right ventricle* may be suspected. However, this echocardiographic sign of discontinuity may

be produced falsely if the transducer is too high on the chest wall, and the three lesions discussed above may be difficult to distinguish by echocardiography alone.

The echocardiogram may also be used to determine the position and size of each ventricle, the presence of the ventricular septum, and the thickness of the septum and the left ventricular free wall, as well as to indicate the adequacy and velocity of motion of different parts of the ventricular wall. Size and motion of mitral and tricuspid valves can often be detected, and atrial size can be shown. Abnormal structures like vegetations on the aortic valve or atrial myxomas can often be demonstrated. Finally, certain characteristic echo patterns may be used to identify certain specific lesions.

LEFT VENTRICULAR FUNCTION. Echocardiographic measurements of changes in left ventricular dimensions have been used to assess ventricular function.

Unfortunately, with single-crystal transducers several assumptions must be made regarding the ventricular morphology, and statistical regression analysis must be used to provide standards for ventricular volumes in systole and diastole. With these measurements, however, an estimate of the ejection fraction can be obtained even in the infant. The rate of change of the echocardiographic dimensions from diastole to systole can be obtained directly from the echocardiogram by relating these diameters to the duration of systole as measured from the point of closure to opening of the mitral valve. This measurement has been termed the mean circumferential fiber shortening diameter, or VCF. These measurements give some information as to how well the ventricle is contracting, but they have not been extensively investigated. Echocardiographic measurements of the duration of systole correlate closely with those measured by phonocardiography and carotid pulse recordings. Right-sided time intervals have also been measured by echocardiography in pediatric patients, and they appear to correlate closely with pulmonary arterial pressure recordings. A noninvasive method is therefore available for measurement of systolic time intervals in the pediatric age range and even in small infants, when carotid pulse tracings may be difficult to record.

NEW ASPECTS. Recent developments in ultrasound techniques have allowed the actual display of cross sections through the heart and great vessels in much the same way as the angiocardiogram demonstrates cardiac structure and function. Horizontal and sagittal time sections in the B mode are now available for echocardiographic analysis. The images are created in two ways. The first uses multiple crystals that are aligned close to each other and display their echo signals simultaneously. When these are placed together, the composite view is displayed on an oscilloscope screen and the images may be recorded on videotape. The images give a real time impression of cardiac structure. Another technique is to use a single crystal that is vibrated through an arc on the chest wall by a motor at a rapid rate, and the sweep is displayed on a screen and recorded on videotape as with the multiple-crystal apparatus. These images give vertical, horizontal, or oblique cuts through various chambers in the heart, so that an accurate image can be obtained providing anatomic and physiologic information. Unfortunately, only a few prototype models have been produced, and they are not yet generally available. With refinement of design we can look forward to extensive and valuable noninvasive diagnosis in pediatric cardiology.

SPECIFIC LESIONS. ATRIAL SEPTAL DEFECTS. There are no direct ways of observing atrial septal defects echocardiographically, but right ventricular diastolic volume overload creates a characteristic echocardiographic pattern. Other conditions causing the same hemodynamic disturbances, such as partial or total anomalous pulmonary venous drainage, pulmonic regurgitation, and tricuspid regurgitation, give rise to the same echocardiographic findings. In these conditions an increase in the diastolic dimension of the right ventricle is noted, and the ventricular septum moves paradoxically (Fig. 16). Normally the ventricular septum behaves as though it were part of the left ventricle, narrowing the minor axis of the left ventricular dimension in systole (Fig. 13). With right ventricular diastolic

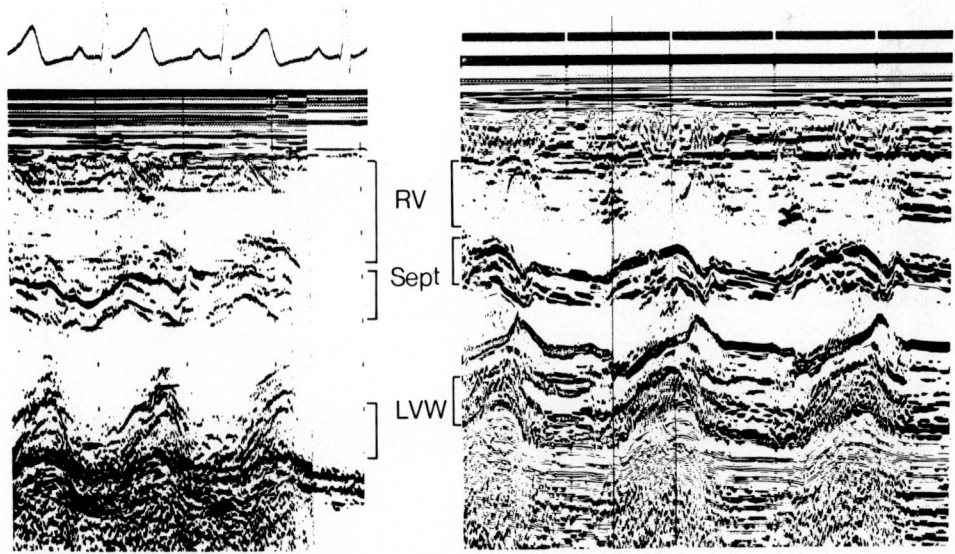

FIG. 16. Echocardiograms from 2 patients with atrial septal defects. Note that the septum (Sept.) moves forward in systole (left) or stays flattened (right). This paradoxic septal motion is found in patients with other forms of right ventricular diastolic overload. The echogram on right has lines indicating onset and termination of systole. See text for details LVW, left ventricular wall.

overload the ventricular septum behaves as though it were part of the right ventricle and moves forward in systole instead of backward.

Two types of abnormal septal motion have been described (Fig. 16): in type A the septal echo moves anteriorly during systole; in type B the anterior motion is less exaggerated, and the echo signal moves more nearly horizontally. Care must be taken to ensure that this abnormal motion is recorded from positions 1 or 2 (Fig. 13), because the upper part of the septum may move paradoxically in normal subjects. Paradoxic septal motion has been recorded in left-to-right shunts when pulmonary flow is more than 1.3 times systemic flow. The type of paradoxic relationship is not dependent on the magnitude of the shunting and is not invariably present even in larger shunts.

VENTRICULAR SEPTAL DEFECTS. Echocardiographic detection of a ventricular septal defect is not common unless the defect is immediately below the aorta or pulmonary artery, or when the defect is extremely large, as in single ventricle, when the ventricular septum is not identified at all. Usually, however, the ventricular septal defect is not identified, and one must rely on the hemodynamic consequences to infer the magnitude of the size of the shunt; these consequences are similar to those seen in patent ductus arteriosus.

PATENT DUCTUS ARTERIOSUS. With large left-to-right shunts absolute left atrial size is increased, and the increase correlates well with the magnitude of the left-to-right shunt. For premature infants with significant ductal shunting, a ratio (left atrial size at end of ventricular systole over aortic size at the same point) has been computed to assess the size of the shunt (Fig. 17). Normal infants have an LA/Ao ratio of less than 1.15:1. In premature babies with ductal shunts that require surgical ligation, the ratios are usually greater than this. Other possible causes of left atrial enlargement must be considered. Measurement of the velocity of shortening

of the internal ventricular diameter (VCF) is helpful in differentiating left atrial and left ventricular enlargement due to left-to-right shunts from those conditions associated with poor myocardial function. Other findings in ventricular or aortopulmonary left-to-right shunts include increases in the left ventricular internal dimensions in diastole and systole.

ENDOCARDIAL CUSHION DEFECTS. Various echocardiographic patterns have been described in endocardial cushion defects. In ostium primum atrial septal defects

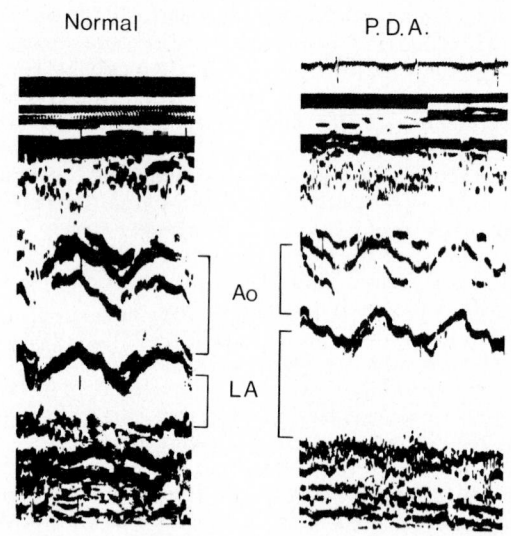

FIG. 17. Two echocardiograms demonstrating the relative sizes of the left atrium and the aorta. On the left is an echogram from a premature infant without cardiac disease (normal). On the right is the echogram of a premature infant with a large left-to-right shunt due to a patent ductus arteriosus. Measurements of aortic and left atrial size are made at the point of maximum anterior excursion of the aortic root echo signals.

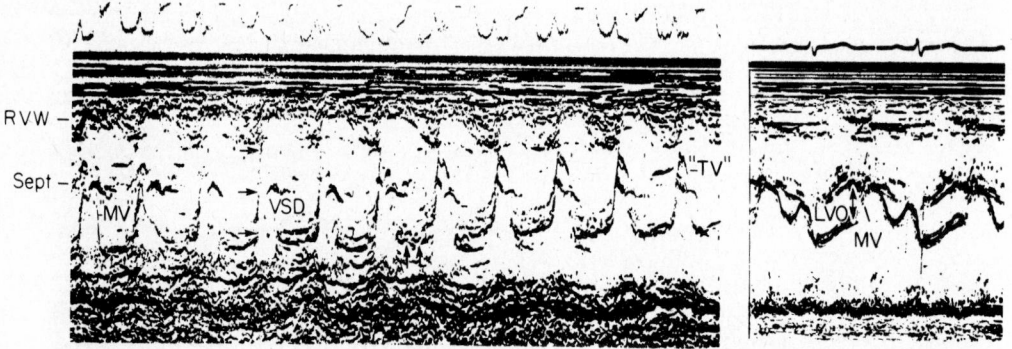

FIG. 18. Left. Complete form of endocardial cushion defect. Note that the mitral portion of the common atrioventricular valve (MV) seems to pass to a forward position as sweep passes toward the right. A large atrioventricular valve signal through the area of the VSD is seen; on the right the echo signal arising from the anterior common leaflet resembles that from the normal tricuspid valve. The appearance of the atrioventricular valve echo marching through the ventricular septum is characteristic of a common atrioventricular valve. RVW, right ventricular wall. Right. Note encroachment of anterior mitral valve leaflet (MV) echo signal on the echo from the ventricular septum. This region is the left ventricular outflow tract (LVO). This finding has been described in ostium primum and more complex endocardial cushion defects.

the findings may be identical to those seen in secundum atrial septal defects; in addition, diastolic apposition of the mitral valve to the septum has been described (Fig. 18). With more complex forms of endocardial cushion defects the anterior diastolic motion from the posterior position of the atrioventricular valve is seen to pass through the ventricular septal echo into the anterior ventricle.

HYPOPLASTIC LEFT AND RIGHT HEART COMPLEXES. In hypoplastic left heart complexes the echocardiogram has provided a noninvasive means for diagnosis (Fig. 19). Large right heart structures are noted, but they are not specific. The echo from the aortic root must be defined for positive diagnosis; it has an extremely narrow diameter, which is less than half that normally noted in the newborn. The left ventricle may not be identified, but when it is the chamber is small, and if echo signals are recorded from the mitral valve they are of low amplitude and have bizarre configurations.

TRICUSPID ATRESIA. In tricuspid atresia the right ventricular cavity varies in size, depending on the presence or absence of a ventricular septal defect. The right ventricular cavity in the usual form of tricuspid atresia is small, and the tricuspid valve echo cannot be recorded; careful searching is necessary to be positive that no tricuspid valve is present. In pulmonary atresia with intact ventricular septum and a small right ventricle, the findings are similar, except that the tricuspid valve is identified.

The echocardiogram is thus a very useful tool for excluding certain clinical diagnoses. For example, if either tricuspid or pulmonic atresia is included in the differential diagnosis of a cyanotic newborn infant, and echocardiographic examination reveals a tricuspid valve, a pulmonic valve, and normal ventricular and great vessel relationships, other causes for cyanosis will have to be sought.

VALVAR AORTIC STENOSIS. In valvar aortic stenosis varying findings have been reported. With a bicuspid aortic valve the diastolic echo, which normally lies in the center of the aortic root echo, may be eccentric. The finding of a bicuspid aortic valve does not in itself indicate aortic stenosis; it is frequently noted in patients with aortic coarctation without aortic stenosis. Multiple diastolic echoes have been reported in aortic stenosis (Fig. 20), but they have also been observed in normal valves. Valve leaflets that have calcified have dense echoes, but calcification is rare in children. The left ventricle is thickened in patients with aortic stenosis, and the cavity size is usually within normal limits, although if aortic or mitral regurgitation supervenes, left ventricular enlargement may be noted.

SUBVALVAR AORTIC STENOSIS. In subvalvar aortic stenosis a narrowing of the echoes in the aortic outflow area may be identified. Aortic valve motion may be disturbed by altered flow patterns induced by the subvalvar obstruction (Fig. 21). The aortic valve is frequently seen to open normally and then close abruptly in the midportion of systole, with the echo signal from the valves staying in a partially closed position for the duration of systole. In sweeping from the mitral valve through the aortic valve, an area of narrowing in the subvalvar region is sometimes seen.

FIG. 19. Echographic sweep in a patient with mitral and aortic atresia and a hypoplastic left ventricle. No mitral valve or left ventricular cavity could be recorded. The tricuspid valve echo (TV) arises anterior to the hypoplastic aorta, which is 5 mm in diameter (Ao). Posterior to the aorta the left atrium (LA) is seen.

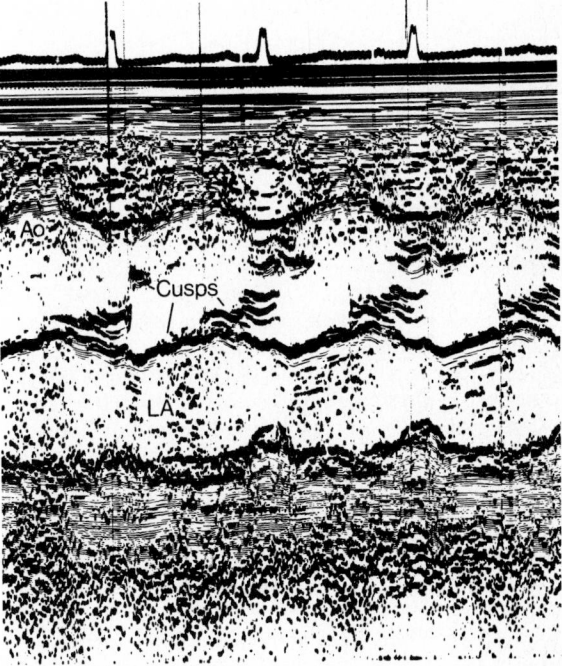

FIG. 20. Aortic echo recorded in a patient with valvar aortic stenosis due to a bicuspid aortic valve. Within the aortic root (Ao) multiple cusp echoes are recorded from the aortic valve cusps (cusps). The diastolic echoes are located in an eccentric position, suggesting a bicuspid valve.

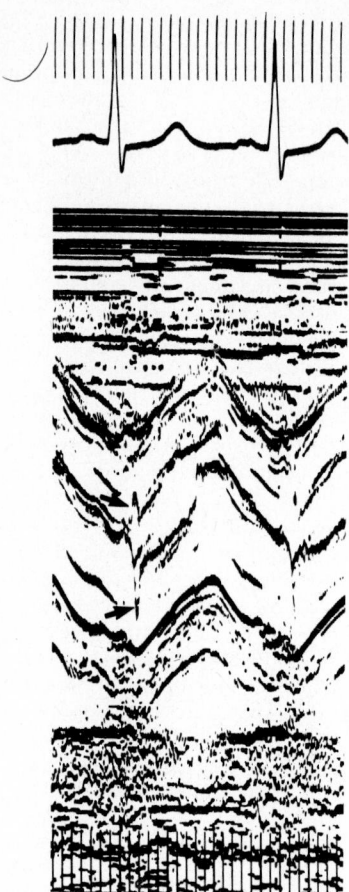

FIG. 21. Echogram of a patient with subvalvar aortic membrane producing stenosis. Note that the aortic leaflet echoes (arrows) show the leaflets opening fully, but moving to a semiclosed position due to alterations of the hemodynamics related to flow. See text for details.

ASYMMETRIC SEPTAL HYPERTROPHY. The classic finding in asymmetric septal hypertrophy (idiopathic hypertrophic subaortic stenosis, IHSS) is a systolic anterior motion of the mitral valve. The mitral valve bulges forward in systole and even comes into contact with the septal echoes for some part of systole (Fig. 22). This systolic anterior motion (SAM) of the mitral valve is not present in some subjects with IHSS, but it can be produced by methods that precipitate outflow tract obstruction, such as inhalation of amyl nitrite or the Valsalva maneuver. The mitral valve diastolic e–f slope is also diminished considerably in this condition, reflecting a decrease in left ventricular compliance. Asymmetric septal hypertrophy (ASH) has been found to be an important pathologic and echocardiographic feature of this lesion. The septum is thicker than normal; it contracts poorly and does not significantly increase its thickness in systole. The ratio of the diastolic thickness of the septum to that of the left ventricular free wall is > 1.3:1. Care must be taken to ensure that the echocardiographic beam passes directly perpendicular to the wall of the ventricular septum before interpreting these

findings. The finding of ASH appears to be the unifying link in understanding the genetic transmission of this disease. Asymmetric septal hypertrophy is found not only in those patients affected with myopathy but also in 50 percent of their relatives; the abnormal septal thickening appears to segregate as if it were an autosomal dominant condition. It is now recommended that echocardiography be performed as a screening procedure to detect this abnormality in the relatives of patients affected with IHSS. The finding of ASH does not indicate that these subjects necessarily will develop overt cardiomyopathy, but rather it brings attention to those that are genetic carriers of this trait. Abnormally thickened ventricular septal echoes have also been described in conditions associated with right ventricular hypertrophy, endocardial fibroelastosis, mitral regurgitation, and hypertrophy of the left ventricle not associated with cardiomyopathy, especially in young patients. The aortic valve motion recorded in patients with obstruction to the left ventricular outflow in IHSS may have a biphasic motion similar to that found in fixed valvar or subvalvar aortic obstruction; the aortic valve may also open early in systole and then close partially, but it tends to reopen, so that late closure is not as prominent as in fixed subvalvar obstruction. The reopening of the aortic valve is exaggerated by the use of amyl nitrite and the Valsalva maneuver.

Fixed subvalvar obstruction and asymmetric hypertrophy may occur concurrently. It is thus good practice to administer amyl nitrite to all patients with subvalvar aortic stenosis to assess whether there is associated systolic anterior mitral movement.

SUPRAVALVAR AORTIC STENOSIS. By sweeping farther up the ascending aorta from the aortic valve, supravalvar narrowing may be detected in supravalvar aortic stenosis (Fig. 23). Care must be taken to ensure that the sweep occurs through the major axis of the aortic diameter and not eccentrically; otherwise, false narrowing may be produced.

AORTIC REGURGITATION. The regurgitant jet from the aortic valve may cause vibration of the anterior mitral leaflet and ventricular septum. This is not a constant finding and does not indicate the severity of regurgitation. With severe aortic regurgitation, left ventricular dimensions are increased. In aortic incompetence resulting from Marfan's syndrome, aortic root dilatation may be noted in addition.

MITRAL STENOSIS. The echocardiographic pattern of the mitral valve in mitral stenosis is distinctive (Fig. 24). Mitral valve opening is delayed, but it occurs abruptly at the d point, which is coincident with the recording of the opening snap. Since there is no rapid ventricular filling phase and the atrioventricular pressure gradient is maintained throughout diastole, the normal mid-diastolic oscillations of the valve are not seen. The valve motion away from the chest wall is related to left ventricular filling and movement of the whole mitral valve apparatus away from the chest wall. There is no further reopening of the valve as a result of atrial systole, but in mild mitral stenosis a small a wave may be visible. At end-diastole the mitral valve closes

Amyl Nitrite

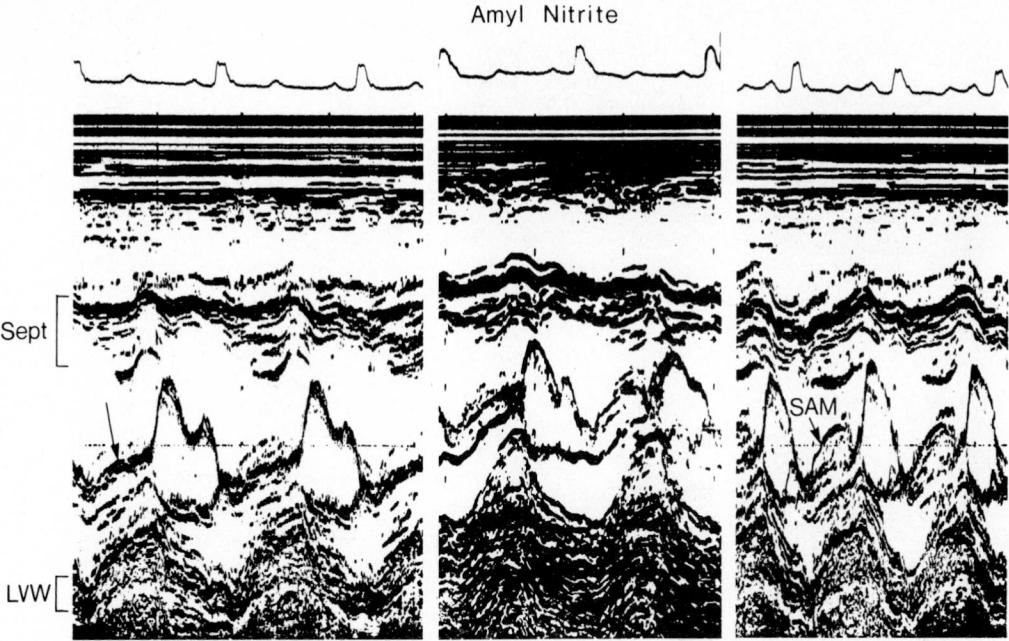

Sept

LVW

SAM

FIG. 22. Echograms from the same strip in a patient with idiopathic hypertrophic subaortic stenosis. Left. At rest the systolic mitral valve echogram shows normal motion (arrow). Center. Small amount of systolic anterior motion (SAM) of the mitral valve toward the ventricular septum in systole with amyl nitrite inhalation. Right. Tachycardia has developed, and SAM (arrow) is more pronounced. From other recordings on this patient that are not shown here the septum was found to be markedly thickened and did not contract significantly, indicating asymmetric septal hypertrophy (ASH).

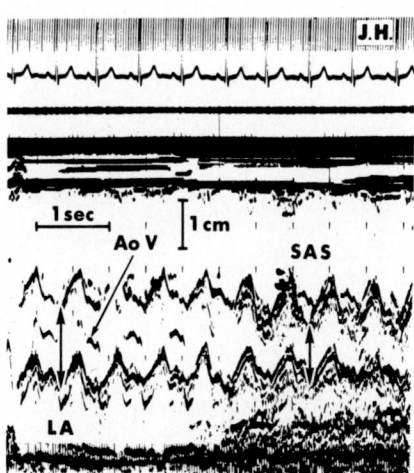

FIG. 23. Echocardiographic sweep up the ascending aorta; from left to right, the aortic valve (AoV) and the area of supravalvar aortic stenosis (SAS) above the aortic valve.

abruptly to the *c* point, coincident with the mitral component of the first heart sound. The echo signals from the mitral valve are stronger than normal and indicate thickening of the leaflet tissue. The normal mitral *e–f* slope is over 60 mm/sec. In adults with acquired mitral stenosis the *e–f* slope is reduced with mild stenosis to 25

to 35 mm/sec, with moderate stenosis to 15 to 25 mm/sec, and with severe stenosis to less than 15 mm/sec. The posterior leaflet is tethered to the anterior leaflet, and the echo signal from the posterior leaflet in diastole moves in the same direction as the anterior leaflet (Fig. 24). A decrease in the *e–f* slope of the anterior mitral leaflet with a normal posterior mitral valve pattern has been seen when there is a decrease in left ventricular filling due to left ventricular failure associated with endocardial fibroelastosis, severe pulmonary hypertension, and IHSS (Fig. 22). In mitral stenosis the left atrial dimension is increased, and with the development of pulmonary hypertension the right-side cavity diameters enlarge. We have noted that in children with parachute mitral valve the features are similar to those of acquired mitral stenosis.

MITRAL VALVE PROLAPSE SYNDROMES. Mitral valve prolapse syndrome, or late-systolic-click systolic-murmur syndrome, which may be associated with atypical chest pain, has become an increasingly common reason for referral for echocardiographic examination. This condition may have several causes in children, but most frequently the syndrome is idiopathic. Various arrhythmias are associated with this condition, and infective endocarditis is an infrequent but important complication. Secondary causes of prolapse are atrial septal defects of the secundum variety, connective tissue disorders such as Marfan's syndrome, Ehlers-Danlos syndrome, mucopolysaccharidoses, and chordal rupture associated with infective endocarditis.

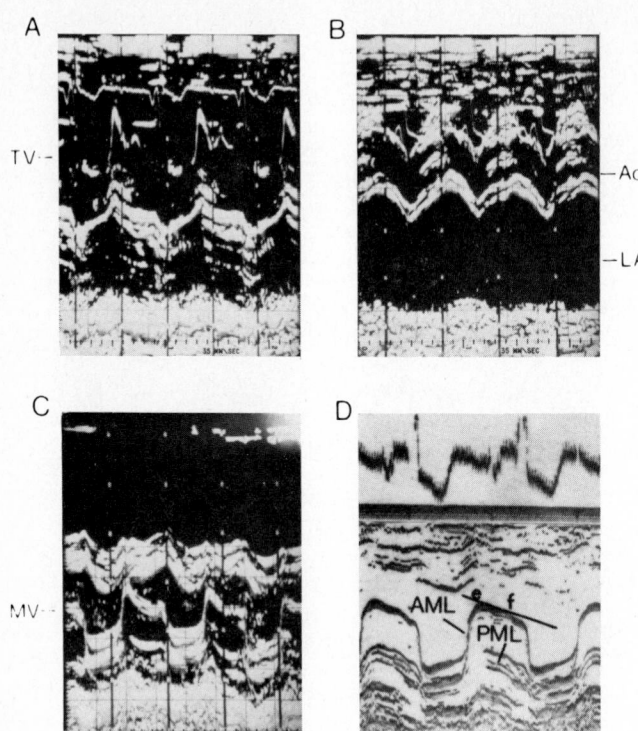

FIG. 24. A, B, and C are from a patient with a parachute mitral valve complex. A. Tricuspid valve (TV). B. Large left atrium (LA) and normal-size aorta (Ao). C. Thickened mitral valve (MV) leaflets with anterior motion of posterior mitral leaflet in diastole. D. Patient with rheumatic mitral stenosis; note the diminished e–f slope of the anterior mitral leaflet (AML) and paradoxic anterior motion of the posterior mitral leaflet (PML).

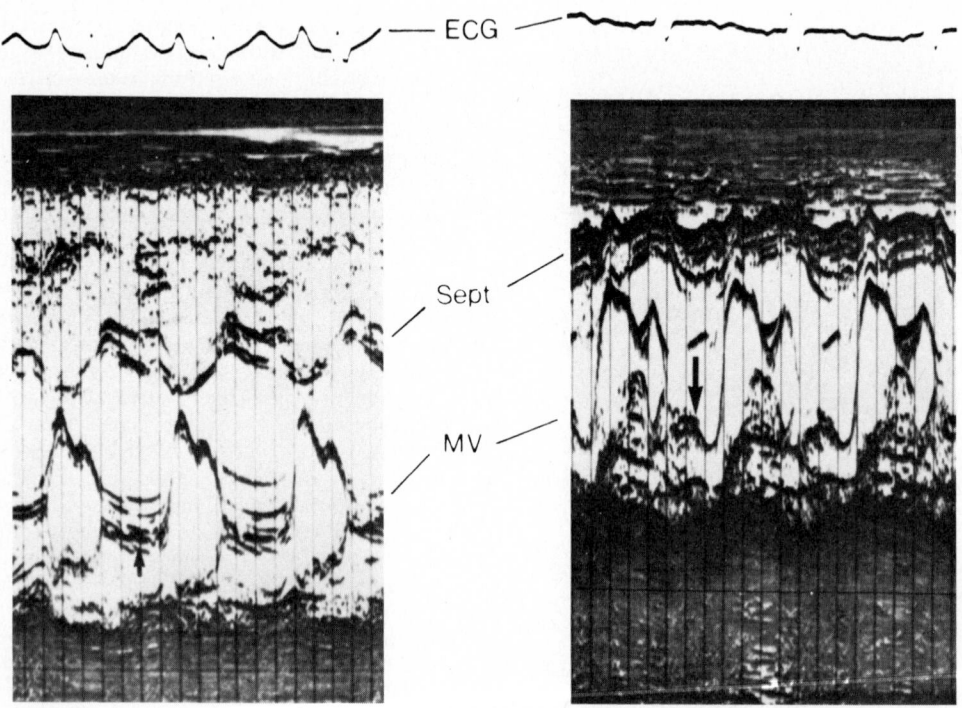

FIG. 25. Two varieties of mitral valve prolapse. Arrows point to the mitral valve prolapsing posteriorly toward the left atrium in systole. On the left the prolapse occurs throughout systole, while on the right the prolapse begins in midsystole.

In the normal systolic position of the mitral valve echo there is a gradual forward movement of the echo lines of the coapted mitral leaflets during systole (compare Figs. 13 and 25). There are several abnormal patterns associated with prolapse. Figure 25 (right panel) shows a normal motion initially, but then a sudden posterior motion of the mitral valve is noted, bulging posteriorly toward the left atrium during midsystole to late systole. This change in motion in some patients coincides with the click that occurs in midsystole or late systole and is related to the abnormal valve motion. In some patients, instead of a forward motion, there is a gradual movement of the entire mitral apparatus toward the left atrium (Fig, 25, left panel). In other patients multiple systolic lines are seen; these are thought to result from the echo beam passing through redundant leaflet tissue. While this sign alone is suggestive of prolapse, it may occur in normal subjects. It is also possible to produce the appearance of pansystolic prolapse if the transducer is placed too high on the chest wall. Careful studies in normal subjects have shown that the echocardiographic demonstration of mild posterior movement is common and may in fact be a normal variant. More severe forms of prolapse, as shown in Figure 25, invariably are associated with valve abnormality. The Valsalva maneuver and amyl nitrite inhalation are useful in demonstrating prolapse of the mitral valve by echocardiography. Sometimes it is not possible to demonstrate the classic echocardiographic features in mild cases in which mitral valve prolapse is suspected from auscultation.

PERICARDIAL EFFUSION.   The echocardiogram is extremely useful in the diagnosis of pericardial effusion (Fig. 26). Because of the different sonic impedances between the tissues of the pericardium, the epicardium, and the fluid, an effusion can be delineated clearly. By suitable damping of the echo signal the effusion may be shown in the potential space between the epicardium and pericardium, which are closely apposed in the normal heart. The presence of pericardial fluid is best assessed with the ultrasonic beam in position 1 or 2 (Fig. 13). Small effusions may be seen only posteriorly, while larger effusions may be seen anteriorly as well. A pattern of partial systolic separation between the echo signals of the epicardium and pericardium and apposition of these in diastole may be observed when effusions are small. Slight systolic separation between the echo signals of the pericardium and epicardium in systole is occasionally seen even in normal subjects; this should not be interpreted as a pericardial effusion.

INFECTIVE ENDOCARDITIS.   In infective endocarditis vegetations as small as 2 mm in diameter have been detected. They produce multiple echocardiographic lines in the region of the valve leaflet echo signals; these lines vary with the phases of the cardiac cycle and have been encountered in mitral and aortic areas. Echocardiography is also helpful in detecting changes in leaflet morphology in patients suspected of having endocarditis. Reports suggest that even after healing the signals in the region of the previous vegetations do not disappear and may be related to scarring of the valve. Serial examination should be done in patients suspected of having endocarditis to evaluate whether there has been any change in valve leaflet motion or structure.

References

Feigenbaum H: Echocardiography. Philadelphia, Lea & Febiger, 1972

Goldberg SJ, Allen HD, Sahn DJ: Pediatric and Adolescent Echocardiography. Chicago, Year Book, 1975

Henry WL, Clark CE, Epstein SE: Asymmetric septal hypertrophy. Circulation 47:225, 1973

Hirschfeld S, Meyer RA, Schwartz DC, Korfhagen J, Kaplan S: Measurement of right and left ventricular systolic time intervals by echocardiography. Circulation 51:304, 1975

Horowitz MS, Schultz CS, Stinson EB, Harrison DC, Popp RL: Sensitivity and specificity of echocardiographic diagnosis of pericardial effusion. Circulation 50:239, 1974

Meyer RA, Kaplan S: Non-invasive techniques in pediatric cardiovascular disease. Prog Cardiovasc Dis 19:341, 1973

Murphy KF, Kotler MN, Reichek N, Perloff JK: Ultrasound in the diagnosis of congenital heart disease. Am Heart J 89:638, 1975

Popp RL, Harrison DC: In Weissler AM (ed): Non-invasive Cardiology. New York, Grune & Stratton, 1974

Sahn DJ, Deely WJ, Hagan AD, Friedman WF: Echocardiographic assessment of left ventricular performance in normal newborns. Circulation 49:232, 1974

——— Allen HP, Goldberg SJ, Solinger R, Meyer RA: Pediatric echocardiography: a review of its clinical utility. J Pediatr 87:335, 1975

Silverman NH, Lewis AB, Heymann MA, Rudolph AM: Echocardiography in patent ductus arteriosus in premature infants. Circulation 50: 821, 1974

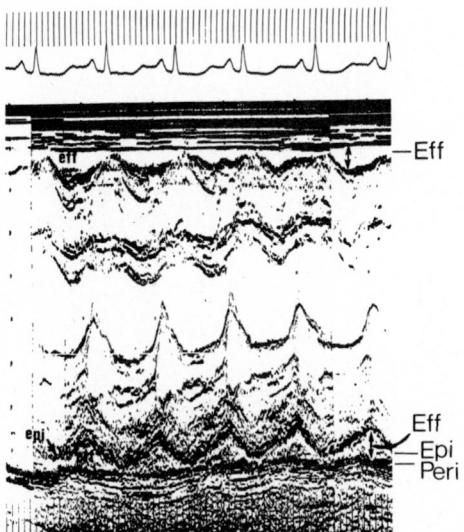

FIG. 26   Echocardiogram of a patient with a large pericardial effusion. Note the echo-free space (Eff) between the chest wall and right ventricular epicardium anteriorly and behind the left ventricular epicardium (Epi) and pericardium (Peri) posteriorly.

ELECTROCARDIOGRAM AND VECTORCARDIOGRAM

JULIEN I.E. HOFFMAN

There are many good texts on electrocardiography, and this section is not meant to replace them. For clear, simple explanations of basic electrocardiography, the books by Grant, Marriott, and Schamroth are recommended, while specific pediatric aspects are covered by Guntheroth and by Cassels and Ziegler.

Normally, electrical depolarization begins in the sinoatrial (SA) node and spreads throughout the atria. Initially three preferential atrial tracts are activated: the anterior, middle, and posterior internodal tracts, the

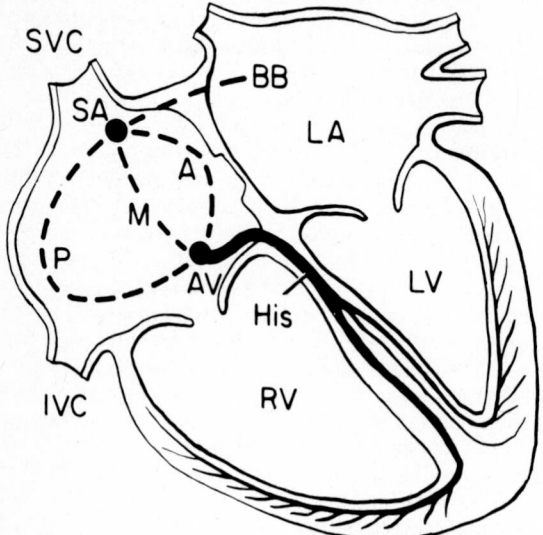

FIG. 27. Diagram of conduction system. SA, sinoatrial node; A, M, and P, anterior, middle, and posterior internodal tracts; and BB, Bachmann's bundle (dashed lines); AV, atrioventricular node; His, bundle of His, dividing into right and left bundles; RV and LV, right and left ventricles; SVC and IVC, superior and inferior venae cava; LA, left atrium.

first of which gives a branch to the left atrium (Fig. 27). From these tracts the atria are activated. The wave of depolarization therefore passes down, to the left and anteriorly, and it generates a potential that is picked up on the body surface as the P wave. A force like this that has both magnitude and direction is termed a vector, and it can be represented by an arrow with direction and magnitude proportional to the force. When the impulse reaches the atrioventricular (AV) node it is delayed, producing the P-R interval and allowing atrial emptying to be completed before ventricular contraction begins. Once the impulse has passed the AV node it moves rapidly down the bundle of His into the right and left branches. As these impulses pass down the septum they activate septal muscle predominantly from the left side, so that the initial ventricular vector passes from left to right, anteriorly and superiorly, and begins the Q wave in lead V_6 or the first part of the R wave in lead V_1 (Fig. 28A). After reaching the apex of the heart the impulse invades the ventricular free walls from endocardium to epicardium and from apex toward the base, thus inscribing the R and S waves; the last part of the heart to be activated is the posterior ventricular muscle just under the AV ring. In adults and older children there is more left than right ventricular muscle, so that the major cardiac vectors point to the left and posteriorly; this produces a tall R wave in V_6 and a deep S wave in V_1. In newborn infants with a thick right ventricle, the major cardiac vectors pass to the right and anteriorly; this produces a dominant R wave in V_1 and a large S wave in V_6. After depolarization has occurred there is slower repolarization that produces the T wave.

The vectors at each point in the cardiac cycle can be drawn as if arising from a common central point; thus they can be represented by a series of arrows fanning

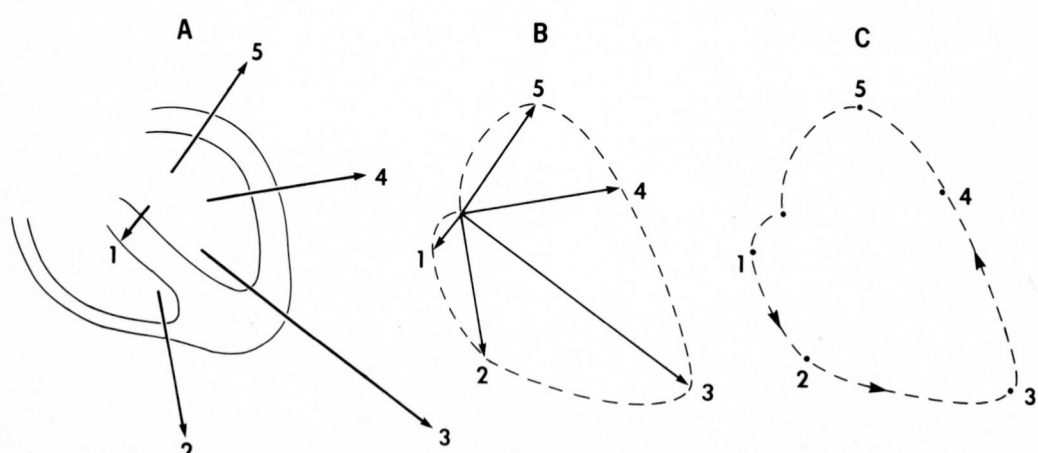

FIG. 28. Normal ventricular depolarization, starting with 1 and ending with 5. A. Section through ventricles with thicker walled left ventricle and thinner walled right ventricle. Arrows are vectors, indicating direction and magnitude of electrical forces at each time. B. Vectors are superimposed on common center, and their tips are joined by a dashed line. C. The dashed line remains to give a vector loop. The vector at any moment would be a line joining the central point to the corresponding part of the loop. The arrows represent the direction of movement of the instantaneous vectors. In practice, direction is indicated by having each dash shaped like a teardrop with the blunt end leading, and the spaces between the dashes occur each 0.0025 sec of the cardiac cycle.

out (Fig. 28B). The ends of the arrows can be joined and the shafts omitted to give a vector loop (Fig. 28C). It is possible to record these vector loops directly by connecting electrodes to the body and recording the voltages between three sets of electrodes at right angles to each other. Thus leads from right to left define an X axis, those from top to bottom define a Y axis, and from those front to back define a Z axis. (A lead may be regarded as a line joining two electrodes or two sets of electrodes.) Simultaneous recording of X and Y axes gives a loop representing the projection of the actual vector loop on the frontal plane of the body (Fig. 29A and B), while simultaneous recording of voltages in the X and Z axes gives the horizontal plane projection of the vector loop (Fig. 29A and B). A third loop, from the Y and Z axes, defines the sagittal plane vector loop, but it adds no new information. Various lead systems have been used, but the one most often used today is the Frank system; the different lead systems give similar patterns but different values of various measurements, so that each must have its own set of standards. In order to record timing, the beam is interrupted each 0.0025 sec, and it usually has a blunt leading edge, so that it is possible to tell which way the vector is moving and at what speed.

The electrocardiogram is a recording of voltage against time that is made on leads to be defined below; it is usually made at a paper speed of 25 mm/sec, with 1mv giving 10 mm of deflection. At any instant the mean vector present can be resolved into two components, one that is parallel to a lead and one at right angles to it. The latter affects both electrodes equally, so that there is no potential difference between them, while the former causes a voltage to appear between the two electrodes. This voltage is proportional to the projection made by the vector on the lead (Fig. 30A). The limb leads (I, II, III, aVr, aVl, aVf) represent the vector in the frontal plane, while the precordial leads essentially represent the vector in the horizontal plane (Fig. 30B); of these, the right chest leads (V_4R, V_3R, V_1, V_2) indicate anteroposterior forces, while the left chest leads (V_5, V_6) indicate left-to-right forces. Remember that there is actually a three-dimensional vector in the heart and that the electrocardiogram and vectorcardiogram merely indicate the projection of that vector on a particular lead or plane, respectively. The electrocardio-

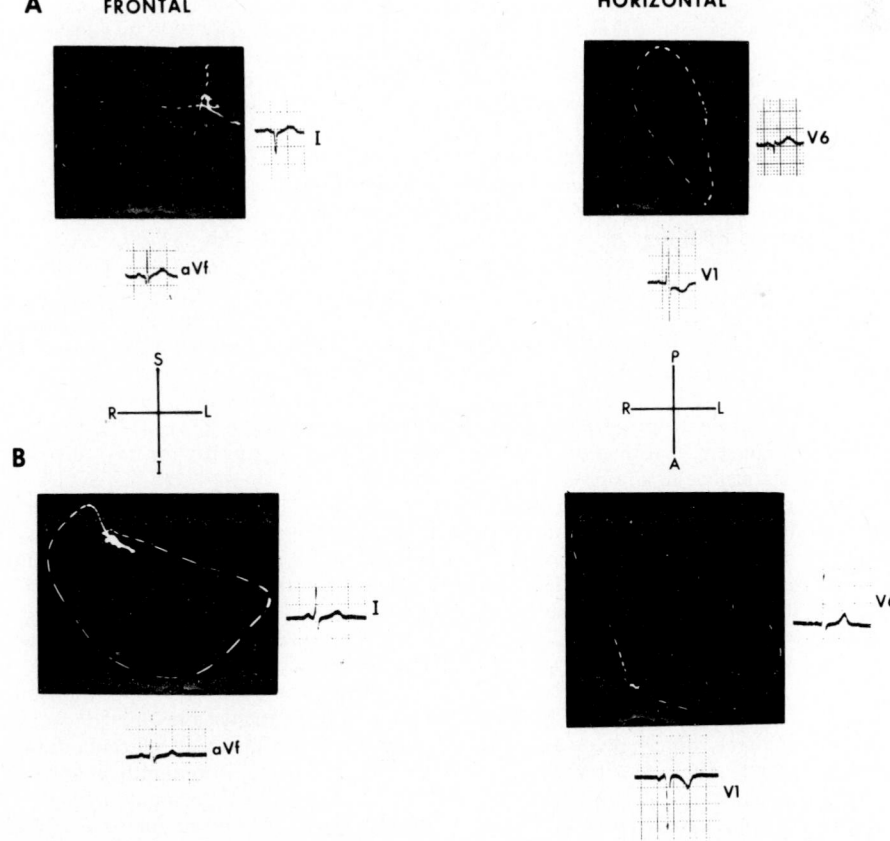

FIG. 29. A. Frontal and horizontal plane vectors of a normal infant 3 weeks old. B. Frontal and horizontal plane vectors of a normal 10-year-old child. Leads I and aVf from the corresponding electrocardiograms are shown in appropriate positions next to the frontal plane loops; similarly, leads V_1 and V_6 are shown next to the horizontal loops.

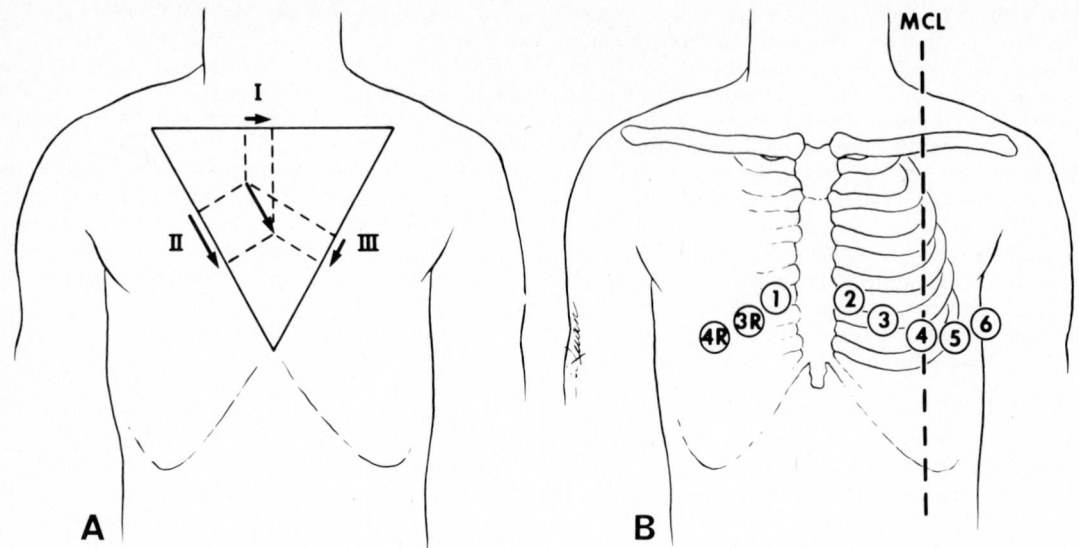

FIG. 30.   A. Einthoven's equilateral triangle is superimposed on the frontal plane of the thorax. A mean QRS vector is shown in the triangle, and its projection on each of the limb leads is obtained by dropping perpendiculars (dashed lines) from the vector to each lead. Note that the angle that the vector makes determines the magnitude of its projection in each lead and that the magnitude is greatest in the lead that is almost parallel to the vector. B. The conventional sites for electrode placement on the thorax (V leads). V_1 and V_2 are in the fourth intercostal space, V_4 is in the fifth space, V_3 is halfway between V_2 and V_4, and V_5 and V_6 are in the fifth space in the anterior and midaxillary lines, respectively. V_3R and V_4R are the right-sided counterparts of V_3 and V_4. These precordial leads lie roughly in the horizontal plane. MCL, mid-clavicular line.

gram is easier to take, and time intervals are more easily measured with it, while the vectorcardiogram gives more precise information about the vector at each moment in the cardiac cycle. Both may be needed.

APPROACH.   It is essential that a routine electrocardiogram include at least one lead (V_3R, V_4R) to the right of V_1 and that if no Q wave is seen in V_6 then leads to the left of V_6 (V_7, V_8) be taken. Once the electrocardiogram has been taken, it should be interpreted with full knowledge of the history, physical examination, drug therapy, and heart size and shape as seen on the chest roentgenogram. It is best to read the electrocardiogram systematically. First measure atrial and ventricular rates and define the rhythm (p. 1387). Then record the P-R interval, QRS duration, and Q-T interval. Measure the frontal plane mean axes of the P waves, QRS complex, and T waves. Finally, look for abnormalities of pattern in the waves and their interconnecting segments and note the voltages of Q, R, S, and T waves.

In general, the electrocardiogram gives valuable information about arrhythmias, hypertrophy of atria or ventricles, electrolyte changes, some myocardial or pericardial infections, and myocardial ischemia and infarction, while there are some specific patterns that occur in certain congenital heart diseases. The electrocardiogram is of no value in diagnosing ventricular dilatation, and it gives little information about myocardial function.

MEASURING QRS AXIS.   To evaluate the mean frontal plane QRS axis the following features must be noted:

1. Lead I runs from the left to the right arm and is arranged electrically so that a deflection passing toward the left arm is positive and a deflection passing away from it is negative (Fig. 31A).

2. Leads II and III are at 60 degrees to each other and to lead I, and they can be superimposed on a common center (Fig. 31B). Note that the lower half of the frontal plane is assigned positive numbers and the upper half negative numbers.

3. Lead aVf runs from the legs up to the heart, and thus lies in the axis +90 to −90 degrees (Fig. 31C). An impulse passing toward the leg thus gives a positive deflection.

4. Leads aVr and aVl pass from the right and left shoulders, respectively, to the heart (Fig. 31D) and their axes are at 60 degrees to each other and to lead aVf. However, because they are unipolar leads, an impulse passing toward either shoulder will give a positive deflection, despite the negative angles associated with the superior ends of the axes in the figure.

5. All six leads may be superimposed on a central point (Fig. 31E) to give axes at 30 degrees to each other.

6. To use this hexaxial reference frame, first decide whether lead I is predominantly positive or negative. In general, this can be determined from the heights of the R and S waves. However, since it is actually area that is being assessed, a tall but narrow R wave might contribute less positivity than a short but wide S wave contributes negativity; if the Q wave is large it should also be included in the assessment. If the result is positive the net vector is passing to the left; if it is negative the net

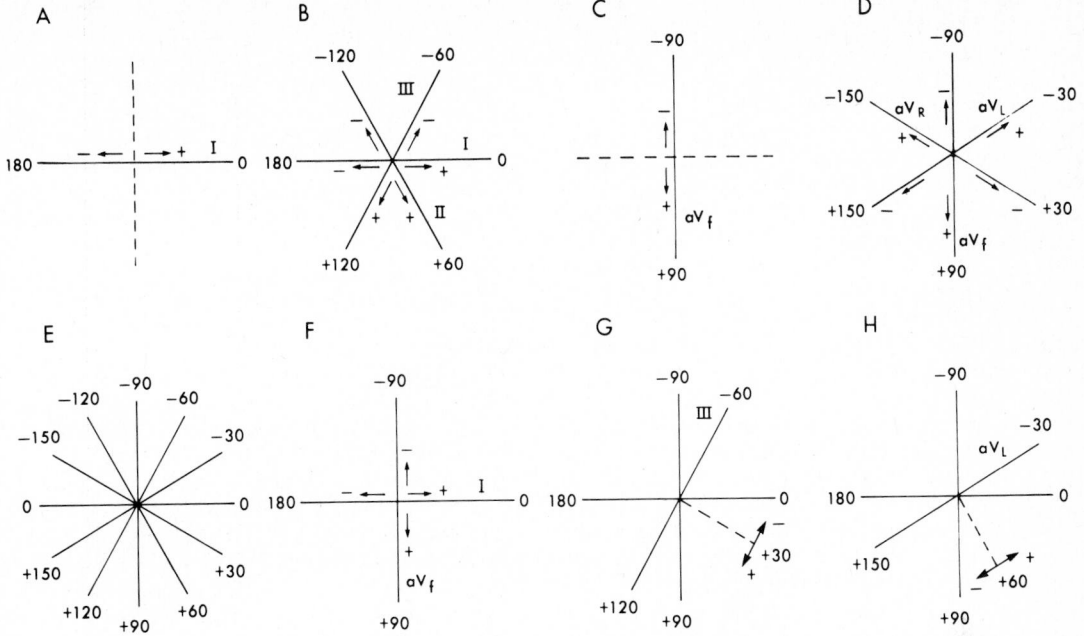

FIG. 31. Measurement of mean frontal plane axes. See text.

vector is passing to the right. If the net voltage is zero (that is, equiphasic R and S complexes) the vector must be passing up at −90 degrees or down at +90 degrees (Fig. 31A).

7. Next examine aVf for its net voltage: if positive, the vector is passing down; if negative, it is passing up; if zero, it is passing directly right or left (Fig. 31C). These two leads can be integrated to assign the vector to one of four quadrants (Fig. 31F). Lead I+, aVf+ indicates the left lower quadrant; lead I+, aVf− indicates the left upper quadrant (left axis); lead I−, aVf+ indicates the right lower quadrant (right axis); lead I−, aVf− indicates the left upper quadrant, sometimes termed the "northwest" quadrant.

8. Once the quadrant is identified, define the axis more closely by referring to the two leads that do *not* pass through that quadrant. Thus if the axis is in the left lower quadrant, refer to leads III and aVl. Consider lead III, which runs from −60 to +120 degrees (Fig. 31G). Any vector greater than +30 degrees will be pointing toward the positive pole of lead III and thus will give a positive deflection in lead III, whereas a negative net voltage in lead III indicates a vector less than +30 degrees. So if lead III is negative, then the QRS vector passes somewhere between +30 and 0 degrees and is commonly measured as halfway between them, or +15 degrees. If lead III is equiphasic, then the axis is +30 degrees. If lead III is positive, then the axis is between +30 and +90 degrees, and now lead aVl should be examined (Fig. 31H). It runs from −30 to +150 degrees, and a vector that is greater than +60 degrees will point away from the left shoulder and thus give a negative deflection, while if the net voltage is positive in aVl the axis must be less than +60 degrees. In this way it

is possible to assign axes of 0, +15, +30, +45, +60, +75, and +90 degrees. Similar descriptions of the angle of the mean QRS axis may be made in the other quadrants by applying the same principles.

9. Occasionally the R and S waves seem to be almost equiphasic in several leads, perhaps in four or in all six. This implies that the QRS vector is mainly perpendicular to the frontal plane and in the frontal plane forms a rough circle, so that there is no true mean axis. This is sometimes termed an indeterminate frontal plane axis. It has no clinical importance except insofar as it prevents the accurate determination of a mean QRS axis.

10. The mean frontal axis of the P and T waves can be calculated in the same way. These measurements are usually easier, since the waves are less complex.

P WAVE. Normally the right atrium is activated before the left atrium, so that the first part of the P wave is right atrial and the last part is left atrial, and forces from both atria make up the middle of the P wave. If there is right atrial hypertrophy the duration of the P wave is not lengthened, although the atrial forces overlap more than normal; however, the P waves become taller and peaked, especially in lead II, and they exceed the normal upper limit of 2.5 mm. In lead V_1, too, there may be a large biphasic P wave. If the left atrium is hypertrophied the initial part of the P wave is unaltered, but the later part is larger and often lasts longer, so that the P waves are wider than normal and bifid with a large second component. Biphasic P waves in V_1 may also be seen.

The normal P frontal plane axis is about +30 to +60 degrees; any marked change from this axis suggests that there is an abnormal focus of atrial activation.

Thus in true mirror-image dextrocardia the P axis is about +120 degrees, giving a negative P wave in lead I, whereas retrograde activation of the atria from a junctional focus gives a P axis of about −30 to −60 degrees; thus P waves are negative in leads II and III.

The P-R interval, from the beginning of the P wave to the onset of the QRS complex, is about 0.10 sec in newborns; it increases to about 0.16 sec at 16 years of age and can be up to 0.21 sec in adults. The interval is slightly shorter at more rapid heart rates at any age.

Q WAVE.   Since the Q wave indicates a septal vector that normally passes to the left anteriorly and superiorly, it is normally present in V_6 and absent in the right chest leads. Absence of the Q wave in left chest leads and its presence on the right may indicate that septal activation is taking place from right to left, either because of left bundle branch block or because of ventricular inversion (corrected transposition of the great arteries). It can also be due to the heart being rotated so that the septum lies in the sagittal plane; the septal vector may then be found by taking leads farther to the right and left of the routine leads. In some patients with very severe right ventricular hypertrophy there may be a qR pattern in the right chest leads, but there will usually be other evidence of right ventricular hypertrophy. Finally, a tiny initial r wave in right chest leads may be missed, especially if the electrocardiogram is recorded by a direct writing instrument.

QRS AND T WAVES.   At birth, with the thick right ventricle of the term infant, the mean QRS axis points anteriorly and to the right, thus giving right axis deviation and large R waves in right precordial leads. The QRS axis shifts to the left in the frontal plane and at about 3 months of age averages +60 to +80 degrees, with a range in normals of +30 to +150 degrees (Fig.

32A). It normally remains in the left lower quadrant throughout life. In the horizontal plane the axis rotates posteriorly until it is pointing leftward at 0 degrees at about 3 months of age and posteriorly at about −45 degrees from age 3 years onward. This explains why with age the R wave decreases in V_1 and increases in V_6, while V_1 shows a large S wave after infancy. In premature infants the right ventricle is not so well developed at birth, so that while premature infants still show right ventricular dominance at birth the QRS vector begins to swing posteriorly and to the left at about 1 month of age; this normal variant has in the past caused overdiagnosis of left ventricular hypertrophy in these preterm infants.

The mean T vector undergoes rapid and marked changes after birth. For the first 12 hours it points to the left and posteriorly and has a frontal plane axis of about +60 degrees; this gives a negative T wave in V_1. Then the T vector rotates anteriorly and to the right, giving a positive T wave in V_1 by 24 hours after birth. It remains anterior for 2 to 5 days (outer limit 7 days) and then moves posteriorly and to the left, so that the T wave again inverts in V_1. The reasons for these rapid changes are not clear. At about 12 years of age the T wave may in some children become upright once again in V_1. T waves normally may be inverted in leads V_5 and V_6 during but not after the first day after birth; they may be inverted normally in V_4 until 5 years of age and in V_3 until 10 years of age. The frontal plane T axis stays at about +60 degrees throughout childhood. Because the T and QRS vectors do not follow the same course in early childhood, the angle between them changes. At birth the frontal plane mean QRS-T angle is about +130 degrees, and it slowly falls until it reaches 30 to 60 degrees by about 3 years of age; there-

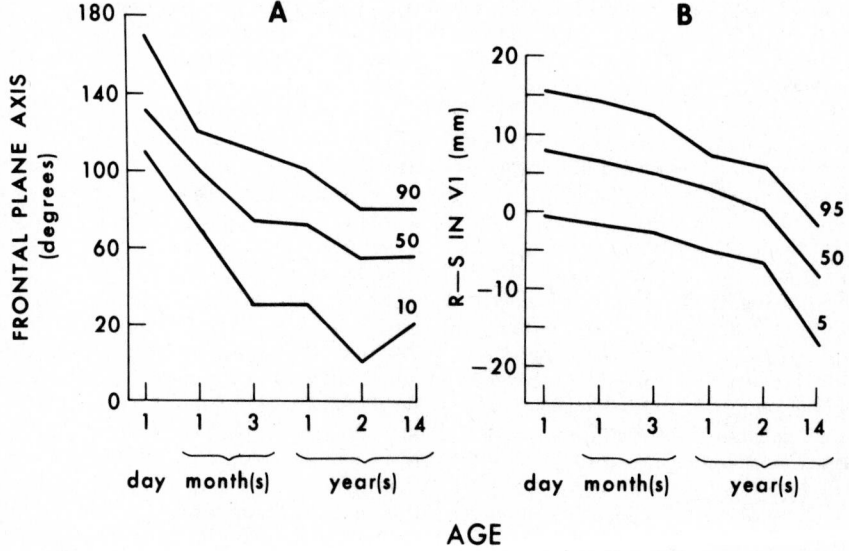

Fig. 32.   A. Normal values for mean frontal plane QRS axis at different ages. Lines show 10th, 50th, and 90th percentiles (data from Naiman and Miller). B. Normal values for the algebraic sum of R and S waves in V_1 at different ages. Lines show 5th, 50th, and 95th percentiles. (Calibration 1 mv = 10 mm. Data from Alimurung et al.)

after it remains under 60 degrees, and any increase suggests that some myocardial abnormality is present.

VENTRICULAR HYPERTROPHY. Ventricular hypertrophy is difficult to diagnose because of the enormous variability of normal standards. Differences in heart position and chest shape can affect how much of the actual cardiac potential is recorded from the body surface, and minor degrees of asynchrony of ventricular depolarization can greatly alter the algebraic sum of the electrical forces at any moment. Because of the wide range of normality it is usually impossible to diagnose slight hypertrophy, especially since the voltages prior to the onset of hypertrophy are seldom known. For example, a child with a 13-mm R wave in V_6 might be in the 50th percentile when normal and with hypertrophy might go to a 20-mm R wave in V_6. Since this value is the 90th percentile for normal children, it would not be possible to diagnose left ventricular hypertrophy if seen for the first time at that second stage. Because of these problems it is necessary to use as much information as possible in attempting to diagnose ventricular hypertrophy; the QRS axis and voltages, abnormal QRS patterns, and P and T wave changes should all be considered. Furthermore, no single sign on its own can be considered reliable; in particular, just an abnormal QRS axis or just a single increased voltage should not lead to the diagnosis if there is no other supportive evidence. This is particularly important since present standards are still based on relatively few normals at any age.

LEFT VENTRICULAR HYPERTROPHY. In infancy, with the increased mass of left ventricular muscle in left ventricular hypertrophy, the mean QRS axis moves to the left and posteriorly. Therefore in the frontal plane the QRS axis moves to between 0 and 90 degrees; an axis less than 60 degrees is uncommon in infancy and should suggest the possibility of left ventricular hypertrophy (Fig. 32A). This leftward shift of the QRS axis increases the R wave and decreases the S wave in V_5 and V_6 and the posterior shift of the QRS axis is shown by decreased R waves and increased S waves in V_1 (Fig. 32B). In older children and adults the QRS axis is normally to the left, posterior, and inferior, so that with left ventricular hypertrophy there is no further axis shift but only an increase in voltage. A left superior frontal axis (0 to −90 degrees) cannot be due to increased inferiorly placed left ventricular muscle and is not the mark of left ventricular hypertrophy, but of a conduction defect.

Without an axis shift to rely on, the diagnosis of left ventricular hypertrophy is based largely on voltage changes. In Figure 32B, if the algebraic sum of R and S waves in V_1 is below the 5th percentile for age, then increased posterior forces are suggested. Increased posterior forces are also suggested separately by R waves below the 10th percentile or S waves above the 90th percentile in V_4R and V_1 (Fig. 33A). The increased left forces are suggested by R waves above the 90th percentile in V_5 and V_6 (Fig. 33B); smaller than normal S waves in V_5 and V_6 are not helpful because

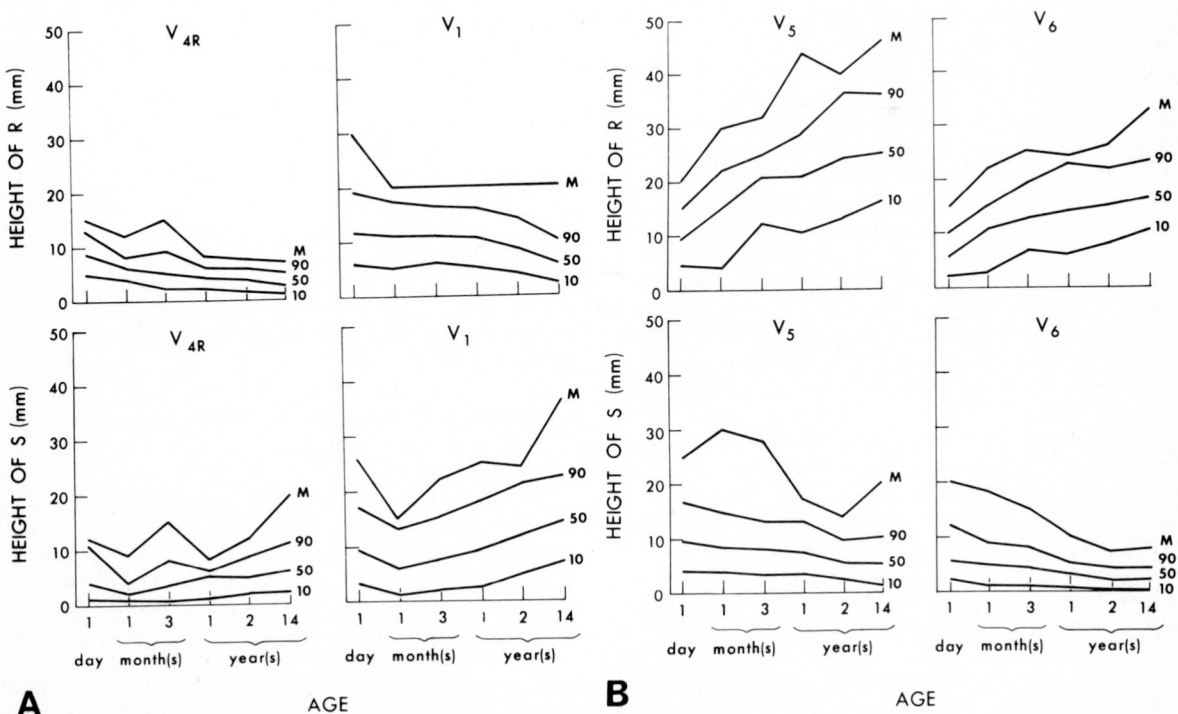

FIG. 33.   Normal values for R and S waves in (A) right and (B) left precordial leads at different ages. Lines represent 10th, 50th, and 90th percentiles and maximum values in data from Naiman and Miller. (Calibration 1 mv = 10 mm.)

they can normally be very small. In addition, since the septum is usually involved in the hypertrophy, there is often a larger than normal Q wave, which when greater than 4 mm is suggestive of left ventricular hypertrophy. T wave changes in the absence of voltage changes do not indicate left ventricular hypertrophy, but if they are associated they suggest either myocardial ischemia, as in severe aortic stenosis, or else what is termed left ventricular strain, which may or may not represent subendocardial ischemia. It is important to note that neither left nor right ventricular hypertrophy can be diagnosed confidently if there is an abnormally wide QRS complex, as occurs in bundle branch block or Wolff-Parkinson-White syndrome.

RIGHT VENTRICULAR HYPERTROPHY. At birth the term infant has a right ventricular wall equal to or slightly thicker than that of the left ventricle and thus, compared to the older child or adult, has physiologic right ventricular hypertrophy. If there is pathologic excessive right ventricular hypertrophy, the mean QRS vector may move farther right and anteriorly, so that frontal plane QRS axes more than the 90th percentile values in Figure 32A suggest right ventricular hypertrophy, provided that there is no conduction defect. This is also true at older ages. The increased anterior and rightward forces produce taller R waves and smaller S waves in right chest leads and smaller R waves and larger S waves in left chest leads (Fig. 33).

In addition to these voltage criteria there are certain patterns that help in the diagnosis. A pure R wave or a qR pattern in the right chest leads is strongly suggestive of pathologic right ventricular hypertrophy, and so is an upright T wave in V_4R and V_1 between 7 days and about 9 years of age.

RIGHT BUNDLE BRANCH BLOCK. If the right bundle is interrupted, as may occur congenitally or at surgery, a predictable change of the electrocardiogram occurs. Septal activation from left to right is unchanged, and then the left ventricle is depolarized to give a force to the left and posteriorly; this force is more marked than usual because the counteracting right ventricular forces have not yet begun. As the left ventricular depolarization is ending, the impulse eventually penetrates the right ventricular muscle and spreads slowly through it to give late-onset slow right and anterior forces. Therefore in right chest leads there is a normal initial r wave followed by a deep S wave and then a tall and wide R′ that brings the QRS duration to over 0.12 sec in adults. (By convention, a deflection under 5 mm is written as a lowercase letter, eg, r, and a deflection over 5 mm is written as a capital letter, eg, R. Also, a second positive deflection is described as r′ or R′.) In left chest leads the pattern is of a qRS type, with a deep and wide terminal S wave. The terminal right and anterior forces, being unopposed by left ventricular forces, are very large and serve to produce a marked right axis shift in the frontal plane.

Variations on this theme in children are important. In the first place, since in the newborn infant the normal QRS duration is about 0.05 to 0.06 sec, it is possible for complete right bundle branch block to widen the QRS but still be under the limit of 0.12 sec that pertains to adults. We have seen complete right bundle branch block with a QRS duration of 0.09 sec. Second, if the child has had a right ventriculotomy there may be a typical right bundle branch block pattern due to cutting of many small terminal conduction fibers in the free wall and not due to any damage to the main right bundle. Finally, many normal children have an rSr′ pattern that is due to a delayed but otherwise normal terminal deflection caused by late depolarization of the posterior part of the right ventricle under the AV groove. This pattern has been termed incomplete right bundle branch block, but in children it usually has nothing to do with conduction changes in the right bundle and its major branches. A similar pattern is also seen in most children with atrial septal defects and in those with mild pulmonic stenosis, but the normal and abnormal causes for the pattern cannot be distinguished on the electrocardiogram.

In some newborn infants there may be a very tall and pure R wave in right chest leads that raises the suspicion of right ventricular hypertrophy. Often close inspection shows a slur or notch on the upstroke of the R wave; with time the slur becomes more marked, a deep notch develops to produce an rR′ pattern, and finally a typical rSr′ pattern develops. In other words, a conduction defect in babies can simulate right ventricular hypertrophy, but absence of other evidence of right ventricular pathology and the evolution of the electrocardiogram will lead to the correct diagnosis.

S-T SEGMENT AND T WAVES. S-T segment and T wave changes other than those related to maturation have similar causes in children and adults. Frequently they are secondary to changes in the QRS complex, such as widening of the QRS complex in conduction abnormalities or an increased QRS amplitude in hypertrophy. These secondary changes of T waves are usually associated with a normal QRS-T angle in the frontal plane. Primary T wave changes are those occurring in the absence of QRS changes, and they may be classified as (1) changes due to electrolyte disturbances; (2) physiologic changes due to local cardiac cooling from drinking iced liquids, anxiety and hyperventilation, postprandial hyperglycemia, and isolated T wave changes; (3) pathologic changes due to drugs, especially digitalis glycosides, myocarditis or pericarditis, cardiomyopathy and degenerative neurologic diseases, and myocardial ischemia. The pathologic changes will be discussed in their respective sections, but the other two groups will be discussed briefly here.

ELECTROLYTE ABNORMALITIES. *Hypocalcemia* lengthens and *hypercalcemia* shortens the Q-T interval. Since normally the Q-T interval varies with heart rate, a rate-independent corrected Q-T interval (Q-Tc) is calculated as the observed Q-T interval divided by the square root of the R-R interval. The normal value is 0.40, with a range of 0.36 to 0.44. A low magnesium level may intensify the effects of low calcium; clinically the long Q-T interval of hypocalcemia in infancy may remain after the calcium level has been restored to normal and improve only after magnesium is given. Other factors can also alter the Q-T interval. Digitalis glycosides and pericarditis may shorten it slightly, and myocarditis and certain genetic syndromes may lengthen it.

A *high serum potassium* level gives high, peaked T waves that are usually clearly abnormal at concentrations above 7 mEq/liter. Higher potassium concentrations not only raise T waves farther, but reduce QRS amplitude, widen QRS duration, and lengthen P-R interval. Above 9 mEq/liter there are usually atrial arrest and very wide QRS complexes that may soon lead to ventricular fibrillation. *Low serum potassium* levels lower T waves, the effect being detectable below 3.5 mEq/liter. As potassium falls more, a U wave appears and the S-T segment becomes depressed.

PHYSIOLOGIC CHANGES. Physiologic changes are important because if they are not appreciated they may lead to the incorrect diagnosis of heart disease, with all the unpleasant consequences of this for the patient. Drinking iced drinks may cool the inferior wall of the left ventricle and cause deep T wave inversion in the left chest leads. Similarly, after heavy meals there can be T wave inversion in left chest leads that some workers associate with hyperglycemia. A history of recent ingestion of food or iced drinks will suggest these causes of T wave changes, and a repeat electrocardiogram while fasting will then show normal T waves.

Anxiety and hyperventilation may also alter T waves. Therefore not only should there be an attempt to assess the patient's anxiety, but an electrocardiogram should be taken with hyperventilation before doing an exercise electrocardiogram so that the effect of hyperventilation by itself can be assessed.

After paroxysmal tachycardias the T waves may be abnormal for several hours or days, perhaps due to transient myocardial ischemia or potassium loss; the T waves usually return to normal, and there is probably no permanent damage.

Two other important normal variants should be considered. Some children and young adults have large upright T waves and elevated S-T segments in precordial or even limb leads, so that pericarditis might be suspected. This change is due to some portions of the ventricle repolarizing early before depolarization of all the muscle is complete. What distinguishes this variant from pericarditis is that here the T waves are very large and do not evolve as they do in pericarditis. The second variant is that of isolated inversion of the T waves in leads over the left ventricular apex, although the T waves are upright in earlier and later leads. This change occurs most often in young males; it can vary from time to time and has no accepted explanation. Like other physiologic T wave changes, this change can usually be returned to normal after oral potassium salts are ingested.

References

Alimurung MM, Joseph LG, Nadas AS, Massell BF: Unipolar precordial and extremity electrocardiogram in normal infants and children. Circulation 4:420, 1951

Cassels DE, Ziegler RF (eds): Electrocardiography in Infants and Children. New York, Grune & Stratton, 1966

Grant RP: Grant's Clinical Electrocardiography: The Spatial Vector Approach. New York, McGraw-Hill, Blakiston, 1970

Guntheroth WA: Pediatric Electrocardiography. Philadelphia, WB Saunders, 1965

Hoffman JIE: The place of electrocardiography in pediatric cardiology. Schweiz Rundschau Medizin 64:816, 1975

——— Primary T-wave changes in children. Schweiz Rundschau Medizin 64:803, 1975

Liebman J: In Moss AJ, Adams FH (eds): Electrocardiography, in Heart Disease in Infants, Children and Adolescents. Baltimore, Williams & Wilkins, p. 183, 1968.

Marriott HJL: Practical Electrocardiography. Baltimore, Williams & Wilkins, 1972

Nadas AS: Pediatric Cardiology. Philadelphia, WB Saunders, 1963

Naimin EP, Miller RA: The normal electrocardiogram and vectorcardiogram in children. In Cassels DE, Ziegler RF (eds): Electrocardiography in Infants and Children. New York, Grune & Stratton, 1966

Schamroth L: An Introduction to Electrocardiography. Oxford, Blackwell, 1971

ARRHYTHMIAS

PAUL STANGER AND JULIEN I.E. HOFFMAN

General Principles

ANATOMY AND PHYSIOLOGY. The heart has specialized cells collected into nodes and tracts (Fig. 27). At the junction of the superior vena cava and right atrium is the sinoatrial (SA) node, which has a rich vagal and sympathetic nerve supply and normally controls heart rate. From the SA node three specialized pathways conduct impulses rapidly to the atrioventricular (AV) node and atrial muscle; these are the anterior, middle, and posterior internodal tracts, the first of which gives off a branch (Bachmann's bundle) to the left atrium. Simultaneously the impulses from the SA node and these tracts spread slowly through atrial muscle from cell to cell like ripples in a pond.

The AV node is near the coronary sinus; it is also innervated by vagal and sympathetic fibers and consists of a mesh of very thin fibers that conduct impulses very slowly. As a result the AV node delays AV conduction, thus giving time for more complete atrial emptying before the ventricles contract. With very rapid atrial rates the AV node limits the number of impulses reaching the ventricles. From the AV node the bundle of His passes into the ventricular septum just behind and below its membranous portion. The bundle of His has large, rapidly conducting fibers and has vagal nerves in only its proximal portion; more distally, there is sympathetic but not vagal innervation of conduction tissue. Near the top of the muscular ventricular septum the bundle of His gives off the compact right bundle branch that has wide fibers and then the left branch bundle that is a diffuse fan of thinner fibers. The peripheral conducting fibers, the Purkinje fibers, ramify just beneath the endocardium, so that the walls of the ventricles are depolarized from within out.

Some people have, in addition to these normal conduction pathways, accessory pathways by which atrial impulses may bypass the AV node and reach the ventricles prematurely. There are three such pathways. The first, the bundle of Kent, is a muscular bridge (or bridges) spanning the AV groove. The other two are specialized conducting fibers; the James fibers bypass the AV node and connect the internodal tracts to the bundle of His; the Mahaim fibers pass from the AV node or His bundle directly to ventricular septal muscle. Each of the accessory pathways may conduct intermittently and in either direction. Anterograde conduction results in early depolarization of the ventricles (*pre-excitation*); retrograde conduction results in rapid re-entry to the atria (Kent and James) or AV node (Mahaim) and may result in initiation of tachyarrhythmias. Note that depolarization and repolarization of atrial and ventricular muscle produce deflections on the surface electrocardiogram but that pacemaker activity and conduction must be inferred from the timing of atrial and ventricular depolarizations (P waves and QRS complexes, respectively).

ELECTROPHYSIOLOGY. If a microelectrode is placed in a cardiac muscle cell the potential between it and an electrode outside the cell is the transmembrane potential. In diastole this potential (the resting potential) is -80 to -90 mv. When the cell is excited there is rapid loss of negativity, which initiates the action potential; after depolarization the cell repolarizes and the resting potential is restored (Fig. 34B). Certain cells have a different pattern, as shown by Figure 34C. Their resting potential starts at about -80 mv, but then automatically becomes more positive. When the potential

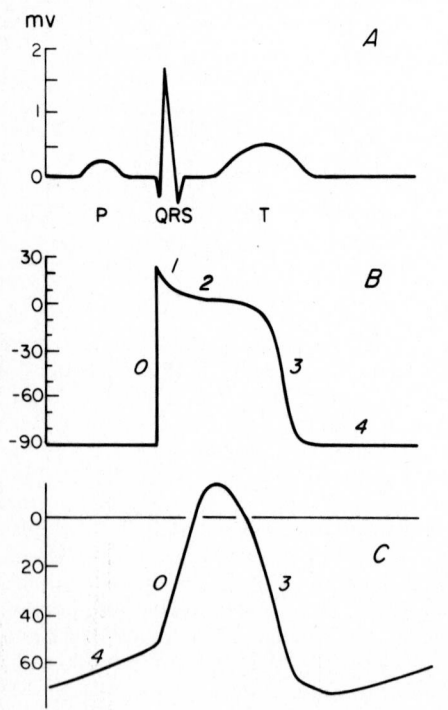

FIG. 34. A. Typical electrocardogram lead II. B. Transmembrane potential of cardiac muscle cell. C. Transmembrane potential of pacemaker cell.

reaches a threshold of about -50 mv the action potential begins spontaneously; thus these cells are called automatic cells and are said to have automaticity. Normally most cardiac muscle cells do not have automaticity; those that do may be found anywhere in the heart, but they are mainly in the SA node, the lower part of the AV node, and the conduction system.

The repetition rate at which groups of automatic cells depolarize depends mainly on the slope of spontaneous depolarization; the more rapid it is the sooner the threshold is reached. This diastolic depolarization rate is increased by catecholamines, by a raised temperature, by decreased extracellular potassium or calcium, or by a fall in tissue pH or oxygen tension; these changes thus tend to increase heart rate. The diastolic depolarization rate and thus automaticity are reduced by vagal stimulation, β-adrenergic blockade, increased extracellular potassium, and drugs like quinidine, procainamide, lidocaine, and diphenylhydantoin. It is the effect of these drugs in reducing automaticity that makes them useful in treating many arrhythmias. It is important to note that different automatic cells have different sensitivities for changes induced by these agents. Thus phenytoin (diphenylphenytoin) increases atrial diastolic depolarization but decreases ventricular diastolic depolarization, and lidocaine has a marked effect on ventricular automaticity but little effect on atrial automaticity.

Normally the discharge rate is highest for automatic cells in the SA node, which is thus the usual pacemaker for the heart. More distal collections of automatic cells (latent pacemakers) have slower diastolic depolarization, the slowest being those in the ventricles. These lower (or ectopic) pacemakers are therefore normally discharged by impulses from the SA node before they can discharge spontaneously, and thus they are normally suppressed by impulses from above. Normally the discharge rate of each pacemaker varies with age (Table 4).

As soon as depolarization is over, cardiac muscle is completely refractory to stimulation, but during repolarization it gradually regains excitability, the period between absolute refractoriness and complete responsiveness being the relative refractory period. A stimulus reaching conduction tissue at this time may be conducted, but at a rate slower than normal. Prolongation of absolute and relative refractory periods occurs with slowing of the ventricular rate, a long R-R interval thus giving a longer refractory period of the second beat. Refractory periods are also prolonged by disease (myocarditis, ischemia) and by some drugs (quinidine, procainamide, propranolol) but not by others (lidocaine, phenytoin).

Basic Features of Arrhythmias

There are three major types of disorders: ectopic impulse formation, abnormal conduction, and fibrillation.

DISORDERS OF ECTOPIC IMPULSE FORMATION. If the SA node discharges abnormally slowly or the impulse from it is not conducted, then an ectopic

TABLE 4. Normal Pacemaker Rates at Various Ages

Pacemaker	Age				
	0–1 month	1 year	5 years	10 years	Adult
SA node	100–180	110–180	60–120	55–110	50–100
AV node	80–90				50–70
Ventricles	50–70				35–50

lower pacemaker, either atrial or more commonly junctional (near the AV node), will take over; if the block is in the AV node or bundle of His, a ventricular pacemaker takes over. In this way lower pacemakers escape from suppression by higher pacemakers. Escape may occur for a single beat or a few beats, or it may result in a permanent lower pacemaker rhythm if the higher pacemaker does not regain control. It should be recognized that escape beats or rhythms indicate abnormality of the higher pacemaker or conduction from it and that the escape is a normal response. An *escape beat* is recognized by its late appearance (longer than normal R-R interval) and evidence of an ectopic focus (abnormal P vector if atrial ectopic, no P wave, or very short P-R if junctional). An *escape rhythm* is characterized by an ectopic rhythm that is slower than a normal sinus rhythm. If P waves are present the atrial rate is slower than the ectopic rhythm, or it is the same rate but with a very short P-R interval (Fig. 35).

The other disorder with ectopic impulse formation is due to premature discharge of a lower pacemaker. One or two of these beats are termed *premature beats* or *extrasystoles,* but three or more in a row are termed *ectopic tachycardia.* If the ectopic focus is in the atrium or near the AV node, then the descending impulse normally reaches the ventricles through the His–Purkinje system, and a normal QRS complex usually occurs. If the ectopic focus is ventricular, then the impulse spreads slowly through muscle cells and produces a wide bizarre QRS complex with T wave polarity opposite to that of the ectopic QRS complex. If the premature beat begins in the right ventricle, then this ventricle is depolarized before the left ventricle, and the QRS pattern resembles that of a left branch block. Conversely, a left ventricular ectopic beat resembles a right bundle branch block. The basic difference between the bundle branch block and the ectopic patterns is that in the former it is only the terminal part of depolarization that is slow, while in the latter the whole QRS complex is slowed and distorted. Often a supraventricular impulse may be conducted aberrantly to the ventricles, giving a wide QRS complex (see below); thus a wide QRS complex is not a sufficient characteristic for diagnosing a ventricular ectopic focus.

With a ventricular premature beat the basic rhythm of the SA node is usually unaltered, so that the first sinus beat after a ventricular extrasystole follows a full compensatory pause; that is, the interval between the sinus beat preceding the extrasystole and the sinus beat following it is twice the normal R-R interval (Fig. 36). With atrial or junctional premature beats, however, the SA node is usually discharged; thus the next sinus beat occurs after an incomplete compensatory pause.

Ectopic tachycardias have QRS complexes like those of the corresponding ectopic beats: usually normal if the focus is supraventricular, almost always widened if it is ventricular, but often widened if there is a supraventricular focus with aberrant conduction. The differentiation between these is discussed below.

The effect of premature beats on atrial P waves depends on the site of the ectopic focus. If it is near the SA node an almost normal P wave and P-R interval occur (Fig. 38); if it is near the AV node, then the mean atrial vector may be directed superiorly, giving inverted P waves in leads II, III, and aVf (Fig. 36B) (p. 1384). Therefore low atrial or high His bundle premature beats give similar P waves, although because of the time taken for retrograde conduction through the AV node to the atria an infranodal pacemaker is more likely to give P waves buried in the QRS complex or following it. If the ectopic focus is ventricular there can be a retrograde P wave after the QRS complex, but often the retrograde impulse is blocked in the AV node and the atrium is activated normally from the SA node. Depending on how premature the ventricular extrasystole is, a normal P wave may follow the QRS complex, may be buried in it, or occasionally may barely precede it.

Premature beats may be due to increased automaticity of an ectopic focus, and they can be due to many causes, including endogenous catecholamines,

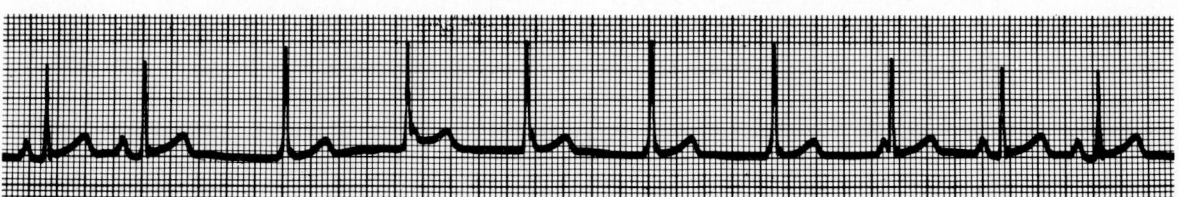

FIG. 35. Junctional escape beats in a healthy 12-year-old boy. The basic rhythm is sinus, and the first two and last two impulses are conducted to the ventricles. Junctional escape beats occur when the sinus rate slows. The notched QRS complex in the escape beats is due to the normal P wave coinciding with the junctional escape beat.

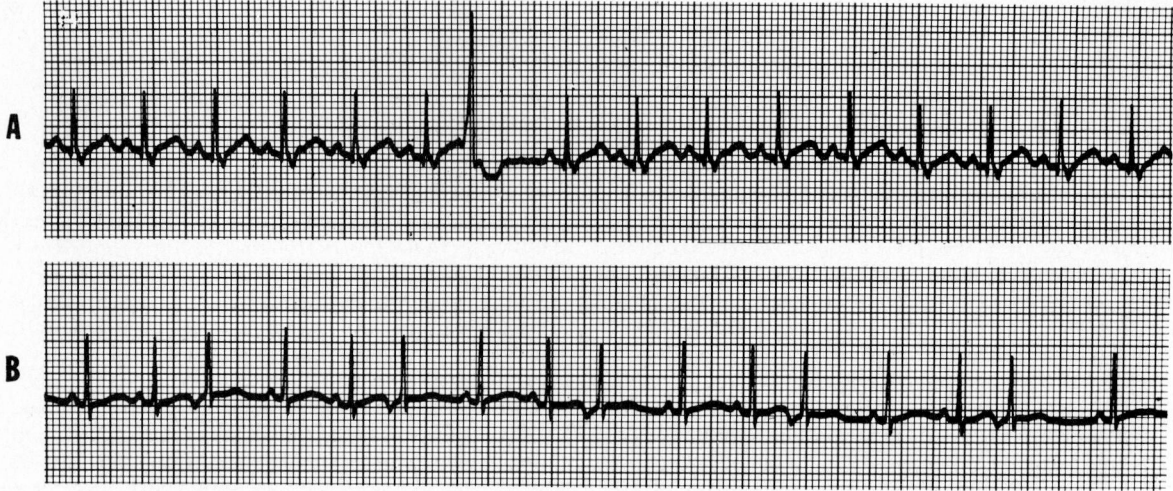

FIG. 36. Compensatory pauses following ectopic beats. A. Premature ventricular ectopic beat followed by a full compensatory pause. B. Premature atrial contractions with incomplete compensatory pauses (3rd, 6th, 9th, and 12th beats) and with a full compensatory pause (15th beat). Both strips are lead II.

drugs, or disease. They may also be due to *re-entry*. For example, if in the ventricle there is a strip of damaged muscle that will not conduct an anterograde impulse but will conduct a retrograde impulse, although at a rate slower than normal, the normal sinus impulse descends and depolarizes the remaining normal muscle, and the wave of depolarization eventually passes slowly retrograde up the abnormal strip that has not been depolarized. By the time the impulse emerges from the abnormal muscle the rest of the muscle is responsive and depolarizes again before the sinus beat stimulates it—a ventricular premature beat. The wave of depolarization does not continue to circulate because the abnormal muscle, having been depolarized, is now refractory to impulses from any direction. The sequence may be repeated to produce bigeminy. Since there is normally slow conduction through the AV node, re-entry through it is thought to explain many types of extrasystoles. If the recirculating wave of depolarization is itself slowed in some other portion of muscle, then the wave may return to the original abnormal muscle strip when it has regained excitability, and a rapid repetitive depolarization (an ectopic tachycardia) will occur. Re-entry is certainly the cause of tachycardia in the Wolff-Parkinson-White syndrome, in which the impulse descends

through the AV node and returns to the atrium through the bundle of Kent.

One specific form of ectopic beat that is more common in ventricles than in atria is *parasystole*. Here the ectopic focus seems to be protected from being discharged by impulses from higher pacemakers; thus it discharges continuously at its own slow rate. If it discharges in the refractory period, then no extrasystole occurs; if it discharges in the ventricle's excitable phase, then there will be a ventricular premature beat. All the premature beats tend to have the same morphology, but there is usually a variable *coupling interval* (that is, a variable interval between the ectopic beat and the preceding normal beat). An even more important criterion of parasystole is that the intervals between ectopic beats are all exact multiples of the shortest interectopic interval.

DISORDERS OF CONDUCTION. Conduction may be delayed or interrupted either by an increase in the refractory period of tissue (pathologic, or primary) or by interference from another impulse that alters the refractory period (physiologic, or secondary). Physiologic factors that affect conduction include *concealed conduction* and *physiologic interference*. When conduction through tissue cannot be detected on the electrocardio-

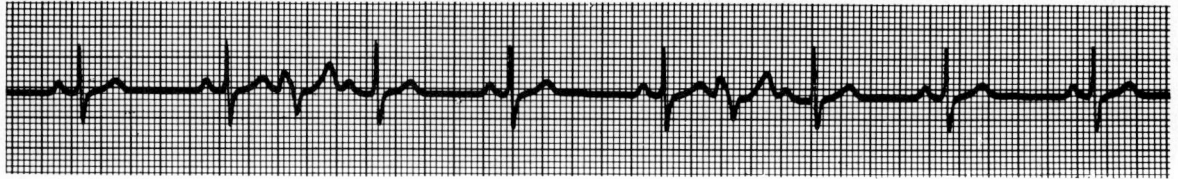

FIG. 37. Interpolated ventricular ectopic beats and concealed conduction. The basic rhythm is sinus and is not altered by the ventricular ectopic beats. Impulses from the ventricular ectopic beats pass retrograde to the AV node. The next sinus beat reaches the AV node before it has fully recovered, and the P-R interval is therefore prolonged after each ectopic beat.

gram, but may be inferred by its effect on conduction of a subsequent impulse, then it is termed concealed conduction. This may be well shown, for example, if there is an interpolated (very early) ventricular premature beat (Fig. 37). The retrograde impulse from the ventricular focus enters the AV node and increases the AV nodal refractory period but does not capture the atrium, which is still refractory from the last beat. The next impulse from the SA node is conducted more slowly than normal through the AV node because it is still partially refractory. The resulting long P-R interval is the evidence for the concealed retrograde conduction.

Interference is shown most simply if there is a very early isolated atrial premature beat. In Figure 38 the ninth P wave is seen on the T wave of the preceding QRS complex, but because the AV node and ventricles are still refractory, the impulse is not conducted. This is physiologic, not pathologic, failure of conduction. A more prolonged episode of physiologic interference may occur if the SA node pacemaker slows or a junctional pacemaker speeds up so that the atria and ventricles beat at roughly similar rates but are controlled by

different pacemakers (Figs. 35 and 39). This is termed *atrioventricular dissociation.* The descending impulse from the SA node does not pass the AV node, which has been made refractory by the retrograde impulse from the ventricle or bundle of His; and in turn this retrograde impulse does not capture the atrium, which has been made refractory by the sinus beat. Failure of the SA node to capture the ventricle is thus not due to an abnormality of conduction but to physiologic effects on refractory periods. An electrocardiogram with this type of interference shows unrelated P waves and QRS complexes with the ventricular rate faster than the atrial rate. Occasionally ventricular and atrial rates are the same, but the P-R interval is too short to diagnose a sinus rhythm; this is termed *isorhythmic dissociation.* Sometimes the interference occurs in the atrium or the ventricle, rather than in the AV node, and then it produces atrial or ventricular *fusion beats,* the latter being more important. Typically a ventricular premature beat has a wide QRS complex. However, if the ventricular premature beat begins while the normal sinus impulse is descending the His–Purkinje system, then some of the ventricle will be depolarized normally and the rest

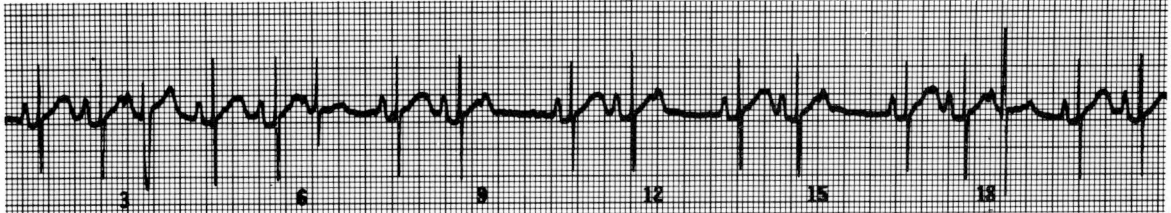

FIG. 38. Premature atrial contractions with varying coupling intervals and the different types of ventricular response. Every third P wave is a premature atrial ectopic beat; however, the interval between the atrial ectopic beat and the preceding QRS complex varies. The 6th and 18th beats are atrial ectopic beats that occur relatively late and reach the ventricles when they have almost completely repolarized; the resulting QRS complex is similar to the normal ventricular complexes. The 9th, 12th, and 15th atrial beats occur early and are not conducted because the impulses reach the AV node and/or ventricles while they are still refractory (interference). The 3rd beat is a premature atrial contraction that is intermediate in timing and shows aberrancy of conduction due to refractoriness of one of the bundle branches.

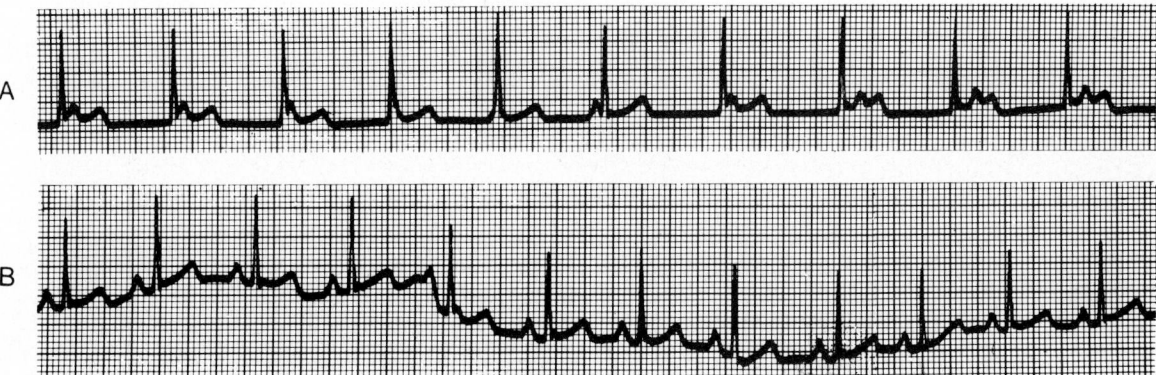

FIG. 39. Atrioventricular dissociation. A. Independent atrial and ventricular contractions with neither depolarizing the other. The atrial rate is slower than the ventricular; consequently the dissociation may be the result of an accelerated junctional pacemaker whose rate exceeds that of the sinus pacemaker. B. Mild exercise speeds up the sinus pacemaker, resulting in conduction to the ventricles and suppression of the junctional pacemaker.

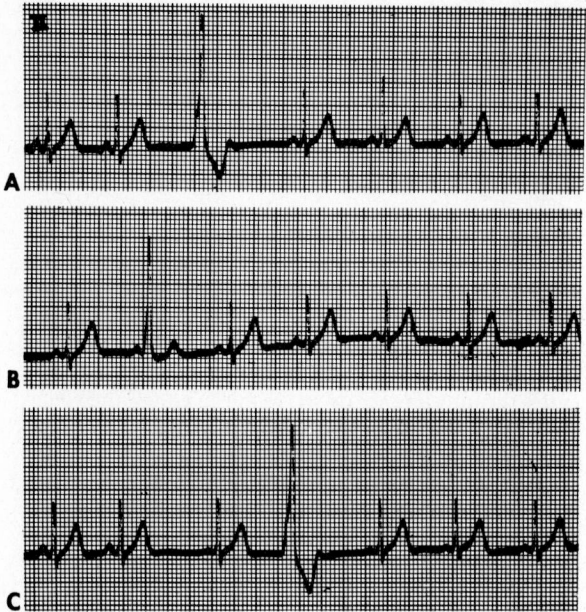

FIG. 40. Ventricular fusion beat. A and C are premature ventricular ectopic beats. B is a fusion beat resulting from a premature ventricular ectopic beat occurring just after the P wave, so that part of the myocardium is depolarized slowly by the ectopic beat and the remainder by the sinus impulse reaching the ventricles via the His–Purkinje system.

slowly; the resulting QRS complex (the fusion beat) will usually be intermediate in form between the normal complex and that due to the ventricular ectopic beat (Figs. 40 and 52).

ABERRANT CONDUCTION. Whenever a supraventricular impulse reaches the AV node or bundle of His in the relative refractory period, the impulse may be transmitted aberrantly because of uneven loss of refractoriness in the AV node or bundle branches. The reasons for the impulse arriving at the AV node or bundle at this time include a premature supraventricular beat, supraventricular tachycardia, or a prolonged Q-T interval of the preceding beat. As a rule the right branch bundle usually takes longer to recover completely because it normally has a longer refractory period than the left bundle. Therefore premature supraventricular beats or tachycardias may be conducted normally to the left ventricle but slowly to the right ventricle, giving the pattern of right bundle branch block and a wide QRS complex (Fig. 38). (About 10 to 20 percent of the time some other pattern of interventricular block is present.) This widening of the QRS complex is particularly important in evaluating tachycardias. The chief features suggesting a supraventricular focus with aberration are that in lead V_1 there will usually be a triphasic complex, most often an rsR', and the initial deflection will be similar to that seen in V_1 when normal beats are present, either in that tracing or in earlier or later ones; similarly, V_6 usually shows a qRs complex. An important point is that a ventricular ectopic focus does not produce triphasic complexes, although a supraventricular focus may at times produce biphasic beats.

AV BLOCK.   If conduction is delayed equally through all parts of the AV node and the bundle of His, then various degrees of AV block occur. If there is merely a long P-R interval, but all beats are conducted, it is a *first-degree AV block* (Fig. 41). If no atrial beats are conducted, so that the ventricles are driven by a bundle of His or a ventricular pacemaker, then there will be normal P waves at one rate and QRS complexes at a slower rate, with usually no fixed relationship between P waves and QRS complexes. This is *complete* or *third-degree AV block* (Fig. 42). If some sinus beats are conducted to the ventricle, but others do not reach it, then there is *second-degree AV block* that takes one of two forms. *Type I second-*

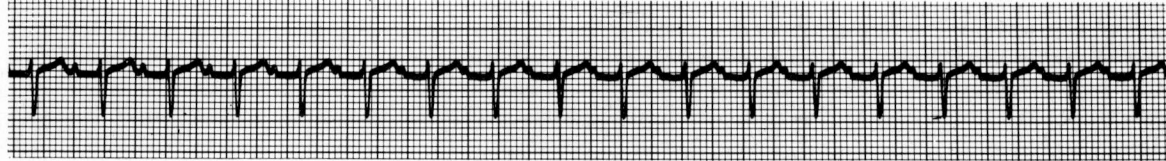

FIG. 41.   First-degree AV block in a newborn infant. The P-R interval is 0.18 sec, which is prolonged for the patient's age and heart rate.

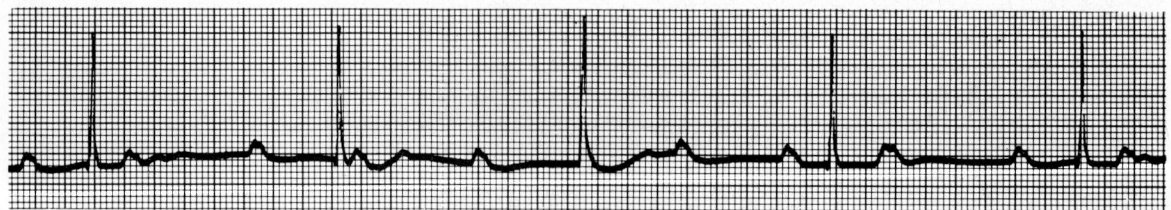

FIG. 42.   Third-degree AV block. The P waves and QRS complexes have no consistent temporal relationship. The atrial rate is 90/minute and the ventricular 38/minute.

degree AV block is characterized by the Wenckebach phenomenon, which is usually due to temporary depression of the AV node. The first atrial impulse of a group of beats is normally conducted, but the next atrial impulse reaches the AV node while it is still partly refractory and thus is conducted more slowly; there is thus a long P-R interval. The next atrial impulse arrives even earlier in the AV nodal refractory period, with an even longer P-R interval as a result. Eventually the atrial impulse reaches the AV node in its absolute refractory period and is blocked, so that no QRS complex follows (Fig. 43). The effect of this on the QRS complexes is to make them occur with progressively shorter R-R intervals, until an unusually long R-R interval indicates that one ventricular complex has dropped out. Two other features are typical of this arrhythmia. The largest increment in P-R intervals is in the second beat after the dropped beat; the first has the shortest P-R interval because the long pause has allowed the AV node to recover. Furthermore, the longest R-R interval is almost always less than two of the short cycles because these contain the cycles with the longest P-R intervals. This feature of progressive shortening of the R-R intervals until a long R-R interval less than two of the shorter R-R intervals occurs is the hallmark that allows the Wenckebach phenomenon to be diagnosed even when P waves are not easily seen.

Type II second-degree AV block occurs when a QRS complex drops out without prior lengthening of the P-R intervals (Fig. 43). This is usually seen with bundle branch block and is due to intermittent block in the remaining conducting bundle. It is less common but more serious than type I second-degree AV block, and it is more likely to lead to complete AV block.

Note that second-degree AV block does not imply a fixed relationship between atrial and ventricular complexes. There may be 2:1 second-degree AV block in which only alternate atrial impulses are conducted to the ventricle; 3:1 second-degree AV block indicates that every third atrial impulse is conducted to the ventricles. There may be higher grades of second-degree block such as 4:1, 5:1, etc; there may be no consistent relationship between the numbers of conducted and blocked atrial impulses.

MYOCARDIAL FIBRILLATION. If there is asymmetric slowing of conduction or shortening of refractoriness, then a stimulus at that time to a region that has repolarized may be conducted at different rates in some directions and may be blocked in others, so that an irregular wave front of depolarization occurs. It takes a tortuous path through the muscle and can return to a region that was formerly refractory but is now excitable. The wave of depolarization can therefore continue, becoming more irregular and leaving behind it refractory cells. Eventually there is a chaotic fragmented contraction that is *fibrillation.*

To produce fibrillation two conditions are needed. First, there must be asymmetric slowing of conduction or shortening of refractoriness, which can be caused by hypoxemia or ischemia, by electrolyte abnormalities, or by many drugs. Second, there must be a premature stimulus like an external electric shock, a premature beat, or tachycardia that occurs very early before all the muscle has repolarized. The fact that an extrasystole can occur so early is itself evidence of decreased refractoriness of some muscle.

If the chaotic rhythm occurs in the atria there is *atrial fibrillation,* which is quite easily provoked, since atrial conduction is normally slow. However, the fibrillation is not sustained unless the atria are enlarged. If the chaotic rhythm occurs in the ventricles there is *ventricular fibrillation;* the vulnerable period in which a shock or ectopic beat can cause fibrillation is at the apex of the T wave.

Diagnosis

Diagnosis of arrhythmias is best made with full knowledge of the history and physical findings and also with all previous electrocardiograms from that patient. The electrocardiogram of the arrhythmia under study should be a routine full electrocardiogram and should also include some very long strips, lasting about 1 minute or more, from leads like II and V_1 that are most likely to show good P waves. Sometimes special leads are required to bring out P waves: for example, a modified CL_1 lead (that is, placing the negative lead near the left shoulder, the positive lead at the fourth right interspace at the right sternal edge, and the ground lead on the right shoulder), or taking the two arm leads and placing them at the upper and lower right sternal edge, or using an esophageal or intracardiac lead.

Once the electrocardiogram is available it should be examined carefully for P waves. These should be inspected for rate, morphology, and mean axis, for P-R

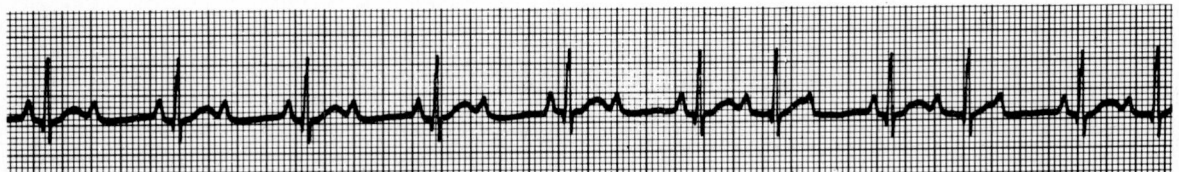

FIG. 43. Second-degree AV block in a patient with digitalis toxicity. The first half of the tracing shows 2:1 AV block. The second portion shows two Wenckebach cycles with progressive lengthening of the P-R interval, until the third atrial beat is not conducted to the ventricles. The 2:1 AV block may also be the result of a Wenckebach phenomenon with a cycle length of only two beats.

intervals and their possible variation, and to find out if the P waves are related to the QRS complex (that is, if they are likely to be the source of the impulse causing the QRS complex). Then the QRS complex should be examined for its rate, rhythm, and morphology.

Some arrhythmias may be diagnosed more easily if the neck veins are also examined. Atrial contractions are absent in atrial fibrillation; flutter waves are seen in atrial flutter, and cannon waves are seen when the atrium contracts while the tricuspid valve is closed, thus indicating coincident atrial and ventricular contraction. Maneuvers that increase AV block (vagal stimuli, injection of procainamide) may slow ventricular rate and allow better definition of atrial and ventricular complexes. They should be performed only while the electrocardiogram is running.

Most arrhythmias can be diagnosed by these means. Sometimes it is necessary to do His bundle recordings at cardiac catheterization to distinguish complex arrhythmias. Sometimes, too, arrhythmias are intermittent, or their informative onset may not be observed. Then it is valuable to make tape recordings continuously for 12 hours or longer and replay them at high speed through some system that allows easy detection of any abnormalities; in this way many obscure arrhythmias may be clarified.

While it is impossible to cover all possible differential diagnoses, it is convenient to discuss certain problems that occur frequently.

REGULAR RHYTHM AT NORMAL RATE. A regular rhythm at normal rate is most likely to be a sinus rhythm, but the electrocardiogram and neck veins should be inspected carefully to exclude atrial tachycardia with 2:1 AV block, atrial flutter with 4:1 AV block, junctional or idioventricular accelerated rhythms, or atrial fibrillation with an independent idioventricular rhythm.

PAUSES. Occasional pauses are most commonly due to nonconducted very early atrial extrasystoles. They can also be due to marked sinus arrhythmia, second-degree AV block, or SA block, as well as to concealed conduction that has made the AV node refractory.

SITE OF ECTOPIC BEAT. If the QRS complex is narrow and normal for that patient, then the ectopic beat is supraventricular. If the P wave is more or less normal in shape and has a normal mean frontal plane vector, then it is an atrial ectopic beat, but if the vector is superior it is a junctional ectopic beat from near the AV node. If the QRS complex is wide there is either a ventricular ectopic focus or a supraventricular focus with aberrant conduction. The differences have been discussed in the section on aberration, but essentially aberration is likely if the beat is triphasic in V_1 and V_6 and resembles a right bundle branch block pattern or if the initial deflections of the wide QRS complex resemble those of the normal beats. Note that if there is an ectopic beat that is not premature, but follows an R-R interval that is longer than normal, then it is an escape beat, and some failure in impulse generation or conduction should be considered.

GROUPS OF BEATS. Bigeminy means that beats occur in pairs. Most commonly this is due to an extrasystole coupled to the previous normal beat, but it can also be due to 3:2 AV block (every third atrial beat not conducted) or to an escape beat that is paired with the next normal beat. Similarly, trigeminy means that there are groups of three beats. These could be two normal and one premature beat, one normal and two premature beats, 4:3 AV block, and so on. Wenckebach periods always produce groups of beats that may be grouped in pairs, triplets, or larger groups.

IRREGULAR RHYTHMS. Occasional irregularities are due either to premature beats or to escape beats, the latter occurring with sinus pauses, blocked atrial premature beats, or second-degree AV block. These are usually easy to differentiate. At times it is difficult to distinguish an atrial fibrillation from a second-degree AV block with Wenckebach periods occurring in a tachycardia where P waves are not easy to find. The diagnosis is made by the characteristic features of Wenckebach periods: progressive shortening of the R-R interval before a long pause, with the longest R-R interval being less than two of the shortest intervals.

TACHYCARDIAS. A rapid heart rate with normal P waves and P-R intervals, and with variations in rate from moment to moment, is a sinus tachycardia. A rapid fixed rate with complete regularity, normal QRS complexes, and either P waves on the T waves or else no clear P waves is probably a supraventricular tachycardia. Vagal stimulation either may cause no change or may cause abrupt reversion to sinus rhythm. A rapid rate, usually fixed and regular, with a wide QRS complex is either a ventricular tachycardia or a supraventricular tachycardia with ventricular aberration or preceding bundle branch block. The diagnosis of a ventricular tachycardia can be made by examining the QRS patterns (see section on aberration), by finding fusion beats, or by noting that the QRS complexes are similar to ventricular ectopic beats found in other electrocardiograms. Vagal stimulation does not affect the arrhythmia. If a slower atrial rhythm is noted from P waves usually deforming the T waves variously from beat to beat, then it is likely that it is a ventricular tachycardia. However, retrograde P waves at the same rate as the ventricles can occur with either junctional or ventricular tachycardias. A rapid supraventricular tachycardia can also be due to atrial flutter with a regular block; this is separated from a plain supraventricular tachycardia by the typical sawtooth flutter waves, although these waves may be seen in only one or two leads. It could also be due to atrial fibrillation, which is detected by slight variations in the R-R intervals. In both these arrhythmias the rate is slowed and the variability is increased by increasing AV nodal block with vagal stimulation or digitalis.

Principles of Treatment

In addition to correct identification of the arrhythmia, proper management of arrhythmias requires attention to four questions:

1. Does the arrhythmia need treatment? In most pediatric patients no treatment is needed. Arrhythmias that require treatment are those that threaten to cause ventricular fibrillation or asystole (eg, ventricular tachycardia, multifocal ventricular ectopic beats) and those in which ventricular rate is too slow or too fast for effective cardiac output. In general the effects of abnormal ventricular rates depend not only on the rates but on how much they differ from the patient's usual rate. Thus a chronically slow ventricular rate of 50 beats per minute is accompanied by ventricular dilatation and hypertrophy and well-maintained cardiac output. On the other hand, a sudden drop from 100 to 50 beats per minute may be poorly tolerated.

2. Can underlying causes be removed? In pediatric patients, particularly neonates, most clinically significant arrhythmias are secondary to apnea, hypoxemia, acidemia, electrolyte disturbances, or drugs such as digitalis or catecholamines.

3. Do secondary effects need treatment? Arrhythmias that reduce cardiac output may cause hypotension and acidemia, which help to maintain the arrhythmia.

4. What specific therapeutic strategy is needed for the arrhythmia? Consider two patients with 2:1 AV block, one with an atrial rate of 260 beats per minute, the other with an atrial rate of 100 beats per minute. The first patient has an adequate ventricular rate of 130 beats per minute, and therapy should be directed at slowing the atrial rate; the AV block should not be treated because it is useful in preventing too many impulses from reaching the ventricles and causing a harmful rapid ventricular rate. In the second patient therapy should be directed to increasing the ventricular rate of 50 beats per minute by improving AV conduction or by pacing the ventricles.

SPECIFIC THERAPIES. BRADYCARDIAS. A slow ventricular rate may be the result of severe sinus bradycardia or arrest or second- or third-degree AV block. The slowing either causes a cardiac output that is too low or allows breakthrough of potentially dangerous ventricular escape beats or tachycardia. Treatment is aimed at increasing ventricular rate by one of several means. *Atropine* (0.01 mg/kg subcutaneously or intravenously) may increase SA nodal discharge rate or accelerate AV conduction, but it does not speed up low ventricular pacemakers, since the vagus does not supply conduction tissue below the bundle of His. *Isoproterenol* (0.05 to 0.5 μg/kg/minute, see p. 1483) may increase pacemaker discharge rates and conductions at any level, but it should be used with caution if there are ventricular arrhythmias as well. Slowed conduction through the AV node, especially if induced by digitalis, may be improved by *phenytoin.* If any therapy is ineffective or contraindicated, then temporary or permanent pacing may be used.

ECTOPIC BEATS AND ECTOPIC TACHYCARDIAS. The arrhythmias with premature beats or tachycardias have abnormalities related to increased automaticity or excitability of cardiac cells or to uneven conduction times that result in re-entry beats. *Vagal stimulation* by any means (carotid sinus massage, baroreceptor reflex to hypertension, anticholinesterase drugs) reduces automaticity and shortens the action potential duration and the effective refractory period of atrial muscle; it also slows atrial and AV nodal conduction and lengthens the refractory period of the AV node. These actions may abolish paroxysmal supraventricular tachycardia, and they decrease ventricular rate in atrial flutter or fibrillation. Because of sparse ventricular innervation, vagal stimulation does not affect ventricular arrhythmias. It should be noted that vagal maneuvers cause a gradual slowing in sinus tachycardia but an abrupt change in supraventricular tachycardias.

Should vagal stimulation fail, the drug of choice for treating atrial arrhythmias is *digitalis* (for dosage see p. 1481). This increases ventricular automaticity and so increases the chances of getting ventricular premature beats and tachycardias, an undesirable effect that explains in part why digitalis is not the drug of choice for treating ventricular arrhythmias. In therapeutic doses both excitability and conduction velocity are depressed. At all doses AV nodal conduction is slowed, so that first the P-R interval lengthens; with larger doses second- or third-degree AV nodal block occurs. Digitalis shortens the action potential duration and the refractory period in atria and ventricles, thus shortening the Q-T interval.

Quinidine and *procainamide* (classed together as group I) decrease myocardial automaticity and excitability. They decrease ventricular conduction velocity and increase action potential duration; as a result there is an increase in the effective refractory period and in the QRS and Q-T durations. They also tend to delay AV nodal conduction, thus increasing the P-R interval or even producing higher degrees of AV block. At times, however, both of these drugs reduce vagal tone and thus can accelerate AV conduction. These drugs also depress myocardial function and can lower blood pressure and cardiac output. Their toxicity, too, is related to myocardial depression, AV block or asystole, or sometimes tachyarrhythmias. From these considerations it is clear that they should be avoided if there is already myocardial depression or impaired AV or intraventricular conduction. They are most useful in abolishing atrial arrhythmias, except those due to digitalis. Quinidine sulfate may be given orally at 6 mg/kg every 2 to 4 hours for three to five doses daily. Procainamide may be given orally at 10 to 15 mg/kg every 4 to 6 hours, intramuscularly at 6 mg/kg every 4 to 6 hours, or intravenously at 2 mg/kg/minute for a maximum of 10 minutes.

Propranolol shares some of the properties of these group I drugs, except that it tends to decrease action potential duration and effective refractory period; thus it does not widen the QRS complex and may decrease the Q-T interval. It is more likely to slow AV nodal conduction than the group I drugs, and thus it should be avoided if there is any AV block. It is capable of abolishing many atrial and ventricular arrhythmias, but it should be used with caution if there is congestive heart failure, since withdrawal of sympathetic drive can be harmful. Conversely, it is the drug of choice for catecholamine-induced arrhythmias. It may be given orally at 0.5 to 1 mg/kg every 4 to 6 hours or intravenously at 0.05 to 0.2 mg/kg.

Lidocaine and *phenytoin* are classed as group II. They decrease automaticity but not excitability; they decrease action potential duration and effective refractory period and increase ventricular and AV nodal conduction velocities. Therefore they do not increase P-R, QRS, or Q-T intervals; in fact, they may decrease the extent of AV block. They do not depress myocardial function, and in toxic doses they cause neurologic but not myocardial toxicity. They are the drugs of choice for ventricular arrhythmias, AV block, and myocardial depression. They are also the drugs of choice for treating digitalis-induced atrial arrhythmias. Lidocaine may be given intravenously at a loading dose of 1 mg/kg and then infused at a rate of 15 to 50 µg/kg/minute. Phenytoin may be given intravenously at 2 mg/kg every 5 to 15 minutes for a maximum of 10 doses or orally at 15 mg/kg on the first day and then 5 to 10 mg/kg once daily.

Caution is needed when extrapolating from pharmacologic effects observed in normal cardiac muscle to diseased muscle. For example, in ischemic heart muscle, lidocaine prolongs conduction and refactoriness, and in fact its effectiveness against some ventricular arrythmias may depend on this action (blocking re-entry) rather than on its depression of excitability. For this reason, selection of the appropriate antiarrythmic agent should be based on experience as well as theory.

Drug therapy is not always successful in abolishing arrhythmias, and there are two other modalities that can be used: electrical therapy and surgical therapy. *Electrical stimulation* by a depolarizing shock (electroversion) is mandatory in ventricular fibrillation and is the method of first or second choice in treating acute tachycardias (paroxysmal atrial or ventricular tachycardias, atrial flutter or fibrillation), especially if they are causing serious cardiovascular difficulties. Appropriately timed electrical shocks with an electrode catheter passed into the heart may make cardiac tissue refractory and thus interrupt re-entrant rhythms. Temporary or permanent electrical pacemaking may drive the heart fast enough to prevent the emergence of ventricular ectopic beats and may abolish or prevent the recurrence of tachycardias (overdrive suppression). If all else fails and the patient suffers from incapacitating arrhythmias (usually tachycardias), surgery can be performed to excise an automatic focus or interrupt a re-entrant pathway.

Specific Arrhythmias

SINUS RHYTHM AND ITS VARIANTS. Rhythms originating in the SA node may be described by the resulting rates: *sinus rhythm* if normal, *sinus tachycardia* if rapid, and *sinus bradycardia* if slow. If there is marked variation of the P-P intervals from beat to beat there is *sinus arrhythmia*. If no modifying terms are used, conduction to the ventricles is assumed to be normal.

SINUS RHYTHM. Sinus rhythm is characterized by a normal atrial rate, normal P waves, and a fairly constant P-P interval. The rate may be influenced by temperature, vagal stimulation, sympathetic stimulation, and catecholamines. Consequently sinus rate can vary with activity, fever, anxiety, drugs, and blood volume. Normal resting sinus rates vary with age (Table 4).

SINUS TACHYCARDIA. Sinus tachycardia is most often due to anxiety or exercise, but it may be due to fever, anemia, hypovolemia, endogenous catecholamine secretion (as in congestive heart failure), hyperthyroidism, and many medications. The rate seldom exceeds 200 beats per minute, even in newborns, and it shows variations with time or activity. The electrocardiogram shows normal P waves. Vagal stimulation gradually slows the heart rate, in contrast to the abrupt slowing that it may cause when there is a paroxysmal supraventricular tachycardia.

SINUS BRADYCARDIA. Sinus bradycardia is physiologic in well-trained athletes, as well as with vagal stimu-

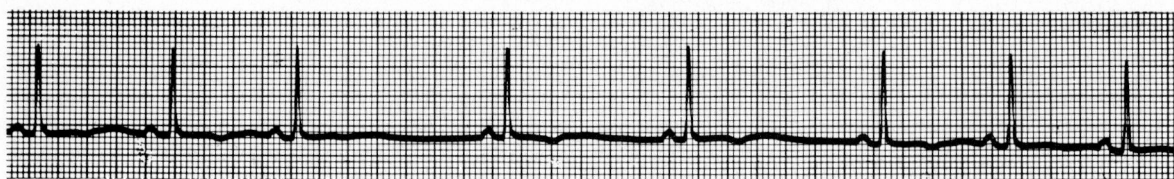

FIG. 44. Sinus arrhythmia. A normal variant in which the sinus rate varies with respiration.

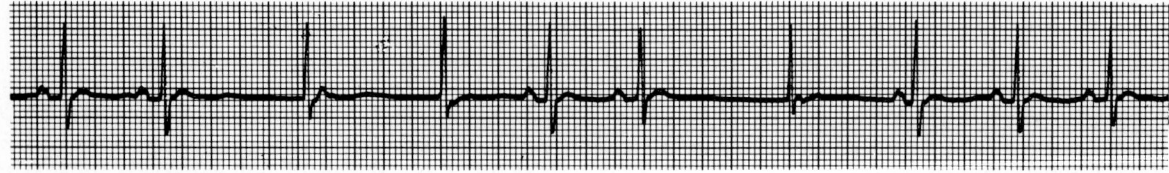

FIG. 45. Sinus arrhythmia with escape beats. This rhythm has also been called wandering pacemaker. During the slow phase of the cycle the sinus rate is less than that of a lower pacemaker. Complexes 3, 4, and probably 7 are junctional escape beats.

lation; it is also seen in pathologic states, including increased intracranial pressure, hypothyroidism, hypoxemia, obstructive jaundice, muscarinic poisoning, vagal effects of digitalis intoxication, and surgical damage to the SA node. It is occasionally seen for no known reason. Note that a slow sinus rhythm without an escape rhythm implies that the lower pacemakers have an even lower discharge rate than the SA node.

SINUS ARRHYTHMIA. Sinus arrhythmia (Figs. 44 and 45) is a normal variant in which the sinus rate varies, usually but not always in phase with respiration; the rate increases with inspiration and slows with expiration. This arrhythmia is usually found when there is good vagal tone with a slow or normal heart rate; it is rare in newborns. During expiration the sinus rate may be sufficiently slowed to allow escape beats from an atrial or junctional pacemaker. Sinus arrhythmia with escape beats has also been called *wandering* or *shifting pacemaker*. The variants of sinus arrhythmia are important only in that they are insignificant and should not be mistaken for serious arrhythmias.

SINUS ARREST. Sinus arrest is a prolonged cessation of SA nodal pacemaker activity for more than two cycles (Fig. 46). With no sinus beats there may be escape beats from a lower pacemaker, but if there are long pauses with no atrial or ventricular activity, then there is failure of the lower pacemakers as well as the SA node.

In *sinoatrial block* (SA exit block) the SA pacemaker is discharging, but occasionally an impulse does not depolarize the atria. This is recognized by pauses that are multiples of a normal P-P interval.

ECTOPIC SUPRAVENTRICULAR RHYTHMS.

Since both atrial and junctional ectopic pacemakers may produce similar QRS complexes and either similarly abnormal P waves or else no visible P waves, they are usually discussed together.

Ectopic atrial rhythm or so-called coronary sinus rhythm is similar to a normal sinus rhythm except for the superior P vector that gives inverted P waves in leads II, III, and aVf (p. 1384). This is a normal variant, and heart rates are normal and may show respiratory variation. It is also common in sinus venosus atrial septal defects and polysplenia syndromes.

ATRIAL PREMATURE BEATS (EXTRASYSTOLES). Atrial premature beats (extrasystoles) are characterized by P waves that occur prematurely; they differ in shape from normal P waves and are followed by a near-normal P-R interval and either a normal or sometimes an aberrant QRS complex (Figs. 36 and 38). In older children there is usually the typical incomplete compensatory pause, but in infants the pause is often complete. Very premature atrial extrasystoles may not be conducted, because the impulse reaches the AV node or ventricles while these are still refractory (Fig. 38). Very early, blocked atrial extrasystoles are the most common cause of an occasional pause in the rhythm. Isolated infrequent atrial extrasystoles are unimportant. They are often seen in newborns and usually disappear by 2 to 6 weeks of age; even if they remain they are usually of no concern. On the other hand, if they are frequent or if there are chaotic atrial rhythms, then therapy is needed to prevent more severe arrhythmias. Multiple atrial

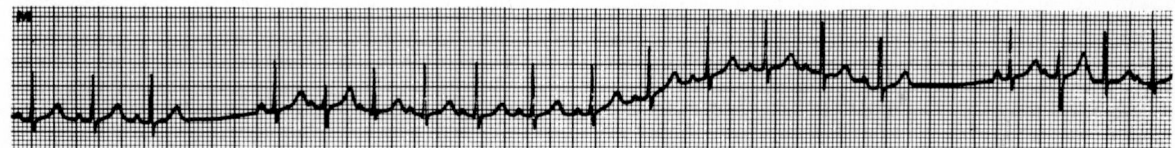

FIG. 46. Sinus arrest. There is cessation of SA nodal activity for more than two cycles. The long pause is terminated by an atrial escape beat with a P wave that is slightly different than those of sinus node origin. The second beat after the long pauses has an abnormal QRS complex due to aberrancy.

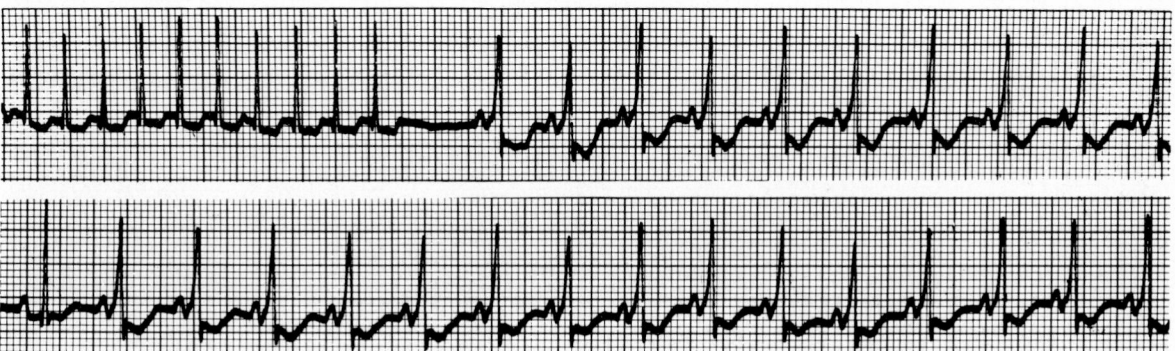

FIG. 47. Supraventricular tachycardia ending abruptly and converting to sinus rhythm with pre-excitation of the Wolff-Parkinson-White type. Note the short P-R interval and the delta wave at the beginning of the QRS complexes when there is sinus rhythm, but not during the tachycardia. The first complex of the second strip shows normal AV conduction.

premature beats often cause transient atrial fibrillation that will not be sustained if the atrium is of normal size.

PAROXYSMAL SUPRAVENTRICULAR TACHYCARDIA. Paroxysmal supraventricular tachycardia is characterized by rapid atrial rates, usually 200 to 300 beats per minute, and usually each beat is conducted to the ventricles (Fig. 47). Initial episodes are most frequent in early infancy, but they can occur at any age and even in utero. Brief episodes may cause no symptoms, although the parents may note mild pallor and a dynamic precordium. Older children may be aware of accelerated heart beats or a feeling of fluttering in the chest. The episodes usually start and end abruptly. Short episodes of tachycardia usually do not harm the patient, but longer episodes (several hours or more) may cause congestive heart failure, particularly in infants. In fact, infants may present in extremis with shock and heart failure, and the tachycardia may not be recognized as being the cause of illness.

Specific causes of the tachycardia are usually not found, although many infants have their initial paroxysm during a respiratory illness. In adolescents and adults, emotional stress, fatigue, excess caffeine ingestion, tobacco, and drugs like amphetamines may precipitate attacks. Underlying congenital heart disease may be present, but it is uncommon. About 5 to 10 percent of patients with paroxysmal supraventricular tachycardias show evidence of ventricular pre-excitation in between the attacks—the *Wolff-Parkinson-White* or *Lown-Ganong-Levine* syndromes (Fig. 47). Patients with the Wolff-Parkinson-White syndrome have one or more bridges of muscle (bundle of Kent) between the atria and ventricles, so that impulses from the atrium can reach the ventricles through two pathways. While the impulse is being delayed in the AV node there is rapid transmission to the ventricles via the bundle of Kent. There is early but slow depolarization of the ventricle adjacent to the bundle of Kent, which produces a short P-R interval and then a slow initial part of the QRS complex—the delta wave. During this slow spread through part of the ventricular muscle the normal activation by the conduction system occurs, and the rest of the ventricles depolarize normally. The two waves of ventricular depolarization meet to produce one form of fusion beat. In the Lown-Ganong-Levine syndrome the premature ventricular excitation is thought to occur

through the James fibers that bypass the AV node; there is thus a short P-R interval, but because ventricular activation takes place through the normal conduction system, there is a normal QRS complex. Both of these syndromes have two AV pathways, one via the AV node and another that bypasses it. In this setting re-entry tachycardias may occur (p. 1388). Note that during the tachycardia the impulse descends through the AV node and re-enters by the abnormal connection; thus the QRS complex is normal, even in the Wolff-Parkinson-White syndrome. Approximately 50 percent of patients with these pre-excitation syndromes have tachyarrhythmias, but only 5 to 10 percent of patients with tachyarrhythmias have these syndromes.

The deleterious cardiac effects of supraventricular tachycardias are caused by the rapid ventricular rates with inadequate ventricular filling due to the short diastole and also to loss of atrial contraction at the right time in the cycle. In addition, there can be myocardial ischemia due to impaired coronary flow; ischemia causes the S-T depression and T wave inversion that are common in the attack. Sometimes supraventricular tachycardia is seen with 2:1 AV block, and then it is usually due to digitalis intoxication (Fig. 48). The effect of digitalis here is to cause the ectopic tachycardia and, by its effect on the AV node, to allow only every second impulse to reach the ventricles. As a result these patients have ventricular rates of about 100 to 150 beats per minute; they may easily be thought to have sinus tachycardia if the alternating blocked P waves are not seen or if the lack of variation of the ventricular rate is not noted. This arrhythmia is important because it may be a prelude to more serious digitalis-induced arrhythmias, including ventricular fibrillation.

Treatment of paroxysmal supraventricular tachycardia is aimed at stopping the present attack and then at preventing future attacks. Treatment of the acute episode depends to some extent on the severity of clinical effects. If the child is not very ill, one should begin by stimulating the vagus. The electrocardiogram should always be recorded before and during vagal stimulation so that there will be a record of the arrhythmia and of vagal effects on it. This can be done mechanically by massaging *one* carotid sinus at a time, by causing gagging with posterior pharyngeal stimulation, by inserting a finger into the anus, by placing a damp cold cloth on

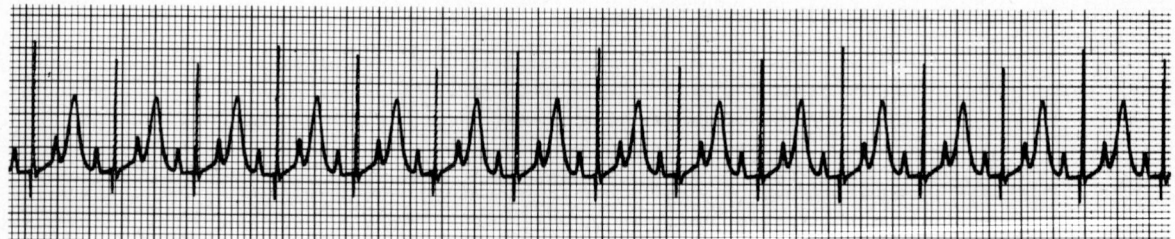

FIG. 48. Paroxysmal atrial tachycardia with 2:1 AV block in a neonate with digitalis toxicity. Although the atrial rate was 240 beats per minute, the ventricular rate was 120 beats per minute, and the patient tolerated the arrhythmia well.

the face and nose, or by placing ice water in the stomach with a nasogastric tube. Eyeball pressure has often been recommended, but it is hazardous and is best avoided. If these simple measures are ineffective, then the vagus can be stimulated by raising the blood pressure suddenly and producing a baroreceptor reflex. To do this, inject methoxamine (Vasoxyl) 0.25 mg/kg intramuscularly or 0.1 mg/kg intravenously or phenylephrine (Neo-Synephrine) 0.02 mg/kg intravenously slowly. The vagus may also be stimulated by giving edrophonium chloride (Tensilon), an anticholinesterase. If this is given rapidly intravenously in a dose of 2 mg for infants, 5 mg for those 1 to 5 years old, and 10 mg for older children, there will be a sudden but temporary vagal stimulation that may stop the attack. Atropine should be available to treat any bronchospasm that might occur, and it is essential to avoid edrophonium if there is a history of asthma.

Digoxin is a well-tested treatment for supraventricular tachycardias in children. It is often successful in stopping the attack even if no other therapy is given, but because it may take some time to act, there is no reason not to try vagal stimulation while digoxin is being absorbed. Furthermore, since digoxin sensitizes the heart to vagal stimulation, repeating the vagal stimulation after digitalization is often successful in stopping a persistent attack.

If the infant is severely ill with shock and heart failure, it is essential to insert an intravenous line for administration of drugs, including sodium bicarbonate to combat acidemia, and to attempt to raise blood pressure with methoxamine or phenylephrine. Simple maneuvers like a precordial blow or carotid sinus massage can be tried, and digoxin should be started. If there is no response, the arrhythmia may be stopped by an electric shock synchronized so that it does not fall in the vulnerable period (cardioversion).

Infants with supraventricular tachycardias may have recurrences for the next 4 to 6 months, and they should be given maintenance treatment for at least 6 months. Children whose tachycardias begin later are more likely to have recurrent attacks for many years. Digoxin is usually the most useful agent for preventing recurrences, but if it is ineffective then propranolol or quinidine may be added. If the patient has ventricular pre-excitation, propranolol is usually the most effective agent in preventing further attacks. Occasionally, other drugs like procainamide or phenytoin may be needed. Some older children have recurrent attacks of supraventricular tachycardia at infrequent intervals with several months between attacks. If the attacks do not cause heart failure and if the patient and family can be reassured, it may be better for them to tolerate the attacks rather than take daily medications to prevent a rare event. On the other hand, occasionally patients have frequent, disabling attacks that do not respond to any form of medical therapy; they may need extensive electrophysiologic investigation and either implantation of an atrial pacemaker to maintain the atrium at a rapid enough rate to suppress the emergence of a lower focus or surgical interruption of anomalous pathways.

ATRIAL FLUTTER. Atrial flutter is characterized by rapid atrial activity, with atrial rates usually between 250 and 350 beats per minute, with a sawtooth configuration of atrial waves (F waves) best seen in leads II, III, and V_1, and with varying degrees of AV block (Fig. 49). The ventricular rate may be regular or irregular; if it is regular the ratio of atrial rate to ventricular rate can range from 2:1 to 8:1, with the 2:1 ratio being seen most often. If there is a reasonable ventricular rate the ar-

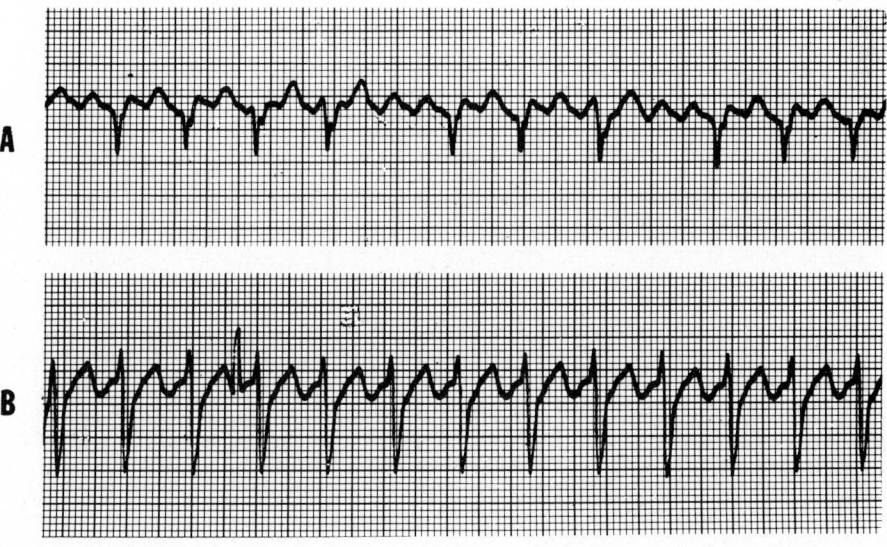

FIG. 49. Atrial flutter. A. Atrial flutter with varying conduction to the ventricles. Note the rapid atrial rate (270 beats per minute) and the sawtooth configuration of the atrial complexes (F waves). B. Tracing obtained from the same patient a few minutes later shows atrial flutter with 2:1 AV block. Every other F wave is buried in a T wave; consequently this arrhythmia might be misinterpreted as a sinus tachycardia.

rhythmia may be tolerated well for a long time, but with rapid ventricular responses severe symptoms can occur. Treatment should initially be with digoxin to increase the AV block and slow ventricular rate; if this does not suffice then propranolol can be added. Sometimes this treatment will cause sinus rhythm to return, but if it does not then the addition of quinidine may abolish the arrhythmia, or else electrical cardioversion may be successful. Atrial flutter is rare in infants and children, and when it is seen it is usually associated with structural heart disease, particularly with dilated atria.

ATRIAL FIBRILLATION.   Atrial fibrillation is also rare in children. It is characterized by disordered atrial activity, and the electrocardiogram shows no P waves, but instead has fine or coarse fibrillatory or f waves (Fig. 50). The ventricular response is very irregular and usually rapid; thus treatment is initially with digoxin to decrease ventricular rate. If the atrium is enlarged then atrial fibrillation may be sustained. To restore sinus rhythm, quinidine may be added, but cardioversion is generally more effective. After sinus rhythm is restored, quinidine may be used to help maintain it. If the atrial fibrillation keeps recurring, it is usually better to leave

it and keep the ventricular rate slow with digoxin; if ventricular rates still rise unduly with exercise, then propranolol may be added.

ECTOPIC VENTRICULAR ARRHYTHMIAS. VENTRICULAR EXTRASYSTOLES. Ventricular extrasystoles may occur infrequently, or they may occur in a fixed ratio with normal beats—bigeminy, trigeminy, quadrigeminy, etc (Figs. 36, 37, 40, and 51). If there is a single ectopic focus, then the coupling interval (that is, the interval between the normal QRS complex and the ectopic one that follows it) is constant or almost constant and the wide QRS complex is uniform in configuration. These *unifocal ventricular extrasystoles* are common in normal adolescents. When the heart rate increases with exercise or anxiety the extrasystoles usually disappear, because the faster sinus rate discharges the ectopic focus before it can produce the premature beat. Alcohol, caffeine, tobacco, fatigue, amphetamines, or other sympathomimetic drugs may increase the frequency of ventricular extrasystoles. In clinically healthy people unifocal ventricular ectopic beats are usually benign. However, if there is evident underlying heart disease, more attention should be paid to these

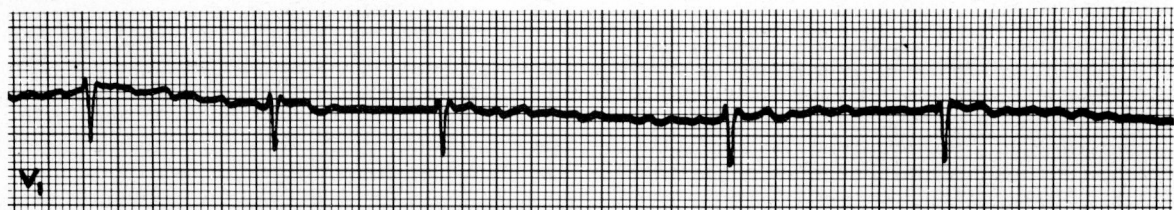

FIG. 50. Atrial fibrillation. The undulating baseline indicates disordered atrial activity. The ventricular response is irregular and slow due to digoxin therapy.

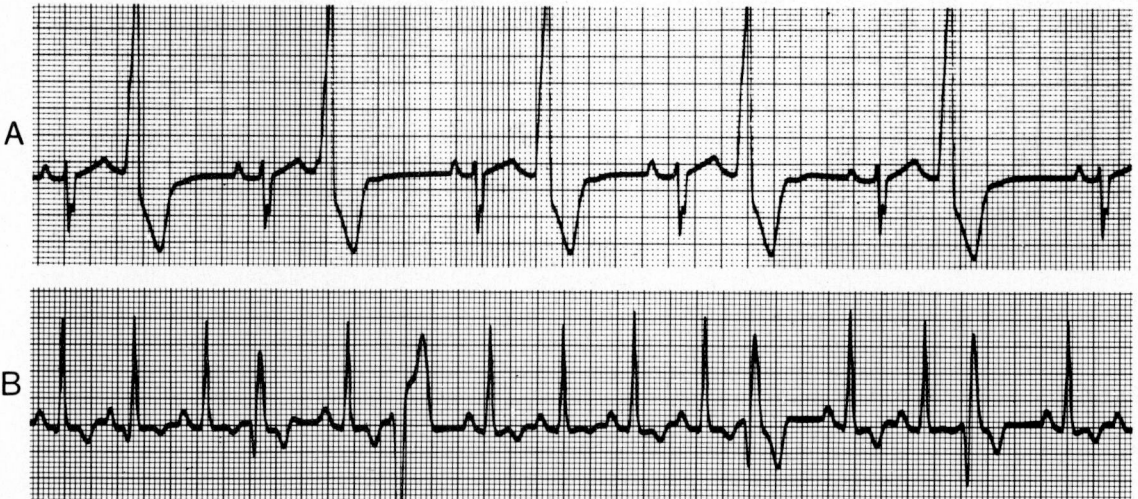

FIG. 51. Ventricular extrasystoles. A. Ventricular bigeminy in which every other beat is a premature ventricular ectopic. The coupling interval is constant, and the ectopic complexes are uniform in configuration. B. Multifocal ventricular ectopic beats. There are at least three different ectopic foci, each having its own coupling interval and QRS pattern.

extrasystoles, especially if they are recent. If the extrasystoles appear in a patient receiving catecholamines or digoxin, they should be regarded as possible signs of toxicity, and the drug dosage should be reduced. Should there be frequent ventricular extrasystoles, particularly if they are known to be of recent onset, cardiac consultation should be obtained in order to exclude underlying heart disease such as mitral valve prolapse, myocarditis, or cardiomyopathy.

More importance should be attached to *multifocal ventricular extrasystoles* (that is, those that have different coupling intervals or varying QRS complexes); these are particularly common in digitalis intoxication in adults, but they are unusual in children. It is possible for a short coupling interval to produce an ectopic beat on the peak of the preceding T wave and thus induce ventricular fibrillation. Paired ectopic beats in which two extrasystoles follow a normal beat are also serious and also demand cardiac consultation. On the other hand, isolated ventricular ectopic beats with uniform morphology but variable coupling intervals may indicate parasystole, which is usually benign. The diagnosis can be confirmed by measuring the interectopic intervals (p. 1390).

VENTRICULAR TACHYCARDIA. Ventricular tachycardia is defined as a series of three or more ventricular ectopic beats, and it usually produces a rapid tachycardia with wide QRS complexes (Fig. 52A). Occasionally the QRS complex may be relatively narrow (Fig. 52B). Often there is AV dissociation, with the P waves occurring less often than the QRS complexes; this may be seen by slight variations of the T waves due to varying superimposition of P waves on them, by a varying intensity of the first heart sound, and by finding cannon waves in the jugular veins. Often, however, there is retrograde capture of the atria, so that there is a 1:1 relationship between atrial and ventricular contraction. The major differential diagnosis is from supraventricular tachycardia with aberrant conduction (p. 1392). Proof of the ventricular origin of the arrhythmia can be obtained if the QRS complexes resemble typical ventricular extrasystoles in previous electrocardiograms or if ventricular fusion beats are seen (Figs. 40 and 52).

Ventricular tachycardia may cause severe symptoms and often may lead to ventricular fibrillation. It should always be treated as an emergency. First, a blow on the precordium can occasionally depolarize the ventricles and stop the ectopic rhythm. If it persists, then cardioversion is effective. Alternatively, lidocaine can be given intravenously at 1 mg/kg over 1 to 2 minutes, or else procainamide intravenously 2 mg/kg/minute for 10 doses, taking care to monitor blood pressure and to

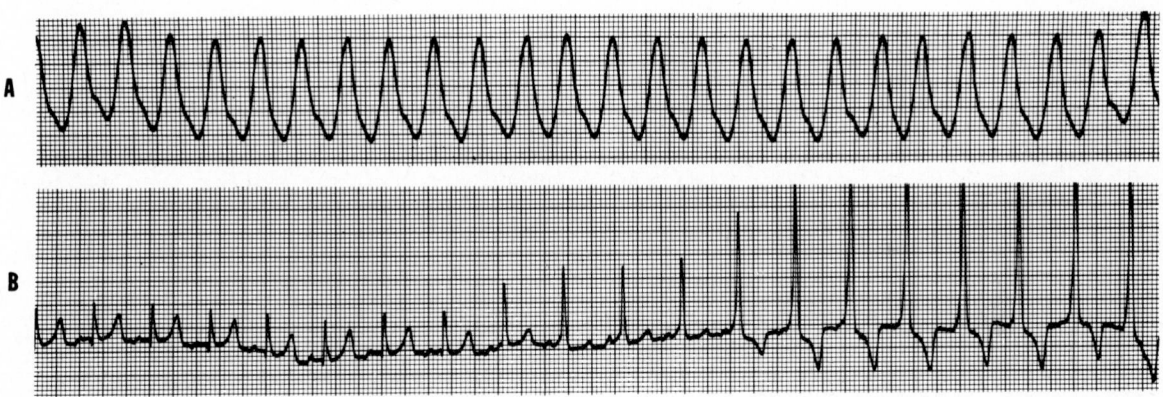

FIG. 52. Ventricular tachycardia. A. Common form of ventricular tachycardia with rapid rate (160 beats per minute) and broad bizarre QRS complexes. B. Ventricular tachycardia with moderately rapid rate (120 beats per minute) and relatively narrow complexes. The sequence of fusion beats at the onset of the arrhythmia clearly identifies it as being ventricular in origin.

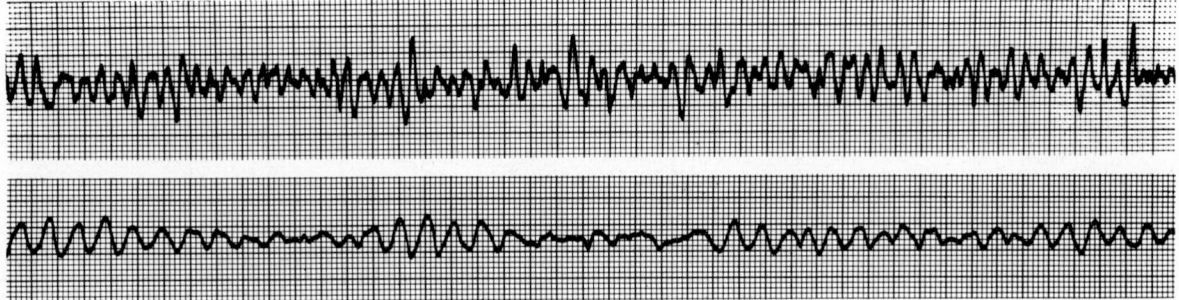

FIG. 53. Ventricular fibrillation may be coarse (A) or undulating (B).

stop should hypotension occur. Phenytoin can also be used, especially if the arrhythmia is due to digoxin toxicity. Future attacks may be prevented with quinidine, propranolol, or phenytoin.

VENTRICULAR FIBRILLATION. Ventricular fibrillation produces a recording with no QRS complexes on it, and there is just a wavy line (Fig. 53); P waves can be present. There is no cardiac output, and cardiopulmonary resuscitation should be commenced while preparations are being made for cardioversion (p. 1499). Occasionally ventricular fibrillation reverts to sinus rhythm spontaneously or after a blow on the precordium, but this change is rare and cannot be relied on.

Ventricular fibrillation is often the terminal event in many illnesses. It may follow hypoxemia, hyperkalemia, digitalis or quinidine intoxication, myocarditis, myocardial infarction, catecholamine infusions, anesthetics, and many drugs. It is also a consequence of other arrhythmias, particularly ventricular tachycardia or multiple multifocal ventricular ectopic beats. It is particularly likely to occur when the ectopic focus discharges in the vulnerable period near the peak of the T wave. Thus it occurs with multifocal premature beats or when the Q-T interval is much prolonged by disease or drugs, especially quinidine used to treat other arrhythmias.

Ventricular fibrillation occurs frequently in two other settings. People with complete (third-degree) AV block have episodes of transient ventricular fibrillation that cause syncope (Adams-Stokes attacks) and indicate the need for artificial pacemakers (p. 1403). Occasionally these attacks occur when the complete heart block is intermittent and is brought on by vagal or other stimuli. Ventricular fibrillation is probably also the cause of the syncope that occurs in the Jervell-Lange-Nielsen and Romano-Ward syndromes. In both of these there is hereditary prolongation of the Q-T interval, and in the first there is congenital deafness. The Q-T interval in these patients may be relatively normal at rest, but it does not shorten when the heart rate speeds up with exercise or anxiety; several of these patients have died suddenly with fright or on hearing an unexpected loud noise. The prolonged Q-T interval is thought to be related to asymmetric sympathetic effects on the heart, and it is thus of importance that some of these patients may be treated by propranolol. Some refractory cases have responded to left stellate ganglionectomy.

ABNORMALITIES OF CONDUCTION. FIRST-DEGREE AV BLOCK. First-degree AV block (Fig. 41) may occur occasionally without any evidence of heart disease; it is sometimes seen when there is congenital heart disease, such as endocardial cushion defect or corrected transposition of the great arteries, and it may also occur with acute infections. It is seen in acute rheumatic fever, diphtheria, and other infections, and its appearance does not necessarily mean that there is a myocarditis. It also occurs with strong vagal stimulation and with digoxin administration. It needs no treatment, but it should be considered carefully to determine if there is an underlying problem and followed to find out if the conduction defect will get worse and produce higher degrees of heart block.

SECOND-DEGREE AV BLOCK. Second-degree AV block (Fig. 43) is almost always due to underlying acute or chronic heart disease and deserves thorough investigation. It does not normally cause symptoms. Occasionally with high-grade block and slow ventricular rates the ventricles may have to be paced or stimulated with sympathomimetic drugs to maintain cardiac output. More often, one should consider whether any drugs that might depress conduction are being given. With type I block, which is usually in the bundle of His or the AV node, atropine abolishes vagal influences and may abol-

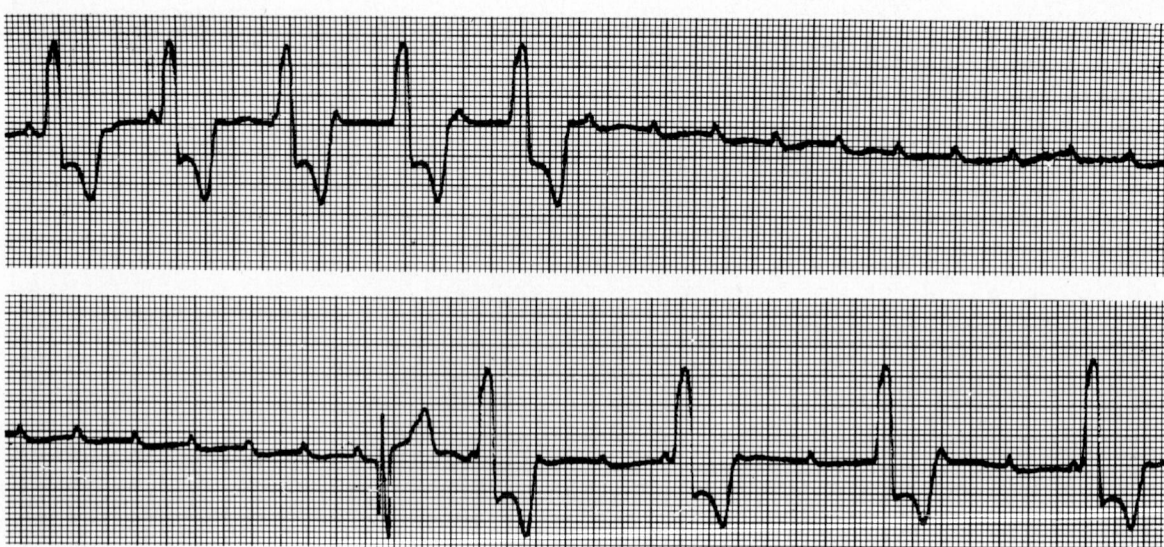

FIG. 54. Adams-Stokes attack in a patient with postoperative third-degree AV block. There was a sudden asystole lasting 6 sec during which the patient fainted.

ish the block. This can be tried if the ventricular rate is too slow. If the patient is on digoxin it should be stopped, and the patient should be treated for digitoxicity (p. 1483).

THIRD-DEGREE (COMPLETE) AV BLOCK. Third-degree (complete) AV block is often congenital and occurs early in childhood. In two-thirds of these children there is no underlying heart disease, while in the remainder there may be a variety of congenital lesions of which the most common is corrected transposition of the great arteries. The block may occur in utero, and there have been instances of cesarean section done because of fetal distress inferred from the slow heart rate. Complete heart block may also follow surgery when patches are placed in the region of the AV node and the bundle of His. Occasionally drugs may cause complete heart block, and it has been seen in digitalis intoxication.

CONGENITAL HEART BLOCK. Congenital heart block may cause no symptoms, with the patients adjusting to the slow rate by increasing stroke volume and by cardiac hypertrophy. They thus have enlarged hearts and may have electrocardiographic signs of hypertrophy; they often have systolic flow murmurs over the base and mid-diastolic flow murmurs over the mitral and tricuspid valves because of the increased stroke volume. The first heart sound varies in intensity because of a varying P-R interval, and there are cannon waves in the jugular veins. Occasionally, atrial sounds may be heard. On the electrocardiogram there are regular P waves at a normal rate, but these will be completely unrelated to the less frequent QRS complexes (Figs. 42 and 54). The QRS complexes are usually narrow and normal, indicating that the pacemaker is high in the bundle of His. Sometimes, especially after surgery, the QRS complexes are wide because the pacemaker is in the ventricles.

Most patients with complete heart block are asymptomatic. Sometimes the ventricular rate is too slow to sustain a cardiac output, and then there will be congestive heart failure. This is treated by implanting a pacemaker, either temporarily or permanently. Sometimes, too, these patients have Adams-Stokes attacks (that is, episodes of syncope due to sudden asystole, Fig. 54), ventricular tachycardia, or ventricular fibrillation. Usually these episodes last between 6 and 60 sec, and then spontaneously the ventricles resume their slow beat, but sometimes the episodes are fatal. The attacks are more common after surgical block than with congenital block and more common with a wide QRS complex than with a narrow QRS complex. Should they occur, then a ventricular pacemaker should be inserted. Isoproterenol at 0.05 to 0.5 μg/kg/minute may be infused to speed the ventricles while preparing to insert the artificial pacemaker.

References

Gelband H, Rosen MR: Pharmacologic basis for the treatment of cardiac arrhythmias. Pediatrics 55:59, 1975

Hoffman BF, Rosen MR, Wit AL: Electrophysiology and pharmacology of cardiac arrhythmias. III. The causes and treatment of cardiac arrhythmias. Am Heart J 89:115, 253, 1975

Kupersmith J: Antiarrhythmic drugs: changing concepts. Am J Cardiol 38:119, 1976

Marriott HJL: Practical Electrocardiography. Baltimore, Williams & Wilkins, 1972

Rosen MR, Wit AL, Hoffman BF: Electrophysiology and pharmacology of cardiac arrhythmias. I. Cellular electrophysiology of the mammalian heart. Am Heart J 88:380, 1974

Schamroth L: The Disorders of Cardiac Rhythm. Oxford, Blackwell, 1971

Wit AL, Rosen MR, Hoffman BF: Electrophysiology and pharmacology of cardiac arrhythmias. II. Relationship of normal and abnormal activity of cardiac fibers to the genesis of arrhythmias. Am Heart J 88:515, 664, 798, 1974

CONGENITAL HEART DISEASES

Introduction

Julien I. E. Hoffman

We do not know how often congenital heart diseases occur in spontaneous abortuses, but some reports suggest that they are frequent. However, many studies show that these diseases occur in about 8 to 10 of 1,000 live-born children. The figures are similar in Sweden, Holland, the United States, and Japan. Good case finding and diagnostic techniques are too recent to determine if there has been a change in incidence over the years. The distributions of various common types of congenital heart diseases at birth are given in Table 5.

ETIOLOGY. Congenital heart diseases are probably due to interaction between genetic predisposition and environmental factors. Sometimes one or other of these predominates.

GENETIC FACTORS. Estimates are that single mutant genes account for 2 percent of congenital heart diseases, while 4 percent are due to gross chromosomal aberrations and the remaining 94 percent are due to multifactorial gene effects.

Single mutant genes (autosomal dominant or recessive or X-linked) almost invariably cause congenital heart disease as part of a complex of abnormalities. The most common of these is Noonan's syndrome (Turner phenotype), in which pulmonic stenosis is the most frequent cardiac lesion; examples of other syndromes with their most common cardiac lesions are Apert's syndrome (coarctation of the aorta), Holt-Oram syndrome (atrial and ventricular septal defects), Duchenne's muscular dystrophy (myocardial degeneration and fibrosis), and Ellis-van Creveld syndrome (single atrium).

Chromosomal abnormalities also cause congenital heart diseases as part of a complex of lesions. Many of these syndromes have a high incidence of congenital heart diseases: for example, cri du chat syndrome (25 percent), XO (Turner's) syndrome (35 percent), trisomy 21 (Down's) syndrome (50 percent), trisomy 13 (90 percent), and trisomy 18 (99 percent). Ventricular septal defects are the most common cardiac lesions in all except Turner's syndrome, which has predominantly coarctation of the aorta.

Multifactorial gene factors are thought to be the basis for most congenital heart diseases and frequently are not associated with lesions elsewhere.

TABLE 5. Incidence and Risk of Recurrence*

Lesion	Incidence/100 Children	Percentage Recurrence Risk
Ventricular septal defect	35–50	6–7 †
Patent ductus arteriosus	10–15	3–4
Atrial septal defect (secundum)	5–10	2.5–3
Endocardial cushion defects	5–10	2.5–3
Coarctation of aorta	6–8	2.5–3
Aortic stenosis	6–8	2.5–3
Pulmonic stenosis	6–8	2.5–3
Tetralogy of Fallot	4–6	2–2.5
Transposition of great arteries	4–6	2–2.5
Pulmonary atresia	1–2	1–1.5
Tricuspid atresia	1–2	1–5
Truncus arteriosus	1–2	1–1.5
Total anomalous pulmonary venous connection	1–2	1–1.5

*This table does not include bicuspid aortic valves, which occur in about 2 to 3 percent of live-born children.
†This is theoretical and higher than the 4.5 to 5 percent actually observed, because the latter does not take into account people whose defects closed spontaneously.

ENVIRONMENTAL FACTORS. Viral Lesions. The rubella embryopathy is often associated with peripheral pulmonic stenosis, patent ductus arteriosus, and sometimes valvar pulmonic stenosis. Other viruses, notably coxsackie viruses, have been thought to cause congenital heart diseases, based on an increased frequency of rising serum titers to this virus in mothers whose infants have congenital heart disease.

Fetal Environment. Women taking lithium salts during pregnancy may have children with congenital heart diseases, with an abnormally high incidence of mitral and tricuspid valve lesions, especially Ebstein's syndrome. There is a suggestion that diabetic women or those taking progesterone in pregnancy have an increased risk of having children with congenital heart diseases. About half the children of alcoholic mothers have congenital heart diseases.

COUNSELING FAMILIES. When a child, especially a first child, is found to have congenital heart disease, the parents frequently have severe guilt feelings and are almost always worried about the risk of occurrence of congenital heart disease in future children. These issues should be discussed openly with the parents, who are often reticent about mentioning them. An explanation of what is known of the causes of congenital heart diseases and reassurance that the parents could not have caused it by acts of omission or commission are arguments that can be used to help allay the parents' guilt feelings. Clearly this approach must be correlated with all the other aspects of giving continued support to parents with chronically ill children.

More specific information can be given about the risk of occurrence of cardiac lesions in future children. If the cardiac lesion is part of a syndrome due to a single gene mutation, then the risk of recurrence of heart disease in future children depends on the specific mutation. In general, autosomal dominant genes will appear in 50 percent of offspring, while autosomal recessive genes will produce disease in 25 percent of offspring. Chromosomal abnormalities have risks of recurrence that vary with the specific chromosomal change in-

volved. Multifactorial inheritance produces a much lower risk of recurrence. If a first-degree relative (sibling, parent) has congenital heart disease, then the risk of the next child having congenital heart disease varies from about 1 percent for rare lesions like truncus arteriosus or pulmonary atresia to about 6 percent for the most common lesion, ventricular septal defect (Table 5). In between are risks of about 3 to 4 percent for patent ductus arteriosus, atrial septal defect, and tetralogy of Fallot. Note that this risk of recurrence is the same if the index case is a sibling or a parent with congenital heart disease. Furthermore, if two first-degree relatives have congenital heart disease, then the risk of heart disease in the next infant is about three times as high as the figures just cited.

This discussion implies that the next child to have congenital heart disease will have the same type as the parent or sibling. In general there is considerable concordance of congenital heart disease in several members of a family, although exceptions do occur.

References

Hoffman JIE: Natural history of congenital heart disease. Circulation 37:97, 1968

Mitchell SC, Korones SB, Berendes HW: Congenital heart disease in 56,109 births. Incidence and natural history. Circulation 43:323, 1971

——— Sellmann AH, Westphal MC, Park J: Etiologic correlates in a study of congenital heart disease in 56,109 births. Am J Cardiol 28:653, 1971

Nora JJ: Multifactorial inheritance hypothesis for the etiology of congenital heart diseases. Circulation 38:604, 1968

LEFT-TO-RIGHT SHUNTS

MICHAEL A. HEYMANN

General Features

In congenital heart defects there may be shunting of blood through an abnormal communication between the pulmonary circulation and the systemic circulation. A shunt from the systemic circulation to the pulmonary circulation is termed a left-to-right shunt, and it allows oxygenated blood to recirculate through the lungs without entering the peripheral arterial circulation. A left-to-right shunt may be present alone or may be associated with right-to-left shunting (bidirectional shunting).

EFFECT ON FETUS. In the presence of defects that are associated with left-to-right shunts after birth, fetal somatic development is apparently unaltered, and blood flow to the fetal organs and placenta is probably normal. However, with certain congenital heart malformations there are within the fetal heart and great vessels alterations in flow patterns that may affect the development of the great vessels. For example, decreased aortic isthmus flow with consequent hypoplasia or even interruption of the aortic isthmus may occur when a significant proportion of left ventricular output is shunted away from the ascending aorta. This could occur in lesions such as endocardial cushion defect, a large ventricular septal defect, or double-outlet right ventricle, particularly if these are associated with subaortic obstruction. Certain congenital heart malformations may also alter the preferential streaming patterns normally found in the heart and so change the composition of blood leaving the heart. Thus with an endocardial cushion defect or large ventricular septal defect the oxygen tension of blood leaving the right ventricle and perfusing the lungs may be higher than that in the normal fetus. This higher oxygen tension may alter the development of the pulmonary resistance vessels, which in turn may affect the clinical features in postnatal life.

FACTORS INFLUENCING LEFT-TO-RIGHT SHUNTS. There are three major interrelated factors that control the amount of left-to-right shunting in the postnatal period: the size of, and therefore the resistance to flow offered by, the abnormal communication between the chambers or vessels; the difference in pressures between the chambers or vessels; the total outflow resistances (including peripheral resistances) of the chambers or vessels. Under certain specific conditions the third factor may not play a role in determining the amount of left-to-right shunting.

After birth the systemic peripheral vascular resistance is normally much higher than the pulmonary vascular resistance, so that systolic pressures in the aorta and left ventricle are much higher than those in the pulmonary artery and right ventricle. If there is a small patent ductus arteriosus or ventricular septal defect, it offers a high resistance to flow through it, so that the left-to-right shunt will be small despite the large pressure difference (Fig. 55A). However, if there is a large communication, then pressures between the left and right ventricles or aorta and pulmonary artery will be equal (Fig. 55B and C), and the magnitude and direction of

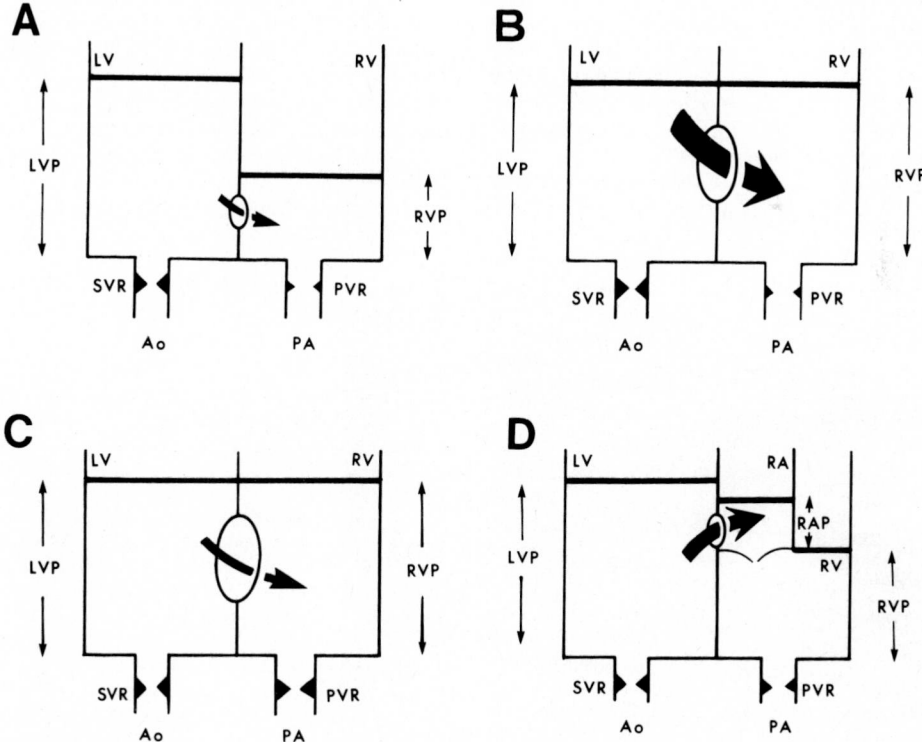

FIG. 55. Diagrammatic representations of the major factors that regulate the magnitude of left-to-right shunting in congenital heart disease. LV, left ventricle; RV, right ventricle; RA, right atrium; Ao, aorta; PA, pulmonary artery; LVP, left ventricular systolic pressure; RVP, right ventricular systolic pressure; RAP, right atrial mean pressure; SVR, systemic vascular resistance; PVR, pulmonary vascular resistance.

shunting will then be determined by the relative outflow resistance of each chamber. If left ventricular outflow resistance is much higher than that of the right ventricle, there will be a large left-to-right shunt (Fig. 55B); if the right ventricular outflow resistance increases and approximates that of the left ventricle or if systemic resistance falls, the left-to-right shunt will be small (Fig. 55C), while if the resistance is higher for the right than for the left ventricle there will be a shunt from right to left. The outflow resistance could be at a distal valve orifice, in a great vessel, in the peripheral resistance vessels, or at any combination of these. In the absence of aortic or pulmonic stenosis the relationship between the pulmonary and systemic vascular resistances will therefore determine the magnitude of shunting. Since systemic vascular resistance is generally high and normally does not change significantly after birth, alteration in pulmonary vascular resistance will be a major determinant in regulating shunting through an aortopulmonary or interventricular defect. This is particularly true in the first several months after birth when the normal progressive fall in pulmonary vascular resistance occurs. On the basis of these considerations, this type of shunting, in which the ratio of pulmonary vascular resistance to systemic vascular resistance determines the shunt, has been termed *dependent* shunting. Left-to-right shunting is also dependent on the ratio of pulmonary vascular resistance to systemic vascular resistance in secundum atrial septal defects, but in these the outflow resistance affects the amount of shunting indirectly. The resistance offered to each ventricle determines its stroke volume and systolic emptying, as well as its wall thickness. The thinner-walled right ventricle empties easily into the low-resistance pulmonary vascular bed in systole. In diastole, if there is a large atrial defect, more blood can enter the distensible right ventricle than the thicker less-distensible left ventricle,

so that there can be a large left-to-right shunt even though atrial pressures may be low and equal.

The second major group of left-to-right shunts is that in which the outflow resistances of the left and right ventricles do not directly affect the magnitude of shunt (Fig. 55D). This type of shunt has a communication between a high-pressure chamber and a low-pressure chamber or vessel, for example, a direct left ventricular to right atrial communication or a systemic arteriovenous fistula. In this group of defects the magnitude of the shunt depends on the size of the communication and the pressure difference between the chambers or vessels involved and not on the pulmonary vascular resistance; this has therefore been termed *obligatory* shunting.

PATHOPHYSIOLOGY.   The exact site of the defect allowing left-to-right shunting determines certain of its specific features; however, many of the clinical features associated with left-to-right shunting are common to several different defects. The major effects depend on the size of the left-to-right shunt and the level at which this shunting occurs, more specifically which ventricle will be the major recipient of the additional blood flow.

In an aortopulmonary left-to-right shunt a portion of left ventricular output leaves the systemic circulation, and pulmonary blood flow is increased by that amount. The resultant greater pulmonary venous return to the left atrium and left ventricle will increase left ventricular diastolic volume and thus increase left ventricular stroke volume and stroke work by means of the Frank-Starling mechanism. Dilatation of the left ventricle elevates left ventricular end-diastolic pressure and left atrial pressure and, if marked, results in left heart failure and pulmonary edema (Fig. 56). The right ventricle does not handle an extra volume load; however, if there is a large communication with pulmonary hypertension

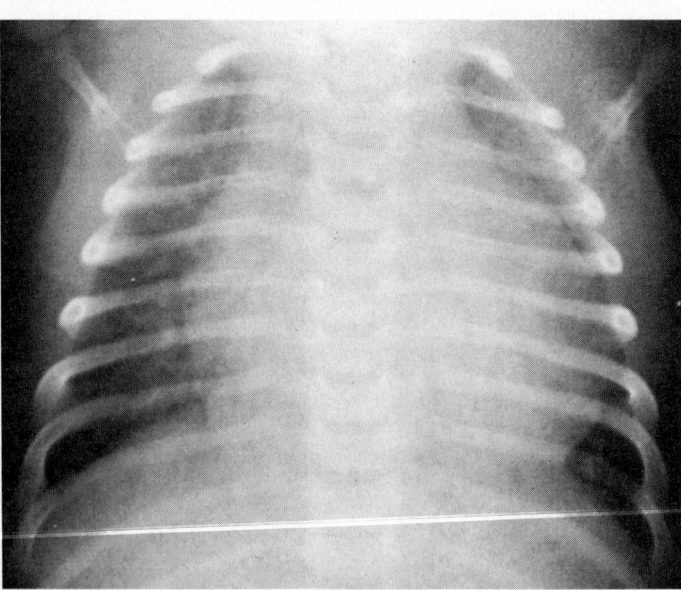

FIG. 56.   Chest roentgenogram in newborn infant with left ventricular failure demonstrating marked cardiomegaly and pulmonary venous congestion, the latter suggested by haziness of the lung fields.

the right ventricle will have a greater pressure load. Similar hemodynamic effects may follow a left-to-right shunt at the ventricular level, with the difference that the right ventricle will also have some volume overload. Left-to-right shunts at the atrial level produce an increased volume load only on the right ventricle, and if there is some outflow obstruction, a moderately increased right ventricular pressure load may also occur. In the group with obligatory shunts volume overloading of both ventricles will occur.

Several physiologic mechanisms are involved in the attempt to maintain adequate myocardial performance and normal systemic output in the face of a left-to-right shunt. In addition to the Frank-Starling mechanism, the sympathetic-adrenal system is important, as is myocardial hypertrophy. There is increased catecholamine release from the adrenal glands, and sympathetic nerve fibers within the myocardium release norepinephrine locally in response to the stress. As a result there are increases in heart rate (chronotropic effect) and in the force of contraction of the myocardium (inotropic effect). This increased sympathetic-adrenal activity is responsible for the rapid heart rates associated with left ventricular failure and also for the excessive sweating often seen in infants with heart failure. These compensatory mechanisms are generally well developed in older children and adults; however, they are not adequately developed in newborn infants, particularly premature infants. In addition, since myocardial structure matures during fetal and neonatal development, premature infants are less capable of handling a volume overload than are mature or older infants. If the increased volume or pressure load on the ventricles persists the muscle fibers will hypertrophy, and the increased amount of contractile protein helps to handle the load without excessive ventricular dilatation or sympathetic stimulation.

The increased workload on the left ventricle will increase myocardial oxygen requirements, mainly because there is more muscle using oxygen. Delivery of oxygen to the myocardium depends on coronary blood flow and the oxygen content of arterial blood. Coronary perfusion to the left ventricle occurs mainly during diastole and depends on the systemic arterial–intramyocardial diastolic pressure difference, as well as on the duration of diastole. Therefore a reduction in arterial diastolic pressure (as in an aortopulmonary communication with a large left-to-right shunt), an increase in left ventricular end-diastolic pressure and therefore subendocardial intramyocardial pressure (as with left ventricular failure), and a reduction in diastolic period (as with tachycardia) are all detrimental to myocardial perfusion and hence oxygen delivery. A low hemoglobin content, as occurs with physiologic anemia in early infancy or after repeated blood sampling during intensive nursery care, also jeopardizes oxygen delivery to the myocardium and may precipitate left ventricular failure.

Anemia places a further demand on the left ventricle to increase systemic output in order to supply adequate oxygen to the entire systemic circulation. Similarly, infections may further stress the left ventricle by increasing tissue oxygen demands and thereby requirements for cardiac output.

Clinically, with a small left-to-right shunt there may be little effect on the heart except for a murmur. If there is a large aortopulmonary or interventricular shunt the left ventricle will become enlarged and hyperactive, the increased precordial activity being generally directly related to the size of the shunt. If there is pulmonary hypertension as well, there may be signs of right ventricular enlargement. With the increased left ventricular output there may be a third heart sound due to rapid left ventricular filling in early diastole and a fourth heart sound due to left atrial hypertrophy. Also, because of the increased pulmonary blood flow and the increased pulmonary venous return to the left atrium, there may be a low-frequency apical mid-diastolic rumbling murmur due to increased diastolic flow across a normal mitral valve. Systolic murmurs related to turbulent flow across the specific defect will be heard. If there is pulmonary hypertension there will be a louder pulmonic valve closure sound (P_2).

On chest roentgenograms left ventricular and left atrial enlargement will be present, and in aortopulmonary communications the ascending aorta, which carries the increased flow, may be dilated. The left atrial dilatation may be quite prominent and may stretch the atrial septum, with resulting incompetence of the valve of the foramen ovale and a left-to-right atrial shunt that may be of clinical significance. Increased pulmonary blood flow will be manifested by prominent dilated main and branch pulmonary arteries extending into the lung fields (Fig. 57). Features of right heart failure may also become evident.

If left ventricular failure should be associated with the left-to-right shunt there may be signs of increased pulmonary venous pressure and pulmonary venous congestion. Clinical pulmonary edema will be indicated by respiratory distress, tachypnea, and rales on auscultation of the lungs. In infancy respiratory distress and sweating are particularly evident during feeding. Slow feeding with frequent breaks due to obvious tiring is common, and poor weight gain due to increased nutritional requirements as well as difficulty with feeding is quite frequent. The pulmonary signs of left ventricular failure are similar to those of bronchiolitis or bronchopneumonia, which may be difficult to differentiate (p. 1560). On chest roentgenogram the pulmonary veins may appear distended, particularly in the perihilar regions. Frank pulmonary edema may also be seen, and there may be edematous septa showing up as horizontal streaks at the lung bases (Kerley B lines) (Fig. 62).

Electrocardiographic evidence of left atrial and ventricular hypertrophy will depend on the duration and magnitude of the shunt. Echocardiographic findings also depend on the magnitude of left-to-right shunting and the degree of heart failure; with aortopulmonary or ventricular shunting increased left atrial and left ventricular cavity diameters are seen (p. 1374).

With an atrial left-to-right shunt the dominant hemodynamic effect will be that of right ventricular volume

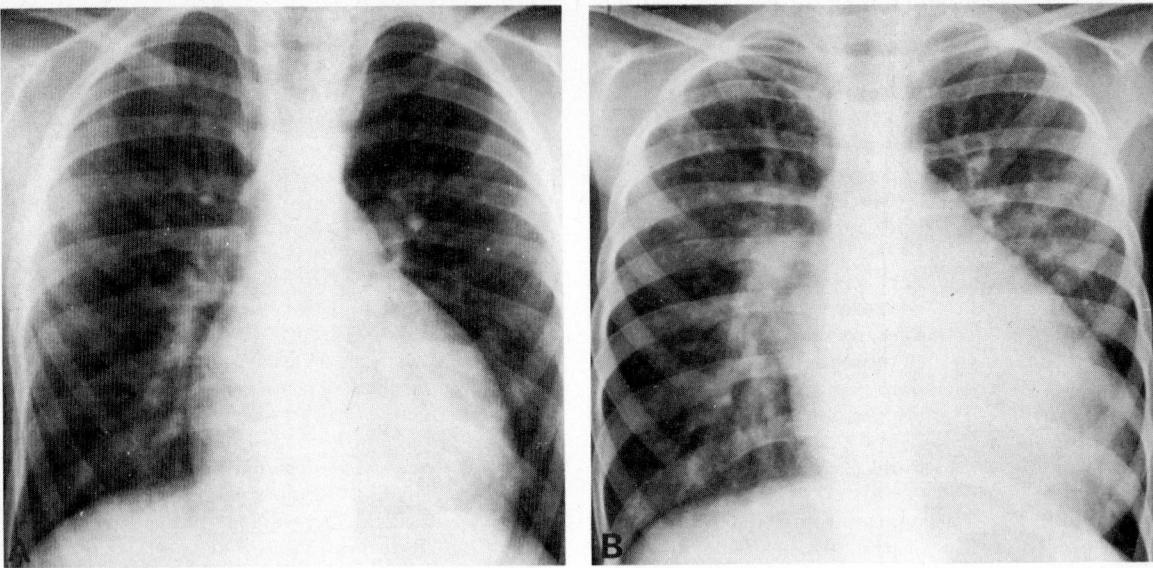

FIG. 57. Chest roentgenograms in (A) a child with a small ventricular septal defect with a moderate left-to-right shunt and (B) a child with a large ventricular septal defect with a large left-to-right shunt and pulmonary arterial hypertension.

overload, but an increase in right ventricular end-diastolic pressure with a subsequent increase in right atrial and systemic venous pressure is not usual. The clinical signs are associated with the increased right ventricular output. Precordial activity is increased, but it is right ventricular in origin (that is, it is generally retrosternal or just to the left of the sternum). Increased flow across the tricuspid valve may result in a low-frequency mid-diastolic murmur heard best at the lower left sternal border. Murmurs are not heard associated with the flow across the atrial septum; however, there is usually a systolic murmur at the base due to the increased flow across the normal pulmonary outflow tract. Commonly the second sound in the pulmonic area is widely split and remains well split throughout the respiratory cycle. On chest roentgenogram the right ventricle is enlarged, and increased pulmonary blood flow will be evident. Electrocardiographic features vary with the different types of atrial communication and will be discussed later. Echocardiograms may also assist in diagnosis (p. 1373).

A combination of both left and right ventricular overload may occur with a shunt from the aorta or left ventricle directly into the right atrium or with a systemic arteriovenous malformation.

EFFECTS ON PULMONARY CIRCULATION.
The normal fall in pulmonary vascular resistance in the immediate postnatal period and the 3 to 6 weeks thereafter is important in determining the magnitude of left-to-right shunting in infants with dependent shunts. Conversely, a left-to-right shunt may have significant effects on the pulmonary circulation. In a patient with a large aortopulmonary or ventricular communication, systemic and pulmonary arterial pressures will be simi-

lar, and because of the persistent high pulmonary arterial pressure the small pulmonary arteries do not undergo their normal postnatal maturational changes. There is some thinning of the medial smooth muscle; however, it does not regress as rapidly nor to the same extent as in normal individuals. Thus, although pulmonary vascular resistance falls rapidly immediately after birth due to the onset of ventilation and subsequent release of hypoxic pulmonary vasoconstriction, there is a slower than normal, later decline of pulmonary vascular resistance. The lowest pulmonary vascular resistance reached is usually delayed some 2 to 3 months, and the actual pulmonary vascular resistance is significantly higher than normal. Infants with large obligatory left-to-right shunts also will have significantly increased pulmonary blood flow and therefore higher than normal pulmonary arterial pressures, because in early infancy the small pulmonary arteries are not distensible; this will also delay the medial smooth muscle regression. Conditions producing hypoxic pulmonary vasoconstriction in the newborn period will markedly retard the regression of the medial muscular layer. This could be associated with many causes, such as high altitude, pulmonary disease, chronic upper airway obstruction, or obstruction of the major airways by dilated pulmonary arteries produced by a large left-to-right shunt (p. 1559). In patients with atrial communications the pulmonary arterial pressure and pulmonary vascular resistance fall normally in the postnatal period, and the small pulmonary arteries undergo the normal regression of medial smooth muscle.

The initial high pulmonary vascular resistance in infants with large left-to-right shunts is associated only with the increased amount of medial smooth muscle.

However, subsequently true pulmonary vascular disease may occur; the first change that occurs is proliferation of the intimal cells with intimal thickening, followed by hyalinization, fibrosis, and eventually thrombosis. The mechanisms involved in producing these intimal changes are probably related to shear stresses, since at high flow and shear rates endothelial cellular damage has been shown to occur. If there is thick medial muscle or vasoconstriction, the velocity of flow through the narrowed lumen will be higher than normal. Blood viscosity also plays a significant role in producing this damage, because shear stresses increase as viscosity rises; therefore, infants who have not only left-to-right shunting with increased pulmonary blood flow but also hypoxemia with a resultant high hematocrit are at even greater risk of developing pulmonary vascular disease. Pulmonary vascular disease may occur in patients with atrial septal defects, but because of the normal muscular regression and the fact that their small pulmonary arteries are thin-walled and easily distensible, the intimal vascular changes are delayed for many years and generally do not occur until the late second or the third decade. The intimal proliferative changes, when well established, with hyalinization and fibrosis, are not reversible by repair of the cardiac defect. As more and more small pulmonary arteries become involved, there is a progressive increase in pulmonary vascular resistance, so that eventually left-to-right shunting will decrease, as will evidence of left ventricular failure. Eventually no left-to-right shunt will remain, and later right-to-left shunting may occur. In severe pulmonary vascular obstructive disease, arteriovenous malformations may develop, and hemoptysis may occur.

ANATOMIC CLASSIFICATION. Left-to-right shunts are classified anatomically by the level at which the systemic and pulmonary circulations communicate (Table 6).

Table 6 Classification of Left-to-Right Shunts

Aorta to pulmonary artery (dependent)
  Patent ductus arteriosus
  Truncus arteriosus communis
  Aortopulmonary fenestration
  Anomalous origin of coronary artery
  Hemitruncus arteriosus
  Lobar sequestration
Aorta to right ventricle (dependent)
  Sinus of Valsalva fistula
  Coronary arteriovenous fistula
Aorta to right atrium or systemic vein (obligatory)
  Systemic arteriovenous fistula
  Sinus of Valsalva fistula
  Coronary arteriovenous fistula
Left ventricle to right ventricle (dependent)
  Ventricular septal defect
  Endocardial cushion defect
Left ventricle to right atrium (obligatory)
  Left ventricular–right atrial communication
  Endocardial cushion defect
Left atrium or pulmonary veins to right atrium (partially dependent)
  Atrial septal defects: incompetent foramen ovale, primum, secundum, sinus venosus
  Partial anomalous pulmonary venous connection

Patent Ductus Arteriosus

PHYSIOLOGY OF CLOSURE. Postnatal closure of the ductus arteriosus is effected by constriction of smooth muscle in the wall of the ductus arteriosus on exposure to an increased oxygen tension. In addition, certain vasoactive substances such as bradykinin or prostaglandins may play some role. In full-term infants functional closure normally occurs within 10 to 15 hours after birth; however, complete anatomic obliteration of the ductus arteriosus is slower and may not be complete until the third postnatal week. Since pulmonary vascular resistance falls as soon as the lungs expand, in the first 10 to 15 hours when the ductus arteriosus is still open a left-to-right shunt through the ductus arteriosus may be present and a murmur may be heard.

The constrictor response of the ductus arteriosus to oxygen is related to gestational age. In fetal lambs at two-thirds of gestation there is a minimal response to an increase in oxygen tension; however, at term the ductus arteriosus will constrict completely when exposed to a high oxygen tension. This lack of response does not represent failure of smooth muscle development, because the ductus arteriosus in an immature animal does respond to vasoactive substances; rather, it represents an inability to respond to the normal stimulus of a rise in oxygen tension.

CAUSES OF PERSISTENT PATENCY. A clinically apparent patent ductus arteriosus may be present in 30 to 40 percent of prematurely born infants under 1,750 g. Although no accurate statistics are available, this would give an incidence of about 8 per 1,000 live births. The mechanisms responsible for continued patency are related to the inability of the ductus arteriosus in immature infants to respond normally to an increased oxygen tension. The incidence of persistent patency of the ductus arteriosus in full-term infants born at high altitude is significantly higher than in those born at sea level, probably because of the lower atmospheric oxygen tension.

Persistent patency of the ductus arteriosus in full-term infants at lower altitudes is generally due to some structural abnormality of the ductus arteriosus itself. No exact cause has been established in most patients; however, maternal rubella in the first trimester of pregnancy is associated with a high incidence of persistent patency of the ductus arteriosus, and rubella virus has been cultured from ductus arteriosus tissue. Persistent patency of the ductus arteriosus has been produced by inbreeding in certain species of dogs and rats.

CLINICAL MANIFESTATIONS IN PREMATURE INFANTS. The clinical features depend on the magnitude of left-to-right shunt through the ductus arteriosus, as well as on the maturity of the infant. Immature infants are less capable of handling a left-to-right shunt than are mature infants, so that in premature infants symptoms begin considerably earlier and with relatively small shunts. Many premature infants who have a patent ductus arteriosus have, in addition, associated idiopathic respiratory distress syndrome. With severe pulmonary disease the pulmonary vascular resistance may be elevated, so that there is at first little or no left-to-right shunt, despite a large patent ductus arteriosus. As the pulmonary disease improves, resistance will fall, left-to-right shunting will increase, and the clinical features of a ductus arteriosus will become evident. In certain premature infants, especially those under 1,000 g, left ventricular failure secondary to a patent ductus arteriosus may be superimposed on the idiopathic respiratory distress syndrome, and these infants are difficult to manage clinically.

In all premature infants with a large patent ductus arteriosus certain clinical features are common. These include widening of the pulse pressure with prominent bounding pulses, marked hyperactivity of the precordium, tachycardia, and often a gallop rhythm. The pulmonic component of the second sound is generally moderately accentuated. A systolic murmur with a fairly typical rough and irregular (or "rocky") quality is usually heard best at the mid-to upper left sternal border. As the shunt increases the murmur becomes longer and may obscure the second sound, but the classic continuous machinery-type murmur described in older patients is not generally heard in premature infants. Some premature infants with large left-to-right shunts through a widely dilated ductus arteriosus may not have even a systolic murmur, due to the lack of turbulent flow through the widely dilated channel. A low-frequency mid-diastolic murmur is unusual in prematures, probably because with an immature myocardium severe failure can occur with only a moderate shunt. Premature infants who do not require ventilatory assistance by positive pressure do develop rales in both lung fields as evidence of their left ventricular failure, but those on positive-pressure ventilation may not manifest rales until left ventricular failure is extremely severe. A fairly consistent finding associated with left ventricular failure in this latter group is a change in ventilatory status. This includes an increase in arterial carbon dioxide tension and a need for higher inspired oxygen concentration, higher continuous positive airway pressure, or higher pressure or rate settings on mechanical ventilators. Additional important features in premature infants with large left-to-right shunts and left ventricular failure are apneic episodes and periods of bradycardia. A further feature of patent ductus arteriosus in premature infants that has been noted recently is the association of necrotizing enterocolitis. It is possible that the intestinal lesion may result from the ductus arteriosus due to left ventricular failure, decreased arterial blood pressure and systemic output and thus reduced blood flow to the bowel.

The electrocardiogram and chest roentgenogram may not be helpful; however, some infants do show increasing cardiomegaly and left ventricular hypertrophy. Echocardiography has become a useful tool in making the differentiation between deterioration due to left ventricular failure with a large left-to-right shunt and that due to primary pulmonary disease. With a large left-to-right shunt through the ductus arteriosus, left atrial diameter is markedly increased by the increased

pulmonary venous return. This does not occur with lung disease alone; the ratio of left atrial diameter to aortic diameter as measured echocardiographically is useful in differential diagnosis (p. 1374).

CLINICAL MANIFESTATIONS IN MATURE INFANTS. The diagnosis of patent ductus arteriosus in full-term infants or older children presents fewer difficulties than in immature infants. Since there is a continuous run-off of blood from the aorta to the pulmonary artery through the ductus arteriosus, the murmur in older infants and children is continuous and has a rumbling, machinery like quality (Fig. 58). If the ductus arteriosus is small, this may be the only abnormal finding. If it is larger, there are additional features related to the increased left ventricular output, the increased pulmonary blood flow, and the manner in which the myocardium is able to handle the extra load.

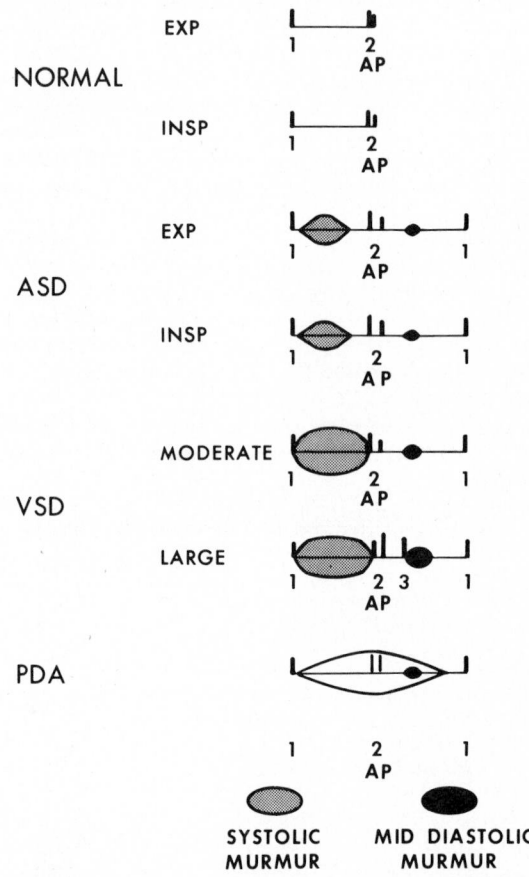

FIG. 58. Diagrammatic representation of the auscultatory findings in normal children and children with atrial septal defect (ASD), ventricular septal defect (VSD), and patent ductus arteriosus (PDA). EXP, at end-expiration; INSP, at end-inspiration; 1, first heart sound; 2, second heart sound; A, aortic component of second heart sound; P, pulmonic component of second heart sound; 3, third heart sound. The continuous murmur of the PDA is indicated by the two curved lines that enclose a clear area. The murmur begins just after S1, reaches a maximal intensity near S2, and dies away in diastole. To qualify as continuous, a murmur must continue from systole into diastole; it need not occupy all of diastole.

The increase in left ventricular output will be associated with tachycardia and an increase in stroke volume that causes a rapid rise in the aortic pulse pressure due to rapid left ventricular ejection and also causes left ventricular hyperactivity. The diastolic run-off through the aortopulmonary communication, plus the peripheral vasodilatation that usually occurs, account for the low diastolic pressure and the collapsing pulse. The increased volume load will lead to enlargement of the left atrium and ventricle, with roentgenographic evidence of dilatation and electrocardiographic evidence of hypertrophy. Since the ascending aorta receives the increased left ventricular output, it is dilated. The increased pulmonary blood flow will be evident from increased vascular markings on the chest roentgenogram and may result in an apical mid-diastolic rumble due to increased flow across the mitral valve. Rapid ventricular filling will be associated with a gallop rhythm. With large left-to-right shunts, left ventricular end-diastolic pressure and left atrial pressure increase, and eventually there may be overt left ventricular failure. If there is a large communication with equal systemic and pulmonary arterial pressures, there will be right ventricular pressure overload manifested by signs of pulmonary arterial hypertension, right ventricular hypertrophy on the electrocardiogram, and eventually right ventricular failure.

DIFFERENTIAL DIAGNOSIS. In premature infants, particularly those under 1,500 g birth weight, there is little chance of clinical findings suggestive of a patent ductus arteriosus being due to some other congenital heart defect. However, in larger premature and full-term infants there are times when a patent ductus arteriosus cannot be differentiated from truncus arteriosus, ventricular septal defect with aortic regurgitation, or arteriovenous fistula. A major problem may occur when there is severe heart failure with a markedly reduced cardiac output; the peripheral pulses may not be bounding, the murmur may be soft and not continuous, and the precordium may not be hyperactive. After appropriate therapy for left ventricular failure the classic physical findings usually reappear.

OUTCOME. In premature infants, if left ventricular failure due to the left-to-right shunt can be controlled by appropriate medical means (p. 1480), spontaneous closure of the ductus arteriosus is frequent. Recent studies of fetal and newborn animals have shown constriction of the immature ductus arteriosus when prostaglandin synthesis has been inhibited by acetylsalicylic acid or by indomethacin. This information has been applied in limited controlled studies in premature infants who are in difficulty from a big patent ductus arteriosus. Indomethacin given in 1 to 3 small doses (0.1 to 0.3 mg/kg) has completely closed the ductus arteriosus in most of these infants. Toxic side effects are uncommon with these doses but have not yet been fully evaluated. More information is needed before this promising therapy can be generally recommended. However, if medical management is unsuccessful or if complications (particularly necrotizing enterocolitis) occur, surgical closure should be performed. In the full-

term infant with a patent ductus arteriosus, spontaneous closure may also occur, but it is less common than in the premature infant. Medical management should be instituted, and at a convenient time surgical closure should be performed. Even if there is no heart failure there are two reasons for considering surgical closure of a patent ductus arteriosus. If there is significant pulmonary hypertension due to a large communication, the danger of the development of pulmonary vascular disease necessitates surgical closure, preferably before 6 to 8 months of age. In the older child with a small patent ductus, surgical closure should still be advised in view of the risk of developing infective endocarditis.

Truncus Arteriosus Communis

Although truncus arteriosus communis produces complete mixing of pulmonary and systemic venous return with a resultant decrease in systemic arterial oxygen tension, cyanosis may not be clinically apparent in early infancy because of a large pulmonary blood flow. Therefore the clinical features may closely simulate other aortopulmonary communications. Certain features, such as increased right ventricular forces, a loud ejection systolic click, a narrow mediastinal shadow compatible with an absent pulmonary artery segment or a right-sided aortic arch on the chest roentgenogram, suggest this diagnosis rather than that of a patent ductus arteriosus. This defect will be discussed in more detail elsewhere (p. 1465).

Aortopulmonary Fenestration

Aortopulmonary fenestration, which is due to failure of formation of the base of the spiral septum, generally produces a large aortopulmonary communication just above the semilunar valves. The pulses are typically bounding or collapsing, like those of a large patent ductus arteriosus. However, the murmur more closely resembles that of a high ventricular septal defect in that it is generally not continuous, it has a rough, often crescendo–decrescendo character, and it is heard maximally along the left sternal border in the third and fourth intercostal spaces. The diagnosis is made by cardiac catheterization and angiocardiography. Surgical closure during cardiopulmonary bypass is corrective.

Anomalous Origin of Left Coronary Artery

In this anomaly the left coronary artery arises from the pulmonary artery, while the right coronary artery arises normally from the anterior aortic sinus and follows a normal course. During fetal life when pulmonary arterial and aortic pressures are similar, myocardial perfusion is normal. However, after birth, when pulmonary arterial pressure falls to its normal low level, blood can flow from the right coronary artery through collateral vessels into the left coronary artery and then into the pulmonary artery. Thus a small left-to-right shunt is produced, and blood destined for the myocardium is diverted to the pulmonary artery through these channels. The portion of myocardium generally involved is the anterolateral wall of the left ventricle.

Generally the presenting features relate to myocardial failure as a result of ischemia or even a frank myocardial infarct, and they usually appear between 2 weeks and 6 months of age. Episodes of restlessness and crying, as if in pain, associated with pallor and sweating have been described in infants with this anomaly, but they are not the usual presenting symptoms. Poor feeding, tachypnea, respiratory symptoms, and other evidence of left ventricular failure are more usual. Severe cardiomegaly is the rule, and mitral insufficiency murmurs are common as a result of dilatation of the mitral valve ring or papillary muscle infarction. Prominent third and fourth heart sounds are also common. The electrocardiogram and vectorcardiogram demonstrate an anterolateral infarction pattern with broad, deep q waves in leads I, aVl, and the left precordium, often associated with persistent S-T segment and T wave changes in these leads. Increased left ventricular forces are also usual. The chest roentgenogram demonstrates cardiomegaly and usually evidence of chronic pulmonary venous congestion. Other conditions that present with many similar findings include endocardial fibroelastosis, myocarditis, and glycogen storage disease involving the heart. Since anomalous origin of the left coronary artery is potentially treatable, this diagnosis needs to be considered whenever there is unexplained left ventricular failure in infancy; it can be confirmed by cardiac catheterization and angiocardiography. Treatment consists of ligation of the anomalous left coronary artery if there is a left-to-right shunt from the right coronary artery into the pulmonary artery. This prevents run-off and thereby permits reasonably good perfusion of the surviving myocardium through the collateral vessels. More recently aortocoronary bypass grafts or reimplantation of the artery into the aorta have been done.

Hemitruncus Arteriosus and Lobar Sequestration

In hemitruncus arteriosus either the left or right pulmonary artery, but more commonly the right, arises abnormally from the aorta. In lobar sequestration a portion of the lung, usually an individual lobe or part of a lobe, gets its arterial blood supply through an abnormal artery arising from the aorta. In both groups the pulmonary artery involved does not communicate with the main pulmonary artery and thereby the right ventricle. The magnitude of flow into the lung or portion of lung is controlled by the pulmonary vascular resistance as well as the resistance offered by the communicating vessel itself. The clinical presentation in children with these lesions will also depend on the magnitude of the shunt and will be very similar to that found with a patent ductus arteriosus. However, the murmur, often continuous in type, may be better heard more laterally or even in the back.

One important additional feature with a hemitruncus is that the normally arising pulmonary artery will be carrying the total right ventricular output, which is the total systemic venous return. Normally this flow is distributed between the two pulmonary arteries, and it is therefore obvious that with a hemitruncus the lung supplied by the single pulmonary artery will in fact be receiving an increased flow. Pressure in the normal pulmonary artery is generally normal, and therefore the risks of subsequent pulmonary vascular disease are similar to those in children with atrial septal defects and a pulmonary blood flow about twice normal. However, if there is an associated left-to-right shunt, blood flow to the normal lung is more than doubled; thus there may be pulmonary hypertension and subsequent pulmonary vascular disease. However, the lung supplied by the abnormally arising vessel is at risk not only from increased flow but also from increased pressure, since this lung is perfused at systemic pressure less the pressure fall offered by the channel itself. If the abnormally arising pulmonary artery is adequately developed, implantation into the main pulmonary artery can be done. If a significant portion of lung is involved in lobar sequestration, a lobectomy is indicated.

Unilateral Absence of Pulmonary Artery

Although this is not a lesion with a left-to-right shunt, it resembles a hemitruncus in some ways. The right or the left pulmonary artery may be congenitally absent, either as an isolated lesion or with other congenital cardiac defects. Absence of the left and right pulmonary arteries has an equal incidence when they are isolated lesions or with most cardiac defects; however, if there is a patent ductus arteriosus, then it is usually the right pulmonary artery that is absent, and in the tetralogy of Fallot it is almost always the left artery that is missing. The lung on the affected side is usually hypoplastic and is supplied by bronchial arteries, so that on chest roentgenogram there is shown a small hemithorax, no hilar pulmonary artery, and often a diffuse reticular pattern of bronchial collaterals. Since ventilation can still take place on that side, there is much wasted ventilation and usually dyspnea on effort.

The chief importance of the lesion is its tendency to produce pulmonary hypertension and pulmonary vascular disease in all except those with the tetralogy of Fallot. Because there is only one pulmonary artery, it receives the total right ventricular output. Therefore, even if there are no other lesions, that lung receives twice its normal blood flow; and if there are left-to-right shunts in addition, it gets more than this. In infancy, before pulmonary arterial muscle has regressed, this increased flow leads to hypertension and can eventually cause severe pulmonary vascular disease, which has been reported in 18 percent of patients with no other lesions and 88 percent of those with cardiac lesions.

Diagnosis is made by angiography. Treatment is directed at repairing the associated defects and avoiding anything that might affect the pulmonary vessels of the normal lung (for example, avoiding living at high altitude or taking contraceptive pills).

Sinus of Valsalva Fistula

Rupture of a sinus of Valsalva into one of the cardiac chambers is secondary to a structural abnormality or weakness in the sinus. Most commonly these changes involve the anterior (right coronary) aortic valve sinus, and subsequent rupture will produce a communication from the right coronary sinus into either the right ventricle or right atrium. Less commonly rupture involves the noncoronary or the left coronary sinus. The aneurysmal dilatation of the sinus that precedes rupture is often related to a ventricular septal defect. Connective tissue disorders such as Marfan's syndrome also may have associated aneurysmal dilatation of the aortic sinuses. Small fistulae may occur after infective endocarditis, but more extensive rupture occurs usually after trauma or spontaneously due to progressive weakening of the sinus. Acute rupture, although more common in young adults, does occur in children. At the time of rupture there is frequently an episode of acute chest pain and dyspnea with sudden onset of a murmur and congestive heart failure; however, a more insidious onset has been described. When rupture occurs into the right ventricle the physical signs will be similar to those of a patent ductus arteriosus, with a loud continuous superficial murmur along the left sternal border, but with the addition of an increased right ventricular volume load. When the rupture occurs into the right atrium this lesion will behave like an obligatory shunt, and the features are those of the patent ductus arteriosus and an atrial shunt combined. Accurate differentiation from other lesions can be made only by cardiac catheterization and angiocardiography. Surgical closure of the fistula can be done with cardiopulmonary bypass.

Coronary Arteriovenous Fistula

In coronary arteriovenous fistula a large fistula generally passes from one of the coronary arteries into the right atrium (either directly or through the coronary sinus) or directly into the right ventricular chamber. Communications with the left ventricle or left atrium are considerably less common. The most common communication is between the right coronary artery and the right ventricle.

The most striking clinical feature is a continuous murmur that is superficial in character and is heard best along the lower left sternal border. The murmur generally is of maximal intensity in diastole and has very high-pitched components. The presence of ventricular hyperactivity and a mid-diastolic rumble will depend on the magnitude of shunting, which is not usually great. A continuous thrill may be palpable. The specific diagnosis depends on cardiac catheterization and angiocardiography. The treatment involves either ligation of the fistulous communication with the coronary sinus or right atrium or specific surgical repair when the communication is with the right ventricular cavity.

Systemic Arteriovenous Fistula

The most common sites for large arteriovenous communications in children are intracranial or hepatic or in the extremities. However, fistulae have been described between internal mammary vessels or other major systemic arteries and their related veins. They may be seen as manifestations of the Rendu-Osler-Weber syndrome, and they also may be traumatic in origin. The most common traumatic varieties are found between renal vessels following needle biopsy of the kidney and in the femoral triangle as a result of needling the femoral vessels.

Since these lesions fall into the group of obligatory left-to-right shunts, the hemodynamic and clinical features will depend on the size of the communication and thus its resistance to flow. The majority of systemic arteriovenous fistulae are not large and therefore do not produce major hemodynamic changes. The exceptions to this are intracranial arteriovenous fistulae, particularly those that involve the great vein of Galen or its tributaries.

Certain clinical manifestations are common to all types of arteriovenous fistulae. These include a systolic or continuous murmur over the site of the fistula, occasionally a pulsatile mass, and the appearance of distended and sometimes pulsatile veins draining the region of the fistula. Increased limb size and swelling may be apparent with peripheral arteriovenous fistulae. Hepatic arteriovenous fistulae generally do not involve one feeder vessel, but are usually hemangiomatous.

Intracranial arteriovenous fistulae generally produce the most severe hemodynamic changes, since they involve vessels of large caliber and the left-to-right shunt is often large. In early infancy they may produce severe congestive heart failure, and they are among the few cardiovascular lesions that produce hydrops fetalis or severe congestive failure in the first days after birth. Clinically they generally present with continuous murmurs over either side of the skull and with bounding carotid pulses and distended jugular veins. The superior vena cava is generally markedly dilated on chest radiograph, and there is significant right and left ventricular volume overload. The peripheral pulses are bounding and even collapsing, unless heart failure is so marked that all pulses except the carotids are feeble. If the shunt is not large, cardiovascular manifestations may be mild, and neurologic sequelae will dominate the clinical picture (p. 1824).

The definitive diagnosis of these lesions is made by cardiac catheterization and angiocardiography. Surgical ligation or excision of the fistula is generally effective, although intracranial fistulae, particularly those involving the great vein of Galen, may also have multiple feeding arteries and may not be operable.

Ventricular Septal Defect

Congenital defects of the interventricular septum are the most common of all congenital heart lesions, accounting for approximately 30 to 50 percent of all patients with congenital heart malformations, excluding patent ductus arteriosus in premature infants; this percentage is equivalent to 3 to 5 of every 1,000 live births. A ventricular septal defect usually occurs as an isolated abnormality, but it may be associated with other congenital cardiac malformations. Although the membranous septum is the most common site, a defect may occur anywhere in the interventricular septum. Defects vary in size from minute openings to almost complete absence of the interventricular septum—a common ventricle. Although fetal development is apparently unaltered with ventricular septal defect, abnormalities of the aorta may occur secondarily, depending on the site of the ventricular communication. Aortic isthmus narrowing is commonly associated with a supracristal or subpulmonic ventricular septal defect, because during fetal life shunting from the left ventricle into the right ventricular outflow and pulmonary artery may occur, thereby decreasing flow across the aortic isthmus.

CLINICAL MANIFESTATIONS. As with all dependent shunts, the clinical course will be dictated by the size of the defect and the rapidity and magnitude of the fall in pulmonary vascular resistance in the early neonatal period. The pathophysiology of left-to-right shunting through a ventricular septal defect is therefore similar to that of a patent ductus arteriosus. In addition, there may be signs of right ventricular volume overload, since the extra volume of the left-to-right shunt passes into the right ventricle before passing into the pulmonary artery.

The systolic murmur of a ventricular septal defect is generally harsh and of the plateau type (Fig. 58). With a small shunt the murmur may be heard only in early systole; however, as the shunt increases the murmur becomes holosystolic in character and ends at the aortic component of the second sound. The intensity of the murmur is not necessarily related to the size of the defect, and in certain instances extremely loud murmurs are heard with hemodynamically insignificant defects (maladie de Roger). Loud murmurs are usually associated with systolic thrills. The murmur is generally heard best at the lower left sternal border, and it radiates throughout the precordium, but maximally toward the subxyphoid area. However, with a high subpulmonic ventricular septal defect the site of maximal intensity may be at the mid-to upper left sternal border, with radiation to the right of the sternum. Occasionally the murmur of a very small defect has a crescendo–decrescendo high-pitched quality and must be separated from an innocent murmur (p. 1363). When the left-to-right shunt is large enough to produce a ratio of pulmonary flow to systemic flow more than 2 to 1, a mid-diastolic rumbling murmur may be audible at and inside the apex, and a third sound may appear. As the shunt increases, precordial activity will increase.

Persistently increased precordial activity with cardiac enlargement in infants and young children often produces significant anterior bulging of the left hemithorax. If the defect is small or medium in size, significant pulmonary hypertension will not be present, and the pulmonic component of the second sound will be either normal or minimally increased in intensity. If there is pulmonary hypertension the pulmonic component of the second sound will be accentuated. With a small or moderate-size shunt the chest roentgenogram will show no increase or a slight increase in left ventricular and left atrial size and pulmonary vascular markings (Fig. 57A). As the volume of shunting increases, cardiac enlargement and pulmonary vascularity will also increase (Fig. 57B), and pulmonary edema may be evident eventually. Since the shunt is at the ventricular level, the ascending aorta will not be dilated as it is in patent ductus arteriosus. The electrocardiogram will be normal if the defect is small; it will show increasing left ventricular hypertrophy as the left-to-right shunt increases, and when there is much right ventricular hypertension, right ventricular hypertrophy will be added. The echocardiogram has the same features as in patent ductus arteriosus (p. 1374), and only with the largest defects are the ventricular septum and anterior aortic root wall separated by a space.

If there is a large left-to-right shunt the clinical signs and symptoms of volume overload and cardiac failure may also be evident. In full-term infants this occurs most commonly between 2 and 6 months of age, but it may occur earlier in premature infants. Although theoretically the left-to-right shunt should generally be greatest between 2 and 3 months of age at the time when pulmonary vascular resistance has dropped to its lowest level, congestive heart failure occurs occasionally in term infants under 1 month of age. It is in these infants that the ventricular septal defect is often associated with significant left-to-right shunting at the atrial level or ductus arteriosus level. In addition, infants who have double-outlet right ventricle with ventricular septal defect are at risk of developing congestive failure earlier than expected. This is probably due to the fact that in fetal life the pulmonary vasculature is perfused with blood that has a higher oxygen tension than normal, and thus they may have an unusually low pulmonary vascular resistance after birth.

The management of an infant with a large ventricular septal defect in whom congestive heart failure is not controllable with the use of digitalis and diuretics is still not settled. Pulmonary artery banding, which will reduce the left-to-right shunt by increasing right ventricular outflow resistance and also reduce the peripheral pulmonary arterial pressure, is still recommended in certain centers. However, since the tendency for spontaneous closure in extremely large defects is less than with smaller defects, it is likely that this group of infants will require subsequent direct closure of the ventricular septal defect. In many institutions primary repair in early infancy is now considered more appropriate. It can be performed in most infants with an acceptably low mortality that is less than the combined mortality of pulmonary arterial banding followed some time later by closure of the defect and removal of the band.

Uncontrollable heart failure is uncommon, and it is more frequent to find a moderate response to medical treatment. Frequently, spontaneous clinical improvement associated with a progressive decrease in the left-to-right shunt occurs after about 6 months of age. This will be manifested by decreasing cardiac hyperactivity and heart size, diminishing intensity and eventual disappearance of the mid-diastolic murmur, decreasing intensity and changing character of the systolic murmur, lessening and then disappearance of tachypnea, and improved appetite and growth. These alterations could be due to one of three events: spontaneous closing of the defect, development of right ventricular outflow obstruction, or development of increasing pulmonary vascular resistance. It is difficult to determine which of these is occurring, and repeated cardiac catheterization may be required to delineate the hemodynamic status.

Several different mechanisms may be responsible for spontaneous closure of a ventricular septal defect. These include growth and hypertrophy of the muscular portion of the defect, formation of a membranous diaphragm (probably due to intimal proliferation), and apposition of the septal leaflet of the tricuspid valve against the defect, which does not generally produce significant tricuspid regurgitation. When the defect is getting smaller the systolic murmur first may increase in intensity, but with progressive decrease in size the murmur becomes softer, and when the defect is extremely small the murmur becomes shorter and acquires a crescendo–decrescendo high-pitched whistling quality that often portends complete closure. Spontaneous closure may eventually occur in up to 50 percent or more of patients, and many of these closures occur within the first year of life. A further 25 percent become smaller, but may not close completely; however, the hemodynamic effects are significantly reduced. Because of these statistics, if the defect seems to be becoming smaller then surgical correction should be delayed in the hope of spontaneous closure.

The clinical differentiation between development of pulmonary vascular disease and right ventricular outflow obstruction due to infundibular hypertrophy may be difficult. In both these changes the left-to-right shunt will be reduced by an increase in outflow resistance of the right ventricle, and both will have clinical and electrocardiographic evidence of right ventricular hypertrophy. However, when a reduction in shunting occurs because the defect is closing spontaneously, right ventricular hypertrophy will decrease. An additional sign that may be helpful in differentiating these three courses is the intensity of the pulmonic component of the second sound. With outflow obstruction or spontaneous closure, pulmonary hypertension will be absent and pulmonary closure will not be accentuated, whereas with pulmonary vascular disease it will become louder and the second sound will be more narrowly split. An early diastolic blowing decrescendo murmur indicative of pulmonic insufficiency may also be heard if there is markedly increased pulmonary vascular resistance. The quality of the systolic murmur usually alters with the development of right ventricular outflow obstruction and takes on the crescendo–decrescendo characteristics of a stenotic murmur. Infundibular pulmonic stenosis associated with a ventricular septal defect has a high incidence (about 25 percent) of right aortic arch; thus a right aortic arch in an infant with a ventricular septal defect and left-to-right shunting should lead one to suspect that infundibular hypertrophy might develop.

Infundibular hypertrophy generally develops fairly rapidly, and there may be only a short period in which the left-to-right shunting is present. Soon thereafter there will be cyanosis, initially on exercise only, but then persistently, and the features of the tetralogy of Fallot can develop (p. 1447). With obstructive pulmonary vascular disease there is often little or no left-to-right shunting and no significant right-to-left shunting for several years. However, generally by 5 to 6 years of age there is increasing cyanosis, particularly during exercise (Eisenmenger syndrome). As severe pulmonary hypertension develops, the main pulmonary artery segment becomes markedly dilated, and the peripheral pulmo-

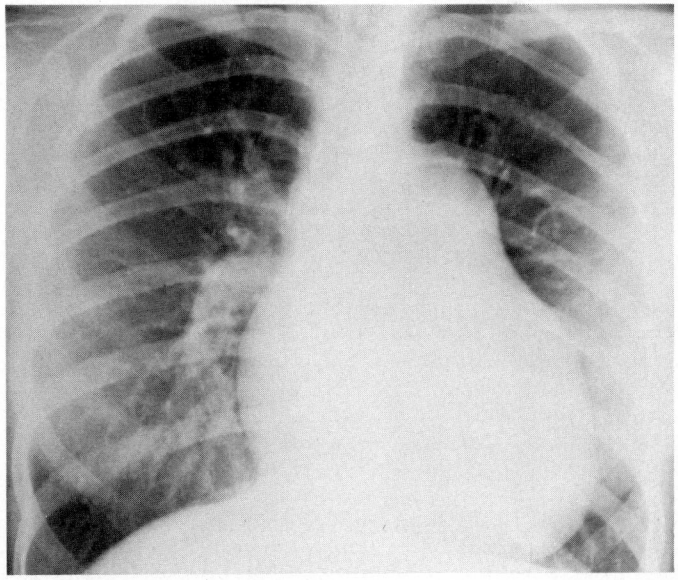

FIG. 59. Chest roentgenogram in a young girl with a ventricular septal defect and pulmonary vascular disease (Eisenmenger syndrome). Marked dilatation of the main pulmonary artery and decreased peripheral vascular markings are shown.

nary vascular markings on the chest roentgenogram decrease (Fig. 59). Obstructive pulmonary vascular disease may progress rapidly in some infants and become irreversible by the age of 12 to 18 months; this should never be allowed to occur. Any doubt as to the cause of any change in clinical status should be investigated by cardiac catheterization, and there is good reason to consider routinely recatheterizing children with large ventricular septal defects at 9 to 12 months of age to detect early pulmonary vascular disease that is not clinically apparent. In those infants who develop right ventricular outflow obstruction the incidence of spontaneous closure of a ventricular septal defect is low, a right-to-left shunt can be further complicated by cerebral thrombosis, embolism, or abscess), and the development of infundibular hypertrophy leads to more difficult surgical repair, so that closure of the defect and infundibular resection, if necessary, should be considered early.

COMPLICATIONS. In several infants in whom there have been significant reductions in left-to-right shunts due to closure of the ventricular septal defects, late systolic clicks have become audible. In these children aneurysmal dilatation of the thin membranous septum that has grown to close the defect has occurred, with bulging of the aneurysm into the right ventricle. A small opening often present at the apex of the aneurysm allows a small left-to-right shunt. Normally the defect closes and the aneurysm slowly shrinks, but rarely it may enlarge progressively.

A number of infants have also developed progressive aortic insufficiency associated with a ventricular septal defect, particularly if it is supracristal. In some instances this has become a very severe complication of the ventricular septal defect. There is generally prolapse of an aortic valve leaflet with dilatation of the aortic valve sinus, and rupture of the aortic sinus or cusp may occur. The development of insufficiency has been attributed to stress on the unsupported aortic valve cusp and perhaps suction on it by the jet of the shunt passing through the defect. Even if there is a small ventricular septal defect, or one that is showing evidence of closure, aortic insufficiency may require surgical closure of the defect to prevent further prolapse.

Infective endocarditis is an additional problem that needs to be considered; it can occur even after spontaneous closure of the defect. If infective endocarditis involves the tricuspid leaflet sealing the ventricular septal defect, rupture may occur, with the production of a direct left ventricular to right atrial communication. Antibiotic prophylaxis should therefore be continued in those children with small defects; whether it should be continued in those in whom spontaneous closure has occurred is uncertain.

In view of the pattern of blood flow in the heart and great vessels of a fetus with a ventricular septal defect and the possibility of the development of aortic arch abnormalities, narrowing of the aortic isthmus or true coarctation should always be considered when an infant with a ventricular septal defect has severe heart failure. Ventricular septal defects are also commonly associated with other forms of congenital cardiac malformations. They are common with corrected transposition, in which systemic atrioventricular valve regurgitation and complete heart block are also frequent. A ventricular septal defect is also present in double-outlet right ventricle, and in the absence of pulmonic stenosis the symptomatology of this combination is the same as that of a ventricular septal defect alone. The differential diagnosis can be suspected from echocardiography and confirmed by cardiac catheterization and angiocardiography. A ventricular septal defect is also always associated with truncus arteriosus communis.

LEVOTRANSPOSITION OF GREAT ARTERIES. Levotransposition (*l*-transposition) occurs when the primitive cardiac tube loops to the left instead of to the right during early development (p. 1355). The anatomic left ventricle comes to be on the right side and connects the right atrium to the pulmonary artery. The anatomic right ventricle receives oxygenated blood from the left atrium and ejects into an anteriorly placed left-sided aorta. There is thus *l*-transposition of the great arteries and inversion of the ventricles, but a normal flow of venous blood to the lungs and arterial blood to the body; hence the designation (physiologically) corrected transposition.

If there are no other lesions, people with this anomaly may live normal lives, but almost all have ventricular septal defects, many have pulmonic stenosis, many have defects of atrioventricular conduction (particularly complete atrioventricular block), and some have an Ebstein-like malformation of the left-sided systemic tricuspid valve that produces left-sided atrioventricular regurgitation. The symptoms and signs will therefore depend on the severity and nature of these associated lesions.

In addition to the murmurs of ventricular septal defects or pulmonic stenosis, these patients characteristically have a loud second heart sound, often single, that is best heard at the upper left sternal border because of the high, left, and anterior position of the aortic valve. The electrocardiogram may show atrioventricular conduction defects, and it will have right- or left-sided hypertrophy as appropriate for the lesions. In about 80 percent of these patients the electrocardiogram will show Q waves in right chest leads and no Q waves on the left, the pattern reflecting the activation of the septum from right to left.

Frequently the chest roentgenogram indicates the diagnosis, because the levoposed aorta produces a straight shoulder on the left heart border (Fig. 60). Echocardiograms also may disclose the abnormal position of the great arteries (p. 1371), as well as another typical anatomic feature, the anteroposterior orientation of the ventricular septum; multibeam systems are more useful than single-beam systems in this respect.

Surgical correction of these lesions is more hazardous than correction of similar lesions without ventricular inversion. The abnormal conduction system increases the risk of surgically produced complete atrioventricular block when a ventricular septal defect is closed. Large coronary arteries often run across the

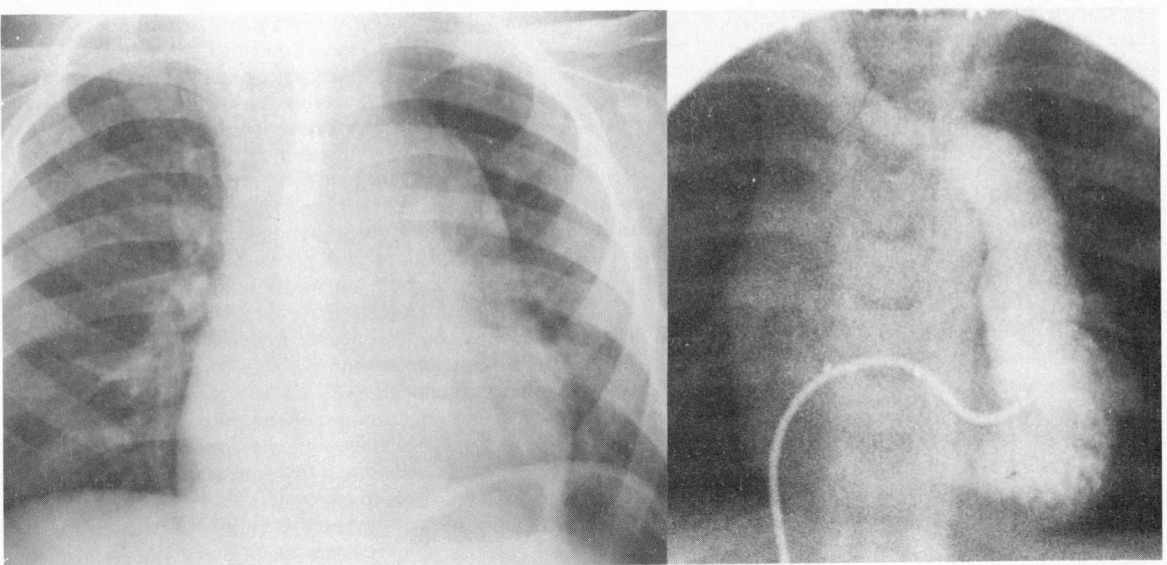

FIG. 60. On the left is the typical chest roentgenogram in corrected transposition, with the filled-in upper left heart border being due to the levoposed aorta, as shown in the angiogram on the right.

outflow tract of the pulmonic ventricle, where an incision would have to be made. The pulmonary artery is very posterior, so that correcting pulmonic stenosis is difficult, particularly because the obstruction is seldom a valvar stenosis, but is more often a subpulmonic fibromuscular narrowing or else a mass of accessory tissue related to the adjacent mitral valve. For these reasons surgery is not advised if patients are doing well. If they deteriorate, then the pulmonary artery may be banded if there is a large left-to-right shunt, or else an aortopulmonary shunt can be done to palliate severe cyanosis. Attempts at complete correction should be done only by a skilled surgeon and only after the risks have been fully assessed.

Atrial Septal Defects

The embryologic development of the atrial septum is discussed on page 1356. Interference with the development of the atrial septum at its lower margin, associated with failure of adequate development of the endocardial cushions, will produce an ostium primum atrial septal defect that has no inferior rim of atrial septal tissue. This lesion is generally associated with abnormalities of the mitral and tricuspid valves (which form from the endocardial cushions), as well as defective formation of the upper portion of the interventricular septum (p. 1356).

A second type of atrial septal defect is the so-called ostium secundum defect. This is a defect in the central portion of the septum in relation to the foramen ovale; it results from inadequate closure of the central hole in the septum primum by the septum secundum and is more appropriately termed a fossa ovalis defect.

A third type of atrial septal defect is the sinus venosus defect, which is located in the superior portion of the atrial septum and generally extends into the superior vena cava. With an abnormal interatrial communication, fetal development is apparently normal. However, it is possible that the preferential streaming patterns found normally in the fetus may be interfered with.

INCOMPETENT (PATENT) FORAMEN OVALE. With the onset of ventilation immediately after birth, pulmonary venous return increases markedly, and left atrial pressure rises. The foramen ovale is therefore normally functionally closed by the membranous valve of the foramen ovale, which is apposed to the crista dividens and the lower portion of the septum secundum. Although functionally closed shortly after birth under normal conditions, the foramen ovale often remains probe-patent. When the pulmonary vascular resistance does not fall normally following birth, the resultant pulmonary hypertension and rises in right ventricular end-diastolic pressure and right atrial pressure are often associated with right-to-left shunting across the foramen ovale. This results in systemic hypoxemia.

In some infants, although the normal atrial pressure relationships occur after birth, the valve of the foramen ovale does not completely cover the foramen, either due to a shortened valve that is incapable of occluding a foramen ovale or due to a foramen ovale that has become enlarged and stretched. This latter occurs in infants in whom left atrial pressure and volume are increased, as with patent ductus arteriosus, ventricular septal defect, or left ventricular outflow obstruction due to aortic stenosis or coarctation. Significant left-to-right shunting may occur through an incompetent foramen ovale when left atrial pressure is high. If the cause of the increased left atrial pressure is relieved, as when a patent ductus arteriosus is closed or aortic coarctation is resected, atrial shunting generally decreases or disappears. In certain congenital heart defects, survival after birth depends on persistent patency of the foramen ovale. These defects include tricuspid and mitral atresia and total anomalous pulmonary venous connection. In aortopulmonary transposition a patent foramen ovale may be the only communication between the systemic and pulmonary circulations. Right-to-left shunting across the foramen ovale is also associated with right ventricular obstructive lesions such as pulmonic stenosis.

OSTIUM SECUNDUM ATRIAL SEPTAL DEFECT. Ostium secundum defects may vary in size from a small defect to one in which only a rim of atrial tissue separates the defect from the atrioventricular valves. Usually ostium secundum defects are isolated lesions, but some may be associated with partial anomalous pulmonary venous connection (usually draining the right lung) or pulmonic stenosis.

The magnitude of left-to-right shunting will be determined by the size of the defect, by the relationship of inflow resistances of the left and right ventricles, and, as discussed previously (p. 1405), by the outflow resistance of each ventricle. Small atrial communications are therefore associated with moderate to small shunts. Large defects are associated with large left-to-right shunts if there is a low inflow resistance of the right ventricle and a low pulmonary resistance. The inflow resistance is related to the distensibility or compliance of each ventricle, and this has been equated to the thicknesses of the respective ventricles. Since after birth the right ventricle soon becomes thinner than the left ventricle, the right ventricle is more easily distended in diastole and thus takes up blood from the right atrium as well as from the left atrium via the defect. The effect of a large shunt at the atrial level is a marked increase in flow through the right atrium and right ventricle. This extra volume load is tolerated well by the right ventricle, since it is handling the increased volume at a low pressure. Therefore cardiac failure is unusual in infancy, and when it occurs it is generally precipitated by either a combination of defects or some other complication.

Infants or children with large atrial septal defects are generally asymptomatic. The increased right ventricular volume load causes precordial hyperactivity, particularly along the left sternal border. The first heart sound is normal, and the second heart sound is characteristically widely split, with absence of the normal respiratory variation in the width of splitting (Fig. 58). Both components of the second sound are of normal intensity. Although fixed splitting of the second sound is a characteristic physical finding in older children, it is important to realize that this sign may not be present, especially in infants or when the communication is only moderately large. Several mechanisms have been invoked to explain the wide splitting; increased right ventricular stroke volume with prolongation of the systolic ejection period and a low pulmonary vascular impedance are those most generally accepted. If there is pul-

monary hypertension, the second sound may be less widely split; this may account for the lack of splitting in early infancy when pulmonary vascular resistance has not fallen to its normal low level. Flow across the atrial septal defect is not associated with a murmur; however, a systolic ejection murmur that is crescendo-decrescendo in type is generally heard at the upper left sternal border and represents increased flow across the right ventricular outflow tract and pulmonic valve. The murmur associated with atrial septal defects can usually be differentiated from innocent pulmonary flow murmurs, whose characteristics are very similar, by the response to the Valsalva maneuver. When intrathoracic pressure is increased, systemic venous return is immediately reduced, with a consequent fall in right ventricular stroke volume under normal circumstances. The intensity of an innocent pulmonary flow murmur will suddenly decrease. However, with a large atrial septal defect the left-to-right shunt across the atrial communication will maintain right ventricular stroke volume for several beats despite the decrease of systemic venous return; thus there is little, if any, change in the intensity of the murmur in the first three to four beats. If the left-to-right shunt is fairly large there is often a rumbling early or mid-diastolic tricuspid flow murmur heard best at the lower left sternal border. Also, a prominent third heart sound often is heard at the lower left sternal border.

The chest roentgenogram (Fig. 61) shows a heart with right atrial and right ventricular enlargement; the outflow region of the right ventricle may also be enlarged. The main pulmonary artery is dilated, and the pulmonary vascular markings are increased. However, the relationship between the prominence of the pulmonary vascularity and the magnitude of left-to-right shunt is not reliable. The electrocardiogram generally shows a right axis deviation with normal atrial complexes and normal atrioventricular conduction. There is right ventricular hypertrophy with a typical rsR' or rSR' pattern in the right precordial leads. The echocardiogram may show paradoxic ventricular septal motion (p.1373). The specific diagnosis can be made only by cardiac catheterization and angiocardiography, and the presence of an abnormally draining pulmonary vein can also be confirmed by these techniques. Radionuclide scanning techniques can be useful in differentiating innocent pulmonary flow murmurs from those produced by an atrial left-to-right shunt. However, a pulmonary scan will indicate the presence of a left-to-right shunt, but not necessarily the specific level at which it occurs.

Under normal conditions right-to-left shunting is unusual in ostium secundum defects. However, with sinus venosus defects there may be right-to-left shunting from the superior vena cava into the left atrium, and mild arterial oxygen desaturation may be found. Infective endocarditis has not been reported in uncomplicated secundum atrial septal defects. Obstructive pulmonary vascular disease may occur, but not usually before the late second or third decade. This will become evident by a decrease in the physical findings associated with the left-to-right shunt and later by right-to-left

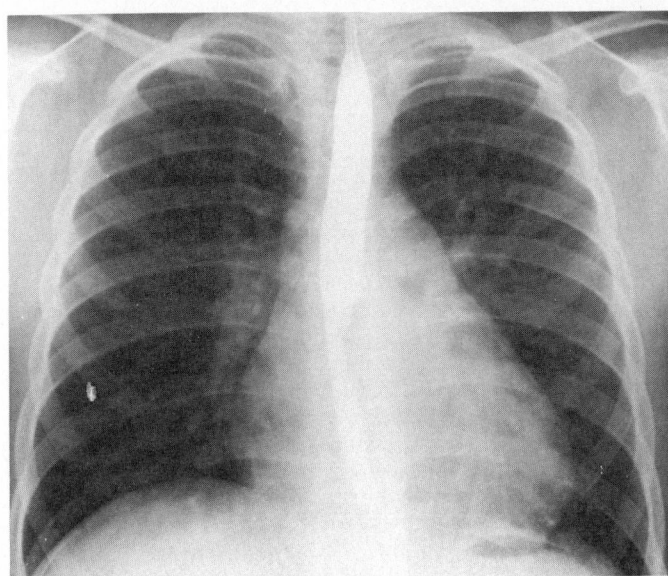

FIG. 61. Chest roentgenogram in a child with ostium secundum atrial septal defect.

shunting. It is concern about the possible development of pulmonary vascular disease that generally leads to surgical closure of the communication. However, atrial arrhythmias, especially atrial fibrillation or flutter (due probably to atrial enlargement), and congestive heart failure may occur in adult life and are added reasons for prophylactic closure of atrial defects in children.

OSTIUM PRIMUM DEFECTS AND ENDOCARDIAL CUSHION DEFECTS. Ostium primum defects and endocardial cushion defects result from arrested or abnormal development of the endocardial cushions in the primitive atrioventricular canal; they range in severity from a small ostium primum atrial septal defect to a complete atrioventricular canal. They may occur as isolated lesions in otherwise normal infants; however, they are often encountered with other congenital abnormalities in syndromes such as trisomy 21 (Down's syndrome), the asplenia or polysplenia syndromes, and the Ellis-van Creveld syndrome.

Fetal somatic development is essentially normal; however, there is a high incidence of secondary hemodynamic alterations in the aorta in this group of lesions. Subaortic outflow obstruction, although often of only minor severity, is common; when associated with the potential obligatory shunt in utero it may result in significant alterations in the patterns of blood flow during fetal life. Therefore aortic isthmus narrowing and juxtaductal coarctation are found in a significant number of infants with this defect. The severity and type of anatomic defect depend on which endocardial cushions are involved and the stage of developmental failure. Since the cushions are involved in the development of both atrial and ventricular septa, as well as the mitral and tricuspid valves, many different combinations of abnormalities in this region are found.

OSTIUM PRIMUM DEFECT. Ostium primum defect is the most benign form of endocardial cushion defect; it

is also termed partial atrioventricular canal defect. The central portion of the atrial septum in the region of the mitral and tricuspid valve rings is absent, and the defect size is variable but usually large. The anterior (or septal) mitral valve leaflet is displaced and commonly is cleft. The tricuspid valve is generally not involved, although a small cleft in the septal leaflet may also be present. The magnitude of the atrial left-to-right shunt in ostium primum defects is controlled by the same mechanisms as in secundum atrial septal defects. The clinical features are similar and include right ventricular hyperactivity, increased pulmonary blood flow, and a widely split second sound. In addition to the right ventricular outflow murmur and the tricuspid mid-diastolic flow murmur, murmurs of mitral and/or tricuspid regurgitation may be present if significant clefts in these valves are present. However, significant regurgitation is unusual, particularly in infancy and early childhood. The electrocardiogram is usually characteristic in that it shows left axis deviation, generally in the −20 to −60 degree range, and right ventricular hypertrophy with an rsR′ pattern in right precordial leads. Chest roentgenographic findings will depend on the magnitude of left-to-right shunt.

COMPLETE ATRIOVENTRICULAR CANAL DEFECT. Complete atrioventricular canal defects are more complicated; they involve failure of development of separate tricuspid and mitral valve rings. In addition to the ostium primum defect, there is a ventricular septal defect in the posterior portion of the interventricular septum, and there are clefts in the septal leaflets of both the tricuspid and mitral valves. The anterior and posterior segments of each septal leaflet are not separated (as in normal development), but join each other through the defect, so that in the most severe form there is a common anterior mitral–tricuspid valve leaflet as well as a common posterior mitral–tricuspid valve leaflet.

The severity of the mitral and tricuspid valve anomaly and the size of the ventricular defect are related to the stage of arrested development of the endocardial cushions; the earlier the defect has occurred, the larger the ventricular septal defect and the more primitive the development of the atrioventricular valves. Although the most severe form may occur as an isolated defect, it may be associated with other complex anomalies such as asplenia or polysplenia syndromes and single ventricle.

The clinical manifestations of the complete form of atrioventricular canal defect are variable, but in general the more severe or primitive the defect, the more marked the clinical manifestations. The ventricular septal defects will behave as any other ventricular septal defect in producing a left ventricular volume load and, if they are large, pulmonary hypertension and associated right ventricular pressure load. The characteristic murmur of a ventricular septal defect will be present, as will a mid-diastolic rumble due to increased pulmonary venous return with increased diastolic flow across the mitral valve. If the cleft in the mitral valve is significant, mitral regurgitation may be present, and an apical pansystolic blowing murmur may be heard. The mid-diastolic rumble will then be further accentuated by the even larger flow across the mitral valve, and left ventricular enlargement will be more prominent. The ostium primum defect portion of the complete canal will present with physical findings similar to those in an isolated atrial septal defect; these include right ventricular volume overload, a tricuspid diastolic flow rumble, and a right ventricular outflow murmur. Should tricuspid regurgitation be present, a pansystolic blowing murmur in the tricuspid area and systolic pulsation of the jugular veins may be evident, and the increased flow across the tricuspid valve will accentuate the mid-diastolic murmur. Both the atrial and ventricular shunts will fall into the dependent category. However, often the cleft in the misplaced mitral valve allows ventricular blood to pass through it and the ostium primum defect to enter the right atrium, so that there is an obligatory left ventricular to right atrial shunt. There may at times be minor right-to-left shunting and mild cyanosis.

Heart failure often occurs by 2 months after birth. However, symptoms may develop very early in infancy if there is an obligatory left ventricular to right atrial shunt or when there is significant atrioventricular valve dysfunction. These symptoms are primarily related to severe congestive heart failure and include tachypnea, sweating, and difficulty with feeding. Systemic cardiac output is generally low, and the infant then has poor pulses, tachycardia, hepatomegaly, and peripheral pallor. Marked cardiomegaly is common (Fig. 56).

As with ostium primum defects, the electrocardiogram shows left axis deviation (superior axis), but in most complete atrioventricular canal defects it is even more negative, in the range -60 to -150 degrees. The frontal plane vector loop is always counterclockwise. The P-R interval frequently is prolonged. The echocardiogram may show the narrowed left ventricular outflow tract due to the displaced mitral valve, and it will also show the mitral and tricuspid valves in continuity across the atrioventricular defect (p. 1371). Ventricular

and atrial hypertrophy will depend on the level of maximal shunting and the amount of atrioventricular valve regurgitation. The left axis deviation is not pathognomonic of an endocardial cushion defect; it also may be found with double-outlet right ventricle, with tricuspid or pulmonary atresia, or even in normal children. The absence of left axis deviation does not exclude the diagnosis of an endocardial cushion defect, although statistically it is strongly against it. The chest roentgenographic findings will again depend on the level of shunting and the amount of atrioventricular valve regurgitation.

Infants with this defect are at high risk of developing obstructive pulmonary vascular disease from severe pulmonary hypertension and a large left-to-right shunt. The management of infants with the more severe forms of endocardial cushion defects depends on the level of major shunting. If this is mainly at the ventricular level, then intractable cardiac failure may be improved by pulmonary artery banding, which will increase the outflow resistance of the right ventricle and thereby decrease the amount of dependent shunting. However, in most infants with complete atrioventricular canal defects the large left ventricular to right atrial shunt or atrioventricular valve regurgitation will be unaffected by pulmonary artery banding. Many infants have poor responses to vigorous medical management, and an attempt at complete surgical correction is often required despite the high risks and relatively poor success rate.

PARTIAL ANOMALOUS PULMONARY VENOUS CONNECTION. Partial anomalous pulmonary venous connection without an associated atrial septal defect is rare. Invariably the anomalous pulmonary veins drain either the complete right lung or a portion of it, and they may connect with the superior vena cava or directly with the right atrium. In addition, there is a specific entity (scimitar syndrome) in which the pulmonary veins from the lower lobe and sometimes the middle lobe of the right lung drain by a common channel into the inferior vena cava. Associated with this is underdevelopment as well as lobar sequestration of that portion of the lung. The chest roentgenogram in scimitar syndrome is typical, and the anomalous vein is generally seen quite easily. The clinical presentation of these lesions resembles that of secundum atrial septal defects, except that the second heart sound is generally normally split. Partial anomalous pulmonary venous connection, when associated with an atrial septal defect, does not generally contribute any specific clinical features.

References

Alzamora-Castro V, Battilana G, Abugattas R, Sialer S: Patent ductus arteriosus and high altitude. Am J Cardiol 5:761, 1960

Askenazi J, Nadas AS: Anomalous left coronary artery originating from the pulmonary artery: report on 15 cases. Circulation 51:976, 1975

Coceani F, Olley PM: The response of the ductus arteriosus to prostaglandins. Can J Physiol Pharmacol 51:220, 1973

Edmunds LH Jr, Gregory GA, Heymann MA, Kitterman JA, Rudolph AM, Tooley WH: Surgical closure of the ductus arteriosus in premature infants. Circulation 48:856, 1973

Freedom RM, White RD, Pieroni DR, Varghese PJ, Krovetz LJ, Rowe RD: The natural history of the so-called aneurysm of the membranous ventricular septum in childhood. Circulation 49:375, 1974

Friedman WF: The intrinsic physiologic properties of the developing heart. In Friedman WF, Lesch M, Sonnenblick EM (eds): Neonatal Heart Disease. New York, Grune & Stratton, 1973, p 21

Heymann MA, Rudolph AM: Effects of congenital heart disease on the fetal and neonatal circulation. Prog Cardiovasc Dis 15:115, 1972

———— Rudolph AM: Control of the ductus arteriosus. Physiol Rev 55:62, 1975

Hoffman JIE: Ventricular septal defect: indications for therapy in infants. Pediatr Clin North Am 18:1091, 1971

———— The normal pulmonary circulation. In Scarpelli EM, Auld PAM, Goldman HS (eds): Pediatric Pulmonary Physiology and Disease. Philadelphia, Lea & Febiger, 1975

———— Abnormal pulmonary circulation. In Scarpelli EM, Auld PAM, Goldman HS (eds): Pediatric Pulmonary Physiology and Disease. Philadelphia, Lea & Febiger, 1977

———— Buckberg GD: Regional myocardial ischemia—causes, prediction and prevention. Vasc Surg 8:115, 1974

———— Rudolph AM: The natural history of ventricular septal defects in infancy. Am J Cardiol 16:634, 1965

———— Rudolph AM, Danilowicz D: Left to right atrial shunts in infants. Am J Cardiol 30:868, 1972

Kitterman JA, Edmunds LH Jr, Gregory GA, Heymann MA, Tooley WH, Rudolph AM: Patent ductus arteriosus in premature infants: incidence, relation to pulmonary disease and management. N Engl J Med 287:473, 1972

Peñaloza D, Arias-Stella J, Sime F, Recavarren S, Marticorena E: The heart and pulmonary circulation in children at high altitudes. Pediatrics 34:568, 1964

Pool PE, Vogel JHK, Blount SG Jr: Congenital unilateral absence of a pulmonary artery. Am J Cardiol 9:706, 1962

Rudolph AM: The changes in the circulation after birth: their importance in congenital heart disease. Circulation 41:343, 1970

———— Congenital Diseases of the Heart. Chicago, Year Book, 1974

———— Heymann MA, Spitznas U: Hemodynamic considerations in the development of narrowing of the aorta. Am J Cardiol 30:514, 1972

REGURGITANT LESIONS

MICHAEL A. HEYMANN

General Features

Regurgitant lesions are those in which blood ejected by either the left or right atrium or ventricle returns to that chamber through an incompetent atrioventricular or semilunar valve. Any one of the four cardiac valves may be involved, and occasionally more than one is regurgitant. Acquired lesions of these valves, particularly after rheumatic carditis, are more common than isolated congenital defects; however, congenital malformations either alone or in combination with other intracardiac abnormalities do occur.

EFFECTS ON FETUS. When an isolated congenital malformation produces regurgitation, fetal somatic development is generally normal, and fetal cardiac output and organ blood flows do not appear to be significantly affected. However, severe tricuspid valve regurgitation has been associated with intrauterine congestive failure and hydrops fetalis.

PATHOPHYSIOLOGY. The physiologic effects and clinical features of a regurgitant lesion are similar to those of a volume load associated with a left-to-right shunt, but with features specific to each regurgitant valve. Significant mitral regurgitation produces left ventricular hyperactivity and dilatation, and the left atrium will be dilated. The first heart sound may be softer than normal. The second sound is normal, or else its pulmonic component is accentuated if there is pulmonary hypertension, and a third heart sound is common. Typically there is a blowing holosystolic murmur maximal at the apex and conducted to the axilla and under the left scapula, although if the regurgitant jet passes through the anterior mitral leaflet the murmur may be better heard along the left sternal border. There is often a mid-diastolic rumbling murmur at the apex due to the increased diastolic flow through the mitral valve. With marked regurgitation there may be left ventricular failure and pulmonary edema. The electrocardiogram and chest roentgenogram reflect the extent of left atrial and ventricular enlargement, as does the echocardiogram.

Aortic regurgitation also causes similar changes in the size and activity of the left ventricle, as seen clinically and by electrocardiogram and chest roentgenogram. However, the aortic component of the second heart sound is usually soft, and the predominant murmur is an early high-pitched blowing decrescendo diastolic murmur heard best along the left and sometimes the right sternal border; the murmur, if soft, is best heard during expiration with the patient leaning forward. If the stroke volume is large there may also be an ejection systolic murmur at the base that resembles the murmur of aortic stenosis. Sometimes there is an apical mid-diastolic rumble at the apex even when there is no mitral valve disease. This is the Austin Flint murmur, and it is thought to be due to fluttering of the mitral valve as it is moved on each side by blood entering the ventricle in diastole through the mitral and aortic valves. Because of the increased forward stroke volume in systole, the ascending aorta and the arch are dilated and unfolded, and this and the low diastolic pressure in the aorta cause marked pulsations of the carotid arteries as well as the typically bounding arterial pulses of marked aortic regurgitation. When the lesion is severe the electrocardiogram may show S-T segment and T wave changes due to subendocardial ischemia caused by poor diastolic coronary perfusion.

Tricuspid incompetence, if marked, causes dilatation and hyperactivity of the right atrium and ventricle. The first and second heart sounds are usually normal, and third and fourth heart sounds may be heard. There is often a holosystolic murmur heard best at the lower left sternal border, although the presence and loudness of this murmur are no guide to the severity of the lesion. In young children with organic tricuspid valve disease the murmur may be low-pitched and rough, but in most it is high-pitched and blowing. The characteristic finding in this lesion is failure of the jugular venous pressure to fall during systole, a sign that precedes the murmur; systolic pulsation of the liver occurs only when there is massive tricuspid regurgitation. Mid-diastolic murmurs may occur, but are not common. The electrocardiogram reveals the right atrial and ventricular enlargement, as does the chest roentgenogram; right atrial enlargement is often very prominent.

Pulmonic regurgitation also makes the right ventricle dilated and hyperactive, but it rarely affects the right atrium. As a rule, the pulmonic component of the second heart sound is absent. The dominant auscultatory finding is a diastolic murmur that starts after the time of pulmonic valve closure and thus begins after aortic valve closure, with a silent gap between them. In organic pulmonary valve lesions the murmur is often low-pitched and rough, while if the cause is pulmonary hypertension the murmur is usually high-pitched and blowing. The electrocardiogram and chest roentgenogram confirm the right ventricular enlargement, and the chest roentgenogram usually shows a dilated main pulmonary artery.

Mitral Valve Regurgitation

Mitral valve regurgitation is usually acquired, although sometimes it occurs with congenital heart diseases and may even be present at birth. The most common cause is rheumatic fever (p. 384). It also often occurs secondary to dilatation of the mitral valve annulus, with left ventricular failure due to pressure or volume loads or myocardial disease; for example, it may occur with endocardial fibroelastosis, anomalous left coronary artery, asphyxia or hypoglycemia, or severe anemia. The added volume overload may exacerbate the left heart failure, and conversely treatment of the heart failure and the basic lesion may reduce or abolish the mitral regurgitation. Infective endocarditis of the mitral valve may either perforate the valve (thereby producing a peculiar high-pitched murmur, the cooing dove murmur) or rupture chordae tendineae. These may also be ruptured by closed chest trauma or myxomatous degeneration. Similarly, the papillary muscle may become infarcted or may rupture, usually with an anomalous left coronary artery, but at times with a pressure load on the left ventricle or with coronary arterial disease. Acute severe mitral regurgitation is often poorly tolerated, so that medical management is frequently inadequate and surgical repair of the lesion is needed. This may involve an annuloplasty or replacement of the valve.

The mitral valve may degenerate in Marfan's syndrome or Hurler's syndrome or may undergo myxomatous degeneration of unknown origin. If there is a left atrial myxoma, the mass may interfere with mitral valve closure and produce mitral regurgitation that often varies with the position of the patient.

Congenital mitral regurgitation is rare, but it may occur because of the abnormal insertion of short, thick chordae tendineae, accessory commissures, or underdevelopment of the valve leaflets. There may be an isolated cleft of the mitral valve, but more often the cleft valve is part of an endocardial cushion defect; the mitral regurgitation adds to the volume load and may produce an obligatory left-to-right shunt (p. 1406). Another congenital lesion that is often associated with apparent mitral regurgitation is *l*-transposition with ventricular inversion (corrected transposition). In this lesion the left-sided (systemic) valve is the tricuspid valve that often shows Ebstein's anomaly and allows left-sided ventriculoatrial regurgitation.

Mitral regurgitation is an important part of idiopathic hypertrophic subaortic stenosis (p. 1430) in which the septal hypertrophy displaces the papillary muscles of the mitral valve leaflets, thus causing traction on the chordae tendineae and leading to mitral regurgitation. This is common and may even dominate the clinical picture.

Prolapsing Mitral Leaflet Syndrome

Prolapsing mitral leaflet syndrome has variously been termed floppy mitral valve, papillary muscle dysfunction, and mitral valve prolapse–click syndrome. Prolapse of one or both of the mitral valve leaflets during systole has been described as a primary condition, as well as in association with myxomatous degeneration of the mitral valve, Marfan's syndrome, Ehlers-Danlos syndrome, myocardial ischemia, and other congenital heart defects, particularly ostium secundum atrial septal defects. When it is present as an isolated lesion there is familial occurrence of the syndrome with an autosomal dominant form of inheritance and also a 2:1 preponderance in females. Most commonly both leaflets of the mitral valve are involved, and least common is involvement of the anterior leaflet alone.

The symptomatology varies; it may include intermittent chest or epigastric pain, easy fatigability, and palpitations. The origin of the chest pain is unexplained. The auscultatory findings are typical and include a nonejection midsystolic click usually followed by a plateau-type late systolic murmur. However, a click without a late systolic murmur or a pansystolic murmur of mitral regurgitation may occur; a musical apical systolic honking or whooping murmur has also been described. The timing of the click corresponds with the point of maximal leaflet prolapse. Both the click and the murmur may vary with the position of the patient, and they are least likely to be heard in the supine position. The click and murmur occur earlier when ventricular volume is reduced during inspiration, as well as in the sitting or erect position, during the Valsalva maneuver, and following inhalation of amyl nitrite. With each of these maneuvers the systolic murmur may become longer but not louder. The opposite happens with squatting: the click is delayed and the systolic murmur shortened. Typical electrocardiographic findings are flattened or inverted T waves in leads II, III, and aVf and the left precordial leads associated generally with S-T depression. T wave inversions in the right precordial leads are more commonly associated with prolapse of both mitral valve leaflets. Premature ventricular contractions are common in these patients, and multiple premature ventricular contractions and even ventricular tachycardia have been reported, especially with exercise. The chest roentgenogram is generally normal. The definitive diagnosis is made either by echocardiography (p. 1377) or by cineangiocardiography at the time of cardiac catheterization. The amount of mitral regurgitation associated with this condition is not usually severe, and surgical correction is not generally indicated. The association with ventricular arrhythmias may lead to subsequent sudden death; however, this is relatively uncommon. Multiple premature ventricular beats should be treated. Prophylaxis against infective endocarditis should be given.

Aortic Root Regurgitation

AORTIC VALVE ABNORMALITIES. A high proportion of patients with valvar aortic stenosis, bicuspid aortic valve, or discrete subaortic stenosis have a minor degree or occasionally an even more significant degree of aortic regurgitation. This may be due to deformity of the valve, or it may follow an episode of infective endocarditis. With a ventricular septal defect, usually the subpulmonic type, muscular support of the normal aortic cusps is often defective, leading to herniation of the right aortic leaflet into the ventricular septal defect. This is progressive and may lead to significant regurgitation. Although it is not strictly aortic valve regurgitation, a moderate degree of truncal regurgitation is fairly common in truncus arteriosus (p. 1465). The murmur is indistinguishable from that of either aortic or pulmonic regurgitation.

SINUS OF VALSALVA ABNORMALITIES. Acute rupture of a sinus of Valsalva generally occurs into the right atrium or right ventricle (p. 1413). However, occasionally rupture may occur into the left ventricle and produce aortic regurgitation. The onset is generally sudden and is usually associated with chest pain and dyspnea. The clinical features are very similar to those of aortic regurgitation; however, a continuous murmur may be heard.

An aneurysm of a sinus of Valsalva without rupture may occur as an isolated lesion, but it is more common in Marfan's syndrome, where there is dilatation of the aortic root. The aortic valve cusp may progressively prolapse, leading eventually to complete disruption of the sinus of Valsalva with severe regurgitation. Acute rupture of the aneurysm or infective endocarditis may also produce regurgitation. Occasionally a tunnel occurs through the muscular portion of the left ventricular outflow region connecting the left ventricular cavity and the aortic root. Both an ejection systolic murmur and a regurgitant diastolic murmur may be present. The diagnosis is by angiography.

Tricuspid Valve Regurgitation

Tricuspid valve regurgitation is common secondary to right ventricular dilatation in many lesions, both congenital and acquired. It is also becoming common for the tricuspid valve to be damaged by infective endocarditis; this may occur even with normal valves in addicts who get intravenous injections of contaminated drugs. A rare cause of acquired tricuspid regurgitation is the carcinoid syndrome.

Tricuspid regurgitation may also occur as part of several congenital lesions. It is relatively common in Ebstein's anomaly (p. 1455). The amount of tricuspid valve regurgitation will depend on the magnitude of malformation and displacement of the tricuspid valve. In the newborn period the usual presentation is that of cyanosis with cardiac enlargement and a murmur of tricuspid regurgitation. However, the presenting signs may be those of tricuspid regurgitation alone. A triple or quadruple rhythm is often present, and a mid-diastolic rumble may be heard at the lower left sternal border. There is an increased incidence of Ebstein's malformation following administration of lithium carbonate for depression during pregnancy.

The tricuspid valve annulus is usually hypoplastic when there is a hypoplastic right ventricle, but at times the formation of the valve may be abnormal and significant tricuspid regurgitation may occur. This is particularly true in pulmonic atresia with an intact interventricular septum (p. 1454). Occasionally the tricuspid valve annulus is normally situated, but the valve leaflets do not form, and only a rim of valve tissue is present. This condition, termed the unguarded tricuspid valve, presents in infancy and may produce right heart failure in utero. It is also frequently associated with atrial arrhythmias.

Isolated congenital tricuspid regurgitation is rare; it may be produced by abnormal chordae tendineae or by an isolated cleft in the tricuspid valve. More commonly a cleft tricuspid valve is associated with an endocardial cushion defect, and the tricuspid regurgitation complicates the left-to-right shunting.

Pulmonic Valve Regurgitation

PULMONARY HYPERTENSION. Pulmonary hypertension, particularly when associated with a dilated main pulmonary artery, may produce varying degrees of pulmonic regurgitation. In the immediate neonatal period pulmonary disease or persistent pulmonary hypertension of the newborn may be associated with pulmonic valve regurgitation, as well as secondary right ventricular dilatation and tricuspid regurgitation. The occurrence of pulmonic valve regurgitation in pulmonary hypertension secondary to pulmonary vascular disease is discussed elsewhere (p. 1439).

ABSENT PULMONIC VALVE. Absent pulmonic valve, a relatively rare condition, is usually associated with a ventricular septal defect and infundibular pulmonic stenosis. The main pulmonary artery and its main branches are generally markedly dilated. The clinical presentation may be that of congestive heart failure or occasionally obstruction of the major upper airways by the enormously dilated main and branch pulmonary arteries. A characteristic rough to-and-fro murmur, described as a sawing-wood murmur, is heard best at the upper left sternal border and is widely transmitted throughout the chest. Occasionally an ejection systolic click is heard; the second sound is single. Inspiratory and expiratory wheezes are often present, and they probably represent obstruction due to compression of the mainstem bronchi by a markedly dilated pulmonary artery. The chest roentgenogram usually shows the enormously dilated pulmonary artery and often severe cardiomegaly. The diagnosis is confirmed by cardiac catheterization and cineangiocardiography. If congestive failure and cyanosis are severe and persistent and the airway obstruction produces major problems, correction of this lesion with insertion of a unicusp valve may produce significant improvement.

OTHER CAUSES.   Isolated congenital incompetence of the pulmonic valve is very uncommon. Rarely a bicuspid pulmonic valve or idiopathic dilatation of the main pulmonary artery may produce significant pulmonic regurgitation. Dilatation of the main pulmonary artery due to valvar pulmonic stenosis is occasionally accompanied by moderate pulmonic regurgitation. More often, pulmonic regurgitation occurs after surgical valvotomy for valvar pulmonic stenosis or after surgical repair of a tetralogy of Fallot.

References

Barlow JB, Pocock WA: The problem of nonejection systolic clicks and associated mitral systolic murmurs: emphasis on the billowing mitral leaflet syndrome. Am Heart J 90:636, 1975

Benzing G III, Schubert W, Hug G, Kaplan S: Simultaneous hypoglycemia and acute congestive heart failure. Circulation 40:209, 1969

Brown OW, De Mots H, Kloster FE, Roberts A, Menashe VD, Beals RK: Aortic root dilatation and mitral valve prolapse in Marfan's syndrome: an echocardiographic study. Circulation 52:651, 1975

Dimich I, Steinfeld L, Litwak RS, Park S, Silvers N: Subpulmonic ventricular septal defect associated with aortic insufficiency. Am J Cardiol 32:325, 1973

Jeresaty RM: Mitral valve prolapse–click syndrome. Prog Cardiovasc Dis 6:623, 1973

Krovetz LJ, Schiebler GL: Cardiovascular manifestations of the genetic mucopolysaccharidoses. Birth Defects 8:192, 1972

Lakier JB, Stanger P, Heymann MA, Hoffman JIE, Rudolph AM: Tetralogy of Fallot with absent pulmonary valve: natural history and hemodynamic considerations. Circulation 50:167, 1974

Nutter DO, Wickliffe C, Gilbert CA, Moody C, King SB: The pathophysiology of idiopathic mitral valve prolapse. Circulation 52:297, 1975

OBSTRUCTIVE LESIONS

MICHAEL A. HEYMANN

General Features

Obstruction to flow due to a congenital abnormality may occur in any part of the pulmonary and systemic vascular systems. However, certain sites are more commonly affected than others, particularly the outflow tracts of each ventricle. The obstruction may be so mild as to produce no significant hemodynamic effects but may still cause certain clinical findings, or else cause total obstruction to flow. Mild or moderate obstruction is called stenosis, whereas complete obstruction is termed atresia. Atresia may occur at either atrioventricular valve, in a semilunar valve, or in the aortic arch. With atresia, blood is diverted from its normal pattern of flow through abnormal pathways in order to maintain systemic or pulmonary blood flow. Since most of these complex lesions involve complete admixture of pulmonary and systemic venous returns, and thus produce

both right-to-left and left-to-right shunting, they will be considered in the section on cyanotic congenital heart disease (p. 1441). When the obstruction is incomplete, blood flow is largely maintained through normal pathways, and the basic anatomy is unaltered. However, in order to maintain a normal output through the area of stenosis, an unusually high pressure proximal to the obstruction is required, which results in an increased pressure load proximal to the obstruction. For example, narrowing of the aorta will produce an increase in left ventricular systolic pressure; with severe obstruction, left ventricular end-diastolic pressure will rise. Left atrial pressure and pulmonary venous pressure will then increase, and pulmonary edema may occur. This then will cause pulmonary hypertension and right ventricular failure, with an increase in systemic venous pressure. Associated with the increased pressure, the chamber of the heart involved will dilate and eventually hypertrophy in order to maintain the pressure load. If this cannot be accomplished, cardiac failure will occur and cardiac output and arterial blood pressure will fall. It is important to remember that although the foramen ovale is functionally closed soon after birth, it may allow shunting between the two circulations in either direction if there is an obstruction distal to the foramen ovale.

PHYSIOLOGIC EFFECTS OF PRESSURE OVERLOAD.   LEFT VENTRICLE.   Following acute obstruction of the left ventricle, systolic pressure rises and stroke volume falls, since the left ventricle cannot instantaneously generate adequate energy to increase its pressure sufficiently to overcome the obstruction. Therefore the residual volume of blood in the ventricle at the end of systole is increased. In the next ventricular diastole the left ventricle fills normally from the left atrium, so that at the end of diastole left ventricular volume is greater than in the preceding beat. The muscle fibers are therefore stretched, and the ventricle contracts more forcibly. Diastolic filling of the left ventricle exceeds stroke volume for several beats; thus there is more ventricular dilatation. Within several beats an equilibrium is reached, and a normal stroke volume is ejected at a higher systolic pressure. As ventricular dilatation occurs, there is an increase in wall tension that is reflected by an increased end-diastolic pressure. Since the relationship of end-diastolic pressure and ventricular volume or fiber length is not linear, at lower levels of end-diastolic pressure there is only a small rise in end-diastolic pressure associated with a marked increase in ventricular volume. At higher levels of pressure there is a disproportionately greater increase in end-diastolic pressure for a lesser increase in volume. As an additional response to acute stress, increased sympathetic activity occurs and produces greater contractile force and rate of ejection, thus shortening systole and lowering end-diastolic pressure.

Most obstructive lesions do not occur rapidly, and therefore compensatory myocardial hypertrophy occurs; the increased muscle mass allows increased cardiac work to be performed with little ventricular dilatation and without greatly increased end-diastolic pressures. However, with severe obstruction even these compensatory mechanisms may fail, and the left ventricle will dilate and end-diastolic pressure will increase.

A further important consideration in the response of the myocardium to increased pressure loads is the ability to provide an adequate oxygen supply. The oxygen requirements of the left ventricular myocardium are related to the systolic pressure generated within the ventricle and the duration of systole (the tension–time index or systolic pressure–time index). As mentioned previously (p. 1407), the amount of oxygen supplied to the myocardium is related to the aortic diastolic pressure, the left ventricular diastolic pressure, the duration of diastole, and the oxygen-carrying capacity of blood perfusing the myocardium. It is apparent, therefore, that with a severe obstruction the oxygen requirements will be significantly increased, but the supply of oxygen may be compromised if there is left ventricular failure with an increase in ventricular diastolic pressure and a diastolic duration shortened by the increased duration of systole and/or tachycardia.

LEFT ATRIUM. Obstruction to outflow from the left atrium due either to abnormalities of the mitral valve apparatus or to left ventricular failure will increase atrial pressure in an attempt to overcome the obstruction or to fill a left ventricle that has an increased diastolic pressure. The left atrium will dilate and hypertrophy.

PULMONARY VEINS. Pulmonary venous pressure will increase with an anatomic obstruction to pulmonary venous return or an increase in left atrial pressure from any cause. With this rise in pulmonary venous pressure there will be increased transudation of fluid through the capillary walls into the interstitial lung spaces, from where it will pass into the alveoli or the lymphatics. Should lymphatic drainage be incapable of removing the increased fluid volume, fluid will accumulate in the interstitial spaces and the alveoli. Capillary permeability will determine the amount of fluid leaving the vascular system when venous pressure is raised. It has been suggested that capillary permeability is greater in infants than in adults and that it is even greater in prematures. If this is so, premature infants may get severe pulmonary edema at much lower pulmonary venous pressures. The fluid accumulation in the alveoli will be clinically apparent as rales and may also interfere with gas exchange, particularly of carbon dioxide, resulting in an increased arterial blood carbon dioxide tension. As fluid accumulation progresses there is lymphatic engorgement that on chest roentgenogram is associated with Kerley B lines, fluid in the major fissures, and eventually frank pleural effusion (Fig. 62). In some infants in whom the diagnosis of congenital lymphangiectasis has been made, subsequent autopsy examination has revealed pulmonary venous obstruction, usually associated with total anomalous pulmonary venous connection.

Frequently an increase in pulmonary vascular resistance is associated with an increased pulmonary venous pressure. The suggested mechanisms that might produce this effect include a decrease in oxygen tension to which the resistance vessels are exposed, with resultant pulmonary vascular constriction, and compression of the resistance vessels by edema fluid. With the increase in pulmonary vascular resistance, pulmonary arterial pressure will rise with a subsequent pressure overload on the right ventricle.

RIGHT VENTRICLE. The responses of the right ventricle to an increased afterload for whatever reason are similar to those described for the left ventricle.

RIGHT ATRIUM. Changes in the right atrium are similar to those in the left atrium. When right atrial pressure rises, systemic venous return is obstructed and systemic venous pressure will rise. Peripheral organs, particularly the liver and spleen, will become congested and enlarged and peripheral edema may result.

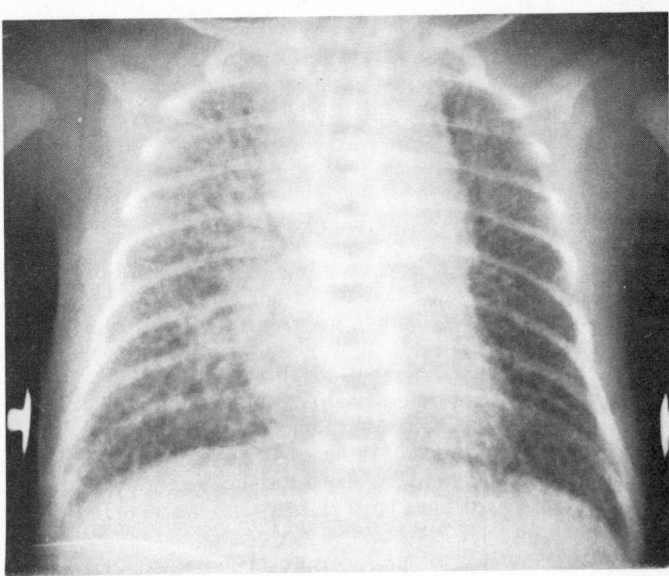

FIG. 62. Pulmonary venous obstruction in an infant with cor triatriatum. Note hazy lung fields obscuring cardiac borders, fluid in horizontal fissure and right pleural cavity, Kerley B lines at bases, and relatively small heart.

CLINICAL FEATURES. The clinical features of pressure overload are determined by the degree and type of compensatory mechanisms invoked. The left ventricular response is manifested by left ventricular hypertrophy, which can be inferred from a slow forceful heave of the left ventricular apex. Hypertrophy by itself does not significantly enlarge the external heart dimensions, for the increased wall thickness may be only a few millimeters; but if there is associated dilatation, the left ventricular apex will be displaced downward and to the left. The heart may or may not show enlargement on a roentgenogram; even if it is not enlarged there may be a slightly more rounded left ventricular contour than is seen normally. There will be no specific changes in the first or second heart sounds, but a third heart sound may appear; if there is systemic hypertension, aortic closure will be loud. Electrocardiography will show increased left inferior and posterior forces. The mean frontal plane QRS axis is normal with pure left ventricular hypertrophy, since an inferiorly placed ventricle with a normal sequence of depolarization does not produce the left superior axis termed left axis deviation.

Left atrial pressure loading may be inferred clinically by hearing a well-marked fourth heart sound, which suggests more forceful contraction by the hypertrophied atrium. Electrocardiographically there may be a widely notched P wave in lead II and in leads V_5 and V_6, and the P wave in V_1 may be enlarged and biphasic or negative. On a chest roentgenogram the typical signs of left atrial dilatation may be seen if the atrium is sufficiently enlarged. An increased pulmonary venous pressure is manifested by change in respiration, which is the cardinal sign of left ventricular failure (p. 1480).

Right ventricular hypertrophy manifests itself by a forceful slow lift felt best along the left sternal border and behind the xiphisternum. If there is associated pulmonary hypertension the pulmonary artery may be felt in systole in the third interspace at the left sternal border, the pulmonic component of the second heart sound will be accentuated, and there may be an ejection systolic click at the base. The right ventricle will appear enlarged on roentgenogram only if dilated; even if the heart is not enlarged the apex may be tipped up. If there is pulmonary hypertension the main pulmonary artery may be enlarged. Electrocardiographically there will be right axis deviation of the mean frontal QRS axis, and the right precordial leads will show tall R waves or perhaps a qR complex; sometimes there may be T wave changes consisting of upright T waves at an age when they should be inverted or deep inversion of the right precordial T waves, described as a strain pattern.

Right atrial pressure loading may reflect itself in a right atrial fourth heart sound, some dilatation of the right atrium on roentgenogram, and tall peaked P waves in leads II and V_1 of the electrocardiogram. Should the systemic venous pressure be elevated, then characteristic enlargement of liver and spleen and edema of the soft tissues may be found. At times the mean venous pressure is not raised, but a large jugular venous *a* wave may be seen.

Raised pulmonary venous pressure is more com-

monly the result of left ventricular failure than of primary obstruction of the left atrium or the pulmonary veins. Similarly, right atrial pressure elevation is usually the result of right ventricular failure. Right ventricular pressure elevation is frequently the result of pulmonary hypertension due to a raised pulmonary venous pressure, which in turn follows left ventricular failure. Since left ventricular pressure overload, as in coarctation of the aorta, can cause a right ventricular pressure overload via a raised pulmonary venous pressure and vascular resistance, it is possible for the clinical picture to be dominated by the right ventricular signs.

Left-sided Obstructive Lesions (Table 7)

PULMONARY VENOUS OBSTRUCTION. Obstruction to pulmonary venous return is generally associated with abnormal connection of the pulmonary veins (p. 1462), although obstruction of normally connected pulmonary veins does occur occasionally. This may be due to external compression by a posterior mediastinal mass or fibrosis or to an intrinsic abnormality in the pulmonary veins. Single or multiple pulmonary veins may be involved. Intrinsic narrowing may be caused by diffuse hypoplasia, by a localized diaphragm, or by narrowing of the pulmonary veins as they enter the left atrium. The clinical presentation includes the signs and symptoms of pulmonary edema and pulmonary hypertension. It can be difficult, particularly in young infants, to differentiate certain forms of chronic pulmonary disease from pulmonary venous obstruction, which should therefore alway be considered if there are refractory pulmonary symptoms and roentgenographic changes.

OBSTRUCTION WITHIN LEFT ATRIUM. *Cor triatriatum* occurs when failure of resorption of the com-

TABLE 7. Classification of Left-sided Obstructive Lesions

Pulmonary venous obstruction
Obstruction within the left atrium
    Cor triatriatum
    Tumor (myxoma)
    Supravalvar stenosing ring
Mitral valve obstruction
    Atresia
    Stenosis
    Parachute mitral valve
Hypoplastic left ventricle
Left ventricular outflow obstruction
    Valvar aortic stenosis
    Bicuspid aortic valve
    Subaortic stenosis: Diffuse
    (idiopathic hypertrophic
    subaortic stenosis), Discrete
    Supravalvar aortic stenosis
Aortic arch obstruction
    Interruption
    Hypoplasia
    Coarctation
Abdominal coarctation
Peripheral systemic arterial stenosis

mon pulmonary vein results in division of the left atrium into upper and lower chambers. The pulmonary veins drain into the proximal chamber, which communicates through an opening, generally restrictive, with the distal portion of the atrium, which in turn is connected to the atrial appendage and the mitral valve. The clinical presentation is essentially the same as in pulmonary venous obstruction. The diagnosis may be made by echocardiography, which may show a membrane in the left atrial cavity; it may be confirmed by cardiac catheterization and more particularly by angiocardiography. Surgical excision of the obstructing diaphragm is curative. An equally uncommon condition producing obstruction within the left atrium is a *supravalvar stenosing ring* associated with a parachute mitral valve, subaortic stenosis, and coarctation. A tumor within the left atrium, usually a *myxoma*, can also produce obstruction within the left atrial chamber, and it generally mimics mitral stenosis; however, since the tumor is often on a pedicle, the obstruction to the mitral valve orifice (and hence the clinical features) may be intermittent.

MITRAL VALVE OBSTRUCTION. The most severe form of mitral valve obstruction is mitral atresia, which is discussed in the section on cyanotic congenital heart disease (p. 1467). Congenital mitral stenosis may occur as an isolated defect or may be associated with other abnormalities such as an atrial or ventricular septal defect, aortic stenosis, coarctation of the aorta, or endocardial fibroelastosis. Congenital malformations of the mitral valve may produce grossly abnormal valve cusps or a valve that appears normal but has fused commissures. Parachute mitral valve, in which the chordae tendineae are all attached to a single papillary muscle, also produces obstruction to flow at the mitral valve level. This may occur as an isolated lesion but, as mentioned above, it is more commonly part of a complex group of abnormalities.

The congenital forms of mitral stenosis are generally severe and present in early infancy with symptoms and physical findings of pulmonary edema; if pulmonary hypertension occurs, severe congestive cardiac failure may supervene. The pulmonic component of the second sound is accentuated, its intensity depending on the severity of pulmonary hypertension. A rumbling apical diastolic murmur with presystolic accentuation is usually present; however, with severe cardiac failure the murmur may not be heard, but may become evident when cardiac failure is controlled. Varying degrees of mitral incompetence may be associated with the stenosis, and there may be an apical blowing murmur of mitral insufficiency. An opening snap of the mitral valve may be heard, but it is not common because the valve is very thick and immobile. Tricuspid regurgitation may also be present if there is severe pulmonary hypertension with right ventricular dilatation. On the electrocardiogram the P waves are broad and notched, suggesting left atrial enlargement, and right ventricular hypertrophy may be present. The chest roentgenogram will show only moderate enlargement of the cardiac silhouette caused by left atrial and possibly right ventricular enlargement. The pulmonary vascular markings will

depend on the severity of obstruction. The specific diagnosis may be made by echocardiography (p. 1376) and should be confirmed by cardiac catheterization and angiocardiography. Medical treatment of severe congenital mitral stenosis with intractable heart failure in infancy and early childhood is usually unsuccessful. Surgical management, because of the marked thickening and deformity of the mitral valve, generally requires the insertion of a prosthetic valve. The prosthetic valve has a limited effective life and repeated insertions may be necessary to adjust for increased flow requirements associated with growth.

HYPOPLASTIC LEFT VENTRICLE. Hypoplastic left ventricle is associated with mitral and aortic atresia, and the left ventricular cavity is a minute slit. There are forms of this defect with severe mitral and aortic stenosis in which the left ventricular cavity is very small. These infants usually present with the features of severe aortic stenosis and succumb within a few weeks.

LEFT VENTRICULAR OUTFLOW OBSTRUCTION. Several congenital cardiovascular malformations produce obstruction to the ejection of blood from the left ventricle. The most common of these is an abnormality of the aortic valve cusps themselves; however, the left ventricular outflow tract may be obstructed by an abnormally situated mitral valve leaflet or papillary muscle, by muscular hypertrophy of the ventricular septum, by a subvalvar fibrous ring, by a thin subvalvar membrane with a small orifice, or by supravalvar aortic narrowing. Since valvar aortic stenosis is the most common form of aortic stenosis, it will be described in detail, and differences associated with other forms of left ventricular outflow tract obstruction will be pointed out.

VALVAR AORTIC STENOSIS. It is rare for congenitally stenotic aortic valves to have three normal leaflets with fusion at the commissures. About 85 percent have bicuspid aortic valves with one small and one large cusp and an eccentric fish-mouth orifice between them. Another 14 percent have no obvious separation into leaflets, so that there is in effect a thick monocusp with an eccentric orifice shaped like a teardrop. The obstruction is due in part to the small orifice left by commissural fusion and in part to thickening and lack of mobility of the valve.

Somatic development is usually normal at the time of birth. If the stenosis has been severe in utero, then blood will have been diverted from the left ventricle, so that it and the ascending aorta are hypoplastic. Because of the high left ventricular pressure, there may be marked endocardial thickening (secondary endocardial fibroelastosis) that probably further impairs left ventricular performance.

PATHOPHYSIOLOGY. With a high systolic pressure and hypertrophy, the left ventricle needs more oxygen and coronary blood flow. If aortic pressure, particularly diastolic pressure, is low and diastole is short, subendocardial blood flow may be inadequate, and subendocardial ischemia may result. This explains the subendocardial necrosis and fibrosis often noted with severe aortic stenosis in infancy. It also explains why exercise in moderately severe aortic stenosis may cause anginal pain and S-T depression or T wave inversion in the left ventricular electrocardiographic leads. Ischemia or ischemic damage may also be responsible for the occasional occurrence of sudden death, almost certainly due to ventricular fibrillation. One other symptom of aortic stenosis is syncope, usually following exertion or prolonged periods of standing. Lesser degrees of stenosis cause left ventricular hypertrophy with no evidence of ischemia at rest or exercise, while the mildest stenotic lesions produce only a murmur with no left ventricular hypertrophy.

After birth, in an infant with severe aortic stenosis, an important factor determining the infant's ability to maintain systemic output is competency of the foramen ovale. If left atrial pressure can rise, left ventricular output will be better maintained due to the higher atrial filling pressure. However, if, as often happens, a left-to-right atrial shunt develops through a large interatrial communication, left atrial pressure may not be sufficient to fill the left ventricle adequately, and left ventricular output cannot be maintained. In either circumstance left ventricular dilatation may be marked, and left ventricular failure occurs. Infants with less severe aortic stenosis are generally capable of maintaining cardiac output and of developing adequate hypertrophy to overcome the effects of the obstruction.

The natural history of aortic stenosis in older infants and children has not been delineated. However, there is evidence that congenital aortic stenosis is usually a progressive disease. As the child grows and cardiac output increases, the valve orifice may not keep pace with increased cardiac output requirements; thus the obstruction becomes relatively more severe, and the pressure difference between the aorta and left ventricle increases. For this reason rapid changes in the severity of aortic stenosis may occur with rapid growth spurts.

CLINICAL FEATURES.   Severe aortic stenosis generally presents in the immediate postnatal period. The physical findings are those of a systolic murmur of variable intensity, depending on the left ventricular output. This systolic murmur is often best heard at the mid-left sternal border in infants; it can be confused with the murmur of ventricular septal defect. If cardiac output is greatly reduced, the murmur may be very soft or may be absent. An ejection click is common. Peripheral perfusion and pulses depend on the degree of failure, but they are generally decreased. Evidence of significant atrial left-to-right shunting with right ventricular hyperactivity is often present. A chest roentgenogram generally shows marked cardiomegaly with severe pulmonary venous congestion. The electrocardiogram is variable, but in many instances it shows increased right ventricular forces; increased left ventricular forces are rarely present in the newborn period. An echocardiogram may show the abnormal aortic valve (p. 1375) and usually demonstrates a dilated, poorly contractile left ventricle.

In older children with aortic stenosis the murmur usually draws attention to the congenital defect. Chest or epigastric pain or syncopal episodes are generally associated with more severe degrees of stenosis and are uncommon presenting symptoms. They may, however, develop in a child who is known to have aortic stenosis and may indicate progression in severity of the stenosis. Many of the physical findings of aortic stenosis correlate roughly with the severity of the stenosis. Left ventricular hypertrophy results in an increased apical impulse. If there has been long-standing severe obstruction from infancy, a left precordial bulge and an apical impulse in the left anterior axillary line may be evident. In children with moderately severe stenosis the systemic arterial pulse is usually normal. In adults, as the stenosis becomes more severe the upstroke of the pulse is slowed and pulse volume is decreased; this sign is uncommon in children, even those with moderately severe stenosis. The first heart sound may be normal or may be soft in severe stenosis, and commonly a systolic ejection click is heard along the left sternal border. Some of the typical auscultatory findings are presented diagrammatically in Figure 63. Due to prolonged left ventricular ejection, the aortic component of the second heart sound is delayed, and the splitting of the second sound therefore narrows. The aortic component is also generally softer than normal. In more severe stenosis, left ventricular ejection is prolonged even more, and the splitting of the second sound may disappear because of superimposition of the aortic and pulmonic components. As severity increases, the aortic component may even follow the pulmonic component, so that the second sound narrows with inspiration and widens with expiration (paradoxic splitting). A prominent apical third sound is frequently heard, and in severe stenosis a fourth sound may also be present. A loud crescendo–decrescendo systolic murmur, generally grade 4-5 in intensity and often associated with a thrill, is characteristic of aortic stenosis. The murmur starts with the first sound and reaches peak intensity early in systole in mild stenosis and later in systole in more severe stenosis. The murmur is usually best heard at the upper right sternal border, and it radiates well into the suprasternal notch and into the neck; but sometimes it is better heard at the upper left sternal border or even the apex. A

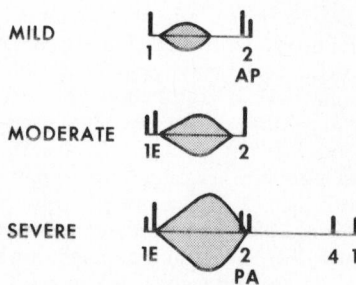

VALVAR AORTIC STENOSIS

FIG. 63.   Diagrammatic representation of the auscultatory findings in valvar aortic stenosis. 1, first heart sound; E, systolic ejection click; 2, second heart sound; A, aortic component of second heart sound; P, pulmonic component of second heart sound; 4, fourth heart sound.

short grade 2-3/6 decrescendo blowing regurgitant murmur occasionally may be heard at the mid-left sternal border.

The electrocardiogram may show left ventricular hypertrophy, but this is a poor index of the severity of the stenosis. T wave flattening or inversion and S-T segment depression in left ventricular precordial leads indicate severe aortic outflow obstruction; these changes may not be present at rest, but may be brought out by graded exercise. The chest roentgenogram occasionally shows left ventricular enlargement, but more often the only abnormal finding is poststenotic dilatation of the ascending aorta (Fig. 64).

It is important to realize that symptoms, physical findings, chest roentgenograms, and electrocardiograms are not reliable in predicting the severity of aortic stenosis. Children with severe stenosis and a large pressure difference between the aorta and the left ventricle may have a benign course and no evidence or minimal evidence of left ventricular stress, whereas some children with only moderately large pressure differences may have more significant physical findings. It is for this reason, and because of the fact that sudden death may occur in children with relatively minor physical findings, that the pressure difference between the aorta and left ventricle and the hemodynamic status should be evaluated by cardiac catheterization.

Cardiac catheterization is mandatory in any child with aortic stenosis who has symptoms, congestive heart failure, or electrocardiographic changes of left ventricular hypertrophy, regardless of whether they are associated with S-T segment and T wave changes. If there is a loud murmur and no evidence of left ventricular hypertrophy, then electrocardiograms should be taken on exercise. S-T segment and T wave changes suggest that the stenosis is severe, and cardiac catheterization is definitely indicated. In patients with a loud systolic mur-

mur, but with a normal electrocardiogram, we strongly recommend cardiac catheterization, since stenosis that is considered severe enough to require surgery may not produce electrocardiographic changes. In a child with a soft systolic ejection murmur and a normal electrocardiogram at rest and during exercise, cardiac catheterization may be delayed, but careful reappraisal of the electrocardiogram, chest roentgenogram, and clinical picture should be made at least annually.

TREATMENT.   Surgery is indicated whenever there is evidence of myocardial ischemia or when there is a very small aortic valve orifice. A valve area of less than 0.65 cm^2/m^2 body surface area is usually associated with a peak systolic pressure drop from left ventricle to aorta of about 70 mm Hg or more, provided that there is a normal cardiac output; this is considered an indication for surgery in most centers. In children, surgery is usually palliative; the valve commissure can be opened to reduce the obstruction, but the surgeon usually does not open the valve orifice up maximally because that might produce massive aortic incompetence. Palliative surgery is life-saving and may produce a good functional result that will last for many years. However, there is a high incidence of restenosis often associated with calcification, and eventually most patients with severe aortic valve stenosis may require valve replacement; if possible, this should be deferred until the patient is fully grown, in order to avoid having to change the valve because of the demands of growth.

BICUSPID AORTIC VALVE. Bicuspid aortic valve is very common; it is estimated to be present in 2 to 3 percent of the population. There is an asymmetric orifice, and the valve may not open fully in systole, but there need not be any obstruction to left ventricular ejection. Bicuspid valves are found in 45 to 75 percent of patients with coarctation of the aorta, but more often they are isolated anomalies. Sometimes they are as-

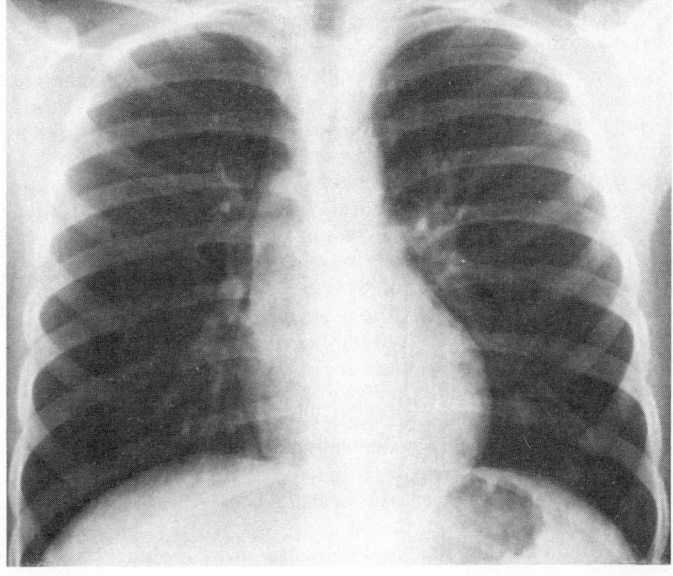

FIG. 64. Chest roentgenogram in a child with valvar aortic stenosis. Dilatation of the ascending aorta at the right upper mediastinum is shown.

sociated with a grade 2-3/6 systolic ejection murmur and click at the right upper sternal border, but often they are not clinically apparent. The diagnosis often may be made by echocardiography (p. 1375).

The importance of bicuspid aortic valves is that they may produce aortic stenosis in later life; middle-aged adults with calcific aortic stenosis usually have congenitally biscuspid aortic valves. The likelihood of late development of calcific aortic stenosis is uncertain, but preliminary data suggest that it may occur in many people with biscuspid aortic valves. Occasionally bicuspid aortic valves are the seat of infective endocarditis; thus if bicuspid aortic valves are diagnosed, suitable prophylaxis against infective endocarditis should be given (p. 1471).

SUBVALVAR AORTIC STENOSIS. Subvalvar aortic stenosis may be due to either a thin membranous diaphragm or a thick fibromuscular obstruction. The aortic valve itself may be thickened and distorted by the high-velocity jet stream passing through the subaortic obstruction. The clinical features are similar to those observed in patients with valvar aortic stenosis, and there are no reliable clinical criteria to differentiate valvar from subvalvar obstruction. However, in the discrete form of subvalvar stenosis a systolic ejection click is heard less commonly, a diastolic regurgitant murmur is heard more commonly, and aortic dilatation (although present in many patients with subaortic stenosis) is less marked than in patients with valvar aortic stenosis. Echocardiography may also be useful (p. 1375). Differentiation between valvar and subvalvar aortic stenosis by cardiac catheterization and angiocardiography is important, since a subvalvar diaphragm is readily removed at surgery with good results. Some children may have subvalvar obstruction from an abnormally placed papillary muscle and displaced mitral valve. This is much more difficult to alleviate surgically, and it may be complicated by mitral regurgitation.

DIFFUSE SUBAORTIC OBSTRUCTION. Diffuse subaortic left ventricular outflow obstruction may be associated with any cause of diffuse hypertrophy of the left ventricle. It occurs in association with valvar aortic stenosis and with certain types of cardiomyopathy such as glycogen storage disease. The most common form, however, is idiopathic. This entity has been called idiopathic hypertrophic subaortic stenosis (IHSS), hypertrophic obstructive cardiomyopathy (HOCM), and asymmetric septal hypertrophy (ASH). The disease is transmitted as a mendelian dominant with variable expression and is usually seen in more than one member of a family. In some families there is a tendency to ventricular arrhythmias and less severe outflow tract obstruction, while in others there is severe obstruction. Many of the physical findings are similar to those in valvar aortic stenosis, but there are certain features that usually distinguish them. A double or triple apical impulse, described as a precordial ripple, is often seen or palpated. The first heart sound may be normal or decreased; systolic clicks are rarely heard. A delayed-onset crescendo–decrescendo systolic murmur, usually of grade 2-4/6 intensity, may best be heard at the middle left to upper right sternal border, and a systolic thrill may be palpable. In some children there is moderate to marked mitral incompetence as well. The second heart sound may be narrow or even paradoxically split. Third and fourth heart sounds are commonly present; diastolic murmurs are unusual. The pulses are unusual in that there is a fast rise, and a bifid carotid pulse may be palpable. Maneuvers that reduce venous return, such as the Valsalva maneuver or assuming an erect posture, often are associated with an increase in the intensity of the systolic murmur; this is explained by a decrease in left ventricular size, with exaggeration of the stenosis. If the patient squats, thereby increasing venous return and peripheral vascular resistance, the murmur decreases in intensity, probably as a result of left ventricular dilatation. All these maneuvers tend to produce opposite effects in valvar aortic stenosis. The chest roentgenogram shows left ventricular enlargement without dilatation of the ascending aorta. The electrocardiogram is also variable, but with severe or moderately severe hypertrophy there are markedly increased left ventricular forces often associated with S-T segment depression and T wave flattening or inversion in the left precordial leads. Deep Q waves in the left precordial leads indicative of septal hypertrophy are more evident than in valvar aortic stenosis. The echocardiogram has been of great help in diagnosing this lesion. It demonstrates the asymmetric septal hypertrophy, and during systole it usually shows anterior movement of the mitral valve, which touches the septum and in part causes the outflow tract obstruction (p. 1376).

The results of treatment in this condition have been variable. Some children respond fairly satisfactorily to administration of β-adrenergic receptor blockers; however, this is generally of only temporary benefit. Surgical excision of the hypertrophied muscle has produced variable results; some children have shown marked improvement, whereas others have not.

SUPRAVALVAR AORTIC STENOSIS. Supravalvar aortic stenosis is a localized or diffuse narrowing that generally occurs in the aorta just above the level of the coronary arteries and the superior annular margin of the sinuses of Valsalva. The coronary arteries usually arise proximal to the obstruction, and after long-term obstruction they become tortuous with thickened medial and intimal layers. Although supravalvar aortic stenosis may occur as an isolated lesion, it is found most commonly in association with idiopathic infantile hypercalcemia (p. 252). In this condition there are mental retardation, peculiar facies, and narrowings of peripheral systemic and pulmonary arteries. The clinical features are generally those of the syndrome of idiopathic infantile hypercalcemia, and the facies and dental development are fairly typical (p. 252). On auscultation the aortic closure sound is frequently accentuated; an ejection click is unusual, and the systolic murmur is best heard at the base and toward the neck. If peripheral pulmonic stenosis is associated, a continuous murmur may be heard in the lateral regions of the chest. Systolic pressure in the right arm is generally higher than that in the left. The chest roentgenogram generally does not show poststenotic dilatation of the ascending aorta. The electrocardiogram shows left ventricular hypertrophy as well as T wave inversion in left chest leads if there is severe stenosis. Echocardiography may demonstrate the supravalvar narrowing (p. 1376). Confirmation of the diagnosis and its severity is best obtained by cardiac catheterization and angiography. If obstruction is severe, the diffuse narrowing can be relieved surgically.

Aortic Arch Obstruction

Obstructive lesions of the aortic arch or proximal portion of the descending aorta may be subdivided into two major groups: diffuse narrowing or interruption of a portion of the aortic arch and localized narrowing, closely related to the attachment of the ductus arteriosus with the aorta; this latter lesion may be associated with a normally developed aortic arch (coarctation of the aorta).

HYPOPLASIA OR INTERRUPTION. In normal fetal life the aortic isthmus (the portion of aorta between the origin of the left subclavian artery and the ductus attachment) conducts only about 10 to 12 percent of the combined output of both the left and right ventricles. This probably accounts for the fact that the aortic isthmus is normally narrower than the descending aorta. In normal full-term infants the diameter of the aortic isthmus is about three-fourths that of the descending aorta; this difference usually disappears by about 6 months of age. Angiographic evidence of a moderate degree of narrowing of the aortic isthmus relative to the ascending or descending aorta in newborns is therefore a normal finding.

Pathologic hypoplasia of the aortic arch (previously called preductal or infantile coarctation) is noted most commonly in the aortic isthmus, but it may occur in other parts of the aortic arch. The most severe form of this lesion is complete interruption of the aortic arch. With rare exceptions, infants with aortic arch interruption of hypoplasia have associated major congenital cardiac defects (for example, a large ventricular septal defect, double-outlet right ventricle, Taussig-Bing anomaly, tricuspid atresia with aortopulmonary transposition, or endocardial cushion defect). In addition, during the newborn period the ductus arteriosus is invariably patent. The reason for these associations is that aortic outflow obstruction associated with these intracardiac lesions may lead to diversion of flow during fetal life, with a consequent reduction in the growth of the aortic arch (p. 1405). The clinical course in infants with these lesions will be dictated by the associated lesions (usually a ventricular septal defect with or without other complicating defects), by the magnitude of right-to-left flow across the ductus arteriosus, and by the degree of obstruction of the aorta.

With complete interruption, descending aortic blood flow is provided only by shunting through the ductus arteriosus. In hypoplasia of the arch, some of the descending aortic blood flow will pass through the aortic arch, the amount depending on the severity of the obstruction and the ability of the left ventricle to overcome the increased afterload. Since there is generally a significant left-to-right shunt across a ventricular septal defect, the normal postnatal fall in pulmonary vascular resistance usually is delayed. Therefore right-to-left shunting into the descending aorta through the patent ductus arteriosus provides descending aortic blood flow and pressure. The magnitude of descending aortic flow therefore depends on the degree of constriction of the ductus arteriosus and the relationship between pulmonary and systemic vascular resistances. Initially, while the ductus arteriosus is well dilated, there may be no arterial blood pressure difference between the upper and lower body. Cyanosis of the toes and feet with normal color of the fingers and hands may be present because of the right-to-left shunt at the ductus arteriosus level. However, with progressive constriction of the ductus arteriosus, the lower body arterial blood pressure falls, and its pulse pressure narrows. The progressive fall in pulmonary vascular resistance after birth will further interfere with the flow of blood across the ductus arteriosus, since flow will preferentially go through the pulmonary circulation rather than to the lower body. Left ventricular myocardial performance, already affected by the increased afterload, is further stressed by this volume load, so that there may be severe left ventricular failure. The time course of these changes is variable. As perfusion to the lower body further decreases, metabolic acidemia may develop, and there may be oliguria or anuria related to inadequate renal blood flow. As the ductus arteriosus constricts, right ventricular failure may also supervene.

In many infants the clinical presentation of these lesions is that of a large left-to-right intracardiac shunt with left-sided failure. In some of these the hypoplasia is not severe, and the arch anomaly is only of secondary importance. In others the arch may be severely hypoplastic or even interrupted, and the diagnosis of aortic arch narrowing or interruption may be made only at the time of cardiac catheterization.

Infants with aortic arch narrowing and an associated intracardiac lesion may respond to medical management. However, surgical repair is indicated if the narrowing is severe or the arch is interrupted. At the time of correction of the aortic arch anomaly, surgical measures to correct or palliate the intracardiac lesion may be necessary.

LOCALIZED JUXTADUCTAL COARCTATION OF AORTA. Several terms, such as postductal or adult-type coarctation, have been applied to this lesion. However, it has become apparent that localized narrowing of the aorta (coarctation of the aorta) is always closely related to the insertion of the ductus arteriosus into the aorta; in fact, the posterolateral shelf that forms the localized narrowing is generally directly opposite the ductus arteriosus. For this reason the term juxtaductal aortic coarctation seems more appropriate. With closure of the ductus arteriosus and growth of the child, the usual concentric obstruction seen in older children and young adults will develop. Unlike the situation with hypoplastic aortic arches, major intracardiac anomalies are not commonly found with isolated coarctation of the aorta; however, there is a high association of this lesion with Turner's syndrome and with bicuspid aortic valve. Other associated abnormalities include aberrant origins of the subclavian arteries, ventricular septal defect, persistent patency of ductus arteriosus, and the group of defects associated with parachute mitral valve (p. 1427). A higher than normal incidence of berry aneurysms of the circle of Willis has also been reported with coarctation of the aorta.

Since the ductus arteriosus is widely patent during fetal life, localized juxtaductal coarctation is unlikely to produce significant alteration in the distribution of blood flow during fetal life, and fetal development is normal. However, in the postnatal period the ductus arteriosus plays an important role in the pathophysiology of juxtaductal coarctation of the aorta. Normally after birth the ductus arteriosus constricts at its pulmonary artery end first, so that although it is functionally closed, an aortic ampulla of the ductus arteriosus persists for several days to several months. There is generally a progressive reduction in the size of the ampulla as the ductus arteriosus constricts progressively toward its aortic end. If there is a juxtaductal aortic coarctation directly opposite the aortic end of the ductus arteriosus, the rapidity of constriction of the ductus arteriosus will significantly affect the clinical presentation during infancy. If the aortic ampulla remains moderately large, flow from the ascending aorta to the descending aorta will not be impeded by the posterolateral shelf, and there will be no clinical evidence of the coarctation. However, as the aortic end of the ductus arteriosus constricts, blood flow will become obstructed. If the posterolateral shelf is large and obstruction develops rapidly, a sudden increase in afterload to the left ventricle will cause left ventricular failure. In this circumstance the clinical presentation is often similar to that of severe aortic stenosis in the neonatal period. Significant left-to-right atrial shunting may occur through a stretched foramen ovale, and when there is severe left ventricular failure all pulses may be weak. However, with improvement in left ventricular function, a significant pressure difference develops between the arms and the legs. Since there has been no obstruction during fetal life and failure has occurred rapidly, collateral circulation is not usually well developed in the newborn. Specific murmurs are not a feature of this lesion in infancy; however, if the ductus arteriosus is still patent, a continuous murmur may be heard at the upper left sternal border. As with aortic stenosis in infancy, the electrocardiogram characteristically shows right axis deviation and right ventricular hypertrophy. The chest roentgenogram shows marked generalized cardiomegaly with pulmonary venous congestion secondary to left ventricular failure. In general, infants who have rapidly developed severe congestive failure due to a coarctation in the neonatal period respond poorly to medical treatment, and surgical excision of the coarctation is frequently required. However, some infants do improve, and their course will be similar to that of the following group.

If the aortic shelf is not very prominent or the ampulla of the ductus arteriosus occludes gradually, aortic obstruction will develop slowly over several weeks or months. Rapid left ventricular failure is less likely, since compensatory mechanisms such as myocardial hypertrophy and development of collateral circulation have time to occur. Collateral anastomoses generally involve the periscapular, intercostal, transverse cervical, and internal mammary arteries. If there are large collateral vessels, only minor pressure differences may be apparent between the ascending and descending aorta at rest; larger differences may be brought out by exercise. Cardiac failure may appear at 3 to 6 months of age as the coarctation becomes more severe. However, if failure does not develop by 6 months of age, it is rare until adult life. In older children the presenting symptoms may be related to significant hypertension in the ascending aorta or to decreased blood flow to the legs during exercise with resultant intermittent claudication. Cerebrovascular accidents associated with hypertension are rare before the age of 7 years. Hypertension in the ascending and descending aorta has been reported in coarctation of the aorta, but the exact mechanism is unclear. Intimal thickening of the coronary arteries may occur. Infective endocarditis is also common with coarctation and most usually involves the aortic wall in the dilated poststenotic segment, but it may occur on the bicuspid aortic valve.

The clinical findings in a child with coarctation of the aorta include easily palpable collateral arteries above the clavicle and over the lateral and inferior scapular margins. The arm pulses are strong, but femoral pulses are decreased and delayed relative to the arm pulses. Since there is a high association of abnormality of one of the subclavian arteries, palpation of both subclavian as well as carotid arteries should be routine. An aberrant right subclavian artery arising below the coarctation gives a low blood pressure in the right arm; the left subclavian artery arises normally, but may be hypoplastic, so that left arm pressures also may be low. Blood pressure measurements in the arm and leg will confirm the palpatory differences. Depending on the severity of the coarctation, the heart may or may not be enlarged and an increased left ventricular impulse palpable. The heart sounds are generally normal; however, with hypertension or an associated bicuspid aortic valve, an ejection systolic click and a third heart sound may be heard. Soft high-frequency continuous murmurs are often audible over the large collateral vessels. A short soft ejection systolic murmur may be heard at the upper sternal area or posteriorly to the left of the spine. The chest roentgenogram (Fig. 65) has several classic features. Cardiac enlargement and left ventricular enlargement depend on the severity of the stenosis. The ascending aorta is often dilated and displaces the superior vena cava to the right. On the left border of the aortic arch and descending aortic shadow the area of poststenotic dilatation below the coarctation and the dilated aortic segment just above the coarctation may be seen as the 3 sign. With barium in the esophagus the dilated and constricted segments may be easily seen on the right aortic margin (the E sign). Notching of the

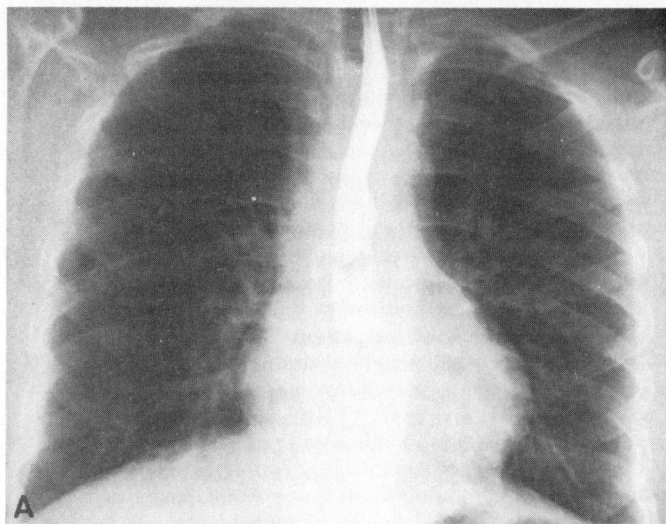

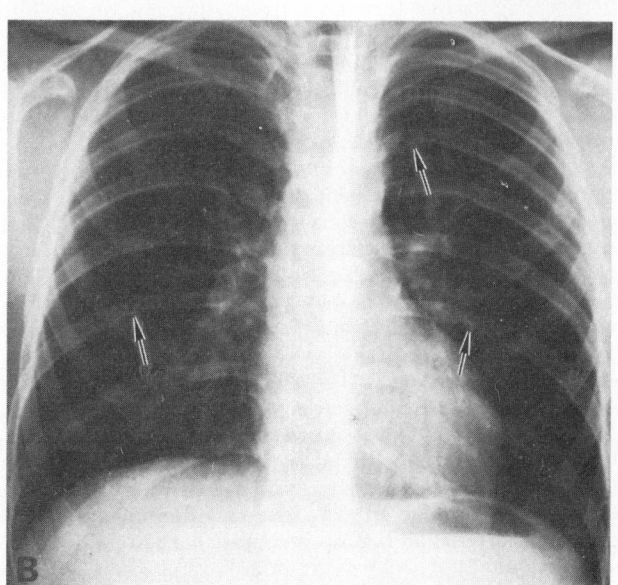

FIG. 65. Chest roentgenograms in 2 children with coarctation of the aorta. The E sign in the barium-filled esophagus and the 3 sign and rib notching are demonstrated.

lower margin of the ribs at about the junction of the middle and medial thirds, due to erosion of the bone by large intercostal arteries, may be seen. The electrocardiogram will demonstrate the degree of left ventricular hypertrophy that has resulted from the obstruction. In older children S-T depression and T wave flattening or inversion in left chest leads may occur.

If the coarctation is not treated, there may be rupture of a berry aneurysm of the circle of Willis, congestive heart failure, infective endocarditis, hypertensive encephalopathy, and also rupture of the aorta; however, the latter has been reported only in adults. For these reasons surgical excision of the coarcted segment with direct anastomosis is recommended. The preferred time for this surgery in children who are asymptomatic used to be 6 to 8 years of age, because even without growth at the site of the suture line the diameter of the aorta is then generally sufficient to provide an adequate channel without significant obstruction even in adults. However, since recoarctation is rare if surgery is done after 2 years of age, many cardiologists now recommend surgery between 2 and 4 years of age to minimize stress on the cardiovascular system.

POSTCOARCTECTOMY SYNDROME. Fever, abdominal pain of varying degree, abdominal distension, nausea, and vomiting may commence 1 to 3 days following surgical repair of aortic coarctation and last for several days. Systemic hypertension is always present. In the most severe forms, infarction of segments of bowel have occurred, but in most children the syndrome is less severe. The exact mechanisms responsible for this complication are unclear. It may be produced by mesenteric arteritis in vessels suddenly perfused with pulsatile flow at pressures higher than those to which they have previously been exposed. The mainstay of treatment is to lower blood pressure with antihypertensive agents.

Other therapy includes fluid and electrolyte maintenance and, if necessary, abdominal decompression by nasogastric suction. Rarely, resection of an infarcted area of bowel becomes necessary.

PSEUDOCOARCTATION.   Increased length of the aortic arch occurs occasionally and causes kinking of the descending thoracic aorta. Murmurs due to turbulent flow across the arch, as well as minor degrees of pressure difference between the arms and the legs, may lead one to suspect a true coarctation of the aorta. The diagnosis is made by cardiac catheterization and angiocardiography. The distal portion of the aortic arch is generally angulated anteriorly in this condition. No specific treatment is usually required although rarely aortic dissection has been reported in adults.

ABDOMINAL COARCTATION.   Obstruction of the lower thoracic or abdominal aorta due to an intrinsic narrowing is considerably less common than the usual form of coarctation of the aorta. Rather than the short segment of constriction seen in juxtaductal coarctation, a long narrow segment is usually present, and one or several major branch arteries of the abdominal aorta usually are involved. The diagnosis is generally suspected when there is a difference between the upper and lower limb pulse volumes and arterial blood pressures without any indication of thoracic collateral arterial circulation or a murmur in the chest. A systolic or continuous murmur is frequently heard over the abdomen and is best heard posteriorly. The diagnosis is confirmed by cardiac catheterization and angiocardiography. Treatment involves surgical removal of the obstructed segment, but this may be difficult, because arterial branches to vital organs may be involved in the coarcted segment.

PERIPHERAL SYSTEMIC ARTERIAL STENOSIS.   Peripheral systemic arterial stenoses may occur in any systemic artery; however, renal artery stenosis is the most common. In the rubella syndrome, peripheral pulmonic stenosis is commonly accompanied by multiple peripheral systemic arterial stenoses, often involving the renal arteries and causing renovascular systemic hypertension.

Right-sided Obstructive Lesions (Table 8)

SYSTEMIC VENOUS OBSTRUCTION.   Obstruction to the superior or inferior vena caval return may be due to an extrinsic lesion such as a mediastinal mass; it may be caused by an intrinsic condition such as thrombosis, or it may occur secondarily to intracardiac surgical procedures such as Mustard's procedure for aortopulmonary transposition. Acute obstruction may present with venous distension and edema of that portion of the body drained by the obstructed vein. However, collateral venous channels generally form rapidly, and these signs soon diminish. Venous collateral channels may be evident superficially. If the inferior vena cava is obstructed above the diaphragm, hepatomegaly that is often severe and splenomegaly may occur.

Congenital interruption of the inferior vena cava occurs commonly in association with cardiac and visceral

TABLE 8. Classification of Right-sided Obstructive Lesions

Systemic venous obstruction
Right atrium
    Tumor (myxoma)
    Thrombus
Tricuspid valve
    Atresia
    Stenosis
Hypoplastic right ventricle
Right ventricular outflow obstruction
    Right ventricular muscle bands
    Subvalvar stenosis: diffuse infundibular, discrete
    Valvar pulmonic stenosis
    Supravalvar pulmonic stenosis
Peripheral pulmonic stenosis
    Single
    Multiple
Pulmonary vascular (arterial) obstruction

malposition. Polysplenia is a common associated finding. Venous drainage is effected through an enlarged azygous system, and there is usually no venous obstruction.

OBSTRUCTION IN RIGHT ATRIUM.   A tumor in the right atrium, generally a myxoma but occasionally an extension of a Wilms' tumor or a hepatic tumor, may produce obstruction to venous return. The clinical presentation usually mimics that of tricuspid stenosis, with intermittent obstruction when there is a myxoma. Right atrial myxomas are far less common than those in the left atrium. Thrombus formation in the right atrium may also produce venous obstruction; this is rare in children.

TRICUSPID VALVE OBSTRUCTION.   The most severe form of tricuspid valve obstruction is tricuspid atresia, which is discussed in the section on cyanotic congenital heart disease (p. 1452). Isolated congenital tricuspid stenosis is rare, and more often underdevelopment of the tricuspid valve and its annulus is associated with underdevelopment of the whole right ventricle. Underdevelopment of the right ventricle (hypoplastic right ventricle) is usually associated with either severe pulmonic stenosis or pulmonary atresia. Whether or not there is an intact ventricular septum, a hypoplastic right ventricle generally presents in infancy with severe cyanosis (p. 1454).

If the interatrial septum is intact, the physical findings of tricuspid stenosis include those of venous obstruction. On auscultation there is usually a mid-diastolic rumbling murmur at the lower left sternal border, a prominent third sound, and in severe stenosis an audible fourth sound. The electrocardiogram may show tall peaked P waves indicative of right atrial enlargement, and the latter may be seen also on the chest roentgenogram.

RIGHT VENTRICULAR OUTFLOW OBSTRUCTION.   As with left ventricular outflow obstruction, right ventricular outflow obstruction may occur at the level of the pulmonic valve or above or below the valve leaflets. Valvar pulmonic stenosis is the most common form of right ventricular outflow obstruction.

VALVAR PULMONIC STENOSIS. In valvar pulmonic stenosis the valve is usually normally formed. In less severe forms there are three normally formed cusps, but the raphae are partly fused, so that the leaflet movement is restricted. In more severe forms there is less clear separation of the cusps, which are thickened to varying degrees and form a dome. Often infundibular hypertrophy, generally as part of the right ventricular hypertrophy, occurs with more severe forms of valvar pulmonic stenosis, and it tends to be progressive, producing a secondary outflow obstruction. With the more severe forms of valvar pulmonic stenosis the valve annulus and even the entire main and major branch pulmonary arteries may be underdeveloped (hypoplastic). In children with Turner's syndrome, particularly Turner's phenotype, there is a high incidence of valvar pulmonic stenosis with thick and myxomatous cusps.

Somatic development is usually normal at the time of birth in infants with pulmonic stenosis. Although the right ventricle is normally the dominant ventricle in the fetus and ejects about two-thirds of the combined ventricular output, total fetal cardiac output probably is maintained in the face of right ventricular outflow obstruction. Systemic venous return probably is diverted across the foramen ovale and is ejected by the left ventricle, which assumes dominance. The wider than normal ascending aorta and aortic isthmus found in infants with severe pulmonic stenosis or pulmonary atresia support this thesis.

With valvar pulmonic stenosis, development of the right ventricle and tricuspid valve in the fetus probably depends on the stage of gestation at which the stenosis occurs. If stenosis develops early in gestation, it is likely that venous return will be diverted across the foramen ovale, with subsequent underdevelopment of the right ventricle and the tricuspid valve. However, if the stenosis occurs later, right ventricular development is more likely to be normal, as it is if there has been marked tricuspid regurgitation.

PATHOPHYSIOLOGY. In pulmonic stenosis the right ventricle requires increased amounts of oxygen and therefore increased coronary blood flow. Currently no information is available as to the exact pressure levels at which right ventricular myocardial ischemia occurs; however, severe pulmonic stenosis is probably required before this becomes a major factor.

After birth, the course of the circulation and the clinical presentation depend on the severity of the pulmonic stenosis and the degree of development of the right ventricular chamber and outflow tract, the tricuspid valve, and the main and branch pulmonary arteries. In severe pulmonic stenosis the right ventricle will be incapable of ejecting the total systemic venous return, and therefore pulmonary blood flow derived from the right ventricle will be diminished. Infants with this form of severe pulmonic stenosis behave as if complete pulmonic atresia were present, and most of the pulmonary blood flow will then have to be provided through either a patent ductus arteriosus or some type of systemic arterial to pulmonary arterial communication.

Although some of the systemic venous return will be ejected by the right ventricle, the rest of the systemic venous return will have to cross the interatrial septum into the left atrium. This is generally through a patent foramen ovale, although true atrial septal defects do occur with pulmonic stenosis. In early infancy obstruction to flow across the interatrial septum is unusual, since the foramen ovale has carried a significant volume of blood in fetal life. However, if the interatrial communication becomes inadequate, systemic output may not be maintained and systemic venous obstruction may occur.

In moderate to moderately severe pulmonic stenosis, adequate pulmonary blood flow may be maintained by the right ventricle when the ductus arteriosus closes. With more severe pulmonic stenosis, the right ventricle may be incapable of maintaining the high pressure required to overcome the obstruction and provide a normal output, and right-sided cardiac failure may therefore develop within a few months after birth. If there is an interatrial communication, right-to-left atrial shunting of moderate to mild degree may occur, with the production of cyanosis. More often, the right ventricle hypertrophies in response to the increased pressure load, and it can usually maintain an adequate output with moderately severe obstructions. Infants with lesser degrees of obstruction are therefore able to maintain normal pulmonary blood flow, and even if they have interatrial communication they have neither right-sided failure nor right-to-left atrial shunting.

Most infants and children with mild or moderate pulmonic stenosis develop and grow normally. Systemic and pulmonary blood flow therefore increases with age, and if the orifice of the obstructed pulmonic valve does not grow, the right ventricular systolic pressure will increase significantly to maintain output. Furthermore, since the normal resting heart rate of an infant is significantly higher than that of an older child, the decrease in heart rate causes stroke volume to increase significantly, and systolic flow across the stenotic valve will be increased commensurately.

CLINICAL FEATURES. Severe pulmonic stenosis presents in the immediate postnatal period and resembles pulmonary atresia. It is discussed on page 1454. In moderately severe pulmonic stenosis during infancy, mild cyanosis may be present if the foramen ovale remains patent. However, if the foramen ovale becomes sealed, the cyanosis will disappear. Right ventricular failure may become evident after about 6 months, but if it does not occur at that time it is generally delayed until young adulthood. When it is present, right ventricular failure will be evidenced by rapid onset of hepatomegaly, prominent pulsatile neck veins (*a*-waves), and a low output state.

The majority of children with moderately severe pulmonic stenosis are asymptomatic and are detected because of the murmur. Many of the physical findings of pulmonic stenosis correlate roughly with the severity of the stenosis. When right ventricular enlargement is produced, a fairly diffuse forceful parasternal impulse along the lower left border of the sternum may be palpable. A systolic thrill is generally palpable at the upper left sternal border in all but the mildest forms. The auscultatory findings are summarized diagrammatically in Figure 66. The first heart sound is usually normal, but may be accentuated. A systolic ejection click is commonly heard along the entire left sternal border, but in patients with severe or progressively increasing stenosis the click either is not heard or becomes softer and may disappear. With progressive development of secondary right ventricular outflow obstruction due to infundibular hypertrophy, an ejection click previously heard may also disappear. The time interval between the Q wave of the electrocardiogram or the first heart sound and the ejection systolic click shortens as the stenosis becomes more severe. The second heart sound is usually moderately soft, and as the stenosis becomes more severe the pulmonic component of the second sound becomes softer and more delayed. Eventually in the most severe forms of pulmonic stenosis the pulmonic component of the second sound may completely disappear. With marked hypertrophy a fourth heart sound is often heard, and with right ventricular failure a third heart sound may be present.

The murmur associated with pulmonic stenosis is a high-frequency ejection systolic murmur of the crescendo–decrescendo type best heard at the upper left sternal border, with radiation to the left infraclavicular area. The intensity of the murmur does not correlate well with the severity of the stenosis; although, it is generally louder in severe stenosis than in very mild stenosis. However, the time during the cardiac cycle at which the intensity is maximal, as well as the duration of the murmur, do correlate well with the severity of the stenosis. As pulmonic stenosis becomes more severe, right ventricular ejection is prolonged; thus with more severe obstruction the peak intensity will be later in systole and the murmur will become longer, until eventually the aortic component of the second sound becomes obscured. During the Valsalva maneuver, as intrathoracic pressure is increased and systemic venous return and right ventricular stroke volume are reduced, the murmur of pulmonic stenosis will decrease immediately un-less there is congestive heart failure or unless there is severe infundibular hypertrophy as well.

The electrocardiogram will show right atrial hypertrophy with peaked P waves. There will also be right ventricular hypertrophy, the amount depending on the severity of the stenosis. Right axis deviation will be present, with the extent of rightward deviation depending to some extent on the amount of right ventricular hypertrophy. The right precordial leads will show tall R waves, and with severe stenosis they may also show T wave inversion and S-T segment depression. If there is no right ventricular conduction delay, there is a rough correlation between the height of the R wave in lead V_1 and the right ventricular systolic pressure; the height of the R wave in millimeters multiplied by 5 is approximately equivalent to the right ventricular systolic pressure in millimeters of mercury. This sign is not reliable in infants.

The chest roentgenogram will show right ventricular prominence with an upturned apex. Again, the magnitude of enlargement will depend on the severity of the stenosis and subsequent development of right ventricular hypertrophy. The main and left pulmonary arteries are prominent due to poststenotic dilatation (Fig. 67). The pulmonary vascular markings are generally within normal limits or may appear slightly diminished.

NATURAL HISTORY.   Some children with moderate degrees of stenosis show little or no change in right ventricular systolic pressure over many years, indicating that the valve orifice has probably enlarged with growth. However, other children have shown a marked increase in right ventricular systolic pressure, suggesting either no growth of the pulmonic valve orifice or development

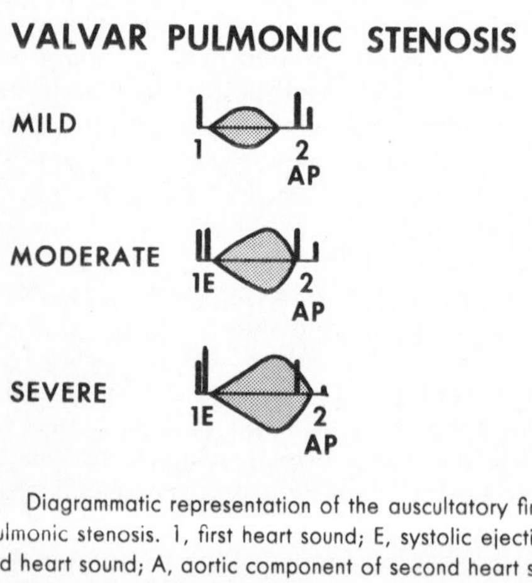

VALVAR PULMONIC STENOSIS

MILD

MODERATE

SEVERE

FIG. 66. Diagrammatic representation of the auscultatory findings in valvar pulmonic stenosis. 1, first heart sound; E, systolic ejection click; 2, second heart sound; A, aortic component of second heart sound, P, pulmonic component of second heart sound.

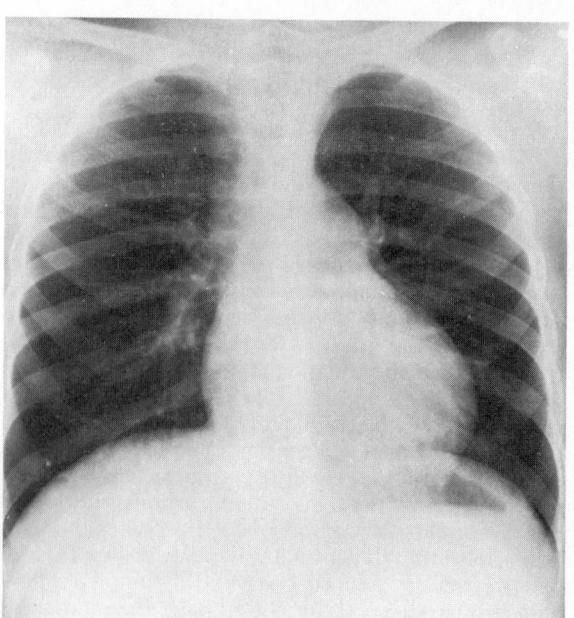

FIG. 67. Chest roentgenogram in a child with isolated valvar pulmonic stenosis. The right ventricle and main pulmonary artery are enlarged; the pulmonary vessels are normal.

of infundibular stenosis or a combination of both. If this should occur, right ventricular end-diastolic pressure will eventually rise, and right heart failure may develop. An additional factor causing right ventricular failure may be the development of inadequate myocardial perfusion. The infundibular stenosis that occurs may be diffuse or may be localized hypertrophy of the crista supraventricularis.

Mild valvar pulmonic stenosis with a small increase in right ventricular systolic pressure may not affect right ventricular output or the right ventricular myocardium significantly. In many instances, with growth of the child there is little or no increase in right ventricular systolic pressure, and minimal right ventricular hypertrophy may occur. The long-term outcome for such types of mild pressure elevation is as yet unknown.

TREATMENT.   Those children with severe stenosis (right ventricular systolic pressure greater than systemic) should undergo pulmonary valvotomy. The majority of children with severe valvar pulmonic stenosis also have infundibular hypertrophy, and there is debate as to whether this should be removed at the time of valvotomy. In general the recommendation is to remove only a distinctly localized area of subvalvar stenosis through the pulmonary artery approach and not to resect a diffusely hypertrophied outflow tract. In most children infundibular hypertrophy retrogresses once the valvar stenosis is relieved. With less severe stenosis (right ventricular systolic pressures less than systemic arterial systolic pressure) the criteria for surgery are not well defined; however, it is believed that a right ventricular systolic pressure of over 60 to 70 mm Hg in children for any prolonged period of time may lead to myocardial damage; thus it is advised that children with these pressures have surgery.

SUBVALVAR PULMONIC STENOSIS.   Isolated diffuse infundibular pulmonic stenosis with a normal pulmonic valve is rare. It is more likely to be associated with a small ventricular septal defect that is not clinically evident or else has closed spontaneously. Obstruction by a discrete subpulmonic fibrous or fibromuscular ring may occur at any level in the right ventricular outflow tract. Obstruction by large aberrant muscular bands that divide the right ventricular cavity into two separate chambers is usually associated with a ventricular septal defect, but it may occur alone.

Diffuse interventricular septal hypertrophy secondary to marked left ventricular hypertrophy may produce a bulging into the right ventricle or outflow tract and thereby produce obstruction (Bernheim effect). Myocardial tumors, particularly those involving the interventricular septum, may also produce right ventricular outflow obstruction. An unusual form of subvalvar pulmonic stenosis occurs in corrected transposition of the great arteries (bulboventricular inversion, *l*-transposition), and although it is generally associated with a ventricular septal defect, it may occur with an intact septum. In this lesion a fibromuscular subpulmonic stenosis usually associated with accessory tissue attached to the right-sided atrioventricular valve (mitral valve) produces the obstruction.

The clinical features of these lesions are similar to those of valvar pulmonic stenosis. However, an ejection click is less commonly heard, and poststenotic dilatation of the pulmonary artery is less prominent or may be absent. The systolic murmur is usually maximal at the third or fourth interspace along the left sternal border. These findings lead one to suspect subvalvar stenosis, and the diagnosis can be confirmed by cardiac catheterization and angiography.

STRAIGHT-BACK SYNDROME AND PECTUS EXCAVATUM.   Straight-back syndrome and pectus excavatum are not obstructive lesions, but they may be mistaken for such lesions. In both conditions the anteroposterior chest diameter is reduced, from behind in the former and from in front in the latter. In straight-back syndrome the right ventricular outflow tract and pulmonary artery lie anteriorly against the sternum. An ejection systolic murmur like that of valvar pulmonic stenosis may be present. Increased right ventricular forces may be evident on the electrocardiogram. The absence of normal thoracic kyphosis and even thoracic lordosis will be evident on the lateral chest roentgenogram. In pectus excavatum a similar systolic murmur may be heard. The murmur may be accentuated by pressure over the sternum, suggesting mechanical origin of the murmur.

SUPRAVALVAR   PULMONIC   STENOSIS. Stenosis of the major pulmonary arteries may occur anywhere along the entire length of the pulmonary arterial tree. Obstruction may be single or multiple and may be produced by a diaphragm or by localized narrowing or may involve more diffuse constrictions. Often there are long hypoplastic segments as well as areas of discrete stenosis.

STENOSIS OF MAIN PULMONARY ARTERY.   In stenosis of the main pulmonary artery (coarctation of the pulmonary artery) a constricting ring usually is present in the main pulmonary artery a short distance distal to the pulmonic valve. This type of stenosis is commonly associated with the rubella syndrome, where it is produced by a thick fibrous ring. In addition, children with peculiar facies and associated supravalvar stenosis without a history of rubella have been reported, and in them a thin supravalvar diaphragm is present. The clinical findings in this condition are similar to those of valvar pulmonic stenosis, but the second heart sound is usually normal. There is also a high incidence of left axis deviation seen on the electrocardiogram. The diagnosis can be made at cardiac catheterization.

PERIPHERAL BRANCH STENOSIS.   In the newborn period a physiologic branch pulmonary arterial stenosis is present, and it accounts for a large number of functional or physiologic murmurs in many newborn infants (p. 1364). True peripheral pulmonary arterial branch stenosis or hypoplasia may occur as an isolated defect or may be associated with underdevelopment of part or all of one lung or with underdevelopment of the right heart (p. 1448). Peripheral pulmonary arterial stenosis is frequently noted in infants with the rubella syndrome, often in association with patent ductus arteriosus. Peripheral branch pulmonary arterial stenosis may also be found in association with other intracardiac congenital heart diseases.

The clinical features are variable and may mimic either valvar pulmonic stenosis or a patent ductus arteriosus. The murmur is generally harsh and systolic and suggestive of pulmonic stenosis, but it usually has wider radiation into the infraclavicular regions (particularly toward the right) and the axillae; occasionally the murmur is continuous. The second heart sound is not consistently altered, and an ejection click may or may not be present. The electrocardiogram shows right ventricular hypertrophy in the more severe cases; in the rubella syndrome, left axis deviation is common. The chest roentgenogram may show right ventricular enlargement and occasionally shows multiple dilated pulmonary artery segments due to poststenotic dilatations. If the peripheral stenosis involves only one lung or one segment of lung, undervascularization of that segment may be evident. These defects are confirmed by cardiac catheterization and angiocardiography. Treatment depends on the severity and the number of stenoses: multiple peripheral lesions well out in the parenchyma of the lung are probably inoperable, but more centrally placed lesions may be relieved surgically.

Increased Pulmonary Vascular Resistance

After about 1 week of age, pulmonary arterial blood pressure is normally low, under 25/12 mm Hg. Any increase in pressure is regarded as pulmonary arterial hypertension, although slight increases are usually not important. To evaluate the causes of pulmonary arterial hypertension, consider first the concept of vascular resistance (R), which is by definition the ratio of pressure drop across a vascular bed to the blood flow through it. For the pulmonary circulation the pressure drop is from the pulmonary artery (P_A) to the pulmonary veins (P_V) and is normally 4 to 10 mm Hg at rest. The flow is the pulmonary blood flow (Q_P), which at all ages is about 3.5 liters/minute for each square meter of body surface area. Thus resting pulmonary vascular resistance is about 1 to 3 mm Hg/liter/minute/m². On exercise in the normal individual, pulmonary blood flow can increase threefold to fourfold with little rise in pulmonary arterial pressure, so that resistance falls to one-third or one-quarter of its resting value; it falls because the small resistance vessels dilate and new vessels are recruited.

The resistance equation $R = (P_A - P_V)/Q_P$ can be rearranged to give $P_A = RQ_P + P_V$, an expression that gives the simplest classification of the causes of pulmonary arterial hypertension. Thus pulmonary arterial pressure (P_A) will rise with an increase in pulmonary vascular resistance, pulmonary blood flow, or pulmonary venous pressure, provided that a rise in one variable does not alter the others. However, an increase in flow normally causes a fall in pulmonary vascular resistance, which tends to prevent a rise in pulmonary arterial pressure. Thus pulmonary arterial pressures are usually normal or only minimally elevated with exercise or with

the large pulmonary flows found when there are large atrial septal defects. Conversely, the high pulmonary arterial pressures seen with large ventricular septal defects (which equalize pressures between the two ventricles) indicate the failure of pulmonary vascular resistance to fall when pulmonary blood flow increases, so that increases in both Q_P and R are responsible for the pulmonary arterial hypertension.

If pulmonary venous pressure rises (for example, due to total anomalous pulmonary venous connection with obstruction, mitral stenosis, or left ventricular failure), then pulmonary arterial pressure rises by about the same amount. Sometimes these patients also have an increased pulmonary vascular resistance (p. 1463), and the pulmonary arterial pressure rises more than pulmonary venous pressure.

The most common causes of pulmonary arterial hypertension are pulmonary venous hypertension from left ventricular failure and increased pulmonary vascular resistance with or without an increased pulmonary blood flow. To analyze pulmonary vascular resistance in more detail, consider the relationship found by Poiseuille for the resistance offered by a glass tube to the steady flow of liquid through it: resistance equals pressure drop across the tube divided by the flow through it, and the value of this ratio (the resistance) = $(8/\pi)$ (l/r^4) (η). That is, resistance depends on a constant $(8/\pi)$, the geometric factor of tube length (l) divided by the fourth power of the radius (r), and the viscosity (η). Although pulsatile blood flow through a vascular bed is not the same as steady flow of water through a glass tube, the factors determining resistance are similar in both, with one major difference: in the lung r does not reflect the cross-sectional area of a single vessel, but is related to the total cross-sectional area of all the resistance vessels.

From this analysis the main causes of an increased pulmonary vascular resistance are noted to be an increase in blood viscosity or a decrease in total cross-sectional area of the resistance vessels; this decreased area may be due to fewer total vessels or else a normal number of vessels but with some or all of them narrowed. The most common cause of increased blood viscosity is a raised hematocrit, as occurs in most children with cyanotic heart disease. As a rough approximation, a rise in hematocrit from about 40 to 70 percent doubles viscosity and hence doubles pulmonary vascular resistance.

A decreased total number of resistance vessels occurs at times with congenital heart diseases (for example, ventricular septal defects) or with congenital lung lesions such as hypoplasia of one lung, emphysema, or cystic changes. If there is a single pulmonary artery, so that all right ventricular output goes to one lung, then in effect the number of vessels available for receiving that output has fallen by about half. The number of vessels can also be reduced postnatally if they are occluded by tumor or blood emboli. This is a common complication in children with hydrocephalus who have a shunt draining cerebrospinal fluid from the brain into the vena cava or right atrium (p. 1756); they may get showers of emboli that can be small or large, sterile or infected, and progressive pulmonary hypertension may compel removal of the shunt.

More commonly the number of vessels is normal, but their luminal diameters are decreased, either by vasoconstriction or by organic changes of the arterial wall that may be permanent. Vasoconstriction can be due to many biologically active agents (for example, serotonin, norepinephrine), but by far the most important cause is alveolar hypoxia, especially if it is potentiated by metabolic acidemia. Some of the major causes in children are as follows: upper airway obstruction (p. 1555); central nervous system depression from many causes, including possibly immaturity as seen in the preterm infant; thoracic cage impairment by obesity (Pickwickian syndrome), neuromuscular diseases, kyphoscoliosis, congenitally small thoracic cage (achondroplasia, Jeune's syndrome), or large diaphragmatic hernia; extensive parenchymal or small airway disease (meconium aspiration, severe bronchiolitis, cystic fibrosis, infections); and high altitude. Most of these lesions cause multiple changes of acid–base balance and blood gases, but the likelihood of pulmonary arterial hypertension and even right-sided congestive heart failure must be considered too. The hypoxic pulmonary vasoconstriction can be reversed by raising alveolar oxygen tension (if possible) or by giving a pulmonary vasodilator like tolazoline hydrochloride (Priscoline). It is important to note that pulmonary arterial hypertension will cause muscular hypertrophy of the pulmonary arterial wall, thereby making it thicker and the lumen narrower. Relief of hypoxic vasoconstriction may not return pulmonary vascular resistance to normal at once because of the residual organic change. However, if pulmonary arterial pressure remains low, the hypertrophied smooth muscle of the media will return to normal over several weeks.

Organic changes in the walls, other than muscular hypertrophy, may have many causes. They occur in a variety of systemic and pulmonary diseases such as collagen diseases and schistosomiasis; the granulomatous lesions due to schistosomal ova are common causes of severe childhood pulmonary arterial hypertension in endemic regions like Puerto Rico, Egypt, and southern Africa. More often these organic changes are due to intimal thickening and fibrosis secondary to large left-to-right shunts with high pulmonary blood flows (p. 1409).

These considerations usually allow the cause of the pulmonary arterial hypertension to be diagnosed, but there are occasional examples where no known cause can be found. For want of a better term, primary or idiopathic pulmonary arterial hypertension is often used. One form of this is a progressive disease, often familial, that eventually causes right heart failure and death; the disease may begin in early childhood or as late as early adult life. On the other hand, there are increasing reports of a syndrome of pulmonary arterial hypertension in the newborn infant. Although causes such as premature closure of the foramen ovale or intrauterine twin–twin transfusion (parabiotic syndrome)

may occasionally cause the syndrome, in most patients no specific cause can be found. This syndrome, often referred to as persistent fetal circulation, is more correctly called persistent pulmonary hypertension of the newborn. Although the infants may be very ill, they can generally be tided over the acute period, after which they apparently recover and develop normally.

CLINICAL MANIFESTATIONS. In infants or children with secondary increases in pulmonary vascular resistance, the underlying pathology may be quite evident. The resultant pulmonary hypertension produced by the increased pulmonary vascular resistance will produce a narrowly split second sound, with the pulmonic component accentuated. In severe pulmonary hypertension the pulmonic component of the second sound will be markedly accentuated; a systolic ejection click is common, and an early diastolic decrescendo blowing murmur of pulmonary regurgitation may be heard. In addition, right ventricular failure (cor pulmonale) may occur with dilatation of the right ventricular cavity and subsequent tricuspid regurgitation, especially in newborn infants. Tricuspid regurgitation may cause a systolic murmur best heard at the lower left sternal border; if the regurgitation is severe, a mid-diastolic flow rumble may be heard, although this is unusual in infants. Right ventricular enlargement may be evident on the chest roentgenogram or electrocardiogram, depending on the duration of the increased pulmonary vascular resistance.

Infants with persistent pulmonary hypertension generally present within the first few hours after birth with fairly severe cyanosis, which may be more marked in the lower body than above because of right-to-left shunting across the ductus arteriosus, tachypnea, acidemia, and a normal chest roentgenogram. Tricuspid regurgitation is commonly present.

Older children with primary pulmonary vascular disease will present with an extremely loud pulmonic component of the second sound that is often palpable at the upper left sternal border. A diastolic regurgitant pulmonic insufficiency murmur is generally heard, and in severe pulmonary hypertension right heart failure may occur. On the chest roentgenogram the pulmonary artery is markedly dilated, and right ventricular as well as right atrial enlargement will be observed. The electrocardiogram also may show right ventricular and right atrial hypertrophy. This condition is progressive and generally fatal.

TREATMENT. In those conditions that produce secondary increases in pulmonary vascular resistance, the underlying disease state should be treated whenever possible. Infants or children with enlarged tonsils and upper airway obstruction and subsequent right heart failure are generally cured by a tonsillectomy and adenoidectomy. Likewise, removal of a retropharyngeal or retrolaryngeal mass will relieve the hypoxia. Underlying pulmonary pathology cannot always be treated, and in diseases such as cystic fibrosis a pulmonary vasodilator such as Priscoline may be advisable. During sleep the rate and depth of respiration normally decrease, so that pulmonary vascular resistance associated with hypoxia will be increased during sleeping hours; pulmonary vasodilator therapy may therefore be most helpful at that time. In infants with persistent pulmonary hypertension of the newborn, supportive therapy, maintenance of electrolytes, and pulmonary vasodilators generally produce good results, albeit after a fairly protracted severe illness.

References

Danilowicz D, Rudolph AM, Hoffman JIE, Heyman MA: Physiologic pressure differences between main and branch pulmonary arteries in infants. Circulation 45:410, 1972

——— Hoffman JIE, Rudolph AM: Serial studies of pulmonary stenosis in infancy and childhood. Br Heart J 37:808, 1975

Daoud G, Kaplan S, Perrin EV, Dorst JP, Edwards FK: Congenital mitral stenosis. Circulation 27:185, 1963

Frank S, Braunwald E: Idiopathic hypertrophic subaortic stenosis. Circulation 37:759, 1968

Friedman WF: The intrinsic physiologic properties of the developing heart. In Friedman WF, Lesch M, Sonnenblick EM (eds): Neonatal Heart Disease. New York, Grune & Stratton, 1973, p 21

Goldberg HP, Glenn F, Dotter CT, Steinberg I: Myxoma of the left atrium. Diagnosis made during life with operative and postmortem findings. Circulation 6:752, 1952

Heymann MA, Rudolph AM: Effects of congenital heart disease on the fetal and neonatal circulations. Prog Cardiovasc Dis 15:115, 1972

Hoffman JIE: The natural history of congenital isolated pulmonic and aortic stenosis. Ann Rev Med 20:15, 1969

——— The normal pulmonary circulation. In Scarpelli EM, Auld PAM, Goldman HS (eds): Pediatric Pulmonary Physiology and Disease. Philadelphia, Lea & Febiger, 1975

Lakier JB, Lewis AB, Heymann MA, et al: Isolated aortic stenosis in the neonate: Natural history and hemodynamic considerations. Circulation 50:801, 1974

Lewis AB, Heymann MA, Stanger P, Hoffman JIE, Rudolph AM: Evaluation of subendocardial ischemia in valvar aortic stenosis in children. Circulation 49:978, 1974

Lucas RV Jr, Varco RL, Lillehei CW, et al: Anomalous muscle bundle of the right ventricle—hemodynamic consequences and surgical considerations. Circulation 25:443, 1962

Roberts N, Moes CAF: Supravalvar pulmonary stenosis. J Pediatr 82:838, 1973

Rowe RD: Maternal rubella and pulmonary artery stenosis. Am J Cardiol 24:318, 1969

Rudolph AM: Congenital Diseases of the Heart. Chicago, Year Book, 1974

——— Heyman MA, Spitznas U: Hemodynamic considerations in the development of narrowing of the aorta. Am J Cardiol 30:514, 1972

Sime F, Banchero N, Peñaloza D, et al: Pulmonary hypertension in children born and living at high altitudes. Am J Cardiol 11:150, 1963

Sinha SN, Kardatzke ML, Cole RB, et al: Coarctation of the aorta in infancy. Circulation 40:385, 1969

Vogelpoel L, Schrire V: Auscultatory and phonocardiographic assessment of pulmonary stenosis with intact ventricular septum. Circulation 22:55, 1960

AORTIC ARCH ANOMALIES

JULIEN I.E. HOFFMAN

Abnormal development of the aortic arches (p. 1359) may produce no symptoms (aberrant right subclavian artery, right aortic arch) or may encroach on the eso-

phagus or trachea and cause dysphagia and airway obstruction. Therefore diagnosis can usually be made by examining the characteristic indentations that the abnormal arteries make on the barium-filled esophagus or the trachea. Physical examination and the electrocardiogram are normal.

Infants with severe obstructions are very ill. Vomiting is frequent, and there is dysphagia, so that feeding is inhibited and weight gain is poor. Wheezing and stridor are often prominent and are made worse by feeding. Frequently the infants hyperextend their heads to reduce tracheal compression.

The most common anomaly is an aberrant right subclavian artery, which occurs when the proximal rather than the distal part of the right fourth arch is absorbed (p. 1359). As a result the right subclavian artery runs posteriorly from the descending thoracic aorta to reach the right arm, passing obliquely up and to the right behind the esophagus and indenting it posteriorly (Fig. 68). This anomaly so rarely causes symptoms that even if it is found in the course of an investigation some other cause of esophageal or respiratory symptoms must be sought.

If the distal fourth arch disappears on the left rather than on the right, there will be a right aortic arch and a mirror-image arrangement of arteries to the arms and head. This is not a cause of symptoms, but the prominent roentgenographic shadow that the arch casts on the right side of the mediastinum may be mistaken for enlarged nodes or a tumor. A right aortic arch is found in about 25 percent of patients with the tetralogy of Fallot and in many with truncus arteriosus.

Most anomalies that cause serious symptoms encircle the esophagus and trachea to form a vascular ring (Fig.

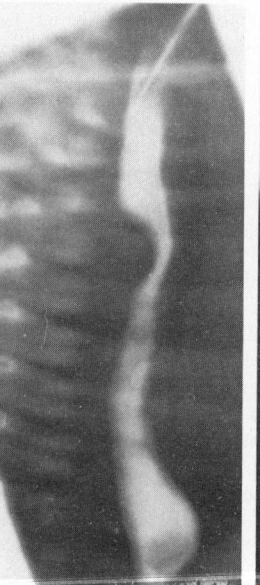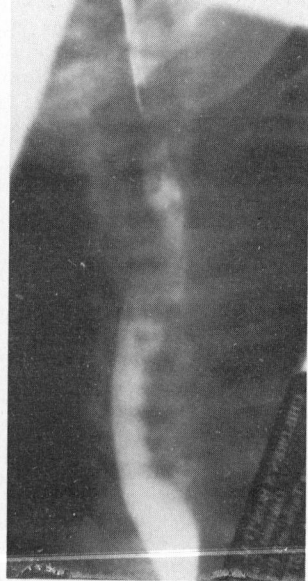

FIG. 68. Lateral (left) and frontal (right) esophagrams in patient with aberrant right subclavian artery. Courtesy of Dr. H. Taybi.

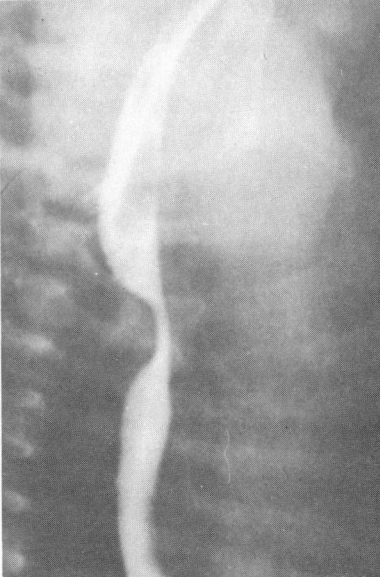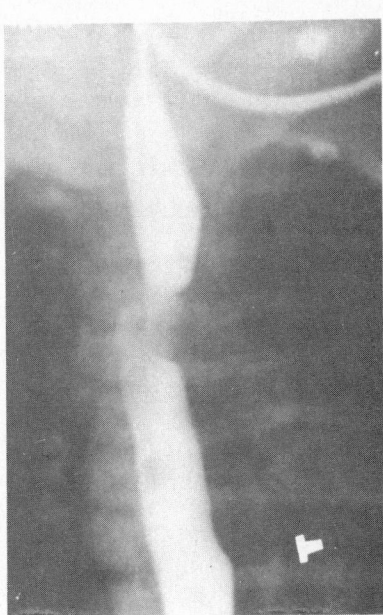

FIG. 69. Lateral (left) and frontal (right) esophagrams in patient with double aortic arch. Note that the esophagus is narrowed in the frontal view and that the right arch is higher than the left arch. *Courtesy of Dr. H. Taybi.*

69). The most common of these is the double aortic arch due to failure of absorption of any part of the embyonic fourth arches. The right and left arches indent the right and left sides of the trachea and the esophagus, and the right arch indents the esophagus posteriorly as it passes to the left behind the esophagus to join the left arch and form the descending aorta. Surgical division of one of the arches, usually the smaller posterior one, opens the constricting ring and is curative.

Almost as common is the right aortic arch that is made into a constricting ring because there is a left-sided patent ductus arteriosus or ligmentum arteriosum. The combination produces indentations on the esophagus and trachea similar to those that occur with a double arch. Surgical division of the ductus or ligamentum is curative.

Occasionally a carotid or innominate artery compresses the anterior margin of the trachea. This may show up on roentgenograms of the tracheal air column or on a tracheogram, but the esophagram is normal. If necessary, the compressing artery can be displaced anteriorly at surgery.

Although it does not form a vascular ring, the anomalous left pulmonary artery also causes airway obstruction. The left pulmonary artery arises from the right pulmonary artery and passes between the esophagus and trachea, compressing the latter. It is the only vascular anomaly to indent only the anterior edge of the esophagus. Surgical reattachment of the left pulmonary artery to the main pulmonary artery relieves the obstruction.

References

Blake HA, Manion WC: Thoracic arterial arch anomalies. Circulation 26:251, 1962

Gross RE, Neuhauser EBD: Compression of the trachea or esophagus by vascular anomalies: surgical therapy in 40 cases. Pediatrics 7:69, 1951

Stewart JR, Kincaid OW, Edwards JE: An Atlas of Vascular Rings and Related Malformations of the Aortic Arch. Springfield, Ill, Charles C Thomas, 1964

RIGHT-TO-LEFT SHUNTS

Milton H. Paul

Certain anatomic and physiologic abnormalities result in some systemic venous blood passing into the systemic arterial circulation without first being oxygenated in the lungs. There is therefore a venous-to-arterial shunt that is usually termed a right-to-left shunt.

Anatomic Classification

RIGHT-TO-LEFT SHUNTS WITH NORMALLY PLACED GREAT VESSELS. For systemic venous blood to bypass the lungs and flow from what is normally a right-sided low-pressure pulmonary circuit to a left-sided high-pressure systemic circuit it is necessary that there be an obstruction to flow on the right side that is distal to an abnormal communication between the two circuits. Thus some venous blood will pass into the aorta through a patent ductus arteriosus if there is a very high resistance to flow through the pulmonary vessels or a severe enough obstruction in the larger pulmonary arteries. These pulmonary vascular obstructions will also cause a right-to-left shunt through a ventricular septal defect, as will severe right ventricular outflow tract obstruction, such as valvar or infundibular pulmonary stenosis or pulmonary atresia (Fig. 70B and C). Finally, a right-to-left shunt through an atrial septal defect or patent foramen ovale will occur with all the above-mentioned obstructions as well as tricuspid

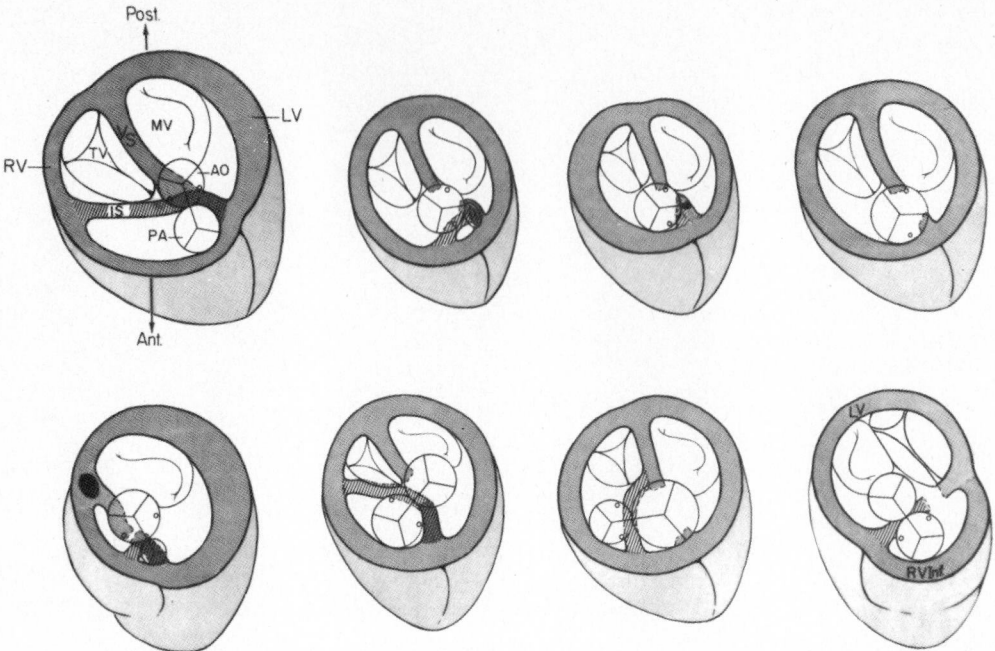

FIG. 70. Schematic diagrams of some relatively frequent forms of cyanotic congenital heart disease; hearts viewed from above, atria (in normal locations) not shown. A. Normal heart. B. Tetralogy of Fallot with infundibular and valvar stenosis. C. Tetralogy of Fallot with pulmonary atresia. D. Truncus arteriosus communis. E. Tricuspid atresia with normally related great arteries. F. Complete *d*-transposition of great arteries. G. Double-outlet right ventricle (Taussing-Bing type). H. Single (left) ventricle malformation with small (right) infundibular outflow chamber with *l*-ventricular loop and *l*-transposition of the great arteries. Ant, anterior; Post, posterior; RV, morphologically right ventricle; RV inf, right ventricle infundibulum; LV, morphologically left ventricle; PA, valve of pulmonary artery; AO, valve of aorta; TV, tricuspid valve; MV, mitral valve; VS, ventricular septum; IS, infundibular septum (cross-hatched).

stenosis or atresia (Fig. 70E). Any lesion that impairs right atrial emptying (right ventricular failure, tricuspid incompetence, Ebstein's malformation of the tricuspid valve) will also cause a right-to-left atrial shunt if there is an interatrial communication.

Tricuspid or pulmonary orifice atresia is an example of *extreme right heart obstruction* (Fig. 70C and E). All the systemic venous blood must pass into the left atrium or ventricle; the systemic venous blood mixes with oxygenated pulmonary venous return, and thus the blood ejected into the aorta is desaturated. Mitral or aortic orifice atresia (hypoplastic left heart syndrome) is an example of *extreme left heart obstruction,* where similarly complete mixing of systemic and pulmonary venous return occurs. All the pulmonary venous return passes from the left to right atrium, where it mixes with the systemic venous return and enters the right ventri._.e and pulmonary artery. The blood that eventually reaches the aorta via a persistent patent ductus arteriosus contains unoxygenated blood and is desaturated. One exception to the requirement for an obstruction is a pulmonary arteriovenous fistula that causes some venous blood to bypass the alveoli.

RIGHT-TO-LEFT SHUNTS WITH ABNORMALLY PLACED GREAT VESSELS. In complete transposition of the great arteries, the aorta arises from the right ventricle and the pulmonary artery from the

left ventricle, so that the systemic venous blood enters the right atrium and ventricle and then passes into the aorta, while the pulmonary venous blood returns to the left atrium and ventricle and then passes back into the lungs from the pulmonary artery (Fig. 70F). For the patient to survive there must be some interchange of blood between the two circuits through a persistent atrial or ventricular septal defect or a patent ductus arteriosus.

Double-outlet right ventricle is a malformation where the pulmonary artery and aorta both arise from the right ventricle; the only outflow from the left ventricle is through the ventricular septal defect, which may be adjacent to either the pulmonary orifice or the aortic orifice. When the pulmonary artery is adjacent to or even overriding a high ventricular septal defect (Taussig-Bing anomaly), the aortic blood flow is derived mainly from the right ventricle (Fig. 70G), and there is significant right-to-left shunting and arterial desaturation. In another common type of double-outlet right ventricle the aorta is placed near the ventricular septal defect, and left ventricular blood streams into the aorta. Here there may be little right-to-left shunting unless there is also severe obstruction to flow on the right side (pulmonary stenosis).

Truncus arteriosus is a malformation in which the septum that ordinarily separates the aorta from the main pulmonary artery has not formed. As a result there is a single large arterial trunk with a single semilunar valve coming off at the base of the heart and overriding a large ventricular septal defect (Fig. 70D). The trunk receives blood from both left and right ventricles, and the mixing of oxygenated and unoxygenated blood results in arterial desaturation.

Total anomalous pulmonary venous connection is a malformation where all systemic and pulmonary venous blood returns to the right atrium, from which some goes normally through the tricuspid valve into the right ventricle, while the rest passes through an atrial septal defect into the left atrium.

Abnormal connection of one or more of the systemic veins to the left atrium is seen occasionally.

Physiologic Mechanisms

When there are large right-to-left shunts the arterial oxygen saturation depends chiefly on the pulmonary blood flow and not on the size of the right-to-left shunt. This occurs because the systemic arterial saturation is determined by how much the almost fully saturated pulmonary venous return (volume of pulmonary blood flow) is diluted by unsaturated systemic venous blood (volume of right-to-left shunt). With the same magnitude of right-to-left shunt a large pulmonary blood flow results in a relatively high arterial oxygen saturation, while a small pulmonary blood flow will give a low arterial oxygen saturation. Since the pulmonary blood flow in these anomalies varies much more than does the amount of right-to-left shunting, the pulmonary blood flow becomes the major determinant of arterial saturation. For this reason many palliative operations for right-to-left shunting lesions are concerned with increasing a diminished pulmonary blood flow rather than reducing any right-to-left shunting. There are four basic physiologic syndromes that patients with right-to-left shunts show, without regard to the precise anatomic lesion.

There may be *massive pulmonary blood flow,* as in transposition of the arteries with a large ventricular septal defect, in tricuspid atresia with a large ventricular septal defect or with transposition of the great arteries, or in truncus arteriosus. Such patients may have very slight systemic arterial oxygen unsaturation and may not even appear cyanotic. Difficulties are due not to hypoxemia but to a torrential pulmonary blood flow and huge volume load on the left ventricle, with resultant left ventricular failure. In this sense the pathophysiology resembles that of a large patent ductus arteriosus or ventricular septal defect. These patients require vigorous medical treatment for heart failure; if that fails, the volume overload of the left ventricle must be reduced by banding the pulmonary artery or by a corrective open heart procedure, if available.

There is a subgroup of these patients with *more moderate pulmonary blood flow* whose systemic arterial oxygen saturation is somewhat lower than that of the previous group and who are usually mildly or moderately cyanotic. However, the desaturation is not severe enough to produce hypoxemic symptoms, nor is the pulmonary blood flow high enough to cause left ventricular failure. These patients may do reasonably well for many years, although they usually have some limitations on exertion. Sooner or later they will need corrective surgery, if it is feasible, or else palliative surgery to permit them to do more than their current pulmonary blood flow allows.

There may be *severely reduced effective pulmonary blood flow* because the venous blood is diverted away from the lungs, as in the tetralogy of Fallot, severe pulmonic stenosis or atresia with intact ventricular septum, and tricuspid atresia or transposition of the great arteries without an adequate intracardiac communication. These patients are markedly desaturated and cyanotic and have symptoms related to severe hypoxemia. Since the supply of oxygen to the tissues is inadequate, these patients, usually infants, are hyperpneic at rest and have a very low stress tolerance. Any exertion increases the cyanosis; feeding may cause fatigue, and thus caloric intake may be seriously compromised. If hypoxemia is severe and prolonged, the infant usually appears quite feeble. Profound metabolic acidemia develops from anaerobic metabolism, because oxygen supply to metabolizing tissues is inadequate. In most patients with metabolic acidemia, reflex hyperventilation lowers arterial carbon dioxide tension and so brings arterial pH to or near normal. Patients with cyanotic heart disease and metabolic acidosis, however, are denied this compensation; although they hyperventilate, such a small amount of blood passes through the lungs that the arterial carbon dioxide tension tends to remain normal, and pH falls markedly. Since anaerobic metabolism increases glycolysis, these infants are also often severely hypoglycemic.

Characteristically, most infants in this group have markedly diminished pulmonary vascular markings on chest roentgenograms; however, in transposition of the great arteries, or rarely in other lesions where there has been an adequate flow through the ductus arteriosus, the lung fields may show fairly normal vascular markings. Usually the heart is small, and enlargement occurs only as a late or terminal event. The combination of severe cyanosis with the roentgenographic findings described indicates that severe disease is present. Further studies should be done *immediately* for two major reasons. If there is metabolic acidemia it must be corrected before more widespread physiologic deterioration occurs; at this stage a wait of even a few hours may be fatal. Even more important in the very young infant, the major portion of the already very low pulmonary blood flow may be coming from the aorta via a precariously patent ductus arteriosus. If it begins to close, as it usually does, hypoxemia will rapidly become worse.

Finally, there is a fourth group in which *pulmonary blood flow is very low because of obstruction to the pulmonary venous return.* In these malformations there is some obstruction to blood flow between the pulmonary veins and the left atrium, as when the pulmonary veins are not connected to the left atrium but rather form a common trunk that drains by various routes into the right atrium.

The trunk is obstructed by being excessively long and narrow or being constricted or extremely compressed or having a stenotic orifice.

These patients are deeply cyanotic because of the low pulmonary blood flow and the right-to-left shunt. In addition, they manifest the effects of a raised pulmonary venous pressure with marked tachypnea and often pulmonary edema. As a result they are very ill, and treatment must be directed toward relieving the pulmonary venous obstruction.

Pulmonary venous obstruction can also occur without anomalous pulmonary venous connections, as in cor triatriatum (stenosis of the common pulmonary vein) or isolated mitral valve stenosis. These malformations do not necessarily have right-to-left intracardiac shunts unless there is severe pulmonary hypertension and a patent ductus arteriosus or a small ventricular septal defect. Obstruction to pulmonary venous drainage also occurs commonly in mitral atresia with too small an interatrial opening.

Clinical Features

The primary physiologic consequence of right-to-left shunting of blood is systemic arterial oxygen desaturation; the clinical result is cyanosis. Cyanosis refers to a dusky, purple blue color due to the presence of an excessive amount of reduced hemoglobin in the circulating blood. It is most readily apparent in superficial capillary-rich sites such as the lips, mucous membranes, and nail beds. The term percentage arterial oxygen saturation refers to the percentage of arterial hemoglobin that is in the form of oxyhemoglobin; normal values range from 94 to 98 percent. Most physicians recognize definite cyanosis at levels of arterial saturation less than 85 percent, but under optimum conditions of appropriate physician color vision, ambient light, patient's skin pigmentation, and circulating hemoglobin, minor degrees of cyanosis at levels of 90 or 91 percent arterial oxygen saturation can be appreciated. Cyanosis is less apparent clinically in patients with severe anemia because the concentration of total circulating reduced hemoglobin in the capillary bed may be severely limited by the anemia. Conversely, apparent cyanosis may occur with normal arterial oxygen saturation when the peripheral circulation is abnormally slow or the hematocrit is so increased as to result in an increased concentration of circulating reduced hemoglobin in the distal capillary beds. This form of peripheral cyanosis is commonly observed in the normal newborn infant and characteristically is limited distally to the hands and feet, with normal color in the proximal portion of the limbs and the lips and tongue. Rarely, excessive transfusion of placental blood at delivery will result in significant neonatal polycythemia, with transient plethora, peripheral cyanosis, and clinical findings of cardiopulmonary strain. Spontaneous improvement generally occurs. Because of the risk of neurologic damage due to polycythemia (p. 179), partial exchange transfusion with plasma or plasma substitutes is indicated if the cardiopulmonary symptoms are significant and persistent or if the early central venous hematocrit is greater than 65 percent.

In addition to cyanosis, which is the specific clinical manifestation of right-to-left shunting of blood, several associated abnormalities are often present in the patient with cyanotic congenital heart disease. Clubbing or hypertrophic osteoarthropathy of the fingers ordinarily does not appear until 1 or 2 years of age in the cyanotic child. Rarely, clubbing may be associated with a noncardiac abnormality such as lung abscess or infective endocarditis, or it may be familial.

Polycythemia with increased hemoglobin and hematocrit is an important consequence of arterial oxygen unsaturation; it represents an adaptation of the hematopoietic system to the anoxic stimulus. The increased oxygen content achieved by this compensatory mechanism is advantageous until the hematocrit reaches levels of about 65 percent, when the effects of the associated high blood viscosity begin to outweigh the advantages of the increased circulating oxyhemoglobin. It is of considerable clinical importance to recognize that hypochromic microcytic anemia should be diagnosed in the severely cyanotic patient who has high erythrocyte counts but relatively normal hemoglobin and hematocrit levels; this anemia can easily be corrected by oral iron administration.

Spontaneous cerebrovascular accidents, particularly in infants, remain a serious and relatively common complication of cyanotic congenital heart disease (2 to 4 percent incidence). The most common manifestation of cerebrovascular accident is the sudden onset of hemiplegia. The increased blood viscosity in severe cyanotic polycythemia may be responsible for cerebral, mesenteric, renal, or pulmonary thromboses. Dehydration may increase the danger of thrombosis, and adequate fluid intake should be maintained, particularly during febrile illnesses and hot weather. Cerebrovascular accidents are the most common, and they generally occur under 2 years of age. Anemia (hypochromic microcytic) in association with hypoxemia has also been implicated as one mechanism for cerebrovascular accidents, probably cerebral infarction, particularly in the infant age group.

Brain abscesses represent a significant complication in patients with venous–arterial shunts, since bacteria normally filtered out in the pulmonary circulation may be shunted directly into the systemic circulation (p. 1869). In contrast to cerebrovascular accidents, which occur most commonly in infants less than 2 years of age, brain abscesses occur most commonly in children over 2 years of age. Symptoms such as persistent headache and a slowly developing neurologic picture also help distinguish this complication from the cerebrovascular accident.

Cyanotic patients with long-standing severe polycythemia may have thrombocytopenia and abnormalities of the soluble coagulation system. Thrombocytopenia is common, particularly in the older patient with long-standing polycythemia, and caution is advised in regard to excessive postoperative bleeding. The fall in platelet count appears to be associated with excessive erythropoiesis and may be due to abnormal platelet physiology or platelet consumption from continuous subclinical thromboses.

The prolonged and severe hypoxemia of cyanotic congenital heart disease frequently results in retarded physical growth that is most strikingly evident in the musculature. Recent studies have suggested that pre-school-age children with prolonged cyanotic heart disease, as a group, may have slightly lower I.Q. scores and perform less well with perceptual motor tasks than children with noncyanotic heart disease.

Medical Therapy

Any patient with severe cyanosis has significant and severe heart disease. Such a patient, particularly the newborn infant or unstable older infant, should be placed into an atmosphere of high oxygen at once, although the limitations of this therapy must be stressed. It is difficult to attain an ambient atmosphere of 100 percent oxygen unless a tight-fitting face mask or head hood is used; allowing oxygen to flow into an Isolette seldom raises the oxygen concentration above 50 or 60 percent, even at flow rates of 10 to 20 liters/minute. The main problem with increasing circulating oxygen in these infants is that because of the small effective pulmonary blood flow the amount of extra oxygen introduced into the body will be very small at best. Furthermore, in the infant with transposition of the great vessels, the hemoglobin that does enter the lungs is almost fully oxygenated, because much of the blood has been recirculating through the pulmonary circuit.

If an infant is very cyanotic, there is little reason to fear that increased ambient oxygen or even hyperbaric oxygen chamber therapy will close the patent ductus arteriosus, since the arterial oxygen tension will not rise much.

Although oxygen therapy should always be employed for the symptomatic severely cyanotic patient with congenital heart disease, the administration of oxygen to an older cyanotic infant or young child with advanced chronic nasopharyngeal obstruction and CO_2 retention due to enlarged tonsillar-adenoid tissue may be dangerous and is contraindicated. The elevated P_{CO_2} can suppress the central nervous system respiratory center, and respiration may stop if it is primarily under peripheral chemoreceptor anoxic drive. At times, provision of a patent orotracheal pathway with positive-pressure respiratory support may be indicated until emergency resection of the obstructive tissue.

In addition, any resultant metabolic acidemia must be treated. Once the arterial pH is known, intravenous infusions of sodium bicarbonate can be given, or TRIS buffer may be used with precautions. Undiluted molar sodium bicarbonate (1 mEq/ml) is generally administered to the neonate intravenously in 5-ml amounts. After each injection, arterial or mixed venous pH should be reassessed so that the time and amount of subsequent injections can be based on the response. Although large total quantities of sodium bicarbonate, involving large injections of water and sodium, may

have to be administered rapidly to the very hypoxic infant, there is little risk of causing congestive heart failure because these infants are often dehydrated. In any event, such a risk must be taken to combat severe metabolic acidemia and its disastrous cardiopulmonary consequences. It must be emphasized that oxygen therapy and treatment of metabolic acidemia are only temporary helpful measures, and as a rule they are used only until surgical palliation or correction can be performed. The infant should also be kept at an optimal temperature (skin temperature about 36.5 C) to minimize oxygen needs. These infants are often so ill that they have acute gastric dilatation, and removal of stomach contents and limitation of oral intake may be necessary to prevent aspiration.

Hypoglycemia is common in these children, because anaerobiasis accelerates glycolysis; thus blood glucose levels should be checked early, and glucose infusions should be given if the levels are low. Hypocalcemia is also common; patients must be monitored for this condition and treated if necessary.

In many forms of cyanotic congenital heart disease the blood supply to the lungs depends entirely or mainly on the ductus arteriosus; as this begins to close, pulmonary blood flow falls, and the patient becomes more hypoxemic and acidemic. Recent studies have shown that infusion of prostaglandin E_1 will dilate such a constricted ductus and permit improved oxygenation and metabolism. The agent is given at a dose of 0.1 μg/kg/minute and is best administered through an aortic catheter with its tip near the ductus arteriosus. The infusion should be continued until surgical relief of the lesion is achieved.

Supportive medical treatment should be aggressively pursued while preparing the infant for surgery and during cardiac catheterization, if indicated. Catheterization and angiographic studies should be undertaken if the diagnosis is not clinically certain regarding anatomic or physiologic facts critical for appropriate decisions about surgical intervention. With transposition of the great arteries, balloon atrial septostomy during the cardiac catheterization procedure provides palliation by enlarging the foramen ovale atrial septal defect.

Surgical Therapy

The surgical procedures employed for palliation or correction in the severely cyanotic infant may be briefly listed: (1) If there is obstruction to the right ventricular outflow tract, such as with isolated severe pulmonary valve stenosis with intact ventricular septum or with the tetralogy of Fallot, it may be possible to widen the pulmonary valve orifice or resect the infundibular obstruction, enlarge the outflow tract, and close a ventricular septal defect, thus increasing the pulmonary blood flow. Whether this can be done depends on the exact anatomy, usually assessed by angiography, and the experience of the surgeon. (2) If a direct attack on the obstruction is not possible, such as with the tetralogy of Fallot with pulmonary atresia or severe hypoplasia, or pulmonary atresia with a minute right ventricle, or tricuspid atresia with a small right ventricle, then pulmonary blood flow can be increased by anastomosing the aorta or subclavian artery or the superior vena cava to a pulmonary artery branch. As an alternative, the ductus arteriosus, if open, can be prevented from constricting for at least some months by subadventitial injection of the ductus with formalin; a thoracotomy is required to do this. In some cardiovascular centers primary intracardiac repair is being undertaken even in neonates, as well as in young infants with the tetralogy of Fallot and severe right ventricular outflow tract obstruction, provided the pulmonary valve annulus and main pulmonary artery branches are of reasonable size; there is a relatively low surgical risk of about 10 percent. Indications and techniques for early primary repair rather than early palliation and late secondary repair are advancing rapidly for several malformations. Arguments in favor of early primary repair are that the risk of one corrective operation is lower than the combined risk of palliation and later correction, the patient and family are spared prolonged anticipatory fears of subsequent corrective surgery, and secondary complications during long-term palliative management are avoided. (3) If there is pulmonary venous obstruction associated with mitral atresia, or systemic venous obstruction associated with tricuspid atresia, or inadequate interatrial mixing in transposition of the great arteries, a larger interatrial communication can be made by partial resection of the atrial septum. (4) Pulmonary venous obstruction associated with total anomalous pulmonary venous connection can be relieved by anastomosing the common pulmonary venous trunk to the left atrium. (5) The functional abnormality in transposition of the great arteries can be completely corrected in young infants after palliative surgery or as a primary repair even in the neonatal period. A large pericardial interatrial baffle is sutured in place to redirect the pulmonary venous return and systemic venous return toward their appropriate circulations.

Differential Diagnosis of Cyanosis

A report of duskiness or blueness in a newborn infant should receive immediate attention, as many of the lesions causing cyanosis may result in rapid deterioration of the infant, even within 1 or 2 hours. The causes of cyanosis are given in Table 9. The differentiation between primary pulmonary disease with right-to-left shunt through the foramen ovale or ductus arteriosus or both and congenital heart disease is often very difficult and is one of the most common problems confronting the pediatrician.

CLINICAL FEATURES. The history of the delivery of the baby and of the prenatal and postnatal periods is often helpful. Cyanotic congenital cardiac lesions are rarely encountered in very premature infants, in contrast to the idiopathic respiratory distress syndrome, which is very common. If the delivery was prolonged and difficult and the infant had a low Apgar score at birth, the possibility of cerebral trauma, intrauterine asphyxia with meconium aspiration, or sepsis

TABLE 9. Causes of Cyanosis in Newborn Infants

Peripheral cyanosis (normal arterial blood oxygen saturation and PO_2)
    Exposure to cold
    Decreased systemic blood flow
    High hemoglobin levels
Abnormal hemoglobin (decreased arterial blood oxygen saturation but normal PO_2)
    Methemoglobinemia
Central cyanosis (decreased arterial blood oxygen saturation and PO_2)
    Physiologic right-to-left shunt
        Pulmonary disease with perfused but unventilated alveoli
        Hypoventilation with perfused but poorly ventilated alveoli: cerebral trauma, depression by drugs, pulmonary disease
    Anatomic right-to-left shunt
        Congenital heart disease with right-to-left shunt of venous blood into systemic arterial system
        Pulmonary arteriovenous fistula
        High pulmonary vascular resistance with right-to-left shunt through a patent ductus arteriosus or patent foramen ovale or both
            Inadequate oxygenation in the lungs (includes all the conditions discussed under Physiologic right-to-left shunts)
            Infections, particularly with group B streptococci and coliform organisms
            High hematocrit levels, associated with increased blood viscosity
            Idiopathic persistent pulmonary hypertension; none of the usual causes of increased pulmonary vascular resistance is recognized

should be considered. A history of maternal infection or of early rupture of the membranes suggests that fetal infection may be responsible for the cyanosis. A history of twitching or convulsions, of stupor or coma, or of flaccidity suggests the probability of cerebral trauma.

Examination of the infant is usually very helpful in differential diagnosis. Peripheral cyanosis is most prominent in the fingers and toes, while the tongue and lips are usually pink. The extremities, manifesting peripheral vasoconstriction, are often cold, pale, and mottled. In the infant with decreased systemic blood flow, pulses are poorly felt and capillary filling is prolonged. Peripheral cyanosis usually disappears when the infant is warmed. Infants with methemoglobinemia often have a slate gray appearance rather than a bluish appearance of the skin and mucous membranes.

The pattern of breathing should be examined carefully. Infants with peripheral cyanosis usually have normal breathing, but if they have developed metabolic acidemia from inadequate systemic perfusion, respiration may be deep but not labored. Infants with polycythemia usually have normal respiration, although a few develop cardiac failure with tachypnea and mild dyspnea. Respiratory distress is unusual in infants with methemoglobinemia; they are quite undisturbed even though severely cyanotic. Airway obstruction, idiopathic respiratory distress syndrome, and other pulmonary disorders almost always are associated with tachypnea and dyspnea, and sternal retraction is often prominent.

The infant with heart disease in which the main disturbance is a large right-to-left shunt often has normal respiration initially, even though he may be markedly cyanosed; when severe hypoxemia and metabolic acidemia develop, breathing becomes very deep and respiratory rate is increased moderately. Congenital heart lesions (such as left-sided obstructive lesions) that are associated with pulmonary edema as well as cyanosis result in both dyspnea and tachypnea. Infants with idiopathic persistent pulmonary hypertension may have normal respirations, but they usually have intermittent tachypnea. Cerebral trauma or infection usually depresses ventilation; these infants often have periods of apnea and thus shallow and sometimes slow breathing. Thus, although breathing patterns are helpful in differential diagnosis, they usually do not provide definitive diagnoses.

Clinical examination of the chest may suggest a diagnosis; the presence of diffuse rales, local absence of air entry, or hyperresonance to percussion may suggest pulmonary disease or pneumothorax. Usually, however, clinical examination of the chest is not very helpful.

The presence of a cardiac murmur does not always indicate structural heart disease. A soft precordial systolic murmur is often heard in infants with persistent pulmonary hypertension and in infants with cardiac failure and cardiomegaly associated with infection or with hypoglycemia and hypocalcemia secondary to hypoxemia and acidemia. Furthermore, in many of the congenital cardiac lesions that are associated with marked cyanosis, such as tricuspid or pulmonary atresia or transposition of the great arteries, murmurs often are not present.

Blood gases and pH should be measured as soon as possible in cyanosed infants, even before the chest roentgenogram and electrocardiogram, as these results are crucial for determining immediate therapy as well as helpful in differential diagnosis. Arterial blood can be obtained most readily within the first 2 to 3 days after birth by umbilical artery catheterization. If this is not possible, needle puncture of a radial, temporal, or femoral artery may be performed.

The actual level of Po_2 is not usually helpful in differential diagnosis, although an arterial blood Po_2 below 20 torr suggests cyanotic congenital heart disease. A normal arterial Po_2 level in a cyanotic infant is indicative either of peripheral cyanosis or of methemoglobinemia. The diagnosis of methemoglobinemia can be confirmed by demonstrating that arterial blood oxygen saturation is reduced even though Po_2 is normal. A Pco_2 level above 45 torr is strongly indicative of lung disease, but an elevated Pco_2 is commonly noted in infants with persistent pulmonary hypertension who do not have overt lung disease. Infants with cyanotic congenital heart lesions rarely have elevated arterial Pco_2 levels, but occasionally Pco_2 is raised above 45 torr in the very sick cyanotic infant who also has severe pulmonary edema. Blood pH may be decreased in infants with either heart or lung disease.

The response of systemic arterial blood Po_2 to 100 percent oxygen administration may be very helpful in differential diagnosis. Since ventilation may be depressed in some infants, it is advisable to perform the oxygen test with assisted ventilation for a period of at least 5 minutes; this can be performed readily by the use of a close-fitting mask and an anesthesia bag. Generally it is believed that in infants with lung disease or alveolar hypoventilation arterial Po_2 increases by at least 15 to 20 torr and usually much more, whereas infants with heart disease and right-to-left shunts do not show a rise of more than 5 to 10 torr with oxygen inhalation. This is usually, but not always, true. Thus a modest increase of about 20 torr in descending aortic Po_2 with 100 percent oxygen administration does not exclude the diagnosis of right-to-left shunting in some forms of cyanotic congenital heart disease where the pulmonary blood flow is not greatly reduced so that the arterial Po_2 may rise moderately.

Since it has become common practice to pass an umbilical arterial catheter in cyanotic infants, most blood gas measurements are made on descending aortic blood. Infants with alveolar hypoventilation often show a marked increase in Po_2 to levels of 300 torr or greater when breathing 100 percent oxygen. In infants with cyanotic congenital heart lesions with markedly reduced pulmonary blood flow (pulmonary atresia) or decreased effective pulmonary blood flow (transposition of the great arteries) the arterial Po_2 may not change or may show only a small rise of 5 to 10 torr. This lack of response of descending aortic Po_2 to 100 percent oxygen inhalation should not be considered uniquely diagnostic of congenital cardiac disease. Neonates with primary pulmonary hypertension and some infants with severe lung disease may show little increase in descending aortic Po_2 with oxygen breathing, but the temporal arterial or right radial blood Po_2 may increase more than 25 torr. In these cases the absence of a significant rise of descending aortic Po_2 is due to the presence of a large right-to-left shunt through the ductus arteriosus.

CARDIAC MALFORMATIONS WITH RIGHT-TO-LEFT SHUNTS

The chest roentgenogram provides the basis for a useful classification of cyanotic heart lesions based on an assessment of pulmonary vascular markings. Furthermore, specific cardiac silhouettes and cardiac size provide important clues (Table 10).

Tetralogy of Fallot

The tetralogy of Fallot is the most common cyanotic heart lesion encountered in patients with cyanotic congenital heart disease who survive beyond infancy. Four structural abnormalities constitute the tetralogy: right ventricular outflow tract stenosis, ventricular septal defect, dextroposition of the aorta, and right ventricular hypertrophy (Figs. 70B and 71). Although these four elements are generally present, there is a wide anatomic variation with resultant physiologic and clinical variations.

MORPHOLOGY. The primary site of obstruction to blood flow is in the infundibulum or outflow tract of the right ventricle (Fig. 71), but other elements of the pulmonary outflow tract are also usually involved, the pulmonary valve being stenotic and the pulmonary arteries hypoplastic. In the most severe form (tetralogy of Fallot with pulmonary atresia, often termed pseudotruncus) the distal infundibular outflow tract and pulmonary valve are atretic and the pulmonary artery and main pulmonary artery branches may be severely hypoplastic or atretic (Figs. 70c and 72). The ventricular septal defect is usually quite large and is located just below the crista supraventricularis and in close proximity to the tricuspid and aortic valves. The aorta arises directly over the ventricular septal defect; the degree of overriding varies greatly and can best be evaluated by angiography. An important anatomic diagnostic feature is the frequent occurrence (about 25 percent) of a right-sided aortic arch.

TABLE 10. Malformations Associated with Pulmonary Blood Flow

Malformations usually associated with decreased pulmonary blood flow
    Tetralogy of Fallot with pulmonary atresia (pseudotruncus)
    Double-outlet right ventricle with pulmonic stenosis
    Transposition of great arteries with pulmonic stenosis and ventricular septal defect
    Single ventricle with pulmonic stenosis
    Pulmonary atresia with intact ventricular septum
    Severe pulmonic stenosis with intact ventricular septum
    Tricuspid atresia
    Ebstein's malformation of the tricuspid valve
Malformations usually associated with increased pulmonary blood flow
    d-Transposition of great arteries; double-outlet right ventricle
    Total anomalous pulmonary venous connection
    Truncus arteriosus
    Hypoplastic left heart syndrome (aortic and mitral atresia)
    Single-ventricle complex
    Tricuspid atresia with transposition of great arteries

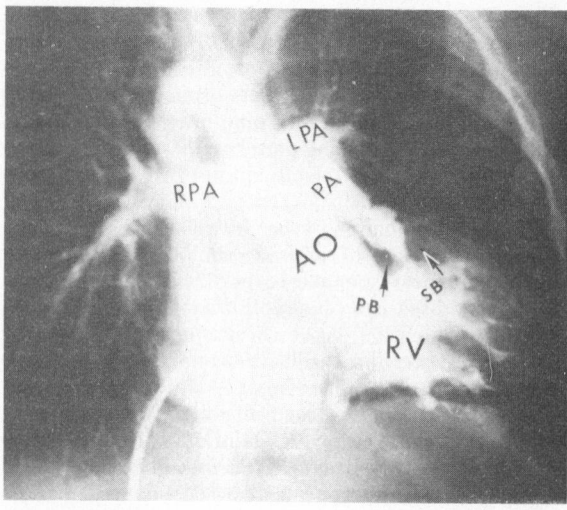

FIG. 71. Angiocardiogram in tetralogy of Fallot; right ventricular (RV) selective injection showing severe infundibular obstruction (arrows) and early filling of aorta (Ao); PA, LPA, and RPA, main, left, and right pulmonary arteries; PB, parietal band; SB, septal band.

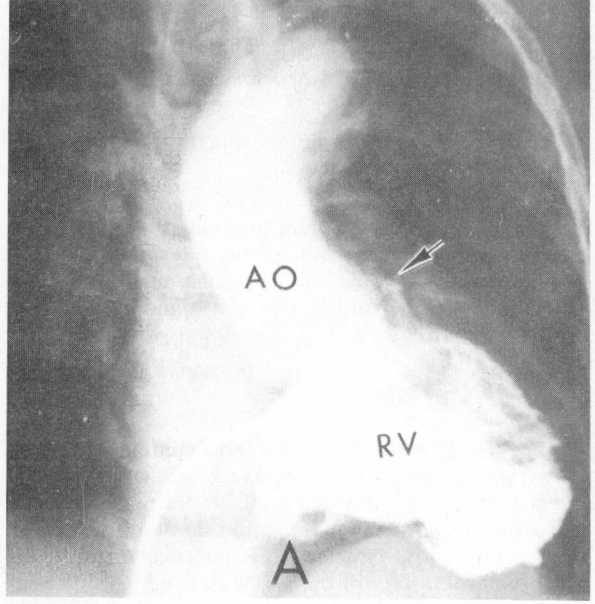

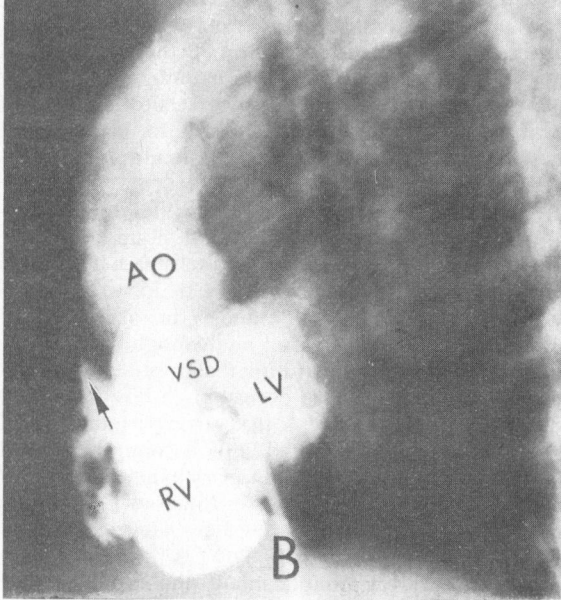

FIG. 72. Angiocardiogram in tetralogy of Fallot with pulmonary atresia. A. Anteroposterior view showing filling of aorta (Ao) from selective right ventricular injection and atretic right ventricular outflow tract (arrow). B. Lateral oblique view showing large ventricular septal defect (VSD) confluent with large overriding aortic orifice.

HEMODYNAMICS.   Right ventricular contraction is unable to eject the entire systemic venous return into the pulmonary vascular bed because of the pulmonary outflow tract obstruction. Varying amounts of venous blood are shunted across the ventricular septal defect and into the aorta, resulting in cyanosis. As a result of the pulmonary outflow tract obstruction the pulmonary artery pressure and pulmonary blood flow are reduced.

Because the ventricular septal defect in the tetralogy of Fallot is usually large, right ventricular peak systolic pressure equals that in the left ventricle and aorta, and the right and left ventricular pressure contours are essentially similar. Rarely the ventricular septal defect is anatomically or functionally small due to apposition of a tricuspid valve leaflet to the defect. Right ventricular pressures will then exceed left ventricular pressures, a finding more commonly noted in patients with severe pulmonary valve stenosis and intact ventricular septum.

The clinical status in the tetralogy of Fallot reflects the magnitude of the pulmonary blood flow, which in turn depends on the anatomic severity of right ventricular outflow tract obstruction, the relative resistances to ventricular outflow imposed by the systemic and pulmonary circulations, and the presence of systemic-to-pulmonary collateral blood supply via bronchial arteries or a persistent patent ductus arteriosus.

Hypertrophy of the crista supraventricularis contributes to the infundibular stenosis and results in formation of an infundibular chamber. Right ventricular obstruction may be relatively fixed, with much fibrosis and permanent narrowing of the outflow tract, or the obstruction may be relatively dynamic and muscular, reflecting various states of contractility of the infundibular musculature.

The acute severe episodes of dyspnea and hypoxemia, termed blue spells, which occur in some infants with the tetralogy reflect a further reduction in the already compromised pulmonary blood flow. The precipitating mechanisms are probably multiple: prolonged crying may result in a decrease in pulmonary blood flow because of the prolonged expirations; functional prolonged constriction of the right ventricular infundibulum will further decrease pulmonary blood flow; decreases in systemic vascular resistance because of immobilization, fever, or spontaneous vasomotor changes will also increase the magnitude of the right-to-left shunt. The fall in systemic vascular resistance associated with peripheral vasodilatation during exercise in the tetralogy of Fallot similarly results in a marked increase in right-to-left shunting.

CLINICAL MANIFESTATIONS.   The clinical findings vary with the severity of the pulmonary stenosis, but few children with the tetralogy of Fallot remain asymptomatic or acyanotic. Cyanosis usually is not present at birth; as long as the ductus arteriosus remains patent there may be adequate pulmonary blood flow. In the symptomatic infant or young child attacks of paroxysmal hyperpnea and increased cyanosis may occur spontaneously or following early morning feedings or prolonged crying. The attacks may last only a few moments and have no significant sequelae; they may be more prolonged and followed by limpness, deep exhaustion, or sleep, rarely they may end in unconsciousness, convulsions, or even death. In the older child, exercise tolerance usually varies in proportion to the severity of the cyanosis. Young children with the tetralogy of Fallot and limited exercise tolerance often adopt a characteristic squatting position after exertion. This maneuver results in an increased arterial oxygen saturation, probably by increasing systemic arterial resistance and decreasing systemic venous return. When right ventricular outflow tract obstruction and ventricular septal defect of the general morphology of the tetralogy of Fallot are present without significant right-to-left shunt, the anomaly is termed acyanotic Fallot.

Without surgical intervention the clinical course and prognosis vary with the severity of right ventricular outflow tract obstruction. Infants with pulmonary atresia usually require some form of palliative surgical intervention in the first few weeks or months of life. Approximately one-third of patients with the tetralogy of Fallot begin to have anoxic spells by 4 or 5 months of age, and many of these infants require surgical intervention quite promptly. These spells may occur even if the children are not cyanotic at rest. The time of onset is often when the children first begin to be cyanotic but have not had time to develop compensatory polycythemia. Some may remain moderately cyanotic, but the frequency of spells diminishes, presumably as a result of the development of bronchial collateral circulation. About one-third of the patients show only modest cyanosis during infancy and are asymptomatic or have infrequent episodes of dyspnea. These children eventually show fatigue on moderate physical exertion and usually show increasing difficulties when school age is reached. A final group of patients shows little or no evidence of cyanosis in infancy or early childhood (acyanotic Fallot). Cyanosis on exertion becomes gradually more manifest as they grow older, but occasionally very rapid clinical change occurs toward the classic severely cyanotic tetralogy.

Major complications associated with this malformation include brain abscess, cerebral thrombosis with hemiplegia, and infective endocarditis. Infective endocarditis is not common in the tetralogy before palliative surgery is performed, but afterward a significant incidence (about 5 percent) has occurred in older children. Prophylactic antibiotic therapy should be administered when surgical procedures involving teeth, throat, ear, and genitourinary tract are undertaken (p. 1471). Growth and development are generally delayed in proportion to the degree of cyanosis.

PHYSICAL FINDINGS.   The heart is not hyperactive, but a right ventricular systolic heave may be present along the lower left sternal border. A systolic thrill may be felt along the lower left sternal border, but is absent in the more severe form of infundibular obstruction and in the tetralogy with pulmonary atresia. The first heart sound usually is accentuated at the lower left sternal border, and in some patients an early systolic ejection sound that is aortic in origin may be heard maximally at the left sternal border and apex. A single loud second heart sound is generally heard corresponding to the aortic valve closure at the left sternal border. When closure of the pulmonary valve is audible, it is delayed and diminished in intensity at the upper left sternal border. In patients with moderate right ventricular outflow tract obstruction the systolic murmur is loud and harsh, stenotic or pansystolic in quality, and is best heard at the mid- or lower left sternal border. The systolic murmur begins early in systole and stops short of the second heart sound; in general, the more severe the obstruction to pulmonary blood flow the shorter the duration of the murmur. In extreme pulmonary outflow tract stenosis or pulmonary atresia, and at the height of a paroxysmal anoxic spell, there may be no murmur or only a very short faint murmur. A faint continuous murmur may be heard over the anterior or posterior chest, particularly in children with pulmonary atresia; this bruit represents flow through enlarged bronchial collateral vessels. Rarely, a significant continuous murmur of persistent ductus arteriosus is heard at the upper left sternal border.

ROENTGENOGRAPHY. The tetralogy of Fallot is characterized by a heart of relatively normal size and poorly vascularized lung fields signifying diminished pulmonary blood flow (Fig. 73). The right ventricular outflow tract and main pulmonary artery segments are usually hypoplastic, resulting in a concavity of the upper left margin of the cardiac silhouette instead of the normal convexity. A characteristic coeur en sabot or boot-

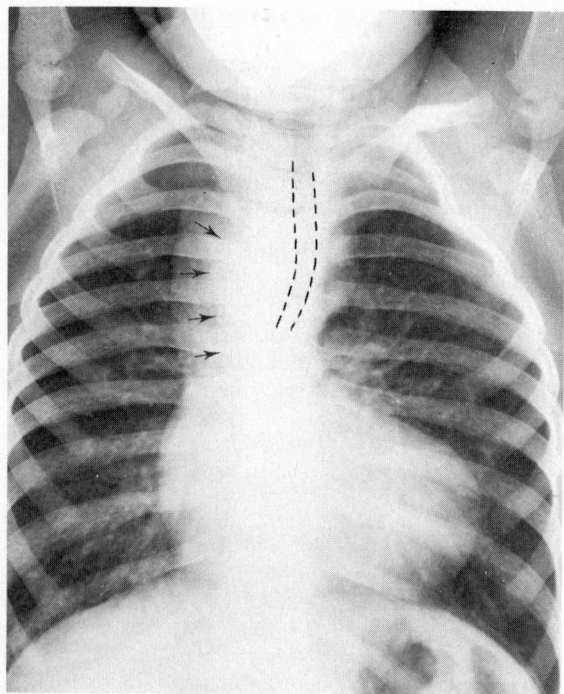

FIG. 73. Chest roentgenogram in tetralogy of Fallot. Arrows indicate right-sided aortic arch and upper thoracic aorta. Dashed lines indicate right-sided aortic indentation on the air tracheogram.

shaped heart may be present, particularly with pulmonary atresia. The ascending aorta is generally large. In about 25 percent of the patients a right-sided aortic arch is present and is easily recognized by observing a right-sided rather than left-sided indentation on the air tracheogram or barium esophagram. The superior vena caval shadow may likewise be displaced to the right. When bronchial collateral circulation is well developed, diffuse fine vascular markings are noted throughout the lung.

ELECTROCARDIOGRAM. In the older infant and child the electrocardiogram shows right axis deviation and right ventricular hypertrophy. In the newborn infant, however, the diagnosis of pathologic right ventricular hypertrophy by electrocardiogram is more difficult because of the normal right ventricular dominance at this age. In the newborn infant a persistent upright T wave in V_1 beyond 5 days of age may constitute the only early evidence of abnormal right ventricular hypertrophy. In the acyanotic tetralogy patient, combined ventricular hypertrophy may be noted at first, with progression into right ventricular hypertrophy as cyanosis develops.

ECHOCARDIOGRAPHY. The echocardiogram will show the thick right ventricular wall and the wide aorta with its anterior wall displaced relative to the septum (p. 1372). However, distinction from truncus arteriosus is difficult unless the pulmonary valve can be seen; this is not always possible, although the cross-sectional echoes given by multibeam systems are better in this respect.

CATHETERIZATION AND ANGIOGRAPHY. In most patients careful evaluation and correlation of the clinical findings, roentgenogram, and electrocardiogram will suffice to establish the diagnosis. A number of other complex cyanotic heart lesions such as transposition or corrected transposition of the great arteries with ventricular septal defect, double-outlet right ventricle, and single ventricle, *when associated with pulmonary outflow tract stenosis*, may mimic the clinical findings of the tetralogy of Fallot. Selective ventricular angiography provides the most useful diagnostic assistance in these problems.

Catheterization substantiates overriding of the aorta by easy passage of the catheter from the right ventricle into the aorta. Right ventricular outflow tract obstruction is confirmed by observing systolic hypertension in the right ventricle and by a drop in systolic pressure as the catheter enters the right ventricular infundibular chamber or pulmonary artery distal to the obstructions. The peak systolic pressures are usually equal in the right ventricle, left ventricle, and aorta. Blood samples provide quantitation of the right-to-left shunt and generally show little significant left-to-right shunting, except in the acyanotic tetralogy.

Selective angiography will demonstrate the anatomy of the outflow tract obstruction in detail, show early filling of the aorta with passage of contrast medium across the ventricular septal defect, and clarify the relationship of the aorta to the ventricular septal defect. It will also evaluate the adequacy of the pulmonary valve annulus and the main pulmonary artery and its branches in regard to corrective surgery and alert the surgeon to any unusual associated cardiovascular malformations. (Figs. 71 and 72).

ASSOCIATED CARDIOVASCULAR ANOMALIES.

Cardiac catheterization and angiography also serve to reveal certain associated cardiovascular anomalies that are difficult to recognize clinically; (1) Atrial septal defects of the secundum type, including patent foramen ovale, should be closed at surgery. (2) Recognition of a persistent left superior vena cava draining into the coronary sinus is important prior to instituting cardiopulmonary bypass. (3) Angiographic delineation of the primary pulmonary artery branches and their relationships to large bronchopulmonary collateral vessels is essential for planning right ventricular outflow tract reconstruction in the tetralogy with pulmonary atresia (Fig. 74). (4) Absence of one pulmonary artery (usually left) may be suspected from the chest roentgenogram, but pulmonary angiography is important because severe unilateral pulmonary branch stenosis may mimic an absent pulmonary artery. (5) Absence of pulmonary valve leaflets is a rare malformation occurring in about 3 to 4 percent of tetralogy of Fallot patients. This is a distinct clinical syndrome characterized by a hyperdynamic heart with a prominent to-and-fro murmur and usually modest cyanosis. Aneurysmal dilatation of the pulmonary artery results in varying degrees of bronchial compression with recurrent pneumonitis or occasionally lobar emphysema. (6) Anomalous coronary artery distribution, or so-called conus coronary, in which the anterior descending artery originates from the right coronary artery and crosses the infundibular area, may constitute a hazard during ventriculotomy.

TREATMENT. *Medical management* is directed primarily toward relief of paroxysmal dyspnea and cyanotic spells and prevention of the complications of right-to-left shunts. An attack of paroxysmal dyspnea may be treated by placing the infant on his abdomen in a knee-chest position or by holding him with the legs flexed upon the abdomen. Oxygen may be administered to lessen the dyspnea and cyanosis. Morphine sulfate (0.2 mg/kg body weight subcutaneously) is especially effective for prolonged or severe attacks. If the spell is protracted and severe and does not respond to the foregoing therapy, metabolic acidosis will ensue, and correction with intravenous sodium bicarbonate or TRIS is essential. Vasopressors can be given either early in the attack or if other therapy fails; methoxamine (Vasoxyl) 0.1 mg/kg intravenously or phenylephrine (Neo-Synephrine) 0.02 mg/kg intravenously will raise systemic resistance and thus increase pulmonary blood flow. If possible, these drugs should be given by continuous intravenous infusion, with the dose being adjusted by monitoring of blood pressure. For continuous infusion the dose of phenylephrine is 2 to 5 μg/kg/minute.

In infancy these attacks may be precipitated by a relative iron deficiency anemia (hypochromic microcytic), and such patients should have iron therapy until the hematocrit reaches more appropriate levels of 60 to 65 percent. Further increase in the hematocrit will result in a marked rise in blood viscosity, with possible resultant impediment to blood flow and risk of cerebral thrombosis.

In some infants, particularly those with a markedly dynamic, muscular right ventricular outflow tract obstruction, oral propranolol (β-adrenergic blocking

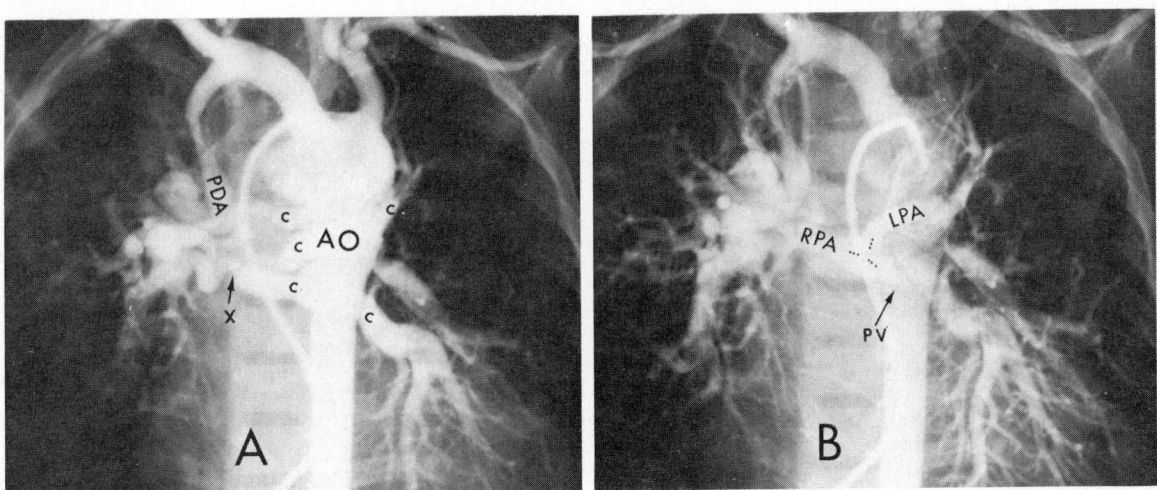

FIG. 74. Angiocardiogram (anteroposterior view) in tetralogy of Fallot with pulmonary atresia and injection into aorta. A. Multiple large bronchopulmonary collateral vessels (c) and patent ductus arteriosus (PDA) providing blood flow to distal pulmonary artery branches; X indicates transition constriction site between bronchial collateral and pulmonary artery vessels. B. Later frames in series showing retrograde filling of small proximal pulmonary artery branches (RPA and LPA) and main pulmonary artery terminating in atretic pulmonary valve (PV).

agent) in doses of 0.5 to 1.0 mg/kg given orally every 6 hours has been effective in preventing or reducing the frequency of paroxysmal dyspneic attacks. Prolonged pharmacologic management with this negative inotropic agent is not advisable, and most cardiologists consider initial surgical therapy preferable.

The indications for *surgery* and the type of surgery to be performed (extracardiac and palliative or intracardiac and corrective) vary with the age of the patient, the anatomic nature of the right ventricular outflow tract obstruction, and the experience of the surgeon. In an infant with severe tetralogy or tetralogy with pulmonary atresia, episodes of paroxysmal dyspnea, persistent deep cyanosis, and failure to gain weight are indications for early surgery.

Infants with the tetralogy of Fallot and a pulmonary outflow tract reasonably adequate in size can have open heart surgical repair of the malformation by highly skilled and experienced surgeons in the first months or year of life with a relatively low operative mortality of about 10 percent. Many infants with severe cyanosis present in the first weeks or months of life with grossly deformed and markedly hypoplastic or atretic right ventricular outflow tracts. This group continues to be palliated in most centers with some form of systemic–pulmonary anastomosis. A systemic-to-pulmonary anastomosis by increasing pulmonary blood flow relieves the cyanosis and hypoxic symptoms and can stabilize the clinical condition for many years. In the neonate an anastomosis of ascending aorta to right pulmonary artery (Waterston-Cooley) is currently the most frequently employed procedure, rather than anastomosis of descending aorta to left pulmonary artery (Potts-Smith-Gibson). In the older infant and child, a subclavian–pulmonary anastomosis (Blalock-Taussig) is preferred whenever it is technically feasible because of the greater difficulty of obliterating an aortic–pulmonary anastomosis at the time of subsequent open heart corrective surgery. Furthermore, a right- or left-sided aortic–pulmonary anastomosis is often too large, with subsequent congestive heart failure or pulmonary hypertension and pulmonary vascular obstructive disease. The subclavian–pulmonary anastomosis is increasingly being employed successfully with special microsuturing techniques in the newborn and young infant. Palliation for the tetralogy of Fallot with shunt operations carries an operative mortality in infants *under 6 weeks of age* of about 20 percent, but by 3 to 6 months of age the mortality for these same procedures is about 5 to 8 percent.

After successful palliation, anoxic spells cease, cyanosis and clubbing diminish, and a machinery-type murmur is heard at the base indicating a functioning systemic–pulmonary anastomosis. The duration of symptomatic relief may be short-lived after a Blalock-Taussig operation, particularly if it is performed during early infancy, because the shunt often is too small. In contrast, the most common complications of the aortic–pulmonary anastomoses are early or persisting congestive heart failure due to an excessively large anastomosis or late development of pulmonary vascular

obstructive pathology due to high pulmonary blood flow and persistent pulmonary hypertension.

The preferred surgical therapy for the tetralogy of Fallot is a single corrective operation with direct relief of the obstruction to the right ventricular outflow tract and closure of the ventricular septal defect, since this obviates the risk of a second-stage procedure for closing a palliative anastomosis and completing the intracardiac repair. Furthermore, there are strong psychologic advantages for both the child and the parents in repairing the cardiac malformation in early infancy and sparing them from continuing anxieties and anticipated future surgical risks.

With the patient's circulation maintained with cardiopulmonary bypass, and sometimes using deep hypothermia, the pathology in the right ventricle is exposed through a right ventricular incision, the infundibular stenosis is resected, coexistent valvar pulmonary stenosis is relieved, and the ventricular septal defect is closed. If the obstruction in the right ventricular outflow tract is not adequately relieved by resection, it may be necessary to enlarge the pulmonary outflow tract by placing a pericardial or plastic patch in the anterior ventricular wall. It may even be necessary to extend the outflow patch across the pulmonary valve annulus into the main pulmonary artery branches to relieve obstruction. Pulmonary valve incompetence usually results, but if there is adequate distal relief of the pulmonary obstruction, a mild regurgitant lesion does not appear to produce serious hemodynamic disturbances. Some surgeons may put in a unicusp homograft or heterograft aortic valve to prevent pulmonic regurgitation.

Repair of tetralogy of Fallot with pulmonary atresia has in recent years been successfully accomplished by inserting a heterograft valve-bearing conduit between the right ventricle and the pulmonary arteries after the ventricular septal defect is closed. Patients with extreme hypoplasia of the distal pulmonary artery bed or with large and bizarre bronchial collateral vessels supporting the pulmonary circulation still present a formidable surgical risk to open heart surgical correction.

TETRALOGY-LIKE LESIONS. Severe pulmonic stenosis with a double-outlet right ventricle, single ventricle, or *l*-transposition of the great arteries with a ventricular septal defect may closely resemble the tetralogy of Fallot. The diagnosis and treatment of the first two are discussed on pages 1462 and 1467. The third entity, which is due to abnormal formation of an *l*-loop in the embryo (p. 1359), may be suspected clinically from its characteristic electrocardiographic, roentgenographic, and echocardiographic features (p. 1416); confirmation may be obtained by catheterization and angiography. Surgical correction is made difficult by the posterior position and abnormal anatomy of the right ventricular outflow tract obstruction (p. 1417) and the high risk of producing complete heart block.

Tricuspid Atresia

Tricuspid atresia, which constitutes 1 to 2 percent of all congenital heart disease in the first year of life, is a much less frequent cause of cyanotic congenital heart disease than transposition of the great vessels (5 to 6 percent) or the tetralogy of Fallot (4 to 5 percent). In tricuspid atresia there is no opening from the right atrium to the right ventricle, and the only outlet from the right atrium for systemic venous blood is an interatrial communication, usually a stretched patent foramen ovale (Fig. 75). Mixing of the entire pulmonary venous and systemic venous return occurs in the left atrium, and consequently systemic arterial oxygen unsaturation will reflect the volume of pulmonary blood flow. Left ventricular output is then distributed directly to the aorta and indirectly (through a ventricular septal defect or patent ductus arteriosus) to the pulmonary vascular bed. Pulmonary blood flow is usually severely diminished in tricuspid atresia because of the small, restrictive size of the ventricular septal defect and the underdeveloped stenotic right ventricular outflow tract. Pulmonary atresia and an extremely hypoplastic right ventricle may be present if there is no ventricular septal defect; pulmonary blood flow will then be derived from the aorta via a patent ductus arterious or bronchial collateral vessels. Increased pulmonary blood flow is encountered less frequently in tricuspid atresia, but it may occur when the ventricular septal defect is large and not restrictive and the pulmonary outflow tract to the right ventricle is well developed or when transposition of the great arteries is present and the pulmonary artery arises directly from the left ventricle.

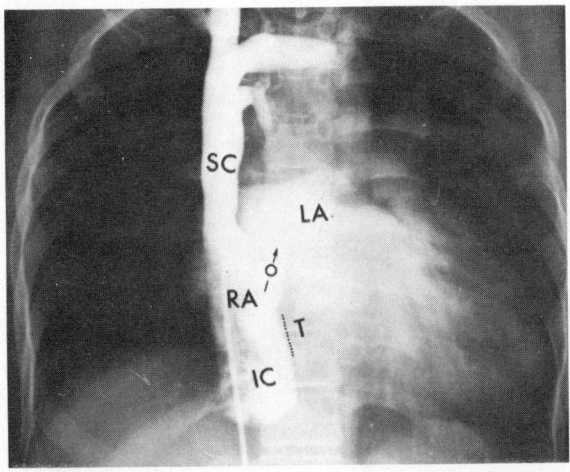

FIG. 75. Angiocardiogram (anteroposterior view) in tricuspid atresia; injection into superior vena cava (SC) showing passage of contrast material from right atrium (RA) to left atrium (LA) through dilated foramen ovale (O). Note site of tricuspid valve atresia (T).

CLINICAL MANIFESTATIONS. Intense cyanosis, dyspnea, and anoxic spells are common symptoms in the infant with tricuspid atresia with diminished pulmonary blood flow. Right heart failure, manifest by hepatomegaly and occasionally by presystolic hepatic pulsations, may occur if right-to-left shunting is ob-

structed at the patent foramen ovale. Clubbing, polycythemia, and occasional squatting, as well as poor physical development, will be apparent in an older infant or child. However, few infants survive beyond six months of age without surgical palliation.

There is usually a harsh systolic murmur, representing the ventricular septal defect and right ventricular infundibular stenosis, audible along the left sternal border. The second heart sound is narrowly split, with a diminished pulmonary component. If the ventricular septum is intact, there may be no significant murmur or only the very faint continuous bruit of a small patent ductus arteriosus. The second heart sound is single.

Infants with tricuspid atresia and persistent large ventricular septal defect or transposition of the great arteries usually show only minimal cyanosis after the newborn period. However, symptoms and signs of congestive heart failure, with tachypnea, dyspnea, excessive perspiration, hepatomegaly, and pulmonary rales, often appear by 3 to 6 weeks of age. The auscultatory findings in these infants are those of a large left-to-right shunt: a long harsh pansystolic murmur along the left sternal border, and a prominent mid-diastolic rumbling murmur at the apex.

The roentgenographic findings in the usual infant with tricuspid atresia include diminished pulmonary vasculature and a heart shape that is often distinctive, with a rounded or apple configuration resulting from deficiency of the right ventricular and pulmonary artery segments. In contrast, the infant with large ventricular septal defect or transposition has increased pulmonary markings, a large cardiac silhouette reflecting left ventricular enlargement, and sometimes findings of pulmonary edema.

The electrocardiographic findings of left superior axis deviation and left ventricular hypertrophy are helpful diagnostic clues for this lesion, since the most prevalent cyanotic heart lesions with diminished pulmonary blood flow (tetralogy) and with increased pulmonary blood flow (d-transposition) usually manifest right axis deviation and right ventricular hypertrophy. Right atrial hypertrophy manifested by prominent peaked P waves in limb lead II is also common, and the P-R interval is often abnormally short. In tricuspid atresia with transposition of the great arteries the QRS axis is usually in the left lower quadrant; occasionally it shows right axis deviation.

The echocardiogram can demonstrate the small right ventricle and the absence of a tricuspid valve, although it may be difficult to exclude various types of single ventricle or even pulmonary atresia; once again the multibeam systems are more useful. In addition, transposition of the great arteries may be disclosed.

Cardiac catheterization will confirm the total right-to-left passage of blood at the atrial level, demonstrate the prominent presystolic contraction waves in the right atrium, and show the right-to-left interatrial pressure gradient. Since the total systemic venous return must pass via the foramen ovale, it is essential that the atrial opening be adequate. Although major obstruction at this site is uncommon, balloon atrial septostomy should be carried out at the time of diagnostic cardiac catheterization in infants under 3 months of age. Angiocardiography demonstrates the sequential opacification of right atrium, left atrium, and left ventricle (Fig. 75) and subsequent opacification of the hypoplastic right ventricular outflow tract if there is a small ventricular septal defect. Demonstration of the pulmonary artery and its branches is provided either directly by the passage of contrast medium from the right ventricle or via a patent ductus arteriosus. The pulmonary artery branches are usually of adequate size for palliative anastomoses in this malformation, in contrast to the relatively high proportion of markedly hypoplastic pulmonary arteries in the severe tetralogy malformation.

MANAGEMENT. The treatment of infants with tricuspid atresia and diminished pulmonary blood flow is surgical and often is urgent. The occurrence of severe anoxic spells in an infant 2 or 3 weeks of age with tricuspid atresia often heralds a closing patent ductus arteriosus and the elimination of the major or only source of pulmonary blood flow. A right- or left-sided aortopulmonary shunt procedure can be performed in most of these very young infants, with about 20 percent surgical mortality. Good 10- to 15-year clinical results have been noted in about two-thirds of the survivors. A palliative shunt operation involving anastomosis between the superior vena cava and the right pulmonary artery (Glenn) has been developed; it has a physiologic advantage over the systemic–pulmonary anastomoses in that it increases pulmonary blood flow by diverting only systemic venous return directly into the pulmonary circulation. Unfortunately, this procedure has a high surgical risk and failure rate for infants less than 6 months of age; in older children excellent initial palliative results have been recorded.

More recently a physiologic corrective procedure (Fontan) has been developed in which the entire systemic venous return is directed to the lungs, and intracardiac mixing of the two circulations is prevented. The right atrium is converted into an outlet to the main pulmonary artery by use of a valve-bearing conduit, and the interatrial communication is closed. A modification interposes a conduit between right atrium and right ventricle and closes the ventricular septal defect, leaving the patient's own pulmonary valve to function in situ. These newer procedures have usually been limited to a subgroup of older children. Although their therapeutic role is yet to be fully assessed, they offer promise of a physiologic correction to several cyanotic congenital malformations that lack a functional pulmonary ventricle.

Infants with tricuspid atresia and transposition of the great arteries with markedly increased pulmonary blood flow can have surgical palliation with pulmonary artery banding to restrict the torrential pulmonary blood flow. The new right atrium to main pulmonary artery diversion procedures (Fontan) can also be used to effect a physiologic correction.

Pulmonary Atresia

Most infants with pulmonary atresia (or severe stenosis) with intact ventricular septum (2 percent of infants

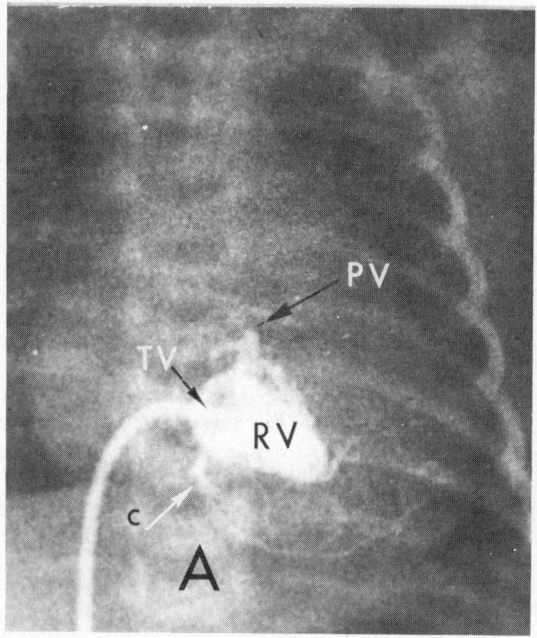 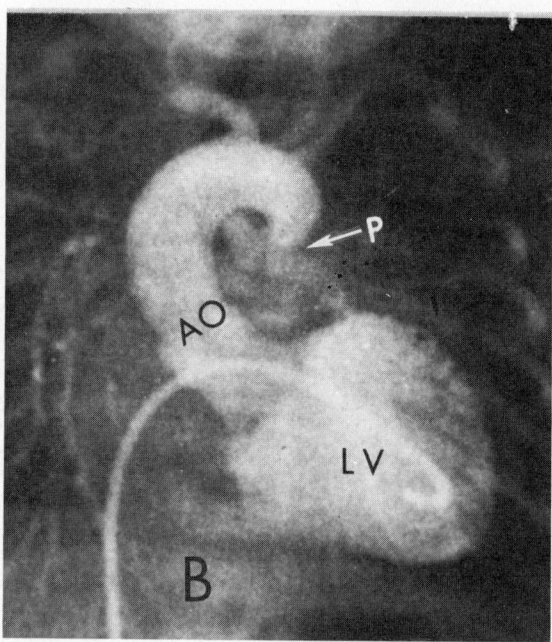

FIG. 76. Angiocardiogram (anteroposterior view) in neonate with pulmonary valve atresia and intact ventricular septum. A. Right ventricular injection showing hypoplastic right ventricular cavity (RV), tricuspid valve (TV), and retrograde filling of coronary arteries (c). B. Left ventricular injection showing relative ventricular chamber sizes (LV and RV) and small pulmonary blood flow derived through patent ductus arteriosus (P).

with congenital heart disease in the first year after birth) have a hypoplastic but thick-walled right ventricle with a markedly hypoplastic tricuspid orifice and valve (Fig. 76). About 15 percent have a right ventricle of normal or large volume, with the tricuspid valve functionally incompetent; intermediate forms between these extremes occur. To some extent the hemodynamics resemble those of tricuspid atresia, since there is no effective outflow from the right ventricle and essentially all the right atrial blood is shunted into the left atrium, left ventricle, and aorta. Occasionally, extreme pulmonary valve stenosis rather than pulmonary valve atresia will be present with a similar pathophysiology. With atresia the pulmonary circulation is sustained primarily through a patent ductus arteriosus (Fig. 77).

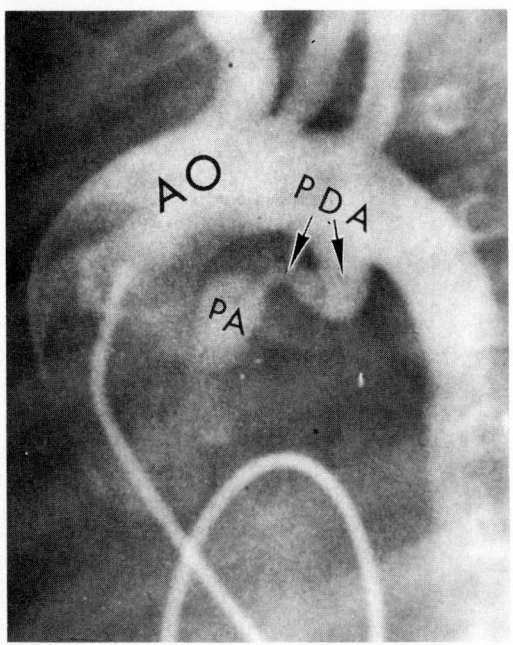

FIG. 77. Angiocardiogram (lateral view) showing long, tortuous, persistent patent ductus arteriosus (PDA) providing tenuous pulmonary blood flow to neonate with pulmonary atresia and intact ventricular septum. PA, pulmonary artery; AO, aorta.

Cyanosis occurs early in the neonatal period, and the clinical status of these infants usually deteriorates rapidly; intense hypoxemia, dyspnea, and early death occur within a few days unless adequate pulmonary blood flow can be provided surgically. Gross cardiac failure occurs in addition, most strikingly in the group with tricuspid incompetence.

If murmurs are heard they are usually quite faint. A soft systolic blowing murmur, probably representing insufficiency of the hypoplastic tricuspid valve, may be heard along the lower left and right sternal borders; a soft continuous bruit of a small patent ductus arteriosus may be heard at the upper left sternal border. The second heart sound at the pulmonary area is single, reflecting only aortic valve closure.

On chest roentgenogram the infant with a markedly reduced tricuspid orifice may show a small heart initially, but progressive cardiomegaly is usual; diminished pulmonary vascular markings are the rule, except in the rare case with a large persistent patent ductus arteriosus. Infants with marked tricuspid insufficiency and large right ventricular volumes have gross cardiomegaly.

On the electrocardiogram left ventricular hypertrophy is commonly noted in the first days or weeks of life, but right ventricular hypertrophy becomes evident as the right ventricular muscle hypertrophies further. In contrast to tricuspid atresia, where there is continuing left ventricular hypertrophy and usually left QRS axis deviation, the infant with pulmonary atresia shows normal or right QRS axis deviation.

An echocardiogram will show the small right ventricle and usually no pulmonary artery. Only if the tricuspid valve is shown can tricuspid atresia be excluded.

Cardiac catheterization will indicate right atrial hypertension, a massive right-to-left interatrial shunt, and right ventricular hypertension, often with peak systolic pressures greater than systemic. A right ventricular selective angiogram will establish the diagnosis by demonstrating the obstruction between the right ventricle and the pulmonary artery, and the size of the ventricular cavity provides important therapeutic criteria. Intramyocardial sinusoids may be noted to fill from the dead-end right ventricular cavity and drain retrograde into the coronary arterial system (Fig. 76A).

Prognosis in this lesion has been generally grim, although increased surgical salvage has occurred in recent years. In the majority of infants with markedly hypoplastic right ventricle and tricuspid orifice, balloon atrial septostomy should be performed at the initial diagnostic cardiac catheterization; then at surgery both a pulmonary valvotomy, if anatomically feasible, and a small systemic–pulmonary anastomosis should be created. The valvotomy permits the right ventricle to eject some blood and may permit some chamber enlargement, while in the interim the anastomosis provides the bulk of increased pulmonary blood flow that is essential for survival. Extreme hypoplasia of the ventricular chamber and a diminutive tricuspid orifice may render the successful distal opening of the pulmonary valve of little value. Infants with severe pulmonary valve stenosis having a small but functionally adequate right ventricular cavity (a criterion that is sometimes difficult to define) require a pulmonary valvotomy only, performed by supravalvar or transventricular approach, and they should not have balloon atrial septostomy.

Ebstein's Anomaly

Ebstein's anomaly is a rare malformation where the tricuspid valve is displaced downward and there is anomalous attachment of the posterior and septal leaflets to the right ventricular wall. The abnormally situated tricuspid valve divides the right ventricle into a proximal "atrial" segment and a distal functional ventricle. This atrialized ventricular segment and the right

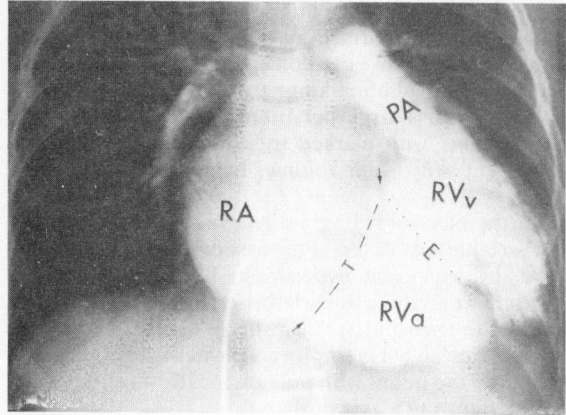

FIG. 78. Angiocardiogram (anteroposterior view) in Ebstein's anomaly of tricuspid valve showing downward displacement of tricuspid valve leaflet attachment (T to E) and division of right ventricle into proximal atrialized segment (RV$_a$) and distal functional ventricular segment (RV$_v$). T, normal tricuspid orifice and valve leaflet level; E, displaced anomalously attached tricuspid valve leaflet level. RA, right atrium; PA, pulmonary artery.

atrium together are usually enormously dilated, and there is evidence of gross tricuspid incompetence (Fig. 78). Hemodynamic abnormalities are related to the extent of the tricuspid regurgitation, to the small size of the remaining functional right ventricle, and to the degree of right-to-left shunting through a patent foramen ovale.

Clinical symptoms vary widely, depending on the extent of the downward displacement of the tricuspid valve. Rarely, in the most severe cases, cardiopulmonary difficulties are prominent in the neonatal period, and death can occur because of massive right heart failure and hypoxemia. Hemodynamic improvement does occur in most infants; it is probably related to the rapid perinatal decrease in the pulmonary vascular resistance. More commonly symptoms are not present in infants with less severe anatomic and physiologic abnormalities. Minimal or modest cyanosis is usually manifest in later childhood, unless the foramen ovale is not patent. Although there frequently is little limitation to activities during childhood, exercise tolerance eventually deteriorates. Attacks of paroxysmal supraventricular tachycardia are common.

On auscultation a characteristic triple or quadruple heart sound rhythm overrides a soft high-pitched systolic murmur of tricuspid regurgitation, and there is a peculiar soft scratchy mid-diastolic murmur at the left sternal border and apex. The second heart sound is usually widely split.

The roentgenographic findings include moderate or marked cardiomegaly, with striking enlargement of the right atrium and usually diminished pulmonary vascular markings. The heart is usually globular (Fig. 79A and B). The electrocardiogram may also be characteristic, usually showing right atrial hypertrophy, prolonged P-R interval, and incomplete or complete right bundle branch block patterns. Pre-excitation patterns (WPW syndrome) are also relatively frequent (about 10 to 15

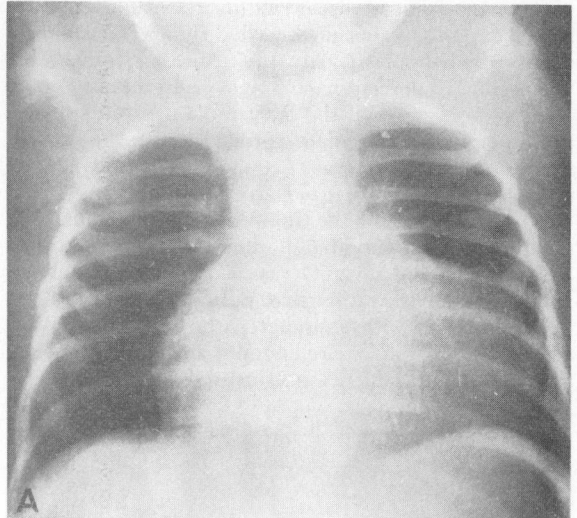

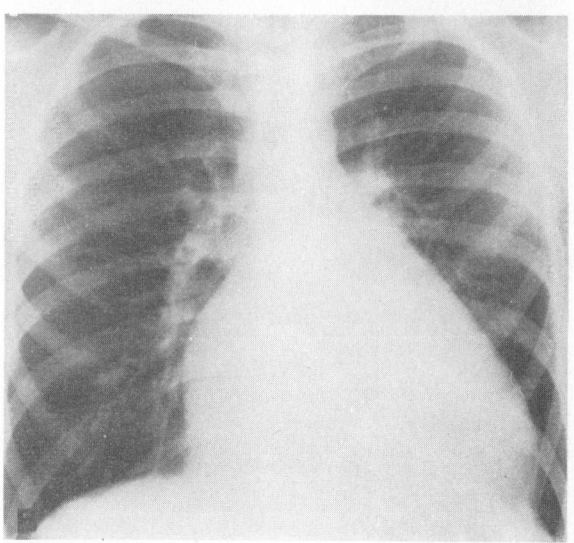

FIG. 79. Roentgenogram showing cardiomegaly, characteristic cardiac silhouette, and diminished pulmonary vascular markings in neonate with Ebstein's anomaly (A) and later at 9 years of age (B).

percent). The echocardiogram is as variable as the spectrum of this lesion. In general the large tricuspid valve is well shown, and tricuspid valve closure is characteristically delayed more than 70 msec after mitral valve closure. Multibeam systems may show the displacement of the tricuspid valve.

Cardiac catheterization, in order to be diagnostic, must demonstrate that a portion of the right ventricle functions as a right atrium because of the abnormal distal displacement of the tricuspid valve leaflets. This atrialization of a portion of the right ventricle is best confirmed by simultaneous intracardiac electrocardiogram–pressure recordings and by detailed angiocardiography. Catheterization is complicated by an increased incidence of induced tachyarrhythmias.

The life expectancy of the patient with Ebstein's anomaly varies widely, depending on the severity of the malformation. The usual cause of death is congestive heart failure in the second or third decade of life. In the child or young adult, the more severe the cyanosis the poorer the prognosis; the onset of florid congestive heart failure suggests death within 4 to 5 years. In the critically ill cyanotic infant it is essential not to confuse Ebstein's anomaly with pulmonary atresia and an intact ventricular septum, lest the infant with Ebstein's anomaly be subjected to surgical pulmonary valvotomy. Conversely, it is equally disastrous to defer surgical intervention in the infant with pulmonary atresia under a mistaken diagnosis of severe Ebstein's anomaly.

Moderate congestive heart failure can be effectively treated with digitalis and diuretics, and disturbing dysrhythmias can usually be controlled pharmacologically. Surgical treatment is seldom necessary in childhood. Surgical maneuvers directed at realigning the tricuspid valve leaflets to their true annulus, resection of redundant atrialized tissue, or placement of a prosthetic tricuspid valve have been attempted. Replacement of the abnormal valve with a prosthesis has been the most successful, but it is associated with a high surgical risk. In deeply cyanotic patients, symptomatic improvement has been observed after anastomosing the superior vena cava to the right pulmonary artery, since this increases pulmonary blood flow while reducing the load on the right ventricle.

Dextrotransposition of Great Arteries

Complete *d*-transposition of the great arteries is one of the most significant cyanotic cardiac lesions of the newborn period. It is the most common cardiac cause of cyanosis in the neonate, and until recently it accounted for the majority of deaths in infants with cyanotic congenital heart disease under 1 year of age. Formerly almost universally fatal, the prognosis has changed dramatically in recent years with the introduction of palliative and corrective procedures.

MORPHOLOGY AND PHYSIOLOGY. Transposition of the great arteries means that the great arteries are abnormally placed across the interventricular septum, and consequently the aorta and pulmonary artery arise from the wrong ventricles (Fig. 70F). Thus the aortic root is abnormally anterior and arises from the right ventricle; the main pulmonary artery is abnormally posterior and arises from the left ventricle (Fig. 80). Since the great vessels arise from the inappropriate ventricles, these relationships can also be termed discordant ventriculoarterial relationships. Concordant relationships mean that the right atrium empties into the right ventricle and the right ventricle into the pulmonary artery, while the left atrium enters into left ventricle and the left ventricle into the aorta. The embryology of these abnormalities is discussed on page 1356.

In complete *d*-transposition of the great arteries the systemic venous return traverses the right atrium and right ventricle and is ejected into the transposed aorta arising from the right ventricle; the pulmonary venous

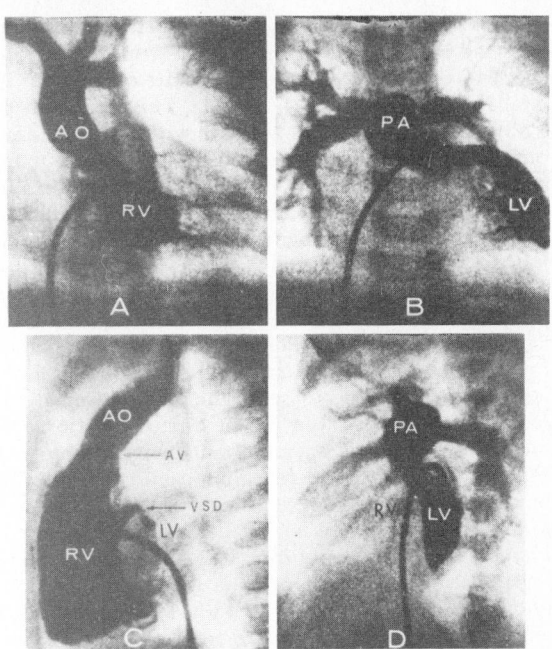

FIG. 80. Selective right (A, C) and left (B, D) ventricular angiograms in infant with transposition of the great arteries and small ventricular septal defect. Top (A, B) are anteroposterior views; bottom (C, D) are lateral views. RV, right ventricle; LV, left ventricle; AO, aorta, PA, pulmonary artery; VSD, ventricular septal defect; AV, aortic valve level.

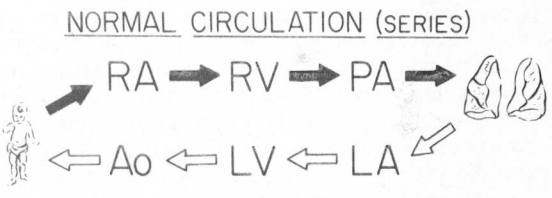

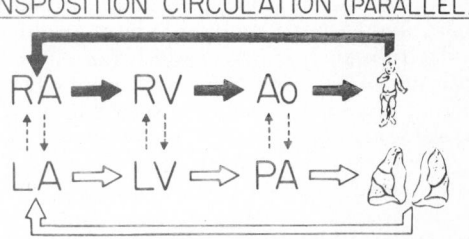

FIG. 81. Circulation pathways with normally related great arteries and with complete transposition of the great arteries. Large open arrows show path of oxygenated pulmonary venous blood; large solid black arrows show path of desaturated systemic venous blood. RA, right atrium; RV, right ventricle; PA, pulmonary artery; LA, left atrium; LV, left ventricle; AO, aorta. Intercirculation shunting of blood (small dashed arrows) at one or more levels is essential for postnatal survival in complete transposition.

return traverses the left atrium and the left ventricle and is ejected back into the lungs via the transposed pulmonary artery. There are thus two separate circulations in parallel instead of in series (Fig. 81). This arrangement is obviously incompatible with life without some anatomic communications to permit oxygenated pulmonary venous blood to enter the systemic circulation and systemic venous blood to enter the pulmonary circulation. In over half the patients with complete transposition the ventricular septum is intact, and intracardiac shunting occurs only through a stretched foramen ovale or rarely a secundum atrial defect. Although a patent ductus arteriosus may be demonstrated in about half of the newborn infants with transposition, it closes functionally and anatomically soon after birth in most patients. A persistent large patent ductus arteriosus is uncommon, but it is an important complication that requires prompt clinical recognition and therapy. Infants with associated large ventricular septal defect have better opportunities for mixing between the two circulations. Left ventricular outflow tract stenosis of varying degrees also may be present; it most often results from a fibrous ridge or collar in the outflow tract of the left ventricle. Common atrioventricular canal, atrioventricular valve atresia, severe pulmonary valve stenosis or atresia, or right aortic arch are rarely present in complete *d*-transposition of the great arteries, but these lesions are commonly associated with the less frequent *l*-transposition malformations or the single-ventricle complexes associated with transposition of the great arteries.

The major physiologic consequences of transposition of the great arteries are severe hypoxemia, metabolic acidemia, and congestive heart failure. The level of systemic arterial oxygen saturation is dependent on the transfer of oxygenated pulmonary venous blood to the systemic circuit, as well as the reciprocal transfer of systemic venous return to the pulmonary circuit. These transfers are a function of the size of the shunting sites: foramen ovale, ostium secundum defect, ventricular septal defect, patent ductus arteriosus, and bronchial collateral circulation. Other important factors, particularly in patients with large ventricular septal defect, are the hemodynamic consequences of moderate pulmonary outflow tract stenosis or increased pulmonary vascular resistance, either of which can effect a greater transfer of left-sided pulmonary venous blood to the right-sided aorta. However, if such pathology is severe it will restrict the pulmonary blood flow and the volume of the oxygenated pulmonary venous return and reduce the systemic arterial oxygen saturation. The existence of the systemic and pulmonary circulatory pathways in parallel instead of in series usually results in high cardiac output levels for both the right and left ventricles, with consequent cardiac dilatation and myocardial failure. Myocardial function can be further compromised by the markedly unsaturated aortic blood flow entering the coronary circulation.

Pulmonary vascular obstructive disease has been observed both by microscopy and by cardiac catheteriza-

tion to be more common and to progress at an unusually rapid rate in infants with transposition of the great arteries and large ventricular septal defect, as contrasted to infants with large ventricular septal defect and normally related great arteries. About 75 percent of all infants with transposition of the great arteries and large ventricular septal defect older than 1 year of age will have developed advanced pulmonary vascular obstructive disease. Early surgical pulmonary artery banding or pulmonary stenosis may protect against the development of pulmonary vascular obstructive disease in this lesion. Histologic studies demonstrate moderate pulmonary vascular disease lesions in many infants with large ventricular septal defect by 3 to 4 months of age. Accordingly, palliative pulmonary artery banding or open heart correction should be considered before this age. Advanced pulmonary vascular obstructive disease has even been observed in about 5 percent of the transposition patients with intact ventricular septum who survive early infancy.

CLINICAL MANIFESTATIONS. Although the clinical course can vary widely as a result of the previously described anatomic and physiologic factors, there are two basic clinical patterns centering about either hypoxemia or congestive heart failure. One extreme is represented by the severely cyanotic, hypoxemic infant who has minimal communication between the pulmonary and systemic circulations—an intact ventricular septum and a limiting patent foramen ovale. The other extreme is represented by the mildly or moderately cyanotic infant with prominent congestive heart failure who has a large communication between the circulations, usually a ventricular septal defect, although occasionally a patent ductus arteriosus.

Most infants with an intact ventricular septum become critically ill the first few days after birth, but if there is a large ventricular septal defect, cyanosis may be slight and congestive heart failure may not become evident until a few weeks after birth. Characteristically, attention is first directed to the infant with inadequate intracardiac mixing by nursery personnel who observe cyanosis in an otherwise apparently healthy infant. A high index of suspicion is needed for early diagnosis; except for persistent cyanosis and progressive hyperpnea in the first days after birth, the infant may appear well developed and hardly distressed, and the chest roentgenogram and electrocardiogram may be deceptively normal in appearance.

On auscultation the second heart sound is usually interpreted as loud and single, but careful auscultation often reveals narrow splitting with a soft distinct pulmonary valve closure. The murmurs are usually unimpressive in the newborn with an intact ventricular septum, but there may be a short grade 2-3/6 ejection systolic murmur at the mid-left sternal border. A loud harsh systolic murmur in a slightly older infant usually indicates a ventricular septal defect or left ventricular outflow tract stenosis. In the former the murmur is pansystolic and maximal along the mid- and lower left sternal border; in the latter the murmur has a more stenotic quality and is maximal at the mid- left sternal border, but with transmission toward the upper right sternal border.

The electrocardiogram may not be helpful in the newborn infant, since it shows right axis deviation and right ventricular hypertrophy of a degree that may be normal for a neonate. After 5 days of age, however, persistence of a positive T wave over the right precordium suggests abnormal right ventricular hypertension. In the older infant with an intact ventricular septum, right atrial hypertrophy and overt right ventricular hypertrophy are present.

The roentgenographic findings can vary from near normal to grossly abnormal. In the newborn the heart is small, but it enlarges over the first 1 to 2 weeks after birth. The pulmonary vascular markings may appear normal or minimally increased initially (Fig. 82A), and only later do the characteristic findings of increased

pulmonary vascularity appear. The classic transposition cardiac silhouette, an egg-shaped or oval heart with a narrow superior mediastinum and small thymic shadow, is highly diagnostic, but it is present early in only about one-third of the newborn infants (Fig. 82B).

Infants with transposition of the great arteries and large ventricular septal defect develop prominent cardiac failure and modest cyanosis, usually at 3 to 4 weeks of age. There is increasing tachypnea, dyspnea, and excessive perspiration. Cyanosis might have increased, but often it is relatively mild because of good circulatory mixing. Pulmonary rales may be heard, and hepatomegaly may be striking. The chest roentgenogram in this group, after the initial newborn period, characteristically shows a larger, more globular heart, with a greater increase of pulmonary vascular markings than is evident in the group with inadequate mixing (Fig. 82C). The electrocardiogram, after the newborn period, charac-

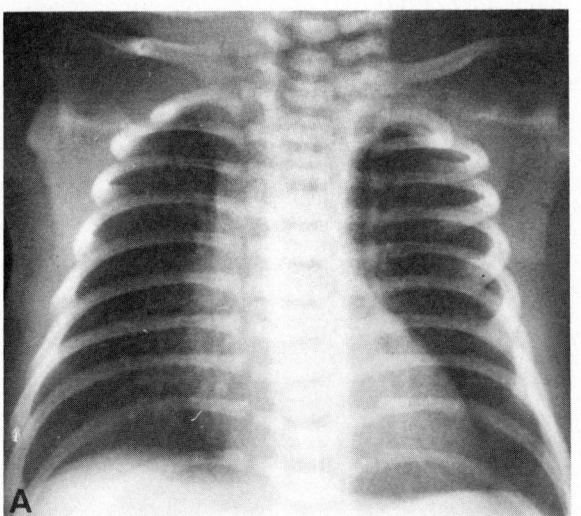
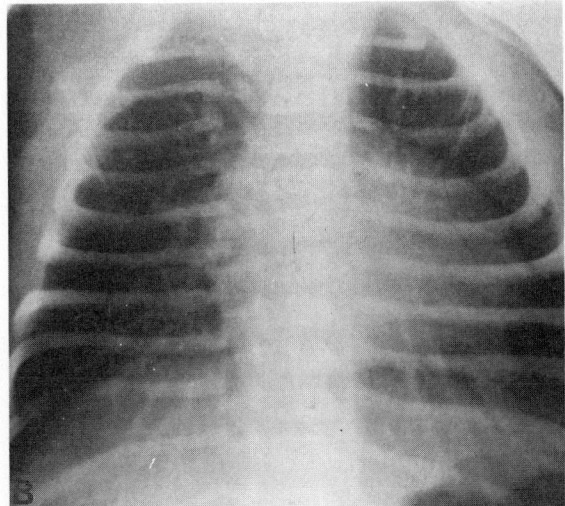
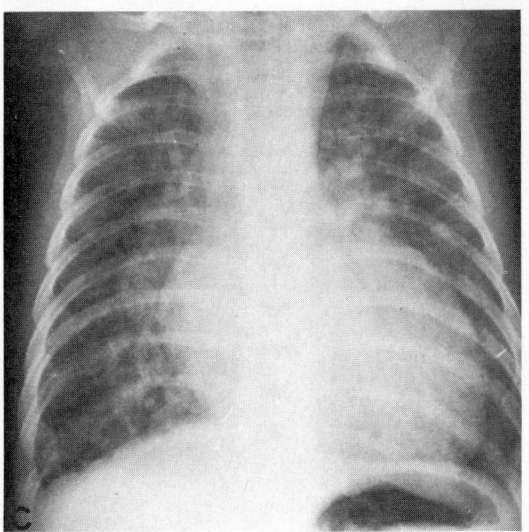

FIG. 82.   Chest roentgenogram in *d*-transposition of the great arteries. A. Infant 1 day old with deceptively normal appearing heart size and pulmonary vascular markings. B. Infant 1 day old with more classic oval-shaped and enlarged heart with slightly increased vascular markings. C. Infant 1 month old with associated large ventricular septal defect showing marked cardiomegaly and pulmonary plethora.

teristically manifests right ventricular or combined ventricular hypertrophy.

Echocardiography, especially with the multibeam system, is useful in the cyanotic newborn infant in showing the normal positions of the great arteries. If valve opening and closure can be shown, then the duration of systole (longer in the pulmonary ventricle) also helps to identify each artery (p. 1371).

Cardiac catheterization and angiography are of value for confirming the diagnosis, establishing the presence of associated lesions, and effecting hemodynamic and clinical improvement by enlarging the interatrial communication with an inflated balloon catheter. Catheterization shows systemic pressure in the right ventricle, and the catheter can easily be manipulated to enter the aorta directly from the right ventricle. The catheter may easily be passed across a foramen ovale into the left atrium and into the left ventricle, and with special maneuvers the pulmonary artery can be entered. Oxygen saturation of the blood in the pulmonary artery is higher than that in the aorta. In the newborn, when the ventricular septum is intact, the left ventricular systolic pressure may equal right ventricular peak systolic pressure, but after a few days left ventricular pressure usually falls to one-half or less of right ventricular pressure unless some left ventricular outflow tract obstruction is present. A pressure gradient across the atrial septum is common, with left atrial pressures exceeding those on the right.

Selective ventricular angiography is diagnostic. Injection into the right ventricle will demonstrate the high anterior position of the aorta arising from the right ventricle, the status of the ventricular septum, and the ductus arteriosus, if it is patent. Selective left ventricular angiography will demonstrate a pulmonary artery arising from the posterior ventricle, the status of the ventricular septum, and any left ventricular outflow tract stenosis (Fig. 80).

Infants with inadequate communications between the circulations should have as little delay as possible in receiving supportive therapy for hypoxemia, metabolic acidemia, and maintenance of body temperature. The diagnosis should be established by cardiac catheterization as soon as possible, and a large interatrial communication should be created by a balloon septostomy procedure (Fig. 83). A balloon catheter may be advanced to traverse the foramen ovale and enter the left atrium, where the balloon is inflated to a diameter of about 15 mm. The catheter and inflated balloon are then abruptly withdrawn into the right atrium and inferior vena caval orifice, thus rupturing the septum primum valve of the fossa ovalis, enlarging the interatrial communication, and providing for more adequate mixing of blood at the atrial level. There is usually an immediate fall in the elevated left atrial pressure, an increase in the systemic arterial oxygen saturation, and a decrease in hyperpnea. Although balloon atrial septostomy is usually successful in stabilizing the infant and promoting survival in the neonatal period, the systemic arterial Po$_2$ sometimes does not maintain the satisfactory levels achieved immediately after the procedure. The Po$_2$ may rise initially to 35 to 45 torr (60 to 75

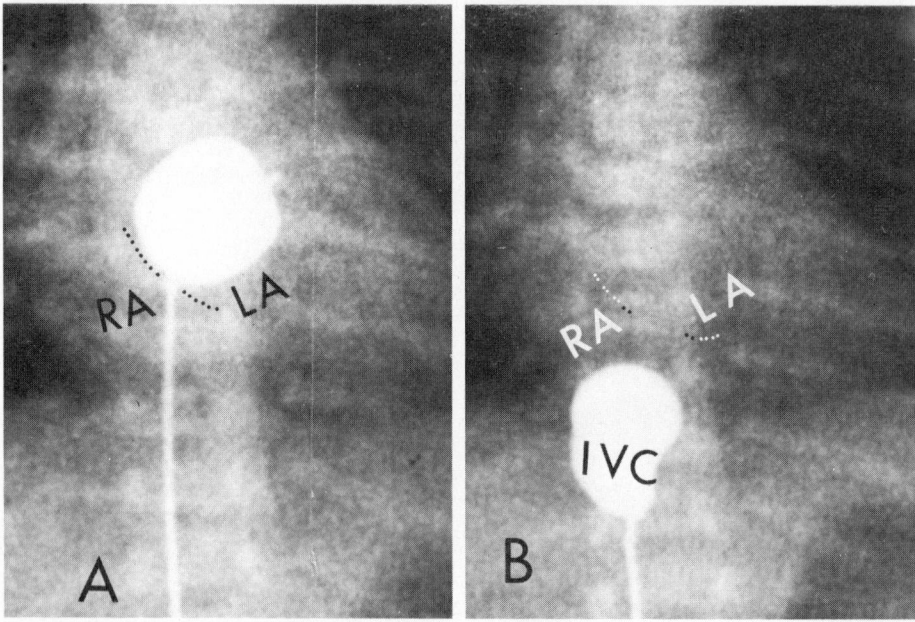

FIG. 83. Creation of large interatrial communication in infant with *d*-transposition of the great arteries by balloon atrial septostomy. A. Catheter in left atrium (LA) with distended balloon immediately before forceful withdrawal through fossa ovalis (dotted line). B. Catheter and balloon in right atrium (RA) and orifice of inferior vena cava (IVC) immediately after being pulled through.

percent oxygen saturation), but then gradually fall over several days to about 25 torr, while the pH remains normal. These infants initially do well clinically, although they remain markedly cyanotic. However, if the arterial Po_2 does not initially rise to a more satisfactory level, surgical palliation is generally performed in the newborn. An atrial septectomy allows for a greater degree of interatrial mixing and a reasonable period of normal growth and development for the infant before corrective surgery must be considered.

Interatrial correction by the Mustard technique, which was first successfully applied in 1964, involves placement of an interatrial baffle of pericardium, which directs systemic venous blood to the mitral valve and posterior left ventricle and pulmonary venous blood to the tricuspid valve and anterior right ventricle. This operation is routinely performed in most infants with transposition of the great arteries and intact ventricular septum by 6 to 9 months of age with a surgical mortality of 10 percent or less. It should not be postponed beyond the age of 1 year because of the evident complications of persistent cyanosis, particularly cerebrovascular accidents. More recently, good initial success has been achieved with the Mustard operation in the newborn period, but wider experience and long-term follow-up are necessary to evaluate this approach.

Clinical improvement after the Mustard operation is dramatic, with disappearance of cyanosis and marked increase in muscular growth, weight gain, and effort tolerance. Late major complications of the extensive atrial incisions and suture lines are atrial arrhythmias, most usually some expression of the so-called sick sinus syndrome, with episodes of atrial tachycardia or flutter alternating eventually with periods of progressively slower junctional rhythms.

In the transposition infant with a large ventricular septal defect, the main problem is one of pulmonary hypertension and the early onset of advanced pulmonary vascular disease. Early pulmonary artery banding by 4 months of age at the latest should be considered, since studies have clearly established that this procedure prevents progression in pulmonary vascular disease. Alternatively, a few centers are currently recommending early open heart corrective surgery with the Mustard operation and closure of the ventricular septal defect, with some increased surgical risk. When advanced pulmonary vascular disease is present in transposition patients with intact ventricular septum, the Mustard procedure is contraindicated, and in transposition patients with large ventricular septal defect, the Mustard procedure with surgical closure of the defect is contraindicated because of high surgical mortality. In the latter group, however, when the defect is not closed, excellent palliation can be achieved from the Mustard procedure with sizable increase in systemic arterial oxygen saturation at a relatively low surgical risk.

Despite the relatively good initial clinical results obtained with the Mustard procedure, cardiologists are concerned about its long-term prospects. Atrial arrhythmias and tricuspid regurgitation are often seen, obstruction to systemic or pulmonary venous drainage

may occur, and the long-term fate of the interatrial baffle is unknown. We are not certain that the right ventricle will perform at systemic pressures for a normal life span. Therefore, several surgical groups have developed methods of channeling left and right ventricular ejection into aorta and pulmonary artery, respectively. The long-term results of these procedures are not yet known.

In the neonate with transposition of the great arteries and persistent large patent ductus arteriosus, the clinical picture is often dominated by signs of congestive heart failure, and cyanosis may not be obvious. After balloon atrial septostomy, many of these infants remain in uncontrollable congestive failure and require urgent surgical closure of the duct. When the duct is surgically ligated there may be an acute malignant phase of cyanosis, and surgical resection of the interatrial septum may also be needed.

TRANSPOSITION OF GREAT ARTERIES WITH PULMONARY STENOSIS. In the infant with transposition of the great arteries and intact ventricular septum, mild or moderate degrees of progressive left ventricular outflow tract stenosis sometimes develop in the subpulmonary region. The degree of obstruction varies extensively, and more advanced degrees of anatomic obstruction should be relieved at the time of the open heart Mustard procedure.

When a ventricular septal defect is present with severe subvalvar left ventricular outflow tract stenosis, the clinical picture may mimic the tetralogy of Fallot. The onset of symptoms may occur at birth, with severe cyanosis and paroxysmal dyspneic spells, and the pulmonary vascular markings on the roentgenogram may be decreased. If the pulmonary stenosis is not severe, cyanosis and clinical symptoms are not as extreme, but they may become so as the infant matures. Selective left ventriculography is needed to define the extent and site of the pulmonary stenosis.

Most centers are performing a systemic–pulmonary artery anastomosis such as the Waterston-Cooley shunt in the extremely cyanotic newborn infant with transposition and severe subpulmonary or pulmonary stenosis or atresia. Intracardiac repair is difficult and should be postponed until late infancy or early childhood. Surgical repair by the Mustard operation, with closure of the ventricular septal defect and direct relief of the left ventricular outflow obstruction, has occasionally been successful, but it is associated with a high mortality, particularly when the outflow tract obstruction is extensive. A more successful surgical procedure consists of repair of the ventricular septal defect with an intracardiac ventricular baffle, so as to connect the left ventricle to the aorta, and then placement of an extracardiac valve-bearing conduit between the right ventricle and the distal stump of the pulmonary artery, so as to completely bypass the severely stenosed left ventricular outflow tract (Rastelli).

Double-Outlet Right Ventricle

Double-outlet right ventricle is a rare lesion that should be classified as a specific malformation representing one of the types of malposition of the great arteries. The lesion is sometimes described as an incomplete or partial transposition complex. Both the aortic and pulmonary valves are positioned over the right ventricle, there is conal tissue below both orifices, and the only outflow from the left ventricle is through the ventricular septal defect, which may be either subpulmonary or subaortic in location. The great arteries appear positioned essentially side by side, although one or the other may be slightly anterior. Subpulmonary infundibular stenosis is a common associated abnormality.

When the pulmonary orifice is related to the ventricular septal defect, the hemodynamics and clinical findings are similar to those of transposition of the great arteries with large ventricular septal defect and pulmonary hypertension. When the aortic orifice is closely related to the ventricular septal defect, there will be little cyanosis, and the clinical findings may be quite similar to those of large ventricular septal defect with pulmonary hypertension. In both these types the natural history, in the absence of significant subpulmonary stenosis, will be dictated by the pulmonary vascular resistance. When there is severe pulmonary outflow tract stenosis, as is commonly found in the type with the aorta related to the ventricular septal defect, the clinical picture may be indistinguishable from the tetralogy of Fallot. In each of these types of double-outlet right ventricular lesions, cardiac catheterization with selective ventricular angiography is essential for establishing the distinguishing morphologic details.

Palliative surgery with a systemic–pulmonary anastomosis to increase pulmonary blood flow has been useful for the management of the young infant with this malformation with severe pulmonary outflow tract stenosis, and pulmonary artery banding has likewise been employed for palliation of the types with marked pulmonary hypertension and increased pulmonary blood flow.

Corrective surgical procedures are becoming increasingly successful for double-outlet right ventricle lesions. In the types where the ventricular septal defect is adjacent to the aorta, correction is done by placing an intraventricular baffle from the defect to the aortic orifice to form an adequate outlet tunnel for left ventricular outflow. Removal of the subpulmonary obstruction is also carried out for the tetralogy type. When the ventricular septal defect is near the pulmonary artery (transposition type), physiologic correction is achieved by directing the left ventricular outflow into the pulmonary artery with closure of the ventricular septal defect and correction of the circulation functionally by the intra-atrial baffle operation (Mustard), as for complete transposition.

Total Anomalous Pulmonary Venous Connection

Total anomalous pulmonary venous connection, which comprises about 2 percent of all congenital heart malformations seen in the first year of life, is characterized by the absence of any direct connection between the pulmonary veins and the left atrium. The pulmonary veins are connected either directly to the right atrium or to various veins draining toward the right atrium, such as right superior vena cava, azygos vein, left innominate vein, coronary sinus, ductus venosus, or various combinations. The pulmonary veins almost always come together to form a common channel that lies behind but separate from the left atrium. This proximity provides the key to successful corrective surgery. The embryologic basis for the malformation is a failure of development of the common pulmonary vein, and consequently an anomalous union occurs between the pulmonary vein plexus of the developing lung buds and one of several systemic venous structures (p. 1358). Three main anatomic types of connection have been described: supracardiac, cardiac, and infracardiac (subdiaphragmatic). About 25 percent of all cases drain from the confluence immediately posterior to the left atrium via a left vertical venous trunk that joins the left innominate vein, and the latter joins the right superior vena cava in normal fashion (Fig. 84). In about 25 percent of the cases the anomalous drainage pathway descends to below the diaphragm to connect usually with the ductus venosus, and the pulmonary venous drainage eventually returns to the heart via the inferior vena cava. In the cardiac type the pulmonary veins may be connected directly to the right atrium or may enter the coronary sinus.

The physiologic and clinical features in an important subgroup of infants with total anomalous pulmonary venous connection are dictated by pulmonary venous obstruction. In the subdiaphragmatic type, severe obstruction to pulmonary venous return is invariably present. Obstruction may result from the length and

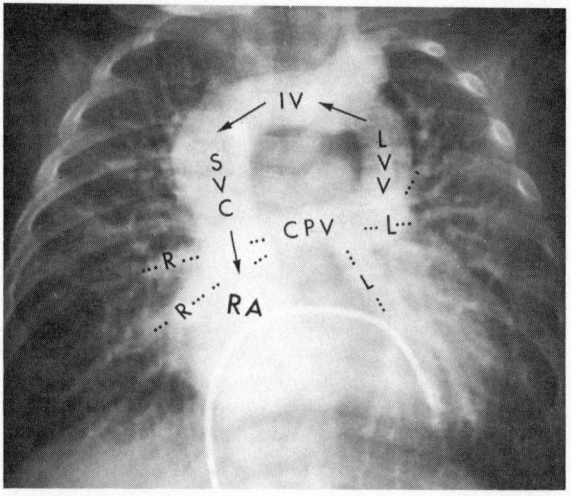

FIG. 84. Angiocardiogram showing abnormal pulmonary venous pathway in supracardiac type of total anomalous pulmonary venous drainage. R and L, right and left pulmonary veins; CPV, common pulmonary vein; LVV, left vertical vein; IV, innominate vien; SVC, superior vena cava; RA, right atrium.

narrowness of the common trunk itself, compression in the esophageal hiatus of the diaphragm, or more often from the constriction that normally occurs in the ductus venosus and the resistance that the total pulmonary venous return faces when it must pass through the portal-hepatic circulation (Fig. 85). Supracardiac drainage pathways also manifest pulmonary venous obstruction, sometimes because of a localized intrinsic constriction, but more frequently because of external compression of the left vertical vein. Compression occurs if the vein passes between the left pulmonary artery anteriorly and the left bronchus posteriorly, rather than taking the usual course that is anterior to the pulmonary artery. Obstruction may also occur with other types of anomalous connection.

Associated intracardiac anomalies occur in about 30 percent of patients with total anomalous pulmonary venous drainage. These anomalies are usually complex lesions such as common atrioventricular canal or transposition or single-ventricle complexes, often with asplenia and polysplenia.

HEMODYNAMICS. All the pulmonary venous blood eventually returns to the right atrium, and there it mixes with the systemic venous return. A variable proportion then passes to the systemic circulation through a stretched patent foramen ovale into the left atrium, ventricle, and aorta and to the pulmonary circulation through the tricuspid valve into the right ventricle and pulmonary artery. Systemic arterial unsaturation is almost always present as a result of the obligatory right-to-left shunting of blood at the atrial level, although rarely streaming of pulmonary venous blood into the left atrium gives normal aortic saturations. The arterial oxygen saturation varies widely, depending on the ratio of pulmonary to systemic blood flow. Since the pulmonary venous blood joins with systemic venous blood at or before the right atrium, the oxygen saturation tends to be similar in all four chambers of the heart and in the two great arteries.

Two hemodynamic and clinical patterns are evident, largely determined by the presence and severity of pulmonary venous obstruction. The majority of infants with supracardiac and cardiac types have high pulmonary blood flow, varying degrees of pulmonary hypertension, and relatively low pulmonary vascular resistance, indicating not much pulmonary venous obstruction. These infants generally survive the first few weeks and months of life, but succumb to severe congestive heart failure during the first year of life unless surgical correction is successful. All infants with the subdiaphragmatic type and about one-third of the infants with the supracardiac type manifest severe pulmonary venous obstruction with severe pulmonary hypertension, restricted pulmonary blood flow, pulmonary venous engorgement, and interstitial pulmonary edema. Pulmonary artery pressures often exceed systemic pressures, and death is common in the first weeks of life if correction is not made. In all types of total anomalous pulmonary venous connection the pressures in the right atrium are invariably higher than those in

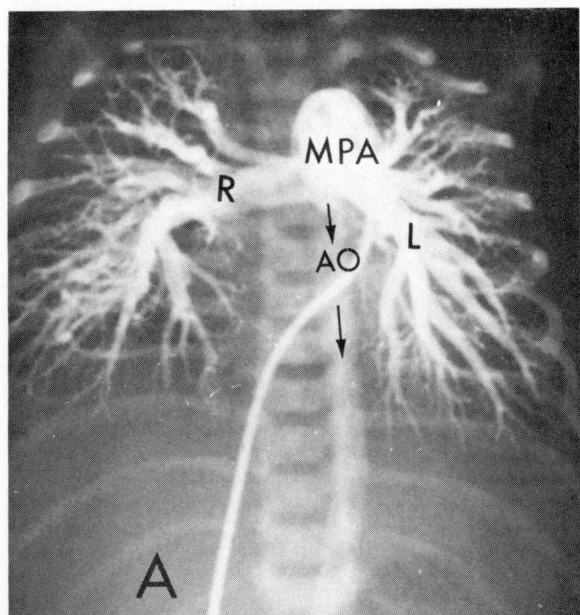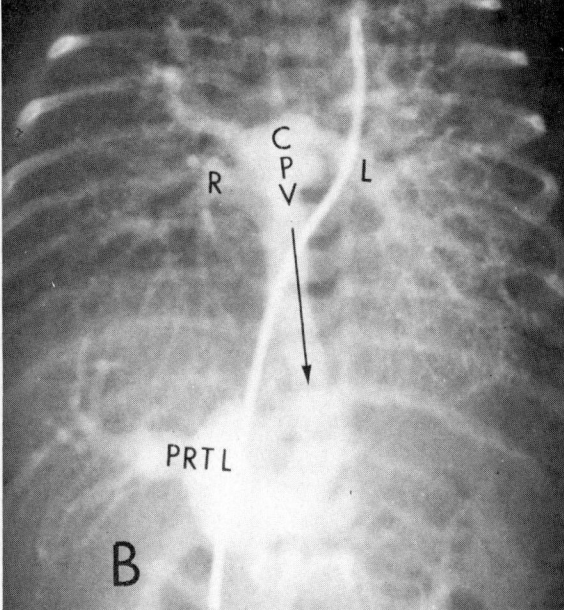

FIG. 85. Angiocardiogram in newborn with infracardiac (subdiaphragmatic) type of total anomalous pulmonary venous drainage. A. Selective injection into main pulmonary artery (MPA) showing prominent right-to-left ductal shunting into descending aorta (AO). B. Delayed pulmonary venous return shows pulmonary veins (R, L) connected to common pulmonary vein (CPV) with descending pulmonary venous channel entering the portal system (PRTL).

the left atrium, and some degree of pulmonary venous obstruction may be ascribed to limitation of flow across the foramen ovale.

CLINICAL FEATURES.   About 80 to 90 percent of all patients develop symptoms early in infancy and manifest tachypnea, congestive heart failure, and failure to thrive. In the group without pulmonary obstruction, cyanosis may be minimal, but cyanosis becomes striking as congestive heart failure progresses. The heart is hyperdynamic, and a quadruple gallop rhythm is frequently heard. A soft ejection systolic murmur is present along the left sternal border, and a mid-diastolic inflow rumble is usually heard at the lower left sternal border and apex. At times a continuous murmur or venous hum may be heard originating from some point in the venous channels.

In the unobstructed group the roentgenographic examination shows marked cardiac enlargement with pulmonary vascular engorgement. A pathognomonic configuration termed figure 8 or snowman may be recognized in the older infant or child, and this silhouette is formed by the dilated left vertical vein, innominate vein, and right superior vena cava sitting astride the dilated heart (Fig. 86).

The electrocardiogram uniformly shows right ventricular hypertrophy and commonly also right atrial hypertrophy. In most patients with this lesion the left atrium is small on the echocardiogram, but the sign is not infallible.

In infants with the obstructed form of total anomalous pulmonary venous drainage there is very early onset of severe dyspnea. The clinical picture is that of rapidly progressive dyspnea, pulmonary edema, cyanosis, and right heart failure. The second heart sound is loud and narrowly split, and a diastolic gallop rhythm may be heard. Murmurs are not prominent, but a soft blowing systolic murmur of tricuspid regurgitation may be heard at the lower left sternal border.

A characteristic chest roentgenogram is associated with pulmonary venous obstruction. The heart is normal or slightly enlarged, and the lung fields show a diffuse, hazy reticulated pattern superficially resembling the ground-glass appearance seen in the respiratory distress syndrome (Fig. 87).

For this severely obstructed group there is uniformly rapid clinical deterioration and early death. Aggressive treatment of hypoxemia and metabolic acidemia should be instituted, cardiac catheterization should be performed, and provision should be made for continuous positive airway pressure while preparations are made for surgical correction with cardiopulmonary bypass. The anomalous pulmonary venous pathway may be identified at cardiac catheterization from the unusual position of the probing catheters, such as in the left vertical vein or common pulmonary vein, and the observation of blood with unusually high oxygen saturation in systemic venous structures such as the coronary sinus, inferior vena cava, or right superior vena cava. Selective pulmonary angiography will usually reveal the anomalous drainage pattern. However, severe pulmonary venous obstruction markedly restricts pulmonary blood flow and slows the pulmonary circulation, and

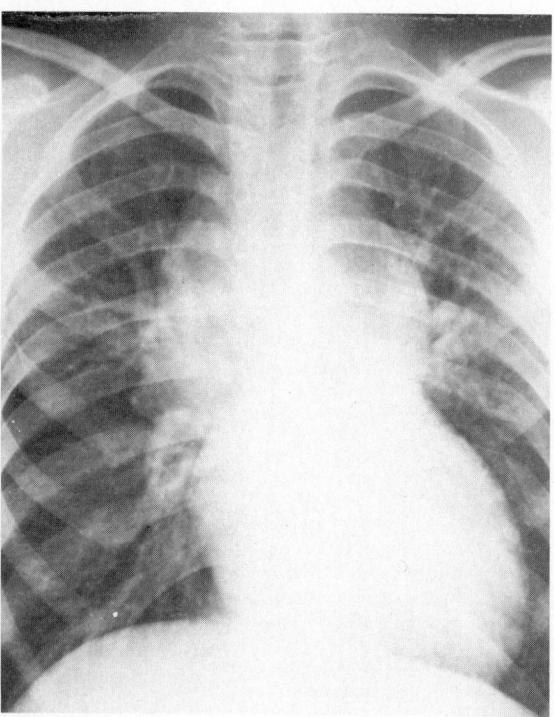

FIG. 86.   Chest roentgenogram showing figure 8 or snowman configuration in total anomalous pulmonary venous drainage due to prominent persistent left vertical vein and dilated right superior vena cava.

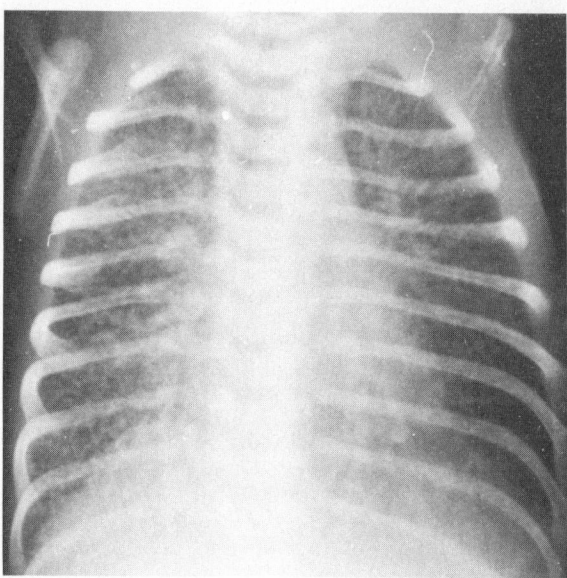

FIG. 87.   Chest roentgenogram in neonate with obstructed subdiaphragmatic type of total anomalous pulmonary venous drainage showing slight cardiac enlargement and characteristic reticulated peripheral lung markings.

under these circumstances the peripheral venous drainage pathways are only very faintly shown.

In the unobstructed type, corrective surgery provides dramatic restoration of the normal circulatory pathways with a modest surgical risk of about 10 to 15 percent under the best circumstances. When severe pulmonary venous obstruction is present, particularly the subdiaphragmatic type, the prognosis remains poor because of continuing high surgical mortality, but prompt referral, aggressive management of metabolic acidemia, and early emergency surgery have been providing increasing success, and excellent long-term results have been achieved.

Truncus Arteriosus

Truncus arteriosus is a rare malformation characterized by the emergence of only a single arterial trunk from the ventricular chambers, and this vessel gives rise directly to the coronary, pulmonary, and systemic circulations. A truncal valve with three or four leaflets overrides a ventricular septal defect, which is always present. The pulmonary arteries generally arise as a single vessel or as two separate vessels from the posterior or lateral wall of the truncus (Fig. 88A). Truncus arteriosus must not be confused with the relatively common lesion tetralogy of Fallot with pulmonary atresia (pseudotruncus). Pseudotruncus is also characterized by a single large vessel, the aorta, which arises from the heart. In pseudotruncus, however, there is a hypoplastic or atretic pulmonary artery attached to the right ventricular outflow region.

HEMODYNAMICS. The right and left ventricles eject blood at a systemic pressure into the common arterial trunk; thus the coronary arteries, pulmonary arteries, and aorta receive a mixture of venous and oxygenated blood at systemic pressure. The pulmonary blood flow is markedly increased in infancy, since there are usually primary pulmonary artery branches of adequate size and the pulmonary vascular resistance is not greatly increased. Consequently cyanosis is minimal, and the hemodynamics as well as the clinical picture are those of a large left-to-right shunt. The pulmonary circulation may be restricted in a few patients by the development of pulmonary vascular obstructive disease or rarely by hypoplastic or stenotic pulmonary arteries arising from the truncus.

Symptoms usually appear in the first weeks or months of life and are consistent with the physiology of a large left-to-right shunt: left heart failure, dyspnea, wheezing, frequent respiratory infections, and poor physical development. In the infant cyanosis is often not apparent or is minimal at rest, since the pulmonary blood flow is markedly increased. The heart is hyperdynamic, and the peripheral pulses are prominent. The second heart sound is loud and single due to the single set of semilunar valves. A prominent systolic click is heard very commonly at the lower and mid-left sternal border. A harsh systolic murmur may best be heard along the mid-left sternal border, and a continuous murmur is heard at the base or lateral chest wall in older infants and children. In newborn or young infants, particularly those with marked congestive heart failure, only a systolic murmur may be heard, which is similar to the findings in some newborn infants with large patent ductus arteriosus. Severe truncal valve incompetence may be suspected from a prominent to-and-fro quality in the murmur.

If the pulmonary blood flow is restricted, either by high pulmonary vascular resistance or by stenotic or hypoplastic pulmonary arteries, the clinical findings are different: cyanosis is more severe, congestive heart fail-

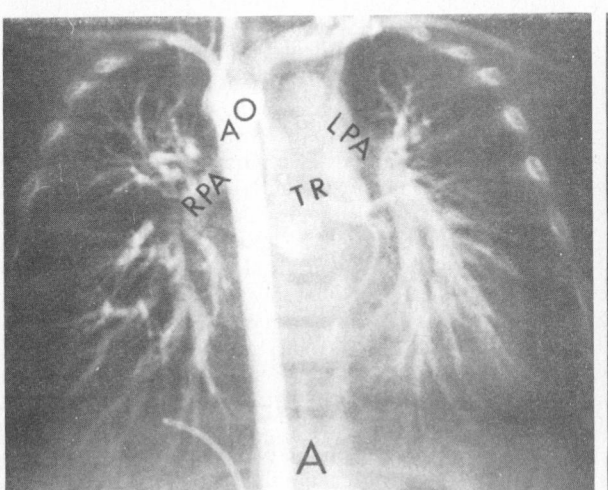
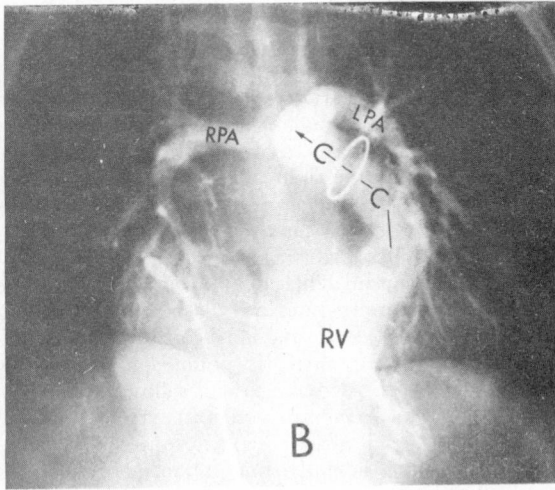

FIG. 88. A. Angiocardiogram (anteroposterior view) in truncus arteriosus showing origin of the pulmonary arteries (RPA, LPA) and aorta (AO) from the truncus (TR). B. Angiocardiogram (anteroposterior view) in truncus arteriosus following corrective surgery with placement of valved conduit (C-C) from right ventricle (RV) to main pulmonary artery and closure of ventricular septal defect.

ure is unusual, only a minimal systolic murmur of short duration and low intensity is heard, and there may be a faint continuous bruit representing bronchial pulmonary collateral flow.

Roentgenographic findings also depend on the size of the pulmonary arteries and the pulmonary blood flow pattern. In most infants there is considerable cardiac enlargement, with increased pulmonary vascular markings; a right aortic arch is common (25 to 30 percent), and the hilar origin of the pulmonary artery may appear superiorly displaced. The electrocardiogram demonstrates right ventricular or combined ventricular hypertrophy, depending on the hemodynamic circumstances. When pulmonary blood flow is decreased, both heart size and pulmonary vascular markings are less prominent. The use of the echocardiogram in diagnosing this and separating it from the tetralogy of Fallot and double-outlet right ventricle has been mentioned (p. 1372).

The diagnosis is best confirmed by catheterization and selective angiography in the ventricular chambers or the truncus vessel; this reveals the common trunk arising from the heart and the origin of the pulmonary arteries from the truncus (Fig. 88A).

The prognosis is variable, depending to a considerable degree on the pulmonary blood flow pattern; most infants die within the first 6 to 12 months from heart failure. Surgical banding of both pulmonary arteries to reduce pulmonary blood flow has been helpful in some infants. Corrective surgery has been developed and widely applied, provided the patient has reached a reasonable size and is free from severe pulmonary vascular obstructive disease: the ventricular septal defect is closed to leave the aorta arising from the left ventricle, the pulmonary arteries are excised from their common truncus origin, and a valved conduit is placed from the free right ventricular wall to the pulmonary arteries (Fig. 88B) to form a new right ventricular outflow tract (Rastelli procedure).

Hypoplastic Left Heart Complex

Hypoplastic left heart complex is a broad term referring to a group of malformations characterized by marked underdevelopment of the entire left side of the heart. In contrast, the right side of the heart is grossly dilated and hypertrophied, with a widely patent ductus arteriosus that delivers blood into the aorta. The specific anatomic abnormalities include underdevelopment of the left atrium and ventricle, stenosis or atresia of the aortic or mitral orifices, and hypoplasia of the ascending aorta. Frequently, aortic and mitral atresia coexist, and the left ventricular cavity is minute or completely obliterated. The material that follows considers primarily this most common and most extreme lesion of the hypoplastic left heart complex group.

The essential hemodynamic abnormality centers about the absence or gross inadequacy of left ventricular function. Pulmonary venous blood is shunted from the left atrium to the right atrium via the patent foramen ovale, and this interatrial communication is often small and restrictive to blood flow, resulting in severe left atrial and pulmonary venous hypertension. The ventricular septum is almost always intact. The right ventricle functions as the systemic ventricle as well as the pulmonary ventricle by delivering blood into the aorta through the widely patent ductus arteriosus. The pulmonary vascular resistance must be high to provide for this systemic function of the right ventricle.

Most infants with hypoplastic left heart complex are acutely ill, with signs of congestive heart failure within the first days or weeks after birth; those with aortic atresia usually succumb within their first few days after birth.

On physical examination there are signs and symptoms of severe right-sided and left-sided heart failure, cyanosis of varying degree, and often a characteristic grayish pallor and poor peripheral pulses, which contrast with hyperdynamic cardiac pulsations. Characteristically the peripheral pulses may diminish and reappear from time to time, which presumably is related to episodes of spontaneous ductus arteriosus closing. The major hemodynamic abnormalities are inadequate maintenance of the systemic circulation and pulmonary venous hypertension. Murmurs are not prominent, but a short soft midsystolic murmur and mid-diastolic rumble may be present. The second heart sound is narrowly split or single and is quite accentuated until clinical deterioration with gross right heart failure is advanced.

The roentgenogram shortly after birth may show only slight enlargement, but with clinical deterioration striking generalized cardiac enlargement and moderately prominent pulmonary vascular markings are noted. Pulmonary venous obstruction may be indicated by hazy lung markings. The electrocardiogram at birth may show normal right ventricular dominance, but if the infant survives a few days right atrial and right ventricular hypertrophy are usual. The echocardiogram can be diagnostic by showing an absent or small aortic root, absent or markedly abnormal mitral valve movements, small posterior ventricle, and large anterior ventricle with prominent, easily identifiable tricuspid valve. These findings are characteristic of an aortic atresia malformation, and taken in conjunction with the clinical picture they should obviate the need for additional invasive diagnostic studies in almost all instances. These infants are critically ill, and intracardiac diagnostic procedures are difficult. Angiocardiography is helpful in detailing the specific anatomic lesions. Injection in the aorta just proximal or distal to the ductus arteriosus will demonstrate the anatomy of the isthmus and the hypoplastic ascending aorta, since flow occurs retrograde to enter the coronary arteries (Fig. 89). A left atrial selective injection shows the size of the chamber, whether or not there is mitral atresia, and the size of the foramen ovale.

Supportive therapy directed at congestive heart failure, hypoxemia, and metabolic acidemia is of only limited benefit, since survival beyond the first days or weeks of life is rare. Because functional closure of the patent ductus arteriosus and restriction to left atrial emptying are the critical physiologic obstructions to the circulatory pathways in this malignant malformation,

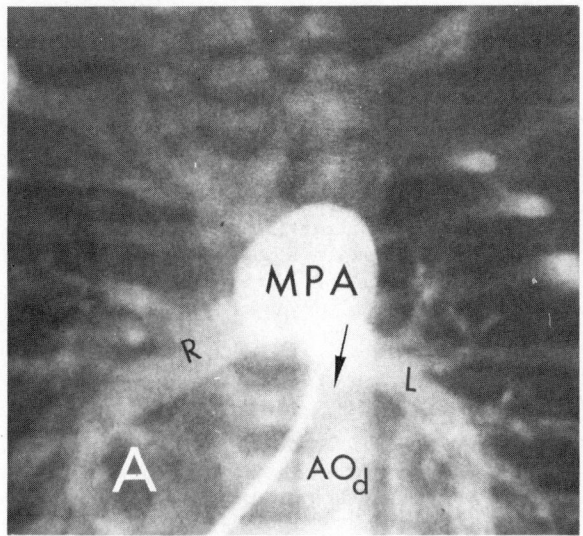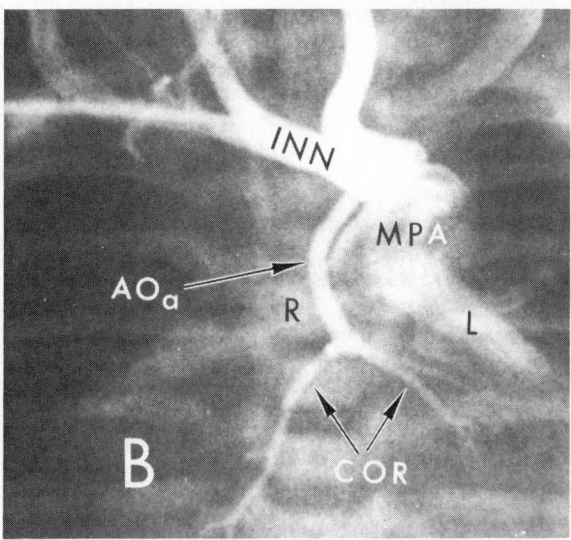

FIG. 89.   Angiocardiogram (anteroposterior view) in hypoplastic left heart complex (age 2 days). A. Injection into pulmonary artery (MPA) shows large right-to-left shunt through patent ductus arteriosus into descending aorta (AOd). B. Injection into region of innominate artery (INN) and aortic arch shows markedly hypoplastic ascending aorta (AOa) with flow to coronary arteries (COR).

palliation is theoretically feasible and has recently been attempted. Surgical creation of an aortic–pulmonary anastomosis, together with surgical atrial septectomy and banding of the main pulmonary artery branches, is a series of formidable procedures in these critically ill infants. The ultimate prognosis in these infants after surgery remains to be seen.

Mitral atresia with a ventricular septal defect is uncommon. If the foramen ovale permits a large left-to-right atrial shunt, the infants may do well, but if the foramen ovale is restrictive there will be pulmonary edema. Palliation by balloon atrial septostomy or surgical atrial septectomy gives good results.

Single Ventricle

A single-ventricle malformation is diagnosed when there is one ventricular chamber that receives both the mitral and tricuspid orifices or a common atrioventricular orifice. About 70 to 80 percent of single-ventricle malformations are derived from an *l*-bulboventricular loop and manifest bulboventricular inversion. These hearts have a single right-sided morphologically left ventricle with absence of the inflow portion of the right ventricle but persistence of a rudimentary left-sided right ventricular outflow chamber. This rudimentary outlet chamber communicates proximally with the single ventricle through a ventricular septal defect (persistent bulboventricular orifice) and distally with an *l*-transposed aorta. The pulmonary artery is posterior and arises from the single ventricle. Transposition (*l*- or *d*-) is present in the majority of single-ventricle malformations, and stenosis or atresia of the pulmonary outflow tract is also common. Complex associated

anomalies are usual, and they include dextrocardia, asplenia, common atrioventricular canal, and total anomalous pulmonary venous connection.

The term common ventricle has been used by some workers to distinguish a rare type of single-ventricle heart that has a well-developed right as well as left ventricular inflow tract; in such a heart the univentricular chamber represents a huge ventricular septal defect.

The hemodynamics and clinical picture vary, depending on the pulmonary blood flow and the associated intracardiac malformations. Cyanosis is always present because of mixing of the pulmonary and systemic venous blood in the single ventricle or, in some cases, the common atrium. When there is significant pulmonary stenosis or atresia, cyanosis may be severe, the heart size may be small, and the pulmonary vascular markings may be diminished.

In contrast, when there is no pulmonary stenosis the clinical and hemodynamic findings are dictated by the relationship between pulmonary and systemic vascular resistances and blood flows. In the infant, and in the older child when pulmonary vascular resistance is low, there will be torrential pulmonary blood flow with marked cardiomegaly and severe congestive heart failure. In the surviving child, increasing pulmonary vascular disease may moderate the excessive flow to the lungs.

With severe pulmonary stenosis the systolic ejection murmur is usually loud; with pulmonary atresia no murmurs are heard. An aortic ejection click may be heard; the second heart sound is usually single and loud. With markedly increased pulmonary blood flow, cyanosis may be quite mild, with the systolic ejection murmur pansystolic, the second heart sound loud and narrowly split, and a third heart sound and short mid-diastolic rumble often present.

The chest roentgenogram will establish the extent of cardiomegaly and pulmonary blood flow; the shape of the heart may be very characteristic and should establish the malformation as a single left ventricle with small rudimentary right ventricular outflow tract associated with *l*-transposition of the great arteries. The rudimentary systemic outflow chamber produces a bulge on the upper left border of the cardiac silhouette, and the ascending aorta is in the *l*-transposition configuration. Echocardiography may also assist in establishing the diagnosis of single ventricle.

The electrocardiogram will be nonspecific, presenting either right or left axis deviation and a precordial QRS pattern suggesting either right, combined ventricular or left ventricular dominance. Large unchanging equiphasic or negative complexes across the precordium should raise a suspicion of single-ventricle malformation.

Cardiac catheterization is helpful in revealing a left-to-right shunt at the ventricular level, identifying the presence of pulmonary or subpulmonary stenosis, measuring the pulmonary vascular resistance, and possibly establishing the anatomic course of the rudimentary small outlet chamber and the position of the aorta. Angiography is essential for establishing the detailed primary and associated malformation diagnoses.

The clinical course and prognosis are generally grave, but palliation and long-term salvage have been effected for infants with decreased pulmonary blood flow by surgically creating either systemic–pulmonary or cavo-pulmonary anastomoses and for infants with increased pulmonary blood flow by pulmonary artery banding. Recently, open heart corrective surgical procedures have been initiated to place a prosthetic septum in such a heart with single ventricle and small outlet chamber and to correct associated defects. These formidable procedures will be significantly aided by the recent recognition in such hearts of grossly abnormal disposition of the cardiac specialized conduction tissue arising from an anterior rather than a normal posterior atrioventricular node and coursing as the bundle of His astride the anterior (conal) septum. Alternatively, a Fontan procedure can be done: a valved conduit connects the right atrium and pulmonary artery, and the single ventricle is left to eject into the aorta.

Pulmonary Arteriovenous Fistula

Occasionally there are fistulae that connect pulmonary artery and vein, bypassing the alveoli. The fistulae may be large and may be single or multiple, or there may be numerous small fistulae scattered throughout the lungs. There may be no other lesions present, but at times the fistulae are part of the Rendu-Weber-Osler syndrome (p. 1203).

The principal findings are cyanosis and clubbing, with rarely a systolic or continuous murmur in the region of a large fistula. The heart is normal clinically, as is the electrocardiogram. There may be telangiectases on skin or mucosa. The chest roentgenogram may show opacities in the lung fields; with large lesions there may be large vessels entering or leaving the mass. Diagnosis is made by cardiac catheterization, which reveals normal pressures but a reduced oxygen saturation in the pulmonary veins, left heart chambers, and aorta. Rarely the fistula connects intercostal arteries and pulmonary veins, and then all left-sided oxgyen saturations are normal. Angiography defines the site, number, and extent of the lesions. Excision of localized lesions, usually with lobectomy, should be done to avoid the risks of polycythemia, brain abscess, or infective arteritis.

Abnormal Systemic Venous Drainage

Rarely the inferior vena cava or a persistent left superior vena cava may connect to the left atrium and produce cyanosis without any other abnormal clinical signs. Diagnosis is made by angiography of these vessels.

DISEASES OF ENDOCARDIUM
JULIEN I.E. HOFFMAN

Acute rheumatic valvulitis is the most important of these diseases; it is discussed on p. 386.

Endocardial Fibroelastosis

Endocardial fibroelastosis is a pathologic condition in which the ventricles or atria are lined by thick white tissue that on microscopy shows marked endocardial and subendocardial fibroelastic proliferation. These changes may be secondary to congenital heart disease or they may be primary.

Secondary fibroelastosis is most often seen in infants with severe obstructive lesions. Thus it may occur in the left ventricle and atrium with severe aortic stenosis or coarctation of the aorta, in the left atrium with mitral atresia and a small foramen ovale, or in the right ventricle with severe pulmonary stenosis or atresia. It is difficult to diagnose the fibroelastosis in addition to the primary lesion, since the latter dominates the clinical picture. However, the fibroelastosis may make cardiac function worse than it would otherwise be, and it may prevent adequate clinical improvement after an apparently successful surgical procedure.

Primary or *idiopathic endocardial fibroelastosis* is a disease of unknown origin that usually occurs in healthy infants under 1 year of age. The disease may appear in small clusters, suggesting an infective origin. Some studies have suggested that there is a viral origin and that associated viral myocarditis may be present. This theory awaits confirmation. Recently, too, many of these infants have been reported to have positive skin reactions to inactivated mumps antigen, implying that there is a specific etiologic relationship. However, this theory is no longer favored, because these infants do not have serologically detectable mumps antibody and because others have found that the skin reaction is not marked enough to be regarded as specific. The endocardial thickening is accompanied by marked myocardial hypertrophy and impaired myocardial function, so that it presents with congestive heart failure. The clinical features are those of any chronic myocardial disorder, as are the radiologic and electrocardiographic features.

The diagnosis can be suspected from these findings, but since it can be proved only at autopsy and since the findings are nonspecific, it is essential to study these children carefully, usually with cardiac catheterization, in order not to miss other lesions. One should never be satisfied with the clinical diagnosis of fibroelastosis. Treatment is symptomatic, with digoxin and diuretics as the mainstays. Most children get worse and die months or years after the onset, but spontaneous remissions have been described occasionally.

Myxomas

Myxomas are benign tumors that are usually pedunculated and usually arise from the atrial septum near the foramen ovale; occasionally they attach elsewhere in the atria or the ventricles. Left atrial myxomas are more common than those in the right atrium. The atrial myxomas may simulate mitral or tricuspid valve disease, since they often prolapse into the valve ring and cause obstruction or incompetence. Less often they embolize to systemic or pulmonary arteries or obstruct pulmonary veins. They may be associated with fever, a raised sedimentation rate, increased gamma globulins, and increased serum antihyaluronidase titers. Diagnosis may be suspected clinically, especially if the mitral or tricuspid murmurs change from time to time or with differences of position. Echocardiography is often useful, and definitive diagnosis is made by demonstrating the filling defect on angiography. Surgical removal is usually successful.

Infective Endocarditis

Originally infective endocarditis was termed acute or subacute bacterial endocarditis, but since many types of micro-organisms cause endocarditis, infective endocarditis has become the preferred term. Some micro-organisms produce an acute severe illness, while others usually cause an insidious subacute process; both usually cause death if they are not treated.

PATHOGENESIS. The micro-organisms usually grow on a part of the heart subjected to abnormal blood streaming and turbulence due to congenital or acquired heart disease. Whenever there is a narrow opening between two parts of the circulation (stenotic or incompetent valve, abnormal communication) there is a high velocity of flow through the opening and considerable eddying and turbulence downstream from the opening. The turbulence predisposes the endocardium to permit growth of micro-organisms. Thus growth may begin on the left ventricular surface of a stenotic mitral valve, the aortic surface of a stenotic aortic valve, the septal leaflet of the tricuspid valve or the right ventricular rim of a ventricular septal defect, the pulmonary arterial end of a patent ductus arteriosus, the venous end of an arterio-

venous fistula, and so on. Growth may also begin where the abnormal jet of blood strikes the opposing endocardium and causes a thickening known as a jet lesion. This dependence on high-velocity streams probably explains why infective endocarditis is more common with small defects than with large defects and why it does not occur with uncomplicated secundum atrial septal defects, across which the velocity of flow is low.

Because of this mechanism the children most likely to have infective endocarditis are those with congenital heart disease; tetralogy of Fallot, especially after a shunt, ventricular septal defect, patent ductus arteriosus, aortic stenosis, and bicuspid aortic valve account for most of the reported cases. Rheumatic heart disease is a much less common cause than it used to be. Occasionally, infective endocarditis develops when there is no apparent underlying heart defect, and then most often there are micro-organisms of unusual type and virulence.

In addition to the cardiac lesion there must also be a portal through which the micro-organisms invade the bloodstream. Any site of localized sepsis can seed organisms into the blood, so that abscesses, osteomyelitis, pyelonephritis, extensive burns, etc, should be treated with special vigor and care in children with heart disease. There are also some specific portals of entry that require special consideration: Normal mouth flora, especially the α-hemolytic streptococci (*Streptococcus viridans*) can enter the bloodstream after extraction or filling of teeth or cleaning and scaling of the teeth by a dental hygienist. Catheterization of the urinary bladder or other genitourinary instrumentation may lead to invasion by enterococci or gram-negative bacilli. After cardiac surgery, particularly if prosthetic patches or valves are inserted, endocarditis may occur; it is commonly due to staphylococci, *Candida,* or diphtheroids. Patients getting hemodialysis through arteriovenous shunts often have infections of the shunts and then may get endocarditis, often with staphylococci or streptococci. Postpartum uterine sepsis may allow invasion by enterococci or gram-negative bacilli. Patients with long-term indwelling venous or right atrial catheters (ventriculoatrial shunts for hydrocephalus, parenteral alimentation) may get infective endocarditis, often with *Staphylococcus epidermidis.* Patients on immunosuppressive therapy may be infected with unusual organisms, as may those getting superinfections after prolonged antibiotic therapy for other diseases. Narcotic addicts who take drugs intravenously may get infective endocarditis, either with *S. viridans* or with unusual micro-organisms, including fungi.

PATHOLOGY. The micro-organisms grow in and on the endocardium to produce rough vegetations that may reach large size, especially in fungal endocarditis. Once the lesion has begun, the growth may extend to adjacent tissues; it may invade the myocardium, perforate the sinuses of Valsalva, erode through the aortic or mitral valves, or rupture chordae tendineae. The vegetations may also break off and embolize.

INCIDENCE. The incidence is not well known, but has been estimated as being from 0.005 to 1 percent per year of the patients at risk of the disease. It is clearly more common in those with repeated exposure, such as narcotic addicts, patients having frequent urinary tract manipulations, and those with poor dental hygiene. The disease is rare under 2 years of age.

BACTERIOLOGY. The most common micro-organisms are *S. viridans* and *Staphylococcus* species, which together account for about 80 percent of infective endocarditis. However, pneumococci, enterococci, *Neisseria, Salmonella,* diphtheroids, *Hemophilus, Candida, Aspergillus, Rickettsia,* and other less common micro-organisms have been described as causing infective endocarditis.

CLINICAL FEATURES. The illness usually begins insidiously, with anorexia, fever, malaise, and weight loss, and hospital admission in children averages 30 days from the onset of the illness. The most common finding is fever in a child who has heart disease. Splenomegaly occurs in 50 to 65 percent and petechiae in 20 to 40 percent. Splinter hemorrhages under the nails, Osler's nodes (red painful intradermal nodes in the pads of fingers or toes), Janeway's spots (painless hemorrhagic spots on the palms and soles), and Roth's spots (fluffy cotton-wool exudates in the retina) are all much rarer today than they used to be. About 20 percent of the patients develop a new murmur or a change in one already known, but in 15 percent no murmurs are present, especially in the early stages.

LABORATORY FINDINGS. A raised erythrocyte sedimentation rate is almost always noted. There is usually a moderate leukocytosis with increased neutrophilia, and anemia is frequent in patients who do not have cyanotic heart disease. Increased numbers of monocytes and histiocytes are common in peripheral blood, but they are nonspecific. There is often hyperglobulinemia and a raised rheumatoid FII factor titer, especially if the disease is over 4 to 6 weeks in duration. Microscopic intermittent hematuria is common.

The mainstay of diagnosis is finding the organisms in blood culture. Venous blood should be taken with good aseptic technique. Ideally 10 ml of blood should be taken on each of six occasions over 12 to 24 hours, and each sample should be put into 100 ml or more of culture medium; a large dilution factor helps to dilute out antibiotics, antibodies, and complement, all of which may inhibit growth of micro-organisms. There is no advantage in waiting for febrile peaks to take blood, and there is evidence that the yield of positive cultures depends more on the total volume of blood taken than on the number of samples. However, it is important to take several different samples; if several bottles grow the organism it is less likely to be a contaminant, but if there is only one culture it may be difficult to evaluate the significance of a growth of an organism like *S. epidermidis.* There is no advantage to taking arterial blood, but occasionally in difficult problems where the organism has not been grown it may help to culture bone marrow or catheterize the pulmonary artery to obtain right-sided blood (if a right-sided endocarditis is suspected). The cultures should be grown aerobically and anaerobically and kept for at least 4 weeks before being considered negative.

PROGNOSIS AND COMPLICATIONS. Infection by a penicillin-sensitive *S. viridans* that is diagnosed early has almost a 100 percent cure rate. However, since many infections are diagnosed late or are due to antibiotic-insensitive organisms, the average mortality rate is about 10 to 25 percent. Death is due most often to congestive heart failure secondary to perforation of mitral or aortic valves, ruptured chordae tendineae, myocardial infarction from coronary embolization, myocardial abscesses, or intracardiac or extracardiac perforations.

Arterial emboli to lungs, brain, spleen, coronary arteries, or kidneys are common. Emboli to large arteries are rare except with fungal endocarditis. Mycotic aneurysms are uncommon, and they and emboli may manifest themselves months or years after the primary infection has been cured.

Neurologic complications are common; they include embolic lesions, rupture of mycotic aneurysms, acute meningitis or meningocerebritis, convulsions, and toxic encephalopathy. Renal involvement is also common. There may be focal embolic glomerulitis or acute or chronic glomerulonephritis, probably due to immune complex disease. Hematuria and proteinuria are thus common, but severe uremia is rare.

MANAGEMENT. It is essential to have a high index of suspicion when any of the features of this disease occur in a susceptible person. Apart from the routine history, physical examination, and laboratory tests, the mainstay of the diagnosis is the blood culture. If the patient is not very ill, there is no good clinical evidence of infective endocarditis, and the illness is of short duration, positive blood cultures or more definite evidence of infective endocarditis should be obtained before starting treatment with antibiotics. There is little risk in delaying treatment for a few days, and the delay may save many patients a prolonged and unnecessary hospital course; most febrile episodes in children with heart disease are short-lived intercurrent infections. On the other hand, if the patient is very ill or the clinical features point strongly to infective endocarditis, the necessary blood cultures should be drawn and treatment begun without waiting for the results. Once they return and antibiotic sensitivities are known, any needed changes can then be made.

The choice of antibiotics depends largely on what organism is suspected. If there is no obvious source or if there has been recent dental manipulation, the likely organism is *S. viridans,* which is usually sensitive to penicillin. Doses and regimes vary, but adequate therapy is obtained by giving 200,000 IU/kg/day of penicillin G intravenously for 5 to 7 days and then 100,000 IU/kg/day intravenously or intramuscularly for the next 3 weeks. The occasional penicillin-resistant *S. viridans* should be treated with the same dosage of penicillin plus streptomycin 50 mg/kg/day intramuscularly for 1 week and then 25 mg/kg/day intramuscularly for 3 weeks.

Staphylococci are often penicillin-resistant; thus they should be treated with methicillin 150 mg/kg/day intravenously for 4 weeks and then cloxacillin 75 to 100 mg/kg/day orally for a total of 6 weeks, or 2 weeks after all abnormal signs have disappeared, whichever is longer. Enterococci are treated with penicillin and streptomycin or, if they are resistant, gentamycin or ampicillin; the latter antibiotics are also most useful for gram-negative infections. Other unusual organisms may need other antibiotics, as determined by sensitivity tests. For all these antibiotics it is useful to determine how bactericidal the serum is by determining what dilution of serum will kill the organisms; a titer of 1:10 is regarded as satisfactory.

Occasionally surgery may be required if there is gross valve destruction with unmanageable heart failure or if infective endocarditis occurs after surgical implantation of a prosthetic patch or valve; infection on prosthetic material usually requires removal of the foreign material before the infection can be controlled.

PROPHYLAXIS. Any infection needs prompt treatment, both for its own sake and to prevent infective endocarditis. Equally important is to give prophylaxis at the time of manipulation of any potentially infected region; this includes dental work and any manipulation of the genitourinary tract or gastrointestinal tract, including catheterization of the urinary bladder. The aim of treatment is to give the recommended antibiotic shortly before the manipulation so that there will be no time to develop resistant organisms and there will be a high blood level during the period of maximal invasion of the blood by micro-organisms. Treatment is then continued for 2 or 3 days, or longer if there is reason to believe that the manipulated region has not healed. Thus for dental work in which *S. viridans* is the likely invader, give either (1) 600,000 IU of procaine penicillin G with 200,000 IU of crystalline penicillin G intramuscularly 1 hour before the procedure and once daily for the next 2 or 3 days or (2) 500 mg penicillin V orally 1 hour before the procedure and then 250 mg every 6 hours for the next 3 days. If the patient is allergic to penicillin or is on continuous penicillin prophylaxis for rheumatic fever, give oral erythromycin 20 mg/kg (in small children) or 500 mg (in adolescents and adults) about 1.5 to 2 hours before the procedure and then half that dose every 6 hours for the next 3 days. For any genitourinary or gastrointestinal manipulation, give the same dose of penicillin or erythromycin as for dental work, but add either (1) streptomycin 40 mg/kg intramuscularly 1 hour before the procedure and once daily for the next 2 days (the maximal dose of streptomycin is 1 g/day) or (2) ampicillin 50 mg/kg orally 1 hour before the procedure and 25 mg/kg every 6 hours for the next 3 days.

References

ENDOCARDIAL FIBROELASTOSIS

Andersen DH, Kelly J: Endocardial fibro-elastosis: I. Endocardial fibro-elastosis associated with congenital malformations of the heart. J Pediatr 41:141, 1956

———— Endocardial fibro-elastosis: II. A clinical and pathological investigation of those cases without associated cardiac malformations, including report of two familial instances. Pediatrics 18:513, 539, 1956

Gersony WM, Katz SL, Nadas AS: Endocardial fibro-elastosis and mumps virus. Pediatrics 37:430, 1966

Manning JA, Keith JD: Fibro-elastosis in children. Prog Cardiovasc Dis 7:172, 1964

MYXOMAS

Van der Hauwaert LG: Cardiac tumours in childhood. In Watson H (ed): Paediatric Cardiology. St Louis, CV Mosby, 1968, p 773

INFECTIVE ENDOCARDITIS

Blumenthal S, Griffiths SP, Morgan BC: Bacterial endocarditis in children with heart disease. Pediatrics 26:993, 1960

Committee Report on Prevention of Bacterial Endocarditis: Circulation 46, 1972 (November).

Johnson DH, Rosenthal A, Nadas AS: A forty year review of bacterial endocarditis in infancy and childhood. Circulation 51:581, 1975

Jones HR, Shekert RG, Geraci JE: Neurologic manifestations of bacterial endocarditis. Ann Intern Med 71:21, 1969

Weinstein L, Rubin RH: Infective endocarditis—1973. Prog Cardiovasc Dis 16:239, 1973

———— Schlesinger J: Treatment of infective endocarditis—1973. Prog Cardiovasc Dis 16:275, 1973

Zakrewski T, Keith JD: Bacterial endocarditis in infants and children. J Pediatr 67:1179, 1965

DISEASES OF MYOCARDIUM

JULIEN I.E. HOFFMAN

The myocardium may be affected by many factors other than increased pressure and volume loads; the most common are infections that either are confined to the heart or are part of a systemic infection. Other less common factors are also discussed in this section. Most of these diseases affect the myocardium diffusely, so that the brunt of the damage is usually borne by the left ventricle, since it is the predominant ventricle after the first few weeks of life. Mild myocardial lesions may be common, but they cannot be diagnosed clinically. More extensive lesions produce one of two main clinical patterns. Acute myocardial damage causes dilatation of the left ventricle or both ventricles, with a low cardiac output and arterial blood pressure and with an increased pulmonary venous pressure and sometimes an increased systemic venous pressure. Therefore there are tachypnea and often rales, tachycardia, an enlarged but quiet heart, soft heart sounds that may have a tic-tac rhythm, usually a gallop rhythm, and either no murmurs or systolic murmurs of mitral or tricuspid incompetence secondary to ventricular dilatation. The chest roentgenogram will show a diffusely enlarged heart and evidence of pulmonary venous congestion and pulmonary edema. The electrocardiogram will show normal or reduced QRS voltages, since there is initially no ventricular hypertrophy, and there are usually S-T segment depression and T wave inversion in the left ventricular leads. If the myocardial lesion is of slow onset and long duration, there will be left ventricular hypertrophy seen both clinically and on the electrocardiogram. In both acute and chronic lesions there may be dysrhythmias.

Acute Myocarditis

Acute rheumatic myocarditis occurs early in an attack of rheumatic fever, usually in the first week. It is almost always accompanied by mitral or aortic valve involvement and sometimes by pericarditis. The clinical features are those of an acute myocardial lesion as outlined above. There may be a prolonged P-R or Q-T interval that is not specific but may be more common in rheumatic fever than in other myocarditides. If there is gross aortic or mitral incompetence it may be difficult to decide if the myocardial lesions or the valvar lesions are the main cause of the heart failure.

Heart failure and marked cardiac dilatation usually respond well to treatment with prednisone (2 mg/kg/day), digoxin, and diuretics. Salicylates should be discontinued, since they may aggravate the heart failure. When the heart failure has gone and the cardiac findings are stable, the steroids should be withdrawn slowly over 1 or 2 weeks to avoid any rebound. Surgical treatment of gross aortic or mitral incompetence may occasionally be necessary if medical treatment fails; even if there is a myocardial component to the heart failure, correction of the mechanical abnormality may be life-saving.

Acute viral myocarditis is usually due to coxsackie viruses or echoviruses, but it is occasionally due to poliomyelitis, mumps, measles, or rubella. There may be outbreaks in infants, who often have associated encephalitis; in older children there may be pleural effusions. The clinical features vary with virulence. At one extreme there may merely be mild S-T and T wave changes in the electrocardiogram, while at the other extreme death may occur only hours after the onset. In between there is a febrile illness that often follows a mild upper respiratory tract infection in the child or a mild viral syndrome in other members of the family. The clinical features are those of acute myocardial damage described above, and occasionally there may be pericarditis or valvulitis. Dysrhythmias are common, especially ventricular premature beats or conduction disturbances. Laboratory tests are compatible with any febrile illness, but there may be an increase in cardio-specific enzymes (isozymes of lactic dehydrogenase and creatine phosphokinase).

Viral myocarditis can be proved only by demonstrating the virus in the myocardium. It can be strongly suspected by isolating the virus from the throat or feces *and* by demonstrating either a fourfold rise in the titer of type-specific neutralizing, hemagglutination-inhibiting, or complement-fixing antibodies or a titer of 1:32 or more of type-specific immunoglobulin-M-neutralizing or hemagglutination-inhibiting antibodies.

Treatment is mainly by prolonged bed rest for 1 to 3 months, depending on the severity of the lesion, together with appropriate treatment for congestive heart failure and dysrhythmias. Steroids, once strongly advocated, are now believed to be contraindicated, since they, as well as exercise, reserpine, and alcohol, have been shown to increase the severity of myocarditis. However, steroids could be used if myocarditis causes acute shock or complete heart block.

Diphtheria exotoxin causes profound myocardial damage by interfering with mitochondrial oxidation. The conduction system is commonly affected, leading to varying degrees of atrioventricular block (including complete heart block), premature beats, ventricular tachycardias, and ventricular fibrillation. Once severe cardiac involvement occurs, the mortality is high, despite therapy; thus it is particularly important to prevent the disease.

Trypanosoma cruzi is a common cause of myocarditis in South and Central America and occurs in the southern United States. It presents often as an acute myocarditis, but often shows more right ventricular dilatation than is noted in viral myocarditis. In the acute stage, parasites may be found in blood films or by culture of blood or bone marrow, and there is a specific complement fixation test.

Chronic Myocarditis

Some viruses and *T. cruzi* may cause chronic interstitial myocarditis in animals and man. There may be chronic cardiomegaly with left or biventricular hypertrophy and congestive heart failure. Dysrhythmias may occur. At autopsy there is diffuse interstitial fibrosis replacing necrotic myocardial cells. It may be difficult to demonstrate the causal organism at this stage.

Endocrine Disorders

Myxedema not only causes bradycardia, low cardiac output, and pericardial effusion, but may cause myocardial degeneration with S-T and T wave changes. Treatment of the hypothyroidism usually reverses the cardiac disability, but there may be residual fibrosis. *Hyperthyroidism* of long standing in adults may cause permanent cardiac damage, but this has not been reported in children. *Pheochromocytoma* may produce left ventricular hypertrophy and heart failure from sustained or paroxysmal hypertension. In addition, high catecholamine blood levels cause subendocardial hemorrhages and myocardial degeneration that may further impair cardiac function. *Congenital adrenal hyperplasia* may produce hyperkalemia and thus affect cardiac function. *Hypoglycemia* may cause cardiac dilatation and congestive heart failure, especially in newborn infants. It should be looked for, particularly in premature infants or those with intrauterine growth retardation, infants of diabetic mothers, and infants with severe cyanotic heart disease. Restoring blood sugar levels usually improves cardiac performance over the next 12 to 24 hours.

Electrolyte Disorders

Low calcium or magnesium levels may occasionally cause cardiac dilatation and heart failure. This is most common in newborn infants, especially premature infants. Clinically there may be hyperactive reflexes, and there may be a long Q-T interval or even atrioventricular block in the electrocardiogram. Infusion of calcium or magnesium usually causes rapid improvement. *Hypokalemia* may occur with malnutrition, vomiting or diarrhea, diuretic or steroid therapy, or hyperaldosteronism. The S-T segments and T waves become depressed, U waves increase in size, and at potassium levels below 2.5 mEq/liter there may be dysrhythmias. Myocardial contraction may be impaired, and susceptibility to digitalis-induced dysrhythmias is markedly increased. *Hyperkalemia,* as seen in renal failure or diabetic acidosis, first causes tall peaked T waves; then the QRS complex widens. At potassium levels above 8 mEq/liter the P-R interval lengthens, and then atrial standstill occurs; at higher levels there may be ventricular tachycardia and fibrillation.

Infiltrative Disorders

Cardiac glycogenosis (Pompe's disease) is a rare autosomal recessive disorder caused by deficiency in α-1,4-glycosidase (p. 731). There is glycogen storage in skeletal and cardiac muscle, with massive ventricular hypertrophy that may even cause outflow tract obstruction. The patients usually present with respiratory tract infections, fevers, and poor growth manifest by 4 to 6 months of age; death from congestive heart failure or infection is usual before 1 year of age. Macroglossia and hypotonia are marked, and limb reflexes are depressed. The electrocardiogram will show a very short P-R interval and enormous QRS complexes. The diagnosis is made by skeletal muscle biopsy. No treatment is known.

Mucopolysaccharidoses may produce myocardial degeneration. The Hurler and Hunter syndromes also cause intimal thickening of the coronary arteries, which causes myocardial ischemia; these two syndromes, as well as the Morquio and Scheie syndromes, also cause valvar regurgitation (p. 1422). *Tuberous sclerosis* may be associated with ventricular rhabdomyosarcomas.

Hemochromatosis is rare as a primary disorder in children, but it is often secondary to repeated blood transfusions in sickle cell anemia, thalassemia, and aplastic anemia. Deposition of hemosiderin may be associated with myocardial fibrosis, which can also be secondary to myocardial ischemia from the anemia. Dysrhythmias are common. *Leukemia* may lead to cardiac infiltration and occasionally cause dysrhythmias. Cardiac disability, however, is usually not of major importance. *Cystinosis* may produce cystine deposits in and degeneration of the myocardium.

Tumors

Rhabdomyosarcoma is often associated with adenoma sebaceum and the neurologic manifestations of tuberous sclerosis. Since the latter usually take several years to appear, the association is rare in early childhood. Dysrhythmias and heart failure usually appear and cause death. Since the lesions are usually multiple, surgery is not often attempted. *Fibromas* are benign ventricular tumors that may produce obstruction to blood flow or dysrhythmias. Surgical removal is possible. *Sarcomas* and angiosarcomas are rare, and they usually cause progressive heart failure and death. *Myxomas.* are discussed under endocardial lesions (p. 1469).

Neurologic Disorders

Friedreich's ataxia may cause murmurs, cardiomegaly, or heart failure, usually in older children and adoles-

cents. There is slowly progressive myocardial fibrosis and hypertrophy; small coronary arteries may become thickened and narrowed, and death may occur from dysrhythmias and heart failure. *Progressive muscular dystrophy* (Duchenne's dystrophy) may cause left ventricular hypertrophy and S-T and T wave changes. While death from heart failure or dysrhythmias may occur, cardiac involvement in this disease is not the usual cause of death. Other forms of muscular dystrophy may also be associated with myocardial changes.

Vascular Anomalies

Coronary embolism is relatively common when there is infective endocarditis, and it may be the cause of death in this disease. *Myocardial ischemic damage* is more likely if there is thickening of the coronary arterial intima with narrowing of the lumen; it is made worse by thrombosis. While the atheromatous lesions seen so often in adults are rare in children, they may occur in homozygous type 2 hyperlipidemia. Other diseases that cause intimal changes and myocardial ischemia are homocystinuria, the Hunter and Hurler syndromes (mucopolysaccharidoses), the vasculitides (systemic lupus erythematosus, polyarteritis nodosa), and the recently described mucocutaneous lymph node syndrome. Coronary occlusion also occurs in the rare syndrome of idiopathic calcification of the coronary arteries. *Congenital lesions* such as anomalous origin of the left coronary artery and coronary arteriovenous fistula may produce ischemia in the region supplied by that artery. All these lesions produce ischemic lesions, the extent of which will vary with the size and number of arteries involved and the amount of collateral formation. There may be cardiomegaly and ventricular hypertrophy, congestive heart failure, dysrhythmias, and often mitral incompetence due to damage to the papillary muscles.

MISCELLANEOUS. *Anemia* that is severe results in myocardial hypoxia, with eventual myocardial necrosis and fibrosis that is most marked in the subendocardial muscle. If there is also hypotension, as in hemorrhagic shock, the subendocardial necrosis may be more marked. *Beri-beri* causes heart failure in areas where malnutrition is still common, particularly in breast-fed infants. Unlike most forms of heart failure in infancy, peripheral edema is striking. Treatment is with thiamine hydrochloride. *Acute nephritis* is a common cause of pulmonary edema and congestive heart failure. The most likely causative factors are hypertension and hypervolemia from fluid retention and overloading, but direct myocardial damage has not been ruled out.

Cardiomyopathy

There are children with left ventricular dilatation and hypertrophy and congestive heart failure who do not appear to have any of the causes listed above. Some of these may be chronic sequelae of viral myocarditis, but others may be due to undiscovered metabolic or other factors. In Africa various forms of cardiomyopathy are common, and regional variations are noted. Viral and nutritional etiologies have been suggested but not proved. The term cardiomyopathy is used to designate this group without implying that they all have a single cause. Treatment is nonspecific, and prognosis is poor.

References

MYOCARDITIS

Ainger LE, Lawyer NG, Fitch CW: Neonatal rubella myocarditis. Br Heart J 28:691, 1966

Bell EJ, Grist NR: Echoviruses, carditis and acute pleurodynia. Lancet 1:326, 1970

Burch GE, Sun SC, Chu KC, Sohal RS, Colcolough HL: Interstitial and coxsackievirus B myocarditis in infants and children: a comparative histologic and immunofluorescent study of 50 autopsied hearts. JAMA 203:1, 1968

Cahill KM: Tropical Diseases in Temperate Climates. Philadelphia, JB Lippincott, 1964

Gore I: Myocardial changes in fatal diphtheria. Am J Med Sci 215:257, 1948

Kibrick S, Benirschke K: Severe generalized disease (encephalohepatomyocarditis) occurring in the newborn period and due to infection with coxsackie virus, group B; evidence of intrauterine infection with this agent. Pediatrics 22:857, 1958

Laranja FS, Dias E, Nobrega G, Miranda A: Chagas' disease. A clinical epidemologic and pathologic study. Circulation 14:1035, 1956

Ledbetter MK, Cannon AB II, Costa AF: The electrocardiogram in diptheritic myocarditis. Am Heart J 68:599, 1964

Lerner AM, Wilson FM: Virus myocardiopathy. Prog Med Virol 15:63, 1973

Morgan BC: Cardiac complications of diphtheria. Pediatrics 32:549, 1963

Roberts WC, Fox SM III: Mumps of the heart. Clinical and pathologic features. Circulation 32:342, 1965

Rosenberg HS, McNamara DG: Acute myocarditis in infancy and childhood. Prog Cardiovasc Dis 7:179, 1964

Saphir O: Non-rheumatic inflammatory diseases of the heart. C. Myocarditis. In Gould SE (ed): Pathology of the Heart. Springfield, Ill, Charles C Thomas, 1960

Spain DM, Bradess VA, Parsonnet V: Myocarditis in poliomyelitis. Am Heart J 40:336, 1950

Wilson FM, Miranda QR, Chason JL, Lerner AM: Residual pathologic changes following murine coxsackie A and B myocarditis. Am J Pathol 55:253, 1969

GLYCOGEN STORAGE DISEASE

Ehler KH, Hagstrom JWC, Lukas DC, Redo SF, Engle MA: Glycogen storage disease of the myocardium with obstruction to left ventricular outflow. Circulation 25:96, 1962

Hohn AR, Lowe CU, Sokal JE, Lambert EC: Cardiac problems in the glycogenoses with specific reference to Pompe's disease. Pediatrics 35:313, 1965

van Creveld S: The clinical course of glycogen disease. Can Med Assoc J 88:1, 1963

MUCOPOLYSACCHARIDOSES

Krovetz LJ, Lorincz AE, Schiebler GL: Cardiovascular manifestations of the Hurler syndrome. Hemodynamic and angiographic observations in 15 patients. Circulation 31:132, 1965

McKusick VA: Heritable Disorders of Connective Tissue. St Louis, CV Mosby, 1972

TUBEROUS SCLEROSIS

Engle MA, Ito T, Ehlers KH, Goldberg HP: Rhabdomyomatosis of the heart: diagnosis during life with clinical and pathologic findings. Circulation 26:712, 1962

TUMORS

van der Hauwaert LG: Cardiac tumours in childhood. In Watson H (ed): Paediatric Cardiology. St Louis, CV Mosby, 1968

NEUROLOGIC DISORDERS

Boyer SH IV, Chisholm AW, McKusick VA: Cardiac aspects of Friedreich's ataxia. Circulation 25:493, 1962

Gilroy J, Cahalan JL, Berman R, Newman M: Cardiac and pulmonary complications in Duchenne's progressive muscular dystrophy. Circulation 27:484, 1963

Ivemark B, Thoren C: The pathology of the heart in Friedreich's ataxia: changes in coronary arteries and myocardium. Acta Med Scand 175:227, 1964

James TN: Observations on the cardiovascular involvement, including the cardiac conduction system, in progressive muscular dystrophy. Am Heart J 63:48, 1962

Manning GW, Cropp GJ: The electrocardiogram in progressive muscular dystrophy. Br Heart J 20:416, 1958

Thilenius OG, Grossman BJ: Friedreich's ataxia with heart disease in children. Pediatrics 27:246, 1961

Zundel WS, Tyler FH: The muscular dystrophies. N Engl J Med 273:537, 1965

COLLAGEN DISORDERS

Brigden W, Bywaters EGL, Lessof MH, Ross IP: The heart in systemic lupus erythematosus. Br Heart J 22:1, 1960

Cathcart ES, Spodick DH: Rheumatoid heart disease. A study of the incidence and nature of cardiac lesions in rheumatoid arthritis. N Engl J Med 266:959, 1962

Cook CD, Wedgewood RJP, Craig JM, Hartmann JR, Janeway CA: Systemic lupus erythematosus. Description of 37 cases in children and a discussion of endocrine therapy in 32 of the cases. Pediatrics 26:570, 1960

Fletcher E, Morton P: Scleroderma heart disease. Br Med J 2:657, 1967

Holsinger DR, Osmundson PJ, Edwards JE: The heart in periarteritis nodosa. Circulation 25:610, 1962

CORONARY ARTERY LESIONS

Askenazi J, Nadas AS: Anomalous left coronary artery originating from the pulmonary artery. Circulation 51:976, 1975

Kato H, Korke S, Yamamoto M, Ito Y, Yano E: Coronary aneurysms in infants and young children with acute febrile mucocutaneous lymph node syndrome. J Pediatr 86:892, 1975

Wesselhoeft H, Fawcett JS, Johnson AL: Anomalous origin of the left coronary artery from the pulmonary trunk: its clinical spectrum, pathology and pathophysiology, based on a review of 140 cases with 7 further cases. Circulation 38:403, 1968

CARDIOMYOPATHY

Harris LC, Nghiem QX: Cardiomyopathies in infants and children. Prog Cardiovasc Dis 15:255, 1972

DISEASES OF PERICARDIUM
JULIEN I.E. HOFFMAN AND PAUL STANGER

GENERAL FEATURES. Pericardial diseases produce pericarditis or pericardial effusion or both; if the effusion makes the pericardium tense and impairs cardiac filling, then there is cardiac tamponade. *Acute pericarditis* is manifested by pain, a friction rub, electrocardiographic changes, and sometimes fever. The pain either is precordial or is referred to the epigastrium, neck, shoulder, or left arm; it may be relieved by leaning forward and made worse by deep inspiration. The friction rub may be heard anywhere on the precordium, but it is most frequent along the left sternal border. The rub has a grating sound like that produced by sandpaper on wood, or it may resemble creaking leather. Often the rub is brought out by firm pressure of the stethoscope on the chest, and it may vary with respiration or posture. It may be soft or loud and is often to-and-fro, or it may have three components. It is always in phase with the heart sounds. The examiner must make sure that the stethoscope does not slip over the skin, particularly over bony prominences, since this may produce a sound much like a friction rub. The electrocardiogram will initially show elevation of the S-T segments in most leads; after about 1 week the S-T segments return to normal and are associated with T wave flattening and inversion in the same leads. These changes may persist for months after the acute lesion has gone. Treatment for each specific lesion is discussed below.

PERICARDIAL EFFUSION. Pericardial effusion distends the pericardium and moves the parietal pericardium away from the heart. As a result the heart is quiet to palpation, the heart sounds are muffled, and there is on percussion an increased area of cardiac dullness with its left border often extending to the left of the apex beat. If there is associated pericarditis there may be a friction rub and the typical S-T and T wave changes, but in addition effusions often produce generalized low QRS voltages and may cause electrical alternans. Radiologically there will be seen a large cardiac silhouette that cannot be distinguished with certainty from cardiac dilatation, although the latter often shows associated pulmonary venous congestion; fluoroscopy does not give added information. The diagnosis of pericardial effusion is best confirmed by echocardiography or scanning the precordium after injection of radiolabeled albumin. These noninvasive methods have largely replaced the use of carbon dioxide and cardiac catheterization to demonstrate an increased gap between the lung and the cardiac chambers.

Cardiac tamponade may occur with relatively little fluid if the pericardium is not distensible or if the fluid accumulates very rapidly. On the other hand, a large effusion can form in a lax pericardium without tamponade. Once the pericardium becomes tense, pressure in the pericardial cavity rises and impairs cardiac relaxation and filling. As a result, ventricular end-diastolic, atrial, and venous pressures rise on both sides of the heart by approximately equal amounts; jugular venous pressure rises, and the liver enlarges. With reduced cardiac filling, the cardiac output and stroke volume fall, so that there is tachycardia, low blood pressure and pulse pressure, and eventually peripheral vasoconstriction, with clammy, cold extremities and reduced skin perfusion. Normally, with inspiration, intrathoracic pressure falls and abdominal pressure rises, so that the systemic venous return increases. With tamponade this increment in venous return cannot be accommodated in the heart; thus the jugular venous pressure rises with inspiration (Kussmaul's sign). Furthermore, with inspiration

the pulmonary venous return and left ventricular output fall for two reasons. The increased systemic venous return distends the right atrium and ventricle, which because of the tense pericardium compress the left atrium and ventricle and reduce their input and thus their output. Second, the tense pericardium acts as a rigid box around the heart, so that when intrathoracic pressure falls on inspiration the pressure gradient from pulmonary veins to left atrium is reduced, and again left-sided filling is reduced. As a result of these mechanisms, inspiration causes aortic blood pressure to fall —the *pulsus paradoxus.* Normally a deep inspiration may drop aortic blood pressure 4 to 8 mm Hg, and any greater fall on deep inspiration is abnormal. To detect this change, place a sphygmomanometer cuff on the arm and determine the blood pressure in the usual way. Then inflate the cuff to just above systolic pressure, and deflate the cuff slowly just until the first Korotkoff sounds appear. Maintain pressure and determine if the sounds disappear with inspiration. If they do, lower cuff pressure at steps of 2 mm Hg and note when the sounds first persist throughout the cardiac cycle. The difference between the two levels is the amount of pulsus paradoxus. This difference is also noted in diastole, but it is easier to measure in systole. This difference in systemic arterial pressures with respiration is not a paradox, but rather an accentuation of the normal changes. A pulsus paradoxus also occurs with airway obstruction, as in asthma, but the pulmonary findings serve to identify this cause.

Although the diagnosis of pericardial effusion may be verified by laboratory tests, the diagnosis of cardiac tamponade can be made only by physical examination; Kussmaul's sign in the jugular veins and the pulsus paradoxus are the crucial criteria. Recently it has been suggested that tamponade can be diagnosed by the degree of compression of the right ventricle determined by echocardiogram. It is important to note that tamponade can occur with a relatively small effusion, so that the size of the heart shadow is of no importance in its diagnosis. Furthermore, patients with enlarged hearts can get an effusion and tamponade that might be interpreted as worsening of heart failure; here, too, pulsus paradoxus will help to make the right diagnosis.

PERICARDIOCENTESIS Pericardiocentesis may be used to remove pericardial fluid for diagnostic study or to decompress the pericardial cavity if there is severe tamponade. Lesser degrees of tamponade may be managed conservatively, provided that the patient can be observed closely during treatment; vital signs should be taken frequently. If tamponade gets worse or if it is severe when the patient is first seen, then fluid should be removed. To do this, have the patient, sedated if necessary, lying at about 45 degrees to the horizontal with the head raised. Clean and sterilize the precordium and apply sterile drapes with full aseptic technique. Infiltrate the skin and subcutaneous tissue with local anesthetic just below the xiphoid process. Connect the patient to the limb leads of an electrocardiograph, and attach the V lead by a sterile connector to a 20 gauge needle on a syringe. (Make sure that the electrocardiograph has been checked to exclude any significant current leakage.)

Start the paper of the electrocardiograph running, insert the needle through the skin just below the xiphoid process, and push it slowly toward the mid-thoracic spine; the needle should be at an angle of about 20 degrees below the perpendicular to the body wall. Attempt to remove fluid with the syringe after each 1 or 2 mm of penetration; as soon as fluid enters the syringe, clamp a hemostat to the needle at the point of entry into the skin to avoid further penetration. If the needle touches the heart, the V lead will show marked S-T elevation because of an injury current; this current is too local to be seen on the usual limb leads. When this injury current is seen, withdraw the needle until the S-T segment returns to normal. Remove the fluid until it ceases to come out easily, and do not try to get more out by moving the needle, as this may injure the heart. If the fluid does not come out, or seems to be thick, refer to a surgeon, who can then remove fluid through a small opening in the pericardium. Pericardiocentesis can be life-saving, but it can also cause dysrhythmias or serious bleeding into the pericardium. It should therefore be done only when there is adequate help available and when complete facilities for resuscitation are present.

CHRONIC CONSTRICTIVE PERICARDITIS.
Chronic constrictive pericarditis is a relatively uncommon sequel to acute pericarditis. It is seen most often after tuberculous or suppurative pericarditis or traumatic hemopericardium and is very rare after acute rheumatic pericarditis. The disease is marked by massive fibrous proliferation that obliterates the pericardial cavity and often calcifies. This produces a chronic tamponade, so that there is gradual development of marked hepatomegaly and ascites, but peripheral edema is less marked. Intestinal venous congestion may cause protein-losing enteropathy and hypoalbuminemia, leading to the wrong diagnosis of liver disease or nephrosis. The heart is quiet to palpation and often is not much enlarged. A prominent early third sound (pericardial knock is common, and it coincides with the rapid fall in jugular venous pressure (steep y descent) when the tricuspid valve opens and blood rushes from the high-pressure right atrium to the relatively indistensible right ventricle. A raised jugular venous pressure with Kussmaul's sign and pulsus paradoxus complete the picture. The diagnosis will be confirmed at cardiac catheterization, and treatment consists of surgical removal of the restricting fibrous tissue. The results are not always good, either because of incomplete removal of the fibrous tissue or because of damage to coronary arteries or diffuse fibrosis extending into the myocardium from the surface. In order to decrease the risk of occurrence of constrictive pericarditis and the risk of operating on it, patients with purulent or tuberculous pericarditis should be referred early for surgical treatment.

INFECTIONS. *Acute rheumatic fever* with extensive pancarditis is less frequent than it used to be in the United States. Pericarditis occurs usually after or with valvulitis and myocarditis, but the friction rub and effusion may mask these other features. Tamponade and constrictive pericarditis are very rare. Treatment is discussed elsewhere (p. 387).

ACUTE NONSPECIFIC PERICARDITIS. Acute nonspecific pericarditis, which is thought to be viral in origin, is an acute pericarditis that often follows a respiratory infection. The pericarditic phase is manifested by fever, malaise, anorexia, and pericardial pain; in infants there are also tachycardia and tachypnea. There is a polymorphonuclear leukocytosis. A pericardial friction rub and effusions are common, and typical electrocardiographic changes are seen. The patients are not usually very ill, and tamponade and constrictive pericarditis are rare. Recovery occurs spontaneously in 2 to 4 weeks. Symptomatic treatment is usually all that is required, but steroids may be needed for the occasional patient with recurrent or unusually severe or long-lasting disease.

PURULENT PERICARDITIS. Purulent pericarditis usually occurs by extension from a septic focus in the lung (pneumonia or empyema), or it may occur with a septicemia or after cardiac surgery. The common organisms are staphylococci, pneumococci, streptococci, *Haemophilus influenzae,* and meningococci. The illness has an acute onset, with a high swinging fever, marked polymorphonuclear leukocytosis, and severe toxicity. Tamponade is common. Intensive treatment with appropriate antibiotics alone has a high mortality. Addition of surgical drainage of the pericardial cavity reduces mortality and decreases the risk of later constrictive pericarditis. Close observation for tamponade is essential. Constrictive pericarditis may follow cure, so that an extended follow-up is necessary.

TUBERCULOUS PERICARDITIS. Tuberculous pericarditis usually complicates tuberculosis elsewhere. It starts insidiously with malaise, anorexia, low-grade fever, and night sweats, and then the typical features of pericarditis develop; there may be an effusion. Diagnosis is by a combination of positive tuberculin test, isolation of tubercle bacilli from pericardial fluid, sputum, or gastric washings, and histologic examination of the pericardium. Antituberculous therapy is effective, but because constrictive pericarditis is a common sequel, some experts advocate early pericardiectomy to avoid having to remove dense fibrous tissue later.

TRAUMA. Hemopericardium occurs after blunt or penetrating trauma, and tamponade may occur rapidly, so that emergency pericardiocentesis may be needed while preparations are made for surgery. Constrictive pericarditis is a common sequel. Tamponade may also occur with bleeding after cardiac surgery, and it must be considered whenever there is a low cardiac output syndrome in the postoperative period.

COLLAGEN DISEASES. In rheumatoid arthritis, pericarditis and high fevers may precede joint involvement. Treatment should be by salicylates first, with steroids reserved for refractory lesions. Systemic lupus erythematosus may have associated pericarditis with effusions and occasionally cardiac tamponade. The effusion may persist after other symptoms disappear with steroid therapy.

UREMIA. Pericarditis and effusions, even with tamponade, may occur with chronic uremia. The diagnosis may be difficult to make because of the cardiomegaly and heart failure in some patients. Futhermore, with longer survival due to hemodialysis or transplantation, constrictive pericarditis has occasionally developed.

CHRONIC ANEMIA. Pericarditis and effusions may be found in sickle cell disease, thalassemia, and congenital aplastic anemia. The mechanism is unknown.

METABOLIC DISORDERS. A pericardial effusion is quite common with myxedema, and it has also been seen in gout.

CONGENITAL HEART DISEASE. Effusions have occasionally been noted with various forms of congenital heart disease and cardiomyopathy. They also occur with anasarca due to liver disease, nephrosis, and congestive heart failure.

MISCELLANEOUS. Pericarditis and effusions may occur after radiation of the chest, with foreign bodies in or near the pericardium, and with the rare tumors that occur there. If effusions after radiation persist beyond 2 to 3 months, a pericardial window may be created surgically to permit drainage.

POSTPERICARDIOTOMY SYNDROME. The postpericardiotomy syndrome may follow any operation in which the pericardium is opened. In different series up to 30 percent of patients have had attacks of acute pericarditis and fever beginning about 3 to 4 weeks (range of 3 days to 6 months) after surgery. There is often a pericardial effusion and sometimes a pleural effusion that need not be on the side of the thoracotomy. There is a mild polymorphonuclear leukocytosis. Theories of etiology include a reaction to blood in the pericardium, an autoimmune response to myocardial tissue, and a viral infection; none has been proved conclusively.

Treatment by bed rest and acetylsalicylic acid (60 mg/kg/day) is usually effective. Once the acute attack is under control, the acetylsalicylic acid can be slowly withdrawn over 6 to 8 weeks; more rapid withdrawal may lead to recurrences, which may occur in 10 to 15 percent of patients in any event. Occasionally steroids may be needed if there is no response to this treatment.

CONGENITAL LESIONS. Congenital pericardial lesions are rare, but they may be important. Localized *pericardial defects* occur most often on the left side, and they may be detected when a spontaneous or induced left pneumothorax also causes a pneumomediastinum. The left atrium can also herniate through the defect, and this may cause chest pain or dysrhythmias. If the defect is larger, so that the left ventricle herniates through, there could be compression of a coronary artery; death from this cause has been reported. The pulmonary artery may herniate and give the appearance of a dilated pulmonary artery. Congenital pericardial cysts or diverticula occur usually on the right side. They are seldom large, but they cause problems of diagnosis.

References

CONGENITAL LESIONS

de Roover P, Maisin J, Laquet A: Congenital pleuro-pericardial cysts. Thorax 18:146, 1963

Duffie ER Jr, Moss AJ, Maloney JV Jr: Congenital pericardial defects with herniation of the heart into the pleural space. Pediatrics 30:746, 1962

Ellis K, Leeds NE, Himmelstein A: Congenital deficiencies in the parietal pericardium. A review with two new cases including successful diagnosis by plain roentgenology. Am J Roentgenol Radium Ther Nucl Med 82:125, 1959

Fowler NO: Congenital defect of the pericardium. Its resemblance to pulmonary artery enlargement. Circulation 26:114, 1962

Hipona FA, Crummy AB Jr: Congenital pericardial defect associated with tetralogy of Fallot. Herniation of normal lung into pericardial cavity. Circulation 29:132, 1964

Tucker DH, Miller DE, Jacoby WJ Jr: Congenital partial absence of the pericardium with herniation of the left atrial appendage. Am J Med 35:560, 1963

PERICARDITIS

Benzing G III, Kaplan SA: Purulent pericarditis. Am J Dis Child 106:289, 1963

Cayler GG, Taybi H, Riley HD Jr, Simon JL: Pericarditis with effusion in infants and children. J Pediatr 63:264, 1963

Engle MA, Ito T: The postpericardiotomy syndrome. Am J Cardiol 7:73, 1961

Fowler NO, Manitsas GT: Infectious pericarditis. Prog Cardiovasc Dis 16:323, 1973

Golinko RJ, Kaplan N, Rudolph AM: The mechanism of pulsus paradoxus during acute pericardial tamponade. J Clin Invest 42:249, 1963

Harvey WP: Auscultatory findings in diseases of the pericardium. Am J Cardiol 7:15, 1961

Liu HY, Garcia R: Acute idiopathic pericarditis. Report of a fatal case with brief review of the literature. Am Heart J 69:677, 1965

Spodick DH: Chronic and Constrictive Pericarditis. New York, Grune & Stratton, 1964

———— Differential diagnosis of acute pericarditis. Prog Cardiovasc Dis 14:192, 1971

Tabatznik B, Isaacs JP: Postpericardiotomy syndrome following traumatic hemopericardium. Am J Cardiol 7:83, 1961

CONGESTIVE HEART FAILURE

JULIEN I.E. HOFFMAN AND PAUL STANGER

Congestive heart failure is a syndrome in which the heart cannot supply enough blood flow to tissues without the compensatory mechanisms causing difficulties.

CAUSES. The major causes of congestive heart failure may be grouped into those with excessive volume or pressure loads and those in which the myocardium cannot function adequately with normal pressure and volume loads. Excessive volume loads occur mainly with large left-to-right shunts, whether or not there are right-to-left shunts as well, but they can also be due to valvar regurgitation or to factors that cause a large increase in cardiac output. Excessive pressure loads are due to obstruction to the circulation and may be classified by the portion of the circulation obstructed. Finally, myocardial factors involve primary or secondary impairment of muscle function due to many different causes.

VOLUME LOADS. For volume loads to cause congestive heart failure there usually must be a large enough left-to-right shunt to cause a volume overload, and the common causes and time of onset of heart failure vary with age. In the premature infant weighing under 1,500 g a patent ductus arteriosus is the most common cause of heart failure (p. 1409), and other forms of structural heart disease are rare. In the larger premature infant a large communication at the ventricular or ductal level may cause early onset of heart failure within the first month after birth, but in term infants these lesions do not usually produce overt heart failure until after the infants are 6 to 8 weeks of age. The reason for this time course in term infants is that with a large defect at ventricular or ductal level it takes longer than normal for the pulmonary vascular resistance to fall; thus as a rule it takes several weeks before the left-to-right shunt becomes large enough to stress the left ventricle. In premature infants, on the other hand, the pulmonary arteries seem less able to constrict, despite their thick muscular walls, so that a large left-to-right shunt can develop early. The times mentioned refer to the onset of overt heart failure; often there is a history of tachypnea and sweating from soon after birth.

Large left-to-right shunts can develop very early and can cause failure even in term infants in certain types of lesions. Endocardial cushion defects commonly cause very early failure, probably because of combinations of atrial and ventricular left-to-right shunts, as well as regurgitation through mitral and tricuspid valves. Other volume loads that can be large even when pulmonary vascular resistance is still high are those through large arteriovenous fistulae, especially in the head, and those due to massive regurgitation at atrioventricular or semilunar valves. When left-to-right shunts are combined with right-to-left shunts in complex anatomic lesions such as truncus arteriosus, transpositions with ventricular septal defects, or tricuspid atresia with transposition, there may also be early onset of heart failure, either because of the added burden of hypoxemia or because there is essentially one ventricle to do the work normally done by two.

Left-to-right shunting at the atrial level alone, as in secundum atrial septal defects, is an unusual cause of congestive heart failure at any age, but occasionally it causes severe difficulty in infants. On the other hand, total anomalous pulmonary venous connection often causes early failure because the venous return may be obstructed and cause pulmonary edema.

PRESSURE LOADS.   Severe aortic stenosis and coarctation of the aorta may cause very severe heart failure within the first month after birth. Both lesions may produce very poor pulses and little murmur, and both may have right ventricular predominance and even a large left-to-right shunt at the atrial level; thus they may be mistaken for right-sided lesions. In addition, these lesions and those with pulmonary venous obstruction, such as cor triatriatum, total anomalous pulmonary venous connection, and mitral atresia, cause pulmonary edema and can easily be mistaken for lung disease.

More commonly in the immediate newborn period there is right-sided congestive heart failure due to severe pulmonary hypertension that may have many causes. It may be secondary to hypoxic lung disease, hypervolemia and polycythemia, premature closure of the foramen ovale or the parabiotic syndrome (intrauterine twin–twin transfusion), or factors as yet unknown.

Frequently these infants are also cyanotic due to a large right-to-left shunt through the ductus arteriosus. Failure from severe pulmonary stenosis is rare.

MYOCARDIAL FACTORS.   While myocarditis and cardiomyopathy can cause heart failure at any age, they are rare in the immediate newborn period, as is endocardial fibroelastosis. Myocardial ischemia due to an anomalous left coronary artery usually causes failure after several weeks or months, when myocardial infarction occurs. What are particularly important in neonates are the nonstructural causes of heart failure. The myocardium can be severely depressed by metabolic abnormalities; severe postpartum asphyxia can cause heart failure, and so can marked hypoglycemia or low calcium and magnesium levels. Severe anemia decreases myocardial oxygen supply and increases cardiac volume work, and so may cause failure at any age. Very slow heart rates (congenital heart block) or paroxysmal tachycardias often cause heart failure in neonates, or occasionally before birth; the tachycardias may be intermittent and thus may be difficult to diagnose until an attack is observed. In the newborn the nonstructural causes of heart failure due to polycythemia, acidemia, asphyxia, or low calcium, magnesium, or glucose should be thought of first, since they urgently require diagnosis and treatment so as to avoid permanent damage.

PATHOPHYSIOLOGY AND SIGNS AND SYMPTOMS.   Most of the clinical features of congestive heart failure can be explained by the side effects of the mechanisms that compensate for excessive loads or myocardial dysfunction. There is dilatation of one or more cardiac chambers, so that the heart is enlarged on clinical and radiologic examination. The heart is not always enlarged in neonates, especially premature infants, either because the ventricles have reduced distensibility or because associated lung disease raises intrathoracic pressure and decreases systemic venous return. The heart also may not be enlarged if there is obstruction to pulmonary venous drainage, as in mitral stenosis or cor triatriatum.

Increased activity of the sympathetic nervous system results from stimulation of the atrial and venous stretch receptors and the aortic and carotid sinus baroreceptors by a reduced aortic blood pressure and pulse pressure. As a result, alpha receptor stimulation decreases flow to the limbs, splanchnic bed, and kidneys, so that the extremities are pale and cold and often have weak pulses and urine output falls. Beta receptor stimulation and increased circulating catecholamines produce tachycardia and also increase myocardial contractility. Also, stimulation of sympathetic cholinergic fibers to the skin causes increased sweating, which is particularly prominent in infants. The sweating is generalized, but may be more marked in the scalp, and it is most prominent during exertion such as crying or feeding. This is in contrast to the normal sweating of many infants, which is exclusively of the scalp and primarily occurs when sleeping.

There are malaise, fatigue, and decreased appetite,

probably related to reduced splanchnic and limb blood flow, venous congestion of the gut, and difficulty in feeding because of tachypnea. Chronic disease may lead to markedly impaired growth and even cachexia. Irritability is often very marked in infants and may be due to sympathetic stimulation, hunger, or marked discomfort.

CARDIAC EDEMA. Patients with congestive heart failure have increased extracellular fluid volume. Initially this is manifest only by weight gain. Further fluid accumulation leads to soft tissue swelling, which because of gravity is most prominent in loose periorbital tissues and over the sacrum after lying down or in the feet and ankles after prolonged standing. With much ankle swelling there may be pitting of the edematous tissue on pressure. Gross fluid excess may produce ascites and pleural effusions. Peripheral pitting edema is less common in infants and young children than in older children and adults, but it is often seen in premature infants.

The basic cause of extracellular fluid volume expansion is decreased renal excretion of sodium with secondary water retention, probably related to increased secretion of antidiuretic hormone. Thus serum osmolality and composition are usually normal in untreated congestive heart failure, although occasionally with very severe failure proportionately more water than sodium is retained and serum sodium concentrations fall (dilutional hyponatremia). More commonly, hyponatremia follows vigorous diuretic therapy and restriction of sodium intake without a corresponding decrease in water.

Three major mechanisms are thought to explain the sodium retention. The first of these is a reduced glomerular filtration rate (GFR), which decreases the total daily amount of sodium and water presented to the tubules and may also lead to absorption of a greater than normal proportion of filtered sodium. The reduced GFR is due to a decreased renal blood flow, and this in turn is due either to a decreased arterial blood pressure or more often to a raised renal vascular resistance; many features of congestive heart failure raise renal vascular resistance, the most important being the generalized sympathetic stimulation that occurs, the increased amount of angiotensin generated (see below), and an increase in renal interstitial pressure because of elevated venous pressures.

Although a decreased GFR is a major mechanism for sodium retention, especially with acute congestive heart failure, it is not always found in chronic heart failure; even when it is found; there is usually a second major cause of sodium retention, namely an increased serum aldosterone concentration. Aldosterone is one of the most powerful of the mineralocorticoids, and it enhances active sodium transport from lumen to blood at the level of the distal convoluted tubules. A raised blood level of any substance can be due to either decreased removal or increased formation, and both factors are responsible for the raised serum aldosterone concentration in congestive heart failure. Aldosterone

is broken down almost entirely in the liver, so that its half-life is markedly prolonged by the reduced hepatic blood flow that occurs with congestive heart failure. In addition, there is up to 50-fold increase in the amount of aldosterone secreted by the adrenals. The increased aldosterone secretion is intimately related to the abnormal renal physiology that occurs in congestive heart failure. Decreased renal blood flow and increased sympathetic stimulation both increase renin secretion from the juxtaglomerular cells. The reduced flow acts either through decreased stimulation of baroreceptors in the renal afferent arterioles or by presenting a reduced sodium load to the macula densa which is stimulated to release renin from the juxtaglomerular cells. The renin acts in the plasma on an α_2-globulin called angiotensinogen to produce angiotensin I, a decapeptide. This in turn is converted to the octapeptide angiotensin II, chiefly by an enzyme in the endothelium of the pulmonary blood vessels. Angiotensin II is thus produced excessively in congestive heart failure, and it promotes sodium retention by at least two mechanisms: it causes renal vasoconstriction and thus reduces glomerular filtration rate, and it acts on adrenal cortical receptors to stimulate aldosterone secretion.

Studies in patients with chronic congestive heart failure who do not appear to show these two main mechanisms of sodium retention indicate that it has other causes. These have been studied in animal experiments, which have shown that there are additional humoral factors that increase sodium reabsorption or decrease sodium excretion; vasoactive peptides and prostaglandin activity may be important. Details are still to be elucidated, but these extra-adrenal sodium-retaining factors are important added causes of cardiac edema.

The pathophysiologic mechanisms that are responsible for sodium retention in congestive heart failure are intensified by exercise. If the heart is unable to increase cardiac output normally with exercise, then renal and hepatic blood flows decrease markedly, venous pressure rises, and sympathetic discharge intensifies. As a result, several factors responsible for increasing sodium and water retention become even more prominent, and extracellular fluid expansion becomes more marked. Conversely, bed rest increases renal and hepatic flow, lowers venous pressure, and decreases sympathetic discharge, thus contributing to increased excretion of sodium and water and helping to relieve the cardiac edema.

VENTRICLES. When the ventricles are affected they dilate, and thus wall tension rises; if distensibility is reduced by disease, the rise is even more marked. The greater wall tension and radius increase the myocardial oxygen consumption and thus may contribute to further myocardial dysfunction. Ventricular dilatation is often associated with a protodiastolic gallop (that is, with an abnormal third heart sound that produces a gallop rhythm). Extreme ventricular dilatation, particularly in neonates, may on occasion lead to mitral or tricuspid regurgitation, which then causes further reduction in forward blood flow and increases in atrial pressures. Ventricular failure may at times cause a pulsus alternans, which is the only direct sign of myocardial dysfunction.

Atria. The atria dilate and later hypertrophy in response to elevated pressures or obstruction at the atrioventricular valves. As a result, there may be a fourth heart sound or presystolic gallop. A more important consequence is that raised atrial pressures cause raised pressures in the veins that drain into the atria, and it is the increased venous pressures that are responsible for many of the cardinal features of congestive heart failure.

PULMONARY VEINS. When the pressure in the pulmonary veins rises, the lungs become stiffer, partly because the veins are distended and partly because of increased interstitial fluid due to increased capillary pressure. As a result, breathing becomes rapid and shallow due to the fall in compliance and to reflex nervous stimuli. A further rise in pressure causing stiffer lungs, or else increased oxygen needs from exertion or feeding, will lead to greater respiratory efforts and greater negative intrathoracic pressures and will produce supracostal, intercostal, and subcostal retractions. There is often orthopnea when there is much pulmonary venous congestion, because pulmonary blood volume increases when people lie flat. Finally, when the capacities of the interstitial space and lymphatic drainage are exceeded, there will be accumulation of fluid in alveoli, with rales and decreased oxygenation. Frank pulmonary edema with blood-stained frothy fluid appearing at the mouth is rare in early childhood.

The raised bronchial venous pressure may be responsible for edema of bronchial mucosa and increased bronchial secretion, thus accounting for the wheezing and rhonchi that are often noted. Mucosal swelling and irritation may also cause a chronic hacking cough.

SYSTEMIC VEINS. Raised right atrial pressure and increased blood volume from fluid retention distend the systemic veins and raise their pressure. The external manifestations of this are hepatomegaly and a raised jugular venous pressure. Because the venous system in infants and young children is very distensible, it is possible to have a marked increase in venous blood volume with marked hepatomegaly but not much increase in venous pressure; this may in part explain why pitting leg edema is uncommon in young children. Further increases in venous pressure may show up on examination of the jugular veins, but the rise may be difficult to detect in babies with short necks or those who are irritable and uncooperative. Renal venous congestion is probably the cause of the proteinuria that is often seen. Other manifestations of a raised systemic venous pressure are splenomegaly and occasionally ascites, which occurs most often with right-sided failure and tricuspid stenosis or incompetence.

DIAGNOSIS. Most patients have evidence of significant underlying heart disease by physical findings, electrocardiogram, and chest roentgenogram, and this plus the signs discussed above usually suffice for the diagnosis. However, certain important points must be remembered:

Most cardiac diseases in childhood affect the left ventricle predominantly; thus most children in heart failure have either isolated left heart failure or biventricular failure. Pure right heart failure is uncommon.

Hepatomegaly is a sign of right heart failure and thus is absent in isolated left heart failure. Therefore absence of an enlarged liver does not exclude heart failure.

In left heart failure the major signs of tachycardia, tachypnea, intercostal retractions, rales, and rhonchi are similar to the findings in pulmonary infections. Furthermore, obstructive airway disease may flatten the diaphragm and cause the liver to descend, thus simulating hepatomegaly, which is the cardinal sign of right heart failure. The differential diagnosis of these two entities may be even more difficult because they may coexist: a pulmonary infection is a common precipitating cause of congestive heart failure in a child with heart disease, while congestive heart failure may predispose to pulmonary infection. The features of an abnormal heart and catecholamine excess (cold sweaty hands) usually serve to make the distinction, but treatment for both diseases may be necessary if a single diagnosis cannot be made with confidence.

TREATMENT. The basic cause of congestive heart failure is usually a structural abnormality that needs surgical correction, but this is almost always best deferred until heart failure has been controlled. Occasionally there are nonstructural abnormalities that can be treated. Thus packed red cells can be given for severe anemia, especially if it is acute. Blood can be removed for marked hypervolemia. Heart failure due to acute rheumatic myocarditis usually responds rapidly to glucocorticoid therapy. Glucose, calcium, or magnesium may be valuable, especially in the newborn, in whom these deficiencies may be the only cause of heart failure. However, in most instances symptomatic therapy is given, the aims of which are to increase tissue oxygen supply, decrease tissue oxygen consumption, correct metabolic abnormalities, remove excess salt and water, and improve myocardial function.

Oxygen supply can be increased slightly by giving the patient cold humidified oxygen, even if there is no cyanosis. The only time oxygen should be avoided or used with caution is in a neonate in whom systemic blood flow depends on a patent ductus arteriosus, as in aortic atresia, coarctation of the aorta, or interrupted aortic arch, since oxygen can induce ductus constriction.

Oxygen consumption can be reduced in several ways: Treat infections and, if necessary, reduce high temperatures. Keep newborn infants warm with an abdominal skin temperature of 36 C to 37 C. Make patients comfortable and reduce the work of breathing by bed rest in the semi-Fowler position; for infants a special cardiac seat is useful. Sedate very irritable infants and children to increase their comfort and reduce oxygen usage. Morphine sulfate at 0.1 mg/kg intramuscularly is effective, especially if there is any pulmonary edema. If it is used, check ventilation and be prepared to assist depressed ventilation.

METABOLIC ABNORMALITIES.   Many children in congestive heart failure have hypoglycemia due to decreased intake and also to increased glycolysis secondary to anaerobic tissue metabolism. If blood glucose is low, it should be raised by slow intravenous infusion of glucose. Calcium and magnesium may be low in neonates, even when heart failure is due to some other cause. Intravenous administration should be employed. Anaerobic metabolism also causes lactic acidemia, with a fall in arterial pH. This will improve after heart failure is controlled, but occasionally with very low pH (below 7.1) the acidemia may need treatment with intravenous sodium bicarbonate or TRIS. These should be given with caution because of the large load of sodium and water that they provide.

CONTROL OF SALT, WATER, AND CALORIE INTAKE.   If the child is very ill, withhold oral feeding until failure has improved. In infants, empty the stomach by nasogastric tube to prevent regurgitation and aspiration, since the stomach is often atonic and dilated. When they are improved, or if they are not very ill when first seen, give a light diet with a low sodium intake. Since low-sodium milk and salt-free foods are unpalatable, they should not be used unless there is no other way of preventing salt and water retention.

Restrict fluid intake initially to 750 ml/m^2/day or 65 ml/kg/day, and increase the quantity as the child improves. However, a few children with chronic congestive heart failure and persistent dilutional hyponatremia may need restriction of fluid intake as the only way to restore serum sodium to normal.

Give *diuretics* to eliminate excess salt and water and prevent their reaccumulation (Table 11).

TABLE 11 Diuretic Therapy

Agent	Route of Administration	Dose
Chlorothiazide (Diuril)	Oral	25–50 mg/kg/day
Hydrochlorothiazide (Hydrodiuril)	Oral	1–2 mg/kg/day
Furosemide (Lasix)	Oral, im, iv	1 mg/kg 1–3 times per day
Spironolactone (Aldactone)	Oral	1–2 mg/kg/day
Triamterene (Dyrenium)	Oral	2–4 mg/kg/day

Other agents such as mercurial diuretics and ethacrynic acid are seldom used now, and they will not be discussed.

Chlorothiazide and hydrochlorothiazide are moderate diuretics that are convenient for long-term therapy. Furosemide is more powerful and acts more quickly if given intravenously; thus it is the agent of choice in severe heart failure when a rapid response is needed. All diuretics should be given orally for smoother action unless the patient is vomiting or needs a rapid diuresis; then intravenous furosemide is the diuretic of choice. These three diuretics all tend to waste potassium, so that serum potassium must be measured periodically,

and potassium supplements may be needed. If possible, these diuretics should be given on alternate days, or else for 4 or 5 days and then stopped for 2 days, in order to allow potassium stores to be replenished. By contrast, spironolactone and triamterene tend to produce mild or moderate diuresis and potassium retention; in fact, they should not be used whenever there is a tendency for potassium retention, as in renal failure, and they usually should not have potassium supplementation. Sometimes one of the first three diuretics is given with one of the last two, so that diuresis is increased but hypokalemia is avoided or minimized. Furosemide should be used with care in neonates, particularly if kanamycin is also being given, since each agent is ototoxic, and the combination may impair hearing. Sometimes peritoneal dialysis may be used to remove excess water and restore electrolyte concentrations to normal.

IMPROVING MYOCARDIAL FUNCTION.   **Digitalis glycosides.**   Digitalis glycosides are the main agents for increasing myocardial contractility. They also slow conduction at the atrioventricular node, thus beneficially lowering ventricular rates in rapid supraventricular arrhythmias, but this effect may also produce heart block when they are given in excess. They slow sinus node pacemaking when there is heart failure, but they are of no value, and are even dangerous, in noncardiogenic sinus tachycardia. Also, they increase automaticity and so can bring on dysrhythmias.

The main preparation used in children today is *digoxin,* because its half-life of 24 to 48 hours is long enough to allow once or twice daily medication and short enough to limit the period of toxicity if an overdose has been given. The other major preparation is *digitoxin,* with a half-life of about 8 days. This has two advantages over digoxin: it is completely absorbed from the gastrointestinal tract, and the long half-life gives a smooth action with once daily dosage. However, if toxicity occurs there is a long period within which dangerous complications can happen. Deslanoside (Cedilanid-D) is a rapidly acting, short-lived preparation that must be given intravenously every 6 hours; it is therefore useful as the initial drug in an emergency, but it should then be replaced by one of the others. The rest of the discussion will be based on digoxin as the preferred agent.

A child with congestive heart failure should be given a digitalizing dose of digoxin with the following considerations: The digoxin should usually be given intramuscularly. Oral medication is too uncertain in the very ill child; the child may vomit, or absorption may be delayed. However, in some mildly affected children oral medication can be given from the onset, while in very sick children with poor muscle perfusion the intravenous route is preferable. If the child has not been taking digoxin for the previous week, calculate a theoretic total digitalizing dose and plan to give it as three divided doses over 8 to 16 hours. From experience the approximate digitalizing doses based on age and weight are known, but these are at best rough estimates that merely avoid gross underdosage or overdosage. If one-half of the digitalizing dose is given initially, one-quarter is given 8 hours later (or even 6 to 4 hours later if the child is still very ill), and the final one-quarter is given as a third dose 8 hours later (or 4 hours later in very ill patients), then toxicity can usually be detected or prevented; it is very unlikely that toxicity will occur after one-half of the digitalizing dose. Also, if there has been no good response, there will usually be time to give added doses of digoxin, since more than 150 percent of the digitalizing dose is seldom needed.

The total *digitalizing dose* intramuscularly is 30 μg/kg (0.03 mg/kg) in premature and small-for-age infants, 60 μg/kg (0.06 mg/kg) in full-term infants up to about 6 months of age, 45 μg/kg (0.045 mg/kg) for infants from 6 months of age to about 2 years, and 30 μg/kg (0.03 mg/kg) after 2 years of age. Full-term infants need more digoxin per unit of body weight and also tolerate higher digoxin levels than do older children and adults. The reasons are not clear, but they may possibly relate to binding to receptors on the muscle cells, since the difference in sensitivity has been noted in isolated muscle strips in a water bath; in addition, infants clear digoxin more rapidly from the blood than do newborns or older children. When the total dosage has been calculated and the fractions to be given at each time have been obtained, always recheck the calculations. Be particularly careful about the decimal point.

Take a routine electrocardiogram if one has not been taken previously. Then give the first dose of digoxin (half the calculated digitalizing dose), and about 2 hours after the dose has been given take a strip of electrocardiogram; the lead with the best P waves, usually lead II, is selected. Since the peak digoxin effect is about 1 to 2 hours after administration, this is the time when signs of digitalis toxicity are most likely to be seen. If there is no contraindication, give the next quarter of the digitalizing dose at the chosen time, and again take an electrocardiogram strip 2 hours later. If again there are no contraindications, give the final quarter dose and once more check the electrocardiogram 2 hours later. (Some people recommend dividing the digitalizing dose into three equal doses because the value of a loading dose is not established and because it reduces the risk of an error in dosage.) If digoxin has to be given intravenously because of an emergency, then the same dosage as used intramuscularly is given.

If there have been signs of toxicity before the full digitalizing dose has been given, then the actual digitalizing dose is less than the total given up to that time. This actual digitalizing dose is what must be used to calculate the maintenance requirements. Similarly, if after giving the calculated dose another one-quarter or one-half of the digitalizing dose has to be given before there is some therapeutic response, then the new total amount is the observed digitalizing dose to be used for calculating the maintenance dosage.

Maintenance dosage is usually one-quarter to one-third of the observed digitalizing dose. It is essential to make sure that the first maintenance dose is not given until about 12 hours after the last of the digitalizing doses; often the maintenance dose is ordered at a fixed time of the day without realizing that this may be only a few hours after the digitalization has been completed. Usu-

ally the maintenance dose is divided in two and given at 12-hour intervals for smoother action and less chance of toxicity. Once the child has begun to improve and can absorb normally, the digoxin can be given orally as elixir of digoxin. Since absorption from the gut is only about 65 to 75 percent complete, the dose must be increased about one-third so that the same amount reaches the tissues. Similarly, when a child who is receiving oral digoxin has to be placed on intramuscular digoxin, the dose must be reduced by about one-third.

Digitoxin is used in the same way as digoxin, but in doses that are exactly half of the digoxin doses. Because of complete absorption from the gut, its oral and intramuscular doses are the same.

If there is a very poor response for which no good cause can be found, the question may be raised of whether that particular patient is really getting enough digoxin. It is then helpful to obtain a digoxin level. In adults the usual therapeutic concentrations of digoxin are under 2 ng/ml blood, and toxicity is commonly seen above that level. In infants, on the other hand, therapeutic levels of digoxin range from 1 to 5 ng/ml (mean 3.5), while toxicity is associated with concentrations over 3 ng/ml. Older children have therapeutic and toxic levels like those of adults.

If the child has been on digoxin recently, it is safest to continue with a calculated maintenance dose and to increase it cautiously, if needed, by small increments. If there is renal failure, then the dosage of digoxin must be reduced to allow for the decreased renal excretion of digoxin.

Since digoxin is removed mainly by renal excretion, its dosage must be reduced when there is renal failure so as to avoid digoxin toxicity. To allow for decreased renal excretion, note that the percentage of digoxin removed each day varies linearly with creatinine clearance and ranges from 34 percent with normal renal function to 14 percent in anuric patients. Therefore, since normal clearance is 100 liters/24 hours/1.73 m^2, percentage daily loss = 14 + (0.2 × creatinine clearance); and to maintain a steady blood digoxin level the daily maintenance dose should be the product of the percentage daily loss and the digitalizing dose. The digitalizing dose itself should be about three-quarters of the usual dose to allow for diminished renal excretion during the time of digitalization.

This formula needs to be modified in two circumstances. The first is that creatinine clearances may not be known at the time digitalization and maintenance are instituted. To deal with this, note that there is a relationship between serum creatinine concentration and creatinine clearance, and this relationship can be combined with the formula relating percentage daily digoxin loss to creatinine clearance. This gives, in adult men, percentage daily digoxin loss = 11.6 + (20/serum creatinine concentration); in adult women, percentage daily loss = 12.6 + (16/serum creatinine concentration); concentrations are in milligrams per 100 ml.

The second problem is that although in young children the percentage daily digoxin loss is the same as in adults, their serum creatinine concentrations and creatinine clearances vary with age. Normal serum creatinine concentrations average about 0.5 mg/100 ml under 5 years of age and increase by 0.1 mg/100 ml each year of age until about 12 years, after which the value remains constant at 1.2 mg/100 ml. As to creatinine clearances, these are about 80 to 100 liters/24 hours/1.73 m^2 in older children and adults and about half these values in newborn and premature infants. The simplest way of allowing for these variations is to estimate percentage daily digoxin loss = 14 + 20 (normal/observed serum creatinine concentrations). The maintenance dose is again this percentage daily loss times the digitalizing dose.

These formulas merely give crude estimates, since other factors affect digoxin levels, and renal function may alter from day to day. The formulas therefore allow selection of initial maintenance dosages that need to be changed according to clinical response, serum digoxin levels, and changes in renal function. Note that digoxin cannot be removed by peritoneal dialysis or hemodialysis, so that patients on dialysis need about 14 percent of the total digitalizing dose for daily maintenance. Note, too, that since digitoxin is metabolized by the liver and has little renal excretion, its dosage is not affected by changes in renal function; it might be the drug of choice.

Digoxin toxicity is serious and common. It is most often due to overdosage (absolute or because of renal failure), but it may be brought on by hypokalemia (often related to marked diuresis), hypomagnesemia, or intravenous calcium injections. Its main features are due to abnormalities of heart rate, conduction, and rhythm.

Marked bradycardia with exaggerated sinus arrhythmia is due to excessive vagal tone. Vagal tone is also partly responsible for some lengthening of the P-R interval, which is frequent as an effect of digoxin and is not itself a sign of toxicity. If the P-R interval becomes more than 50 percent longer than it was before treatment, digoxin toxicity should be suspected. Further depression of atrioventricular conduction may cause second- or third-degree heart block, which are the most common forms of digitalis-induced arrhythmias in infants and small children.

Increased automaticity is shown by ectopic beats (especially ventricular), paroxysmal supraventricular tachycardia with 2:1 atrioventricular block, accelerated junctional pacemaker with atrioventricular dissociation, ventricular tachycardia, or even ventricular fibrillation.

Noncardiac signs of gastrointestinal or neurologic toxicity are uncommon in children. Vomiting may be a sign of toxicity, but it can also be a nonspecific sign of gastric irritation from congestion or swallowed mucus. If there are no other signs of toxicity, a single episode of vomiting does not warrant stopping medication; several episodes indicate the need for a thorough examination, a check of serum digoxin, potassium, and magnesium levels, and probably withdrawal of the digoxin until proof of the absence of toxicity has been given. Infants often spit up after feeding, and this is not a sign of toxicity.

The treatment of digoxin toxicity involves several steps: (1) Discontinue digoxin promptly. (2) Draw blood for serum digoxin, potassium, and magnesium levels. (3) Place patient on a monitor, and also obtain a full electrocardiogram. (4) If toxicity is not severe and serum potassium is normal, merely wait for the digoxin to be excreted. Usually toxicity disappears in 12 to 24 hours. (5) If there is a low serum potassium level, or a normal potassium level but severe digoxin toxicity, then give intravenous potassium, provided that there is good renal function and no second- or third- degree atrioventricular block that might be made worse or prolonged by potassium. Dilute the potassium to under 80 mEq/liter and give it slowly at rates no greater than 0.3 mEq/kg/hour. *Do not give potassium if there is renal failure, a high serum potassium level, or marked atrioventricular block.* (6) If there are atrioventricular block, tachycardias, or ventricular irritability, give phenytoin (Dilantin) at 1 to 2 mg/kg intravenously over 2 minutes. This can be repeated every 5 to 15 minutes until the disturbance disappears or until 10 doses have been given. Monitor arterial blood pressure with each dose, and stop or slow administration if there is hypotension. (7) Propranolol at 0.05 to 0.20 mg/kg intravenously may be given for ventricular extrasystoles or tachycardia. It should be avoided in asthmatics and if there is atrioventricular block. It may also intensify congestive heart failure and so should be used with caution. (8) If there is a slow ventricular rate because of sinus bradycardia or heart block, atropine (0.01 mg/kg intravenously or subcutaneously) should be given. If the slow rate persists, then a ventricular pacemaker should be inserted transvenously, or if that is not possible, transthoracically. Multiple ventricular ectopic beats that cannot readily be controlled by drugs may be suppressed by atrial pacing at a rate rapid enough to prevent discharge of the ectopic focus.

Catecholamines. Catecholamines are powerful boosters of myocardial contractility, and they may help temporarily to alleviate congestive heart failure until more permanent therapy can be established. These agents can be used in any form of congestive heart failure except those due to obstructive lesions. Isoproterenol is the agent most often used. It is convenient to take one ampule of isoproterenol with 1 mg/5 ml and add it to 250 ml of 5 percent dextrose in water to get a final concentration of 4 µg/ml. This dilute solution should be infused with a constant-rate pump at 0.05 to 0.5 µg/kg/minute, beginning with the smaller dose and increasing it until either a beneficial effect is reached or ectopic beats occur. If there are ectopic beats at the lowest dose, reduce the amount given. Once the desired dose has been achieved, it may be necessary to make up more concentrated solutions to avoid giving too much fluid. Norepinephrine can be used in the same way, the usual effective dose being 0.25 to 1 µg/kg/minute. Dopamine has been used recently, and it has the advantage that it may also increase splanchnic and renal blood flow. It may be started at a dose of 5 µg/kg/minute. It is not useful in infants, but may be used in older children.

Any of these agents should be given, if possible, through a separate intravenous line, for two reasons. One is that the infusion will not have to be discontinued to give other intravenous injections or to take blood. The second and more important reason is that an intravenous injection given through the same tubing may push in a bolus of catecholamine and cause ventricular fibrillation. If only one intravenous line can be inserted and must be used for the catecholamine infusion as well as other injections, the line must be cleared of catecholamine before infusing the second substance. This can be accomplished by withdrawing fluid from the line until pure blood enters the syringe, discarding what has been withdrawn, and then administering what is needed through the line.

Vasodilators. Vasodilators such as sodium nitroprusside have been used to lower systemic vascular resistance, increase cardiac output, and reduce congestive heart failure. They have been useful in adults but have not been evaluated in children.

PULMONARY EDEMA. Massive pulmonary edema, with the chest full of rales and blood-stained foam appearing at the mouth, is a rare but serious emergency. The most important aspects of treatment are the following: (1) Positive-pressure respiration with 100 percent oxygen that not only raises the reduced arterial oxygen saturation but also helps to decrease the passage of fluid from blood to alveoli. (2) Morphine at 0.1 mg/kg subcutaneously or intramuscularly, which can be repeated once in 20 to 30 minutes if the patient is still restless and has no respiratory depression. The drug reduces irritability and may have the pharmacologic effect of decreasing venous return and lowering left atrial pressure. (3) Furosemide (Lasix) at 1 mg/kg intravenously to obtain rapid diuresis. (4) Place tourniquets proximally on three limbs and rotate them every 15 minutes so that no limb has a tourniquet on for more than 45 minutes without relief. The tourniquets should be broad and soft so as not to injure the limb and should be applied tightly enough to obstruct venous drainage but not arterial inflow. Ideally, three blood pressure cuffs maintained at pressures of about 40 mm Hg could be used. These tourniquets pool venous blood in the limbs and thus decrease circulating blood volume. (5) If there is evidence of gross congestion, blood volume may be decreased by removing venous blood at 10 to 20 ml/kg. Before doing this, be sure that there is no anemia; if there is anemia and blood must be removed, be prepared to do a partial exchange transfusion with return of a smaller volume of packed red cells than of blood removed. (6) Begin digitalization. (7) If there is no rapid improvement, give aminophylline at 5 mg/kg intravenously over 3 minutes. *Monitor heart rate and blood pressure, and stop if there is bradycardia or hypotension.* (8) Give a catecholamine infusion (see above) if the other measures have not been successful.

References

MECHANISMS

Braunwald E (ed): The Myocardium : Failure and Infarction. New York, HP Publishing, 1974

Edwards JE: Pathology of the failing heart. Prog Cardiovasc Dis 13:1, 1970

Talner NS: Congestive heart failure in the infant: a functional approach. Pediatr Clin North Am 18:1011, 1971

THERAPY

Loggie JMH, Kleinman LI, van Maanen EF: Renal function and diuretic therapy in infants and children. Part II. Part III. J Pediatr 86:657, 825, 1975

DIGITALIS

Beller GA, Smith TW, Abelmann WH, Haber E, Hood WB Jr: Digitalis intoxication. A prospective clinical study with serum level concentrations. N Engl J Med 284:959, 1971

Bigger JT Jr, Strauss HC: Digitalis toxicity: drug interactions promoting toxicity and the management of toxicity. Semin Drug Treat 2:147, 1972

Boerth RC: Decreased sensitivity of newborn myocardium to the positive inotropic effects of ouabain. In Morselli PL, Garattini S, Sereni F (eds): Basic and Therapeutic Aspects of Perinatal Pharmacology. New York, Raven, 1975

Dungan WT, Doherty JE, Harvey C, Char F, Dalrymple GV: Tritiated digoxin. XVIII. Studies in infants and children. Pediatrics 52:561, 1973.

Hayes CJ, Butler VP, Gersony WM: Serum digoxin studies in infants and children. Pediatrics 52:561, 1973

Krasula RW, Pellegrino PA, Hastreiter AR, Soyka LF: Serum levels of digoxin in infants and children. J Pediatr 81:566, 1972

Larese RJ, Mirkin BL: Kinetics of digoxin absorption and relation of serum levels to cardiac arrhythmias in children. Clin Pharmacol Ther 15:387, 1974

Levine OR, Blumenthal S: Digoxin dosage in premature infants. Pediatrics 29:18, 1962

Rogers MC, Willerson JT, Goldblatt A, Smith TW: Serum digoxin concentrations in the human fetus, neonate and infant. N Engl J Med 287:1010, 1972

Seller RH: The role of magnesium in digitalis toxicity. Am Heart J 82:511, 1971

Smith TW, Haber E: Digitalis. N Engl J Med 289:945, 1010, 1063, 1125, 1973

Wagner JG, Yates JD, Willis PW II, Sakmar E, Stoll RG: Correlation of plasma levels of digoxin in cardiac patients with dose and measures of renal function. Clin Pharmacol Ther 15:291, 1974

SYSTEMIC ARTERIAL HYPERTENSION
JULIEN I. E. HOFFMAN AND PAUL STANGER

Hypertension exists when systemic arterial blood pressure is above normal for age (Table 12). Moderate or severe arterial hypertension in children is uncommon and is usually secondary to a detectable underlying cause that may need treatment. In adults most arterial hypertension has no detectable cause and is termed essential or primary. This form of hypertension is common; there were at least 17 million adults with arterial pressures above 160/90 mm Hg in a 1960-1962 nationwide USA survey. Milder forms of essential hypertension may be common at all ages.

Basic Mechanisms

Blood pressure is the product of cardiac output (CO) and peripheral vascular resistance (PR): BP = CO × PR. An increase in cardiac output or peripheral resistance will therefore raise blood pressure as long as the other variable does not fall. Thus a high cardiac output does not cause hypertension in anemia because peripheral resistance falls, but does raise blood pressure with anxiety in which peripheral resistance does not fall.

TABLE 12. Normal Arterial Blood Pressures at Different Ages*

Age	Systolic		Diastolic	
	50th Percentile (mm Hg)	95th Percentile (mm Hg)	50th Percentile (mm Hg)	95th Percentile (mm Hg)
Birth–6 months	80	110	45	60
3 years	95	112	64	80
5 years	97	115	65	84
10 years	110	130	70	92
15 years	116	138	70	95
Adults	120	140	80	90–95

*Adapted from Londe: Clin Pediatr 5:71, 1966; Moss and Adams: Problems of Blood Pressure in Childhood, Springfield, Ill, Thomas, 1962; Zinner et al: N Engl J Med 284:401, 1971.

An increased cardiac output associated with hypertension may occur in two main ways. It may be due to increased sympathetic stimulation, as in anxiety or as part of the response to exercise. It may also occur when ventricular preload is increased by an increased blood volume which may follow excessive infusion of blood or saline, excessive salt intake, decreased water excretion with renal failure, and mineralocorticoid excess. (p.1644). Note that the increased blood volume of congestive heart failure does not cause hypertension because cardiac output is usually reduced.

An increased peripheral resistance associated with hypertension may occur in several ways.

Arteriolar vasoconstriction is caused by stimulation of alpha-adrenergic receptors. This may follow increased sympathetic nerve activity due to cortical or hypothalamic stimulation, stimulation of the medulla oblongata (area postrema) by angiotensin, or increased baroreceptor reflexes. The receptors may also be stimulated by increases in circulating catecholamines, as in pheochromocytoma and neuroblastoma, or they may have added stimulation by increased local catecholamine activity. Thus glucocorticoid excess increases vascular reactivity by inhibiting catechol-ortho-methyl-transferase which normally breaks down some of the norepinephrine liberated by the vesicles in the nerve endings. On the other hand, angiotensin not only stimulates local norepinephrine synthesis but also increases its release from nerve endings on sympathetic stimulation and inhibits its uptake by the vesicles.

The renin-angiotensin system is one of the major regulators of blood pressure. Renin is an enzyme formed chiefly in the juxta-glomerular apparatus, a group of modified smooth muscle cells in the afferent arteriole at its junction with the glomerulus. Once in the blood, renin acts on an alpha-2-globulin known as plasma renin substrate or angiotensinogen that is produced mainly in the liver. From the substrate renin produces a decapaptide known as angiotensin I that has little effect on blood pressure. However, this peptide is changed by a converting enzyme found mainly in the pulmonary endothelium into an octapeptide, angiotensin II, which is the most powerful pressor substance known. It does not last long in the blood because it is broken down by angiotensinases to a heptapeptide (sometimes termed angiotensin III) that has some pressor activity and then to an inactive hexapeptide.

Renin release from the kidney is stimulated by a fall of blood pressure, a decrease in blood volume, a decrease in filtered sodium load in the kidney or stimulation of beta adrenergic receptors. Thus its production and release increase with standing; dehydration; sympathetic stimulation; the administration of diuretics and hypotensive drugs like diazoxide, nitroprusside and hydralazine; and lesions that produce renal ischemia like renal arterial stenosis or some chronic parenchymal renal diseases. Conversely, renin release is reduced by lying down; an increased blood volume or sodium load; and reduced beta sympathetic stimulation with ganglion blockers, propranolol, reserpine, and drugs like clonidine and alpha methyl dopa. For these reasons, renin levels in plasma are usually low whenever blood volume and blood pressure are raised by primary increases in aldosterone or other mineralocorticoids. Although the level of renin is usually the rate limiting factor in the generation of angiotensin, a marked increase in plasma renin substrate, as may occur in women on contraceptive pills, also has been associated with hypertension.

Once an increased renin has produced more angiotensin II, not only is peripheral resistance raised but there is also increased production of aldosterone by the adrenal cortex. Aldosterone increases sodium reabsorption and thus raises blood volume and blood pressure. This increase in turn decreases renin production, and normally these two substances—renin and aldosterone—play a major role in sodium and water balance and thus in blood pressure regulation.

There are some mechanical factors that may increase peripheral resistance. A coarctation of the aorta (p 1431) causes hypertension in the arms. Then, when there has been hypertension of any cause for several weeks or months, the arterioles develop thicker muscular walls and in some instances the sodium content of the arterial wall rises. The thicker walls by themselves decrease lumen width and so increase peripheral resistance; even if all arteriolar tone is abolished the resistance still will not be as low as in normal vessels. The increased sodium content may make the arterioles more reactive to many stimuli. If the walls are thick and the lumens narrow, a further small decrease in lumen width will produce an exaggerated rise in peripheral resistance because resistance is inversely related to the fourth power of the radius.

There are several vasodilators that are normally produced in the body. These include bradykinin, kallikrein, prostaglandins and certain neutral lipids that are formed in the renal medulla. Decrease in these could raise peripheral resistance, although whether this plays a part in any of the hypertensive syndromes in man has not been established.

Measurement of Blood Pressure

The first time a subject is seen, the blood pressure should be measured in both arms and at least one leg; thereafter measurement in one arm is adequate as long as the pulses all feel equal and there is no radiofemoral delay. To measure pressure in the arm the subject should be resting and relaxed and in a quiet room, either sitting or supine. Place the arm at heart level and apply a cuff firmly to the upper arm so that the brachial artery is in the center of the rubber bag within the cuff. The rubber bag must be wide enough to cover two-thirds of the length of the upper arm and long enough to cover three-fourths of the arm circumference. Feel the brachial pulse and inflate the cuff until the pulse disappears, then deflate the cuff and note the pressure at which the pulse reappears. After about 15 sec reinflate the cuff to about 30 mm Hg above the palpatory systolic pressure, place the stethoscope on the brachial artery, and deflate the cuff at 3 to 5 mm Hg per second. The first Korotkoff sounds indicate the systolic pressure. The sounds become louder, suddenly muffle, and finally disappear; current studies indicate that the point of muffling is a better estimate of diastolic pressure than the point of disappearance, which is occasionally much too low. Repeat the measurements twice to determine variability; often the third pressure is the lowest because the subject is more relaxed. Record the pulse rate with each measurement, because tachycardia increases blood pressure and denotes an unrelaxed state.

Leg pressures are measured with the subject prone so that the stethoscope can be placed on the popliteal artery. The rubber bag should cover two-thirds of the thigh length and three-fourths of its circumference; thus the cuff is usually larger than the arm cuff for that subject.

In infants, blood pressure may be difficult to obtain by this method of auscultation or even by palpation; it can then be measured by ultrasonic (Doppler) devices. If these devices are not available, then flush pressures can be measured even though they have less accuracy. To obtain these, the hand or foot should be vasodilated by placing it in warm water or by rubbing. Then apply a cuff to wrist or ankle, lift the extremity above heart level, and squeeze the hand or foot to drain blood out of the limb. Inflate the cuff above the estimated systolic pressure, deflate it at about 5 mm Hg per second and have another observer indicate when the blanched hand or foot suddenly flushes. The child should be quiet while the test is being done, and the test should be repeated until the end point is clearly defined and the results are consistent. The flush pressure is somewhere between systolic and diastolic arterial pressure and is useful for gauging major deviations from normal and comparing arm and leg pressures when coarctation of the aorta is suspected. For the latter, connecting two cuffs with a **Y** connector and obtaining simultaneous arm and leg measurements is particularly useful.

Effects of Hypertension

Long-standing hypertension produces disability and death by causing congestive heart failure or degenerative vascular diseases of the brain, kidneys, or heart. In adults it is the most common cause of congestive heart failure and is the precursor of almost all cerebral vascular accidents. By causing renal arteriolar damage, it contributes to renal failure, and it is one of the major risk factors in coronary artery disease, especially in women.

Long-term studies indicate that there is no particular level of blood pressure above which complications occur, but rather that each elevation of pressure above the normal mean systolic and diastolic pressures adds to the risk of developing cardiovascular disease. These studies have also shown that a raised systolic pressure is as harmful as a raised diastolic pressure. All these cardiovascular complications are uncommon in children, unless the pressures are extremely high. Nevertheless, since mild hypertension may cause these complications and may begin in childhood, recording the blood pressure and assessing any elevations must be considered an important part of any pediatric examination.

Causes of Hypertension

The approach to diagnosing the cause of hypertension is based on knowing the possible underlying causes, most of which can be diagnosed by history, physical examination, and a few simple tests. Occasionally, more extensive investigations are required.

Hypertension is often wrongly diagnosed due to the use of too small a blood pressure cuff. This error is detected by repeating the measurement with the correct cuff. For some patients, particularly obese patients, there may not be a suitable cuff available, or there may be doubt about the elevated blood pressure reading obtained. When adequacy of cuff size is questioned, a good estimate of systolic blood pressure can be made by placing the cuff around the forearm and measuring systolic pressure in the radial artery by palpation.

Anxiety and tachycardia elevate pressure above its normal resting level. Therefore the subject should be resting and as calm as possible, and a record of the heart rate and the appearance of anxiety should accompany the blood pressure reading. If the pressure is high under these circumstances, repeat it later when the subject is calmer. Some authorities believe that subjects whose pressures rise excessively with stress and anxiety (labile hypertension) are more likely to develop fixed hypertension in later life.

Coarctation of the aorta is readily diagnosed by finding a pressure difference between arms and legs, absent or weak and delayed femoral arterial pulses, and the other typical features of this lesion.

Some children have systolic hypertension associated with a large stroke volume and usually a low diastolic pressure. This may occur with very slow heart rates due to sinus bradycardia or complete heart block. It may also happen when there is a rapid runoff of blood from the aorta, as in a large patent ductus arteriosus or arteriovenous fistula, aortic incompetence, and occasionally thyrotoxicosis. All of these are readily diagnosed by their distinctive physical signs.

Lead poisoning is common in slum areas with old, peeling, leaded paint on the walls. By the time there is hypertension there will also be a history of pica, colic, and constipation. Occasionally there will be features of a peripheral neuropathy or encephalopathy, anemia, or stippled red cells, as well as glycosuria, increased urinary porphyrins, and increased blood or urinary lead concentrations.

Central nervous system disorders may be associated with hypertension. They include lesions causing a raised intracranial pressure, encephalitis, and diencephalic lesions, all of which have clincial features that draw attention to the primary disease. Hypertension is also noted after intracranial surgery.

Hypervolemia and hypernatremia may cause hypertension, usually in patients receiving intravenous therapy, but occasionally in patients with excess mineralocorticoids.

Hypertension may be an incidental finding in a variety of acute disorders, including acute intermittent porphyria, poliomyelitis, Guillain-Barré syndrome, gonadal dysgenesis, familial dysautonomia, mercury toxicity, amphetamine overdose, burns, preeclampsia, Stevens-Johnson syndrome, leukemia, and hypercalcemia. These disorders present with their own specific findings, and the hypertension usually requires no further investigation unless it persists once the primary disorder has been cleared up.

All the above causes of hypertension usually are diagnosed by history, physical examination, and specifically indicated laboratory tests (for example, lead levels, brain scan). Elaborate investigation for the hypertension is usually not indicated. This may also be true for the hypertension due to endocrine or renal disorders, which will be discussed next, but it is in these groups that at times extensive investigations for the cause of the hypertension will be needed.

ENDOCRINE DISORDERS. **Excess Catecholamines.** Tumors such as pheochromocytoma and neuroblastoma produce excess norepinephrine, epinephrine, and sometimes dopamine. Pheochromocytomas may cause paroxysmal or sustained hypertension, sweating, hypermetabolism, hyperglycemia, and glycosuria (p. 1661). About one-third to one-half of patients with neuroblastomas have hypertension, but by this stage the tumors usually present with calcified abdominal or thoracic masses. If needed, urinary catecholamines and their metabolites can be measured, and there is a simple screening test (p. 1661).

Giving large doses of reserpine or α-methyldopa in-travenously may release norepinephrine and cause marked but transient hypertension.

There may be supersensitivity to normally circulating catecholamines. This has occurred when foods containing much tyramine (aged cheeses, pickled herring, some red wines or beers) are taken while the subject is on monoamine oxidase inhibitors for example tranylcypromine (Parnate) or phenelzine sulfate (Nardil). It also occurs if decongestants with sympathomimetic amines are taken by a person being treated with reserpine or α-methyldopa.

Sometimes small children taking decongestants with sympathomimetic amines may have hypertension during the treatment.

Excess Mineralocorticoids. Patients with aldosterone-secreting tumors or hyperplasias of the adrenals may develop hypertension. This is usually associated with hypernatremia, hypokalemia, metabolic alkalosis, increased plasma volume, a low and fixed plasma renin level, and increased aldosterone secretion rates. Serum electrolytes provide a fairly good screening test for this disorder, and they can be followed by measurement of peripheral renin levels after 2 hours in the erect position. Persistent low renin levels then indicate the need for the more time-consuming and expensive measurements of aldosterone concentrations or secretion rates and tests to determine if aldosterone can be suppressed by giving a high salt intake and dexamethasone.

There may be hypertension in some types of adrenogenital syndrome, those due to 11β- and 17α-hydroxylase deficiencies. The former tend to have virilization and hyperkalemia with hyponatremia; the latter often have hypokalemic alkalosis. The hypertension is associated with increased fluid and sodium retention due to overproduction of desoxycorticosterone. There are also hypertensive patients with overproduction of 18 hydroxydesoxycorticosterone.

Hypertension has been described with ingestion of vast amounts of licorice which contains a mineralo corticoid-like substance.

Excess glucocorticoids. These might be given as therapy for various diseases, so that blood pressure should be checked frequently in those on high steroid dosage.

Hypertension occurs in Cushing's syndrome. These patients usually have the typical cushingoid facies, buffalo hump, obesity, striae, hyperglycemia and polycythemia so that routine measurements of 17-ketosteroids in an otherwise asymptomatic hypertensive patient without Cushingoid features are not justified.

Sex Hormones. Girls taking oral contraceptives may develop hypertension, but it is reversible if the agent is stopped. Testosterone administration may also cause blood pressure to rise.

RENAL DISORDERS. Any type of renal parenchymal or vascular disease can cause hypertension. Acute glomerulonephritis usually has oliguria, hematuria with red cell casts, and a history of preceding streptococcal infection. Creatinine and blood urea are raised, while their clearances are decreased (p. 1643). Chronic glomerulonephritis with renal failure is a common cause of hypertension. There may be polyuria or oliguria with urine of low specific gravity containing excess protein and casts, as well as other evidence of chronic renal failure (p. 1268). Pyelonephritis, acute or chronic, may cause hypertension. The diagnosis is simple if there are pyuria and bacteriuria, but it is difficult in the chronic stages (p. 1249). Renal vascular diseases are being reported more commonly in children. There could be a congenital stricture or compression of the renal artery, an arteriovenous fistula, aneurysm, thrombosis, or fibromuscular dysplasia of the renal artery.

ESSENTIAL HYPERTENSION.   By definition, essential hypertension can be diagnosed only when other causes of hypertension are absent. Its specific features will be discussed later.

Approach to Diagnosis

Hypertension in children, as in adults, runs the twin perils of neglect and overinvestigation. While it is important to diagnose the cause of hypertension and treat any significant hypertension, it is equally important to avoid misdiagnosing or mislabeling a patient as hypertensive when in fact the pressures are either normal or merely transiently elevated. Overdiagnosis leads to unnecessary, expensive, and at times risky tests, and false labeling may have serious consequences when the subject applies for a job or for life insurance.

One way of approaching the diagnostic problem is to decide whether the hypertension is mild, moderate, or severe and plan the methods of investigation accordingly. At one end of the scale are those whose pressures are at or just above the 95th percentile values given in Table 12. They deserve a thorough history, including a family history, and physical examination. A routine urinalysis should be done, and serum electrolyte, urea, and creatinine measurements may be made. What is important is that if no abnormalities are revealed at this stage, further intensive investigations are not needed; rather, repeat the blood pressure measurements some weeks later. If it is no higher, merely continue to observe at intervals. Mild hypertension does not need treatment as a matter of urgency, especially in children, and elaborate studies to identify its cause are not warranted.

At the other extreme are those patients with severe hypertension, which is manifested by one or more of the following features: blood pressures that are very high (greater than 180 mm Hg systolic or 110 mm Hg diastolic) or are increasing rapidly; localizing neurologic signs, focal or generalized seizures, marked irritability, isolated facial nerve palsy; blurred vision, severe headaches, papilledema, retinal hemorrhages or exudates, constriction of retinal arteries; severe back or abdominal pain; congestive heart failure, pulmonary edema, left ventricular hypertrophy; decreasing renal function; abdominal or renal masses or bruits. When any of these features is present, the patient should be admitted to hospital at once, and investigations to elucidate the cause should be begun. It may be necessary to reduce the blood pressure to prevent serious complications,

and this is dealt with elsewhere (p 1489).

When the blood pressures are significantly elevated, but not to very high levels, and no other signs of severity are present, then an ordered sequence of investigations should be done. This should include a thorough history, including a family history, a thorough physical examination, with special emphasis on the correct taking of blood pressures in arms and legs, palpation of the abdomen for masses, auscultation of the epigastrium and renal angles for bruits, detection of any of the cardiac lesions referred to previously as well as assessment of left ventricular hypertrophy, and examination of the fundi. Some screening laboratory tests are in order, including urinalysis (looking specifically for specific gravity and formed elements), urine culture, routine blood count, serum electrolytes, urea, and creatinine, and measurement of urinary catecholamines and their metabolites (if pheochromocytoma or neuroblastoma is suspected).

If these tests do not give a diagnosis, then it is likely that there is an endocrine (mineralocorticoid excess) cause or else a renal cause that might well be renovascular disease. These considerations lead to the following procedures:

A flat plate of the abdomen should be taken for renal size or for calcification. This is followed by a rapid-sequence intravenous urogram (that is, one in which films are taken 30 sec and 1, 2, 3, and 5 minutes after injection of the contrast material). If there is unilateral renal artery obstruction, then there will be a delay in excretion on that side, which will show up late. Because of the reduced renal blood flow and glomerular filtration, the contrast material will eventually be more concentrated on the abnormal side, and thus the later films will show up more densely on that side. A decreased clearance on one side may also be shown by the ^{131}I-orthoiodohippurate renogram, in which there is delayed uptake and excretion rate on the abnormal side detected by scanning. More recently, injection of technetium-labeled albumin intravenously has allowed the distribution of the intra-arterial label to the kidneys to be followed, so that any decreased blood supply to one side may be detected.

Plasma renin may be measured before getting out of bed in the morning and again after being erect for 2 hours and perhaps being placed on a low sodium diet; each institution has its own method of doing these tests and its own standards, so that the person making the measurements should be consulted about the details. Aldosterone may also be measured. Finally, renal vein renins may be measured at catheterization, and renal arteriography might be done. Since these are the most invasive and the most expensive steps of the investigation, they should not be done without good cause or before consultation with experts in the field.

Treatment of Hypertension

If the cause cannot be removed, or while awaiting definitive treatment, it may be necessary to lower the blood pressure with drugs. Most information about

TABLE 13. Main Sites of Action of Hypotensive Drugs

Main Site (and Basic Mechanism) of Action	Drugs
Central sympathetic nervous system (depression)	Methyldopa, clonidine, barbiturates
Sympathetic ganglia (blockade)	Trimethaphan camsylate, mecamylamine hydrochloride
Postganglionic adrenergic nerves (depression)	Guanethidine, bretylium, debrisoquin
Adrenergic nerve endings (catecholamine depletion)	Reserpine
α-Adrenergic receptors (blockade)	Phentolamine, phenoxy-benzamine
β-Adrenergic receptors (blockade)	Propranolol
Arteriolar smooth muscle (relaxation)	Hydralazine, diazoxide, diuretics, nitroprusside, minoxidil
Body sodium, extracellular fluid volume (decreased)	Thiazides, furosemide, spironolactone, triamterene

drug therapy comes from studies in adults, but there is no reason to think that there will be major differences in children.

PRINCIPLES OF DRUG THERAPY. Hypotensive drugs may work at one or more levels in the body to lower cardiac output or cause systemic arterial vasodilatation (Table 13). Often the primary action is partly or completely counteracted by compensatory changes; for example, vasodilatation may cause a rise in heart rate and cardiac output that returns pressure to its former value, and this may also happen if a fall in cardiac output causes reflex vasoconstriction. Furthermore, reduction in blood volume with a diuretic usually produces a rise in renin secretion. On the other hand, decreasing renin production and lowering blood pressure may lead to sodium retention, increase in blood volume and thus restoration of blood pressure to its former value. Therefore if blood pressure is not effectively lowered by moderate doses of a drug it is best to add another drug with a different mode of action. Not only does this lower blood pressure more effectively, but the unwanted side effects are minimized by keeping the dose of each drug relatively low. When treating chronically it is important to start on low doses of drugs and increase the dose only after 3 to 7 days. This reduces the chances of incurring severe hypertension or severe side effects.

EMERGENCY TREATMENT. Hypertensive emergencies are those with very high blood pressures or with any of the features discussed on p. 1488. If it is decided that the blood pressure should be lowered rapidly within a few hours, then the following agents are available.

Phentolamine (Regitine) at 0.02 to 0.1 mg/kg intravenously may be given if there is any reason to think that there might be a pheochromocytoma. This agent will reduce blood pressure rapidly if it is due to excess circulating catecholamines, but it will have little or no effect on other causes of hypertension.

Diazoxide (Hyperstat) at 5 mg/kg may be given by rapid intravenous injection without diluting the contents of the vial. This agent may produce direct smooth muscle relaxation within minutes, and it is not likely to lower the blood pressure too much. The effect may last for about 12 hours. The drug has not yet been cleared for use in children by the Federal Drug Administration, although approval is expected.

Hydralazine (Apresoline) at 0.15 mg/kg acts within 10 minutes given intravenously and within 20 to 30 minutes intramuscularly. The maximum effect occurs within about 2 hours, and the dose can be adjusted at 4-to 6-hour intervals, depending on the response. This agent does not usually cause hypotension and does not depend on body position for its action. It may have a disadvantage in producing reflex tachycardia, which may be harmful if there is heart failure.

Reserpine (Serpasil) may be added to the hydralazine at a dose of 0.02 mg/kg intramuscularly. It can be repeated at 4- to 6-hour intervals and increased up to 0.07 mg/kg if necessary. Its main disadvantages are that it takes 2 to 3 hours to act, it may produce nasal congestion that can be dangerous in small infants who are nose breathers, and it can cause somnolence that interferes with the clinical assessment of the patient.

Methyldopa (Aldomet) can be used intravenously at a dose of 10 mg/kg. It takes 1 to 2 hours to act and does produce some sedation, although not as much as reserpine.

If a very rapid fall in blood pressure is needed and is not obtained with the above agents, it is necessary to infuse slowly intravenously either *trimethaphan camsylate* (Arfonad) or *sodium nitroprusside*. The starting doses of these are 50 to 150 μg/kg/minute and 2 to 3 μg/kg/minute, respectively, and the infusion rate or concentration should be raised or lowered as indicated. Both of these will produce very rapid and controllable falls in blood pressure, but they need continuous or frequent monitoring of arterial blood pressure. Since there is considerable venous pooling with these agents, they have marked postural effects and work best if the patient is not completely horizontal. Furthermore, putting the patient erect while the infusion is being given should be done with caution. Sodium nitroprusside is the easier to use of the two drugs; the effect of trimethaphan lags several minutes behind a change in dose so that the correct infusion rate is more difficult to control.

Trimethaphan has the disadvantages of any ganglion blocker of producing paralytic ileus and urinary retention in some patients, and it cannot be used for more than 48 hours without losing effect. Sodium nitroprusside is converted to thiocyanate ions, which can cause toxicity (predominantly neurologic and psychologic changes and gastrointestinal upsets) if allowed to reach concentrations over 12 mg/100 ml blood; with long infusions blood levels must be monitored.

CHRONIC THERAPY. Since therapy of chronic hypertension may need to go on for many years, even for life, it is essential to be sure that therapy is needed and then to commence with simpler forms before going on to more powerful and more complex drug treatment.

Reduction of weight, a prudent diet, and regular exercise may all help in selected people. Salt intake should be restricted, provided it does not impair food intake.

Psychotherapy to help the patient deal with stresses may be of great value. It is possible that biofeedback techniques will become useful.

Sedative drugs like barbiturates or benzodiazepines (Valium) can be very helpful, provided that they are used with usual precautions about excessive sedation and the risk of addiction.

The next addition is to give diuretics, usually thiazides. These have effects in reducing salt and water and thus reducing blood volume, but they may also have some direct effect in lowering pressure. Chlorothiazide (Diuril) at 25 to 50 mg/kg/day or hydrochlorothiazide (Hydrodiuril) at 1 to 2 mg/kg/day can be used and may be all that is needed in mild hypertension. Better diuresis, if needed, may be obtained with oral furosemide 1 to 3 mg/kg/day. These diuretics should be given in divided doses twice daily in order to provide the best hypotensive effect. The second dose of the day should be given relatively early in the evening so that nocturnal diuresis does not inconvenience the patient. For this reason chlorthalidone (0.5-1.5 mg/kg/day) has been advocated since it can be given once daily. These diuretics cause little change in renal blood flow, and furosemide may actually increase it; they can therefore be used when there is moderate renal failure. These drugs act by lowering blood volume and also by decreasing vascular reactivity. When used over long periods they tend to cause potassium depletion, hyperglycemia and hyperuricemia, none of which is usually severe. Potassium loss can be avoided with potassium supplements or by adding either spironolactone (1-2 mg/kg/day) or triamterene (2-4 mg/kg/day) which retain potassium; in fact, the latter two drugs must not be given if there is renal failure to avoid producing hyperpotassemia. Spironolactone is the diuretic of choice when there is marked aldosterone excess and is not effective if aldosterone is low. Triamterene works independently of aldosterone but is not by itself a powerful diuretic.

It is important to note that the hypotensive effects of these diuretics can be overcome if salt intake is high, and there is a tendency for people to increase their salt intake when they take these diuretics. Therefore, they should be advised to avoid salty foods and not to add salt when food is brought to the table. Salt restriction is particularly important in renal hypertension in which sodium excretion is often markedly impaired and in which an increased blood volume is often a major factor in the hypertension.

If diuretics alone do not control hypertension there is a wide choice of drugs that can be added. Whatever else is used, however, should be combined with a diuretic because most of the other agents tend to increase blood volume which thus nullifies their hypotensive effects. There is no set regime for adding drugs and different patients may need different combinations. The main agents in use will be presented briefly.

There are two agents that act predominantly at the central nervous system level to reduce sympathetic outflow. Alpha methyldopa given orally 10-50 mg/kg once daily is often used. In addition to its central action it also replaces norepinephrine in the storage granules of the vesicles and acts as an inefficient neurotransmitter. It has a major disadvantage in males of reducing libido and preventing ejaculation. The other drug is clonidine (Catapres) that has been used extensively in adults but not much in children. It is given 4 times daily for a total dose of 5-25 µg/kg/day. Like alpha methyldopa it lowers peripheral resistence, decreases renin production and does not lower renal blood flow. Because of their central actions both of these drugs produce sedation and drowsiness that may become less troublesome after several weeks of treatment. If the drugs are stopped suddenly there may be sympathetic overactivity and severe rebound hypertension that may limit their use in unreliable patients.

Ganglion blocking agents like trimethaphan camsylate, pentolinium, and mecamylamine act by venous pooling of blood and lowering of cardiac output. They therefore give significant postural hypertension and, being unselective, may cause problems with many organ systems. They are therefore less used now than formerly.

Several drugs affect the formation, storage and release of norepinephrine in the storage granules of the post-ganglionic sympathetic nerve endings. Guanethidine has been used extensively in adults but less often in children. It blocks the release of norepinephrine from nerve endings and may lower their content of norepinephrine; it also has the advantages of not crossing the blood brain barrier and thus not producing sedation and depression and of being given once a day in a dose of 0.15-3 mg/kg. However, it often has severe side effects—postural hypotension, diarrhea and failure of ejaculation—that limit its usefulness. Bethanidine and debrisoquin have similar actions with fewer side effects; they are used in England but not yet released for use in the United States. Reserpine is also a member of this group. It acts primarily by depleting the storage granules of norepinephrine and also has a central effect. In a dose of 0.01 mg/kg/day the drug may be effective in lowering blood pressure but because of the risk of mental depression, nasal congestion, diarrhea, and increases in gastric acidity and renin it has lost favor.

Alpha adrenergic blockers have limited usefulness. Phentolamine (0.02-0.1 mg/kg) is used to test for the possibility of increased circulating catecholamines as the cause of the hypertension, and phenoxybenzamine, which is better for chronic administration, is used to prepare patients with pheochromocytomas for surgery. These agents, too, are used in treating the rebound hypertension due to alpha methyl dopa or clonidine withdrawal. Beta adrenergic blockers like propranolol have been used extensively in Europe and even in the United States, although they have not yet been released for general use by the FDA. They work best in those patients with high renin levels, and may be combined with other agents to prevent reflex tachycardia. The usual dose range is 0.25-1 mg/kg/day given in four divided doses.

Finally, there are drugs that act directly on smooth muscle, the two most often used being hydralazine and minoxidil. Hydralazine given by mouth 4 times daily for a total daily dose of 1.5-3 mg/kg is well tolerated without much postural hypotension. It increases renal blood flow but also increases renin production. In high doses it produces a syndrome that resembles lupus erythematosus. Because the sympathetic nervous system is not depressed by this drug, the hypotension it produces often causes reflex tachycardia that not only tends to raise cardiac output and thus blood pressure but may be unacceptable if patients are in heart failure. Therefore this drug is often combined with those that lower heart rate (clonidine, propranolol, reserpine). Minoxidil, given 4 times daily in a total dose of 0.25-0.5 mg/kg/day has recently been used experimentally and has been very effective. Its effects are similar to those of hydralazine and its major side effect is the production of severe hypertrichosis.

Renovascular Hypertension

Renovascular disease causing hypertension is uncommon in children but it should still be considered seriously in investigating significant hypertension. There may be congenital arterial strictures or renal arteriovenous malformations; compression of the renal artery by masses; renal artery aneurysm or thrombus; fibromuscular dysplasia of the wall; and arteriosclerotic plaques, although these latter are almost all in adults. The site of obstruction may be in the main renal artery or in some of its intrarenal branches. The effect of obstruction from any cause is to decrease total or regional renal blood flow and thus to stimulate renin release.

Stenosis of a renal artery may cause a murmur best heard in the epigastrium. Unilaterally reduced renal flow may cause atrophy on that side, with a discrepancy in renal size on abdominal roentgenograms. The reduced flow is also the basis of the radiolabeled hippurate excretion test and rapid-sequence urogram. Both tests show reduced early clearance of indicator by the abnormal kidney, but some late concentration by the abnormal side because of the reduced glomerular filtra-

tion rate with normal tubular reabsorption on that side. Unfortunately, these tests may be unreliable if there is bilateral renovascular disease.

Once there is strong suspicion that there may be renovascular disease, and if the hypertension is high enough to warrant further investigation, then renal arteriography should be done. In order to show up regions of narrowing, it is essential for the test to be done by experienced radiologists, who will make sure that all the proper views are taken. When a renal arterial obstruction is found, it is essential to prove that it is physiologically significant. Passage of the catheter beyond the stenosis and a recording of a large pressure difference indicates that the obstruction is important, but this cannot always be done. If not, then renin levels should be obtained from both renal veins; if the concentration on one side is two or three times higher than on the other, it is likely that a renal obstruction on that side is significant. There are problems of interpretation of this test, such as allowing for dilution of the renal vein blood with blood from gonads or adrenals and assessing bilateral stenoses. At times, bilateral renal biopsies may be helpful. Nevertheless, the combination of renal size, excretory urograms, renal arteriograms, and renal vein renins will serve to make the diagnosis in about 95 percent of patients.

The treatment of the lesion depends on the degree of hypertension and the type of obstruction. Surgery is required for extrinsic obstructions by masses, but the decision is not as clear for other lesions. Since surgery has some risk to the patient, it should not be done for mild hypertension. If surgery is warranted, it might involve plastic repair of the artery if it is accessible, heminephrectomy if the lesions are confined to one part of the kidney, removal of the kidney and reimplantation in the pelvis to avoid having to reconstruct a difficult ostial stenosis, or occasionally nephrectomy. The decision to do any of these depends on the site, severity, and accessibility of the stenotic lesions, as well as on the size of the patient's vessels. In most children the blood pressure will return to normal after surgery, but this is by no means guaranteed. Nevertheless, with severe hypertension and clear-cut evidence of renal artery obstruction and renal ischemia, surgery is usually indicated.

Essential Hypertension

Typically, essential hypertension is a disorder that is recognized in the third decade and progresses slowly over many years. Recent studies emphasize not only the strong familial incidence of essential hypertension but also that young children of hypertensive parents have pressures that are at the upper limits of normal. In some instances these children's pressures remain at the upper limits of normal and rise with age, and it might be these people who in the third decade have pressures recognized as being above a threshold level and thus are diagnosed as having essential hypertension. If this is true, it indicates that children whose pressures are at or above the 95th percentile may indeed have early pathology and that statistical normality and physiologic normality must be dissociated.

Whether the cause of essential hypertension is genetic or environmental or a mixture of both is still not known, and in fact we do not know if this is a single disease or merely a syndrome common to many different diseases. Laragh and his colleagues have shown that adults with essential hypertension have a variety of combinations of high, normal, and low renin and aldosterone concentrations, so that they are different physiologically even if not etiologically. Similar studies have not yet been reported in children.

Essential hypertension is diagnosed on the basis of a family history and the exclusion of other causes of hypertension. In adults there is some evidence that lowering blood pressure by various means can reduce the cardiovascular complications of hypertension, even if it is fairly mild. However, probably no one would use medications to treat children with mild essential hypertension, since the long-term effects of the available drugs are not known. Probably the wisest course would be use of preventive measures like eliminating causes of stress, avoiding obesity and smoking, taking regular exercise, and eating a prudent diet. Medications should, however, be used if blood pressure is high or if there are signs that it is causing damage.

References

GENERAL

Biglieri EG, Stockigt JR, Schambelan M: Adrenal mineralocorticoid hormones causing hypertension. In Laragh JH (ed): Hypertensive Manual: Mechanisms, Methods and Management. New York, Yorke, 1974

Burton AC: The criterion for diastolic pressure—revolution and counter revolution. Circulation 36:805, 1967

Frohlich ED, Tarazi RC, Dustan HP: Re-examination of the hemodynamics of hypertension. Am J Med Sci 257:9, 1969

Guyton AC, Coleman TG, Fourcade JC, Navar LG: Physiologic control of arterial pressure. Bull NY Acad Med 45:811, 1969

Hypertension and hypertensive heart disease in adults: United States 1960–1962 (data from the National Health Survey). Public Health Service Publication 1000, Series 11-13. Washington, DC, USPHS, 1966

Kannel WB, Castelli WP, McNamara PM, Sorbie P: Some factors affecting morbidity and mortality in hypertension. Milbank Mem Fund Q 47:116, 1969

Laragh JH, Baer L, Brunner HK, et al: Renin, angiotensin, and aldosterone system in pathogenesis and management of hypertensive vascular disease. Am J Med 52:633, 1972

Lieberman E: Essential hypertension in children and youth: a pediatric perspective. J Pediatr 85:1, 1974

Loggie JMH: Hypertension in children and adolescents. 1. Causes and diagnostic studies. J Pediatr 74:331, 1966

Londe S: Blood pressure in children as determined under office conditions. Clin Pediatr 5:71, 1966

McLaughlin GW, Kirley RR, Kemmerer WT, de Lemos RA: Indirect measurement of blood pressure in infants using Doppler ultrasound. J Pediatr 79:300, 1971

Moss AJ, Adams FH Jr: Problems of Blood Pressure in Childhood. Springfield, Ill, Charles C Thomas, 1962

——— Adams FH Jr: Index of indirect estimation of diastolic blood pressure. Muffling versus complete cessation of vascular sounds. Am J Dis Child 106:364, 1963

Page I: The mosaic theory of arterial hypertension—its interpretation. Perspect Biol Med 10:326, 1967

Paul O, Ostfeld AM: Epidemiology of hypertension. Prog Cardiovasc Dis 8:106, 1965

Sokolow M, Werdergar D, Kam HK, Hinman AT: Relationship between level of blood pressure measured casually and by portable recorders and severity of complications in essential hypertension. Circulation 34:279, 1966

Stockigt JR, Collins RD, Noakes CA, Schambelan M, Biglieri EG: Renal vein renin in various forms of hypertension. Lancet 1:1194, 1972

Tarazi RC, Dustan HP: Plasma volume and chronic hypertension. Relationship to arterial pressure levels in different hypertensive diseases. Arch Intern Med 125:835, 1970

Zinner SH, Levy PS, Kass EH: Familial aggregation of blood pressure in childhood. N Engl J Med 284:401, 1971

RENOVASCULAR

Coran AG, Schuster SR: Renovascular hypertension in childhood. Surgery 64:672, 1968

Gifford RW Jr, Poutasse EH: Renal vascular hypertension: diagnosis and treatment. Prog Cardiovasc Dis 8:141, 1965

Sinaiko A, Najarian J, Michael AF, Mirkin BL: Renal autotransplantation in the treatment of bilateral renal artery stenosis: relief of hypertension in an 8 year old boy. J Pediatr 82:409, 1973

TREATMENT

Bourne HR, Melmon K: Guides to the pharmacologic management of essential hypertension. Pharmacology for Physicians, 5:1, 1971

Frolich ED: Hypertension 1973: treatment—why and how. Ann Intern Med 78:717, 1973

Koch-Weser J: Hypertensive emergencies. N Engl J Med 290:211, 1974

Majid PA, Meeran MK, Benaim ME, Sharma B, Taylor SH: Alpha- and beta-adrenergic receptor blockade in the treatment of hypertension. Br Heart J 36:588, 1974

Pettinger WA, Mitchell HC: Minoxidil—an alternative to nephrectomy for refractory hypertension. N Engl J Med 289:167, 1973

Taguchi J, Freis ED: Partial reduction of blood pressure and prevention of complications in hypertension. N Engl J Med 291:329, 1974

Zacest R, Gilmane E, Koch-Weser J: Treatment of essential hypertension with combined vasodilatation and beta-adrenergic blockade. N Engl J Med 286:617, 1972

ATHEROSCLEROSIS

JULIEN I.E. HOFFMAN

Atherosclerosis is a fibrofatty degeneration of the intima and media of vessels, especially arteries. As a result of these changes, arteries are narrowed and blood supply to organs is reduced; secondary thrombosis may further reduce flow. While any organ can be affected, the major changes occur in the aorta and the coronary, cerebral, iliac, and femoral arteries. In the United States coronary atherosclerosis and cerebral vascular disease account for about 30 percent and 12 percent, respectively, of all deaths; they are major causes of disability and death in middle-aged and even young adults. Since almost all coronary arterial disease and much cerebral vascular disease is atherosclerotic, it is clear that atherosclerosis is a major cause of death and disability in the United States; in fact, this is true of all Western industrialized countries. While the manifestations of atherosclerosis usually occur after childhood, there is much evidence to suggest that the atherosclerotic process starts in childhood or that habits acquired in childhood predispose to the development of atherosclerosis in later life.

Of the two main types of atherosclerosis, that in cerebral arteries is predominantly due to hypertension, and it may be common in communities where coronary arterial disease is rare. Hypertension has been discussed (p. 1484), and the remainder of this section will concentrate on coronary arterial disease.

ANATOMY AND PATHOLOGY. In the fetus the coronary arteries have a very thin intima, a thick internal elastic lamina, and a media with delicate smooth muscle and a few elastic fibers. Just after birth the intima thickens, the internal elastic lamina fragments, smooth muscle cells in longitudinal bundles appear between the fragments, and eventually a patchy musculoelastic layer forms between the intima and the media. Fibroblasts proliferate in the intima, and by 6 months there is diffuse fibrous thickening of the intima. These changes may vary in degree for genetic reasons; for example, in Israel the intimal thickening of infancy is more marked in Ashkenazi Jews than in Yemenite Jews or Bedouin. With normal aging, smooth muscle cells and extracellular matrix gradually increase within the intima.

Beyond infancy, the earliest focal lesions are fatty streaks: thin, yellow, slightly raised streaks due to accumulation of fatty droplets inside intimal cells (foam cells). These fatty streaks appear in the aorta in the first decade and in the coronary arteries at the end of the second decade, but their role as precursors of atherosclerotic plaques is uncertain, because they are found in equal numbers in countries with high and low incidences of coronary arterial disease. Definite atherosclerotic lesions include the fibrous plaques, which are raised white lesions due to focal accumulation of intimal, lipid-containing smooth muscle cells. Later these plaques contain much collagen, and they form a cap covering a deeper deposit of extracellular lipid and cellular debris. Still later in some people there may be calcification, cell necrosis, or hemorrhage into the plaque. The plaques are eccentrically placed in the wall and are almost always confined to the extramural coronary arteries.

PATHOGENESIS. The atherosclerotic plaque is a nonspecific response to arterial injury. The growth of smooth muscle in the intima probably comes from muscle that migrates from the media; this has been shown in monkeys after endothelial damage has been produced. The mechanism may be stimulation of muscle migration and division by plasma proteins and lipoproteins that leak into the intima; it is of interest that muscle growth is more marked when the monkeys are hypercholesterolemic. Plasma lipoproteins, like many substances, can diffuse into the arterial wall. The very low density (prebeta) and low-density (beta) lipoproteins contain a protein (apoprotein B) that reacts with a mucopolysaccharide (dermatan sulfate) in the arterial wall, so that the lipoprotein does not pass readily into the lymph or back into the blood. The lipoprotein complexed with mucopolysaccharide appears to be degraded in situ. These intimal smooth muscle cells produce collagen and elastic fibers and also take up or metabolize cholesterol. The increased lipid in the plaques is mainly cholesterol or its esters, and it may be

produced locally and not be adequately regulated or removed, or else it may enter from the blood; the last of these is probably the major mechanism. Endothelial injury also encourages microthrombi, which may be incorporated into the intima and eventually form typical plaques.

ETIOLOGY. Any explanation for coronary atherosclerosis should account for its varied features, including the rapid increase in prevalence of coronary arterial disease in this century in industrialized Western countries without a comparable increase in fat intake, the rapid but temporary decrease in its prevalence in Europe during World War II, the lesser incidence in women under 55 years of age, the risk factors that have been established, and on the other hand, the fact that about 20 percent of people with clinical coronary arterial disease have none of the known risk factors, although even these have higher blood lipid levels than are found in underdeveloped countries.

The main risk factors are smoking, hypertension, and hyperlipidemia; with very low lipid levels the other risk factors are not of great importance. Inadequate exercise, mental stress, diabetes mellitus, and consumption of soft water are other associations that might be important. Many of these factors are common to affluent industrial societies. The move from manual labor in the country to sedentary work behind a city desk has increased mental stress and decreased the amount of heavy exercise. A better standard of living has caused increased consumption of expensive animal fats and refined carbohydrates, leading to obesity and hyperlipoproteinemia. Finally, treating water to make it soft is again a modern refinement.

There is a strong familial association with coronary arterial disease that may come about for many reasons. Basic intimal thickness may be genetically determined, as found in the studies in Israel, and this could make arterial occlusion easier in some people than in others. Some families have genetically inherited hyperlipoproteinemias that account for some coronary atherosclerosis and especially for some premature coronary disease, although these do not account for the majority of cases. Diabetics have more coronary arterial disease, as do hypertensives, so that again a strong familial association would be expected. Finally, families tend to share common environments that may be factors in causing coronary arterial disease.

PREVENTION. Without knowing the specific causes of the disease, we cannot institute definite programs for preventing it. Nevertheless, enough is known about some of the major risk factors to allow us to make recommendations that are likely to reduce the prevalence of coronary arterial disease greatly.

Because of the strong familial association, a pediatric history should include questions about diabetes mellitus, hypertension and coronary arterial disease, sudden death, xanthomata, or raised blood cholesterol levels in parents or close relatives. Any positive responses indicate the need for careful assessment of factors that could promote coronary atherosclerosis.

Physical exercise should be encouraged; it is important for many other reasons as well. Isometric exercises are not adequate for prevention of coronary atherosclerosis. On the other hand, there is evidence that 20 to 30 minutes of strenuous exercise two to three times a week may have as much protective effect against coronary atherosclerosis as more intensive exercise regimes.

Smoking should be discouraged, especially cigarettes. Not only will this markedly decrease the risk of getting premature coronary arterial disease, but it should also decrease the risk of getting pulmonary emphysema and carcinoma of the lung.

There should be an attempt to modify life styles to reduce the tensions of daily living. Clearly this is more easily said than done, but there is no reason not to attempt it.

The major controversy today centers around the importance of hyperlipidemia and the need to modify diet in a major fashion. Reduction of cholesterol and saturated fats in the diet is suggested by the close association of high blood cholesterol and triglyceride levels with an increased incidence of premature coronary arterial disease, both in individuals and in communities. This is particularly true of those with genetic hyperlipidemias, and in these individuals lowering of blood cholesterol may cause disappearance of xanthomas and even a decrease in intermittent claudication. Finally, there is the excess cholesterol in the atherosclerotic plaques, experimental evidence of greater plaque formation in hypercholesterolemic monkeys, and some suggestion that dietary lowering of cholesterol can reverse atherosclerotic lesions in animals.

Before going to major revisions of the usual diet, it is important to remember that the requirements for cholesterol and fatty acids in growing human children have not been fully worked out, that some of the correlations with coronary arterial disease suggest that the association with high blood lipids may be complex, and that dietary modifications may be expensive and not as a rule well accepted by people unless they clearly relieve some acute distress. Because of these uncertainties, it is worth attending to all the other preventive measures and then recommending dietary changes for select groups. These are, first of all, those with genetic hyperlipidemias, and secondly those with a family history of premature coronary or peripheral arterial disease, xanthomas, or high blood cholesterol levels. Whether dietary changes should be made in otherwise healthy children with no family history of coronary arterial disease is not yet known, and authorities differ on their recommendations. However, a prudent diet that does not impose excessive restrictions can be safely recommended to anyone.

The decision to alter diet to reduce cholesterol levels is made more difficult because we do not know what a normal value is. In the United States and in England, cord blood has serum cholesterol concentrations of 70 to 80 mg/100 ml, with a standard deviation of about 20 mg/100 ml. By 4 months of age the mean values vary from 110 to 175 mg/100 ml in different series, being highest in breast-fed babies. From 1 year to 14 years of age, serum cholesterol is independent of age and has mean values in different series of 161 to 182 mg/100 ml, with a standard deviation of about 35 mg/100 ml. There are also normal values for various lipoprotein fractions (Table 14). These are the normal values in Western societies, but in rural Mexico the total blood cholesterol between the ages of 5 and 14 years was 100 mg/100 ml, with only 4 per cent of the children having levels over 140 mg/100 ml. It is possible, but not proven, that the higher values in our society are associated with greater predisposition to premature coronary arterial disease.

If because of a high serum cholesterol or a bad family history dietary changes are needed, they should be made only after several determinations of serum lipids have been made to determine if the levels are constant and what the baseline values are. Because of variability of diet and growth needs in infancy and early childhood, there is seldom any purpose to modifying diet for patients under 5 years of age, at which time myelination is almost complete. After that a prudent diet should be given, unless the combination of a genetic hyperlipidemia with very high serum lipid levels makes more energetic measures necessary. The total calorie intake should be adjusted so that there is a normal but not excessive weight gain, and it is essential to emphasize to parents that an overweight baby is not a healthy one. To decrease cholesterol the number of eggs in the diet should be reduced, and organ meats and fatty meats should be avoided. Skim milk and margarine should be substituted for whole milk and butter, and intake of whole-milk cheeses should be reduced (cottage cheese is a good source of protein with little fat or cholesterol). Such dietary changes are probably best and most easily made for the whole family, to whom the importance of the changes should be repeatedly explained. With a bad family history of premature coronary arterial disease it is possible to get cooperation from the family, although continued reinforcement will be necessary. Once again, whether these changes should be made in people not at such high risk is not known at the present time.

If hyperlipoproteinemia does not respond to dietary changes and is severe enough to warrant added drug therapy, several drugs are available, although none is ideal. It is essential to define the type of hyperlipoproteinemia (p.734), because the drugs have specific actions. Thus clofibrate (Atromid) at a dosage of 1 to 2 g daily lowers the VLDL component of lipoproteins and thus is most effective in types III, IV, V, and perhaps IIb; it is therefore not often needed in children. It may increase the LDL fraction, so that serial measurements of various lipoprotein factors must be made. For type II abnormalities, cholestyramine resin given at a dosage of 250 to 800 mg/kg/day to heterozygotes and 0.5 to 1.5 g/kg/day to homozygotes has been useful, as has Colestipol; FDA approval for their use must be obtained. An alternative drug is p-aminosalicylic acid at 150 mg/kg/day. Nicotinic acid at 25 to 75 mg/kg/day and dextrothyroxine have also been used. Most of these drugs have significant side effects, and patient compliance tends to fall off with time. Therapy should therefore not be given without good cause; if it is given, the

TABLE 14. Suggested Normal Limits of Plasma Lipid and Lipoprotein Cholesterol Concentrations*

Age (years)	Total Cholesterol (mg/100 ml)	Triglyceride (mg/100 ml)	LDL Cholesterol (mg/100 ml)	HDL Cholesterol (mg/100 ml)
Birth (cord blood)	50–95	10–65	20–45	30–55
1–19	120–230	10–140	50–170	30–65 (boys) 30–70 (girls)

From Levy and Rifkind: Am J Cardiol 31:547, 1973.

patients should be seen frequently and given much encouragement. Treatment of hypertension is important, although, as pointed out (see p. 1490), this is seldom warranted in the pediatric age group.

References

Darmady JM, Fosbrooke AS, Lloyd JK: Prospective study of serum cholesterol levels during first year of life. Br Med J 2:685, 1972

Fomon SJ: Infant Nutrition. Philadelphia, WB Saunders, 1974

Glueck CJ, Fallat RW, Tsang R: Hypercholesterolemia and hypertriglyceridemia in children. Am J Dis Child 12:569, 1974

Golubjatnikov R, Paskey T, Inhorn SL: Serum cholesterol levels of Mexican and Wisconsin school children. Am J Epidemial 96:36, 1972.

Lverius PH: The interaction between human plasma lipoproteins and connective tissue glycosaminoglycans. J Biol Chem 247:2607, 1972.

Kannel WB, Dawber TR: Atherosclerosis as a pediatric problem. J Pediatr 80:544, 1972

Kwiterovich PO Jr, Levy RI, Frederickson DS: Neonatal diagnosis of familial type-11 hyperlipoproteinemia. Lancet 1:118, 1973

Lauer RM, Connor WE, Leaverton PE, Reiter MA, Clarke WR: Coronary heart disease risk factors in school children: the Muscatine study. J Pediatr 86:697, 1975

Levy RI, Rifkind BM: Diagnosis and management of hyperlipoproteinemia in infants and children. Am J Cardiol 31:547, 1973

Mishkel MA: Neonatal plasma lipids as measured in cord blood. Can Med Assoc J 111:775, 1974

Mitchell SC, Blount SG Jr, Blumenthal S, Jesse Mj, Weidman WH: The pediatrician and atherosclerosis. Pediatrics 49:165, 1972

Owen GM, Kram KM, Garry PJ, Lowe JE Jr, Lubin AH: A study of nutritional status of preschool children in the United States, 1968–1970. Pediatrics 53:597, 1974

Ross R, Glomset JG: Atherosclerosis and the arterial smooth muscle cell: proliferation of smooth muscle is a key event in the genesis of the lesions of atherosclerosis. Science 180:1332, 1973

Slack J: Ischaemic heart-disease and familial hyperlipoproteinemia. Lancet 2:1380, 1969

Strong JP, McGill HCJ: The pediatric aspects of atherosclerosis. J Atheroscler 9:251, 1969

COMMON MANAGEMENT PROBLEMS

PAUL STANGER AND JULIEN I.E. HOFFMAN

Once heart disease has been diagnosed, day-to-day management is needed for the many minor problems and questions that arise. This is true not only of the common minor heart lesions but also of those major lesions that have had surgery or will need surgery in the future.

EFFECTS OF ALTITUDE. With increasing height above sea level the atmospheric oxygen tension falls, and therefore so does the alveolar oxygen tension and the oxygen tension and saturation of pulmonary venous blood (Table 15). Up to 3,000 feet there is no noticeable effect on oxygenation of blood in the lungs, at 5,000 feet saturation falls slightly, and above 8,000 feet there is a substantial fall in pulmonary venous oxygen saturation. Therefore patients with cyanotic heart disease should probably live at altitudes below 5,000 feet so that there will be no further compromise of oxygen delivery to the body. Whether they should be allowed to go temporarily to high altitudes (for example, when the family goes skiing) depends mainly on the severity of their disease. Those who are tolerating their lesion well should be allowed to try the higher altitudes, but they should be warned to return to lower altitudes quickly if they become at all distressed. An exception to this is children with the tetralogy of Fallot, who are at risk of having hypoxemic spells; they should avoid high altitudes until after surgical treatment to increase pulmonary blood flow. Any patient with significant pulmonary hypertension due to pulmonary vascular disease should avoid altitudes over 3000 feet, especially if the patient is actively exercising, because the reduced al-

TABLE 15. Effects of Altitude

Atmosphere			Alveolar Oxygen Tension (torr)*		Pulmonary Venous Oxygen Saturation (%)	
Altitude (feet)	Total Pressure (torr)	Oxygen Tension (torr)	Acute	Acclimatized	Acute	Acclimatized
0	760	159	110	110	98	98
3000	681	143	92	89	94	95
5000	632	132	78	82	93	94
8000	565	118	66	68	89	90
11000	503	105	54	60	80	86
14000	446	93	44	52	70	80

The alveolar values are approximate, since they depend on metabolism, ventilation, and the alveolar–arterial oxygen difference. With acclimatization and chronic hyperventilation, the alveolar oxygen rises.

veolar oxygen tension may increase pulmonary vaso-constriction. However, patients with large left-to-right shunts usually have no difficulty at high altitudes, and in fact any pulmonary vasoconstriction that altitude causes will reduce the left-to-right shunt and produce some mild improvement. It has been noted that children with large ventricular septal defects seldom have pulmonary flows as large in Denver (5,200 feet above sea level) as at sea level.

Similar considerations apply to flying in commercial aircraft. These are pressurized to the equivalent of 7,000 to 8,000 feet above sea level, which could be hazardous for children who are deeply cyanotic. All commercial aircraft are required to have a supply of oxygen, and this can be made available to the patient. However, the airlines will not take responsibility for the patient and will at times request approval of the flight by the patient's physician before permitting it. It is important to note that signs of distress during flight may not be cardiac in origin. Distress, especially during descent, may be the result of aerotitis; this can be avoided by having the infant feed and swallow during ascent and descent and also by not flying during or just after an upper respiratory tract infection.

CEREBRAL COMPLICATIONS. Patients with cyanotic heart disease are at risk of developing cerebral vascular accidents or brain abscesses; the former is most common under 2 years of age, and the latter is rare under 18 months of age. Each of these complications occurs more often with greater arterial desaturation and more cyanosis. Thrombosis usually presents rapidly, with seizures or paralysis, usually a hemiparesis; brain abscess has a more insidious onset marked by headaches, low-grade fever, personality changes vomiting, and occasionally seizures or paralysis.

Cerebral thrombosis may occur in two settings. When the hematocrit is over 65 the blood becomes very viscous and is more likely to clot. However, cerebral thromboses may be even more frequent in very cyanotic children who have relatively low hematocrits. These children have marked arterial desaturation, but because of iron deficiency they have an inappropriately low hematocrit that may be only about 45 to 55. Their tendency to have cerebral vascular accidents may be ascribed to one of two causes: iron deficiency may damage endothelial cells, or the hypoxemia may damage brain tissue, causing edema and thus slowing flow. It is therefore important in any cyanotic child to check repeatedly at least the hematocrit and hemoglobin. If their ratio is greater than 3:1, then the red cell count and the appearance of the red cells on a smear should be checked so that iron deficiency can be detected and treated. Should the hematocrit rise to very high levels (and this sometimes follows iron therapy), then that is itself an indication for surgery. If this cannot be done, the hematocrit should be reduced by periodic removal of whole blood; if the volume removed is large, it should be replaced with an equal amount of albumin solution. Reduction of the hematocrit to about 60 to 65 not only may reduce the risk of thrombosis but will also increases the oxygen

delivery to tissues by lowering blood viscosity. Before removing red cells, however, it is essential to exclude relative iron deficiency.

Cerebral vascular accidents can occur spontaneously, but they are more likely if oxygen requirements are raised by fever or if blood viscosity is increased further by dehydration due to vomiting and/or diarrhea. Therefore in cyanotic patients these ailments need prompt treatment. Another precaution required in the adolescent cyanotic girl is to avoid the use of oral steroid contraceptives, since these have been associated with an increased incidence of cerebral thromboses.

FEBRILE ILLNESSES. It is a rare child who does not have febrile illnesses, and children with heart disease are no different from others in this respect. However, if the child has heart disease, there are more than the usual number of things to think about. If the child has cyanotic heart disease, then the possibility of a high fever causing cerebral thrombosis must be considered, as well as the possibility that the fever is due to a brain abscess. In a child with a large left-to-right shunt, the chest should be carefully examined both clinically and by roentgenography, since these children have an increased incidence of pneumonitis. Furthermore, congestive heart failure may be precipitated or made worse by a fever of any origin because of the increased oxygen requirements that ensue. These children may need increased medications or even hospitalization at these times. If the child has had recent cardiac surgery, the postpericardiotomy syndrome (p 1477) and the post-pump syndrome due to infection with cytomegalovirus must be considered.

All febrile children known to have heart disease must be assessed carefully to exclude infective endocarditis (p 1469). However, it is important not to start treatment for infective endocarditis without good cause, otherwise almost all children with heart disease will be treated unnecessarily for what will usually prove to be an intercurrent infection. In general, infective endocarditis does not present with sudden onset of fever. Therefore a child who has heart disease and is seen at the onset of an acute febrile illness is likely to have one of the common causes of fever and should be investigated and treated like any child of the same age. The use of antibiotics without a specific diagnosis, just because the child has a heart lesion, is unwarranted.

There is often confusion about the need for and timing of blood cultures in these children. In some febrile children, blood cultures should be obtained very early, but this should be based on the patient's age, the severity of the illness, and its specific signs and symptoms, and not on whether there is an associated cardiac lesion. If the fever persists without obvious cause for more than 1 to 3 days, it is then advisable to obtain blood cultures to exclude infective endocarditis (p 1469). Under some circumstances, however, blood cultures should be taken at the onset of fever. Stenotic or bicuspid aortic valves are common sites of infective endocarditis; valve destruction by infection may be early and devastating, and systemic embolization from an infected aortic valve is common. Therefore blood cultures should be taken early if a patient with a known aortic valve lesion becomes febrile. Prompt action is also needed if a patient has had a valve replaced with a prosthetic, heterograft, or homograft valve, because once an infection becomes established on foreign material it may be impossible to cure with antibiotics.

ANTIBIOTIC PROPHYLAXIS. It is important to insist that prophylaxis be given against infective endocarditis, especially at times of dental treatment. In general, oral penicillin prophylaxis is more likely to be accepted than injections (p 1471). The dental treatment to be covered includes extractions, scaling and cleaning of the teeth by a dental hygienist, and most drilling to prepare cavities for filling. In addition, fitting of braces and major readjustments to braces require penicillin prophylaxis. However, the frequent minor readjustments that are made should probably not be accompanied by penicillin, because then there would be the risk of colonizing the mouth with penicillin-resistant organisms. For these reasons, too, the decision to start orthodontic treatment in children with heart disease should be made carefully, and minor unimportant orthodontic procedures should probably be avoided. However, corrective procedures in children may reduce the amount of dental care needed later and thus reduce the risk of infective endocarditis then. Decisions must be individualized; a child may be more handicapped by having buckteeth than by having mild pulmonic stenosis. Other oral procedures, such as tonsillectomy, or oral trauma also require prophylaxis, as does gastrointestinal or urinary tract surgery (p 1471).

Children who have had rheumatic fever should take penicillin prophylaxis for many years (p. 387) to prevent recurrences and cardiac damage. Either intramuscular Bicillin once monthly or daily oral penicillin can be used. The intramuscular injection ensures that the agent is given, whereas individual oral doses can be forgotten; but it is uncomfortable and may cause reactions. An even greater difficulty is persuading people who feel entirely well to take medication for several years. They therefore need frequent assurances of the importance of the prophylaxis, and it must be emphasized that this implies prevention, not that they are ill.

EXERCISE RESTRICTIONS. Exercise increases oxygen consumption, cardiac output, heart rate, and systemic blood pressure and thus increases cardiac work. This by itself is no reason to restrict children with most types of heart disease. In the first place, most children with cyanotic heart disease or left-to-right shunts will restrict themselves because they become dyspneic with fatigue or effort, and there is no reason to think that they come to any harm as a result. The decision to restrict exercise is more difficult when patients have obstructive lesions: aortic or pulmonic stenosis, coarctation of the aorta, or systemic or pulmonic hypertension. If the stenosis is severe it will probably come to early surgery and may no longer be a problem; however, the vascular lesions or milder stenotic lesions are more difficult to manage, because with exercise there

may be no symptoms despite potentially dangerous and damaging levels of pressure. Management is difficult and is best left to the cardiologist. The following are some of the considerations.

In all but the mildest of obstructive lesions, exhausting exercise should be avoided. This includes competitive sports and team sports in which the children may feel obliged to play as hard as possible and may forget their restrictions. In patients with mild or moderate obstructive lesions examining the effects of different levels of exercise of the circulation may prove useful. Thus an exercise study in patients with moderate systemic hypertension or mild coarctation of the aorta (usually post surgery) will allow determination of arm blood pressures and any electrocardiographic changes that ensue. At normal cardiac outputs, the arm pressures may not be high, but with an exercise-induced increase in cardiac output significant hypertension may develop. If there is no excessive hypertension nor ischemic S-T changes with exercise, then normal exercise may probably be allowed safely; competitive sports should still be avoided. With aortic stenosis the electrocardiogram is a useful but not infallible guide to how much can be done. If there are any ischemic S-T changes at any exercise level, that patient should probably undergo surgery; however, normal electrocardiographic patterns do not completely exclude subtle ischemic damage, so that it is probably always wise to avoid severe exercise with this lesion.

Pulmonic stenosis is more difficult to evaluate. If it is mild there will probably be no electrocardiographic changes with exercise. The only guide is to measure the right ventricular pressures during exercise at cardiac catheterization; presumably, if after this there is no indication for surgery, then strenuous, noncompetitive exercise can be permitted.

If there is severe pulmonary hypertension without a communication between the two circulations (primary pulmonary hypertension or residual severe pulmonary vascular disease after closure of a ventricular septal defect or a ductus arteriosus), then all levels of exercise should be avoided. An increase in cardiac output will produce severe right ventricular hypertension and can cause acute right ventricular failure and death.

Exercise restriction may be needed in some children who have had their lesions repaired surgically. Those with obstructive lesions have already been discussed. Some of those who have had ventriculotomies, especially for repairs of a tetralogy of Fallot, have been shown to have bursts of ventricular tachycardia with exercise, and since these could give rise to ventricular fibrillation, it is advisable to evaluate the electrocardiographic responses to exercise before deciding how much exercise can be allowed.

Resumption of normal activity after cardiac surgery can take place when the patient feels well enough. As a rule the incisions in the chest wall, vessels, or heart are well healed after about 2 to 4 weeks, and the child can return to school then. However, a median sternotomy may take about 2 months for firm union, so that vigorous exercise or activity that could lead to bumping the chest, such as falling off a bicycle, should be avoided for at least 2 months. After certain procedures (for example, correction of a tetralogy of Fallot or the Fontan procedure for tricuspid atresia) patients may have moderate congestive heart failure for some months. For a while after such procedures their activity should be restricted.

If a child has acute rheumatic fever but no clinical carditis, normal activity can be resumed once the pain and fever have disappeared, usually after 5 to 7 days. If there is mild carditis as manifested by a soft mitral or aortic murmur, then a longer period of bed rest is needed, at least 10 to 15 days, in order to ensure that there is no progressive deterioration. It is pointless to wait for the murmur to disappear, since it may never do so. In both these groups, too, the erythrocyte sedimentation rate is not a good guide to the course of the illness; the rate may in some people remain high until the patient gets up, and only then may the rate fall. On the other hand, if there is severe carditis as shown by marked cardiomegaly or congestive heart failure, the patient should be kept at rest for several weeks, until the heart size either returns to normal or is at least stable.

CHEST PAIN. Chest pain is an uncommon symptom of cardiac disease in children, but it does occur occasionally. Usually a careful history and physical examination will serve to make the diagnosis, but at times chest roentgenograms, electrocardiograms, or echocardiograms may be needed.

The most common cause of chest pain is musculoskeletal, related to exertion; reproduction of the pain on movement and local tenderness are often present, and the history of the type of pain and its position, radiation, and causation is enough for the diagnosis. Other types of chest wall pain may be related to skeletal abnormalities, such as scoliosis, or occasionally to costochondritis.

Pain due to pleurisy or pericarditis is usually associated with fever; it is of acute onset and has specific physical findings (p.1474). Esophageal or gastric pain may be referred to the chest.

Chest pain due to anxiety, with or without hyperventilation, is also frequent. There may be local tenderness over the cardiac apex, and this may represent muscle tenderness due to the underlying heart beat. At other times the pain may have no definite pattern or may resemble angina pectoris; there is often a history of recent death of a member of the family or a close friend from a myocardial infarct.

Arrhythmias are another cardiac cause of chest pain, or more likely chest discomfort or cardiac awareness. The patient may have a fluttering or turning sensation, and this may be associated with pallor, sweating, and anxiety.

Pericardial defects or coronary artery abnormalities are rare causes of chest pain.

Cardiac pain that is ischemic in type (angina pectoris) does occur when there is severe aortic stenosis, pulmonic stenosis, or pulmonary hypertension without

shunt. The pain usually follows effort; it is restrosternal and gripping in character and is rapidly relieved by rest. The associated signs of the cardiac lesion are present. Similar pain may occur with hypertrophic subaortic stenosis, which again has specific features (p 1430); echocardiography is of particular value in making the diagnosis. The one cardiac lesion that can cause chest pain and not be very obvious on examination is prolapse of the mitral valve. The typical physical findings of this lesion are an apical midsystolic click followed by a late systolic murmur of mitral incompetence. At times the physical findings are not typical, and then an echocardiogram is of great help in making the diagnosis (p 1377).

SYNCOPE. Syncope is not a common feature of heart disease, but if the symptom occurs, certain forms of heart disease should be excluded. Severe aortic stenosis or severe pulmonary hypertension without a shunt may lead to syncope, usually during or just after exertion; the physical findings will be obvious for each lesion. Acute obstruction of the mitral valve orifice by a mobile left atrial myxoma is a rare cause of syncope; as a rule this will have specific physical signs and echocardiographic features (p 1469). More common cardiac causes are arrhythmias. Children with congenital complete atrioventricular block may faint (Adams-Stokes attacks), and these attacks are more common with surgically produced heart block. Less obvious are the sudden bouts of bradycardia or tachycardia that occur in those with the so-called sick sinus syndrome. The syndrome is rare in children unless there has been atrial surgery, either to close an atrial septal defect or to correct transposition of the great arteries with the Mustard procedure.

PSYCHOLOGIC SUPPORT. Any child who has heart disease is probably worried about it, as are the parents and possibly the siblings. Insofar as is possible, the anxieties of these people should be elicited and support should be given.

Fear of sudden death is common, but sudden death is rare in most forms of childhood heart disease; reassurance can validly be given. If there is a very sick infant who requires a great deal of care, it is common for the siblings to be neglected, and even for marriages to break up. While the pediatrician is not necessarily the best person to counsel the family on these issues, he should certainly be aware of the problems and attempt to ease them.

Older children are apt to be concerned about differences that set them apart from their peers; clearly this is accentuated if they are restricted. Thus it is important to look for these problems, attempt to discuss them with the child and the parents, and avoid unnecessary restrictions.

In adolescents, marriageability and the ability to have children are often matters of great concern. Reassurance can usually be given to patients with mild or treated heart disease. It should be noted however, that their children will be at greater than normal risk of also having congenital heart disease (p 1403). Most girls with severe cyanotic heart disease are infertile; if one does become pregnant, her health will usually not be compromised. The one group for whom pregnancy is contraindicated is the group with severe pulmonary hypertension without a ventricular septal defect or a ductus arteriosus. To allow pregnancy to continue to term almost always results in maternal death; thus contraception (other than oral steroids) or sterilization is mandatory.

Employment restrictions are similar to those for exercise. A separate problem that is of considerable concern even in patients with minimal cardiac abnormalities is their inability to obtain life insurance at normal premiums, if at all. At present, most insurance companies will sell life insurance at normal premiums if a small or medium-size patent ductus arteriosus had been closed surgically, but they are reluctant to do so for any other lesions. Since the companies make the rules, it is difficult to change them, especially since they tend to weight the chances in their own favor. It is perhaps worth emphasizing to the patients that this is not an indication that they are seriously ill, but rather that it illustrates the excess caution of the insurance companies.

RESUSCITATION
Julien I.E. Hoffman

Resuscitation for actual or impending circulatory or respiratory arrest should always be done when the arrest occurs unexpectedly or when no one in attendance is familiar with the patient's illness. If a patient is dying uncomfortably from an incurable disease, the decision might have been made in advance not to institute heroic procedures, but a decision of such importance should not be made during an emergency by people unfamiliar with the patient.

Circulatory arrest stops cerebral blood flow and thus is soon followed by respiratory arrest, while when respiration stops there is soon cardiac arrest from hypoxemia. Therefore, in practice, both systems often need simultaneous attention.

CIRCULATORY ARREST. The term circulatory arrest strictly refers to complete circulatory arrest, but since this may be preceded by a period of extremely low cardiac output, the two entities will be considered together. The common causes of circulatory arrest are as follows: (1) Respiratory failure causing hypoxia, acidemia, or hypercarbia. Sudden improved ventilation with rapid fall is carbon dioxide may also cause ventricular fibrillation. (2) Vagal stimulation (for example, with tracheal intubation, extubation, or suction), rectal examination, pulling on eye muscles or peritoneum at surgery. Hypoxemia increases the sensitivity of the heart to vagal stimulation. (3) Very rapid dysrhythmias due to heart disease, drugs, cardiac catheterization, or angiography, or else for no known reason. The syndromes with long Q-T intervals (p 1402) or complete heart block (p 1403) often caused cardiac arrest. (4) Hypotension and metabolic acidosis due to trauma, hemorrhage, sepsis, anaphylaxis, postoperative or metabolic disorders. (5) Massive blood transfusions,

especially with cold blood. (6) Drugs, especially digitalis, quinidine, rapid potassium infusion, local or general anesthetics. (7) Electric shock, faulty artificial cardiac pacemaker. (8) Pericardial tamponade. (9) Massive air embolism.

RESPIRATORY ARREST. Respiratory arrest is due to airway obstruction, central nervous system depression, mechanical factors that prevent adequate lung expansion, and severe parenchymal disease.

Acute Airway Obstruction. Nasal obstruction is important in neonates and small infants who might not have learned to breathe through their mouths. It may be due to a number of causes: (1) choanal atresia, tumors or polyps, or gross mucosal swelling from inflammation, allergy, or reserpine. (2) Oropharyngeal obstruction from a large tongue, glossoptosis in the Pierre Robin syndrome, or the tongue falling back in comatose patients; cysts and tumors; peritonsillar abscess or very large tonsils; angioneurotic endema. (3) Laryngeal obstruction from laryngomalacia, epiglottitis, tumors, or edema. (4) Tracheal obstruction from extrinsic masses, including vascular rings; stenosis or atresia; or rarely from inflammatory exudates. (5) Bronchial obstruction from foreign bodies, aspirated blood or vomitus, fluid (drowning, pulmonary edema), excess mucus, marked bronchospasm, inflammatory exudate.

Central Nervous System Depression. Central nervous system depression may be due to trauma, drugs and poisons, electric shock, cerebral edema, infections, tumors, severe hypoxemia, or hypercarbia.

Mechanical Impairment of Ventilation. Mechanical impairment of ventilation may be caused by neuromuscular paralysis of the chest wall or diaphragm, including postoperative phrenic nerve damage, Gross chest wall trauma with a flail chest, or Restriction of ventilation due to bilateral tension pneumothorax, massive pleural effusion, or large diaphragmatic hernia.

Extensive Parenchymal Disease. Extensive parenchymal disease may occur, with loss of ability to transfer oxygen and carbon dioxide between air and blood.

PATHOPHYSIOLOGY. Cardiopulmonary arrest causes hypoxia and carbon dioxide retention. The tissues begin to metabolize anaerobically and produce hydrogen ions and lactic acid, so that tissue and blood pH fall markedly. Continued arrest then leads to cell death, with the brain being affected permanently before other organs. Complete circulatory arrest for 4 minutes may cause irreversible brain death.

DIAGNOSIS. Diagnosis must be made clinically as soon as cardiopulmonary arrest is suspected. The clinical features are as follows: (1) Weak or absent pulses and heart sounds, or marked bradycardia or tachycardia. Note that there may be venous (atrial) waves in the neck even if there is ventricular fibrillation. (2) Poor or absent chest movements and breath sounds. However, good chest movement does not mean that alveolar ventilation is effective. (3) Loss of consciousness and dilatation of the pupils, both of which soon follow cardiopulmonary arrest. (4) Cyanosis or pallor, depending on whether ventilation stops before the circulation or not, or if there are specific causes of skin vasoconstriction such as hemorrhage or hypercarbia. Presence or absence of capillary refill is not a useful sign. It is essential that at this stage no time be wasted in taking blood pressure or an electrocardiogram, and too much time should not be spent trying to feel pulses or listen for breath sounds. Rather, commence resuscitation and then carry out these procedures at leisure.

TREATMENT. The aims of therapy are initially to ventilate, maintain a circulation, and correct metabolic abnormalities. Once these are being done, attention can be paid to the underlying causes.

GENERAL. If possible, send for help, since cardiorespiratory arrest cannot be managed adequately by one person. Ideally three or four people should manage the problem, and one of these or one other person should be designated to organize the activities and take notes of what is done.

Ventilation. First clear the upper airways of any solid material with the fingers or suction, if available. Then extend the neck slightly (the patient is usually supine) with a rolled towel under the shoulders. It is important not to overextend the neck, especially in infants, since this might stretch and thus narrow the trachea.

Keep the tongue forward so that it does not block the glottis. To do this either insert an oral airway or else pull the jaw forward with the fingers behind the angles of the mandible.

Ventilate the patient with a light-fitting face mask and bag, or else by mouth-to-mouth breathing after pinching the nose closed. (In small infants place your mouth over the infant's nose and mouth.) Inflate the patient's lungs enough to give good movements and breath sounds, especially at the apices. After inflation, remove your mouth and allow the patient's lungs to deflate. Inflate the lungs 20 to 40 times per minute in neonates and 15 to 20 times per minute for older children and adults; inflation must be synchronized with cardiac massage. Begin inflation with room air and change to 100 percent oxygen as soon as possible.

If the stomach becomes distended, aspirate the air from it with a nasogastric tube. Slight alterations in the position of the head may reduce the amount of air forced into the stomach. Compression of the epigastrium may also prevent distension.

Endotracheal intubation should not be done until some ventilation has been given and the patient seems better oxygenated. Then it can be done provided the person inserting the tube is experienced in doing so. If the attempted intubation is unsuccessful, do not persist for too long; continue ventilating the patient and then try to intubate again once there is better oxygenation.

Circulation. On rare occasions asystole or rapid tachycardia may revert to normal sinus rhythm after 2 to 4 hard thumps have been given on the precordium. Sudden elevation of the legs to increase venous return and distend the heart may also start the heart beating again. If these simple measures do not work, then external cardiac massage is essential.

If the patient is a small infant, place your hands behind the thorax to support it and push on the sternum with your thumbs. Compress the midsternum and not the lower sternum, since the heart is relatively higher in the chest in the newborn, and try to push the sternum about two-thirds of the way toward the spine. Try to maintain a regular compression rate of 80 to 120 per minute and synchronize so that there are 3 or 4 beats for each inflation of the lungs.

Older patients should be lying on a firm support, either a bed board or else the floor. Place the heel of the hand on the lower sternum and compress it about 60 to 80 times per minute; synchronize each 4 or 5 beats with one inflation. The force required is that which will produce an adequate circulation; excessive force can fracture ribs and rupture the liver. Usually the arm needs to be stiff so that your full weight can be swung over it. Try to push slowly in for about 0.5 sec and then allow 0.5 sec rest so that the ventricles can refill; a short, sharp push does not usually give an adequate cardiac output. The best evidence of improved circulation is return of normal skin color and decrease in pupillary size (provided the patient is not on drugs that will alter the pupil size). Feeling the pulse is usually difficult because of the rhythmic shaking of the patient by the cardiac massage.

When ventilation and circulation are under control, an electrocardiogram can be taken to determine what rhythm is present; while recording, stop the cardiac massage transiently to avoid artifacts. This recording will indicate whether there is asystole, ventricular fibrillation, severe bradycardia, or tachycardia, and further specific therapy will need to be given according to what is found.

If external massage fails and the patient is in hospital, consult the surgical team to decide if open chest cardiac massage is feasible. It is certainly more effective than external massage in producing peripheral perfusion. Furthermore, open chest cardiac massage does not produce the very high systemic and pulmonary venous pressures than can occur when the chest is being compressed.

Metabolic Changes While ventilation and cardiac massage are being done, another person should insert an intravenous line, either through a cutdown in the leg or else with a percutaneously introduced catheter. Merely inserting a needle into a peripheral vein should be avoided, unless there is no alternative, because of the risk that it will come out with the movements of the patient. Then give sodium bicarbonate at 3 to 5 mEq/kg body weight over 2 to 4 minutes, because there will almost certainly be a metabolic acidemia. Once the alkali has been given, take arterial blood gases and use the results to determine further alkaline therapy. Some fluid should be infused, and either Ringer's lactate or 5 percent dextrose in water is suitable at the onset. They can be changed (for example, to plasma or blood) once a firm diagnosis leads to a specific course of action.

SPECIFIC TREATMENT. Asystole. If the heart does not beat after simple mechanical maneuvers, epinephrine should be given. Dilute epinephrine to 1 mg/10 ml by adding 1 ml of 1:1000 epinephrine from the ampule to 9 ml of saline, and give 1 ml/10 kg of this dilute mixture; this is equivalent to 10 μg/kg. It is best to give the epinephrine intravenously rather than by direct intracardiac injection, since the latter may damage coronary arteries; however, intracardiac injection may be tried as a last resort. If the heart does not start beating, give more sodium bicarbonate and repeat the epinephrine. If the heart still does not beat, insert a pacemaker transthoracically.

Ventricular Fibrillation. If ventricular fibrillation is present, first attempt to improve oxygenation and combat acidemia before using electrical defibrillation. Then rub electrode jelly in firmly enough to produce local erythema at two sites—the lower right sternal border and the posterior axillary line at the level of the cardiac apex. The erythema lowers skin impedance so that most of the current will flow through the thorax, and the two sites specified will place the bulk of the ventricles between the two electrode paddles.

Disconnect the electrocardiograph from the patient by pulling out the patient cable. Set the energy level of the defibrillator to about 2 to 3 joules/kg (watt-sec/kg). (If the ventricular fibrillation is due to digoxin toxicity, start at lower settings.) Then press electrode paddles of appropriate size firmly on the prepared sites. Make sure that you are holding the insulated parts of the paddles and that no one is touching the patient or the bed, and discharge the defibrillator.

After the shock, continue cardiac massage while someone plugs the patient cable back into the electrocardiograph. Then stop massage briefly while a strip of electrocardiogram is taken. If ventricular fibrillation persists, continue cardiac massage, give more sodium bicarbonate, increase the energy level, and repeat the shock. If this is still ineffective, give intravenous epinephrine, which sometimes makes defibrillation effective. If the first electrocardiographic strip shows sinus rhythm, but this rapidly reverts to ventricular fibrillation, repeat the defibrillatory sequence once or twice and give more sodium bicarbonate; resumption of cardiac contraction may wash out metabolites from tissues and thus cause ventricular fibrillation again. If sinus rhythm does not persist, give propranolol at 0.1 mg/kg intravenously and repeat the shock. If sinus rhythm returns and persists, make sure that there is an effective heart beat by feeling the pulse. A normal electrocardiogram does not guarantee an adequate cardiac output.

Other Arrythmias. For treatment of other arrhythmias see page 1394.

Hypotension. Cardiopulmonary arrest may cause hypotension, probably by venous pooling. As a result, perfusion is impaired, and this may perpetuate the cardiac difficulty. As a first step, raise the legs, and if necessary apply elastic bandages to them. If blood pressure does not return to normal and perfusion remains poor, give blood or plasma expanders, or else titrate the blood pressure with intravenous infusion of metaraminol (Aramine) or norepinephrine (Levophed). Sometimes hypotension reflects poor myocardial contractility, which may improve with norepinephrine or dopamine (p 1483) or calcium, which can be given as 10 percent calcium chloride or gluconate at a dose of 0.2 ml/kg intravenously and may be repeated until a maximum of 2 ml/kg has been given.

STOPPING RESUSCITATION. It is important to realize that as long as the pupils are not widely dilated and unreactive there is a chance for the patient to recover; thus resuscitation attempts should not be abandoned too soon. There have been occasional reports of people who survived after 4 to 8 hours of continuous cardiac massage. On the other hand, there is no point in prolonging the maneuvers if there is no chance for survival. Furthermore, often the heart beat returns to normal and the patient is ventilated mechanically, but consciousness does not return. The decision to cease resuscitation is difficult, and it should be made only after consultation among all people concerned with the patient's care and with full understanding of the legal aspects in any particular state or country. In general, recovery will not take place if for at least 24 hours there are no spontaneous respirations, no voluntary or reflex movements, widely dilated pupils that do not respond to light, and a flat EEG, provided that the patient is not hypothermic and is not under the influence of massive amounts of sedative drugs. If it is known that resuscitation began very late, so that severe cerebral damage had almost certainly occurred, resuscitation may be stopped after a shorter period without improvement.

Reference

Stephenson HE Jr: Cardiac Arrest and Resuscitation, 4th ed. St Louis, CV. Mosby, 1974

CHAPTER 28

The Lung

WILLIAM H. TOOLEY, *Associate Editor*

DEVELOPMENT OF THE LUNG AND THE ONSET OF RESPIRATION

WILLIAM H. TOOLEY

After birth, the lungs assume the function of oxygen and carbon dioxide exchange, which, in fetal life, is performed by the placenta. In order for the newborn infant to survive, he must inflate his lungs and provide a large enough area of contact between capillaries and gas to effect the gas transfer needed to subserve metabolic needs. Whether he will be viable depends largely on the state of development reached by the lungs at the time of birth.

LUNG GROWTH

At 28 days postconceptional age the lung begins as a bud on the embryonic gut. This bifurcates to form the rudimentary main stem bronchi which grow into the surrounding mesenchyma. These solid tubes grow and

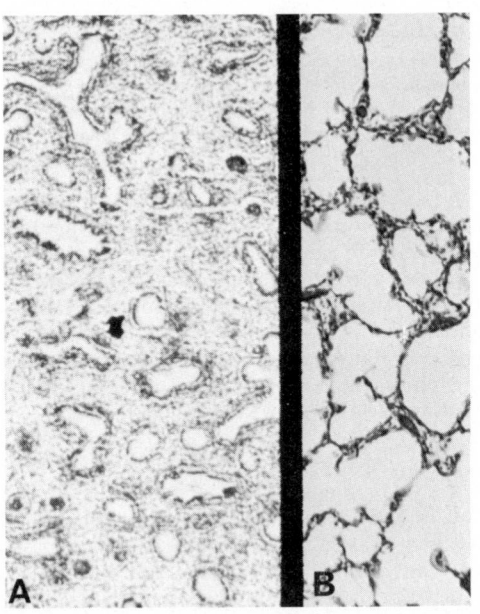

FIG. 1. **A.** The lung, of a fetus of 20 weeks gestation, distended and fixed with 10 cm H_2O pressure. The airways are canalized. The tissue between the airways is a loose mesenchyme with few blood vessels (X250 magnification). **B.** The lung of an infant born after a 30-week gestation and who lived 4 days, distended and fixed with 10 cm H_2O pressure. The interalveolar septa are thin and contain many capillaries. The total surface area is large (X250 magnification).

divide until the 16th week, at which time there are 20 generations of bronchi. This period is called the *glandular stage* of development. At about 16 weeks the primitive airways begin to canalize. The *canalicular stage* of development lasts from the 16th to about the 24th week (Fig. 1). Vascularization of the lung proceeds more slowly than the development of the primitive airways. The pulmonary artery appears at about 10 weeks, and its branches follow the developing bronchi. The first capillaries can be identified in the middle part of the canalicular phase of the development. The end of the canalicular phase is heralded by a rapid proliferation of capillaries into the mesenchyma. This event is accompanied by the development of alveolar ducts on the terminal bronchioles. This *alveolar stage* of development continues until birth.

From the point of view of lung function, a fetus is potentially viable when the canalicular stage of development is complete. However, the timing of the end of the canalicular period of development and the beginning of the alveolar period is variable so that no absolute minimum number of weeks in utero can be said to be necessary for neonatal survival. On average, alveolar ducts surrounded by capillaries appear at 26 weeks, and alveoli and alveolar capillaries appear at about 30 weeks. However, these changes can begin as early as 22 weeks or as late as 28 weeks. Lung development can be hastened by administration of glucocorticoids and probably by stress, and it is probable that the length of the alveolar stage of development can be shortened from 14 to 1 or 2 weeks. By 26 weeks gestation, most fetuses can live for a while outside the uterus, although the surface area for gas transfer may be relatively small and inadequate to sustain life if metabolic needs are high. The appearance of the lung of a 26-week fetus who did not breathe is shown in Figure 2A, and is compared with a lung of a 27-week fetus who lived for 3 days in Figure 2B. Note the relatively thick interalveolar septa and the small number of capillaries in the nonbreathing fetus. Following birth, the interalveolar septa become thin and there is an increase in the number of capillaries. These morphologic features of the lung of the 26-week fetus may evolve in 3 to 4 days to the appearance shown in Figure 2B.

DEVELOPMENT OF PULMONARY SURFACTANT

At the same time that alveolar ducts appear and the number of capillaries is rapidly increasing, there is a change in the appearance of the epithelial cells lining the airways. Early in the canalicular phase, the airways

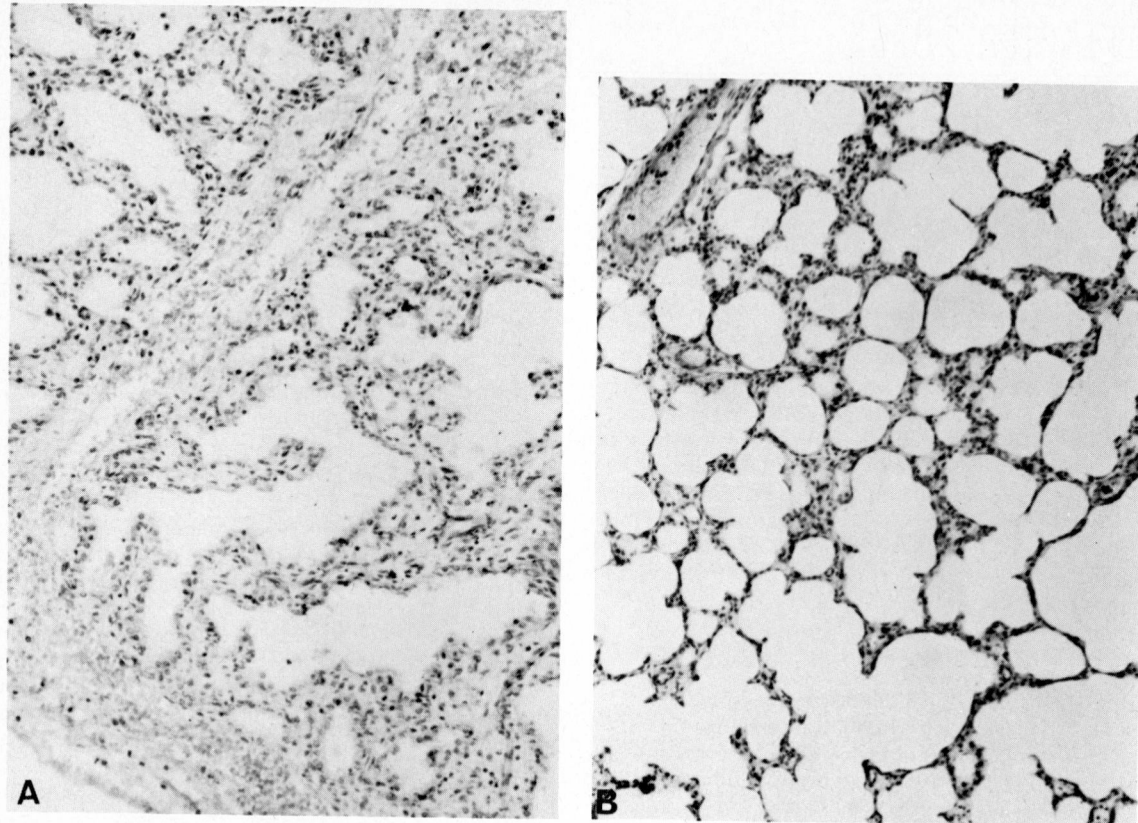

FIG. 2.   A. The lung from a fetus of 26 weeks who did not breathe, distended and fixed with 10 cm H_2O pressure. Note the thick interalveolar and interlobular septa and the relatively few capillaries. The total surface area is larger than the lung in Fig 1. but smaller than that in B (X300 magnification). **B.** The lung of a newborn infant, born after 29 weeks gestation, who breathed for several days and died of an intracranial hemorrhage. The fixation and magnification are the same as in Figure 2A. The interalveolar septa are thinner and the total surface area is larger than the lung in 2A.

are lined with large suboidal cells which are filled with glycogen. At about 18 weeks some of the epithelial cells are vacuolated and contain cytoplasmic inclusion bodies, *the alveolar epithelial type II cells.* The arrival of these cells occurs at the same time that pulmonary surfactant appears in extracts of lung tissue. Type II cells synthesize pulmonary surfactant and store it in their cytoplasmic inclusion bodies. The time of appearance of the type II cells varies and they may be present as early as 16 weeks or not appear until as late as 20 weeks gestation.

Von Neergaard first called attention to the importance of surface tension in the lung. He pointed out that most of the retractile force of the lung achieved during inflation is due to a high surface tension. Subsequently, Pattle noted that the bubbles in pulmonary edema were very stable and persisted for many hours. Later, Clements showed that the material forming these bubbles had a low surface tension when layered on a surface and compressed, and a relatively high surface tension when allowed to spread over a larger surface area. In the lung, the behavior of this surface active materials augments

passive expiration (high surface tension when lung surface area is large) and stabilizes the lung at low volumes (low surface area when lung surface area is small). The newborn infant's lung must have pulmonary surfactant to remain air-filled at end-expiration. When it is absent, progressive diffuse atelectasis occurs in the hours after birth. This causes the clinical syndrome of Hyaline Membrane Disease (p. 1519).

LUNG FLUID

The lung is fluid-filled from the beginning of the canalicular phase until the completion of fetal development. The lung secretes this liquid at the rate of about 2 to 4 ml/kg/minute in the lamb. It is an ultrafiltrate and its composition changes very little during gestation, except for potassium which doubles in concentration from 4 to 9 mEq/l during the last 2 weeks of gestation (Table 1). The development of a significant gradient for potassium between plasma and lung fluid is in marked contrast to the other electrolytes for which the gradients remain the same throughout gestation. The increase in

TABLE 1. Plasma and Tracheal Fluid Electrolytes in Fetal Lambs From 120 to 150 Days Gestation

Electrolyte	Plasma	Tracheal Fluid
Sodium, mEq/liter	146	148
Chloride, mEq/liter	110	153
Total calcium, mg/ 100 ml	12	2
Magnesium, mg/100 ml	2	< 0.5
Bicarbonate, mEq/liter	27	2
Total protein, mg/100 ml	4	< 0.06
pH	7	6.23

Term is 150 days in the lamb. Note the gradients for chloride, calcium, and bicarbonate. These suggest an active electrolyte pump. There is no potassium gradient between plasma (4 mEq/liter) and lung liquid until 2 weeks before term when the tracheal fluid concentration rises to 9 mEq/liter (see text).

potassium flux parallels the increase in the amount of surfactant in lung liquid which occurs near term, and is probably another reflection of the increased secretion of alveolar cells. During fetal life some of the liquid is swallowed and some moves into the amniotic cavity. That which reaches the amniotic cavity carries along surfactant so that analysis of amniotic fluid for surfactant can be done to predict whether an infant has mature lungs or runs the risk of developing hyaline membrane disease. At term, there is about 20 to 25 ml/kg body weight of lung fluid in the lung, which must either be expelled during delivery of the chest or absorbed after delivery.

THE FIRST BREATH

After the head is delivered, the thorax is compressed as it passes through the birth canal and some intraalveolar fluid is expelled. After delivery of the thorax, when the chest cage resumes its previous volume, air is pulled into the upper airway and increases the volume of the airways. This triggers a strong inspiratory effort (Head's paradoxical reflex, see below). This first inspiratory effort must be large enough to overcome the viscous resistance to movement of the intrapulmonary liquid and the resistive forces to air movement imposed by the tissue and surface tension. The greatest resistance to the aeration of the fetal lungs is the surface tension of the lung liquid. The pulmonary surfactant in the lung liquid of the mature infant lowers the surface tension between it and the advancing column of air. In the absence of surfactant, the pressure to inflate the smallest units of the lung is high since it is proportional to the surface tension. The force needed to inflate the respiratory bronchioles also depends upon the size of the bronchiolar unit, the smaller the radius of curvature the greater the force. Thus, in keeping with the Laplace relationship ($P = 2 \, ST/r$, where P is distending pressure; ST, surface tension; and r, the radius of curvature), the pressure required to inflate the lung is a function of lung size and presence or absence of surfactant. As a consequence, prematurely born infants require higher pressures to inflate their lungs than do infants born at term.

Following the initial inflation of the lung, the intraalveolar lung fluid moves into the interstitial space and is partially absorbed by the capillaries and partly removed by the lymphatics in the first hours of life. Delay in absorption of lung fluid will interfere with respiratory gas transfer and cause respiratory distress. The inflation of the normal newborn lung after birth is complete within a very few breaths, and most of the alveoli are expanded within the first hour of life. The newborn's lung volume is 25 ml/kg by an hour of age, and increases very little more during the first weeks of life.

Because the initial aeration of the lung requires a large effort, its success depends on the infant's ability to produce a high transpulmonary pressure. At the time of delivery, the infant is exposed to a large number of stimuli that will promote gasping, including cold, light, noise, increased force of gravity, as well as a rapidly rising hydrogen ion and falling oxygen tension. All of these stimuli work through the nervous system, and their effect will be blunted if the infant is depressed by trauma or drugs. In addition to an adequate stimulus to breathing, the pressure an infant can create will be determined by the stability of his chest wall and the strength of the muscles of inspiration. The prematurely born infant has a compliant chest cage, which makes diaphragmatic function inefficient. This limits the infant's ability to generate a large transpulmonary pressure. Following aeration of the lung, pulmonary vascular resistance falls, pulmonary blood flow increases, left atrial pressure rises, and the foramen ovale closes. With the completion of aeration of the lungs, and with the establishment of the usual adult pattern of circulation, the infant is able to meet his metabolic needs if he is not unduly stressed and if the lungs can remain gas-filled during subsequent respiratory cycles. Failure to expand the lung adequately at birth, or to prevent atelectasis following birth causes increasing respiratory distress.

LUNG FUNCTION

Measurements of the lung volumes and the mechanics of respiration have been made on infants born as early as 28 weeks after conception, and with birth weight as little as 1,000 grams. Lung compliance is larger in term infants than in infants born prematurely. In both prematurely born and term infants, lung compliance increases in the days following birth by 20 to 40 percent, but this is less in the prematurely born infant than in the term infant (Table 2). This age-dependent change in the elastic properties of the lungs suggests that newborn infants have a variable amount of atelectasis which can be abolished with successive respirations, excess lung water which decreases in the first days of life, and/or lung tissue which changes in quality after ventilation with air begins.

The volume of the airways of the newborn infant is relatively large and, during quiet breathing, the fraction of each tidal volume required to clear the respiratory dead space (Vd/VT) is 0.45 in the very prematurely born infant, compared with 0.35 in the term infant and

Table 2. Anatomic Dead Space to Tidal Volume Ratio (V_D/V_T) and Lung Compliance Divided by the Lung Volume at Which It Was Measured, (Specific Compliance, CL/FRC) for Infants Born Prematurely and at Term, and Adults

	Prematurely Born Infants		Term Infant	Adult
	BW < 1,500 g	BW > 1,500 g		
V_D/V_T	0.45	0.40	0.35	0.30
CL/FRC				
(ml/cm H_2O/ml)	0.03 → 0.04	0.04 → 0.05	0.050 → 0.055	0.06

Two values are presented for CL/FRC for infants; the first was obtained during the first 24 hours of life and the second in infants over 24 hours of age. Specific compliance is lower in prematurely born infants than in those born at term and increases in the days following birth in infants of all birthweights (data from Chu J, Cotton EK, Klaus MH, Sweet AY, Tooley WH: Pediatrics 40(2):709,1967).

0.30 in the adult. The airways of the prematurely born infant are about twice as compliant as those of mature infants or adults. Because of a relatively large respiratory dead space, the preterm infant must use a greater proportion of his tidal volume to ventilate the airways than the term infant or the adult. By itself, this would decrease respiratory efficiency; however, in the preterm infant, the relatively large airways impose less resistance to breathing than would airways with a smaller

dead space volume. Thus, while infants may have to increase gas flow in order to increase the minute volume of respiration and compensate for a large dead space ventilation, this extra ventilation can be achieved without so great an increase in the work of breathing as would be necessary if the airways were smaller.

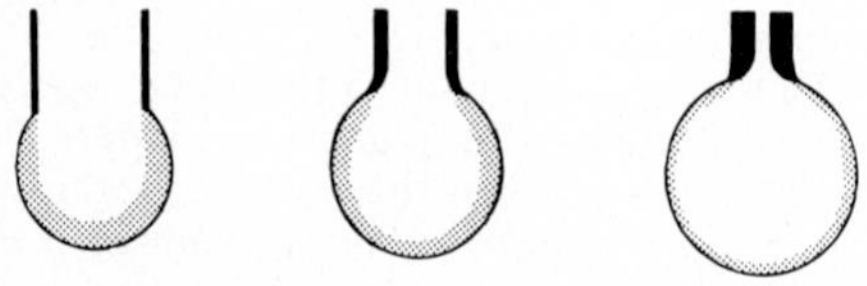

Bibliography

Avery ME, Mead J: Surface properties in relation to atelectasis and hyaline membrane disease. Am J Dis Child 97:517, 1959

Avery ME: In Fomon SJ (ed): Normal and abnormal respiration in children. Report 37th Ross Conferences on Pediatric Research, Columbus, Ohio, 1961

Chu J, Clements JA, Cotton EK, et al: Neonatal pulmonary ischemia. Pediatrics (Suppl) 40:709, 1967

Chu JS, Dawson P, Klaus M, Sweet AY: Lung compliance and lung volume measured concurrently in normal full-term and premature infants. Pediatrics 34:525, 1964

Clements JA: Surface tension of lung extracts. Proc Soc Exp Biol Med 95:170, 1957

Cook CD, Cherry RB, O'Brien D, Karlberg P, Smith CA: Studies of respiratory physiology in the newborn infant. I. Observations of normal premature and ful-term infants. J Clin Invest 34:975, 1955

Gruenwald P: Surface tension as a factor in the resistance of neonatal lungs to aeration. Am J Obstet Gynecol 53:996, 1947

Karlberg P, Cherry RB, Escardo FE, Koch G: Respiratory studies in newborn infants. II. Pulmonary ventilation and mechanics of breathing in the first minutes of life, including the onset of respiration. Acta Paediatr 51:121, 1962

Karlberg P, Adams FH, Guebelle F, Wallgren G: A'teration of the infant's thorax during vaginal delivery. Acta Obstet Gynecol Scand 41:223, 1962

Klaus M, Tooley WH, Weaver KH, Clements JA: Lung volume in the newborn infant. Pediatrics 30:III, 1962

Mescher EJ, Platzker ACG, Ballard PL, et al: Ontogeny of tracheal fluid, pulmonary surfactant, and plasma corticoids in the fetal lamb. J Appl Physiol 39:1020, 1975

Reid L: The embryology of the lung. In De Reuck AVS, Porter R (eds): Ciba Foundation Symposium: Development of the Lung. Churchill, London, 1967

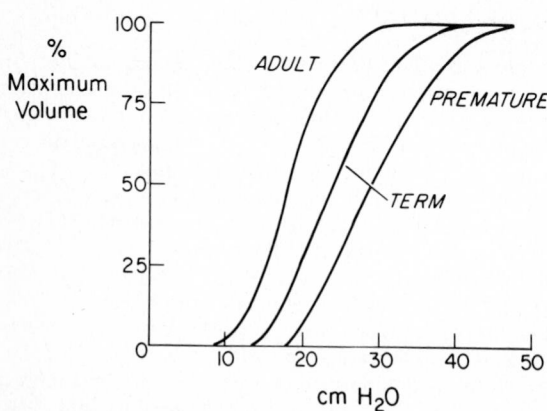

FIG. 3. Schematic representation of the airways and acini in infants born prematurely and at term, compared to the adult. As the lung grows the airway becomes relatively thicker and the lumen smaller. As a consequence V_D/V_T and airway compliance decrease with increasing maturity. The walls of the alveoli and the alveolar ducts become thinner and more compliant with growth so that more of each breath can be accommodated by these structures.

FIG. 4. The approximate pressures required for inflation of airless lungs from a premature infant of birthweight about 1,500 g, an infant born at term, and an adult. Pressures of about 20, 15, and 10 cm H_2O are needed to initiate inflation, and pressures of about 40, 30, and 20 cm H_2O are required to completely inflate the lungs of prematurely born infants, infants born at term, and adults, respectively.

CARDIOPULMONARY CARE OF THE NEWBORN INFANT AT BIRTH

GEORGE A. GREGORY

About 10 percent of newborn infants are unable to make a successful cardiopulmonary adaption to extrauterine life and cannot expand their lungs spontaneously, begin rhythmic respiration, and alter their circulation from the fetal to the adult pattern. These infants require resuscitation.

ASSESSMENT OF THE INFANT AT BIRTH

The Apgar Score

Dr. Virginia Apgar proposed this system for evaluation of the newborn; it provides an easy measure of the degree of intrapartum stress. In it, a score of 0, 1, or 2 is assigned at 1 and 5 minutes after birth for each of five variables described below and in Table 3. A score of 4 or less at 1 minute is associated with a high incidence of hyaline membrane disease and death, while a score of 8 to 10 indicates an excellent chance for survival.

HEART RATE. The normal heart rate at birth is between 120 and 160 beats/minute. Rates below 100 usually indicate asphyxia. The Apgar score assigns a score of 0 for no detectable heart beat; 1 for a heart rate less than 100/minute; and 2 for a rate of 100/minute or more.

RESPIRATORY EFFORT. Normal infants gasp at birth, make deep respiratory efforts within 30 sec, and have sustained respiration at a frequency of 30 to 60/minute by 90 minutes after delivery. Apnea or slow or irregular breathing occur with severe acidosis, asphyxia, fetal infections, central nervous system damage, or depression of respiratory drive due to drugs, such as barbiturates and tranquilizers given to the mother. No respiratory effort receives a score of 0; irregular respiration a score of 1; sustained rhythmic respiration a score of 2.

MUSCLE TONE. Normal infants move all extremities actively immediately after birth. Those who fail to move or have poor muscle tone are usually asphyxiated, depressed by drugs, or have had the central nervous system traumatized. If the infant is limp, he gets a score of 0; some flexion of the extremities a score of 1; active movement a score of 2.

REFLEX IRRITABILITY. The normal response to inserting a catheter through a nostril into the posterior pharynx is a grimace, cough, or sneeze. Absence of response rates a 0 score; a grimace alone a score of 1; a grimace, cough, or sneeze a score of 2.

COLOR. The infant's skin is blue in color at birth but becomes pink with the onset of effective ventilation. Most infants have pink bodies and lips but cyanotic hands and feet (*acrocyanosis*) by 90 sec after birth. Generalized cyanosis after 90 sec occurs with low cardiac output, methemoglobinemia, polycythemia, cyanotic congenital heart disease, and pulmonary diseases, such as hyaline membrane disease, aspiration of blood or meconium and airway obstruction, hypoplastic lungs, and diaphragmatic hernia. Most infants who are pale at birth have peripheral vasoconstriction caused by asphyxia, hypovolemia, or severe acidosis. Some infants with hemolytic disease may have anemia severe enough to cause pallor, and this is often associated with edema (hydrops fetalis). Respiratory alkalosis (as might occur with too vigorous assistance to ventilation), excessive heating, magnesium or acute maternal alcohol ingestion, or infusion may cause marked vasodilation and striking peripheral plethora. Plethora also occurs in infants who are hypervolemic because of a large placental transfusion; these infants contract their vascular volume during the first few hours after birth and become polycythemic and cyanotic as their blood concentrates. A pale or blue baby receives a score of 0; acrocyanosis a score of 1; uniform pinkness a score of 2.

RESUSCITATION

Someone skilled in the technical aspects of resuscitation of the newborn must evaluate and, when necessary, treat each newborn infant. If delivery is premature or asphyxia is suspected because of naternal history or signs of fetal distress, two persons are needed—one expands the lungs and begins ventilation, the other catheterizes umbilical vessels, supports the circulation, and treats acidemia and other abnormalities. Table 4 presents the disorders in which asphyxia at birth may be expected (see also p. 167). Each delivery room should have the equipment listed in Table 5 and prior to each birth one member of the delivery room staff must check each item's performance.

TYING THE UMBILICAL CORD. The time after delivery, when the umbilical cord should be ligated, depends on the infant's respiratory efficiency, gestational age, and presence of intrapartum stress. Hypovolemia and shock may occur if the umbilical cord is clamped before there has been an adequate transfusion of blood from placenta to infant. These conditions are worsened by maternal hypotension, fetal asphyxia, and clamping the cord before the first breath. On the other hand, delayed clamping of the cord or stripping blood from the cord into the baby's circulation may produce hypervolemia

Table 3. The Apgar Scoring System

SCORE	0	1	2
Heart rate	Absent	Less than 100/min	More than 100/min
Respiratory effort	Absent	Slow, irregular	Good, crying
Muscle tone	Limp	Some flexion of extremities	Active motion
Reflex irritability (in response to catheter in nose)	Absent	Grimace	Cough or sneeze
Color	Blue, pale	Body pink, extremities blue (acrocyanosis)	Completely pink

Each sign is evaluated individually and scored from 0 to 2 at both 1 and 5 minutes of life. The final Score at each time is the sum of the individual scores. (From Apgar V: Curr Res Anesthesiol 32:260, 1953).

Table 4. Disorders That Commonly Cause Intrapartum Asphyxia

Maternal Conditions

Diabetes
Hypertension
Toxemia
Maternal treatment with
  reserpine, lithium
  magnesium
  ethyl alcohol
  β-adrenergic drugs
Abnormal estriol levels
Anemia (hemoglobin less
  than 10 g/100 ml)
Blood group isoimmunization
  with high levels of bili-
  rubin present in amniotic
  fluid
Abruptio placenta
Placenta previa
Antepartum hemorrhage
Previous prenatal death
Narcotic, barbiturate,
  tranquilizer, or psychedelic
  drug use
Ethyl alcohol intoxication

Conditions of Labor and Delivery

Forceps delivery other than low elective
Vacuum extraction delivery
Breech or other abnormal presentation
  and delivery
Cesarean section
Prolonged second stage of labor
Prolapsed umbilical cord
Maternal hypotension
Sedative or analgesic drugs given intra-
  venously within 1 hour of delivery or
  intramuscularly within 2 hours of
  delivery

Fetal Conditions

Multiple births
Polyhydramnios
Meconium-stained amniotic fluid
Abnormal heart rate or rhythm
Acidosis (fetal scalp capillary blood)
Decreased rate of growth (uterine size)
Premature delivery
Amniotic fluid surfactant test negative or
  intermediate within 24 hours of delivery

Table 5. Resuscitation Equipment Required in Each Delivery Room*

Infrared heater with servo control mechanism for maintaining body temperature

Suction— bulb syringe
          wall suction with adjustable pressure

Electrocardiographic monitor and ECG electrodes

Laryngoscope with blade sizes 00 to 1

Endotracheal tubes Cole type (Fr sizes 8, 10, 12, 14)

End-hole suction catheters (Fr sizes, 3, 5, 8)

Oral airways, sizes 00 to 1.0

Umbilical vessel catheterization tray
The performance of this equipment must be checked before each delivery.

and cause tachypnea, delayed absorption of lung fluid, pulmonary edema, and an increased work of breathing. Infants born following uncomplicated pregnancies, labor, and delivery and who appear well at birth should be held at the level of the placenta until they cry and the umbilical arteries stop pulsating before the umbilical cord is tied. If the infant is limp and makes no respiratory effort, suction the nose and mouth and then clamp the cord, without milking it, as soon as the baby is born. After drying and placing the baby on a resuscitation platform, again briefly suction the mouth and nose before proceeding.

APGAR SCORES OF 8 TO 10 AT 1 MINUTE OF AGE. Most liveborn infants are in this group and after airway suctioning seldom require additional resuscitation unless they are very small or have had unusual intrauterine stress. However, all infants require careful reevaluation at 5 minutes of age because some who are apparently normal at birth hypoventilate and develop asphyxia after the stimulation of birth ceases. Regardless of the 5-minute Apgar score, all infants must be observed carefully for 2 to 12 hours after delivery until they have demonstrated that they have successfully adapted to extrauterine life.

APGAR SCORES OF 5 TO 7 AT 1 MINUTE OF AGE. These infants are midly asphyxiated but usually respond to oxygen and vigorous drying with a towel. *Do not slap them on the buttocks.* If the infant does not have sustained rhythmic breathing after stimulation, continue stimulation while blowing oxygen over the nose and mouth.

APGAR SCORES OF 3 TO 4 AT 1 MINUTE OF AGE. These infants usually respond to ventilation with bag and mask. If they do not begin to breathe rhythmically, or their Apgar score is 5 or less at 5 minutes of age, they should have their tracheas intubated, the lungs ventilated, and be treated as indicated below.

APGAR SCORES OF 0 TO 2 AT 1 MINUTE OF AGE. These infants are severely asphyxiated and require immediate ventilation and may require cardiac massage and circulatory support. If ventilation with mask and bag is not immediately successful, the trachea must be intubated and the lungs expanded and ventilated with 60 to 80 percent oxygen. Examination of the apices of the chest for equal expansion will indicate whether ventilation is adequate. This is a better sign than auscultation because bilateral breath sounds do not assure bilateral ventilation, since breath sounds are well transmitted in a small chest. When ventilation is adequate, the heart rate will rise and cyanosis disappear, unless there is a profound metabolic acidosis. Measurement of arterial pH, P_{CO_2}, and P_{O_2} is the only reliable method of assessing the adequacy of ventilation. The pressure needed with the first breaths, to expand the lungs, may be 30 to 40 cm H_2O; after expansion adequate ventilation generally requires less than 20 cm H_2O.

TRACHEAL INTUBATION. This is best accomplished with the head in a neutral position, not flexed or extended (Fig. 5). With the laryngoscope held with the first finger and thumb of the left hand, grasp the chin firmly with the second and third fingers. The small finger of the left hand compresses the hyoid bone and moves the anterior larynx of the infant posteriorly to expose the vocal cords. Insert the endotracheal tube about 2 cm below the glottis and expand the lungs gently with an anesthesia bag at a rate of 20 to 50 breaths per minute. If the arterial P_{O_2} rises above 100

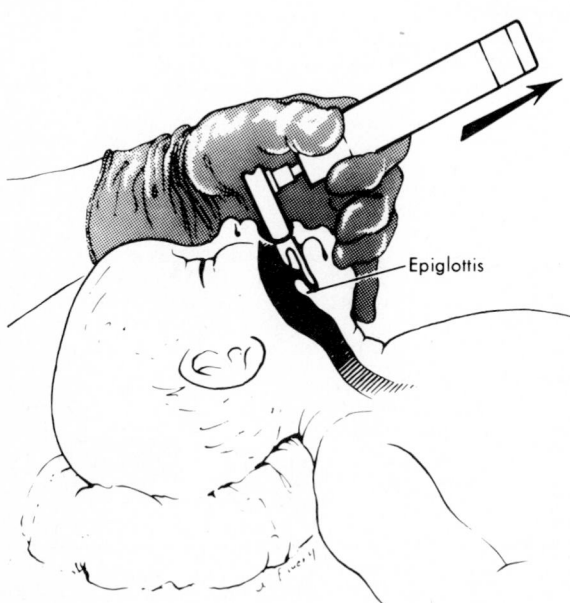

Epiglottis

FIG. 5. Laryngoscopy technique. (From Gregory GA: In Schnider S, Moya F (eds): The Anesthesiologist, the Mother and the Newborn. Baltimore, Williams and Wilkins, 1974)

torr, the inspired oxygen must be lowered to keep it in the range of 50 to 80 torr. During laryngoscopy, monitor the heart rate and rhythm, because dysrythmias and bradycardia are common.

TRACHEAL SUCTIONING. Sixty percent of the infants born with meconium staining of their amniotic fluid have meconium below the vocal cords. Those with particulate meconium in the amniotic fluid require immediate tracheal suctioning before ventilation. Remove the meconium by using the endotracheal tube as a straw, sucking on the tube while withdrawing it from the trachea. If meconium is retrieved, repeat the procedure until none is obtained, and then gently expand the lungs.

VASCULAR RESUSCITATION

When depression is severe and the infant fails to respond immediately to ventilation, the resuscitator should insert an umbilical arterial catheter to measure blood gases, pH, and blood pressure and to administer drugs. The technique of umbilical vessel catherization is described on p. 168. In most instances ventilation alone increases pulmonary blood flow by raising arterial P_{O_2} and pH and lowering pulmonary vascular resistance. However, some severely depressed infants have severe acidosis and/or hypovolemia and require expansion of blood volume and correction of acidosis.

CORRECTION OF ACIDOSIS. Respiratory acidosis is corrected by increasing alveolar ventilation, by either improving the patient's own ventilation or providing assisted ventilation. Marked metabolic acidosis may require treatment with sodium bicarbonate. If ventilation is adequate, the infusion of sodium bicarbonate will quickly raise the pH and relieve the intense vasoconstriction that usually accompanies acidosis and, when the circulating blood volume is low, can cause hypotension (Fig. 6). If the Apgar score is 5 or less at 5 minutes despite oxygen, stimulation, and assisted ventilation, sodium bicarbonate ($NaHCO_3$), 2 or 3 mEq/kg body weight, can be given though an umbilical arterial catheter at the rate of 1 mEq/kg/minute. Before the infusion, blood must be obtained for measurement of pH and for oxygen and carbon dioxide tensions. *Ventilation must be assisted during the time $NaHCO_3$ is administered* since, if ventilation is inadequate, arterial P_{CO_2} will rise. Following the initial infusion, additional alkali may be needed if there is marked metabolic acidosis. If the arterial pH is less than 7.1 and is primarily due to metabolic acidosis, correct one-quarter of the base deficit with $NaHCO_3$ (mEq $NaHCO_3$ to be infused = ¼ [0.6 × body weight in kg × base excess]. If the pH is 7.1 or greater, continue assisted ventilation and repeat blood gas and pH measurements in 5 minutes. With adequate ventilation, cardiac output usually improves, the blood pH spontaneously rises above 7.20, and no additional alkali is required. Hypertonic sodium bicarbonate may cause hepatic necrosis if given into the portal circulation, so infusion into a catheter in the umbilical vein should be avoided unless the catheter tip is in the inferior vena cava.

VOLUME EXPANSION.   Prematurely born infants who are asphyxiated in utero may have an inadequate circulating blood volume at birth. Because most of them are acidotic and have peripheral vasoconstriction, initially they may have normal arterial blood pressures. However, the vascular capacity enlarges as the pH rises, and the circulating blood volume may no longer be adequate and the arterial and central venous blood pressures fall. This sequence of events is illustrated in Figures 6 and 7. Hypovolemia may be missed if the measurement of vascular pressures is not part of the resuscitation routine.

Hypovolemia is diagnosed when arterial and central venous pressures and pulse volume are low, skin color

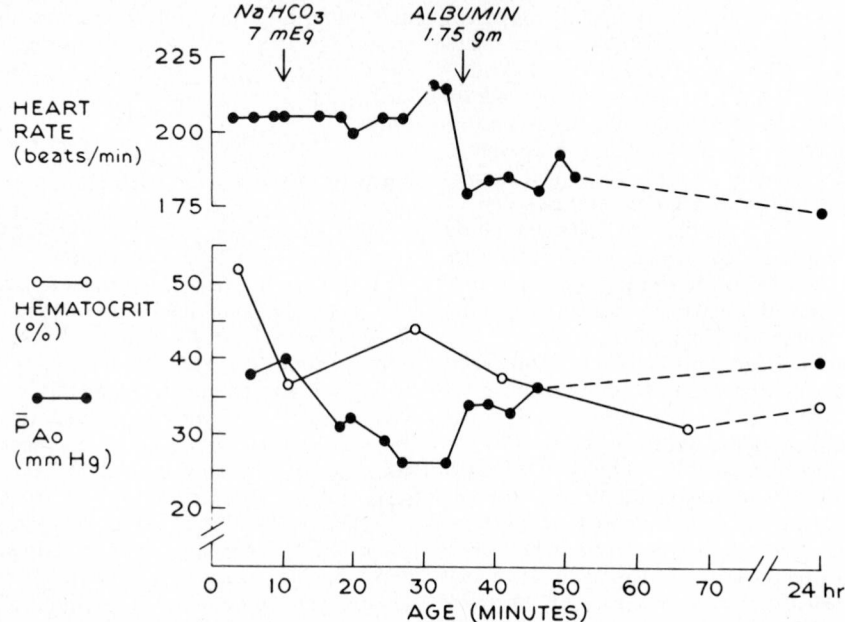

FIG. 6.   The effects of sodium bicarbonate (NaHCO₃) on mean aortic blood pressure (PaO), heart rate, and hematocrit. Hypotension and tachycardia occurred following the treatment of acidosis. These are signs of hypovolemia, which were initially masked by the vasoconstriction caused by the acidosis. The drop in hematocrit and rise in blood pressure with the infusion of NaHCO₃ suggest that the blood volume was transiently increased. However, a sustained drop in hematocrit and a normal heart rate and blood pressure required the infusion of albumin.

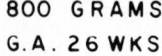

800 GRAMS

G.A. 26 WKS

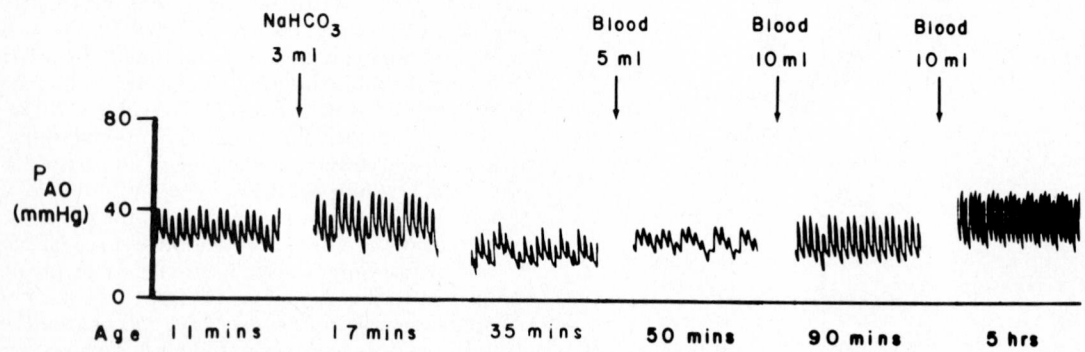

FIG. 7.   Aortic blood pressure (PaO) during the first 5 hours after birth in an 800-g infant born after a 26-week gestation. After initial ventilation and correction of metabolic acidosis, arterial blood pressure was 30/10 torr and varied markedly with respiration. After receiving 25 ml of blood (about 35 percent of the infant's blood volume), the aortic pressure was normal. (From Kitterman JA, Phibbs RH, Tooley WH: Pediatr Clin North Am 17:895, 1970)

is pale, and capillary filling is slow. Arterial blood pressure should be measured continously, directly from an umbilical artery, or it can be measured indirectly with a Doppler system. Normal values for intra-arterial pressure during the first 12 hours are shown in Figure 27, p.165. If the mean arterial pressure is more than 2 SD below the average, the infant is hypotensive and in most cases has hypovolemia. The hypotension can be profound (Fig. 7). Intrathoracic venous pressures (right or left atrial) are also useful for the diagnosis of hypovolemia. Normally, right and left atrial and inferior vena cava pressures are 3 to 8 cm H_2O above atmospheric pressure at end-expiration. If they are less than 3 cm H_2O above atmospheric pressure, circulating volume depletion should be suspected.

The treatment of hypovolemia is blood volume expansion. When the physician has advance notice of the premature delivery of a potentially asphyxiated and possibly hypovolemic infant, O-negative low titer blood should be crossmatched against the mother so that it can be given at birth if necessary. This is particularly important when there has been antepartum hemorrhage. Until blood is available, the blood volume can be expanded with plasma, 10 ml/kg body weight, or albumin, 1 g/kg body weight mixed with 10 ml/kg body weight physiologic saline or Ringer's lactate solution. Often these infusions must be followed by additional volumes of blood; the volumes of blood and fluid required to bring intravascular pressure, pulse, and perfusion to normal may be very large (Fig. 7).

Infants with an overexpanded vascular capacity (as with the intense vasodilation that occurs with infusion of alcohol or magnesium into the mother or with excessive heating with a heat lamp) may also have hypotension, and in them volume expansion must be done cautiously. Most of these infants will have blood pressure below the normal range even after they receive large volumes of fluid. If their peripheral perfusion (as judged by capillary filling) is normal, they are adequately ventilated, and do not develop a metabolic acidosis, *they should not be treated with volume expanders.* Their blood pressures will rise as the effect of the vasodilator wears off and their vascular capacity decreases.

The other causes of hypotension include pneumothorax and pneumomediastinum, so it is prudent to

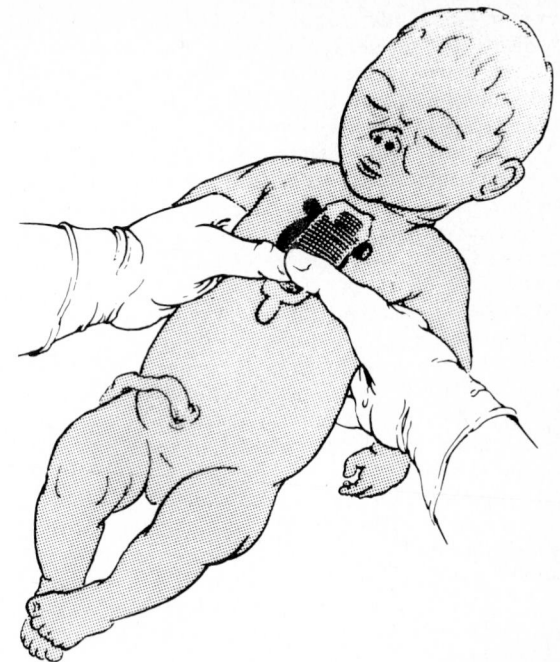

FIG. 8. Closed chest cardiac massage. For simplification, ventilation of the infant is not shown. (From Gregory GA: In Schnider S, Moya F (eds): The Anesthesiologist, The Mother and The Newborn. Baltimore, Williams and Wilkins, 1974)

obtain a film of the chest as soon after birth as possible if an infant has signs of shock. Large air leaks may cause hypotension by reducing the return of venous blood to the heart and decreasing cardiac output. Hypoglycemia, a blood glucose under 20 or 30 mg/100 ml in preterm and term infants, respectively, and hypocalcemia may also depress the myocardium, reduce cardiac output, and cause hypotension.

CARDIAC MASSAGE. If the heart rate is less than 100 beats/minute and does not increase to normal with stimulation and ventilation, closed chest cardiac massage must be done at a rate of 100 chest compressions per minute. To do this place your fingers behind the infant's chest to support the back, and your thumbs over the junction of the lower and middle third of the

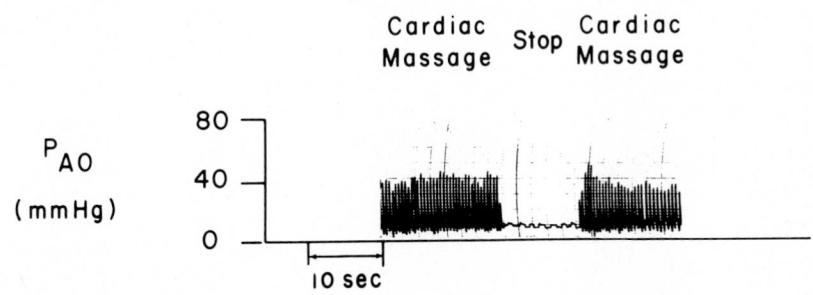

FIG. 9. Aortic blood pressure (Pao) during cardiac massage. (From Kitterman JA, Phibbs RH, Tooley WH: Pediatr Clin North Am 17:895, 1970)

sternum (Fig. 8), then compress the sternum two-thirds the distance to the vertebral column. The effectiveness of cardiac massage should be monitored by arterial blood pressure, as measured via an umbilical arterial catheter, and by an electrocardiogram. An arterial systolic pressure of approximately 80 torr at 100 compressions per minute will maintain a diastolic blood pressure of 15 to 20 torr, which is probably adequate for coronary perfusion (Fig. 9). While performing cardiac massage, ventilate the infant at a frequency of about 40 breaths a minute.

Throughout resuscitation, an infant must be warm. Cooling increases pulmonary vascular resistance and oxygen consumption. After resuscitation, carefully observe the severely depressed infant, who often is irritable and may have involuntary muscular movements, which are often due to electrolyte abnormalities. Since many of these infants have hypoglycemia, hypokalemia, and hypocalcemia in the first days after birth, we have usually given them 10 percent glucose, 2 mEq KCl/kg/24 hours and 200 mg/kg/24 hours of calcium gluconate for the first 24 to 48 hours. It is important to follow severely depressed infants for several years in order to document their neuromuscular and intellectual development.

Bibliography

Apgar V: A proposal for a new method of evaluation of the newborn infant. Curr Res Anesth 32:260, 1953

Apgar V, James LS: Further observations on the newborn scoring system. Am J Dis Child 104:419, 1962

Drage JS, Berendes H: Apgar scores and outcome of the newborn. Pediatr Clin North Am 13:635, 1966

James LS, Weisbrot IM, Prince CE, et al: The acid-base status of human infants in relation to birth asphyxia and onset of respiration. J Pediatr 52:379, 1958

Eckenhoff JE: Some anatomic considerations of the infant larynx influencing endotracheal anesthesia. Anesthesiology 12:401, 1951

Gregory GA: Resuscitation of the newborn. Anesthesiology 43:225, 1975

Gregory GA, Gooding C, Phibbs RH, Tooley WH: Meconium aspiration in infants, a prospective study. J Pediatr 85:848, 1974

Gunther M: The transfer of blood between baby and placenta in the minutes after birth. Lancet 1:1277, 1957

Kitterman JA, Phibbs RH, Tooley WH: Aortic blood pressure in normal newborn infants. Pediatr Clin North Am 17:895, 1970

Kitterman JA, Phibbs RH, Tooley WH: Catheterization of umbilical vessels in newborn infants. Pediatrics 44:959, 1969

Oh W, Lind J, Gessner IH: The circulatory and respiratory adaptation to early and late cord clamping in newborn infants. Acta Pediatr Scand 55:17, 1966

Oh W, Wallgren G, Hanson VS, et al: The effects of placental transfusion on respiratory mechanics of normal term infants. Pediatrics 40:6, 1967

THE CONTROL OF BREATHING

JUNE P. BRADY
JOHN G. BROOKS

During the early months of life there are important changes in an infant's ability to reflexly increase ventilation. Compared to the adult, the newborn infant has a relatively greater ventilatory requirement but a less effective system of respiratory function and control. This discrepancy is exaggerated by premature birth. The newborn infant's relatively greater oxygen consumption (4 to 6 ml/kg/minute compared to 3 to 4 ml/kg/minute in the adult) and his lower serum buffering capacity necessitate greater ventilation to maintain a normal arterial Po_2 and pH. Immaturity of both peripheral and central nervous system influences the control of breathing in early life. At birth there is incomplete myelination of peripheral nerves, which may prolong nerve conducting time, and there is relatively sparse integration of some central nervous system pathways, which may contribute to instability of respiratory drive.

The immaturity of the chest wall, airways, and lung parenchyma is of major significance in the ventilatory responsiveness of the newborn baby. Adequate ventilation requires relatively more work in the infant than in the adult because of differences in parenchymal and airway anatomy. The thicker interalveolar septa and a deficiency of surfactant in the newborn infant increase the amount of transpulmonary pressure needed for lung inflation. The relatively greater compliance of conducting airways compared to terminal airspaces leads to a large portion of each breath being used to expand the conducting airways, and a higher dead space to tidal volume ratio than in the adult. This further increases the minute ventilation requirements in the newborn. There are no true alveoli at birth so that there is a relative deficit in both quantity and quality of alveolar-capillary surface for gas exchange.

Newborn infants also have compliant chest walls, which limit their ability to generate the negative intrathoracic pressures required to inflate their relatively stiff lungs. This, and the relatively weak respiratory muscles, can be especially marked handicaps for prematurely born infants. Absence of alveolar pores for collateral ventilation, poor chest wall support, small respiratory units, and, in some premature newborns, inadequate surfactant all contribute to the development of atelectasis and increase the work of breathing.

The newborn infant's airway is vulnerable to obstruction, and this also may interfere with effective ventilation. Newborn infants have relative micrognathia, and the base of the tongue is posterior. This and the higher level of the larynx and epiglottis make the posterior pharyngeal airway narrow and easy to obstruct. In some infants flexion of the neck or lying in the supine position may cause some degree of upper airway obstruction. In addition, most infants are obligate nose breathers until 2 to 3 months of age, and many will not attempt to breathe through the mouth when the nose is obstructed.

CHEMICAL CONTROL

The chemical control of respiration is mediated by peripheral chemoreceptors, the carotid and aortic bodies which are primarily sensitive to hypoxemia, and the central medullary chemoreceptor which is most sensitive to hydrogen ion concentration and responds to changes in arterial Pco_2 (Fig. 10).

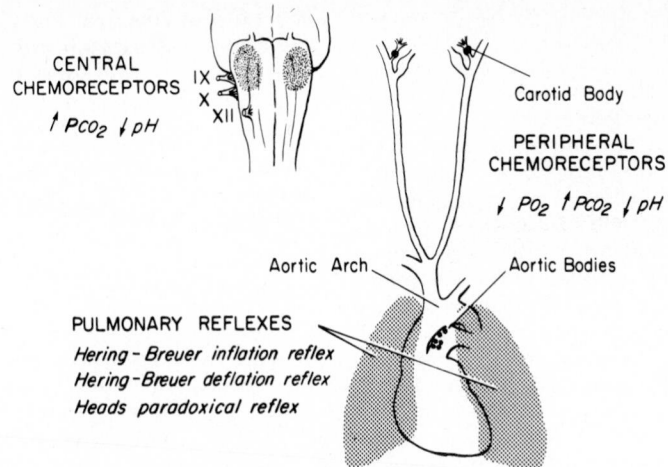

FIG. 10.   Schematic diagram of heart, lungs, and dorsal medulla, showing major sites of pulmonary and cardiovascular chemoreceptors and central chemosensitive areas in the medulla.

The peripheral chemoreceptors are present in the fetus, both anatomically and functionally, by the seventh month of gestation. They appear less sensitive in the fetus than after birth, requiring greater falls in arterial Po_2 to stimulate respiratory effort. The hypoxic ventilatory response can be evaluated by administering either hyperoxic or hypoxic inspiratory gas mixtures. Both methods produce biphasic ventilatory responses in newborns. The typical newborn response to breathing 100 percent oxygen is a 20 to 40 percent decrease in ventilation over the first minute, primarily due to a decrease in respiratory frequency, followed by an increase in ventilation to 10 to 30 percent above control values by the end of the third minute. The initial decrease probably reflects elimination of some normal hypoxic ventilatory stimulation. Rigatto and Brady found no significant effect of gestational age (32 to 37 weeks) or of postnatal age (2 to 26 days) on the ventilatory response to hyperoxia, although there was a trend toward more prolonged respiratory depression in more mature infants.

In both full-term and premature newborns, hypoxic inspired gas (12 to 15 percent oxygen) produces a 10 to 20 percent increase in minute ventilation during the first minute followed by a decrease to 10 to 20 percent below control values by the third minute (Fig. 11). There is a trend toward a greater hyperventilation phase with increasing gestational age. At about 10 days after birth in the full-term and by 18 days in the prematurely born, breathing an hypoxic gas mixture causes sustained hyperventilation. This change in response may be due to changes in pulmonary function or closure of the fetal circulatory channels rather than any alteration in chemoreceptors or in the neural reflex system.

Both hyperoxia and hypoxia can produce irregular respiratory patterns. In many premature infants an abrupt change from 15 to 21 percent or 21 to 100 percent inspired oxygen will result in intermittent respiratory pauses, usually self limiting, with resumption of a

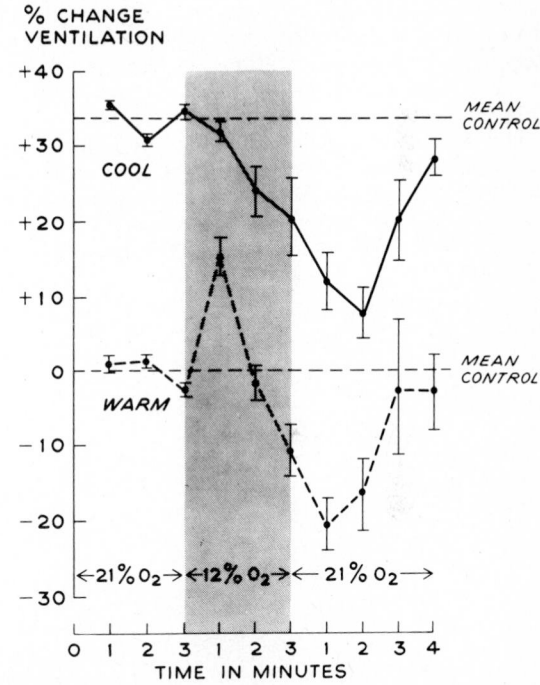

FIG. 11.   The effect of cooling the environment on the ventilatory response to hypoxia in 10 normal term infants. Note that ventilation is significantly increased in the cool environment compared with the warm (thermoneutral) environment. When hypoxia is present, the initial hyperventilation, but not the secondary hypoventilation, is abolished. (From Ceruti E: Pediatrics 37:566, 1966)

regular rhythm after several minutes. Mild, chronic hypoxemia may cause periodic breathing in some premature infants.

Almost all newborns respond to inspired CO_2 concentrations of 0.5 to 6.5 percent with an increase of minute ventilation, or at least an increase in the work of breathing. Newborn infants have a low resting arterial P_{CO_2} (32 to 36 torr) compared to the adults (38 to 42 torr) which indicates that they have a lower CO_2 threshold. There is no significant difference in CO_2 sensitivity between the infant born at term and the adult, when the response is standardized for body weight. Rigatto and Brady found no significant effect of gestational age (32 to 37 weeks) or postnatal age (2 to 27 days) on CO_2 threshold in prematures; however, they did demonstrate an increase in CO_2 sensitivity with increasing gestational age. There is a good correlation between CO_2 sensitivity and lung compliance in newborns, so it is not clear whether the increasing sensitivity with increasing age is due to changing lung mechanics or to neural maturation, since both occur simultaneously during the neonatal period. CO_2 sensitivity is depressed by morphine and probably during active or rapid eye movement (REM) sleep (Fig. 12).

Cool environmental temperatures (25 to 28 C) cause a 30 to 40 percent increase in minute ventilation in full-term newborns, presumably to meet the infant's increased oxygen needs. When given 12 percent oxygen in nitrogen to breathe, such cool infants immediately hypoventilate, with no transient hyperventilation. Cooling does not affect the ventilatory response to CO_2 in normal full-term infants.

The pulmonary stretch receptors located throughout most of the conducting airways and the chest wall intercostal muscle spindle receptors both respond to mechanical deformation and influence respiratory drive (see Table 6). The pulmonary stretch receptors re-

Table 6. The Location, Stimulus, Afferent Pathway, and Effect on Respiratory Drive of the Respiratory Mechanoreceptors

	Stretch Receptors	Chest Wall Receptors
Location	Conducting airways	Intercostal muscle spindles
Stimulus	↑ Lung volume	↑ Respiratory load
Afferent pathway	Vagus	Intercostal nerves
Effect on respiratory drive	↓	↑

spond to increases in transpulmonary pressure (usually due to increases in lung volume); the afferent pathway is the vagus and the response is respiratory inhibition. This is the Hering-Breuer inflation-inhibition reflex and may be important in controlling respiratory rate in newborn infants (Fig. 13). This reflex is very active by 36 to 38 weeks of gestation and is probably active much earlier. Its presence can be demonstrated for several weeks after a full-term birth and several months after a premature birth but cannot be demonstrated in normal conscious adults within the normal tidal volume range. The decline in the Hering-Breuer reflex after a month of age may be due to a simultaneous increase in lung compliance, since decreases in lung compliance appear to sensitize the pulmonary stretch receptors.

The chest wall mechanoreceptors are stimulated by an increase in respiratory work load; the dorsal branches of the intercostal nerves carry the afferent impulses. The response to this stimulus is an increase in respiratory muscle power. This important reflex can be evaluated by measuring the inspiratory effort generated when the airway is transiently occluded. Bodegard demonstrated that newborn infants of about 31 weeks gestational age may *decrease* their inspiratory effort when the

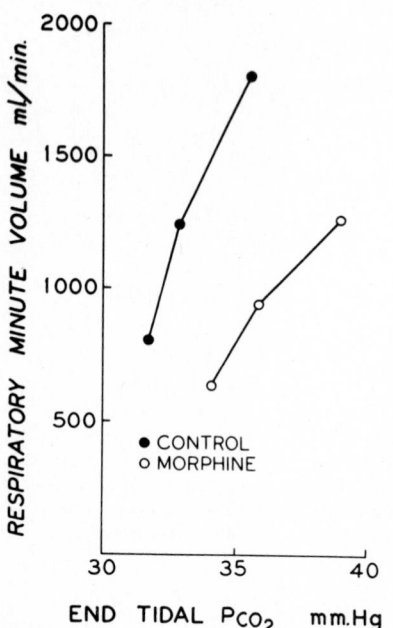

FIG. 12. Effect of morphine on the CO_2 response curve of 4 normal term infants. Note that the curve is depressed and shifted to the right after the administration of morphine. (Redrawn from Way WL: Clin Pharmacol Thera 6:454, 1965)

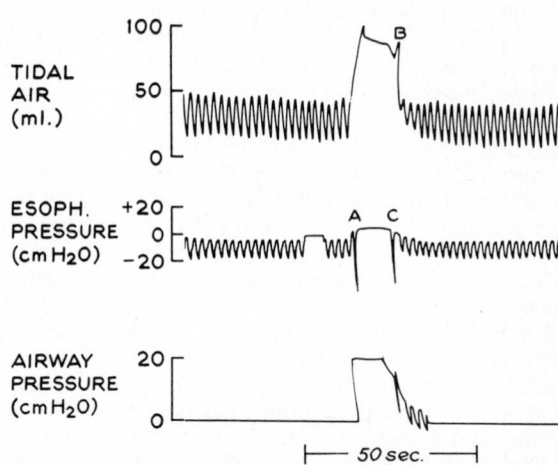

FIG. 13. The Hering-Breuer and Head's paradoxic reflexes in a full-term infant, 25 hours old. Inflation of the lungs by positive pressure produces gasp (A) followed by apnea (A-C). When the airway pressure drops, there is a second gasp (B) and resumption of normal breathing. (From Cross KW et al: J Physiol (London) 151:551, 1960)

airway is occluded, while normal full-term newborn infants will nearly double their inspiratory effort to overcome an airway occlusion. Others have shown that a small number of full-term newborns, particularly during REM sleep, will make little or no apparent effort to inspire when cellophane is placed over the nose and mouth. This phenomenon may reflect the activity of some naso-oral apnea-inducing receptors.

ABNORMALITIES OF CONTROL OF RESPIRATION

Apnea (cessation of breathing for 10 sec) is one of the most common problems of infants born after less than 34 weeks gestation who are more than 4 days of age. It tends to occur after feeding, with a bowel movement, with overheating, or during sleep, and usually begins

Table 7. Causes of Apnea in the Newborn Infant

Pathologic Causes

Infection
    Neonatal pneumonia (with or without hypoxemia),
       sepsis (from any cause), meningitis
Respiratory distress
    Severe hyaline membrane disease, moderate
       hyaline membrane disease with hypoxemia,
       pulmonary hemorrhage, pulmonary dysmaturity
       syndrome
Metabolic
    Hypoglycemia, hypocalcemia, hypernatremia
Cardiovascular
    Shock, patent ductus arteriosus with congestive
       heart failure, polycythemia
Central nervous system
    Seizures, intracranial hemorrhage, bilirubin
       encephalopathy
Maternal drugs
    Morphine, magnesium sulfate
Maternal drug withdrawal
    Heroin, methadone

Physiologic Causes (Uncommon except in premature)

Sleep
Feeding
Bowel movement
Increase in environmental
    temperature
Mild hypoxemia

after a period of periodic breathing during expiration. In the first 4 days after birth, it is usually a grave sign, but it may indicate major disease at any time. The causes of neonatal apnea are listed in Table 7.

Periodic breathing consists of regular and repeated episodes of breathing of less than 30 sec, followed by respiratory pauses longer than 2 sec (Fig. 14). It can be induced by mild hypoxemia and is often abolished by breathing oxygen or carbon dioxide. Infants with periodic breathing often have a reduction in minute ventilation, an increase in both arterial and alveolar carbon dioxide, and a decrease in arterial and alveolar oxygen tensions.

TREATMENT.   Periodic breathing is of no significance unless it is associated with recurrent periods of apnea, requiring stimulation and ventilatory assistance to initiate breathing. Cardiorespiratory monitors allow early recognition of the apneic spell before severe hypoxemia occurs. In some instances raising the inspired oxygen by 1 or 2 percent (ie, from 21 to 23 percent) may stimulate respiration and prevent apnea. However, high levels of oxygen are contraindicated in the *healthy* preterm infant, unless there are frequent measurements of arterial Po_2 so that it is kept at 60 to 80 torr. Recently, it has been shown that the application of a continuous positive airway pressure with a mask decreases the number and severity of apneic spells. This suggests that infants with periodic breathing may be breathing near their residual volume, which promotes atelectasis, increases respiratory work, and causes hypoxemia and hypercarbia. Theophylline has been reported to reduce periodic breathing and apnea, but its usefulness is uncertain. If theophylline is used, frequent determinations of its levels in serum must be made.

SUDDEN INFANT DEATH SYNDROME (SIDS)

Each year about 10,000 infants (1 per 300 to 400 live births) die without apparent cause between 1 week and 1 year of age (see also p. 831). Usually they appear healthy when last observed alive and are found dead in their cribs in the morning (hence the alternate terms *crib death* and *cot death*). At postmortem examination, the only regularly noted abnormalities are petechiae on the intrathoracic structures and a minor amount of intra-

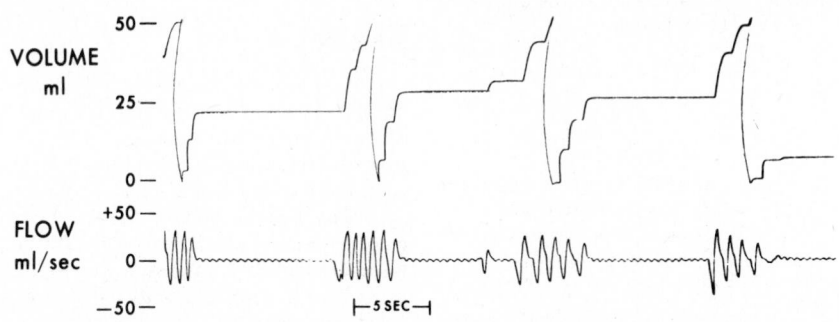

FIG. 14. Tracing of respiratory volume and flow from a 13-day-old, 1,600 g, preterm infant. Note periods of breathing (5 sec) with periods of apnea (8 sec). (From Rigatto H, Brady JP: J Appl Physiol 32:423, 1973)

alveolar fluid. Some of the infants have a mild degree of laryngeal inflammation, but apparently not enough to obstruct the airway.

The risk of death from SIDS is greatest in infants born prematurely, twins, siblings of infants who have died of SIDS, and infants from poor families. Deaths are most likely to occur in winter months, are more common in cold than in temperate climates, and may increase in number after several days of cold weather. These observations have suggested that SIDS may be related to respiratory tract infections or hyperemia of mucous membranes (the consequence of keeping infants in dry, heated rooms on cold winter days). Repeated efforts to isolate a virus from these infants have failed and only subtle traces of viral disease (the laryngeal inflammation) have been found at autopsy.

Obstruction of the upper airway and/or disordered control of respiration, particularly during sleep, are the most likely causes of SIDS. Infants are obligatory nose-breathers and, when the nasopharynx becomes occluded, some nose-breathing infants may not breathe through their mouths. Some sleeping infants with occlusion of the upper airway make vigorous respiratory efforts but do not struggle or awaken. About half of the infants in REM sleep do not struggle, cry, or attempt to breathe through their mouths for at least 25 sec after occlusion of the nose. The infant with a partially or completely obstructed upper airway may create a markedly subatmospheric intrathoracic pressure as he or she attempts to breathe, and this might explain the intrathoracic petechiae and pulmonary edema. These observations support the possible role of upper airway obstruction with inflammation, edema, or mucus as the initiating event in some infants, particularly in the infant with little drive to respiration from hypercarbia or hypoxemia. As noted above, most newborn infants do not have well-developed peripheral chemoreceptor reflexes, and both central and peripheral chemoreceptor reflexes may be attenuated in some infants in the first months of life. The frequency and length of breath-holding spells increase in infants in the first year of life during REM sleep, and airway obstruction is often exaggerated during REM sleep. At this time the most reasonable explanation for SIDS would combine some disorder of respiratory control, perhaps transient in nature, with mild-to-moderate respiratory obstruction at an age when the infant is a nose-breather and is having increasingly long periods of REM sleep.

Bibliography

CHEMORECEPTORS

Krauss AM, Klain DB, Waldman S, Auld PAM: Ventilatory response to carbon dioxide in newborn infants. Pediatr Res 9:46, 1975

Rigatto H, Brady JP, Verduzco RT: Chemoreceptor reflexes in preterm infants: I. The effect of gestational and postnatal age on the ventilatory response to inhalation of 100% and 15% of O_2. Pediatrics 55:604, 1975

Rigatto H, Brady JP, Verduzco RT: Chemoreceptor reflexes in preterm infants: II. The effect of gestational and postnatal age on the ventilatory response to inhaled carbon dioxide. Pediatrics 55:614, 1975.

MECHANORECEPTORS

Bodegard G, Schwieler GH, Skoglund S, Zetterstrom R: Control of respiration in newborn babies: I. The development of the Hering-Breuer inflation reflex. Acta Pediatr Scand 58:567, 1969

Bodegard G, Schwieler GH: Control of respiration in newborn babies: II. The development of the thoracic reflex response to an added respiratory load. Acta Pediatr Scand 60:181, 1971

Cross KW, Klaus M, Tooley WH, Weisser K: The response of the newborn baby to inflation of the lungs. J Physiol 151:551, 1960

Olinsky A, Bryan MH, Bryan AC: Influence of lung inflation on respiratory control in neonates. J Appl Physiol 36:426, 1974

Olinsky A, Bryan MH, Bryan AC: Response of newborn infants to added respiratory loads. J Appl Physiol 37:190, 1974

SLEEP

Hathorn MKS: Analyses of the rhythm of infantile breathing. Br Med Bull 31:8, 1975

SUDDEN INFANT DEATH SYNDROME

Cross KW, Lewis SR: Upper respiratory tract obstruction and cot death. Arch Dis Child 45:211, 1971

Shaw EB: Sudden unexpected death in infancy syndrome. Am J Dis Child 116:115, 1968.

Steinschneider A: Prolonged apnea and the sudden infant death syndrome: Clinical and laboratory observations. Pediatrics 50:646, 1972

Swift PG, Emery JL: Clinical observations on responses to nasal occlusion in infancy. Arch Dis Child 48:947, 1973

CONGENITAL OBSTRUCTION OF THE RESPIRATORY TRACT

JOSEPH A. KITTERMAN

Obstruction to respiratory gas flow may occur at any location in the respiratory tract and, in most cases, constitutes a serious emergency. Although some obstructions are incompatible with life, diagnostic efforts should be vigorous in all infants with respiratory obstruction so that correctable lesions can be adequately treated before death or irreversible brain damage occurs secondary to asphyxia.

In addition to careful physical examination, diagnostic studies may include passage of a nasal catheter, direct laryngoscopy, bronchoscopy, contrast studies of larynx, trachea, and bronchi, and cineangiography of intrathoracic vessels.

CHOANAL ATRESIA

Congenital obstruction of the posterior nares (choanae) is a relatively common anomaly that is twice as frequent in females as males. In 90 percent of cases the obstruction is bony, and in the others it is membranous. Although several familial cases have been reported, it is not considered a genetic defect. Associated anomalies are frequent, especially congenital heart defects, gastrointestinal obstructions, and coloboma iridis. Unilateral choanal atresia usually causes no difficulties in the newborn period.

Bilateral choanal atresia causes severe distress immediately after birth, which is relieved by opening the infant's mouth. Since most newborn infants are obligate nose-breathers, asphyxia occurs unless the infant's mouth is kept open. The diagnosis is made by the inability to pass a flexible plastic catheter (size 8 Fr) through either nostril into the pharynx. Immediate treatment is to maintain the infant's mouth open with an oropharyngeal airway or a feeding nipple with a large hole cut in the tip. Definitive treatment consists of surgical excision of the obstructing bony plate. Postoperative regrowth of tissue with resultant obstruction can be prevented by inserting plastic tubes through the nose from the anterior nares to the pharynx. Survival depends upon early recognition to prevent asphyxia and the severity of any associated anomalies. Follow-up studies of patients have shown that they have normal growth of facial bones, palate, and paranasal sinuses and that they have a normal sense of smell.

PIERRE ROBIN ANOMALY

This condition consists of micrognathia and glossoptosis, with or without associated cleft palate. Respiratory obstruction occurs when the tongue falls against the posterior pharyngeal wall during inspiration and is held there by the marked negative pressure in the lower pharynx caused by the inspiratory effort. Signs of obstruction are usually accentuated when the infant is supine or asleep. In rapid eye movement (REM) sleep, relaxation of the muscles in the posterior pharynx may allow the tongue to almost completely occlude the larynx. Cor pulmonale may result secondary to chronic alveolar hypoxia. Feeding is a major problem because of the respiratory obstruction and also the cleft palate, when present.

Several methods of treatment have been suggested. These include maintaining the infant in the prone position, an elastoplast cap to support the head when the infant is prone, glossopexy to keep the tongue held forward, and a flexible, indwelling nasoesophageal tube to prevent respiratory obstruction by avoiding development of marked negative pressure in the lower pharynx during inspiration. In severe cases only a tracheostomy will prevent continued obstruction with hypoventilation, pulmonary hypertension, congestive heart failure, and death. Feedings are accomplished by gavage or through a gastrostomy. With adequate nutrition, the infant's mandible usually grows to normal size, thus relieving the cause of the respiratory obstruction, and after 2 to 4 years the tracheostomy can be closed.

LARYNGEAL OBSTRUCTION

Several anomalies of the larynx may cause complete or partial respiratory obstruction. With the latter, there is stridor and, in some cases, an absent voice. Direct laryngoscopy can establish the diagnosis in most cases.

Atresia of the larynx is rare and is incompatible with life because of complete respiratory obstruction.

LARYNGEAL WEBS. Supraglottic webs are caused by portions of the false vocal cords, which remain fused together during development. Glottic webs result from fusion of a portion of the true cords. Subglottic webs are found in association with deformities of the cricoid cartilage. In some cases, the webs may be incised under direct laryngoscopy, but more extensive surgery is often necessary.

Cysts of the larynx may cause severe obstruction and an absent voice; in some cases, they are pedunculated and cause intermittent obstruction, and diagnosis may be very difficult, requiring direct laryngoscopy under general anesthesia. Excision of the cysts is necessary. A thyroglossal duct cyst at the base of the tongue may cause laryngeal obstruction; in these cases, symptoms are more severe with the infant supine.

Most *tumors of the larynx* are papillomas, which require resection. Other tumors are rare and include hemangiomas, lymphangiomas, and sarcomas (see p. 1554).

Paralysis of the vocal cords may be unilateral or bilateral. With the former, there is stridor and a weak cry; on laryngoscopy the affected cord is seen to lie flaccid in the midline. The causes include *Erb's palsy*, with right vocal cord paralysis and cardiovascular anomalies, mediastinal tumors, or thoracic surgery when the left cord is involved. With bilateral vocal cord paralysis, the cry sounds normal, but there is severe stridor; this condition is associated with birth injury, cerebral agenesis, and meningomyelocele.

Although not due to congenital factors, laryngeal obstruction may occur in newborn infants after removal of an endotracheal tube used for treatment of respiratory insufficiency. The most common cause is laryngeal edema, which becomes evident in the first few hours after the endotracheal tube has been removed. Because of the small size of an infant's larynx, a small amount of edema may cause severe obstruction. Treatment should include intermittent nebulization of racemic epinephrine and frequent measurements of arterial blood gases to detect progressive retention of carbon dioxide. In severe cases reinsertion of the endotracheal tube may be necessary; adrenal corticosteroids should be given for 24 hours before the endotracheal tube is again removed and should be continued for 2 to 3 days. In some infants, progressive obstruction due to subglottic stenosis may develop after removal of an endotracheal tube. This can be avoided in most cases by using a soft Portex tube without a wide shoulder and by ensuring the tube is not too large, as evidenced by a small leak around the tube at the larynx.

TRACHEAL AND BRONCHIAL OBSTRUCTIONS

Tracheomalacia is discussed on p. 1558.

Tracheal agenesis is a rare condition in which the larynx is hypoplastic, the trachea is absent, and the bronchi communicate with the esophagus. The diagnosis should be considered when respiratory distress occurs immediately after birth and the trachea cannot be intubated despite adequate visualization of the larynx. Death usually occurs shortly after birth due to respiratory insufficiency. Associated cardiovascular and gastrointestinal anomalies are common.

Other tracheal anomalies causing respiratory obstruction are also rare; they include stenosis, webs, diverticula, and thickened cartilaginous rings.

Obstructive bronchial lesions include agenesis (which may be associated with a fluid filled bronchogenic cyst) and stenosis. Stenosis of a mainstem bronchus may cause unilateral obstruction; successful resection of such lesions has been accomplished.

CARDIOVASCULAR CAUSES OF RESPIRATORY OBSTRUCTION

VASCULAR RING.　Anomalous vessels in the thorax may cause respiratory obstruction due to compression of the trachea or bronchi (see also p. 1440). Symptoms may begin shortly after birth or may not be apparent for several months.

Anomalies that have been shown to cause respiratory obstruction include double aortic arch, right aortic arch with left patent ductus arteriosus or ligamentum arteriosum, anomalous left common carotid artery, and anomalous left pulmonary artery arising from the right pulmonary artery. Anomalous right subclavian artery almost always passes behind the esophagus; it may cause dysphagia but does not cause respiratory obstruction. In patients in whom aberrant vessels cause respiratory obstruction, an exact anatomic diagnosis should be made before operative correction is attempted. This usually requires cineangiography and may require contrast studies of the tracheobronchial tree.

OBSTRUCTION ASSOCIATED WITH ACYANOTIC CONGENITAL HEART DISEASE.　In infants with acyanotic heart disease, respiratory obstruction may occur due to pulmonary hypertension or an enlarged left atrium (see also p. 1559). With pulmonary hypertension, the usual sites of obstruction are the superior aspect of the left mainstem bronchus, which may be compressed by the left pulmonary artery, and the intermediate bronchus (at its junction with the right middle lobe bronchus), which may be compressed by the right pulmonary artery. Left atrial enlargement may compress the left mainstem bronchus.

Such cases of obstruction will result in atelectasis if there is complete obstruction, or overinflation if there is partial obstruction; the latter situation is an unusual cause of congenital lobar emphysema, which is discussed elsewhere.

In addition, massive cardiomegaly may obstruct the left mainstem bronchus or left lower bronchus and lead to atelectasis of the entire left lung or left lower lobe, respectively.

In all these cases the respiratory obstruction is a secondary effect and treatment should be directed toward the primary cardiac lesion. In some cases bronchial compression by cardiovascular structures may be an important cause of respiratory complications after cardiac surgery.

OTHER CAUSES OF RESPIRATORY OBSTRUCTION. Congenital goiter and cystic hygroma present as obvious masses in the neck and rarely may cause tracheal obstruction. Intrathoracic tumors rarely cause respiratory obstruction; when they do, therapy and prognosis depend upon the specific tumor present.

Bibliography

Altman RP, Randolph JG, Shearin RB: Tracheal agenesis: recognition and management. J Pediatr Surg 7:112, 1972

Chang N, Hertzler JH, Gregg RH, Lofti MW, Brough AJ: Congenital stenosis of the right mainstem bronchus. Pediatrics 41:739, 1968

Dennison WM: The Pierre Robin Syndrome. Pediatrics 36:336, 1965

Flake CG, Ferguson CF: Congenital choanal atresia in infants and children. Ann Otolaryngol 73:458, 1964

Gregory GA: Respiratory care of newborn infants. Pediatr Clin North Am 19:311, 1972

Gross RE, Neuhauser EBD: Compression of the trachea or esophagus by vascular anomalies. Pediatrics 7:69, 1957

Hobolth N, Buchmann G, Sandberg LE: Congenital choanal atresia. Acta Pediatr Scand 56:286, 1967

Lewison MM, Lim DT: Apnea in the supine position as an alerting symptom of a tumor at the base of the tongue in small infants. J Pediatr 66:1092, 1965

Mattila MHK, Suutarinen T, Sulamaa M: Prolonged endotracheal intubation or tracheostomy in infants and children. J Pediatr Surg 4:674, 1969

Pruzansky S, Richmond JB: Growth of mandible in infants with micrognathia. Am J Dis Child 88:29, 1954

Stanger P, Lucas RV, Edwards JE: Anatomic factors causing respiratory distress in acyanotic congenital cardiac disease. Pediatrics 43:760, 1969

Stern LM, Fonkalsrud EW, Hassakis P, Jones MH: Management of Pierre Robin Syndrome in infancy by prolonged nasoesophageal intubation. Am J Dis Child 124:78, 1972

Swenson O: Pediatric Surgery, 3rd ed. Appleton-Century-Crofts, New York, 1900, p 1417

Warkany J: Congenital malformations. Year Book Publishers, Chicago, 1971, p 1309

Zumbro GL, Treasure RL, Geiger JP: Respiratory obstruction in the newborn associated with increased volume and opacification of the hemithorax. Ann Thor Surg 18:622, 1974

ACUTE RESPIRATORY DISTRESS SYNDROMES

DELAYED ABSORPTION OF FETAL LUNG FLUID

RICHARD D. BLAND

An essential step for extrauterine adaptation is the displacement of intraalveolar fluid by air and the absorption of excessive pulmonary interstitial fluid into the vascular system. This transition is remarkably brief in most newborn infants, facilitating exchange of oxygen and carbon dioxide within minutes of birth. In some infants, however, the process is delayed, producing the clinical and radiographic features of *delayed absorption of fetal lung liquid* sometimes called *transient tachypnea of the newborn* or *wet lung disease*.

CLINICAL FEATURES.　In 1966, Avery and associates described the clinical and radiographic features of 8 babies with transient tachypnea of the newborn, a condition they attributed to delayed absorption of fetal lung liquid. All of the infants they described were delivered at term, and only one by cesarean section. However, subsequent reports have stressed the increased incidence of this condition in infants born prematurely, by cesarean section, or following vaginal birth with breech presentation. It is more common in males than in females and is characterized by the early onset of an elevated respiratory rate, ranging from 60 to 160/minute, sometimes with retractions of the chest wall, grunting on expiration, and, occasionally, mild cyanosis, which can be relieved by increasing environmental oxygen. Auscultation of the lungs usually reveals clear breath sounds, with no rales or rhonchi. The symptoms usually disappear within 4 days after birth. Most infants with transient tachypnea have hypoproteinemia, suggesting that reduced intravascular colloid osmotic pressure may contribute to the delay in absorption of lung fluid. The differential diagnosis includes hyaline membrane disease, pneumothorax and pneumomediastinum, congestive heart failure, aspiration of meconium, or bacterial pneumonitis, airway obstruction, and diaphragmatic hernia. The radiographic features usually distinguish these other causes of acute respiratory distress.

RADIOGRAPHIC APPEARANCE. Figure 15 is a chest radiograph from a newborn infant with delayed absorption of fetal lung liquid. The characteristic features include prominence of the pulmonary vascular markings, particularly toward the hilar regions, hyperaeration of the lungs, flattening and depression of the diaphragmatic domes, widening of the interlobar fissures, and a cardiac silhouette slightly larger than normal. There may be fluid in the pleural spaces.

PATHOPHYSIOLOGY. Interpretation of the pathophysiology of delayed absorption of lung fluid originates for the most part from observations made on fetal and neonatal lambs delivered by cesarean section. Though some fetal lung fluid may be removed from the mouth by compression of the thorax during the course of a vaginal delivery, most of it appears to be absorbed

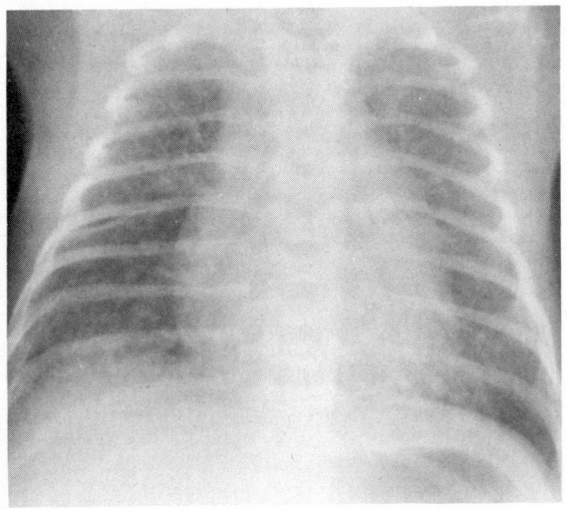

FIG. 15. Chest radiograph of an infant with delayed absorption of fetal lung liquid (transient tachypnea of the newborn). Note thickening of the interlobar fissure on the right, the bilateral prominence of the pleura, and the prominent perihilar vascular markings, all of which suggest the presence of excessive fluid in the lungs. The cardiac shadow is slightly enlarged.

via the pulmonary circulation and lymphatics. After breathing starts, there is a steady decline in lung water over the first 72 hours, most of it within 6 hours of birth. During this time, fluid distends the loose interlobular perivascular, peribronchial, and subpleural tissue spaces. Simultaneously, lymphatics become engorged as they transport up to 40 percent of the alveolar fluid to the systemic venous system. The remainder of the fluid presumably is absorbed directly by the pulmonary vasculature. Boston and his coworkers (1965) found a threefold increase in lung lymph flow in mature fetal lambs following the onset of ventilation, compared to a doubling of flow in the immature fetus. This difference in fluid clearance may account for some of the early respiratory distress of prematurely born infants. Fluid removal from the alveolar space and airways after birth can be delayed by antenatal asphyxia or hypervolemia (where an increase in the hydrostatic pressure in the pulmonary microcirculation favors movement of fluid out of the capillaries into the interstitial space).

TREATMENT. Unless the infant has immature lungs and develops hyaline membrane disease, absorption of fetal lung fluid usually is complete by 24 hours afterbirth and the symptoms disappear. An increased concentration of inspired oxygen may be required to maintain a normal Pao_2. Usually no other therapy is usually required.

Bibliography

DELAYED ABSORPTION OF LUNG FLUID

Adams FH, Yanagisawa M, Kuzela D, Martinek H: The disappearance of fetal lung fluid following birth. J Pediatr 78:837, 1971

Aberne W, Dawkins MJR: The removal of fluid from the pulmonary airways after birth in the rabbit, and the effect on this of prematurity and prenatal hypoxia. Biol Neonat 7:214, 1964.

Avery ME, Gatewood OB, Brumley G: Transient tachypnea of newborn. Possible delayed resorption of fluid at birth. Am J Dis Child 111:380, 1966

Humphreys PW, Normand ICS, Reynolds EOR, Strang LB: Pulmonary lymph flow and the uptake of liquid from the lungs of the lamb at the start of breathing. J Physiol 193:1, 1967

Karlberg P, Adams FH, Geubelle F, Wallgren G: Alteration of the infant's thorax during vaginal delivery. Acta Obstet Gynecol Scand 41:223, 1962

Kuhn JP, Fletcher BD, DeLemos RA: Roentgen findings in transient tachypnea of the newborn. Radiology 92:751, 1969

Sundell H, Garrott J, Blankenship WJ, Shepard FM, Stahlman MT: Studies on infants with type II respiratory distress syndrome. J Pediatr 78:754, 1971

HYALINE MEMBRANE DISEASE

WILLIAM H. TOOLEY

Hyaline membrane disease is the most common cause of severe, acute respiratory distress in the first days after birth and occurs in about 1 percent of newborn infants. It is also the most common cause of death in the neonatal period. Until about 1970, 50 percent of infants with this form of respiratory distress died. However, in recent years, improved methods of treatment have decreased mortality markedly, so that in many centers for newborn infant care, 80 to 90 percent of infants with hyaline membrane disease survive.

Hyaline membrane disease occurs mainly in infants born prematurely. It is the clinical expression of an immature lung, with small respiratory units that inflate with difficulty and do not remain gas-filled between respiratory efforts. This behavior is, in part, due to an inadequate amount of pulmonary surfactant. When surfactant is absent, the surface tension at the interface of gas and alveolar wall is high, and the lung tends to become progressively atelectatic. The infant has increasingly labored breathing, and perfusion of nonventilated areas of lung causes cyanosis.

One to 4 days following birth an immature lung can mature and develop thin-walled respiratory units that retain gas at end-expiration; when this occurs the signs and symptoms of respiratory distress subside. However, during this interval, lung damage may occur from the combined effects of ischemia, oxygen, and the high pressures used to assist ventilation, thereby prolonging the respiratory distress for many days or weeks.

Pathology

Hochheim, in 1903, provided the original description of the morphologic features of hyaline membrane disease. He noted membranes lining the walls of respiratory units in the lungs of many prematurely born infants who died during the first days of life. He called them myelin and postulated that they were caused by the aspiration of amniotic fluid.

At postmortem examination, the lungs from infants with hyaline membrane disease are very firm and airless. Atelectasis is striking on gross inspection. Even when the lungs are inflated before fixation, only the airways and a few alveolar ducts are air-filled (Fig. 16). Diffuse atelectasis characterizes the microscopic picture; in addition, many of the dilated terminal bronchioles and alveolar ducts have a lining of homogeneous hyaline-staining material (Fig. 17). These are the hyaline membranes, which are plasma clots composed of fibrin, other blood products, and cellular debris. The small pulmonary arterioles appear to be constricted, and there is appreciable congestion of pulmonary capillaries

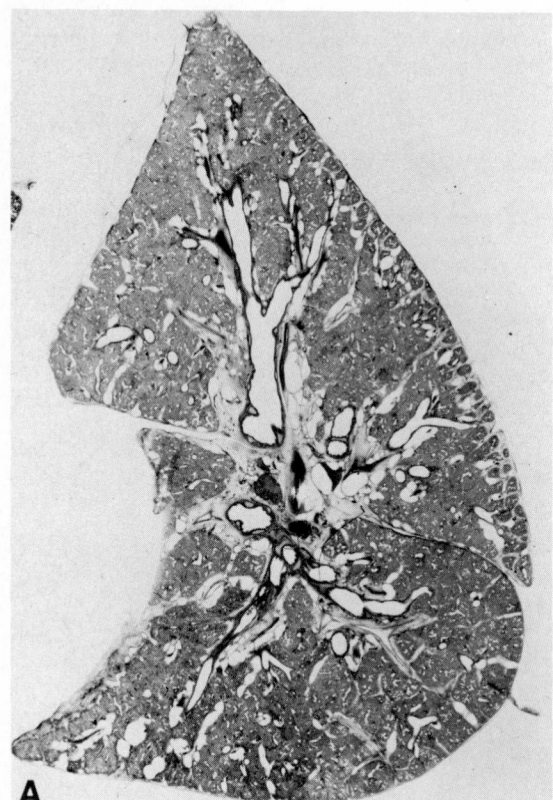
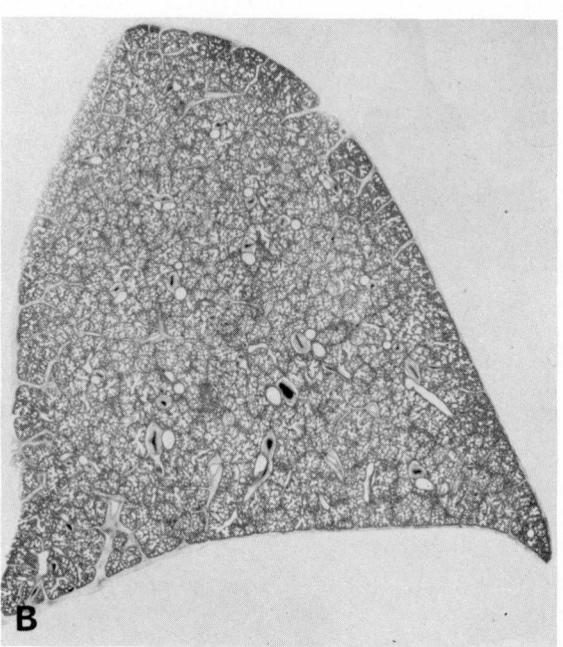

FIG. 16.   A. Longitudinal section of the left lung of a 1,560-g infant, born after a 30-week gestation, who died at 60 hours of age with hyaline membrane disease. The lung was expanded with air to a pressure of 40 cm H_2O, then deflated to 10 cm H_2O and fixed with the bronchus clamped. The airways are distended, and a few of the respiratory bronchioles are overinflated. Most of the alveolar ducts and alveoli are airless. **B.** Cross section of the left upper lobe of a 1,420-g infant, born after a 29-week gestation, without lung disease, who died at 1 week of age with a sudden, massive intraventricular hemorrhage. Inflation and fixation were identical to those used for the lung in Figure 16A. Almost all of the alveolar ducts are air-filled and the airways are not overdistended.

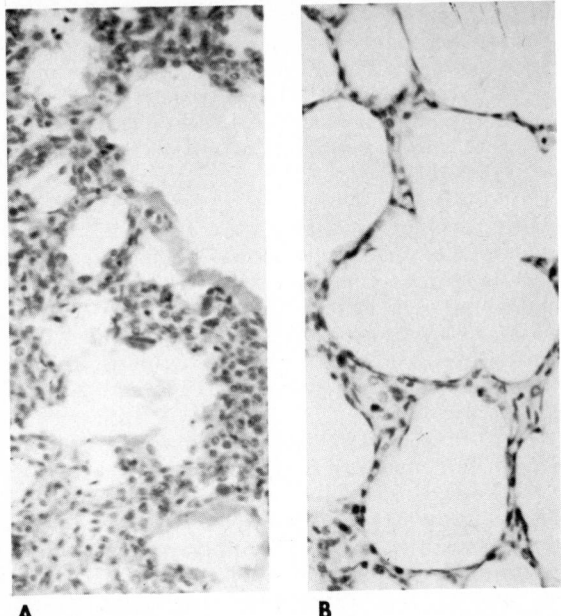

FIG. 17. **A.** Lung shown in Figure 16A at X100 magnification. Some of the alveolar ducts are inflated, but there are no alveoli. The interstitial tissue appears crowded, but no inflammatory cells are present. The homogeneous staining material lining the walls of the alveolar ducts are the hyaline membranes. **B.** Lung shown in Figure 16B at X100 magnification. The interstitial tissue is thin. Although there are no true alveoli in this section, the total surface area is large; particularly compared to the lung in Figure 17A.

and veins; in some cases the alveoli and hyaline membranes contain red cells. The intrapulmonary lymphatics are dilated, particularly those in the septa and around small airways and vessels.

If death occurs after several days, numerous macrophages engulf the intraalveolar material, with fragmentation of hyaline membranes. Electron microscopic studies show degeneration of epithelial and endothelial cells and ruptures of basement membranes. Dead cells and cell fragments enter the airspaces and become incorporated in the hyaline membranes.

When inflated with air, the lungs accept only 10 to 20 percent of the gas accommodated by normal lungs. After full expansion, as the distending pressure is decreased, the amount of gas retained at each pressure is a smaller proportion of the maximum gas volume than in the normal lung. This indicates that retractive forces are high in the air-filled lung with hyaline membrane disease. When distended with liquid, there is less difference in the pressure-volume relationships between the normal lung and the lung with hyaline membrane disease. This behavior was explained when Avery and Mead reported that extracts of lungs of infants dying with the disease did not have a low surface tension when studied with a Wilhelmy balance. The surface tension/surface area characteristics of extracts of lung with and without hyaline membrane disease are shown in Figure 18. Additional support for inadequate surfactant in this disease is the decreased amounts of phospholipids found in lung tissue, especially the disaturated lecithin characteristic of pulmonary surfactant.

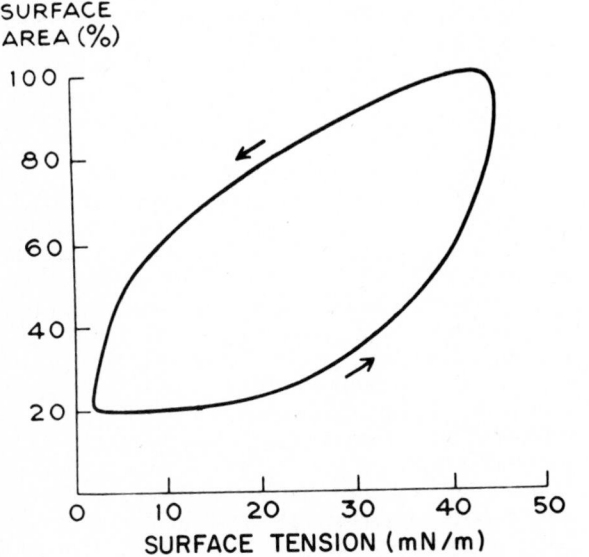

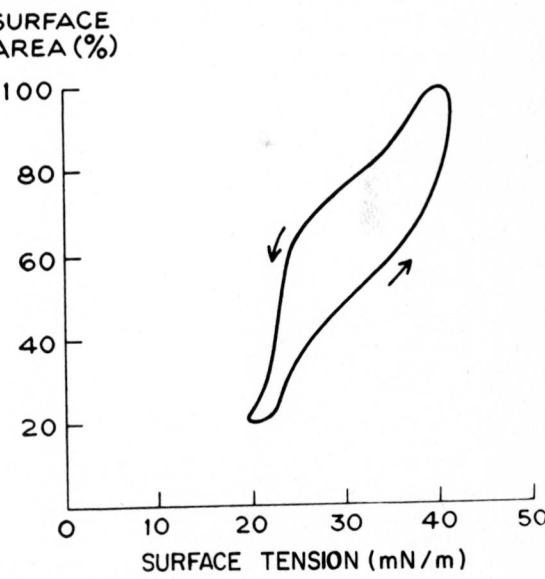

FIG. 18. Surface tension/surface area diagrams of extracts of lung from an infant with hyaline membrane disease (right) and a lung from an infant with normal lungs (left). These were obtained from a modified Wilhelmy surface tension balance in which surface tension is continuously recorded as the surface area of the lung extract is reduced and increased. When the surface area is reduced to 20 percent (equivalent to a lung changing from total lung capacity to residual volume) the surface tension of the extract from the lung with hyaline membrane disease is 20 milli Newtons per meter (20mN/m), a high tension, which, if present at the surface of the alveolus, would favor atelectasis. The surface tension at 20% surface area for extracts of normal lungs is 6 mN/m.

Clinical Features

Some infants with hyaline membrane disease fail to expand their lungs at birth even with vigorous inspiratory efforts, and have respiratory distress from the first minutes after birth. Others inflate their lungs initially but develop progressive atelectasis and increasingly labored breathing in the first few hours. The most characteristic clinical feature is an expiratory complaint or grunt; this noise is the result of a prolonged expiratory effort against a partially closed glottis. It is usually preceded by a strong inspiratory effort, with intrathoracic pressure well below atmospheric pressure. However, during the prolonged expiration, intrathoracic pressure is maintained above atmospheric pressure (Fig. 19). Infants do not grunt with every breath, but those with severe disease grunt most frequently. Grunting respiration is probably an effort to increase or maintain a lung volume that is adequate for respiratory gas exchange. When not grunting, infants with hyaline membrane disease have small tidal volumes and a rapid respiratory rate. Apneic periods and irregularities of respiratory rhythm are common as the work of breathing increases and the infants tire.

The large negative intrathoracic pressures generated by the infant as he attempts to inflate his lungs are reflected in retractions of the soft tissues of the chest cage. These are particularly notable in very small preterm infants because of the compliant chest wall. In severe cases, the lower sternum may be pulled in by the forceful contraction of the diaphragm. Since the chest wall is so compliant and since an infant breathes primarily with his diaphragm, the negative pressures generated during inspiration result in what has been

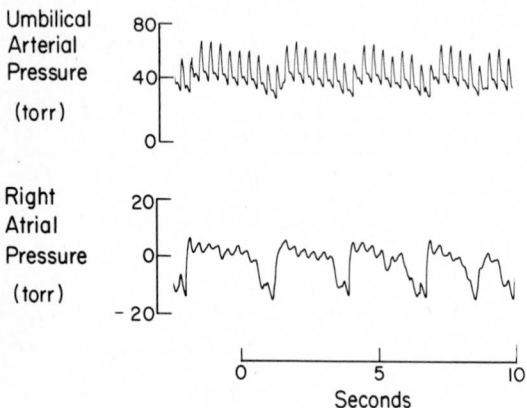

FIG. 19. Aortic blood pressure from an umbilical arterial catheter and right atrial pressure from an umbilical venous catheter in an infant with hyaline membrane disease who was grunting with each breath. With inspiration the right atrial pressure drops to 18 torr (mm Hg) below atmospheric pressure, reflecting the increased force required to expand the lung. During the prolonged expiration, or grunt, the atrial pressure is 4 torr above atmospheric pressure as a result of forcefully expiring against a partially closed glottis. The arterial pressure and pulse pressure decrease as the grunt continues, suggesting that the cardiac output is falling. The pattern of these vascular pressure changes is identical to that seen during Valsalva's maneuver.

called *paradoxic breathing.* The descent of the diaphragm increases lung volume in a cephalocaudad direction and encroaches on the abdominal cavity; thus, with inspiration, chest circumference becomes smaller and the abdominal circumference increases. There is flaring of the alae nasae during inspiration as respiration becomes more labored.

Cyanosis is an early sign and, as the atelectasis progresses, may be present even when an infant breathes 100 percent oxygen. Blood perfusing nonaerated areas of the lung (intrapulmonary shunting), venous blood entering the arterial circuit by way of the foramen ovale and ductus arteriosus (extrapulmonary shunting), and alveolar hypoventilation cause the cyanosis. Infants with rapidly increasing cyanosis often require assisted ventilation.

When using blood from an umbilical arterial catheter to judge oxygenation, it is well to keep the catheter tip in the lower aorta. If the catheter is above the diaphragm, its tip may enter the pulmonary artery by way of the ductus arteriosus. Blood withdrawn from this site will have a lower oxygen tension than arterial blood, and its use to guide treatment may lead to the delivery of unnecessarily high concentrations of oxygen to the infant.

Percussion of the chest is usually of no diagnostic help, except in the presence of a pneumothorax. Breath sounds are diminished in intensity and have a harsh, tubular quality. Occasionally there are fine rales, particularly in those infants born by cesarean section, who may have excessive lung liquid. Wheezing does not occur during the acute phase of the disease.

As the lungs become more difficult to ventilate, the work of breathing increases, and arterial carbon dioxide tension rises. At the same time hypoxemia increases, with accumulation of lactic acid as a result of anaerobic metabolism. With the development of acidosis, potassium leaves the cells and its concentration in serum may rise, in some instances to very high levels.

Many of these infants have systemic hypotension, peripheral pallor, slow capillary filling, and hypothermia; some are hypovolemic. In most cases the circulatory disturbances seem to be caused by hypoxemia and acidosis. Cardiac output may be low or normal but, as arterial oxygen tension falls and carbon dioxide rises, cardiac output is redistributed and blood flow to skin, kidney, and gut decreases. Diminished renal blood flow may cause renal shutdown. In all infants with hyaline membrane disease, urine output is low during the first days after birth. Peripheral edema is present in many cases. Reduced mesenteric blood flow may account, in part, for the ileus that often accompanies the disease. Another consequence of slow blood flow and pooling is increased hemolysis and jaundice. In small premature infants with low serum albumin, the indirect bilirubin may be high enough to require exchange transfusion. Occasionally, there is thrombocytopenia, prolonged thrombin and prothrombin times, and decreased fibrinogen. These signs of disseminated intravascular coagulation reflect the severity of the shock.

In mild to moderate cases, respiration becomes increasingly difficult for about 48 hours, but after 72 hours of age, grunting and retractions decrease and improvement is rapid. Recovery is usually heralded by diuresis. During this phase, a large amount of potassium may be excreted and the resulting hypokalemia may prolong the ileus and delay recovery. Clinical improvement is accompanied by a rapid fall in pulmonary vascular resistance and a rise in systemic arterial pressure. In some infants, particularly the least mature, with birthweights less than 1,500 g, this may permit development of a large shunt from the aorta through the ductus arteriosus to the pulmonary artery. In these infants recovery may be interrupted 4 to 5 days after birth by the development of congestive heart failure and pulmonary edema. The ductus usually closes spontaneously with conservative medical treatment of cardiac failure, but in some instances operative ligation may be necessary (see section on ductus arteriosus Chap 27, p. 1409). Recently, it has been shown that prostaglandin synthetase inhibitors, such as indomethacin given orally or rectally, may effectively close the ductus arteriosus.

Infants with more severe disease, which requires assisted ventilation, may have a more protracted course; but even in such cases, the amount of positive pressure needed to effect adequate ventilation is usually less after 72 hours. Thereafter, recovery may slow because of additional lung injury caused by treatment with oxygen and assisted ventilation. A prolonged course and the development of chronic respiratory distress is most common in infants who have had recurrent pulmonary air leaks (see below).

PULMONARY FUNCTION. Respiratory rate is rapid, and tidal volumes are small. Minute volume is usually increased; but since more than half of every breath is dead space ventilation, alveolar ventilation is low. Lung volume is low and tends to decrease during the first 48 hours after birth in infants who are not being treated with positive pressure ventilation. Lung compliance is very low, and airway resistance is increased, causing an appreciable increase in the work of breathing.

The relation of ventilation to perfusion is very abnormal. Some areas of the lung are ventilated but have little blood flow. This is presumably caused by ventilation of the dilated small airways and accounts for the large difference between alveolar and arterial carbon dioxide tensions. Other areas of the lung have little ventilation but a large blood flow, which accounts for much of the arterial desaturation. The rest is due to shunting of blood from right to left through the foramen ovale and ductus arteriosus. The relative contribution of the intra- and extrapulmonary shunts to the cyanosis probably varies from infant to infant and from time to time in the same infant. In most cases, the ductal component is small.

RADIOLOGIC FEATURES. The usual radiographic appearance of the lungs in infants with hyaline membrane disease is shown in Figure 20. There is a diffuse reticulogranular pattern of increased density, which is usually uniform in distribution but occasionally more marked in the bases or on one side. This represents miliary atelectasis. Lung volume is small and even radiographs taken after a maximal inspiration rarely show the diaphragm to be below the 8th to 9th interspace. The bronchial tree is clearly outlined by air against the poorly aerated lung (air bronchogram). The

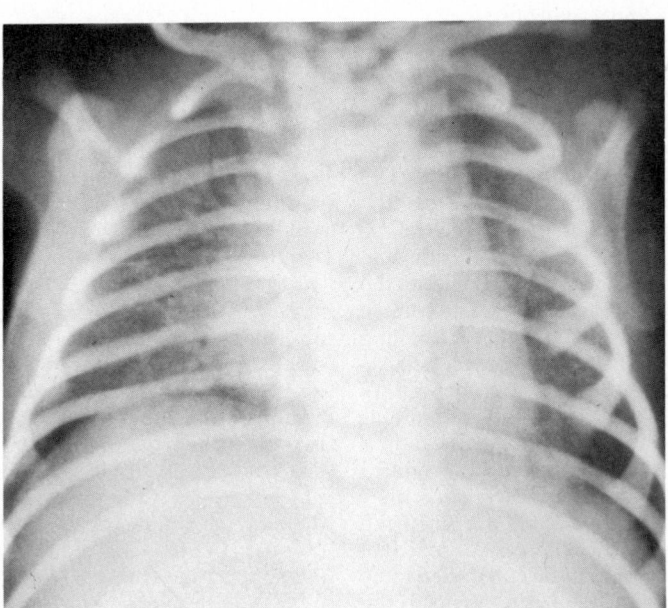

FIG. 20. Chest radiograph of an infant with hyaline membrane disease. The diaphragm is at the 7th interspace and there are fine reticulogranular patterns of density in both lung fields and bilateral air bronchograms.

heart is usually normal in size, although it often appears large because of the large thymic shadow and decreased lung volume.

This typical picture of diffuse atelectasis can be affected by treatment. Infants breathing against a positive airway pressure (see below) may have well-aerated lungs without air bronchograms. Infants with very severe disease, on the other hand, may be unable to expand their lungs at all and have totally opaque radiographs in which even the heart borders are obscured. Later in the course of the disease, pulmonary edema or pulmonary hemorrhage may distort the typical radiologic appearance.

PATHOGENESIS. The primary problem in hyaline membrane disease is atelectasis. This develops in small preterm infants from three interrelated factors: small respiratory units, a weak chest cage, and an amount of pulmonay surfactant that is inadequate to cover the internal surface of the lung.

In the adult, the alveolar diameter is about 200μ, in the term infant 100μ, and in the preterm infant 75μ. The diameter of the alveolar ducts and respiratory bronchioles of the prematurely born infant is also relatively smaller than that of infants born at term. Since the respiratory units are sharply curved, they should be governed by the Laplace relationship, which states that the pressure difference, P, across a curved surface needed to maintain a given radius, r, is inversely proportioned to the radius and directly related to the surface tension, ST; $(P = 2ST/r)$. The small respiratory units of the preterm infant require a greater force to inflate and a relatively larger transpulmonary pressure at end-expiration to keep them from deflating than those of the infant born at term. Infants born prematurely may not be able to create these pressures because their chest walls are weak and compliant.

The immature infant has a poorly supported chest cage and, during inspiration as the diaphragm descends, the chest wall is pushed in as intrathoracic pressure becomes negative. This inability to fix the lateral dimensions of the chest cage limits the amount of negative intrathoracic pressure that can be produced (Fig. 21). In addition, the highly compliant chest wall of the immature infant does not resist as well as that of the more mature infant the natural tendency of the lungs to collapse, so that at end-expiration the volume of the lungs and thorax tends to approach the residual volume of the lung. Incomplete initial inflation and a small lung volume at end-expiration both promote atelectasis.

Despite these handicaps, some prematurely born infants can inflate their lungs and acquire a stable surface area sufficient for the gas transfer required to meet their metabolic needs. The adaptation of these infants to extrauterine life, even with an inefficient chest cage, must depend on the structural development of the lung, with the appearance of alveoli and accumulation of sufficient surfactant to cover the alveolar surface. Synthesis and storage of surfactant begins at about 16 weeks of gestation, and lung homogenates have high concentrations of surfactant by 20 weeks. However, it does not reach the surface of the lung until later, appearing in amniotic

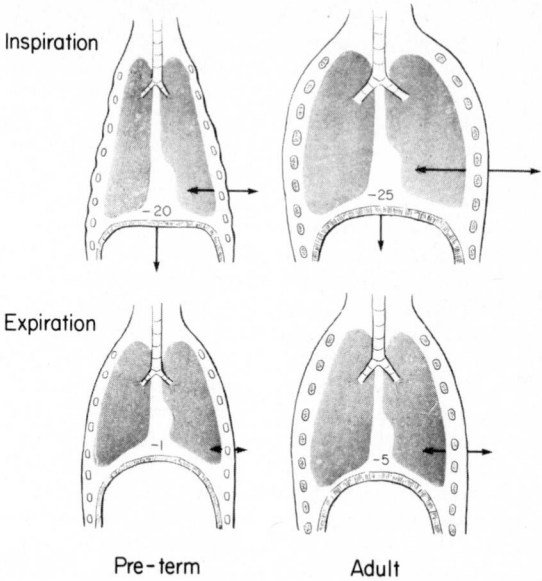

CHEST WALL IN PRE-TERM INFANT AND ADULT

Inspiration

Expiration

Pre-term   Adult

FIG. 21. The chest cage of a preterm infant is compared with the chest cage of an adult during inspiration and expiration. In the adult with a fixed or expanding lateral chest diameter, contraction and descent of the diaphragm enlarges the chest cage. When the diaphragm contracts in the preterm infant, the lateral diameter of the chest wall tends to be pushed inward and narrows so that the increase in volume of the chest cage is less than in the adult. At end-expiration, the chest wall does not resist the tendency of the lung to reach residual volume and the resting volume of the lung and thorax tends to approach the residual volume of the lung. In contrast the adult has a lung volume at end-expiration which is about 50 percent greater than the residual volume of the lung.

fluid between 28 and 38 weeks of gestation, as shown in Figure 22 and discussed below. Factors that control the secretion of surfactant are unknown, but secretion starts at about the same time as alveolar development begins. The variation in time of appearance of surfactant is evidence that the lung matures at different rates in different individuals. This explains why some infants with a gestational age of less than 30 weeks do not acquire hyaline membrane disease, while other infants with a longer gestation may do so.

PREDISPOSING FACTORS. There are several important factors, besides premature birth, which predispose newborn infants to hyaline membrane disease. The condition is twice as common in males as in females at every gestational age. It frequently follows delivery by cesarean section, particularly if this is done before labor has begun. Infants of diabetic mothers are five times more likely to develop hyaline membrane disease than infants of nondiabetic mothers, with the same gestational age, sex, and mode of delivery.

Asphyxia increases the possibility that an immature infant will develop hyaline membrane disease. At each gestational age, infants with Apgar scores below 8 at 5 minutes of age are more likely to have the disease than infants of the same gestational age with Apgar scores of

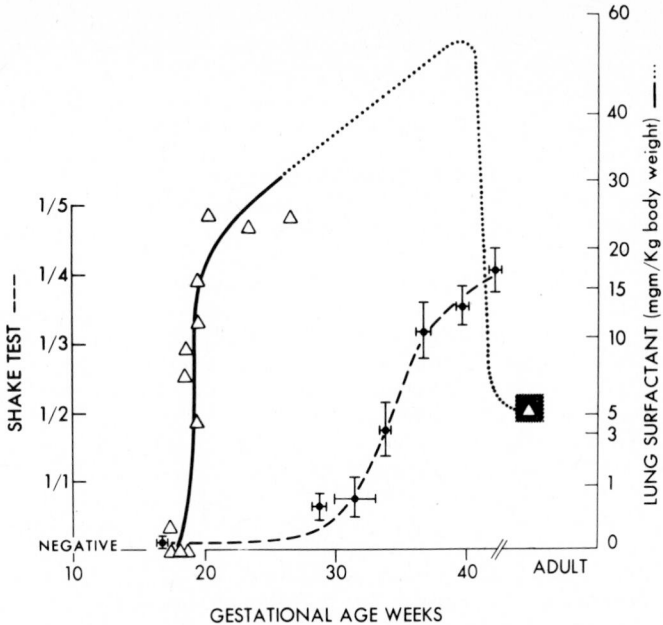

FIG. 22. The relation between gestational age and surfactant in homogenates of whole lung (open circles and solid line) and gestational age and surfactant in amniotic fluid as judged by the shake test (see text, broken line and solid dots). By 22 weeks gestation there is more than 10 times as much surfactant per gram of fetal lung than in the adult lung. However, surfactant is usually not detected in amniotic fluid until after 30 weeks gestation and cannot be demonstrated in dilute amniotic fluid until 35 to 36 weeks gestation.

8 or above. That asphyxia may be associated with atelectasis in the neonatal period is not surprising, since depressed asphyxiated infants may not be able to make sufficiently vigorous initial inspiratory efforts to inflate the lungs fully at birth. Furthermore there is good evidence that acidosis interferes with production of surfactant. The likelihood of hyaline membrane disease is also increased by hypo- or hypervolemia, antepartum hemorrhage, and shock. Hypovolemia can occur when there is rupture of the umbilical cord at birth, bleeding from the cut cord, or sequestration of blood in the placenta just before the cord is cut. Hypervolemia occurs when an excessive amount of placental blood is transferred to the infant at the time of birth. This may cause congestive heart failure, delay absorption of fetal lung liquid, and limit the capacity of the lung for gas. The consequent increase in intraalveolar and interstitial fluid decreases lung compliance and increases the work of breathing. These factors also promote progressive hypoxemia and hypercarbia.

PREDICTION. Because fluid moves from the fetal lung into the amniotic cavity and transports suspended surfactant from the alveoli, the concentration of this material in amniotic fluid reflects its availability at the alveolar surfaces and thus the potential stability of the alveolar structure and risk of hyaline membrane disease. Gluck and associates pioneered the use of phospholipid analysis in amniotic fluid to predict the likelihood of hyaline membrane disease before birth. They noted that the proportion of different phospholip-

ids in amniotic fluid changed with gestation: the concentrations of lecithin and sphingomyelin are equal in midgestation, but after 34 to 36 weeks there is twice as much lecithin as sphingomyelin; this change parallels the maturation of the lung. Their work led to the widespread use of the lecithin-sphingomyelin (L/S) ratio for prediction of hyaline membrane disease.

To avoid the use of relatively costly phospholipid analyses, a rapid and simple method has been devised for the estimation of pulmonary surfactant in amniotic fluid. This is the *foam stability* or *shake* test described by Clements and associates. The rationale of this test is based on the ability of pulmonary surfactant to form highly stable surface films that can support the structure of a foam for relatively long periods. Since other substances in amniotic fluid, such as proteins, bile salts, or salts of free fatty acids, can also form a stable foam, these are excluded from the surface films by the nonfoaming competitive surfactant ethanol. At a surface tension of 29 mN/meter corresponding to a volume fraction of 47.5 percent ethanol, only double-chain phospholipids compete effectively for the surface film. Fortunately, the foam formed with unsaturated species breaks down in a few seconds whereas that formed by saturated phosphatidylcholine of the kind that predominates in pulmonary surfactant can be observed for several hours at room temperature. Mixing amniotic fluid with an equal volume of 95 percent ethanol poises the system so as to reveal the pulmonary surfactant in it when it is shaken with air to generate a foam. To make the test semiquantitative, tube dilutions are prepared in ratios of 1:1, 1:1.3, 1:2, 1:4, and 1:5. This technique permits some interpolation between the extremes of positive and negative tests (Fig. 22).

By testing amniotic fluid for the presence of surfactant using the L/S ratio or the shake test, the chance that an unborn fetus will develop hyaline membrane disease can be assessed.

PREVENTION. Since the disease is associated with incomplete development of the lung at the time of birth, premature delivery should be delayed, where possible, at least until the lung is mature, as judged by analysis of amniotic fluid for surfactant. Delivery has been delayed on some occasions by the infusion of alcohol and more recently by β-adrenergic stimulating agents. If premature delivery cannot be avoided, an effort can be made to accelerate lung maturation. In 1972 Liggins and Howie reported that administration of betamethasone to women in premature labor at least 2 days prior to delivery significantly reduced the incidence of respiratory distress in infants born at a gestation of less than 32 weeks. This observation is consistent with experimental studies that have shown that glucocorticoids accelerate lung maturation in fetal rabbits and lambs (Fig. 23). Currently, at many institutions, women with threatened premature delivery of an infant whose lungs are immature receive glucocorticoids. After birth, however, glucocorticoid treatment of infants *with* hyaline membrane disease is contraindicated, since it does not affect the course of the disease and may be associated with an increased incidence of intracranial hemorrhage.

TREATMENT. The newborn infant at high risk of developing hyaline membrane disease (eg, infants born prematurely, infants of diabetic mothers, or infants subjected to marked asphyxia during delivery) should be resuscitated vigorously. This should include expansion of the lungs with positive pressure if spontaneous respiratory efforts do not completely expand the lung, and assisted ventilation with a mixture of oxygen and air if there is hypercarbia and/or hypoxemia (see resuscitation, p. 1507). Measurement of arterial and, when possible, central venous pressures is necessary for judging the adequacy of the circulation during the early neonatal period and to detect hypo- or hypervolemia. When hypovolemic infants are asphyxiated, arterial and central venous pressures may be normal or slightly elevated immediately after birth, as a reflection of marked vasoconstriction. When asphyxia is treated adequately, however, the resistance may decrease and the capacitance vessels may dilate, lowering arterial and central venous pressures below normal levels. Since hypovolemia often predisposes to hyaline membrane disease, the circulatory volume should be increased to normal by the infusion of a volume expander, preferably albumin or blood. Since hypervolemia may also cause respiratory distress, increasing the blood volume of a premature infant by stripping the cord is contraindicated.

If, despite efforts to prevent atelectasis, an infant has respiratory distress, the hypoxemia, hypercarbia, acidemia, hyperkalemia, and inadequate circulating volume that may occur must be treated, while the infant is kept in a warm, neutral thermal environment. *The*

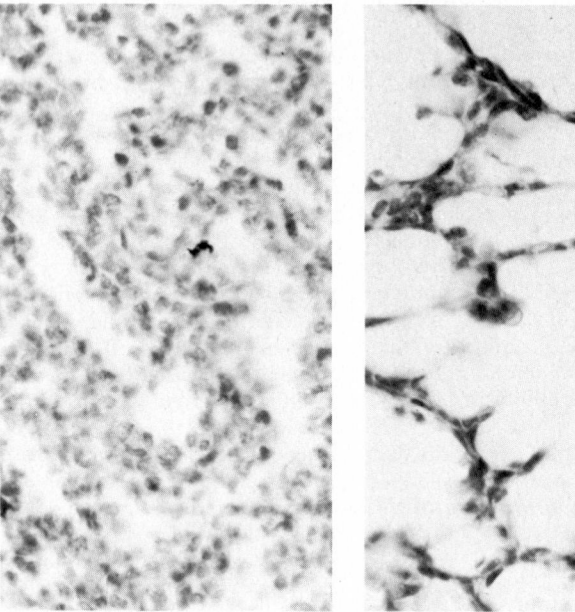

FIG. 23. Lungs from a pair of twin lambs delivered by cesarean section after a 128-day gestation and killed at birth. The lungs were distended with formalin at 10 cm H_2O pressure and fixed. The twin whose lung is at the right received 10 mg betamethasone 48 hours before delivery. The other twin (lung at left) was untreated.

environmental oxygen should be kept just high enough to maintain the arterial oxygen tension between 50 and 70 torr. If the arterial carbon dioxide tension rises above 60 torr, the infant's ventilation should be assisted. Once ventilation is adequate, severe metabolic acidemia (pH < 7.20 and a base deficit > 10 mEq/liter) should be corrected by the infusion of sodium bicarbonate. This, in addition to the intravascular infusion of 10 percent glucose (60 to 80 ml/kg/24 hours), usually will correct hyperkalemia. After the asphyxia is corrected, hypokalemia and hypocalcemia may occur, so that both potassium (2 mEq/kg/day) and calcium (calcium gluconate 200 mg/kg/day) should be added to the intravascular infusion. If the arterial and central venous pressures are low in the early course of the disease, and if peripheral circulation is inadequate, as judged by poor capillary filling, the circulating volume should be increased with either a solution of 5 percent salt poor albumin and normal saline or blood until intravascular pressures are normal. The many variables affected by hyaline membrane disease are interrelated and must be frequently measured throughout the course of the illness.

Since progressive atelectasis is the central characteristic of hyaline membrane disease, direct treatment requires distension of the lung. If the infant is depressed at birth and cannot make vigorous inspiratory efforts on his own, the lung should be inflated with 30 cm H_2O for 3 to 5 sec. If, after vigorous resuscitation, an infant develops progressive atelectasis and cannot maintain an arterial oxygen tension above 50 torr while breathing 60 to 80 percent oxygen, the application of a continuous intrapulmonary distending pressure may be required to overcome the high surface tension forces. Figure 24 illustrates the effect of such pressure on a lung without surfactant. When surfactant is absent, surface tension at end-expiration is high and, with each expiration, some respiratory units become airless and all tend to become smaller. A continuous positive airway pressure (CPAP) opposes the high surface tension, augments inspiration, and impedes expiration. With this system, breathing is spontaneous and, with successive respirations, respiratory units become larger until they are stabilized. When infants treated with CPAP develop hypercarbia (CO_2 above 60 torr) or apnea, mechanical ventilation with a continuous pressure of 4 to 7 cm H_2O during expiration is necessary. CPAP may be

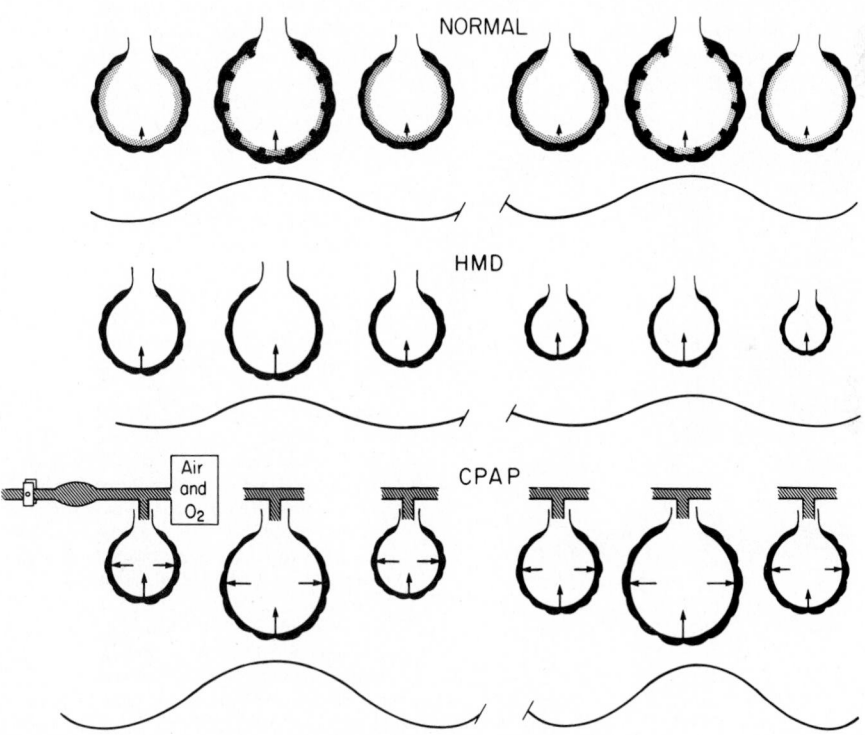

FIG. 24. At end-expiration in the normal lung, surfactant (the stippled zone at the surface of the model alveolus) is tightly packed and surface tension at the interface between alveolar gas and the alveolar wall is low, so that pulmonary units remain inflated. With inspiration, surfactant is spread over a larger area, which allows some nonsurface active material to reach the surface and surface tension rises. With repeated respiratory cycles respiratory units do not change in size. Surfactant is absent in the lungs of infants with hyaline membrane disease (HMD) and surface tension at end-expiration is high. In these infants respiratory units tend to become smaller with each successive expiration, until they are airless. Continuous positive airway pressure (CPAP) applied through an endotracheal tube opposes the high surface tension and, with successive respirations, respiratory units become larger until they reach a stable volume.

applied via an endotracheal tube, mask, nasal prongs, or head box. The lungs may also be distended by applying a continuous negative pressure around the chest as suggested by Chernick.

Upon application of CPAP, arterial oxygen tension usually rises sharply. As airway pressure increases, there is little change in arterial or central venous pressures, provided that airway pressure is not elevated too much. It would appear that most of the pressure applied to the lung is not transmitted to the central circulation. One of the most striking results of applying CPAP to the infant with hyaline membrane disease is the ability to maintain arterial oxygen tension between 50 and 70 torr with inspired oxygen concentrations between 40 and 50 percent. The increase in aeration of the lung with CPAP is shown dramatically in Figure 25. In most infants treated with CPAP, the amount of pressure required to maintain the Pao_2 between 50 and 70 torr abruptly decreases at about 72 hours of age, and shortly thereafter assisted ventilation can be stopped.

COMPLICATIONS. Complications of hyaline membrane disease occur most frequently in the smallest infants and are probably related to the degree of maturity. The most frequent complications include pulmonary air leaks, patent ductus arteriosus, intraventricular hemorrhage, and chronic lung disease. They are discussed in detail elsewhere.

OUTCOME. Eighty to 90 percent of the infants with hyaline membrane disease survive and most of the survivors have normal lungs by 1 month of age. However, a few develop persistent respiratory distress and may require an increased inspired oxygen for many weeks (p. 1536). Most of the survivors have normal intellectual development when compared with infants of the same gestational age without hyaline membrane disease.

Bibliography

Avery ME, Mead J: Surface properties in relation to atelectasis and hyaline membrane disease. Am J Dis Child 97:517, 1959

Campiche M, Prod'hom S, Gautier A: Etude au microscope electronique du poumon de prématurés morts en détresse respiratoire. Ann Paediatr 196:81, 1961

Chernick V: Hyaline membrane disease—therapy with constant lung-distending pressure. N Engl J Med 289:302, 1973

Chu J, Clements JA, Cotton EK, et al: Neonatal pulmonary ischemia. Pediatrics (Suppl) 40:709, 1967

Clements JA: Surface phenomena in relation to pulmonary function (Sixth Bowditch Lecture). Physiologist 5:11, 1962

Clements JA, Platzker AC, Tierney DF, et al: Assessment of the risk of the respiratory distress syndrome by a rapid test for surfactant in amniotic fluid. N Engl J Med 286:1077, 1972

deLemos RA, Shermeta DW, Knelson JH, Kotas R, Avery ME: Acceleration of appearance of pulmonary surfactant in the fetal lamb by administration of corticosteroids. Am Rev Resp Dis 102:459, 1970

Gitlin D, Craig JM: The nature of the hyaline membrane in asphyxia of the newborn. Pediatrics 17:64, 1956

Gluck L, Kulovich MV, Borer RC, et al: Diagnosis of the respiratory distress syndrome by amniocentesis. Am J Obstet Gynecol 109:440, 1971

Gregory GA, Kitterman JA, Phibbs RH, Tooley WH, Hamilton WK: Treatment of idiopathic respiratory distress syndrome with continuous positive airway pressure. N Engl J Med 284:1333, 1971

Grunwald P: Surface tension as a factor in the resistance of neonatal lungs to aeration. Am J Obstet Gynecol 53:996, 1947

Hochheim K: Ueber einige Befunde in den Lungen von Neugeborenen und die Beziehung derselben zur Aspiration von Fruchtwasser. Pathol Anat Arb, Berl, 421, 1903

Karlberg P, Cook CD, O'Brien D, Cherry RB, Smith CA: Studies of respiratory physiology in the newborn infant: observations during and after respiratory distress. Acta Paediatr 43 (suppl 100): 397, 1954

Lauweryns JM, Claessens S, Boussau WL: The pulmonary lymphatics in neonatal hyaline membrane disease. Pediatrics 41:917, 1968

Liggens GC: Premature delivery of foetal lambs infused with glucocorticoids. J Endocrinol 45:515, 1969

Liggens GC, Howie RN: A controlled trial of antepartum glucocorticoid treatment for prevention of the respiratory distress syndrome in premature infants. Pediatrics 50:515, 1972

Merritt TA, Farrell PM: Diminished pulmonary lecithin synthesis in acidosis: Experimental findings as related to the respiratory distress syndrome. Pediatrics 57:32, 1976

Nelson NM: On the etiology of hyaline membrane disease. Pediatr Clin North Am 17:943, 1970

Platzker ACG, Kitterman JA, Mescher J, Clements JA, Tooley WHL: Surfactant in the lung and tracheal fluid of the fetal lamb and acceleration of its appearance by dexamethasone. Pediatrics 56:556, 1975

Reynolds EOR: Hyaline membrane disease. Am J Obstet Gynecol 106:780, 1970

Robert MF, Neff RK, Hubbell JP, Taeusch HW, Avery ME: Association between maternal diabetes and the respiratory distress syndrome in the newborn. N Engl J Med 294:357, 1976

Stahlman M, Blankenship WJ, Shepard FM, et al: Circulatory studies in clinical hyaline membrane disease. Biol Neonate 20:300, 1972

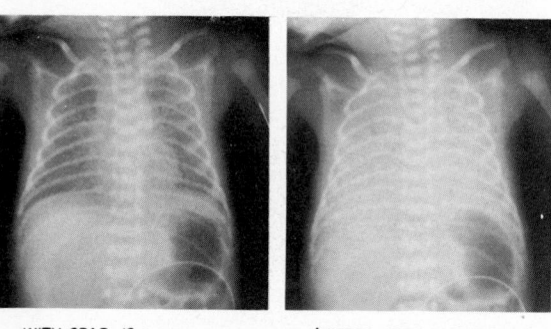

WITH CPAP 10 torr   1' AFTER CPAP REMOVED

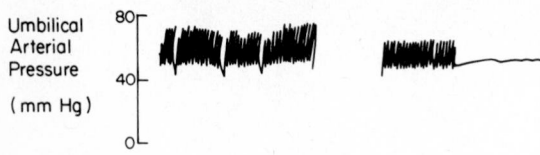

Umbilical Arterial Pressure (mm Hg)

Blood from Umbilical Arterial Catheter			
$F_I O_2$	0.45	0.45	
P_{O_2}	80	25	torr
pH	7.32	7.28	
P_{CO_2}	48	52	torr

FIG. 25. Chest radiographs, aortic blood pressure, pH, and blood gases in an infant with hyaline membrane disease during spontaneous breathing (left) and 1 minute after CPAP was temporarily removed (right). The marked fall in arterial oxygen tension from 80 to 25 torr parallels the rapid development of atelectasis shown in the radiograph.

MECONIUM ASPIRATION

GEORGE A. GREGORY

Meconium staining of amniotic fluid occurs in 10 percent of all births and meconium aspiration accounts for 1.8 percent of all perinatal deaths. Most of the infants who aspirate meconium are born at term, few are premature, and only those with intrauterine growth retardation weigh less than 2,000 g. The mortality of meconium-stained infants is twice that of nonstained infants.

CLINICAL FEATURES. Approximately 60 percent of infants born with meconium stained amniotic fluid have meconium in their tracheas. If they breathe before it is removed, it obstructs airways and leads to respiratory distress. Signs and symptoms of respiratory insufficiency increase in the first hours after birth, with intercostal and sternal retractions, expiratory grunting, and progressive cyanosis. Hypercapnia occurs late in the disease. The lung has a low compliance and there is mismatching of ventilation and perfusion. Lung compliance of infants who had meconium aspiration was noted to be 58 percent of normal on day 1, increasing to 88 percent of normal by day 3. In most the symptoms become less after the first 24 to 48 hours, unless large quantities of meconium have been aspirated. Hyperventilation with respiratory alkalosis is common during the first week after birth, even after arterial oxygen tension and the chest roentgenogram have become normal. The incidence of pneumothorax and/or pneumomediastinum in meconium-stained infants is nearly 10 times that of those without staining.

RADIOGRAPHIC APPEARANCE. The chest roentgenogram is characterized by patchy infiltrates and pulmonary fluid (Fig. 26). The pulmonary fluid usually disappears within 24 hours, but the patchy infiltrates may persist for days.

PATHOGENESIS. Meconium is the breakdown product of swallowed amniotic fluid, fetal hair, gastrointestinal secretions, and mucosal cells sloughed from the

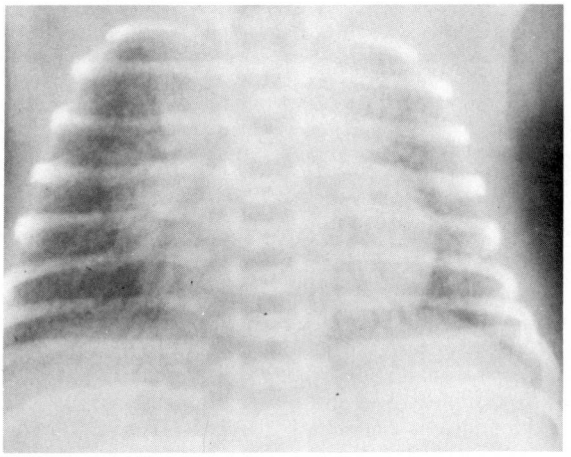

FIG. 26. A typical roentgenogram of meconium aspiration. Note the patchy infiltrate, fluid in the minor fissure, and air bronchograms. There may also be fluid in the costophrenic angles.

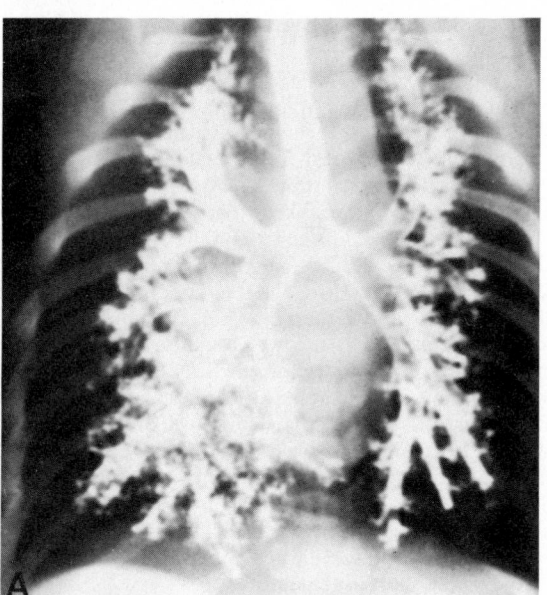
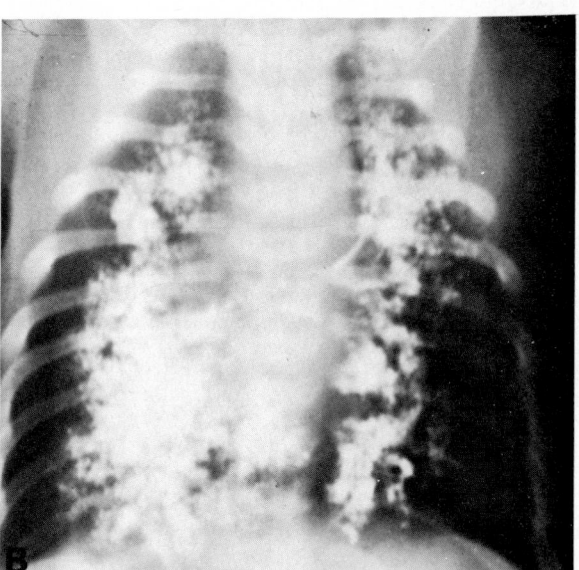

FIG. 27. **A.** Roentgenogram of a puppy at 1 minute after birth when meconium mixed with tantalum had been instilled in the airways before birth. Note that the meconium-tantalum mixture is primarily in large airways. **B.** Film taken 30 minutes later. Note that the meconium-tantalum mixture has been cleared from the major airways and alveoli. Removal of the meconium-tantalum from the major airways will prevent the alveolarization of the meconium-tantalum mixture.

gut wall itself. During the first two trimesters of pregnancy, the quantity of meconium in the gut is small, but in the last third of pregnancy the volume in the gut increases rapidly. Asphyxia or other stress increases gut motility and causes expulsion of meconium into the amniotic fluid. Amniotic fluid with meconium can then be aspirated into the lungs during normal fetal breathing or during fetal gasping stimulated by asphyxia. With the onset of air breathing, aspirated meconium, which is mainly in the major airways (Fig. 27A), is drawn into the lung periphery where it obstructs small airways and alveoli (Fig. 27B). It may partially or totally occlude some airways so that the aeration of the lung is nonuniform. Those respiratory units where airways are partially obstructed enlarge and may rupture into the interstitial tissue, leading to interstitial airleaks, pneumomediastinum, and pneumothoraces. The presence of meconium in the airway appears to cause persistence of the high pulmonary vascular resistance of fetal life. The mechanism for this is not known.

TREATMENT.   Treatment of meconium aspiration begins in the delivery room, with careful removal of oropharyngeal and tracheal meconium. To do this, an endotracheal tube should be inserted and suction applied with one's mouth as the tube is removed. This is done *only* if the child is born following particulate or *pea soup* meconium staining. If significant amounts of meconium are removed from the trachea, this procedure is repeated a second time. Then, the lungs are expanded *gently* with positive pressure and oxygen. The heart rate should be monitored continously during suctioning, as bradycardia may occur occasionally. In the nursery, percussion of the chest and hourly postural drainage for the first 8 hours after birth may be useful in removing any meconium remaining in the lung. Severe cases of meconium aspiration may require mechanical ventilation for hypoxemia and carbon dioxide retention.

In some cases of meconium aspiration, pulmonary vascular resistance is high and blood shunts from the pulmonary artery to the aorta through the ductus arteriosus, as demonstrated by a difference in the Pao_2 between the temporal and umbilical arteries (Table 8). Pulmonary vascular resistance can often be decreased by an infusion of tolazoline into the venous circulation. An initial bolus of 1 to 3 mg/kg is given intravenously over 5 minutes. If umbilical arterial Pao_2 rises, a continuous infusion of tolazoline at 2 to 5 mg/kg/hour should be given. The drug must be tapered slowly over

1 to 5 days. Tolazoline is a potent peripheral vasodilator, which may cause marked hypotension if the infant is somewhat hypovolemic. If hypotension does occur blood volume must be expanded immediately with blood, plasma, or saline. When tolazoline is stopped and vascular capacity decreases, a phlebotomy may be required.

Bibliography

Fujikura T, Klionsky B: The significance of meconium staining. Am J Obstet Gynecol 121:45, 1975

Gooding C, Gregory GA, Tabor P, Wright RR: An experimental model for the study of meconium aspiration of the newborn. Radiology 100: 137, 1971.

Gregory GA, Gooding C, Phibbs RH, Tooley WH: Meconium aspiration in infants, a prospective study. J Pediatr 85:848, 1974

Steele RW, Metz JR, Bass JW, Dubois JJ: Pneumothorax and pneumomediastinum in the newborn. Radiology 98:629, 1971

PULMONARY HEMORRHAGE

JOSEPH A. KITTERMAN

Pulmonary hemorrhage is found in 9 percent of autopsies of newborn infants, and its incidence is 1 in 1,000 live births. The bleeding may be alveolar, interstitial, or a combination both; grossly, it usually involves more than one-third of the lungs. Concurrent bleeding at other sites is common, particularly the central nervous system and within the abdomen.

CLINICAL FEATURES.   Pulmonary hemorrhage occurs most commonly with first pregnancies, toxemia of pregnancy, after prolonged rupture of membranes, and breech or cesarean delivery. Neonatal factors associated with pulmonary hemorrhage include infection, cold injury, congenital heart disease, kernicterus, Rh isoimmunization, clotting abnormalities, and asphyxia. Recent reports emphasize the frequent association with assisted ventilation for hyaline membrane disease. Infants usually rapidly develop respiratory distress and cyanosis and have blood fluid oozing from the nose, mouth, or endotracheal tube. The radiographic appearance of the lungs is variable and may include scattered linear or nodular densities or complete opacification.

PATHOPHYSIOLOGY.   Although the pathogenesis is not definitely known, Cole and her associates have shown that the bloody fluid is actually hemorrhagic pulmonary edema; it has a lower hematocrit than blood and a higher concentration of small proteins than plasma. They postulate that these infants have asphyxia, which causes left ventricular failure, raising pulmonary capillary pressure and increasing filtration of plasma; finally, bleeding into the interstitial space occurs. Contributing factors may include clotting abnormalities, lung damage, and conditions favoring increased plasma filtration from lung capillaries (eg, low plasma proteins, high alveolar surface tension).

TREATMENT.   Besides treatment of underlying abnormalities, therapy should include tracheal suction and positive pressure ventilation, which may help control bleeding. When blood loss is large, immediate infusion of blood or volume expanders may be necessary to adequately support the circulation.

Table 8. Effect of Tolazoline on Arterial Po_2 (torr) Following Meconium Aspiration in 2 Infants Breathing 100 percent Oxygen

Patient	a	b
Before Tolazoline		
Temporal artery	156	200
Umbilical artery	25	32
After Tolazoline		
Temporal artery	160	200
Umbilical artery	155	196

Bibliography

Ahvenainen EK, Call JD: Pulmonary hemorrhage in infants; a descriptive study. Am J Pathol 28:1, 1952

Chessells JM, Wigglesworth JS: Haemostatic failure in babies with Rhesus isoimmunization. Arch Dis Child 46:38, 1971

Cole VA, Normand ICS, Reynolds EOR, Rivers RPA: Pathogenesis of hemorrhagic pulmonary edema and massive pulmonary hemorrhage in the newborn. Pediatrics 51:175, 1973

Esterly JR, Oppenheimer EH: Massive pulmonary hemorrhage in the newborn. I. Pathologic considerations. J Pediatr 69:3, 1966

Fedrick J, Butler NR: Certain causes of neonatal death. IV. Massive pulmonary hemorrhage. Biol Neonate 18:243, 1971

Mann TP, Elliott RIK: Neonatal cold injury due to accidental exposure to cold. Lancet 1:229, 1957

Rowe S, Avery ME: Massive pulmonary hemorrhage in the newborn. II. Clinical considerations. J Pediatr 69:12, 1966

Trompeter R, Yu VYH, Aynsley-Green A, Roberton NRC: Massive pulmonary haemorrhage in the newborn infant. Arch Dis Child 50:123, 1975

IDIOPATHIC PERSISTENT PULMONARY HYPERTENSION OF THE NEWBORN

DANIEL L. LEVIN

Persistent pulmonary hypertension of the newborn may be associated with diseases of known etiology, such as central nervous system abnormalities that cause hypoventilation; infection, particularly Group B β-hemolytic streptococcus pneumonia; polycythemia; upper airway obstruction, eg, micrognathia; pulmonary parenchymal disorders, eg, meconium aspiration; or congenital heart disease, eg, ventricular septal defect. Another form of persistent pulmonary hypertension, which is not clearly associated with any of these known etiologic mechanisms, has been recognized recently. This is sometimes called *persistent fetal circulation, persistent pulmonary vascular obstruction, progressive pulmonary hypertension, persistent fetal cardiopulmonary circulatory pathway,* or *persistent transitional circulation.*

CLINICAL FEATURES. Infants with idiopathic persistent pulmonary hypertension are usually full-term, although some are preterm, and are otherwise normal. Many, but not all, have a history of maternal diabetes, drug use, or preeclampsia. Signs of intrapartum asphyxia usually are not noted. Shortly after birth, they are cyanotic, tachypneic or, in some cases, apneic, and have a systolic murmur.

They always have marked hypoxemia, hypercarbia, and acidemia, and frequently have hypocalcemia and hypoglycemia. They have marked intercostal and sternal retractions and usually have grunting respirations. They resemble infants with hyaline membrane disease. Untreated, their hypoxemia may become extreme and, despite assisted ventilation with high pressures, some infants rapidly worsen and die. In the survivors, the respiratory distress decreases after 3 to 5 days; thereafter, the infants rapidly return to normal.

Simultaneous samples of temporal or right radial and umbilical arterial blood oxygen are sometimes helpful in making the diagnosis, if there is a large right-to-left shunt through the patent ductus arteriosus. The infants should breathe oxygen when these samples are obtained in order to maximize the difference in oxygen tensions. Cardiac catheterization and cineangiography reveal anatomically normal hearts with poor ventricular function and mitral, tricuspid, and/or pulmonic valvar insufficiency.

RADIOLOGIC FEATURES. Despite the severe respiratory distress, the lungs are well expanded and appear normal on chest roentgenogram. The pulmonary vessels are of normal size, but the heart is usually enlarged.

PATHOGENESIS. The etiology is unknown. Theoretically, it might be associated with any of the following: a genetically determined primary increase in pulmonary arterial smooth muscle; chronic intrauterine stress, resulting in secondary or overwork hypertrophy of pulmonary arterial smooth muscle; a genetically or functionally related decrease in the total number of pulmonary arterial resistance vessels, which would result in a decrease in the cross-sectional area of the pulmonary vascular bed; an increased availability of a pulmonary vasoconstrictive substance before or after birth (eg, angiotensin II), or a decreased availability of a vasodilatory substance at birth (eg, bradykinin). Infants with a structural decrease of the cross-sectional area of the pulmonary vascular bed would have a prolonged clinical course, while the duration of illness in infants with an increased amount of pulmonary arterial smooth muscle might be several days. Transient imbalance of circulating vasoactive agents would also have a short course.

TREATMENT. Hypothermia, hypocalcemia, and hypoglycemia should be promptly diagnosed and treated, since they may have direct adverse effects on pulmonary arterial and/or myocardial muscle. Oxygen and sodium bicarbonate should be given as needed for hypoxemia and metabolic acidosis. Most of the infants require assisted ventilation with continuous positive airway pressure and mechanical ventilation. In those cases where assisted ventilation cannot oxygenate the arterial blood and prevent the development of metabolic acidosis, pulmonary vasodilatation may be attempted with pharmacologic agents. Tolazoline (Priscoline), an α-receptor blocker, is a potent pulmonary and systemic vasodilator that is often helpful in this condition. Ideally, it should be given in a bolus of 0.5 to 1.0 mg/kg over 15 to 30 sec directly into the pulmonary artery beyond the origin of the ductus arteriosus. When this is not possible, it may be given into the right-sided chambers of the heart or intravenously into a vein in the head or arms. Delivery from these sites will make delivery to the pulmonary vessels more likely. After the bolus is injected, there is often a prompt increase in oxygenation in the descending aorta and a decrease in the temporal/umbilical arterial blood oxygen tension difference. Since tolazoline often is delivered to the systemic vascular bed through the ductus arteriosus, systemic blood pressure must be measured and hypotension treated with volume expansion, when it occurs. A continuous intravenous infusion of tolazoline at a rate of 2 to 5 mg/kg/hour is usually necessary after the bolus to maintain pulmonary vasodilation. After 48 hours, the dose may be decreased if improvement has persisted. Rapid cessation of tolazoline may be followed by a return of the high pulmonary vascular resistance. Isoproterenol, another potent pulmonary vasodilator, has also been successfully used intravenously at a rate of 0.1 µg/kg/minute. When mechanical ventilation and pulmonary vasodilators do not effect adequate arterial oxygen, the infants may benefit from muscle paralysis with curare. Curare probably is effective because it increases chest wall compliance and eliminates struggling, both of which make ventilation more efficient. Also, there is evidence that curare may be a histamine releaser and, in man, histamine is a pulmonary vasodilator.

OUTCOME. Thirty-nine patients with persistent pulmonary hypertension of the newborn, unassociated with disease of known etiology, have been reported. Thirty-one improved or recovered completely within 1 to 14 days after birth. One patient survived after a prolonged course of more than 16 weeks. Seven patients died after a course of days to months. Death was usually due to pulmonary insufficiency or intracranial hemorrhage. In our experience, only 1 of 11 patients died. Aggressive management may be responsible for survival in these critically ill infants. Although survivors appear to be perfectly normal, the relationship of these events in the newborn period to the onset of primary pulmonary vascular obstruction in older children and adults is not known.

Bibliography

Bauer CR, Tispuras D, Fletcher BD: Syndrome of persistent pulmonary vascular obstruction of the newborn. Roentgen findings. Am J Roentgenol 120:285, 1974

Brown R, Pickering K: Persistent transitional circulation. Arch Dis Child 49:883, 1974

Burnell RH, Joseph MC, Lees MH: Progressive pulmonary hypertension in newborn infants. Am J Dis Child 123:167, 1972

Gersony WM, Duc GC, Sinclair JC: "PFC" syndromes (persistence of the fetal circulation). Circulation 40:87, 1969

Levin DL, Cates L, Newfeld EA, Muster AJ, Paul MH: Persistence of the fetal cardiopulmonary circulatory pathway: survival of an infant after a prolonged course. Pediatrics 56:58, 1975

Rudolph AM, Paul MH, Sommer LS, Nadas AS: Effects of tolazoline hydrochloride (priscoline) on circulatory dynamics of patients with pulmonary hypertension. Am Heart J 55:424, 1958

Siassi B, Goldberg SJ, Emmanouilides GC, Higashino SM, Lewis E: Persistent pulmonary vascular obstruction in newborn infants. J Pediatr 78:610, 1971

Neonatal Pneumonia due to β-Hemolytic Streptococcus B Group

William H. Tooley

Escherichia coli and *Staphylococcus aureus,* until recent years, were the most common organisms causing pneumonia in newborn infants. However, in the past decade, the group B streptococcus (*Streptococcus agalactiae*) has become the principal agent responsible for severe neonatal infections—2 to 3 cases per 1,000 live births. About one-half of these infants develop a fulminating pneumonia in the first day of life, which has a greater than 75 percent mortality. One of the clinical characteristics displayed by infants with this infection is progressive respiratory distress, which often cannot be distinguished from that associated with hyaline membrane disease.

CLINICAL FEATURES. Infants born both at and before term are candidates for infection with group B streptococcus. Delivery is often, but not always, preceded by early rupture of the fetal membranes and, occasionally, mothers have fever and other signs of infection. Infected infants rapidly become sick, and most have onset of symptoms within the first 6 hours after birth. In one series of 8 infants all were dead within 26 hours.

Severe respiratory distress is the hallmark of this disease, with expiratory grunting, intercostal and sternal retractions, tachypnea, and progressive cyanosis. Within hours of the onset, hypoxemia and hypercarbemia are usually so marked and pulmonary blood flow so low that ventilation must be supported mechanically. Despite very high inspiratory and end-expiratory pressures, respiratory gas exchange cannot be effected. This clinical picture is similar to that in infants with persistent pulmonary hypertension. At the same time, systemic blood pressure falls, the peripheral circulation decreases, and the infants develop metabolic acidosis. These are the clinical signs of shock. Pulmonary air leaks with pneumothoraces and pneumomediastinum are common. Despite vigorous support of ventilation and circulation, hypoxemia and shock usually cannot be reversed and the infants die.

Cultures of tracheal secretions and blood always grow group B streptococcus. Characteristically, there is a peripheral leukopenia, as leukocytes are sequestered in the lung. Thrombocytopenia, prolonged thrombin and prothrombin times, and decreased fibrinogen are common and, within 12 hours of the onset of symptoms, most of these infants are bleeding from the lung and most mucous membranes. These evidences of disseminated intravascular coagulation are probably secondary to the infant's profound shock.

RADIOGRAPHIC FEATURES. Two types of radiographs are seen in group B streptococcus. About half of the affected infants, usually those with lowest birth weight, have findings similar to those of infants with hyaline membrane disease. Their lungs have a fine, diffuse, granular opacification against which the bronchi are sharply outlined (air bronchogram). The edge of the diaphragms and the border of the heart are hazy and the volume of the lungs appears slightly reduced. The thymus is usually small. The uniformity of the process suggests that the lungs were infected in utero by blood-borne organisms. Other infants have patchy infiltrates in their lungs, usually most marked in the bases. Occasionally, there is fluid in the fissures and costophrenic angle. This pattern is similar to aspiration pneumonitis and suggests that these infants inhaled the streptococcus at birth.

PATHOGENESIS. The lungs of infants dying with β-hemolytic streptococcus group B pneumonia are filled with organisms, particularly if death occurs in the first day of life. The lungs are heavy, and only some of the alveolar ducts are filled with air. There are sheets of intraalveolar and interstitial polymorphonuclear leukocytes. These sequestered white cells apparently account for the peripheral leukopenia. The constricted small pulmonary arterioles are consistent with the clinical finding of pulmonary hypoperfusion. Hyaline membranes are prominent and line the dilated alveolar ducts. There is often diffuse, marked interstitial hemorrhage. In those sections where there are few organisms, leukocytes look exactly like those from lungs of infants dying with hyaline membrane disease.

TREATMENT. The organisms are sensitive to penicillin and if infants with pneumonia are to survive, prompt treatment with antibiotics is essential. Combined treatment with penicillin G (100,000 units/kg/day) and kanamycin (15 mg/kg/day) is recommended. Oxygen, up to 100 percent, may be required to treat cyanosis; and assisted ventilation, with inspiratory pressures as high as 60 cm H_2O, has been used to effect adequate transfer of oxygen and carbon dioxide. Often, improved arterial oxygenation can only be achieved after curarization and continuous infusion of a vasodilator (isoproterenol, 0.1 μg/kg/minute, or tolazoline, 2 to 5 mg/kg/hour).

Bibliography

Ablow RC, Driscoll SG, Effmann EL, et al: A comparison of early-onset group B streptococcal neonatal infection and the respiratory-distress syndrome of the newborn. N Engl J Med 294:65, 1976

Franciosi RA, Knostman JD, Zimmerman RA: Group B streptococcal neonatal and infant infections. J Pediatr 82:707, 1973

Howard JB, McCracken GH: The spectrum of group B streptococcal infections in infancy. Am J Dis Child 128:815, 1974

McCracken GH: Group B streptococci: the new challenge in neonatal infections. J Pediatr 82:703, 1973

Quirante J, Ceballor R, Cassady G: Group B β-hemolytic streptococcal infection in the newborn. I. Early onset infection. Am J Dis Child 128:659, 1974

PULMONARY AIR LEAKS

GEORGE A. GREGORY

Pulmonary air leaks are relatively common and frequently cause serious problems in newborn infants. There are several types. The most common is air within the pleural space (pneumothorax). However, air may also collect in the mediastinal space (pneumomediastinum), within the pericardial sac (pneumopericardium), in the interstitial spaces of the lungs (pulmonary interstitial emphysema), or extend into the peritoneal cavity (pneumoperitoneum).

INCIDENCE. Among infants born at term, a spontaneous pneumothorax occurs in 1.3 percent of infants born vaginally and 2 percent of those delivered by cesarean section; the incidence is highest among preterm infants. Pneumomediastinum occurs in 0.25 percent of infants. Air leaks are much more common in infants

with lung disease, and occur in 10 percent of infants born through meconium. With hyaline membrane disease, the incidence of pneumothorax ranges from 5 percent in mild cases, who require no ventilatory assistance, to 35 percent among the most severely ill, who receive the most vigorous assisted ventilation.

CLINICAL FEATURES. The clinical signs of pulmonary air leaks depend on the size and location of the gas accumulation. With pulmonary interstitial emphysema, there is progressive overexpansion and there may be decreased movement and breath sounds on the affected side. Shift of mediastinal structures to the contralateral side may occur. Progressive hypercarbia and hypoxia are common.

Pneumomediastinum is a cause of severe respiratory distress only in exceptional cases and is often an unexpected radiographic finding. Subcutaneous emphysema of the neck, face, and chest frequently occurs, and Hamman's sign (a crunching sound heard over the heart) may be present. If air extends below the diaphragm to cause pneumoperitoneum, the abdomen becomes distended and tympanitic. This condition must be differentiated from a perforated viscus.

BILATERAL TENSION PNEUMOTHORAX

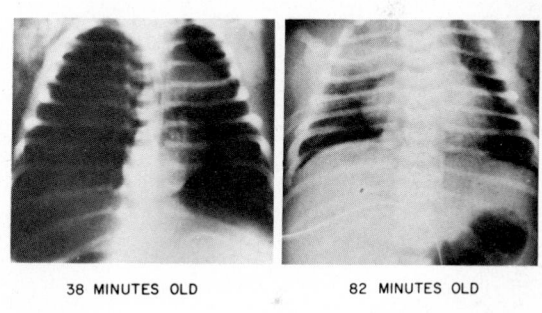

38 MINUTES OLD   82 MINUTES OLD

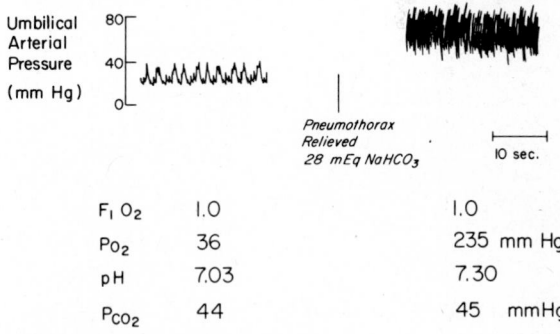

Umbilical Arterial Pressure (mm Hg)

Pneumothorax Relieved 28 mEq $NaHCO_3$

10 sec.

$F_I O_2$	1.0	1.0
P_{O_2}	36	235 mm Hg
pH	7.03	7.30
P_{CO_2}	44	45 mmHg

FIG. 28. Bilateral tension pneumothorax occuring at birth in a 3,200 g infant born after a 41-week gestation. Note both chest cavities are filled with air, the lung is compressed, the heart is small, and marked hypotension and bradycardia are present. There are marked hypoxemia, acidosis, and failure of respiratory compensation for metabolic acidosis. These are signs of impeded venous return and low cardiac output. After removal of intrapleural air the lung re-expanded, and the heart size, arterial blood pressure, blood gases, and heart rate were normal.

With pneumothorax, the degree of lung collapse depends upon the compliance of the lung. With compliant lungs, there is marked collapse, as shown in Figure 28. With severe lung disease, the lung does not completely collapse despite a large accumulation of gas as in Figure 29.

With a small pneumothorax, signs are mild; there may be only slight tachypnea and retractions. With increasing severity of pneumothorax, the infant develops severe respiratory distress with agitation, tachypnea, retractions, and cyanosis; the onset is often sudden. Hypoxia is secondary to atelectasis of the affected lung, and hypercarbia is due to decreased ventilation. In the most severe cases with tension pneumothorax, there

may be apnea and even cardiac arrest. The compliant chest wall of the small infant allows the affected side of the chest cage to overexpand and bulge outward, and breath sounds may be decreased on the affected side. This latter sign is often absent despite a large pneumothorax, especially in small infants, because breath

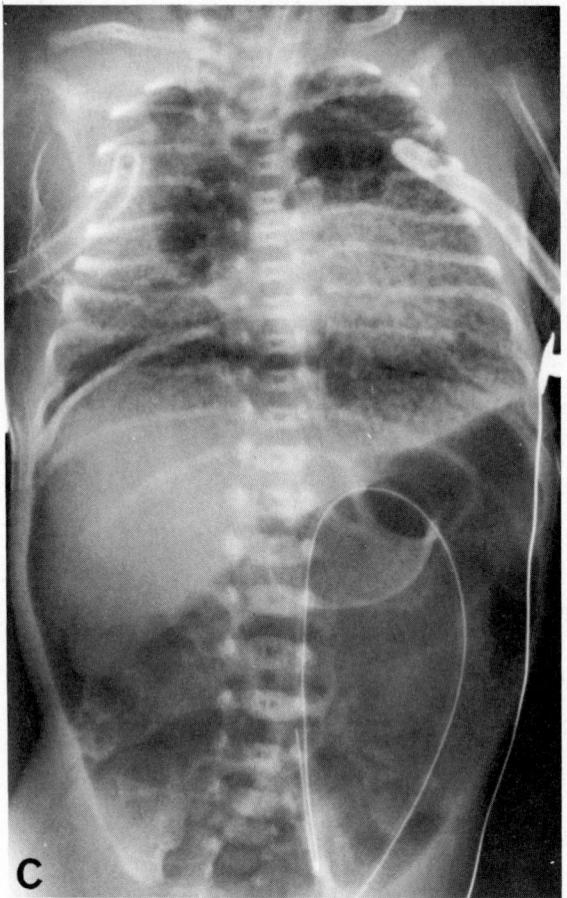

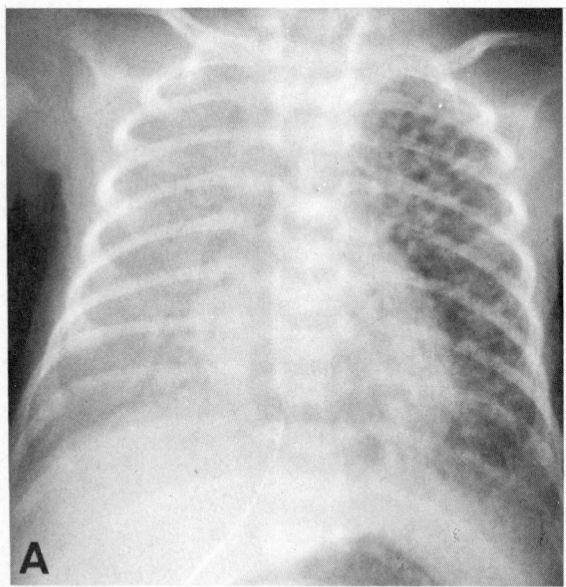

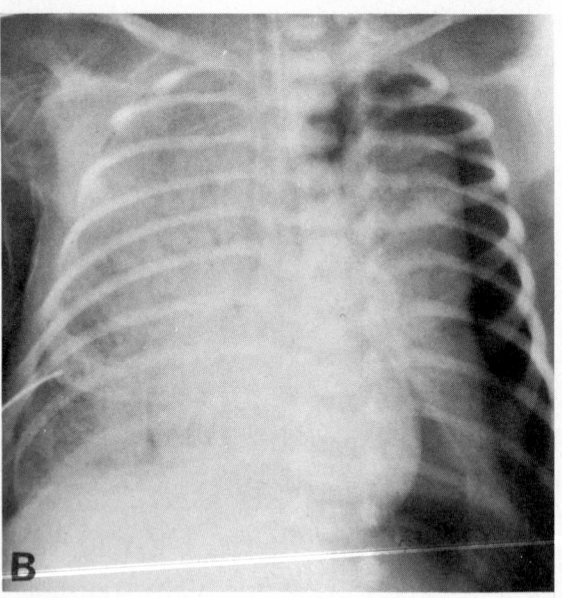

FIG. 29.   A. Severe hyaline membrane disease in a 1,500 g, 31-week gestation infant. The infant's trachea is intubated and he is being ventilated with high inspiratory pressures. Despite this the right lung is poorly ventilated. The coarse reticular pattern of the left lung is characteristic of interstitial air. An umbilical venous catheter with its tip in the right atrium is present. **B.** The same infant 2 hours later. There is a left pneumothorax. Note that the left lung is not collapsed; this is typical of the stiff lung of hyaline membrane disease. There is air in the mediastinum and probably in the pericardial sac. There is now interstitial air in the right lung. The right atrial catheter has been removed. **C.** The same infant 24 hours later. There are two chest tubes decompressing bilateral pneumothoraces. There is interstitial air in both lungs. The mediastinal air has lifted the thymus off the heart, a typical "sail sign," and has advanced into the neck (subcutaneous emphysema) and into the peritoneum producing a pneumoperitoneum. Note the sharply outlined peritoneal cavity (football sign) and liver. There is also a subpleural collection of air at the base of the right lung. An umbilical arterial catheter is present with its tip at T4-5. Ventilation pressure was lowered in this infant, after which the air absorbed. He survived and at 2 years of age appears normal.

sounds are easily transmitted throughout the chest from the nonaffected side. There may be shift of the mediastinum with the trachea, cardiac impulse, and heart sounds shifted toward the nonaffected side. With a tension pneumothorax the air in the pleural space is under increased pressure. This increased intrathoracic pressure decreases venous return to the chest, and cardiac output falls and peripheral venous congestion occurs. There is arterial hypotension, a narrow pulse pressure, shock, and metabolic acidosis (Fig. 28). Most infants will die if the pneumothorax is not decompressed.

RADIOGRAPHIC FEATURES. The characteristic picture of interstitial emphysema is a coarse reticular pattern with fine lines of radiolucency extending out from the hilum parallel to blood vessels and airways (Fig. 29). With pneumomediastinum there may be free air in the neck and axilla and the thymus may be elevated producing a striking silhouette (sail sign) as shown in Figure 29.

Radiologic diagnosis of pneumothorax is usually simple, unless the gas leak is small. The diagnosis is best made during expiration; this decreases the quantity of air within the lung, makes the lung parenchyma more radiodense, and increases the contrast between lung and the air-filled pleural space. A pneumothorax is uniformly translucent and has no lung markings. The air collection is usually superior to the lung; therefore, with the patient supine, a cross table lateral radiograph may be necessary to detect it, particularly with noncompliant lungs, as in hyaline membrane disease, which do not readily collapse. With a tension pneumothorax the diaphragm is depressed and the heart and trachea are deviated to the nonaffected side. With bilateral tension pneumothoraces or with severe pneumopericardium, the heart appears small due to obstruction of venous return to the heart.

PATHOPHYSIOLOGY. Air enters the interstitial spaces of the lung via a tear in the alveolar wall and then moves toward the hilum through loose peribronchial and perivascular tissue. If a substantial amount of air enters the interstitial spaces and remains there, the lung becomes overexpanded, stiff, and difficult to ventilate because of the interstitial emphysema. This occurs most commonly in small preterm infants, probably because they have loosely bound interstitial tissue, making it easy to form new air channels. In some cases the air extends along the peribronchial and perivascular tissues and collects in the mediastinum, from which it may dissect up into the neck or down into the peritoneal cavity (Fig. 29). In most cases, the air escapes through a pleural tear into the pleural cavity to form a pneumothorax. Pulmonary interstitial emphysema often precedes pneumothorax, as shown in Figure 29.

TREATMENT. If spontaneous pneumothorax occurs in an otherwise healthy infant with normal arterial blood gases and vital signs and the pneumothorax is estimated to occupy less than 20 percent of the chest cavity, close observation is usually all that is required. Resorption of extra pulmonary intrathoracic gas may be accelerated by breathing oxygen for 1 to 2 hours. This creates a gradient for nitrogen between the extrapulmonary, intrathoracic gas and the blood, thus facilitating nitrogen resorption. *This method of treatment should not be used in newborn infants because of the possibility that hyperoxemia may cause retrolental fibroplasia.*

If there is acute onset of respiratory distress, hypoxemia, hypercarbia, and hypotension, immediate decompression of the pneumothorax is mandatory. A 22 to 25 gauge needle, connected to a three-way stopcock and a large syringe is inserted through the pleura in the second intercostal space at the midclavicular line, and the gas should be evacuated. While this may be lifesaving, it seldom relieves the pneumothorax permanently and therefore is usually not definitive treatment. In addition, this procedure may in itself produce a pneumothorax in a substantial number of cases when no pneumothorax existed prior to the insertion of the needle. Following emergency decompression with needle and syringe, a chest radiograph should always be done. Accumulations of intrapleural air that occupy more than 20 percent of the thoracic cavity should be treated with thoracostomy, by inserting a large bore chest tube into the pleural space through the second intercostal space at the midclavicular line or in the midaxillary line at the fourth intercostal space. The tube should then be connected to an underwater suction at a pressure of 15 to 25 cm H_2O below atmospheric. When there has been no evidence of gas leak for 8 hours, discontinue suction but leave the chest tube connected to underwater seal for an additional 8 hours without clamping the tube. If there is no further evidence of pneumothorax at that time, the chest tube can be removed.

Treatment of pneumomediastinum is seldom necessary. However, if it becomes tense and obstructs venous return, a needle can be inserted substernally and gas evacuated with a syringe. Similarly it is rare that pericardial air needs to be evacuated; but when there is obstruction to venous return, evacuation of the pericardium by inserting a needle below the xyphoid process and directing its tip toward the heart will restore the circulation to normal. Interstitial emphysema will usually disappear if the positive pressure used for ventilation is decreased. In rare instances, air will accumulate below the pleura and compress the underlying lung without breaking into the intrapleural space. These subpleural accumulations can be evacuated by needle aspiration under fluoroscopic control, or very rarely they may require incision after open thoracotomy. Pneumoperitoneum requires no direct intervention and this air will quickly be absorbed when the mediastinal air leak, from which the air came, has been sealed.

Bibliography

PULMONARY AIR LEAKS

Chernick V, Avery ME: Spontaneous alveolar rupture at birth. Pediatrics 32:816, 1963

Gregory GA, Gooding C, Phibbs RH, Tooley WH: Meconium aspiration in infants—a prospective study. J Pediatr 85:848, 1974

Hall RT, Rhodes PG: Pneumothorax and pneumomediastinum in infants with idiopathic respiratory distress syndrome receiving CPAP. Pediatrics 55:493, 1975

Lubchenco LO: Recognition of spontaneous pneumothorax in premature infants. Pediatrics 24:996, 1959

Macklin CC: Transport of air along sheaths of pulmonic blood vessels from alveoli to mediastinum: clinical applications. Arch Intern Med. 64:913, 1939

Steele R, Metz JR, Bass JW, DuBois JJ: Pneumothorax and pneumomediastinum in the newborn. Radiology 98:629, 1971

PERSISTENT RESPIRATORY DISTRESS SYNDROMES

RICHARD D. BLAND

WILLIAM H. TOOLEY

Until recent years, chronic lung disease in infancy was a rarity. With the development of improved methods to care for infants born prematurely, persistent respiratory distress syndromes have become more common. Prolonged respiratory distress is most often associated with the healing phase of severe hyaline membrane disease. This type of chronic lung disease also occasionally follows aspiration of blood or meconium, pulmonary hemorrhage, and severe neonatal pneumonia. These conditions and hyaline membrane disease may damage lung tissue, and while the lungs heal, their clinical and morphologic features are similar. This group of diseases, which we call *chronic lung disease following neonatal lung injury*, is also known as *bronchopulmonary dysplasia*.

Persistent respiratory distress is seen also in some small preterm infants, without any preceding lung injury. In these infants respiratory distress usually starts at the end of the first or during the second week after birth. Wilson and Mikity first described the condition in 1960, and it is often called the *Wilson-Mikity syndrome*. However, we prefer the term *pulmonary dysmaturity syndrome*, which was suggested by Baghdassarian, Avery, and Neuhauser, for what is apparently the same condition. Krauss, Klain, and Auld recently described a third condition in infants born very prematurely which they called *chronic pulmonary insufficiency of prematurity*. However, since it appears to be associated with progressive atelectasis, we have given it the term *late diffuse atelectasis in prematurely born infants*.

CHRONIC LUNG DISEASE FOLLOWING NEONATAL LUNG INJURY (BRONCHOPULMONARY DYSPLASIA)

This form of persistent respiratory distress usually follows severe hyaline membrane disease treated with prolonged endotracheal intubation, mechanical ventilation, and a high inspired oxygen concentration. There is disagreement regarding its primary cause, with advocates for oxygen toxicity, mechanical injury, chronic infection and late manifestations of severe hyaline membrane disease itself, which are allowed to develop by effective therapy. It is probable that the lungs of the infant with severe hyaline membrane disease are further damaged by all three—oxygen, trauma, and infection—and that they all contribute to the cellular proliferation characteristic of the early stages of the condition.

CLINICAL FEATURES. Most infants with chronic lung disease following neonatal lung injury are born prematurely and, shortly after birth, they acquire symptoms of pulmonary disease with cyanosis, tachypnea, retractions of the chest wall, expiratory grunting, and nasal flaring. Infants with this condition usually have received more than 60 percent oxygen for a day or more and have had ventilatory assistance with continuous positive airway pressure. This form of persistent respiratory distress develops in infants with the most severe acute disease, which has required treatment with high inspiratory and end-expiratory pressures. Many have had interstitial air leaks and pneumothoraces.

After the acute phase of the disease, usually about a week after birth, the infant's clinical condition improves, and oxygen tensions of arterial blood can be maintained with lower concentrations of inspired oxygen. However, for some, the improvement is transient and their condition often deteriorates in the second week in association with the development of a large left-to-right shunt through the ductus arteriosus. When this induces pulmonary edema (see p.1539), the lungs become less compliant, the work of breathing increases, and the infants hypoventilate, increasing arterial CO_2 tension. Closure of the ductus arteriosus, either spontaneously or by surgical or medical management, may lessen respiratory distress, but for some infants subsequent recovery is slow.

In all infants who develop chronic lung disease, with or without the complication of a patent ductus and pulmonary edema, retractions of the chest wall continue and sometimes become worse than during the acute phase of the disorder. Recurrent rales occur commonly, and the infants require increasing concentrations of inspired oxygen to maintain adequate tissue oxygenation. The lungs become hyperinflated, the chest is hyperresonant, and the anterior-posterior diameter of the chest increases, sometimes accompanied by inward deformity of the lower sternum (pectus excavatum). Intermittently, respiratory distress worsens, hypoxemia and hypercarbemia occur, and episodes of apnea and bradycardia may develop.

Symptoms in surviving infants resolve slowly over several weeks. In some, healing may require months to 2 to 3 years. The majority of infants are asymptomatic by 2 years, and only one of our survivors has had signs or symptoms of lung disease after 5 years. During this prolonged course of healing, pulmonary hypertension and congestive heart failure may develop, nutrition may be inadequate, and growth may be delayed.

RADIOGRAPHIC FEATURES. Northway, Rosan, and Porter reported radiographic findings in infants with hyaline membrane disease treated with prolonged assisted ventilation and high concentrations of oxygen. They described a sequence of changes, which they divided into four stages. In stage I (period of acute respiratory distress) there is a generalized granular pattern, with increased lung density and prominent

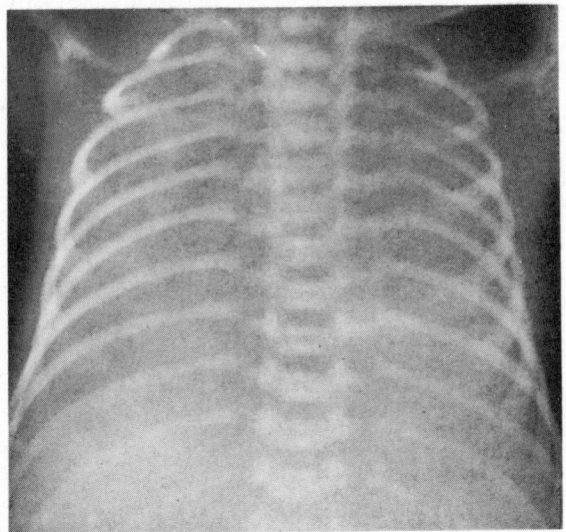

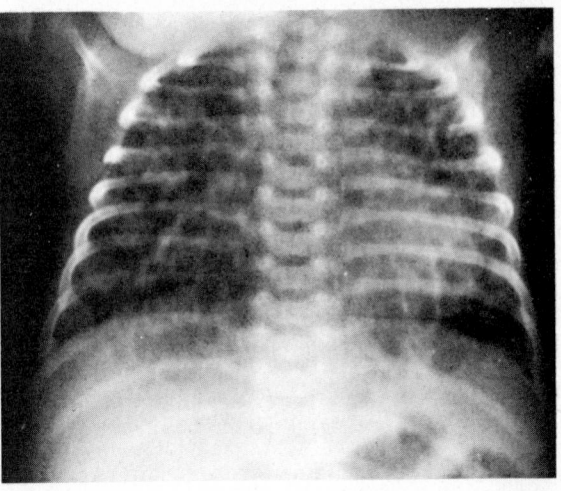

FIG. 31.   The third stage of chronic lung disease following neonatal lung injury. The chest radiograph reveals bilateral patchy densities interspersed with areas of increased lucency. The diaphragm is flattened, and there is evidence of pulmonary hyperinflation.

FIG. 30.   Chest radiograph showing the early stage of chronic lung disease, during the healing phase of hyaline membrane disease, in which there is almost complete opacification of both lungs, obscuring the heart borders and outline of the diaphragm. This picture is consistent with generalized atelectasis and accumulation of interstitial fluid.

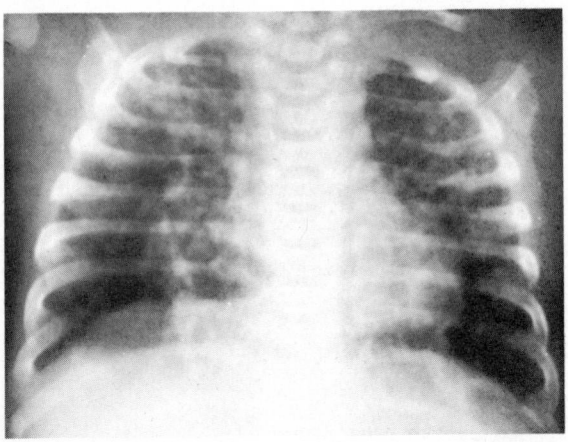

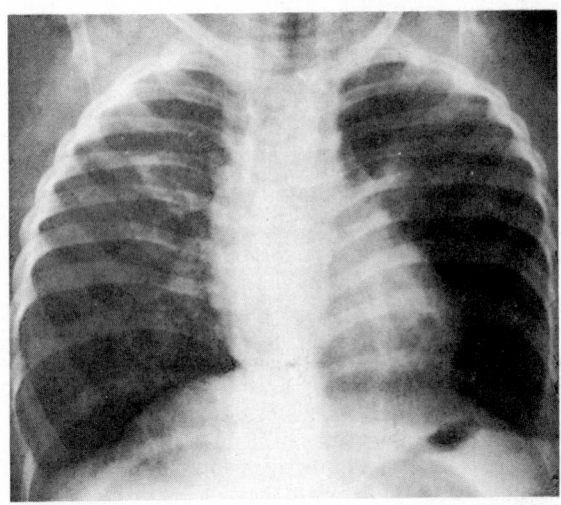

FIG. 32.   Chest radiograph of the fourth stage of chronic lung disease, demonstrating hyperlucency of the lower lobes, diffuse bilateral densities, and slight cardiomegaly.

FIG. 33.   Radiographic abnormalities persist at 2 years of age in an infant with chronic lung disease following prolonged mechanical ventilation with supplemental oxygen for severe hyaline membrane disease. There is bilateral hyperlucency, with increased perihilar markings, depression of the diaphragm, and hyperexpansion of the chest wall. The hyperinflation is most marked in the bases of the lung.

bronchial air shadows (air bronchograms) (see Fig. 20). In stage II, from 4 to 10 days of age, there may be almost complete opacification of both lungs (Fig. 30). This opacification is consistent with accumulation of extravascular lung fluid and atelectasis. From 10 to 20 days of age, bilateral irregular densities appear, combined with small areas of radiolucency (stage III). This picture is consistent with nonhomogeneous ventilation, a mixture of over- and underinflated areas (Fig. 31), similar to that seen in the *pulmonary dysmaturity syndrome* (see below). In stage IV, there is cardiomegaly and hyperlucency in the lower lobes (Fig. 32). Thereafter,

the hyperinflation, streaky densities, and prominent perihilar markings persist for many months. The radiographic picture suggests emphysema and fibrosis (Fig. 33). In our experience radiographic abnormalities were present at 2 years of age in 25 percent of surviving infants with hyaline membrane disease, whom we treated with continuous positive airway pressure or assisted ventilation with positive end-expiratory pressure.

PATHOLOGY.   During the first 2 to 3 days of hyaline membrane disease, the most prominent pathologic findings in the lungs are fibrin clots (hyaline membranes) lining dilated alveolar ducts, increased interstitial fluid, dilated lymphatics, and diffuse atelectasis (see hyaline membrane disease, p. 1519). The airway mucosa appears almost normal at this stage, with only mild metaplasia of the bronchiolar lining and minimal disturbance of ciliated epithelial cells and mucous glands. During this early exudative phase, there is moderate-to-severe vascular congestion and the lungs are heavy, sometimes hemorrhagic.

At 4 to 10 days, hyaline membranes persist but may be fragmented. The interalveolar septa are necrotic, the air spaces coalesce, and the microvascular basement membranes widen. The perivascular and interlobar tissue distends with fluid, and there are prominent pulmonary lymphatics. There are many macrophages in the intra- and interalveolar spaces; in addition, there is often necrosis of the airway mucosa, with squamous metaplasia and eosinophilic exudate on the mucosal surface.

Between 10 and 40 days, the exudate regresses and the number of macrophages, alveolar epithelial cells, plasma cells, and fibroblasts increases. There are fewer hyaline membranes and the alveolar epithelium appears disorganized. Bronchial and bronchiolar mucosal hyperplasia and metaplasia are notable, alveolar macrophages and histiocytes enter the airways, and overdistended alveolar ducts are interspersed between areas of cellular proliferation and atelectasis.

After the first month, smooth muscle surrounding airways hypertrophies, producing further hyperinflation. The pulmonary vessels increase in number, with development of medial hypertrophy and scattered fibrosis. There are many new capillaries, which often are widely separated from the alveolar epithelium and airspaces. Lymphatics remain prominent and tortuous within the widened interstitial tissue spaces. The peribronchiolar and periarteriolar lymphatics are particularly prominent, often appearing large enough to compress the airways and vessels.

TREATMENT.   Since so many infants with this condition have a history of receiving high concentrations of oxygen, every effort must be made to reduce the inspired oxygen concentration to below 50 percent as quickly as possible. Recent reports suggest that the early use of continuous positive or negative pressure, particularly without an endotracheal tube, may reduce the incidence of chronic changes following hyaline membrane disease.

A limited salt and water intake is desirable, since pulmonary edema is a prominent feature of the early stages of persistent respiratory distress after hyaline membrane disease. Digitalis is of little or no benefit and, because of intermittent disturbances in potassium balance, its use may be dangerous.

In some cases potent diuretics appear to reduce pulmonary infiltrates and improve gas exchange. We have found that intravenous or intramuscular furosemide (1 to 2 mg/kg body weight) may be particularly beneficial in these infants when they have a sudden deterioration associated with rales and carbon dioxide retention.

Continued diuretic therapy may be helpful in reducing the accumulation of interstitial fluid in severe cases.

All these infants must be observed closely for signs and symptoms of respiratory infection, which may lead to further lung damage and delay healing. The use of continuous antibiotic therapy, however, has not yielded any benefit and may, in fact, predispose to infection with organisms difficult to treat.

PULMONARY DYSMATURITY SYNDROME (WILSON-MIKITY SYNDROME, CYSTIC EMPHYSEMA)

CLINICAL FEATURES.   This syndrome occurs mostly in infants with birthweight below 1,500 g who are less than 30 weeks gestation. They usually have no respiratory distress during the first week after birth, but there is often a history of birth asphyxia and antepartum maternal hemorrhage. The onset is insidious, with progressive tachypnea, intercostal retractions, and cyanosis. Symptoms are usually mild and intermittent during the first 1 to 2 weeks. Cough, wheezing, and feeding difficulties develop after 2 to 3 weeks, with increasing signs of respiratory insufficiency. Apnea may ensue, requiring ventilatory assistance and increased concentrations of inspired oxygen. These infants have arterial hypoxemia, respiratory acidosis, low lung volumes and compliance, increased expiratory flow resistance, and an increase in the work of breathing. In some, osteoporosis and stress fractures occur near the posterior rib angles.

RADIOGRAPHIC FEATURES.   The chest roentgenogram initially shows a bilateral, diffuse reticularity, within which are scattered small, hyperlucent patches, producing a "bubbly" appearance (Fig. 34). There is generalized hyperaeration during this stage of the dis-

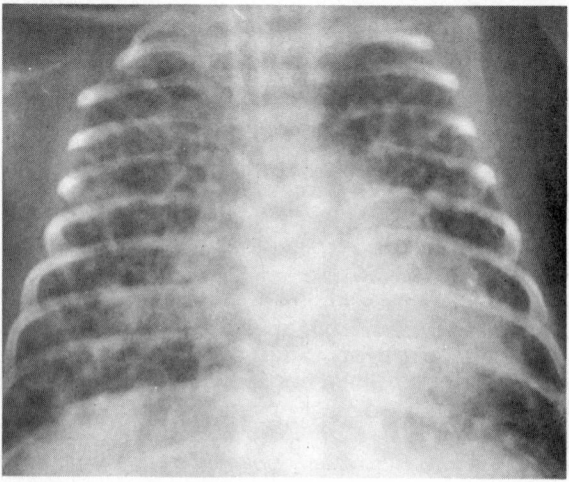

FIG. 34.   Typical radiographic features of the pulmonary dysmaturity syndrome include bilateral streaky lung densities with patches of hyperlucency, producing a bubbly appearance.

ease. In some cases the picture is preceded by hazy densities in both lung fields. By 6 weeks, the radiographic picture changes to one of bilateral, coarse streaks radiating from the hilar region, more in the upper than the lower lobes. With further progression, the lucent foci enlarge and coalesce, with flattening of the diaphragms and overexpansion of both lungs. These findings are similar to stage IV abnormalities in the Northway classification for chronic lung disease following neonatal lung injury. In most cases the chest roentgenogram become normal within 4 to 11 months.

PATHOLOGY. Hodgman and associates described the lungs after death as hyperinflated and bulky, with a mixture of collapsed and overdistended alveoli but no cellular proliferation; scattered fibrosis and vascular proliferation were noted late in the disease. In many cases the right ventricle was hypertrophied. Late in the disease, the clinical, radiologic, and morphologic features are indistinguishable from those in chronic lung disease following lung injury.

TREATMENT. In the chronic stage, treatment includes increased oxygen, vitamin supplements, and adequate nutrition. Chronic pulmonary edema is unusual, unless the infant has required prolonged assisted ventilation with a mechanical ventilator. When pulmonary edema is present, treatment is similar to that in chronic disease following hyaline membrane disease.

LATE DIFFUSE ATELECTASIS IN PRETERM INFANTS (CHRONIC PULMONARY INSUFFICIENCY OF PREMATURITY)

This condition characteristically develops in very small, prematurely born infants who initially appear to have normal lungs. During the first week, they develop progressive atelectasis, hypoxemia, and increasing respiratory distress. A likely explanation of this phenomenon is the immature infant's compliant chest cage, which at end-expiration does not expand and opposes the retractive force of the lung, so that the functional residual capacity of the lung decreases with successive expirations. Many of these infants compensate for this with frequent sighs, which reexpand their small and atelectactic airspaces. Some of them apparently cannot maintain an adequate lung volume with sighing and develop progressive atelectasis. As lung volume decreases, intrapulmonary shunts occur, producing progressive cyanosis. Apnea is a common feature, often requiring ventilatory assistance. If these infants require endotracheal intubation and mechanical ventilation, lung injury may occur, comparable to that following hyaline membrane disease. The chest roentgenogram is characterized by reduced lung size and a diffuse parenchymal haziness early in the disease. Later, particularly if the infants are treated with mechanical ventilation, there may be secondary lung injury, making it difficult to differentiate this condition from chronic lung disease following hyaline membrane disease.

TREATMENT. In the early stage, intermittent expansion of the lungs with mask and bag or by stimula-tion may be helpful. Some infants may require lung distention by application of a continuous positive or negative airway pressure. The prognosis is good.

Bibliography

Baghdassarian OM, Avery ME, Neuhauser EBD: A form of pulmonary insufficiency in premature infants. Pulmonary dysmaturity? Am J Roentgenol 89:1020, 1963

Berg TJ, Pagtakhan RD, Reed MH, Langston C, Chernick V: Bronchopulmonary dysplasia and lung rupture in hyaline membrane disease: influence of continuous distending pressure. Pediatrics 55:51, 1975

Butterfield J, Moscovici C, Berry C: Cystic emphysema in premature infants, a report of an outbreak with the isolation of type 19 ECHO virus in one case. N Engl J Med 268:18, 1963

Campiche M, Jaccottet M, Juillard E: La pneumonose à membranes hyalines. Observations au microscope éléctronique. Ann Paediatr 199:74, 1962

Hodgman JE, Mikity VG, Tatter D, Cleland RS: Chronic respiratory distress in the premature infant. Wilson-Mikity syndrome. Pediatrics 44:179, 1969

Krauss AN, Klain DB, Auld PAM: Chronic pulmonary insufficiency of prematurity (CPIP). Pediatrics 55:55, 1975

Moylan FMB, O'Connell KC, Todres ID, Shannon DC: Edema of the pulmonary interstitium in infants and children. Pediatrics 55:783, 1975

Northway WH Jr, Rosan RC, Porter DY: Pulmonary disease following respiratory therapy of hyaline membrane disease. Bronchopulmonary dysplasia. N Engl J Med 276:358, 1967

Northway WH Jr, Rosan RC: Radiographic features of pulmonary oxygen toxicity in the newborn: bronchopulmonary dysplasia. Radiology 91:49, 1968

Rhodes PG, Hall RT, Leonidas JC: Chronic pulmonary disease in neonates with assisted ventilation. Pediatrics 55:788, 1975

Shepard FM, Johnson RB, Klatte EC, Barke H, Stahlman M: Residual pulmonary findings in clinical hyaline membrane disease. N Engl J Med 279:1063, 1968

Wilson MG, Mikity VG: A new form of respiratory distress in premature infants. Am J Dis Child 99:489, 1960

PULMONARY EDEMA

RICHARD D. BLAND

In the lung, as in other organs, fluid and protein flow continuously out of the blood into the interstitial space and return to the vascular system, either directly across the microvascular endothelium or through an extensive network of lymphatic channels. Pulmonary edema develops when the net outward flow from the pulmonary circulation exceeds the clearance capacity of the lymphatics.

Initially, fluid accumulates in the loose connective tissue of the lung interstitium, beneath the pleura, between lobes, and surrounding airways and vessels. In the early stages of edema, most of the extravascular fluid gravitates to the dependent portions of the lung, where the intravascular hydrostatic pressure is highest. When the capacity of the interstitium is exceeded, fluid moves abruptly into the airspaces, pulling protein across the normally solute-restrictive alveolar epithelium. The lungs become boggy and congested, fluid distends the lymphatics, lung compliance and vital capacity fall, and gas exchange is impaired.

Figure 35 illustrates schematically forces that determine fluid balance in the lung. As described by Starling in 1896, the movement of liquid across the semipermeable capillary endothelial membrane is governed by the difference between (a) hydrostatic pressure within the vessel and in the surrounding interstitium, and (b) colloid osmotic pressure of plasma protein molecules inside the vessel and those in the extravascular space. Other contributory variables are permeability of the microvascular membrane to plasma proteins, tissue forces originating from changes in transpulmonary pressure, and surface tension of the alveoli, which in turn affects interstitial hydrostatic pressure.

Pulmonary edema is a frequent pathologic finding in infants who die from a variety of cardiorespiratory disorders, including congenital heart disease, hyaline membrane disease, upper airway obstruction, and chronic lung disease. Excessive accumulation of lung fluid also occurs in disorders of the central nervous system, hydrops fetalis, and endotoxic shock and in association with the sudden infant death syndrome.

Most cases of pulmonary edema in the newborn period are attributable to increased pulmonary microvascular pressure, usually from left ventricular failure. This may be precipitated by a large placental transfusion; *stripping* of the umbilical cord at birth; excessive infusions of blood, colloid, or crystalloid solutions; asphyxia; or cardiac decompensation in cases of congenital heart disease(p.1407) or myocardial diseases (p.1471).

Low plasma colloid osmotic pressure, resulting from hypoproteinemia, also may produce disturbances in lung fluid clearance and predispose infants to pulmonary edema. Guyton and Lindsay found that by halving the intravascular colloid osmotic pressure of dogs, they could produce pulmonary edema at a left atrial pressure less than half that required to cause edema in the presence of a normal plasma protein concentration. Reduced levels of plasma proteins are particularly prevalent among prematurely born infants; large infusions of protein-free fluids may depress the plasma protein level further and thereby predispose infants to pulmonary edema.

Pattle suggested that an abnormally high surface tension at the air–liquid interface of terminal airspaces might be expected to lower lung interstitial pressure, resulting in extravasation of fluid and protein from the vascular space. This might explain the pulmonary edema found in the early phase of the respiratory distress syndrome. A similar explanation has been invoked to explain the pulmonary edema sometimes associated with upper airway obstruction in which substantial increases in transpulmonary pressure may lower interstitial hydrostatic pressure and precipitate increased movement of fluid and protein out of the circulation. Warren and associates found, in dogs, that inspiratory obstruction produced a substantial rise in lung lymph flow; this has been attributed to changes in filtration pressure.

Other experimental work suggests that the pulmonary microvascular endothelium of the fetus and newborn is more permeable to protein molecules than in the adult. Damage to the capillary membrane by excessive concentrations of inspired oxygen or by endotoxemia associated with infection may further disrupt normal lung fluid balance.

The usual clinical manifestations of pulmonary edema in infancy are tachypnea, retractions of the chest wall, flaring of the alae nasae, grunting, tachycardia, hepatomegaly, oxygen dependence (cyanosis), and feeding intolerance. Compression of small airways by

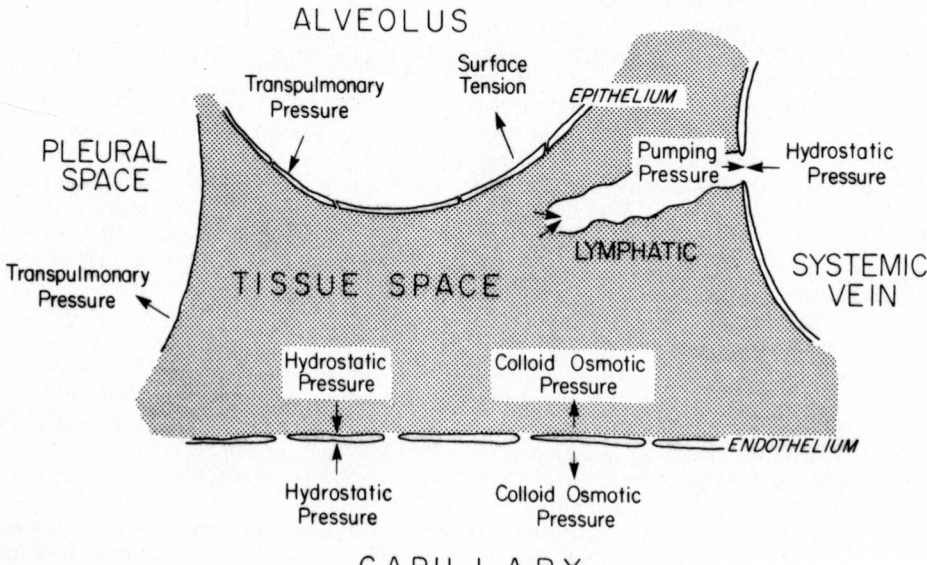

FIG. 35.   Schematic drawing of the lung, demonstrating the various forces that move fluid in and out of the interstitial tissue space.

tissue fluid may produce expiratory wheezing. Progressive decompensation leads to gasping respirations, apnea, peripheral vasoconstriction, and bradycardia. With alveolar flooding, there may be moist rales in addition to blood-tinged or grossly bloody orotracheal secretions. Ventilatory failure, with insufficient oxygen delivery to tissues, will result in combined metabolic and respiratory acidemia.

Unfortunately, in most cases, the diagnosis of pulmonary edema is difficult before the onset of overt physical signs of respiratory distress. Cardiovascular causes should be considered (p. 1477). The chest roentgenograms may demonstrate diffuse, bilateral infiltrates, particularly in the peripheral and basilar areas, with prominent vascularity and cardiomegaly. Fluid in the interlobar fissures and pleural space also may be present. With alveolar flooding, this picture may progress to a diffuse, bilateral haziness, with air bronchograms, and obliteration of the cardiac silhouette.

In the late stages of alveolar edema, the diagnosis may be confirmed by analysis of the lung effluent collected from the airway. The fluid usually has a protein concentration at least half of that in plasma. The secretions contain more albumin than globulin, which is evidence that molecular sieving occurs in the vascular endothelium.

Treatment includes restriction of fluid and sodium equivalent to insensible losses, digitalis for cardiogenic pulmonary edema (p. 1481), diuretics, and supplemental oxygen to maintain a normal arterial partial pressure of oxygen. Chlorthiazide, 10 mg/kg, two to four times a day, or, in severe edema, furosemide, 1 mg/kg intravenously, usually produces a satisfactory diuresis. If diuretics are required over an extended period of time, potassium supplements must be given. In light of recent evidence that furosemide displaces bilirubin from albumin, this potent diuretic should be withheld from infants with appreciable hyperbilirubinemia. In the acute stages of pulmonary edema, intramuscular morphine sulfate, 0.1 to 0.2 mg/kg, may be beneficial but must be given with caution because of its potential depressant effect on ventilation. If these measures are not successful in achieving substantial improvement, ventilatory support with continuous positive airway pressure may be useful. In cases of respiratory failure, mechanical ventilation with positive end-expiratory pressure should be utilized. Cardiac lesions should be treated appropriately with, if indicated, surgery.

Bibliography

Cole VA, Normand ICS, Reynolds EOR, Rivers RPA: Pathogenesis of hemorrhagic pulmonary edema and massive pulmonary hemorrhage in the newborn. Pediatrics 51:175, 1973

Guyton AC, Lindsay AW: Effect of elevated left atrial pressure and decreased plasma protein concentration on the development of pulmonary edema. Circ Res 7:649, 1959

Haddy FJ, Campbell GS, Visscher MB: Pulmonary vascular pressures in relation to edema production by airway resistance and plethora in dogs. Am J Physiol 161:336, 1950

Pattle RE: Properties, function, and origin of the alveolar lining layer. Proc R Soc London 148:217, 1958

Staub NC: Pathogenesis of pulmonary edema. Am Rev Resp Dis 109: 358, 1974

Staub NC: Pulmonary edema. Physiol Rev 54:679, 1974

Visscher MB, Haddy FJ, Stephens G: The physiology and pharmacology of lung edema. Pharmacol Rev 8:839, 1956

Warren MF, Peterson DK, Drinker CK: The effects of heightened negative pressure in the chest, together with further experiments upon anoxia in increasing the flow of lung lymph. Am J Physiol 137:641, 1942

CONGENITAL PULMONARY LYMPHANGIECTASIS

Richard D. Bland

Congenital dilatation of the lung lymphatics, first described by Virchow in 1856, is a rare disorder that usually produces respiratory failure and death within the first few days after birth. In most cases it occurs either as a primary developmental anomaly or as a consequence of obstruction to pulmonary venous drainage or left ventricular outflow. Rarely, it may present as part of a generalized form of lymphangiectasis, in which pulmonary involvement is less severe and is associated with a better prognosis for survival.

CLINICAL FEATURES. Males are affected more often than females. About one-third of the infants with this condition have been born prematurely, and over one-half have had other major congenital malformations. Symptoms of cyanosis and severe respiratory distress usually begin at birth, and the infants have increasing respiratory distress and usually die within days or weeks. In cases of prolonged survival, the clinical features are overexpanded lungs, recurrent wheezing, and alveolar hypoventilation, producing hypoxemia and hypercapnia, with eventual pulmonary hypertension and cor pulmonale. Congenital dilatation of the lymphatics should be considered in the differential diagnosis of respiratory distress syndrome, aspiration pneumonitis, pulmonary hemorrhage, and fulminant pneumonia. Chronic lung disease, pulmonary edema, and cystic fibrosis must be distinguished from lymphangiectasis in those who survive beyond the newborn period.

Characteristic radiographic findings in this condition are hyperaeration, with a depressed diaphragm, diffuse nodular infiltrates, and a bilateral reticular appearance of the lungs. Bullous changes may develop if survival is prolonged, and rupture of an air-filled cyst may produce a pneumothorax. At autopsy, the lungs are large, firm, inelastic, and heavy, with gross dilatation and tortuosity of the subpleural, perivascular, and interlobar lymphatic channels. Cut sections of lung reveal fluid-filled, irregularly shaped cysts, and a considerable amount of fibrous tissue. The right side of the heart is usually hypertrophied, and there is a high incidence of total anomalous pulmonary venous connection (p. 1462) and hypoplasia of the left heart, among infants with lymphangiectasis. Several cases have been described in association with agenesis of the spleen. There is no effective therapy for this condition; cardiac catheterization should be performed in suspected cases to rule out remediable causes of pulmonary venous obstruction. Temporizing measures may include administration of supplemental oxygen, digoxin, and diuretics.

Bibliography

CONGENITAL PULMONARY LYMPHANGIECTASIS

Ekelund H, Palmstierna S, Ostberg G: Congenital pulmonary lymphangiectasis. Acta Paediatr Scand 55:121, 1966

Felman AH, Rhatigan RM, Pierson KK: Pulmonary lymphangiectasis, observations in 17 patients and proposed classification. Am J Roentgenol 116:548, 1972

France NE, Brown RJK: Congenital pulmonary lymphangiectasis. Report of 11 examples with special reference to cardiovascular findings. Arch Dis Child 46:528, 1971

Fronstin MH, Hooper GS, Besse BE, Ferreri S: Congenital pulmonary cystic lymphangiectasis, case report and review of 32 cases. Am J Dis Child 114:330, 1967

Noonan JA, Walter LR, Reeves JT: Congenital pulmonary lymphangiectasis. Am J Dis Child 120:314, 1970

PATENT DUCTUS ARTERIOSUS AND PULMONARY EDEMA

JOSEPH A. KITTERMAN

In term infants, the ductus arteriosus constricts shortly after birth in response to the postnatal rise in arterial oxygen tension (Pao$_2$). In small preterm infants, persistent patency of the ductus arteriosus is common and occurs in up to 40 percent of infants of birth weight 1,750 g or less; two-thirds of these may develop pulmonary edema and congestive heart failure. The clinical features, differential diagnosis, and management of this condition are discussed in Chapter 27, page 1411.

Bibliography

DesLignenes S, Larroche JC: Ductus arteriosus. I. Anatomical and histological study of its development during the second half of gestation and its closure after birth. II. Histological study of a few cases of patent ductus arteriosus in infancy. Biol Neonat 16:278, 1970

Griffin AJ, Ferrara JD, Lax JO, Cassels DE: Pulmonary compliance: an index of cardiovascular status in infancy. Am J Dis Child 123:89, 1972

Kitterman JA, Edmunds LH, Gregory GA, et al: Patent ductus arteriosus in premature infants: incidence, relation to pulmonary disease and management. N Engl J Med 287:473, 1972

McMurphy DM, Heymann MA, Rudolph AM, Melmon KL: Developmental changes in constriction of the ductus arteriosus: responses to oxygen and vasoactive agents in the isolated ductus arteriosus of the fetal lamb. Pediatr Res 6:231, 1972

Powell ML: Patent ductus arteriosus in premature infants. Med J Austral 2:58, 1963

DIAPHRAGMATIC HERNIA

GEORGE A. GREGORY

JOSEPH A. KITTERMAN

Diaphragmatic hernia is a condition in which failure of normal fetal development of the diaphragm results in intrusion of abdominal contents into the thorax. It occurs in approximately 1 per 2,000 births.

EMBRYOLOGY. During the 8th to 10th week of fetal life, the diaphragm forms, dividing the coelomic cavity into its abdominal and thoracic components. The transverse septum grows backward to join the dorsal mesentery of the foregut, to form the central portion of the diaphragm; pleuroperitoneal folds develop and extend laterally and posteriorly to complete the diaphragm. The folds are initially membranous and, later, are reinforced by muscle fibers derived from cervical myotomes. The posterior part of the diaphragm is usually the last to close, the left closing later than the right. When open it forms a triangular defect, the foramen of Bochdalek, the site of the Bochdalek hernia, the most common type of diaphragmatic hernia. Failure of fusion of the central and lateral portions of the diaphragm results in a retrosternal defect, the foramen of Morgagni. This is an uncommon site for diaphragmatic hernias, as is the esophageal hiatus. The incidence of the various types of hernia is shown in Table 9.

TABLE 9. Incidence of Congenital Diaphragmatic Hernia

Type	Number	Percent
Bochdalek	69	59.5
Morgagni	3	2.6
Hiatus hernia	16	13.8
Short esophagus	11	9.5
Eventration	17	14.6
Total	116	100.0

(From Baffes: Pediatric Surgery. Year Book Med. Publishers, Chicago, 1969)

While the diaphragm is forming, the midgut rapidly elongates into the umbilical pouch. About the 10th week of gestation the midgut rotates and returns to the abdominal cavity; if the diaphragm has not formed completely, the gut may enter the thoracic cavity. The gut may also enter the thorax if the diaphragm is complete but has poor muscular development, as in eventration of the diaphragm. Failure of the esophagus to elongate early in fetal life may prevent descent of the stomach into the abdominal cavity.

When the gut enters the chest it occupies space that normally would be occupied by lung and causes an arrest in lung growth on the ipsilateral side; growth is also decreased in the contralateral lung, but not as severely. On the ipsilateral side, the number of airways and alveoli are markedly reduced. The pulmonary artery at the hilum is appropriate for the size of the lung but too small for the size of the infant. The amount of muscle in small pulmonary vessels is greater than normal. These factors probably explain why these infants have a marked increase in pulmonary vascular resistance.

DIAGNOSIS depends on the type of hernia present. *Foramen of Morgagni* hernias are infrequent and usually contain a true sac. The signs are more often of bowel obstruction and seldom of respiratory embarrassment. Symptoms may not occur until later in life. Diagnosis often is made incidentally on chest radiograph. If bowel obstruction or respiratory embarrassment occurs, immediate surgical repair is mandatory. Those which do not cause symptoms may not need repair. With *eventration of the diaphragm*, the severity of clinical signs depends on the size of eventration. Those which are large may cause considerable respiratory embarrassment and require repair. *Formen of Bochdalek hernias* are the most common and most often cause respiratory embarrassment. Their presence in the thoracic cavity interferes with lung function and growth, manifested as cyanosis and respiratory distress in the immediate neonatal period. With the onset of respiration, the negative intrathoracic pressure tends to fill the intrathoracic gut with swallowed gas. As the gut dilates ventilatory difficulty increases. Prompt diagnosis and treatment are necessary to prevent death.

PHYSICAL EXAMINATION. The infant is tachypneic and the abdomen is scaphoid. When pulmonary vascular resistance is high and there is a right-to-left shunt through the ductus arteriosus, differential cyanosis may be present; the head is pink, but the lower body is blue. The affected side of the chest is dull to percussion before the gut fills with air and tympanic afterwards. Breath sounds may be absent. Bowel sounds are rarely heard in the chest. Heart tones are displaced contralaterally.

The diagnosis is confirmed by chest and abdominal radiographs, which show the intestine, and often the stomach, within the thorax and a paucity of gas in the abdominal cavity (Fig. 36). It is rarely necessary to give radiopaque materials to diagnose diaphragmatic hernia, although occasionally it is necessary to differentiate diaphragmatic hernia from lung cysts and other congenital anomalies.

TREATMENT. As soon as the diagnosis is suspected, a catheter should be inserted into an umbilical artery for measurement of blood gases, pH, and blood pressure. Shock and hypotension may be present if large amounts of fluid accumulate within the gut lumen after birth. Due to right-to-left shunting through the ductus arteriosus, P_{O_2} in the descending aortic blood may be lower than that in the right radial or temporal artery. Because of inadequate alveolar ventilation, arterial P_{CO_2} is often elevated above 70 torr; if P_{CO_2} is markedly increased, the trachea should be intubated and ventilation assisted at rapid rates and small tidal volumes to decrease the likelihood of pneumothorax. Surgery to remove the gut from the thoracic cavity often is required before blood gases and pH will improve. During surgery, the lung should be expanded gently but *under no circumstances should one try to inflate the hypoplastic lung to its expected normal size.* This will cause a pneumothorax, often on the *normal side,* and is often the cause of death after successful surgery. Bilateral thoracotomy tubes should be left in place to an under water seal for several days.

During the postoperative period, the baby may have difficulty in breathing due to a distended abdomen, poor diaphragmatic function, and lung hypoplasia. Therefore, ventilation almost always needs support. This usually can be accomplished with continuous positive airway pressure, if hypercarbia is not present. If arterial carbon dioxide tension is more than 60 torr, mechanical ventilation with positive end-expiratory pressure should be continued. The positive end-expiratory pressure helps to reduce atelectasis and improve oxygenation.

Because of fluid losses into the intestinal lumen, thoracic cavity, abdominal cavity, and via gastric suction, the infant may become hypovolemic and hypotensive

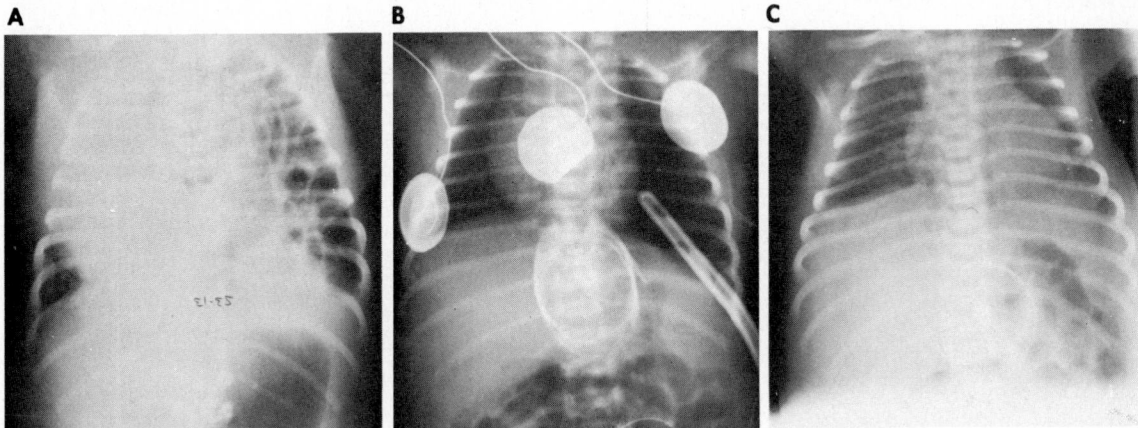

A   **B**   **C**

FIG. 36. **A.** 2-hour-old infant with a Bochdalek hernia. Note the bowel filled with air in the left chest, the displacement of the heart into the right chest, the marked atelectasis of the right upper lung, and the gas-filled stomach. The functional residual capacity was 8.5 ml/kg or 30 percent of that predicted. **B.** Immediately after surgery. Note that the bowel has been returned to the abdominal cavity, the left thorax is filled with air, and the lung is not seen. The heart and mediastinum have been relieved. The infant was being treated with 6 torr continuous positive airway pressure. Functional residual capacity was 14 ml/kg or 50 percent of predicted. **C.** On postoperative day 21, the left chest is filled with lung. Functional residual capacity was 21.5 ml/kg or 80 percent of that predicted. This increase in functional residual capacity is too great to have occurred except by expansion of a severely atelectatic left lung. This suggests that the bowel entered the left chest late in gestation.

and require large volumes of blood, colloids, and electrolyte solutions to maintain an adequate circulation. Once intestinal motility has become adequate, oral feedings can be started and the parenteral fluids discontinued. Usually these infants eventually are able to maintain adequate ventilation on their own, and the affected lung expands; thus early diagnosis and therapy are mandatory.

Bibliography

Baffes TG: Diaphragmatic hernia. In Mustard WT, Ravitch MM, Snyder WH Jr, et al (eds): Pediatric Surgery. Year Book Medical Publishers, Chicago, 1969

deLorimier AF, Tierney DF, Parker HR: Hypoplastic lungs in fetal lambs with surgically produced congenital diaphragmatic hernia. Surgery 62:12, 1967

Kitagawa M, Hislap A, Boyden EA, Reid L: Lung hypoplasia in congenital diaphragmatic hernia. A quantitative study of airway, artery and alveolar development. Br J Surg 58:342, 1971

RESPIRATORY FUNCTION AND PULMONARY DISEASE IN OLDER INFANTS AND CHILDREN

WILLIAM H. TOOLEY
HERMAN W. LIPOW

Respiration is the sequence of physical and chemical steps needed to supply oxygen for oxidative metabolism and to remove carbon dioxide formed in energy-producing reactions. The lungs and circulation subserve this process. The lungs consist of a distribution system (the airways) and millions of small sacs (alveoli) with a large surface area where the exchange of oxygen and carbon dioxide between air and blood is accomplished by diffusion across a thin barrier composed of alveolar and capillary walls (the parenchyma). Movement of gas in and out of the lungs is effected by the contraction and relaxation of the diaphragm and the intercostal and abdominal muscles, which increase and decrease the volume of the thorax.

THE AIRWAYS

Defective structure, foreign bodies, tumors, and inflammation can decrease the internal diameter of the airway and obstruct the flow of gas. Since the signs, symptoms, physiologic consequences, and principles of treatment for all airway obstructions are similar regardless of the proximate cause, the general problem of airway blockage will be considered before detailing particular diseases.

Anatomy

The nose, pharynx, larynx, and the upper part of the trachea which is outside the thorax (extrathoracic airway) are considered to be the upper airway. The lower airway includes the lower part of the trachea, the bron-

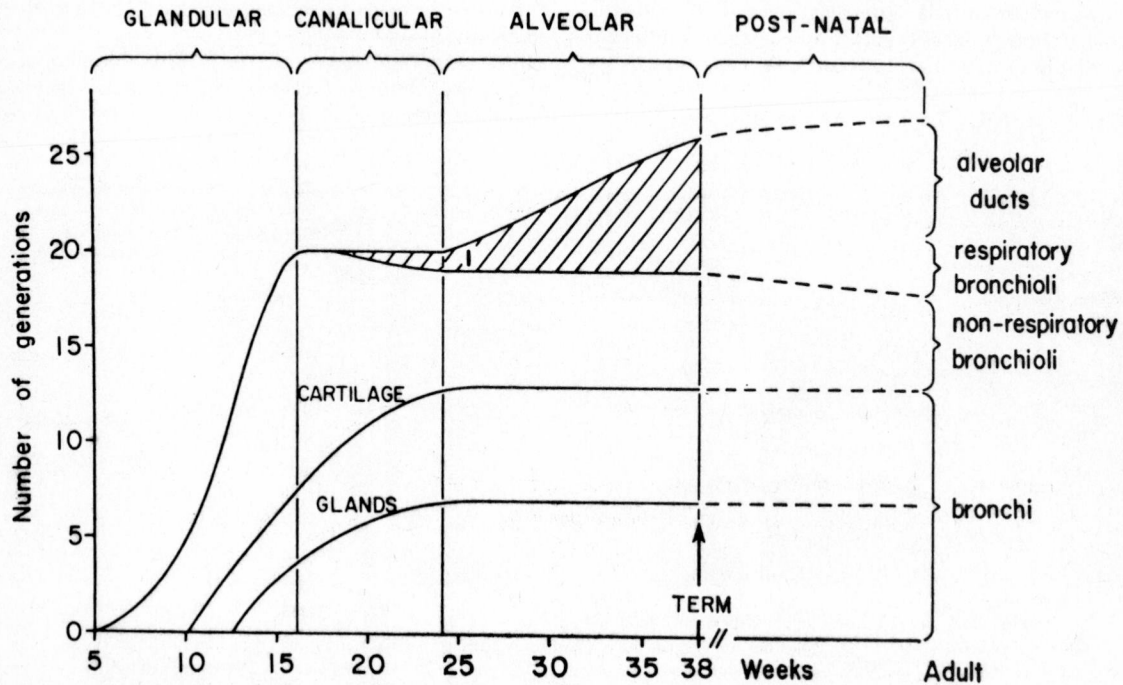

FIG. 37. Diagrammatic representation of the development of the bronchial tree. Lobar bronchi appear at the 6th week of gestation; by 16 weeks, all nonrespiratory airways are present. Most respiratory airways appear between 16 and 40 weeks. Bronchial cartilage appears at 10 weeks, and by 24 weeks is present in 13 generations of bronchi. Bronchial glands appear at 13 weeks and are present in the first seven generations by the 24th week of gestation. (From Reid L: Scientific Foundations of Paediatrics. Courtesy of Wm Heinemann, Ltd)

chi, and their subdivisions to the level of the respiratory bronchioles (intrathoracic airway).

The airways, alveoli, and blood vessels develop at different rates. Reid has summarized the pattern of lung growth (Fig. 37):

1. The bronchial tree is developed by the 16th week of intrauterine life;
2. Alveoli develop after birth, increasing in number until the age of 8 years, and in size until growth of the chest wall finishes with adulthood;
3. The pre-acinar vessels (arteries and veins) follow the development of the airways, the intra-acinar follow those of the alveoli.

The airways receive their blood supply from vessels derived from the third and fourth embryonic aortic arches: the larynx from the external carotid (third arch); the extrathoracic trachea from the subclavian (fourth arch); and the lower airway from the aorta (fourth arch) via the bronchial arteries. The motor nerves of the larynx come from the recurrent branches of the vagus and the sensory nerves from the superior laryngeal branch of the vagus. Sympathetic and parasympathetic fibers supply the entire lower airway.

Squamous cells line the larynx; equal numbers of ciliated columnar and goblet cells line the trachea, bronchi, and larger bronchioles; and ciliated cuboidal cells and occasional goblet cells line the smaller bronchioles. There are numerous mucous glands in the submucosal and muscular layers of the trachea and bronchi, but not in the smaller bronchi. The bases of the cilia are covered with a serous fluid, and their free ends extend into a mucous sheet that coats the entire tracheobronchial tree.

Three single and three paired articulated cartilages, which are connected by elastic tissue and muscles, make up the framework of the larynx. The muscles operate upon the paired cartilages, widening and narrowing the opening of the larynx into the lower pharynx. The dorsal ends of the cartilaginous crescents, which support the trachea and bronchi, are connected by muscle and connective tissue. These rings of muscle and cartilage are irregular and may split or fuse, particularly at the carina, whose framework may be membranous or cartilaginous. In the medium- and small-sized bronchi only fragments of cartilage remain, and the muscle forms a loose sheath that operates independently of the cartilage. In the bronchioles, muscle bundles spiral in helical turns and are proportionately thicker than in the larger airways.

The cartilage, other supporting structures, and glandular tissue are present at all ages, but the amount, strength, and distribution vary with growth. The ciliated cells are well developed at birth, but there are few goblet cells and mucous glands in the bronchi. After the first few months, goblet cells increase rapidly in number; the mucous glands increase in number and size and are abundant by 1 year of age. Growth in the cross-sectional area and tissue mass for the subdivision of the airway are not uniform. The rate of increase in diameter of the trachea and bronchi is accelerated in the early

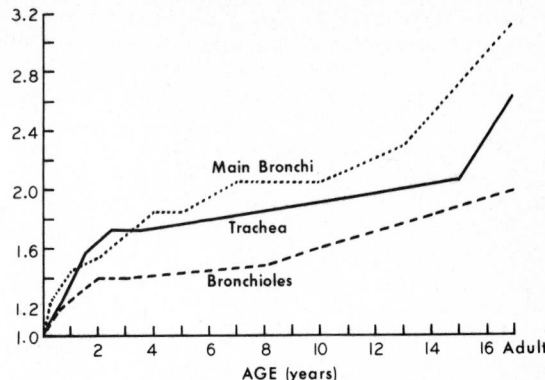

FIG. 38. The relative change in diameter of the principal components of the airway plotted against age. The diameter of the trachea doubles at about 15 years; that of the bronchi at 6 years. After an increase in diameter of 40 percent by 2 years, the bronchioles grow slowly, and in adult life are twice the diameter at birth. (From Engel: Lung Structure, courtesy of Charles C Thomas)

years and during puberty, whereas after an initial growth spurt, the bronchiolar diameter increases slowly (Fig. 38). From birth to the completion of growth, the weight of the lungs and the total lung capacity increase twentyfold, while the airway diameters increase only two- to threefold. In the newborn, the trachea and bronchi have relatively little cartilage, elastic tissue, connective tissue, or muscle and the ratio of the diameter of the lumen to wall thickness is large. The muscle is thin in the smaller airways in the neonatal period and enlarges only slightly in the first year, but after the fourth year, it increases in thickness in proportion to the growth of the lungs. From birth to 15 years, the diameter of large bronchioles doubles, the thickness of their walls triples, and the amount of supporting tissue increases four- or fivefold (Fig. 39).

Function

The airway warms or cools, moistens, and purifies incoming air, and protects the lung against foreign bodies. It regulates the resistance to gas flow and its own

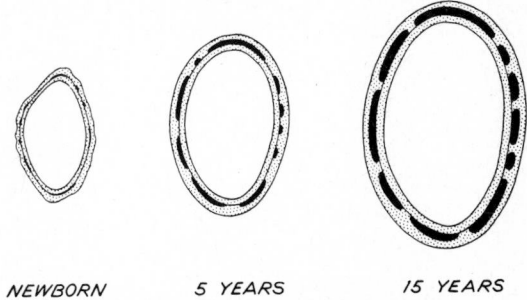

NEWBORN   5 YEARS   15 YEARS

FIG. 39. Diagrammatic representation of a large bronchiole at three ages. With growth, muscle, as depicted by the thick black lines within the wall, increases in amount and thickness. The diameter of the lumen and the ratio of wall thickness to luminal diameter also increase.

volume by altering the width of its lumen. By regional changes in resistance, the amount of gas going to different regions of the lungs can be varied. This provides less ventilation to those regions with a small blood flow, thus matching ventilation to perfusion.

The large and vascular surface of the nose and pharynx adds water and changes the temperature of inspired air to body temperature. During quiet breathing, even at extremes of environmental temperature and humidity, air is at body temperature and saturated with water when it reaches the larynx. When air flow is increased and cold, hot, or dry air is breathed, or when breathing is through an endotracheal or tracheotomy tube, temperature and humidity control are shared by the trachea and bronchi. Most large particles are blocked by nasal hairs, caught on the tortuous nasal passages, or carried by mucus into the pharynx and swallowed. Aspiration of food, foreign bodies, and mucus is prevented by closure of the larynx. Smaller particles settle on the airway's mucus blanket, which is constantly moved upward toward the pharynx by the cilia and keeps the alveoli free of almost all foreign matter. The propulsion of mucus is so rapid that it moves the length of the airway in a few hours. The airway in newborn and young infants is well adapted for air conditioning. However, the scarcity of mucus-producing elements may interfere with production of the mucus blanket, make the surface of the airway more susceptible to infection, and deprive the alveoli of some of their protection from bacteria and other foreign material. On the other hand, the hazard of clogging or blocking small passages because of excess production of mucus is reduced. Mucus does, however, block the small airways of some infants, as in cystic fibrosis.

Since there is little exchange of gas between the lumina of the airways and blood, their volume is respiratory dead space. For efficiency, dead space must be substantially smaller than the volume of each respiration (the tidal volume). In older children and adults, the ratio of dead space to tidal volume is about 0.3; ie, two-thirds of the volume of each breath reaches the alveolar ducts and alveoli, and one-third is left behind to fill the airway (anatomic dead space). In the premature baby this ratio is about 0.5; in the full-term baby and young infant, about 0.4 (Table 10). The relatively large volume of the airway is a disadvantage to the infant and requires movement of proportionally more gas in and out of the lungs each minute (minute volume). However, since the lumina are comparatively wide, the work of breathing is not excessive.

The pressure of a gas is determined by the number of molecules present in a given volume. When the diaphragm contracts and the thorax enlarges, the volume of the lungs increases, the intrapulmonary gas expands, and its concentration of gas molecules decreases. The pressure within the lungs is then less than at the mouth, and since gas moves from regions of relatively high to relatively low pressure, inspiration occurs. The volume of air that moves along the airway in a given period of time (flow) is approximately proportional to this pressure difference and to the radius of the airway raised to the fourth power, and inversely proportional to the length of the airway and the viscosity of the gas. Of these factors, the pressure change and width of the airway can vary the most. For example, doubling the pressure will double the flow, while if the pressure is constant and the radius doubled, this will increase flow 16 times. If the airway is small, the pressure difference must be large to sustain a given flow, and the work of breathing will be great. The strength of the muscles of inspiration and the capacity of the thorax to enlarge will limit the extent to which intrapulmonary pressure will fall below atmospheric pressure. The maximal pressure difference that the newborn can achieve is about 100 cm H_2O during inspiration and about 150 cm H_2O during expiration (maximal inspiratory and expiratory pressures). These transient pressure gradients are almost as large as in the adult (Table 10).

Respiratory maneuvers alter the airway diameter. During inspiration the pressure in the intrapleural space is less than atmospheric. With inspiration, the larynx and extrathoracic trachea tend to collapse, since their intraluminal pressures are less than those in the surrounding tissues; the intrathoracic trachea, bronchi, and bronchioles dilate, since their intraluminal pressures are higher than the pressure in the surrounding lung. The tendency of the extrathoracic airway to collapse and the intrathoracic airway to dilate with inspiration is greater when support is weak, as in the first years of life (Fig. 40). The dilation of most of the intrathoracic airway with inspiration increases the dead space and accounts, in part, for the infant's large dead space to

TABLE 10. Respiratory Function

	New-born	5	10	15	Adult
			Age (yr)		
Frequency (breaths/min)	30	24	20	16	12
Tidal volume (ml)	20	100	225	375	450
Dead space (ml)	8	35	75	125	150
Minute volume (ml/min)	600	2,400	4,500	6,000	6,000
Dead space/tidal volume	0.4	0.35	0.33	0.33	0.33
Alveolar ventilation (ml/min)	360	1,560	3,000	4,200	4,200
Maximal inspiratory pressure (cm H_2O)	100		100		125
Maximal expiratory pressure (cm H_2O)	150		200		250
Maximal inspiratory flow (liter/min)	8	75	160	325	400
Maximal expiratory flow (liter/min)	10	110	210	400	500

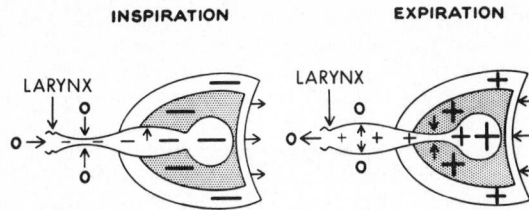

INSPIRATION   **EXPIRATION**

FIG. 40. The pressures along the airway and in the lung and intrapleural space during inspiration and expiration are represented by the size of the minus and plus signs. Atmospheric pressure is indicated by 0. The size of the arrows point out the magnitude of forces. The thin outline of the infant's airway indicates weak support. With inspiration, there is a gradual change from atmospheric pressure at the mouth to subatmospheric pressure in the alveoli. The extrathoracic trachea tends to collapse, since the pressure is less in the lumen than in the surrounding tissue, while the intrathoracic airway dilates. With expiration, pressure gradually changes from atmospheric in the alveoli to atmospheric at the mouth. The intrathoracic airway tends to collapse and the extrathoracic trachea tends to dilate. In the infant whose airways are weak and poorly supported, these phenomena may be marked.

tidal volume ratio. In order to maintain a given minute volume when the larynx is partially obstructed, the flow of air across the obstruction is rapid, the pressure in the trachea below the obstruction is significantly less than atmospheric, and the tendency of the extrathoracic trachea to collapse is exaggerated (Fig. 41).

Conversely, during expiration, tissue elasticity and surface tension of the distended alveoli generate pressures above atmospheric, so that gas flows from the alveoli up the airways to the mouth. As the inspiratory muscles relax, intrapleural pressure rises, tending to compress the intrathoracic airways. Cartilage in the wall of the airway makes it less compliant and resistant to compression.

Accelerated airflow past a bronchiolar obstruction, as in acute bronchiolitis, causes a significant pressure drop across the obstruction, thus increasing the difference between pressures in the airway and surrounding tissue, tending to compress the poorly supported bronchi. These mechanical consequences of respiration affect the trachea and bronchi more than the bronchioles,

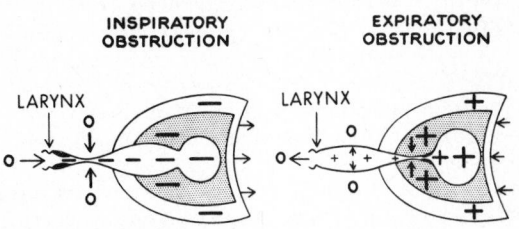

**INSPIRATORY   EXPIRATORY
OBSTRUCTION   OBSTRUCTION**

Fig. 41. When the upper airway is obstructed by a foreign body, mucus, or inflammation, the transtracheal pressure gradient is large during inspiration and the tendency of the trachea to collapse is exaggerated. With obstruction of the smaller airways, the transbronchial pressure gradient is large and the forces which tend to collapse the larger bronchi increase. When, as in the infant and small child, the cartilaginous, muscular, and elastic support is weak, the collapse of the trachea and large bronchi may significantly add to the obstruction.

since the latter are supported in part by the elastic network of the pulmonary parenchyma (Figs. 40 and 41).

The trachea and bronchi are also actively narrowed by contraction of their muscles, which pull together the dorsal ends of the cartilaginous crescents. These muscles are small and weak in the infant and young child; however, during this time the cartilages are also weak so that, as in the adult, muscular contraction narrows the larger airways. Contraction of the spirally oriented muscle fibers reduces the diameter of the bronchioles without decreasing their length. Since the bronchioles are relatively large (Fig. 38) and have few muscle bundles (Fig. 39) in the first years of life, their potential for constriction during this period is proportionally less than in the adult.

In summary:

The chance of obstruction of the infant's airway by mucus may be reduced because of the small amount of glandular tissue in the infant's airway but as a result, his lungs may be more susceptible to infection. However, the absolute cross section of the airway in infants and children is smaller than that in adults and hence more easily occluded by small amounts of foreign bodies, mucus, and debris. The small diameter of the young child's bronchi may predispose him to diseases that cause obstruction, such as bronchiolitis and asthma. By 1 year, the lining of the airway resembles that of the adult.

The airway is proportionally larger in the infant and young child than in the older child and adult. This causes a proportional increase in the respiratory dead space and minute volume, but a proportional decrease in the work of breathing.

The infant and child are able to increase and decrease intrapulmonary pressure to nearly the same extent as the adult. Since they are capable of creating large pressure differences, maximal breathing maneuvers may cause obstruction during the first years of life at a time when the airways have little structural support. This may aggravate the obstruction in diseases like laryngitis (by causing inspiratory collapse of the extrathoracic trachea) and bronchiolitis (by causing the large intrathoracic airways to collapse).

Bronchiolar muscle is sparse at birth and increases in bulk throughout the first 5 years. Since the infant's small airways have little muscle, and since the ratio of wall thickness to diameter is relatively less than in adults, obstruction due to active reduction in diameter is limited. However, a little reduction in size by contraction of these muscles may obstruct the young child's bronchi, as in asthma. This inability to constrict may impair regional regulation of ventilation and result in a disproportionately large amount of ventilation in areas of the lung with reduced pulmonary blood flow (wasted ventilation or dead space).

Obstruction

SIGNS AND SYMPTOMS. **Anxiety and Restlessness.** The inability to breathe with ease creates anxiety. A decrease in oxygen (hypoxemia) and an accumulation of carbon dioxide (hypercarbia) in arterial blood accentuate this feeling. Restlessness, agitation, and vigorous respiratory efforts may accompany this sensation of strangulation and be the first signs of hypoxemia. The fatigued infant with obstruction and labored breathing who suddenly becomes more active may not be improving; he may be much worse and his increased activity may be a sign of respiratory failure.

CYANOSIS.   When obstruction is marked, even maximal respiratory efforts cannot deliver sufficient oxygen to the alveoli to saturate arterial blood. As the young child increases his respiratory efforts, his airway collapses and obstruction is increased; this further reduces ventilation and augments hypoxemia. When the child is anemic, significant hypoxemia may be present without cyanosis. Also, the degree of cyanosis is difficult to estimate when there is peripheral vasoconstriction, as in shock and acidosis; hence, cyanosis may not be a good index of hypoxemia under these circumstances and arterial blood gases must be measured.

RESPIRATORY SOUNDS.   Abnormal breath sounds that occur with obstruction are influenced by the depth of breathing, the velocity of airflow, the position of the patient, and the size and location of the obstructed airway. They are a composite of the vibrations produced by the movement of air. The pitch of breath sounds depends upon the size of the orifices or the diameter of the tube; the smaller the orifice or tube, the higher the pitch. The intensity of breath sounds varies with the velocity of airflow, an increase in tidal volume or rate of flow accentuating them.

Masses at the base of the tongue and in the posterior pharynx cause a gargling or snoring sound. Breathing through an obstruction of the larynx produces a relatively high-pitched, harsh noise called *stridor*. Since laryngeal obstruction is augmented during inspiration and reduced during expiration, laryngeal stridor is predominantly inspiratory. Masses at the base of the tongue and in the anterior pharynx are more likely to obstruct the larynx and cause stridor when the patient is on his back. An obstruction of the extrathoracic trachea creates noises of somewhat higher pitch during inspiration. The sounds of obstruction of the intrathoracic trachea and bronchi are predominantly expiratory. Partial blockage of the smaller airways hinders the inflow and outflow of gas. Wheezes are heard during inspiration but are more prominent during expiration.

COUGH.   A cough is an explosive expiration. After a deep inspiration the glottis is closed and the muscles of expiration contract, compressing the lung and raising intrapulmonary pressure above atmospheric pressure. The glottis then opens and gas is expelled at a rapid rate. A cough may be voluntary or reflex. The cough reflex is initiated by the irritation of subepithelial mechanoreceptors in the trachea and bronchi. These cough receptors may be activated by dusts, chemicals, inflammation, or mucus. Rapid changes in airway volume with deep breaths stimulate other nerves in the wall of the airway and start another cough reflex. A cough, started by local irritation, will rapidly change the caliber of the airway and produce additional coughs.

The infant and child have well-developed cough reflexes. A series of coughs following one inspiration is called a paroxysm and is common in pertussis and cystic fibrosis. When foreign bodies and excess mucus are present, coughing is useful. However, the high intrathoracic pressures created during active expiration in the young child may collapse and obstruct the flabby airways. When there is no mucus or debris to be expelled, coughing may be harmful and suppression of the cough reflex helpful.

HYPERINFLATION.   Since disease of the lower airway obstructs expiration more than inspiration, more gas enters than leaves the lung, and the volume of the lung at the end of expiration (functional residual capacity) enlarges. When overinflated, the chest is tympanitic on percussion, the anterior-posterior diameter of the chest is large, and the lungs appear radiolucent. The term *emphysema* is frequently used to describe this type of overdistension. However, emphysema implies an irreversible process, and its use should be limited to degenerative disease characterized by irreversible breakdown of alveolar septa, decrease in pulmonary elastic tissue, and atrophy of bronchial walls. The enlargement of the lungs in asthma and bronchiolitis is *reversible* and should be called hyperinflation.

HEMOPTYSIS.   In most instances, blood in the upper airway comes from the oropharynx and esophagus. However, erosion of the airway by injury or inflammation, as occurs with foreign bodies or inflammation, may cause bleeding.

PAIN.   Tissue damage from trauma or inflammation stimulates nerve endings by increasing tissue tension or releasing chemical agents. Irritation of the trachea and bronchi causes pain, which can be abolished by vagotomy. Only the larynx, trachea, and major bronchi have sensory innervation; these nerves are probably present and functioning from birth.

Foreign bodies in the larynx and extrathoracic trachea cause continuous sharp pain in the anterior neck. Inflammation or foreign bodies in the intrathoracic trachea and large bronchi cause substernal sharp or aching pain, which is increased with coughing. The pain is usually referred to the ipsilateral anterior chest wall and helps to localize the process. Pain caused by injury to the airway is usually increased by deep breaths.

RETRACTIONS.   The nonrigid parts of the chest wall tend to balloon out when intrathoracic pressure is high and to retract when it is subatmospheric. Retraction of the sternum and suprasternal and intercostal spaces occurs during normal respiration in the small infant. In the older infant and child with a stronger chest wall, retractions reflect the large negative intrapleural pressures created during inspiration through an obstructed airway, or those necessary to inflate a stiff or airless lung.

SECRETIONS.   Inflammation and the inhalation of particulate foreign matter, such as smoke, dusts, milk, or blood, increase the secretory activity of the mucous glands and goblet cells. The secretions are swept toward the mouth either by the action of the cilia or by coughing. Secretions clean the airway, but if abundant they may block it. The infant's airways are small, and although the production of mucus may not be large, the likelihood of obstruction is great.

CIRCULATORY CHANGES. The circulatory changes with obstruction vary with the magnitude of the respiratory effort and the degree of asphyxia. An increase in the depth and rate of breathing and anxiety causes tachycardia. Asphyxia may cause peripheral vasoconstriction, hypertension, and bradycardia or tachycardia depending upon the duration. Hypoxemia and acidosis impair myocardial function and increase pulmonary vascular resistance, and thus right ventricle pressure and work. With chronic upper airway obstruction, as with greatly enlarged tonsils, pulmonary hypertension and cor pulmonale may occur. Coughing raises the mean intrathoracic pressure, decreases venous return to the heart, lowers cardiac output, and may cause syncope. Prolonged coughing, as in pertussis, may raise the pressure in the superior vena cava, frequently resulting in subconjunctival hemorrhages and, rarely, bleeding into the central nervous system.

RESPIRATORY ACIDOSIS AND DEHYDRATION. Severe airway obstruction impairs the elimination of the carbon dioxide formed by tissue metabolism. The $Paco_2$ (partial pressure of carbon dioxide in arterial blood) and the carbonic acid and hydrogen ion (H^+) concentrations rise and the pH falls. H^+ enters cells, potassium ions (K^+) leave, and the plasma K^+ and urinary excretion of K^+ increase, thus causing depletion of total body potassium. The kidneys respond to respiratory acidosis by increasing the tubular reabsorption of bicarbonate (HCO_3^-). The resulting increase in plasma HCO_3^- is "compensating" in the sense that the degree of acidosis is lessened. When the child's airway obstruction is removed or the ventilation assisted, the $Paco_2$ falls, pH rises, K^+ reenters cells, and its concentration in plasma falls. However, a rapid decrease in $Paco_2$, when the plasma HCO_3^- concentration is high, may cause alkalosis. This may be striking if large amounts of additional HCO_3^- have been given. The low total and circulating K^+ impairs the renal excretion of HCO_3^- and delays the correction of alkalosis. An abnormally high plasma HCO_3^- and pH may complicate the child's recovery in three ways: respiration is depressed and the time necessary to lower $Paco_2$ to normal is prolonged; apnea may follow discontinuation of assisted ventilation; and alkalosis may produce, as part of tetany, laryngeal spasm and bronchial constriction.

Many children with obstructive airway disease have inadequate fluid intake and may lose weight because of a reduction in total body water, causing the circulating blood volume to decrease. Hypovolemia, acidemia, and hypoxemia constrict the vessels of muscle, skin, and kidney, thus decreasing the blood flow to these tissues. Hypoxemia and a regional reduction in perfusion decrease oxidative metabolism and increase lactic acid production. As a consequence, an additional load of metabolic acidosis is present in most of these patients.

DIAGNOSTIC PROCEDURES. LARYNGOSCOPY AND BRONCHOSCOPY. Visualization of the airway by laryngoscopy is useful in diagnosis of airway obstruc-

tion and is an essential procedure for the removal of foreign bodies. Laryngoscopy is not difficult. Bronchoscopy in infants and children requires great skill and must be done under general anesthesia, which suppresses coughing. The procedure irritates the upper airway, increases mucus production, and adds upper airway obstruction to lower airway disease. Premedication and atropine decrease bronchial secretion, relax bronchial smooth muscle, and may prevent postinstrumentation laryngospasm. Careful suctioning and postural drainage following bronchoscopy are essential.

RADIOGRAPHY, BRONCHOGRAPHY, FLUOROSCOPY. In children, anteroposterior and lateral films of the neck, while the arms are down and the back of the head is up and the neck extended, and posteroanterior films of the chest will show the shape of the air-filled larynx, trachea, or major bronchi and may reveal the sites of obstruction or distortion. Compression or exaggerated dilation of these structures with respiratory maneuvers can be determined with fluoroscopy; cinefluoroscopy is particularly useful, since the film can be viewed in slow motion.

If films and cinefluorography do not indicate the type and location of the obstruction, contrast material may be placed in the airway for visualization. An aqueous solution of propyliodone (Dionosil) is thick enough to cling to the walls of the airway, is rapidly removed by ciliary action, and is not very irritating. However, only small amounts should be injected, since an excess of Dionosil will occlude rather than outline the airway.

Most of the methods for the introduction of contrast material require general anesthesia. This has the disadvantages of suppressing the cough reflex and prohibiting spontaneous respiratory maneuvers. More recently we have used powdered tantalum aerosol, as described by Nadel and associates. It is nonirritating, does not obstruct, is rapidly cleared, and outlines the small airways with great clarity (see Fig. 27).

BLOOD GASES, pH, ELECTROLYTES. The pH, Pco_2, HCO_3^-, and other electrolytes in blood drawn from a vein, that drains a poorly perfused area of the body may reflect only severe regional hypoxemia and acidemia. Measurements of $Paco_2$ and pH in venous blood do not indicate the efficiency of ventilation. An accurate assessment of ventilation, acid-base regulation, and electrolyte changes that accompany acidosis and hypoxemia requires the analysis of arterial blood. Depending upon the age of the child, one of four sampling sites are usually available. In the young infant with a small amount of scalp tissue, the temporal artery is easily palpated and entered with a 23- or 24-gauge needle, as described by Schlueter. In older infants and children, after local infiltration with 1 percent lidocaine, the femoral, brachial, or radial artery can be punctured with a 20-gauge needle. When a sample directly from an artery is unobtainable, arterialized capillary blood can be used. Warming a heel of an infant or a finger of an older child accelerates local blood flow so that the pH and Pco_2 of capillary and arterial samples are almost the same. Arterialized capillary Po_2 may be lower than that of arterial blood, and must be interpreted with caution. In newborns the acrocyanosis makes arterialized capillary blood gas measurements unreliable. In any child with peripheral vasoconstriction or shock, arterial samples must be obtained to gain accurate information concerning ventilatory status.

MICROBIOLOGIC SAMPLES. The identification of specific infectious agents includes appropriate sampling, isolation in culture, and presence of antibodies in the blood.

Organisms cultured from nasopharyngeal material may be responsible for upper but not for lower airway disease. There are numerous procedures for obtaining samples from the lower airway: collection of sputum; irritation of the larynx with a swab to provoke a cough; aspiration through a tracheal catheter, with or without tracheal lavage using normal saline; and direct puncture of the lung through the chest wall. This last procedure has been recommended by Klein in three groups of children: the critically ill child in whom a specific etiologic diagnosis is of major importance to guide antimicrobial therapy; the child who has deteriorated while on therapy and in whom an etiologic agent is not available from the usual upper respiratory tract culture; and the child with pneumonia complicated by underlying disease or drugs that limit normal host-defense mechanisms. In these circumstances the advantages of having a specific diagnosis are greater than the small risk from pneumothorax. Meticulous attention to the details of technique, as outlined by Klein, will minimize complications.

PULMONARY FUNCTION TESTS. Numerous tests of function are available for assessing airway obstruction and the associated physiologic abnormality. The $Paco_2$ and Pao_2 indicate whether ventilation is adequate and are essential for evaluation of the severity of the illness and effectiveness of treatment. The measurement of dead space, functional residual capacity, the maximal volume of gas that can be expelled from the lungs by forceful effort after a maximal inspiration (vital capacity), resistance to gas flow through the airway (airway resistance), maximal flow rates, maximal flow-volume curves, and maximal inspiratory and expiratory pressures all aid in establishing the diagnosis and in the objective evaluation of therapy.

Simple spirometry, easily done in the office or at the bedside, allows the physician to quantify vital capacity (a measure of volume) and forced inspiratory and expiratory air flow. With these simple measurements of lung volume and air flow, the physician can recognize the two main groups of physiologic dysfunction in children with pulmonary problems: obstructive lung disease and restrictive lung disease.

Children with obstructive lung disease have a spirometric pattern indicating obstruction to air flow on either expiration, inspiration, or both, while the lung volumes may be normal, low, or high. Children with restrictive lung disease have a reduced lung volume due to loss of lung tissue or decreased chest wall movement. Air flow is frequently normal, but can be low unless it is related to lung volume, since most tests of flow are dependent on the volume available to generate the flow (volume-dependent measurements). Table 11 shows typical patterns of simple pulmonary function in lung disease.

Comroe and associates give a lucid and detailed description of these and other pulmonary function tests. Polgar and Promadhat have surveyed previously reported pulmonary function testing in children and provide normal values for most pulmonary function tests. Summary curves for lung volumes and peak flow rates are shown in Figure 42.

TREATMENT. The removal of obstruction and the maintenance of adequate ventilation are the primary goals of treatment. When a foreign body causes the obstruction, it is removed by aspiration; tumors, cysts, and other masses that occlude or compress the airway are excised. With other types of obstruction, one or more of the following may be required.

TRACHEAL INTUBATION AND TRACHEOSTOMY. Marked narrowing of the larynx by structural anomalies, spasm, or inflammation must be bypassed by introducing an endotracheal tube or by performing a tracheostomy; occasionally these procedures are also necessary for the adequate performance of positive pressure breathing devices.

Tracheostomy has many complications: dislodgment of the tube during spasms of coughing; dissection of air into the subcutaneous tissue of the neck and mediastinum; pneumothorax; and the difficulty of decannulation. For laryngeal bypass during acute obstruction, the widespread availability of nonirritating endotracheal

Table 11. Patterns of Simple Pulmonary Function Testing in Lung Disease

	Obstructive Disease		Restrictive Disease
	Intrathoracic lesions (expiratory obstruction)	Extrathoracic lesions (inspiratory obstruction)	
Lung volume			
Vital capacity	↓	N	↓
Residual volume	↑	N	↓ or N
Total lung capacity	N	N	↓
Flow			
Expiration	↓	N or ↓	N or ↑
Inspiration	N	↓	N or ↓

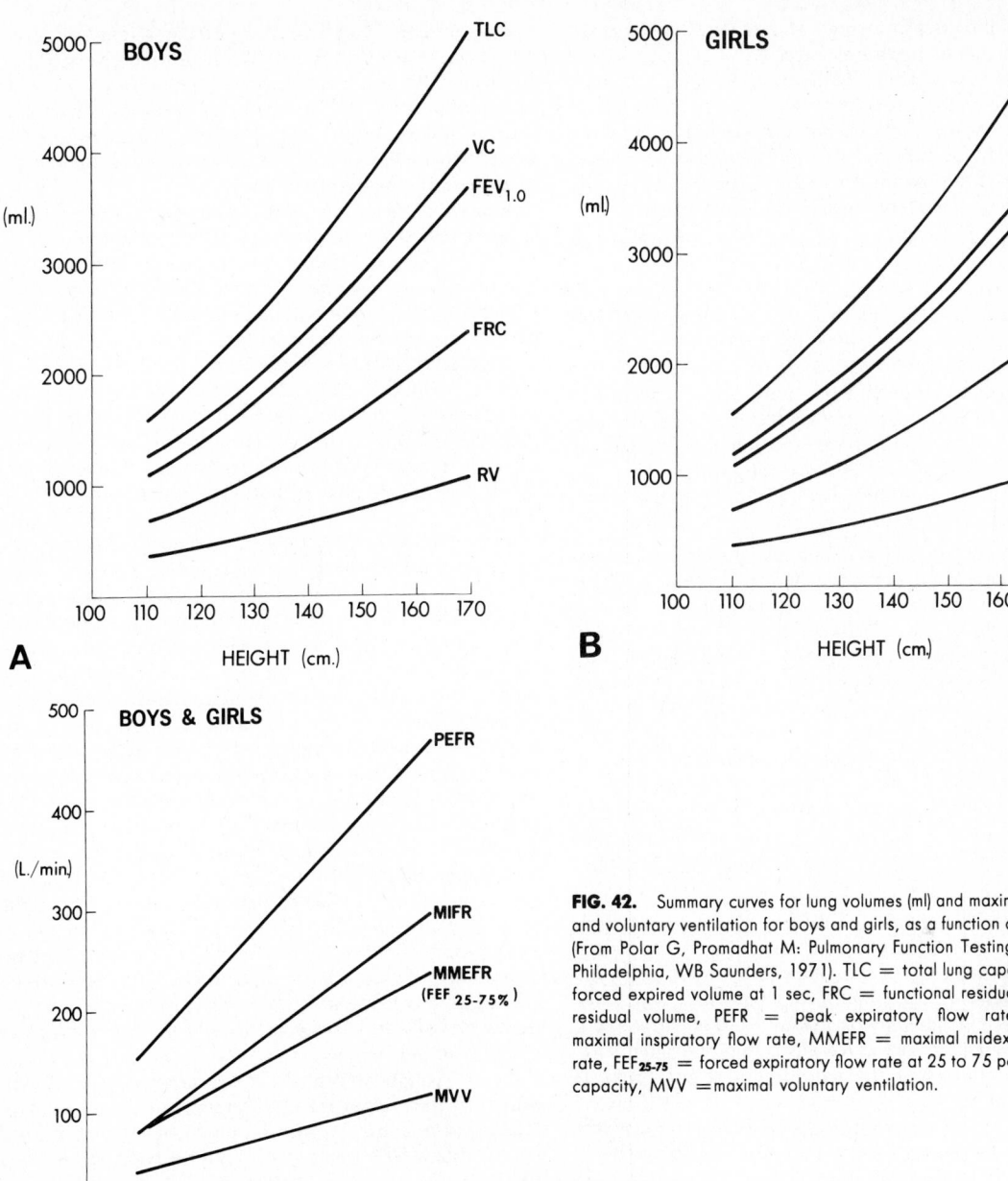

FIG. 42. Summary curves for lung volumes (ml) and maximal flow rates and voluntary ventilation for boys and girls, as a function of height (cm). (From Polar G, Promadhat M: Pulmonary Function Testing in Children. Philadelphia, WB Saunders, 1971). TLC = total lung capacity, FEV$_1$ = forced expired volume at 1 sec, FRC = functional residual capacity, E residual volume, PEFR = peak expiratory flow rate, MIFR = maximal inspiratory flow rate, MMEFR = maximal midexpiratory flow rate, FEF$_{25-75}$ = forced expiratory flow rate at 25 to 75 percent of vital capacity, MVV = maximal voluntary ventilation.

tubes has led to tracheal intubation instead of tracheostomy. Choice of nasotracheal versus oral-tracheal passage of the tube is a matter of personal preference. If tracheal intubation is unsuccessful, tracheostomy must be done.

Tracheostomies and endotracheal tubes impair the cleansing action of the mucous lining of the airway, make coughing difficult, and eliminate the filtering and air conditioning provided by the nose and the pharynx. Management must include the warming and moistening of inspired air and frequent suctioning of the trachea and bronchi. Suctioning removes air as well as particulate matter. This reduces lung volume and promotes atelectasis. The lung should be reexpanded by a series of inflations after each episode of suctioning.

Tracheostomy and endotracheal intubation may be lifesaving and should not be delayed when upper airway obstruction is severe and progressive.

MANAGEMENT OF SECRETIONS.   When irritated, the epithelium of the airway releases large quantities of mucus, which entraps foreign bodies and debris. If the amount of mucus does not exceed the capacity of the cilia to clear the airway, this reaction helps to maintain the patency of the bronchial tree. When production is too great, mucus adds to the obstruction; when too little, foreign bodies and inflammatory exudate block the airway. If the mucus is too thick, the cilia have difficulty moving it and the mucus stream is slowed.

Coughing. Coughing accelerates the movement of accumulated mucus, and cough reflexes should not be depressed except when there is little mucus to be evacuated. Codeine (0.3 mg/kg repeated three to four times a day) suppresses the cough reflexes but also depresses respiration. Drugs like dextromethorphan (0.3 mg/kg repeated three to four times a day) are just as effective antitussive agents, do not depress respiration, and are not addictive. Mild exercise, change in position, and deep breaths may initiate coughing. They also make coughing more effective by freeing aggregations of mucus from the bronchial walls.

Postural Drainage. Gravity speeds the flow of mucus from the upper lobe bronchi when the patient is sitting or standing. By varying the position of the chest in relation to the mouth, drainage of other major bronchi can also be facilitated by gravity. Pounding the chest wall with cupped hands over the area being drained, followed by vibrating the chest wall, as outlined by Waring, significantly improves the removal of secretions from the airway. The use of postural drainage is particularly useful for removing localized intrabronchial obstructions. When mucous obstruction is generalized, the child should be placed for 5 to 10 minutes in each position necessary for optimal drainage of the major bronchi.

Alteration of the Viscocity of Mucus. Parasympatholytic drugs decrease secretory activity and ciliary motion and increase the viscosity of the mucus blanket. Antihistaminics are weakly parasympatholytic and have the same action. These drugs may be useful in upper airway disease, but in lower airway disease, they should be restricted to control of the irritation that accompanies bronchoscopy.

To prevent mucus from drying, the larynx and the trachea should be kept warm and moist when airflow is rapid, as it is in all obstructive diseases. Mouth breathing is frequently present in patients with airway obstruction, bypassing the normal humidification mechanism of the nasal passages and increasing the tendency to thickened mucous secretions. Numerous vaporizers and croup tents are available to add moisture to the inspired gases. When the mucus produced is thick, tenacious, or crusted, it is more easily expelled by coughing and moved by cilia if it is moistened by inhaling an aerosol with droplets of suitable size for deposition in smaller airways (about 5μ). The effectiveness of our current mist tents and aerosol treatments to accomplish this has been challenged by recent studies with aerosols of technetium-labeled water administered to children with cystic fibrosis. More studies are needed before dogmatic recommendations can be formulated.

Expectorants. The use of potassium iodide or glyceryl guaiacolate for expectorant action has been disappointing in most patients. The best way to maintain normal viscosity of mucus is to assure adequate hydration. Ample oral fluid should be encouraged in patients with airway obstruction and intravenous fluids used if oral intake is inadequate.

Mucolytic Agents. Among other agents whose action is said to decrease the viscosity of mucous secretions are crystalline trypsin, desoxyribonuclease, streptokinase, hyaluronidase, lysosyme, acetylcysteine, and pimetine hydrochloride. Some of these drugs are effective in fibrin lysis, others split disulfide bonds, but only lysozyme clearly dissolves normal mucus. There is no convincing evidence that any of them affect the thick secretions of chronic airway diseases, such as bronchiectasis. Some, if not all, irritate the mucosa, cause smooth muscle constriction, and increase obstruction. Their use in pediatric pulmonary patients is very limited.

BRONCHODILATORS. The normal tone of the smooth muscle of the airways is under control of the autonomic nervous system and represents a balance of parasympathetic (cholinergic) effects that cause bronchoconstriction and sympathetic (adrenergic) effects that induce bronchodilation. In individuals with normal lungs, the inhalation of bronchodilator aerosol decreases airway resistance by about 25 percent.

The importance of increased activity of the parasympathetic limb of the autonomic nervous system in bronchospastic conditions is currently under active investigation, but parasympathetic pharmacologic blocking agents are not available for clinical use at this time.

Bronchodilation through adrenergic stimulation is useful in all lower airway diseases where the normal tone is increased (bronchoconstriction) by irritation with foreign bodies, dust, chemicals, cold air, and inflammation. Drugs that relax bronchial smooth muscle can be given orally, subcutaneously, intramuscularly or intravenously or introduced locally to the respiratory tract as an aerosol.

Acute bronchospasm is relieved most easily by subcutaneous injection of 1:1,000 epinephrine (0.02 ml/kg). It is rapid in action (3 to 5 minutes) but short in duration and may be repeated at 20-minute intervals for two to three doses, if necessary, Bronchospasm may be relieved by inhalation of a bronchodilator, such as an aerosol; epinephrine, racemic epinephrine, isoproterenol, isoetharine, and many other sympathomimetic compounds are effective by this route.

The selective action of some sympathomimetic (adrenergic) compounds in producing primary bronchodilation with minimal cardiac stimulation has been explained on the basis of different types of adrenergic receptors, with those having primarily bronchodilator action being labeled β_2 receptors. Over the past 10 years, a group of new dilator compounds has been developed, which appears to have predominantly β_2 activity. Terbutaline has been released recently for use in the United States, and Salbutomol may be available shortly.

Ephedrine and theophylline (as aminophylline or other salts) also have been useful in producing bronchodilation. Use of ephedrine is limited due to its central nervous system excitatory effect; this has led to combining it with theophylline and sedatives in an attempt to achieve optimal bronchodilation without overstimulation. Recent studies favor the use of theophylline (or its salts). Doses of 5 to 6 mg/kg/6 hours, orally or by slow intravenous infusion over 30 minutes, produce optimal therapeutic levels in most patients (10 to 20 μg/100 ml). Monitoring serum theophylline levels is now practical and should lead to more effective schedules in difficult patients. Some patients metabolize theophylline more rapidly and may need doses as high as 10 mg/kg/6 hours to maintain adequate blood levels.

ANTI-INFLAMMATORY AGENTS.   Corticosteroids, in pharmacologic doses, suppress the reactivity of connective tissue to injury, inhibit fibroblast formation, probably reduce the constriction of bronchial smooth muscle by histamine, and reduce edema. Their anti-inflammatory action could benefit most forms of obstruction associated with inflammation. Maximum action of hydrocortisone requires 4 to 6 hours. Antibiotics should also be given when it is used in conditions in which bacterial infection may be present. Inflammation is a more important cause of obstruction in the young infant than is bronchoconstriction. The anti-inflammatory action of cortisone is particularly useful for minimizing the reduction in the lumen of the airway in this age group. Hydrocortisone (about 8 mg/kg/day in divided doses) or equivalent doses of other corticosteroids, for 4 to 7 days, may be indicated in many acute obstructive conditions.

OXYGEN.   When hypoxemia is present, increasing oxygen concentration in inspired gas will reduce anxiety and the forceful inspiratory or expiratory efforts that augment obstruction, decrease the work of breathing, decrease pulmonary vascular resistence, and improve cardiovascular function. An inspired oxygen concentration of 30 to 100 percent may be necessary to bring Pao_2 to normal levels.

There are several methods for delivering oxygen to children, the choice depending upon the amount needed. A tent has a large volume and many leaks, and even at high flow rates, an oxygen concentration of 40 percent is rarely achieved; oxygen flowing at 4 to 5 liters/minute, through a 4 to 5-liter plastic hood placed over the infant's head will produce a concentration of close to 100 percent; oxygen flowing through a nasal catheter into the nasopharynx at 4 liters/minute will provide a concentration of about 50 percent; the inspired gas may be 100 percent if a tightly fitting oxygen mask, with a reservoir bag is used. Since cold, dry oxygen is irritating, it should be warmed and moistened, regardless of the mode of delivery.

In infants and children with chronic airway obstruction and incipient hypercapnia, oxygen breathing may depress respiration and aggravate respiratory acidosis. Frequent arterial blood gas measurements are required when oxygen therapy is initiated in this situation. On the other hand, the improved oxygenation may lead to

a decrease in pulmonary vasoconstriction, resulting in greater pulmonary blood flow to some units that have been ventilated but not perfused. This increases elimination of carbon dioxide even though total ventilation may be decreased. Oxygen therapy in infants with acute airway obstruction usually causes a fall in $Paco_2$ by reducing anxiety and decreasing forceful respiration. In any event, since the prompt use of mechanical respirators can correct hypoventilation, oxygen should not be witheld from any child with severe hypoxemia.

Normal adults breathing 100 percent oxygen for prolonged periods of time may develop tracheobronchitis, fatigue, and vomiting. Although limiting the inspired oxygen concentration to 50 percent usually eliminates the likelihood of oxygen toxicity, the possibility that it may occur with 100 percent oxygen should not preclude its use when necessary. Atelectasis is more apt to occur if the gas trapped behind an obstruction of the lower airway is 100 percent oxygen rather than 80 percent nitrogen. However, as the child recovers, spontaneous deep breaths and sighs are usually sufficient to correct this.

MECHANICAL VENTILATION.   Infants and children with severe airway obstruction must be watched carefully for the onset of respiratory failure, and mechanical ventilation initiated promptly if cardiopulmonary arrest is to be avoided. Recent technologic advances in endotracheal tubes, models of mechanical ventilators available, and pharmacologic preparations for sedation and muscular paralysis have made mechanical ventilation easier, safer, and more likely to be successful. Despite these improvements, mechanical ventilation of infants and children remains an exacting, time-consuming, and difficult undertaking, and should be done only in special intensive care units that are well organized and fully staffed by nurses and physicians experienced in managing respiratory failure. Reliable blood gas measurements, available around the clock, are an absolute necessity to the success of mechanical ventilation. Excellent descriptions of mechanical ventilation and the organization of a Pediatric Intensive Care Unit have been published by Downes and Jones.

Bibliography

AIRWAY ANATOMY AND FUNCTION

American Physiological Society: Washington DC, Handbook of Physiology, Sec 3. Fenn WO, Rahn H (eds): Respiration. Baltimore, Williams & Wilkins, 1964, Vol. I, II

Avery ME: The Lung and Its Disorders in the Newborn Infant. WB Saunders, Philadelphia, 1974, p 3

Bucher U, Reid L: Development of the mucus-secreting elements in human lung. Thorax 16:219, 1961

Butler, J, Caro CG. Alcala R, DuBois AB: Physiological factors affecting airway resistance in normal subjects and in patients with obstructive respiratory disease. J Clin Invest 39:584, 1960

Comroe JH Jr: Physiology of Respiration. Chicago, Year Book Publishers, 1965

Cudmore RE, Emery JL, Mithal A: Postnatal growth of the bronchi and bronchioles. Arch Dis Child 37:481, 1962

Engel S: Lung Structure. Springfield, Ill., Charles C Thomas, 1962

Pride NB, Permutt S, Riley RL, Bromberger-Barnea R: Determinants of maximal expiratory flow from the lungs. J Appl Physiol 23:646, 1967

Reid L: Growth and development of the respiratory system, In Davis JA, Dobbings J (eds): Scientific Foundations of Paediatrics. Philadelphia, WB Saunders, 1970, p 220

Scammon RE: The respiratory system. In Abt IA (ed): Pediatrics, Vol 1. 1st ed. Philadelphia, WB Saunders, 1923, pp 335-352

von Hayek H: The Human Lung. New York, Hafner, 1960

Walker JEC, Wells RE Jr: Heat and water exchange in the respiratory tract. Am J Med 30:259, 1961

Weibel E: Morphometry of the Human Lung, New York, Academic Press, 1963

DIAGNOSIS AND TREATMENT FOR OBSTRUCTION

Avery ME, Galina M, Nachman R: Mist therapy. Pediatrics 39:160, 1967

Bierman CW, Pierson WW: The pharmacologic management of status asthmaticus in children. Pediatrics 54:245, 1974

Briscoe WA, DuBois AB: The relationship between airway resistance, airway conductance and lung volume in subjects of different age and body size. J Clin Invest 37:1279, 1958

Comroe JH Jr, Forester RE II, DuBois AB, Briscoe WA, Carlsen F: The Lung, 2nd ed. Year Book Publishers, Chicago, 1962

Connolly NM: Dosage of oral salbutamol in asthmatic children. Arch Dis Child 46:869, 1971

Davis RH, Beren AV, Galant SP: Capillary pH of blood gas determinations in asthmatic children. J Allergy Clin Immunol 56:33, 1975

DeMuth GR, Howatt WF, Hill B: The growth of lung function. Part V. Forced flow rates. Pediatrics 35:200 (Suppl), 1965

Downes JJ, Fulgencio T, Raphaely RC: Acute respiratory failure in infants and children. Pediatr Clin North Am 19:423, 1972

Engström L, Karlberg P, Kraepelien S: Respiratory studies in children. I. Lung volumes in healthy children 6-14 years of age. Acta Paediatr Scand 45:277, 1956

Heliesen PJ, Cook CD, Friedlander L, et al.: Studies of respiratory physiology in children. I. Mechanics of respiration and lung volumes in 85 normal children 5 to 17 years of age. Pediatrics 22:80, 1958

Jones RS, Owen-Thomas JB: Care of the Critically Ill Child. Edward Arnold, London, 1971

Klein JO: Diagnostic lung puncture in the pneumonias of infants and children. Pediatrics 44:486, 1969

Leegaard J. Fjulsrud S: Terbutaline in children with asthma. Arch Dis Child 48:222, 1973

Marshall R: The physical properties of the lungs in relation to the subdivisions of lung volume. Clin Sci 16:507, 1957

Milner AD, Ingram D: Bronchodilator and cardiac effects of isoprenaline, orciprenaline and salbutamol aerosols in asthma. Arch Dis Child 46:502, 1971

Nadel JA, Wolfe WG, Graf PD, et al: Powdered tantalum: a new contrast medium for roentgenographic examination of human airways. N Engl J Med 283:281, 1970

Nolke AC: Severe toxic effects from aminophylline and theophylline suppositories in children. JAMA 161:693, 1956

Pierson WE, Bierman CW, Stamm SV, Van Arsdel PP Jr: Double-blind trial of aminophylline in status asthmaticus. Pediatrics 48:642, 1971

Polgar G, Promadhat V: Pulmonary Function Testing in Children: Techniques and Standards. WB Saunders Co, Philadelphia, 1971

Radford EP Jr, Ferris BG Jr, Kriete BC: Clinical use of a nomogram to estimate proper ventilation during artificial respiration. N Engl J Med 251:877, 1954

Schlueter MA, Johnson BB, Sudman DA, et al: Blood sampling from scalp arteries in infants. Pediatrics 51:120, 1973

Waring, WW: Diagnostic and therapeutic procedures. In Kendig EL (ed): Disorders of the Respiratory Tract in Children, Vol 1. WB Saunders Co, Philadelphia, 1972, p 97

Weinberg MM, Bronsky A: Evaluation of oral bronchodilator therapy in asthmatic children. J Pediatr 84:421, 1974

Weng T-R, Levison H: Standards of pulmonary function in children. Am Rev Resp Dis 99:879, 1969

SPECIFIC DISEASES CAUSING OBSTRUCTION

William H. Tooley
Herman W. Lipow

INSPIRATORY OBSTRUCTION (EXTRATHORACIC LESIONS—UPPER AIRWAY OBSTRUCTION)

The extrathoracic airways tend to narrow during inspiration and dilate during expiration (p. 1590). Obstruction of the extrathoracic airway causes intraluminal pressure distal to the obstruction to fall more during inspiration, which accentuates the inspiratory narrowing. Inspiratory stridor, hoarseness, and suprasternal and intracostal retractions are the signs of partial obstruction of the larynx and extrathoracic trachea. If the obstruction is severe, agitation, cyanosis, acidosis, and circulatory collapse also occur.

LARYNGOMALACIA (CONGENITAL LARYNGEAL STRIDOR). This is a relatively common condition in young infants in which laryngeal obstruction occurs as an inadequately supported epiglottis or redundant aryepiglottic folds are sucked into the glottis during inspiration. As inspiratory effort increases, the larynx below the temporarily obstructed glottal opening narrows, increasing the obstruction.

Most infants with congenital laryngeal stridor continue to thrive despite the noisy breathing, and their cry is of normal intensity and pitch. It is unusual to have cyanosis, difficulty in feeding, inadequate weight gain, cough, or other signs of respiratory distress. The stridor is maximal when the infant is supine with the neck flexed, and minimal or absent when prone with the head hyperextended. Congenital laryngeal stridor is almost always a benign condition. However, any infant who has persistent stridor should be examined carefully for the presence of more serious causes of obstruction, such as laryngeal webs, cysts, or masses at the base of the tongue or in the hypopharynx.

LARYNGEAL WEB. (see p. 1517). This usually presents with partial or complete respiratory obstruction in the newborn. In some instances, symptoms may not be severe in the newborn, and intermittent obstruction occurs due to swelling of the web.

TRAUMA. Vocal cord paralysis following birth injury, local surgery, or other injury and dislocation of the cricothyroid or the cricoarytenoid articulations at birth or later may lead to marked inspiratory obstruction.

TUMORS. Teratoma of the tonsil and nasopharyngeal angiofibromas are encountered rarely. Laryngeal papillomas and fibroleiomyomas, and leiomyomas and adenocarcinomas occur in childhood and may result in airway obstruction. These tumors require surgical excision. Subglottic hemangiomas may be associated with superficial hemangiomas on other parts of the torso. Signs and symptoms are intermittent, depending upon the degree of vascular engorgement. They tend to fill when the infant is crying. No voice changes may be present, as they rarely involve the cords. Hydrocortisone may result in striking improvement. Tracheostomy is often necessary.

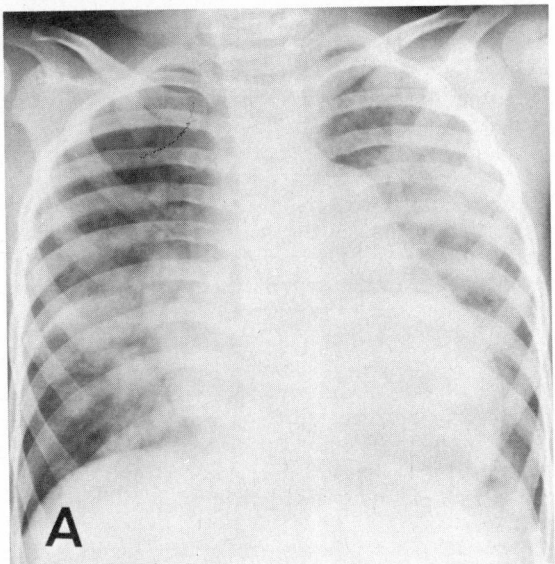

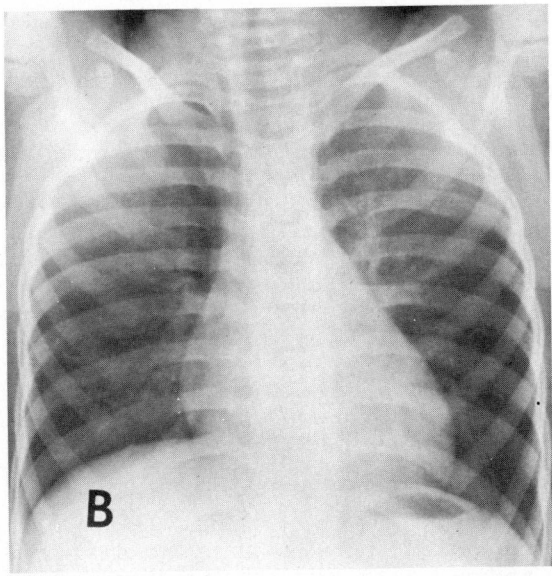

FIG. 43. **A.** Chest radiograph of 2.5-year-old child showing gross cardiomegaly and pulmonary edema secondary to chronic upper airway obstruction. **B.** Follow-up chest roentgenogram at 4 years of age. Adenoidectomy performed at 2.5 years of age. Heart size and lung fields are now normal.

OBSTRUCTION BY ENLARGED TONSILS AND ADENOIDS.

The syndrome of chronic upper airway obstruction, hypoventilation, and cor pulmonale was first recognized in 1965 by Menashe, Farrehi, and Miller. Grossly enlarged tonsils and adenoids cause inspiratory obstruction and noisy breathing that is accentuated when the child is supine, is sleeping (particularly after sedation), or has acute tonsillitis. The obstruction can be so marked and the work of breathing so great that they begin to hypoventilate, particularly during

sleep, develop cyanosis, and have hypercarbia, pulmonary hypertension, and congestive heart failure. They may present with gross edema, dyspnea, and a large heart on chest roentgenogram (Fig. 43A). The acute congestive failure responds temporarily to vigorous treatment with diuretics, oxygen, and digitalis but cure is achieved only when the tonsils and adenoids are removed surgically (Fig. 43B). This condition is one of the few absolute indications for adenotonsillectomy. The adenoidal enlargement in some of these children has recently been associated with milk allergy.

COMPRESSION BY EXTERNAL MASSES. Cystic masses, such as cystic hygroma and lingual cysts and oropharyngeal abscesses may obstruct the glottis. Thyroglossal duct cysts and thyroid adenomas may obstruct the trachea. These must be removed surgically.

METABOLIC DISORDERS. Rickets with tetany or other metabolic problems associated with hypocalcemia or alkalosis promote laryngeal constriction and obstruction of the upper airways. This laryngospasm responds dramatically but transiently to intravenous calcium gluconate, and allows time to investigate the basic metabolic problem and to institute more definitive treatment.

INFLAMMATION. THE CROUP SYNDROME. Croup is an acute clinical syndrome with inspiratory stridor, barking or brassy cough, and, usually, hoarseness. The course varies from a mild illness lasting 3 to 4 days (usually viral in etiology) to a fulminating acute epiglottitis that may lead to total airway obstruction and death in less than 6 hours (usually due to *H. influenza* type B, p. 444). The croup syndrome is a conscientious pediatrician's nightmare; the early signs and symptoms may be deceptively mild, but change rapidly and become life-threatening in a few hours. For this reason, all children with croup syndrome must be followed closely and the potential seriousness of the disorder appreciated by parents. A helpful classification in approaching the croup syndrome has been suggested by Cramblett: acute epiglottitis; acute laryngotracheobronchitis; spasmodic croup; and diphtheritic croup.

Acute Epiglottitis. This is an infection of the larynx, with rapid swelling of the epiglottis and increasing inspiratory difficulty. It is almost always caused by *H. influenzae* type B and requires early and aggressive treatment. The child with acute epiglottitis is usually over 3 years of age. In contrast to a child with viral laryngotracheobronchitis, there is usually no history of an antecedent upper respiratory infection. The onset is frequently acute, with inspiratory stridor that progresses over a period of 4 to 12 hours to almost total airway obstruction. Usually, fever and other signs of systemic toxicity are present.

In patients seen early, when auscultation reveals good air exchange over the lung fields in spite of stridor, a cautious examination of the posterior pharynx (carefully not touching the wall of the pharynx with the tongue blade) will reveal a grossly edematous epiglottis just beyond the base of the tongue. This swollen epiglottis has been described as resembling a bright red, inflamed raspberry and is diagnostic of *H. influenzae* epiglottitis. Once the tip of the swollen epiglottis is visualized, the examination of the pharynx should be stopped; any further manipulation of the inflamed epiglottis may cause complete laryngeal obstruction.

After obtaining blood for culture, treatment of the early or mild case includes immediate infusion of intravenous ampicillin (400 mg/kg/day) or chloramphenicol (100 mg/kg/day) and provision of oxygen and cool mist. The child should be placed in an intensive care unit for monitoring of pulse, respiration, and arterial pH and blood gases.

In children with severe obstruction who are seen later in the course of the disease, auscultation reveals poor air exchange over the lung fields. The child tends to remain in a sitting position with his chin extended and may complain of pain in his throat on swallowing; secretions tend to pool and drooling is common. As the obstruction progresses, stridor may decrease as breathing becomes shallow and rapid. At this stage, the child is too ill to be moved for radiologic investigation. If radiographic confirmation of the epiglottal swelling is felt to be necessary for diagnosis, a portable soft tissue film may be taken at the bedside.

The child who shows signs of increasing fatigue, increasing heart rate or hypercapnia should have an airway established either by endotracheal tube or tracheostomy. This should be done as rapidly as possible, preferably in the operating room. Experience with the use of small endotracheal tubes (usually 0.5 to 1.0 mm smaller than appropriate for age and size) and intensive antibiotic therapy has been very encouraging. Endotracheal intubation may be difficult and should be done by an experienced physician. Tracheostomy may be the treatment of choice for those who are more experienced with the procedure; however, most surgeons prefer to perform the tracheostomy after the airway is secured by an endotracheal tube or bronchoscope. Many physicians argue that once the child has been intubated, the reason for tracheostomy no longer exists. The average time of endotracheal intubation, after starting appropriate antibiotics, has been 2 to 3 days; in one series, it was 12 to 14 hours. The incidence of postintubation complications appears to be less than after tracheostomy.

Acute Laryngotracheobronchitis (Viral Croup) is the most common croup syndrome encountered in pediatric practice. It usually occurs in the winter months, when viral respiratory infections have their peak incidence. The child is usually between 6 months and 3 years of age and often has had a diffuse upper respiratory infection for 2 to 3 days before inspiratory stridor develops. The infection spreads to the lower respiratory tract, with varying degrees of involvement of the larynx, trachea, and bronchi. With swelling of the subglottic area, inspiratory stridor develops. Low grade fever may be present, but the child usually does not appear very ill. On cautious examination of the posterior pharynx, the epiglottis is found to be moderately red and generally edematous but fails to show the gross swelling of acute epiglottitis. The obstruction in acute laryngotracheobronchitis is primarily subglottic in location. A variety of viruses has been isolated from the airway secretions; the principal agents are parainfluenza, influenza, adenovirus, and respiratory syncytial virus.

Treatment consists of cool mist, oxygen, bed rest, and adequate hydration. Oropharyngeal suctioning should be done cautiously, since stimulation of the posterior pharynx may cause reflex laryngeal and bronchial constriction. If signs of severe obstruction develop, treatment with intermittent positive pressure aerosol of racemic epinephrine (2.25 percent) nebulized with 100 percent oxygen, and gradually increasing the pressure (to 20 to 25 cm H_2O), as recommended by Adair and associates, has frequently provided dramatic relief. This may need to be repeated frequently for the first few hours. Intubation or tracheostomy is rarely necessary. Sedation is best avoided or used very cautiously. Arterial pH and blood gases are helpful in guiding treatment.

Spasmodic Croup. Acute spasmodic croup (acute spasmodic laryngitis) refers to a distinctive clinical entity of acute attacks of inspiratory stridor that tend to occur suddenly in the evening or night, last several hours, and then subside only to recur during the following few nights.

Characteristically, the child is between 1 and 3 years of age, awakens with a barking, metallic cough and marked inspiratory stridor. Fever is absent and, although the child may have had a mild upper respiratory infection preceding the attack, examination of the posterior pharynx reveals minimal signs of inflammation. An element of acute adductor spasm of the cords has been suspected, possibly triggered by a mild viral illness or allergy. Recurrent episodes are not uncommon.

The degree of inspiratory obstruction can be striking, with retractions of the supraclavicular and substernal areas. Exposing the child to steam in a closed bathroom in which a hot shower is running may bring relief in a few minutes. If the child fails to improve and is taken to a hospital emergency room, exposure to the cool night air enroute frequently breaks the attack before the hospital is reached. Treatment with an aerosol of racemic epinephrine, administered by intermittent positive pressure as described under Acute Laryngotracheobronchitis, will terminate the attack.

Diphtheritic Croup. Diphtheria must be considered in the differential diagnosis of every child with acute infectious croup. A history of completed immunizations for diphtheria is almost enough to rule out the diagnosis. Typically, a child with diphtheritic croup has been ill for 3 to 4 days, looks toxic, and has a serous or serosanguinous nasal discharge. Examination of the posterior pharynx may reveal a gray-white membrane over the tonsils, with possible extension to the uvula; occasionally, this membrane is limited to the larynx, making the diagnosis extremely difficult.

Treatment requires the immediate administration of diphtheria antitoxin and pencillin or erythromycin (see Diphtheria, Chap 12 p. 435).

Expiratory Obstruction (Intrathoracic Lesions—Lower Airway Obstruction)

Figure 44 shows some of the mechanisms that cause obstruction. Foreign bodies, inflammation, or edema may occlude the airway. In addition, the child's poorly supported large airways collapse normally during forced expiration (Fig. 40), as with crying, and when expired gas flow is accelerated in order to pass a partially occluded segment of the large bronchi. If the lumina of the smaller airways narrow, gas flow accelerates through the small bronchi, pressure differences across the walls of the larger bronchi increase, and the force tending to buckle the walls is greater (see Fig. 41).

After complete obstruction of an airway, there is absorption of gas distal to the blockage. Depending upon the location of the block, atelectasis may include a respiratory bronchiole and its alveolar ducts and alveoli, or a mainstem bronchus and the whole lung. Usually

pulmonary blood flow to the occluded unit decreases within 24 hours. Initially, the involved segment of the lung is small and, in some instances, such as asthma, may remain so. In patients with blockage due to a foreign body, after a few days the atelectatic area may enlarge as it fills with mucus. Deprived of blood flow and the cleansing action of the cilia and mucous lining, infection flourishes. Abscesses may form, or chronic inflammation may slowly erode and destroy the wall of the airway, causing bronchiectasis. Weeks after occlusion, blood flow increases through the atelectatic segment and the mucus becomes absorbed.

Partial obstruction causes air trapping. If the obstruction is generalized as in asthma, bronchitis, or bronchiolitis, there will be uniform hyperinflation. If the obstruction is localized, the lung distal to the obstruction will expand, and occasionally cystic lesions develop and may become infected.

In all of these conditions, if the bronchus is less

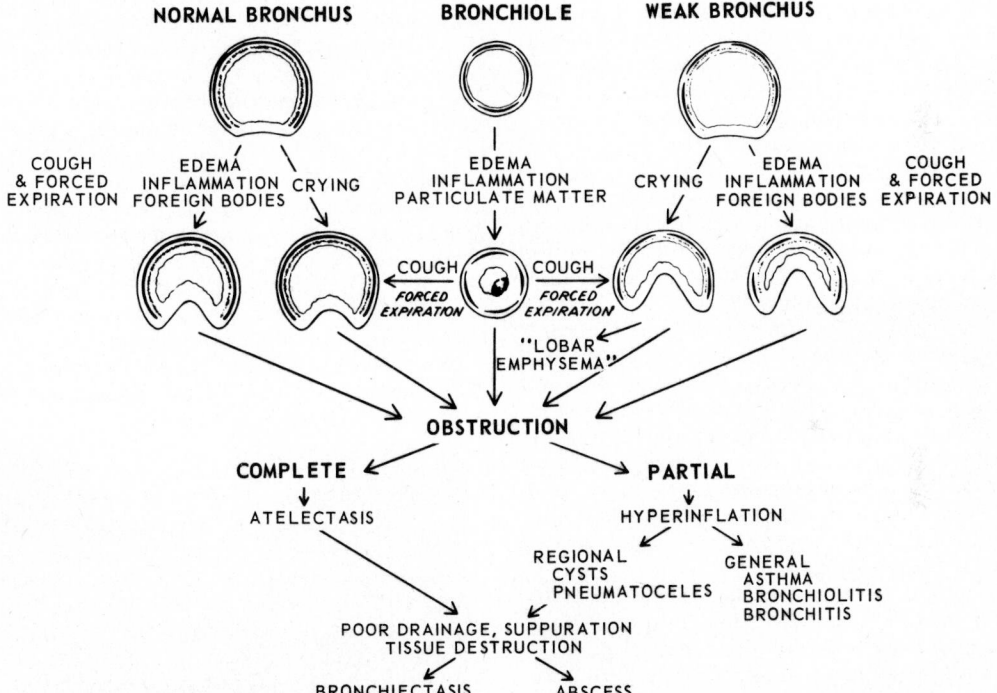

FIG. 44. A scheme showing some of the factors that cause obstruction and the consequences of the obstruction. The child's bronchus has proportionately little intrinsic support (normal bronchus). Segments of all of the bronchi in some children may be particularly weak (weak bronchus). Partial occlusion of the bronchioles increases the velocity of gas flow and provokes coughing; the pressure differences across the wall of the bronchi becomes greater and the bronchial walls buckle. The weak bronchus buckles more than the normal one. Crying and primary bronchial occlusion also invaginate the walls of the bronchi. Obstruction is either complete or partial—if complete, the lungs become atelectatic; if partial, the lung becomes hyperinflated. A small, weak segment of bronchus may collapse with forced or even expiration and overdistend a lobe or smaller subdivision of the lung, causing idioopathic lobar emphysema. Asthma, bronchiolitis, and bronchitis, partially occlude most of the airway structures and cause generalized hyperinflation. If a bronchiole is partially blocked, cystic dilatation of the structures distal to the block may occur, producing cysts or pneumatoceles. If these become infected, abscesses may form. Areas of the lung with partially or completely obstructed airways drain poorly and become infected. If the process is long standing, suppuration and bronchiectasis may develop.

sturdy than normal because of regional anomalies, delayed maturation, or destructive processes, expiratory obstruction is accentuated.

ASPIRATION OF FOREIGN BODIES

In a review of over 1,000 cases of endobronchial foreign bodies, Hollinger lists the following as most common: bones (20 percent), hardware (15 percent), nuts (14 percent), coins (14 percent), and safety pins (11 percent). When the trachea, major bronchi, and their subdivisions divide, one of the two divisions is larger. The angle of take-off of the smaller branch is more acute than that of the larger. Large inspired particles tend to follow the path of the larger subdivisions and lodge in the lower lobe of the right lung. In the infant with diaphragmatic breathing, the lumina of the ventral and lateral bronchi are narrow, while the basilar bronchi are wide. As a consequence, foreign bodies most frequently occlude the superior, lateral, and basilar segments of the right lower lobe; they involve the basilar and lateral segments of the left lower lobe less often.

Inspiration distributes small particles in a random manner. Large foreign bodies block large airways and cause acute respiratory distress, with either atelectasis or localized hyperinflation, depending upon whether the occlusion is complete or partial. There is an explosive onset of coughing and dyspnea. Hemoptysis, purulent sputum, fever, and leukocytosis develop if the foreign body lacerates the airway or if there is infection. If there is partial obstruction and overdistension, the unit may rupture, causing mediastinal emphysema or pneumothorax. Foreign bodies rarely erode into the interstitial space to produce mediastinal emphysema. If the foreign bodies are radiopaque, they are easily diagnosed and can be removed by bronchoscopy. Nuts and other nonopaque materials are less easily diagnosed. Peanuts, pumpkin seeds, and popcorn often cause partial obstruction. Infants who have inhaled these items often present with acute respiratory distress, hyperinflation of the ipsilateral lung with shift of the mediastinum to the contralateral side. *Small children should not be given nuts, pumpkin seeds, or popcorn.*

Smaller foreign bodies block small bronchi, and a mild cough may be the only symptom. However, if not treated, fever, cough with the production of purulent sputum, and other symptoms of pulmonary suppuration occur. Indeed, these are often the first indication of a previous aspiration. Inhaled vegetable matter is particularly likely to produce a local inflammatory reaction and distal infection with abscess formation. Even after foreign bodies are removed, patients may have cough, excessive bronchial secretions, residual bronchial inflammation, and, rarely, endobronchial granulation with more or less permanent obstruction.

Barbed grass heads (timothy grass heads) are an especially troublesome problem. They anchor themselves to the wall of the airway, causing a marked local inflammatory reaction. They are not easily coughed up or moved by ciliary action and remain in the bronchi until removed by bronchoscopy. Some have such acute barbs that respiratory movements may carry them

through the bronchus into the parenchyma toward the pleura and create bronchopleural fistulas.

Roentgenographic diagnosis of nonradiopaque foreign bodies may be facilitated by inspiratory, expiratory, and lateral decubitus views of the chest. The recent development of an operating infant bronchoscope, which contains a magnifying lens system, has significantly improved the endoscopist's ability to remove aspirated foreign bodies.

STRUCTURAL DEFECTS

TRACHEOBRONCHOMALACIA.
The intrathoracic airways narrow during expiration. The degree of narrowing is limited by cartilage and other supportive tissue in the larger airways and by the elastic matrix of peripheral lung parenchyma. Since the large airways of normal infants do not have much cartilage, they are particularly likely to be compressed during forced expiration. Some infants have marked delays in the development of the supportive structure of large airways, and airway obstruction during respiratory maneuvers may become severe. The classification of infants with collapsing airways is based on the anatomic area involved —*tracheomalacia, tracheobronchomalacia,* or *bronchomalacia.* The symptoms include wheezing, respiratory distress, hyperinflation of both lungs or varying portions of one lung or its individual lobes, depending upon the site and extent of the collapsing segment. Symptoms are increased with respiratory infections. As some children with localized defects of the lower trachea or the major bronchi become older, the segments become more stable and the symptoms improve. In others, the flabby airways persist and are associated with recurring episodes of infection and hyperinflation.

Campbell and Williams have described a group of children who have a generalized deficiency of bronchial

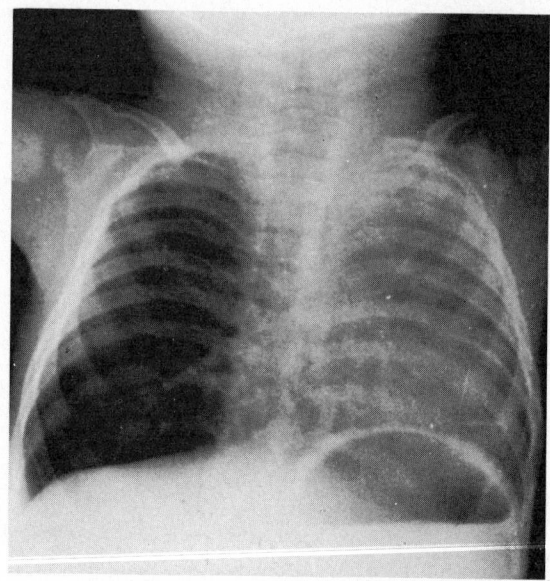

FIG. 45. Chest radiogram showing hyperinflation of the right lung with mediastinal shift to the left.

cartilages in the fourth to eighth generation of bronchi. These children have wheezing, cough, and recurrent pulmonary infections from early infancy and tend to develop bronchiectasis and pulmonary hypertension at an early age.

LOBAR EMPHYSEMA. This condition may present as an acute respiratory emergency. Tachypnea, retractions, and cyanosis usually appear in the newborn period, but the onset of symptoms may be insidious and become most marked at 2 to 3 months. There is hyperinflation localized to one lung, lobe, or segment, which compresses adjacent lung tissue and pushes the mediastinum to the contralateral side (Fig. 45). Histologically, the lung has distended alveoli, ruptured intraalveolar septa, and large cavitations. Often there is fibrosis of the remaining intraalveolar tissue, which may represent healing of concurrent or intercurrent inflammation. External pressure by anomalous vessels, cysts, or tumors, may be responsible. Stanger and associates point out that compression of a bronchus by a distended pulmonary artery or the left atrium may cause this syndrome. Some cases are probably due to intrinsic weakness of a small segment of the airway (Fig. 46), while others appear to be due to a generalized disorder of growth of the segment or lobe.

In cases where symptoms are severe and the condition appears life-threatening, surgical removal of the obstructed segment and hyperinflated pulmonary tissue is mandatory. When symptoms are less marked, oral or inhaled bronchodilators may be useful in long-term management.

TRACHEAL STENOSIS. There were 23 cases of

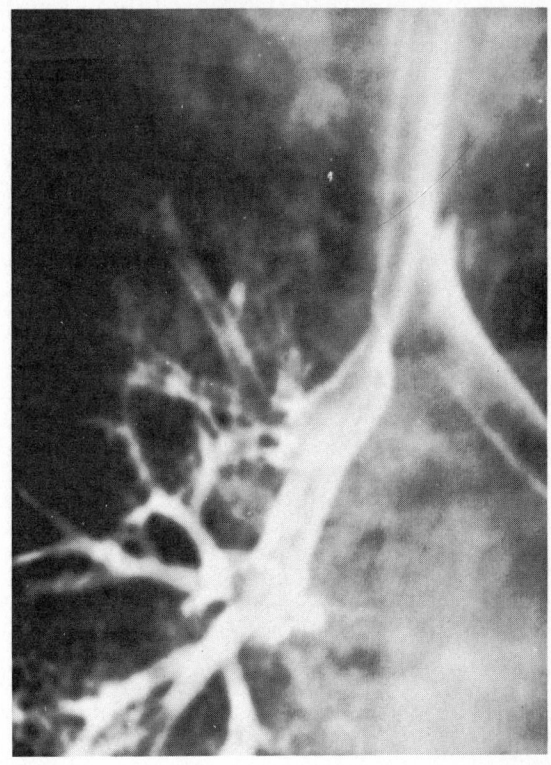

FIG. 46. Cinebronchiogram of same patient as shown in Fig 45; a small segment of the right mainstem bronchus, just below the carina, is narrow on forced expiration.

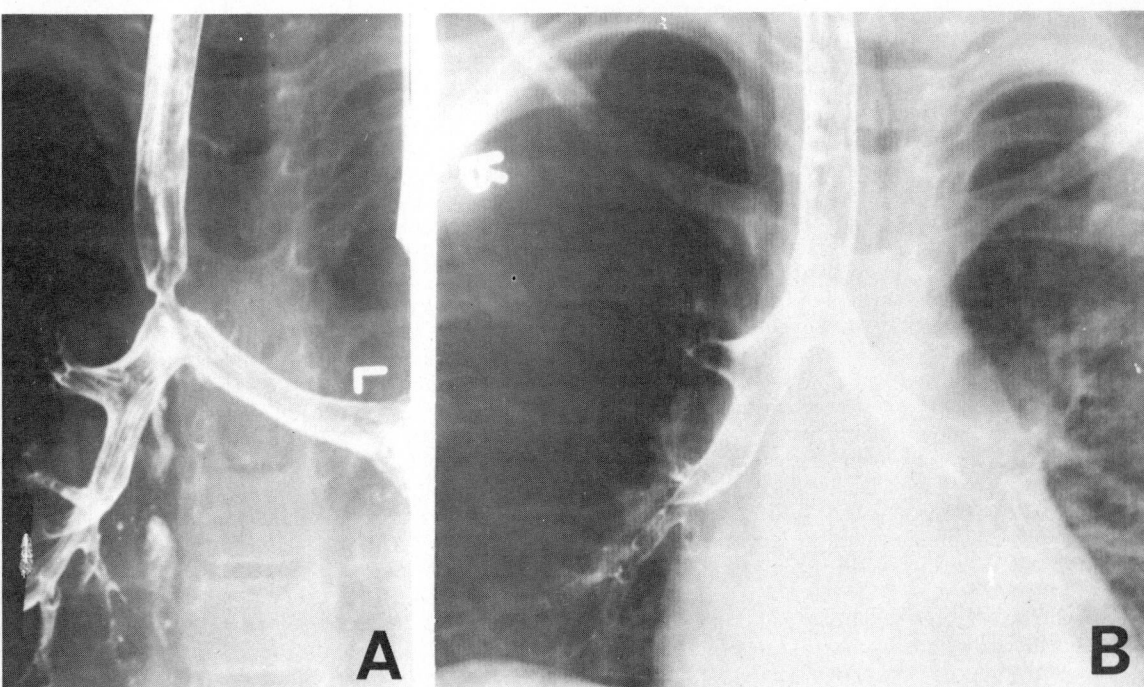

FIG. 47. Tracheal stenosis. **A.** Tantalum tracheogram showing marked tracheal stenosis just above the carina. **B.** Repeat tantalum tracheogram 4 months after surgical excision of stenotic area. Tracheal lumen is normal.

this anomaly reported by 1957: 12 were caused by regional absence of the membranous part of the trachea, with the tracheal cartilages forming a complete small ring; the rest were associated with absent or incomplete cartilaginous rings. Inspiratory stridor occurs with extrathoracic stenosis; inspiratory and expiratory stridor accompany intrathoracic stenosis. The symptoms are present from birth. If there is a cartilaginous ring and the stenotic segment is short, it should be excised (Fig. 47). Regional areas of weakness due to cartilaginous insufficiency become strengthened by stiffening as the infant grows and obstruction disappears.

TUMORS AND EXTERNAL COMPRESSION

External compression of the trachea or major bronchi by tumors, cysts, or vascular anomalies may cause partial or complete obstruction.

BRONCHIAL ADENOMAS AND PAPILLOMATA. Bronchial adenomas are rare in childhood. They may arise from either the cells of the mucous glands of the bronchus or the cells lining the excretory ducts of these glands. Two histologic types are defined. The carcinoid type (90 percent), resembling the carcinoid tumors of the small bowel but without symptoms of the carcinoid syndrome, has been reported in children. The cylindromatous type (10 percent) is made up of cuboidal or flattened epithelial cells, closely resembles mixed tumors of the salivary gland, and has a 40 percent chance of malignancy.

Papillomata of the trachea and bronchi have been recorded in 23 children. They are frequently multiple, tend to be attached by a pedicle, and oscillate during inspiration and expiration. Dyspnea and stridor are common. Secondary obstructive changes, with obstructive emphysema, atelectasis, pneumonia, and bronchiectasis, may occur when papillomata are in the distal parts of the tracheobronchial tree.

Cysts arising in bronchial walls or lymphatic tissue are more common. These may occur in any part of the lung but are most common in the posterior mediastinum. Adenomas and cysts usually cause wheezing, repeated episodes of infection, and hemoptysis. If they obstruct a large airway, they cause dyspnea, retractions, and cyanosis. Adenomas usually obstruct bronchi but may occlude the trachea. In bronchial adenoma, respiratory symptoms are typically relieved by flexing the neck and are aggravated by hyperextension. Cysts, because of their posterior placement, ordinarily cause anterior displacement and compression of the major bronchi or trachea. Bronchial adenomas and cysts should be removed surgically.

VASCULAR ANOMALIES. Stridor, wheezing, and intermittent pulmonary infections may be caused by extrinsic compression of the trachea or bronchi by vascular anomalies such as double aortic arch, which is most common (see p. 1440). Prolonged compression of the trachea or bronchus by vascular or other extrinsic masses may produce permanent softening of the airway segment, which may continue to collapse during expiration after surgery. Therefore, surgical correction of these anomalies is best done early in life if the infant is symptomatic.

BRONCHIOLITIS. Bronchiolitis is a disease of infants and young children, most commonly seen in winter and spring and often occurring in epidemics. After a period of upper respiratory tract infection, lasting one to several days, there is an abrupt onset of accelerated respiratory rate and intercostal and subcostal retractions, associated with the rapid development of hyperinflation of the lungs. In addition, infants with bronchiolitis have tachycardia, cyanosis, increase in pulmonary vascular resistance, and, occasionally, right heart failure. In a review of 1,230 cases, Heycock reports a 5.5 percent overall mortality, but most large series report a mortality of under 1 percent.

The walls of the small bronchi and bronchioles are thick and infiltrated with inflammatory cells; the lumina are often completely occluded with leukocytes and debris. There is also inflammation and partial occlusion of the medium-sized bronchi, and this probably is responsible for most of the expiratory obstruction. Almost all cases of bronchiolitis are due to viral infection. Holdaway and associates, in a study of 211 infants with acute bronchiolitis, isolated respiratory syncytial virus from 59 percent, and from only 1.4 percent of an equal number of control infants. Adenovirus was found in another group of infants. No convincing correlation with bacteria cultured from the nasopharynx and bronchiolitis has been found.

There is a marked obstruction to expiration with gas trapping. Functional residual capacity increases and vital capacity decreases. Lung compliance also decreases as the lung is overdistended. Late in the disease, the patient may hypoventilate and develop respiratory acidosis and hypoxemia. Although infants with bronchiolitis frequently appear very ill early in the disease, they often improve in 12 to 24 hours and are almost always better after 48 hours.

Determining the correct treatment for infants with bronchiolitis is complicated by difficulty in differentiating them from infants with severe asthma or bacterial bronchopneumonia. They should be treated in intensive care units, with continuous electronic monitoring of heart rate and respiration and intermittent measurements of arterial pH and blood gases. Almost all infants with bronchiolitis have hypoxemia and require treatment with moist oxygen in concentrations of 30 to 40 percent. Although mild hypercapnia is not uncommon, increasing inspired oxygen does not depress the respiratory drive in these infants. They should be given sufficient intravenous glucose and saline solutions to restore and maintain adequate hydration. Since the young infant has little bronchiolar muscle, bronchodilators are not very effective. However, some asthmatic patients with bronchiolitis improve after intravenous bronchodilators, such as aminophylline, but its effects must be monitored carefully; if no definite improvement is noted, it should not be continued. Corticosteroids have been recommended, but several studies show no benefit from their routine use. If used at all, they should be reserved for desperately ill infants with gross respiratory failure. A small number of infants develop progressive respiratory failure and may require mechanical ventilation.

ASTHMA. Asthma is characterized by paroxysmal attacks of wheezing, dyspnea, and cough (see also p. 346). These episodes are frequently preceded by symptoms of mild upper respiratory tract infection. Occasionally, respiratory distress is severe, the retractions and tachypnea become more marked, and there may be a rapid deterioration in the patient's condition, with a precipitous fall in Pao_2 and a dramatic rise in $Paco_2$.

The child with asthma has extremely sensitive airways, which contract vigorously when exposed to a wide variety of airborne or ingested allergens; to respiratory tract infections; to inhaled physical, chemical, or thermal irritants; and during exercise and emotional disturbances.

Bronchoconstriction is caused by the local release of chemical mediators (histamine, slow-reacting substances, etc.) within the lung, which also cause edema of the bronchial walls and increased secretion of mucus by the bronchial glands. Leukocytes, predominantly eosinophils, surround the bronchi, invade their walls, and appear in the lumen. Recent research suggests that reflex bronchoconstriction, mediated by the parasympathetic fibers of the vagus nerve, may account for some of the bronchoconstriction in all asthmatics, and may be responsible primarily for asthma in an occasional individual; investigations in dogs show that this reflex can be blocked by atropine. The relative importance of this finding in clinical asthma awaits further study.

The edema, mucopurulent material, and muscular constriction reduce the size of the bronchial lumen and increase resistance to airflow. The larger airways tend to collapse during forced expiration, and the combination of large and small airway obstruction leads to air trapping and hyperinflation of the lungs. As the lungs become larger, the vital capacity decreases and the work of breathing increases. Maldistribution of inspired gas causes hypoxemia to develop early in a severe asthmatic attack. As the episode progresses, alveolar ventilation decreases and $Paco_2$ begins to rise.

The air trapping, hyperinflation of the lungs, and uneven distribution of inspired gas in asthma are usually reversible with aggressive therapy. Asymptomatic children with asthma can have significant airway obstruction between acute attacks, and it is possible that prolonged airway obstruction may lead to irreversible pulmonary damage.

The comprehensive approach to the allergic child is covered on p. 338. The physician must provide more than only emergency care during the acute asthmatic episode. The parent and child must know how to avoid contact with known precipitating factors and the importance of early treatment of acute attacks with bronchodilators. Prompt administration of oral bronchodilators can stop an episode of wheezing; if they are ineffective, the child should inhale a bronchodilator aerosol or be given injections of epinephrine.

If symptoms continue to worsen, respiratory failure must be suspected and the child should be hospitalized so that vital signs can be monitored frequently. An initial arterial blood sample for oxygen and carbon dioxide tensions and a chest radiograph should be obtained. The child should be placed in 30 to 40 percent humidified oxygen and given intravenous fluids at about 1.5 times the calculated maintenance volume. Bronchodilation should first be attempted with intravenous aminophylline (theophylline ethylenediamine) with a loading dose of 5 to 7 mg/kg given over 15 minutes (unless the child has been receiving aminophylline prior to hospital entry, in which case the initial dose must be reduced, usually to half the recommended dose). The aminophylline level should then be maintained by the constant infusion of 1 mg/kg/hour or intermittent infusions of 4 to 6 mg/kg every 4 to 6 hours.

The periodic inhalation of aerosols of β-adrenergic catecholamines in saline, with oxygen as the carrier gas, usually without positive pressure, can often effect bronchodilation until aminophylline and hydration exert their effects. Isoproterenol is short acting and, if the pulse rate is below 160/min, may be used as frequently as every 1 to 2 hours. Metaproterenol, Salbutamol, and Terbutaline are longer acting and may be given every 4 to 6 hours.

Metabolic acidemia due to dehydration and poor peripheral perfusion, and respiratory acidemia may be marked. Since acidemia increases pulmonary vascular resistance and also causes disturbances in K^+ distribution, pH should not be allowed to fall below 7.25. If the acidemia is metabolic and the child has a normal or low $Paco_2$, or is having ventilatory assistance, 1 to 2 mEq/kg sodium bicarbonate should be used with caution, if there is respiratory acidemia, as it may further depress ventilation. Frequent Pao_2 and $Paco_2$ measurements are necessary during treatment; overenthusiastic correction of the intial acidemia can result in troublesome alkalemia once the patient's ventilation begins to improve.

If the child shows evidence of hypercapnia, has had steroids recently, or has required steroids for previous attacks, intravenous hydrocortisone should be given in doses of 4 mg/kg every 4 hours (or equivalent doses of methylprednisolone or dexamethasone).

If ventilation decreases and $Paco_2$ rises above 55 torr, an infusion of isoproterenol should be started while continuously monitoring heart rate and electrocardiogram. The concentration of isoproterenol used should be 1 μg/kg/ml (ie, the concentration for a 15-kg child should be 15 μg/ml). Begin with 0.1 μg/kg/minute (0.1 ml/minute of the solution) administered with a calibrated infusion pump. If there is no effect, double the rate of infusion every 20 minutes while carefully monitoring heart rate and electrocardiographic form until the $Paco_2$ begins to fall. The usual dose of isoproterenol required is 0.1 to 3.5 μg/kg/minute, with an average of 0.7 μg/kg/minute. When $Paco_2$ begins to decrease, the isoproterenol is continued at the same rate until normal $Paco_2$ is achieved. The average duration of isoproterenol infusion is 48 hours, but ranges from 17 hours to 6 days. If the child develops tachycardia but no arrhythmia, the infusion should be slowed to keep the heart rate at or below 180/minute. If arrhythmia occurs, the isoproterenol must be stopped. Since the biologic half-life of isoproterenol is about 2 minutes, the arrhythmia will usually disappear quickly; when the rhythm returns to normal, intravenous isoproterenol can be restarted, using a smaller dose.

The patient with severe hypercapnia on admission to the hospital or with increasing CO_2 retention, and with a $Paco_2$ greater than 70 torr, should be intubated and mechanically ventilated. Morphine should be given immediately before intubation to decrease anxiety and discomfort. Since the lungs have decreased compliance, a volume ventilator is usually required and muscular paralysis with curare may be needed to achieve synchronization of the patient with the ventilator. The details of this procedure have been well described by Downes and his associates.

When the acute attack is controlled, bronchodilation with oral aminophylline or isoproterenol should be continued for at least 1 to 3 weeks. Prevention of subsequent attacks depends largely on educating the patient and his parents of the importance of a continuing program of avoiding environmental allergens and early use of bronchodilator treatment. (See p. 338 for details of allergic management.)

BRONCHIECTASIS. Bronchiectasis, or dilatation of the bronchus, occurs whenever secretions accumulate and distend a bronchus. Inflamed bronchi clear mucus slowly; an irritated bronchus produces an excess of mucus and bronchodilation ensues. Bronchi also dilate after obstruction by a foreign body or a mucous plug, as the alveoli surrounding them become airless and collapse; the bronchi and supporting structures remain normal and return to normal size when the disease process is resolved. However, if a mucus-dilated bronchus becomes infected, the bronchial wall may be damaged permanently and thus impair bronchial mucus clearance and promote continued local infection and permanent dilatation. In the absence of better terms, these two conditions are called *reversible bronchiectasis* (or pseudobronchiectasis, a confusing term) and *irreversible bronchiectasis.*

The terms used by radiologists to describe variations in the appearance of bronchi on bronchograms suggests a more detailed classification and understanding of bronchiectasis than actually exists. Terms such as tubular, cylindrical, fusiform, saccular, or cystic are rarely helpful in planning management. Even saccular bronchiectasis after post-traumatic bronchial stenosis, often thought to be the hallmark of irreversible bronchiectasis, can disappear completely after the stenotic segment is repaired surgically.

Bronchiectasis is a chronic inflammatory disease that produces a more or less continuous cough and is often accompanied by intermittent fever, hemoptysis, and signs of pneumonia. The chest is enlarged, and rales of various types are heard diffusely throughout the lungs. Clubbing of the fingers is common. Children with extensive bronchiectasis fatigue easily, and have reduced exercise capacity and delayed physical growth. Bronchograms show widely dilated bronchi (Fig. 48).

Bronchiectasis is usually associated with chronic

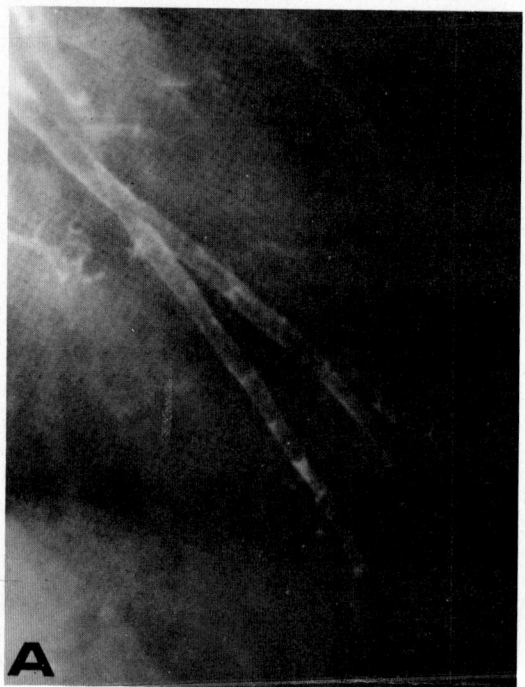
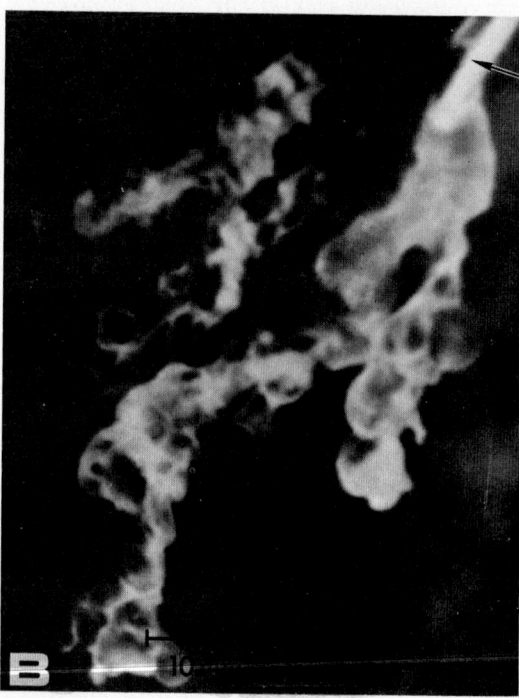

FIG. 48. **A.** Normal left lower lobe bronchi outlined with tantalum. **B.** The same patient's right lower lobe bronchi outlined with tantalum, showing the dilation of the bronchi characteristic of bronchiectasis. (Courtesy of Dr. JA Nadel)

purulent inflammation and destruction of the walls of the bronchi. Complete or partial obstruction decreases bronchial drainage and increases the infection. Atelectasis and abscess formation are usual when obstruction is complete; when obstruction is partial, there is regional hyperinflation.

Twenty percent of the reported cases begin under 1 year and 75 percent prior to 5 years of age. This early onset suggests that some infants may be predisposed to ectasia because of the narrow lumina and weak structure of the bronchi.

Children with advanced bronchiectasis frequently have a large total lung capacity, large functional residual capacity, and a small vital capacity. There is an increase in airway resistance and a decrease in flow rates, particularly forced expiratory flow. Ventilation and pulmonary perfusion are unevenly distributed. Some areas of the lung may have little ventilation and a large blood flow; this causes inadequate oxygenation, resulting in a decreased Pao_2. Other areas of the lung receive little blood flow and may be relatively well ventilated; this tends to increase the respiratory dead space, decrease the ventilatory efficiency, and increase the work of breathing.

Allergic children with severe asthma and excessive production of airway mucus probably constitute the largest group of patients who tend to develop localized dilation of the airways. This type of bronchiectasis is almost always reversible and surgery for bronchiectasis in asthmatic children should never be considered before a trial of aggressive medical management. Atelectasis of the right middle lobe, accompanied by *cylindrical bronchiectasis*, often occurs in allergic children; this also is almost always reversible. Removal of the right middle lobe may *cure* the bronchiectasis, but almost never improves the allergic pulmonary disease. With comprehensive medical treatment, the bronchial changes in the right middle lobe almost always will revert to normal within a few years.

We consider the diagnosis of *right middle lobe syndrome* to be unsatisfactory as it suggests that the disease is specific to the right middle lobe. Right middle lobe infiltration or atelectasis is almost always associated with asthma, cystic fibrosis, presence of a foreign body, or other more general pulmonary problems. Attention to the treatment of the basic disease state is most important and surgical removal of the right middle lobe is rarely justified or helpful. Foreign bodies in a bronchus almost always promote recurrent infections and structural damage. They must be removed by bronchoscopy, if the patient does not cough them out spontaneously. In localized destructive bronchiectasis following foreign body aspiration or extensive infarction, surgical removal of the involved lobe can be curative.

Before the wide used of antibiotic therapy, bacterial infection of a bronchus obstructed with mucus was common. Irreversible bronchiectasis often developed after infection with measles, whooping cough, or bacterial pneumonias, or with aspiration of foreign bodies. Use of antibiotics has decreased the incidence of bronchiectasis dramatically. Children with cystic fibrosis or those with immunoglobulin deficiency have a great tendency to develop irreversible bronchiectasis, and most children with bronchiectasis encountered now have one of these conditions; bronchiectasis appears gradually after recurrent pulmonary infections.

Treatment consists of aerosol or systemic bronchodilation followed by a vigorous program of postural drainage. Specific infections are treated with antibiotics; prolonged antibiotic therapy may be necessary to suppress chronic infection. Since both diseases lead to progressive widespread involvement of the lung, a surgical approach to the bronchiectasis is not justified, except in the case of large localized lung abscesses.

CYSTIC FIBROSIS

Cystic fibrosis is the most common cause of chronic suppurative lung disease in children. Although we do not know its cause and have no cure, early diagnosis and comprehensive treatment can slow the development of respiratory failure and extend the duration and quality of life of children and adults with cystic fibrosis. The disease was first recognized as a separate entity by Fanconi in 1936. Anderson described the clinical and pathologic features and considered it to be a rare pancreatic disorder affecting young infants that was uniformly fatal; they called it cystic fibrosis of the pancreas. Farber later pointed out the generalized nature of the disease, with involvement of all the mucus-secreting glands, and suggested the name *mucoviscidosis*. When di Sant'Agnese demonstrated the consistent involvement of sweat and salivary glands as well, it became evident that cystic fibrosis is a generalized disease affecting many and perhaps all exocrine glands. While the name cystic fibrosis for this disease is historically based, it does not indicate the basic pathology; however, it is widely accepted and should continue to be used until we have a better understanding of the basic abnormality.

DEFINITION. Cystic fibrosis is an inherited disorder of generalized dysfunction of the exocrine secretory glands. The concentrations of sodium and chloride in sweat are markedly elevated. Mucus-producing glands throughout the body secrete organic products with abnormal physicochemical behavior; these secretions tend to precipitate in the duct lumina and obstruct the flow of secretions. Almost all of the clinical manifestations of cystic fibrosis are secondary to these two abnormalities. Patients with cystic fibrosis frequently have involvement of multiple organ systems, including the lungs, pancreas, liver, intestines, sweat glands, nasal sinuses, salivary glands, and male and female genital tracts. The full spectrum of this disease can be appreciated from Table 12.

GENETICS AND PREVALENCE. Cystic fibrosis is transmitted as a mendelian recessive disorder. Both parents must be carriers (heterozygotes) and the affected child is homozygous. Most investigators believe that a single mutant allele causes the disease, but the presence of multiple alleles at different loci cannot be excluded. Theoretically, 1 in 4 siblings are affected, and a greater incidence in any family is thought to be a chance distribution. Any couple who has produced a child with cystic fibrosis faces a 25 percent chance of

Table 12. Pathophysiology, Clinical Manifestations, and Complications in Various Organs Involved in Cystic Fibrosis

Organ Involved	Secretory Dysfunction	Clinical Manifestations	Complications
Sweat glands	Elevated concentration of sodium and chloride in sweat	Hyponatremia, hypochloremia	Heat prostration shock
Intestine			
Newborn	Viscid meconium	Meconium ileus with intestinal obstruction	Meconium peritonitis
Older child and adults	Inspissated mucofecal masses (intestinal sludging)	Partial intestinal obstruction with severe cramping pains	Intestinal obstruction Intussusception
Pancreas	Inspissation and precipitation of pancreatic secretions causing obstruction of pancreatic ducts	Absence of pancreatic enzymes causing malabsorption of food and fatty, bulky stools	Hypoproteinemia, iron deficiency anemia, vitamin K deficiency and rectal prolapse, and/or insulin deficiency.
Liver	Insulin deficiency Inspissation and precipitation of bile in biliary system	Glucose intolerance Focal biliary cirrhosis; shrunken "hob-nail" liver	Diabetes mellitus Portal hypertension with esophageal varices and hematemesis
Salivary glands	Inspissation and precipitation of secretions in small ducts of submaxillary and sublingual salivary glands	Mild patchy fibrosis of salivary glands	None
Paranasal	Viscid mucus	Retention of mucus. Clouding on sinus roentgenograms	Mucopyoceles with nasal deformity or orbital cavity extension
Nose	Nasal polyps	Obstruction to nasal airflow	None
Lungs	Viscid mucus in bronchioles and bronchi	Obstruction of bronchioles causing bronchiolectasis, bronchiectasis, and chronic suppurative lung infection	Hemoptysis, pneumothorax, cor pulmonale
Reproductive tract			
Males	Viscid genital tract secretions during embryologic development, causing failure of formation of normal wolffian duct structures.	Sterility	None
Females	Distension of the endocervical epithelial cells with cytoplasmic mucin	None proved; ? decreased fertility	Polypoid cervicitis while taking oral contraceptives

having another affected child with each pregnancy, regardless of how many affected or unaffected children they have had in the past.

The differences in prevalence of cystic fibrosis in various racial groups is striking. The disease has been reported in almost all racial groups, but the highest incidence, approximately 1 in 2,500 live births, is in Caucasian families of central European background. In Sweden the incidence is only about 1 in 7,500 births, while in American Blacks, it is estimated to occur in 1 in 12,000 births. It is much less common in persons of Asian ancestry, and rare in American Indians.

PATHOLOGY. Morphologic changes in cystic fibrosis are almost all secondary to obstruction of the ducts of the mucus-secreting organs throughout the body. The extent of the damage tends to be proportional to the mucus component of the secretions, and the length and tortuosity of the duct system involved. The physicochemical abnormality that causes the mucus obstruction still is not known.

The altered function of the exocrine sweat glands is the most consistent abnormality encountered in patients with cystic fibrosis, but no morphologic or histochemical change has been described. Sweat produced at the bottom of the glands is approximately isotonic both in normal persons and in patients with cystic fibrosis. In normal children, the sodium and chloride are largely reabsorbed during flow along the duct to the skin surface, resulting in sweat that is markedly hypotonic (under 40 mEg/liter sodium and chloride). In patients with cystic fibrosis, sodium and chloride are less well reabsorbed as the sweat traverses the sweat duct on its way to the skin surface; the electrolyte concentrations in surface sweat remain closer to isotonic values, in the range of 60 to 130 mEq/liter.

The pancreas most frequently shows characteristic structural changes in cystic fibrosis. Microscopically, the ducts are blocked by inspissated eosinophilic material; the epithelial lining is flattened and the ducts are dilated, sometimes appearing cystlike. With time, a diffuse fibrosis and leukocytic infiltration develops and eventually the pancreas is replaced by fatty tissue. These changes are usually well developed at birth, but varying degrees of pancreatic involvement occur, and pancreatic insufficiency may not develop until some time after birth. Although the islets of Langerhans are not intrinsically affected, as pancreatic fibrosis progresses the number of β cells decrease and may result in glucose intolerance and glycosuria.

The salivary glands may be similarly affected, but

fibrosis is much less marked, probably because the saliva does not contain irritating proteolytic enzymes.

The liver may develop focal obstructive lesions resulting from bile-containing mucous plugs, and these changes are called *focal biliary cirrhosis*. With time, the adjacent portal areas tend to become fibrosed and grossly distort the hepatic lobule, leading to multilobular biliary cirrhosis. The liver is described as "hobnailed" with multiple large clefts, but sufficient intact liver substance remains to sustain almost normal hepatocellular function. Advanced changes in the liver occur in less than 5 percent of patients with cystic fibrosis and, when present, may lead to portal vein obstruction, portal hypertension, esophageal varices, and gross hematemesis.

The lungs appear grossly normal at birth, although the mucus-producing epithelial cells that line the small bronchi are distended. The initial physiologic dysfunction is an expiratory bronchiolar obstruction secondary to partial mucous occlusion of the lumen; hyperinflation of the lungs is common. Mucous stasis lends itself to early bacterial infection and produces bronchiolitis, bronchitis, and finally destructive changes in the bronchial walls, which lead to bronchiolectasis, bronchiectasis, peribronchitis, and pulmonary fibrosis. The chronic suppurative infection of the lower airway is difficult to control because of the impaired ability of the lungs to clear mucus and infected debris from the distal airway. As the disease progresses, the larger airways are involved, with increasing obstruction to airflow; localized abscess formation and recurrent episodes of bacterial pneumonia (alveolitis) are common. A natural consequence of the airway obstruction is marked hypoxemia secondary to severe ventilation–perfusion inequality. Pulmonary hypertension develops frequently, with resultant right ventricular hypertrophy, cor pulmonale, and congestive heart failure.

The reproductive organs are commonly involved; females show distension of the epithelial cells of the cervical glands with mucin, and in males the mesonephric derivatives (epididymis, vas deferens, and seminal vesicles) are generally abnormal, presumably as the result of abnormal secretions early in fetal life. The normal pathway for passage of spermatozoa is absent and results in sterility in most males, despite the fact that normal spermatogenesis has been observed.

CLINICAL MANIFESTATIONS.   The wide variety of clinical manifestations secondary to obstruction of mucus-secreting glands and elevated sweat chloride levels is shown in Table 12. The remarkable variation in age at the onset of symptoms severe enough to lead to diagnosis has not been emphasized sufficiently in the past. A few children with cystic fibrosis may show normal growth and development in the first decade, then develop pulmonary disease sometime in the second decade. Retrospectively, symptoms of mild-to-moderate malabsorption may have been present but ignored by the child and his parents.

The original description of cystic fibrosis as an infant disease is valid for perhaps 50 percent of children with the disease. This includes symptoms of malabsorption (large, foul-smelling, fatty stools) present almost from birth, poor weight gain, and early onset of a persistent, dry, hacking paroxysmal cough, and multiple bouts of pneumonitis in the first year. Many children who develop pulmonary symptoms in the first few years may have no evidence of pancreatic insufficiency, and malabsorption may become evident only after pulmonary pathology is well advanced. Conversely, a severe malabsorptive state in infancy may antedate the onset of pulmonary symptoms by many years. Since it is a genetically determined disease, it is difficult to understand why involvement of various organs occurs at different ages.

The sweat gland abnormality is the one exception to the variations described. The elevated concentrations of sodium and chloride in sweat are always present from birth. This accounts for the great reliance placed on measurement of sweat electrolytes for the diagnosis of cystic fibrosis. Because of the large amounts of sodium and chloride in sweat, these patients are prone to develop severe hyponatremia and hypochloremia with excessive sweating. They may present with shock and extremely low serum electrolytes (sodium below 120 mEq/liter); this occurs most often in hot humid weather. With severe hyponatremia, patients with cystic fibrosis are not able to decrease the concentration of sodium and chloride in their sweat, and thus conserve body salt. This susceptibility to heat prostration must be recognized and oral salt supplements offered during times of profuse sweating.

PULMONARY MANIFESTATIONS.   The earliest symptom of pulmonary involvement is cough due to the retained tenacious mucous secretions. Initially, this produces bronchiolitis and, later, bronchitis. Cough may be severe and unproductive and frequently the diagnosis of pertussis is considered because of the persistent and paroxysmal nature of the cough. As the disease progresses, mucus production increases and coarse rales are present on auscultation of the chest.

In infants, widespread bronchiolar involvement commonly is accompanied by wheezing. Widely distributed fine inspiratory rales as well as coarse rhonchi may be heard. Hyperinflation of the chest is almost always present, with an increase in the anterior-posterior diameter of the thorax. As the process continues, bronchiectatic changes develop in the airway, with increasing mucopurulent secretions and productive cough (Fig. 49).

Patchy areas of atelectasis or collapse of a lobar segment, particularly the right upper lobe, is common. Maldistribution of ventilation and atelectatic areas may lead to hypoxemia. The lungs gradually develop diffuse suppuration involving almost the entire pulmonary parenchyma. With prolonged survival, pneumothorax or massive hemoptysis occurs with increasing frequency. Pulmonary hypertension, cor pulmonale, and congestive heart failure may develop as pulmonary changes become more severe. Respiratory insufficiency with hypercapnia and severe hypoxemia is a frequent terminal event.

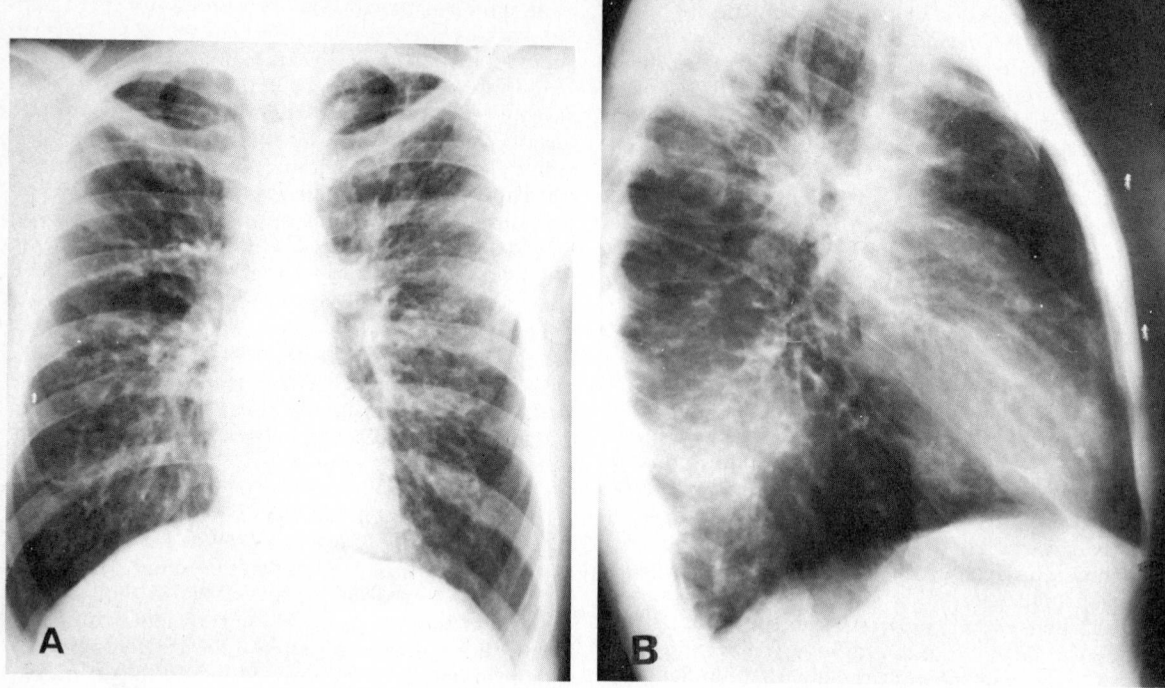

Fig. 49. Chest roentgenograms (posterior-anterior and lateral views) of 22-year-old male with cystic fibrosis, showing advanced pulmonary fibrosis and bronchiectasis.

GASTROINTESTINAL MANIFESTATIONS (see Chap 22 p. 993). *Meconium ileus,* the earliest manifestation of cystic fibrosis, is present as birth in 10 to 15 percent of cases. Meconium, the normal content of the intestinal tract at the time of birth, fails to undergo digestion and softening because of the lack of adequate pancreatic enzymes in the bowel. Normal meconium consists primarily of carbohydrates, but in infants with cystic fibrosis it has a high protein content and is abnormally viscid so that passage by normal bowel peristalsis is difficult. Abdominal distension may be present at birth or may begin within the first 12 hours as air is swallowed into the gastrointestinal tract. The clinical picture is similar to other types of lower small bowel obstruction. A typical roentgenogram of the abdomen shows dilated proximal loops of small bowel and a reticular pattern in many segments of the distal bowel that contain air mixed with meconium, causing a "spongy" appearance. Occasionally, the small bowel may perforate in utero, resulting in meconium peritonitis and intraabdominal calcifications. The failure of meconium to move beyond the ileocecal valve in utero results in a "pencil-like" microcolon that has the capacity to expand once the ileal impaction is removed or dissolved.

Until quite recently, the only successful treatment was surgical removal of the inspissated meconium, usually followed by temporary ileostomy. Gastrografin, a contrast agent with a very high osmolality, has been successfully used as an enema to wash out the bowel and promote passage of the sticky meconium. It appears worthy of trial before committing the infant to surgery (details of the technique have been published by Noblett).

MALABSORPTION. Most patients have little or no pancreatic enzymes entering the duodenum at the time of birth. The stools are abnormal, tend to be bulky, unduly frequent, and have a penetrating "cheesy" odor. The stools may appear pale or greasy and, as the amount of fat in the child's diet increases, a ring of oil around the stool deposit may be visible on the diaper. Typically, the infant has a ravenous appetite. If he takes a cow's milk formula, he may compensate for his incomplete absorption of fat and protein by ingesting large volumes of milk and other foods. Infants who are breastfed or on a soybean formula have a lower protein intake and are more likely to develop hypoproteinemia and edema in the first 6 months after birth. Even on the high protein intake of cow's milk, most of these infants fail to gain adequately.

Symptoms from deficiency of fat-soluble vitamins were more common before vitamin-enriched milks and vitamin supplements were used widely. Vitamin K deficiency, with prolonged prothrombin time and subcutaneous bleeding, is observed occasionally. Vitamin D deficiency rickets is very rare, for reasons that have not been clearly explained.

Rectal prolapse, which may be the first symptom, is due to wasting of perirectal supporting tissues, secondary to malnutrition. Every child with rectal prolapse should have a sweat chloride determination to rule out cystic fibrosis; with adequate dietary treatment and pancreatic enzyme therapy, rectal prolapse invariably resolves without need for surgery.

Focal biliary cirrhosis rarely gives rise to clinical manifestations, although prolonged neonatal jaundice has been reported. With diffuse multilobar biliary cirrhosis, liver involvement is still patchy and liver function tests are almost always within normal limits, even late in the course of the disease. Portal vein obstruction develops in a small percentage of patients, leading to esophageal varices and episodes of gross hematemesis. Occasionally, splenomegaly and hypersplenism are encountered.

Glucose intolerance and glycosuria occur as pancreatic fibrosis and fatty replacement lead to a decrease in the number of β cells in the pancreas and limited insulin production. Abnormal glucose tolerance curves and glycosuria may be present for prolonged periods, with little tendency to develop ketonemia or frank diabetic ketoacidosis. This diabetic state usually can be controlled with small injections of insulin.

Some patients seem to have difficulty with *inspissation* of small bowel contents; the "sludged" material appears to act as the leading point for ileocecal intussusception. Usually, this occurs in children under 12 years of age and requires hydrostatic or surgical reduction. Intermittent intussusception that resolves spontaneously may be more common than has been realized, and may be responsible for attacks of severe cramping abdominal pains. Older patients may develop recurrent attacks of severe crampy abdominal pain that are disabling; others develop a large hard fecal bolus in the ascending colon, which may be palpable for many months on abdominal examination. Recurrent abdominal cramps due to inspissation of ileal contents and persistent fecal bolus have been labeled *meconium equivalent syndromes.* However, this term adds little to our understanding of the disease process, and the conditions are better classified as "sludge" complications. Small oral doses of acetylcysteine may provide dramatic relief to some patients with intestinal "sludging."

Roentgenograms of the *paranasal sinuses* consistently show clouding, but attacks of acute sinusitis are rare. Very rarely, mucopyoceles develop in the ethmoidal sinuses, extend into the orbital cavity, and result in proptosis, or they extend beyond the ethmoidal sinuses and result in a deformity of the lateral nasal bridge and surrounding structures. These mucopyoceles respond well to surgery. Nasal polyps develop in a significant number of patients, and if nasal obstruction occurs, polypectomy is indicated even though the polyps have a strong tendency to recur.

DIAGNOSIS. The diagnosis of cystic fibrosis must be considered in any chronically ill infant or child who has gastrointestinal symptoms suggestive of malabsorption, accompanied by recurrent pulmonary infections. The diagnosis is also suggested by meconium ileus, prolapse of the rectum, intussusception, inadequately explained hyponatremia, nasal polyps, proptosis, and recurrent severe cramping abdominal pains. Early diagnosis is important if rapid progress of destructive changes in the lungs is to be avoided.

Determination of the levels of sodium and chloride in the sweat (sweat test) will quickly establish or rule out the diagnosis permanently. Elevated values for sodium and chloride in a sample of sweat collected after pilocarpine iontophoresis are virtually diagnostic. The sweat test is positive in 98 to 99 percent of children with cystic fibrosis. Although elevated sweat electrolytes (sodium and chloride) have been reported with untreated adrenal insufficiency, glycogen storage disease, pitressin-resistant diabetes insipidus, and occasionally other metabolic diseases, none of these is likely to be confused with cystic fibrosis.

SWEAT TEST. This must be performed by personnel who perform the test frequently; a minimum of 100 tests a year maintain the high degree of technical proficiency needed for reliable results. Cystic fibrosis is a potentially lethal disease and since the diagnosis hinges almost entirely on the accuracy of the sweat test, nothing less than complete reliability is acceptable; definitive sweat testing is not an office procedure.

The sweat test is carried out in three stages: stimulation of the sweat glands; collection of the sweat sample; and analysis of the sweat. The stimulation is best obtained by pilocarpine iontophoresis over a 5 to 6 minute period. This method is painless and works well in all age groups. After stimulation, sweat over the next 30 minutes can be either collected directly on preweighed gauze pads or allowed to accumulate on the skin under a rubber ring covered with plastic, after which it is aspirated into capillary tubes, then analyzed for chloride by titration and for sodium by flame photometry. Electrical conductivity of the sweat can be substituted for the sodium determination. Electrical conductivity is suitable as a screening procedure or can be used as a secondary check on sweat chloride values in place of sweat sodium determination. Measurement of electrical conductivity should never be used alone for the definitive diagnosis of cystic fibrosis.

A satisfactory sweat chloride report must contain the following information: weight (or volume) of sweat collected; a minimum of 50 mg (50 μl) are necessary for accurate testing; chloride concentration in milliequivalents per liter and either sodium concentration in milliequivalents per liter or electrical conductivity values. With a known adequate volume and two separate tests for sweat electrolytes, the physician can be comfortable in accepting or rejecting the diagnosis of cystic fibrosis. If the test is positive, it should be repeated on another day before definitely making the diagnosis. Details of the standards and procedures for sweat testing are available without charge from the Cystic Fibrosis Foundation, 3379 Peachtree Road, N.E., Atlanta, Georgia 30326.

Children with cystic fibrosis have levels of sodium and chloride above 60 mEq/liter; normal children under 14 years of age usually have values below 40 mEq/liter. Levels of sweat sodium and chloride tend to rise gradually with age; some normal older teenagers and adults have sweat sodium-chloride levels in the range of 60 to 80 mEq/liter, diminishing the value of the sweat test in older individuals. A value of over 100 mEq/liter sodium and chloride is probably diagnostic, even in adults.

Unaffected siblings and parents of patients with cystic

fibrosis have sweat electrolyte values within the normal range. This establishes the fact that carriers (heterozygotes) do not have elevated sweat chlorides. When one child in the family is diagnosed as having cystic fibrosis, sweat electrolytes should be determined on all other siblings. It is not unusual to discover a healthy sibling with elevated sweat electrolytes who has not yet developed significant gastrointestinal or pulmonary symptoms. This child will become symptomatic as the disease progresses and can be treated very early.

The direct-reading ion-specific chloride electrodes, which may be applied directly to the skin after iontophoresis, have received considerable attention. In our experience, the presently available electrodes have not proved to be consistently reliable in routine clinical testing, and we do not recommend them at this time.

Tests for pancreatic function, such as duodenal drainage and measurements of enzyme activity, are rarely performed at the present time for the routine diagnosis of cystic fibrosis.

TREATMENT.   The great increase over the last 30 years in length of survival of patients with cystic fibrosis attests to the success of current treatment programs. Over half of the patients now live well into the second decade. About 20 percent survive beyond 15 years of age and a number to the mid-twenties. Treatment programs are oriented to alleviating symptoms rather than to altering the basic disturbance; many aspects of treatment remain controversial because of difficulties in gathering acceptable scientific evidence of their efficacy.

No other disease in pediatrics demands more of the parents in the way of time, personal physical involvement, and constancy of effort, than cystic fibrosis. The demands of the treatment program drastically alter the life style of the entire family. As the disease progresses and the use of medications increases, the costs could be beyond the capacity of all but the wealthy, but the costs are often shared by the community through insurance programs, Crippled Children's Services, and other specially funded programs.

The first step in starting a newly diagnosed child on a treatment program involves the education of the parents about the nature and course of the disease. Repeated conferences are required to impart necessary information and to establish rapport and confidence between physician and parents, which is required for successful treatment. Physicians who are experienced and comfortable in the treatment of children with cystic fibrosis can present a positive, optimistic approach. They can convey the feeling that much can be done to help the child and, at the same time, are honest about their inability to cure or even permanently prevent the progression of the disease. Most children respond dramatically to a well-organized treatment program and can return to a normal active life for long periods of time.

Parents must be aware of the spectrum of the severity of the disease. They should know that some children do well with little treatment, and others with severe involvement do poorly in spite of maximal efforts by the physician and the parents. Unless these facts are discussed at the start, many parents develop almost crippling guilt feelings if their child's clinical status begins to deteriorate. Genetic counseling in simple terms should be given to the parents soon after the diagnosis is established. If the parents are uncertain about having other children, it is well to suggest that they wait a year or two before making a final decision. This gives them time to establish a good treatment program for their child and gain a better understanding of the disease. Some parents react to the diagnosis by deciding on immediate sterilization for themselves. This should be discouraged in young couples who are just beginning to have their families. It is not possible to know the effect of future scientific discoveries on cystic fibrosis, so that contraception is probably a better decision in the immediate postdiagnostic period. Prenatal diagnosis of cystic fibrosis by amniocentesis has not been developed yet, but may be available in the future.

Each treatment program should be individually designed to treat presenting signs and symptoms. The treatment program is best discussed on the basis of the organ system involved.

SWEAT ELECTROLYTE LOSSES.   Generous salting of the food may compensate for the large amounts of sodium and chloride lost through sweating. As soon as the child reaches an age when he can manipulate his own salt shaker, he can usually be left to regulate his own salt intake. During hot weather, particularly in a humid environment, most children will need salt supplements in the form of sodium chloride tablets. A dose of 1 to 2 g of extra sodium chloride spread through the day is usually adequate.

PANCREATIC ENZYME DEFICIENCY.   Patients with diminished pancreatic function need treatment with pancreatin (whole pancreas of animal origin) containing the pancreatic enzymes necessary for digestion. Untreated, a large percentage of the total caloric intake is undigested, with resultant poor growth and large stools. The intake of food may be extremely large to compensate for the caloric losses. With the introduction of oral pancreatin, digestion improves markedly, absorption increases, and the child's hunger is satisfied on a more reasonable caloric intake. Although it may also be necessary to limit the ingestion of fatty foods, to return the stool pattern to near-normal, no routine attempt should be made to change the child's basic diet. To place the child on a diet completely different from that of his family can have serious psychologic and emotional consequences and should not be undertaken lightly.

Pancreatic enzymes (Viokase and Cotazyme) are available as powder, tablets, and capsules. While it should be given in concentrated doses as medicine, the powder may be folded into cold sweet fruits or jams to improve the taste. It should not be sprinkled over milk or other foods. Optimal doses vary widely, and must be titrated individually. Most infants require between one-quarter and 1 teaspoon with each feeding; older children may require 2 to 10 tablets or capsules with each meal. Extra pancreatin with midafternoon or prebedtime snacks is usually desirable. Not uncommonly, adolescents and young adults require less pancreatin than children in their years of rapid growth. Fat-soluble vitamins (A,D,E,K) may not be absorbed adequately, so that twice the recommended daily dose of water-soluble vitamins should be added (see also p. 194).

PULMONARY INFECTION.　Progression of pulmonary disease still accounts for the eventual death of most patients with cystic fibrosis. Not being able to change the basic process of inspissated mucus in the small airways, treatment is directed at the infection that always develops in the obstructed airways. The aggressive use of antibiotics and respiratory physiotherapy to help the patient cough out his secretions are the essentials of treatment. Since potent antibiotics have been developed, the threat of a rapidly spreading and uncontrolled pneumonia, which could overwhelm the lungs, has almost disappeared. The present threat is a low-grade simmering infection that slowly leads to local destruction of alveoli and airways, pockets of chronic suppurative bronchiectasis, and increasing interference with gas exchange.

No treatment program currently available is permanently successful in preventing these changes. There is no conclusive evidence, in our opinion, that continuous antibiotics in a young infant or child with a clear chest on physical examination, or anything else currently available, will prevent or modify the occurrence or progression of pulmonary changes of cystic fibrosis. Continuous antibiotic treatment may even hasten the emergence of antibiotic-resistant strains of bacteria, and thus more than offset any potential benefits.

All children, including those with cystic fibrosis, develop respiratory tract infections throughout infancy. For the child who is known to have cystic fibrosis, we start antibiotic therapy early during the infection, even though it is thought to be of viral origin. Recent studies suggest that viral infections may interfere with some immune mechanisms and decrease the patient's ability to handle bacterial infections. The well-recognized tendency of patients with cystic fibrosis to show rapid progression of pulmonary disease during the acute infective episodes also justifies aggressive utilization of respiratory physiotherapy to increase drainage of purulent secretions. The child is placed in a position that promotes gravity drainage of the involved areas of the lung and the chest wall is clapped with the cupped hand, followed by vibration and supervised coughing. The rales in the chest may clear slowly. Antibiotics and respiratory physiotherapy are continued for 3 to 4 weeks and then stopped until the next infection occurs.

As the pulmonary disease progresses, permanent bronchiectatic changes result in persistent coarse rales, even after weeks of aggressive treatment with antibiotics and physiotherapy. A low-grade infection is constantly present in the airways. At this stage, respiratory physiotherapy, with clapping, vibration, and drainage of involved lung segments, must be continued on at least a twice daily basis.

The clinician then develops a new set of criteria for initiating or continuing antibiotic therapy. Decreased appetite, decreased energy for play and other physical activities, weight loss or lack of continued weight gain, increased cough and sputum production, and possibly a low-grade fever are symptoms that might suggest an increase in the pulmonary infection. Then, antibiotic treatment in full therapeutic doses is started and continued for at least 3 weeks.

The lower respiratory tract of a patient with cystic fibrosis will have been colonized with *Staphylococcus aureus,* almost from the beginning. After a variable period of time, the lungs of almost all patients become colonized with Pseudomonas, which probably is harbored in the lungs permanently. This Pseudomonas infection is amazingly benign in most patients with cystic fibrosis and may be present on every culture of sputum over a period of more than 10 years.

Physicians oriented to treating bacterial infections of the lungs with a view to eradicating all the organisms have difficulty adjusting to the treatment programs necessary for managing patients with cystic fibrosis and advanced pulmonary disease. Long-term oral antibiotic treatment of chronic suppurative lung infections, with the goal of suppressing infection, is often extremely effective in keeping the patient in good health and able to pursue a meaningful life, even though organisms are not eradicated.

Choice of antibiotics for treatment will vary widely, but penicillinase-resistant penicillins and cephalosporins frequently prove valuable for staphylococcal infectons. Once Pseudomonas is established in the respiratory tract, the effectiveness of oral antibiotics is more limited. Sulfonamides, tetracyclines, trimethoprin with sulfamethoxazole, and chloramphenicol are often helpful clinically, even when in vitro studies suggest that Pseudomonas is not sensitive to these antibiotics. If chloramphenicol is used, frequent blood counts are required to detect hematologic abnormalities, although they are rare. Optic neuritis and peripheral neuritis are also encountered with long-term chloramphenicol therapy, but are usually reversible if the drug is stopped when symptoms first occur.

In patients with advanced pulmonary disease, acute or subacute exacerbations may require hospitalization and intensive treatment with intravenous antibiotics in high doses. Cultures of sputum and antibiotic sensitivity testing should be done, but antibiotic therapy can be started even before sensitivities are available. Methicillin and other penicillinase-resistant penicillins combined with gentamicin are currently used for intravenous therapy until the results of sensitivity studies become available.

Adolescents and Young Adults with Cystic Fibrosis

Pediatricians are accustomed to examining children, explaining programs to parents, and expecting parents to implement treatment programs. The adolescent patient with cystic fibrosis frequently resists the continued dependence on his parents imposed by the complicated treatment program. Attempts by the physician to work through the parents to intensify the treatment program are usually doomed to failure. The approach most likely to be successful is the building of a strong personal relationship between the physician and the adolescent, making the adolescent responsible for his own treatment program in every way possible. Many compromises with what the physician may consider the ideal program may be necessary. Without this personal approach, it is possible that the adolescent or young adult may make a bid for independence and choose to totally ignore his disease and abandon his treatment program. This may reduce survival considerably.

Bibliography

INSPIRATORY OBSTRUCTION (EXTRATHORACIC LESIONS)

Boat TF, Polmar SH, Whitman V, et al: Hypersensitivity to cow milk in young children with pulmonary hemosiderosis and cor pulmonale secondary to nasopharyngeal obstruction. J Pediatr 87:23, 1975

Campbell JS, Wiglesworth FW, Latarroca R, et al: Congenital subglottic hemangiomas of the larynx and trachea in infants. Pediatrics 22:727, 1958

Cayler GG, Johnson EE, Lewis BE, et al: Heart failure due to enlarged tonsils and adenoids. Am J Dis Child 118:708, 1969

Cox MA, Schiebler GL, Taylor WJ, Wheat MW, Krovetz LJ: Reversible pulmonary hypertension in a child with respiratory obstruction and cor pulmonale. J Pediatr 67:192, 1965

Holinger PH, Johnston KC, Schild JA: Congenital anomalies of the tracheobronchial tree and of the esophagus; diagnosis and treatment. Pediatr Clin North Am 9:1113, 1962

Levin DL, Muster AJ, Packman LM, et al: Cor pulmonale secondary to upper airway obstruction. Cardiac catheterization, immunologic and psychometric evaluation in nine patients. Chest 68:166, 1975

Menashe VD, Farrehi C, Miller M: Hypoventilation and cor pulmonale due to classic upper airway obstruction. J Pediatr 67:198, 1965

CROUP SYNDROME

Adair JC, Ring WH, Jordan WS, Elwyn RA: Ten year experience with IPPB in the treatment of acute laryngotracheobronchitis. Anesthesiol Analg 50:649, 1971

Battaglia JD, Lockhart CH: Management of acute epiglottitis by nasotracheal intubation. Am J Dis Child 129:334, 1975

Cramblett, HG: Croup (epiglottitis, laryngitis, laryngotracheobronchitis). In Kendig EL (ed): Disorders of the Respiratory Tract in Children. Vol 1. WB Saunders Co, Philadelphia, 1972, p 209

Jones RS: The management of acute croup. Arch Dis Child 47:661, 1972

Milko DA, Marshak G, Striker TW: Nasotracheal intubation in the treatment of acute epiglottitis. Pediatrics 53:674, 1974

Newth CJL, Levison H, Bryan AC: The respiratory status of children with croup. J Pediatr 81:1068, 1972

Tos M: Nasotracheal intubation in acute epiglottiditis. Arch Otolaryngol 97:373, 1973

EXPIRATORY OBSTRUCTION
(INTRATHORACIC LESIONS—LOWER AIRWAY OBSTRUCTION)

Aspiration

Clery AP, Ellis FH Jr, Schmidt HW: Problems associated with aspiration of grass heads (inflorescences). JAMA 171:1478, 1959

Bloomer WE: Trauma to the chest. In Lindskog GE, Liebow AA, Glenn WWL (eds): Thoracic and Cardiovascular Surgey with Related Pathology. Appleton-Century-Crofts, New York, 1962, pp 26-29

Holinger PH, Andrews AH Jr, Anison GC: Pulmonary complications due to endobronchial foreign bodies. Illinois Med J 93:19, 1948

Inhaled foreign bodies. Br Med J 5440:943, 1965

Jewett TC, Butsch WL: Infection from timothy grass. J Thorac Cardiovasc Surg 50:124, 1965

Structural Defects, Tumors, and External Compression

Brooks JW: Tumors of the chest. In Kendig EL (ed): Disorders of the Respiratory Tract in Children, Vol 1. WB Saunders Co, Philadelphia, 1972, p 377

Brünner S, Poulsen PT, Vesterdal J: Cysts of the lung in infants and children. Acta Paediatr Scand 49:39, 1960

Campbell JS, Wigelsworth FW, Latarroca R, Wilde H: Congenital subglottic hemangiomas of the larynx and trachea in infants. Pediatrics 22:727, 1958

DeLuca FG, Wesselhoeft CW, Frates R: Congenital lobar emphysema documented by serial roentgenograms. J Paediatr 82:859, 1973

Derrick JR, Stoeckle H: Bronchial obstruction secondary to an aberrant pulmonary artery. Am Dis Child 99:830, 1960

Fishman L: Papilloma of the trachea. J Thorac Cardiovasc Surg 44:264, 1962

Henderson R, Hislop A, Reid L: New pathological findings in emphysema of childhood. 3. Unilateral congenital emphysema with hypoplasia and compensatory emphysema of the contralateral lung. Thorax 26:195, 1971

Levin SJ, Adler P, Scherer RA: Collapsible trachea (tracheomalacia). a non-allergic cause of wheezing in infancy. Ann Allergy 22:20, 1964

Litt RE, Mencia LF, Altman DH: Congenital stenosis of the right mainstem bronchus. Am J Roentgenol 89:1017, 1963

Mustard WT, Trimble AW, Trusler GA: Mediastinal vascular anomalies causing tracheal esophageal compression and obstruction in children. Can Med Assoc J 87:1301, 1962

Neches WH, Williams RL, McNamara DG: Pulmonary angiographic findings in infantile lobar emphysema. Am J Dis Child 123:171, 1972

Opsahl T, Berman EJ: Bronchiogenic media cysts in infants: case report and review of the literature. Pediatrics 30:372, 1962

Pontius RG: Bronchial obstruction of congenital origin. Am J Surg 106:8, 1963

Sloan H: Lobar obstructive emphysema in infancy removed by lobectomy. J Thorac Surg 26:1, 1953

Soderlund S, Robertson B, Borlenghi R: Infantile lobar emphysema. Acta Paediatr Scand 159(suppl):89, 1965

Stanger P, Lucas RV Jr, Edwards JE: Anatomic factors causing respiratory distress in acyanotic congenital cardiac disease: special reference to bronchial obstruction. Pediatrics 43:760, 1969

Van Epps EF, Davies DH: Lobar emphysema. Am J Roentgenol, 73:375, 1955

Weisel W, Lepley D: Tracheal and bronchial adenomas in childhood. Pediatrics 28:394, 1961

Williams HE, Landau LI, Phelan PD: Generalized bronchiectasis due to extensive deficiency of bronchial cartilage. Arch Dis Child 47:423, 1972

BRONCHIOLITIS

American Academy of Pediatrics, Committee on Drugs: Should steroids be used in treating bronchiolitis? Pediatrics 46:640, 1970

Connolly C, Field CMB, Glasgow JFT, et al: A double blind trial of prednisolone in epidemic bronchiolitis due to respiratory syncytial virus. Acta Paediatr Scand 58:116, 1969

Downes JJ, Wood DW, Striker TW, Haddad C: Acute respiratory failure in infants with bronchiolitis. Anesthesiology 29:426, 1968

Elderkin FM, Gardner PS, Turk DC, White AC: Aetiology and management of bronchiolitis and pneumonia in childhood. Br Med J 2:722, 1965

Heycock JB, Noble GC: 1230 cases of acute bronchiolitis in infancy. Br Med J 2:879, 1962

Holdaway D, Romer AC, Gardner PS: The diagnosis and management of bronchiolitis. Pediatrics 39:924, 1967

James JA: Dexamethasone in croup, a controlled study. Am J Dis Child 117:511, 1969

Leer JA Green JL, Heimlich EM, et al: Corticosteroid treatment in bronchiolitis, a controlled collaborative study in 297 infants and children. Am J Dis Child 117:495, 1969

Phelan PD, Williams HE: Sympathomimetic drugs in acute viral bronchiolitis. Their effect on pulmonary resistance. Pediatrics 43:493, 1969

——— Stocks JG: Management of severe viral bronchiolitis and severe acute asthma. Arch Dis Child 49:143, 1974

Radford M: Effect of salbutamol in infants with wheezing bronchitis. Arch Dis Child 50:535, 1975

Reynolds EOR, Cook CD: The treatment of bronchiolitis. J Pediatr 63:1205, 1963

Reynolds EOR: Bronchiolitis. In Kendig EL (ed): Disorders of the Respiratory Tract in Children, Vol 1. WB Saunders Co, Philadelphia, 1972, p 223

Wohl MEB, Stigol LC, Mead J: Resistance of the total respiratory system in healthy infants and infants with bronchiolitis. Pediatrics 43:495, 1969

Wright FH, Beem MO: Diagnosis and treatment: management of acute viral bronchiolitis in infancy. Pediatrics 35:334, 1965

ASTHMA

Bierman CW, Pierson WE: The pharmacologic management of status asthmaticus in children. Pediatrics 54:245, 1974

Bocles JS: Status asthmaticus. Med Clin North Am 54:493, 1970

Chai H, Newcomb RW: Pharmacologic management of childhood asthma. Am J Dis Child 125:757, 1973

Downes JJ, Fulgencio T, Raphaely RC: Acute respiratory failure in infants and children. Pediatr Clin North Am 19:423, 1972

Editorial: Intravenous aminophylline. Lancet 2:950, 1973

Engström I: Respiratory studies in children. XI. Mechanics of breathing, lung, volumes and ventilatory capacity in asthmatic children from attack to symptom-free status. Acta Paediatr Scand (Suppl 155): 1964

Kraepelien S: Respiratory studies in children. IV. The effect of bronchodilator drugs on the lung volumes in symptom-free asthmatic children. Acta Paediatr Scand 47:547, 1958

Maselli R, Casal GL, Ellis EF: Pharmacologic effects of intravenously administered aminophylline in asthmatic children. J Pediatr 76:777, 1970

McFadden ER, Lyons HA: Serial studies of factors influencing airway dynamics during recovery from acute asthma attacks. J Appl Physiol 27:452, 1969

Middleton E Jr: The anatomical and biochemical basis of bronchial obstruction in asthma. Ann Intern Med 63:695, 1965

Pierson WE, Bierman CW, Kelley VC: A double-blind trial of corticosteroid therapy in status asthmaticus. Pediatrics 54:282, 1974

Rackemann FM, Edwards MC: Asthma in children. N Engl J Med 246:815, 1952

Tooley WH, DeMuth G, Nadel JA: The reversibility of obstructive changes in severe childhood asthma. J Pediatr 66:517, 1965

Wood DW, Downes JJ, Leeks HI: A clinical scoring system for the diagnosis of respiratory failure. Preliminary report on childhood status asthmaticus. Am J Dis Child 123:227, 1972

——— Downes JJ, Scheinkopf H, Leeks HI: Intravenous isoproterenol in the management of respiratory failure in childhood status asthmaticus. J Allergy Clin Immunol 50:75, 1972

Yu DYC, Galant SP, Gold WM: Inhibition of antigen-induced bronchoconstriction by atropine in asthmatic patients. J Appl Physiol 32:823, 1972

BRONCHIECTASIS

Avery ME, Riley MC, Weiss A: The course of bronchiectasis in childhood. Bull Hopkins Hosp 109:20, 1961

Becroft DMO: Bronchiolitis obliterans, bronchiectasis and other sequelae of adenovirus type 21 infection in young infants. J Clin Pathol 24:72, 1971

Drapanas T, Siewers R, Feist JH: Reversible post-stenotic bronchiectasis. N Eng J Med 275:917, 1966

Field CE: Bronchiectasis. Third report on a follow-up study of medical and surgical cases from childhood. Arch Dis Child 44:551, 1969

Fleshman JK, Wilson JF, Cohen JJ: Bronchiectasis in Alaskan native children. Arch Environ Health 17:517, 1968

Glauser EM, Cook CD, Harris GBC: Bronchiectasis: a review of 187 cases in children with followup pulmonary function studies in 58. Acta Paediatr Scand (supp 165):1, 1966

Iacocca VF, Sibinga MS, Barbero GJ: Respiratory tract bacteriology in cystic fibrosis. Am J Dis Child 106:315, 1963

Kjellman B: Prognosis and lung function in children with bronchial asthma and recurrent pneumonia. Acta Paediatr Scand 61:197, 1972

Nemir RL: Bronchiectasis. In Kendig EL (ed): Disorders of the Respiratory Tract in Children, Vol 1. WB Saunders Co, Philadelphia, 1972, p 268

Williams HE, Landau LI, Phelan PD: Generalized bronchiectasis due to extensive deficiency of bronchial cartilage. Arch Dis Child 47:423, 1972

CYSTIC FIBROSIS

Andersen DH: Cystic fibrosis of the pancreas and its relation to celiac disease. Am J Dis Child 56:344, 1938

di Sant'Agnese PA, Talamo RC: Pathogenesis and physiopathology of cyctic fibrosis of the pancreas. N Engl J Med 277:1287, 1343, 1399, 1967

Handwerger S, Roth J, Gorden P, et al: Glucose intolerance in cystic fibrosis. N Engl J Med 281:451, 1969

Huang N (ed): Guide to Drug Therapy in Patients with Cystic Fibrosis. Cystic Fiborsis Foundation, 3379 Peachtree Road, NE, Atlanta, Georgia 30326

Matthews LW, Boershuk CF, Stern R, et al: Comprehensive and preventive treatment of cystic fibrosis. In Fundamental Problems of Cystic Fibrosis and Related Diseases. Intercontinental Medical Book Corporation, New York, 1973, p 303

Noblett HR: Treatment of uncomplicated meconium ileus by gastrografin enema: a preliminary report. J Pediatr Surg 4:190, 1969

Schwachman H, Redmond A, Khaw KT: Studies in cystic fibrosis: report of 130 patients diagnosed under 3 months of age over a 20-year period. Pediatrics 46:335, 1970

——— Khaw KT: Cystic fibrosis. In Shirkey HC (ed): Pediatric Therapy, 4th ed. CV Mosby Co, St Louis, 1972, p 573

Taussig LM, Kattwinkel J, Friedewald WT, di Sant'Agnese PA: A new prognostic score and clinical evaluation system for cystic fibrosis. J Pediatr 82:380, 1973

Williams HE, Phelan PD: Cystic fibrosis. In Respiratory Illness in Children. Blackwell Scientific Publications, Oxford, 1975, p 216

THE PARENCHYMA

WILLIAM H. TOOLEY
HERMAN W. LIPOW

Anatomy

The parenchyma includes the respiratory bronchioles, alveolar ducts, alveoli, pulmonary capillaries, lymphatics, and their interstitial supporting tissue. The respiratory bronchioles, which have a somewhat greater diameter than the terminal bronchioles, divide into alveolar ducts from which numerous alveoli protrude. These structures, which are nourished by the pulmonary arterial circulation, probably have no nerve supply, but the smooth muscle in the walls of the respiratory bronchioles and surrounding the openings of the alveoli reacts to locally applied stimuli.

Ciliated and nonciliated cuboidal cells line the respiratory bronchioles. This epithelium is continuous with the flat, nonciliated cells lining the alveolar ducts and alveoli. The nuclei of the alveolar lining cells lie in depressions in the capillary walls and are widely spaced, occupying only about one-tenth of the surface of the alveoli. Their cytoplasmic attenuations cover the remainder of the surface. There are no mucous cells in the respiratory bronchioles. However, a deposit resembling mucus, which is continuous with an acellular layer covering the alveolar cell cytoplasm, covers the respiratory bronchiolar epithelium.

Just as the lumen of the bronchioles is continuous with the alveoli, the supporting elements of the bronchiolar tree are continuous with the framework of the alveoli. Helical turns of smooth muscle proceed from the terminal bronchioles to surround the respiratory bronchioles. The muscle mass gradually decreases as the blind ends of the alveolar ducts are approached, and residual strands of smooth muscle terminate by forming rings around the mouths of the alveoli. The loose interstitial tissue between respiratory bronchioles contains many small lymph vessels and small divisions of pulmonary arteries and veins. Elastic, collagen, and reticular tissue also course through the interstitial space between the parenchymal structures and tend to localize at the mouths of the alveoli. The collagen fibers form wavy bundles when the lung is at a small volume, but are pulled straight when the lung is expanded and limit the volume to which the lung can be inflated. Expansion of the lung stretches the elastic and reticular fibers. At the end of inspiration these fibers return to their original length, facilitating expiration.

There is a large amount of interstitial tissue in the lung of the newborn. It is composed principally of vascular tissue, elastic and collagen tissue being present in proportionately smaller amounts than in the adult lung. Elastic fibers increase in number and size until about 4 years of age when their distribution and concentration are similar to those in the adult lung. The elastic tissue in the lung of the newborn has different staining qualities from mature elastic tissue, so that there may be a qualitative as well as quantitative distinction. The staining characteristics of elastic tissue change little in the first months, but by 1 year of age they are similar to the adult.

The lung is divided into four primary volumes and four capacities, each of which includes two or more primary volumes (Fig. 50).

Volumes

Tidal volume (TV) is the volume of gas inspired or expired during each respiratory cycle.

Inspiratory reserve volume (IRV) is the maximal amount of gas that can be inspired after a normal inspiration.

Expiratory reserve volume (ERV) is the maximal amount of gas that can be expired after a normal expiration.

Residual volume (RV) is the volume of gas remaining in the lungs at the end of a maximal expiration.

Capacities

Total lung capacity (TLC) is the amount of gas in the lung at the end of a maximal inspiration.

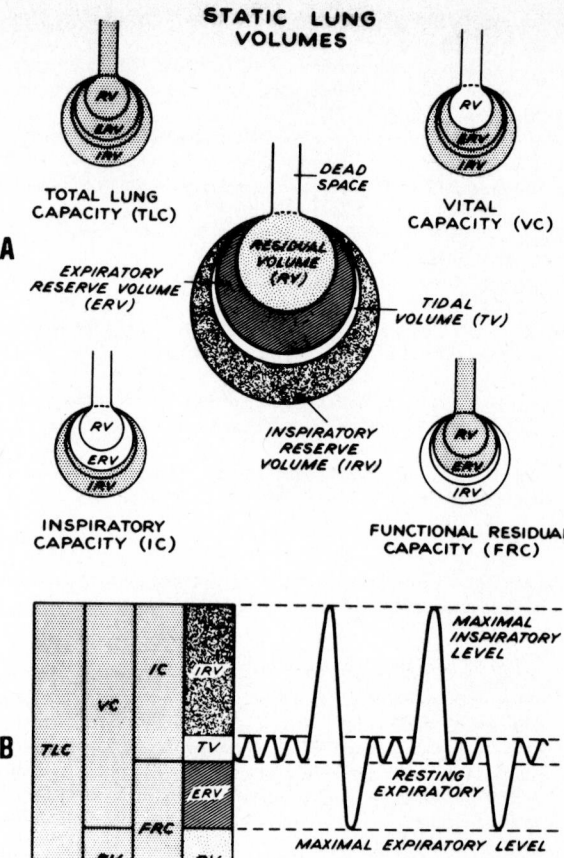

FIG. 50. A. The large central diagram illustrates the four primary lung volumes and their approximate magnitude. The outermost line indicates the greatest size to which the lung can expand; the innermost circle (residual volume) indicates the volume that remains after a maximal expiration. The shaded areas in the smaller diagrams represent the four lung capacities. **B.** Lung volumes as they appear on a spirogram tracing; shading in the vertical bar next to the spirogram tracing corresponds to that in the central diagram. The relation of the lung capacities to the spirogram are also indicated. (From Comroe et al: The Lung, 2 ed. Courtesy of Year Book Publishers.)

Vital capacity (VC) is the maximal volume of gas that can be expelled from the lungs by forceful effort following a maximal inspiration.

Inspiratory capacity (IC) is the maximal volume of gas that can be inspired after a normal expiration (resting expiratory level).

Functional residual capacity (FRC) is the volume of gas that remains in the lungs at resting expiratory level.

The lung grows by increasing the size and number of alveoli. Dunhill calculated that there are 24 million alveoli at birth, 250 million at 4 years, and 296 million in the adult. These figures suggest that lung growth may be due principally to generation of new units in infancy; but in childhood growth is probably the result of an increase in size of units, since their diameters continue to increase until adulthood. Lung growth is alinear with respect to age, but from infancy to adulthood the size of the lung is proportional to body height, and the relative sizes of the primary lung volumes and capacities are the same at all ages: the residual volume is approximately 25 percent, the functional residual capacity approximately 40 percent, and the tidal volume during normal respiration about 8 percent of the total lung capacity.

Function

The parenchyma permits exchange of carbon dioxide and oxygen between air and blood and maintains a barrier between gas and liquid which prevents undissolved gas from entering the interstitial space and fluid from entering the alveolar lumina. Phagocytosis and the mouthward movement of the acellular alveolar lining prevent the accumulation of foreign material.

The amount of oxygen and carbon dioxide exchanged depends upon the volume of fresh air reaching the alveoli each minute (ventilation), the difference between their partial pressures in alveolar gas and capillary blood, the alveolar surface area, the amount and distribution of pulmonary blood flow, and the depth of the tissue separating blood and gas.

VENTILATION. The amount of air reaching the alveoli is determined by *the dead space, the resistance to gas flow, the resistance of the lung to deformation, the size of the lung, the work capacity of the respiratory system,* and *reflexes* which increase or decrease the respiratory drive. When the tissue is rigid and resists deformation, it has a high elasticity or a low compliance; compliance is the change in volume effected by a given change in intrapleural pressure and is expressed as liters per centimeter of water. The amount of force needed to increase the lung volume depends upon the resistance of the tissue and the surface tension of the internal surface of the lung. The alveolar surface has a low surface tension when its area is small, as when the lung is at its functional residual capacity (FRC), but surface tension rises rapidly when, during inspiration, the area of surface is expanded. The low surface tension at FRC tends to keep the alveoli from collapsing when the distending pressure is low and prevents atelectasis; the relatively high tension that develops during inspiration is the major part of the tissue resistance that must be overcome during respiration. At the end of inspiration, about two-thirds of the lung's elastic recoil is provided by surface tension forces and one-third by tissue elastic recoil. Since the young infant and child exert maximal inspiratory forces equivalent to the adult (Table 10), change in volume is governed by lung size, tissue composition, and surface tension. When the lung is small, the change in volume for a given pressure change will be small. The lung of the newborn has a compliance of 0.006 liter/cm H_2O and a vital capacity of 200 ml (Table 13). The compliance is small when compared with the child or adult, but when it is divided by the FRC at which it was measured, it is 0.06 liter/cm H_2O/liter at all ages. This is called specific compliance and makes it possible to compare lung compliance measurements in patients of different size. The vital capacity is about twice the FRC in infancy and adulthood. Although the amount and composition of tissue elements alter with growth, the elasticity of the lungs does not seem to be affected. It is probable that in normal lungs the alveolar lining, which is apparently the same at all ages, is the predominant determinant of lung elasticity. When airway resistance, FRC, the chest wall, and inspiratory force are normal, the vital capacity is a good index of lung compliance.

ALVEOLAR-PULMONARY CAPILLARY OXYGEN AND CARBON DIOXIDE PRESSURE DIFFERENCE. The larger the differences in partial pressure between the air and blood phase, the more gas is exchanged; thus, maximum flux occurs when the partial pressure of oxygen is high in the alveolus and low in precapillary blood; the opposite is true of the partial pressure of carbon dioxide. When ventilation is greater than normal, partial pressure of oxygen in the alveoli is high and that of carbon dioxide is low, whereas when ventilation is too low, the reverse is true. When cardiac output is diminished, or when the uptake of oxygen and production of carbon dioxide by the body's tissues are increased, the partial pressure of oxygen is low and the partial pressure of carbon dioxide is high in blood entering the pulmonary capillaries. Conversely, when cardiac output is excessive or tissue oxygen uptake and carbon dioxide production are small, partial pressure of oxygen in precapillary blood is high and that of carbon dioxide is low. At high altitude the partial pressure of oxygen in the alveoli is low.

ALVEOLAR SURFACE AREA. The normal adult lung has a surface area of about 80 m^2 or approximately

TABLE 13. Ventilation

	Newborn	5 yr	10 yr	15 yr	Adult
Compliance (liter/cm H_2O)	0.006	0.045	0.075	0.15	0.18
Compliance/FRC (liter/cm H_2O/liter)	0.06	0.06	0.06	0.06	0.06
Vital capacity (ml)	200	1,300	2,300	4,000	5,000
Functional residual capacity (FRC) (ml)	100	750	1,250	2,500	3,000
Diffusion capacity for carbon monoxide (ml/min/mm Hg pressure of CO_2)	1.5	7.5	15	25	30

1 m²/kg. The surface area of the lung in the newborn is 4 m², also about 1 m²/kg. Alveolar surface area appears to remain proportional to body size throughout childhood. It is not, however, proportional to metabolic requirements. The relatively large oxygen uptake of the infant requires an increase in total ventilation.

PULMONARY BLOOD FLOW. Venous return to the heart and the magnitude of right-to-left shunt determine total pulmonary blood flow. Cardiac output and pulmonary blood flow increase when either oxygen utilization, ventilation, or both increase, and when arterial oxygen tension is low. Ventilation and pulmonary blood flow are controlled by reflexes that can increase or decrease ventilation and cardiac output depending upon the amount of gas exchange needed. Changes in airway and vascular resistance are caused by alterations in the pH and oxygen tension of local tissue: when the pH or oxygen tension is low, small airways dilate and pulmonary arterioles constrict; when the pH or oxygen is high, airways constrict and pulmonary arterioles dilate. These reactions tend to match regional ventilation and blood flow and lead to an increase or decrease in ventilation to areas where blood flow is high or low, and an increase or decrease in perfusion to areas where ventilation is large or small. Thus, when regional blood flow is reduced suddenly, carbon dioxide tension in the alveoli and surrounding tissue falls, the pH of the tissue rises, the bronchioles constrict, and ventilation to this region decreases. These mechanisms maintain partial pressures of 100 and 40 torr, respectively, for oxygen and carbon dioxide in arterial blood during periods of widely varying metabolic demands and activity.

DIFFERENCE BETWEEN ALVEOLAR GAS AND CAPILLARY BLOOD. Carbon dioxide diffuses readily; in normal infants, children, and adults its partial pressure is only 1 to 2 torr higher in arterial blood than in the alveoli. Oxygen diffuses less easily; when the partial pressure of alveolar oxygen is 100 torr, pulmonary venous oxygen partial pressure depends upon the length of time blood is in the pulmonary capillaries and exposed to alveolar gas and upon the depth of tissue between gas and blood. In normal adults, the difference in partial pressure of oxygen between alveolar gas and arterial blood is less than 10 torr; in infants it is greater. This difference may be due to several factors: rapid blood flow through short capillaries, proportionally large amounts of interstitial tissue in the infant, uneven distribution of ventilation and perfusion, or intrapulmonary right-to-left shunts. The large amount of loose interstitial tissue in the infant may be increased further with pulmonary edema and inflammation, which markedly widen the diffusion distance. In infants, children, and adults the uptake of carbon monoxide from the alveoli has been used to measure diffusion capacity. In the newborn it appears low; in older children, as in adults, it is closely related to total lung capacity (surface area) (Table 13).

THE BARRIER FUNCTION OF THE PARENCHYMA. Alveolar cells and their protoplasmic processes delimit the interstitial space and, by regulating their permeability, keep tissue fluid from entering the alveoli. With maximal breaths and hypoxia, the cells are attenuated and diffusion distance is decreased; also the alveolar walls are more permeable to fluids and red blood cells. In the young infant, when undissolved gas enters the interstitial space, it can easily dissect between loosely supported vessels and airways toward the hilum and periphery. This process probably explains why pneumomediastinum, interstitial emphysema, and pneumothorax are common in infancy and childhood.

Diagnostic Procedures

BIOPSY. Biopsies of the lung or of regional lymph nodes are often necessary to diagnose localized or diffuse parenchymal disease. Biopsies are particularly useful in sarcoidosis and other granulomatous conditions and in unusual chronic diseases due to hypersensitivity or infection. Our most common indication for lung biopsy is a continuing and life-threatening pulmonary infection in an immunodeficient or immunosuppressed child who has failed to improve after adequate antibiotic treatment for the usual type of pulmonary infection. Infections due to *Pneumocystis carinii*, aspergillus, candida, and other opportunistic infections usually require lung tissue for definitive diagnosis. There are several techniques for obtaining lung tissue for histologic examination: open lung biopsy, percutaneous needle biopsy, high-speed drill trephine biopsy, and transbronchial biopsy. In the pediatric age group, there has been inadequate experience with all of these techniques, except open lung biopsy, to recommend them.

Although open lung biopsy is more difficult for the child, it is relatively safe, with almost no mortality and a low morbidity; it also has the advantage of allowing study of tissue that is superior to that obtained with other techniques. Lung biopsy is quite a common procedure in our institution. We inflate the lung with an intrapulmonary pressure of 10 cm H_2O, place two clamps across the segment to be biopsied, cut between the clamps, and immediately place the clamped specimen in a rapidly penetrating fixative. This procedure usually preserves the architecture of the lung as it is during life. In 105 open lung biopsies reviewed by Gaensler and associates, there were one operative death and two major complications.

The fatty tissue overlying the scalenus anticus muscle in the neck usually contains a number of small lymph nodes into which lymph drains from the lungs. Daniels recommended the removal and examination of these nodes for the diagnosis of malignant and nonmalignant pulmonary lesions such as sarcoidosis, tuberculosis, silicosis, and histoplasmosis. Complications are rare, but pneumothorax due to puncture of the apical pleura, hemidiaphragmatic paralysis following accidental section of the phrenic nerve, air embolism, hemorrhage, and infection occur occasionally.

PULMONARY FUNCTION TESTS. Diseases of the lung parenchyma may decrease lung volume, increase the amount of tissue between alveoli, partially or completely occlude bronchioles, and interrupt the pulmonary circulation. Depending on the type and distribution of the process, there will be decreases in vital capacity, lung compliance, pulmonary diffusion capacity, and partial pressure of oxygen in arterial blood, but increases in dead space ventilation and partial pressure of carbon dioxide in arterial blood. Comroe and his associates have described in detail the various types of pulmonary function tests that may be useful in parenchymal diseases.

Since the maximal inspiratory force is constant in childhood (Table 10), an increase in tissue elasticity or a decrease in lung volume will also decrease vital capacity, so that in those cases where compliance is low, vital capacity will also be reduced. Vital capacity maneuvers are easily performed with a spirometer, which can also be used for measuring inspiratory and expiratory flow rates (Fig. 50). It is the most useful single test for evaluating the stiffness of the lung. In most children the efficiency of gas exchange and the quality of lung tissue can be determined by measuring vital capacity and partial pressure of oxygen and carbon dioxide in arterial blood at rest and during exercise.

Radioactive nuclide scanning is an important method for assessing ventilation and perfusion in children. Radiographs of the chest after injection of radioactive xenon into an antecubital vein show the gross distribution of perfusion. The uniformity with which radioactivity disappears indicates how well respiratory units are ventilated.

Bibliography

Chehreh MN, Young RC Jr, Viaene H, Ross CW, Scott RB: Spirometric standards for healthy inner-city Black children. Am J Dis Child 126: 159, 1973

Comroe JH Jr, Forster RE, DuBois AB, Briscoe WA, Carlsen: The Lung, 2nd ed. Year Book Publishers, Chicago, 1962

————: Physiology of Respiration. Year Book Medical Publishers, Chicago 1974

Cook CD, Hamann JF: Relations of lung volumes to height in healthy persons between the ages of 5 and 38 years. J Pediatr 59:710, 1961

DeMuth GR, Howatt WF: The growth of lung function. Part III. Pulmonary diffusion. Pediatrics 35:185, 1965

Dunhill MS: Postnatal growth of the lung. Thorax 17:329, 1962

Gaensler EA, Moister MVB, Hamm J: Open-lung biopsy in diffuse pulmonary disease. N Engl J Med 270:1319, 1964

Godfrey S, Kamburoff PL, Nairn JR: Spirometry, lung volumes and airways resistance in normal children 5-18 years. Br J Dis Chest 64:15, 1970

Hewitt CJ, Hull D, Keeling JW: Open lung biopsy in children with diffuse lung disease. Arch Dis Child 49:27, 1974

Polgar G, Promadhot V: Pulmonary Function Testing in Children: Techniques and Standards. WB Saunders Co, Philadelphia, 1971

Weng TR, Levison H, Wentworth P, et al: Open lung biopsy in children. Am Rev Resp Dis 97:673, 1968

————Levison H: Standards of pulmonary function in children. Am Rev Resp Dis 99:879, 1969

DISEASES CAUSING REDUCTION OF THE PARENCHYMA

WILLIAM H. TOOLEY
HERMAN H. LIPOW

Reduction in Parenchyma Because of Absence of Tissue

AGENESIS OF THE LUNG. In the embryo the respiratory system begins as a median ventral diverticulum of the foregut, from which the epithelium and glands of the trachea, bronchi, and alveoli originate. This diverticulum grows into the mesoderm on the ventral surface of the foregut, which provides mesenchymal support, and divides into two lung buds. Each bud contains one tube, or bronchus, which divides dichotomously, until there are usually 18 generations at birth. Inhibition or aberrations in the sprouting of the bronchial tree may produce complete absence of bronchi and parenchyma (agenesis or aplasia) or underdeveloped lung, varying in degree from conditions in which the bronchus is present as a small outpocketing of the trachea to small lungs with normal architecture (hypoplasia). Absence of both lungs or of one lobe is very rare; agenesis of one lung is more common.

Valle, in a review of 120 cases of unilateral pulmonary aplasia, found that symptoms are usually present from birth, but occasionally the condition is asymptomatic. There is labored breathing, cyanosis, and cough. The thorax is usually symmetric, but there may be some scoliosis. Breath sounds from the aplastic lung are absent or bronchial in quality. The mediastinum shifts toward the affected side, and there is overinflation of the contralateral lung. Chest roentgenograms show a dense, homogeneous shadow with narrowing of the intercostal spaces. The appearance resembles massive atelectasis, and this is usually the initial diagnosis. In about one-third of the 73 cases described by Oyamada and associates, there were other congenital anomalies. This condition is compatible with life and may not produce symptoms.

HYPOPLASIA OF THE LUNG. Hypoplasia of the lung may be primary or secondary to a reduction in intrathoracic volume, as occurs with congenital diaphragmatic herniation. In the 24 cases of congenital diaphragmatic hernia described by Roe and Stephens, there were 10 hypoplastic lungs. In the primary cases not associated with thoracic space-occupying masses, the pulmonary artery is small and the hypoplasia may be due to failure of bronchial branching or secondary to hypoplasia of the pulmonary artery.

The signs and symptoms of a hypoplastic lung may be minimal. The involved hemothorax tends to be smaller than the contralateral side. Breath sounds can be normal or diminished. Recurrent pulmonary infections may be frequent. Ventilation and perfusion radionuclide lung imaging provide a valuable noninvasive technique for detecting this disorder but definitive diagnosis is by bronchography and pulmonary angiography.

LOBECTOMY AND PNEUMONECTOMY. Segmental resections and the removal of lobes or whole lungs are done for a variety of reasons in childhood. When the excision is done for localized diseases, such as cysts and aspiration of foreign bodies with atelectasis, there is usually no residual disease in the remaining parts of the lung. When a localized area of a generalized pulmonary disease, such as tuberculosis or bronchiectasis, is removed, the remaining lung may still be diseased. In these patients there is usually a slight decrease in lung volume, an increase in resistance to airflow, and overdistension of the remaining units.

Reduction in Parenchyma Because of Space-Occupying Lesions

CYSTS OF THE LUNG. There are a number of conditions in which sharply defined fluid- or air-filled cysts with definite walls are found within the lung. About one-third of all reported cases have been in children.

Pulmonary cysts in children often produce no symptoms. However, if they are large and compress adjacent airways, they may cause coughing, wheezing, and other evidences of obstructive airway disease. If they markedly reduce the amount of pulmonary tissue available for gas exchange, there will be cyanosis, a decrease in vital capacity, and a decrease in maximal expiratory flow rates. Some cysts are secondary to obstruction of an airway, as previously noted. These may become very large and require surgical excision. Other cysts (pneumatoceles) result from purulent, particularly staphylococcal, pneumonias. These lesions are rarely large, are almost always asymptomatic, and do not require surgical excision. They usually regress spontaneously. However, cysts are occasionally found when there is no evidence of preceding obstruction or infection. These are probably congenital, since they commonly appear in children under 1 year of age and, when removed, there is no pathologic evidence of inflammation of the bronchi, vessels, or alveoli. The high incidence in some ethnic groups, as reported by Baum and associates, suggests that some may be inherited. If congenital cysts are large and infected and cause symptoms, they should be removed. If they are small and not infected, they should be observed.

CONGENITAL CYSTIC ADENOMATOID MALFORMATION OF THE LUNG. These are hamartomas or non-neoplastic, tumorlike malformations with abnormal mixtures of pulmonary tissues. Kwittken and Reiner reviewed 32 cases. In the involved lung there are large numbers of cystic terminal respiratory structures that communicate with each other and are lined with pseudostratified ciliated columnar epithelium or respiratory cuboidal epithelium. There is an increase in elastic tissue, polypoid configuration of the mucosa, and, commonly, mucogenic cells lining the alveoli There is usually no cartilage present and no evidence of inflammation.

These structures usually cause severe respiratory distress and cyanosis, beginning at a few days or weeks of age. Chest roentgenograms show an increase in the size of the affected lobe, with areas of radiolucency. About one-half of the affected newborns are hydropic, and there is a history of polyhydramnios in 20 percent of the cases. Since these lesions are large, prompt diagnosis and surgical excision are required.

ACCESSORY LOBES AND SEQUESTERED LUNG. Accessory lobes (extralobar sequestration) are small, usually located in the inferior portion of the left thorax, and are often associated with diaphragmatic defects. They may or may not have a communication with the bronchial tree. The blood supply may be from the bronchial arteries but more commonly small arteries from the aorta nourish the accessory lobe. They are usually asymptomatic, but if there is a bronchial connection, they may become infected and bronchiectasis may develop.

Sequestered lung segments are cystic intrapulmonary lesions that have no direct communication with the bronchial tree and receive their blood supply from the systemic circulation. They are usually asymptomatic and are diagnosed incidentally roentgenographically. However, respiratory distress may occur in the newborn because a sequestered lobe interferes with ventilation of the remaining normal lung.

PULMONARY TUMORS. Most of the intrathoracic tumors of childhood are in the mediastinum. Few cases of benign intrapulmonary tumors, such as fibromas, lipomas, and hemangiomas, have been reported. They are usually small and asymptomatic. Intrapulmonary malignant tumors, such as neuroblastomas, sarcomas, lymphoblastomas, ganglioneuromas, and endotheliomas, are somewhat more common.

Primary bronchogenic carcinoma of the lung is rare. Anderson reviewed 16 cases of carcinoma of the lung in children of 10 months to 14 years of age; all were adenocarcinomas or undifferentiated carcinomas and occurred with equal frequency in both sexes. As with all malignancies of childhood, carcinomas of the lung grow rapidly and metastasize early; all of the patients reported by Anderson died.

PULMONARY ARTERIOVENOUS FISTULAS. Large channels connecting a branch of the pulmonary artery to a pulmonary vein may be congenital or due to trauma. Purriel and Muras reviewed 170 cases; 37 percent were children. In 75 percent of those diagnosed as adults, symptoms were present prior to the age of 15 years; 14 percent had symptoms from infancy.

In some cases, arteriovenous fistulas are asymptomatic and are discovered accidentally. In about 85 percent there is clubbing of the fingers and toes, cyanosis, and polycythemia; many patients have hemoptysis. A bruit is often present. A radiograph of the chest shows one or several large, irregular, lobulated densities in the mid or lower portion of the lung.

About 70 percent of patients with arteriovenous fistulas have cutaneous telangiectases. Telangiectases are small localized arteriovenous capillary connections that are actually tiny AV fistulas. They form groups of ruby-red lesions in the skin of the face and body and on the lips, and may occur in all organs of the body. When they bleed they cause hemoptysis, hematuria, and gastrointestinal hemorrhage. Telangiectases are inherited. Hodgson and his colleagues found 129 cases of hereditary hemorrhagic telangiectasia (often called Rendu-Osler-Weber syndrome) in one family with 330 members; 15 percent of these 129 cases had AV fistulas. Since most pulmonary AV fistulas are one manifestation of hereditary telangiectasia, they should always be looked for when cutaneous telangiectases are present. When pulmonary AV fistulas cause symptoms, they should be removed.

CONGENITAL PULMONARY LYMPHANGIECTASIS (CONGENITAL DILATION OF THE PULMONARY LYMPHATICS). This rare condition is a generalized disease of the lung, causing cysts in the subpleural and interlobular connective tissue, which are rarely more than 10μ in diameter. There is abundant connective tissue in the septa, which appears to be embryonic.

Noonan and associates reviewed 45 cases and found that pulmonary lymphangiectasis occurs as part of a generalized lymphangiectasis, secondary to pulmonary venous obstruction in congenital cardiac lesions, or as a primary developmental defect of the lung. No abnormalities outside the lungs were present in 30 of the 45 cases reviewed.

Reduction in Parenchyma Because of Inflammation

Inflammation of the lung parenchyma may involve the alveolar spaces primarily, as in bacterial pneumonias, or be confined principally to the interalveolar (interstitial) tissues, as in viral pneumonia and pulmonary hypersensitivity diseases.

THE BACTERIAL PNEUMONIAS. Hospitalization for bacterial pneumonias has declined during the past three decades. Early treatment of respiratory infections with antibiotics is probably the principal cause of this reduction in incidence. However, particularly in the winter months, bacterial pneumonias continue to be an important cause of severe illness.

As described by McCracken and Eichenwald, the defense mechanisms of the respiratory tract are extraordinarily efficient in preventing infection of the lungs. The defense mechanisms include: the epiglottal reflex, which prevents aspiration of infected secretions; ciliary action, which serves to clear the respiratory epithelium of aspirated microorganisms; the cough reflex, which propels foreign material out of the lower tract; the mucous blanket of the respiratory tract, to which airborne organisms adhere; the lymphatics, which drain the terminal bronchi and bronchioles; and phagocytic cells that normally line the alveoli.

Viral infections are the common events that disturb these defense mechanisms, and frequently precede the development of bacterial pneumonia by a few days.

The acute primary bacterial pneumonias have many common features. Their distribution is typical of pulmonary infections due to inhalation, and they usually locate in one or more of the following lobes or segments: the middle lobe, the lingula, the posterior and anterior segments of the upper lobes, or the superior segments of the lower lobes. As lobes or segments become consolidated and airless, the vital capacity decreases and the work of breathing increases—reflected in young infants and children by intercostal *retractions* and *flaring* of the alae nasae. The vital capacity and lung compliance are usually lower than would be predicted from the extent of consolidation. These changes are probably the result of congestion and an increase in parenchymal rigidity in the apparently normal areas of the lung. When the lung is extremely stiff, or if inspiration is inhibited by pleurisy and pain, the patient is unable to maintain an adequate ventilation, and oxygen tension falls and carbon dioxide tension rises in arterial blood. Blood which continues to flow through consolidated areas of the lung cannot be oxygenated, which adds to the arterial desaturation.

Patients with bacterial pneumonia should be placed in bed and ensured adequate fluid intake (at least 100 to 120 ml/kg/day for infants). When cyanosis is present, oxygen should be provided by tent or nasal catheter. Aspirin or acetaminophen usually reduces the agitation and apprehension associated with fever and the discomfort caused by pleurisy. If pleuritic pain is severe, codeine (0.3 mg/kg body weight, every 4 to 6 hours) should be given. Codeine will slightly depress the respiratory center, but by reducing splinting of the chest wall, it allows deeper breaths and often permits an increase in ventilation.

PNEUMOCOCCAL PNEUMONIA. The pneumococcus rarely causes a primary infection, but usually invades the lung after the respiratory tract has been damaged by an unrelated viral or chemical agent. Initially, pneumococcal pneumonia is characterized by a rapidly mounting inflammatory edema and exudation of serum and red blood cells into the alveoli. Quickly, within 24 to 48 hours, the alveoli are filled with fibrin, leukocytes, red cells, and large numbers of pneumococci (red hepatization).

The onset of pneumococcal pneumonia is abrupt, with fever, chills, chest pain, and dyspnea. These symptoms are usually preceded by an upper respiratory infection. Cough, which produces blood-tinged sputum, is present early but may disappear with lobar consolidation. The child appears acutely ill, with tachypnea, tachycardia, and limited depth of respiration. There is dullness to percussion over the affected segment of the lung, breath sounds are diminished, and bronchial breathing and pleural friction rubs may be heard. Rales are not heard until later in the course of the disease. Small, sterile, pleural effusions are common, and empyema may be a late complication. Thoracentesis may be necessary to distinguish between these two complications.

Penicillin is the specific treatment for pneumococcal pneumonia. Although there are reports of successful use of oral preparations, we prefer procaine penicillin G, 50,000 units/kg administered intramuscularly, once daily, for uncomplicated cases. Treatment should continue for at least 2 days after the patient's temperature becomes normal. Erythromycin or a cephalosporin may be given to those children who are allergic to penicillin. Although sterile effusions may persist for several weeks, they usually resolve without treatment. Complicating empyemas require closed-suction drainage.

The pneumococcus does not produce a true exotoxin, and the antigen of the polysaccharide capsule does not cause tissue necrosis. Consequently, there is usually no residual lung damage following pneumococcal pneumonia.

STREPTOCOCCAL PNEUMONIA. Pneumonia caused by Group A hemolytic streptococci usually follows one of the childhood exanthemata, particularly rubeola, varicella, and scarlet fever. The streptococcus first invades the upper respiratory tract. Local inflammatory reaction may block lymphatic vessels, after which there is retrograde extension of the infection through the lymphphatics to the bronchi, lung parenchyma, and pleural surface. In the early stage most of the inflammatory reaction is often interstitial and resembles that of interstitial pneumonias caused by viruses or pleuropneumonialike organisms. The small bronchi may become partially obstructed if there is peribronchiolar inflammation. Distal to the obstruction, poorly ventilated, hyperinflated regions of the parenchyma may become the site of abscess or pneumatocele formation. In other cases there is a rapid accumulation of edema fluid in the interstitial spaces, which enters the alveoli. The interstitial spaces and the bronchial walls are infiltrated with leukocytes, and there is shedding of the alveolar epithelium. During the healing phase of streptococcal pneumonia, the intraalveolar edema fluid, red blood cells, fibrin, and other debris may coalesce and produce hyaline membranes.

Streptococcal pneumonia characteristically follows the sudden onset of sore throat, with hoarseness, fever, chest pain, cough, and marked respiratory distress. The child appears acutely ill. Leukocytosis is usually present. There is dullness to percussion over the affected lung. If an effusion is present and if the pneumonia is localized to a segment or lobe, crepitant rales and pleural friction rubs are usually heard. A radiograph of the chest may show segmental involvement, diffuse peribronchiolar densities, or effusion; the findings may resemble those in interstitial pneumonia caused by viruses, or the purulent pneumonias with abscess formation and pneumatoceles seen with staphylococcal lung infections. In addition to abscess formation the most common complication is empyema. Less commonly, pericarditis, peritonitis, systemic streptococcal disease, and purpura fulminans occur.

Large doses of intravenous or intramuscular penicillin G (100,000 units/kg/day or more) are necessary to treat streptococcal pneumonia effectively. The clinical response, the decrease in the white cell count, and the disappearance of the streptococcus may proceed slowly after penicillin therapy is initiated; 3 to 4 weeks of treatment may be required. Empyema requires closed-suction drainage.

STAPHYLOCOCCAL PNEUMONIA. Although now less frequent than pneumococcal, β-hemolytic streptococcus Group B, or viral pneumonias, staphylococcal pneumonia may be serious and tends to progress rapidly. Unless treated early and vigorously, infants with staphylococcal pneumonia are prone to develop pneumatocele, pneumothoraces, and empyema. The organisms first produce a diffuse inflammation in one or more segments of the lung, which may early—and deceptively—resemble pneumonitis of viral etiology. The right lung is more often affected than the left. Inflamed bronchi become partially occluded and pneumatoceles are formed beyond the obstruction. The bacteria grow rapidly and produce a necrotizing toxin, which causes tissue destruction. Microabscesses form around small bronchi and in pneumatoceles. Pneumatoceles and abscesses extend toward the pleural space and frequently rupture into it, causing empyema and pneumothorax.

Staphylococcal pneumonias are usually characterized by the rapid development of fever, tachypnea, dyspnea, tachycardia, and cyanosis. The onset is often preceded by an upper respiratory infection for which antibiotics have been given. The child with staphylococcal pneumonia may be lethargic or irritable and usually appears acutely ill. Ileus and abdominal distension are common. The physical signs reflect the progress of the disease. There may be evidence of inflammation and consolidation, hyperinflation if pneumatoceles are large, pneumothorax, or pleural effusions. The chest roentgenogram may show a lobar distribution of radiodensities, effusion, or pneumothorax; most characteristic are discrete areas of overinflation and distinct pneumatoceles.

When staphylococcal pneumonia is suspected, diagnostic procedures must be done quickly and treatment with methicillin (50 to 75 mg/kg/6 hours, intravenously) started immediately. If cultures from blood or empyema fluid reveal a staphylococcus that is sensitive to penicillin G, then methicillin should be stopped and penicillin G started (25,000 to 50,000 units/kg/6 hours, intravenously), as methicillin is potentially nephrotoxic.

Pneumothorax, which occurs in the first or second day of the disease, must be decompressed, but large pneumatoceles may resemble a pneumothorax so that caution must be exercised not to enter a pneumatocele inadvertently, causing a pneumothorax and inducing an empyema. Pneumatoceles are part of the healing process and are seen 3 to 4 days after treatment has begun. If empyema is present, it must be treated promptly by closed-suction drainage. Surgical decompression is most urgent in infancy.

Huxtable, Tucker, and Wedgwood, in a study of 22 children who had recovered from staphylococcal pneumonia, noted complete radiologic resolution in 19 and only minimal residua in 3. All had normal exercise tolerance and growth following recovery.

HAEMOPHILUS INFLUENZAE PNEUMONIA. The incidence of pneumonia due to *H. influenzae* type B in infants and young children appears to be increasing; this is possibly due to lower levels of circulating anti-*H. influenzae* antibody in the adult population. Although cultures of the upper respiratory tract of healthy children often grow nonencapsulated strains of *H. influenzae*, most extensive pneumonias due to Hemophilus are caused by encapsulated *H. influenzae* type B organisms.

The distribution may be either focal (lobar pneumonia) or disseminated (bronchopneumonia). Pathologically, the lungs show areas of inflammation infiltrated with polymorphonuclear leukocytes, with destruction of the bronchial and bronchiolar epithelium. Edema extending into the interstitial areas may be striking.

Clinical presentation with lobar distribution may be almost indistinguishable from pneumococcal pneumonia, although the onset may be more insidious. The bronchopneumonic variety may mimic acute bronchiolitis in the early stages, but increasing interstitial edema, producing a "shaggy" appearance on roentgenograms, should alert the physician that a bacterial infection must be considered.

The treatment of choice has been ampicillin (100 to 200 mg/kg/day, intravenously or intramuscularly). The recent appearance of strains of *H. influenzae* type B, resistant to ampicillin, makes chloramphenicol the drug of choice if the patient's response to ampicillin is unsatisfactory.

FRIEDLANDER'S BACILLUS (KLEBSIELLA PNEUMONIAE) PNEUMONIA. Although *Klebsiella pneumoniae* are found in the respiratory and gastrointestinal tracts in about 5 percent of healthy children, it is rarely the cause of pneumonia in infants and children. Occasional epidemics of *Klebsiella pneumoniae* in newborn nurseries have been described. Cases in older children are more likely to occur if they are debilitated or after treatment with mist therapy or as secondary invaders after prolonged endotracheal intubation. The clinical picture is indistinguishable from other varieties of pneumonia, but the presence of copious, thick, purulent secretions should suggest the diagnosis. Older children are prone to develop pulmonary abscesses and cavitation (pneumatoceles). Bacteremia and empyema are common. The mortality rate is high.

Friedlander's bacillus does not respond to the antibiotics used to treat most pulmonary infections in childhood (ampicillin and penicillinase-resistant penicillins). Kanamycin and gentamicin are the drugs of choice.

THE MYCOTIC INFECTIONS. There are two types of pulmonary infections caused by fungi: infections in children with normal host resistance exposed to indigenous fungi. The symptoms produced by most of these infections are mild (often diagnosed as flu-like illness) and self-limiting and rarely require treatment. Histoplasmosis and coccidioidomycosis are examples. The second type of infection occurs in children with diminished immunologic competence either due to a basic immunodeficiency disorder or secondary to immunosuppressive therapy (as in leukemia, neoplasms, or organ transplant patients). Fungi are ubiquitous, usually noninvasive, and result in widespread pulmonary disease only in immunologically compromised hosts. Candida and aspergillus are the primary offenders (see also, p. 610, 619).

HISTOPLASMOSIS. Primary infection of the lung with *Histoplasma capsulatum* is very common in endemic areas and usually produces no symptoms. Occasionally, histoplasmosis is a disseminated systemic infection. Rarely, an acute rapidly progressing pulmonary inflammation occurs and is associated with fever, anorexia, malaise, tachypnea, tachycardia, and rales. Chest roentgenograms show enlargement of the hilar nodes with perihilar parenchymal opacities. In children the chronic progressive form of pulmonary histoplasmosis is rare. The only effective treatment for disseminated or progressive pulmonary histoplasmosis is intravenous amphotericin B. This frequently must be continued for many months, possesses great toxicity, and should be used only by physicians experienced in its use.

COCCIDIOIDOMYCOSIS. Primary infection of the lungs with *Coccidioides immitis* is also very common in endemic areas, especially in arid regions of the southwest United States, Mexico, and other parts of Central America. Many of these have a low-grade fever, minimal lung involvement, and erythema nodosum, typical of *valley fever*. Occasionally, there is a progressive primary lung inflammation or dissemination that must be treated vigorously. Serologic testing for coccidioidal precipitins and complement fixing antibodies are the most sensitive methods of following the response to treatment. The only effective treatment is intravenous administration of amphotericin B, usually for many months, until there is evidence of definite serologic improvement. Toxic reactions, including renal damage, are common and require very close monitoring (see p. 617 for details of amphotericin therapy).

ASPERGILLUS. Aspergillus species are widely distributed in soil, decaying vegetable matter, and bird droppings. Aspergilli, particularly *A. fumigatus,* are commonly found in the sputum of patients with chronic pulmonary disease. These may be harmless, saprophytic commensals and may not be responsible for the pulmonary disease. The spectrum of pulmonary disease produced by aspergilli is broad and depends on the nature of the exposure, the immunologic status of the subject, and whether there is preexisting lung disease. The clinical entities include:

Asthma. In atopic subjects, the spores may act as allergens and precipitate acute asthmatic attacks.
Allergic bronchopulmonary aspergillosis. This is characterized by recurrent fevers, migratory pulmonary lesions, eosinophilia, expectoration of mucous plugs containing aspergillus mycelia, and bronchial damage.
Aspergillomas (fungal balls). These are saprophytic masses of aspergilli that grow in previously existing bronchiectatic cavities, such as occur in cavitary histoplasmosis or tuberculosis.
Invasive aspergillosis with acute pneumonia. This occurs most often in immunologically deficient children but has been reported by Strelling and associates in apparently normal children. This disease should not be diagnosed without a lung biopsy demonstrating tissue invasion.

Treatment with intravenous amphotericin B (1 mg/kg/day) is the only effective therapy and must be continued for at least 1 month until signs of improvement are seen (see p. 617 for details of amphotericin therapy). Localized aspergillomas should be excised if the remainder of the lung is normal or treated with local instillations of amphotericin B, as described by Ramirez.

ACTINOMYCOSIS. A chronic mycotic infection that tends to be suppurative and forms abscesses and sinus tracts in the cervicofacial area is actinomycosis. Pulmonary infections are not uncommon in adults. In children actinomycosis is rare. The clinical picture is that of chronic pulmonary infection with cough, sputum, fever, dyspnea, hemoptysis, and weight loss. Multiple abscesses may be present; extension into the pleural cavity or pericardium or involvement of the ribs and subcutaneous tissues with sinus formation is common. Anaerobic cultures are necessary to grow the organism, but the diagnosis can be strongly suspected by finding *sulfur granules* in the pus from a draining sinus. The treatment of choice is massive doses of penicillin (10 million units/day) intravenously, for 4 to 6 weeks, followed by oral penicillin for a minimum of 6 months, as outlined by Riley.

NOCARDIOSIS. This chronic and suppurative disease resembles actinomycosis. Abscesses and sinuses are less common, however, and in children the lung is often involved. It may occur as a complication of immunodeficiency disease, such as fatal granulomatous disease. There is persistent cough, intermittent septic fever, hepatosplenomegaly, and progressive pulmonary insufficiency. Treatment with sulfadiazine or a combination of trimethoprin and sulfamethoxazole has been effective in the early stages of this disease. Localized abscesses, when they occur, should be drained.

BLASTOMYCOSIS, CRYPTOCOCCOSIS, CANDIDIASIS, SPOROTRICHOSIS. Blastomyces, cryptococcus, and candida have all caused pulmonary inflammation in children, and for these amphotericin B and 5-fluorocystosine, although toxic, are the only effective agents. Sporotrichum has been identified occasionally as the organism responsible for chronic pulmonary inflammation. This infection responds to some extent to therapy with potassium iodide, but again amphotericin B is probably the drug of choice.

Bibliography

DISEASES CAUSING REDUCTION IN PARENCHYMA BECAUSE OF ABSENCE OF TISSUE

Booth JB, Berry CL: Unilateral pulmonary agenesis. Arch Dis Child 42:361, 1967

Chatrath RR, Shafie ME, Jones RS: Fate of hypoplastic lungs after repair of congenital diaphragmatic hernia. Arch Dis Child 46:633, 1971

Cook CD, Bucci G: Studies of respiratory physiology in children. IV. The late effects of lobectomy on pulmonary function. Pediatrics 28:234, 1961

deLorimer AA, Tierney DF, Parker HR: Hypoplastic lungs in fetal lambs with surgically-produced congenital diaphragmatic hernia. Surgery 62:12, 1967

Ferencz C: Congenital abnormalities of pulmonary vessels and their relation to malformations of the lung. Pediatrics 28:993, 1961

Filler J: Effects upon pulmonary function of lobectomy performed during childhood. Am Rev Resp Dis 89:801, 1964

Giammona ST, Mandelbaum I, Battersby JS, Daly WJ: The late cardiopulmonary effects of childhood pneumonectomy. Pediatrics 37:79, 1966

Oyamada A, Gasul BM, Holinger PH: Agenesis of the lung. Report of a case, with a review of all previously reported cases. Am J Dis Child 85:182, 1953

Roe BB, Stephens HB: Congenital diaphragmatic hernia and hypoplastic lung. J Thorac Surg 32:279, 1956

SPACE-OCCUPYING LESIONS

Anderson AE: Bronchogenic carcinoma in young men. Am J Med 16:404, 1954

Caffey J: On the natural regression of pulmonary cysts during early infancy. Pediatrics 11:48, 1953

Hodgson CH, Burchell HB, Good CA, Clagett OT: Hereditary hemorrhagic telangiectasia and pulmonary arteriovenous fistula. N Engl J Med 261:625, 1959

Javett SN, Webster I, Braudo JL: Congenital dilatation of the pulmonary lymphatics. Pediatrics 31:416, 1963

Klein ZL: An accessory lobe of the lung in a newborn. Pediatrics 45:118, 1970

Kwittken J, Reiner L: Congenital cystic adenomatoid malformation of the lung. Pediatrics 30:759, 1962

Laurence KM: Congenital pulmonary lymphangiectasis. J Clin Pathol 12:62, 1959

Noonan JA, Walters LR, Reeves JT: Congenital pulmonary lymphangiectasis. Am J Dis Child 120:314, 1970

Pearl M: Sequestration of the lung. Am J Dis Child 124:706, 1972

Pinney CT, Salyer JM: Bronchopulmonary sequestration. J Thorac Surg 33:791, 1957

INFLAMMATION

The Bacterial Pneumonias

Gourlay RH: Staphylococcal pneumonia and empyema in infants and children. Can Med Assoc J 87:1101, 1962

Huxtable KA, Tucker AS, Wedgwood RJ: Staphylococcal pneumonia in childhood. Long-term follow-up. Am J Dis Child 108:262, 1964

Kevy SV, Lowe BA: Streptococcal pneumonia and empyema in childhood. N Engl J Med 264:738, 1961

McCracken G, Eichenwald H: Bacterial pneumonia. In Vaughan VC, McKay RJ (eds): Textbook of Pediatrics. WB Saunders, Philadelphia, 1975, p 969

Middlekamp JN, Purkerson ML, Burford TH: The changing pattern of empyema thoracis in pediatrics. J Thorac Cardiovasc Surg 47:165, 1964

Ravitch MM, Fein R: The changing picture of pneumonia and empyema in infants and children. JAMA 175:1039, 1961

Riley HD, Bracken EC: Empyema due to *Hemophilus influenzae* in infants and children. Am J Dis Child 110:24, 1965

Smith MHC: Pneumococcal pneumonia. In Kendig EL Jr (ed): Disorders of the Respiratory Tract in Children, 2nd ed. WB Saunders, Philadelphia, 1972

Witt RL, Hamburger M: The nature and treatment of penumococcal pneumonia. Med Clin North Am 47:1257, 1963

Mycotic Infections

Blattner R: Pulmonary aspergillosis in children. J Pediatr 70:139, 1967

Paul FM: Two cases of thoracic actinomycosis in children. Arch Dis Child 38:276, 1963

Peabody JW, Seabury JH: Actinomycosis and nocardiosis. A review of basic differences in therapy. Am J Med 28:99, 1960

Pepys J (ed): Pulmonary aspergillosis. In Hypersensitivity Diseases of the Lungs Due to Fungi and Organic Dusts. S Karger, New York, 1969, p 20

Ramirez RJ: Pulmonary aspergilloma—endobronchial treatment. N Engl J Med 271:1281, 1964

Ridgeway NA, Whitcomb FC, Erickson EE, Law SW: Primary pulmonary sporotrichosis. Am J Med 32:153, 1962

Riley HD: Systemic mycosis in children. Curr Problems Pediatr 2:12, 3:1, 1972

Slavin RG, Laird TS, Cherry JD: Allergic bronchopulmonary aspergillosis in a child. J Pediatr 76:416, 1970

Strelling MK, Rhaney K, Simmons DAR, Thomson J: Fatal acute pulmonary aspergillosis in two children of one family. Arch Dis Child 41:34, 1966

Tesh RB, Shacklette MH, Diercks FH, Hirschl D: Histoplasmosis in children. Pediatrics 33:894, 1964

Ziering WH, Rockas HR: Coccidioidomycosis. Long term treatment with amphotericin B of disseminated disease in a three month old baby. Am J Dis Child 108:454, 1964

DISEASES CAUSING INTERSTITIAL INJURY

WILLIAM H. TOOLEY

HERMAN H. LIPOW

Viral and certain parasitic infections, chemical irritants, allergic reactions, and some diseases of unknown origin cause an interstitial inflammation. The reaction may be acute, with histamine release, which causes bronchospasm and pulmonary edema; or it may be subacute, with the accumulation of round cells and the formation of granulomas in the interstitial areas. After injury of this type there is a proliferation of fibroblasts, and healing is often accompanied by fibrosis.

The signs, symptoms, and pathophysiology of these diseases vary, depending upon the localization of the inflammation. Figure 51 displays some of the possible sites of interstitial infiltration. If the process is confined to the boundary between alveoli and capillaries, the lung will be stiff, vital capacity reduced, the pulmonary diffusion capacity low, and there will be desaturation of arterial blood with exercise or, in severe cases, at rest. Such localization and pure *alveolar-capillary block* probably does not occur. Infiltration about small airways produces the signs and symptoms of airway obstruction, with a decrease in vital capacity, a decrease in expiratory flow rates, and an increase in the work of breathing. When inflammation surrounds the pulmonary vessels, vital capacity may be normal but diffusion capacity will be low, and the apparent physiologic dead space will be large. Most interstitial diseases of the lung affect the alveolar-capillary boundary and the peribronchial and perivascular spaces, causing signs, symptoms, and physiologic changes that are a combination of those seen in alveolar-capillary block and obstruction of the airways and pulmonary vessels.

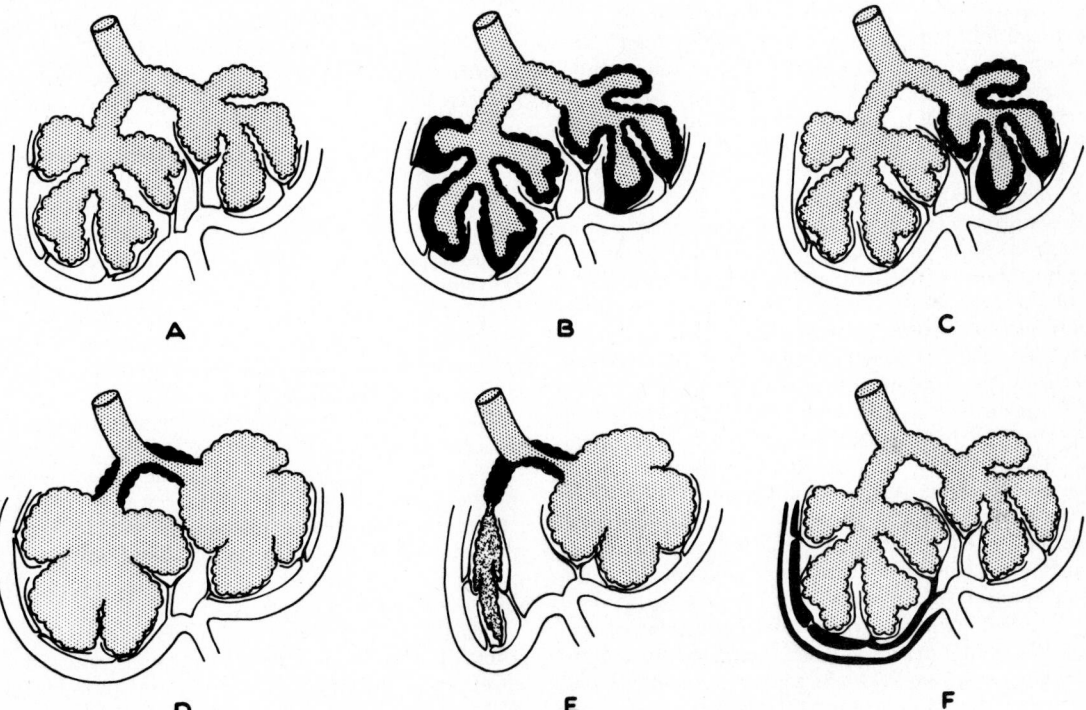

FIG. 51. A schematic representation of the possible sites of interalveolar inflammation. **A.** Normal portion of lung with a narrow space between the alveolar and capillary walls and uniform distribution of both ventilation and blood flow. **B.** An inflammatory process spread out evenly between the alveoli and pulmonary capillaries—lung volume, vital capacity, lung compliance, and diffusion capacity are low; there is arterial desaturation with exercise; the distribution of ventilation and perfusion is uniform. **C.** Part of the lung is normal and part is affected—again lung volume, vital capacity, lung compliance, and diffusion capacity are low; there is arterial desaturation, but in this instance the distribution of ventilation and perfusion is not uniform. **D.** An inflammatory reaction surrounding all the small bronchi—lung volume is large, vital capacity low, and diffusion capacity normal; there may be arterial desaturation with exercise; the distribution of ventilation and perfusion is uniform. **E.** Peribronchial inflammation partially occluding some small airways, causing hyperinflation and completely occluding other small airways producing atelectasis. Lung volume may be normal or low; vital capacity and lung compliance are low; diffusion capacity is normal when related to the volume of lung ventilated, but is low in absolute terms. There is arterial desaturation at rest and with exercise; the distribution of ventilation and perfusion is not uniform. **F.** Only the perivascular area of the parenchyma is involved. Lung volume, vital capacity, and lung compliance are normal; diffusion capacity is low. The apparent physiologic dead space is large; there is arterial desaturation with exercise, and there may be some at rest; the distribution of ventilation is uniform, but the distribution of perfusion is not uniform.

Infections

THE VIRAL PNEUMONIAS. Many viruses can cause pneumonia in infants and children. These include respiratory syncytial virus, parainfluenza viruses, adenoviruses, rhinoviruses, and influenza viruses. Varicella and rubeola viruses may also produce widespread pneumonia, particularly in immunologically compromised patients.

Viral infections of the lungs tend to produce inflammation in the interalveolar areas (interstitial spaces) but, if severe, may involve the alveolar sacs. They are characterized by the sudden onset of tachypnea, nonproductive cough, substernal discomfort, low-grade fever, and malaise after several days of an upper respiratory tract or exanthematous infection. The pharynx is reddened, and there is a slight nasopharyngeal mucous discharge. There may be dullness over the lung, diminished breath sounds, and fine, crepitant rales. Often, however, there are no physical signs of lung disease, even though diffuse perihilar and parenchymal infiltrations are seen on roentgenograms.

No specific therapy is available. Treatment includes rest, adequate fluid intake, and aspirin. If airway obstruction is present, bronchodilators and the other measures outlined previously for diseases of the airway should be used. If there is cyanosis or significant hypoxemia, oxygen should be given.

The mortality rate is low, but convalescence is often prolonged. Some infections, particularly in young infants, may cause extensive damage and, if not fatal, may require one or more years for healing. Bronchiolitis obliterans with adenovirus infections is an example.

PSITTACOSIS-ORNITHOSIS PNEUMONIA. The responsible organism, previously regarded as a large virus, is now classified with the Chlamydia group. The signs and symptoms of the infection are indistinguishable from those associated with other viral infections of the lung. A history of contact with birds, particularly caged birds, should suggest the diagnosis. Treatment with tetracyclines in children over 8 years, or penicillin in younger children, may shorten the duration of the illness.

Q FEVER. *Coxiella burnetii*, a rickettsial organism, causes an acute pneumonitis characterized by infiltration of the peribronchiolar and perivascular spaces with plasma cells and lymphocytes. The disease is endemic in sheep and it frequently is transmitted to sheep handlers. The disease usually begins with severe headache, which is followed by the gradual onset of chills, fever, malaise, nonproductive cough, and substernal chest pain. The clinical and radiographic picture is similar to other viral infections of the lung. The diagnosis of Q fever requires the demonstration of rising serum antibodies or recovery of *C. burnetii* from the patient's blood, urine, or sputum after careful intraperitoneal inoculation into guinea pigs. The organism is very contagious, and extreme care must accompany the handling of the specimens in the laboratory. Serologic testing includes complement fixing antibodies and agglutinins and, in most clinical situations, is the accepted method of establishing the diagnosis. The clinical

course is self-limited, lasting up to 3 weeks; mortality is low. *C. burnetii* is susceptible to chloramphenicol and tetracycline in vitro, but the in vivo response is not impressive.

MYCOPLASMA PNEUMONIAE (EATON AGENT) PNEUMONIA. The pleuropneumonialike organisms (PPLO) cause an acute interstitial pneumonitis. After about a 2-week incubation period, the onset of symptoms is usually gradual but may be abrupt, with malaise, generalized aches, and a paroxysmal nonproductive cough. There are few physical findings, but rales are usually heard at the bases of the lung late in the disease. As in the viral pneumonias, the absence of physical signs is in contrast to the radiographic appearance of marked perihilar densities and diffuse, mottled, parenchymal infiltrations. A specific diagnosis can be established by culturing *Mycoplasma pneumoniae* from sputum or blood, although this is technically difficult. In addition, serum from these patients contains a macroglobulin that, in an environment of 0 to 10 C, agglutinates human type 0 red cells (cold agglutination).

Treatment of mycoplasma pneumonitis with either erythromycin or tetracycline has been reported to shorten the febrile course of the disease in adults, but not in children.

THE PARASITIC PNEUMONIAS PNEUMOCYSTIS CARINII PNEUMONIA. *Pneumocystis carinii* pneumonia occurs in immunosuppressed infants and children and debilitated infants. Originally described as an infection in premature infants, occurring sporadically and occasionally in epidemics, it is now recognized frequently in children of all ages with primary immune deficiency disorders, and in patients receiving immunosuppressive drugs for lymphoreticular malignancies or organ transplantation.

The organism *Pneumocystis carinii* is ubiquitous and has not been grown in vitro. It is thought by most investigators to be a protozoon, although recent electron microscopic studies have suggested it may be a fungus. Three separate attacks in a patient with hypogammaglobulinemia, reported by Richman and associates, suggest that reactivation of a latent pulmonary infection is probable.

Typically, the first symptom is unexplained low-grade fever followed by nonproductive cough in the absence of upper respiratory tract symptoms. Vomiting and diarrhea are common, and older children usually complain of pain in the anterior part of the chest or substernal region. Over a period of 1 to 4 weeks, the child develops increasing tachypnea and cyanosis, and appears acutely ill. Auscultatory findings may be surprisingly few, but areas of fine crepitant rales may be present, particularly after coughing. A chest roentgenogram, in the early stages of the disease, shows a bilateral perihilar interstitial haziness, progressing to diffuse linear shadows that radiate toward the periphery. In moderately advanced pneumonia, there are generalized irregular patches of consolidation, surrounded by areas of increased translucency. Bilateral diffuse consolidation is apparent in advanced pneumonia. Mediastinal and hilar adenomegaly are not present.

As Pneumocystis cannot be grown in vitro, diagnosis

rests on demonstrating the organism by Giemsa and silver stains in material obtained from the lung by tracheal aspiration, tracheal lavage, transtracheal biopsy through a bronchoscope, needle aspiration of the lung, or open lung biopsy. We have found open lung biopsy to be the safest and most reliable way of making the diagnosis rapidly in critically ill children. Recent advances in serologic testing offer promise that indirect methods of diagnosis may be possible.

All children with *Pneumocystis carinii* are more comfortable when breathing oxygen. If started early, specific treatment with pentamidine isothionate intramuscularly (obtainable from the Center for Infectious Disease Control, Atlanta, Georgia 30333) results in a cure rate of over 60 percent. Current reports suggest that a combination of oral pyrimethamine and sulfadiazine, or trimethaprin with sulfamethoxazole, may be as effective.

TOXOCARA CANIS PNEUMONITIS (VISCERAL LARVA MIGRANS). Infestation with *T. canis* usually occurs in children under 4 years of age with a history of pica. The parasite is swallowed, invades the intestine, and is carried by the portal circulation to the liver. In 7 of 17 cases reported by Snyder, there was pulmonary involvement. The disease is characterized by recurrent fever, cough, lassitude, anorexia, and weight loss. There is usually hepatomegaly. Eosinophilia of greater than 30 percent is a constant feature of the disease. The chest film shows a diffuse, parenchymal infiltration, and occasionally miliary nodules similar to those seen in miliary tuberculosis. The organism can be identified directly only by liver or lung biopsy. Treatment with thiabendazole (50 mg/kg for 3 to 5 days) has been shown to kill encysted larvae. Corticosteroids may be used for the relief of severe symptoms.

FILARIA PNEUMONITIS (TROPICAL EOSINOPHILIA). Tropical eosinophilia is a common cause of pneumonitis in India and some areas of Central America and Southeast Asia. Most of the cases are in children under 10 years of age. The disease is characterized by diffuse interstitial edema and interalveolar infiltration of eosinophils.The onset is insidious with a low-grade fever, hacking dry cough, wheezing, and nocturnal respiratory distress. Rales may be heard at the bases of the lungs. Chest films show diminished translucency with an increase in hilar markings. The eosinophil count is always elevated to at least 2,500 cells/mm^3. Treatment with diethylcarbamazine (4 mg/kg, 3 times a day for 5 days) is usually successful.

Chemical Pneumonitis

HYDROCARBON PNEUMONITIS (see also p. 795). The inhalation of hydrocarbon into the lungs causes widespread inflammatory reaction characterized by extensive filling of the alveoli with blood-tinged edema fluid. Bilateral pulmonary infiltrates are seen on roentgenogram, and fever, shortness of breath, and hypoxemia are usually present. Hydrocarbons are still widely present in the home environment of many children, although the exact products change with time.

Kerosene (paraffin) was a frequent offender in the past, as were some of the furniture polishes (Old English and Red Cedar particularly). In the suburbs in the United States charcoal lighter fluid has replaced kerosene as the major offender.

Considerable controversy over the route of hydrocarbon entry to the lungs persisted for many years, but current evidence favors direct aspiration of hydrocarbons into the trachea as the most significant pathway. The low viscosity of hydrocarbons allow these substances to flow from the hypopharynx into the larynx. As a consequence, vomiting or gastric lavage may permit increased aspiration and is not recommended. With less extensive aspiration, the onset of pulmonary inflammation may not be evident for 12 to 24 hours. If the child is seen shortly after ingestion, it is important to observe him carefully for 24 to 48 hours before deciding that his lungs are not involved.

Treatment is mainly supportive. Fever and dyspnea may last up to 2 weeks in severe cases, but with oxygen, respiratory physiotherapy to help clear secretions, adequate fluid and caloric intake, and antibiotics for secondary bacterial infection, most children will recover completely. After the first week it is not uncommon for pneumatoceles to develop in areas of extensive consolidation. These cysts do not rupture and should be treated conservatively. Steroids given early and in large doses have been recommended, but there is no convincing evidence that they alter the course of the disease. Counseling parents on the potential dangers of the common household substances must be a regular part of well child care. *Volatile hydrocarbon,* if kept in the house, should be kept out of the reach of children, preferably in locked cupboards.

SILO-FILLERS' DISEASE. Lowry and Schuman described an acute pneumonitis in adults following exposure to freshly filled silos, but it has also occurred in children. The disease is caused by inhalation of nitrogen dioxide. The interalveolar septa become edematous, widened, and filled with an accumulation of mononuclear cells and fibroblasts; the alveolar epithelium becomes hyperplastic. At the time of exposure, cough and dyspnea occur, followed by several days of no symptoms. There is then an abrupt onset of chills, fever, dyspnea, cyanosis, and cough, with rales throughout the lungs. Radiologically there is diffuse pulmonary infiltration. Corticosteroids have been used in treatment. However, the course is usually fulminating and mortality is high.

PARAQUAT LUNG. Paraquat, a bipyridylium compound, is a potent weed killer. It is highly toxic for man, and death is due to respiratory failure that develops a few days to 2 weeks after ingestion. Paraquat is corrosive and, if ingested, results in immediate painful lesions of the mouth and esophagus. Renal excretion causes tubular damage, with azotemia and hematuria.

The pulmonary lesion is secondary to systemic absorption, not pulmonary aspiration, and occurs after cutaneous absorption.The basic lung lesion is a proliferative bronchiolitis and alveolitis, with pulmonary hemorrhage causing intraalveolar hyaline membranes and fibrosis. Gas exchange is impaired early; gas transfer, as measured by carbon monoxide diffusion, is helpful in quantitating the degree of damage. No effective treatment is known. General supportive measures and forced osmotic diuresis to increase excretion have been recommended. Experimental data in animals suggest that breathing high concentrations of oxygen may increase the pulmonary toxicity.

PNEUMONITIS FROM OTHER CHEMICALS. Many chemicals, if inhaled in high concentrations, may cause acute interalveolar edema and mononuclear infiltration with sudden onset of cough, substernal pain, and cyanosis. Prolonged exposure to lower concentrations of the same agents may cause a chronic interstitial pneumonitis, characterized by interalveolar granuloma formation similar to that seen in sarcoidosis. Organic compounds, such as shellac, gum arabic, and polyvinylpyrrolidone (a macromolecular substance found in hair spray), and inorganic substances, such as beryllium, mercury vapors, and chlorine, may cause this reaction. Corticosteroids reduce the inflammatory process and may prevent fibrosis.

Interstitial Pneumonitis due to Hypersensitivity

HYPERSENSITIVITY LUNG DISEASE. The reactions of the body to various stimuli mediated through humoral and cellular reactions are classified as immune responses. Deficient or impaired immunologic reaction may lead to recurrent or progressive pulmonary infections (see p. 304). Occasionally the immunologic reaction (allergies, hypersensitivity reactions) cause noninfectious inflammation and disease of the lungs. Gell and Coombs divide these into four types: type I (IgE-dependent, immediate hypersensitivity response); type II (tissue-specific antibody, cytotoxic); type III (immune-complex disease, intermediate hypersensitivity reaction); and type IV (cell-mediated, delayed hypersensitivity (see p. 330). Probably all four types of reactions, and other types yet to be delineated, are involved in varying combinations to produce the spectrum of hypersensitivity lung disease. Few diseases are clearly the result of only one type of response. Asthma, due to the inhalation of extrinsic antigens, appears to be a type I, immediate reaction, and Goodpasture's disease is type II.

HYPERSENSITIVITY TO INHALED ORGANIC MATERIAL (EXTRINSIC ALLERGIC ALVEOLITIS). In some sensitized children the inhalation of organic dust may produce an acute interstitial inflammation of the lungs. These children usually are not atopic but have specific serum precipitins. The acute pneumonitis is caused by the organic dust reacting with the precipitins and was called extrinsic allergic alveolitis by Pepys. These type III immune-complex reactions begin 3 to 6 hours after inhalation, peak in 6 to 8 hours, and begin to subside by 24 hours.

Campbell reported an acute pneumonitis in farm workers following exposure to moldy hay (*farmers'*

lung). The inflammation is subacute, with accumulations of lymphocytes, plasma cells, epithelioid cells, and Langhans' giant cells, which widen the interstitial space. An identical reaction occurs in some individuals following exposure to pigeons (*pigeon breeders' lung*), maple-bark (*maple-bark strippers' disease*), redwood tree bark, and moldy sugar cane bark (*bagassosis*). In farmers' lung, the specific antigen is hay mold; in pigeon breeders' lung, pigeon feathers and droppings; in maple-bark strippers' disease, the fungus *Cryptostroma corticale;* in redwood tree exposure, the redwood fungus of the species *Graphium;* and in bagassosis, sugar cane mold. Farmers' lung has been reported in children, but maple-bark strippers' disease or bagassosis have not as yet. However, Stiehm and associates reported pigeon-breeders' lung in children and it is likely that these and similar parenchymal diseases of hypersensitivity are common causes of pneumonitis in childhood. Recently, pulmonary hypersensitivity associated with the inhalation of pancreatin powder has been reported in exposed parents while mixing pancreatin powder in the food to be administered to children with cystic fibrosis.

Acute, subacute, and chronic stages have been distinguished in these diseases, but usually one stage merges imperceptibly into the next. Acute episodes begin several hours after exposure and are characterized by dyspnea, fever, and chest pain. Physical findings are minimal and consist only of a few moist rales and occasional wheezes. Chest radiographs are normal. If exposure to the antigen continues, there is severe dyspnea, nonproductive cough, cyanosis, and the chest film shows a diffuse, fine, mottled infiltration, usually most marked in the lower part of the lungs; there is a marked reduction in vital capacity and diffusion capacity, and arterial desaturation at rest, exaggerated with exercise. Hypergammaglobulinemia with elevation of the IgG, IgM, and IgA fractions is common, but serum complement is normal.

Diagnosis can be strongly supported by the demonstration of specific precipitins in the serum. Intradermal injection of a specific antigen may cause erythema and induration, beginning in 3 to 6 hours and reaching a maximum intensity at 6 to 8 hours. However, many of the antigens are locally irritating to normal subjects and a positive test should be followed by precipitin tests for serum antigens.

Since pulmonary fibrosis may develop if inhalation challenge continues, vigorous treatment is desirable. Immediate removal of the specific antigen from the patient's environment is mandatory. If pulmonary disease is extensive, treatment with corticosteroids (prednisone 1 to 2 mg/kg/day for 1 to 2 months) will usually result in rapid disappearance of the signs and symptoms and radiologic abnormalities.

Sarcoidosis (See also p. 1230)

Sarcoidosis is a generalized disease of unknown cause, which may affect the lungs, eyes, skin, lymph nodes, liver, and other tissues. In the lung there are interalveolar, peribronchiolar, and periarteriolar granulomas characterized by nests of epithelioid cells and Langhans' giant cells surrounded by a thin wall of lymphocytes. The granulomas are rarely necrotic and never show central caseation. Diffuse infiltration of the interalveolar space with mononuclear cells precedes the formation of granulomas. The periarteriolar granulomas are relatively vascular and are often surrounded with hyalinelike material. This stage of the disease resembles polyarteritis nodosa. Late in the disease the granulomas may be replaced by fibroblasts and fibrous tissue.

The onset of sarcoidosis is insidious, with anorexia, fatigue, lethargy, and weight loss. There may be a dry, hacking cough with mild dyspnea. Physical findings related to the lung are usually minimal. The presence of the disease in other organs is responsible for most of the symptoms—particularly the eyes, with iritis, uveitis, and keratitis; the parotid gland, with uveoparotid fever; and the kidneys, with acute glomerulonephritis. The serum globulins, particularly the a_2 globulins, are elevated, serum albumin is low, and occasionally there is hypercalcemia. Initially, the chest film shows enlargement of hilar nodes, followed by a diffuse pulmonary infiltration after weeks or months. Pulmonary function testing frequently shows restrictive lung disease with reduced lung volumes without airways obstruction. Diagnosis is best made by scalene node or lung biopsy.

Spontaneous remissions of sarcoidosis occur in most patients. Long-term therapy with corticosteroid should be reserved for children with extensive pulmonary involvement and dyspnea, or involvement of the eye, central nervous system, or myocardium. Criteria for steroid treatment have been detailed by the Committee on Therapy of the American Thoracic Society (1971). Corticosteroids (Prednisone 1 to 2 mg/kg/day for 1 month, followed by alternate-day therapy for 3 to 6 months) may be necessary to control the inflammatory process.

Interstitial Pneumonitis of Unknown Etiology

There is no completely satisfactory clinical or pathologic classification for a group of children with subacute and chronic interstitial pneumonitis; this reflects our lack of knowledge regarding the etiology and natural course of these diseases. A workable classification based on current understanding includes: diffuse interstitial pulmonary fibrosis; desquamative interstitial pneumonitis; pulmonary hemosiderosis; collagen diseases; and other diseases.

DIFFUSE INTERSTITIAL PULMONARY FIBROSIS (HAMMAN-RICH SYNDROME; FIBROSING ALVEOLITIS). This disease is characterized by an infiltration of inflammatory cells in the interalveolar septa with variable fibrous tissue proliferation. Since the report of Hamman and Rich of several cases of diffuse interstitial fibrosis of the lung, the clinical syndrome and characteristic pathology have been well defined. It is undoubtedly not a specific disease but probably represents the endstage of chronic interstitial pneumonitis.

The clinical manifestations vary. Usually, there is gradual onset of a dry, irritating cough and breathlessness, which progresses over a period of weeks or, less commonly, months. Limited exercise tolerance and weight loss appear and tachycardia is striking. Fine crepitations may be heard over the lung bases but, more commonly, the lungs are clean on auscultation. Cyanosis occurs early during exercise, and later at rest. Clubbing of the fingers and toes is common. The disease tends to follow a relentless course over a period of months to 2 years. Cor pulmonale and right-sided heart failure develop terminally. Most children die of respiratory failure, usually precipitated by an intercurrent respiratory infection. In the early stages chest roentgenograms may be normal, but as the disease progresses, a diffuse granular infiltration appears. Other patients may show infiltrates that have been described as linear, nodular, and confluent. As more fibrosis develops, the densities assume a linear appearance, that is, coarse and strandlike.

Pulmonary function tests show a reduced vital capacity, decreased compliance, reduced diffusion capacity, and usually no increase in airway resistance. Hypoxemia is present at rest and increases markedly with exercise.

At autopsy the lungs are firm and rubbery and sink in water. Most of the interalveolar space is occupied by dense fibrous tissue, but there are usually scattered areas of chronic inflammation.

Treatment of this disease with corticosteroids is usually unsuccessful, since only those parts of the lung that show chronic penumonitis without fibrosis might be expected to resume normal function. Oxygen and other supportive measures may provide temporary improvement. The poor prognosis in pulmonary fibrosis emphasizes the importance of using corticosteroids in the earlier stages of proliferative interstitial pulmonary disease to prevent permanent damage. Immunosuppressive drugs have been of value in some adults, but their use in children has not been reported.

DESQUAMATIVE INTERSTITIAL PNEUMONITIS. This may be a relatively common pathologic change in chronic lung disease in childhood. The disease may occur in young infants, with symptoms starting at 1 to 2 months of age. Tachypnea is the first symptom, progressing to cyanosis while breathing room air. Nonproductive cough and weight loss are common, but fever is not noted. Clubbing may occur early and become severe. Rales are rarely heard. In advanced cases the chest roentgenogram shows a ground-glass appearance at the bases, with large ill-defined densities at the hilar and posterior portions of the lungs.

The microscopic lesions in the lung are characterized by massive proliferation and desquamation of innumerable granular pneumocytes (type II alveolar lining cells) that fill the alveoli and some bronchioles. There is usually relatively minor interstitial infiltration of lymphocytes, eosinophils, and plasma cells.

Most cases respond to steroid treatment, usually with stabilization and sometimes by remission of clinical and roentgenographic changes, but Barnes and associates reported a 2-month-old infant who failed to respond to corticosteroids or azathiaprine. We have followed a child in whom the disease first appeared at 3 years of age; she showed mild improvement with steroid therapy, but responded dramatically to chloroquine, administered at 6 years of age.

PULMONARY HEMOSIDEROSIS. This is an uncommon disease characterized by recurrent or persistent intra-alveolar hemorrhage. This causes an abnormally large amount of hemosiderin in the lung tissue and a secondary iron deficiency anemia. Pulmonary hemosiderosis begins in infancy and childhood, the youngest reported patient being 4 months of age. The cause of this disease is unknown; structural defects in the alveolar capillary bed, allergy to milk proteins, autoimmune processes, and genetic factors have all been implicated. Patients with pulmonary hemosiderosis may be classified clinically as:

1. Idiopathic pulmonary hemosiderosis;
2. Associated with other diseases: cow's milk hypersensitivity (Heiner's syndrome), glomerulonephritis (Goodpasture's syndrome), and myocarditis;
3. Secondary pulmonary hemosiderosis: with primary cardiac disease, with collagen vascular disease, and with hemorrhagic disease.

The typical clinical picture consists of episodes of dyspnea, cough, hemoptysis, and often pallor. Fever, wheezing, and widespread rales may accompany the acute attack. Anemia, leukocytosis, and an elevated sedimentation rate are usually present, and chest roentgenograms may show mottled shadows in the perihilar region, and diffuse speckling in the more peripheral portions of the lung fields.

Sometimes bleeding into the alveoli is occult and chronic iron deficiency anemia with pallor is the single initial finding. The course may be chronic, but more often it is characterized by recurrent acute episodes, sometimes associated with gross hemoptysis or melena.

The recurrent pulmonary bleeding leads to the widespread deposition of hemosiderin in the interstitial portions of the lung, frequently followed by extensive fibrosis. The course is unpredictable and about 50 percent of the patients die within 5 years of the onset of illness. The usual cause of death is respiratory insufficiency from massive intrapulmonary hemorrhage.

Diagnosis is made by finding extensive iron-laden macrophages (siderophages) in sputum or tracheobronchial washings. In patients with unexplained pulmonary disease accompanied by iron deficiency anemia, the finding of siderophages in early morning gastric aspirates is presumptive evidence of pulmonary hemosiderosis. Open lung biopsy is diagnostic; the findings include alveolar epithelial hyperplasia, large numbers of siderocytes, varying amounts of interstitial fibrosis, and sclerotic vascular changes. Because of the risks involved, lung biopsy should not be considered essential for diagnosis in all cases. Needle aspiration biopsy of the lung has been recommended, but serious complications have followed this procedure and we prefer open lung biopsy if the diagnosis remains obscure.

Most cases of pulmonary hemosiderosis have no obvious cause and are considered idiopathic.

Hypersensitivity to cow's milk appears to be the inciting trigger in a group of patients described by Heiner. In addition to the typical clinical picture described above, these children had unusually high titers of serum precipitins to multiple constituents of cow's milk, positive intradermal skin tests to various cow's milk proteins, chronic rhinitis, recurrent otitis media, and growth retardation. The symptoms improved when cow's milk was removed from the diet, and returned with reintroduction of milk. A few children without multiple precipitins in their serum have improved clinically on a milk-free diet. A 1-month trial of a milk-free diet is probably indicated in any child with pulmonary hemosiderosis. Recently, Boat and colleagues have reported a group of infants with high titers of milk precipitins, pulmonary hemosiderosis, and cor pulmonale secondary to nasopharyngeal obstruction due to enlarged adenoids. Improvement followed 5 to 21 days after initiation of a milk-free diet.

Pulmonary hemosiderosis associated with *acute membranous or proliferative glomerulonephritis (Goodpasture's syndrome)* is clinically indistinguishable from idiopathic pulmonary hemosiderosis. This is primarily a disease of young adults and is rarely encountered in children. The clinical picture is usually initiated by pulmonary involvement with hemoptysis and iron deficiency anemia. The glomerulonephritis tends to be progressive, and hypertension and renal failure are common. The pulmonary disease has cleared rapidly in a few patients following bilateral nephrectomy but has remained unchanged in others (see also Chap 26, p. 1277).

Pulmonary hemosiderosis with associated myocarditis is encountered occasionally, and the myocardial disease may be minimal or extensive. It is often difficult to determine if the pulmonary hemosiderosis is primary or secondary to the cardiac involvement.

Intrapulmonary bleeding is seen in the clinical course of collagen vascular disease and occasionally may be the presenting symptom. Hemorrhagic disorders, including anaphylactoid purpura, have presented a picture indistinguishable from idiopathic pulmonary hemosiderosis.

Treatment of pulmonary hemosiderosis involves packed red cell transfusions for severe anemia and oral iron therapy. Corticosteroids seem to limit acute bleeding episodes but probably have little effect on the long-term progress of the disease. Immunosuppressant drugs (Azathiaprine) have been reported to help some patients. A trial on a milk-free diet in young infants and children is probably worthwhile.

Collagen Diseases

The collagen diseases involve many organ systems and include polyarteritis nodosa, rheumatoid arthritis, lupus erythematosus, scleroderma, dermatomyositis, and rheumatic fever. The cellular pattern of the pulmonary lesions in these conditions is similar and resembles the changes in interstitial tissue of other organs. In the initial stages there is an accumulation of mucopolysaccharides, water, and granular eosinophilic material in the interstitial spaces, which widens the interalveolar septa. Lymphocytes, monocytes, and plasma cells invade the interstitial space, particularly the peribronchiolar and periarteriolar regions. Later, there is a proliferation of fibroblasts and the formation of fibrous tissue.

When the collagen diseases involve the lung, the principal signs and symptoms are dyspnea, cyanosis, nonproductive cough, clubbing of the fingers, and occasional basilar rales. Chest roentgenograms show a nonspecific, diffuse parenchymal infiltration. The vital capacity, lung compliance, and arterial oxygen saturation are usually reduced. The use of corticosteroids (Prednisone 1 to 2 mg/kg/day) may be successful in the treatment of the pulmonary manifestations of collagen disease when the interstitial inflammation is acute. However, corticosteroids are of little value in the later stages when there is widespread fibrosis.

The lungs are involved in more than half the cases of systemic lupus erythematosus. The lesions tend to be proliferative and usually respond well to corticosteroids. Chloroquine may increase the effectiveness of steroid therapy.

Scleroderma usually affects the lung. Progressive sclerotic involvement of the muscles of the chest wall may limit respiration and cause hypoventilation, but this is not the main source of the respiratory insufficiency. When the lungs are involved, there is a diffuse, interstitial fibrosis, which may thicken the alveolar walls and obliterate the alveoli or partially obstruct small airways, overdistend alveoli, and cause cysts. The pulmonary blood vessels may be encased in collagenous sheaths that obliterate their lumina.

Other Diseases

PULMONARY ALVEOLAR PROTEINOSIS. This is a rare chronic disease of the lung in which there is an intraalveolar deposition of PAS-positive proteinaceous material rich in lipids. The condition is characterized by dyspnea associated with a cough, which is productive of yellow sputum, fatigue, and weight loss. Physical examination may reveal a few scattered rales and, rarely, clubbing of the fingers and toes. Chest radiographs show a fine, diffuse perihilar, radiating, feathery, or vaguely nodular density similar to that seen in pulmonary edema.

Definitive diagnosis requires open lung biopsy. Immunodeficiency states have been found in some patients with pulmonary alveolar proteinosis, possibly explaining the coincidence of bacterial and fungal infections that occur with this disease.

The clinical picture and histologic appearance of the lung in some patients are similar to those with desquamative interstitial pneumonitis. Corticosteroids and pulmonary lavage have been recommended, but there is little evidence that they change the progressive pulmonary involvement in children, which usually leads to death from respiratory failure within a year from the onset of the disease.

PULMONARY ALVEOLAR MICROLITHIASIS. This is a rare disease in which small deposits of calcium carbonate slowly fill the lungs. In roentgenograms, the lungs are stippled with fine foci of calcium densities concentrated in the central segments and the bases. The apices and lateral segments are spared. Microscopically, the alveoli are filled with microcalculi with no reaction in the interstitial tissue. Serum concentrations of calcium and phosphorus are always normal. The patients are usually without symptoms early in the course of the disease. As the disease progresses pulmonary insufficiency and right heart failure appear. There is no known treatment.

LIPID PNEUMONIA. This is a chronic pulmonary disease, that follows the aspiration of fats or oils. The use of oily nose drops was responsible for most of the reported cases. Lately, this condition has become increasingly rare, since the risk of using oily nose drops has become generally appreciated.

The pathologic changes depend to some extent on the type of oil aspirated. Fats that have a high content of free fatty acids cause an intense, acute inflammatory reaction in the lung, which may result in localized abscesses or areas of gangrene. More characteristic is the picture produced by bland oils, such as mineral oil. These cause an outpouring of mononuclear phagocytes, which absorb the oil until they are filled with fine droplets, giving them a foamlike appearance. These cells then enter the interalveolar septa and are carried up the lymphatics to the hilar lymph nodes. There is a proliferation of alveolar epithelium, and occasional interalveolar giant cells are formed.

The onset of the condition is insidious. Often there are no symptoms, the condition being discovered accidentally on roentgenography. There may be a dry, unproductive cough, tachypnea, and weight loss. Physical examination may show nothing abnormal, or there may be signs typical of bronchitis or pneumonitis. Chest roentgenograms show radiodensities of a nonspecific nature. The prognosis of uncomplicated lipid pneumonia is good. There is no specific therapy.

Bibliography

INTERSTITIAL PNEUMONITIS CAUSED BY INFECTIOUS AGENTS

Clyde WA, Denny FW Jr: The etiology and therapy of atypical pneumonia. Med Clin North Am 47:1201, 1963

Clyde W, Denny FW Jr: Mycoplasma infections in childhood. Pediatrics 40:669, 1967

Deamer WC, Zollinger HU: Interstitial "plasma cell" pneumonia of premature and young infants. Pediatrics 12:11, 1953

Drew WK, Finley TN, Mintz L, et al: Diagnosis of *pneumocystis carinii* pneumonia in children with cancer: diagnosis and treatment. JAMA 230:713, 1974

Johnson HD, Johnson WW: *Pneumocystis carinii* pneumonia in children with cancer. JAMA 214:1067, 1970

Richman DD, Zamvil L. Remington JS: Recurrent *pneumocystic carinii* pneumonia in a child with hypogammaglobulinemia. Am J Dis Child 125:102, 1973

Snyder CH: Visceral larva migrans. Pediatrics 28:85, 1961

Walzer PD, Schultz MG, Western KA, et al: *Pneumocystis carinii* pneumonia and primary immune deficiency diseases of infancy and childhood. J Pediatr 82:416, 1973

Wang JJ, Freeman AI, Gaeta JF, et al: Unusual complications of pentamidine in the treatment of *pneumocystis carinii* pneumonia. J Pediatr 77:311, 1970

Wright HT: Acute respiratory infections. Curr Probl Pediatr 5:49, 1974

PARAQUAT

Bullivant CM: Accidental poisoning by paraquat: report of 2 cases in man. Br Med J 1:1272, 1966

INTESTINAL PNEUMONITIS CAUSED BY CHEMICAL AGENTS

Bergeson PS, Hales SW, Lustgarten MD, et al: Pneumatoceles following hydrocarbon ingestion. Am J Dis Child 129:49, 1975

Bratton L, Haddow JE: Ingestion of charcoal lighter fluid. J Pediatr 77:633, 1975

Daeschner CW Jr, Blattner RJ, Collins VP: Hydrocarbon penumonitis. Pediatr Clin North Am: 243, Feb 1957

Eade NR, Taussig LM, Marks MI: Hydrocarbon pneumonitis. Pediatrics 54:351, 1974

Haggerty RJ: Toxic hazards: furniture polish. N Engl J Med 260:835, 1959

Hatthes FT, Kirschner R, Yow MD, et al: Acute poisoning associated with inhalation of mercury vapor. Report of four cases. Pediatrics 22:675, 1958

Jiminez JP, Lester RG: Pulmonary complications following furniture polish ingestion, report of 21 cases. Am J Roentgenol 98:323, 1966

Lesser LI, Weens HS, McKey JD: Pulmonary manifestations following ingestion of kerosene. J Pediatr 23:352, 1943

Lowry T, Schuman LM: Silo-filler's disease—a syndrome caused by nitrogen dioxide. JAMA 162:153, 1956

Lund JS, Feldt-Rasmussen M: Accidental aspiration of talcum (report of a case in a 2 year old). Acta Pediatr Scand 58:255, 1969

Olson ET: Occurrence of silo-filler's disease in children. J Pediatr 64:724, 1964

Park S, Giamonna S: Toxic effects of tear gas on an infant following prolonged exposure. Am J Dis Child 123:245, 1972

Pearlman ME, Finkler JF, Creason JP, et al: Nitrogen dioxide and lower respiratory illness. Pediatrics 47:391, 1971

INTERSTITIAL PNEUMONITIS DUE TO HYPERSENSITIVITY

Banaszak EF, Thiede WH, Fink JN: Hypersensitivity pneumonitis due to contamination of an air conditioner. N Engl J Med 283:271, 1970

Bergner A, Bergner RK: Pulmonary hypersensitivity associated with pancreatin powder exposure. Pediatrics 55:814, 1975

Campbell JM: Acute symptoms following work with hay. Br Med J 2:1143, 1932

Emanuel DA, Wenzel FJ, Bowerman CI, et al: Farmer's lung: clinical, pathologic, and immunologic study of twenty-four patients. Am J Med 37:392, 1964

Emanuel DA, Wenzel FJ, Lawton BR: Pneumonitis due to *Cryptostroma corticale* (maple-bark disease). N Engl J Med 274:1413, 1966

Gell PGH, Coombs RRA: Classification of allergic reactions responsible for clinical hypersensitivity and disease. In Gell PGH, Coombs RRA (eds): Clinical Aspects of Immunology, 3rd ed. Blackwell Scientific Publications, Oxford, 1900,

Hughes WF, Mattimore JM, Arbesman CE: Farmer's lung in an adolescent boy. Am J Dis Child 118:777, 1969

McCombs RP: Diseases due to immunologic reactions in the lungs. N Engl J Med 286:1186, 1245, 1972

Parish WE, Pepys J: The lung in allergic disease. In Gell PGH, Coombs RRA (eds): Clinical Aspects of Immunology, 3rd ed. Blackwell Scientific Publications, Oxford, 1900,

Pepys J: Hypersentivity diseases of the lungs due to fungi and organic dusts. S Karger, New York, 1969.

SARCOIDOSIS

Beier FR, Lahey ME: Sarcoidosis among children in Utah and Idaho. J Pediatr 65:350, 1964

Committee on Therapy, American Thoracic Society: Treatment of sarcoidosis. Am Rev Resp Dis 103:433, 1971

Kendig EL: The clinical picture of sarcoidosis in children. Pediatrics 54:289, 1974

McGovern JP, Merritt DH: Sarcoidosis in childhood. Adv Pediatr 8:97, 1956

Mitchell DN, Scadding JG: Sarcoidosis—state of the art. Am Rev Resp Dis 110:774, 1974

Morse SI, Cohn ZA, Hirsch JG, Schaedler RW: The treatment of sarcoidosis with chloroquine. Am J Med 30:779, 1961

Siltzbach LE, Greenberg GM: Childhood sarcoidosis—a study of 18 patients. N Engl J Med 279:1239, 1968

DIFFUSE INTERSTITIAL PULMONARY FIBROSIS (HAMMAN-RICH)

Bradley CA III: Diffuse interstitial fibrosis of the lungs in children. J Pediatr 48:442, 1956

Brown CH, Turner-Warwick M: The treatment of cryptogenic fibrosing alveolitis with immunosuppressant drugs. Q J Med 40:289, 1971

Hamman L, Rich AR: Acute diffuse interstitial fibrosis of lungs. Bull Hopkins Hosp 74:177, 1944

Talner NS, Howatt WF, DeMuth GR, et al: The syndrome of alveolar-capillary block. Pediatrics 27:227, 1961

DESQUAMATIVE INTERSTITIAL PNEUMONITIS

Barnes SE, Godfrey S, Millward-Sadler GH, Roberton NRC: Desquamative fibrosing alveolitis unresponsive to steroids and cytotoxic therapy. Arch Dis Child 50:324, 1975

Buchta RM, Park S, Giammona ST: Desquamative interstitial phenomena in a 7-week old infant. Am J Dis Child 120:341, 1970

Gaensler EA, Godd AM, Prowse CM: Desquamative interstitial pneumonia. N Engl J Med 274:113, 1966

Liebow AA, Steer A, Billingsley JG: Desquamative interstitial pneumonia. Am J Med 39:369, 1965

————Desquamative interstitial pneumonia. In Kendig EL (ed): Disorders of the Respiratory Tract in Children, Vol 1. WB Saunders, Philadelphia, 1972, p 325

Rosenow EC, O'Connell EJ, Harrison EG Jr: Desquamative interstitial pneumonia in children. Am J Dis Child 120:344, 1970

IDIOPATHIC PULMONARY HEMOSIDEROSIS

Allue X, Wise MB, Beaudry PH: Pulmonary function studies in idiopathic pulmonary hemosiderosis in childhood. Am Rev Resp Dis 107:410, 1973

Boat TF, Polmar SH, Whitman V, et al: Hyperreactivity to cow milk in young children with pulmonary hemosiderosis and cor pulmonale secondary to nasopharyngeal obstruction. J Pediatr 87:23, 1975

Cooper AS: Idiopathic pulmonary hemosiderosis. N Engl J Med 263:1100, 1960

Gilman PA, Zinkham WH: Severe idiopathic pulmonary hemosiderosis in the absence of clinical or radiologic evidence of pulmonary disease. J Pediatr 75:118, 1969

Heiner DC, Sears JW, Kniker WT: Multiple precipitins to cow's milk in chronic respiratory disease. Am J Dis Child 103:40, 1962

Irvin JM, Snowden PW: Idiopathic pulmonary hemosiderosis. Am J Dis Child 93:182, 1957

Soergel KH, Sommers SC: Idiopathic pulmonary hemosiderosis and related syndromes. Am J Med 32:499, 1962

COLLAGEN DISEASE

Baker LA, David D: Pulmonary manifestations of collagen diseases. Med Clin North Am 43:145, 1959

Brinkman GL, Chaikof L: Rheumatoid lung disease: report of a case which developed in childhood. Am Rev Resp Dis 80:732, 1959

Dubowitz LMS, Dubowitz V: Acute dermatomyositis presenting with pulmonary manifestations. Arch Dis Child 39:293, 1964

Goldring D, Behrer MR, Brown G, Elliott G: Rheumatic pneumonitis. Part II. Report on the clinical and laboratory findings in twenty-three patients. J Pediatr 53:547, 1958

Martel W, Abell M, Mikkelson WM, Whitehouse WM: Pulmonary and pleural lesions in rheumatoid disease. Radiology 90:641, 1968

Meisin AG, Rothfield N: Systemic lupus erythematosus in childhood. Pediatrics 42:37, 1968

Melam H, Patterson R: Periarteritis nodosa. Am J Dis Child 121:424, 1971

Ziff M, Esserman P, McEwen C: Observations on the course and treatment of systemic lupus erythematosus. Arthritis Rheum 1:332, 1958

PULMONARY ALVEOLAR PROTEINOSIS

Bhagwat AG, Wentworth P, Conen PE: Observations on the relationship of desquamative interstitial pneumonia and pulmonary alveolar proteinosis in childhood: a pathological and experimental study. Dis Chest 58:326, 1970

Colon AR Jr, Lawrence RD, Mills SD, O'Connell EJ: Childhood pulmonary alveolar proteinosis. Am J Dis Child 121:481, 1971

Danigelis JA, Markarian B: Pulmonary alveolar proteinosis including pulmonary electron microscopy. Am J Dis Child 118:871, 1969

Ramirez J: Pulmonary alveolar proteinosis, treatment by massive bronchopulmonary lavage. Arch Intern Med 119:147, 1967

Rosen SH, Castleman D, Liebow AA: Pulmonary alveolar proteinosis. N Engl J Med 258:1123, 1958

Wilkinson RH, Blanc WA, Haystrom JWC: Pulmonary alveolar proteinosis in three infants. Pediatrics 41:510, 1968

LIPID PNEUMONIA

Balakrishan S: Lipoid pneumonia in infants and children in South India. Br Med J 4:329, 1973

Bromer RS, Wolman IJ: Lipoid pneumonia in infants and children. Radiology 32:1, 1939

Goodwin TC: Lipoid cell penumonia. Am J Dis Child 48:309, 1934

Laughlen GF: Studies on pneumonia following nasopharyngeal injections of oil. Am J Pathol 1:407, 1925

PULMONARY ALVEOLAR MICROLITHIASIS

Balikian JP: Pulmonary alveolar microlithiasis: report of five cases with special reference to roentgen manifestations. Am J Roentgenol 103:509, 1968

Caffrey PR, Altman RS: Pulmonary alveolar microlithiasis occurring in premature twins. J Pediatr 66:758, 1965

Clark RB, Johnson FC: Idiopathic pulmonary alveolar microlithiasis. Pediatrics 28:650, 1961

Rotem Y, Solomon M, Hertz-Frankenhuis M: Pulmonary alveolar microlithiasis. Ann Pediatr 201:4, 1963

CHEST WALL DISEASES

ROBERT H. GREGG

The Chest Wall

Air moves in and out of the lung in response to changes in the intrathoracic pressure, which, in turn, follow changes in intrathoracic volume. The volume changes are initiated by the chest wall and the diaphragm, working as a unit. In addition to its respiratory function, the chest wall serves an obvious protective function.

THE RIB CAGE. The motion of the rib cage has been carefully studied in adult man but not in children. In the adult, the principal and probably only motion is at the point of articulation with the spine, around the axis of the neck of the rib. Because the ribs slope downward and forward, this motion raises the sternum and increases the anteroposterior diameter of the rib cage (Fig. 52), most evident in the upper six ribs. Rotation of the heads of the seventh to tenth ribs results in slight depression of the lower sternum, but these ribs effectively increase the intrathoracic volume by increasing the lateral diameter of the chest.

The angle of the rib neck and the course and curvature of the ribs, which account for this effect, are not easy to visualize without a three-dimensional model. Such a model can be improvised by making a semicircle with the thumb and forefinger, with the thumb representing the head of the rib at the articulation with the spine and the tip of the forefinger representing the sternal end of the rib. The ribs slope downward and forward, so the head of the rib at the spine (the thumb) is higher than the sternal end (the finger). Rotate the

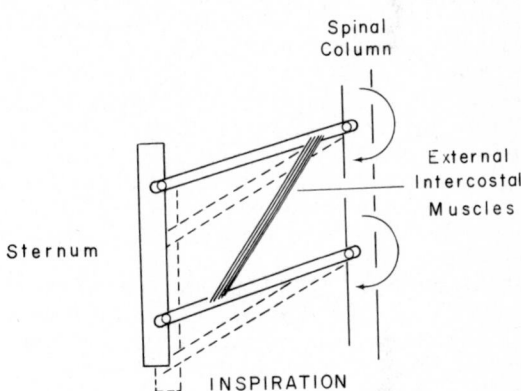

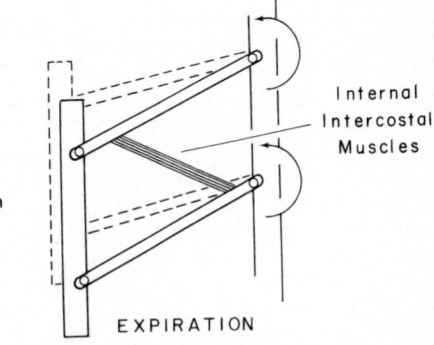

FIG. 52. Action of the upper ribs and the intercostal muscles. Inspiration: Contraction of the external intercostal muscles elevates the ribs and sternum and increases the anterior-posterior diameter of the chest. Expiration: With expiration the sternum decends and with forced expiration the internal intercostal muscles contract. (Modified from Fenn: Sci Amer 202:142, 1960.)

semicircle on the thumb tip around the long axis of the distal phalanx of the thumb, and note that the motion raises and lowers the "sternal" end of the model, and represents the motion of the upper ribs.

The Respiratory Musculature

DIAPHRAGM. The diaphragm is the most important of the respiratory muscles, and its action accounts for approximately two-thirds of the tidal exchange during quiet breathing. As the diaphragm contracts, the central portion moves downward like a piston. The pistonlike descent is limited by increasing intraabdominal pressure. At this point, the diaphragm retains its domed shape, and many of its muscle fibers are in a nearly vertical direction along the chest wall. As contraction continues, upward traction is exerted on the costal margin, enlarging the rib cage. In addition, the increased intraabdominal pressure probably results in a direct upward force on the rib cage, so that diaphragmatic action causes both a pull from above and a push from below on the rib margins. The term *diaphragmatic* or *abdominal breathing* usually applied to newborn infants has little meaning, since the relative expansion of the chest and abdomen depends more on the compliance of these structures than on which muscles are active.

INTERCOSTAL MUSCLES. The external intercostals, which contract during quiet inspiration, slant downward and forward between the ribs. When they contract, they raise the ribs (Fig. 52). The internal intercostals, which are active only during forced expiration, run in the opposite direction; when they contract, the ribs are forced downward and the thoracic volume is decreased.

MECHANICS OF THORACIC MOTION. Inspiration is always an active process; the work is done by the diaphragm and the external intercostals. During quiet breathing, only small pressure changes are required, and the energy consumed is only a small fraction of the basal metabolic needs. When forceful inspiration is required, there is augmented contraction of the diaphragm and external intercostals, and accessory muscles of inspiration are used. The most important of these are the sternocleidomastoid and the strap muscles of the neck. Additional chest expansion can be achieved by extension of the trunk. This mechanism is used when ventilatory needs are great. In patients with extreme respiratory distress, the platysma becomes active. Its contraction is ineffectual in increasing ventilation, but it does distort the mouth with each breath, causing the ominous sign called *fishmouthing*.

Quiet expiration is passive, powered only by the elastic recoil of the lung. During forceful expiration the internal intercostals contract (Fig. 52). In cases of severe expiratory obstruction or increased ventilatory needs the musculature of the abdominal wall is also used. These muscles increase the intraabdominal pressure and push the diaphragm up. In addition, they decrease intrathoracic volume by flexing the trunk and by pulling the lower costal margins toward the midline. These are strong muscles capable of sustaining an in-

traabdominal and, hence, intrathoracic pressure of 100 torr. A transient rise to 200 or 300 torr occurs with vigorous coughing and is a necessary part of this protective reflex.

In children with acute illnesses, which cause cough or expiratory obstruction, muscular cramps often cause pain and tenderness of the abdominal wall; the presenting symptom may be abdominal pain. In children with chronic respiratory obstruction or cough, the abdominal wall musculature is often visibly and palpably hypertrophied.

CHANGES WITH GROWTH. The chest wall of the infant differs in several anatomic respects from that of an older child or adult. The wall is much more compliant and flexible, the shape is more nearly round, and the ribs have a more horizontal course. These anatomic differences impose no apparent functional handicap, although diaphragmatic paralysis does not seem to be tolerated as well in infancy as in the adult.

The rounded shape of the chest present at birth changes rapidly to the flattened ellipse found in older children and adults. The lateral diameter of the chest increases more rapidly than the anterior-posterior dimension. The ratio of the antero-posterior to lateral diameter is 0.93 at birth and 0.78 at 1 year of age and approaches the value of 0.69 found in older children by the age of 2 years.

Neuromotor Diseases that Impair Ventilation

A decrease in ventilatory capacity occurs when the nerve supply of any of the respiratory muscles is lost or these muscles are unable to respond to neural stimulation. Neuromotor weakness limits the ability of the respiratory musculature to expand the thorax. This is easily quantitated by measuring vital capacity but, since a large reserve of ventilatory capacity is present normally, small losses of effective muscle strength do not interfere with normal ventilation. The first clinical symptom of respiratory weakness is decreased force in coughing, since a large increase in intrathoracic pressure is necessary for effective coughing. When the cough is weak, secretions may accumulate and cause atelectasis.

If the disability becomes more severe, an increased effort is required to maintain tidal volume at the normal level, and the patient finds it easier to breathe rapidly and shallowly. Rapid, shallow breathing, without occasional deep breaths or sighs, leads to the development of focal areas of atelectasis, and the compliance of the lungs decreases. As the lungs become more stiff, expansion is even more difficult, tidal volume decreases further, alveolar hypoventilation occurs, and the carbon dioxide tension of blood increases. Hypoventilation and a physiologic right-to-left shunt in the atelectatic areas decrease oxygen tension in arterial blood.

The child becomes anxious and frightened and has an increased blood pressure and pulse rate; cyanosis and mental confusion are late signs. The diagnosis can be confirmed by arterial blood gas analysis. Slowly progressive ventilatory failure can be difficult to diagnose. Initially, attention may be drawn away from the respiratory tract, since chronic hypoxemia may cause pulmonary hypertension and right-sided heart failure, polycythemia, or even symptoms suggestive of neurasthenia. However, a careful history, physical examination, and arterial blood gas analysis should identify the organ system primarily involved.

POLIOMYELITIS. Respiratory paralysis caused by poliomyelitis is now uncommon in immunized populations. Respiratory paralysis occurs during the acute phase of infection, either while the patient is febrile or shortly after the fever subsides. The extent of paralysis is spotty and asymmetric, so that no single pattern of breathing can be expected. The diaphragm is often involved, either partially or completely. Intercostal muscle paralysis is apt to be incomplete, since innervation of these muscles is randomly distributed. The physiologic changes common to other forms of respiratory paralysis are noted.

MANAGEMENT. Management of the acutely ill patient with respiratory failure poses a complex and often rapidly changing series of problems, which severely tax the ingenuity and judgment of the physician even if he is experienced in handling such cases. If severe impairment of respiratory muscle function alone is present, the tank respirator is indicated. It should be used when signs of respiratory decompensation are progressive and vital capacity reaches less than 50 percent of normal. For children, respiratory rates up to 30/minute with pressures of $+3$ to -12 or -15 cm H_2O, and for adults rates of 18/minute with pressures of $+3$ to -18, are recommended, but these must be adjusted to the individual case. Weaning from the tank respirator should begin within several days. The chest (cuirass) respirator and the rocking bed are useful adjuncts during the weaning period but are inadequate for handling acute stage of respiratory failure. In cases of bulbar involvement, with central respiratory failure and obstruction due to pooling of bronchotracheal secretions, continuous O_2 inhalation, postural drainage, and removal of secretions with a suction apparatus generally suffice. If these measures fail to keep the airway clear, a high tracheostomy is indicated. This procedure is also necessary if abductor paralysis of the vocal cords develops, or if there are repeated bouts of pulmonary atelectasis requiring tracheal aspiration and bronchoscopy. Adequately humidified O_2 is given through the tracheostomy tube in concentrations of 40 to 60 percent, although emergencies may necessitate 100 percent for brief periods. Positive pressure respiration through a cuffed tracheostomy tube may be substituted for the tank respirator in patients requiring artificial respiration. The tank respirator is contraindicated in bulbar poliomyelitis unless a tracheostomy has been performed so that adequate suctioning of secretions can be carried out.

GUILLAIN-BARRÉ SYNDROME. Respiratory paralysis occurs occasionally in this syndrome and is the usual cause of death in fatal cases. This condition is now probably more common than respiratory paralysis due to poliomyelitis. The onset of respiratory paralysis is gradual, often insidious, and difficult to detect in the early stages. The paralysis usually follows an ascending path and involves the intercostals before the diaphragm. Symmetric involvement is the rule in this illness, in contrast to the spotty paralysis of poliomyelitis. Complete recovery is expected in the Guillain-Barré syndrome (see p. 1864). The respiratory care is similar to that presented for poliomyelitis.

PROGRESSIVE INFANTILE SPINAL ATROPHY (WERDNIG-HOFFMAN SYNDROME). Progressive loss of anterior horn cells, leading to paralysis of respiratory and other musculature, is the hallmark of this lethal disease of infancy and early childhood. Death usually occurs before 5 years of age from ventilatory failure and intercurrent pneumonia. The intercostal muscles are severely involved, whereas diaphragmatic function is comparatively well preserved, giving the affected child a characteristic appearance. During inspiration, the chest wall collapses and the upper abdomen protrudes markedly, producing a see-saw or paradoxic pattern of breathing (Fig. 53). The child's cry is weak, and his cough is feeble and ineffective. As the disease progresses, the chest gradually becomes flattened in the anteroposterior diameter. This flattening, usually symmetric, is a particularly striking finding, since normal children of this age have a rounded chest. Long-term mechanical support of respiration is not recommended since recovery cannot occur. However, short-term respiratory support during an acute infection might be used, even though the course of the disease cannot be changed.

SPINAL CORD INJURY. Cord transections are an infrequent cause of childhood respiratory paralysis. A high cervical transection causes paralysis of both diaphragms and the intercostals, and is incompatible with prolonged survival. Transection between C5 and D1 will permit continued diaphragmatic function but will result in intercostal paralysis. With the diaphragm active and the intercostals paralyzed, the chest collapses

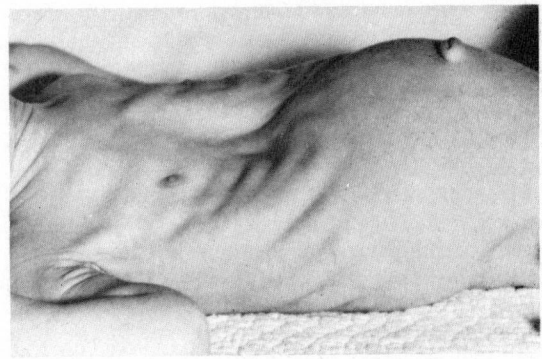

FIG. 53. A child with advanced infantile spinal atrophy during an inspiratory effort. Note that the diaphragm has descended and is distending the abdomen but the absence of effective intercostal muscle contraction has allowed the chest to collapse partially. The anterior-posterior diameter is decreased. From Dekabon: Neurology of Infancy, 1959. Courtesy of The Williams & Wilkins Co.)

and the abdomen protrudes on inspiration, as seen with infantile spinal atrophy.

DIAPHRAGMATIC PARALYSIS. Paralysis of one leaf of the diaphragm is noted occasionally in the newborn infant, particularly after difficult breech deliveries. If the phrenic nerve has been subjected to a stretch injury, the paralysis may be temporary; if actual avulsion of the roots of nerves from C3, 4, and 5 has occurred, the paralysis is permanent. Injuries of the brachial plexus are commonly associated with phrenic nerve injuries and are caused by the same type of birth trauma. Diaphragmatic paralysis may also occur as a rare complication of pneumonia, or following damage to the phrenic nerve during cardiac surgery.

When one leaf of the diaphragm is paralyzed, it moves higher in passive response to subatmospheric intrapleural pressure. After prolonged denervation, the muscle fibers atrophy and the diaphragmatic leaf moves still higher. After atrophy, when the diaphragm is inert and flaccid, paradoxic motion occurs quite regularly; on fluoroscopic examination, the diaphragm moves up with inspiration and down with expiration. Also the mediastinum may shift away from the paralyzed side on inspiration. These abnormal motions may be absent if some muscle tone remains or the paralysis is incomplete.

On physical examination there is an increased flaring motion of the lower costal margin on the involved side. This increase in motion on the paralyzed side is caused either by the absence of the diaphragmatic contraction that normally opposes this flaring motion or by a compensating increase in intercostal activity. The normal protrusion of the epigastrium, which occurs when the diaphragm contracts and descends, is not seen. The combination of abnormal and asymmetric movements of the epigastrium and the rib margins should suggest the diagnosis.

The loss of function resulting from diaphragmatic paralysis is variable. Healthy adults and older children tolerate complete paralysis of one leaf of the diaphragm without distress, and some newborn infants with diaphragmatic paralysis are also asymptomatic. However, most infants with paralysis of one diaphragmatic leaf have symptoms, and several deaths have been attributed to it. If respiratory distress does occur and the diaphragm is high and moves paradoxically and there is a mediastinal shift, surgical plication of the paralyzed leaf may be of benefit.

EVENTRATION OF THE DIAPHRAGM. A defect in the diaphragmatic muscle, allowing limited protrusion of abdominal contents into the thoracic cavity, is called an eventration. Small eventrations are minor anomalies but, when all of the muscle of one leaf of the diaphragm is missing, the remaining membrane is elevated and moves paradoxically. In this severe form of eventration, the functional handicap is the same as that seen in diaphragmatic paralysis of long duration, and it is often impossible to differentiate between the two conditions. Surgical repair of these defects is rarely required in older children. Occasionally in the newborn infant, an extremely large eventration may closely resemble a congenital diaphragmatic hernia, may cause severe respiratory symptoms, and does require surgical intervention.

MUSCULAR DYSTROPHY. Respiratory failure caused by muscular dystrophy occurs late in the course of the disease, most often involving adolescent or young adult patients. Patients with the myotonic form of muscular dystrophy may have a nearly normal vital capacity, even when alveolar hypoventilation and hypercapnea are present. This unusual combination of findings might be expected in this disease, since loss of the muscle's ability to relax precedes muscular atrophy. In the nonmyotonic forms of muscular dystrophy, seen more often in childhood, vital capacity and maximum voluntary ventilation are markedly reduced. Arterial oxygenation is maintained only by increased effort and by decreasing metabolic needs through inactivity.

MYASTHENIA GRAVIS. Myasthenia gravis can cause ventilatory failure at any age. In the usual form of this disease, ventilatory failure occurs only after ptosis and generalized weakness have been present for a prolonged period.

A transient form of myasthenia gravis sometimes occurs in newborn infants whose mothers have the disease. Respiratory failure may result in the infant's death a few hours after birth; if the infant can be kept alive with proper drug therapy and respiratory support, recovery occurs within a few weeks.

Structural Abnormalities of the Thorax

ROBERT H. GREGG

Some structural abnormalities of the thorax have only cosmetic significance. Others may limit thoracic motion; if the limitation is severe, alveolar hypoventilation can occur.

PECTUS EXCAVATUM. Pectus excavatum is a funnel-shaped depression of the anterior thorax caused by posterior displacement of the lower sternum. This common, often familial, deformity is usually inconspicuous or absent at birth, but develops over a period of months or years, for unknown reasons.

The physiologic importance of pectus excavatum has been the subject of much debate, but the objective data now available suggest that it is rarely, if ever, a cause of pulmonary disability. Small decreases of about 10 percent in total lung capacity, vital capacity, and maximum voluntary ventilation are found in children with this defect. Similar minor disturbances are noted in adults with pectus excavatum, so it is unlikely that there is a progression of symptoms with age. Surgical repair of the deformity has not resulted in improved pulmonary function.

Several findings in pectus excavatum are superficially suggestive of cardiac disease. The heart is displaced to the left by the sternum and may appear to be enlarged on an anterior-posterior roentgenogram. The change in cardiac position is also responsible for electrocardiographic abnormalities. A parasternal systolic murmur is heard in most children with pectus excavatum. Despite these findings cardiac catheterization is not apt to demonstrate any hemodynamic abnormality and should not be undertaken without compelling indication. However, recent studies of cardiac output during exercise in the upright position do suggest that the maximal cardiac output is limited in children with pectus excavatum, and improvement did occur after surgical correction of the deformity. These studies give credence to the suggestion of improved exercise tolerance after surgical repair.

Surgical repair of pectus excavatum is usually undertaken when the cosmetic defect is considered important enough to justify the procedure, but should be done only rarely before the deformity becomes stable at 3 to 4 years of age, since some improve spontaneously. Improved exercise tolerance may occur as a result of repair, but most children with pectus excavatum do not require any treatment. The operative procedure should carry little risk and the cosmetic results are usually acceptable.

A funnel chest is sometimes an acquired abnormality. Persistent sternal depression develops in children who have respiratory tract obstruction or parenchymal disease of the lung, requiring forceful inspiratory efforts that result in retractions of the sternum for a prolonged period. This is most apt to occur in young infants who have a soft, compliant thoracic wall. If the obstruction is relieved or the lung disease clears, the sternal depression will disappear rapidly in the infant but more slowly in the older child.

PECTUS CARINATUM. The "pigeon breast" deformity is less common than pectus excavatum and has not been as well studied. There is no evidence that this deformity causes cardiopulmonary disabilities, and treatment, if any, should be based on the need for cosmetic repair.

THORACIC DEFORMITY DUE TO BONE DYSPLASIA. In several forms of generalized bone dysplasia the thorax is small and causes neonatal asphyxia when the abnormality is severe. The interrelationships of this group of diseases are not clear. Achondroplasia is not included. This condition causes nasal obstruction and hence some respiratory distress, particularly in the newborn infant, but the chest is probably not abnormally small.

ASPHYXIATING THORACIC DYSTROPHY OF JEUNE. Is now being recognized quite frequently. Children with this genetically determined condition have a small, bell-shaped thorax, and at postmortem examination, somewhat small lungs as well. Respiratory insufficiency may occur in the newborn period or in association with intercurrent infections in older infants. The affected children seem to improve with age and growth; if they survive infancy, their respiratory limitations may decrease. Other features of this illness are polydactyly, dysplasia of the pelvis, short stature, and sometimes an unusual and severe form of renal disease (Fig. 54).

Similar thoracic deformities are seen in *chondroectodermal dysplasia*, or the Ellis-van Creveld syndrome, another form of generalized bone dysplasia and

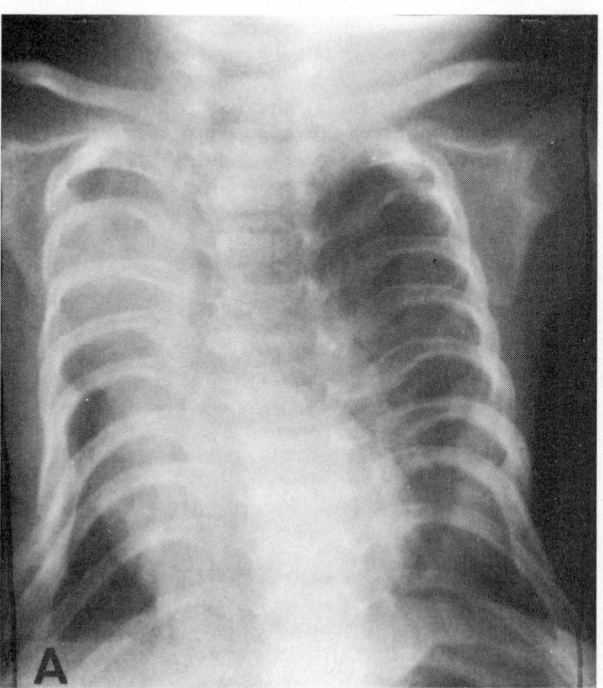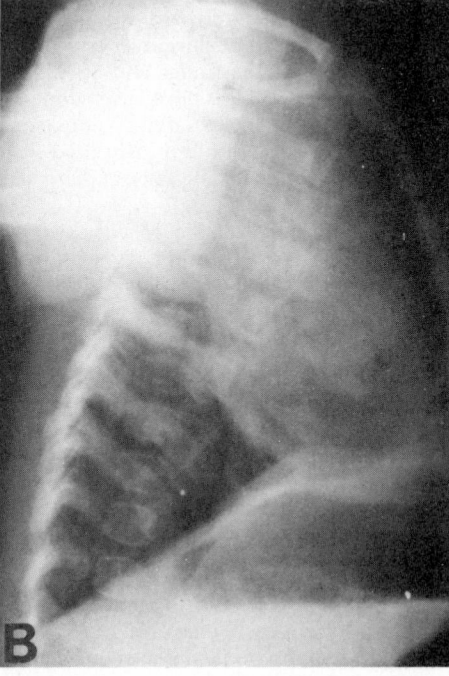

FIG. 54. Roentgenograms of newborn infant with more severe reduction in chest volume due to thoracic dystrophy of Jeune. Note the bell-shaped chest,

dwarfism. The distal portions of the extremities are foreshortened more than the proximal segments. The nails are dystrophic, and the teeth and hair are hypoplastic. The thorax is small and bell-shaped, much like that described in patients with the thoracic dystrophy of Jeune. Since these children seem to improve with age, sternal splitting procedures to increase intrathoracic volume have been recommended, but there is little experience with them.

Thanatophoric dwarfism causes neonatal death (thanatophoric = death-bringing) from asphyxia. The chest is tiny, rigid, and bell-shaped, a combination that produces inadequate aeration of the lung. Although the general body configuration suggests an extreme form of achondroplasia, thanatophoric dwarfism is a distinct entity. Some of the neonatal deaths attributed to achondroplasia may, in fact, be caused by this disease.

ACHONDROPLASIA. Children with the usual heterozygotic form of achondroplasia do not have a disproportionately small thorax. However, the rare instances of homozygotic achondroplasia resemble thanatophoric dwarfism in that these babies have tiny chests and early respiratory failure (see Chap 32, p. 2006).

ACHONDROGENESIS. Achondrogenesis is characterized by micromelic dwarfism and a small chest. Most such infants are stillborn or die from asphyxia soon after birth (see Chap 32, p. 2006).

OTHER CONGENITAL ANOMALIES OF THE THORAX. The sternum is formed by midline fusion of paired sternal bands. A *failure of fusion* of the upper portion of the sternum leaves the mediastinum covered only by skin and subcutaneous tissue, which moves paradoxically with respiration. The absence of supporting bone allows this area to be forced inward with inspiration and to protrude with expiration. Surgical repair is advised to protect the upper mediastinum and to improve the child's appearance. Repair is most easily done in young infants. Severe defects of sternal fusion expose the heart (ectopia cordis), are often associated with other major cardiovascular malformations, and are usually fatal.

Occasionally, *congenital absence of portions of ribs* leaves an area of the chest wall unsupported by bone; such areas move paradoxically with respiration, much like the sternal cleft defects. Children who have large defects that cause functional disability are candidates for surgical repair. However, in most instances the bone defects are small, the children are asymptomatic, and surgical correction is unnecessary.

KYPHOSCOLIOSIS. The chest may be deformed by forward angulation (kyphosis) or lateral curves (scoliosis of the spine). These are relatively common in childhood and result from neuromuscular disease, vertebral anomalies, neurofibromatosis, and from unknown causes. These deformities become progressively more severe with growth and tend to stabilize after growth ceases. Patients with early onset of kyphoscoliosis and persistent progression of the deformity develop cardiopulmonary handicaps; their total lung volume and vital capacity are reduced. Lung compliance is also reduced, probably because of uneven ventilation, focal atelecta-

sis, and the inability to take occasional deep breaths. The chest wall remains surprisingly compliant in children but becomes abnormally rigid in early adult life. These changes increase the work of respiration and lead to rapid, shallow breathing, which minimizes energy expenditures but results in alveolar hypoventilation. The carbon dioxide tension of arterial blood increases and arterial oxygen tension decreases. Oxygen tension is further decreased by a shuntlike effect in atelectatic areas. The hypoxemia causes constriction of the pulmonary arterioles, increased pulmonary arterial pressure, and right ventricular hypertrophy. Cardiopulmonary failure and death occur in the late stages of this progression.

If cardiopulmonary failure is to be prevented, treatment must be started in childhood when the severity of this deformity increases most rapidly. Braces and casts may slow or halt the progression of idiopathic scoliosis, but surgical correction is usually required for those cases due to congenital abnormalities or to asymmetric paralysis. In addition to close orthopedic supervision, vital capacity and other pulmonary functions should be measured regularly. A decreasing vital capacity is an ominous sign, since values under 60 percent of the expected normal are associated with eventual cardiopulmonary failure. Surgical correction of the deformity slows or halts the deterioration in pulmonary function, with a gratifying improvement after prolonged follow-up. The prolonged immobilization required in the postoperative period is surprisingly well tolerated.

OBESITY AND CARDIOPULMONARY FAILURE (PICKWICKIAN SYNDROME). An accumulation of fat on the chest wall acts like a binder, limiting expansion and squeezing the chest enough so that lung volume at end-expiration is reduced. This reduction in volume allows some lung units to close, which in turn causes loss of compliance of the lung itself. This loss of compliance in both the lung and the chest wall greatly adds to the work of breathing. Further, a shunt effect occurs where the airways have closed, causing hypoxemia.

These handicaps are well tolerated by most obese persons, but some progress to hypoventilation, cyanosis, plethora, cor pulmonale, periodic breathing, and somnolence (the Pickwickian syndrome). Why only some obese patients develop this syndrome is incompletely understood; the degree of obesity is not the only factor. Nocturnal upper airway obstruction (snoring) is a critical additive in some instances and abnormal function of the respiratory center may play some role. In extreme cases, artificial ventilation may be needed but weight reduction is essential for improvement.

CONNECTIVE TISSUE DISEASES THAT AFFECT THE CHEST WALL. Rheumatoid spondylitis, infrequent in children, may, in its severe form, cause complete immobility of the spine and the rib cage. The chest becomes fixed in a position of partial inspiration, so that functional residual volume is increased and vital capacity is decreased. When the thorax is rigid the diaphragm becomes solely responsible for ventilation, but this causes no major pulmonary disability.

PROGRESSIVE SYSTEMIC SCLEROSIS (SCLERODERMA). This condition may be associated with a rapid respiratory rate, breathlessness, and a decrease in compliance of the lungs. Since the soft tissues become rigid, it has been suggested that the primary loss of compliance is in the chest wall, ie, a "hidebound" chest. This suspicion is not substantiated by careful studies which demonstrate that parenchymal involvement of the lung itself is the principal abnormality causing a loss of pulmonary compliance (p. 1587).

TRAUMA. Multiple fractures of the ribs or costal cartilages from crushing chest trauma may cause a *flail* chest. The rib cage loses its rigidity and its ability to function as the framework for the respiratory bellows. Chest wall motion becomes paradoxic; the crushed section collapses on inspiration and bulges on expiration. Although the chest wall of a child is resilient and resistant to trauma, crush injuries do occur when the injuring force is large. Adequate ventilation often requires continuous positive pressure respiratory assistance. The positive pressure inflates the lungs and the inflated lung serves as an internal splint for the crushed chest wall. Contusion of the lung, causing a fluffy shadow on the roentgenogram, may occur in the absence of rib fractures.

Pleural Diseases

Robert H. Gregg

Pleural disease may restrict ventilation in two ways: collection of fluid or air in the pleural space may compress one or both lungs; or scarring of the pleura, following hemothorax or empyema, may envelop the lung in a rigid fibrous coating that severely limits expansion. The ventilatory restriction in pleural disease is often marked, even when the roentgenographic abnormality is not striking.

EMPYEMA. Empyema was once frequent and usually followed pneumonococcal pneumonia. It is now infrequent but may be a complication of staphylococcal, streptococcal, or *H.influenzae* pneumonia. Staphylococcal empyema, the most severe type, and *H.influenzae* empyema occur most often in infants under 1 year of age; streptococcal empyema is more common in older children. The onset of major symptoms is abrupt, particularly in infants. The babies are usually seriously ill at the time they are first seen and appear gray, lethargic, tachypneic, and anxious. The nostrils flare with inspiration and an expiratory grunt is almost always present. The physical signs of empyema are easily recognized. The chest is dull to percussion throughout the involved side, and breath sounds are diminished on that side.

Whenever purulent fluid accumulates in the pleural space, it should be removed promptly. Occasionally, it is possible to evacuate thin and watery pleural fluid by thoracentesis, but catheter drainage of the intrapleural space is the preferred method. The catheter should be placed in a dependent position and connected to a water-sealed drainage system. The mechanics of the drainage system require careful and continuous attention, since the catheters often become obstructed by thick pus or may drain only a small and loculated portion of the pleural cavity. Inadequate or delayed drainage may leave purulent material in the pleural space, and permanently restrict motion of the lung and thorax. The fibrous scar can be successfully removed surgically by a decortication procedure; however, if the diagnosis can be made early in the course of the illness, and antibiotics and pleural drainage used properly, decortication procedures are rarely needed.

Pneumothorax occurs frequently in staphylococcal pneumonia and empyema, usually in the first day or two of hospitalization. A sudden increase in respiratory distress or rapid deterioration of the child's condition should suggest this possibility. Prompt removal of the trapped air by needle aspiration may be helpful momentarily, but in all such cases a catheter should then be inserted through the anterior chest wall into the pleural space and connected to a closed drainage system.

HEMOTHORAX. Collections of blood in the pleural space are usually caused by trauma. Blood is mildly irritating to the pleural surfaces and is not completely absorbed. If the blood is not removed, pleural scarring and fibrothorax follow.

SPONTANEOUS PNEUMOTHORAX. Four of five cases of spontaneous pneumothorax occur in older boys. The cause of these air leaks is not always known, but minor congenital anomalies of the lung are sometimes present and must always be suspected. A history of a cough or vigorous exercise sometimes, but not always, precedes the event; some episodes begin during sleep or quiet breathing.

Spontaneous pneumothorax usually does not cause serious illness. Sudden chest pain or discomfort occurs at the onset, and is the usual reason for seeking medical care. Dyspnea, if present, is not severe. No active treatment is required, early recovery can be expected, and recurrence is unlikely. A reversible Horner's syndrome occasionally accompanies left-sided pneumothorax. However, the condition is not always so benign. Collapse of the lung on the involved side may be complete, air in the pleural space may be trapped under pressure, the contralateral lung becomes compressed, and venous return to the heart may be impeded. Death may occur if the trapped pleural air is not removed promptly. Aspiration of air from the pleural cavity by thoracentesis will provide effective relief if no further air leak occurs, but in cases of tension pneumothorax a continuing leak is to be expected and the pleural air should be removed through a catheter inserted into the pleural cavity and connected to water-sealed drainage.

If a patient has recurrent episodes of pneumothorax, a thoracotomy should be performed in order to resect the source of air leak if it can be identified, and/or obliterate the pleural space. Either procedure should be effective in preventing further recurrences.

CHYLOTHORAX. A leak in the thoracic duct, or in the major lymph channels of the mediastinum which transport fat absorbed from the gut, allows chyle to accumulate in the intrapleural space. Lymph that leaks from the lungs or pleura is clear, and does not contain the fat characteristic of chyle. Chylothorax may occur after thoracic surgery, mediastinal tumors, or major trauma, but is most frequent in the neonatal period. Birth trauma is probably an important factor in these cases.

Chylothorax may not appear for several days or weeks after birth or after trauma. In these instances, the initial chyle leak may be into the mediastinal tissues, with delayed rupture into the pleural space. The clinical manifestations are those of any hydrothorax. As the pleural fluid gradually increases in volume, respiratory distress becomes more severe.

The chyle leak usually stops spontaneously and abruptly after an unpredictable interval of several days, weeks, or months. Thoracentesis and a diet based on casein and medium chain triglycerides should be tried, since the latter are transported through the portal circulation and not through the thoracic duct. Prompt clearing following the use of such a diet has been reported often.

When other methods fail the thoracic duct should be ligated and the pleural space obliterated. Such procedures are usually successful.

Bibliography

POLIOMYELITIS

Affeldt JE: Neuromotor paralysis. In Fenn WO, Rahn H (eds): Handbook of Physiology, Vol 2, Sec. 3, Respiration. Washington, DC, Am Physiol Soc, 1965, p 1509

Ferris BG, Mead J, Whittenberger JL, Saxton GA: Pulmonary function in convalescent poliomyelitis patients. III. Compliance of lungs and thorax. N Engl J Med 247:390, 1952

Spencer WA: Treatment of Acute Poliomyelitis. Charles C Thomas, Springfield, Illinois, 1954

SPINAL CORD LESIONS

Sandor F: Diaphragmatic respiration: a sign of cervical cord lesion in the unconscious patient ("horizontal paradox"). Br Med J 1:465, 1966

MUSCULAR DYSTROPHY

Kilburn KH, Egan JT, Sieker HO, Heyman A: Cardiopulmonary insufficiency in myotonic and progressive muscular dystrophy. N Engl J Med 261:1089, 1959

DIAPHRAGMATIC PARALYSIS

Ahmed S, Gill B: Nonoperative management of post-thoracotomy diaphragmatic paralysis in two neonates. Austral Paediatr J 11:81, 1975

Bishop HC, Koop CE: Acquired eventration of the diaphragm in infancy. Pediatrics 22:1088, 1958

McCredie M, Lovejoy FW, Kaltreider NL: Pulmonary function in diaphragmatic paralysis. Thorax 17:213, 1962

Riley EA: Idiopathic diaphragmatic paralysis, a report of 8 cases. Am J Med 32:404, 1962

Shifrin N: Unilateral paralysis of the diaphragm in the newborn infant due to phrenic nerve injury, with and without associated brachial palsy. Pediatrics 9:69, 1952

MYASTHENIA GRAVIS

Bundy S: Genetic study of infantile and juvenile myasthenis gravis. J Neurol Neurosurg 35:41, 1972

Namba T, Brown SB, Grob D: Neonatal myasthenia gravis. Report of 2 cases and review of literature. Pediatrics 45:488, 1970

Sivanesaratnam V and Lee EL: Myasthenia gravis in pregnancy and in newborn infant. Austral NZ J Obstet Gynecol 15:111, 1975

PECTUS EXCAVATUM

Ben-Menachem Y, O'Hara AE, Kane HA: Paradoxical cardiac enlargement during inspiration in children with pectus excavatum; a new observation. Br J Radiol 46:38, 1973

Fink A, Rivin A, Murray JF: Pectus excavatum. An analysis of twenty-seven cases. Arch Intern Med 108:427, 1961

Orzalesi MM, Cook CD: Pulmonary function in children with pectus excavatum. J Pediat 66:898, 1965

Reusch CS: Hemodynamic studies in pectus excavatum. Circulation 24:1143, 1961

THORACIC DYSTROPHY

Hanissian AS, Riggs WW Jr, Thomas DA: Infantile thoracic dystrophy—a variant of Ellis-van Creveld syndrome. J Pediatr 71:855, 1967

Hull D, Barnes ND: Children with small chests. Arch Dis Child 47:12, 1972

Jeune M, Beraud C, Carron R: Dystrophie thoracique asphyxiante de caractère familial. Arch Franc Pediatr 12:886, 1955

Kohler E, Babbitt DP: Dystrophic thoraces and infantile asphyxia. Radiology 94:55, 1970

Maroteaux P, Lamy M, Robert JM: Le nanisme thanatophore. Presse Med 75:2519, 1967

Pirnar T, Neuhauser EBD: Asphyxiating thoracic dystrophy of the newborn. Am J Roentgenol 98:359, 1966

THORACIC ANOMALIES

Bernhardt LC: Bifid sternum. J Thorac Cardiovasc Surg 55:758, 1968

Ravitch MM: Atypical deformities of the chest wall—absence and deformities of the ribs and costal cartilages. Surgery 59:438, 1966

KYPHOSCOLIOSIS

Bergofsky EH: Quantitation of the function of respiratory muscles in normal individuals and quadriplegic patients. Arch Phys Med 45:575, 1964

———Turino GM, Fishman AP: Cardiorespiratory failure in kyphoscoliosis. Medicine 38:263, 1959

Caro CG, DuBois AB: Pulmonary function in kyphoscoliosis. Thorax 16:282, 1961

Cook CD, Barrie H, DeForest BA, et al: Pulmonary physiology in children. III. Lung volumes, mechanics of respiration and respiratory muscle strength in scoliosis. Pediatrics 25:766, 1960

Makley JT, Herndon CH, Inkley S, et al: Pulmonary function in paralytic and non-paralytic scoliosis before and after treatment. J Bone Joint Surg (Br) 50A:1379, 1968

Westgate HD, Moe JH: Pulmonary function in kyphoscoliosis before and after correction by the Harrington instrumentation method. J Bone Joint Surg (Br) 51:935, 1969

PICKWICKIAN SYNDROME

Barrera F, Reidenberg MM, Winters WL: Pulmonary function in the obese patient. Am J Med Sci 254:785, 1967

Cayler GG: Cardiorespiratory syndrome of obesity (Pickwickian syndrome) in children. Pediatric 27:237, 1961

Cherniak RM: Management of cardiopulmonary disorders in the obese patients. Mod Treatm 4:1162, 1967

Finkelstein JW, Avery ME: The Pickwickian syndrome, studies on ventilation and carbohydrate metabolism. Case report of a child who recovered. Am J Dis Child 106:251, 1963

CONNECTIVE TISSUE DISEASE

Bowden DH, Favara BE, Donohue JL: Marfan's syndrome: accelerated course in childhood associated with lesions of mitral valve and pulmonary artery. Am Heart J 69:96, 1965

Travis, DM, Cook CD, Julian DG, et al: The lungs in rheumatoid spondylitis, gas exchange and lung mechanics in a form of restrictive pulmonary disease. Am J Med 29:623, 1960

SCLERODERMA

Adhikari PK, Bianchi FA, Boushy SF, Sakamoto A, Lewis BM: Pulmonary function in scleroderma. Its relation to changes in chest roentgenogram and in the skin of the thorax. Am Rev Resp Dis 86:823, 1962

TRAUMA

Brewer LA: The management of crushing injuries of the chest. Surg Clin North Am 48:1279, 1968

EMPYEMA

Béchamps GJ, Lynn HB, Wenzel JE: Empyema in children; review of Mayo Clinic experience. Mayo Clin Proc 45:43, 1970

Hendren WH, Haggerty RJ: Staphylococcic pneumonia in infancy and childhood. JAMA 168:61, 1958

Hertzler JH, Miller AE, Tuttle WM: Present concepts in the treatment of empyema in children. AMA Arch Surg 68:838, 1954

Simmons EM, Sauer P, Alkadi A, MacKenzie JW, Almond CH: Review of nontuberculous empyema at University of Missouri Medical Center, 1957-1961. J Thorac Cardiovasc Surg 64:578, 1972

Smith PL, Gerald B: Empyema in childhood followed roentgenographically: Decortication seldom needed. Am J Roentgen 106:114, 1969

Stiles, QR, Lindesmith GG, Tucker BL, Meyer BW, Jones JC: Pleural empyema in children. Ann Thorac Surg 10:37, 1970

Wise MB, Beaudry PH, Bates DV: Long-term follow-up of staphylococcal pneumonia. Pediatrics 38:398, 1966

PNEUMOTHORAX

Neonatal pneumothorax, Lancet 2:1304, 1973

Chernick V, Reed MH: Pneumothorax and chylothorax in neonatal period. J Pediatr 624, 1970

Cran IR, Rumball CA: Survey of spontaneous pneumothoraces in the Royal Air Force. Thorax 22:462, 1967

Renert WA, Berdon WE, Baker DH, Rose JS: Obstructive urologic malformations of fetus and infant; relation to neonatal pneumomediastinum and pneumothorax. Radiology 105:97, 1972

Stradling P, Poole G: Conservative management of spontaneous pneumothorax. Thorax 21:145, 1966

Yu VYH, Liew SW, Robertson NRC: Pneumothorax in newborn; changing pattern. Arch Dis Child 50:449, 1975

CHYLOTHORAX

Lichter L, Hill GL, Nye ER: The use of medium-chain triglycerides in the treatment of chylothorax in a child. Ann Thorac Surg 5:352, 1968

Maloney JV Jr, Spencer FC: The nonoperative treatment of traumatic chylothorax. Surgery 40:121, 1956

McKendry JBJ, Lindsay WK, Gerstein MC: Congenital defects of the lymphatics in infancy. Pediatrics 19:21, 1957

Randolph JG, Gross RE: Congenital chylothorax. AMA Arch Surg 74:405, 1957

CHAPTER 29

Endocrine System

MELVIN M. GRUMBACH, *Associate Editor*

NEURAL AND ENDOCRINE COMMUNICATIONS

RICHARD J. WURTMAN

Mammals have three kinds of cells that mediate communications between organs: neurons, neuroendocrine transducers, and glandular cells. Neurons receive and transmit information at the synapse, which is a specific anatomic locus with a characteristic appearance. Neuroendocrine transducers have a synaptic input, but they transmit their signals via the circulation. Glandular cells lack synapses and use the blood stream as the source of their input and the medium for their secretions.

The transmission of signals across synapses is mediated by a well-described process: a specific neurotransmitter substance, such as acetylcholine or nor-epinephrine that is stored within a characteristic subcellular vesicle is released into the synaptic cleft from the presynaptic cell. The neurotransmitter then diffuses across a short distance to reach a specialzed receptor zone on the postsynaptic cell, where it alters the flux of specific ions. This causes a change in electrical potential within the postsynaptic neuron and alters the probability that an action potential will be generated and a nerve impulse propagated. Nearly all the compounds thought to function as neurotransmitters have similar chemical characteristics; they are low-molecular-weight water-soluble amines and possibly amino acids. Moreover, they are rapidly inactivated by physical and chemical processes, such as enzymatic transformation or reuptake into their cells of origin. Their concentrations in the blood tend to be very low.

Hormonal signals, in contrast, are transmitted via the bloodstream. The array of chemicals used by the body as hormones is far broader than the current list of probable neurotransmitters; furthermore, the hormones seem to lack common chemical characteristics. Thus insulin is water-soluble, while progesterone is highly nonpolar; thyroxine is a low molecular weight amino acid, while thyroid-stimulating hormone (TSH) appears to be a large glycoprotein; epinephrine is cleared rapidly from the circulation by enzymatic transformation or uptake into sympathetic nerve endings, whereas cortisol persists in the blood for relatively long periods. The specific anatomic locus on or in the receptor cell at which a hormone acts has yet to be identified, but it almost certainly lacks the well-defined structural features of the postsynaptic membrane. Similarly, no characteristic electrical response seems to exist in hormone-responsive cells analogous to the ion fluxes and potential changes observed in the postsynaptic neuron. One can usually tell within seconds whether a given neuron has received and responded to a neurotransmitter; considerably more time is required to determine whether a thyroid cell has responded to circulating TSH.

Perhaps the most characteristic difference between transmission of signals by neurotransmitters and transmission by hormones lies in the techniques used by these communication systems to achieve "privacy." Nervous systems obtain privacy by anatomic means, with a given neuron apparently transmitting signals only to the small number of cells with which it makes synapses, or to cells lying within a few hundred angstroms of its terminal boutons. Thus, even though the particular chemical signal (eg, ácetylcholine) emitted when a specific neuron fires might be capable of stimulating billions of neurons within the brain, only hundreds actually respond, because only hundreds actually receive quanta of the neurotransmitter.

Communication systems that utilize the circulation to transmit signals attain privacy by biochemical means. A given signal may be distributed by the blood to every cell in the body; however, because the signal is coded, only the relatively small number of cells able to perform the decoding operation can obtain the information. The high degree of specificity attainable by hormonal communication systems is well illustrated by the physiologic regulation of the thyroid gland. TSH, the input to this organ, is carried by the circulation to every organ in the body; thyroxine, its output, is distributed in essentially the same volume. Only the thyroid gland, however, appears capable of responding to the information present in circulating TSH levels, while the heart, the liver, and most other organs show biochemical responses to circulating thyroxine.

NEUROENDOCRINE TRANSDUCER CELLS. The conversion of neural signals to hormonal signals is accomplished by neuroendocrine transducer cells. These cells are apparently stimulated by the same neurotransmitter substances as neurons. Their output signals exhibit all the variety typical of hormones: epinephrine is water-soluble, while melatonin is relatively nonpolar; renin is a high molecular weight protein, while epinephrine and melatonin are low molecular weight derivatives of single amino acids. The output signals (the releasing factors or hypophysiotropic hormones) emitted by hypothalamic transducer cells, which mediate the neural control of the anterior pituitary, apparently act only on this single target organ. In contrast, oxytocin, a hormonal signal emitted by the paraventricular nucleus, carries instructions to both the uterus and the myoepithelium of the mammary glands.

Demonstration that a given cell functions as a neuroendocrine transducer requires two types of evidence. The cell must be shown by electron microscopy to receive a direct innervation, and it must be demonstrated that the cell's ability to secrete its hormone under appropriate physiologic conditions is impaired on interruption of this innervation. With these criteria, at least five groups of cells have been shown to be neuroendocrine transducers: (1) The *chromaffin cells* of the adrenal medulla respond to a sympathetic cholinergic input by releasing the hormone epinephrine. (2) The *parenchymal cells* of the mammalian pineal organ respond to a sympathetic noradrenergic input by synthesizing and releasing the hormone melatonin. (3) The *cells of the supraoptic and paraventricular hypothalamic nuclei* respond to noradrenergic and/or cholinergic inputs by releasing the hormones vasopressin and oxytocin. (4) *Hypothalamic cells* secrete releasing factors and release-inhibiting factors or hormones into the pituitary portal circulation under the influence, in part, of noradrenergic, dopaminergic, or serotoninergic input.(5) The *juxtaglomerular cells* of the mammalian kidney respond to a sympathetic noradrenergic input by releasing renin into the bloodstream. The list of neuroendocrine transducers will probably continue to expand. Whenever it can be demonstrated that the brain influences secretion of a hormone from a peripheral organ (eg, insulin from the pancreas), a prima facie case is made for the participation of a neuroendocrine transducer in the secretory process.

References

Reichlin S: Neuroendocrinology, In Williams RH (ed): Textbook of Endocrinology. Philadelphia, WB Saunders, 1974, p 774

Wurtman RJ: Neuroendocrine transducer cells in mammals. In Schmitt FO (ed): The Neurosciences: Second Study Program. New York, Rockefeller Univ Press, 1970

HORMONE ACTIONS
Alfred M. Bongiovanni

There are three main chemical classes of hormones: polypeptides, steroids, and amines. The hypothalamic hormones are generally small polypeptides, the tropic hormones are complex polypeptides and glycoproteins, and the hormones of the end organs are usually smaller molecules, either steroids or amines, and are often associated with specific binding proteins in the plasma following their release. Although these binding proteins were first thought to serve the all-important function of transport to responsive tissues, it now appears that the much smaller unbound moiety is the active moiety.

In general, hormones act at the cellular level by their effects on membranes, genes, and enzymes; these are usually interrelated. The effects on membranes are many; they include alterations in permeability to a variety of substances and activation of constituents within the membrane that secondarily influence a number of intracellular events. Certain hormones (steroids and thyroid hormones) are transported to a nuclear site, where they modify gene expression. The effects on enzymes include increased synthesis, interconversion between active and inactive forms of the enzyme molecule, and effects on substrate (such as translocation to the vicinity of the enzyme), ionic concentration, and cofactors.

At the cellular level, two patterns of interaction with the hormone are now recognized. The first, exemplified by epinephrine and a number of peptide hormones, involves reaction of the hormone with the cellular membrane to stimulate a nucleotide cyclase system. This then converts adenosine triphosphate (ATP) to cyclic adenosine-3',5'-monophosphate (cAMP). The second pattern, observed with certain steroid hormones, entails the entry of the hormone into the cell. It then is bound to a specific cytoplasmic receptor protein characteristic of the cell, which in turn becomes attached to a region of the nucleus and influences specific RNA synthesis.

MEMBRANE RECEPTORS. On cell membranes of certain tissues there are receptor sites with specific structural complementarity for individual hormones and drugs. Adrenocortical cell membranes thus contain receptors for ACTH that do not react with glucagon or catecholamines, whereas there are receptors in cardiac cells for catecholamines but not for ACTH. Following such attachment, there is activation of adenyl cyclase, which leads to the formation of cAMP, the so-called second messenger. Sometimes calcium is regarded as the second messenger because the hormone receptor on the membrane permits increased entrance of this cation into the cell, probably as a primary event, with subsequent efflux of Ca^{++} from mitochondria and activation of the nucleotide cyclase. The cAMP activates a protein kinase by its binding to a regulatory subunit, which ordinarily restrains the catalytic activity of the enzyme. This cAMP-dependent protein kinase catalyzes the transfer of phosphorus from ATP to certain enzymes that are thus activated (or sometimes inactivated). Other cAMP effects seem to be independent of a protein kinase. In *Escherichia coli*, for example, a protein receptor of cAMP is not associated with a kinase. This complex binds to DNA in such a way that there is an increase in the formation of specific mRNA. Sometimes the major event following hormone–membrane binding and adenyl cyclase activation is substrate translocation. The major effect of ACTH on adrenal cells may be to promote the entrance of cholesterol into mitochondria, which is Ca^{++}-dependent, rather than to exert an effect directly on steroidogenic enzymes. The specificity of the ultimate response depends on the presence of receptors complementary for the hormone on the cell membrane and the inherent mechanisms within the differentiated cell capable of the specific response.

A number of hormones are associated with such cellular membrane receptors, for example, angiotensin, vasopressin, parathormone, growth hormone, prolactin, gonadotropins, oxytocin, some prostaglandins, and insulin; but not all (eg, insulin) are associated with activation of adenyl cyclase. The specificity of membrane receptors is such that membrane particles from appropriate cells have been employed successfully in competitive binding systems for the accurate and highly selective measurement of hormones. Cyclic nucleotides, other than cAMP, eg, guanosine-3′,5′-monophosphate (cGMP), are important in some cells; often the action of cGMP is antagonistic to that of cAMP.

INTRACELLULAR RECEPTORS. With the work of Jensen it became recognized that some hormones, including the steroids and thyroid hormones, enter cells freely. They do not bind to components of the outer membrane, and they are subsequently bound to the nuclei of these cells, where they influence gene expression and result in initiation or acceleration of specific mRNA synthesis. The sequence of events has been studied most thoroughly with estrogens, testosterone, and glucocorticoids. Vitamin D (which is sometimes considered as hormone) probably follows a similar scheme. This concept entails the rapid and free entry of the hormone into cells, where in its specific end organ it becomes bound to a specific protein receptor in the cytosol. Prior to migration and attachment to the nucleus, "activation" of the complex occurs, which appears to involve disaggregation into subunits. This altered unit then becomes bound to a limited number of nuclear acceptor sites *as a unit*. These nuclear sites may be limited in function, or there may be a large number of different nuclear sites (eg, glucocorticoids are known to influence the synthesis of a large number of hepatic enzymes). It sometimes appears that the hormone itself must undergo an intracellular alteration before it can reach the nucleus. Thus, in some tissues, testosterone must first be reduced to its dihydro form, which binds to the cytosol receptor and is then bound to nuclei after the administration of testosterone. Whether this also applies to the thyroid hormone is not entirely clear at present. The evidence indicates that both triiodothyronine and thyroxine are significantly bound to nuclei. Vitamin D_2 undergoes hydroxylation of carbons 25 and 1 by liver and kidney, respectively, before it is bound by a cytoplasmic receptor in gastrointestinal cells. Thereafter, by a similar course of events, these cells synthesize a calcium-transporting enzyme.

The studies of O'Malley using the chick oviduct system provide an elegant model of this sequence of events. The synthesis of ovalbumin by tubular gland cells of the oviduct is stimulated by estrogen, and progesterone stimulates avidin synthesis by the goblet cells. After estrogen, there is an increase in RNA polymerase activity, which results from the exposure of previously repressed regions of the DNA template. With the production of avidin, under the influence of progesterone, there is a change in template activity of isolated chromatin prior to the appearance of this specific protein product. The evidence points to an effect at the transcriptional level. These events appear to be related to the binding of the steroid cytoplasmic receptor protein complex to specific chromatin regions of the nucleus.

References

Bitensky MW, Gorman RE: Chemical mediation of hormone action. Ann Rev Med 23:263, 1972

Jensen EV, DeSombre ER: Estrogen–receptor interaction. Science 182:126, 1973

Lefkowitz RJ: Isolated hormone receptors. N Engl J Med 288:1061, 1973

O'Malley BW, Schrader WT: The receptors of steroid hormones. Sci Am 234:32, 1976

Sutherland EW: Studies on the mechanisms of hormone action. Science 177:401, 1972

ANTERIOR PITUITARY
Robert M. Blizzard

The pituitary gland was at one time termed the master gland and was considered to have physiologic importance out of proportion to its small size (500 to 600 mg in the adult). Recently it has been realized that this important structure does not function autonomously and that many influences are exerted on it by the nervous system and peripheral endocrine glands. Consequently, functions and diseases of the anterior pituitary must be considered in relation to the normal and abnormal physiology of other organs or organ systems.

Interrelationships of Hypothalamus and Anterior Pituitary

The anterior pituitary (adenohypophysis) is derived from an outpouching of the stomodeum (Rathke's pouch). The posterior pituitary (neurohypophysis) originates from the infundibular process of the diencephalon. When these two structures meet, the anterior wall of Rathke's pouch thickens to form the pars distalis of the anterior pituitary. The posterior wall of Rathke's pouch forms the pars intermedia between the pars distalis of the anterior lobe and the posterior lobe (pars nervosa). The infundibular stem connects the hypothalamus and the pars nervosa. Paired extensions of the pars distalis form a cuff tissue, the pars tuberalis, which surrounds the infundibular stalk. In Figure 1, for purposes of clarity, the pars tuberalis is drawn only on the anterior surface of the infundibular stem. Occasionally the migratory tract of the adenohypophysis fails to obliterate completely, and cysts are formed within the sella turcica. These may grow into the suprasellar area. Cysts filled with tumor cells are called craniopharyngiomas.

The hypothalamus, which is located directly above the pituitary, has no efferent neural fibers to the anterior pituitary, but several neural tracts traverse from centers in the hypothalamus through the neural stalk into the neurohypophysis or pars nervosa. The median eminence of the hypothalamus, a broadening at the cephalic end of the hypophyseal stalk, lies proximally above the pars tuberalis and probably plays a direct role as intermediator between the hypothalamus and the anterior pituitary. Various neurohumoral substances produced in hypothalamic centers enter the capillary

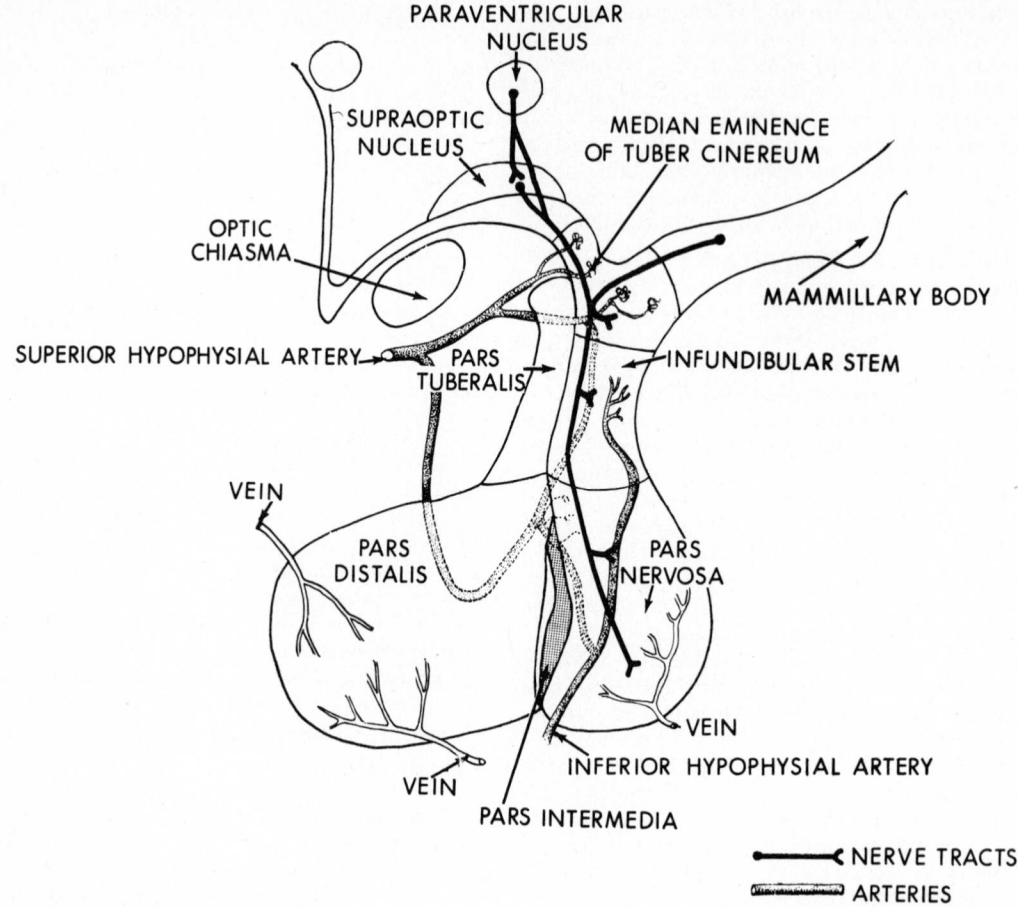

FIG. 1. Interrelationships of hypothalamus and pituitary, including arterial blood supply (which does not supply the anterior pituitary). The blood supply of the anterior pituitary (not shown) is completely venous in origin. The portal venous system originates in the median eminence and transports neurohumoral secretions from the hypothalamus to the anterior pituitary. [Adapted from Crosby, Humphrey and Luer: *In* Wilkins (ed): *The Diagnosis and Treatment of Endocrine Disorders in Childhood,* 3rd ed, 1965. Courtesy of Charles C Thomas.]

plexus of the portal system in the median eminence and are conveyed to the anterior pituitary by the portal veins.

There are hypothalamic releasing factors for all the hormones of anterior pituitary origin. In addition, there are hypothalamic inhibiting factors for growth hormone and prolactin and possibly for melanocyte-stimulating hormone; none has been identified for the gonadotropic hormones, ACTH, or thyrotropin. Occasionally, hypothalamic centers such as those for appetite, thirst, and sleep are involved in hypothalamic lesions, and symptoms related to disturbances of these centers may accompany manifestations of pituitary dysfunction.

The optic chiasm lies directly anterior to the infundibular stalk, and visual disturbances, especially bilateral hemianopia, often result when a pituitary tumor extends out of the sella and compresses the chiasm.

The blood supply of the anterior pituitary is all of venous origin, in contrast to the situation with the posterior pituitary, the median eminence of the hypo-thalamus, and the hypothalamus, which are supplied by the superior and inferior hypophyseal arteries. The portal veins of the anterior lobe originate in the median eminence and the upper and lower portions of the infundibular stem. Thus the origin of the blood supply is located to receive neurohumors, which are transmitted downstream to the anterior lobe. Since some of these vessels originate below the diaphragma sellae (a membranous diaphragm covering the sella, through which the infundibular stem penetrates), stalk sections performed above the diaphragm may be only partially effective in producing decreased pituitary function. However, coagulation of the distal stalk usually produces complete necrosis and pituitary dysfunction.

Hormones of Hypothalamus

In the hypothalamus there are releasing hormones for the gonadotropins (FSH and LH), thyroid-stimulating hormone (TSH), growth hormone or somatotropin

(STH), melanocyte-stimulating hormone (MSH), and prolactin (PRL). The gonadotropin-releasing hormone (LRH) is a decapeptide that has been identified, synthesized, and administered on an experimental basis. There probably is only one LRH that stimulates the release of both FSH and LH. Thyrotropin-releasing hormone (TRH), a tripeptide, also has been isolated and synthesized. Its administration causes the release of TSH and PRL; this is a secondary action, as it is not the primary prolactin-releasing hormone. Growth hormone or somatotropin-releasing factor (SRF) has been extracted from rat hypothalami, but its peptide structure is not yet known. A factor inhibiting the release of growth hormone (termed somatostatin) has been characterized and synthesized. It has 14 amino acids, and it significantly decreases the release of growth hormone to many of the usual stimuli, such as arginine, insulin, and exercise. It also inhibits the release of TSH when TRH is administered, but it does not affect PRL release in this instance. Somatostatin release inhibiting factor (SRIF) also has the unique quality of inhibiting the release of glucagon and insulin at the pancreas.

Corticotropin-releasing factor has not been characterized chemically, but there is a large body of evidence to support its presence in the hypothalamus and its role in the regulation of adrenocorticotropin (ACTH). Vasopressin has corticotropin releasing factor activity. Prolactin secretion is under the control of prolactin-release inhibiting factor (PRIF) and possibly a prolactin releasing factor (PRF) in addition to TRH. The structures of these compounds have not been identified, but the existence of PRIF in the hypothalamus is unequivocal.

The releasing factors are under dopamine and serotonin control and also under control of the adrenergic nervous system to a significant extent. For example, propranolol, a β-adrenergic blocking agent, enhances and augments the release of growth hormone in response to provocative stimuli. In contrast, phentolamine, an α-adrenergic blocking agent, inhibits the release of growth hormone from the usual stimuli.

Hormones of Anterior Pituitary

There are many cell types in the adenohypophysis, and each probably produces its own hormone. Initially the cell types were divided into chromophobes, eosinophils, and basophils; however, with refinement of staining techniques at least seven cell types are now identifiable (Fig. 2). The eosinophils (acidophils) or alpha cells produce STH and prolactin. The basophils have been subcategorized as β_1, β_2, Δ_1, and Δ_2 cells. ACTH is produced by β_1 cells, thyrotropin by β_2 cells, LH by Δ_1 cells, and follicle-stimulating hormone (FSH) by Δ_2 cells. Chromophobes have been subdivided into γ, β_3, and primordial (stem) cells. Presumably the β_3 cells, like the β_1 cells, produce ACTH.

Homeostatic regulation of production or secretion of pituitary hormones is controlled by several factors: circulating hormones of the peripheral endocrine glands, stress, and in some instances circulating levels of non-hormonal substances such as blood sugar, whose concentration affects STH release.

Secretion of many tropic hormones is controlled by feedback mechanisms, and the amount secreted is inversely related to the concentration of the circulating hormones produced by the peripheral endocrine glands. In primary hypothyroidism, for example, TSH is secreted in excess. Conversely, with exogenous administration of thyroxine or triiodothyronine in complete replacement dosages, the pituitary is put at rest via hypothalamic and pituitary suppression, and there is no further release of TSH. Similarly, with primary hypogonadism the gonadotropins are excreted in excess; exogenous administration of large amounts of estrogen or testosterone suppresses their release. Normally the levels of circulating cortisol and ACTH are inversely related in a similar manner.

Pituitary hormones may be inhibited by excesses of certain peripheral hormones, even though the tropic hormones are not directly responsible for the production of peripheral hormones; for example, excess hydrocortisone may inhibit growth hormone. Also, excessive production of certain tropic hormones may result from deficiences of peripheral hormones for which they are not directly responsible; excessive prolactin and gonadotropin secretions have resulted from deficiency of thyroid hormone. These relationships have been termed overflow stimulation.

Stress apparently functions independently of the feedback mechanisms. Surgical stress, for example, is associated with increased ACTH output, even though circulating levels of hydrocortisone may be elevated. Similarly, stress induced by intravenous administration of Piromen, a *Pseudomonas* polysaccharide, results in increased secretion of cortisol and ACTH; Piromen also causes STH release. Circulating blood sugar levels affect the circulating level of human growth hormone (somatotropin). The levels increase with hypoglycemia and decrease with hyperglycemia. Intracellular glucose levels may actually be the controlling agent, since exercise and 2-desoxyglucose also are stimuli for increasing the concentration of growth hormone in serum.

The metabolic actions of the pituitary hormones are multiple. Growth hormone, which has been isolated from human and simian pituitaries, is an unbranched polypeptide with a molecular weight of approximately 21,500 daltons; it is metabolically active in man and certain other mammals. Unfortunately growth hormone obtained from nonprimates is not metabolically active in the human because of structural differences. Pituitary glands of all ages contain growth hormone at a concentration of 4 to 10 percent of dry weight.

Administration of growth hormone to hypopituitary dwarfs causes rapid growth of the skeletal system, usually without a proportionate increase in skeletal maturation. This relationship between linear growth and skeletal maturation contrasts markedly with the increase in linear growth that occurs with testosterone treatment but that is accompanied by a proportionately greater rate of increase in skeletal maturation. In association with growth, nitrogen, calcium, potassium,

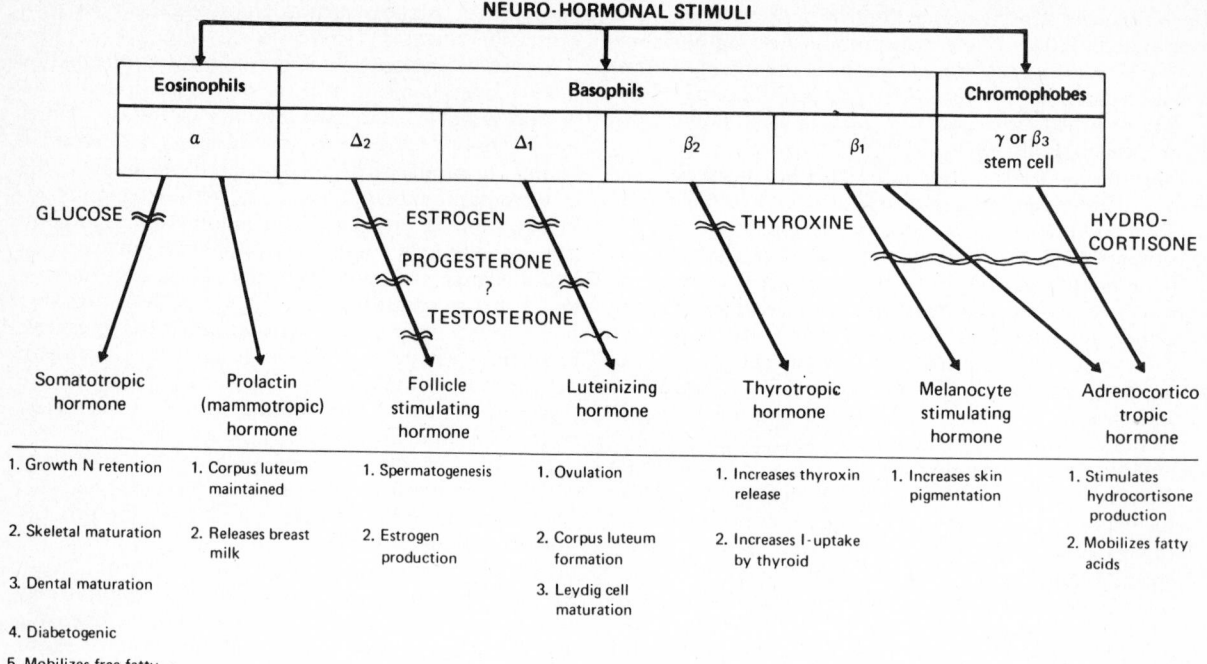

FIG. 2. Hormones produced by the anterior pituitary and their effects.

and phosphorus are retained. Concentrations of serum urea and other nonprotein nitrogens fall, and free fatty acids are mobilized from fat.

Growth hormone also has an action on carbohydrate metabolism. Individuals with growth hormone deficiency may have hypoglycemia, which improves when STH is given despite an increase in insulin output in response to a glucose load. If increased insulin cannot be produced, as in a patient with diabetes mellitus, the administration of growth hormone can produce ketonemia and hyperglycemia.

Prolactin from human pituitaries has been chemically separated from growth hormone. One preliminary report suggests that ovine prolactin administered to hypophysectomized animals has some metabolic actions similar to those of STH; another suggests that ovine prolactin administered to growth hormone deficient humans acts in a manner similar to STH. Because of its limited supply, the metabolic effects of human prolactin have not been studied in man. Other actions are listed in Figure 2. Prolactin inhibits ovulation and probably accounts for the anovulatory period following pregnancy with suckling.

The gonadotropins (LH and FSH), ACTH, and TSH act primarily on their respective peripheral endocrine glands. MSH is closely related chemically to ACTH; it causes increased pigmentation, and as with ACTH, its production is inhibited by hydrocortisone or cortisone.

LABORATORY MEASUREMENTS OF PITUITARY FUNCTION

The development of immunoassay techniques has permitted direct measurement of nanogram amounts of all the pituitary hormones. The ready availability of growth hormone immunoassays in many hospital and commercial laboratories simplifies the evaluation of the short child when growth hormone deficiency is suspected (Table 1). Since STH concentrations are very variable during the day, specific stimuli are used to release growth hormone before serum is drawn for assessment of the STH concentration.

Exercise stimulation is a good screening test. This is done by fasting the patient for 4 hours, then drawing serum. After exercise, either by climbing stairs or by jogging 20 minutes, a second specimen of blood is drawn. The patient then rests prone for 20 minutes, and a third specimen is drawn. The growth hormone concentration is stable even at room temperatures for 2 or 3 days.

Another stimulatory test is the infusion of 10 percent arginine monochloride (0.5 g/kg body weight) over a 30-minute period, with serum specimens drawn at 0, 15, 30, 45, and 60 minutes; this is followed immediately with intravenous injection of insulin (0.075 IU/kg). Serum specimens are then drawn at 15, 30, 45, and 60 minutes. Absence (< 6.0 ng/ml) of significant response

TABLE 1. Laboratory Determinations of Pituitary Hormones by Direct and Indirect Means

	Blood		Urine		Reserve
	Direct	*Indirect*	*Direct*	*Indirect*	
Growth Hormone	Immunoassay	Somatomedin or sulfation factor	0	0	Immunochemical in blood with insulin, arginine, L-dopa, glucagon, and/or exercise stimulation
TSH	Immunoassay Bioassay	^{131}I uptake of thyroid gland; serum thyroxine (T4), triiodothyronine (T3), and free T4 and T3	0	0	TRH stimulation
ACTH	Immunoassay Bioassay	Cortisol levels	0	17-OHCS excretion 17-KS excretion	Metyrapone Insulin
FSH	Immunoassay	0	Immunoassay Bioassay	Sperm count	Clomiphene stimulation LRH stimulation
LH	Immunoassay	Testosterone	Immunoassay Bioassay	Testosterone	Clomiphene stimulation LRH stimulation
PRL	Immunoassay Bioassay	0	0	0	TRH stimulation

in either the fasting or the stimulated state is very suggestive of STH deficiency. Some normal individuals release STH only with one of these stimuli, so that STH deficiency cannot be diagnosed unless there is failure to respond to two or more stimuli. Random samples of serum may be obtained 3 to 4 hours postprandially, or with deep sleep. Levodopa may be given orally in doses of 9 to 10 mg/kg body weight, and blood specimens being drawn at 0, 30, 60, and 90 minutes. Glucagon at doses of 15 μg/kg also may be given, with blood being drawn at 0, 30, 60, 90, and 120 minutes. Measurements in urine are not useful because STH is not excreted in significant quantities.

Direct measurement of gonadotropins is also possible by bioassay, but urinary gonadotropin determinations, as currently measured by most clinical laboratories, represent a summation effect of FSH and LH. Normal values for adults of premenopausal age are 6 to 52 mouse units per 24 hours (approximately 2 mouse units equals 1 rat unit).

Small amounts of gonadotropins are produced before adolescence, and they can be measured by immunoassay in both serum and urine, but usually not by bioassay techniques, since the quantities excreted are very small. Increased quantities appear normally at approximately 9 to 10 years of age in both boys and girls, and they increase with each stage of sexual development until adulthood. Then values in males and females are essentially similar, except in females during the ovulatory (midcycle) peak and postmenopausally, when the values increase very significantly.

Usually, direct measurement of pituitary gonadotropins in serum and urine is of limited value until adolescence. Children do not excrete sufficient gonadotropins prior to that time to differentiate hypopituitarism from constitutional delayed adolescence. However, there are specific instances when measurements of either serum or urinary gonadotropins can be helpful in the evaluation of children: At the time of expected adolescence in tall eunuchoid boys with sexual infantilism, they assist in differentiating gonadotropin deficiency from primary testicular failure; in the former the values will be preadolescent, and in the latter they will be either elevated or at normal adolescent levels. This measurement is also of value in differentiating the syndrome of gonadal dysgenesis (Turner's syndrome) from hypopituitarism in sexually immature females. Patients with gonadal dysgenesis or primary ovarian failure will have increases over preadolescent values, particularly of FSH, even in infancy. In contrast, patients with hypopituitarism or constitutional delayed adolescence have preadolescent values.

Administration of clomiphene citrate stimulates release of gonadotropins in sexually mature individuals, but not in preadolescent or early adolescent children. Therefore its usefulness as a measure of gonadotropin reserve in children is limited.

Intravenous administration of LRH at doses of 3 μg/kg will cause release of LH and FSH within 30 to 120 minutes. Serum samples should be drawn at 0, 30, 60, 90, and 120 minutes and evaluated for the capacity of the pituitary to release LH and FSH secondary to administration of the releasing hormone. However, this test is of limited use in the differentiation of hypothalamic hypopituitarism from lesions of the pituitary itself, as some patients with hypothalamic deficiency of LRH as the cause of hypogonadotropic hypogonadism and eunuchoidism require repeated doses or prolonged infusions of LRH before a rise in LH and FSH can be elicited by an acute LRH challenge. LH values should increase by increments of 10 to 120 mU/ml over the base value. The LH rise in children is strikingly less than that in pubertal children and adults.

TSH also is measured by radioimmunoassay techniques; normal values are 0 to 10 μU/ml. Values are elevated in compensated or uncompensated primary hypothyroidism in the first 24 hours after birth, and with ingestion of certain goitrogenic agents over a prolonged period. TRH can be given at a dose of 7 μg/kg intravenously to test TSH reserve, with blood being drawn at 15, 30, 45, and 60 minutes. Individuals who have hypothalamic defects leading to TSH deficiency (third-degree hypothyroidism) exhibit significantly increased TSH concentrations, but those with TSH deficiency secondary to pituitary lesions do not (second-degree hypothyroidism). Patients with thyrotoxicosis or those receiving large amounts of thyroid hormones do not release TSH with this stimulus, as the thyroid hormone blocks TSH release even with TRH administration. In the absence of excessive thyroid hormone, a failure in response is indicative of a pituitary lesion.

A radioimmunoassay technique for measuring ACTH has been described but is not yet widely available for clinical studies. Bioassays measuring the concentrations of 17-hydroxycorticosteroids (17-OHCS) or corticosterone in adrenal vein blood of hypophysectomized dogs and rats, respectively, after injection of plasma have been used as research techniques to measure ACTH. These bioassay methods are tedious and are not sufficiently sensitive to measure the hormone in the plasma of normal nonstressed individuals. However, extraction of plasma and testing by these methods have made it possible to determine that in the normal individual the concentration of ACTH is 0.11 to 0.25 mU/100 ml. These values correlate with the diurnal variation of plasma 17-OHCS.

Some clinics still must depend on indirect measurements of pituitary function to determine if an abnormality exists. Indirect tests often are still used when evaluating TSH production. However, the accessibility of TSH radioimmunoassays is rapidly causing the indirect procedures to be replaced. Patients with hypopituitarism frequently have low or low normal T$_4$, free thyroxine, and ^{131}I uptake, even in the absence of clinical hypothyroidism. When these values are low, differentiation of primary thyroid disease from pituitary insufficiency can be made by administering 5 to 10 U of TSH every day for 2 to 3 days and repeating the uptake and the chemical T$_4$ determination. A patient with primary hypothyroidism will not respond with increased values, whereas one with hypothyroidism secondary to hypopituitarism will have appreciable rises in these parameters. The normal responses to standard dosages must be determined for each laboratory; thus no specific normal values are given here. Clinicians are urged to use the direct measurement of TSH in preference to these indirect, less precise, less specific, more expensive, and time-consuming techniques.

ACTH function is usually evaluated by indirect techniques. The excretion of cortisol metabolites, 17-OHCS, or 17-ketogenic steroids (17-KGS) may be of assistance, as patients deficient in ACTH often excrete subnormal amounts (normal values must be determined for each laboratory). However, some patients with partial hypopituitarism excrete normal amounts of 17-OHCS or 17-KGS, but they cannot increase the secretion of ACTH in response to iatrogenically induced low serum concentrations of cortisol. Serum concentrations of cortisol can be reduced and ACTH reserve can be measured by giving metyrapone (SU 4885), an 11-hydroxylase steroid blocker. One then determines whether the urinary 17-OHCS or 17-KGS are appreciably increased. Normally these values double or triple as a result of increased ACTH secretion because of increased excretion of compound S (11-deoxy-17-hydroxycorticosterone), a cortisol precursor secreted when 11-hydroxylation of the steroid nucleus does not occur. Failure of the 17-OHCS or 17-KGS to rise normally, providing ACTH injection produces a significant increase of 17-OHCS or 17-KGS, rules out primary adrenal disease, and is indicative of an abnormality in the hypothalamus or pituitary. The 17-ketosteroids (androgen metabolites) can also be measured,

but since androgens normally are not synthesized before puberty, this is of little value in children unless one is looking for excessive excretion.

Tolerance tests related to carbohydrate metabolism may be used as indirect measurements of STH and ACTH production by the pituitary; however, their usefulness has decreased with the availability of direct methods for evaluating pituitary function for STH. The glucose tolerance test (GTT) frequently is diabetic in character when excessive STH or ACTH is present. Hypoglycemic unresponsiveness at the 4th and 5th hour following a glucose tolerance test is frequent when STH or ACTH is deficient.

Growth hormone also can be measured indirectly; somatomedin or sulfation factor activity will reflect STH-like activity on cartilage. There are apparently three different somatomedins (A, B, and C). C is apparently the one that best reflects the STH-like activity in serum. The serum of STH-deficient humans and animals has decreased activity, whereas serum activity is increased in acromegalic individuals, who produce excessive STH. Injection of somatomedin into hypophysectomized animals or humans increases somatomedin activity. As yet, little is known about the variability with age.

HYPOPITUITARISM

Theoretically, hypopituitarism can arise as an idiopathic or organic entity, with deficiency of either single or multiple tropic hormones in either instance. Lesions

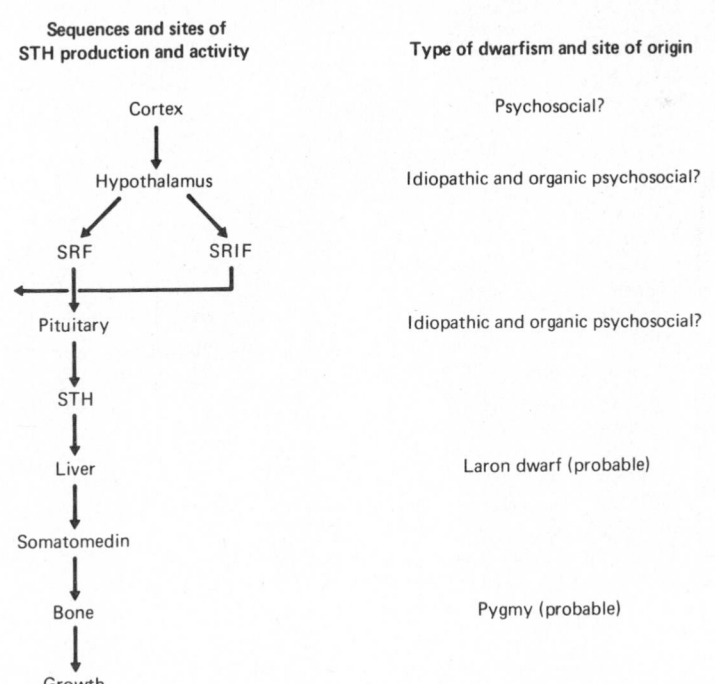

FIG. 3. Sites of probable origin of various types of hypopituitary and hypopituitarylike syndromes. SRF, somatotropin-releasing factor; SRIF, somatostatin; STH, somatotropin or growth hormone.

can occur in the hypothalamus or the pituitary. Relative growth hormone deficiency can also occur because of inability to generate somatomedin or from production of a somatotropin that is biologically inactive although measurable by immunoassay. Occasionally, growth hormone deficiency occurs secondary to an inhibition of tropic hormone release resulting from emotional disturbances, termed psychosocial dwarfism. Prolonged suppression of the pituitary by exogenously administered hormones (eg, hydrocortisone) also can produce iatrogenic hypopituitarism. The possible sites of defects in somatotropin production or action are shown in Figure 3. Each of these theoretic entities will be considered individually.

Idiopathic Hypopituitarism

No anatomic defect is demonstrable to account for deficiencies of tropic hormones. Idiopathic hypopituitarism is probably more common than hypopituitarism of organic origin. Although all the tropic hormones may be deficient, commonly only somatotropin is involved; other tropic hormones are deficient in about 50 percent of patients with STH deficiency. Consequently the presenting complaint of the child with idiopathic hypopituitarism is nearly always short stature. Hypopituitarism should be suspected in any child who grows less than 5.0 cm/year after 2 years of age and in whom there is no explanation for the growth failure. Occasionally patients with isolated gonadotropin deficiency will present at adolescence with sexual infantilism and normal stature. Isolated deficiencies of ACTH or TSH have been reported only rarely.

Idiopathic hypopituitarism is believed to have a hypothalamic origin. This has been demonstrated by administering TRH and observing TSH release in patients who have both STH and TSH deficiencies. Such individuals almost invariably release TSH secondary to TRH stimulation, which indicates that the defect is in the release of hormones and not in the production of TSH. In at least one such instance STH was identified in the pituitary of an STH-deficient patient. To unequivocally establish this in relation to patients who have only isolated growth hormone deficiency, the growth hormone releasing factor, when available, will have to be administered to determine whether growth

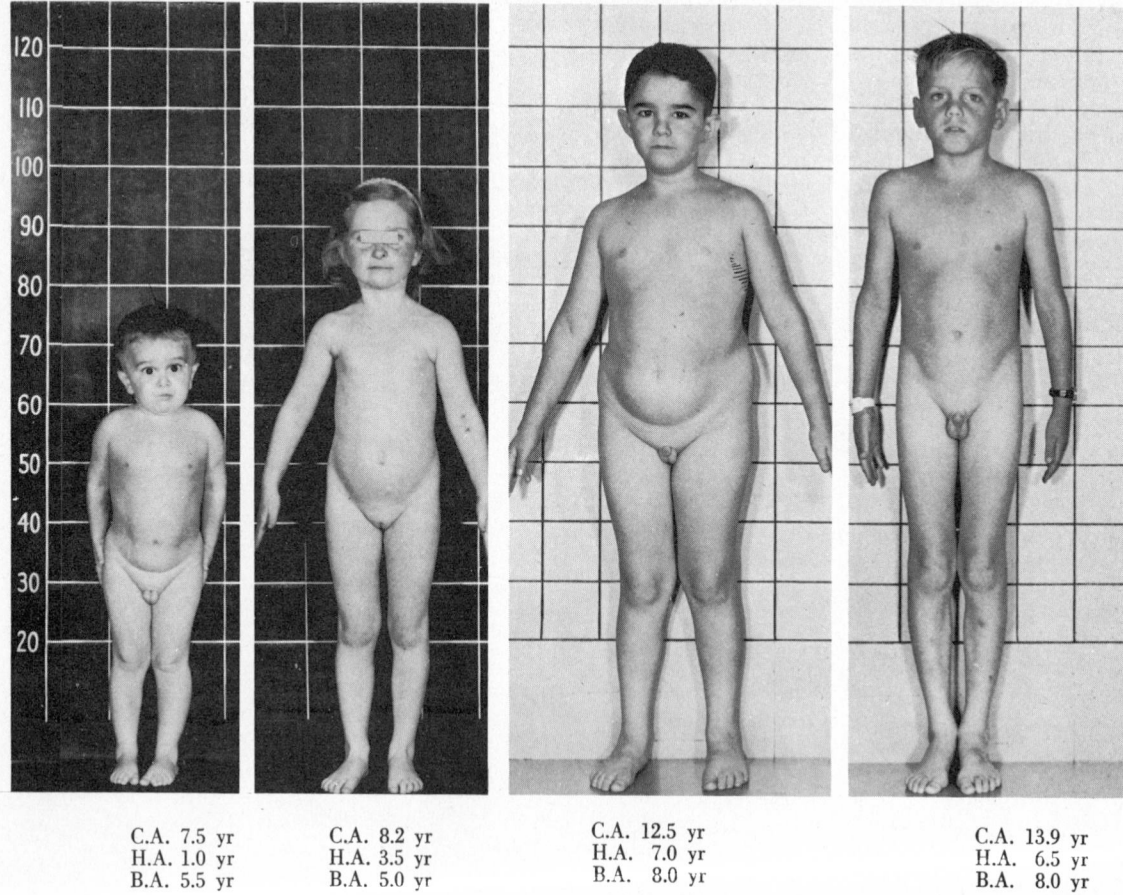

C.A. 7.5 yr	C.A. 8.2 yr	C.A. 12.5 yr	C.A. 13.9 yr
H.A. 1.0 yr	H.A. 3.5 yr	H.A. 7.0 yr	H.A. 6.5 yr
B.A. 5.5 yr	B.A. 5.0 yr	B.A. 8.0 yr	B.A. 8.0 yr

FIG. 4.   Variability of body contours in patients with idiopathic hypopituitarism. Third patient from left has isolated growth hormone deficiency.

hormone is released from the pituitary secondary to this stimulus. Patients with primary hypopituitarism would not be expected to release STH with this stimulus.

As noted in Figure 3, a few patients may have an inability to generate somatomedin even in the presence of endogenous or exogenous STH. Laron dwarfs, who have immunochemically measurable hormone but low somatomedin levels, probably have this defect, although the possibility has not been excluded that they may produce an immunologically active but biologically inactive hormone. These patients appear to be STH-deficient, but they have normal or high levels of STH; treatment is ineffective. Pygmies have normal STH and somatomedin levels, but they fail to grow; it has been postulated that they have end-organ resistance to somatomedin.

Growth retardation occurs before the age of 12 months in about 30 percent of patients with idiopathic hypopituitarism. The eruption of the primary dentition is often delayed, but delayed eruption of the secondary teeth is even more common. The body appearance is constant, in that all the patients appear much younger than their actual ages. However, the body contours are exceedingly variable (Fig. 4). Frequently, although not invariably, there is adiposity of the trunk with flabby musculature covered with so-called baby fat. Sexual infantilism often persists into adult life; occasionally, gonadotropins are produced in late adolescence, and secondary sexual characteristics then develop. Diabetes insipidus does not occur in idiopathic hypopituitarism, and skull radiographs and visual fields are normal. Only 1 patient of more than 100 in our clinic, initially diagnosed as having idiopathic hypopituitarism, subsequently developed a demonstrable organic lesion. However, this patient did not have skull radiography until central nervous system symptoms occurred. If skull films had been obtained, organic hypopituitarism might have been diagnosed earlier.

Diagnosis is made using the studies outlined in the laboratory section (p. 1604) and in Table 2. Skeletal age is usually, but not always, markedly delayed. There is less than 6.0 ng/ml of growth hormone (depending on laboratory norms) in serum after stimulation by exercise, arginine, insulin-induced hypoglycemia, and administration of L-dopa or glucagon. If the urinary method is used, the metyrapone test is abnormal in those with accompanying ACTH deficiency. ACTH reserve also can be assessed by determining the change in plasma corticol concentration during the insulin tolerance test or by the rise in plasma 11-deoxycortisol (compound S) after intravenous or oral administration of metyrapone.

The ^{131}I uptake and serum thyroxine determinations may be low normal or slightly low in some patients. Measurements of gonadotropins by bioassay are of little value in diagnosing this entity, as these are not usually measurable in the preadolescent; measurement by immunoassay also is of limited value, as both normal and hypopituitary children have only small amounts of immunoreactive gonadotropins in their serum and urine. However, occasionally a patient with hypopituitarism will have such low values that there is no question that gonadotropin deficiency will be present at adolescence. The test is of distinct value when Turner's syndrome is suspected. A patient with Turner's syndrome will have high FSH, even at 4 to 5 years of age, whereas one with hypopituitarism will have normal to low values.

Carbohydrate function studies are abnormal in about 65 percent of patients with STH deficiency. In our experience, 40 percent of these patients who are tested with an oral GTT have chemically reactive hypoglycemia at the 4th or 5th hour. Many have diabetic peaks, with a rapid drop to hypoglycemic levels; 60 percent of patients have been insulin-sensitive.

An approach to the differential diagnosis of children with short stature is presented in Table 2. The more obvious causes of short stature, such as renal, cardiac, and skeletal disease as well as malabsorption, which simulate growth hormone deficiency, are discussed below and on page 111.

Idiopathic hypopituitarism is usually sporadic; however, a small proportion of cases are due to a mutant gene. Over 63 families with 193 affected members have been observed; approximately 50 percent of these families have had gonadotropin deficiency in association with growth hormone deficiency. Prognosis must be guarded for the occurrence of this disease in subsequent offspring of parents who have had a child with hypopituitarism.

Treatment consists of desiccated thyroid (1 to 2 grains/day) or thyroxine (100 to 200 μg/day) for those who have thyroid deficiency and cortisone (15 to 25 mg/m^2/day in divided doses) for those who have hypoglycemia. Thyroid should never be administered without cortisone unless the metyrapone response is normal. At the age of 15 to 16 years testosterone can be given to males, and estrogen plus testosterone can be given to females (testosterone may be needed in small doses in females to induce growth of sexual hair). Human growth hormone has been administered to a number of patients with growth hormone deficiency, and normal growth or supernormal growth rates have been obtained without toxicity. This is in contrast to the minimal response obtained when growth hormone, in comparable amounts, is given to patients with other types of dwarfism. However, 5 to 10 percent of these patients develop antibodies to growth hormone, which interferes with subsequent growth. This hormone should be more readily available in the future, thus making it possible for hypopituitary patients to achieve normal heights. The hypoglycemia, when present, also can be controlled with growth hormone.

A growth hormone releasing factor may be identified and synthesized soon; its synthesis would be easier than that of growth hormone, and it would greatly facilitate the treatment of hypopituitary patients, particularly those whose inability is in releasing rather than synthesizing the hormone.

Specific Gonadotropin Deficiency

Patients with specific gonadotropin deficiency must be differentiated from those with primary hypogona-

TABLE 2. Differential Diagnosis of Children With Short Stature

	Hypothyroidism	Constitutional Delay	Hypopituitarism	Primordial Dwarfism	Gonadal Dysgenesis	Psychosocial Dwarfism
Family history	Occasionally	Often	Occasionally	Occasionally	None	Occasionally
Birth weight	Normal	Normal	Normal	Often low	Often low	Normal
Hypoglycemia	None	None	At times	Rarely	Normal	Normal
Dental eruption	Delayed	Minimally delayed	Delayed	Normal	Normal	Normal or delayed (1+)
Facial features	Cretinoid or myxedematous	Slightly immature	Juvenile	Normal, progeroid, or pinched	Normal or peculiar to condition	Juvenile
Dwarfing	Minimal to marked	Minimal to moderate	Minimal to marked	Moderate to marked	Moderate	Minimal to marked
Sexual development	Infantile (usually)	Delayed	Infantile (50%)	Normal	Infantile, except sexual hair	Infantile
Body structure	Chubby	Normal	Normal	Subcutaneous tissue often decreased	Normal or peculiar to condition	Normal, chubby, or slender
Ratio of upper to lower segment	Immature	Slightly immature	Normal	Normal	Normal	Normal
Bone age	Delayed (1-4+)	Delayed (1-2+)	Delayed (2-4+)	Normal or delayed (1-2+)	Normal or delayed (1+)	Normal or delayed (1-3+)
Insulin sensitivity	Normal	Normal	Often present	Normal	Normal	Often present
Buccal smear	Normal	Normal	Normal	Normal	80% chromatin− 20% chromatin+	Normal
Thyroxine	Usually low	Normal	Often low normal or low	Normal	Normal	Usually normal or occasionally low
^{131}I uptake	Usually low	Normal	Often low normal or low	Normal	Normal	Usually normal or occasionally low
Metyrapone	Normal	Normal	Often abnormal	Normal	Normal	Often abnormal
Growth hormone	Often abnormally low	Normal	Abnormal	Normal	Normal	Often abnormal

dism, in whom urinary and blood gonadotropins are elevated at adolescence. Delayed release of gonadotropins in otherwise normal adolescent males can occur as late as 18 years of age; this can be differentiated from specific gonadotropin deficiency only by observations into adult life. Females rarely have such prolonged delayed adolescence.

Hyposmia or anosmia is commonly associated with gonadotropin deficiency; this familial entity (Kallmann syndrome) occurs more frequently in males. Treatment of males consists of replacement with testosterone. Injections of chorionic gonadotropin are effective, but its use is more expensive and less practical. Females are treated with estrogen and progesterone. Human menopausal gonadotropin is available to induce fertility in those patients whose gonads will respond.

ISOLATED ACTH AND TSH DEFICIENCIES. Isolated ACTH and TSH deficiencies are extremely rare. The 17-OHCS excretion increases with ACTH administration in patients with ACTH deficiency, but not in those with adrenal insufficiency. Determinations of plasma cortisol can be used for the differentiation instead of the 17-OHCS excretion. Infusions of ACTH are given over a 4- to 6-hour period, with a maximum dose of 25 IU. Blood is drawn for plasma cortisol determinations at 0, 2, 4, and 6 hours. Clinically, pigmentation and symptoms of salt loss are usually found in the adrenal-insufficient patient, in contrast to the ACTH-deficient patient.

Patients who have apparent thyroxine deficiency and who are suspected of having TSH deficiency should have TSH measured. Those with primary hypothyroidism will have elevations of TSH, in contrast to patients with secondary hypothyroidism, who will have low TSH values. TRH can be given to determine whether the inability to release TSH results from a pituitary or hypothalamic defect (p. 1606).

Organic Hypopituitarism

Of the many causes of organic hypopituitarism, the most common is craniopharyngioma (see page 1601 for embryologic development). In our clinic, 70 percent of patients with organic hypopituitarism have had craniopharyngiomas. In others the lesions have included suprasellar undifferentiated carcinoma, aberrant pinealoma, germinoma and chromophobe adenoma. Occasionally hypopituitarism arises from a basal skull fracture with interruption of the hypophyseal–venous portal system. Congenital malformations and other lesions of the hypothalamus may be responsible. Tuberous sclerosis, Hand-Schüller-Christian disease, encephalitis (particularly of the Economo type), hamartomas, and Recklinghausen's neurofibromatosis have all been implicated. However, hamartomas are more prone to produce sexual precocity, and neurofibromatosis is more commonly associated with somatic overgrowth.

The presenting complaints of patients with organic hypopituitarism are usually those related to visual dis-

turbances and central nervous system disease, rather than those related to growth disturbances or hypoglycemia, which are the common presenting complaints of patients with idiopathic hypopituitarism. In a recent study only 3 of 19 patients with organic hypopituitarism were of normal size; they were the youngest patients in the group.

The age of onset is variable, and signs and symptoms, which can occur as early as the first year, include evidences of idiopathic hypopituitarism, visual disturbances, headache, vomiting, and/or diabetes insipidus. The latter occurs in 20 to 35 percent of reported cases, but it may be obscured if there is associated ACTH deficiency and consequent cortisol deficiency. Administration of cortisone or related steroids uncovers the diabetes insipidus, probably because of the enhancing effect of cortisol on the clearance of free water in the renal tubule. Diabetes insipidus does not occur in idiopathic hypopituitarism. With lesions involving the hypothalamus, dysfunction of the hypothalamus, as reflected by poikilothermy, hypersomnia, obesity, or autonomic or uncinate epilepsy may be noted.

Radiologic examination of the skull is of great assistance in differentiating organic and idiopathic hypopituitarism; usually, gross abnormalities are noted. The most common pathology is calcification in the sella or suprasellar area, particularly with craniopharyngiomas, 80 percent of which have calcification. Frequently with craniopharyngioma there is destruction of the clinoid processes and flattening of the sella caused by pressure exerted from above. In contrast, adenomas of the pituitary produce a large expanded sella. If calcification is not present and there are no sellar changes in a patient with hypopituitarism and central nervous system symptoms, one must suspect internal hydrocephalus or a glioma in the area of the chiasm or third ventricle, which may produce the same symptoms.

The evaluation of endocrine function is as indicated on page 1604 and in the discussion of idiopathic hypopituitarism (p. 1608). Therapy must be directed toward hormonal replacement and toward surgical or radiation treatment of the space-occupying lesion, if one is present.

Psychosocial Dwarfism (See also p. 217)

Patients with emotional deprivation simulating idiopathic hypopituitarism, or psychosocial dwarfism, have been described. These children are rejected emotionally by their parents, who are almost uniformly psychologically disturbed. The signs and symptoms include short stature, polyphagia, polydipsia, polyuria (in spite of ability to concentrate urine), encopresis, gorging and vomiting, shyness, and temper tantrums. Skeletal development is usually delayed to the same severe extent as height for age. I.Q. levels have been less than 90 in most but not all of these children.

We have observed 25 proven cases; 6 of 11 children tested with both arginine monochloride and insulin failed to respond with a significant increase in STH concentration. Low serum thyroxine level or ^{131}I uptake is uncommon. Fifteen of these 25 children have been more than 10 percent underweight for height. Caloric malnutrition may be a factor in some but not all such patients. Psychosocial dwarfism may be difficult to differentiate from idiopathic hypopituitarism by clinical and laboratory examination. While the bizarre history is very helpful, the diagnosis can be proved only by removing the patient from the adverse environment and observing more rapid growth. In a favorable environment the mean growth rate of 25 patients was 6.6 inches/year during the first few months.

Iatrogenic Hypopituitarism

The term iatrogenic hypopituitarism refers to suppression of the pituitary and peripheral endocrine glands after administration of exogenous hormones, particularly cortisol and similar steroids. Continuous treatment with cortisol for periods of more than 2 to 4 weeks may be associated with absent or diminished adrenal response to administration of metyrapone. Patients who have received cortisol or cortisol-like steroids for 30 days or longer may have circulatory collapse when subjected to surgical or infectious stress. When this happens, oral cortisone (50 to 100 mg/m^2/day) should be given during periods of stress for 1 year following cessation of prolonged glucocorticoid therapy. If intramuscular treatment is used, the dosage is 25 to 50 mg/m^2/day.

HYPERPITUITARISM

Eosinophilic adenomas, the rarest of all pituitary tumors in childhood, lead to gigantism during childhood and superimposed features of acromegaly in late childhood and adulthood. These children usually present as problems of overgrowth; headaches are common. Initially the growth is symmetric, but with progression of the disease there is coarsening and thickening of the features, prognathism, kyphosis, and wide spacing of the teeth. The onset of sexual development is either at the usual time or late, but it progresses slowly, and hypogonadism eventually occurs; epiphyseal fusion occurs late. Muscular weakness and thyroid deficiency may also ensue.

Serum chemistries may be of some assistance. Hyperglycemia, a diabetic glucose tolerance test, and an elevated serum phosphorus level are all compatible with hypersomatotropism. Growth hormone is increased in all samples of serum, and it persists with glucose infusion, in contrast to the absence of growth hormone in the serum of normal individuals receiving glucose. Somatomedin levels are increased in patients with acromegaly. The visual fields usually are not affected, but if they are affected, alterations occur late in the course of the disease. Skull radiographs often show a slightly enlarged sella. Tufting of the phalanges may be demonstrated by roentgenography. The bone age is only minimally advanced, if at all.

Both chromophobe and basophilic adenomas have been associated with Cushing's syndrome of the adrenal hyperplasia type; both types of cells produce ACTH. Most of these tumors have been detected after subtotal or total adrenalectomy for treatment of the adrenal hyperplasia. Hyperpigmentation in association with Cushing's disease or after adrenalectomy for its treatment is highly indicative of an ACTH-secreting pituitary adenoma (Nelson's syndrome) even in the absence of sellar enlargement. Recent data suggest that nearly all cases of adrenal hyperplasia (Cushing's disease) may be of pituitary origin and therefore may possibly be related to adenomas. Occasionally the pituitary lesion is a carcinoma, and metastases may occur. Symptoms related to the central nervous system or visual tracts occur very late in these patients, and sellar enlargement occurs late, as does visual field abnormality. Exceptions do occur, particularly with tumors that grow rapidly.

Treatment of pituitary tumors is usually directed toward relieving the central nervous system and visual problems. However, the hyperfunction that sometimes occurs with eosinophilic, chromophobe, or basophilic adenomas may require treatment. With tumors that produce hypopituitarism, surgical removal is required to prevent visual deterioration. Craniopharyngiomas and cystic chromophobe adenomas that produce hypopituitarism are resistant to radiotherapy. Prior to surgery the patient must be given cortisone intramuscularly (100 mg/m^2/day) for 2 to 3 days. Postoperatively, 25 mg/m^2/day in divided doses should be given for several days, or continuously if the anterior pituitary is destroyed. Thyroid hormone may be required subsequently. Diabetes insipidus frequently results and requires treatment (p. 1617). Unfortunately, removal of cystic tumors is often incomplete, so that further observation is very important; repeat surgery may be necessary.

Tumors associated with hyperfunction are less likely to damage the optic chiasm, but they are also treated surgically when optic atrophy, papilledema, or limitation of visual fields is present. External irradiation frequently is beneficial with eosinophilic adenomas that do not affect the optic tracts. The total irradiation given through multiple portals should not exceed 4,500 roentgens, or cerebral necrosis and vascular damage may occur. Transsphenoidal removal of pituitary anomalies is now a feasible procedure. Individuals who have enlargement of the sella but no extension above the diaphragma sellae can benefit from a transsphenoidal approach. The morbidity following removal of the pituitary transsphenoidally is minimal, in contrast to surgical hypophysectomy. Radioactive gold and yttrium have also been implanted into the sella; preliminary reports in adults suggest that this may be a satisfactory form of treatment of eosinophilic adenoma. Treatment with cyclotron irradiation or cryosurgery also has been effective in some cases. Somatostatin decreases the amount of growth hormone in blood, but it has short activity and therefore is not useful for chronic therapy; however, a long-acting somatostatin preparation may be forthcoming. Further follow-up studies of the results of the various types of treatment are necessary.

The same forms of treatment have been utilized in managing pituitary tumors that produce Cushing's disease. External irradiation to the pituitary with similar doses has been used extensively in the past to control the symptoms of Cushing's disease with adrenal hyperplasia, but with only minimal success. For this reason subtotal or usually total adrenalectomy has been performed. If hyperpigmentation subsequently occurs in spite of adequate cortisone replacement, or if the sella is noted by periodic tomograms to be increasing in size, then irradiation, surgery, or cryotherapy must be considered. Surgery is indicated if the visual fields are affected. Either cryosurgery or irradiation is probably preferable; otherwise, pellet implantation with radioactive gold or yttrium or treatment with the cyclotron is superior to cobalt irradiation.

Functional Hyperpituitarism

Certain lesions or pathologic entities in some obscure way stimulate or simulate overactivity of the hypothalamic–pituitary axis, particularly in their association with excessive growth. Gliomas of the optic tract, often associated with neurofibromatosis, may extend into the hypothalamus; sometimes they are accompanied by somatic overgrowth instead of growth failure, but without gross evidence of acromegaly or excessive production of TSH, ACTH, or STH. Occasionally patients with neurofibromatosis without detectable intracranial tumor also present with overgrowth. In these patients, bone age is normal, and the tufting or other features of the acromegalic patient do not develop.

Patients have been reported who have mental retardation of apparent congenital origin, features simulating those of the acromegalic, and excessive growth during the first 4 to 5 years of childhood. After that time the growth parallels the normal curve. These patients with cerebral gigantism have advanced bone age, and they mature early, although they do not have true sexual precocity as it is ordinarily defined. With true sexual precocity the bone age continues to advance rapidly out of proportion to linear growth, and sexual maturation occurs early. In cerebral gigantism the skeletal age advances proportionately to the acceleration in linear growth, and sexual maturation occurs only 1 to 2 years before the expected time. The mechanisms involved are unknown.

Beckwith's syndrome is characterized by mental retardation, hepatomegaly, large body stature, hypoglycemia in early infancy, and mental retardation. It can be differentiated from cerebral gigantism and acromegaly by the associated visceromegaly and hypoglycemia.

Obesity has been considered to be associated with functional hyperpituitarism, since many obese children are overgrown, have a 1- to 2-year advancement of skeletal age, and frequently mature sexually more rapidly than nonobese children. Thyrotoxicosis and Marfan's syndrome are also associated with overgrowth and must be differentiated from acromegaly or true hyperpituitarism. Occasionally one observes overflow stimulation of the pituitary; in some patients with chronic primary hypothyroidism of long duration, the sella is enlarged. This is believed to result from excessive TSH production and pituitary hyperplasia, which occurs because of thyroxine deficiency. At times sexual precocity and galactorrhea also occur, and there is excessive gonadotropin and prolactin secretion in addition to excessive TSH.

References

Besser GM, Mortimer CH: Hypothalamic regulatory hormones: a review. J Clin Pathol 27:173, 1974

Brasel JA, Wright JC, Wilkins L, Blizzard RM: An evaluation of 75 patients with hypopituitarism beginning in childhood. Am J Med 38:484, 1963

————— Review of findings in patients with emotional deprivation. In Gardner LI, Amacher P (eds): Endocrine Aspects of Malnutrition; Marasmus, Kwashiorkor, and Psychosocial Dwarfism. Santa Ynez, Calif, Kroc Foundation, 1973

Ciba Collection of Medical Illustrations. Embryologic Development of the Pituitary. Boston, Little, Brown, 1965

Costom BH, Grumbach MM, Kaplan SL: Effect of thyrotropin-releasing factor on serum thyroid-stimulating hormone, an approach to distinguishing hypothalamic from pituitary forms of idiopathic hypopituitary dwarfism. J Clin Invest 50:2219, 1971

Daughaday WH: The adenohypophysis. In Williams RH (ed): Textbook of Endocrinology. Philadelphia, WB Saunders, 1974

Foley TP, Owings J, Hayford JT, Blizzard RM: Serum thyrotropin responses to synthetic thyrotropin-releasing hormone in normal children and hypopituitary patients. A new test to distinguish primary releasing hormone deficiency from primary pituitary hormone deficiency. J Clin Invest 51:431, 1972

Goodman HG, Grumbach MM, Kaplan SL: Growth and growth hormone. II. Comparison of isolated growth-hormone deficiency and multiple pituitary hormone deficiencies in 35 patients with idiopathic hypopituitary dwarfism. N Engl J Med 278:57, 1968

Hall K, Luft R: Growth hormone and somatomedin. Adv Metab Disord 7:1, 1974

Harris GT, Donovan BT: The Pituitary Gland, vols 1–3. Berkeley, Univ California Press, 1966

Heald FP, Hung W (eds): Endocrinology of Adolescence. New York, Appleton-Century-Crofts, 1970

Lovinger RD, Kaplan SL, Grumbach MM: Congenital hypopituitarism associated with neonatal hypoglycemia and microphallus: Four cases secondary to hypothalamic hormone deficiencies. J Pediatr 87:1171, 1975

Powell GF, Brasel JA, Blizzard RM: Emotional deprivation and growth retardation simulating idiopathic hypopituitarism. I. Clinical evaluation of the syndrome. N Engl J Med 276:1271, 1967

Raiti S (ed): Human Growth Hormone Research. DHEW Publication (NIH) 74-612. Bethesda, NIAMDD, NIH, 1974

Rasmussen H: Organization and control of endocrine systems. In Williams RH (ed): Textbook of Endocrinology. Philadelphia, WB Saunders, 1974

Sotos JF, Dodge PR, Muirhead D, Crawford JD, Talbot NB: Cerebral gigantism in childhood. A syndrome of excessively rapid growth with acromegalic features and a non-progressive neurologic disorder. N Engl J Med 271:109, 1964

Van Wyk JJ, Underwood LE, Hintz RL, Clemmons DR, Voina S, Weaver RP: The somatomedins: a family of insulin-like hormones under growth hormone control. Recent Prog Horm Res 30:259, 1974

Wilkins L: The Diagnosis and Treatment of Endocrine Disorders in Childhood and Adolescence, 3rd ed. Springfield, Ill, Charles C Thomas, 1965

PRIMARY DISTURBANCES OF WATER HOMEOSTASIS

William E. Segar

PHYSIOLOGY OF WATER HOMEOSTASIS

The volume and the tonicity of body fluids are maintained within remarkably narrow limits by a variety of highly sensitive mechanisms. If body water homeostasis is to be maintained, daily renal water excretion must equal water intake less extrarenal water losses. Water intake is regulated by thirst; renal water loss is determined primarily by intrarenal mechanisms and by the action of antidiuretic hormone (ADH) on the renal concentrating system.

The neurohypophyseal system, which is responsible for the synthesis, storage, and release of ADH, consists of the supraoptic and paraventricular hypothalamic nuclei and the neurohypophyseal tract. This is comprised of axons originating from these nuclei and terminating in the pars nervosa or posterior lobe of the pituitary gland, where the hormone, an octapeptide, is stored. By electron microscopy the hormone is seen to be in the nerve cell bodies bound to an intraaxonal protein carrier termed neurophysin, and it moves by axoplasmic streaming down the axons to terminate in the posterior lobe. ADH is probably released into the circulation in an unbound form, and release is dependent on impulses arising in the supraoptic nuclei and propagated down the axon to the posterior pituitary. The origin of ADH in these anterior hypothalamic structures explains why extirpation or destruction of the posterior lobe does not in itself result in permanent diabetes insipidus.

In the absence of ADH, maximal water diuresis develops, with urine osmolality usually being less than 100 mOsm/kg; in the adult 10 liters/day or more of urine may be excreted. When ADH levels are high, urine osmolality may exceed 1,200 mOsm/kg. The normal daily urine solute load of an adult may be excreted in less than 500 ml of urine. Thus the mechanisms that regulate ADH release from the posterior pituitary are important for the maintenance of body water homeostasis. The release of ADH is governed primarily by the effective intravascular fluid volume and by osmolality of the extracellular fluid. However, pain, stress, emotional factors, and certain drugs also may stimulate release of ADH from the hypothalamic–neurohypophyseal system. During periods of hypotension, baroreceptors located in the aorta, carotid sinus, and carotid bodies also participate in the regulation of ADH release.

The experiments of Verney provided the initial evidence that release of ADH is controlled by the plasma concentrations of solutes, to which cells of the hypothalamus are either partially or completely impermeable. His studies in dogs documenting the inhibition of water diuresis after intracarotid infusion of hypertonic saline, as well as those of Arndt and Gauer demonstrating induction of water diuresis after intracarotid infusion of water in the unanesthetized dog, provided evidence of an osmoreceptive area in the distribution of the carotid artery, probably the anterior hypothalamus. More recently, Dunn and associates, using a sensitive and specific radioimmunoassay for plasma arginine vasopressin, have demonstrated that the intraperitoneal injection of hypertonic saline, which has no effect on blood volume and which increases plasma osmolality, results in a progressive rise in plasma ADH levels.

Several years before Verney's studies, Peters proposed the concept that the fullness of the intravascular space is sensed by the organism and that the contraction of this space leads to antidiuresis, whereas expansion results in diuresis. Gauer and Henry concluded that the so-called volume receptor is located within the capacitance vessels of the thorax. The work of several investigators suggests that the left atrium is the likely site. Johnson and coworkers demonstrated that physiologic changes in left atrial pressure in the anesthetized dog are inversely related to blood ADH levels in the absence of alterations in renal hemodynamics or plasma osmolality. Segar and Moore showed that the blood ADH level changes rapidly with change in position or environmental temperature—procedures that alter the distribution of blood within the vascular compartment despite constancy of plasma osmolality. The rapidity of change in blood ADH concentration in these circumstances indicates a great sensitivity and a prime functional role for the volume receptor in the regulation of ADH release. Although osmotic and volume stimuli work synergistically under most physiologic conditions, their relative influence on ADH release has not been clarified completely. The available information suggests an increasingly important effect for the osmoreceptor as plasma osmolality rises above 290 mOsm/kg, with little or no effect when plasma tonicity is less than 285 mOsm/kg. On the other hand, the volume receptor appears to influence ADH release to some degree at all levels of left atrial filling. Impulses reaching the hypothalamus via the left vagus, at normal degrees of left atrial stretch, tonically inhibit ADH release. However, when left atrial stretch is decreased, cessation of inhibition occurs, and ADH is released into the plasma. This latter reflex is abolished by left vagotomy.

When the concentration of ADH in the blood is less than 1 μU/ml, dilute urine is elaborated; with a blood concentration of 4 μU/ml or more, urine is maximally concentrated. During periods of shock, anesthesia, or dehydration, the blood ADH concentration may increase to 10 μU/ml or more. The blood ADH concentration can be considered normal or abnormal only in reference to the state of hydration and the body fluid tonicity of the patient. A value of 0 μU/ml is normal in the hydrated prone subject, but it is not normal if the subject is dehydrated or hypertonic or is standing. A value of 4 μU/ml is normal in the dehydrated or hypertonic patient, but abnormal (or inappropriate) if the patient is overhydrated or hypotonic.

The half-life of ADH in man is approximately 7 minutes. During periods of prolonged antidiuresis, nearly continuous release of ADH must occur. Once released from storage in the posterior pituitary, ADH is carried to the kidney, where it exerts its only significant physiologic effect. While in the blood, ADH is dialyzable and ultrafilterable from plasma, indicating an absence of protein binding.

Urine formation begins with the passage of the ultrafiltrate of plasma through the glomerular membrane. This filtrate is isosmotic, and most of it (perhaps 60 to 70 percent) is reabsorbed passively, accompanying the active reabsorption of sodium as the fluid passes through the proximal tubule. As the filtrate moves through the loop of Henle, it first becomes more concentrated as water moves from the lumen into the hypertonic medullary interstitium near the tip of the loop. It is then diluted, with sodium being extruded and water retained, as the fluid moves up the ascending limb. Therefore the fluid entering the distal convolution is hypotonic. Thus far, the mechanisms for diuresis and antidiuresis are the same.

During water diuresis, little water is reabsorbed as the filtrate passes through the distal convolution and collecting duct, but because sodium reabsorption continues, a dilute urine results. During antidiuresis the presence of ADH produces a marked increase in the permeability to water of the tubular epithelium, so that equilibrium of the filtrate with interstitial fluid occurs. Because the collecting ducts pass through the zone of marked interstitial fluid hypertonicity in the inner medulla and papillae, the fluid entering the renal pelvis becomes highly concentrated. In man a urine concentration of 1,200 to 1,400 mOsm/kg may be reached. Higher concentrations are achieved by other mammals.

The action of ADH on cellular permeability has been studied experimentally on toad bladder, a membrane with characteristics similar to those of the renal tubular epithelium. ADH has been shown to increase cellular permeability by making the membrane responsive to bulk flow. The nature of these membrane changes and the means by which they are induced remains unclear. Recent evidence does indicate that the action of vasopressin is mediated by release of cyclic adenosine -3',5'-monophosphate (cAMP) and that injection of cAMP into the renal artery of an experimental animal produces antidiuresis, as would the injection of vasopressin; cAMP is present in human urine, and its excretion increases following injection of vasopressin. The fact that most children with nephrogenic diabetes insipidus have decreased amounts of cAMP in their urine and have neither a biochemical nor a physiologic response to vasopressin administration suggests that the basic defect in their disease is an abnormality in cAMP metabolism in the renal tubular cells.

THIRST. Although thirst is a physiologic function of obvious importance, it has received relatively little critical study, and the factors regulating thirst in man remain poorly understood. Thirst is a cortical or conscious sensation. Specific nuclear centers exist in the ventromedial and anterior hypothalamus for the integration of various signals altering water ingestion. Subcortical and cortical connections of these centers are required for transforming a need for water into appropriate behavior. Both local and systemic factors contribute to regulation of the sensation of thirst. Among the most important local factors are dryness of the mucous membranes which produces the sensation of thirst, and fullness of the stomach which inhibits this feeling. Systemic factors also contribute to regulation of thirst: isotonic expansion of the body fluid inhibits thirst, while hypertonicity produces thirst. Isotonic dehydration and hypovolemia, particularly hypovolemia following acute hemorrhage, produce intense thirst. Indeed, intense thirst in a well-hydrated patient should suggest a diminished intravascular volume. Certain drugs alter thirst, and psychologic factors affect it profoundly. Since several areas of the hypothalamus play significant roles in the regulation of thirst, certain central nervous system lesions may alter it. Ablative lesions of the preoptic nucleus, ventromedial nucleus, anterior hypothalamus, and subcommissural organ cause adipsia, while similar lesions in the basal tuberal region cause polydipsia. Polydipsia can also be produced by stimulation of several of the hypothalamic nuclei with a weak electric current or by certain drugs.

Although a variety of stimuli can direct a person with an intact central nervous system and no psychologic abnormalities to increase water intake above that usually consumed, there seems to be no physiologic mechanism available to man to signal him to reduce fluid intake below normal. This is significant in the pathogenesis of several hyponatremic states.

DIABETES INSIPIDUS

Diabetes insipidus is an uncommon disease characterized clinically by polyuria and polydipsia. Two forms of diabetes insipidus are encountered in children: true ADH deficiency and a familial X-linked form in which blood ADH levels are increased (nephrogenic diabetes insipidus). The former responds satisfactorily to administration of exogenous ADH; the latter is refractory to this therapy.

CLINICAL MANIFESTATIONS. Polyuria and polydipsia are the main clinical manifestations of diabetes insipidus. Urine volume may exceed 10 liters/day in the adult or 300 to 400 ml/kg/day in the infant. The onset of symptoms is frequently abrupt. In the alert, conscious adult or older child these symptoms may be little more than an inconvenience. In the younger child disturbances in sleep and activities are more serious. If the child is able to meet increased water requirement by increasing water intake, no additional symptoms are noted. However, if the patient is very young or is incapacitated or unconscious, dehydration will develop rapidly. Hyperpyrexia occurs, and because the urine is hypotonic, hypernatremia develops. Either hyperpyrexia or hypernatremia or both may cause severe or fatal injury to the central nervous system.

The osmolality of the urine of the patient with diabetes insipidus is usually less than 150 mOsm/kg; specific gravity is 1.001 to 1.005. The urine may become isotonic (or rarely hypertonic) during periods of dehydration if the glomerular filtration rate is decreased markedly as a result of hypovolemia. The serum sodium concentration and osmolality are usually normal or slightly elevated in children with uncomplicated diabetes insipidus. During dehydration, both may increase to pathologic concentrations.

ADH-Deficient Diabetes Insipidus

ADH-deficient diabetes insipidus may be classified as primary or secondary, depending on the presence or absence of underlying disease. A specific cause for ADH deficiency cannot be found in approximately one-third of all patients. Of these patients, more commonly infants and children than adults, the majority must be classified as having an idiopathic form. A familial form of primary diabetes insipidus that follows a mendelian dominant pattern of inheritance does occur, but it is rare. Unfortunately, the cause of diabetes insipidus may be difficult to ascertain. Unless the family history is diagnostic, the diagnosis of primary or idiopathic diabetes insipidus must remain suspect until careful observations for 5 to 10 years fail to demonstrate evidence of a neoplasm or histiocytosis.

Secondary diabetes insipidus may result from any lesion that damages the neurohypophyseal system. Trauma, either accidental or neurosurgical, is a major cause. Infections, tumors (particularly craniopharyngiomas, pituitary adenomas, and pinealomas), Hand-Schüller-Christian disease, and in rare cases metastatic neoplasms or degenerative diseases of the central nervous system also can be causes. When secondary diabetes insipidus is produced as a result of trauma or a neurosurgical procedure, a triphasic clinical course often follows. Initially there is a period of diuresis and, presumably, ADH deficiency. Antidiuresis ensues after a few days. Severe hyponatremia may occur if water intake is not curtailed during this so-called interphase period. The interphase phenomenon is believed to be due to the uncontrolled release of ADH from damaged neurohypophyseal tracts. Finally, persistent diabetes insipidus follows a few days later, once ADH stores are exhausted.

ADH-Resistant Diabetes Insipidus

ADH-resistant (nephrogenic) diabetes insipidus is a genetically determined disorder that is clinically similar to diabetes insipidus. The renal tubular cells of these patients apparently are insensitive to ADH, and a hypotonic urine is excreted despite normal or high blood ADH levels. Polyuria and polydipsia result. The disease may be present from birth. These infants require very high daily water intakes (300 to 500 ml/kg/day). Dehydration may develop with extreme rapidity. Hyperpyrexia and failure to thrive are common complications. The biochemical mechanisms involved in this disorder are discussed elsewhere (p. 1314).

PRIMARY POLYDIPSIA

The ingestion of water in excess of that required to maintain normal water balance should be termed primary polydipsia. Polydipsia is the result of a physiologic or psychologic thirst drive. Traditionally it has been assumed that primary polydipsia is a psychogenic entity, and it has been called compulsive water drinking. Although primary polydipsia can occur as a result of serious behavior disturbance, and thus properly be classified as psychogenic polydipsia, it is now recognized that pathologic lesions of the hypothalamus also may cause excessive thirst, producing the syndrome termed neurogenic polydipsia. Because the hypothalamic regions regulating thirst and those concerned with ADH production are contiguous, diabetes insipidus can coexist with primary polydipsia. Primary (neurogenic) polydipsia also may mimic diabetes insipidus in a patient with a known hypothalamic lesion. Each patient with polydipsia must have a comprehensive neurologic examination, and often a psychologic examination, before the condition can be classified as neurogenic or psychogenic.

DIFFERENTIAL DIAGNOSIS. Because polyuria and polydipsia can result from true diabetes insipidus, from hypothalamic damage that alters thirst but not ADH release (neurogenic polydipsia), from nephrogenic diabetes insipidus, or from psychogenic polydipsia (see below), various diagnostic procedures are needed to determine the cause of these symptoms. The urine osmolality will be low (<270 mOsm/kg) in each instance. The serum osmolality may be normal (275 to 290 mOsm/kg) or slightly increased in diabetes insipidus or nephrogenic diabetes insipidus, but it will be normal or slightly low in primary polydipsia.

A water-deprivation test will often differentiate diabetes insipidus from primary polydipsia. Fluid should be withheld until the patient has lost 3 to 5 percent of body weight. The patient with diabetes insipidus will suffer a rapid weight loss, and urine will remain hypotonic. The patient with primary polydipsia will lose weight more slowly, and urine osmolality will increase as dehydration occurs. Constant surveillance during the period of water deprivation is essential to avoid the effects of severe dehydration and to prevent surreptitious water intake. The physician should be aware of certain pitfalls in this test. A patient with diabetes insipidus may produce a hypertonic urine (>300 mOsm/kg), despite the lack of ADH, if the glomerular filtration rate is decreased significantly as a result of severe dehydration. Chronic overhydration will result in a diminished capacity to concentrate urine because of washout of solute from the renal medullary interstitium, so that a patient with primary polydipsia may not demonstrate an increase in urine osmolality of the magnitude expected in response to water deprivation. Furthermore, because such a patient may be significantly overhydrated initially, a weigh loss of 5 percent may be insufficient to produce underhydration. Physical examination will indicate if the water-deprivation test should be continued until a weight loss of more than 5 percent is achieved. The response of the kidney to water deprivation may be impaired by diseases such as interstitial nephritis, pyelonephritis, hypercalcemia, and chronic potassium deficiency. Usually a slightly hypertonic urine is produced in each of these states.

Once it has been determined that the patient cannot produce a hypertonic urine despite dehydration, his response to exogenous ADH (vasopressin) should be tested. A patient with nephrogenic diabetes insipidus will exhibit no response, while one with diatebes insipidus will show an increase in urine osmolality. Either aqueous or long-acting vasopressin tannate in oil can be used. Aqueous vasopressin can be administered for 1 hour by slow intravenous infusion (5 μU/minute), or vasopressin tannate in oil can be given intramuscularly (5 U). Prompt diminution in urine minute volume and an increase in urine osmolality can be expected in the former test; in the latter the overnight urine specimen and the next three urine specimens should be examined for increased osmolality. The use of long-acting vasopressin tannate in oil is potentially hazardous. Should the patient have primary polydipsia and continue to drink excessively, hyponatremia and central nervous system symptoms may be produced following vasopressin administration. This complication may also arise when a child with previously untreated diabetes insipidus is first given vasopressin. The patient who is conditioned to a large fluid intake may not decrease his fluid intake despite his diminished need for water and even despite his inability to excrete the water load. If the patient's urine volume decreases after vasopressin administration, his fluid intake should be monitored until he has "learned" of this decreased need for water.

TREATMENT. Reduction of the solute load by restricting the protein and salt content of the diet will ameliorate polyuria in either true or nephrogenic diabetes insipidus. This is usually necessary only for patients with nephrogenic diabetes insipidus, and one must then be certain that the diet provides the calories and essential nutrients needed for normal growth. An adequate supply of water must always be available for the child with either form of the disease. Diuretics, particularly chlorothiazide, were shown by Crawford and associates to produce a slight but significant increase in urine solute concentration in children with nephrogenic diabetes insipidus. The mode of action of these drugs is uncertain, but if urine osmolality is increased from 100 to only 200 mOsm/kg, the urine volume and the need for water are decreased by half.

Commercial preparations are available for effective treatment of diabetes insipidus. The short half-life of aqueous vasopressin precludes its use therapeutically. However, the suspension of vasopressin tannate in peanut oil (5 U/ml) is a satisfactory drug; 0.5 to 1.0 ml intramuscularly will provide relief of symptoms for 24 to 72 hours. The injection should be repeated when symptoms recur. The ampule must be warmed and vigorously shaken before use.

A lysine vasopressin nasal spray is available, as is vasopressin powder snuff. Both of these preparations have the disadvantage of short duration of action and ineffectiveness with upper respiratory infections; with the snuff, chronic inflammation of the nasal mucous membranes is a frequent occurrence. However, clinical trials are in progress to assess a long-acting analogue, desaminocys[1]-D-arg[8]-vasopressin (DDAVP). When ad-ministered in aqueous solution by nasal insufflation, it is effective for 8 to 24 hours.

Diabetes insipidus is difficult to manage in comatose patients, in those who are recovering from neurosurgical procedures, and in other circumstances in which the patient's thirst drive is not available to aid in the regulation of water intake. These patients can be managed readily by daily injection of 5 U or more of vasopressin tannate in oil and, if hydration is satisfactory, by administration of about 80 percent of the normal maintenance fluid intake. Body weight, urine volume, and serum sodium or osmolality should be monitored daily. More vasopressin is needed when body weight decreases, serum sodium increases, and urine volume is large. If weight increases, serum sodium decreases, and urine volume is low, too much water is being given. The patient is receiving an inadequate fluid intake if serum sodium increases as weight decreases despite a small urine volume.

In addition to appropriate medical or surgical therapy, patients with neurogenic polydipsia must be taught to restrict fluid intake. Psychogenic polydipsia is evidence of a complex emotional disturbance, and psychiatric therapy is usually necessary.

EXCESSIVE ADH RELEASE

Inappropriate ADH Secretion

A variety of disease states, including malignant tumors (particularly bronchogenic carcinoma), acute and chronic pulmonary disease (such as tuberculosis, bronchopneumonia, and status asthmaticus), hypothyroidism, and disorders of the central nervous system (such as meningitis, head injuries, encephalitis, Guillain-Barré syndrome, acute intermittent porphyria, and brain tumors) may be accompanied by hyponatremia and production of hypertonic urine, despite absence of any evidence indicative of hypovolemia and despite normal renal and adrenal function. These diseases have been termed the syndrome of inappropriate ADH secretion. Blood ADH levels are increased, resulting in an inability to elaborate other than a hypertonic urine. The combination of maximal renal conservation of water (due to persistently high blood ADH levels) and a normal fluid intake leads to water retention and dilutional hyponatremia. In these circumstances, efforts to correct the hyponatremia by sodium administration are usually futile; water restriction, on the other hand, results in gradual correction of the disturbance in serum sodium concentration.

In most cases the cause for the increased blood ADH level, and therefore for the hyponatremia, can be determined. Certain malignant tumors apparently synthesize a peptide similar to or identical with ADH, because in such cases high ADH levels are found on bioassay or radioimmunoassay of the plasma. Analysis of the tumor reveals an extremely high content of ADH or ADH-like substances. ADH levels return to normal after effective treatment of the malignancy. Patients who have bronchopneumonia, status asthmaticus, emphysema, or chronic obstructive pulmonary disease or who are receiving positive-pressure ventilatory assistance may exhibit hyponatremia and increased blood ADH levels. In these cases the decreased filling of the left atrium, which is due to increased resistance of blood flow through the pulmonary bed, is the apparent cause of the elevation of the plasma ADH level. The blood ADH level decreases promptly, and diuresis ensues if ventilatory assistance is discontinued or if the underlying pulmonary disease is treated adequately. Because patients with this group of pulmonary diseases may have elevated blood ADH levels, fluids must be administered to them with caution. This is particularly true of patients who have status asthmaticus or of those who are receiving ventilatory assistance where the provision of normal amounts of water, orally or intravenously, may result in hyponatremia and the associated symptoms of water intoxication. Should hyponatremia occur in these circumstances, water intake must be curtailed. Once the patient recovers from the acute disease, or once ventilatory assistance is discontinued, diuresis will ensue and the serum sodium concentration will return to normal.

Cerebral Salt-Wasting

Hyponatremia occasionally may occur with central nervous system lesions if the hypothalamic regions concerned with ADH production are stimulated by the pathologic process. However, a different pathogenesis for the syndrome of cerebral salt-wasting is more frequent. Patients with severe central nervous system disease or with conditions characterized by paralysis, such as the Guillain-Barré syndrome, lie motionless in bed. The blood will pool in the dependent portions of the vascular compartment if periodic muscular contractions do not aid its return to the chest. Left atrial filling decreases, ADH release occurs, and the persistently increased blood ADH level combined with a normal fluid intake produces hyponatremia. If the legs of the patient are wrapped with an elastic bandage, or if the foot of the bed is raised, blood return to the chest is enhanced; increased filling of the left atrium results in inhibition of ADH release, and a prompt diuresis ensues. Occasionally the cause of the increased ADH production cannot be determined, or if it is known it cannot be corrected. Water restriction is the preferred method of treatment of the hyponatremia caused by inappropriate or unwanted high circulating levels of ADH. The administration of hypertonic saline solutions is usually futile unless combined with diuretic therapy. The latter approach requires careful continuous clinical and laboratory monitoring of the hyponatremic state; simple water restriction, although slower, is safe.

Lithium salts also can interfere with the renal concentrating mechanism. Some patients receiving lithium have developed polydipsia and polyuria refractory to vasopressin. Lithium is believed to exert this action by inhibition of the adenylcyclase system in the renal medulla. If this action occurs in a reproducible manner,

lithium may prove to be a useful drug for rapid treatment of the hyponatremia associated with the syndrome of inappropriate ADH. It should not be used in patients with nephrosis or cirrhosis, where hyponatremia is accompanied by hypovolemia.

Other Conditions

Increased blood ADH levels occur in all hypovolemic states. The blood ADH is high in shock, in the nephrotic syndrome, in cirrhosis, and in other diseases characterized by hypoproteinemia and edema. Pain and anesthesia cause ADH release, and high blood ADH levels are observed following surgical procedures. The blood ADH level may remain increased for 7 to 10 days after cardiac surgery, and because a dilute urine cannot be elaborated during this period, hyponatremia will develop unless water intake is decreased to 50 to 70 percent of maintenance level. Since physicians now are aware of this phenomenon, postoperative intravenous fluid administration is restricted routinely. However, once oral feedings are begun, these restrictions may be relaxed. Hyponatremia can then develop if the patient, unaware of his inability to dilute urine and experiencing no diminution of thirst, resumes his "normal" fluid intake.

Vincristine, which is used in the treatment of childhood leukemia and certain malignant diseases, also may cause hyponatremia. Available evidence suggests that vincristine has a specific effect on the central nervous system that results in ADH release. Blood ADH levels are elevated following vincristine administration, and hyponatremia results if the patient receives an excessive fluid intake. The hyponatremic state is corrected by water restriction.

Hypodipsia is an uncommon condition characterized by chronic hypernatremia and hyperosmolality; it occurs in patients in whom the sensation of thirst is diminished or absent. Destructive lesions of the hypothalamus are the usual cause of this syndrome, although hypodipsia with serum hyperosmolality may occur in children with occult hydrocephalus or microcephaly. Hypodipsia has been produced experimentally in animals by ablative lesions of the hypothalamus. Rarely, destructive hypothalamic lesions cause both diabetes insipidus and hypodipsia. All patients with hypodipsia should be given complete neurologic examination. Treatment consists of appropriate measures to ensure that the patient consumes an adequate amount of water daily.

References

Andersson B, Cale CC, Sundsten JW: Thirst. In Wayner MJ (ed): Thirst in the Regulation of Body Water. New York, Pergamon, 1964

Arndt JO, Gauer OH: Diuresis induced by water infusion into the carotid loop of unanesthetized dogs. Pfluegers Arch 282:301, 1965

Bartter FC, Schwartz WB: The syndrome of inappropriate secretion of antidiuretic hormone. Am J Med 42:790, 1967

Berliner RW, Bennett CM: Concentration of urine in the mammalian kidney. Am J Med 42:777, 1967

Bode HH, Crawford JD: Nephrogenic diabetes insipidus in North America—the Hopewell hypothesis. N Engl J Med 280:750, 1969

Bower BF, Mason DM, Forsham PH: Bronchogenic carcinoma with inappropriate antidiuretic activity in plasma and tumor. N Engl J Med 271:934, 1964

Crawford JD, Kennedy GC, Hill LE: Clinical results of treatment of diabetes insipidus with drugs of the chlorothiazide series. N Engl J Med 262:737, 1960

Dashe AM, Cramm RE, Crist CA, Habener JF, Solomon DH: A water deprivation test for the differential diagnosis of polyuria. JAMA 185:699, 1963

De Wardener HE: Polyuria. J Chronic Dis 11:199, 1960

Dunn FL, Brennan TJ, Nelson AE, Robertson GL: The role of blood osmolality and volume in regulating vasopressin secretion in the rat. J Clin Invest 52:3212, 1973

Fitzsimons JT: The hypothalamus and drinking. Br Med Bull 22:232, 1966

Gauer OH, Henry JP: Circulatory basis of fluid volume control. Physiol Rev 43:423, 1963

Johnson JA, Moore WW, Segar WE: Small changes in left atrial pressure and plasma antidiuretic hormone titers in dogs. Am J Physiol 217:210, 1969

Jones NF, Barraclough MA, Barnes N, Cottom DG: Nephrogenic diabetes insipidus—effects of 3,5, cyclic-adenosine monophosphate. Arch Dis Child 47:794, 1972

Leaf A: Membrane effects of antidiuretic hormone. Am J Med 42:745, 1967

——— Coggins CH: The Neurohypophysis. In Williams RH (ed): Textbook of Endocrinology. Philadelphia, WB Saunders, 1974, p 938

Peters JP: Body Water: The Exchange of Fluid in Man. Springfield, Ill, Charles C Thomas, 1935

Randall RV, Clark EC, Bahn RC: Classification of the causes of diabetes insipidus. Mayo Clin Proc 34:299, 1959

Robinson AG: DDAVP in the treatment of central diabetes insipidus. N Engl J Med 294:507, 1976

Sawyer WH: Neurohypophyseal hormones. Pharmacol Rev 13:225, 1961

Schwartz WB, Bennett W, Curelop S, Bartter FC: A syndrome of renal sodium loss and hyponatremia probably resulting from inappropriate secretion of antidiuretic hormone. Am J Med 23:529, 1957

Segar WE, Moore WW: The regulation of antidiuretic hormone release in man I. Effects of change in position and ambient temperature on blood ADH levels. J Clin Invest 47:2143, 1968

Share L: Vasopressin, its bioassay and the physiological control of its release. Am J Med 42:701, 1967

Smith HW: Salt and water volume receptors: an exercise in physiologic apologetics. Am J Med 23:623, 1957

Stevko RM, Balsley M, Segar WE: Primary polydipsia—compulsive water drinking: report of two cases. J Pediatr 73:845, 1968

Verney EB: The antidiuretic hormone and the factors which determine its release. Proc R Soc Lond [Biol] 135:25, 1947

White MG, Fetner CD: Treatment of the syndrome of inappropriate secretion of antidiuretic hormone with lithium carbonate. N Engl J Med 292:390, 1975

Wolf AV: Thirst, Physiology of the Urge to Drink and Problems of Water Lack. Springfield, Ill, Charles C Thomas, 1958

ADRENAL CORTEX

CLAUDE J. MIGEON

PHYSIOLOGY

Anatomy, Embryology, Chemical Content

The adrenal glands are located on the upper poles of the kidneys, embedded in the perirenal adipose tissue. Each weighs 4 to 6 g. Extraglandular nodules of adrenocortical tissue are frequently found. In the female they are usually located near the ovaries in the broad ligaments. In the male they can be located in or near the testes or along the cord. Tumors located in extraglandular tissue have been reported in the lower pole of the kidney. The existence of these extraglandular nodules and their location are related to the embryonic development of these glands from a common adrenogenital ridge.

The adrenal gland is composed of two elements: the medulla, which is ectodermal in origin, and the cortex, which arises from the mesonephros. The cortex of the adrenal gland comprises about 90 percent of the volume of the gland. An arterial subcapsular plexus sends small arterial twigs to the medulla of the adrenal gland, with capillary loops going to the cortex. The blood returns to the sinus of the outer zone of the cortex and then to the central vein of the gland. The anatomy of the blood circulation in the gland is thought to play an important role in the secretion of medullary and cortical hormones. Cortical hormones must go through the medulla before they reach the general circulation, with the high concentration of the cortisol permitting activation of the methyltransferase required for the conversion of norepinephrine into epinephrine in the medulla. Conversely, the high concentrations of epinephrine in the venous system may influence the secretion of adrenocortical hormones. The presence of longitudinal muscle bundles in the wall of the central vein is a unique feature. It is of interest that few if any nerve fibers are seen in the adrenal cortex.

Histologically, three distinct zones can be seen in the cortex; from without in, they are the zona glomerulosa, zona fasciculata, and zona reticularis. Their respective volumes in the adult subject are 15, 75, and 10 percent of the cortex. By electron microscopy the cells of the zona glomerulosa are seen to have large nuclei, moderate amounts of mitochondria, and dense endoplasmic reticulum, while the cells of the zona fasciculata contain a large amount of lipid but very few mitochondria and light endoplasmic reticulum. The compact cells of the zona reticularis have few lipid globules and abundant mitochondria and endoplasmic reticulum, as well as microvilli.

The adrenal cortex arises in fetal life from an outgrowth of the coelomic mesothelium, as do the gonads and the liver. However, other tissues such as red cells also contain enzymes capable of metabolizing such steroids as ketosteroid reductase. After the adrenal cortex has differentiated from the gonadal tissue, it is invaded by sympathetic neural elements that shortly thereafter differentiate into chromaffin cells. This takes place during the 7th or 8th week of fetal life. In the 3-month-old embryo the adrenal glands are about as large as the kidneys, and at birth they weigh 8 to 9 g, representing 0.5 percent of the body weight, in contrast to 0.0175 percent in the adult (Fig. 5). The adrenal cortex of the human fetus consists almost exclusively of specific cells forming a large fetal zone. The remarkable size of the fetal adrenal is due to this tissue. During the first 3 weeks after birth the fetal zone undergoes cell resorp-

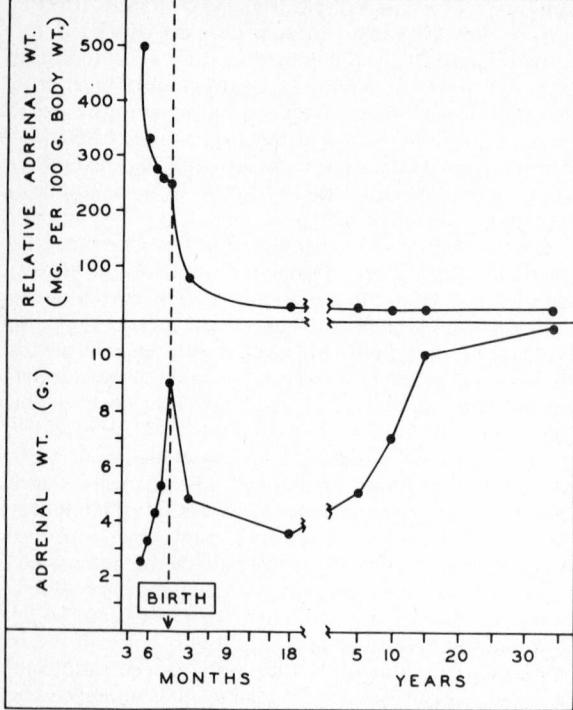

FIG. 5. Absolute and relative weights of adrenal glands in man from fetal life to adulthood. (Data from Spector: Handbook of Biological Data, 1956. Courtesy of W.B. Saunders.)

tion that results in a 50 percent decrease in adrenal weight.

The cytoplasm of adrenocortical cells, particularly those of the zona fasciculata, contain lipid droplets. To-

tal lipids represent 20 percent of the wet weight of a gland and are mainly cholesterol and phosphatides. The cholesterol is in great part esterified, and it arises both from the blood circulation and from local synthesis. In the newborn the lipids represent only 4 percent of the wet weight of a gland.

The cells of the adrenal cortex do not store the steroids, and minimal amounts of hormones are found in the gland. However, more than 50 compounds have been isolated from adrenal extracts. Ascorbic acid, in its reduced state, is found in high concentration in the adrenal cortex. Its role in steroid biogenesis remains unclear. Vitamins A and B$_2$ are also present in relatively large concentrations.

The adrenal cortex also contains numerous enzymes. The concentrations of coenzyme A, which is required for cholesterol synthesis, are the highest in the body except for those found in liver. Enzymes necessary for the transformation of cholesterol to pregnenolone and then to the various steroid hormones are also present. Their distributions in the cells will be described later. The enzymatic system of the pentose monophosphate shunt is much more active than the triose phosphate pathway. Acid phosphatase activity is located mainly in the zona reticularis, while alkaline phosphatase activity is restricted to capillary walls. Of special importance is the adenylcyclase activity associated with the cell membrane. It is through this enzyme that activation of steroid biogenesis by adrenocorticotropic hormone (ACTH) takes place. Some β-glucuronidase and arylsulfatase activities are also present in the adrenocortical tissue.

Biosynthesis of Adrenocortical Hormones

CHOLESTEROL AND PREGNENOLONE. Bloch demonstrated that administration of radioactive

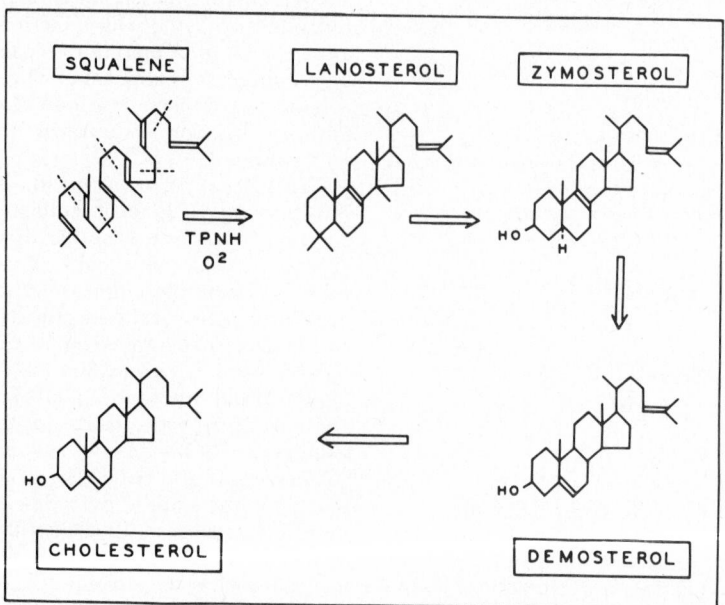

FIG. 6. Biosynthesis of cholesterol from squalene.

cholesterol to a pregnant woman resulted in the excretion of tagged pregnanediol in urine. Since then, it has been well demonstrated that perfusion of adrenal glands or incubation of adrenal slides with labeled cholesterol and acetate results in the formation of radioactive steroids. Although cholesterol is well established as a precursor of steroid hormones, it is not clear how much is extracted from the blood and how much is actually formed from acetate in the adrenal cells.

Acetate is first activated by coenzyme A, and after several steps mevalonic acid is formed. The condensation of six molecules of the dimethylallyl pyrophosphate results in the formation of a 30-carbon compound called squalene, which after cyclization, removal of 3 carbons, reduction of several double bonds, and hydroxylation of carbon 3 gives rise to cholesterol (Fig. 6). The steps that result in the formation of pregnenolone from cholesterol have not been elucidated completely. It is thought that following hydroxylation of carbon 20 and 22, a desmolase removes the six extra carbons (Fig. 7).

VARIOUS STEROIDS FROM PREGNENOLONE. A 3β-hydroxysteroid dehydrogenase, requiring a diphosphopyridine nucleotide and an isomerase, transforms pregnenolone to progesterone (Fig. 8). The biosynthesis of cortisol from progesterone requires the action of three NADPH-dependent hydroxylases and molecular oxygen. The 17α- and 21-hydroxylases are associated with the microsomal fraction of adrenals, while the 11β-hydroxylase is located in the mitochondria. NADPH is the first element in a chain of electron transfer that includes a flavoprotein, a nonheme iron-containing protein, and cytochrome P-450 and results in formation of activated oxygen. Under normal conditions the order of these hydroxylations is 17α-, 21-, and 11β-hydroxylation. In cases of genetic deficiency of one of these enzyme systems, however, the other will proceed.

An 18-hydroxylase and dehydrogenase are required for the synthesis of aldosterone from corticosterone. The 17α-hydroxylation of pregnenolone or progesterone and the removal of the side chain will result in formation of dehydroisoandrosterone and 4-androstene-3,17-dione, respectively. Since the aromatization of ring A of 4-androstene-3,17-dione and the loss of carbon 19 will bring out the formation of estrogens, one can see that the adrenal and gonadal steroids appear to follow similar pathways of biosynthesis, each gland specializing in the production of a certain group of compounds.

CORTISOL SECRETION. ACTH controls the secretion of cortisol. The stimulating effect of ACTH appears to be at the level of the conversion of cholesterol to pregnenolone. The membranes of adrenal cells possess specific receptors for ACTH. The binding of ACTH to its receptor enables adenylcyclase to promote the formation of cyclic adenosine -3′,5′- monophosphate (cyclic AMP) from adenosine triphosphate (ATP). Cyclic AMP can activate a number of enzyme precursors, among them cholesterol esterase, which makes free cholesterol available for steroidogenesis. ACTH has also been shown to accelerate the transport of amino acids into adrenal cells; this could result in increased formation of enzymes such as 20- and 22-hydroxylases. Another model for the mode of action of ACTH involves activation of the phosphorylase enzyme and stimulation of the pentose monophosphate shunt, which in turn results in formation of NADPH, the cofactor necessary for electron transfer during hydroxylation. The secretion of ACTH by the anterior part of the

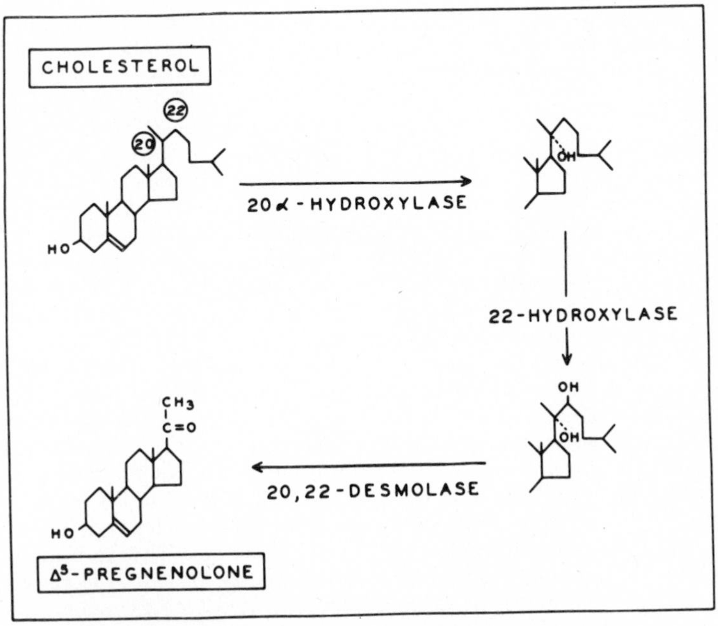

FIG. 7. Biosynthesis of Δ^5-pregnenolone from cholesterol.

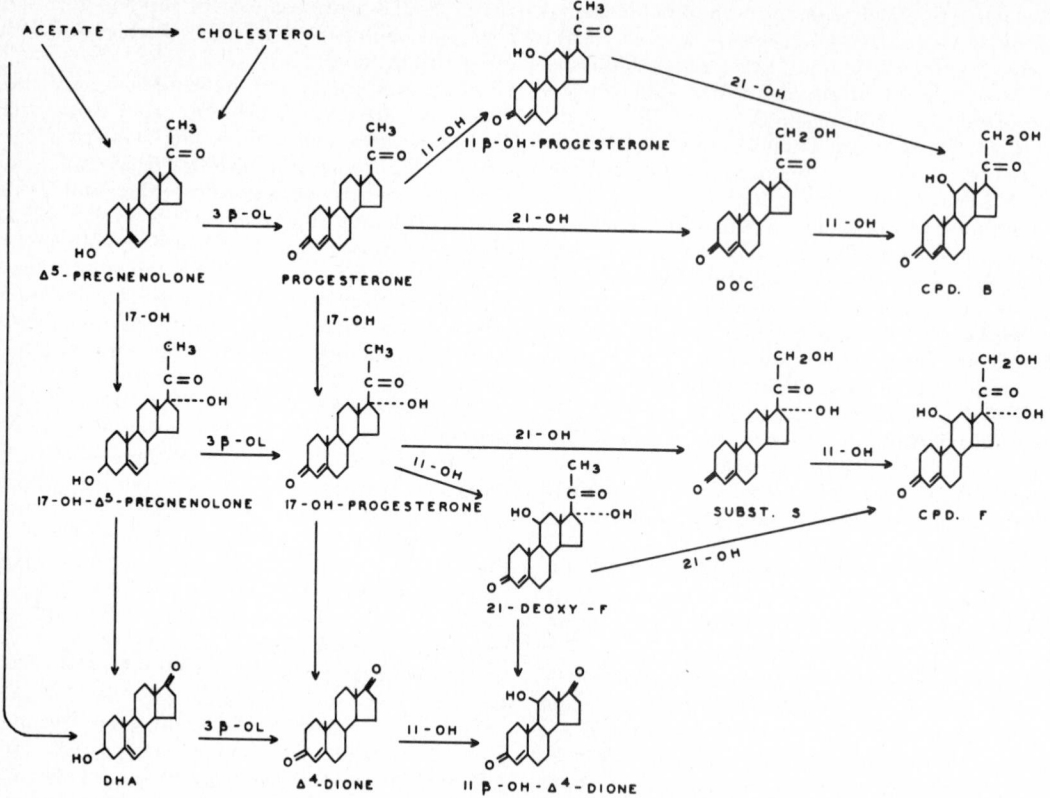

FIG. 8. Biosynthesis of adrenocortical steroids from pregnenolone in normal subjects. Progesterone is the precursor of corticosterone (Cpd B) and aldosterone, whereas 17-hydroxyprogesterone is the precursor of cortisol (Cpd F). Cleavage of the side chain of the 17-hydroxylated 21-carbon steroids results in formation of androgens, dehydroisoandrosterone (DHA), Δ^4-androstenedione (Δ^4-dione), and 11β-hydroxy-Δ^4-androstenedione.

pituitary gland is controlled by the corticotropic-releasing factor (CRF) from the hypothalamus. Although many hypothalamic releasing factors have now been identified, CRF remains to be characterized and synthesized.

Physiologically, the levels of unbound cortisol in plasma control the rate of secretion of pituitary ACTH. When the cortisol concentrations decrease in the peripheral circulation, an increased secretion of ACTH tends to correct this situation by increasing adrenal secretion. Conversely, high levels of cortisol will block ACTH secretion. This blocking effect also can be obtained by administration of biologically active glucocorticoids. However, when prolonged administration of such drugs is stopped, pituitary function may not recover immediately. The mechanism by which plasma cortisol levels control ACTH secretion is not clearly understood at present, but its action on both the hypothalamus and the pituitary gland is involved.

The hypothalamic-pituitary-adrenal axis is also influenced by the biologic clock. Secretions and plasma levels of ACTH and cortisol increase markedly in the early hours of the day (about 4 A.M.) and reach a maximum between 6 and 10 A.M. Then the levels decline throughout the afternoon and reach their lowest values in the evening and night. Young children, like adults, show this diurnal variation, and 2- to 18-month-old infants have higher plasma cortisol in the morning.

ALDOSTERONE SECRETION. The major regulator of aldosterone secretion by the cells of the zona glomerulosa is the renin–angiotensin system. Other factors, such as ACTH and potassium, play smaller roles in the control of aldosterone levels. Renin is an enzyme formed in the juxtaglomerular apparatus of the kidney; on its release in the circulation it will cleave angiotensin I from the renin substrate, a plasma globulin arising from the liver. Angiotensin I is a decapeptide that will be transformed into an octapeptide (angiotensin II) by the converting enzyme in the lung. Angiotensin II, like ACTH, appears to have a specific receptor on the membrane of the glomerulosa cells. However, it is not known how it activates aldosterone secretion. ACTH increases aldosterone secretion within 1 to 2 hours, but after 24 to 48 hours of administration, the aldosterone levels return to normal. This may be related to the fact that other steroids with some salt-retaining activity, such as cortisol and corticosterone, are also produced in large amounts and result in an increased blood volume, which in turn suppresses the renin-angiotensin-aldosterone system.

Adrenocortical Hormones and Their Metabolism

Although many steroids have been isolated from adrenal extracts and from adrenal perfusates, only a few compounds have been identified in the adrenal venous blood of man.

HORMONES SECRETED. The main glucocorticoids are cortisol and corticosterone, their secretion rates in adults being about 20 and 2 mg/day, respectively. The rate of secretion of aldosterone and its precursors, desoxycorticosterone and 18-hydroxycorticosterone, is approximately 100 µg/24 hours each, on a normal sodium diet. The adrenal androgens include dehydroisoandrosterone and its sulfate, androstenedione, as well as its 11β-hydroxylated derivative. Small amounts of estrogen, progesterone, and 17-hydroxyprogesterone are also secreted.

CIRCULATING HORMONES. When the steroids reach the general circulation, they are mostly bound to plasma proteins. Cortisol is bound by a specific α-globulin called transcortin, or corticosteroid-binding globulin. At 37 C normal plasma binds approximately 94 percent of cortisol; a small fraction of cortisol is loosely bound to albumin. Although transcortin has a great affinity for cortisol, its capacity is limited to about 25 µg/100 ml plasma. It is of interest that transcortin-bound cortisol is physiologically inactive. Even though other steroids may be bound to transcortin, in the presence of normal levels of plasma cortisol they are displaced and carried almost entirely by albumin. The red blood cells contribute, to a small extent, to the transport of some steroids in blood.

BODY DISTRIBUTION. Steroid hormones distribute themselves very rapidly into the various body compartments, particularly into the extracellular fluid (Fig. 9). Thoracic duct lymph contains transcortin at a concentration 90 percent of that in plasma. This suggests that, at least in the case of cortisol, the steroid-binding protein is circulating from the blood to the extracellular space; it also explains why the volumes of distribution of cortisol and other steroids are much greater than the blood volume. Steroids can easily penetrate the cells of the body; however, only target cells for a given steroid will retain the hormone, because their cytosol contains a specific receptor. There are about 10,000 binding sites per cell.

The present concept of steroid hormone action is that the steroid receptor complex is translocated in the nucleus, where it finds a specific acceptor site on chromatin. This, in turn, induces formation of mRNA, which eventually is translated into a protein (p. 1601). Cortisol induces many enzymes, whereas aldosterone has a much more selective role on the kidney cell. The half-life of cortisol is about 60 minutes, and its metabolic clearance rate is 150 ($\pm$ 30 SD) liters/m^2/24

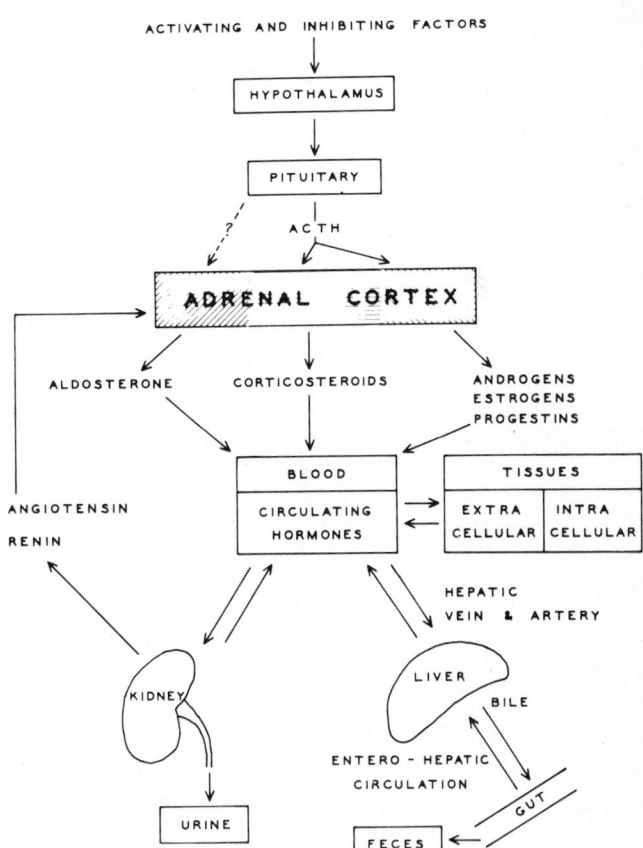

FIG. 9. General metabolism of adrenocortical steroids.

hours in the morning. Clearance in the evening and night is only 60 percent of that observed in early morning.

LIVER METABOLISM. Liver cells are important targets of cortisol action. In addition, the liver extracts most steroids from the circulation where they are rapidly metabolized; Figure 10 shows the various transformations that can take place in the cortisol molecule. The conjugation of the 3-hydroxyl group is very important, since under normal conditions large fractions of the steroids are excreted in a conjugated form. Compounds with a 3α-hydroxyl group are mainly conjugated with glucuronic acid, whereas steroids with Δ^5-3 β-hydroxyl configuration are conjugated mainly with sulfuric acid. After passage through the liver, steroids are either returned to the circulation via the hepatic vein or excreted by the bile into the intestine, where they can be reabsorbed from the intestine to undergo enterohepatic circulation. The contributions of these two phenomena vary with the steroids under consideration. Only 5 percent of a dose of cortisol is excreted by the bile, and little of it is reabsorbed from the intestine. The other glucocorticoid of man, corticosterone, is excreted by the bile to the extent of 20 percent of a given dose, while progesterone and estrogens are involved in enterohepatic circulation to an even greater degree.

EXCRETION. Major fractions of the steroids are excreted by the kidney, while the balance is excreted in the feces. For cortisol, 95 percent of an administered dose is recovered in urine, while recovery is 80 percent for estrogens and androgens. A small fraction of a dose is excreted in urine in unconjugated form.

Tests of Adrenocortical Function

GLUCOCORTICOSTEROID SECRETION. Various clinical tests such as fasting blood glucose and glucose tolerance might suggest hyposecretion or hypersecretion of glucocorticosteroids (Table 3). In the intravenous glucose tolerance test a prolonged hypoglycemic response may be seen in primary or secondary hypoadrenocorticism, while a curve of the diabetic type is often observed in Cushing's syndrome. The insulin tolerance test is dangerous in children with hypoglycemia and should not be carried out if hypoadrenocorticism is suspected. The eosinophil test is unreliable as an index of adrenal secretion.

PLASMA CORTISOL. Plasma cortisol levels can be determined accurately on an ethanolic extract of a 20-μl plasma sample using a competitive protein binding assay or radioimmunoassay. Because of a marked diurnal variation of the levels, it is important to collect control plasma specimens at a standard time, usually 8 A.M. Using a constant-withdrawal pump (3 ml/hour) and a nonthrombogenic catheter it is possible to collect successive 30-minute samples of blood and to determine the 24-hour profile of plasma cortisol concentrations.

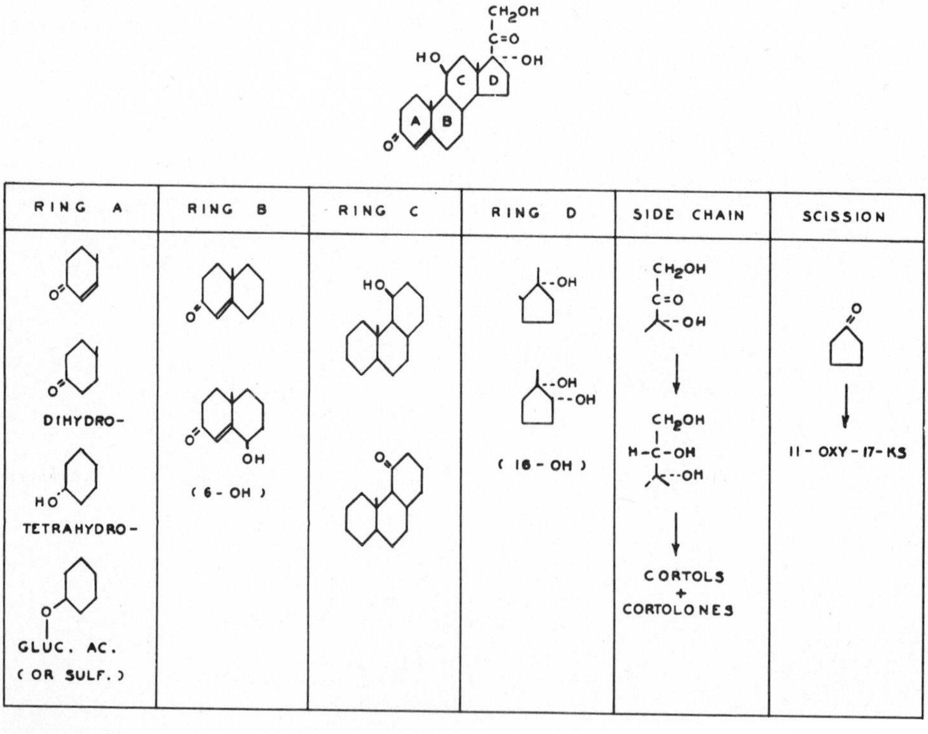

FIG. 10. Transformations of cortisol during its metabolism. Reduction of the -Δ^4-3-ketone in ring A, followed by conjugation of the 3-hydroxyl group, is the most important transformation. 6-Hydroxylation of ring B is important during the newborn period. (From Migeon: J Pediatr 55:280, 1959.)

URINARY 17-HYDROXYCORTICOSTEROIDS. The technique of Glenn and Nelson or its modifications remain the most reliable methods of measurement of urinary 17-hydroxycorticosteroids (17-OHCS). Normal values are 3.0 ($\pm$ 1.0 SD) mg/m^2/24 hours.

URINARY FREE CORTISOL. Approximately 0.5 percent of the cortisol produced is excreted unchanged in urine. Unbound plasma cortisol, in contrast to transcortin-bound steroid, can be excreted by the kidney. Since only unbound cortisol is biologically active, urinary free cortisol reflects well the glucocorticoid activity, and its measurement is helpful in evaluating adrenocortical status (Table 3).

CORTISOL SECRETION RATE. The cortisol secretion rate is obtained from the following formula: secretion rate = dose administered/(SA metabolite $\times$ t), where the dose is the total amount of tritiated cortisol injected (usually 0.25 to 1.0 μCi), SA metabolite is the specific activity of any one of the specific urinary metabolites of cortisol (tetrahydrocortisol, allotetrahydrocortisol, or tetrahydrocortisone), and t is the period of time of urine collection. The values of secretion corrected for body surface area in normal subjects of all ages are in the same range, except for young infants. The total body radiation resulting from the test is less than 10 μrad.

ADRENAL CAPACITY (ACTH) TESTS. A 6-hour infusion of 25 USP units of Acthar gel will give maximal stimulation of cortisol secretion. This test can be helpful in determining the cause of Cushing's syndrome (p. 1645). Intravenous injection of 0.25 to 1.0 mg of synthetic 1,24-ACTH (cortrosyn) results in submaximal levels of plasma cortisol 120 minutes after the injection. In patients suspected of primary hypoadrenocorticism, an absence of response of urinary 17-OHCS on the intramuscular ACTH test is pathognomonic of Addison's disease.

ACTH RESERVE OF PITUITARY GLAND. Metyrapone (Metopirone) has the property of being able to inhibit the 11-hydroxylase of the adrenal cortex. This results in a decreased secretion of cortisol and a lowering of its plasma levels. In order to compensate, the normal pituitary secretes a greater amount of ACTH, which stimulates steroid secretion by the adrenal. Because of the 11-hydroxylase block, a cortisol precursor that lacks the 11 oxygen (compound S) is produced in great quantities. Its urinary metabolites are measured as 17-OHCS. In the normal subject, administration of metyrapone results in increased excretion of urinary 17-OHCS, whereas in the patient with deficient ACTH secretion there will be no increase (Table 3). This test is usually carried out after an intramuscular ACTH test has eliminated the possibility of primary adrenal insufficiency.

PITUITARY SUPPRESSION. Pituitary suppression tests are based on homeostatic regulation of pituitary ACTH secretion by the level of plasma free cortisol. The administration of a potent glucocorticosteroid, such as dexamethasone, will suppress ACTH secretion and result in a decrease in urinary 17-OHCS. This test is important in differentiating Cushing's syndrome from simple obesity and in determining the pathogenesis of Cushing's syndrome (p. 1645).

ANDROGEN SECRETION. Various clinical signs (such as size of phallus and prostate, pigmentation and stippling of the scrotum, presence of pubic, axillary, and facial hair, and deepening of the voice) will suggest secretion of androgens in the prepubertal male. In the female an enlarged clitoris, deepening of the voice, and signs of hirsutism raise the possibility of abnormal androgen production.

URINARY 17-KETOSTEROIDS. Table 4 shows the range of normal values obtained with this test. The values are physiologically low prior to puberty. In this age group it is particularly important to correct the results for unspecific pigments by applying an Allen correction.

FRACTIONATION OF URINARY 17-KETOSTEROIDS. An approximation of the amount of dehydroisoandrosterone present in urine can be obtained by using the rather nonspecific method of Allen, Hayward, and Pinto. If this compound represents more than 50 percent of the total 17-ketosteroids and if no suppression is obtained in the 17-ketosteroid suppression test, the presence of an adrenal tumor is strongly suggested. In congenital adrenal hyperplasia due to a 3β-ol-dehydrogenase defi-

TABLE 3. Tests Related to Glucocorticosteroid Secretion (Mean $\pm$ SD)

Test	Values
Resting levels	
Plasma cortisol	8 a.m. 11 $\pm$ 2.5 μg/100 ml; 8 p.m. 3.5 $\pm$ 1.5 μg/100 ml
Urinary 17-OHCS (glucuronides)	3.0 $\pm$ 1.0 mg/m^2/24 hours
Urinary free cortisol	From 25 to 75 μg/m^2/24 hours
Cortisol secretion rate	12 $\pm$ 3 mg/m^2/24 hours
Adrenal capacity	
IV test: 25 USP U Acthar over 6 hours	Plasma cortisol: 40 $\pm$ 5 μg/100 ml at 6 hours
IV test: 1 mg 1,24-ACTH stat	Plasma cortisol: 32 $\pm$ 4 μg/100 ml at 2 hours
IM test: 20 U/m^2 Acthargel every 8 hours for 3 days	Urinary 17-OHCS = 85 $\pm$ 15 mg/m^2/24 hours
ACTH capacity of pituitary gland	
Oral metyrapone: 300 mg/m^2 every 4 hours for 24 hours	Urinary 17-OHCS increase > 9 mg/m^2/24 hours
IV Metyrapone: 35 mg/kg (max, 1 g) over 4 hours	Plasma S 5.9 $\pm$ 1.5 μg/100 ml at 5 hours
Pituitary suppression test	
Low-dose dexamethasone: 1.25 ng/m^2/24 hours (in 3 divided doses) for 3 days	Urinary 17-OHCS < 1 mg/m^2/24 hours
High-dose dexamethasone: same with 3.75 mg/m^2/24 hours	Same

TABLE 4. Measurement of Total Urinary 17-Ketosteroids

Hormones measured	Unconjugated and conjugated neutral 19-carbon steroids with a 17-ketone (Zimmermann reaction)
Limitations	Does not measure biologically active androgenic hormones, but rather their metabolites; only fractions of the metabolites are excreted as urinary 17-ketosteroids (about one-third for testosterone).
Normal values (mg/24 hours)	First few weeks of life = up to 2 mg 1 month to 5 years = 0.5 mg or less 6–8 years = 1.0 to 2.0 mg Puberty = progressive increase to adult levels Normal adult males = 7 to 17 mg Normal adult females = 5 to 15 mg

ciency, the relative amount of dehydroisoandrosterone is also increased, but both total urinary 17-ketosteroids and dehydroisoandrosterone will be depressed to normal values in the glucocorticoid suppression test (Table 5).

URINARY 17-KETOSTEROID SUPPRESSION TEST. Dexamethasone is administered at a dosage of 1.25 mg/m²/24 hours (given in three equal portions at 8-hour intervals, for 7 to 10 days. This test is used in patients who have greater than normal urinary excretion of 17-ketosteroids and clinical symptoms suggesting the adrenogenital syndrome (Table 5).

PLASMA ANDROGENS. Androstenedione has limited biologic activity, but its peripheral conversion gives rise to testosterone. In women, in contrast to men, it contributes more than 50 percent of the total production of testosterone. Dehydroisoandrosterone and its sulfate are also secreted by the adult cortex. Their biologic significance is not clear. The high concentrations of dehydroisoandrosterone sulfate in plasma (Table 6) are in large part due to its prolonged half-life.

ALDOSTERONE SECRETION. The study of serum electrolytes and the study of sweat and saliva sodium–potassium ratios are of great importance in the diagnosis of syndromes involving disturbance of the electrolyte-regulating factor.

PLASMA ALDOSTERONE. Aldosterone can be measured in plasma by radioimmunoassay. The levels follow a circadian variation similar to that of cortisol, although not as marked. In addition, plasma aldosterone concentrations show rapid changes in relation to body position (Table 7). The effects of changes in electrolyte intake occur more slowly. For this reason studies of aldosterone on low or high sodium uptake must be carried out only on the 4th to 5th days of a given diet. During the first year after birth plasma values are high, but they decline toward adult levels shortly thereafter.

URINARY ALDOSTERONE. About 10 percent of the aldosterone produced is excreted in urine as the 3-oxo glucuronide conjugate of aldosterone; after hydrolysis at pH 1.0 the freed aldosterone can be measured by radioimmunoassay.

ALDOSTERONE SECRETION RATE. The aldosterone secretion rate (ASR) is determined as is the rate for cortisol. Following administration of 1 μCi of tritiated aldosterone, the specific activity of 3-oxo conjugate of aldosterone in urine is determined. The ASR is relatively constant throughout life, except for the slightly lower values during the first 2 weeks after birth. The fact that plasma aldosterone levels are high during the first year of life and then decrease to adult values can be explained by the fact that the ASR is the same at all ages, with the clearance rate corrected for body size being only slightly higher (about 1.5 times) than that of adults.

PLASMA RENIN ACTIVITY. Plasma renin activity (PRA) is determined by bioassay, and its levels are expressed in nanograms of angiotensin II formed per milliliter of plasma per hour. Radioimmunoassays are also available. This determination is of great importance in the work-up of hypertensive patients.

ESTROGEN AND PROGESTIN SECRETION. In female infants and children prior to puberty, the best and simplest test of estrogenic activity is study of the vaginal smear, using the special stain devised by Shorr. Pink cells with pyknotic nuclei are typical of full estronization. The method of Brown for the fractionation of urinary estrogens also is quite reliable. However, values obtained in children are often difficult to interpret. Radioimmunoassays for measurement of estradiol in plasma are available. Similarly, values of urinary excretion of pregnanediol in children are not very helpful. Plasma progesterone levels determined by radioimmunoassay may be more informative.

In congenital adrenal hyperplasia (CAH) due to 21-hydroxylase deficiency, 17α-hydroxyprogesterone is produced in large amounts by the adrenal cortex, and one of its main urinary metabolites is pregnanetriol (Fig. 11). 17α-hydroxyprogesterone also can be measured accurately in plasma (Table 6) using specific radioimmunoassays.

Adrenocortical Hormone Action

It is now accepted that steroids can readily penetrate any cell of the body and can just as readily move out of a cell. Only target cells that have differentiated so that they contain in their cytosol a specific receptor protein for a specific steroid can retain such steroid. The complex steroid–receptor is then translocated into the nucleus when it finds its specific acceptor on the chromatin. This, in turn, initiates the formation of new mRNA, which is then translated into newly formed proteins, usually enzymes. Cortisol is known to induce a large number of enzymes, particularly in the liver. The net effect of enzyme induction in the liver cell results in gluconeogenesis. The way cortisol increases surfactant in fetal lung is also probably related to enzyme induc-

TABLE 5. Adrenocortical Disorders With Increased Excretion of Urinary 17-KS

	Androsterone	DHA-S	11-Oxygenated 17-KS	Suppression of 17-KS in Suppression Test
Congenital adrenal hyperplasia				
Simple virilizing form	3+*	In proportion to total 17-KS	2+	Yes
Salt-losing	3+	same	2+	Yes
Hypertensive	3+†	same	—	Yes
3β-o1-dehydrogenase deficiency	—	3+	—	Yes
Lipoid hyperplasia (20,22-desmolase system defect)	—	—	—	Low control
17-hydroxylase deficiency	—	—	—	Low control
Virilizing adrenal tumor	1+	3+	N	No
Feminizing adrenal tumor	N to 2+	N to 2+	N	No
Cushing's syndrome				
Bilateral hyperplasia	1+	1+	1+	Partial
Adrenal adenoma	—	—	1+	Often low control
Adrenal carcinoma	1+ to 3+	1+	1+ to 3+	No

N = normal levels; — = lower than normal; 1+ to 3+ = higher than normal.
† Mainly etiocholanolone.

TABLE 6. Concentrations (Mean ± SD) of Androgens and 17-Hydroxyprogesterone in Plasma (ng/100 ml)*

	Adult Males	Adult Females	Pregnant Females	Females at Delivery	Umbilical Cord	Prepubertal Children (< 7 years)
Testosterone	559 ± 151	48 ± 14	114 ± 38	134 ± 72	46 ± 24	11.5 ± 4.5
Androstenedione	114 ± 21	180 ± 58	249 ± 82	387 ± 176	126 ± 58	21 ± 12
Dehydroisoandrosterone	553 ± 178	534 ± 157	363 ± 233	1016 ± 806	203 ± 139	39 ± 28
Dehydroisoandrosterone sulfate (μg/100 ml)	126 ± 34	113 ± 28	—	38 ± 20	91 ± 37	6.0 ± 4.5
17-OH-progesterone	95 ± 30	60 ± 20	230 ± 30*	660 ± 60*	2220 ± 280*	35 ± 25
		270 ± 60				

* Data from Tulchinsky and Simmer: J Clin Endocrinol Metab 35:799, 1972.

TABLE 7. Aldosterone Concentration in Plasma (ng/100 ml) of Normal Subjects on Diets Low, Normal, and High in Sodium Content (Mean ± SD)

Body Posture	Low (< 17 mEq)	Normal (ad lib)	High (ad lib + 150 mEq)
Supine	16.7 ± 7.1	2.1 ± 1.0	1.6 ± 1.0
Standing	32.6 ± 19.0	11.3 ± 6.5	4.5 ± 3.5

tion. However, the numerous other actions of cortisol have not yet been clearly explained, such as suppression of inflammatory and immune reactions, effects on muscle, adipose, and blood cells, etc (p. 1652). Aldosterone also has been shown to induce the formation of a protein in kidney cells that plays a major role in sodium transport.

Adrenocortical Function at Various Stages

PREGNANCY. There is an increase in transcortin concentration in plasma that is probably related to the increased estrogen production. This results in a greater binding capacity for cortisol and a progressive rise in plasma levels of total cortisol. The unbound cortisol is also elevated, thus suggesting the presence of a mild state of hyperadrenocorticism during pregnancy. The increased transcortin concentrations probably explain the prolonged half-life of cortisol that is observed in pregnant women. At the same time, cortisol secretion rate corrected for body surface area is slightly but significantly decreased.

Progesterone, which is produced in large amounts during pregnancy, has been shown to have a mild natriuretic effect. The increases in plasma renin activity, plasma aldosterone level, and aldosterone secretion rate observed in pregnant women would be the response of the renin-angiotensin-aldosterone system to the salt-losing tendency evoked by progesterone. Unlike cortisol, aldosterone does not have a specific binding protein and is loosely bound in blood. Furthermore, its binding to plasma proteins does not increase and its metabolic clearance rate does not change during pregnancy.

FETAL LIFE. The fetal adrenal contains steroids, including cortisol, aldosterone, and androgens. It is also well known that in cases of congenital adrenal hyperplasia, masculinization of the external genitalia of the female fetus is due to an abnormal production of androgens by the fetal adrenal. Since this sexual differentiation takes place during the third to fourth month of pregnancy, the fetal pituitary–adrenal axis, including the capacity of the fetal adrenal to secrete steroids must be functional at that stage of fetal life. However, in vitro experiments have shown that the fetal cortex is deficient in 3β-hydroxysteroid dehydrogenase, which results in relatively large secretion of Δ^5-3β-hydroxysteroids

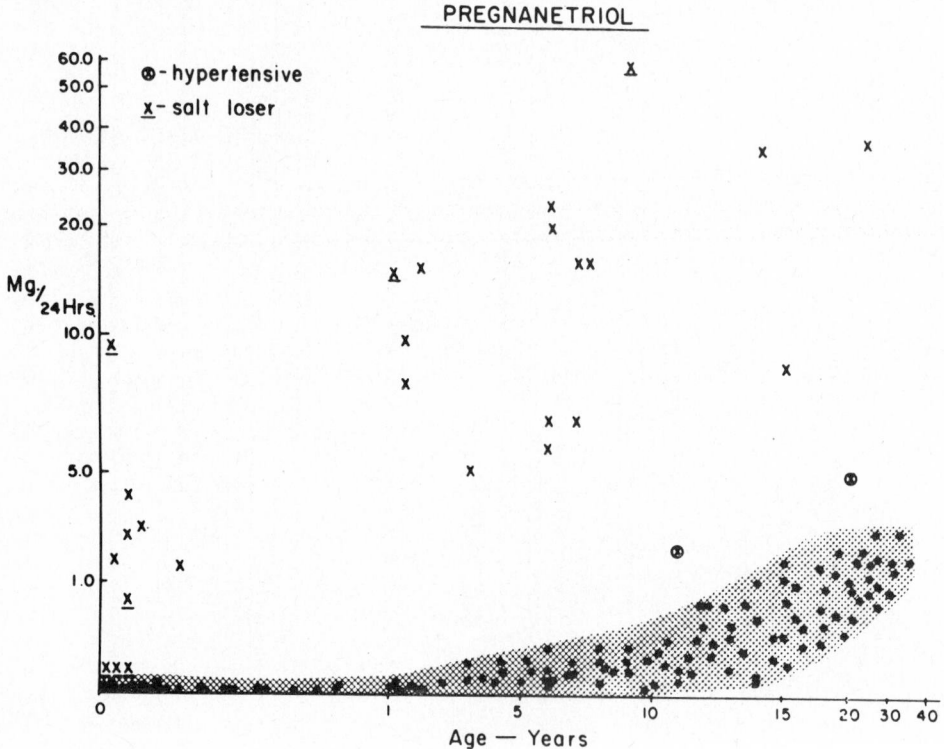

FIG. 11. Urinary excretion of pregnanetriol in normal subjects (black dots in shaded area) and in patients with CAH (×). (From Bongiovanni and Eberlein: Metabolism 10:917, 1961.)

such as pregnenolone, dehydroisoandrosterone, 16α-hydroxydehydroisoandrosterone, and their sulfates. In contrast, the placenta is rich in 3β-hydroxysteroid dehydrogenase and sulfatase, and it will metabolize the fetal steroids to the corresponding Δ^4-3-ketones. Progesterone is then returned to the fetal adrenal, which can then carry out the final steps of steroidogenesis. 16α-hydroxydehydroisoandrosterone is the precursor of fetal estriol, which explains why a drop in maternal excretion of estriol reflects fetal distress.

Tagged cortisol administered to the mother can cross the placenta but, at equilibrium, maternal levels are 18 times higher than those in cord plasma; it has been estimated that the mother contributes 25 percent of the total fetal cortisol. Radioactive aldosterone also can be transferred from mother to fetus, the maternal concentrations being 1.25 to 2 times higher than those in the cord. However, the endogenous aldosterone concentration of the fetus is about 2 times higher than that of the mother; the mother contributes 20 to 40 percent of fetal aldosterone near term.

DELIVERY, BIRTH AND NEONATAL PERIOD. Labor and vaginal delivery produce a further elevation of the level of cortisol in maternal plasma, due in part to an increase in cortisol secretion by the adrenal cortex and in part to a slower clearance rate of the steroid. On the other hand, the early stages of the surgical procedure in elective cesarean section (ie, until delivery of the infant) do not produce any noticeable increase in the plasma level of cortisol in the mother.

At birth, term infants delivered by elective cesarean section have plasma cortisol concentrations of 4 to 11 μg/100 ml, these values being 5 times lower than those of their mothers. Of interest is the fact that newborn infants have similar cortisone and cortisol levels. Infants delivered vaginally have, like their mothers, higher levels of cortisol at birth. It must be noted that transcortin concentration is low at birth as compared with adult values; this could result in proportionately high levels of unbound, and hence biologically active, cortisol. Aldosterone levels in cord plasma are about 1.5 times higher than those of maternal plasma. A low-sodium diet and/or diuretic administration during pregnancy can result in a tripling of the plasma aldosterone levels in both maternal and cord blood; the aldosterone concentration remains elevated for at least 72 hours in the infant.

During the first week after birth the plasma aldosterone concentrations are similar to those of adults. However, after that, and up to 1 year of age, levels are significantly higher than those found at any other age. After the first weeks of life the aldosterone secretion rates are similar at all ages, ranging from 40 to 120 μg/24 hours, but they are somewhat lower during the first weeks.

During the neonatal period, plasma levels of cortisol tend to be low. However, a normal rise is obtained after administration of ACTH. In infants born by vaginal delivery, cortisol secretion rates corrected for body surface area are slightly higher than adult values; after 8 days of age the rates are more comparable to those of adult subjects. Preterm infants delivered by the vaginal route and infants delivered by elective cesarean section have similar secretion rates.

The rates of metabolism of cortisol in the neonate and the adult are quite different. In infants the half-life of cortisol in plasma is twice that observed in normal adults. This is due to a slower rate of reduction of ring A of the molecule. In addition, conjugation with glucuronic acid is also much slower. In spite of this the infant can excrete a dose of cortisol in its urine at a rate that is not much different fron that of the adult.

Plasma androgens (Table 6) and urinary 17-ketosteroid levels (Table 4) are relatively elevated in the newborn infant but they fall to low values after 1 month. These changes parallel the involution of the fetal zone of the adrenal cortex.

PUBERTAL PERIOD. During childhood, cortisol secretion, corrected for body surface area, is similar to that of adult subjects, but adrenal androgen secretion is low and the urinary 17-ketosteroids are mainly 11 oxygenated androsterone and etiocholanolone, which probably arise from the metabolism of cortisol. At puberty the pituitary secretion of gonadotropins triggers the secretion of estrogens and progesterone by the ovary and of testosterone by the testis. In addition, the adrenal cortex in both males and females starts to produce androgens, which are excreted as dehydroepiandrosterone, androsterone, and etiocholanolone, thus accounting for the rather sharp elevation in urinary 17-ketosteroid excretion occurring at the time of puberty. The mechanism that triggers the secretion of adrenal androgens at puberty is not known. In premature pubarche, adrenal maturation occurs prematurely and in the absence of gonadal maturation (p. 1718).

Hypothalamic-Pituitary-Adrenal Axis

HOMEOSTATIC REGULATION. Plasma concentrations of unbound cortisol and of aldosterone control their own rates of secretion, the former directly at the hypothalamic–pituitary level, the latter indirectly at the juxtaglomerular apparatus through changes in electrolytes and blood volume. In hypothyroidism or liver disease the half-life of cortisol is prolonged, and a temporary increase in cortisol concentration in plasma results in a decreased ACTH secretion. Eventually, normal levels of cortisol will be maintained by a cortisol secretion rate slower than normal. In hyperthyroidism, on the other hand, the half-life of cortisol is short, and in order to maintain normal levels of cortisol in the circulation, the secretion rate is faster than normal. Hemorrhage, a low-sodium diet, or a high-potassium diet may result in an increase in aldosterone secretion. Body posture also can bring about rapid changes in plasma aldosterone levels.

STRESS. A large variety of circumstances termed stress can be responsible for an increase in adrenocortical secretion secondary to an increased ACTH output. It is thought that ACTH secretion is under the control of corticotropin-releasing factor (CRF) formed in the hypothalamus, which reaches the pituitary gland via the capillary loops of the portal vessels of the hypophysis. The secretion of CRF is itself under neural control. Surgery, trauma, acute illness, emotional stress, pyrogen, insulin, and many other stimuli can increase adrenal function. Some of these factors, such as surgery, induce not only an increased secretion of cortisol but also a longer half-life of this steroid. Some stresses, such as surgery, are also accompanied by increased aldosterone secretion.

DIETARY FACTORS. In anorexia nervosa the pituitary glands appear to produce less ACTH than normal. On the other hand, acute and complete starvation can result in adrenal hypertrophy. Obesity related to overeating is often accompanied by increased rates of secretion of cortisol. Vitamin deficiencies have been reported to affect adrenal function in experimental animals, but little information is available on this effect in man. Electrolyte composition of the diet influences aldosterone secretion. A low-sodium diet first results in a negative sodium balance with a decrease in total blood volume. Only then will the rate of secretion of aldosterone increase in an attempt to reestablish the homeostatic balance.

INHIBITORS.   Dichlorodiphenyldichloroethane (DDD) and related compounds such as o,p'-DDD can produce destruction of cells of the inner cortex of the adrenal. This substance has been used in the treatment of adrenocarcinoma with some interesting results, but the drug is often badly tolerated. Amphenone B (1,1-bis[p-aminophenyl]-1-methylpropanone) increases the size of the adrenal but reduces its secretion. Both Amphenone B and o,p'-DDD have unspecific effects and seem to decrease the activity of most of the adrenocortical enzymes. Aminoglutethimide can affect both thyroid and adrenal function. In the adrenal cortex it appears to block 20α-hydroxylation, and thereby it inhibits the transformation of cholesterol to pregnenolone. Cyanoketone, a steroid derivative, presumably inhibits the 3β-hydroxysteroid dehydrogenase system, thus blocking the formation of progesterone and other Δ⁴-3-ketosteroids. Metyrapone blocks 11β-hydroxylation; other inhibitors have been found to block both 17- and 18-hydroxylation. In addition to direct effects on enzymes involved in the biosynthesis of hormones, certain steroid derivatives, such as spironolactone, are aldosterone antagonists at the kidney level. Their effect is related to their ability to compete for the aldosterone receptors in the cytosol on the target cells. Progesterone and 17-hydroxyprogesterone appear to have similar properties and therefore are considered as mild salt-losing hormones.

HYPOADRENOCORTICISM

Primary adrenal failure is the main cause of hypoadrenocorticism. However, adrenal cortical insufficiency can also occur secondary to decreased ACTH secretion by the pituitary gland. In rare cases a transient hypoadrenocorticism appears to be related to end-organ unresponsiveness to normal production of adrenocorticoid hormones (Table 8).

TABLE 8. Classification of Syndromes of Hypoadrenocorticism

Primary
  Hypoadrenocorticism of the neonatal period
    Congenital hypoplasia of adrenals
    Bilateral adrenal hemorrhage of the newborn
    Congenital adrenal hyperplasia
      21-hydroxylase deficiency
      11β-hydroxylase deficiency
      17α-hydroxylase deficiency
      3β-hydroxysteroid dehydrogenase deficiency
      Deficiency of enzymes prior to Δ⁵-pregnenolone
    Congenital deficiency of 18-hydroxylase or 18-dehydrogenase
    Congenital adrenocortical unresponsiveness to ACTH
  Adrenal crisis of acute infection
  Chronic hypoadrenocorticism (Addison's disease)
Secondary to insufficient ACTH secretion
  Hypopituitarism (idiopathic or pituitary tumor)
  Cessation of glucocorticoid therapy; removal of unilateral cortisol-producing adrenal tumor
  Anencephaly
  Infants born to steroid-treated mothers
  Respiratory distress syndrome
  Inanition, anorexia nervosa
Secondary to end-organ unresponsiveness
  Transient unresponsiveness of kidney to sodium-retaining hormones

Primary Hypoadrenocorticism

NEONATAL HYPOADRENOCORTICISM.

APLASIA OR MARKED HYPOPLASIA OF ADRENAL GLANDS.   Children with aplasia or marked hypoplasia of the adrenal glands present in acute shock, with extreme tachycardia and eventual vascular collapse. The skin is cold and clammy; central and peripheral cyanosis is present. It is difficult to differentiate this abnormality from septicemia, intracranial hemorrhage, or pulmonary infection; it is impossible to differentiate it from adrenal hemorrhage. It has been suggested that the condition may be recognized by the presence of low maternal estriol and a fetus with a normal head size, the latter differentiating this condition from the anencephalic infant. This disease may be sporadic or familial, but sex-linked recessive inheritance is more usual. In most of the cases reported the diagnosis was made at autopsy.

ADRENAL HEMORRHAGE.   Children with massive adrenal hemorrhage present with acute shock due to blood loss and adrenal insufficiency. There is usually a mass palpable in the flank. This disorder occurs most often in large male infants who have had traumatic delivery. It should be differentiated from renal vein thrombosis, where there is gross hematuria; in adrenal hemorrhage the hematuria is microscopic. In renal vein thrombosis the intravenous pyelogram shows no excretion of dye on the affected side, while in adrenal hemorrhage the kidney excretes normally but is displaced downward, and its upper calices are flattened. The cases of unilateral hemorrhage do not show symptons of adrenal insufficiency, but they may show shock from blood loss. Patients who have survived bilateral adrenal

TABLE 9. Inherited Disorders of Adrenal Cortex With Their Respective Enzyme Deficiencies and Resulting Steroid Patterns

	Enzyme Deficiency	Cortisol	Aldo sterone	Androgens	Renin Activity
Congenital adrenal hyperplasia					
Simple virilizing	Partial 21-OH	N*	+	+ +	+
Salt-losing	More complete 21-OH	−	−	+ +	+
Hypertensive	11-OH	− (S++)	− (DOC+)	+ +	−
17-OH deficiency	17-OH	− (B++)	− (DOC+)	−	−
Lethal	3β-o1-dehydrogenase	−	−	+ + as DHA	+
Lethal	Prior to Δ⁵-pregnenolone	−	−	−	+
Deficiency of 18-hydroxylase or 18-dehydrogenase	18-OH or 18-dehydrogenase	N	− (B+)	N	
Adrenal unresponsiveness to ACTH	ACTH-activated enzymatic systems	−	N	?	N

* N, normal secretion; +, increased secretion; −, decreased secretion; S, compound S; DOC, deoxycorticosterone; B, corticosterone; DHA, dehydroisoandrosterone.

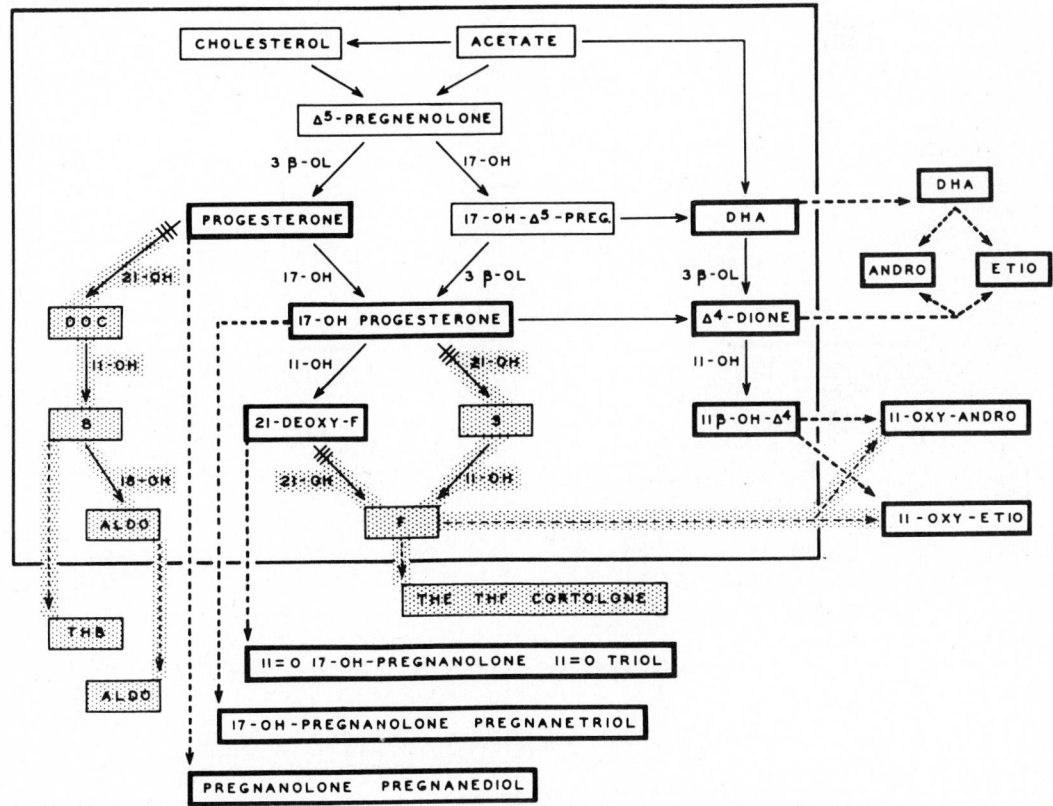

FIG. 12. Biosynthesis of adrenocorticosteroids in salt-losing form of CAH (marked 21-hydroxylase deficiency). Steroids inside large rectangle indicate adrenal biosynthesis, while compounds outside rectangle indicate urinary metabolites. Shaded boxes indicate secretion of steroids that are situated after the enzymatic deficiency and are decreased or absent; heavy boxes indicate that steroids prior to block are increased. Decrease in cortisol secretion results in increased output of ACTH and, as a consequence, elevated secretion of androgens and cortisol precursors. There is also a decrease or absence of of aldosterone secretion, which explains the salt loss. [From Migeon: In Cooke RE (ed): The Biological Basis of Pediatric Practice, 1968, Courtesy of McGraw-Hill.]

hemorrhage often do not show saltwasting, which may be due to regeneration of the subcapsular zona glomerulosa. As the hemorrhage resolves, it leaves a residual calcification that may be visible 3 to 4 weeks later and may persist for life.

CONGENITAL ADRENAL HYPERPLASIA.   Congenital adrenal hyperplasia is an inherited inborn error in metabolism. There are several forms of the syndrome, each of which is due to a specific enzyme deficiency (Table 9). In each of these forms one of the enzymes involved in the biosynthesis of cortisol is defective. Because of decreased cortisol secretion, there is hyperproduction of ACTH by the pituitary, which in turn leads to adrenal hyperplasia. The simple virilizing form and the salt-losing form are by far the more frequent.

Enzyme Deficiencies and Patterns of Steroid Secretion.   In the simple virilizing form a partial 21-hydroxylase deficiency is compensated for by an increase in ACTH output, so that the cortisol secretion is close to normal (Fig. 12). At the same time, the increased ACTH secretion produces a massive elevation of androgens and cortisol precursors, some of which, such as progesterone and 17-OH-progesterone, have a salt-losing tendency. This tendency, however, is well compensated by an increase in aldosterone secretion. In the salt-losing form, the 21-hydroxylase deficiency is almost complete, thus resulting in absence of both cortisol and aldosterone. The

only steroids increased by the elevated ACTH output are the androgens and the steroids with salt-losing tendencies. The hypertensive form is characterized by an 11-hydroxylase deficiency (Fig. 13). Compound S and deoxycorticosterone (DOC), the respective precursors of cortisol and aldosterone, are secreted in large amounts, the latter being responsible for the hypertension. In 17-hydroxylase deficiency cortisol cannot be synthesized, but an increased output of corticosterone compensates almost entirely. In the normal adrenal, DOC is a corticosterone precursor and is under angiotensin control in the zona glomerulosa, while in the zonae fasciculata and reticularis it is also a corticosterone precursor but is under ACTH control. In the 17-hydroxylase deficiency, the DOC secretion controlled by ACTH is increased, resulting in some degree of hypertension. As in 11-hydroxylase deficiency, the elevated blood DOC levels decrease the formation of renin–angiotensin and hence decrease aldosterone secretion. Finally, the 17-hydroxylase deficiency is also present in the gonads; since this enzyme is necessary for the formation of androgens and estrogens, these patients lack gonadal hormones.

The 3β-hydroxysteroid dehydrogenase deficiency (Fig. 14) results in an almost complete absence of all adrenal steroids. The only compounds prior to the enzymatic block that are produced in large amounts are

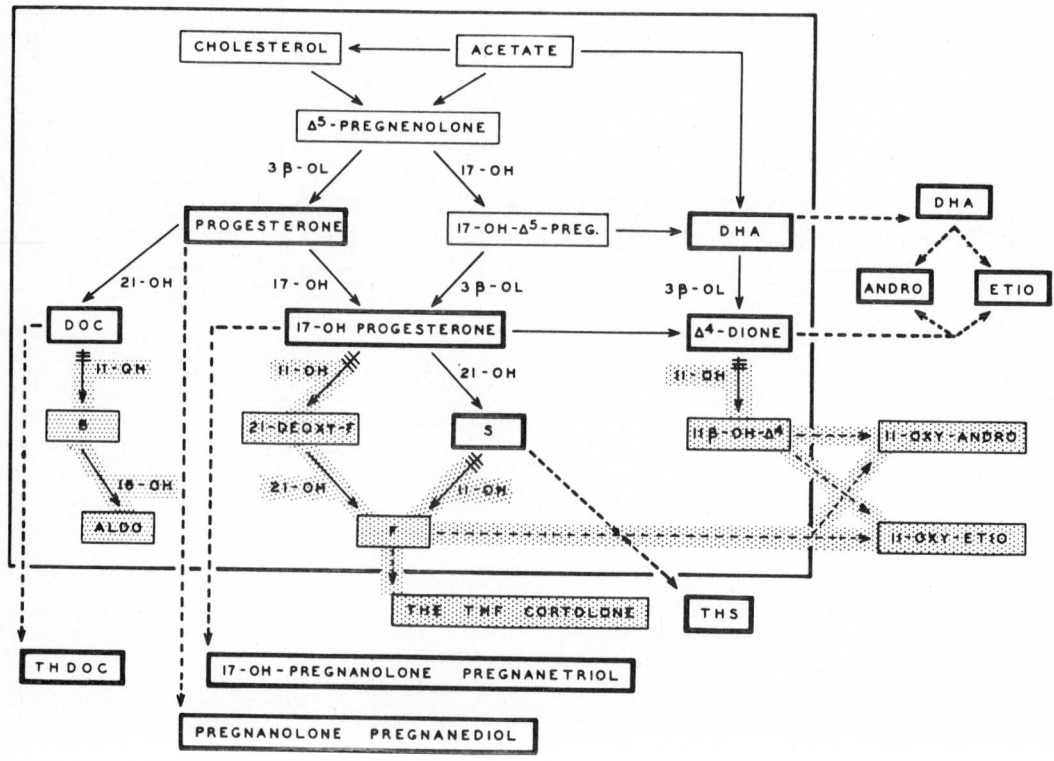

FIG. 13.   Biosynsthesis of adrenocortical steroids in patients with CAH due to 11-hydroxylase deficiency (hypertensive form). Metabolites found in increased amount in urine (outside large rectangle) are THS, tetrahydrodeoxycorticosterone (THDOC), derivatives of progesterone, 17α-hydroxyprogesterone, and 11-deoxy-17-ketosteroids.

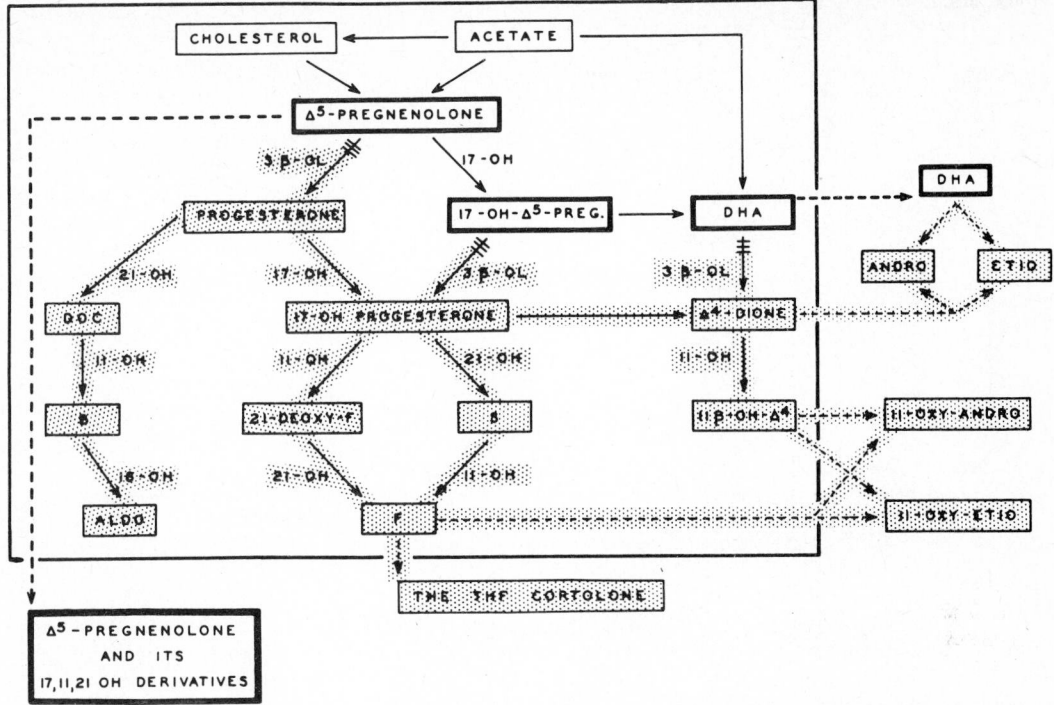

FIG. 14. Biosynthesis of adrenocorticosteroids in form of CAH due to a deficiency of 3β-hydroxysteroid dehydrogenase. In this form of the syndrome, aldosterone and cortisol secretions are decreased markedly, and only Δ⁵-steroids are produced in large amounts. [From Migeon: In Cooke (ed): The Biological Basis of Pediatric Practice, 1968, Courtesy of McGraw-Hill.]

pregnenolone, its 17-hydroxy derivative, and dehydroisoandrosterone, an androgen with little biologic activity. As in the instance of 17-hydroxylase deficiency, the 3β-hydroxysteroid dehydrogenase enzyme system is also deficient in the gonads of these patients. In its complete form, this deficiency does not appear to be compatible with life; it is thought to be due to the fact that the same enzyme system is involved in other vital processes.

In a limited number of patients a deficiency of one of the enzymes necessary for the formation of pregnenolone from cholesterol has been reported, including the 20-hydroxylase, 22-hydroxylase and 20,22-desmolase. These deficiencies are referred to as lipoadrenal hyperplasia. These forms also appear to be lethal when the deficiency is complete. In a group of 150 patients with congenital adrenal hyperplasia seen at the Pediatric Endocrine Clinic of the Johns Hopkins Hospital, 55 percent had the non-salt-losing form, 37 percent had the salt-losing form, 6 percent had the hypertensive form, and 2 percent had a deficiency of 3β-hydroxysteroid dehydrogenase or a deficiency of an enzyme prior to pregnenolone.

Symptomatology and Diagnosis. This is a congenital disease, and the deficient production of cortisol starts during fetal life. In the simple virilizing, salt-losing, and hypertensive forms, the excessive secretion of adrenal androgens in the female fetus causes masculinization of the external genitalia, with enlargement of the clitoris and a variable degree of labioscrotal fusion (p. 1697). In some cases the fusion may be so extensive that the external genitalia may be mistaken for those of a cryptorchid male with or without hypospadias (Fig. 15). However, the genital ducts and gonads of these females remain perfectly normal. In the male, the increased secretion of fetal adrenal androgens is not noticeable at birth except for excessive pigmentation of the external genitalia in some cases. In the other forms (deficiency of 3β-hydroxysteroid dehydrogenase, enzymes prior to pregnenolone, 17-hydroxylase) the same enzyme system is also deficient in the fetal testes, and it interferes with the fetal secretion of testosterone and with the normal masculinization of the external genitalia. As a result such a male infant may appear to have female external genitalia or a small phallus with perineal hypospadias.

The acute adrenal crisis of the salt-losing form is due to the absence of secretion of aldosterone. However, the low cortisol production coupled with excessive output of steroids with salt-losing tendency contributes to the acute crisis. It usually occurs on the fifth to seventh day after birth, with an increase in serum potassium often being the first abnormality of serum chemistry. These infants have poor appetites and fail to gain weight. An excessive loss of sodium eventually results in severe water loss and marked dehydration; cardiovas-

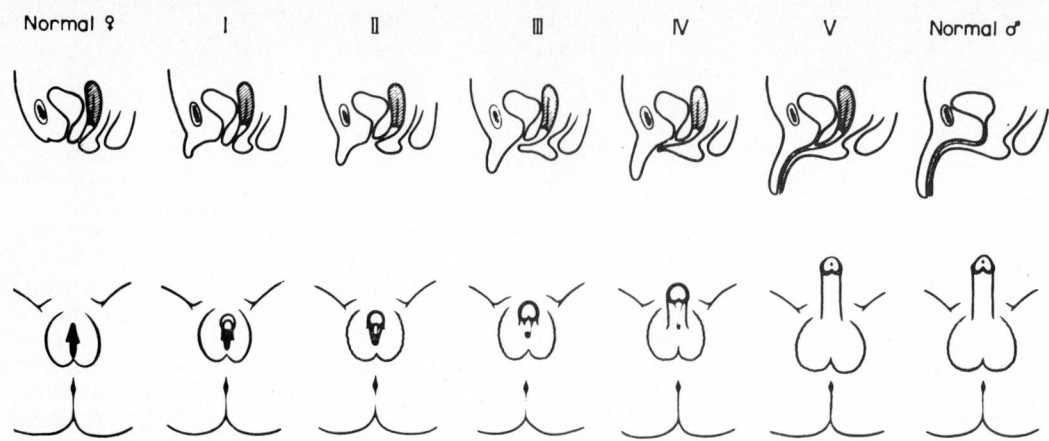

FIG. 15. Genital configuration in female pseudohermaphroditism due to CAH, compared with normal males and females. In type I, the only abnormality is enlargement of the clitoris; in type II, partial labioscrotal fusion; in type III, funnel-shaped urogenital sinus at posterior end of shallow vulva; in type IV, very small urogenital sinus situated at base of enlarged phallus; in type V, penile urethra. (From Prader: Helv Paediatr Acta 13:5, 1958.)

cular collapse occurs, and in some cases sudden cardiac arrest due to hyperkalemia is the cause of death. A somewhat similar clinical picture is observed in pyloric stenosis, but the hypokalemic alkalosis that accompanies this disorder contrasts with the low sodium, chloride, and bicarbonate levels and the elevated potassium levels of congenital adrenal hyperplasia. The abnormalities of the external genitalia in girls will remind the physician of the possibility of CAH. However, in infant boys the lack of abnormality of the genitalia will make the diagnosis more difficult. The history of neonatal death of previous siblings with a similar syndrome of dehydration should alert one to the probability that one is dealing with CAH. The finding of elevated urinary excretion of 17-ketosteroids and pregnanetriol along with a very marked increase in plasma 17-hydroxyprogesterone will confirm the diagnosis. The tendency toward salt loss appears to be less marked after the first 2 or 3 years of life, and a number of adult patients do not require mineralocorticoid therapy. However, it does not disappear completely, as the patients cannot adequately sustain a prolonged low-sodium diet. A similar crisis will take place in the rare cases of 3β-hydroxysteroid dehydrogenase deficiency and deficiency of one of the enzymes prior to pregnenolone.

As mentioned earlier, the salt-losing tendency of the simple virilizing form is compensated by an increase in plasma renin activity and a secretion of aldosterone above normal levels. In both the 11- and 17-hydroxylase deficiencies the decrease in aldosterone secretion is due to the increased DOC secretion.

Later on in life, progressive virilization occurs in the 21- and 11β-hydroxylase deficiencies. It includes the early appearance of pubic and axillary hair followed by the appearance of facial hair and increased total body hair, deepening of the voice, acne, and frequent phallic erections. Concurrently, rapid somatic growth, in-

creased musculature, and accelerated epiphyseal development are noted. Although the patients are taller than normal during early childhood, abnormally short adult stature results because of premature closure of the epiphyseal disks. Increased secretion of adrenal androgens is also responsible for the low gonadotropin secretion in postpubertal patients. This results in absence of menses in girls and small size of testes in boys; however, there are exceptions, and menses and spermatogenesis are present in a few untreated patients.

Patients with complete deficiency of 3β-hydroxysteroid dehydrogenase or one of the enzymes prior to pregnenolone would not be expected to demonstrate sexual maturation at the time of puberty; however, since these patients die in early infancy, this assumption has not been verified. Of interest is the fact that a few male patients who have had partial deficiency and have survived have shown some virilization at puberty. In the 17-hydroxylase deficiency there is partial or complete absence of secretion of gonadal hormones, and therefore no pubertal development is observed.

The pseudohermaphroditism of baby girls and the abnormal external genitalia of baby boys must be differentiated from the various kinds of intersexes. The study of the buccal smear and sex chromosome complement will establish the chromosomal sex of the patient. In addition, the study of urinary and plasma steroids will establish the abnormal pattern of hormone secretion. Macrogenitosomia praecox in boys must be differentiated from sexual precocity, either idiopathic or due to an intracranial lesion. The determination of gonadotropins will show normal adult levels in true precocious puberty and usually low levels in CAH. In addition, the study of plasma androgens will show a predominance of androstenedione over testosterone in CAH patients, whereas in precocious puberty testosterone levels are 4 to 10 times greater than those of androstenedione as expected in normal adult male subjects. In all patients (except those with a deficiency of 17-hydroxylase or of one of the enzymes prior to pregnenolone) the urinary excretion of 17-ketosteroids is increased for age. This increase must be demonstrated in order to make a positive diagnosis. The differential diagnosis of elevated urinary 17-ketosteroids is presented in Table 5; the dexamethasone test of suppression of urinary 17-ketosteroids differentiates adrenal hyperplasia from virilizing adrenal tumors. Patients with 21 and 11-hydroxylase deficiencies also have increased secretion of urinary pregnanetriol and to a lesser degree pregnanediol; however, excretion of urinary pregnanetriol is often low very early in life because of the fact that newborns have low glucuronyl transferase activity and because laboratory methods for urinary pregnanetriol measure only glucuronide conjugates. In order to alleviate this problem, it is possible to measure plasma 17-hydroxyprogesterone, the precursor of urinary pregnanetriol. In affected patients with 21-hydroxylase deficiency this compound will be greatly elevated.

With a deficiency of 3β-hydroxysteroid dehydrogenase, urinary pregnanetriol and plasma 17-hydroxyprogesterone are not elevated. Instead, large amounts of Δ^5 compounds, such as pregnenolone and its 17-, 11-, and 21-hydroxy derivatives (Fig. 14), will be detected.

The lack of secretion of any steroid when there is a deficiency in an enzyme prior to pregnenolone makes the laboratory diagnosis extremely difficult. Measurement of precursors of pregnenolone are not routinely available. A genetic male (XY karotype) with salt loss and abnormal external genitalia will make one think of the diagnosis. On the other hand, in a genetic female the external genitalia will be normal, and it will be difficult to demonstrate an abnormally low steroid secretion, since normal newborns have physiologically low steroid excretion and plasma levels. An absence of response to the ACTH test is helpful in such patients. Aldosterone secretion will be increased in the simple virilizing form, but decreased in all the other forms of CAH. Renin activity will be increased in both partial and complete 21-hydroxylase deficiency, and low in both 11- and 17-hydroxylase deficiencies.

Genetics of Congenital Adrenal Hyperplasia.   Although the number of female tends to be greater than the number of male patients, study of affected siblings shows that the apparent difference in frequency is probably due to the greater difficulty in recognizing the disorder in males. CAH is due to an autosomal recessive gene that manifests itself only on the homozygote. From data collected 20 years ago in the state of Maryland on 21-hydroxylase deficiency, it was calculated that the disorder occurred in at least 1 of 67,000 births and that the incidence of the gene in the general population was at least 1 in 128 individuals. These values were probably underestimated; data collected later in Switzerland and in the United States suggest a much higher incidence of the disease and suggest that the gene frequency may be 1 in 35 individuals.

Despite a few reports to the contrary, an affected sibship presents only one form of the disease, often with the same degree of severity. In the past, attempts to detect heterozygotes have been unsuccessful. More recently, studies with an acute ACTH test (intravenous injection of synthetic 1,24-ACTH and blood collection 30 to 60 minutes after injection) have shown a greater increase of plasma level of 17-hydroxyprogesterone in heterozygotes than in random individuals.

CONGENITAL DEFICIENCY OF 18-HYDROXYLASE OR 18-DEHYDROGENASE.   These patients present a salt-losing syndrome early in life, but in contrast to the salt-losing form of CAH, female patients have normal external genitalia, and in both sexes the urinary excretion of 17-ketosteroids and pregnanetriol is normal. In some cases the salt-losing tendency is not marked, and failure to thrive is the major symptom. A deficiency of 18-dehydrogenase results in a block in the biosynthesis of aldosterone. Such patients have been found to have low aldosterone secretion rates, along with increased secretion of 18-hydroxycorticosterone, corticosterone, and to a lesser extent DOC. Because these precursors of aldosterone have some salt-retaining properties, their increased secretion may tend to compensate partially for the deficient production of aldosterone. It is of interest to note that affected patients have an increased concentration of plasma renin, thus demonstrating that they have a partial lack of mineralocorticoids. One of the main urinary metabolites of 18-hydroxycorticosterone is 18-hydroxy-THA (3α, 18,21-trihydroxypregnane-11,20-dione), a compound that gives the Porter-Silber reaction and therefore is measured along with the urinary 17-hydroxycorticosteroids (17,21-dihydroxy-20-ketones). For this reason, it has been suggested that laboratory diagnosis of the syndrome could be made on the basis of an increase in total Porter-Silber steroids, which would be further increased by sodium deprivation, not significantly suppressed by dexamethasone administration, but brought down to normal levels by salt and deoxycorticosterone acetate (DOCA) therapy. However, such criteria would not apply if the enzymatic block were at the level of the 18-hydroxylase instead of the 18-dehydrogenase.

CONGENITAL ADRENOCORTICAL UNRESPONSIVENESS TO ACTH.   The defect in the syndrome of familial congenital adrenocortical unresponsiveness to ACTH may be located either at the level of the ACTH receptor site of the membrane of adrenal cells or at the level of the enzymatic system that is activated by ACTH in order to increase steroid biosynthesis (Table 10). As a consequence, cortical secretion is impaired, resulting in feeding problems and failure to thrive sometimes with hypoglycemic episodes. The skin hyperpigmentation probably is related to increased secretion of ACTH. Aldosterone secretion is normal, and there is no abnormality of serum electrolytes. Recent reports suggest variability in the clinical picture. In some patients the adrenal cortex has been found to be markedly atrophic, probably because of lack of stimulation by ACTH.

ADRENAL CRISIS OF ACUTE INFECTION.   In 1894 Voelcker described a syndrome characterized by

TABLE 10. Main Characteristics of Congenital Adrenocortical Unresponsiveness to ACTH

Positive clinical	Feeding problems; hypoglycemic episodes; skin hyperpigmentation
Negative clinical	No sodium depletion; blood pressure and serum electrolytes normal; PPD, histoplasmin tests negative; no adrenal antibodies
Laboratory	Low cortisol secretion; no increment under ACTH; normal aldosterone secretion; normal increment under low-sodium diet
Pathology	Atrophic adrenal cortex; normal glomerulus; atrophic fasciculata reticularis
Pathogenesis	Defect in ACTH receptor site or in ACTH-dependent system involved in cortisol biosynthesis
Genetics	Autosomal recessive; X-linked patterns (?)

severe shock that evolved rapidly into coma and death, with fulminating purpura and bilateral adrenal hemorrhage. Later on, this syndrome was recognized to be related to meningococcemia, and Waterhouse and Friderichsen made comprehensive reviews of the literature. Meningitis may or may not be present; very often the petechial rash progresses rapidly and coalesces, resulting in large ecchymoses. At the same time, the pulse becomes rapid, blood pressure falls, respiration is labored, and the skin is cyanotic and cold; hyponatremia may be masked by hemoconcentration. The course of the disease toward coma and death can be extremely rapid. A similar adrenal crisis can also occur, although more rarely, with pneumococcal, streptococcal, and diptheritic infection. It must be emphasized that the adrenal hemorrhage is purely a pathologic diagnosis and that one cannot be certain about the anatomy of the adrenal cortex of a living patient. For this reason Lanman has suggested that the clinical term fulminating meningococcemia be used for those patients with meningococcal infection who show signs of shock and/or severe hemorrhagic lesions and that the term the Waterhouse-Friderichsen syndrome (fulminating meningococcal infection with adrenal hemorrhages) be used for those fatal cases demonstrating both the clinical syndrome and adrenal hemorrhages at autopsy.

CHRONIC HYPOADRENOCORTICISM (ADDISON'S DISEASE). Limited hypoplasia or hemorrhage of the adrenal glands in an infant may leave sufficient cortex to provide a limited amount of hormones, so that adrenal insufficiency may appear several months or years later, often at the time of a minor infection. Or the hemorrhage may be replaced by calcium deposit, so that at the time of overt chronic adrenal insufficiency, calcified adrenals will be noted radiologically. Symptoms of chronic adrenal insufficiency can appear if the adrenal cortex is damaged by infection or by any destructive process. Until recently, tuberculosis of the adrenal glands was the most frequent etiologic factor. However, with the decrease in incidence of this infection, other factors have been incriminated, such as histoplasmosis, various types of mycosis, metastatic tumors, and amyloidosis. In some cases no etiologic factor can be found . At autopsy the adrenal glands may be small, and a lymphocytic infiltration may replace the cortex, thus suggesting that adrenal destruction is related to an autoimmune process. Familial incidence of Addison's disease might be explained on the basis of a genetic sensitivity to autoimmunization; an alternative explanation might be that the adrenal cortex produces an abnormal product on a genetic basis that is primarily responsible for adrenal destruction, while the formation of circulating antibodies is secondary to this destruction.

In a survey of 118 patients with idiopathic Addison's disease, 67 had Addison's disease only, while 51 had Addison's disease plus another disorder. Adrenal antibodies were found in 31 percent of the patients with only Addison's disease and in 71 percent of the Addisonian patients with associated disorders. Addison's disease may be associated with idiopathic hypoparathyroidism, hypothyroidism, diabetes, and pernicious anemia; such associations are thought to represent examples of polyglandular autoimmune diseases. Among the 51 patients who presented with Addison's disease and an associated disorder, the most frequent associated disorder was thyroid disease, followed by hypoparathyroidism and diabetes. Thyroid disorders were found mainly in adults, while hypoparathyroidism was found mainly in children. Of the 118 patients with idiopathic Addison's disease 64 percent had an associated disorder either diagnosed as such or with only

TABLE 11. Familial Aggregation of Patients With Addison's Disease and Other Endocrine Disorders

Groups	Age at Onset	Sex (M:F)	Familial	Homo-geneous	Associated Disorders
Addison's alone	Early	20:6	Mendelian recessive	yes	None by definition
Addison's alone	Late	11:5	No	No	No; some will become Schmidt's
Schmidt's; Addison's + diabetes and/or thyroid	Late	12:21	Mendelian recessive	No	Yes by definition
Hypoparathyroidism and Addison's	Early	16:15	Mendelian recessive	Yes	P.A. *Monilia*
Hypoparathyroidism without Addison's	Early	1:11	?	Yes	P.A. *Monilia*
Hypoparathyroidism alone	Early	7:18	No	No	None

positive antibodies. Chronic moniliasis also can accompany Addison's disease and its associated disorders.

Pedigree studies in affected families have shown a significantly greater clinical similarity among patients within families than among unrelated persons. This suggests that there are several syndromes distinct in origin and in characteristics, some apparently determined genetically in a pattern compatible with autosomal recessive inheritance (Table 11). The clinical picture of Addison's disease is that of chronic, progressive debilitating illness with gastrointestinal disorders and skin hyperpigmentation. However, an acute adrenal crisis can occur and often is precipitated by infection, trauma, or surgical procedure that brings about more muscular weakness and general worsening of the gastrointestinal signs, with a fall in blood pressure, abdominal pain, and acute dehydration. The dehydration can produce hemoconcentration, which may mask the drop in serum concentration of sodium and chloride. The levels of nonprotein nitrogen and hematocrit can be useful in determinging the degree of hemoconcentration and in interpreting the sodium and chloride levels.

The diagnosis of Addison's disease is often difficult to establish, because states of dehydration and gastrointestinal disorders are encountered frequently in young children. Low serum sodium and chloride levels are observed often in pediatric practice, including the syndrome of salt-losing kidney. Elevated levels of serum potassium can occur shortly before death from any cause, and red cell hemolysis must be eliminated as a cause of high potassium concentration. Furthermore, prolonged infusions of glucose may lower the serum potassium level to a normal value.

Skin pigmentation can be a helpful sign in diagnosis, but it must be distinguished from the pigmentation found in other disorders (von Recklinghausen's disease, some drug poisonings, hemochromatosis). Limited destruction of the adrenal tissue may be completely asymptomatic, and calcification of the adrenal glands may be an incidental finding on an x-ray of the abdomen. The occurrence of normal adrenal function, despite extensive bilateral adrenal calcification, must mean that enough adrenal tissue has remained functional to cover the needs of these children.

Several degenerative syndromes have been reported to be associated with hypoadrenocorticism. In most of them the etiology of the adrenal insufficiency is poorly understood. Primary familial xanthomatosis with adrenal calcification early in life produces a clinical picture of malnutrition, failure to thrive, and hepatosplenomegaly. All patients die before 1 year of age. At autopsy the main finding is an excessive accumulation of normally esterified cholesterol in almost all organs, including the brain. The characteristic adrenal calcification is not clearly explained. A study of families presenting with this syndrome suggests an autosomal recessive inheritance of the disorder. Diffuse cerebral sclerosis, as described by Schilder, can be associated with adrenal insufficiency (adrenal leukodystrophy); neurologic and endocrine symptoms appear in a dissociated fashion, although the adrenal insufficiency is usually present early in childhood. Studies on cultured fibroblasts have shown abnormal cholesterol uptake and accumulation. All patients have been males, often with affected siblings and affected maternal uncles and cousins. Therefore it seems that this syndrome is an X-linked defect.

Hypoadrenocorticism Secondary to Deficient ACTH Secretion

HYPOPITUITARISM. Idiopathic panhypopituitarism is characterized by a deficient secretion of all tropic hormones normally secreted by the anterior part of the pituitary gland; the function of the posterior part usually is normal. Growth hormone deficiency results in dwarfism, and gonadotropin deficiency is responsible for the sexual infantilism. The secretion of thyroid-stimulating hormone (TSH) is also deficient, but the symptoms of hypothyroidism are usually mild. Despite ACTH deficiency, the symptoms of hypoadrenocorticism are often minimal. Although the cortisol secretion rate in panhypopituitarism can be significantly decreased, the plasma concentration of cortisol often reaches near-normal levels, probably due to the fact that hypothyroidism results in prolongation of the half-life of cortisol.

Symptoms of hypoglycemia are not rare, and many patients have decreased excretion of water load, which can be corrected by cortisol administration. Hypersensitivity to insulin is observed, and for that reason insulin tolerance tests in connection with growth hormone assay must be supervised carefully. The symptoms of hypoadrenocorticism may appear in some patients only at times of medical or surgical stress. Because ACTH has little effect on the homeostatic regulation of aldosterone secretion, no alteration of electrolytes is observed in patients with hypopituitarism. In some patients the idiopathic hypopituitarism does not involve all tropic hormones, and only one or two of them are deficient, although rare cases of isolated ACTH deficiency have been reported.

Pituitary tumors, particularly craniopharyngiomas, can produce tropic hormone deficiency involving ACTH. Surgical removal of such tumors often is followed by worsening of the pituitary hormone deficiencies, which can be further complicated by a deficiency of antidiuretic hormone.

About one-half of patients with idiopathic hypopituitarism have abnormal responses to the oral metyrapone test. However, most patients respond normally to the intravenous metyrapone test, as well as to the insulin and piromen (bacterial pyrogen) tests. Therefore the oral metyrapone test does not appear to measure the full capability of the hypothalamic–pituitary unit to respond to stress. Furthermore, the fact that stimulation of ACTH output can be obtained during acute tests does not prove that it can be sustained in conditions of prolonged stress. We therefore believe that steroids during major infection, trauma, or surgery seem prudent in subjects who have abnormal responses to the oral metyrapone test. Organic hypopituitarism, in contrast to the idiopathic form, will often result in severe impairment of ACTH secretion and will require cortisone replacement therapy.

CESSATION OF GLUCOCORTICOID THERAPY. The administration of cortisol-like compounds suppresses the secretion of pituitary ACTH, and as a consequence the adrenal cortex becomes atrophic. After cessation of glucocorticoid therapy, normal ACTH secretion is not resumed immediately. With rare exceptions the following general rules can be stated:

If a patient has received large doses of glucocorticoid for a short period of time (less than 1 month) or small doses (less than replacement level) for any period of time, it is possible to assume that he will present little or no pituitary–adrenal insufficiency when terminating therapy.

When patients have received continuously large doses of glucocorticoids for a period longer than 1 month, it must be assumed that most have pituitary–adrenal insufficiency, the duration of which is variable and is not necessarily related to dosage or length of treatment. Recovery will be achieved within 6 weeks in about half of the subjects, and in almost all of them after 6 months.

Intermittent treatment every other day, or 3 days on and 4 days off every week, can be advantageous, particularly if it results in administration of a smaller dose of glucocorticoid when compared with the dose necessary with continuous therapy. It may also result in less frequent absence but not complete absence of pituitary–adrenal insufficiency when treatment is stopped.

Slow tapering of the dosage will help to decrease the occurrence of cortisol insufficiency.

Although it is perhaps too sensitive, the oral metyrapone test remains a satisfactory method of determining the return to normal of the hypothalamic-pituitary-adrenal axis.

Pituitary–adrenal insufficiency after cessation of glucocorticoid therapy can be dangerous at the time of stress. Therefore steroid therapy for conditions of stress is recommended in patients who have negative responses to the oral metyrapone test or who have stopped therapy for less than 6 months.

Unilateral adrenal tumors resulting in Cushing's syndrome produce cortisol in an autonomous fashion without requiring ACTH activation. The high levels of circulating cortisol tend to suppress ACTH secretion by the anterior part of the pituitary gland, and the contralateral adrenal becomes atrophic. Removal of such a tumor without supportive therapy can result in severe symptoms of hypoadrenocorticism due to cortisol deficiency.

ANENCEPHALY. In anencephaly the adrenal glands at birth are markedly reduced in size and lack the fetal zone; it has been suggested that absence of pituitary tissue is the cause of this adrenal atrophy. Of 3 anencephalic infants in whom cortisol secretion was determined during their periods of survival, 2 had normal secretion, and one had a low value. It is very rare that the pituitary tissue is completely absent, and remnants of the gland might be the reason for the normal cortisol values found in some cases.

STEROID-TREATED MOTHERS. Infants born of steroid-treated mothers theoretically would be expected to present with hypoadrenocorticism shortly after birth, since cortisol can cross the placenta from the mother to the fetus during pregnancy. However, a review of 260 pregnancies, during which pharmacologic doses of cortisone or its analogues had been administered for variable periods of time, showed that only one infant was suspected of having adrenocortical insufficiency, and even in this child it was not documented adequately. There has also been a report of a neonatal death attributed to steroid therapy and secondary adrenal atrophy. However, the cortisol secretion rates of 8 infants born of steroid-treated women were found to be in the range observed for normal newborn babies.

Studies with tagged steroids have shown that cortisone and prednisone administered to mothers are rapidly transformed into the biologically active hormones cortisol and prednisolone, respectively; the maternal concentrations of these two steroids are about four times greater than those of cortisone and prednisone, respectively. At equilibrium the concentrations of tagged cortisol and prednisolone in cord plasma represented 7.5 to 11 percent of the corresponding maternal concentrations. In contrast, the cord concentrations of the steroids that were not biologically active (cortisone and prednisone) were similar to those of the mothers. Similar results were obtained when tagged cortisol and prednisolone were administered to mothers. This phenomenon may be related to the presence of an active 11β-hydroxysteroid dehydrogenase in the placenta that can convert maternal cortisol into fetal cortisone. The fact that maternal cortisol is largely bound to transcortin, whereas cortisone is only loosely bound to albumin, may also contribute to the distribution of the two steroids on both sides of the placenta.

Thus the suppression of fetal ACTH is theoretically possible, but it would take a much higher maternal dose than is usually employed. Nevertheless, infants born to mothers receiving steroids should be observed for signs and symptoms of hypoglycemia that may be caused by cortisol deficiency. If the blood levels of true glucose fall below 30 mg/100 ml, glucose infusion in amounts sufficient to maintain normal concentration should be the first and only therapeutic measure. In any event, no mineralocorticoid deficiency is to be expected, since ACTH has little influence on aldosterone secretion.

Hypoadrenocorticism Secondary to End-Organ Unresponsiveness

Several infants have been reported with a transient salt-losing syndrome that did not respond to salt-retaining hormones. They failed to gain weight, had poor appetite, and developed hyponatremia despite normal adrenocortical function tests, including normal or elevated aldosterone excretion. The urinary loss of salt and sweat electrolytes did not respond to administration of adrenocortical steroids; the only effective treatment was salt supplementation. Spontaneous remission occurred in all patients at 15 to 24 months of age. This syndrome may be due to a temporary unresponsiveness to salt-retaining hormones that affect both the sweat glands and the kidneys.

Treatment

Treatment of adrenal insufficiency should be based on physiologic replacement of the hormone or hormones that are absent. In the acute adrenal crisis there may be deficiencies of both cortisol and aldosterone, as well as marked dehydration. In the immediate newborn period it is usually possible to maintain the infant on salt and fluid replacement while the appropriate 24-hour urine specimen is collected for diagnostic purposes. We recommend that during the first hour of therapy the patient receive 20 ml/kg of isotonic saline in 5 percent glucose or 20 ml/kg of the following mixture: one-third sodium lactate (1/6), two-thirds 0.85 percent sodium chloride, and dextrose to make a 5 percent solution. The advantage of this last mixture is that it will correct the acidosis, whereas isotonic saline alone will not. At the end of the first hour, if the blood pressure is satisfactory and the patient's vital signs are stable, the intravenous solution should be continued to deliver 60 ml/kg over the next 24 hours. If at the end of the first hour the infant has not improved and the blood chemistry has not changed, the use of DOCA (1 mg intramuscularly) is indicated. The DOCA will not interfere with measurement of urinary 17-ketosteroids, 17-hydroxycorticosteroids, or pregnanetriol, but it will give a mineralocorticoid effect. In the newborn period this regimen has usually been sufficient for the treatment of acute crises. If the patient shows further deterioration, the use of hydrocortisone is indicated. We prefer the sodium succinate salt (Solu-Cortef) given as a 50-mg bolus intravenously. An additional 25 mg should be placed into the intravenous maintenance solution. If the patient shows further decompensation, plasma (10 ml/kg) instead of other intravenous fluids

may be used. The 24-hour fluid requirement will be from 80 to 120 ml/kg body weight. Sympathomimetic agents such as phenylephrine hydrochloride (Neo-Synephrine), *l*-norepinephrine bitartrate (Levophed), and epinephrine have, rarely, been used in the treatment of acute adrenal insufficiency during the neonatal period.

The use of morphine, barbiturates, or other sedatives is contraindicated. Potassium should not be added to any intravenous fluids. There is also danger of administration of too much intravenous fluid and/or salt along with large amounts of mineralocorticoids, since this can result in pulmonary edema, cardiac failure, and hypernatremia.

MAINTENANCE THERAPY. The doses of both hormones must be individualized to the patient's needs. Close attention must be given to weight gain or loss, serum electrolytes, and blood pressure. Overtreatment is characterized by hypertension, rapid weight gain, and elevated serum sodium. Undertreatment is characterized by failure to thrive, with weight loss and dehydration, elevated serum potassium with decreased serum sodium, and hypotension. The family must be aware that the patient will require medication for the rest of his life. The only exceptions are the rare patients with end-organ unresponsiveness who require only added salt for the first 2 to 3 years of life. The patient should be identified as one who requires glucocorticoid and/or mineralocorticoid replacement by a Medic Alert bracelet or amulet. The family should also be aware that there will be an increased need for glucocorticoid at times of stress, whether medical or surgical.

REPLACEMENT OF GLUCOCORTICOIDS. Cortisol is the drug of choice for replacement of glucocorticoid action in adrenal insufficiency. It is the major physiologic glucocorticoid secreted by the adrenal cortex, and it contributes to sodium retention, whereas synthetic preparations do not (Table 12). During childhood the dosage of cortisol may be better regulated than dosages of synthetic preparations that have greater potency.

TABLE 12. Potency of Various Oral Steriod Preparations as Related to Cortisol and DOCA

Generic Name	Trade Names	Glucocorticoid Effect Equivalent to 100 mg Cortisol Given Orally	Na Retention Effect Equivalent to 1 mg DOCA (im)
Cortisol (hydrocortisone)	Hydrocortone, Cortef	100	20
Cortisone	Cortone	125	20
Δ^1-cortisol (prednisolone)	Meticortelone, Delta-Cortef	20	50
Δ^1-cortisone (prednisone)	Deltasone, Meticorten, Delta-Dome	25	50
6α-CH₃-Δ^1-prednisolone (methylprednisolone)	Medrol	15 (20*)	No effect*
16-OH-9α-fluoro-prednisolone (triamcinolone)	Aristocort, Kenacort	10 (20*)	No effect*
6α-fluoro-16α-CH₃-Δ^1-prednisolone (paramethasone)	Haldrone	(10*)	No effect or salt loss*
9α-fluoro-16α-CH₃-prednisolone (dexamethasone)	Gammacorten, Decadron, Hexadrol, Deronil	1.5 (3.75*)	No effect*
9α-fluoro-16β-CH₃-prednisolone (betamethasone)	Celestone	(3*)	No effect or salt loss*
Aldosterone	Not commercially available	300	0.1–0.04
9α-fluorocortisol acetate	Florinef Acetate	6.5	0.1
Deoxycorticosterone acetate	Percorten, Doca	0	1.0 (im)

* Values estimated by pharmaceutical companies.

TABLE 13. Treatment of Adrenocortical Insufficiency During Maintenance and Stress

	Maintenance (mg/day)	Stress (mg/day)
Cortisol replacement		
Oral cortisol (1/3 dose, tid)	$25/m^2$	$75/m^2$
Intramuscular cortisol	$12.5/m^2$	$37.5/m^2$*
Intravenous cortisol sodium succinate (Solu-Cortef)	—	50–100†
Aldosterone replacement		
DOCA pellets/subcut	125–250 every 9–12 months	If pellets present, no additional therapy
Oral 9α-fluorocortisol acetate	0.05–0.10	0.05–0.10
Intrasmuscular DOCA	—	1*

* Intramuscular therapy is given if patient cannot retain oral preparations.
† If oral therapy has not been retained for more than 12 hours.

As noted earlier, the physiologic secretion of cortisol (mean $\pm$ SD) is 12.1 ± 2.9 mg/m²/24 hours. A daily intramuscular injection of 12.5 mg of cortisol to a child with a body surface area of 1 m² will therefore be replacement therapy (Table 13). Cortisol acetate is usually given as a single injection at a dose three times the daily requirement every third day. In general, no correction in dosage is made for the fact that 10 percent of the weight of cortisol acetate is due to the acetyl group. However, if cortisone acetate is used, replacement is made on the basis of 16 mg/m²/24 hours. If it is not practical to administer intramuscular injections, cortisol can be given orally; it is reabsorbed rapidly from the gastrointestinal tract. Because of the short half-life of this steroid in plasma (60 minutes) and also because of a partial inactivation of the hormone by gastric acidity, the maintenance daily dose of oral cortisol must be approximately twice the physiologic production (25 mg/m²/24 hours) and must be fractionated (one-third of the daily dose every 8 hours, or at mealtimes). During the first 18 months of life we prefer to use the intramuscular route, thus eliminating the variable gastric absorption of oral preparations. Furthermore, infants regurgitate easily, which may result in loss of oral medication.

REPLACEMENT OF MINERALOCORTICOIDS. Aldosterone is presently not available for human therapy in the United States; DOCA, a biosynthetic precursor of aldosterone with significant mineralocorticoid action, is used. Since the secretion rates of children after 2 weeks of age are not significantly different from those of adults, the daily dose of DOCA is 1 mg (sometimes 2 mg) intramuscularly for all patients. The intramuscular DOCA may be replaced by oral 9α-fluorocortisol acetate (Florinef), 0.05 to 0.10 mg as a single daily dose. It is important to note that mineralocorticoid treatment will be effective only if salt is administered simultaneously. Most prepared infant formulas are low in salt, and oral salt supplementation may be needed until solid foods are introduced into the diet (one-fifth teaspoon of salt or about 18 mEq sodium to the formula, once each day).

We implant DOCA pellets in infant patients who require mineralocorticoid, especially in those who have a tendency to regurgitate. We usually implant two 125-mg pellets and replace them after 9 to 12 months; the pellets are reabsorbed slowly and provide a constant level of mineralocorticoid activity. However, following the initial implantation there may be variable absorption. Patients may need 1 mg of DOCA intramuscularly on the day following implantation. Other patients may have increased reabsorption of the DOCA, with salt and water retention, which will best be handled by a low-sodium diet; if this is not successful, one of the pellets may have to be removed.

CONDITIONS OF STRESS. The adrenal responds to stress with a markedly increased secretion of cortisol; in the patient with adrenal insufficiency this stress response is absent. Therefore, additional cortisol must be provided; if it is not, the patient may manifest symptoms of acute adrenal insufficiency.

Minor infections with low-grade fever may not require any increase in medication. Moderate stress requires a doubling of the dosage, whereas major infections or surgery need a tripling of the dosage. In infants this is done by giving a daily injection of twice or three times the maintenance dose. It is important to return to maintenance levels as soon as possible to avoid the problems of overtreatment, with poor growth and symptoms of Cushing's disease.

If possible, the child should be in the hospital for at least 2 days prior to surgery. The dosage of intramuscular cortisol should be tripled (37.5 mg/m²/24 hours) and given as a single injection on each of the 2 days prior to and on the day of surgery. If DOCA pellets are implanted, no additional mineralocorticoid will be necessary. For patients on oral mineralocorticoid replacement, this should be continued up to the day of surgery, and 1 mg of DOCA intramuscularly should be given on the day of surgery. Intramuscular therapy should be continued during the days immediately after surgery. It may be decreased on the fourth day, and replacement may be resumed by the fifth or sixth postoperative day, as summarized in Table 14.

When emergency surgery is indicated, the patient cannot be prepared in the above manner. Then the patient should receive an intramuscular dose of cortisone (37.5 mg/m²) and an immediate dose of 50 mg cortisol hemisuccinate prior to anesthesia. In addition, 50 mg of Solu-Cortef should be given during surgery

TABLE 14. Treatment of Adrenocortical Insufficiency at Time of Surgery

| | Elective Surgery | | Emergency Surgery | | |
Days to Surgery	IM Cortisol (mg/m²/day)	IM DOCA (mg/day)*	IM Cortisol (mg/m²/day)	IV Solu-Cortef (mg/day)	IM DOCA (mg/day)*
−2	37.5–50	0.05–0.10			
−1	37.5–50	0.05–0.10			
Preanesthesia	37.5–50	IM DOCA 1	37.5–50	50 (stat);	
During surgery				(continuous infusion of 50 mg during surgery and recovery)	
+1	37.5–50	1	37.5–50		1
+2	37.5–50	1	37.5–50		1
+3	37.5–50	1	37.5–50		1
+4	25–37.5	1	25–37.5		1
+5	Resume replacement therapy		Resume replacement therapy		

* If pellets, no additional DOCA necessary. Do not use if patient is on oral Florinef.

and recovery, added to the intravenous fluids. After this time intramuscular cortisol will have its full glucocorticoid effect.

ADJUSTMENT TO ADRENAL INSUFFICIENCY.
ADRENAL CRISIS OF NEONATAL PERIOD. Vigorous therapy must be instituted rapidly; otherwise the infant may die within 24 to 72 hours after the appearance of the first symptoms of adrenal insufficiency. Fluid and electrolyte replacement must be carried out immediately, and serial studies of serum electrolytes, along with clinical evaluation of the state of dehydration, must guide the therapy. If these measures are sufficient to maintain the patient, it will be important to establish the diagnosis and particularly to collect several 24-hour urine specimens for steroid analysis. In many cases it is not possible to make a differential diagnosis in the newborn period, and steroid replacement therapy must be started with the idea of withdrawing it later on for specific diagnosis.

After the second or third day, when the patient shows signs of rehydration, the salt intake should be brought back to normal while intramuscular doses of cortisol and DOCA are reduced to maintenance levels. If the diagnosis of salt-losing adrenal hyperplasia has already been established, implantation of DOCA pellets is recommended.

The rare patients in whom adrenal aplasia or hemorrhage has been recognized, and who survive the neonatal crisis, will require treatment for the rest of their lives, like addisonian patients. However, those with adrenal hemorrhage should in later childhood have an evaluation of adrenal status to determine if there has been any return of function.

CONGENITAL ADRENAL HYPERPLASIA. In the salt-losing form of this disorder it is obvious that treatment must be started at the time of the adrenal crisis and must be continued thereafter. This would also apply to patients with a deficiency in 3β-hydroxysteroid dehydrogenase and in enzyme defects prior to pregnanolone. In the simple virilizing form and in the 11-hydroxylase deficiency, best results are obtained when treatment is started prior to 1 year of age. With proper therapy such children will grow normally, will not show any signs of virilization, and will develop sexually at the physiologic age. The hypertension of the 11-hydroxylase deficiency will also be under control.

In females with masculinized genitalia, a simple surgical procedure can be carried out before 1 year of age that will correct the problem. The correction is more difficult in patients in whom the masculinization has resulted in a penile urethra, with the vagina opening posteriorly in the "urethra." Treated patients are capable of reproducing. If the mate is unaffected, all their children will be heterozygotes. However, if the mate is a heterozygote, then the couple will have a 50 percent chance of producing homozygous children. In order to maintain regular menses and fertility, experience has shown that cortisol replacement therapy must be adequate and must result in urinary 17-ketosteroids of less than 6 mg/24 hours. Maintenance therapy should not be changed during pregnancy, but during labor and delivery cortisol treatment should be increased.

If treatment is started late in life, the rapid growth and virilization can be checked, but the bone age may be so advanced as to result in stunting of ultimate height. In addition, gonadal maturation (with spermatogenesis in boys, ovulatory menstrual cycles in girls) will occur if treatment is begun when the bone age is that at which physiologic puberty would be expected.

Cessation of treatment results in recurrence of virilization, with intractable acne and amenorrhea. Unfortunately, one of the major problems with these patients is the difficulty encountered with therapeutic compliance. The patients and their parents require psychologic counseling at various stages of their development in order to reinforce the need for compliance and to explain the specifics of the disorder. An exception to what has been said is the rare patient with 17-hydroxylase deficiency who does not develop normal gonadal function at puberty despite replacement cortisol therapy. Treatment with gonadal steroids will be required to obtain normal secondary sex characteristics.

18-HYDROXYLASE AND 18-DEHYDROGENASE DEFI-CIENCY. These patients are also characterized by an adrenal crisis during the neonatal period; because of the enzymatic block, they are unable to produce normal secretion of aldosterone, but they have hypersecretion of corticosterone, which has some salt-retaining activity. For this reason the crisis tends to be less dramatic than that of the salt-losing form of CAH. Nevertheless, they often require emergency fluid and electrolyte replacement therapy. For maintenance purposes, these patients need either intramuscular DOCA or oral 9α-fluorocortisol. It must be noted that these patients do not require cortisol treatment, as secretion of this steroid is normal.

CONGENITAL ADRENOCORTICAL UNRESPONSIVENESS TO ACTH. The adrenal crisis of this condition is also more insidious and less striking than that in the salt-losing form of CAH. In these patients there is no problem with water and electrolyte metabolism; the only deficient hormone is cortisol, which results in hypoglycemic episodes requiring administration of glucose. The long-range treatment for these patients is cortisol replacement.

MENINGOCOCCEMIA. There is some difference of opinion on the need for administering cortisol as preventive or supportive therapy to patients with meningitis and meningococcemia who show no obvious signs of adrenal insufficiency. This infection is accompanied by an increase in cortisol secretion and cortisol concentration in plasma. The question of whether the increment of cortisol is sufficient for the stress situation can be answered only by therapeutic tests. Presently available data suggest that clear-cut beneficial effects have not been established.

On the other hand, patients with fulminating meningococcemia and bilateral adrenal hemorrhages have low levels of plasma cortisol. It would appear that adrenal hemorrhages result in a loss of cortisol secretion; therefore, if such patients are to be saved, they should receive replacement therapy. Animal studies suggest that cortisone treatment during endotoxemia is detrimental and increases the chances of development of a generalized Shwartzman reaction. This dilemma could be the cause of the poor results obtained in fulminating meningococcemia with adrenal hemorrhages, whether steroids are administered or not. A pessimistic view would be that the occurrence of adrenal hemorrhages is a sign that the infectious process has gone beyond any helpful therapeutic measure and that only earlier specific antibiotic treatment can prevent shock and death. Early administration of antibiotics is certainly of the utmost importance, but cortisol therapy should be instituted when shock appears. On the basis of experimental data, Lillehei and his colleagues have suggested the administration of pharmacologic amounts of intravenous cortisol along with generous volumes of plasma: 0.5 to 1.0 g intravenously in one injection followed by a constant infusion of a total of 50 mg/kg body weight. At the present time such a therapeutic trial seems to be worthwhile, but its efficacy needs to be proved.

ADDISON'S DISEASE. Patients with chronic hypoadrenocorticism often come to medical attention for the first time during an acute adrenal crisis (Table 15). At that time they will require cortisol hemisuccinate added to intravenous fluid treatment for the first 24 to 48 hours, along with simultaneous injections of daily doses of intramuscular cortisol (three times the replacement level) and DOCA (1 to 2 mg). As the patient improves, the cortisol dosage should be brought to a maintenance level, and the intramuscular DOCA should be replaced by oral 9α-fluorocortisol acetate (0.05 to 0.1 mg). All the various rules relating to cortisol treatment mentioned earlier apply to these patients, particularly the increase of dosage during conditions of stress and the shift to intramuscular preparations of cortisol and DOCA when the patients are unable to receive oral therapy.

Patients with familial xanthomatosis with adrenal calcification or diffuse cerebral sclerosis with adrenal insufficiency experience progressive deterioration of adrenal function and eventually require both glucocorticoid and mineralocorticoid replacement. At that time they can be considered as having Addison's disease.

ADRENAL INSUFFICIENCY SECONDARY TO ACTH DEFICIENCY. Patients with hypopituitarism do not have any impairment of aldosterone secretion. Approximately one-half of these patients have entirely normal cortisol secretion; the rest of them may have normal secretion under basal conditions but may not be able to increase and sustain their cortisol levels during stress. For these

TABLE 15. Symptoms of Addison's Disease as Related to Various Steroid Deficiencies

Symptoms related to deficient secretion of aldosterone
  Hyperkalemic acidosis: Na, Cl,-HCO$_3$$^-$ levels are low; K level is elevated
  Cardiovascular disorders
    Hypotension
    Decreased size of heart
    ECG low voltage and T wave changes
    Decreased blood volume
  Gastrointestinal disorders
    Anorexia
    Nausea
    Vomiting
    Diarrhea
    Salt Craving
  Muscular weakness, asthenia, weight loss
Symptoms related to deficient secretion of cortisol
  Disturbance of carbohydrate metabolism
  Fasting hypoglycemia; insulin hypersensitivity
  Marked secondary hypoglycemia following intravenous glucose tolerance test
  Gastrointestinal disorders
  Decreased gastric acidity
Symptoms related to deficient secretion of androgens
  Lack of protein anabolism
  Decreased axillary and pubic hair and libido
Symptoms related to increased secretion of pituitary ACTH and increased plasma MSH. Skin pigmentation localized to nipples, genitalia, creases of the palms, mucosa, areas exposed to friction
  Generalized, with areas of vitiligo

TABLE 16. Mode of Steroid Withdrawal in a Child of 1 m² Body Surface Area

	Oral Cortisol (mg/day)
Therapeutic dose	200
Days 1–3	100
Days 4–6	50
Days 7–9 (replacement level*)	25
Days 10–19	12.5
Days 20–29	6
Day 30	0

* Oral replacement level 25 mg/m² /24 hours.

reasons such individuals require steroid treatment at the time of surgery or during acute infection. In patients in whom deficiencies of both thyroid and adrenal function have been demonstrated, thyroid hormone replacement therapy should not be started by itself: it might produce symptoms of acute adrenal insufficiency. Cortisol replacement, therefore, should be started prior to or at the same time as thyroid replacement therapy. In patients with both posterior and anterior hypopituitarism, symptoms of diabetes insipidus often appear only after cortisone therapy.

Long-term steroid treatment should not be stopped abruptly. However, the therapeutic dosage can be decreased fairly rapidly until it reaches a level corresponding to one-half the daily maintenance dosage. Then subsequent decreases may be made more slowly (Table 16). ACTH administration is of no practical value, since exogenous ACTH will suppress endogenous production; thus the patient will be in the same condition 3 to 4 days after exogenous ACTH is stopped as before it was started. Six weeks after cessation of therapy about one-half of these patients will have recovered, and almost all of them after 6 months. To be certain that recovery has occurred, a metyrapone test can be carried out. If the response is abnormal, or if the test is not done, it is prudent to give cortisol therapy for surgery or any other major stress during the first 6 months after withdrawal.

When a unilateral adrenal tumor that produces cortisol is removed, the patient must be treated like an addisonian patient undergoing elective surgery. Following removal of the tumor the patient should be treated as if he has been withdrawn from prolonged cortisol therapy. Theoretically, a purely virilizing adrenal tumor should not require cortisol administration at the time of tumor removal, since it would be expected that the contralateral adrenal would be producing normal amounts of cortisol. However, it is probably safer to treat these patients.

Generally, no adrenal steroid treatment is needed in anorexia nervosa or in inanition. Infants exposed to increased steroids in utero should be observed for hypoglycemia. If it is present, intravenous glucose should be given at an initial dose of 25 percent dextrose, followed with a 10 percent maintenance solution, but the use of steroids is not indicated.

HYPERADRENOCORTICISM

Hyperadrenocorticism can involve any of the hormones secreted by the adrenal cortex, either singly or in combination. Depending on the predominance of a specific steroid, this condition can be categorized as follows (Table 17): Cushing's syndrome is characterized by an increased secretion of cortisol; adrenogenital syndrome is related to elevated output of androgens; feminizing syndromes are characterized by high secretions of estrogens; hyperaldosteronism is due to an abnormal production of aldosterone. In each of these syndromes the secretion of other steroid hormones can be increased concurrently.

Cushing's Syndrome

ETIOLOGY. Abnormally elevated cortisol secretion results in the clinical picture of Cushing's syndrome. This syndrome is rare in infancy and childhood as compared with its frequency in adulthood. There are two main causes for the syndrome. The first is an increase in ACTH production with bilateral adrenal hyperplasia. This can be related either to a chromophobe adenoma or to multiple microadenomas of the pituitary gland. More frequently it is related to abnormal cortisol–ACTH homeostatic regulation. Certain tu-

TABLE 17. Classification of Hyperadrenocorticism

Syndrome	Etiology	Hormonal Dysfunction			
		Androgens	*Corticosteroids*	*Aldosterone*	*Estrogens*
Cushing's syndrome	Bilateral adrenal hyperplasia	+ or N*	+++	N	N or +
	Unilateral adrenal adenoma	– or N	+++	?	?
	Unilateral adrenal carcinoma	+ to +++	+++	?	?
Adrenogenital syndrome	Congenital adrenal hyperplasia				
	Non-salt-losing	+++	– or N	N to +	+
	Salt-losing	+++	–	–	+
	Hypertensive	+++	+++ (Cpd S)	+ (DOC)	+
	Virilizing adrenal tumor	+++	N	N	+
Feminizing tumor	Adrenal tumor	N to +	N	N	+ to +++
Primary hyperaldosteronism	Adrenal tumor	N	N	+ to +++	N

* N = normal levels; – = lower than normal levels; + to +++ = higher than normal levels.

mors arising in tissues other than the pituitary gland can secrete a variety of hypophyseal hormones, including ACTH. In such cases the ectopic ACTH stimulates the adrenal cortex, which becomes hyperplastic. The second cause of Cushing's syndrome is an adrenal tumor, either a benign adenoma or a highly malignant carcinoma.

Among adults, slightly more than half of the cases of Cushing's syndrome are due to increased secretion of pituitary ACTH related to abnormal homeostatic regulation, while the rest of the cases are due about equally to ectopic ACTH, adrenal adenoma, and carcinoma. In infancy and early childhood most of the cases of Cushing's syndrome are due to malignant adrenal tumors. After 8 years of age the frequency of the various etiologic factors is somewhat similar to that found among adults, except for the ectopic ACTH syndrome, which remains rare.

CLINICAL MANIFESTATIONS. The symptoms of Cushing's syndrome due to an adrenal tumor are similar to those due to bilateral adrenal hyperplasia. Most of the symptomatology can be explained on the basis of increased cortisol secretion (Table 18). Cortisol is known to accelerate gluconeogenesis; in this fashion it increases protein catabolism, resulting in a negative nitrogen balance, manifested by a definite retardation of body growth. There is also a marked decrease in muscle mass, with resulting muscular weakness. The increased protein catabolism also may be responsible for the capillary friability and the thinning of the skin, resulting in the formation of ecchymoses and striae, respectively. Another result of the increased gluconeogenesis produced by increased cortisol secretion is abnormality of carbohydrate metabolism. A few patients may have fasting blood glucose levels above the normal range, with intermittent glycosuria. More frequently, a patient will have normal blood glucose concentration but will show a diabetic curve in the glucose tolerance test. Excessive secretion of cortisol also has profound

---

TABLE 18. Symptoms of Cushing's Syndrome Related to Hypersecretion of Cortisol

Increased protein catabolism with negative nitrogen balance
  Muscular weakness
  Retarded growth in children
  Capillary friability and ecchymosis
  Skin friability and purple striae
  Osteoporosis
  Pathologic fractures
Disturbances of carbohydrate metabolism
  Diabetic glucose tolerance curve, glycosuria, and diabetes
Increased fat depot
  Total fat depot
  Trunk fat depot
  Cervical fat pad
  Moonface
  Plethora
Electrolyte disturbance with increased blood volume
  Hypertension
  Weakness
  Peripheral edema
Mental disturbances

---

effects on fat metabolism; it results in the obesity that is characteristic of the syndrome. The obesity is localized specifically in the trunk, particularly the abdomen. Deposition of adipose tissue in the facial area results in the characteristic moon facies. Cortisol also has a marked effect on electrolyte metabolism, promoting sodium retention and potassium loss. Hypertension and increased blood volume often are observed, but hypernatremia with hypokalemic alkalosis is rare. Not only does Cushing's syndrome result in retardation of bone development, but also it produces osteoporosis. In general, patients maintain normal calcium levels but tend to have low phosphorus concentrations. Involution of lymphoid tissue also is due to the increased cortisol secretion; in infants it results in characteristic involution of the thymus. Decreased numbers of circulating lymphocytes and eosinophils and increased numbers of polymorphonuclear neutrophils and erythrocytes are characteristic of Cushing's syndrome. Some patients manifest signs of increased androgen secretion, particularly hirsutism and acne. In addition, a few patients may show some degree of breast development.

LABORATORY DIAGNOSIS. The main abnormality in Cushing's syndrome is increased secretion of cortisol. Adrenocortical tumors which produce this syndrome are ACTH-independent. In contrast, bilateral adrenal hyperplasia is under ACTH control. Therefore the various diagnostic tests of endocrine function should be directed toward proving that the cortisol secretion is increased and that secretion is either dependent or independent of ACTH stimulation. The funcional status of the adrenal cortex can be evaluated with great precision, and the final diagnosis of Cushing's syndrome will rest with the laboratory.

Since approximately one-third of the cortisol secreted appears in urine as 17-OHCS, the measurement of urinary 17-OHCS excretion is helpful for the diagnosis. Normal children and adults have values of 3 ± 1 mg/m^2/24 hours (mean $\pm$ 1 SD), and urinary 17-OHCS excretion greater than 6 mg/m^2/24 hours must be considered as abnormal. In simple obesity, however, values above the upper limit of normal may be obtained in one-fourth of patients. No obese patient has values over 10 mg/m^2/24 hours, but a few with Cushing's syndrome may have values as low as 7 to 10 mg/m^2/24 hours. Subjects with values in this range must be studied carefully by additional tests.

Physical stress (fever, infection, surgery) as well as emotional stress can increase secretion of cortisol and urinary excretion of 17-OHCS. Therefore the urine collection must be made at a time when there is no such stress. Care must be taken to assure completeness of the collection. Finally, certain drugs can invalidate the determination of urinary 17-OHCS concentrations because of their interference with the metabolism of cortisol or with the method of measurement.

Since free urinary cortisol excretion is a reflection of plasma cortisol concentration, and particularly of the unbound fraction, this assay is particularly useful in detecting adrenal hyperactivity. In Cushing's syndrome, whatever its etiology, plasma cortisol levels are elevated, and their diurnal variation tends to be abolished or minimized. However, the use of 8 A.M. and 8 P.M. levels for the purpose of diagnosis may be unreliable because of large fluctuations in concentration in normal subjects and in some patients with Cushing's syndrome. Normal subjects have a cortisol secretion rate of 12 $\pm$ 3 mg/m^2/24 hours (mean $\pm$ 1 SD). Obese subjects have increased cortisol secretion rates; in a group of 31 obese patients 24 had values below 21 mg/m^2/24 hours (mean $\pm$ 3 SD), and 7 had values between 21 and 27 mg/m^2/24 hours. In contrast, 40 patients with Cushing's syndrome had cortisol secretion rates that were not less than 30 mg/m^2/24 hours, except in one case.

Although the technique of the assay for serum ACTH concentration is complicated and usually is not available routinely, a low level of ACTH along with a high cortisol secretion rate is characteristic of an autonomous adrenal tumor. In contrast, inappropriately high ACTH levels will be found in cases of adrenal hyperplasia.

The excretion of urinary 17-ketosteroids (17-KS) is increased moderately to markedly in all patients with Cushing's syndrome, except those with adrenal adenoma, in whom the excretion tends to be decreased or normal. The highest values are in patients with adrenal carcinoma. The 11-oxygenated 17-KS are increased markedly in absolute quantity, as well as in proportion of total urinary 17-KS. The amount of dehydroepiandrosterone also might be increased, but it usually represents a normal percentage of the total neutral steroids.

Tests of ACTH stimulation and dexamethasone suppression are helpful in differentiating primary adrenal tumors from other causes of Cushing's syndrome. When Cushing's syndrome is due to an adrenal carcinoma, the basal cortisol levels are elevated, but they do not change during an intravenous ACTH infusion over 6 hours. In adrenal adenoma and bilateral adrenal hyperplasia there is usually a hyperresponse or, less commonly, a normal response.

In the low-dose dexamethasone suppression test, patients with Cushing's syndrome show minimal or no suppression of urinary 17-OHCS on the third day of suppression. On the third day of high-dose suppression there is still no change in urinary 17-OHCS of patients with adrenal adenoma or carcinoma. In contrast, patients with bilateral adrenal hyperplasia due to abnormal homeostatic regulation show marked decreases of their urinary 17-OHCS.

DIAGNOSIS. The diagnosis of Cushing's syndrome is based on the clinical symptoms of hypercortisolemia and on the laboratory demonstration of an increase in cortisol secretion, either accompanied or not accompanied by an increase in androgen secretion.

When it occurs in infancy or early childhood, the clinical picture of Cushing's syndrome is so characteristic that it can hardly be missed. At that time of life Cushing's syndrome is usually due to malignant carcinoma, and the patients often are seen when metastases have already extended into several organs. Congenital hemihypertrophy of the body has been associated with adrenocortical neoplasms in 6 patients, one of whom had Cushing's syndrome.

Later on in childhood, Cushing's syndrome must be differentiated from obesity. In a few children the symptoms of increased cortisol secretion are minimal, and the main complaint is growth delay. Iatrogenic Cushing's syndrome must also be recognized: inquiries must be made about steroid therapy in children with allergy or eczema; then the problem is to determine the pathogenesis of the syndrome. The tests of ACTH stimulation and dexamethasone suppression will help in determining whether an adrenal tumor is present. It is also desirable to know the location and size of the tumor, as it may help in selecting the surgical approach. On occasion, an x-ray of the abdomen will show calcification of certain areas of the tumor. Tomograms may be helpful in revealing the shadow of the suprarenal mass. A pyelogram may demonstrate a downward displacement of a kidney by a tumor mass. Aortography has been reported to be helpful in outlining adrenal tumors; in certain instances the results can be interpreted easily, but they can also be misleading, particularly on the left side, where a shadow may be due to a spleen or an abnormally located pancreas. Unfortunately, none of these procedures is helpful in diagnosing bilateral adrenal hyperplasia.

TREATMENT. *Adrenal carcinoma* producing Cushing's syndrome is usually very malignant, and the long-range prognosis is poor. However, if the tumor is removed prior to its spread to other organs, cure may be effected in a few cases, and in a few others there may be remission of several years prior to recurrence. In the period that follows surgery, radiation therapy to the general area of the tumor is often given as a preventive measure against recurrence. When metastases are present (often to the lungs and bones), treatment with *o, p'*-DDD may give temporary remission; however, this drug can also produce undesirable side effects, such as nausea and anorexia.

The *adrenal adenoma* offers the best opportunity for a complete cure. After its surgical removal the patient will present with hypoadrenocorticism secondary to suppressed ACTH secretion and should receive glucocorticoid therapy. The mode of steroid withdrawal is shown in Table 16, and follow-up should be similar to that for patients after cessation of glucocorticoid therapy. Usually 6 months post-surgery the subject is entirely normal and the contralateral adrenal gland provides the full steroid requirement.

In *bilateral adrenal hyperplasia* the primary defect is at the level of the hypophysis, whether or not a pituitary tumor is present. Therefore, therapy should be directed toward the pituitary gland. Radiation of the sella turcica can give good remission in adults. Unfortunately, growth hormone-producing cells are rather sensitive to x-rays, and this problem must be considered in growing children. Recently, drugs that modulate the neuroendocrine system such as cyproheptadine (Periactin) have been tried in the treatment of Cushing's syndrome due to bilateral adrenal hyperplasia. Early short-term success will need to be confirmed, but this general therapeutic approach seems very promising. At the present time, total adrenalectomy is preferred, the patients then being treated as individuals with Addison's disease. Under replacement therapy, ACTH and MSH production remain above normal, and patients often have variable degrees of skin hyperpigmentation. In some children pituitary tumors have developed, and the possibility of this distressful complication must be considered when total adrenalectomy is contemplated.

All patients submitted to surgery for either removal of a unilateral tumor or total adrenalectomy should receive the treatment outlined in Table 14 for adrenocortical insufficiency at time of surgery.

Adrenogenital Syndrome

Adrenogenital syndrome is characterized by symptoms of virilism and increased protein anabolism caused by hypersecretion of adrenal androgens. As defined, the syndrome includes virilizing adrenal tumors and congenital adrenal hyperplasia (CAH), particularly the simple virilizing form (partial 21-hydroxylase deficiency), the salt-losing form (complete 21-hydroxylase deficiency), and the hypertensive form (11β-hydroxylase deficiency). The other forms of CAH (deficiencies of 17-hydroxylase, 3β-hydroxysteroid dehydrogenase, and enzyme defects prior to pregnenolone) do not result in symptoms related to increased secretion of androgenic steroids. Since the basic disorder in CAH is a deficiency of one of the enzymes necessary to the biosynthesis of cortisol, its symptoms, diagnosis, and treatment have been discussed in the section on hypoadrenocorticism.

Virilizing adrenal tumors are rare, even though they are the most frequent type of adrenal tumor in children. The fact that the number of cases occurring in girls is twice that reported in boys is probably related to the fact that the clinical manifestations are more obvious in female subjects. Virilizing tumors of the adrenals can develop at any period of life; a few have been reported to occur as early as the first year. However, there are no reports of tumors arising during fetal life and almost none occurring immediately after birth. This is of help in differentiating them from CAH.

PATHOLOGY. When tumors are examined macroscopically, it often is difficult to decide whether one is dealing with a carcinoma or an adenoma. Furthermore, the clinical evolution does not always parallel the pathologic appearance of the tumor. An adrenocortical carcinoma tends to be larger and to have greater vascularization; in advanced cases malignancy is evidenced by local invasion of the kidney or by metastases to the lung, liver, or other organs. These tumors are often heterogeneous, presenting areas of cyst formation, hemorrhage, necrosis, and sometimes calcification.

CLINICAL MANIFESTATIONS. In the female these tumors cause hirsutism and virilization. The appearance of pubic hair is often the first sign. Clitoral enlargement also may attract attention initially. However, in contrast to patients with CAH, those with viriliz-

ing tumors have no labial fusion. Usually no breast development takes place, and the menses do not appear at the usual pubertal age.

Virilizing adrenal tumor in the prepubertal boy produces macrogenitosomia praecox and hirsutism without testicular maturation (Fig. 16). The penis and prostate can be enlarged to adult size, and pubic and axillary hair are present. In almost all patients the testes remain small and immature, contrasting with the obvious signs of virilism. This lack of testicular development is similar to that seen in CAH, but it is in contrast to the gonadal maturation found in isosexual precocious puberty of idiopathic origin. However, it must be noted that in a few patients with virilizing adrenal tumor the testes have been larger than expected for age.

In both girls and boys, muscles are extremely well developed, and there is rapid statural growth with marked advance in osseous maturation. This results in early closure of the epiphyses, and the patient does not achieve full growth. Mental age is usually at the level of chronologic age.

DIAGNOSIS. The diagnosis of virilizing adrenal tumors is made on clinical signs and symptoms, along with markedly increased urinary 17-KS (50 percent or more DHA) that are not suppressed during dexamethasone administration. The tumor is rarely palpable, but

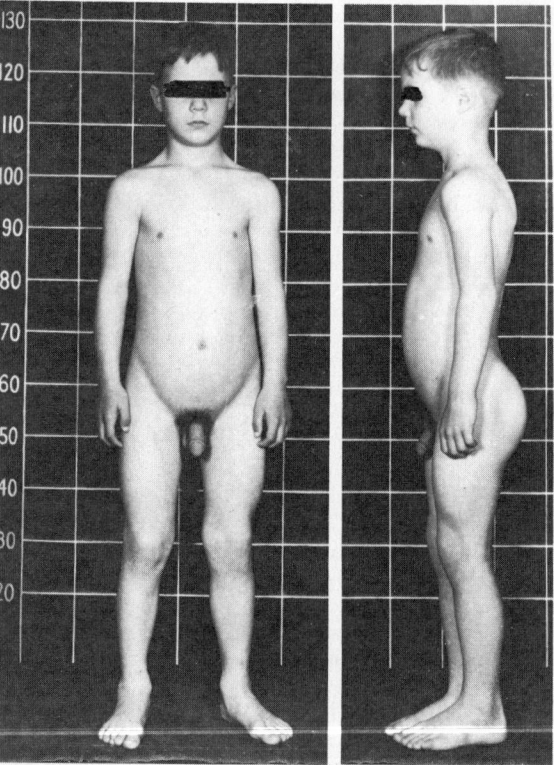

FIG. 16. Virilizing adrenal tumor in a boy 4 years 9 months of age; height age 8 years, bone age 12 years; 17-KS, 106 to 504 mg/24 hours (more than 90 percent as DHA).

often one can find a kidney pushed downward by the adrenal adenoma or carcinoma. The tumor often may be visualized by radiologic examination, particularly when combined with tomography and/or an intravenous pyelogram, and, if necessary, arteriography. In the differential diagnosis, virilization due to androgens of either adrenal or gonadal origin must be considered. In young girls with CAH the labial fusion characteristic of the masculinization of the external genitalia will contrast with the absence of fusion in adrenal tumors. In males, virilism due to CAH may not become evident until some time after birth, and in rare instances not until the age of 3 or 4 years. In both males and females the great excess of urinary pregnanetriol and 17-KS that return to normal levels during a dexamethasone suppression test will help in making the diagnosis.

Certain ovarian tumors (arrhenoblastoma, hilar cell tumors, adrenal-rest tumors) can produce virilizing symptoms. These tumors are very rare in girls prior to puberty; a careful gynecologic examination often reveals their presence. The urinary 17-KS are usually moderately increased.

In boys, a *Leydig cell tumor* of the testis will produce symptoms of masculinization. The testicular tumor and the small size of the contralateral testis will help in making the diagnosis. Urinary 17-KS can be quite elevated and are not suppressed during a dexamethasone test.

A few *hepatomas* have been observed to produce large amounts of an LH-like hormone that activates testicular Leydig cell function; this results in virilization of the patient. An enlarged liver and high gonadotropin titers are characteristic of this condition. Such hepatomas are highly malignant.

Idiopathic sexual precocity in boys is due to early maturation of the hypothalamus–pituitary. The findings of serum gonadotropins and steroid excretion that are normal for a pubertal child will be in contrast with the low gonadotropins and elevated steroid excretion of virilizing adrenal tumors. *Premature pubarche* in boys or girls will also easily be diagnosed on the basis of low gonadotropins, low plasma androgens (except for an increase in DHA sulfate toward adult levels), and low urinary steroid excretion (p. 1722).

In *Cushing's syndrome,* especially when due to an adrenal carcinoma, the excretion of urinary 17-KS can be markedly elevated. In the late stage of development of such tumors, DHA may constitute a large proportion of the androgens. Neither the 17-KS nor the urinary DHA is suppressed in the dexamethasone suppression test. In such patients the clinical symptoms of increased cortisol secretion along with increased excretion of urinary 17-OHCS will help in differentiation from purely virilizing adrenal tumors.

HORMONAL ABNORMALITIES. In almost all patients the total neutral 17-KS in urine are greatly elevated (Table 5), but it must be remembered that there can be extreme variability of levels from day to day. The elevation of the urinary 17-KS is due in great part to a marked increase of DHA, which represents 50 percent or more of the total urinary 17-KS. DHA is excreted mostly as an ester sulfate. In addition, 7- and 16α-hydroxy derivatives of DHA are also excreted in large amounts. Among 21-carbon steroids, great quantities of compounds with a 5–6 double bond (pregnenolone, 17-hydroxypregnenolone, and their derivatives) are found in urinary extracts. The plasma concentration of DHA sulfate (DHAS) in children with virilizing adrenal tumors can be very elevated, reaching values of 1 to 3 mg/100 ml of plasma. Unconjugated DHA also is found in increased concentration; however, it is 1,000 times less than that of its sulfate. The study of simultaneous concentrations of androgens in peripheral and adrenal vein plasma has permitted the conclusion that DHA and DHAS are secreted by adrenal tumors.

In contrast with CAH, virilizing adrenal tumors show no suppression of plasma androgens or urinary 17-KS during a dexamethasone suppression test. Furthermore, ACTH administration has no effect on the steroid output of the tumor, thus demonstrating that secretion by the tumor is not ACTH-dependent. The large secretion of sulfate conjugates could be related to a decreased cholesterol esterase activity. Patients with virilizing tumors and normal subjects metabolize DHA differently, a much larger amount of DHAS being excreted in the urine of the patients. In patients with virilizing adrenal tumors the urinary excretion of cortisol metabolites is normal, despite the marked increase in DHAS. In rare cases a slight elevation of urinary 17-OHCS has been reported, due mainly to the tetrahydro derivatives of compound S. Children with virilizing adrenal tumors have never shown any abnormality of serum electrolytes, and aldosterone secretion has been reported to be normal in the few cases in which it was determined.

TREATMENT. The tumor should be excised carefully without cutting the capsule. When metastases are present, efforts should be made to remove them as completely as possible, since this may prolong the patient's life; when they are widespread and cannot be removed surgically, radiotherapy and chemotherapy should be used. There is no consensus as to the effectiveness of radiotherapy, but in view of the fact that adrenal tumors with metastases are extremely malignant, it seems justified to use this treatment. Chemotherapy (aminoglutethimide, *o,p'*-DDD) can also be attempted.

Virilizing adrenal tumors do not produce excessive amounts of cortisol. For this reason the contralateral gland secretes cortisol normally; therefore it seems unnecessary to administer glucocorticoids prior to, during, and after ablation of such tumors. However, it is probably safer to do so.

Whereas adrenal carcinoma, which produces Cushing's syndrome, has a great tendency to recur and metastasize, tumors that produce pure virilism generally grow more slowly, have less tendency to recur, and often have a very good prognosis.

After surgery, patients should be checked frequently by thorough clinical examination and steroid determinations. A reappearance of symptoms or increased urinary 17-KS will suggest local recurrence.

Feminizing Adrenal Tumors

Feminizing adrenal tumors are very rare; probably no more than a dozen cases have been reported in children. They may be a variant of virilizing adrenal tumors.

PATHOLOGY. These feminizing tumors can be either adenomas or carcinomas, but their general appearance and their histology are similar to those of the virilizing tumors. The fact that many patients have survived many years following surgery would suggest that the tumors, if malignant, usually are not markedly so.

CLINICAL MANIFESTATIONS. In addition to the gynecomastia, which will bring male patients to medical attention, there is rapid growth, and height and bone age are markedly advanced. The penis and testes are normal in size for age, while pubic hair may or may not be present. Because some of these tumors produce not only estrogens but also androgens, the prostate may be somewhat enlarged for a prepubertal child. Feminizing tumors in girls result in manifestations similar to those found in isosexual precocious puberty, including enlargement of breast, appearance of pubic hair, estrogenization of the labia minora and of the vaginal smear, vaginal bleeding, and advanced bone age and height age (Fig. 17). In some patients there is a concomitant increase in androgen secretion, which results in slight enlargement of the clitoris as well as increased muscular development.

DIAGNOSIS. The diagnosis of feminizing adrenal tumors in children often can be difficult, particularly in girls. The finding of increased urinary estrogen excretion along with increased urinary excretion of 17-KS

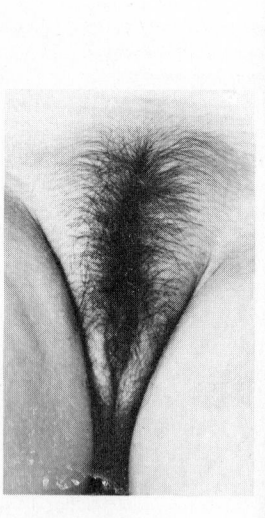
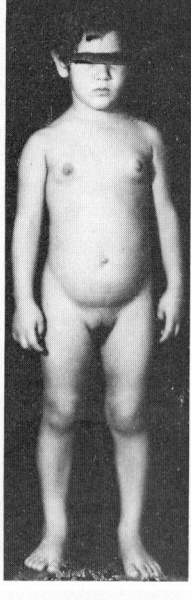

FIG. 17. Feminizing and masculinizing adrenal tumor in a girl. Labia and vagina are feminized; pubic hair is present, but there is no clitoral enlargement. There was an encapsulated right adrenal tumor. Age 3 years 3 months; height age 4 years; bone age 6 years; 17-KS, 21 to 30 mg/24 hours.

and DHA that does not respond to a dexamethasone suppression test is the key to the diagnosis. In girls, premature thelarche (early breast development without menstruation or pubic hair) and idiopathic isosexual precocity must be ruled out, although the fact that these two conditions occur much more frequently than feminizing adrenal tumors should not result in failure to recognize a tumor. Elevated excretion of 17-KS and low levels of gonadotropins favor the presence of adrenal tumor, while normal pubertal excretion of 17-KS and elevation of LH level, as observed at the time of adolescence, suggest idiopathic sexual precocity. In premature thelarche both 17-KS and LH levels are low. In boys the differential diagnosis is mainly that of gynecomastia. Transient gynecomastia of moderate degree often occurs physiologically at the time of puberty. Since puberty is accompanied by a certain increase in excretion of urinary 17-KS and sometimes urinary estrogens, the differentiation from feminizing tumors, which present with only moderately increased steroid excretion, can be very difficult. In contrast to boys undergoing pubertal development, whether at the proper age or precociously, patients with feminizing adrenal tumors have no testicular enlargement. A normal suppression of urinary 17-KS during a suppression test also helps to rule out an adrenal tumor. Gynecomastia may appear following administration of certain drugs (reserpine, meprobamate, digitalis) or inadvertent ingestion of estrogen-containing products. A diligent search for a history of ingestion of such compounds will help in making this differential diagnosis. Gynecomastia can occur in patients with malnutrition or liver disease, but these disorders usually can be diagnosed easily. It also has been reported occasionally in patients with diabetes or thyrotoxicosis; again, the clinical manifestations of these endocrinopathies usually are obvious. Feminizing adrenal tumors that develop in boys after puberty result in decreased testicular size and libido, in addition to gynecomastia. The hypogonadism with the gynecomastia of Klinefelter's syndrome is accompanied by increased gonadotropin levels.

HORMONAL ABNORMALITIES. Whether determined by bioassay or chemical techniques, urinary estrogens are elevated in all patients, as compared with norms for age and sex. However, in most patients the values are not greatly different from those expected in adult women, including the relative amounts of estrone, estradiol, and estriol. Although the main characteristic of feminizing adrenal tumors is an increase in excretion of estrogen production, there is also in most patients an increase in androgen secretion. The increase in urinary 17-KS may be marked (Table 5). In some patients DHA represents more than 50 percent of the total 17-KS excreted, and there is no decrease of DHA in urinary 17-KS during a dexamethasone suppression test. In children with feminizing adrenal tumors the urinary excretion of 17-OHCS is normal, and so is their aldosterone secretion. Although in most patients the urinary excretion of pregnanetriol is normal, there is often a slight to moderate elevation in pregnanediol excretion.

TREATMENT. The tumor should be removed as soon as the diagnosis is established. Pure feminizing tumors, like virilizing adrenal tumors, do not significantly alter cortisol secretion; however, it might be safer to protect the patient from acute adrenal crisis by glucocorticoid administration during surgery. The rare tumors that occur in children are less malignant than those observed in adults; most of the patients survive surgery by more than 5 years.

Hyperaldosteronism

In 1955 Conn described a syndrome of arterial hypertension, polyuria resistant to antidiuretic hormone, and muscle weakness with hypokalemic alkalosis. The syndrome was termed primary aldosteronism and was found to be due to an adrenal tumor secreting excessive amounts of aldosterone. The syndrome is encountered more frequently in females and is a disorder of adulthood, since fewer than 10 affected children have been reported. Prior to 1955, and before the structure of aldosterone was known, it had been established that syndromes in which edema was present resulted in increased urinary excretion of salt-retaining hormone. It is now understood that blood volume is one of the factors that control aldosterone secretion; when intravascular volume is decreased because of edema or ascites, secondary hyperaldosteronism develops. Other disorders involving hyperaldosteronism are the Bartter syndrome and dexamethasone-suppressible hyperaldosteronism.

BARTTER SYNDROME. The Bartter syndrome is characterized by hypertrophy of the juxtaglomerular apparatus of the kidneys, increased plasma renin activity, increased aldosterone secretion with hypokalemic alkalosis, and impairment of urinary concentrating ability. However, the blood pressure is persistently normal. Another important feature of the syndrome is growth failure. The pathophysiology of the syndrome is based on unresponsiveness of the arteries to the vasoconstrictive property of renin, resulting in a decrease in the effective blood volume and a compensatory increase in renin secretion with secondary hyperaldosteronism. Elevated renin levels would not produce hypertension because of the arterial unresponsiveness, while elevated aldosterone levels would result in hypokalemia, the electrolyte imbalance being itself the cause of the failure to grow normally. However, a primary abnormality of the juxtaglomerular apparatus has also been suggested.

PRIMARY HYPERALDOSTERONISM. The clinical picture of the syndrome of primary hyperaldosteronism can be related entirely to the hyperaldosteronism. One of the main features is increased blood pressure, both diastolic and systolic, related to an increase in blood volume, which itself is due to the hypernatremia. Despite the hypertension, there are usually only minimal eye signs, and peripheral edema is exceptional. The second important manifestation is hypokalemia, which results in marked muscle weakness with various types of paresthesias and sometimes unusual types of periodic paralysis. The chronic hypokalemia also may be responsible for the nocturnal polyuria and the resulting polydipsia. Persistent frontal headaches also are frequent. The patients usually have normal cortisol secretion and no other steroid abnormalities. The increased aldosterone secretion results in low renin levels.

The clinical diagnosis is based on the hypertension, the low serum potassium, and the polyuria that fails to respond to antidiuretic hormone. Patients on a normal sodium diet have high aldosterone secretion and low renin levels. A high-sodium diet or administration of DOCA will fail to suppress the increased aldosterone secretion. The main diagnostic problem is to differentiate primary hyperaldosteronism from secondary hyperaldosteronism. An increase in plasma renin activity, with resulting increased aldosterone secretion, is a physiologic mechanism for the maintenance of serum electrolyte concentrations and extracellular fluid volume. It will occur in conditions resulting in sodium loss, potassium retention, or decrease in blood volume. Sodium loss occurs with administration of diuretics. There is also sodium loss during diarrhea or excessive sweating. Sodium-losing nephritis and renal tubular acidosis can result in sodium loss. During edema (nephrosis, congestive heart failure) or ascites (cirrhosis of the liver) there is a decrease in blood volume, which will result in elevated aldosterone secretion; blood loss has a similar effect. Secondary hyperaldosteronism can be found in patients with malignant hypertension, hypertension due to unilateral renal disease, and sometimes with essential benign hypertension. In all these conditions hyperaldosteronism is accompanied by elevated plasma renin activity and angiotensin levels. This contrasts with the low activity observed in primary hyperaldosteronism.

Tumors that produce primary hyperaldosteronism are not malignant, and their surgical removal will in most cases cure the hypertension. The main exception is, of course provided by the patients in whom permanent renal damage is present. Because aldosterone-secreting adenomas are small in size, they cannot be visualized prior to surgery; therefore a bilateral exploration is necessary. Since these patients have normal cortisol–ACTH homeostatic regulation, there is no need for cortisol therapy during or after surgery. It must be noted that some patients have done well for a period of time when treated with a low-sodium diet and/or spironolactone. A certain number of patients with primary hyperaldosteronism have been reported to present with bilateral adrenal hyperplasia. It is possible that these patients had a syndrome similar to that reported by Sutherland and associates and by other investigators in which the hypertension and increased aldosterone secretion were relieved by dexamethasone administration.

References

ADRENAL CORTEX

Beitins IZ, Bayard F, Ances IG, Kowarski A, Migeon CJ: The metabolic clearance rate, blood production, interconversion and transplacental passage of cortisol and cortisone in pregnancy near term. Pediatr Res 7:509, 1973

Christy NP (ed): The Human Adrenal Cortex. New York, Harper & Row, 1971

Dorfman RI (ed): Steroid Hormones. Amsterdam, North Holland, 1975

Johannisson E: The foetal adrenal cortex in the human. Its ultrastructure at different stages of development and in different functional states. Acta Endocrinol [Suppl 130] 1968

Gardner LI: Endocrine and Genetic Diseases of Childhood, 2nd ed. Philadelphia, WB Saunders, 1975

Liddle GW, Melmon KL: The Adrenals. In Williams RH (ed): Textbook of Endocrinology, 5th ed. Philadelphia, WB Saunders, 1974

Migeon CJ: Cortisol production and metabolism in the neonate. J Pediatr 55:280, 1959

Villee DB: The development of steroidogenesis. Am J Med 53:533, 1972

Visser HKA: The adrenal cortex in childhood. 1. Physiological aspects. 2. Pathological aspects. Arch Dis Child 41:113, 1966

Wilkins L: The Diagnosis and Treatment of Endocrine Disorders in Childhood and Adolescence, 3rd ed. Springfield, Ill, Charles C Thomas, 1965

HYPOADRENOCORTICISM

Baulieu EE, Peillon F, Migeon CJ: Adrenogenital Syndrome. In Eisenstein AB (ed): The Adrenal Cortex. Boston, Little, Brown, 1967

Biglieri EG, Herron MA, Brust N: 17-Hydroxylation deficiency in man. J Clin Invest 45:1946, 1966

Black J, Williams DI: Natural history of adrenal hemorrhage in the newborn. Arch Dis Child 48:183, 1973

Blizzard RM, Albert M: Hypopituitarism, hypoadrenalism and hypogonadism in the newborn infant. J Pediatr 48:782, 1956

Bongiovanni AM: Disorders of adrenocortical steroid biogenesis (the adrenogenital syndrome associated with congenital adrenal hyperplasia). In Stanbury JB, Wyngaarden JB, Fredrickson DS (eds): The Metabolic Basis of Inherited Disease, 3rd ed. New York, McGraw-Hill, 1972

——— Root AW: The adrenogenital syndrome. N Engl J Med 268:1283, 1342, 1391, 1963

——— The adrenogenital syndrome with deficiency of 3β-hydroxysteroid Dehydrogenase. J Clin Invest 41:2086, 1962

Burton BK, Nadler HL: Schilder's disease: abnormal cholesterol retention and accumulation in cultivated fibroblasts. Pediatr Res 8:170, 1974

Camacho AM, Kowarski A, Migeon CJ, Brough AJ: Congenital adrenal hyperplasia due to a deficiency of one of the enzymes involved in the biosynthesis of pregnenolone. J Clin Endocrinol Metab 28:153, 1968

Cheek DB, Perry JW: A salt wasting syndrome in infancy. Arch Dis Child 33:252, 1958

Childs B, Grumbach MM, Van Wyk JJ: Virilizing adrenal hyperplasia: a genetic and hormonal study. J Clin Invest 35:213, 1956

Crocker AC, Vawter GF, Neuhauser EBO, Rosowsky A: Wolman's disease: three new patients with recently described lipidosis. Pediatrics 35:627, 1965

David R, Golan S, and Drucker W: Familial aldosterone deficiency: enzyme defect, diagnosis and clinical course. Pediatrics 41:403, 1968

Degenhart HJ, Visser HKA, Boon H, O'Doherty NJ: Evidence for deficient 20α-cholesterol-hydroxylase activity in adrenal tissue of a patient with lipoid adrenal hyperplasia. Acta Endocrinol 71:512, 1972

Grumbach MM, Van Wyk JJ: Disorders of sex differentiation. In Williams RH (ed): Textbook of Endocrinology, 5th ed. Philadelphia, WB Saunders, 1974, p 423

Kelch RP, Kaplan SL, Biglieri EG, Daniels GH, Epstein CJ, Grumbach MM: Hereditary adrenocortical unresponsiveness to adrenocorticotropic hormone. J Pediatr 81:726, 1972

Kenny FM, Preeyasombat C, Spaulding JS, Migeon CJ: Cortisol production rate. IV. Infants born of steroid-treated mothers and of diabetic mothers: infants with trisomy syndrome and with anencephaly. Pediatrics 37:960, 1966

Kowarski A, Finkelstein JW, Spaulding JS, Holman GH, Migeon CJ: Aldosterone secretion rate in congenital adrenal hyperplasia. J Clin Invest 44:1505, 1965

Lanman JT: Adrenal steroids in meningococcemia. J Pediatr 46:724, 1955

Lee PL, Plotnick LP, Kowarski A, Migeon CJ (eds): Treatment of Congenital Adrenal Hyperplasia: A Quarter of a Century Later, Baltimore, University Park Press, 1976

Loras B, Baour F, Bertrand J: Exchangeable sodium and aldosterone secretion in children with congenital adrenal hyperplasia due to 21-hydroxylase deficiency. Pediatr Res 4:145, 1970

Migeon CJ, Kenny FM, Hung W, Voorhess ML: Study of adrenal function in children with meningitis. Pediatrics 40:163, 1967

——— Kenny FM, Kowarski A, et al: The syndrome of adrenocortical unresponsiveness to ACTH. Report of six cases, Pediatr Res 2:501, 1968

New M, Peterson RE: Aldosterone in childhood. Adv Pediatr 15:111, 1968

Postel-Vinay MC, Alberti GM, Ricour C, Limal JM, Rappaport R, Royer P: Pseudohypoaldosteronism: persistence of hyperaldosteronism and evidence for renal tubular and intestinal responsiveness to endogenous aldosterone. J Clin Endocrinol Metab 39:1038, 1974

Raine DN, Roy J: A salt-losing syndrome in infancy. Arch Dis Child 37:548, 1962

Ulick S, Gantier E, Vetter KK, Markello JR, Yaffe S, Lowe CV: An aldosterone biosynthesis defect in a salt-losing disorder. J Clin Endocrinol Metab 24:669, 1964

Visser HKA, Cost WS: A new hereditary defect in the biosynthesis of aldosterone: urinary C_{21}-corticosteroid pattern in three related patients with a salt losing syndrome, suggesting an 18-oxidation defect, Acta Endocrinol 47:589, 1964

Wilkins L, Gardner LI, Crigler JF Jr, Silverman SH, Migeon CJ: The control of hypertension with cortisone, with a discussion of variations in the type of congenital adrenal hyperplasia and report of a case with probable defect of carbohydrate regulating hormones. J Clin Endocrinol Metab 12:1015, 1952

——— The Diagnosis and Treatment of Endocrine Disorders in Childhood and Adolescence, 3rd ed. Springfield, Ill, Charles C Thomas, 1965.

CUSHING'S SYNDROME

Bergenstal DM, Hertz R, Lipsett MB, Moy RH: Chemotherapy of adrenocortical cancer with o,p'-DDD. Ann Intern Med 53:672, 1960

Cushing H: The basophil adenomas of the pituitary body and their clinical manifestations (pituitary basophilism). Bull Johns Hopkins Hosp 50:137, 1932

Liddle GW: Tests of pituitary-adrenal suppressibility in the diagnosis of Cushing's syndrome. J Clin Endocrinol Metab 20:1539, 1960

——— Givens JR, Nicholson WE, Island DP: The ectopic ACTH syndrome. Cancer Res 25:1057, 1965

Lindsay AE, Migeon CJ, Nugent CA, Brown H: The diagnostic value of plasma and urinary 17-hydroxycorticosteroid determinations in Cushing's syndrome. Am J Med 20:15, 1956

Migeon CJ, Green OC, Eckert JP: Study of adrenocortical function in obesity. Metabolism 12:718, 1963

Nelson DH, Meakin JW, Thorn GW: ACTH-producing pituitary tumors following adrenalectomy for Cushing's syndrome. Ann Intern Med 52:560, 1960

Nugent CA, Nichols T, Tyler FH: Diagnosis of Cushing's syndrome: single dose dexamethasone suppression test. Arch Intern Med 116:172, 1965

Wilkins L: Adrenal disorders. I. Cushing's syndrome and its puzzles. Arch Dis Child 37:1, 1962

VIRILIZING ADRENAL TUMORS

Allen WM, Hayward SJ, Pinto A: A color test for dehydroisoandrosterone and closely related steroids of use in the diagnosis of adrenocortical tumors. J Clin Endocrinol Metab 10:54, 1950

Fraumeni JE, Miller RW: Adrenocortical neoplasms with hemihypertrophy, brain tumors, and other disorders. J Pediatr 70:129, 1967

Goldstein AE, Rubin SW, Askin JA: Carcinoma of adrenal cortex with adrenogenital syndrome in children: complete review of the literature and report of a case with recovery in a child eight months of age. Am J Dis Child 72:563, 1946

Lipsett MB, Wilson H: Adrenocortical cancer: steroid biosynthesis and metabolism evaluated by urinary metabolites. J Clin Endocrinol Metab 22:906, 1962

Loras B, Migeon CJ: Metabolism of 7-^{3}H-dehydroisoandrosterone in patients with virilizing adrenal tumors. Steroids 7:459, 1966

Saez JM, Rivarola MA, Migeon CJ: Studies of androgens in patients with adrenocortical tumors. J Clin Endocrinol Metab 27:615, 1967

Wilkins L, Ravitch MM: Adrenocortical tumor arising in the liver of a three-year-old boy with signs of virilism and Cushing's syndrome: report of a case with cure after partial resection of the right lobe of the liver. Pediatrics 9:671, 1952

FEMINIZING ADRENAL TUMORS

Fontaine R, Sacrez R, Klein M, et al: Puberte precoce avec developpement des seins chez un garçon porteur d'une tumeur de la surrenale. Arch Fr Pediatr 11:417, 1954

Gabrilove JL, Sharma DC, Wotiz HH, Dorfman RI: Feminizing adrenocortical tumors in the male: a review of 52 cases including a case report. Medicine 44:37, 1965

Mosier HD, Goodwin WE: Feminizing adrenal adenoma in a seven year old boy. Pediatrics 27:1016, 1961

Snaith AH: A case of feminizing adrenal tumor in a girl. J Clin Endocrinol Metab 18:318, 1958

Wilkins L: A feminizing adrenal tumor causing gynecomastia in a boy of five years contrasted with a virilizing tumor in a five-year-old girl: classification of seventy cases of adrenal tumor in children according to their hormonal manifestations and a review of eleven cases of feminizing adrenal tumor in adults. J Clin Endocrinol Metab 8:111, 1948

PRIMARY HYPERALDOSTERONISM

Bartter FC, Pronove P, Gillo JR, MacCardle RC: Hyperplasia of the juxtaglomerular complex with hyperaldosteronism and hypokalemic alkalosis. Am J Med 33:811, 1962

Biglieri EG, Slaton PE Jr, Kronfield SJ, Schambelan M: Diagnosis of an aldosterone-producing adenoma in primary aldosteronism: an evaluative maneuver. JAMA 201:510, 1967

Conn JW, Rovner DR, Cohen EL: Normal and altered function of the renin-angiotensin-aldosterone system in man: application in clinical and research medicine. Ann Intern Med 63:266, 1965

Davis WW, Newcome HH Jr, Wright LD, Hammond WG, Easton J, Bartter FC: Bilateral adrenal hyperplasia as a cause of primary aldosteronism with hypertension, hypokalemia and suppressed renin activity. Am J Med 42:642, 1967

Grim CE, McBryde AC, Glenn JF, Gunnells JC Jr: Childhood primary aldosteronism with bilateral adrenocortical hyperplasia: plasma renin activity as an aid to diagnosis. J Pediatr 71:377, 1967

Kelch RP, Connors MH, Kaplan SL, Biglieri EG, Grumbach MM: A calcified aldosterone-producing tumor in a hypertensive, normokalemic, prepubertal girl. J Pediatr 83:432, 1973

Sutherland DJA, Ruse JL, Laidlaw JC: Hypertension, increased aldosterone secretion, and low plasma renin activity relieved by dexamethasone. Can Med Assoc J 95:1109, 1966

ADRENAL STEROID THERAPY

ALFRED M. BONGIOVANNI

Great therapeutic advances in the management of adrenocortical insufficiency were made following the isolation, characterization, and synthesis of the natural steroids. Currently, steroids usually are used in amounts far exceeding the endogenous secretion of the adrenal gland under any circumstances, and they are used for conditions other than primary insufficiency. The therapeutic objectives are often associated with the recognized antiinflammatory action of excessive amounts of the hormones.

Cortisol (compound F, hydrocortisone) may be regarded as the principal secretory product of the adrenal cortex. When administered alone, it is able to satisfy most of the requirements for survival in the face of adrenal insufficiency. It is the major compound for controlling pituitary–adrenal homeostatic regulation. The mechanisms that regulate secretion and release of adrenocorticotropin (ACTH) are sensitive to the concentration of circulating cortisol and do not seem to respond to mineralocorticoids, androgens, or estrogens of adrenal origin. Cortisol and its many natural and synthetic analogues possess the antiinflammatory and related pharmacologic properties that have found such extensive application in pediatric practice.

Normally the adrenal cortex secretes approximately 12 mg of cortisol per square meter of body surface per day. This quantity is the replacement dose of exogenous cortisol required for normal maintenance in the absence of adrenocortical function; for pharmacologic action a far greater amount is required.

The favorable responses of many disorders to the administration of pharmacologic amounts of corticosteroids may be related to their antiinflammatory action, although in most instances the rationale is not clear. Thus the use of steroids is to be regarded as empirical, since the basic causes of the diseases that respond are not removed or altered, although the clinical manifestations may be controlled. With treatment, it is hoped that the inciting factor will become exhausted and that in due course the steroid therapy can be discontinued without return of clinical disease; this is not common. Sometimes the etiologic agent is recognized, and steroids are used to prevent certain undesirable sequelae of specific therapy. For example, in tuberculous meningitis, steroids may be given concurrently with antituberculous drugs to minimize damage to the central nervous system resulting from inflammation.

Many diseases of childhood respond favorably to steroids; however, steroids should not be the first choice for therapy in all conditions known to respond (eg, in treatment of hypoglycemia, steroids are being supplanted by diazoxide). Table 19 lists some conditions in childhood for which steroids have been used with temporary or lasting success.

ACTIONS. The glucocorticoids increase the rate of synthesis of hepatic enzymes involved in carbohydrate and amino acid metabolism. These are compounds resembling cortisol, with a Δ^4 ketone group, a 17 side chain, and 17- and 11-hydroxyl groups. Their effects are most notable after administration of glucocorticoids in vivo. Among the enzymes of carbohydrate metabolism that are increased are glucose-6-phosphatase, fructose-1,6-diphosphatase, phosphoenolpyruvate carboxykinase, and pyruvate carboxylase. The

TABLE 19. Some Conditions Treated With Pharmacologic Doses of Glucocorticoids

Aregenerative anemia	Lupus erythematosus
Asthma	Nephrotic syndrome
Atopic dermatitis	Renal transplant rejection
Cerebral edema	Rheumatic fever with carditis
Diffuse pulmonary fibrosis	Rheumatoid arthritis
Prevention of hyaline membrane disease (prenatal therapy)	Septic shock
Hypercalcemia	Serum sickness, anaphylaxis
Infections (tuberculosis, typhoid, meningococcemia, viral*)	Stevens-Johnson syndrome
Leukemia	Thrombocytopenic purpura
	Ulcerative colitis
	Uveitis, iritis, keratitis

Under special circumstances and with appropriate antibiotics when available.

enzymes concerned with amino acid metabolism that increase are tryptophan pyrrolase and various transaminases, including tyrosine, alanine, glutamate-pyruvate, threonine dehydrase, and serine dehydrase. Certain of the latter enzymes, by causing diversion of the amino acid pool from other peripheral tissues, may partly account for the so-called catabolic effects in muscle and bone, as well as increased alkaline phosphatase in human leukocytes and HeLa cells in tissue culture. The glucocorticoids induce precocious development of intestinal alkaline phosphatase, invertase, and retinal glutamine synthetase in embryos of several species; they also stabilize lysozymes against various labilizing agents such as vitamin A and ultraviolet irradiation, possibly through some action on the lipid of lysosomal membranes. The prevention of the rupture of these membranes avoids the release of acid hydrolases contained within the organelle that not only digest cell contents but further perpetuate inflammatory response by attacking extracellular protein. This theory would explain, in part, the etiology of some collagen diseases wherein the denaturation of the native constituents of the injured cells and surrounding tissue is thought to provoke an injurious autoimmune response.

Although there are several other explanations for the antiinflammatory action of corticoids, there is as yet no unified concept. It could be that suppression of the inflammatory response by steroids is nonspecific. Inhibition of response has been noted against a wide variety of injuries that have no clear common basis. The effect is apparently local and requires an adequate concentration of steroid in the vicinity of the injured cells. Furthermore, steroids inhibit the increased permeability of the endothelium and the exudation of cells that normally characterize inflammation, so that local tissue reaction and swelling are minimized. Fibroblastic activity and thus localization and scarring are blocked.

Actions other than the antiinflammatory effects, such as induction of hepatic enzymes and cytolysis of small lymphocytes (T cells) and thymocytes, are now understood somewhat better. These tissues contain specific cytoplasmic receptors for glucocorticoids; these receptors are necessary for the action of the steroid in these cells. The cytoplasmic receptor–steroid complex is in some manner activated (allosteric transformation) and then transported as a unit to a nuclear receptor site. This is believed to be a portion of chromatin that is active in the transcription of specified events. In the lymphocyte the consequences are diminution of glucose and amino acid transport into the cell, glucose phosphorylation, and thymidine incorporation. Leukemic lymphoblasts, which contain the cytoplasmic receptors, are susceptible to cytolysis in response to steroids, whereas resistant cells no longer contain the receptors. In hepatocytes a similar sequence of events induces the synthesis of those enzymes indicated above. Steroids seem to induce anomalous hydroxylation of

TABLE 20. Effects of Large Doses of Adrenocortical Steroids

Clinical Manifestations	Basic Mechanisms
Hyperglycemia ("diabetes") and hyperamino-acidemia	↑Hepatic gluconeogenic enzymes and amino acid transferases ↑Gluconeogenesis Insulin resistance Hyperglucagonemia
Growth failure, osteoporosis, muscle wasting	↓Amino acid incorporation into protein ↓Growth hormone (variable) ↓Somatomedin synthesis ↓Entrance of glucose into cells
Hypertension, hypernatremia, hypokalemia	Variable Na retention and K loss ↑Epinephrine sensitivity (dose-dependent)
Fat redistribution, buffalo obesity, hyperlipidemia	Extremities: ↓glucose into fat cells, ↓lipogenesis Truncal fat: ↑lipogenesis
Osteomalacia, hypocalcemia	Antagonizes vitamin D metabolism, ↓calcium absorption
Impaired resistance to infection, inflammation	↓Vascular permeability, ↓white cell function, stabilizes lysozymes
Secondary adrenocortical insufficiency	Suppresses hypothalamus and pituitary
Peptic ulcer	↑Gastric HCl and pepsin, mucus
↓Delayed hypersensitivity and allograft rejection	↓Lymphocytes (T cells) and eosinophils
Miscellaneous effects not well understood: euphoria, benign intracranial hypertension, thromboembolism	

vitamin D into an inactive metabolite, with resultant relative vitamin D deficiency.

Some of the basic actions of steroids and their related clinical effects are listed in Table 20. Certain fundamental mechanisms produce the antiinflammatory and other desirable results; however, many of the consequences are unwelcome. Some of the newer synthetic steroids mitigate certain of these unwanted effects, but it has not been possible to eliminate toxic effects completely. Salt and water retention is less marked and is even reversed with some synthetic analogues; however, even with cortisol this activity has not been very marked or consistent. Under some circumstances (eg, nephrosis) cortisol or cortisone will produce diuresis despite some mineralocorticoid activity. Throughout the period of intensive treatment with large doses, diminished incorporation of amino acids into protein (except in the liver) and occasional suppression of growth hormone can lead to virtual growth arrest in the child. Gluconeogenesis, as well as diminished peripheral utilization of glucose, produces variable degrees of hyperglycemia and glycosuria. Sometimes this may be the expression of latent diabetes. The diminished inflammatory reactions, which are desirable for control of many diseases, also can be a disadvantage, since intercurrent infections may overwhelm the child if they go unrecognized or if they are not susceptible to available antibiotics. Further, peptic ulcer, an uncommon complication of steroid treatment in childhood, may not be recognized.

DRUGS AND DOSAGE. Many natural and synthetic glucocorticoids are available, some with very potent antiinflammatory activity, which usually parallels their gluconeogenic action. Variations in potency depend not only on the basic biologic activity but also on the rate of disposition. The details of several widely used drugs are shown in Table 21. The unnatural compounds are less susceptible to those hepatic enzymes that reduce and conjugate the natural compounds, so that their duration of action is longer, as shown by the plasma half-life. Their frequency of administration may thus be less than that of cortisol. Although the biologic half-life is based on hypothalamic–pituitary suppression, this also often corresponds to the duration of antiinflammatory activity. While cortisol at 12 mg/m²/day (or equivalent amounts of other steroids) is the physiologic quantity normally secreted, some 10-fold greater amounts are needed for the initiation of treatment in most disorders. This should be reduced to the minimal effective dose within as short a time as possible and should be discontinued as quickly as possible. Dosages will vary with the disease, its severity, and individual response, but treatment is often a matter of trial and error. Recommendations are found in the discussion of specific diseases elsewhere in this text.

Adrenocorticotropin (ACTH) is rarely used now. It stimulates the adrenal cortex to produce a variety of steroids, some of which are undesirable and are more likely to induce sodium retention and potassium loss. The newer synthetic steroids avoid these effects. In some quarters, however, ACTH is favored on the basis that the concomitant secretion of adrenal androgens is of benefit in promoting growth; this is not well proven. Its main usefulness is diagnostic, for the assessment of adrenocortical function.

Steroids have been widely used in the treatment of a

TABLE 21. Relative Potencies of Glucocorticoids*

Compound	Anti-inflammatory	Na-Retaining	Plasma Half-Life (min)	Biologic Half-Life (hr)	Forms
Cortisol (hydrocortisone)	1	1	90	8	Oral: 10-, 20-mg tablets; 10 mg/ml suspension (ester) IM: 5, 50 mg/ml Local: 1%, 2.5% ointment IV: phosphate and hemisuccinate
Cortisone acetate	0.8	0.8	90	8	Oral: 5-, 25-mg tablets IM: 25, 50 mg/ml
Prednisone and prednisolone (1-ene cortisone, 1-ene cortisol)	4.0	0.8	200	12–36	Oral: 1-, 2.5, 5.0-mg tablets IM: 25 mg/ml (prednisolone acetate) IV: prednisolone phosphate Local: several forms
Triamcinolone (9α-fluoro-16α-hydroxyprednisolone)	5.0	0	200+	12–36	Oral: 1-, 2-, 4-, 16-mg tablets; syrup (diacetate) 5 mg/5 ml IM: 25 mg/ml (diacetate) Local: various
Dexamethasone (9α-fluoro-16α-methylprednisolone)	25	0	300+	36–54	Oral: 0.5-, 0.75-mg tablets; 0.5 mg/5 ml elixir IM: 4 mg/ml (also for IV)
9α-Fluorocortisol	15	125	?	?	Oral: 0.1-mg tablets, used only as mineralocorticoid Local: various

* Potencies as compared to cortisol. Biological half-life based on duration of hypothalamic–pituitary suppression.

variety of infections. In the few well-controlled studies there has been little evidence that such treatment exerts any direct benefit. In the opinion of some, the indications are the following: to control the severe constitutional symptoms of infection, as in typhoid and some viral diseases; to suppress acute and chronic inflammation in order to minimize damage to vital tissues; for cardiovascular effects, ie, increased cardiac output and diminished peripheral resistance and shock. The reputed advantage of megadoses in the treatment of gram-negative sepsis remains controversial. However there is evidence of benefit in tuberculous meningitis, mumps orchitis, and pericarditis, as well as in the prevention of postherpetic neuralgia. Some infections are worsened by steroids; these include staphylococcal infection, tuberculosis, varicella, herpes zoster and simplex, variola, and cytomegalovirus infections, candidiasis, cryptococcosis, and pneumocystis infection. The hazards, however, appear to be minimal if steroids are given in short courses of a few days and if appropriate antibiotics also are used against the etiologic agent.

Steroids may adversely affect infections by the following means: suppression of inflammatory and localizing processes, suppression of delayed hypersensitivity, suppression of intracellular mechanisms for disposal of ingested foreign material by phagocytes, suppression of the ability of the reticuloendothelial system to clear the bloodstream of foreign particles, diminished interferon synthesis, interference with fibroplastic proliferation and healing, and suppression of antibody formation (rarely observed except on prolonged huge dosages).

There is rapid absorption of steroids after oral administration, with a peak blood level occurring within 30 minutes. Following intramuscular administration the rate of absorption is very slow and variable; blood levels may be sustained for 2 to 4 days, depending on the form of steroid and the dosage. Oral doses are larger than parenteral doses because oral administration leads to inactivation of some portion of the dose by the liver and because of the rapid absorption and excretion. The intramuscular route has been favored by those who believe that sustained, moderately elevated levels are more effective than the variable high peaks that occur with oral treatment. However, recent evidence indicates that sporadic high levels are equally effective and are attended by fewer side effects.

At present there is a tendency to administer the daily dosage by mouth only once a day on alternate days, or even every 3 to 4 days. Under these circumstances the dosage must be determined by trial and error. Generally the amount necessary is not less than a full dose for a single day; if given on alternate days, more may be necessary. Significant adrenocortical suppression does not seem to occur with this type of administration. Intravenous preparations of steroids should be used for acute emergencies only, and only temporarily; depending on the dose, the blood level may remain significantly elevated up to 24 hours. If the indications for steroid administration are clear, it is well to administer the calculated dose intramuscularly as well as intravenously; thus the steroid level will remain sustained following depletion of the intravenous drug.

PRECAUTIONS. The clinical consequences of the steroid hormones administered in large quantities are listed in Table 20. Some of these are unavoidable, such as the redistribution of fat that produces the buffalo type of obesity and the moonface (Fig. 18). In assessing the effects of treatment in patients with diseases that require pharmacologic doses, the absence of some manifestations of Cushing's syndrome would suggest inadequate treatment. Even these signs may be minimized by intermittent treatment. With the newer steroids, the action on water and mineral metabolism, which is rarely marked even with cortisol, is virtually absent (Table 21). It is unnecessary to restrict sodium during treatment, especially in the presence of disease accompanied by anorexia. It is difficult enough to feed the child without reducing the palatability of the diet. Hypertension occurs rarely, unless the disease itself is associated with an elevated blood pressure, in which case it may rise further. Additional potassium is rarely required, particularly when the appetite is good and the intake of food is adequate.

The risk of disguised infection at the start of therapy or acquired infection thereafter cannot be exaggerated. Intercurrent infections are often masked, and a high index of suspicion must be maintained at all times. In areas where tuberculosis is prevalent, or in children from groups known to be susceptible to tuberculosis, it is advisable to rule out its presence by the tuberculin test and/or chest radiography. The presence of infection does not contraindicate the use of steroids where the basic disease is serious and is known to be responsive. However, appropriate and adequate antimicrobial therapy should be administered simultaneously. Although the routine use of broad-spectrum antibiotics is not advised throughout the period of steroid therapy, suitable antibiotics should be given on the smallest provocation. Exposure to some infectious diseases for which there are no effective antibiotics (eg, chickenpox) is cause for concern. At such times it is a good rule to reduce the dosage of steroids to approximately three times the physiologic replacement dose. This amount is adequate for the stress of possible superimposed infection and more than enough to prevent adrenal crisis,

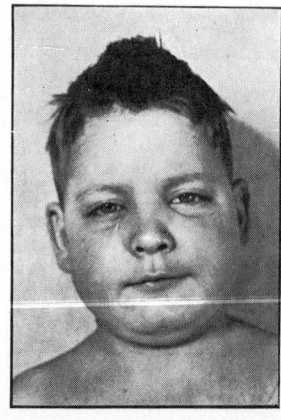

FIG. 18. Moonface following treatment of rheumatic fever with ACTH.

but not so great as to arrest the natural defenses. After the infection subsides, higher doses may be resumed.

Glycosuria and moderate hyperglycemia do not necessarily denote true diabetes mellitus, and they are not occasions to discontinue therapy. In true diabetes mellitus there is a retarded elevation in serum pyruvate and lactate following glucose ingestion, which may be corrected by insulin. This is not the case in normal subjects treated with glucocorticoids, although blood levels of citrate and α-ketoglutarate remain unchanged and suggest an inhibition of pyruvate utilization. If the basis for steroid therapy is sound, treatment should be continued; if true diabetes mellitus is present, adequate doses of insulin should be added to the regimen. For reasons detailed previously, it may be advisable to administer a modestly increased amount of vitamin D unless hypercalcemia is present initially.

The most troublesome problem in children undergoing chronic treatment with steroid hormones is growth arrest. Following cessation, after continuous treatment for up to 2 years, there will be resumption of growth at a rapid pace to compensate for the temporary arrest. If treatment has to be continued for many years, growth failure and arrest of osseous maturation can become relatively severe. Large doses of human growth hormone administered throughout the period of treatment may overcome the growth retardation, but this hormone is not available in sufficient supply to meet the demand. Concomitant administration of anabolic-androgenic hormones may restore growth and maturation, but further investigation is required before definite recommendations can be made. The use of anabolic steroids would also prevent osteoporosis and cessation of osseous maturational advancement. As noted previously, intermittent administration of steroids seems to produce less growth arrest.

Among the other complications of steroid therapy with large doses are proximal muscle wasting, euphoria, ocular hypertension with glaucoma, posterior subcapsular cataracts, osteoporosis, aseptic bone necrosis due to fat emboli, diminished radioactive iodine uptake by the thyroid (as well as thyroxine and thyroxine-binding globulin), increased renal excretion of iodine, pancreatitis, and nodular panniculitis (after discontinuation or dosage reduction). Benign intracranial hypertension (pseudotumor cerebri) (p. 1819) is sometimes a complication of treatment, especially during the period of dosage reduction in childhood, but in other circumstances it is a useful agent in reducing or preventing cerebral edema after trauma or surgery.

CONTRAINDICATIONS. There are few contraindications in life-threatening or crippling diseases that are known to respond to steroid therapy. While concurrent diseases, such as infection or peptic ulcer, may require direct treatment, they will not necessarily contraindicate the use of steroid hormones. However, under such circumstances steroid therapy may be deferred. The complications of steroid therapy prohibit their use in trivial disorders or in conditions shown to respond to other more innocuous measures. Their use in serious illness, in which they are known to be ineffective, should be resisted.

WITHDRAWAL. Continuous administration of steroid hormones, in amounts equivalent to or greater than the normal production rate, leads to suppression of ACTH secretion and to temporary adrenal atrophy and unresponsiveness. After this, recovery of adrenal function is gradual and is related to the duration of steroid therapy. When used only for several days, even large doses do not lead to significant suppression of adrenocortical function, except under most unusual circumstances.

Abrupt withdrawal following short courses of treatment is usually without consequence. If treatment with large doses has been continued for more than 2 weeks, there is some risk of adrenocortical insufficiency following abrupt withdrawal; therefore the steroids should be reduced gradually in order to permit restoration of adrenocortical function, which may not begin until the dosage falls below the physiologic level. The initial withdrawal can proceed by large (25 percent) reductions in dosage every 5 to 6 days until the physiologic amount is reached. Then it is well to substitute cortisol or cortisone in equivalent dosage if more potent steroids were used at the start. With these compounds it is easier to reduce dosage by small gradations, since they are natural substances, and they will be more effective in preventing adrenal insufficiency. Thereafter, reduction should be continued by 25 percent each week until the steroid is completely withdrawn. More rapid withdrawal is permissible only if the child is in the hospital and under constant surveillance. The use of ACTH to restore adrenocortical function during withdrawal is not recommended.

During withdrawal of steroids the child must be watched for signs of adrenocortical insufficiency or recurrence of the disease for which they were given. Rarely, disturbances may occur that resemble or are identical with collagen diseases, even though the initial disturbance was not in this category. Lupus-like states and arteritis also have been described, and muscle pain and weakness are common. It is sometimes difficult to distinguish the effects of withdrawal from those of the original condition. If either becomes prominent, it may be necessary to raise the dosage moderately and proceed with reduction at a slower pace.

References

Baxter JD, Forsham PH: Tissue effects of glucocorticoids. Am J Med 53:573, 1972

Dale DC, Petersdorf RG: Steroids in infectious disease. Med Clin North Am 57:1277, 1973

Dluhy RG, Lauler DP, Thorn GW: Pharmacology and chemistry of adrenal glucocorticoids. Med Clin North Am 57:1155, 1973

Melby JC: Systemic corticosteroid therapy: pharmacology and endocrinologic consideration. Ann Intern Med 81:505, 1974

ADRENAL MEDULLA AND SYMPATHETIC NERVOUS TISSUE
Mary L. Voorhess

The adrenal medulla and the sympathetic nerves and ganglia are derived from neural crest ectoderm. Some crest cells migrate from the neural tube and differentiate to become neuroblasts, which in turn give rise to ganglion cells. Aggregations of these cells form sympathetic ganglia, which then become linked to make sympathetic trunks. Other crest cells are transformed into chromaffin cells. These move to the anlage of the adrenal cortex, penetrate its substance, and eventually comprise the adrenal medulla. Chromaffin cells also are found in the para-aortic region. Their largest mass is in the organ of Zuckerkandl adjacent to the origin of the inferior mesenteric artery. These extraadrenal chromaffin tissues exert an adrenergic effect during fetal life and infancy. Subsequently that function is assumed by the chromaffin cells of the adrenal medulla. Rarely, ectopic rests of neural crest tissue are found in other sites in the chest and abdomen.

CATECHOLAMINES

SYNTHESIS.   Catecholamine synthesis takes place within the sympathetic nerve endings, in the chromaffin tissue, and in brain and other sites where neural crest tissue is found. The main physiologic pathway for formation of the catecholamines is via dopamine, norepinephrine, and epinephrine (Fig. 19). The conversion of tyrosine (obtained from the circulation) to dopa takes place in the cytoplasm of the adrenergic cell. It is the rate-limiting step, so that inhibition of tyrosine hydroxylase results in decreased production of catecholamines. Synthesis of dopamine from dopa also occurs in the cytoplasm, where large amounts of dopa decarboxylase are found. Then the dopamine must be transported

actively into granules within the cytoplasm of adrenal medullary cells and in sympathetic nerve endings. The enzyme dopamine β-hydroxylase then transforms dopamine to norepinephrine. Part of the newly formed norepinephrine remains stored in the granules, and the rest is discharged into the cytoplasm of the adrenergic cell. Catecholamine synthesis terminates at this step, except in the adrenal medulla and selected other tissues. There the enzyme phenylethanolamine-N-methyl transferase (PNMT) is present to N-methylate the norepinephrine to epinephrine. This enzyme appears to be dependent on adrenal glucocorticoids for its activity. Thus there is an intimate relationship between medulla and cortex within the adrenal gland.

The control of synthesis depends primarily on nervous and chemical stimuli that influence the rate of turnover of catecholamines. When the concentration of cytoplasmic norepinephrine falls, the feedback inhibition of tyrosine hydroxylase is reduced and synthesis increases. Compounds such as α-methyltyrosine, which inhibit tyrosine hydroxylase, decrease the rate of synthesis.

Dopamine constitutes about 50 percent of the catecholamine content of sympathetic nervous tissue; the remainder is norepinephrine. Epinephrine is present in insignificant amount because methyl transferase is present in very small quantities. However, epinephrine accounts for 60 to 80 percent of the catecholamines in the adrenal medulla, the rest being norepinephrine. Small amounts of norepinephrine and epinephrine are secreted continuously, but most is released in pulses in response to specific stimuli. Circulating epinephrine

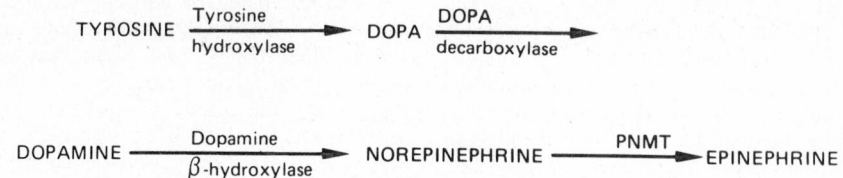

FIG. 19.   Primary physiologic pathway for catecholamine synthesis; PNMT, phenylethanolamine-N-methyl-transferase.

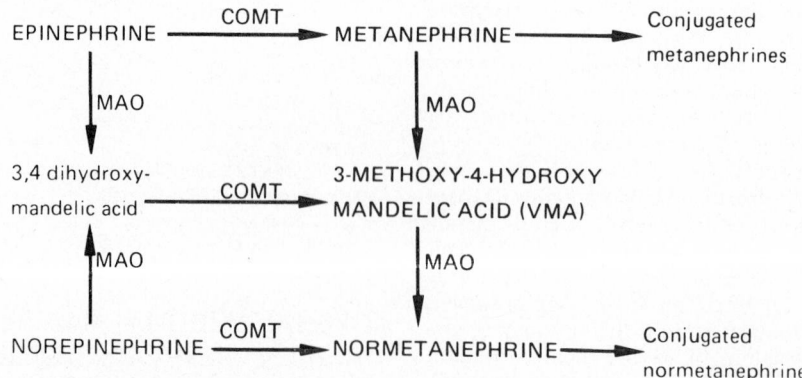

FIG. 20.   Major pathway for metabolism of circulating norepinephrine and epinephrine. COMT, catechol-o-methyl transferase; MAO, monoamine oxidase.

comes almost solely from the adrenal medulla, whereas sympathetic nerve endings are the major source of norepinephrine in blood.

INACTIVATION. Cytoplasmic granules play a role in the synthesis of catecholamines, but the uptake and storage of norepinephrine and epinephrine within granules of the sympathetic nervous tissue and the adrenal medulla also are important mechanisms in biologic inactivation. Each compound is stored separately in granules with adenine nucleotide (mostly ATP), protein, lipid, and water and is released on signal into the circulation, mainly by exocytosis. The discharge of catecholamine can be selective, so that epinephrine may be released without concomitant release of norepinephrine or vice versa. After the compound has acted on the effector site, it is metabolized by plasma enzymes and then excreted unchanged in the urine or taken up across the neuronal membrane into the storage granule.

The major pathway for the metabolism of circulating norepinephrine and epinephrine in man is demonstrated in Figure 20. The enzyme catechol-*o*-methyl transferase plays the principal role by *o*-methylating both medullary hormones; monoamine oxidase is less important. The biologically inactive compounds metanephrine, normetanephrine, and 3-methoxy-4-hydroxymandelic acid (VMA) are clinically important end products. Similar enzyme systems are involved in degradation of dopamine to its primary metabolite, homovanillic acid (HVA).

ASSAY OF CATECHOLAMINES AND METABOLITES. Measurement of plasma catecholamine levels is difficult, and most procedures require 10 to 20 ml of plasma per sample, so that determinations have limited application in clinical pediatrics. When the sensitive and specific double-isotope dilution method is used, resting catecholamine concentrations of 0.12 to 0.52 μg/liter are found in healthy humans. Patients with pheochromocytomas may have an increase of 10-fold or more.

Quantitation of catecholamines and metabolites in urine is performed by many clinical laboratories. A number of analytic methods having varying sensitivity and specificity are used; so results must be interpreted carefully based on the normal range of each particular laboratory. It is important to remember that the daily output of the compounds increases with age (Table 22). Because there is a diurnal pattern to catecholamine excretion and because creatinine output often varies from day to day, analysis of 24-hour urine specimens is preferable. However, expression of VMA, normetanephrine and metanephrine, and HVA excretions in terms of micrograms of metabolite per milligram of creatinine can be used to differentiate normal children from those with tumors of neural crest origin.

PHYSIOLOGICAL EFFECTS. The biologic activities of norepinephrine and epinephrine are thought to result from chemical interaction between the amine and a specific receptor site within the target organ that leads to a change in the intracellular concentration of cyclic AMP. Two types of hypothetical catecholamine receptors (α and β) have been postulated. In general, activation of α receptors is excitatory, and activation of β receptors is inhibitory. However, there are exceptions: stimulation of α receptors in the gut relaxes the muscle, and stimulation of β receptors in the myocardium is excitatory. Norepinephrine is the most potent excitatory catecholamine and has low activity as an inhibitor; epinephrine is relatively potent as both an excitor and an inhibitor of smooth muscle. Endogenous epinephrine is an important hormone in metabolic processes, but it has little effect on cardiovascular reactions except in severe stress.

Norepinephrine stimulates α receptors and evokes generalized constriction of arterioles and venules, which results in a rise in systolic and diastolic blood pressure and reflex bradycardia. Epinephrine affects both α- and β-adrenergic responses. It increases heart rate, cardiac conduction rate, and ventricular contractility, relaxes bronchial musculature, promotes glycoge-

TABLE 22. Daily Urinary Excretion of Catecholamines and VMA at Various Ages*

Age	Dopamine (μg/24 hours)	Norepinephrine (μg/24 hours)	Epinephrine (μg/24 hours)	VMA (μg/24 hours)
Birth to 1 year				
Range	17.7–99	5.4–15.9	0.1–4.3	169–1,350
Mean	60.9	10.6	1.3	569
SD	± 24.3	± 3.4	± 1.2	± 309
1–5 years				
Range	48.3–217.2	8.1–30.8	0.8–9.1	465–2,200
Mean	124.1	18.8	3.2	1348
SD	± 40.7	± 7.0	± 2.7	± 443
6–15 years				
Range	79.9–364.7	19.0–71.1	1.3–10.5	1,050–3,740
Mean	169.3	37.4	4.8	2373
SD	± 72.6	± 16.6	± 2.4	± 698
Over 15 years				
Range	170.9–377.0	34.4–87.0	3.5–13.2	2,050–4,250
Mean	249.1	50.7	7.1	3192
SD	± 74.9	± 15.7	± 3.3	± 669

* *From Voorhess: Pediatrics 39:252, 1967.*

nolysis in liver and skeletal muscle with subsequent increase in blood sugar, stimulates glucagon secretion, inhibits insulin secretion to further raise blood glucose, and acts on adipose tissue to produce release of free fatty acids. Despite these important actions of norepinephrine and epinephrine, the adrenal medulla is not necessary for life. There is no evidence of adrenal medullary insufficiency after total bilateral adrenalectomy.

Knowledge is expanding rapidly concerning the importance of dopamine in the physiologic functioning of the peripheral nervous system. Specific dopamine receptors have been identified, and the amine is known to be widely distributed throughout the body. It appears to play a role in the regulation of the renin–angiotensin system, as well as in postural adaptation mechanisms. It increases renal blood flow and glomerular filtration rate, induces sodium diuresis, and is important in the control of gastrointestinal motility. Indeed, dopamine is more than just a precursor of norepinephrine and epinephrine in the sympathoadrenal system.

DISEASES

In the pediatric age group the most commonly described abnormalities of the adrenal medulla and sympathetic nervous tissue are neoplasms, ie, pheochromocytoma, neuroblastoma, and ganglioneuroma. These tumors are usually associated with increased urinary excretion of catecholamines or their metabolites or both. Their measurement in urine is an important aid in diagnosis and in follow-up care of children with neoplasms of neural crest origin. Abnormalities of catecholamine excretion have also been found in such disorders as familial autonomic dysfunction, idiopathic hypoglycemia, and malignant melanoma.

Neuroblastoma

Neuroblastoma is a common malignant neoplasm of infancy and childhood that develops from the immature and undifferentiated neuroblasts of neural crest ectoderm. It can be found wherever sympathetic nervous tissue is located, but most often it arises from the left or right adrenal gland or along the sympathetic chain in the abdomen or chest. The tumor metastasizes early to lymph nodes, liver, bone marrow, and skeleton. In about 66 percent of cases, widespread disease is present at the time of diagnosis. Sometimes, before a primary lesion is evident, retro-orbital, skin, or skeletal metastases herald its presence.

Neuroblastoma is a disorder of early life, and it may appear at any time from birth to 6 years of age, with a peak incidence before 3 years of age. Initial diagnosis in late childhood is rare; at that time it is associated with a poor prognosis. Neuroblastoma occurs in about 1 in 10,000 live births, with a slight preponderance in males. Familial cases have been reported, but the mode of inheritance is not clear.

Grossly, a neuroblastoma may be smooth and rounded or nodular. When extensive hemorrhage and necrosis occur, it is cystic and red to violet in color. The tumor is generally soft and friable. Although encapsulated early, it soon invades surrounding tissue; metastases may be so extensive that the primary site cannot be identified. Microscopically the neuroblastoma is composed of sheets of small cells, with deeply staining nuclei and sparse cytoplasm. The cells contain many mitotic figures, and often there is blood vessel invasion; in some areas the cells form rosettes.

Neuroblastoma has the highest spontaneous regression rate of any malignancy in man, which suggests a host immune defense against the tumor. Patterns of organ involvement (such as liver metastases) that usually are associated with fatal outcome in other malignant diseases do not have such a grave prognosis in neuroblastoma. There has been lymphocyte-mediated inhibition of neuroblastoma cells and serum-mediated blocking of lymphocyte cytotoxicity. Further, a positive relationship exists between lymphocytic infiltration of neuroblastoma and survival, and increased lymphoblasts may be observed in the bone marrow of patients whose ages and tumor stagings are correlated with good prognosis. In addition to spontaneous regression, neuroblastomas have the ability to differentiate and mature into ganglioneuroblastomas, ganglioneuromas, and even neurofibromas. The mechanisms responsible for this phenomenon are not known, but patients with more mature tumors have a better survival rate.

CLINICAL FEATURES.   The most frequent presenting complaint is an abdominal mass that often is found on routine examination. Sometimes the neuroblastoma appears to fill the retroperitoneal cavity, particularly with sudden enlargement following blunt trauma to the abdomen and extensive hemorrhage into the tumor. Occasionally the first indication of disease will be metastatic lesions that cause unilateral periorbital swelling, with ecchymosis and proptosis, a cervical mass, or subcutaneous nodules. In early stages the patient will have little systemic evidence of malignancy, but in advanced cases irritability, anorexia, weight loss, fever, bone pain, and anemia will be prominent features. There can be paresis of the lower extremities when a tumor arises from dorsal root ganglia or extends intraspinally from the retroperitoneal space and compresses the spinal cord. Some children have hypertension; rarely, a child may have paroxysmal attacks of flushing, pallor, tachycardia, and perspiration similar to those seen in someone who harbors a pheochromocytoma. An unexplained association has been reported between acute cerebellar ataxia, opsoclonia, atactic conjugate movements of the eyes, and occult neuroblastoma.

DIAGNOSIS.   When neuroblastoma arises from the adrenal medulla, an intravenous pyelogram will show lateral and downward displacement of the ipsilateral kidney, with preservation of the normal caliceal pattern. A tumor originating from the paravertebral sympathetic ganglia will often displace the ureter laterally (Fig. 21). Extension of disease along the paravertebral spaces into the thorax, or the presence of tumor in the posterior mediastinum, usually can be identified on

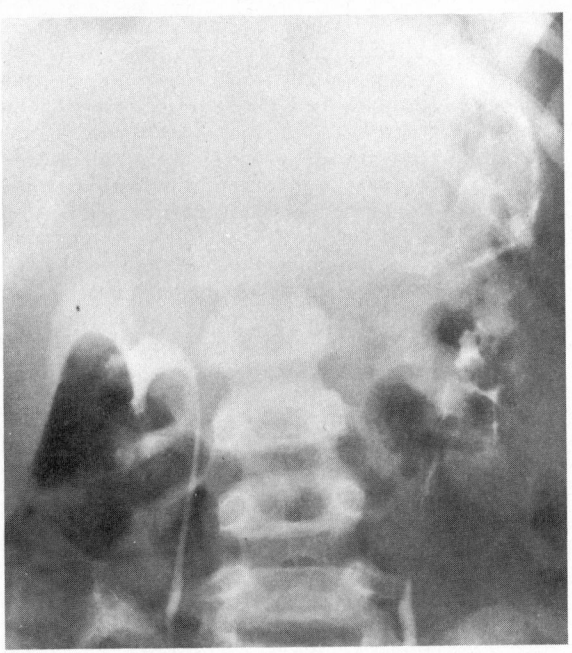

FIG. 21. Intravenous pyelogram showing lateral displacement of left kidney by a large calcified suprarenal mass. (Courtesy of Dr. A. Berne.)

chest radiographs. Flecks of calcium may be visible within tumors of neural crest origin, but their absence has no diagnostic significance. Myelography should be performed promptly whenever there is paresis of the extremities, loss of bladder control, or other evidence suggesting encroachment of tumor on the spinal cord. Emergency decompression is necessary to prevent permanent nerve damage. The physician should look for neoplastic cells in bone marrow aspirate when skeletal survey (including skull and long bones) fails to reveal evidence of osseous metastases. Bone, liver, and brain scans also are important in delineating the extent of disease. In selected cases, angiography of the inferior vena cava and aorta and pedal lymphangiography may be indicated. Since the extent of disease is important in staging of the tumor, choosing the method of therapy, and determining the prognosis, detailed radiologic and isotope studies of patients usually are indicated.

Measurement of urinary excretion of catecholamines and their metabolites is the most specific aid to preoperative diagnosis. Abnormally high levels of dopamine, HVA, norepinephrine, normetanephrine, VMA, and other metabolites are found in the urine of most patients. The pattern varies in different individuals, but determination of output of HVA and VMA is sufficient for diagnosis in most cases. Many laboratories are unable to perform quantitative analyses of these compounds; thus screening tests for urinary VMA excretion have been developed. However, it is important to understand their limitations. A negative screening test does not rule out the presence of neuroblastoma, because 15 to 20 percent of children with this tumor

have normal urinary excretion of VMA. Furthermore, false-positive tests, intermediate reactions, and false-negative tests have been reported. The screening procedures have their greatest value in follow-up care of patients with neuroblastoma whose quantitative VMA levels are high prior to therapy. Definitive diagnosis depends on histologic identification of the tumor tissue.

DIFFERENTIAL DIAGNOSIS. Wilms' tumor, Ewing's tumor, lymphoma, sarcoma, and leukemic infiltrate of bone can mimic neuroblastoma. However, patients with these malignancies do not excrete abnormally large amounts of catecholamines and metabolites in their urine. Both pheochromocytoma and neuroblastoma are capable of synthesizing catecholamines, but the clinical manifestations of these two disorders usually permit the physician to differentiate one from the other. Most patients with neuroblastoma excrete dopamine, norepinephrine, and their metabolites, while those with pheochromocytoma excrete norepinephrine, epinephrine, and their metabolites. Much larger quantities are excreted by patients with pheochromocytoma.

STAGING. The clinical course of neuroblastoma depends in part on the pattern of organ involvement. The following staging was developed to assist in evaluating the efficacy of treatment regimens and in estimating the prognosis:

Stage I. Stage I tumors are confined to the organ or structure of origin.

Stage II. Stage II tumors extend beyond the organ or structure of origin but do not cross the midline. Regional lymph nodes on the ipsilateral side may be involved.

Stage III. Stage III tumors extend beyond the midline; regional lymph nodes may be involved bilaterally.

Stage IV. Stage IV features remote disease involving the skeleton, parenchymatous organs, soft tissue, and distant lymph node groups.

Stage IV-S. Stage IV-S includes patients who would otherwise be stage I or II, but who have remote disease confined to liver, spleen, or bone marrow and who have no radiographic evidence of bone metastases on complete skeletal survey.

TREATMENT. Surgery, radiation therapy, and chemotherapy are used in various combinations to treat patients with neuroblastoma. The treatment of choice is surgical removal of localized tumor. Most patients, however, have metastatic spread at the time of diagnosis, which makes total excision impossible. Some surgeons excise as much neoplasm as possible and use postoperative radiation to the tumor site for control of local disease. Incomplete removal of primary neuroblastoma does not jeopardize survival, as it does in Wilms' tumor. Other workers stage the disease, biopsy the tumor, and await results of combination radiation therapy and chemotherapy before considering surgical removal. Dramatic shrinkage of tumor often occurs, since the neuroblastoma is remarkably sensitive to radiation therapy and chemotherapy. The cobalt 60 unit is preferred for irradiation, and doses of 2,500 to 3,000 rads in 3 to 4 weeks usually are effective.

Treatment with a variety of chemotherapeutic drugs used alone or in combination usually results in subjective and objective evidence of response. The two best agents continue to be cyclophosphamide and vincristine. These two drugs have different mechanisms of action and different toxic manifestations, so that an additive tumor effect can be obtained without increasing the risk of therapy. The primary toxicity of cyclophosphamide is bone marrow depression and cystitis. Vincristine sulfate causes neuromuscular side effects.

There is lack of agreement about the value of chemotherapy in patients with localized disease who can be treated by surgery and radiation therapy. Some physicians refrain from chemotherapy in such cases. Others prescribe cyclophosphamide, hoping to control any potential metastases that might develop following release of malignant cells into the blood or the lymphatic system. In these cases a suitable regimen is cyclophosphamide 10 mg/kg/day orally for 7 to 10 days every month for 1 year. Patients with bone marrow involvement and disseminated disease should be given chemotherapeutic agents. Even though treatment usually leads to little improvement in overall survival, it is helpful in palliation of disease. The outcome is similar whether the drugs are used concurrently, sequentially, or on an alternate-week basis. One regimen consists of vincristine 1.5 mg/m^2/2 weeks intravenously, alternating at weekly intervals with cyclophosphamide 300 mg/m^2/2 weeks orally or intravenously. This course of therapy lasts at least 12 weeks. Another schedule consists of cyclophosphamide 10 mg/kg/5 days intravenously and vincristine 0.05 mg/kg intravenously on days 1, 14, and 21. This course is repeated every 28 days as long as there is a therapeutic response. When other drugs fail, daunomycin, adriamycin, actinomycin D, and corticosterone have been used. Before beginning treatment, current medical literature should be consulted for recommendations regarding chemotherapeutic programs. Careful attention must be given to drug dosage, duration of therapy, and natural history of the disease, because the immune response of a patient with neuroblastoma appears to play a role in recovery, and most chemotherapeutic agents depress the immune response. Overtreatment should be avoided.

PROGNOSIS AND FOLLOW-UP. There has been little change in overall survival despite vigorous efforts over the past 15 years. The younger the patient the more favorable the outlook. The expectation of cure is best in patients less than 1 year of age whose diseases are stage I, II, or IV-S. A 2-year survival rate of 92 percent in infants less than 12 months of age with stage I and II disease and a 90 percent survival rate in those with stage IV-S have been reported. Survival of children with widespread disease who are more than 2 years of age at diagnosis is very low (3 percent). Patients with tumors arising from thoracic and pelvic ganglia have a much better prognosis than those with neuroblastoma of the adrenal medulla. Girls seem to fare better than boys. The overall survival rate in most series is about 30 to 35 percent. The child usually can be regarded as cured if there is no disease 2 years after treatment has been completed; unfortunately, some patients may have a recurrence after an interval of 8 to 10 years.

Serial determinations of urinary excretion of catecholamines and their metabolites are helpful in monitoring the response to therapy and should be an integral part of care. Response to therapy is accompanied by a decrease in excretion to normal rates; the presence of residual tumor or recurrence of disease is indicated by abnormally high levels of the various compounds. Serial measurements of VMA output may be used to follow those patients who had abnormally high excretion of the compound before treatment was started. However, it is a less sensitive indicator of tumor function than analysis of levels of dopamine, HVA, or norepinephrine.

Long-term complications of radiation therapy may develop in survivors. Radiation nephritis, bone growth abnormalities, and secondary bone tumors may become manifest many years later. The gonads of young infant girls who receive radiation therapy to the pelvis must be protected to prevent future disturbances in sexual maturation.

Ganglioneuroblastoma

Neuroblastomas have the capacity to mature and differentiate into ganglioneuroblastomas. These are tumors composed of neuroblasts and mature ganglion cells. The etiology of this maturation phenomenon is unknown; it appears to occur predominantly in neuroblastomas of extraadrenal sites and in a higher proportion of girls than boys. Usually the tumor is quite well encapsulated, so that surgical resection is possible. The cure rate of children with ganglioneuroblastoma is much higher than for those with neuroblastoma. Those tumors comprised primarily of mature ganglion cells with few neuroblasts are associated with a better prognosis. If maturation is related to host immune defenses, it is important that pathologists carefully search for ganglion cells in the tumor tissue. If they are present, treatment should be planned carefully in order to prevent depression of immune mechanisms. In most cases, surgical excision, without subsequent radiation therapy or chemotherapy, is sufficient. Ganglioneuroblastoma cannot be differentiated from neuroblastoma by biochemical analysis. Patients with either tumor have an abnormally high urinary output of catecholamines and metabolites. Measurements of these compounds before and after treatment are helpful not only for diagnosis but also for following the response to therapy.

Ganglioneuroma

Current knowledge suggests that a ganglioneuroma is a neuroblastoma that has undergone complete differentiation into a benign neoplasm composed of mature ganglion cells. It is a well-encapsulated tumor that is usually found along the sympathetic chain in the posterior mediastinum or the abdomen. Surgical excision is the treatment of choice. The author has not found a pure ganglioneuroma associated with abnormally high urinary catecholamine excretion, except when accompanied by the syndrome of chronic diarrhea.

Syndrome of Diarrhea and Neural Tumor

Chronic diarrhea with failure to thrive, malar flush, skin rash, persistent cough, abdominal distension, and hypokalemia may occur in association with tumors of neural crest origin. Bowel movements are generally foul-smelling, frequent, and watery and do not respond to medical therapy. Symptoms usually begin at 8 to 24 months of age and continue relentlessly until the tumor is removed surgically; then the diarrhea ceases. Ganglioneuroblastoma and ganglioneuroma are much more commonly associated with this syndrome than is neuroblastoma. The output of catecholamines and metabolites is abnormally high before the tumor is removed; then it falls to normal with successful therapy. The etiology of the diarrhea is not known, but there is a definite relationship between watery stools and tumor; it has been suggested that the tumor secretes a factor that may be similar to vasoactive intestinal peptide (VIP). It is of interest that the diarrhea does not always reappear with recurrence of tumor. When total excision of the tumor is not possible, adrenocorticosteroid therapy has been effective in controlling the diarrhea.

FAMILIAL NEUROBLASTOMA, GANGLIONEUROBLASTOMA, AND GANGLIONEUROMA. Neuroblastomas appear to occur in two forms: hereditary and nonhereditary. Several families have been described wherein more than one individual has had a tumor of neural crest origin. Close relatives of affected children should be examined for evidence of neurocutaneous syndromes, hypertension, neurofibromatosis, and other findings suggestive of nervous system dysfunction. When an abnormality is discovered, determinations should be made of urinary excretion of catecholamines and metabolites in search of an occult tumor.

Pheochromocytoma

The pheochromocytoma most commonly arises from chromaffin cells of the adrenal medulla, but it may be found throughout the body wherever chromaffin tissue is located. In both children and adults the tumor involves the right adrenal medulla more often than the left. However, in children, many more tumors are bilateral or multiple. They may vary in size from tiny nodules to the size of large lemons. It is difficult to determine by histologic criteria whether pheochromocytomas are malignant or benign. The cells of innocent tumors often look malignant and invade veins, but most tumors are benign. There is a 3:2 preponderance in the male, and often there is familial transmission as an autosomal dominant trait. The onset of symptoms may begin as early as a few weeks of age, but most cases have been diagnosed between 6 and 14 years of age. The tumor may be present in association with such neurocutaneous syndromes as neurofibromatosis and Lindau-von Hippel disease. Medullary carcinoma of the thyroid and pheochromocytoma (Sipple syndrome)

have been reported in several families (p. 1690), and recently parathyroid adenomas or hyperplasia have been associated with the disorder. The tumor also has been found in patients with Cushing's syndrome.

SYMPTOMS AND SIGNS. The symptoms are caused by the large amounts of circulating norepinephrine and epinephrine that are produced by the tumor. Hypertension is present in all cases of functioning pheochromocytoma, and it is more often sustained than paroxysmal in children. The systolic blood pressure may reach levels over 250 mm Hg, with a corresponding increase in diastolic pressure. Cardiac enlargement and hypertensive retinopathy may be found in long-standing cases. Headache, tachycardia, profuse sweating, nausea and vomiting, and visual disturbances are frequently present. The child often has an anxious expression and appears pale and weak; he may complain of palpitations and abdominal pain. Sometimes these findings occur in paroxysmal attacks that take place from several times daily to once every month or so. Rarely, abdominal massage over the periadrenal area will provoke an attack by causing liberation of catecholamines from the tumor. Polydipsia and polyuria occur more commonly in children than in adults. Weight gain may be poor; sometimes growth failure is pronounced. The extremities may be cool, with a peculiar reddish blue discoloration, and edema of the tip of the nose and fingers has been reported. There may be severe constipation.

DIAGNOSIS. The most specific aid to diagnosis of pheochromocytoma is the finding of abnormally high levels of norepinephrine, epinephrine, and/or normetanephrine, metanephrine, and VMA in urine. Very rarely is there normal excretion of both the catecholamines and their metabolites in the presence of a functioning tumor. The pattern of excretion varies from patient to patient, depending on the size of the tumor and the rate of synthesis and turnover of catecholamines. However, the total urinary catecholamine excretion is usually more than 300 μg/24 hours when a pheochromocytoma is present. In children the predominant catecholamine excreted is norepinephrine, in contrast to the case with adults, in whom both epinephrine and norepinephrine outputs are high. In children a benign pheochromocytoma can be associated with abnormally elevated dopamine and HVA excretion, thus negating the value of these tests for biochemical differentiation of malignant and benign tumors.

Since most children with pheochromocytoma have abnormally high urinary excretion of VMA and/or metanephrine and normetanephrine, measurement of these compounds in 24-hour urine specimens is a satisfactory screening test for its presence. However, quantitative excretions of these metabolites may be similar in children with neuroblastoma and in those with pheochromocytoma, whereas levels of catecholamines, per se, usually are much higher in patients with pheochromocytoma.

Catecholamine excretion can be measured while a patient is being treated with reserpine, thiazides, guanethidine, and ganglionic blocking agents. Quinidine, tetracyclines, bilirubin, and α-methyldopa are among the compounds that interfere with fluorometric determination of norepinephrine and epinephrine. Fruits and vanilla-containing foods can result in falsely high levels of VMA.

The use of pharmacologic tests to establish the diagnosis of pheochromocytoma has been largely replaced by measurement of catecholamines. False-positive or false-negative results can occur with phentolamine (Regitine), tyrosine, and histamine tests. Intravenous histamine may provoke a serious hypertensive episode by causing the discharge of large amounts of norepinephrine and epinephrine from storage sites. Pharmacologic testing of children should be reserved for those in whom repeated measurements of catecholamines and metabolites are normal and suspicion of a pheochromocytoma still is high.

Albuminuria, glucosuria, hyperglycemia, increased metabolic rate, and abnormal adrenal cortical function have been reported in some children with pheochromocytoma, but these findings are of little value in establishing the diagnosis.

Intracranial neoplasms, particularly those arising from the posterior fossa, may cause hypertension and mimic the clinical features of pheochromocytoma; astrocytoma, medulloblastoma, and hemangioblastoma are among the tumors reported to cause this picture. However, most affected patients excrete normal amounts of catecholamines and metabolites in their urine.

The familial medullary thyroid carcinoma syndrome in its fullest expression, in addition to pheochromocytoma, thyroid tumors, and hyperparathyroidism, includes mucosal neuromas, intestinal ganglioneuromatosis, marfanoid habitus, pectus excavatum, and poorly developed musculature. The pheochromocytoma may be nonfunctioning under normal circumstances and may release excessive catecholamines only during stressful situations, with serious consequences. When there is a family history of the Sipple syndrome, pheochromocytoma, or such clinical findings as noted, one must suspect multiple tumors of neuroectodermal origin.

LOCALIZATION OF TUMOR. Preoperative localization of the tumor is difficult. Chest radiographs may reveal a paravertebral or posterior mediastinal mass. Tumors arising from the adrenal medulla may be defined by intravenous pyelography and tomography. Retroperitoneal infusion of carbon dioxide, arteriography, and venography are useful in selected cases, but they are not recommended as routine tests because they are associated with a low but definite incidence of complications. Hypertensive crises may be avoided during these procedures by pretreatment with α-adrenergic blocking agents. Often the site of the tumor cannot be found before surgical exploration; since more than one pheochromocytoma may be present, the entire abdominal cavity should be explored.

Determination of plasma catecholamine concentration at different sites during catheterization of the inferior or superior vena cava may be helpful when the tumor cannot be located by other means. The results must be interpreted with great care; multiple tumors, intermittent secretion of catecholamine by a single pheochromocytoma, blood flow patterns in the various vessels, and other factors may raise or lower catecholamine concentration.

TREATMENT. Excision of the tumor should be carried out as soon as the child has been prepared for surgery. Hypertension must be controlled preoperatively. This usually is accomplished by use of an α-adrenergic blocking agent such as phentolamine (Regitine) or phenoxybenzamine hydrochloride (Dibenzyline). Phentolamine, a short-acting drug, is particularly effective for intravenous use when precise control of blood pressure is necessary. The oral preparation may cause gastric distress and must be given every 4 to 6 hours; thus it is not as convenient a medication as Dibenzyline, which is administered orally every 12 hours. If symptoms of catecholamine excess persist, the addition of β-adrenergic blocking agents may be beneficial. Some patients with pheochromocytoma have reductions in blood volume and total red cell mass. Identification and correction of hypovolemia should be carried out preoperatively and during surgery. Otherwise, shock may develop after removal of tumor because of the sudden decrease in pressor amines with profound vasodilatation.

During induction of anesthesia and manipulation of the tumor, careful observation for hypertensive crisis is necessary. At these times intravenous phentolamine is a suitable agent for controlling marked blood pressure elevation; β-adrenergic blocking agents such as propranolol are useful in controlling cardiac arrhythmias.

When operating on a child with pheochromocytoma, a transabdominal approach is preferred because of the high incidence of bilateral adrenal tumors and multiple tumors. Rarely, an intravenous infusion of norepinephrine is needed to support blood pressure for 24 to 36 hours following surgery; however, blood pressure may remain elevated for several days after removal of a tumor. When a bilateral adrenal pheochromocytoma is excised, hydrocortisone should be administered to prevent adrenocortical insufficiency.

Several days after removal of a tumor, 24-hour urinary excretions of catecholamines and metabolites should be measured to be certain that all functioning tumor has been removed. In those cases where surgical excision is impossible, or where malignant pheochromocytoma with metastases is present, the tyrosine hydroxylase inhibitor α-methyltyrosine may be effective in controlling symptoms of excessive pressor amine production.

FOLLOW-UP. Continued follow-up care of children with pheochromocytoma is important, not only because the tumor may recur years later but also to observe for thyroid medullary carcinoma. Furthermore, families of children with pheochromocytoma should be evaluated, particularly when multiple tumors are found in the patient. Besides the history and physical examination, a screening diagnostic study includes 24-hour urine for VMA determination and measurement of serum calcium, phosphorus, phosphatase, calcitonin, and histaminase; medullary carcinomas of the thyroid produce calcitonin and the enzyme histaminase. However, there may be a span of many years between appearance of the various components of the Sipple syndrome; usually thyroid carcinoma develops before pheochromocytoma.

References

Bolande RP: The neurocristopathies. A unifying concept of disease arising in neural crest maldevelopment. Hum Pathol 5:409, 1974

Cameron SJ, Doig A: Cerebellar tumors presenting with clinical features of pheochromocytoma. Lancet 1:492, 1970

D'Angio GJ, Evans AE, Koop EC: Special pattern of widespread neuroblastoma with a favourable prognosis. Lancet 1:1046, 1971

Engelman K, Portnoy B, Lovenberg W: A sensitive and specific double-isotope derivative method for the determination of catecholamines in biological specimens. Am J Med Sci 255:259, 1968

Evans AE, D'Angio GJ, Randolph J: A proposed staging for children with neuroblastoma. Cancer 27:374, 1971

Frier DT, Tank ES, Harrison TS: Pediatric and adult pheochromocytomas. A biochemical and clinical comparison. Arch Surg 107:252, 1973

Gitlow SE, Mendlowitz M, Wilk EK, Wilk S, Wolf RL, Bertani LM: Excretion of catecholamine catabolites by normal children. J Lab Clin Med 72:612, 1968

———Pertsemlidis D, Bertani LM: Management of patients with pheochromocytoma. Am Heart J 82:557, 1971

Hellström KE, Hellström I: Immunity to neuroblastomas and melanomas. Ann Rev Med 23:19, 1972

Keiser HR, Beaven MA, Doppman J, Wells S Jr, Buja LM: Sipple's syndrome: medullary thyroid carcinoma, pheochromocytoma and parathyroid disease. Ann Intern Med 78:561, 1973

Leikin S, Evans A, Heyn R, Newton W: The impact of chemotherapy on advanced neuroblastoma. J Pediatr 84:131, 1974

Sawitsky A, et al: Vincristine and cyclophosphamide therapy in generalized neuroblastoma. Am J Dis Child 119:308, 1970

Starling KA, Sutow WW, Donaldson MH, Land VJ, Lane DM: Drug trials in neuroblastoma. Cancer Chemother Rep 58:683, 1974

Swift PGF, Bloom SR, Harris F: Watery diarrhoea and ganglioneuroma with secretion of vasoactive intestinal peptide. Arch Dis Child 50:896, 1975

Thorner MO: Dopamine is an important neurotransmitter in the autonomic nervous system. Lancet 1:662, 1975

Voorhess ML: Neuroblastoma-pheochromocytoma: products and pathogenesis. Ann NY Acad Sci 230:187, 1974

Wilson LMK, Draper GJ: Neuroblastoma, its natural history and prognosis. Br Med J 3:301, 1974

Wong KY, Hanenson IB, Lampkin BC: Familial neuroblastoma. Am J Dis Child 121:415, 1971

THYROID

JUDSON J. VAN WYK AND DELBERT A. FISHER

The mammalian thyroid gland evolved from the primitive gut into an endocrine organ capable of concentrating iodine and manufacturing and secreting iodothyronines. The most primitive thyroid gland is the subpharyngeal exocrine gland of the larval lamprey. This gland, under pituitary control, concentrates iodide and synthesizes hormone. The hormone precursors are secreted into the pharynx, where intestinal enzymes hydrolyze the thyroglobulinlike protein to release thyroxine. After metamorphosis the gland becomes an endocrine gland; the duct closes and the thyroprotein is stored and digested within the gland. This series of events in the lamprey probably recapitulates the pattern of evolution of the vertebrate thyroid gland from an iodide-concentrating organ much like a salivary gland into an endocrine gland.

The function of the thyroid gland is to concentrate iodide from the blood and return it to peripheral tissues in a hormonally active form. Triiodothyronine (T_3) and thyroxine (T_4), the principal thyroid hormones, are amino acids bearing, respectively, three and four iodine atoms per molecule (Fig. 22). The concentration of hormonal iodine available to the tissue is highly critical, since this governs the rate of tissue respiration and many other metabolic processes, including those concerned with growth and maturation. To maintain this level within permissible limits in those vast areas of the earth where iodine is scarce, the individual's body must husband iodine and protect against hormonal excess when iodine is in abundance.

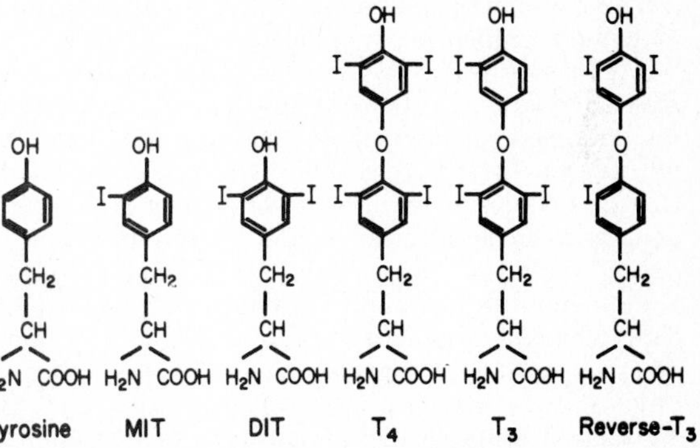

FIG. 22. Structures of thyroid hormone precursors tyrosine, monoiodotyrosine (MIT), and diiodotyrosine (DIT) and of the major iodothyronines thyroxine (T4), triiodothyronine (T3), and reverse T3.

IODINE AND THYROID HORMONE METABOLISM

Fate of Dietary Iodine

The distribution and fate of ingested iodine have been carefully documented with the use of ^{131}I tracers. Iodine is absorbed quantitatively from the upper gastrointestinal tract. After reaching the bloodstream it is distributed within the extrathyroidal iodide space, which has the approximate dimensions of the extracellular space. This space is being cleared constantly of inorganic iodide by two competitive processes: excretion by the kidneys and transport into thyroid cells. The extent of thyroid iodide uptake is governed by the number of functioning thyroid cells and, more particularly, by the efficiency of the active transport mechanism in the basilar membrane of these cells; this iodide concentrating mechanism, often referred to as the iodide pump, confers on the thyroid its unique ability to concentrate iodide to many times its level in plasma.

As long as intrathyroidal iodide ions remain in reduced form, they are in reversible equilibrium with serum iodide and can diffuse back into the circulation as serum levels fall. Normally, however, once iodide has entered the thyroid gland it is very rapidly incorporated into organic compounds and is no longer in equilibrium with serum iodide. The proportion of administered ^{131}I accumulated by the thyroid gland in organic form is governed by the capacity of the iodide pump, the rate of conversion of iodide into organic compounds, and the rate of renal excretion. Iodide is excreted largely in urine via glomerular filtration; 1 to 2 percent may be excreted in sweat under basal conditions, and this fraction may increase to as much as 7 to 9 percent with severe sweating. Although there is continuous secretion of iodide by the salivary and digestive glands, normally all but a negligible proportion is reabsorbed, and there is no substantial fecal excretion of iodide.

Biosynthesis of Thyroid Hormones

The steps in synthesis and release of thyroid hormones are graphically summarized in Figures 23, 24. These include the following: iodide trapping by the thyroid gland; organification of trapped iodide; coupling of the iodotyrosines monoiodotyrosine (MIT) and diiodotyrosine (DIT) to form iodothyronines (T3 and T4); storage of thyroid hormones in follicular colloid; endocytosis of colloid droplets and hydrolysis of colloid thyroglobulin to release MIT, DIT, T3, and T4; and deiodination of MIT and DIT and intrathyroidal recycling of the iodotyrosine iodine.

IODIDE CONCENTRATING MECHANISM. The transport of iodide across the cell membrane into the thyroid follicular cell is the first and rate-limiting step in thyroid hormone biosynthesis. The other major substrate for hormone synthesis, tyrosine, has not been found to be rate-limiting, even in patients with phenylketonuria, where tyrosine becomes an essential amino acid. Under normal circumstances the thyroid iodide pump generates a thyroid/serum (T/S ratio) concentration gradient of 30 to 40-fold; this gradient can reach several hundredfold when the thyroid gland is stimulated by a low-iodine diet, by thyrotropin-stimulating hormone (TSH), by a variety of thyroid-stimulating immunoglobulins such as long-acting thyroid stimulator (LATS) in Graves' disease, or by drugs that impair the efficiency of hormone synthesis. Other tissues such as the salivary glands, gastric mucosa, mammary glands, ciliary body, choroid plexus, and placenta also are capable of concentrating iodide against a gradient. However, these tissues are not capable of organifying inorganic iodide.

Iodide concentrated or pumped by the thyroid follicular cell is oxidized rapidly and bound in organic form, so that less than 1 percent of the total thyroidal iodine is present as inorganic iodide. However, the iodide pump mechanism can be isolated from the organification process by blocking organification with one of the antithyroid drugs such as propylthiouracil or methimazole. In this way the transport mechanism

within the plasma membrane has been studied and characterized. The capacity for iodide accumulation is 1 to 5 mmoles/g wet weight of thyroid. The pump requires oxygen and functions optimally at 37 C and at a pH approximating 7.0. High-energy phosphate bonds supply the necessary energy. The membrane-bound, Mg^{++}-activated, ouabain-sensitive, Na^{+}-K^{+}-dependent ATPase system also appears to be essential. TSH stimulates iodide transport through a sequence of increased cyclic AMP formation and RNA and protein synthesis. Certain anions that are themselves accumulated by the thyroid are capable of competitively

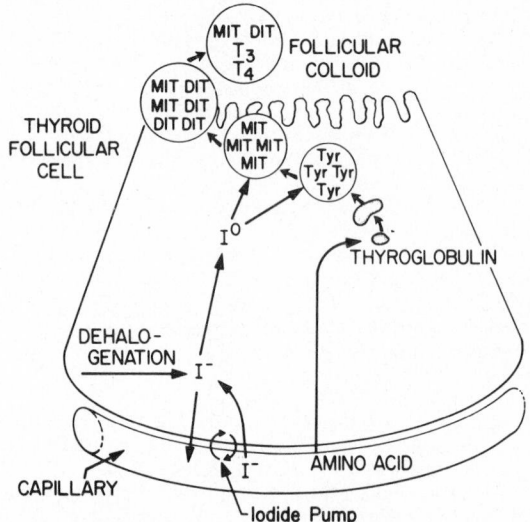

FIG. 23. Steps in synthesis of thyroid hormones, including iodide trapping, thyroglobulin synthesis, iodide organification, and iodotyrosine coupling.

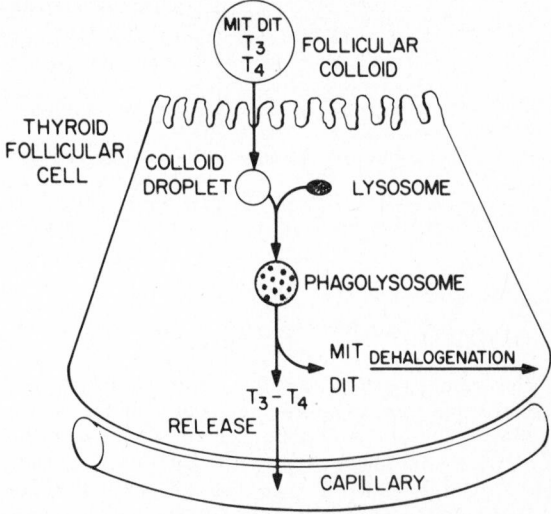

FIG. 24. Steps in thyroid hormone secretion, including endocytosis, formation of phagolysosomes, thyroglobulin hydrolysis, iodotyrosine deiodination, and hormone release.

inhibiting iodide transport. These, in order of increasing potency, include bromide (Br^-), nitrite (NO_2^-), thiocyanate (SCN^-), selenacyanate ($SeCN^-$), fluoroborate (BF_4^-), and perchlorate (ClO_4^-). The existence of familial goiter, with a specific inability to concentrate iodide, indicates that the iodide-concentrating mechanism is under genetic control. In addition to control by TSH, iodide transport is stimulated by a low-iodine diet, a mechanism that provides a measure of thyroidal self-regulation.

ORGANIFICATION OF TRAPPED IODIDE. Organification of iodide involves two processes: oxidation of iodide and iodination of thyroglobulin. Thyroglobulin is the essential substrate for organification and is the major protein component of thyroid colloid. It is an iodinated glycoprotein with a molecular weight approximating 650,000 daltons and a sedimentation coefficient of 19.4 (19S). It is composed of two 12S subunits, each of which is composed of two to four peptide chains. The iodine content of thyroglobulin depends on dietary iodine. MIT, DIT, T3, and T4 are present within the protein molecule as iodoaminoacyl residues that can be cleaved by proteolytic enzymes. The tyrosine residues, which are the iodine acceptors of thyroglobulin, form about 3 percent of the weight of the protein, and about two-thirds of these are spatially oriented to be susceptible to iodination.

Thyroglobulin is synthesized on ribosome-studded membranes of the follicular cell; it migrates in the cisternae of the endoplasmic reticulum to the Golgi apparatus, and finally to vesicles near the apical cell membrane, where exocytosis into follicular lumen occurs. Iodination of tyrosyl residues occurs after thyroglobulin synthesis, probably at or near the apical cell membrane adjacent to the colloid space.

Thyroid hormone biosynthesis begins with oxidation of iodide to an active intermediate (perhaps I^0 or I^+), followed by iodination of thyroglobulin-bound tyrosyl residues to form the iodotyrosines MIT and DIT (Fig. 23). These processes are very rapid, with the half-time of incorporation of iodide into protein being of the order of 2 minutes. Both steps are catalyzed by a thyroid peroxidase enzyme system. Thyroid peroxidase is a membrane-bound heme protein that requires peroxide and an acceptor, which in the normal thyroid gland is thyroglobulin, but can be albumin or other peptides or proteins. The hydrogen peroxide may be provided by one or more of several flavoprotein enzyme systems.

In addition to catalyzing the formation of iodotyrosines, thyroid peroxidase probably also catalyzes the coupling of iodotyrosines within the thyroglobulin molecule to form T3 and T4 (Fig. 23). DIT and MIT couple, with loss of an alanine side chain, to form T3; DIT plus DIT couple to form T4. The mechanism is not known. The relative proportions of T3 and T4 formed depend on the amount of available iodide and the extent of thyroglobulin iodination. Low-iodine diets increase the MIT/DIT ratio and increase T3 synthesis; high-iodine diets decrease the MIT/DIT ratio and favor T4 synthesis. Normally the thyroid gland contains about 0.5 mg thyroglobulin for 1 g of gland; 70 percent

TABLE 23. Thyroid Weights for Various Ages*

Age (years)	Average Thyroid Weight (g)
Birth	1.5
1	2.5
5	6.1
10	8.7
15	15.8
Adult	20.0

* From Handmaker and Lowenstein (eds): Nuclear Medicine in Clinical Pediatrics, 1975. Courtesy of Society of Nuclear Medicine.

of the iodoprotein is iodotyrosine, and the remainder is iodothyronine, with a T4/T3 ratio of 10/1 to 20/1. Normal thyroid gland weight versus age is shown in Table 23. As a rule of thumb, the thyroid gland weight is equivalent to chronologic age until the adult weight is achieved at 20 years, ie, the gland weighs 5 g at 5 years, 10 g at 10 years, and 20 g at 20 years.

The complexity of the organification reaction suggests the possibility that one of several defects might occur to impair function of the system; in fact, several presumably genetically mediated defects have been described. Patients with these defects are goitrous, either euthyroid or hypothyroid, and discharge iodide from their thyroid glands during the perchlorate discharge test. The defects can be classified as follows: (1) absent or abnormal peroxidase leading to impaired enzyme activity; (2) abnormal peroxidase with impaired binding for the hematin prosthetic group; activity is restored in vitro with an excess of hematin; (3) deficient organification of iodide with normal peroxidase activity, perhaps due to defective H_2O_2 generation; associated with deafness (Pendred's syndrome); (4) deficient organification of iodide with normal peroxidase, which may be a consequence of defects in H_2O_2 generation or deficient substrate for iodination.

Whenever the ability to oxidize iodide is selectively impaired, TSH secretion is increased, the pool of organic iodine is reduced, and the thyroid gland tends to undergo hyperplasia. When radioiodine is administered to such patients, thyroid uptake reaches an early peak followed by a fall due to diffusion of iodide back into the bloodstream and/or rapid turnover of the small organic iodine pool (Fig. 25). Normally, thyroid radioiodine uptake peaks at 24 to 48 hours, whereas in these patients uptake may peak before 6 hours. If the organification defect is complete, thyroidal radioactivity falls at a rate that parallels the decrease in plasma radioactivity via renal excretion. Administration of potassium perchlorate ($KClO_3$), 0.5 g orally 1 to 2 hours after the dose of radioiodine, will lead to rapid displacement of the nonorganified iodide within the thyroid cell (Fig. 25). This perchlorate discharge test is a useful method for detecting an organification defect from any cause.

DIGESTION OF THYROGLOBULIN AND SECRETION OF THYROID HORMONES. Thyroglobulin is stored in colloid after iodination and coupling have occurred at the cell–colloid apical membrane interface. Before release (Fig. 24), the colloid must first

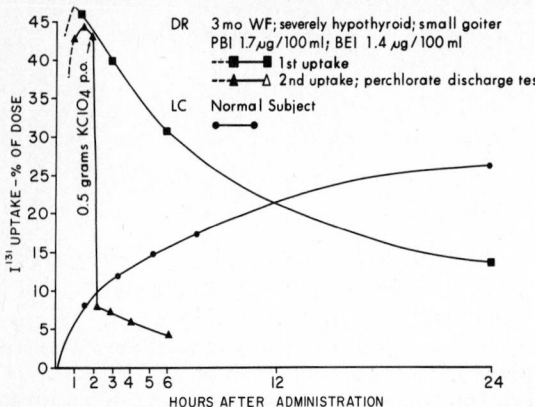

FIG. 25. Effect of peroxidase defect on kinetics of radioiodine uptake in 3-month-old cretin. Because of hypothyroid state and resultant hypersecretion of TSH, the patient had developed a goiter and markedly increased thyroid radioiodine uptake. This peaked early (1 to 2 hours), and discharge was evident by 3 and 6 hours, in contrast to the uptake pattern in normal subjects. Lack of organic binding of radioiodine is reflected by abrupt and marked decrease in thyroid radioactivity during second uptake study after administration of potassium perchlorate.

be ingested by the follicular cell (the process of endocytosis). The ingested thyroglobulin is then enzymatically hydrolyzed, and the free hormones are released to the bloodstream. This process of hormone secretion is under the control of TSH. Within a few minutes after administration of TSH, large pseudopods can be observed at the apical cell surface. These ingested colloid droplets fuse with apically streaming proteolytic hormone containing lysosomes to form phagolysosomes, wherein thyroglobulin hydrolysis occurs. The free MIT, DIT, T3, and T4 within the phagolysosomes are then released into the follicular cell. Since the series of events can be stimulated by dibutyryl cyclic AMP, as well as by TSH, it is believed that cyclic AMP mediates the TSH stimulation of thyroid hormone release.

DEIODINATION OF IODOTYROSINES AND INTRATHYROIDAL RECIRCULATION OF IODIDE. After enzymatic digestion of thyroglobulin, T3 and T4 are released and diffuse from the thyroid follicu-

lar cell into thyroid capillary blood. The MIT and DIT released are largely if not totally deiodinated under the influence of an iodotyrosine dehalogenase. This microsomal enzyme is stimulated by flavine adenine nucleotides in the presence of reduced nucleotide adenosine diphosphate (NADPH). The significance of this enzyme is best illustrated by patients who manifest goitrous hypothyroidism due to congenital iodotyrosine dehalogenase deficiency. These patients develop severe iodine deficiency via loss of thyroidal iodotyrosines in blood and urine; about 50 percent of the total iodine ingested daily can be lost in the urine as iodotyrosine in this condition. Moreover, supplementation of the diet of such patients with iodine allows complete reversal of the goiter and the hypothyroidism. Most, if not all, of the MIT-DIT is deiodinated, and the iodide thus generated enters the intracellular iodide pool and is reutilized or recycled through the organification process for new hormone synthesis.

Thyroid Hormones In Blood

Both T3 and T4 are found in blood, associated with plasma proteins after direct secretion by the thyroid gland. The thyroid gland is the sole source of T4, but most of the T3 in blood is derived from nonglandular sources via monodeiodination of T4 in peripheral tissues. The concentration of T4 in human blood is 50 to 100 times greater than that of T3. The concentrations of both are relatively constant in the steady state. The mean T4 level approximates 8 μg/100 ml in the adult, ranging from 5 to 13.5 μg/100 ml; the mean T3 concentration approximates 130 ng/100 ml and ranges from 50 to 220 ng/100 ml. Average values relative to age are shown in Table 24.

Both hormones exist in blood, bound reversibly and competitively to transport proteins. These include thyroxine-binding interalpha globulin (TBG), thyroxine-binding prealbumin (TBPA), and albumin. The binding reactions are nearly complete, so that the euthyroid steady-state concentrations of free T4 and free T3 approximate 0.03 percent and 0.30 percent, respectively, of the total hormone concentrations. Absolute mean free T4 and T3 concentrations in adults approximate 2.4 and 0.260 ng/100 ml, respectively. TBG, which has

TABLE 24. Normal Values for Serum Thyroid Hormone Concentration Versus Age*

Age	T4 (μg/100 ml)	T3 (ng/100 ml)	Reverse T3 (ng/100 ml)	TBG (mg/100 ml)
Cord Blood	12.7 (3.4)[†]	50 (18)	150 (50)	5.4 (2.4)
24 hours	16.2 (2.4)	419 (160)	165 (58)	5.0 (1.4)
7 days	14.1 (2.1)	—	55 (26)	4.9 (1.3)
6 weeks	11.7 (2.2)	163 (24)	40 (10)	—
3–12 months	10.4 (2.2)	—	—	—
1–6 years	9.9 (1.8)	168 (27)	—	—
6–10 years	8.7 (1.8)	161 (25)	—	—
10–16 years	7.4 (1.8)	144 (45)	—	4.0 (0.7)
16–20 years	7.7 (1.8)	—	—	—
Adult	8.1 (1.7)	130 (43)	41 (10)	3.4 (0.7)

Data adapted from Fisher: J Pediatr 82:1, 1973; Chopra: J Clin Invest 33:583, 1974; Fisher: unpublished.
[†] *Values expressed as mean ± SD; all values represent radioimmunoassay methods.*

TABLE 25. Predicted Values of Plasma Total T3 and T4 Concentrations in Human Adult and Their Distribution Among Binding Proteins in Absence of One of Protein Species

Condition	Mean Concentration T3 (ng/100 ml)	Mean Concentration T4 (µg/100 ml)	Percentage with T3 TBG	Percentage with T3 Alb	Percentage with T3 TBPA	Percentage with T4 TBG	Percentage with T4 Alb	Percentage with T4 TBPA
Normal	120	8.0	46	1	53	67	20	13
Absent TBG	70	5.3	—	2	98	—	59	41
Absent TBPA	120	6.7	46	—	54	83	—	17
Absent albumin	60	7.3	98	2	—	77	23	—

the lowest plasma concentration of the several binding proteins (1 to 3 mg/100 ml in the adult), binds about half of the total T3 and 70 percent of T4. TBPA, with a plasma concentration of 10 to 20 mg/100 ml, binds only about 1 percent of T3 and 20 percent of T4. Albumin, with a concentration several thousandfold greater (2 to 5 g/100 ml) binds about half of the T3 and only about 10 percent of the T4. The significance of the several binding proteins is shown more clearly in Table 25, where the predicted effects of deletion of one of the binding protein species are shown. It is clear that, quantitatively, TBG is the most important carrier protein for T4. TBG and albumin seem equally important for T3 binding. The presence of hormone-binding proteins in plasma increases the effective capacity of plasma for

hormone storage and provides the organism with a rapidly exchangeable hormone pool in blood. The concentrations of carrier proteins vary with age. TBG levels are higher in prepubertal children than in adults, and they decrease at the time of puberty to values comparable to those in adults. Reciprocal changes are observed in TBPA binding (Fig. 26).

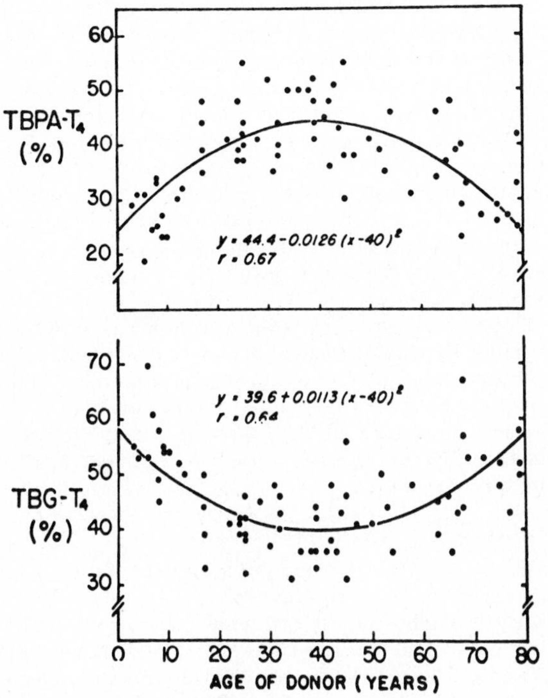

Distribution Of Thyroid Hormones

Thyroid hormones are distributed to all body tissues in differing proportions. In all tissues the distribution into cells is a nonlinear process dependent on blood and interstitial fluid protein binding, physical properties of capillary and cell membranes, and intracellular binding processes. Two major extravascular pools of T3 and T4 probably exist, one in which plasma–tissue interchange is rapid (chiefly liver, kidney, and lung) and one in which exchange is slow (chiefly skeletal muscle and skin). An additional pool with an intermediate exchange rate has been suggested (chiefly gut and bone). Peak T4 concentrations after single pulse doses of labeled hormone occur in these quasi-anatomic (rapid, intermediate, and slow) pools in minutes, hours, and days, respectively. Total body T4 distribution has been estimated as follows: 22 percent in plasma, 31 percent in fast tissues, 44 percent in slow tissues, and about 3 percent in intermediate tissues.

The transcapillary exchange of T4 with liver interstitial fluid occurs as a T4–protein complex. The exchange of T4 with extrahepatic tissues occurs predominantly in the form of free hormone rather than protein-bound hormone. Thus the current concept is that free T4 is the physiologically significant moiety with regard to the tissue effects of thyroid hormones.

Metabolism Of Thyroid Hormones

Deiodination is the major pathway of thyroid hormone metabolism in man; about 80 percent of the hormonal iodine is removed from the thyroxine rings and either excreted in urine (and to a small extent in sweat and saliva) or reutilized (Fig. 27). The first step in metabolism probably is monodeiodination of T4 either to T3 or to reverse T3. Monodeiodination of the beta or phenyl hydroxyl ring produces T3 (Fig. 22). T3 has three to four times the metabolic potency of T4, whereas reverse T3 is largely inactive metabolically. Thus beta-ring deiodination may be of much greater metabolic significance than alpha-ring deiodination. Under normal circumstances both T3 and reverse T3

FIG. 26. Percentage binding of tracer concentrations of thyroxine to thyroxine-binding prealbumin (TBPA) and thyroxine-binding globulin (TBG) in serum of euthyroid subjects of various ages. The best-fit regression equations and the parabolic curves that they generate are shown (X, age of patient); *r* values are coefficients of correlation in linear relationships between TBPA–T4 and TBG–T4 and values for $(X-40)^2$. For both correlations $p < 0.01$. (From Braverman et al: J Clin Invest 45:1273, 1966.)

In figure: $y = 44.4 - 0.0126(x-40)^2$, $r = 0.67$ (TBPA-T4)

$y = 39.6 + 0.0113(x-40)^2$, $r = 0.64$ (TBG-T4)

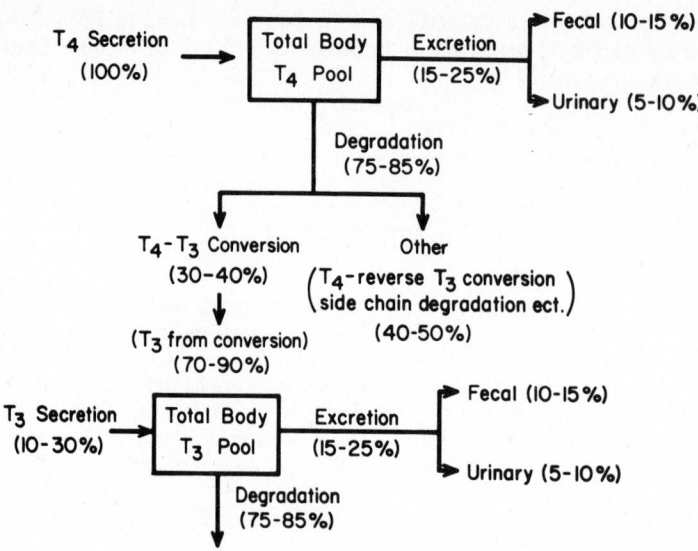

FIG. 27.   Quantitative pattern of thyroid hormone metabolism in euthyroid adult. [Adapted from DiStefano and Fisher: In Hershman and Bray (eds): Pharmacology of the Thyroid Gland, 1975. Courtesy of Pergamon Press.]

probably are produced at approximately similar rates.

Both T3 and reverse T3 diffuse rapidly from tissue to interstitial fluid to plasma. Significant amounts of T3 and small amounts of reverse T3 are synthesized and released by the thyroid gland, so that the circulating levels of these hormones reflect both secretion and peripheral production. From 70 to 90 percent of circulating T3 is derived from peripheral conversion and 10 to 25 percent from the thyroid gland; values for reverse T3 probably are 96 to 98 percent and 2 to 4 percent, respectively (Fig. 27). Under certain circumstances, such as in the fetus and in the euthyroid sick patient, beta-ring monodeiodination is reduced and alpha-ring monodeiodination is unchanged or increased, so that circulating levels of T3 are decreased and reverse T3 concentrations are increased. The opposite may be true in Graves' disease.

The alanine side chain of the alpha (tyrosyl) ring of the hormones also is subject to degradative reactions, including transamination, deamination, and decarboxylation. Pyruvic acid analogues and small amounts of lactic acid analogues have been observed in urine and bile; these have minimal biologic activity. The acetic acid analogues found in tissue, bile, and urine may have some activity, albeit reduced. The extent of these reactions, relative to deiodination, has not been adequately quantified. Another route of metabolism is formation of protein-bound material containing iodine derived from the beta ring of the molecule. This iodoprotein has been reported in a variety of tissues and in plasma. Tissue iodoprotein may account for as much as 5 to 10 percent of tissue organic iodine.

Thyroid Hormone Excretion

Thyroid hormones are excreted in urine and stool in both free and conjugated forms. The conjugation reactions involve both glucuronide and sulfoconjugation. Although both reactions occur in a variety of tissues, glucuronide conjugation occurs mainly in liver via microsomal glucuronyl transferase. Ethereal sulfoconjugation is most prominent in extrahepatic tissues, particularly in kidney. The patterns of conjugation of T3 and T4 differ markedly, in contrast to their similarity with respect to deiodination. Probably this is due to the different tissue locations of the glucuronide and sulfoconjugation systems. T4 is glucuronide-conjugated in the liver, and nearly all of it is excreted in bile; T3 seems to be predominantly sulfoconjugated in kidney and other tissues, where it is produced via monodeiodination.

Fecal excretion of thyroid hormones is somewhat variable, depending on hepatic function and biliary flow rate, intestinal luminal contents (such as dietary components, bacteria, drugs, and binding proteins), and physical attributes of the intestinal tract. Normally, however, 10 to 15 percent of T3 or T4 is excreted via the gut (Fig. 27).

Control Of Thyroid Function

Pituitary TSH is the major determinant of the level of activity of the thyroid. Removal of the pituitary causes thyroid atrophy, but thyroid cellular integrity and function are maintained at basal levels. Thus TSH functions as a tropic hormone. However, in addition to maintaining thyroid size and probably influencing thyroid gland growth during infancy and childhood, TSH stimulates all stages of thyroid iodine metabolism. The mechanism of this stimulation is not entirely clear, but it is known that TSH interacts with thyroid follicular cells by binding to a specific receptor site on the outer side of the thyroid follicular cell plasma membrane and activating the membrane-bound adenylate cyclase. Adenylate cyclase catalyzes the transformation of ATP to cyclic AMP, which then mediates the TSH effects on iodide trapping and oxidation, iodothyronine synthesis, colloid endocytosis, and hormone secretion. The molecular mechanism by which cylic AMP mediates these manifold effects is still obscure.

TSH secretion is in turn influenced by secretion of thyrotropin-releasing factor or hormone (TRH) from the hypothalamus (Fig. 28). TRH, a small tripeptide molecule, is secreted by hypothalamic neuroendocrine cells into the pituitary portal system for transport to the anterior pituitary. Here TRH, via cell membrane receptor → adenylate cyclase → cyclic AMP, stimulates TSH synthesis and release by pituitary thyrotrope cells. Thyroid hormones also can act on the thyrotrope cells to inhibit the TRH effect. This inhibitory effect is not immediate, but requires several hours, since it requires thyroid hormone stimulation of new protein synthesis. Thus TRH and TSH act to stimulate thyroid hormone synthesis and release. The thyroid hormones, in turn, feed back at the pituitary level to inhibit the TRH effect. When the titer of circulating thyroid hormones increases, the TRH effect is inhibited, serum TSH falls, and thyroid hormone release is inhibited. Conversely, decreased levels of thyroid hormones allow an uninhibited effect of TRH, increasing TSH secretion so that thyroid hormone secretion is increased. Under normal circumstances TRH may function to provide a more or less tonic stimulus for pituitary TSH secretion on which feedback control is superimposed. It is not clear what

determines the tonic level of TRH secretion or the set point of the system by the hypothalamus (Fig. 28).

Serum TSH can readily be measured by using radioimmunoassay techniques. Normal values range from undetectable to 10 μU/ml. Values in primary hypothyroidism nearly always exceed 20 μU/ml and may range to 10 to 20 times that amount. This measurement is the most sensitive test available for primary hypothyroidism.

Synthetic TRH is available for testing purposes and is useful in the differential diagnosis of thyroid disorders. Intravenous injection of TRH at 7 μg/kg body weight normally increases serum TSH concentrations 5 to 40 μU/ml within 30 minutes. An increased response suggests hypothyroidism or decreased thyroid reserve. An absent response in a patient with high or high-normal total and/or free T4 and/or free T3 concentrations suggests hyperthyroidism. An absent response in a patient with low thyroid hormone levels suggests pituitary insufficiency. Finally, a normal or more sustained response in a patient with low thyroid hormone concentrations suggests hypothalamic disease.

Actions Of Thyroid Hormones

The effects of thyroid hormones are widespread. They influence growth and development, oxygen consumption and heat production, nerve function, and metabolism of lipids, carbohydrates, proteins, nucleic acids, vitamins, and inorganic ions, and they have important effects on other hormone actions. The free hormones penetrate the cell membrane, bind to specific cytosol T4- or T3-binding proteins, and are transported to exert their effects on mitochondria and effects within the nucleus. The earliest effect of the hormone, which is manifest within minutes, is an effect on mitochondrial oxidative phosphorylation. A small dose of T4 increases oxygen utilization in hypothyroid mitochondria without depressing the efficiency of phosphorylation; thus the rate of transformation of immediately available energy is increased. Large doses produce uncoupling, with depressed phosphorylation. These effects are correlated with the presence of increased amounts of the hormone in the mitochondria.

Thyroid hormones exert their most important effects on the nucleus. The hormones are transported to the nucleus, where they bind to chromosomal nonhistone protein and activate the transcription process.

T4 and/or T3, via direct stimulation of nuclear genome activity, stimulate synthesis of nuclear RNA and cytoplasmic protein synthesis. Calorigenesis also is stimulated via synthesis of mitochondrial enzymes and structural elements. Thus thyroid hormones influence nearly all cells by directly stimulating mitochondrial activity and indirectly augmenting mitochondrial calorigenesis by increasing the mass of functioning mitochondria. In addition, various tissues and cell functions are stimulated in specific ways by varying patterns of genome activation and protein synthesis to account for the multiple physiologic actions of thyroid hormones. In addition to calorigenesis, these include stimulation

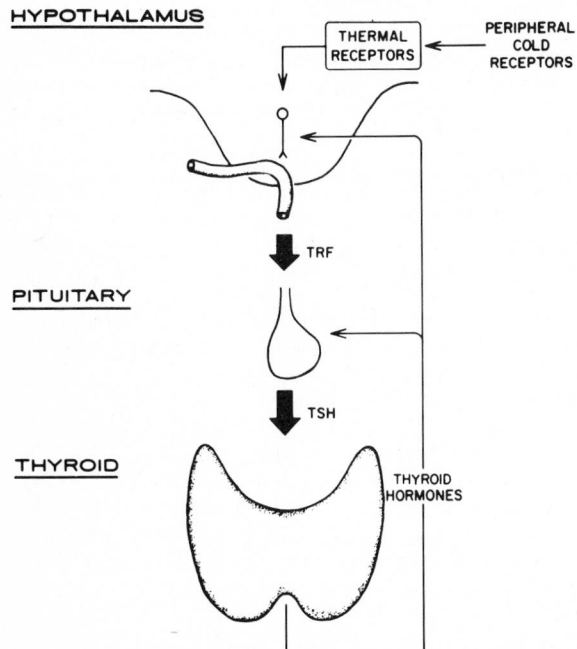

FIG. 28. Hypothalamus-pituitary-thyroid axis. Secretion of TSH is regulated by hypothalamic TRF (or TRH) and negative-feedback influence of thyroid hormones.

of growth and development of various tissues at critical periods (including the central nervous system and skeleton), regulation of water and ion transport, regulation of cholesterol and fat metabolism, and stimulation of protein metabolism, to name a few.

One of the interesting effects of thyroid hormones is to potentiate the actions of catecholamines; increased catecholamine effects are prominent manifestations of the hyperthyroid state. These effects are manifest in the face of normal or lowered circulating concentrations of catecholamines. The β-adrenergic effects such as tachycardia, tremor, and lid lag can be blocked in hyperthyroid subjects by propranolol, a β-receptor blocking agent. But propranolol does not alter thyroid function or the basal level of cellular activity.

FETAL AND NEWBORN THYROID FUNCTION

Fetal Thyroid Function

The thyroid gland anlage in the human fetus is first visible in the 16- to 17-day embryo. By 31 to 32 days the gland consists of a bilobed mass of proliferating cells ventral to the trachea in the lower neck. By 70 to 75 days the gland can accumulate radioiodine and synthesize hormone, and extracellular stored colloid is visible by 12 weeks. The fetal pituitary is identifiable histologically at 10 to 11 weeks, and it contains TSH by 12 weeks. However, fetal serum TSH, T4, T3, free T4, and free T3 concentrations are either undetectable or very low before midgestation. Thus, although it is largely differentiated and apparently capable of function by 10 to 12 weeks, the fetal pituitary–thyroid system functions at a hypopituitary level before 20 weeks.

Despite this secondary (pituitary) hypothyroid state in the fetus, placental transfer of TSH or of thyroid hormones is minimal. Little maternal–fetal transfer of labeled T4 occurs during gestation; the marked maternal–fetal gradients of serum TSH, free T4, and free T3 during the first half of gestation, and the fetal–maternal TSH and free T4 gradients thereafter, are consistent with experiments that indicate limited placental transport of these hormones. Thus, either embryogenesis and early fetal growth are not thyroid-hormone-dependent or these events are sensitive to very low thyroid hormone concentrations.

Between 18 and 24 weeks of gestation there is a progressive increase in pituitary TSH content and concentration and a progressive increase in fetal serum TSH concentration. By 24 weeks, mean fetal serum TSH levels consistently exceed paired maternal serum concentrations; this fetal–maternal TSH gradient is maintained to term. The observation that fetal thyroid radioiodine uptake and fetal serum T4 and free T4 concentrations increase in parallel suggests a coincident increase in TSH effect on the fetal gland. Thus there appears to be an abrupt stimulation of TSH synthesis and secretion at midgestation. The temporal correlation of these events with maturation of the hypothalamic and pituitary portal blood vascular system suggests that this stimulation represents hypothalamic-pituitary maturation and results from hypothalamic

stimulation of the anterior pituitary thyrotrope, presumably mediated by augmented secretion of TRH. The midgestation increases in fetal pituitary growth hormone and FSH and LH concentrations and in fetal serum growth hormone, FSH, and LH levels support this view and suggest that other hypothalamic anterior pituitary control systems also become operative at this time.

Between midgestation and term, fetal serum TSH concentrations remain relatively high; levels at 24 to 35 weeks are 5.2 to 20 μU/ml, with a mean of about 9 μU/ml. These increased levels stimulate a progressive increase in fetal serum T4 during the second half of gestation. There also is a progressive increase in serum TBG concentrations during this time, but the concomitant increase in free T4 indicates a progressive saturation of protein binding sites. Taken together, these data suggest a progressive increase in fetal T4 secretion during the last trimester of pregnancy. This view is supported by studies of serum T4 concentrations and production rate measurements in fetal sheep during the last trimester. Total and free T4 concentrations in fetal ovine serum consistently exceed maternal values during the last trimester, and the mean T4 production rate (40 μg/kg/day) exceeds the maternal rate (5.6 μg/kg/day) about eightfold. The observed lack of placental transfer of labeled T4 or T3 in these studies and the marked fetal-to-maternal gradient of free T4 indicate that placental T4 transfer is minimal. This conclusion is further supported by the observation that when the fetal sheep is thyroidectomized, serum T4 concentrations fall within 3 to 5 days to unmeasurable levels, and fetal serum TSH concentrations increase markedly. The sheep studies substantiate the human data and indicate minimal placental transfer of thyroid hormones or TSH, autonomy of fetal pituitary–thyroid function, and a high rate of fetal T4 secretion during the last trimester.

FETAL TRIIODOTHYRONINE DEFICIENCY. Serum T3 concentrations are low in both the human fetus and the sheep fetus throughout gestation. Kinetic studies using labeled hormones in fetal sheep have shown a low mean T3 production rate and a high T4/T3 production ratio, thus suggesting a state of T3 deficiency. Recent studies of human fetal serum suggest a similar state of T3 deficiency. In contrast to T3, reverse T3 levels are high in fetal serum of both humans and sheep, and reverse T3 production rates are high in fetal sheep. The fact that fetal thyroidal T3 and reverse T3 content is low suggests that secretion of both hormones is minimal in utero. Thus most of the circulating T3 and reverse T3 in the fetus must be derived from monodeiodination of T4. The high reverse-T3/T3 production ratio suggests that enzymatic beta ring T4 monodeiodination is markedly reduced in the fetus while alpha ring T4 monodeiodination is normal or even increased.

Newborn Thyroid Function

With parturition, the newbon infant is transformed from a state of chemical T3 deficiency to chemical T3 thyrotoxicosis. After birth, serum TSH concentrations

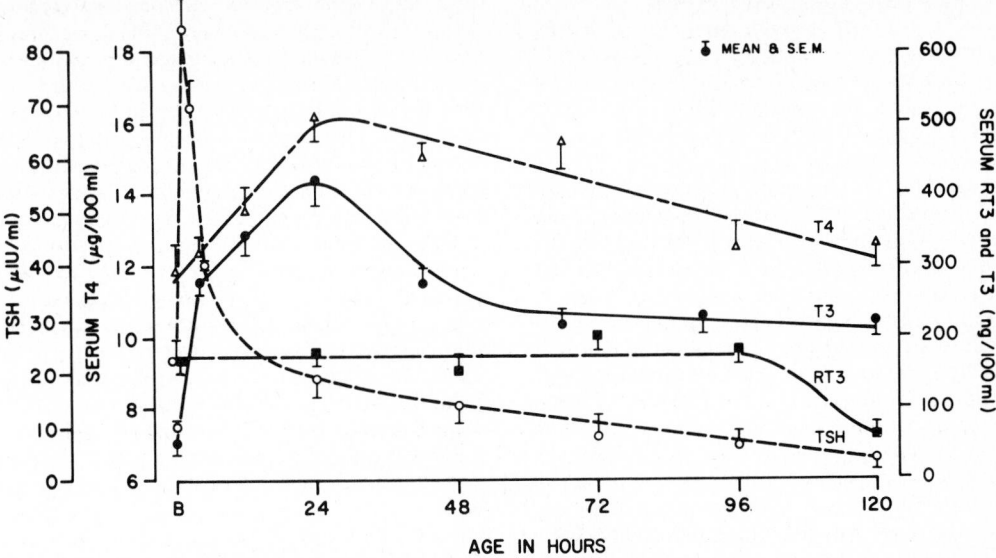

FIG. 29. Patterns of secretion of TSH, T4, T3, and reverse T3 in 4 newborns.

increase rapidly to a mean peak level of 86 μU/ml by 30 minutes. Serum T4 and free T4 levels increase briskly from cord blood values of 11.9 μg/100 ml and 2.9 ng/100 ml, respectively, to peak values of 16.2 μg/100 ml and 7 ng/100 ml by 24 to 48 hours (Fig. 29). Even more striking increases in serum T3 and free T3 concentrations are observed, from cord values of 50 ng/100 ml and 146 pg/100 ml to peak values of 419 ng/100 ml and 1,260 pg/100 ml at 24 hours. TBG concentrations, in contrast, remain unchanged at levels approximating 5.0 mg, and the high levels of serum reverse T3 only gradually decrease to adult values during the first week (Fig. 29).

The mechanisms responsible for these changes are not yet clear. The early (60-minute) increase in serum T3 levels appears to be due, at least in sheep, to a marked increase in the rate of beta-ring monodeiodination of T4. This and the early catecholamine response, as well as the consequent augmentation of nonshivering thermogenesis in the newborn lamb, are triggered by cutting the umbilical cord. The later and more gradual increases in serum T4 and T3 values, which peak at 24 hours, probably are due to increased thyroidal secretion mediated by the TSH surge. The mechanism of the TSH surge remains to be clearly defined. Data indicate that body cooling in the newborn augments serum TSH and T4 levels relative to control values in infants kept in warm environments.

The physiologic significance of the resulting hyperthyroid state also remains speculative. Thyroid hormones are known to augment catecholamine-mediated mobilization of fatty acid from body fat stores and catecholamine-mediated nonshivering thermogenesis.

Congenital Hypothyroidism

Cretinism is an ancient term that has long been used in Europe to describe a form of imbecility and dwarfism

that was common in areas of endemic goiter. The implications of this term are vague, and the trend is to deemphasize the end result and apply this designation to any individual with a congenital deficiency in thyroid secretion dating from birth. An etiologic classification of cretinism is provided in Table 26.

TABLE 26. Etiologic Classification of Cretinism

Endemic cretinism
Embryonic errors in development (thyroid dysgenesis)
  Thyroid aplasia (athyrotic cretinism)
  Thyroid dysplasia
    Ectopic remnant in pathway of descent (cryptothyroidism)
    Rudimentary thyroid in normal location
Inborn errors of thyroid function (goitrous cretinism, familial cretinism)
  Defective TSH molecule or thyroidal responsiveness to TSH
  Failure to concentrate iodide
  Peroxidase system defects
    Absent or abnormal peroxidase
    Abnormal hematin binding
    Pendred's syndrome (defective H_2O_2 generation?)
    Normal peroxidase (defective H_2O_2 generation? absent receptor?)
  Iodotyrosine deiodinase defect
  Defects of thyroglobulin metabolism
    Coupling defect
    Iodoprotein secretion defect
    Defective thyroglobulin synthesis
  Defective peripheral response to thyroid hormone

Endemic Cretinism

Although it has largely been eliminated from North America, endemic goiter persists in many areas of the world. Iodine deficiency, dietary goitrogens, and endemic pockets of heritable defects in thyroid metabolism all have been implicated as etiologic factors. The frequency of goiter in populations where goiter is endemic varies widely, but it may exceed 50 percent. Goiter is infrequent in the newborn; the peak incidence is observed at 11 to 14 years of age. Defects in development that have been related to endemic goiter include: deaf-mutism, diplegia, squint, mental deficiency, dwarfing, and hypothyroidism. Whether these are acquired in utero is not clear.

Two syndromes of endemic cretinism exist. One, which is characterized by mental deficiency and/or deaf-mutism, sometimes with neuromuscular disorders but without hypothyroidism, has been described in New Guinea. The second, reported from the Congo, is a form of thyroidal hypoplasia leading to hypothyroidism that begins in utero or in early infancy and is associated with dwarfing and mental deficiency resembling those seen in sporadic cretinism. These syndromes have been referred to as nervous endemic cretinism and myxedematous endemic cretinism. Both types have been observed in several endemic goiter areas, and they may occur in the same area. Their combined incidence varies from 1 to 6 percent of infants in endemic goiter areas. The pathogenesis is not understood, but both forms can be eliminated by iodine prophylaxis.

Errors In Embryologic Development

Errors in embryologic development (thyroid dysgenesis) may be responsible for either complete absence of thyroid tissue (thyroid aplasia) or anomalous differentiation of the gland (thyroid dysplasia). Athyrotic children have no detectable uptake of ^{131}I in the neck, and they develop severe clinical manifestations of hypothyroidism in early infancy. Most infants with thyroid dysgenesis have some residual functioning thyroid tissue. In many instances this tissue is located ectopically in the pathway of descent from the base of the tongue; more rarely, aberrant tissue is located laterally. These thyroid rests are small and are incapable of responding to stimulation by TSH. It has been suggested, on the basis of thyroid scanning results, that 60 to 80 percent of infants with thyroid dysgenesis have some residual functioning thyroid tissue. Thyroid dysgenesis associated with significant amounts of such residual tissue and delayed onset of hypothyroidism has been referred to as cryptothyroidism.

The cause of the embryologic defects in cretinism is not clear. Cretins are usually free of the multiple somatic anomalies that characterize other syndromes associated with mental retardation. Although there is a slightly increased tendency for cretinism to recur in subsequent children born to mothers who have given birth to one such child, the distribution does not follow any mendelian pattern of inheritance. A number of instances have been recorded in which identical twins were discordant for athyrotic cretinism, and there have been occasional instances in which a mother has given birth to more than one cretinous infant; this suggests that a maternal factor may play a role. Blizzard found antithyroid antibodies in 29 percent of a series of 121 mothers who have given birth to one or more cretins. These antibodies cross the placenta and remain in the blood of the baby for several months after birth. How-

ever, thyroid damage has not been demonstrated following the passive transfer of such antibodies, and active immunization of pregnant animals has not produced any fetal thyroid dysfunction, even when extensive damage has been produced in the mother's gland. Although these antibodies are probably not themselves the cause of cretinism, they do suggest that an autoimmune process in the mother may be associated with arrested development of the fetal thyroid gland.

One possibility is that lymphocytes of mothers with autoimmune thyroid disease traverse the placenta and produce a delayed hypersenstivity reaction in embryonic thyroid tissue. Goldsmith and associates recently reported a family with autoimmune thyroid disease involving at least 3 members of two generations. Congenital, partially reversible, nongoitrous hypothyroidism occurred in 6 third-generation offspring of one mother. The authors postulated placental transfer of a thyroid suppressive agent, perhaps microsomal antibody.

Inborn Errors Of Thyroid Function

Stanbury demonstrated that cretinism may result from inheritance of a metabolic error in thyroidal iodine metabolism or thyroid hormone synthesis. Several defects have been proposed, although in some the specificity of the findings is questionable. A classification of possible or proven defects is included in Table 26, and defects in thyroid hormone synthesis are displayed graphically in Figure 30. The mode of inheri-

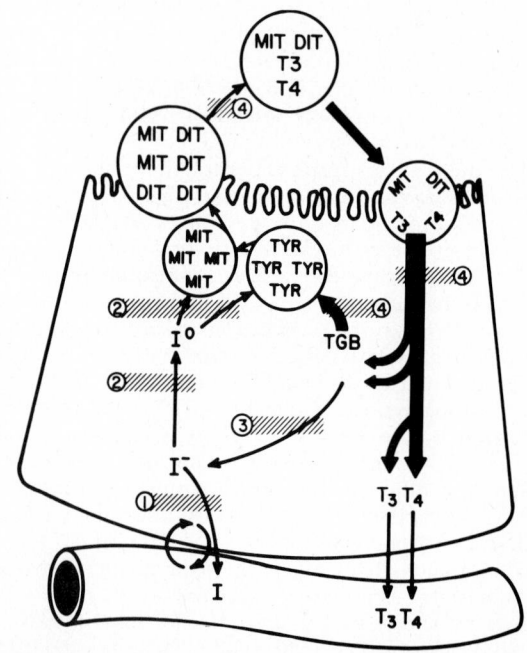

FIG. 30. Graphic representation of sites of defects in thyroid hormone synthesis involved in goitrous hypothyroidism: 1, iodide trapping; 2, peroxidase system; 3, iodotyrosine deiodination; 4, thyroglobulin synthesis or metabolism.

tance has usually proved to be that of a simple autosomal recessive trait. The clinical manifestations of cretinism due to a biochemical defect are similar to those arising from an embryologic error in development, apart from the familial incidence and propensity for affected individuals to develop large goiters; the term goitrous cretinism has been applied to these patients, but the term is misleading, since thyroid enlargement is delayed for months or years in 60 to 80 percent of patients and may be absent altogether. Presumably, similar but less severe errors in synthesis may produce goiters that first make their appearance in later childhood or adulthood; such patients may remain euthyroid or may develop only mild hypothyroidism.

DEFECTIVE TSH METABOLISM.   Hypothalamic (TRH) or pituitary (TSH) deficiency may occur as an isolated defect or in association with other hypothalamic or pituitary hormone deficiencies. Thyroidal unresponsiveness to TSH has been postulated by Stanbury to explain the thyroid function abnormalities in an 8-year-old child with the appearance of cretinism who had signs in infancy. There was no goiter, thyroidal radioiodine uptake was low normal, serum TSH was high, and there was no thyroidal response to exogenous TSH, but there was good response to exogenous thyroid hormone.

FAILURE TO CONCENTRATE IODIDE.   Several patients have been described with hyperplastic thyroid glands but only minimal uptake of radioactive iodide (2 to 11 percent at 24 hours). The thyroid glands were enlarged twofold to fourfold, and the patients were clearly hypothyroid. Other iodine-concentrating tissues (salivary glands, gastric mucosa) also failed to concentrate iodide from the circulation, so that the low salivary/serum radioiodine concentration ratio is a useful diagnostic point. Lugol's solution will correct the hypothyroidism by increasing the serum iodide to high levels and increasing the intrathyroidal inorganic iodide concentration via diffusion. One drop daily is an adequate dose. The defect in this disorder is not known.

PEROXIDASE SYSTEM DEFECTS.   The first of the defects described by Stanbury was attributed to a deficiency of the peroxidase enzymes necessary to oxidize thyroidal iodide to iodine. Due to long-standing stimulation by TSH, radioactive iodide is concentrated at an accelerated rate in such a gland. Since the ^{131}I remains in reduced form, the thyroidal radioactivity falls at a rate that parallels the clearance of plasma ^{131}I by renal excretion. The administration of thiocyanate or perchlorate to such patients is followed by a precipitous fall in thyroid radioactivity (Fig. 25).

The association between familial goiter and deafmutism was first reported in 1896 by Pendred, an English country practitioner. In 1960 Fraser and associates reported 113 such cases in 72 families, with a distribution conforming to an autosomal recessive mode of inheritance. In these families goiter was found to have an obligatory association with nerve deafness. A positive perchlorate discharge test was found in affected individuals. In most instances affected individuals were euthyroid or only mildly hypothyroid, and the discharge

of radioactivity following perchlorate was less complete than in severe cretins with this defect. Thus the deafness could not be attributed to intrauterine hypothyroidism. The goiters tended to recur following partial thyroidectomy unless full replacement dosages of thyroid hormone were administered.

More recently, a number of patients have been described with mild hypothyroidism and only partial discharge of radioiodine following perchlorate administration. In one patient who was studied carefully the thyroid gland was found to contain no peroxidase activity, but activity could be restored by adding hematin, the noncovalently bound prosthetic group of the peroxidase. In contrast with these patients with deficient thyroid peroxidase activity, at least two groups have been described with goitrous hypothyroidism and positive perchlorate discharge results in the presence of normal peroxidase activity. These include patients with associated nerve deafness (Pendred's syndrome) as well as those without cranial nerve VIII involvement. The peroxidase system abnormality in these patient groups is not known.

A positive perchlorate discharge result also has been reported in patients with absent or defective thyroglobulin, thus suggesting that absence of a normal protein receptor might be involved. Another possibility involves a defective mechanism for hydrogen peroxide generation.

IODOTYROSINE DEIODINASE DEFECT.   Deficiency of the iodotyrosine dehalogenase enzyme can produce a hereditary defect causing either cretinism or a less severe form of familial goiter. Failure to deiodinate thyroid MIT and DIT as they are released from thyroglobulin leads to severe iodine wastage as these iodotyrosines are excreted in urine. Iodotyrosine deiodinases are present in both thyroid cells and in peripheral tissues. Cretins with this defect are severely deficient in both the thyroidal and peripheral enzymes, but less severe hypothyroidism has been described in goitrous patients in whom only the thyroidal enzyme is lacking. Mildly reduced activity of the peripheral deiodinase systems may occur in association with myxedema, but thyroid hormone therapy corrects this promptly. The presence of this defect can be detected by direct enzymatic studies of thyroid tissue. The more usual test, which measures only the integrity of the peripheral deiodinase enzymes, is to administer ^{131}I-labeled diiodotyrosine and determine the chemical form of the radioactivity excreted in the urine. Normally more than 90 percent of the urinary radioactivity is recovered in the form of iodide; patients with this defect excrete mostly unchanged ^{131}I-labeled diiodotyrosine. It is possible to treat such patients by administering large amounts of iodine, but it is simpler and more efficacious to treat with thyroid hormone itself.

DEFECTS OF THYROGLOBULIN METABOLISM.   The coupling defect, the iodoprotein secretion defect, and defective thyroglobulin synthetic defects probably comprise a spectrum of abnormalities. Coupling of iodotyrosines is a complex chemical transformation that is poorly understood. It may be catalyzed by the peroxidase enzyme system, and it requires the presence of normal thyroglobulin. A number of possible defects may lead to similar functional abnormalities, so that the defects are difficult to distinguish. A coupling enzyme defect could evoke glandular hyperplasia, increased thyroglobulin turnover, and decreased glandular thyroglobulin stores. Under these circumstances, alternative substrates for the organification reaction might result in release of increased quantities of iodoalbumin or other iodoproteins. An abnormal perchlorate discharge also might occur, as well as abnormal ratios of iodotyrosines to iodothyronines within the gland. A coupling defect could be caused by absent or abnormal thyroglobulin. The abnormality could be so minimal that only the spatial orientation of the tyrosyl residues is altered. An abnormal receptor for the peroxidase enzyme or a separate coupling enzyme deficiency also could exist. A number of patients have been described with findings suggestive of impaired thyroglobulin synthesis or abnormal thyroglobulins; most of these patients were observed to secrete iodoalbumin.

DEFECTIVE PERIPHERAL RESPONSE TO THYROID HORMONES. Another defect that has been suggested is a specific inability of peripheral cells to utilize T4. Several patients have been alleged to require unusually large dosages of thyroid hormone to correct hypothyroidism, but there has been insufficient documentation to prove a primary defect in peripheral utilization. However, Refetoff and associates have described a familial syndrome, in 3 siblings with deaf-mutism, stippled epiphyses, retarded skeletal age, goiter, and greatly elevated levels of serum T4, free T4, and free T3, but normal plasma TSH. Growth rate, metabolic rate, and intelligence were normal. Kinetic studies indicated that the glands were secreting about five times the normal amount of thyroxine daily. Administration of 1,000μg/day of T4 or 375 μg/day of T3 produced little or no metabolic effects. Thyroxine was shown to enter the cells, and mitochondrial metabolism was normal. As the patients matured, the plasma T4 tended to return to normal levels, the epiphyses closed, and the goiters disappeared. Thus, although the patients were clearly refractory to the metabolic effects of thyroid hormone, clear evidence of hypothyroidism was lacking. The mechanism for the refractoriness remains to be defined.

Thyroid Hormones In Growth And Development

Normal somatic growth and development, normal growth and maturation of the central nervous system, and normal puberty are dependent on adequate supplies of thyroid hormones. Animals thyroidectomized in the neonatal period grow more slowly than normal, and body size lags progressively. Bony tissues remain immature because of delayed growth of long bones, delayed epiphyseal maturation, retarded skull growth, and marked retardation of skull suture closure. In addition, nitrogen retention is reduced, metabolic rate is low, and levels of function of most body organ systems are subnormal. Thyroid hormone deficiency present from birth also leads to marked delay in central nervous system development. Growth and arborization of nerve cells are delayed, axodendritic interaction and connectivity are reduced, vascularization and myelination proceed at subnormal rates, and irreversible mental retardation occurs if treatment is delayed. The period of central nervous system thyroid hormone dependency extends to 2 to 3 years of age in the human infant. The onset of hypothyroidism after this time does not produce mental deficiency.

The situation in utero, however, is not entirely clear. The observations that the placenta is essentially impermeable to thyroid hormones and that the newborn hypothyroid infant appears clinically euthyroid imply that fetal growth and development are not dependent on thyroid hormone. It is now conceded that this is so for somatic and linear bone growth; the hypothyroid newborn is longer and heavier than his normal counterpart, even though bone maturation is usually delayed. Although the critical period of thyroid hormone dependency for central nervous system growth and maturation in man begins in late fetal life and extends to 2 years after birth, it is not clear to what extent it is important for intrauterine brain development. Replacement therapy with thyroid hormone will minimize mental retardation when begun within 3 months after birth in human cretins.

CLINICAL FEATURES. Most infants with congenital hypothyroidism are born with little or no clinical evidence of thyroid hormone deficiency. Thus detection based on signs and symptoms usually is delayed 6

TABLE 27. Frequencies of Some Signs and Symptoms of Congenital Hypothyroidism*

	0–3 Months	4–6 Months	7–24 Months
Symptoms			
Constipation	65[†]	48	59
Feeding problems	60	61	35
Lethargy	55	48	31
Respiratory (signs and/or symptoms)	30	13	1
Signs			
Umbilical hernia	68	65	44
Enlarged, protruding tongue	65	91	100
Facies	25	91	100
Neonatal jaundice	28	17	15
Hoarse cry	23	30	21

* Adapted from Raiti and Newns: Arch Dis Child 46:692, 1971.
† Values recorded as percentages of patients.

to 12 weeks or longer. Table 27 shows the incidences of some of the common symptoms and signs of hypothyroidism versus age. It is clear that the classic signs, including the characteristic facies, enlarged protruding tongue, and the growth and developmental retardation, evolve progressively during the first several months of life (Fig. 31). Therefore early clinical diagnosis must be based on a high index of suspicion regarding nonspecific symptoms and signs. Although many of the signs of hypothyroidism may be blunted in the newborn period, the diagnosis should be considered in those who maintain subnormal temperatures, exhibit excessive circulatory mottling, fail to nurse properly, or exhibit respiratory distress with feeding. The diagnosis should also be suspected in newborns who are inactive, who cry frequently, who are unduly constipated, or who have persistent unexplained jaundice or an enlarged posterior fontanelle. The classic facies in older cretins is due to accumulation of myxedema in the subcutaneous tissues and in the tongue. The thickened tongue becomes protuberant, and the infant develops increasing difficulty in nursing and handling salivary secretions. The cry is hoarse because of myxedema of the vocal cords. More prolonged hypothyroidism also leads to marked muscular hypotonia and mental torpor. An umbilical hernia and the characteristic potbelly are due to muscular hypotonia involving both the smooth muscles of the gut and striated muscle of the abdominal wall. The deleterious effects of prolonged hypothyroidism on the heart and circulation may be marked. There usually is relative bradycardia and diminished pulse pressure. The cardiac silhouette may be enlarged due to myxedematous infiltration or to pericardial effusion. The electrocardiogram may show low voltage and a prolonged conduction time. As a consequence of inadequate perfusion of peripheral tissues, the extremities are cool and may exhibit extreme pallor and circulatory mottling.

Markedly hypothyroid infants exhibit numerous metabolic deficits. Insensible water loss is greatly diminished due to the lowered basal metabolic rate. The glomerular filtration rate is markedly impaired, and inappropriate secretion of antidiuretic hormone has been described. As a result of these changes, administration of forced feedings or intravenous fluids may lead rapidly to water intoxication and hyponatremia. The conjugation and excretion of drugs are markedly impaired, thereby causing these patients to be exquisitely sensitive to small amounts of such drugs as barbiturates and narcotics. The conjugation of bilirubin is also impaired, thus accounting for prolonged neonatal jaundice. Carotenemia and hypercholesterolemia are further indications of the hypothyroid state, although in young untreated cretins the serum cholesterol is not strikingly elevated. Vitamin D intoxication has been encountered with dosages only moderately in excess of daily requirements. Most cretins are moderately anemic and fail to respond to iron. Reticulocytosis follows institution of thyroid treatment.

LABORATORY DIAGNOSIS. Recent data in a number of species, including man, have indicated that placental transfer of thyroid hormones is markedly lim-

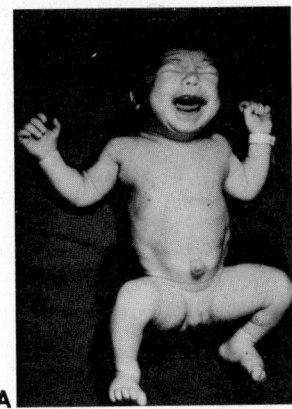

A

C.A.	3 mo
H.A.	Newborn
B.A.	< Birth
PBI	1.3 µg/100 ml

^{131}I Uptake   < 1%

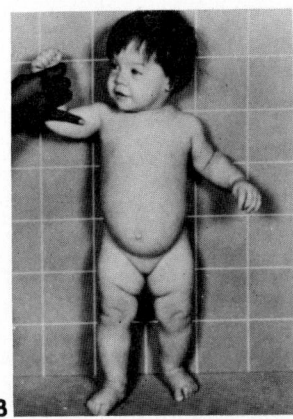

B

14 mo

10 mo

4 mo

2.2 µg/100 ml

4% ; No response to TSH

Thyroid Scan: Single ectopic focus

FIG. 31. Clinical picture of cretinism depends more on severity of hypothyroidism than on, etiologic mechanism. Infant **A** had severe peripheral skin mottling, muscular hypotonia, umbilical hernia, and myxedema. Infant **B** had a functioning thyroid remnant that delayed diagnosis for over 1 year.

ited. With this information and the recent development of highly sensitive and specific radioimmunoassay systems for measurement of thyroid hormones and TSH using small volumes of blood, newborn screening for hypothyroidism has become feasible. Dussault and associates in Quebec adapted the T4 radioimmunoassay technique to the measurement of T4 in the same filter paper blood spots used for phenylketonuria screening and detected 7 cretins in a study of 50,000 newborns. The cost was about $4,000 per hypothyroid infant detected. The screening and follow-up were accomplished within 6 weeks, at which time hypothyroidism had been suspected in only 1 of the 7 infants. Klein and associates have used the TSH radioimmunoassay to measure TSH in cord blood; they detected 1 cretin in a preliminary study of 4,000 infants.

These data confirm that T4 values are low and TSH concentrations high in newborns with hypothyroidism. The incidence of 1 hypothyroid infant in about 7,000 newborns in these studies is in good agreement with earlier epidemiologic estimates of 1 in 5,000 to 1 in 10,000 births. In the past it was thought that 60 to 80 percent of infants with congenital hypothyroidism had significant amounts of residual functioning thyroid tissue that might delay diagnosis, but the results of Dussault and associates suggest that this tissue is not extensive enough to delay diagnosis, since most of the expected infants were detected at birth.

Cretinism also can be diagnosed by measurement of serum T4 and TSH concentrations in individual cord blood samples or blood samples collected during the neonatal period in suspicious cases. A cord serum T4 of 6.0 μg/100 ml or less by radioimmunoassay, with a TSH in excess of 100 μU/ml, is diagnostic. After 3 days a serum T4 less than 5 μg/100 ml with a serum TSH in excess of 20 μU/ml is diagnostic. Cord serum T3 values measured by radioimmunoassay are not useful in diagnosis of hypothyroidism at birth. However, values of less than 70 ng/100 ml are suggestive of hypothyroidism after 2 to 3 days. TBG screening is not necessary if serum TSH values are elevated, but a low T4 by itself is not sufficient for diagnosis; a low T3 resin uptake result and/or low free thyroxine concentration or TBG measurement are necessary to exclude a low serum TBG for any reason. A serum TSH measurement is the most sensitive test for primary hypothyroidism, and it should be conducted in any patient with a low T4 value.

Secondary hypothyroidism is more difficult to diagnose. A low T4 and a low T3 resin uptake (with a low corrected T4 result), or a low free T4 concentration, indicates hypothyroidism rather than a low TBG concentration. A normal or low TSH resulting under these circumstances suggests secondary rather than primary hypothyroidism. This can be confirmed with a TRH stimulation test. If there is a subnormal TSH response to TRH, a diagnosis of pituitary hypothyroidism is in order. If the peak level of TSH after TRH is normal (not increased), hypothalamic TRH deficiency can be inferred.

TREATMENT. Treatment of hypothyroidism requires administration of exogenous thyroid hormone. A number of thyroid preparations are available. Thyroid USP is a dried and powdered preparation of porcine and/or bovine thyroid gland. Thyroglobulin is the final purified product of porcine thyroid gland. Synthetic preparations of Na-l-thyroxine and Na-l-triiodothyronine are available alone or mixed in a 4:1 ratio of T4:T3. Potency ratios are thyroid USP 120 mg; thyroglobulin 120 mg; Na-l-thyroxine 100 μg (0.1 mg); and Na-l-triiodothyronine 25 μg (0.025 mg). All these preparations are suitable for replacement therapy. However, Na-l-thyroxine is favored because it is more uniform in potency than the natural preparations. Absorption is more reliable, and it produces normal serum levels of both T4 and T3, the latter because of peripheral conversion.

The best guide to adequacy of therapy is periodic measurement of circulating levels of T4 and TSH; during the initial stages of treatment a T3 determination also may be of value. The history and physical examination are important in follow-up, but mild hypothyroidism or hyperthyroidism cannot always be excluded in this way. Using thyroid USP or Na-l-thyroxine, the serum T4 should be adjusted to the mid normal range, at which time the serum TSH level and T3 levels should be normal (<7 μU/ml and 70 to 250 ng/100 ml, respectively).

For markedly hypothyroid infants the usual starting dose of Na-l-thyroxine is 15 μg/kg/day; 2 to 3 weeks are usually required to observe the maximal effects from a constant dosage. Hayek and associates have shown that intramuscular thyroxine in three daily doses of 100 μg raise levels of serum T4 and lower TSH within 3 to 4 days, at which time oral maintenance doses of 50 to 100 μg T4 or equivalent will maintain normal levels of serum T4. This approach supplies the nervous system with adequate thyroid hormone more rapidly. The risk of cardiac arrhythmia is minimal when therapy is begun early. If the hypothyroidism is prolonged 6 months or longer, initial treatment should be started more slowly.

Adequate dosage in the first year ordinarily ranges between 75 and 100 μg Na-l-thyroxine. Persistent manifestations of bradycardia, circulatory mottling, inactivity, hoarse cry, or constipation or delay in the relaxation phase of deep tendon reflexes are indication to increase the dosage. The enlarged tongue may not disappear for many months in the presence of otherwise adequate therapy. The growth rate should be accelerated markedly after initiation of therapy; the growth deficit usually is restored by 9 to 24 months, depending on the age and degree of dwarfism existing at the beginning of treatment. Supplemental vitamins should be prescribed to meet the increased requirements during the period of catch-up growth. Bone age is a sensitive index of thyroid deficiency and may suggest inadequate dosage when other signs of hypothyroidism have been obliterated.

Overtreatment produces such pathologic signs as tachycardia, excessive nervousness, disturbed sleep patterns, and other findings suggesting thyrotoxicosis. Excessive dosages over a longer period produce osteoporosis, premature synostosis of cranial sutures, and undue advancement of bone age. Rapid shedding of lanugo and, in older infants, devitalized scalp hair are normal consequences of treatment and do not indicate a need to reduce the dosage.

Acquired Juvenile Hypothyroidism

Etiology

Hypothyroidism may develop at any age in previously normal individuals; it is more common in females than in males. The onset is usually insidious, and in most cases the gland undergoes atrophy; usually no precipitating cause can be identified. A high proportion of such individuals have circulating antithyroid antibodies, and the hypothyroidism is probably the end result of an autoimmune process (p. 1682). In a few instances, acquired juvenile hypothyroidism may be attributed to some goitrogenic agent, or it may occur as a late manifestation of an inborn error of thyroidal biosynthesis.

The complex interaction of genetic factors, sexual predisposition, and environmental goitrogens is demonstrated by the 13-year-old girl illustrated in Figure 32. When a small asymptomatic goiter was found at age 8, she was placed on 30 drops of Lugol's solution daily. The immediate slowing of her growth curve that followed this therapy dated the onset of hypothyroidism to this point, although overt signs of myxedema developed insidiously and were not recognized for another 4 years. Genetic studies revealed a marked predisposition to goiter, apparently inherited as an autosomal dominant trait with greater expression in the female. A distinctive biochemical abnormality in this family was the presence of circulating iodopeptides. Some of these in-

dividuals were also excessively sensitive to iodine and developed myxedema rapidly with moderate doses. A number of close relatives of the proband had been subjected to multiple thyroidectomies. Circulating antithyroid antibodies were found in these patients, and the histologic picture of their thyroid glands resembled that of Hashimoto's thyroiditis.

The frequency with which acquired hypothyroidism is associated with juvenile diabetes mellitus suggests more than coincidence. In 4 out of 10 such patients followed at the University of North Carolina Pediatric Endocrine Clinic, hypothyroidism preceded the onset of diabetes by 9 months to 2 years, whereas in 6 others hypothyroidism followed the onset of diabetes by 6 months to 5 years. Many of these patients had elevated titers of antithyroid antibodies, thus suggesting an autoimmune basis for the thyroid component of their illness. A similar immunologic mechanism has been suggested as the basis for some cases of diabetes. In one family, 3 of 4 siblings were afflicted with both diseases.

DIAGNOSIS. The most useful aid in the recognition of acquired hypothyroidism in childhood is a serial record of growth performance. Usually a number of years elapse between the onset of hypothyroidism and the emergence of classic signs of myxedema. However, if growth records are available, the onset of hypothyroidism can readily be documented by progressive downward deviation from a previously normal growth channel. Weight tends to increase, and in most instances weight for age is proportionately greater than height for age (Fig. 33).

The possibility of thyroid deficiency should be con-

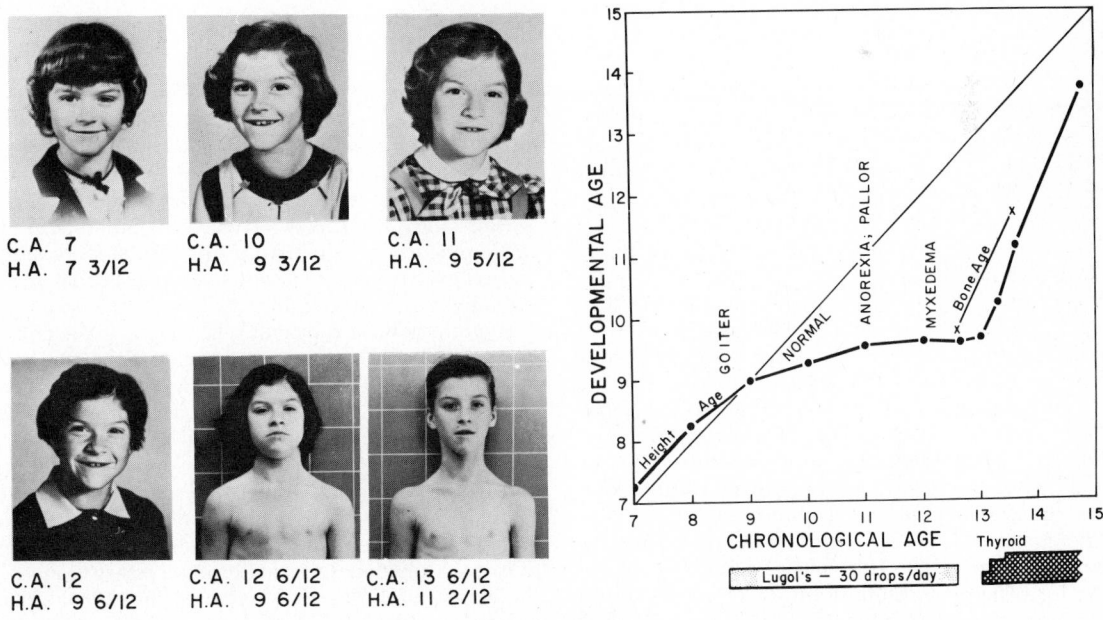

FIG. 32. Patient with familial goiter who developed hypothyroidism shortly after institution of treatment with Lugol's solution. This patient is discussed in text. C.A., chronologic age; H.A., height age.

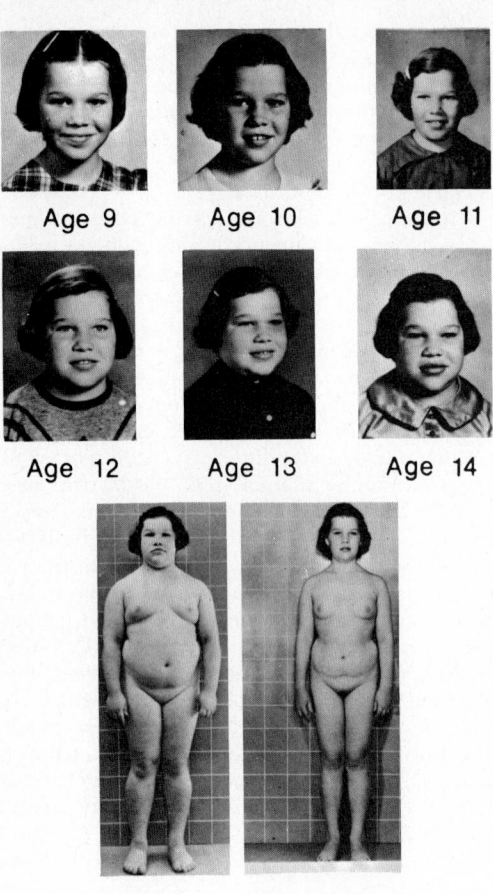

Age 9   Age 10   Age 11

Age 12   Age 13   Age 14

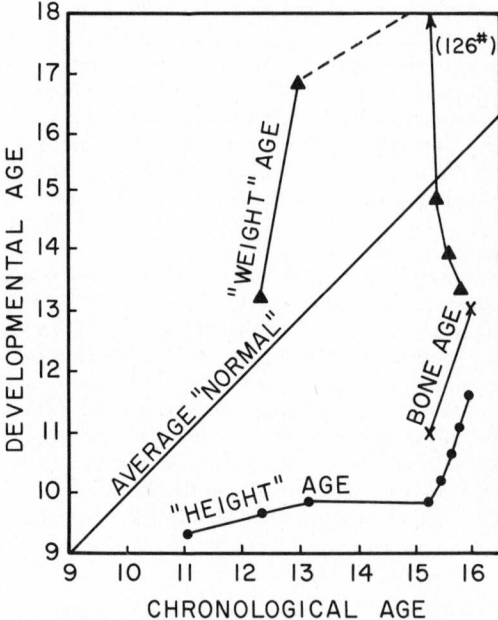

FIG. 33. Evolution of hypothyroidism in 15-year-old girl is illustrated by serial photographs and growth measurements obtained from school records. Height record suggests that thyroid function began to fail between 9 and 10 years, but the full clinical picture of myxedema required several years to emerge.

sidered in any child who is not growing normally. A dwarfed child who is underweight for his stature is less likely to be hypothyroid than in the reverse circumstance. The retardation of bone age in hypothyroidism almost always equals or exceeds the retardation in linear growth. This finding also is present in other forms of dwarfism and is by no means pathognomonic of hypothyroidism.

Hypothyroidism is frequently suspected in obese, sluggish individuals. It should be emphasized, however, that the stature of most obese children is above the 50th percentile for age, and skeletal maturation also is advanced. In contrast, children with untreated hypothyroidism are retarded in both height and bone age, unless the thyroid deficiency is of very recent onset. Thyroid function studies are not usually indicated in obese children with advanced stature.

The effects of hypothyroidism on the cardiovascular system produce some of the most useful clues to the diagnosis. The precordium is unusually quiet, and the pulse pressure is diminished. Circulatory mottling, pallor, and cool extremities are often striking. Brown pigmentation over the neck, knees, and elbows is often mistaken for caked dirt. Although the skin and hair are dry, these alterations are often subtle and are of little

diagnostic value; occasionally there is marked loss of hair. The thyroid-deficient patient usually exhibits slowing of the deep tendon reflexes, with a greatly delayed relaxation phase; this can be observed best by percussion of the Achilles tendon with the child kneeling on a chair. Since the speed of reflexes is modified by the autonomic tone at the time of the test, anxiety, drugs, and other extrathyroidal influences may render the results invalid as an indicator of thyroid function.

Hypothyroidism is usually a lifelong disease, and the diagnosis should always be supported with tests of thyroid function before treatment is instituted. With adequate treatment the child will be restored to full physical normality, and the original diagnosis will inevitably be challenged. Minimal documentation should consist of measuring plasma cholesterol, thyroxine (or thyroxine iodine), TSH, and antithyroid antibodies. With the improvement shown in other laboratory tests of thyroid function, it is usually unnecessary to measure the uptake of radioactive iodine by the thyroid gland. However, such studies are of great value in delineating biosynthetic errors and ectopic location of the thyroid gland and in differentiating primary from secondary hypothyroidism.

In recent years the measurement of plasma TSH concentration by radioimmunoassay has proved to be the most sensitive indicator of primary hypothyroidism. In normal children the TSH levels range from below detectability to about 10 μU/ml; in mild hypothyroidism these levels are considerably elevated and in more severe cases may reach values to 20 to 30 times that.

Before undertaking treatment it is important to discriminate between primary hypothyroidism and that secondary to hypopituitarism. An elevated TSH level establishes that the disease originates in the thyroid rather than the pituitary gland. Theoretically it should be possible to differentiate primary from secondary hypothyroidism by measurement of thyroid uptake of radioactive iodine before and after administration of TSH. The thyroid gland of a child with primary hypothyroidism is already under maximal endogenous TSH stimulation, and it fails to respond to administration of additional TSH. In hypopituitarism the administration of TSH usually results in a marked increase of ^{131}I uptake. A common procedure is to administer two intramuscular injections of bovine thyrotropin (5 USP units each) 48 hours and 24 hours before the second iodine uptake test. Unfortunately, about one-third of the children in our clinic with proven hypopituitarism have, for unknown reasons, failed to respond to TSH, even after more prolonged stimulation. Whenever secondary hypothyroidism is suspected, it is mandatory that other pituitary deficiencies be sought by a complete set of pituitary function studies, including provocative tests of growth hormone secretion (see p.1604) and plasma response of TSH to administration of TRH. Skull radiographs and visual field examinations should be performed to exclude the presence of a pituitary tumor.

PRECOCIOUS SEXUAL DEVELOPMENT AND JUVENILE HYPOTHYROIDISM. The sexual development of most hypothyroid children is retarded to the same extent as retardation of skeletal maturation. This is not invariable, since over 50 children with long-standing primary hypothyroidism have now been described with precocious menstruation and breast development and galactorrhea. The genital tract shows evidence of marked estrogen stimulation, and the ovaries are often markedly enlarged and cystic. In the male this syndrome is associated with excessive enlargement of the penis and testes. Most of these patients lack sexual hair, and bone age is retarded in keeping with hypothyroid state. In many the sella turcica is enlarged. When the hypothyroid state is alleviated, the manifestations of sexual precocity regress, and normal puberty ensues when the general level of maturity has progressed appropriately. In some instances the sella turcica has become smaller in size after the institution of substitution therapy, thus demonstrating that the previously enlarged pituitary fossa was secondary to compensatory hyperplasia of the pituitary rather than to a primary pituitary adenoma. In 1960 it was postulated by Van Wyk and Grumbach that the apparently inappropriate sexual development in such patients is due to an overlapping secretion of gonadotropins and prolactin along with the expected hypersecretion of TSH. The mechanism of this phenomenon has been partially cla-

rified by the finding that the hypothalamic thyrotropin-releasing hormone (TRH) stimulates the pituitary to secrete both prolactin and TSH and that hyperprolactinemia as well as elevated TSH levels accompany long-standing primary hypothyroidism. Following the initiation of adequate substitution therapy with thyroid hormone, levels of both TSH and prolactin return to normal. Although this explains the galactorrhea, the mechanism of the excessive gonadal stimulation remains unclear, since by bioassay, urinary gonadotropic hormones usually are not elevated. The explanation of the gonadal stimulation may be found in the molecular overlap that exists between the TSH, LH, and FSH molecules. All three glycohormones share a common alpha subunit, but they differ in their beta subunits, which confer their respective hormonal specificities. Detailed analysis of these hormones and their respective subunits in the plasma of these patients should shed light on which tropic hormones are responsible for the gonadal stimulation.

TREATMENT. Substitution therapy in older children with hypothyroidism should follow the same guidelines outlined for the treatment of cretinism. Most children respond well to a dose of L-thyroxine equivalent to about 100 μg/m^2 body surface. However, the response of the hypothyroid child to even a small amount of hormone is so dramatic that there is a temptation to provide less than full replacement dosages. Parents are frequently alarmed by an initial rapid weight loss, excessive shedding of hair, and increased assertiveness of previously passive children. These complaints usually are not supported by direct evidence of thyrotoxicity, and they disappear with continued treatment. Following institution of treatment, the hypothyroid child resumes growth at a rate greater than normal, the period of so-called catch-up growth; indeed, accurate serial height measurements provide the best assurance that the dosage provided is adequate. Excessive dosage is marked by disproportionate advancement in skeletal age, which should be avoided, since this will hasten the closure of epiphyses and shorten the ultimate stature attained.

Goiter and Transient Hypothyroidism in Newborns

ETIOLOGY. The presence of a goiter at birth usually is due to ingestion of goitrogenic substances by the mother. Infants with cretinism due to an inborn error of metabolism may have a palpable thyroid gland, but only rarely is this sufficiently enlarged to be visible or to threaten respiration. Infants with severe peroxidase deficiencies are more prone to have large neonatal goiters than are those with other hereditary defects. In areas of endemic goiter, congenital goiter is a frequent cause of neonatal death by asphyxiation.

In the United States the most frequent and serious cause of neonatal goiter is maternal ingestion of large dosages of iodides during pregnancy (Fig. 34), usually prescribed as expectorants in asthma or for treatment of maternal thyrotoxicosis. There is convincing evidence that iodides potentiate those goitrogenic sub-

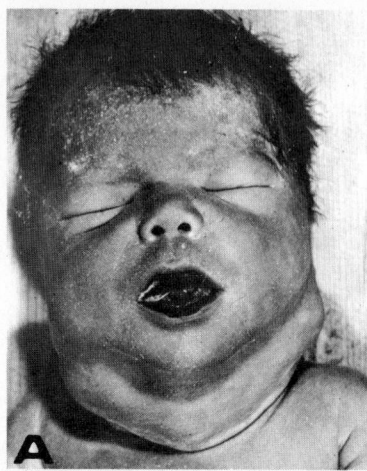

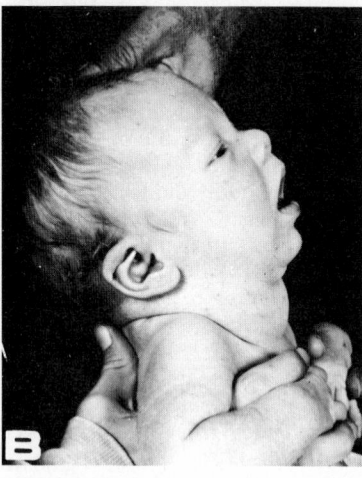

FIG. 34. Iodide goiters in newborns. The mothers of all 4 infants suffered from asthma and received medication containing iodides during their pregnancies. A. Full-term infant who died of asphyxiation 18 minutes after birth. B. Infant 1 month of age who survived, but who may have incurred mild brain damage. PBI was 18 μg/100 ml and BEI was 4.6 μg/100 ml. (From Galina, Avnet, and Inhorn: N. Engl. J Med 267:1124, 1962.)

stances that act by inhibiting peroxidase enzymes. Many drugs given to patients with asthma are complex formulations containing a variety of substances that might potentially influence thyroid function. The mothers of these children often have taken iodide for many years without developing large goiters and have been euthyroid during pregnancy. The unusual sensitivity of the fetus to iodides is probably caused by the great capacity of the fetal gland to concentrate this element during the latter period of pregnancy. However, since many women take comparable dosages of iodides during pregnancy without apparent harm to their babies, it is suspected that the severely affected infants may have some additional predisposing abnormality. Other goitrogens that have caused neonatal goiter are the thioureas, sulfonamides, and hematinic preparations

containing cobalt. The thyroid glands of these babies usually exhibit extreme hyperplasia. Neonatal goiters due to propylthiouracil are rare unless exceptionally large dosages are given to the mother with thyrotoxicosis. The dosage of the drug appears to be a more critical factor than the mother's thyroidal status.

TREATMENT. Neonatal goiter due to maternal ingestion of goitrogenic substances is usually of short duration and disappears spontaneously. It may be necessary to interrupt breast feeding, as the thiourea drugs and iodides are secreted in breast milk. If hypothyroidism is present or if the goiter is sufficiently large to cause dyspnea, it is advisable to provide full substitution therapy with thyroid hormone to achieve immediate euthyroidism and more rapid shrinkage of the gland. For this purpose, T3 may be the drug of choice because of its more rapid onset of action. Iodides are contraindicated, since they make the gland more firm and may aggravate tracheal compression. If respiratory obstruction is severe, tracheal decompression must be carried out by surgical resection of the thyroid isthmus. In these babies, tracheostomy alone is hazardous, and any attempt to carry out this procedure usually ends fatally. Infants with large goiters at birth are often hypothyroid during intrauterine life, as well as transitorily following birth. Permanent mental damage may have been inflicted in such babies even though a euthyroid state has been quickly achieved in the newborn period.

GOITER IN CHILDHOOD AND ADOLESCENCE

Simple Goiter

Simple thyroid enlargement is usually a response to compensatory stimulation by pituitary thyrotropic hormone. TSH is secreted whenever the level of circulating thyroid hormone falls, regardless of the cause.

Iodine Deficiency and Endemic Goiter

On a worldwide basis the most common cause of thyroid enlargement is endemic goiter. Although it has been demonstrated that iodine deficiency is the principal cause, there is no simple linear relationship between the iodine content of the soil or water and the incidence of thyroid enlargement. In some areas, particularly those that are isolated, it is believed that the pattern of the endemic goiter is modified by genetic abnormalities due to inbreeding or by goitrogenic agents in the water or diet. Recently, the concept that pollution of water supplies might be an important etiologic factor has been revived.

Simple goiter still is common, even in regions where iodine is plentiful or where the diet has been fortified by iodized salt. The possibility that a relative degree of iodine deficiency is responsible for some instances of goiter in nonendemic regions is difficult to exclude, since the requirement for iodine is moderately increased during adolescence and pregnancy and greatly increased in patients with certain types of errors in thyroidal biosynthesis. The presence of iodine deficiency should be suspected in any euthyroid goitrous individual with an abnormally high thyroidal uptake of [131]I. Indeed, results of iodine kinetic studies in iodine deficiency closely resemble those in hyperthyroidism.

If iodine deficiency is suspected, it can be corrected by the provision of iodized salt. The time-honored practice of administering Lugol's solution for the treatment of goiter is irrational and frequently harmful. Each drop of Lugol's solution contains approximately 8,000 μg of elemental iodine, an amount more than 50 times the daily requirement. Such massive dosages have an inhibitory effect on thyroidal biosynthesis and may provoke hypothyroidism in susceptible patients.

As judged by ^{131}I kinetic studies, iodine deficiency is a rare cause of goiter along the eastern seaboard and probably in other parts of the United States. Studies of urinary iodine excretion have revealed average values as high as 325 μg/day in regions of the United States, in contrast to values in the range of 100 μg/day in Western Europe and below 50 μg/day in most regions of endemic goiter. Since the accumulation of a tracer dose of ^{131}I is reciprocally related to the daily inorganic iodine consumption, regional differences in iodine intake are also reflected in the "normal" [131]I uptake values. The 24-hour ^{131}I uptake in apparently healthy children on the eastern seaboard is frequently about 10 to 20 percent, whereas in Europe uptakes of 30 to 50 percent are more characteristic. In iodine-deficient areas of South America, uptakes of 80 percent are common in euthyroid nongoitrous subjects.

Pittman demonstrated that in Alabama between 1959 and 1968 average normal values of ^{131}I uptake decreased from 28.6 to 15.4 percent. This was attributed to a tripling of the average daily consumption of inorganic iodides, primarily as a consequence of adding iodates to white bread.

Exposure To Goitrogenic Agents

Any food or drug that interferes with thyroid hormone synthesis is a potential cause of goiter. A partial list of such agents is given in Table 28. However, in only

TABLE 28. Some Goitrogenic Agents

Anions
   Iodine (in large amounts)
   Perchlorate
   Thiocyanate
Cations
   Cobalt (in certain hematinic preparations)
   Arsenic salts
   Lithium salts
Drugs
   Propylthiouracil
   Methimazole
   p-Aminosalicylic acid
   Aminoglutethimide
   Phenylbutazone
Naturally occurring substances
   Goitrin (1,5-vinyl-2-thiooxazolidone) (present in cabbage and other
     members of the genus *Brassica*)
   Soybeans (not soybean milk as presently prepared)

a small proportion of the patients presenting with simple goiter is it possible to identify a known goitrogen. Dietary goitrogens are particularly difficult to identify, since they may reach the subject through a devious route. Clements demonstrated a great increase in the incidence of goiter in Tasmanian school children after the introduction of a new forage crop of the genus *Brassica*. He was able to relate this to the presence of a goitrogenic agent in the milk of cows fed on this crop.

It is our impression that excessive intake of iodine is becoming an increasingly common cause of goiter. In some instances the source of this iodine has been traced to chronic medication with cold remedies and antiasthmatic drugs, but more commonly the source of exposure cannot be found. High levels of inorganic iodide inhibit thyroid function in the same manner as do thiourea goitrogens. Peroxidase is inhibited, and there is a shift to the left in the intrathyroidal iodoamino acids, with increases in the ratios of iodotyrosines to iodothyronines and of MIT to DIT. Furthermore, high levels of iodides potentiate the effects of other drugs that by themselves are only weakly goitrogenic. For these reasons it is a matter of considerable concern that many communities have recently begun to substitute iodine for chlorine to purify public water supplies.

Hashimoto's Struma

Hashimoto's struma (chronic thyroiditis, lymphadenoid goiter, autoimmune thyroiditis) was defined in 1912 when Hashimoto described 4 patients with goiters that on biopsy were characterized by diffuse infiltrations of plasma cells and lymphocytes, fibrosis, parenchymal atrophy, and eosinophilic degeneration in some of the acini. The disease has a marked predilection for females. Although it was once thought to occur only rarely before adolescence, it is being diagnosed increasingly in younger children. The onset is usually insidious, with no history of painful thyroid gland enlargement or fever. Occasionally patients, particularly those in adolescence, transiently experience tachycardia, nervousness, and other signs suggestive of thyrotoxicosis, but exophthalmos is not present. The thyroid gland is usually irregularly enlarged and firm, with accentuation of the normal lobular architecture. Not infrequently the goiter gives rise to the sensation of local pressure and difficulty in swallowing. Lymph nodes are often enlarged, especially the lymph nodes along the cervical chain and the delphian node above the isthmus.

The course of Hashimoto's struma, if left untreated, is variable. In some patients the gland undergoes atrophy, and the patient presents with acquired myxedema without any recognized period of compensatory hypertrophy. More frequently the gland slowly undergoes progressive enlargement, with maintenance of the euthyroid state for long periods of time. However, myxedema may ensue at any time.

Although the exact mechanism remains undetermined, it is likely that the histologic picture in the thyroid glands of patients with Hashimoto's struma is due to an autoimmune reaction of the delayed hypersensitivity type. Similar lesions have been produced experimentally by immunizing animals with thyroid extracts from the same or different species or by infusing lymphocytes from previously sensitized animals.

A characteristic feature of Hashimoto's struma is the presence of circulating antithyroid antibodies. Antibodies directed to at least four different components of the thyroid gland have been described: those directed to thyroglobulin, a colloid component other than thyroglobulin, thyroid microsomes, and thyroid nuclei. The prevalence of such antibodies is dependent on the patient's age and the nature of the detection system employed. Children and adolescents tend to have lower titers than older patients, and their levels may remain undetectable with the usual clinical tests. Even in adults with biopsy-proven Hashimoto's struma, up to 10 percent fail to display elevated titers, as judged by the tanned red cell hemagglutination technique (which is commonly used to measure antibodies directed against thyroglobulin). However, with the use of specific radioactive competitive binding assays for antimicrosomal and antithyroglobulin antibodies, the incidence of elevated titers approaches nearly 100 percent in adults with biopsy-proven disease; whether this concordance will apply equally well in children remains to be seen.

The presence of antithyroid antibodies should not be considered a definitive diagnostic test for Hashimoto's struma. If sufficiently sensitive techniques are used, antithyroid antibodies are also universally present in untreated Graves' disease, and there is growing evidence that the two diseases are different manifestations of a similar pathogenetic process. A markedly increased prevalence of antithyroid antibodies is also found in patients with other autoimmune diseases, such as rheumatoid arthritis, Addison's disease, hypoparathyroidism, and pernicious anemia. The prevalence also is increased in patients with juvenile diabetes mellitus. These antibodies may be present even though the patient lacks any demonstrable abnormality of thyroid size or function. Hall found an increased prevalence of autoimmune antibodies in close relatives of affected individuals and concluded that the disease is due to a basic genetic defect either in the thyroid gland itself or in the immune mechanism.

The frequent association of Hashimoto's struma with antithyroid antibodies and other types of thyroid disease in close relatives is well established. Evidence that autoimmune thyroid disease is attributable to an inherited defect of the immune system, rather than being secondary to a primary abnormality in the thyroid gland itself, is derived from a number of studies employing advanced immunologic methodology. Using a sensitive leukocyte migration-inhibition test, Volpé has demonstrated that blood from virtually all patients with Hashimoto's struma and Graves' disease contains a population of thymus-dependent (T) lymphocytes sensitized against the particulate portion of thyroid cells (microsomes and cell membranes). Volpé has postulated that whereas all individuals develop such sensi-

tized T lymphocytes in a random fashion, in normal individuals the proliferation of clones of these cells is prevented by the normal operation of the immunologic surveillance system. A genetically determined defect in the surveillance system is therefore postulated in patients with autoimmune thyroid disease. The postulated defect would necessarily require a relatively high degree of specificity, since a generalized defect in surveillance would be accompanied by all of the manifestations seen in children with thymic aplasia.

Unsuppressed clones of T lymphocytes sensitized against thyroidal components could explain those histologic features of autoimmune thyroiditis that are suggestive of a cell-mediated immune response and also the presence of humoral antibodies directed at various thyroidal components. Although the latter antibodies are produced by B rather than T lymphocytes, it is currently believed that the interaction of T and B lymphocytes plays a crucial role in the elaboration of immunoglobulins by the latter cells. This hypothesis is compatible with the random emergence of autoimmune thyroid disease in a genetically predisposed population.

Although Hashimoto's struma was originally defined in terms of a specific histologic picture, and more recently in terms of specific immunologic abnormalities, the presence of this disorder may be suspected on the basis of characteristic thyroid function tests. A common finding is an abnormally large discrepancy between the PBI and the thyroxine iodine concentration due to excessive quantities of iodinated protein in the circulation. The thyroidal uptake of ^{131}I is exceedingly variable and by itself is of little diagnostic value. In some patients defective oxidation of iodide within the thyroid can be demonstrated by an abnormal discharge of radioactivity following administration of perchlorate.

One of the characteristics of this disorder is unusual sensitivity to iodides. This can be demonstrated by the iodide suppression test. In normal patients and in those with goiter from other causes, 2 mg of stable iodide reduce the 24-hour ^{131}I uptake by less than 50 percent. In one study of patients with Hashimoto's thyroiditis the average suppression was 77 percent (range 46 to 95 percent).

The abnormal sensitivity of patients with Hashimoto's thyroiditis to iodides has raised the question whether excessive iodine intake may play some etiologic role. Thyroid enlargement with a histologic picture similar to that of Hashimoto's struma has been produced experimentally in dogs by a diet with a high iodine content. Hashimoto's struma is rare in iodine-deficient areas with endemic goiter, whereas in many parts of the country the incidence of Hashimoto's struma has risen sharply and has paralleled the greatly increased intake of iodine already mentioned. While such observations are highly provocative, excess iodide ingestion fails to explain the familial pattern and immunologic abnormalities that are characteristic of the human disease. However, it can no longer be doubted that iodide therapy is contraindicated in the treatment of patients with this disorder.

Adolescent Goiter

The term adolescent goiter has no etiologic meaning, since the incidence of all types of goiter rises abruptly in the years preceding the onset of puberty, particularly in girls. The reasons for this are not known, although the initiation of gonadal and pituitary hormone secretions may be responsible. Estrogens are known to affect thyroid function by increasing the T4 binding capacity of plasma and by other means that are less well understood. Females are also more susceptible to all kinds of autoimmune disease than are males. The concept that more thyroid hormone is required to meet the so-called increased metabolic needs of adolescence is probably without foundation, since, when expressed on either a weight or surface-area basis, caloric expenditure is greater in boys than in girls, and in both sexes it decreases during adolescence. An increased glomerular filtration rate of iodide has been shown to occur during adolescence, and this would increase susceptibility to iodine deficiency unless balanced by a proportionate increase in rate of thyroidal uptake.

Familial Goiter

The most common finding in goitrous children has been, in our experience, a family history of goiter. In many children with a strong family history of thyroid disease, detailed tests of thyroid function fail to reveal identifiable defects. The genetic pattern in such families is suggestive of an autosomal dominant mode of transmission, with greater expression in the female, and Hashimoto's struma is a common finding. Most of the biosynthetic abnormalities that have been identified in patients with goitrous cretinism have also been associated with less severe forms of goiter that develop in postnatal life. Pendred's syndrome and deiodinase deficiencies have followed an autosomal recessive mode of inheritance.

TREATMENT OF SIMPLE GOITER. Simple enlargement of the thyroid, particularly if it is mild, often remains asymptomatic for many years or may regress spontaneously even without therapy. However, many patients who develop nodular goiters in the third, fourth, and fifth decades have a history of mild diffuse thyroid enlargement during childhood or adolescence. Nodular goiters in such patients may have developed from recurring episodes of hyperplasia and involution. This suspicion provides the rationale for treating those patients in whom pressure symptoms or cosmetic considerations provide insufficient grounds for undertaking long-term therapy.

Appropriate treatment for most types of goiter consists of providing full substitution therapy with desiccated thyroid, L-thyroxine, or L-triiodothyronine. The dosages employed are the same as those used for treating primary hypothyroidism. After several years have elapsed, the need for continuing treatment should be reevaluated by withdrawing the medication for a period of several months.

In those patients whose glands mainly exhibit hyperplasia, regression to normal size is often dramatic following institution of adequate replacement therapy. However, in Hashimoto's struma there may be little visible response to treatment, particularly if there is much fibrosis and scarring, but even in these patients full substitution should be continued indefinitely to inhibit further TSH stimulation. Iodides are contraindicated in most forms of simple goiter.

Lingual Goiter and Thyroglossal Duct Cysts

A number of children with ectopic thyroid glands first come to attention because of an enlarging mass at the base of the tongue or along the course of the thyroglossal duct (p. 1663). Surgical excision of a lingual thyroid is often undertaken because of progressive enlargement with attendant dysphagia and irritation from trauma. The enlargement may occur at any age, but it commonly is accelerated shortly before adolescence. In most, if not all, cases the lingual thyroid is the only functional thyroid tissue present, and its enlargement represents a compensatory phenomenon for impending hypothyroidism. Provision of complete substitution treatment usually causes the goiter to shrink sufficiently that surgery can be avoided. Full substitution must be continued for life.

Severe hypothyroidism occasionally follows surgical removal of what has been presumed to be a thyroglossal duct cyst (Fig. 35). As with lingual thyroids, masses high in the neck often prove to be the only functional thyroid

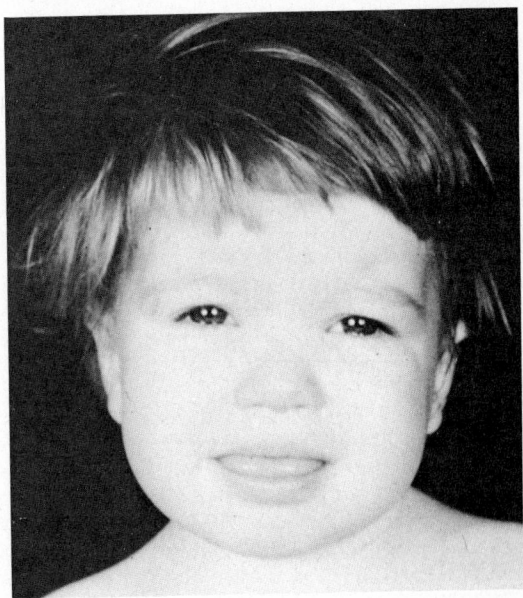

FIG. 35. Infant 19 months of age who became severely hypothyroid after a thyroglossal duct cyst was removed at 12 months of age. Note puffy face, pallor, and large tongue. (From Strickland, Macfie, Van Wyk, and French: JAMA 208:207, 1969.)

tissue present. In some cases, enlargement of the mass is correlated with failing thyroid function prior to surgery. Such patients may be considered to have mild forms of thyroid dysgenesis. In these patients the ectopic thyroid remnant has sufficient capacity to enlarge and function for the patient to be maintained in a euthyroid state for some time after birth, and cretinism does not occur. We have seen 6 children in whom such thyroglossal cysts proved to be the sole functioning thyroid tissue; in 5 of them the error was not recognized until growth had slowed and symptoms of hypothyroidism had appeared. For this reason it is prudent to perform ^{131}I uptake study with scan prior to surgical removal of a midline mass in the neck of a young child. If the mass accumulates iodine, surgery usually can be avoided by placing the child on full substitution doses of thyroid hormone.

Subacute Thyroiditis

Subacute thyroiditis is a self-limited inflammation of the thyroid that usually follows an upper respiratory illness. A few patients have been identified with mumps virus and others with cat-scratch fever. It is likely that a variety of viral agents may be responsible for this condition. In contrast to the situation with other thyroid disease, the incidence is the same in both sexes. The onset is accompanied by fever and pain that may occur locally or may be referred to the angles of the jaws. The thyroid gland is exquisitely sensitive to palpation. The inflammation may persist for a number of weeks, but it usually resolves spontaneously.

Symptoms usually can be controlled by large doses of acetylsalicylic acid or, in severe cases, corticosteroids. Suppressive dosages of thyroid hormone may also give symptomatic relief. The level of serum thyroxine may occasionally become elevated, and mild symptoms of thyrotoxicosis may develop during the acute phase. Most patients do not develop antithyroid antibodies, but recover normally, with no residual defect in thyroid function. Subacute thyroiditis may sometimes be difficult to distinguish from acute purulent thyroiditis. We have observed several children with purulent abscesses due to nonhemolytic streptococci; they required antibiotic therapy and surgical drainage.

JUVENILE THYROTOXICOSIS

Thyrotoxicosis in childhood and adolescence (Graves' disease) occurs almost exclusively as a consequence of diffuse thyroid hyperplasia, rather than hyperfunctioning nodules. Girls are afflicted approximately six times as often as boys. Although the disease is not uncommon in preschool children and rarely may begin in infancy, there is a sharp increase in incidence as children approach adolescence.

ETIOLOGY. This disease has some genetic basis, since a high proportion of patients come from families in whom thyrotoxicosis has occurred in a parent, grandparent, uncle, or aunt. A prevalent opinion is that both Graves' disease and Hashimoto's struma arise randomly in a genetically predisposed population. The concordance rate for Graves' disease in monozygotic twins has been reported as 30 to 60 percent; in dizygotic twins it has been reported as 3 to 9 percent. Family studies have disclosed that a high percentage of near relatives have circulating antithyroid antibodies; in these individuals there is an increased incidence of both Graves' disease and Hashimoto's struma. Data concerning the mendelian pattern of inheritance of this trait are conflicting. Based on pedigree analyses in Denmark, Bartels suggested that the predisposition to Graves' disease is inherited as a simple autosomal recessive trait with greater penetrance in the female. Others have postulated an autosomal dominant mode of inheritance, and yet others have attempted to explain the predilection for females on the basis of X-linked inheritance. However, a more probable explanation for the increased frequency in females is that estrogenic hormones may play a potentiating role, since many autoimmune disorders occur with greater frequency in the female during the reproductive years and are accentuated during pregnancy.

For many years Graves' disease was believed to have psychosomatic origins, since the onset of the hyperthyroid state sometimes follows some type of psychic trauma; in some instances this association is striking. According to this hypothesis, neural factors would release excessive quantities of TSH from the pituitary gland, but this has been disproved by the observation that most patients with Graves' disease have either greatly diminished or undetectable levels of TSH in plasma. If stress plays an initiating role in the onset of thyrotoxicosis, it must be by some other mechanism, possibly by hypersecretion of glucocorticoid hormones that affect immunologic responses.

Evidence that Graves' disease arises from an intrinsic abnormality within the thyroid gland itself is based on certain peculiarities of iodine metabolism that are characteristic of this disorder. Werner has shown that in thyrotoxicosis the uptake of ^{131}I by the thyroid gland is not suppressed by administration of T3, whereas administration of similar doses to normal individuals results in a fall of more than 40 percent. Administration of stable iodide to patients with Graves' disease produces a greater than normal inhibition of both ^{131}I uptake and hormonal release from the gland.

Substantial progress toward an understanding of Graves' disease has come from the demonstration by Purves and Adams, by McKenzie, and by Kriss that the plasma of many patients with Graves' disease contains a substance with thyroid-stimulating properties that differs from normal thyrotropin. When injected into mice, this material, known as long-acting thyroid stimulator (LATS), has a much more prolonged action than normal thyrotropic hormone. LATS has now been isolated in relatively pure form from the blood of thyrotoxic patients and has been identified as a 7S gamma globulin. The origin of this presumed antibody is in lymphoid tissue, and in vitro cultures of lymphocytes from thyrotoxic patients yield substantial quantities of LATS. During incubation with ^{14}C-labeled amino acids added to such lymphocyte cultures, the radioactive label is incorporated into 7S globulins with LATS activity. This material has been shown to bind to cytoplasmic microsomes in thyroid cells, but not to cells from other organs. LATS stimulates adenylate cyclase in thyroid cell membranes in a manner similar to TSH. In other biochemical variables, as well, LATS mimics the action of TSH. Papain digestion of LATS liberates a shorter-chain peptide that has a much briefer action on the thyroid, more nearly like that of pituitary TSH.

A causal role for LATS in the genesis of the hyperthyroid state has been disputed on the basis that these thyroid-stimulating antibodies are undetectable by the mouse bioassay in up to 30 percent of patients with classic untreated Graves' disease. However, nearly 100 percent of such patients can be shown to have thyroid-stimulating immunoglobulins by more sensitive in vitro tests on human thyroid tissue, in which LATS antibodies mimic the action of TSH. Among the responses reported are stimulation of colloid droplets in human thyroid slices, stimulation of adenylate cyclase in thyroid cells or membranes, and competition of LATS with ^{125}I-TSH for binding to the thyroid receptor on cell membranes. The results of the latter test leave little doubt about the central role of specific immunoglobulins in the pathophysiology of Graves' disease.

The production of these humoral antibodies by B lymphocytes is in all probability a secondary response to a cell-mediated immune reaction requiring involvement of T lymphocytes in a manner similar to that postulated for Hashimoto's struma (p. 1681). Cell cultures of lymphocytes from patients with Graves' disease produce immunoglobulins only after stimulation with phytohemagglutinin. Since the latter substance stimulates only T cells (which are incapable of secreting immunoglobulins), it may be inferred that cell-mediated as well as humoral immune mechanisms are involved in the genesis of the thyrotoxic state. Large gaps remain in our knowledge of how these autoimmune processes are initiated and perpetuated, and such knowledge is essential before fully rational and specific modalities of therapy can be developed.

CLINICAL FEATURES. The onset of thyrotoxicosis usually is insidious, with a period of increasing nervousness, palpitation, and increased appetite. Extreme weight loss occurs in some patients, but not infrequently this is prevented by development of a voracious appetite. Rarely, children, especially adolescents, actually show a weight increase with the onset of the disease. There is a tendency for thyrotoxic children to be in the upper percentile channels for height. Except for exophthalmos and other eye signs, the symptoms of thyrotoxicosis are nonspecific and for prolonged periods may be mistaken for some other condition. Behavior abnormalities, declining school performance, and nervous instability frequently dominate the clinical picture, and often the patient is initially referred to a guidance clinic or psychiatrist. In other patients cardiovascular signs are more prominent, and attention is focused on a cardiac murmur or decreased exercise tolerance.

Most of the signs and symptoms of Graves' disease

are similar to those produced by a hyperactive sympathetic nervous system; therefore they can be fully simulated by anxiety, fright, or acute illness. Even in patients in whom tachycardia is not impressive, the pulse pressure is widened and the precordium overactive. Underlying heart disease is difficult to exclude in the presence of cardiomegaly, ejection murmurs, precordial thrill, and gallop rhythms. Other signs of sympathetic overactivity are tremor, increased skin temperature, excessive perspiration, rapid tendon reflexes, and emotional lability. Even the increased basal metabolic rate may be mediated through a hyperactive sympathetic nervous system. It is sufficient only to recall that the highest metabolic rates encountered clinically are not in thyrotoxic patients but in those harboring pheochromocytomas.

The size of the thyroid gland is highly variable, and the development of a goiter may escape notice in a patient whose gland is only slightly enlarged. A better appreciation of thyroidal size and consistency can be gained if the patient is examined in the supine position with the neck thrust forward by hyperextension (Fig. 36). Bimanual palpation during swallowing and during digital displacement of each lobe delineates the thyroid from other structures. Tracings of the two-dimensional projection of the gland, outlined by skin pencil, provide a valuable method of recording serial changes.

The characteristics of the thyroid to be noted on physical examination are size, uniformity, and consistency. The presence of a bruit or thrill provides some indication of the degree of hyperplasia, but it has no specific diagnostic value. During phases of active hyperplasia the thyroid typically has a resilient bulging characteristic that is lost as recovery takes place.

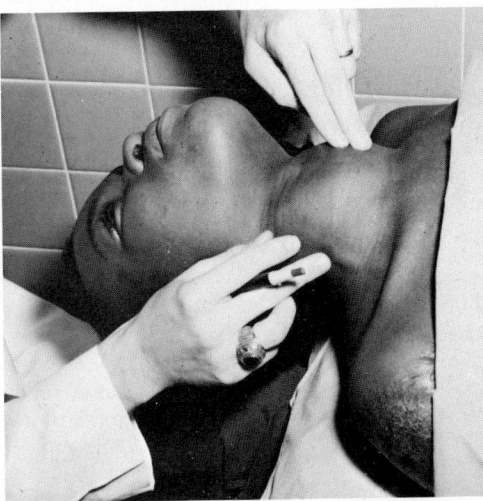

FIG. 36. Preferred method of palpating thyroid gland. Neck is hyperextended over end of examining table. Lobular outline and consistency are then easily determined by bimanual palpation. Gland is outlined by skin pencil and transcribed on transparent paper. Serial records of thyroidal size and consistency provide one of the best methods for following the progress of the disease.

EYE SIGNS. Severe ophthalmopathy is much less common in children with Graves' disease than in older individuals, and malignant exophthalmos is virtually unknown. The eye findings in this disease may be grouped as those due to sympathetic hyperactivity and those due to specific pathologic changes in the orbit. Those due to sympathetic hyperactivity give the appearance of a stare, owing to retraction of the upper lid and a wide palpebral aperture. There is also a lag in the descent of the upper lid on downward gaze, as well as infrequent blinking and absence of forehead wrinkling on upward gaze. The eyes frequently present a glazed appearance. These findings, to a large extent, parallel the severity of the disease and disappear as the patient is rendered euthyroid.

In addition, there are changes in the orbit that are more specific for Graves' disease and are accounted for by infiltrations of mucopolysaccharides, lymphocytes, and edema fluid within the ocular muscles, lacrimal glands, and retro-orbital fat. These changes lead to exophthalmos, ophthalmoplegia, chemosis of the conjunctiva, pain, swelling, and irritation. Although the inflammatory changes usually improve with treatment of the hyperthyroid state, some degree of exophthalmos tends to remain after recovery from the disease.

UNUSUAL FINDINGS. Accumulations of mucopolysaccharides in skeletal muscles and pretibial myxedema are findings that are particularly likely to occur in patients with severe exophthalmos and in individuals with dependent edema or previous trauma to their legs. Pretibial myxedema is rare in children. Occasionally a patient with severe untreated hyperthyroidism may present with profound muscle weakness and a history of collapse that occurs suddenly with attempts to walk or get out of bed. Severe muscular wasting is present in some, but not all, of these patients. It is likely that this degree of myopathy is not due to the thyrotoxicosis itself but is a secondary consequence. Patients with severe long-standing thyrotoxicosis become depleted of B-complex vitamins. Pyridoxine deficiency has been demonstrated in such patients by the finding that they respond to a tryptophan load by excreting abnormally large quantities of xanthurenic acid; this is corrected by administering pyridoxine. These and other unusual features that are sporadically present in thyrotoxicosis are probably secondary consequences of a long-standing hypermetabolic state rather than direct results of increased thyroxine levels.

GRAVES' DISEASE AND HASHIMOTO'S STRUMA. Occasionally patients are encountered who have histologic and laboratory findings characteristic of Hashimoto's struma but who exhibit mild to severe thyrotoxicosis and resistance to thyroidal suppression by T3. As in uncomplicated Graves' disease, the iodine suppression test is positive. The somewhat whimsical terms Hashitoxicosis and Toximoto's disease have been applied to these patients. These terms may serve a useful purpose in underscoring the points of similarity between the two disorders and stimulate further search for fundamental mechanisms common to both. Combined treatment with PTU and thyroid hormone, as outlined for treatment of thyrotoxicosis, is probably the preferable form of management for this group of patients.

LABORATORY DIAGNOSIS. The diagnosis of hyperthyroidism usually can be made on clinical grounds, and laboratory confirmation can be limited to the determination of plasma thyroxine content. Determinations of the plasma T3 concentration and free T4 level may be helpful in some patients. With rare exceptions, the concentration of serum TSH is low, and TSH response to TRH administration is absent or limited.

Determination of radioactive iodine uptake by the thyroid gland rarely is used by itself as a diagnostic method for thyrotoxicosis; measurements at 1, 3, and 6 hours more reliably discriminate between hyperthyroid and euthyroid patients than do 24-hour measurements. The principal use of radioactive iodine uptake measurements is in the T3 suppression test, which is used to indicate independence from pituitary control. This test may be of great help in diagnosing those patients whose chief findings are goiter and nervousness but who lack eye findings and other clear signs of hyperthyroidism. T3 is given for 8 days at a dosage of 100 μg daily; ^{131}I uptake is determined both before and at the completion of this treatment. In normal individuals and in those with simple goiter, the second iodine uptake should fall by at least 50 percent, whereas in Graves' disease the suppression is less marked.

TREATMENT. Treatment of thyrotoxicosis must be directed toward reducing the secretory rate of thyroid hormones and, if possible, blunting the toxic effects produced by high circulating levels. Three principal methods are available for reducing thyroid secretions: subtotal ablation with radioactive iodine, subtotal thyroidectomy, and blocking thyroid hormone biosynthesis by means of drugs.

TREATMENT WITH RADIOACTIVE IODINE. In terms of ease, cost, efficacy, and short-term safety, there is no doubt that treatment with ^{131}I is superior. The potential hazards of radioactive iodine are induction of permanent hypothyroidism, thyroid cancer, leukemia, and genetic damage. The magnitude of these risks in childhood is unknown, and estimates have varied widely. Until very recently the prevailing practice in most centers had been to use ^{131}I only in the rare cases where other forms of therapy could not be used or would carry an increased risk. Since the introduction of radioactive iodine, there has been a perceptible lessening of fears concerning harmful late side effects. For this reason many clinics are now using ^{131}I more liberally in the treatment of thyrotoxicosis in childhood. The reasons for taking a more cautious approach are as follows:

Late development of primary hypothyroidism after ^{131}I therapy has occurred in every series of patients studied, regardless of the dosage employed. The extent of this complication is only now being recognized, since hypothyroidism often does not develop until some years have elapsed. It is estimated that 50 percent of patients treated with ^{131}I will be hypothyroid within 10 years, and a large majority within 20 years. Thus prolonged medical follow-up and the eventual requirement of lifelong medication cannot be avoided with this mode of treatment.

Radioactive iodine has now been used therapeutically *in adults* for a sufficient length of time that fears of inducing thyroid carcinoma have been largely alleviated. This is less so in children. It has been well demonstrated that thyroid glands of young animals are much more susceptible to induction of thyroid carcinoma by ionizing radiation than those of older animals. Radiation to the neck in infancy has been incriminated as the principal cause of thyroid cancer in children, whereas this is infrequent in adults. Finally, several children treated with ^{131}I have been reported with the late development of thyroid nodules; in at least one instance the histologic diagnosis was that of carcinoma.

Following administration of therapeutic doses of ^{131}I, gross abnormalities have been described in the chromosomes of white blood cells; the implications of this finding are uncertain. The development of leukemia *in adults* following ^{131}I treatment of thyrotoxicosis is no more frequent than in the population at large. Since the number of children treated with therapeutic dosages of ^{131}I is relatively small, it is impossible to be certain that children will not develop leukemia more frequently than adults. In all probability, the risk of leukemia is sufficiently low that it would not by itself constitute a contraindication.

Available reports provide no evidence that fetal malformations occur more frequently in the offspring of women previously treated with ^{131}I than in infants of other women. However, an increased number of mutant genes of the recessive variety can be determined in a statistical sense only after several generations have elapsed. Therefore the risk of genetic damage to an individual whose entire reproductive life still lies ahead cannot be ascertained directly. However, if the bladder is emptied frequently after therapeutic dosages of ^{131}I, the gonadal radiation dose should not exceed that from many routine radiographic techniques.

It has been the practice in most clinics to reserve the use of ^{131}I for treatment of thyrotoxicosis in older adolescents who fail to follow a medical regimen and who cannot be adequately prepared for surgical thyroidectomy. However, this is a group of patients who also often prove unreliable in taking thyroid substitution therapy after development of hypothyroidism. Several such patients have indeed become myxedematous and have failed to return to the clinic for follow-up supervision.

SUBTOTAL SURGICAL THYROIDECTOMY. With proper preparation of the patient for surgical thyroidectomy, the immediate operative mortality has been all but eliminated. With proper surgical management, most patients achieve satisfactory remission, and requirements for intensive medical follow-up are less rigorous than in those patients treated exclusively by pharmacologic agents. However, the incidence of hypoparathyroidism following subtotal thyroidectomy is still appreciable, and this serious complication may require lifelong treatment. Unless an adequate amount of thyroid tissue is removed, a satisfactory remission may not be achieved, or there may be a late recurrence. In the large Mayo Clinic series reported by Hayles and associates, recurrences were encountered in 28 percent of 196 surgically treated patients. The average interval between surgery and relapse was 8 years, and in 3 patients relapses occurred more than 25 years later. When hyperthyroidism recurs in a surgical remnant, secondary operations are fraught with an increased hazard of injuring the recurrent laryngeal nerves or removing the parathyroid glands. If, on the other hand, sufficient thyroid tissue is removed to guarantee against such recurrences, the incidence of postoperative hypothyroidism is greatly increased. In some series the incidence of permanent hypothyroidism after subtotal thyroidectomy has approached 50 percent.

MEDICAL MANAGEMENT. Definitive medical management with antithyroid drugs is inefficient, since a prolonged period is required to render the patient euthyroid, and close supervision by the physician is necessary for a period of years. Even in those patients treated successfully a permanent remission is sustained in not more than 60 to 70 percent. Although the surgical complications are avoided, a small percentage of patients are hypersensitive to propylthiouracil or methimazole and develop either skin rashes or a sufficient degree of leukopenia to require discontinuation of the drug. These reactions are usually mild, and they disappear when the drug is withdrawn. Rarely a patient will develop a lupus-like syndrome.

The choice of therapy in thyrotoxicosis must be individualized, taking into consideration any coexisting illnesses, the quality of thyroid surgery available, and the socioeconomic factors that play such a large role in determining the success of a prolonged medical regimen. The choice between subtotal thyroidectomy and definitive long-term medical therapy is usually best deferred for several months, since the initial management is the same, and in any event surgery is contraindicated until after the patient has been rendered euthyroid.

In severely toxic patients the β-adrenergic blocking agent propranolol has proved to be of great value in controlling many of the manifestations of Graves' disease. This agent has largely supplanted the use of such other antiadrenergic drugs as guanethidine, reserpine, and α-methyldopa. Propranolol produces both subjective and objective improvement in palpitation, excessive sweating, tremor, hyperactive reflexes, lid lag, and stare. However, its more impressive effects are in reducing the cardiac manifestations, which include tachycardia, elevated pulse pressure, and shortened circulation time. Since there is substantial evidence that thyroid hormones have a direct effect on myocardial contractility apart from those mediated through the autonomic nervous system, it is not surprising that the increased cardiac contractility is not immediately diminished following acute administration of β-adrenergic blocking agents. However, controlled studies after more prolonged administration have not been reported. Propranolol has no effect on thyroid function per se, nor on exophthalmos.

β-Adrenergic blockade is of particular value in the initial treatment of severely thyrotoxic patients in the long interval before specific antithyroid drugs become effective. Although propranolol by itself should never be considered adequate preoperative preparation for subtotal thyroidectomy, it has proved of great value in hastening the preparation of patients who have not been optimally suppressed on antithyroid medication. Propranolol has in some instances proved life-saving in critically ill patients in thyroid storm or in neonates with congenital thyrotoxicosis. Propranolol is potentially dangerous in those with established cardiac failure or arrythmias. The drug is usually given at a dosage of 10 to 30 mg orally every 6 hours (adult dose), depending on the response of the patient. In critically ill patients it may be given with caution intravenously (0.1 mg/kg) using constant electrocardiographic monitoring.

In the United States, propylthiouracil and methimazole are the antithyroid drugs most commonly used. Both are reducing agents that act in the thyroid by inhibiting oxidation of iodide and thereby blocking synthesis of thyroid hormones. In addition, propylthiouracil reduces the conversion of T4 to T3 at the periphery. They do not block the release of thyroid hormones into the circulation nor the effect of TSH on the iodide pump. There is always a lag between institution of antithyroid therapy and achievement of a euthyroid state, since the biosynthetic block is not complete and the stores of preformed hormone must be discharged first. The rapidity of response to therapy correlates best with the initial size of the thyroid gland, rather than with the degree of thyrotoxicity. Those patients with a small gland and rapid thyroidal turnover usually exhibit marked improvement in a few weeks, whereas in those with very large glands a satisfactory euthyroid state may not be achieved for many months.

The initial dosage of propylthiouracil varies from 300 to 600 mg daily (175 mg/m^2 or 5 mg/kg) in dosages spaced at 6- or 8-hour intervals. The dosage of methimazole is about one-tenth that of propylthiouracil. If these dosages are continued after the patient becomes euthyroid, the gland will enlarge further because of the added stimulation by pituitary thyrotropic hormone. This compensatory enlargement can be averted by titrating the dosage of antithyroid drug downward. Since this manipulation of dosage requires careful supervision of the patient at frequent intervals, many clinics continue dosages of propylthiouracil as high as 300 to 400 mg/day for the duration of the illness and prevent the development of hypothyroidism and thyroid enlargement by adding thyroid hormone to the regimen as soon as the patient becomes euthyroid. T 3 is particularly useful for this purpose, since it does not itself contribute to the PBI or thyroxine concentration. With T3 dosages of 50 to 100 μg/day, the serum thyroxine level in adequately controlled patients on this combined regimen should be depressed well into the range usually associated with severe hypothyroidism. Should the patient develop renewed symptoms of thyrotoxicosis with a low serum T4 level, the dosage of exogenous T3 can be lowered safely; however, renewed thyrotoxicosis with a normal or elevated serum T4 level suggests that the antithyroid drugs either are not being taken regularly or are being prescribed at too low a dosage.

Serious toxic reactions to propylthiouracil are rare, but they may occur at any time in the course of therapy. Drug-induced leukopenia is often difficult to assess, since even without therapy patients with Graves' disease are prone to exhibit leukopenia and relative lymphocytosis. It is less important to obtain blood counts at frequent intervals than to ensure that the patient has a prompt hematologic investigation with every infection or unexplained fever. In those rare instances where severe granulocytopenia is attributable to medication, corticosteroids often induce prompt improvement in the blood picture. Although in some instances treatment can be resumed with methimazole, cross-reactions are common. In such patients, surgery should be carried out after obtaining as complete a remission as possible with Lugol's solution and propranolol. Sodium perchlorate at a dosage of 500 mg every 6 hours may be used as an alternative to Lugol's solution, but several fatal cases of aplastic anemia have occurred with this drug.

Skin rashes occur in about 5 percent of patients treated with propylthiouracil or methimazole early in the course of therapy, but they disappear when the drug is withheld. Often these rashes are mild and can be controlled with antihistamine drugs. As the patients becomes euthyroid, the propensity toward allergic phenomena becomes less marked. Patients who are markedly hypersensitive to propylthiouracil and/or methimazole should receive alternative forms of therapy, as indicated previously. We have observed several children on prophythiouracil who developed protracted hepatitis of unusual severity. In these patients it was impossible to ascertain whether this occurrence was a chance coincidence or was attributable to the drug or to underlying Graves' disease.

After all signs of thyrotoxicosis have disappeared, the best prognostic guide in judging when to discontinue therapy has been a marked diminution in the size of the thyroid and a loss of the resilient bulging quality that characterizes the hyperplastic gland. We do not discontinue therapy at less than 2 years. In many instances treatment has been continued for 3 to 4 years before the gland has lost its hyperplastic character.

Although it is not known whether management of thyrotoxicosis with antithyroid drugs has any influence on the fundamental disease process, it does permit the patient to remain euthyroid and in good health until such time as the disease has spontaneously run its course. When it is judged safe to discontinue therapy, propylthiouracil and T3 are reduced in stepwise fashion over a period of 4 to 6 months. Although a mild rebound in thyrotoxic symptoms often occurs after discontinuation of therapy, most patients settle down spontaneously and remain euthyroid without the need for reinstituting treatment.

Prior to the introduction of thiourea goitrogens in the treatment of thyrotoxicosis, it was customary to prepare patients for surgery by administering Lugol's solution. Large dosages of inorganic iodine not only block hormone biosynthesis but also inhibit the release of preformed hormone and render the gland less vascular. The effect on thyroidal status is more prompt than that of the thiourea goitrogens. Unfortunately, an iodine blockade can be maintained for only a limited period of time before escape occurs, and a fully euthyroid state is often not achieved. Therefore the use of inorganic iodine is now reserved for severely toxic patients with impending thyroid storm and for the immediate preoperative preparation of patients who are about to undergo subtotal thyroidectomy. In others, iodides may complicate long-term medical management by interfering with the involution of the gland.

THYROTOXICOSIS OF NEWBORNS

Rarely, thyrotoxicosis occurs in infants born to mothers with Graves' disease. Unlike the situation with classic Graves' disease, the sex incidence is equally distributed between males and females. Such infants usually exhibit exophthalmos. With rare exceptions, the disorder is self-limited and disappears spontaneously within about 3 months. The suggestion that neonatal Graves' disease is passively transmitted by maternal immunoglobulins is supported by the finding of LATS activity in the plasma of most of these infants. It is significant that 7S gamma globulins traverse the placenta, whereas normal thyrotropin does not. Occasionally the course of neonatal thyrotoxicosis is different from that described in that it persists for a much longer period of time and has the rest of the characteristics that are typical of classic Graves' disease. The etiology of this form of neonatal hyperthyroidism cannot be explained by passive placental transmission of maternal antibodies, but it could arise from maternal transmission of sensitized T lymphocytes that simulate the early appearance of the disease in a genetically predisposed infant.

Infants with neonatal thyrotoxicosis are threatened by asphyxiation by tracheal compression as well as by the thyrotoxic state itself. We have observed 1 infant with permanent distortion of her orbits and another who died in thyroid storm 48 hours after birth. The premature synostosis of cranial sutures in some of these infants is directly attributable to high levels of thyroid hormone, since a similar association has been reported in cretins treated with excessively high dosages of thyroid hormone. Although the disease is self-limited, treatment should be based on the same principles governing the management of other forms of Graves' disease and should be guided by the urgency of the problem. In severe cases, propylthiouracil, pro-

pranolol, and vigorous supportive measures are indicated. Iodides should be used only in the most severe cases, since the thyroid-blocking action is of limited duration, and high thyroidal iodine levels blunt the response to propylthiouracil.

THYROID NEOPLASMS IN CHILDHOOD AND ADOLESCENCE

A thyroid neoplasm should be suspected whenever a child is found to have a solitary mass with a consistency differing from that of the rest of the thyroid gland. A solitary nodule during the first two decades of life has a much greater chance of being malignant than those in older age groups. The incidence of cancer in children with thyroid nodules has been estimated to be 20 to 52 percent. The ratio of females to males among children with thyroid cancer is only 2:1, in contrast to the much higher predominance of females with thyroid enlargement from other causes. Nodular enlargement in the male is somewhat more likely to be cancerous than in the female.

CLASSIFICATION. A classification of thyroid neoplasms is shown in Table 29. Fifty percent or more of solitary thyroid nodules during childhood prove to be cystic lesions or benign adenomas. Hyperfunctioning adenomas are exceedingly uncommon during the first two decades of life. Well-differentiated carcinomas account for well over 90 percent of the malignant lesions in this age group. Further classification of well-differentiated carcinomas into papillary and follicular adenocarcinomas has received much more emphasis than is warranted, at least in children. If sufficient tissue sections are examined, most well-differentiated carcinomas will contain both histologic pictures, and management and prognosis are roughly similar for both types.

Other malignant tumors of the thyroid gland during

TABLE 29. Thyroid Neoplasms in Childhood and Adolescence*

Benign adenoma
  Fetal or embryonal
  Follicular
  Papillary
  Hyperfunctioning adenoma
Malignant tumors
  Well-differentiated adenocarcinoma
    Papillary or papillary–follicular
      Encapsulated or occult sclerosing
      Invasive
    Follicular
      Encapsulated
      Invasive
  Medullary carcinoma (from parafollicular cells)
  Undifferentiated (anaplastic, small cell, spindle cell, giant cell)
  Infiltrations and metastases from tumors arising elsewhere
    (lymphoma, sarcoma, metastatic carcinoma)

* Adapted from Thomas: In Sabiston (ed): Textbook of Surgery, Vol 1, 10th ed, 1972. Courtesy of W.B. Saunders.

childhood are accounted for by medullary carcinoma arising in the parafollicular cells, poorly differentiated thyroid carcinoma, and tumors such as lymphomas and metastatic carcinomas arising in other tissues. The prognosis in these tumors is much worse than in well-differentiated adenocarcinoma of the thyroid, and hence it is important to establish a tissue diagnosis as early as possible and design the treatment accordingly. Well-differentiated carcinomas have little tendency to become undifferentiated neoplasms.

ETIOLOGY. In experimental animals, thyroid neoplasia can be induced by ionizing radiation or by any influence that leads to prolonged stimulation by thyrotropic hormone. These factors are often synergistic, since in the presence of TSH stimulation, a smaller dose of radiation is required to induce neoplasia than in its absence. Thyroid tumors can be induced far more readily by irradiation in young animals than in older ones.

A frequent predisposing cause for development of thyroid cancer in children and young adults is irradiation of the thyroid gland during infancy and childhood. In Winship's series of 364 children with thyroid cancer, 80 percent had histories of prior radiotherapy. In most instances this had been administered during early infancy to the upper mediastinum and neck for control of "enlarged" thymus glands. Cancer also occurred following irradiation of hypertrophied tonsils and adenoids in older children and adolescents. The average time between the irradiation and the recognition of the tumor was 10.9 years. Adults who receive similar types of irradiation are less prone to develop subsequent thyroid cancer, but such cases are now being recognized with increasing frequency.

HORMONAL MANIFESTATIONS OF MEDULLARY CARCINOMA. Medullary carcinomas arising in the parafollicular or C cells of the thyroid gland are being recognized with increasing frequency. They have a distinctive histologic picture, with large deposits of amyloid situated among sheets of pleomorphic epithelial cells. Although many sporadic cases of medullary carcinoma have been described, at least half of them occur in kindreds with a number of afflicted individuals and are apparently inherited as an autosomal dominant trait. Many of these familial cases are associated with pheochromocytoma, parathyroid adenoma, mucosal neuromas, a marfanoid habitus, and neurofibromas. Some also are associated with ectopic secretion of ACTH and serotonin. The common feature of all these tumors is a neuroectodermal origin. Those with mucosal neuromas usually have a distinctive appearance, with protruding, thick, and often bumpy lips and occasionally prognathism.

The distinctive feature of medullary carcinoma is excessive secretion of calcitonin. Although calcitonin levels are invariably elevated in patients with palpable tumors, this tumor can be detected in children before the development of a palpable mass by calcitonin stimulation tests following administration of intravenous calcium or pentagastrin. Using the pentagastrin stimulation test, Hennessy and associates were able to identify medullary carcinoma in 4 prepubescent children of affected parents and remove the thyroid at a time when the tumor was only a few millimeters in size and could only be identified histologically. Since pentagastrin stimulation tests require only a few minutes to perform and can easily be done as an office procedure, they should be carried out at regular intervals on all children of affected parents.

DIAGNOSIS. Children with Hashimoto's struma frequently have a firm irregular gland with marked accentuation of the normal lobular pattern. However, the characteristic picture associated with this clinical condition is such that differentiation from a neoplasm is rarely difficult for a physician experienced in thyroid palpation. Open surgery of such a gland can usually be avoided by confirming the clinical impression with a needle biopsy and by demonstrating regression following administration of suppressive doses of thyroid hormone.

A scan of the neck following administration of ^{131}I or ^{99m}Tc is rarely decisive in the diagnosis of thyroid nodules during childhood, except in the rare case of a hyperfunctioning nodule. In such patients the nodule is said to be hot, whereas uptake of radioactivity in the rest of the gland is suppressed. Most other thyroidal neoplasms fail to accumulate iodine (cold nodules); however, failure to accumulate ^{131}I or ^{99m}Tc does not distinguish between benign and malignant lesions. Scanning the neck with ultrasound is of value in distinguishing cystic lesions and neoplasms from normal thyroid tissue neoplasms, since these lesions have a considerably different density than surrounding normal thyroid architecture. In most instances, however, pathologic examination is required for definitive diagnosis.

TREATMENT. Since solitary nodules occur rarely in childhood, and because a high percentage prove to be malignant, it is recommended that every child with such enlargement be submitted to simple removal of the affected lobe. No further surgery is necessary if the mass proves to be a cystic lesion or benign adenoma. Since well-differentiated carcinomas are prone to involve multifocal sites in the thyroid gland, total lobectomy should be carried out on the side of origin, and as much of the contralateral lobe should be excised as is compatible with preservation of the parathyroid glands and recurrent laryngeal nerves. Although accessible regional nodes should be removed, a mutilating neck dissection is rarely warranted. It is important that, following surgery, the patient be maintained on full substitution dosages of exogenous thyroid hormone to protect the gland from any further stimulation by thyrotropic hormone. Use of therapeutic dosages of ^{131}I following surgery is of no proven benefit in patients with well-differentiated thyroid carcinoma. On the other hand, whole body scans following administration of ^{131}I may be of value in the rare patient in whom distant metastases are suspected.

About three-fourths of all thyroid cancers have spread to regional lymph nodes by the time the initial diagnosis is made. However, the aggressiveness of the initial operation should be dictated more by the natural history of that particular cell type than by other considerations. Although every effort should be made to spare the parathyroid glands, permanent hypoparathyroidism is a common sequel to surgery for thyroid neoplasms. Consideration should be given to autotransplantation of parathyroid glands in cases where removal is necessary or where it occurs inadvertently. The treatment of hypoparathyroidism is discussed elsewhere (p. 248).

PROGNOSIS. The prognosis in children with well-differentiated thyroid cancer is far better than in most other types of childhood cancer. The course is usually an indolent one, with long periods in which there is little progression. In most instances, spread is confined to regional lymph nodes, with little tendency to metastasize by the blood. In a series of 54 patients with the diagnosis of well-differentiated carcinoma made before the age of 21 years, Buchwalter and associates were unable to demonstrate any difference in life expectancy when compared with a normal population of similar age. Since spread to the lymph nodes had occurred prior to surgery in most of these patients, the excellent prognosis may be related more to the biologic nature of this form of cancer than to total removal of all cancerous cells at the initial operation. Mortality in thyroid carcinoma during childhood and adolescence is primarily accounted for by the relatively uncommon instances of medullary carcinoma and undifferentiated carcinoma. In these cases more radical surgery combined with radiation or cancer chemotherapy is fully justified.

References

GENERAL

Gluck L: Modern Perinatal Medicine. Chicago, Year Book, 1975

Ingbar SH, Woeber KA: The Thyroid Gland. In Williams WH (ed): Textbook of Endocrinology. Philadelphia, WB Saunders, 1974

Means JH, DeGroot LJ, Stanbury JB: The Thyroid and Its Diseases, 3rd ed. New York, McGraw-Hill, 1963

Werner S, Ingbar SH: The Thyroid: A Fundamental and Clinical Text, 3rd ed. New York, Harper & Row, 1971

IODINE AND THYROID HORMONE METABOLISM

Braverman L, Ingbar S, Sterling K: Conversion of thyroxine (T_4) to triiodothyronine (T_3) in athyreotic human subjects. J Clin Invest 49:855, 1970

Dumont JE: The action of thyrotropin on thyroid metabolism. Vitam Horm 29:287, 1971

Greer MA, Solomon DH (eds): Handbook of Physiology, Vol 3 The Thyroid. Washington DC, American Physiological Society, 1974

Harrison TS: Adrenal medullary and thyroid relationships. Physiol Rev 44:161, 1964

Hershman JM, Bray GA (eds): Pharmacology of the Thyroid Gland. Oxford, Pergamon, 1975

McQuillan MT, Trikojus VM: Thyroglobulin. In Gottschalk A (ed): Glycoproteins, Their Composition, Structure, and Function. New York, Elsevier, 1972, p 926

Odell WD, Wilber JF, Utiger RD: Studies of thyrotropin physiology by means of radioimmunoassay. Recent Prog Horm Res 23:47, 1967

Pittman JA, Dailey GE, Beschi RJ: Changing normal values for thyroidal radioiodine uptake. N Engl J Med 280:1431, 1969

Samuels HH, Tsai JS: Thyroid hormone action. Demonstration of similar receptors in isolated nuclei of rat liver and cultured GH cells. J Clin Invest 53:656, 1974

Taurog A: Thyroid peroxidase and thyroxine biosynthesis. Recent Prog Horm Res 26:189, 1970

Wolff J: Iodide concentrating mechanism. In Berson SA (ed): Methods in Investigative and Diagnostic Endocrinology, Vol 1. Amsterdam, North Holland, 1972, p 115

FETAL AND NEWBORN THYROID FUNCTION

Chopra IJ, Sack J, Fisher DA: Circulating 3,3'5'-triiodothyronine (reverse T3) in the human newborn. J Clin Invest 55:1137, 1975

Ehrenberg A, Phelps D, Lam R, Fisher DA: Total and free thyroid hormone concentrations in the neonatal period. Pediatrics 53:211, 1974

Fisher DA, Dussault JH, Lam RW: Serum and gland triiodothyronine in the human fetus. J Clin Endocrinol Metab 36:397, 1973

——— Hobel CJ, Garza R, Pierce CA: Thyroid function in the preterm fetus. Pediatrics 46:208, 1970

——— Odell WD: Acute release of thyrotropin in the newborn. J Clin Invest 48:1670, 1969

——— Burrow GN (eds): Perinatal Thyroid Physiology and Disease, Vol 3. Kroc Foundation Series. New York, Raven, 1975

Greenberg AH, Czernichow P, Reba RC, Tyson J, Blizzard RM: Observations on the maturation of thyroid function in early fetal life. J Clin Invest 49:1790, 1970

Grumbach MM, Kaplan SL: Fetal pituitary hormones and the maturation of central nervous system regulation of anterior pituitary function. In Gluck L (ed): Modern Perinatal Medicine. Chicago, Year Book, 1974, p 247

Shepard TH: Onset of function in the human fetal thyroid: biochemical and radioautographic studies from organ culture. J Clin Endocrinol Metab 27:945, 1967

Stern L, Lees MH, Leduc J: Environmental temperature, oxygen consumption and catecholamine excretion in newborn infants. Pediatrics 36:367, 1965

Van Herle AJ, Young RT, Fisher DA, Uller RP, Brickman CH: Intrauterine treatment of a hypothyroid fetus. J Clin Endocrinol Metab 40:474, 1975

CONGENITAL HYPOTHYROIDISM

Choufoer JC, Van Rijn MH, Querido A: Endemic goiter in western New Guinea. II. Clinical picture, incidence and pathogenesis of endemic cretinism. J Clin Endocrinol Metab 25:385, 1965

DeLange F, Costa A, Ermans AM, Ibbetson HK, Querido A, Stanbury JB: A survey of the clinical and metabolic patterns of endemic cretinism. In Stanbury JB, Kroc RL (eds): Human Development and the Thyroid Gland, Relation to Endemic Cretinism. New York, Plenum, 1972, p 175

Dussault JH, Coulombe P, Laberge C: Preliminary report on a mass screening program for neonatal hypothyroidism. J Pediatr 86:670, 1975

Ehrenberg A, Omori K, Menkes JH, Oh W, Fisher DA: Growth and development of the thyroidectomized ovine fetus. Pediatr Res 8:783, 1974

Fisher DA, Sack J: Thyroid function in the neonate: possible approaches to newborn screening for hypothyroidism. In Fisher DA, Burrow G (eds): Perinatal Thyroid Physiology and Disease. New York, Raven, 1975, p 197

Fraser GR, Morgans WE, Trotter W: The syndrome of sporadic goiter and congenital deafness. Q J Med 29:279, 1960

Galina MP, Avnet NL, Einhorn A: Iodides during pregnancy, an apparent cause of neonatal death. N Engl J Med 267:1124, 1962

Goldsmith RE, McAdams AJ, Larsen PR, MacKenzie M, Hess EV: Familial autoimmune thyroiditis: maternal–fetal relationship and the role of generalized autoimmunity. J Clin Endocrinol Metab 37:265, 1973

Greenberg AH, Najjar S, Blizzard RM: Effects of thyroid hormone on growth, differentiation and development. In: Handbook of Physiology, Vol 3, The Thyroid. Washington, DC, American Physiological Society, 1974, p 377

Hayek A, Maloof F, Crawford JD: Thyrotropin behavior in thyroid disorders of childhood. Pediatr Res 7:28, 1973

Hetzel BS: Similarities and differences between sporadic and endemic cretinism. In Stanbury JB, Kroc RL (eds): Human Development and the Thyroid Gland: Relation to Endemic Cretinism. New York, Plenum, 1972, p 119

Holt AB, Cheek DB, Kerr GR: Prenatal hypothyroidism and brain composition in a primate. Nature 243:413, 1973

Klein AH, Agustin AV, Foley TP: Successful laboratory screening for congenital hypothyroidism. Lancet 2:77, 1974

Klein A, Meltzer S, Kenny F: Improved prognosis in congenital hypothyroidism treated before age three months. J Pediatr 81:912, 1972

Little B, Meador CK, Cunningham R, Pittman JA: Cryptothyroidism, the major cause of sporadic athyreotic cretinism. J Clin Endocrinol Metab 25:1529, 1965

McGirr EM, Hutchinson JH: Dysgenesis of the thyroid gland as a cause of cretinism and juvenile myxedema. J Clin Endocrinol Metab 15:668, 1955

Penfold JL, Simpson DA: Premature synostosis, a complication of thyroid replacement therapy. J Pediatr 86:360, 1975

Raiti S, Newns GH: Cretinism: early diagnosis and its relation to mental prognosis. Arch Dis Child 46:692, 1971

Refetoff S, DeGroot LJ, Bernard B, DeWind LT: Studies of a sibship with apparent hereditary resistance to the intracellular action of thyroid hormone. Metabolism 21:723, 1972

Smith DW, Blizzard RM, Wilkins L: The mental prognosis in hypothyroidism of infancy and childhood: a review of 128 cases. Pediatrics 18:1011, 1957

Stanbury JB: Familial goiter. In Stanbury JB, Wyngaarden JB, Fredrickson DS (eds): The Metabolic Basis of Inherited Disease, 3rd ed. New York, McGraw-Hill, 1972, p 223

Tolley D: The inherited errors of the thyroid system. In Hershman JM, Bray GA (eds): Pharmacology of the Thyroid Gland. Oxford, Pergamon, 1975, p 0000

GOITER AND TRANSIENT HYPOTHYROIDISM IN NEWBORNS

Boyle JA, Thompson JA, Murray PC, Fulton S, Nicol J, McGirr EM: Phenomenon of iodide inhibition in various states of thyroid function with observations on one mechanism of its occurrence. J Clin Endocrinol Metab 25:1255, 1965

Braverman LE, Ingbar SH, Vagenakis AG, Adams L, Maloof F: Enhanced susceptibility to iodide myxedema in patients with Hashimoto's disease. J Clin Endocrinol Metab 32:515, 1971

Carpenter CCJ, Solomon N, Silverberg SG, et al: Schmidt's syndrome (thyroid and adrenal insufficiency), including 10 instances of coexistent diabetes mellitus. Medicine 43:153, 1964

Chamberlain JL: Thyroid enlargement probably induced by cobalt: a report of three cases. J Pediatr 59:81, 1961

Falliers CJ: Goiter and thyroid dysfunction following the use of iodides in asthmatic children. Am J Dis Child 99:428, 1960

Gordin A, Saarinen P, Pelkonen R, Lamberg BA: Serum thyrotrophin and the response to thyrotrophin-releasing hormone in symptomless autoimmune thyroiditis and in borderline and overt hypothyroidism. Acta Endocrinol 75:274, 1974

LeBoeuf G, Bongiovanni AM, Steiker DD, Eberlein WR: Immunologic and thyroid function studies in euthyroid children with goiter. J Pediatr 58:477, 1961

Rallison ML, Kumagi LF, Tyler FH: Goitrous hypothyroidism induced by amino-glutethimide, anticonvulsant drug. J Clin Endocrinol Metab 27:265, 1967

Rallison M, Dobyns BM, Keating FR, Rall JE, Tyler FH: Occurrence and natural history of thyroiditis in children. J Pediatr 86:675, 1975

Van Wyk JJ, Grumbach MM: Syndrome of precocious menstruation and galactorrhea in juvenile hypothyroidism: an example of hormonal overlap in pituitary feedback. J Pediatr 57:416, 1960

Volpé R, Row VV, Webster BR, Johnston MW, Ezrin C: Studies of iodine metabolism in Hashimoto's thyroiditis. J Clin Endocrinol Metab 25:593, 1965

Vought RL, London WT, Stebbing GET: Endemic goiter in northern Virginia, J Clin Endocrinol Metab 27:1381, 1967

HYPERTHYROIDISM

Buchanan WW, Alexander WD, Crooks J, et al: Association of thyrotoxicosis and autoimmune thyroiditis. Br Med J 1:843, 1961

Dunn JT, Chapman EM: Rising incidence of hypothyroidism after radioactive-iodine therapy in thyrotoxicosis. N Engl J Med 271:1037, 1964

Elasa LJ, Whittemore R, Burrow GN: Maternal and neonatal Graves' disease, JAMA 200:250, 1967

Galaburda M, Rosman NP, Haddow JE: Thyroid storm in an 11-year-old boy managed by propanolol. Pediatrics 53:920, 1974

Grossman W, Robin NI, Johnson LE, Brooks HL, Selenkow HA, Dexter L: Effects of beta blockade on the peripheral manifestations of thyrotoxicosis. Ann Intern Med 74:875, 1971

Hayek A, Chapman EM, Crawford JD: Long term results of I[131] treatment of thyrotoxicosis in children. N Engl J Med 283:949, 1970

Hayles AB, Kennedy RL, Beahrs OH, Woolner LB: Exophthalmic goiter in children. J Clin Endocrinol Metab 19:138, 1959

Hermann HT, Quarton GC: Physiological changes and psychogenesis in thyroid hormone disorders. J Clin Endocrinol Metab 25:327, 1965

Hollingsworth DR, Mabry CC, Eckerd J: Hereditary aspects of Graves' disease in infancy and childhood. J Pediatr 81:446, 1972

Hung W, Wilkins L, Blizzard R: Medical therapy of thyrotoxicosis in children. Pediatrics 30:17, 1962

Lamki L, Row VV, Volpé R: Cell-mediated immunity in Graves' disease and in Hashimoto's thyroiditis as shown by the demonstration of migration inhibition factor (MIF). J Clin Endocrinol Metab 36:358, 1973

Lipman LM, Green DE, Snyder NJ, Nelson JC, Solomon DH: Relationship of long-acting thyroid stimulator to the clinical features and course of Graves disease, Am J Med 43:486, 1967

McKenzie JM: Neonatal graves' disease, J Clin Endocrinol Metab 24:660, 1964

Mori T, Kriss JP: Measurements by competitive binding radioassay of serum anti-microsomal and anti-thyroglobulin antibodies in Graves' disease and other thyroid disorders. J Clin Endocrinol Metab 33:688, 1971

Mukhtar ME, Smith BR, Pyle GA, Hall R, Vice P: Relation of thyroid-stimulating immunoglobulin to thyroid function and effects of surgery, radioiodine, and antithyroid drugs, Lancet 1:713, 1975

Onaya T, Kotani M, Yamada T, Ochi Y: New in vitro tests to detect the thyroid stimulator in sera from hyperthyroid patients by measuring colloid droplet formation and cyclic AMP in human thyroid slices. J Clin Endocrinol Metab 36:859, 1973

Saxena KM, Crawford JD, Talbot NB: Childhood thyrotoxicosis: a long term perspective. Br Med J 2:1153, 1964

Sheline GE, Lindsay S, Bell HG: Occurrence of thyroid nodules in children following therapy with radioiodine for hyperthyroidism. J Clin Endocrinol Metab 19:127, 1959

Smith CS, Howard NJ: Propanolol in treatment of neonatal thyrotoxicosis. J Pediatr 86:1046, 1973

Thomson JA, Riley ID: Neonatal thyrotoxicosis associated with maternal hypothyroidism. Lancet 1:635, 1966

Volpé R, Farid NR, von Westarp C, Row VV: The pathogenesis of Graves' disease and Hashimoto's thyroiditis. Clin Endocrinol (Oxf) 3:239, 1974

Werner SC, Spooner M: A new and simple test for hyperthyroidism employing L-triiodothyronine and the 24 hour I[131] uptake method. Bull NY Acad Med 31:137, 1955

THYROID NEOPLASMS IN CHILDHOOD AND ADOLESCENCE

Buckwalter JA, Thomas CG Jr Freeman JB: Is childhood thyroid cancer a lethal disease? Ann Surg 181:632, 1975

Hennessy JF, Wells SA Jr, Ontjes DA, Cooper CW: A comparison of pentagastrin injection and calcium infusion as provocative agents for detection of medullary carcinoma of the thyroid. J Clin Endocrinol Metab 39:487, 1974

Khairi MRA, Dexter RN, Burzynski NJ, Johnston CC Jr: Mucosal neuroma, pheochromocytoma and medullary thyroid carcinoma:multiple endocrine neoplasia, Type 3. Medicine 54:89, 1975

Raventos A, Winship T: The latent interval for thyroid cancer following irradiation. Radiology 83:501, 1964

Rimoin DL, Schimke RN: Genetic Disorders of the Endocrine Glands. St Louis, CV Mosby, 1971, p 134

Thomas CG Jr: Nodular goiter and benign and malignant neoplasms of the thyroid. In Sabiston DC (ed): Textbook of Surgery, Vol 1, 10th ed.Philadelphia, WB Saunders, 1972 p 631

PARATHYROID GLANDS

SEE P. 246.

PINEAL ORGAN

RICHARD J. WURTMAN

The mammalian pineal organ is a *neuroendocrine transducer*. Like the adrenal medulla, the supraoptic nucleus of the hypothalamus, the releasing factor cells in the median eminence, and the juxtaglomerular apparatus, the pineal converts an input of neuronal signals to a hormonal output. Pineal parenchymal cells receive nerve impulses from sympathetic neurons whose cell bodies lie outside the cranial cavity in the superior cervical ganglia. They respond to these impulses by synthesizing and secreting a family of hormones, the methoxyindoles, of which the prototype is melatonin (*N*-acetyl-5-methoxytryptamine). Melatonin synthesis is controlled by environmental lighting, which acts via the retina. In rats, exposure to darkness stimulates melatonin synthesis, while light suppresses it. Melatonin is secreted into the blood or cerebrospinal fluid and apparently acts on the brain to influence several physiologic processes that share a tendency toward time-dependence (ie, they vary cyclically or with age); these include onset of puberty, ovulation, and sleep. Considerable information is available about the factors that control pineal function; much less is known about the uses to which the body puts melatonin and other pineal secretions.

EVOLUTION OF MAMMALIAN PINEAL.
The mammalian pineal is a vastly different organ from the pineals (or epiphyses) of such lower vertebrates as the frog. The frog pineal is a true third eye. It responds directly to light waves by generating nerve impulses, which it transmits to the brain via pineal nerves. The mammalian organ has lost any direct photosensitivity, and it neither generates impulses for transmission to the brain nor receives them from the brain. The biochemical activity of the mammalian pineal continues to be influenced by environmental lighting, but indirectly. Light impinging on the retina generates nerve impulses that travel along the optic nerves to the optic chiasm.

Just behind the chiasm a small bundle of accessory optic fibres leaves the main optic tract to run in the medial forebrain bundle of the lateral hypothalamus. These fibers feed into a multisynaptic pathway that extends through the brainstem and down the spinal cord, ultimately reaching the cell bodies of neurons that send presynaptic fibers to the superior cervical ganglia. Postsynaptic fibers from these ganglia enter the pineal and transmit signals directly to the pineal parenchymal cells. The points at which their terminal boutons impinge on pinealocytes satisfy many of the morphologic criteria for synapses. In the rat, a nocturnal species, a shining light on the retina *decreases* the number of sympathetic nerve impulses reaching the pineal. The effects of light on the neural input to the pineal may be opposite in diurnally active animals.

Another important difference between frog and mammalian pineals concerns the uniqueness of the ability to synthesize melatonin. In mammals, only pineal and retinal cells contain the enzyme hydroxyindole-*o*-methyl transferase (HIOMT), which catalyzes melatonin biosynthesis; only the pineal has been shown to be able to synthesize melatonin from its circulating precursor, tryptophan. In frogs, HIOMT is widely distributed throughout neural structures. One can conclude that, with evolution, the pineal has changed from an organ that converts an input of environmental lighting into an output of neurotransmitter substances (released at synapses within the brain) to one whose input is a sympathetic neurotransmitter and whose output is a circulating hormone. The particular neurotransmitter released by the sympathetic nerves in the pineal is norepinephrine. The mechanism by which this substance enhances melatonin synthesis involves a so-called second messenger, cyclic AMP.

LIGHT, PINEAL FUNCTION, AND BIOLOGIC RHYTHM.
If rats are kept in a lighted environment, the activity of HIOMT (the enzyme that synthesizes melatonin) declines markedly, and melatonin synthesis and secretion probably show parallel declines. An environment of darkness causes HIOMT activity to increase manyfold. Because the environment in which most mammals live is characterized by light and dark periods during each 24-hour day, melatonin synthesis is also rhythmic, and the pineal provides the rest of the body with a circulating time signal. In rats, melatonin synthesis is least toward the end of the daily light period, and it rises sharply with the onset of darkness. In humans, melatonin excretion is also greatest between 11 P.M. and 7 A.M.

The discoveries that melatonin is the pineal output (or one of the pineal outputs) and that the synthesis of this compound normally varies within a 24-hour rhythm have given physiologists new and relatively fruitful ways of examining pineal function. The question "What do pineal hormones do?" can now be rephrased as "What other organs in the body respond to changes in melatonin secretion?" The answer to this question has been sought in two ways. In one approach, scientists have examined the effects of administered melatonin on neuroendocrine functions, while others have tried to determine which light-dependent and time-dependent phenomena in the body are altered when the source of melatonin, the pineal, is removed.

If melatonin is administered chronically to young rats, they experience a delay in gonadal growth and a subsequent disturbance in the ovulatory cycle, as indicated by changes in the vaginal estrous cycle. Melatonin implants in certain brain regions, such as the median eminence and the midbrain, block the rise in pituitary levels of luteinizing hormone (LH) that follows castration; hence the pineal hormone might produce part of its gonadal effects by interfering with gonadotropin secretion from the pituitary. 5-Methoxytryptophol, another compound produced uniquely in the pineal through the action of HIOMT, also influences pituitary gonadotropin levels when implanted in the brain. Unlike melatonin, this compound acts primarily on follicle-stimulating hormone (FSH) secretion. It is possible that the mammalian pineal produces a family of hormones that influence gonadal function and that are chemically unique in that they are methoxyindoles, synthesized through the action of HIOMT. Recent studies suggest that the pineal may also synthesize characteristic biologically active peptides such as arginine vasotocin.

Since HIOMT acts to convert hydroxyindoles, which enter the brain with some difficulty, to methoxyindoles, which have free access to the brain, and since melatonin implants in the brain modify pituitary gonadal function, it is generally held that the locus at which melatonin acts in producing its neuroendocrine effects resides within the brain. This hypothesis is supported by evidence that melatonin injections alter the levels of serotonin (believed to be a neurotransmitter substance) in the hypothalamus and midbrain and that the pineal hormone can induce changes in the electroencephalogram and in behavior that resemble sleep.

When most birds and mammals are blinded, or when they are exposed to continuous light or darkness, marked changes are observed in the timing of gonadal maturation and in subsequent ovulatory cycles. Blind humans exhibit a significant acceleration of menarche; blind rats show the opposite response. Hamsters kept in continuous darkness show a pronounced atrophy of the gonads; this effect is blocked by pinealectomy, which suggests that it is mediated by dark-induced changes in secretion of melatonin or some other pineal hormone. Gonadal maturation is accelerated in most avian species by exposure to artificial long days (ie, days in which light is presented for at least 14 hours). The stimulatory effect of light on the Japanese quail is blocked by removing the pineal; hence in this species the pineal must normally *stimulate* gonadal maturation. The two procedures of exposing a rat to continuous light and removing its pineal produce comparable increases in ovarian weight. The effects of the procedures are not additive, thus suggesting that both operate by depressing the amount of an inhibitory pineal substance (melatonin) that acts on the neuroendocrine axis.

Very little information is available about the role of the pineal in producing the 24-hour rhythms observed in glandular secretion and other functions (eg, body temperature, urine production). The pineal could provide the rhythmic signal that generates rhythms in functions such as adrenocortical secretion. More likely, it might serve to modify the phasing of an intrinsic rhythm.

HUMAN PINEAL AND DISEASE. Heubner, a German pathologist, first noted that certain pineal tumors were associated with precocious puberty in young boys; he postulated that the pineal normally secretes a hormone that suppresses the onset of sexual maturation, that tumors that destroy the pineal remove this brake, and that precocious puberty soon follows. Pineal tumors composed of cells that resemble true pinealocytes might be expected to cause a delay in sexual maturation or an inhibition of gonadal function. This correlation has, in fact, been observed in a small number of patients.

This thesis has not been confirmed, inasmuch as no pineal substance that inhibits gonad function has been shown to be present in the body fluids of normal prepubertal children or absent in children with precocious puberty induced by destructive pineal tumors. Melatonin or a related methoxyindole appears to be a good candidate for Heubner's inhibitory hormone. However, no assays are currently available for measuring melatonin or its chief metabolites in clinical material; thus this hypothesis has not yet been tested. It should be noted that diencephalic tumors unrelated to the pineal can also lead to precocious puberty; thus it is possible that some, if not all, of the gonadal sequelae of pineal tumors result not from changes in the secretion of pineal hormones but from pressure exerted by the tumor on other brain areas. This pressure hypothesis fails to explain the correlation between the endocrine effects of a given tumor and its histologic appearance. Most cases of pineal tumors associated with precocious puberty in the male have involved pineal teratomas, which secrete an LH-like hormone, while true pinealomas composed of cells that resemble pinealocytes have more commonly caused a delay in sexual maturation. Tissue samples from 2 children with parenchymal pinealomas and delayed pubescence were found to synthesize large amounts of melatonin in vitro. Progress in evaluating the role of the human pineal in health and disease might be expected to accelerate now that good assays are finally available for the melatonin levels in human body fluids.

Human pineal organs typically show radiologically observable calcification by the end of the second decade of life. Microscopically identifiable calcification may be noted soon after birth. The etiology and physiologic significance of pineal calcification remain obscure. Pineal calcification does not alter the activity of any pineal enzyme yet examined, and it probably has no effect on the ability of the pineal to synthesize its characteristic indolic hormones.

References

Lynch HJ, Wurtman RJ, Moskowitz MA, Archer MC, Ho MH: Daily rhythm in human urinary melatonin. Science 187:169, 1975

Wurtman RJ, Axelrod J, Kelly DE: The Pineal. New York, Academic, 1968

ABNORMALITIES OF SEX DIFFERENTIATION

MELVIN M. GRUMBACH

The terms hermaphroditism and intersexuality are generally applied to individuals with gonads of one or both sexes and some degree of ambisexual differentiation of the accessory sexual structures. Depending on the morphology of the gonad, patients with these congenital abnormalities have been described as male pseudohermaphrodites (when testes are present), female pseudohermaphrodites (when ovaries are present), or true hermaphrodites (when both testicular and ovarian tissue can be identified). This definition does not include postnatal virilization or feminization, or such psychiatric disorders as homosexuality and transvestism. Some important human sexual anomalies that may be grouped together are characterized by absent or defective gonads and, in many instances discrepancy between nuclear sex chromatin pattern and somatic sexual development. Examples of the latter are to be found in the syndrome of gonadal dysgenesis (Turner's syndrome) and in a congenital testicular disorder, seminiferous tubule dysgenesis (Klinefelter's syndrome). Chromosomal aberrations are found in this interesting group of gonadal anomalies. Abnormalities of sex differentiation are not especially rare; estimates of incidence, where available, are discussed with the specific disorders.

HUMAN SEX DIFFERENTIATION

The human embryo is potentially a bisexual organism equipped with gonadal and genital primordia capable of differentiating in either a masculine or a feminine direction. It is now well accepted that the sex of the zygote at fertilization is established by a chromosomal mechanism that results in an unequal balance of sex-determining genes. Evidence adduced from detection of abnormal sex chromosome constitution in man indicates that the Y chromosome has potent male determiners [which appear to be identical with, or linked to, the gene coding for the histocompatibility antigen HY (male)] and induces testicular differentiation of the primordial bipotential gonad, whereas with rare exceptions, two X chromosomes are required for the differentiation of human ovaries. The embryonic gonad is the first structure to emerge from the indifferent stage. During the seventh week of gestation, testicular differentiation occurs; however, ovarian differentiation does not begin until about 11 or 12 weeks, when oogonia are first transformed into oocytes. The bipotential primordial germ cells—progenitors of oogonia and spermatogonia—arise from an extragonadal site, migrate to the urogenital ridge, and implant themselves in the primitive undifferentiated gonad. This earliest sex differentiation is followed by sex-specific development of the genital ducts and subsequently the urogenital sinus and external genitalia. Although the embryo possesses a male and a female set of duct primordia, normally only the homologous pair develop completely, whereas the opposite set retrogress and persist as vestigial structures. In the male the wolffian ducts form the vas deferens, epididymis, and seminal vesicles; in the female the müllerian ducts differentiate into the fallopian tubes, the uterus, and the upper portion of the vagina. The urogenital sinus and the anlage of the external genitalia are neutral primordia that give rise to homologous structures in the male and the female. These homologous structures include the clitoris and penis, the labia majora and scrotum, the labia minora and corpus spongiosum that encloses the penile urethra, and the paraurethral glands and prostate.

The role of the gonad in embryogenesis of the accessory sex structures has been clarified by the fetal castration experiments of Jost and other embryologists and by analysis of abnormalities of sex differentiation in man. These studies support the concept of an inherent tendency of the fetus to develop along female lines irrespective of chromosomal sex in the absence of fetal testes and their morphogenetic hormones. The fetal testicular morphogenetic hormones seem essential for differentiation of male sex structures and for retrogression of the female ducts. The fetal testicular secretions are of two types: a macromolecule (the müllerian duct inhibitory factor) secreted by the Sertoli cell that acts locally and leads to ipsilateral regression of the müllerian (female) ducts and testosterone (secreted by the fetal Leydig cells), which induces male development of the urogenital sinus and external genitalia and stimulates growth of the wolffian (male) ducts. Testosterone promotes male differentiation of the somatic sex structures by two mechanisms. It acts directly and probably ipsilaterally on the wolffian duct to bring about differentiation of the epididymis, vas deferens, and seminal vesicle. On the other hand, it is the prohormone for dihydrotestosterone, which is formed by enzymatic reduction in the target tissue—the urogenital sinus and external genitalia. Dihydrotestosterone is the hormone that induces masculinization of the urogenital sinus, with formation of the prostate and male-type urethra, and masculinization of the primordia of the external genitalia to cause differentiation of the penis, penile urethra, and scrotum (Fig. 37). Whereas a functioning fetal gonad is not a prerequisite for development of a female genital system, exposure of the female fetus to androgenic hormones can arrest female differentiation of the urogenital sinus and external genitalia and induce masculinization of the lower genital tract.

A schematic representation of the present concept of sex determination and differentiation is shown in Figure 37. Intrinsic or extrinsic factors that adversely affect any of the stages of these mechanisms may lead to anomalies of sexual structure. These factors include the following: a sex chromosome abnormality arising in the ovum or sperm of the parent or in the zygote following fertilization that affects gonadogenesis, as in the syndrome of gonadal dysgenesis (Turner's syndrome) and seminiferous tubule dysgenesis (Klinefelter's syndrome); a mutant gene, as in the feminizing testis form of male pseudohermaphrodism that leads to end-organ resistance to testosterone and other androgens in fetal and postnatal life; translocation of sex-determining genes involving too minute an amount of chromosomal

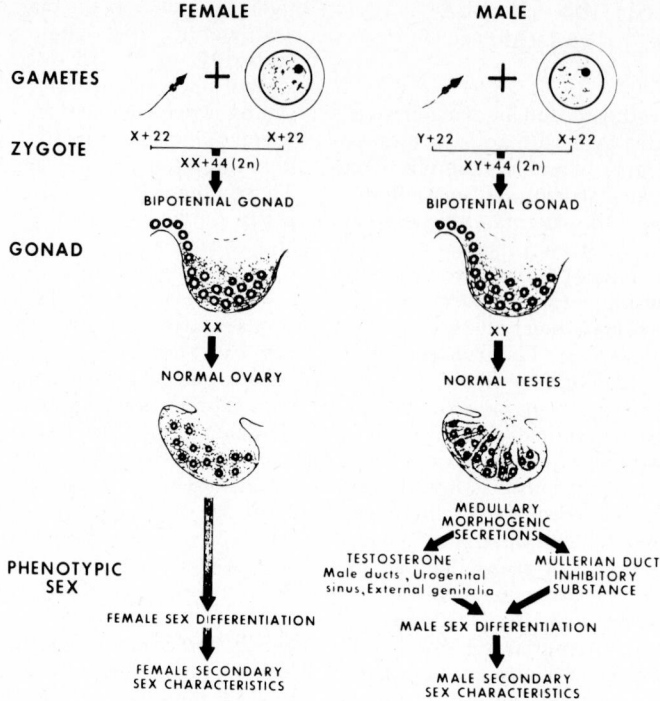

FIG. 37. Diagrammatic scheme of human sex determination and differentiation.

material to be visible by light microscopy (eg, between a Y chromosome and an X chromosome or an autosome), which may be a cause of true hermaphroditism; exposure of the fetus at a critical stage to inappropriate sex hormones that modify the sex-specific differentiation of the derivatives of the urogenital sinus and the primordia of the external genitalia, as in the form of female pseudohermaphroditism caused by congenital virilizing adrenal hyperplasia; undefined genetic or environmentally determined abnormalities in the differentiation of the primordial genital tract.

SEX CHROMATIN PATTERN: BARR BODY AND FLUORESCENT Y.   The discovery by Barr and his associates of a sexual dimorphism in nuclear structure provided a relatively simple method for indirectly assessing chromosomal sex. In the female a proportion of somatic interphase nuclei contain focal masses of chromatin now known as sex chromatin. The sex chromatin is usually a planoconvex, not infrequently bipartite, mass that measures about 1 μ in diameter and is typically located against the inner surface of the nuclear membrane. In specimens from male subjects it is rare to find more than a few percent of nuclei that contain a mass of chromatin simulating the sex chromatin. Reliable techniques have been developed for detecting the sex chromatin pattern using such accessible tissues as skin, buccal or vaginal mucosa, and leukocytes. The oral smear method is preferred by many workers because of its simplicity and reliability. Preparations of good technical quality are essential to avoid errors of interpretation. In buccal smears from normal

females the proportion of chromatin-positive cells in well-preserved nuclei is not less than 25 percent in our experience. However, some workers have observed a decreased frequency of chromatin-positive nuclei in buccal smears of newborn females in the first 2 days after birth.

The sex chromatin mass seen in somatic cells of normal females arises from a large part of one of the two X chromosomes in each cell. The two X chromosomes in female diploid somatic cells exhibit striking morphologic and functional differences. One X chromosome is in a highly condensed (heteropyknotic) state in interphase, visible as sex chromatin; it completes DNA synthesis later than any other chromosome in the complement, and the action of genes located on the precociously condensed segments is suppressed. The other X chromosome, the single X chromosome in male somatic cells, is in a highly extended (isopyknotic) state during interphase; it completes DNA replication with most of the complement and is genetically active. This discordant behavior of the two homologous X chromosomes in female somatic cells serves as a mechanism of dosage compensation. The inactivation of much of the genic activity of all but one X chromosome in individuals with X polysomy minimizes the phenotypic expression of the extra X chromosome or chromosomes in somatic cells. In X chromosome polysomy, more than one sex chromatin body is visible. With rare exceptions, the maximum number of sex chromatin bodies found in a diploid somatic nucleus is one less than the number of X chromosomes in the sex chromosome complex (Fig.

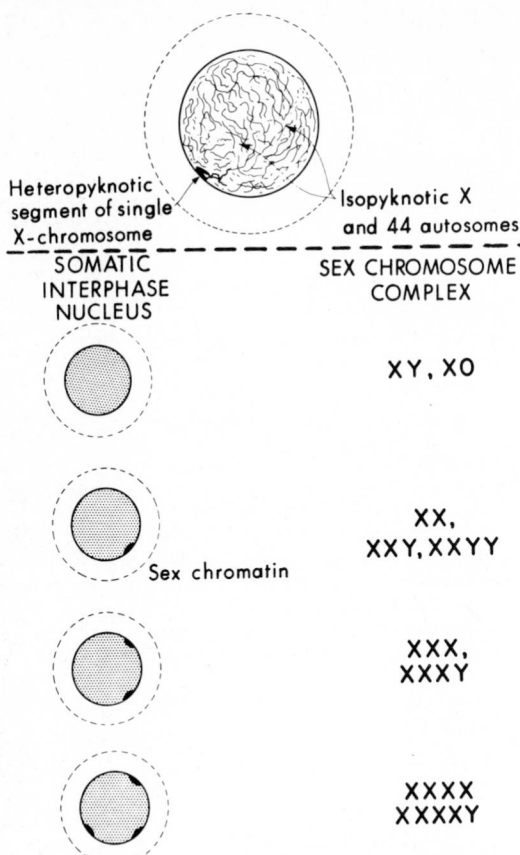

Heteropyknotic segment of single X-chromosome

Isopyknotic X and 44 autosomes

SOMATIC INTERPHASE NUCLEUS

SEX CHROMOSOME COMPLEX

XY, XO

Sex chromatin

XX, XXY, XXYY

XXX, XXXY

XXXX XXXXY

FIG. 38. Relationship of sex chromosomes to sex chromatin. Upper portion of diagram illustrates heteropyknotic X chromosome that forms sex chromatin body in a female interphase nucleus. Other X chromosome and autosomes are largely in an extended (isopyknotic) state and give rise to particulate chromatin. Lower diagram shows correlation between maximum number of sex chromatin bodies in diploid interphase nuclei and number of X chromosomes in sex chromosome complement, with number of sex chromatin bodies being one less than number of X chromosomes. In presence of certain sex chromosome mosaicism of XO/XX type, for example, XO cell line often leads to lowering of chromatin-positive cells below normal range for females. (From Grumbach and Morishima: Acta Cytol 6:46, 1962.)

38). The size of the sex chromatin body is altered by certain structural abnormalities of the X chromosome. An abnormally large sex chromatin body has been associated with a large X chromosome, an X isochromosome composed of two long arms of the X but lacking a short arm. Small sex chromatin bodies may be found in individuals who have a deletion of the short or long arm of an X chromosome or a ring X chromosome. When there is a structurally abnormal X chromosome, the sex chromatin body is formed by the anomalous X chromosome and not the normal X chromosome.

Recently, a staining method for identification of the human Y chromosome has been reported. Quinacrine hydrochloride, an acridine derivative, produces intense fluorescent staining of the distal part of the long arm of the Y chromosome in metaphase preparations, in interphase nuclei including cells from the buccal mucosa, and in Y-bearing sperm. Diploid nuclei, which contain two Y chromosomes (eg, XYY and other double Y karyotypes), have two fluorescent Y chromosomes.

CLASSIFICATION

The problem of classification of hermaphrodism has not been entirely resolved. Table 30 contains a classification that is convenient for clinical use. It is important to emphasize that such terms as female pseudohermaphroditism and male pseudohermaphroditism describe a heterogeneous group of disorders that have in common certain morphologic characteristics.

Female Pseudohermaphrodism

Individuals with female pseudohermaphrodism have ovaries, female ducts, and varying degrees of masculine differentiation of the urogenital sinus and external genitalia. The sex chromatin pattern is positive (female). The syndrome illustrates well the complexity of pathogenetic factors that may result in similar malformations. Table 31 contains a classification according to etiology.

The most common cause of female pseudohermaphrodism is congenital virilizing adrenal hyperplasia; it accounts for approximately one-half of all patients with ambiguous external genitalia. This disorder (p. 1632) is caused by an inborn error of adrenocortical biosynthesis that results in relative deficiency of hydrocortisone production, increased secretion of ACTH, and relative excess of androgenic hormones and other steroids. There are six types, of which the defect in 21-hydroxylation is by far the most common. The mode of inheritance is an autosomal trait. The minimum incidence has been estimated at 1 in 15,000 live white births. At birth the external genitalia are, as a rule, conspicuously abnormal. The degree of masculinization can be judged by the size of the clitoris and the completeness of labioscrotal fusion, which determines the size of the urogenital sinus (Fig. 39). The phallus is invariably enlarged, often approximating the size of a penis (Figs. 40 and 41). It is generally bound in chordee, behind which a perineal hypospadias is situated. In rare cases the urethra extends to the tip of the phallus (Fig. 42). Commonly the labia majora have the appearance of a bifid scrotum. Within the perineal opening of the urogenital sinus lie the orifices of the vagina and the urethra. Greater or lesser degrees of fusion of the labioscrotal folds result in a perineal opening that varies in size from that of a small urethralike opening to a relatively normal female introitus with a separate urethra and vagina (Fig. 39).

The appearance of the external genitalia is not specific, and the genital abnormality may be indistinguishable from that found in other forms of hermaphrodism with bilateral cryptorchidism. The feature that sets this disorder apart from all other varieties of hermaphroditism is the secretion of excessive quantities of adrenal

TABLE 30. Classification of Anomalous Sexual Development*

Condition	Distinguishing Features
DISORDERS OF GONADAL DIFFERENTIATION	
Seminiferous tubule dysgenesis (Klinefelter's syndrome)	Usually attributable to anomalous sex chromosomes; karyotype, X chromatin, and Y bodies variable. Differentiation of genital ducts, external genitalia, and hormonal sex concordant with gonadal histology. Frequently associated with mental retardation and somatic abnormalities.
Syndrome of gonadal dysgenesis and its variants (Turner's syndrome)	
Familial and sporadic XX and XY gonadal dysgenesis and their variants	
True hermaphrodism	
Other forms	
FEMALE PSEUDOHERMAPHRODISM	
Congenital virilizing adrenal hyperplasia	X-chromatin-positive; XX karyotype. Ovaries and internal ducts normal female. External genitalia may range from mild clitoral hypertrophy to simulant cryptorchid male.
Androgens and synthetic progestogens transferred from maternal circulation	
Malformations of intestine and urinary tract	
Other teratologic factors	
MALE PSEUDOHERMAPHRODISM	
Testicular unresponsiveness to hCG and LH (?)	X-chromatin-negative; XY karyotype. Testes only; some authors exclude dysgenetic testes due to chromosomal anomalies from this group, but for clinical consideration this category is regarded as belonging in the group of ambiguous genitalia due to dysgenetic male pseudohermaphrodism. Genital ducts are usually male. External genitalia vary in appearance from mild hypospadias to structures simulating female genitalia, attributable to insufficient production of testosterone by fetal testes during period of sex differentiation and defects in response of target tissues to androgen.
Inborn errors of testosterone biosynthesis	
Errors affecting synthesis of both corticosteroids and testosterone (variants of congenital adrenal hyperplasia)	
Cholesterol 20α-hydroxylase deficiency (congenital lipoid adrenal hyperplasia)	
3β-hydroxysteroid dehydrogenase deficiency	
17α-hydroxylase deficiency	
Errors primarily affecting testosterone biosynthesis	
17,20-desmolase (lyase) deficiency	
17β-hydroxysteroid oxidoreductase deficiency	
Defects in androgen dependent target tissues	
End-organ insensitivity to androgenic hormones	
Complete syndrome of testicular feminization	
Incomplete syndrome of testicular feminization	
Inborn Error in testosterone metabolism	
Male pseudohermaphrodism with normal virilization at puberty	
5α-reductase deficiency (familial perineal hypospadias with ambiguous development of urogenital sinus and male puberty; pseudovaginal perineoscrotal hypospadias)	
Less severe forms of hypospadias	
Dysgenetic male pseudohermaphroditism	
X-chromatin-negative variants of syndrome of gonadal dysgenesis (eg, XO, XY; XYp−)	
Incomplete form of familial XY gonadal dysgenesis	
Associated with degenerative renal disease	
Defect in synthesis, secretion, or response to müllerian duct inhibitory factor	
Female genital ducts in otherwise normal men (uteri herniae inguinale)	
Maternal ingestion of estrogens or progestogens	
Other forms	
UNCLASSIFIED FORMS OF ABNORMAL SEXUAL DEVELOPMENT	
In males	Heterogeneous group of disorders of uncertain cause. Some may be variants of other forms of intersexuality. Sex chromosomes, however, are presumably normal, and ambiguity of genitalia is not usually a prominent feature.
Cryptorchidism	
Anorchia (vanishing-testes syndrome)	
Familial forms of primary hypogonadism and gynecomastia (Rosewater syndrome)	
In females	
Absence or anomalous development of uterus and fallopian tubes	
Congenital absence of vagina; Rokitansky-Küstner syndrome	

Modified from Grumbach and Van Wyk: In Williams RH (ed): Textbook of Endocrinology, 1974. Courtesy of W.B. Saunders.

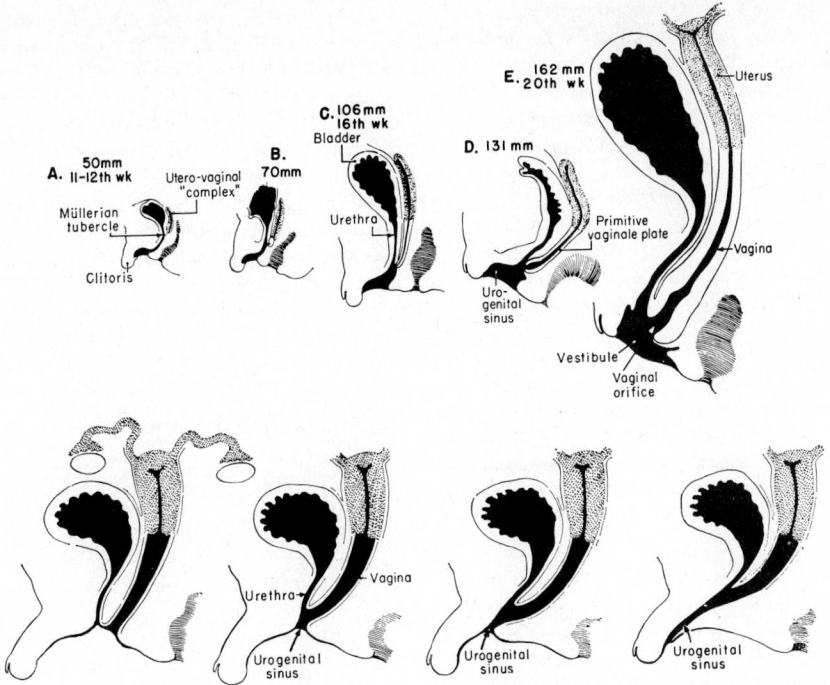

FIG. 39. Development of female pseudohermaphrodism. Upper diagrams show sequence of differentiation of female accessory sex structures. Note gradual descent of uterovaginal complex (adapted from Koff). To modify the differentiation of the urogenital sinus, especially the urethral groove, it seems that androgens must act on the female fetus before the 13th week of gestation, although enlargement of the clitoris can be induced at later stages. Lower schematic diagram illustrates variations in degree of masculinization of urogenital sinus and external genitalia in androgen-induced female pseudohermaphroditism. (From Grumbach and Ducharme: *Fertil Steril* 11:157, 1960.)

TABLE 31. Classification of Female Pseudohermaphrodism

Androgen-induced
  Fetal source
    Congenital virilizing adrenal hyperplasia
    Virilism only (defective adrenal 21-hydroxylation—compensated)
    Virilism with hypertension (defective adrenal 11-hydroxylation)
    Virilism with salt-losing syndrome (defective adrenal 21-hydroxy-
      lation—uncompensated)
  Maternal source
    Virilizing ovarian or adrenal tumor
    Iatrogenic
      Testosterone and related steroids
      Certain synthetic oral progestins and rarely stilbestrol
  Undetermined source
Other teratogenic factors
  Nonhormonal disturbances in differentiation of urogenital structures

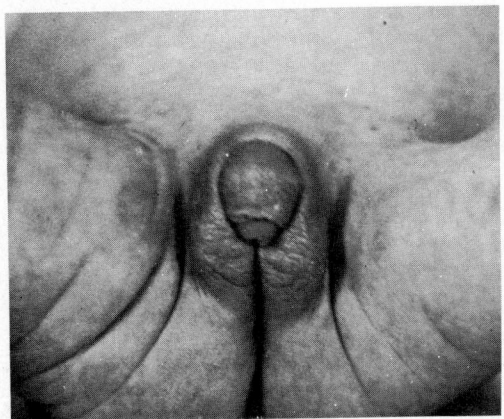

FIG. 40. External genitalia in 2-week-old female pseudohermaphrodite with congenital adrenal hyperplasia. Enlarged phallus, bound in chordee, overlies funnel-shaped orifice of urogenital sinus. Labioscrotal folds have appearance of bifid scrotum.

androgen. The urine contains 17-ketosteroids and, in patients with defective 21-hydroxylation, pregnanetriol in greater amounts than are found in any of the other forms of abnormal sex differentiation. (In normal infants the excretion of 17-ketosteroids during the first 2 weeks may be as high as 2.5 mg/day, later diminishing to less than 1 mg/day.) The concentration of plasma 17-hydroxyprogesterone is strikingly elevated in patients with 21-hydroxylase deficiency (both salt-losers and non-salt-losers), and its determination provides a useful diagnostic test. High plasma 17-hydroxyprogesterone values are found in affected newborn infants, in whom this determination can lead to rapid detection. In older children signs of virilization, rapid growth, and

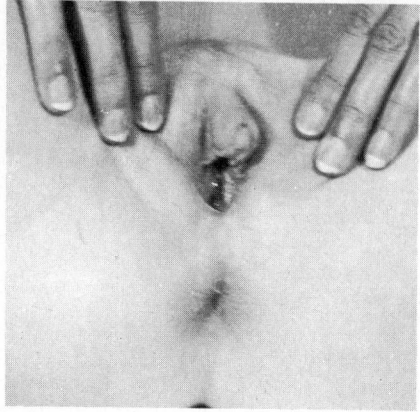

FIG. 41. Enlargement of clitoris without fusion of labioscrotal folds in 4-year-old female with congenital adrenal hyperplasia. Hypertrophy of clitoris was noted at birth. Separate vaginal and urethral orifices were identified by inspection. Note also sparse pubic hair.

accelerated skeletal development are present (Fig. 42). The three main forms of congenital virilizing adrenal hyperplasia that have been associated with female pseudohermaphrodism are listed in Table 31; other forms of congenital adrenal hyperplasia not accompanied by virilization or with minimal virilization of the female fetus have been described (p. 1632). With rare exceptions, affected pedigrees have exhibited only one form of the disorder.

Less frequent are forms of androgen-induced female pseudohermaphrodism caused by placental transfer of androgens from the mother. In rare instances a virilizing ovarian or adrenal tumor existing in the mother during pregnancy results in partial masculinization of the external genitalia of the female fetus. More frequently the maternal source has been therapeutic: administration of steroids with androgenic activity during pregnancy. In several instances testosterone or a testosterone analogue has been administered during pregnancy. Comparable cases have been associated with administration of certain oral semisynthetic progestins, such as 17α-ethynyltestosterone (Lutocylol, Pranone, Nugestoral), 17α-ethynyl-19-nortestosterone (Norlutin), norethynodrel (Enovid), and medroxyprogesterone acetate, to pregnant women in an effort to control habitual or threatened abortion. Fusion of the labioscrotal folds and formation of a urogenital sinus occur when androgen has been administered before the 13th week of gestation, but enlargement of the clitoris may follow androgen treatment of the mother at any time during pregnancy. In rare cases diethylstilbestrol, an estrogen, has been suggested as a possible fetal masculinizing agent. Recently, maternal ingestion of stilbestrol and related synthetic estrogens during pregnancy has been associated, in adolescents and young adult females, with a much increased risk of clear cell adenocarcinoma of the vagina and cervix and vaginal adenosis.

Another distinct and rare type of female pseudoher-

maphrodism is not caused by androgen excess. Associated developmental anomalies of the urinary tract and cloaca may be present and there may be absence of a fallopian tube or an ovary and a poorly developed uterus. There may be atresia of the rectum or rectovaginal fistula. Stenosis of the urethra may cause urinary retention in early infancy.

In individuals with nonadrenal female pseudohermaphrodism mistaken for cryptorchid males, the correct sex diagnosis may not be appreciated until gynecomastia and recurrent "hematuria" due to menstruation appear at adolescence. No sexual development occurs before puberty, at which time female secondary sexual characteristics appear.

Male Pseudohermaphrodism

Individuals in this group have testes, variable degrees of ambisexual development of the genital ducts or the urogenital sinus and external genitalia or both, and chromatin-negative nuclei (Fig. 43). The morphology of the seminiferous tubules is usually abnormal, but frequently Leydig cells appear at the age of puberty. The appearance of the external genitalia varies from that of a normal female to that of a male, with a penile urethra and either bilateral or unilateral cryptorchidism. Commonly there is perineal hypospadias. The testes may be located inside the abdomen, sometimes in the position of ovaries, in the inguinal region, or in the labioscrotal folds.

Male pseudohermaphrodism occurs in a heterogeneous group of disorders that have in common failure of the fetal testis to bring about complete masculinization of the somatic sex structures or impaired end-organ responsiveness to fetal testicular secretions. With advances in our understanding of etiologic mechanisms, the classification of disorders in this group of intersexes has been simplified (Table 30). It is convenient to categorize male pseudohermaphrodites who are incompletely masculinized because of a defect in testicular differentiation as dysgenetic male pseudohermaphrodites. In such patients the gonadal defect is usually due to an anomaly of the sex chromosomes (eg, XO/XY mosaicism or a structural abnormality of the Y chromosome) or, less frequently, to a mutant gene that leads to defective gonadogenesis (incomplete form of familial XY gonadal dysgenesis). It is in these forms that a variable degree of differentiation of the müllerian ducts is often found. In these and other patients with dysgenetic testes, the failure of the internal and external genitalia to undergo full male differentiation correlates quite well with the incomplete testicular differentiation.

Many male pseudohermaphrodites have an XY sex chromosome constitution and relatively normal embryonic differentiation of their testes. In such patients, defective male development of the somatic sex structures is a consequence of failure of the normally differentiated fetal testis to overcome the inherent tendency to feminize the derivatives of the urogenital sinus and the external genitalia. This failure may arise from the insensitivity of the fetal testis to chorionic gonadotropin and

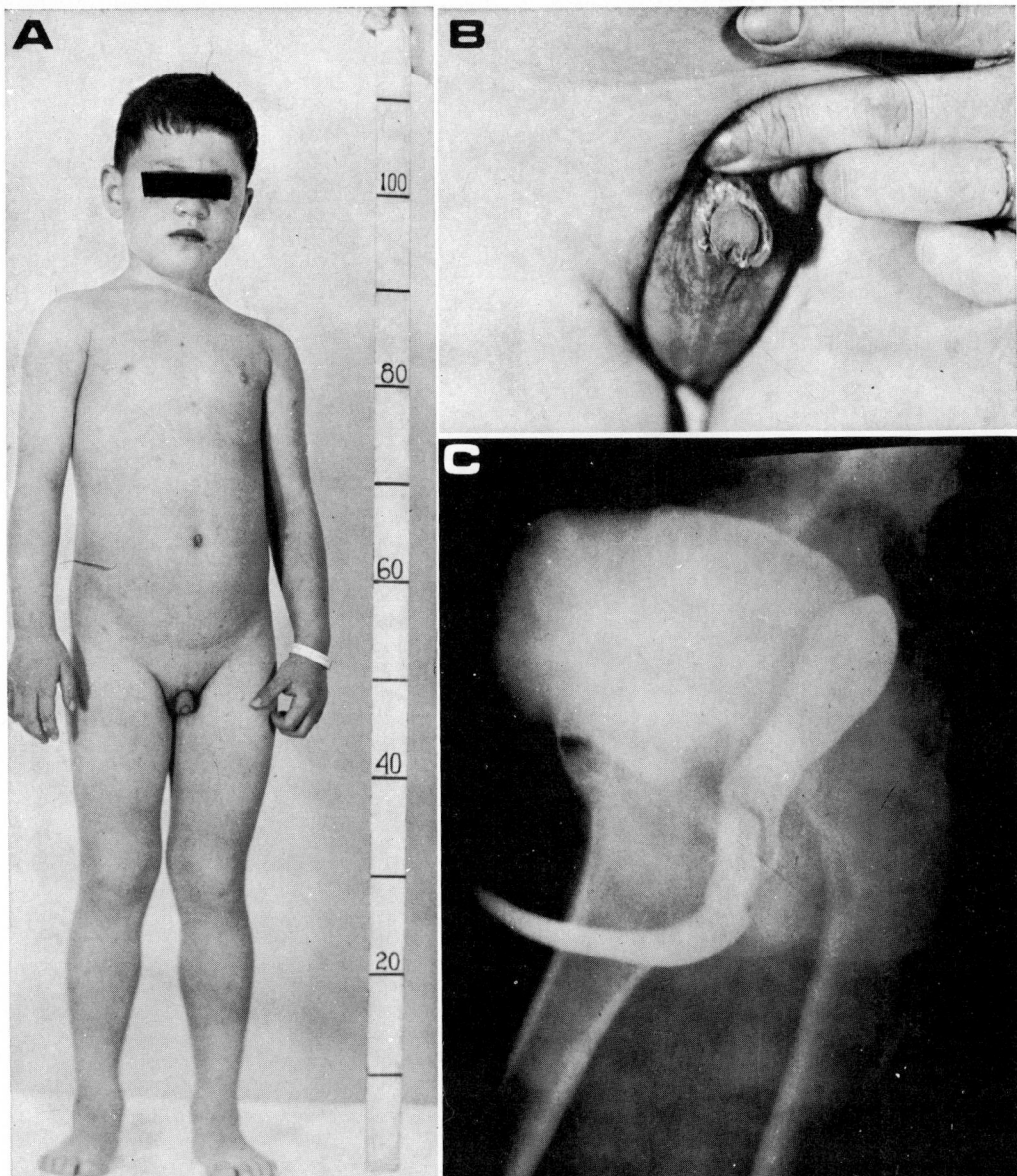

FIG. 42. A. Female pseudohermaphrodite 45 months old with congenital adrenal hyperplasia and penile urethra, reared as male. Height 112 cm (+2.5 SD), bone age 8 years, urinary 17-ketosteroids 11.5 to 13.8 mg/day, and pregnanetriol 3 to 4 mg/day. Sex chromatin pattern was positive. B. Appearance of external genitalia. C. Urethrogram shows urogenital sinus and distended vagina. Some contrast medium also entered bladder. (From Grumbach and Ducharme: *Fertil Steril* 11:157, 1960.)

fetal pituitary LH, from inborn errors in testosterone biosynthesis by the fetal testis, or from failure of the target tissues to respond normally to testosterone stimulation; all of these categories are hereditary disorders arising from a single mutant gene. In none of these forms is development of müllerian derivatives (fallopian tube, uterus) found. A rare form is due to lack of synthesis or secretion of the müllerian duct inhibitory factor or an end organ that is unresponsive to this fac-

tor. Here both müllerian duct derivatives (fallopian tubes and uterus), as well as wolffian duct development, are found, whereas the external genitalia are usually male. The classification of male pseudohermaphrodism outlined in Table 30 is according to this scheme.

INBORN ERRORS OF TESTOSTERONE BIO-SYNTHESIS. Figure 44 illustrates the major pathways in testosterone biosynthesis; each step is associated with an enzymatic defect inherited as an

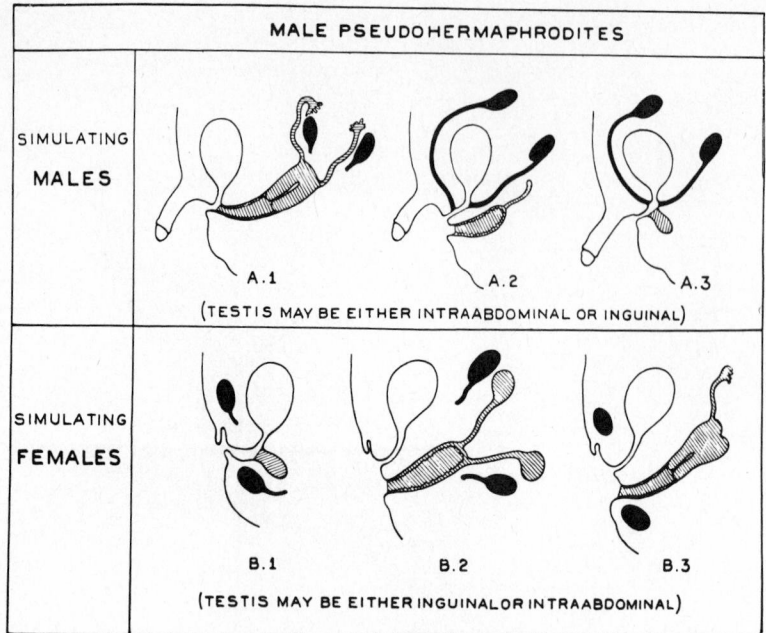

FIG. 43. Common anatomic findings in male pseudohermaphrodites. Black structures are testes, derivatives of wolffian ducts. Cross-hatched areas include derivatives of müllerian ducts and female urogenital structures.

Enzymatic deficiencies in the biosynthetic pathways to TESTOSTERONE

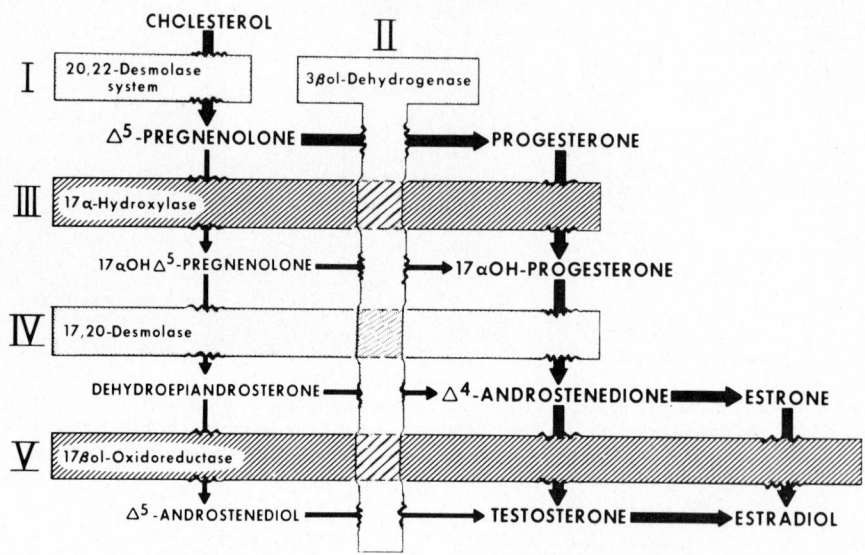

FIG. 44. Enzymatic deficiencies in biosynthetic pathways to testosterone.

autosomal recessive trait that results in incomplete masculinization of the urogenital sinus and/or external genitalia but not differentiation of müllerian duct structures. The sex chromosome constitution is XY. Steps I, II, and III are associated with errors in synthesis of both corticosteroids (cortisol and aldosterone) and testosterone biosynthesis (p. 1620).

ERRORS AFFECTING SYNTHESIS OF BOTH CORTICOSTEROIDS AND TESTOSTERONE (VARIANTS OF CONGENITAL ADRENAL HYPERPLASIA). 20,22-DESMOLASE COMPLEX DEFECT (MALE PSEUDOHERMAPHRODISM, SEXUAL INFANTILISM, ADRENAL INSUFFICIENCY). This is a defect at an early step in the biosynthetic pathway of all C_{21}, C_{19}, and C_{18} steroids that results in enormous accumulations of lipid in the cells of both the adrenal cortex and gonads, severe adrenal insufficiency, and death in early infancy if it is untreated. The excretion of urinary 17-ketosteroids and glucocorticoids is low. Males exhibit pseudohermaphrodism, including a blind vaginal pouch, undescended testes, and with a severe defect, female external genitalia. In several instances the defect in the desmolase complex has been localized at the 20 α-hydroxylation step.

3B-HYDROXYSTEROID DEHYDROGENASE DEFICIENCY (MALE PSEUDOHERMAPHRODISM AND ADRENAL INSUFFICIENCY). This is a rare form of adrenal hyperplasia that produces salt loss (due to aldosterone deficiency) and a defect in cortisol and sex steroid secretion. Males are incompletely masculinized. The presence of high urinary 17-ketosteroids associated with elevated urinary dehydroepiandrosterone and other 3β-hydroxysteroids is diagnostic.

17A-HYDROXYLASE DEFICIENCY (MALE PSEUDOHERMAPHRODISM, SEXUAL INFANTILISM, HYPERTENSION AND HYPOKALEMIC ALKALOSIS). These patients have impaired synthesis of 17α-hydroxyprogesterone and 17α-hydroxypregnenolone and their products (androgens, estrogens, and cortisol). Increased secretion of corticosterone and deoxycorticosterone leads to hypokalemic alkalosis and hypertension # in the presence of low plasma renin levels. Excretion of urinary 17-ketosteroids is low. Affected males are incompletely masculinized and may appear to be phenotypic females.

ERRORS PRIMARILY AFFECTING TESTOSTERONE SYNTHESIS. 17,20-DESMOLASE DEFICIENCY. These patients have ambiguous external genitalia and inguinal or intra-abdominal testes. At puberty, incomplete masculinization may occur; gynecomastia has not been described. If the diagnosis is made in infancy, these patients can be reared as males and treated with testosterone to induce male secondary characteristics and phallic growth.

17B-HYDROXYSTEROID OXIDOREDUCTASE DEFECT. In this defect, patients have female or ambiguous external genitalia, inguinal testes, male duct development, and progressive virilization at puberty, usually with concomitant breast development. Levels of androstenedione and estrone are strikingly elevated because their conversion to testosterone and estradiol is impaired. The usual testosterone/androstenedione ratio is reversed in peripheral and spermatic vein blood at puberty and in affected prepubertal patients stimulated with human chorionic gonadotropin. These patients must be distinguished from those with the incomplete feminizing testes syndrome, who exhibit a similar phenotype but not a similar sex steroid pattern.

END-ORGAN INSENSITIVITY TO ANDROGENIC HORMONES. SYNDROME OF FEMINIZING TESTES (TESTICULAR FEMINIZATION). This syndrome is a relatively common and well-defined form of male pseudohermaphrodism; more than 100 cases have been reported. These patients are genetic males; their sex chromosome constitution is XY. They have testes, which are usually located in the inguinal canal or in the labial folds. Because these patients present a normal female appearance, the diagnosis is often not suspected. The occurrence of multiple cases within a family is frequent, and family pedigrees and other genetic studies suggest that the condition is transmitted by a sex-linked recessive gene. The external genitalia are female in configuration; occasionally the clitoris is slightly enlarged and the labioscrotal folds are partially fused. Characteristically there is a blind vaginal pouch. The development of the genital ducts is variable, but the uterus is absent or rudimentary. At puberty, estrogenic steroids secreted by the testes bring about feminization of body habitus, development of breasts, and estrinization of vaginal mucosa, but menstruation fails to occur. The testes also secrete testosterone, and at puberty the concentration of plasma testosterone is usually within the normal range for males. However, there is lack of response of the appropriate end organs, both genital and somatic, to androgens in the fetus and at puberty, which leads to the female differentiation of the urogenital sinus and external genitalia and to the feminization at puberty. The hypothalamic feedback mechanism similarly lacks normal sensitivity to testosterone, which leads to elevated serum LH levels but usually a normal serum FSH concentration. Castration leads to a fall in urinary estrogens and testosterone, a rise in both FSH and LH, and menopausal symptoms. In the majority of cases, pubic and axillary hair is absent or sparse, a manifestation of the impaired response to androgen of the hair follicles that give rise to sexual hair. In the classic form of the syndrome, administration of large amounts of testosterone does not induce either masculinization or an appropriate degree of protein anabolism. Recent evidence suggests that the underlying defect is an absent or defective target cell receptor (either cytoplasmic or nuclear) for dihydrotestosterone.

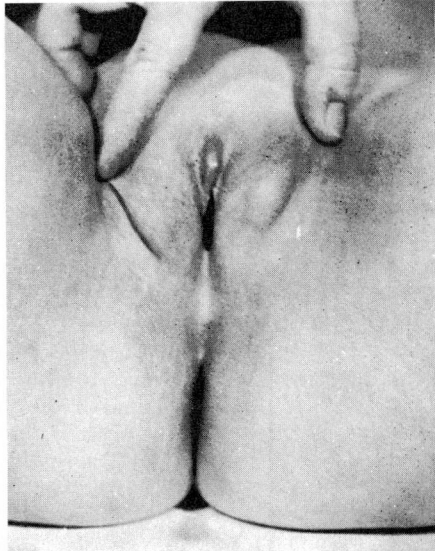

FIG. 45. External genitalia in 5-year-old patient with male pseudohermaphrodism. Note labial masses; at operation they proved to be testes. (From Grumbach and Barr: Recent Prog Horm Res 14:255, 1958.)

During childhood the discovery of a testis in an inguinal or labial hernia is usually the only clue to the diagnosis in the absence of a familial history (Fig. 45). The diagnosis should be considered in an adolescent girl with primary amenorrhea in the presence of otherwise female secondary sexual characteristics, especially when associated with absence of sexual hair and unilateral or bilateral hernial masses. There is a propensity for the testes to undergo neoplastic transformation, and orchidectomy is recommended by late adolescence.

INCOMPLETE VARIANTS. There are patients with similar patterns of inheritance in whom the findings are similar but are clinically distinct. These patients, while they exhibit breast development at puberty, undergo variable degrees of masculinization. Often there is clitoral enlargement at birth and even labioscrotal fusion. They show only partial resistance to testosterone. The defect, while at the end organ, may involve any site between the binding of dihydrotestosterone by the cytoplasmic receptor and the activation of synthesis of specific messenger RNA at the level of the genome.

MALE PSEUDOHERMAPHRODISM WITH NORMAL VIRILIZATION AT PUBERTY. The preceding categories of male pseudohermaphrodism can be attributed to defective androgen biosynthesis or defective end-organ response, but there are other familial forms of male pseudohermaphrodism in which virilization occurs at puberty; in these patients the secretion of testosterone is normal. The karyotype is uniformly XY, and only male genital ducts are present. As with other forms of male pseudohermaphrodism, these encompass the full spectrum of external sexual ambiguity, extending from those with only mild hypospadias and a normal-size phallus to individuals more closely resembling females, with minimal clitoral enlargement and incomplete masculinization of the urogenital sinus. One form has recently been defined—a target cell defect in 5α-reductase. Other forms may be related to differences in site and degree of an end-organ defect in the action of androgen.

5α-REDUCTASE DEFECT (FAMILIAL PERINEAL HYPOSPADIAS WITH AMBIGUOUS DEVELOPMENT OF UROGENITAL SINUS AND MALE PU- BERTY, PSEUDOVAGINAL PERINEOSCROTAL HYPOSPADIAS). These patients have an XY karyotype, normally differentiated testes, male internal genital ducts, and ambiguous external genitalia. At birth the phallus is usually small and hypospadiac. There is persistence of the urogenital sinus with a blind vaginal pouch; in severe cases separate vaginal and urethral orifices are present. Recent studies indicate that these patients have a deficiency of 5α-reductase at the target cell, with impaired enzymatic transformation of testosterone to its active hormone (dihydrotestosterone) at these end organs. The disorder is transmitted as an autosomal recessive trait. At puberty, these patients masculinize, and the phallus enlarges; in addition, there is growth of axillary and pubic hair, and in at least some cases there is male sex identity. Acne, facial hair, and temporal recession of the hairline are absent or minimal. The findings in these patients suggest that male differentiation of the urogenital sinus and external genitalia is mainly effected by dihydrotestosterone and not testosterone, while differentiation of male genital ducts is mediated primarily by testosterone.

DYSGENETIC MALE PSEUDOHERMAPHRODISM. Male Pseudohermaphrodism as Variant of Syndrome of Gonadal Dysgenesis. A highly diverse phenotype has been described in patients with XO/XY mosaicism or structural abnormality of the Y chromosome. The appearance may range from sexually infantile phenotypic females, with or without somatic anomalies of Turner's syndrome and with bilateral streak gonads, through patients with variable degrees of masculine differentiation of the external genitalia, urogenital sinus, and genital ducts, to those who have virtually normal male differentiation of the genital tract. In some patients a dysgenetic testis is present on one side and a streak gonad on the other. Short stature and the somatic anomalies of Turner's syndrome are inconstant features. Removal of the dysgenetic testes is necessary because of their increased tendency to develop malignant tumors.

Incomplete Form of Familial XY Gonadal Dysgenesis. These XY patients are of normal stature and do not exhibit the stigmata of Turner's syndrome. The testes are dysgenetic, and there are usually both müllerian and wolffian duct derivatives; the external genitalia are ambiguous. The gonads exhibit varying degrees of dysgenetic testicular differentiation, and some degree of virilization occurs at puberty. Gonadotropins are elevated. The defective testes should be removed because of the risk of neoplastic transformation. These patients are variants of familial XY gonadal dysgenesis, which is transmitted as an X-linked recessive or sex-limited autosomal dominant trait. Both the complete form, which has a female phenotype, and the incomplete form may occur in the same pedigree.

True Hermaphrodism

This group of intersexes is composed of individuals who have both an ovary and a testis or, more commonly, in whom one or both gonads are ovotestes. Although this disorder is rare, more than 300 cases have been reported, including two affected sibships in which a single gene mutation may be the cause. The sex chromatin pattern may be negative or positive; a preponderance of chromatin-positive cases has been observed. Development of the accessory sexual structures is highly variable. Three-fourths of these patients have been reared as males, but they have variable degrees of hypospadias. Cryptorchidism and inguinal hernias that contain a gonad or vestigial uterus and fallopian tube are present in 50 percent of cases. Predominantly masculine or feminine maturation occurs at puberty. A sex chromosome abnormality has not been demonstrated in most patients with true hermaphrodism. Usually, an XX sex chromosome constitution has been found, although mosaicism is not readily excluded as a possibility. Recently, XX true hermaphrodites were shown to have HY antigen which may explain the differentiation of testicular tissue. In a few instances sex chromosome abnormalities have been detected, such as XX/XY chimerism (which is thought to arise by double fertilization of a binucleate ovum or by fusion of two independently fertilized zygotes) and XX/XXY mosaicism. The occurrence of this syndrome in patients with an XX or XY karyotype suggests an environmental factor that disrupts gonadogenesis or a translocation of sex-determining genes during spermatogenesis in the father, eg, translocation of male-determining genes from the Y chromosome to the X chromosome or an autosome. The positive HY (male) antigen in XX patients supports this contention. Some of these patients are potentially fertile, and when it is possible, after deciding on the sex of rearing, an attempt should be made to preserve the appropriate gonad or gonadal segment, especially if any ovary is present in the mesosalpinx or a testis is attached to its exocrine ducts in the scrotum. However, there is an increased risk of gonadal neoplasms.

Gonadal Dysgenesis

The typical form of the syndrome of gonadal dysgenesis (*Turner's syndrome, gonadal dysplasia, ovarian agenesis, Bonnevie-Ullrich syndrome*), first delineated by Turner in 1938, is characterized by a female phenotype, short stature, sexual infantilism, streak gonads, and a diversity of associated somatic anomalies (Fig. 46); these features are a consequence of the X chromosome monosomy (XO karyotype) of these individuals. The most common associated congenital malformations include atypical facies, broad shieldlike chest, low hairline over the nape of the neck, webbed neck (in about 40 percent), congenital lymphedema of the extremities, especially the hands and feet (30 percent), coarctation of the aorta (20 percent), cubitus valgus, short fourth metacarpal (50 percent), high arched palate, a variety of skeletal anomalies, hypoplastic nails, microthelia, and

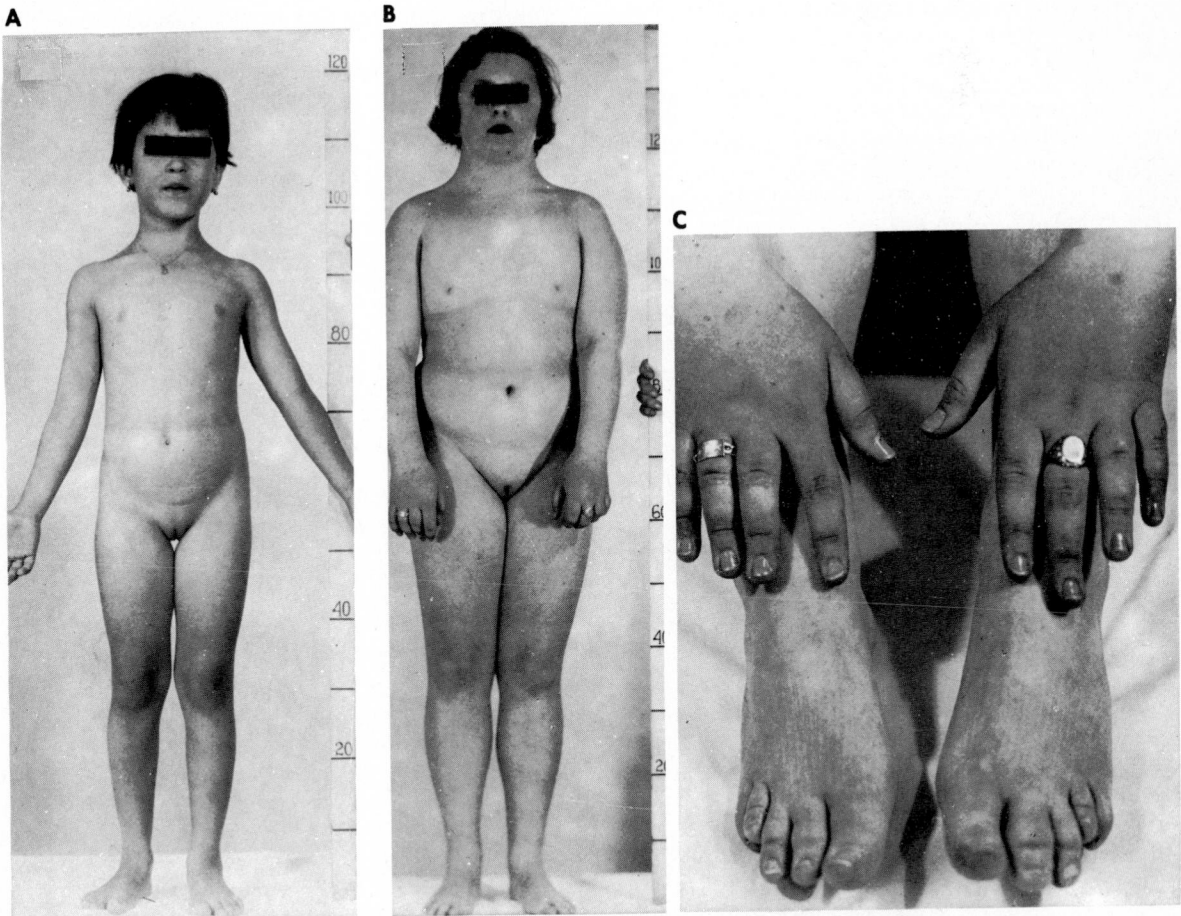

FIG. 46. Two patients with syndrome of gonadal dysgenesis, chromatin-negative somatic nuclei, and 45,XO karyotype. A. Age 9 years, 11 months. Short stature was the complaint. B. Age 15½ years; classic aspect of Turner's syndrome. C. Hands and feet of patient on the right, illustrating useful clinical signs of conspicuous shortening of fourth digits due to underdevelopment of metacarpals and metatarsals, puffiness over dorsum of digits between interphalangeal joints, convexity of nails, and prominence of pulp of finger beyond tip of fingernail.

cutaneous (pigmented nevi and predisposition to keloid formation), ocular, otitic (tendency for recurrent otitis media, perceptive hearing loss), and renal (most commonly horseshoe kidney) abnormalities (50 percent). A small proportion of patients are mentally defective; deficits of space–form recognition and directional sense are common despite a normal intelligence quotient. Skeletal maturation is normal or mildly delayed before puberty. Diminished mineralization of the hands, feet, and elbows is common.

The habitus is usually typical; it consists of a short stocky build, broad chest, short neck, and small mandible. Increased numbers of pigmented nevi are frequently found. No true gonad is present; in each mesosalpinx there is a ridge of connective tissue devoid of any germinal elements. These individuals develop none of the secondary sexual characteristics caused by secretion of estrogen at puberty, but in contrast to the situation with hypopituitary dwarfs, sexual hair does appear. Very rarely some degree of feminization occurs at puberty, and in one instance fertility has been described. During adolescence the serum FSH and LH concentrations and the excretion of urinary gonadotropins rise to castrate levels; elevated levels of serum FSH are frequently detectable in infancy and early childhood. Chromatin-negative nuclei have been found in about 80 percent of cases. This latter finding, in association with the characteristic features of the syndrome, especially lymphedema and loose folds of skin about the nape of the neck (Bonnevie-Ullrich syndrome), provides a

method for establishing the diagnosis as early as the neonatal period (Fig. 47). Pleural effusion may occur in the newborn.

Intrauterine growth retardation is common. There is increased prevalence of twinning, but familial cases are exceedingly rare. About 5 percent of spontaneous abortions are estimated to have an XO karyotype. It is estimated that about 1 percent of all zygotes are XO, but less than 5 percent survive to term. The mortality rate is increased in infancy.

The prevalence of chromatin-negative phenotypic females in surveys of newborn nurseries is 0.37 per 1,000; in comparison, the frequency of XXX newborn females is 1.2 per 1,000, and the frequency of newborn chromatin-positive phenotypic males is 2.07 per 1,000.

The typical sex chromosome abnormality in chromatin-negative cases, first described by Ford and associates, is an XO sex chromosome constitution with a diploid chromosome number of 45. The monosomic X sex chromosome complement may arise as a consequence of meiotic nondisjunction during gametogenesis in one parent or from loss of a sex chromosome (either the X or Y) during an early cleavage division of the zygote.

Other sex chromosome abnormalities have been described, all of which represent a less than complete absence of a second sex chromosome. The variable deficiency of the sex chromosomes is associated with a highly diverse modification of the classic XO phenotype. These clinical variants of the syndrome of gonadal

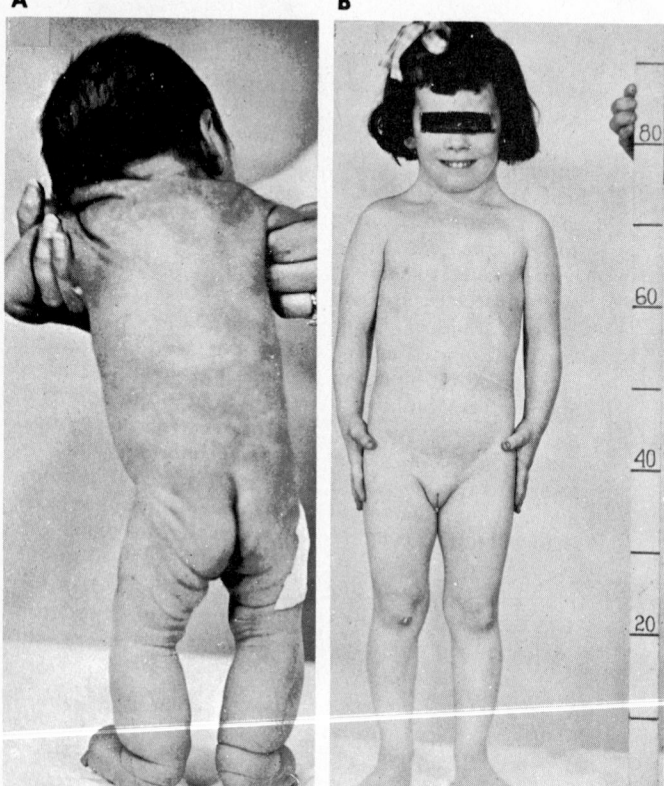

A   **B**

FIG. 47. Patient with syndrome of XO gonadal dysgenesis, features of Bonnevie-Ullrich syndrome, negative sex chromatin pattern, and XO karyotype. A. Appearance at age 7 days. Note massive edema of distal parts of lower extremities, puffiness of hands, and loose folds of skin over nape of neck. Dressing covers site of skin biopsy. B. Age 4 years. Note broad chest and microthelia. (From Grumbach and Barr: *Recent Prog Horm Res* 14:255, 1958.)

dysgenesis are found in patients with sex chromosome mosaicism involving an XO cell line (such as XO/XX, XO/XX/XXX, and XO/XY mosaicism) or a structural abnormality of an X or Y chromosome such as a long arm isochromosome X (XXqi), an X or Y chromosome deletion, or a ring X or Y chromosome. Structural abnormalities of the sex chromosomes are commonly associated with XO mosaicism owing to loss of the heteromorphic chromosome from some cells (eg, XO/XXqi, XO/X ring X).

Sex chromosome mosaicism involving an XO cell line and structural abnormalities of the X or Y chromosome usually modifies the phenotypic expresssion of the classic form of the syndrome of gonadal dysgenesis associated with an XO karyotype. The modifications of the typical Turner phenotype in the variant forms of the syndrome are toward a more normal phenotype, and they may involve all or any of the following aspects of the disorder: gonadal differentiation and function, stature, and associated somatic stigmata. In the chromatin-positive variants associated with XO/XX or XO/XX/XXX mosaicism, normal stature may be achieved, a variable degree of ovarian function (including ovulation) may be found, and the associated somatic anomalies may be absent or minimal. In other cases with the same type of mosaicism the phenotype is indistinguishable from that of the XO individual. In these forms of sex chromosome mosaicism the sex chromatin pattern is positive, but a diminished proportion of chromatin-positive cells is often found. When a diploid cell line containing more than two X chromosomes is present, multiple sex chromatin bodies are usually found in some of the chromatin-positive cells. The X long arm isochromosome X individuals have a positive sex chromatin pattern with larger Barr bodies, and the phenotype does not depart from the typical form, even though such somatic anomalies as lymphedema of the extremities, webbed neck, and coarctation of the aorta are rare in these individuals. In patients with a deletion of the short arm of the X (XXp−), short stature and typical stigmata are found. However, several patients studied by the author exhibited well-developed female secondary sex characteristics and had dysfunctional menstrual bleeding. Patients with an XO/X ring-X karyotype usually have short stature and associated somatic anomalies, but they may menstruate.

XO/XY mosaicism is associated with a diverse phenotype (see male pseudohermaphrodism). The karyotype may be associated with a variable degree of testicular differentiation, leading in some cases to ambisexual development of the external genitalia and in others to a virtually normal male phenotype.

Therapy is directed toward correction of remediable congenital anomalies and sexual infantilism. In phenotypic females with elevated urinary gonadotropin, treatment with estrogen should be initiated at about 13 years of age, continuously for 2 to 4 months, and then cyclically for 3 out of 4 weeks, to bring about the development of feminine secondary sexual characteristics and estrogen-withdrawal bleeding. In addition, it is useful to administer an oral progestin during the last 5 days of estrogen therapy. Gonadectomy is recommended in XO/XY and related forms of mosaicism because of the increased risk of gonadal neoplasm.

XY GONADAL DYSGENESIS. The term XY gonadal dysgenesis has been applied to phenotypic females who have an XY karyotype, streak gonads, sexual infantilism, and normal or tall stature and who lack the somatic stigmata of Turner's syndrome. The prevalence of gonadal neoplasms such as seminoma and gonadoblastoma is significantly increased. Familial occurrence is common and in some sibships an affected sibling has had male pseudohermaphrodism with dysgenetic testes and ambiguous external genitalia (p. 1704). The reported pedigrees suggest X-linked recessive or sex-linked autosomal dominant inheritance.

FAMILIAL XX GONADAL DYSGENESIS. These are phenotypic females with normal stature, sexual infantilism, bilateral streak gonads, normal female external and internal genitalia, primary amenorrhea, elevated gonadotropins, low values of serum and urinary estrogens, and XX karyotypes. The habitus is often eunuchoid, and the somatic anomalies associated with XO gonadal dysgenesis are absent or minimal. Families in which multiple siblings are affected are not uncommon, and the transmission is consistent with autosomal recessive inheritance. In some families the gonadal defect is associated with sensorineural deafness. In sporadic cases the disorder is rarely recognized before puberty.

MALE TURNER'S SYNDROME. Phenotypic males with so-called male Turner's syndrome have been described who have short stature, webbed neck, certain other somatic anomalies that occur in Turner's syndrome, and hypoplastic and frequently undescended testes. The similar appearance of these males to phenotypic females with the syndrome of gonadal dysgenesis had suggested that the origins of Turner's syndrome in males and females were similar. However, with few exceptions, this is not so.

A few phenotypic males with this syndrome have a sex chromosome abnormality, such as XO/XY or XO/XYY, and represent a variant of all typical form of gonadal dysgenesis; in almost all other cases the karyotype has been XY. These XY cases form a heterogeneous group, quite likely of diverse origin, and ought not to be considered the female counterpart of XO gonadal dysgenesis. Many of the cases previously considered as male Turner's syndrome are examples of the syndrome described next.

XX AND XY TURNER PHENOTYPE (NOONAN'S SYNDROME, PSEUDO-TURNER SYNDROME, ULLRICH SYNDROME). Among the group of phenotypic males with features of male Turner's syndrome, a distinctive entity has been described that has led to the recognition of its counterpart in the female and its differentiation from the syndrome of gonadal dysgenesis. These patients often have characteristic facies: ptosis, antimongoloid palpebral slant, broad flat nose, webbed neck, short stature, high arched palate, and malformed ears (Fig. 48). Congenital heart disease (most commonly atrial septal defect and /or

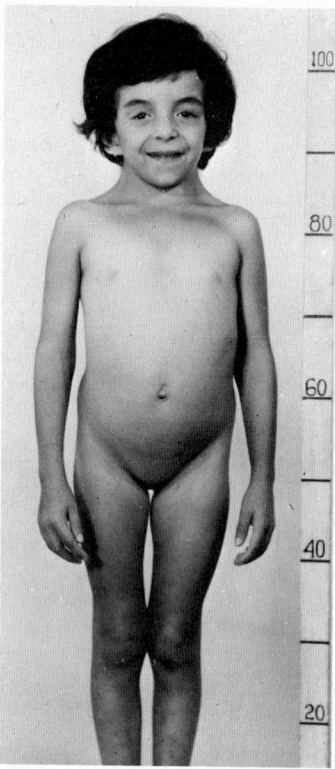

FIG. 48. Phenotypic 8-year-old female with syndrome of webbed neck, ptosis, congenital heart disease, short stature, and hypogonadism showing triangular facies, prominent brow, hypertelorism, antimongoloid slant of palpebral fissures, broad apex nasi, low-set ears, pectus excavatum. Height 106.2 cm (height age 4 years 4 months). Pulmonic stenosis was present. XX/46 karyotype. (From Grumbach and Barr: *Recent Prog Horm Res* 14:255, 1958.)

pulmonic stenosis, but not coarctation of the aorta) is a cardinal but not invariable feature. Pectus excavatum, cubitus valgus, and impaired mental development are frequent associated findings. In males, one or both testes may be undescended. Germinal cell aplasia or hypoplasia of the testis is common, and usually there is evidence of androgen deficiency. Functioning ovaries are present in affected females. In both sexes the karyotype is normal, and gonadal differentiation is consistent with the chromosomal and phenotypic sex. Familial cases consistent with autosomal dominant transmission have been described.

Seminiferous Tubule Dysgenesis

The most common human sex chromosomal aberration, an XXY karyotype, is associated with the sex-chromatin-positive form of seminiferous tubule dysgenesis (Klinefelter's syndrome). This disorder, a common cause of primary hypogonadism in the male, is characterized by male phenotype, by small, firm defective testes (measuring less than 3.0 cm in length), and in affected adults by azoospermia and sterility. During or after puberty the variable features of gynecomastia

and androgen deficiency with signs of eunuchoidism are present in about one-half of cases. Excretion of urinary gonadotropin is elevated. Cryptorchidism is infrequent. These patients tend to grow tall, the characteristic feature being the disproportionately long legs, which may be detected before puberty. Epiphyseal fusion is usually not delayed, and osseous development follows the male pattern. The diagnosis should be suspected in a long-legged adolescent boy with small, firm testes, gynecomastia, and poorly developed male secondary sex characteristics. The incidence of subnormal intelligence is increased; about 0.8 percent of males in institutions for the mentally defective are chromatin-positive. Behavior disorders, mental disease, mongolism, and, in adults, chronic pulmonary disease, varicose veins, and mild diabetes mellitus also occur with increased infrequency in this disorder.

INCIDENCE. In surveys of newborn infants, 30 of 14,526 male infants were found to be chromatin-positive, or approximately 1 in 500 males. Among 18 chromatin-positive male infants in whom karyotype analyses were reported by Maclean and associates, 12 showed an XXY sex chromosome constitution, 1 had an XXYY sex chromosome complex, and 5 were XY/XXY mosaics. Since the XY cell line may have a beneficial effect, some of the XY/XXY mosaics are potentially fertile.

The histopathology of the testis is variable. In one chromatin-positive premature infant the testicular morphology was normal. The prepubertal testis shows a diminished number of germ cells. With the onset of puberty, and in association with the action of pituitary gonadotropins, the characteristic testicular defect is evident: hyalinization and atrophy of seminiferous tubules, absence of peritubular elastic tissue, aggregation and pseudoadenomatous groupings of Leydig cells, and occasional tubules lined by Sertoli cells. Rarely, spermatogenesis is seen in isolated tubules.

The typical sex chromosome aberration, first described by Jacobs and Strong and by Ford and associates, is an XXY sex chromosome constitution and a diploid chromosome number of 47. The XXY karyotype can arise from meiotic nondisjunction of the sex chromosomes during parental gametosgenesis or from mitotic nondisjunction in an early division of the fertilized zygote. Evidence for both of these mechanisms exists. The mean maternal age is increased in chromatin-positive seminiferous tubule dysgenesis (but not as advanced as in mothers of infants with mongolism). This observation is consistent with a meiotic error occurring during oogenesis, giving rise to an XX ovum in some cases. The maternal age effect in chromosome errors appears to be a consequence of the long dormant diplotene stage (late prophase) of human ova from birth to ovulation. Studies of X-linked genetic markers (such as color blindness, the Xg^a blood group antigen, and glucose-6-phosphate dehydrogenase activity) in informative pedigrees indicate a maternal origin of both X chromosomes in some XXY patients. This may be a consequence of meiotic nondisjunction during oogenesis or mitotic nondisjunction in the zygote. In others, the nondisjunction occurs during spermatogenesis, probably at the first meiotic division, and the Y and one of the two X chromosomes are of paternal origin. The extra X chromosome is estimated to arise from the father in 40 percent of cases.

Other sex chromosome anomalies are less commonly found in this disorder. These include XX/XXY and XY/XXY mosaicism, an XX karyotype, and an XXXY sex chromosome complex; in this latter form radioulnar synostosis is a useful clinical sign. As mentioned previously, the XY cell line may have an ameliorating effect, and some patients with this form of mosaicism have been fertile.

OTHER VARIANT FORMS. Additional clinical features have been characteristic of certain variants of the XXY karyotype. XXYY individuals, as a group, are taller and more long-legged than XXY patients, and quite consistent dermatoglyphic patterns have been described. Most of these patients are severely retarded mentally. Xg^a blood analyses indicate that the XXYY male is the result of successive errors in the first and second meiotic divisions in spermatogenesis and fertilization of an X ovum by an XYY-bearing sperm.

In addition to severe mental retardation, the XXXXY cases studied have had a variety of associated malformations. The typical phenotypic features, while not pathognomonic, include the following: a variety of skeletal abnormalities (6 of 9 patients had radioulnar synostosis and short in-curved fifth digits); hypoplastic external genitalia and very small (commonly undescended) testes exhibiting prepubertal testicular dysgenesis; typical facies in many patients including prognathism, epicanthal folds, hypertelorism, strabismus, broad flat nose, and malformed ears; and severe mental deficiency. A variety of other anomalies, including congenital heart disease, cleft palate, and microcephaly, may be present. The extra X chromosomes in XXXXY males are of maternal origin. The finding of three sex chromatin bodies in the buccal smear is strong evidence in support of the diagnosis. In a few instances sex chromosome mosaicism has been found.

TREATMENT. The testicular lesion is irreversible. If androgen deficiency is present at adolescence, treatment with male sex hormone is effective. The gynecomastia is not affected by hormonal treatment, and mastectomy may be necessary in some patients for cosmetic reasons.

XYY SYNDROME. This sex chromosome anomaly occurs in about 1 in 500 male births. A large unselected group of XYY males has not yet been studied, and our present knowledge is limited to surveys in selected populations such as prison inmates and to isolated case reports. The phenotype is male; small numbers of patients with undescended testes and less often hypogonadism have been described. Tall stature and severe acne are common characteristics of the XYY individuals detected in prison surveys. Impulsiveness and criminal and psychopathic behavior are associated with this syndrome, but the frequency of aberrant behavior among XYY males is not known. Some XYY males have normal physique and exhibit normal behavior. Two

fluorescent Y chromatin masses are present in a high proportion of nuclei in quinacrine-stained buccal smears.

DIAGNOSIS OF ABNORMALITIES OF SEX DIFFERENTIATION

In infants with ambisexual development it is of greatest importance to establish a diagnosis as soon after birth as possible, not only for psychologic and social reasons but also because of the dangers inherent in failure to recognize the salt-losing form of congenital adrenal hyperplasia (p. 1632). Table 32 lists the conditions that should alert the physician to consider an anomaly of sex.

Ambiguous or incomplete masculinization of the external genitalia is a cardinal feature of intersexuality, and this diagnosis should be excluded before such an infant is regarded as a cryptorchid hypospadic male. The appearance of the external genitalia may be highly variable; in some instances the phallus resembles a large clitoris. Usually, however, there is some fusion of the labioscrotal folds and only a single perineal orifice. The presence of a palpable gonad in a labioscrotal fold or in the groin is a strong point against the diagnosis of female pseudohermaphrodism. As indicated in Table 30, the appearance of the external genitalia in some forms of intersexuality is not ambiguous. In male pseudohermaphrodites with the feminizing testes syndrome, the external genital structures are female (Fig. 45), whereas female pseudohermaphrodites in whom the orifice of the urogenital sinus is located at or close to the tip of the phallus (Fig. 42) have the appearance of cryptorchid males. Seminiferous tubule dysgenesis and the typical form of the syndrome of gonadal dysgenesis are not associated with anomalous development of the external genitalia. The diagnosis of the syndrome of feminizing testes should be suspected in the phenotypic females with a firm mass in the inguinal region or labium majus. In instances in which a previous sibling or a relative has an abnormality of sex differentiation, the external genitalia of a newborn infant should be examined with special care, and additional tests should be performed even if the external genitalia

TABLE 32. Features Suggesting an Anomaly of Sex

In infancy
  Ambiguous appearance of external genitalia
  Phenotypic male with cryptorchidism, especially if phallus is small
  Phenotypic female with mass in groin or labium majus
  Affected sibling with sexual anomaly
  Phenotypic female with prominent edema of distal parts of extremities and loose folds of skin over nape of neck
After infancy
  Short female, especially with features of gonadal dysgenesis
  Adolescent boy with small testes, especially if associated with gynecomastia
  Primary amenorrhea in adolescent girl associated with breast development and sparse or absent pubic and axillary hair

are normal, depending on the nature of the disorder in the affected individual. Phenotypic female infants with prominent edema of the hands and feet and loose folds of skin over the nape of the neck may have the syndrome of gonadal dysgenesis (Bonnevie-Ullrich syndrome).

Table 33 summarizes the diagnostic procedures of value to the physician in the differential diagnosis of an infant with ambiguous external genitalia or in whom for other reasons an abnormality of sex is suspected.

Female pseudohermaphodism must be distinguished from other forms of intersexuality in which there is bilateral cryptorchidism. The configuration of the external genitalia is not a distinctive feature. The history may reveal other siblings affected with congenital virilizing adrenal hyperplasia, signs of progressive virilization, or evidence of dehydration, vomiting, and collapse suggestive of an addisonianlike electrolyte disorder. The mother and the obstetrician should be queried concerning hormones administered during pregnancy.

The detection of chromatin-positive nuclei quickly limits the diagnostic possibilities to some form of female pseudohermaphrodism or to true hermaphrodism with undescended gonads. Twenty four hour specimens of urine should be examined for total 17-ketosteroids and, when possible, for pregnanetriol and 17-ketogenic steroids. In virilizing adrenal hyperplasia these steroids are excreted in increased amounts, but not always in the first weeks of life; when there is a defect in 21-hydroxylation, the plasma 17-hydroxy-progesterone concentration is strikingly elevated, even at 1 day of age. Laparotomy is a superfluous diagnostic procedure in this disorder. Serum electrolyte concentrations should be measured in any infant in whom adrenal hyperplasia is suspected.

Chromatin-positive patients who have normal values for urinary steroids may be either true hermaphrodites or nonadrenal female pseudohermaphrodites, a distinction that can be made after laparotomy and gonadal biopsy. However, those patients are no longer subjected to surgical exploration whose mothers were treated during pregnancy with hormones implicated as potential fetal masculinizing agents. It is sometimes advisable to inject a radiopaque contrast medium into the single perineal orifice to outline the urogenital sinus under fluoroscopic examination when separate urethral and vaginal orifices cannot be identified by inspection. An intravenous pyelogram is of value for detection of anomalies of the urinary tract in non-androgen-induced forms of female pseudohermaphroditism.

TABLE 33. Steps in Diagnosis of Intersexuality in Infancy

History: family history, pregnancy (hormones), crises, virilization
Inspection
Palpation of inguinal region and labioscrotal folds and rectal examination
Oral mucosal smear—sex chromatin pattern; karyotype—sex chromosome constitution
Excretion of 17-ketosteroids and pregnanetriol; serum 17-hydroxyprogesterone
Provisional diagnosis

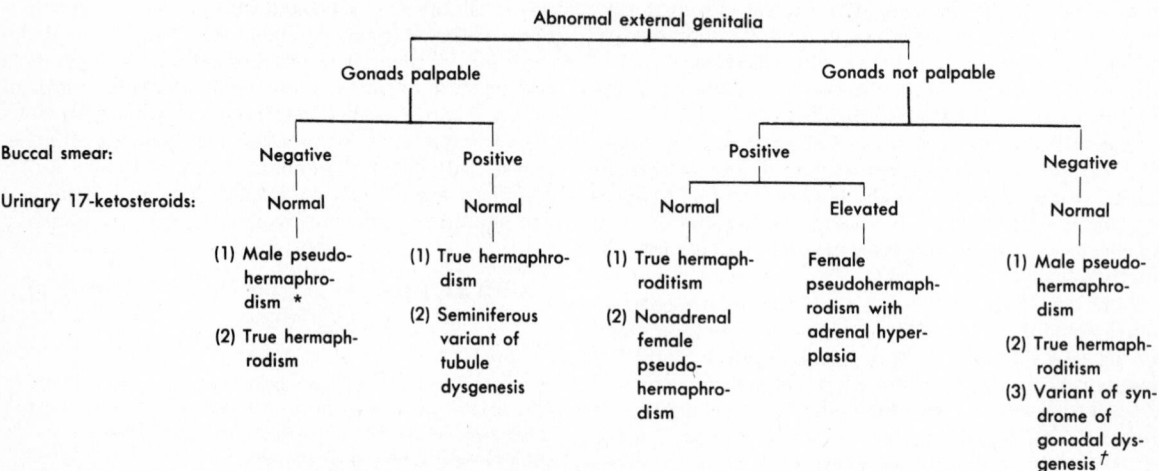

"Vaginogram" (urogenital sinus): selected cases
Endoscopy, laparotomy, gonadal biopsy: restricted to suspected male pseudohermaphrodites, true hermaphrodites, and selected instances of nonadrenal female pseudo-hermaphrodism

* Excretion of 17-ketosteroids is increased in male pseudohermaphrodites who have congenital adrenal hyperplasia due to a defect in 3β-hydroxy dehydrogenase.
† In variants of the syndrome of gonadal dysgenesis the appearance of the external genitalia may be normal.

Chromatin-negative individuals with abnormal external genitalia may be either male pseudohermaphrodites (including a variant of the syndrome of gonadal dysgenesis) or true hermaphrodites. Exploratory laparotomy and bilateral gonadal biopsy are necessary for a definitive diagnosis. Prior to operation, the anatomic findings should be defined by fluoroscopic and radiographic studies after injection of radiopaque material into the hypospadiac orifice, as well as by urethroscopic examination.

MANAGEMENT

The responsibility of the physician lies in the recognition of ambisexual development, especially in the infant. Early diagnosis and skillful management obviate many of the serious psychologic and social problems of the patients and his parents, as well as the difficult decisions that may face the physician when the diagnosis is incorrect or the selection of sex is indecisive or is delayed until childhood. It is during the period before the child has established a gender role that a carefully considered decision must be made as to the sex most suitable for the subject with a disorder of sex differentiation and, if indicated, the assigned sex changed accordingly. The following discussion concerns the classic forms of intersexuality; ambisexual differentiation of the genital tract does not occur in the typical forms of gonadal dysgenesis and seminiferous tubule dysgenesis.

If the diagnosis proves to be female pseudohermaphrodism, the infant should be reared as a female irrespective of the appearance of the external genitalia. In female pseudohermaphrodism associated with congenital adrenal hyperplasia, corticosteroid therapy should be administered to prevent virilization and accelerated development. The genital defect is readily corrected by appropriate surgical procedures, which should be performed during the first 12 months after birth. Since female pseudohermaphrodites have ovaries, fallopian tubes, and uterus, they are potentially fertile.

In male pseudohermaphrodites the basis for deciding on the sex of rearing is largely determined by the morphology of the external genitalia and the facility with which these structures can be surgically adapted to those of either a male or a female. It is desirable, whenever possible, to assign the sex of rearing in accordance with gonadal and chromosomal sex; however, these latter two variables are not absolute guides. In some male pseudohermaphrodites, for example in a patient with an exceedingly hypoplastic phallus or with predominantly female external genital structures, as in the syndrome of feminizing testes, the genitalia cannot possibly be reconstructed to function as male organs. In most instances it is preferable to recommend that individuals with inadequate male external genitalia be reared as females. The studies of Wilkins and associates and of Money and the Hampsons indicate the feasibility and importance of assigning such patients to the sex that conforms to the genital morphology, although this may be contrary to gonadal and chromosomal sex. The

decision, once made, should be firmly adhered to. Since many of these individuals are sterile, it is difficult to justify assignment of sex or change of sex in later childhood solely on the basis of potential fertility. Alteration of assigned sex is even less justifiable if this potentiality cannot be realized because of anatomic factors or serious psychologic difficulties.

The assignment of sex in true hermaphrodism is based on the morphology of the external genitalia and gonads. If the external genitalia are inadequate for a functional male, the individual should be raised as a female, and testicular tissue should be removed. In instances in which the ambiguity of the genital structures is such that the individual could be reared, following plastic surgical procedures, as a male or a female, weight in the selection of sex should be given to whether the ovarian or testicular elements are better developed and to the potential for fertility; the gonad contrary to the selected sex should be removed.

The age at which gender role and sexual orientation become firmly established in childhood is uncertain. From their studies, Money and associates suggest that this generally occurs between 1.5 and 2.5 years of age. Contrary to former opinion, psychosexual orientation does not appear to be instinctive and automatic, based on a single factor such as chromosomal sex, gonadal sex, or hormonal sex, but is a result of growing up and of all the experiences this implies. An important aspect of management is the physician's role in relieving parental apprehension and misconceptions and in providing them with practical guidance. The parents should have a part in the decision after they have been provided with an explanation of the findings in terms of the bipotential character of the fetal genital tract and of the incomplete development of the sexual organs in their child. It is especially important to reassure the parents that their child is not half boy and half girl and that the anomalous development does not lead to homosexuality or transvestism. Serious psychologic disturbances may result from attempts to change the sex of rearing during childhood after a gender role has been established. In general, such alterations should not be recommended in childhood after the age of 18 to 36 months. The rare exceptions in which after careful consideration it is decided to change the sex of rearing (eg, instances in which the child feels uncertain about his or her gender role) require the concurrence and assistance of a psychiatrist and provisions for extended counseling of the patient and the parents.

The question of gonadectomy is a difficult one. The decision to remove the gonads should be based on the type of secondary sexual development to be expected at puberty, bearing in mind the form of male pseudohermaphrodism with feminizing testes and the risk of malignant changes in later life. The latter consideration is not of importance in childhood or adolescence; however, in rare instances a malignant tumor of the gonad has been found before the age of puberty in patients with intersexuality. When gonadectomy is performed, it is important that the parents be advised of the need for appropriate hormonal therapy at the age of puberty.

References

Bardin CW, Bullock LP, Sherins RJ, Mowszowicz I, Blackburn WR: II. Androgen metabolism and mechanism of action in male pseudohermaphroditism: a study of testicular feminization. Recent Prog Horm Res 29:65, 1973

Bongiovanni AM: In Stanbury JB, Wyngaarden JB, and Fredrickson DS (eds): The Metabolic Basis of Inherited Disease, 3rd ed. New York, McGraw-Hill, 1972, p 587

Carpentier PJ, Potter EL: Nuclear sex and genital malformation in 48 cases of renal agenesis, with especial reference to nonspecific female pseudohermaphrodism. Am J Obstet Gynecol 78:235, 1959

Conte FA, Grumbach MM, Kaplan SL: A diphasic pattern of gonadotropin secretion in patients with the syndrome of gonadal dysgenesis. J Clin Endocrinal 40:670, 1975

Court Brown WM, Harnden DG, Jacobs PA, Maclean N, Mantle DJ: Abnormalities of the sex chromosomes complement in man. Med Res Counc Spec Rep Ser (Lond) 1964, p 305

————Males with an XYY sex chromosome complement. J Med Genet 5:341, 1968

Federman D: Abnormal Sexual Development—A Genetic and Endocrine Approach to Differential Diagnosis. Philadelphia, WB Saunders, 1967

Ferguson-Smith MA: Karyotype—phenotype correlations in gonadal dysgenesis and their bearing on the pathogenesis of malformations. J Med Genet 2:142, 1965

French FS, Van Wyk JJ, Baggett B, Easterling WE, Talbert LM, Johnston FR: Further evidence of a target organ defect in the syndrome of testicular feminization. J Clin Endocrinol 26:493, 1966

Grumbach MM, Ducharme JR: The effects of androgens on fetal development: androgen-induced female pseudohermaphrodism. Fertil Steril 11:157, 1960

————Ducharme JR, Moloshok RE: On the fetal masculinizing action of certain oral progestins. J Clin Endocrinol 19:1369, 1959

————Morishima A, Liu N: A distinctive clinical entity simulating Turner's syndrome in boys and girls associated with congenital heart disease, appropriate gonadal differentiation, and a normal sex chromosome constitution. J Pediatr 67:966, 1965

————Morishima A, Taylor JH: Human sex chromosome abnormalities in relation to DNA replication and heterochromatinization. Proc Natl Acad Sci USA 49:581, 1963

————Van Wyk JJ: Disorders of sex differentiation. In Williams WH (ed): Textbook of Endocrinology, 5th ed. Philadelphia, WB Saunders, 1974, p 423

Hamerton JL: Human Cytogenetics, Clinial Cytogenetics, Vol 2. New York, Academic, 1971

Imperato-McGinley J, Guerrero L, Gautier T, Peterson RE: Steroid 5α-reductase deficiency in man: an inherited form of male pseudohermaphrodism. Science 186:213, 1974

Jones HW Jr, Scott WW: Hermaphroditism, Genital Anomalies and Related Endocrine Disorders, 2nd ed. Baltimore, Williams & Wilkins, 1971

Jost A: Problems of fetal endocrinology: the gonadal and hypophyseal hormones. Recent Prog Horm Res 8:379, 1953

————A new look at the mechanisms controlling sex differentiation in mammals. Johns Hopkins Med J 130:38, 1972

Klinger HP, Ludwig KS: A universal stain for the sex chromatin body. Stain Technol 32:235, 1957

Lewis VG, Ehrhardt AA, Money J: Genital operations in girls with the adrenogenital syndrome. Subsequent psychologic development. Obstet Gynecol 36:11, 1970

Lyon MF: Sex chromatin and gene action in the mammalian X-chromosome. Am J Hum Genet 14:135, 1962

————X-chromosome inactivation and developmental patterns in mammals. Biol Rev 47:1, 1972

Maclean N, Harnden DG, Court Brown WM, Bond J, Mantle DJ: Sex-chromosome abnormalities in newborn babies. Lancet 1:286, 1964

————Mitchell JM, Harnden DG, A survey of sex chromosome abnormalities among 4514 mental defectives. Lancet 1:293, 1962

McKusick VA: On the X-Chromosome of Man. American Institution of Biological Sciences, 1964

Money J, Hampson JG, Hampson JL: Hermaphroditism: recommendations concerning assignment of sex, change of sex and psychologic management. Bull Johns Hopkins Hosp 97:284, 1955

————Hampson JG, Hampson JL: Sexual incongruities and psychopathology: the evidence of human hermaphroditism. Bull Johns Hopkins Hosp 98:43, 1956

————Psychologic evaluation of the child with intersex problems. Pediatrics 36:51, 1965

————Ehrhardt AA: Man and Woman, Boy and Girl: The Differentiation and Dimorphism of Gender Identity from Conception to Maturity. Baltimore, Johns Hopkins Univ Press, 1972

Moore KL (ed): The Sex Chromatin. Philadelphia, WB Saunders, 1966

Morishima A, Grumbach MM: The interrelationship of sex chromosome constitution and phenotype in the syndrome of gonadal dysgenesis and its variants. Ann NY Acad Sci 155:695, 1968

Noonan JA: Hypertelorism with Turner phenotype, a new syndrome with associated congenital heart disease. Am J Dis Child 116:373, 1968

Overzier C: Intersexuality. New York, Academic, 1963

Paulsen CA, Gordon DL, Carpenter RW, Gandy HM, Drucker WD: Klinefelter's syndrome and its variants: a hormonal and chromosomal study. Recent Prog Horm Res 24:321, 1968

Pearson PL, Borrow M, Vosa CG: Technique for identifying Y chromosomes in human interphase nuclei. Nature 226:78, 1970

Rimoin DL, Schimke RN: Genetic Disorders of the Endocrine Glands. St Louis, CV Mosby, 1971

Scully RE: Gonadoblastoma, a review of 74 cases. Cancer 25:1340, 1970

Walsh PC, Madden JD, Harrod MJ, Goldstein JL, MacDonald PC, Wilson JD: Familial incomplete male pseudohermaphroditism, type 2. N Engl J Med 291:944, 1974

Wilkins L: Masculinization of female fetus due to use of orally given progestins. JAMA 172:1028, 1960

————The Diagnosis and Treatment of Endocrine Disorders in Childhood and Adolescence, 3rd ed. Springfield, Ill, Charles C Thomas, 1965

NORMAL PUBERTAL DEVELOPMENT

HOWARD E. KULIN

SOMATIC CHANGES. Puberty is characterized by an increase in growth rate and the appearance of striking somatic sex differences. The onset of these changes actually antedates the appearance of secondary sex characteristics by a few years. Thus sexual maturation is a considerably longer process than can be ascribed to the period of visible changes induced by marked increments in gonadal hormones. In contrast to the situation with boys, increases in body fat in girls become manifest at 7 years of age, with continued acceleration, so that girls have twice as much fat at 16 years of age as their male counterparts.

Total body water reflects lean body mass, which is primarily made up of muscle and skeletal tissues. At 9.5 years of age, total body water increases significantly in boys and signals the onset of more rapid growth in lean body mass. Muscle mass in boys doubles between the ages of 10 and 17 years, and skeletal mass doubles between ages 12 and 16 years. In fact, during adolescence the male exceeds the female in body measurements, except in hip width and body fat (p. 109).

The changes in growth of body constituents during puberty are, of course, most impressively reflected by increments in height and weight. The age of initiation of the adolescent growth spurt precedes the onset of secondary sex characteristics by approximately 1 year in boys and girls. The onset and progression of puberty appear to bear some relationship to weight; menarche occurs somewhat earlier in obese girls, and sexual development is delayed by malnutrition. The decrease in the age of menarche observed over the past century, which has been associated with an increase in body size for a given age, is apparently related to improved general health and nutrition and other socioeconomic factors.

Marshall and Tanner have described the changes of puberty by a rating scale for pubic hair, male genital stages, and breast development (Figs. 49, 50, and 51). Pubic hair for boys and girls can be rated as follows: stage 1, prepubertal, with no true pubic hair; stage 2, sparse growth of long, slightly pigmented hair; stage 3, hair becomes darker, coarser, and more curled and begins to spread over pubic symphysis; stage 4, hair is adult in character but not in distribution, without spread to medial surface of thighs; stage 5, adult. Marked individual variations may occur in the pattern of pubertal development regarding both onset and duration of pubic hair, breast development, and genital stages. A boy with midpubertal genital development, for instance, may have no pubic hair or nearly adult amounts and yet may fall within the range of normal. Despite this variability, knowledge of the mean time of onset and duration of various pubertal stages (Tables 34 and 35) will provide the physician with a reliable index of suspicion regarding abnormalities of sexual maturation. Skeletal age varies less than chronologic age for most pubertal events, and it remains an excellent predictor of pubertal onset.

The very first sign of pubertal development in boys (enlargement of testicular size) occurs only about 6 months later than the first change in girls, which is usually breast development. Thus the timing of the onset of the pubertal process may be similar for boys and girls, in contrast to the progressive development of secondary sexual characteristics (Table 34). Pubic hair, for instance, appears about 1.5 years later in boys than in girls, and peak height velocity is reached almost 2 years later in boys than in girls. Peak height velocity in girls occurs before menarche, which in turn takes place approximately 2.5 years after the first signs of breast development. In each sex it takes about 4.5 years from the first appearance of secondary sex characteristics to adult configuration (Table 35).

HORMONAL MODULATION. While the secretory products of the hypothalamic-pituitary-gonadal axis are the primary modulators of the somatic changes that appear during puberty, other hormones also play

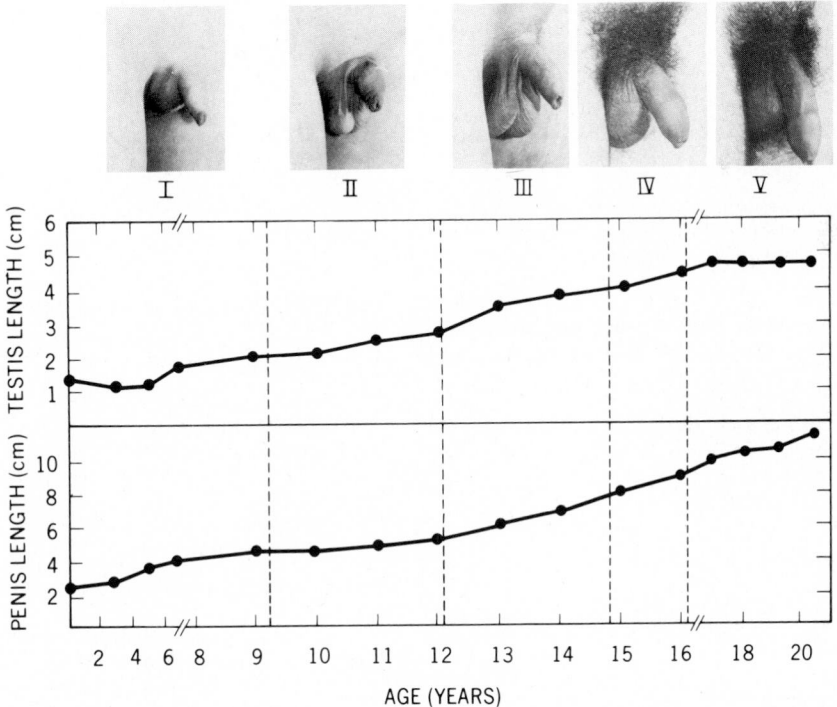

FIG. 49. Genital development in boys: stage I, prepubertal; stage II, enlargement of testes, appearance of scrotal reddening, and increase in scrotal rugations; stage III, increase in length and, to a lesser extent, breadth of penis, with further growth of testes; stage IV, further increase in size of penis and testes and darkening of scrotal skin; stage V, adult.

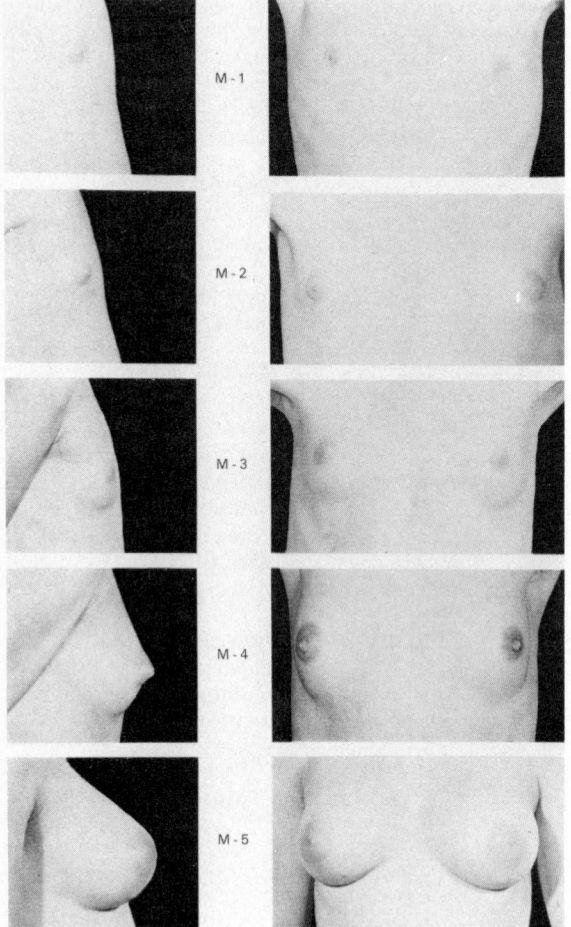

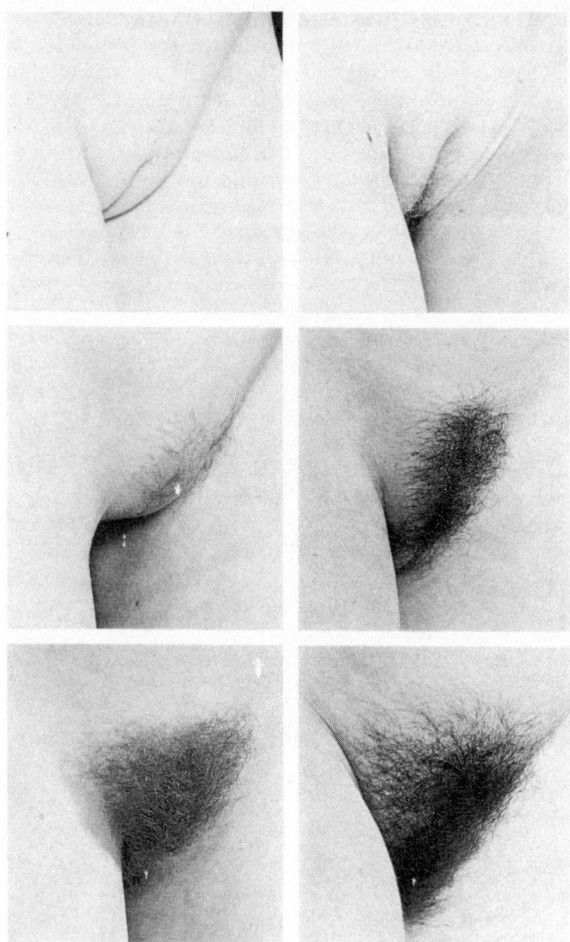

FIG. 50. Breast development in girls: stage I, prepubertal; stage II,-budding; stage III, appearance of small adult breast; stage IV, areola and papilla form a secondary mound; stage V, adult.

FIG. 51. Stages of appearance of pubic and labial hair in girls (stage I, prepubertal; Stage V, adult).

TABLE 34. Patterns of Pubertal Development in Boys and Girls for the British Population*

Interval	Mean (years)[†]
From breast bud to onset of pubic hair	0.5
From breast bud to peak height velocity	1.0
From breast bud to menarche	2.3
From breast bud to adult pubic hair	3.1
From breast bud to adult breast	4.5

From Marshall and Tanner: Arch Dis Child 44:291, 1969; 45:13, 1970.
[†] *SD for each event is approximately 1 year. American standards are 6 to 12 months earlier for girls and 2 to 6 months earlier for boys.*

TABLE 35. Duration of Pubertal Stages in Girls*

Pubertal Event	Mean Age of Onset	
	Boys	Girls
Breast development[†]	—	11.2
Testicular enlargement	11.6	—
Pubic hair development	13.4	11.7
Peak height velocity	14.1	12.1
Menarche	—	13.5
Adult pubic hair configuration	15.2	14.4
Adult-type breast	—	15.3

From Marshall and Tanner: Arch Dis Child 44:291, 1969; 45:13, 1970.
[†] *There is great individual variation in the length of these stages, eg, a period of 1 to 5 years may elapse from onset of breast development to menarche and still fall within the normal range.*

a role. In particular, growth hormone appears to be necessary to realize the full growth-promoting effects of some gonadal steroids. Boys deficient in growth hormone exhibit a growth spurt when exposed to testosterone, but to a lesser degree than in the presence of growth hormone. While changes in growth hormone

production with age have been described, the adolescent growth spurt appears to be independent of these variations.

Thyroxine levels do not change with puberty, but

there is a permissive action in terms of maximal linear growth. Thyroid hormone appears to act as a primary stimulant to skeletal maturation; the delayed bone age resulting from thyroxine deficiency may be associated with delays in neuroregulation of pubertal onset. Primary hypothyroidism in children may also be associated with an increase in gonadotropins and prolactin, as well as the characteristic elevation of thyroid-stimulating hormone (TSH); precocious puberty with a relatively delayed bone age may occur paradoxically.

A change in adrenal production of weakly androgenic substances, as represented by an increase in excretion of urinary 17-ketosteroids, is a well-known pubertal event. The primary circulating adrenal androgens are dehydroepiandrosterone (DHEA) and its sulfate; these hormones have now been assayed during the course of puberty. The role of adrenal androgens in causing the pubertal growth spurt, particularly in girls, remains controversial; however, they have an important effect on the development of pubic and axillary hair in girls. Estrogens may play an important part in the augmented production of 17-ketosteroids that accompanies puberty, but the precise cause of the rise in adrenal androgens remains unknown. The significant somatic changes (eg, increments in lean body mass and height acceleration), which precede by a year or more the appearance of secondary sexual characteristics, could be the results of adrenal steroids or a subliminal increase in production of gonadal hormones.

Glucocorticoid excess, either endogenous or exogenous, is almost invariably associated with a decrease in rate of growth and a delay in pubertal onset. These effects appear to be mediated at end-organ sites as part of the catabolic effects of these drugs. When glucocorticoids are used in the therapy of disease states that in themselves may delay growth, the delay in the pubertal process may be marked and prolonged.

GONADAL FUNCTION.   Although the testis increases significantly in size in the several years prior to onset of puberty, testosterone levels appear to remain constant at less than 20 to 30 ng/100 ml (in boys and girls) throughout childhood. Depending on assay sensitivity, testicular size may increase outside of the prepubertal range without a significant change in measurable testosterone. A testicular length of more than 2.5 cm is consistent with early pubertal development, the change being due primarily to the tubular constituents of the gonad. Once testosterone levels begin to rise in boys, they do so relatively rapidly. However, many androgen-mediated changes, such as the pubertal growth spurt, occur in the presence of relatively low testosterone levels. There is great variability between pubic hair development and plasma testosterone, and even with advanced stages of pubic hair development in the male, testosterone measurements may be within the adult female range. During puberty in the male, circulating testosterone increases more than 20-fold (Fig. 52).

The prepubertal testis may be easily stimulated when exposed to the appropriate tropin. Human chorionic

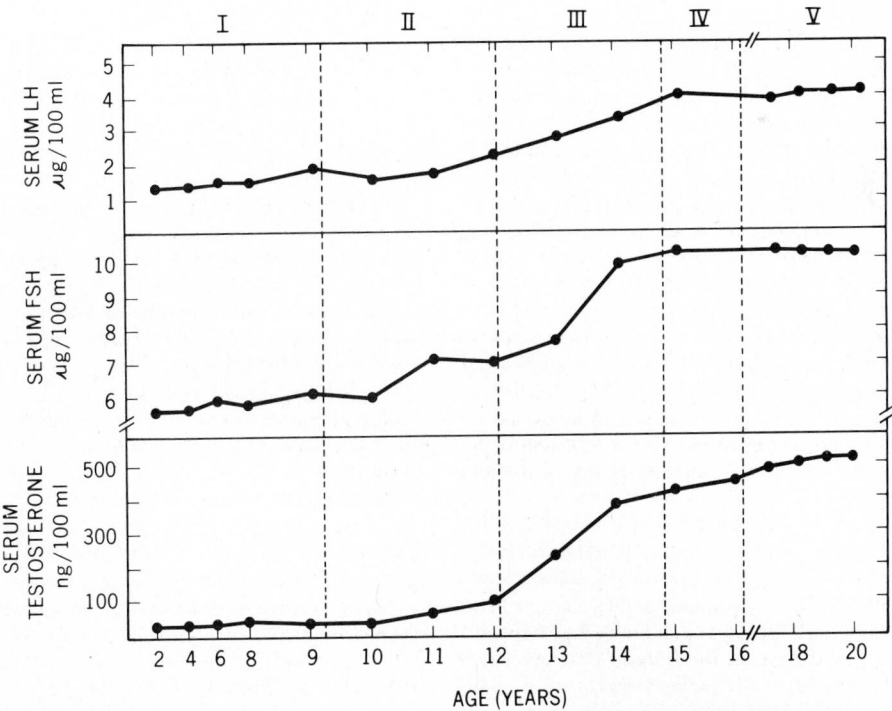

FIG. 52. Blood gonadotropin and testosterone levels in boys. [From Faiman and Winter: In Grumbach, Grave, and Mayer (eds): The Control of the Onset of Puberty, 1974. Courtesy of John Wiley & Sons.]

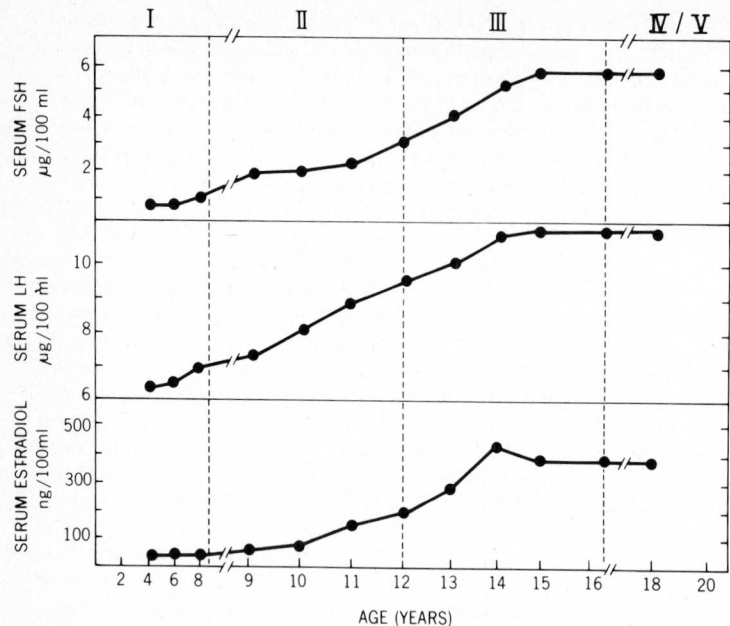

FIG. 53. Blood gonadotropin and estradiol levels in girls in relation to stages of breast development. [From Faiman and Winter: In Grumbach, Grave, and Mayer (eds): The Control of the Onset of Puberty, 1974. Courtesy of John Wiley & Sons.]

gonadotropin (HCG), a luteinizing hormonelike substance, causes a prompt increase in measurable testosterone; administration of this material can aid in the assessment of testicular function even before the onset of puberty. The pubertal testis is highly responsive to HCG stimulation even within 24 to 48 hours. The capacity to secrete testicular androgen is not a limiting factor in the onset of male puberty.

While the prepubertal ovary exhibits rather dramatic changes in terms of histologic development and regression of follicles (presumably gonadotropin-induced), measurable differences in circulating 17β-estradiol (E$_2$) beween boys and girls are not detectable before 7 or 8 years of age; blood levels of this most active gonadal estrogen are less than 10 pg/ml before the onset of puberty. Studies utilizing urethral cytology, however, support a decidedly different estrogen milieu between the sexes, even in childhood. By age 10 years, levels of E$_2$ in girls exceed those in boys by approximately twofold. Then there is a steady rise in estradiol concentration throughout puberty (Fig. 53), with wide individual fluctuations manifest by the time menarche occurs. A small but significant increase in estradiol also occurs in the male as a result of both testicular secretion and the peripheral conversion of other hormones (eg, testosterone) to estrogens.

The prepubertal ovary, like the testis, can be stimulated when exposed to the appropriate stimulus, and ovulation can be induced by exogenous gonadotropin.

PITUITARY SECRETION. Prolactin levels change little during childhood and adolescence. There has been no convincing demonstration in the human that prolactin plays a role in the onset of sexual maturation. The gonadotropins are the key hormones in this regard, and both follicle-stimulating hormone (FSH) and luteinizing hormone (LH) have been quantified in blood and urine of prepubertal children.

There are no sex differences in the levels of gonadotropins during much of childhood, although FSH levels do appear greater in girls than in boys in the first 2 years. Gonadotropin secretion may reach a nadir at 3 to 5 years of age, after which levels steadily increase. As puberty approaches, FSH appears to increase somewhat more rapidly than LH and attains adult levels before LH.

Levels of serum gonadotropin in the adult are only twofold to fourfold greater than in the child, with considerable variation. Results adapted from a longitudinal study are shown in Figures 52 and 53. On the other hand, striking increments in urinary excretion of FSH and LH have been detected during puberty, so that adults excrete about 30 times as much LH and 10 times as much FSH as prepubertal children (Fig. 54); if related to body size, this difference, is reduced to eightfold for LH and threefold for FSH.

The hypothalamic releasing hormone LRF (LRH), which is instrumental in the control of LH and FSH, has now been synthesized and administered to children. The pituitary gland responds to this tropin with a prompt release of LH and FSH, indicating that hypophyseal function is not a limiting factor in the onset of puberty.

NONHORMONAL MODULATION. Almost all nonhormonal factors that influence growth in general have an effect on the timing and progression of the pubertal process. These influences may operate by directly decreasing hormone production, thus advancing unknown neural mechanisms, or by direct effects on end organ tissue (eg, bone) itself. Genetic contributions play an important role in the onset of puberty, as do such diverse factors as nutrition, geography, altitude, and underlying systemic disease. The latter factor may be particularly important, and a careful search for conditions involving heart, kidney, and gas-

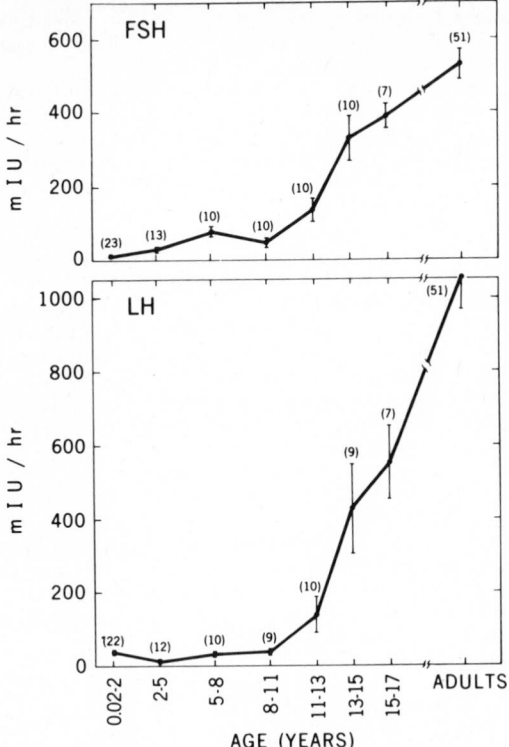

FIG. 54. Radioimmunoassay results (X ± SEM) of FSH and LH in acetone concentrates made from timed urine collections in children and adults mIU/hour). Numbers of subjects (male and female) are listed for each of the age groups in parentheses. (From Kulin et al: J Clin Endocrinol Metab 40:783, 1975.)

trointestinal tract must be considered in the evaluation of any patient with a significant delay in pubertal onset. The complexities of environmental and/or psychologic factors are evident in various deprivation syndromes and in anorexia nervosa. Certainly caloric factors are operative in causing pubertal delay in such conditions, but so are other ill-defined psychic processes.

MECHANISMS OF PUBERTAL ONSET AND PROGRESSION. While the precise neurochemical process leading to onset of puberty remains unknown, a number of physiologic events, primarily relating to gonadotropin control mechanisms, have been recognized. Both the pituitary and hypothalamus are involved in these changes. Gonadotropin secretion is episodic in nature because of the pulsatile release of endogenous LRF. Episodic LH release has been considered a pubertal phenomenon; this is one reason that a single blood measurement of FSH and LH may have only limited diagnostic value in children and adolescents. Increased amounts of LH during sleep have been detected in the blood and urine of pubertal children. The increase in absolute magnitude of sleep-associated LH secretion also produces elevations in nocturnal testosterone levels in boys. These nocturnal elevations in testosterone may cause the first visible somatic changes of puberty.

FEEDBACK RELATIONSHIPS. Negative feedback is the homeostatic control mechanism that allows gonadal steroids to maintain a given level of FSH and/or LH. Elimination of the gonadal product will cause a release from negative feedback and a consequent increase in pituitary hormones; similarly, an increase in gonadal secretions will suppress FSH and LH.

There are several lines of evidence that suggest the existence of negative feedback in the prepubertal child. Most important is the fact that elevated levels of gonadotropins have been detected in children without gonads, a clinically useful finding in the evaluation of patients suspect for gonadal dysgenesis. Another interesting observation bearing on negative feedback is the fact that prepubertal boys with unilateral cryptorchidism have larger scrotal testes than normal controls. This finding suggests that a decrease in gonadal secretory products in such individuals causes a secondary rise in gonadotropins and further stimulation of the remaining scrotal testis. Finally, when estrogen or drugs with estrogen-like activity have been administered to prepubertal children, considerably smaller amounts of these substances are required for depression of gonadotropins in children as compared with adults. These observations indicate that negative feedback is present before puberty and operates at a highly sensitive level.

A change in the sensitivity of this negative-feedback system occurs during sexual maturation in man. The adult-type interaction is attained only in midpuberty or late puberty as levels of gonadotropins and gonadal steroids increase. The major site of negative-feedback control is at the hypothalamus, but the pituitary is also involved.

A second important interaction between gonad, hypothalamus, and pituitary gland is that referred to as positive feedback. This type of interaction exists when gonadal hormones further stimulate the hypothalamic–pituitary axis to secrete additional amounts of gonadotropins, especially LH. This form of feedback is integral to the ovulatory process in normal menstruating women, in whom rising levels of estrogen precede the sharp midcycle burst of LH that causes the release of the ovum from the appropriately ripened follicle (Fig. 55). This rise in estrogen from the maturing follicle is the trigger for ovulation and induces the ovulatory LH surge by means of positive feedback. An artificial reproduction of these events has been carried out by administration of exogenous estrogen early in the course of the menstrual cycle; when given at this time, a prompt rise in LH follows administration of estrogen to mature women. On the other hand, prepubertal girls will not diplay such a rise in LH when exposed to similar levels of circulating estrogen. With further progression of puberty, positive feedback does become manifest, presumably somewhat late in the process of sexual maturation. Recent evidence indicates that there is a pituitary component as well as a hypothalamic component to the process of positive feedback.

TESTS THAT ASSESS MATURITY OF HYPOTHALAMIC-PITUITARY-GONADAL   AXIS.
While a great deal may be learned from measurement

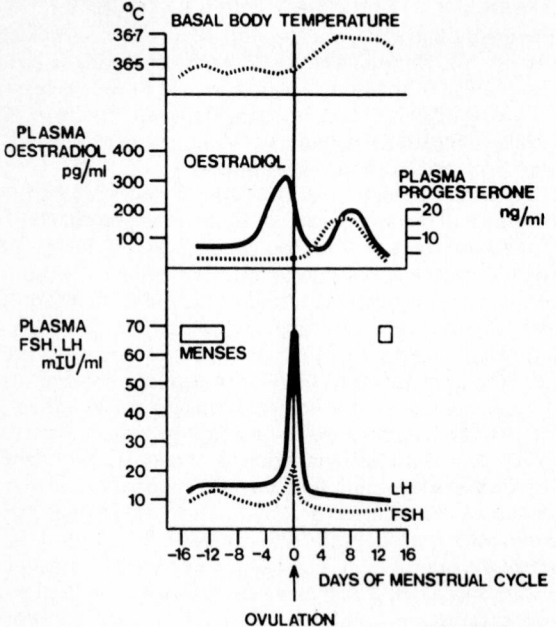

FIG. 55. Hormonal events of the menstrual cycle. Note that rising estradiol levels precede the midcycle surge of LH, an example of positive feedback. (From Visser: Arch Dis Child 48:169, 1973.)

of the concentration of serum FSH, LH, testosterone, and estradiol, a single time point has limited value in terms of an ongoing process like puberty. Significant hormonal increments over several months are the most reassuring laboratory evidence of normal pubertal progression. Frequent sampling to assess the nature of periodic LH release or to detect circadian rhythms may be useful, but it is difficult to perform in children. Timed urine collections provide a convenient means of obtaining specimens for gonadotropin radioimmunoassay.

There is no specific provocative test for LRF release in children. In adults, clomiphene citrate can be used for such a purpose, but a stimulatory response to this drug does not become manifest until midpuberty evolves. At present, administration of LRF or LRH may be one of the most useful tests in pubertal staging: with acute intravenous administration of LRF the magnitude of the rise in LH may reflect the level of endogenous releasing hormone.

It should be borne in mind that no available tests can supplant the careful history and physical examination coupled with knowledge of the normal pattern and progression of secondary sex characteristics. Few physiologic processes remain so complex (and mysterious) as the interactions involved in sexual maturity—physical, psychologic, and hormonal.

References

Blizzard RM, Thompson RG, Baghdassarian A, Kowarski A, Migeon SJ, Rodriguez A: The interrelationship of steroids, growth hormone, and other hormones on pubertal growth. In Grumbach MM, Grave GD, Mayer FE (eds): The Control of the Onset of Puberty. New York, Wiley, 1974

Boyar RM, Rosenfeld RS, Kapen S, et al: Human puberty. Simultaneous augmented secretion of luteinizing hormone and testosterone during sleep. J Clin Invest 54:609, 1974

Cheek DB: Body composition, hormones, nutrition, and adolescent growth. In Grumbach MM, Grave GD, Mayer FE (eds): The Control of the Onset of Puberty. New York, Wiley, 1974

Conte FA, Grumbach MM, Kaplan SL: A diphasic pattern of gonadotropin secretion in patients with the syndrome of gonadal dysgenesis. J Clin Endocrinol Metab 40:670, 1975

Faiman C, Winter JSD: Gonadotropins and sex hormone patterns in puberty. In Grumbach MM, Grave GD, Mayer FE (eds): The Control of the Onset of Puberty. New York, Wiley, 1974

Grumbach MM, Roth JC, Kaplan SL, Kelch RP: Hypothalamic-pituitary regulation of puberty in man: evidence and concepts derived from clinical research. In Grumbach MM, Grave GD, Mayer FE (eds): The Control of the Onset of Puberty. New York, Wiley, 1974

Hopper BR, Yen SSC: Circulating concentrations of dehydroepiandrosterone and dehydroepiandrosterone sulfate during puberty. J Clin Endocrinol Metab 40:458, 1975

Kulin HE, Grumbach MM, Kaplan SL: Changing sensitivity of the pubertal gonadal hypothalamic feedback mechanism in man. Science 166:-1012, 1969

———— Bell PM, Santen RJ, Ferber AJ: Integration of pulsatile gonadotropin secretion by timed urinary measurements: an accurate and sensitive 3-hour test. J Clin Endocrinol Metab 40:783, 1975

Marshall WA, Tanner JM: Variations in patterns of pubertal changes in girls. Arch Dis Child 44:291, 1969

———— Tanner JM: Variations in the pattern of pubertal changes in boys. Arch Dis Child 45:13, 1970

———— Interrelationships of skeletal maturation, sexual development and somatic growth in man. Ann Hum Biol 1:29, 1974

Reiter EO, Kulin HE, Hamwood SM: The absence of positive feedback between estrogen and luteinizing hormone in sexually immature girls. Pediatr Res 8:740, 1974

Ross GT, Cargille CM, Lipsett MB, et al: Pituitary and gonadal hormones in women during spontaneous and induced ovulatory cycles. Recent Prog Horm Res 26:1, 1970

Visser HKA: Some physiological and clinical aspects of puberty. Arch Dis Child 48:169, 1973

Zachman M, Prader A: Anabolic and androgenic effect of testosterone in sexually immature boys and its dependency on growth hormone. J Clin Endocrinol 30:85, 1970

SEXUAL PRECOCITY AND SEXUAL INFANTILISM

Robert P. Kelch

The time of onset and subsequent course of hormonal and physical changes during puberty are highly variable and are influenced by many factors, such as genetic endowment, chronic illness, nutritional and socioeconomic status, and geography (eg, altitude). Breast budding in girls and testicular enlargement with reddening and thinning of the scrotum in boys are usually the first signs of sexual maturation (p. 1713). The appearance of secondary sex characteristics before 8 years of age in girls and 9 years in boys should be considered precocious. Puberty is considered to be delayed if physical changes are not apparent before 13 years in girls and 14 years in boys. Puberty should also be considered delayed if more than 5 years have elapsed between the first physical signs of puberty and the onset of menarche in girls or the completion of genital growth in boys.

It is necessary for the physician to be aware of the detailed studies of progression of physical changes during puberty reported by Marshall and Tanner (p. 1713). Growth velocity reaches a nadir just before the onset of pubertal development. Maximum growth velocity occurs in early puberty in girls (before menarche), while in boys maximum growth velocity occurs in midpuberty or late puberty, approximately 2 years later than in girls. The average time between breast budding and menarche is 2.5 years in the United States; the average age at menarche is 12.5 to 13 years. Finally, menstrual cycles are often irregular and anovulatory for the first 6 to 12 months. Normal serum gonadotropin and sex steroid values for children of different ages are discussed elsewhere (p. 1716).

Recent technical advances have allowed precise measurement of pituitary and steroid hormones in serum as well as urine samples and have increased our understanding of the hormonal changes that occur during puberty. A highly sensitive negative-feedback system between the immature gonads (ovaries or testes) and the hypothalamus and pituitary is operative in the prepubertal child. This system appears to develop during late fetal life. Nonetheless, significant sex differences in the negative-feedback system have been demonstrated in prepubertal children. For example, infant girls have greater concentrations of serum gonadotropins and estradiol (LH and FSH) than boys and girls over 2 years of age; prepubertal girls release more FSH than prepubertal boys or adult men when challenged with synthetic luteinizing hormone releasing factor (LRF), and infant males have greater concentrations of serum testosterone than infant females.

Two major changes in the regulation of gonadotropin secretion seem to occur during puberty. First, the set-point of the hypothalamic–pituitary axis increases gradually. Thus greater concentrations of sex hormones (testosterone, estradiol, progesterone, etc) are required to suppress the secretion of LH and FSH. Second, the potential for a positive-feedback response to rising concentrations of circulating estrogens appears around midpuberty. The positive-feedback system is responsible for the midcycle surge of LH and FSH and subsequent ovulation in the sexually mature female. The sites and mechanisms of these feedback systems are still incompletely understood.

Isosexual Precocious Development

Clinically it is useful to distinguish between isosexual and heterosexual precocious development. Isosexual refers to development that is consistent with the phenotypic sex of the individual, whereas physical changes consistent with those of the opposite sex are considered heterosexual. Tables 36 and 37 summarize the differential diagnosis of isosexual and heterosexual precocious development.

Precocious pubertal development is much more common in girls than in boys. The most common final diagnosis in girls is idiopathic precocious puberty. Approximately 85 percent of cases of sexual precocity in girls and 35 percent in boys can be attributed to premature maturation of the hypothalamic-pituitary-

TABLE 36. Differential Diagnosis of Isosexual Precocity

Neurogenic precocious puberty
Idiopathic precocious puberty
    Sporadic (most common form in females)
    Familial (only males affected in most pedigrees)
Central nervous system disorders
    Tumors
    Congenital anomalies
    Postinflammatory
    Trauma
    Syndromes: McCune-Albright, neurofibromatosis, tuberous sclerosis, Russell-Silver
Gonadal tumors
    Ovarian: granulosa-theca cell tumor, granulosa-luteal cell cysts
    Testicular: Leydig cell tumor, adrenal rest tumor
Adrenal disorders
    Congenital adrenal hyperplasia (in boys)
    Adenomas and carcinomas: virilizing (in boys), feminizing (in girls)
Exogenous sex steroids or treatment with HCG
Gonadotropin-secreting tumors
    Chorioepithelioma
    Teratoma
    Hepatoblastoma (boys only)
Primary hypothyroidism—severe
Incomplete sexual precocity
    Premature thelarche
    Premature adrenarche

TABLE 37. Differential Diagnosis of Heterosexual Precocious Development

Girls
    Congenital adrenal hyperplasia
    Androgen-producing tumors: adrenal adenoma or carcinoma, ovarian arrhenoblastoma, teratoma
    Exogenous androgens
    Idiopathic hirsutism
Boys
    Adolescent gynecomastia
    Estrogen-producing tumors: adrenal adenoma or carcinoma, teratoma
    Exogenous estrogens

gonadal axis. Despite the high incidence of idiopathic precocious puberty, clinicians must diligently search for evidence of the other conditions outlined in Table 37. In boys the increased chance of finding an organic etiology for sexual precocity demands an even more aggressive diagnostic approach.

As with most clinical conditions, a thorough history and physical examination usually point toward the correct diagnosis. Specific questions should be asked to elicit any history of recent growth acceleration, behavior changes, central nervous system trauma, or infections (eg, previous meningitis or encephalitis), as well as any history of use of facial creams or oral, parenteral, or topical medications or a history of similar precocious development in parents or siblings. Familial precocious puberty has been reported several times, but it has been limited almost exclusively to males.

Physical examination must include a thorough neurologic examination with funduscopic and gross visual field examinations when the child is old enough. It is necessary to measure and maintain a record of height, weight, head circumference, arm span, sitting height, breast diameter in girls, and phallic length and width and the longest diameter of each testis (excluding epididymis) in boys. Examination of the skin for hyperpigmentation (congenital adrenal hyperplasia), "coast of Maine" (McCune-Albright) or "coast of California" café au lait spots (neurofibromatosis), carotenemia, dryness and coolness (hypothyroidism), and sebaceous gland activity may provide useful diagnostic findings. In both sexes, early signs of androgen secretion are indicated by the presence of comedones over the nose and in the external ear and oiliness of the facial skin. Breasts, genitalia, and sexual hair development should be assessed in detail. Galactorrhea is unusual, but its presence is suggestive of primary hypothyroidism or a pituitary or hypothalamic tumor. Bimanual abdominal and rectal examination is mandatory to assess uterine development or to detect adnexal masses; sedation or anesthesia may be necessary in younger patients to ensure an adequate examination.

When significant sexual precocity is detected, the initial diagnostic evaluation should include radiographic evaluation of the skull (detailed views of the optic foramina in cases with visual defects or suspected neurofibromatosis) and hands for bone age determinations, 24-hour urinary 17-ketosteroid excretion, serum LH, FSH, testosterone (in boys), and estradiol (in girls) determined by radioimmunoassay, and serum thyroxine concentration. Because of the significant overlap of normal values between prepubertal children and adults, single determinations of serum gonadotropins frequently are not diagnostic. Nonetheless, because of the cross-reactivity of chorionic gonadotropins and LH, the radioimmunoassay technique frequently will detect the presence of the rare gonadotropin-producing tumor. Although they are less sensitive, urinary pregnancy tests will also detect chorionic gonadotropin activity. Urinary gonadotropin determinations by bioassay are not useful in most cases; radioimmunoassay determinations of urinary LH and FSH may be more useful, although this technique is not readily available. Further diagnostic evaluation will depend on the observed results and the sex of the patient.

Children with idiopathic precocious puberty will typically have normal skull radiographs, advanced bone age (often greater than height age), urinary 17-ketosteroid excretion appropriate for the degree of pubertal development, and serum gonadotropins and sex steroid concentrations in the broad pubertal range. However, their clinical courses are highly variable. Girls will usually show breast development, sexual hair, development of labia minora and majora, and in due course, periodic menstruation. If untreated, ovulation occurs in some very young girls with precocious puberty, and pregnancies have been reported. Boys will display phallic enlargement, testicular enlargement, and progressive signs of androgen secretion: pubic and axillary hair, acne to a variable degree, facial hair, and emissions. Often, however, the rate of progression of sexual maturation is unpredictable and does not follow the normal

pattern. Many children with precocious puberty have been followed for extended periods of time and have led normal lives as adults. Although significant manifestations of disease of the central nervous system are usually absent, there is increased incidence of abnormal electroencephalographic tracings.

Isosexual precocity in girls may also be secondary to tumors of the central nervous system or to estrogen secretion by ovarian or adrenal tumors. Testing with LRF may be helpful diagnostically, since recent studies indicate that patients with idiopathic precocious puberty have augmented responsiveness. Brain scans are of limited value, but computerized axial tomography is a promising noninvasive procedure. Pneumoencephalography or carotid arteriography should be reserved for cases with historical or physical evidence of central nervous system abnormalities. The Russell-Silver syndrome is characterized by intrauterine growth retardation, subnormal growth velocity, triangular facies, clinodactyly, simian creases, increased prevalence of structural abnormalities of the genitourinary tract, and in some patients skeletal asymmetry. The McCune-Albright syndrome is more common in females and is associated with polyostotic fibrous dysplasia and prominent areas of skin pigmentation, usually unilateral and generally on the same side as the osseous lesions. Patients with neurofibromatosis may harbor a glioma in or around the hypothalamus, which may lead to an increased, or more commonly decreased, pituitary function.

Various central nervous system tumors, malignant and benign, may impinge on ventral hypothalamic areas and activate the centers that control gonadotropin secretion. The classic example of a benign tumor is the hamartoma of the tuber cinereum. These tumors rarely damage the hypothalamus; they generally have secondary effects on other parts of the central nervous system and usually are asymptomatic, except for sexual precocity. Nonparenchymatous tumors of the pineal gland also may cause sexual precocity in boys, while parenchymatous tumors are associated with delayed sexual development.

Nearly all estrogen-producing ovarian tumors are palpable on bimanual abdominal-rectal examination. They are usually unilateral, smooth, firm, and encapsulated. Histologically they are either granulosa-theca cell tumors or cysts; at times there is luteinization of the cyst. Granulosa-theca cell tumors generally grow rapidly, but usually are benign. Approximately 30 percent are malignant, but accurate statistics are not available. It may be difficult to differentiate small ovarian tumors because of the overlap in laboratory values. For example, at times urinary and serum estrogens may be only slightly elevated, and serum and urinary gonadotropins may be present in normal amounts. Treatment of ovarian tumors is primarily surgical and usually involves unilateral ovariectomy. The presence of an adnexal mass requires surgical exploration. Small or moderate-sized ovarian cysts are sometimes palpable in girls with idiopathic precocious puberty. These are usually bilateral and may recur after careful excision. These cysts are probably the result of the precocious release of gonadotropins; care must be taken to avoid surgical trauma to the remaining ovarian tissue.

Feminizing adrenal tumors are rare and often difficult to recognize. Frequently they also secrete excessive amounts of adrenal androgens, and hence 17-ketosteroid excretion is increased. Intravenous pyelography may be helpful in cases where an adrenal adenoma or carcinoma is a distinct possibility. Adrenal scans performed with administration of radioiodinated cholesterol before and after dexamethasone suppression may also prove useful as further experience is acquired with children. Adrenal venography or arteriography should be performed only by highly skilled personnel and when the index of suspicion is great.

In boys, true precocious puberty, whether idiopathic or secondary to a structural abnormality of the central nervous system, must be differentiated from excessive androgen production alone. The most common cause of excessive androgen production is congenital adrenal hyperplasia (non-salt-losing form of 21-hydroxylase deficiency). Examination of the external genitalia will usually distinguish between these possibilities. Boys with precocious puberty will have bilateral testicular enlargement, testes 2.5 to 3.0 cm or more in the longest diameter, and skeletal age and 17-ketosteroid excretion appropriate for the degree of pubertal development. Boys with androgen excess alone usually have small, prepubertal-size testes, despite advanced genital development and often more striking advancement of skeletal age and 17-ketosteroid excretion.

Unfortunately, there are rare exceptions to this rule. Occasionally boys with congenital adrenal hyperplasia will have testicular enlargement because they really have entered into puberty or because of bilateral hyperplasia of adrenal rests in the testes. Leydig cell (interstitial cell) tumors, while rare, are usually unilateral and palpable. Although many of these are benign, metastases have been reported years after removal of a primary tumor. Most boys with Leydig cell tumors have been under 6 years of age. Detailed studies of individual plasma sex steroids and urinary 17-ketosteroids have assisted in the differentiation from adrenal lesions. In instances of Leydig cell tumors, the urinary 17-ketosteroids are usually metabolites of testosterone, and the principal circulating androgen is testosterone, whereas adrenal androgen-producing lesions secrete primarily dehydroepiandrosterone and its sulfate.

Adrenocortical tumors, adenomas, or carcinomas can occur in either sex at any time in life. Adrenal tumors are exceedingly rare in earliest infancy and are not an important consideration in the differential diagnosis of neonatal sexual ambiguity. These tumors are usually unilateral and may be associated principally with the secretion of excessive quantities of androgens. Urinary 17-ketosteroids are strikingly elevated in most cases, sometimes reaching levels in excess of 50 mg/day. Glucocorticoid suppression tests and intravenous pyelography are the most useful diagnostic studies. In some cases the contralateral adrenal gland may be atrophic secondary to glucocorticoid secretion by the tumor. Thus when unilateral adrenalectomy is planned, the patient should receive stress doses of glucocorticoids to prevent the possibility of acute adrenal insufficiency. Surgical removal of adenomata is usually curative, but adrenal carcinomas are usually rapidly fatal.

In both boys and girls, gonadotropin-producing tumors are rare. These neoplasms arise in an extrapituitary site; gonadotropin-producing tumor of the pituitary gland is essentially unknown as a cause of sexual precocity. Chorioepitheliomas are the classic gonadotropin-producing tumors. They may occur in any part of the body, even within the cranial cavity. Generally they are highly malignant. Hepatoblastoma may produce a chorionic-gonadotropin-like hormone and cause sexual precocity in boys. Testicular biopsy will reveal Leydig cell hyperplasia. Hepatomegaly may be present, but without evidence of gross hepatic functional disturbance. Teratomas may occur in the gonads or retroperitoneum or anywhere along the median or paramedian line from the base of the skull to the sacrococcygeal region. They are often benign and may secrete chorionic gonadotropins.

Because the source of androgen excess frequently is not obvious, adrenal gland suppression with glucocorticoids, such as oral dexamethasone (1.25 mg/m^2 /day in four equal doses), may be necessary. When evaluating adrenal androgen secretion by determination of 17-ketosteroid excretion, suppression should be carried out for at least 4 to 5 days because of the slow clearance rate of circulating adrenal androgens. In addition, urinary pregnanetriol should be measured before and at the end of dexamethasone suppression. Pregnanetriol is the urinary metabolite of 17-hydroxyprogesterone, the steroid hormone that is increased strikingly in patients with congenital adrenal hyperplasia due to 21-hydroxylase deficiency. Increased but suppressible urinary 17-ketosteroids and pregnanetriol will confirm the diagnosis of congenital adrenal hyperplasia. Incomplete suppression of 17-ketosteroids but marked suppression of pregnanetriol suggests that the patient already has entered into puberty. Strikingly increased and nonsuppressible 17-ketosteroid excretion suggests the presence of an androgen-producing tumor, most likely adrenal in origin. If the baseline urinary 17-hydroxycorticosteroids are elevated, suppression with a higher dose of dexamethasone (3.75 mg/m^2/day in four equal doses) for an additional 2 days would be necessary to differentiate between an adrenal tumor and Cushing's disease. Cushing's disease is rare in children, and the effects of excess glucocorticoid (obesity, striae, hypertension, moon facies, and poor growth) should be apparent clinically.

Boys with bilateral testicular enlargement, appropriate urinary 17-ketosteroid, serum testosterone, and gonadotropin values for the degree of pubertal development, and normal urinary pregnananetriol excretion probably have true precocious puberty. If there is no obvious reason for precocious development (eg, positive family history in brother, previous central nervous system infection or inflammation), and even if there are no discernible neurologic abnormalities, a computerized axial tomographic brain scan should be performed, and pneumoencephalography should be considered to rule out the possibility of a hypothalamic tumor. This recommendation is given despite the inoperable nature of most tumors associated with precocious puberty.

In both sexes, severe primary hypothyroidism has been associated with sexual precocity. Galactorrhea is a common finding in affected females. The precocious development in primary hypothyroidism appears to be secondary to inappropriate secretion of pituitary gonadotropins, and the galactorrhea appears to be a consequence of increased secretion of prolactin in the presence of severe thyroid hormone deficiency.

The term incomplete sexual precocity should be limited to children who have only a single manifestation of sexual development. The precocious development of breast tissue has been termed premature thelarche, while precocious appearance of sexual hair is designated premature adrenarche or pubarche. In the past these conditions were thought to be the result of increased end organ sensitivity to sex hormones. However, considerable evidence now indicates that the concentrations of sex hormones are elevated in many of these patients, thus suggesting precocious but often unsustained secretion of ovarian or adrenal sex steroids.

Premature thelarche must be differentiated from neonatal hyperplasia of the breast, which can occur in either sex and generally subsides spontaneously within a few weeks or months. Obviously, no treatment is necessary for this type of neonatal breast enlargement. Typically, girls with premature thelarche present between 6 months and 2 years of age, but precocious breast development alone can occur at any time during the first 8 years. Breast development can be slight; it often regresses after several months to a year, but it may remain for long periods of time, even until the normal onset of puberty. Usually there is no history of accelerated growth, and bone age and 17-ketosteroid values are normal or only minimally increased for age.

Premature adrenarche is more common in girls between 5 and 8 years of age. Their growth velocity may be increased, and bone age is usually slightly advanced. Urinary 17-ketosteroids and plasma dehydroepiandrosterone are often in the early pubertal range, and comedones and axillary sweating and hair may be present in addition to pubic hair. This condition must be differentiated from an adrenocortical tumor or congenital adrenal hyperplasia. Determinations of urinary pregnanetriol or serum 17-hydroxyprogesterone will usually differentiate premature adrenarche from mild forms of virilizing congenital adrenal hyperplasia. Skeletal maturation usually does not progress as rapidly as in idiopathic precocious puberty or in virilizing adrenal disorders. Serum gonadotropins may be slightly elevated in girls with premature thelarche and normal in girls with premature adrenarche. However, single determinations of serum or urinary gonadotropins are of little clinical usefulness because of the wide range of normal values.

Appropriate therapy for sexual precocity demands a precise diagnosis. Tumors of the central nervous system, adrenal glands, or gonads require a joint medical-surgical approach. Patients with congenital adrenal hyperplasia should be placed on replacement doses of glucocorticoids as discussed elsewhere (p. 1639). Usually only replacement doses of thyroid hormone are necessary in severe primary hypothyroidism associated with sexual precocity. Only reassurance and close follow-up are required in the management of most patients with premature thelarche and premature adrenarche. Their evaluation in most instances should not be extensive. *Breast biopsies should never be performed* in girls with premature development of breast tissue.

The most important aspect of treatment of the precociously developing child is detailed supportive counseling. Parents should be advised to respond to their child in a manner appropriate to chronologic age and not in relation to physical appearance; similar advice must be given to teachers and other school personnel. Parents, especially fathers, often have a great deal of difficulty relating to a physically precocious child, and they must be taught to accept the normal caresses and physical contact appropriate for the child's chronologic age. Unfortunately, many parents physically shun their child, and the child, in turn, interprets this as frank rejection. The parents must be told that the physically precocious child does not have heightened heterosexual interest and activity beyond that appropriate for chronologic age.

The medical treatment of precocious puberty is unsatisfactory and difficult to evaluate. Several drugs have been used with variable success: medroxyprogesterone acetate (Provera), an ethinyl analogue (Danazol), cyproterone acetate, and chlormadinone. None of these compounds has controlled sexual precocity and accelerated osseous maturation without significant side effects, and treatment with any of them must be considered investigational at the present time. Provera has been the most widely used compound; it is a progestational steroid that decreases gonadotropin secretion, but it has significant glucocorticoid actions. Adrenal suppression and even Cushing's syndrome have resulted when Provera has been given parenterally in large doses chronically. Provera also has produced chromosomal alterations in testicular germ cells. Although this drug controls menses and frequently causes regression of breast tissue, it has not altered the rapid growth rate or bone maturation appreciably. Danazol has definite anti-gonadotropic activity in humans, but its inherent androgenic activity limits its clinical usefulness. Cyproterone acetate, an antiandrogen, has not been used in this country, but it has no major advantage over Provera. Very little is known about the efficacy of chlormadinone, which is a progestational steroid. Antagonists to the hypothalamic hormone LRF are being developed, and theoretically they could provide a more specific and effective means of therapy.

Medical intervention should be considered when menarche has occurred or seems imminent in a child in whom this would produce significant psychologic trauma. Patients with rapidly progressive precocious puberty may be given Provera (5 to 10 mg/day orally). Adrenal suppression with this dosage is minimal, and menses and breast development are arrested. In general, patients who have tumors or structural abnormalities of the central nervous system respond poorly. In many patients with idiopathic precocious puberty, the waxing and waning course makes it difficult to assess any mode of therapy. Since ultimate height is not increased by currently available drugs, treatment is indicated only to lessen the psychologic trauma associated with sexual precocity.

HETEROSEXUAL PRECOCIOUS DEVELOPMENT

Heterosexual precocious development (virilization of a girl or feminization of a boy) is a relatively uncommon complaint after the newborn period (Table 37). The diagnostic approach is similar to that for isosexual precocity, but special attention must be given to the possibility of a sex-hormone-producing tumor. Arrhenoblastoma of the ovary is a rare lesion that leads to virilization in the young female. Laboratory findings resemble those of Leydig cell tumors of the testis.

Some young girls develop moderately generalized hirsutism, without other signs of an endocrine disorder. This is often constitutional or familial, but it is a distressing occurrence in our culture. Urinary 17-ketosteroid excretion may be slightly elevated. These patients must be differentiated from those with mild forms of congenital adrenal hyperplasia. Medical treatment is not indicated, but reassurance and depilatory creams or electrolysis for cosmetically unacceptable facial hair can be advised. Some of these girls may be in the early stages of polycystic ovarian disease, the Stein-Leventhal syndrome, although most of them do not develop the other components of this syndrome.

Gynecomastia is a very common finding during male adolescence. The overall incidence is estimated at approximately 40 percent, with a peak prevalence at 14 years of age. In most cases it is mild and transitory and is noticed only during a careful physical examination. Severe gynecomastia is uncommon and in many cases is accompanied by obesity. The differential diagnosis includes Klinefelter's syndrome and estrogen-producing tumors. A thorough physical examination should suggest Klinefelter's syndrome (eunuchoid body habitus, incomplete masculinization, and small firm testes). Estrogen-producing tumors also cause testicular atrophy; they may be palpable if they are testicular in origin, but estrogen-producing Leydig cell tumors occur only after adolescence. Diagnostic studies in severe cases of gynecomastia should include buccal smear, serum gonadotropins, and total urinary estrogens. Weight reduction, reassurance, and time may be the only therapy necessary. When the patient is especially disturbed by his appearance, a reduction mammoplasty should be performed by a skilled plastic surgeon.

In all instances of sexual precocity clinicians must search diligently for possible exposure to sex steroids.

Poor control of manufacturing processes has led to contamination of vitamin capsules and other medications with potent estrogens. Estrogens are widely used in human medicine, and unfortunately they are incorporated into some facial skin creams. A child can develop significant breast enlargement secondary to the estrogenic hormone in the mother's facial cream, acquired through maternal fondling and kissing. A helpful clinical sign is the presence of very darkly pigmented nipples. This is a frequent side effect of synthetic estrogens, especially stilbestrol.

DELAYED ADOLESCENT DEVELOPMENT

In contrast to precocious sexual development, delayed adolescent development is a much more common complaint in boys than in girls. A careful history and physical examination with precise body measurements and assessment of sexual maturation is mandatory, with special attention to clues suggestive of chronic illness, hypopituitarism, hypothyroidism, hyposmia or anosmia, Turner's syndrome, or Klinefelter's syndrome. Table 38 lists the causes of delayed adolescent development, based primarily on whether the serum gonadotropins are normal or increased. The basic laboratory evaluation should include urinalysis, complete blood cell count, sedimentation rate, lateral skull radiographs to evaluate the pituitary fossa, bone age determination, and serum thyroxine measurement. Girls with short stature and delayed development should have a buccal smear performed during initial evaluation.

Serum gonadotropins, especially FSH, are increased

TABLE 38. Differential Diagnosis of Delayed or Incomplete Adolescent Development

Normal or low serum gonadotropin values
  Constitutional delayed adolescence
  Hypopituitarism, idiopathic or acquired
    Multiple pituitary tropic hormone deficiencies
    Isolated deficiencies: gonadotropins (Kallman syndrome), growth hormone
  Chronic illness
  Hypothyroidism
  Congenital anomalies: absent uterus and/or vagina, imperforate hymen
Increased serum gonadotropin values
  Gonadal dysgenesis (Turner's syndrome)
  Klinefelter's syndrome
  Bilateral gonadal failure: traumatic, infectious, postsurgical, post-irradiation, idiopathic (empty-scrotum or vanishing-testes syndrome)
Miscellaneous conditions
  Prader-Willi syndrome
  Laurence-Moon-Biedl syndrome
Testicular feminization (complete and incomplete)
del Castillo syndrome
Steroidogenic enzyme deficiencies (adrenal and gonadal): cholesterol desmolase complex, 3β-hydroxysteroid dehydrogenase, 17α-hydroxylase, C17, 20-desmolase, 17β-hydroxysteroid oxidoreductase
Myotonic dystrophy

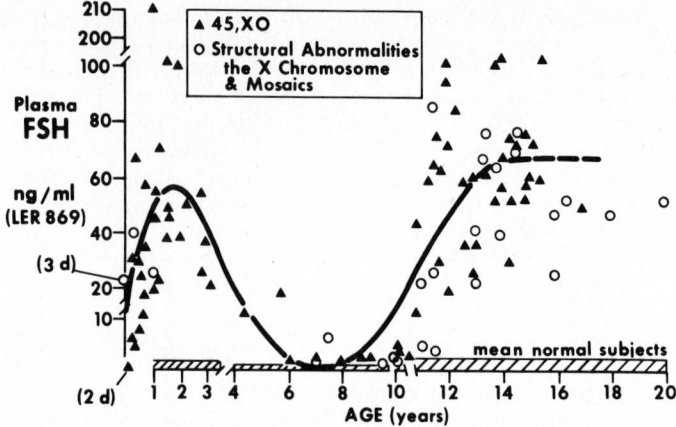

FIG. 56. Gonadotropin secretion in patients with gonadal dysgenesis. Triangles indicate patients with 45,X karyotype. Circles designate patients with X chromosome mosaicism and /or structural abnormalities of X chromosome. Curve is a polynomial regression plot of data. Hatched lines indicate mean plasma FSH values in normal females. (From Conte, Grumbach, and Kaplan: J Clin Endocrinol Metab 40:670, 1975.)

significantly in children with primary hypogonadism who are 12 years of age or older. They are also slightly increased in younger hypogonadal children, but there is some overlap with the normal range between 3 and 11 years (Fig. 56). Although most laboratories can detect a statistically significant difference between hypopituitary patients and prepubertal children, problems arise in attempting to differentiate between normal and pathologically low serum gonadotropin levels by a single determination.

The most common final diagnosis for adolescents with delayed development and serum gonadotropins within the broad normal range is constitutional delayed adolescence. Typically the patient is a healthy but short boy with moderately retarded bone age and a lifelong history of short stature. Frequently his father or brothers also developed slowly and may not have achieved full adult height until after 20 years of age. Because of the failure of many clinicians to recognize the earliest signs of sexual maturation in males, many boys are unnecessarily referred for endocrine evaluations. Such patients can be reassured about their normalcy when early testicular and phallic enlargement and reddening and thinning of the scrotum are noted on repeat evaluation at 6-month intervals; greater masculinization will eventually become apparent. Thus the physical examination is extremely important, since undue concern and laboratory evaluation only increase anxiety and hinder the patient's psychosocial development.

Hypopituitarism is not a common cause of delayed adolescent development, but it must be kept in mind, especially in patients with severe short stature (more than 3 standard deviations below the mean for chronologic age), immature doll-like facies, truncal pudginess, small hands and feet, and small external genitalia (p. 1608). Perhaps the most difficult condition to eliminate is isolated gonadotropin deficiency. When this condition is associated with hyposmia or anosmia it is called Kallman syndrome. However, olfaction may be normal,

it may occur in females as well as males, and at times it is associated with such facial defects as cleft lip and palate. In the past, only time could reliably separate isolated gonadotropin deficiency from constitutional delayed adolescence, but recent studies indicate that an intravenous LRF stimulation test can usually make the correct diagnosis. Patients with isolated gonadotropin deficiency and bone age in excess of 12 years typically either will fail to respond or will have a blunted immature-type LH response. However until additional longitudinal studies confirm these findings, repeat follow-up evaluation remain necessary.

Chronic illness of almost any nature will delay growth and sexual development. Some common conditions are sickle cell disease, diabetes mellitus, cyanotic congenital heart disease, chronic connective tissue diseases, anorexia nervosa, and regional enteritis.

Congenital anomalies of the müllerian system usually cause incomplete sexual development (amenorrhea). They should be sought in any girl who has not menstruated within 5 years of the onset of breast development.

Turner's syndrome (gonadal dysgenesis) is by far the most common cause of delayed development associated with increased serum gonadotropins. These girls present with short stature and primary amenorrhea. The buccal smear is chromatin-negative in most patients. However, approximately 20 percent of girls with gonadal dysgenesis have positive buccal smears because of the presence of mosaicism or a structurally abnormal X chromosome. Even if the buccal smear is positive, chromosome analysis should be performed on girls with increased gonadotropins and sexual infantilism. This condition is discussed elsewhere (p. 1705).

Patients with Klinefelter's syndrome seldom come to a pediatrician because of delayed sexual maturation. They are normal in height but have eunuchoid body habitus. Adrenarche occurs at the normal time, and hence they may have a female-type pubic hair pattern.

Gynecomastia becomes more apparent late in adolescence and during adulthood. The most important physical finding is testicular atrophy. The testes are small (usually less than 2.5 cm in diameter) and firm. The buccal smear reveals a positive chromatin pattern consistent with the most common karyotype: 46,XXY (p. 1708).

Bilateral gonadal failure has many possible etiologies, but it is an uncommon condition. However, the so-called vanishing-testes syndrome deserves further discussion. Patients with this syndrome have a normal 46,XY karyotype and masculine-appearing external genitalia. However, the testes are not palpable, and normal male puberty does not occur. Presumably both testes became atrophied or were destroyed at some time after fetal differentiation of the external genitalia. Stimulation with chorionic gonadotropin is useful to determine whether some abdominal testicular tissue is present. However, in the face of elevated serum FSH and LH, it is unlikely that this would be the case. Although the risk of surgery may equal the risk of possible malignant degeneration, these boys probably should undergo an exploratory laparotomy to detect and remove gonadal tissue. At the same time, prosthetic testes can be placed in the scrotum.

The miscellaneous conditions listed in Table 38 are all rare. Patients with the Prader-Willi syndrome are characterized by obesity, short stature, hypogonadism, small hands and feet, mental retardation, and infantile hypotonia. Bilateral cryptorchidism and a small flat scrotum are characteristic. The phallus appears quite small in childhood, and as the obesity progresses the phallus seemingly disappears. Their primary defect has not been defined precisely, but there is evidence to suggest abnormal hypothalamic function. There is usually a blunted response or a failure to respond to intravenous administration of synthetic LRF. Females as well as males can be affected, and glucose intolerance is common. The etiology is unknown, and most cases have been sporadic.

The Laurence-Moon-Biedl syndrome is characterized by retinitis pigmentosa, polydactyly, obesity, and hypogonadism. The hypogonadotropic hypogonadism occurs in most affected males and in approximately one-half of the affected females. This condition seems to be inherited as an autosomal recessive, with marked intrafamily variability.

Testicular feminization secondary to end-organ insensitivity to androgens and defects in testosterone biosynthesis (eg, 17α-hydroxylase and 17β-hydroxysteroid oxidoreductase deficiency) are forms of familial male pseudohermaphrodism; deficiencies in the female can lead to amenorrhea (p. 1703).

Patients with the del Castillo syndrome (Sertoli cell syndrome) have germinal cell aplasia and moderately increased serum FSH, but they are normally virilized.

Postpubertal seminiferous tubule sclerosis and cataracts occur in males with chronic muscular dystrophy. A wide variety of genetic disorders can be associated with cryptorchidism or abnormal gonadal function.

Whenever possible, therapy for delayed adolescent development should be directed at its cause. Patients with gonadal failure or proven gonadotropin deficiency require replacement therapy with sex steroids. If the age of the patient permits, the dosage of sex steroids should be gradually increased to full replacement over approximately 2 years, in an attempt to mimic the normal course of pubertal changes. In girls, conjugated estrogens (Premarin 0.3 mg/day orally) or their equivalent can be gradually increased to full replacement. When vaginal spotting occurs, cyclical therapy should be begun 21 or 25 days per month. In boys, intramuscular testosterone enanthate, 100 mg/month initially with increases up to 300 mg every 3 to 4 weeks, is effective. However, some adolescent males prefer oral medications such as methytestosterone (25 to 50 mg/day orally), fluoxymesterone (Halotestin, 2 to 10 mg/day orally), or testosterone propionate (10 mg/day orally). Boys with constitutionally delayed growth should be reassured that they are normal and will develop without intervention; however, when there is no evidence of significant masculinization by 14 to 15 years of age and emotional well-being is adversely affected, short-term treatment with androgens may be wise. Androgens can be given orally or intramuscularly for 3 to 6 months without significant adverse effects on adult height. This often produces enough masculinization to alleviate anxiety and social pressures and seems not to have any deleterious effect on ultimate height. In rare cases short-term therapy with low-dose estrogens is used for girls with markedly delayed development; usually reassurance and a padded brassiere are sufficient.

UNDESCENDED TESTES

An undescended testis is one that has failed to descend to its normal scrotal position by 1 year of age; if palpable, it cannot be brought manually into the upper part of the scrotum. Cryptorchid testes are located along the pathway of descent, whereas ectopic testes are not. Undescended testes may be unilateral or bilateral; if unilateral, the right testis is more commonly affected. Differentiation between an undescended testis and a retractile testis is often difficult. By definition, retractile testes can be brought manually into the bottom of the scrotum. Examination of the patient while he is sitting with his legs crossed "Indian style" is a useful maneuver. As mentioned, numerous genetic disorders are associated with testicular malfunction or maldescent; hence special attention should be paid to the presence of other physical abnormalities.

The treatment of undescended testes is often vigorously debated, despite the absence of clearcut data. Controlled prospective studies have not been performed to determine the optimal time of surgical intervention and whether treatment with chorionic gonadotropin is of benefit. The approach to these patients depends on the degree of involvement. Patients with unilateral or bilateral palpable but undescended testes may be given a 6-week course of HCG, 1,000 IU intramuscularly three times per week; numerous dosage schedules have been proposed, both higher and lower. In the prospective study by Sudman, a shorter course of

HCG treatment caused descent in 31 percent of patients with palpable testes.

Treatment with HCG will not cause the descent of nonpalpable (abdominal) testes. When no testicular tissue can be palpated, a 3-day course of HCG (2,000 IU/day intramuscularly) with measurement of serum testosterone on the fourth day, may be used to determine the presence of abdominal testes. The risk of surgical intervention may equal the risk of malignant degeneration of abdominal testes. Nonetheless, an attempt at surgical correction should be performed before the patient starts school. If the testicles cannot be brought into a palpable location, they probably should be removed. Testicular prostheses should be offered, and replacement therapy with androgens should be started at about 12 years of age. Careful biopsies should be performed to assess testicular histology at the time of orchiopexy. This approach is not universally agreed on, and some clinicians feel that bilateral abdominal testes are best left for future endocrine function.

MICROPENIS.   Occasionally boys are brought to the physician because of the small size of the phallus. Usually the penis is within the normal range in size, although embedded in suprapubic fat. Only reassurance and dietary restriction are necessary in most instances. Rarely is the penis truly hypoplastic. Then the clinician must look carefully for signs of hypopituitarism, Prader-Willi syndrome, and other dysmorphic disorders. Micropenis and hypoglycemia in a newborn male infant are cardinal features of congenital hypopituitarism. Short-term parenteral testosterone therapy may be beneficial in infancy or early childhood, but it should be prescribed cautiously and by an experienced physician. Topical testosterone cream has been reported to be of significant benefit in the preoperative preparation of patients with congenital hypospadias.

References

Barnes ND, Cloutier MD, Hayles AB: Central nervous system and precocious puberty. In Grumbach MM, Grave GD, Mayer FE (eds): The Control of the Onset of Puberty. New York, Wiley, 1974, p 213

Beas F, Zurbrugg RP, Leibow SG, Patton RG, Gardner LI: Familial male sexual precocity: report of the eleventh kindred found, with observations on blood group linkage and urinary c$_{19}$-steroid excretion. J Clin Endocrinal Metab 22:1095, 1962

Camacho AM, Williams DL, Montalvo JM: Alterations of testicular histology and chromosomes in patients with constitutional sexual precocity treated with medroxyprogesterone acetate. J Clin Endocrinal Metab 34:279, 1972

Faiman C, Winter JSD: Gonadotropins and sex hormone patterns in puberty, clinical data. In Grumbach MM, Grave GD, Mayer FE (eds): The Control of the Onset of Puberty. New York, Wiley, 1974, p 32

Grumbach MM, Roth JC, Kaplan SL, Kelch RP: Hypothalamic-pituitary regulation of puberty: evidence and concepts derived from clinical research. In Grumbach MM, Grave GD, Mayer FE (eds): The Control of the Onset of Puberty. New York, Wiley, 1974, p 115

Guthrie RD, Smith DW, Graham CB: Testosterone treatment for micropenis during early childhood. J Pediatr 83:247, 1973

Jenner MR, Kelch RP, Kaplan SL, Grumbach MM: Hormonal changes in puberty: IV. Plasma estradiol, LH, and FSH in prepubertal children,

pubertal females, and in precocious puberty, premature thelarche, hypogonadism , and in a child with a feminizing ovarian tumor. J Clin Endocrinal Metab 34:521, 1972

Kaplan JG, Moshang T Jr, Bernstein R, Parks JS, Bongiovanni AM: Constitutional delay of growth and development: effects of treatment with androgens. J Pediatr 82:38, 1973

Kulin HE, Reiter EO: Delayed sexual maturation, with special emphasis on the occurrence of the syndrome in the male. In Grumbach MM, Grave GD, Mayer FE (eds): The Control of the Onset of Puberty. New York, Wiley, 1974, p 238

Liu N, Grumbach MM, deNapoli RA, Morishima A: Prevalence of electroencephalographic abnormalities in idiopathic precocious puberty and premature pubarche: bearing on pathogenesis and neuroendocrine regulation of puberty. J Clin Endocrinol Metab 25: 1296, 1965

Loop JW: Precocious puberty. Pneumoencephalography demonstrating a hamartoma in the absence of cerebral symptoms. N Engl J Med 271:409, 1964

Lovinger RD, Kaplan SL, Grumbach MM: Congenital hypopituitarism associated with neonatal hypoglycemia and microphallus: four cases secondary to hypothalamic hormone deficiencies. J Pediatr 87:1171, 1975

Marshall WA, Tanner JM: Variations in pattern of pubertal changes in girls. Arch Dis Child 44:291, 1969

———— Tanner JM: Variations in the pattern of pubertal changes in boys. Arch Dis Child 45:13, 1970

Myers RP, Kelalis PP: Cryptorchidism reassessed: is there an optimal time for surgical correction? Mayo Clin Proc 48:94, 1973

Rimoin DL, Schimke RN: The Gonads. In Genetic Disorders of the Endocrine Glands. St Louis, CV Mosby, 1971, p 258

Root A, Steinberger E, Smith K, Steinberger A, Russ D, Somers L: Isosexual pseudoprecocity in a 6-year old boy with a testicular interstitial cell adenoma. J Pediatr 80:264, 1972

Rosenfield RL: Plasma 17-ketosteroids and 17-beta-hydroxysteroids in girls with premature development of sexual hair. J Pediatr 79:260, 1971

Sadeghi-Nejad A, Kaplan SL, Grumbach MM: The effect of medroxyprogesterone acetate on adrenocortical function in children with precocious puberty. J Pediatr 78:616, 1971

Van Wyk JJ, Grumbach MM: Syndrome of precocious menstruation and galactorrhea in juvenile hypothyroidism: an example of hormonal overlap in pituitary feedback. J Pediatr 57:416, 1960

Winter JSD, Taraska S, Faiman C: The hormonal response to HCG stimulation in male children and adolescents. J Clin Endocrinol Metab 34:348, 1972

OVARIES
GRIFF T. ROSS

Disorders of ovarian function from birth to puberty are rare and are likely to present clinically in one of three ways: failure to grow, with or without musculoskeletal malformations; abnormalities of initiation and progression of pubescence; vaginal bleeding, either temporally or quantitatively abnormal. In addition to their association with primary ovarian disorders, these clinical problems may result from abnormalities in urogenital differentiation during fetal life or from postnatal functional abnormalities of pituitary adrenals.

To distinguish among these etiologic alternatives, with minimal cost to the patient, the physician must understand the normal prenatal and postnatal interactions among the components of the hypothalamic-pituitary-ovary-genital axis. These interactions on the pituitary, the adrenal, prenatal and postnatal sexual differentiation, and puberty are detailed elsewhere in this chapter. Here the emphasis will be on the ovaries.

Prepubertal Ovarian Growth And Development

Beginning in the second month of fetal life, primordial germ cells in the ovarian anlage undergo mitotic division to produce millions of oogonia. Around the fifth month of fetal life, some of these oogonial cells enter the prophase of the first meiotic division and become invested with a layer of cells called granulosa cells, which are separated from surrounding stromal cells by a lamina basalis. Stromal cells outside but immediately adjacent to and surrounding the lamina basalis are referred to as thecal cells. These complexes, consisting of an oocyte and granulosa cells surrounded by a lamina basalis and theca cells, are called primordial follicles. These are embedded in stroma, which consists of supportive cells, some hormonally responsive cells called interstitial cells, blood vessels, and lymphatic spaces. Proliferation of germ cells stops prior to birth when all those present have become incorporated into primordial follicles.

Around the seventh month of fetal life, cohorts of the primordial follicles begin to mature. When maturation begins, granulosa cells first become cuboid in shape, then begin to proliferate. Granulosa cell proliferation is followed by differentiation of the theca cells into layers, of which the inner is called theca interna and the outer theca externa. As the follicle continues to enlarge, accumulation of fluid among the granulosa cells marks the formation of an antrum, the hallmark of graafian follicles. Throughout the period prior to antrum formation, the oocyte progressively enlarges, but it achieves its maximal volume while the follicle continues to enlarge. Follicular maturation is evident in ovaries of all newborn infants and has advanced to the point of antrum formation in about 50 percent of cases.

For unknown reasons, growth is initiated in only a small fraction of follicles present, and prior to menarche all follicles in these cohorts undergo a degenerative process called atresia. Atresia is characterized by death of the oocyte and granulosa cells, which disappear and leave only a residue of scar tissue and stromal cells. As a result of atresia in successive cohorts, the number of primordial follicles progressively declines from millions at birth to hundreds of thousands just prior to the first ovulation, followed by menses.

The mass of the ovaries increases from a few hundred milligrams at birth to 10 to 15 g by the time of sexual maturity. This increase in mass results from an expanding stroma and a progressive increase in maximal size achieved by maturing follicles prior to undergoing atresia.

Hormonal stimulation is required for follicular maturation. Preantral follicle growth depends on stimulation of mitosis in granulosa cells by estrogen produced in response to gonadotropins, so that the occurrence of follicular growth and maturation prior to puberty implies that gonadotropins are being secreted by the pituitary and estrogen is being synthesized by the prepubertal ovary. Moreover, once a follicle has begun to mature, continued stimulation by gonadotropins is required to maintain viability, and withdrawal of stimulation results in atresia. Occurrence of follicular growth and atresia in the prepubertal ovary, then, implies that pituitary gonadotropin secretion must wax and wane prior to the first ovulation. Indeed, 28- to 40-day cyclic increments and decrements in urinary gonadotropin excretion have been shown to occur in premenarchal, prepubertal girls. The excretory patterns of these gonadotropins in first morning urine specimens from prepubertal girls are similar to those seen in such specimens collected from postmenarchal girls. A relationship between these cyclic variations in gonadotropin secretion and ovarian steroid hormone secretion is implied but remains to be demonstrated by measurements of both steroids and gonadotropins in aliquots of the same specimens.

Normal Ovarian Function Prior to and During Pubescence

There are at least two products of normal ovarian function: sex steroid hormones and oocytes. These result from follicular maturation, which requires stimulation by pituitary hormones, including gonadotropins and possibly prolactin. As noted, all follicles in cohorts maturing prior to the first ovulation undergo atresia, so that ovarian function during this period relates exclusively to secretion of sex steroid hormones. Prior to menarche, ovarian function is reflected in the effects of sex steroid hormones on target tissues.

Sex steroid hormones secreted by maturing follicles act at several loci. First, estrogens, androgens, and progestogens act within the ovary to regulate growth and atresia of follicles responding to gonadotropins. Outside the ovary these substances act both on anterior pituitary cells, which secrete gonadotropins and prolactin, and on the hypothalamus, which secretes hypophysiotropic hormones that either stimulate or inhibit secretion of pituitary hormones. Studies of ovarian morphology and serum and urinary gonadotropin levels suggest that these hypothalamic-pituitary-ovarian interactions begin during gestation and continue throughout life.

In addition to hypothalamic and pituitary sites, estrogens, androgens, and progestogens stimulate proliferation and growth of vascular, muscular, and epithelial components of the gonaducts, external genitalia, and breasts, irrespective of the genetic sex of the individual. Sex steroid hormones also act on osseous tissues to stimulate linear growth, which is accelerated just prior to menarche. These effects are manifest clinically in a sequence of changes that begins with breast budding and appearance of pubic hair and culminates with menarche. These pubertal changes can be accomplished initially by administration of estrogen and subsequently with a combination of estrogens with a progestagen.

Normative values for age at onset of puberty and rates of progression of changes, including age at menarche, vary from population to population and are modified by socioeconomic factors and such diseases as diabetes and obesity. Marshall and Tanner have described five stages of breast and pubic hair development, ranging from Stage 1 (prepubertal) to Stage 5 (mature) (p. 1714). These data are useful in answering three questions in relation to the onset and progression of pubertal changes reflecting ovarian function in girls: Is pubertal development within normal limits for age? Once initiated, is development of breasts and pubic hair proceeding at a normal rate? Are breasts and pubic hair developing synchronously and in the proper temporal relationship to accelerated linear growth and to menarche? Normal age at menarche for girls in the United States ranges from 9 to 16 years (mean 12.6 years). The most important determinant of age at first menses appears to be body weight; girls whose weight exceeds that of their peers by more than 30 percent menstruate earlier, on the average.

ABNORMAL OVARIAN FUNCTION PRIOR TO AND DURING PUBESCENCE

Precocious Puberty

Disease processes associated with premature isosexual or heterosexual development of puberty have been discussed (p. 1719). When the pathophysiologic basis of sexual precocity or pseudopuberty is primarily ovarian, the disease is likely to be serious, and although this is rare, it must be eliminated from consideration. It is important to make the distinction between benign and potentially life-threatening disorders. Once the possibility of a life-threatening basis for the disorder is eliminated, it is feasible to temporize without further diagnostic or therapeutic intervention.

Follicular cysts occur frequently in ovaries of newborn and prepubertal girls. Rarely, one of these cysts will secrete significant quantities of estrogen, with resultant premature stimulation of development of secondary sexual characteristics, including vaginal bleeding. These cysts are associated with palpable enlargement of the ovaries, and they must be examined surgically in order to eliminate the remote possibility of functioning ovarian tumors, which occur (rarely) in prepubertal children. One also must rule out neoplasms that involve the floor of the third ventricle or the hypothalamic area, those that secrete gonadotropins that stimulate sex steroid hormone secretion, and tumors of the adrenals that secrete either androgens or estrogens (p. 1719).

Delayed Puberty and Primary Amenorrhea

Failure of initiation or progression of puberty is the basis for seeking medical advice more frequently than for premature sexual development. The physician must understand the sequence of events and the range of variation that can occur during normal pubescence (p. 1712). In evaluating patients with delay in onset of puberty, it is convenient to distinguish, from information obtained during the initial interview with the patient and her parents, whether the onset of puberty is normal or minimally delayed or is clearly delayed. When these distinctions are made at the outset, the constellations of signs and symptoms and characteristics of certain syndromes dictate a series of logical choices and sequences of diagnostic maneuvers. Some clinicians prefer to obtain a battery of tests on the first encounter with every

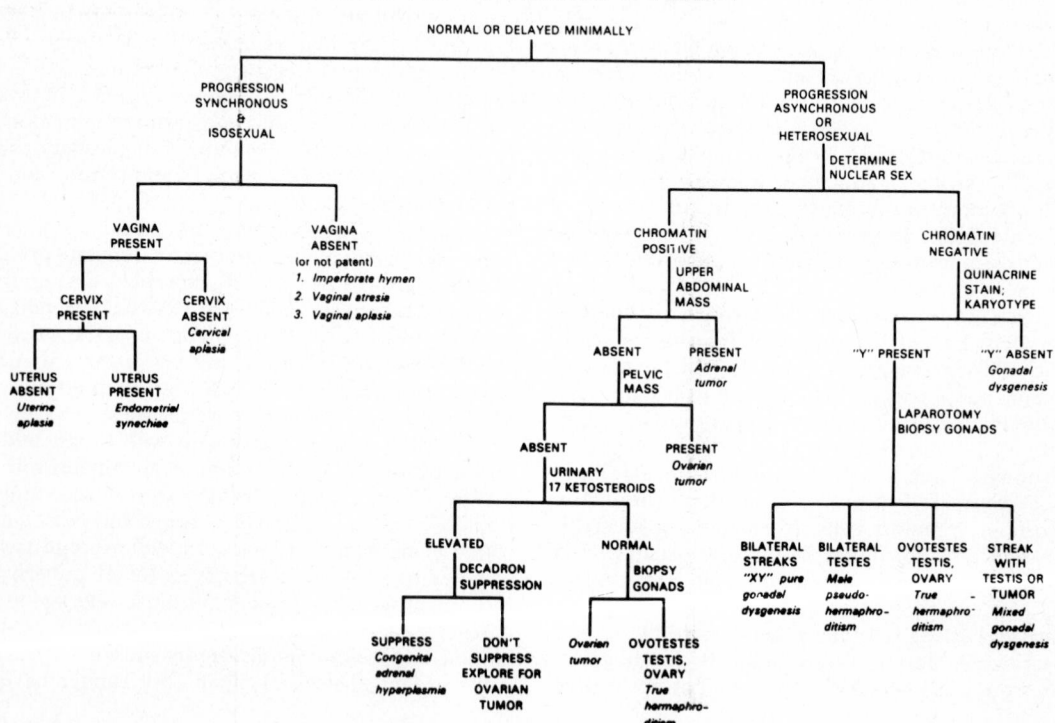

ONSET AND PROGRESSION OF PUBERTY

patient, using the results of these screening tests as the basis for further evaluation. Such an approach may result in more extensive testing than is required for every patient, but pragmatic considerations sometimes may make this the least expensive alternative. The sequence in which the tests are done may vary, depending on the

ease with which certain tests can be obtained and the time required to obtain results. Figure 57 may facilitate recall of constellations of signs and symptoms and emphasize the tests that are essential for definitive diagnosis.

Some examples will illustrate the usefulness of such

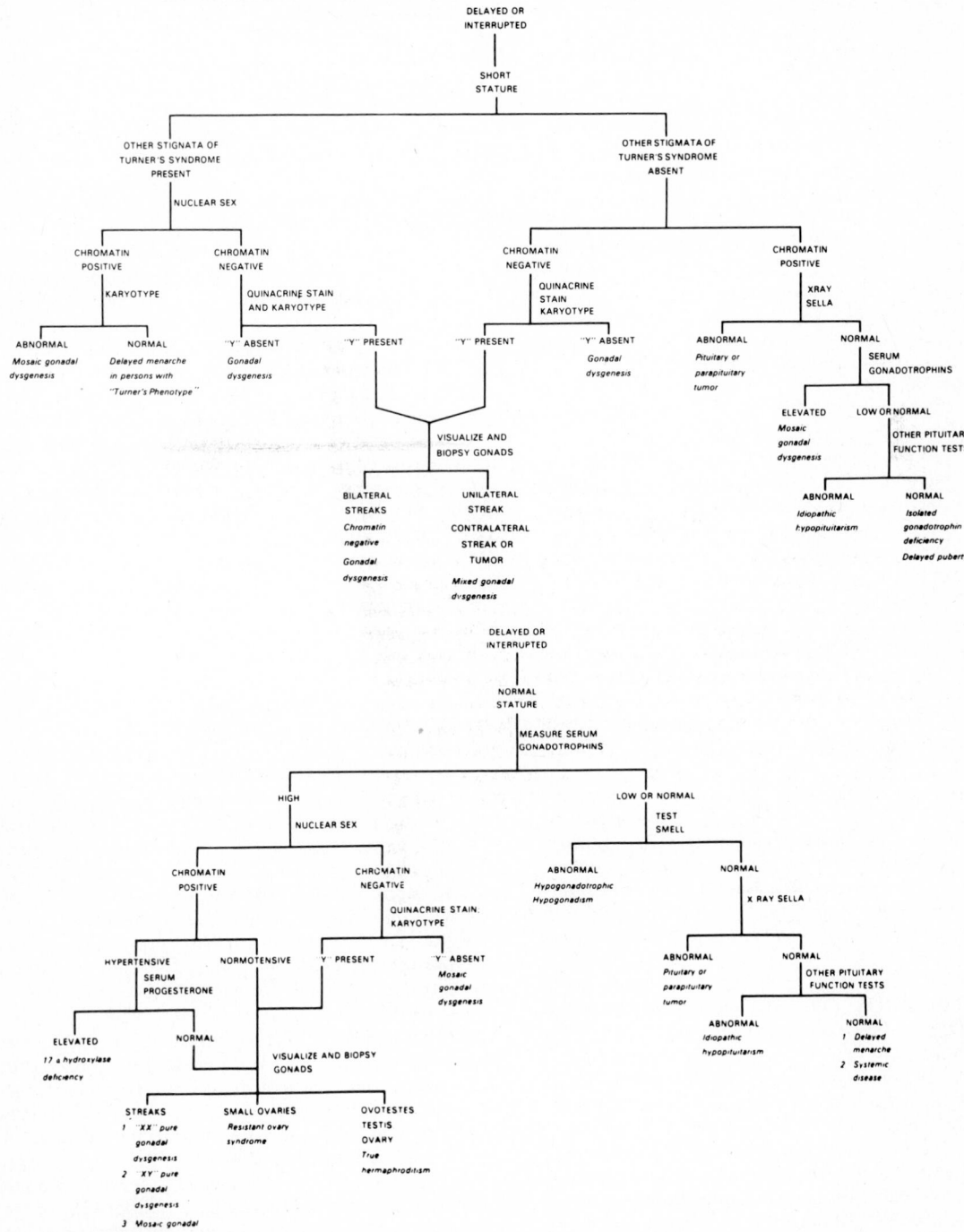

FIG. 57. Constellations of signs and symptoms and tests for definitive diagnosis in primary amenorrhea and delayed puberty.

a chart. For instance, primary amenorrhea associated with normal onset, normal synchronous isosexual progression of secondary sexual maturation, and patent vagina with cervix but no uterus should suggest the rare entity called uterine aplasia. For this syndrome a large battery of tests, including measurements of hormones in blood and urine, provides no essential information for diagnosis.

Appearance of secondary sexual characteristics at an appropriate age associated with signs of virilization, chromatin-positive nuclear sex, and upper abdominal mass should lead to suspicion of an adrenal tumor. Elevated urinary 17-ketosteroid secretion constitutes a useful clue to the correct diagnosis. A skull radiograph for delineating the sella turcica will provide no essential information for either diagnosis or treatment.

ASSOCIATED WITH NORMAL ONSET AND ISOSEXUAL PROGRESSION.

Synchronous and isosexual progression of puberty with delayed onset of menses is pathognomonic of an abnormality in development of the müllerian duct derivatives. When a vagina is present, one should look for a cervix; if a cervix is present, the possibility of uterine aplasia, a rare disorder, should be considered. Normal development of the vagina and uterus may occur in the rare syndrome of congenital absence of the cervix.

If the vagina is absent or not patent, one should consider the possibilities of an imperforate hymen, vaginal atresia, or vaginal aplasia, in order of increasing severity. The correction of these disorders requires plastic repair. Since ovarian function in these persons is usually normal, then the endometrium, if present, responds appropriately to ovarian estrogen and progestagen; but lack of egress through the vagina leads to spillage of menstrual fluid into the abdomen and pelvis, and the fluid contains viable endometrium. This ectopic endometrium is also hormonally responsive and forms endometriomas, which are commonly associated with cyclic abdominal pain and masses that can be palpated rectally.

The *androgen insensitivity syndrome* in phenotypic females with XY sex chromosome constitution is another cause of primary amenorrhea. This X-linked disorder, characterized by bilateral testes, female phenotype, absent uterus, female secondary sex characteristics (breast development, feminine habitus), but absent or sparse pubic and axillary hair, is discussed on p. 1703.

ASSOCIATED WITH NORMAL ONSET BUT ASYNCHRONOUS OR HETEROSEXUAL PROGRESSION.

Evaluation of such a patient is somewhat more complex. The first step is to determine the genetic sex of the patient. Quinacrine staining for a Y sex chromosome should be done in patients with chromatin-negative nuclear sex. If no evidence is found of a Y chromosome, a clinical diagnosis of gonadal dysgenesis should be entertained. However, quinacrine staining is not inevitably effective in delineating the presence or absence of a Y sex chromosome, so that the karyotype should be determined in order to make the distinction between a 45,X sex chromosomal constitution and a 45,XY sex chromosomal constitution.

In patients in whom quinacrine staining indicates the presence of a Y chromosome, a laparotomy should be performed and gonadal tissue biopsied. If bilateral streaks are discovered, XY "pure" gonadal dysgenesis is diagnosed. Bilateral testes are diagnostic of incomplete male pseudohermaphrodism. In some, one may find ovotestes, or a testis and an ovary, diagnostic of true hermaphrodism. A streak gonad (one side with a contralateral testis or gonadal tumor) is diagnostic of dysgenetic male pseudohermaphrodism, and gonadal tissue should be removed.

On the initial screening of chromatin-positive individuals, an upper abdominal mass should be sought. The presence of such a mass is suggestive of an adrenal tumor, and appropriate studies should be done. If no abdominal mass is found, a careful examination should be made for a pelvic mass; if a pelvic mass is found, surgical exploration is indicated to rule out the possibility of an ovarian neoplasm. If neither a pelvic mass nor an abdominal mass is found, measurement of urinary 17-ketosteroid excretion may be useful. Virilizing signs associated with normal urinary 17-ketosteroid excretion and neither a pelvic mass nor an abdominal mass in a person with chromatin-positive nuclear sex who has been raised as a girl should lead to a gonadal biopsy. Gonadal biopsy makes it possible to distinguish true hermaphrodism from sclerocystic ovaries and ovarian tumors that might function sufficiently to virilize the patient and yet not be palpable on pelvic, rectal, or abdominal examination. Sclerocystic ovaries, sometimes referred to as polycystic ovaries, have been found on pelvic exploration of girls developing signs of androgen excess during pubescence. This syndrome, although rare, should be considered in the differential diagnosis of primary amenorrhea associated with heterosexual progression of puberty.

When 17-ketosteroid excretion is elevated in a person with chromatin-positive nuclear sex, an attempt should be made to determine whether the secretory process can be suppressed with an exogenous glucocorticoid hormone, such as dexamethasone. Failure of glucocorticoid to suppress urinary 17-ketosteroid secretion is suggestive of an ovarian source of androgens. In contrast, when 17-ketosteroid excretion is suppressed, an ACTH-dependent adrenal source of excess androgen should be considered, and appropriate studies should be done to distinguish congenital adrenal hyperplasia with impaired glucocorticoid synthesis from Cushing's syndrome due to adrenal cortical hyperplasia with excessive glucocorticoid secretion.

ASSOCIATED WITH SHORT STATURE.

In those patients with delayed onset of pubescence or in whom progression of the process is interrupted, an initial distinction may be made on the basis of stature. Among persons with short stature one should seek for the stigmata of Turner's syndrome. If these are absent, nuclear sex should be determined. Those with chromatin-positive nuclear sex should have radiographs of the sella turcica. If these are abnormal, further evaluation should be undertaken for pituitary or parapituitary tumors, with the help of a colleague in neurosurgery.

Serum gonadotropins should be measured if sella

radiographs reveal no abnormality in a person with short stature, no other stigmata of Turner's syndrome, and chromatin-positive nuclear sex. If serum gonadotropins are low or normal, idiopathic hypopituitarism is the most probable diagnosis. Greater than normal levels of serum gonadotropins for chronologic age would be consistent with a diagnosis of chromatin-positive gonadal dysgenesis without the stigmata of Turner's syndrome, probably associated with sex chromosomal mosaicism.

For persons with short stature and chromatin-negative nuclear sex, quinacrine staining and determination of the karyotype are indicated. If there is no evidence of a Y chromosome, the diagnosis of chromatin-negative gonadal dysgenesis without other stigmata of Turner's syndrome is made, and no further diagnostic evaluation is necessary. In contrast, if a Y chromosome is found, one should visualize and biopsy the gonads. Bilateral streaks are consistent with a diagnosis of chromatin-negative gonadal dysgenesis, and a unilateral streak with contralateral testis is diagnostic of dysgenetic male pseudohermaphrodism.

In the population of patients with short stature and other stigmata of Turner's syndrome who are chromatin-negative, it is important to establish whether a Y sex chromosome is present. As noted earlier, this requires a karyotype when quinacrine staining reveals no evidence of a Y body. When a Y chromosome is found, visualization and biopsy of the gonads should be undertaken to minimize the risk of neoplastic degeneration in dysgenetic gonads in genetic males.

Absence of other stigmata of Turner's syndrome in a person with delayed puberty and short stature does not eliminate the diagnosis of gonadal dysgenesis, and appropriate additional studies are indicated. In those with chromatin-negative nuclear sex, procedures to be followed are no different than for patients with other stigmata of Turner's syndrome,

The constellation of delayed puberty, short stature without other stigmata of Turner's syndrome, and chromatin-positive nuclear sex is still consistent with gonadal dysgenesis. However, sella radiographs should be helpful in identifying those in whom this syndrome results from a pituitary or parapituitary tumor for which a karyotype is not essential. If the sella turcica is normal in both anteroposterior and lateral projections, measuring serum gonadotropins is useful to distinguish primary gonadal disease from primary pituitary or hypothalamic disease. In persons suspected of having idiopathic pituitary or hypothalamic disease, provocative tests are indicated to stimulate or inhibit other pituitary hormone secretion.

ASSOCIATED WITH NORMAL STATURE.
High serum gonadotropins suggest some ovarian disease that results in failure of sex steroid hormone secretion. Determining nuclear sex distinguishes chromatin-positive from chromatin-negative groups and eliminates the need for determining the karyotype in the chromatin-positive group. The combination of hypertension and increased serum progesterone levels is diagnostic of a very rare variety of congenital adrenal hyperplasia due to deficiency of the enzymes responsible for the 17α-hydroxylation of progesterone, a critical step in the biosynthesis of glucocorticoid hormones by the adrenals, and of testosterone and estradiol by the ovaries. In view of the essential role of estrogens in preantral follicle growth and development of secondary sexual characteristics, it is not surprising that follicular maturation is inhibited and sexual infantilism is present and is usually severe.

The gonads should be visualized and biopsied in normotensive persons with normal stature, high serum gonadotropins, and chromatin-positive nuclear sex, as well as in those with chromatin-negative nuclear sex associated with a 46,XY karyotype. No gonadal biopsy is required when a 46,XX or mosaic karyotype without an XY or other Y-bearing cell line has been found. The finding of bilateral streak gonads in a person with chromatin-positive nuclear sex is consistent with a diagnosis of 46,XX gonadal dysgenesis, but it does not eliminate gonadal dysgenesis with sex chromosomal mosaicism. The presence of ovotestes with testis or ovaries or both is diagnostic of true hermaphrodism. Small ovaries containing primordial follicles in a person with high serum or urinary gonadotropin, chromatin-positive nuclear sex, sexual immaturity, and primary amenorrhea are diagnostic of the resistant ovary syndromes. Persons with this constellation are identified with increasing frequency, and a gonadal biopsy is critical for the diagnosis.

Delayed puberty in a person with normal stature and low or normal serum gonadotropins should lead the physician to suspect a hypogonadotropic syndrome. The demonstration of anosmia or hyposmia distinguishes the variants of the Kallman syndrome, sporadic or familial, with or without midline defects, from other hypogonadotropic states. In the absence of hyposmia or anosmia, skull radiographs will aid in diagnosis of a pituitary or parapituitary tumor.

EXCESSIVE VAGINAL BLEEDING

A presenting complaint of perimenarchal girls may be excessive vaginal bleeding, recurring irregularly. Whether the pathophysiologic basis for the disease is at the ovarian or hypothalamic–pituitary level of the axis remains to be determined. However, follicular maturation that terminates in atresia, rather than ovulation, in premenarchal girls is associated with ovarian secretion of sufficient hormone to stimulate growth of extraovarian estrogen-dependent target tissues, including the endometrium. Since ovulation does not occur, ovarian progesterone secretion is inconsequential, so that the endometrium is responding to estrogen only. Either failure to maintain estrogen production (estrogen withdrawal) or sustained continuous production of estrogen that fails to suppress gonadotropin secretion by the hypothalamic–pituitary unit may result in acute or chronic vaginal bleeding sufficient to cause hypovolemia and anemia. Similar problems may be encountered during initiation of estrogen replacement therapy in girls with gonadal dysgenesis. In either event, once local causes of bleeding such as polyps or vaginal lesions have been excluded, bleeding usually can be controlled by administration of estrogens and progestogens over a period sufficient to allow for correction of anemia. Once anemia is corrected, steroid hormone replacement can be withdrawn, with the expectation that cyclic events will be resumed without further difficulty.

References

Barnes ND, Cloutier MD, Hayles AB: The central nervous system and precocious puberty. In Grumbach MM, Grave GD, Mayer FE (eds): The Control of the Onset of Puberty. New York, Wiley, 1974, p 213

Canales ES, Zarate A, Castelazo-Ayala L: Primary amenorrhea associated with polycystic ovaries. Endocrine, cytogenetic and therapeutic considerations. Obstet Gynecol 37:205, 1971

Eberlein WR, Bongiovanni AM, Jones IT, Yakovic WC: Ovarian tumors and cysts associated with sexual precocity. J Pediatr 57:484, 1960

Ein SH, Darte JMM, Stephens CA: Cystic and solid ovarian tumors in children: a 44-year review. J Pediatr Surg 5:148, 1970

Grumbach MM, Van Wyk JJ: Disorders of sex differentiation. In Williams RH (ed): Textbook of Endocrinology. Philadelphia, WB Saunders, 1974, p 423

Jenner MR, Kelch RP, Kaplan SL, Grumbach MM: Hormonal changes in puberty: IV. Plasma estradiol, LH and FSH in prepubertal children, pubertal females and in precocious puberty, premature thelarche, hypogonadism, and in a child with a feminizing ovarian tumor. J Clin Endocrinal Metab 34:521, 1972.

Jones GS, Moraes-Ruehsen M: A new syndrome of amenorrhea in association with hypergonadotropism and apparently normal ovarian follicular apparatus. Am J Obstet Gynecol 104:597, 1969

Kraus FT, Neubecker RD: Luteinization of the ovarian theca in infants and children. Am J Clin Pathol 37:389, 1962

Marshall WA, Tanner JM: Variations in pattern of pubertal changes in girls. Arch Dis Child 44:291, 1969

Morris JML, Scully RE: Endocrine Pathology of the Ovary. St Louis, CV Mosby, 1958

Ober WB, Bernstein J: Observations on the endometrium and ovary in the newborn. Pediatrics 16:445, 1955

Polhemus DW: Ovarian maturation and cyst formation in children. Pediatrics 11:588, 1953

Potter EL: The ovary in infancy and childhood. In Grady HG, Smith DE (eds): The Ovary. Baltimore, Williams & Wilkins, 1963, p 11

Ross GT: Gonadotrophins and preantral follicular maturation in women. Fertil Steril 25:522, 1974

———— Vande Wiele RL: The ovaries. In Williams RH (ed): Textbook of Endocrinology. 5th ed Philadelphia, WB Saunders, 1974, p 368

Sigurjonsdottir TJ, Hayles AB: Precocious puberty, a report of 96 cases. Am J Dis Child 115:309, 1968

Sizonenko PC, Burr IM, Kaplan SL, Grumbach MM: Hormonal changes in puberty. II. Correlation of serum luteinizing hormone and follicle stimulating hormone with stages of puberty and bone age in normal girls. Pediatr Res 4:36, 1970

Winter JSD, Faiman C, Hobson WC, Prasad AV, Reyes FI: Pituitary-gonadal relations in infancy. I. Patterns of serum gonadotropin concentrations from birth to four years of age in man and chimpanzee. J Clin Endocrinol Metab 40:545, 1975

Zacharias L, Wurtman RK, Schatzoff M: Sexual maturation in contemporary American girls. Am J Obstet Gynecol 108:833, 1970

CHAPTER 30

Nervous System

SIDNEY CARTER AND ARNOLD P. GOLD, *Associate Editors*

DIAGNOSIS OF NEUROLOGIC DISEASE

SIDNEY CARTER AND ARNOLD P. GOLD

Children with neurologic disorders comprise a significant portion of pediatric practice. Approximately 30 percent of all children admitted to an active teaching hospital either have primary neurologic disease or suffer from nervous system involvement secondary to other systemic conditions. Consequently it is advantageous to the pediatrician to understand the fundamentals of good neurologic diagnosis and to be aware of developmental changes in the nervous system.

Neurologic diagnosis is dependent on the evaluation of the patient's history, the performance of a careful and detailed neurologic examination, and the utilization of appropriate ancillary procedures. This permits localization of a lesion to one or more areas of the nervous system. This localization is of primary importance in making a correct etiologic diagnosis because neurologic disorders have a predilection for specific areas of the nervous system. Thus the astute clinician attempts to answer two simple but important questions: Where? and What? Ideally, an answer should also be found to a third question: Why?

EVALUATION OF HISTORY

A detailed chronologic history is the initial guide to localization and differential diagnosis.

OBTAINING HISTORICAL DATA. Historical data should be obtained from both parents and, when possible, the child; even the preschool child may supply invaluable diagnostic information. However, the initial history should be obtained in the absence of the child, for the infant may be a source of distraction to the parents and the physician, and the older child may understand to some extent but may misinterpret historical facts and as a result suffer emotional trauma. Also, the presence of the child may limit the freedom of the parents to relate a detailed and accurate history. Historical information from other sources, such as school records, medical reports, and observations by friends and relatives, may be invaluable.

IMPORTANCE OF CHRONOLOGIC DOCUMENTATION. Chronologic presentation of the clinical manifestations will frequently suggest localization and etiology. The rate of onset is important; diagnosis may be suggested by the rapidity with which the symptoms become evident. Thus vascular disease may be a valid diagnosis when hemiplegia appears suddenly, while a subacute or insidious evolution of hemiparesis is more characteristic of neoplasia. It is also important

to know whether the symptoms are progressive, static, or regressive. Diagnosis of progressive lesions is largely dependent on the age of onset and the rate of evolution. For example, GM_2 gangliosidosis (Tay-Sachs disease) characteristically has its onset in early infancy and rapidly progresses to death in 2 to 3 years, while Friedreich's ataxia usually appears at 5 to 10 years and slowly evolves for many years. In static lesions, which account for two-thirds of neurologic disorders of childhood, diagnosis must not be obscured by the fact that despite the nonprogressive nature of such lesions, maturation of the nervous system may cause either improvement or worsening. Thus in some cases of cerebral palsy, ataxia improves with age, while the hydrocephalus secondary to aqueductal stenosis becomes more marked, even though the disease itself is not progressive.

EVALUATION OF SYMPTOMS AND SIGNS

Certain manifestations by themselves suggest neurologic involvement, while others incriminate the nervous system only indirectly. The more important symptoms and signs and their relationships to localization and etiologic diagnosis are described here.

GASTROINTESTINAL COMPLAINTS. Although the physician's attention is most often focused on possible local causes, it is most important, and at times life-saving, to be aware of the multiple neurologic entities that may be the basis for altered gastrointestinal function. Feeding problems, vomiting, and abdominal pain may be symptomatic of neurologic disorders.

Feeding problems include difficulties with sucking and/or swallowing that result from brainstem (bulbar) dysfunction. Newborns (especially prematures) may exhibit sucking and swallowing difficulties as a result of physiologic immaturity of the nervous system or as a result of maternal oversedation during delivery, but lesions in the nervous system should always be suspected. Sucking and swallowing problems may be the earliest manifestations of diffuse brain involvement, as in cerebral palsies; the symptoms may diminish and disappear with age. Other conditions that may produce these problems are subdural hematoma, neonatal myasthenia gravis, congenital defects of the motor nuclei of the brainstem (Möbius syndrome), familial dysautonomia, and myotonic dystrophy. The appearance of sucking and swallowing problems in the infant and older child usually implies a progressive disorder of the nervous system. Consideration should be given to infectious processes such as bulbar poliomyelitis, brainstem tumors, subacute necrotizing encephalomyelopathy

TABLE 1. Normal Age for Attainment of Major Developmental Milestones

Age	Motor	Language	Adaptive Behavior
4–6 wk	Head lifted from prone position and turned from side to side	Cries	Smiles
4 mo	No head lag when pulled to sitting from supine position Tries to grasp large objects	Sounds of pleasure	Smiles, laughs aloud, and shows pleasure to familiar objects or persons
5 mo	Voluntary grasp with both hands Plays with toes	Primitive sounds: "ah goo"	Smiles at self in mirror
6 mo	Grasps with one hand Rolls prone to supine Sits with support	Range of sounds greater	Expresses displeasure and food preferences
8 mo	Sits without support Transfers objects from hand to hand Rolls supine to prone	Combines syllables: "baba, dada, mama"	Responds to "No"
10 mo	Sits well Creeping Stands holding Finger–thumb apposition in picking up small objects		Waves "bye-bye," plays "patty-cake" and "peek-a-boo"
12 mo	Stands holding Walks with support	Says 2 or 3 words with meaning	Understands names of objects Shows interest in pictures
15 mo	Walks alone	Several intelligible words	Requests by pointing Imitates
18 mo	Walks up and down stairs holding Removes clothes	Many intelligible words	Carries out simple commands
2 yr	Walks up and down stairs by self Runs	2- to 3-word phrases	Organized play Points to some parts of body

(Leigh's disease), and degenerative disorders resulting from abnormal storage of lipid and glycogen.

Vomiting may be due to direct or indirect involvement of the vomiting center in the brainstem. Persistent vomiting in the absence of an overt cause should always raise the question of increased intracranial pressure. In the absence of increased pressure, one should suspect tumors of the third and fourth ventricles, disease of the brainstem, seizure variants, or labyrinthitis.

Abdominal pain that is acute and persistent may be the result of radicular involvement secondary to polyneuritis, spinal cord tumors, or complication of a lumbar puncture, while chronic or recurrent abdominal pain with or without vomiting may be the sole manifestation of an epileptic state. Abdominal pain due to acute intermittent porphyria or lead colic is rarely observed in pediatric patients.

DELAYED DEVELOPMENT. Developmental milestones mark the achievement of an expected physiologic function, including motor performance, language development, and adaptive behavior. Studies of large numbers of normal children have established age levels at which these various functions should be attained. Individual variations are common, and Table 1 presents only an approximation of normal development.

While delay in the acquisition of a specific function may imply an impaired nervous system, it is a possible that this is physiologic. However, multiple or global delay usually signifies an underlying nervous system disorder of the static type. Delay in the acquisition of many or all of the milestones usually indicates diffuse involvement of the brain with mental retardation or a severe form of cerebral palsy. Delays in any one of the three areas of development are indicative of specific disorders. Delayed *motor function* occurs in cerebral dysfunction or in disorders of muscle, spinal cord, or peripheral nerves. *Speech* fails to develop normally with brain disorders or with peripheral hearing loss. Poor *adaptive behavior* usually implies a diffuse disturbance of the brain, but it can occur with psychosocial disturbances.

MACROCEPHALIA. Head circumference must be measured at every examination to determine whether the head is increasing in size faster than is normal. Head circumference greater than normal may be a manifestation of a familial trait; if it is pathologic it is the result of alterations in one or more of the four cranial compartments: the ventricles, the brain, the meninges, and the skull and scalp. Abnormal head enlargement may be due to any condition with obstructed flow of cerebrospinal fluid, since this causes enlarged ventricles with hydrocephalus. Head enlargement occurs when the brain substance is increased, as in congenital megalencephaly or certain metabolic and degenerative disorders. It is also noted when brain substance is decreased, as in hydranencephaly and porencephaly, but excessive fluid accumulates; this may also result from accumulation of fluid in the subdural space. Changes in the membranous bone of skull, as in cleidocranial dysostosis or achondroplasia, as well as scalp involvement by cephalhematoma may result in head enlargement.

MOTOR DISTURBANCES. Disturbances in motor function may be manifested as muscle weakness, ataxia, or abnormal involuntary movements. They may be evident from early infancy as a delay in development of motor milestones. At a later age they may appear as a loss or disturbance of voluntary motor activity. *Muscle weakness* may result from upper or lower motor neuron disturbances. Upper motor neuron lesions of the brain involving the motor cortex or its outflow cause total or partial spastic paralysis of the extremities of the opposite side. Such lesions may be either congenital fixed defects or acquired disturbances due to tumors, vascular insults, or degenerative disease. With fixed lesions the weakness does not increase, and it may actually improve by compensatory mechanisms. In acquired lesions the sudden appearance of a hemiparesis suggests vascular disease, while a slowly developing weakness implies a tumor or degenerative disorder. Additional clinical features indicative of upper motor neuron disease are exaggerated deep tendon reflexes and the pathologic extensor plantar sign (Babinski reflex) on the involved side. Lower motor neuron disturbances are characterized by a flaccid muscle weakness; they result from involvement of muscle, peripheral nerve, or anterior horn cells. In primary muscle disorders, such as muscular dystrophy, the weakness is greatest in the large girdle muscles. Symmetric involvement of the nerve trunks, as in polyneuritis, also causes diffuse weakness, but the distal musculature of the hands and feet is involved more than proximal girdle musculature. In anterior horn cell disease the weakness may be symmetric or asymmetric, involving isolated muscle groups. Lower motor neuron disease is further characterized by atrophy, by the presence of a normal plantar response, and by hypoactive deep tendon reflexes or absence of deep tendon reflexes.

Ataxia results from involvement of the cerebellum and its pathways. Unsteadiness of voluntary movements may be due to a congenital defect of the cerebellum (ataxic form of cerebral palsy); this condition is characterized by poor balance during sitting and standing and the development of unsteady gait and hand function. Acquired forms of ataxia may be either acute or insidious in onset. Acute ataxia occurs with intoxications, exanthems (particularly varicella), and nonspecific infections (acute cerebellar ataxia); or it may be episodic in nature, as in vertiginous epilepsy or vestibular neuronitis. Slowly developing ataxia may be observed with increased intracranial pressure, cerebellar and brainstem tumors, heredodegenerative disorders (as in ataxia-telangiectasia and Friedreich's ataxia), and some inborn errors of metabolism (such as Hartnup disease).

Abnormal involuntary movements may be psychogenic in origin, as in tics, or they may be the result of extrapyramidal dysfunction, as manifested by chorea, athetosis, dystonia, tremor, and ballismus. *Tics* or *habit spasms,* the most common abnormal movements, are characterized by isolated repetitions such as winking, grimacing, twisting the neck, and shrugging the shoulders. More complex tic phenomena may have associated vocalizations, such as coughing, barking, and clearing the throat; when the vocal component is manifested as obscene language it is called Gilles de la Tourette's disease.

Chorea is characterized by sudden, irregular jerky movements that may involve any group of skeletal muscles, including the face. Chorea may occur in rheumatic fever (Sydenham's chorea), encephalitis, hypoparathyroidism, and occasionally lupus erythematosus. The movements of *athetosis* are slow and writhing and mainly affect the muscles of the extremities; they may be accompanied by choreiform movements (choreoathetosis). Athetosis is a manifestation of kernicterus and congenital defects of the brain.

Dystonia is characterized by involuntary sustained spasms of the muscles of the neck, trunk, and extremities that result in abnormal posture. Dystonic movements may be manifestations of dystonia musculorum deformans, some forms of encephalitis, and birth defects; they may be associated with rigidity in hepatolenticular degeneration (Wilson's disease). Dystonia is most commonly seen in children as an idiosyncrasy to phenothiazines. *Tremor* of basal ganglial origin occurs at rest, while the cerebellar form of tremor becomes evident in volitional movements. It is seen in its most benign form as familial or essential tremor and in its severe form in the wing-beating tremor of Wilson's disease.

DISTURBANCES IN SENSATION. Pain, burning, tingling, and numbness are manifestations of sensory disorders. Episodic sensory disturbances may be the only manifestations of a focal seizure or of hypoparathyroidism. Persistent sensory phenomena are seen in the polyneuropathies. Dysautonomic children, interestingly, have a raised pain threshold, and a congenital indifference to pain has also been noted in a few children.

VISUAL LOSS. Sudden loss of vision is a manifestation of retrobulbar or optic neuritis, while transient impairment in visual function may be seen in seizure disorders or migraine. It is difficult to detect the onset of gradual visual loss, since children tend to be uncomplaining and parents unobservant; however, it may become evident when the child is observed holding books closer to his face, sitting nearer to the television set, or bumping into objects. It is difficult to detect a decrease in the field of vision in young children.

OCULAR DISORDERS. Diplopia follows rapid development of extraocular muscle paresis and its presence is rarely mentioned by children with long-standing eye muscle dysfunction. Nonparalytic *strabismus* is seen with extraocular muscle imbalance and often is a manifestation of nonprogressive lesions of the brain. Paralytic squint most commonly results from third and sixth cranial nerve involvement. A turning in of one or both eyes may occur with any condition causing increased intracranial pressure. Brainstem gliomas and myasthenia gravis also give rise to a variety of extraocular muscle palsies. *Nystagmus,* exhibited as rhythmic, wiggling, jerky, or pendular oscillations of the eyeball, is associated with disorders of the eye, brainstem, and cerebellum. A searching type of nystagmic movement occurs in the blind. Pendular oscillations are most often ocular in origin, as in spasmus nutans and congenital forms of nystagmus. Vertical nystagmus is almost always a manifestation of brainstem dysfunction, while the horizontal variety may indicate either brainstem or cerebellar pathology. Both vertical and horizontal nystagmus frequently result from drug intoxication with barbiturates or hydantoins. Opsoclonia, a bizarre type of nystagmus, is characterized by coarse, irregular, nonrhythmic but conjugate eye movements in all directions of gaze. It often occurs in the syndrome of acute cerebellar ataxia with an occult neoplasm. *Ptosis* may be permanent or intermittent, and in some forms it may be altered by the movements of the jaw (Marcus Gunn syndrome). Permanent ptosis is seen congenitally and follows lesions of the third cranial nerve. The ptosis of myasthenia gravis is intermittent and is least evident on awakening; it increases with fatigue and is most marked at the end of the day. When associated with miosis and enophthalmos (Horner's syndrome), ptosis is a manifestation of impaired sympathetic function. Exophthalmos, when bilateral, usually signifies an endocrinopathy, while unilateral protrusions are most often secondary to retrobulbar tumors, optic nerve gliomas, or disease of the cavernous sinus.

HEARING LOSS. Defective hearing of peripheral origin may be secondary to kernicterus, trauma, exanthems (most commonly mumps), tumors of the brainstem, drugs, or otologic disorders. Some children with intact peripheral pathways have apparent hearing loss; it is assumed that they have impairment of the central connections of hearing (receptive aphasia). Often the first clue to an early hearing loss is failure to develop normal speech patterns.

SPEECH DISORDERS. Defective speech may arise from impaired hearing or expressive difficulties. Delay in the acquisition of speech patterns or faulty development of speech patterns may be the first sign of fixed or progressive lesions of the brain, while loss of previously acquired speech is indicative of hearing disorders or degenerative disease of the brain.

POOR SCHOOL PERFORMANCE. Problems in learning are often related to visual or hearing defects. They may also be the result of unrecognized seizure states (particularly petit mal) or of progressive degenerative diseases. Specific learning disabilities, most commonly reading difficulties, are often seen in children with the syndrome of minimal brain dysfunction. Poor school performance may be the first indication of mild mental retardation.

PERSONALITY CHANGES. Personality changes often develop at some time during the course of neoplastic diseases, especially when the tumor involves the temporal lobe, and during the course of infections and degenerative and metabolic disorders. Hyperactivity (or less commonly apathy) is a frequent manifestation of nonprogressive brain lesions.

HEAD TILT. Head tilt is most commonly associated with tumors of the cerebellum or brainstem. Head tilt may result from local irritation of the cervical musculature or from ocular or central nervous system pathology.

FACIAL WEAKNESS. Asymmetry of the face during crying or a complete lack of facial expression in a child is an indication of facial weakness. In the neonatal period this condition may be secondary to congenital anomalies such as facial nuclear aplasia (Möbius syndrome) and partial muscular hypoplasia (Hofnagel syndrome), or it may be acquired as the result of facial nerve compression. The older child may demonstrate a peripheral facial weakness from Bell's palsy, polyneuritis, brainstem gliomas, or mastoid disease. Rarely there may be a progressive hemiatrophy of the face that includes the facial muscles. Facial weakness limited to the lower half of the face (upper motor neuron paresis) may accompany a hemiparesis secondary to a brain lesion.

CONVULSIONS. In the newborn infant, convulsions may be due either to developmental or acquired lesions of the brain or to metabolic disorders such as hypoglycemia, hypocalcemia, hypomagnesemia, or pyridoxine dependency. Rarely they may be a manifestation of maple syrup urine disease. Seizures during the neonatal period may be confused with apneic or cyanotic spells. In children less than 2 years of age, seizures not associated with fever are usually due to structural defects of the brain. Febrile convulsions may be associated with extracranial infections, or they may be the earliest manifestations of meningitis. Breath-holding spells are common in this age group and may be accompanied by convulsive phenomena. Focal motor seizures in children of this age group do not have the same significance as in adults. Often these focal spells will vary from side to side, and unless they persistently recur on one side, they are usually not related to a specific brain lesion. Petit mal seizures rarely occur before 2 years of age.

HEADACHES. Headaches are relatively common in childhood. Undue irritability in young children may be an indication of recurrent or persistent headache. Older children may have headaches that are related to increased intracranial pressure from any cause or to migraine, tension, trauma, or systemic disease. These painful episodes may precede, may follow, or may be the only manifestation of convulsions.

VERTIGO. Evaluation of vertigo is very difficult and depends on the ability of the child to describe this subjective phenomenon. Vestibular neuronitis results in paroxysmal episodes of vertigo, and seizures may present only as vertiginous attacks. Vertigo may also be a symptom of Meniere's disease, but this is rare in childhood.

COMA. Coma in any age group is a perplexing and life-threatening problem. A careful history is invaluable in ascertaining the underlying pathology. Coma is commonly caused by drug intoxication, trauma, and postictal states and less frequently by meningitis, encephalitis, cerebrovascular accidents, and metabolic disorders.

NEUROLOGIC EXAMINATION

The neurologic examination is essential to determination of nervous system involvement and localization of the site of the pathologic process. Specific etiologic diagnosis may be made from a detailed history combined with a thorough neurologic examination. For example, localization of a lesion to the brainstem is indicated by the presence of multiple cranial nerve palsies, ataxia, and pyramidal tract signs. If the history shows slow progression, the lesion may be diagnosed as a probable tumor.

The *general pediatric examination* is of vital importance in neurologic diagnosis. The head should be carefully measured and auscultated for intracranial bruits. Transillumination of the skull in the infant may indicate the presence of a subdural fluid collection, hydrocephalus, or hydranencephaly. Certain skin lesions are helpful in neurologic diagnosis; depigmented nevi may be the initial cutaneous manifestations of tuberous sclerosis; later the child may develop the more classic adenoma sebaceum. Café au lait spots suggest neurofibromatosis, and port-wine facial hemangiomas often signify encephalotrigeminal angiomatosis (Sturge-Weber-Dimitri syndrome). Midline skin defects, patches of hair, or hemangiomata may be associated with underlying defects of the spinal cord and brain.

In the *neurologic examination* observation of the child may provide many clues to disturbed neurologic function. Successful observation depends on the ingenuity of the examiner in obtaining the cooperation of the child. Ideally the evaluation should be performed in a leisurely manner, and at all times a nonthreatening atmosphere should be carefully staged, perhaps with the child seated in his mother's lap. At some time during the examination the child must be completely undressed. Painful or difficult parts of the examination should be reserved until the end. Examination of the newborn may be difficult because the infant can offer no cooperation; it is further complicated by the possibility that abnormal findings may be a reflection of an immature nervous system rather than transient or permanent defects.

NEUROLOGIC EXAMINATION OF NEONATES

M. RICHARD KOENIGSBERGER AND JOHN M. DRISCOLL

Neurologic examination of the neonate is helpful in establishing gestational age as well as in delineating neurologic dysfunction. At the present time neurologic examination and neurophysiologic techniques provide the most accurate means of assessing gestational age in

TABLE 2. Changes in Muscle Tone at Various Gestational Ages

	24 weeks	28 weeks	32 weeks	34 weeks	37 weeks	41 weeks
Posture	Lateral decubitus	Total extension (hypotonia)	Total extension; slight tone lower extremities	Lower extremities flexed, extended upper extremities (froglike)	Sometimes total flexion; sometimes froglike	Total flexion
Recoil	0	0	Slight in lower extremities	Good in lower extremities, none in upper extremities	Slow in upper extremities	Good in upper extremities
Motility	Slow, global	Slow, extensive		Raises pelvis		Little, Jerky
Popliteal Angle	180°	180°	150°	120°	90°	90°
Heel to Ear	No resistance	No resistance	Slight resistance	Difficult	Almost impossible	Impossible
Scarf maneuver	No resistance	No resistance	No resistance	Slight resistance	Fair resistance	Difficult
Neck						
Extensors	0	0	Slight	Fair	Good	Good
Flexors	0	0	0	0	Slight	Fair

TABLE 3. Changes in Reflexes at Various Gestational Ages

	24 Weeks	28 Weeks	32 Weeks	34 Weeks	37 Weeks	41 Weeks
Moro	Barely apparent	Complete (exhaustable)	Complete	Complete	Complete	Complete
Grasp	Feeble	Fair	Solid	Solid	May pick up infant	As before
Root	Minimal (must reinforce)	Good (with reinforcement)	Good (no reinforcement)	Good	Good	Good
Suck	0	Improving	Present	Strong (synchronous with swallow)	As before	As before
Superciliary tap (McCarthy)	?	Inconstant	Present	Present	Present	Present
Pupillary Response	0	0	Present	Present	Present	Present
Trunk elevation (redressment)	0	0	0	Slight	Good trunk on hips	As before
Automatic walk	0	0	0	Minimal	Fair on toes	Good on heels
Crossed extension	0	Slight withdrawal	Withdrawal	Withdrawal	Withdrawal extension	Withdrawal extension adduction
Cry	Feeble (exhaustible)	Brief, high-pitched	Good	Good	Good	Good

newborn infants. Assessment of gestational age is important in distinguishing between infants who are small for gestational age and those who are born prematurely (p. 155).

The central nervous system matures at a fairly constant rate that is not particularly influenced by premature delivery. Consequently a 4-week-old infant that was born at 32 weeks gestation will demonstrate the same neurologic features as a 1-day-old baby born at 36 weeks gestation. Thus in the normal infant an assessment of actual postconceptual age can be made no matter when the examination is performed. By means of neurologic examination or electroencephalogram gestational age can be established with an accuracy of about 14 days. Careful measurement of peripheral nerve motor conduction velocities allows assessment to within about 10 days.

Abnormal neurologic findings in infants are usually nonspecific. Since a specific diagnosis usually cannot be made, the baby can be considered to be definitely or suspiciously abnormal neurologically. One of the limitations of the neonatal neurologic examination is that rapid changes in tone and reflexes occur during the first 2 days, and there is considerable fluctuation from moment to moment and day to day in the infant's state of alertness. Thus tone and most reflexes are more brisk in the awake infant than in the somnolent infant. Thus ideally the examination should be performed an hour before the next scheduled feeding. Reliance on a single sign as an absolute index of gestational age or neurologic abnormality is unwise, and corroboration with other findings is advised. Many infants show improvement of abnormal neurologic findings in the first few weeks, but this does not necessarily indicate an ultimate good prognosis.

The examination should be done systematically. An initial observation of the infant's posture and movements in the supine position is helpful in gauging gestational age (p. 156). Changes in muscle tone and reflexes at various gestational ages are shown in Tables 2 and 3. The resting supine posture progresses from total extension of upper and lower extremities at less than 31 to 32 weeks to complete flexion at 36 to 40 weeks gestation. In full-term infants flexed arms and extended legs (abnormal tone discrepancy) have been correlated with subsequent neurologic abnormality. Flexion of the extremities on one side with contralateral extension may indicate hemiparesis or a tonic neck response.

Spontaneous movements may be difficult to classify. Tremulousness may be seen in normal and abnormal babies. High-frequency tremors of small amplitude may be benign, but low-frequency high-amplitude tremors and shaking of the extremities suggest hypercalcemia, hypoglycemia, or drug withdrawal. Writhing movements beyond 36 weeks gestation arouse suspicion of basal ganglia disease (kernicterus). Clonus suggests the presence of a neurologic lesion causing spasticity. Slower, more rhythmic clonic movements in the extremities or the face may represent seizures.

The head should be inspected for vault deformity and craniofacial disproportion. The sutures and fontanelles should then be palpated while feeling for cephalhematomas and defects in the skull. The head should be measured, auscultated for bruits, and transilluminated in total darkness.

EYES. Although a newborn does not usually follow light, the head and eyes may remain fixed on the light stimulus when the body is rotated. If they are not totally blind newborns will at least compress their eyelids when a bright light is directed at them, whether their eyes are open or closed. The earliest sign of visual impairment may be pendular nystagmus characterized by equal to-and-fro movements of the eyes. The eyelids of a 24-week fetus do not open, but by 28 weeks all infants completely open their eyes. Persistent palpebral fissure asymmetry suggests ptosis or contralateral facial peresis. The pupils are small (1 to 2 mm diameter) and react slowly to light at 31 to 34 weeks gestation; after 34 weeks they react briskly. The presence of cataracts should be noted. Eye movements are conjugate in most premature and full-term infants. Disconjugate movements do not necessarily imply central nervous system injury, but they warrant careful follow-up. To distinguish a paralytic from a nonparalytic strabismus, the infant should be rotated slowly in the vertical position with the head tilted 30 degrees toward the examiner.

During rotation the eyes normally will move toward the side to which the infant is spun. After two 360-degree turns a slow movement of the eyes away from the direction of rotation will occur unless there is a paralytic strabismus or the vestibular apparatus is not functioning.

Direct fundoscopy is best performed while the infant is sucking on a pacifier, because an infant often keeps his eyes open during sucking. If the examination is difficult the pupils should be dilated pharmacologically and lid retractors should be used. The disc is usually quite pale. A search should be made for hemorrhages and choreoretinitis in the periphery. A few small (1 to 3 mm) flame hemorrhages may be normal in the newborn, but more extensive and numerous flame or subhyaloid hemmorrhages suggest bleeding into the subdural or subarachnoid space. If necessary for complete visualization of the peripheral fundus, indirect ophthalmoscopy should be employed.

FACE. A glabellar tap performed by gently striking the glabella (forehead) with the fingertip, or a similar percussion over the eyebrow (McCarthy reflex), should cause a reactive blink of the eyes. At 30 to 34 weeks gestation the blink response is asymmetric and variable, but after 34 weeks it is bilateral, symmetric, and constant. During crying, asymmetric movement or flatness of one nasolabial fold and incomplete eyelid closure suggest homolateral seventh nerve involvement. Differentiating upper and lower motor neuron lesions of the seventh nerve can be difficult, as infants do not readily wrinkle their foreheads. The presence of a forceps mark on the affected side suggests lower motor neuron etiology, while a homolateral hemiparesis supports an upper motor neuron disorder. Unilateral ptosis may be congenital or familial. Its presence in association with a miotic pupil indicates an acquired Horner's syndrome. Bilateral ptosis demands further work-up for neuromuscular disease.

BULBAR MUSCULATURE. Crying, sucking, swallowing, and gagging are mediated mainly by the bulbar musculature. With normal pulmonary function a newborn of 32 weeks gestation can sustain a strong cry. A high-pitched or hoarse cry suggests diffuse cortical disease, if difficult intubation has been excluded. Sucking is present to a variable degree from 28 weeks gestation. At 32 weeks sucking should be strong, and at 34 weeks it is usually synchronized with swallowing, thus allowing the infant to be bottle-fed. The rooting reflex is elicited by gently stimulating the corners of the baby's mouth; the head is turned toward the stimulated side. It may be helpful to reinforce this reflex by holding the neck of the infant up slightly. After 32 weeks gestation this reinforcement is not necessary. A depressed rooting reflex is often associated with poor sucking. The gag reflex and movements of the tongue should also be evaluated. True tongue fasciculations usually indicate anterior horn cell disease, but normal movements of the tongue are often incorrectly interpreted as fasciculations.

NECK MUSCLES. The neck extensors are best inspected with the infant held in a sitting position. The facility with which the chin is raised away from the chest should be assessed. It should be fairly well developed by 34 weeks and well developed at 36 weeks. For evaluation of the neck flexors one should observe flexion of the head as the infant is brought to the sitting position from the supine position while held by the hands. The head starts to follow the trunk at 36 weeks, and at full term it will remain in the plane of the trunk for a few seconds. The Moro response appears at 28 weeks or younger, but it may not be obtained consistently until 32 weeks gestation. It is provoked by any maneuver that produces a rapid extension of the neck muscles. As noted in Table 3, a complete Moro reflex (extension of the arms followed by flexion and simultaneous spread of the fingers) is present after 32 weeks gestation. Depression of the Moro response may be due to generalized central nervous system depression, while consistent asymmetry suggests plexus injury or direct trauma to the limb with the diminished response.

If the neck is slowly rotated 90 degrees and maintained in that position, a tonic neck reflex may result with the infant supine. The extremities toward which the chin points extend, while the extremities on the side of the occiput are held in flexion (fencing position). This is not an abnormal response in the first 2 months of life, but it can be deemed suspicious if the tonic neck posture is maintained spontaneously and continuously.

UPPER EXTREMITIES. The recoil of the extremities is tested by extending the arms at the elbows, holding for a count of three, and releasing. At 36 weeks gestation the return to flexion is slow, but as the infant approaches term the recoil becomes much more vigorous. A consistent asymmetry of response may denote a focal deficit. The *scarf maneuver* is performed by drawing the arm of the infant across the chin toward the opposite shoulder. This maneuver meets with increasing resistance after 34 weeks gestation. Upper brachial plexus palsy (Erb's palsy) results in decreased resistance. The *grasp reflex* produced by palmar stimulation from the ulnar side may be present early. With advancing gestation there is spread of the response up the arm, including flexion at the elbow, so that at 36 weeks gestation some infants can be lifted off the bed.

TRUNK. Superficial reflexes (abdominal and cremasteric) are variable in the neonatal period and are of no help in gauging gestational age. The anal reflex should be tested if cord injury is suspected. Stimulation of the anal mucosa should result in contraction of the anal orifice. If the examiner is not certain of the response, rectal tone should be tested. Urinary incontinence in the neonate, particularly in the male, can be tested by grasping the infant under the arms and holding him erect; constant dribbling will result if there is sphincter incontinence. Trunk tone can be tested by searching for trunk elevation (trunk righting). This is elicited by holding the infant with his legs vertical and his trunk leaning forward 45 degrees and then stimulating the soles of his feet. By 37 to 38 weeks gestation the infant will pull his trunk to the vertical position upon stimulation.

LOWER EXTREMITIES. Differences in spontaneous motility and recoil between the legs should be noted. The *popliteal angle* is the greatest angle that can be measured in the popliteal fossa when the leg is extended at the knee with the pelvis fixed in place; the angle decreases from 180 degrees at 28 weeks to 90 degrees or less at term. The heel-to-ear maneuver, in which the examiner attempts to approximate the infant's heel to the head with the trunk fixed, also meets with increased resistance as gestational age increases. The *crossed extension reflex*, which is induced by excitation of the sole of the foot with the leg held firmly in extension, produces a response of the opposite lower extremity with three successive and distinct components: withdrawal, extension, and adduction. Withdrawal is seen at 34 weeks, withdrawal and extension are seen at 37 weeks, and the complete response of withdrawal, extension, and adduction is seen at 40 weeks. Knee jerks are usually brisk in the newborn. Ankle jerks are usually obtainable and are best elicited with the infant in the prone position. Two to three beats of either knee or ankle clonus are not unusual in the normal newborn infant. Automatic walking is performed by grasping the neonate under the arms, tilting him slightly forward, and bringing his feet in contact with a firm surface. The normal baby takes a few steps starting at 34 weeks gestation. This reflex may be absent in a severely depressed infant or in an infant with spinal cord disease. The Babinski response is very variable in the neonate, but it should be apparent if there is a marked difference in the responses of the right and left sides.

NEUROLOGIC EXAMINATION OF INFANTS AND OLDER CHILDREN

SIDNEY CARTER AND ARNOLD P. GOLD

The purpose of the neurologic examination in the infant and the older child is to localize a lesion or lesions to a particular area of the nervous system. It must be emphasized that the infant's level of development can modify the findings and the significance of this evaluation. For example, the presence of an extensor plantar reflex (the Babinski response) can be physiologic at 6 months of age, whereas such a finding in the older child is almost always pathologic. Since the cooperation of the infant cannot be gained, a detailed evaluation of sensation and cerebellar function is not possible.

Mental status cannot be formally evaluated in infancy, but it can be assessed from responses to the environment and accomplishments at a given age. The normal infant smiles at 4 to 6 weeks, shows awareness of familiar objects or persons by smiling or laughing aloud at 4 months, expresses displeasure or preferences and holds arms out to be picked up at 6 months, responds to "No" at 8 months, and performs imitative behavior (waves "bye-bye," plays "patty-cake" and "peek-a-boo") at 10 months. After the age of 1 year the infant's intellectual abilities can be tested with more precision.

The infant understands names of objects and shows an interest in pictures at 12 months, requests by pointing and carries out more complex imitative behavior at 15 months, follows simple commands at 18 months, and is able to participate in organized play and point to body parts at 2 years.

There is a close correlation between the development of speech and future intellectual function. Normal hearing and intellect are prerequisites for the development of language. The normal infant cries at birth, produces sounds of pleasure at 4 months, makes primitive sounds ("ah, goo") at 5 months, increases the range of sounds at 6 months, and combines syllables ("baba, dada, mama") at 8 months. In the second year of life the infant says two or three words with meaning at 12 to 15 months, uses many intelligible words at 18 months, and forms two- to three-word sentences at 2 years. Future problems with articulation can be suspected even in the very young infant. The neonate who has difficulty with sucking or swallowing, or the older infant who drools excessively or has difficulty with chewing are at risk of developing speech problems.

Examination of the cranium includes measurement of head circumference, determination of fontanelle size, percussion, auscultation and transillumination of the cranium, and inspection for cranial asymmetries and abnormal ridging. The head circumference must be measured at each examination with a steel tape and plotted on the appropriate head circumference chart. The fontanelle should be measured for size and tension. Not only are changes in head circumference of importance, but cranial asymmetries and ridging may indicate premature closure of a suture (craniosynostosis). The crack-pot percussion note in the older infant indicates separation of the sutures secondary to increased intracranial pressure or skull fracture. Auscultation of the skull reveals a soft bruit in about half of normal infants. Pathologic bruits, which may indicate cerebral vascular malformations or increased intracranial pressure, are loud, sonorous, and synchronous with systole. Transillumination of the cranium in the young infant may reveal a thin cortical mantle, such as with hydrocephalus, hydranencephaly, cerebral atrophy, or porencephaly; or it can be diagnostic of subdural fluid collections. Transillumination must be performed in a darkened room after a suitable period of dark adaptation. A flashlight fitted with a rubber adapter is the most common source of light, but more elaborate apparatus is available commercially. All areas of the cranium must be systematically scanned. Normally there is a 2-cm halo around the adapter in the frontoparietal area, and this gradually decreases to 1 cm in the occipital area. A wider area of transillumination is usually abnormal. Fresh or recent subdural hematomas may decrease the halo, whereas old collections that are largely devoid of blood increase the halo. A localized increase in the size of the halo in the occipital region suggests a Dandy-Walker malformation, and a generalized lighting-up of the cranium is seen with hyranencephaly or severe hydrocephalus.

Motor functions can best be tested by observing the infant perform voluntary movements (Table 1). The young infant should move all four extremities actively, symmetrically, and equally. During the first year there are drastic changes in motor functions in that relatively nonfunctioning neonates gradually progress toward purposeful prehension, sitting ability, and independent locomotion. Prehension and purposeful movements in the upper extremities change with chronologic age. At 3 to 4 months the hands are normally open and there is midline hand play. At 5 to 7 months the infant should reach for and grasp objects; at this age the child should be able to remove a cloth covering his face with either hand. At 10 months a pincer grasp involving apposition of thumb and index fingers should become evident and should be associated with purposeful hand function. Motor function in the trunk and lower extremities likewise shows significant change with age. Head control in the prone position is usually acquired at 1 month of age, and at 4 months the head should no longer lag when the infant is lifted from the supine position. The infant should turn from supine to prone at 4 to 6 months and in the opposite direction about 2 months later. The ability to sit when placed should be attained at 6 to 7 months; most infants sit alone at 8 months. Crawling on hands and knees and standing with support should be evident at 10 months, standing alone should be possible at 12 to 13 months, and walking unassisted should be established before 15 months.

The inability of a child to perform these activities at the expected ages may be a reflection of motor impairment, maturational delay, or mental retardation. Muscle tone is a valuable indication of motor function. Increased muscle tone or spasticity is reflected by tightness of muscle groups when they are passively stretched. In the upper extremities such muscle tightness can be noted by the degree of resistance to extension and supination of the forearm, representing increase in tone in the biceps and pronator muscles. In the lower extremities spasticity is demonstrated by tightness in the hip flexors, the hamstrings, and the gastrocnemius-soleus group of muscles. Decrease in muscle tone is evidenced by hyperextensibility of affected muscle groups. Spasticity is a reflection of upper motor neuron lesions, best exemplified by cerebral palsy. In contrast, decrease in muscle tone is usually associated with lower motor neuron lesions and is typically seen in Werdnig-Hoffmann disease.

Evaluation of *reflex activity* is an important part of the neurologic examination. The normal infant demonstrates Moro, grasping, rooting, and sucking reflexes until about 4 months of age. Failure to develop these reflexes, their premature loss before the age of 4 months, or their persistence after this time is a significant indication of neurologic dysfunction. The asymmetric tonic neck reflex is elicited by rotating the infant's head to either side; this results in extension of the arm and leg on the side toward which the face is rotated and flexion of the limbs on the side of the occiput. Partial tonic neck reflexes may be observed in normal infants until the age of 6 months. Obligatory and persistent tonic neck reflexes are pathologic at any age. After 8 months of age the parachute response may give invaluable information. To elicit this response the infant is suddenly brought head down toward a horizontal surface; normally there is extension of the arms with spreading of the fingers as if to check the fall.

Evaluation of *deep tendon reflexes* is an integral part of any neurologic examination. These are always present and equal, but in the newborn the triceps and ankle jerks may be difficult to elicit. In upper motor neuron disease the deep tendon reflexes are exaggerated and are usually associated with an extensor plantar response (Babinski sign). In lower motor neuron disease they are either diminished or absent and are associated with a normal plantar response. Overflow of the knee jerk to include adduction of both thighs may be observed normally in infants up to 6 months of age, but is abnormal after that time. Sustained ankle clonus is pathologic in infancy and childhood.

Superficial abdominal and cremasteric reflexes have limited clinical significance. They are frequently absent in upper motor neuron lesions. The plantar response may be physiologically extensor until 18 months. After that time an extensor response (Babinski sign) is usually indicative of upper motor neuron disease.

Examination of the *cranial nerves* is difficult in infants; it requires both patience and ingenuity. The first cranial nerve cannot be evaluated in the young child. The second cranial nerve is examined by testing visual activity and visual fields and by careful fundoscopy. The third, fourth, and sixth cranial nerves mediate eye movements and pupillary responses; they are tested by noting conjugate movements in all directions of gaze. Abnormal findings include eye muscle palsies, nystagmus, bizarre eye movements, and absence or inequality of pupillary responses. The corneal reflexes can be tested accurately at any age; they indicate the integrity of the first branch of the fifth or trigeminal nerve. Facial movements should be observed under all states of activity, including crying. Involvement of the facial nerve can occur in both upper and lower motor neuron disorders. Upper motor neuron lesions of the facial nerve are characterized by inability to move the corner of the mouth on the involved side while crying or smiling, with the ability to wrinkle the forehead and close the eye on that side being preserved. In lower motor neuron disease (nuclear and infranuclear involvement of the facial nerve) all muscles of the face and forehead are involved. Hearing should be tested by observing the response to sound: in early infancy there is eye blinking; by 3 to 4 months there is turning of the head and eyes in the direction of the stimulus. The gag reflex, a function of the ninth and tenth cranial nerves, is normally present at any age. The tongue should be examined as it lies in the mouth for atrophy and fasciculations, such as are seen with hypoglossal nuclear involvement in Werdnig-Hoffmann disease. Tremulous movements of the tongue in a crying child are frequently misinterpreted as fasciculations.

The funduscopic examination and the response to pinprick (sensory examination) should be delayed to the end of the examination. The child's responses to pinpricks applied to various parts of the body should be noted, as evidenced by withdrawal of the stimulated area and by facial grimacing or crying; withdrawal alone may be a reflection of spinal automatism rather than sensory perception.

Neuro-ophthalmologic examination of the infant and older child is discussed on p. 1746.

ANCILLARY PROCEDURES

SIDNEY CARTER AND ARNOLD P. GOLD

Additional diagnostic procedures should be carefully planned, and maximum information should be obtained from each study. Increasing knowledge in the field of electrophysiology and improved radiologic techniques have made available a variety of new diagnostic aids. Many of these tests are highly specialized and require expert interpretation.

RADIOGRAPHIC STUDIES. Plain radiographs of the *skull* are indicated in all children suspected of having intracranial disease or head trauma. Routine films include anteroposterior, posteroanterior, stereolateral, and base views. In special circumstances films of the optic foramina and mastoids as well as laminagrams may be necessary. Plain radiographs may show evidence of increased intracranial pressure, such as suture diastasis, erosion of the posterior clinoids, and deepening of the sella turcica. The so-called beaten-silver appearance may be normal and by itself is not evidence of increased intracranial pressure. Radiographs can also reveal premature closure of sutures, fractures, skull tumors, or unilateral cerebral atrophy (Dyke-Davidoff-Masson syndrome). Intracranial calcifications may be seen after infections with toxoplasmosis, cytomegalic inclusion disease or chronic brain abscesses, and in association with tumors, vascular malformations, neuroectodermal dysplasias, and metabolic disorders. Calcification of the pineal gland is rare in childhood.

Radiographs of the *spine* are indicated following trauma and when there is a suggestion of an underlying congenital anomaly or a tumor is suspected. They may also have diagnostic significance in certain metabolic disorders, such as Morquio's disease or Hurler's disease. Anteroposterior and lateral views should be taken routinely.

Contrast studies are radiographic procedures that include air encephalography, cerebral arteriography, and myeolography and should be performed only in the presence of specific indications. *Air encephalography* (Fig. 1) is indicated primarily in children suspected of having mass lesions or in those with progressive neurologic disorders associated with increased intracranial pressure. Most epileptic children and those with nonprogressive conditions, including mental retardation, cerebral palsy, and abnormal behavior accompanied by learning disabilities, should not be subjected to this procedure. In the case of increased intracranial pres-

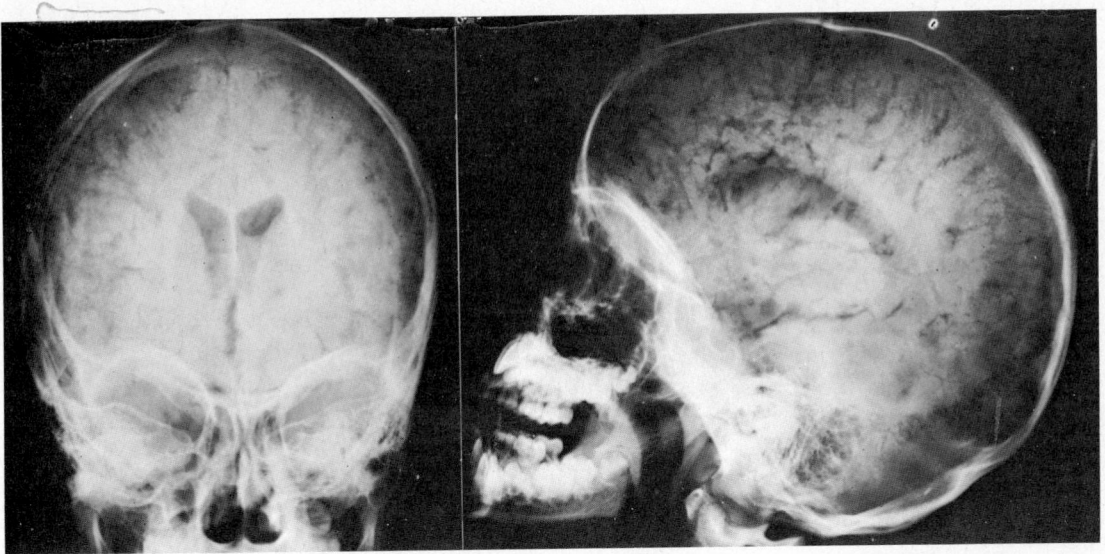

FIG. 1.   Normal pneumoencephalogram in a 5-year-old girl.

sure, air is introduced directly into the ventricles (ventriculography). In most situations, however, air introduced via the lumbar subarachnoid space (pneumoencephalography) is adequate and is preferable for suspected brainstem and optic chiasm tumors. *Cerebral arteriography* (Fig. 2) is a method of visualizing the vessels of the brain after injecting a radiopaque substance into a major artery; it is best utilized when a focal lesion, rather than a diffuse lesion, is suspected. The primary indications for cerebral arteriography include vascular malformations, subdural hematoma, cerebral hemisphere tumors, and pseudotumor cerebri. *Myelography* is a method of visualizing the spinal canal after the introduction of a radiopaque substance into the spinal subarachnoid space. The prime indication for this procedure is suspected intraspinal tumor.

Computer-assisted tomography (CT scan, EMI scan, Fig. 3) is a unique noninvasive radiologic technique that utilizes a narrow x-ray beam to scan the patient's head in a linear fashion. The scans are then analyzed by computer, and pictures of the skull and its contents are obtained. The procedure is very helpful in diagnosis of intracranial mass lesions, in delineation of orbital contents, and in definition of ventricular size and shape. It may obviate the need for air encephalography or arteriography in some instances.

LUMBAR PUNCTURE.   Examination of the *cerebrospinal fluid* is the single most useful ancillary procedure in the evaluation of neurologic disease; it is mandatory when infection of the central nervous system is suspected, and it may be useful in evaluating undiagnosed disease of the central nervous system. Lumbar puncture is also justified in all children with increased intracranial pressure with suggestive evidence of infection of the central nervous system; it is contraindicated in the presence of increased intracranial pressure un-

related to infection or when there is cutaneous infection at the site of the projected lumbar puncture.

Maximum information is obtained when cerebrospinal fluid pressure is measured, the fluid is analyzed for cellular, protein, and sugar contents, and a serologic examination is performed. Sedation and local anesthesia are important adjuncts to obtaining reliable pressure measurements with the child in a relaxed state in a lateral recumbent position. The pressure normally varies between 50 and 180 mm of water and is accurate only when measured with a water manometer. Rate of flow is a crude method of estimating pressure and may be misleading. Jugular compression or formal cuff manometrics should be utilized when a spinal cord lesion is suspected.

Normal fluid is clear and colorless, but in the newborn, xanthochromic coloring is common. Hemorrhagic fluid may signify either a traumatic lumbar puncture or hemorrhage in the central nervous system. Differentiation is possible by collection of fluid in three tubes and examination of the supernatant after centrifugation. Hemorrhagic fluid due to a traumatic lumbar puncture will show a progressive decrease in the number of red blood cells in the three consecutive tubes, and the supernatant will be colorless; hemorrhagic fluid due to hemorrhage in the central nervous system will show no change in the three tubes, and the supernatant will be xanthochromic.

The cell count of the fluid must be determined immediately; normally it does not exceed 5 white blood cells per cubic millimeter. If more than this number are present, a disorder in the central nervous system is suspected. Crenated red blood cells do not by themselves necessarily indicate previous hemorrhage. Protein content is normally 10 to 15 mg/100 ml in the lateral ventricles and up to about 40 mg/100 ml in the lumbar

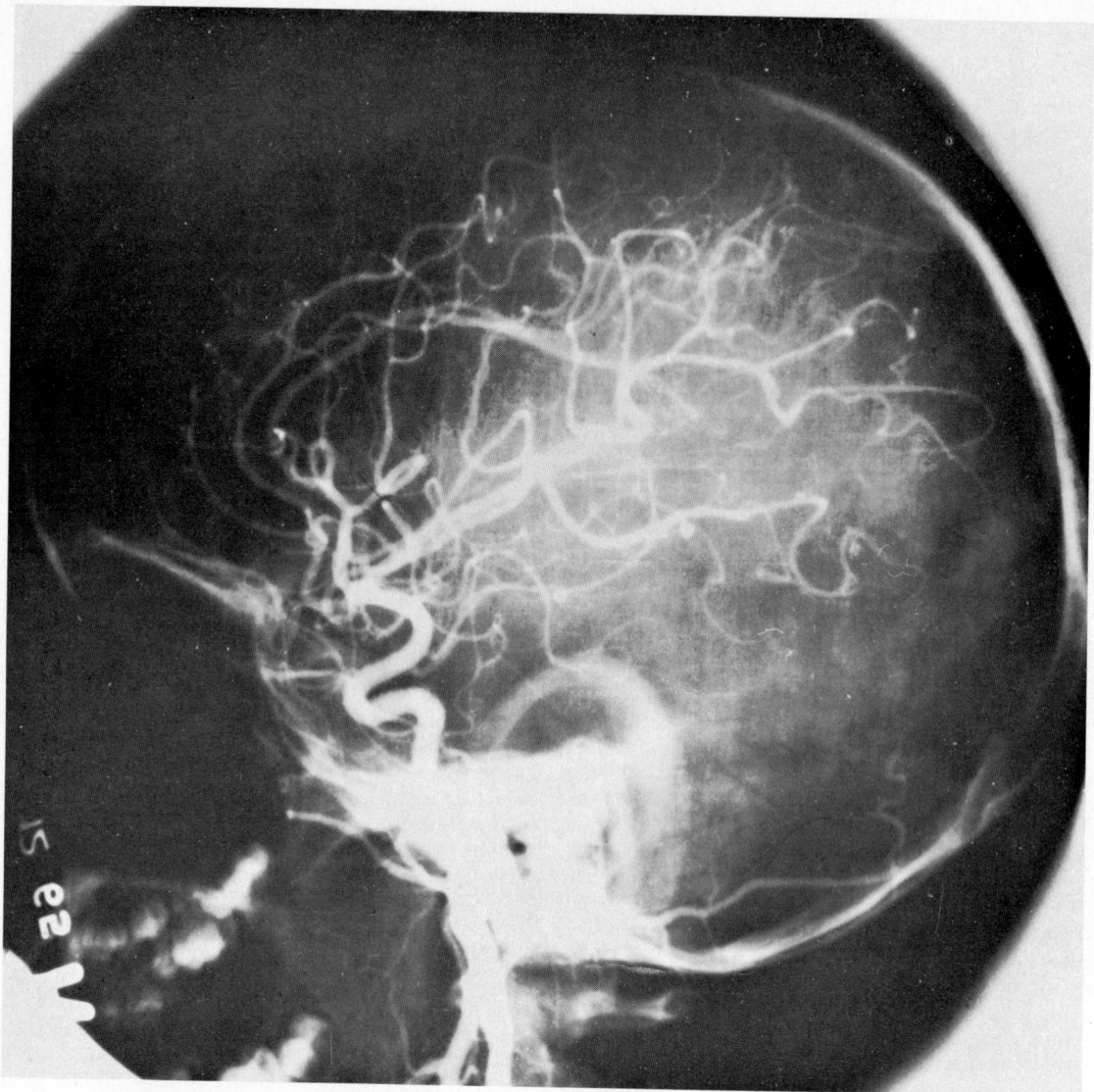

FIG. 2. Normal carotid arteriogram

subarachnoid space. Newborn infants of both low and normal birth weight normally have protein concentrations of 75 to 125 mg/100 ml. Sugar content of cerebrospinal fluid is generally two-thirds of the blood sugar, and its diagnostic value is enhanced when simultaneous determinations are performed. A significant decrease in glucose concentration is seen in hypoglycemic states, bacterial and fungal infections of the central nervous system, and neoplastic meningeal infiltrations. When indicated, the fluid can be analyzed for gamma globulin or enzyme concentrations. Millipore techniques for obtaining and identifying cells may be invaluable in identification of some intracranial tumors.

SUBDURAL PUNCTURE. Subdural puncture should be performed in all infants suspected of having subdural hematoma or effusions and in those with unexplained macrocephaly; it is contraindicated in the presence of scalp infections. Cerebrospinal fluid may inadvertently be obtained at the time of the puncture and misinterpreted as a subdural fluid collection. True subdural fluid has either a xanthochromic discoloration or, when colorless, a protein content considerably higher than that of lumbar subarachnoid fluid.

ELECTRODIAGNOSTIC PROCEDURES. *Electroencephalography* (EEG) is a relatively simple and innocuous procedure. Pediatric electroencephalography requires familiarity with developmental changes in order to properly interpret deviations from the norm (Fig. 4). Electroencephalography has its greatest use as a diagnostic aid in seizure disorders and suspected space-

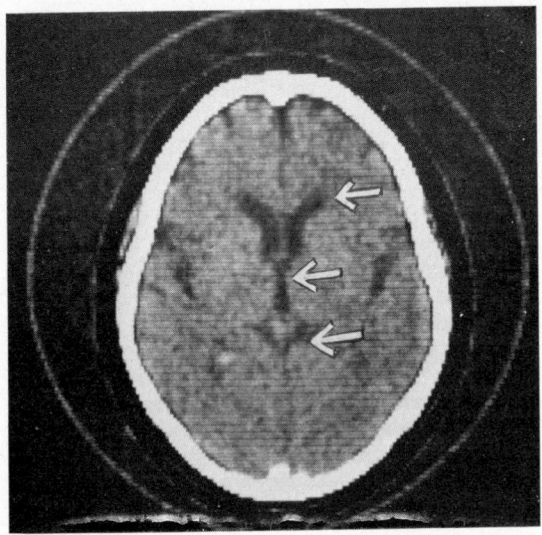

FIG. 3. Normal CAT (computerized axial tomography) (CTT or EMI scan) at the level of the third ventricle; upper arrow, lateral ventricle; middle arrow, third ventricle; lower arrow, quadrigeminal plate cistern. (Courtesy of Dr. S. Hilal.)

occupying lesions. It is also useful in monitoring the progress of encephalitis and head injury. *Electromyography* and nerve conduction studies are useful in determining the site of pathology in neuromuscular disorder. Electromyography aids in differentiating between primary muscle disease and disorders of neural origin. Nerve conduction studies may be of value in differentiating peripheral nerve disorders from anterior horn cell disorders.

ECHOENCEPHALOGRAPHY. Echoencephalography is a procedure in which high-frequency sound recordings are used to establish the shift of midline structures secondary to subdural hematomas and hemispheric mass lesions. More recently it has been useful in the determination of ventricular size (echoventriculography).

RADIOISOTOPE BRAIN SCANS. Brain scans utilize radioiodinated serum albumin (RISA) or mercury- or technetium-labeled compounds in the localization of intracranial lesions such as neoplasms, abscesses, and vascular malformations. Intrathecal RISA can be utilized in the evaluation of hydrocephalus; the presence of radioactivity in the ventricular system indicates abnormal cerebrospinal fluid flow and absorption.

PSYCHOLOGIC TESTS. Psychologic tests can be valuable in the documentation of organic brain dysfunction and in delineation of intellectual potential. Projective tests may show evidence of personality disturbance. These procedures should not be repeated frequently, but at properly spaced intervals they can be useful in differentiation of static and progressive encephalopathies.

References

Amiel-Tison C: Neurological evaluation of the maturity of newborn infants. Arch Dis Child 43:89, 1968

Baker HL Jr, Campbell JK, Houser DW, et al: Computer assisted tonography of the head, an early evaluation. Mayo Clin Proc 49:17, 1974

Beintema DJ: A Neurological Study of Newborn Infants. Clinics in Developmental Medicine, No 28. London, Spastics International Medical Publications, William Heinemann, 1968

Brazelton TB: Neonatal Behavioral Assessment Scale. Clinics in Developmental Medicine, No 50. London, Spastics International Medical Publications, William Heinemann; Philadelphia, JB Lippincott, 1973

Dreyfus-Brisac C: The electroencephalogram of the premature infant. World Neurology 3:1, 1962

Egan D, Illingworth RS, MacKeith RC: Developmental Screening 0–5 Years. Clinics in Developmental Medicine, No 30. London, Spastics International Medical Publications, 1969

Illingworth RS: An Introduction to Developmental Assessment in the First Year. Little Club Clinics in Developmental Medicine, No 3. London, National Spastics Society, 1962

Kistler PJ, Hochberg IH, Brooks BR, Richardson EP Jr, New PFJ, Schnur J: Computerized axial tomography: clinicopathologic correlation. Neurology (Minneap) 25:201, 1970

Koenigsberger MR: Judgment of fetal age. I. Neurologic evaluation. Pediatr Clin North Am 13:823, 1966

Paine RS, Oppe TE: Neurological Examination of Children. Clinics in Developmental Medicine, No 20, 21. London, National Spastics Society, 1966

Prechtl H, Beintema D: The Neurological Examination of the Full Term

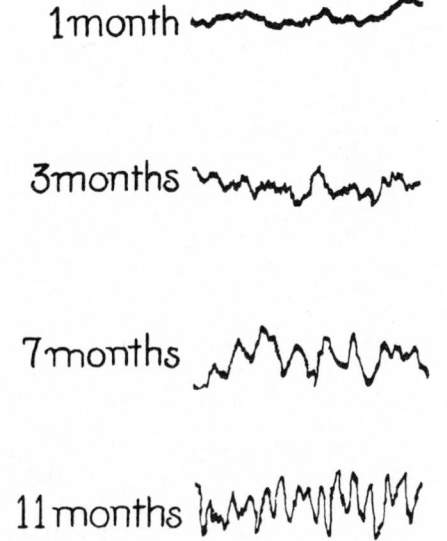

FIG. 4. Electroencephalograms of a normal infant at various ages illustrating the development of the fundamental rhythm. (From Lindsay: J Gen Psychol 19:285, 1938.)

Newborn Infant. Little Club Clinics in Developmental Medicine, No 12. London, National Spastics Society, 1964

Schlagenhauff RE, Mazurowski J, Smith BH: Echoencephalography in neurologic diagnosis. NY State J Med 67:1035, 1967

Thomas JA, Chesni Y, Saint-Anne Dargassies S: The Neurological Examination of the Infant. Little Club Clinics in Developmental Medicine, No 1. London, National Spastics Society, 1960

THE NEURO-OPTHALMOLOGIC EXAMINATION OF THE CHILD (SEE ALSO P. 1963)

MYLES M. BEHRENS

VISUAL EXAMINATION. The technique of visual examination depends on the child's age. In the older child visual acuity can be tested with a letter of number chart. The "E" or picture chart with isolated figures may be necessary in nonreading children. Finger counting and, in the younger child, finger mimicking may be used: extended fingers are roughly of 20/200 object size and the distance can be varied to assess visual acuity. It is normally about 20/200 at one year, 20/70 at two years and 20/20 by three years.

An infant is best examined when alert, eg hungry and seated, and may be tested at first with both eyes open to avoid annoyance by monocular occlusion. Recognition and following of a human face, bottle, toy or light can be tested. Response to an optokinetic tape or drum, threat stimulus, or to bright light are means of assessing low vision.

Formal visual field examination is usually not feasible until seven to ten years of age, but careful confrontation visual field testing can be relied upon to elicit most visual field defects. Visual fields can be analyzed by asking the child to count or mimic fingers presented in the right and left halves of the field simultaneously or to point to the hand which appears clearer. In the infant consistent preference for objects presented on one side upon such simultaneous bilateral stimulation suggests hemianopic defect. This is homonymous, ie of retrochiasmal origin, if present with both eyes open. Monocular temporal hemianopic field defect can be found even without cooperation in fixation by testing temporally beyond the child's full lateral gaze even with both eyes open.

All chiasmal compressive lesions causing visual defect, however minimal, are accompanied by temporal hemianopic dimming of red objects of any size. This can be easily detected on monocular confrontation testing.

Optic nerve defect, most typically central scotoma or altitudinal defect respecting the horizontal meridian nasally, can also be sought on confrontation. Other parameters of optic nerve dysfunction, beyond visual acuity and field, include the comparitive brightness of light or of a red object in the two eyes as well as the perception of color test plates.

PUPILS. The demonstration of a relative afferent pupillary defect (the Marcus-Gunn pupillary phenomenon) by the swinging flashlight test provides objective corroboration of unilateral optic nerve dysfunction and is essential for that clinical diagnosis. It is not present with nonorganic visual loss, simple strabismic or refractive amblyaopia, opacities in the media, or minor retinal pathology.

The pupils constrict less to light stimulation of an eye with optic nerve conduction defect than to stimulation of the normal eye. A flashlight held just beneath the visual axis is swung back and forth from eye to eye with the child fixing his gaze, if possible, on a distant object in dim illumination. Normally both pupils constrict when the light reaches either eye, after briefly opening as the light swings past the nose. Dilation or lack of constriction as the light reaches either eye indicates relative afferent pupillary defect. The pupils remain equal in size regardless of the nature of any afferent defect. This may not be appreciated if examination of one eye at a time is required by poor cooperation. Therefore either pupil can be observed although one generally observes the one illuminated. If there is an efferent defect, as in third nerve palsy, the normal pupil can be watched at all times.

In a child with bilateral visual impairment, diminished pupillary reactivity to light is important evidence of pregeniculate pathology. Since several factors affect pupil size, including alertness and the extent of near reaction, one must make sure that any constriction seen is reproducably due to the applied light stimulus.

Anisocoria prompts consideration of third nerve palsy, but if it is isolated, without motility disturbance or ptosis, there is almost invariably another benign explanation. The main considerations are a tonic, or "Adie's" pupil and topical atropine effect. The former is due to a ciliary ganglion lesion, usually idiopathic, posttraumatic or postinflammatory, eg postvaricella. It is usually unilateral with dilated pupil reacting with only sectoral constriction to light as seen on slit lamp examination and barely evident grossly—if at all. There is often a more extensive though slow, or "tonic," near response and demonstrable denervation supersensitivity (constricting to 2.5 percent Methacholine (mecholyl) or dilute pilocarpine). Topical atropine effect may last several weeks and is proved by failure of the pupil to constrict to one drop of 1 percent pilocarpine; this may also occur with evident iris sphincter rupture following contusion of the eye or with synechial adhesions after iritis.

Horner's syndrome is suggested by mild anisocoria with normal pupil reactivity. The anisocoria is more evident in the dark or with excitement than when the pupils are small. Physiologic (central) anisocoria is similar although more uniform throughout the range of pupillary size and is infrequent in children. In Horner's syndrome there is generally partial narrowing of the palpebral fissure from above and below ("upside down" ptosis). When congenital there is alteration in iris color.

FUNDUS EXAMINATION. Aids to ophthalmoscopy include *dilation* (with mydriatic, eg phenylephrine 10 percent, and/or cycloplegic, eg tropicamide 1 percent; a *lid speculum,* particularly in the young infant (with instillation of anesthetic drop first); and *sedation,* eg chloral hydrate orally or rectally, with *anesthesia* only occasionally required. Indirect ophthalmoscopy provides a large stereoscopic field but direct ophthalmoscopy ordinarily will suffice. Refractive error can be roughly estimated by the ophthalmoscopic lens setting required, more precisely by retinoscopy. Opacities in the media can be seen by focusing with high plus lens.

Optic atrophy is indicated by pallor and decreased vascularity of the optic nerve head. The disc in early infancy may be normally pale, especially in the premature, where there is often vasoconstriction as well. Both are exacerbated by lid squeezing of a speculum on the globe.

Certain forms of optic atrophy must be distinguished, eg secondary atrophy (after papilledema or papillitis), and glaucomatous cupping as well as anomalies, eg coloboma and optic nerve hypoplasia. The hypoplastic optic nerve head is small, usually with a peripapillary halo, which corresponds to the expected size of the disc. Narrowing of retinal artery calibre must be sought as an early sign of retinal degeneration, although early in congenital Leber's amaurosis the fundus may be normal.

The macula is 2 1/2 disc diameters temporal to the disc, and is best examined simply by allowing the child to look directly at the light. Here there are no retinal vessels and usually, but not necessarily, a central foveal dot light reflex is seen. It is this area which, when surrounded by lipid laden ganglion cells, will appear as a cherry red spot, or brown in the darkly pigmented patient. Similarly there may be splotchy pigmentation as well as narrowed arterioles in other cerebromacular degenerations. Some granularity of the pigment epithelium may be normal.

Early findings in *papilledema* include *venous engorgement* with loss of spontaneous venous pulsation —its presence indicates only normal intracranial pressure at that instant and is usually but not always present in the normal; hyperemia of the disc with engorgement of fine vessels; and blurring or *edema of the nerve fiber layer* at the disc magins (initially above and below, and nasally before temporally). There may also be *hemorrhages* in the nerve fiber layer as well as microinfarcts, or cotton wool spots, *retinal wrinkling* often concentric to the disc margin and *choroidal folds* between the disc and macula. There may be retinal wrinkles in that region, with elevation of the macula as well as *exudates* or edema residues, which may form a partial star figure. Some visual loss may be due to such macular disturbance rather than the ischemic involution to secondary atrophy which is generally accompanied by a loss of disc color as well as narrow arterioles and usually preceded by subjective obscurations. Simple papilledema is unaccompanied by visual loss beyond enlargement of the blind spot. *Optociliary shunt vessels* on the disc occasionally appear as a sequel to chronic central retinal venous obstruction in chronic papilledema; they can be seen as large central retinal venous branches which stop abruptly at the disc margin entering the choroid.

Other causes of a blurred or elevated disc must be distinguished from true papilledema. In the small crowded hyperopic-type disc the full complement of nerve fibers passes through a smaller opening resulting in blurred margins and relatively more vascularized appearance with veins appearing relatively fuller, but without the aforementioned stigmata of dilated fine vessels or edematous clouding of the nerve fibre layer.

Elevated disc anomalies, often due to buried drusen, must be distinguished. The drusen or small nodules which glow on adjacent illumination tend to appear particularly near the edge of the disc in the second or third decade with the development of visible nerve fiber loss and arcuate field defects. Occasionally hemorrhage occurs. In the young child the nodules are generally not appreciated. The parents should be examined, since this condition is often hereditary. Such elevated disc anomalies lack the characteristics of papilledema described above; in particular, the vessels can be clearly seen on the surface, unobscured by edema, and the central part of the disc is often highest rather than the early elevation at the disc margins characteristic of papilledema.

Causes of true disc edema other than increased intracranial pressure may be occasionally encountered, eg ischemic as in juvenile diabetes or cyanotic heart disease, as well as in diabetic or hypertensive retinopathy and of course in optic neuritis, where there is visual loss.

OCULAR MOTILITY.   Ocular motility disorders are best analyzed by testing the subsystems of ocular motor control separately. The examination should begin with observation of the child at rest for abnormal spontaneous eye movements, eg nystagmus, which will be discussed later. *Following (pursuit)* of a slowly moving object is tested horizontally and vertically. The degree of smoothness may be assessed. It becomes jerky (or saccadic) in various circumstances including cerebellar and basal ganglia disturbances, as well as sedative and anticonvulsant drug therapy. Gaze evoked nystagmus can be appreciated, if present, and the range of eye movement gauged (including testing in the cardinal positions.

Saccades, or rapid eye movements, are elicited horizontally and vertically by command or attraction toward objects. Abnormal overshoot or oscillation on return to the primary position indicates ocular dysmetria.

Convergence is tested by bringing an accommodative target, eg small picture, toward's the child's nose. Pupillary constriction and accommodation are associated.

Vestibular function can be tested, when necessary, by doll's head maneuver, caloric injection (with the head raised at a 30 degree angle while supine for testing horizontal movements), or by rotation, eg with an infant held upright with head tipped forward. The last two should produce nystagmus rather than just tonic deviation in the alert state. The direction of the nystagmus is indicated by the mnemonic *COWS* (cold opposite, warm same).

Bell's phenomenon, usually an upward divergent movement of both eyes on forced lid closure, may be tested. In some posterior-midcerebral hemisphere lesions there is deviation of the eyes to the opposite side instead.

Some supranuclear disorders involve specific control subsystems. In *congenital ocular motor apraxia* the child is unable to turn his eyes voluntarily to the side and substitutes head thrust past the object, the eyes swinging fully to the opposite side and achieving fixation in that position and holding it as the head slowly moves back so the eyes end up in the primary position. This disorder with its striking head thrusts in infancy generally subsides in the second decade to virtual normalcy.

With the Sylvian aqueduct syndrome, as in pine- aloma, there is loss of upgaze with convergence-retraction nystagmus replacing vertical saccades. There is often associated impaired pupillary response and occasionally lid retraction, or "sunsetting."

OCULAR MUSCLE IMBALANCE (STRABISMUS). In strabismus the eyes are improperly aligned. The corneal reflections of a fixation light are not centered in each pupil. In the ordinary nonparalytic, or concomitant type, the malalignment is present to the same degree in all directions of gaze.There is no diplopia due to ready suppression of one image in the young child. If strabismus is paralytic (eg due to *sixth nerve paresis*), it is more evident on gaze to the side of the paretic muscle. The deviation is greater when the paretic eye is fixing than when the normal eye is fixing. The older child would complain of diplopia. This would be greatest in the direction of action of the muscle involved and may prompt a head turn to minimize the deviation.

Duane's retraction syndrome may resemble sixth nerve paresis with limited abduction, but on adduction retraction of the globe results in narrowing of the palpebral fissure. This is generally due to congenitally aberrant innervation and not accompanied by diplopia. *Functional spasm of the near response* can also cause esotropia with complaint of diplopia and/or blurred vision. The hallmarks are the associated miosis, often induced myopia, and fluctuation in the degree of deviation.

With a *third nerve palsy* there is marked ptosis. The eye is deviated out unless the sixth nerve is also involved. There is limited adduction, elevation, and depression. The pupil may or may not be involved; if so it is mid-dilated and fixed, or at least sluggish, to light. If sluggish to light but not significantly dilated, one might consider a superimposed Horner's Syndrome. If the fourth nerve is intact, on attempt to look down there is intortion of the globe, readily seen by watching conjuctival blood vessels nasally. With an isolated *fourth nerve paresis* there is hyperdeviation of the involved eye with diplopia maximal on down gaze, especially down to the opposite side, with a tortional element as well. There is often tilt of the head toward the opposite shoulder in attempt to minimize this.

Proptosis is better appreciated from above than in front. An exophthalmometer is useful for measurement. A difference of 2 mm or less may be insignificant, due to normal asymmetry; and lax muscles, as in third nerve palsy, may also allow up to this amount of proptosis. A wider fissure may reflect proptosis, lid retraction, or orbicularis weakness (eg seventh nerve paresis). An early sign of the last is diminished blinking. Injection of

the globe can be observed and bruit listened for over gently closed lids, eg in carotid-cavernous fistula.

In analyzing malalignment of the eyes one must consider not only concomitant and paralytic strabismus, but also defect of the myoneural junction, the muscle itself, and mechanical factors in the orbit. The first of these, eg *myasthenia gravis*, often has associated ptosis which can be demonstrated to increase with fatigue on sustained upgaze. Occasionally lid quivering or twitch are elicited especially upon return from gaze down to the primary position. Anticholinesterase drugs would be expected to reverse the ptosis as well as to enhance ocular movement. In myasthenia gravis the ptosis and limitation of ocular motility are usually asymmetric. When symmetric, chronic progressive external ophthalmoplegia must be distinguished, as in the Kearns-Sayre syndrome.

The *traction test* is a valuable indicator of mechanical limitation. It is easily performed in the older child by instilling topical anesthetic and applying a cocainized swab to a rectus muscle insertion, which if necessary may be grasped with forceps; and, with the child looking in the desired direction, attempt is made to push the eye in the same direction. If this is not possible the traction test is positive for mechanical limitation, as in orbital fracture or congenital adherence syndrome. Such mechanical limitation may also occur in thyroid ophthalmopathy and inflammatory orbital pseudotumor. This latter spectrum of disorders also includes ocular myositis, where there may be painful and limited movement with injection and tenderness of involved muscles.

NYSTAGMUS Nystagmus is an involuntary rhythmic oscillation of the eyes, which is generally conjugate and of equal amplitude, although occasionally disconjugate as in the Sylvian aqueduct syndrome and occasionally dissociated in amplitude as in internuclear ophthalmoplegia. The amplitude may be fine or coarse and the velocity rapid or slow. The oscillations may be pendular or jerk.

Nystagmus of infancy is most commonly due either to congenital or early visual deprivation or to primary motor defect which is usually hereditary.

Sensory deprivation nystagmus is not present at birth but develops after several months in the absence of normally developing foveal function as in albinism. It is pendular, although appearing jerky to the side. When visual loss is severe, it may be quite coarse and irregular.

Congenital motor nystagmus is a jerk nystagmus to either side of a quite position or a pendular nystagmus which becomes jerky to the sides. It is present at birth although it may not be noted immediately. Because it is generally minimal in one position, which may be eccentric, a head turn is often adopted for a maximal acuity. There may be partially compensatory head oscillation on fixation effort. The nystagmus generally remains horizontal on upgaze and decreases on convergence.

Spasmus nutans is an entity consisting of a triad of nystagmus, head nodding and head tilting, any one or two of which may be present without the others. The nystagmus may be distinguished from congenital nystagmus on occasion only by its later onset (most commonly toward the end of the first year) and its resolution, usually by 3 or 4 years. In spasmus nutans the nystagmus is usually more rapid and usually asymmetric. It may appear monocular although fine nystagmus may often be appreciated in the other eye on ophthalmoscopy. Similar monocular nystagmus is occasionally due to unilateral refractive or strabismic amblyopia or optic nerve pathology.

Horizontal and vertical *gaze evoked* (first degree) *nystagmus* is usually due to sedative and anticonvulsant drugs. Otherwise it suggests posterior fossa pathology. It must be distinguished, sometimes with difficulty, from extreme end gaze physiologic nystagmus. The latter is often present horizontally although not vertically, decreases on returning a few degrees from the extremes of gaze, often appears to "fatigue" and may be greater in the abducting eye. If jerk nystagmus is present in the primary position (second degree) horizontally or if there is a rotary component one can usually assume that the vestibular system is involved.

Downbeating nystagmus in the primary position, often present in other positions as well and particularly marked on lateral gaze and down to the sides, is often indicative of cervicomedullary junction pathology, eg Arnold-Chiari malformation or platybasia. *Ocular bobbing* which occurs in the setting of total horizontal positive gaze palsy is easily distinguished. It is irregular and not rhythmic and the initial movement is downward with slow return.

Upbeating nystagmus in the primary position may indicate anterior cerebellar vermis involvement when coarse and increasing on upgaze, and medullary pathology when fine and increasing on downgaze.

Seesaw nystagmus is a vertically disconjugate form of nystagmus, wherein there is elevation with intortion of one eye and simultaneous depression with extortion of the other eye. It is often seen with bitemporal hemianopia, ie chiasmal lesions of varied etiology, but may be present on a congenital basis without such field defect.

Other ocular oscillations occur with cerebellar system disease, eg acute cerebellar ataxia, usually together with ocular dysmetria described earlier: *ocular flutter*, bursts of conjugate horizontal oscillation; *opsoclonus*, chaotic multidirectional conjugate saccades; *fixation instability*, eg small irregular "square wave jerks" away from and back to center.

PRENATAL AND DEVELOPMENTAL DEFECTS

BRAIN

WILLIAM DeMyer

Abnormal Head Size

Abnormal head size warns of an abnormal brain. A small head is termed *occupying most of the intracranial space,*

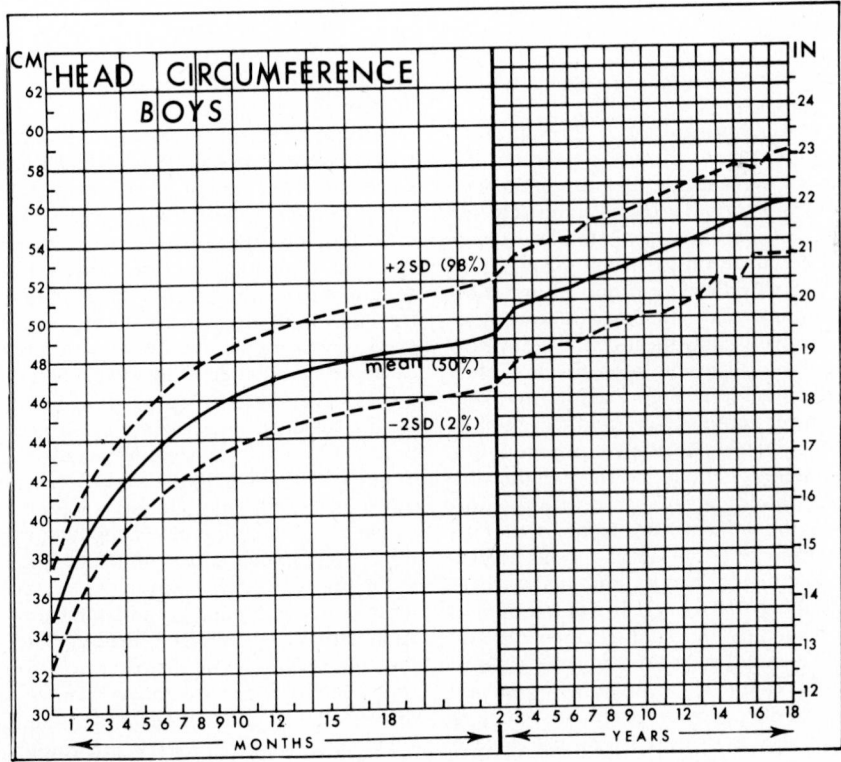

FIG. 5A. Graph of head circumference in boys from birth to 18 years of age. (From Nellhaus: Pediatrics 41:106, 1968.)

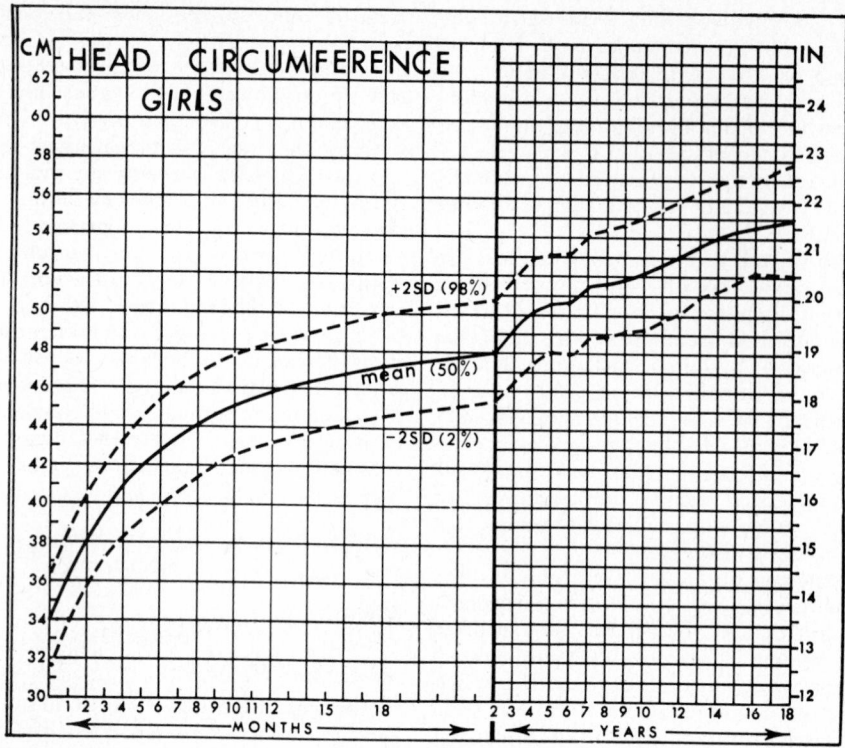

FIG. 5B. Graph of head circumference in girls from birth to 18 years of age. (From Nellaus: Pediatrics 41:106, 1968.)

or it may be huge and heavy, a condition termed *megalencephaly*.

Early recognition of abnormal head size requires accurate serial measurements of the occipitofrontal circumference (OFC) of every infant, beginning at birth (Fig. 5). Deviations from normal growth can be detected readily. A difference of more than two standard deviations (2 SD) from the mean raises strong suspicion of a brain disorder, while a difference of more than 3 SD clearly indicates an abnormal brain. Since microcephaly and megalocephaly involve statistical concepts of normality, head circumference may deviate 2 SD or slightly more in some normal children. Before assuming that a boderline measurement implies an abnormal brain, one should evaluate other factors. Relationships among the child's head circumference, body weight, height, and chest circumference should be compared with the normal limits, as should the same measurements of parents and siblings. A neurologic examination should be performed and a developmental history obtained.

Once microcephaly or macrocephaly has been identified, the forms of therapy and family counseling and the prognosis will depend on diagnosing the type of cerebral lesion and its cause. The history, pedigree, and physical examination may provide diagnostic clues to heredofamilial disorders or distinct malformation syndromes. If the child has a peculiar facies, it is useful to consult an atlas of malformation syndromes, such as those compiled by Holmes and associates, by Bergsma, and by Smith. The head should be transilluminated in

all infants (p. 1741). Focal lesions such as encephaloceles, porencephaly, subdural fluid accumulations, or atrophic lesions of the cerebral wall may show restricted transillumination. With extreme thinning or destruction of the cerebrum, as in hydranencephaly, the whole cranium will light up. Every infant with an abnormal OFC should have skull radiographs and usually an electroencephalogram. Chromosome studies, nuclear sexing, and dermatoglyphic prints are useful if the patient has multiple somatic anomalies or if an intersex syndrome is suspected. If a degenerative, biochemical, or heredofamilial disorder is suspected, blood chemistry, urine, and cerebrospinal fluid should be examined. In the absence of evidence of increased intracranial pressure, which may require ventriculography, or evidence of subdural fluid accumulations, which may require subdural tap, lumbar puncture should be considered. If a pneumoencephalogram is indicated, the cerebrospinal fluid examination should be deferred, since previous lumbar puncture may permit subdural leakage of cerebrospinal fluid and cause collapse of the subarachnoid space, thus making introduction of air difficult. Exact definition of an anatomic brain lesion frequently requires specialized neuroradiologic procedures, such as radioisotope brain scanning, computerized axial tomography, pneumoencephalography, ventriculography, and angiography (p. 1742).

MICROCEPHALY. Aside from the situation in craniosynostosis, microcephaly is always secondary to microncephaly. A severe degree of microcephaly implies a prenatal, perinatal, or early postnatal lesion. Almost any noxious agent can limit the brain size of the developing embryo or fetus. In experimental animals microcephaly may result from many teratogens, such as vitamin deficiency or excess, drugs, or irradiation. In man common causes of reduced brain size include maternal illnesses and infections, malnutrition, drug ingestion, chromosomal errors and hereditary factors, and disorders of implantation and placentation. Thus microcephaly itself provides no clue as to its cause. The mother should be questioned about the pregnancy and delivery; a history of infertility or pregnancy wastage is common, and sometimes the pedigree discloses a distinct mendelian pattern.

In some microcephalics the brain, although small, has a fairly normal internal and external configuration. Others may have malformations or destructive lesions with symmetrically or asymmetrically dilated ventricles. Mi-

crocephalics are usually mentally defective and may have cerebral palsy and seizures. In many instances the combination of microcephaly with other clinical or laboratory findings permits a specific etiologic diagnosis.

MEGALOCEPHALY. The most common cause of megalocephaly is increased intracranial pressure with hydrocephalus. The cerebral wall thins as the head enlarges and brain weight, exclusive of intraventricular fluid, is normal or reduced. A rarer cause of megalocephaly is megalencephaly, an abnormally large and heavy brain. Megalencephaly may be a primary malformation with huge gyri, either of simple pattern or with polymicrogyria. It may be sporadic or may be associated with neurofibromatosis, tuberous sclerosis, myelomeningocele (Chiari malformation), or achondroplasia. The brain is large in pituitary gigantism, but not in acromegaly; it is also large in the syndrome of cerebral

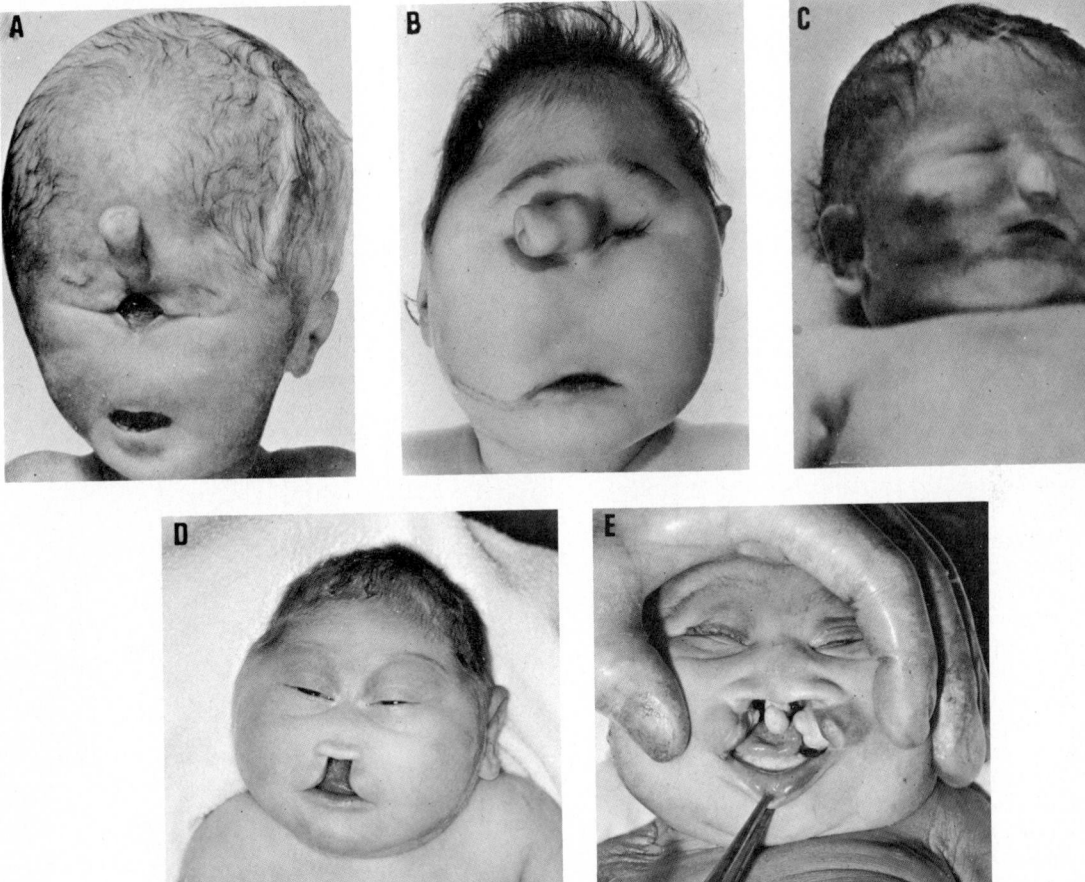

FIG. 6. Diagnostic facies of holoprosencephaly. A. Cyclopia. Notice the proboscis attached above the orbit. (From Potter: Pathology of the Fetus and Newborn . Courtesy of Year Book Medical Publishers.) B. Ethmocephaly. (Courtesy of Dr. P. Fluery.) The proboscis has migrated down between the orbits, which are separated but show hypotelorism, as do C, D, and E. C. Cebocephaly. The proboscis has migrated to the normal location for the nose. The single nostril leads into a cul-de-sac. D. With median cleft lip. Rudimentary nares and a nasal cavity are present. The nasal septum is lacking. *E.* With hypoplastic intermaxillary segment (philtrum-premaxillary anlage). A rudimentary nasal septum is present.

gigantism, in which no endocrine defects have been identified. Patients with primary megalencephaly are often mentally deficient and may have motor deficits and seizures. Secondary megalencephaly is due to accumulation of abnormal metabolic products and includes the infantile form of amaurotic idiocy, gargoylism, spongy degeneration of the white matter, and some of the leukodystrophies such as metachromatic leukodystrophy and Krabbe's disease. A large brain from cerebral edema or from neoplasms is not considered as megalencephaly.

In hydrocephalus with increased pressure the head enlarges rapidly, the fontanelles bulge, the sutures split, and there may be papilledema. These features usually are absent in primary megalencephaly, but may occur in secondary megalencephaly. If the megalocephalic patient has no evidence of increased pressure or neurologic deficits, the OFC of siblings and parents should be measured. If other family members have enlarged heads without neurologic deficits, the condition is benign familial megalencephaly, and further diagnostic procedures are not necessary. If it is not familial, further investigation is indicated. Studies should include skull radiography, electroencephalography, subdural taps, computerized axial tomography, air contrast studies, and in some cases cerebral arteriography.

Median Facial Defects and Holoprosencephaly

The holoprosencephalies (arhinencephaly) are a teratologic series of defects of graded severity characterized by median malformations of the face and brain (Fig. 6). They are due to total or partial failure of the prosencephalon to undergo median cleavage into cerebral hemispheres or to form lobes. This holistic prosencephalon or holoprosencephalon has a single-chambered ventricle and usually lacks olfactory bulbs and tracts. Median facial anomalies consist of orbital hypotelorism in combination with a flat nose or proboscis and oral deformities, such as a median cleft of the lip and palate. Some of these patients have trigonocephaly (sharply pointed, keel-shaped forehead), and almost all are microcephalic. The crista galli, ethmoid, vomer, nasal, and premaxillary bones are absent or hypoplastic. The unity of the median faciocerebral defects is explained by the role of prechordal mesoderm, which normally gives rise to the median facial bones; prechordal mesoderm is absent or hypoplastic in holoprosencephaly. Furthermore, by embryonic induction this mesoderm determines not only the differentiation of the ectoderm as neural tissue but also its morphogenesis into lobated hemispheres.

According to the pattern and the severity of median facial anomalies, at least five types of facies can be recognized that are pathognomonic and predict the malformed brain. These are shown in Figure 6 arranged in order of decreasing severity. At the less severe end of the spectrum, where absence of the olfactory bulbs and tracts is the only brain abnormality, the face may have no obvious median defects; some of these subjects are eunuchoids. The clinical diagnosis can be made from the pathognomonic facies, which are strikingly similar in all patients. Orbital hypotelorism, as measured on posteroanterior skull radiographs, is essential for diagnosis, but one or more of the other median facial defects must be present to distinguish the hypotelorism of holoprosencephaly from other conditions with microcrania. In categories A through D the brain volume is often much smaller than the intracranial space, thus permitting transillumination of the head. The electroencephalogram records little or no electrical activity over the areas of transillumination, but elsewhere shows repetitive seizure discharges.

The cause of holoprosencephaly is unknown; most reported cases are regarded as sporadic, but familial cases occur. Some have 13–15 trisomy and often have multiple extracephalic malformations such as polydactyly. Others, with 46 chromosomes, have few or no extracephalic anomalies. The face predicts the malformed brain irrespective of karyotype or extracephalic anomalies.

Median Cleft Face Syndrome

The stereotyped, stylized facies of holoprosencephaly should not be confused with another pattern of median facial defects: the median cleft face syndrome, which consists of frontal meningoencephalocele, orbital hypertelorism, bifid nose, and median cleft of the lip (Fig. 7). In spite of the grotesque facies, these patients

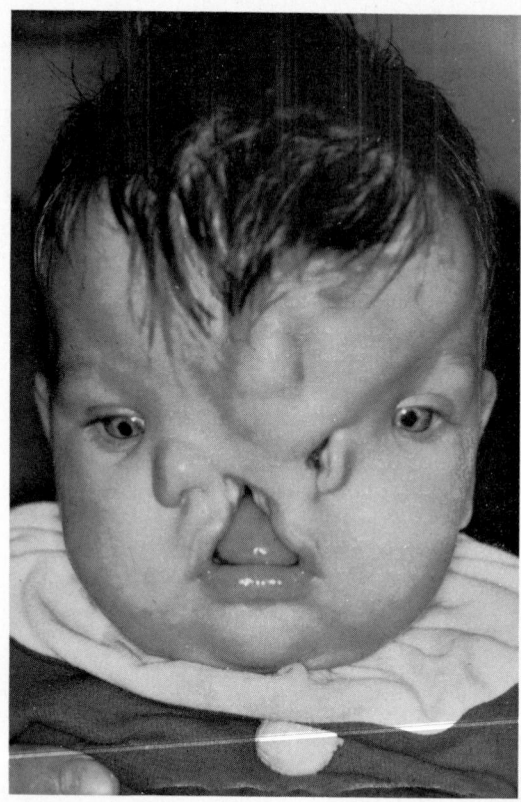

FIG. 7. Typical facies of median cleft face syndrome, consisting of median cleft lip, bifid nose, hypertelorism, and frontal encephalocele.

often are mentally normal or only mildly retarded. These patients also can be arranged into a teratologic series of defects of graded severity, the least severe of which is a simple median notch in the nose or upper lip.

Hydranencephaly

Hydranencephaly is a congenital malformation in which the cerebral hemispheres either are missing or have huge, complete symmetric defects in the cerebral wall because of intrauterine destruction, malformation, or possibly severe increased intracranial pressure during fetal life. The skull and scalp are well formed, thus distinguishing hydranencephaly from anencephaly, encephaloceles, and other dysraphic lesions. Most cases are sporadic.

In contrast to the situation with holoprosencephaly, most patients have no facial or extracephalic malformations. Thus the disorder may not be suspected until the infant fails to show psychomotor progress, has seizures, or manifests spastic quadriplegia; most patients die in infancy, but some survive several years. The head may be small or normal, and in some instances it may enlarge rapidly. In young infants the head always transilluminates brightly. An air bubble placed through the anterior fontanelle can be traced around the inner table of the skull on radiographs. Arteriograms show attenuated vessels. In hydranencephaly the electroencephalogram shows little or no electrical activity, except over local remnants of cortex. In hydrocephalus with preserved cortex, where the head transilluminates brightly because of the extremely thin cerebral wall, the electroencephalogram shows generalized activity.

Agenesis of Corpus Callosum

The corpus callosum is a large bundle of nerve fibers that connect the cortex of one cerebral hemisphere with the other. It is formed as the axons from cortical neurons of each cerebral hemisphere reach the midline, decussate, and grow to the opposite cerebral cortex. There the fibers synapse with the cortical areas that are mirror images of their own areas of origin. As these fibers accumulate at the midline they form the corpus callosum. Agenesis or hypoplasia of the corpus callosum occurs if the fibers fail to grow out, are destroyed, or are prevented from crossing. When the fibers reach the midline and fail to decussate, they pile up along the ventricular wall.

Although experimental studies have shown that the corpus callosum normally mediates interhemispheric transfer of information (and also may mediate interhemispheric propagation of some seizure discharges), there is no characteristic neurologic deficit or bedside test for agenesis. The diagnosis can be made only by radiologic contrast procedures. If simple nondecussation of the corpus callosum fibers is the sole brain lesion, the individual may lead a relatively normal life. More commonly agenesis of the corpus callosum is associated with other malformations, such as heterotopias, holoprosencephaly, or destructive lesions; the neurologic deficits reflect these associated brain lesions.

Most cases of agenesis of the corpus callosum are discovered incidentally when air contrast procedures are performed to elucidate a neurologic problem such as mental deficiency, epilepsy, or cerebral palsy. In the pure cases of agenesis of the corpus callosum the ventricular shadows in posteroanterior pneumoencephalograms have a pathognomonic bat-wing outline. In other cases of agenesis or hypoplasia of the corpus callosum a single cerebral ventricle may be present.

HYDROCEPHALUS

JOSEPH RANSOHOFF AND FRED EPSTEIN

Hydrocephalus is a pathologic condition characterized by an increased volume of cerebrospinal fluid (CSF) that either is or has been under increased pressure. Almost without exception the fluid accumulates in the ventricular system as a result of distal obstruction to normal CSF circulation. When the condition develops prior to fusion of the cranial sutures, it produces enlargement of the head, which may reach extreme proportions. Hydrocephalus attracted the attention of the early physicians, and it was well described by Hippocrates. Although modern theories are based largely on the classic studies of Dandy and Blackfan, concepts concerning the physiology of CSF have undergone considerable modification.

CSF CIRCULATION. Anatomically the CSF pathways can be divided into the ventricular system and the subarachnoid spaces. The paired lateral ventricles lie within each cerebral hemisphere and connect via the foramina of Monro to the midline third ventricle; this in turn connects via the aqueduct of Sylvius with the midline fourth ventricle of the posterior fossa. Along the floor of each lateral ventricle, in the roof of the third ventricle, and in the roof and lateral recesses of the fourth ventricle lies an outpouching of highly vascularized pia mater with a modified ependymal covering called the choroid plexus. The subarachnoid space lies between the arachnoid membrane, which follows the inner surface of dura mater, and the pial membrane, which hugs the contour of the brain and spinal cord surfaces. In certain areas, especially at the base of the brain, the subarachnoid space is enlarged into lakes or cisterns (cisterna magna, basalis, chiasmatis). The ventricular system connects with the subarachnoid spaces via the medial foramen of Magendie at the outlet of the fourth ventricle and the lateral foramina of Luschka. Along the large venous sinuses in the dura, outpouchings of arachnoid villi form a unidirectional valvular system composed of a labyrinth of small tubules that establish open connections between the subarachnoid spaces and the venous channels.

It is generally accepted that CSF is formed mainly within the ventricular system, approximately 60 percent from the choroid plexus and 40 percent from the brain. The active transport of fluid from the blood to the CSF compartment is primarily a function of the choroid plexus. The forces required for this secretory bulk flow are not completely understood, but they probably involve an energy-dependent solute pump with an osmotically coupled solvent (or water) flow.

In an overall sense the circulation of CSF is a unidirectional flow from the ventricular system to the posterior fossa foramina and into the cisterns and subarachnoid spaces. A significant percentage of the fluid is reabsorbed into the bloodstream via the arachnoid villi in the venous sinuses. The generating force for this flow is in part derived from the arterial pulsation of the choroid plexuses and perhaps that of other large arteries at the base of the brain. In addition, absorption is probably also dependent on the CSF pressure being greater than the intracranial venous pressure.

PATHOGENESIS. There are three possible mechanisms for the development of hydrocephalus: (1) obstruction of the CSF pathways within the ventricular system (eg, foramen of Monro or aqueduct of Sylvius) or in the subarachnoid pathways (eg, tentorial incisura) with secondary dilation of the channels proximal to the site of obstruction; (2) defective absorption of CSF through the arachnoid villi; (3) choroid plexus tumors that rarely may result in overproduction of CSF with secondary dilatation of the ventricular system and all the subarachnoid pathways. Various types of hydrocephalus have been described, such as communicating, noncommunicating, obstructive, and nonobstructive. With rare exception all neonatal hydrocephalus is obstructive. The term noncommunicating hydrocephalus implies that the obstruction is in a strategic location and can thus prevent egress of spinal fluid from the ventricular system, eg, aqueductal stenosis. Communicating hydrocephalus implies that the spinal fluid escapes from the ventricles but that the extracerebral pathways along the basal cisterns are not patent, in which case the obstruction is extraventricular. Perhaps it would be preferable to discard all of these older terms in favor of more accurate descriptions of the site and nature of obstruction, such as intraventricular or extraventricular.

ETIOLOGY. The three major causes of hydrocephalus are neoplasms, congenital malformations, and post-traumatic or postinflammatory lesions. Neoplasms are seldom encountered in the neonatal period, but they may develop at any time thereafter. The most common neoplasms of infancy and childhood that produce hydrocephalus are gliomas located in the third ventricle, in the periaqueductal region, or in the fourth ventricle and the cerebellum.

Developmental anomalies that produce hydrocephalus include spina bifida with meningomyelocele, which often is associated with the Arnold-Chiari type II hindbrain malformation. In this malformation there is elongation of the lower brainstem and caudal displacement of the fourth ventricle into the upper cervical canal. At the inferior tip of the fourth ventricle there is a small knuckle of medulla, which suggests a buckling effect at this site. This impaction of the posterior fossa structures down through the foramen magnum with associated adhesive arachnoidal thickening and subsequent blockage of the CSF pathways may finally result in ventricular dilatation. Stenosis of the aqueduct of Sylvius or forking of the aqueduct often produces early severe hydrocephalus. It may be congenital, but it can also appear secondary to progressive periaqueductal gliosis, with symptoms and signs occurring at any age during childhood or even in adults. Overgrowth of fibrillary subependymal neuroglia may constrict or even occlude what apparently was once a normal aqueduct. Congenital septa or membranes occluding the outlets of the fourth ventricle (Dandy-Walker syndrome) have occasionally been described. A huge cyst may develop in the posterior fossa displacing the cerebellar hemispheres to either side, resulting in dysgenesis of the cerebellar vermis and associated elevation of the tentorium.

Probably the most frequent cause of hydrocephalus is postinflammatory or post-traumatic obstruction of the basilar cisterns and associated subarachnoid pathways, particularly in the region of the tentorium. There may be intracranial bleeding at the time of birth or meningitis in the perinatal or neonatal period that may go unrecognized. These may lead to progressive fibrosis of the arachnoidal pathways at the base of the brain, eventually resulting in obliteration of the extraventricular circulation and absorption of CSF. Cysticercosis, toxoplasmosis, and other parasitic infections occasionally may produce ventricular or subarachnoid obstruction.

These obstructions produce secondary changes in the brain. Pressure from the distended ventricles leads to progressive thinning of the brain, with the white matter suffering greater loss or demyelinization than the gray. The layer of brain surrounding the ventricles, or the cortical mantle, is sometimes no more than 5 to 6 mm thick, and the ependyma of the ventricle and the pia may actually be in contact. Marked ventricular dilation may result in rupture of the septum pellucidum. When very extensive ventricular enlargement is present, the brain resembles a large sac, and at times there may be areas of cortical rupture into the subarachnoid space that form external CSF fistulas. Attenuation of the dural venous sinuses, as well as atrophy of the choroid plexuses, has been seen in these extensive lesions. In less severe cases there is only flattening of the convolutions, and atrophic changes in ganglion cells may be observed microscopically. With this degree of enlargement of the head the bones are often thinned, the fontanelles are enlarged, and the suture margins are widely separated.

CLINICAL MANIFESTATIONS. In many cases of congenital hydrocephalus the infant dies in utero; in other cases the process may be so far advanced before birth that cesarean section may be necessary before delivery is possible. In the majority of cases nothing unusual may be observed at birth, or the head may be only slightly larger than normal. In the early weeks of life it may be discovered that the head is increasing in size at an abnormal rate and the fontanelles are enlarging. The eyes may assume a staring expression, with sclera visible above the cornea (sunset sign), and the infant may have difficulty in holding up his head. Scalp veins may be prominent, and the forehead may appear to overhang the eyes. There is disproportion between the large size of the cranial vault and the normal size of the face. As a rule the capacity of the head to expand with increased intracranial pressure protects the eyes. Although the orbits may be shallow and the globes depressed in relation to the slits, vision usually remains unimpaired, and the eyegrounds fail to show evidence of papilledema. In severe chronic cases optic atrophy may be found. Neurologic examination may show no abnormalities except for delayed ability to hold up the head and other developmental limitations that can be explained entirely by the abnormal weight of the cranium. In some children spasticity may be observed, while others may show ataxic phenomena. In the child with decompensating hydrocephalus, signs of increased intracranial pressure may be observed, with vomiting, lethargy, and failure to gain weight.

DIAGNOSIS. In the classic case of far-advanced hydrocephalus characterized by large head, distended scalp veins, downward deviation of the eyes, and retarded motor milestones there is no need for reference to charts of head circumference or other aids, for the diagnosis is obvious. However, in cases not so far advanced the diagnosis may be more difficult to establish. Although comparison of the head size (occipitofrontal circumference) with the normal range is of value, repeated careful observations of the rate of head growth are of paramount importance. Regular measurements of the anterior fontanelle are useful, since active hydrocephalus does not occur in conjunction with a closing fontanelle. If the fontanelle is enlarging from month to month, additional investigations are warranted. Roentgenograms of the skull will confirm the disproportion between the facial bones and the enlarged vault

and may show thinning of the bone and widening of the cranial sutures.

Careful transillumination of the head in a darkened room may disclose the presence of porencephalic cysts, hydranencephaly, or elevation of the tentorium secondary to a posterior fossa cyst (Dandy-Walker syndrome). A large subdural effusion as a cause of an enlarging head must always be considered; it can be ruled out by careful subdural taps. Papilledema suggests a neoplastic cause for the hydrocephalus. Macrocephaly may result from conditions other than hydrocephalus.

The conclusive diagnosis of hydrocephalus may be made by ventriculography, pneumoencephalography, and computerized axial tomography. For ventriculography a variable amount of air is injected into one ventricle; it distributes itself throughout the ventricular system. Subsequent roentgenograms disclose whether the ventricles are enlarged, whether communication exists between the ventricular system and the subarachnoid spaces, the thickness of the cortical mantle, and the precise location of the obstructing lesion (Fig. 8). Occasionally a pneumoencephalogram is performed in which air is injected via the lumbar route to more accurately outline the fourth ventricle and cisterns of the posterior fossa. Recently computerized axial tomography has been utilized in diagnosing hydrocephalus; this noninvasive technique provides an excellent picture of the entire ventricular system. In addition, the etiology of the hydrocephalus may often be inferred with accuracy (Fig. 9). Since the advent of computerized axial tomography, the need for air contrast studies has diminished.

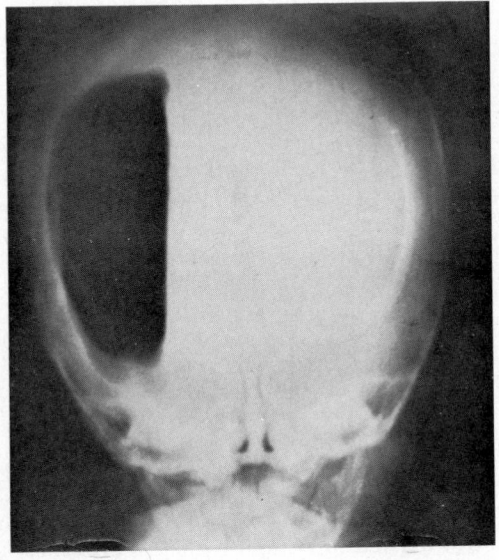
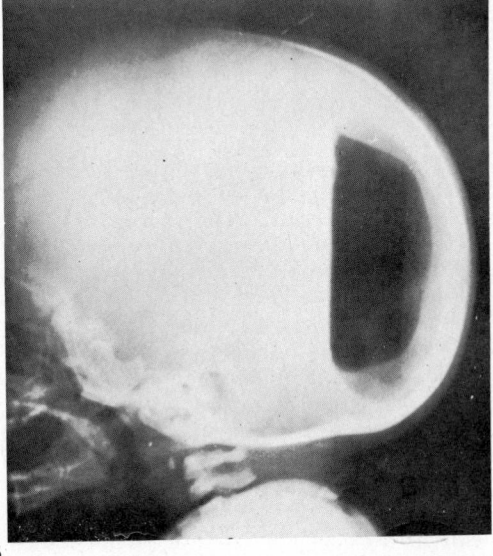

A   **B**

FIG. 8.   Bubble ventriculogram demonstrating advanced hydrocephalus. *A.* Anteroposterior view with left side of head down, showing fluid level in dilated right ventricle. *B.* Lateral view with brow down, showing posterior extent of lateral ventricles.

TREATMENT. Evaluation of any medical or surgical therapy must be made against the background of the rate of spontaneous arrest and the physical and mental states of the survivors. Although some cases of hydrocephalus do arrest spontaneously, with active and progressive hydrocephalus surgery offers a better prognosis for survival and intellectual development. Therapeutic success depends on careful individualized treatment of each infant.

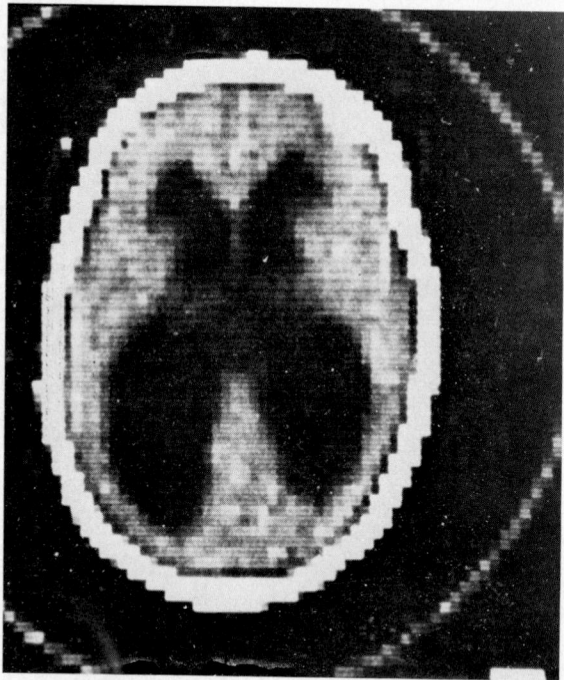

FIG. 9. Computerized axial tomography showing severe hydrocephalus.

In 1918 Dandy devised an operation to attempt to reduce total volume of spinal fluid produced by partially removing the choroid plexus. This procedure is now rarely performed because the morbidity and mortality are considerable and the long-term results are no better than with shunting procedures.

With the development of inert plastics that are well tolerated by the body, shunting procedures have achieved great popularity. While no single shunt is invariably successful or applicable to all patients, satisfactory results are frequently obtained. The so-called universal shunting procedures drain the lateral ventricles and are applicable to all types of hydrocephalus; draining the lumbar subarachnoid space is helpful only when the ventricles communicate with the spinal subarachnoid space.

As early as 1908 attempts were made to channel CSF into the great veins and into the heart. Development of competent silicone valves allowing unidirectional flow finally led to a successful bypass from the cerebral ventricle into the right atrium via the jugular vein. The valve is placed either along the course of the tube system or in the cardiac end. Experience has shown that in order to avoid thrombosis the vascular end of the shunt must lie freely in a large moving pool of blood. Therefore in this type of shunt periodic visualization of the cardiac end of the tubing in the growing infant must be carried out to prevent retraction of the shunt from the right atrium and thrombosis of the jugular vein. It may be wise to carry out elective revision in hope of maintaining function rather than to wait for signs of active hydrocephalus and then attempt revision. This type of shunt mechanism is not without complications, the most frequent being infection, particularly with *Staphylococcus albus.* Frequently there is no evidence of infection in any other part of the body. However, children with chronic *Staphylococcus albus* infection may have hepatosplenomegaly and anemia. A low-grade fever is also not uncommon. Despite all methods of parenteral antibiotic therapy, including intrathecal injection, the bacteremia can almost never be cleared unless the entire shunt is removed and replaced with a new sterile shunt mechanism.

Pulmonary hypertension may also be encountered; it is believed that microemboli arising from the right atrium embolize to the lungs and occlude the small pulmonary arteries, resulting in this diffuse pulmonary vascular obstructive disease. This may progress to right heart failure. If the silastic tubing breaks off into the vascular pathways, the fragments may lodge in the heart in trabeculae of the right ventricle, or pass into the parenchyma of the lung. The silastic tubing may also become disconnected and migrate into the cerebral ventricle. This is not a serious complication, and the lost tubing can remain in the ventricle without producing any neurologic deficit.

If a kidney is sacrificed the ureter can be used to accept a plastic or silicone rubber tube to drain the CSF from the ventricle or subarachnoid space, the CSF then being excreted with the urine. As the body loses the CSF, salt depletion may become a problem, and urinary infection may lead to secondary meningitis. CSF has been shunted into the peritoneal and pleural cavities; they are sterile areas from which the fluid can be absorbed into the general circulation. Difficulties have arisen from occlusion of the tubing due to pleural or omental reaction or due to the inability of the cavity to absorb the fluid as rapidly as it accumulates. However, these procedures have been employed successfully in many patients.

As a rule, a child who has an open myelomeningocele at birth and associated hydrocephalus is not shunted primarily into the vascular system, in spite of negative cultures from his ventricular fluid. A peritoneal shunt is first employed; if necessary, this can be converted later in life to a vascular or pleural shunt. Thus many different procedures are currently utilized in the treatment of hydrocephalus. The choice of operation depends on the site of obstruction to the flow of CSF as well as on the experience of the group undertaking therapy. No operation is foolproof, and all require meticulous follow-up care for the life of the child.

LOW-PRESSURE HYDROCEPHALUS. In the past decade numerous reports have appeared defining a syndrome of occult or low-pressure hydrocephalus. The characteristic picture occurs in adults, and the findings are disabling dementia with psychomotor retardation, often associated with ataxia and incontinence. This syndrome is rarely observed in children and is most frequently encountered as a complication of posterior fossa surgery. These chronically symptomatic patients are reported to have a normal CSF pressure (180 mm H_2O or less). Pneumoencephalography reveals a communicating type of hydrocephalus without air being found over the convexities of the brain. RISA cisternography also confirms the diagnosis of an incisural block and probably is even more accurate in establishing the correct diagnosis. The underlying mechanism may be trauma, subarachnoid hemorrhage, or arachnoiditis secondary to infection. Shunting procedures utilizing low-pressure valves have often resulted in remarkable restoration of neurologic functions. The best results have been in patients in whom an episode of subarachnoid bleeding has occurred, with secondary fibrosis of the subarachnoid space resulting in hydrocephalus.

Choroid Plexus Papilloma

Choroid plexus papilloma has been found in the newborn, but it occurs most frequently in the first 2 years of life. This rare tumor arises most commonly in the lateral ventricle, rarely in the third ventricle, and occasionally in the fourth ventricle, with extension into the cerebellar-pontine angle. Its clinical course is insidious, but may be sudden in onset, with intraventricular hemorrhage or with associated sudden increase in intracranial pressure due to obstruction of one of the intraventricular foramina. The intraventricular location of this tumor results in the overproduction of CSF, with subsequent enlargement of the ventricular system as well as the subarachnoid pathways.

The tumor is histologically benign, with a characteristic papillary architecture, its stroma being composed of vascularized connective tissue; it must be distinguished from the papillary ependymoma that also presents as an intraventricular tumor but whose stroma is mainly composed of fibrillary neuroglia. It is rarely malignant but will invade local neural structures, losing the normal papillary architecture and showing obvious mitosis. The diagnosis is made from the clinical picture as well as by careful complete ventriculography in which all aspects of the ventricular system are well seen. When the benign tumor is totally removed, the prognosis is excellent and the hydrocephalic condition arrested.

CLOSURE DEFECTS OF NEURAL PLATE

KENNETH SHULMAN AND KENNETH SHAPIRO

Developmental defects of the central nervous system arise from embryologic derangements of migration, diverticulation, vascular development, and midline closure. The entities presented in this section have in common a defect in midline closure of the neural tube. Varying locations and expressions of this defect, plus other associated anomalies, produce the different clinical entities described below.

Embryologically the central nervous system develops from a thickening of ectoderm referred to as the neural plate. With proliferation of cells, the neural plate invaginates to form the neural groove. Closure of this groove in the midline produces the neural tube. This midline fusion begins in the mid-dorsal region and then extends toward the anterior and posterior neuropores. Fusion is delayed at the neuropores, so that the neural tube communicates with the amniotic cavity until the end of the fourth week, when neural tube closure is complete. Segmentation of the neural tube is accompanied by separation of the surrounding mesoderm into somites. The mesoderm comes to lie completely around the neural ectoderm and separates it from the ectoderm that becomes the skin. The mesodermal segments give rise to the skull and vertebral column, as well as the meninges and blood vessels of the brain and spinal cord. Defects in midline closure give rise to cranium bifidum when confined to the region of the anterior neuropore; spina bifida may follow from defective closure at any level.

Cranial Anomalies

ANENCEPHALY. The incidence of this catastrophic malformation ranges from 0.1 to 6.7 per 1,000 births, making it the most common central nervous system malformation incompatible with life. Epidemiology varies from area to area, with the highest prevalence rates occurring in the British Isles and low rates occurring in Africa, Asia, and South America. Anencephaly is six times more common in whites than in blacks. The incidence is three to seven times higher in female fetuses and prematures. The concordance rate in twins is low, with the incidence in identical twins approaching that in fraternal twins. The mother often has hydramnios, and the diagnosis of anencephaly can be made prepartum by radiography of the abdomen. Usually the fetus is either stillborn or dies a few minutes after birth; rarely a fetus may survive a few days.

The pathology ranges from complete absence of the central nervous system (with open cranium and vertebral canal and all bones of the skull vault and vertebral lamina being unfused) to the less severe defect known as hemicrania, in which the bones of the posterior skull vault and the brainstem and cerebellum are present. The brain remnant is pervaded with a highly vascularized stroma and covered with a thin membrane, continuous with hair-bearing skin. Choroid plexus and ependyma are usually found in the brain remnant. With poor development of the central nervous tissue the posterior lobe of the pituitary and the hypothalamus are also absent, as are the ganglion cells of the retina. The anterior pituitary is usually normal, and the thyroid, although often deficient in cells, is usually of a mature character. Adrenal atrophy is usually seen and is explained by absence of trophic hormones in the defective hypothalamus. Other abnormalities commonly found with anencephaly are poorly lobated lungs, a large thymus, and a high arched palate. Spina bifida accompanies anencephaly in 9 to 30 percent of cases reported.

Pathogenetic theories focus on several mechanisms. Some authors believe that anencephaly results from nonclosure of the neural tube; others invoke a reopening of the previously closed neural tube or damage to the prosencephalon and its overlying mesoderm and ectoderm. That the brain vesicles may develop and undergo secondary infarction due to an insufficient blood supply during the third to fifth week of fetal life is suggested by Vogel's finding that the major arteries do not penetrate the areas of the cerebral malformation, but rather are replaced by a number of abnormal branches arising from the internal carotid arteries. Alternatively, this vascular anomaly may be secondary to abnormal brain development. Experimentally it has been found that teratogenic agents must be applied early (shortly after gastrulation) to cause anencephaly in the mouse. The cephalic end of the neuropore remains open, but the cerebral hemispheres and striatum develop and then necrose before histogenesis of the cortex has occurred.

Management of anencephaly necessitates early detection so that pregnancy can be interrupted. Pregnancies at risk include those occurring in mothers with one or more children with neural tube defects, those complicated by hydramniotic abdomen, and those with low estriol excretion. Since the normal fetal adrenal system plays a major role in estrogen metabolism during pregnancy, one should suspect the adrenal atrophy that is associated with anencephaly when confronted with low estriol excretion in a pregnancy with a living fetus. Various other modalities have been employed to confirm the suspicion of the anencephalic fetus (p. 126). Ultrasonic investigation has enjoyed success in carefully selected cases. Amniocentesis with assay for elevated levels of amniotic α-fetoprotein has identified fetuses with neural tube defects, thus permitting safe termination of pregnancy. In pregnancies not terminated iatrogenically, the anencephalic fetus is usually born prematurely and presents no obstetric difficulty. Neurosurgical treatment, of course, is not indicated.

CRANIUM BIFIDUM AND ENCEPHALOCELE. The term encephalocele has found wide neurosurgical usage to describe all cystic masses associated with midline cranial closure defects (cranium bifidum); the term encompasses cranial meningocele and cranial meningoencephalocele. Whether brain is present within a cystic enlargement is not apparent before surgery, and more precise terminology is therefore not necessary. The occult form of closure defect, which is rare and is not of major surgical interest, could be termed cranium bifidum occulta. In the authors' series of cases referred for neurosurgical care, encephaloceles have occurred at one-tenth the frequency of spina bifida cystica. The incidence of encephalocele has been estimated at 1 in 3,000 to 10,000 live births. Occurring with greatest frequency in the occipital regions of the skull, the encephalocele is in the midline or slightly removed to one side. Those found at the anterior extreme of the skull present as nasal, nasopharyngeal, or naso-orbital masses.

Occipital encephaloceles vary in size from small pedunculated masses to those equal in size to the cranial cavity. The base is usually small and well covered with hairless skin. Those lesions with wider bases are more apt to contain brain tissue, and in the posterior encephalocele there is a correlation between the amount of brain tissue within the sac and the associated anomalies of the residual brain in the cranial cavity. The most frequently associated secondary condition is hydrocephalus. Thus with a sizable occipital encephalocele one may perform a bubble ventriculogram either prior to encephalocele repair or after encephalocele repair and before discharge to assess the CSF pathways (Fig. 10). However, no exact relationship exists between the size of the encephalocele and its contents. In some cases skin may cover the entire sac; in other cases exposed brain or dura may occur at the tip of the lesion, making repair of the encephalocele an urgent matter. Transillumination with a high-intensity light is often useful in showing the contents of the sac. Skull roentgenograms will show the bone defect and its relation to cranial sutures and major intracranial venous sinuses.

Surgical repair of most posterior encephaloceles is indicated in the newborn period to close over any communication through a skin defect with brain and meninges, to remove the mass so that the child can be handled by nurses and the mother, to replace the contents into more normal surroundings, and to prevent secondary skin breakdown over large encephaloceles that might lead to infection and death. Surgery is well tolerated in the face-down position if care is taken to maintain the infant's temperature and to replace blood judiciously during the procedure.

Two factors appear to have the most prognostic significance. The presence of recognizable brain tissue in the sac enables one to predict either that the child will not survive or that survival will be complicated by severe mental retardation with significant neurologic deficits such as blindness (occipital cortex) and incoordination (cerebellum). The long-range care and prognosis will also depend heavily upon success or failure in effectively managing hydrocephalus.

Anterior encephaloceles are uncommon, except in Mon-

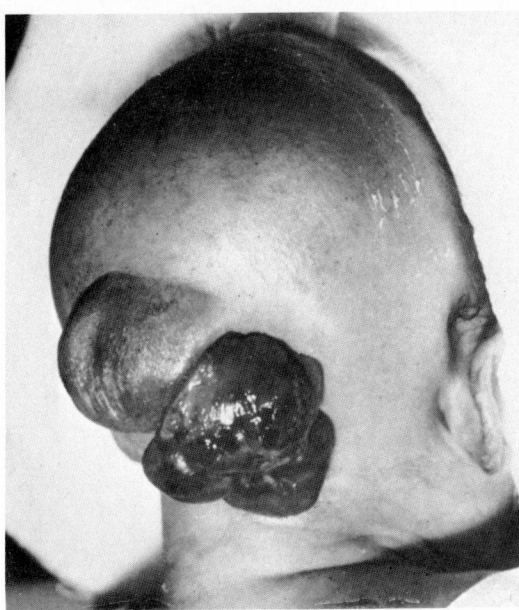

FIG. 10. Newborn showing poorly covered encephalocele containing brain tissue.

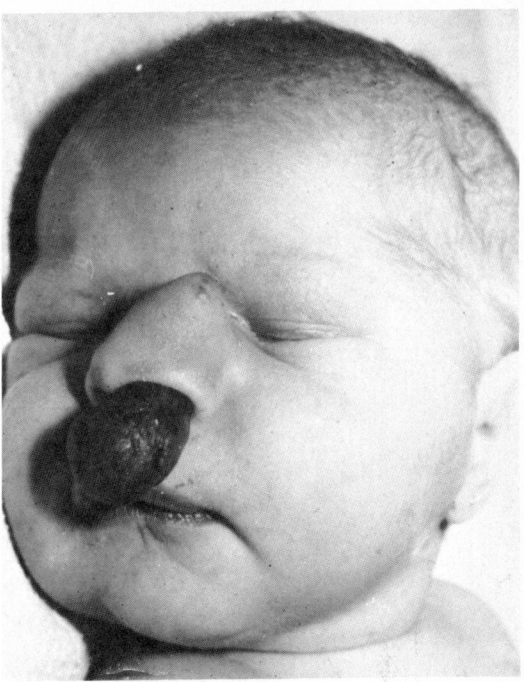

FIG. 11. Large nasal encephalocele in a newborn prior to repair by craniotomy plus nasal excision.

golian races, in which they may constitute a majority of encephaloceles. Their locations may be nasofrontal, nasoethmoidal, naso-orbital, or basal. As contrasted with occipital encephaloceles, their diagnosis may be more difficult, especially the lesions that extend into the nose and that may erroneously be called polyps and be biopsied, thus leading to catastrophic intracranial infection (Fig. 11). Encephaloceles at the nasal-orbital-cranial junction are obvious, but do not lend themselves to easy technical repair, since they are often associated with other craniofacial anomalies. The incidence of either hydrocephalus or significant associated brain anomalies is lower than with occipital encephaloceles.

Nasofrontal encephaloceles should be treated by frontal craniotomy, with excision or replacement of intracranial contents, dural repair, and an attempt to fill the bony defect. Naso-orbital lesions, in which there is less risk of infection, should be repaired during the first year of life by a neurosurgeon and ophthalmic or plastic surgeon to achieve the best possible orbital alignment and cosmetic result (Fig. 12).

SPINAL ANOMALIES

SPINA BIFIDA. Derangements in neural tube closure coupled with derangements of germ cell layers give rise to the broad clinical spectrum of midline closure defects of the vertebral column known as spina bifida. The neural plate defect is held responsible for the neurologic involvement in spina bifida, for the elements

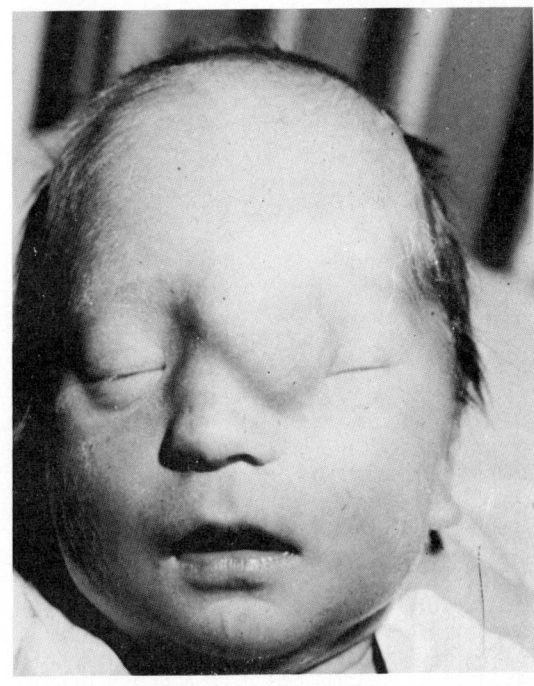

FIG. 12. Naso-orbital encephalocele in newborn (left).

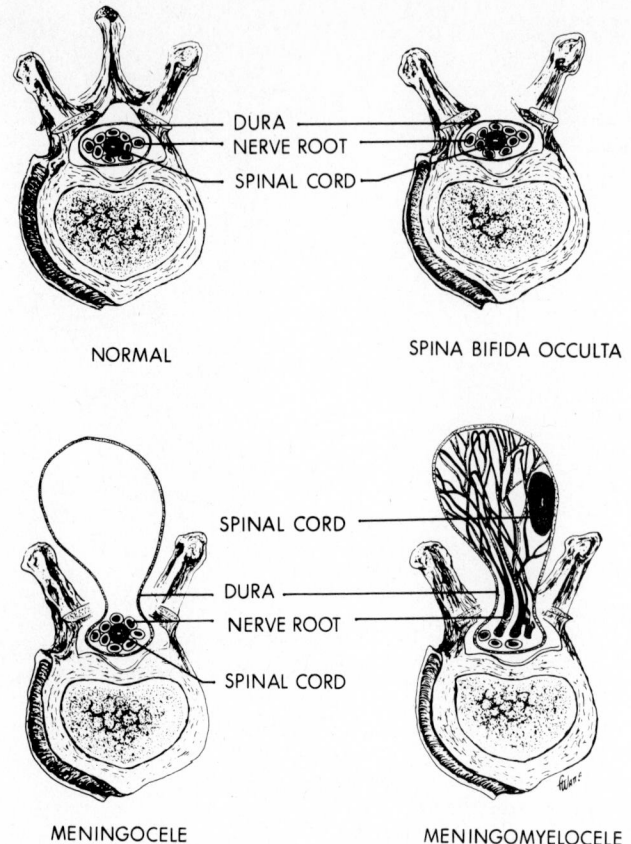

NORMAL

SPINA BIFIDA OCCULTA

MENINGOCELE

MENINGOMYELOCELE

FIG. 13. The varieties of spina bifida.

of the nervous system arising from epithelial ectoderm (peripheral roots and ganglia) are often spared in this entity. The clinical spectrum comprises the occult form of spina bifida, which is found in 10 percent of routine spine radiographs, and the cystic forms of spina bifida (Fig. 13). Although many names, such as myelodysplasia, myeloschisis, spinal dysraphism, meningocele, and meningomyelocele, have been applied to the cystic forms, it would seem that only the last two terms need be retained.

SPINA BIFIDA OCCULTA.   This form of spina bifida, which is rarely symptomatic, occurs with greatest frequency in the fifth lumbar and first sacral vertebral segments. Often a cutaneous or subcutaneous abnormality, such as a tuft of hair, angioma, lipoma, or skin dimple, accompanies the bony defect. In a small number of children with the defect, neurologic difficulty will occur when the child is growing rapidly and the spinal cord is called upon to ascend. In such children the symptoms may be based on an underlying cord abnormality, such as dilatation of the central canal (hydromyelia), a splitting of the cord (diastematomyelia), or an associated

congenital tumor such as a lipoma or dermoid at the end of the cord that fixes it in the infantile position. The neurologic deficit resulting from such lesions manifests as muscle weakness leading to gait disturbance or sensory loss resulting in trophic ulcers. Loss of sphincter control is not uncommon, and a child who was once toilet trained may become incontinent. Pain is usually not a feature. It is important to obtain spine roentgenograms in children with these signs, and if a defect is noted myelography should be performed. A good neurosurgical result may be expected if the lesion can be explored and removed early or if tension on the nerve roots of the cauda equina can be relieved by section of the filum terminale. Preventive surgery in these lesions is usually not indicated, unless they are associated with a low spinal diastematomyelia.

SPINA BIFIDA CYSTICA.   As with anencephaly, the geographic distribution and incidence of spina bifida cystica (meningocele and meningomyelocele) vary widely in countries populated by Caucasians of similar backgrounds; for instance, there is a reported incidence of 4.2 per 1,000 live births in Ireland, 2.8 per 1,000 in

Buckinghamshire, and 1.5 per 1,000 in southeastern England. The lower socioeconomic groups seem to be more affected. Laurence made etiologic inquiries in 179 families, and no evidence of any abnormal exogenous influence on pregnancy, such as infection, x-rays, drugs, or diet, could be elicited. It is possible, however, that prenatal insults sustained during the first month of gestation may have been overlooked. In most series the incidence of meningomyelocele in other children in the same family has been very high (approaching 7.8 percent); furthermore, the incidence of other congenital anomalies has been high (2.4 percent). Thus there is a considerable risk of abnormal children in subsequent pregnancies in these families.

MENINGOCELE. Meningocele is defined as a cystic lesion in the midline of the back that contains only meninges or perhaps meninges and nerve roots and is free of central nervous tissue, is well covered with skin, and is unassociated with neurologic deficit. When this definition is used, meningoceles comprise about 10 percent of all cases of spina bifida cystica. When such lesions have been excised and examined pathologically, the sacs of a number of them that on clinical and gross pathologic examination had been thought to be meningoceles have been found to contain nerve roots and spinal cord. Thus they would have to be classified as meningomyeloceles. Meningoceles have similar frequencies of occurrence in the cervical, the thoracic, and the lumbar spines. The incidence of spina bifida cystica is much higher in the lumbar region; thus the chance of a lesion in the cervical or thoracic region being a meningocele is greater. Associated cord abnormalities may result in neurologic deficit, but it is implied in the concept of meningocele that there is no progressive neurologic symptomatology. Thus there is no need to close the sac, which has good skin covering, in the newborn period. It is advocated that the sac be closed electively after the age of 3 months. By that time a child who is destined to develop hydrocephalus will have done so, and treatment of hydrocephalus may be indicated prior to repair of the meningocele.

MENINGOMYELOCELE. In meningomyelocele the neural ectoderm that develops into the spinal cord and nerve roots appears to have failed to separate from the epithelium, resulting in a sac containing CSF, incompletely formed meninges, and malformed spinal cord. Usually the neural plate that has failed to close is exposed in the center of the sac as a reddened, weeping area, the stroking of which may provoke involuntary movements of the legs. The sac often leaks in utero or ruptures at birth, so that cerebrospinal fluid drains freely, and it is distinctly unusual to have anything resembling normal skin covering the mass. The leakage of the CSF, with the threat of ascending meningitis, makes immediate surgical closure of the defect imperative. Meningomyelocele is most common in the lumbosacral region. In addition to the exposed dysplastic neural plate, the spinal cord above the defect often shows abnormalities such as hydromyelia, diastematomyelia, or syrinx formation. Rarely meningomyelocele may present ventral to the vertebra as a pelvic mass that gives rise to symptoms of bowel obstruction.

By definition, some neurologic deficit will be present in the limbs and cutaneous areas below the mass. In sacral meningomyeloceles below the exit of the lumbosacral plexus the lower extremities may be normal, but there is loss of sphincter control and sensory loss in the saddle area. Such loss may be detected in the newborn by dribbling of urine during crying and inability to initiate a urinary stream in the male. A child with a lumbosacral meningomyelocele usually has reasonably good movements at the hips and knees, but presents with paralyzed ankles and inverted feet held in an equinovarus position. If the mass is thoracolumbar the legs may be flaccid and the lower abdominal musculature poorly developed, so that the abdomen is protuberant; the hips will be congenitally dislocated, and there will be sphincter involvement.

The leaking meningomyelocele sac may undergo some recovery and repair, stimulated at least partly by granulation tissue response to superficial infection. This inflammatory fibrosis leads to scarring and may impair function of those nerve roots involved in the scar formation. This possible loss of function and the real danger of ascending infection if the sac is not closed suggest that back closure of the infant with myelomeningocele be performed as soon as possible after birth in those patients who are to be treated aggressively. This rationale for early back closure in selected patients is generally accepted. There is currently a controversy regarding the possible improvement afforded by early surgery and the selection of patients for surgery. Improved function after back closure on the day following birth has been reported, but these results have not been verified. It is probable that the reported improvement reflected return of intrinsic function that was lost because of trauma to the meningomyelocele during birth, rather than the effects of early surgery.

The paralysis associated with meningomyelocele is a basic part of the disease; the most serious complication is hydrocephalus. This results from malformations in the brain, most commonly the Arnold-Chiari hindbrain malformation with partial or complete occlusion of the Sylvian aqueduct, and from obliteration of the subarachnoid pathways by ascending secondary infections.

Modern treatment has significantly altered the prospects for survival of children with meningomyelocele. Several articles have reviewed the results of a program in England of early meningomyelocele sac closure and aggressive management of hydrocephalus and the accompanying orthopedic and urologic complications of the disease. Although the results in large children's centers in the United States are not quite comparable, the available reports indicate that despite massive effort and outlay of resources to provide definitive care for each child there results a group of patients who are severely handicapped, who depend on the hospital for repeated admissions, and who never achieve either physical or psychologic independence. In reviewing his own data Lorber has identified criteria that exclude from treatment those infants whose survival would be associated with severe mental and physical handicaps. The criteria are advanced hydrocephalus at birth, complete paralysis below the upper lumbar segments, severe kyphoscoliosis, and gross congenital anomalies or major birth injuries. Two or more of these adverse criteria present at birth would indicate that the child should not be treated but should be given only supportive care. If the back heals spontaneously, further treatment may be indicated based upon the desires of the parents. Such selection of patients for treatment permits a concentration of resources for developing a comprehensive program for surveillance and management of the complications of myelomeningocele. Children are best followed in a multidisciplinary birth defects center where urologic, orthopedic, and neurosurgical care is available. Such comprehensive programs enable 80 percent of the children selected for aggressive treatment to reach 3 years of age, with normal developmental quotients in 60 percent of survivors.

The higher incidence of spina bifida in families where there is already an affected child makes informed family planning and genetic counseling mandatory for these high-risk families. The role of intrauterine investigation of unborn siblings in such families awaits clarification.

DIASTEMATOMYELIA. In diastematomyelia the spinal cord is divided into two halves, each of which may undergo modification of structure. It is most common in the lumbar and midthoracic areas. The two cords are separated by a fibrous or bony spicule that can often be seen on roentgenograms. Each half of the divided cord

has its own pial investment, but the arachnoid and dura may be shared. The different rates of elongation of the spinal cord and vertebral column may cause increasing pressure on the spinal cord, which is tethered at the spur. This may lead to progressive neurologic symptoms that usually develop at about 4 years of age or later. Prophylactic surgery is thus indicated in children with diastematomyelia in the low thoracic or lumbar area in order to prevent the development of neurologic symptoms. In older children with lesions at a higher level, where the ascent of the cord is not so great, operations are not required unless progressive neurologic symptoms develop. Myelography is indicated prior to surgery. The operative results are generally good; if there is uncertainty exploratory laminectomy is warranted, because there is little risk of harming the patient with careful surgery.

DERMAL SINUS. Dermal sinus tracts may occur at any site along the spinal axis, but they are most common in the lumbosacral area. Developmentally they result from failure of the neural ectoderm to separate from the skin ectoderm, with a sinus tract covered by epithelial tissue leading down to or through the dura. There may or may not be a spina bifida occulta on roentgenography. Sinuses should be looked for in all children with recurrent unexplained meningitis. If a sinus tract is found it should be excised, with prior preparations being made for laminectomy and intradural exploration in case they prove necessary. When possible, sinus tracts should be excised prior to infection, for once infection has taken place the gross scarring around the intradural contents of the sinus increases the difficulty of the surgery.

In additon to spinal dermal sinuses, cranial dermal sinuses may occur at any place in the midline of the skull, but most commonly in the occipital region. They appear as defects in the midline of the occipital bone that are directed obliquely and have hyperostosis around the bone edges (Fig. 14). Prophylactic excision of such sinus tracts is indicated to prevent intracranial suppuration and abscess formation. It is advisable to study the child with pneumoencephalography prior to excision of the sac to determine whether there is intracranial extension, which should be dealt with if it is found. A normal air study does not rule out intracranial extension; this is because the brain and cyst are formed and developed over the same period of time, so that the cerebral tissue is not displaced by the cyst but merely fails to develop in the region.

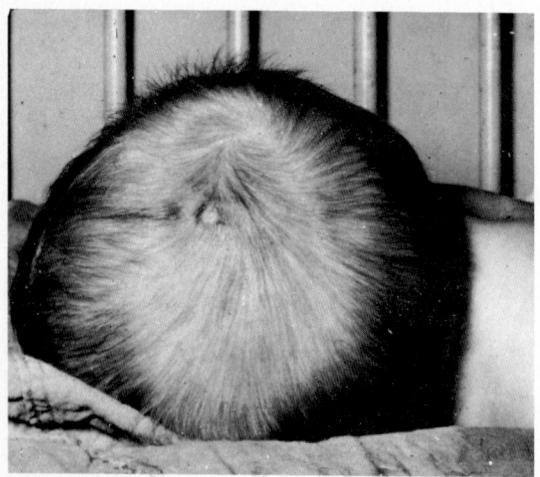

FIG. 14. Occipital dermal sinus with head shaved and sinus readily apparent

References

ABNORMAL HEAD SIZE

Baum J, Searls D: Head shape and size of pre-term low-birthweight infants. Dev Med Child Neurol 13:576, 1971

Bergsma D: Birth Defects: Atlas and Compendium. Baltimore, The National Foundation—March of Dimes, Williams & Wilkins, 1973

DeMyer W: Technique of the Neurologic Examination: A Programmed Text, 2nd ed. New York, McGraw-Hill, 1974

Illingworth R, Eid E: The head circumference in infants and other measurements to which it may be related. Acta Paediatr Scand 60:333, 1971

Nellhaus G: Head circumference from birth to eighteen years. Pediatrics 41:106, 1968

O'Neill EM: Normal head growth and the prediction of head size in infantile hydrocephalus. Arch Dis Child 36:241, 1961

———— Minimal rates of head growth in the first four months of life. Arch Dis Child 37:415, 1962

Sjögren I, Engsner G: Transillumination of the skull in infants and children. Acta Paediatr Scand 61:426, 1972

MICROCEPHALY

Baron J, Youngblood L, Siewers M, Medearis D Jr: The incidence of cytomegalovirus, herpes simplex, rubella, and toxoplasma antibodies in microcephalic, mentally retarded, and normocephalic children. Pediatrics 44:932, 1969

Chase H, Dabiere C, Welch N, O'Brien D: Intra-uterine undernutrition and brain development. Pediatrics 47:491, 1971

Pryor H, Thelander H: Abnormally small head size and intellect in children. J Pediatr 73:593, 1968

Winick M, Rosso P: Head circumference and cellular growth of the brain in normal and marasmic children. J Pediatr 74:774, 1969

MEGALOCEPHALY

DeMyer W: Megalencephaly in children. Clinical syndromes, genetic patterns and differential diagnosis from hydrocephalus. Neurology 22:634, 1972

Ford F: Diseases of the Nervous System in Infancy, Childhood and Adolescence, 5th ed. Springfield, Ill, Charles C Thomas, 1966

MEDIAN FACIAL DEFECTS AND HOLOPROSENCEPHALY

Currarino G, Silverman F: Orbital hypotelorism, arhinencephaly, and trigonocephaly. Radiology 74:206, 1960

DeMyer W: Classification of cerebral malformations. Birth Defects 7:78, 1971

Yakovlev P: Pathoarchitectonic studies of cerebral malformations. III. Arhinencephalies (holotelencephalies). J Neuropathol Exp Neurol 18:22, 1959

Zingesser L, Schechter M, Medina A: Angiographic and pneumoencephalographic features of holoprosencephaly. Am J Roentgenol Radium Ther Nucl Med 97:561, 1966

MEDIAN CLEFT FACE SYNDROME

DeMyer W: The median cleft face syndrome. Neurology 17:961, 1967

HYDRANENCEPHALY

Halsey J, Allen N, Chamberlin H: The morphogenesis of hydranencephaly. J Neurol Sci 12:187, 1971

Poser C, Walsh F, Scheinberg L: Hydranencephaly. Neurology 5:284, 1955

AGENESIS OF CORPUS CALLOSUM

Carpenter MB: Agenesis of the corpus callosum. A study of 18 cases diagnosed during life. Neurology 4:200, 1954

Loeser J, Alvard E, Jr: Agenesis of the corpus callosum. Brain 91:553, 1968

HYDROCEPHALUS

Adams RD, Fisher CM, Hakim S, Ojemann RG, Sweet WH: Symptomatic occult hydrocephalus with "normal" cerebrospinal fluid pressure. A treatable syndrome. N Engl J Med 273:117, 1965

Ambrose J: Computerized x-ray scanning of the brain. J Neurosurg 40:679, 1974

Aylett MJ: Spina bifida in general practice. Practitioner 211:75, 1973

Bering EA Jr: Circulation of the cerebrospinal fluid, demonstration of the choroid plexuses as the generator of the force of flow of fluid and ventricular enlargement. J Neurosurg 19:405, 1962

Bruce AM, Lorber J, Shedden WIH, Zachary RB: Persistent bacteraemia following ventriculo-caval shunt operations for hydrocephalus in infancy. Dev Med Child Neurol 5:461, 1963

Dandy WE, Blackfan KD: Internal hydrocephalus, an experimental, clinical and pathological study. Am J Dis Child 8:406, 1914

Davson H: Physiology of the Ocular and Cerebrospinal Fluids. Boston, Little, Brown, 1956

Farmer TW: Pediatric Neurology. New York, Paul B Hoeber, 1964

Foltz EL, Shurtleff DB: Five year comparative study of hydrocephalus in children with and without operation (113 cases). J Neurosurg 20:1064, 1963

Friedman S, Zita-Gozum C, Chatten J: Pulmonary vascular changes complicating ventriculovascular shunting for hydrocephalus. J Pediatr 64:305, 1964

Lange SA: The effects of prolonged cerebrospinal fluid shunting on the developing skull and brain. Dev Med Child Neurol 16:219, 1974

Laurence KM: The natural history of hydrocephalus. Lancet 2:1152, 1958

Lin JP, Goodkin R, Tong E, Epstein FJ, Vinaguerra E: Radioiodinated serum albumin (RISA) cisternography in the diagnosis of incisural block and occult hydrocephalus. Radiology 90:36, 1968

McLaurin RL: Infected cerebrospinal fluid shunts. Surg Neurol 1:191, 1973

Matson DD: Clinical classification and evaluation of hydrocephalus. In Fields WS, Desmond MM (eds): Disorders of the Developing Nervous System. Springfield, Ill, Charles C Thomas, 1961

———— Neurosurgery in Infancy and Childhood, 2nd ed. Springfield, Ill, Charles C Thomas, 1969

Pudenz RH, Russel FE, Hurd AH, Shelden CH: Ventriculoauriculostomy: a technique for shunting cerebrospinal fluid into the right auricle. J Neurosurg 14:171, 1957

Scarff JE: Treatment of hydrocephalus: a historical and critical review of methods and results. J Neurol Neurosurg Psychiatry 26:1, 1963

Selverstone B: Studies of the Formation and Absorption of the Cerebrospinal Fluid Using Radioactive Isotopes. Ciba Foundation Symposium on the Cerebrospinal Fluid. Boston, Little, Brown, 1958, p 147

Strenger L: Complications of ventriculovenous shunts. J Neurosurg 20:219, 1963

CLOSURE DEFECTS OF NEURAL PLATE

Badell Ribera A, Swinyard CA: Rehabilitation of Children with Spina Bifida Cystica. Exerpta Medica International Congress Series No 76, September 1964, p 180

Brock DJH: Prenatal diagnosis of anencephaly through maternal serum-alphafetoprotein measurement. Lancet 2:923, 1973

Dale AJD: Diastematomyelia. Arch Neurol 20:309, 1969

Doran PA, Guthkelch N: Studies in spina bifida cystica (general survey and reassessment of the problem). J Neurol Neurosurg Psychiatry 24:331, 1961

Laurence KM, Tew BJ: Natural history of spina bifida cystica and cranium bifidum cysticum. Major central nervous sytem malformations in South Wales, Part IV. Arch Dis Child 46:127, 1971

Lorber J: The prognosis of occipital encephaloceles. Dev Med Child Neurol [Suppl] 13:75, 1966

———— Results of treatment of myelomeningocele. Dev Med Child Neurol 13:279, 1971

———— Early results of selective treatment of spina bifida cystica. Br Med J 4:201, 1973

Mealey J Jr, Dzennis AJ, Hockey AA: The prognosis of encephaloceles. J Neurosurg 32:209, 1970

Nakano KK: Anencephaly: a review. Dev Med Child Neurol 15:383, 1973

Sharrard WJW, Zachary RB, Lorber J, Bruce AM: A controlled trial of immediate and delayed closure of spina bifida cystica. Arch Dis Child 38:18, 1963

Shulman K, Ames M: Results of intensive treatment of fifty consecutive children born with myelomeningocele. NY State J Med 68:2656, 1968

Smith GK, Smith ED: Selection for treatment in spina bifida cystica. Br Med J 4:189, 1973

STATIC ENCEPHALOPATHIES

SIDNEY CARTER AND ARNOLD P. GOLD

Chronic nonprogressive cerebral dysfunction results from various causes and produces a variety of clinical syndromes, and the clinical picture is dependent on the site and extent of the lesion and on gestational age at the time of its occurrence. The developing nervous system is more susceptible to insults occurring during the first trimester of pregnancy. Cerebral palsy results from involvement of motor areas of the brain. Mental retardation usually follows diffuse cerebral involvement, but small lesions occurring early in gestation may interfere with normal cerebral maturation, with resulting intellectual deficit. Impairment of the senses of sight and hearing follows involvement of certain areas of the brain and their pathways. Convulsions most commonly result from cortical lesions. Speech disturbances may be a reflection of diffuse cerebral involvement or a focal lesion involving the speech area. Behavioral disorders and learning disabilities have less well defined anatomic localization. These syndromes may occur as isolated clinical phenomena or in any combination. Spastic diplegia may be the only manifestation of cerebral palsy; however, mental deficit, seizures, impairment of vision and/or hearing, or behavioral disturbances may accompany this motor deficit. These defects of cerebral function can be the result of well-recognized anatomic or biochemical lesions, but in many impaired children the cause may not be apparent. Prenatal factors affecting the developing nervous system are both endogenous and exogenous. The fetus may be affected by faulty implantation of the ovum, chromosomal anomalies, infections, trauma, radiation, and toxic substances. Later in pregnancy maternal toxemia and diabetes may produce damage to the nervous system. Anoxia and trauma are the most commonly encountered causative factors in the perinatal period. In the postnatal period infections, inborn errors of metabolism, trauma, toxins, and vascular disease are often incriminated.

Today children with chronic nonprogressive lesions of the brain are being recognized with increasing frequency. More prevalence studies are needed, but available figures illustrate the magnitude of this common pediatric problem. It is estimated that 1 of 1,000 infants born live will be severely retarded, 3 of 1,000 moderately retarded, and 25 of 1,000 mildly retarded. In the United States 5.5 million individuals have some degree of retardation; cerebral palsy affects approximately 400,000 children. Approximately 5 percent of all children will have one or more seizures. The incidences of organically induced behavioral disturbances and specific learning disabilities are not known, but these conditions greatly outnumber any of the other clinical syndromes.

MINIMAL BRAIN DYSFUNCTION

Many different terms have been applied to children with deviant behavior or specific learning disabilities or both. The terms employed include the Strauss syndrome, choreiform syndrome, minimal cerebral palsy, minimal cerebral damage, minimal cerebral dysfunction, organic reaction syndrome, nonmotor brain damage, and chronic brain syndrome, as well as the brain-injured child and the hyperkinetic child; they have a common feature in suggesting organicity as a basis for the observed clinical manifestations. The term minimal brain dysfunction appears to be satisfactory in that it implies impaired cerebral function without implicating specific areas of the brain. This diagnosis is used in describing children with normal or nearly normal intellect who demonstrate abnormal behavior patterns or specific learning disabilities or both.

CLINICAL MANIFESTATIONS.   The clincial syndrome is variable, and the manifestations may change with age. Deviant behavior, learning disabilities, speech disorders, and poor coordination are the most common presentations. The behavioral patterns most frequently encountered are those relating to hyperactivity, but hypoactivity or even normal behavior can be seen. Hyperkinetic behavior is often evidenced in infancy as restlessness, irritability, and poor sleep patterns. Overactive behavior in the older child is without direction and is purposeless; it shifts from moment to moment. The hyperkinesis fluctuates; it is most marked when the child is confronted with new or stressful situations, and it is often diminished in familiar settings. Overactivity tends to diminish spontaneously at about 12 years of age and in most instances is significantly modified by 15 years. Less frequently the behavior may be manifested by hypoactivity, in which the child is placid and retiring.

Behavioral changes closely related to the hyperactivity include a short attention span, irritability, low frustration threshold, impulsivity, distractibility, and social immaturity. Short attention span is characterized by difficulty in focusing and maintaining attention on a given task, with inability to eliminate the distraction produced by minimal or trivial auditory, visual, or tactile stimuli. Impulsivity and distractibility are contributing factors. The shortened attention is variable and may be replaced by perseveration. During these periods there is rigidity of behavior, with an abnormal preoccupation for a single object or detail and a resistance to change and failure to respond appropriately to changing stimuli. Emotional lability may be prominent, and the affective response may inappropriately change from one moment to another. The frustration threshold is often low, and insignificant conditions can provoke uncontrollable rage, unintentional aggressive outbursts, and temper tantrums. Social function is usually at a level below chronologic or mental age; this social immaturity may manifest as a preference for playing with children of a younger age.

Specific learning problems unrelated to intellectual potential or deviant behavior are additonal features of the minimal brain dysfunction syndrome. Impaired perceptual performance (auditory and/or visual) results in academic difficulties primarily involving reading and mathematical concepts. Specific reading disability (dyslexia) implies that the inability to read is unrelated to mental retardation, sensory impairment, inadequate schooling, poor motivation, or developmental lag. Either the child cannot read or reading is below age level and may be complicated by mirror reading. Some children also have an inability to write or to spell properly. They often demonstrate mirror writing or letter reversals and may be unable to distinguish *p* from *q, b* from *d, n* from *u,* and *w* from *m.* In some children there is inadequate ability to calculate. Many of these children are ambidextrous, which is attributed to failure to develop cerebral dominance. Difficulties with abstract concepts are a common feature of the syndrome and are more evident with increasing age. During the early school years learning is at a relatively concrete level, with little demand on abstract ideation. This disability may further complicate the difficulties in learning encountered by many of these children, or it may be the initial educational problem that is encountered by some who have previously been successful at the concrete level by use of rote.

Language difficulties are common; some children remain nonverbal, but more commonly there is delay in the development of speech patterns. Once speech patterns are established there may be problems in the formation of phrases and sentences and a prominent tendency to preserve more immature modes of expression. Speech may be characterized by paucity or misuse of words and by poor articulation. The flow of expressive language may be either slow and hesitant or explosive. Coordination is frequently impaired, and these children are often clumsy and awkward. Muscular fine coordination is poor and is initially demonstrated by difficulties with buttoning, zippering, or tying shoelaces. Subsequent manifestations may be seen in the manipulation of scissors, by inability to color within a figure or draw a straight line, and eventually by poor handwriting. More gross incoordination is evident in delay in learning to hop, skip, ride a bicycle, and catch a ball. Social incompetence and peer rejection result in secondary emotional symptoms characterized by aggression, destruction, withdrawal, and fantasy life.

Neurologic examination characteristically reveals a paucity of gross abnormalities, but minimal subtle signs are usually present. Gait may be lumbering and awkward. After 5 years of age there may be impaired ability to hop, and after 7 years there may be difficulty in walking. Examination of the motor system reveals impairment of rapid alternating movements, choreiform activity of extended fingers, and occasional tightness of various muscle groups, including hamstrings, posterior tibials, and pronators. Not uncommonly there is a right–left confusion and a failure to establish handedness. The deep tendon reflexes may be asymmetric, but the plantar responses are usually physiologic. Eye muscle imbalance of the convergent or divergent types is commonly observed; it tends to diminish with age. Poor speech patterns are often associated with drooling and inability to perform rapid lateral tongue movements.

LABORATORY FINDINGS. There are no specific laboratory studies to confirm the clinical diagnosis. Electroencephalograms are not in themselves diagnostic; they may be normal or may show abnormalities of organization with voltage and frequency changes or even multispike and spike and wave activity. Plain radiographs of the skull are usually normal. Pneumoencephalography and cerebral arteriography are contraindicated.

Psychologic testing is the most helpful ancillary procedure in that it supplies further evidence to support the concept of impaired cerebral function and provides an esimate of intellectual potential. Signs of organicity include discrepancy between high verbal and low performance scales that may be as great as 40 points, scatter on the subtests, and, above all, perceptual difficulties on the Bender Visual Motor Gestalt Test. Deviant perceptual performance is manifested by difficulty in copying forms and designs that are often correctly identified orally. There may be rotation or reorientation of the major axis of the figure. Difficulties with number concepts and abstract ideation may also be noted.

DIAGNOSIS. There is no isolated finding that is diagnostic of this clinical syndrome. Diagnosis can be accomplished only by combining the historical data with the results of the examinations. Differential diagnosis must include variants of the normal and psychiatric disturbances. Many normal children show a hyperactivity that is more readily controlled and is unassociated with short attention span, low frustration tolerance, or distractibility. Psychiatric disorders that may require differentiation include some neuroses, the character disorders, and certain psychoses. Not uncommonly the child with minimal brain dysfunction may present with prominent emotional manifestations. These apparently functional phenomena usually result from frustrations produced by learning disabilities and the excessive demands made by parents, peers, and teachers. Many physicians, including some psychiatrists, incorrectly interpret these secondary manifestations as primary emotional phenomena.

TREATMENT. A sound therapeutic program includes family counseling, a dynamic educational program, and medication to improve behavior. Family counseling is of primary importance. Explanation of the physical nature of the disability not infrequently relieves parental anxiety and guilt. The family must be made to accept the handicap. Unnecessary pressures should be eliminated and realistic goals formulated; a structured environment with consistent discipline and demands should be established. The family physician is often most effective in providing adequate parental guidance, but a seriously disturbed parent–child relationship may require psychiatric assistance.

Educational planning depends on the nature of the disability and the intellectual endowment. Adequate school placement is difficult to obtain even in the most sophisticated community. Some children can be maintained in a regular class supplemented by a resource program, while others require special class placement. All too often the neurologically impaired class is a heterogeneous group made up of children with differing learning problems and intellectual abilities. Ideally the class should be small in size, limited to children with similar intellectual endowments and learning problems, and directed by a teacher trained in remedial education. Efforts should be made to minimize distraction and competition. Emphasis should be placed on individual performance and the use of concrete teaching aids. In some instances residential placement may be desirable for both the child and family.

Drug therapy is unpredictable, and the effectiveness of a particular agent may diminish with time. Four groups of compounds have been particularly effective: amphetamines, methylphenidates, phenothiazines, and diphenylmethane derivatives.

AMPHETAMINES. Dextroamphetamine sulfate (Dexedrine) is the most effective amphetamine. The apparent paradoxic effect of this drug is most frequently observed in children demonstrating barbiturate-induced hyperactivity. Dexedrine is administered in doses of 2.5 to 30 mg/day given half after breakfast and half after lunch. Initially 2.5 mg is given, and this is gradually increased on succeeding days until the desired clinical effect is observed or until toxic reactions become prominent. The undesirable side effects that usually necessitate discontinuance of this compound are either increased hyperactivity with irritability and emotional lability or, more rarely, marked lethargy. When prescribing the drug the physician should inform the parents that there is difficulty with sleep for the first 3 to 4 nights and anorexia that generally improves spontaneously in a few weeks. These effects are usually not severe enough to warrant discontinuation of the compound. Amphetamine sulfate (Benzedrine) has pharmacologic activity similar to that of Dexedrine and is prescribed in similar doses. Occasionally a child will show a poor response to one compound, and the other will be effective.

METHYLPHENIDATES. Methylphenidate hydrochloride (Ritalin) is often effective in children with hyperactivity. The response is similar to that observed with the amphetamine group, and in therapeutic doses Ritalin is less likely to result in sedation, lethargy, anorexia, and insomnia. After an initial trial with 5 mg orally, the school-age child requires 5 mg three times daily; if necessary this is further increased to a total daily dose of 60 mg. The side effects are similar to those of the amphetamines, and when they occur they are managed in similar fashion. High doses (in excess of 30 mg/day) prescribed over a prolonged period may result in growth retardation.

PHENOTHIAZINES. Thioridazine (Mellaril) is the most effective and least toxic of the phenothiazine group of agents for management of the hyperkinetic behavior syndrome. A preschool child generally requires 10 mg three to four times a day and an older child 25 mg two to four times a day. Toxic reactions are rarely seen, but they may include extrapyramidal disorders, pigmentary retinopathy with night blindness, leukopenia, and agranulocytosis. These side effects are indications for prompt discontinuation of the drug. Specific treatment of extrapyramidal complications is discussed under basal ganglia diseases (p. 1925). Chlorpromazine (Thorazine) is often effective in controlling the acutely agitated child, but it has limited value in long-term management of the hyperkinetic child. Thorazine is usually given in dosages of 20 to 80 mg/day, but up to 300 mg/day may be necessary to achieve the desired results. Extrapyramidal reactions or jaundice as complications of therapy are rarely observed in children. Drowsiness, nasal congestion, dryness of the buccal mucosa, and postural hypotension are infrequent side effects, and their presence is not an indication for discontinuing the drug. Increased sensitivity to light may be so marked in some children that the drug cannot be tolerated. Other phenothiazines have limited usefulness in the hyperkinetic child because of relatively low therapeutic value or high incidence of toxic side effects. Specifically, prochlorperazine (Compazine) should not be prescribed in the pediatric age group because of the relatively high frequency of extrapyramidal involvement with this drug.

DIPHENYLMETHANE DERIVATIVES. Diphenhydramine hydrochloride (Benadryl) is occasionally effective, especially in anxious children with repetitive motor activities such as tics, head banging, and body rocking. The preschool child generally requires 10 mg three to four times a day, and after 6 years of age 25 mg three times daily may be necessary. Lethargy is a frequent minor side effect with this compound, and if it is disturbing it can be controlled by the addition of 2.5 to 5 mg of dextroamphetamine. Other drugs that may be effective in certain children include pemoline (Cylert) and haloperidol (Haldol). Caffeine and even coffee have been shown to have therapeutic benefit in a small group of hyperactive children. Dietary measures, including the elimination of food additives, are currently being evaluated.

References

Birch HG (ed): Brain Damage in Children: The Biological and Social Aspects. Baltimore, Williams & Wilkins, 1964

Chalfant JC, Scheffelin MA: Central processings dysfunctions in children. NINDS Monograph No 9. Bethesda, Md, US Public Health Service, 1969

Clements SD: Minimal brain dysfunction in children. NINDB Monograph No 3. Public Health Service Publication No 1415. Washington, DC, US Public Health Service, 1964

Cruickshank WM: The Brain-injured Child in Home, School, and Community. Syracuse, Syracuse University Press, 1967

Eisenberg L: Behavior modification by drugs: III. The clinical use of stimulant drugs in children. Pediatrics 49:709, 1972

——— The management of the hyperkinetic child. Dev Med Child Neurol 8:593, 1966

Millichap JG: Drugs in the management of minimal brain dysfunction. Ann NY Acad Pediatr 205:321, 1973

Paine RS: Minimal chronic brain syndromes in children. Dev Med Child Neurol 4:21, 1962

Sapir SG, Nitzburg AC: Children with Learning Problems. New York, Brunner/Mazel, 1973

Schain RJ: Neurology of Childhood Learning Disorders. Baltimore, Williams & Wilkins, 1972

——— Reynard CL: Observations on effects of a central stimulant drug (methylphenidate) in children with hyperactive behavior. Pediatrics 55:709, 1975

Strauss AA, Lehtinen L: Psychopathology and Education of the Brain-Injured Child. New York, Grune & Stratton, 1947

Touiven BCL, Prechtl HFR: The Neurological Examination of the Child with Minor Nervous Dysfunction. Clinics in Developmental Medicine No 38. London, William Heinemann, 1970

Wender PH: Minimal Brain Dysfunction in Children. New York, Wiley, 1971

MENTAL RETARDATION

Lawrence T. Taft and Herbert J. Cohen

Mental retardation is a major health, education, and social problem throughout the world. Its effects are often profound and devastating to the child and to his family. It is therefore essential that all physicians have an understanding of this important area of concern. Mental retardation is associated with many syndromes and diseases. Traditionally individuals have been labeled as being mentally retarded if their performance has fallen two standard deviations below the mean on a standardized psychologic test. However, different psychologic tests measure different aspects of cognitive functioning, and the tests are not culture-free. A low intelligence quotient may not always be a reliable indicator of intellectual incompetence. Performance on intelligence tests, in certain cases, can be significantly changed by a modification of the environment, by test preparation, by test familiarity, and by improved motivation. The primary concern with the individual who performs poorly on standardized intelligence tests is whether he is able to adapt and successfully compete in society. Tests that measure cognitive abilities do have some predictive value in determining future adaptation to society's demands. However, these demands are quite variable. A child with a low intelligence quotient (IQ) may be considered handicapped in some settings and not in others.

Because of changing conceptions of what constitutes retardation, the American Association on Mental Deficiency (AAMD) recently published a new manual on mental retardation that defined the condition as follows: "Mental Retardation refers to significantly subaverage general intellectual functioning existing concurrently with deficits in adaptive behavior, and manifested during the developmental period." In the child with mild intellectual deficit, mental retardation may be unrecognized until the start of schooling, since at that time his behavior must conform to stricter standards and his intellectual competence in selected areas is first challenged. At the completion of schooling the same individual may once again fade into the general population and, freed of academic demands, function competitively with his peers. Because of variations in societal pressures, mental retardation is reported more frequently during the school years than at any other developmental stage; and some individuals identified at this time are probably not intrinsically retarded. Even those who are retarded will be less likely to be identified after their school years are over.

Adaptive difficulties can exist in individuals who function at any level on standardized psychologic tests. It is erroneous to assume that the tests used to classify a specific population as retarded automatically absolve individuals who score slightly above that level from being functionally handicapped. In addition, learning disabilities and educational failure can occur even when an individual is of normal or superior intelligence.

CLASSIFICATION AND ETIOLOGY. It is convenient to define the degree of mental retardation as mild, moderate, severe, or profound. Many professionals continue to regard an IQ between 70 and 80 on standard tests as indicative of functioning at borderline levels of intelligence, although this classification is no longer used by the AAMD. Mild retardation is equated with an IQ between 50 and 70 and indicates that the individual is both educable and trainable. In general, most children in this category can reach a third- to fifth-grade level of academic achievement, and if there are no major associated handicaps they may be independent in activities of daily living. Prognostically the majority of this group, especially those functioning at the upper end of the range and without severe emotional problems, can be expected to achieve relative independence in adult life. They should be able to work as unskilled or semiskilled laborers and be able to assume family responsibilities. Moderate mental retardation implies that the individual will have very limited academic achievements but will be able to benefit from special education and training in self-care activities. The moderately retarded individual, who is not considered educable but is considered trainable, may learn to read and write at a primer or first-grade level. Vocational placement is usually limited to employment in a sheltered workshop, and supervised care is necessary. Individuals with severe mental retardation (IQ below 35) usually acquire no formal academic skills, and special intensive programming may be required to acquire skills in the activities of daily living. Closely supervised care is generally required. The profoundly retarded (IQ less than 20) have very limited potential for acquiring self-care skills and usually require institutional care or very carefully monitored living arrangements.

It is useful to classify individuals with intellectual handicaps in the two subgroups of those with true mental defects (biologic) and those with functional mental retardation. Retardation in those with true mental defects may be due to either structural or metabolic brain defects. However, the degree to which an individual will be retarded cannot be predicted on the basis of knowing the nature of the biologic defect. Although such an individual is not able to perform within the normal range on formal psychologic testing even when he is functioning at his highest level, the diagnostic label alone does not tell whether retardation will be mild or severe. A prime example is Down's syndrome, which includes persons functioning at all IQ levels from profound to very mild retardation, although most individuals with Down's syndrome are moderately retarded. In contrast, functional retardation implies that affected individuals have the capacity to perform within the normal range but are unable to do so because of such factors as emotional disturbance, deprivation, cultural disadvantage, discrimination, or educational handicap (Fig. 15).

Adequate anatomic and etiologic classifications for causes of mental retardation are not available, since pathogenesis and neuropathology have generally not been correlated with clinical manifestations. In addition, conditions associated with brain damage or maldevelopment (eg, absence of the corpus callosum) may not always be associated with mental retardation. Many conditions etiologically associated with mental retardation in one individual may cause cerebral palsy, epilepsy, learning disability, or some combination of these in other individuals. Although several hundred conditions are now known to be associated with the occurrence of mental retardation, in the vast majority of persons with mild retardation no single etiologic factor can be identified, and a comprehensive evaluation including physical and neurologic examinations and biochemical and cytogenetic studies usually fails to demonstrate the presence of clear-cut cerebral pa-

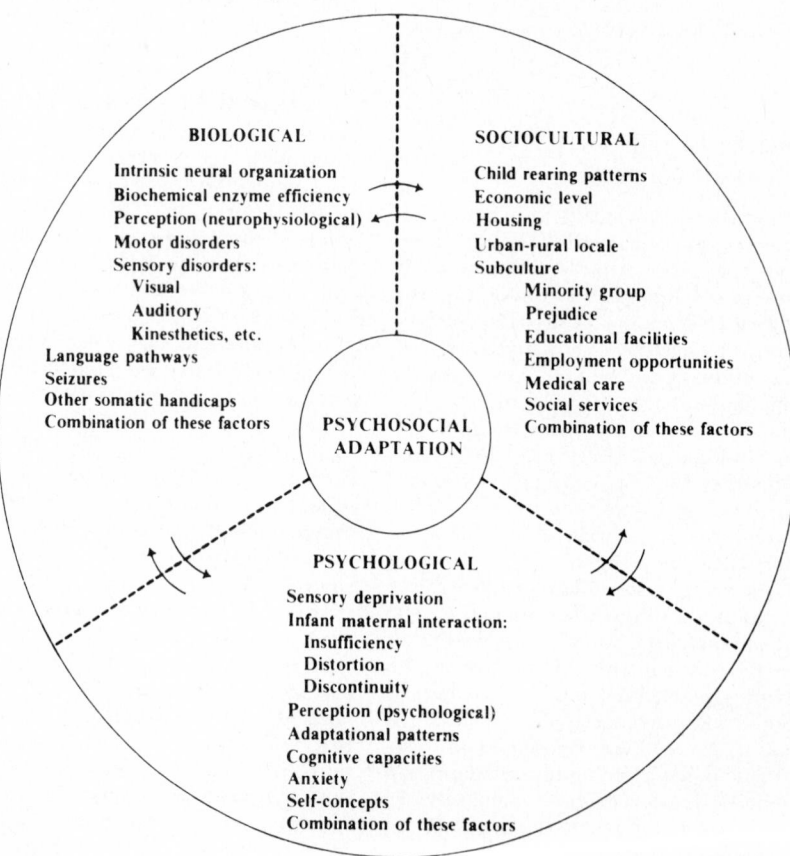

FIG. 15. Interacting factors in abnormal development. (Courtesy of Dr. J. B. Richmond.)

thology. Table 4 gives a broad outline of some of the determinants of mental retardation and other developmental disabilities; these are described elsewhere in the text. Biochemical disorders associated with mental retardation are shown in Tables 5 and 6.

INCIDENCE AND DISTRIBUTION. Mental retardation is believed to occur in approximately 3 percent of the population, although the frequency is estimated to be higher in urban settings. Overall, about 75 percent of retardation is mild, 20 percent moderate, and only 5 percent severe or profound. There are marked variations in this distribution that are associated with chronologic, cultural, and socioeconomic factors, with the prevalence of mild retardation being highest in the lower socioeconomic groups. In contrast, moderate retardation and severe retardation are distributed more evenly among all socioeconomic classes. This finding has created considerable controversy as to whether biologic factors or social (experiential) factors play the major role in causing mild mental retardation. Severe deprivation, protein malnutrition, and environmental factors have all been demonstrated to cause diminished rate and level of learning and subsequent subnormal mental functioning. Recent studies of adopted Korean children who suffered severe nutritional deficiencies in the first 18 months of life have revealed that their subsequent intellectual development has been normal; Winick has suggested that this is because these children were not returned to their former poor environment after correction of their nutritional deficits but were raised in a generally adequate nutritional, social, and educational milieu (the United States). A high frequency of retardation among the lower socioeconomic classes has suggested that polygenic or multifactorial hereditary patterns are important. Roberts has demonstrated that mildly retarded individuals have siblings with lower IQ's than the siblings of more severely retarded individuals. Studies of twins have generally supported the view that heredity is of major importance in determining eventual intelligence. However, the phenotypic expression of any genotype may also depend on environmental factors, and recent data appear to reinforce this view. It is probable that there are certain biologic determinants of behavior and that external stimuli modify their expressivity and vary the degree or type of responsiveness. In general, the long-standing nature-versus-nurture controversy has demonstrated only that each has a role and that many factors may operate in a relatively covert manner. The absence of clearly demonstrable central nervous system pathology in a given individual may simply reflect the lack of refinement of our clinical diagnostic tools, and many subtle abnormalities in function may go undetected.

PRESENTING FEATURES. The presence of mental retardation may be suspected either by the recognition of a specific syndrome with its overt anomalies or by a developmental lag. Down's syndrome is a classic example of the former and is usually recognized at birth, as are most cases where multiple anomalies are present. Retardation manifested only by delay in development without obvious physical anomalies is usually diagnosed at a later age. Severe mental retardation is manifested in the first year of life by marked lag in motor and adaptive behavior. However, in the presence of motor retardation only, the diagnosis of mental retardation must be made with caution, and other causes of the motor delay should be sought. A child with moderate retardation is usually delayed in motor and adaptive behavior in early infancy but may not be sufficiently deviant from the norm to arouse suspicion unless speech development is also significantly delayed. As stated earlier, mild retardation is often unrecognized until school age, when the child is in direct competition with youngsters of normal mental capacity.

Mild retardation may be identified by developmental screening examinations. The presence of high-risk factors (Table 4) should alert the physician that certain infants and children require careful developmental evaluation. For infants and toddlers developmental tests such as the Denver Developmental Screening Examination or the more complete Gesell or Bayley scales are useful in this regard (p. 37 and p. 1786). Although these tests cannot define a child's future intelligence, they do have reasonable predictive value in identifying mental subnormality; if they are performed sequentially they can be useful indicators of rate of development over a period of time, which gives a better indication than a single spot check. While physicians should be aware of the nature and scope of various quick tests, they should be cautious in attempting to administer them as office screening devices and should recognize that a thorough knowledge of normal growth and development is of paramount importance in assessing aberrant development.

ROLE OF PHYSICIAN. The physician's primary responsibility in the case of the retarded child is to examine the patient and identify any specific etiologic and pathologic entities that are known to cause mental subnormality. A complete diagnostic evaluation should be performed on a child with symptoms of maldevelopment as soon as the problem is recognized. Although remediable conditions are not common, there are a few treatable conditions in which early institution of therapy can produce favorable results. In addition, attention to coexisting remediable conditions is of value in enhancing developmental potential. Early diagnosis and intervention are important in treatable conditions such as phenylketonuria, cretinism, and other metabolic disorders, in conditions where surgery can alter the course of the disease (as in subdural hematoma or hydrocephalus), and in heritable disorders, where subsequent births of similarly affected children may be prevented. In addition to his important role in diagnosis and in providing general medical care for retarded children and adults, the physician may have a key role as a counselor to the family. Frequently the physician is the person who communicates the fact of the child's retardation to the family, and he is frequently seen as the

TABLE 4. Biologic Factors in Causation of Mental Retardation

Prenatal Occurrence

  Genetically determined

    Chromosomal anomalies
      Autosomes: nondysfunction (trisomies), translocations, deletion or partial deletion of chromosome material, mosaicism

    Sex chromosome anomalies

    Effects of abnormal genes:
    Homozygous genes producing identifiable recessive disorders of
    metabolism of: amino acids, lipids (leukodystrophies, lipidoses, etc), carbohydrates (galactosemia, mucopolysaccharidoses), purines
        (hyperuricemia)

    Heterozygous genes: carrier states (phenylketonuria, Tay-Sachs disease, etc), dominant disorders (some anencephalies, osteogenesis
        imperfecta)

    X-linked recessive disorders

    Unknown causation: identifiable syndromes of unknown etiology

  Deleterious intrauterine influences

    Maternal illness, infection, nutritional deficiency, hormonal imbalance, etc

    Teratogens: material drug ingestion, including alcohol, antimetabolites, nicotine, quinine, etc; environmental toxins; radiation,
        therapeutic, and other

    Uterine disease, malformations, dysfunction

    Multiple pregnancy

    Placental dysfunction, malimplantation

    Isoimmunization

    Trauma: foreign body inserted in uterus; direct blow or accident *Intrapartum and Neonatal Occurrence*

  Associated with trauma and/or hypoxia

    Prolonged labor due to malpresentation of fetus; cephalopelvic disproportion; uterine inertia, etc

    Placental abnormalities: placenta previa, abruptio placentae, etc

    Umbilical cord prolapse, torsion, around neck, etc

    Maternal hypotension: hemorrhage, anesthesia

  Neonatal sepsis

  Asphyxia neonatorum

  Kernicterus

Postnatal occurrence

  Anoxia (drowning, plastic bag over head, etc)

  Cerebrovascular accidents: hemorrhage, thrombosis, embolism

  Degenerative diseases: leukodystrophies, Tay-Sachs disease, etc

  Encephalopathies: postimmunization, associated with common childhood infections, secondary to toxins; "metabolic," eg, hypoglycemia

  Endocrine causation: eg, thyroid

  Head trauma: falls, auto accidents, child abuse

  Infections of CNS: meningitis, encephalitis

  Nutritional deficiencies

  Poisons and environmental toxins: lead ingestion, carbon monoxide, other contaminants of food, water, air

  Space-occupying lesions: neoplasms, abscesses, subdural hematoma

  Anatomic factors: premature synostosis, hydrocephalus

TABLE 5. Biochemical Disorders Often Associated with Mental Retardation and Elevated Blood Amino Acids[*]

Disease	Amino Acid Increased in Blood	Clinical Features
Phenylketonuria	Phenylalanine/ohydroxy-phenylacetic acid, other phenolic acid compounds in urine)	Mousy odor, eczema, seizures
Homocystinuria (vitamin B$_6$-sensitive and B$_6$-insensitive forms)	Methionine (homocystine in urine)	Dislocated lenses, malar flush, generalized osteoporosis, thromboembolic phenomena
Histidinemia	Histidine	Retarded speech development, articulatory defects
Maple syrup urine disease	Alloisoleucine, isoleucine, leucine, valine	Maple syrup odor of urine; hypertonia, seizures
Prolinemia type II	Proline (proline, hydroxy-proline, glycine in urine)	Association with seizures; mental retardation
Glycinemia, nonketotic	Glycine	Seizures, spasticity, opisthotonos
Lysinemia, persistant	Lysine	Growth failure, absence of secondary sex characteristics
Hyperammonemia type I (carbamylphosphate synthetase deficiency)	Glycine, glutamine	Episodic vomiting, irritability, lethargy, coma, seizures, hyperammonemia
Hyperammonemia type II (ornithine transcarbamylasse transferase deficiency)	Glutamine (plus orotic acid in urine)	As above, with hepatomegaly, SGOT hyperammonemia
Citrullinemia	Citrulline	Attacks of vomitting post-absorptive hyperammonemia
Argininemia	Arginine (arginine, cystine, lysine, and ornithine in urine)	Spastic diplegia, seizures, hyperammonemia
Argininosuccini aciduria	Argininosuccinic acid	Seizures, hepatomegaly, vomiting, coma, intermittent ataxia, abnormal hair, postprandial hyperammonemia
Lesch-Nyhan syndrome (hypoxanthine-guanine phosphoribosyl transferase deficiency)	Serum urate elevated (urinary uric acid excretion increased)	Self-multilation, choreoathefosis, spasticity

[*] *Adapted from Richmond JB: Mental Retardation. Courtesy of the American Medical Association.*

ultimate authority in deciding what is "best" for the child and the family (p. 17).

PHYSICAL FINDINGS. The presence of congenital stigmata such as abnormalities of head shape, peculiar facies, and anomalies of ears, eyes, or mouth may provide clues that fetal maldevelopment has occurred. A host of abnormal findings may be due to chromosomal defects or to first trimester teratogenic influences on the fetus. A search for skin lesions such as adenoma sebaceum, vitiligo, and café au lait spots may provide important diagnostic clues in certain diseases such as tuberous sclerosis. The presence of organomegaly should lead to the suspicion of a lipid or carbohydrate storage disease. Careful eyeground examination can rule out the optic atrophy, macular abnormalities, and pigmentary degeneration that are found in certain diseases of the central nervous system and the chorioretinitis that is associated with congenital toxoplasmosis, cytomegalic inclusion disease, or rubella. Metabolic disorders such as cretinism or mucopolysaccharidosis may be suspected if the child has coarse facial features. Unusual body odor or urinary odor may suggest an amino-aciduria. Constipation is a common finding in cretinism. Short stature is a frequent nonspecific

TABLE 6. Biochemical Disorders Associated with Mental Retardation Characterized by Increased Urinary Amino Acids, but Little or No Increase in Blood Concentrations*

Disease	Amino Acid in Excess in Urine	Some Additional Clinical Features
Cystathioninuria	Cystathionine	Features inconstant, may be a benign disorder of metabolism (?)
Hartnup's disease	Specific pattern of amino-aciduria (monoamino-monocarboxylic amino acids)	Pellagrous rash, intermittent ataxia, short stature

Qualitative Screening Tests of Urine†

Test	Phenyl-ketonuria	Homo-cystinuria	Histidin-emia	Maple Syrup Urine Disease	Galactosemia (Transferase and Kinase Deficiency)	Hurler's Disease
Ferric chloride and/or buffered dip stick	+	−	+	−	−	−
2,4-dinitro-phenythydrazine	+	−	±	+	−	−
Cyanide-nitro-prusside	−	+	−	−	−	−
Benedict's (reducing substance)	−	−	−	−	+	−
Glucose oxidase test	−	−	−	−	−	−
Acid albumin turbidity	−	−	−	−	−	+
Spot tests: toluidine blue Alcian blue	−	−	−	−	−	+

Adapted from Richmond JB: Mental Retardation. Courtesy of the American Medical Association.
† These are simple screening tests for urine that can be done for older children in the office. However, blood screening tests, such as the Guthrie for elevated phenylalanine level in PKU, may be the preferred screening procedure, especially in the newborn.

finding in mentally retarded persons, both institutionalized and noninstitutionalized. Not infrequently, complete investigations into known causes of short stature prove unrevealing. In these patients brain damage is assumed to be etiologically related to dwarfed stature, but the pathophysiologic mechanism is unknown. Short stature has also been reported as a consequence of emotional deprivation in otherwise normal individuals.

It is important to measure the child's head size at regular intervals. Graphs of normal values are available for premature and full-term infants and older children. A head circumference of three standard deviations or more from the mean should always be investigated. Head circumferences two standard deviations from the mean should be regarded with suspicion, especially if the circumference is out of proportion as compared with the child's percentiles for height and weight. In most cases of malnutrition, especially when this occurs after 1 year of age, the head will grow at a relatively normal rate and will appear relatively large in comparison to body size. Microcephaly at birth suggests the possibility of prenatal infections (eg, rubella, toxoplasmosis, cytomegalic inclusion disease, herpes), Paine's sex-linked recessive microcephaly with amino-aciduria, chromosomal aberration, or fetal maldevelopment of unknown origin. When head circumference is normal at birth but there is subsequently a slow rate of growth, the physician should suspect perinatal brain damage, metabolic disorder (eg, phenylketonuria), degenerative brain disease, or rubella, cytomegalic inclusion disease, toxoplasmosis, or herpes acquired in utero. There is increasing evidence that maternal addiction to drugs (especially alcohol and heroin) may result in microcephaly and other deficits. The importance of a careful history cannot be overemphasized in such cases.

Additional laboratory investigation should be done only when indicated by the findings on clinical examination. Specific biochemical studies (blood and/or urine) may be advisable; these are delineated in Tables 5 and 6. Also, confirmatory serologic tests for toxoplasmosis, cytomegalic inclusion disease, rubella, and herpes, as well as examination of the spinal fluid, may at times be indicated. Skull x-rays should be performed on microcephalic or retarded children, since identification of cerebral calcifications, although uncommon, may assist in detecting previously undiagnosed cases of cytomegalic inclusion disease, toxoplasmosis, or tuberous sclerosis. Brain scans, angiograms, pneumoencephalograms, or ventriculograms are rarely needed or even appropriate. In most cases of mental retardation an electroencephalogram is of little specific diagnostic help, although abnormalities associated with localized lesions such as subdural hematomas, as well as infantile spasms or petit mal status, have occasionally been identified by means of an electroencephalogram. Such conditions require early and specific treatment. However, the electroencephalogram is often overused or misused in the assessment of the disabled child.

The deaf child may present with a clinical picture suggestive of retardation, and appropriate hearing tests should be made to exclude this possibility. The very young deaf child is often characterized as a quiet baby, but care should be taken to evaluate hearing even in babies who do vocalize, as even profoundly deaf infants will do so in the early months.

Cytogenetic studies are normal in most cases, except where Down's syndrome or other chromosomal disorders are present. Karyotypes should be selectively performed when there are physical stigmata or a family history to suggest a chromosomal disorder. Such studies can confirm the clinical diagnosis and prove of value for future family planning. With the introduction of banding and similar techniques, abnormalities are being found in repeat karyotypes on individuals previously believed to have normal chromosomes.

PSYCHOLOGIC AND SOCIAL EVALUATION. A comprehensive assessment of any child with developmental delay should always include a careful clinical psychologic evaluation. It is common practice to use patterns of functioning on standard psychologic tests to help differentiate environmentally deprived, genetically deficient, and organically impaired patients. Psychometric testing performed in a one-to-one setting by an experienced psychologist can be helpful in determining the extent to which emotional factors, sensory impairments, and perceptual problems are limiting learning capacity. Such testing can be helpful not only in defining the patterns of disability but also in delineating areas of strength, so that prescriptive and remedial teaching and treatment can be based on maximum utilization of all available skills (p. 1785).

The results of psychologic tests are influenced by the child's attitude toward the tester and the testing, by his familiarity with test situations, by his level of anxiety in a strange and demanding setting, and by the general environment in which he has developed. Although the psychologist can competently evaluate some of these factors, a psychiatrist and social worker can be of great assistance in this regard. In the presence of suspected behavior aberrations that may depress intellectual function, a psychiatric evaluation should be performed. Children with infantile autism or childhood psychosis may appear retarded, but actually they may have considerable intellectual potential. The child who is hallucinating and whose thinking is heavily involved with fantasy may not perform up to his intellectual potential. The same is true of the overanxious child or the inhibited child. A psychiatric examination may be useful in determining the importance of emotional factors and their influence on intellectual functioning. A social worker may be extremely helpful in clarifying the family's attitude toward the retarded or handicapped child. An understanding of family dynamics, sibling and extended family relationships, and the family's economic situation is essential in formulating appropriate recommendations, and the family may more readily give this important information to a social worker than to a physician. There are many situations in which the social worker can communicate with the family more effectively than can the physician. Continuing social service contact with the families of retarded children is also most useful after completion of the diagnostic evaluation; here the social worker may provide help to the family in a variety of ways, including counseling and referral to appropriate community resources and other supportive services.

In many areas centers have been established to evaluate children with suspected mental retardation. These diagnostic centers have an interdisciplinary staff, usually including a pediatrician or pediatric neurologist, psychiatrist, psychologist, social worker, educational consultant, and nurse. Often speech, occupational, and physical therapists are also included. The team approach is useful in delineating all factors affecting the function of the referred patient; it is especially helpful in cases that present complex diagnostic problems. However, the full team approach appears unnecessary in straightforward cases where the diagnosis, treatment, and prognosis are obvious and where, provided he is willing to take the time to do so, a physician with knowledge of community resources for the retarded may well be able to handle the problem effectively without referral to a major diagnostic and treatment center.

TREATMENT. Since the causes of mental retardation are complex and multifactorial, there is no single therapeutic approach that is universally applicable to all individuals with this condition. It is clear, however, that the major approach to mental retardation is nonmedical and must emphasize provision of education, habilitation, social and recreational services, adequate housing arrangements, and vocational training. Nevertheless, the physician's role is important not only as a provider of health care but as a consultant to the staffs of generic and voluntary agencies that provide needed services for the mentally retarded.

Mental retardation due to apparently treatable metabolic disorders (eg, phenylketonuria) is rare. There are a few currently known disorders where a relatively uncomplicated procedure, such as dietary change, may produce a major change in the course of the disease. Conditions such as hydrocephalus that may cause mental retardation if untreated can be corrected by neurosurgical procedures. With early treatment the results are generally favorable. The need to identify curable conditions accurately and promptly is of obvious importance, but it is essential to stress that therapeutic recommendations in complex multifactorial cases of mental subnormality must be based on a thorough understanding of the relative importance of the organic, psychologic, genetic, and environmental components in producing the intellectual deficiency.

The parents must be given a practical and meaningful interpretation of the child's problems and behavior, along with an understanding of the anticipated changes in function and behavior that will occur with maturation. The concept of a static condition with changing manifestations related to developmental progression is often difficult to convey and is not always clearly grasped by parents, physicians, and other professionals dealing with the retarded individual. While physicians must be forthright in indicating when the prognosis is poor, they must also be cautious in prognosticating when the eventual outcome is uncertain. The need for periodic reevaluation in order to assess a child's progress should be stressed. If the physician can be candid with the family and yet convey with compassion and sympathy his genuine concern about their child, the tendency to shop for other opinions will be minimized.

EDUCATIONAL PROGRAMS. Until recently there were in many parts of the country few educational resources for the retarded, although some communities have long provided a wide range of special education classes. The increasing availability of schooling has been stimulated by the activities of parent organizations and others who over the years have led the movement to mandate appropriate schooling for all children. Just as classes of various types have been established, many sophisticated tests have been developed that assess the nature of learning disabilities and perceptual or intersensory integrative functions in the retarded, as well as

social, adaptive, behavioral, and prevocational skills for all ages and for various degrees of disability. These diagnostic procedures may be carried out by a psychoeducational consultant on the staff of a diagnostic clinic or school system, and they can be useful in developing an educational prescription in collaboration with the teacher and others (p. 1802). It must be stressed that whatever the remedial techniques applied success in a particular child is usually dependent on the child's basic abilities or disabilities, as influenced by the interest, attitude, and enthusiasm of the instructor, the motivation and cooperation of the child, the degree of structuring in the program, and the amount of time allotted for instruction, which often is related to class size. The difficulty of determining the relative importance of each of these variables has complicated the task of assessing the true worth of many of the special educational techniques that are currently being utilized.

SOCIAL AND RECREATIONAL NEEDS. Since the early 1960s there has been increasing openness in discussing mental retardation and handicapping conditions in general and increasing emphasis on so-called normalization. Nevertheless, the retarded child is still often rejected by his chronologic peers, by society in general, and even by his siblings and other family members. Yet, like any other child, he has social and recreational needs that are frequently unmet. In school he is socially isolated along with other children with similar problems, and meaningful social relationships with normal models are rare. Retarded children and adolescents desperately need after-school, weekend, and other social and recreational programs, and these are unavailable in many communities.

BEHAVIOR MODIFICATION. The past decade has witnessed an expansion of interest in techniques such as operant conditioning that are being utilized to teach the severely and profoundly retarded new skills such as toileting, dressing, feeding, and grooming, as well as modification or elimination of undesirable or self-destructive behavior. These methods train or condition via a system of rewards and punishments using positive and negative reinforcement and have produced improvements in gross functioning and in achieving a modicum of independence in daily living in some moderately to severely retarded and emotionally disturbed children. Similar techniques applied to certain mildly retarded children appear to have produced successful results in improving learning and behavior under controlled conditions. The advantages of these techniques are that they identify goals and objectives in treatment, they foster careful treatment planning, they necessitate close observation and monitoring, and they can be administered by relatively unskilled personnel after appropriate training. Many people have misgivings about negative reinforcement, which could lead to abuse, as well as ethical concerns about the dehumanizing aspects of the entire methodology.

MEDICATION. Drug treatment in mentally retarded children has been confined to the use of appropriate medications to treat specific symptoms in selected patients. No medication has yet been demonstrated to improve overall mental functioning in retarded children. Certain drugs have been useful in treating concomitant medical problems, with resultant improvement in overall functioning of the retarded child. Thus occasionally a child with petit mal status may appear retarded and/or autistic, but when diagnosed by electroencephalography and effectively treated with appropriate anticonvulsants may show a dramatic improvement in intellectual functioning. Equally dramatic results have been reported in a few individuals with psychomotor seizures. A substantial number of children with "minimal brain damage" who are very hyperactive and have a short attention span appear to function as mildly retarded children. Some of these children improve markedly when treated with amphetamines or methylphenidates.

The retarded child with significant emotional problems may also benefit from drug treatment. A high anxiety level stemming from feelings of frustration, from recurrent failure, and from a sense of rejection may have adverse effects on the academic performance of any child, especially the brain-damaged child, whether he functions in the retarded range or not. A child of this type may benefit from tranquilizers such as the phenothiazines, and the effective dosage level may be quite variable. With a decrease in the level of anxiety, concomitant improvement in intellectual functioning may occur. However, it should be pointed out that drug therapy in brain-damaged, hyperactive, anxious, or emotionally disturbed children merely permits the expression of the underlying intellectual potential and has no direct effect in improving intelligence per se.

VOCATIONAL TRAINING.   The majority of those with mild retardation appear to function well among the general population. Although academic failure increases the probability of unemployment, factors other than intelligence level, such as psychologic and social adjustment, often have a significant determining role in this regard. In an increasingly complex technological society the labor market for unskilled workers is shrinking, and job openings for mildly mentally retarded individuals are becoming more scarce. Thus vocational training for semiskilled or repetitive jobs, in which some retarded individuals show greater perseverance than the nonretarded, is essential. Failure in a vocational placement may be related to factors such as associated personality disorder, speech defect, motor problem, or cosmetic defect. Motivational factors are also important in determining ultimate success. Failures experienced in early childhood often lead to loss of initiative and fear of competing. Zigler has shown how important motivational reinforcement may be in helping a young person who is mentally retarded achieve at a higher level. It is important to emphasize that the value of investment in vocational training for the mildly retarded and the physically handicapped has been demonstrated. It decreases dependency and increases employability and productivity and the likelihood of long-range economic self-sufficiency. The imponderable values, such as enhancing one's sense of self-worth, dignity, etc, are not as readily demonstrated, but they are becoming increasingly important issues to advocacy groups.

For moderately and severely retarded persons there are limited opportunities for competitive employment. Although it has been possible to train severely retarded people to complete complex tasks by breaking down the chore into numerous steps and teaching these in a separate sequential manner, there is little likelihood that these or other training techniques will permit employment anywhere other than in a sheltered workshop that receives governmental or voluntary agency subsidies.

EARLY INTERVENTION.   There is growing enthusiasm for early identification and treatment programs for very young mentally retarded or otherwise disabled children. Several treatment approaches are now being utilized that stress methodologies such as education by parents (teaching parents how to work with their child and what to expect of their child), modeling (having a parent or child imitate the techniques of the teacher), or direct stimulation and training or manipulation of the child. While most of these approaches appear to produce short-term gains for many retarded children, there is concern that they do not have long-term positive results, and that they may, particularly in the parent-education model, exacerbate the parent's feelings of guilt, inadequacy, and ambivalence toward the child, and that they may have undesirable effects if the child receives so much early stimulation that there results an increase in later aberrant behavior. Overall, the most impressive and consistent results suggest that retarded children who are enrolled in early treatment programs display improved social skills and increased motivation to participate in activities, thus reflecting their true potential rather than actually improving in intellectual ability.

RESIDENTIAL CARE.   One of the most difficult decisions facing the physician who cares for a retarded child is whether to suggest that the family consider placement of their child in residential care outside of his own home. Surveys of institutions that care for retarded children indicate that the majority of residents fall within the range of moderately to severely retarded. In general, the child who is more severely handicapped, more deformed, more stigmatized, or more in need of physical care and supervision will be suggested for referral for residential care earlier. The stress and hardship of caring for such a child at home cause considerable physical and emotional drain on the parents, particularly the mother, who usually assumes most of the burden.

When dealing with parents of a young infant with multiple deformities or Down's syndrome, where the prognosis is relatively clear, the role of the pediatrician or family physician as a counselor to the family is often compromised by what the obstetrician and others may already have told the parents. If the pediatrician is the first to inform the parents of the diagnosis, his approach may be more flexible. A complete exposition of the diagnosis and its implications during the first interview may overwhelm most parents, even those who indicate a preference for full disclosure of all aspects of the problem. Sensitive and detailed discussion is necessary to enable the family to work through the sense of grief and loss, and if possible both parents should be participants in visits that are extended over a period of time, so that the implications can be fully explored. It is important for the physician to avoid imposing his personal beliefs and prejudices on parents who are grappling with decisions that can have long-range social, emotional, and financial implications for the entire family. The physician should make it clear that even when residential placement is desired by the parents it is often difficult to arrange; appropriate, acceptable facilities may not be readily available at a cost the parents can afford. Most states have ceased to construct large institutions for the retarded, and this trend toward deinstitutionalization, coupled with development of a range of community services for the preschool and school-age group and diminution of the social stigma of having a retarded child, has considerably diminished the pressures for early residential placement. Given these options, most parents prefer to care for their retarded infant or young child at home. The physician may offer advice on these matters, particularly if he is well acquainted with the family's social dynamics and has some knowledge of community resources. However, he should not make the final decision about home care versus residential placement. If he is not well acquainted with the range of educational and other services that are available, it is his obligation to refer the family to an agency or organization that can be of help to them. Organizations such as the local affiliates of the National Association for Retarded Citizens and other voluntary agencies are often helpful in supplying this information to both the physician and the family. Finally, when the physician does advise the family on the question of residential placement, he should consider the total effect of the retarded child on this particular family, and he should be aware that residential placement does not eliminate or erase the problems engendered by having a retarded family member. Once he has done his part in providing information and needed insight, the physician can best help the family by being supportive of their decision.

In situations where the parents of a mildly or moderately retarded child have maintained the child at home with the help of community programs, new strains may arise as adolescence approaches. As with the normal adolescent, behavior problems may increase and the child may become more difficult to manage, even as social, vocational, and recreational opportunities for this age group are less readily available. Concern arises regarding the child's incipient sexuality that is often manifested as fear of sexual abuse of the naive female or unwarranted concern about sexual aggressivity in the retarded male. As a result, parents of retarded children often reconsider or first consider the idea of residential placement. This is particularly true if the parents are advanced in age and are concerned about who will care for the child after they are gone.

As noted previously, during the last decade we have seen the growth and development of a variety of community mental retardation programs as the crowded, remote, and often dehumanizing institutions of the past have given way to more enlightened approaches. These changes not only have provided the impetus for expansion and development of a large variety of day programs and services for children and adults who remain in their own homes in the community but also have fostered development of alternative types of residential care. This has paralleled a strong movement to deinstitutionalize, to arrange for people formerly placed in large institutions to return to their communities of origin. The emphasis in all of these programs has been on normalization, the provision of as normal a living, educational, and working environment as possible. The types of alternative living arrangements in the community include small hostels, halfway houses, group homes, foster care, clusters of apartments, and in some cases independent living with either very limited supervision or no supervision. Community care has been promoted by effective advocacy programs that have through legal and political pressures enabled the retarded to utilize generic (education, social, and health) services from which they previously were often excluded. This approach, plus the increased public awareness of the problem, is bringing about a revolution in the management, care, and treatment of the mentally retarded.

SEX EDUCATION AND CHILDBEARING. One of the most sensitive issues to deal with is sex education for mentally retarded adults and prevention of unwanted pregnancies. Until recently there were few formal sex education programs, and a primary means of avoiding pregnancies was by legislating mandatory sterilization. Surgical sterilization of the mentally retarded is still permitted by statute in some states, even without the consent of the individual, although this is becoming less prevalent following a number of recent court decisions on the ethical and legal issues involved. The question of true informed consent for sterilization from an individual who is retarded presents considerable problems involving the right to be sterilized and the right not to be sterilized if sterilization is not desired. Increasing public concern about violations of the rights of all citizens has engendered notable caution in regard to sterilization, abortion, and other aspects of medical care for the retarded and other disabled citizens.

Despite popular misconceptions and public concerns, unwanted pregnancies among the institutionalized population and those in supervised community care are relatively uncommon. This is related to such factors as the general absence of promiscuity among the retarded, the increased use, acceptance, and availability of birth control measures including intrauterine devices and the pill, and the increasing availability of sex education, which can be successfuly taught through creative new methods of instructing mentally retarded people of almost all levels of functioning in the utilization of these preventive techniques. While the liberalization of abortion laws has facilitated easier termination of unwanted pregnancies, the complex medical, legal, and ethical issues alluded to previously make it essential to deal with each case individually. The physician must bear in mind the relative infrequency of genetically transmitted mental retardation in the total spectrum of mental retardation and consider carefully the needs and desires of mildly retarded persons who may wish to marry and even bear children versus the needs of such children and of the larger society.

DOWN'S SYNDROME

Genetic conditions that are associated with mental retardation are discussed in Chapter 8. The most common of these conditions is Down's syndrome, which will be discussed here. This entity was first described by Langdon Down in 1866. In 1959 Lejeune and his associates reported that the syndrome was associated with a consistent cytologic anomaly—the presence of an excess of chromosomal material derived from one of the pairs of the G group. Originally it was thought that the extra chromosome was number 21, but recent evidence indicates that it is the number 22 chromosome. However, by convention Down's syndrome is still called trisomy 21. Karyotypic analysis has revealed that the majority of patients with Down's syndrome have 47 chromosomes with a trisomy of chromosome 21. The underlying genetic mechanism for this event is nondisjunction. A small percentage of individuals with Down's syndrome have a structural chromosomal abnormality (translocation) with a total chromosome number of 46. Translocations occur because of centric fusion of two chromosomes, which most commonly involves chromosomes 21 and 15. However, translocations involving chromosomes 21 and 25 have been reported.

There are individuals who have been found to be mildly or moderately affected whose cells karyotypically are mixtures of normal cells and cells trisomic for chromosome 21. This condition is called mosaicism and results either from nondisjunction in early cell division of a normal zygote or from loss of a chromosome in a developing trisomic zygote.

The correlation of Down's syndrome with maternal age has long been recognized. The trisomy 21 anomaly is encountered with increasing frequency in older mothers, while the rarer translocation anomaly is seen in younger mothers. There also appears to be some increased risk of Down's syndrome when mothers are very young. However, the birth of a child with trisomy 21 may occur at any maternal age, and because most children are born to mothers between the ages of 18 and 30 years, a considerable proportion of those with Down's syndrome will be born to mothers in this age range.

The etiology of the cytogenetic disturbance as-

sociated with Down's syndrome remains unknown. The increased incidence of Down's syndrome with increasing maternal age has led to the theory that the oocyte deteriorates with advancing age. This deterioration may simply be an aging factor, or it may be related to the increased exposure to deleterious environmental factors (ie, radiation, virus, etc) that occurs with time. The virus of infective hepatitis has been suspected, but this has not been proved. Thyroid autoantibodies are more common in mothers of babies with Down's syndrome than in controls.

CLINICAL FINDINGS. Infants with Down's syndrome are usually recognized at birth, and they become more easily recognizable during infancy and childhood (Fig. 16). With adulthood and early maturity the diagnostic features are less clearly discernible, and the adult with Down's syndrome may be perceived as a retarded person without specific etiology. Trisomy 21 and trans-

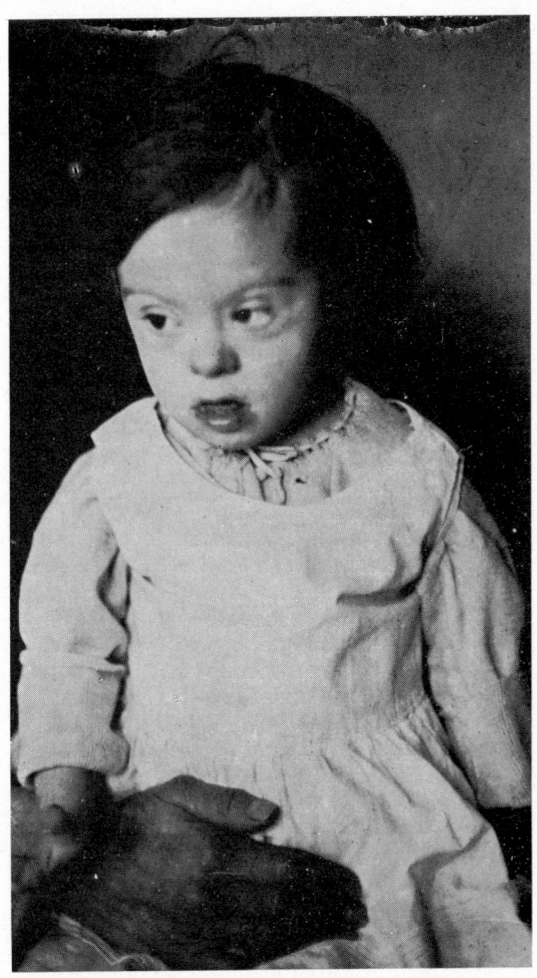

FIG. 16. Girl 4 years of age with Down's syndrome showing characteristic facies.

location are clinically indistinguishable. However, the features are less typical in mosaicism, and normal intellect has been reported in some cases. The clinical features are listed in Table 7. The most frequently reported findings eyes, are hypotonia, flat occiput, clinodactyly, upward-slanting, epicanthal folds, large tongue, and single midpalmar crease (simian line). Cardiac lesions are present in 10 to 15 percent of infants with Down's syndrome, the most frequent being endocardial cushion defects.

TABLE 7. Clinical Features in Down's Syndrome*

Head	Microcephaly; *flat occiput;* brachycephaly
Eyes	*Inner and outer epicanthal folds slanted upward and outward;* bilateral speckling of iris (Brushfield's spots) around limbic area; strabismus; refractive error; cataracts in early adulthood
Ears	*Simple or aberrant helix formation;* low set
Nose	Usually small with flattened bridge
Mouth	Tongue large and fissured; *nasopharynx small* (causes mouth breathing); abnormal morphology and frequent absence of teeth
Neck	Short; occasional webbing
Hands	*Stubby, distal triradius; radial loop on digit IV and ulnar loops of all other digits;* digital loop between digits IV and V; *incurved short 5th fingers (clinodactyly) with single crease; single four-finger-breadth midpalmar crease (simian line) (usually bilateral)*
Feet	Short and stubby; widespread 1st and 2nd toes; deep crease leading distally from angle of 1st and 2nd toes; distinctive dermatoglyphics
Abdomen	*Protuberant; umbilical hernia; duodenal atresia;* megacolon; microcolon
Skin	Dry; decreased elasticity
Heart	*Septal defects;* pulmonary stenosis; aortic stenosis
Genitalia	Male—testes undescended; small penis Female—labia minora underdeveloped; menopause early
Pelvis	Iliac wings large and flared; *iliac index measured on x-ray is decreased*
Neurologic	*Hypotonia,* normoreflexia; poor fine and gross coordination
Speech	Voice is usually low-pitched and raucous; speech has infantile omissions and substitutions

The more common clinical features are italicized.

PATHOLOGY. Although extensive neuropathologic changes have been observed, both the gross and microscopic abnormalities are variable. Myelination of white matter, immature differentiation of ganglion cells, and abnormal embryonic cell piles are all fairly common findings. Signs of maldevelopment and malfunction have been reported in the thyroid, pituitary, adrenal, and thymus glands.

INTELLIGENCE. It is important to note that in individuals with Down's syndrome intelligence is variable; the curve of levels of intelligence is a bell-shaped distribution, with the median in the lower range of mild to the upper range of moderate mental retardation. The number and severity of physical features indicative of Down's syndrome do not predict the level of intelligence, and it is not possible to predict whether any given newborn will be mildly, moderately, or severely retarded as growth and development proceed. It has been reported that the rate of intellectual development decreases as the patient gets older; this may reflect central nervous system degeneration related to premature aging or a possible arrest in psychologic and social capacities.

DEVELOPMENT. Many infants with Down's syndrome give the appearance of developing within the lower range of normal in the first few weeks of life, which often leads to unfounded parental optimism. However, in most cases all aspects of development will have slowed by the end of the first year, and the acquisition of motor and verbal skills is generally delayed. Almost all individuals with Down's syndrome ambulate by 3 to 4 years of age, while over 90 percent develop simple language by 5 years of age. This is often limited to single words or short phrases. There is increasing evidence that language deficits are relatively more severe than motor problems. The aging process is rapid, and cataracts and arteriosclerosis are frequent complications in early adult life. A rapid metabolic turnover has been implicated as a possible cause for this phenomenon.

LABORATORY FINDINGS. Laboratory investigations have yielded inconsistent findings, including the following reported abnormalities: decreased serum serotonin levels; increased serum gamma globulin levels with decreased serum albumin, low serum calcium, and decreased acid and alkaline phosphatase levels; decreased level of pseudocholinesterase and elevated serum β-aminoisobutyric acid levels. Thyroid function studies have given conflicting results.

TREATMENT. There is no specific medical treatment for this condition. Although many drugs have been tried in attempts to improve functioning, vitamins, special diets, and thyroid medication have not proved useful; while use of 5-hydroxytryptophan or L-tryptophan has been reported to increase muscle tone, these drugs have been disappointing over prolonged trials.

PROGNOSIS. Individuals with Down's syndrome who are functioning within the mild-to-high-moderate range of mental retardation can be educated to elementary-school levels of accomplishment. Although many can be employed in sheltered workshops, very few, if any, become independent in the community. Their obvious physical characteristics often lead to stigmatization and add to their problem in being accepted, even when their abilities permit them to compete vocationally. Although some may die in infancy or early childhood as a result of associated severe congenital anomalies (eg, congenital heart disease, duodenal atresia), the average lifespan is no longer as markedly shortened as it once was. At one time death as a result of respiratory and other infections was a common early occurrence, but most individuals with uncomplicated

Down's syndrome now survive to the fourth or fifth decade. Death in the middle years is believed to be related to rapid aging processes. Leukemia occurs three times as frequently as in normal children.

GENETIC COUNSELING. It is desirable to obtain chromosome studies on all children with Down's syndrome, especially if the mother is under 35 years of age at the time of birth. The occurrence of trisomy 21 in an infant, with a normal karyotype in the mother, suggests that the risk of trisomy 21 in subsequent pregnancy is low. In contrast, a mother over 35 years of age, even if she has a normal karyotype, runs a risk of recurrence that is six times as great. It is generally accepted today that any pregnant woman age 35 years or older should be offered the option of prenatal diagnostic studies.

If the propositus is found to have mosaicism or a translocation anomaly, chromosome studies should be performed on both parents and on any siblings. A phenotypically normal individual may be a carrier of the translocation. Appropriate genetic counseling on recurrence risks can then be offered by the physician. Down's syndrome has been noted in association with Klinefelter's syndrome. XXY trisomy has been reported in 6.25 percent of males with Down's syndrome in a survey performed soon after birth, but in only 0.35 percent of older males with Down's syndrome. The reported difference in relative frequencies may mean that the combination increases the patient's risk of a shortened lifespan. Down's syndrome has also been reported in association with XXX, Turner's syndrome, and trisomy D. Of particular interest are the reports of Down's syndrome in patients with siblings who have another type of trisomy (XXY, trisomy E, XXX). This association may reflect a familial predisposition toward chromosomal errors, or they may be purely chance happenings.

References

Allen PC: The retarded citizen: victim of mental and legal deficiency. Maryland Law Forum 2:4, 1971

Bergsma D: Birth Defects: Atlas and Compendium. Baltimore, Williams & Wilkins, 1973

Birch HG, Richardson SA, Baird D, Horokin G, Illsley R: Mental Subnormality in the Community. Baltimore, Williams & Wilkins, 1970

Carter CH: Handbook of Mental Retardation Syndromes, 2nd ed. Springfield, Ill, Charles C Thomas, 1971

Conley RW: The Economics of Mental Retardation. Baltimore, Johns Hopkins University Press, 1973

Crome L, Stern J: Pathology of Mental Retardation. Edinburgh, Churchill and Livingstone, 1972

de la Cruz FF, la Veck GD: Human Sexuality and the Mentally Retarded. New York, Brunner/Mazel, 1973

Eisenberg L: Behavioral manifestations of cerebral damage in children. In Birch HG (ed): Brain Damage in Children: The Biological and Social Aspects. Baltimore, Williams & Wilkins, 1963

Frankenburg WK, Dodds JB: The Denver Developmental Screening Test. J Pediatr 71:181, 1967

Grossman H (ed): Manual on Terminology and Classification in Mental Retardation. Baltimore, Garamond Predemark, 1973

Holmes LB, Moses HW, Halldorsson S, et al: Mental Retardation: An Atlas of Diseases with Associated Physical Abnormalities. New York, Macmillan, 1972

Laufer MW, Denhoff E: Hyperkinetic behavior syndrome in children. J Pediatr 50:463, 1957

Masland RL, Sarason B, Gladwin T: Mental Subnormality. New York, Basic Books, 1958

Mental Retardation. A Family Crisis. The Therapeutic Role of the Physician. GAP Vol V, Report No 56. New York, Group for the Advancement of Psychiatry, 1963

Nawas M, Braun S: The use of operant techniques for modifying the behavior of the severely and profoundly retarded. Ment Retard 8:18, 1970

Pediatrician and the Child with Mental Retardation. Committee on Children with Handicaps, Evanston, American Academy of Pediatrics, 1971

Richmond JB, Tarjan G, Mendelsohn RS (eds): Mental Retardation—A Handbook for the Primary Physician. Chicago, AMA, 1974

Smith DW: Recognizable Patterns of Human Malformation. Philadelphia, WB Saunders, 1970

Tarjan G: Sex: a tri-polar conflict in mental retardation. Presented at the Joseph P. Kennedy, Jr., Foundation International Symposium on Human Rights. Retardation and Research. Washington, DC, Oct 1971

CEREBRAL PALSY

NEILS L. LOW

Cerebral palsy is the name given to a group of diverse nonprogressive syndromes affecting the brain and manifesting themselves as impairment in motor function; the term is usually limited to conditions that are presumed to have had their onset either before birth or during the first few years of life. Since its clinical manifestations as well as its causes are variable, cerebral palsy is not a specific medical diagnosis; it may include mental retardation, learning disabilities, and seizures, in addition to the motor deficit.

ETIOLOGY. Both genetic and acquired factors may be responsible for these syndromes. The acquired causes usually result in damage to the fetal central nervous system during the early gestational period, and they may be related to faulty implantation of the ovum or to diseases of the mother. Extreme nutritional deficiencies, infections, injuries, toxins, and radiation can interfere with the developing fetal brain and lead to permanent motor defects.

During the perinatal period a rapid succession of events occurs that may damage the brain and result in cerebral palsy. Prematurity is one of the most common associated conditions, and it predisposes the neonate to asphyxia and cerebral hemorrhage. In certain instances prematurity may result from pre-existing abnormalities, and it may be difficult to determine whether the brain damage is the result or the cause of prematurity. Between 20 and 25 percent of children with cerebral palsy have birth weights less than 2,500 g. Pathologic studies indicate that the most common mechanism leading to brain injury is asphyxia. Multiple births are also frequently associated; these neonates are often of low birth weight and are born prematurely. Asphyxia seems to be an important factor, especially in the second-born twin.

Another factor is the birth process, which possibly may cause venous stasis involving primarily the deep-draining veins, with resultant hemorrhage from microscopic extravasation or actual rupture of these vessels. These vascular complications are often the result of asphyxia. Full-term, small-for-age neonates are also particularly prone to cerebral palsy. The recent establishment of regional intensive care units for newborns and premature infants is likely to reduce the incidence of sequelae to neonatal disease.

Kernicterus from neonatal hyperbilirubinemia is recognized as one of the causes of the athetoid type of cerebral palsy. In such children nerve deafness, paresis of upward gaze, or mental retardation may occur. This condition has become less common because of the judicious use of exchange transfusions and, above all, because of administration of gamma globulin containing a high titer of anti-D antibody (RhoGAM) to RH-negative unsensitized mothers. In the postnatal period infections such as meningitis or encephalitis may damage the brain. Marasmus and dehydration with subsequent venous thrombosis are occasionally causative factors. Arterial occlusions occurring before or after birth may lead to infantile hemiplegia.

PATHOLOGY. Gross malformations, regardless of basic origin, are found in about one-third of autopsied cerebral palsy children. In the other two-thirds the changes, often microscopic, may be primarily cortical or subcortical. The cortical lesions are characterized by laminar degeneration, fallout of neurons, and cortical atrophy with narrowing of gyri and widening of sulci. The subcortical defects consist of atrophy of white matter and gliosis in the deep central structures, sometimes with cyst formation. The cortical changes are significantly more common in the group acquiring their complications postnatally, and the subcortical abnormalities are more frequent in conjunction with perinatal complications. Patients with athetosis, the aftereffect of kernicterus, show symmetric demyelination of the globus pallidus and the subthalamic nucleus.

CLINICAL CLASSIFICATION. The various syndromes are classified according to the predominant clinical manifestations. The classification given in Table 8 is descriptive and simple.

TABLE 8. Clinical Classification of Cerebral Palsy

Spastic cerebral palsy
  Spastic hemiplegia
  Spastic tetraplegia
  Diplegia
    1. Spastic
    2. Atonic
  Spastic paraplegia
  Monoplegias and triplegias
Dyskinetic cerebral palsy
  Athetosis
  Other forms
Ataxic cerebral palsy
Mixed syndromes

SPASTIC CEREBRAL PALSY. The spastic types of cerebral palsy are due to involvement of the upper motor neurons and are characterized by increased tone of the involved musculature, exaggeration of the deep tendon reflexes, clonus, abnormal reflexes (extensor plantar response), and a tendency to contractures (Fig. 17).

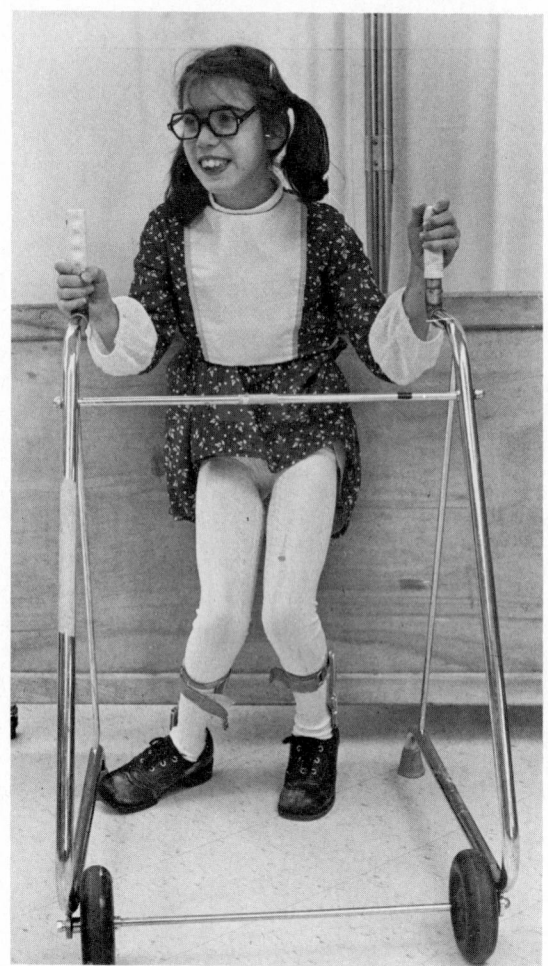

FIG. 17. Typical standing posture in spastic diplegia. (Courtesy of Dr. M. H. Levy.)

Hemiplegia. Hemiplegia implies that both extremities on one side are involved; the upper extremity is usually more severely affected than the lower. In addition to increased deep tendon and periosteal reflexes in the involved arm and leg, there usually is some weakness of the peripheral muscles, especially dorsiflexors at the wrist and the ankle, and the forearm supinators. Because of this weakness and the tendency to contracture, the upper extremity tends to be kept flexed at the elbow, wrist, and fingers. In mildly affected children the handicap may not be apparent while the patient rests in a sitting or standing position, but walking and especially running accentuate the abnormal position. In the mildest cases spasticity may be elicited by supination of the previously outstretched pronated arm, which will produce flexion of the elbow on the involved side.

The child with spastic hemiplegia characteristically walks more on the toes than on the heel, with a resultant circumduction of the affected leg in order to compensate for the apparent lengthening. Mildly affected children appear to have a normal gait; they walk well on tiptoes, but are unable to walk on the affected heel with the toes elevated. This functional asymmetry may be enhanced by running. Further evidence of a mild hemiplegia may be obtained from an examination of the child's shoes: the unaffected side shows normal heel wear, while the involved side has a scuffed toe and a relatively unworn heel. The signs of upper motor neuron involvement are often elicited in the paretic extremities. Characteristically there is increased tone, with tightness of the adductors of the thigh, the hamstrings, and the posterior calf muscles. This results in an inability to fully abduct the thigh, to extend the leg at the knee, and to dorsiflex the foot. The involved extremities, especially the upper, may be shorter in length and have reduced muscle volume. In addition to the weakness, the involved hand may show cortical sensory impairment with inability to discriminate objects (astereognosis). This is best demonstrated by placing familiar small objects in the child's hand and having them identify them without the aid of vision. Useful function can rarely be attained in the presence of such a deficit. There may be evidence of a central facial weakness and a homonymous hemianopsia.

Tetraplegia. The designation tetraplegia or quadriplegia is used when spasticity involves all four extremities to approximately the same degree. The clinical manifestations described above are present symmetrically, or nearly so, on both sides. Tightness of the hip adductors and the hamstring muscles (knee flexors) is usually more marked in this condition than in hemiplegia. A few children with spasticity in all extremities have more involvement of the arms than the legs. Some clinics use the term double hemiplegia in these instances. Children with equal involvement of all four extremities may manifest pseudobulbar palsy. Speech is dysarthric, swallowing is impaired, and lingual protrusion and palatal movement are restricted, but the gag reflex is usually present. These clinical manifestations are the result of bilateral involvement of the corticobulbar fibers.

Spastic Diplegia. Spastic diplegia is characterized by greater involvement of the lower limbs than the upper limbs. The demarcation between tetraplegia and diplegia is not always clear; it frequently depends on individual judgment regarding degree of involvement of the upper and lower extremities. The child with typical spastic diplegia is frequently the result of a premature birth; he may be recognized by clinical signs of spasticity in the lower extremities and relatively mild abnormal findings in the upper limbs. In the young child the

arms and hands may appear free of involvement, with only careful reexaminations later demonstrating slight findings such as weakness of dorsiflexors of the wrist or abnormal posturing when running.

Atonic diplegia is an unexplained variant of this form of cerebral palsy. It is characterized by marked delay in all motor milestones, decreased tone of the musculature of the lower extremities with increased range of passive movement, normal or increased deep tendon reflexes, and mental retardation. The presence of deep tendon reflexes differentiates atonic diplegia from anterior horn cell disease and peripheral nerve disease. A characteristic sign is flexion of the hips when the child is suspended upright under the arms (Foerster's sign). Atonic diplegia is a stage in the development of the affected child; as the child becomes older hypertonicity usually supervenes and the hyperextensibility disappears. Because of this developmental change this diagnosis usually can be made only in children between 6 months and 4 years of age.

Spastic Paraplegia. Spastic paraplegia refers to involvement of both legs but complete sparing of the upper extremities. Paraplegia is most often due to spinal cord pathology and only rarely results from brain disease. The differentiation between diplegia and paraplegia may be difficult, since hand involvement in diplegia may not be readily evident. Paraplegia, like spastic diplegia, is characterized by adduction spasms of the thighs that lead to a scissoring gait, a tendency to flexion contracture at the knees, and a tightening of the heel cords (Achilles tendons) with resulting toe gait.

Monoplegias and Triplegias. Monoplegias and triplegias are rare conditions involving one and three extremities, respectively. In triplegia one arm is usually the limb that is spared.

DYSKINETIC CEREBRAL PALSIES. Dyskinesia implies an impairment of volitional activity by uncontrolled and purposeless movements that disappear during sleep. These movement disorders are often related to lesions of the basal ganglia. The most common type is athetosis, which is characterized by relatively slow, wormlike, writhing movements usually involving all four extremities, as well as the face, the neck, and to a lesser degree the trunk. A child may display a similar pattern for years, but the clinical picture may vary somewhat with age. When the movements have a jerky component they resemble chorea, and the term choreoathetosis is used. The abnormal movements are less apparent when the patient is relaxed, and they increase under stress or tension. During various periods of the natural life cycle of this form of cerebral palsy, abnormal movements, rigidity, and dystonia may be seen, but these variations do not justify a separate classification with arbitrary definitions and separations. Athetosis is usually symmetric, but some degree of asymmetry may occur. Athetosis involving only one extremity or part of an extremity is exceedingly rare. Because of the continuous movements of extremities and trunk, hypertrophy of some muscles is common, especially around the neck and in the paravertebral area. The athetosis due to kernicterus often has associated nerve deafness and paresis of upward gaze.

ATAXIC CEREBRAL PALSY.   The ataxic variety of cerebral palsy is characterized by ataxic phenomena from early childhood and a lack of progression of the disease. It is related to a static lesion of the cerebellum or its pathways. Involved children have a wide-based gait and have difficulty in turning rapidly; they perform fast repetitive movements poorly and show decomposition on the finger-to-finger and finger-to-nose pointing tests. Any evidence of progression, foot deformity, abnormal sensory findings, or familial history of ataxia would exclude the diagnosis of this form of cerebral palsy. The ataxic type has the best prognosis for functional improvement.

MIXED FORMS.   Clinical manifestations of more than one type of cerebral palsy may be present in some children. The combination of spasticity and athetosis is seen most frequently, and ataxia and athetosis may be found. Although it may be difficult to separate the features of multiple involvement, the clinical phenomena in a child with a mixed form are characteristically the summation of the findings of both types involved.

ASSOCIATED CONDITIONS.   Children who have motor disabilities that fall within the definition of cerebral palsy may have additional syndromes. The most common of these are seizure disorders and mental retardation. The frequency of convulsions in children with cerebral palsy is difficult to assess, but about 25 to 35 percent of all children with cerebral palsy have epilepsy. Seizures are more common in the postnatally acquired forms of cerebral palsy. They are present in over 40 percent of children with hemiplegia and are less common in the other spastic varieties. Dyskinetic children have less than a 1 in 10 chance of developing convulsions, and ataxic patients have less than a 1 in 20 chance. Seizures may be evident in early infancy, but they are more frequent between 2 and 6 years of age. In some patients the onset may be delayed until the second decade. Varied seizure patterns such as infantile spasms, grand mal, focal, multifocal, and psychomotor are seen. The type of seizure may be related to age of onset.

The prevalence of mental retardation has variously been reported to be as low as 25 percent and as high as 75 percent, but these figures are meaningful only when the type of cerebral palsy is considered. The incidence is highest in the mixed group, less in the spastic type, still lower in athetosis, and least in ataxia. Nevertheless, individuals with a severe movement disorder may be extremely handicapped by their physical disability and lack of control of tongue, swallowing, and hand movements; they may be unable to function adequately even if they are highly intelligent. Intelligence is statistically lower when cerebral palsy is associated with a seizure disorder. Aside from speech delay in mental retardation, cerebral palsy may be associated with a variety of speech disorders, including different degrees and expressions of aphasia, articulatory disturbances, apraxias, and abnormalities of rhythm.

Attention to visual handicaps is particularly important because of the high incidence of strabismus, refractive errors, and visual field defects. Visual perceptual problems are commonly encountered in children with cerebral palsy. Deafness is uncommon except in children with athetosis due to kernicterus. Peripheral hearing loss (hypacusis) must be differentiated from lack of response to speech and other auditory stimuli in children who are not deaf (central hearing loss or dysacusis).

INCIDENCE.   The differences in incidence among the various series reported are so great that no true frequency can be given. Most reports from the United States give a higher birth incidence than is reported in the European literature. The most extensive survey throughout an entire country was made by Hansen in Denmark. He found an incidence of 1.3 per 1,000 births. This study also revealed that the birth incidence and the frequency of cerebral palsy in Denmark were on the increase at that time. Of all children with cerebral palsy, approximately 70 percent are spastic, 15 percent athetotic, and 5 percent ataxic; the remaining 10 percent have more than one type, most often spasticity with athetosis. In the Cerebral Palsy Clinic of the Columbia-Presbyterian Medical Center in New York City the incidence of athetosis and ataxia has been decreasing over the last 20 years. Most spastics have either hemiplegia (40 to 45 percent) or diplegia (35 percent); monoplegia and triplegia are rare forms.

LABORATORY DATA.   The common laboratory tests such as urinalysis, blood count, and sedimentation rate do not contribute to the diagnosis and differential analysis of the cerebral palsies. Roentgenograms of the skull should be done routinely. Asymmetries may be seen in hemiplegic children, and relative microcephaly is not uncommon, but usually the films are normal. Electroencephalography cannot be used as a diagnostic tool to differentiate cerebral palsy from other neuropathologic conditions. Clearly abnormal electroencephalograms are common in all types of cerebral palsy whether seizures are manifestly present or not. The most common electroencephalographic abnormality is spike seizure discharge. Asymmetries may occur with or without seizure discharges.

COURSE AND PROGNOSIS.   By definition, cerebral palsy is the result of a static lesion of the brain that cannot be cured and does not progress; however, the clinical picture can change with time. Spasticity may not become apparent until late in the first year of life. Children with spasticity manifest a tendency to contracture, and without proper management the handicap may increase. Untreated spastics who once could walk with or without aids have been known to become chairbound or bedridden. Frequent seizures may disable some children, and the associated repeated asphyxia may further reduce their intelligence. Apparent improvement may be seen in some nonretarded children with the athetotic or ataxic varieties of cerebral palsy.

TREATMENT.   The management of children with cerebral palsy varies with the child's age, the type and severity of involvement, the presence or absence of seizures, and the degree of intellect. It is important that none of these aspects be regarded as an isolated factor requiring treatment; the whole child and his family must be properly cared for, including social and educational factors (p. 1801).

The motor aspects can be modified to a certain degree. Spastic children develop contractures, and this tendency can be counteracted by surgical and nonsurgical means. Tendons that are tight can be stretched by passive and active exercises. The intervention of a physical or occupational therapist can frequently produce beneficial results. Stretching exercises can be made more effective with certain mechanical devices. Examples of such devices are short leg braces with adjustable stops to prevent footdrop or toe-walking. This type of brace is sometimes used only at night to keep the foot dorsiflexed during sleeping hours. The Benesh Brace Boot (by Markell) prevents the patient's heel from slipping up within the shoe. Stretching the tight adductors of the thighs can be accomplished at night by a so-called **A** frame that separates the legs during resting hours. Various splints can be used to prevent contracture of wrist flexors, finger flexors, and thumb adductors. A variety of orthopedic procedures have been devised for the correction of contractures that do not respond to medical measures. Deformity alone is rarely an adequate indication for surgery; specific functional improvement should be expected to result from an operative procedure before it is chosen. Athetosis and other forms of dyskinesia are affected only slightly, if at all, by exercises and appliances. In general, braces are contraindicated in athetosis.

Medications have frequently been unsuccessful in reducing spasticity or influencing the abnormal movements of cerebral palsy. Diazepam (Valium) will ameliorate spasticity and athetosis in some children in whom emotional tension contributes to the severity of the clinical manifestations. Dantrolene sodium (Dantrium), a new hydantoin derivative, has been shown to produce relaxation of skeletal muscle by an effect beyond the myoneural junction and directly on the muscle itself. The dosage in children should be started at 1/mg/kg twice daily and increased very gradually until good results are obtained, but the dose should not exceed 100 mg four times a day. The management of seizures requires the daily use of anticonvulsants.

Significant mental retardation makes treatment a more difficult problem. Given two children with very similar physical handicaps, better results can be expected in the child with normal or near-normal intelligence than in the retarded child. The best results can be obtained when parents and the child can actively cooperate in treatment. Other ancillary methods of treatment can reduce the individual child's handicap; these include speech therapy for children with difficulties in verbal communication and early correction of visual handicaps. Psychotherapy may occasionally be of value in some children; it is of more benefit in helping the family adjust to the handicapped child. School placement must be individualized, just as are other forms of management. If the child is not retarded and the physical handicap is not severe, regular school placement is indicated. Special classes should be recommended only if the child is unable to perform adequately in a normal setting. Where available, classes for physically handicapped children of normal intellect or for the retarded should be recommended. Institutional care may become advisable for children who cannot be managed at home because of physical, social, or emotional factors affecting them or the family.

References

Christensen E, Melchior J: Cerebral Palsy—A Clinical and Neuropathologic Study. Clinics in Developmental Medicine No 25. London, National Spastics Society, 1967

Ellis E: The Physical Management of Developmental Disorders. Clinics in Developmental Medicine No 26. London, National Spastics Society, 1967

Gold AP, Carter S: Treatment of cerebral palsy. In Conn HF (ed): Current Therapy. Philadelphia, WB Saunders, 1969

Hagberg B, Sanner G, Steen M: The dysequilibrium syndrome in cerebral palsy. Acta Paediatr Scand [Suppl 226] 1972, p 1

Heimer CB, Cutler R, Freedman AM: Neurological sequelae of premature birth. Am J Dis Child 108:122, 1964

Low NL, Downey JA: Cerebral Palsy. In Downey JA, Low NL (eds): The Child with Disabling Illness. Philadelphia, WB Saunders, 1974

Malamud N, Itabashi HH, Castor J, Messinger HB: An etiologic and diagnostic study of cerebral palsy. J Pediatr 65:270, 1964

Perlstein MA, Hood PN: Infantile spastic hemiplegia. I. Incidence. Pediatrics 14:436, 1954

———— Hood PN: Infantile spastic hemiplegia. III. Intelligence. Pediatrics 15:676, 1955

———— Hood PN: Etiology of postnatally acquired cerebral palsy. JAMA 188:126, 1964

EDUCATION OF HANDICAPPED CHILDREN

SELMA G. SAPIR AND BERNICE M. WILSON

Recent scientific and medical discoveries combined with better medical care have succeeded in mitigating some of the more damaging effects of many childhood diseases. Accompanying this diminution in serious childhood illnesses has been a corresponding increase in chronic problems of a type that not all physicians are accustomed to seeing. These include behavioral, social, and cognitive problems that cause difficulty in school and at home and interfere with optimal learning. Such problems are complex and multifactorial and are related to economic, social, and environmental forces, all of which impinge on the growing child and tend to exaggerate his biologic weaknesses. Grossman has defined learning disorders as "anything which interferes with the student's learning. . . . Mental retardation, perceptual handicaps, neurological dysfunction, immaturity, emotional problems, behavioral difficulties, sociocultural disadvantages, and a host of other problems are all considered as learning disorders."

As federal and state laws are enacted to establish screening, identification, or intervention programs for high-risk children, physicians will find themselves consulted by schools, organizations, and parents who need guidance. Parents may be confused by controversies and specialized viewpoints within the field and by sensationalized articles in the lay press. At the same time, schools will increasingly ask physicians to help formulate treatment plans for children who cannot cope in the classroom.

Many modern social patterns of industrialization and family living are antithetical to optimal child growth and development. Young children need opportunities to explore in a secure supportive environment, but instability, noise, crowding, and social isolation decrease opportunities for developmental experiences and create tensions for families at all socioeconomic levels; poverty compounds all such problems. In addition, poor children are at greater risk of malnutrition due to lack of adequate nutrients in the diet and to ignorance of nutritional values even when a wider selection of food is available. The relationship of poor nutrition to impaired development is well known. Birch said that "poor children are not merely born into poverty, they are born *of* poverty, and are thus at risk of defective development even before their births."

The learning process is inextricably intertwined with personality development; school is the child's work. If the child is unable to learn he begins to perceive himself as being in some way defective, and unless he receives encouragement at home and in school he may give up or react with hostility and defiance; ie, failure to learn breeds a low self-image, which in turn inhibits the child from daring and caring to try again.

Like all children, handicapped children can learn and do learn, at a pace and in a manner related not only to their individual endowment and maturational patterns but also to the environment. There is a continuum of learning problems from the most severe (as in the case of the profoundly mentally retarded and/or physically impaired) to the child with a fairly normal but uneven developmental pattern. In order to learn, all children need stability and sound educational approaches, but the normal child may surmount adverse home and school conditions that may overwhelm the child with problems. Many damaged children cannot function except in a well-organized and structured setting in which they can learn to cope in their own style. It is important that professionals try to understand the underlying problems and acknowledge individual differences in children.

Diagnostic labeling in an attempt to help children may in fact be counterproductive, as it offers no solutions and encourages neglect of individual differences and variations in style and pace of learning. A sophisticated variation of such labeling is the practice of compartmentalizing children into deficit categories

(visual-motor or auditory-linguistic) and remediating on the basis of the alleged deficit. While such refined systems diagnosis and treatment can sensitize a teacher to special needs, they can also, like labeling, lead to a fragmented sterile view of the child that obscures rather than illuminates. The essential requisite for helping children to learn, especially handicapped children, is a humane, clear, nonpressured educational setting. If the teacher can further be helped to perceive the child's learning style and pace, it may be possible to guide the child into finding his own best compensatory mechanisms for learning. Specialists have found that it is possible for a child to use alternate sensory pathways to overcome weaknesses in functioning.

It is self-evident that learning is enhanced if opportunity for success is built into the task. Learning theorists believe that some frustration also enhances learning. Handicapped children often live with so much frustration that they tend to lose hope and begin to see themselves as being unable to satisfy themselves or others. When they are helped to succeed, no matter how simple the task, they are willing to attempt the next more complex step.

It is far easier to delineate problems than areas of healthy functioning. It is also easier for educators to develop programs that correct for specific deficits rather than to restructure the entire teaching and learning process. In such situations the child is often treated as if he were the cause of the problem, thus reaffirming his negative self-image. Skilled educational specialists choose from many specific programs those aspects that are appropriate for a particular child, utilizing methods that make maximum use of his skills while strengthening weak areas. If the adult (parent or teacher) provides the necessary tools, opportunities, and supports for continuing progress, as well as a humane, respectful, nonpressuring atmosphere, the child will find courage to explore new avenues of learning.

SUPPORT FOR PARENTS.   Working supportively and collaboratively with the parents of a handicapped child is crucial to physicians, teachers, and others who hope to succeed in aiding the child. No one is fully prepared to be the parent of a handicapped child, and parents may react with intense feelings of grief equivalent to those that result from the death of a loved one. They may also react with outward expressions of hostility, especially to those who have conveyed the bad news. The manner in which parents are involved and told about a diagnosis seems to have a lasting impact upon their later attitudes and ability to deal with the child's problems. Thus attempts to be helpful to parents are often complicated by the complexity of individual parental differences and by possible previous negative experiences with other professionals in relation to their child.

After learning that they have a handicapped child, many parents may shop for a more favorable diagnosis before eventual acceptance. Olshansky's concept of chronic sorrow as a normal reaction to a tragic situation that cannot be overcome is useful in understanding acceptance. Indeed, he questions whether acceptance is necessarily positive and suggests that it may merely mean acceptance of the professional's view of things. If hostility and shopping are recognized as phases in a normal process, it is easier for those dealing with parents to maintain an understanding and supportive relationship with them.

Grief reactions are frequently mingled with anxiety, denial, estrangement, and guilt and may be confused with rejection and other individual stress responses. The response of each parent is based on past experience; the strengths, weaknesses, and attitudes of each individual determine the manner of adapting to the situation and responding to support or to offers of help.

Professionals should not too hurriedly seek to eliminate signs of grief and denial and unrealistic expectations; parents have a lifetime in which to deal with the situation on a day-to-day basis, and it may be unnecessarily cruel to immediately deny them hope by insisting on viewing matters realistically. Clear acknowledgement of the validity of their feelings will engender a feeling of relief and provide possibilities for insight. It may also be useful to let parents know that they may go through various phases as a normal part of coming to grips with a difficult situation.

When a teacher, physician, or other professional becomes concerned about a child's development, the parents must be included in discussions of that concern, even if a full assessment has not been completed. They may have concerns of their own that have not been articulated, and they may react with relief that others agree with them. The initiation of a full-scale diagnostic assessment will then focus the diffuse anxiety that the parents have experienced in regard to the child.

SUPPORT FOR CHILD.   Parents tend to look to the pediatrician as an expert without whose advice they hesitate to embark on any new program for their child. While the pediatrician does focus on the child, he is often as guilty as many other professionals of consulting with colleagues, talking to parents, and implementing plans without ever talking directly to the child himself about how he feels, how he sees himself, and what he wishes and fears for himself. Yet the child is probably one of the most important sources of information about the true nature of his problems. Most handicapped children are aware that they are different, and they may be acutely aware of their failures and inability to please the important adults in their lives. They often see themselves as being severely impaired, and they can be extremely frightened and insecure. The reluctance of adults (parents, teachers, or physicians) to talk with them honestly about their problem tends to make them feel even more ashamed and confused. They attempt to cope in ways that are not appropriate to the situation but are in keeping with their temperament and personality (withdrawal, flight, perseveration, acting out, clownishness, denial), which may catch them up in a circular process of failure, estrangement, and further

unacceptable behavior. Energy is thus diverted, and little is left for learning.

Depending on his age and intellectual ability, the problem may be discussed directly with the child; even very young children often have surprisingly accurate perceptions of the true situation. It is useful to ask the child what he understands about the difficulties he is experiencing at home and in school; some children will talk freely and reveal considerable insight, while others will have fearful and distorted notions that must be dispelled. Honest acknowledgment of the problem usually brings great relief to the child. The loneliest children are those who cannot communicate with others, especially their loved ones, about their problems. Some children are reluctant to share their feelings, experiences, and perceptions with others. Very often a child has learned defensive maneuvers against onslaughts to his self-esteem, privacy, and autonomy. Other children try to shield their loved ones from what they consider to be the truth about themselves (their perceived inadequacy) and may even see their handicap as something that keeps the family united. It is difficult for such children to give up these roles.

Many children, when handled with respect, can be encouraged to share with the physician, although they may draw the line at opening communication with parents and teachers. Their reasons for self-protection and secrecy may be complex and variable. They may be quite correct in their assessment of their own situation as requiring caution. Many professionals inadvertently give the impression that they are on the side of the parents. Yet it is important that the teacher, psychologist, and physician be seen by the child as people who listen and care. The child and the parents must be convinced that to this particular adult the child is an important person to be respected and an autonomous being with a major role in his own life.

Psychoeducational Evaluation

When a child is referred for counseling because of school problems, the physician should keep in mind that a thorough psychoeducational evaluation by a qualified psychologist is useful. If this has not been performed through the educational system, the physician may wish to refer the child for such studies to an appropriate group or individual. The psychoeducational evaluation will explore the child's skills in reading, writing, and arithmetic, his ability to use these skills in complex ways, and his own perception of his performance. It includes information on the intellectual, perceptual (visual, auditory, motor, and integrative abilities), language, and emotional development of the child, as well as his achievement level in educational tasks.

The individual diagnostic work-up should reveal the child's skill level and his point of breakdown and should provide an analysis of errors, information on his style of learning, and a review of his functioning and behavior in reading, writing, and arithmetic, thus enabling the examiner to observe the learning processes used. When complete, such an evaluation can help in planning matters as broad as the decision about school or residential placement or as specific as size or type of class or reading approach that will be most helpful to the child.

Frequently a psychoeducational evaluation will already have been completed by the time the child and parents are referred to the physician, but in some cases the testing will have been done at a much earlier time, and in others it will have been limited in scope or improperly interpreted. In particular, stretching the age ceiling of tests or using them for children or problems for which they were not designed tends to invalidate the results. The physician needs to be able to evaluate the report and the child in the light of the child's current problems and life situation. The possible dramatic effect of the process of psychologic testing on a child must not be overlooked: he may see it as supportive, as offering some hope, as providing helpful insights into his own abilities and disabilities; or it may confirm his fears that there is indeed something very wrong with him. The physician should remember that excessive testing can be harmful to children; thus if the information is incomplete or questionable, further testing can be restricted to those specific areas about which more information is needed. Retesting with the same test instrument before a 6-month lapse is invalid because of the practice effect. Verification of test data can often be obtained by using play materials, drawings, and other nonthreatening media.

Where it is impossible to obtain anything but school reports, particularly group-standardized paper-and-pencil intelligence and achievement tests, the physician must be aware of the inadequacy of such tests (Table 9 lists commonly used tests). In the areas of intelligence and language, poor children or minority children are often penalized by particular items on many tests that are outside their experience. Physically handicapped children also may test poorly because of their motor problems rather than because of an intellectual deficit. Group tests in particular are likely to unfairly penalize handicapped children who may not be able to hold a pencil, keep their place on the paper, compete in the presence of others, sort materials readily, or even organize themselves for testing. If the child cannot read he obviously will obtain a lower intelligence quotient (IQ) score on a test in which he has to read the tasks. In some cases the form of the test rather than its content prevents a child from showing his true abilities and achievement level. A child with visual-motor problems may not complete the requirements for timed responses; he may have the capacity but may need more time than a nonhandicapped child.

TABLE 9. Commonly Used Psychologic Tests

Purpose	Test	Age Range	Scope and Value	Limitations
Developmental Infant Scales				
To measure infant's general ability	Bayley Scales of Infant Development (Bayley N: Psychological Corp) or	2–30 mo	Preferred infant test; most useful as indicator of current development levels	As with all infant scales, heavily weighted with motor items, which limits predictive accuracy
	Cattell Infant Intelligence Scale (Cattell P: Psychological Corp)	3–30 mo	Easy to administer, shorter than Gesell	Normative data not as thorough as Bayley
To measure infant and child development	Gesell Developmental Scales (Gesell et al: Psychological Corp)	4 wk to 6 yr	A useful standardized procedure for observing and evaluating behavior	Questionable predictive value
Early Identification and Screening Tests				
	Boehm Test of Basic Concepts (Boehm A: Psychological Corp)	3–6 yr	All these tests are useful as suggestive indicators of possible dysfunction. All can be given readily by school or health personnel after brief familiarization with methodology. They have some value, particularly if repeated at a later date, to show if development is progressing.	This is often misused by educators, nurses, and others who assume greater than actual validity. These are *screening* tests, and if they arouse suspicion the child should be fully and completely evaluated by standard battery. If misused they can provide fallacious IQ and lead to premature and often misleading information.
	Denver Developmental Screening Test (Frankenburg W: Ladoca Project Publishing Foundation; Mead Johnson)	0–6 yr		
	Meeting Street School Screening Test (Crippled Children and Adults of Rhode Island, Inc)	4–6 yr		

TABLE 9. Commonly Used Psychologic Tests (cont.)

Purpose	Test	Age Range	Scope and Value	Limitations
Early Identification and Screening Tests (cont.)				
	Sapir Developmental Scale (Sapir G: Brunner/Mazel)	3–6 yr		
	Vane Kindergarten Test (Clinical Psychology Publishing)	4–6 yr		
Intellectual Evaluation				
To assess the child's present intellectual level by providing an intelligence quotient, with other indicators depending on the particular test	McCarthy Scales of Children's Abilities (McCarthy D: Psychological Corp)	2.5–8.5 yr	Yields general cognitive index as indicator of child's present level of intellectual functioning; made up of enjoyable and appropriate tasks; utilizes information from play and games to ascertain child's natural abilities	Test requires sophisticated examiner with solid knowledge of child development
	Standford-Binet Intelligence Scale (Terman L, Merrill H: Houghton, Mifflin)	2 yr to adult	Yields mental age and intelligence quotient; the oldest intelligence test; well known and used frequently	No differentiation of strengths and weaknesses through subtests; requires careful interpretation of responses; by 6 years is heavily weighted with verbal items and highly correlated with school achievement; may penalize child for cultural differences or learning problems
	Wechsler Intelligence Scale for Children (WISC)	5 yr to 15 yr 11 mo	All 3 assess intelligence and yield a verbal IQ and a full scale IQ. The availability of subtests whose scoring and content make it possible for compare intertest and intratest variability is helpful diagnostically. Discrepancies between verbal and performance IQ's and subtest variability may indicate greater potential than overall scores indicate, or point to specific areas of dysfunction	Requires skilled interpretation and a task analysis approach; performance tests may be testing other than performance skills, as they may require inner language for responses; observations of behavior, verbalizations and analysis of items are often more revealing than test scores
	Wechsler Intelligence Scale for Children Revised (WISC-R)	6 yr to 16 yr 11 mo		
	Wechsler Preschool and Primary Scale of Infant Intelligence (WIPPSIE) (Wechsler D: Psychological Corp)	3 yr to 6.5 yr		
Language Evaluation				
To evaluate expressive and receptive language: to analyze communicative skills and deficiencies; and to diagnose language disorders.	Examining for Aphasia (Eisenson J: Psychological Corp)	Primarily for impaired adolescents and adults; can be used at all ages.	Can be used more broadly than test title indicates; provides opportunity to investigate many academic skills and fundamental language ability. Test is simple to administer and provides a profile of strengths and weaknesses. It may be used selectively, with examiner administering only relevant portions.	Norms are only on general age limits; subtests are not normed, so that it requires skilled interpretation

(Continued)

TABLE 9. Commonly Used Psychologic Tests (cont.)

Purpose	Test	Age Range	Scope and Value	Limitations
Language Evaluation (cont.)				
	Illinois Test of Psycholinguistic Abilities (ITPA) (Kirk S A, McCarthy J J and Kirk W: Univ. Illinois Press.	2 yrs 4 mo to 10 yrs 3 mo	Sets out to analyze various levels of communication and language organization and to delineate specific abilities and disabilities for remediation. Yields a psycholinguistic age (PLA). Test provides an opportunity for	Commonly used but has questionable overall value, reliability or validity; confusing to interpret and difficult to administer
	Peabody Picture Vocabulary Test (PPVT) (Dunn LH: American Guidance Service)	2.5–18 yr	Effective test of receptive language, especially for children with speech and motor impairment	Although it yields a verbal IQ, its use for this purpose is not justifiable, as it measures only one function (receptive language), and intelligence tests should measure many cognitive abilities
	Raven Progressive Matrices (Raven JC: Psychological Corp)	3–6 yr (Form Board) 6 yr and above (Book Form)	Said to measure conceptual thought processes in a perceptual field, without use of expressive language; interesting and nonthreatening test that resembles use of visual analogies	The test task is highly complex, involves several modes of functioning, and is therefore difficult to use in defining discrete problems
Perceptual Evaluation				
To assess motor proficiency in areas of fine and gross motor activities, visual motor functioning, kinesthetic and tactile perception; auditory discrimination; spatial relationships; sensory integrative processes; etc	Auditory Discrimination Test (Wepman J: Western Psychological Services)	Normed for 5–8 yr (may be used for older children)	Examines ability to detect likenesses and differences in pairs of words presented auditorily, a very important function because of central role of auditory processes to reading	Test is gross measure that is difficult to analyze; does not tap fine problems of auditory perception, sequencing, and integration; lack of attention may distort results
	Bender Visual Motor Gestalt Test (Bender L: Psychological Corp)	4 yr to adult	To assess visual motor functioning in relation to maturation; an important test that is not threatening, is easy to administer, and offers much information about the individual in addition to specific visual motor functioning (for which developed); helpful in testing visual perception, motor processing, intersensory integration, and compensatory mechanisms	Deceptively simple; often used and abused by unqualified people; open to overinterpretation
	Developmental Test of Visual Motor Integration (Beery KE: Follett Publishing)	2 yr 10 mo to 15 yr 11 mo	Used to assess visual motor performance in individual or group; interesting if compared with Bender, as does not require ability in spatial organization	Much less useful than Bender diagnostically
	Goldman-Fristoe-Woodcock Test of	4 yr to adult	Used to assess speech sound discrimination in both quiet	Not as well known as Wepman test

TABLE 9. Commonly Used Psychologic Tests (cont.)

Purpose	Test	Age Range	Scope and Value	Limitations
Perceptual Evaluation (cont.)				
	Auditory Discrimination (Goldman R, Fristoe M, Woodcock RW: American Guidance Service)		and noisy environments; this feature is of value, as is provision of training procedures	
	Harris Test of Lateral Dominance (Harris AJ: Psychological Corp)	7 yr to adult	Simple, clear, well-chosen, easily administered test of lateral dominance in eye, hand, and foot	Relationship of lateral dominance to learning problems remains unsubstantiated and controversial
	Frostig Developmental Test of Visual Perception (Frostig M, LeFever W, Whittlesey O: Consulting Psychologists Press)	4 to 8 yr	Pioneering effort to predict learning problems from visual perceptual dysfunction; sets out to explore eye motor coordination, figure-ground discrimination, constancy of shape perception, and spatial discrimination and relationships; useful if given individually to observe approach and style in dealing with processes	Questionable validity as predictor of academic success or as basis for grouping in class; many tasks on test are influenced by factors other than those specified; analysis is difficult; no scientific basis for assumption that ability to perform on this test is necessary precursor to reading
	Osoretsky Test of Motor Proficiency (Doll EA: American Guidance Service)	4 to 16 yr	Measures gross and fine motor proficiency and gives insight into child's motor performance	No evidence that motor abilities alone relate to possible learning problems; value in educational planning doubtful
	Perceptual Survey Rating Scale (Kephart WC: Chas E Merrill Publishing)	4–7 yr	Reveals areas of strength and weakness in perceptual motor performance; can suggest games and activities to improve functioning	Value in relation to education limited
	Southern California Sensory Integration Tests (SCSIT) (Ayres J: Western Psychological Services)	4–10 yr	Determines status of sensory integrative processes and various perceptual skills; can become part of physician's informal battery of tests; requires little verbal response	Unproven assumptions relating integration of somatic sensations to academic performance; some directions difficult to follow; underlying theory somewhat questionable
	Visual Retention Test (Benton A: Psychological Corp)	8 yr to adult	Test claims to assess visual perception, visual memory, and visual constructive abilities, and provides an excellent manual	Doubtful if diagnosis of stated functions can be made on basis of this test alone
Emotional Evaluation				
To assess and evaluate various aspects of adjustment, personality structure, ego strength, self-image, etc	Children's Apperception Test (CAT) (Bellak L, Bellak S: Psychological Corp) and Thematic Apperception Test (TAT) Murray HA: Psychological Corp)	3–10 yr 4 yr to adult	These tests are excellent in the hands of an expert. They help to assess the adjustment pattern of the subject, including fears, hopes, defense mechanisms, and ego strengths	Like Rorschach, need expert and experienced interpretation; usually given as adjunct to Rorschach

(Continued)

TABLE 9. Commonly Used Psychologic Tests (cont.)

Purpose	Test	Age Range	Scope and Value	Limitations
Emotional Evaluation (cont.)				
	Rorschach Psycho-diagnostic Plates (Rorschach H: Psychological Corp)	3 yr through adulthood	Used to evaluate personality structure, ego strengths, and reality testing; interpretation is highly complex; very useful in hands of skilled psychologist	Highly subjective interpretation; unless well acquainted with person administering test, physician should be cautious in accepting results uncritically
	Figure Drawings Draw-A-Person Test (Machover K: Chas C Thomas.)	All ages	Figure drawings, an important part of any battery, are easy to administer, usually nonthreatening to the child, and helpful in establishing rapport. Drawings can lead to verbal expressions of feelings and reveal of great deal regarding self-image, level of cognitive and emotional development, adjustment to family and environment, and intellectual ability.	Interpretation must be related to good knowledge of child development and normal patterns of expression
	Family Drawings			
	Goodenough-Harris Drawing Test (Harcourt Brace Jovanovich)			
	House-Tree-Person Test (Buck JN: Western Psychological Services)			

The significance of group achievement tests is often misunderstood. They should be viewed in the frame of reference for which they were developed: to provide a general survey of a total school population, not an individual score. Their original objective was to determine if entire school systems were teaching skills their designers deemed important. There is a high level of chance error in the individual score, so that reporting scores in units other than percentile or rank order is inappropriate. In fact, the individual child's score may be poorly related to his actual capacities, and his so-called grade score will not necessarily be his functional or instructional level.

Ideally a psychoeducational evaluation of a child with deficits should encompass the child's total functioning in his environment. If there are educational problems as a result of deficits, the child will have difficulty emotionally and socially as well as cognitively. The evaluation will lead to the formulation of a treatment plan that is not only sensible educationally but that will allow for improvement of the child's self-image and better relationships with others. The evaluation will include information on the child's overall development, such as his cognitive (intellectual) strengths and weaknesses, his visual, auditory, tactile, and kinesthetic patterns and organization, his temperamental style and pace, his ability to attend, concentrate, and focus, and his body awareness and alertness. It will also provide a picture of the child's perceptual integration, the oral and written language he uses, the language he understands, his level of frustration tolerance, his ways of relating to others, and his degree of organization or disorganiza-

tion. The psychologist must keep in mind the child's situation, including the degree of support and empathy afforded at home and in school, the degree of honest communication, the opportunities for successful completion of tasks and for autonomous functioning, and the clarity of expectations, as well as the position of the handicapped child in the family and his relationships with family members. These are all important to a real understanding of his needs and functions. When a child fails, the examiner must analyze the nature of the task and the reason for the failure. An excellent diagnostic method is to attempt to teach the child something on which he has previously failed, using a variety of approaches and exploring the limitations of his educability on that test material. The psychologist also needs to be aware of the impact of the test situation and his own personality on the performance of the child. Also, a child who has a minor illness such as a cold or who has not breakfasted or whose sleep was interrupted for any reason may test poorly. In all testing, *processes* are more important than *products*. A good psychoeducational evaluation depends on understanding what areas need to be explored, not on simply reporting test after test. The skilled psychologist who is familiar with a battery of tests will use those most applicable and informative in a given situation and will know how to utilize all or part of a given test.

TESTING.   Although technically it is not within the purview of the psychoeducational diagnostician, testing of very young children (from birth to 3 years old) has profound implications if it becomes a part of the labeling process that decides the educational course from the earliest years. *Infant testing* has been carefully standardized through studies on large populations. Among the tests frequently used are the Gesell, Cattell, and Bayley scales of infant development, as well as such screening tests as the Denver Developmental Screening Test. By using data from infant research and clinical experience with special populations, psychologists are becoming increasingly aware of the prelanguage and early cognitive development of infants and are becoming better able to assess children's patterns of development in these areas. A careful evaluation may reveal discrepancies between the child's prelanguage and language development and his gross and fine motor skills and point to potential developmental difficulties. In addition, characteristics of infant behavior patterns, including the level of activity, degree of irritability, and threshold of responsiveness, provide an increasingly sensitive framework within which to evaluate a young child's interaction with his environment.

It is imprecise and often impossible to predict later intelligence on the basis of infant developmental scales, most of which are heavily weighted with motor items, whereas tests given to older children are constructed to measure acquired skills and academic performance and are dependent largely on verbal competency. However, the fact that infant scales do not consistently predict later IQ need not preclude their use. They provide one means of assessing the child's efficiency in various functional areas, and if they are cautiously interpreted they may be helpful in developing programs for management or therapy.

Preschool testing has also burgeoned in recent years; this has been particularly obvious in the proliferation of early identification screening scales for children from 2 to 6 years of age. This has in part been in response to the concern of educators and parents about ever-increasing numbers of children failing in school, as well as in response to the findings of biomedical research directed to high-risk children. Development of programs for preschool children (2 to 5 years) such as Head Start and day care, with curricula that stress early intervention for children classified as possibly having learning problems, and enactment of educational laws requiring early screening and intervention have stimulated the search for a quick, reliable, useful, culture-free test that can be given to large numbers of children.

The content of the screening tool depends on its author's frame of reference. The tests currently in use attempt to define the child's strengths and weaknesses and focus on the remediation of deficit areas. The scales theoretically enable an examiner to provide a prescription for the teacher or remedial specialist. In general the assumptions of these tests are highly questionable, in that they suggest that the scale will be able to predict those children who will experience failure in school, that they have tapped the functions that are the cause of the learning problem, and that the teacher will understand the prescription and the suggested remedial procedures. Since validation of these assumptions is not yet available, caution is advised in accepting the premises of any currently available screening tests.

INTELLECTUAL ASSESSMENT. When assessing the school-age or preschool child, a diagnosis of intellectual capacity is an essential component of a psychoeducational evaluation. It is obviously important to distinguish between a child with an organic defect and one whose learning problems mask normal or superior ability. This can be quite difficult, because the child with severe learning difficulties may function far below his actual intellectual potential. Moreover, because many tests are based on reading ability, and the learning-disabled child is generally retarded in reading, the measured IQ may be low. This may reflect not only learning, language, and memory deficits but also defeatist attitudes learned from past failures, rather than true lack of intellectual capacity. In such cases test results cannot stand alone as the basis for diagnosis and remedial planning. In some cases IQ scores have risen markedly with appropriate educational, social, and environmental changes.

The psychologist who seeks a differential diagnosis of mental retardation must look for signs of brightness, alertness, language or conceptual skills, or sense of humor that might give clues to a higher potential. Obviously the psychologist must have a thorough knowledge of normal development and functioning before he can diagnose abnormal development. A good method for searching out hidden potential is to attempt to teach a child some tasks he has failed to master to see how much he can learn under optimal circumstances. Particular care must be taken not to underestimate the intellectual potential of children with obvious brain damage, as in the case of children with cerebral palsy whose physical handicaps and perceptual difficulties may mislead one into a diagnosis of mental retardation and assignment of an inaccurate label that may persist through life. A careful psychoeducational evaluation of the specific strengths and deficits of the child is much more important than any label and can lead to development of a teaching strategy in which strengths can be utilized in a carefully designed program to help overcome weaknesses.

INTELLIGENCE TESTS. Many standardized individual and group tests are currently being used (Table 9). The individual intelligence tests most frequently administered are the Wechsler Intelligence Scale for Children (WISC), the Wechsler Preschool and Primary Scale of Intelligence, and the Stanford-Binet Intelligence Scale. The appropriate WISC is generally the preferred test, as it is believed to have diagnostic value. It is organized to yield a verbal IQ, a performance IQ, and a full-scale IQ (calculated on the basis of both the verbal and performance scores). Each major section is divided into six subtests that are intended to tap specific areas of intellectual functioning. In spite of this attempt to separate out specific functions, a task analysis approach reveals that many of the subtests involve skills other than, or in addition to, those that the test is intended to measure. Many of the performance items, for example, require a great deal of inner language; failures may represent language dysfunctions rather than the perceptual motor deficits they are meant to reveal. Cultural differences may also invalidate results, especially where idiomatic or experiential differences make the questions difficult for the test subject to understand. Large differences between verbal and performance scores and intertest score variations are indicators of uneven cognitive development and suggest greater potential than the overall score reveals. In*tra*test discrepancies (failure on easy items and success on difficult ones within an individual subtest) may indicate high anxiety or distractibility. In general, in*ter*-test variability suggests uneven cognitive development, while in*tra*test variability tends to be more indicative of emotional factors.

The diagnostic value of the WISC test may be greatly diminished by the standard method of averaging subtest scores to obtain a total IQ. For obvious reasons this approach should be viewed with great caution. For example, a child may receive a standard score of 15 on the Similarities section of the test (which requires ability to deal with verbal abstractions, and for which 10 is the average score) and a score of 5 on the Arithmetic section. If the total score is averaged to yield a 10 (100 IQ), this average score in no way relates to the way this particular child performs; it tells us nothing of his excellence in one area requiring real intellectual ability or his deficits in another area, and in fact it distorts the information that has been obtained. Therefore such a scoring method will not add to the teacher's armamentarium in devising an approach to the learning behavior of a specific child, unless she has access to the raw data.

Observation of behavior and of verbalizations and a task analysis of items is often more revealing than test scores. Interpretation of responses is essential; a simple recounting of scores is not useful. In fact, incorrect responses may sometimes offer greater insight into intellectual processes than correct ones if the examiner inquires into the way in which the child arrived at the erroneous answer.

LANGUAGE EVALUATION. Language development and the way in which language is used must be a major component of a good psychoeducational evaluation. For the purpose of this discussion, language will be defined as the ability to deal with any and all types of symbols (on a continuum from such nonlinguistic symbols as traffic lights to such linguistic symbols as words and sentences, all of which have arbitrary meanings assigned to them) and to use them in such a way as to carry on thinking processes and expressive and receptive communication. Evaluation of language is most difficult because of the complicated relationships between receptive and expressive language and thought processes. Norms are lacking for age-appropriate language behavior, except in the most simplistic terms and in relation to discrete areas of language.

Whenever we consider language development, we must do so in the larger cultural framework in which cultural semantic differences have a large role in determining how individuals use language. Semantic complexities only add to those already mentioned and are not pathologic. The critical period of language development occurs before the age of 3 years, and early language dysfunction is an important diagnostic indicator.

Problems may become evident in infancy when there is inadequate response to verbal stimuli or later when the child shows delay in speech, does not understand, or has difficulty expressing himself. Questions about early language functioning are crucial to understanding later developmental and educational difficulties.

Communication, both expressive and receptive, includes verbal and nonverbal aspects. Oral expressive language must be considered in terms of number of words used, syntactical relationships, and accuracy of vocabulary. Receptive language can be assessed only in terms of the nature of the response to the spoken or written language of others. Orderly development of syntactical structure requires gradual acquisition of a usable vocabulary. At first the child uses simple words, and gradually he understands increasing numbers of different words that he begins to put together in short phrases and then sentences. He makes a syntactical distinction between representations, such as the difference in meaning between "Dog sees" and "See dog." Disturbances in distinguishing syntactical relationships have significant bearing on later academic functioning in language areas

Cognitive thinking depends on the capacity for inner speech, which according to Luria is the "controlling factor in man's conscious action." Disturbance in behavior, as well as hyperactivity, may be related to poorly developed or disorganized inner language (conceptual thought processes). Conceptual development proceeds from concrete thinking to visual imagery to symbolization. In the normally developing child there is great overlapping of these stages, with fluid movement up and down these three areas depending on the difficulty of the task. This fluidity persists at all ages; even a person of great intellect, when asked to attempt a difficult abstract task, may need to move to a more concrete order of thinking to resolve the problem. For example, a person with high abstract ability but poor directional sense, on coming out of a subway in a neighborhood where he is unfamiliar with his surroundings, may step down in his thinking to the lower order of visual imagery and try to visualize which way the subway was going in order to orient himself. If this method does not work he may become even more concrete in his thinking and turn his body in the direction the train was going. Some handicapped children may be unable to shift in this way because of a neurologic disability or because they tend to cling to an earlier learned response as a defense against feelings of inadequacy. Both normal and handicapped children and adults may proceed in a concrete, rigid manner, and may tend to repeat what has been successful in the past and expect familiar responses to solve new problems. This tendency to perseveration is frequently seen with certain types of brain damage and with some emotional disorders.

Because of the dynamic network of interacting forces, few guidelines for language evaluation have been developed. Evaluations should attempt to clarify differences among disorders in receptive and expressive language, syntax, and level and flexibility of conceptual thinking, so that it is possible to understand what the child is experiencing and to determine how best to communicate with him and teach him.

LANGUAGE TESTS. The most common tests in use at the present time are the Illinois Test of Psycholinguistic Abilities (ITPA), the Peabody Picture Vocabulary Test (PPVT), and Eisenson's "Examining for aphasia" test. Although the ITPA is very popular because it seems to offer an analysis of complex language functions, the psycholinguistic age and profiles can be useful only when integrated with other diagnostic procedures. Reference to specific examples of actual test responses can be most useful, as some sections offer the child an opportunity for expression of his individual language style. For example, in the subtest on verbal expression the child is handed an object like a ball and asked to tell all about it. If an 8-year-old boy tries to describe the ball by saying "to bounce, to throw, to hit" and, in spite of much prompting by the examiner, shows he is not able to shift his thinking to other attributes like color, shape, and physical characteristics, this could be interpreted as a paucity of verbal expressive ability, or more likely an index of some difficulty in shifting categories. Unfortunately, despite its popularity, the ITPA is not valid for children above the age of 10 years. It has questionable validity for children from lower socioeconomic groups or from families who do not use standard English. Its administration and scoring procedures are complex and allow many opportunities for examiner error; the titles of some of the subtests can be very misleading, and they are often used to test abilities other than those specific to the authors' intent.

The PPVT is a useful test of receptive language; if used in a nonstandardized way it can provide helpful information about reception and expression of words and sentences, including concrete and abstract concepts. Although Eisenson's test "Examining for aphasia," was developed primarily for adolescents and older children, it has the advantages of comprehensive examination and ease of interpretation, and it can be useful for all ages.

PERCEPTUAL FUNCTIONING. Another essential aspect of a psychoeducational evaluation is the assessment of perceptual functioning. Children with neurologic or developmental deficits and other learning-related problems often have difficulty in visual, auditory, kinesthetic, and tactile functioning and/or in integrating these functions. Children between the ages of 4 and 7 years use perceptual-motor functioning as a primary mode, and there is later a shift in emphasis to more cognitive levels. Residual perceptual deficits may be discernible at any age level and may interfere with thinking and learning processes, although many individuals seem to devise their own unique modes for overcoming and mastering such deficits. While an appraisal of perceptual functioning is an integral part of an evaluation, the capacity to adjust suggests that perceptual training programs are not always necessary, nor are they the optimal means of educating the child with perceptual deficits.

One of the most important and widely used tests in this area is the Bender Visual Motor Gestalt Test, which was devised to assess visual-motor functioning in relation to maturation. This test is simple to administer, but it may be gravely misinterpreted by unqualified people and should only be used selectively as part of a total evaluation. Bender standardized the designs for the age range from 4 years to adulthood to serve as a developmental test in which perception and reproduction of the Gestalt figures may vary according to the growth pattern and maturation of the individual and his organic or functional pathology. This test is an important part of any battery because in skilled hands it can serve many purposes. It is nonthreatening to children and is easy to administer; it can be given in a short time and yields valuable information about many areas of functioning, including level of development in visual-motor perception, organizational ability, ability to form gestalts out of discrete forms, and temperament and personality. It offers clues to overall functioning through observations on how the child holds a pencil, which hand he uses, the direction in which he copies, and the nature of verbalizations, and it assists in differential diagnosis between the brain-injured, mentally retarded, emotionaly disturbed, and learning-disabled. Innumerable other tests of perceptual functioning are also in use, including those of Frostig, Beery, Wepman, and Ayres. All have some value, but none is perfect. Each of them can do more harm than good when misused.

EMOTIONAL FACTORS AND PROJECTIVE TESTS. A psychoeducational evaluation does not ordinarily include projective testing, except for figure drawings, unless there is serious concern about emotional factors. Most projective tests, including the Rorschach, are dependent upon the interpretive skill of the examiner; to preclude distortion they should be done only by a psychologist with much experience in the interpretation of such tests.

Unlike other projective tests, figure drawings are part of almost every psychoeducational evaluation, because they give information on developmental levels and intellectual functioning of the child. They are easy to administer and extremely informative, and they often form a bridge to verbal exchange with the child.

While drawings may be used in different ways, some aspects of each test can be particularly helpful. The draw-a-person-test measures self-image; the house-tree-person-test compares self-image to one's adjustment to the natural world and to human and social environment; family drawings are used to assess the child's perception of his role in the family. The Goodenough-Harris drawing test measures intellectual ability. In analyzing projective aspects of drawings the interpreter must be aware that while a subject depicts only those physical and psychologic aspects that are part of his self-concept, he also taps primitive feeling levels not accessible in other language. Moreover, a subject may not draw himself but rather an ego ideal or other significant person in his life. Drawings may thus reveal aspects of cognitive functioning within the context of emotions, body image, and overall self-perception. If these are interpreted with care and sensitivity, they can be a valu-

TABLE 10. Commonly Used Tests of Academic Abilities

Tests	Comment
Individual Gilmore Oral Reading Test (Harcourt Brace Jovanovich.) Gray Oral Reading Tests (Bobbs-Merrill) Informal Reading Inventory (any publisher's graded reading series) Standardized Oral Reading Paragraphs (Gray C: Bobbs-Merrill)	Any of these reading tests can, in the hands of an experienced educational diagnostician, give important information on level, errors, and their significance
Trial Lessons for the Virtual Non-reader (Harris A, Roswell F: Clinical Diagnosis of Reading Disability. J Psychol 36:323, 1953)	A simple and pragmatic way to investigate a child's response to various reading approaches—visual, linguistic, phonic, visual motor, or kinesthetic
Wide Range Achievement Test (WRAT) (Jastak J, Bijou S, Jastak S: Psychological Corp)	Used to quickly assess academic skills, kindergarten to 12th grade, the WRAT yields a grade equivalent score that is a rough approximation of skills. It is useful for screening purposes over time, but is inaccurate at early levels.
Group California Achievement Tests (CTB/McGraw-Hill) Durrell Analysis of Reading Difficulty (Harcourt Brace Jovanovich) Gate-MacGinite Reading Readines Tests and Gates-MacGinite Reading Tests (Teachers College Press) Iowa Tests of Basic Skills(Houghton Mifflin) Metropolitan Reading Test (Harcourt Brace Jovanovich.) Murphy-Durell Reading Readiness Analysis (Harcourt Brace Jovanovich.)	All group tests tend to penalize some children. They can provide distorted results. They are clearly surveys that should be interpreted as indicators that further investigation is needed. It should be understood that the student with a learning disability may be penalized for other than specified reason.
Pre-reading Screening Procedures (Slingerland C: Educators Publishing Service) Stanford Achievement Tests Stanford Diagnostic Arithmetic Test (Harcourt Brace Jovanovich)	These do provide some specific information that can be helpful to teachers
Slingerland Screening Tests for Identifying Children with Specific Language Disability (Slingerland B: Educators Publishers Service)	Useful screening test of perceptual processes within three modalities (auditory, visual, kinesthetic), but lacks examination of conceptual processes

able adjunct to a psychoeducational or medical assessment.

Other commonly used tests of academic ability are listed in Table 10.

EDUCATIONAL PROGRAMS

Many issues relating to the education of handicapped children remain controversial. Changes in philosophy, programming, and educational methodology have been rapid and have caused confusion and controversy. How these crucial issues are viewed will determine how the learning-disabled child is defined, how his deficits are conceptualized, and on what basis remediation is predicated.

Some years ago, as a reaction to the earlier failure of diffuse, ill-defined general teaching programs, techniques were offered to remedy specific areas of weakness and impairment. Educators began to talk of prescriptive teaching and to view children as a collection of isolated skills, often losing sight of the whole child in the process. More recently, perhaps in reaction to the overemphasis on a host of different types of special classes in the past 15 to 20 years, a vogue seems to be developing favoring "mainstreaming." As always in the initiation of any educational "solution" there are concomitant dangers in the loss of options for different children and the use of labels to designate vastly different approaches. Mainstreaming is well intended; its objective is normalization of educational experiences as far as this is possible. Unfortunately, for many children the effect is akin to throwing a nonswimmer into the middle of a rapidly flowing river. In order to make an appropriate decision for a child, one must take into consideration myriad factors, such as severity and type of impairment, family patterns and needs, the child's self-image and emotional strength, and available resources and quality of educational support systems that can be offered. Also the needs of the child may change with age and development. An examination of the educational environment itself in relation to the existing needs of the child should take precedence over a particular model.

When considering an educational program for a child, it is important to bear in mind certain methodologic questions, including whether specific cognitive factors can be isolated in such a way that they can be assessed and can provide a basis for curriculum planning. Such a presumption is the foundation of the notion of prescriptive teaching, but there is some question that such fractionating is possible or fruitful. It would seem more valuable to analyze the tasks as well as the child. It is also important to ask whether teachers should teach to the strengths or correct the weaknesses of children. On a broad conceptual level one must teach through the child's strengths, but this does not preclude using measures to deal with deficits.

The child should be encouraged to become an active collaborator in trying to overcome his own weaknesses by developing an awareness of his problems and utilizing any effective compensatory mechanisms. Often the child can be helped to use good conceptual skills (for example, to consciously tackle a difficult perceptual problem). Such mobilization of the child's strengths would seem to be effective both for training where a skill is lacking and for building self-confidence and problem-solving ability. Many educators believe that it is more important to teach the processes of thinking and the means of seeking data rather than to teach the child an assortment of facts. Early learning experiences must be structured in a way that enables children to discover and integrate knowledge about the world. Cognitive functioning proceeds through developmental stages, in each of which the organism and the environment interact in a natural sequence. The environment allows for appropriate developmental learning, from which the child will build a cognitive structure on which he can achieve age-appropriate intellectual mastery. The accumulation of facts alone will not accomplish this.

An optimal environment will enable the child to develop feelings of competence and self-esteem as he masters the necessary cognitive and social skills and learns to use them in effective interaction with people and in work. Furthermore, the ingredients of ego strength and the associated competence must be fostered by the school and must be appropriate to the child's developmental stage. In the developmental interaction approach of Shapiro and Biber, "The school also promotes the integration of functions, rather than, as is more often the case, the compartmentalization of functions. Thus, the school supports the integration of thought and feeling, thought and action, the subjective and the objective, self-feeling and empathy with others, original and conventional forms of communication, spontaneous and ritualized forms of responses. . . .

Generally stated, it is the goal of the school to minimize the gap between capacity and performance by providing an environment that allows and encourages children to do what they are capable of. . . . It is a basic tenet of the Developmental-Interaction approach that the growth of cognitive functions—acquiring and ordering information, judging, reasoning, problem solving, using systems of symbols—cannot be separated from the growth of personal and interpersonal processes—the development of self-esteem and a sense of identity, internalization of impulse control, capacity for autonomous response, relatedness to other people. . . . Educational goals are conceived in terms of developmental processes, not concrete achievements."

Skills must be taught as they are needed, on a continuum and in an integrated way, so that reading, writing, perceptual, and conceptual skills can be seen as a unified whole. Emphasis should be placed on a scheme that fosters thinking processes and encourages the development of strategies that will be effective regardless of the circumstances.

Where there is a deficit in perceiving, it is not possible to train the individual as though he were at an earlier overall stage of development. Obviously, when dealing with a multilevel developmental function of great complexity, simplistic thinking is often ineffective. A child 12 years old who has a visual perceptual discrimination problem cannot be taught in the same way as the normal 4 or 5 year old child. Many of the current programs do not take such factors into account, nor do they recognize that the mere presentation of an interesting worksheet or exercise is not necessarily teaching. Many handicapped children become very frustrated at the introduction of new material; it must be carefully presented, with timing and pacing appropriate to the individual child. Stinchcombe coined the phrase "developmental pressure" to describe the educational task of providing a balance between experiences that help to consolidate the child's understanding and those that provide desirable growth-inducing challenge.

Many remedial programs have been developed in recent years, each with its adherents and its critics, each with some measure of success or failure. Some of the programs that are widely acclaimed promise instant success; others are more circumspect. Many that depend on special hardware and commercial materials have become large business ventures that utilize sophisticated advertising techniques to sell their programs and products. They often find a ready market, for as apprehension about the increasing numbers of school failures grows, it is only natural that educators and institutions begin to seek panaceas. Almost all of these special programs are luxuries in terms of expenditure and efficient use of time, but many have components that can be helpful in a particular case. Very few of the programs have been properly researched over a sufficient period of time with different types of populations, and the manner in which they are used often has evolved from a misinterpretation of what was intended by the conceptualizers. The effectiveness of any program depends upon the sensitivity, the concern, and the knowledge of child development of the professionals who employ it, and the specific training method is sometimes its least important component.

One of the basic misconceptions about each of the programs is that it will be good for all children, which is unlikely since all children behave differently, have different levels of cognitive and emotional development, and process information uniquely. Each program tends to focus on a specific narrow field, and the underlying assumption is that this field is most closely related to the learning process. Yet it should be obvious that sound educational ideas apply not only to handicapped children but to all children everywhere. The criteria for selection of programs must follow universal pedagogic principles and must meet the needs of each individual child.

Mann and Phillips question the value of assessing and trying to remedy specific areas and subareas of functioning and malfunctioning in perception, intellective performance, communication, etc. They are concerned with the widespread uncritical acceptance of many evaluative tools such as the Illinois Test of Psycholinguistic Ability, the Frostig Test of Visual Perception, the Ayres Space Test, and others that claim to develop potentialities and remedy inadequacies. They express the view that these tests and programs "hold some disturbing portents for special education: in their often facile extrapolation of unsettled and controversial experimental and theoretical issues into educational and clinical dicta and practice; in their establishment of techniques of uncertain and, at best, limited validity, as prime diagnostic and treatment instruments; in their seeming disregard of the handicapped child as a unitary, though complex, organism, in their approach to him as a collection of discrete and isolated functions."

As already indicated, many of the educational programs currently in use are aimed at remedying specific deficits, and therefore they tend to be limited in scope and purpose. In general the major educational hurdle is reading, and reading problems remain paramount as the major factor in school failure, with arithmetic, language, and handwriting difficulties all contributing to the defective learning process in some children.

READING PROGRAMS. Many methods have been developed to teach reading (decoding words) at the earliest levels. The successful reader uses a complex processing system integrating many sensory channels and thought processes. While some learn primarily by looking and others by listening, many utilize a combination of sensory modalities. Not only is it necessary to translate a visual symbol into an auditory symbol, or auditory into visual, but it is also necessary to anticipate the next thought or phrase and to be sure it fits acceptably into the syntactical structure. A reading program must be considered in terms of the needs of each child. In order to be successful any program should take into consideration whether the child processes information

in wholes or in parts, which sensory channel is his primary channel, and what his particular personality needs and interests are. The *experiential approach* is considered to be successful for most children because its material is taken from their own activities and experiences, thus providing highest motivation and interests. Reading ability grows out of particular experiences and is enhanced by classroom exercises and other activities.

Commercial reading programs and reading systems are commonly used because they are readily available, completely packaged, and easily utilized. They lend themselves to large-group learning and provide manuals that offer many suggestions. Some of these programs rely on the *whole-word sight method,* which is claimed to be fast and efficient. In contrast, in most *phonetic systems* (Sullivan: Words in Color, Lippincott,) letters are each taught by their individual sounds, not their names, and children have to learn how to blend sounds. Many children never master this necessary skill. The *linguistic phonemic method* (Stern: Structural Reading) follows the theoretical phonemic structure of the language more closely and is in accord with psycholinguistic principles. Psycholinguists say that since consonants are not separated from vowels when spoken, the artificial separation in reading programs can only confuse. Therefore the consonant is always taught in conjunction with its vowel, and the child concentrates on making words by changing the endings. If this program is used strictly as suggested, children look only at the ends of words and pay little attention to beginnings; this contrasts with the phonic programs where they tend to look only at beginnings. On the other hand, the *linguistic spelling systems* (Science Research Associates, and Charles C. Merrill) teach the child the names of the letters, not their sounds. As words are identified by their letters in left-to-right progression, the child begins to realize that the words have the same letters at the end, and therefore rhyme. In each of the last three systems the child needs to concentrate on the decoding process. The requirement to read stories is even more difficult (especially for children who have good language and poor perceptual ability), because the words are all similar, both in the way they sound and in the way they look, and yet there is little meaning in the story.

Research financed by the U.S. Office of Education comparing first-grade reading methods throughout the country concluded that it is impossible to meet the needs of all children by any one method and that the most important element in any reading program is the teacher. If reading can be taught by the method most appropriate for a particular child by a teacher sensitive to his problems and needs, it can almost always be a successful and pleasurable experience. Too often reading is presented as if it were something quite alien and is taught in isolation with no relevance to the developmental stage of the child.

ARITHMETIC PROGRAMS. It is not surprising that many children with and without learning problems have difficulty with numerals and arithmetic operations. Stumbling blocks impeding mastery of arithmetic for learning-disabled children and for children whose cultural backgrounds may not have exposed them to arithmetic concepts include difficulty in linking visual memory of form, direction, and sequence to meaningful concepts, difficulty in writing numbers and in organization, problems in abstraction, and confusion in the language area of mathematics. The so-called new math, with its increased abstract terminology (such as associative, commutative, etc), its horizontal presentation of simple arithmetic operations, and its rejection of memory drill, may have created many problems especially for handicapped children. New math may necessitate remedial math. The memory facility stage lasts from 3 to 8 years of age and is never again as efficient; the loss of memory experiences during that period may never be retrieved later. Many of the new developmental series of math workbooks have formats that present difficulties in organization for handicapped children because of their problems with direction and sequence.

Some children who have severe problems with reading and/or writing may be very strong in math and may merely need help in organization and in the writing of numbers. Some may even be superior in all phases of arithmetic computation and concepts. Many young children are helped by the use of appropriate manipulative materials and real experiences, which are then translated into numbers. Older dyslexic children may be quite capable of mastering algebraic concepts but may not have memorized the multiplication tables. Many handicapped children are at a concrete level and need three-dimensional aids to assist them in computation. These are available from many commercial sources, and selections can be based on personal preference, cost, and content of the curriculum. In addition, there are programs that are built and organized to be comprehensive, individualized, and concrete, such as the *structural arithmetic programs* (Stern, Gould and Stern) based on the tenets of Gestalt psychology. The method is excellent, but it must be utilized intact and must be continued for several years for maximum realization of its goals, ie, mastery of arithmetic computation and development of mathematical thinking. The revised edition of the text suggests many remedial activities for use with children having trouble with specific concepts, but the necessary materials are expensive, although virtually indestructible. Also, teachers must have a good understanding of mathematics and should take at least a short training course in the use of this method.

Cuisenaire programs (Davidson) use the Cuisenaire rods, which are very versatile and can be adapted for a multitude of uses, permitting a great deal of flexibility and creativity on the part of the teacher. There are no lesson plans or guides, but teachers can use the rods in a variety of ways. The program extends from kindergarten through high school, with many ordering possibilities that can be the basis for selection of other texts, games, and resource materials. In addition to the rods

and activity cards, there are series of workbooks available. The value of the program depends on how it is applied and the nature of the teaching, since the rods can be used as a separate program or as supplementary materials. Instructions are clear, and the rods attractive. There are many workshops at which teachers may become more facile in their use. The size of the rods and the way they are organized make them difficult for the young handicapped child to explore, but they provide a suitable support system for the older child to use in his problem-solving, thus reducing the stigma of using "babyish crutches." The lack of grade designation makes them a useful resource for the older child who has difficulty.

LANGUAGE PROGRAMS. In the middle elementary years and continuing through junior and senior high school, the child with persistent learning problems faces an increasing amount of frustration and failure. Problems in language and thought, which are often the cause of the disability, are usually undetected in the young child and become a severe obstacle to his performance in later years. As the level of academic work becomes more abstract and requires a higher order of language organization, the child finds himself in more and more trouble. Although there is a plethora of materials for perceptual motor organization, there is a dearth of them for thinking and writing processes. There are language skill boxes with materials that limit themselves to the development of a thinking skill, such as finding the main idea or making inferences. These offer a very poor solution to the problems of organizing the child's thinking and helping him decide how and where to begin.

It is not uncommon to find remedial teachers working with children in the fourth, fifth, and sixth grades still using the same materials that the child used in earlier grades. Even when different readers and workbooks are used, failure is likely if children are forced to use the same methods. The content of the material must be appropriate, methods must ensure success, and reading miscues must be understood as thinking miscues. Where there is difficulty with word finding, syntax, or concepts, specific help should be provided. The developmental level of the child who is 11 or 12 years old or older precludes the use of methods that are appropriate for a younger child. Sometimes it is necessary to present materials in somewhat concrete ways, but this can be done with experiences that are appropriate to the child's developmental stage. For example, a cooking experience in which the child is encouraged to write down each step as he proceeds with his cooking can help with his organizational problems in writing. This allows for integration of the concrete experience with the thought processes that involve words, measurement concepts, logical sequences, and inferences.

Every teacher should accommodate not only to the cognitive level but also to the physical and psychologic levels of the youngster. At each stage of development children have different priorities, and a wise teacher makes the most of the child's interests. The adolescent years are a time of self-doubt and introspection for all. The language-disabled student is even more vulnerable because of years of failures and humiliations of varying severity. The adolescent especially needs a teacher who is sensitive to his academic efforts and to the convergent forces within him. He needs the respect of the adults around him in order to find the strength to acknowledge his learning problems and accept language therapy.

LANGUAGE THERAPY. The disabled student usually has acquired some of the elements of reading and writing, but they are often fragmented and confused. The language therapist must reorganize past language experiences and structure new learning into sequential steps in order to assure success. Older children can make learning leaps once they grasp concepts. Experiences should be provided to enable the student himself to formulate the rules. Cognitive understanding of the function and structure of English speech patterns should be acquired according to simple generalizations discovered by the student himself. Emphasis should be placed on the orderliness of the language once derivations and structure are understood. Often a student is amazed to find out how much he already knows. Oral language is always used as a precursor to written language. The teacher should help him to put his knowledge into an organized frame of reference wherein he uses his oral language as a basis for both reading and writing skills. In reading the student should be encouraged to anticipate the author's words, to guess and to check. He will discover that in many cases he can guess the author's exact wording; in other cases he may finish the thought even more skillfully than the author himself.

For many learning-disabled children the most persistent and troubling school problem is organizing and writing reports. Two important teacher-based factors contribute to these problems: one is the increase in demands in the higher grades for report-writing, note-taking, notebook organization, and creative writing; the other is the increasing assumption on the part of teachers that students in the upper elementary grades, junior high school, and high school have already developed the necessary skills to accomplish these assignments. This is a mistaken assumption. Many older students have received little instruction or poor instruction in the functional application of these organizing and writing skills. The learning-disabled student has additional problems when faced with the stringent demands of higher education.

The teacher can help the student in many ways. Teachers should state their expectations exactly, so that the student will know how to start an assignment. Assignments must be very specific. While the normal student can slide by when faced with questionable educational practices, the handicapped student will be felled by them. All students must be taught to write twice; revising is part of writing. One problem in rewriting and editing is the difficulty that handicapped students have in self-monitoring, ie, they often cannot find their own errors, and they need understanding and concrete instruction in this skill. Success depends on support from the teacher as well as effort from the student. The teacher must understand the cognitive, physical, and psychologic needs and characteristics of the student, as well as the appropriateness of teaching strategies within that context.

Language training programs based on the *Illinois Test of Psycholinguistic Abilities* (Kork, McCarthy, and Kirk) have become the basis for several remedial and developmental language programs that are being extensively used in schools at this time. Attempts to apply the ITPA principles to large-scale language programs have been reviewed in many studies in the past 10 years, and the consensus is that these programs are not generally efficacious in remedying language deficits. On the other hand, the *Peabody language development kits* (Dunn, Lim, and Smith: American Guidance Service, 1966) are designed to supplement the classroom language program; they are appropriate for all types of children up to 10 years of age, and they assist in building vocabulary and developing a sense of sentence structure, relationships, and reasoning ability. It is a flexible program that emphasizes overall language development and requires active involvement by the teacher; it may well succeed because it is not as doctrinaire as some others.

CONTROVERSIAL PROGRAMS. There are in vogue a number of controversial therapies that purport to help handicapped children learn. New ideas are reported constantly in newspapers and magazines. Many parents of handicapped children continually seek out and try any new suggestion that might in some way improve the functioning of their children; frequently they turn to a professional for guidance.

There are a number of therapy programs based on the assumption that by stimulating specific sensory input channels or exercising specific motor patterns one can retrain or improve the functioning of a part of the central nervous system. Well known among these programs are sensory integration training (Ayres), motor patterning (Doman-Delacato), programs for development of visual perception (Frostig), and optometric therapy. At this writing there are insufficient objective data to evaluate these techniques and little evidence to substantiate their claims. These therapies may be of value to a particular child with some special deficit, but physicians and other professionals should consider carefully before recommending such treatment over other options.

The *Ayres program of sensory integration* is based on Ayres' view that "a sensory integrative approach to treating learning disorders differs from any other procedures in that it does not teach specific skills such as matching visual stimuli, learning to remember a sequence of sounds, differentiating one sound from another, drawing lines from one point to another, or even the basic academic material. Rather, the objective is to enhance the brain's ability to learn how to do these things. If the brain develops the *capacity* to perceive, remember, and motor plan, the ability can then be applied toward mastery of all academic and other tasks, regardless of the specific content. The objective is modification of the neurological dysfunction interfering with learning rather than attacking the symptoms of the dysfunction." Her methodology includes tactile, vestibular, and other proprioceptive stimulation through rubbing, swinging, spinning, and other motor activities, as well as efforts to establish hand dominance and lateralization of cerebral function. Little research has been done to validate the results of this program, and little evidence has been offered to suggest that any such intervention programs will change brain processes or mechanisms. It is possible that by participating in the program some children may gain added control over their motor and perceptual activities and therefore build some self-esteem.

The *Frostig program for development of visual perception* (Follett Publishing) claims to train visual perception of all children in kindergarten and first grade and to be useful as a remedial program for any child with impaired visual perceptual development. The program includes exercises (body movements and manipulations) that in conjunction with worksheet activities allegedly strengthen functions such as visual motor coordination, figure-ground perception, perceptual constancy, perception of position in space, and perception of spatial relationships. It includes a teacher's guide that can provide excellent suggestions for developmental activities with the young child and a selection of stencils for production of prescribed worksheets. The worksheets follow a tight perceptual skills sequence whose value is questionable, since a child's functioning is not normally lock-stepped but flows and changes from activity to activity and is integrated throughout a range of various developmental levels. Moreover, the natural milieu of children under 6 years old is not two-dimensional worksheets, but the world of movement and objects. There is no consistent research evidence that training on this program leads to improved reading readiness or more competency in reading achievement, although there is consistent evidence that it improves scores on the Frostig tests. The practice of deferring reading instruction until after completion of the Frostig program, as is followed in some schools, is totally unwarranted. Furthermore, the training program is age-specific and should only be considered for use with children under 8 years of age. It must also be evaluated in terms of the effort and time it requires, which might better be spent on other school activities. The fractional approach will train the child in specific skills, but there is little transfer; one must question whether such training is worthwhile.

The *Doman-Delacato* approach is based on the writings of Temple Fay, and others who believed that phylogeny recapitulates ontogeny and that skills must be learned in a sequence that is logical and that is essential to adequate functioning. Where dysfunction exists this program requires regression to an earlier stage, followed by complex motor patterning procedures requiring many participants and countless hours of effort. As in the other programs discussed, research data are lacking for an objective evaluation.

The importance of *nutrition* and its effects on the central nervous system have recently received much attention. Nutrition cannot be ignored. There have been findings in underdeveloped countries that without adequate diets cognitive levels are seriously impaired. Some have suggested that learning disabilities are influenced by nutritional factors such as chemical additives and excessive carbohydrate intake. Nutritional influences on learning problems are being carefully researched, but it will take a number of years before any data will be available. Until such time, caution is recommended. The indiscriminate prescription of massive doses of vitamins, food supplements, and special diets is probably not a wise course.

Neither the families of children with learning problems nor the professionals who work with them can depend on any simple or magic cures. Unless new treatments can (under controlled conditions) reveal substantial changes in growth and competence of children, they should not be considered. Psychoeducational evaluation, chemotherapy (when prescribed and monitored by the physician), and sound educational treatment, although all very time-consuming, offer the greatest promise and have been the most productive measures.

EDUCATING CHILDREN WITH MBD. The concept of "brain damage" had its first impact on the educational scene with the publications of Strauss and Lehtinen in 1947, and later Kephart and others. Emphasis on the syndrome of brain injury or organic brain dysfunction increased as physicians became aware of a population without frank brain damage but with a definable syndrome, and educators and school psychologists began to recognize increasing numbers of children with uneven cognitive development and learning and behavior difficulties. At the same time, parents began to exert pressure to develop suitable educational programs for children who, despite apparently normal intelligence, were having severe problems in school. Children were described along a continuum from seemingly normal with reading problems to profoundly disabled with many dysfunctions, with at least 50 different names being employed to describe the syndrome. Attempts to integrate the disciplines of education, medicine, and behavioral science were unsuccessful because of the difficulties of definition. Everyone writing on the subject seemed to have different designations and theories, and tremendous effort and controversy preceded the refinement of a definition.

In 1966 a task force on terminology and identification of the child with minimal brain dysfunction was co-sponsored by the National Society for Crippled Children and Adults and the National Institute of

Neurogical Diseases and Blindness of the National Institutes of Health. The task force concluded: "The term 'minimal brain dysfunction syndrome' refers to children of near average, average or above average general intelligence with certain learning or behavioral disabilities ranging from mild to severe which are associated with deviations of function of the central nervous system. These deviations may manifest themselves by various combinations of impairment in perception, conceptualization, language, memory and control of attention, impulse or motor function. Similar symptoms may or may not complicate the problems of children with cerebral palsy, epilepsy, mental retardation, blindness or deafness." By 1968 the National Advisory Committee to the Bureau of Education for the Handicapped, U.S. Office of Education, had added its definition: "Children with specific learning disabilities exhibit a disorder in one or more of the basic psychological processes involved in understanding or in using spoken or written language. These may be manifested in disorders of listening, thinking, talking, reading, writing, spelling or arithmetic. They include conditions which have been referred to as perceptual handicaps, brain injury, minimal brain dysfunction, dyslexia, developmental aphasia, etc. They do not include learning problems which are due primarily to visual, hearing or motor handicaps, to mental retardation, emotional disturbance or to environmental deprivations." The U.S. Department of Health, Education, and Welfare, in its terminology in *Minimal Brain Dysfunction in Children,* listed the 10 most commonly cited characteristics of the condition: hyperactivity; perceptual motor impairments; emotional lability; general coordination deficits; disorders of attention (short attention span, distractibility, perseveration); impulsivity; disorders of memory and thinking; specific learning disabilities in reading, arithmetic, writing, and spelling; disorder of speech and hearing; equivocal neurologic signs and electroencephalographic irregularities.

In view of the multiplicity of characteristics and the enormous variability of presenting features, it is important to use caution in labeling a child as having minimal brain dysfunction (MBD). Each child has his own particular set of clinical manifestations, and their number, severity, and degree of deviation from the norm determine use of the MBD label. According to Gallagher and Bradley, "Children with learning disabilities are defined in varying ways but are often identified as children with specific defects in processing information or properly interpreting information from their environment. Such a problem would be revealed by developmental imbalances *within* the individual child. The key indication of trouble is wide variations and fluctuating strengths and weaknesses of this child against his own developmental norms." The major significance of learning disability in Western culture is related to the value placed not only on the acquisition of knowledge and skills but also on social adjust-

ment and peer group relationships, all of which are impaired in MBD. Learning disability is the most serious problem affecting school-age children at the present time, and it is far more prevalent in boys than in girls. It is subject to difficulty in diagnosis and disagreement regarding management; all too often its remediation has become involved with fads.

As there has been confusion in definition and description, so has there been in treatment and educational programming. It is only natural that as a new field emerges much trial and error must occur. The general educational principles and methods described earlier are applicable to the education of the child with MBD. However, it should be remembered that while most schools pay lip service to individualization and respect for the individual, children who do not fit into the routine of the curriculum are often labeled as problems. Mechanistic thinking mandates that all children be ready for school at the same time; if they are not, then individual programs should hurry them up and enable them to succeed. In practice this is not the case. Education presently uses terms like open classrooms, team teaching, and nongrading, all of which would seem to be excellent for most children and for MBD children in particular. These terms imply availability of meaningful and individual activities that should encourage the development of skills in all children. In fact, pupils in many open classrooms are left to flounder on their own, nongrading may become departmentalization that fragments the child and increases his sense of failure, and team teaching may signify double-size classes with noncooperating teachers.

The goal of all education, and more significantly for the MBD child, is a precise match between the cognitive style of the learner and the cognitive demands of the task. The child must be permitted to discover his own best learning processes and thus become his own diagnostician. For example, the child may know or may need to learn, that he needs slow pacing and repetition of directions. He may require one-to-one tutoring for a time and may also require structure, order, and a skilled teacher. Given these, the outlook is often good.

Current educational policies are focused on mainstreaming children by placing them in regular classes and providing special services within a school learning resource center and/or by utilizing itinerant teachers. In theory this would appear to be an excellent policy for those minimally handicapped, but its success or failure will depend on the quality of the programs. There is no basis for thinking that every school will have a large number of well-trained personnel who can offer MBD children an adequate support system. A successful support system must be predicated on individualization of a program and availability of personnel. Parents and professionals will have to monitor programs and make repeated demands for more qualified staff and money to furnish more services. For the child with more severe impairments mainstreaming is likely to be deleterious or inappropriate, and alternate modes may be needed.

Children with severe physical disabilities related to cerebral palsy and other orthopedic handicaps may continue to require special classes, as will some of the mentally retarded.

EDUCATING CHILDREN WITH CEREBRAL PALSY. As previously indicated, cerebral palsy encompasses a group of nonprogressive diverse motor deficits that originate in early life, and their clinical features are very variable.It is only within the last 25 years that specific attention has been given to the education of the child with this condition. Cerebral palsy appears to have increased in incidence in highly developed countries, perhaps because of medical advances that save the lives of premature and seriously ill infants who might previously have died. The cerebral palsy continuum ranges from the mildest hand tremor that only an experienced eye can detect to the most severe physical handicap of complete paralysis. As the condition may affect not only motor functioning but also higher order processes of perception, speech, and thinking, its complexity among children and the variability of disabilities in each child are its chief characteristics. It may also be associated with mental retardation, seizure disorders, visual and auditory impairment of all degrees, and other medical problems. The range and variability of dysfunction make examination, planning, and treatment very difficult, and prognosis must be deferred while rate of development and acquisition of skills are carefully and periodically reviewed.

As with all major disabilities, the development of educational and rehabilitation services for children with cerebral palsy began with parents seeking treatment for their children that was not provided by public school or health facilities. There are at present some 350 organizations involved in the education and rehabilitation of the child with cerebral palsy and generally affiliated with the United Cerebral Palsy Associations and the Easter Seal Association for Crippled Children and Adults.

The problems that arise in the care of the child are bewildering and endless; concerns regarding his development and possible future and the impact of his condition on his family cannot be underestimated. Many of these children go through their early years socially isolated. Their daily lives are complex, with hours of therapy and travel to treatment centers. Throughout the early years many parents retain the subconscious hope that cerebral palsy will respond to active treatment. If the degree of handicap is moderate to severe, these years are filled with various treatment programs and evaluations. Periodic progress reports are read selectively, with positive features maximized and negative features minimized. Since many children with cerebral palsy seem like younger children because of their small stature, their social immaturity from lack of experiences, and their delayed motor and language skills, parents tend to view them as being simply slow in growing up.

True awareness of the extent and permanence of their handicapping condition with all its ramifications (social problems, vocational difficulties, lack of independent living skills) may not occur until the onset of adolescence. In fact, the phrase the critical years is often applied to suggest this as the time child and family will need their greatest support and assistance from professionals and from the community. The adolescent may react to this new awareness in either of two equally disastrous ways: he may withdraw his effort, or he may frantically put forth maximum effort to little avail. The usual adolescent frustrations cannot be worked out through sports, endless telephone conversations, dancing, or club work. In some cases the normal desire for privacy cannot be respected because of the necessity for assistance with dressing or toileting. This can be an almost intolerable period for all concerned; parents must give up their secret wishes for a normal child with a normal future. While these critical years cannot be escaped, they can be made more bearable by sensitive and understanding physicians and educators.

Because of the nature of cerebral palsy and the complexity and range of its symptomatology, the individual with this condition presents a real challenge to the educator. Whenever it is possible, regular school placement is desirable. However, diagnosis for the purpose of educational planning is sometimes difficult. Motor impairment, bizarre movements, and language deficits often result in a misdiagnosis of mental retardation. Obviously any plan must take into consideration the particular constellation of physical, perceptual, behavior, and cognitive patterns of each child; but built into each plan must be the awareness that periodic reevaluation is essential, as the abilities and needs of the child change with growth and development.

The major educational patterns and needs of some children may be most like those of the mentally retarded, while others may have patterns and needs similar to those of children with minimal brain dysfunction. Various degrees and types of language impairment necessitate different kinds of remediation. Speech therapy alone may suffice for some, while a specialized language program may be needed for others who have difficulty in organizing sentences, and communication boards may be needed for those who are unable to use speech at all. The content of the board depends on age and specific interests and on the intellectual, perceptual, and educational levels of the child for whom the board is developed. The use of language boards, sign language, or other communication methods that are used with the child should be imparted to the famiy so that there may be carryover into the home.

Motor impairments require physical education programs and sometimes such specialized equipment as specially adapted typewriters, head pointers, individually modified wheelchairs, tape recorders, earphones, and other electronic devices. It is often desirable to include physical therapy and other treatment modalities in the school day. It is obvious that careful scheduling is necessary in order to provide this without removing the able student from important classwork.

EDUCATING MENTALLY RETARDED CHILDREN

BLUMA B. WEINER

Since midcentury there have been important changes in the treatment and education of persons who are called mentally retarded. The momentum of the human rights movement and civil rights movement has reached this group; the concepts of zero reject, mainstreaming, and normalization are guiding social and political efforts to decentralize and humanize their care and make them potential participants as well as recipients in our society. The impact of these efforts has rippled out in every direction and has affected every helping profession. The pediatrician is in a strategic position to provide helpful information and counsel to parents, to the lay community, and to his professional colleagues.

Mental retardation is regarded by many educators as the equivalent of lowered capacity for functioning in the standard school situation; it is often thought of as slowness or an inability to keep up with age peers. The condition is more complicated than such a simplistic observation suggests. While it has been customary to indicate the degree of developmental, adaptive, and intellectual deficit by classifying individuals as mildly, moderately, severely, or profoundly retarded, educators have used the words educable and trainable as gross but convenient terms to differentiate two groups: those who are perceived to be capable of achieving a useful level of literacy and socioeconomic independence (educable) and those who are perceived to be incapable of such attainments but who are able to learn self-help skills and perform useful tasks in a protected situation (trainable). Until very recently the severely to profoundly retarded, who have been presumed incapable of learning to any useful degree, have not entered the purview of public schooling. However, as a result of right-to-education rulings in federal courts and pressures by parents it is becoming commonplace to find developmental centers for this group in local and county special education systems.

Experiences during the past 20 years suggest that categorization as either educable or trainable tends to limit flexibility in program planning, especially for moderately and severely retarded children. Any child with a significant degree of developmental and/or learning disorder requires a thoughtful individual description rather than a label. The process of defining should be allied with the processes of treatment and teaching, and labeling should not be used to exclude a child from service or opportunity. Weiner employs the concept of dimensions of educability and presents an array of developmental areas that parallel and elaborate the conventional nursery and elementary school curriculum. She suggests observations on an appropriate assortment of experiences based on level, rate, and range of learning as a better basis for educational decisions and predictions than the unitary terms educable and trainable. It is important that physicians and others recognize that education of the moderately to severely retarded is a valid concept, provided that education is not narrowly construed as providing only academic training in reading, computation, etc. If, instead, education is viewed as preparation for the fullest and most effective functioning possible for the individual, the needs of the mentally retarded child can be placed in a realistic framework, and an educational plan appropriate to his abilities can be developed.

There are several aspects of the development of mentally retarded children that at various times in their lives generate particular concern. On the whole, these features correspond to the developmental tasks postulated by Erikson and by Havighurst. Parental anxiety is heightened by prolongation of the time required for their attainment and by the possiblity or probability that some of these tasks will never be achieved in the fullest sense. Initially there is concern about mastering the basic tasks related to body functions. Programs that serve severely and profoundly retarded children of preschool age must work on techniques for eliciting postural responses and controls, easing feeding difficulties, attending to various stimuli, and learning to trust adults. Programs for severely and moderately retarded children of primary age extend these efforts into the areas of teaching conventional behaviors of toileting, feeding, dressing, grooming, and getting along with other children. Language delay and articulation difficulties need special attention and training efforts, as do activities to improve general body coordination and eye–hand coordination. Accumulated evidence suggests that the incidental learning of even moderately and mildly retarded children is inefficient and requires that parents and teachers work systematically to help the children associate ideas and form concepts.

There may be a combination of global delay and specific difficulties in acquiring the abstract skills needed for reading, writing, and arithmetic, and therefore the same use of diagnostic and prescriptive teaching is needed for the retarded as for other disabled children. Instruction geared to the idiosyncrasies of the individual is essential. The retarded child should have access to a wide range of growth-promoting experiences. The basic orientation of his curriculum should be developmental: his teachers should attend to the strengthening of abilities that are already evident and the stimulation of the precursors of functions that are embryonic or latent. Instruction should be paced rather than pushed. Techniques of behavior analysis and precision teaching should be instituted where they are most appropriate. They are especially applicable in enabling a child to establish self-help skills and control his own activity.

Retarded children, like other children, need help in recognizing and expressing their feelings. They also require specific provisions to help them recognize and respond appropriately to the feelings expressed by others. They need help in social interaction with other children and with adults and assistance in learning the conventional behaviors regarding person and property. With increasing years and physical maturation, the social demands for acceptable behaviors become more pressing. Instruction and supervision must be increasingly responsive to changing needs without becoming irrational, disrespectful, and coercive. In essence, the principle of normalization should be taken to heart by every adult who works with retarded children. They should be assisted in every possible way to come into contact with the world about them and to share in the common experiences of childhood, and their educational experiences should be as comprehensive and meaningful as possible.

References

Birch HG, Gussow JD: Disadvantaged Children: Health, Nutrition and School Failure. New York, Grune & Stratton, 1970

Grossman HJ: Forward: symposium on learning disorders. Pediatr Clin North Am 20:541, 1973

SUPPORT FOR PARENTS

Freeman RD: Review of medicine in special education. The crisis of diagnosis: need for intervention. J Special Education 5:389, 1971

Olshansky S: Chronic sorrow: a response to having a mentally defective child. Social Casework 43:191, 1962

Solnit AJ, Stark MH: Mourning and the birth of a defective child. Psychoanal Study Child 16:523, 1961

PSYCHOEDUCATIONAL EVALUATION

Ayres AJ: Patterns of perceptual-motor dysfunction in children: a factor analytic study. Percept Mot Skills 20:335, 1965

Bellak L, Adelman C: The Children's Apperception Test (CAT). In Rabin AI, Haworth MR (eds): Projective Techniques with Children. New York, Grune & Stratton, 1960

Bender L: A Visual Motor Gestalt Test and Its Clinical Use. Research Monograph 3. New York, American Orthopsychiatric Association, 1938

Buck JN: The House-Tree-Person Technique. Los Angeles, Western Psychological Service, 1966

Eisenson J: When is language delay childhood aphasia? Delivered at 1975 International Conference, Association for Children with Learning Disability, New York, Feb 28, 1975

Kephart NC: Slow Learner in the Classroom. Columbus, Ohio, Charles Merrill, 1964, p 120

Koppitz EM: The Bender Gestalt Test for Young Children. New York, Grune & Stratton, 1964

Luria AR: The origin and cerebral organization of man's conscious action. In Sapir SG, Nitzburg AC (eds): Children with Learning Problems. New York, Brunner/Mazel, 1973, p 109

Myklebust HR: Development and Disorders of Written Language. New York, Grune & Stratton, 1965

Newcomer P, Hare B, Hammill D, McGettigan J: Construct validity of the ITPA. Except Child 40:509, 1974

Wepman J: Auditory discrimination, speech and reading Elementary School J 60:325, 1960

EDUCATIONAL PROGRAMS

Ayres J: Sensory Integration and Learning Disorders. Los Angeles, Western Psychological Services, 1974

Biber B: A developmental-interaction approach: Bank Street College of Education. In Parker R (ed): Pre-Schools in Action, 2nd ed. New York, Allyn & Bacon, 1975

Carman R, Adams WR: Study Skills: A Student's Guide for Survival. New York, Wiley, 1972, p 144

Chall J: Learning to Read: The Great Debate. New York, McGraw-Hill, 1967

Davidson J: Using the Cuisenaire Rods—A Photo/Text Guide for Teachers. New Rochelle, NY, Cuisenaire, 1969

Delacato CH, Doman G: Diagnosis and Treatment of Speech and Reading Problems, Springfield, Ill, Charles C Thomas, 1964

Jacobs, JN, Wirthlin LD, Miller CB: A follow-up evaluation of the Frostig Visual Perception Training Program. Educ Leadership 26:169, 1968

Kirk SA, Kirk WD: Psycholinguistic Learning Disabilities: Diagnosis and Remediation. Chicago, University of Illinois Press, 1971

Kuntz J: Modern Mathematics Made Meaningful: An Introductory Kit for Teachers. New Rochelle, NY, Cuisenaire

Mann L, Phillips W: Fractional practices in special education: a critique. Except Child 33:311, 1967

Montessori, M: The Montessori Method, New York, Schocken Books, 1964.

Sapir S: Learning disability and deficit-centered classroom training. In Hellmuth J (ed): Cognitive Studies, Vol 2. New York, Brunner/Mazel, 1972

Shapiro E, Biber B: The education of young children: a developmental-interaction approach. Teachers College Record 74:55, 1972

Stinchcombe AL: Environment, the cumulation of events. Harvard Educ Rev 39:511, 1969

Strunk W Jr, White EB: The Elements of Style. New York, Macmillan, 1972

White R: Motivation reconsidered: the concept of competence. Psychol Rev 66:297, 1959

EDUCATING CHILDREN WITH MBD

Clements SD: Minimal Brain Dysfunction in Children: Task Force I, National Institute of Neurological Disease and Blindness, Monograph 3. Washington, DC, US Department of Health, Education and Welfare, 1966, p 10

Gallagher JJ, Bradley RH: Early identification of developmental difficulties. In Gordon I (ed): Early Childhood Education. Chicago, University of Chicago Press, 1972

National Advisory Committee on Handicapped Children: Special Education for Handicapped Children, Toward Fulfillment of the Nation's Commitment, 1st Annual Report, Jan 31, 1968

Sapir S: Sex differences in perceptual motor development. Percept Mot Skills 22:987, 1966

———— Wilson B: Patterns of developmental deficits. Percept Mot Skills 24:1291, 1967

Strauss AA, Kephart NC: Pscychopathology and Education of the Brain Injured Child, Vol 2. New York, Grune & Stratton, 1958

———— Lehtinen L: Psychopathology and Education of the Brain Injured Child, Vol 1. New York, Grune & Stratton, 1948

Sutherland RL: Preface. In Smith BK (ed): Your Non-learning Child. Boston, Beacon Press, 1968

EDUCATING CHILDREN WITH CEREBRAL PALSY

Aphonic Communication for Those with Cerebral Palsy: A Guide for the Development and Use of a Conversation Board. United Cerebral Palsy Association, New York, NY

McDonald ET, Schultz AR: Communication boards for cerebral palsied children. J Speech Hear Disord 38:73, 1973

EDUCATING MENTALLY RETARDED CHILDREN

Dittman LA: The Mentally Retarded Child at Home, Children's Bureau Publication 37. Washington, DC, US Department of Health, Education, and Welfare, 1959

Erikson EH: Childhood and Society, 2nd ed. New York, WW Norton, 1963

Havighurst RJ: Developmental Tasks and Education, 3rd ed. New York, Longmans Green, 1972

Kirk SA, Karnes MB, Kirk WD: You and Your Retarded Child, New York, Macmillan, 1955

Weiner BB: Curriculum development and the dimensions of educability. Educ Therapy 2:79, 1969

Wolfensberger W: The Principle of Normalization in Human Services. Toronto, National Institute for Mental Retardation, York University, 1972

TUMORS OF THE CENTRAL NERVOUS SYSTEM

ABE M. CHUTORIAN

BRAIN TUMORS

Brain tumors are second only to leukemia as a cause of neoplasia in children. While they are exceedingly rare in the first year of life, their frequency remains fairly constant during each succeeding year. Some series indicate a significantly higher incidence of medulloblastomas and ependymomas in males, but otherwise there are no striking differences in sex incidence.

Important differences exist between children and adults in regard to both type and location of tumors. Gliomas account for 75 percent of intracranial neoplasms in children, compared with 45 percent in adults. In children 50 to 60 percent of brain tumors are infratentorial (cerebellar, fourth ventricular, and brainstem), whereas in adults they are chiefly supratentorial. Finally, 75 percent or more of brain tumors in children occur in the midline (third and fourth ventricle, optic chiasm, and brainstem). Many of the differences are accounted for by the high incidence of astrocytomas and medulloblastomas in children. The former arise predominantly, and the latter almost exclusively, in the posterior fossa. Also, craniopharyngiomas and optic gliomas primarily affect children, whereas meningiomas, pituitary adenomas, acoustic neurinomas, and metastatic tumors occur chiefly in adults.

Many intracranial neoplasms in children can only be treated palliatively. It is also frequently impossible to differentiate on clinical grounds, or even following contrast radiographic studies, between those that can and those that cannot be totally extirpated. Furthermore, many relatively slowly growing neoplasms that cannot be totally removed may be associated with prolonged survival in the absence of severe neurologic deficit. For these reasons specific diagnosis and appropriate treatment are eminently worthwhile.

CLINICAL MANIFESTATIONS. When a child presents with manifestations of increased intracranial pressure plus focal neurologic deficit, the possibility of brain tumor should be given serious consideration. In the following discussion of symptoms and signs an attempt is made to emphasize early factors that should alert the physician to the possibility of a cerebral neoplasm. Early diagnosis can often lead to effective therapy and a good prognosis.

INCREASED INTRACRANIAL PRESSURE. The classic symptoms and signs of increased intracranial pressure are headache, vomiting, diplopia, papilledema, enlarged cranium, and, late in the course, lethargy and somnolence.

Headache. Headache in children is rarely of localizing value, and there is usually nothing to distinguish the headache associated with brain tumor from that encountered in other illnesses. Perhaps the most important feature is that headache associated with tumor tends to remit and exacerbate. Presumably the remissions are associated with transient accommodation of increased intracranial pressure by ventricular dilation or spread of cranial sutures. Headache may be absent for considerable periods of time. An intermittent headache that recurs with increasing frequency and severity, that occurs after a prolonged period of recumbency at night or on arising in the morning, and that is exacerbated by coughing or straining at stool should arouse suspicion of increased intracranial pressure. In younger children the only manifestations may be marked irritability or constipation due to reluctance to strain at stool. With rare exceptions headache tends to occur frontally or occipitally but is not of localizing value; it is seen with equal frequency in supratentorial and infratentorial tumors.

Cranial Enlargement. When neoplasms arising in midline structures begin their growth early in life, obstructive hydrocephalus will occur; it cannot readily be differentiated from hydrocephalus due to other causes.

Vomiting. Vomiting is variable and intermittent in character and tends to occur on arising; it may or may not be associated with a headache. It may be an irritative phenomenon in the absence of increased intracranial pressure early in the course of posterior fossa neoplasms. It may be difficult to delineate the cause of the vomiting, but its recurrent nature should suggest an intracranial cause.

Diplopia and Strabismus Double vision is the result of a sixth nerve palsy. This is a nonspecific finding of increased intracranial pressure and does not have localizing value. Diplopia may not be apparent despite the presence of paralytic strabismus, since suppression of binocular vision by central or peripheral mechanisms occurs rapidly in children. Hence it is more common for a parent to report a tendency on the part of the child to tilt the head to one side or to turn the head laterally to view objects near the central field of vision in compensation for some degree of abducens paresis and associated internal strabismus. Another mechanism of suppression of binocular vision involves partial closure of one eye, which may be interpreted as involuntary ptosis until each eye is examined separately while the other is covered.

Papilledema. Papilledema is not always present, but it may be the only sign that intracranial pressure is elevated. Thus it is especially important to obtain adequate visualization of the fundi in the presence of unexplained vomiting and headache. Optic atrophy is unusual as a result of increased intracranial pressure early in the course of neoplasms arising distant from the optic chiasm. Optic atrophy may result from direct chiasmatic compression or infiltration (eg, craniopharyngioma, chiasmal glioma) or from chronic increased intracranial pressure where gliosis of the optic nerve prevents the development of edema.

Differentiation of papilledema from pseudopapill-edema and papillitis (optic neuritis) is important. In pseudopapilledema the blind spot may be normal in size, and it is usually possible to detect frank or buried drusen at some point along the disk margin. In papillitis there is acute loss of vision, as well as pain on ocular movement, with central or paracentral scotomas on visual field plots.

FOCAL NEUROLOGIC SIGNS. Focal neurologic signs of localizing significance may occur with or without manifestations of increased intracranial pressure.

Nystagmus. Nystagmus on fixation of gaze within the range of binocular vision is of particular importance in connection with intracranial neoplasms. However, its localizing value is limited, for any lesions involving cerebellovestibular pathways in the same location may produce nystagmus. Furthermore, unilateral cerebellar hemisphere lesions may produce bilateral manifesta-tions by compression across the midline, while lesions located entirely within the brainstem may produce nys-tagmus that is indistinguishable from that due to cere-bellar lesions. If there are coarse movements on deviation of the eyes in one direction and either fine rapid nystagmus or no nystagmus on gaze in the oppo-site direction, the lesion is very apt to be on the side to which coarse nystagmus occurs. Nystagmus may also be produced by increased intracranial pressure and by many drugs, including phenobarbital and diphenyl-hydantoin. The presence of true vertigo in association with nystagmus indicates peripheral labyrinthine dis-turbance; in children it is rarely associated with neo-plasia.

As a rule, pendular nystagmus on forward gaze with marked visual deficit occurs in the first 2 years of life and may be associated with peripheral or cortical blind-ness, congenital optic atrophy, or tumors in the chias-matic region. It is also seen as a congenital phenomenon, in which case it may be unilateral or bilat-eral, without defective vision. Vertical nystagmus im-plies intrinsic brainstem disease, but may be produced by lesions causing brainstem compression or by drugs. A paretic ocular muscle may undergo nystagmoid movements when moving the globe in the direction of its major action.

Opticokinetic nystagmus is a normal phenomenon encountered in following a moving object such as a rotating drum. Diminution or absence of this phenome-non in one direction implies a lesion of the contralateral parietal lobe; hence it is frequently but not always as-sociated with hemianopia.

Impaired Vision. The visual fields and acuity of young children are notoriously difficult to measure accurately. It is therefore mandatory for the physician to vigorously pursue the diagnostic evaluation of visual deficit in a child. Unless there is clearly full refractive correction of defective vision, which is rarely documented in younger children, the possibility of a lesion within or in the neighborhood of the optic nerves, chiasm, tracts, or radiations must be kept in mind. For reasons that are not entirely clear, fully one-third of children with optic gliomas, and not infrequently children with cranio-pharyngiomas, have their visual deficits at least partially corrected with lenses for varying periods before the diagnosis is made.

Visual field defects, generally bitemporal hemia-nopia, may be seen in optic atrophy without neoplasia, but more often they are a reflection of chiasmal com-pression by craniopharyngioma, chiasmal glioma, teratoma, or other tumors of the chiasmal area. Homo-nymous defects in the visual field may be seen with any lesion involving the optic pathways behind the chiasm.

Cranial Neuropathy. Cranial nerve involvement oc-curs as one of the first symptoms in 20 to 25 percent of children with brain tumor. Abducens paresis occurs with increased intracranial pressure, but it is of no local-izing value.

Supranuclear palsies are manifested chiefly by in-volvement of facial musculature or the tongue or as pseudobulbar palsies. In a supranuclear facial paresis the muscles of the forehead are spared, and orbicularis oculi muscles are *relatively* intact. Supranuclear lesions involving pathways to the hypoglossal nuclei result in weakness of the tongue, with deviation to the contralat-eral side, but the atrophy and fasciculations characteris-tic of a nuclear lesion are absent. In pseudobulbar palsy, although swallowing and handling of secretions may be impaired, the gag reflex and movements of the uvula are intact, thus differentiating this from bulbar palsy.

Nuclear palsies (eg, bulbar palsy) occur with brain-stem tumors, in which case multiple cranial nerves are usually involved. Differentiation from the intrinsic cranial neuropathies encountered in poliomyelitis, polyneuritis, meningitis, and other conditions such as myasthenia gravis does not usually present any diffi-culty. In brainstem gliomas the pyramidal tracts and cerebellar outflow pathways are almost invariably in-volved, giving rise to characteristic symptoms and signs.

The cranial nerves may be involved in infranuclear palsy anywhere along their course within the brainstem or along the base of the brain to their destinations. Nasopharyngeal carcinomas, chondrosarcomas, rhab-domyosarcomas, lymphosarcomas, and chordomas are the neoplasms that characteristically involve multiple cranial nerves successively in their extramedullary course. They do not commonly have sufficient bulk early in their course to produce other signs and symp-toms by compression of the base of the brain or brain-stem.

Head Tilt. Abnormal posturing of the head is seen with extraocular muscle paresis, particularly of the su-perior oblique muscle. Lesions of the pathway from the flocculonodular lobe of the cerebellum to the vestibular nuclei may produce head tilt, with the occiput tilted toward the side of the lesion. However, nuchal rigidity with some degree of head tilt occurs in association with posterior fossa neoplasms as a result of either traction on the dura and lower cranial nerves or displacement of the cerebellar tonsils. In the latter instance the head tilt is not of localizing value. Posterior fossa tumors abut-ting on the ventricular or subarachnoid spaces may pro-duce cerebrospinal fluid pleocytosis and an elevated protein content, which in association with nuchal rigidity may lead to a diagnosis of meningitis. The normal sugar and bacteriologic studies will militate against this diagnosis, but on occasion the difficulty of diagnosis is compounded by the presence of low-grade fever and, in the case of extensive subarachnoid seeding of a tumor such as medulloblastoma, by a fall in cerebrospinal fluid sugar.

Personality Change.   Personality change is hardly to be considered specific to intracranial neoplasia. However, nonspecific changes such as irritability, apathy, emotional lability, pallor, and fatigue may be early symptoms of brain tumor in children. Their presence should alert the physician to the possibility of such a lesion.

Ataxia.   Incoordination of the axial musculature is frequently referred to as titubation. Ataxia caused by cerebellar neoplasm involves the axial musculature when the tumor is vermian or midline. Cerebellar hemisphere tumors produce ataxia in the ipsilateral extremities. False localization is not uncommon because of contrecoup effects or simultaneous involvement of the midline and hemispheral structures. Ataxia is a common manifestation of brainstem gliomas due to involvement of the cerebellar pathways. The unsteadiness in such instances may be axial and/or of the extremities.

Ataxia by itself is not a valuable localizing sign. It may be seen in aqueductal insufficiency, presumably as a result of transmission of increased intracranial pressure to cerebellar pathways anywhere from the frontal lobes to the brainstem. Unilateral incoordination may result from a frontal lobe, thalamic, or cerebellar hemisphere neoplasm, and it may not be possible on clinical grounds to ascertain the source. Ataxia may also be caused by proprioceptive defects produced by lesions of the peripheral nerve root or posterior column. In this instance the ataxia is aggravated by eye closure. Other causes of ataxia include degenerative, metabolic, and infectious central nervous system disorders. So-called acute cerebellar ataxia is characterized by its relatively acute onset and course and by the absence of increased intracranial pressure (p. 1940).

Focal Pyramidal Deficit.   Slowly progressive upper motor neuron lesions are usually first manifested in children by subtle changes of handedness, posture, and dexterity that are often overlooked until the appearance of frank paralysis or marked spasticity. Examination usually reveals a combination of increased deep tendon reflexes, altered superficial reflexes, and Babinski reflexes and some degree of spasticity. Frank weakness may be manifest, but a tendency to disuse or abnormal postures of the suspected extremity often occur. The acuteness of onset of a lesion helps to differentiate congenital, vascular, traumatic, and toxic lesions from neoplastic causes. Since pyramidal deficit implies a cerebral, brainstem, or spinal cord lesion, the presence of parietal lobe phenomena is helpful in ascertaining the site of the lesion. If the child is old enough to cooperate, testing for corticosensory discriminations, visual field defects, and optikokinetic nystagmus may be helpful. Although pyramidal tract deficit is rare in association with cerebellar tumors or neoplasms in the

chiasmatic area, it is encountered occasionally when there is brainstem compression and/or infiltration.

Seizures.   Generalized psychomotor and focal motor or sensory seizures may be the initial symptoms of cerebral hemisphere neoplasms in children. The seizures may persist for years before the diagnosis becomes evident. Seizures in the pediatric age group are more likely the result of static lesions or metabolic factors. Seizures are considered an unusual manifestation of posterior fossa tumors. Ictus infratentorialis refers to the intermittent decerebrate posture observed in some children with posterior fossa neoplasms or other lesions. The best evidence indicates that such episodes are due to interruption of vermian or anterior lobe cerebellar stimuli to reticular nuclei. When accompanied by cyanosis, respiratory irregularity, and alteration of consciousness, impending cerebellar herniation through the foramen magnum may be suspected. The occurrence of convulsions in children with medulloblastoma is most readily explained by the presence of cerebral hemisphere tumor implants.

HYPOTHALAMIC AND ENDOCRINE DYSFUNCTION. Tumors giving rise to disturbances of hypothalamic and endocrine function include craniopharyngiomas, optic and other gliomas, anterior third ventricular dermoids, teratomas, and ectopic or metastatic pinealomas. It is peculiar that the manifestations differ so significantly among the different tumor types despite the large bulks and the apparently similar compressive effects of the different lesions. Thus the occurrence of sexual and somatic infantilism is the rule in craniopharyngioma, but this is uncommon in chiasmal glioma. Any sexual abnormality in chiasmal glioma is apt to involve sexual precocity, with the same being true of pineal tumors and teratomas. The diencephalic syndrome of infancy is characterized by emaciation and recurrent vomiting in a euphoric, alert baby. The lesion is usually an astrocytoma arising in the anterior third ventricle. The syndrome characteristically occurs before the tumor has produced macrocephaly or other manifestations of raised intracranial pressure. All tumors in the hypothalamic region share the propensity to produce early and progressive optic atrophy due to involvement of the optic chiasm.

DIAGNOSTIC PROCEDURES.   Ancillary procedures of value in the diagnosis of brain tumors include skull radiography, electroencephalography, echoencephalography, radioisotope brain scanning, cerebrospinal fluid analysis (pressure, cells, protein, sugar, enzymes, and Millipore filtration for identification of tumor cells), intracranial contrast radiography (pneumoencephalography, ventriculography, and cerebral angiography), and computerized transverse axial tomography. Computerized transverse axial tomography has major advantages over other radiologic techniques in the diagnosis of brain tumors of childhood because tumors can be localized without the risk of invasive techniques. Their diagnostic value is often enhanced by the use of intravenous contrast material. Also, computerized scanning can provide information concerning the solid, semisolid, or frankly cystic character of all or part of the localized mass lesion. The method is many times more sensitive than conventional radiologic procedures and can distinguish very small differences in tissue density.

TREATMENT. Specific therapy includes surgery, roentgen therapy, chemotherapy, and drugs employed to reduce increased intracranial pressure. Surgical and roentgen therapy are discussed separately for the individual tumors. Chemotherapy remains a palliative procedure of limited value in the treatment of intracranial tumors in children. Current experimentation with the use of intracarotid or intrathecal chemotherapy is not sufficiently well advanced for it to be recommended routinely. Remissions of variable duration following the use of sequential intravenous vincristine or intrathecal methotrexate have been reported. The chief indication for such treatment at present is clinical relapse following maximal permissible surgery and radiotherapy for glioblastoma, ependymoma, and medulloblastoma. The prophylactic potential of chemotherapy has not been adequately explored. Immunotherapy is also gaining as an experimental therapeutic modality.

The use of adrenocorticosteroids for the relief of increased intracranial pressure in children with brain tumor is recommended in selected cases. Dramatic results are sometimes obtained, and symptoms of increased intracranial pressure associated with edema are improved in most patients. Variable but significant improvement of focal neurologic deficit has also been observed. Adrenocorticosteroids are particularly indicated when increased intracranial pressure occurs during roentgen therapy or when decompressive surgery either has already been performed or for various reasons is being avoided. In older children dexamethasone (4 to 8 mg intravenously) may be given, followed with 2 mg intramuscularly four times daily for several days. Attempts to taper and discontinue the drug over a period of 1 to 2 weeks should be made. Corticosteroid therapy is of value postsurgically as well as preoperatively in selected cases. Patients who develop sterile meningitis (which is often accompanied by a significant febrile reaction) following either posterior fossa surgery or communication of a cystic lesion with the ventricular subarachnoid space may show striking remission of cerebrospinal fluid pleocytosis, hypoglycorrhachia, fever, and meningeal signs after corticosteroid administration. Bacterial infection should be ruled out prior to such therapy. The value of steroid therapy in patients with neoplasms of the posterior fossa must be weighed against the increased risk of intestinal ulceration in these children. In more acute situations demanding urgent treatment of increased intracranial pressure, parenteral urea or mannitol should be used and may be life-saving. The combined use of dexamethasone and mannitol tends to prevent the rebound of pressure that is characteristic following the use of urea and to a lesser extent following the use of mannitol.

METASTATIC INTRACRANIAL TUMORS. Cerebral metastatic disease in childhood is rare, accounting for only about 6 percent of tumors. Wilms' tumor and embryonal rhabdomyosarcoma are the most common, followed by neuroblastoma. Central nervous system dysfunction is preceded by pulmonary metastases in all cases.

TUMORS OF THE CEREBELLUM

Astrocytoma

Approximately 25 percent of all brain tumors in children are cerebellar astrocytomas. The highest incidence is from 5 to 8 years of age, but no age group is excepted.

CLINICAL MANIFESTATIONS. The symptoms and signs in this group are not sufficiently distinctive to differentiate them accurately from other posterior fossa neoplasms. They include signs and symptoms of increased intracranial pressure, ataxia predominating in or confined to one side in the case of a cerebellar hemisphere astrocytoma, nystagmus that is sometimes of localizing value, and head tilt. Within this symptom complex there is considerable variation. Thus a cystic astrocytoma confined to one hemisphere may produce ipsilateral intention tremor and ataxia before any other phenomena become evident, or it may result in signs of impending herniation of the cerebellar tonsils, with pyramidal deficit due to brainstem compression and possibly impairment of vision due to chronic papilledema. Cerebellar astrocytoma in children is insidious in onset, slow in progression, and relatively benign in outlook. However, the variation in duration of symptoms is quite great. The majority of patients have symptoms for 2 to 7 months prior to diagnosis, some even for several years; this contrasts sharply with the situation with medulloblastoma, where the majority are symptomatic less than 2 months prior to diagnosis.

DIAGNOSIS. Papilledema and spread of cranial sutures are commonly seen on roentgenograms. Tumor calcification is rare. Occasionally local occipital rarefaction of bone, or enlargement of the opening that admits the occipital emissary vein, will suggest the presence of a slowly growing cerebellar astrocytoma. Ventriculography will establish the location of the tumor, but not its type, which is established at the time of suboccipital craniotomy. Brachial and vertebral angiography, which delineate the posterior fossa circulation, have limited value in diagnosis of posterior fossa mass lesions; they are most helpful in patients whose cerebellar deficit is so minimal that doubt exists as to the location of the neoplasm. Radioisotope brain scanning tends to be less reliable for localization of posterior fossa tumors because of high uptake of isotope by the occipitocervical musculature and the lateral sinuses. These studies are not required routinely and are being replaced by computerized tomography, which provides more detailed information concerning the actual location of solid and cystic portions of the tumor (Fig. 18).

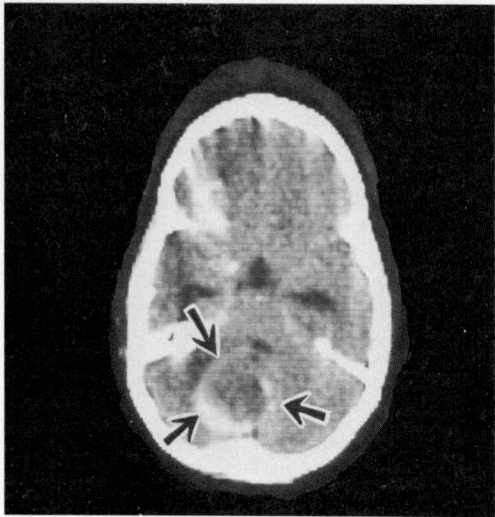

FIG. 18. Cystic astrocytoma in left cerebellar hemisphere in an 11-year-old boy (CAT scan). Note the lucency of the mass that replaces much of the left cerebellar hemisphere and the dense ring provided by the collection of intravenously injected contrast material. The fourth ventricle is collapsed anterior to the mass. (Courtesy of Dr. S. Kreps and Dr. Hilal.)

THERAPY AND PROGNOSIS. In about one-third of cases the tumor is entirely within one cerebellar hemisphere. Often the tumors are mainly cystic, but in some cases solid tissue surrounds a small cyst. In many cases the tumor can be removed totally, with eminently successful results.

The solid midline astrocytomas tend to extend deeply toward cerebellar peduncles, the aqueduct of Sylvius, and the brainstem. Therefore the surgical results are far less satisfactory than with the cystic tumors, but years of freedom from symptoms may follow decompression and partial extirpation. Partly because of their inherently slow growth and protracted development there is no proof that the growth of these tumors is altered by radiotherapy, which is therefore frequently withheld, especially following removal of a cystic cerebellar hemisphere astrocytoma. However, there is definite evidence that radiotherapy does affect astrocytomas of the brainstem and of the optic nerve and chiasm, which are similar histologically to many cerebellar astrocytomas. Of 150 patients with cerebellar astrocytoma treated at Columbia-Presbyterian Medical Center in New York, 93 had subtotal tumor excision and irradiation, with an average interval of 7 years to the time of tumor recurrence. In other series in which radiotherapy was not given, subtotal removal alone was associated with recurrence after an average interval of 3 years. Thus radiotherapy is recommended if it is believed that tumor tissue has been left behind after surgery. Postoperative intravenous fluids are rarely required after 24 to 48 hours, but during this period it is advisable to provide normal maintenance water and electrolytes. Following removal of a cerebellar astrocytoma the cerebellar deficit is characteristically aggravated, and ataxia and tremor are more pronounced. Symptoms improve progressively over several weeks or months, and although symptoms may persist, they are rarely disabling. Postoperative hydrocephalus secondary to aseptic inflammatory changes in the meninges occurs occasionally.

Medulloblastoma

Medulloblastoma is the most common posterior fossa tumor in children, comprising about 40 percent of the total. The male-to-female incidence ratio is 3 to 2, and the peak age range is from 3 to 5 years.

CLINICAL MANIFESTATIONS. The symptoms and signs of medulloblastoma are similar to those of cerebellar astrocytoma; however, its onset is typically more acute, and despite its short history the complete picture of an advanced posterior fossa neoplasm is more apt to be encountered. The signs are more characteristic of a midline cerebellar neoplasm (ie, early obstructive hydrocephalus and prominent ataxia of axial musculature). Seizures are rare with medulloblastomas, their occurrence reflecting cerebral implantation of tumor. Similarly, in advanced cases extensive seeding of a tumor along the subarachnoid space may produce the picture of a polyneuropathy, with loss of tendon reflexes, root pain, paresthesias, and cranial nerve involvement. The course is rapid and the outlook is poor.

DIAGNOSIS. Roentgenograms show cranial suture spread and features of increased intracranial pressure. Ventriculograms show dilated lateral and third ventricles, but the fourth ventricle is not usually seen because of obstruction of the aqueduct. The indications for angiography and the limitations of brain scanning are as described for astrocytomas. Computerized axial tomography accurately discloses the midline origin of these neoplasms and their solid rather than cystic character. Medulloblastomas tend to seed their actively growing cells throughout the subarachoid space. Tumor implants become a source of further seeding. A

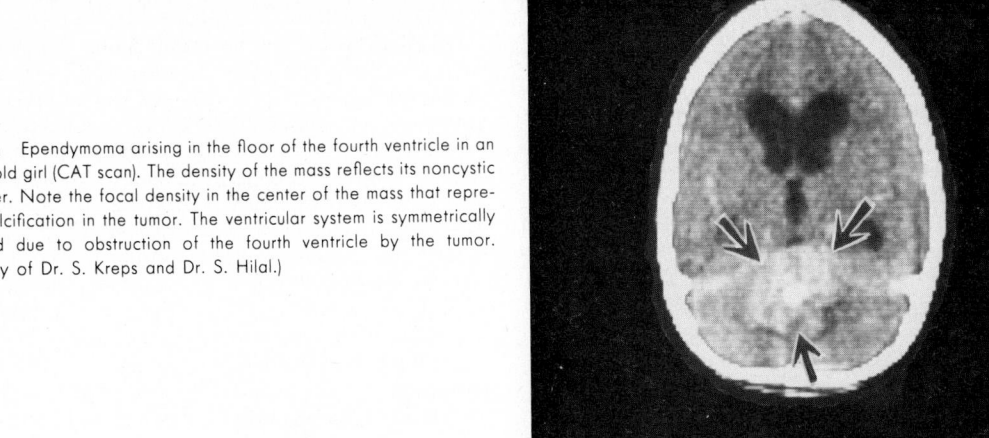

FIG. 19. Ependymoma arising in the floor of the fourth ventricle in an 8-year-old girl (CAT scan). The density of the mass reflects its noncystic character. Note the focal density in the center of the mass that represents calcification in the tumor. The ventricular system is symmetrically enlarged due to obstruction of the fourth ventricle by the tumor. (Courtesy of Dr. S. Kreps and Dr. S. Hilal.)

diagnosis of recurrence or seeding of medulloblastoma can be made in some cases by detecting tumor cells in Millipore filtrates of cerebrospinal fluid.

THERAPY AND PROGNOSIS. Since medulloblastoma cannot be differentiated with certainty from other cerebellar neoplasms without a tissue diagnosis, all patients should have a craniotomy. The tumor is characteristically bulky, and considerable portions must be removed in order to reestablish free flow of cerebrospinal fluid through the fourth ventricle; it is never possible to extirpate the tumor completely. The tumor is highly radiosensitive. Because of the strong proclivity of the neoplasm to seed tumor cells through the neuraxis, radiotherapy is initially routinely directed to the entire neuraxis. The outlook is poor; 70 percent of patients do not live more than 3 years. Newer techniques in radiation therapy are resulting in somewhat longer survivals. The use of chemotherapy was discussed previously (p. 1807).

Tumors of the Fourth Ventricle

Ependymoma

Ependymoma is the third most frequent infratentorial neoplasm, accounting for approximately 10 percent of all posterior fossa tumors in children. There is a preponderance of males (2 to 1) and a relatively early age of onset. Clinically these tumors resemble medulloblastomas more than astrocytomas. Choroid plexus papillomas and other lateral ventricle ependymomas are far less frequent. The duration of symptoms is intermediate between that of medulloblastoma and that of astrocytoma, as is the outlook for survival. The average duration of symptoms prior to diagnosis is 2 to 3 months.

The point of attachment of the tumor is almost always the floor of the fourth ventricle (which is frequently filled with tumor), and obstructive hydrocephalus occurs early. However, the ependymoma is more likely than other posterior fossa tumors to be associated with repeated vomiting as the earliest manifestation, which is due to direct stimulation of emetic centers underlying the site of origin of the tumor. On rare occasions the tumor arises in one of the lateral recesses of the fourth ventricle and grows out into the cerebellopontine angle, producing combined ipsilateral selective cranial nerve involvement and cerebellar signs, which in the adult would more likely signify an acoustic neuroma or cerebellopontine angle meningioma. Otherwise the symptoms and signs are the same as in other posterior fossa neoplasms, as described previously. Ependymomas may extend intraspinally from the posterior fossa and may even seed to more distant sites in the subarachnoid space, but this is less likely than in medulloblastoma. Consequently radiotherapy is not routinely directed to the entire neuraxis.

DIAGNOSIS. Most children with ependymomas show cranial suture separation and other signs of increased intracranial pressure. Microscopically ependymomas show extensively distributed flecks of calcium, but this is not usually seen on roentgenography. The diagnosis is more likely to be confused with that of subacute meningitis than is the case with the other posterior fossa tumors. Ventriculography is being replaced by computerized axial tomography for diagnosis (Fig. 19), but final confirmation must be made from histologic examination of tissue at craniotomy.

THERAPY. Ependymomas are inseparable from vital structures in the floor of the fourth ventricle. Therefore surgery is limited to the bulk of the tumor beyond the floor of the ventricle and is aimed chiefly at reestablishing free circulation of cerebrospinal fluid. X-ray therapy should be directed to the posterior fossa after surgery. Comments on chemotherapy have been made in the introductory treatment section (p. 1807).

PROGNOSIS. The immediate postoperative mortality is not high if the surgeon avoids excessive manipulation and dissection. In the rare cerebellopontine angle tumor, total excision is theoretically possible but is not usually achieved. Survival beyond the postoperative period is variable and is generally intermediate in duration between that with medulloblastoma and that with astrocytoma. Survival thus varies from several months to 10 years or longer, usually lasting several years.

TUMORS OF THE BRAINSTEM

Brainstem Gliomas

Brainstem gliomas occur almost exclusively in children, although no age group is exempted; they constitute approximately 10 percent of all intracranial tumors in children. The average age of onset is 6.5 years. The duration of symptoms is typically 3 to 5 months, but it may be considerably longer or shorter.

CLINICAL MANIFESTATIONS. Brainstem glioma presents with one of the most characteristic clinical pictures found among the tumors, but unfortunately it is one of the least amenable to therapy, except of a transient and palliative nature. The onset of neurologic symptoms and signs is usually insidious, and increased intracranial pressure is frequent, except as a late manifestation. Because of its location this tumor is likely to interfere early with function of cranial nerve nuclei, pyramidal tracts, and cerebellar pathways, giving rise to a characteristic triad:

CRANIAL NERVE NUCLEI. Isolated cranial nerve deficit may occur early, but later multiple involvement is the rule. Although any cranial nerve nucleus may be affected, the most common are VII, 90 percent; IX and X, 80 percent; V (sensory), 60 percent; and VI, 55 percent. Since the tumor (astrocytoma or less often glioblastoma) is infiltrative in nature, skip lesions are common, and bilateral involvement of different cranial nerves is the rule. Paresis of conjugate gaze, the most important sign localizing the lesion within the brainstem, occurs in more than half of the patients.

PYRAMIDAL TRACTS. Signs of pyramidal tract involvement occur in 80 to 90 percent of cases, but they may be masked by the more prominent ataxic manifestations or may present chiefly as subtle changes in gait, handedness, or posture of an extremity. Hemiparesis is associated with hyperreflexia and usually a Babinski response; bilateral reflex changes are frequent, and rarely weakness of all extremities is seen.

CEREBELLAR PATHWAYS. Most children have truncal and extremity ataxia that indicates involvement of corticopontocerebellar fibers coursing through the brainstem. Horizontal nystagmus is present in almost one-third of the patients.

Occasionally nuchal rigidity and urinary retention confuse the picture. Papilledema occurs at some time in approximately one-third of the patients. Sensory deficits are uncommon, and basal ganglia manifestations such as tremor and choreoathetosis are rare.

DIAGNOSIS. Cerebrospinal fluid pressure, cell count, protein, and sugar are all normal. Rarely, impingement on the leptomeninges will produce a low-grade pleocytosis and elevated cerebrospinal fluid protein. Plain radiographs of the skull are usually normal. If intracranial pressure is believed to be normal, pneumoencephalography should be performed. The typical findings include posterior and upward displacement of the aqueduct of Sylvius and the fourth ventricle, which is best seen in the lateral view. Computerized axial tomography has definite diagnostic value.

THERAPY. Craniotomy is seldom, if ever, indicated in patients with brainstem gliomas. The diagnosis is usually clear from the clinical picture and the pneumoencephalogram, and radiotherapy should be instituted. However, survival with radiotherapy averages about 12 months. Most patients improve significantly 3 to 6 weeks after beginning therapy, with incomplete clearing of cranial nerve palsies, pyramidal signs, and ataxic phenomena. The degree of improvement varies greatly, and relapse may be expected, usually within 6 months; occasionally survival with useful function may extend to several years or longer.

TUMORS OF THE THIRD VENTRICLE

Tumors of the third ventricle include pinealomas, colloid cysts, and hypothalamic gliomas. The last produces the diencephalic syndrome of infancy. Suprasellar and chiasmatic tumors, which by virtue of their origin in the region of the anterior of the third ventricle may closely mimic the signs and symptoms of third ventricle tumors, are discussed separately (p. 1814).

Pinealomas

Pinealomas comprise less than 2 percent of all gliomas. About one-third occur in children less than 15 years of age, with an average onset at 10 to 11 years of age; 80 percent are found in males.

CLINICAL MANIFESTATIONS. The classic localizing sign of a pinealoma is paralysis of upward gaze (Parinaud's syndrome), the first manifestation of which may be bilateral ptosis. This finding is indicative of pressure on the superior colliculi, above which the pineal gland protrudes. The inferior colliculi may also be involved, with the production of bilateral hearing loss. However, these signs have also been produced in the absence of tumor by increased intracranial pressure in the pineal area. A further distinctive but uncommon syndrome is macrogenitosomia praecox. Other neurologic manifestations of pineal tumors are nonspecific. Increased intracranial pressure is produced by early obstruction of the aqueduct of Sylvius, which lies close beneath the colliculi. Ataxia, nystagmus, and nuchal rigidity occur in many of these patients, and pyramidal deficit results from pressure on the long tracts in the brainstem.

DIAGNOSIS. Calcification of the pineal gland, particularly if it is unusual in character or extensive, is sufficiently uncommon in children to suggest the diagnosis in the presence of the typical clinical picture. In the past ventriculography was necessary to demonstrate the extent of the lesion, but now computerized axial tomography provides superior delineation of the presumed site of origin of the tumor, as well as its character and the degree of obstructive hydrocephalus produced.

TREATMENT. The infiltrative nature of pineal tumors precludes surgical removal. Shunting of cerebrospinal fluid (if possible, by the Torkildsen procedure) is usually indicated, followed by deep roentgen therapy.

PROGNOSIS. Symptoms may be expected to abate following therapy, with freedom from recurrence averaging 2 to 5 years, after which time a second course of radiotherapy may be considered. Occasionally a patient will enjoy many years of freedom from recurrence.

Colloid Cyst

Colloid cysts are rare; they arise in the anterior part of the third ventricle, possibly from remnants of the paraphysis, and produce symptoms by occluding the foramina of Monro. Most patients are diagnosed in adult life, but half of them have had intermittent symptoms for as long as 10 years or more and clearly have had onset of symptoms in childhood.

The characteristic syndrome involves sudden severe headache, vomiting, and stupor, especially in association with changes in position that cause the tumor to completely occlude the foramina of Monro. Since occlusion may be intermittent, the symptoms may remit and exacerbate and may be induced by flexion of the head and neck. Some patients present with nonlocalized symptoms and signs of increased intracranial pressure, others have paroxysmal symptoms severe enough to lead to stupor or loss of consciousness, and a few undergo progressive dementia as a result of slowly progressive hydrocephalus. Endocrine symptoms have not been prominent. Transient glycosuria has been noted, especially during acute attacks. Scattered instances of obesity, weight loss, polyuria, polyphagia, and acromegaly have occurred.

Prognosis after surgical removal of the cyst is good, with most patients surviving up to about 15 years of age; headache and visual symptoms are relieved. About 20 percent of these patients die suddenly, and occasionally an asymptomatic colloid cyst may be noted at autopsy after death from unrelated cause.

Diencephalic Syndrome

The diencephalic syndrome is a rare symptom complex in young infants that usually begins at 2 to 5 months of age and is associated with a glioma of the hypothalamus. The most striking features of the syndrome are the preservation of alertness and the presence of euphoria in the face of marked emaciation. Emaciation is universal, and unusual alertness, wiry vigor, and hyperkinesis are common. Vomiting is usually present but is frequently mild; it does not account for the virtual absence of subcutaneous fat. Optic atrophy and associated nystagmus, usually of the combined searching and oscillatory type, are common in view of the proximity of the tumor to the optic chiasm. Excessive diaphoresis, polyuria, and tremor are variable symptoms. Some cranial enlargement may occur, but usually the head appears enlarged because of the wasted trunk and extremities. Acute peptic ulceration and gastric hemorrhage may occur.

The occurrence of emaciation and undue alertness in infants with hypothalamic tumor, rather than the growth retardation and obesity that are more commonly associated with neoplasms of this region in older children, is unexplained. Marked emaciation does occur occasionally in older children with hypothalamic tumors, and it is not necessarily restricted to gliomas. The diagnosis is confirmed by pneumoencephalography, which because of the open fontanelle can safely be performed even in the presence of optic atrophy and in unusual instances of suspected hydrocephalus. Plain radiograms of the skull are not helpful, and the cerebrospinal fluid protein content is usually normal.

Because of the location of the neoplasm, surgical excision is impossible, and only roentgen therapy can be offered. The prognosis for long-term survival is poor, with death usually occurring between 10 months and 2 years of age. Exceptional cases show a more striking response to radiotherapy and do well for many years.

THALAMIC TUMORS

Cerebral tumor is generally not considered in the differential diagnosis of extrapyramidal signs and symptoms in children. However, basal ganglia tumors have been reported in children, and a syndrome similar to parkinsonism may occur, with tumors involving both thalami. The frequency of tumors in this location in childhood is greater than the number of reported cases would suggest.

A rhythmic alternating tremor of one extremity is the common finding. Other manifestations include athetosis, torsion spasm, posturing, rigidity, and bradykinesia. A thalamic tumor in a child is more likely to masquerade as a cerebellar or cerebral tumor. Thus a tremor indistinguishable from that produced by a cerebellar neoplasm or hemiparesis of varying degree may be the earliest or sole manifestation of a thalamic tumor in children. Despite profound hemiplegia associated with thalamic tumors in children, sensation may be completely intact. Signs and symptoms of increased intracranial pressure are common, since the thalami form the major portion of the walls of the third ventricle.

These tumors are mainly astrocytomas and glioblastomas, and because of their inaccessible location the outlook is poor. Occasionally a cystic astrocytoma may be treated by partial excision and aspiration of the cyst followed by radiotherapy with a surprising number of years of remission.

Tumors of the Cerebral Hemispheres

It has been generally stated that infratentorial tumors tend to predominate in children. However, experience in some large medical centers, including our own, indicates an approximately equal incidence of supratentorial and infratentorial neoplasms. In general, about one-third of supratentorial tumors in children are gliomas of the cerebral hemispheres. There is no striking difference in age or sex incidences. Half of the patients fall into the group between 7 and 11 years of age.

CLINICAL MANIFESTATIONS. Personality changes, a difficult symptom to document, is the most common early manifestation of a cerebral hemisphere tumor in a child. In retrospect, irritability and/or listlessness virtually always antedate the more specific symptoms and signs that precipitate neurodiagnostic study. Headache or vomiting or both occur early in 80 or 90 percent of patients. However, headache without vomiting is much more common than in posterior fossa or midline supratentorial tumors (distal to midline channels of cerebrospinal fluid communication and to medullary vomiting centers). The diagnostic value of this symptom is related to the child's ability to verbalize.

Motor weakness occurs in over one-third of these patients. Focal pyramidal deficit is common and presents as spasticity, hyperreflexia, and extensor plantar response in the absence of demonstrable weakness. Motor weakness may reveal itself in subtle fashion by change of handedness, reluctance to use an extremity, or unilateral abnormal posturing of the extremities on walking or performing other routine activities of daily living. Convulsions have been present in 38 percent of these patients studied at Columbia-Presbyterian Medical Center; in half of these the convulsions have been generalized. The seizures have frequently been of mixed types, with 80 percent having either focal or psychomotor attacks. It is of interest that one-third of these children with seizures and cerebral hemisphere tumors have had convulsions for 3 to 10 years prior to diagnosis.

Severe papilledema is unusual, but some degree is present in most patients at the time of diagnosis. Aside from focal pyramidal deficit, other focal signs such as sensory deficit, visual field defects, and aphasic phenomena are rarely encountered, probably because of the large proportion of patients too young to cooperate reliably. The use of devices to detect defects in opticokinetic nystagmus in children with parietal lobe tumors may increase the prevalence of this finding.

False localizing signs, particularly those ascribed to defects in cerebellar pathway function, have been discussed earlier. The findings on neurologic examination in children with cerebral hemisphere tumors are at times so sparse that a midline neoplasm or pseudotumor cerebri is suspected.

DIAGNOSIS. Ancillary studies are especially important in these patients because it is usually possible to localize the tumor precisely without resorting to ventriculography. The differential diagnosis includes space-occupying lesions of the hemisphere, such as subdural hematoma or hygroma, brain abscess, and rarely

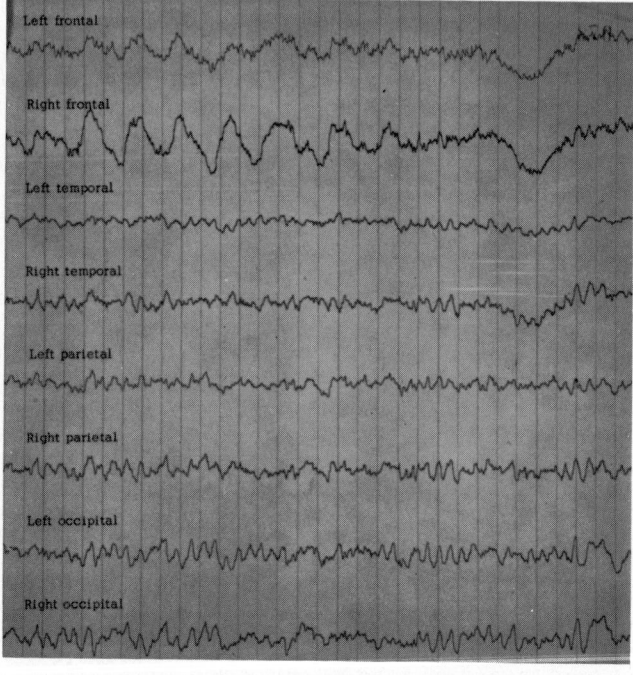

FIG. 20. Electroencephalogram showing a right frontal slow wave focus associated with an underlying astrocytoma.

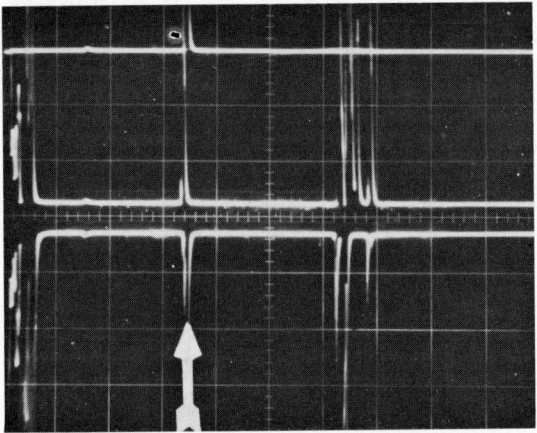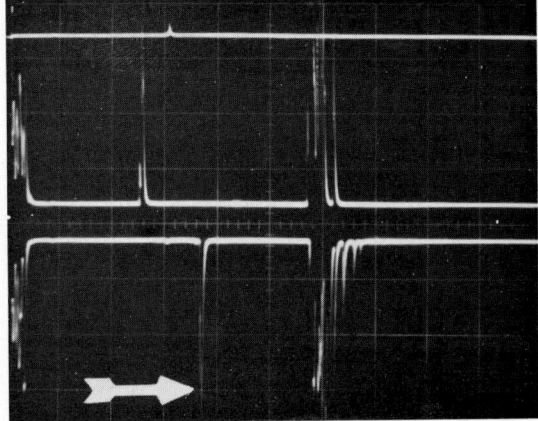

FIG. 21. Left. Normal echoencephalogram. Arrow indicates that midline structures are in normal position. Right. Abnormal echoencephalogram. Arrow indicates 10-mm shift of midline echoes from left to right, in this case because of a large left parietal lobe glioma in a 6-year-old boy.

hydatid cyst or tuberculoma. On occasion, acute or subacute encephalitis, particularly herpes simplex encephalitis, will preferentially involve the temporal lobe, producing signs and symptoms of an expanding lesion within this structure. On rare occasions a porencephalic cyst communicates with the subarachnoid space in ball-valve fashion, so that a subarachnoid collection of fluid accumulates progressively and acts as a mass lesion. In contradistinction to the case with midline or posterior fossa neoplasms, in which the electroencephalogram shows nonspecific generalized dysrhythmia especially in the occipital region, the electroencephalogram may be of definite localizing value in cerebral hemisphere tumors. The most consistent abnormality is focal high-amplitude slowing, although this is not diagnostic of a cerebral neoplasm (Fig. 20). The electroencephalogram is abnormal in over 90 percent of supratentorial tumors in children and is of localizing value in 75 percent. When the cerebral cortex is involved, localizing value approaches 90 percent.

Brain scanning for focal collection of radioisotope is diagnostic in almost 90 percent of cerebral hemisphere neoplasms, as compared with only 60 percent of posterior fossa neoplasms. Sequential scanning provides valuable information concerning tumor recurrence or extension following subtotal excision and/or radiotherapy. Technetium is currently favored for sequential scanning because of lower radiation exposure. Plain radiograms of the skull are helpful in localization when tumor calcification (approximately 10 percent) or local bony erosion is evident. The majority of patients show suture spread or other evidence of increased intracranial pressure. The skull radiogram is normal in 25 to 30 percent of children with cerebral hemisphere gliomas.

Echoencephalography may help to detect shifts of midline cerebral structures created by unilateral space-occupying lesions (Fig. 21). It is particularly useful in

children, in whom the pineal gland is rarely calcified. Ultrasound is deflected by structures in the region of the third ventricle, and distance from the left and right sides of the cranium can be measured. Shifts of more than 2 mm (considered to be the upper limit of normal) occur in at least 75 percent of cerebral hemisphere tumors.

When signs of increased intracranial pressure are absent, lumbar puncture may be performed; it may reveal some increase in cerebrospinal fluid pressure or protein content. Cerebrospinal fluid enzymes (eg, transaminase, lactic dehydrogenase, phosphohexose isomerase) may be elevated; these findings are not specific. Computerized axial tomography has become the procedure of choice to localize and define the lesion, and now air contrast studies are not often done (Fig. 22). However,

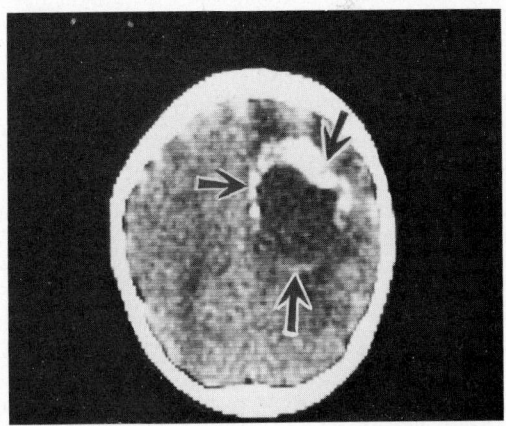

FIG. 22. Right frontoparietal cystic astrocytoma with calcified rim in a 9-year-old boy (CAT scan). Note the lucent center representing the cystic component and the increased density of the calcium surrounding the cyst. (Courtesy of Dr. S. Kreps and Dr. S. Hillal.)

percutaneous cerebral angiography may be useful to delineate the vascular supply to a neoplasm; this may be important in planning the surgical approach.

TABLE 11. Pathology of 104 Verified Cerebral Hemisphere Tumors

Type of Tumor	Number
Astrocytoma (pure and mixed)	46
Solid 30	
Cystic 16	
Glioblastoma	13
Ependymoma	8
Meningioma	6
Sarcoma	5
Oligodendroglioma	4
Ganglioglioma	4
Malignant teratoma	2
Metastatic neuroblastoma	2
Choroid plexus papilloma	2
Miscellaneous	12

TREATMENT AND PROGNOSIS. Treatment and its outcome depend largely on the histology of the tumor, although in general the results are disappointing. The histologic types encountered in 104 verified cerebral hemisphere tumors at the Columbia-Presbyterian Medical Center are outlined in Table 11; they will not be discussed separately. Astrocytoma is the leading cerebral hemisphere tumor. It is far less commonly cystic than the cerebellar astrocytoma, and only occasionally does it present as a mural nodule in a large cyst. The tumor is so infiltrative that complete surgical excision is rarely if ever achieved, but several years of remission can be achieved in many children. The location of the tumor dictates the extent of surgical excision possible. A tumor in the motor and speech areas of the dominant cerebral hemisphere does not readily lend itself to surgical intervention, whereas a tumor in one frontal lobe can be attacked more radically. Anticonvulsant medication is routinely recommended postoperatively for children with cerebral hemisphere neoplasms and should be continued indefinitely.

TUMORS OF THE OPTIC NERVE AND CHIASM

Almost all tumors of the optic nerve and chiasm are gliomas (astrocytomas), and over 95 percent occur in children. Meningiomas of the dural sheath of the optic nerve are rare in children; their incidence is only 5 percent of that of optic nerve gliomas. At the Columbia-Presbyterian Medical Center between the years 1940 and 1964, 5 percent of 1,124 intracranial tumors in children under 16 years were optic nerve gliomas. Symptoms first presented under 2 years of age in 33 percent and under 6 months of age in 10 percent. However, the diagnosis is characteristically delayed for 1 year to several years after onset.

CLINICAL MANIFESTATIONS. Diminished visual acuity is a very common presenting feature, but children will tolerate occult visual deficit for long periods. Exophthalmos is a particularly early and frequent (96 percent) sign when the tumor is confined to one optic nerve, although 20 percent of patients with chiasmal gliomas also have some degree of proptosis. Nystagmus is related chiefly to the presence of severe visual deficit prior to 4 years and especially prior to 2 years of age. Increased intracranial pressure is present only when the chiasm is involved and a large tumor has occluded the foramina of Monro. Multiple café au lait spots, the most common manifestation of neurofibromatosis, are present in approximately 25 percent of these children. Strabismus, when encountered, is not paretic in type, but relates to defective fixation of a poorly seeing eye. Optic atrophy is an invariable finding. It may be confined to one optic nerve, despite early involvement of the chiasm.

DIAGNOSIS. The differential diagnosis of optic nerve tumor includes other tumors of the orbit, particularly neurofibroma and less frequently meningioma and retinoblastoma. The diagnosis can be made on clinical and radiologic criteria in most cases without resorting to tissue diagnosis. The most important differential points are that in optic glioma proptosis is of mild degree, it occurs in a straightforward axis with little lateral or vertical displacement of the globe, and it is associated with a significant degree of optic atrophy and visual defect. Other orbital tumors producing proptosis lead to protrusion that is more marked and is more bizarrely positioned, all in the presence of remarkable preservation of vision and usually absence of optic atrophy.

Chiasmal gliomas may be confused with other tumors in this area: craniopharyngiomas, teratomas, dermoids, ectopic pinealomas, colloid cysts of the third ventricle, and hypothalamic gliomas. The skull radiograms characteristically show enlarged optic foramina and a typical deformity of the anterior clinoids in chiasmal gliomas (Fig. 23). Helpful clinical features include multiple café au lait spots and the characteristic but not invariable absence of diabetes insipidus and growth retardation in children with chiasmal gliomas. About 5 percent of children with chiasmal gliomas show endocrine changes; if they are present they usually include precocious puberty.

Over 25 percent of children with optic gliomas are followed for 1 to 3 years after the onset of visual defects, strabismus, or nystagmus before the diagnosis is established. The optic disk pallor is often ascribed to congenital optic atrophy. For unexplained reasons, some children show improvement of visual acuity with appropriate refraction. Because of their age it is difficult for the ophthalmologist to be sure that full correction has been achieved. It is thus important, when disk pallor of any degree is present or when visual defect is not fully corrected by refraction, to obtain skull radiographs with views of the optic foramina and sella turcica.

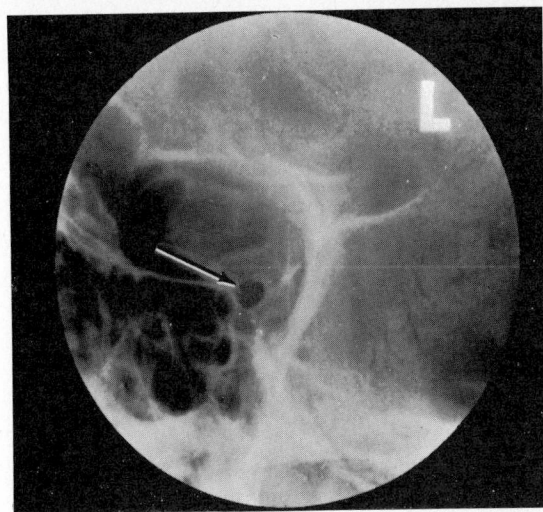

A

FIG. 23.   Orbital and intracranial right optic nerve glioma in a 14-year-old boy. The normal left optic (A) canal is oval and is 5 mm in diameter. The right optic canal (B) is enlarged to a circular lumen 11 mm in diameter with intact cortical margin.

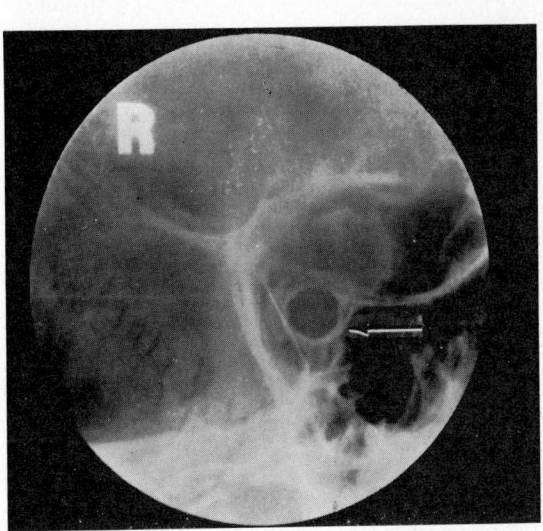

B

In addition to measurement of visual fields and acuity, careful examination of the fundi, and radiographic examination, intracranial pneumography is useful in diagnosis. In the presence of a chiasmal glioma, pneumoencephalography will reveal a filling defect in the anterior portion of the third ventricle, which is invaginated by the optic chiasm. Intracranial involvement of a single optic nerve may also be detected by intracranial pneumography, but it may be missed by this study if the chiasm is not involved. Computerized axial tomograms are of more limited value for the detection of small chiasmal lesions due to the proximity of such lesions to the dense bony structures of the anterior portion of the middle fossa. However, the intraorbital portion of an intracranial tumor such as the optic glioma may be displayed to great advantage.

TREATMENT.   If it is suspected that an optic nerve glioma is confined to a single optic nerve, a combined transcranial operation with unroofing of the orbit, preferably performed jointly by a neurosurgeon and an ophthalmologist, is indicated even if pneumography fails to reveal intracranial extension. In this manner the tumor can be completely resected. It is almost always possible to preserve the globe, which subsequently serves as an excellent natural prosthesis and moves reflexly in conjugate fashion directed by the eye with useful vision. Chiasmal gliomas cannot be totally resected and are best treated by radiotherapy. It may be possible to partially resect a chiasmal glioma in order to reestablish cerebrospinal fluid communication when the foramina of Monro are obstructed, but more commonly ventricular shunting is indicated as an adjunct to radiotherapy. Transient diabetes insipidus may occur after surgery in this region, and it requires careful replacement therapy.

PROGNOSIS. Patients with proptosis seem to do well, regardless of whether the chiasm is involved. Undoubtedly this is because proptosis reflects origin of a very slowly growing tumor in the optic nerve. The prognosis is variable. Many patients do well, but in others in whom a biopsy shows identical histologic features the course is rapid, with death occurring within 1 year. Patients with gliomas confined to the optic nerve can be completely cured in almost every instance. More than 80 percent of those who have done poorly have had increased intracranial pressure at the time of diagnosis; however, as many as one-third of patients with chiasmal gliomas who have experienced long-term survival with useful vision have also had increased intracranial pressure when diagnosed. The majority of patients with chiasmal gliomas treated with radiotherapy may be expected to survive with little or no neurologic deficit and with useful vision for many years. One patient with a chiasmal glioma has survived 30 years without evidence of clinical relapse following biopsy of the lesion and radiotherapy.

CRANIOPHARYNGIOMA

The incidence of craniopharyngiomas is only slightly higher than that of all optic nerve gliomas, but it is much greater than that of chiasmal gliomas, with which they may occasionally be confused. From 5 to 10 percent of all intracranial tumors in children are craniopharyngiomas. The majority of the children seen for the first time are 7 to 12 years of age.

CLINCAL MANIFESTATIONS. The cardinal signs and symptoms of craniopharyngioma are increased intracranial pressure, visual defects, and endocrine and hypothalamic dysfunction. Increased intracranial pressure is due to upward extension of the tumor and obstruction of one or both foramina of Monro. The signs and symptoms are not distinctive, but occasionally optic atrophy prevents the occurrence of papilledema. Almost always, however, papilledema and disk pallor are both present at the time of initial diagnosis. Visual acuity is usually diminished considerably due to chiasmatic compression and optic atrophy. Visual field defects are common and variable in type, but since the tumor is in the midline, the typical finding is bitemporal hemianopia. In very young, dull, or inarticulate children it may not be possible to document the type or extent of visual deficit. Diminished pituitary activity may result in growth retardation and sexual infantilism. Clinical manifestations of hypothyroidism are not to be expected preoperatively. While these children tend to tire easily and may be hypotensive, obesity of the female type is more common than cachexia, and florid panhypopituitarism is distinctly rare. Diabetes insipidus is uncommon, but it may occur before surgical extirpation. Other evidences of hypothalamic involvement include growth retardation, somnolence, obesity, hypothermia or hyperthermia, hypertension or hypotension, inappropriate secretion of antidiuretic hormone, and alarming changes in vital signs. However, with the exception of somatic and sexual infantilism, these phenomena present more often as postoperative complications.

DIAGNOSIS. About 75 percent of children with craniopharyngiomas show diffuse flecks of calcification in the sella or suprasellar region in skull radiograms. Enlargement of the sella is present in 50 percent, and more than half show nonspecific signs of increased intracranial pressure. When calcification is absent, films of the optic foramina should be obtained to study the anterior clinoids for evidence of a chiasmal glioma. Other less common tumors in this region include teratomas, dermoids, colloid cysts, and hypothalamic gliomas. Calcification may occur in dermoid tumors and teratomas, but it is rare in the others. Computerized axial tomography is especially helpful in the diagnosis of calcific lesions that occasionally escape plain tomography; if it is diagnostic it may avoid the need for ventriculography. Cerebral angiography may be helpful to the neurosurgeon by indicating displacement of major vessels in the surgical field. It is essential to document the extent of endocrine disturbance. The urine osmolality, serum electrolytes, and preoperative blood pressure require special attention so that optimal correction may be made preoperatively. Bone age is determined by radiograms of the hemiskeleton or of the hand and wrist. Other endocrine functions may be estimated by the various tests of anterior and posterior pituitary, thyroid, and adrenal function; postoperative comparison can be made when the condition stabilizes so that optimal replacement endocrine therapy can be instituted. The visual fields and acuity should be carefully plotted, preoperatively and after stabilization postoperatively, to permit comparison on subsequent examination for detection of recurrence.

TREATMENT. Regardless of the results of endocrine study, cortisone should be given preoperatively and during surgery; it has become the single most important factor in the marked increase in immediate postoperative survival and in the increase in the number of patients capable of having radical tumor removal. An average dose of cortisone is 50 mg on the evening prior to surgery and 50 mg on the morning of surgery. Approximately 100 mg of cortisone are given intravenously during surgery. On the first postoperative day 100 mg of cortisone are administered, thereafter tapering the dose by 25 mg daily to a maintenance level of approximately 15 mg daily.

Gross total excision of the tumor can be accomplished in over 50 percent of patients. These tumors are encapsulated and are almost always cystic to some extent. They may be located within the sella or entirely beyond the diaphragm of the sella in the pituitary stalk. The tumor capsule may adhere inseparably to the anterior cerebral or internal carotid vessels, the optic chiasm, or the hypothalamus. In such cases only partial excision is possible, and recurrence is invariable. However, dramatic remission of symptoms and restoration of vision may be achieved simply by aspiration of the oily fluid from a large cyst that has compressed surrounding structures.

The tumors, being squamous epitheliomas, are relatively radioresistant, but it is believed that radiotherapy may retard at least the rate of reaccumulation of cyst fluid. In the immediate postoperative period symptoms of diabetes insipidus may be severe, and careful attention to water and electrolyte balance is essential. For the first few days replacement of water and electrolytes (p. 262) is generally advisable without the use of vasopressin, because the immediate effects of surgery wane and diabetes insipidus is invariably lessened. If vasopressin is necessary the aqueous parenteral preparation may be used every 6 hours. When the stable level of diabetes insipidus is determined, it is treated as described elsewhere (p. 1617). Cortisone and thyroid replacement are often necessary, particularly when a radical tumor excision has been performed. Details of treatment are described elsewhere (p. 1611). If it is available, human growth hormone may reestablish normal growth curves in those with retarded growth. Normal pubescence may also be achieved by appropriate hormonal therapy, and even reproduction may be secured with the use of human chorionic gonadotropin. Visual fields and acuity and periodic skull radiographs should be checked regularly to detect recurrence in patients who have had excision.

PROGNOSIS. Children treated prior to 1950 almost uniformly failed to survive. The long-term results in children treated more recently are considerably more promising. Even when total tumor excision is not possible, recurrence may not be evident for many years, although it may occur in less than a year. Repeated partial excision of solid tumor and capsule and cyst aspiration may keep such patients alive and functioning well for many years. Unfortunately, visual deficit often mounts with each insult, and the risk of postoperative morbidity and mortality is compounded.

Tumors of the Spinal Cord

Intraspinal tumors in infants and children are far less common than intracranial tumors, the ratio being approximately 1 to 5. Meningiomas and neurofibromas, which are relatively common in adults, are rarely encountered in children. Intraspinal lipomas, dermoid and teratoid tumors, neuroblastomas, and intramedullary gliomas are the common intraspinal neoplasms in children. About 20 percent are benign dermoids or lipomas of congenital origin. Gliomas and sarcomas each account for 20 percent of the total. Neuroblastomas comprise 5 to 10 percent. Early diagnosis of intraspinal tumors in children is essential because (1) irreversible neurologic deficit may occur when diagnosis is delayed, even if the neoplasm is benign; (2) intramedullary gliomas may sometimes be excised totally or may respond dramatically to radiotherapy; (3) the lipoma, dermoid, and teratoid groups (benign varieties of extramedullary tumors) may be associated, even after only partial excision, with prolonged relief.

CLINICAL MANIFESTATIONS. DISTURBANCE OF GAIT AND POSTURE. Disturbances of gait and posture are the most frequent symptoms of intraspinal tumors; when they are present an intraspinal neoplasm should always be considered. These changes may be due to weakness, spasticity, or compensatory posture to avoid pain. The most frequent disturbance of posture is a reluctance to flex the trunk; it may be present before frank neurologic deficit is detectable. There may be prominent paraspinal muscle spasm, a particularly important sign in the nonverbal or inarticulate child. The child with a cervical intramedullary glioma characteristically has flaillike drooping of the shoulders and reduced swing of the arms due to segmental anterior horn cell involvement. Other abnormalities of gait depend upon the extremity involved and changes of tone and power.

PAIN. Pain is a commom symptom that occurs as an initial complaint in about 50 percent of children with intraspinal tumors. In the young child pain may be manifested by irritability and postural guarding. Older children frequently describe the pain as being accentuated by coughing, sneezing, or straining, as well as by flexion of the neck or trunk or extension of the lower extremities.

WEAKNESS. Weakness is evident on initial examination in about 60 percent of children with intraspinal tumors. Functionally this may be evident only as a limp, easy fatigability, or reduced activity of one or more extremities. There is a flaccid paresis at the level of the lesion, below which the extremities are spastic. The weakness may be of the flaccid type below the level of the lesion when spinal shock occurs, as in rapidly evolving cord compression from neuroblastoma or other metastatic lesions.

REFLEX CHANGES. Deep tendon reflexes may be decreased within the limited segments occupied by tumor due to encroachment on anterior horn cells, while hyperactive reflexes and extensor plantar responses are expected below the level of the lesion. In spinal shock deep tendon reflexes are absent. Thus in intramedullary neoplasms of the cervical cord, diminished reflexes, and loss of tone in the upper extremities are commonly associated with spasticity, hyperreflexia, and extensor plantar responses in the lower extremities. Absence or diminution of reflexes in the lower extremities is suggestive of a lesion of the cauda equina. An absent anal reflex is additional evidence of sacral cord or root involvement.

IMPAIRED BLADDER OR BOWEL FUNCTION. Bowel and bladder function may be impaired by involvement of descending tracts or by segmental loss of innervation in lumbosacral lesions. The result may be either a spastic low-capacity bladder with frequency of urination or a distended atonic bladder with dribbling of urine. Laxity of the rectal sphincter and a diminished anal reflex with regressive bowel or bladder function are valuable objective signs. Loss of sensation in the saddle area is a less reliable sign in children.

SENSORY IMPAIRMENT. Although sensory examination is often difficult and unreliable in children, careful testing may be rewarding even in infants. Changes in facial expression may help to fix the level of a spinal cord lesion. Although sensory complaints are rare, sensory deficits may be demonstrated in one-third of children with intraspinal tumors. Absence or diminution of sweating below the level of the lesion is a valuable sign in young children.

CUTANEOUS AND SKELETAL CHANGES. Cutaneous or subcutaneous lesions may indicate an underlying neoplasm. Multiple café au lait spots in a child with spinal cord symptoms suggest the diagnosis of neurofibroma. Rarely a single café au lait spot may mark the site of the tumor. A subcutaneous lipoma, nevus flammeus, dimple, sinus, or tuft of hair in the dorsal or lumbosacral region may be an innocent dermal anomaly; however, if such a lesion is associated with neurologic signs, the possibility of an underlying neoplasm of the lipomatous, dermoid, or teratoid type should be considered. Scoliosis may be a local manifestation of an intraspinal tumor or may be associated with neurofibromatosis even in the absence of any intraspinal tumor. However, an intraspinal tumor should be excluded in all patients with neurofibromatosis and scoliosis.

MISCELLANEOUS SIGNS. Occasionally opsoclonus with polymyoclonia or cerebellar ataxia may be the only signs suggesting the possibility of an occult intraspinal ganglioneuroma or neuroblastoma.

LABORATORY STUDIES. Lumbar puncture is valuable in the diagnosis of spinal cord neoplasm, but it should always be preceded by radiographs of the vertebral spine. With suspected spinal cord lesions, fluid pressure should always be measured carefully. The fluid may be slightly discolored or frankly xanthochromic; cell count and sugar content are usually normal. Metastatic seeding (leptomeningeal sarcomatosis or carcinomatosis) may produce an increase in cells and a marked reduction in sugar content; when these findings are associated with nuchal rigidity, bacterial meningitis may be suspected. Cerebrospinal fluid protein is usually increased with spinal cord tumors; with complete subarachnoid block the protein content is markedly elevated and there is an associated deep yellow discoloration (Froin's syndrome).

Radiographs of the spine show bone changes in about two-thirds of children with intraspinal tumors. Two significant findings are widening of the interpedicular space and erosion of the pedicles. Myelography definitively establishes the level of the lesion and its intramedullary or extramedullar location. Computerized axial tomographic scanning has been used successfully to diagnose spinal cord lesions, but not yet as effectively as for intracranial lesions.

DIFFERENTIAL DIAGNOSIS. The differential diagnosis of intraspinal tumors includes congential defects (eg, diastematomyelia), vascular malformations, tumors of the bony spine, and degenerative diseases.

TREATMENT. Therapy is largely dependent on the location of the tumor. Surgical extirpation is feasible for some extramedullary lesions; occasionally partial removal and rarely total removal of an intramedullary tumor is possible. Decompressive laminectomy may give symptomatic relief. Radiation therapy is utilized for inoperable tumors and as a supplement for radiosensitive mass lesions removed subtotally. Corticosteroid therapy may be of vital benefit both in reducing cord edema associated with radiation therapy and prior to surgical decompression.

References

TUMORS OF THE CENTRAL NERVOUS SYSTEM

Abramson N, Raben M, Cavanagh P: Brain tumors in children: analysis of 136 cases. Radiology 112:669, 1974

Ambrose J: Computerized x-ray scanning of the brain. Neurosurgery 40:679, 1974

Aron BS: Twenty years' experience with radiation therapy medulloblastoma. Am J Roentgenol Radium Ther Nucl Med 105:37, 1969

Bailey P, Buchanan DN, Bucy PC: Intracranial Tumors of Infancy and Childhood. Chicago, University of Chicago Press, 1939

Banna M, Hoare RD, Stanley P, Till K: Craniopharyngioma in children. Pediatrics 83:781, 1973

Bloom HJG, Wallace MB, Henk JM: The treatment and prognosis of medulloblastoma in children. Am J Roentgenol Radium Ther Nucl Med 105:43, 1969

Bouchard JJ: Radiation Therapy of Tumors and Diseases of the Nervous System. Philadelphia, Lea & Febiger, 1966

Bryan P: CSF seeding of intra-cranial tumours: a study of 96 cases. Clin Radiol 25:355, 1974

Cheek WR, Taveras JM: Thalamic tumors. J Neurosurg 24:505, 1966

Chutorian AM, Schwartz JF, Evans RA, Carter S: Optic gliomas in children. Neurology 14:83 1964

Davidoff LM: Some considerations in the therapy of pineal tumors. Bull NY Acad Med 43:537, 1967

Fokes EC, Earle KM: Ependymomas: clinical and pathological aspects. J Neurosurg 30:585, 1969

French LA: The use of steroids in the treatment of cerebral edema. Bull NY Acad Med 42:30, 1966

Gawler J, Du Boulay GH, Bull JWD, Marshall J: Computer-assisted tomography (EMI scanner). Its place in investigation of suspected intracranial tumours. Lancet 2:419, 1974

Hammill JF, Carter S: Brain Tumors in Childhood. Practice of Pediatrics. Hagerstown, Md, WF Prior, 1966

Lassman LP, Pearce GW, Gang J: Effect of vincristine sulfate on the intracranial gliomata of childhood. Br J Surg 53:9, 1966

Low NL, Correll JW, Hammill JF: Tumors of the cerebral hemispheres in children. Arch Neurol 13:547, 1965

McFarland D, Horwitz H, Saenger E: Medulloblastoma—a review of prognosis and survival. Br J Radiol 42:198, 1969

Markesbery WR, McDonald JV: Diencephalic syndrome. Am J Dis Child 125:123, 1973

Matson DD: Neurosurgery of Infancy and Childhood, 2nd ed. Springfield, Ill, Charles C Thomas, 1969

Millichap JG, Bickford RG, Miller RH, Backus RE: The EEG in children with intracranial tumors and seizures. Neurology 12:239, 1962

Newton WA Jr, Sayers MP, Samuels LD: Intrathecal methotrexate therapy for brain tumors in children. Cancer Chemother Rep 52:527, 1968

Panitch HS, Berg BO: Brain stem tumors of childhood and adolescence. Am J Dis Child 119:465, 1970

Peirce CB: The efficacy of radiation therapy in the treatment of tumors of the brain and brain stem. Clin Neurosurg 10:195, 1964

Sayers MP: Surgery and chemotherapy of brain tumors in children. Prog Exp Tumor Res 17:414, 1972

Shapiro WR: Chemotherapy of primary malignant brain tumors in children. Cancer 35:965, 1975

Smith CE, Long DM, Jones TK, Levitt SH: Experiences in treating medulloblastoma at the University of Minnesota Hospitals. Radiology 109:179, 1973

Tamaka K, Ito K, Wagai I: The localization of brain tumors by ultrasonic techniques (a clinical review of 111 cases). J Neurosurg 23:135, 1965

Vannucci RC, Baten M: Cerebral metastatic disease in childhood. Neurology 24:981, 1974

SPINAL CORD TUMORS

Coxe WS: Tumors of the spinal canal in children. Am Surg 27:62, 1961

Greenwodd J Jr: Intramedullary tumors of the spinal cord; followup study after total surgical removal. J Neurosurg 20:665, 1963

Haft H, Ransohoff J, Carter S: Spinal cord tumors in children. Pediatrics 23:1152, 1959

Matson DD, Tachdjian MO: Intraspinal tumors in infants and children. Review of 115 cases. Postgrad Med 279, 1963

Rand RW, Rand CW: Intraspinal Tumors of Childhood. Springfield, Ill, Charles C Thomas, 1960

Slooff JL, Kernahan JW, MacCarty CS: Primary Intramedullary Tumors of the Spinal Cord and Filum Terminale. Philadelphia, WB Saunders, 1964

Wyburn-Mason R: The Vascular Abnormalities and Tumors of the Spinal Cord and Its Membranes. London, Henry Kimpton, 1944

PSEUDOTUMOR CEREBRI

Melvin Greer

Pseudotumor cerebri refers to a neurologic syndrome characterized by increased intracranial pressure unassociated with focal signs of neural impairment, convulsions, alterations in mentation, or cerebrospinal fluid (CSF) changes. The signs and symptoms may otherwise be the same as those seen with any intracranial mass or hydrocephalus. The course is benign and the prognosis is usually good. Impairment of visual acuity as a consequence of persistent intracranial hypertension is the major problem.

ETIOLOGY. Pseudotumor cerebri is a syndrome of intracranial hypertension in which the cause and pathogenesis are often not apparent. Absence of convulsions and the presence of normal mental state argue against cerebral edema as the causative mechanism. Intrathecal injections of radioiodinated serum albumin suggest that a defect in CSF absorption is the underlying factor. In any given patient it is essential to consider the common causes of increased pressure: neoplasm, infection, congenital malformation, hematoma, and degenerative and toxic states. A common cause of pseudotumor cerebri in children is obstruction of the intracranial venous drainage, often secondary to chronic mastoiditis and occlusion of the major draining lateral sinus (otitic hydrocephalus). Less commonly, obstruction of the sagittal sinus follows traumatic skull fracture or invasion by metastatic neuroblastoma. Superior vena caval obstruction may occur after surgery or from an intrathoracic mass. The intracranial venous system is dilated, CSF absorption is impaired, and increased pressure results.

Hormonal aberrations have been implicated in children with pseudotumor cerebri following corticosteroid therapy, in girls entering menarche, and in obese adolescent females. Hypoparathyroidism and hypophosphatasia have also been implicated. Pseudotumor cerebri has been recognized with severe iron-deficiency anemia associated with excessive menstruation in adolescent females. In infants, chronic vitamin A intoxication or ingestion of massive amounts of vitamin A after a prolonged deficiency may cause the syndrome. However, signs such as fever, dehydration, diarrhea, irritability, and lethargy in infancy would indicate a toxic encephalopathy rather than a deficiency or excess of vitamin A. Infectious, toxic, or metabolic encephalopathies may produce a wide spectrum of signs ranging from disturbed mentation and seizures to minimal signs of neural dysfunction. The latter group may be confused with pseudotumor cerebri. Fevers from any cause (eg, roseola infantum) are often associated with a bulging fontanelle; this has been termed meningism. Pseudotumor cerebri has also been noted in afebrile infants on tetracycline therapy for several days, in patients on nalidixic acid therapy, and in children with Sydenham's chorea, Aldrich's syndrome, galactosemia, and closed head trauma. In malnourished children, including those with cystic fibrosis, improvement in nutritional state leads to a temporary state of intracranial hypertension that presumably reflects a state of catch-up brain growth.

CLINICAL MANIFESTATIONS. The presenting complaints include headache, nausea, vomiting, dizziness, blurred vision, and diplopia. The symptoms are intermittent and commonly exist for weeks. The child's apparent well-being is often striking in view of the florid papilledema and abducens nerve paresis that reflect the generalized increased pressure. There are no consistent signs of neurologic dysfunction, although mild un-steadiness of gait has often been described.

LABORATORY FINDINGS. Suture diastasis or erosion of the dorsum sellae seen on skull radiography confirms the presence of intracranial hypertension. The electroencephalogram, echoencephalogram, and brain scan are normal. Historical evidence suggesting mastoiditis or other diseases known to be related to intracranial hypertension calls for specific laboratory investigations such as mastoid radiographs and determination of serum calcium, phosphorus, alkaline phosphatase, and vitamin A levels.

DIAGNOSIS. Carotid angiography (venous phase) may demonstrate intracranial venous sinus obstruction and at the same time exclude ventricular dilation. If arteriography does not define a sinus obstruction, a mass lesion, or ventricular dilation, pneumoencephalography may show narrowing of the air-filled ventricles. Ventriculography has often been employed by neurosurgeons as a diagnostic study of choice. In the presence of a mass lesion there is risk of cerebellar herniation and brainstem compression following pneumoencephalography; however, the more benign vascular study followed by air encephalography via the lumbar route lessens the trauma and risk attending ventricular puncture under general anesthesia in children.

TREATMENT. Therapy is specific for children whose intracranial hypertension is caused by lateral sinus obstruction (mastoidectomy, antibiotics), hypoparathyroidism (calcium, vitamin D), anemia of menstruation (iron, transfusion), drug intoxication (drug withdrawal), or possible adrenocortical insufficiency following cessation of corticosteroid therapy (reinstitution of corticosteroids). In those children for whom no specific therapy is available, treatment must be supportive. It is assumed that the illness in these instances is self-limiting. Indeed, in about one-half of such children the intracranial hypertension subsides spontaneously after air encephalography. The risk of blindness from persistent intracranial hypertension necessitates some treatment to reduce the pressure in those patients in whom spontaneous recovery is not immediate. This can be accomplished by serial lumbar punctures. Corticosteroids, carbonic anhydrase inhibitors, and intravenous or oral hyperosmolar agents such as glycerol have been used to lower intracranial pressure; however, a response to these measures has not been proved. In a small number of children neither repeated spinal taps nor drugs have been effective in maintaining normal intracranial pressure. It is always advisable to repeat neuroradiologic studies if the symptoms and signs persist for more than 3 months. If intracranial pressure is still elevated, surgical treatment may be warranted. Spinal shunting (lumboperitoneal) is much preferred to the crude subtemporal decompression procedure, since the latter entails a postoperative risk of temporal lobe trauma and seizures.

References

Beller AJ: Benign post-traumatic intracranial hypertension. J Neurol Neurosurg Psychiatry 27:149, 1964

Bercaw BL, Greer M: Transport in intrathecal ^{131}I RISA in benign intracranial hypertension. Neurology 20:787, 1970

Bray PF, Herbst JJ: Pseudotumor cerebri as a sign of "catch-up" in cystic fibrosis. Am J Dis Child 126:78, 1973

DeLevie M, Nogrady MB: Rapid brain growth upon restoration of adequate nutrition causing false radiologic evidence of increased intracanial pressure. J Pediatr 76:523, 1970

Feldman MH, Schlezinger NS: Benign intracranial hypertension associated with hypervitaminosis A. Arch Neurol 22:1, 1970

Fields JP: Bulging fontanel: a complication of tetracycline therapy in infants. J Pediatr 58:74, 1961

Greer M: Benign intracranial hypertension. I. Mastoiditis and lateral sinus obstruction. Neurology 12:472, 1962

——— Benign intracranial hypertension. II. Following corticosteroid therapy. Neurology 13:439, 1963

——— Benign intracranial hypertension. IV. Menarche. Neurology 14:569, 1964

——— Benign intracranial hypertension. VI. Obesity. Neurology 15:382, 1965

——— Benign intracranial hypertension (pseudotumor cerebri). Pediatr Clin North Am 14:819, 1967

——— Management of benign intracranial hypertension (pseudotumor cerebri). Clin Neurosurg 15:161, 1968

Hooper R: Hydrocephalus and obstruction of the superior vena cava in infancy. Pediatrics 28:792, 1961

Johnston I: Reduced CSF absorption syndrome. Lancet 2:418, 1973

Rose A, Matson DD: Benign intracranial hypertension in children. Pediatrics 39:227, 1967

Weisberg LA: The syndrome of increased intracranial pressure without localizing signs: a reappraisal. Neurology 25:85, 1975

CEREBROVASCULAR DISEASES

Arnold P. Gold, James F. Hammill, and Sidney Carter

Cerebrovascular diseases include those morbid processes, either primary or secondary, that involve the blood vessels of the brain. A comprehensive survey of this pediatric problem has recently been completed by the Subcommittee for Strokes in Children of the Joint Committee for Stroke Facilities. Vascular disease in children may be divided into two categories: a small group of conditions in which the cause can be defined (Table 12) and a much larger group of conditions in which, despite detailed investigation, the etiology is obscure. Modern technologic advances, including cerebral blood flow studies, improved cerebral ateriography, and computerized axial tomography (CAT), have contributed much to diagnosis and therapy.

Cerebrovascular accidents are most frequent in the elderly, but they are not infrequent in children. Cerebrovascular diseases account for about 5 percent of admissions to the average university pediatric neurology service and are present in 10 percent of pediatric autopsies. Congenital heart disease is a well-identified risk factor and may be associated with emboli or with arterial or venous thromboses. Contributing factors in-

TABLE 12. Classification of Cerebrovascular Disease

Occlusive Vascular Disease
  Dural sinus and cerebral venous thrombosis, associated with:
    Meningitis
    Infections of face, ears, or paranasal sinuses
    Dehydration and /or hyperosmolarity
    Debilitating states (marantic)
    Metastatic neoplasms, eg, neuroblastoma
    Congenital heart disease
    Lead encephalopathy
    Sturge-Weber-Dimitri syndrome (trigeminal enceph-
      aloangiomatosis)
  Arterial thrombosis
    Idiopathic or spontaneous, associated with:
      Dissecting cerebral aneurysm
      Arteriosclerosis (progeria)
      Cyanotic congenital heart disease
      Cerebral arteritis
        Acute infectious diseases
        Granulomatous (Takayasu's disease)
        Syphilis
      Collagen diseases
        Polyarteritis nodosa
        Lupus erythematosus
      Blood dyscrasias: sickle cell disease, polycythemia, throm-
        botic thrombocytopenia
      Trauma to the carotid or cerebral arteries
      Complications of arteriography
      Extra-arterial diseases
        Retropharyngeal abscess
        Mucomycosis
        Tumours of the base of the skull
        Craniometaphyseal dysplasia
    Metabolic
      Homocystinuria
      Diabetes mellitus

Occlusive Vascular Disease (cont.)
  Cerebral embolism, associated with:
    Atrial fibrillation or other arrhythmias
      Rheumatic heart disease
      Congenital heart disease, right-to-left shunt
      Coronary thrombosis
    Acute or subacute bacterial endocarditis
    Infarcted necrotic placental tissue
    Air: complications of cardiac, neck, or thoracic surgery
    Septic: pneumonia or lung abscess
    Fat: complications of fractures of long bones
    Tumor

Intracranial Hemorrhage (includes intracerebral and subarachnoid)
  Arteriovenous malformation or angioma
  Intracranial aneurysm
  Trauma
    Cavernous sinus fistula
    Subdural hemorrhage
    Epidural hemorrhage
  Blood dyscrasias
    Leukemia
    Thrombocytopenic purpura
    Aplastic anemia
    Hemophilia
    Anaphylactoid purpura
  Hypertension
  Liver disease
  Complications of anticoagulant therapy
  Intracranial neoplasms
  Deficiency syndromes
    Vitamin B_1 deficiency (Wernicke's encephalopathy)
    Vitamin C deficiency (scurvy)
    Vitamin K deficiency (hemorrhagic disease of the newborn)
  Toxic or infectious encephalopathy

clude polycythemia, iron-deficiency anemia, dehydration, and congestive heart failure. Infants and young children with congenital cardiac lesions with right-to-left shunts have a 5 percent risk of hemiplegia, whereas the risk is only 2 percent in those with left-to-right shunt lesions. Ten percent of patients with the tetralogy of Fallot have cerebrovascular accidents, and 25 percent of all autopsied cardiac cases have evidence of cerebrovascular occlusion.

Hematologic disorders are also important predisposing factors in cerebrovascular accidents. Spontaneous cerebral hemorrhage that involves primarily cerebral white matter is found in about 50 percent of leukemic patients at necropsy. Intracranial hemorrhage occurs in 2.2 to 7.4 percent of children with hemophilia, but in only 1 percent of those with idiopathic thrombocytopenic purpura. Other hematologic disorders such as sickle cell disease and thrombotic thrombocytopenic purpura may be associated with cerebrovascular complications.

Trauma is an important risk factor, with concussion or head injury occurring in approximately 3 percent of children during the first 7 years of life. In this age group ateriovenous malformations are ten times as common as intracranial aneurysms and are the most common cause of primary subarachnoid hemorrhage.

OCCLUSIVE VASCULAR DISEASE

Arterial or venous occlusion deprives the brain of oxygen, with resultant necrosis (encephalomalacia) of tissue. If death does not result, a process of repair occurs over several months, with the formation of an astrocytic or fibroblastic scar. The ischemic area, or infarct, is the nonspecific final result of any type of occlusion; however, the changes in the blood vessels or surrounding brain may be quite specific. Thus arteriosclerosis of progeria, vascular changes in granulomatous arteritis (Takayasu's disease), and the lesions associated with blood dyscrasias may each produce characteristic anatomic changes.

Cerebral Venous and Dural Sinus Thrombosis

Obstruction of venous drainage may lead to cerebral edema and hemorrhagic infarction of the brain. In some cases thrombosis of venous sinuses may not cause any gross cerebral lesion because effective cerebral venous anastomoses may permit adequate venous drainage. Venous occlusion most commonly occurs after pyogenic infections of the face, mouth, mastoids, or leptomeninges or in association with dehydration, debilitating and cachectic states, trauma, sickle cell disease, or polycythemia. Less frequently it is noted in Sturge-Weber-Dimitri syndrome, lead encephalopathy, metastatic neoplasia, or thrombotic thrombocytopenia.

CLINICAL MANIFESTATIONS. The clinical picture of venous thromboses is related to extent of involvement, rapidity of occlusion, and nature of the primary disease. Common manifestations include increased intracranial pressure, focal motor deficits, seizures, altered states of consciousness, and signs of circulatory stasis. Lateral sinus occlusion may result in pseudotumor cerebri (p. 1819). If focal signs develop recovery may be slow and there may be residual hemiparesis, seizures, or mental retardation. Superior sagittal sinus thrombosis is suggested by alternating hemiplegias and multifocal seizures. Signs of circulatory stasis may be pathognomonic for involvement of a specific vessel. Cavernous sinus thrombosis is characterized by exophthalmos of the homolateral eye, palpebral and conjunctival edema, and involvement of the third, fourth, fifth (first two branches), and sixth cranial nerves. Lateral sinus thrombosis may be accompanied by painful swelling in the mastoid region. Occlusion of the superior sagittal sinus may result in venous distension over the scalp and eyelids.

LABORATORY FINDINGS. There is often a moderate polymorphonuclear leukocytosis and an elevated erythrocyte sedimentation rate. CSF findings depend on the pathologic process. Unless there is an associated infection, the fluid, which may be under increased pressure, is usually clear and colorless with little or no pleocytosis. The Tobey-Ayer test, while not always reliable, may be of some value in the diagnosis of lateral sinus thrombosis. Compression of the jugular vein on the affected side produces no rise in CSF pressure, while compression on the normal side produces a prompt rise in pressure. The electroencephalogram may be normal or diffusely slow in the presence of increased intracranial pressure, or it may show marked abnormalities of a focal nature. Skull radiographs may be normal or may show signs of increased intracranial pressure and mastoid disease. The site and extent of the thrombosis can often be confirmed by evaluating the venous phase of a carotid arteriogram.

Arterial Thrombosis

Cerebral arterial thromboses produce variable clinical pictures that depend on the rapidity of occlusion, the collateral circulation, and the maintenance of systemic blood pressure. Arterial occlusion usually occurs in a previously healthy child, but it may be a complication of certain systemic diseases (Table 12).

CLINICAL MANIFESTATIONS. The clinical features depend on the cause and the vessel involved. *Acute infantile hemiplegia* characteristically appears in the first 2 years after birth. Unexplained or idiopathic hemiplegia is uncommon after the age of 5 years. The previously well child may suddenly develop fever, have a series of convulsions, and be left with a hemiplegia that may partially clear. Cortical hemisensory loss, hemianopia, and aphasia may also be associated. Recurrent focal motor seizures that are often resistant to anticonvulsants may complicate the subsequent course. When the child is seen years after onset the involved extremities may be short, atrophic, and spastic. Arterial thrombosis may result in either cerebral hemiatrophy with a small head circumference or cerebral porencephaly with resultant macrocephaly. Seizures at the onset of the hemiparesis are more common in children under the age of 2 years; they herald a poor prognosis for seizures and hemiplegia as well as intellect and behavior.

LABORATORY FINDINGS. CSF analysis during the acute episode is usually normal, but a slight leukocytic pleocytosis may be found a few weeks later. Electroencephalograms, which occasionally are normal, may be characterized by a slow-wave focus over the involved area. In the early phase skull radiographs are normal, but later the effect of cerebral hemiatrophy or porencephaly may be seen. Cerebral atrophy may be associated with thickening of the cranial vault, over-development of the frontal and ethmoid sinuses, and elevation of the petrous pyramid of the temporal bone on the involved side. Porencephaly is suggested by bulging and thinning of the cranial vault on the affected side and cephalofacial disproportion. Arteriography may demonstrate the arterial occlusion, and air contrast studies may show cerebral atrophy or a porencephalic cavity or fistula. On angiography primary cerebral arterial thrombosis can be classified into the following five groups:

EXTRACRANIAL CAROTID OCCLUSIVE DISEASE. Trauma is the most common cause of occlusion of the cervical carotid artery. External trauma results in compression of the internal carotid artery against the transverse process of C-2. Internal trauma results from penetration of the paratonsillar region by a pointed object. Characteristically carotid artery occlusion results in seizures and/or hemiparesis after a latent period of 1 to 24 hours. Congenital stenosis, retrograde thrombosis, and fibromuscular dysplasia also may affect the extracranial portion of the internal carotid artery in children, resulting in hemiplegia, seizures, behavior problems, and/or learning disability. Fibromuscular dysplasia is often associated with similar lesions in the renal artery. Residual hemiparesis is observed in most children with this disorder.

BASAL OCCLUSIVE DISEASE WITHOUT TELANGIECTASIA. This group of diseases (Fig. 24) and the following group affect the arteries at the base of the brain, including the supraclinoid portion of the internal carotid artery, the origins of the anterior and middle cerebral arteries, and the basilar artery. The occlusion may be associated with congenital lesions such as large porencephalic cysts in the neonatal period or acquired conditions such as acute infantile hemiplegia. It is usually unilateral, and recurrences are rare. The medial members of the group of striate arteries are

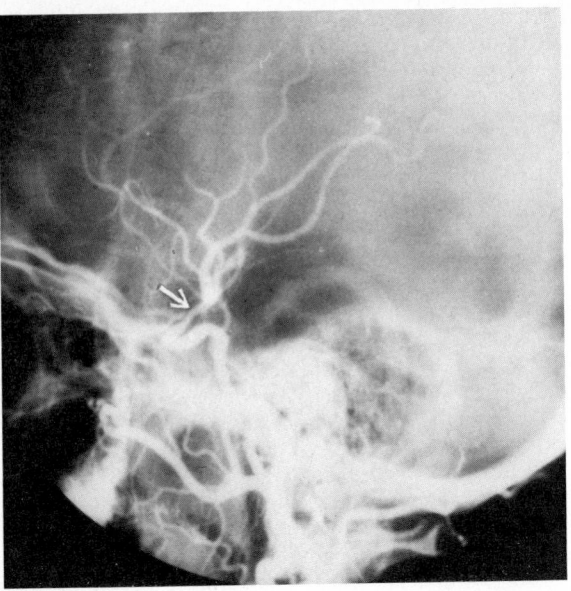

FIG. 24. Basal occlusive vascular disease without telangiectasia. Lateral view of cerebral arteriogram. Arrow is at occlusion of the internal carotid artery. (Courtesy of Dr. S. Hilal.)

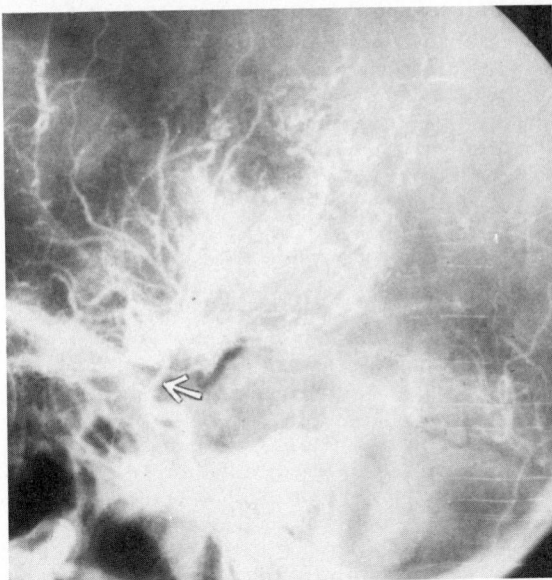

FIG. 25. Basal occlusive vascular disease with telangiectasia (Moyamoya disease). Lateral view of cerebral arteriogram. Arrow is at the site of occlusion, and above is the prominent telangiectasia. (Courtesy of Dr. S. Hilal.)

most commonly involved, and this explains the greater motor weakness in the arm than in the leg. Vasculitis, tumor encasement, and radiation therapy have been implicated as specific etiologic factors. Prognosis for this condition is good, because most children do not develop seizures, learning disabilities, or behavior problems, and in only a few cases is there residual hemiparesis.

BASAL OCCLUSIVE DISEASE WITH TELANGIECTASIA. This condition, which is often referred to as Moyamoya disease (Fig. 25), is characterized by basal occlusive disease with prominent telangiectatic collaterals in the region of the basal ganglia and around the corpus callosum. The condition is more common in girls and has a higher incidence in children of Japanese ancestry. Headache prior to the onset of the hemiplegia is common; there may be multiple episodes with unilateral or bilateral involvement and a clinical picture of alternating hemiplegia. Exacerbations and remissions are common, but usually a persistent motor deficit develops. Long-term prognosis is poor; most children develop moderately severe hemiparesis, and many have epilepsy; in adult life there may be a rare occurrence of sudden subarachnoid hemorrhage.

DISTAL BRANCH OCCLUSION OVER THE CONVEXITY. Primary occlusion resulting from changes in the vessel wall may be a complication of diabetes mellitus, sickle cell disease, intravenous drug abuse, and the neurocutaneous syndromes. Leptomeningeal artery occlusions can be secondary to trauma, tumor encasement, or cerebral abscesses. Clinically the child usually presents with hemiplegia alone,

and often the motor deficit improves. Seizures (at the onset or subsequently) are unusual, and this form of arterial occlusion does not result in intellectual or behavior problems.

SMALL ARTERY DISEASE. Periarteritis nodosa and homocystinuria may affect the small perforating striate arteries. In periarteritis nodosa the cerebral arterial lesions are usually bilateral, and other organ systems (particularly the kidneys and heart) may be affected. Children with these conditions usually have a poor prognosis, as there may be a persistent motor deficit, bilateral or alternating hemiparesis, and associated epilepsy and intellectual deficit.

Cerebral Embolism

Cerebral arteries may be occluded by emboli from an organized thrombus or by bacteria, air, fat, or tumor. The middle cerebral artery or one of its branches is the vessel most frequently occluded. Cerebral embolic phenomena in childhood are usually of cardiac origin and occur in cyanotic congenital cardiac lesions and rheumatic valvular disease. Arrhythmias favor mural thrombus formation, and subsequent dislodgment may produce emboli. Emboli also may result from the vegetations of bacterial endocarditis or from neck and thoracic surgery. In the neonate cerebral emboli may originate from liberated infarcted placental tissue. Arterial air embolism has been encountered with greater frequency since the advent of cardiopulmonary bypass. Fat embolism is usually associated with fractures of long bones.

CLINICAL MANIFESTATIONS. Cerebral embolism is characterized by acute onset without significant prodromata, but premonitory symptoms of headache, vomiting, and lassitude may occur. Convulsions, transient loss of consciousness, and headache may be observed initially; focal neurologic findings depend on the cerebral artery occluded. Transient blindness is the most characteristic manifestation of air embolism.

Fat embolism has a typical clinical picture. Between 12 and 48 hours after fracture of a long bone, fever, respiratory distress, and blood-tinged sputum are noted. Within a few hours neurologic manifestations, petechial hemorrhages in the skin, fat in the retinal vessels, and free fat droplets in the urine appear.

LABORATORY FINDINGS. A moderate polymorphonuclear leukocytosis is common. CSF analysis and skull radiographs are usually normal. Electroencephalograms most commonly show a persistent slow-wave focus over the involved areas.

INTRACRANIAL HEMORRHAGE

Intracranial hemorrhage results in extravasation of blood into one or more of the following: brain, ventricles, and subarachnoid, epidural, and subdural spaces. Trauma is the most frequent cause of hemorrhage; it may result from rupture of a vascular malformation or aneurysm, or it may be associated with infectious, toxic, metabolic, or neoplastic conditions (Table 12). Despite the varied causes, the clinical manifestations of the various hemorrhages are similar, and etiologic delineation is further complicated by the presence of blood in the CSF. Proper management is largely dependent on knowledge of the specific cause.

Subarachnoid hemorrhage is characterized by signs and symptoms of increased intracranial pressure and meningeal irritation. The onset is usually dramatic, with severe headache, vomiting, loss of consciousness, and convulsions. Fever, which is often a misleading feature, may be prominent, and systemic hypertension is not uncommon. Evidence of meningeal irritation is an early clinical manifestation, with nuchal rigidity and Brudzinski and Kernig signs. The child with intracerebral bleeding may have blood in the subarachnoid space, in which case these features may also be associated with focal neurologic deficit. In children who survive subarachnoid bleeding, secondary hydrocephalus may develop from partial obliteration of the subarachnoid space. In the neonate the findings are nonspecific and may include apathy or restlessness, cyanosis or pallor, bulging of the fontanelles, respiratory distress, convulsions, high-pitched cry, vomiting, poor sucking, and an exaggerated or absent Moro reflex.

Children with intracranial hemorrhage may show polymorphonuclear leukocytosis with cell counts higher than $20,000/mm^3$, and transient hyperglycemia, albuminuria, and glycosuria. The electroencephalographic changes with subarachnoid hemorrhage are similar to those seen in closed head injury; the tracing is diffusely abnormal, with generalized slow-wave activity that disappears as the clinical state of the child improves. Blood in the CSF is the most conclusive evidence of intracranial bleeding. This must be clearly differentiated from the hemorrhage due to traumatic lumbar puncture. Failure of the fluid to clear in successive test tubes or a xanthochromic supernatant in a hemorrhage older than 2 hours is diagnostic of bleeding antedating the puncture. Usually the fluid is under increased pressure, the protein content is elevated, and white cells are in proportion to red cells.

Vascular Malformations

Primary subarachnoid hemorrhage in children is most commonly due to vascular anomalies and rarely to intracranial aneurysms. The vascular malformations may be traumatic or infectious, but are usually congenital. Arteriovenous malformations occur most frequently in two forms: deep midline (the area drained by the great vein of Galen) and hemispheric (the area supplied by major branches of the internal carotid artery).

DEEP MIDLINE ARTERIOVENOUS MALFORMATION. The malformation involving the galenic system is a direct anastomosis between major cerebral arteries, most commonly the posterior cerebral or the superior cerebellar artery and the great vein. There is marked enlargement of the vein, with formation of a midline aneurysm that not infrequently compresses and displaces the aqueduct, the third ventricle, and the quadrigeminal plate.

The clinical manifestations depend on the size of the shunt and the age at which symptoms first appear. The symptomatic newborn infant has a shunt of arterial blood into the venous circulation of such magnitude that it results in early congestive heart failure. In infancy, if less blood is shunted, cardiomegaly may be present but no cardiac failure is evident. Hydrocephalus is the most prominent feature as the distended vein of Galen displaces and compresses the aqueduct of Sylvius. An important sign in this age group is an intracranial bruit. The older child has a still smaller shunt, and dilation of the vein of Galen is only moderate. There is neither cardiovascular dysfunction nor hydrocephalus, but headaches and episodes of subarachnoid hemorrhage are common. Because of the small size of the shunt, an intracranial bruit is rarely heard.

Laboratory findings are variable and depend on the magnitude of the arteriovenous shunt. In the neonate marked cardiomegaly is usually noted on chest roentgenogram, but in older infants only mild enlargement is noted. The electrocardiogram may show combined ventricular hypertrophy in the neonate and left ventricular hypertrophy in older infants. The CSF is usually under increased pressure and may show evidence of recent or old hemorrhage. Increased oxygen tension in jugular venous blood is an important simple diagnostic test. Skull roentgenograms may show evidence of increased intracranial pressure in the younger child. Air contrast studies may suggest a malformation of a vein of Galen by demonstrating a posterior midline mass displacing the aqueduct downward. Cerebral angiography is the definitive diagnostic tool; it demonstrates a midline collection of contrast material outlining the vein of Galen.

HEMISPHERIC MALFORMATION. Hemispheric malformation involving branches of the internal carotid artery is most frequently found over the convexity of the brain in the territory of the middle cerebral artery. The lesion consists of an enlarged feeding artery and a mass of dilated tortuous veins. The onset of clinical manifestations is most commonly in late childhood or in adolescence, but cardiac failure may occur in the neonate. The child may complain of periodic migrainoid headaches for many years, but diagnosis is frequently not made until acute onset of subarachnoid hemorrhage. The child with a hemispheric malformation may complain of a localized pulsatile sound in the head, and a pathologic bruit may be heard on auscultation. The cardinal clinical manifestations are related to the site of the malformation. Involvement of branches of the middle cerebral artery is characterized by clinical manifestations referable to the motor cortex with focal motor or sensory and generalized seizures followed by transient postictal paralysis that gradually becomes a permanent lateralizing sign. Parietal lobe involvement is suggested by contralateral sensory seizures and hemisensory deficit involving position, stereognosis, discrimination, and localization of tactile stimuli and body image. Posterior fossa malformations produce signs of cerebellar dysfunction and evidence of increased intracranial pressure.

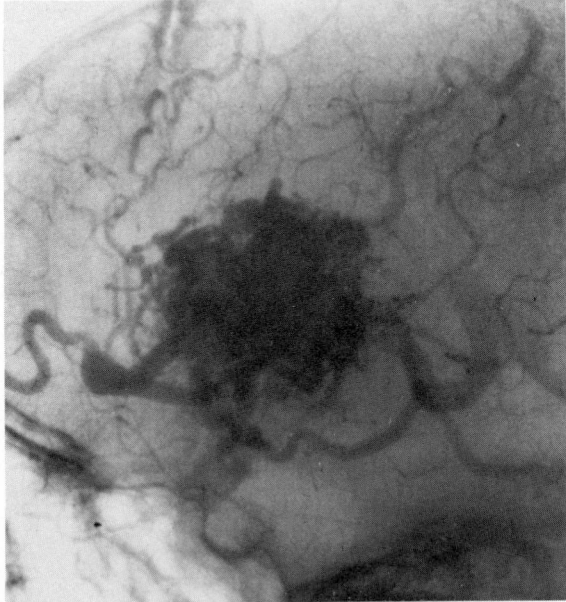

FIG. 26. Hemispheric vascular malformation. Arteriovenous malformation in left parietal lobe in a child with refractory seizures and a reading disability.

Skull roentgenograms, electroencephalograms, and CSF analysis are often normal; special studies are usually required. Visual fields may demonstrate a homonymous hemianopia. Radioisotope studies may show abnormal uptake. The diagnosis can be confirmed only by cerebral angiography (Fig. 26).

Traumatic Arteriovenous Fistula

Traumatic arteriovenous fistula can occur only in the region of the cavernous sinus where the internal carotid artery and the venous sinus are in juxtaposition. Following trauma there develops a classic clinical picture of pulsating exophthalmos, intracranial bruit, and involvement of the first two branches of the trigeminal nerve (facial sensory loss and diminished corneal reflex) and the oculomotor, trochlear, and abducens nerves (dilated and fixed pupil, diplopia, and extraocular muscle palsies). A carotid angiogram is usually diagnostic, with demonstration of the cavernous sinus during the arterial phase.

Intracranial Aneurysm

Ruptured saccular aneurysms are a rare cause of subarachnoid hemorrhage in children. Coarctation of the aorta, polycystic kidney disease, and generalized connective tissue disease are associated with intracranial aneurysms. Many cases go unrecognized because the aneurysm more commonly involves the bifurcation of the smaller peripherally placed arteries. The aneurysm in the child may be of giant size, and if it is unruptured it may produce signs and symptoms by mass effect. If the posterior circulation is involved with a giant aneurysm, progressive brainstem compression with cranial nerve involvement is usually observed.

Clinical manifestations are due to direct pressure of the aneurysm on surrounding structures or to hemorrhage from rupture. The onset is often dramatic and without warning, and death may result from massive bleeding into the subarachnoid space. Intracortical hemorrhage may give rise to focal neurologic signs that are dependent on the areas involved. Unless the aneurysm is occluded by a thrombus, its presence can often be demonstrated by cerebral angiography. Early angiography is indicated, except in the presence of coma with fluctuating vital signs.

Arteriovenous Malformation of the Spinal Cord

Vascular malformations of the spinal cord usually become symptomatic in childhood and are most commonly localized to the middle or lower thoracic and upper lumbar spinal cord. When the child is symptomatic he often complains of acute pain at the approximate site of the vascular lesion, and this is associated with signs and symptoms of subarachnoid hemorrhage. Subsequently the spinal cord is involved, with motor weakness and impaired sphincter function. A segmental cutaneous angioma at the level of the major feeding artery and the discovery of a paravertebral bruit may be useful clinical clues. Diagnosis is accomplished by selective spinal segmental angiography.

Diagnosis and Treatment

Differential diagnosis must distinguish the various types of cerebrovascular lesions from other conditions involving the central nervous system, such as brain tumor, abscess, trauma, epilepsy, and meningitis. A rational therapeutic program must take into consideration the pathologic process and resultant altered function. Nonspecific therapy consists of fluids to prevent dehydration, antibiotics to combat infection, anticonvulsants to control seizures, and anticoagulants to prevent extension of thrombus, when indicated. Increased intracranial pressure secondary to cerebral edema may be managed by the induction of mild hypothermia and the use of corticosteroids and/or urea.

Venous and dural sinus thromboses are managed by strict control of fluids and electrolytes and by antibiotics and anticonvulsants, when indicated. Mastoidectomy with decompression of the lateral sinus may be indicated when the dural sinus is involved. Repeated, often daily, lumbar punctures may be necessary to reduce the pressure, but if they are ineffective a lumboperitoneal shunt may be required to preserve vision. Arterial thromboses are treated symptomatically. Anticoagulation is contraindicated. The only indication for vascular surgery is thrombosis of the extracranial portion of the internal carotid artery. The management of arterial emboli is mainly symptomatic; anticoagulation may be used to prevent the formation of future emboli.

With arteriovenous malformations, severe cardiac failure should be treated with digitalis and diuretics. Surgery is hazardous, but it offers the only possibility for cure. It may be indicated if the vascular lesion is accessible, even when the vascular malformation involves the dominant hemisphere. Extirpation without resulting neurologic deficit would suggest that the arterial supply to the arteriovenous malformation is sometimes independent of the blood supply to the cerebral structures. Recently some malformations that could not be surgically resected have been successfully treated by percutaneous embolization techniques in which feeding arteries are occluded by embolization with silastic (silicone rubber) spheres. Lesions most amenable to successful embolization are those supplied by the leptomeningeal branches of the middle cerebral artery, as well as arteriovenous malformations in the diencephalon and posterior thalamus.

Intracranial aneurysms are best managed by surgery, even in the young child. The occurrence of a secondary hemorrhage following rapidly after the initial subarachnoid hemorrhage is suprisingly uncommon in children, and for this reason conservative management is indicated until the child is in an optimum condition to tolerate surgery.

References

GENERAL

Classification and outline of cerebrovascular diseases. Neurology 8: 395, 1958

Gold AP, Challenor YB, Gilles FH, et al: Report of joint committee for stroke facilities. IX. Strokes in children (Part 1). Stroke 4:834, 1973; (Part 2). 4:1007, 1973

CEREBRAL VENOUS AND DURAL SINUS THROMBOSIS

Gold AP: Abnormalities of the venous sinuses, vein of Galen aneurysms, cavernous sinus fistula, and cavernous sinus thrombosis. In Goldensohn E, Appel SH (eds): Scientific Approaches to Clinical Neurology. Philadelphia, Lea & Febiger, 1976

Kalbag RM, Wolff AL: Cerebral Venous Thrombosis with Special Reference to Aseptic Thrombosis. London, Oxford University Press, 1967

Portnoy BA, Herion JC: Neurological manifestations in sickle cell disease with review of the literature and emphasis on the prevalence of hemiplegia. Ann Intern Med 76:643, 1972

ARTERIAL THROMBOSIS

Banker BQ: Cerebral vascular disease in infancy and childhood: 1. Occlusive vascular diseases. J Neuropathol Exp Neurol 20:127, 1961

Carter S, Gold AP: Acute hemiplegia in infancy and childhood. Pediatr Clin North Am 14:851, 1967

Davie JC, Coxe W: Occlusive disease of the carotid artery in children. Arch Neurol 17:313, 1967

DeVivo DC, Farrell FW Jr: Vertebrobasilar occlusive disease in children: a recognizable clinical entity. Arch Neurol 26:278, 1972

Harwood-Nash DC, McDonald P, Argent W: Cerebral arterial disease in children. An angiographic study of 40 cases. Am J Roentgenol Radium Ther Nucl Med 111:672, 1971

Hilal SK, Solomon GE, Gold AP, Carter S: Primary cerebral arterial occlusive disease in children. Part I. Acute acquired hemiplegia. Radiology 99:71, 1971

——— Solomon GE, Gold AP, Carter S: Primary cerebral arterial occlusive disease in children. Part II. Neurocutaneous syndromes. Radiology 99:87, 1971

Houser OW, Baker HL Jr: Fibromuscular dysplasia and other uncommon diseases of the cervical carotid artery: angiographic aspects. Am J Roentgenol Radium Ther Nucl Med 104:201, 1968

Ouvrier RA, Hopkins IJ: Occlusive disease of the vertebro-basilar arterial system in childhood. Dev Med Child Neurol 12:186, 1970

Shillito J Jr: Carotid arteritis: a cause of hemiplegia in childhood. J Neurosurg 21:540, 1964

Solomon GE, Hilal SK, Gold AP, Carter S: Natural history of acute hemiplegia of childhood. Brain 93:107, 1970

Tyler HR, Clark DB: Cerebrovascular accidents in patients with congenital heart disease. Arch Neurol Psychiatry 77:483, 1957

CEREBRAL EMBOLISM

Wells CE: Cerebral embolism: the natural history, prognostic signs, and effects of anticoagulation. Arch Neurol Psychiatry 81:667, 1959

INTRACRANIAL HEMORRHAGE

Amacher AL, Drake CG: Cerebral artery aneurysms in infancy, childhood and adolescence. Child's Brain 1:72, 1975

Chalgreen WS: Neurologic complications of the hemorrhagic disease. Neurology 3:126, 1953

Gold AP: Cerebral arteriovenous malformations. Dev Med Child Neurol 15:84, 1973

——— Ransohoff J, Carter S: Vein of Galen malformation. Acta Neurol Scand [Suppl I] 1964, p 40

Holden AM, Fyler DC, Shillito J: Congestive heart failure from intracranial arteriovenous fistula in infancy. Pediatrics 49:30, 1972

Levine OR, Jameson AG, Nellhaus G, Gold AP: Cardiac complication of cerebral arteriovenous fistulas. Pediatrics 30:563, 1962

Lewis IC, Philpott MG: Neurological complications of Schönlein-Henoch syndrome. Arch Dis Child 31:369, 1956

Matson DD: Intracranial arterial aneurysms in childhood. J Neurosurg 23:578, 1965

Patel AN, Richardson AE: Ruptured intracranial aneurysms in the first two decades of life. J Neurosurg 35:571, 1971

Sedzimer CB, Robinson J: Intracranial haemorrhage in children and adolescents. J Neurosurg 38:269, 1973

Silverstein A: Intracranial bleeding in hemophilia. Arch Neurol Psychiatry 3:141, 1960

Zeller RS, Chutorian AM: Vascular malformations of the pons in children. Neurology 25:776, 1975

DIAGNOSIS AND TREATMENT

Carter S, Gold AP: Status epilepticus. In Smith CA (ed): The Critically Ill Child: Diagnosis and Management. Philadelphia, WB Saunders, 1972

Gold AP, Carter S: Pediatric neurology. In Shirkey HC (ed): Pediatric Therapy, 4th ed. St Louis, CV Mosby, 1972

———— Challenor Y: Cerebrovascular disease in children. In Downey JA, Low NL (eds): The Child with Disabling Illness: Principles of Rehabilitation. Philadelphia, WB Saunders, 1974

TRAUMA TO THE NERVOUS SYSTEM

JAMES F. HAMMILL

Among children in the United States, accidental injuries are by far the most serious threat to life. Trauma results in 100,000 deaths per year, of which 15,000 are children; more than half of these are due to motor vehicle accidents in which the child is a passenger or pedestrian. Deaths from trauma in the age group from birth to 14 years exceed the combined fatalities from infection, malignancy, and cardiovascular-renal disease.

Forty percent of all trauma cases in childhood involve head injuries, either alone or combined with other injuries. The peak age incidence is in the second year of life, with males outnumbering females 2 to 1. Peak seasonal incidence is in the spring and summer months during the late afternoon and early evening hours. The mortality rate is about 0.5 percent. Head injuries may affect the scalp, the skull, or the nervous system alone or in combination. Most injuries involving the nervous system are simple concussion or mild contusion, and there is usually complete recovery without complications. Some, however, may be more serious, or even life-threatening; these require careful analysis and management.

SCALP INJURIES

Lacerations

Scalp injury is usually due to blunt trauma; however, the resulting wound is usually a smooth linear cut due to the unyielding surface of the bone over which the blow occurs. Wounds of the skin layer are usually separated only minimally, owing to fixation by the underlying fibrous tissue septa. When the galea is involved the wound will gape, particularly if it is in a transverse direction. Bleeding is quite marked because of the rich anastomotic blood supply of the scalp and the limited contraction-retraction ability of the vessels firmly anchored in the dense connective tissue layer. Consequently, large lacerations heal quite well, and infection rarely occurs unless there is gross contamination or tissue destruction. However, infections of the skull and intracranial contents present serious hazards; they invariably result from poor initial handling. Such wounds are best treated by primary closure, but if the child's condition prohibits immediate handling, this can be delayed for 8 to 12 hours without significant increase in risk of infection.

Hematoma and Cephalohematoma

Hematomas in the dense connective tissue layer of the scalp are common, but because of the density of the tissue they are usually not very large and absorb within 2 to 3 days. Galeal laceration permits bleeding from above to permeate the subgaleal loose connective tissue layer and may result in rapid extensive swelling of enormous proportions, since there is no limiting membrane to prevent its spread.

Bleeding beneath the pericranium is most common in the incompletely ossified and highly vascular skull characteristic of the first 2 years of life. These collections are restricted by the pericranial suture line attachment; they occur most often in the parietal area and are known as cephalohematomas (Fig. 27). On palpation, subgaleal and subpericranial hematomas may be confused with an underlying depressed fracture. Subgaleal collections of partially clotted blood may develop a soft center surrounded by an indurated ring, which may be mistaken for a rim of bone about an area of skull depression. The

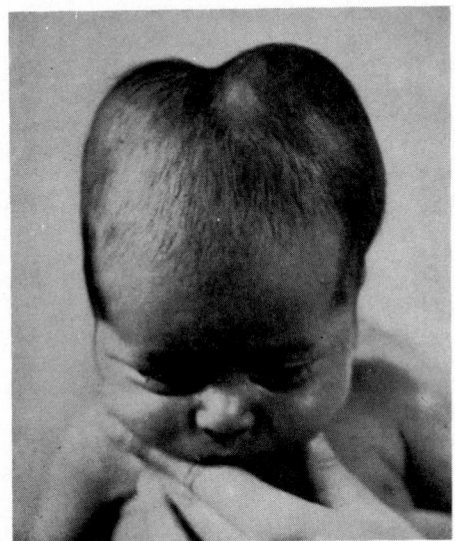

FIG. 27.   Cephalohematoma involving both parietal bones in an infant 13 days old.

pericranial fibrous suture attachment demarcating cephalohematomas is also commonly confused with a depressed skull fracture. Fracture sites (depressed or linear) underlying hematomas require radiographic examination to clarify the diagnosis.

The larger hematomas are absorbed in 2 to 4 weeks. When cephalohematomas persist, pericranial proliferation occurs with the production of bony callus; ultimately a thin layer of bone may be formed in the involved area. Only rarely is there calcification of an entire nonabsorbed hemorrhagic area. Aspiration or open evacuation of hematomas is contraindicated, as the partially clotted blood is difficult to aspirate and the risk of infection is great. In the infant cephalohematomas may be large enough to cause anemia and mild jaundice. Collections of CSF that are termed subgaleal or subepicranial hydromas may occur over linear skull fractures when there is a meningeal tear. They are usually less extensive and softer than hematomas and have a less well defined ring of induration. When the fluid is not mixed with blood, transillumination is greater than in the case of hematomas, and the mass may be noted to fluctuate with coughing and straining. These collections subside spontaneously with healing of the underlying dural tear. If the collection is large or if it persists beyond 4 to 7 days, the swelling may be reduced by lumbar puncture. Pressure dressings do not hasten absorption of hematomas and hydromas, and they may contribute to skin breakdown and infection.

Craniocerebral Trauma

The human head may withstand tremendous force and yet maintain both skull and cerebral integrity. The position of the head at impact, suture patency, and degree of movement at the craniospinal junction are important variables. Blood pressure may reach 150 percent of normal or even higher in an attempt to compensate for increased intracranial pressure and maintain cerebral circulation.

Shock rarely occurs on a purely neural basis; it is usually due to blood loss from associated extracerebral injuries. Neural shock may occur with extensive and irreversible cerebral damage; this is an ominous prognostic sign. In the acute postconcussive phase of experimental cerebral injury, cerebral edema may increase brain volume more than 5 percent within minutes and produce marked bradycardia

Mass movement of intracranial contents with the injury results in contusion at the point of impact and at some distance from it. Subarachnoid and intracerebral bleeding may occur. Subdural bleeding results when blood vessels between the brain and meninges are torn; this usually occurs because the cortical bridging veins enter the dural-encased superior longitudinal sinus. Extradural hematomas may result from disruption of extradural veins or arteries.

Transient unconsciousness after injury reflects a sudden physiologic block at the brainstem level. The brainstem reticular formation has an alerting function, mediating sensory input to higher centers. Following trauma this formation may enter an absolutely refractory state, recovery from which directly correlates with return to consciousness. This mechanism is the most common cause of the transient concussion picture and is due to increased cervicocranial mobility after impact that permits transmission of increased angular acceleration and shear strains to the entire brain but particularly the brainstem. Animals with the head relatively fixed can sustain a head injury force double that usually resulting in concussion.

Skull Fractures

Skull fractures may involve the vault or base and may be of the simple linear or of the diastatic (abnormal suture separation occuring at the time of impact) type, simple depressed, comminuted, or ping-pong or pond variety. They may occur as isolated manifestations of head trauma, but more often they are associated with underlying cerebral injury. Simple linear and diastatic fractures are of little immediate significance other than to indicate the force of the blow and the point of maximal impact. Over 80 percent of all skull fractures are of this type, and the parietal area is involved five times more frequently than other regions. Diastatic fractures have the same medicolegal significance as a fracture line, and they most often involve the lambdoid suture. A separation of the lambdoid suture wider than 1.5 mm, particularly at several points in its course, is usually considered abnormal, as is a coronal suture spread of more than 2 mm.

The cranial vault is less calcified in infants less than 1 year old, and it has greater elasticity of its inner and outer tables. Both tables may be displaced inward without an actual break occuring, thus producing the ping-pong or pond fracture. Fractures of the base of the skull may be indicated by bilateral orbital ecchymoses in anterior fossa lesions and by retroauricular ecchymosis (Battle's sign) with tympanic membrane discoloration in involvement of the petrous bone in the middle fossa. Otorrhea and rhinorrhea imply basilar skull fracture and are potentially of more serious consequence because of the risk of infection. Post-traumatic collection of intracranial air in any of the meningeal spaces (aerocele) or the ventricular system (pneumoencephalocele) implies fractures through the paranasal sinuses.

LABORATORY DATA AND DIAGNOSIS. Skull radiographs are the essential aid to diagnosis. There is seldom an emergency indication for films, since films rarely add to management of the immediate problem and are best delayed until the child's condition permits optimal radiographic study of the skull and of all suspected areas of trauma. A skeletal survey to detect areas of multiple osseous injury is essential in infants, but may also be indicated in older children. If CSF drainage from the nose is suspected, the presence of glucose will confirm its origin, since nasal secretions have negligible amounts of glucose.

TREATMENT. Simple linear fractures without underlying damage do not require treatment other than analgesics for headache and irritability. It should be made clear to the parents that a simple skull fracture is of little concern and is not an indication to restrict activities. A repeat skull radiograph is recommended after 3 months to demonstrate union; if union is not progressing, films should be repeated at intervals of 3 months to detect possible complications such as leptomeningeal cyst. Fractures usually heal in 6 to 12 months.

Pond fractures usually do not require surgical elevation. Rarely an underlying defect of cerebral cortex may result in a lack of brain growth and failure of the skull depression to elevate; a 3-month period of observation will determine this (Fig. 28). Fractures depressed more than 0.5 cm should be elevated to avoid the formation of undesirable cerebromeningeal cicatrices with the attendant danger of focal neurologic defect and seizures. Early surgery is indicated, as it is in all compound and comminuted skull fractures.

Basal skull fractures resulting in rhinorrhea or otorrhea require hospitalization. The child should be maintained in a semiupright position; plugging or irrigation of the involved orifices is contraindicated. The use of prophylactic antibiotics and chemotherapy is controversial; however, in the presence of a demonstrated CSF leak, therapy is comparable to that for undiagnosed bacterial meningitis (p. 422). Spontaneous cessation of CSF drainage may occur. If flow persists beyond a week, surgical repair should be considered, as the danger of meningitis is overwhelming. This hazard remains as long as fistulous patency exists, and it may result in repeated infections, diffuse arachnoiditis, and secondary hydrocephalus. Traumatic aerocele, if persistent, is also an indication for operative intervention. Intracranial air tends to be rapidly absorbed. If radiographs at 48- to 72-hour intervals show persistence or increased collection of air, surgery should not be delayed. In cases of rhinorrhea, coughing and sneezing may produce increased drainage and may actually permit air to enter the intracranial cavity. Accentuation of headache under these circumstances may be the result of delayed intracranial air collection and may be documented by repeat radiographs. Suppression of coughing and sneezing is indicated in all patients with post-traumatic otorrhea or rhinorrhea.

A late sequela of a linear fracture in young children is a leptomeningeal cyst, or more accurately a growing skull fracture. This results from dural laceration, projection of the arachnoid membrane into the fracture site with brain herniation and produces bone erosion of the overlying skull over a period of months or years. The late onset of focal seizures, increased intracranial pressure, focal neurologic signs, and occasionally visible and palpable skull deformity should suggest this complication. Skull radiographs are diagnostic (Fig. 29), revealing an area of erosion over a prior fracture site. Growing skull factures are usually in the parietal area and should be suspected when the initial fracture line is wide or is associated with a subepicranial hydroma.

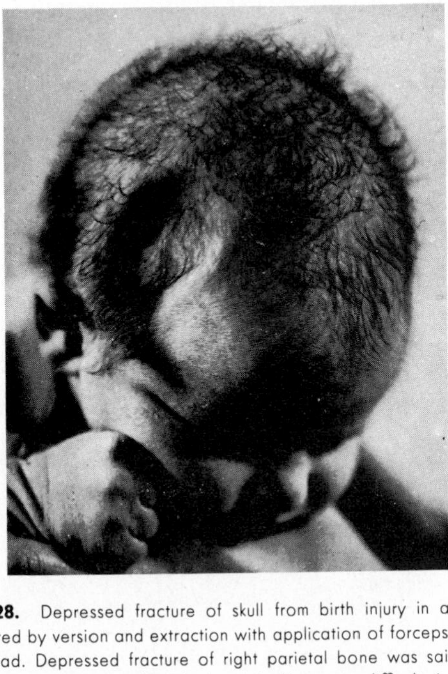

FIG. 28. Depressed fracture of skull from birth injury in an infant delivered by version and extraction with application of forceps to trailing head. Depressed fracture of right parietal bone was said to be related to abnormality of mother's pelvis. There was difficulty in resuscitation and cyanosis during the first few hours, with right internal strabismus but no signs of increased intracranial pressure. Patients made complete recovery without operation and was physically and mentally normal at age 5.5 years.

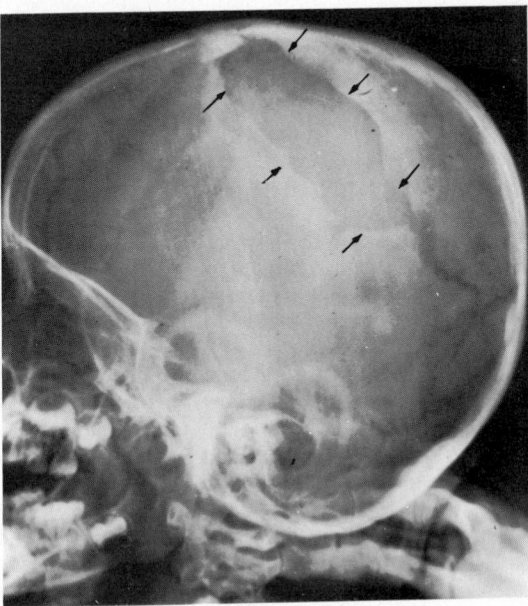

FIG. 29. Leptomeningeal cyst showing large area of parietal skull erosion 8 months after a simple linear fracture

Extradural Hematoma

Extradural hematoma refers to bleeding between the skull and dura usually from a tear in the middle meningeal artery due to a temporal bone fracture; it may also result from extradural vessels. As the skull matures, vessels in this location are firmly embedded in bony grooves and are more vulnerable to damage by fractures. Children less than 2 years of age rarely sustain extradural hemorrhage, as these vessels are less adherent to the calvarium. Because of the greater elasticity of the young skull, damage of this type may exist without radiographic demonstration of fracture.

The typical clinical syndrome is apparent during the first 12 to 24 hours after initial injury. The child may be rendered briefly unconscious by the original trauma, then regain awareness, and after a period of several hours lapse into coma with signs of increased intracranial pressure, hemiplegia, and at times focal seizures. An equal number of children present without a lucid interval; these progressively merge from a moderate initial lethargy or stupor into a state of profound coma.

There is no mechanism for the absorption of an extradural hemorrhage, and its increasing mass rapidly raises intracranial pressure, with a progressive hypertension and bradycardia. Later respirations become slow and irregular, and hypotension and tachycardia develop terminally. The suddenly increased intracranial pressure may cause early third cranial nerve compression on the affected side, with a fixed dilated pupil. Subhyaloid hemorrhages, which are mobile collections between the retina and the overlying subhyaloid membrane, may occur; they may change shape and position with head movement. In young children a fracture line may be absent or not visible, suture diastasis may be the only evidence of trauma, and the lucid interval may be absent. The syndrome usually runs a course of 6 to 12 hours in adults, but may extend from 24 to 96 hours in children because of the greater incidence of venous bleeding rather than arterial bleeding. Either type is more commonly associated with anemia in children than in adults.

Extradural hemorrhage is the most lethal complication of head injury, with a mortality rate in untreated cases of 100 percent and in operatively treated cases of almost 50 percent. Untreated cases seldom survive more than 2 to 3 days. Treatment demands immediate diagnosis and definitive surgery. Local conditions or the patient's critical status may preclude detailed evaluation and necessitate immediate surgery on clinical grounds. However, skull radiography, echoencephalography, arteriography, and computer-assisted tomography (EMI scan) should be considered in less urgent cases.

Prognosis for survival and neurologic integrity is directly proportional to the patient's preoperative status and duration of unconsciousness. Under optimal conditions complete recovery without residua may be expected.

Subdural Hematoma

In contrast to the infrequent occurrence of extradural hematomas in children and their relative rarity in patients less than 2 years of age, subdural hematomas are common, with approximately 85 percent occurring in children 1 year of age or less. The syndrome may present acutely (within 3 days), subacutely (within 4 to 20 days), or chronically (after 20 days), as dated from the presumed time of trauma. Hemorrhage is venous, and blood collects in the potential space between dura and arachnoid. It arises from laceration of veins bridging the area from the cortex to the superior longitudinal sinus, or less often from venous bleeding associated with cerebral laceration or an actual venous sinus tear. Such collections in children are bilateral in 80 percent of cases. These hemorrhages seldom absorb and tend to become encapsulated by dural proliferation.

In infancy the clinical picture often consists of gradually increasing intracranial pressure, with an enlarging head, bulging fontanelle, anemia, seizures, irritability, vomiting, and failure to thrive. The relative frequencies of signs and symptoms are indicated in Table 13. In young children the diagnosis can be made by subdural puncture through the lateral recess of a patent anterior fontanelle. This must be performed bilaterally. When the diagnosis has been established, repeated daily aspirations of 50 ml or more of subdural fluid from alternate sides, within the limits of patient tolerance and ease of flow, may be made. This technique attempts to empty the subdural space and permit cortical reexpansion to obliterate it. If after 10 to 14 days this regimen has not been effective, it is unlikely that further attempts will be sussessful. Inability to tap the subdural space "dry" may be due to absolute enlargement of the cranial cavity by the hematoma to such a degree that the brain cannot reexpand to fill it, failure of expansion due to membrane formation about a chronic hematoma, sceondary cerebral atrophy, a fistula from the subarachnoid into the subdural space, or continued bleeding. Surgical drainage, craniotomy with membrane removal, or a shunting procedure will be necessary. Careful attention must be directed to preventing or correcting anemia, hypoproteinemia, and electrolyte abnormali-

TABLE 13. Frequencies of Signs and Symptoms of Subdural Hematomas

Signs	Frequency (%)
Anemia	70
Seizures	65
Vomiting	50
X-ray signs of increased pressure	50
Enlarged head	40
History of trauma	40
Retinal hemorrhages	40
Hyperirritability	35
Bulging fontanelle	35
Focal neurologic defect	35
Slowed development	20
Skull fracture	20

ties during the period of therapy. Subdural hematomas in older children require surgical drainage and seldom reaccumulate after operation.

Negative findings from subdural punctures do not absolutely rule out subdural collections. The exploring needle may not enter the fluid lake, or viscous compartmented liquid may preclude withdrawal. Evidence of increasing intracranial pressure, focal seizures, and deterioration in general neurologic status and level of consciousness should alert one to the problem. Electroencephalography may reveal marked unilateral or bilateral cortical depression over subdural collections, but electroencephalograms are often normal or nonspecific. Cerebral angiography and computer-assisted tomography (Fig. 30) are the best diagnostic tests to indicate the presence and extent of subdural collection; they should be considered if the condition is suspected.

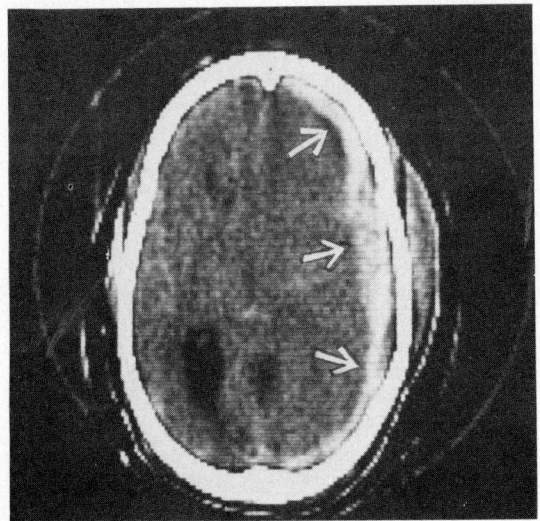

FIG. 30. Large subdural hematoma (CAT scan). There is a large hematoma in the subdural space on the right side extending from the midline of the frontal bone to the midline of the occipital bone covering the entire convexity of the right cerebral hemisphere. Fresh blood, as usual, is radiodense, and the hematoma appears as a white band under the calvarium. Another component of the hematoma is seen on the outside of the skull in the subcutaneous tissues in the right temporal area. (Courtesy of Dr. S. Hilal.)

Treatment is usually successful when the diagnosis is made early, before cerebral atrophy and a fixed neurologic deficit have occurred. Post-traumatic lacerations of the arachnoid membrane resulting in CSF collections in the subdural space, termed subdural hygromas, present the same general clinical picture and problems as subdural hematomas.

Concussion

Closed head injuries make up the largest group of cases of craniocerebral trauma. The term implies no more injury to the underlying bone than a linear fracture. The simplest type of head trauma is cerebral concussion. Following a sudden head blow, transient loss of consciousness occurs, but is followed by full recovery without sequelae. More prolonged unconsciousness, often associated with some evidence of focal neurologic defect and varying degrees of amnesia, implies a cerebral contusion or laceration. Children with either injury often vomit and later are pale and apathetic or quite irritable. Overwhelming cerebral stimuli may result in convulsions. This is especially common in young children and does not necessarily imply severe brain damage or a high risk of future convulsions. Transient loss of vision may also be noted after concussion; although this may be disturbing it is usually benign. In cases of simple concussion or mild contusion the child should be examined carefully with attention to gross evidence of skull fracture and associated damage to viscera and bones. Recording of vital signs and observation until full recovery of consciousness is mandatory. In most cases the child will have recovered partially by the time he is seen and, other than pallor, irritability, and bruises, will have few signs on examination. These children are best managed at home, provided the parents can cooperate in noting the youngster's pupillary equality, level of responsiveness, and general motor power. Arousal of the patient every 2 hours to determine the level of awareness and other signs is advisable for 12 to 24 hours after injury.

Cerebral Contusion and Laceration

Severe degrees of head injury or prolonged unconsciousness require hospitalization to evaluate the extent of injury and the need for specific therapy. Immediate attention must be given to airway maintenance, treatment of shock and fractures, control of hemorrhage, prevention of fat embolization, or care of splenic rupture, lung perforation, aspiration, atelectasis, or rarer complications such as disseminated intravascular coagulation and acute respiratory distress syndrome.

Evaluation of the head injury requires a detailed history, with particular regard to the time sequence of events. Examination should include precise evaluation of the individual's level of consciousness and content of verbalizations and performance: Is the child irritable, agitated, confused, disoriented, confabulatory, amnesic, or completely unresponsive? Is there a response to sound and pain stimuli? Is it appropriate or purposeless?

Hospitalization is recommended to assess the course and intelligently anticipate and treat complications. All pertinent items must therefore be clearly recorded to afford any examiner or consultant the comparative analysis that is the essential feature in the management of head injury patients. Pupillary size and reaction, observed extraocular movements, findings from examination of the fundi, symmetry of facial movement (either spontaneous or with pain stimulus), corneal responses, gag reflex, spontaneous or induced limb movements, tonus, deep tendon reflexes, and response to plantar stimulation should be listed, in addition to vital signs, evidence of meningeal irritation, and a description of any discharge from ears or nose; also the scalp and skull should be examined carefully.

CSF studies are of limited value in cases of head injury, and their routine use cannot be justified. However, when there is suspicion of concurrent meningitis, lumbar puncture is clearly indicated. In the acute post-traumatic period a spinal tap has little differentiating value, since intracortical, subdural, or extradural hematomas may be characterized by either clear or bloody fluid. An elevated CSF pressure is usual after any significant degree of cerebral contusion, whether there has been a post-traumatic subarachnoid hemorrhage or not. In the latter instance, headache and meningeal discomfort may be relieved by the withdrawal of CSF after the patient's general condition has been stabilized for 72 hours or more.

Meningeal signs are often delayed for 8 to 24 hours after subarachnoid hemorrhage. This type of bleeding is common and is not a serious complication apart from the fact that it produces discomfort and prolongs convalescence. Rarely, obstruction to the CSF pathway may develop after bleeding into the subarachnoid space caused by obstruction at the incisura; this is often temporary, but post-traumatic hydrocephalus may result, necessitating a shunting procedure. Depending on the degree of cerebral damage, the child may not regain full consciousness for a period ranging from hours to several weeks. During this time supportive care may be complicated by problems of nutrition and electrolyte balance, restlessness, seizures, respiration, fever, bladder care, and otorrhea or rhinorrhea.

Patients remaining unconscious for any significant period of time may present a problem in fluid balance secondary to post-traumatic diabetes insipidus, paradoxic antidiuretic hormone excretion, and varied degrees of hyponatremia or hypernatremia. Fluid intake and urinary output should be recorded in conjunction with weight and serum electrolyte determinations until intake and output return to normal. Restlessness, increasing stupor, and seizures may result from gross electrolyte imbalance, usually on the basis of failing to recognize an increased thirst or by iatrogenic water intoxication. As soon as feasible, nutrition and fluid balance should progress from intravenous to nasogastric feedings and finally to normal oral feeding. Post-traumatic diabetes insipidus is usually transient, but may require a period of Pitressin therapy, either by injection or as snuff. A number of children have a brief vasodepressor shocklike reaction to Pitressin tannate in oil and initially are best treated with an aqueous Pitressin preparation.

An irritable, lethargic-stuporous state characterizes many injured patients. Depressant drugs of the barbiturate or phenothiazine groups are best avoided in the acute period after injury. Diazepam (Valium), 2 to 4 mg intramuscularly or orally every 4 to 6 hours as needed, is safe, as is paraldehyde 2 to 4 ml via the same routes. Bladder drainage, adequate hydration, loose restraints about wrists and ankles, boxing gloves for older children, and a well-padded crib or bed rails may be necessary to calm and protect the disturbed patient.

Convulsions, other than at the time of the initial impact, demand suppressant therapy. This usually implies an initial phenobarbital or paraldehyde regimen in conjunction with diphenylhydantoin (Dilantin) therapy. Dosages, routes of administration, and management of convulsive status are described in detail elsewhere (p. 1848). The appearance of generalized or focal seizure phenomena may reflect the presence of a subdural or intracortical hematoma; however, convulsions are seldom the only manifestations in such cases, and they most often reflect underlying cortical contusion and laceration rather than a specific vascular complication.

Maintenance of a clear respiratory passage by proper positioning, suction, oropharyngeal airway, endotracheal intubation or tracheostomy is essential. Tracheostomy should be an elective procedure and preferably should be performed on a previously inserted endotracheal tube. In cases of severe brain damage with impaired gag and cough mechanisms, tracheostomy is an initial step in management to prevent aspiration, atelectasis, and pneumonia. In the young child requiring respiratory aid, a properly positioned high tracheostomy with a tube of maximal caliber is essential.

Significant temperature elevations in the absence of infection occur after head injury. However, even in cases with post-traumatic subarachnoid hemorrhage the temperature rarely exceeds 39 C unless there is severe cortical and brainstem involvement. The patient in the latter category is usually in profound coma and may demonstrate marked temperature variations with elevations above 40 C. In these cases, if the patient is unresponsive to aspirin and sponging, the use of hypothermia may be considered with the temperature maintained at 33 to 35 C in an effort to decrease cerebral and general metabolic requirements in a situation of probable hypothalamic damage.

Urinary care may become a problem either because of continued soiling with resultant skin irritation and breakdown or because of periodic retention. The usual techniques (diaper, urinary collection bag, or catheter) may be utilized. Should an indwelling catheter be necessary, prophylactic antibiotics will not be effective in preventing infection in the absence of scrupulous aseptic catheter technique and bladder irrigation.

Varying degrees of cerebral edema occur after head injury. It may be restricted to the contused, lacerated area, or it may become generalized and present a picture of markedly increased intracranial pressure, focal neurologic signs, and seizures. Differentiation from hematoma formation or active intracranial bleeding is often impossible. The diagnosis is most frequently made retrospectively after clot or hemorrhage has been ruled out. General supportive care is all that is usually needed, but in critical situations efforts to decrease brain bulk by intravenous urea or mannitol may be of value. Hyperosmolar substances of this type produce a marked diuresis and a decrease in cerebral bulk by dehydration. A bladder catheter should be inserted whenever these compounds are used, and electrolyte balance should be carefully followed. Urea is given in an intravenous dose of 1.0 to 1.5 g/kg body weight. Mannitol is infused as a 20 percent solution in a dose of 2 to 3 g/kg. Rebound swelling occurs with either compound, and therapy may be needed over several days. There is no conclusive evidence that hypothermia is beneficial in the management of cerebral edema; however, efforts to maintain normothermia in the febrile patient may be of value. A more effective means of treating cerebral edema is with the use of steroids. Dexamethasone (Decadron), 4 to 16 mg daily for 3 days and gradually decreasing thereafter, is the drug of choice. Therapy of this type is best accomplished in specialized treatment units where the necessary equipment and nursing personnel are available.

Intracortical hematomas are usually small; large solitary post-traumatic collections are uncommon. Surgically significant hematomas are often clinically indistinguishable from extradural or subdural collections. Increasing intracranial pressure and progressive focal neurologic signs may result from an intracerebral clot in the absence of the more common hematomas. Diagnosis requires ancillary studies. The most valuable investigation is computer-assisted tomography; it is noninvasive and can clearly differentiate varied fluid collections from cerebral edema as well as aid in precise localization. Many hematomas resolve without the need for surgical intervention; however, with increasing neurologic deficit and intracranial pressure and with ancillary evidence of progressive displacement, surgery should be considered.

Sequelae of Craniocerebral Trauma

Combinations of fixed neurologic defects may exist after brain injury, but they are usually self-evident. The less predictable sequelae are seizures, organic mental changes, and post-traumatic syndrome.

SEIZURES. Post-traumatic seizures are most often generalized rather than focal, but they may be of any type other than petit mal. The incidence of persistent convulsive phenomena after head injury is unknown, and it would be extremely difficult to determine. The severity of the injury, the duration of unconsciousness, the occurrence of early seizures other than at the time of impact, and the serial electroencephalographic patterns are of some value in analyzing the problem.

Penetrating depressed fractures have a residual seizure incidence of 30 to 60 percent, particularly if they are associated with periods of unconsciousness greater than 24 hours and the presence of convulsions during the acute phase. Children surviving subdural, extradural, or intracortical hematomas have a similar late seizure potential. A normal electroencephalogram with absence of paroxysmal or focal abnormalities 3 months after injury tends to make post-traumatic epilepsy less likely than when such discharges exist. A progressively worsening tracing is quite suspect; however, a delay of months to a year or more in the development of any electrical abnormality may be seen in patients who have

or will subsequently develop seizures. Gross irregularity of the electroencephalogram may be present after head trauma in a perfectly normal child, and at times the tracing may appear relatively normal in the presence of frank focal neurologic defect. Nevertheless, a tracing should be obtained after significant head trauma as a baseline in cases with or without seizures concomitant with the acute episode. Unfortunately the electroencephalogram is often of little help and may be actually misleading in predicting the chances of epilepsy developing after any given injury.

In closed head injuries late epilepsy occurs in less than 5 percent of cases. The seizures may present from 3 months to 4 years or more after injury, with the peak incidence occurring at 6 to 18 months. Previously controlled seizure states in known epileptics may be exacerbated after head injury, although analysis of such groups has revealed no consistent pattern.

Convulsive phenomena during the acute episode will usually result in the patient being placed on anticonvulsant therapy, which should be maintained for at least a 2-year period of freedom from seizures before gradual withdrawal of the drug. The appearance of the electroencephalogram at this time bears little relationship to the occurrence of subsequent convulsions, either with or without medication. Some authorities think that a paroxysmal or focally abnormal electroencephalogram after injury is in itself an indication for prolonged anticonvulsive drug therapy. This remains a controversial point.

ORGANIC MENTAL SYNDROMES. Self-limited memory defects and minor personality changes may be noted after head injury. Persistent frank organic dementia is uncommon in children, as is intellectual defect; with severe and extensive injuries, particularly in infancy, psychomotor retardation may be seen.

POST-TRAUMATIC SYNDROME. The problem of general sequelae following head injury (the post-traumatic syndrome) is less common in children than in adults; however, it does occur. The symptoms tend to vary somewhat from those in the adult (headache, irritability, and postural vertigo). They are more commonly in the realm of enuresis, disturbances of sleep pattern, episodically aggressive behavior, and decline in school performance. How much of this is due to organic rather than primarily psychologic factors is difficult to state. Symptomatic management with sedatives, tranquilizers, and sometimes psychotherapy may be needed. Investigation as to the presence of typical or fragmentary convulsive phenomena may be profitable, and improvement may be noted after the institution of anticonvulsive therapy.

A commonsense attitude toward general care during the acute phase is extremely important. Overhospitalization, gratuitous unfounded remarks about possible future brain damage, and prolonged litigation correlate highly with the incidence of post-traumatic behavior dysfunction. The physician must maintain an attitude of expectancy for return to normal function, both with the parents and the child. The avoidance of oversolicitous and unnecessary limitation of school, play, and social activities will ameliorate a common factor in the etiology of the post-traumatic reaction syndrome.

Group statistical studies tend to indicate that children with behavior and mental defects are more prone to head injury and more prone to display sequelae than mentally stable individuals.

INJURIES TO THE SPINAL CORD

Trauma to the vertebral column and spinal cord constitutes less than 5 percent of childhood injuries. The enclosure of the spinal cord in a bony canal is of great protective value; however, the mobility of the cervical spine and enlargement of the spinal cord at this level make it the single most common area of spinal injury at all ages. Dislocation may occur without fracture and may result in a neural defect well beyond what might be inferred from the seemingly minimal osseous-ligamentous disturbance. The additional support given the thoracic vertebrae by the trunk, and the smaller size of the spinal cord in this area, are further protective factors that can only be overcome by excessive force. The pelvis gives additional support to the lumbar spine; however, as the spinal cord ends at the second lumbar vertebra in the older child, there is somewhat less protection of the lower thoracic and upper lumbar areas.

In infancy, birth injury is the most common cause of spinal cord trauma; it is most likely to occur with forceful breech extraction with spinal hyperextension. Birth injuries of this type may also be seen with cephalic presentation or with version maneuvers, cephalocervical angulation, or unusual traction. The majority of these injuries result in cord transection in the midcervical to upper thoracic area. Those resulting in high cervical lesions involve the cervicomedullary junction and are seldom compatible with life.

In older children trauma may be indirect, as in whiplash injuries where the spine is either hyperextended or flexed beyond its normal range. Direct trauma resulting in crush injuries to the spine and its contents is less common and is most often due to impact secondary to falls from a considerable height. The general pathology of spinal cord injury varies from complete severance to contusion and compression.

DIAGNOSIS.   Cord injuries in the newborn period may be suspected in any case of difficult extraction necessitating considerable force. Resuscitation may be difficult; there may be intercostal paralysis, retracted thorax, prominent abdomen, diaphragmatic respiration, and weak cry. The child is usually noted to have flaccid, abducted, and motionless lower extremities. Sensory evaluation is difficult, but a level of decreased response may be detected compatible with the usual midcervical to upper thoracic area of pathology. Because of the site of injury, only upper extremity movements may be noted, with shoulder and forearm motions but little else. In this areflexic spinal shock stage, respiratory, urinary, and skin infections are common and often fatal. Hyperreflexia may occur subsequently with mass reflex upon stimulation, resulting in

total flexion in the involved areas that may be misinterpreted as functional return.

If the baby survives, the late picture depends on the site and severity of the lesion. Whether the patient's paraplegia assumes a position of flexion, extension, flaccidity, or spasticity depends on the completeness and extent of the spinal cord defect. A sharply demarcated level is uncommon, since the defect is more often of such longitudinal extent as to cover many segments and preclude the development of spasticity. Intercurrent infection, whether acute or chronic, will delay the development of spasticity or decrease its extent. Early bladder function tends to manifest itself as an overflow with constant dribbling, while later automatic function occurs with reflex emptying upon distension to a moderate volume.

Laboratory evaluation should include spinal radiographs, which are usually normal, although fracture or subluxation may be detected. A number of normal variations of the cervical spine in childhood (pseudodislocation, hypermobility, etc) often make radiologic interpretation difficult and are causes of interpretive error. The CSF is usually bloody and has an increased protein content. The diagnosis is often self-evident, but it may at times be confused with neonatal asphyxia, intracranial injury, congenital defects, or progressive infantile spinal muscular atrophy.

MANAGEMENT.   The neonate requires immediate airway attention, oxygenation, suction, and meticulous skin, bladder, and bowel care. Antibiotics may be of value if long-term catheterization is required; they should be given early with evidence of any acute infection. Myelography and surgery are not indicated; they decrease survival potential and in no way enhance recovery. Survivors usually have normal intelligence; they can use their upper extremities fairly well, but they rarely ambulate or even sit without support. Early in life urinary and rectal sphincter control may be adequate; however, as the child grows older, surgery may be required to maintain adequacy of function. Surgical procedures may also be indicated for the orthopedic problems.

Trauma to the spinal cord of older children presents many similar problems; however, immediate management tends to be more definitive, the initial goal being safe, rapid transportation of the patient to where he will receive definitive care. Injury in this group is more likely to be complicated by damage to the vertebral column. It is of paramount importance that the patient be handled in such a manner that additional injury to the cord is not produced by improper posture or undue mobility of the vertebrae at the level of injury. Other bodily injuries may also have occurred, and judgment must be exercised for their proper care in keeping with the demands of the spinal cord injury. The patient must be so placed on the litter as to maintain the normal cervical and lumbar lordosis and to prevent movement that might cause additional injury. Intravenous fluids, intranasal oxygen, and urethral catheterization are often invaluable adjuncts in the initial management of spinal cord injuries. During the early stages the patient must not be given anything by mouth nor strong sedatives or any drugs that would mask neurologic changes.

Open injuries must be treated surgically. Closed cord injuries may require either surgical or nonsurgical treatment. Unwise surgery in patients with cervical injury may be fatal, and indications for surgery must be appraised with great care.

The cervical spinal cord is typically injured by a fracture, a dislocation, or a fracture-dislocation of one or more vertebrae. Severe injury above the level of the fifth cervical cord segment is rarely compatible with life. The radiograms may show marked crushing of the bodies, fragmentation of the pedicles, laminae, and spines, and such dislocation that facets are locked entirely out of position. Under no condition whatsoever must the grave error be made of trying to reduce such dislocation anywhere in the cervical spine by closed manipulation. In most severe lesions of the vertebrae there will be a complete transverse physiologic loss of cord function, often at one or more segments above the uppermost visible vertebral injury. In other instances the vertebral lesions demonstrated roentgenologically will be minimal in comparison with the marked neurologic loss. There are no means of knowing whether an early spinal cord injury is due to contusion, with physiologic interruption and anatomic preservation, or whether the lesion is one of frank anatomic discontinuity. Closed injuries to the cervical cord with evidence of vertebral dislocation are best treated by placing the patient on a firm mattress or special frame and applying continuous traction to the slightly extended head. The vertebrae will in most instances relocate in almost normal alignment within 24 to 36 hours. Serial lateral bedside-portable radiograms will demonstrate progress of the restitution. Occasionally spinal puncture may also be done to follow the manometric effect of the closed decompression. Traction should be maintained for at least 6 weeks.

Immediate decompressive laminectomy for the injured cervical cord is attended by severe morbidity and high mortality, but there are two instances when it is proper to operate early: (1) when the state of the patient was initially one of incomplete loss of cord function, and hours or days later increasing loss of function appears; (2) when at any time after the injury (immediately or days later) good radiographs show clearly that a bone fragment rests upon the cord in such a way that traction could not or has not relieved its pressure. The possibility of a mass of centrally extruded intervertebral disk substance as a result of injury must not be overlooked.

The thoracic segments of the vertebral column form a relatively rigid mass. The thoracic vertebral canal is the narrowest of all parts of the canal, and the spinal cord throughout its thoracic extent has a less rich blood supply than at either the cervical or lumbar level. Spinal cord injury at this level is usually the result of direct severe trauma and carries a poor prognosis. All these factors must be considered in the early care of closed injuries to this area. Cord compression will almost invariably reveal total block of the flow of CSF. The value of surgical decompression is highly variable.

As with injury at the thoracic level, dislocation of one lumbar vertebral body under another, wedging of a body with kyphosis, or fracture of the posterior arches calls for immediate decompressive laminectomy. Injury of the conus medullaris (T-12 to L-1 vertebral levels) is of grave significance. Below that level the delicate filaments of the cauda equina may be badly torn and attenuated, the injury being associated with considerable subarachnoid hemorrhage.

The long-term care and rehabilitation of patients with spinal injuries provide a challenge that is often best met in a special center or unit geared to this type of care. Extensive efforts to reestablish bowel and bladder function will be needed, as will attention to such considerations as skin integrity, nutrition, late syndromes of pain, spasms, autonomic dysfunction, genitourinary complications, psychiatric problems, and programs of education and training.

PERIPHERAL NERVE INJURIES

Injuries to the peripheral nervous system are not common in childhood. Those seen early in life are usually due to damage of the brachial plexus or sciatic nerves. The spinal roots of the fifth cervical through the first thoracic nerves form the brachial plexus. These roots are poorly stabilized at birth, and traction damage is rarely transmitted to the spinal cord. Injuries to infants result in almost pure root syndromes, as contrasted to the more distal involvement and diffuse damage seen with injuries in older children and adults. Recovery is better in children than in adults in regard to both spontaneous resolution and surgical results.

Etiologically, any force changing the normal relationship of arm, shoulder, and neck may result in plexus injury. Birth trauma is the most common cause. The plexus has points of fascial fixation to the first rib medially and the coracoid process of the scapula laterally. Abduction of the arm stretches the nerves under and against the coracoid, resulting in stretch, avulsion, or compression of the lower plexus. Lateral deviation of the head and shoulder depression stretch the nerves over and against the first ribs, resulting in similar damage to the upper plexus. Traction injuries of these types may occur with breech or cephalic deliveries.

Upper plexus root injuries (Erb-Duchenne type) are the most common. The shoulder sags, the arm hangs limp in internal rotation, and the wrist is pronated, reflecting paralysis of spinati, deltoid, biceps, brachioradialis, and extensor carpi radialis muscles, and often rhomboids, serratus, and levator scapulae as well. The deep tendon reflexes of the involved extremity are usually lost, but it is unusual to be able to demonstrate a sensory defect. Treatment requires that the deformity be overcome to prevent posterior subluxation of the humeral head from the glenoid fossa. The arm should be placed in abduction and external rotation by a brace or by pinning a towel over the wrist and fixing it to the mattress in the desired position. A full range of motion of the shoulder by passive exercises should be performed daily. Well over 80 percent of these patients will have complete recovery within 3 months. Anomalous plexus configuration may include the fourth cervical root, or trauma may be transmitted to this level resulting in phrenic nerve damage and ipsilateral diaphragmatic paralysis, which is rarely a problem unless significant bilateral injury has occurred.

Lower plexus root injuries (Klumpke-Dejerine type) show more sensory and vasomotor involvement, with paralysis of the flexors and extensors of the forearm and the intrinsic muscles of the hand. Marked involvement of the first thoracic root results in cervical sympathetic damage and Horner's syndrome, often with delay of normal pigmentation of the ipsilateral iris. The deep tendon reflexes are usually intact, with a poor grasp response. Sensory changes involve the ulnar side of the hand and forearm. Dependent edema and cyanosis are common. Treatment involves splinting the forearm and wrist in a neutral position, with passive range-of-motion exercises. The majority of cases completely recover within 3 to 6 months, although the overall prognosis is not as favorable as in the upper plexus lesions (Fig. 31).

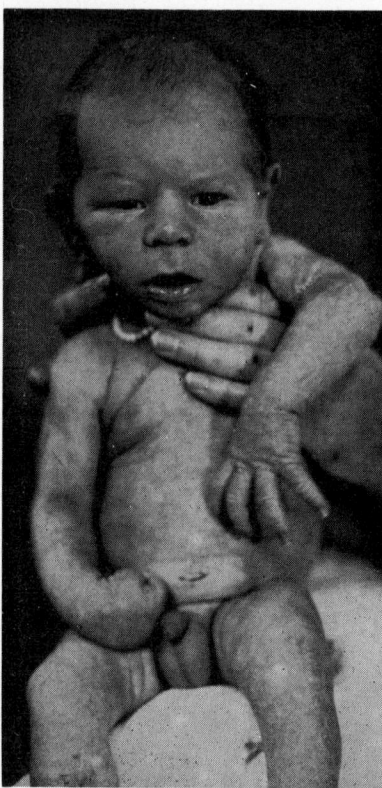

FIG. 31. Brachial plexus injury to an infant 12 days old. Involvement of the upper, middle, and lower trunks of the right brachial plexus, combined with right enophthalmos, a component of Horner's syndrome.

Injuries to the brachial plexus in older children are usually of mixed upper and lower plexus types. If they are due to traction and hyperabduction the prognosis

may be good, although at this age the usual cause is severe trauma, which often results in root avulsion or a degree of hemorrhage and scarring that precludes functional recovery. Direct plexus surgery is consistently unprofitable. In cases with persistent defects, orthopedic procedures to stabilize joints in favorable positions and tendon transplantation, where feasible, are the only available treatments.

The peripheral nerves in the upper extremity may be involved alone or in varied combinations, due usually to direct laceration trauma or severe injuries with combined osseous-vascular-neural damage. Compression neuropathies are uncommon in childhood.

Serratus anterior palsy due to involvement of the long thoracic nerve (nerve of Bell) is usually a result of pressure on the shoulder or excessive forceful activity with the arms elevated. It is most frequently seen in prepuberal athletic boys in association with baseball pitching, weight lifting, or carrying heavy loads. The scapula becomes winglike with horizontal forward pressure of the arms, and there is weakness in lifting and arm elevation due to impaired scapula fixation. Treatment should provide full functional recovery, although some residual scapular winging may persist. Activities possibly associated with the lesion should be discontinued. During the first week the weight of the shoulder may be removed from the scapula by a simple arm sling, but this is often not necessary unless the paralysis is total or there is considerable discomfort. Range-of-motion exercises, then more active shoulder strengthening maneuvers, are the only measures indicated.

The axillary or circumflex nerve that innervates the deltoid and teres minor muscles is usually injured only in association with anterior dislocations of the shoulder, particularly when associated with fractures of the greater tuberosity of the humerus. The axillary nerve winds around the surgical neck of the humerus and may be injured by fractures in this location. Injury to the nerve is detected by inability to abduct the arm to the horizontal position and a zone of hypoesthesia of the lower posterior deltoid area. Therapy is that of the primary injury, and with rare exceptions full neural recovery can be anticipated.

Radial nerve injury is most commonly a result of fracture through the middle third of the humerus with neural stretch or contusion. The triceps muscle may not be involved, but there is marked weakness of the brachioradialis and the extensors of the wrist and fingers (wristdrop). Sensation is lost in an area between index finger and thumb on the dorsum of the hand. In the acute state it is impossible to tell whether the nerve has been lacerated or severed. Therefore, where feasible, open reduction of the fracture and nerve repair are reasonable considerations. Later, electrical testing will give information as to whether there is anatomic continuity of the nerve. Where permanent residua exist in spite of all efforts, tendon transplantation gives quite effective wrist, finger, and thumb extension.

The ulnar nerve may be lacerated along its course in the forearm near the wrist or in conjunction with fractures as it passes behind the medial epicondyle of the humerus at the elbow. The epiphysis of the medial epicondyle does not fuse to the humerus until late adolescence and is particularly prone to avulsion. The ulnar nerve may be contused at the time of injury or compressed later by scar formation. Sensory loss involves the fifth and ulnar half of the fourth digits and extends along the medial side of the palm to the lower forearm. Weakness may involve the interossei, lumbricales, and hypothenar muscles, as well as the adductor pollicis, the flexor carpi ulnaris, and the deep flexor of the fourth and fifths digits, resulting in defects in spreading the fingers, adducting the thumb, flexing the fourth and fifth digits at the distal interphalangeal joints, and poor opposition of the fifth finger. Treatment is that of the primary injury. Surgical intervention depends on how nearly intact the nerve is, as determined by clinical and electrical studies, and can consist of suturing or grafting the involved nerve.

The median nerve may be damaged similarly as the ulnar and is often injured with it. In addition to the more common laceration injury, there may be damage in anterior dislocation fractures at the elbow or wrist. There is sensory loss on the palmar surface of the hand that involves thumb, index, and middle fingers, the radial half of the ring finger, and the radial surface of the palm. Weakness of the pronators of the forearm, the long flexors of the fingers, and the short adductor and opponens of the thumb is the major motor defect. Therapeutic considerations are similar to those in cases of ulnar palsy.

Peripheral nerve injuries involving the lower extremities almost exclusively involve the sciatic nerve and its branches. It is the largest nerve in the body, and at the knee it divides into the tibial and common peroneal nerves. Iatrogenic trauma secondary to intramuscular injections is the leading cause of sciatic neuropathy in infancy. Lesions of this type are also seen in older children and adults. The normal course of the sciatic nerve in the hollow midway between the ischial tuberosity and the greater trochanter under cover of the gluteus maximus muscle varies greatly. This fact, taken together with the small size of the infant gluteal mass and the potential neurotoxicity of many antibiotics, makes it unwise to utilize this area for intramuscular injections. Intragluteal injections are contraindicated in infancy and should be used in older children with extreme caution. The anterolateral compartment of the thigh and the deltoid areas are safer and always preferable. Complete sciatic lesions produce total foot paralysis and loss of leg flexion. There is a flail footdrop, an absence of ankle jerk, and a sensory loss below the knee involving the entire leg except for its medial aspect.

The tragedy of nerve injury in infancy is accentuated by the residua of short, small extremities due to lack of stimulation of the muscular-tendon movement that is essential to bone growth. All cases of sciatic palsy must be carefully evaluated with a view toward surgery, although high lesions rarely show complete recovery and are usually associated with marked permanent disability.

The peroneal nerve is vulnerable to pressure neuropathy as well as other injury. It descends from the popliteal fossa to a superficial position on the lateral aspect of the leg, passing posterior to the head of the fibula. Injury here results in sensory loss over the dorsum of the foot and anterolateral surface of the leg, with weakness of the dorsiflexors and evertors of the foot and toes. The tibial nerve descends deep in the calf, rounds the posterior aspect of the medial malleolus, and enters the foot. It innervates the muscles controlling plantar flexion of the foot and toes and the intrinsic muscles of the foot. Sensory loss is usually confined to the sole. Combined peroneal and tibial nerve injuries often occur. Treatment is similar to that described for ulnar nerve injuries.

CRANIAL NERVE INJURIES

Trauma to the cranial nerves is seldom an isolated occurrence; it usually reflects more diffuse craniocerebral injury. The olfactory nerve is frequently torn as its filaments pass from the subfrontal area of the brain through the cribriform plate. The defect is rarely complete and is usually asymptomatic. If severe anosmia persists, distortion of taste is the presenting complaint. Trauma to the optic nerve occurs in association with orbital fracture, but it may be seen with cerebral contusion and hemorrhage into the nerve sheath. Injury to the chiasmal area is uncommon. The hypothalamus and brainstem usually receive the brunt of injury in this region, with resulting fatality.

The most common cranial nerve injuries are those involving the third, fourth, sixth, seventh, and eighth nerves. Laceration of the carotid artery in its cavernous sinus position due to fractures or transmitted trauma may result in a carotid-cavernous fistula (p.1825). Damage to the oculomotor nerves is more common, and permanent or transient dysfunctions of the extraocular muscles occur more frequently in the pediatric age group than in the adult.

Fractures through the petrous portion of the temporal bone may damage the facial nerve. Paralysis may be immediate or delayed. Neonatal facial paralysis may follow forceps extraction or may reflect unusual positions in utero. Immediate treatment is directed to corneal protection. Damage to the nerve distal to the geniculate ganglion may be associated with blood behind the tympanic membrane and a conductive hearing loss. Injury central to the ganglion tends to be associated with labyrinthine dysfunction and a pattern of sensorineural hearing loss, implying a level of injury that is not amenable to direct therapy. In all other instances evaluation and management are aimed at the functional state of the nerve. Electrodiagnostic tests to follow and determine the degree of degeneration and estimate anatomic continuity of the nerve are not infallible; however, when there is evidence of neural degeneration, careful evaluation should be made and consideration should be given to operative intervention. Surgical decompression and/or nerve graft, where feasible, give the best results. Hypoglossal facial anastomosis and plastic procedures to enhance facial symmetry are less satisfactory, but at times they offer the only possible approach to the problem.

Fractures through the base of the skull, direct blows on or near the ear, or extravasation of blood from subarachnoid hemorrhage may affect both vestibular and auditory components of the eighth cranial nerve, as well as cause direct damage to the labyrinth, cochlea, or middle car. Post-traumatic neural deafness has a relatively poor prognosis for full recovery. Labyrinthine dysfunction as evidenced by postural vertigo and increased sensitivity to motion is usually transient.

References

Baker H Jr, Campbell JK, Houser OW, Reese DF, Sheedy PF, Holman CB: Computerized assisted tomography of the head. Mayo Clin Proc 49:17, 1974

Caveness WE, Walker AE (eds): Head Injury Conference Proceedings. Philadelphia, JB Lippincott, 1966

Clinical Neurology: Proceedings of the Congress of Neurological Surgeons, Vol 19. Baltimore, Williams & Wilkins, 1972

Dillon H, Leopold RL: Children and the post-concussion syndrome. JAMA 172:86, 1961

Drayer BP Poser CM: Disseminated intravascular coagulation and head trauma. JAMA 231:174, 1975

Griffith JP, Dodge PR: Transient blindness following head injury in children. N Eng J Med 278:648, 1968

Haymaker W, Woodhall B: Peripheral Nerve Injuries, 2nd ed. Philadelphia, WB Saunders, 1953

Hjern B, Nylander I: Acute head injuries in children. Acta Paediatr Scand Suppl 152:1, 1964

Jennett WB, van de Sande J: EEG prediction of post-traumatic epilepsy. Epilepsia 16:251, 1975

Lauer B, Ten Broeck E: Battered child syndrome: review of 130 patients with controls. Pediatrics 54:67, 1974

Leech PJ: Conservative and operative management for cerebrospinal-fluid leakage after closed head injury. Lancet 1:1013, 1973

Lende RA, Erickson TC: Growing skull fractures of childhood. J Neurosurg 18:479, 1961

Low NL, Correll JW: Head pain due to leptomeningeal cysts. Br J Surg 53:971, 1966

Mealey J Jr: Pediatric Head Injuries. Springfield, III, Charles C Thomas, 1968

Selby I: Skull fractures in infants. Acta Chir Scand 122:30, 1961

Shelness A, Seymour C: Children as passengers in automobiles: the neglected minority on the nation's highways. Pediatrics 56:271, 1975

Shrays GG: Cervical spine injuries: association with head trauma. Am J Roentgenol Radium Ther Nucl Med 118:670, 1973

PAROXYSMAL DISORDERS

DORA CHAO, SIDNEY CARTER, AND ARNOLD P. GOLD

EPILEPSY

Epilepsy is as old as the human race. The ancient Greeks and Romans looked upon epilepsy as a sacred disease, a curse by the gods. Although this was disputed by Hippocrates, the misconception persisted through the ages. Even today many epileptics and their families suffer from social prejudice and stigma. The period of scientific inquiry and social enlightenment began in the middle of the nineteenth century when Hughlings Jackson theorized that fits were caused by occasional, excessive, and disorderly discharge in the cerebral gray matter. Scientific advances that have led to an understanding of the disorder include (1) development of modern neurology, neuroanatomy, neuropathology, neuroradiology, and neurophysiology; (2) development of electroencephalography; (3) advances in drug therapy; (4) development of surgical treatment of focal epilepsy; (5) recent development of neurochemistry, electron microscopy, and electroneurophysiology, which have brought research on seizure mechanisms to the cellular level. Despite these developments the clinician still has the age-old problem of adequate care and treatment of epileptic patients.

There is no accurate survey of the incidence of epilepsy in the United States, but it has been estimated to occur in 0.5 to 1.0 percent of the population. In children it is a major problem, and about 5 percent of children have had a seizure at some time in their lives, if only in association with fever. Today, however, medical therapy is 50 to 60 percent effective. Increased understanding and acceptance by the public have also brought improvement in the social and economic outlook for the epileptic patient and his family.

DEFINITIONS.   The word *epilepsy* has its origin in Greek and means to lay on or to seize. A seizure (an attack, a fit, a spell) is an episode of cerebral dysfunction produced by abnormal, excessive neuronal discharge occurring in the brain that may be caused by a variety of conditions. A seizure is a symptom, not a disease. Its manifestations depend on the location of the discharge and its spread. Thus it may manifest as a change in the state of consciousness, an abnormal sensory experience, disordered motor activities (tonic or clonic contractions), or disturbances of vegetative, intellectual, and behavioral functions. When seizures become recurrent, the condition is termed epilepsy. Gibbs and Lennox defined epilepsy as a paroxysmal cerebral dysrhythmia. They emphasized not only the abnormal rhythms but also their paroxysmal occurrence as the essential features of the epileptic dysfunction. The term *convulsion* implies generalized or widespread abnormal motor activity as a prominent component in an epileptic attack. Not all convulsions are epileptic in nature, and many types of epilepsy do not have a convulsive element. A *prodrome* consists of symptoms that appear hours or days before the onset of the actual seizure. For example, on the basis of past experience the family might recognize that a seizure is habitually heralded by the child becoming whiny, anorexic, and irritable. An *aura* is the subjective sensation or experience that habitually precedes an epileptic attack and is frequently recognized by the patient as immediate warning of an impending seizure. Physiologically, an aura is the beginning of the abnormal neuronal discharge; hence it may be a helpful sign for localization of the epileptogenic focus. Ictus is derived from Latin and means a sudden attack. The adjective *ictal* means pertaining to an attack. Preictal and postictal refer to the time immediately before and shortly after a seizure; interictal refers to the interim between attacks.

Classification

Until recently four systems of classification were in general use: clinical, anatomic, electroencephalographic, and etiologic. This is inevitable, because epilepsy is only a symptom of many disease conditions of diverse functional disturbances. A new classification combining clinical seizure type, electroencephalographic expression, anatomic substrate, etiology, and age was proposed by the Vienna Congress of the International League Against Epilepsy.

CLINICAL CLASSIFICATION. This is the oldest and most widely used system. Some of the terms are apt because the pattern of attack is simple; for example, lapse or absence, akinetic or drop seizure, and massive myoclonic (jackknife) spasms. Some other terms are more ambiguous and require further definition because the seizure patterns are complex and cannot be characterized by a simple descriptive term or phrase; for example, minor motor seizure is a misnomer because minor gives a false implication in relation to the severity of the symptoms and the usually grave prognosis. These criticisms notwithstanding, classification by seizure pattern is meaningful and useful when used with other systems of classification. The major seizure types are:

Generalized convulsions (major motor)
  Tonic-clonic (grand mal)
  Tonic
Focal seizures
  Focal motor
  Focal sensory
  Frontal adversive
  Occipital
  Inhibitory
  Temporal lobe
Petit mal
Minor motor
  Akinetic
  Myoclonic
  Infantile spasms
Psychomotor epilepsy
Autonomic epilepsy (convulsive equivalent seizures)
Miscellaneous

ANATOMIC CLASSIFICATION. Hughlings Jackson first introduced an anatomic classification, with such terms as uncinate fits and rhinencephalis seizures. This concept of focal origin of seizure discharge has led to extensive studies of functional anatomy of the brain. The advent of electroencephalography, including cortical and depth electrography, has allowed this anatomic knowledge to be applied to management of epilepsy in humans at the time of surgery. It is thus logical and necessary for the neurosurgeon to classify seizure symptoms on an anatomic basis. The anatomic terms have become more or less identified with certain clinical epilepsies; for example:

Centrencephalic seizures: Grand mal epilepsy,
                            Petit mal epilepsy
Diencephalic epilepsy   Convulsive equivalent
  (thalamic-   syndrome
  hypothalamic):   (autonomic epilepsy)

Focal cortical seizures
  Temporal lobe epilepsy: Psychomotor epilepsy
  Frontal lobe epilepsy: Adversive seizures,
                            Jacksonian epilepsy
  Parietal lobe epilepsy: Focal sensory seizures
  Occipital lobe epilepsy: Visual sensations.

It should be noted that the anatomic classification is still not perfect, and some designations (eg, temporal lobe) need additional definition (see psychomotor epilepsy).

ELECTROENCEPHALOGRAPHIC CLASSIFICATION. The electroencephalogram (EEG) provides a pictorial record of cerebral activity reflected at the cortex in electrical terms. In the course of its clinical application many specific patterns have been found to correlate to varying degrees with the clinical types of epilepsy. Some of the well-known examples of EEG patterns follow (Fig. 32).

Three-per-second spike-and-wave dysrhythmia is the classic EEG abnormality found in genetic epilepsy of the pure lapse or petit mal type. However, it also occurs in patients who have grand mal attacks only or who have both types of attack.

Paroxysmal polyspike-and-wave dysrhythmia is closely correlated with myoclonic jerks.

Paroxysmal or continuous slow-spike and slow-wave dysrhythmia is generally associated with diffuse encephalopathy. The seizures are chiefly akinetic or myoclonic, with or without generalized convulsion. The EEG pattern was referred to as petit mal variant by Lennox, and the clinical picture has borne such names as minor motor seizures, atypical petit mal, myokinetic epilepsy, and the Lennox syndrome.

Hypsarhythmia is a continuously abnormal EEG pattern characterized by high-voltage, poorly organized slow- and sharp-wave activity mixed with bursts of irregular spikes and polyspike-and-wave activity showing poor interhemispheric correlation. It is found in 90 percent of children with massive myoclonic spasms.

Fourteen- and six-per-second positive spike dysrhythmia occurring in the drowsy state or during light sleep is believed to arise from diencephalic nuclei and/or the limbic system; it is often found in children with seizure equivalent. Recently it has been observed in 15 to 55 percent of apparently normal school children, with a peak age incidence at 12 years. Although these observations suggest an age dependence and have raised doubt regarding its pathologic significance, its frequent concordance (with or without other EEG abnormalities) with vegetative dysfunctions and post-traumatic, post-breath-holding, choreic, and migraine syndromes remains an intriguing finding.

Focal (or *multifocal*) *discharges* may arise from an epileptogenic focus (or foci) in the cerebral cortex or subcortical centers. The clinical seizure symptoms depend on the functional attributes at the site of discharge and the manner of spread. Focal seizures may escalate into generalized convulsions. The so-called temporal lobe is the most common site of epileptogenic discharge (Fig. 33). Sometimes a primary lesion located elsewhere may

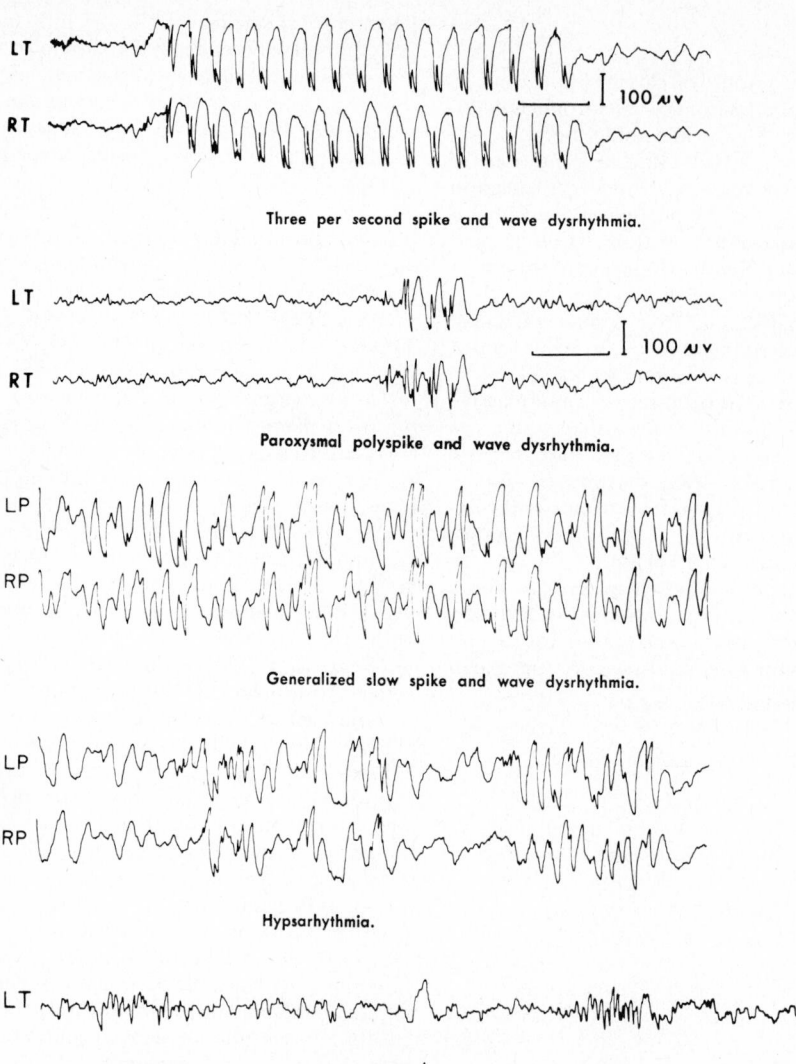

FIG. 32. Abnormal electroencephalographic patterns in various types of convulsive disorders.

activate the temporal regions remotely. The concordance between temporal lobe focus and psychomotor epilepsy is about 60 percent. On the basis of correlative studies, certain EEG terms have been used interchangeably with clinical terminology. This is not justified because the correlation is rarely perfect.

ETIOLOGIC CLASSIFICATION. The epilepsies may be divided into two general groups: genetic and symptomatic. The genetic epilepsies are characterized by the absence of a demonstrable structural lesion of the brain, the tendency to spontaneous cerebral dysrhythmia being genetically inherited. In contrast, the symptomatic epilepsies are associated with metabolic disorders or organic pathology of the brain acquired through developmental error, injury, or disease. In some cases symptomatic and genetic epilepsy may occur concomitantly.

GENETIC EPILEPSY. The etiologic role of heredity, first implicated by Hippocrates, has been established by extensive studies of epileptic families and relatives.

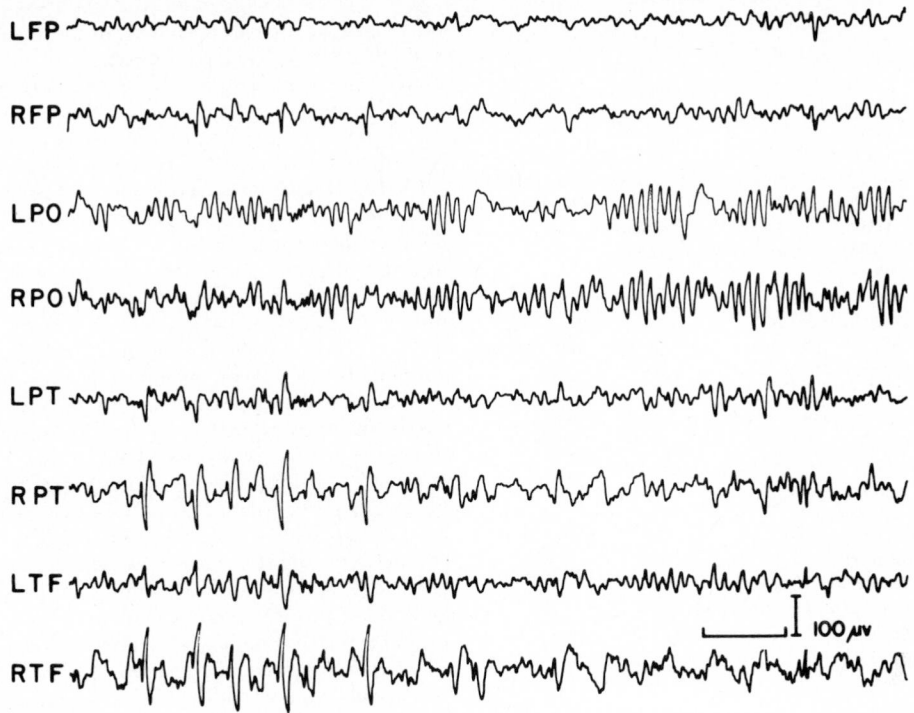

FIG. 33. Temporal spike focus.

Both Conrad and Lennox found that when epilepsy occurred in monozygous twins both twins were affected in about 85 percent of cases, whereas in dizygous twins both were affected in only 3 percent and 15.9 percent of their cases, respectively. EEG studies of the epileptic families led them to suggest that cerebral dysrhythmia underlying epileptic diathesis was inherited as a mendelian dominant factor. These observations were confirmed by Metrakos and Metrakos, who demonstrated further that the EEG trait and the clinical seizure of genetic epilepsy usually manifest at the age of 5 to 12 years. The seizure manifestation is either generalized convulsion or pure petit mal or a combination of the two, often with myoclonic components. In 4 to 8 percent of epileptics a hereditary factor seems involved. Even when there is no overt epilepsy, a low seizure threshold may be evidenced by paroxysmal spike-and-wave or polyspike-and-wave dysrhythmia occurring spontaneously or by activation from sleep, intermittent photic stimulation, or hyperventilation. The risk of producing epileptic offspring is 2 to 4 percent.

SYMPTOMATIC OR ACQUIRED EPILEPSY.   The causes of symptomatic epilepsies are diverse. A structural or metabolic cerebral lesion develops and serves as the focus of epileptogenesis. This process may be localized or diffuse, static or progressive, traumatic or inflammatory, neoplastic or degenerative, vascular or allergic. Some of the etiologic factors are listed in Table 14.

Pathogenesis

The common denominator in the pathology of epileptogenic diseases is a structural or a metabolic disturbance in the brain giving rise to seizure discharge. A typical epileptogenic cortical scar consists of a central zone, in which no nerve cells survive, and an intermediate zone, in which the surviving cells are diminished in number and are undergoing different phases of degeneration. An intermediate zone also intervenes between a tumor or other structural lesion and the normal surrounding tissue. In either case the blood supply to the intermediate zone is compromised, and the degenerating cells are more excitable. It is these unstable cells that constitute the epileptogenic focus.

Regardless of etiology and pathology of the cerebral lesions, the pathophysiology of seizure discharge is the same. The basic mechanism appears to be prolonged depolarization with consequent hyperactive and hypersynchronous discharge from abnormal neurons. Such epileptic discharge may be circumscribed, or it may spread and thus activate distant neurons, causing them to become secondarily or in some instances independently epileptogenic. The biochemical basis of epileptic discharge remains incompletely understood. Experimental studies with epileptogenic cortex from animals and human patients suggest that the production and maintenance of such discharge involves an accumula-

TABLE 14. Etiologic Factors Associated with Epilepsy

Prenatal Factors

    Genetic
        Genetic epilepsy
        Inborn errors of metabolism
            Carbohydrate: glycogen storage disease, hypoglycemia
            Protein: phenylketonuria, maple syrup urine disease
            Fat: cerebral lipidoses, leukodystrophies
        Heredofamilial diseases: myoclonus epilepsy
    Congenital structural anomalies
        Porencephaly
        Vascular malformations
        Neurocutaneous syndrome
        Developmental defects of brain
    Fetal infections
        Viral encephalopathy: rubella, cytomegalic inclusion disease
        Protozoan meningoencephalitis: toxoplasmosis
    Maternal diseases
        Toxemia of pregnancy
        Chronic renal disease
        Diabetes mellitus
        Radiation during pregnancy
        Drug usage and drug intoxication
        Trauma

Perinatal Factors

    Trauma
    Hypoxia
    Jaundice
    Infection
    Prematurity
    Drug withdrawal

Postnatal Factors

    Primary infection of central nervous system
    Infectious diseases of childhood with encephalopathy (eg, measles, mumps)
    Head trauma
    Circulatory diseases
        Vascular anomalies
        Occlusive diseases: arterial, venous
        Hemorrhage
        Hypertensive encephalopathy
    Toxic encephalopathy
        Thallium
        Lead
        Convulsogenic drugs: INH, steroids
    Allergic encephalopathy
        Immunization reactions
        Drug reactions
    Physical and metabolic encephalopathies
        Fever and febrile convulsions
        Anoxia and hypoxia
        Prolonged convulsions with cyanosis
        Electrolyte disturbance
        Acute porphyria
        Hypoglycemia
        Hypocalcemia
        Hypomagnesemia
        Hyponatremia and hypernatremia and others
        Pyridoxine deficiency or dependency
    Degenerative diseases of the brain
    Tumors

tion of excess acetylcholine or other excitatory substance and an increased membrane permeability, with an increase in intracellular sodium ions and depletion of intracellular potassium ions. Systemic metabolic disturbances such as hypoglycemia, hypocalcemia, anoxia, hypocapnia, and pyridoxine deficiency are believed to exert their influence on these basic factors.

TRIGGERING MECHANISM. Most epileptic attacks appear suddenly and fortuitously without apparent immediate cause. On the other hand, many seizures do seem to occur under the influence of a triggering factor. The onset of these seizures may be cyclic and thus may suggest a periodically recurring triggering mechanism, or onset may be provoked in an erratic manner. In the cyclic group the hormonal factors related to menstrual period, menarche, and menopause are conspicuous examples. In the induced seizures the provoking agents are diverse. They may be nonsensory or sensory. Among the nonsensory group are hyperthermia, hyperventilation, metabolic disorders, physical stress, sleep deprivation, and emotional disturbances. The sensory triggers may be visual (eg, photogenic, television, reading), auditory (musicogenic), vegetative, tactile, and proprioceptive. They may be spontaneous normal sensory stimuli of daily life or unexpected sensory experiences (startle reaction), and at times they may be self-induced. In the latter group hyperexcitable brainstem structures provide the pathologic substrate for escalation of normal startle reactions to epileptic seizures.

AGE FACTOR. Epilepsy is much more common in children than in adults. In genetic epilepsy the appearance and disappearance of the clinical seizures and the electrical dysrhythmia are age-dependent. Thus pure petit mal attacks and the three-per-second EEG pattern have a peak incidence between 4 and 10 years and tend to disappear by the end of adolescence.

Seizures that occur before 2 years of age suggest a metabolic disorder or an underlying structural defect of the brain. Newborn infants are more likely to have poorly organized movements (twitching, trembling, or shaking) than a bona fide tonic-clonic convulsion. They often have apneic or blue spells, limp or stiff spells, and vasomotor changes with flushing, pallor, and clamminess. Such seizure discharges probably originate mostly in subcortical structures; as the cortex develops, more differentiated types of seizure patterns become evident.

Seventy-five percent of structural growth of the brain occurs in the first 2 years of life. Generally speaking, the younger the child and the more immature the brain, the more susceptible it is to injury, and the more far-reaching the resultant functional disorganization.

Seizure Types

GENERALIZED CONVULSIONS. Generalized convulsions are the most common type of seizure in childhood. In the genetic type of epilepsy the seizure discharge is believed to originate in centrencephalic structures and to spread rapidly to both cerebral hemispheres with immediate loss of consciousness and generalized convulsions. As a rule there is no aura preceding the onset and no localizing neurologic sign following the attack. In contrast, the symptomatic type may be associated with an aura and/or a postictal phenomenon that suggest a focal origin of the generalized seizure. With the rapid spread of the seizure discharge from the epileptogenic focus, the memory of the aura may be obscured. This is especially true in children.

The classic grand mal attack is usually precipitous in onset. Typically the eyes roll up or to one side, the pupils dilate, and the face becomes flushed or pale. Consciousness is quickly lost, and the entire body is seized by a tonic spasm. There is often a sharp cry, and if the child is standing he falls heavily to the ground. With the tonic spasm, respiration is arrested and the child becomes cyanotic. After a period of 10 to 30 sec the tonic phase gives way to generalized clonic jerking lasting from 1 to 5 minutes or longer. Breathing is resumed but is labored. There may be profuse perspiration and salivation and involuntary bladder and bowel evacuation, and the tongue may be bitten. Gradually the attack diminishes in severity; the muscle contractions become less violent and finally cease. If the duration of the attack is short, the child may recover his senses quickly and show little or no aftereffect. More commonly, however, he remains stuporous and sinks into postictal sleep lasting an hour or more. When he awakens he may have headache, generalized fatigue, and restlessness for a variable period. Postictally, transient neurologic deficits may be present, and these sometimes may be of significance in the diagnosis of a focal lesion.

STATUS EPILEPTICUS. Grand mal seizures may occur in series without consciousness being regained between attacks. This condition is known as status epilepticus. It may be induced by sudden withdrawal of anticonvulsant medication, or it may be incident to intercurrent infection or without known cause. If not treated promptly and effectively, the status may persist for many hours or days, with development of serious sequelae or even death. Transient postictal signs and symptoms include aphasia, ataxia, and mental sluggishness. Persistent symptoms and signs may develop, indicating that irreversible brain damage has occurred as a result of prolonged cellular hypoxia. Status epilepticus should therefore be treated as a medical emergency.

TONIC SEIZURES. Tonic seizures are seizures in which the patient's body stiffens, with increased tonicity of the entire musculature, and consciousness is lost. Such attacks arise when the midbrain is primarily involved in the seizure discharge.

FOCAL SEIZURES. When the initial event of a seizure consistently indicates a local origin in some part of the brain, the epilepsy is focal epilepsy. The epileptic discharge may originate at any level of the nervous system. It may remain localized or may spread across the midline to the opposite side and become generalized.

Focal discharging lesions may be transient in young children. The significance of focal seizures in young children is not the same as in older children or adults. Not infrequently the focal attack may vary from side to side, giving rise to multifocal epilepsy.

FOCAL MOTOR SEIZURES. Focal motor seizures may manifest as involvement of one entire side of the body simultaneously (hemiconvulsion) or may be limited to one extremity and/or the face. Jacksonian epilepsy is one that originates in one part of the motor cortex and spreads to involve the rest of the motor strip. The common points of onset are the thumb, the face, and the toe —structures having relatively large cortical representation. The orderly spread of the electrical discharge is reflected in the classic march that was described by Jackson 100 years ago. Jacksonian seizures frequently escalate into grand mal attacks. Following a seizure there may be transient paresis or paralysis lasting minutes or hours. This phenomenon, known as Todd's paralysis, is believed to result from a localized neuronal exhaustion. When Todd's paralysis becomes progressively longer in duration, or when the weakness persists during the interictal periods, one should suspect a progressive lesion. Epilepsia partialis continua refers to local convulsive movements of a continuous type, when a discharge maintains itself at a certain point continually.

FOCAL SENSORY SEIZURES. In focal sensory seizures (somatic sensory seizures) numbness and tingling are the usual sensations; these seizures arise from the sensory cortex. The abnormal sensations may also proceed in a march and at times may spread to the motor area with resultant motor seizures.

FOCAL ADVERSIVE SEIZURES. Focal adversive seizures consist of turning of the head, eyes, and trunk away from the side of the cerebral lesion, with loss of consciousness. The seizure discharge is generally located in the prefrontal area, but other areas such as the occipital and temporal cortex may give rise to such attacks.

OCCIPITAL SEIZURES. Seizure discharges in the visual cortical areas produce simple visual impressions, such as dimness of vision, seeing shadows and clouds in front of the eyes, or a transient blindness.

INHIBITORY SEIZURES. With inhibitory seizures (ictal paralysis) the epileptic discharge, even from the motor areas, may produce inactivation or paralysis instead of excitation or motor activity.

TEMPORAL LOBE (PSYCHOMOTOR) EPILEPSY AND DIENCEPHALIC (CONVULSIVE EQUIVALENT) EPILEPSY. These are the most common types of seizures of focal origin in childhood; they will be discussed on (p.1845).

PETIT MAL. In their pure form, absence or lapse attacks are characterized by episodes of abrupt, momentary loss of consciousness accompanied by cessation of voluntary activities. The child has a blank expression and stares into space. The duration of each attack rarely exceeds 5 to 15 sec. Just as abruptly the child recovers his senses and resumes his activity as if no interruption had occurred. Typically there is no aura and no postictal disturbance. In 60 to 70 percent of patients myoclonic jerks may occur. The common forms are slow rhythmic blinking of the eyes and rhythmic jerking of the head, arms, or trunk. The child rarely falls or loses bladder control. While having a petit mal attack, some children may perform semipurposeful motor acts such as snapping the fingers, patting movement, or walking around or in circles. These have been termed petit mal automatism.

The frequency of absence attacks varies widely, from an occasional attack to hundreds per day. Attentiveness in work or play diminishes the number of attacks; idleness, fatigue, excessive hydration, emotional stress, menstruation, overventilation, and photic stimulation tend to increase the frequency. When attacks occur in close succession for a prolonged period of time, mental function is continually impaired and the child remains dazed and confused. The sudden obtunding of mental function may lead to a false impression of degenerative or toxic encephalopathy. This is known as petit mal status. It may be ushered in by a febrile illness, an emotional upset, or a menstrual period, or it may occur without obvious cause. The occurrence of petit mal status seldom affects the ultimate prognosis.

The age of onset of pure petit mal epilepsy is usually at 4 to 10 years of age. The incidence is slightly higher in girls than in boys (6 to 4). The child's physical and mental development is usually unaffected, and the neurologic findings are entirely normal. The attacks tend to decrease with time, and in about 50 percent of patients they completely disappear in the late teens; however, they may persist into adult life. About one-third to one-half of patients with petit mal may have grand mal seizures. In these patients the petit mal seizures usually make their appearance first.

The EEG abnormality of absence attacks is characteristic. Bursts of generalized bilaterally synchronous three-per-second spike-and-wave complexes appear, usually against a background of normal activity. Short bursts of such activity may not be accompanied by an overt clinical seizure but may be associated with subtle impairment of mental efficiency. Bursts lasting longer than 5 seconds are often accompanied by clinical attacks.

MINOR MOTOR SEIZURES.   AKINETIC ATTACKS. Akinetic attacks are also known as drop fits. Postural tone is controlled by a balanced discharge of facilitory and inhibitory impulses from the reticular formation in the upper brainstem. Drop seizures are believed to result from a sudden increase of inhibitory discharges that transiently overwhelms the influence of the facilitory center and leads to sudden loss of postural tone. The muscles involved may be limited to the neck, giving rise to head bobbing or more generally resulting in collapse of the body. The attacks are so abrupt and unexpected that the patient and parents are caught unprepared, and significant injury may result.

Although akinetic attacks have been seen in genetic petit mal epilepsy, the majority of such attacks occur in patients with symptomatic epilepsy. The children affected are much younger than the genetic group. The nodding seizures appear when the infant is able to assume sitting position, and the drop seizures occur when the child is able to get about. The frequency may be as high as several hundred seizures a day. Severe physical injuries are common, and there is constant danger to life. The cause is frequently unknown, but in many cases the history may strongly implicate diffuse encephalopathy incident to past infections due to measles, other viral agents, immunization antigens, toxins, residua from tuberculous meningitis, or tuberous sclerosis. The EEG may show continuous runs of generalized slow spike and 1.5 to 2-per-second slow waves. Various degrees of brain damage are frequently present, as evidenced by mental retardation and neurologic abnormalities such as a Babinski sign, unequal deep tendon reflexes, abnormal muscle tone, apraxia, and incoordination. As a rule the course is protracted, with the seizures subsiding slowly and the EEG reverting gradually to a slow dysrhythmia. The child may become a slow learner or frankly retarded.

MYOCLONIC EPILEPSIES.   Myoclonus is a phenomenon of clonic spasms of an isolated muscle or groups of muscles. Neither term necessarily implies epilepsy, although in some epileptic disorders myoclonus is a prominent symptom. Physiologically, myoclonus is believed to occur because of sudden release from inhibitory control of motor centers in the midbrain, the brainstem, or the spinal cord. The uninhibited discharge from these centers may spread to high structures, which may influence the myoclonus but are not essential in its occurrence. A variety of pathologic conditions may produce myoclonus, particularly those with diffuse involvement of the brain.

Clinically, myoclonic seizures may occur in genetic epilepsies in association with petit mal or grand mal attacks. More severe myoclonic seizures are not uncommon in symptomatic epilepsies incident to nonprogressive and progressive diffuse encephalopathies. That these myoclonic phenomena are epileptic in nature is attested to by the presence of cerebral dysrhythmia. There are four types:

Myoclonic Seizures in Genetic Epilepsies.   Slow rhythmic jerks of the eyelids, the neck, or the arms are seen in 60 to 70 percent of children with absence attacks. These jerks do not alter the course or prognosis of the pure petit mal epilepsy. The EEG is that of the absence pattern. Some patients with genetic epilepsy may have mixed seizures of myoclonic and grand mal attacks. The myoclonic seizures usually antedate the grand mal attacks by months or years. They tend to come on in the morning, causing the child to fall or to drop things without alteration of consciousness. Sometimes the parents may mistake these episodes for mere carelessness or teenage clumsiness, only to realize their true nature when a long train of myoclonic jerks merges into grand mal attacks. The EEG may reveal paroxysmal multiple spike, slow wave, and normal background activity.

Myoclonic Seizures in Nonprogressive Diffuse Encephalopathies. The incidence in this group is highest between 2 and 6 years of age. Although the cause is often unknown, symptoms and signs of brain damage are almost always present, and a past history of undiagnosed infection or reaction to immunization may be obtained. Sometimes a history of childhood infectious disease among siblings may be a significant clue that the patient has had a subclinical infection by the same etiologic agent. The myoclonus may occur alone or in association with akinetic attacks or grand mal seizures. In some cases the myoclonus may be no more than a shudder or quick jerks of the eyes, which may be unnoticed by the parents, or it may be more gross and widespread. The jerks are usually arrhythmic. The EEG frequently shows generalized multiple spike-and slow-wave dysrhythmia. The course may be protracted, with gradual improvement and subsidence of seizures in 2 years or more. Some degree of mental subnormality and residual neurologic deficit is quite common.

Myoclonic Seizures in Progressive Diffuse Encephalopathies. Severe or moderate myoclonus is a prominent feature in the middle stages of subacute sclerosing panencephalitis (inclusion body encephalitis) and in neuronal storage diseases. The attacks are usually diffuse. The EEG may show periodic succession of high-voltage complexes that are synchronous in all leads with the myoclonic jerks. Treatment is ineffective. The underlying disease runs a protracted course with uniformly bad prognosis.

Familial Myoclonus Epilepsy of Unverricht. This is a relatively rare heredofamilial degenerative disease first described by Unverricht. The onset occurs in childhood or at puberty and is marked by increasingly severe, arrhythmic myoclonic attacks involving chiefly the trunk and limb muscles. As the disease progresses, dementia, ataxia, and spasticity appear, and the myoclonus tends to diminish and disappear with the onset of generalized rigidity. Bulbar palsy and deepening stupor lead to death in 10 to 20 years. Pathologically, Lafora bodies having acid mucopolysaccharide reactions have been demonstrated in the ganglion cells of cerebellar and subcortical nuclei.

MASSIVE MYOCLONIC SPASMS. Massive myoclonic spasms (infantile spasms, massive spasms, lightning seizures, jackknife seizures) are peculiar to infants and occur in diffuse encephalopathies. The seizures may occur in apparently normal infants or in infants obviously defective since birth. The cause is unknown in about one-half of cases; in the remainder a history of cerebral insult occurring during gestation, birth, or infancy may be obtained. The nature of the cerebral insult may be a developmental anomaly, intrauterine factors of placental and maternal origin, birth trauma, anoxia, phenylketonuria, tuberous sclerosis, postnatal head injury, meningoencephalitis of bacterial or viral origin, and toxic or allergic encephalopathies. More recently there has been a growing belief that the basic disturbance responsible for epileptogenesis may be biochemical rather than structural, although its exact nature remains to be elucidated.

Massive myoclonic spasms are not uncommon in infantile epilepsy, which is second in incidence only to grand mal seizures. The peak incidence is between the ages of 3 and 6 months, although it has appeared as early as 1 day after birth; onset after the age of 2 years is uncommon. There is no significant difference in sex incidence.

The attacks may occur singly, but more often they occur in a series of successive episodes. Each attack is characterized by sudden, forceful myoclonic contractions involving the musculature of the trunk, the neck, and the extremities. In the flexor type the patient adducts and flexes his limbs, drops his head, and doubles upon himself, much like closing a jackknife. In the extensor type the neck is extended, the arms spread out, and the body bent backward in a manner aptly described as spread-eagle. A cry or grunt may accompany the more severe attacks. The infant may grimace or laugh or appear fearful during or after the attack. Individual attacks are momentary in duration, never exceeding 1 minute; the frequency varies from several to hundreds per day. In 90 percent of cases the EEG shows a characteristic pattern known as hypsarhythmia; the severity of the electrical disturbance generally correlates with the severity of seizures.

The natural course of massive myoclonic spasms is protracted. After a period of months or years the spasms may gradually diminish in frequency and severity and then cease. Occasionally they give way to focal seizures, grand mal seizures, or minor motor seizures. The sequelae of brain damage are permanent. With the onset of the seizures, development either is arrested or regresses. As the attacks persist, mentality and motor functions continue to deteriorate. Ultimately 10 to 15 percent of the children succumb; of the surviving, more than 90 percent are mentally retarded.

PSYCHOMOTOR EPILEPSY. The incidence of psychomotor epilepsy is highest between ages 3 and 6 years and becomes much lower after the age of 12 years. The seizure discharge usually originates in the temporal lobe, which comprises the gray matter of the Sylvian fissure, the insula, the uncus, the amygdala, and the hippocampus, in addition to the three lateral temporal convolutions. In a series of 250 cases a temporal lobe EEG focus was found in 60 percent. Atrophic lesions due to birth injury, postnatal trauma, febrile convulsions in infancy, and thrombotic and infectious meningoencephalopathies are far more common than expanding lesions.

Prodromal symptoms of irritability or gastric upset may precede the onset of a seizure by hours or days. Sleep is a common precipitant. An aura of fear, gastric sensation, buzzing in the ear, or bad odor may usher in the attack. An infant who cannot express himself may hold up his hands to his ears or to the epigastrium with a facial expression of fear, pain, or alarm. The seizures are characteristically of brief duration, lasting from 0.5

to 10 minutes. Consciousness is often impaired but is rarely completely lost. The most common motor symptoms are drawing or jerking of the mouth and face, usually opposite to the side of the discharge. Aphasia or dysphasia may be present if the discharge originates from the dominant side. The eyes may stare in a searching manner. There may be tonic posturing or a desire to urinate. Coordinated but inappropriate movements may be performed repeatedly in a stereotyped manner (automatism), common examples being clutching, fumbling, kicking, walking or running in circles, swallowing, smacking, chewing, licking, and spitting. Pill-rolling, athetoid, or flinging movements are less common. Inhibitory seizures with loss of tone (limpness) or arrest of motion (freezing) may occur. Affective expressions such as laughing or crying are not unusual. Psychical symptoms such as forced thinking, rage, illusions, or hallucinations are rare in children. Chronic behavior disorder may be present. When the attack is over there may or may not be postictal sluggishness or sleep. Amnesia of the attack is the rule.

AUTONOMIC EPILEPSY OR SEIZURE EQUIVALENT SYNDROME. This syndrome may be defined as an entity of epilepsy characterized by paroxysmal attacks of autonomic disturbances with or without associated seizures of other types and with or without disorders of other cerebral functions. The syndrome occurs in children of all ages, with peak incidence at 6 to 7 years. Boys predominate by a ratio of 2 to 1. A history of birth injury, postnatal head trauma, encephalopathies, or prenatal injury, with occurrence descending in the order named, may be elicited in 40 to 50 percent of these children. A family history of epilepsy is present in 20 to 30 percent of the patients.

The most common symptoms are headache and abdominal pain. The headache may be severe or mild, diffuse or ill-defined, and almost never hemicranial. The abdominal pain, which also varies in severity and may be accompanied by nausea, vomiting, and other visceral symptoms, has been diagnosed as an acute surgical emergency and has led to unnecessary laparotomy. Unexplained diarrhea may suddenly appear. Other symptoms that have been observed include profuse salivation, thermal disturbances, various vasomotor symptoms, unexplained fits of rage, uncontrollable laughter, syncopal episodes, and sudden collapse with complete limpness. The seizures generally last for minutes and rarely for hours. More than three symptoms should be present in recurrent attacks before the diagnosis can be considered. Overexertion, anxiety, and sleep are the usual precipitants. Nearly half of these children may have other types of epilepsy; psychomotor seizures, grand mal, and limp attacks are the most common. It is probable that these seizure discharges originate in or near the hypothalamus. Autonomic symptoms may also be produced by discharge from the insular and the orbitofrontal regions.

OTHER NONEPILEPTIC ICTAL PHENOMENA. An EEG may sometimes reveal abnormal activities in children with no overt seizures but with behavior or personality disorders. Besides focal abnormalities, generalized bilateral synchronous paroxysmal activity may be present. Similar findings may be recorded in children with aphasia, learning problems, and sleep disturbances. That an ictal discharge plays an important role in the mechanism of the disorder in such cases is supported by the fact that a good response to anticonvulsant therapy is sometimes obtained.

Diagnostic Evaluation

The first step in the study of a child who has a convulsion is to document its occurrence. Every effort should be made to obtain a description of the seizure, particularly premonitory symptoms, loss of consciousness, convulsive movements, duration of the attack, and state of the patient following the attack. Breath-holding spells in infants may simulate convulsive seizures. In breath-holding spells there is always a precipitating factor, usually an injury or some emotional disturbance that results in violent crying and ends suddenly in respiratory apnea; cyanosis appears before loss of consciousness and convulsive movements (p. 1856).

The second step is to determine whether the seizure is associated with an organic lesion of the central nervous system or a metabolic disturbance. Every child who has had a convulsion should be subjected to thorough study, including skull radiographs, EEG, and blood chemistry.

HISTORY TAKING. Frequently a good history provides essential evidence for the diagnosis. The frequency of attacks may increase with passage of time in untreated cases of petit mal but remain stationary in psychomotor and convulsive equivalent seizures. The duration of the attack is pertinent. Absence attacks seldom exceed 30 sec in duration, whereas psychomotor seizures often last several minutes. The time of occurrence may be of value; early morning attacks or episodes recurring after a meal suggest the possibility of hypoglycemia. Factors tending to precipitate seizures, such as bright light, television, flickering light, loud noise, overbreathing, emotional disturbance, physical fatigue, hunger, menstruation, and fever, should be ascertained so that appropriate measures may be taken to diminish their influence. A detailed prenatal and perinatal history should be obtained to elicit potential high-risk factors (Table 14, p. 1842). In infancy and childhood, head injury, untoward reaction to immunizations, and infections are significant. Febrile convulsions are also important. A detailed developmental history should be obtained. Headache, abdominal pain, restless sleep, and behavior disorders are frequent minor symptoms. Their persistence after commencement of epilepsy treatment may indicate that medication is not sufficient. Symptoms referable to speech, vision, fine skills, and higher mental functions are also of relevance; their progressive deterioration is often a bad omen. A detailed exploration of the family history for epilepsy should be made. The type, dosage, and duration of previous medication and the patient's response are important data helpful in planning treatment.

EXAMINATION. The child should be observed carefully for general behavior, for motor and mental development, and for subtle seizure activity that may not have been evident to the parents.

NEUROLOGIC EXAMINATION. A complete examination, as described earlier in this chapter, should be performed with special consideration of signs that may point to the etiologic factors listed in Table 13. Some examples are: a large head may suggest hydrocephalus, subdural hematoma, or intracranial mass, while a small head may indicate cerebral atrophy; dilated scalp veins may indicate increased intracranial pressure; a skull bruit suggests a vascular anomaly; and skin depigmentation indicates adenoma sebaceum. A careful funduscopic examination may reveal a cherry-red spot that suggests cerebral lipidosis or papilledema that indicates increased intracranial pressure, optic atrophy, or chorioretinitis.

GENERAL PHYSICAL EXAMINATION. A detailed examination is important because it may provide indications of a cause of symptomatic epilepsy. Examples include the presence of hypertension, which may cause encephalopathy, and cerebral abscess, which may be associated with cyanotic congenital cardiac lesions. Also, hepatosplenomegaly may suggest lipidoses. If the history suggests petit mal seizures, hyperventilation for 3 minutes may sometimes induce an attack.

LABORATORY EXAMINATION. The diagnostic impression derived from the history and physical examination should determine which laboratory tests should be performed.

EEG. Of the various ancillary studies the EEG is the most informative, and it frequently provides the only objective evidence of cerebral disorder in seizure patients. It is also helpful in differentiating diffuse encephalopathies from localized lesions. Serial studies may indicate whether the lesion is static or progressive. As discussed above, although certain specific EEG patterns correlate closely with certain seizures, a diagnosis should not be based on the EEG alone when it does not conform with the clinical picture. Electrocorticography and depth electrode recordings are highly specialized procedures to be carried out only when precise localization of an epileptogenic lesion is required prior to surgical exploration.

Radiographic Studies. Radiographic examination of the skull occasionally provides unique information. Asymmetry of the cranium with unilateral thickening of the vault, elevation of the sphenoid and petrous ridges, and increased development of the sinus cells is indicative of a cerebral hemiatrophy. Asymmetry associated with localized thinning and bulging of the vault may suggest an underlying expanding lesion such as porencephalic cyst. Increased intracranial pressure may be reflected by sellar changes and separation of sutures.

Abnormal calcifications may help localize the cerebral lesion and provide a clue to its nature. More specific procedures such as computerized axial tomography, cerebral angiography, and air studies are indicated when there is a possibility of a vascular or neoplastic lesion. Echoencephalography and brain scan may also be helpful.

Other Tests. Lumbar puncture and examination of the CSF are of particular value when cerebral tumor or progessive degenerative or inflammatory disease is suspected. A complete blood count and urinalysis should be routine tests; it is particularly important to obtain them before drug therapy is instituted. Sickle cell preparations should be done when indicated. Other studies that may be performed when indicated include urinary amino acid, urinary sediment and cytomegalic inclusion and metachromatic bodies, urinary porphobilinogen, and urinary phenylpyruvic acid test. Serum calcium and phosphorus determinations as well as a fasting blood sugar should be performed routinely.

Differential Diagnosis

The child with episodic disturbances in his state of consciousness may have a seizure disorder, syncope, migraine, or functional disorder. In the epileptic patient it is essential to determine whether the attacks are associated with underlying organic or metabolic disorder (symptomatic) or are of undetermined cause (unknown).

UNDETERMINED ETIOLOGY. There is often a family history of similar seizures or febrile convulsions. Grand mal seizures usually have an onset between 2 and 16 years of age, and petit mal seizures usually begin between 4 and 16 years. The seizures present with an absence, as generalized tonic-clonic convulsions, or as myoclonus or rarely akinetic episodes, but there are no focal features. Intelligence is usually normal, and physical findings are normal. The EEG typically shows bilateral three-per-second spike-and-wave or synchronous paroxysmal slow dysrhythmia.

SYMPTOMATIC ETIOLOGY. Space-occupying lesions should always be considered when there are focal seizures and focal EEG abnormalities. If the seizures are refractory to drug therapy or if symptoms or signs progress, additional studies may be necessary. Temporal lobe tumors may grow slowly and simulate idiopathic epilepsy. Degenerative and infectious encephalopathies are often associated with other symptoms and signs such as regression of mentation and speech, change in personality, visual complaints, and headache. EEG changes are often progressive, as in conditions such as subacute sclerosing panencephalitis or cerebral lipidosis. Convulsions may occur at the time of *craniocerebral trauma* or shortly there after, and these impact seizures usually have a benign prognosis. The convulsions that occur weeks to months after a head injury are usually indicative of cerebral contusion with subsequent scarring and not infrequently are followed by recurring seizures. Recurring convulsions can be a

TABLE 15. Etiology of Neonatal Seizures

Congenital malformation: agenesis of the corpus calosum, porencephaly, hydranencephaly, vascular anomalies, heterotopias and microgyria

Trauma at birth: hypoxia, intracranial hemorrhage

Infections: generalized sepsis, bacterial meningitis, viral meningoencephalitis, congenital toxoplasmos, congenital syphilis

Metabolic: hypoglycemia, hypocalcemia, hypomagnesemia, pyridoxine deficiency, pyridoxine dependency

Toxic and electrolyte: hypernatremia, hyponatremia, narcotic withdrawal, uremia, hyperbilirubinemia

reflection of *metabolic disturbances* such as hypoglycemia, hypocalcemia, hypomagnesemia, or abrupt changes in sodium concentration.

Neonatal seizures are invariably symptomatic (Table 15). Prompt recognition of etiology is essential, as many are secondary to treatable disorders. Convulsions in the newborn may be a reflection of generalized sepsis, neonatal tetany, symptomatic hypoglycemia, or hypomagnesemia. The neonate born to the heroin-addicted mother may be jittery or may actually convulse for hours to days after birth. The appearance of these symptoms may be delayed as long as 2 weeks in those infants born to mothers receiving methadone. Tumors rarely cause seizures in the newborn period.

Epilepsy must be distinguished from other paroxysmal phenomena including syncope (p. 1857), migraine (p. 1858), and hysteria. Older children from 6 to 16 years of age may have episodes of hysteria that simulate epileptic attacks because of anxiety or other psychologic causes; neurologic examination and EEG usually show no abnormality.

Course and Prognosis

The course and prognosis vary with the nature and severity of the underlying disease. The prognosis of the *epilepsies of undetermined etiology* is generally good. Pure petit mal attacks tend to diminish in frequency with age, and by adolescence they disappear in about 50 percent of patients; the outcome is favorable even in cases with petit mal status. Grand mal seizures generally respond to medical therapy and tend to disappear after the age of 20 years. Mixed grand mal and petit mal seizure pattern is more difficult to control.

Of the *symptomatic epilepsies*, post-traumatic and focal epilepsies have a favorable prognosis. About 50 to 65 percent of psychomotor seizures are difficult to control. Every effort should be made to gain control of seizures as soon as possible, because delay may result in a discrete EEG focus giving way to mirror foci and subsequently more diffuse abnormalities. In such cases the seizures may be more complex, protracted, and refractory to anticonvulsants. As a consequence the patient's intellect may be adversely affected. Other acquired epilepsies, including massive myoclonic, minor motor, and mixed types, are difficult to treat, but the result is not unrewarding. Most children in this category have other manifestations of brain dysfunction; institutional care may be indicated for a few. Age is not as important as the pathologic nature of the cerebral lesion in determining prognosis. The history of duration of seizures is important. Severe convulsions with cyanosis lasting more than 30 minutes may cause brain damage, and prolonged anoxia may be fatal. The prospect of successful treatment is diminished if symptoms have been long-standing. Also, recurrent bouts of status epilepticus generally indicate a poor prognosis.

Serial EEGs are helpful as a general guide in prognosis. The prognosis is better if the EEG shows progressive improvement and finally normalizes. Generally the EEG reverts to normal before seizures arrest; in some cases the EEG abnormality persists for a long time, but the child remains well. One should not attempt to "treat" the EEG. Progressive worsening of EEG calls for reevaluation.

The attitude of the family, relatives, school authorities, and schoolmates may have an important influence on the child's own reaction toward his illness. The physician can play an important role in obviating these influences by thoughtful counseling.

Management

Three aspects of management of the epileptic child should be considered: specific therapy of the seizure, overall management of the child as a person, and counseling of the parents. It is important to recognize the chronicity of the disorder and the recurrent nature of the paroxysms. Relapses may occur in a child who is apparently under good control, particularly at the time of puberty. Thus medication should be continued for 3 to 4 years after the attacks have been arrested; if relapse occurs drug therapy should be reinstituted for an additional 2 to 3 years.

DRUG THERAPY.   With proper choice and dosage of drugs appropriate to the seizure type, about 60 percent of all epileptic attacks can be satisfactorily controlled. Phenobarbital was introduced in 1912; it remains the best anticonvulsant among the barbiturates. The introduction of diphenylhydantoin (Dilantin) in 1936 marked the beginning of modern drug therapy for epilepsy, and in 1944 trimethadione (Tridione) proved its specific usefulness for petit mal. Since then large numbers of new drugs have been added. Barbituric acid derivatives with less sedative action than phenobarbital include mephobarbital (Mebaral), metharbital (Gemonil), and primidone (Mysoline). Phenylethylmethylhydantoin (Mesantoin) and ethotoin (Peganone) are newer hydantoin drugs. The succinimides (Milontin, Celontin, Zarontin) are valuable in petit mal and psychomotor seizures. Many drugs that do not have a primary anticonvulsive action have proved useful. Among these is acetazolamide (Diamox), which has an inhibitory action on brain carbonic anhydrase. Some tranquilizing agents have antiseizure properties. Chlordiazepoxide hydrochloride (Librium) is a weak antiepileptic agent, but two of its analogues are more effective: diazepam (Valium) is now the drug of choice for all types of status epilepticus; nitrazepam (Mogadon) is widely and successfully used in Europe and South America for minor motor seizures. Carbamazepine (Tegretol), which is chemically related to imipramine hydrochloride (Tofranil), a drug for trigeminal neuralgia, has been used in major motor and psychomotor epilepsies. The amphetamines and the antimalarials also have their places in the antiepileptic armamentarium. Adrenal steroids and ACTH preparations have produced some dramatic results in massive myoclonic and minor motor seizures. The indications, dosages, and toxic reactions of the drugs used are shown in Tables 16 and 17.

GENERAL PRINCIPLES. Some drugs are broad-spectrum drugs (Dilantin, phenobarbital, Diamox), and others more specific (Tridione, Celontin, Zarontin) in their antiepileptic activity. The selection of the most effective drug or drugs for each individual patient requires judgment and experience. Some general guidelines follow: A prime factor in successful therapy is choice of the most effective drug, which depends on correct identification of the clinical seizure type. Use one drug at a time, and give it a fair trial before deciding it is ineffective. Increase dosage to tolerance and give it for a reasonable period of time. A combination of two or more drugs may be required, especially for mixed seizures. Give each addition or deletion thoughtful consideration until a satisfactory regimen is found. Give adequate dosage. Young children can tolerate comparatively large doses of anticonvulsants. Adjust doses to be consistent with growth. The duration of therapy should be prolonged; early termination of medication may be followed by relapse. A safe rule is to continue the medication for at least 3 or 4 years after the last attack. Weaning from medication should always be gradual, with stepwise reduction of dosage and withdrawal of one drug at a time. Complete control of symptoms may not be achieved in every patient. It is better to have a functional child with satisfactory control than complete control at the expense of drug toxicity. Sometimes a drug, or a combination of drugs, may activate instead of

TABLE 16. The Drugs of Choice for the Various Seizure Types (in Order of Preference)

Generalized (major motor), focal, psychomotor, and convulsive equivalent epilepsy
 Dilantin
 Phenobarbital or Mebaral
 Mysoline
 Mesantoin
 Celontin
 Phenurone
 Bromides
Petit mal
 Zarontin
 Tridione
 Valium
 Diamox
 Milontin
 Aralen
Minor motor
 ACTH or adrenal corticosteroids
 Mogadon
 Ketogenic diet
 Zarontin, Tridione, Valium, and Celontin
 Dexedrine
 Meprobamate
 Gemonil
Status epilepticus
 Valium (iv)
 Sodium pentobarbital (iv)
 Sodium phenobarbital (iv or im)
 Paraldehyde (iv, im, or rectal)
 Volatile anesthetics

suppress the seizure activity. This may also occur with excessive doses of anticonvulsants. Antacids may interfere with the absorption of anticonvulsants, particularly Dilantin. Conversely, some drugs interfere with metabolism of anticonvulsants, thus producing drug toxicity (eg, isoniazid given with Dilantin). Therapeutic drug levels (Table 18) should be obtained at regular intervals; they are available for Dilantin, phenobarbital, Mysoline, Zarontin, Tegretol, and bromides. These determinations are particularly valuable in establishing the reliability of daily drug intake, in identifying the child who abnormally metabolizes the compound, and in establishing an effective therapeutic dose. Factors that trigger or aggravate seizures should be prevented or controlled; these include fever, constipation, allergic states, emotional upset, frustration, physical exhaustion, and premenstrual edema.

SPECIFIC ANTICONVULSIVE THERAPY. Grand Mal. Most grand mal seizures, regardless of cause, respond well to Dilantin or phenobarbital or both. It is wise to use only one drug at the beginning. Phenobarbital is the first choice, but it may cause hyperactivity and irritability in young children and sluggishness in children of school age. Mephobarbital (Mebaral) is also an effective barbiturate and is usually well tol-

TABLE 17. Anticonvulsants for Childhood Epilepsy

	Indications	Dosage 0-1 Year	Dosage 5 Years	Dosage 12 Years and Up	mg/kg/day	Toxicity
Aralen (chloroquine)	Petit mal*	60 mg, 1-2 times per day	200 mg per day	400 mg per day	15-20	Bleaching of hair, blurring vision
Bromides	Same as Dilantin	250-500 mg daily	500 mg, 2-3 times daily	500 mg 4-6 times daily	50-100	Drowsiness, skin rash, mental dullness, toxic psychosis
Celontin (methsuximide)	Psychomotor,* minor motor†	75 mg, 2-3 times daily	150 mg, 3 times daily	300 mg, 2-3 times daily	15-20	Drowsiness, ataxia, skin rash, rare aplastic anemia
Dexedrine (dextroamphetamine)	Petit mal	1.25 mg, 2-3 times daily	5 mg, 2 times daily	10 mg, 2-3 times daily	0.25-0.75	Restlessness, irritability, sleeplessness
Diamox (acetazolamide)	Petit mal,* all types†	125 mg, 3 times daily	250 mg, 3 times daily	250 mg, 4 times daily	15-30	Anorexia, paresthesia, drowsiness, polyuria, hyperpnea, headache
Dilantin (diphenylhydantoin)	Generalized, psychomotor, focal	20 mg, 3-4 times daily	50 mg, 3 times daily	100 mg, 3-4 times daily	3-8	Gum hypertrophy, ataxia, diplopia, nystagmus, rash, fever, nausea, vomiting, hirsutism
Gemonil (metharbital)	Minor motor*	25 mg, 4-6 times daily	50 mg, 4-6 times daily	100 mg, 3-4 times daily	5-15	Rare drowsiness
Librium (chlordiazepoxide)	Same as phenobarbital	15 mg, 4-5 times daily	32 mg, 3-4 times daily	100 mg 3-4 times daily	2-8	Drowsiness, irritability, rash
Mebaral (mephobarbital)	Minor motor	—	—	30-150 mg per day		Nausea, lethargy, dizziness
Meprobamate (Equanil, Miltown)	Petit mal,* minor motor†	200 mg, 2-3 times daily	200 mg, 3-5 times daily	400 mg, 2-3 times daily	20-40	Drowsiness, hyperactivity
Mesantoin (phenylethylmethyl hydantoin)	Same as Dilantin	25 mg, 3-4 times daily	50 mg, 3-4 times daily	100 mg, 4-6 times daily	4-10	Rash and fever, leukopenia and agranulocytosis, ataxia
Milontin (phensuximide)	Petit mal,* minor motor†	50 mg, 4-5 times daily	250 mg, 3-4 times daily	500 mg, 3-6 times daily	20-40	Nephrotoxic (slightly)
Mogadon (nitrazepam)	(not available in USA)					
Mysoline (primidone)	Same as Dilantin	50 mg, 3-4 times daily	125 mg, 2-3 times daily	250 mg, 4-6 times daily	12-25	Drowsiness, ataxia, skin rash
Paradione (paramethadione)	Same as Tridione					
Paraldehyde (paracetaldehyde)	Status epilepticus	1 ml, im or iv; 2 ml, rectally	3ml, im or iv; 6 ml, rectally	3-6 ml, iv; 8 ml, im		Unpleasant odor, drowsiness
Peganone (ethotoin)	Same as Dilantin		500 mg, 2-4 times daily	1,000 mg, 3-4 times daily		Same as Dilantin except for hirsutism and gum hypertrophy
Phenobarbital (5-ethyl-5-phenyl-barbituric acid)	Same as Dilantin,* minor motor†	15 mg, 3-4 times daily	30 mg, 2-3 times daily	60 mg, 2-3 times daily	1-5	Drowsiness, skin rash, and fever, hyperirritability in infants
Phenurone (phenacemide)	Psychomotor	125 mg, 3-4 times daily	250 mg, 4-6 times daily	500 mg, 4 times daily	20-35	Hepatotoxic, leukopenia, agranulocytosis, rash, irritability, and mental derangement
Tridione (trimethadione)	Petit mal,* minor motor†	25 mg, 4-6 times daily	150 mg, 4-6 times daily	300 mg, 4-6 times daily	20-50	Rash, leukopenia and agranulocytosis, nephrosis, photophobia, irritability
Valium (diazepam)	Status epilepticus*	1-2 mg, iv	5 mg, iv	10 mg, iv	Slow injection, 1-2 mg/min	Drowsiness, ataxia
	Minor motor, petit mal	1 mg, 1-3 times daily	2 mg, 1-3 times daily	5 mg, 1-3 times daily		
Zarontin (ethosuximide)	Petit mal,* minor motor†		250 mg, 2-3 times daily	250 mg, 3-4 times daily	20-50	Drowsiness, skin rash, gastric upset, rare aplastic anemia

*Primary indication.
†Secondary indication.

TABLE 18. Optimal Levels of Common Anticonvulsive Drugs in Children

Drug	Optimal* Levels (µg/ml)
Diphenylhydantoin	10–20
Phenobarbital	20–40
Primodone	8–12
Ethosuximide	60–100

* These levels have been reported to provide adequate seizure control in most patients.

erated by children. Mephobarbital is metabolized to phenobarbital, and in equivalent doses its effect is half that of phenobarbital; the effective dose is therefore twice that of phenobarbital. Dilantin is the second drug of choice, and frequently it is necessary to use a combination of both drugs.

All these drugs may cause toxic symptoms from overdosage or idiosyncrasy. Fever, morbilliform rash, and even exfoliative dermatitis may develop, in which case the drug should be discontinued. Sometimes, after the symptoms clear, smaller dosage may be tolerated in a new trial. Other common toxic reactions from Dilantin overdosage are cerebellar signs (usually reversible), nausea, vomiting, and irritability (more common in infants). The more subtle symptoms of headache, dizziness, and mental depression often are not recognized as idiosyncrasy or mild toxicity to Dilantin, and they may lead to suspicion of disease of the central nervous system, psychoneurosis, or even brain tumor. Most of these symptoms are reversible. More severe forms of idiosyncrasy to Dilantin include the development of Stevens-Johnson syndrome, lupus erythematosus, and lymphadenopathy simulating lymphoma. These are urgent indications to stop Dilantin therapy immediately. Recent reports have indicated that Dilantin, Mysoline, and phenobarbital, alone or combined, may cause subnormal serum folate levels. Whether megaloblastic anemia reversible by folic acid therapy occurs in children requires further study. Gum hypertrophy occurs in about 50 percent of children on Dilantin therapy; it is not a contraindication to its use. Firm massage of the gums may alleviate this side effect. Excessive hair growth is also common in young children, but this is generally reversible after the drug is discontinued. Mesantoin is more toxic than Dilantin and may produce neutropenia or aplastic anemia; periodic blood counts are indicated when this agent is used.

Primidone (Mysoline) is a satisfactory anticonvulsant; the desired dose should be built up gradually, lest the child become oversedated. Mysoline may cause irritability, anorexia, and lethargy, but it is generally well tolerated by children. Metharbital (Gemonil), a weaker anticonvulsant, is almost devoid of side effects and can be used as an adjunctive drug.

If the initial seizure (febrile or nonfebrile) is witnessed and is found to be unduly prolonged (10 min-

utes or more), it should be controlled by the use of intravenous sodium phenobarbital. In such circumstances an infant under the age of 1 year may require 0.06 to 0.1 g, a child between the ages of 2 and 5 years, 0.12 to 0.2 g, and the older child, up to 0.3 g.

Status Epilepticus. Status epilepticus is a medical emergency requiring immediate treatment, as it has a mortality of 5 to 10 percent. An open airway must be maintained and oxygen administered if cyanosis is present. The convulsions must be stopped and recurrence prevented by effective medication. The specific anticonvulsants should always be given intravenously in amounts large enough to stop seizure activity quickly. A common error is the frequent use of small aliquots of anticonvulsants with resultant toxicity but continued status. Recently diazepam (Valium) has superseded the barbiturates and paraldehyde as the drug of choice for the treatment of status epilepticus. The drug is given by slow intravenous injection at a rate not exceeding 1 mg/minute. For infants the optimal single dose is 1 to 2 mg, for young children 2 to 5 mg, and for older children 5 to 10 mg. The response of the patient to intravenous therapy with diazepam may be monitored by EEG, if it is available, and the injection may be stopped promptly as electrical and clinical arrest of the seizure becomes evident. The majority of cases will respond favorably to one injection. If symptoms recur a second or even third injection may be required at 20- to 30-minute intervals. Diazepam has been found to be safe and less toxic than barbiturates or paraldehyde with respect to respiratory and cardiovascular depression. It should be borne in mind that diazepam potentiates barbiturates. This form of therapy has also been used for petit mal status and epilepsy partialis continua. The focus of depressive action is believed to be in the brainstem reticular system. The next drug of choice is sodium phenobarbital administered intravenously in the doses outlined above. If respiration is depressed, paraldehyde is preferred. This is an effective agent and is given intravenously as a dilute solution of 4 ml in 100 ml of 0.25-N NaCl with 5 percent glucose solution. Untoward side effects of paraldehyde are respiratory distress and acute cardiac failure; if used judiciously in a dilute solution, these complications are rare. It can also be given rectally with a wide margin of safety. Volatile anesthetic agents including vinyl ether or chloroform may be useful in controlling status, especially when it is difficult to give medications by the intravenous route. Concomitant with the acute emergency therapy, long-acting drugs, preferably phenobarbital or diphenylhydantoin, should be given by the intramuscular route.

Focal Cortical Epilepsy. Focal seizures respond favorably to the same drugs used in grand mal attacks. Multifocal seizures are less easy to control.

Psychomotor Seizures. Dilantin is the drug of choice, and it may be combined with phenobarbital. Methsuximide (Celontin) is useful in some children; its side effects include drowsiness, anorexia, skin rash, fever, and occasionally neutropenia. In some instances Celontin has proved to be more effective than Dilantin. Tegretol has recently proved to be very effective in some children with psychomotor epilepsy. Because of the possible toxic action on the liver and bone marrow, phenacemide (Phenurone) has not been widely used in the treatment of psychomotor epilepsy.

Pure Petit Mal Absence. Ethosuximide (Zarontin) is the drug of choice in the treatment of petit mal attacks. Untoward reactions include anorexia, abdominal pain, drowsiness, and occasional skin rash. Aplastic anemia has been reported rarely. Trimethadione (Tridione) is also a relatively specific drug for petit mal. A common cause of failure is timidity in prescribing high dosage. Monthly blood counts should forewarn of the possibility of neutropenia; as the neutrophil count drops to $1,600/mm^3$ reduction of dosage or change of medication should be considered seriously. Skin rash with fever is also an indication to stop Zarontin or decrease the dosage. The nephrotic syndrome is an indication to discontinue Tridione. Lupus erythematosus is an uncommon complication of both Tridione and Zarontin therapy. Other less important side effects are photophobia, drowsiness, and eosinophilia. Acetazolamide (Diamox), either alone or combined with Tridione, is effective. In a rare patient in whom none of the foregoing drugs brought relief, the antimalarial agent chloroquine (Aralen) has proved useful. The side effects are visual disturbances (lacrimation, blurred vision, ptosis, and strabismus), skin sensitivity, and occasional peripheral neuropathy. All these symptoms, except the retinopathy, are reversible. Periodic examination of the visual field is mandatory, since visual field defects precede the onset of retinitis, and at this stage the eye lesions are still reversible.

Myoclonic Epilepsy. Myoclonic epilepsy is more difficult to manage than pure petit mal attacks. The drug of choice is Celontin, which may have dramatic effect. Next choices are Valium, Tridione, Diamox, and meprobamate. Corticosteroids or corticotrophins may be effective in some resistant cases. The myoclonic epilepsy seen in degenerative diseases is resistant to drugs.

Minor Motor Seizures. *Akinetic seizures* are notoriously difficult to control. In a few patients beneficial results may be obtained from Valium, Celontin, Tridione, Zarontin, or Diamox. In some cases a trial of ACTH therapy is highly recommended. With severe drop seizures children often sustain bruises of the face and eyes or even fractures of teeth or skull. Wearing a padded football helmet may prevent or minimize such injuries. The ketogenic diet may be the most effective form of treatment for this type of seizure, but this requires the full cooperation of the child and the family.

Massive myoclonic spasms are very resistant to the usual anticonvulsants. ACTH is the drug of choice. The efficacy of ACTH or steroid therapy appears to depend on the underlying cause of the spasms and the promptness and intensity of the medication. The earlier and the more intensive the therapy, the better the response.

The seizures may be controlled or abated in 50 percent of cases. The mental impairment, however, is much less affected by any type of therapy. We recommend that Acthar gel be given intramuscularly in two divided doses daily according to the following schedule: 40 IU/day for 2 weeks, 30 IU/day for the third week, and 20 IU/day for the fourth week, followed by 20 IU/day for 3 days and 10 IU/day for a further 3 days. Proper precautions of steroid therapy should be closely followed (p. 1654). The sleeplessness and irritability that are often seen during the second or third week of therapy may be counteracted by oral or rectal chlorpromazine.

Convulsive Equivalent (Autonomic) Epilepsy. The majority of these patients can be successfully treated with anticonvulsive drugs. Dilantin, alone or in conjunction with Diamox, is most satisfactory. Diamox alone may sometimes be effective. Meprobamate, Mebaral, and Tridione may also be useful.

DIETARY TREATMENT. The ketogenic diet was introduced as a form of antiepileptic treatment by Wilder in 1921. Since the advent of modern anticonvulsant drugs, the need for dietary therapy has become limited to selected patients in whom drugs have utterly failed or have had to be discontinued because of intolerance or idiosyncrasy. The diet is most effective in patients with akinetic seizures. The ketogenic diet is more expensive than ordinary meals, and its preparation requires intelligence and care. Rigid control must be enforced lest the effectiveness be diminished or lost; thus it should be prescribed only for selected children. The parents must have complete understanding and must be willing to cooperate fully. It is used most readily in children 2 to 5 years of age; young infants may not tolerate the high fat content; older children may rebel and refuse to take the diet. Retarded or brain-damaged children may not cooperate in finishing their meals and may accept carbohydrate foods offered inadvertently.

Preferably the child should be hospitalized for the initiation of the dietary regime, which should be preceded by a period of total starvation (3 to 4 days) during which only water is given. If this is successful the child is so hungry that he is ready and willing to eat what is served. The ketosis induced by the starvation is maintained as long as the dietary regime is not broken. Even minor infringement such as consuming a small amount of carbohydrate may diminish the effectiveness of the diet drastically. Like drug therapy, the diet should be continued for 2 to 3 years. In weaning from the diet, the proportion of fat should be decreased gradually over a period of weeks, lest sudden reversion of ketosis precipitate a convulsive attack. The basic requirement of a ketogenic diet is to provide sufficient protein and calories for growth and maintenance with a ratio of fat to protein–carbohydrate of 4 to 1 by weight. The diet has been described in detail by Livingston and by Keith.

SURGICAL TREATMENT. With the development of refined diagnostic techniques, surgical treatment of certain types of focal epilepsy has become effective. This therapeutic approach requires a competent and experienced team such as is usually available only in large medical centers. Indications for surgical therapy are clear in patients with progressive lesions of the brain (tumor, abscess, hematoma, and vascular malformation). For chronic epilepsy due to static or atrophic lesions the primary treatment is medical, and surgery should be considered only when drug, dietary, and other therapeutic measures have failed after adequate trial.

The indication for surgery is limited further to cases in which clinical and laboratory studies clearly point to a well-localized lesion in a surgically accessible site in one cerebral hemisphere. Bilateral, diffuse, or subcortical lesions are contraindications, as are the genetic epilepsies. The general status of the patient, the physical and mental deficits other than epilepsy, and the disability that may be anticipated following surgical intervention should be carefully evaluated before it is recommended. When surgery is indicated, exact cortical localization of the epileptogenic focus or foci must be accomplished through clinical and special radiographic and electrographic studies carried out preoperatively as well as during the operation.

A number of effective procedures have been developed, such as local excision, total lobectomy, and hemispherectomy. The tendency has been toward wider excision of tissues surrounding the epileptogenic focus. In competent hands the surgical mortality is 1 to 2 percent; complete control or marked improvement is obtained in more than 50 percent of properly selected cases.

PATIENT MANAGEMENT. The epileptic child should be treated as a person, not a case. It should be reemphasized that epilepsy is only a symptom of an underlying disease that may exhibit other symptoms of equal or more serious import. The child may have emotional problems, either because of his seizures or because of poor schoolwork secondary to cerebral dysfunction. In addition, as the child grows into adolescence and young adulthood, educational, social, and economic problems arise and demand solution. The physician should provide suggestions and direction. Generally speaking, the epileptic child should be encouraged to live as normal a life as is consistent with safety. If the seizures are under good control, such physical exercises as riding a bicycle, jumping rope, roller skating, and swimming (under supervision) may be permitted; if the child is able, certain competitive sports may also be allowed. Except for patients on the ketogenic diet, dietary and fluid restrictions play no role in the management of epilepsy.

Although petit mal seldom affects the intellect, the same assurance may not be given for all genetic epilepsies, especially when the seizures are prolonged and numerous. Symptomatic seizures are often associated with brain damage; in addition to their seizures, these children also may have mental, motor, or speech deficits. These difficulties may in turn lead to secondary emotional disorders, and such children should receive special assistance to overcome their handicaps.

PARENT COUNSELING. It must be realized that all parents need counseling and reassurance. They may have prejudices about their child's affliction, have a sense of guilt or shame, and be worried, anxious, fearful, or even hostile. They may have shopped around without a clear idea of what the real trouble is or what the future holds for the child. The strain on their emotional and economic resources may threaten the welfare of the entire family. Clearly it is the obligation of the physician to enlighten, to reassure, to answer questions, and to help solve secondary problems. The parents should be apprised of the diagnosis, treatment plan, and prognosis. As they come to understand the nature of the condition and what to expect, they will be in a better position to carry on the care of their child without unduly dislocating their family life. The importance of this to the total welfare of the epileptic child cannot be overstated. Wisely carried out, parent counseling is a small investment in terms of time and effort on the part of the physician, that can pay huge dividends as the family's fears and uncertainties are allayed through an understanding of the definitive diagnosis and plan of treatment.

FEBRILE CONVULSIONS

Convulsive disorder can be divided into two major categories: the acute sporadic and the chronic paroxysmal. The first group includes the febrile convulsions of infancy and childhood. By definition, febrile convulsions are provoked by hyperthermia associated with an acute illness of extracranial origin. Acute convulsions associated with intracranial diseases of infectious, toxic, metabolic, vascular, and neoplastic origin are also classified in the first group. Although febrile convulsions are the most common seizure disorders in childhood, their exact incidence is not known. It is estimated to be about 5 percent. They commonly occur at 6 months to 3 years of age, with a peak incidence at 18 months. The incidence is slightly greater in boys, and there is a high familial incidence (about 30 percent) as well as a high incidence of other epileptic disorders (about 15 percent) that suggest the importance of genetic predisposition.

DIAGNOSIS. The most common cause of febrile convulsions is acute upper respiratory infection. The suddenness of the rise in temperature appears to be more important than the final temperature reached, and the threshold for convulsion differs in individual patients. In an infant with fever and convulsions, the diagnosis of benign febrile convulsion should not be made without excluding other causes, particularly intracranial infections such as meningitis. When febrile convulsion is diagnosed with reasonable assurance, benign (or typical) should be differentiated from nonbenign (or atypical) febrile seizure; this is important in management and prognosis. Any child presenting with a febrile convulsion deserves a careful work-up and a planned follow-up. Laboratory studies should include examination of the CSF, measurement of blood glucose, calcium, and phosphorus, radiographs of the skull, and an EEG.

Benign febrile convulsions most commonly occur in neurologically normal children between 6 months and 3 years of age. Criteria that may be helpful in differentiating benign febrile convulsions from nonbenign convulsions are a positive family history of febrile convulsions, an abrupt rise in temperature to over 39.5 C inciting a generalized convulsion seldom longer than a few minutes in duration, no neurologic abnormality after the attack, and normal laboratory studies, including EEG. In contrast, children with *nonbenign* febrile convulsions often have a lowered seizure threshold that may be related to a preexisting but subclinical condition such as prematurity or birth trauma. In these cases fever acts as a trigger, and the convulsive episodes are more prone to be repetitive, with lowering degree of fever each time and finally with no fever at all. In this group should also be included those children who were neurologically normal but who sustained brain insult during their first febrile convulsion. Helpful criteria in identifying the nonbenign group are asymmetric or focal seizure with or without Todd's paralysis, seizures lasting longer than 30 minutes, repeated seizures during one febrile illness, presence of neurologic deficits before, during, or after the seizure, persistent and significant EEG abnormalities, and onset of seizures before 6 months or after 3 years of age. The EEG should not be recorded too soon after a seizure, but preferably a week after the initial attack. A single examination is of little assistance in prognosis; serial studies should be performed in children with recurrent febrile convulsions. Abnormal EEGs are found in about 25 percent of children with febrile convulsions, and 10 percent show definite epileptiform activity.

PROGNOSIS. Febrile convulsions are not necessarily benign. The child may experience subsequent febrile seizures, develop afebrile seizures (epilepsy), or manifest signs of underlying brain dysfunction. Children with *recurrent febrile seizures* have an increasing risk of further febrile convulsion with each additional attack; there is a 35 percent recurrence after the first seizure, 47 percent after the second, and 60 percent after the third. In a longitudinal study of *recurrent afebrile seizures* covering the ages 15 to 22 years, Livingston found that the incidence of chronic epilepsy was 2.9 in the benign group and 97 percent in the nonbenign group. Psychomotor epilepsy has been found to occur more frequently in children with a history of benign febrile convulsions.

The question of the possibility of *brain damage* and mental retardation as sequelae of febrile convulsions cannot be easily answered, since carefully planned, long-term follow-up studies are lacking. Of the overall febrile convulsion group, the incidence of mental retar-

dation has been reported as 6 to 8 percent and behavior disorder as 10 percent. It is unknown what proportions of these belong to the benign and nonbenign groups of febrile convulsions. In our experience, subtle changes of brain function are more common than obvious mental retardation; these include behavior disturbance, speech disorder, learning deficiencies, and autonomic dysfunctions. The latter may manifest as sleep disturbance and visceral, sensory, vasomotor, or other autonomic seizure equivalents. Fortunately many of these symptoms tend to improve and even disappear with maturation of the central nervous system.

TREATMENT. Treatment of febrile convulsions should be directed at controlling the convulsions with maintenance anticonvulsants, lowering the fever, and treating the underlying infection. There is a difference of opinion as to the value of long-term prophylactic anticonvulsant therapy. The difficulty in distinguishing the benign from the nonbenign febrile convulsion and in identifying the complications that may result from a seizure has prompted us to recommend that all children be treated with daily phenobarbital in a dose of 5 mg/kg body weight; a blood level between 16 μg/ml and 30 μg/ml should be maintained until the child is 5 to 6 years of age.

References

GENERAL

Chao D, Druckman R, Kellaway P: Convulsive Disorders of Children. Philadelphia, WB Saunders, 1958

Jasper HH, Ward AA, Pope A: Basic Mechanisms of the Epilepsies. Boston, Little, Brown, 1969

Jeavons PM, Bower BD: Infantile Spasms: A Review of the Literature and a Study of 112 Cases. Clinics of Developmental Medicine No 15. London, William Heinemann Medical Books, 1964

Lagos JC: Seizures, Epilepsy and Your Child. New York, Harper & Row, 1974

Lennox-Buchthal MA: Febrile convulsions : A reappraisal. Electroencephalogr Clin Neurophysiol [Suppl 32], 1973

Livingston S: Comprehensive Management of Epilepsy in Infancy, Childhood and Adolescence. Springfield, Ill, Charles C Thomas, 1972

——— Living with Epileptic Seizures. Springfield, Ill, Charles C Thomas, 1963

Millichap JG: Febrile Convulsions. New York, Macmillan, 1968

Penfield W, Jasper HH: Epilepsy and the Functional Anatomy of the Human Brain. Boston, Little, Brown, 1954

Robb P: Epilepsy: a review of basic and clinical research. NINDB Monograph No 1, US Public Health Service Publication No 1357. Washington, DC, US Department of Health, Education and Welfare, 1965

Rodin EA: The Prognosis of Patients with Epilepsy. Springfield, Ill, Charles C Thomas, 1968

Schmidt RP, Wilder BJ: Epilepsy. Philadelphia, FA Davis, 1968

Sibley HH: Diagnosis and treatment of epilepsy: overview and general principles. Pediatrics 53:529, 1974

Tower DB: Neurochemistry of Epilepsy. Springfield, Ill, Charles C Thomas, 1960

CLASSIFICATION

Brown JK, Cockburn F, Forfar JO: Clinical and chemical correlates in convulsions of the newborn. Lancet 1:135, 1972

———— Convulsions in the newborn period. Dev Med Child Neurol 15:823, 1973

Craig WS: Convulsive movements occurring in the first 10 days of life. Arch Dis Child 35:336, 1960

Evans JH: Post-traumatic epilepsy. Neurology 12:665, 1962

Fowler M: Brain damage after febrile convulsions. Arch Dis Child 32:67, 1957

Friedlander WJ: Epilepsy. Am J Psychiatry 120:674, 1964

Gastaut H, Caveness WF, Landolt H, et al: A proposed international classification of epileptic seizures. Epilepsia 5:297, 1964

Gold AP: Psychomotor epilepsy in childhood. Pediatrics 53: 540, 1974

Jennett B: Early traumatic epilepsy. Arch Neurol 30:349, 1974

Lennox W G, Gibbs EL, Gibbs FA: Inheritance of cerebral dysrhythmia and epilepsy. Arch Neurol Psychiatry 44:1155, 1940

Marson CA: A newly proposed classification of epileptic seizures: neurophysiological basis. Epilepsia 6:275, 1965

Volpe J: Neonatal seizures. N Engl J Med 289:413, 1973

CLINICAL

Bray PF: Temporal lobe epilepsy syndrome. Pediatrics 29:612, 1962

Chao D: Seizures in infancy and early childhood. Med Clin North Am 42:399, 1958

———— Sexton JA, Pardo LS: Temporal lobe epilepsy in children. J Pediatr 60:686, 1962

———— Taylor FM, Druckman R: Massive spasms in infancy and childhood. J Pediatr 50:670, 1958

Charlton MH, Yahr MD: Long-term follow-up of patients with petit mal. Arch Neurol 16:595, 1967

Debiolley D: Petit mal variant or Lennox syndrome. Electroencephalogr Clin Neurophysiol 23:282, 1967

Epstein MH, O'Connor JS: Destructive effects of prolonged status epilepticus. J Neurol Neurosurg Psychiatry 29:251, 1966

Frantzen E, Lennox-Buchthal M, Nygaard A: Longitudinal EEG and clinical study of children with febrile convulsions. Electroencephalogr Clin Neurophysiol 24:197, 1968

Gastaut H, Roger J, Soulayrol R, et al: Childhood epileptic encephalopathy with diffuse slow spike-waves (otherwise known as "petit mal variant") or Lennox syndrome. Epilepsia 7:139, 1966

Gibberd, FB: The prognosis of petit mal. Brain 89:531, 1966

Hammill JF, Carter S: Febrile convulsions. N Engl J Med 274:563, 1966

Lennox WG: Significance of febrile convulsions. Pediatrics 11:341, 1953

Livingston S: Infantile febrile convulsions. Dev Med Child Neurol 10:374, 1968

Lombroso CT, Lerman P: Breathholding spells (cyanotic and pallid infantile syncope). Pediatrics 39:563, 1967

Meyer A, Beck E, Shepherd M: Unusually severe lesions in the brain following status epilepticus. J Neurol Neurosurg Psychiatry 18:24, 1955

Rogina V, Serafetinides EA: Epilepsy and behavior disorder in patients with generalized spike and wave complexes. Electroencephalogr Clin Neurophysiol 14:376, 1962

Steinschneider A, Ginsberg T, George ED, Lipton EL: Febrile convulsions. Neurology 14:362, 1964

Swanson PD, Luttrell CN, Magladery JW: Myoclonus. Medicine 41: 339, 1962

Walsh O: Unusual presentations of epilepsies. Pediatrics 53: 548, 1974

Yanai N: Febrile convulsions in children. Dev Med Child Neurol 10:255, 1967

TREATMENT

Bell DS: Dangers of treatment of status epilepticus with diazepam. Br Med J 1:159, 1969

Borofsky LC, Louis S, Kutt H: Diphenlhydantoin in children: pharmacology and efficacy. Neurology 23:967, 1973

Carson MJ: Treatment of minor motor seizures with nitrazepam. Dev Med Child Neurol 10:772, 1968

Carter S, Gold AP: Seizures in childhood. N Engl J Med 278:315, 1968

———— Gold AP: Care of the critically ill child: management of status epilepticus. Pediatrics 44:732, 1969

Chao D: Overall management of the epileptic child. Med Clin North Am 42:461, 1958

———— Drug therapy in paroxysmal disorders. Pediatr Clin North Am 10:3, 1963

Eadie MJ, Tyrer JH: Anticonvulsant Therapy. London, Churchill-Livingstone, 1974

Faer O, Kastrup KW, Nielsen, EL: Melchoir JC, Thorn I: Successful prophylaxis of febrile convulsions with phenobarbital. Epilepsia 13: 279, 1972

Gallagher BB, Baumel IP, Mattson RH, Woodbury SG: Primidone, diphenylhydantoin and phenobarbital: aspects of acute and chronic toxicity. Neurology 23:145, 1973

Gold AP, Carter S: Pediatric neurology. In Shirkey HC (ed): Pediatric Therapy. St Louis, CV Mosby, 1972

Hammill JF, Carter S: Febrile convulsions. N Engl J Med 274:563, 1965

Hooshmand H: Toxic effects of anticonvulsants: general principles. Pediatrics 53:551, 1974

Keith HM: Convulsive Disorders in Children with Special Reference to Treatment with Ketogenic Diet. Boston, Little, Brown, 1963

Kutt H: The use of blood levels of antiepileptic drugs in clinical practice. Pediatrics. 53:557, 1974

Livingston S: Diagnosis and treatment of childhood myoclonic seizures. Pediatrics 53:542, 1974

———— Berman W: Participation of epileptic patients in sports. JAMA 244:236, 1973

———— Berman W, Pauli LL: Anticonvulsant drug blood levels. JAMA 232:60, 1975

Lombroso CT: The treatment of status epilepticus. Pediatrics 53:536, 1974

McLaurin RL: Epilepsy and contact sports: factors contraindicating participation. JAMA 225:285, 1973

Monson RP, Rosenberg L, Hartz SC, Shapiro S, Heinonen OP, Slone D: Diphenylhydantoin and selected congenital malformations. N Engl J Med 289:1049, 1973

Nicol CF, Tutton JC, Smith BH: Parenteral diazepam in status epilepticus. Neurology 19:332, 1969

Nygaard Jensen O, Vendeline Olesen O: The Clinical Importance of Folic Acid in Patients Treated with Anticonvulsant Drugs. International Congress Series 193. Amsterdam, Excerpta Medica, 1969, p 260

Penfield W, Paine K: Results of surgical therapy of focal epileptic seizures. Can Med Assoc J 73:515, 1955

Peterson WG: Clinical study of Mogadon, a new anticonvulsant. Neurology 17:878, 1967

Reynolds EH, Miller CG, Matthews DM: Anticonvulsant therapy, folic acid and vitamin B_{12} metabolism and mental symptoms. Epilepsia 7:261, 1966

Woodbury DM, Penry, JK, Schmidt RP: Antiepileptic Drugs. New York, Raven, 1972

NONEPILEPTIFORM PAROXYSMAL DISORDERS OF CHILDHOOD

ABE M. CHUTORIAN

The nonepileptiform paroxysmal disorders are a heterogeneous group identified chiefly by two clinical features: a propensity for the disorders to affect the patient as more or less dramatic paroxysms, with the interictal state being normal, and a finding of nonepileptiform pathogenesis. In some instances consciousness is affected (eg, breath-holding, syncope, narcolepsy), while in others only a subjective experience may signal the occurrence of a paroxysm (eg, migraine). In yet other instances both a unique subjective experience and related outward manifestations occur (eg, paroxysmal vertigo with ataxia). The resemblance of these disorders to unusual forms of epilepsy may be impressive. Therefore differentiation from epilepsy is often required as part of the diagnostic process or therapeutic-diagnostic process. Thus it should be emphasized that in addition to performing those ancillary studies that may be pertinent to the suspected nonepileptiform paroxysmal disorder, the physician often requires evidence of a negative character that indicates the absence of epileptic features. This evidence is derived from two sources: from a nonparoxysmal electroencephalogram (EEG) and from the absence of a therapeutic response to anticonvulsive medication. Since neither of these features is sufficient to rule out epilepsy entirely, in unusual instances the physician must be content to manage the patient empirically, with a provisional diagnosis based on the clinical and ancillary diagnostic features and on the response or absence of response to certain therapeutic compounds. This need for an empiric approach is increased by our ignorance of the apparently varied pathogeneses of most of these disorders. The anatomic and physiologic bases of these conditions are in some instances hypothetical and in others entirely speculative.

These disorders will be discussed under the following headings: breath-holding attacks; syncope; paroxysmal headache (migraine, headache and epilspey, functional headache); cyclic vomiting (occult abdominal epilepsy, abdominal migraine, recurrent acetonemic vomiting); benign paroxysmal vertigo; paroxysmal torticollis, tortipelvis, and retrocollis; disorders of wake–sleep cycle; cranial neuralgia; and paroxysmal disorders due to specific structural and metabolic abnormalities.

BREATH-HOLDING ATTACKS

The common phenomenon of breath-holding in early childhood is foremost among the nonepileptiform disorders that raise the question of epilepsy in differential diagnosis. This is due in part to the characteristic loss of consciousness and in part to the occurrence in a minority of these children of incontinence or generalized rhythmic muscular contractions indistinguishable (although of briefer duration) from those that occur in a grand mal seizure. Estimates of the frequency of breath-holding attacks range to more than 5 percent of the childhood population, with the peak incidence being at 2 to 3 years of age. The disorder rarely affects infants less than 6 months or children more than 6 years of age, but apparently authentic neonatal cases have been described. The sexes are affected equally. A history of breath-holding attacks in the early childhood of

a near relative is obtained in more than one-fourth of the cases. The view that the breath-holding spell is a form of syncope is supported by the tendency in later life toward more typical syncopal episodes in 10 to 20 percent of individuals previously subject to breath-holding.

There are two varieties of breath-holding, the features of which overlap considerably. In the more common cyanotic type, crying occurs after a physical or emotional insult that precipitates fear, anger, or frustration. The cry is dramatically suspended by apnea, and in all but the more trivial or abortive episodes rigidity and opisthotonos occur in association with central cyanosis. After a brief period of opisthotonos, loss of body tone occurs, following which there is either instant restoration of full awareness or a brief period of relative inactivity (occasionally a period of sleep), but never the severe depression of sensorium that may be seen after a grand mal seizure. The various stages rarely last more than 10 to 15 sec (usually only 5 sec or less), so that the entire attack consists of stages that telescope into one another over an entire period of 10 to 60 sec. Episodes lasting longer than 1 minute should be suspect, but in rare instances episodes culminate in several seconds of clonic rhythmic generalized muscular contractions indistinguishable from those of a generalized epileptiform seizure, save for the relative brevity of this activity. However, rhythmic muscular contractions are more apt to occur in the final phase of the second or pallid variety of breath-holding attack. The interepisodic EEG is normal, and anticonvulsive drugs do not prevent the attacks.

In the pallid type of breath-holding spell the child responds to an unexpected painful stimulus with sudden apnea and loss of consciousness. The other features of the attack do not differ appreciably from those described for the cyanotic type of attack, and the attack may or may not involve opisthotonos and seizure activity before it terminates. Occasionally urinary incontinence occurs, but it is not the rule.

It seems that although the features of pallid and cyanotic breath-holding spells overlap considerably, the pallid group includes a large number of children with a hypersensitive oculocardiac reflex, as judged by the response to ocular compression. The latter response includes cardiac slowing and asystole, synchronous EEG slowing, and anoxic seizure activity. The seizure activity tends to correlate with the duration of cardiac asystole and the associated EEG slowing, but many children with breath-holding attacks are resistant to the occurrence of these features even when cardiac asystole is relatively prolonged. The similarities of the pallid and cyanotic types of attack are greater than their differences. Indeed, a significant minority (20 percent) have both types. A similar number suffer from only pallid episodes, but the majority have cyanotic attacks that follow crying.

The various mechanisms involved in the attack have been postulated to culminate in cerebral ischemia, either on the basis of apnea, hypocapnea, and cerebral vasoconstriction in the crying phase or on the basis of reduced cardiac output secondary to respiratory spasm or asystole. A uniformly favorable outlook for spontaneous cessation of the attacks should be given to the parents of an affected child, despite the exceedingly rare experience with fatality allegedly based on aspiration or permanent asystole. Subsequent syncopal episodes occur in a significant minority. Severe psychologic disturbance in both the affected child and the involved parents may be seen when attacks are frequent and the parents believe that failure to intervene may result in fatality. The child is actually conditioned to a higher frequency of apneic episodes by the vicious cycle of crying and parental permissiveness.

The frequency of attacks varies from several in a year to multiple weekly episodes; an intermediate frequency is the rule. The prognosis is not altered by the duration or frequency of attacks, nor does the response to treatment depend on these variables. A tendency to recurrent syncopal episodes is occasionally seen in older children who were subject in earlier childhood to breath-holding spells.

Curiously, although atropine and similar compounds theoretically should benefit the child subject to pallid attacks, these drugs have been said to benefit both types of attacks. Some clinicians believe that anticonvulsive drugs are helpful despite the nonepileptiform character of the disorder, but this is doubtful. In general, the efficacy of drug therapy is poorly documented; hence medication cannot be routinely recommended.

SYNCOPE

Loss of consciousness and muscle tone of brief duration (syncope) is a physiologic phenomenon that occurs under certain more or less extreme conditions affecting emotion, temperature, and posture. The more common situations that may evoke syncope in any healthy child, but that tend to do so as a recurrent phenomenon in certain children prone to syncope, include formal religious services and prolongation of the erect posture in a warm, poorly ventilated environment. Whether the mechanism is similar in the apparently spontaneous episodes of some otherwise apparently normal children is uncertain.

The characteristic features of syncope include loss of muscle tone and consciousness for less than a minute, followed by rapid restoration of awareness, in contradistinction to the postictal depression that follows an epileptiform attack. In some instances a syncopal attack terminates in a brief series of generalized muscle jerks, evidently on the basis of cerebral anoxia, such as occasionally occurs in uncomplicated breath-holding attacks.

Syncopal episodes can occur as seizure equivalents in some epileptic patients. The concurrence of other more clearly epileptiform attacks in such patients, or the occurrence of paroxysmal abnormalities in their ictal or interictal EEGs, as well as their responses to anticonvulsive drugs, help to distinguish the seizure equivalent episodes from the apparently spontaneous episodes of syncope.

Hyperventilation, a recurrent manifestation of anxiety in some children, may lead to syncope, presumably on the basis of hypocapnea and cerebral ischemia. This maneuver is combined with the Valsalva maneuver in the "messhall trick" to produce syncope in normal individuals and has been prevented in such experimental subjects by both hyperbaric oxygen and acetazolamide.

The occurrences of cough (tussive) syncope and of micturition syncope require attention. In the former, a child with chronic pulmonary disease (usually asthma) or with pertussis tends to undergo a syncopal attack following a bout of coughing, very probably on the basis of cerebral ischemia as in breath-holding, possibly due to the combined mechanisms of hypoxia and reduced cardiac return associated with respiratory spasm (Valsalva). Micturition syncope appears to involve reduced cardiac return associated with both postural hypotension and splanchnic vascular stasis following rapid bladder decompression, as it tends to occur in individuals who harbor a systemic illness and arise from sleep to micturate.

The differential diagnosis includes a variety of cardiac disorders such as cyanotic congenital heart disease; spells may occur particularly in the tetralogy of Fallot. Certain disorders of cardiac rhythm, some not signalled by the presence of either cyanosis or cardiac murmur, must be considered, particularly those involving cardiac conduction defects. These include the syndrome of ophthalmoplegia plus (Kearns-Sayers), in which retinitis, ophthalmoplegia, short stature, and various neuromuscular manifestations (especially ataxia) are associated with prolonged Q-T interval, fainting, and sudden death. Similar episodes occur in a syndrome of prolonged Q-T interval associated with autosomal recessive congenital deafness. Thus an EKG, optimally combined with exercise if needed, should be obtained in children with recurrent syncope. Syncope also may occur in children with aortic stenosis (p. 1428) and in some with primary pulmonary vascular disease.

The typical child with recurrent uncomplicated syncope suffers attacks that are triggered by sudden fear, anger, or other strong emotion. Some of these children, like those with breath-holding spells, have a sensitive oculocardiac reflex. Indeed, some were subject to breath-holding attacks in earlier childhood. Vasovagal syncope occurs rarely as a troublesome symptom in childhood on the basis of uncomplicated postural hypotension.

The child with recurrent syncope who particularly merits special attention with a view to specific diagnosis and therapy is the child with spontaneous episodes, ie, those that occur without the provocation of sudden postural, tussive, micturitional, or other physical or emotional stimuli. Occasionally one must be content to manage such children empirically, with the knowledge that specific diagnostic or therapeutic measures are of no avail.

PAROXYSMAL HEADACHE

Paroxysmal headaches in children are as a rule migrainous, psychogenic, or epileptiform. Psychogenic headache is usually nonparoxysmal; indeed, it is suspected when the affected individual complains that the headache is constant over a period of many weeks or months.

MIGRAINE. The largest and most frequently cited study of children with headache is that of Bille in 1962. Since Scandinavians may be particularly prone to vascular cephalgia, the incidence (4 percent) found in that study of the school population between 7 and 15 years of age is perhaps greater than in the United States. Nevertheless, the disorder is relatively common and possibly surpasses in incidence all of the other paroxysmal disorders combined.

Animal and human experimentation has yielded a good deal of information about the pathogenesis of migraine, although studies of the biochemical events associated with attacks of migraine and the interictal state have not yielded uniform results. It appears that the disorder is inherited in autosomal dominant fashion, with variable penetrance and expression. A child thus endowed genetically may or may not suffer subsequent attacks of headache, depending on a multitude of precipitating events. Emotional factors are often of extreme importance and are commonly encountered in children striving for perfection. Certain dietary factors appear to be important in other individuals. Recently hotdog headaches have been documented to occur in migraine-prone patients due to the nitrates used in preserving the red color of such luncheon meats. Others have implicated the tyramine content of yellow cheese and the oxalate in chocolate. Migraine with vomiting may occur in some children as a result of hyperammonemia and in others as a result of sensitivity to dietary oxalate. All of this suggests that when attacks of migraine are severe and frequent, an elimination diet is worthy of consideration as both a diagnostic and therapeutic measure.

Whatever the triggering mechanism, the first phase of the migraine cycle is characterized by spasm of the affected cephalic and intracranial vasculature, during which time the prodrome may occur. Although a visual prodrome of scotomata or scintillomata in one visual field is relatively common in adult migraine, it seems to be quite uncommon in children, who tend to deny a prodrome. Occasionally the prodrome is detected by an observant parent in the form of pallor, nonspecific malaise, or irritability. The prodrome is usually brief, lasting perhaps a few minutes.

Following vascular spasm there is hyperdilatation of the affected vasculature, during which time pulsatile or throbbing headache occurs as a result of stretching of the pain-sensitive structures investing the outer walls of the arteries, whose caliber increases following each systolic ejection. As a rule, this period lasts several hours or longer and is associated with considerable pain. The child often withdraws to a darkened room and resents any external stimulus such as movement or noise. The child may escape into sleep, often waking to vomit, usually within an hour of the onset of headache. Occasionally, repeated vomiting occurs. After several hours the child awakes greatly improved and may be able to function normally. Uncommonly, incapacitating headache may persist longer than a day in a single attack. Although generalized headache is more typical in childhood migraine than in adult migraine, focal onset or persistent local headache particularly affecting the frontotemporal area is the rule.

There is no consensus on the minimum symptomatology necessary for the designation of migraine. In children, who are less apt to have the more classic features of migraine than are adults, a combination of two or more of the following features is necessary for the diagnosis: typical migraine in a parent or sibling; one-sided headache (usually supraorbital, frontal, or frontotemporal); vomiting with the attack; and a visual prodrome. In a child the occurrence of a paroxysm of severe headache may in itself suggest the diagnosis. It must be remembered, however, that vascular headache of this type can be mimicked by such disorders as hypertension and intracranial vascular malformations. Although it is rare, pheochromocytoma typically gives rise to paroxysms or crises of hypertensive headache in which adrenergic symptoms, particularly diaphoresis, are prominent. The possiblity of an intracranial vascular malformation is increased when attacks of headache are persistently confined to the same side; the possibility is decreased when the headaches are reported to occur on either side. Occasionally, but not typically, patients with migraine have all of their paroxysms of headache confined to one side, and families are encountered in which this phenomenon occurs in parent and child. A history of this kind, when obtained, is as confirming as the random occurrence of right- or left-sided hemicranial pain. Concern for a space-occupying lesion is aroused by the occasional incidence of hemiplegic or ophthalmologic migraine in which the ischemic phase of the vascular cycle underlying migraine is sufficiently severe to produce hemisensory and/or hemiparetic signs or oculomotor paresis. Fortunately these uncommon manifestations are usually reversible.

Cluster headaches, migrainous neuralgia, and Horton's syndrome are interchangeable terms applied to a rare disorder involving attacks of excruciating unilateral pain of brief duration (often only 15 to 30 minutes) typically beginning nocturnally and associated with lacrimation and nasal congestion on the affected side, often together with ptosis and miosis. The term cluster headaches is applicable because of the tendency for attacks to recur frequently for several days or weeks and then remit for several months.

Although some children who are believed to have had benign paroxysmal vertigo of childhood subsequently are said to develop migraine, a history of paroxysms of vertigo in children with migraine is extremely uncommon. The occurrence of vertigo, ataxia, and other signs or symptoms of brainstem dysfunction can on rare occasions be ascribed to basilar artery migraine in children, a far less common manifestation of migraine in comparison to migraine affecting the more cephalad vasculature. The headache that follows the ischemic prodrome in these patients is likely to be occipital.

Certain confusional states, acute ophthalmoplegic syndromes, and even post-traumatic syndromes have been ascribed to migraine, but the classification in these instances, if the more typical features of migraine are lacking, cannot be accepted without serious reservation. Whether paroxysms of apparent autonomic dysfunction such as pallor, nausea, abdominal discomfort, and cyclic emesis that occur in a significant minority of children with migraine are vasogenic and hence are migraine equivalents, is unknown. Attempts have been made to link epilepsy with migraine, for the most part unsuccessfully, but there is consensus that some relationship, however obscure, exists. Similarities include EEG abnormalities, the association of autonomic (particularly gastrointestinal) dysfunction, the occurrence of a significantly greater incidence of epilepsy in near relatives of migraine sufferers (5 to 10 percent), and the alleged response to diphenylhydantoin in some children with apparently typical migraine. Headache is recognized as an epileptiform ictal or postictal phenomenon. Differentiation between migraine and headache as a seizure equivalent may at times be difficult.

Laboratory studies in migraine are not generally helpful. Serotonin, epinephrine, histamine, bradykinin, and other substances have been implicated, but not in a clear-cut fashion. Cerebral circulation studies are of academic interest rather than of diagnostic importance. Although abnormal EEGs appear to occur in at least a significant minority, the problems inherent in headache classification as well as in EEG interpretation cast doubt on the validity of the reported incidence and character of abnormal EEGs (incidence ranging up to 70 percent).

The prognosis is variable. Permanent sequelae from ischemic cerebral episodes are uncommon. It seems that children with more frequent and severe attacks are less likely to have an early remission, but in general the disorder is either greatly improved or resolved in over half of affected children by puberty.

Treatment of migraine requires recognition of the multiple factors involved. Emotional factors are of prime importance in some and of little or no importance in others. Dietary factors have been mentioned previously, but for the most part they have not been studied systematically in children with migraine and hence are of unknown statistical importace. Ergotamine and caffeine (Cafergot) are effective when administered early in the attack when prodromal symptoms are under way. The frequent denial of prodrome by children, the occurrence of attacks when medication is inaccessible (a liability not shared by adults, whose medication is self-administered), and the occurrence of sufficiently frequent attacks in some youngsters to render the repeated use of Cafergot inadvisable limit the usefulness of the drug. Administration of methysergide malleate (Sansert) as prophylactic therapy should be reserved for patients refractory to other modalities of therapy. The relatively high incidence of side effects and the occasional occurrence of retroperitoneal, pleural, or cardiac valvular fibrosis from prolonged therapy seriously limit the use of Sansert, but use of the drug for periods limited to 6 months or less avoids the more serious complications. Propranolol is clearly effective in adults, but systematic studies in children are lacking. Anticonvulsants such as diphenylhydantoin, phenobarbital, and Tegretol have been useful in some patients.

HEADACHE AND EPILEPSY. Headache following generalized seizures is common and may be quite severe. It is usually generalized, lasting a few minutes to a few hours, and may be pulsatile, which suggests a vascular component in the pathogenesis. Less frequently, headache may be associated with psychomotor seizures or may occur as a seizure equivalent. In the latter instance the diagnosis may be suspected if other varieties of paroxysmal symptomatology occur (such as syncope, abdominal discomfort, vomiting, pallor, and diaphoresis) or if frank seizures occur at other times. However, on occasion headache is the only epileptiform symptom. The diagnosis must then be based on the EEG, on the ictal as well as the interictal record, if possible, and on the response to anticonvulsive medication. Although the most common features of presumptive epileptiform headache in children include the brevity of the attack (usually less than 1 hour) and the association of lethargy and abdominal discomfort, it must be remembered that lethargy and gastrointestinal symptoms are also encountered in many children with migraine. Both focal and generalized headaches occur as seizure equivalents, and since some children with migraine benefit from phenobarbital or diphenylhydantoin and may even have EEG abnormalities, the diagnostic confusion is considerable. For these reasons the physician who suspects a child of having headache as a seizure equivalent, even when the EEG and the response to medication are suggestive, must take particular care not to label the youngster epileptic on the basis of the headache alone.

FUNCTIONAL HEADACHE. Headache is a symptom of depression in some children and malingering in others, and in yet others it appears to be a hysterical manifestation. Particularly troublesome is the conscious or unconscious recognition by a minority of children who genuinely suffer from migraine that secondary gain may accrue from more frequent headaches, in the form of sympathy, attention, and withdrawal from competition. Moreover, children with migraine are not exempt from depression; indeed, they are to some extent prone to suffer from this mood state. However, depression is not typically associated with migraine, and children who suffer from depression are more apt to have nonmigrainous headache.

In general, children with functional headache have nonmigrainous headache; that is, their headaches are more apt to be generalized, nonpulsatile, and constant or frequent rather than paroxysmal and infrequent. As a rule the headaches are vaguely described and do not obviously appear to be causing severe discomfort. They are, moreover, commonly associated with complaints of dizziness and visual blurring, although it is usually not possible to obtain an accurate impression of the true nature of these complaints. When secondary gain from the complaint of functional headache is evident, counseling of the parents and child often suffices therapeutically. In other instances formal psychologic support is advisable.

CYCLIC VOMITING

Cyclic vomiting refers to recurrent, spontaneous, paroxysmal vomiting of variable duration, with comparatively long asymptomatic intervals and absence of symptoms and signs pointing to disease of a specific organ or system. The diagnosis should be made with confidence only after exclusion of the infections and metabolic and structural disorders that may cause intermittent vomiting and that are often associated with more or less specific historical, clinical, and laboratory features. The differential diagnosis includes a multitude of conditons, including hypoglycemia, hyperammonemia, organic acidosis, pylorospasm, familial dysautonomia, and gastrointestinal or central nervous system disturbances. Brain tumors are capable of causing vomiting that remits and exacerbates because of intermittent relief of raised intracranial pressure by ventricular dilatation and cranial suture diastasis. Even when the more specific diagnostic categories are excluded, a number of disorders remain that appear to be quite unrelated in pathogenesis. These include occult abdominal epilepsy, abdominal migraine, and cyclic vomiting of undetermined nature, often termed recurrent acetonemic vomiting. The last of these is the most distinctive of the syndromes and the one most often signified when the designation cyclic vomiting is applied.

OCCULT ABDOMINAL EPILEPSY. Children suffering from abdominal seizure equivalents have their attacks on the basis of paroxysmal cerebral discharge. Although accurate incidence figures are difficult to obtain, it seems that only a minority (perhaps 25 percent) of the children who have abdominal seizures suffer from frank seizures of the more classic type. Another 25 percent or more have other paroxysmal symptoms, including syncopelike attacks, headache, and episodic autonomic dysfunction such as pallor, flushing, tachycardia, or diaphoresis. Abdominal epilepsy should be suspected when the attack is of brief duration (usually 30 minutes or less) and lethargy is associated. Vomiting occurs in a minority. The diagnosis is supported by a paroxysmal ictal (if not interictal) EEG, as well as by a response to anticonvulsive therapy. Diphenylhydantoin tends to be more effective than barbiturates.

ABDOMINAL MIGRAINE. In this obscure and somewhat controversial disorder the criteria for diagnosis should ordinarily include a family history of more typical migraine, subsequent evolution into more typical migraine, or complaint of headache during the attack of abdominal pain and vomiting, and the symptoms should be responsive to antimigrainous therapy. These attacks may last several hours or longer. The more protracted episodes may mimic recurrent acetonemic vomiting. At the first sign of an attack, half of a Cafergot suppository may be inserted rectally, and this dose may be repeated if necessary in 30 minutes. The oral or sublingual preparations may be preferred in older children if they can be taken before vomiting obviates this route. Sansert may be effective prophylactic therapy when attacks are frequent and severe. Recent indications that hyperammonemia and oxalate play a role in the precipitation of abdominal migraine in some children constitute a possible rational basis for dietary therapy.

RECURRENT ACETONEMIC VOMITING. In cyclic vomiting of undetermined nature the vomiting tends to be frequent and severe, with rapid progression to prostration and a tendency to early ketosis. Minor infection often acts to trigger the attacks, which usually last several hours to several days. Marked lethargy and inactivity are typical during the attacks. A tendency to recurrent dehydration in some children makes parenteral fluid therapy advisable from the onset. There is a curious tendency for the cyclic attacks of vomiting to occur punctually, as if by schedules, with the episodes being separated by an asymptomatic interictal period of weeks or months.

Treatment is symptomatic, with emphasis on early nutrition to prevent starvation ketosis and relapse. Sedatives and antiemetics may be helpful. Anticonvulsants are not beneficial. The possible identity of cyclic vomiting with abdominal migraine in some children prompts attention to recent claims for the efficacy of either low-protein or low-oxalate diets. Children responsive to the former diet may have a tendency to hyperammonemia demonstrable by loading tests or by the finding of a relative deficiency of ornithine transcarbamylase. The low-oxalate diet may be effective in children who are prone to precipitation of ketosis by oxalate (high-oxalate foods include oranges, chocolate, cocoa, tea, and rhubarb).

BENIGN PAROXYSMAL VERTIGO

Benign paroxysmal vertigo, a relatively uncommon disorder, occurs in early childhood, with onset ranging between 1 and 7 years of age and only rarely beginning after the age of 3 years. The affected child is normal interictally and lacks all of the features that may be encountered in symptomatic vertigo of either central nervous system or vestibular origin, except for abnormal caloric (Hallpike) vestibular function testing. The striking feature of an attack is ataxia of gait associated with vertigo. The ataxia is often masked by sudden immobility, apparently due to fear of aggravating the sense of uncontrolled motion induced by the vertiginous experience. The child often closes his eyelids in an apparent attempt to abolish the visual phenomena accompanying vertigo. Another impressive feature of an attack is its extreme brevity, as a rule lasting only 1 to 2 minutes or less and only very rarely longer. The more articulate child 2 or 3 years old is able to describe a rotational experience, with or without the aid of gestures; although gripped by fear during the first few attacks, the child demonstrates intact mentation and speech. There is no postictal fatigue, drowsiness, or depression. Tinnitus and hearing loss are uniformly absent. Occasionally associated symptoms or signs include pallor, nausea and vomiting, nystagmus, and intercurrent catarrhal signs.

Episodes may occur as frequently as several times weekly, but more typically they occur at intervals of 1 week to several weeks or less often. The brevity of each attack and the relative infrequency thus obviate any pressing need for an effective therapeutic regimen other than parental reassurance. Dimenhydrinate (Dramamine) appears to be useful in the prevention of attacks, but this has not been documented in a controlled study. The drug should therefore be used when attacks are sufficiently frequent and disturbing to warrant a therapeutic trial.

As already indicated, abnormal Hallpike caloric tests are the only positive laboratory feature of the disorder, the pathogenesis of which is unknown. Evidence supports a reversible vestibular lesion rather than a brainstem or even more central disorder, because directional preponderance is absent and canal paresis is typical on caloric testing. These terms are easily defined and are based on the finding that cool water injected into the patent external auditory canal produces nystagmus, the quick component of which is directed to the opposite side, and that warm water similarly injected causes nystagmus directed toward the injected side. Canal paresis exists when the appropriate labyrinth is underresponsive to stimulation (when the duration of nystagmus to both cool and warm water in one ear is less than in the other ear). Directional preponderance occurs when the duration of nystagmus in one direction (the sum of responses to cool water in one ear and warm water in the other ear) is significantly greater than in the other direction. This is believed to occur more typically when the lesion is in the central nervous system, ie, in the vestibular nuclei of the brainstem or their connections. There is reason to believe that central and peripheral lesions cannot be completely separated on the basis of these tests. The audiogram, skull radiograph, and EEG are normal in benign paroxysmal vertigo.

The differential diagnosis includes psychomotor epilepsy, vestibular neuronitis, and vestibulogenic epilepsy. Vertigo as a manifestation of psychomotor epilepsy is usually overshadowed by the more typically epileptiform features of the attack. Thus some impairment of mentation or speech is the rule in psychomotor seizures, either ictally or postictally; the attacks are of longer duration, and automatisms are frequent. Moreover, the EEG (particularly with the aid of nasopharyngeal leads and activating procedures) is likely to be abnormal and the response to anticonvulsive therapy evident. Vestibular neuronitis, typically a disorder of older children or adults, is usually characterized by a more or less protracted subacute illness. It is precipitated by infection rather than by a recurrent paroxysmal disorder and is often associated with directional preponderance on caloric testing.

The outlook is for complete cessation of attacks within 1 year or at most a few years. There may possibly be a proclivity for future migraine in a minority of patients, but this is not clear. Dimenhydrinate may prevent episodes, but the efficacy of the drug remains in question because of the natural tendency to spontaneous remission.

PAROXYSMAL TORTICOLLIS, TORTIPELVIS, AND RETROCOLLIS

In the peculiar disorder of torticollis an otherwise normal infant (usually female) inexplicably begins to tilt her head to the left or right side for a variable period of less than 1 hour or as long as 2 weeks. These bouts of torticollis may be accompanied by or interspersed with episodic tortipelvis or retrocollis, the latter posture particularly tending to occur on vertical suspension, the former at any time. Episodes decrease in frequency with maturation; at the peak frequency there may be several days to a few weeks of freedom from torticollis between attacks. The recurrent paroxysms usually disappear by 2 years of age, but occasionally persist for several years. The pathogenesis is unknown.

During an attack the affected child is usually quite comfortable and may or may not resist passive attempts to abolish the abnormal head posture. Occasionally severe vomiting occurs at the onset of an attack or during an attack. The ambulatory child may be ataxic during an attack, but nystagmus, eye closure, and reports of subjective vertigo do not occur. The tendency to vomit varies from occasional episodes to severe and frequent projectile emesis that interferes with nutrition during infancy. As a rule the vomiting ceases before 1 year of age, while the episodes of torticollis usually recur for considerably longer. Thus there is a characteristic lack of direct relationship between the torticollis and vomiting in regard to the chronology of the individual attacks as well as the persistence of the condition. However, notable exceptions do occur, in which severe paroxysms of vomiting occur with the onset of torticollis.

Some of these children who are apparently normal interictally share with the children who have benign paroxysmal vertigo a tendency to abnormal vestibular function as tested by Hallpike caloric studies. However, it would appear that the majority of children with this disorder have normal caloric studies and lack evidence of vertigo. Since some of the children with paroxysmal torticollis may have impaired hearing, which suggests a peripheral lesion affecting the cochlear and vestibular complex, a similar pathogenesis has been suggested. However, pathologic evidence is lacking in both of these very benign disorders. Therefore one must rely on the signs and symptoms, which reflect a striking difference in the clinical profiles of the two disorders. Aside from the occasional depression of response to caloric stimulation, laboratory studies (including gastrointestinal barium series, EEG, and contrast roentgen studies of the brain and spinal cord) are unrevealing.

Experimental lesions in the peripheral vestibular apparatus, in the vestibular nuclei of the brainstem, and in the flocculonodulus of the cerebellum can cause torticollis, dysequilibrium, and abnormal caloric studies, but they do not provide a convincing model for the paroxysmal disorder in infants and children. Differential diagnosis of torticollis requires consideration only on the occasion of the first episode, as recurrent paroxysms of head tilt are not seen in the other disorders. The systemic causes include hiatus hernia, cervical adenopathy, soft tissue injury, retropharyngeal abscess, and cervical spine dislocation. Neurogenic causes are trochlear palsy, spasmodic torticollis, dystonia, cerebellar and brainstem lesions, and paroxysmal torticollis.

There is no known effective therapy, although theoretically dimenhydrinate should have some merit. Reassurance as to the ultimate disappearance of the symptoms ought to suffice, particularly since the majority of patients outgrow the disorder by the time they are 2 years old.

DISORDERS OF WAKE–SLEEP CYCLE

In recent years research has greatly expanded in the field of sleep electroencephalography. Therefore it is no surprise that current concepts regarding disorders of the wake–sleep cycle should have evolved in relation to an understanding of the psychologic and physiologic correlates of the various stages of sleep. It has been suggested that somnambulism and night terrors would more appropriately be termed disorders of arousal, since they arise out of slow-wave sleep (stages 3 and 4) that is associated with body movement, intense autonomic activation, relative nonreactivity to external stimuli, amnesia for intercurrent events, and no dream recall. In night terrors and somnambulism the attack, although initiated out of stage 4 sleep, takes place during an EEG stage approaching light sleep or wakefulness.

NARCOLEPSY, CATAPLEXY, SLEEP PARALYSIS, AND HYPNAGOGIC HALLUCINATIONS. Narcolepsy is an uncommon syndrome of childhood; it tends to occur in young adults. Narcolepsy consists of a sudden, episodic irresistible urge to sleep. It is often associated with episodic abrupt loss of muscle tone in response to strong emotion (cataplexy) and occasionally with inability to move in the transitional period between the sleeping and waking states (sleep paralysis) or with auditory or visual hallucinations occurring at a similar time (hypnagogic hallucinations).

Possibly fundamental to the pathophysiology of this disorder is a disturbance of the sleep cycle manifest in a majority of affected individuals by transition from the awake state to stage 1 and thence to rapid-eye-movement (REM) sleep, without passing through the normal four stages of non-rapid-eye-movement (NREM) sleep. The EEG documentation of this phenomenon has been supplemented by demonstration that a therapeutically active monoamine oxidase inhibitor (imipramine) tends to obliterate REM sleep and that this drug is therapeutically effective against cataplexy. The narcoleptic attack varies in duration from less than 1 minute to more than 1 hour, but the less common associated symptoms are typically brief. The disorder usually occurs spontaneously, without antecedent illness or accompanying signs of physical or emotional abnormality. Occasionally it appears to be symptomatic of a nonspecific substrate of organic cerebral dysfunction.

Analeptic drugs, including methamphetamine and methylphenidate, are frequently effective when taken daily to prevent the occurrence of attacks of sleep, and recently imipramine has proved to be equally effective against cataplexy. A combination of the two drugs has been tolerated and proved effective in the prevention of both narcolepsy and cataplexy. Still more recently, phenelzine and methysergide, the former a REM sleep suppressant and the latter an NREM sleep suppressant, have proved effective in refractory narcolepsy. The toxic potential of these drugs contraindicates their routine use in narcolepsy.

No consistent personality pattern or emotional disturbance seems to be associated with somnambulism. Distinction of the disorder from nocturnal psychomotor epilepsy is achieved by a negative sleep EEG supplemented by nasopharyngeal recording and, if necessary, by absence of a therapeutic response to diphenylhydantoin.

The prognosis is excellent, with the disorder waning in frequency with maturation and usually ceasing within a few years of its onset. When frequent, prolonged, or complex attacks occur, treatment with tranquilizers or with imipramine may be effective, although controlled studies of their efficacy are lacking.

NIGHT TERRORS.   The incidence of night terrors in children varies from 1 to 3 percent, with the group 5 to 7 years of age being chiefly affected. Boys are more often affected. Occasionally night terrors persist into adult life. Somnambulism accompanies night terrors in perhaps one-third of the cases. Night terrors occur during stage 3 and stage 4 slow-wave sleep. The episode is aptly named because the affected child, who is interictally normal, is characteristically seized with stark terror during the attack and cannot be consoled or reasoned with for several minutes, during which time the vocal and autonomic manifestations of extreme fear are seen. The eyes of the child are open but unseeing. Verbalization is minimal and perseverative. The episode begins with loud, piercing screams, the child being in a state characterized by motility, often somnambulism, and intense autonomic discharge (tachycardia and increased respiratory amplitude); after a duration of 1 to 3 minutes there is rapid return to sleep, with amnesia for the episode. The nightmare, on the other hand, occurs in REM sleep; autonomic accompaniments are slight, and recall is often accurate.

Diphenylhydantoin may be tried in the less typical or very frequent attacks, although the large majority of children having night terrors do not appear to have nocturnal psychomotor epilepsy, as indicated by EEG sleep recording and by absence of response to anticonvulsive medication. Parental reassurance usually suffices, since attacks are usually brief and infrequent and the disorder is outgrown with maturation. Both diazepam and imipramine have been useful in more troublesome cases, but controlled studies are lacking.

CRANIAL NEURALGIA

Cranial (trigeminal and glossopharyngeal) neuralgias are relatively common disorders of adult life, but are exceedingly rare in childhood. They are of unknown etiology in the majority of affected adults, but occasionally a symptomatic case is encountered where the affected cranial nerve is the site of an irritative lesion (such as a neoplasm) or a demyelinating or postsurgical cicatricial lesion. The rarity of cranial neuralgia in children should prompt an even greater suspicion of an underlying disorder than in adults. In trigeminal neuralgia any of the three facial areas supplied by the branches of the trigeminal nerve may be affected and may experience transitory, lancinating paroxysms of exquisite pain, usually occurring frequently and at times being triggered by certain volitional or automatic facial movements. When the maxillary or mandibular division is severely affected, and paroxysms of pain are triggered by chewing, a severely affected patient may choose chronic hunger and malnutrition, thus testifying to the severity of the pain experienced in this disorder. Pharyngeal or glossopharyngeal neuralgia has occurred as a rare complication of tonsillectomy and adenoidectomy of childhood. The paroxysms of pain in this instance either occur spontaneously or are triggered by swallowing. Diphenylhydantoin is effective in some patients as prophylactic therapy, the pain being too frequent and transitory to constitute an indication for analgesic therapy. Carbamazepine (Tegretol) provides more effective therapy, but it has greater toxicity. Surgical therapy, ranging from local injection of drugs or thermal agents through nerve section, is available for the most refractory cases.

STRUCTURAL AND METABOLIC PAROXYSMAL DISORDERS

A number of disorders are associated with attacks of autonomic dysfunction, weakness, or ataxia, with or without interictal residua of the underlying disorder. The differential diagnosis and treatment of these disorders are discussed in the appropriate sections of this text.

AUTONOMIC DYSFUNCTION. Paroxysmal symptoms of autonomic dysfunction, with or without stupor or frank seizures, may occur on the basis of both fasting and postprandial hypoglycemia. In the typically affected child the interictal examination is physically and biochemically normal, but the glucose tolerance test shows an abnormally high peak less than 1 hour after glucose loading and an abnormal nadir at 3 hours, in association with drowsiness, diaphoresis, pallor, and hunger (p. 728). Insulin assays after glucose loading in these children tend to show appropriate responses and suggest that reactive hypoglycemia in children may not be prediabetic. Paroxysms of autonomic dysfunction are also seen in children with familial dysautonomia, including hyperthermic crises, pallor, mottling and diaphoresis, vomiting, and bronchospasm.

PAROXYSMAL WEAKNESS. When cerebral symp- toms and signs are lacking in children with paroxysmal weakness, attention should be directed to the brainstem, spinal cord, and lower motor neuron, despite the infrequency of these sites as sources of paroxysmal disorders. Vascular malformations of the brainstem typically cause recurrent attacks of brainstem malfunction that are often sufficiently dramatic to suggest a vascular accident, but at times they produce only subtle signs, among which weakness due to pyramidal deficit is included. More often than not ataxia, vertigo, or ophthalmoplegia is added to the picture, thus suggesting the anatomic site affected. Arteriovenous malformations of the spinal cord may also cause exacerbating and remitting weakness, usually with signs of segmental and pyramidal deficit that point to the site of ischemic spinal cord dysfunction. Occasionally paroxysms of weakness are due to inborn errors of muscle metabolism. Typically painless episodes of this type occur in familial and symptomatic hypokalemic and hyperkalemic myopathy, while episodes of weakness associated with muscle cramps and occasionally with myoglobinuria are encountered in McAardle's disease. Paroxysmal myoglobinuria occurs on the basis of other metabolic defects as well. Weakness also waxes and wanes, tending to occur in more or less severe paroxysms in myasthenia gravis.

EPISODIC ATAXIA. As previously indicated, vertigo is typically associated with ataxia and may be seen in children with a variety of paroxysmal disorders affecting the vestibular apparatus or its connections with the nervous system. Ataxia occasionally occurs as a paroxysmal symptom in disorders affecting the cerebellum or its connections. Hartnup's disease, in which a variety of symptoms may occur, including mental deficiency and dermal eruptions, is associated with episodic ataxia. A rare familial disorder has been described in which episodic ataxia recurs in relation to nonspecific infections, and sporadic cases of recurrent ataxia with apparently trivial occipital head injury have been seen.

References

Rabe EF: Recurrent paroxysmal nonepileptic disorders. Curr Probl Pediatr 4:1, 1974

BREATH-HOLDING ATTACKS

Livingston S: Disorders simulating epilepsy. In Comprehensive Management of Epilepsy in Infancy, Childhood and Adolescence. Springfield, Ill, Charles C Thomas, 1972

SYNCOPE

Farmer TW: Convulsive disorders, syncope, and headache. In Farmer TW (ed): Pediatric Neurology. New York, Harper & Row, 1975
Hooshmand H: Apneic seizures treated with atropine: report of a case. Neurology 22:1217, 1972
Katz RM: Cough syncope in children with asthma. J Pediatr 77:48, 1970
Lyle CB, Monroe JT, Flinn DE, Lamb LF: Micturition syncope: report of 24 cases. N Engl J Med 265:982, 1961
Wennevold A, Kringelbach J: Prolonged Q-T interval and cardiac syncopes. Acta Paediatr Scand 60:239, 1971

HEADACHE

Basser LS: The relation of migraine and epilepsy. Brain 92:285, 1969

Bille B: Migraine in school children. A study of the incidence and short term progress and a clinical, psychological and encephalographic comparison between children with migraine and matched controls. Acta Paediatr Scand [Suppl] 51:136, 1962

Dugan MD, Locke S, Gallagher RJ: Occipital neuralgia in adolescents and young adults. N Engl J Med 267:1166, 1962

Farguhar HG: Abdominal migraine in children. Br Med J 2:1082, 1956

Ferry PC: Diagnosis and office management of headaches in children. Clin Pediatr 11:195, 1972

Friedman AP: Migraine headache: part I. JAMA 222:1399, 1972

Froelich WA, Carter CC, O'Leary JL, Rosenbaum HE: Headache in childhood: electroencephalographic evaluation of 500 cases. Neurology 10:639, 1960

Gold AP, Chutorian AM, Carter S: Migraine allied head pains in children. In Friedman AP, Harms E (eds): Headaches in Children. Springfield, Ill, Charles C Thomas, 1967

Graham JR: Methysergide for prevention of headache: experience in 500 patients over 3 years. N Engl J Med 270:67, 1964

Holguin J, Fenichel G: Migraine. J Pediatr 70:290, 1967

Kashiwagi T, McClure JN Jr, Wetzel RD: Headache and psychiatric disorders. Dis Nerv Syst 33:659, 1972

Russell A: The implications of hyperammonemia in common disorders, including migraine (part II). Mt Sinai J Med NY 40:723, 1973

Slatter KH: Some clinical and EEG findings in patients with migraine. Brain 91:285, 1968

Weber RB, Reinmuth OM: The treatment of migraine with propranolol. Neurology 22:366, 1972

Whitehouse D, Pappas JA, Excala PH, Livingston S: Electroencephalographic changes in children with migraine. N Engl J Med 276:23, 1967

CYCLIC VOMITING

Chao D, Sexton JS, Davis SD: Convulsive equivalent syndrome of childhood. J Pediatr 64:499, 1964

Douglas EG, White PT: Abdominal epilepsy—a reappraisal. J Pediatr 78:59, 1967

Hoyt CS, Strickler GB: A study of 44 children with the syndrome of recurrent (cyclic) vomiting. Pediatrics 25:775, 1960

Millichap JG, Lombroso CT, Lennox WG: Cyclic vomiting as a form of epilepsy in children. Pediatrics 15:705, 1955

Papatheophilou R, Jeavons PM, Disney ME: Recurrent abdominal pain: a clinical and electroencephalographic study. Dev Med Child Neurol 14:31, 1972

BENIGN PAROXYSMAL VERTIGO

Basser LS: Benign paroxysmal vertigo of childhood (a variety of vestibular neuronitis). Brain 87:141, 1964

Chutorian AM: Benign paroxysmal vertigo of childhood. Dev Med Child Neurol 14:513, 1972

Koenigsberger MR, Chutorian AM, Gold AP, Schvey MS: Benign paroxysmal vertigo of childhood. Neurology 20:1108, 1970

PAROXYSMAL TORTICOLLIS

Chutorian AM: Benign paroxysmal torticollis, tortipelvis and retrocollis of infancy. Neurology 24:366, 1974

Snyder CH: Paroxysmal torticollis in infancy. A possible form of labrynthitis. Am J Dis Child 117:458, 1969

DISORDERS OF WAKE–SLEEP CYCLE

Anders TF, Weinstein P: Sleep and its disorders in infants and children: a review. Pediatrics 50:312, 1972

Broughton RJ: Sleep disorders: disorders of arousal. Science 159:1070, 1968

Fisher C, Kahn E, Edwards A, Davis DM: A psychophysiologic study of nightmares and night terrors. I. Physiological aspects of the stage 4 night terror. J Nerv Ment Dis 157:75, 1973

Glick B, Schulman D, Turecki S: Diazepam (Valium) treatment in childhood sleep disorders, a preliminary investigation. Dis Nerv Syst 32:565, 1971

Kales A, Jacobson A, Paulson MJ, Kales JD, Walter RD: Somnambulism: psychophysiological correlates. I. All-night EEG correlates. Arch Gen Psychiatry 14:586, 1966

————Kales J: Evaluation, diagnosis and treatment of clinical conditions related to sleep. JAMA 213:2229, 1970

————Paulson MJ, Jacobson A, Kales JD: Somnambulism: psychophysiological correlates. II. Psychiatric interviews, psychological testing and discussion. Arch Gen Psychiatry 14:595, 1966

Mack JE: Nightmares and Human Conflict. Boston, Little, Brown, 1970

Wyatt RJ, Fram DH, Buchbinder R, Snyder F: Treatment of intractable narcolepsy with a monoamine oxidase inhibitor. N Engl J Med 285:987, 1971

Wyler AR, Wilkus RJ, Troupin AS: Methysergide in the treatment of narcolepsy. Arch Neurol 32:265, 1975

Zarcone V: Medical progress: narcolepsy. N Engl J Med 288:1156, 1973

CRANIAL NEURALGIA

Ekbour KA, Westerberg CE: Carbamazepine in glossopharyngeal neuralgia. Arch Neurol 14:595, 1966

Hassler R, Walker AE: Trigeminal Neuralgia. Philadelphia, WB Saunders, 1970

PAROXYSMAL DISORDERS

Chutorian AM, Koenigsberger R: Myopathies associated with specific metabolic disorders. In Brenneman's Practice of Pediatrics, Vol IV. Hagerstown, Md, Harper & Row, 1972

————Koenigsberger R: Miscellaneous Disorders of Muscle. In Brenneman's Practice of Pediatrics, Vol IV. Hagerstown, Md, Harper & Row, 1972

————Nicholson JF, Killian P: Reactive hypoglycemia in children. Trans Am Neurol Assoc 98:64, 1973

PERIPHERAL NEUROPATHIES
Niels L. Low

Acute Polyneuritis

The peripheral nervous system may be affected by toxic agents, inflammatory diseases, and metabolic disorders of known and unknown causes. Diseases of peripheral nerves are classified as acute, chronic, or recurrent neuropathies. Single nerve involvement is termed mononeuritis; disease of multiple peripheral nerves or cranial nerves or both is called polyneuritis. Synonyms for acute polyneuritis are polyneuropathy, polyradiculoneuropathy, infectious neuronitis, schwannitis, and Guillain-Barré syndrome.

ETIOLOGY. Table 19 lists some of the known causes of the neuropathies, but in the vast majority of patients the cause is unknown. Since polyneuropathy of unknown origin is frequently preceded by an infection, it is commonly called postinfectious polyneuritis. However, etiologic delineation can be established in some cases, and it is of primary importance because of the possible therapeutic implications. Among the specific

TABLE 19. Etiology of Neuropathies*

	Acute	Chronic
Infections (eg diphtheria)	+	−
Post infections	+	−
Toxic		
Tick paralysis	+	−
Thallium, lead, mercury	+	+
Post immunization	+	+
Dilantin	−	+
Antimetabolic drugs	+	+
Collagen vascular diseases	−	+
Metabolic diseases		
Diabetes mellitus	+	+
Avitaminosis (B_1, B_6)	+	+
Porphyria	+	+
Traumatic	+	+
Heredofamilial diseases	−	+
Charcot-Marie-Tooth		
Dejerine-Sottas		
Tangier (alphalipoproteinemia)		
Bassen-Kornzweig (abetalipopro- teinemia)		
Retsum		
Metachromatic leukodystrophy		
Globoid cell leukodystrophy		
Unknown etiolgy	+	+

* Adapted from Chutorian AM: Lower motor neuron diseases. In: Brennemann-Kelley's Pediatrics, 1975. Courtesy of Harper & Row.

bacterial and viral agents known to produce this condition is diphtheria, with its particular affinity for the ninth and tenth cranial nerves that leads to impairment of gag, swallow, and phonation functions. Infectious mononucleosis, rubeola, rubella, coxsackievirus, and other viral infections have been known to produce the clinical picture of polyneuritis. Metabolic disorders such as diabetes and toxins such as lead may produce neuropathy; this is common in adults but rare in children. There is strong suggestion that sickle cell disease may predispose to lead neuropathy, as this condition has been reported in S-S and S-C disease (p. 1149). Mercury and other heavy-metal toxins are also etiologic factors; thallium toxicity should be considered when the paresis is associated with alopecia and optic atrophy.

Tick paralysis is an uncommon form of very acute and overwhelming polyneuropathy that appears to be due to a toxin released by the wood tick during feeding on the human host; it may cause respiratory muscle paralysis that can be fatal. Removal of the tick results in immediate and full recovery; thus it is important to search carefully for ticks, especially in the region of the head and neck in children, in cases where such exposure may have occurred. Trauma may cause a neuropathy, as is seen in the brachial plexus as a complication of childbirth (Erb's palsy); this occurs in neonates but is uncommon in older children.

PATHOLOGY. The earliest changes in the peripheral or cranial nerves are edema and early disintegration of myelin and axis cylinders. Phagocytosis and proliferation of Schwann cells occur later; macrophages

with myelin inclusion are seen in patients who die late in the disease. Polyneuroradiculitis, an involvement of the roots of cranial nerves and the ventral roots along the spinal axis, is common. The degree of elevation of cerebrospinal fluid (CSF) protein and the presence of meningeal signs are apparently related to the extent of root involvement.

CLINICAL MANIFESTATIONS. Polyneuritis has the same incidence for both sexes. A respiratory or gastrointestinal infection frequently precedes the disease by a few days to 2 weeks. The clinical picture is usually characterized by acute ascending motor paralysis, motor and sensory findings of peripheral nerve distribution, and cranial nerve involvement. Muscle weakness normally precedes sensory symptoms, but paresthesia in hands and feet may be the initial complaint. Weakness, usually first apparent in the lower extremities, may manifest as a quadriparesis from the onset.

Motor Manifestations. Paresis may remain mild; more commonly it becomes profound. It is usually ascending and symmetric in distribution, and the distal parts of the extremities are more severely affected than the proximal muscle groups. The muscle weakness is of the flaccid type. With involvement of the intercostal nerves, respiratory weakness of varying severity occurs. Atrophy of the skeletal muscles in the affected areas tends to occur early, especially in the intrinsic muscles of the hands and in the calves.

Cranial Nerves. Any motor nerve from the third to the twelfth may be involved, with resultant paresis in the corresponding muscles. Bilateral facial nerve paresis occurs in over one-third of affected children; unilateral facial weakness is less common. Involvement of the ninth and tenth nerves has potentially serious consequences because of impaired gag, swallow, and cough functions. Other cranial nerves are rarely involved, but complete ophthalmoplegia may occur. Papilledema is occasionally observed; it is unrelated to CSF pressure, but is often associated with an elevated CSF protein content.

Autonomic System. Postural hypotension in some children is due to impairment of the preganglionic nerves in the ventral roots, with subsequent reduction of vasoconstriction. Absent or reduced sweating in the involved areas is presumably due to a similar process. The mechanism leading to the arterial hypertension that is occasionally observed is unclear.

Sensation. Paresthesias or impaired sensation or both are common findings, but they may be absent. Position sense is the most frequently impaired sensory modality, followed by vibration, pain, and touch in descending order of frequency.

Reflexes. The deep tendon reflexes are usually absent, but incomplete loss may occur. Loss of reflexes usually correlates with the degree of weakness. Abdominal and cremasteric reflexes may also disappear early in the disease process.

Bladder and Bowel Dysfunction. Urinary incontinence or retention may occur transiently. Constipation is common, due to weakness of the abdominal muscles as well as the difficulty of defecating in the recumbent positon. Fecal incontinence with absent anal reflex is uncommon.

Meningeal Signs.   Slight nuchal pain and rigidity are commonly observed, but they may occasionally be severe. Positive Kernig and Brudzinski signs are found in a moderate number of children.

LABORATORY FINDINGS.   Most children with acute polyneuritis have normal peripheral blood count, urinalysis, and sedimentation rate. The CSF should always be examined in a suspected case of polyneuropathy. CSF pressure is usually normal; cell count also is usually normal, but a pleocytosis of 50 to as many as 300 white blood cells per cubic millimeter does not exclude the diagnosis. CSF protein is elevated in about 75 percent of cases; usually it is mildly increased, but levels of 400 mg/100 ml have been encountered. Protein usually is slightly increased during the first 1 to 2 weeks; it reaches a peak at about 4 weeks and then gradually declines over several more weeks. The frequent observation of normal cell count and elevated protein was first described by Guillain, Barré, and Strohl, and polyneuritis is often called the *Guillain-Barré syndrome*. Because these findings are not always present, it is probably wise not to use that eponym. The CSF sugar should always be in the normal range. Electrical testing is a useful ancillary procedure. Electromyography may show fibrillations and positive potentials; on contraction of the muscle, abnormalities of the motor unit characteristic of denervation may be evident. The conduction velocity of the motor nerve is usually decreased, and the chronaxy values are elevated; the decreased nerve conduction time is diagnostic of peripheral nerve disease. The flare reaction on the skin obtained by scratch or intradermal injection of histamine may be absent.

DIAGNOSIS.   When a child presents with muscle weakness associated with loss or reduction of tendon reflexes, acute polyneuritis should be suspected whether or not there are sensory changes. Tests for diphtheria and infectious mononucleosis should be performed. Appropriate serologic tests for viral infections should be made. Diabetes should be excluded, and a detailed history should be taken regarding possible exposure to toxins such as mercury, lead, and thallium; a suspicious history should be supported by laboratory tests as indicated. Primary disease of muscle and of the anterior horn cells of the spinal cord may give a clinical picture that simulates polyneuritis. Muscular dystrophy is differentiated by its slow development and its tendency to involve proximal rather than distal musculature. Polymyositis may be difficult to distinguish, but the deep tendon reflexes are usually retained. Electromyography and nerve conduction studies are of the greatest value in distinguishing muscle disease from peripheral nerve disease. Infantile spinal muscular atrophy (Werdnig-Hoffmann disease), which is characterized by muscle weakness secondary to anterior horn cell

disease, is distinguished from polyneuropathy by early age of onset, progressive course, tongue involvement, and absence of sensory findings.

COURSE AND PROGNOSIS.   The clinical course is variable. Paresis may be very insidious in onset, but it is usually progressive and tends to reach a peak within 7 to 10 days. Approximately one-half of patients show clinical improvement by the end of the second week of the illness; the period necessary for complete recovery varies from 2 to 18 months. Muscle strength returns much more rapidly than tendon reflexes. Complete recovery without residua is the most common result. With proper management and detailed attention to respiratory complications, mortality should be rare.

MANAGEMENT.   A therapeutic program should recognize the multiple etiologies and correct or remove known factors. General supportive or symptomatic care is essential to achieve maximum rehabilitation; this should include complete bed rest, adequate hydration and nutrition, skillful nursing care, prevention of contractures and deformities, and intermittent catheterization when there is urinary retention. Analgesics may be required for pain resulting from root involvement. Assisted ventilation is crucial in the presence of severe respiratory difficulties. Physiotherapy is essential in all phases of the disease; early in the course it should be limited to proper positioning and passive range-of-motion exercises, and later an active program of exercises, gait training, and bracing should be employed. Overexertion and fatigue should be avoided until full recovery has been achieved. Corticosteroids have been recommended in the acute stage, but there is no good evidence that they alter the course significantly.

CHRONIC AND RECURRENT POLYNEUROPATHIES.   Occasionally a child will develop polyneuropathy with a long, protracted chronic course leading to progressive atrophy and severe disability over a number of years. The cause of this form of chronic disease of the peripheral nervous system is unknown. Other children suffer from repeated attacks of acute polyneuritis with incomplete recovery between attacks; the residual signs tend to increase with each exacerbation. It is not known whether the chronic and the recurrent types are the same disease or separate entities. Patients with idiopathic chronic or relapsing polyneuritis often benefit from treatment with adrenocorticosteroids; if an initial 4-week trial results in improvement, the steroids may be indicated for months or years. If the response to steroids is inadequate or if the child becomes steroid-dependent, other immunosuppressive agents such as azathioprine (Imuran) (3 mg/kg/day) may be tried.

SPECIAL CLINICAL ENTITIES.   The *chronic hypertrophic polyneuropathy of Dejerine-Sottas* is a familial disease of dominant inheritance characterized by the onset in childhood of slowly progressing weakness and sensory phenomena in the distal parts of the extremities. The disease is usually fatal by the second or third decade. The typical pathologic findings are axonal destruction and proliferation of Schwann cells leading to thickened, palpable peripheral nerves. These changes may be diffuse along the entire length of a nerve or they may be of nodular or intermittent distribution.

Charcot-Marie-Tooth disease (peroneal muscular atrophy) is a familial disease with an autosomal dominant mode of inheritance. It involves predominantly the lower parts of the legs and the small muscles of the hands. The clinical spectrum is variable: sometimes only the peripheral nerves are affected; in other cases the cord and probably even the muscles may be involved. Peroneal atrophy progresses more slowly than in Dejerine-Sottas disease. The differential diagnosis of Charcot-Marie-Tooth disease and the various hereditary forms of spinal degenerative disease may be difficult and at times impossible. One form may gradually change into another in a given patient, and both forms may be seen in different members of a given family. No specific therapy is available for this condition; steroids are of no benefit.

Progressive involvement of peripheral nerves is not uncommon in periarteritis nodosa; less frequently it is seen in lupus erythematosus. Peripheral nerve involvement may accompany several hereditary metabolic disorders, as seen in Chediak-Higashi syndrome (p. 325), acanthocytosis (p. 1919), Tangier disease (p. 1919), Refsum's syndrome (p. 1918), metachromatic leukodystrophy (p. 1912), globoid cell leukodystrophy (Krabbe's disease) (p. 1912), and porphyria (p. 756). Certain antimetabolites (Vincristine) and anticonvulsants (Dilantin) can also result in chronic disturbance of peripheral nerve function. Heredofamilial neuritis with brachial predilection is characterized by recurrent painful neuropathy involving the shoulders and arms. The facial appearances of involved persons are conspicuously similar. The disease has a dominant inheritance and does not tend to progress to chronic disability.

CRANIAL NERVE PALSIES

Cranial nerve palsies may occur with polyneuritis and are commonly noted in acute poliomyelitis. They may be manifestations of other diseases, and they are characteristic of brainstem tumors. Facial weakness may be due to primary muscle disease; myasthenia gravis typically manifests itself in weakness of the extraocular muscles. Isolated impairment of one or both abducens nerves is usually secondary to increased intracranial pressure, but occasionally its involvement is benign. The third, fourth, fifth, and sixth cranial nerves may be involved in diseases such as thrombosis, injury, or tumor in and around the cavernous sinus.

Isolated peripheral facial weakness may be present from birth or may be acquired. If it is congenital it may be one of the manifestations or the only manifestation of Möbius' syndrome. Acquired facial palsy may be present from birth and may result from forceps pressure on the facial nerve; in such patients full recovery can be expected. Isolated, acquired neuritis of the seventh

cranial nerve is called *Bell's palsy.* The clinical signs of Bell's palsy are obliteration of the nasolabial fold on the affected side, a pulling of the corner of the mouth to the opposite (stronger) side, incomplete closure of the eyelid, and inability to wrinkle the forehead on the affected side. Retroauricular pain may be present, and taste may be impaired over the anterior two-thirds of the ipsilateral side of the tongue. The cause is unknown in most instances, but the palsy frequently follows mild respiratory infections. Association with purulent otitis media, acute mastoiditis, or parotitis is uncommon. Herpes zoster, syphilis, and sarcoidosis are rare causes. If there is no specific cause, recovery within a few weeks to several months can be expected in the vast majority of cases. It has not been established whether treatment with ACTH, adrenocorticosteroids, or surgical decompression is helpful.

References

ACUTE POLYNEURITIS

Adler K: Tick paralysis. Can Med Assoc J 94:550, 1966

Dunn HG, Buckler WSJ, Morrison GCE, Emory AW: Conduction velocity of motor nerves in infants and children. Pediatrics 34:708, 1964

Erenberg G, Rinsler SS, Fish BG: Lead neuropathy and sickle cell disease. Pediatrics 54:438, 1974

CHRONIC AND RECURRENT POLYNEUROPATHIES

Low NL, Downey JA: Lower Motor Neuron Diseases. In Downey JA, Low NL (eds): The Child with Disabling Illness. Philadelphia, WB Saunders, 1974

Tasker WG, Chutorian AM: Chronic polyneuritis of childhood. J Pediatr 74:699, 1969

Taylor RA: Heredofamilial mononeuritis multiplex with brachial predilection. Brain 83:113, 1960

Tooth HH: The Peroneal Type of Progressive Muscular Atrophy. London, HK Lewis, 1886

CRANIAL NERVE PALSIES

Boone PC: Bell's palsy. Acta Neurochir (Wien) 7:16, 1959

Evans PR: Nuclear agenesis. Arch Dis Child 30:237, 1955

Henderson JL: The congenital facial diplegia syndrome. Brain 62:381, 1939

FOCAL INFECTION OF THE CENTRAL NERVOUS SYSTEM

PETER W. CARMEL

Focal infections of the central nervous system (CNS) are potentially life-threatening and are capable of producing severe neurologic deficits. Modern antibiotic therapy has somewhat reduced the peril from these infections, but there remains a very significant mortality and morbidity. Further prevention of death and reduction of sequelae are not likely to be achieved by new antibiotics or by wider use of antibiotics. Progress will come only from more rapid and accurate diagnosis and earlier institution of rational therapy.

Infections of the CNS are secondary complications rather than primary illnesses. Focal sepsis may be due to penetrating trauma, extension along tissue planes from paracranial or paraspinal infective foci, or hematogenous or metastatic spread from distant infections. Treatment of the primary infective site must be carried out along with therapy for the CNS infection. A diligent search for primary infection sites will reveal the source in almost 90 percent of cases.

Infections can be located in any portion of the brain, spinal cord, or meninges. Brain abscesses may range in size from miliary foci to large encapsulated structures containing 80 ml of purulent material. Subdural empyema initially flows freely in the subdural space, but tends to become loculated; encapsulated subdural abscesses may be found on both the medial and lateral surfaces of the cerebral hemisphere or at the base of the brain. Epidural abscesses are usually relatively small collections, often consisting of a granulomatous mass.

Neurologic deficits from focal infections may be caused by the mass effect of the abscess, as well as by surrounding brain edema, venous stasis, arterial occlusion, and direct compression of cranial or spinal nerves. An important advance in therapy has been the use of steroids to control edema and decrease the mass effect of the abscess. Steroid therapy is used when neural deficits are present, despite the theoretic masking of further inflammatory changes.

CRANIAL EPIDURAL ABSCESS

Purulent collections in the epidural space usually develop by direct extension from surrounding bony structures. They typically follow chronic infections of frontal, sphenoid, or mastoid sinuses, otitis, or dental abscess. Dental, otologic, or neurosurgical procedures may spread or introduce infection into the epidural space. Fractures of the skull under open lacerations may allow bacteria direct access to this space.

Symptoms are usually mild. The local site may be painful and tender; there may be headache, low-grade fever, and slight elevations of white blood cell count and erythrocyte sedimentation rate. Neurologic deficits are slight, and often they are entirely lacking. These infections are frequently discovered only during investigation of the primary site. Infection in the epidural space can affect blood flow in the transverse or sigmoid dural sinuses, which can be compressed by the epidural mass or thrombosed by infection in the sinus wall. Obstruction of a major dural sinus is a cause of benign increased intracranial pressure (pseudotumor cerebri) (p. 1819).

Skull radiographs will indicate infection at the primary focus in most cases, and osteomyelitis of the skull may suggest epidural suppuration. Less frequently, changes associated with chronically increased intracranial pressure will be seen. CSF pressure may be normal or elevated, and CSF chemical and cellular values are usually normal. The EEG and brain scan can be abnormal, but they rarely accurately localize the infected site. Epidural abscess must be distinguished from other forms of intracranial infection. The absence of focal neurologic findings and the absence of an identifiable infection site on skull films suggest the diagnosis. Angiography may be needed to rule out other septic processes.

Antibiotic therapy is always required. Some epidural infections will not require surgery; however, if a mass lesion is identified it must be drained promptly. At operation all chronically infected granulation tissue should be removed, as well as any infected overlying bone. For management of pseudotumor cerebri see page 1819.

CRANIAL SUBDURAL EMPYEMA

Subdural infection accounts for nearly one-fifth of intracranial abscesses. Despite antibiotic therapy the mortality rate still remains over 40 percent. It most frequently follows inadequate antibiotic treatment of a prior infection. In older children subdural empyema is often associated with otorhinologic infection, while in infants it is usually a sequela of poorly treated meningitis with an infected effusion. Subdural empyema may also follow trauma, intracranial surgery, and hematogenous seeding of the subdural space.

When paranasal sinus infection is followed by severe headache, alteration of consciousness, fever, meningeal signs, and frontal or orbital swelling, it is clear that the infection has entered the subdural space. Purulent material may spread widely in the subdural space, causing focal or hemispheric neurologic signs. Intracranial pressure is usually elevated, and infants may present with fever and an enlarging head. Seizures are not infrequent signs. In an infant with prior meningitis, any new focal or hemispheric deficit, change in level of consciousness, or spreading of sutures ought to suggest the possibility of subdural empyema. An enlarging head in a postmeningitic infant may be due to subdural empyema, subdural effusion, or postmeningitic hydrocephalus. Contrast studies or special procedures are usually required to differentiate these conditions. Pus along the falx between the cerebral hemispheres may be overlooked when convexity collections are drained; this has been responsible for recurrent infections and accounts for the high mortality associated with subdural empyema.

Computerized transaxial tomography (CTT scan) has proved to be valuable in localizing purulent collections. The CTT scan also identifies areas of cerebritis and cerebral edema that appear as avascular regions on angiography and may be misinterpreted as intracerebral abscess. The CTT scan will usually resolve this problem.

Treatment of subdural empyema should be by early and definitive drainage coupled with intensive appropriate antibiotic therapy. The purulent cavity must be opened widely and cleaned. Loculated pockets of infected material usually located along the falx, posterior parietal convexity, and base must be sought out and removed. Adequate drainage may not be possible through burr holes, and wide craniotomy may be necessary. Some surgeons advise irrigation of the space via indwelling drains for several days postoperatively. Systemic steroids will reduce the underlying cerebral edema. Dexamethasone (Decadron) at a dosage of 0.25 mg/kg/day in divided doses should be given.

The infection is most likely due to streptococci or a microaerophilic or anaerobic organism. Subdural infections following penetrating wounds or surgical operations are likely to be caused by staphylococci or gram-negative organisms. The organism should be identified from material obtained at surgery. Therapy with high doses of penicillin should be initiated pending return of sensitivity tests. Dilute solutions of penicillin may be used to irrigate the subdural space directly; however, care must be taken because of the epileptogenic potential of cortically applied penicillin. Bacitracin (2,000 IU/ml), which is less neurotoxic than penicillin, is an alternative. Intrathecal gentamycin has been used effectively against intracerebral and intraventricular gram-negative organisms. Antibiotic therapy is usually continued for several weeks. However, chronic sinus or bone infection may require prolonged treatment extending to several months. Antibiotics for prolonged treatment should be chosen for their ability to penetrate bone as well as to cross the blood-brain and blood-CSF boundaries.

BRAIN ABSCESS

In 1893, MacEwen demonstrated that abscess of the brain is a surgically curable disease, with only 1 of his 19 patients succumbing to infection. However, most contemporary reports cite overall mortality rates of 30 to 45 percent for all forms of therapy and operative mortality rates of 20 to 40 percent. While the introduction of antibiotics has resulted in dramatic improvement of therapy in meningitis and some focal forms of intracranial infection, this has not been the case for children with brain abscess.

The incidence of brain abscess is difficult to determine, but it is probably between 2 and 3 per 10,000 general hospital admissions. A preponderance of males has been noted in most large series. Brain abscess is rarely found in infants under 1 year of age; but the incidence rises rapidly thereafter, and nearly one-third of all cases are in the pediatric age range.

The main causes of brain abscess are extension from otorhinologic infection, hematogenous or metastatic spread from distant infection, hematogenous or metastatic spread in cyanotic children due to cardiac anomalies or pulmonary arteriovenous malformation, brain penetration by a foreign body or surgery, and extension into the brain from infection in scalp, bone, or meninges. In about 6 percent of cases the primary source cannot be detected. Extension to brain from paranasal, mastoid, or ear infections has been reported in many series as the most common cause of brain abscess. However, the incidence from otorhinologic sources has fallen markedly since the introduction of antibiotics,

and metastatic abscess is now more common in children. Metastatic abscesses usually originate in either the heart or the lungs, although osteomyelitis, renal infection, or skin abscess can be the primary source. Chronic pulmonary abscesses are a more frequent source than acute lung infections, and abscess is more likely to follow subacute than acute bacterial endocarditis.

A frequent associated factor in children with brain abscess is cyanosis, due either to congenital heart disease or to pulmonary arteriovenous shunting. Postmortem studies indicate that brain abscesses are found in 0.4 percent of deaths from all causes, while in patients with congenital heart disease the incidence may be as high as 6 percent. The incidence of brain abscess in all children with congenital cyanotic heart disease is 2 to 3 percent. Children with right-to-left intracardiac shunting are deprived of the phagocytic filtering action of the pulmonary capillary bed, and their cerebral circulation is subject to recurrent bacteremia. These children also are likely to have focal encephalomalacia due to hypoxia and decreased cerebral blood flow caused by the increased viscosity of polycythemia. The coincidence of an area of recent infarct and bacteremia will predispose to abscess formation. A relationship has been shown to exist between the severity of hypoxemia and the development and prognosis of brain abscess in these patients. Children with low oxygen saturation levels are more likely to develop and succumb to brain abscess than those with higher oxygen saturation levels. Since brain abscess is rare in infants, complete surgical correction of cyanotic cardiac defects before the age of 2 years would probably virtually eliminate brain abscess in these children. Palliative surgery will alleviate hypoxemia but will not remove the hazard of brain abscess.

PATHOPHYSIOLOGY. Abscess formation within the brain starts with an area of cerebritis surrounding an infective focus. Within a few days the center of the area liquefies and necroses and becomes surrounded by edematous, friable brain. Necrotic and edematous regions blend without clear demarcation. Encapsulation of the abscess usually starts at 10 to 14 days, but it may extend outward in several directions to form daughter abscesses. In traumatic foreign-body wounds the abscess often spreads along the penetration tract. Thickening of the wall, liquefaction of the cavity contents, edema of surrounding brain, and encephalitis all contribute to the mass effect of the lesion.

SIGNS AND SYMPTOMS. The initial symptoms of brain abscess are more likely to be related to its intracranial mass effect than to the infectious nature of the illness. Lethargy, anorexia, and vomiting are usually noted, and older children often complain of headache. Occassionally there may be a distinct period of cerebritis or meningitis preceding abscess formation. Focal or grand mal seizures may be the first indication of cerebral involvement and may lead to discovery of previously unnoticed neurologic deficits. Fever may be mild, and almost half of these children are afebrile on hospital admission, although they often give a history of recent febrile illness. Brain abscesses are usually rapidly progressive, and the duration of symptoms is often less than a week and seldom more than a month. The children are often lethargic or comatose, with signs of increased intracranial pressure by the time they are admitted to hospital. Specific neurologic deficits depend on the area of involvement and may include hemiparesis, sensory impairment, and visual field abnormalities. Posterior fossa abscess will cause ataxia, dysmetria, and cranial nerve palsies.

DIAGNOSIS. A moderate leukocytosis and an elevated erythrocyte sedimentation rate may be noted. Skull radiographs often indicate a chronic otorhinologic infection, and occasionally there is evidence of mass effect or increased intracranial pressure. Slowing of the EEG over the affected hemisphere is seen in two-thirds of cases, but often it is not focal. If there is evidence of increased intracranial pressure or intracranial structure shift, lumbar puncture is contraindicated. The information obtained from the CSF of patients with brain abscess is usually nonspecific; it often does not demonstrate the causative organism, and there may be risk of fatality in obtaining the CSF. Angiography is used to define the location of the abscess. The ring sign (a dense circle of vessels surrounding a radiolucent center), which is associated with well-walled-off abscesses, is found in less than one-third of cases. More typically, signs of midline vessel shift accompanying an avascular mass effect, without a surrounding zone of hyperemia, are found. Angiography may fail in diagnosis during the early stage of cerebritis or when there are multiple abscesses. Cerebral angiography carries an increased risk in children with severe cyanotic heart disease.

Radionuclide brain scanning has proved to be extremely sensitive in diagnosis; practically all abscesses greater than 1 cm in diameter produce positive scans. Radionuclide scanning is particularly helpful in delineating multiple abscesses, which are often not shown by angiography. Experience with use of the CTT scan is still limited, but it is clearly a significant advance in the diagnosis of these lesions and in the evaluation of therapy (Fig. 34). Complex clinical developments during the postoperative course in these patients may be clarified by CTT scan without the use of invasive techniques. Ventriculography is not often used now, and pneumoencephalography is contraindicated because of risk of brain herniation.

THERAPY. An intracerebral abscess may act as a rapidly expanding intracranial mass around which massive cerebral edema may develop. Secondary midbrain and brainstem compression due to herniation of the uncus can lead to coma and death in a very short time. Therefore therapy is aimed at decreasing the intracerebral pressure and mass effect. Until definitive therapy can be instituted, dexamethasone should be given in large doses, and osmotic agents such as urea or mannitol may reverse the more severe symptoms briefly.

Several techniques have been devised for operative

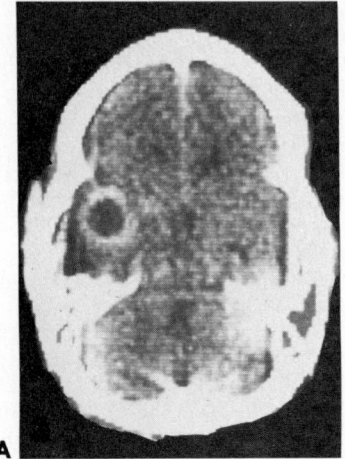

A

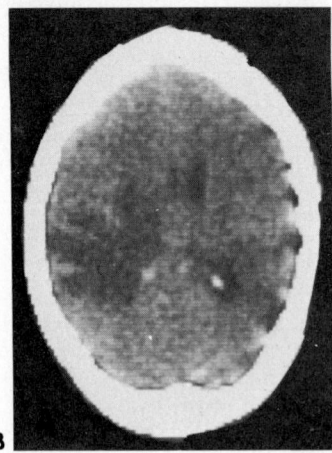

B

FIG. 34. A. CAT scan of teenage girl with left temporal brain abscess. She had a dental infection drained 1 month earlier, followed by 5 days of oral tetracycline therapy. Oral antibiotics were again given when the patient became febrile 2 weeks later. At time of study she was lethargic and aphasic and had a right hemiparesis. The dark area reflects edema of the left temporal lobe and basal ganglia region. The left ventricle is compressed and shifted to the right. **B.** CAT scan after injection of contrast material (the plane of this cross section is immediately ventral to that shown in A). An area (ring) of hyper vascularity around the wall of the abscess is clearly seen. Following total excision of the abscess, neurologic deficits slowly cleared, and the patient fully recovered. Culture of the abscess contents failed to grow an organism.

treatment of abscesses, and selection of a procedure will depend on the condition of the patient, abscess location, and degree of abscess encapsulation. The clinical condition at the time of operation is a more important factor in determining result than is the choice of operative therapy. Decompression of mass effect is the primary goal of surgery.

Aspiration of the abscess through a burr hole is preferable for severely ill children, for known multiple abscesses, or for abscesses with thin or poorly developed walls. After irrigation of the abscess contents, contrast material is often instilled into the cavity to aid in continued evaluation and reaspiration. Thorium dioxide (Thorotrast) was once widely used, but it is no longer available because of potential radiation hazard; suspensions of barium can be used . Availability of the CTT scan to localize the abscess may make instillation of contrast material unnecessary. Most abscesses require two or three further aspirations in the postoperative period, with multiple taps needed occasionally. Catheter drainage of the abscess over several days may also be carried out. This allows frequent irrigation of the cavity to remove further infected material. Antibiotic solutions can be used for irrigation, but systemically administered antibiotics will usually achieve adequate levels within the abscess.

Total excision of the abscess should be attempted if the abscess is single and well encapsulated, if it is not underlying a primary cortical area, and if the patient is not deeply obtunded or moribund. Excision has the advantages of effective immediate decompression of the mass and decreased risk of recurrence from remaining infected material or spillage. It may be delayed until aspiration and a period of antibiotic and steroid therapy allow shrinkage of the cavity and formation of a thick capsule, thus facilitating total excision.

Massive intravenous antibiotic therapy is required intraoperatively and for at least several weeks thereafter. Penicillin is most commonly used, but best results are achieved with combinations of agents. Therapy can be altered as soon as sensitivity testing has been performed on the purulent material obtained at operation. It must be stressed that antibiotic therapy alone is rarely adequate treatment of cerebral abscess, and decompression is almost always required. Anticonvulsants should be given to all patients with supratentorial purulent lesions for at least 2 years following surgery. Seizures are frequent preoperatively, occurring in almost 50 percent of cases.

PROGNOSIS. Mortality rates for brain abscess are largely related to the time of diagnosis and the number of lesions. If proper diagnosis is delayed until the child is obtunded or comatose, mortality is 65 to 90 percent; in children with multiple abscesses, mortality rates are as high as 80 percent. Recent introduction of more sophisticated diagnostic techniques that will permit earlier recognition may improve the situation.

SPINAL ABSCESS

Pyogenic abscesses of the spine are rare in children. Infection may occur in any of the intraspinal planes, but most commonly in the epidural space. Subdural empyema and intramedullary spinal abscess are very rare. Infection of the spinal epidural space may be metastatic, via the veins of Batson's plexus, or may be by direct extension from spondylitis or lung or perirenal infections. Spinal abscesses are most frequent in the lumbar and thoracic regions. Occasionally a congenital dermal

sinus, usually in the pilonidal region, will lead to spinal infection.

Spinal infections in children are generally more acute than those in adults, and symptoms may progress very rapidly; sometimes only a few hours elapse between onset of symptoms and paraplegia. The initial complaint is usually backache with well-defined localization of tenderness; as the lesion expands, root signs appear, and there is sharp unilateral or bilateral girdling pain at the level of the abscess. Sensory deficits and weakness of the legs appear, and gait difficulty, loss of sphincter control, and finally paraplegia follow in rapid order. Since chances for recovery after total loss of leg, bladder, and bowel function are small, early diagnosis and surgical decompression are of great importance.

Laboratory examination usually reveals leukocytosis and elevated erythrocyte sedimentation rate. Spinal radiographs may show local spondylitis or paraspinal soft tissue mass. The CSF shows pleocytosis, elevated protein levels, and decreased glucose. Unless the abscess is penetrated by the spinal needle, cultures are negative. If the diagnosis of spinal abscess is considered, myelography is the definitive diagnostic study and should not be delayed. Lumbar puncture should be deferred until simultaneous contrast study can be arranged, since myelography may not be feasible if the lumbar sac has been decompressed by recent lumbar puncture. When lumbar myelography is not feasible, a lateral C-1 to C-2 percutaneous approach may be used.

Differential considerations include tumors and transverse myelopathy. The latter condition is more common in children than spinal abscess and may closely mimic its symptoms. Contrast study is needed in any event to define the pathology. If an epidural or subdural collection is demonstrated, surgery should follow without delay. Decompressive laminectomy, removal of the purulent material, and copious irrigation should be carried out. Antibiotic irrigation has been recommended, but the spinal epidural space is well perfused by systemically administered antibiotics.

References

Anagnostopoulos DI, Gortvai P: Intracranial subdural abscess. Br J Surg 60:50, 1973

Baker CJ: Primary spinal epidural abscess. Am J Dis Child 121:337, 1971

Beller AJ, Sahar A, Praiss I: Brain abscess; review of 89 cases over a period of 30 years. J Neurol Neurosurg Psychiatry 36:757, 1973

Black P, Graybill JR, Charache P: Penetration of brain abscess by systemically administered antibiotics. J Neurosurg 38:705, 1973

Butler IJ, Johnson RT: Central nervous system infections. Pediatr Clin North Am 21:649, 1974

Coonrod JD, Dans PE: Subdural empyema. Am J Med 53:85, 1972

Editor: Subdural suppuration. Lancet 2:1299, 1972

Farmer TW, Wise GR: Subdural empyema in infants, children and adults. Neurology 23:254, 1973

Fischbein CA, Rosenthal A, Fischer EG, Nadas AS, Welch K: Risk factors for brain abscess in patients with congenital heart disease. Am J Cardiol 34:97, 1974

Fraser RA, Ratzan K, Wolpert SM, Weinstein L: Spinal subdural empyema. Arch Neurol 28:235, 1973

French LA, Chou SN: Treatment of brain abscesses. In Thompson RA, Green JR (eds): Advances in Neurology. New York, Raven, 1974

Galbraith JG, Barr VW: Epidural abscess and subdural empyema. In Thompson RA, Green JR (eds): Advances in Neurology. New York, Raven, 1974

LeBeau J, Criessard P, Harispe L, Redondo A: Surgical treatment of brain abscess and subdural empyema. J Neurosurg 38:198, 1973

Samson DS, Clark K: A current review of brain abscess. Am J Med 54:201, 1973

Wilkins RH, Goree JA: Interhemispheric subdural empyema: angiographic appearance. J Neurosurg 32:459, 1970

ENCEPHALITIS

HORACE L. HODES

Encephalitis may be caused by a variety of infectious agents including protozoa, fungi, bacteria, and viruses. The present discussion will be confined largely to the last group. Viral encephalitides are of two general types. In primary encephalitis there is direct invasion of the central nervous system by the virus, the pathologic changes being those of inflammation and neuronal injury. In secondary encephalitis the infecting virus is not recoverable from the nervous system, with some indirect mechanism apparently being responsible; the pathologic changes in this type of encephalitis are predominantly those of perivascular demyelination. A similar demyelinating process sometimes occurs in association with active immunization with viral antigens, notably after vaccination against smallpox and rabies.

Primary Viral Encephalitis

The virus-caused primary encephalitides in man include von Economo's disease (virus not isolated) and the arthropod-borne encephalitides (St. Louis encephalitis, Western equine encephalitis, Eastern equine encephalitis, Venezuelan equine encephalitis, Japanese encephalitis,* Russian spring-summer encephalitis, and Murray Valley encephalitis or Australian X disease). The viruses causing primary encephalitis in man include mumps virus, herpes simplex virus, and the virus of infectious mononucleosis. Poliovirus, coxsackievirus, and echovirus, as well as rabies and lymphocytic choriomeningitis viruses, belong in this group, but they are discussed in Chapter 12. The pathologic picture is in general similar for all the agents listed. Neuronal injury is apparent early in the disease, with varying degrees of degeneration and necrosis of neurons and supporting cells being observed, followed by inflammatory changes. Neuronophagia, proliferation of glia, and perivascular infiltration with polymorphonuclear and mononuclear cells are seen. Areas of hemorrhage and necrosis in the ground substance of the gray and white matter are common, and cellular infiltration of the meninges is the rule. Specific changes are seen in some of these infections, such as the Negri bodies of rabies. The viruses of Japanese encephalitis and Russian spring-summer encephalitis exhibit a particular tendency to attack the Purkinje cells of the cerebellum, whereas the related equine and St. Louis encephalitis viruses do not; usually it is not possible to make an etiologic diagnosis from the pathologic changes.

The clinical picture is also nonspecific. The onset of symptoms may be gradual, following a prodromal illness resembling influenza. In other instances evidences of central nervous disorder appear with explosive suddenness. There may be fever, headache, and meningeal signs (stiff neck, Kernig and Brudzinski signs). Ataxia may be conspicuous. The sensorium is variably affected. There may be drowsiness and lethargy followed by stupor and coma, or the patient may be excited, irritable, confused, or disoriented. Muscular twitchings, tremors, and convulsions may occur. Often there are bulbar symptoms: paralysis of the ocular or facial muscles or the muscles of deglutition. Respiration is commonly affected, becoming jerky or irregular. Profound variations in blood pressure and marked hyperthermia may occur. Involvement of the spinal cord may be revealed by paralytic and sensory disturbances or by loss of sphincter control. In infants the onset is usually sudden, and they are generally more severely affected than adults.

The blood commonly shows a moderate polymorphonuclear leukocytosis of 10,000 to 15,000 cells per mm^3. The spinal fluid is under pressure and shows some elevation of protein and a pleocytosis (20 to 600 cells, mostly mononuclear); however, it may be quite normal. Glucose concentration is normal or slightly elevated, and chloride is not affected. The EEG shows widespread cerebral disturbance, with irregular, slow, high-voltage complexes replacing the normal patterns.

Laboratory studies have shown that inapparent infections are common with all of the viruses listed above. The ratio of apparent infections to inapparent infections is highest with Eastern equine virus (1 to 18) and lowest with Japanese virus (1 to 500). In some inapparent cases it seems probable that infection gives rise to mild constitutional symptoms, but there is no evidence of invasion of the central nervous system.

The greater severity of the symptoms with Eastern equine encephalitis is notable; the fatality rate is higher, and permanent sequelae in the form of mental retardation, palsies, and convulsive disorders are more frequent. Such sequelae are also common in Japanese encephalitis, in contrast to the Western equine and St. Louis virus infections. However, clinical differentiation of the various types of encephalitis is impossible; this must be accomplished by recovery of virus or by antibody studies.

Primary encephalitis must be differentiated from a number of other conditions that affect the central nervous system. Helpful information may be gained by a careful history. If there is a history of pica, lead poisoning is a strong possibility, and other evidences of this

---

* Originally designated Japanese B encephalitis.

condition should be sought, particularly stippling of the red cells, lead lines in the bones, and the presence of an excess of lead in the plasma. The spinal fluid in lead encephalopathy is characterized by a relatively mild pleocytosis but a greatly increased concentration of protein. If there is a history of swimming in (or perhaps falling into) stagnant water that may have been contaminated by animals, leptospirosis should be kept in mind. Tuberculous meningitis is readily confused with viral encephalitis. Evidence of tuberculosis elsewhere is important, particularly if the subject is an infant. Moderate decreases in glucose and chloride in the spinal fluid are characteristic of tuberculous meningitis, as contrasted with viral encephalitis. Occasionally a low-grade bacterial meningitis will cause diagnostic difficulty, especially a mild meningococcal infection that may have been unrecognized. Such cases may present a predominantly lymphocytic reaction and a reduced sugar level in the spinal fluid. Brain abscess may cause confusion at times; a history of preceding otitis media or of purulent meningitis may be helpful. Brain tumor may be a cause of difficulty, particularly when symptoms appear abruptly, as may occur with pontine tumors. A pleocytosis of the spinal fluid may be observed with medulloblastoma; the mononuclear cells are not readily differentiated from lymphocytes unless a cell block is made.

The development of flaccid paralysis points to poliomyelitis, although this has been observed in coxsackie virus infections. Clinical evidence of mumps can also suggest the nature of the cerebral process, but by and large the identification of the agent rests with the virus laboratory. Recovery of virus from the blood is practical only with Russian encephalitis; recovery from the spinal fluid is practical only with mumps virus and coxsackie virus infections. A more practical procedure is demonstration of a rising antibody titer in the blood or spinal fluid during convalescence: Two specimens should be secured, one early in the disease and another 2 or 3 weeks later. Specific information can be obtained from neutralizing antibodies, hemagglutination-inhibiting antibodies, or complement-fixing antibodies, the last-named being the most useful.

Therapy for this group of infections is symptomatic. Sedation is often needed. When coma or bulbar symptoms are present, frequent aspiration may be needed to keep an open airway; tracheotomy may be necessary to remove secretions effectively. When tube feeding proves to be necessary, the danger of aspiration pneumonia must be borne in mind. Respiratory paralysis may require the use of mechanical devices to assist respiration. Marked hyperthermia may be relieved by cold packs or by placing the patient on a hollow rubber mattress through which a cooled solution is circulated. Hypothermia has been employed in treating patients critically ill with viral encephalitis; its value is difficult to establish because of the variable course of these infections. Anticonvulsants should be given if there are seizures. In some types, such as mumps encephalitis, complete and relatively rapid recovery is the rule. In other types a variable percentage of patients exhibit residual damage. The specific types of primary encephalitis will now be considered.

VON ECONOMO'S DISEASE. Von Economo's disease (encephalitis lethargica, epidemic encephalitis type A) was almost certainly caused by a virus, but a causative agent was never isolated. In 1917 it was well described by von Economo in Vienna. The disease appeared in the United States in 1918, and up to 1926 it occurred in many parts of the world; but no new cases have been observed since that time. Nothing is known about the spread of the infection. Most cases were observed in the winter and spring months, particularly in young adults, but all ages were affected.

The disease affects only the central nervous system. Lesions are most conspicuous in nuclear masses such as the cranial nerve nuclei in the substantia nigra, globus pallidus, and subthalamic nuclei, and the medulla and pons. The white matter is rarely affected.

The clinical features include fever, headache, oculomotor palsies, and somnolence. Occasionally CSF pleocytosis is noted early in the disease. Sequelae are frequent and include parkinsonism, sleep reversal, and serious personality changes and mental abnormalities that may result in severe dementia. Lesions in the region of the pituitary and hypothalamus have been known to cause obesity, diabetes insipidus, or sexual precocity. The immediate mortality is 20 to 40 percent, the ultimate mortality being considerably greater because of the progressive nature of the disease. Not more than 25 percent of patients are well after 3 years, and even fewer make a complete recovery.

The diagnosis is easy if typical symptoms are present and an epidemic is in progress, but it can be difficult if this is not the case. The progressive nature of the disease and the characteristic late symptoms are important features. Late cases may strongly resemble the post-traumatic syndrome. Unless a clear history of a previous acute episode is obtained, the diagnosis cannot be made with confidence.

Treatment is purely symptomatic. If there is excitement or choreiform movement, sedatives are indicated. Residual behavior disorders may require special treatment (p. 1764).

ARTHROPOD-BORNE VIRAL ENCEPHALITIDES. The arbovirus encephalitides include Eastern equine encephalitis, Western equine encephalitis, Venezuelan equine encephalitis, St. Louis encephalitis, Japanese encephalitis, Murray Valley encephalitis, and Russian spring-summer encephalitis. The viruses are related and are now considered to be members of a single family, named togaviruses. The family is divided by antigenic differences into two genera: group A and group B. Eastern and Western equine and Venezuelan viruses are group A viruses; the others listed above are in group B. Togaviruses contain a single strand of RNA; they have a lipid coat (*toga,* coat) and are inactivated by lipid solvents.

The encephalitides caused by the various togaviruses have many features in common. They all occur in epidemic as well as sporadic form, with epidemics reaching their peaks during the summer. Reservoirs of the virus exist among wild and domestic mammals and birds. The infection is transmitted by arthropod vectors, which usually become infected by feeding on the blood of birds, in which viremia is more prolonged than in mammals. The viruses have a similar host range among laboratory animals; all produce fatal encephalomyelitis in mice. They are similar in size and produce similar pathologic changes in the central nervous system, primarily by direct invasion of neurons. Outbreaks of St. Louis encephalitis and Western and Eastern equine encephalitis have occurred in many parts of the United States.

St. Louis encephalitis was first observed in Illinois in 1932; larger epidemics occurred the following year in St. Louis and Kansas City. Since then the disease has been observed sporadically, as well as in local outbreaks in western Canada and many parts of the United States. In 1964 a severe outbreak occurred in eight states; Texas and New Jersey were the most seriously affected. Reservoirs of the St. Louis virus infection exist in both mammals and domestic birds, but wild birds are the main reservoir. Cox demonstrated the presence of St. Louis virus infection in horses, but the horse, like man, is a dead-end host. Two vectors are concerned in its transmission. It has been found that in chickens and in wild birds various mites transmit the infection from bird to bird, inducing a long-standing viremia without encephalitis. Mites can also transmit the infection to their own offspring; thus a large reservoir in birds is readily maintained. However, bird mites do not bite mammals, and transmission to mammals is accomplished by mosquitoes, particularly *Culex tarsalis* and *C. pipiens*. Prophylaxis consists in measures for mosquito control and avoidance.

Serologic surveys have shown that many persons have antibody against the St. Louis virus, although they have had no obvious illness. Therefore it is clear that it produces several hundred inapparent infections for each case of encephalitis; the same is true of the other group B togaviruses.

Western equine encephalitis is in most respects similar to the St. Louis type. In 1930 Meyer first recognized the infection in horses in California, the first human cases being described in 1938. Outbreaks have been observed in California, Washington, Montana, Saskatchewan, Manitoba, the Dakotas, Nebraska, and Texas. The disease is observed among horses, but there appears to be a bird reservoir. The infection has been found in mites from chickens, blackbirds, and tropical birds; it appears that they transmit the virus from bird to bird, transmission from bird to mammal being by mosquitoes, chiefly *C. tarsalis*.

Western equine encephalitis virus causes a less severe disease than does Eastern equine encepalitis virus, and most patients recover completely from Western equine encephalitis. The Western equine virus frequently causes clinically inapparent infection or an abortive illness with fever and headache that is not followed by encephalitis.

Eastern equine encephalitis was first discovered in horses by Ten Broeck in 1933, the first human cases being recognized in 1938 in Massachusetts. Both in horses and in man the disease is exceptionally severe, with a high mortality and a strong probability of residual damage among survivors. In the 1947 Louisiana epidemic 3,700 horses and mules died of this infection. Ten human cases were observed, nine of them in children, of whom seven died. Outbreaks of the disease among horses have occurred in the East, South, and Midwest, as well as in the Caribbean, Panama, and Brazil. In some of these epidemics the disease has developed in humans; in others antibodies to the virus have been found in man. Recovery of virus from mites and lice on chickens and also wild birds suggests that birds are the main reservoir for this virus; commercially bred pheasants seem to be particularly susceptible. Mosquitoes are apparently responsible for transmission from bird to mammal as well as from bird to bird. *C. malnura* is regarded as the most important vector, although evidence from the 1959 New Jersey epidemic pointed toward *Aedes sollicitans*.

Venezuelan equine encephalitis virus infects horses as the primary host. When the virus is transmitted to man it usually causes only mild systemic symptoms; severe encephalitis is rare. The Venezuelan virus caused a very large epidemic of encephalitis among horses in the southwestern part of the United States in 1971. During this outbreak many humans suffered a mild disease without encephalitis. The virus is found over a wide geographic area, including Florida, the southwestern United States, Mexico, Central America, and the northern part of South America. The reservoir of the virus has not been found, and the vector that transmits the virus has not been determined.

Prophylactic vaccines have been developed for Western and Eastern equine encephalitides; they are recommended for horses and mules in infected areas and have been used in persons closely exposed to these viruses in the laboratory. They are not recommended for general use. Greater reliance may be placed on mosquito control.

Japanese encephalitis, although not yet reported in this country, has been recognized in eastern Asia since the end of the nineteenth century. It is found in Japan, Taiwan, Korea, eastern China, and Indonesia, and outbreaks have been observed as far west as India and as far east as Guam. In the Okinawa epidemic of 1945, infection was demonstrated in horses; pigs and other domestic animals were also incriminated as reservoirs. However, it is probable that nesting wild birds, especially those of the heron family, are the most important source of infection for the mosquito vectors and for subsequent spread of the disease to man. Many species of mosquitoes have been shown to be capable of transmitting the infection. Japanese encephalitis is generally a more severe disease than St. Louis encephalitis; it has a higher fatality rate (about 10 percent), and permanent neurologic damage is reported in 30 to 40 percent of cases.

A Japanese encephalitis vaccine made by formalin

inactivation of virus cultivated in chick embryos has been used for children in Japan. The vaccine was reported to have been successful, but a similar vaccine did not prove to be effective for American army personnel stationed in the Far East.

Australian X disease, an epidemic form of encephalitis, was first recognized in Australia in 1917. This disease has been renamed Murray Valley encephalitis. The virus that causes this form of encephalitis is closely related to Japanese encephalitis virus.

Russian spring-summer encephalitis is another anthropod-borne disease that is caused by a similar virus. This disease, transmitted by a wood tick, occurs in eastern Russia and Siberia. Domestic animals and rodents serve as reservoirs for the virus. Human cases occur chiefly among forest workers who have been bitten by ticks.

MUMPS MENINGOENCEPHALITIS. Mumps virus is probably the most common cause of encephalitis in the United States and Canada. Pleocytosis in the CSF occurs in 30 to 50 percent of mumps patients, but only 5 to 10 percent show clinical evidence of meningoencephalitis. Meningoencephalitis may be the only clinical manifestation of mumps. A large proportion of patients with so-called aseptic meningitis have infection with mumps virus.

In most cases the picture is that of a primary encephalitis; virus is present in the nervous system and can be recovered from the spinal fluid. The symptoms, although often marked, nearly always clear completely; they are largely meningeal, with little evidence of brain involvement. The nervous manifestations tend to occur at the height of the parotitis; rarely a secondary type of encephalitis develops after mumps in which pathologic changes resemble those of measles and other postinfectious encephalitides, the outstanding change being perivascular demyelination. In such cases the symptoms are encephalitic rather than meningeal. Paralysis, particularly of the cranial nerves, may develop; it is sometimes permanent. The rare fatalities occur in this type. Symptoms of drowsiness, coma, or excitement or the presence of paralytic manifestations do not in themselves indicate a grave prognosis, and complete recovery may occur. Cranial nerve recovery is usually complete; however, when deafness develops it is likely to be permanent, but unilateral. CSF pressure is generally increased, and there is a pleocytosis of 50 to 500 cells, mostly lymphocytes. The protein is only moderately increased, and the sugar is normal or slightly elevated.

Diagnosis offers little difficulty when parotitis or orchitis is present; when these are absent the diagnosis is often in doubt. A history of exposure to mumps is helpful. An important differential point between mumps and poliomyelitis is the character of the spinal fluid. Early in poliomyelitis the cells in the spinal fluid may be predominantly polymorphonuclear, with lymphocytes predominating at a later stage; in mumps the cells are predominantly mononuclear from the start. The laboratory diagnosis of mumps is considered elsewhere, as is the prophylaxis of the disease. Convalescent gamma globulin from mumps patients has been employed in

therapy, as have steroids, but evidence that they are of value is unconvincing.

HERPES SIMPLEX ENCEPHALITIS. Both type 1 and type 2 herpes simplex viruses cause encephalitis, which may occur at any age. In the newborn, type 2 is more often the cause of encephalitis than is type 1. Beyond the newborn age, nearly all cases of herpes simplex encephalitis are caused by the type 1 virus. Herpes simplex encephalitis is relatively common as a sporadic encephalitis. It has been estimated that 4,000 cases occur each year in the United States; about 25 percent involve children or adolescents. Herpes simplex encephalitis usually occurs in individuals who have had no previous infection with herpes simplex virus, but it has occurred in people who have had previous herpes infection. Lesions are found chiefly in the cortex but also in the hypothalamus, medulla, pons, and caudate nucleus. There is widespread evidence of neuronal injury, with necrotic changes particularly in the cortical gray matter. Perivascular accumulations of lymphocytes and mononuclear cells are found; proliferation of oligodendroglia may be present, and there may be petechial hemorrhages. Spherical or elongated acidophilic inclusion bodies similar to those seen in other tissues may be found in the nuclei of ganglion cells of the cortex. The meninges may be intensely infiltrated with lymphocytes and mononuclear cells.

The symptoms are both meningeal and encephalitic. Headache and fever are common; there may be convulsions and delirium leading to stupor and coma and perhaps death. Cranial nerve palsies may occur. A focal variant with unilateral temporal lobe predilection may mimic a neoplasm; ancillary studies may confirm the presence of a mass lesion. The CSF may be normal or may show a mononuclear pleocytosis of 50 to 600 cells, an increase in protein, and no reduction in glucose.

In the absence of other manifestations of herpes the diagnosis can be made only by biopsy, by recovery of herpes virus from the spinal fluid, or by demonstration of a rise in complement-fixing antibody in convalescence. The mortality is high and the sequelae serious.

In 1970 Juel-Jensen reported that the antimetabolite cytosine arabinoside (Cytarabine) had brought about "dramatic recovery" in 5 patients with severe forms of generalized *herpes virus hominis* infection and that the same result had been obtained in a man with early simian herpes virus encephalitis; cytarabine was given intravenously once daily for 5 days. Subsequent treatment of a number of patients with human herpes simplex virus encephalitis with cytosine arabinoside produced variable results. Since the drug has toxic effects on the hematopoietic system and may be immunosuppressive, it has been replaced by adenosine arabinoside (Ara-A). The effectiveness of Ara-A in herpes encephalitis and its toxicity have not been established; controlled studies are now in progress.

INFECTIOUS MONONUCLEOSIS. Neurologic complications of infectious mononucleosis have been reported since 1931 in the English and American literature. The clinical picture may be that of the Guillain-Barré syndrome, or there may be a meningoencephalitis with mononuclear pleocytosis in the spinal fluid. Bulbar symptoms are often present. Recovery is the rule, but permanent damage may occur; a few fatalities have been reported. Diagnosis depends on the presence of nervous symptoms in association with other symptoms of infectious mononucleosis, a typical blood picture, and a positive heterophile antibody test (p. 539). Mumps, herpes, and the arthropod-borne encephalitides can be excluded by complement-fixation tests, and coxsackie virus and echo virus can be excluded by failure to recover them from spinal fluid or feces that have been inoculated into suckling mice or tissue cultures.

Postinfectious Encephalitis

Many acute infectious diseases, particularly those of viral origin, are followed by an acute encephalitis characterized by diffuse demyelination of the brain and spinal cord. Postinfectious encephalitis is also called secondary encephalitis, allergic encephalitis, and acute demyelinating encephalitis. It is most commonly seen following measles, but it may occur after chickenpox, rubella, smallpox, and vaccinia; some cases associated with mumps fall into this category. Similar involvement of the nervous system may occur after vaccination with antigens of various types. The incidence of postvaccination encephalitis is higher after antirabies vaccination than after other commonly employed antigens.

Injury to the nervous system is not attributable to the presence of the infectious agent. Virus cannot be demonstrated in the nervous tissue when the disease is at its height; furthermore, the symptoms usually develop gradually during convalescence. Many theories have been advanced to explain this type of encephalitis. The most satisfactory one postulates a primary asymptomatic injury to the nervous system, with the production of altered chemical substances that then act as antigens. Antibodies to these substances are then formed that react not only against this material but also with unaltered nerve cell constituents; the available evidence indicates that myelin may be involved in this reaction. This theory is supported by the experimental production of postinfectious and postimmunization encephalitis in monkeys by repeated injections of homologous and heterologous nerve tissue. Occasionally symptoms of central nervous system disease begin early in the course of a primary infection. In these cases it is possible that encephalitis results from direct action of the virus on the central nervous system.

MEASLES ENCEPHALITIS. The incidence of measles encephalitis following measles varies considerably from outbreak to outbreak, ranging from 1 in 600 to 1 in 3,000 cases of measles. In our own experience the incidence has been about 1 case of encephalitis for every 1,200 cases of measles. Measles encephalitis is more likely to occur in children suffering from severe attacks of measles than in those with mild cases. Although no accurate statistical data are available, it appears that the incidence of encephalitis following modified measles is much lower than that following the natural disease.

PATHOLOGY. The brain is usually congested, with a few petechial hemorrhages over the cortex. The characteristic lesion is perivascular demyelination with phagocytosis of lipid material by the microglia; myelin sheaths of the nerve fibers in the affected areas are destroyed. In the center of each demyelinated area there is generally a small, distended vein that shows endothelial and adventitial thickening. The axis cylinders are not affected early, but in long-standing cases secondary degeneration of these structures may be present. About the margins of the demyelinated areas there is usually proliferation of the astrocytes and glial fibers. The gray matter is usually less severely involved than the white matter, but evidences of neuronal degeneration may be found. The distribution of lesions is not uniform; they are most common in the brain, the spinal cord, or the cerebellum.

SYMPTOMS. In rare instances symptoms of encephalitis begin at the height of the measles eruption or even during the prodromal period, but they may be delayed as long as 2 weeks after the appearance of the rash; usually they develop 4 to 6 days after the appearance of the exanthem, when the fever has fallen and the rash has begun to fade. The temperature rises again and may rapidly reach a peak of 40 C. Headache, vomiting, and stiffness of the neck are common. In some severe cases convulsions are the initial symptoms; in others there is gradually deepening drowsiness, followed by stupor and coma. Evidences of bulbar involvement may be present, such as irregularities in the rhythm and rate of respiration and difficulty in swallowing. Death may occur within a few days of onset. In some instances consciousness returns gradually, in others quite suddenly. The period of coma may vary from 12 hours to more than 3 weeks. After consciousness is regained, neurologic examination may be entirely normal; in other cases monoplegia, paraplegia, or hemiplegia of the upper motor neuron type may be noted. Mental confusion, disorientation, loss of memory, and speech disturbances may be present. Changes in personality are quite common. Nystagmus, ataxia, and loss of muscle tone pointing to involvement of the cerebellum are sometimes seen. In a small proportion of cases the nervous symptoms are due entirely to changes in the spinal cord. These patients may show the picture of transverse myelitis or of ascending myelitis without involvement of the pons, medulla, or cerebrum. Paraplegia, loss of sphincter control, and changes in the reflexes are common findings.

DIAGNOSIS. The symptoms of central nervous system disease appearing during convalescence from a typical case of measles usually make the diagnosis of measles encephalitis apparent. Confusion arises chiefly in those cases in which nervous symptoms accompany the febrile rise that immediately precedes or coincides with the appearance of the measles eruption. These symptoms usually disappear promptly, in contrast to measles encephalitis, in which they commonly persist for more than 24 hours. In case of doubt, lumbar puncture should be performed. In about 80 percent of cases of measles encephalitis, an increase of CSF protein concentration and a mononuclear pleocytosis are found.

TREATMENT. There is no specific treatment for measles encephalitis. Convalescent serum and gamma globulin have been used without demonstrable benefit. Some authors have employed steroids with what they have considered to be favorable results, but others could not confirm that they produced any benefit. Hypothermia has been used with variable results. Good general care is important. Particular attention should be paid to providing adequate fluids and nutrition when the patient is unable to swallow because of paralysis of the pharyngeal muscles or because he is comatose; intravenous administration of fluids or tube feeding may be required. Care should be taken to avoid aspiration, and assisted ventilation should be provided as indicated. It should be emphasized that the course of measles encephalitis is strikingly unpredictable, and no child's condition should be regarded as hopeless so long as life persists.

PROGNOSIS. About 10 percent of patients with measles encephalitis die in the acute phase of the disease. However, the general tendency is toward recovery; many patients whose conditions appear hopeless in the beginning recover completely. We have seen complete recovery in patients comatose for more than a month; unfortunately, about 20 percent suffer permanent damage. The sequelae range from minor changes in personality to complete dementia and generalized paralysis. Weakness of one or more extremities, hemiplegia, and paraplegia may occur, and epilepsy may develop. Cerebellar ataxia, nerve deafness, and permanent injury to the optic nerves are less fequent. Lesions in the region of the pituitary may lead to precocious puberty and other endocrine disturbances.

ENCEPHALITIS WITH VARICELLA, RUBELLA, AND SMALLPOX. Encephalomyelitis resembling the encephalomyelitis that follows measles may occur in association with *varicella* (p. 519). The symptoms generally begin 2 to 14 days after appearance of the rash, but rarely neurologic symptoms may precede the eruption. The incidence of encephalitis is much lower than with measles. Cerebellar symptoms are relatively more common than with measles; the course tends to be milder, and the prognosis is better. The mortality rate is low, and complete recovery is likely. Rarely, mental defects, spastic paraplegia, and monoplegia have been noted. Encephalitis is extremely rare in *rubella* (p. 580). The symptoms begin some days after the acute phase. Complete recovery is the rule, but a few fatal cases have been reported. Encephalitis associated with *smallpox* is similar to measles encephalitis. The incidence of neurologic symptoms does not appear to be related to the severity of the smallpox. Death may result, but survivors usually recover completely, or very nearly so. There is no specific treatment.

POSTVACCINATION ENCEPHALITIS. Enceph-alitis following vaccination against *smallpox* (p. 591) was first reported in 1907. This complication has been encountered most frequently in England, Ger-

many, Austria, and The Netherlands and less frequently in the United States. During the spring of 1947 roughly 4 million people in New York City were vaccinated against smallpox. It was believed that approximately 45 cases of encephalitis could be attributed to vaccination, an incidence of about 1 per 1,000,000 vaccinations. The pathologic features of postvaccination encephalitis are similar to those that occur with measles. Symptoms usually appear 10 to 11 days after vaccination, but they may be seen as early as 2 days and as late as 25 days after vaccination. The disease is very rare in children under 1 year of age and appears to be less common in persons who have been vaccinated previously. The onset is generally abrupt. Its clinical course and neurologic and laboratory findings are similar to those of measles encephalitis, with the possible exception that involvement of the spinal cord is more common in postvaccination encephalitis.

Encephalitis following vaccination against *rabies* is a form of demyelinating encephalomyelitis caused by hypersensitivity to the nervous tissue present in the vaccine. The incidence of neurologic sequelae following rabies vaccination has variously been reported to be 1 in 50 to 1 in 85,000. The vaccine most often used in the United States contains fixed rabies virus, which has been cultivated in embryonated duck eggs and inactivated by β-propiolactone. The duck egg vaccine contains much less nervous tissue than the previously available vaccines, which were made from the spinal cords of infected rabbits. The use of duck egg vaccine has greatly reduced the incidence of encephalitis following rabies vaccination but has not completely eliminated it. Along similar lines, attempts have also been made to reduce the neuroantigenicity of rabies vaccine by cultivating the virus in the nervous tissue of immature animals. In 1937 Hodes and Webster made an effective antirabies vaccine by propagating rabies virus in embryo mouse brain and inactivating the virus by ultraviolet light. At the present time a rabies vaccine from suckling mouse brain is in use in Latin America and in France, and a vaccine from suckling rat brain is used in the U.S.S.R.

The clinical symptoms are similar to those of measles encephalitis, except that cord symptoms are more frequent; sometimes only a transverse myelitis is seen. The onset usually occurs 10 to 20 days after vaccination is begun; it may be abrupt or gradual. Paresthesia and pain in the extremities may be noted, followed by motor weakness, usually in the limbs; bladder function may be impaired. Bulbar symptoms may occur early; in other instances an ascending Landry type of paralysis has been observed. The spinal fluid is sometimes normal, but it may show a mild pleotosis with an excess of protein. About 15 percent of the cases have been fatal, but recovered patients rarely show residual damage, and only occasionally do paralytic phenomena persist.

PERTUSSIS ENCEPHALOPATHY. The brain may be affected in several ways by pertussis. Occasionally, massive hemorrhages may occur in the brain substance or in the meninges; their cause is not clear, but they may be due to damage to vessels or due to congestion resulting from paroxysms of coughing. Inflammatory lesions in the cortex have been described, and rarely extensive atrophy of the cerebral cortex due chiefly to loss of neurons has been seen. Whether this is to be regarded as a result of toxic encephalopathy or of disturbances of cerebral circulation is still uncertain.

The clinical manifestations are quite variable. Convulsions are the most common and usually the first symptoms of involvement of the brain; rarely tetany has been observed. The convulsions may cease promptly and leave no sequelae, or the child may remain in a state of stupor and exhibit general muscular rigidity or hemiplegia. Tremors, loss of vision, mental defects, and paralysis may occur, and meningeal symptoms may be encountered, usually with a lymphocytosis in the CSF. The cases followed by generalized cerebral atrophy present a fairly typical picture: After a series of convulsions the child becomes comatose and remains unconscious for periods of weeks or months. There is progressive rigidity of all the muscles that may reach extraordinary intensity. All cortical functions seem to be abolished, and death may be long deferred.

PERTUSSIS VACCINATION ENCEPHALO-PATHY. Central nervous system damage may occur following the use of bacterial vaccines and antitoxins, in a manner similar to that described for viral vaccines. Administration of typhoid vaccine or tetanus antitoxin has on rare occasions been followed by lesions of the brain, spinal cord, and peripheral nerves. Similar results have been observed following vaccination against pertussis. In 1948 Byers and Moll described 15 infants who had suffered convulsions and severe brain injury following such vaccination. The symptoms of central nervous system involvement began 20 minutes to 72 hours after injection of the vaccine; convulsions, irritability, drowsiness, and coma were observed. These explosive reactions occurred after the first as well as the second and third immunizing injections. CSF showed an increase in protein concentration in most cases and a mononuclear pleocytosis. The eventual outcome was grave; of 12 patients observed for a long period, only 1 patient recovered completely. The remaining children suffered from various combinations of cerebral palsy, continuing convulsive seizures, cortical atrophy, and mental retardation.

The pathogenesis of the encephalopathy associated with pertussis vaccination is not clear. It is impossible to conceive of an allergic or hyperimmune antigen-antibody type of reaction occurring so abruptly after the first injection of vaccine. Toxic filtrates and endotoxins from *Hemophilus pertussis* have produced fatal encephalopathy in animals. The incidence of pertussis vaccination encephalopathy is so low that there is no doubt regarding the wisdom of continuing mass pertussis immunization programs. However, past experience suggests that pertussis immunization should not be continued if an injection of the vaccine is followed by very high fever, drowsiness, convulsions, or any other symptoms referable to the central nervous system.

References

ENCEPHALITIS

Cramblett HG, Stegmiller H, Spencer C: California encephalitis virus infections in children. Clinical and laboratory studies. JAMA 198: 108, 1966

Ford FR: Diseases of the Nervous System in Infancy, Childhood, and Adolescence, 4th ed. Springfield, Ill, Charles C Thomas, 1959

Hodes HL: Common types of encephalitis in children. NY State J Med 50:2277, 1950

Neal JB, et al: Epidemic Encephalitis: Etiology, Epidemiology and Treatment. Reports of the Matheson Commission, New York, Columbia University Press, 1929, 1932, 1939

———— Encephalitis: A Clinical Study. New York, Grune & Stratton, 1942

ARTHROPOD-BORNE VIRAL ENCEPHALITIDES

Casals J: Arboviruses. In Maramorosch K, Kurstak E (eds): Comparative Virology. New York, Academic, 1971, p 307

MUMPS MENINGOENCEPHALITIS

Lennette EH, Caplan GE, Magoffin RL: Mumps virus infection simulating paralytic poliomyelitis; a report of 11 cases. Pediatrics 25:788, 1960

HERPES SIMPLEX ENCEPHALITIS

Florman AL, Mindlin RL: Generalized herpes simplex in an eleven-day-old premature infant. Am J Dis Child 83:481, 1952

Haymaker W: Herpes simplex encephalitis in man, with a report of 3 cases. J Neuropathol Exp Neurol 8:132, 1949

POSTINFECTIOUS ENCEPHALITIS

Ferraro A: Pathology of demyelinating diseases as an allergic reaction of the brain. Arch Neurol Psychiatry 52:443, 1944

Morgan IM: Allergic encephalomyelitis in monkeys in response to injection of normal monkey nervous tissue. J Exp Med 85:131, 1947

Rivers TM, Schwentker FF: Encephalomyelitis accompanied by myelin destruction experimentally produced in monkeys. J Exp Med 61:689, 1935

MEASLES ENCEPHALITIS

Appelbaum E, Dolgopol VB, Dolgin J: Measles encephalitis. Am J Dis Child 77:25, 1949

Ford FR: Diseases of the Nervous System in Infancy, Childhood, and Adolescence, 4th ed. Springfield, Ill, Charles C Thomas, 1959

Hamilton PM, Hanna RJ: Encephalitis complicating measles; a report on 241 cases collected from the literature and on 44 additional cases. Am J Dis Child 61:483, 1941

Haymaker W, Smadel J: The Pathology of the Viral Encephalitides. Washington, US Army Medical Museum, 1943

Hodes HL: Encephalitides and postinfectious encephalopathies. In McIntosh R, Hare CC (eds): Neurology and Psychiatry in Childhood, Vol 34. Baltimore, Williams & Wilkins, 1954

———— Common types of encephalitis in children. NY State J Med 50:2277, 1950

Karelitz S, Eisenberg M: Measles encephalitis; evaluation of treatment with ACTH and adrenal corticosteroids. Pediatrics 27:811, 1961

Litvak AM, Sands IJ, Gibel H: Encephalitis complicating measles, report of 56 cases with follow-up studies in 32. Am J Dis Child 65:265, 1943

Spragins M, Shinners BM, Rochester B: Measles encephalitis; clinical and electroencephalographic study. Pediatrics 5:599, 1950

ENCEPHALITIS WITH VARICELLA, RUBELLA, AND SMALLPOX

Boughton CR: Varicella zoster in Sydney. II. Neurological complications of varicella. Med J Aust 2:444, 1966

Davison C, Friedfeld L: Acute encephalomyelitis following German measles. Am J Dis Child 55:496, 1938

Wilson RE, Ford FR: The nervous complications of variola, vaccinia and varicella, with a report of cases. Bull Johns Hopkins Hospital 40:337, 1927

Zimmerman HM, Yannet H: Nonsuppurative encephalomyelitis accompanying chickenpox. Arch Neurol Psychiatry 26:322, 1931

POSTVACCINATION ENCEPHALITIS

Hodes HL, Lavin GI, Webster LT: Antirabic immunization with culture virus rendered avirulent by ultraviolet light. Science 86:447, 1937

Greenberg M, Appelbaum E: Postvaccinal encephalitis: a report of 45 cases in New York City. Am J Med Sci 216:565, 1948

Plotkin SA, Clark HF: Prevention of rabies in man. J Infect Dis 123:227, 1971

PERTUSSIS ENCEPHALOPATHY

Byers RK, Moll FC: Encephalopathies following prophylactic pertussis vaccine. Pediatrics 1:437, 1948

SLOW VIRUS INFECTIONS

MICHAEL KATZ

Conventionally, virus infections have been considered short-term infections, with the resulting disease appearing suddenly after a defined incubation period of several days to several weeks and also terminating quickly, either in good health or in death. Rarely, acute viral infections may leave lifelong sequelae, such as deafness after mumps or paralysis after poliomyelitis. The concept of slow virus infections is relatively new, having first been proposed in 1954 by Bjorn Sigurdson in Iceland. In its current version this concept holds that there are host–virus interactions that develop on a scale of years rather than weeks. The host suffers no symptoms during the very long incubation period, but once the disease has developed, its course is relatively rapid and is usually fatal. Thus slow virus infections are distinguished from chronic infections in that the latter are characterized by remissions and exacerbations.

According to Sigurdson's postulate, all of the stages of virus–cell interactions known to take place in conventional infections also occur in the slow infections, but the time scale is stretched. Although this may not be entirely correct, there is at present no definitive explanation of the pathogenesis of slow virus infections that would apply in all instances. Thus the characteristic features of these infections are the extraordinarily long incubation period and the almost invariable course of relentless deterioration usually leading to death. Currently, slow virus infections are divided into those caused by unconventional and conventional agents.

The unconventional agents are responsible for a group of conditions known as spongiform encephalopathies. These diseases have incubation periods ranging from 18 months to 4 years; their pathologic hallmark is vacuolization of the gray matter, resulting in status spongiosus; there is negligible inflammatory reaction. Although the agents themselves have not been isolated, infection can be achieved by inoculation of tissue homogenates of affected animals into other animals. Experimental studies based on in vivo infection have revealed that the infectious agents are quite resistant to heat and radiation and to chemical agents such as fat solvents and proteolytic and nucleolytic enzymes. The agents are also quite small, ranging from 7 nm to 27 nm in diameter. The current concept is that they contain small quantities of nucleic acids that are tightly bound to cell membranes and that this association protects the nucleic acids from damage. The major example of a spongiform encephalopathy is scrapie in sheep. The only two human diseases in this category are quite rare: kuru and Jakob-Creutzfeldt disease.

Kuru has been known to occur only in the highlands of New Guinea, in the Fore people, among whom the disease is endemic. Until the mid-1960s kuru in adults showed predominance among women; children of both sexes were equally affected. Recently the incidence of kuru has been on the decrease, and the sex differential has virtually disappeared. The earliest symptoms of kuru are unsteadiness of gait, which evolves into ataxia. There are also personality changes leading to euphoria in some victims. Ultimately the victim becomes unable to walk and simply lies down and awaits death. Most victims of kuru die within 6 months of the onset of symptoms, usually from pneumonia. Few laboratory tests have been carried out on the afflicted individuals. Notably, CSF is normal. Pathologic changes are limited to gray matter, which shows astrocytosis, loss of neurons, and vacuolization.

The mode of transmission is uncertain, but it has been possible to transmit kuru experimentally to chimpanzees by inoculating them with brain homogenates of kuru victims. Intracerebral and extracerebral parenteral inoculation resulted in kuru after an incubation period of 18 months to 4 years. Transmission through the oral route has not been successful thus far. In view of its transmission by inoculation, it is possible that kuru in its natural setting has been transmitted during the process of ritual cannibalism, but probably only through contact of abraded skin with diseased tissues, rather than through ingestion. The relationship to cannibalism is supported circumstantially by the concomitant decrease in kuru and the decrease in cannibalism.

Jakob-Creutzfeldt disease has a worldwide distribution, but it is rare. It has not been described in children. Pathologically it resembles kuru, and like kuru it has been transmitted to chimpanzees. There is no known therapy for either of these two diseases.

Slow virus infections due to *conventional viruses* probably result from an unusual host–virus relationship, and this in turn may be a consequence of an ineffective host response to the infectious organism resulting in tolerance of the infection, either because it occurred at a time when the host was temporarily immunoincompetent or because of a genetically dependent specific immunoincompetence of a particular host. Another possibility is that the agents may have become altered either before or during the process of infection. Thus they may be different in some respect and may be capable of developing a defective infection that is primarily intracellular and persistent, despite the presence of adequate host immunologic defense mechanisms.

Two human diseases attributed to slow infections with conventional agents are subacute sclerosing panencephalitis (SSPE), and progressive multifocal leukoencephalopathy (PML). Isolation of viruses in vitro from patients with these diseases has been difficult; it has been accomplished by establishing cell cultures from tissues and cocultivating them with human or simian tissue culture lines.

SSPE is a disease of children and young adults, with an incidence of approximately 0.1 per 100,000 population. It has an insidious onset, with gradual impairment of the intellect and unusual behavior. Seizures begin early and are typically myoclonic. These evolve into sustained myoclonic seizures; the patient lapses into coma and becomes spastic and decorticate. The EEG has a characteristic burst–suppression pattern. The CSF has an increased concentration of gamma globulin. Death often is a result of an intercurrent bacterial infection. The course is variable, but most patients die within 2 years of the onset of symptoms. Rare long-term remissions have been reported. There is a strong etiologic association of SSPE with measles virus. All patients have elevated titers of serum and CSF measles antibodies.

Histologically the brain and spinal cord show involvement of both gray and white matter, with perivascular cuffing, gliosis, and RNA-containing intranuclear inclusion bodies in the neurons and oligodendroglial cells. There is substantial loss of neurons. Electron microscopic studies reveal nuclear and cytoplasmic accumulations of structures resembling nucleocapsids of paramyxovirus. In a number of cases a measleslike virus has been identified from explants of SSPE brain tissues.

SSPE predominantly affects boys. Epidemiologic studies have shown that SSPE patients tend to have had measles early in life, before the age of 2 years. There is suggestive evidence that the disease incidence is higher in rural than in urban areas. No definitive association between SSPE and administration of the live attenuated measles virus vaccine has been shown; it has not yet been possible to determine whether measles vaccine programs have reduced the incidence of SSPE.

It has not been possible to identify an immune defect in SSPE patients, although specific failure of cell-mediated immunity and the presence of a circulating inhibitor of cell-mediated immunity have been suggested. Viruses isolated from SSPE patients can be distinguished by their in vitro behavior from standard measles viruses, but not sufficiently so to consider them different viruses. The distinctions that have been observed could well have resulted from their prolonged residence in and adaptation to the brain tissue, which may have rendered them neurotropic. At the present time pathogenesis of SSPE remains obscure. There is no effective therapy.

PML is a rare degenerative demyelinating disease of the brain characterized by the development of bizzare giant astrocytes. It usually occurs in debilitated patients who are affected by a multisystem disease such as a lymphoma and who are therefore immunoincompetent. PML has been invariably fatal. It has not been reported in children. In all instances in which the affected brain tissue has been examined under the electron microscope, it has been noted to contain structures resembling papovaviruses. Recently papovaviruses have been found in brain tissues of patients with PML. One of the isolated viruses (the JC agent) appears to be a new papovavirus not previously described; others have the characteristics of simian virus 40. Another new papovavirus (the BK virus) has been isolated from the urine of patients who underwent renal transplantation. None of these immunosuppressed patients developed clinical PML, nor has the BK virus been isolated from any case of PML. It seems to be a ubiquitous agent, since antibodies to it are prevalent in most populations tested.

There are many diseases that possibly may be slow virus infections. Among them, multiple sclerosis (MS) figures most prominently. A viral etiology of MS has been postulated on epidemiologic grounds. Serologic studies have suggested association between MS and measles and vaccinia viruses, but this has not been proved. Although consistent isolation of virus from MS brains has not been experienced, a report of isolation of a parainfluenza 1 virus from two human patients with MS is intriguing. Its etiologic relationship to the basic disease is yet to be established. There has been speculation on a priori grounds that epilepsia partialis continua, Alzheimer's disease, and some collagen diseases (notably lupus erythematosus) may be examples of slow virus infections.

References

Gibbs CJ Jr, Gajdusek DC: Biology of kuru and Creutzfeldt-Jakob diseases. In Zeman W, Lennette E (eds): Slow Virus Diseases. Baltimore, Williams & Wilkins, 1974

Hotchin J (ed): Slow Virus Diseases. Progress in Medical Virology, Vol 18. Basel, Karger, 1974

―――― Persistent and Slow Virus Infections. Monographs in Virology, Vol 3. Basel, Karger, 1971

Hunter GD: Scrapie, a prototype slow virus infection. J Infect Dis 125: 427, 1972

Katz M: Measles and central nervous system diseases; a critical appraisal. Med Microbiol Immunol 160:247, 1974

Koprowski H, ter Meulen V: Multiple sclerosis and parainfluenza 1 virus. J Neurol 208:175, 1975

Preble OJ, Youngner J: Temperature sensitive viruses and the etiology of chronic and inapparent infections. J Infect Dis 131:467, 1975

Sell KW, Ahmed A, Strong DM: Plasma and spinal fluid blocking factor in SSPE. N Engl J Med 288:215, 1973

ter Meulen V: Pathogenic aspects of measles virus infections. Med Microbiol Immunol (Berl) 160:165, 1974

―――― Katz M, Müller D: Subacute sclerosing panencephalitis, A Review. Curr Top Microbiol Immunol 57:1, 1972

Weiner LP, Narayan O: Progressive multifocal leukoencephapathy. In Thomas RA, Green JR (eds): Advances in Neurology. New York, Raven, 1974, p 87

Wolfgram F, Ellison GW, Stevens JG, Andrews TM: Multiple Sclerosis, Immunology, Virology, and Ultrastructure. UCLA Forum in Medical Sciences No 16. New York, Academic, 1972

DISEASES OF THE MUSCLES

J. Gordon Millichap

Clinical disorders of muscle may involve primarily the muscle fiber, or they may be secondary to disease that occurs in other organs. In myopathies such as progressive musclular dystrophy and polymyositis, the pathology is centered largely in the muscle, whereas in polyneuritis and progressive spinal muscular atrophy (Werdnig-Hoffman disease), muscle dysfunction is secondary to lesions in the nerve and spinal cord. In both, hypotonia, weakness, atrophy, and contracture of muscles are the chief clinical manifestations.

The diagnosis of myopathy depends principally on the clinical features, but valuable additional information may be obtained from muscle biopsy, electromyography, nerve conduction velocities, radiographs of the soft tissues, and biochemical tests. Examples of the histologic and electrical changes characteristic of certain myopathies are shown in Figures 35 and 36. Muscle biopsy is most reliable when the specimen is taken in the early stages of disease from muscle that is not completely atrophied. It may be helpful in the differentiation of polymyositis from muscular dystrophy; in addition it reflects the characteristic muscle changes due to lower motor neuron diseases. Electromyography is of particular value in the distinction of neuropathic from myopathic disorders. Decrease in nerve conduction velocity indicates peripheral nerve rather than anterior horn cell disease as a cause of neuropathic atrophy.

The interpretation of muscle histology and electromyography without reference to the clinical findings is sometimes difficult, and the occasional limitations of these methods of investigation must be recognized when diagnosis and prognosis are assessed.

Limp Infant Syndrome

The limp infant (floppy child) syndrome is a term now used to describe all infants who have weak and hypotonic muscles, an increased range of joint movement or contracture, and various degrees of flaccid paralysis. In some infants hypotonia is marked and paresis is slight, whereas in others muscular paralysis is profound. The symptoms may be obvious at birth or may present in late infancy. The prognosis is variable and depends on the underlying disease. The disease may progress rapidly, and death may ensue early. But in some cases progression is slow; in others the disease becomes arrested and recovery may be partial or even complete. This clinical picture may be produced by various diseases with primary lesions in the cerebrum, cerebellum, spinal cord, peripheral nerve, neuromuscular junctions, or the muscle itself. Most commonly it is due to a degeneration or malformation of the anterior horn cells of the spinal cord (Werdnig-Hoffman disease). The differential diagnosis of the limp infant syndrome is outlined in Table 20.

In those cases described by Oppenheim that were characterized by improvement, the pathology was not

TABLE 20. Differential Diagnosis of Limp Child Syndrome*

Cerebral Diseases (Atonic Diplegia)
 Cerebral malformations
 Cerebral damage from hypoxia
 Cerebral birth injury
 Mongolism
 Metabolic (Lowe's syndrome, hypophosphatasia, rickets, hypercalcemia)
 Familial dysautonomia
Spinal Cord Diseases
 Infantile spinal muscular atrophy (Werdnig-Hoffmann)
 Poliomyelitis
 Spinal and birth injury
Peripheral Nerve Disease
 Polyneuritis
Neuromuscular Junction Disorders
 Developmental
  Congenital hypotonia?
 Metabolic
  Myasthenia gravis
Muscle Disorders
 Myopathies
  Infantile muscular dystrophy
  Arthrogryposis multiplex congenita
  Central core disease
  Nemaline myopathy
 Other conditions
  Glycogen storage disease of muscle
  Polymyositis

Adapted from Grinker, Bucy, and Sahs

recorded; the clinical picture and course correspond most closely to those of benign congenital hypotonia and universal muscular hypoplasia.

Benign congenital hypotonia is the term coined by Walton for a form of early amyotonia that characteristically improves with time and in which the muscle fibers may appear universally small for age but usually show no structural abnormality. The infant is limp and hypotonic at birth; the deep tendon reflexes may be absent or depressed, but respiration is rarely affected. Sitting and walking are delayed; yet muscular wasting is not profound, and the eventual development is essentially normal.

Congenital universal muscular hypoplasia is a rare disorder described by Krabbe in which all skeletal muscles are small and weak but otherwise normal. Deep tendon reflexes are normal or depressed. Changes of dystrophy or neurogenic atrophy of muscle are absent on histologic examination. The condition is nonprogressive.

Congenital or *infantile muscular dystrophy* is sometimes familial and is characterized by weakness that involves principally the proximal muscle groups; it is present at or soon after birth and progresses at varying rates, but in most cases slowly. The muscles are atrophied and hypotonic; all movements may be performed, although feebly. The deep tendon reflexes are depressed or absent. Contractures of limb muscles tend to appear late, with equal involvement of the intercostals and diaphragm. The pharyngeal muscles are not involved, and dysphagia is not a symptom of the disease.

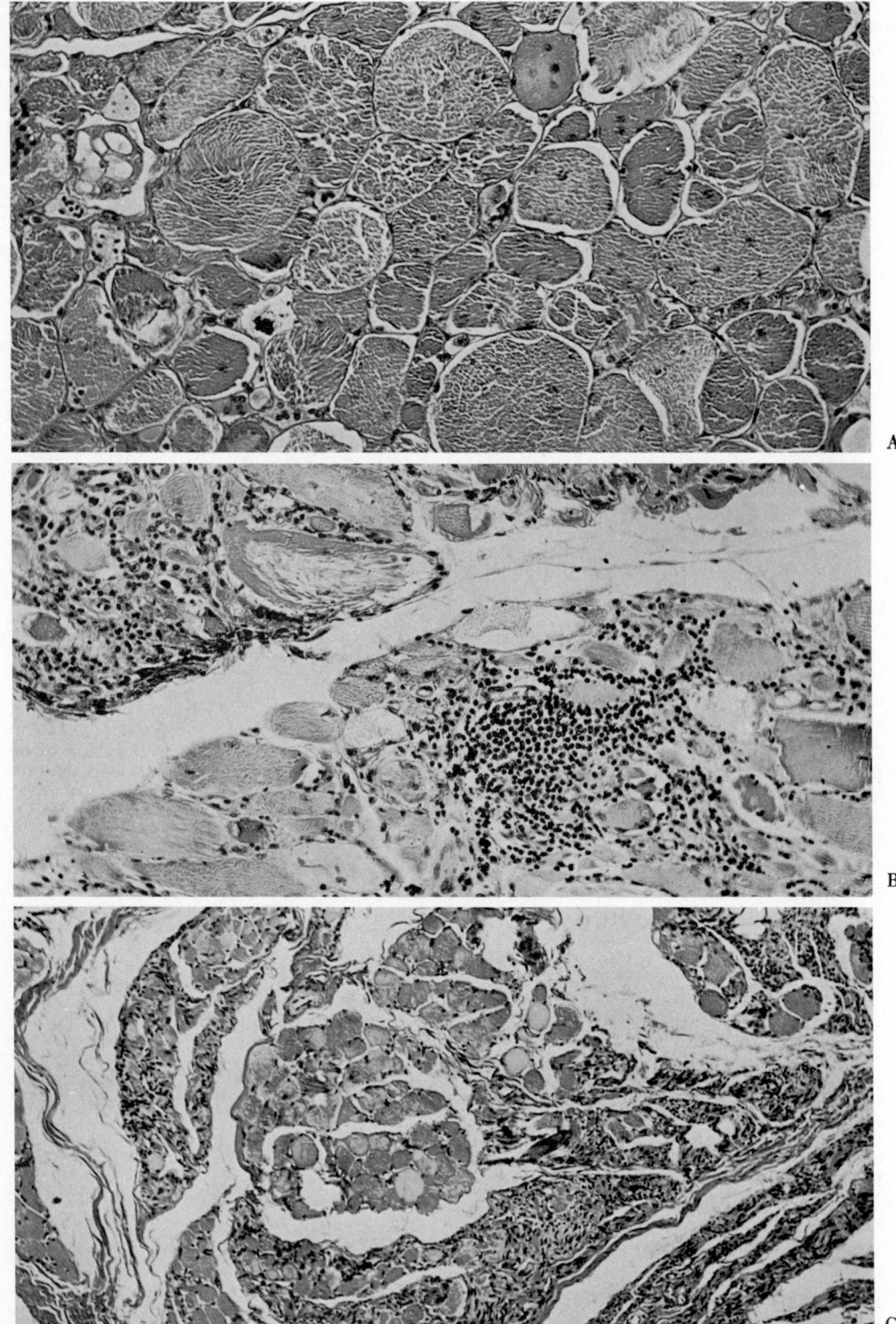

FIG. 35. A. Progressive muscular dystrophy. Section of muscle showing degeneration and variability of size of muscle fibers. **B.** Polymyositis. Section of muscle showing atrophy of fibers and infiltration with inflammatory cells. **C.** Infantile spinal muscular atrophy (Werdnig-Hoffmann disease); section of muscle showing groups of small atrophic fibers mixed with groups of normal fibers. (Courtesy of Dr. Raymond D. Adams.)

FIG. 36. Electromyograms in neuromuscular disease. Electric activity of quadriceps femoris muscle detected with a needle electrode inserted into the muscle and recorded by photographing the trace of a double-beam cathode-ray oscilloscope on moving film. The lower beam of the oscilloscope traced a timing signal of 100 Hz. On the upper beam an upward deflection indicated a change of voltage in the negative direction at the tip of the needle electrode. A pair of records is shown for each patient. The upper record of each pair was obtained from the resting muscle; the lower record of each pair was obtained during voluntary contraction of the muscle. Amplification of the signal in the upper record of each pair is five times the amplification of the signal in the lower record. Calibrations are in millivolts and are the same for each pair of records.

Normal Infant. Upper record, no electric activity in the resting muscle. Lower record, numerous motor-unit action potentials during voluntary contraction.

Infantile Spinal Muscular Atrophy. Upper record, fibrillation potentials in the resting muscle. Lower record, greatly reduced number of motor-unit action potentials. A large, single motor-unit action potential recurs in the range of the needle electrode.

Progressive Muscular Dystrophy. Upper record, no electric activity in the resting muscle. Minimal electric activity may occasionally be observed. Lower record, numerous motor-unit action potentials during voluntary contraction. These are shorter in duration and lower in amplitude than normal.

Dermatomyositis. Upper record, fibrillation potentials in the resting muscle. This is a much more common occurrence in polymyositis than in progressive muscular dystrophy. Lower record, numerous motor-unit action potentials during voluntary contraction. These are shorter in duration and lower in amplitude than normal. (Courtesy of Dr. E. H. Lambert.)

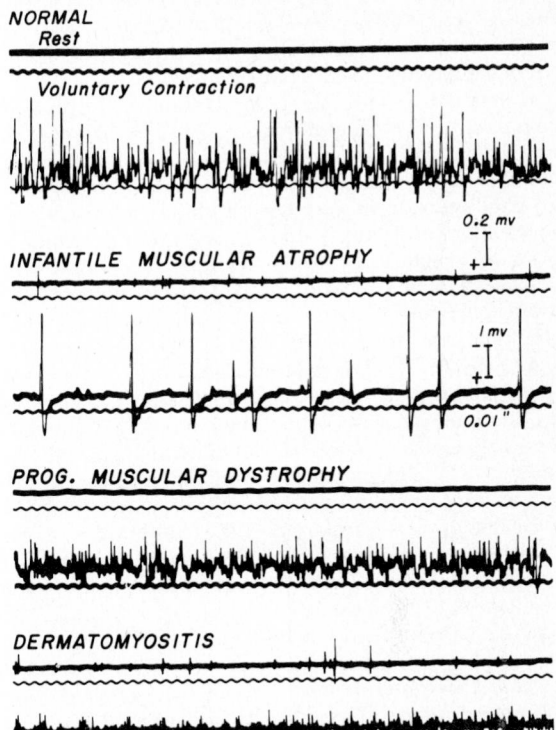

EMG in INFANTS and CHILDREN

NORMAL
Rest

Voluntary Contraction

0.2 mv

INFANTILE MUSCULAR ATROPHY

1 mv

0.01"

PROG. MUSCULAR DYSTROPHY

DERMATOMYOSITIS

The diagnosis rests on the histologic appearance of the muscle (Fig. 35) and on the clinical course. Soft tissue radiographs may demonstrate severe wasting of muscles and thus aid in the differentiation of this disorder from benign congenital hypotonia.

Central core disease is a nonprogressive myopathy that is present at or shortly after birth: it involves proximal muscle groups and is said to cause distinctive histologic appearance of the muscle. Shy and Magee described 5 patients with this disorder in three generations of a family. Sitting and walking were delayed, and although all patients were ambulatory, running and climbing stairs were never performed without difficulty. Deep tendon reflexes were active, and the muscles supplied by cranial nerves were spared. On biopsy examination of muscles, a central core of closely set myofibrils with an amorphous appearance and altered staining qualities was interpreted as a characteristic feature of the disease.

Nemaline myopathy is another rare, nonprogressive congenital myopathy that may be distinguished only by muscle biopsy. Engel and associates have reported female patients (ages 4 and 16 years) with mild weakness and wasting of proximal muscles that on histologic examination show rod-shaped structures in the fibers. Myotubular and mitochondrial myopathies are two of the more recently described congenital myopathies. They may present the classic features of the limp infant syndrome. Diagnosis is possible only by muscle biopsy.

CONGENITAL DEFECTS OF MUSCLE

SKELETAL MUSCLE. Single muscles or groups of muscles occasionally fail to develop. Most frequently the pectoralis major, particularly the lower sternocostal portion, is deficient. Congenital absence of muscles is clearly evident when the hands are pressed together while the elbows are abducted. Other muscles that may fail to develop include the trapezius, serratus anticus, and quadratus femoris.

Defects of skeletal muscles may occur together with other congenital abnormalities. Agenesis of the pectoral muscle is sometimes associated with malformation of a rib, a defect of the mammary gland, and scoliosis. Congenital absence of abdominal muscles is most frequently seen in boys. There are concomitant genitourinary anomalies including enlargement of the bladder, dilation of the ureters, hydronephrosis, and cryptorchidism. The weakened abdominal wall is deeply furrowed; defecation and coughing are hampered, and death from pulmonary complications often occurs in early infancy.

CRANIAL MUSCLES. Congenital ptosis due to weakness of the levator palpebrae may occur as an isolated anomaly without involvement of other muscles supplied by the oculomotor nerve. In some cases muscular dystrophy or myasthenia gravis has developed in later life, and a primary myopathy affecting the levator muscle has seemed a more likely explanation than a lesion involving the third cranial nerve of its nucleus. In the rare jaw-winking phenomenon of Marcus Gunn, the ptosed eyelid is elevated when the mouth is opened or when the jaw is moved from side to side.

Congenital facial diplegia, or Möbius' syndrome, is characterized by bilateral weakness of the facial muscles and the external rectus muscles of the eyes. It may occur alone or may be associated with congenital malformations of the extremities. The condition is recognized soon after birth and has been explained as either a primary hypoplasia of cranial nerve nuclei or a primary deficiency of the muscles derived from the first two branchial arches. A dysgenesis of both neural and muscle tissue may occur concomitantly in some cases.

CLUBFOOT.   The abnormal posture of the foot and ankle in the relatively common deformity of clubfoot (talipes) is usually plantar flexion (talipes equinus); less frequently it may be dorsiflexion (talipes calcaneus), inversion and adduction (talipes varus), or eversion and abduction (talipes valgus). Two-thirds of these children are males, and the condition may be familial. The anterior tibial and peroneal muscles are atrophic and may be replaced by adipose tissue. The mechanism of the muscular atrophy and antenatal contracture has not definitely been determined, but occasionally the amyoplasia is secondary to a developmental defect of the anterior horn cells of the spinal cord or peripheral nerves. The disorder is discussed from an orthopedic and therapeutic standpoint elsewhere (p. 1989).

TORTICOLLIS.   Torticollis (wryneck), a deformity associated with shortening and fibrosis of the sternomastoid muscle, is discussed elsewhere (p. 1861).

ARTHROGRYPOSIS MULTIPLEX.   Arthrogryposis multiplex congenita, also known as amyoplasia congenita or myodystrophia fetalis deformans, is characterized by deformity and rigidity of the extremities, with the infant having the appearance of a wooden doll (Fig. 37). The limbs may be fixed in almost any position, but most often the arms are rotated inward and extended at the elbows, with forearms pronated and hands flexed. Usually the lower extremities are flexed at the hips and externally rotated, the knees are either partly flexed or extended, and the feet are in equinovarus. The small limbs contrast with the unusually large and fusiform joints. The muscles are weak and hypotonic, and the tendon reflexes are absent. The skin and subcutaneous tissues are thickened, wrinkled, and flabby. Other congenital abnormalities are sometimes associated.

Fixation of joints is the most distinctive and constant clinical feature, but the underlying pathology is varied and may involve the spinal cord, muscles, or joints. When the disorder is associated with congenital muscular dystrophy, a characteristic posture of flexion at the hips and knees and adduction of the legs has been observed. When contractures are due to a primary defect in the anterior horn cells of the spinal cord or nerve roots, an attitude of extension and abduction of the legs is more frequent. Orthopedic treatment may effect

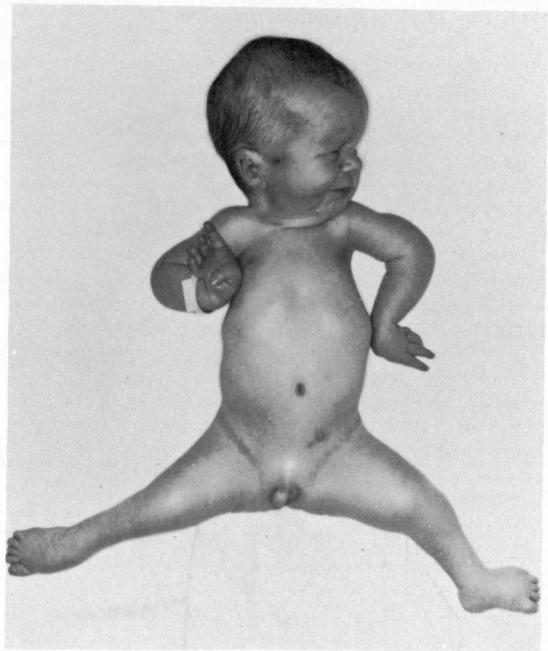

FIG. 37.   Arthrogryposis multipled congenita of the neuropathic type in an infant with unusual fixed postures.

some improvement in posture, but little or no change in muscle power is to be expected.

CONGENITAL MUSCULAR HYPERTROPHY.   Congenital muscular hypertrophy may result from a variety of causes. In the syndrome described by De-Lange there is generalized symmetric muscular hypertrophy, hypertonia, and an increase in muscle power. The head is small or deformed, and the neck is usually retracted. Infants affected are mentally deficient and survive for only a few months. A congenital lesion of the brain consisting of polygyria, microgyria, and multiple cystic cavities has been described in some cases. In the Debré-Semelaigne syndrome there is an associated thyroid deficiency (cretinism). In a third variety of congenital muscular hypertrophy there are macroglossia and cardiomegaly in addition to the hypertrophied skeletal musculature. Some infants with omphaloceles may have an associated muscular hypertrophy as well as macroglossia and hypoglycemia (Beckwith's syndrome).

MUSCULAR DYSTROPHIES

Progressive muscular dystrophy is a primary degenerative disease of skeletal muscles of unknown cause that is characterized by muscular weakness and wasting. Three major groups, which are clinically and genetically distinct, are recognized. These are the pseudohypertrophic, facioscapulohumeral, and limb girdle types.

The *pseudohypertrophic dystrophy* of Duchenne is a rapidly progressive myopathy that usually begins in early childhood; it has a strong familial incidence and occurs predominantly in males (Fig. 38). It is transmitted as a

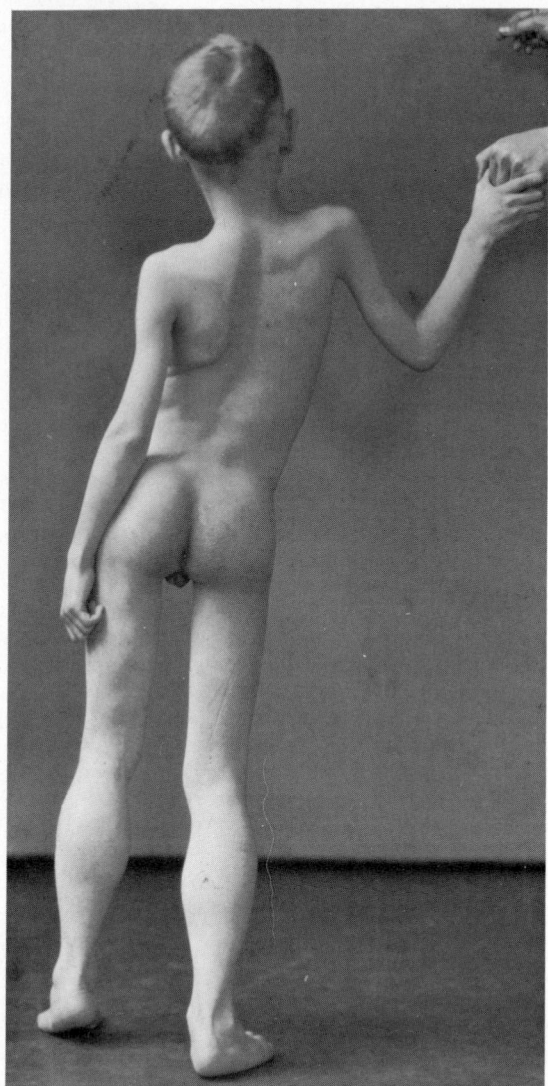

FIG. 38. Progressive muscular dystrophy, Duchenne type. A boy 10 years of age with weakness and atrophy of the proximal musculature, pseudohypertrophy of the calves and buttocks, scoliosis, lordosis of the lumbar spine, and a tendency to walk on the toes. (Courtesy of the Mayo Clinic, Rochester, Minn.)

cles. Muscles of the shoulder girdle become involved after 3 to 5 years. The deep tendon reflexes are usually depressed or absent; rarely they are hyperactive in the early stages of the disease. Positive Babinski signs and other evidence of an associated upper motor neuron lesion have been reported rarely. Pseudohypertrophy affects the calf muscles in 80 percent of cases; it is uncommon in the hamstrings and gluteal muscles and involves the deltoid and triceps muscles rarely. Contracture and wasting of the muscles lead to atrophy and deformity of the skeleton, and obesity is a common complication of the resultant immobility. A moderate degree of mental retardation is not unusual. The progressive nature of the disease is evidenced by the rarity of survival beyond the age of 20 years.

The *Becker variant* of pseudohypertrophic muscular dystrophy begins at a later age and has a slower rate of progression; survival into late adult life is not uncommon. The *facioscapulohumeral dystrophy* of Landouzy and Dejerine is a slowly progressive myopathy that may begin at any age from early childhood until adult life; it is sometimes familial and affects male and female with equal frequency. It is usually transmitted by an autosomal dominant (rarely by an autosomal recessive) gene. Inability to close the eyes completely may be noted from early childhood, and pouting of the lips and immobility of facial expression characterize the myopathic facies. The first symptoms usually include drooping of the shoulders, with difficulty in raising the arms above the head; they generally occur between 6 and 20 years of age. The deep tendon reflexes are depressed or absent in affected muscles. Weakness of the lower limbs is often delayed for 20 to 30 years, and pseudohypertrophy of muscles is uncommon. The disease may become arrested for prolonged periods, and most patients remain active and have a normal life expectancy. Contractures and skeletal deformities develop less frequently and are less prominent than in the Duchenne form.

Limb girdle muscular dystrophy commences late in the first decade or in the second or third decade. It progresses more slowly than the Duchenne type but more rapidly than the facioscapulohumeral type. It is usually transmitted as an autosomal recessive trait and only occasionally as a dominant. Those cases that begin with muscular weakness in the shoulder girdle are traditionally classified as juvenile scapulohumeral muscular dystrophy of Erb. Those in which the pelvic girdle and thigh muscles are first affected are examples of the atrophic pelvifemoral dystrophy of Leyden and Möbius. The course of the disease, although relatively slow, nevertheless leads to severe disablement and a shortened life expectancy. Pseudohypertrophy is rare, but prominence of the deltoid and gluteal musculature commonly occurs as a compensatory physiologic hypertrophy in the early stages of the disease.

Other less common forms of muscular dystrophy include *Gower's type,* in which the distal rather than the proximal limb muscles are affected first, and dystrophic ophthalmoplegia, which is very slowly progressive and is limited to the levators of the eyelids and the external ocular muscles. In the ophthalmoplegic type, ptosis of

sex-linked recessive trait. The most common presenting symptoms are slowness and clumsiness in walking and running and a tendency to fall frequently. Sitting, standing, and walking are delayed, and often there is difficulty in climbing stairs. Muscular weakness always begins in the muscles of the pelvic girdle and is responsible for a waddling gait. The method of rising from the floor by "climbing up the legs" (Gower's sign), although not a pathognomonic sign, is characteristic and results from weakness of the lumbar and gluteal muscles (Fig. 38). The foot assumes a talipes equinovarus position, and the patient tends to walk on his toes, owing to weakness of the anterior tibial and peroneal mus-

the eyelids, which is the first symptom, may present at any age from infancy to adult life and is associated later with weakness of lateral and vertical movements of the eyes. A history of similar symptoms in the family is obtained in half the cases.

In about 10 percent of patients with progressive muscular dystrophy the electrocardiogram shows nonspecific abnormalities. Cardiomegaly is not uncommon, and cardiac failure due to cardiomyopathy may cause sudden death. Determination of certain serum enzymes may be a useful diagnostic aid. Elevated enzyme levels are observed only during the period when muscles are actively undergoing change; late in the disease enzyme levels are often normal. A marked increase of creatine kinase activity in the serum has been reported in patients with the Duchenne type of muscular dystrophy and in their female relatives (heterozygotes), and lesser degrees of abnormal activity occur in patients with other types of dystrophy. Also, elevations of glutamic oxaloacetic transaminase and aldolase are observed. Reduction in the transformation of creatine to creatinine, the most constant biochemical abnormality, reflects only a decrease in total effective muscle mass and is not pathognomonic of dystrophy. Administration of vitamin E is followed by a reduction in creatinuria, but it does not result in objective improvement of muscle function.

In treatment, physical rehabilitation may help to maintain residual function. Frequent but not violent activity is advisable, and all limb joints should be moved regularly, both actively and passively, through a full range to prevent contractures. Confinement to bed must be avoided. When possible, school attendance or occupation with tasks and hobbies should be encouraged. Supportive attitudes by physician and parents are important in the psychologic management.

MYOTONIAS

CONGENITAL MYOTONIA. Congenital myotonia (Thomsen's disease) is an anomaly of muscular contraction manifested by muscular spasms or cramps and hypertrophy. It may present during infancy, early childhood, or adolescence and is inherited as a mendelian dominant or occasionally as a recessive factor. Muscular contraction is strong, but relaxation is delayed and normal motor function is impeded. The infant may be slow to stand and walk. The disease may affect most of the skeletal muscles, but it seldom involves the muscles of respiration or swallowing. Muscular hypertrophy, especially prominent in the lower limbs, may also affect the upper limbs and face, producing a herculean appearance. Percussion of the surface of the muscle results in a sustained contraction and localized dimpling. Muscles of the thenar eminence, forearm, and tongue are especially susceptible. Tendon reflexes are normal or slightly exaggerated. On shaking hands, the patient's grip is relaxed slowly and awkwardly in a manner pathognomonic of myotonia; after tight closure, the eyes are opened slowly. With repetition of muscular effort, movement becomes more rapid, and relaxation following contraction is more prompt.

Symptoms of myotonia are relieved by quinine, calcium, and procaine amide; they are exacerbated by cold.

DYSTROPHIA MYOTONICA. Dystrophia myotonica (myotonic dystrophy) is a steadily progressive, familial disease in which a myopathy is complicated by myotonia. Cataracts, baldness, and testicular atrophy are frequently associated, and mental retardation is not uncommon. The disease is usually transmitted as a mendelian dominant, and the phenomenon of anticipation is observed: the children are affected at an earlier age than the parent was, and they are more likely to exhibit the fully developed syndrome. The syndrome of congenital dystrophia myotonica differs from the adult form by the appearance of symptoms immediately after birth, the associated congenital physical defects including talipes, a tented upper lip, and a greater incidence of mental retardation.

Muscular weakness and wasting may begin at any age. The symptomatic infant has difficulty in sucking because of bilateral facial weakness. Muscle weakness, hypotonia, and delay in attaining motor milestones are other manifestations during infancy. Rarely, pure myotonia may be the only feature of this disorder in early childhood. In contrast to most myopathies, the distal rather than proximal muscles of the limbs are affected primarily. The tendon reflexes are often depressed or lost. Ptosis of the eyelids and weakness and atrophy of the facial muscles may be early manifestations; in the older child, wasting of the sternomastoids and the development of a swan-neck posture occur later. Weakness of laryngeal and pharyngeal muscles is apparent later in the monotonous and nasal character of the voice and the dysphagia. Myotonia does not involve all skeletal muscles, but is particularly evident in the hands, face, and tongue. Acrocyanosis is indicative of changes in peripheral blood vessels. Cardiomyopathy is evidenced by electrocardiographic changes (p. 1472). Electromyography is useful in confirming the diagnosis. Quinine and procaine amide control the myotonia to some extent, but otherwise treatment is of no avail.

PARAMYOTONIA. Paramyotonia, a syndrome of myotonia, is usually restricted to the tongue; it spreads to involve the muscles of the face and extremities only on exposure to cold. Unlike dystrophia myotonica, paramyotonia is not progressive and is not complicated by muscular wasting; it differs from myotonia congenita in its lack of hypertrophy and its restricted involvement of muscles. The disorder is inherited through a single autosomal dominant gene and is not transmitted by unaffected members of a family. Drager reported a family with 30 members affected. These patients complained of cramping of the muscles of the face in cold weather and slurred speech associated with stiffness of the tongue after drinking cold liquids. Weakness of the extremities may occur in some attacks and may be associated with elevation of serum potassium. The relation of paramyotonia to familial hyperkalemic paralysis is discussed elsewhere (p. 1888).

MYOSITIS

INFECTIOUS MYOSITIS. Acute suppurative myositis may occur with bloodstream infection or in association with infectious arthritis. Staphylococci and streptococci are the most common causative organisms. Gas gangrene due to *Clostridium perfringens* develops only in traumatized or necrotic muscle. Tuberculous infection in striated muscle may be due to local extension from a neighboring joint or cold abscess or rarely may result from hematogenous dissemination.

Trichinosis is the most frequent parasitic infection of muscle in the Western Hemisphere; cysticercosis commonly involves muscle in infected patients in India and other Asiatic countries. *Toxoplasma* may invade muscle but causes no specific symptoms; the demonstration of the protozoan parasite in a biopsy of muscle is sometimes of value in the diagnosis of acquired toxoplasmosis.

POLYMYOSITIS. Polymyositis is an acute, subacute, or chronic disorder of muscle characterized by symmetric weakness predominant in the shoulder and pelvic girdles. Polymyositis is associated with cutaneous lesions in dermatomyositis (p. 379) and may also occur in scleroderma or rheumatoid arthritis. Muscular pain, tenderness, atrophy, and depression of deep tendon reflexes are inconstant and appear late in the course. Dysphagia occurs in more than half the patients. The electromyographic and histologic abnormalities are characteristic but not pathognomonic of the disease. Nonspecific clinical features include fever, arthralgia, loss of weight, Raynaud's phenomenon, edema, and heliotrope erythema of the eyelids and face. Leukocytosis, an elevated erythrocyte sedimentation rate, and sometimes eosinophilia are noted. High levels of creatinuria and of creatine phosphokinase and aldolase in the serum are indicative of persistent activity of the disease.

Most cases are related to the collagen diseases, but some may result from unknown toxic and metabolic factors. In the absence of skin and joint involvement, the acute forms of the disease may bear a close clinical resemblance to idiopathic myoglobinuria, while chronic forms may resemble progressive muscular dystrophy. The differentiation from muscular dystrophy (Table 21) is often difficult but is important in prognosis and therapy. Some patients with polymyositis improve or recover spontaneously, but treatment with corticosteroids is advisable in those with progressive weakness.

MYOSITIS FIBROSA. Generalized myositis fibrosa is a slowly progressive disease that begins in early life and is characterized by replacement of muscle with fibrous connective tissue. The muscles are firm and woody to palpation; their elasticity is lost. In the final stages movement becomes impossible. The sternomastoids and the muscles of the legs, neck, chest, and back are among those first affected. With the development of muscular contractures the joints become fixed in abnormal postures. Myositis fibrosa is sometimes classed as a chronic progressive form of dermatomyositis, since the histologic changes in the muscle may be similar to those of polymyositis. A therapeutic trial of corticosteroids should be considered.

MYOSITIS OSSIFICANS. Generalized progressive myositis ossificans is a rare disease of unknown cause characterized by the formation of soft, fluctuant, or hard swellings in the interstitial tissue of the muscle and related structures. The masses are of variable size and shape and consist at first of fibrous tissue, often with subsequent formation of bone; they sometimes shrink before ossification occurs. Usually they are painless, but the overlying skin is often reddened and occasionally ulcerated. The disease generally begins before 10 years of age, and the muscles of the neck and back are affected first. The swellings develop spontaneously or follow minimal trauma; they appear in succession over a period of months or years. The muscle fibers are not involved primarily, but undergo atrophy and destruction secondary to pressure and inactivity as a result of disease in the interstitial tissue. Congenital anomalies, the most frequent of which is underdevelopment of the great toes or thumbs, are associated in about 75 percent of cases. The prognosis is grave, and survival beyond puberty is rare. Treatment is usually ineffectual, although it is claimed that remissions have been induced by corticosteroids. Generalized myositis ossificans must be differentiated from a localized traumatic form and from calcinosis universalis, in which calcium is deposited in the subcutaneous tissues.

METABOLIC MYOPATHIES

FAMILIAL PERIODIC PARALYSIS. Familial periodic paralysis is characterized by intermittent at-

TABLE 21. Differential Diagnosis of Polymyositis and Duchenne Muscular Dystrophy*

Clinical Features	Polymyositis	Duchenne Muscular Dystrophy
Sex incidence	females > males	males only
Rate of progress	rapid	slow
Muscular weakness	symmetric and proximal	proximal
Dysphagia	common	unknown
Muscular atrophy	mild	marked
Pseudohypertrophy	rare	common
Muscle pain and tenderness	common	uncommon or rare
Deep tendon reflexes	absent, normal, or brisk	depressed or absent
Muscle biopsy	inflammatory cell infiltration	no inflammatory cells
Dermatomyositis, scleroderma, or rheumatoid arthritis	sometimes associated	not associated
Spontaneous remission	occasional	never
Response to cortisone	remission	none

*Adapted from Walton and Adams: Polymyositis, 1958. Courtesy of E. & S. Livingstone.

tacks of flaccid paralysis with complete absence of deep tendon reflexes and electrical inexcitability of the muscles. The onset is usually before puberty, and attacks may recur for years. The sexes are affected equally. An attack generally begins with weakness in the muscles of the back and pelvic girdle, and flaccidity gradually spreads to involve the lower limbs, shoulder girdle, upper limbs, and neck. The respiratory muscles and muscles innervated by the cranial nerves are usually spared. Dysphagia may occur in severe attacks, and death, although rare, has been reported. Smooth muscle is not affected, but cardiac enlargement and a slow and irregular pulse are present in some cases. Attacks may occur at any time, but most commonly during sleep or inactivity. They may be preceded and accompanied by excessive perspiration and thirst and are precipitated by ingestion of excess carbohydrate, exposure to cold, muscular exertion followed by inactivity, or injection of insulin or epinephrine. Attacks usually last 2 to 3 hours, but they may persist as long as 7 days. Recovery is gradual and usually complete, although slight weakness may persist. The presence of vacuoles in muscle is characteristic.

The paralysis is associated with hypokalemia but is not related to the absolute concentration of serum potassium. The fall in the level of serum potassium is not reflected in an increased urinary excretion, but may be related to a shift of potassium from the blood to the cells of the muscles and liver. An abnormal degree of binding of potassium by large protein molecules may occur. In some cases attacks have been preceded by an increase in the urinary excretion of aldosterone and retention of sodium. An abrupt fall in the level of potassium in serum and urine has been observed. As the attack subsides there are diuresis of sodium, an increase in the urinary excretion of potassium, and a return to normal of the level of aldosterone in the urine. Attacks appear to be precipitated by retention of sodium and may be prevented by restriction of dietary sodium. Potassium chloride is given for the treatment of acute attacks. The prognosis is excellent, and the episodes becomes less frequent and less severe in adult life.

HYPOKALEMIC PARALYSIS.   The association of low serum potassium levels and weakness or paralysis of skeletal muscles may occur in diabetic acidosis, in Addison's disease following the administration of excess deoxycorticosterone (DOCA), and in some cases of renal insufficiency. Complete paralysis, as observed in familial periodic paralysis, is rare. The more usual findings are diffuse muscular weakness and apathy, with delirium, coarse muscular twitching, and tetany. The electrocardiogram is of value in the differentiation of hypokalemia and hyperkalemia (p. 1387).

HYPERKALEMIC PARALYSIS.   Muscular weakness and elevated levels of serum potassium may occur in patients with renal insufficiency (especially after the administration of potassium), in untreated Addison's disease, and in crush syndrome and hemolytic reactions. The onset and evolution of paresis are rapid, and the distribution resembles that of familial periodic paralysis. The legs, trunk, and arms are affected in an ascending sequence. The administration of 5 to 15 g of potassium by mouth to healthy individuals will often produce paresthesia, but muscular weakness is exceptional.

HEREDITARY EPISODIC ADYNAMIA.   As described by Gamstorp, hereditary episodic adynamia is characterized by attacks of spontaneously abating paralysis that affect particularly the muscles of the extremities and the trunk and are generally accompanied by an elevation of the serum potassium. The disease is inherited through a single autosomal dominant gene with complete or almost complete penetrance. The incidence is the same in both sexes.

The onset of episodic symptoms is usually before the age of 10 years. Attacks invariably occur during rest that follows exertion and at least once a week; they last at most 1 hour. The extent and severity of the paresis vary from slight weakness of a single extremity to severe states in which the patient is unable to turn over or sit up. Respiration is seldom involved, and the muscles innervated by cranial nerves are affected only mildly. Deep tendon reflexes may be weak or absent, and Chvostek's sign is sometimes positive during attacks. Percussion myotonia may be elicited, and the disease is more troublesome in cold, damp weather. The clinical manifestations of adynamia episodica resemble those of paramyotonia. The term adynamia episodica hereditaria should be retained for those patients who, in response to a small dose of potassium, have elevated serum levels and react with muscular weakness, regardless of the presence of myotonia.

As a general rule, paresis is accompanied by an increase in the level of serum potassium without change in the urinary excretion of potassium. Electrocardiographic changes are consistent with hyperkalemia. Attacks may be precipitated by oral administration of potassium in doses insufficient to produce symptoms in normal persons. Symptoms are prevented by glucose, with or without insulin, administered before or simultaneously with a provocative dose of potassium. Acetazolamide administered orally, calcium administered intravenously, an intake of food (especially bread), or gentle exercise may shorten the duration of attacks, but the symptoms abate spontaneously. Improvement occurs and attacks are less frequent after 30 years of age.

MYOHEMOGLOBINURIA.   Myohemoglobin may appear in the urine spontaneously and without known cause, or it may appear following crush injuries, extreme muscular activity, or ingestion of eels or fish poisoned by resinous waste products of factories (Haff disease). In the cryptogenic cases (Meyer-Betz) paroxysmal attacks of myohemoglobinuria are associated with weakness or paralysis of skeletal muscles. The onset of illness is usually sudden and is sometimes accompanied by nausea, fever, and vomiting. The affected muscles are swollen and painful. The disease may be familial, may occur at any age, and may vary greatly in severity. The patient may die from uremia or respiratory paralysis in the first attack or may recover and suffer repeated episodes of muscle weakess. Cardiac and smooth muscles are unaffected. The diagnosis of myohemoglobinuria is established by electrophoresis or spectroscopic examination; it may be suspected in a patient who shows no evidence of hemolytic anemia when the urine is dark and who gives a positive reaction for occult blood in the absence of red blood cells. Serum enzymes are markedly elevated.

GLYCOGEN MYOPATHIES. Of five different types of glycogen storage disease, two (types II and V) have significantly increased amounts of glycogen in the skeletal muscle associated with weakness. They are discussed in detail in Chapter 14.

TYPE II. Clinically, cardiomuscular glycogen disease (Pompe's disease) closely resembles Werdnig-Hoffman disease in that the child often is asymptomatic at birth and manifests progressive hypotonia, areflexia, and muscle weakness after a few months. Macroglossia and cardiomegaly are additional features. The infant usually dies by 1 year of age from cardiac or respiratory failure. The late infantile type of the disease closely resembles Duchenne's pseudohypertrophic muscular dystrophy.

TYPE V. The symptoms of McArdle's disease begin in childhood and occur only after moderately severe exercise. Muscular weakness, stiffness, and painful cramps develop with effort and disappear rapidly with rest. Between attacks the physical examination is normal, including deep tendon reflexes.

TYPES I, III, AND IV. In type I (von Gierke's disease) skeletal muscle is not involved. Types III and IV, rare varieties, involve primarily the liver, as well as the myocardium and skeletal muscles to a lesser extent.

Disorders of muscles may occur with many endocrine diseases. Morphologic changes are usually slight or absent, and a derangement of some enzyme system necessary for contraction of muscle has been invoked to explain the muscle weakness. A chronic form of myopathy has been reported in hyperthyroidism, and an acute thyrotoxic myopathy that sometimes progresses to a form of bulbar paralysis may also occur. Treatment of the hyperthyroidism alleviates the muscle weakness. Thyrotoxicosis and myasthenia gravis may occur concomitantly, but their association is unexplained. About 5 percent of all patients with myasthenia gravis developed thyrotoxicosis at some time during their illness, and an inverse relationship is occasionally observed. Symptoms of myasthenia may be aggravated by administration of antithyroid drugs and alleviated on their withdrawal. The frequency of abnormalities of the thymus gland and the occurrence of focal collections of small lymphocytes, or lymphorrhages, in striated muscles in both myasthenia gravis and thyrotoxicosis point to some common factor in etiology.

Hypothyroidism may be complicated by true generalized hypertrophy of muscles. The Debré-Semelaigne syndrome, characterized by enlarged muscles, weakness, early fatigue, and slowness of movements, is one of the clinical manifestations of cretinism. The symptoms are relieved by thyroid medication. In hyperparathyroidism, symmetric weakness, fatigability, and atrophy of limb muscles, with discomfort on muscular effort, are prominent symptoms, usually of neuropathic origin, which may be related to the disorder of calcium metabolism. Hypopituitarism is associated with muscle weakness and atrophy. Flexion contractures of the

limbs observed in Addison's disease may be related to an excessive accumulation of sodium in the tendons and their consequent shortening. The deformities have been relieved following treatment with ACTH.

MYASTHENIA GRAVIS

Myasthenia gravis is characterized by undue weakness and fatigue following maintained contraction of voluntary muscles, with a tendency to recovery with rest. Ocular movements, facial expression, mastication, deglutition, and speech are affected primarily. Muscles of the neck, trunk, and limbs may be involved, and respiratory embarrassment occurs in severe cases. Cardiac and smooth muscles are spared. The disease may develop at any age, but in children the first symptoms occur most commonly at or soon after birth or puberty. Three forms of myasthenia gravis of infancy and childhood are distinguished: neonatal transient form, neonatal persistent (or congential) form, and juvenile myasthenia gravis. Myasthenic symptoms may occur with diseases other than myasthenia gravis, such as muscular dystrophy, polymyositis, ocular myopathy, and thyrotoxicosis.

Neonatal transient myasthenia occurs in infants born to mothers with the disease. The majority of infants of myasthenic mothers are unaffected, with symptoms developing in only 10 to 20 percent. There is no correlation between the severity of the infant's symptoms and the duration or severity of the mother's illness and her treatment during pregnancy. At birth or within a few hours thereafter the infant becomes limp, his cry and movements are feeble, he is unable to suck, and his swallowing and breathing are impaired. Muscular weakness and hypotonia are generalized and symmetric, and the Moro and deep tendon reflexes are absent or depressed. External ophthalmoplegia and ptosis are infrequent.

A newborn infant of a myasthenic mother whose previous pregnancy resulted in a neonatal death of undetermined cause should be carefully observed for signs of myasthenia. The diagnosis is established by the intramuscular or intravenous injection of edrophonium chloride (Tensilon) in a dose of 1 mg or neostigmine methyl sulfate 0.1 to 0.2 mg. Symptoms should be relieved almost immediately (Fig. 39). In moderate and severe cases, and especially those with bulbar symptoms, a positive Tensilon test should be followed by continuous therapy with anticholinesterase drugs. In the milder forms of the disorder the infant may recover completely without specific therapy, but treatment must be instituted immediately should respiratory difficulty, choking, dysphagia, or inability to suck supervene.

Pyridostigmine bromide (Mestinon) and neostigmine bromide (Prostigmin) have a less rapid but more prolonged effect than Tensilon and may be effectively used in treatment. Mestinon is preferred because it is less toxic, having fewer muscarinic side effects. The required dosage differs in each patient and must be adjusted according to the individual response. The following have been found satisfactory as initial doses, to be given every 4 hours at the time of each feeding.

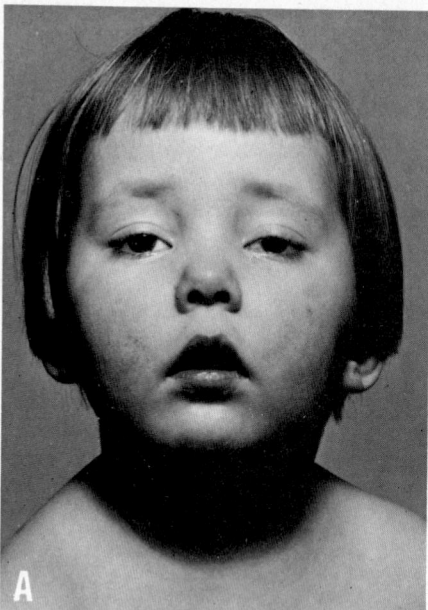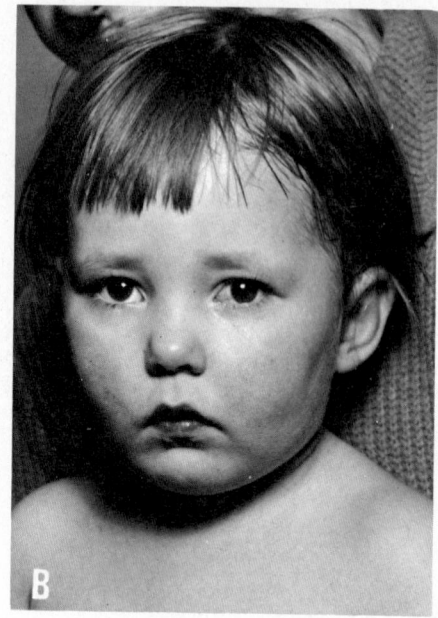

FIG. 39. A. 3-year-old girl with myasthenia gravis. Ptosis, bilateral and asymmetric, was most marked at the end of the day and was not apparent on waking. A right-sided exophoria was variable in degree. **B.** After Tensilon (5 mg intravenously) the ptosis cleared within 30 sec, and the benefical response lasted about 10 minutes. The patient was treated with regular doses of Mestinon, 7.5 mg three times a day.

Oral doses: Mestinon bromide, 5 mg (5 drops of syrup of Mestinon, containing 60 mg/4 ml); Prostigmin bromide, 1 mg. Parenteral preparations are approximately 30 times as potent as the oral. Intramuscular dose: Prostigmin methyl sulfate, 0.05 to 0.1 mg. When a dosage level sufficient to relieve bulbar symptoms has been determined, further increments in dosage are unnecessary and may be hazardous.

Overdosage with anticholinesterase medication (cholinergic crisis) is manifested by the following signs: increase in muscle weakness and worsening of respiratory difficulty and dysphagia after each dose of drug, muscular fasciculations, and prominent muscarinic side effects, which include excessive salivation, vomiting, diarrhea, pallor, sweating, and bradycardia. Tensilon, 0.05 ml (0.5 mg) given intravenously, will cause a mild and transient exacerbation of cholinergic weakness and may be used to differentiate the crisis due to excessive medication and that associated with a worsening of myasthenia. Atropine may be administered for anticholinesterase overdosage. The oronasopharyngeal secretions should be suctioned repeatedly, and oxygen should be administered when indicated. After the first week of treatment, gradual withdrawal of medication may be attempted. If symptoms increase, the original dosage should be reinstituted, and the effects of withdrawal will be observed again after 2 to 3 days. The duration of the illness is short, and the natural course is from a few hours to 7 weeks. With efficient therapy recovery should be complete.

Congenital myasthenia gravis occurs in infants born to mothers who are unaffected by the disease. In contrast to the transient neonatal type, involvement of bulbar musculature is unusual, and generalized muscle weakness is not severe. Ptosis that is relieved by sleep is the most common presenting sign, and external ophthalmoplegia and diplopia occur frequently during childhood and later life. Other less common symptoms include weakness of the facial muscles and limbs, a weak and nasal voice, and some difficulty in chewing and swallowing. A family history of myasthenia in brothers, sisters, and cousins is occasionally obtained. In contrast to the late form, congenital myasthenia affects both sexes equally and is rarely complicated by acute myasthenic crises; symptoms are only moderately severe, but they are persistent. Ophthalmoplegia is largely resistant to anticholinesterase medication, and complete remission of the disease is rare.

In *juvenile myasthenia gravis* the onset may be in early childhood, but in the majority of cases symptoms begin after 10 years of age. The disease is occasionally familial; before puberty females are affected six times more frequently than males. The most common first symptom is intermittent and asymmetric ptosis, which later becomes bilateral. Weakness of the legs following exertion such as swimming, generalized muscle weakness, and nasal voice also occur as frequent initial symptoms. Facial weakness, difficulty in chewing and swallowing, ophthalmoplegia, and diplopia are less common at the onset, but they frequently develop later. In young children, walking may be delayed, and gait is awkward and interrupted by frequent stumbling. Older children are incapable of sustained activity; they tire easily and their shoulders droop. As the disease progresses, muscles weakened by use take longer to recover, and some additional exertion or intercurrent infection may precipitate a paralytic failure of the respiratory musculature.

The primary lesion in myasthenia gravis is believed to involve defective transmission of impulses at the neuromuscular synapse, the exact nature of which is unknown. The motor nerve fibers conduct normally, and the response of skeletal muscle to direct stimulation is normal. The neuromuscular block and the symptoms of myasthenia are similar to those of curare poisoning, and an abnormal metabolite with a curarelike action has been postulated as a possible factor in etiology. Other theories of the mechanism of the neuromuscular block include a deficient synthesis of acetylcholine due to overactivity of the enzyme cholinesterase or an abnormal structure of the synapse.

The general character of myasthenia gravis is suggestive of an endocrine or metabolic disorder. The onset often occurs at puberty, and remission or relapse is frequently associated with menstruation, pregnancy, or changes of thyroid function. At autopsy the central and peripheral nervous systems show no gross or microscopic abnormalities; focal collections of small lymphocytes (lymphorrhages) present in affected skeletal muscles cannot be considered causative. That the thymus may play a significant role in the mechanism of myasthenia is suggested by the coincidence of thymic hyperplasia in 50 percent of cases and the apparent beneficial effect of thymectomy in some patients. It has been suggested that myasthenia is an autoimmune disease in which the thymus reacts against protein antigens in the motor end plate. Thymoma has been found in almost one-third of the reported cases in adults, but it is rare in childhood.

The differential diagnosis includes bulbar poliomyelitis, diphtheritic paralysis, polyneuritis, intracranial tumor, and hyperthyroidism. The initial illness is commonly misdiagnosed as hysteria or laziness. Diagnosis may be confirmed by intravenous injection of Tensilon (Fig. 39), which relieves the presenting symptoms within a few minutes. In children weighing up to 34 kg, the dose is 0.2 ml (2 mg); in those over 34 kg, 0.5 ml (5 mg) may be given. If Prostigmin is employed, the intramuscular dose is 0.25 to 1.0 mg of Prostigmin methyl sulfate, depending on the weight or surface area of the child. The patient should be examined for signs of improvement at 5- or 10-minute intervals for a period of 45 minutes, and atropine may be required for the relief of muscarinic side effects.

Treatment with anticholinesterase drugs should be instituted and controlled as outlined for neonatal myasthenia. Mestinon should be given orally in initial trial doses of 5 to 10 mg at intervals of 2 to 4 hours, or Prostigmin in doses of 1 to 5 mg orally. Ambenonium chloride (Mytelase) is prescribed occasionally; it causes less bronchial secretion than do other anticholinesterase drugs, and its use may be indicated in patients with respiratory paralysis. Five milligrams of Mytelase chloride are equivalent to 15 mg of Prostigmin bromide or 60 mg of Mestinon bromide. Prednisone or corticotropin, in gradually increasing doses on alternate days, may be of benefit to patients with severe generalized myasthenia gravis who are not satisfactorily controlled by anticholinesterase medication. This type of treatment should be administered only in refractory cases and in a respiratory intensive care unit.

Thymectomy may be followed by improvement and sometimes by complete remission. It is considered of particular value in young female patients who have had the disease for less than 5 years and is indicated especially in patients with generalized muscle weakness and bulbar symptoms resistant to pharmacologic agents.

The prognosis in children is variable, but it is relatively good compared with that in adults. The case fatality rate is about 5 percent. The course is generally prolonged, and complete remission following drug therapy or thymectomy may be expected in less than 25 percent of cases up to 6 years from onset; complete remission after this time is rare. Ptosis and ocular palsies are often refractory to treatment; relapse and failure of response to medication are frequently related to systemic or upper respiratory infection and to menstruation.

References

DISEASES OF THE MUSCLES

Adams RD, Denny-Brown D, Pearson CM: Diseases of Muscle. A Study in Pathology, 2nd ed. New York, Paul B Hoeber, 1962

Swaiman KF, Wright FS: Neuromuscular Diseases of Infancy and Childhood. Springfield, Ill, Charles C Thomas, 1970

Walton JN (ed): Disorders of Voluntary Muscle. Boston, Little, Brown, 1964

———— Nattrass FJ: On the classification, natural history and treatment of myopathies. Brain 77:169, 1954

LIMP INFANT SYNDROME

Batten FE: The myopathies or muscular dystrophies; critical review. QJ Med 3:313, 1910

Dubowitz V: The Floppy Infant. Clinics in Developmental Medicine No 21. London, National Spastics Society, 1969

Greenfield JG, Cornman T, Shy GM: The prognostic value of the muscle biopsy in the "floppy" infant. Brain 81:461, 1958

Tizzard JPM: Neuromuscular disorder of infancy. In Walton JN (ed): Disorders of Voluntary Muscle. Boston, Little, Brown, 1964, p 369

Turner JWA: Relationship between amyotonia congenita and congenital myopathy. Brain 63:163, 1940

Walton JN: The limp child. J Neurol Neurosurg Psychiatry 20:144, 1957

MUSCULAR DYSTROPHIES

Jackson CE, Carey JH: Progressive muscular dystrophy; autosomal recessive type. Pediatrics 28:77, 1961

Milhorat AT: The diagnosis of muscular dystrophy. Am J Phys Med 35:103, 1955

Pearce JMS, Pennington RJ, Walton JN: Serum enzyme studies in muscle disease. Part II. Serum creatine kinase activity in muscular dystrophy and in other myopathic and neuropathic disorders. J Neurol Neurosurg Psychiatry 27:96, 1964

Walton JN: Muscular dystrophy and its relation to the other myopathies. Res Publ Assoc Res Nerv Ment Dis 38:378, 1959

Zellweger H, Hansen JW: Slowly progressive X-linked recessive muscular dystrophy (type IIIB). Arch Intern Med 120:525, 1967

MYOTONIAS

Adams RD, Denny-Brown D, Pearson CM: Diseases of Muscle, A Study in Pathology, 2nd ed. New York, Paul B Hoeber 1962

Bastron JA: Myotonia and other abnormalities of muscular contraction arising from disorders of the motor unit. Res Publ Assoc Res Nerv Ment Dis 38:534, 1959

Dodge PR, Gamstorp I, Byers RK, Russell P: Myotonic dystrophy in infancy and childhood. Pediatrics 35:3, 1965

Dyken PR, Harper PS: Congenital dystrophia myotonica. Neurology 23:465, 1973

MYOSITIS

Barwick DD, Walton JN: Polymyositis. Am J Med 35:646, 1963

Eaton LM: The perspective of neurology in regard to polymyositis, study of 41 cases. Neurology 4:245, 1954

Riley HD Jr, Christie A: Myositis ossificans progressiva. Pediatrics 8:753, 1951

Rowland LR: Muscular dystrophies, polymyositis and other myopathies. J Chronic Dis 8:510, 1958

Vignos PF Jr, Goldwyn J: Evaluation of laboratory tests in diagnosis and management of polymyositis. Am J Med Sci 263:291, 1972

METABOLIC MYOPATHIES

Conn JW, Fajans SS, Louis LH, Streeten DHP, Johnson RD: Intermittent aldosteronism in periodic paralysis. Lancet 1:802, 1957

Danowski TS, Tarail R: Potassium metabolism and dysfunction of the nervous system associated with hyper- and hypokalemia. Res Publ Assoc Res Nerv Ment Dis 32:372, 1953

Engel WK: Muscle biopsies in neuromuscular diseases. Pediatr Clin North Am 14:963, 1967

Gass H, Cherkasky M, Savitsky N: Potassium and periodic paralysis. Medicine 27:105, 1948

McArdle B: Metabolic myopathies. Am J Med 35:661, 1963

Patten BM, Bilezikian JP, Mallette LE, Prince A, Engel WK, Aurbach GD: Neuromuscular disease in primary hyperparathyroidism. Ann Intern Med 80:182, 1974

Rowland LP, Fahn S, Hirschberg E, Harter DH: Myoglobinuria. Arch Neurol 10:537, 1964

Shy GM: Some metabolic and endocrinological aspects of disorders of striated muscle. Res Publ Assoc Res Nerv Ment Dis 38:274, 1959

Wyllie WG, Watkins AG: Periodic familial paralysis. Proc R Soc Med 41:861, 1948

MYASTHENIA GRAVIS

Brunner NG, Namba T, Grob D: Corticosteroids in management of severe, generalized myasthenia gravis: effectiveness and comparison with corticotropic therapy. Neurology 22:603, 1972

Keynes G: The results of thymectomy in myasthenia gravis. Br Med J 2:611, 1949

Millichap JG, Dodge PR: Diagnosis and treatment of myasthenia gravis in infancy, childhood and adolescence; a study of 51 patients. Neurology 10:1007, 1960

Osserman IE: Myasthenia Gravis. New York, Grune & Stratton, 1958

Rowland OP, Hoefer PFA, Aranow H Jr: Myasthenic syndromes. Res Publ Assoc Res Nerv Ment Dis 38:548, 1959

Schwab RS, Viets HR: Myasthenia gravis. Res Publ Assoc Res Nerv Ment Dis 38:624, 1959

Seybold ME, Drachman DB: Gradually increasing doses of prednisone in myasthenia gravis: reducing the hazards of treatment. N Engl J Med 290:81, 1974

Simpson JA: An evaluation of thymectomy in myasthenia gravis. Brain 81:112, 1958

Wyllie WG, Bodian M, Burrows NFE: Myasthenia gravis in children. Arch Dis Child 26:457, 1951

PROGRESSIVE GENETIC-METABOLIC DISEASES OF THE CENTRAL NERVOUS SYSTEM

ISABELLE RAPIN

The change in the title of this section (from "The Degenerative and Demyelinating Diseases of the Nervous System" in the 15th edition) reflects significant advances toward an understanding of the pathogenesis of at least some of the relentlessly progressive neurologic diseases of children. A few, such as subacute sclerosing panencephalitis and progressive multifocal leukoencephalopathy, have been shown to be due to infection with slow viruses. It is likely that multiple sclerosis, which may start with a bout of optic neuritis in a child, may be triggered by an infectious process that sets up an immunologic reaction in the nervous system of hosts with a particular predisposition. Others, such as Parkinson's disease, probably have multifactorial etiologies where genetic predisposition and environmental factors interact.

The majority of conditions discussed here are known, or are assumed, to be genetic in origin. They are still called progressive in order to indicate our continuing lack of effective treatment for most of them. With progress toward identification of metabolic blocks or enzymatic defects, rational and effective therapy becomes a realistic prospect. As will be emphasized in the subsection on the sphingolipidoses, the pediatrician has a strong responsibility to refer any child suspected of having a genetic-metabolic disease to an appropriate center for precise diagnosis, since this is an absolute requirement for further progress and for genetic counseling.

GENETIC DIAGNOSIS.   Some diseases, such as Tay-Sachs disease, can be diagnosed by amniocentesis (p. 129) and thus prevented by selective abortion. The need for genetic counseling for many disorders will be discussed. The complex moral and ethical questions relating to genetic screening, intrauterine diagnosis and abortion, and genetic counseling have been reviewed elsewhere (p. 292). Nevertheless, the availability of genetic screening and intrauterine diagnosis enables families to make rational decisions regarding future offspring, provided they have been informed of the options and risks involved. Discussion of the cost–benefit ratio of mass screening for a variety of diseases is beyond the scope of this section, but it will considered for several diseases.

TISSUE DIAGNOSIS.   The need to resort to biopsy to establish an exact diagnosis is becoming less frequent. Biopsies are no longer justified for those diseases for which enzymatic diagnosis is available. Liver biopsy to measure copper content is still considered essential for diagnosing Wilson's disease. Skin and muscle biopsies may show characteristic inclusions in ceroid lipofuscinosis, a group of diseases for which there is as yet no enzymatic test. Bone marrow examination is benign and may be helpful in screening a child for lysosomal disorders such as Gaucher's disease, Niemann-Pick disease, mucopolysaccharidosis, and mucolipidosis, but it rarely provides a definitive diagnosis. Rectal biopsy is rarely justified today because it provides so few neurons for examination that only limited morphologic studies are possible and chemical study is virtually precluded.

Cerebral biopsies are never justified unless they are carried out in a center with adequate skills in neuropathology, histochemistry, electron microscopy, and, ideally, neurochemistry to enable maximum information to be obtained. Studies to be performed should be planned in advance. Properly carried out, there has been no mortality and a low morbidity in children; temporary worsening of seizures with transient hemiparesis has occurred in a few children with preexisting convulsive disorders. Brain biopsies are justified to diagnose diseases for which there are no enzymatic or biochemical tests when parents wish to have a definite diagnosis for genetic purposes or to plan for the future of the child; spongy degeneration of the brain, Alexander's disease, neuroaxonal dystrophy, and atypical ceroid lipofuscinosis are examples. Biopsy is not always diagnostic; this is a particular problem if an inadequate sample of white matter is obtained, especially in leukodystrophies. A specific diagnosis is not often made from biopsy in infants with seizures and mental retardation in whom there are no clues for a specific lesion; indiscriminant use of biopsies in such cases must be questioned.

The ethical questions involved in performing cerebral biopsies on children with advanced neurologic disease primarily for the purpose of increasing knowledge about the disease are subject to much debate. Such a decision cannot be made lightly; it must be discussed at length with the parents and with the appropriate research review committees. Nevertheless, brain biopsy has made contributions to an understanding of the pathogenesis and course of several diseases. The place of such studies needs to be reevaluated frequently, and the possibility of obtaining the same information by other means, such as metabolic studies of fibroblasts in tissue culture, of autopsy material, or of animal models, should be considered.

STATIC VERSUS PROGRESSIVE DISEASE. It is easy to determine that a disease is progressive when its

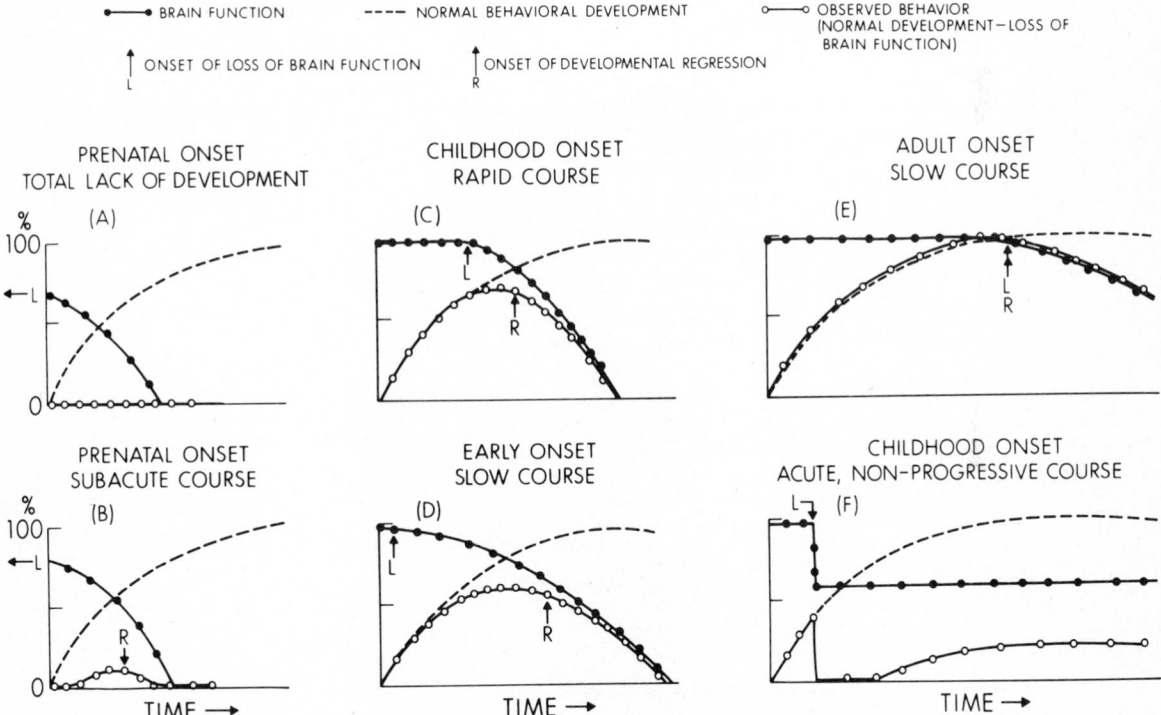

FIG. 40. Theoretical curves to show the possible effects of a progressive illness on behavior, depending on time of onset and rapidity of its course (A–F). The curve depicting observed behavior (solid line with open circles) is the resultant of the difference between the curves indicating expected development (dash line) and brain function (dash line and circles). A. Prenatal onset; damage at birth so advanced that no development is observed, suggesting a severe static encephalopathy. B. Prenatal onset; damage at birth somewhat less severe. Development is minimal and markedly delayed, but does appear to be taking place initially. C and D. Onset at birth; less acute course. E. Onset in adulthood. Note in B, C, D that loss of milestones (R) may not appear until months or years after onset of illness, which will therefore not appear progressive unless it is realized that deceleration of development or developmental standstill implies deteriorating function. When a progressive disease starts after adolescence (E), loss of function should be less delayed and the disease recognized as progressive virtually from its start. A severe static lesion acquired postnatally (F) may produce total regression acutely, but development may be expected to resume until the time of puberty.

course is rapid and the patient's previously acquired skills deteriorate; it becomes more difficult in very slowly progressive diseases where the deterioration may be insidious. Detection of slowly progressive diseases that start in infancy may be extremely difficult because neurological development may advance so rapidly in infancy that acquisition of milestones is delayed, rather than not being attained at all. If the disease starts prenatally the infant may fail to acquire any milestones and therefore may appear to have a static deficit (Fig. 40A and B). In normal infants, development often progresses sporadically, with periods of several weeks during which the infant appears to have reached a plateau. Prolongation of such plateaus may be the only thing noted initially in a progressive disease (Fig. 40C and D). The acquisition of new developmental milestones by no means excludes the existence of a progressive disease; infants with Tay-Sachs disease learn to smile, respond, and reach for objects; yet ganglioside storage is noted in fetuses. Symptoms will not be apparent if the disease impairs the function of a system that has not yet come into use: cerebellar dysfunction will not be noted in an infant who does not yet attempt to hold his head erect or reach for objects; dementias may not be evident until the time that children usually begin to play or speak.

Figure 40 illustrates that unless development is plotted as a curve and its slope compared to the norm, the existence of a progressive disease may pass unnoticed until such a time as failure to achieve obvious milestones such as walking or language can no longer be attributed to slowness. Early in the course of progressive genetic diseases, erroneous diagnoses of fixed encephalopathy or cerebral palsy may have disastrous consequences if the parents are reassured that the child's neurologic problem is adventitous and they then proceed to have other children. The pediatrician should be reluctant to make a diagnosis of cerebral palsy or mental retardation in children with motor signs and developmental delays in the absence of a documented prenatal or perinatal cause. Signs such as optic atrophy, nystagmus, tremors, floppiness, unusual features, organomegaly, myoclonus, or intractable seizures should suggest that the child probably has an evolving disease. Table 22 has been prepared as a guide to diagnosis based on the salient clinical features of various diseases.

TABLE 22a. Diagnostic Features of Progressive Genetic-Metabolic Diseases in Relation to Age of Onset

Onset in Infancy

With Organomegaly: Mucopolysaccharidoses I-H, II-A, IV, VI, VII; mucolipidoses II (I cell disease); fucosidosis, infantile variant; mannosidoses (mild); GM₁-gangliosidosis, infantile variant; GM₃-gangliosidosis; Gaucher's disease; Niemann-Pick disease; Farber's disease (mild); cerebrohepato renal syndrome (Zellweger); galactosemia; glyogenosis type I (Pompe)

With joint and/or bony abnormalities: mucopolysaccharidoses, all but type III (Sanfilippo) early; mucolipidosis II (I cell), III; fucosidosis, infantile variant; Faber's disease; cerebrohepato renal syndrome

With floppiness: GM₁-gangliosidosis, infantile variant; Tay-Sachs disease; Niemann-Pick disease, infantile variant; Farber's disease; fucosidosis, infantile variant; ceroid lipofuscinosis, infantile (Finnish) variant; spongy degeneration (neck especially); cerebrohepatorenal syndrome; trichopoliodystrophy; Leigh's syndrome; neuroaxonal dystrophy (note: floppiness suggests cerebellar, anterior horn cell, peripheral nerve, or muscular involvement)

With abnormal movements: Lesch-Nyhan syndrome; infantile Hallervorden-Spatz syndrome

With myoclonus and/or prominent seizures: GM₁-gangliosidosis; GM₁-gangliosidosis; Krabbe's disease; ceroid lipofuscinosis; sudanophilic leukodystrophy with meningeal angiomatosis; cerebrohepato-renal syndrome; trichopoliodystrophy; glioneuronal dystrophy; amino-acidurias; tuberous sclerosis (hypsarythmia)

With increased tone: Krabbe, Gaucher, Pelizaeus-Merzbacher; glioneuronal dystrophy (Alper); Sjögren-Larsson Hallervorden-Spatz; Lesch-Nyhan; trichopoliodystrophy; spongy degeneration

With mental deficiency or dementia: MPS I (Hurler); mucolipidosis II, IV; gangliosidoses; Krabbe; Niemann-Pick; Farber; Pelizaeus-Merzmacher (connatal type); ceroid lipofuscinosis (Finnish variant); spongy degeneration) cerebrohepatorenal syndrome; trichopoliodystrophy; Sjögren-Larsson; incontinentia pigmenti; neuroaxonal dystrophy

Onset in Preschool Age

With organomegaly: MPS III (Sanfilippo), mild; Niemann-Pick type D (Nova Scotia variant); metachromatic leukodystrophy with sulfatase deficiency; Chediak-Higashi

With joint and/or bony abnormalities: MPS III; mucolipidoses I (I cell), III; fucosidosis (juvenile variant); Cockayne

With hypotonia: CM₁-gangliosidosis, late infantile variant; GM₂-gangliosidosis, late infantile variant; metachromatic leukodystrophy, late infantile variant; neuroaxonal dystrophy; ceroid lipofuscinosis, late infantile (Jansky-Bielschowsky)

TABLE 22a. Diagnostic Features of Progressive Genetic-Metabolic Diseases in Relation to Age of Onset (cont.)

Onset in Preschool Age (cont.)

With abnormal movements: familial (essential) tremor; Lesch-Nyhan syndrome

With ataxia: metachromatic leukodystrophy; neuroaxonal dystrophy; late infantile ceroid lipofuscinosis; late infantile GM$_1$-gangliosidosis; Leigh's syndrome; Pelizaeus-Merzbacher, classic type; Niemann-Pick type D (Nova Scotia variant)

With myoclonus and/or prominent seizures: GM$_1$-and GM$_2$-gangliosidoses (late infantile variants); MPS III (Sanfilippo); metachromatic leukodystrophy with multiple sulfatase deficiency; atypical hyperuricemia responding to allopurinol; tuberous sclerosis; neurofibromatosis (occasionally); linear nevus sebacceous; Nevus unius lateralis; Sturge-Weber; Niemann-Pick type D

With increased tone: GM$_1$- and GM$_2$-gangliosidoses (late infantile variants); metachromatic leukodystrophy; Pelizaeus-Merzbacher

With dementia or mental deficiency: mucopolysaccharidosis III (Sanfilippo); fucosidosis; mannosidosis; apartylglucosaminuria; gangliosidoses; metachromatic leukodystrophy; ceroid lipofuscinosis; Pelizaeus-Merbacher (classic type); Marinesco-Sjögren syndrome; Leigh's syndrome; Alexander disease; Cockayne disease; xeroderma pigmentosum with multiple endocrine deficiencies

Onset in School Age or in Adolescence

With organomegaly: Niemann-Pick, some juvenile variants; juvenile nonneuropathic Gaucher's disease; Wilson's disease (not always)

With joint and/or bony changes: MPS I-H/S; MS II, mild form

With abnormal posture and/or movements: Adult (chronic) GM$_2$-gangliosidosis; juvenile GM$_2$-gangliosidosis; MPS II (Sanfilippo), inconstant; juvenile Niemann-Pick with vertical ophthalmoplegia; juvenile Pelizaeus-Merzbacher; juvenile ceroid lipofuscinosis (Batten-Spielmeyer-Vogt-Sjögren); Hallervorden-Spatz, classic type; Huntington's Chorea: Wilson's disease; dystonia musculorum deformans; juvenile parkinsonism; Gilles de la Tourette; ataxia-telangiectasia; familial calcification of the basal ganglia; hypoparathyroidism and pseudohypoparathyroidism; xeroderma pigmentosum with endocrine dysfunction

With ataxia: Friedreich's ataxia; other variants of spinocerebellar degeneration; vitamin B$_{12}$deficiency; ataxia-telangiectasia; xeroderma pigmentosum; Refsum's disease; abetalipoproteinemia; adrenoleukodystrophy (Shilder's disease); cerebrotendinous xanthomatosis; juvenile spongy degeneration; juvenile ceroid lipofuscinosis; sea blue histiocyte syndrome; Wilson's disease; GM$_2$-gangliosidosis, juvenile and adult (chronic) variants; Niemann-Pick disease, some juvenile variants; juvenile metachromatic leukodystrophy; juvenile Krabbe; Lafora disease; dyssynergia cerebellaris myoclonica (Ramsey-Hunt); Unverricht-Lundborg disease; Leber's syndrome; Usher's syndrome; Chediak-Higashi; Lindau-von Hippel (with cerebellar hemangioblastoma); cherry-red spot myoclonus syndrome

With increased tone: spinocerebellar degenerations; familial spastic paraplegia; Hallervorden-Spatz; Huntingon's chorea; dystonia musculorum deformans; juvenile parkinsonism; juvenile Pelizaeus-Merzbacher; adrenoleukodystrophy; ataxia-telangiectasia; juvenile metachromatic leukodystrophy; juvenile GM$_2$-gangliosidosis; juvenile Krabbe; juvenile ceroid lipofuscinosis; MPS VI (cord compression); SSPE (note: see note to Table)

With dementia: Huntington's chorea; MPS III (Sanfilippo); juvenile GM$_2$-gangliosidosis; metachromatic leukodystrophy, juvenile variant; juvenile Krabbe; juvenile ceroid lipofuscinosis; adrenoleukodystrophy; juvenile Pelizaeus-Merzbacher; Hallervorden-Spatz, classic type; juvenile spongy degeneration; Lafora disease; pseudohypoparathyroidism (mental deficiency); xeroderma pigmentosum with endocrine dysfunction; SSPE; some spinocerebellar degenerations

With psychosis: acute intermittent prophyria

With seizures and/or myoclonus: Lafora disease; dyssynergia cerebellars myoclonica; Unverricht-Lundborg; cherry-red spot myoclonus syndrome; juvenile GM$_2$-gangliosidosis; juvenile metachromatic leukodystrophy; adrenoleukodystrophy; MPS III (Sanfilippo); juvenile ceroid lipofuscinosis (Batten-Speilmeyer-Vogt); atypical ceroid lipofuscinosis; SSPE; Huntington's chorea; hyppoparathyroidism and pseudohypoparathyroidism; tuberous sclerosis; acute intermittent porphyria

TABLE 22b. Diagnostic Features of Progressive Genetic-Metabolic Diseases in Relation to Clinical and Laboratory Manifestations

Skin Anomalies

Pigmented lesions: neurofibromatosis (café au lait spots, freckles, moles); tuberous sclerosis (depigmented spots, chagrin patches, adenoma sebacceum); neurocutaneous melanosis (giant hairy nevi); polyostotic fibrous dysplasia (large melanotic nevi with irregular edges); incontinentia pigmenti (pigmented swirls); xeroderma pigmentosum (freckles)

(Continued)

TABLE 22b. Diagnostic Features of Progressive Genetic-Metabolic Diseases in Relation to Clinical and Laboratory Manifestations (cont.)

Skin Anomalies (cont.)

Vascular lesions: Sturge-Weber; Wyburn-Mason (facial angioma inconstant); cutaneous spinal angiomatosis; disseminated neurocutaneous angiomatosis; ataxia-telangiectasia; leukodystrophy with meningeal angiomatosis (cutis marmorata universalis)

Discrete eruptive lesions: infantile Niemann-Pick (xanthomas, inconstant); fucosidosis, juvenile variant (angiokeratoma); Fabry's disease (angiokeratoma, belly, groins, buttocks especially); tuberous sclerosis (adenoma sebaceum, butterfly area); linear nevus sebaceous; nevus unis lateralis; incontinentia pigmenti (early stages, bullous, verrucous)

Hyperkeratotic lesions (ichthyosiform):   Refsum's disease; Sjögren-Larsson syndrome; trichopoliodystrophy (seborrheic dermatitis)

Discoloration of skin: Adrenoleukodystrophy (melanosis of adrenal insufficiency); Hallervorden-Spatz (melanosis, late inconstant); Niemann-Pick, infantile (brownish yellow); Farber's disease (brownish); Chediak-Higashi (partial albinism); trichopoliodystrophy (hypopigmentation)

Change in skin texture: MPS II (Hunter) (focal thickening in scalpular region); MPS IV (Morquio) (loose); GM_1-gangliosidosis (infantile) (loose, edematous); GM_3-gangliosidosis (loose); fucosidosis, infantile (thickened); tuberous sclerosis (chagrin patches); neurofibromatosis (localized hypertrophy and redundancy); Cockayne syndrome (thin, atrophic); xeroderma pigmentosum (thin, atrophic scarred)

Cutaneous neoplasms: tuberous sclerosis (molluscum pendulum, subungual fibromas); neurofibromatosis (fibromas, neurofibromas); neurocutaneous melanosis (melanomas); xeroderma pigmentosum (cutaneous carcinomas, melanomas)

Subcutaneous nodules: Neurofibromatosis; Farber's disease (periarticular); cerebrotendinous xanthomatosis (Achilles tendon)

Actinic changes, premature aging: xeroderma pigmentosum; Cockayne symdrome; ataxia-telangiectasia

Abnormality of sweating: Fabry's disease (decreased); fucosidosis, juvenile variant (decreased); fucosidosis, infantile variant (increased)

Hair Abnormality

MPS I, II, IV (hirsutism); GM_1-gangliosidosis, infantile variant (hirsutism of face); trichopoliodystrophy (pale, twisted, beaded, brittle, frayed ends); Chediak-Higashi (pale); ataxia-telangiectasis (premature graying); Cockayne (premature graying); progeria (premature graying)

Eye Abnormalities

Corneal opacity: MPS, all types, except Hunter; mucolipidosis II (inconstant); mucolipidosis III, IV; Fabry (slit-lamp only); Wilson's disease (Kayser-Fleischer ring); xeroderma pigmentosum (exposure kiratitsis)

Lens opacity: mannosidosis (slight); Wilson's disease (sunflowercataract, inconstant); cerebrotendinous xanthomatosis; Marinesco-Sjögren syndrome; galactosemia; Lowe's oculocerebrorenal syndrome

Glaucoma: MPS I (Scheie); Sturge-Weber (on same side as angioma)

Cherry-red spot: Tay-Sachs, types B, O, and AB; G_{M1}-gangliosidosis (infantile only) in 50% of cases; infantile Niemann-Pick disease in 50% of cases; metachromatic leukodystrophty with multiple sulfatase deficiency; Farber's disease (inconstant ?); cherry-red spot myoclonus variant of ceroid lipofuscinosis (CRS may fade); mucolipidosis I (not all variants)

Pigmentary degeneration of retina: ceroid lipofuscinosis, except adult (Kufs) and atypical types; MPS I-H, I-S, II (adult variant), III; abetalipoproteinemia (Bassen-Kornzweig); Refsum's disease (night blindness); Usher's syndrome (night blindness); juvenile spongy degeneration; Hallervorden-Spatz (not always); Kearns-Shy syndrome; Cockayne disease (note: eventually leads to optic atrophy and blindness)

Optic atrophy: All diseases with pigmentary degeneration of retina; Tay-Sachs disease; G_{M1}-gangliosidosis; Metachromatic leukodystrophy; Krabbe's disease; Pelizaeus-Merzbacher disease; adrenoleukodystrophy; spongy degeneration; glioneuronal dystrophy (Alper); neuroaxonal dystrophy; Leigh's disease (inconstant); olivepontocerebellar atrophy; Leber's disease; Freidreich's ataxia and other spinocerebellar degenerations (inconstant); polyostotic fibrous dysplasia; neurofibromatosis with optic glioma, other chronic brain tumors

Ophthalmoplegia (usually incomplete):   abetalipoproteinemia; ataxia-telangiectasia (oculomotor apraxia); Leigh's disease; infantile Gaucher; Niemann-Pick variant with vertical ophthalmoplegia

Nystagmus: GM_1-gangliosidosis; metachromatic leukodystrophy; Krabbe's disease; Pelizaeus-Merzbacher (very striking in classic type); Leigh's syndrome; Chediak-Higashi; spinocerebellar degenerations; neuroaxonal dystrophy (note: nystagmus in the primary position of gaze is present in most young children with poor vision)

TABLE 22b. Diagnostic Features of Progressive Genetic-Metabolic Diseases in Relation to Clinical and Laboratory Manifestations (cont.)

Eye Abnormalities (cont.)

Abnormal vessels: ataxia-telangiectasis, conjunctival; Fabry's disease, conjunctival and retinal

Visual loss without retinal findings: Lafora disease

Increased Intracranial Pressure

MPS I, II, VI, VII (due to hydrocephalus): Alexander's disease (hydrocephalus); mannosidosis; adrenoleukodystrophy; neoplasms in neurofibromatosis, tuberous sclerosis, Lindau-von Hippel; neurocutaneous melanosis
(hydrocephalus, melanomas); incontinentia pigmenti (rarely hydrocephalus)

Unusual Facies

All the MPS, except MPS III (Sanfilippo) early; mucolipidosis II; aspartylglucosaminuria (AGU); mannosidosis;
fucosidosis, infantile (inconstant); infantile GM_1-gangliosidosis; GM_3-gangliosidosis; cerebrohepato
renal syndrome; trichopoliodystrophy; Cockayne syndrome; polyostotic fibrous dysplasia; Sturge-Weber;
linear nevus sebaceous

Growth Anomalies

Dwarfing: MPS, all types except III (Sanfilippo); Mannosidosis; fucosidosis, juvenile type; Cockayne
syndrome; xeroderma pigmentosum (with endocrine dysfunction); ataxia-telangiectasia; Marinesco-
Sjögren syndrome; Lesch-Nyhan (note: all severe encephalopathies of early life lead to malnutrition
and stunted growth)

Failure to thrive: Wolman's disease; Niemann-Pick, infantile variant;
Cockayne syndrome; abetalipoproteinemia (Bassen-Kornzweig); cerebrohepatorenal syndrome (Zellweger);
trichopoliodystrophy (see note above)

Cardiovascular Pathology

Cardiomyopathy and/or conduction defect: Friedreich's ataxia (early); atypical spinocerebellar degenerations
(inconstant); Refsum's disease; abetalipoproteinemia (late); fucosidosis, infantile variant;
glycogenosis type I (Pompe); tuberous sclerosis (hamartomas)

Valvular pathology: mucopolysaccharidosis, most types

Coronary artery disease: Fabry's disease; Cockayne syndrome

Cerebrovascular disease (strokes): Fabry's disease; infantile Gaucher; trichopoliodystrophy; sudanophilic
leukodystrophy with meningeal angiomatosis; Cockayne syndrome

Other Visceral Involvement

Lung infiltrates: Niemann-Pick (several variants); Gaucher, juvenile nonneuropathic form; tuberous
sclerosis (honeycomb lesions)

Renal: Fabry's disease (renal failure); Lesch-Nyhan (stones); tuberous sclerosis (phakomas, cystadenomas)
cerebrohepatorenal syndrome (cysts); Lindau-von Hippel (polycystic kidneys); metachromatic leuko
dystrophy (no clinical signs); mucopolysaccharidoses (no clinical signs); GM_1-gangliosidosis (no clinical
signs); mucolipidosis (no clinical signs)

Gastrointestinal: abetalipoproteinemia (malabsorption); Wolman's disease (malabsorption); metachromatic leukodystrophy (nonfunctioning gallbladder); fucosidosis, infantile (nonfunctioning gallbladder);
neurofibromatosis (tumors of the gastric and/or intestinal wall); cerebrohepatorenal syndrome
(cirrhosis); Niemann-Pick, infantile (jaundice); Wilson's disease (cirrhosis)

Enlarged nodes: Farber's disease; Niemann-Pick; nonneuropathic Gaucher; Chediak-Higashi; ataxia-telangiectasisia
(lymphomas)

Enlarged tonsils: Tangier disease (orange)

Endocrine dysfunctionj: adrenoleukodystrophy (adrenal insufficiency); Wolman's disease (adrenal calcification);
dysplasia (precocious puberty in girls); neurofibromatosis (pheochromocytoma, precocious puberty);
xeroderma pigmentosum (gonadal hypoplasia) (not all families)

Hernias: mucopolysaccharidoses; mucolipidoses, type II mostly

Abnormal Skull

Macrocephaly: Tay-Sachs disease (after age 1½ years); spongy degeneration) Alexander's disease (megalencephaly
and/or hydrocephalus); MPS I, II, VI, and VII (hydrocephalus)

(Continued)

TABLE 22b. Diagnostic Features of Progressive Genetic–Metabolic Diseases in Relation to Clinical and Laboratory Manifestations (cont.)

Abnormal Skull (cont.)

Thickened skull: MPS III (Sanfilippo); aspartylglucosaminuria (AGU); polyostotic fibrous dysplasia

Microcephaly: Krabbe's disease; infantile variant of ceroid lipofuscinosis; incontinentia pigmenti; glioneuronal dystrophy (Alper); neurosaxonal dystrophy; Cockayne disease; hypophosphatasia (cranio synotosis with osteoid in sutures)

Intracranial calcification: tuberous sclerosis; familial calcification of basal ganglia; hypo parathyroidism and pseudohypoparathyroidism; Sturge-Weber syndrome ("trolley tracks"); Cockayne disease; intrauterine infection; phakomatoses with intracranial neoplasms

Hearing Loss

MPS I (Hurler); MPS II (Hunter); MPS III (Sanfilippo); MPS IV (Morquio) mucolipidosis I (inconstant); metachromatic leukodystrophy with multiple sulfatase deficiency; adrenoleukodystrophy; neurofibromatosis with bilateral acoustic neurinomas; polyostotic fibrous dysplasia (Albright); trichopoliodystrophy; Cockayne syndrome; Refsum's disease; Usher's syndrome (profound, congenital); Sjögren-Larsson syndrome; atypical spinocerebellar degenerations; Leigh's syndrome (inconstant); xeroderma pigmentosum (inconstant); neuroaxonal dystrophy

Compression of Spinal Cord

Neurofibromatosis with intraspinal neurofibromas; MPS IV (Morquio); MPS VI (Maroteaux-Lamy); Lesch-Nyhan (occasionally); dystonia musculorum deformans (occasionally)

Kyphosis and/or Scoliosis

Freidreich's ataxia and other spinocerebellar degenerations; ataxia-telangiectasia; abetalipoproteinemia; dystonia musculorum deformans; MPS (all types); mucolipidosis II and III; Cockayne syndrome; neuro fibromatosis (note: all advanced encephalopathies and conditions leading to severe motor signs or immobility can produce a scoliosis)

Foot Deformities

Freidreich's ataxia and other spinocerebellar degenerations; Hallervorden-Spatz syndrome; dystonia weakness of intrinsic muscles will result in foot and hand deformities)

Neuropathy

Mucopolysaccharidoses, entrapment neuropathy in types I, II, VI, mucolipidoses I and III; metachromatic leukodystrophy; Fabry's disease (painful); infantile Krabbe; infantile Niemann-Pick; neuroaxonal dystrophy; Refsum's disease; Tangier disease; abetalipoproteinemia; Lévy-Roussy syndrome; Leigh's syndrome (not always) spongy degeneration (mild, inconstant); acute intermittent porphyria; ataxia-telangiectasia; Chediak-Higashi (inconstant)

Increased Spinal Fluid Protein

Metachromatic leukodystrophy; Krabbe; Farber's disease; Refsum's disease; adrenoleukodystrophy (inconsistant); acute intermittent porphyria (inconstant); Friedreich's ataxia (inconstant); atypical spinocerebellar ataxia (inconstant)

Predilection for Jewish Children

Classic Tay-Sachs disease (type B only); juvenile Gaucher's disease; Niemann-Pick disease ? (infantile type only); mucolipidosis IV ?; spongy degeneration; dystonia musculorum deformans (recessive type); dysautonomia

Sex-linked Recessive Inheritance

MPS II (Hunter) (both types); Pelizaeus-Merzbacher (late infantile; infantile?); trichopoliodystrophy; adrenoleukodystrophy (Schilder's disease); Fabry's disease; Lesch-Nyhan syndrome; Alexander's disease ? ; Leber's disease ?

MUCOPOLYSACCHARIDOSES

The mucopolysaccharidoses (see also p. 751) are disorders of glycoprotein and lipoprotein breakdown that affect virtually all body tissues, including the nervous system, to a variable extent.

BIOCHEMISTRY.   The mucopolysaccharides are complex glycoproteins that are particularly actively synthesized in connective tissue. Different tissues synthesize different species of mucopolysaccharides, which in part accounts for the variability of symptoms among the various disorders. Mucopolysaccharides are made up of a linear protein backbone to which long chains with repeating carbohydrate units are attached, usually to serine by xylose and two galactoses (trisaccharide linkage). To this linkage is attached a long chain of repeating disaccharide units, consisting of a uronic acid and an amino sugar for most mucopolysaccharides (galactose and amino sugar for keratan sulfate). Most, but not all, repeating units are sulfated, and the site of attachment and number of sulfates per unit vary. Two types of lysosomal enzymes appear to be deficient in the mucopolysaccharides: sulfatases, which cleave sulfate residues from the carbohydrate moieties, and exoglycosidases, which break the bonds between successive hexose units. The classifications used here are those proposed by McKusick.

LYSOSOMAL DISORDERS. The mucopolysaccharidoses, sphingolipidoses, and other neuronal storage diseases are considered to be lysosomal disorders. Lysosomes are membrane-bound intracellular organelles that contain acid hydrolases—enzymes that facilitate the catabolism of complex molecules that are products of the cell's metabolism (autophagy) or products of exogenous materials taken up by the cell. In lysosomal storage diseases the deficiency of one hydrolase results in a block in catabolism and the accumulation of undigested materials in greatly distended lysosomes. There materials usually include not only the one substrate that cannot be degraded but other more distantly related compounds. Nonspecific secondary increases or decreases of other lysosomal hydrolases are quite common in lysosomal storage diseases. For example, a nonspecific severe decrease of β-galactosidase is found in many of the mucopolysaccharidoses. The concentrations of hydrolases differ in various tissues; thus lack of a particular hydrolase will have different consequences in different tissues. For example, virtually no histologic abnormalities are noted in extracerebral tissues in Tay-Sachs disease.

ENZYMES IN LYSOSOMAL DISEASES. It is thought that most storage diseases are not due to complete failure to synthesize the enzyme protein but rather to mutation of a structural or regulatory gene that results in the synthesis of an inactive enzyme. Several allelic mutations may occur, and they may result in the synthesis of several different deficient enzymes that can often be separated by properties such as temperature stability, electrophoretic mobility, substrate affinity, and pH optimum. When two diseases that are clinically and genetically distinct appear to have an identical enzymatic defect, such as Hurler's disease and Scheie's disease, subtle differences between enzymes must be sought. In general, variants of diseases with less severely deficient enzymatic activity tend to start later in childhood and to run a slower course.

TISSUE CULTURE AND CORRECTIVE FACTORS. One of the advances that had a profound effect on the elucidation of the mucopolysaccharidoses was the discovery by Danes and Bearn in 1965 that fibroblasts of patients with mucopolysaccharidosis exhibit a pink metachromasia in tissue culture when stained with toluidine blue and that this metachromasia is due to an accumulation of excess mucopolysaccharides in their cytoplasm. A series of metabolic studies was then undertaken, and in 1968 Fratantoni and associates made the crucial observation that when fibroblasts from patients with Hurler's disease and patients

with Hunter's disease are grown together in a mixed culture, neither shows the expected metachromasia and neither accumulates radiolabeled sulfated compounds as each does when grown independently. They extended these observations to other mucopolysaccharide disorders and showed that this correction was due to factors secreted by the fibroblasts into the culture medium. Fibroblasts and urine from normal individuals were found to contain these corrective factors, which later were shown to be active enzyme proteins that enter the cells, replace the missing enzyme activity, and enable normal catabolism of the accumulated mucopolysaccharides to take place. This cell system was used to investigate the various mucopolysaccharide syndromes. It can be stated with confidence that 2 patients whose fibroblasts cross-correct each other are suffering from different diseases with different enzyme defects. Fibroblasts of individuals heterozygotic for each of the autosomal recessive mucopolysaccharide genes are metachromatic in tissue culture and thus are not easily distinguished from those of homozygotes. Detection of heterozygotes by demonstrating levels of enzyme activity intermediate between those of normals and those of homozygotes appears to be possible.

DISORDERS AFFECTING MULTIPLE HYDROLASES. Fibroblasts isolated from patients with mucolipidosis, or I cell disease (a disease resembling a mucopolysaccharidosis but without the mucopolysacchariduria), are characterized by severe intracellular deficiency of multiple hydrolases and marked excess of these hydrolases in the culture medium. Enzyme synthesis could not be deficient in these cells, and currently I cell disease is considered to be related to deficient enzymatic uptake into lysosomes.

The following subsections provide a brief description of the mucopolysaccharidosis (MPS) syndromes that particularly affect the nervous system; those that do not have significant neurologic manifestations are discussed in Chapter 14. The differentiating features are presented in Table 23.

MPS TYPE I (A-L-IDURONIDASE DEFICIENCY). At least three syndromes can be attributed to a deficiency of α-L-iduronidase. MPS type I-H, or Hurler's disease, is one of the most common and severe of the MPS syndromes. MPS type I-S, or Scheie's disease, is one of the least severe and is genetically, if not enzymatically, distinct. Total urinary mucopolysaccharides are normally less than 15 mg/24hours (approximately 90 percent chondroitin sulfate, 8 percent heparan sulfate, 1 percent dermatan sulfate, 1 percent keratan sulfate and hyaluronic acid). In MPS total excretion usually exceeds 100 mg/24 hours. Dermatan sulfate and heparan sulfate are increased in both syndromes, with dermatan sulfate exceeding heparan sulfate by a ratio of 2 to 1 in most patients with type I MPS. Both heparan sulfate and dermatan sulfate are stored in the viscera; both contain L-iduronic acid, which explains why the deficiency of α-L-iduronidase (which cleaves L-iduronic acid from the adjacent amino sugar) results in a catabolic block and the accumulation of both. When grown together in tissue culture, skin fibroblasts of patients with MPS type I-H and MPS type I-S do not cross-

TABLE 23. Mucopolysaccharidoses: Differential Features*

Type	Enzymatic Defect	Urinary MPS†	Death (years)	Dwarfing	Skeletal Anomalies	Abnormal Facies	Cloudy Corneas	Hearing Loss	Organomegaly	Heart Disease	Mental Retardation	Other CNS Signs	Other Features
I Hunter	α-L-iduronidase	H,D	<10	+++	+++	+++	+++	++	+++	+++	+++	Hydrocephalus	Hypertrichosis, hernias, stiff joints
I Scheie	α-L-iduronidase	H,D	>40	±	±	±	+++ (peripheral)	±	±	±	0	Entrapment neuropathies	Retinitis pigmentosa, wide mouth
I-H/S	α-L-iduronidase	H,D	Adult	+	++	++	+++		++	+	±	Hydrocephalus, entrapment neuropathies	Stiff joints
II Hunter, severe form	Sulfoiduronidosulfatase	H,D	10–20	++	++	++	0	+++	+	±	+	Hydrocephalus	*Sex-linked recessive*, nodular skin, hirsutism
II Hunter, mild form	Sulfoiduronidosulfatase	H,D	>60	±	±	±	0	++	±	±	0	Entrapment neuropathies	*Sex-linked recessive*, nodular skin, retinitis pigmentosa
III Sanfilippo A	Heparan sulfate sulfaminidase	H	10–20+	0	+	±	0	++	+	+	+++	Varied	Retinal degeneration, thick skull, stiff joints
III Sanfilippo B	N-acetyl-α-d-glucosaminidase	H	10–20+	0	+	±	0	++	+	+	+++	Varied	Retinal degeneration, thick skull, stiff joints

Type	Enzymatic Defect	Urinary MPS†	Death (years)	Dwarfing	Skeletal Anomalies	Abnormal Facies	Cloudy Corneas	Hearing Loss	Organo-megaly	Heart Disease	Mental Retarda-tion	Other CNS Signs	Other Features
IV Morquio (? 2 types)	Chondroitin sulfate, N-acetyl hexo-samine 6-sulfate sulfatase	K	Adult	+++	+++	±	++	++	±	++	0	Cord compression	Lax joints, atlanto-occipital dislocation
VI Maroteaux-Lamy, severe form	Arylsulfatase B (chondroitin sulfate, N-acetyl galacto-samine, 4-sulfate sulfatase)	D	>20	++	++	++	++ (peripheral)	+	±	++	0	Cord compression, entrapment neuropathies, hydrocephalus	Coarse metachromatic granules in WBC joints
VI Maroteaux-Lamy, mild form	?	D	Adult	+	+	±	±			+	0	Cord compression, entrapment neuropathies	Coarse metachromatic granules in WBC
VII β-Glucuronidase deficiency (? 2 types)	β-Glucuronidase	D? K-S?	?	++	++	+	±		+		++	Hydrocephalus	Metachromatic granules in WBC, puffy hands and feet, hernias

*0 = absent; ± = inconsistent; + = mild; ++ = moderate; +++ = severe; blank = no data.
†H = heparan sulfate, D = dermatan sulfate, K = keratan sulfate, K-S = chondroitin 4 and / or 6 sulfate.

correct each other; by this criterion the two corrective factors (enzymes) are identical.

MPS TYPE I-H (HURLER'S DISEASE). MPS type I-H, an autosomal recessive disorder, has no racial predilection. The phenotype is quite constant, and the majority of patients can be identified at a glance (see Fig. 17, p. 753). Signs and symptoms appear during the first year and are progressive, with death before the age of 10 years, usually from cardiac involvement. Mental retardation is severe in most cases, especially in patients who develop hydrocephalus because of leptomeningeal thickening or the formation of an arachnoidal cyst. Most children learn to walk, but few speak. Seizures are not a feature of the illness. Diffuse corneal opacity is progressive and eventually leads to severe visual loss, in some cases complicated by retinal degeneration. Conductive hearing loss is common. While patients grow rapidly during the first year of life, bony deformities lead to severe dwarfing by 3 years, although hands and feet tend to remain disproportionately broad and thick. A lumbar gibbus appears before 1 year, and impaired joint mobility with periarticular swelling and claw hands develops. Hepatomegaly and abdominal distension are severe. Umbilical and inguinal hernias, diffuse hypertrichosis, and bushy eyebrows are characteristic features. The facies becomes grotesque, with frontal bossing, hypertelorism, coarse lips, enlarged tongue, open mouth, and constant rhinorrhea. The teeth are peg-shaped and widely spaced, and they erupt late. Respiratory infections are common. The heart enlarges progressively; valvular disease and coronary occlusion by stored MPS in the adventitia are frequent causes of death.

Characteristic changes that may be seen radiographically occur in most bones; they include a J-shaped or enlarged sella, beaked wedge-shaped lumbar vertebrae at the apex of the gibbus, wing-shaped tapering ilia, distended peg-shaped metacarpals, spatulate ribs, genu valgum, coxa vara, and many others. Tests for mucopolysacchariduria, metachromatic granules in white blood cells and in plasma cells in the bone marrow, and metachromasia of cultured fibroblasts are helpful. The definitive test is the demonstration of α-L-iduronidase deficiency in skin fibroblasts or other tissues. A nonspecific but marked and consistent decrease in β-galactosidase is also found.

The characteristic pathologic feature is the presence of innumerable clear vacuoles in enlarged gargoyle cells, which may be parenchymal cells (such as hepatocytes) or connective tissue cells (such as fibroblasts or macrophages) (Fig. 41A). Storage occurs in virtually all tissues and results in severe organomegaly or distortion, as in bone. Marked increase in collagen accompanied by fibrosis may occur, as in heart valves and periarticular tissues. In the brain, perivascular spaces are distended by mucopolysaccharide-filled perithelial cells. Neurons are ballooned by pleomorphic glycolipid inclusions, with relatively few mucopolysaccharide inclusions. Ultrastructural examination reveals characteristic membrane-bound inclusions consisting of stacked membranes grouped into prominent transverse bands (zebra bodies) or granulomembranous amorphous

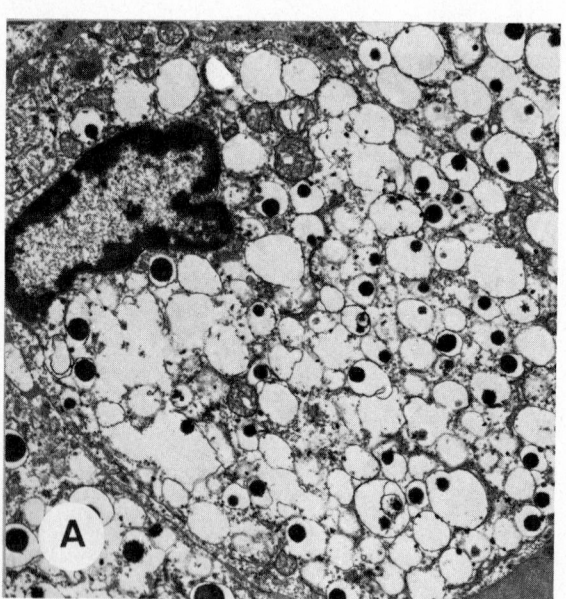
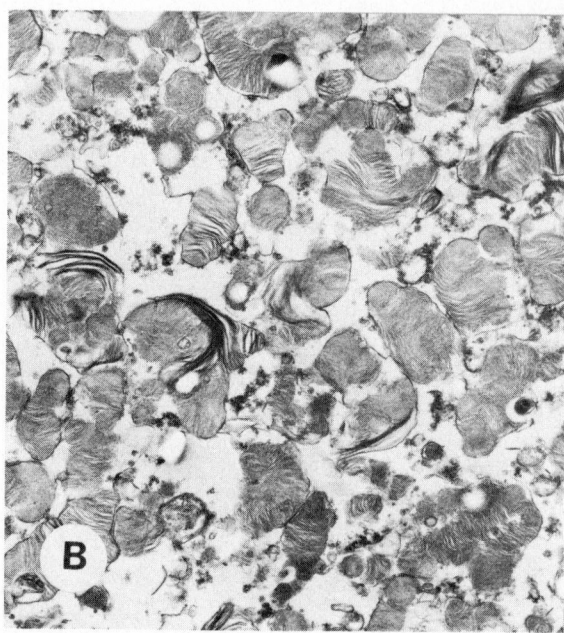

FIG. 41. Hurler's disease A. Endothelial cell from the spleen showing numerous membrane-bound clear vacuoles in the cytoplasm, presumably filled with soluble mucopolysaccharide (electronmicrograph, X11,000) B. Neuron from the cerebral cortex filled with Zebra bodies, stacked membranes, and other inclusions (X21,000). (Courtesy of Dr. K. Suzuki.)

deposits (Fig. 41B). No specific treatment is available. Corneal grafts are usually unsuccessful because they become clouded. Shunting to relieve hydrocephalus has been performed in some children and perhaps should be used more frequently to retard the dementia.

MPS TYPE I-S (SCHEIE'S DISEASE). MPS type I-S (formerly MPS type V), which at this time cannot be distinguished from Hurler's disease by enzymatic criteria, is quite different clinically and is the least severe of the MPS syndromes. It is also autosomal recessive and about one-fifth as frequent as Hurler's disease. The patients are not dwarfed and do not demonstrate the grotesque facies of other MPS syndromes, but they have a characteristic broad mouth. They develop cloudy corneas (which may spare the center of the cornea and therefore may not interfere with vision for many years), retinal pigmentary degeneration, and eventually glaucoma. Compression neuropathies leading to carpal tunnel syndromes and clawing of the hands are common. Aortic regurgitation has been described in several patients. Intelligence is usually unaffected, and bony changes are quite unimpressive. Life expectancy is uncertain, but some patients have reached adulthood and have had normal children.

Diagnosis is based on the urinary excretion of dermatan sulfate and heparan sulfate in the proportion 70:30 and the demonstration of a lack of α-L-iduronidase activity. Therapy is symptomatic; corneal grafts have been attempted, but clouding of the graft is likely to occur. Genetic counseling and information regarding the probability of visual and cardiac handicaps are in order.

MPS TYPE I-H/S. Patients with MPS type I-H/S are thought to be heterozygous for both the I-H and I-S genes. Their phenotype is intermediate between those of patients with Hurler's disease and patients with Scheie's disease. They are not severely dwarfed, but they do have bony deformities, grotesque facies, corneal clouding, claw hands, and decreased joint mobility. They survive at least into their twenties and are not severely demented. One of these patients developed an arachnoidal cyst and evidence of hydrocephalus. The defect in these patients' fibroblasts is corrected by neither the Hurler nor the Scheie corrective factor. They have a deficit in α-L-iduronidase.

MPS TYPE II (HUNTER'S SYNDROME, L-IDURONOSULFATE SULFATASE DEFICIENCY). Hunter's syndrome is inherited as a sex-linked recessive trait. The nervous system is less severely affected than in MPS Type I; the syndrome is discussed further in Chapter 14. There is a defect in L-iduronosulfate sulfatase, which cleaves the sulfate group from sulfated iduronic acid in the terminal position. Both dermatan sulfate and heparan sulfate have sulfated iduronic acids in terminal positions; therefore both accumulate and are excreted in the urine.

MPS TYPE III (SANFILIPPO'S SYNDROME). MPS type III, or Sanfilippo's syndrome (see also p. 752), which presents clinically as a single phenotype, has recently been found to exist in at least two forms with genetic heterogeneity. All patients excrete large amounts of heparan sulfate in the urine, but cross-cor-

rection studies in cultured fibroblasts indicate two different enzymatic defects. In one group (Sanfilippo A) the patients are deficient in heparan sulfate sulfamidase, an enzyme that cleaves a sulfate group linked to the amino group of glucosamine. Patients in the other group (Sanfilippo B) are deficient in N-acetyl-α-D-glucosaminidase, which cleaves N-acetyl-α-D-glucosamine groups from heparan sulfate. The reason patients with Sanfilippo's disease do not excrete excessive dermatan sulfate is that the amino sugar involved is N-acetylgalactosamine, not glucosamine as is the case in heparan sulfate.

SANFILIPPO A AND B. Both forms of Sanfilippo's disease are transmitted as autosomal recessive traits. These children appear normal at birth, and they walk and speak at a normal age. Behavior deteriorates during the preschool years. Dementia becomes evident soon thereafter and progresses rapidly. By 10 to 12 years of age these children are essentially mute, but they remain ambulatory for several more years and show only mild somatic anomalies, although hearing loss is common by midchildhood. They may develop mild dorsal gibbus, some limitation of joint mobility (particularly claw hands), and stiff gait. Mild hepatomegaly is common. While most have no cardiac involvement, severe involvement of the heart valves can occur. The facies coarsens during the second decade and eventually resembles that of the other MPS syndromes. Only the second dentition is affected. The neurologic signs that have been reported include seizures, mild athetosis and tremors, and progressive spastic diplegia. Death usually occurs at the end of the second decade, but it may occur earlier.

Urinary excretion of heparan sulfate and characteristic clusters of metachromatic granules in lymphocytes suggest the diagnosis, which can be confirmed by appropriate enzymatic tests. According to Kresse, detection of heterozygotes is possible in type A, and findings in cultured amniotic cells indicate that intrauterine diagnosis will be possible. Storage of both mucopolysaccharide and glycolipid and distended lysosomes are seen in most organs, including the brain. No therapy is available beyond management of the severe behavior abnormality and family counseling.

MPS TYPE IV (MORQUIO'S DISEASE). McKusick has suggested that two variants of MPS type IV may exist, one with keratanuria and one without. A deficit of the enzyme chondroitin sulfate N-acetylhexosamine sulfate sulfatase has recently been found. This deficit confirms the diagnosis made from the distinct clinical and radiographic findings.

Although these children appear normal at birth, a lumbar gibbus and mild hepatosplenomegaly may be noted in infancy and may suggest Hurler's disease. Early development is normal. At 2 to 3 years awkward gait, flaring ribs, or growth failure may develop. A slit-lamp examination may reveal the corneal haze that usually becomes dense by the end of the second decade, when hearing loss is also likely. Bony abnormalities become severe, and growth ceases completely after 6 to 7 years, leading to severe dwarfing. The patient has a prominent pectus carinatum and thoracic kyphosis. The joints are misshapen, but excess laxity of the joints leads to instability. The hips and knees are severely affected; coxa valga and eventual disappearance and dislocation of the femoral head are common. Severe genu valgum, flat feet, and a crouching posture develop. Hyperlaxity of ligaments and anomalies of the odontoid process lead to the life-threatening complication of cord compression by atlanto-occipital dislocation and luxation of the odontoid peg. Most children with this syndrome develop a spastic paraparesis, which may become a paraplegia or tetraplegia, with urinary retention. Sudden death from intubation for surgery or from hyperextension of the neck during a fall, or even during sleep, has occurred in several cases.

The facies may show only minor abnormalities, although snuffy breathing and an open mouth are common. The teeth are widely spaced and have defective enamel. Mild hirsutism, loose skin, and telangiectasias have been described. Respiratory failure caused by the spinal and chest deformities is common. Many patients have aortic regurgitation. Radiographs show distinctive changes, especially in the spine. In the early stages the thoracic vertebrae have an ovoid shape, which is later replaced by severe platyspondyly. The ilium is flared and is constricted above the acetabulum. Phalanges, metacarpals, and metatarsals are widened and have tapering ends. Tubular bones are widened and deformed.

In therapy, supportive care and correction of deformities are in order. Particular attention must be given to the stability of the spine; if surgical therapy is undertaken, attention must be given to the dangers of hyperextending the neck during intubation. Adequate hearing aids, educational and vocational opportunities, and supportive counseling are essential for these intellectually intact patients. This disorder is inherited as an autosomal recessive, and females have a somewhat better prognosis than males.

MPS TYPE V. The former designation MPS type V has been changed to MPS type I-S (Scheie's disease) (p. 1903).

MPS TYPE VI (MAROTEAUX-LAMY SYNDROME). MPS type VI, an autosomal recessive disorder, is characterized by severe bony deformities and retention of normal intelligence. The children excrete predominantly dermatan sulfate in the urine. Preliminary reports suggest that there may be a deficiency of arylsulfatase B in the severe form of this syndrome, but details of the biochemical disorder remain to be worked out. Two forms of the disease are known, and according to McKusick, cross-correction between them suggests that they are not allelic.

MPS TYPE VI-A (SEVERE FORM). These children manifest bony deformities in early life and resemble children with Hurler's disease, except for their more benign course and preserved intelligence. They may develop hydrocephalus and require shunts; like patients with MPS type IV they run the risk of sudden cord compression or death from cervical spine subluxation. Most suffer from a progressive spastic paraparesis, presumably on a spinal cord basis. They also suffer from entrapment neuropathies and the carpal tunnel syndrome. They have corneal clouding that is often more dense at the periphery. Other features are similar to those of MPS type I (p. 1899).

The diagnosis is based on the finding of particularly coarse metachromatic inclusions (Alder-Reilley bodies) that are found in 100 percent of their neutrophils and 50 percent of their lymphocytes, on the fact that they excrete dermatan sulfate, and on the characteristic radiographs. Treatment is symptomatic; genetic counseling is mandatory, and it will be facilitated when definitive enzymatic tests become available.

MPS TYPE VI-B (MILD FORM). Several adults have been described who excrete predominantly dermatan sulfate and have radiographic findings similar to, but milder than, those of MPS type VI-A. They are not intellectually affected; corneal clouding is slight and dwarfing is mild, but entrapment neuropathies and cord compression due to cervical or odontoid dislocation may occur.

MPS TYPE VII (B-GLUCURONIDASE DEFICIENCY). Patients with increased urinary excretion of chondroitin-4-sulfate and chondroitin-6-sulfate and decreased activity of the enzyme β-glucuronidase in the white cells have not been classified. Severe cases have presented in infancy with features of Hurler's disease (p. 1899).

MUCOLIPIDOSES

The term mucolipidoses was proposed by Spranger and Wiedemann to encompass those disorders that are characterized by storage of both polysaccharides and glycolipids. They share many features with the MPS syndromes, except that mucopolysacchariduria is not a feature. Spranger and Wiedemann included GM_1 gangliosidosis, the MLD variant with multiple sulfatase deficiency, fucosidosis, mannosidosis, three syndromes named mucolipidosis I (lipomucopolysaccharidosis or Gal+ disease), mucolipidosis II (I cell disease), and mucolipidosis III (pseudo-Hurler polydystrophy), Farber's disease (ceramidase deficiency), and aspartylglucosaminuria. GM_1 gangliosidosis, the MLD variant, and Farber's disease are discussed in the section on the sphingolipidoses (p. 1906). Table 24 summarizes the differential features of these disorders.

MUCOLIPIDOSIS I (GAL+ DISEASE). Mucolipidosis I is an autosomal recessive disorder with mild Hurler-like symptoms, moderate mental retardation, and metachromatic inclusions in fibroblasts and white blood cells. There is increased β-galactosidase activity (hence Gal+ disease) and other hydrolases in the liver.

MUCOLIPIDOSIS II (I CELL DISEASE). Mucolipidosis II, an autosomal recessive disorder, is characterized by intracellular deficiency of multiple hydrolases that appear in great excess in serum, urine, spinal fluid, and fibroblast culture medium. High levels in the plasma of arylsulfatase A hexosaminidase and β-glucuronidase suggest the diagnosis, especially if they are associated with a deficiency of β-galactosidase in skin fibroblasts. The disease presents with the features of Hurler's disease without mucopolysacchariduria

TABLE 24. Mucolipidoses: Differential Features

	Enzymatic Defect	Storage	Death (years)	Dwarfing	Skeletal Anomalies	Abnormal Facies	Cloudy Corneas	Skin	Organomegaly	Heart Disease	Mental Retardation
I Gal+	?	?	Adult	±	±	±	0		±	+	++
II I cell, infantile type	Multiple hydrolases ↑ extracellularly ↓ intracellularly	?	<8	+++	+++	+++	±	Tight, rough	++	++	+++
II I cell, juvenile type	Same	?	Adult	±	±	±	±		+	+	±
III Pseudo-Hurler dystrophy	Same	?	Adult	++	++	±	+			+	±
IV	?	?	?	0	0	0	+++	0	0	0	+++
Aspartylglucosaminuria	Aspartylglucosaminidase	?	Adult	+	+	++	0				++
Mannosidosis	α-Mannosidase	Mannose-containing glycolipids and glycoproteins	Childhood	+	+	+	0		±		+
Fucosidosis, infantile	α-Fucosidase	Fucose-containing glycolipids and glycoproteins	<6	0	+	±	0	Thick	+	+	+++
Fucosidosis, chronic	α-Fucosidase	Same	20	0	+	+	0	Angiokeratoma			++
MLD-MSD*	Multiple sulfatases	Sulfatides + MPS	<12	±	+	+	0	Ichthyosis	+		++
GM_1-gangliosidosis, infantile variant	β-galactosidase A, B, C	GM_1-ganglioside oligosaccharides	2	++	++	+++	0	Thick, rough	++	+	+++
GM_1-gangliosidosis, late infantile variant	β-galactosidase B and C ?	GM_1-ganglioside oligosaccharides	10	0	±	±	0	0	0	0	+++
Farber's disease	Ceramidase	Ceramide, GM_3-ganglioside, and MPS	2 (? rarely adolescence)	0	+	0	0	Subcutaneous nodules	±		++

*Metachromatic leukodystrophy, multiple sulfatase deficiency

(p. 1899) and striking refractile nonmetachromatic inclusions in fibroblasts (inclusion cells or I cells).

MUCOLIPIDOSIS III (PSEUDO-HURLER DYSTROPHY). Mucolipidosis III, an autosomal recessive disorder, is characterized by early and severe restriction of joint mobility, dwarfing, and hip dysplasia. Facial abnormalities and mental retardation are mild or absent, and patients have prolonged survival.

ASPARTYLGLUCOSAMINURIA. Aspartylglucosaminuria, a progressive autosomal recessive disorder, has recently been recognized in Finland as one of the more common causes of mental retardation in patients with coarse features. The diagnosis can be made from excessive amounts of aspartylglucosamine in the urine. A deficiency of aspartylglucosaminidase has been found in homozygotes and intermediate values in heterozygotes. These children, who appear normal at birth, progressively develop a characteristic facies, with thick lips and broad nose with anteverted nostrils. Mental deficiency, which is present from early life, progresses slowly and in adults is often complicated by episodes of agitation and psychotic behavior. Hypotonia, clumsiness, and defective speech are often presenting symptoms. Bony changes consist of thickening of the skull, thinning of the cortex of the long bones, and flattening of the vertebrae. Lymphocytes and bone marrow histiocytes are vacuolated. Biopsies show large clear lysosomal inclusions in hepatocytes and in kidney glomerular and tubular epithelium. Smaller and darker inclusions are noted in the liver and neurons. Specific chemical abnormalities have yet to be defined.

MANNOSIDOSIS. Children with mannosidosis have coarse features, slight hepatosplenomegaly, and psychomotor retardation. After 2 years growth slows, the tongue enlarges, and lumbar kyphosis and prominent forehead develop. The corneas are clear, but there are mild opacities in the lens. Urinary excretion of mucopolysaccharides is at the upper limit of normal; IgG is low, and IgM and IgA are virtually absent. Vacuolization of lymphocytes has been striking in all reported cases. The enzymatic defect, profound deficiency of α-mannosidase, leads to accumulation of mannose-containing oligosaccharides. There is no increase in mucopolysaccharides or glycolipids in liver or brain. Deficiency of α-mannosidase A and B can be demonstrated in cultured skin fibroblasts.

FUCOSIDOSIS. Two variants of fucosidosis have been described: an infantile variant with features of mucopolysaccharidoses and a juvenile variant resembling Fabry's disease. They seem to be due to drastic reduction of the enzyme α-L-fucosidase, which cleaves fucose from various glycopeptides and oligosaccharides. The infantile variant appears to be inherited as an autosomal recessive trait and becomes clinically evident before 2 years of age. These children lose developmental milestones and become hypotonic and later spastic and decorticate. They may have some features of mucopolysaccharidoses (Table 23), thick skin with abundant sweating, an enlarged heart, and mild hepatosplenomegaly. Their gall bladders become nonfunctional, and sweat electrolytes are elevated. Vacuolated

lymphocytes are seen, but not mucopolysacchariduria. Death occurs between 3.5 and 5 years of age. The juvenile (chronic) variant also becomes evident in infancy and early childhood, with regression in developmental milestones and the appearance of anhydrosis and punctate skin lesions resembling the angiokeratoma seen in Fabry's disease. Coarse facial features without corneal clouding, bony lesions, and dwarfism reminiscent of Morquio's disease develop. These children are totally disabled before school age, but they usually survive into their twenties.

SPHINGOLIPIDOSES

The sphingolipidoses are disorders of metabolism that are due to a block in the catabolism of complex lipid molecules because of lack of activity of a specific lysosomal enzyme (acid hydrolase). This results in accumulation of the nondegradable compound in lysosomes, which become massively distended. The distended lysosomes may interfere with the function of the cell, or they may leak or burst and release their hydrolytic enzymes into the cell cytoplasm and thus damage or kill the cell. Other consequences of the metabolic derangement may be production of abnormal membranes that alter the electrophysiologic properties of neurons or accumulation of a toxic product of intermediary metabolism that interferes with cellular function.

The symptoms and signs of a particular metabolic disorder depend on the tissue in which the blocked metabolic pathway is most active and on the rate of turnover of the involved compounds. Some pathways (eg, myelin formation and turnover) are not active until the last trimester of gestation. Myelination proceeds rapidly during the third trimester of gestation and the first 2 years of life, then slows down during childhood and adolescence. The concentrations of enzymes required for myelin turnover are very low until just before myelination starts. In the adult, myelin is very stable and turns over very slowly. Thus in Krabbe's leukodystrophy (galactosylceramide lipidosis), lack of cerebroside β-galactosidase blocks the breakdown of cerebroside, a major component of myelin; it produces almost no histologic lesions in the brain of a fetus, but it becomes clinically apparent some months after birth and is incompatible with survival for more than 1 to 2 years. In general, the more complete the metabolic block and enzyme deficiency, the earlier the illness becomes apparent and the more severe its course.

PREVENTION AND GENETIC COUNSELING. Perhaps the most encouraging development concerning these diseases is the ability to detect affected heterozygote carriers, make an intrauterine diagnosis, and abort affected fetuses, thus sparing families from bearing a second child whom they will helplessly have to watch regress and die. For rare disorders with no ethnic predilection, genetic counseling and monitoring of pregnancies at risk are limited to those families who have already produced an affected homozygous child (or hemizygous in the case of a sex-linked recessive

SCHEMATIC PATHWAYS FOR SPHINGOLIPID CATABOLISM

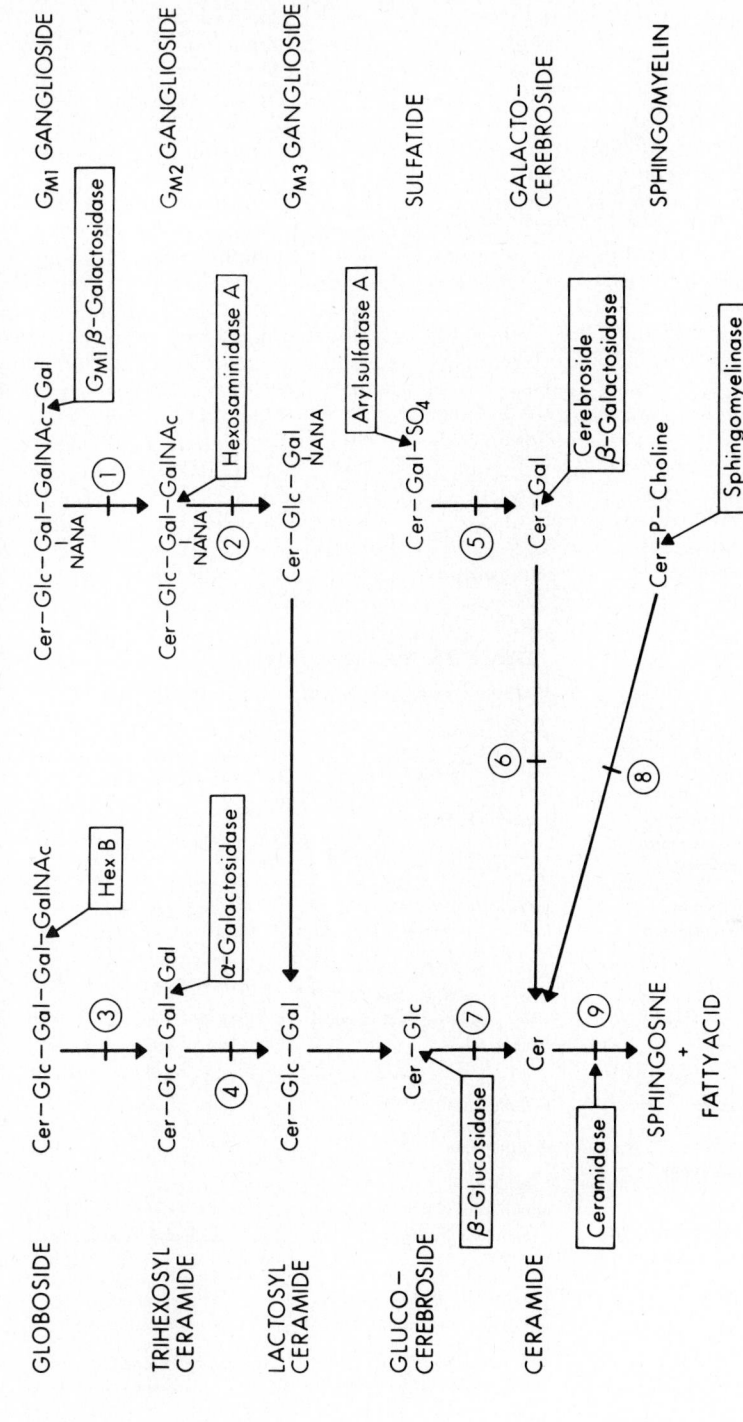

FIG. 42. Simplified diagram of the catabolism of the sphingolipids. The trivial names of the compounds are indicated in capital letters. The name of the hydrolase involved at each step is indicated in the box, and the arrow points to its site of action. The pathways for removal of NANA (N-acetylneuraminic acid) to form the asialo derivatives of the gangliosides are omitted for the sake of clarity. Hexosaminidase A and β-galactosidase are also active against these asialo derivatives. The numbers refer to the disease that results from a catabolic block at the indicated site: 1. GM_1-gangliosidosis; 2. Tay-Sachs disease; 2 and 3. Sandhoff's disease; 4. Fabry's disease; 5. metachromatic leukodystrophy; 6. Krabbe's disease; 7. Gaucher's disease; 8. Niemann-Pick disease; 9. Farber's disease. Note: Lactosylceramidosis is not indicated, as there is some doubt of its existence. GM_3-gangliosidosis is not included because only a single case has been reported, and the disease may be the result of a synthetic enzymatic deficit.

disorder). Screening whole populations becomes a practical possibility in the case of illnesses that have a striking ethnic predilection and for which there is a convenient, reliable, and inexpensive screening test. The best example is Tay-Sachs disease. Screening of Ashkenazi Jewish groups is currently taking place. The costs in terms of anxiety for individuals who are discovered to be heterozygote carriers will have to be weighed against the advantages of preventing the birth of even one affected child to a couple when both are carriers. It has been suggested, for instance, that screening be delayed until a couple is contemplating starting a pregnancy, in order not to add to the psychologic stresses that accompany the choosing of a mate.

CHEMISTRY. The sphingolipids are compounds of sphingosine, a long-chain (usually 18 carbons) amino alcohol. The amino group at the second carbon of sphingosine is substituted with the acyl group of a long-chain fatty acid, producing the neutral compound ceramide. A wide variety of oligosaccharides, single sugars, phosphate esters, and other polar groups may be attached to the first-carbon hydroxyl group of sphingosine. The ceramide end of sphingolipids is hydrophobic, and the polar group hydrophilic. Sphingolipids are important constituents of cell membranes.

Gangliosides are glycosphingolipids in which one or more sialic acids are attached to the sugar moiety. N-Acetylneuraminic acid (NANA) is the sialic acid that occurs in human gangliosides. Gangliosides that have lost their sialic acid side chain through the action of a neuraminidase are referred to as asialogangliosides or ceramide oligohexosides. These, as well as the corresponding ganglioside, accumulate in the gangliosidoses.

Figure 42 illustrates the major sphingolipids and in schematic form shows the main pathway for their catabolism. Catabolism occurs through a series of hydrolases acting on the terminal group of each sphingolipid compound. Most sphingolipidoses have been shown to be due to lack of a single specific catabolic enzyme, with resultant accumulation of the compound that cannot be broken down. Table 25 summarizes the known disorders of sphingosine metabolism, the sphingolipid stored, and the enzymatic deficiency.

GM$_1$ GANGLIOSIDOSIS. GM$_1$ gangliosidosis (β-galactosidase deficiency) is an autosomal recessive disorder in which at least two forms are recognized: an infantile form (generalized gangliosidosis or neurovisceral lipidosis) with prominent visceral storage and a late infantile or juvenile variant in which clinical mani-

TABLE 25. Sphingolipidoses*

Disease	Enzyme Activity Deficient	Compounds Stored
1. GM$_1$-gangliosidosis (neurovisceral lipidosis)	β-galactosidase	GM$_1$-ganglioside, asialo GM^1, oligosaccharides (in viscera)
2. GM$_2$-gangliosidosis (Tay-Sachs disease and variants)	Hexosaminidase A	GM$_2$-ganglioside, asialo GM$_2$
3. GM$_2$-ganglioside variant (Sandhoff disease)	Hexosaminidase A and B	GM$_2$-ganglioside, asialo GM$_2$, globoside (in the viscera)
GM$_3$-gangliosidosis?	UDP-N-acetyl-galactosaminyl transferase?	? mild increase GM$_3$? lack of higher gangliosides
4. Fabry disease	α-Galactosidase	Trihexosylceramide
5. Metachromatic leukodystrophy	Arylsulfatase A	Sulfatide
Metachromatic leukodystrophy-multiple sulfatase deficiency	Arylsulfatase A, B, C, steroid sulfatase	Sulfatide and mucopolysaccharides
6. Krabbe disease	Cerebroside β-galactosidase, Psychosine β-galactosidase	Galactosyl ceramide (galactocerebroside)
7. Gaucher disease	β-Glucosidase, Psychosine β-glucosidase	Glucosyl ceramide (glucocerebroside)
8. Niemann-Pick disease	Sphingomyelinase	Phosphoryl choline ceramide (sphingomyelin)
9. Farber disease	Ceramidase	Ceramide

The numbers correspond to the enzymatic blocks in Fig. 42.

festations are limited to the nervous system. The disease results from a deficiency of the enzyme β-galactosidase, which cleaves galactose in the terminal position from GM_1 ganglioside and from some mucopolysaccharides and glycoproteins (Fig. 42). In these compounds galactose is attached either to N-acetylglucosamine (GM_1) or N-acetylglucosamine (keratan sulfate).

GM_1 is the main monosialoganglioside in the brain. Levels of GM_1 and its derivative asialo-GM_1 (produced by removal of the neuraminic acid side chain) are markedly elevated in the nervous system and in the viscera, especially in the liver, where its level is 20 to 50 times normal. Oligosaccharides similar to keratan sulfate also accumulate in the viscera in amounts that are comparable to those seen in the mucopolysaccharidoses and that are 50 times greater than the amount of GM_1 ganglioside. GM_1 gangliosidosis is closely related to the mucopolysaccharidoses, since they are characterized by storage of glycolipids and mucopolysaccharides, and GM_1 gangliosidosis is considered by some writers to be a mucolipidosis.

INFANTILE GM_1 GANGLIOSIDOSIS. Infantile GM_1 gangliosidosis (neurovisceral lipidosis) is manifest at birth, and its course is more rapid and more severe than that of either Tay-Sachs disease or Hurler's disease, with both of which it shares some features. Soon after birth these infants are hypotonic and weak; they suck poorly and gain weight slowly. Their faces show frontal bossing, large low-set ears, and increased distance between nose and upper lip. They have a downy hirsutism over the face. Hypertrophy of the gingiva (especially the maxilla) and macroglossia are constant features. The corneas are clear, but 50 percent of these children develop a cherry-red spot at the macula. Peripheral edema is usually noted. Development is slow, and the children do not achieve independent sitting or crawling, although some may learn to reach for objects. Strabismus, horizontal nystagmus, and convulsions appear, accompanied in some cases by exaggerated response to sound (so-called hyperacusis). By 6 months hepatomegaly and slight enlargement of the spleen become apparent, as well as stiffness of the joints, dorsolumbar kyphosis, thickening and coarsening of the skin, and atrophy of intrinsic hand muscles with claw deformities of the hands. The infants are apathetic and eventually become decerebrate and unresponsive to their environment. Frequent respiratory infections or cardiac arrhythmias lead to death before the age of 2 years.

Laboratory tests reveal vacuolated lymphocytes and foamy histiocytes in the bone marrow, but these are not as prominent as in Niemann-Pick disease or Gaucher's disease. Urinary excretion of oligosaccharides similar to keratan sulfate is excessive, but the usual screening tests for mucopolysacchariduria may miss this finding. After the age of 6 months radiographs show characteristic beaking of vertebral bodies at the apex of the kyphosis, swelling of the long bones at midshaft, and in early life, periosteal new bone formation cloaking the ribs and long bones. The skull resembles that seen in Hurler's disease and may have a J-shaped sella.

Definitive diagnosis no longer requires biopsies. It can readily be made from blood or cultured fibroblasts, which show a deficiency of the enzyme β-galactosidase. Detection of heterozygote carriers (whose enzyme levels are intermediate between those of homozygotes and normals) and intrauterine diagnosis are possible. Differential diagnosis includes infantile Gaucher's disease and Niemann-Pick disease, which run a similar course and have organomegaly but do not show the prominent bony abnormalities of infantile GM_1 gangliosidosis. I cell disease (mucolipidosis II) has similar bony changes but less severe organomegaly. Tay-Sachs disease presents later and lacks evidence of visceral involvement. Hurler's disease has a much more protracted course and less rapidly progressive neurologic signs. Children with Krabbe's disease are spastic earlier than those with GM_1 gangliosidosis. All of these disorders can be tested for with specific enzymatic assays.

Neurons throughout the central nervous system and myenteric plexus are markedly ballooned. The nucleus and Nissl substance are displaced to the periphery of the cell. Electron microscopy reveals multiple membranocytoplasmic bodies within lysosomes consisting of concentric lamellae usually surrounding a granular core. Neuronal dropout, demyelination, and gliosis explain the brain atrophy that is usually quite prominent in infants who survive to 2 years. The viscera contain large numbers of foamy histiocytes and vacuolated parenchymal cells. Typically, epithelial cells of the renal glomeruli are swollen with similar storage vacuoles. Storage in the kidney is typical of GM_1 gangliosidosis and Fabry's disease. No treatment is available.

LATE INFANTILE GM_1 GANGLIOSIDOSIS. Late infantile GM_1 gangliosidosis appears to be genetically distinct from the infantile variant. Clinical manifestations are limited to the nervous system and usually appear at 1 to 3 years of age. Abnormal development and muscle weakness may be noted in early infancy. The fundi may be normal or may show optic atrophy late in the course; the corneas are clear, there is no organomegaly, and bony changes are usually absent. The earliest findings are usually unsteadiness of gait and ataxia, followed by hypotonia and increased deep tendon reflexes. Speech becomes dysarthric and eventually is lost. Rapidly progressive dementia with seizures and a spastic quadriplegia with evidence of anterior horn cell disease develop. The usual cause of death is pneumonia. Laboratory tests are nonspecific. Definitive diagnosis rests on the demonstration of decreased activity of β-galactosidase in blood or cultured fibroblasts. The pathology is similar to that of the infantile variant. Therapy is limited to supportive care and the use of anticonvulsants. Genetic counseling can be based on the detection of heterozygote carriers. Intrauterine diagnosis is possible.

GM_2 GANGLIOSIDOSIS. GM_2 gangliosidosis (Tay-Sachs disease) was the first of the sphingolipidoses to be identified clinically, but it soon became apparent that other forms of GM_2 ganglioside existed.

GM_2 TYPE B. GM_2 type B (infantile variant), or Tay-Sachs disease, is an autosomal recessive disorder with a marked ethnic predilection for Ashkenazi Jews. Gene frequency among them has been estimated to be 1 in 25 to 1 in 30, compared to 1 in 300 in non-Jews. The disease has complete penetrance in the homozygote, and the heterozygote carrier shows no manifestation of the disease. The incidence of the disease is 1 in 8,000 live births among Jews, and each year 100 to 200 infants are born with the disease in the United States.

These infants appear normal at birth, and the diagnosis is rarely suspected before 6 months of age; mothers who have had a previous child with Tay-Sachs disease may note that startle reflex to sound and slight hypotonia may be present soon after birth. The infants learn to smile and reach for objects, but do not learn to sit or crawl. So-called hyperacusis (a myoclonic jerk reaction to sound) is constant finding, as is the cherry-red spot at the macula. This is due to thickening of the retina because of storage of ganglioside in ganglion cells around the macula, which contains no cells and appears red by contrast with the white halo surrounding it. Soon thereafter the babies become floppy and weak, but have hyperactive reflexes, clonus, and extensor plantar responses. Abnormal eye movements, apathy, and loss of developmental milestones lead by the second year to a stage where the infants lie in a frog position, with little spontaneous movement and little regard for the environment. Seizures and myoclonus make their appearance, but they usually subside by about 2 years, as does the hyperacusis. Eventually the infants become decorticate, but floppy; they need tube feeding, have difficulty with secretions, and appear blind. Head circumference enlarges progressively above the 90th percentile from 1 to 3 years, after which it stabilizes. Death is due to intercurrent infection, usually pneumonia. The infants have no organomegaly and no deformities other than those due to their neurologic disability; in early stages they are frequently described as having a doll-like ap-

pearance, perhaps because of mild facial weakness, decreased activity, translucent skin, and long eyelashes.

The diagnosis may be strongly suspected on clinical grounds, especially in a Jewish infant without organomegaly who has mixed upper and lower motor neuron signs, myoclonus to sound, and a cherry-red spot. Diagnosis is confirmed by the finding of an absence of hexosaminidase A in serum, white cells, or skin fibroblasts. Results are expressed as the ratio of hexosaminidase A to hexosaminidase B, since total hexosaminidase varies greatly. It is no longer justified to perform rectal or brain biopsies to arrive at a diagnosis. Niemann-Pick disease and GM_1 gangliosidosis, which may also have a cherry-red spot, can be excluded by the organomegaly and other clinical features, as well as on enzymatic grounds.

Figure 43A shows the classic appearance of the grossly ballooned neurons that are found throughout the brain, cerebellum, and spinal cord. The cytoplasm is filled with pale homogeneous-appearing material that pushes the nucleus and Nissl substance to a corner of the cell. With the electron microscope this material can be shown to be made up of membrane-bound membranocytoplasmic bodies with regular concentric dark and pale lamellae that usually surround a granular core (Fig. 43B). These organelles are greatly distended lysosomes. The nucleus and other organelles usually appear normal. Astrocytes and pericytes contain much smaller dense inclusions. A massive increase in fibrous astrocytes is thought to be the reason for the megalencephaly that is characteristic of the illness at midcourse and that may increase brain weight by 50 percent. Late in the course of the illness there is intense demyelination of the white matter to a degree comparable to that noted in the leukodystrophies. Storage is also evident in

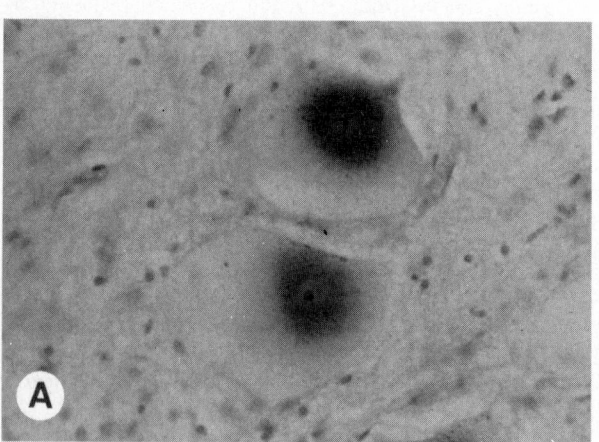

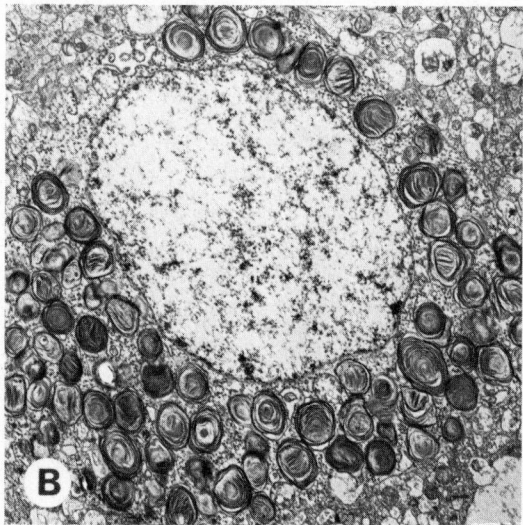

FIG. 43. Tay-Sachs disease. A. Anterior horn cells of the spinal cord, grossly ballooned by ample storage material pushing the nucleus and Nissl substance to the periphery (Nissl stain, X400). B. Neuron in the cerebral cortex filled with concentric membranous cytoplasmic bodies (MCB). (electronmicrography X9,000). (Courtesy of Dr. K Suzuki.)

autonomic neurons and has been the basis for tissue diagnosis by rectal biopsy.

A massive increase in GM_2 ganglioside in the brain is the hallmark of the illness; GM_2 content is increased in the viscera, but to a much smaller degree. Total hexosaminidase (an enzyme capable of cleaving both N-acetylgalactosamine and N-acetylglucosamine from artificial substrates) may be normal or increased, but the ratio of hexosaminidase A to hexosaminidase B is greatly decreased. This deficiency is present in all tissues and in the tears and has been found in amniotic cells and fetal tissues. Heterozygotes have an intermediate percentage of hexosaminidase A to total hexosaminidase. Semiautomated methods have been developed for population screening.

No therapy is available. The outlook for an effective treatment appears dim in view of the histologic and chemical evidence of significant storage found in 20-week fetuses. The ability to detect heterozygotes and abort affected fetuses provides an effective means of prevention. Even if the birth of a first child with Tay-Sachs disease cannot always be prevented, the birth of a second affected child need never occur except in families who refuse an abortion on religious or ethical grounds. Counseling for all family members should be mandatory.

GM_2 TYPE O. GM_2 type O (infantile variant), or Sandhoff disease, cannot be distinguished on clinical grounds from classic Tay-Sachs disease(with the single exception that the patients are not Jewish). These patients do not have organomegaly, and their symptoms and the course of the illness are identical to those in Tay-Sachs disease. They can be distinguished on enzymatic grounds, because they are lacking in both A and B components of hexosaminidase. Vacuolated histiocytes are found in all organs; but they are not nearly as prevalent as in Niemann-Pick disease or Gaucher's disease.

NONINFANTILE GM_2 GANGLIOSIDOSIS WITH PARTIAL DEFICIENCY OF HEXOSAMINIDASE A. At least 15 cases of noninfantile GM_2 gangliosidosis with an associated partial deficiency of hexosaminidase A have been reported. The clinical picture does not appear to be uniform. In 7 children the illness became apparent before 2 years of age and led to death before 10 years. All of the children were severely demented. Ataxia, spasticity, and seizures were noted in most. The fundi showed variable abnormalities or were normal. In 8 children the onset occurred after 4 years of age and extended at least into adolescence.

FABRY'S DISEASE. Fabry's disease (trihexosylceramide lipidosis) is the only sphingolipidosis known to be inherited as a sex-linked recessive trait. The hemizygous males manifest serious disease, but heterozygous females have milder symptoms. Female carriers of the Fabry trait have two clonal populations, one with normal enzyme activity, the other with severe deficiency. Prenatal diagnosis may be made by enzyme determination in cultured amniotic cells. Fabry's disease is a systemic illness characterized by widespread storage of trihexosylceramide, which cannot be catabol-

ized because of deficiency of the enzyme trihexosylceramide-α-galactosidase (Fig. 42). The main source of trihexosylceramide appears to be globoside from senescent erythrocytes. The disease is a visceral lipidosis with prominent skin and renal manifestations. It affects the peripheral nervous system directly and the central nervous system mainly through the effects of glycolipid storage in the walls of blood vessels. There is minor storage in small neurons of the posterior horns, dorsal root ganglia, brainstem nuclei, basal ganglia, and hypothalamus, as well as in autonomic ganglia.

HEMIZYGOUS MALES. The disease usually becomes manifest in late childhood or adolescence, but it may be delayed until adult life. Presenting symptoms are brief lancinating pains in the limbs, especially the feet and hands, often precipitated by changes in temperature and accompanied by paresthesias and in some cases abdominal crises. Anhydrosis and unexplained episodes of hyperpyrexia are common. Characteristic skin lesions can usually be found in children, but they become florid in adults; innumerable telangiectatic, purpuric, hyperkeratotic lesions of the size of pinheads appear, mostly between the umbilicus and the knees, with a predilection for the groin, buttocks, and scrotum. Similar lesions are common in the mouth. Although the disease derived its name (angiokeratoma corporis diffusum universale) from skin lesions, they are not always present. Renal involvement is a major feature of the illness. In children asymptomatic proteinuria is the rule; in some cases hyposthenuria and polyuria may resemble vasopressin-resistant diabetes insipidus. In the earliest stages, examination of urinary sediment with a polarized light will reveal Maltese crosses, thus reflecting the excretion of excess glycolipid arising from desquamated renal tubular cells filled with glycolipid. Renal involvement eventually leads to hypertension, azotemia, and renal failure, usually in the third or fourth decade. Ocular lesions are of two types: tortuous conjunctival, and to a lesser degree, retinal vessels with sausagelike dilatations, and haziness of the cornea due to glycolipid deposits. Corneal lesions have been seen by slit-lamp examination in early childhood.

Neurologic symptoms and signs are of several types. The painful crises and paresthesias are thought to be due to peripheral neuropathy and involvement of small cells in dorsal root ganglia and posterior horns of the cord. Involvement of the autonomic nervous system explains the abdominal crises, nausea, vomiting and diarrhea, hypohydrosis, and hyperthermia. Storage in blood vessel walls can result in infarction presenting as a focal neurologic deficit (such as hemiparesis, aphasia, seizure, hearing loss, or labyrinthine dysfunction) or may lead to a frank cerebral hemorrhage. The neuropathy may result from involvement of the vasa nervorum. Others signs may include articular lesions that are most likely vascular in origin. Necrosis of the femoral head and swelling of terminal interphalangeal joints are characteristic. Involvement of the lungs may be manifest by wheezing and dyspnea. Endocrine signs such as growth retardation, acromegaly, and delayed puberty may be due to sphingolipid storage in the pituitary or hypothalamic involvement. Cardiac failure may be the consequence of myocardial involvement or of coronary artery disease.

HETEROZYGOUS FEMALES. Mothers and sisters of males with Fabry's disease have more limited symptoms. Corneal opacity is the most common sign. Skin lesions are usually subtle or absent. All other symptoms are also less severe. While life expectancy is longer than in males, increasing symptoms develop, and patients tend to die of renal or cardiac complications.

Widespread deposition of trihexosylceramide can be demonstrated, predominantly in endothelial, perithelial, and smooth muscle cells of blood vessels, and to a lesser degree in histiocytes. Lipid deposits are prominent in the cornea, glomeruli, and tubules of the kidney, cardiac muscle fibers, autonomic neurons, and Schwann cells; storage cells can be found in the bone marrow. The stored material appears as refractile crystalline deposits that show birefringence with typical Maltese crosses. Blood vessel walls in all organs, including the central nervous system, show extensive storage in all cell layers, which leads to occlusions and large and small areas of infarction. The demonstration of deficient trihexosylceramide-α-galactosidase in skin fibroblasts, plasma, leukocytes, or tears proves the diagnosis.

Symptomatic relief of the lightening pains has been achieved with diphenylhydantoin. Attempts at enzyme therapy have included infusions of plasma and purified enzyme. While significant reductions in levels of trihexosylceramide have been achieved, they have been transient. The possibility that renal transplantation may achieve the goal of providing a new undamaged kidney and a source of active enzyme is an interesting consideration. Genetic counseling is extremely important for members of the mother's family and for sisters and daughters of affected males. Heterozygotes can now be detected.

METACHROMATIC LEUKODYSTROPHY. Metachromatic leukodystrophy (sulfatide lipidosis) includes a group of autosomal recessive disorders that result from an accumulation of sulfatide (ceramide galactose sulfate) and a relative decrease in cerebroside in the myelin of the central nervous system and peripheral nerves, in the kidney, and to a lesser degree in other organs. Failure to catabolize sulfatide to cerebroside is attributed to deficient cerebroside sulfatase activity in lysosomes, usually measured as arylsulfatase A activity (Fig. 42). Arylsulfatase A activity is profoundly deficient in white cells, skin fibroblasts, urine, cultured amniotic cells, kidney, liver, brain, and other tissues in this disease. Four clinical subtypes of metachromatic leukodystrophy (MLD) are recognized. Thus far, except for type 4 (multiple sulfatase deficiency metachromatic leukodystrophy, MSD-MLD), it has not been possible to distinguish enzymatically between late infantile, juvenile, and adult variants, which appear to be distinct on clinical and genetic grounds. Type 4 is distinct in that arylsulfatase A, B, and C are decreased, as are several steroid sulfatases; pathologically, in addition to sulfatide accumulation in myelin, there is also ganglioside in neurons and mucopolysaccharide in liver and brain.

The *late infantile variant* is the most common type. It manifests during the second year with motor weakness, clumsiness, and ataxia. The muscles are hypotonic, especially in the legs, and tendon stretch reflexes are sluggish. Characteristically nerve conduction velocities are prolonged and CSF protein is elevated. Within 1 to 2 years dulling of intellect, nystagmus and optic atrophy, dysarthria, loss of language, and spasticity with absence of reflexes lead to a decorticate vegetative state. Seizures, if they occur at all, are a late symptom. Death occurs from intercurrent illness, usually between the ages of 4 and 8 years. The *juvenile variant* starts at 5 to 10 years of age and runs an essentially similar, although more protracted, course. The *adult variant* usually is diagnosed after death in a psychiatric hospital, with a previous diagnosis of schizophrenia or organic dementia and manifestations that have progressed over many years to a deteriorated state with movement disorder, seizures, neuropathy, and terminal vegetative state. The *MSD-MLD variant* becomes manifest in late infancy when developmental milestones are not achieved; rapid regression with ataxia, spasticity, and seizures supervene. These children have flared ribs, pigeon breast or pectus excavatum, widened phalanges, and ichthyosis of the skin. Some features of the mucopolysaccharidoses may be noted. These children excrete excess mucopolysaccharide and sulfatide in their urine (Table 24).

Austin has demonstrated the presence of metachromatic granules in the urine. Quantitative estimates of sulfatide excretion and arylsulfatase A activity can now be made. Arylsulfatase A activity in leukocytes or skin fibroblasts is drastically reduced in all affected patients. Successful intrauterine detection of an affected fetus by drastically reduced levels of arylsulfatase A activity in cultured amniotic cells has been reported. There is a loss of myelin sheaths and oligodendroglia in the brain, with accumulation of spherical granular masses within macrophages around blood vessels and free in the tissue. Electron microscopy shows granular and lamellar inclusions within neurons, glial cells, and Schwann cells, changes in the density of myelin lamellae, and thickening of the cristae of Schwann cell mitochondria. Metachromatic granules are found in the epithelial cells of the kidney tubules and the mucosa of the gall bladder. No effective therapy has yet been described.

GLOBOID CELL LEUKODYSTROPHY. Globoid cell leukodystrophy (galactosylceramide lipidosis, Krabbe's disease) is an autosomal recessive disorder of early infancy that is identified by characteristic globoid cells and mononucleated and polynucleated phagocytes that infiltrate the white matter. The disease is considered a leukodystrophy because there is virtually total disappearance of myelin in the brain. A profound deficiency of the enzyme galactocerebroside-β-galactosidase, which cleaves galactose from cerebroside (galactose ceramide) has been demonstrated in all tissues of affected children (Fig. 42); the disease is, in fact, a galactocerebroside storage disease, even though the amount of cerebroside in the brain is not increased.

Heterozygote carriers, whose enzymatic activity in white blood cells and skin fibroblasts is intermediate, have been detected, and the affected fetus can be recognized by amniocentesis.

The vast majority of these infants are normal at birth; before the age of 6 months there is the onset of characteristic irritability and periods of inconsolable crying. The child may run unexplained fevers and is hypersensitive to light and sound, which may precipitate tonic spasms. Development slows and developmental milestones are lost. Tone may be increased; tendon stretch reflexes are usually present. After several months the child develops retraction of the head and assumes a decerebrate or decorticate posture of the limbs; there is markedly increased tone. Reflexes cannot always be elicited. The infant is usually out of contact with his environment; he may appear blind with nystagmus, although not all of these infants show optic atrophy. Seizures, myoclonus, and autonomic crises with increased sweating and hyperpyrexia are common. Finally, the infant becomes immobile and unresponsive, and death occurs at 2 to 3 years from infection. Clinical findings are summarized in Table 24. Laboratory tests show increased spinal fluid protein and slow nerve conduction velocities. Enzymatic diagnosis provides a definitive answer.

Differential diagnosis includes subacute encephalopathies that become manifest below the age of 1 year. They include the following: spongy degeneration, where the head is large and the spinal fluid protein normal; connatal Pelizaeus-Merzbacher disease, which has a slower course and characteristic oscillations of the eyes, but in which CSF protein and nerve conduction velocities are normal; neuroaxonal dystrophy, which also has a neuropathy, but normal spinal fluid protein and a less acute course.

The late infantile and juvenile variants have their onset at 2 to 5 years of age, and the age at death is 3 to 8 years. The course of these variants is more insidious, and diagnosis may be confused with a demyelinating disorder akin to multiple sclerosis, postinfectious encephalomyelitis, or Schilder's disease. Hemiparesis, spastic gait, ataxia, and visual loss are common presenting complaints. Nerve conduction velocities are usually normal, as is the spinal fluid. Later, blindness, dementia, and sometimes seizures become evident. Enzyme levels in these children are as low as in the infants.

The pathology of this disorder is characterized by severe loss of myelin in the brain, affecting particularly recently myelinated tracts; there is almost total loss of oligodendroglial cells in demyelinated areas, and there are numerous mononuclear or multinucleated globoid cells in the white matter. Severe degenerative changes and perineurial fibrosis are common in advanced cases. The characteristic ultrastructural feature of the disease is the accumulation of twisted tubules within the cytoplasm of globoid cells; the tubules are similar to those seen in Gaucher's disease, where there is an accumulation of glucose cerebroside. No therapy is available beyond supportive measures and anticonvulsants. Genetic counseling is essential, since detection of heterozygotes and prenatal diagnosis by amniocentesis are possible.

GAUCHER'S DISEASE.   Gaucher's disease (glucosylceramide lipidosis), an autosomal recessive disorder, is the most frequent of the lipidoses, especially in its chronic, visceral, non-neuropathic form, that may go on for years and in some patients does not affect life span. An acute neuropathic form of the disease occurs in infants. There is no admixture of the two variants within one family. A third variant occurs in childhood and produces a chronic effect on the nervous system. The disease is characterized by storage of glucocerebroside (glucosylceramide) in the reticuloendothelial system, particularly in the spleen (Fig. 42). Glucosylceramide is a product of the degradation of gangliosides (mostly from brain and other tissues, including leukocytes) and globoside (derived mainly from senescent erythrocytes). A specific catabolic enzyme, cerebroside β-glucosidase, is lacking in this disease; the enzyme cleaves glucose from ceramide and is found in spleen, liver, white blood cells, skin fibroblasts, and brain. Heterozygote carriers can be detected by enzyme levels, and intrauterine diagnosis of the infantile variant has been accomplished.

CHRONIC NON-NEUROPATHIC (ADULT) FORM.   Lack of involvement of the nervous system is a sine qua non for the diagnosis of chronic non-neuropathic (adult) form of Gaucher's disease. It is discussed in detail on page 749. The illness is more common in Ashkenazi Jews, and it may start in childhood or may be delayed until adult life. Splenic enlargement is the main feature and may be accompanied by signs of hypersplenism, especially thrombocytopenia; usually the liver is also enlarged, and the bones, lungs, lymph nodes, and skin may be involved. Diagnosis is usually made by bone marrow examination, which shows characteristic Gaucher cells; acid phosphatase levels in the blood are elevated. Cerebroside β-glucosidase activity in white cells and other tissues is diminished. Enzyme activity is not totally absent in the adult form, in contrast to the infantile variant, in which it is absent. The course of the illness is variable, with age at death varying from childhood to late middle age. Splenectomy may be indicated.

ACUTE NEUROPATHIC FORM.   Infantile Gaucher's disease (acute neuropathic form) has no striking predilection for Ashkenazi Jews. It has a subacute onset that may occur from birth to 1 year of age, and it leads to death before the age of 2 years. These infants have protuberant abdomens with markedly enlarged spleens and dramatically enlarged livers. Difficulty in sucking and swallowing, weight loss, and developmental regression soon become evident. Cranial nerve involvement is striking; in addition to dysphagia it includes strabismus, facial weakness, and stridor. The infants become markedly spastic or rigid, they hold their heads retracted in opisthotonos, and they have increased reflexes. Late in the illness they may become flaccid and weak, presumably reflecting involvement of anterior horn cells. Some develop seizures. Vision is usually preserved, and the fundi do not show a cherry-red spot or optic atrophy. The infants eventually become totally indifferent to their environment and usually die of pneumonia.

Diagnosis is usually made by finding Gaucher cells in the bone marrow. Acid phosphatase levels are elevated in the blood. Cerebroside β-glucosidase is drastically reduced in white cells, fibroblasts, and other tissues. The differential diagnosis includes Niemann-Pick disease, where cherry-red spots may be found and where foamy cells rather than Gaucher cells are found in the bone marrow. Lymphocytes may be vacuolated; acid phosphatase is not elevated, and sphingomyelinase deficiency can be demonstrated. Infants with neurovisceral lipidosis (infantile GM_1 gangliosidosis) have coarse features, cherry-red spots, and bony anomalies. The enzyme defect is a ganglioside β-galactosidase. The mucopolysaccharidoses have a much more chronic course and characteristic bony and ocular changes. Glycogen storage disease and galactosemia can be diagnosed definitively chemically and are associated with liver enlargement rather than splenomegaly.

Pathologically the Gaucher cell is a macrophage stuffed with glucocerebroside. It is a very large cell (20 to 100 μ) whose nucleus has been pushed to the periphery and whose cytoplasm is filled with fibrils that give it the appearance of crumpled silk. The Gaucher cell is clearly distinct from the foamy cells seen in Niemann-Pick disease and most other lipidoses. With the electron microcsope, tubular helical structures can be seen within lysosomes that resemble the configuration taken by pure glucocerebroside molecules. They are also very similar to the helical tubules seen in Krabbe's disease, which are made up of galactocerebroside. Gaucher cells are seen in most organs (eg, spleen, liver, lymph nodes, bone marrow) and in the adventitia of blood vessels. They may obstruct capillaries and produce infarcts in bones, lungs, and elsewhere. In the infantile variant they are very prominent around cerebral blood vessels of the leptomeninges, in the cortex, and especially in the deep white matter. The neurologic findings are due not to neuronal storage but to neuronal loss; myelin is normal.

JUVENILE (SUBACUTE) NEUROPATHIC FORM.

Patients with the juvenile (subacute) neuropathic form of Gaucher's disease with visceral glucocerebroside storage develop neurologic signs in childhood or adolescence.

It is doubtful that any specific therapy, other than preventing the birth of a second affected infant by intrauterine diagnosis and abortion, will be available for the infantile variant. Significant fetal pathology may be found in Tay-Sachs disease, Niemann-Pick disease, GM_1 gangliosidosis, and Krabbe's disease, indicating that storage starts early in pregnancy. Even though at birth it has not reached a stage advanced enough to be clinically evident, it seems doubtful that therapy started postnatally will be effective, especially in those diseases where enzyme activity would need to be delivered across the blood-brain barrier. The outlook is more favorable in the chronic non-neuropathic form of the disease, where diagnosis is possible before severe tissue destruction has taken place. Recently intravenous infusion of purified glucocerebrosidase in two patients, one with non-neuropathic Gaucher's disease and one with a juvenile neuropathic form, decreased the glucocerebroside content of liver and red cells for several days. It is hoped that this approach may be developed into a therapeutically meaningful tool. Genetic counseling, identification of heterozygote carriers, and monitoring of pregnancies at risk are most important preventive steps, especially in families with the infantile form of the illness.

NIEMANN-PICK DISEASE.

Niemann-Pick disease (sphingomyelin lipidosis) and its variants are presumably autosomal recessive genetic diseases characterized by an increase in sphingomyelin (ceramide phosphorylcholine) and free cholesterol content of various tissues, notably the spleen. The infantile form is known as Niemann-Pick disease; it is the most frequent and most severe form and accounts for 75 percent of cases of sphingomyelin lipidosis. Brady and associates have demonstrated a deficiency of sphingomyelinase activity (an enzyme that cleaves phosphorylcholine from ceramide) in infants with Niemann-Pick disease (Fig. 42). Lesser degrees of deficiency have been found in some, but not all, of the other patients with foam cells and increased visceral sphingomyelin.

INFANTILE FORM.

In the infantile form of Niemann-Pick disease infants become symptomatic soon after birth, with failure to thrive, abdominal distension, and progressive hepatosplenomegaly. The skin often has a brownish yellow tinge. Liver function tests usually remain adequate until late in the course, although jaundice has been reported. Hypersplenism is unusual. Lymph nodes may become diffusely enlarged and rarely xanthomatous. Skin eruptions appear. Bony changes are mild. Diffuse haziness or patchy infiltrates in the lungs occurs in most infants. Apathy, hypotonia, and dulling of intellect become apparent before 1 year of age. Slow nerve conduction velocities denote a neuropathy. About half of these infants develop macular cherry-red spot. Seizures are infrequent, and the myoclonic response to sound so characteristic of Tay-Sachs disease is not seen. Death in marasmus, or because of an infection, usually occurs before the age of 2 years.

The condition is diagnosed by finding vacuolated lymphocytes in the peripheral blood and foamy macrophages in the bone marrow or liver; it is confirmed by the demonstration of decreased sphingomyelinase activity in white blood cells or cultured fibroblasts. Increased sphingomyelin can be demonstrated in the liver and in the urine, although false positives may occur in the presence of a urinary tract infection. Nonesterified cholesterol is also increased, but to a lesser degree, and this is thought to be a secondary defect. Prenatal diagnosis of Niemann-Pick disease on cultured amniotic cells is possible, as is detection of heterozygote carriers on cultured skin fibroblasts. There is some predilection of infantile Niemann-Pick disease for Ashkenazi Jews, but this is not as striking as for Tay-Sachs disease.

VISCERAL FORM WITH DECREASED SPHINGOMYELI-NASE ACTIVITY SPARING THE CENTRAL NERVOUS SYSTEM. Asymptomatic splenomegaly or hepatosplenomegaly has been found to be due to sphingomyelin storage in patients ranging from infancy to old age. On radiography these patients usually show striking opacities in the lungs, but they may not be symptomatic.

SUBACUTE OR JUVENILE NEUROPATHIC SPHINGOMYELIN LIPIDOSIS. A number of patients have been described who do not develop signs of illness until 1 year to several years after birth. Motor symptoms may include ataxia, choreoathetosis, gait abnormality, and dysarthria; progression varies, but some die before 10 years of age. Hepatosplenomegaly is variable in severity. Inclusion in this group depends on the demonstration of increased amounts of sphingomyelin and cholesterol in the spleen. It is thought unlikely that this type is homogeneous and represents a single syndrome.

NOVA SCOTIA VARIANT (VISCERAL AND NEUROPATHIC). A variant of sphingomyelin lipidosis has been described in a genetic isolate from Nova Scotia. These children have hepatosplenomegaly from early infancy, and many develop jaundice early. Mental dullness or dementia, a tabetic gait, and progressive convulsive disorder lead to severe deterioration and death within months or a few years. Foam cells predominate in the spleen, bone marrow, and nodes, but the liver is usually fibrotic. Lipid storage in the brain and loss of Purkinje cells in the cerebellum are characteristic. Sphingomyelinase activity has been normal in some cases and somewhat decreased in others.

SEA-BLUE HISTIOCYTE SYNDROME. Silverstein described patients with hepatosplenomegaly and thrombocytopenia whose bone marrow and spleen contained numerous granulated histiocytes that stained bright blue with Wright-Giemsa stain. Increased amounts of sphingomyelin were found in the viscera. Lung infiltrates, perimacular retinal changes, and a neurologic disorder characterized by ataxia, dementia, and seizures have occurred in some, but not all, of these patients. Fibroblasts in culture produce many sea-blue histiocytes whose granulations are thought to be ceroid.

Splenomegaly, with or without hepatomegaly, and demonstration of foam cells in the bone marrow and in other viscera are strongly suggestive of sphingomyelin lipidosis. Gaucher cells can be distinguished from Niemann-Pick histiocytes by their morphologic appearance. Lack of cardiomegaly and the severe splenomegaly rule out glycogen storage disease type II; galactosemia is excluded by lack of cataracts and lack of galactose in the urine. Bony changes are less severe than in the mucopolysaccharidoses, and the corneas are not cloudy. Seizures are much less dramatic than in the gangliosidoses. In older children and adults with atypical neurologic abnormalities, especially ataxic, choreoathetotic, and dystonic syndromes, a bone marrow biopsy should be performed. Definite diagnosis depends on demonstrating depressed levels of sphingomyelinase activity in white blood cells, cultured fibroblasts, or cultured amniotic cells. This assay requires the use of radioactive natural substrates and is available in a few centers (eg, Dr. R.O. Brady at NIH).

Ubiquitous foam cells (macrophages filled with lipid droplets and in some cases ceroid) are found in the spleen, liver, bone marrow, lymph nodes, lung alveoli, tonsils, thymus, endocrine glands, and perivascular spaces of the brain. They are birefringent and are filled with droplets measuring 20 to 90 μ that give them a foamy or mulberry appearance. The cells stain with fat stains and are periodic-acid-Schiff-positive (PAS-positive) and positive for acid phosphatase. Those that contain ceroid have a green autofluorescence. Cells that stain blue green with Wright-Giemsa stain have been given the name sea-blue histiocytes. Neurons are ballooned and on electron microscopy are shown to contain membranous structures resembling the membranous cytoplasmic bodies of the gangliosidoses. There is also neuronal dropout, gliosis, and some demyelination. Neurons of the myenteric plexus and histiocytes of the rectal wall show a storage process. No specific therapy is available. Splenectomy has been carried out in some patients who have had hypersplenism as their primary clinical symptom. Supportive therapy and genetic counseling are essential.

FARBER'S LIPOGRANULOMATOSIS. Farber's lipogranulomatosis (ceramide lipidosis), an extremely rare storage disease, is characterized by the accumulation of ceramide in subcutaneous nodules and viscera and may be due to a deficiency in the activity of the enzyme ceramidase, which cleaves ceramide into sphingosine and a fatty acid (Fig. 42). Most reported cases have been infants with involvement of the central nervous system. It has also been classified as a mucolipidosis (Table 24). Soon after birth infants have periarticular swellings, especially in the small joints of the hands and feet. Nodules may be noted on the eyelids, spine, and face, and also on the larynx. Hypotonia, loss of reflexes, and paucity of movement reflect involvement of anterior horn cells; swallowing difficulty reflects involvement of bulbar neurons. Spinal fluid protein is sometimes elevated. Death occurs before the age of 2 years. The granulomatous nodules show foam cells, histiocytes, and chronic inflammatory cells and are similar to those in the histiocytoses. Joint synovial membranes are thickened. No therapy is known.

LEUKODYSTROPHIES

The term leukodystrophy implies a specific abnormality in the laying down or maintenance of myelin. This may very well be the case in diseases such as galactosylceramide lipidosis (Krabbe's disease) and sulfatide lipidosis (metachromatic leukodystrophy) in which two main components of myelin (sulfatide and cerebroside) accumulate and in which the composition of myelin is abnormal. It has not yet been possible to show that myelin has an abnormal composition in diseases such as Pelizaeus-Merzbacher disease or adrenoleukodystrophy, which are characterized pathologically by a severe deficiency of myelin formation or a breakdown of myelin to neutral fat (cholesterol esters) along the usual pathways of myelin catabolism (orthochromatic sudanophilic demyelination). Recent evidence suggests that a systemic defect in sterol metabolism may be present in adrenoleukodystrophy.

Active myelination starts in the third trimester of pregnancy and progresses from the cord upward; it is most active during the first 2 years of life, then tapers off during childhood. The composition of myelin is not stable throughout life; it changes during fetal life and childhood before reaching adult values. The timetable for changes in the various components of myelin varies. The activities of various enzymes also change over time. In adults myelin constituents continue to turn over, but at a low rate, so that myelin is quite stable chemically. Leukodystrophies presumably arise from deficiencies in normal myelin formation, or the laying down of unstable myelin. Leukodystrophies of early life tend to be more acute than those of later childhood. The term describes the pathology, but it has no etiologic validity. Thus subacute sclerosing panencephalitis (previously classified among the leukodystrophies) is now known to be due to a slow viral infection. As metabolic entities become defined, diseases are being removed from the category of leukodystrophies and classified according to their chemical pathology; Krabbe's disease and metachromatic leukodystrophy are now defined as sphingolipidoses; maple syrup urine disease and phenylketonuria, which are characterized pathologically by the laying down of abnormal myelin, are now classified with the amino-acidurias. No satisfactory classification of the leukodystrophies is possible. Table 26 lists conditions frequently subsumed under the term leukodystrophy.

SUDANOPHILIC LEUKODYSTROPHIES. Only a brief review of the various subtypes of sudanophilic leukodystrophies will be presented, since their validity is in question.

Infants with *connatal (infantile) sudanophilic leukodystrophy with diffuse lack of myelin* are abnormal from birth or soon after and die in infancy or early childhood. Inheritance is probably autosomal recessive; symptoms include striking nystagmus, which is often rotatory and chaotic, and a movement disorder, with later development of progressive spasticity and optic atrophy. Many of these infants develop seizures, and scoliosis is common. They do not have organomegaly, cloudy corneas, cataracts, or skin lesions. There are no laboratory findings that enable one to make a diagnosis. The brain is diffusely atrophic, including the brainstem, cerebellum and spinal cord; myelin is almost totally lacking, but peripheral myelin is intact.

Classic cases of *Pelizaeus-Merzbacher disease* involve males, and this disorder is considered to have a sex-linked recessive pattern of inheritance. The onset may be early, as in the connatal type, or it may be delayed until early childhood. The course of the illness is protracted, and while some children have died before 5 years, most survive to the third decade or later. The symptoms are similar to those in the infantile variant,

TABLE 26. LEUKODYSTROPHIES

Type	Enzyme Activity Deficient	Remarks
Sphingolipidoses		
Krabbe's disease	Cerebroside β-galactosidase	Storage of galactosyl-ceramide (cerebroside)
Metachromatic leukodystrophy	Arylsulfatase A	Storage of sulfatide (cerebroside sulfate)
Adrenoleukodystrophy (sex-linked Schilder's disease)	?	? disorder of sterol metabolism
Sudanophilic leukodystrophy (Pelizaeus-Merzbacher and variants)	?	?
Sudanophilic leukodystrophy with associated features		
Cockayne disease	?	Premature aging, deafness, dwarfing
With meningeal angiomatosis	?	?
Amino-acidurias		
Phenylketonuria	Phenylalanine hydroxylase	Defective myelination
Maple syrup urine disease	Branched-chain keto acid decarboxylase	Defective myelination
Spongy degeneration	?	Chronic edema in protoplasmic astrocytes and within myelin lamellae

but the patients are less demented. They eventually develop optic atrophy, and in some cases seizures. Death is usually due to malnutrition and intercurrent illness. Pathology is similar to that in the infantile type.

The *adult type* is rare and encompasses an ill-defined group.

There are *transitional* and *unclassified types* that start in infancy, with the patients surviving to the end of the second decade. Subtotal loss of myelin is seen, more severe than in classic Pelizaeus-Merzbacher disease. Cases have been sporadic, and both sexes have been involved; the course is similar to that of the classic cases. The diagnosis of connatal and classic Pelizaeus-Merzbacher disease can be made on clinical grounds. Adult cases are usually not diagnosed until post mortem. No therapy is available except for supportive therapy and treatment of seizures. Genetic counseling should be offered to those families where the sex-linked recessive pattern of inheritance is obvious.

COCKAYNE'S SYNDROME. Cockayne's syndrome, a rare autosomal recessive disease, is characterized by dwarfism, microcephaly, premature aging, photodermatitis, bony changes, intracranial calcification, deafness, blindness due to a pigmentary degeneration of the retina, corneal opacity, and a neurologic disorder reflecting a sudanophilic demyelination similar to that found in Pelizaeus-Merzbacher disease. Because many signs overlap with those of other diseases (eg, progeria, xeroderma pigmentosum) and multiple systems are involved, the possibility of linked polygenic inheritance has been raised. A single disorder of lipid metabolism affecting multiple tissues cannot be dismissed as the cause.

These children are normal at birth and do not show signs until the end of the first year. Failure to grow eventually leads to cachectic dwarfism; scoliosis and flexion deformities of the limbs may develop. Bone age remains normal, and endocrine function, including gonadal function, may be preserved. There is no loss of hair (in contrast to progeria), but the beaked nose, hypotelorism, and severe cachexia are quite similar. Microcephaly reflects severe brain atrophy due to loss of myelin. These children are unduly sensitive to sunlight; they develop a red scaling rash in exposed areas followed by scarring and hyperpigmentation. They do not sweat. Ocular lesions include keratitis, irregular pupils, failure of lacrimation, and progressive punctate pigmentary degeneration of the retina leading to blindness and optic atrophy. Characteristically the pupils respond slowly to mydriatics. Limb and gait ataxia, nystagmus, and choreoathetosis are noted much more often than spasticity. Weakness and muscle atrophy probably reflect a peripheral neuropathy due to segmental demyelination. The course of the illness is slow; some children have survived into the fourth decade, although others have died in childhood. No treatment is available.

Patchy sudanophilic demyelination of the white matter in the centrum semiovale, brainstem, and cerebellum is characteristic. Islands of preserved myelin without preservation of U fibers, as well as sparing of axis cylinders, are constant features. Severe brain atrophy reflects diffuse atrophy of the white matter, including the pons and brainstem. Perivascular mineral concretions containing calcium and iron are most striking in the basal ganglia and cerebellum; they can often be seen on radiographs. No specific abnormality of cerebral lipids has been found. All lipids are decreased with the exception of cholesterol esters, which are increased, as in other sudanophilic leukodystrophies.

LEUKODYSTROPHY WITH MENINGEAL ANGIOMATOSIS. Families have been described in which infants presented with intractable seizures in infancy, myoclonus, progressive dementia, and increased tone with increased reflexes, terminating in coma and death between 2 and 4 years of age. The EEGs were grossly abnormal, and diffuse angiomatosis of the leptomeninges, loss of neurons in the deep nuclei, brainstem, and cerebellum and extensive orthochromatic demyelination of the white matter and long tracts were noted at autopsy. There is no explanation for the coincidence of the angiomatosis and the demyelination.

OTHER DISORDERS OF LIPID METABOLISM

ADRENOLEUKODYSTROPHY. Adrenoleukodystrophy (sex-linked Schilder's disease) was until recently thought to be a primary demyelinating disease of childhood akin to disseminated sclerosis. It is characterized by widespread demyelination of the cerebral white matter, starting occipitally and spreading frontally, sparing the subcortical U fibers. Recently Schaumburg and associates have found adrenal lesions at autopsy in most cases of Schilder's disease, whether or not the patients had adrenal insufficiency during life. They suggest that most cases diagnosed as Schilder's disease were adrenoleukodystrophy, which they postulate to be due to a systemic disorder of sterol metabolism or long-chain fatty acids that affects the adrenal glands, the brain, the interstitial cells of the testes, and Schwann cells. Recent evidence from fibroblast tissue culture supports this hypothesis.

The signs and symptoms of neurologic and adrenal involvement may proceed independently. Male relatives of patients with adrenoleukodystrophy have died of Addison's disease without neurologic signs, and many patients with adrenoleukodystrophy have had no clinical evidence of adrenal involvement. The disease presents most often in boys of school age, with cortical visual loss, intellectual apathy, and an atactic-spastic gait disturbance. Spasticity progresses until the patient lies in a decorticate state. Involuntary movements do not occur, and seizures occur late. Focal neurologic signs, optic atrophy, increased intracranial pressure, and hearing loss may make the differential diagnosis from a neoplasm or multiple sclerosis difficult. Melanoderma, maximum in skin folds, may become evident at any time during the illness. The child usually expires either from an adrenal crisis or in a vegetative state 6 months to 5 years after the first symptoms. The spinal fluid pressure may be elevated and protein and gamma globulin content mildly increased. Skull radiographs may show split sutures; EEGs may be normal initially or may show focal or diffuse slowing or paroxysmal discharges.

The most striking pathologic finding is extensive sudanophilic demyelination of the white matter, which usually spreads forward from the occipital region. Electron microscopy demonstrates pathognomonic lipid lamellae, similar to those in the adrenals and testes. The adrenal cortex is atrophic. Granular eosinophilic swelling of cells in the zona reticularis and the inner portion of the fasciculi are attributed to exaggerated ACTH stimulation. The pathognomonic cell is large, with a striated cytoplasm, and contains intracytoplasmic lamellae and lamellar lipid profiles that appear to contain a free 3β-hydroxysterol; the lamellae are birefringent. Inflammatory changes are noted in the brain and adrenal.

Steroid replacement therapy is indicated in all patients during the stress of intercurrent illness and in children with evidence of adrenal insufficiency; however, it does not change the course of either the adrenal or the neurologic illness. Appropriate supportive care, anticonvulsive therapy, and symptomatic therapy must be offered. Equally important, genetic counseling must be provided because of the high risk run by male relatives of the mother.

CEREBROTENDINOUS XANTHOMATOSIS. Cerebrotendinous xanthomatosis (cholestanol storage disease) is an autosomal recessive disorder characterized by storage of cholestanol (dihydrocholesterol) rather than cholesterol in the brain. The basic enzymatic deficit remains to be described. The disease usually becomes manifest in midchildhood or adolescence; its course is prolonged, with death in the fifth decade. The patients usually present with borderline intellect or an insidious dementia, followed by ataxia, spasticity, juvenile cataracts, and tendon xanthomas, most often starting in the Achilles tendon. Later, dysarthria, distal muscle atrophy, and loss of position and vibration sense develop. Serum cholesterol and lipid profile are usually normal, which differentiates this disease from type II and type III hyperlipoproteinemia. Cholestanol is increased in the plasma.

The xanthomas consist of a dense accumulation of birefringent crystals within granulomas. Loss of granular and Purkinje cells, demyelination of long tracts in the brainstem and spinal cord, and in some cases granulomas in the basal ganglia have been found. Increased levels of free and esterified cholestanol have been found in cerebellum and cerebrum, as well as in the tendinous xanthomas. Free cholestanol may replace cholesterol in myelin, since it is increased in frontal white matter.

WOLMAN'S DISEASE. Wolman's disease (cholesterol ester and triglyceride storage disease) is a rare autosomal recessive lipid storage disease of infancy related to deficient activity of acid lipase, which degrades triglycerides and cholesterol esters. Extensive storage of cholesterol esters and triglycerides in macrophages of liver, spleen, bone marrow, lymph nodes, adrenals, and intestinal mucosa is noted. In the brain, lipid storage is noted in the choroid plexus, leptomeninges, and endothelial and perithelial cells. Lipid storage in neurons, in particular Purkinje cells and glial cells, may occur, and sudanophilia of the white matter may be present. A diagnosis can be made by rectal biopsy, which demonstrates severe sudanophilic storage in neurons of the myenteric plexus.

These infants develop severe vomiting, diarrhea, abdominal distension, and occasionally jaundice soon after birth. Failure to thrive, anemia, vacuolated lymphocytes, hepatosplenomegaly, and calcification of the adrenal glands are noted. There is a progressive decrease in alertness and activity, but no seizures. Death usually occurs by 6 months of age. Vacuolated lymphocytes, foam cells in the bone marrow, hepatosplenomegaly, and failure to thrive may suggest the diagnosis of Niemann-Pick disease, but radiographic evidence of adrenal calcification is pathognomonic of Wolman's disease. Chemical analysis of biopsy material and enzymatic assay confirm the diagnosis and enable one to rule out glycogen storage disease, galactosemia, and other malabsorption syndromes. There is no effective therapy.

REFSUM'S DISEASE. Refsum's disease (phytanic acid storage disease, heredopathia atactica polyneuritiformis) is an autosomal recessive disorder that presents with small pupils, gait ataxia in childhood, and progressive night blindness; in early adult life constricted visual fields and hearing loss develop. There is insidious motor and sensory neuropathy, with particular impairment of position and vibration sense, followed by signs of autonomic dysfunction and sudden death in early middle age, presumably due to cardiac dysfunction. These patients have storage of phytanic acid, (a 20-carbon fatty acid derived from chlorophyll) in the viscera that results from a defect at the first step of catabolism of phytanic acid—the α-oxidation of the terminal carboxyl group. Heterozygotes can be detected by demonstration of somewhat elevated levels of phytanic acid in the plasma and a reduced rate of phytanic oxidation in fibroblasts in tissue culture.

Refsum's disease is the only lipid storage disease where effective therapy (a diet poor in phytol and phytanic acid) can be offered. It is essential to consider the diagnosis in any patient with atypical spinocerebellar degeneration and chronic neuropathy. Night blindness is almost always present and should suggest the diagnosis.

The characteristic findings include retinitis pigmentosa, peripheral neuropathy, cerebellar ataxia, and high spinal fluid protein. Signs usually develop in childhood. Nerve deafness, anosmia, pupillary abnormalities, cataracts, and ichthyosis are found in most patients. Congenital abnormalities of the bones of the hands and toes and epiphyseal dysplasia may occur. Nonspecific ECG abnormalities, including conduction defects, may explain the sudden death that has been reported as early as 7 years. The course is generally progressive, with unexplained remissions and periods of exacerbation that occur postpartum or following intercurrent illnesses. Intellectual deterioration and seizures do not occur. Pes cavus, areflexia, muscle weakness and wasting, loss of proprioception, and ataxia may suggest a spinocerebellar ataxia of the Friedreich type, but dramatically slowed nerve conduction velocities and spinal fluid protein elevation reflect the neuropathy. Diagnosis rests on the demonstration of excess phytanic acid in the plasma and urine and lack of α-oxidation of phytanic acid by cultured skin fibroblasts.

There is an interstitial neuritis with some loss of axons and demyelination. Neuronal loss is mild, and storage is not present. Therapy consists in providing a diet that excludes dairy fat, ruminant fat, and chlorophyll. Remission of some neurologic symptoms occurs when phytanic acid levels drop in the blood. Exacerbations usually reflect inadequate dietary control. In some cases a liquid synthetic formula free of phytanic acid has been particularly effective.

TANGIER DISEASE.　Tangier disease is a rare autosomal recessive disorder characterized by storage of cholesterol esters in liver, spleen, lymph nodes, tonsils, thymus, cornea, intestinal mucosa, skin, and peripheral nerves. The diagnosis is suggested by the finding of large yellow orange tonsils filled with foam cells in a child or an adult and absence of high-density lipoproteins (α lipoproteins) in the plasma, with very low cholesterol and increased triglyceride levels. The basic enzymatic defect is unknown. The course is slow, with a fluctuating mixed peripheral neuropathy or with slowly progressive distal neuropathy with pain and temperature loss, distal muscle atrophy, oculomotor weakness, ptosis, and stabbing pains. Loss of position and vibration sense occurs much later. Nerve conduction velocities are slow.

ABETALIPOPROTEINEMIA.　Abetalipoproteinemia (Bassen-Kornzweig syndrome) is a rare autosomal recessive disorder that presents with malabsorption of fat, acanthocytosis, retinitis pigmentosa, and atactic neuropathic symptoms in addition to the abetalipoproteinemia. It should be considered in the differential diagnosis of patients with spinocerebellar degenerations. Cholesterol, phospholipids and triglycerides, chylomicrons, and β and pre-β lipoproteins (very low density lipoproteins and low-density lipoproteins) are absent from the plasma; only high-density lipoproteins are demonstrable, and only at low levels. It is thought that there may be a fundamental deficit of the apoprotein (carrier protein) for low-density lipoproteins. Consequently chylomicrons will not be transported across the intestinal mucosa into the plasma, and long-chain triglycerides cannot be removed from cells. Linoleic acid is deficient. Malabsorption involves fat-soluble vitamin A and vitamin E. Low vitamin E levels may favor abnormal lipid peroxidation in the central nervous system and may explain the excess ceroid described in the cerebral cortex and myocardium.

Patients present in infancy with steatorrhea, abdominal distension, and disturbed growth. Retinitis pigmentosa develops by 5 to 10 years of age, with impaired dark adaptation, decreased visual acuity, and constricted visual fields. The neurologic deficit, which mimics Friedreich's ataxia or Refsum's disease, consists of an atactic gait, areflexia, loss of proprioception, and cerebellar signs. Muscle wasting, kyphoscoliosis, impaired eye motility, ptosis, facial weakness, decreased sensation for pain and temperature, and Babinski signs appear later. The patients develop scoliosis and signs of cardiomyopathy and may expire in childhood or not until the fourth decade. The spinal fluid protein is usually normal; nerve conduction velocities are prolonged.

Jejunal biopsy is pathognomonic. The mucosal villi are of normal thickness. Lipid droplets (triglycerides) are present in many mucosal cells, but there is no lipid in the villous core or lacteals. Acanthocytes with long spiny excrescences are frequent in peripheral blood smears. A low-fat diet is essential to minimize the malabsorption. Medium-chain triglycerides can be used as a supplemental source of calories. Parenteral vitamin A administration apparently improves the night blindness but does not prevent development of retinitis pigmentosa.

CEROID LIPOFUSCINOSES.　The diseases grouped as ceroid lipofuscinoses are characterized histologically by the accumulation in swollen neurons of autofluorescent lipopigments in abnormal cytosomes. In this sense they fall within the category of neuronal storage diseases and lysosomal disorders, but no storage has been demonstrated chemically and no deficit in an acid hydrolase has been discovered. The basic metabolic defect is still unknown, but it may be related to peroxidation of fatty acids. Both ceroid and lipofuscin accumulate in lysosomes in the brain of a patient with ceroid lipofuscinosis; both are insoluble in the usual fat solvents. Several variants have been described; the following classification must be considered quite tentative.

INFANTILE VARIANT.　The infantile (Finnish) variant is an autosomal recessive syndrome and is the most common of the progressive encephalopathies of early childhood in Finland. These infants appear normal until about 8 months of age; delay in motor and intellectual development and visual loss herald the onset of the disease. Hypotonia and ataxia of the trunk and limbs progress rapidly. There is no evidence of neuropathy or of visceral storage. By 2 years the infants are virtually blind; the fundi show widespread retinal atrophy with macular degeneration, optic atrophy, and unreactive pupils. Myoclonic jerks are prominent. While the EEG may show some paroxysmal activity early in the course, it becomes progressively slower and lower voltage, and by 3 years it is usually isoelectric. Microcephaly with a thickened skull is almost invariably present and reflects extreme atrophy. Death supervenes by 3 to 10 years of age.

Laboratory tests are not helpful, with the exception of the early extinction of the electroretinogram and the persistently isoelectric EEG by age 3 years. Differential diagnosis from the sphingolipidoses of early childhood can be made easily on clinical and enzymatic grounds.

LATE INFANTILE VARIANT.   The late infantile variant (Bielschowsky-Jansky disease) has clinical features similar to those of the infantile type and also has a rapid course, but it starts at 2 to 4 years of age. The electroretinogram is abnormal early in the course and later becomes extinguished; giant visual- and somatosensory-evoked potentials can be recorded in the plain EEG with slow rates of stimulation, but the visual-evoked response disappears when blindness is complete. The EEG is characterized by frequent bursts of 2.5- to 4-Hz slow waves and atypical spikes and waves. The disease is autosomal recessive. It should be considered in preschool children with severe drop attacks that do not respond to anticonvulsants or ketogenic diets. An abnormal electroretinogram and giant visual-evoked responses are helpful in making the diagnosis.

JUVENILE VARIANT.   The juvenile variant (Spielmeyer-Sjögren disease), which is autosomal recessive, has a rather stereotyped and much longer course than the other variants. A rapidly progressive retinal degeneration starts at 5 to 8 years of age; the fundi show macular degeneration, optic atrophy, attenuated vessels, and black corpuscles in the periphery of the retina. Dementia, seizures, and motor findings may not appear until the teenage years and may vary in severity. A disturbance of speech is characteristic: the children speak very rapidly with syllable repetitions and poorly modulated voice. They develop motor apraxia (eg, they may be unable to get out of a chair or start walking without being pushed). Eventually they walk with a stooped posture and small festinating steps. Dystonic features, dysmetria, fine tremors of the face, and hyperactive reflexes are common. Progressive dementia and motor deterioration occur, with death in the late teenage years. The EEG shows dysrhythmic high-voltage discharges before the onset of seizures, which vary in frequency and severity. Seizures can usually be controlled with anticonvulsants, although some patients tolerate diphenylhydantoin poorly. The electroretinogram is abnormal in the early stages, but giant responses characteristic of the late infantile variant are not present.

ADULT VARIANTS.   The adult vairant known as *Kufs's disease* presents with seizures, myoclonus, cerebellar ataxia, and progressive dementia, but without retinal degeneration. In the *myoclonic variant* with cherry-red spot, myoclonic jerks are common, evoked responses are large, and the red spot may be noted in adolescence.

Brain atrophy may be extreme in the infantile group, but it varies in severity in older patients. Neuronal dropout is marked, particularly in the cortex, where astrocytes and macrophages may be the only cells left. Ceroid and lipofuscin storage is noted in histiocytes in skin, muscle, viscera, and the myenteric plexus. Diagnosis can be made from skin, muscle, or rectal biopsy.

Supportive treatment, adequate educational placement, anticonvulsants, and eventually total nursing care are required. Genetic counseling is essential; most of these disorders can be assumed to be autosomal reces-

sive, with a high risk of recurrence among siblings and virtually no risk in collaterals or descendants. Intrauterine diagnosis is not available at this time.

DISEASES OF ASTROCYTIC PATHOLOGY

SPONGY CNS DEGENERATION.   Spongy degeneration of the central nervous system (Van Bogaert-Bertrand type, Canavan's disease) is an autosomal recessive disorder that has a predilection for northern Ashkenazi Jews and is one of the more common progressive encephalopathies of infancy. The hallmark of the disease is a severe chronic edema that in the cortex affects protoplasmic astrocytes. In the white matter it appears to spread from the extracellular space rather than from the oligodendroglia. The demyelination is secondary, and the spongy degeneration does not appear to be a primary leukodystrophy. There is a marked increase in the water content of white matter, which has the composition of a plasma filtrate. At this time the diagnosis, which can be strongly suspected on clinical grounds, can be confirmed only by brain biopsy.

Most children appear normal at birth, but they usually do not achieve normal head control. Accelerated head growth is evident by 6 months of age, when psychomotor development slows before it later regresses. Generalized hypotonia is superseded during the second year by spasticity, with decorticate posture, although the head remains floppy. Opisthotonic crises may develop from auditory, visual, and tactile stimuli. Vision fails and optic atrophy develops, usually after the age of 2 years. Head growth decelerates, seizures develop, and paroxysmal episodes of sweating, hyperthermia, vomiting, and hypotension occur terminally. Death usually supervenes by 4 years. The EEG is normal initially; later it may slow and show paroxysmal features. CSF is usually normal. The disease may be evident at birth; the infant is floppy and lethargic and has difficulty sucking and swallowing; death occurs within a few weeks. Some infants dying of arginosuccinic acidemia, maple syrup urine disease, and hyperglycinemia have been found to have striking spongy changes in their brains. A juvenile variant starting at age 5 years, with survival into late adolescence, has been described. It is characterized by a progressive cerebellar syndrome, dementia, loss of vision, optic atrophy, and spasticity. Pigmentary degeneration of the retina may lead to an erroneous diagnosis of juvenile ceroid lipofuscinosis.

Brain weight is increased because of the severe cerebral edema that affects the deeper layers of the cortex and superficial layers of the white matter in the early stages. As the disease progresses, sponginess spreads to the brainstem, cerebellum, and spinal cord, involving long tracts as well as subcortical nuclear masses. Later, neuronal loss becomes severe in the cerebrum and cerebellum as vacuolation spreads to all layers of the now atrophic cortex. The ventricles become markedly dilated as more white matter is destroyed. The vacuoles in the deep layers of the cortex often appear to surround neurons and small vessels. They are due to massive swelling of protoplasmic astrocytes whose cytoplasm is watery and whose abnormal processes contain bizarre, grossly elongated mitochondria. In the white matter the vacuoles occupy the extracellular space and are seen within the myelin lamellae. In advanced cases, there is severe myelin destruction and gliosis.

The presence of an enlarged head since early infancy in a hypotonic baby who later develops spasticity, a decorticate posture, optic atrophy, and seizures is quite characteristic. Head enlargement does not develop until late in the second year in Tay-Sachs disease, and these infants have the characteristic macular cherry-red spot, evidence of anterior horn cell disease, early myoclonus, and pathognomonic decrease in hexosaminidase A. Alexander's disease also has megalencephaly, and its course may be similar to that of spongy degeneration. Therapy is limited to treatment of seizures and supportive care. Genetic counseling should be offered to the parents.

ALEXANDER'S DISEASE. Alexander's disease is a rare disorder of early childhood characterized clinically by a large head, mental retardation, spasticity, and in some cases seizures developing in the first year. Hydrocephalus is due to obstruction of the aqueduct of Sylvius. Most of these children have died between 2 and 8 years of age. No treatment is known. This disease is unique pathologically and is characterized by the widespread deposition of hyaline eosinophilic deposits in the footplates of astrocytes in the subpial and subependymal layers of the brain and spinal cord and around blood vessels. The material deposited resembles neurokeratin. The only means of making a definitive diagnosis during life is by brain biopsy.

DISEASES INVOLVING CATIONS

HEPATOLENTICULAR DEGENERATION. Hepatolenticular degeneration (Wilson's disease), an autosomal recessive disease, is important because an effective therapy is available, and treatment of still asymptomatic homozygotes will prevent the development of symptoms and signs for many years, possibly indefinitely. In any child with unexplained liver disease, hepatosplenomegaly, subacute infectious hepatitis, or juvenile cirrhosis, and in any child with an acquired movement disorder, ataxia, or atypical behavior, the condition should be suspected; at the minimum the patient's serum ceruloplasmin should be measured.

While it is clear that the disease is due to a positive copper balance despite increased excretion of copper in the urine, the fundamental enzymatic defect is still unknown. Deposition of copper in abnormal concretions in liver, brain, and kidney produces functional alterations of these organs and explains the signs and symptoms. The diagnosis rests on the demonstration of low ceruloplasmin levels (less than 20 mg/100 ml) and high levels of hepatic copper (more than $250\mu g/g$ dry weight), each of which is present in about 95 percent of these patients. Inconstant findings may include increased urinary excretion of copper (more than 100 $\mu g/24$ hours), decreased fecal excretion of copper, low serum uric acid, and increased urinary excretion of uric acid and amino acids. Copper incorporation into ceruloplasmin is greatly reduced. The Kayser-Fleischer ring is pathognomonic of WWilson's disease and is always present in patients who have signs of neurologic dysfunction, but it may be absent in children who have only hepatic evidence of the disease.

The frequency of the disease is estimated to be 1 in 200,000 individuals, with a carrier frequency of 1 in 200. Detection of heterozygotes is possible but is not clear-cut. Carriers never develop clinical signs; yet their ceruloplasmin levels may be lowered and their hepatic copper concentrations may be higher than normal. They incorporate copper into ceruloplasmin at a reduced rate. Normal infants have high concentrations of hepatic copper and low levels of ceruloplasmin, so that neonatal and intrauterine diagnosis is not possible. Pregnancy, estrogen administration, thyrotoxicosis, infections, cancer, and biliary cirrhosis may increase ceruloplasmin levels. They may be decreased in normal infants under the age of 6 months, in infants with sprue and nephrosis, and in infants with anemia and malnutrition. It is crucial to determine whether an individual (usually a sibling of a patient known to have Wilson's disease) is an asymptomatic homozygote who should be treated forthwith or a heterozygote who should not. Most heterozygotes do not have ceruloplasmin levels below 20 mg/100 ml, elevated nonceruloplasmin serum copper, and increased excretion of copper.

Clinical Findings. Diagnosis is obvious when there is evidence of both hepatic and neurologic dysfunction. However, signs and symptoms are variable, spontaneous exacerbations and remissions are common, and the severity of hepatic and neurologic dysfunction varies independently and widely between patients. Age of onset ranges from below 6 years to the fifth decade. Liver disease is more common in children, and neurologic dysfunction is more likely in adults.

Liver disease manifests with unexplained jaundice, hepatomegaly, and abnormal liver function tests and may occur as young as 3 years of age. Quite often the disease is clinically silent until subacute liver failure and jaundice, ascites, spider angiomata, and weakness develop; it may lead to coma and death within a few weeks. If the diagnosis of Wilson's disease is not considered, it may be missed even if an autopsy is performed, since the pathology is not pathognomonic and since not all patients who die of liver failure have Kayser-Fleischer rings. More chronic liver disease may manifest itself by hepatomegaly or a shrunken liver, with signs of portal hypertension. Pregnancy tends to improve the manifestations of Wilson's disease. Hepatic coma and ascites are infrequent, except late in the stage of hepatic decompensation.

Neurologic Signs. Two main syndromes have been recognized. In older patients cerebellar signs may predominate, the course of the illness is prolonged, and prognosis and response to therapy are favorable. Characteristic findings include resting and intention tremors, a flapping tremor of the hands and shoulders brought out by abducting the arms and holding the forearms horizontal in front of the body (wing beating), irregular oscillations of the eyeballs, infrequent blinking, and atactic unsteady gait. These patients may not be able to dress, drink out of a cup, or light a cigarette. They may be quite dysarthric. This variant is referred to as the pseudosclerotic variant (because of resemblances to multiple sclerosis). In adolescents and young adults a dystonic variant is more likely to occur. It is characterized by a frozen face with an almost pathognomonic retracted upper lip, athetoid or choreic movements, dystonia, often asymmetric posture of the limbs with the wrist in flexion and hand fisted, and rather frequent myoclonus. Seizures, including focal seizures, have been reported. At times the signs may be so asymmetric as to present as a dystonic hemiparesis. These juvenile cases may have a less favorable prognosis because cavitation of the basal ganglia may develop and produce irreversible signs.

Psychiatric signs may range from inattentiveness and behavior disorders to severe personality changes with a schizophrenic picture. These signs are thought to be due to storage of copper in the cortex as well as in the basal ganglia. The psychiatric signs and many of the neurologic signs are reversible with copper chelating therapy. Even patients who have been bedridden and unable to walk, dress, speak, or feed themselves have made substantial, if not total, recoveries. Samples of the patient's handwriting or his ability to draw a spiral are sensitive means of following a patient's progress. Neurologic signs may vary and may in fact increase at the onset of therapy. Improvement may be delayed and quite slow, but it can be anticipated with confidence in all but the most severely affected patients.

Other signs include the Kayser-Fleischer ring, which is pathognomonic of the illness and is always present in patients with neurologic signs; it may be totally reversible by chelation. It is most prominent at the inferior and superior margins of the limbus (Fig. 44, color plate 3) and does not interfere with vision. It is easy to see with the naked eye in patients with light-colored irises, especially if a narrow beam of light from a flashlight is shone tangentially to the cornea. In patients with dark irises, or very early in the course of the disease, slit-lamp examination is required. Sunflower cataracts similar to those noted in patients with copper foreign bodies in the eye may be seen in some patients. A bluish discoloration of the lunulae of the fingernails (azure lunula) is seen occasionally. Bony changes consisting of wedging of thoracic vertebrae, foci of osteochondritis dissecans, osteoporosis, poor healing of fractures, and osteoarthritis have been described in advanced cases, and the episodes of hyperpyrexia, abdominal pain, and headache remain unexplained.

Pathology.   Histologic findings on liver biopsy are suggestive but not pathognomonic of the disease. They include lipid droplets in hepatocytes, increased glycogen in the nuclei of hepatocytes, condensation of mitochondria with indistinct cristae and amorphous inclusions, and fibrosis of the portal spaces. Eventually liver necrosis ensues, and the histologic picture is similar to that seen in other hepatic processes that lead to liver destruction. There is no storage of copper in Kupffer cells. In the brain the most striking pathology is found in the caudate nucleus and putamen, which may appear shrunken or even cavitated and have a brownish color. Neuronal dropout and gliosis may be severe. Alzheimer type II astrocytes, which have large vesicular nuclei with one or more nucleoli, are numerous in the striatum. In the thalamus, globus pallidus, zona reticulata of the substantia nigra, but usually not in the striatum, one may find Opalski cells that are characteristic of Wilson's disease. These large rounded cells, thought to be histocytes, have a foamy cytoplasm that stains light pink with Nissl's stain.

Differential Diagnosis.   Ceruloplasmin blood levels should be obtained in all patients with acquired movement disorders, atactic syndromes, or schizophrenialike psychosis. If levels are above 43 mg/100 ml Wilson's disease is virtually excluded, while if they are below 20 mg/100 ml the diagnosis becomes very likely. Examination for a Kayser-Fleischer ring and measurement of 24-hour urinary excretion of copper (below 100 μg/24 hours in normals) will usually clarify the diagnosis. Rarely it will be necessary to perform a liver biopsy for histology (including electron microscopy) and measurement of copper content (below 100 μg/g dry weight in normals, usually above 250 μg/g in patients with Wilson's disease).

Treatment.   Therapy consists of decreasing the copper content of the diet, decreasing intestinal absorption of copper by binding it in the gut, and chelating copper stores from the tissues. To achieve a low-copper diet, chocolate, cocoa, nuts, mushrooms, liver, brain, shellfish, molasses, and broccoli should be excluded. Copper binding in the gut may be accomplished by administering 40 mg of potassium sulfide with each meal. For chelation the drug of choice is D-penicillamine (the DL-form produces pyridoxine deficiency and is more likely to result in side effects), 1 to 4 g/day in divided doses. While this drug is usually well tolerated, significant side effects may include fever, nausea, skin rashes, lymphadenopathy, iron-deficiency anemia, leukopenia, thrombocytopenia, optic neuritis, a lupuslike syndrome, and the nephrotic syndrome. Side effects almost always subside if the drug is discontinued and then is reintroduced very gradually in slowly increasing doses. Occasionally steroids may be used for a few days to increase tolerance. Weekly doses of ferrous sulfate and multivitamins (in particular pyridoxine) are administered preventively. Penicillamine markedly increases urinary excretion of copper, which may reach 7 mg/24 hours (5 percent of total body copper). It appears to act by releasing copper from ceruloplasmin and albumin, which permits its excretion by the kidneys. The amount of copper excreted is much higher at the start of therapy than later, when it may not exceed 1 mg/24 hours. Lesser amounts suggest the need for increasing the dose of penicillamine.

Genetic counseling and thorough investigation of all siblings of patients with Wilson's disease are in order as soon as the diagnosis is established. Asymptomatic homozygote siblings should be treated indefinitely to avoid symptoms.

CEREBROHEPATORENAL SYNDROME. Cerebrohepatorenal syndrome (Zellweger's syndrome) is a lethal condition of infancy characterized by profound hypotonia, cirrhosis of the liver, renal cysts, minor skeletal anomalies, a characteristic facies, failure to thrive and develop, seizures, and death before 6 months of age. The diagnosis can be strongly suspected on the basis of the facial features: frontal bossing, hypertelorism, epicanthal folds, long upper lip, and pursed mouth. The children suck poorly, fail to gain weight, and tend to be jaundiced. A characteristic laboratory finding is an increase in serum iron and serum iron binding capacity. No therapy is available.

TRICHOPOLIODYSTROPHY. Trichopoliodystrophy (kinky hair disease), a sex-linked recessive disorder described by Menkes, is due to a defect in the release of copper from epithelial cells of the gut, with resulting generalized copper deficiency. It is fatal within the first 3 years of life. It is important that it be recognized early, since it is possible that early replacement therapy may be effective. These infants have low levels of hepatic and serum copper, low ceruloplasmin, and impaired activity of copper-containing or copper-dependent enzymes, among them cytochrome oxidase, monoamine oxidase, ascorbic acid oxidase, and tyrosinase. Signs and symptoms can be explained by interference with energy metabolism, with the synthesis of melanin, myelin, elastin, and perhaps collagen and various proteins.

These infants are frequently born prematurely. Hypothermic episodes and lethargy may be noted soon after birth, but the infants generally appear normal for the first weeks of life. They may achieve early developmental milestones such as visual fixation and smiling. The first sign of the disease may be failure to thrive or seizures. The infants have characteristic hair that is poorly pigmented, sparse, and wiry. Under the microscope it appears twisted (pili torti), beaded (monilethrix), and brittle, with frayed nodular ends (trichorrhexis nodosa). The facies may be distinctive, with pudgy cheeks, small chin, horizontal twisted eyebrows, little facial expression, and hypopigmented skin. The infants are usually hypotonic and do not appear to see or hear well; microcysts of the iris and seborrheic dermatitis may be noted.

Seizures and/or myoclonus may be a major problem and respond poorly to anticonvulsants. The EEG is abnormal, often multifocal or hypsarhythmic. The electroretinogram is also abnormal and suggests poor rod function. Visual- and auditory-evoked responses may be extinguished, reflecting the poor response to visual and auditory stimuli. A variety of neurologic abnormalities have been encountered. Spasticity with increased reflexes supervenes but does not become extreme. The children make little further developmental progress and lose the few milestones they have achieved. They are susceptible to infection and have poor temperature regulation; eventually they require tube feeding. They usually expire before the age of 3 years.

Radiographic findings resemble those seen in scurvy and infantile copper deficiency. There is metaphyseal spurring and irregularity and in some cases periosteal new bone formation. Angiography reveals extreme tortuosity and irregularity of systemic and cerebral arteries. The ventricular system may be enlarged because of loss of white matter, and subdural hematoma may complicate the severe brain atrophy. Low ceruloplasmin levels and low serum copper levels confirm the diagnosis.

Widespread degenerative changes are noted in the systemic and intracranial arteries. The brain and cerebellum show severe and diffuse neuronal loss, with areas of focal necrosis, perhaps reflecting the severe vascular involvement.

Copper supplementation has been attempted in these infants; less than 1 percent of orally administered copper is absorbed per 24 hours. Administration of large doses does increase serum copper levels, but it may or may not increase ceruloplasmin; intravenous administration of copper raises ceruloplasmin levels. It is too soon to know whether this mode of therapy will have any value in the very young infant.

FAMILIAL CALCIFICATION OF BASAL GANGLIA. Skull radiographs may reveal bilaterally symmetric calcification of the basal ganglia and dentate nuclei in a variety of situations. The most common are hypoparathyroidism and pseudohypoparathyroidism, where seizures, raised intracranial pressure, extrapyramidal signs, and psychiatric disturbances may lead to an erroneous diagnosis of a mass lesion. They are also characteristic of Cockayne's syndrome and are present, although not dense enough to be seen on plain radiographs, in Hallervorden-Spatz syndrome (p. 1917). Fahr's disease is a condition in which calcification of the basal ganglia is found in several family members. The significance and pathogenesis of the deposition of calcium (hydroxyapatite) in these nuclei is unknown. It may be noteworthy that they contain an excess of manganese, since manganese may have an affinity for the basal ganglia.

Diseases Involving Carbohydrate Metabolism

SUBACUTE NECROTIZING ENCEPHALOMYELOPATHY. Subacute necrotizing encephalomyelopathy (Leigh's syndrome) is most common in infancy and early childhood. It involves the brainstem and usually other parts of the nervous system to a variable degree. The pathology resembles that of thiamine deficiency (Wernicke's encephalopathy). It is probably caused by several different but related disorders of intermediary carbohydrate metabolism; recently a deficiency of cerebral thiamine triphosphate has been noted. The syndrome is inherited as a recessive, but is more common in males. Signs of the illness appear before the age of 1 year in over 50 percent of these patients, and by 2 years in 90 percent. The course is remitting, with acute exacerbations, usually precipitated by infection. Death may occur in a few days, but more commonly after several weeks or months.

Diagnosis is difficult because the illness presents in many different ways. Its hallmark is brainstem dysfunction, including respiratory irregularity and failure, difficulty in swallowing, dysarthria, facial weakness, hearing loss, extraocular palsies, ptosis, rolling eye movements, nystagmus, ataxia, and spasticity. Recurrent vomiting and lethargy may rapidly lead to coma. Episodic sighing respiration, sobbing without crying, and rapid irregular breathing are more common than in other diseases affecting the brainstem. Some infants are floppy because of peripheral neuropathy or myopathy. Many are mentally retarded. Failure to thrive may be a prominent feature. Blindness due to optic atrophy has been reported. The disease may develop suddenly in a previously normal child or may progress very slowly and present clinical and skeletal features strongly reminiscent of Friedreich's ataxia. Seizures are prominent in some patients but absent in many others.

Urine of patients with Leigh's syndrome contains an inhibitor of the enzyme thiamine pyrophosphate adenosine triphosphate phosphotransferase. This enzyme is responsible for the synthesis of cerebral thiamine triphosphate, which is deficient in the brain of patients with Leigh's syndrome. The presence of the enzyme inhibitor in the urine is diagnostic of Leigh's syndrome. It is present in obligate heterozygotes as well as affected patients, but disappears after prolonged treatment with high doses of thiamine. Blood pyruvate and lactate levels may be increased, but there is no change in lactate–pyruvate ratio. Blood alanine may be high, and metabolic acidosis may develop, partly from lactic acidosis, but also from a defect of renal tubular reabsorption of bicarbonate. These findings have suggested a block in pyruvate metabolism.

The presence in the urine of the inhibitor of the enzyme thiamine pyrophosphate has made diagnosis much easier. Thiamine deficiency can usually be excluded on the basis of the history and by the finding of normal levels of thiamine in the urine of children with Leigh's syndrome. Anticonvulsant toxicity and alcohol intoxication should be ruled out. Brainstem glioma, acute cerebellar ataxia, metachromatic leukodystrophy, neuroaxonal dystrophy, ataxia-telangiectasia, brainstem encephalitis, basilar artery migraine, Friedreich's ataxia, and Refsum's disease may be considered in some children. Late-onset methylmalonic-aciduria also produces an intermittent ataxia, as do Hartnup's disease and intermittent branched-chain ketoaciduria, but examination of the urine for amino acids will readily exclude them.

The characteristic feature is a spongy degeneration of the neuropil, with proliferation of capillaries and precapillaries. In more advanced lesions necrosis of the tissue and demyelination occur, with relative sparing of axons and neuronal cell bodies. Lesions have a predilection for subependymal regions of the medulla and pons, mesencephalon, diencephalon, and around the lateral ventricles. In contrast to thiamine deficiency (Wernicke's encephalopathy), lesions are less likely to be hemorrhagic, and the mamillary bodies and hypothalamus are often spared. Lesions are found in the spinal cord and often are of different ages.

Thiamine in pharmacologic doses has been effective occasionally. It has been suggested that derivatives of thiamine, such as thiamine propyldisulfide (which, unlike thiamine, enters cells by diffusion rather than by active transport), may be more effective, provided the content of thiamine in spinal fluid reaches 70 to 80 μg/100 ml. This may not be achieved, even with several grams of thiamine per day. Lipoic acid has been recommended at a dosage of 0.7 mg/kg intramuscularly three times a week; this agent is involved with thiamine pyrophosphate in the pyruvate decarboxylase reaction. Avoidance of high carbohydrate intake seems indicated, as exacerbations may follow especially high carbohydrate intake. In a disease characterized by an exacerbating and remitting course, the evaluation of any therapy is extremely difficult. Symptomatic treatment of acidemia, dehydration, and respiratory difficulty is indicated. Genetic counseling is in order. Heterozygote carriers may perhaps be distinguished from homozygotes on the basis of the thiamine pyrophosphate adenosine triphosphate phosphotransferase inhibitor 24-hour urine assay.

LAFORA'S DISEASE. Lafora's disease (progressive myoclonus epilepsy), an autosomal recessive disorder, is characterized by seizures, reflex and action myoclonus, progressive dementia, and cerebellar signs. It occurs most often in the second decade and leads to death in 2 to 10 years. Lafora bodies are diagnostic. They consist of round inclusions in neurons and their processes and have staining properties that suggest they are carbohydrate polymers; they also are found in liver, muscle, and myocardium. The cause of the disease is unknown, and no definitive therapy is available.

Seizures or myoclonus may be the presenting symptom. The myoclonus may consist of rapid, asynchronous, asymmetric jerks that involve only a small part of a muscle or massive myoclonic jerks that cause the patient to fall. The myoclonus becomes incapacitating and may be precipated by movement, touch, and light stimuli. The myoclonic jerks are not well correlated with the spikes in the EEG, which is diffusely slow throughout the course of the illness. Evoked responses to light or nerve stimulation are grossly increased. A series of myoclonic jerks may culminate in seizures, but consciousness may not be lost. The seizures respond better to anticonvulsants than the myoclonic jerks, which are quite resistant. Intravenous diazepam may suppress both seizures and myoclonus temporarily.

Dementia may be heralded by behavior abnormalities or psychosis; it is a rapidly progressive organic brain syndrome that may be delayed for several years after the onset of the myoclonus. Patients become atactic and are more likely to be hypotonic than spastic. Terminally the patients become totally incapacitated and demented; death may be hastened by myocardial involvement. The spinal fluid is normal. There are no diagnostic tests short of liver, muscle, or brain biopsy that enable one to make a definitive diagnosis. Differential diagnosis includes subacute sclerosing panencephalitis, late infantile ceroid lipofuscinosis, Unverricht-Lundborg disease, and ceroid lipofuscinosis with cherry-red spot and myoclonus.

The Lafora inclusions are pathognomonic and occur only in neurons, axons, and dendrites in the brain. They usually have a dense core and a lighter halo and measure 3 to 40 μ. The inclusions stain blue with hematoxylin; they are PAS- positive and are thought to contain a glucose polymer (polyglycosan) with very little protein. They are readily digested by diastase and amylase, thus confirming their similarity to starch and glycogen. Neurons may appear atrophic and may contain excess lipofuscin. The white matter appears normal, and gliosis is not prominent. Inclusions are found in the liver and result in ballooning of hepatocytes in skeletal muscle and in the myocardium. With the electron microscope Lafora bodies may be seen to be composed of a dense granular core with fine, irregular, loosely packed filaments in the periphery. They are not membrane-bound in neurons. The chemical pathology of the disorder is unknown. Therapy is limited to symptomatic treatment of the seizures (which respond fairly well to anticonvulsants) and of the myoclonus (which is resistant to most drugs except intravenous diazepam). A trial of 5-hydroxytryptophan seems justified.

DISEASES OF BASAL GANGLIA INVOLVING NEUROTRANSMITTERS

HUNTINGTON'S DISEASE. Huntington's disease, which has an autosomal dominant inheritance with complete penetrance and a low rate of spontaneous mutation, usually runs its course in middle age and is characterized by various behavior aberrations, a relentlessly progressive movement disorder, and dementia. In 5 percent of cases the disease starts in childhood; it is four to five times more likely for the fathers of these children to be choreic than the mothers. The illness is invariably fatal after a course of 10 to 15 years. Its pathogenesis is still unknown. The gene frequency is estimated to be 1 in 10,000 individuals, and Huntington's chorea accounts for at least 1 percent of all patients hospitalized for mental illness.

Clinical manifestations in children are quite different from those in adults. Whereas chorea (with a characteristic dancing gait) and dementia are the hallmarks of the disease in adults, seizures, rigidity, and dementia characterize the illness in children. Misdiagnosis in children is common unless it is known that one of the parents has chorea. Rigidity associated with dementia that may lead to mutism sometimes suggests the diagnosis of autism or catatonia. In adolescents depression and suicidal tendencies are quite common. The age of onset in children

ranges from 3 to 9 years; average age at death is 12 years. No specific tests are available to confirm the diagnosis, but atrophy of the head of the caudate nucleus noted on computerized axial tomography scan or on air encephalography may be helpful although unnecessary if a positive family history is obtained.

Any neurologic or psychiatric illness in a child of a choreic parent should be considered Huntington's disease until proven otherwise. Sydenham's chorea, Gilles de la Tourette's disease, and Wilson's disease always enter into the differential diagnosis. It is especially important to rule out Wilson's disease, since it is a treatable condition.

The hallmark of the illness is loss of small neurons, with severe gliosis in the caudate nucleus and putamen. In children severe gliosis of the globus pallidus without conspicuous neuronal loss may account for the rigidity. Diffuse cortical neuronal dropout is present in both children and adults.

Drugs like physostigmine (which is cholinergic), reserpin (which depletes dopamine), and postsynaptic dopaminergic blocking agents like the phenothiazines have had limited and unpredictable effects. Anticholinergic drugs and L-dopa are contraindicated because they may worsen the movement disorder.

DYSTONIA MUSCULORUM DEFORMANS. Dystonia is a genetic disease of the nervous system in which no one pathologic lesion has consistently been demonstrated. The course of the illness is variable; some patients progress over a period of months or years; others stabilize or even improve spontaneously. Age of onset also varies; rarely it may start in the first year, but it usually presents at 5 to 15 years. The findings are quite varied, even in the same family; they may consist of writer's cramp or isolated spasmodic torticollis, or the child may be bent and twisted and totally disabled. There are no seizures and no reflex changes; the face is often spared, and intellect and personality are remarkably preserved. The disease is often mistakenly considered psychogenic.

A dominant form of the illness had been recognized for some time. Recently a recessive form with a predilection for Ashkenazi Jews has been identified. The recessive form tends to start earlier, almost always before the age of 15 years; it tends to involve the limbs rather than the axial musculature and to progress rapidly to severe or total disability.

Dystonia refers to the sustained contraction of agonist and antagonist muscles. This may result either in a fixed posture or in a disorder of movement that becomes evident with attempts to move. A classic mode of presentation is the semilunar foot, which is held in equinovarus position as soon as walking is attempted. In advanced cases severe hypertrophy of affected muscles may occur, and a radicular syndrome from arthritic changes in the cervical spine may accompany spasmodic torticollis. Although the movements disappear in sleep, children whose posture is fixed day after day eventually develop contractures and disuse atrophy. Sustained dystonia may be very painful, and children lose weight and may develop decubitus or spontaneous fractures.

Dystonia of abdominal muscles may interfere with eating, as swallowing and chewing become very difficult; speech becomes totally unintelligible.

The differential diagnosis includes Wilson's disease, the side effects of the major tranquilizers, congenital athetosis due to kernicterus or neonatal asphyxia, Huntington's disease, Sydenham's chorea, atypical ceroid lipofuscinosis, and Hallervorden-Spatz syndrome. Dystonia may occur following encephalitis or brain injury.

All the treatments offered are purely empiric; L-dopa is of no value, but carbamazepine may be helpful. Cryothalamotomy has been effective in relieving symptoms; in some patients the relief is permanent, and in others dystonia recurs. Multiple lesions may be needed, and patients run a significant risk of becoming severely dysarthric and developing corticospinal deficits. It should not be offered to children who are not severely disabled.

JUVENILE PARKINSONISM.   Parkinsonism, which is characterized by rigidity, bradykinesia or akinesia, and tremor at rest, usually occurs in middle adult life; it is rare in children. As in the adult, it may respond to L-dopa.

FAMILIAL (ESSENTIAL) TREMOR.   Essential tremor is inherited as an autosomal dominant trait. The tremor may start at any age, including childhood; it is benign, but may produce difficulties at school because of poor handwriting. It should not be confused with more serious tremors having their origin in the basal ganglia or cerebellum. Essential tremor is a postural tremor, as opposed to parkinsonian tremor, which is a tremor at rest, and cerebellar tremor, which becomes worse during voluntary movements. Children will rarely require treatment; propranolol, a β-adrenergic blocking agent, is reported to be the drug of choice for those adults who require therapy.

GILLES DE LA TOURETTE'S SYNDROME. Gilles de la Tourette's syndrome (multiple tic disease) is presumed to have its origin in the basal ganglia. Pediatricians should be aware of the syndrome, particularly since an effective therapeutic agent (haloperidol) is now available. It usually starts before the age of 12 years, with the child developing multiple tics. These usually begin in the shoulders and the face, but eventually may involve all parts of the body; they consist of blinking, twitching, grimacing, jerking movements. The movements are usually repetitive and have a semipurposeful character, and they can usually be suppressed momentarily. They are made worse by psychic tension, and they disappear in sleep. The muscles of respiration and swallowing become involved, so that throat clearing, coughs, snorts, hiccups, or other noises are made. In advanced cases coprolalia, swearing, spitting, and elaborate gestures may appear. Multiple tics with any respiratory component are considered sufficient for the diagnosis. The illness is chronic and often persists into adult life. No other signs of neurologic or psychiatric illness develop, and there is no risk for developing convulsive disorders or psychoses.

The disease is about three times as common in males as in females. It is thought to be a disorder of biogenic amine metabolism. Several drugs that are thought to influence biogenic amine metabolism can precipitate ticlike syndromes, in particular the phenothiazines and L-dopa. Methylphenidate and dextroamphetamine can precipitate Gilles de la Tourette's syndrome, and l-dopa can increase the tics in patients with the syndrome. Details of the neurochemical basis of the illness are unknown, but it is tempting to speculate that increased levels of dopamine may be important. Haloperidol and the phenothiazines are thought to act by blocking dopamine receptors, while methylphenidate blocks the reuptake of dopamine in presynaptic terminals, thereby increasing the amount of dopamine at the synapse and stimulating the dopaminergic postsynaptic neurons.

Shapiro recommends titrating the dose of haloperidol against the end point of symptom relief and the occurrence of incapacitating side effects. The starting dosage is 0.5 mg twice a day, and it is increased progressively until the desired effect is obtained. Large dosage, even up to 200 mg, may be required initially, and the routine use of antiparkinsonian agents (ie, benztropine 0.5 to 1.0 mg/day) may be necessary. Marked improvement is usually obtained within 1 month, and improvement is maximum within 18 months. The dosage of haloperidol is then reduced slowly, and after 18 months sustained improvement can be attained with a dosage of 4 mg/day or less.

DISORDERS OF PURINE METABOLISM

LESCH-NYHAN SYNDROME.   The Lesch-Nyhan syndrome (see also p. 691) is a sex-linked recessive disorder of early childhood characterized clinically by choreoathetosis, compulsive self-mutilation, a variable degree of mental retardation, and growth failure. Markedly increased urinary excretion of uric acid may lead to nephrolithiasis, gout, and renal failure. The primary enzymatic defect is a profound lack of activity of hypoxanthine guanine phosphoribosyltransferase (HGPRT). Lowering the serum uric acid level with allopurinol prevents the renal and articular manifestations of the disease, but has no effect on the neurologic signs. The neurologic manifestations appear to be caused by biochemical rather than structural derangements. The usual cause of death, which occurs in childhood or adolescence in untreated boys, is renal failure.

These children appear normal at birth; motor milestones are delayed, and choreoathetoid movements involving the hands, feet, and face develop within a few months. Self-mutilation consisting of compulsive biting of the fingers and lips usually starts at about 2 years of age. Some children bang their heads; irritability and unprovoked rages are common. A calming effect can be obtained by applying splints or wrapping the hands. Dental appliances may be necessary to prevent grotesque damage to the mouth, and the teeth may even have to be extracted. Muscle tone is usually increased, with scissoring; the abnormal movements, spasticity, and dystonic posture preclude ambulation. The cranial nerves are unimpaired except for dysarthria. Opisthotonic crises of great severity can be precipitated by stressful situations or agitation; they can result in cervical subluxation. Intellectual function is variable, but it is not always severely affected. Some children who have been kept out of institutions and have been prevented from mutilating themselves have been educable and have developed pleasant personalities, but they tend to have unprovoked aggressive outbursts. Nephrolithiasis occurs in young children. In advanced cases gouty arthritis, tophi, renal failure, and megaloblastic anemia occur.

The diagnosis is suggested by levels of serum uric acid over 6 mg/100 ml. Increased excretion of uric acid (more than 25 mg/kg of body weight in 24 hours) and increased ratio of uric acid to creatinine (normal range at 4 years is 0.4:1.7) are excellent screening tests. The diagnosis rests on demonstration of the absence of, or very low levels of, HGPRT in red cells, with normal or elevated adenine phosphoribosyltransferase activity. Prenatal diagnosis is possible and is based on lack of incorporation of radioactive hypoxanthine into cultured amniotic cells from affected male fetuses. A partial deficiency of HGPRT has been found in boys who have presented with juvenile gout, renal stones, and sometimes mental retardation, mild spastic quadriparesis, dysarthria, cerebellar ataxia, and seizures. Neurologic signs have been present only in patients with 0.5 percent or less of normal HGPRT activity in erythrocytes. A 24-hour determination of urinary uric acid excretion should probably be included in screening batteries for obscure neurologic syndromes, since high uric acid excretion has been associated with bizarre neurologic presentations, and allopurinol has produced dramatic improvement. Allopurinol is the drug of choice to reduce plasma uric acid levels and prevent nephrolithiasis, renal damage, and gouty arthritis. The initial dosage is 2.5 mg/kg/day; it is then titrated by the amount of uric acid excreted in the urine and the serum uric acid level. Allopurinol inhibits the activity of hypoxanthine xanthine oxidase.

DISEASES OF PORPHYRIN METABOLISM (SEE ALSO P. 756)

ACUTE INTERMITTENT PORPHYRIA. Acute intermittent porphyria is a rare autosomal dominant genetic disorder of heme biosynthesis. It is rare in children and is more common in females. Severe colicky abdominal pain is a cardinal sign. A rapidly progressive polyneuropathy, with or without sensory deficit or paresthesias, may result in flaccid tetraparesis and respiratory paralysis. Involvement of cranial nerves and the bulbar musculature is common. The neuropathy is usually completely reversible, and recovery over a period of several weeks can be anticipated. An acute psychosis, in some cases resembling schizophrenia, may develop, although psychiatric symptoms are less common in children. Delirium, coma, and focal or generalized seizures have been reported. All these changes are reversible. Autonomic dysfunction may present as tachycardia, hypertension, fever, dysuria, or urinary retention. Drugs, particularly barbiturates, may precipitate attacks of porphyria.

The most helpful diagnostic test is demonstration of elevated levels of the porphyrin precursors Δ-aminolevulinic acid and porphobilinogen in the urine during acute attacks. A partial deficiency of the enzyme uroporphyrinogen I synthetase is found in liver, erythrocytes, and skin fibroblasts of patients with acute intermittent porphyria. Treatment is mainly symptomatic during acute attacks.

DISEASES OF IMMUNE DEFICIENCY

ATAXIA-TELANGIECTASIA. Ataxia-telangiectasia, an autosomal recessive disease, is characterized by progressive cerebellar ataxia starting in infancy, progressive oculocutaneous telangiectasias, proneness to sinopulmonary infection, and defective humoral and cellular immunity. Ataxia presents in infancy, when sudden myoclonic jerks may occur, especially during voluntary movements. Oculomotor apraxia is more characteristic than nystagmus; the child has difficulty with horizontal deviation of the eyes. Ocular telangiectasias are usually evident by 6 years of age; later, telangiectasias appear on the eyelids, pinnas, neck, supraclavicular region, and antecubital and popliteal fossae. In older children, graying of the hair and dryness, thinning, and irregular pigmentation of the skin in areas exposed to sunlight suggest premature aging. Basal cell carcinomas may develop. By the second decade dystonic postures of the hands and feet that suggest involvement of the basal ganglia and athetotic movements dominate the picture. By the third decade evidence of spinal cord involvement includes loss of position and vibration sense, atrophy of intrinsic muscles of the hands and feet, and spasticity of the limbs. Skeletal deformities are not as marked as in Friedreich's ataxia. Scoliosis and kyphosis develop late. Cranial nerve involvement is reflected by the oculomotor apraxia, dysarthria, drooling, swallowing difficulty, and expressionless face.

Sinopulmonary infections are common, manifesting as chronic middle ear disease, repeated pneumonia, and bronchiectasis. Severe thymic hypoplasia is a constant feature of this illness. The thymus contains neither germinal centers nor Hassall corpuscles, and the adenoids, tonsils, lymph nodes, and even the spleen may be hypoplastic. Humoral immunologic deficiency is due to hypogammaglobulinemia with decreased IgA and/or IgE levels (p. 318). Patients with ataxia-telangiectasia have a dramatically increased incidence of malignant neoplasms, most notably lymphomas. Endocrine dysfunction is another frequent feature of this illness; ovarian aplasia or hypoplasia is quite frequent in girls; hypogonadism is less striking but does occur in males. Insulin-resistant diabetes mellitus has been reported in some patients who have survived to early adult life.

The lesion in the nervous system is not vascular, but primarily damage to neurons. The cerebellar cortex is severely atrophic because Purkinje cells, granular cells, and basket cells drop out. Aneuploidy and giant cell formation may be found in several organs, including the anterior pituitary; they are thought to reflect a tendency to chromosomal breakage and atypical cellular proliferation. Infections should be treated actively, and prophylactic antibiotics may be indicated. Surveillance for malignancies is essential. Support of the child and the family and genetic counseling are important aspects of their care.

CHEDIAK-HIGASHI SYNDROME. The Chediak-Higashi syndrome is an autosomal recessive disorder characterized by partial oculocutaneous albinism, increased susceptibility to infection, and the presence of large lysosomelike granules in many tissues including polymorphonuclear phagocytes and melanocytes. Splenomegaly and hypersplenism, hepatomegaly, and lymphadenopathy are common. Most patients die within their first two decades. Nystagmus and photophobia occur because of the ocular albinism. Peripheral neuropathy occurs frequently in older children and adolescents, with areflexia, footdrop, weakness, and sensory loss. It is one of the conditions that produce the picture of spinocerebellar degeneration.

DISEASES WITH DYING-BACK PHENOMENA

SPINAL AND SPINOCEREBELLAR DEGENERATIONS.
The hallmark of these disorders is degeneration of the most distal portions of axons, progressing slowly toward the nerve cell body. The most striking pathology is a tract degeneration or a neuropathy, while loss of nerve cell bodies is less marked. Demyelination is not thought to be due to primary involvement of Schwann cells or oligodendroglia, but to a dying-back process of axons. Certain tracts are involved selectively, while others are unaffected (system degeneration). All of these disorders are genetic; some, like autosomal recessive Friedreich's ataxia, are clearly defined by their clinical symptomatology and their distinctive pathology. Greenfield's monograph provides a detailed description of the spinocerebellar degenerations.

Friedreich's ataxia is the classic form of this disease. It is inherited as an autosomal recessive trait and presents in childhood or adolescence. It runs its course over less than a decade and is associated with a cardiomyopathy that is a frequent cause of death. The first sign is usually an atactic gait; later, ataxia of the hands, dysarthria, and nystagmus appear. Typically the deep tendon reflexes are absent, but the plantar response is extensor. Sensory examination reveals loss of position and vibration sense, first in the feet, then progressing to involve the hands. The characteristic Friedreich foot has a high arch, with hammer toes and tight heel cords. Scoliosis or kyphoscoliosis is almost invariably present, and gross chest deformities may occur. The heart is enlarged, and dysrhythmias and conduction defects are common. Anginal pain and pericarditis may occur, but they are rare. The electrocardiogram reflects diffuse or focal myocardial damage, as well as ventricular enlargement. The spinal fluid protein may be mildly elevated. Pathologic examination reveals atrophy, demyelination, and severe gliosis of the posterior columns and spinocerebellar

tracts, and to a lesser degree the lateral corticospinal tracts. The cells in Clarke's column that give rise to the dorsal spinocerebellar tract degenerate, as do the dorsal root ganglion cells that give rise to the fibers of the ascending sensory pathways in the posterior columns. Degeneration tends to be most marked in the lower thoracic and lumbar cord. No treatment is available. *Dominant spinocerebellar degeneration* is similar to the recessive variant, but usually is less severe. *Dominant spinocerebellar degeneration with chronic neuropathy (Lévy-Roussy syndrome)* starts in early childhood and resembles Friedreich's ataxia, but has an associated amyotrophy of muscles below the knee and in the hands and forearms. *Marinesco-Sjögren syndrome* is an autosomal recessive trait manifested by a slowly progressive atactic syndrome, with nystagmus appearing in early childhood, weakness and distal muscle atrophy in the legs in late adolescence, cataracts in infancy or early childhood, slow development and mental retardation, and small stature. Pathologically the disorder is characterized by severe cerebellar atrophy. *Spinocerebellar syndromes with blindness or deafness or both* have been reported in many families.

PHAKOMATOSES AND OTHER NEUROCUTANEOUS SYNDROMES

The term phakomatosis is applied to a variety of neurocutaneous syndromes, most of which have a dominant pattern of inheritance; in some there is a tendency toward the development of neoplasms. The lesions are embryonal in origin, but their pathogenesis is not understood. In the dominant syndromes the penetrance of the gene appears to be high, but the phenotypic expressivity is so variable as to render detailed genetic study quite difficult. Table 27 lists some of the disorders that are considered to be phakomatoses. Neurofibromatosis and tuberous sclerosis are common disorders whose prevalence is underestimated because of their variable expressivity, which involves many organ systems.

TUBEROUS SCLEROSIS. Tuberous sclerosis (adenoma sebaceum, epiloia, Bourneville's disease, Pringle's disease) is inherited as a dominant autosomal trait, the expression of which is dependent on the presence or absence of a modifying gene. This accounts for the marked variability of expression noted in clinical practice (Fig. 45, colorplate 4).

The full syndrome is characterized by seizures, mental deficiency, and adenoma sebaceum, with foci of intracranial calcification, particularly in the periventricular region, although they may be scattered throughout the hemispheres. The seizures are most often infantile spasms in the young child and the grand mal type in the older child. In the full syndrome mental deficiency is generally severe. However, intellectual capacity may be normal or near normal. The characteristic skin lesions (fibroangiomatous nevi) have been mislabeled adenoma sebaceum; the sebaceous glands are only involved secondarily. Fibroangiomatous nevi may be present during the first year of life, but they usually are not noted until the age of 4 or 5 years. These

TABLE 27. Neurocutaneous Syndromes

	Genetics	Skin	Other
Predominantly neuroectodermal phakomatoses			
Neurofibromatosis (von Recklinghausen's disease)	Autosomal dominant	Café au lait spots, multiple tumors	Multiple neoplasms of CNS and PNS; disorder of cell migration, bony lesions, and other anomalies
Tuberous sclerosis	Autosomal dominant	Depigmented spots, adenoma sebaceum, etc	Tubers in brain (calcified); disorder of cell migration (seizures, mental retardation)
Predominantly vascular phakomatoses			
Sturge-Weber syndrome (encephalo-trigeminal angiomatosis)	Not genetic ?	Facial angioma	Occipital angioma, "trolley track" calcification, mental retardation, seizures, glaucoma?
Lindau-von Hippel syndrome (oculocerebellar hemangio-blastomatosis)	Autosomal dominant	—	hemangioblastoma of cerebellum, retina; cysts in other organs
Other pigmented neurocutaneous syndromes			
Neurocutaneous melanosis	Not genetic	Giant nevi	Melanosis of meninges, hydrocephalus, malignant melanoma
Albright's syndrome (polyostotic fibrous dysplasia)	Not genetic	Café au lait patches	Polyostotic fibrous dysplasia; precocious puberty in females; mental retardation
Incontinentia pigmenti (Bloch-Sulzberger)	X-linked dominant ?	Bullous-verrucous pigmented skin lesions (swirls)	Disorder of cell migration? (mental retardation, seizures); ocular lesions
Linear nevus sebaceous	Not genetic	Linear nevus sebaceous of face or elsewhere	Mental retardation, seizures (focal deficit)
Other vascular neurocutaneous syndromes			
Wyburn-Mason syndrome	Not genetic	Angiomas of facial structures (inconstant)	Cirsoid aneurysm of retina and base of brain
Cutaneous spinal angiomatosis (Cobb)	Not genetic	Hemangioma over back	Hemangioma of cord
Ataxia-telangiectasia	Autosomal recessive	Telangiectasia of conjunctiva and face, gray hair	Cerebellar-dystonic syndrome; immune deficiency; neoplasms
Leukodystrophy with meningeal angiomatosis	Autosomal recessive	Cutis marmorata universalis	Sudanophilic leukodystrophy; angiomatosis of meninges
Miscellaneous neurocutaneous syndromes			
Sjögren-Larsson syndrome	Autosomal recessive	Ichthyosis	Spastic diplegia; mental retardation; leukodystrophy
Refsum's disease (phytanic acid lipidosis)	Autosomal recessive	Ichthyosis	Night blindness neuropathy; ataxia; hearing loss
Xeroderma pigmentosum	Autosomal recessive	Extreme sensitivity to light, skin carcinomas	Mental retardation; ataxia; speech defect; endocrinopathies
Cockayne syndrome	Autosomal recessive	Actinic dermatitis; progeric changes; gray hair	Microcephaly; dwarfism; eye anomalies; calcification of basal ganglia

lesions take the form of discrete pink or yellowish papules, principally on the face in the butterfly distribution on the bridge of the nose, the malar prominences, and along the nasal-labial folds. They may also occur on forehead, neck, and trunk. Individual lesions remain static, gradually growing redder and eventually becoming brownish. They do not itch, nor do they suppurate; this distinguishes them from acne vulgaris and seborrheic dermatitis. Other skin lesions consist of raised plaquelike flesh-colored lesion, which may be found anywhere on the body, and shagreen patches, which are slightly pigmented and raised and resemble coarse-grained leather. Fibromas of the scalp are seen on occasion, as are areas of depigmentation. The latter may be one of the earliest ectodermal manifestations of tuberous sclerosis. The subungual fibroma, a flesh-colored sessile growth emerging from the groove of the nailbed, is characteristic. Several retinal lesions may be observed. Small, flat, white or yellowish phakoma or spots may occur on or close to the optic nerve head. A second lesion is a raised cluster of translucent white tissue in the fundus. Systemic involvement may include multiple small fibroadenomas of the kidney, rhabdomyoma of the heart, and myomas of the uterus and vagina. Lesions in the lung may produce a honeycomb effect, and polycystic kidneys have been noted.

The brain contains many small firm sclerotic nodules (tubera), chiefly in the cortex. They may project into the ventricle, causing deformities that can be detected by pneumoencephalography (Fig. 45, colorplate 4). Hydrocephalus with increased intracranial pressure may develop as a result of one of these masses blocking the ventricular system. These nodules contain giant-sized haphazardly arranged cells. Adjacent to these collections of giant glial cells may be found degeneration of nerve cells and fibers and often cavity formation. Dense astrocytic gliosis is also seen.

The diagnosis can be established on the basis of the triad of seizures, mental deficiency, and adenoma sebaceum. Radiographs often show intracranial calcifications and small cystic lesions in the distal phalanges of the hands and feet. Treatment is entirely symptomatic.

NEUROFIBROMATOSIS. Neurofibromatosis (von Recklinghausen's disease) is inherited as an autosomal dominant trait with marked variability of expression; while the characteristic pathology consists of neurofibromas of the peripheral, spinal, and cranial nerves, meningiomas and gliomas of the spinal cord and brain do occur. The condition includes the following manifestations: multiple soft tumors beneath the skin (fibroma molluscum), multiple tumors situated along nerve trunks (neurofibromas), and pigmentation of the skin. Varying degrees of mental deficiency may occur. The peripheral neurofibromas are found along the course of nerve trunks, subcutaneous nerves, and cranial nerves. The auditory nerve is very frequently involved. The optic nerve is a frequent site of astrocytoma and less commonly meningioma. Within the spinal cord ependymomas, astrocytomas, and diffuse gliomas are seen. Pheochromocytomas are seen in the adult age group.

Clinically, a common sequence is excessive pigmentation during infancy, with the characteristic superficial skin lesions making their appearance in childhood or puberty; individual lesions grow slowly, with puberty and pregnancy apparently exercising an accelerating effect. Siblings, parents, and other members of the family often show the typical skin lesions. These cutaneous manifestations may take two forms: café au lait spots and pigmented nevi (Fig. 46, colorplate 4). The pigmented nevi appear at an earlier age and are in no way different from common moles, but they are numerous. The café au lait lesions are fewer in number and tend to be distributed along the paths of the cutaneous nerves. They are oval in outline, with the long axis parallel to the nerve.

The tumors may be confined to the subcutaneous tissues or may be predominantly within the bony confines of the central nervous system. The most common histologic lesion is the benign neurilemoma. Fibromas are also present, and sarcomatous degeneration may occur in the adult. When the tumors occupy bone they produce localized areas of rarefaction, or they may give rise to thickening or excessive linear growth of the long bones. Involvement of the spine may produce scoliosis, and orbital wall defects may result in pulsating exophthalmos. Pendulous masses of fibrous tissue and skin, which are characteristic of the adult form of neurofibromatosis, are rare in children.

Neurofibromatosis must be differentiated from tuberous sclerosis. In the former the lesions tend to involve the peripheral outflow of the central nervous system, whereas in tuberous sclerosis the lesions are central. Mental deficiency is much more frequent with tuberous sclerosis. Epilepsy may occur in both, but it is very common in tuberous sclerosis and relatively rare in neurofibromatosis.

A great variety of signs and symptoms may occur in neurofibromatosis, depending on the location of the lesions. Optic nerve tumors within the orbit may lead to progressive exophthalmos with optic atrophy. Astrocytomas of the third ventricle and hypothalamus may result in the symptom complex of diabetes insipidus, adiposity, and genital maldevelopment or precocious puberty. The lesions may present as intramedullary tumors of the spinal cord. In some families bilateral acoustic nerve tumors may be the prominent feature, with few skin manifestations. Congenital anomalies such as spina bifida, pes cavus, rib anomalies, and vertebral anomalies may be associated. Radiographic studies may reveal large scalloped neural foramina in the spine, scoliosis, or enlarged optic foramina if optic nerve tumors are present. With auditory nerve tumors an enlarged internal auditory canal may be apparent. The diagnosis is best made on the basis of the nature of the cutaneous manifestations and evidence of multiple peripheral nerve lesions.

Therapy is surgical removal of the offending neurofibromas, but no definitive cure can be expected owing to the multiple nature of the lesions. Surgery should be carried out only when a particular lesion becomes a major symptomatic problem for the patient.

ENCEPHALOTRIGEMINAL ANGIOMATOSIS. Encephalotrigeminal angiomatosis (Sturge-Weber-Dimitri syndrome) includes a port wine vascular nevus (often in the distribution of the first division of the trigeminal nerve), convulsions (often focal and involving the contralateral side), contralateral hemiparesis, and occasionally homonymous hemianopsia. Ipsilateral intracranial calcifications are found by x-ray. These calcifications are characteristically in paired lines, often called trolley tracks (Fig. 47). Increased intraocular ten-

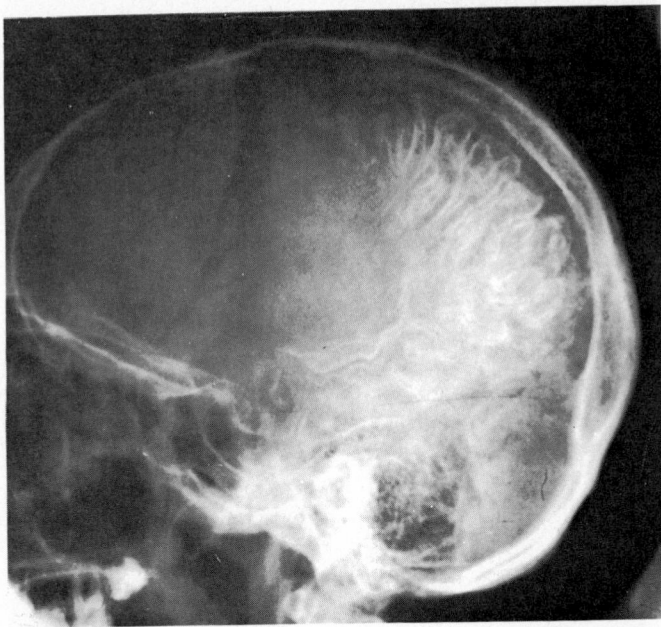

FIG. 47. Encephalotrigeminal angiomatosis. Skull x-ray showing characteristic intracranial calcification.

sion may be caused by angiomatous involvement of the uveal tract and may give rise to enlargement of the involved globe. About two-thirds of the children with this condition are mentally retarded, and more than 50 percent have convulsive disorders. A hemiparesis is less common. There is great variability in the severity of the individual symptoms, and one or another may be missing entirely. Hemangiomas may be found in parts of the body other than the face, and rarely in the fundi.

The intracranial lesion is angiomatous and involves the meninges in the area supplied by the first division of the trigeminal nerve and sometimes also the superficial vessels occupying the sulci over the convexity, particularly in the occipital and parietal regions. This may cause atrophy of the underlying brain tissue, and the degenerative changes in cerebral tissue just below the gyral surface are frequently followed by the characteristic calcifications. The demonstration of intracranial calcifications limited to the convexity of the brain and showing the characteristic gyral pattern is almost pathognomonic. The diagnosis is usually made from the physical findings alone.

The differential diagnosis should include the Wyburn-Mason syndrome, in which telangiectasia or hypertrophic angiomas may appear on the face. However, in this condition there is the constant association of cirsoid angioma of the retina and mesencephalic aneurysmal angiomas. The syndrome of Van Bogaert-Divry is a combination of diffuse cortical meningeal angiomatosis in which dementia, severe convulsive disorder, pyramidal and extrapyramidal motor symptoms, and congenital poikiloderma with multiple telangiectasia are found. Therapy is symptomatic, although early surgical intervention has been successful occasionally.

LINDAU-VON HIPPEL DISEASE. Lindau-von Hippel disease, an autosomal dominant syndrome, does not become symptomatic before late adolescence or early adult life. The key features are hemangioblastomas of the cerebellum and the retina. They usually present as cerebellar neoplasms with increased intracranial pressure and few localizing signs. The lesions are readily diagnosed by brain scans and posterior fossa angiograms. Visceral lesions include cystic lesions of the kidney, pancreas, and epididymis, as well as pheochromocytoma and hypernephroma.

NEUROCUTANEOUS MELANOSIS. Neurocutaneous melanosis is a sporadic disorder characterized by giant pigmented nevi of the skin associated with melanosis of the leptomeninges. The nevi are usually dark and often hairy; they may occupy a large area of the trunk in a bathing suit or cape distribution. They tend to originate from the posterior midline and to follow a dermatome distribution. Multiple smaller nevi may be scattered over the rest of the body. Melanosis of the leptomeninges, often with pigmentation of parenchymal areas of the brainstem or cerebellum, is present in most of these children. Hydrocephalus may occur because of CSF obstruction by benign melanotic cells or because of malignant transformation, which is common. Malignant transformation of the skin lesion may also take place. Increased CSF protein, increased melanin content of the CSF, and recovery of melanoblasts from the CSF suggest malignancy. Convulsive disorders and mental retardation may occur in this syndrome even in the absence of hydrocephalus or malignant transformation.

POLYOSTOTIC FIBROUS DYSPLASIA. In polyostotic fibrous dysplasia (Albright's syndrome) the complete syndrome includes fibrous dysplasia of multiple bones, large pigmented cutaneous nevi with irregular margins ("coast of Maine") that may be limited to one side of the trunk, and precocious sexual development, especially in females. The syndrome is not considered to be genetic (p. 2015). Primary neurologic features of the syndrome include mental deficiency, epilepsy, and headaches.

INCONTINENTIA PIGMENTI. Incontinentia pigmenti (Bloch-Sulzberger syndrome) is characterized by congenital skin lesions with mental retardation (in at least one-third of patients) and ocular pathology. The syndrome is much more common in females than in males. Skin lesions show three stages of development; the infant may be born with the lesions at any of the stages, or they may appear soon after birth. Erythematous bullous lesions first appear on the trunk or the limbs. The bullae rupture, ooze, and crust, and the lesions then become verrucose. Later the verrucae clear, leaving discrete and confluent areas of hyperpigmentation that have a linear swirled or marbled appearance. The lesions fade gradually. Dystrophy of the hair, nails, and teeth, disordered sweating, and areas of alopecia may persist to adult life. The ocular findings include frequent strabismus, optic atrophy, opacities of the cornea and lens, an abnormal pattern of pigmentation of the choroid and retina, pseudogliomas, and microphthalmia. Symptomatic treatment of the child and genetic counseling are in order.

LINEAR NEVUS SEBACEOUS; NEVUS UNIUS LATERALIS. Linear nevus sebaceus is a sporadic syndrome in which congenital, slightly raised yellowish verrucose skin lesions associated with orange yellow or dark brown plaques with a waxy surface occur, mainly on the middle of the face. They may be quite extensive and are frequently associated with mental retardation and seizures. They consist of hyperkeratosis of the epidermis, hyperplasia of the sebaceous glands, and abortive hair follicles within the dermis. The skin lesions may degenerate into basal cell carcinomas, and early removal for prophylactic and cosmetic reasons has been advocated.

Nevus unius lateralis consists of a much less striking unilateral linear array of papules that are light to dark brown and are present at birth or develop during the first year. They consist of hyperkeratosis, papillomatosis, and acanthosis of the epidermis, while the dermis and subcutaneous tissues are not affected. Mental retardation, seizures, and hemiparesis are less frequent than with linear nevus sebaceus, but occur in about 25 percent of these children. Eye anomalies are rare.

WYBURN-MASON SYNDROME. Wyburn-Mason syndrome (Bonnet-Dechaume-Blanc syndrome) is characterized by unilateral cirsoid vascular anomalies of the retina associated with an intracranial arteriovenous anomaly involving the mesencephalon and base of the brain. Unilateral exophthalmos, enlarged facial draining veins, or a facial angioma may occur. Neurologic signs include hemiparesis, ataxia, cranial nerve anomalies, and visual field defects; less commonly there may be sensory symptoms due to thalamic involvement or hydrocephalus due to obstruction of the aqueduct of Sylvius. Mental retardation and seizures may occur. Episodes of subarachnoid hemorrhage leave sequelae of variable severity. Angiography will reveal the extent of the intracranial and orbital pathology and their close relationship.

CUTANEOUS-SPINAL ANGIOMATOSIS. A capillary hemangioma of the skin on the back may be associated with an angiomatous anomaly of the underlying leptomeninges and cord. The anomalies lie in the same metamere and may affect the muscles or the vertebrae, with the development of a scoliosis. The symptoms of spinal cord involvement may occur in childhood or adolescence or may be delayed until adult life.

SJÖGREN-LARSSON SYNDROME. Sjögren-Larsson syndrome, a rare autosomal recessive condition, is characterized by a congenital nonbullous ichthyosiform erythroderma. A spastic diplegia usually is apparent from early life, and most children are moderately to severely intellectually deficient. It may be related to Refsum's disease.

XERODERMA PIGMENTOSUM. Xeroderma pigmentosum is an autosomal recessive disorder characterized by failure to repair epidermal DNA damaged by ultraviolet light because of lack of the functional form of the ultraviolet-specific endonuclease. Clinical manifestations include severe actinic dermatitis, with marked blistering and freckling of the unexposed skin, which becomes severely atrophic and hyperkeratotic. Innumerable squamous and basal cell carcinomas, and sometimes melanomas, develop. Death usually occurs in childhood or early adult life from the malignancies or from increased susceptibility to infection. Failure to grow, hypogonadism, microcephaly, intellectual deficit, and a progressive neurologic syndrome with ataxia, spasticity, choreoathetosis, and progressive hearing loss may be associated.

NEUROAXONAL DYSTROPHIES. Hallervorden and Spatz have described a progressive familial disease that starts in midchildhood and is characterized by gait abnormality, stiffness of the legs, foot deformity, movement disorder, dysarthria, and dementia, with death occurring in 10 to 15 years. At autopsy these patients have brown iron-containing pigmentation of the globus pallidus and zona reticulata of the substantia nigra, loss of myelin in the globus pallidus, and peculiar axonal swellings (so-called spheroids) in the central nervous system.

Infantile neuroaxonal dystrophy is an autosomal recessive condition manifesting before the age of 1 year with a combination of upper and lower motor neuron signs leading to profound floppiness, loss of pain sensation starting in the legs, atonic bladder, nystagmus, and late development of optic atrophy. Most of these patients die within 4 to 5 years. Pathology shows numerous spheroids in areas of high neuronal density. The condition must be differentiated from metachromatic leukodystrophy, spongy degeneration, ceroid lipofuscinosis, and various lipidoses, mucopolysaccharidoses, and gangliosidoses.

DEMYELINATING SCLEROSES

In contrast to the leukodystrophies, the demyelinating scleroses are myelinoclastic and pathologically multifocal, perivenous, and inflammatory. The absence of a familial distribution of cases further tends to distinguish these diseases from the familial leukodystrophies. Etiology is obscure; the concept of an autoimmune response to some component of myelin seems most tenable. Demyelinating diseases can be further separated into the diffuse and disseminated forms. Schilder's disease represents the diffuse demyelinating scleroses. The disseminated demyelinating scleroses include acute and chronic multiple sclerosis, acute necrotizing hemorrhagic leukoencephalitis, and the acute disseminated encephalomyelitides that follow infection and immunization procedures. Neuromyelitis optica and the concentric sclerosis of Balo are probably subtypes of the disseminated form of acute multiple sclerosis.

ACUTE DISSEMINATED ENCEPHALOMYEL-ITIDES. Acute disseminated encephalomyelitides occur following rubella, rubeola, variola, varicella, and the influenza syndrome. Immunization against variola, rabies treatment, and rarely pertussis immunization may be followed by an acute episode of disseminated encephalomyelitis. Signs of an acute encephalitis with evidence of multiple sites of central nervous system involvement are associated with an elevation of spinal fluid protein and a lymphocytic pleocytosis in the spinal fluid. Fever, convulsions, stupor, ocular palsies, dysarthria, paraplegias, and cerebellar ataxia, together with urinary and fecal incontinence, may occur in various combinations. Severe forms of the disorder will leave permanent neurologic deficits. About 15 percent of all cases are fatal. There is no specific therapy. Unlike other forms of disseminated sclerosis, recurrences are rare.

ACUTE NECROTIZING HEMORRHAGIC LEUKOENCEPH-ALITIS. Acute necrotizing hemorrhagic leukoencephalitis (Hurst's disease) is a fulminating and usually fatal disease that follows minor upper respiratory infection. Pathologically one or more large hemorrhagic and necrotic foci of demyelination are found in brain, spinal cord, and brainstem. Presenting signs and symptoms depend on the site of the lesion or lesions. Headache, fever, and signs of meningitis are present. Cerebrospinal fluid protein is elevated, and up to several hundred leukocytes may be present. These cells are predominantly neutrophilic, in contrast to the lymphocytic pleocytosis of the acute disseminated encephalomyelitides. No specific form of therapy is available.

MULTIPLE OR DISSEMINATED SCLEROSIS. Multiple sclerosis is relatively rare in children, but it can occur in the first decade. The diagnosis is based on the occurrence of multiple attacks and evidence of multiple sites of neurologic involvement. Preferential sites of involvement are segmental portions of the brainstem, spinal cord, and cerebellum. Cerebral symptoms are uncommon. In order of frequency, one encounters motor weakness of the extremities, retrobulbar neuritis, paresthesias, diplopia, disturbance of balance, and bladder difficulties. Mild increases in cells and protein in spinal fluid may be noted. Pathologically the findings consist of scattered areas of demyelination; the gray matter is usually spared. The disease occurs sporadically, and between attacks the symptoms may clear partially or even completely. Over a period of years there is a tendency for slow, progressive neurologic disability.

NEUROMYELITIS OPTICA. Neuromyelitis optica (Devic's disease) is more common in children. Neuropathologically, it is similar to multiple sclerosis. The disease is characterized by the association of transverse myelitis and bilateral optic neuritis. These may develop simultaneously or one after the other. Visual loss is severe and is usually accompanied by inflammation of the nerve head. Involvement of the spinal cord produces a complete transverse myelitis; however, it may be disseminated. On pathologic examination some cases show the classic lesions of multiple sclerosis. Others may show subacute or acute necrotizing hemorrhagic myelitis. In some cases large confluent plaques of demyelination may occur within the cerebral hemispheres; these patients have an elevation of spinal fluid protein and a mononuclear pleocytosis. Recovery may be quite rapid and may be complete in several weeks. Some cases are associated with permanent residua, and those that fall in the classification of subacute necrotic myelopathy are usually fatal. Management is entirely symptomatic.

BALO'S CONCENTRIC SCLEROSIS. Balo's concentric sclerosis has many of the histopathologic features of multiple sclerosis, but the lesions are primarily confined to the cerebral white matter. The distinguishing features are the occurrence of alternate concentric bands of destruction and preservation of myelin.

References

Bergsma G (ed): Enzyme therapy in genetic diseases. National Foundation. Birth Defects; Original article series 9 1973

Blackwood W: Cerebral biopsy. In Vinken PJ, Bruyn GW (eds): Handbook of Clinical Neurology, Vol 10. Leucodystrophies and Poliodystrophies. New York, American Elsevier, 1970, p 680

Nelson JS: Rectal biopsy in the diagnosis of pediatric neurological disorders. Dev Med Child Neurol 16:831, 1974

O'Brien JS, Okada S, Fillerup DL: Tay-Sachs disease: prenatal diagnosis. Science 172:61, 1971

Veath RM: Ethical issues in genetics. Prog Med Genet 10:223, 1974

MUCOPOLYSACCHARIDOSES

Danes BS, Bearn AG: Hurler's syndrome: demonstration of an inherited disorder of connective tissue in cell culture. Science 149:987, 1965

——— Bearn AG: Hurler's syndrome: a genetic study of clones in cell culture with particular reference to the Lyon hypothesis. J Exp Med 126:509, 1967

Dorfman A, Matalon R: The mucopolysaccharidoses. In Stanbury JB, Wyngaarden JB, Fredrickson DS (eds): The Metabolic Basis of Inherited Disease, 3rd ed. New York, McGraw-Hill, 1972, p 1218

Fratantoni JS, Hall CW, Neufeld EF: Hurler and Hunter syndromes: mutual correction of the defect in cultured fibroblasts. Science 162:570, 1968

Groover RV, Burke EC, Gordon H, Berdon WE: The genetic mucopolysaccharidoses. Semin Hematol 9:371, 1972

Hers HG, van Hoof F: Lysosomes and Storage Diseases. New York, Academic, 1973

Kolodny EH: Clinical and biochemical genetics of the lipidoses. Semin Hematol 9:251, 1972

McKusick VA: The nosology of the mucopolysaccharidoses. Am J Med 47:730, 1969

——— Heritable Disorders of Connective Tissue, 4th ed. St Louis, CV Mosby, 1972, p 521

Neufeld EG: The biochemical basis of mucopolysaccharidoses and mucolipidoses. Prog Med Genet 10:81, 1974

Sloan HR, Fredrickson DS: GM_2 gangliosidoses: Tay-Sachs disease. In Stanbury JB, Wyngaarden JB, Fredrickson DS (eds): The Metabolic Basis of Inherited Disease, 3rd ed. New York, McGraw-Hill, 1972, p 614

Stumpf D, Neuwelt E, Austin J, Kohler P: Immunological studies of arylsulfatase A in normals and in metachromatic leukodystrophy. Trans Am Neurol Assoc 96:80, 1971

Tateson R, Bain AD: GM_2 gangliosidoses: consideration of the genetic defect. Lancet 2:612, 1971

Wiesmann U, Neufeld EF: Scheie and Hurler syndromes: apparent identity of the biochemical defect. Science 169:72, 1970

MPS TYPE I

Aleu FP, Terry RD, Zellweger H: Electron microscopy of two cerebral biopsies in gargoylism. J Neuropathol Exp Neurol 24:304, 1965

Bach G, Friedman R, Weissman B, et al: The defect in the Hurler and Scheie syndromes: deficiency of α-L-iduronidase. Proc Natl Acad Sci USA 60:2048, 1972

Berman ER, Vered J, Bach G: A reliable spot test for mucopolysaccharidoses. Clin Chem 17:886, 1971

Groover RV, Burke EC, Gordon H, Berdon WE: The genetic mucopolysaccharidoses. Semin Hematol 9:371, 1972

Matalon R, Dorfman A: Hurler's syndrome, an alpha-L-iduronidase deficiency. Biochem Biophys Res Commun 47:959, 1972

Rezvani I, Collipp PJ, DiGeorge AM: Evaluation of screening tests for urinary mucopolysaccharides. Pediatrics 52:64, 1973

MPS TYPE III

Berman ER: Diagnosis of metabolic eye disease by chemical analysis of serum, leukocytes, and skin fibroblasts. Birth Defects (in press)

Danks DM, Campbell PE, Cartwright E, et al: The Sanfilippo syndrome, clinical, biochemical, radiological, haematological and pathological features of nine cases. Aust Paediatr J 8:174, 1972

Dekaban AS, Patton VM: Hurler's and Sanfilippo's variants of mucopolysaccharidosis. Cerebral pathology and lipid chemistry. Arch Pathol 91:434, 1971

Harper PS, Laurence KM, Parkes A, et al: Sanfilippo A disease in the fetus. J Med Genet 11:123, 1974

Kresse H: Mucopolysaccharidoses III A (Sanfilippo A disease): deficiency of a heparan sulfamidase in skin fibroblasts and leucocytes. Biochem Biophys Res Commun 54:1111, 1973

Moser, HW, O'Brien JS, Atkins L, et al: Influence of normal HL-A identical leukocytes in Sanfilippo disease type B. Arch Neurol 31:329, 1974

MPS TYPE IV

Berman ER: Diagnosis of metabolic eye disease by chemical analysis of serum, leukocytes, and skin fibroblasts. Birth Defects (in press)

Gilles FH, Deuel RK: Neuronal cytoplasmic globules in the brain in Morquio's syndrome. Arch Neurol 25:393, 1971

Matalon R, Arbogast B, Justile P, et al: Morquio's syndrome: deficiency of a chondroitin sulfate N-acetylhexosamine sulfate sulfatase. Biochem Biophys Res Commun 61:759, 1974

MPS TYPE VI

Peterson DI, Bacchus H, Seaich L, Kelly TE: Myelopathy associated with Maroteaux-Lamy syndrome. Arch Neurol 32:127, 1975

MPS TYPE VII

Benson PF, Dean MF, Muir H: A form of mucopolysaccharidosis with visceral storage and excessive urinary excretion of chondroitin sulphate. Dev Med Child Neurol 14:69, 1972

Sly WS, Quinton BA, McAlister WH, Rimoin DL: Betaglucuronidase deficiency: report of clinical, neurological and biochemical features of a new mucopolysaccharidosis. J Pediatr 82:249, 1973

MUCOLIPIDOSES

Arstila AU, Palo J, Haltia M, et al: Aspartylglucosaminuria. I. Fine structural studies on brain, liver and kidney. Acta Neuropathol (Berl) 20:207, 1972

Aula P, Näntö V, Laipio ML, Autio S: et al: aspratylglucosaminuria: deficieney of aspartylglucosaminidase in cultured fibroblast of patients and their heterozygous parents. Clin Genet 4:297, 1973

Autio S, Visakarpi JK, Järvinen H: Aspartylglucosaminuria (AGU). Further aspects of its clinical picture, mode of inheritance and epidemiology based on a study of 57 patients. Ann Clin Res 5:149, 1973

Berman ER, Livni N, Shapira E, et al: Congenital corneal clouding with abnormal systemic storage bodies: a new variant of mucolipidosis. J Pediatr 84:519, 1974

Blank E, Linder D: I-cell disease (mucolipidosis II): a lysosomopathy. Pediatrics 54:797, 1974

Hickman S, Neufeld EF: A hypothesis for I-cell disease: defective hydrolases that do not enter lysosomes. Biochem Biophys Res Commun 49:992, 1972

Kenyon KR, Sensenbrenner JA: Mucolipidosis II (I-cell disease): ultrastructural observation of conjunctiva and skin. Invest Ophthalmol 10:555, 1971

Kohn G, Livni N, Beyth Y: Prenatal diagnosis of mucolipidosis IV by electronmicroscopy. Pediatr Res 9:314, 1975

Leroy JG, DeMars RI: Mutant enzymatic and cytological phenotypes in cultured human fibroblasts. Science 157:804, 1967

——— Spranger JW, Feingold M, et al: I-cell disease: a clinical picture. J Pediatr 79:360, 1971

Melham R, Dorst JP, Scott CI, McKusick VA: Roentgen findings in mucolipidosis III (pseudo-Hurler polydystrophy). Radiology 106:153, 1973

Merin S, Livni N, Berman ER, Yatziv S: Mucolipidosis IV: ocular, systemic, and ultrastructural findings. Invest Ophthalmol 14:437, 1975

Öckerman PA: Mannosidosis. In Hers HG, van Hoof F (eds): Lysosomes and Storages Diseases. New York, Academic, 1973, p 291

Patel V, Watanabe I, Zeman W: Deficiency of alpha-L-fucosidase. Science 176:426, 1972

Spranger JW, Weidemann HR: The genetic mucolipidoses; diagnosis and differential diagnosis. Humangenetik 9:113, 1970

Taber P, Gyepes MT, Philippart M, Ling S: Roentgenographic manifestations of Leroy's I-cell disease. Am J Roentgenol Radium Ther Nucl Med 118:213, 1973

Taylor HA, Thomas GH, Miller CS, et al: Mucolipidosis III (pseudo-Hurler polydystrophy): cytological and ultrastructural observations of cultured fibroblast cells. Clin Genet 4:388, 1973

van Hoof F: Fucosidosis. In Hers HG, van Hoof F (eds): Lysosomes and Storage Diseases. New York, Academic, 1973, p 277

Wiederschain GYA, Kolibaba LG, Rosenfeld EL: Human alpha-L-fucosidosis. Clin Chim Acta 46:305, 1973

SPHINGOLIPIDOSES

Ellis WG, Schneider EL, McCulloch JR, et al: Fetal globoid cell leukodystrophy (Krabbe's disease). Pathological and biochemical examination. Arch Neurol 29:253, 1973

Hers HG, van Hoof F: Lysosomes and Storage Diseases. New York, Academic, 1973

Kuhr MD: Doubtful benefits of Tay-Sachs screening. N Engl J Med 292:371, 1975

Stanbury JB, Wyngaarden JB, Fredrickson DS: The Metabolic Basis of Inherited Disease, 3d ed. New York, McGraw-Hill, 1972

Suzuki K, Suzuki K: Disorders of sphingolipid metabolism. In Gaull GE (ed): Biology of Brain Dysfunction, Vol 2. New York, Plenum, RC 386. 633 1973, p 1

Vinken PJ, Bruyn GW (eds): Handbook of Clinical Neurology, Vol 10, Leucodystrophies and Poliodystrophies. New York, American Elsevier, 1970

Volk BW, Aronson SM (eds): Sphingolipids, Sphingolipidoses and Allied Disorders. New York, Plenum, 1972

GM₁ GANGLIOSIDOSIS

Booth CW, Gerbie AB, Nadler HL: Intrauterine detection of GM₁ gangliosidosis, type 2. Pediatrics 52:521, 1973

Landing BH, Silverman FN, Craig MM, et al: Familial neurovisceral lipisodis. Am J Dis Child 108:503, 1964

Lowden JA, Cutz E, Conen PE, et al: Prenatal diagnosis of GM₁-gangliosidosis. N Engl J Med 288:225, 1973

O'Brien JS: GM₁ gangliosidosis. In Stanbury JB, Wyngaarden JB, Fredrickson DS (eds): The Metabolic Basis of Inherited Disease, 3rd ed. New York, McGraw-Hill, 1972, p 639

———— Ho MW, Veath ML, et al: Juvenile GM₁ gangliosidosis. Clinical, pathological, chemical and enzymatic studies. Clin Genet 3:411, 1972

Okada S, O'Brien JS: Generalized gangliosidosis: beta-galactosidase deficiency. Science 160:1002, 1968

Suzuki Y, Crocker AC, Suzuki K: GM₁ gangliosidosis. Correlation of clinical and biochemical data. Arch Neurol 24:58, 1971

Wolfe LS, Senior RG, Ng Ying Kim NMK: The structure of oligosaccharides accumulating in the liver of GM₁ gangliosidosis, type 1. J Biol Chem 249:1828, 1974

GM₂ GANGLIOSIDOSIS

Aronson SM, Myrianthopoulos NC: Epidemiology and genetics of the sphingolipidoses. In Vinken PJ, Bruyn GW (eds): Handbook of Clinical Neurology, Vol 10, Leucodystrophies and Poliodystrophies. New York, American Elsevier, 1970, p 556

Bach G, Suzuki K: Heterogeneity of human hepatic N-acetyl-β-D-hexosaminidase A activity toward natural glycosphingolipid substrates. J Biol Chem 250:1328, 1975

Brett EM, Ellis RB, Haas L, et al: Late onset GM₂-gangliosidosis. Clinical, pathological, and biochemical studies on 8 patients. Arch Dis Child 48:775, 1973

Dreyfus JC, Poenaru L, Svennerholm L: Absence of hexosaminidase A and B in a normal adult. N Engl J Med 292:61, 1975

Hultberg B: N-acetyl hexosaminidase activities in Tay-Sachs disease. Lancet 2:1195, 1969

Kaback MM, Zeigler RS, Reynolds LW, Sonneborn M: Approaches to the control and prevention of Tay-Sachs disease. Progr Med Genet 10:103, 1974

Kolodny EH: Clinical and biochemical genetics of the lipidoses. Semin Hematol 9:251, 1972

Korey SR, Gonatas J, Stein A: Studies in Tay-Sachs disease III. Biochemistry. A. Analytic and metabolic aspects. B. Catabolism of gangliosides and related compounds. J Neuropathol Exp Neurol 22:56, 1963

O'Brien JS, Okada S, Chen A, Fillerup DL: Tay-Sachs disease: detection of heterozygotes and homozygotes by serum hexosaminidase assay. N Engl J Med 283:15, 1970.

———— Okada S, Fillerup DL, et al: Tay-Sachs disease: prenatal diagnosis. Science 172:61, 1971

Okada S, O'Brien JS: Tay-Sachs disease: generalized absence of a beta-D-N-acetyl hexosaminidase component. Science 165:698, 1969

Samuels S, Korey SR, Gonatas J, et al: Studies on Tay-Sachs disease. IV. Membranous cytoplasmic granules in infantile amaurotic idiocy. J Neuropathol Exp Neurol 22:81, 1963

Sandhoff K, Harzer K, Wässler W, Jatzkewitz H: Enzyme alterations and lipid storage in three variants of Tay-Sachs disease. J Neurochem 18:2469, 1971

Schneck L, Amsterdam D, Brooks SE, et al: The Tay-Sachs disease fibroblast model: failure to respond to exogenous hexosaminidase A. Pediatrics 52:221, 1973

Sloan HR, Fredrickson DS: GM₂ gangliosidoses: Tay-Sachs disease. In Stanbury JB, Wyngaarden JB, Fredrickson DS (eds): The Metabolic Basis of Inherited Disease, 3rd ed. New York, McGraw-Hill, 1972

Suzuki Y, Suzuki K: Partial deficiency of hexosaminidase component A in juvenile GM₂ gangliosidosis. Neurology 20:848, 1970

Tateson R, Bain AC: GM₂ gangliosidoses: consideration of the genetic defects. Lancet 2:612, 1971

Volk BW, Schneck L, Adachi M: Clinic, pathology and biochemistry of Tay-Sachs disease. In Vinken PJ, Bruyn GW (eds): Handbook of Clinical Neurology, Vol 10, Leucodystrophies and Poliodystrophies. New York, American Elsevier, 1970, p 385

FABRY'S DISEASE

Brady RO, Gal AE, Bradley RM, et al: Enzymatic defect in Fabry's disease: ceramide-trihexosidase deficiency. New Engl J Med 276:1163, 1967

———— Uhlendorf BW, Jacobson CB: Fabry's disease: antenatal detection. Science 172:174, 1971

Clarke JTR, Guttman RD, Wolfe LS, et al: Enzyme replacement therapy by renal allotransplantation in Fabry's disease. N Engl J Med 287:1215, 1972

Del Monte MA, Johnson DL, Cotlier E, et al: Diagnosis of Fabry's disease by tear alpha-galactosidase A. N Engl J Med 290:57, 1974

Mapes CA, Anderson RL, Sweeley CC, et al: Enzyme replacement in Fabry's disease, an inborn error of metabolism. Science 170:987, 1970

Sweeley CC, Klonsky B, Krivit W, Desnick RJ: Fabry's disease: glycosphingolipid lipidosis. In Stanbury JB, Wyngaarden JB, Frederickson DS (eds): The Metabolic Basis of Inherited Disease, 3rd ed. New York, McGraw-Hill, 1972, p 663

METACHROMATIC LEUKODYSTROPHY

Austin JH: Metachromatic form of diffuse sclerosis. I. Diagnosis during life by urine sediment examination. Neurology 7:415, 1957

———— Studies in metachromatic leukodystrophy. XII. Multiple sulfatase deficiency. Arch Neurol 28:258, 1973

———— Armstrong D, Shearer L. McAfee D: Metachromatic form of diffuse cerebral sclerosis. VI. A rapid test for the sulfatase A deficiency in metachromatic leukodystrophy (MLD) urine. Arch Neurol 14:259, 1966

Percy AK, Kaback MM: Infantile and adult-onset metachromatic leukodystrophy. Biochemical comparisons and predictive diagnosis. N Engl J Med 285:785, 1971

Suzuki Y, Mizuno Y: Juvenile metachromatic leukodystrophy: deficiency of an arylsulfatase A component. J Pediatr 85:823, 1974

———— Suzuki K, Chen GC: Isolation and chemical characterization of metachromatic granules from a brain with metachromatic leukodystrophy. J Neuropathol Exp Neurol 26:537, 1967

GLOBOID CELL LEUKODYSTROPHY

Crome L, Hanefeld F, Patrick D, Wilson J: Late onset globoid cell leucodystrophy. Brain 96:841, 1973

Dunn HG, Lake BD, Dolman CL, Wilson J: The neuropathy of Krabbe's infantile cerebral sclerosis (globoid cell leucodystrophy). Brain 92:329, 1969

Ellis WG, Schneider EL, McCulloch JR, et al: Fetal globoid cell leukodystrophy (Krabbe disease). Pathological and biochemical examination. Arch Neurol 29:253, 1973

Hagberg B, Kollberg H, Sourander P, Åkesson HO: Infantile globoid cell leukodystrophy (Krabbe's disease). A clinical and genetic study of 32 Swedish cases (1953–1967). Neuropaediatrie 1:74, 1969

NERVOUS SYSTEM

Suzuki K, Suzuki Y: Galactosyl ceramide lipidosis: globoid cell leukodystrophy (Krabbe's disease). In Stanbury JB, Wyngaarden JB, Fredrickson DS (eds): The Metabolic Basis of Inherited Disease, 3rd ed. New York, McGraw-Hill, 1972, p 760

GAUCHER'S DISEASE

Brady RO, Kanfer JN, Shapiro D: Metabolism of glucocerebrosides. II. Evidence of an enyzmatic deficiency in Gaucher's disease. Biochem Biophys Res Commun 18:221, 1965
———Pentchev PG, Gal AE, et al: Replacement therapy for inherited enzyme deficiency. Use of purified glucocerebrosidase in Gaucher's disease. N Engl J Med 291:989, 1974
Fredrickson DS, Sloan HR: Glucosylceramide lipidoses: Gaucher's disease. In Stanbury JB, Wyngaarden JB, Fredrickson DS (eds): The Metabolic Basis of Inherited Disease, 3d ed. New York, McGraw-Hill, 1972, p 730
Gonzalez-Sastre F, Pampols T, Sabater J: Infantile Gaucher's disease: a biochemical study. Neurology 24:162, 1974
Patrick DA: A deficiency of glucocerebrosidase in Gaucher's disease. Biochem J 97:17c, 1965
Raghavan SS, Mumford RA, Kanfer JN: Deficiency of glucosylsphingosine: beta-glucosidase in Gaucher disease. Biochem Biophys Res Commun 54:256, 1973
Schneider EL, Ellis WG, Brady RO, et al: Infantile (type II) Gaucher's disease: in utero diagnosis and fetal pathology. J Pediatr 81:1134, 1972

NIEMANN-PICK DISEASE

Brady RO, Kanfer JN, Mock MB, Fredrickson DS: The metabolism of sphingomyelin. II. Evidence of an enzymatic deficiency in Niemann-Pick disease. Proc Natl Acad Sci USA 55:366, 1966
Crocker AC: The cerebral defect in Tay-Sachs disease and Niemann-Pick disease. J Neurochem 7:69, 1961
——— Farber S: Niemann-Pick disease: A review of eighteen patients. Medicine 37:1, 1958
Dacremont G, Kint JA, Cocquit G: Niemann-Pick disease. N Engl J Med 289:592, 1973
Fredrickson DS, Sloan HR: Sphingomyelin lipidoses: Niemann-Pick disease. In Stanbury JB, Wyngaarden JB, Fredrickson DS (eds): The Metabolic Basis of Inherited Disease, 3rd ed. New York, McGraw-Hill, 1972, p 783
Lachman R, Crocker A, Schulman J, Strand R: Radiological findings in Niemann-Pick disease. Radiology 108:659, 1973
Neville BGR, Lake BD, Stephens R, Sanders MD: A neurovisceral storage disease with vertical supranuclear ophthalmoplegia, and its relationship to Niemann-Pick disease: a report of nine patients. Brain 96:97, 1973
Oppenheimer DR, Norman RM, Tingey AH, Aherne WA: Histological and chemical findings in juvenile Niemann-Pick disease. J Neurol Sci 5:579, 1967
Savitzky A, Rosner F, Chodsky S: The sea-blue histiocyte syndrome, a review: genetic and biochemical studies. Semin Hematol 9:285, 1972
Schneider EL, Ellis WG, Brady RO, et al: Prenatal Niemann-Pick disease: biochemical and histologic examination of a 19-gestational week fetus. Pediatr Res 6:720, 1972
Silverstein MN, Ellefson RD, Aherne EJ: The syndrome of the sea-blue histiocyte. N Enlg J Med 282:1, 1970

FARBER'S LIPOGRANULOMATOSIS

Samuelsson K, Zetterstrom R: Ceramides in a patient with lipogranulomatosis (Farber's disease) with chronic course. Scand J Clin Lab Invest 27:393, 1971

LEUKODYSTROPHIES

Powers JM, Schaumburg HH: Adreno-leukodystrophy (sex-linked Schilder's disease). Am J Pathol 76:481, 1974
Percy AK, McKhann GM: The biochemistry of myelin and the leukodystrophies. In Vinken PJ, Bruyn GW (eds): Handbook of Clinical Neurology, Vol 10, Leucodystrophies and Poliodystrophies. New York, American Elsevier, 1970, p 134

SUDANOPHILIC LEUKODYSTROPHIES

Seitelberger F: Pelizaeus-Merzbacher disease. In Vinken PJ, Bruyn GW (eds): Handbook of Clinical Neurology, Vol 10, Leucodystrophies and Poliodystrophies. New York, American Elsevier, 1970, p 150
Tyler HR: Pelizaeus-Merzbacher disease. A clinical study. Arch Neurol Psychiatry 80:162, 1958

COCKAYNE'S SYNDROME

Guzzetta F: Cockayne-Neill-Dingwall syndrome. In Vinken PJ, GW Bruyn (eds): Handbook of Clinical Neurology, Vol 13, Neuroretinal Degenerations. New York, American Elsevier, 1972, p 431
Seitelberger F: Pelizaeus-Merzbacher disease. In Vinken PJ, Bruyn GW (eds): Handbook of Clinical Neurology, Vol 10, Leucodystrophies and Poliodystrophies. New York, American Elsevier, 1970, p 150

ADRENOLEUKODYSTROPHY

Blaw MD: Melanodermic type leukodystrophy (adrenoleukodystrophy). In Vinken PJ, Bruyn GW (eds): Handbook of Neurology, Vol 10, Leucodystrophies and Poliodystrophies. New York, American Elsevier, 1970, p 128
Burton BK, Nadler HL: Schilder's disease: abnormal cholesterol retention and accumulation in cultivated fibroblasts. Pediatr Res 8:170, 1974
Powers JM, Schaumburg HH: Adreno-leukodystrophy (sex-linked Schilder's disease). Am J Pathol 76:481, 1974
Schaumburg HH, Richardson EP, Johnson PC, et al: Schilder's disease, sex-linked recessive transmission with specific adrenal changes. Arch Neurol 27:458, 1972
——— Powers JM, Raine CS, Suzuki K, Richardson EP: Adrenoleukodystrophy. A clinical and pathological study of 17 cases. Arch Neurol 32:577, 1975
Suzuki K, Grover WD: Ultrastructural and biochemical studies of Schilder's disease. I. Ultrastructure. J Neuropathol Exp Neurol 29:392, 1970
Valenstein E, Rosman NP, Carter AP: Schilder's disease: positive brain scan. JAMA 217:1699, 1971

CEREBROTENDINOUS XANTHOMATOSIS

Menkes JH, Schimschock JR, Swanson PD: Cerebrotendinous xanthomatosis. The storage of cholestanol within the nervous system. Arch Neurol 19:47, 1968

WOLMAN'S DISEASE

Burke JA, Schubert WK: Deficient activity of hepatic acid lipase in cholesterol ester storage disease. Science 176:309, 1972
Raafet F, Hashemian MP, Abrishami MA: Wolman's disease: report of two new cases with a review of the literature. Am J Clin Pathol 59:490, 1973

REFSUM'S DISEASE

Nevin NC, Cumings JN, McKeown F: Refsum's syndrome. Heredopathia atactica polyneuritiformis. Brain 90:419, 1967
Refsum S: Heredopathia atactica polyneuritiformis. Acta Psychiatr Scand [Suppl 38] 1946, p 1
Richterich R, Moser H, Rossi E: Refsum's disease (heredopathia atactica polyneuritiformis): an inborn error of lipid metabolism with storage of 3,7,11,15-tetra-methyl hexadecanoic acid. A review of clinical findings. Humangenetik 1:322, 1965
Steinberg D: Phytanic acid storage disease: Refsum's syndrome. In Stanbury JB, Wyngaarden JB, Fredrickson DS (eds): The Metabolic Basis of Inherited Disease, 3rd ed. New York, McGraw-Hill, 1972, p 833

TANGIER DISEASE

Fredrickson DS, Gotto AM, Levy RI: Familial lipoprotein deficiency (abetalipoproteinemia, hypobetalipoproteinemia, and Tangier disease). In Stanbury JB, Wyngaarden JB, Fredrickson DS (eds): The Metabolic Basis of Inherited Disease, 3rd ed. New York, McGraw-Hill, 1972, p 493

Haas LF, Austad WW, Bergin JD: Tangier disease. Brain 97:351, 1974

ABETALIPOPROTEINEMIA

Fredrickson DS, Gotto AM, Levy RI: Familial lipoprotein deficiency (abetalipoproteinamia, hypobetalipoproteinemia, and Tangier disease). In Stanbury JB, Wyngaarden JB, Fredrickson DS (eds): The Metabolic Basis of Inherited Disease, 3rd ed. New York, McGraw-Hill, 1972, p 493

Schwartz JF, Rowland LP, Eder H, et al: Bassen-Kornzweig syndrome: deficiency of serum β-lipoprotein. Arch Neurol 8:438, 1963

CEROID LIPOFUSCINOSES

Beckerman BL, Rapin I: Ceroid-lipofuscinosis. Am J Ophthalmol 80:73, 1975

Carpenter S, Karpati G, Andermann F: Specific involvement of muscle, nerve, and skin in late infantile and juvenile amaurotic idiocy. Neurology 22:170, 1972

DalCanto MC, Rapin I, Suzuki K: Neuronol storage disorder with chorea and curvilinear bodies. Neurology 24:1026, 1974

Greene JG: Neurophysiological studies in Batten's disease. Dev Med Child Neurol 13:477, 1971

Hagberg B, Haltia M, Sourander P, et al: Polyunsaturated fatty acid lipidosis—infantile form of so-called ceroid lipofuscinosis. I. Clinical and morphological aspects. Acta Paediatr Scand 57:495, 1974

Rapin I, Katzman R, Engel J Jr: Cherry red spots and progressive myoclonus without dementia; a distinct syndrome with neuronal storage. Trans Am Neurol Assoc 100:39, 1975

Santavuori P, Haltia M, Rapola J: Infantile type of so-called neuronal ceroid-lipofuscinosis. Dev Med Child Neurol 16:644, 1974

Svennerholm L, Hagberg B, Haltia M, et al: Polyunsaturated fatty acid lipidosis. II. Lipid biochemical studies. Acta Paediatr Scand 64:489, 1975

Zeman W: Studies in the neuronal ceroid-lipofuscinoses. J Neuropathol Exp Neurol 33:1, 1974

——— Siakotos AN: The neuronal ceroid-lipofuscinoses. In Hers HG, van Hoof F (eds): Lysosomes and Storage Diseases. New York, Academic, 1973, p 519

SPONGY CNS DEGENERATION

Adachi M, Schneck L, Cara J, Volk BW: Spongy degeneration of the central nervous system (van Bogaert and Bertrand type; Canavan's disease). A review. Hum Pathol 4:331, 1973

Canavan M: Schilder's encephalitis periaxialis diffusa. Report of a child aged sixteen and one-half months. Arch Neurol Psychiatry 25:299, 1931

Sacks O, Brown WJ, Aguilar MJ: Spongy degeneration of white matter. Canavan's sclerosis. Neurology 15:165, 1965

Silberman J, Dancis J, Feigin I: Neuropathological observations in maple syrup urine disease. Arch Neurol 5:351, 1961

Suzuki K: Peripheral nerve lesion in spongy degeneration of the central nervous system. Acta Neuropathol (Berl) 10:95, 1968

ALEXANDER'S DISEASE

Schreier H, Rapin I, Davis J: Familial megalencephaly or hydrocephalus? Neurology 24:232, 1974

WILSON'S DISEASE

Bearn AG: Wilson's disease. In Stanbury JB, Wyngaarden JB, Fredrickson DS (eds): The Metabolic Basis of Inherited Disease, 3rd ed. New York, McGraw-Hill, 1972, p 1033

Denny-Brown D: Hepatolenticular degeneration (Wilson's disease). Two different components. N Engl J Med 270:1149, 1964

O'Reilly S, Strickland GT, Weber PM, et al: Abnormalities in the physiology of copper in Wilson's disease. I. The whole-body turnover of copper. Arch Neurol 24:385, 1971

Sternlieb I, Scheinberg IH: Prevention of Wilson's disease in asymptomatic patients. N Engl J Med 278:352, 1968

——— van den Hamer CJA, Morell AG, et al: Lysosomal defect of hepatic copper excretion in Wilson's disease (hepatolenticular degeneration). Gastroenterology 64:99, 1973

CEREBROHEPATORENAL SYNDROME

Passarge E, McAdams AJ: Cerebro-hepato-renal syndrome. A newly recognized hereditary disorder of multiple congenital defects, including sudanophilic leukodystrophy, cirrhosis of the liver, and polycystic kidneys. J Pediatr 71:691, 1967

TRICHOPOLIODYSTROPHY

Ashkenazi A, Levin S, Djaldetti M, et al: The syndrome of neonatal copper deficiency. Pediatrics 52:525, 1973

Bucknall WE, Haslam RHA, Holtzman NA: Kinky hair syndrome: response to copper therapy. Pediatrics 52:653, 1973

Danks DM, Cartwright E, Stevens BJ, Townley RRW: Menkes' kinky hair disease: further definition of the defect in copper transport. Science 179:1140, 1973

——— Stevens BJ, Campbell PE, et al: Menkes' kinky-hair syndrome. An inherited defect in copper absorption with widespread effects. Pediatrics 50:188, 1972

Grover WD, Scrutton MC: Intravenous copper therapy in trichopoliodystrophy. Neurology 24:367, 1974

Lott IT, DiPaolo R, Schwartz D: Copper metabolism in the steely-hair syndrome. N Engl J Med 292:197, 1975

Menkes JH, Alter M, Steigleder M, et al: A sex-linked recessive disorder with retardation of growth, peculiar hair, and focal cerebral and cerebellar degeneration. Pediatrics 29:764, 1962

FAMILIAL CALCIFICATION OF BASAL GANGLIA

Babbitt DP, Tang T, Dobbs J, Berk R: Idiopathic familial cerebrovascular ferrocalcinosis (Fahr's disease) and review of differential diagnosis of intracranial calcification in children. Am J Roentgenol Radium Ther Nucl Med 105:352, 1969

SUBACUTE NECROTIZING ENCEPHALOMYELOPATHY

Blass JP, Kark RAP, Engel WK: Clinical studies in a patient with pyruvate decarboxylase deficiency. Arch Neurol 25:449, 1971

Brunette MG, Delvin E, Hazel B, Scriber CR: Thiamine-responsive lactic acidosis in a patient with a deficient low-Km pyruvate carboxylase activity in liver. Pediatrics 50:702, 1972

Gruskin AB, Patel MS, Linshaw M, et al: Renal function studies and kidney pyruvate carboxylase in subacute necrotizing encephalomyelopathy (Leigh's syndrome). Pediatr Res 7:832, 1973

Lonsdale D, Faulkner WR, Price JW, et al: Intermittent cerebellar ataxia associated with hyperpyruvic acidemia, hyperalaninemia and hyperalaninuria. Pediatrics 43:1025, 1969

Murphy JV, Craig LJ, Glew RH: Leigh's disease: biochemical characteristics of the inhibitor. Arch Neurol 31:220, 1974

Pincus JH: Subacute necrotizing encephalomyelopathy (Leigh's disease): a consideration of clinical features and etiology. Dev Med Child Neurol 14:87, 1972

Pincus JH, Cooper JR, Murphy JV, et al: Thiamine derivatives in subacute necrotizing encephalomyelopathy. Pediatrics 51:716, 1973

Shapira Y, Cederbaum SD, Cancilla PA, et al: Familial poliodystrophy, mitochondrial myopathy, and lactate acidemia. Neurology 25:614, 1975

LAFORA'S DISEASE

Neville HE, Brooks MH, Austin JH: Studies in myoclonus epilepsy (Lafora body form). IV: Skeletal muscle abnormalities. Arch Neurol 30:466, 1974

van Heycop ten Ham MW: Lafora disease: a form of progressive myoclonus epilepsy. In Vinken PJ, Bruyn GW (eds): Handbook of Clinical Neurology, Vol 15, The Epilepsies. New York, American Elsevier, 1974, p 382

van Woert MH, Sethy VH: Therapy of intention myoclonus with I-5-hydroxytrytophane and a peripheral decarboxylase inhibitor MK 486. Neurology 25:135, 1975

HUNTINGTON'S DISEASE

Barbeau A, Chase TN, Paulson GW (eds): Huntington's Chorea (1872–1972). Advances in Neurology, Vol 1. New York, Raven, 1973

Haerer AF, Currier RD, Jackson JF: Hereditary nonprogressive chorea of early onset. N Engl J Med 276:1220, 1967

Klawans HL Jr, Paulson GW, Ringel SP, Barbeau A: Use of L-dopa in the detection of presymptomatic Huntington's chorea. N Engl J Med 286:1332, 1972

Markham CH, Knox JW: Observations on Huntington's chorea in childhood. J Pediatr 67:46, 1965

DYSTONIA MUSCULORUM DEFORMANS

Cooper IS: Involuntary Movement Disorders. New York, Harper & Row, 1969

Ebstein RP, Freeman LS, Lieberman A, et al: A familial study on serum dopamine-β-hydroxylase levels in torsion dystonia. Neurology 24:684, 1974

Eldridge R: The torsion dystonias: literature review and genetic and clinical studies. Neurology 20 [Suppl 11]:1, 1970

Marsden CD, Harrison MJG: Idiopathic torsion dystonia (dystonia musculorum deformans). A review of 42 patients. Brain 97:793, 1974

Wooten GF, Eldridge R, Axelrod J, et al: Elevated plasma dopamine-β-hydroxylase activity in autosomal dominant torsion dystonia. N Engl J Med 288:284, 1973

Zeman W, Dyken P: Dystonia musculorum deformans. In Vinken PJ, Bruyn GW (eds): Handbook of Clinical Neurology, Vol 6, Diseases of the Basal Ganglia. New York, Wiley, 1968, p 517

FAMILIAL (ESSENTIAL) TREMOR

Larsson T, Sjögren T: Essential tremor. A clinical and genetic population study. Acta Psychiatr Neurol Scand [Suppl 144] 36:1 1960

Morgan MH, Hewer RL, Cooper R: Effect of the beta adrenergic blocking agent propranolol on essential tremor. J Neurol Neurosurg Psychiatry 36:618, 1973

Winkler GF, Young RR: Efficacy of chronic propranolol therapy in action tremor of the familiar, senile or essential varieties. N Engl J Med 290:984, 1974

GILLES DE LA TOURETTE'S SYNDROME

Cooper JR, Bloom FE, Roth RH: The Biochemical Basis of Neuropharmacology, 2nd ed. New York, Oxford Univ Press, 1974

Shapiro AK, Shapiro E, Wayne HL: The treatment of Gilles de la Tourette's syndrome with haloperidol: review of 34 cases. Arch Gen Psychiatry 28:92, 1973

——— Shapiro E, Wayne HL, et al: Tourette's syndrome: summary of data on 34 patients. Psychosom Med 35:419, 1973

Sweet RD, Bruun RD, Shapiro AK: Dopamine and Gilles de la Tourette's syndrome. Neurology 24:388, 1974

——— Solomon G, Wayne H, et al: Neurological features of Gilles de la Tourette syndrome. J Neurol Neurosurg Psychiatry 36:1, 1973

ACUTE INTERMITTENT PORPHYRIA

Marver HS, Schmid R: The Porphyrias. In Stanbury JB, Wyngaarden JB, Fredrickson DS (eds): The Metabolic Basis of Inherited Disease, 3rd ed. New York, McGraw-Hill, 1972, p 1087

Peters HA, Cripps DJ, Reese HH: Porphyria: theories of etiology and treatment. Int Rev Neurobiol 16:301, 1974

Whitelaw AGL: Acute intermittent porphyria in childhood. A neglected diagnosis? Arch Dis Child 49:404, 1974

ATAXIA-TELANGIECTASIA

Ammann AJ, Hong R: Autoimmune phenomena in ataxia telangiectasia. J Pediatr 78:821, 1971

Hecht F, McCaw BK, Koler RD: Ataxia-telangiectasia—clonal growth of translocation lymphocytes. N Engl J Med 289:286, 1973

McFarlin DE, Strober W, Waldmann TA: Ataxia telangiectasia. Medicine 51:281, 1972

Sedgwick RP, Boder E: Ataxia-telangiectasia. In Vinken PJ, Bruyn GW (eds): Handbook of Clinical Neurology, Vol 14, The Phakomatoses. New York, American Elsevier, 1972, p 267

SPINAL AND SPINOCEREBELLAR DEGENERATIONS

Alter M, Talbert OR, Croffead G: Cerebellar ataxia, congenital cataracts, and retarded somatic and mental maturation. Report of cases of Marinesco-Sjögren syndrome. Neurology 12:836, 1962

Greenfield JG: The Spino-Cerebellar Degenerations. Oxford, Blackwell, 1954

Konigsmark BW, Weiner LP: The olivopontocerebellar atrophies. A review. Medicine 49:227, 1970

Landis DMD, Rosenberg RN, Landis SL, et al: Olivopontocerebellar degeneration: clinical and ultrastructural abnormalities. Arch Neurol 31:395, 1974

PHAKOMATOSES AND OTHER NEUROCUTANEOUS SYNDROMES

Alexander GL: Sturge-Weber syndrome. In Vinken PJ, Bruyn GW (eds): Handbook of Clinical Neurology, Vol 14, The Phakomatoses. New York, American Elsevier, 1972, p 223

Canale DJ, Bebin J: Von Recklinghausen disease of the nervous system. In Vinken PJ, Bruyn GW (eds): Handbook of Clinical Neurology, Vol 14, The Phakomatoses. New York, American Elsevier, 1972, p 132

De Recondo J, Haguenau M: Neuropathologic survey of the phakomatoses and allied disorders. In Vinken PJ, Bruyn GW (eds): Handbook of Clinical Neurology, Vol 14, The Phakomatoses. New York, American Elsevier, 1972, p 19

Donegani G, Grattarola FR, Wildi E: Tuberous sclerosis. Bourneville disease. In Vinken PJ, Bruyn GW (eds): Handbook of Clinical Neurology, Vol 14, The Phakomatoses. New York, American Elsevier, 1972, p 340

Fox H: Neurocutaneous melanosis. In Vinken PJ, Bruyn GW (eds): Handbook of Clinical Neurology, Vol 14, The Phakomatoses. New York, American Elsevier, 1972, p 414

Grossman M, Melman KL: Von Hippel-Lindau disease. In Vinken PJ, Bruyn GW (eds): Handbook of Clinical Neurology, Vol 14, The Phakomatoses. New York, American Elsevier, 1972, p 241

Kissel P, Dureaux JB: Cobb syndrome: cutaneomeningospinal angiomatosis. In Vinken PJ, Bruyn GW (eds): Handbook of Clinical Neurology, Vol 14, The Phakomatoses. New York, American Elsevier, 1972, p 429

Lecuire J, Dechaume JP, Bret P: Bonnet-Dechaume-Blanc syndrome. In Vinken PJ, Bruyn GW (eds): Handbook of Clinical Neurology, Vol 14, The Phakomatoses. New York, American Elsevier, 1972, p 260

Lovejoy FH Jr, Boyle WW Jr: Linear nevus sebaceous syndrome: report of two cases and a review of the literature. Pediatrics 52:382, 1973

McLennan JE, Gilles FH, Robb RM: Neuropathological correlation in Sjögren-Larsson syndrome. Oligophrenia, ichthyosis and spasticity. Brain 97:693, 1974

O'Doherty N: Bloch-Sulzberger syndrome. Incontinentia pigmenti. In Vinken PJ, Bruyn GW (eds): Handbook of Clinical Neurology, Vol 14, The Phakomatoses. New York, American Elsevier, 1972, p 213

Regan JD, Setlow RB, Kaback MM, et al: Xeroderma pigmentosum: a rapid sensitive method for prenatal diagnosis. Science 174:147, 1971

Robbins JH, Kraemer KH, Lutzner MA, et al: Xeroderma pigmentosum. An inherited disease with sun sensitivity, multiple cutaneous neoplasms, and abnormal DNA repair. Ann Intern Med 80:221, 1974

Rosman NP, Pearce J: The brain in multiple neurofibromatosis (von Recklinghausen's disease): a suggested neuropathological basis for the associated mental defect. Brain 90:829, 1967

Sjögren T, Larsson T: Oligophrenia in combination with congenital ichthyosis and spastic disorders. Acta Psychiatr Neurol Scand [Suppl 113] 1957, p 1

Van Tilburg W: Fibrous dysplasia. In Vinken PJ, Bruyn GW (eds): Handbook of Clinical Neurology, Vol 14, The Phakomatoses. New York, American Elsevier, 1972, p 163

Vinken PJ, Bruyn GW (eds): Handbook of Clinical Neurology, Vol 14, The Phakomatoses. New York, American Elsevier, 1972

NEUROAXONAL DYSTROPHIES

Defendini R, Markesbury WR, Mastri AR, Duffy PE: Hallervorden-Spatz disease and infantile neuroaxonal dystrophy. J Neurol Sci 20:7, 1973

Dooling EC, Schoene WC, Richardson ED Jr: Hallervorden-Spatz syndrome. Arch Neurol 30:70, 1974

Gilman S, Barrett RE: Hallervorden-Spatz disease and infantile neuroaxonal dystrophy. J Neurol Sci 19:189, 1973

Wigboldus JM, Bruyn GW: Hallervorden-Spatz disease. In Vinken PJ, Bruyn GW (eds): Handbook of Clinical Neurology, Vol 6, Diseases of the Basal Ganglia. New York, Wiley 1968, p 604

DEMYELINATING SCLEROSES

Gall JC Jr, Hayles AB, Siekert RG, Keith HM: Multiple sclerosis in children. A clinical study of 40 cases with onset in childhood. Pediatrics 21:703, 1958

Low NL, Carter S: Multiple sclerosis in childhood. Pediatrics 18:24, 1956

Multiple Sclerosis and the Demyelinating Diseases. Res Publ Assoc Res Nerv Ment Dis Vol 28, 1950

NERVOUS SYSTEM DISORDERS SPECIFIC TO CHILDREN

Arnold P. Gold and Sidney Carter

Spasmus nutans, familial dysautonomia, and acute cerebellar ataxia are rare disorders specific to children.

Spasmus Nutans

Spasmus nutans (head nodding) characteristically presents with a triad of signs: intermittent nystagmus, head nodding, and tilting of the head. The condition is self-limited, generally disappearing by 3 years of age. The syndrome has its onset in infancy, most often between the ages of 4 and 16 months. There is no particular sex incidence, but it is more common in blacks; the cause is unknown. Spasmus nutans is seen more frequently during the winter months. Nystagmus may be the initial sign. It is often either unilateral or more marked in one eye and is characterized by rapid movements of small amplitude in any direction. The abnormal eye movement disappears on covering the eyes and during sleep. The head nodding, which may occur in any direction, is typically slow and inconstant, with a series of nods usually lasting but a few seconds. This movement is increased by placing the child in a vertical position and is abolished when the child is supine. Head tilt is the least common finding and is often a compensa-

tory posturing for the impaired vision secondary to the nystagmus. Spasmus nutans must be differentiated from congenital nystagmus, which tends to be familial and to involve both eyes and fails to improve with time. When head movement is present it is in the same direction as the nystagmus. The condition is self-limited, and there is no specific therapy.

Familial Dysautonomia

Ralph E. Moloshok

Familial dysautonomia (Riley-Day syndrome) is transmitted as an autosomal recessive and occurs particularly in Ashkenazi Jews. It presents with diffuse disturbance of the nervous system, but autonomic dysfunction predominates. Features that have been present in all cases are reduced or absent tear production during crying, postural hypotension, coldness of the hands and feet, excessive perspiration (usually with transient blotching of the skin with excitement or during eating), relative indifference to pain, and emotional lability. Muscular coordination is impaired, as is manifested by difficulty in swallowing and chewing during infancy, prolonged drooling, dysarthria, and delay in reaching the milestones of motor development. There is general retardation of body growth, and pubescence is usually delayed. Scoliosis occurs in about half of the children who have survived past the age of 10 years. Deep tendon reflexes may be hypoactive, or often they may be absent. Impairment of autonomic homeostasis is manifested by erratic regulation of body temperature, with hypothermia, particular during infancy, and periods of unexplained hyperpyrexia. Hypertension may occur with excitement or in association with febrile crises, while other patients are unable to maintain the upright position because of severe postural hypotension. Corneal anesthesia and defective lacrimation predispose to ulceration and scarring, with impaired vision.

Severe life-threatening episodes are experienced in the course of the disease. Acute pulmonary crises occur as a result of bronchial hypersecretion, aspiration, and bronchopneumonia. Periodic bouts of intractable vomiting may be associated with bizarre self-destructive schizoid behavior. Severe hyperpyrexia may be accompanied by hypertension and diminished renal function or by a convulsive state. In a few instances sudden death has followed a shocklike state. Cardiac arrest and shock have been experienced during anesthesia.

The cause of this syndrome is unknown. An inborn error of metabolism affecting synthesis of a neurohumoral transmitter substance has been postulated. Anatomic findings include a marked reduction in the number of unmyelinated fibers in sural nerve biopsies. Reduced numbers of neurons in autonomic ganglia and dorsal root ganglia and a marked diminution in sensory axons in the tongue have been found. Defects in catecholamine metabolism include a uniform elevation of the ratio of homovanillic acid (a product of dopamine metabolism) excreted in the urine as compared with vanillylmandelic acid (a product of epinephrine and norepinephrine metabolism). A reduced plasma activity of dopamine β-hydroxylase, which converts dopamine to norepinephrine, has also been described. However, further studies suggest that these abnormalities in catecholamine metabolism are secondary to a cholinergic defect with a deficit in acetylcholine synthesis or release and its effect on synaptic function.

A valuable diagnostic test is the response to the intradermal injection of 0.02 ml of a 1:10,000 dilution of histamine. The reaction of denervation is observed in patients with dysautonomia. Normally a wheal about 1 cm in diameter is produced, surrounded by a red flare 3 to 5 cm in diameter. The flare is dependent on an axon reflex along sensory fibers; it has been uniformly absent in patients with dysautonomia. Hypersensitivity to the intravenous infusion of norepinephrine is another diagnostic feature in patients with dysautonomia, in whom a rise in blood pressure greater than 50 mm Hg is seen. While the normal pupil does not respond to the intraconjunctival instillation of a 2.5 percent solution of methacholine, in dysautonomia miosis occurs. The absence of taste buds on the tongue, which is similarly a reaction of denervation, provides an objective anatomic diagnostic sign. Physiologic studies of respiration in dysautonomic children have revealed a relative insensitivity to hypoxia and to elevated carbon dioxide levels in the blood.

Prognosis for life must be guarded, as death from these acute crises has occurred in about 25 percent of known cases, especially during the early years of life. The survivors have been handicapped by psychomotor difficulties, although with increasing age adaptation to stress appears to improve.

Treatment is principally symptomatic. Guidance for the parents in the management of difficult behavior patterns in these children is most important. Vomiting attacks can often be controlled by the use of chlorpromazine in combination with phenobarbital. The administration of bethanechol (Urecholine) to a small group of children with familial dysautonomia has been reported to have a favorable effect on some of the manifestations of this syndrome. There was an increase in eye moisture, a reduction in gastric distension and vomiting, and improvement in esophageal motility and bladder control. Corneal complications have been decreased with the use of artificial tears and protective glasses or soft contact lenses. If general anesthesia is necessary, careful monitoring of blood pressure and blood gases should be provided. Due to the lack of appropriate response to hypoxia and hypercapnia, diving and underwater swimming are contraindicated. Inasmuch as these children adjust poorly to environmental change and stress, a stable routine of daily activity may prove helpful. The use of tranquilizing drugs has been of benefit to some children.

ACUTE CEREBELLAR ATAXIA
STUART WEISS

Acute cerebellar ataxia, an unusual neurologic syndrome peculiar to children, is characterized by sudden or subacute onset of ataxia of trunk and extremities and ocular movement without other neurologic involvement or systemic symptoms. Complete recovery occurs within a few weeks or months in a high percentage of patients. Children of both sexes between the ages of 1 and 4 years are most often affected, but older children may be involved.

A history of preceding upper respiratory or gastrointestinal disturbance is sometimes obtained, but most children develop ataxia without prior illness. Some authors consider acute cerebellar ataxia to be a transient sensitivity or inflammatory reaction of the cerebellum or cerebellar tracts to a viral or systemic illness, but others regard the syndrome as a viral cerebellitis, especially in the few severely involved patients. Occasionally inborn errors of protein metabolism have been discovered in children with acute ataxia. Recurrent acute ataxia, often precipitated by minor infections, has been inherited in several families as a mendelian dominant. Recently some children with acute cerebellar ataxia have been shown to have neuroblastomas.

The major clinical feature of the syndrome is the rapid development of truncal ataxia with a lesser degree of extremity ataxia, which is less marked in the arms than in the legs. In the more severely involved child there may be complete inability to support the body in a sitting position or keep the head erect. Muscles of the trunk and extremities are hypotonic. Often an irregular jerky tremor of the head and body is present. Some children with severe ataxia may also develop jerky irregular ocular activity with volitional eye movement (ocular dysmetria); others may develop involuntary darting multidirectional conjugate ocular movement (opsoclonia), and a few develop nystagmus with rhythmic fast–slow components. These abnormal eye movements may be associated with myoclonic jerks. Isolated cranial nerve involvement, particularly the facial and less often the vagus, may occur in association with cerebellar ataxia. A specific viral infection (poliovirus 1) has been documented as the etiologic factor in the latter patients. Vague systemic abnormalities such as lethargy, irritability, photophobia, and mild nuchal rigidity may accompany the neurologic deficit.

Most laboratory studies are normal. Occasionally a mild mononuclear pleocytosis is noted in spinal fluid, but protein is normal. In a few children viral cultures have grown poliovirus 1 and echoviruses 6 and 9. Antibodies to *Mycoplasma pneumoniae* have been demonstrated in several patients.

A variety of diagnostic possibilities should be considered in a child with acute cerebellar ataxia. Posterior fossa tumors may produce ataxia abruptly. This ataxia is usually asymmetric in the degree of involvement of extremities and is associated with evidence of increased intracranial pressure, cranial nerve palsies, head tilt, and nystagmus with preponderance in one direction. Acute truncal ataxia without fever or meningism has been the initial clinical manifestation of *Hemophilus* or meningococcal meningitis. Classic acute ataxia in the course of varicella is of sufficiently frequent occurrence to be recognized, and it has been reported with rubella, rubeola, mumps, typhoid fever, and infectious mononucleosis. Acute ataxia associated with myoclonic jerking and opsoclonus may be the initial manifestation of an occult neuroblastoma. Acute ataxia with a photosensitive pellagralike skin rash occurs with Hartnup's disease. Urinary screening for indican and indole acetic acid and characteristic blood and urinary chromatographic patterns of amino acids indicate this diagnosis in suspected patients. Leigh's syndrome also may cause ataxia (p. 1923). Drugs such as diphenylhydantoin and barbiturates, or inhalation or ingestion of DDT or lindane, may cause ataxia as an early sign of toxicity. Lead ingestion and thallium poisoning produce ataxic syndromes that may not be readily reversible.

Most patients with acute cerebellar ataxia experience a rapid recovery of extremity coordination and gait stability within periods of 1 week to 6 months. Some have persistent neurologic deficit, with ocular dysmetria, truncal and extremity ataxia, and lesser degrees of intellectual impairment. However, even in this group of patients gradual improvement has taken place over periods of several years. There has been some correlation between the severity of the initial neurologic manifestations of the disease and a less favorable prognosis. The occurrence of abnormal eye movements (ocular dysmetria and opsoclonus) has been associated with poor or slow recovery from the ataxia. A number of such children are left intellectually impaired.

In the absence of a specific treatable cause of the syndrome, therapy of acute cerebellar ataxia is symptomatic, being directed toward maintenance of fluid and nutritional requirements, nursing supervision for general body care, and physical rehabilitation after the acute phase of illness is past. The child should be kept at bed rest until the active progression of ataxia has ceased. Bed sides and rails should be protected with padding, as the children are often irritable and may strike their atactic extremities against metal bed surfaces. Barbiturates or other sedatives should be used judiciously if the irritability or agitation is sufficiently severe to exhaust the child. Active intervention with ACTH therapy is indicated in any child (usually an infant) who presents with opsoclonus, myoclonic jerks, and ataxia. Attempts at standing or walking the child should be withheld until the ataxia has sufficiently improved to avoid injurious falls. In patients with unusually severe and persisting problems in balance, football helmets may be worn during rehabilitation.

References

SPASMUS NUTANS

Herrman C: Head shaking with nystagmus in infants; a study of sixty-four cases. Am J Dis Child 16:180, 1918

Norton EWD, Cogan D: Spasmus nutans; a clinical study of twenty cases followed two years or more since onset. Arch Ophthalmol 52:442, 1954

FAMILIAL DYSAUTONOMIA

Aguayo AJ, Nair CPV, Bray GM: Peripheral nerve abnormalities in the Riley-Day syndrome. Arch Neurol 24:106, 1971

Axelrod FB, Nachtigal R, Dancis J: Familial dysautonomia: diagnosis, pathogenesis and management. Adv Pediatr 21:75, 1974

Brunt PW, McKusick VA: Familial dysautonomia. Report of genetic and clinical studies with a review of the literature. Medicine 49:343, 1970

Pearson J, Budzilovich G, Finegold MJ: Sensory, motor and autonomic dysfunction: the nervous system in familial dysautonomia. Neurology 21:486, 1971

Riley CM: Familial dysautonomia. Adv Pediatr 9:157, 1957

Smith AA, Dancis J: Current concepts; familial dysautonomia. N Engl J Med 274:207, 1966

ACUTE CEREBELLAR ATAXIA

Blass JP, Kark AP, Engel WK: Clinical studies of a patient with pyruvate decarboxylase deficiency. Arch Neurol 25:449, 1971

Hill W, Sherman H: Acute intermittent familial cerebellar ataxia. Arch Neurol 18:350, 1968

King G, Schwartz GA, Slade HW: Acute cerebellar ataxia. Pediatrics 21:731, 1958

Lasater GM, Jabbour JT: Acute ataxia of childhood: a summary of fifteen cases. Am J Dis Child 97:61, 1959

Lonsdale D, Faulkner WR, Price W, Smeby RR: Pyruvic acidemia with hyperalaninemia: vitamin B dependency. J Pediatr 74:827, 1969

Schwartz JF: Ataxia in bacterial meningitis. Neurology 22:1071, 1972

Weiss S, Carter S: Course and prognosis of acute cerebellar ataxia in children. Neurology 9:711, 1959

CHAPTER 31

The Eyes

LEONARD APT AND WILLIAM L. GAFFNEY, *Associate Editors*

This chapter will consider conditions involving the eyes that are likely to be encountered by the pediatrician. He must be able to recognize and treat common ocular and adnexal inflammations and attend to minor trauma and superficial foreign bodies. Most other ocular diseases should be referred to an ophthalmologist. For a more complete discussion of pediatric ocular disease, standard ophthalmology texts should be consulted (see References).

EXAMINATION OF THE EYE

Some estimation of visual acuity and a systematic detailed examination of the eye are important parts of every pediatric physical examination. An orderly sequence should be employed in which attention is directed to the ocular adnexa and to the exterior and interior of the globe. A careful history, including family history of ocular disease, should accompany each examination, since many pediatric ocular conditions (eg, strabismus) have a familial or hereditary basis. The examination is especially difficult in infants. Any attempt to separate the lids produces a forceful closure of the lids and a pronounced Bell's phenomenon; the pupils are small and the fissures narrow. Lid retractors (fashioned from paper clips or metal retractors made for this purpose), sedation, a pacifier, and colorful noisy toys may be helpful; sometimes an assistant may be required. Occasionally general anesthesia is necessary for an adequate examination of the fundus and other structures.

Visual Acuity

An ocular examination should begin with an attempt at an assessment of visual acuity, regardless of the child's age. Some idea of visual acuity in infants can be gained from the subject's ability to fix upon and follow a light or interesting object. Each eye should be tested separately. A newborn may show transitory monocular fixation. By the age of 4 to 6 weeks he should be able to follow a light or large object held close to the face over a short range. Failure to do so by 6 to 8 weeks of age (unless premature) may be a sign of mental impairment or may indicate decreased vision. By the age of 3 months the infant can follow an object or light over a wide range. Opticokinetic nystagmus (OKN) can be elicited with a rotating striped drum in 50 to 75 percent of normal newborns and even in some preterm infants. The presence of OKN indicates a visual acuity approximately equivalent to 20/670 on the Snellen chart. Pupillary reactions to direct light depend on functioning

retina and optic nerve, but can be present with cortical blindness. Startle reflexes can be a gross test of visual function. After 7 to 8 weeks of life an object brought swiftly toward the eyes will elicit blinking. Unilateral visual loss in a young child may be discovered by covering one eye. If the child loses interest or cries, but is attentive when the other eye is covered, vision is probably decreased in the first eye. By the age of 3 to 4 years a more precise determination of acuity is possible through use of the Snellen Illiterate E chart or standardized easily recognizable pictures. The pinhole test may be used in still older children. A pinhole should improve visual acuity if it is decreased due to a refractive error. Failure to improve visions with a pinhole indicates a cause for poor vision other than a refractive error, such as an opacity of the ocular media or retinal disease. Visual acuity at birth is approximately 20/400, but it gradually increases until age 4 to 5, when the normal child has an adult-level visual acuity of 20/20.

Electrophysiologic tests have become useful in the diagnosis of infantile organic blindness, since they permit differentiation between retinal and cortical causes. The electroretinogram (ERG) and electro-oculogram (EOG) record electrical responses to light at the retinal level, and the visual evoked response (VER) does the same at the cortical level. In cortical blindness the ERG response is normal, but the VER is absent.

Color Vision

Color vision screening is important because color vision deficiencies may lead to learning difficulties in school. Even though there is no suitable treatment for color vision deficiency, parents and teachers can help children in adjusting to this condition. Color blindness is usually partial and is nearly always of the red–green deficiency type. It occurs in 7.5 percent of white males and 4 percent of black males, while only 0.6 percent of all girls are affected, thus reflecting a sex-linked recessive inheritance. Pseudoisochromatic tests such as the Ishihara test may be used for detection of color blindness in children by having them trace or identify the numbers.

External Examination

External examination should begin with an estimate of any forward protrusion (exophthalmos)or retraction (enophthalmos) of the globe. Any enlargement (buphthalmos) or smallness (microphthalmos) of the globe should be noted. The newborn eye is 75 percent adult size which it reaches by the eighth year of life. The position and function of the lids are evaluated. Any drooping of the upper lids (ptosis) is due to a weakness of the levator muscle. Frequent blinking of the lids is usually without cause, but it is a common concern of parents. Refractive error, blepharitis, and conjunctivitis should be ruled out as etiologies. If a foreign body is suspected, the lid should be everted and inspected. The upper lid may be everted by having the child look down, then grasping the lashes and pulling the lid forward while placing an applicator approximately 1 cm above the lid margin and pressing down on the lid. Sterile fluorescein solution may be instilled if a corneal foreign body or abrasion is suspected. The palpebral and bulbar conjunctiva is carefully inspected for injection, follicles, or discharge. Conjunctival injection (bright red color and involving large superficial vessels lying in the conjunctiva), which is usually associated with conjunctivitis, should be distinguished from ciliary injection (violet color and involving fine, deep perilimbal vessels), which connotes corneal or intraocular disease. The cornea is inspected for clouding, scarring, ulceration, or vascularization, and its diameter is appraised. Photophobia frequently accompanies diseases of the cornea such as phlyctenular and interstitial keratitis. Light sensitivity may also be a sign of congenital glaucoma, acute iritis, or ocular albinism. Following evaluation of the anterior chamber and iris, the pupil is inspected. Leukokoria or white pupillary reflex can be caused by a number of intraocular diseases, but is most often secondary to cataract, retinoblastoma, retrolental fibroplasia, or nematode endophthalmitis. It is urgent to refer every patient with leukokoria to an ophthalmologist because of the possibility of a retinoblastoma.

Intraocular Pressure

The accurate measurement of intraocular pressure requires a tonometer. Tactile tensions are highly unreliable. If glaucoma is suspected in infants and young children, tonometry must be carried out under general anesthesia.

Extraocular Muscles

The action of the extraocular muscles and ocular alignment can be tested with a light and occluder. Gross alignment of the eyes may be checked by holding a pocket flashlight in front of the patient's eyes and observing the corneal light reflex (Hirschberg test). If the eyes are aligned the light reflex will be in the same position in each eye. If the light reflex is displaced temporally in one eye, an inward deviation or esotropia exists. If the light reflex is positioned nasally in one eye, an outward deviation or exotropia is present. The cover test is a more accurate method of studying ocular alignment. The patient is asked to look at an object while one eye is covered with an occluder. If the opposite (uncovered) eye makes a movement to pick up fixation, it is not straight, and the direction of the corrective movement indicates the type of deviation. The other eye is similarly tested. The cardinal positions of gaze can then be

checked to detect any paralysis of movement in a certain direction of gaze. The six extraocular muscles and their corresponding fields of action are: *medial rectus*, inward: *lateral rectus*, outward: *superior rectus*, upward, when eye is rotated outward: *inferior rectus*, downward, when eye is rotated outward; *superior oblique*, downward, when eye has been rotated inward; *inferior oblique*, upward, when eye has been rotated inward.

Visual Fields

In young children visual fields can be examined grossly by using large lights or objects in the confrontation method. Reliable testing with the tangent screen or perimeter can be done after the age of 5 or 6 years.

Ophthalmoscopy

Adequate ophthalmoscopy of the fundus requires pupillary dilatation. There should be no reluctance to use mydriatics because acute glaucoma does not occur in children. One drop of 2.5 percent phenylephrine (Neo-Synephrine) or 1.0 percent tropicamide (Mydriacyl), or both, in each eye will give safe and satisfactory pupillary dilatation in 15 to 20 minutes in infants and children of all ages. Cycloplegics (Cyclogyl, atropine) are unnecessary unless refraction by retinoscopy is to be performed. Toxic reactions to atropine are common in children and may even be fatal, especially in children with brain damage and mongolism. Ten percent phenylephrine should be avoided in infants and young children, as it can cause dangerous elevations of blood pressure after ocular administration. In some cases direct ophthalmoscopy may be impossible because of eye movements, and it may be necessary to use indirect ophthalmoscopy and even general anesthesia to study ocular fundi.

References

Apt L: Diagnostic Procedures in Pediatric Ophthalmology. Boston, Little, Brown, 1963.
——— Gaffney WL: Toxicity of ophthalmic drugs used in the management of childhood strabismus. In Leopold IH (ed): Ocular Therapy, Vol VIII. St Louis, Mosby, 1975
Arena JM (ed); Davison's Compleat Pediatrician, 9th ed. Philadelphia, Lea & Febiger, 1969.
Carr RE, Gowas P: Clinical electroretinography. JAMA 198:173, 1966
Ellis RP: Eye. In Kempe CH, Silver HK, O'Brien D (eds): Current Pediatric Diagnosis and Treatment, 3rd ed. Los Altos, Calif, Lange Medical, 1974
Kiff RD, Lepard C: Visual response of premature infants. Arch Ophthalmol 75:631 1966
Scheie HG, Albert DM: Adler's Textbook of Ophthalmology, 8th ed. Philadelphia, WB Saunders, 1969
Thuline HC: Color blindness in children. The importance and feasibility of early recognition. Clin Pediatr 11:295, 1972

DEVELOPMENTAL ANOMALIES OF THE GLOBE

Anomalies of the entire eye are common in stillbirths and rare in viable infants. They usually reflect a total body metabolic defect of genetic origin. However, there are also acquired prenatal causes, including drugs (thalidomide, aminopterin), toxins (organic mercury compounds), infectious agents (rubella, toxoplasmosis), and radiation or radiomimetic agents.

Failure of development of the primary optic vesicle results in *anophthalmos*. Although this term implies complete absence of an eye, some vestige usually can be located in the orbit. Fusion of the two optic vesicles produces *cyclopia,* the single median eye famed in antiquity. It is always associated with severe cranial and systemic abnormalities and is the result of a highly lethal autosomal recessive gene. *Microphthalmos,* or small eye, is frequently bilateral and is associated with other ocular defects such as cataract, aniridia, hyperopia. It is inherited as an autosomal trait, either dominant or recessive, and also occurs in multiple syndromes, con-

genital toxoplasmosis, and congenital rubella. Whenever microphthalmos is discovered, a search should be made for other abnormalities.

Defective closure of the optic fissure produces a *coloboma.* Typically a coloboma is bilateral and is located inferiorly or inferonasally, and it involves the iris and produces a keyhole defect. It may, however, involve the lens, ciliary body, choroid, retina, and optic nerve, with either slight or severe damage to vision. Characteristically it appears in the fundus of the eye as a white area with heavily pigmented edges extending from below the disc to the ora serrata. Inheritance is irregularly autosomal dominant.

Chromosomal Disorders

All major chromosomal observations are associated with significant eye abnormalities. Table 1 lists those eye deformities reported with major chromosomal defects.

References

Apt L, Gaffney WL: Congenital eye abnormalities from drugs during pregnancy. In. Leopold IH (ed): Ocular Therapy, Vol VII. St Louis , Mosby, 1974

Duke-Elder S: Normal and abnormal development. Congenital deformities. In System of Ophthalmology, Vol III, Part 2. St Louis, Mosby, 1964

Friedman T: Hereditary eye disease and prenatal diagnosis. Ann Ophthalmol 6:271, 1974

Geeraets WJ: Ocular Syndromes, 2nd ed. Philadelphia, Lea & Febiger, 1969

Ginsberg J, Bove K: Ocular pathology of trisomy 13, Ann Ophthalmol 6:113, 1974

———— Bove K, Nelson R, Englender GS: Ocular pathology of trisomy 18. Ann Ophthalmol 3:273, 1971

Keith CG: Chromosomal disorders and their ocular manifestations. In Sorsby A, Miller S (eds): Modern Trends in Ophthalmology, Vol 5. London, Butterworth, 1973

Mann I: Developmental Anomalies of the Eye. Philadelphia, JB Lippincott, 1958

TABLE 1. Chromosomal Aberrations and Their Eye Deformities

Chromosome Defects	Eye Manifestations
Trisomy 13–15 (trisomy D, Patau's syndrome)	Microphthalmia, coloboma (uvea and optic nerve), cataract, retinal dysplasia, intraocular cartilage
Trisomy 18 (E syndrome)	Microphthalmia, cataract, coloboma (uvea and optic nerve), corneal opacities, small or oblique palpebral fissures, ptosis, epicanthus, hypertelorism
Trisomy 21 (Down's syndrome, mongolism)	Cataract, peripheral iris hypoplasia, Brushfield's spots in iris, keratoconus, high myopia, strabismus, nystagmus, short round palpebral fissures slanting upward, epicanthus, hypertelorism
Deletion of short arm of chromosome 4	Iris deformities, strabismus, epicanthus, exophthalmos, absence of medial half of eyebrow
Partial deletion of short arm of chromsome 5 (cri-du-chat syndrome)	Strabismus, epicanthus, hypertelorism
Deletion of long arm of chromsome 18	Optic atrophy, funduscopic abnormalities, nystagmus, hypertelorism, epicanthus, strabismus
Deletion of short arm of chromosome	Ptosis, flat nasal bridge, hypertelorism, epicanthus, strabismus
XXXXY syndrome (Greig syndrome)	Optic atrophy, strabismus, bilateral VI nerve palsy, epicanthus, hypertelorism, deformities (lids, brows, fissures)
XO syndrome (Turner-Albright syndrome)	Corneal opacities, cataract, deficient retinal pigment, blue sclera, strabismus, nystagmus, mild exophthalmos, hypertelorism, epicanthus, ptosis

THE LIDS
Congenital Anomalies

Palpebral colobomas usually appear as a triangular notch in the upper lid, less often in the lower lid. They occur in the upper lid in association with epibulbar dermoids in Goldenhar's syndrome. Their appearance in the lower lid suggests Franceschetti's syndrome.

Blepharophimosis is a bilateral and symmetric decrease in size of the palpebral fissure. Inherited as an autosomal dominant trait, it may be associated with other lid anomalies, including ptosis. Children with Waardenburg's syndrome may have this defect.

A common anomaly of the lids is *epicanthus,* a bilateral vertical semilunar fold arising in the upper lid, extending down the side of the nose to the lower lid, and covering the normal inner canthus. It is similar to the racial characteristic of mongols and many Orientals and is a constant finding in trisomy 21 (Down's syndrome).

It is also found in normal subjects as a familial characteristic and in infants with flat nasal bridges. In these infants it creates an illusory appearance of convergent strabismus (pseudostrabismus). As the bridge of the nose becomes formed with development of the face, the folds usually disappear, with resolution of the pseudostrabismus.

In *entropion* the lid margins are turned in, causing the cilia to rub against the cornea (trichiasis). Surgery is necessary if corneal damage ensues. Rarely the lid margins may turn out (*ectropion*).

The most common anomaly of the eyelids is congenital *ptosis* or drooping of the upper lid. Usually unilateral, but frequently bilateral, congenital ptosis is secondary to defective development or absence of the levator muscle. It is often inherited as an autosomal dominant trait. Ptosis may occur alone, or it may be associated with weakness of the superior rectus muscle on the same side, since both the levator muscle and superior rectus muscle are derived from the same mesodermal anlage. Acquired causes of ptosis include birth trauma, third nerve palsy, Horner's syndrome, and local tumor such as hemangioma. The child may raise his eyebrow using his frontalis to lift the lid. In bilateral ptosis he may also tip his head backward. Cosmetic surgery is usually deferred until the age of 4 or 5 years. However, if ptosis interferes with vision, surgery is performed earlier to avoid amblyopia. Surgical correction of ptosis involves either resection of the levator muscle or, in those cases with no levator function, suspension of the lid from the brow with fascia lata.

A peculiar form of ptosis occurs in the *jaw-winking* or *Marcus Gunn phenomenon.* An anomalous connection between the external pterygoid muscle and the levator muscle leads to elevation of the ptotic lid when the mouth is opened or when the jaw is moved to the side opposite the ptosis. This condition usually does not require surgery.

Replacement of the meibomian glands by a second row of lashes is termed *distichia.* The abnormal row of lashes usually rubs against the cornea and must be removed by electrolysis or surgery.

Dermoid cysts arise from ectodermal remnants cut off from the surface. They lie along cranial sutures, most often in the lateral part of the upper lid, occasionally in the median portion of the upper lid and in the lower lids. Their consistency is rubbery or hard, the overlying skin is free and unattached, and they contain secretions of the epithelial glands lining the cyst. Traumatic rupture of the cyst may release these secretions into surrounding tissues and result in severe inflammation. For this reason and for cosmesis these cysts should be excised surgically at an early age.

Lid Infections

BLEPHARITIS. Blepharitis is a common chronic and recurrent inflammation of the lid margins associated with redness, scaling, burning, irritation, loss of lashes, and keratoconjunctivitis. There are four basic types: staphylococcal, seborrheic, mixed, and angular. The first three types account for over 90 percent of cases.

Staphylococcal blepharitis is characterized clinically by hard and tenacious collarettes or scales at the base of the lashes; occasionally, there are ulcers or pustules or both on the lid margins and an associated conjunctivitis and keratitis. Smears show gram-positive cocci with polymorphonuclear leukocytes, and cultures are positive for pathogenic *Staphylococcus aureus.*

Seborrheic or *squamous blepharitis* presents with greasy, easily removed scales and associated seborrhea of the scalp and brow. Conjunctivitis and keratitis are usually absent. Eyelid margin scrapings frequently show a round gram-positive budding yeast form (*Pityrosporon ovale*), which is not considered a causative agent. Mixed types of blepharitis are common, as staphylococcal infection usually complicates seborrhea of the lids.

Angular blepharitis is a type of squamous blepharitis caused by *Haemophilus duplex* (diplobacillus of Morax-Axenfeld) that is typified by minimal scaling and inflammation of the skin and mucocutaneous borders of the angles of the lids. Large gram-negative diplobacilli with no leukocytes are seen on eyelid scrapings. For the successful treatment of blepharitis, scales should be removed from the eyelid margin twice daily with a cotton-tip applicator soaked in water or baby shampoo. Hot moist compresses may help loosen scales. Antibiotic ointments (bacitracin, Neosporin, sulfacetamide, tetracycline) are rubbed into the lid margins three or four times a day. Local corticosteroids have been used in combination with antibiotic agents to reduce the hypersensitivity reaction that may accompany the infection. Skin staphylococci should be controlled by the daily use of a hexachlorophene-containing soap, and seborrhea of the scalp should be treated with appropriate shampoos. Resistant cases may require the administration of oral antibiotics or staphylococcal toxoid. In angular blepharitis, zinc sulfate is effective in a 0.25 to 0.50 percent solution, as well as the broad-spectrum antibiotics.

Parasitic infestation of the lids by the crab louse (*Pediculus pubis*) or head louse (*Pediculus capitis*) causes inflammation and itching of the lid margins. The lice, along with their ova (nits), may be seen attached to the lashes or brows. Treatment consists of removing the parasites and their ova from the lashes with forceps, followed by the application of 3 percent ammoniated mercury ointment or eserine ointment four times a day for 1 week. Other areas of infestation such as the scalp must be treated simultaneously with a delousing preparation. Clipping the hair and lashes may hasten recovery.

HORDEOLUM. *External hordeolum* is the common sty, a pyogenic infection (usually staphylococcal) of the ciliary follicle and its associated sebaceous glands along the lid margin. Susceptible individuals may have recurrences. The lesion begins as a circumscribed swelling at the lid margin, progresses to suppuration, and finally ruptures with resolution of pain and tenderness. Treatment consists of warm moist compresses applied for 20 minutes several times a day and the application locally of an antistaphylococcal ointment. The sty should not be squeezed. Occasionally it may be necessary to incise the sty to allow drainage of the pus. For recurrent sty, treatment with staphylococcal toxoid or vaccine or an autogenous vaccine has been recommended.

Internal hordeolum is an acute pyogenic infection of a meibomian gland. The area of localized redness, swelling, and suppuration presents on the conjunctival surface of the lid corresponding to the location of the gland. Spontaneous rupture is less frequent than with the external sty, but the treatment is the same.

CHALAZION. A chalazion is a chronic lipogranuloma caused by retention of secretions of a meibomian gland. Clinically there is a slow-growing firm round mass in the tarsus unaccompanied by pain or tenderness, unless there is a secondary purulent infection. It may resorb spontaneously, but it frequently requires incision by an ophthalmologist and evacuation through the conjunctival surface of the lid.

References

Allen JH: Blepharitis marginalis. In Bellows JC (ed): Contemporary Ophthalmology. Baltimore, Williams & Wilkins, 1972

Apt L: The eye. In Gellis SS, Kagan BM (eds): Current Pediatric Therapy, Vol 6. Philadelphia, WB Saunders, 1973

Thygeson P: Complications of staphylococcic blepharitis. Am J Ophthalmol 68:446, 1969

THE CONJUNCTIVA

Congenital Anomalies

With the exception of pigmentation, anomalies are rare. Congenital *melanosis oculi* is an inherited unilateral disorder characterized by hyperpigmentation of the conjunctiva and sclera. There also may be increased pigmentation in the uveal tract and periorbital skin (nevus of Ota). Malanosis oculi is not accompanied by any functional disorder of the eye, but malignant melanomas may arise in later life.

Structural anomalies ranging from abnormal folds and bands to complete absence of the conjunctiva occur infrequently. Dermolipoma, angioma, and lymphangioma are uncommon.

Inflammatory Diseases of the Conjunctiva

OPHTHALMIA NEONATORUM. Acute conjunctivitis in the newborn may be due to a chemical irritant, such as 1 percent silver nitrate instilled as the Credé prophylaxis against gonococcus, or to a bacterial or infectious agent acquired during delivery. Knowing the time of onset of the conjunctivitis is helpful in the diagnosis: silver nitrate conjunctivitis occurs in the first 12 to 24 hours after birth and disappears spontaneously in 3 to 4 days; bacterial conjunctivitis occurs within 2 to 5 days after birth and viral conjunctivitis within 5 to 10 days. Appropriate bacteriologic and microscopic studies are essential in identifying the specific etiologic agent.

SILVER NITRATE CONJUNCTIVITIS. Silver nitrate conjunctivitis is the most common cause of ophthalmia neonatorum today. It is a sterile inflammation characterized by moderate hyperemia of the conjunctiva, minimal discharge, and edema of the lids. Because of its irritating nature, silver nitrate is being replaced in some hospitals by antibiotics (tetracycline, chloramphenicol, erythromycin) with equally good results. Silver nitrate irritation requires no specific treatment except on occasion local antibiotics to treat secondary infection. Permanent residual damage to the eye is rare.

BACTERIAL CONJUNCTIVITIS. Bacterial conjunctivitis due to *Neisseria gonorrhoeae* is a hyperacute purulent conjunctivitis requiring prompt diagnosis and treatment. Typically there is bilateral involvement, with marked edema of the lids, chemosis, deep red conjunctivae, and copious discharge of pus. Conjunctival scrapings show intraepithelial gram-negative diplococci. In the absence of proper and immediate therapy, corneal involvement, with ulceration, perforation, panophthalmitis, and even septicemia, may occur. With adequate treatment most cases clear up completely in 1 to 4 days. Since the advent of the routine instillation of silver nitrate or antibiotics in the eyes of infants immediately after birth, blindness from gonococcal conjunctivitis has become a rarity, occurring in less than 0.03 percent of infants born in the United States. Treatment of gonorrheal conjunctivitis in the newborn should begin immediately and should consist of (1) topical chloramphenicol, tetracycline, or erythromycin every 1 to 2 hours, (2) systemic antibiotics for 5 days as penicillin G 30,000 units or ampicillin 50 mg/kg body weight or erythromycin ethyl succinate 5 mg/kg body weight injected intramuscularly every 12 hours, (3) frequent irrigation of the conjunctival sac with isotonic sodium chloride solution, and (4) cycloplegics in cases with corneal involvement.

In addition to gonococcus, any common bacterial pathogen may produce a neonatal conjunctivitis that has less propensity for corneal involvement. *Staphylococcus*, pneumococcus, *Streptococcus*, *Pseudomonas*, and coliform bacteria have all been implicated. The same topical antibiotic preparations used for gonorrheal conjunctivitis may be used with excellent results. *Pseudomonas* infections, especially in premature infants, are particularly serious. A *Pseudomonas* infection of the conjunctiva or cornea may rapidly progress to an orbital cellulitis, panophthalmitis, and even death from septicemia. Treatment should consist of frequent instillations of gentamicin, colistin, or polymyxin B. Systemic carbenicillin or gentamicin therapy may be needed.

VIRAL CONJUNCTIVITIS. *Inclusion blennorrhea* (inclusion conjunctivitis) is the most common neonatal viral conjunctivitis. The causative organism is a large atypical virus (*Chlamydia oculogenitalis*) belonging to the psittacosis/lymphogranuloma venereum/trachoma group of viruses. It is resistant to silver nitrate prophylaxis. Clinically there is acute swelling and redness of the lids, with a profuse mucopurulent exudate in one or both eyes. The conjunctiva of the lower tarsus and fornix is most markedly involved. Giemsa-stained scrapings from the conjunctiva of the lower lid usually show numerous basophilic granular intracytoplasmic inclusions in epithelial cells. Inclusion blennorrhea in the newborn responds well to topical tetracycline or sulfacetamide preparations, although the response is not as rapid as in gonococcal conjunctivitis.

Herpes simplex acquired from the mother's infected genital tract (type 2, genital herpes) may on occasion produce conjunctivitis, keratitis, cataracts, and chorioretinitis with or without disseminated systemic disease. It may occur between the second and sixteenth days of life (p. 536).

ACUTE CATARRHAL CONJUNCTIVITIS. Also known as acute mucopurulent conjunctivitis or epidemic pink-eye, acute catarrhal conjunctivitis is a highly contagious infection caused by pathogenic *Staphylococcus*, pneumococcus, *Haemophilus influenzae*, Koch-Weeks bacillus (*Haemophilus aegyptius*, *Haemophilus conjunctivitidis*), and *Streptococcus*. The bulbar conjunctiva is intensely injected, while the tarsal conjunctiva usually shows a mild papillary reaction giving it a velvety appearance. Marginal keratitis may be present (marginal catarrhal ulcers), particularly in staphylococcal infections. Petechial hemorrhages of the conjunctiva are most common with pneumococcal and Koch-Weeks bacillus infections. The infection heals spontaneously in several weeks if left untreated, although a chronic catarrhal conjunctivitis may persist. Treatment should consist of frequent instillation of antibacterial drugs such as bacitracin, neomycin, erythromycin, or sulfacetamide. Cultures and antibiotic sensitivities should be obtained and the appropriate antibiotic used if clinical respose is poor. Precautions should be taken to avoid spread to other sites or to other people, but the eyes should not be patched. Corticosteroids should be avoided.

CHRONIC CATARRHAL CONJUNCTIVITIS. Chronic conjunctivitis may follow an acute attack of any of the aforementioned agents, but it is usually due to *Staphylococcus* or Morax-Axenfeld diplobacillus. Typically the patient reports burning, foreign-body sensation, and eye strain, all of which are more bothersome at night or in the morning. The palpebral conjunctiva is primarily affected with mild papillary injection, and discharge is slight and mucoid. Associated conditions are blepharitis, keratitis (superficial punctate keratitis, marginal infiltrates, ulcers), recurrent sties, and loss of cilia. A number of factors contribute to the chronic nature of the inflammation, including poor hygiene, irritants, allergic factors, and seborrhea. Treatment is essentially the same as for acute catarrhal conjunctivitis, except that attention must be turned to eliminating any of these contributing factors. Any associated blepharitis must be treated by the methods outlined previously; the eye must be carefully checked for a foreign body, and any inflammation in the lacrimal sac must be treated.

ACUTE FOLLICULAR CONJUNCTIVITIS. Follicular conjunctivitis is characterized by the production of follicles that are foci of hyperplastic lymphoid tissue located in the subconjunctival tissue of the lids and fornices. Follicles do not appear in the conjunctiva before the third month of life, but subsequently they are prevalent even in noninfected children. They appear as grayish round elevations with avascular centers. The causes of acute follicular conjunctivitis include (1) inclusion conjunctivitis, (2) trachoma, (3) adenovirus conjunctivitis (epidemic keratoconjunctivitis and pharyngoconjunctival fever), (4) primary herpes simplex keratoconjunctivitis, and (5) Newcastle disease conjunctivitis.

Inclusion blennorrhea in the newborn was discussed previously under ophthalmia neonatorum (p. 1947). The infection in children and adults seems to arise as a result of autoinoculation of the eyes by the patient from his own infected genitourinary tract. Eye-to-eye transmission is rare. The infection is no longer acquired by swimming in contaminated pools, probably because of widespread use of chlorination. The conjunctivitis is similar to that occuring in newborn infants, except that follicles are a prominent feature. Differentiating points from adenovirus infection are (1) a profuse mucopurulent discharge that usually sticks the lids shut during the night (unlike adenovirus conjunctivitis, in which the scanty exudate almost never does) and (2) conjunctival scrapings that show a large number of polynucleated neutrophils (unlike adenovirus conjunctivitis, in which exudate is dominated by mononuclear cells). Preauricular adenopathy and corneal involvement (epithelial keratitis and marginal and subepithelial infiltrates) may occur. The acute inflammatory stage usually lasts for several weeks, and without treatment it may progress to a chronic keratoconjunctivitis lasting a year or more. Associated clinical problems include nongonococcal urethritis in males, chronic vaginitis in prepubertal females, and Reiter's syndrome. Unlike the neonatal infection, inclusion blennorrhea in the older child and adult responds poorly to topical tetracycline or sulfacetamide, but excellent results are obtained with full systemic doses of tetracycline given for 3 to 6 weeks.

Trachoma is the greatest cause of impaired vision and blindness in the world. It occurs sporadically in all parts of this country, but in certain localities it is endemic, notably in the reservations of the American Indians and in the Mexican-American population of California, particularly in families from or still living in rural areas. In endemically infected populations, trachoma usually starts in childhood and is associated with annual epidemics of bacterial conjunctivitis. The virus belongs to the psittacosis/lymphogranuloma venereum group of agents known as *Chlamydia*. In the early acute stage trachoma is a follicular conjunctivitis with follicles on the upper tarsal conjunctiva and upper limbus. A superficial keratitis of the upper half of the cornea with associated pannus occurs. Secondary bacterial infection is common. Intracytoplasmic inclusion bodies can be found in epithelial scrapings; they are indistinguishable from the ones found in inclusion blennorrhea, but are fewer in number. The virus may be isolated in the laboratory in the yolk sac of embryonated eggs. The acute stage is followed by a period of low-grade inflammation lasting for years. During this time scarring of the cornea, conjunctiva, and lid can develop. Eventually evidence of inflammation subsides, and cicatricial complications including entropion, trichiasis, dacryostenosis, and keratitis sicca lead to further corneal scarring, ulceration, and visual loss. The conjunctivitis in trachoma can be treated effectively with a combination of local and systemic sulfonamides or tetracycline. Corticosteroids reactivate the virus and are contraindicated.

Epidemic keratoconjunctivitis is an acute contagious disease of the conjunctiva and cornea caused most often by adenovirus type 8. Epidemics may occur by spread from contaminated fingers, tonometers, and eye solutions. There is rapid onset of a severe acute follicular conjunctivitis, with lacrimation, chemosis, and preauricular adenopathy. Both eyes are usually involved, since the infection is easily spread from one eye to the other. Systemic signs are absent except very rarely in infants. Discharge is usually minimal and either watery or mucopurulent. The exudate contains both mononuclear cells and polymorphonuclear cells, but no inclusions. In infants the infection may be pseudomembranous in type. Initially there is a diffuse epithelial keratitis. After approximately 10 days subepithelial infiltrates may develop in the central cornea. The round corneal opacities are nearly pathognomonic. They usually resolve slowly over a period of months without scarring, but occasionally they persist up to 2 years. Treatment consists of local sulfonamide or broad-spectrum antibiotic drugs to prevent secondary bacterial infection. No drug is known to inhibit the virus specifically. Isolation precautions should be taken, because the disease is highly contagious up to 14 days after onset.

Pharyngoconjunctival fever is encountered more often in children than in adults and is characterized by a self-limited acute follicular conjunctivitis that lasts 10 to 14 days, as well as fever, malaise, pharyngitis, and preauricular and cervical lymphadenopathy. The disease is usually caused by adenovirus type 3. In most instances superficial punctate corneal opacities develop, but they disappear without sequelae as the conjunctivitis subsides. The highly contagious disease is spread by direct contact or indirectly through contaminated swimming pools (even though chlorinated) and causes epidemics in the later summer months. Children may spread the infection to adults. The only therapy is isolation precautions and topical antibacterial eye medication to prevent secondary bacterial infection.

In *herpetic keratoconjunctivitis* the primary attack of herpes simplex may have an associated follicular conjunctivitis involving one or both eyes, along with the mouth, nose, lids, and skin. Vesicular eruptions in the skin or mucous membranes precede the acute follicular conjunctivitis. Corneal involvement consists of a dendritic epithelial ulceration associated with decreased corneal sensitivity. Conjunctival scrapings show primarily mononuclear cells and giant multinucleated epithelial cells characteristic of herpes simplex. Treatment consists of frequent instillation of 0.1 percent solution of idoxuridine, cycloplegics, and broad-spectrum antibiotics to prevent secondary bacterial infection. Corticosteroids are contraindicated.

Newcastle disease conjunctivitis is contracted by children who play with infected fowl. The virus causes an acute follicular conjunctivitis resembling pharyngoconjunctival fever but with no keratitis.

CHRONIC FOLLICULAR CONJUNCTIVITIS. Chronic follicular conjunctivitis in children can be subdivided into the Axenfeld type, the epidemic type, and the toxic or reactive type. The reactive type occurs as a result of a toxic stimulus rather than from a primary disease of the conjunctiva. Except for Parinaud's oculoglandular conjunctivitis, the chronic follicular conjunctivitides do not have preauricular lymphadenopathy.

Axenfeld's follicular conjunctivitis is found solely in children; it occurs epidemically and, on occasion, sporadically in orphanages. The findings include large follicles with minimal hyperemia and exudate. Corneal involvement does not occur. Healing is spontaneous in 18 months to 2 years. The etiologic agent is unknown, but conjunctival scrapings show a predominance of mononuclear cells, thus suggesting a viral etiology.

Epidemic chronic follicular conjunctivitis has been reported in small epidemics in California and Arizona. The characteristics are (1) follicles most numerous in the fornices, (2) epithelial keratitis superiorly, occasionally with a micropannus, (3) minimal discharge without characteristic cytology, and (4) spontaneous healing in a few months without scarring.

Reactive follicular conjunctivitis due to drugs is limited to the miotics (eserine, pilocarpine, diisopropyl fluorophosphate) and to idoxuridine. The conjunctivitis is considered toxic or irritative rather than allergic, since follicular hypertrophy does not occur in allergic conditions. Trachomalike scarring of the cornea and micropannus may occur in cases that are neglected. If the drug is discontinued, follicular hypertrophy and conjunctival inflammation rapidly disappear.

Molluscum contagiosum keratoconjunctivitis is considered a toxic or reactive type of chronic follicular conjunctivitis because the viral infection is limited to the skin. Umbilicated molluscum papillae or nodules located on the eyelid margins discharge toxic desquamated material into the conjunctival sac, producing a reactive follicular conjunctivitis. An associated epithelial keratitis is frequent. Treatment involves removing the lesion from the lid margin by surgery or by cauterization.

Parinaud's oculoglandular conjunctivitis is a unilateral follicular conjunctivitis caused by one or more granulomas involving the palpebral conjunctiva and associated with marked preauricular and cervical lymphadenopathy, malaise, and fever. Causative agents include any of the granulomatous diseases such as syphilis, sarcoidosis, tuberculosis, and tularemia. A gram positive bacillus *Leptotrichia buccalis,* is also a common cause; it produces severe follicular hypertrophy that may mask the underlying granuloma. Still other causes include cat-scratch disease and lymphogranuloma venereum.

Recovery usually occurs spontaneously after several months. Specific chemotherapy and antibiotics should be given.

Folliculosis is quite common in children. In general, the conjunctiva of a child is much more reactive than that of an adult. Folliculosis may represent part of a generalized lymphoid hyperplasia or may occur secondary to a localized condition such as chronic dacryocystitis. Folliculosis is usually unaccompanied by discharge or erythema and is asymptomatic. It disappears with growth of the child or when a primary cause, if any, is removed.

EXANTHEMATOUS CONJUNCTIVITIS. Many of the childhood exanthems such as measles, chickenpox, and smallpox may be accompanied by an acute catarrhal conjunctivitis. No specific treatment is necessary unless secondary bacterial infection or corneal involvement occurs.

Keratoconjunctivitis is a characteristic and constant finding during the acute stage of measles. Ocular involvement may precede the skin eruption. A pecular swelling of the plica semilunaris (Meyer's sign) and Koplik's spots on the caruncle and semilunar fold may occur during the period of incubation. In debilitated children, secondary bacterial infection of the cornea with ulceration and perforation is common. Small papular lesions may occur on the lid margins and the conjunctiva of children with chickenpox. Superficial or deep keratitis may complicate the infection, but it usually resolves spontaneously. Idoxuridine (IDU) therapy may have some value in corneal epithelial involvement. In the preeruptive stage of smallpox, a catarrhal conjunctivitis often appears about the fifth day and clears up readily. Pustules are rarely found in the eye.

Vaccinal conjunctivitis may occur from autoinoculation or inoculation from a contact. In a patient with little or no immunity, serious corneal damage can occur. Symblepharon, entropion, and trichiasis may result from lid margin involvement. Specific treatment is very effective if given early in the infection. Local treatment consists of idoxuridine 0.1 percent every 1 to 2 hours around the clock and continued for a week or longer after the inflammation has subsided. Vaccine immune globulin (VIG) administered intramuscularly in doses of 0.3 cc produces prompt improvement of lesions in generalized vaccinia. This drug is indicated in patients with lid and conjunctival involvement, because rapid clearing of lid lesions may decrease the risk of corneal involvement. Topical or systemic VIG is probably contraindicated in established vaccinal keratitis, as the agent may aggravate the keratitis and produce more extensive stromal lesions.

MEMBRANOUS CONJUNCTIVITIS. Membranous and pseudomembranous conjunctivitis may occur in diphtherial and streptococcal infection or in severe conjunctivitis from any cause. A membrane forms on the conjunctiva from exudate; it can be stripped off easily without bleeding (pseudomembrane), or it can be tightly adherent to the conjunctiva, leaving a raw, bleeding surface when removed from the underlying epithelium (membrane). True membranous conjunctivitis may result in severe damage to the conjunctiva

and cornea, but fortunately this inflammation is rare today.

MUCOCUTANEOUS OCULAR DISEASES. The mucocutaneous ocular diseases such as erythema multiforme, Stevens-Johnson syndrome, and Reiter's syndrome produce a mild to severe keratoconjunctivitis that is followed in some cases by marked loss of visual function. In Stevens-Johnson syndrome a lack of tears, symblepharon, corneal ulcer, and corneal perforation may occur, while in Reiter's disease scleritis, interstitial keratitis, and hypopyon uveitis may complicate the course. Because of the seriousness of the ocular complications, it is advisable to have an ophthalmologist treat the ocular aspects of these diseases.

ALLERGIC FORMS OF CONJUNCTIVITIS. The conjunctiva, like other epithelial tissues, may develop a local hypersensitivity to a specific allergen. All of the changes encountered in simple allergic reactions may occur in the conjunctiva. In acute cases there is sudden vascular dilation with marked chemosis that disappears with removal of the irritant. In chronic cases cellular infiltration and newly formed connective tissue follow. Eosinophils usually are present in conjunctival scrapings, and basophils are also seen. Lymphoid hypertrophy with follicle formation usually does not occur in immunologic or allergic conjunctivitis. Allergic conjunctivitis can be divided into four basic types: atopic, drug sensitivity, vernal, and phlyctenular.

Simple allergic or atopic conjunctivitis is an immediate type of hypersensitivity in a patient with a history of atopy. It is caused primarily by pollens (hay fever), animal hair, fungi, dusts, and ingestion of some foods. A hyperemic reaction of the tarsal and bulbar conjunctiva is produced, accompanied by edema of the conjunctiva and lids and profuse lacrimation with itching. Itching is usually far more conspicuous than in infectious conjunctivitis. There may be a scant, stringy discharge containing a variable number of eosinophils.

Treatment consists of removing the offending allergen if possible, desensitization to the allergen, and symptomatic relief with the use of local vasoconstrictors, astringents, antihistamines, and corticosteroids. Corticosteroids should be used only when other agents fail to control the allergic reaction. They should be used in the minimum amount needed to control the reaction and for the shortest time possible. Cataracts and glaucoma have been seen in children and adults who have used topical corticosteroids indiscriminately for the treatment of allergy.

Local drug sensitivity may produce a similar reaction in the conjunctiva. Sensitivity to drugs occurs usually after repeated instillations and is most common with atropine and neomycin. Once developed, this sensitivity lasts indefinitely and is often associated with cutaneous sensitivity to the drug (positive patch test). Treatment consists of removal of the offending agent and local use of corticosteroids for symptomatic relief.

Vernal conjunctivitis or spring catarrh is a bilateral chronic recurrent inflammation characterized by large pale flat-topped papillae in the upper palpebral conjunctiva giving the typical cobblestone appearance. The papilla may abrade the cornea, causing ulceration and opacification. Papillary hypertrophy is less often observed in the limbal region as gray elevated lesions. It occurs during spring and summer and is primarily a disease of childhood, occurring most frequently in boys from 5 to 15 years of age. A familial history of allergy is usual, but identification of specific allergens has been unsuccessful. Symptomatic treatment consists of topical vasoconstrictors, topical and oral antihistamines, and soluble topical corticosteroid drops. Cold packs and ice-cold saline lavage are very soothing. In severe cases systemic corticosteroids are required. Disodium cromoglycate shows some promise as a second-line drug to corticosteroids. Beta radiation, cryoablation, or surgical removal of giant papillae may be needed in severe cases, but recurrence of the papillae is usual. Desensitization to allergens has not been helpful. In some cases change to a cool climate can lead to improvement.

Phlyctenular conjunctivitis is characterized by one or more small, hard, red elevated nodules surrounded by hyperemic vessels and appearing most commonly at the limbus and on the bulbar conjunctiva. Microscopically the phlyctena is a subepithelial collection of lymphocytes. The apex of the phlyctena ulcerates and subsequently heals, but on occasion the disease can spread onto the adjacent cornea, with opacification and pannus formation. With involvement of the cornea there is severe photophobia, profuse lacrimation, and blepharospasm. The child may hide his eyes from all light, and it may be difficult to pry the lids open to examine the cornea. The disease is thought to be a hypersensitivity reaction to foreign proteins, such as those from the tubercle bacillus and *Staphylococcus.* Contributing factors are malnutrition, poor hygiene, and debilitation from systemic disease. Interestingly, it is more common in girls. Treatment should be directed at improving diet and personal hygiene. A topical steroid or a steroid-antibiotic combination is effective in treating the disease and any secondary infection that may be present. Cycloplegics are indicated to relieve photophobia when corneal disease is present. Careful search should be made for a systemic disease such as tuberculosis.

SUBCONJUNCTIVAL HEMORRHAGE. Subconjunctival bleeding from a capillary of the bulbar conjunctiva is common. Multiple causes are known, including mild trauma, violent coughing, sneezing, or vomiting, acute conjunctivitis (particularly pneumococcal), acute septicemia, malaria, blood dyscrasias, scurvy, and purpuric diseases; or it may be spontaneous (idiopathic). The appearance is quite alarming to most parents; thus reassurance is necessary. The blood is usually completely absorbed in 1 to 2 weeks.

General Remarks about Therapy

In young children medication in ointment form may be easier to instill with less chance of overdosage. In the older child it is desirable to use drops during the day, which do not interfere with vision, and ointment at bedtime. Local eye anesthetics should never be prescribed for home use, as they delay corneal healing, and injury to the anesthetized eye may occur inadvertently.

Antibiotics are used routinely in the treatment of conjunctivitis, but it is good practice to determine the causative agent and its sensitivity to specific antibiotics. The tendency to administer antibiotics indiscriminately to all external inflammations may result in the development of host sensitization and resistance to the organism. A word of caution is necessary about the use of corticosteroids in conjunctivitis: Although they are highly effective in the allergic types, they are generally contraindicated in bacterial and viral inflammations. They may cause exacerbations of the disease, particularly in herpes simplex infections. Combinations of antibiotics and steroids do not altogether remove this danger.

References

Apt L: The eye. In Gellis SS, Kagan BM (eds): Current Pediatric Therapy, Vol 6. Philadephia, WB Saunders, 1973

Burns RP, Rhodes DH Jr: Pseudomonas eye infections as a cause of death in premature infants. Arch Ophthalmol 65:517, 1961

Ellis PP, Winograd LA: Ocular vaccinia. Arch Ophthalmol 68:56, 1962

Fedukowicz HB: External Infections of the Eye. New York, Appleton, 1963

Hales RH: Glaucoma induced by careless use of steroids. J Pediatr Ophthalmol 10:206, 1973

Harbin T, Curren RE: Gonococcal conjunctivitis. Ann Ophthalmol 6:221, 1974

Locatcher-Khorazo D, Seegel BC: Microbiology of the Eye. St Louis, Mosby, 1972

Schusterman M: Inflammations of the conjunctiva. In The Eye of Childhood. Staff, Toronto Hospital for Sick Children: Chicago, Year Book, 1967

Thygeson P: Follicular conjunctivitis. In Bellows JC (ed): Contemporary Ophthalmology. Baltimore, Williams & Wilkins 1972

———— Dawson CR: Trachoma and follicular conjunctivitis in children. Arch Ophthalmol 75:3, 1966

———— Trachoma Manual and Atlas. Public Health Service Publ. 541, Rev 1960

THE CORNEA
Congenital Anomalies

The most common congenital anomalies of the cornea are those associated with defects in transparency. The causes of congenital corneal opacification are listed in Table 2.

Size variation includes the cornea being abnormally small (less than 10 mm at birth or 11 mm at 1 year of age). This condition is termed *microcornea* and can occur in an otherwise normal eye, but it is usually associated with a number of other ocular abnormalities such as microphthalmia, hyperopia, anterior segment dysgenesis, coloboma, and cataract. A frequent complication is glaucoma, and in cases with elevated pressure the cornea may be hazy, due to edema, and the globe may be enlarged (*buphthalmos*). An abnormally large cornea (*megalocornea*) has a diameter at birth greater than 12 mm. True megalocornea is inherited as a sex-linked recessive (rarely autosomal dominant) and is unaccompanied by anterior chamber angle anomalies or by glaucoma. Enlargement of the cornea as part of buphthalmosin congenital glaucoma should be easily differentiated. Megalocornea is also associated with oculocerebrorenal syndrome (Lowe's syndrome), osteogenesis imperfecta, and Marfan's syndrome.

TABLE 2. Differential Diagnosis of Congenital Corneal Opacities

1. Congenital iridocorneal adhesions
2. Corneal leukoma
3. Congenital hereditary corneal dystrophies
4. Cornea plana
5. Mucopolysaccharidoses (I, IV, V, VI)
6. Cystinosis
7. Intrauterine infection (rubella, syphilis, others)
8. Congenital glaucoma
9. Melanosis corneae
10. Anterior embryotoxon (arcus juvenilis)
11. Posterior embryotoxon (Axenfeld's anomaly)
12. Riegers' syndrome (mesodermal dysgenesis)
13. Trisomy 18 syndrome
14. XO syndrome (Turner-Albright)
15. Fabry-Anderson syndrome
16. Pachyonychia congenita (Jadassohn-Lewandowski syndrome)
17. Lowe's syndrome (oculocerebrorenal syndrome)
18. Birth trauma
19. Chemical (silver nitrate) burns
20. Vitamin A deficiency

Congenital dermoids of the cornea occur rarely and may involve a portion of the cornea or in severe cases the entire cornea. The limbal type is most common. These tumors are composed of fatty and fibrous tissue covered by epidermal rather than conjunctival epithelium, and they may contain hair and sweat glands and subaceous glands. They may occur as isolated anomalies or with cri-du-chat syndrome and oculoauriculovertebral dysplasia (Goldenhar's syndrome).

Therapy of Corneal Disease

Diseases of the cornea usually require prompt examination and treatment by an ophthalmologist. Even minor corneal injury or infection can lead to serious ocular complications, including blindness. The pediatrician must learn to recognize the signs and symptoms of corneal disease so that prompt referral may be made. Patients with corneal disease usually have photophobia, tearing, blepharospasm, decreased vision, pain, circumlimbal hyperemia (ciliary injection), corneal opacity, and often a history of trauma. Treatment of corneal disease will not be thoroughly detailed here, as this should be performed by an ophthalmologist.

Corneal Inflammations: Keratitis

SUPERFICIAL PUNCTATE KERATITIS. Inflammation of the epithelium of the cornea is a frequent accompaniment of many types of conjunctivitis, particularly the staphylococcal type. It may, however, be secondary to drugs, exposure, or trichiasis. Fine punctate infiltrates are seen in the central superficial portion of the cornea with slit-lamp magnification. Superficial erosions may occur. Treatment is directed at the underlying cause.

HERPES SIMPLEX KERATITIS. Dendritic keratitis due to the herpes simplex virus is probably the most important corneal disease leading to loss of vision in the United States. Its incidence and severity have increased with the widespread use of local and systemic corticosteroids. The disease begins with a dendritic superficial epithelial ulcer (best outlined with fluorescein) and associated decreased corneal sensitivity. These may accompany a primary herpetic infection of the skin or mucous membranes, in which case an accompanying follicular conjunctivitis is frequent; or the disease may occur during febrile attacks of any origin or under conditions that lower general resistance. It usually begins in the center of the cornea as a small row of vesicles that break down and leave a linear defect. The infected epithelium is destroyed, forming an irregular branching ulcer. This may clear over the course of 3 weeks, leaving no trace (but frequently recurring); or particularly when topical corticosteroids have been used it may affect the deeper layers of the cornea and produce an interstitial disciform opacity. There may be an associated anterior uveitis. Subjectively there is pain, lacrimation, photophobia, and decreased vision. Multinucleated giant cells may be seen in epithelial scrapings. Typical herpes simplex keratitis may appear in the newborn at birth or shortly thereafter. Presumably it is acquired transplacentally or by the ascending route across the fetal membranes.

Treatment of superficial keratitis consists of debridement of the involved epithelium and frequent instillation of the antimetabolite idoxuridine (IDU). IDU inhibits viral synthesis by becoming incorporated into viral DNA, instead of thymidine. Other promising agents that are not yet commercially available include trifluorothymidine, adenosine arabinoside (ARA), and interferon. With stromal involvement IDU is much less effective. Corticosteroids are contraindicated in the epithelial form of the disease, since they accelerate the spread of the viral infection, but they may be used in conjunction with IDU in the stromal form to reduce the toxic or hypersensitive response to the virus or virus products. Cycloplegics, antibiotics, conjunctival flaps, or penetrating keratoplasty may be required.

HERPES ZOSTER KERATITIS. Herpes zoster may infect the ophthalmic division of the fifth cranial nerve; zoster keratitis occurs in about 40 percent of patients so affected. Keratitis and conjunctivitis usually occur during the acute phase of the skin eruption. Corneal involvement may begin as a coarse superficial punctate keratitis, progress to combined epithelial and subepithelial lesions, and finally develop a large nummular stromal opacity. Corneal sensation is reduced or absent. Iritis always accompanies the keratitis, but it can occur alone. Iritis can be severe, with hypopyon, glaucoma, and hyphema. The incidence of herpes zoster is highest in patients over 40 or under 14 years of age. Its presence in children should raise suspicion of an underlying lymphoma or leukemia.

Cautious use of topical corticosteroids in conjunction with cycloplegics relieves the keratitis and iritis in herpes zoster. Systemic steroids are probably contraindicated because of deaths reported of children who developed varicella while receiving steroid therapy.

BACTERIAL CORNEAL ULCERS. Corneal ulcers may be identified by placing a drop of sterile fluorescein solution or moistened ophthalmic strip (Fluor-I-Strip) in the conjunctival sac and observing the intense green staining of the ulcer. To determine the etiology of a corneal ulcer, scrapings (gram and Giemsa stains), cultures, and sensitivity tests should be performed.

Marginal ulcers are usually sterile and secondary to a hypersensitivity or toxic reaction of the cornea to bacterial infection (usually *Staphylococcus* Koch-Weeks) of the conjunctiva or eyelid. Treatment is directed at the underlying conjunctivitis, while topical corticosteroids are used to heal the ulcer.

Central corneal ulcers are a serious ocular emergency and require intensive treatment. They frequently develop after trauma or during topical corticosteroid therapy. There is an intense purulent reaction in and around the ulcer, giving it a white appearance. It may spread quickly into deeper corneal layers, and without treatment it may cause perforation. A sterile hypopyon is frequently associated. There is some variation in incidence of types of bacterial corneal ulcers according to geographic location and climate, but the most commonly cultured pathogens are *Diplococcus pneumoniae, Pseudomonas aeruginosa, Moraxella liquefaciens,* and *Staphylococcus aureus. Pseudomonas* is the most virulent organism; it produces a rapid and fulminating destruction of the cornea. Antimicrobial treatment should be instituted immediately after smears and cultures of the ulcer are done. Occasionally general anesthesia is required in young children for proper examination of the eye and adequate performance of debridement, scrapings, and cultures. Broad-spectrum local antibiotics should be used until the studies reveal the antimicrobial drug of choice. Cycloplegics, analgesics, and sedation are frequently helpful.

FUNGAL KERATITIS. As a result of more widespread use of local corticosteroids and antibiotics, the incidence of keratomycosis has increased in recent years. Fungi infect the cornea following damage to the epithelium from trauma or inflammation. Numerous species of fungi, many saprophytic, have been isolated. The organism may be undetected in scrapings and culture. The diagnosis should be considered in any persistent, slowly progressive corneal ulceration. Medical treatment consists of local antifungal agents such as copper sulfate, nystatin, amphotericin, and pimaricin.

INTERSTITIAL KERATITIS. Most cases of interstitial keratitis appear between the ages of 5 and 15 years, although it may occur as early as 1 year. It is most often due to congenital syphilis; saddle nose, deafness, and Hutchinson's teeth may be seen. The bilateral keratitis begins as a delicate zone of opacities in the middle layers of the stroma. There is pericorneal injection and edema of the epithelium followed by vascularization of the posterior two-thirds of the corneal stroma. The cornea assumes a ground-glass appearance with orange-red areas (salmon patches) due to the vascularization. The subjective symptoms are decreased vision, intense photophobia, lacrimation, and pain. An associated uveitis is common. The reaction begins to regress after several months, with residual deep scarring and ghost vessels in the stroma. *Treponema pallidum* is not found in the cornea during the acute stage, although it may be recovered subsequently from the anterior chamber. Both the narrow angle form and the chronic open angle form of glaucoma may occur in later years. Antisyphilitic medication has little effect on the course of the disease. Local steroids and cycloplegics provide symptomatic relief. In cases with severe corneal scarring, penetrating keratoplasty may be performed after the inflammation has been quiescent for a period of years. Other causes of interstitial keratitis include acquired syphilis, tuberculosis, leprosy, parasites (onchocerciasis, malaria), mumps, influenza, lymphogranuloma venereum, herpes simplex, herpes zoster, and phlyctenular disease.

Xerophthalmia (Xerosis)

Dryness of the conjunctiva and cornea may result from the following diseases: (1) keratitis sicca secondary to decreased lacrimal gland secretion, (2) exposure keratitis following seventh nerve palsies and exophthalmos, (3) neuroparalytic keratitis resulting from loss of fifth nerve innervation, (4) familial dysautonomia (Riley-Day syndrome), in which there is congenital absence or deficiency of tears, (5) Stevens-Johnson syndrome and benign mucous membrane pemphigoid, which destroy conjunctival mucous glands, and (6) avitaminosis A. Treatment of corneal drying and exposure consists of frequent instillations of artificial tears (methyl cellulose, polyvinyl alcohol, normal saline) and bland ointment, soft contact lenses, moisture-retaining goggles, and tarsorrhaphy.

Systemic malnutrition with avitaminosis A produces a lackluster appearance of the conjunctiva and cornea and Bitot's spots. The latter are small, white or creamy, foamy patches lying on the conjunctiva near the limbus in the palpebral aperture. In severe cases progressive corneal keratinization causes complete loss of vision, and keratomalacia with necrosis and infection may result in loss of the eye. Treatment consists of a nutritious diet and large doses of Vitamin A.

Metabolic Disorders of the Cornea

Corneal clouding occurs as a local manifestation of systemic *mucopolysaccharidosis* (p. 751). Hurler's syndrome or gargoylism is the best known of these disorders. On clinical, biochemical, and genetic grounds these have been grouped into six entities. Four of the six have corneal clouding: Hurler's syndrome (I), Morquio's syndrome (IV), Scheie's syndrome (V), and Maroteaux-Lamy syndrome (VI). Hunter's syndrome (II) and Sanfilippo's syndrome (III) do not have macroscopic clouding. The clinical findings and the urinary mucopolysaccharide excretion pattern distinguish the foregoing corneal dystrophies from other causes of corneal clouding. Patients with these dystrophies are poor candidates for corneal transplantation.

Arcus juvenilis results from the deposition of lipids in the periphery of the cornea. The arcus tends to appear during the early teenage years and remains confined to the peripheral cornea; thus it does not affect vision. It is most frequent in type II familial and type III familial hyperlipoproteinemia.

In *cystinosis* crystals of cystine are deposited on the

superficial cornea and conjunctival epithelium. Visible by slit-lamp examination, the corneal signs may be the first evidence of cystine storage. Diagnosis may be made by biopsy of the conjunctiva.

Hepatolenticular degeneration (Wilson's disease) is a congenital inborn error of copper metabolism (p. 1921). An associated Kayser-Fleischer ring of the cornea is pathognomonic and may be the first sign of the disease. It contains copper and appears as a greenish golden annular opacity lying just inside the limbus in the deep layers of the cornea. Visible initially only with the slit-lamp, it later becomes denser and broader and can be detected with the naked eye.

Superficial deposition of calcium in the cornea, or *band keratopathy*, occurs less commonly in children than in adults. It may occur as part of a systemic disorder that produces hypercalcemia (hyperparathyroidism, vitamin D intoxication, sarcoidosis, and renal failure). Band keratopathy is a frequent complication of keratitis, uveitis, glaucoma, and alkali burns of the cornea. It may accompany juvenile rheumatoid arthritis, discoid lupus erythematosus, gout, tuberous sclerosis, and ichthyosis. Treatment consists of preliminary curettage of the epithelium, followed by the application of a chelating agent such as EDTA. Improvement in vision may be dramatic, and the procedure can be repeated as often as necessary.

Keratoconus

Keratoconus is a corneal ectasia that is more common in females; it usually begins at puberty, but occasionally starts in childhood. It is usually bilateral, but asymmetric. Its etiology is unknown, but it probably has a hereditary basis. The patient initially complains of a reduction in vision. At this early stage a keratometer or retinoscope is necessary to make the diagnosis. The condition may then progress slowly over many years or reach a point of arrest and become stationary. Acute relapses (hydrops) may occur. In more advanced stages the cone-shaped cornea is easily seen, along with indentation of the lower lid by the cornea (Munson's sign). Treatment involves the use of spectacles until the astigmatism becomes severe, at which time contact lenses can be worn. Eventually even contact lenses may not correct the vision, and a corneal transplant or thermokeratoplasty becomes necessary. However, this point is hardly ever reached in childhood or adolescence. Keratoconus occurs with some regularity with atopic dermatitis, Marfan's syndrome, Down's syndrome, Ehlers-Danlos syndrome, vernal catarrh, congenital cataract, blue sclera, aniridia, and retinitis pigmentosa.

References

Allen HF: Current status of prevention, diagnosis and management of bacterial corneal ulcers. Ann Ophthalmol 3:235, 1971

Aronson SB, Elliott JH: Ocular Inflammation. St Louis, Mosby, 1972

Cogan DG, Kuwabara T: Ocular pathology of cystinosis. Arch Ophthalmol 63:51, 1960

DeVoe A: Corneal disorders in children. In Symposium on the Cornea. New Orleans Academy of Ophthalmology. St Louis, Mosby, 1972

Friewald MJ: Prevention of complications of herpes zoster ophthalmicus with special reference to steroid therapy. Eye Ear Nose Throat Mon 46:444, 1967

Goldberg MF, Maumenee AE, McKusick VA: Corneal dystrophies associated with abnormalities of mucopolysaccharide metabolism. Arch Ophthalmol 74:516, 1965

———— von Noorden GK: Ophthalmologic findings in Wilson's hepatolenticular degeneration. Arch Ophthalmol 75:162, 1966

Grayson M, Keates RH: Manual of Diseases of the Cornea. Boston, Little, Brown, 1969

Hutchinson DS, Smith RE, Haughton PB: Congenital herpetic keratitis. Arch Ophthalmol 93:70, 1975

Laibson PR: Herpes simplex. Annual review. Cornea and sclera. Arch Ophthalmol 83:637, 1970

Venkataswamy G: Ocular manifestations of vitamin A deficiency. Br J Ophthalmol 51:854, 1967

Walsh FG, Murray RG: Ocular manifestations of disturbances in calcium metabolism. Am J Ophthalmol 36:1657, 1953

Zimmerman LE: Keratomycosis. Surv Ophthalmol 8:1, 1963

THE SCLERA

Blue Sclera

The normal sclera of young infants, being relatively thin by comparison with that of adults, is often mistaken for the true congenital anomaly of blue sclera. But most infants, by the end of the first year, show the normal porcelain white color of the sclera. The anomaly of blue sclera is secondary to persistent thinning and alteration in the structure of the sclera, which allows the pigmented choroid to show through and gives the sclera a blue appearance. Blue sclera occurs in disorders of connective tissue such as osteogenesis imperfecta, Ehlers-Danlos syndrome, craniofacial dysostosis (Crouzon's disease), Marfan's syndrome, Hallerman-Streiff syndrome, and pseudohypoparathyroidism.

Scleritis and Episcleritis

Inflammation of the sclera and episclera (the thin layer of vascular elastic tissue between the conjunctiva and sclera) is infrequent and has much the same etiology and therapy as uveitis. These disorders may be a manifestation of a systemic disease—most commonly one of the so-called collagen diseases, particularly adult rheumatoid arthritis. Juvenile rheumatoid arthritis is more often associated with uveitis than with scleritis. Scleritis is a constant finding in Felty's syndrome and may be so severe as to cause scleromalacia perforans. Still other causes include mumps, syphilis, tuberculosis, sarcoidosis, and gout.

Episcleritis is manifested as a localized purplish nodular area over which the conjunctiva moves easily. It is recurrent and benign. Scleritis is a deeper, more diffuse, and more severe inflammation that may cause thinning and perforation of the sclera. Both scleritis and episcleritis may produce severe ocular pain and are often associated with uveitis. Treatment should be directed at specific therapy of any systemic condition present. Topical corticosteroids and cycloplegics will make the eye more comfortable. Nonsteroid anti-inflammatory agents such as aspirin, oxyphenbutazone (Tandearil), and indomethacin (Indocin) have been used with some success. Treatment is suppressive until a natural remission occurs.

References

Lyne AF, Pilkeathley DA: Episcleritis and scleritis. Arch Ophthalmol 80: 171, 1968

McKusick VA: Heritable Disorders of Connective Tissue, 3rd ed. St Louis, Mosby, 1966

Maumenee AE: Ocular manifestations of collagen diseases. Arch Ophthalmol 56:557, 1956

Ostriker PJ, Ostriker M, Lasky MA: Keratitis and scleritis associated with Felty's syndrome. Arch Ophthalmol 58:858, 1955

Swan JW, Penn RF: Scleritis following mumps. Am J Ophthalmol 53:366, 1962

THE LACRIMAL APPARATUS

Dacryostenosis

Dacryostenosis, or congenital obstruction of the nasolacrimal duct, is manifested in the newborn by tearing (epiphora) and may be observed as early as the first week of life. Contrary to a widely held belief, most newborns do secrete tears in the first week of life. Obstruction of the nasolacrimal duct is usually unilateral and secondary to failure of spontaneous atrophy of the thin membrane that separates the lower ostium of the duct and the inferior nasal meatus. Other causes include clogging of the duct with epithelial debris, a stricture of the bony canal, or a redundancy of the nasal mucosa at the lower opening of the duct into the nose.

As a consequence of the obstruction, a mucocele may form in the lacrimal sac. Examination will show a fluctuant swelling in the region of the tear sac. Transillumination demonstrates distension of the sac with clear fluid, and pressure on the sac may cause regurgitation of straw-colored fluid from the puncta. If the obstruction resolves the mucocele subsides rapidly. Continued obstruction leads to stagnation and infection. Recurrent or chronic conjunctivitis and dacryocystitis may occur, accompanied by a purulent discharge through the puncta. Dacryocystitis is caused by the common gram-positive pyogenic bacteria. It produces a tender swelling in the region of the lacrimal sac and erythema and swelling of the overlying skin and lids. Treatment with hot compresses and local or systemic antibiotics usually overcomes the acute infection. Untreated or recurrent cases may go on to abscess formation, with rupture through the skin and establishment of a draining sinus. Cicatricial scarring of the lacrimal sac with obliteration of the lacrimal passages is a troublesome consequence of chronic infection.

Conservative treatment of dacryostenosis consists of massage of the lacrimal sac followed by instillation of a broad-spectrum antibiotic drop (not ointment) four to six times a day. The proper technique of massage is as follows: Firm pressure with the index finger is applied in a posterior medial direction on and behind the anterior lacrimal crest over the lacrimal sac. A reflux of pus or mucus may be observed through the puncta.

If the obstruction persists after an adequate trial of conservative treatment, then gentle probing under general anesthesia by an ophthalmologist should be performed. In order for probing to be successful, it should not be postponed beyond 6 months, and it should be done earlier if acute dacryocystitis develops. A single irrigation and probing of the nasolacrimal system is usually sufficient, although occasionally it must be repeated. If the nasolacrimal duct cannot be opened by probing, a dacryocystorhinostomy may be performed to restore lacrimal drainage into the nose.

Dacryoadenitis

Acute dacryoadenitis presents clinically with pain and fullness over the lacrimal gland, edema and redness of the temporal half of the upper lid and conjunctiva, possible mucoid or purulent discharge, and orbital cellulitis. There may even be diplopia and restricted movement of the globe if the orbital lobe of the gland is involved. With eversion of the lid, the gland can be seen to be enlarged and inflamed. Frequently an associated systemic infection is the cause, including mumps, infectious mononucleosis, syphilis, gonorrhea, influenza, or an exanthem. Local causes are staphylococci, trachoma, and herpes zoster. Treatment consists of appropriate systemic work-up, local cultures, and cytology, followed by antibiotics (if indicated), heat, and analgesia.

Chronic dacryoadenitis is frequently bilateral. The lacrimal gland is enlarged and indurated, producing a swelling in the upper temporal half of the upper lid. No discharge or inflammatory signs are present. Sarcoidosis is the most frequent etiology, but other causes include trachoma, tuberculosis, syphilis, and Mikulicz's syndrome. Treatment is directed at the underlying systemic disease.

Familial Dysautonomia

Congenital deficiency or absence of tearing and corneal hypesthesia or anesthesia are consistently present in familial dysautonomia or Riley-Day syndrome (p. 1939). Complications include corneal drying, with the formation of erosion, ulceration, and scarring. Mecholyl chloride (2.5 percent eye drops) will usually cause miosis in patients with familial dysautonomia, but not in normal eyes—a response consistent with parasympathetic denervation. Treatment is directed at protection of the cornea with artificial tears and bland ointments. Moisture chambers (airtight goggles), tarsorrhaphy, and soft contact lenses have also been used.

References

Apt L, Cullen BF: Newborns do secrete tears. JAMA 189:95, 1964

Ffooks OO: Dacryocystitis in infancy. Br J Ophthalmol 46:422, 1962

Howard RO: Familial dysautonomia (Riley-Day syndrome). Am J Ophthalmol 64:392, 1967

Jones BR: The clinical features and etiology of dacryoadenitis. Trans Ophthalmol Soc UK 75:435, 1955

Riley CM, Day RL, Greeley DM, Langford WS: Central autonomic dysfunction with defective lacrimation: report of five cases. Pediatrics 3:468, 1949

Viers ER: Lacrimal disorders in infants and children. In Apt L (ed): Diagnostic Procedures in Pediatric Ophthalmology, Boston, Little, Brown, 1963

——— Disorders of the nasolacrimal apparatus in infants and children. J Pediatr Ophthalmol 3:32, 1966

CONGENITAL GLAUCOMA

Congenital (infantile, developmental) glaucoma is an elevation of the intraocular pressure that manifests at birth or shortly thereafter. When glaucoma becomes evident after 3 years of age, it is termed juvenile glaucoma. The signs and symptoms of juvenile glaucoma are identical to those of adult open angle glaucoma and need not be elucidated here.

Congenital glaucoma is transmitted as an autosomal recessive characteristic. Two-thirds of the patients are males, but sex linkage is not common in the inheritance pattern. Most cases are bilateral and are apparent at or shortly after birth. The increase in intraocular pressure results from an interference with outflow of aqueous humor from the anterior chamber angle caused by developmental anomalies in the angle structures. There may be maldevelopment or absence of the trabecula, abnormal insertion of the longitudinal ciliary body muscle onto the trabecula, and a membrane (Barkan's membrane) covering the angle structures. With impairment of the passage of fluid out of the eye, intraocular fluid volume and pressure increase, distending the coats of the eye and producing the clinical picture of congenital glaucoma.

Although congenital glaucoma is rare, the threat to vision is serious, and the prognosis is poor unless it is promptly recognized and treatment is given. The cardinal symptom of congenital glaucoma is photophobia. This light sensitivity may be so extreme that an infant may shield his eyes from bright light by hiding his head in a pillow. Usually there is associated blepharospasm and tearing, which may lead to the mistaken diagnosis of dacryostenosis and conjunctivitis. The characteristic signs are bilateral increased intraocular pressure (usually worse in one eye), edema and slight congestion of the conjunctiva, corneal haziness due to edema, increased diameter of the cornea (greater than 11 mm in the newborn or 12 mm in the first year of life), linear white opacities in the cornea (tears in Descemet's membrane), deep anterior chamber, and cupping and atrophy of the optic nerve. Because of the distensibility of an infant's eye in the first 3 years of life, enlargement of the globe may occur, and thus the name *buphthalmos* (ox eye) is sometimes given to the disease. Unilateral enlargement of the globe from high myopia (quiet eye with no corneal haze and normal intraocular pressure) and megalocornea (sex-linked disorder occuring in males and not associated with an elevation of intraocular pressure) must be differentiated. In addition, any of the other causes of corneal opacity in infants (Table 2) must be considered.

Usually the diagnosis can be made from the signs and symptoms, but examination of the eyes and measurement of the intraocular pressure under general anesthesia is mandatory. The normal infantile intraocular pressure under general anesthesia, in our experience, ranges between 8 and 18 mm Hg, and a pressure over 22 mm Hg is characteristic of glaucoma.

Early surgical treatment is essential and may be done at the time of the initial examination under anesthesia. Medical therapy with the usual glaucoma drugs (miotics, epinephrine, Diamox) is rarely of value. The surgical procedure of choice is either goniotomy or trabeculotomy. In both cases an opening is made in the trabecular meshwork to allow aqueous humor to drain from the eye. Occasionally the procedure must be done several times to obtain an adequate opening. In over 75 percent of the cases surgery is successful in controlling the intraocular pressure.

Congenital glaucoma must be differentiated from secondary forms of glaucoma that occur in infants and children. Usually some abnormal tissue in the anterior chamber angle is obstructing the outflow of aqueous. The causes are multiple; they include aniridia, spherophakia, microcornea, rubella, Lowe's syndrome (oculocerebrorenal), Sturge-Weber syndrome, Recklinghausen's disease, Lindau-von Hippel disease, Marfan's syndrome, mesodermal dysgenesis (Riegers' anomaly), Pierre Robin syndrome, Hallerman-Streiff syndrome, and Ullrich's syndrome. In addition, other causes of elevated intraocular pressure must be recognized, including trauma (hyphema, lens dislocation), uveitis (intraocular inflammation, polyarthritis), retinoblastoma (leukokoria, shallow anterior chamber), corticosteroid treatment (history of steroid intake), retrolental fibroplasia, and juvenile xanthogranuloma of the iris.

The prognosis in congenital glaucoma depends on the age at onset (the earlier the onset, the worse the prognosis), the amount of myopia induced by enlargement of the eye, corneal scarring, damage to the optic nerve, and lens opacification or other injury to the eye secondary to surgical trauma. Frequently the more severely involved eye becomes divergent, less often esotropic, and it may be amblyopic. Usually one eye can be controlled and can maintain satisfactory visual acuity.

References

Alfano JE: Steroid induced glaucoma simulating congenital glaucoma. Am J Ophthalmol 78:501, 1974

Kolker AE, Hetherington J JR: Becker-Shaffer's Diagnosis and Therapy of the Glaucomas. St Louis, Mosby, 1970

Radtke ND, Cohan BE: Intraocular pressure measurement in the newborn. Am J Ophthalmol 78:501, 1974

Shaffer RN, Weiss DI: Congenital and Pediatric Glaucomas. St Louis, Mosby, 1970

THE LENS

Abnormalities of Size, Shape, and Position

Microphakia (spherophakia) is a small spherical lens that is prone to subluxation. Pupillary block glaucoma may occur secondary to anterior subluxation. Eyes containing spherophakic lenses are highly myopic. This lens anomaly may be inherited as an autosomal recessive trait, or it may occur in congenital rubella, homocystinuria, hyperlysinemia, Marfan's syndrome,

Weill-Marchesani syndrome, Lowe's syndrome, and Alport's syndrome. Abnormalities of lens shape may change the refractive properties of the lens to such an extent that extraction is indicated even though the lens is clear; most commonly seen are coloboma, lenticonus (anterior or posterior conical protrusion), and umbilication (central depression).

Ectopia lentis refers to subluxation or complete dislocation of the lens. The rim of the lens may be seen crossing the pupil, and the iris is tremulous (iridodonesis). In cases of anterior dislocation, acute pupillary block glaucoma may result. Ectopia lentis may occur in a wide variety of ocular and systemic syndromes or it may be inherited as an isolated abnormality. Superior dislocation of the lens is found in 79 percent of eyes with Marfan's syndrome. This subluxation occurs late; frequently it is not detected until the fourth or fifth decade. Inferiorly dislocated lenses are the most frequent ocular complication of homocystinuria, occurring in nearly 90 percent of such patients. The ectopia is detected early in life, and almost one-third eventually luxate into the vitreous or the anterior chamber. Although the ectopic lenses in homocystinuria are frequently cataractous, lens extraction under general anesthesia should be avoided, since fatal thromboembolic complications may occur during or shortly after surgery. Other conditions in which ectopia lentis is less often present include Frenkel's syndrome (ocular contusion), Riegers' anomaly, spherophakia, Ehlers-Danlos syndrome, Weill-Marchesani syndrome, dwarfism, oxycephaly, the mandibulofacial dysostoses, sulfite oxidase deficiency, and hyperlysinemia.

Cataract

A cataract is any opacity of the crystalline lens. Most congenital cataracts are present at birth, but frequently they are not discovered until some time during the first year of life. The terms congenital cataract and infantile cataract are thus used synonymously. The degree of opacity varies widely from a small dot to total clouding of the lens, and although congenital cataracts are usually stationary, they may progress in severity during childhood. Congenital lens opacities account for 11.5 percent of blindness in preschool children and are a common cause of amblyopia.

Congenital cataracts may be classified according to type (partial or complete) or etiology. Partial cataracts (nuclear, anterior, or posterior polar, lamellar, or zonular) involve the central portion of the lens, leaving the peripheral zone clear. With the ophthalmoscope one sees a dark central opacity surrounded by a clear rim of cortex through which the red reflex is seen. Complete or total cataracts may be present from birth or may result from the progression of partial cataracts. There is complete opacification of the lens, which creates a dense white pupillary reflex.

Approximately 25 to 50 percent of congenital cataracts cannot be classified as to etiology. Of those in which an etiology is established, *hereditary* or *familial* forms are most common. Cataracts inherited in an autosomal dominant manner are usually nuclear in type. In most other cases the cataract is associated with other ocular anomalies or systemic disease.

Intrauterine infection with rubella is the most frequent single disease causing congenital cataracts. The cataract is either nuclear or complete, unilateral or bilateral, and is characterized by the retention of nuclei (and virus) within the fetal nucleus of the lens. Microphthalmos, spherophakia, iris atrophy, and poor development of the dilator muscle of the iris are often present. Other intrauterine infections that may cause cataracts are toxoplasmosis, cytomegalic inclusion disease, and syphilis.

A host of *endocrine disorders* and *inborn errors of metabolism* may produce cataracts. In galactosemia, galactose fails to metabolize normally. Initially the lens takes on an oil-droplet appearance, and later a nuclear or zonular cataract develops. These opacities are reversible if appropriate dietary measures are taken early in life. Homocystinuria, tetany (with hypocalcemia), diabetes mellitus, Wilson's disease, and Lowe's syndrome are just a few of the other metabolic etiologies.

Intraocular disease may produce a cataract (congenital glaucoma, uveitis) or lead to an erroneous diagnosis of cataract (leukokoria due to retrolental fibroplasia, persistent hyperplastic primary vitreous, retinal dysplasia, retinoblastoma). The presence of a cataract should alert the examining physician to the possibility of coexistence of other ocular diseases or congenital ocular anomalies.

Other causes of congenital cataracts include *trauma* (severe birth trauma, chronic head banging), *prematurity*, *drugs* (corticosteroids), *ionizing radiation, chromosomal aberrations* (trisomies 13–15, 18, 21, Turner's syndrome), and a number of *systemic disorders*. Patients with cerebral palsy, mental deficiency, and other neurologic abnormalities may have cataracts, presumably on the basis of prenatal or postnatal hypoxia. For a complete list of etiologies, the references at the end of this section should be consulted.

The prognosis and the management of congenital cataracts will depend on the morphology of the lens opacities, whether they are unilateral or bilateral, and their association with other ocular defects or systemic diseases. Children with bilateral and complete cataracts fail to receive foveal stimulation during the critical first 3 to 4 months of visual development. As a result, ocular nystagmus develops. Surgery should be performed on at least one eye before the age of 4 months in order to avoid nystagmus and irreversible amblyopia. Children with a unilateral complete cataract almost invariably develop profound amblyopia even after surgery. The only possibility of obtaining useful vision is early surgical removal of the cataract (before 6 months), early contact lens fitting, and occlusion therapy of the phakic eye. It is not universally accepted that surgical removal of a unilateral cataract is indicated, but if it is to be done, it should be done early in life.

The best visual prognosis is in patients with bilateral

partial cataracts. In many cases the clear peripheral zone allows a retinal image to be formed in each eye. Nystagmus does not develop, there is little or no amblyopia, and the functional result of surgery is often good at whatever age it is done. The use of mydriatics or the performance of an optical iridectomy may allow surgery to be delayed until the age of 4 to 6 years, when visual acuity can be accurately tested. If distance visual acuity is less than 20/60, then surgery may be done. However, near or reading vision may be satisfactory in spite of poor distance acuity, and in these cases it is advisable to delay surgery as long as possible. Unilateral partial cataracts frequently lead to amblyopia, so that the visual outcome after surgery is not as favorable as with bilateral partial lens opacities.

Rubella cataracts present a particularly difficult management problem. The postoperative complication rate is high (50 percent of cases compared to 5 percent for uncomplicated congenital cataract surgery), possibly because of the severe uveitis that may develop. This uveitis is presumably secondary to the release of live virus contained in the lens into the eye. As a result, some surgeons prefer to do preliminary optical iridectomies early in life and defer cataract aspiration until the age of 18 months, when there is less chance of live virus being present. Other surgeons claim less discrepancy between the postoperative complication rates for rubella and nonrubella cases. In children with bilateral complete cataracts, one eye probably should be done at an early age, in the hope that some useful vision may be salvaged despite the risks. Surgery on the second eye is then performed, based on the results and complications encountered with the first eye.

In general, conservatism is indicated in the surgical removal of congenital cataracts. The long-term prognosis is always guarded; only rarely is a visual acuity level of 20/20 reached. In addition, there is a high incidence of late retinal detachment.

References

Cross HE, Jensen AD: Ocular manifestations in the Marfan syndrome and homocystinuria. Am J Ophthalmol 75:405, 1973

Francois J: Congenital Cataracts. Springfield, Ill, Charles C Thomas, 1963

Merin S, Crawford JS: The etiology of congenital cataracts. Can J Ophthalmol 6:178, 1971

Prestley GD, Stinson IW, Sidbury JB: Homocystinuria. Am J Ophthalmol 66:884, 1968

Roy FH: Ocular Differential Diagnosis, 2nd ed. Philadelphia, Lea & Febiger, 1975

Scheie HG, Schaffer DB: Congenital cataracts. In Symposium on Surgical and Medical Management of Congenital Anomalies of the Eye. Transactions of the New Orleans Academy of Ophthalmology. St Louis, Mosby, 1968

———— Schaffer DB, Plotkin SA, Kertesz ED: Congenital rubella cataracts. Arch Ophthalmol 77:440, 1967

Sheppard RW, Crawford JS: The treatment of congenital cataracts. Surv Ophthalmol 17:340, 1973

Wolff SM: The ocular manifestations of congenital rubella. J Pediatr Ophthalmol 10:101, 1973

THE UVEA

Congenital Anomalies

The uveal tract, comprising the iris, ciliary body, and choroid, is the pigmented and vascular layer of the eye. The common defect, *coloboma,* is described under Developmental Anomalies of the Globe, (p. 1945). Anomalies may include two or more pupils in one eye (*polycoria*), abnormality in the shape of the pupil (*dyscoria*), or location of the pupil to one side of center of the iris (*corectopia*). Unequal pupils (*anisocoria*) is an autosomal dominant trait present in about 25 percent of normal individuals. Persistent pupillary membrane remnants are extremely common (80 percent of individuals). The persistence of an intact pupillary membrane in premature infants may be related to oxygen therapy.

Aniridia is a bilateral hypoplasia of the iris inherited as an autosomal dominant trait. It is associated with cataracts, aplasia of the macula, hypoplasia of the optic nerve, glaucoma, nystagmus, ectopia lentis, and high refractive errors. Aniridia (usually a sporadic form) may occur with Wilms' tumor (p. 1346) or other congenital defects, particularly genitourinary anomalies in boys. In both affected males and females there is an increased incidence of microcephaly, mental retardation, and deformities of the pinna; less commonly there may be skull or craniofacial dysmorphism, umbilical and inguinal hernias, and hypotonia.

A difference in color of the two irides (heterochromia) may be inherited as an autosomal dominant trait or may be secondary to a number of disorders, including congenital Horner's syndrome, iris atrophy secondary to iritis, Waardenburg's syndrome, hemifacial atrophy of Romberg, and status dysraphicus.

Albinism (p. 678) is an inborn error of metabolism caused by a deficiency of the enzyme tyrosinase. No trace of this enzyme is detectable in the uveal melanocytes of complete albinos. The most striking ocular findings are in the iris, choroid, and retina. The iris is thin and devoid of pigment, which allows the red fundus reflex to be transmitted through the pupil and translucent iris. The choroid has little or no pigment. Retinal pigment granules are pale and few in number. The macula is hypoplastic or aplastic. The patients have poor vision, photophobia, pendular nystagmus, and myopia or astigmatism. One form of albinism, ocular albinism, is confined to the eye and is inherited as a sex-linked recessive trait. Therapy of albinotic eyes includes tinted spectacles and contact lenses; in the newborn, pinhole contact lenses are designed to reduce intraocular illumination, and theoretically they allow the macula to develop normally. Further experience is needed with this therapeutic approach.

Uveitis

Inflammation of the uveal tract occurs less often in children than in adults, but it is more serious in that it more often leads to blindness. In a pathologic study, uveitis was the third most common cause (7 percent) of enucleation in pediatric patients. Uveitis is in many respects a different disease in children than in adults. More often in children it is low-grade and chronic, with few outward signs. Children under the age of 10 years do not generally have pain, redness, and photophobia. In fact, they are usually referred to an ophthalmologist not because of symptoms of uveitis but for the complications of amblyopia, band-shaped keratopathy, cataracts, or glaucoma. In all suspected cases of uveitis a slit-lamp examination and indirect ophthalmoscopy by an ophthalmologist are essential.

The fundamental problem in uveitis is its causation. In relatively few cases can a specific organism or allergen be incriminated. Uveitis has been subdivided into two forms: granulomatous and nongranulomatous. In the former it is believed that the uveal tissue is actively invaded by specific organisms; the latter is considered to be an allergic response to an antigen that may have been elaborated locally or at a remote site. These distinctions are not hard and fast, and in many cases they are difficult to make. A more useful and clinically practical classification of uveitis is one that emphasizes the site of involvement: anterior uveitis (iritis, iridocyclitis, cyclitis), posterior uveitis (choroiditis), and diffuse uveitis (panuveitis).

Anterior uveitis is rarely ever acute in children—usually only following trauma. A chronic and very low grade anterior uveitis has been found in approximately 17 percent of children with juvenile rheumatoid arthritis, usually the monoarticular type. Band-shaped keratopathy has been identified in the past with this form of uveitis, but it may occur in any chronic anterior uveitis of childhood. The most common form of uveitis in children is *chronic cyclitis (peripheral uveitis)*. The usual onset is at 6 to 10 years of age, and unlike the anterior uveitis associated with juvenile rheumatoid arthritis, which is more frequent in girls, chronic cyclitis is much more common in boys. In chronic cyclitis there are cells and opacities in the anterior and inferior vitreous. Occasionally snowball-like opacities may form in the deep vitreous. A white exudate (snowbank) may form over the peripheral retina and pars plana inferiorly. Indirect ophthalmoscopy is required to see these changes. This cyclitis may be active for months to years and may burn out during the teenage period. The nematode *Toxocara canis* may produce a similar chronic cyclitis in children. Other less common causes of anterior uveitis in children are sarcoidosis, syphilis, herpes simplex, herpes zoster, and Behçet's syndrome.

The two most frequent causes of *posterior uveitis* in children are toxoplasmosis and toxocariasis. Tuberculosis is not an important etiologic factor in the production of uveitis today. Toxoplasmosis retinochoroiditis may occur in three forms. One-third of the cases are congenital, with healed, densely pigmented chorioretinal scars in both eyes. Usually the macula is involved in one eye only. Two-thirds of the cases have recurrent retinochoroiditis with active satellite lesions arising within or adjacent to healed chorioretinal scars. Occasionally the retinochoroiditis is acquired, in which case no healed scars are present. Recent evidence suggests that the *Toxoplasma* organism may be acquired from eating raw meat or from the feces of household cats. Pregnant women are advised to avoid taking on a new pet cat; if a cat is already present in the household, a pregnant woman should not dig in the garden if there is any likelihood that cat feces may be buried in the area. Posterior uveitis due to *Toxocara* (visceral larva migrans), a common nematode larva of puppies and kittens, is acquired in children by ingestion of soil contaminated with *Toxocara canis* or *cati* ova. The initial infection occurs in young children age 2 to 3 years, with ocular involvement appearing several years later; 75 percent of patients are males. Typically there is a unilateral white solitary granuloma of the retina close to the optic disc and macula. There may be signs of peripheral uveitis, and endophthalmitis or retinal detachment may occur.

Diffuse uveitis is rare in children. Vogt-Koyanagi-Harada syndrome is a severe bilateral uveitis with exudative retinal detachment associated with pleocytosis, ringing in the ears and hearing loss, alopecia, and vitiligo. Sympathetic ophthalmia is a very rare but tragic consequence of perforating ocular injury. Following a perforating injury involving the uveal tract of one eye, severe bilateral granulomatous uveitis may develop. It has been suggested that sympathetic ophthalmia is due to autosensitivity to uveal pigment, but this hypothesis remains unproved. The onset in the sympathizing eye may follow the injury by 2 weeks or several years and is insidious, with slight irritative symptoms and mild evidence of uveitis. Once sympathetic inflammation has developed, removal of the exciting eye may prove unavailing. However, the formerly almost hopeless prognosis has been markedly improved by the use of corticosteroid therapy. Corticosteroids cannot prevent the disease, but they may suppress the inflammation and thus preserve some vision.

One important intraocular cause of simulated uveitis is retinoblastoma. Ciliary injection, keratic precipitates, iris nodules, and hypopyon, together with a limited visualization of the fundus, may lead to a misdiagnosis of uveitis. Fortunately the tumor, with its characteristic pinkish cream color and blood vessels on the surface, can usually be seen in the posterior segment of the eye. The demonstration of intraocular calcification (present in 75 percent of cases of retinoblastoma) by x-ray can also be helpful in the differentiation.

Current treatment of uveitis consists of topical mydriatics and cycloplegics, corticosteroids, antibiotics, and chemotherapeutic agents. Topical corticosteroids are effective for anterior uveitis, but posterior uveitis requires their injection under Tenon's capsule or retrobulbar or systemic administration. Corticosteroids may have to be given for many months or years to suppress the uveitis. Alternate-day oral therapy, if effective, reduces steroid complications. Sulfonamides and pyrimethamine (Daraprim) are recommended for acute toxoplasmosis retinochoroiditis. Anti-inflammatory drugs such as aspirin and indomethacin may have some limited value in uveitis. Antimetabolite drugs have been used with some success in severe, recalcitrant cases of chronic uveitis and sympathetic ophthalmia. There is no effective treatment for ocular infection by *Toxocara*.

References

Apt L, Sarin LK: Causes for enucleation of the eye in infants and children. JAMA 181:948, 1962

Brown DH: Ocular Toxocara canis. J Pediatr Ophthalmol 7:182, 1970

Fraumeni JF Jr, Glass AG: Wilms' tumor and congenital aniridia. JAMA 206:825, 1968

Giles CL: Anterior uveitis in children. Arch Ophthalmol 70:770, 1963

Haicken BN, Miller DR: Simultaneous occurrence of congenital aniridia, hamartoma, and Wilms' tumor. J Pediatr 78:497, 1971

Kaufman HE, Witmer R, Kimura SJ, Gordon DM: Uveitis in children. In Turtz A (ed): Proceedings of the Centennial Symposium Manhattan Eye, Ear, and Throat Hospital, Vol 1. Ophthalmology. St Louis, Mosby, 1969

Mazow ML: Diagnosis and management of uveitis and complications in children. J Pediatr Ophthalmol 10:167, 1973

Piper RC, Cole CR, Shadduck JA: Natural and experimental ocular toxoplasmosis in animals. Am J Ophthalmol 69:662, 1970

Richards WW: Retinoblastoma simulating uveitis. Am J Ophthalmol 65:427, 1968

Schlaegel TF Jr: Essentials of Uveitis. Boston, Little, Brown, 1969

THE RETINA

Congenital Anomalies

Coloboma of the retina has been described elsewhere (p. 1945). *Congenital retinal fold* results from a mass of connective tissue near the lens equator. As the globe enlarges, a fold develops that extends from the disc to the equator of the lens. Congenital detachment of the retina can result. This condition is inherited as a recessive trait, occurring most often in one eye of full-term infants.

Persistent hyperplastic primary vitreous (PHPV) is a unilateral eye abnormality caused by a failure of regression of the tunica vasculosa lentis. A white fibrous mass incorporated in long ciliary processes extending to the periphery persists behind a cataractous lens. The eye is usually microphthalmic. The retina is formed normally, but is detached by adherence to the retrolental mass. The abnormality is found in full-term infants. The subsequent development of secondary glaucoma and the cosmetic disfigurement associated with this abnormality frequently lead to evisceration or enucleation.

Retinal dysplasia may occur as an isolated uniocular abnormality, but the complete retinal dysplasia syndrome has been identified with the trisomy 13–15 chromosome aberration (Table 1). The syndrome is characterized by bilateral congenital malformations of the eyes, severe anomalies of the brain, heart, and other viscera (which are usually incompatible with life), and other visible abnormalities such as harelip, cleft palate, and polydactylia. Retinal dysplasia is associated in these cases with colobomas of the iris, ciliary body, and cho-

roid, as well as microphthalmos, cataracts, and PHPV. A characteristic feature of the syndrome is an island of cartilage contained within a mass of fibrous connective tissue passing through the coloboma of the ciliary body of the iris.

Norrie's disease is a rare sex-linked recessive hyaloideoretinal dysplasia that causes bilateral congenital blindness. The eyes may be small, normal, or large in size. The anterior chamber is shallow and the iris is atrophic. The retina is totally detached and gliotic. In time, corneal and lenticular opacities develop, the retina becomes a mass of vascularized connective tissue, and the eyes shrink. The affected children may be mentally retarded and deaf.

Retinoblastoma

Retinoblastoma is a congenital malignant tumor composed of embryonal retinal cells. It is the most common intraocular tumor of infancy and childhood and is second only to malignant melanoma of the uvea among all intraocular tumors. Increasing numbers of cases have been reported in the past three decades due to an increased mutation rate and a falling mortality rate. The current incidence is 1 in 15,000 live births. The tumor is always congenital and may be present at birth. Seventy percent of cases are discovered before the age of 3 years, and presentation after the age of 6 years is rare. Careful examination of both eyes is essential, because approximately 30 percent of patients have bilateral tumors. Males and females are equally affected, except for a rare diffuse infiltrating form of the tumor that is more common in boys and appears between the ages of 6 and 11 years.

Most cases are sporadic. Of the sporadic tumors, 10 to 20 percent are secondary to a germinal mutation in one parent who is free of the disease. These children usually have bilateral tumors and may transmit the disease to 50 percent of their offspring. The remaining sporadic cases are unilateral and are due to a somatic mutation in the retina of the affected infant that cannot be transmitted. Familial occurrence is associated with the autosomal dominant mode of inheritance. Penetrance is approximately 80 percent, so that generations may be skipped. Inherited cases are invariably bilateral, and survivors transmit the disease to 40 percent of their offspring, with 10 percent becoming symptomless carriers. When retinoblastoma occurs in one child with healthy parents, the chance of further children being affected is 6 percent. If two retinoblastomatous children are born to the same parents, one parent must be a carrier; so a strong possibility exists that subsequent children will have the tumor. Retinoblastoma has been reported in association with partial deletion of the long arm or ring of the D (13–15) group chromosome.

Retinoblastoma frequently has a multifocal origin from the retina and shows a facility to seed other ocular tissues through the vitreous or subretinal fluid. Grossly the tumor is pinkish white or cream colored and often nodular. Histologically the tumor is composed of tightly packed undifferentiated retinoblasts that may show variable degrees of differentiation toward rods and cones (rosettes and fleurettes). The blood supply is invariably inadequate, and patchy necrosis and degeneration with calcium deposition are characteristic. The demonstration of intraocular calcium on x-ray is an important diagnostic sign, because it is uncommon in children's eyes in any other condition.

The clinical characteristics depend on the stage of growth of the tumor at the time of its discovery. When the tumor is small and at the posterior pole of the eye, the initial sign may be strabismus secondary to impairment of vision. Therefore every young pediatric patient with strabismus should have a careful ophthalmoscopic examination. As the tumor grows in size, a creamy white pupillary reflex (*cat's eye* or *leukokoria*) develops, and the mass may be visualized easily. At this stage the lesion is far advanced. In endophytic growths the tumor is seen in front of the retina, while in exophytic growths the retina is lifted up by the tumor and lies detached over it. Further growth leads to secondary glaucoma, buphthalmos, uveitis, and endophthalmitis. Unusual presentations include heterochromia, spontaneous hyphema, unilateral pupillary dilatation, orbital cellulitis, and proptosis.

Several diagnostic points are worth emphasizing. Usually the eye harboring a retinoblastoma is white and of normal size for age, and the anterior chamber is of normal depth. Transillumination of the eye will reveal a solid tissue mass. Calcium is usually demonstrable on x-ray. Ultrasonography may be helpful when visualization of the fundus is impaired. Optic foramen x-rays may show enlargement due to extension of the tumor along the optic nerve. An anterior chamber diagnostic tap may be helpful, either to identify tumor cells or to measure the characteristically elevated aqueous lactic dehydrogenase concentration. Finally, delayed cutaneous hypersensitivity response to membrane extract of retinoblastoma may be a useful diagnostic test for patients in whom the diagnosis is uncertain.

A number of conditions may be misinterpreted as retinoblastoma. In retrolental fibroplasia a bilateral white reflex in the pupil may be present, but there is also a history of prematurity and oxygen administration; the globes are frequently small and the anterior chambers shallow. No calcium is present. Persistent hyperplastic primary vitreous may suggest retinoblastoma; however, this diagnosis is usually excluded by an experienced ophthalmologist's familiarity with the appearance of the embryonic mass, the lack of calcium, its occurrence in a microphthalmic eye, and the presence of a cataract. Endophthalmitis with granuloma formation due to *Toxocara canis* or *Toxoplasma gondii* may suggest retinoblastoma. Coats' disease, retinal dysplasia, and organization of the retina following hemorrhage may require consideration.

Retinoblastoma has a predilection for invasion of the optic nerve, and by extension it may reach the subarachnoid space and the brain. Intracranial extension is the most common cause of death. Local spread may also occur into the choroid, the orbit, and the lymphatics. Hematogenous metastases to bone (skull, ribs, humerus) are frequent; metastases to viscera and muscles occur less often.

The prognosis in retinoblastoma patients has improved over the past 20 years due to improved methods of diagnosis and earlier discovery of tumors. If the tumor is unilateral and small and the eye is promptly enucleated, there is a 90 percent chance of survival. Once the tumor has extended into the optic nerve, the cure rate decreases to approximately 50 percent. Extension into the cranium or orbit or heavy infiltration into the choroid are grave prognostic signs. Spontaneous regression has been reported, but it is rare; it usually occurs in one of a bilateral pair of tumors and is thought to be secondary to a host immunologic response. A recent study indicates that bilateral retinoblastoma survivors may be more likely to develop another primary malignant neoplasm than other cancer patients.

The usual treatment of unilateral retinoblastoma is immediate enucleation, with removal of as much of the optic nerve as possible. Small discrete tumors in one eye have been treated with photocoagulation, radiation, and implantation of radon seeds with varying success. The fellow eye must be checked at 3- to 4-month intervals throughout childhood. In bilateral cases the eye with the more advanced tumor is enucleated, and the fellow eye is treated with radiation and chemotherapy (usually triethylenemelamine, TEM) if less than a third of the retina is involved. When the lesion is so advanced in both eyes that radiation has little to offer for conservation of vision, bilateral enucleation is performed.

Retrolental Fibroplasia

In the early 1950s the toxic effect of oxygen therapy in premature infants was first discovered. This was a striking example of an iatrogenic disease yielding to intensive investigation. The control of oxygen therapy in premature babies led to a decline in this condition, but in the past decade the more liberal use of oxygen in the treatment of respiratory distress syndrome and in the endeavor to prevent cerebral palsy has resulted in an increase in cases of retrolental fibroplasia. Any concentration of oxygen in excess of that in air carries the risk of producing retrolental fibroplasia. Close surveillance of premature infants is necessary, with frequent periodic arterial oxygen tension values as a guide. Although oxygen appears to be the major factor in the pathogenesis of retrolental fibroplasia, other contributory elements requiring further research may be present. The disease has been encountered occasionally in both premature and full-term infants who have not been exposed to oxygen.

The first signs of retinopathy are the obliteration of developing retinal vessels in the temporal retina caused by a high ambient concentration of oxygen. This vascular obliteration is followed by a profuse neovascularization with exudation during the relative anoxia that results from return of the infant with its now avascular retina to normal atmospheric conditions. Most of the cases spontaneously regress at the stage of neovascularization. In 25 percent of cases, a progressive cicatricial phase ensues, with retinal folds, retinal detachment, vitreous strands, and extension of the fibrovascular process into the vitreous. The disc, vessels, and macula are often dragged temporally by the vitreoretinal scarring. Retinal detachment repair may be required at an early age to prevent progression of the detachment. Severe cases progress to the formation of a dense white mass lying behind the lens and total blindness. Eyes with extensive retinopathy are typically small, with shallow anterior chambers. Strabismus, pendular nystagmus, and myopia are frequent.

Retinal Detachment

The most common causes of retinal detachment in children are trauma, high myopia, cataract extraction, retinal dialysis, and retrolental fibroplasia. It is important that the retina be examined in all young patients after blunt injury because of the possibility of a long latency period between trauma and detachment and the inability of children to give a history of decreasing vision. Retinal detachments are more common in certain systemic diseases, including Marfan's syndrome, Waardenburg's syndrome, Ehlers-Danlos syndrome, and Pierre Robin syndrome.

Coats' disease is an unusual cause of uniocular retinal detachment and leukokoria in young males. It is characterized by telangiectases of the retinal vessels associated with massive white or yellow exudate and hemorrhages. A total retinal detachment may occur with cataract, glaucoma, and phthisis bulbi. The etiology is unknown, but some cases have been associated with hypogammaglobulinemia.

Retinitis Pigmentosa

Pigmentary degeneration of the retina is a form of abiotrophy in which the retinal neuroepithelium and pigment layer degenerate. It is inherited as an autosomal or sex-linked recessive, but only 50 percent of cases have a family pattern of inheritance. Characteristic symptoms are nyctalopia (night blindness), delayed dark adaptation, and constriction of the visual field leading to total blindness. In a well-developed case the appearance of the fundus is typical. The vessels are attenuated and the disc is pale. Bone-corpuscle-shaped pigment is scattered throughout the fundus near blood vessels. Posterior subcapsular cataracts occur in time. The electroretinogram (ERG) is severely depressed or absent. In early cases abnormalities in the ERG may precede visible changes in the fundus. As a rule, incapacity does not develop until early adulthood, but signs and symptoms may appear early in childhood. When the onset occurs in childhood the prognosis is poor, and no treatment is effective. Retinitis pigmentosa may occur in a number of neurologic syndromes including Laurence-Moon-Biedl syndrome, Refsum's syndrome, progressive external ophthalmoplegia, myotonic dystrophy, and Cockayne's syndrome.

A number of other conditions may produce a pigmentary disturbance of the retina in the form of punctate, bone-corpuscular, or heaped-up masses of pigment. These disturbances are termed pseudoretinitis pigmentosa or secondary retinitis pigmentosa. Included in this group are infections (syphilis, rubella, cytomegalic inclusion disease, influenza virus), obstetric trauma, radiotherapy, drugs (phenothiazines, chloroquine), trauma, vascular occlusion, mucopolysaccharidoses, Leber's congenital amaurosis, Waardenburg's syndrome, Vogt-Spielmeyer disease, and cystinosis.

Rubella retinitis requires special comment because of its frequent occurrence in congenital rubella along with microphthalmia, glaucoma, cataracts, and nystagmus. It is usually bilateral and more advanced in one eye. The fundus shows a diffuse salt-and-pepper pigmentary mottling. The retinitis is inactive at birth, and little or no progression occurs. The effect on visual acuity caused by these pigmentary changes is difficult to estimate because of the other ocular abnormalities that impair vision. Visual acuity seems to be unaffected in most cases, and color vision, visual fields, and ERG are normal.

Lipidoses

The general medical aspects of the lipidoses have been discussed elsewhere (p. 747), and only the main ocular manifestations will be presented here. The sphingolipidoses are inherited cerebroretinal degenerations due to inborn errors of lipid metabolism. They lead inevitably to blindness and dementia, followed by death. The sphingolipidoses occur in three familial forms: gangliosidoses, sphingomyelinoses, and cerebrosidoses.

The *gangliosidoses* are autosomal recessive disorders characterized by the accumulation of gangliosides in the ganglion cells of the retina. There have been five gangliosidoses described. The most common form is Tay-Sachs disease (infantile amaurotic familial idiocy, GM_2—gangliosidosis—type 1), in which there is decreasing vision, strabismus, and characteristic ophthalmoscopic findings. These consist of a white area in the macular region approximately two disc diameters in size with a small red central area (cherry red spot). The white area is produced by swelling of the ganglion cells of the ganglion layer of the retina associated with ganglioside accumulation. The central macula is devoid of ganglion cells, and thus the contrasting red coloration. With time, retinal degeneration and optic nerve atrophy occur, with blindness. The other gangliosidoses with later onset in life show salt-and-pepper pigment degeneration of the retina and macula instead of a cherry red spot.

Sphingomyelinosis (Niemann-Pick disease) involves the reticuloendothelial and nervous systems. Sphingomyelin accumulates in the ganglion cells of the retina, producing a cherry red spot in 25 to 50 percent of cases. Decreasing vision, strabismus, and optic atrophy likewise can occur.

Cerebrosidoses are a group of rare familial disorders that may involve the nervous system. In the pediatric form of Gaucher's disease, strabismus is common, and a cherry red spot in the macula has been described on occasion. In older children and adults, large yellow-brown wedge-shaped pingueculas with their bases at the cornea may be seen.

Various other systemic disorders of lipid metabolism may produce retinal degeneration in children. Fabry's angiokeratomatosis is characterized by dilated tortuous retinal vessels, retinal hemorrhages, and a cherry red spot in the macula. Farber's disease (disseminated lipogranulomatosis) produces a fine pigmentary retinopathy and a cherry red spot in the macula. The leukodystrophies may on occasion also exhibit a cherry red spot in the macula.

Phakomatosis

Several congenital syndromes are characterized by the formation of hamartomas involving multiple tissues, primarily the eyes, nervous system, and skin. These syndromes are collectively referred to by ophthalmologists as the phakomatoses (p. 1928).

Tuberous sclerosis (Bourneville's disease) may be present early in life with solitary or multiple astrocytic hamartomas (gliomas) of the retina. These white tumors may take one of two forms: a flat plaquelike growth or a nodular mulberrylike mass. These tumors extend locally in the retina only. Associated ocular findings may include *drusen* of the optic nerve, glioma of the optic nerve, angioid streaks, and lens or corneal opacities.

Neurofibromatosis (Recklinghausen's disease) may have similar gliomas in the retina and optic nerve. In addition, nodular neurofibromata may be present in the orbit, lids, conjunctiva, iris, or choroid. Secondary glaucoma, ptosis, proptosis, and optic atrophy may result.

Angiomatosis retinae (Lindau-von Hippel angiomatosis) is an angioblastic retinal hamartoma that is frequently bilateral. The yellow retinal tumor is supplied by a large tortuous artery and vein. Its presence leads to hemorrhage, exudation, retinal detachment, and secondary glaucoma. Some eyes have been saved by photocoagulation of the tumor before retinal detachment occurs.

Sturge-Weber syndrome (encephalofacial angiomatosis) may have angiomatous tumors in the conjunctiva, iris, and choroid. Glaucoma is almost inevitable, and retinal detachment may occur.

References

Arentsen JJ, Welch RB: Retinal detachment in the young individual: a survey of 100 cases seen at the Wilmer Institute. J Pediatr Ophthalmol 11:198. 1974

Binder PS: Unusual manifestations of retinoblastoma. Am J Ophthalmol 77:674, 1974

Boniuk M (ed): Ocular and Adnexal Tumors. St Louis, Mosby, 1964

Egerer I, Tasman W, Tomer TL: Coats' disease. Arch Ophthalmol 92:109, 1974

Ellsworth RM: Practical management of retinoblastoma. Trans Am Ophthalmol Soc 67:462, 1969

Holmes LB: Norrie's disease: X-linked syndrome of retinal malformation, mental retardation, deafness. J Pediatr 79:89, 1971

Howard RO, Breg WR, Alber DM, Lesser RL: Retinoblastoma and chromosome abnormality. Arch Ophthalmol 92:490, 1974

Patz A: Retrolental fibroplasia. Surv Ophthalmol 14:1, 1969

Ramirez LD, de Buen S: Clinical and pathologic findings in 100 retinoblastoma patients. J Pediatr Ophthalmol 10:12, 1973

Reese AB: Tumors of the Eye, 2nd ed. New York, Harper & Row, 1963
——— Straatsma BR: Retinal dysplasia. Am J Ophthalmol 45:199, 1959

Tasman W (ed): Retinal Diseases in Children. New York, Harper & Row, 1971

Wolff SM: The ocular manifestations of congenital rubella. J Pediatr Ophthalmol 10:101, 1973

NEURO-OPHTHALMOLOGY

Congenital Anomalies of Optic Nerve

Hypoplasia of the optic disc is a rare anomaly always associated with severe amblyopia. The optic disc is one-half to one-third normal size and is pale with blurred margins. The central retinal vessels are large in comparison with the small nerve head. Hypoplasia is usually an isolated developmental defect, but it may occur with microphthalmos or in association with widespread brain malformations. Ingestion of quinine by the mother during the first weeks of pregnancy has been implicated in the production of optic nerve hypoplasia.

Optic nerve pits are congenital, and the stationary dark gray holes are usually on the temporal side of one disc. The involved optic nerve is larger than normal. The pits are important clinically in that they may produce arcuate scotomas and macular edema with permanent loss of central vision.

Drusen (hyaline bodies) of the optic nerve are white or yellow translucent spheres lying in front of the lamina cribrosa, especially on the nasal side of the optic disc. They may elevate the nerve head, thus simulating papilledema. In young children they may be inconspicuous, but within one to two decades the drusen become visible on the disc surface as shiny, refractile bodies that glow with indirect light. In adulthood visual field defects may appear and progress slowly. Central visual acuity is usually not affected. Drusen are found predominantly in blond white children and never occur in Orientals or blacks. They have been described with retinitis pigmentosa, tuberous sclerosis, angioid streaks, and meningiomas, but usually they are not associated with other ocular or nervous system disease. Some cases are hereditary (irregular dominant).

Besides optic nerve drusen, two other congenital anomalies may produce an elevation of the disc. Moderate to severe hyperopia in children associated with excessive glial tissue on the nerve head, or persistent hyaloid remnants on the optic disc, may produce an anomalous elevation of the nerve head. Both of these anomalies may be distinguished from true papilledema by the presence of a central cup and the absence of edema, exudate, hemorrhage, venous dilatation, or visual field defect.

Medullated nerve fibers are extremely common developmental anomalies occurring in 0.3 to 0.4 percent of eye patients. In this anomaly, myelinization fails to stop at the lamina cribrosa and appears on the optic disc and in the retina as patches of glistening white fibers with feathered edges. The medullated fibers may surround the optic disc and simulate papilledema. Less frequently they appear as isolated patches in the peripheral retina where they may be confused with retinal exudate or chorioretinitis. Relative scotomas may occur, but visual acuity is usually not affected. Medullated nerve fibers occur more frequently in males, and they are associated with myopia, oxycephaly, and neurofibromatosis.

Papilledema

Papilledema is a swelling of the optic nerve head due to an increase in intracranial pressure. It is characterized by an elevation of the optic papilla, with blurring of the disc margins, obliteration of the physiologic cup, venous congestion, loss of venous pulsations, splinter hemorrhages distributed radially around the disc margins, and edema of the adjacent retina producing an enlarged blind spot on visual field testing. Vision is rarely affected; when it is affected it is usually only after the swelling has persisted for months. It differs from papillitis (optic neuritis) by the absence of inflammatory signs (cells in the vitreous), centrocecal scotoma, and pain with movement of the eye. Both papilledema and papillitis may be confused with pseudopapilledema, in which an elevation of the disc is secondary to drusen or excessive glial tissue on the disc surface. Conditions that characteristically produce papilledema in children are tumors (craniopharyngiomas, cerebellar medulloblastoma), head injuries, hydrocephalus, central nervous system infections (Guillain-Barré syndrome, meningitis), and pseudotumor cerebri.

Pseudotumor cerebri (meningeal hydrops, benign intracranial hypertension) occurs most often in overweight young to middle aged females, but it can occur in infants and children. Symptoms are headache and diplopia (secondary to sixth nerve palsy). Occasionally visual field defects or decreased vision develop. Although papilledema is evident, the ventricles are either normal in size or small, as seen on pneumoencephalography. Presumably there is an obstruction to outflow or an increased secretion of cerebrospinal fluid. Specific causes in children include thrombosis of the lateral and sagittal sinuses from dehydration or otitis media and mastoiditis (particularly on the right side), Cushing's or Addison's disease, corticosteroids, tetracyclines, and vitamin A intoxication. Most cases, however, are idiopathic. The prognosis is usually good, with spontaneous resolution and no sequelae. In 25 percent of patients an intracranial tumor is discovered in later years; so periodic neurologic follow-up is indicated.

Optic Neuritis

Optic neuritis refers to both *papillitis* (apparent on the nerve head) and *retrobulbar neuritis* (involvement of the nerve behind the globe). It is characterized by profound loss of central vision, pain on movement of the eye, centrocecal scotoma, depressed color vision, and afferent pupillary defect.

Optic neuritis in children may result from inflammation in contiguous structures or from systemic infection. Optic neuritis secondary to meningoencephalitis is most common in children; it accounts for most of the cases of bilateral optic neuritis in the first decade of life. The optic nerves may be involved by spread from orbital abscesses, cellulitis, and foci of infection in the teeth, tonsils, and sinuses. Optic neuritis may occur in infective diseases that are more prevalent in childhood, such as measles, chickenpox, mumps, pertussis, poliomyelitis, and in other communicable diseases not especially confined to children, such as infectious mononucleosis, Asiatic influenza, and smallpox. Usually the optic neuritis appears 1 to 2 weeks after the onset of the infectious illness and resolves completely. Occasionally, marked loss of vision results, with partial or complete atrophy of the nerve. Syphilis was once a common cause of optic neuritis. Ascending polyneuritis (Guillain-Barré) may be accompanied by optic neuritis. Behçet's disease is characterized by the triad of relapsing ulcers of the mouth and genitalia, chronic uveitis with hypopyon, and optic neuritis.

The optic neuritides due to demyelinating disease in children usually fall into the class of diffuse sclerosis. *Multiple sclerosis* (disseminated sclerosis) can occur at a young age, but rarely occurs under the age of 10 years. Unlike multiple sclerosis, the diseases under the heading of diffuse sclerosis tend to involve the cerebral hemispheres. They include Schilder's disesase and various leukodystrophies. *Schilder's disease* (encephalitis periaxialis diffusa) may occur with optic neuritis in the first few decades of life. It has a rapid, often fatal, course. The *leukodystrophies* are inborn errors of metabolism, usually beginning in childhood. They are similar to Schilder's disease. Optic atrophy is frequent, but a definite history of optic neuritis is often absent. *Devic's disease* (opticomyelitis) is an acute bilateral optic neuritis associated with paraplegia and incontinence. In children it may run a rapid, severe, even fatal, course. It may be a manifestation of demyelinating disease, or it may be inflammatory in origin.

Other causes of childhood neuritides include intraocular inflammation (choroiditis, retinitis), drugs (chloroquine, chloramphenicol), toxins (methyl alcohol, lead), metabolic diseases (diabetes, anemia, pellagra, beriberi), and glioma of the optic nerve.

The treatment of optic neuritis with corticosteroids is controversial. Although steroids may hasten the return of vision in some patients, there is no proof that they change the ultimate visual prognosis.

Optic Atrophy

Optic atrophy indicates a permanent loss of function of part or all of the optic nerve. There is pallor or the nerve head due to decreased vascularity and gliosis.

The optic nerve head of the normal infant is paler than that of the adult; therefore a diagnosis of optic atrophy and blindness in the infant should be made only when one is very sure of the findings. *Kestenbaum's sign* may be a reliable indicator of optic atrophy. Normally, approximately ten arterioles cross the margin of the disc, but Kestenbaum consistently noted less than seven in optic atrophy.

The causes of optic atrophy in childhood are summarized in Table 3. The most common cause is an expanding lesion of the orbit—frequently glioma of the optic nerve. This diagnosis should be suspected in a child exhibiting unilateral optic atrophy, exophthalmos, and x-ray evidence of an enlarged optic foramen. Optic nerve gliomas are most common in the first decade, particularly in girls. They grow slowly and do not metastasize, but they can involve the chiasm to produce a gourdlike deformity of the sella turcica. Their treatment is controversial; it may consist of surgical excision, irradiation, or simply observation, depending on the specific case.

Hereditary forms of optic atrophy have a characteristic spontaneous and often sudden loss of vision to 20/200 or less with bilateral central scotomas. Thereafter, vision deteriorates only slightly and rarely is lost completely. *Leber's optic atrophy* may develop at any age, but it usually begins in the late teens or early twenties. It is inherited as a sex-linked recessive trait and may be associated with hereditary ataxia. True congenital optic atrophy is a rare defect transmitted as a dominant trait in which signs of optic atrophy are present at birth.

Ocular Motor Nerves

THIRD AND FOURTH NERVES. Congenital palsies at the third cranial nerve are rare. More commonly there is selective paresis of the levator and superior rectus muscles together. Children with congenital fourth nerve palsies (superior oblique muscle) may develop a head tilt that compensates so well for the ocular motor paralysis that the cause of torticollis may not be realized. Some patients have reportedly undergone tenotomies of the sternocleidomastoid muscle under the mistaken impression that the neck muscles were at fault. The fourth cranial nerve is easily damaged by closed head trauma, because it comes off the brainstem dorsally and can be pressed against the tentorium.

SIXTH NERVE. Sixth nerve palsies are quite common and are of special interest in children. They are characterized by inability to turn the eye out beyond the midline, diplopia, and head turn toward the side of the palsy. Frequent causes are purulent meningitis, increased intracranial pressure, skull fractures, intracranial neoplasm (particularly pontine glioma), and viral infections. Postinfectious sixth nerve palsies develop 7 to 21 days after a viral upper respiratory illness and nearly always resolve within 10 weeks. If a sixth nerve palsy follows a cold or other viral illness, diagnostic studies for tumor should be deferred. A special cause of abducens palsy follows middle ear infections or mas-

TABLE 3. Optic Atrophy in Childhood

1. Hereditary optic atrophy
   X-linked type, Leber's disease
   Dominant type
   Recessive type
   Congenital type
2. Developmental defect with cerebral palsy, other neurologic defects
3. Hydranencephaly, craniostenosis (oxycephaly), hydrocephalus
4. Heredodegenerative diseases of children
   Bielschowsky's disease
   Tay-Sachs disease
   Metachromatic leukodystrophy
   Spongy degeneration of brain
   Infantile neuronal axial dystrophy
5. Glioma, optic nerve
6. Intracranial tumors: craniopharyngioma, glioma, meningioma, pinealoma, cerebellar medulloblastoma
7. Multiple sclerosis, Devic's disease, diffuse sclerosis
8. Acute viral illness
9. Syphilis
10. Charcot-Marie-Tooth disease
11. Hyperparathyroidism, osteopetrosis
12. Toxins, plumbism
13. Idiopathic disease

toiditis (Gradenigo's syndrome): an osteitis of the petrous pyramid develops, producing diplopia, facial pain (fifth nerve involvement), and deafness. Duane's syndrome is a simulated sixth nerve palsy caused by anomalous innervation to the extraocular muscles. On attempted abduction, there is cocontraction of the medial and lateral rectus muscles that prevents abduction of the eye past the midline. Abducens palsy (more often on the left) may occur transiently in the newborn due to birth trauma or other factors. Full recovery of function within 6 weeks is the rule.

Moebius syndrome is a curious anomaly that combines palsies of several cranial nerves. A bilateral and asymmetric seventh nerve paralysis creates a mask face, with open drooling mouth and eyelids that do not close completely. Esotropia (sixth nerve), ptosis (third nerve), deafness (eighth nerve), and corneal anesthesia (fifth nerve) may also occur less often. Presumably the etiology is a nuclear aplasia in the brainstem. Other associated anomalies include webbed neck, fingers, and toes, supernumerary digits, and mental retardation.

Pontine gliomas are the most frequent cause of multiple bulbar palsies in childhood. All of the ocular motor nerves can be affected, as well as nerves five, six, and eight. Vertical nystagmus and cerebellar ataxia are frequent, but signs of increased intracranial pressure such as papilledema are late.

Motility Disorders Secondary to Brainstem Lesions

Parinaud's syndrome results directly from lesions in the vicinity of the upper midbrain (near superior colliculi) or indirectly from conditions that elevate the pressure in the third ventricle. The characteristic signs are paralysis of upward gaze, a less marked weakness of downward gaze, poor convergence and accommodation, retraction nystagmus with attempted upward or downward gaze, failure of the pupil to react to light with preservation of reaction to near, and lid retraction (Collier's sign). The most common causes of this syndrome include pinealoma, internal hydrocephalus, third ventricle tumor, aqueduct stenosis, trauma, encephalitis, syphilis, and congenital defect.

Skew deviation is any vertical imbalance of the eyes (a hypertropia or elevation of one eye above the other) not due to an extraocular muscle or nerve lesion. Brainstem contusion and posterior fossa tumor or wound are frequent causes. The low eye is often, although not invariably on the side of the lesion.

Ocular motor apraxia is a loss of lateral gaze following movement. The child turns his head until his eyes pick up fixation. An overshoot of the head occurs, followed by a jerk of the head back and a characteristic blink of the eyes. The site of the underlying lesion is unknown. The congenital form of this disorder tends to subside during the first and second decades (head thrust becomes much less prominent). Affected children may be otherwise normal or may have other neurologic diseases such as hydrocephalus and mental and physical retardation. Interestingly, ocular motor apraxia occurs in the vertical plane in ataxia-telangiectasia.

Nystagmus

Nystagmus consists of involuntary rhythmic to-and-fro movements of the eyes of either the pendular or the jerk type. *Pendular nystagmus* is composed of to-and-fro oscillations that are equal in rate. *Jerk nystagmus* has two phases: a slow drifting phase in one direction followed by a rapid recovery jerk in the opposite direction. By convention, the direction of the rapid recovery movement is used to designate the direction of the jerk nystagmus. For discussion purposes, childhood nystagmus may conveniently be divided into four main types: ocular, congenital, neurologic, and opticokinetic.

Ocular nystagmus is pendular in type and is secondary to some impairment in vision early in life (before 2 years) that prevents the development of normal fixation reflexes. Causes can include congenital anomalies of the optic nerves (hypoplasia, optic atrophy), bilateral failure of macular development (albinism, aniridia, high myopia, total color blindness), or congenital opacities of the cornea or lens. A loss of central vision after the age of 2 years results in the development of irregular searching movements of the eyes, but no true nystagmus; central visual loss after the age of 6 years is not accompanied by nystagmus. Latent nystagmus is a special form of ocular nystagmus elicited only by covering one eye. Since monocular visual acuity is much poorer than binocular visual acuity, a child with latent nystagmus may do poorly on school vision tests unless binocular as well as monocular vision is tested.

Congenital nystagmus may be pendular or jerky. Usually it is pendular over a narrow range of gaze and jerky elsewhere. Congenital nystagmus is present at birth, but it is not commonly detected before the age of 2 to 3 months (when fixation and conjugate movements develop). The nystagmus may be horizontal (most common), vertical, or rotary, or a combination of these, and it is invariably bilateral. Although hereditary cases have been described, most cases are sporadic and of unknown etiology. Frequently there is a position of gaze in which the nystagmus is greatest and one in which it is least (optimum position). The child may develop a head turn to take advantage of the eye position with least nystagmus. When the position of least nystagmus is in extreme gaze with a marked head turn, surgery can be done to reset the muscles on the eyes (move the eyes in the direction of the head turn) and put the optimum position in a more favorable viewing position. Congenital nystagmus is characteristically variable. It can be quite violent in association with excitement or stress, and it may be absent when the child is relaxed or sedated. Almost invariably there is some visual impairment, but near vision may be remarkably good. A child should not be discouraged from holding reading material close to the eyes or in an eccentric position, since he may achieve quite good near vision in this manner. His early education should be fostered and encouraged, because as the child becomes older his nystagmus will tend to decrease and his educational achievements may be unlimited.

Neurologic nystagmus includes a number of forms of acquired nystagmus that are usually jerky in type and secondary to lesions in the vestibular apparatus, the cerebellum, or the brainstem. Peripheral vestibular disease (labyrinthine) produces horizontal and rotary nystagmus with vertigo. Vestibular nuclear lesions produce horizontal, rotary, or vertical nystagmus, with the fast phase toward the diseased side. Brainstem lesions often cause vertical nystagmus. Cerebellar lesions are associated with jerk nystagmus to the same side as the lesion.

Ocular myoclonus or dancing-eye syndrome is an unusual form of nystagmus that follows encephalitis. Bilateral intermittent bursts of high-frequency to-and-fro jerks (no slow phase) are the same frequency in all cases (100 oscillations per minute). Mainly horizontal, these jerky movements persist during sleep.

Opsoclonus consists of bizarre, chaotic conjugate eye movements in young patients following an acute febrile illness, or in unconscious patients with encephalitis or brainstem disease. The to-and-fro oscillations are irregular and nonrhythmic in both horizontal and vertical directions. An awake individual may have to close his eyes to reduce the awareness of ocular movement. Truncal ataxia may be associated. The illness usually clears spontaneously in a few weeks to months if there is no major underlying disease. Opsoclonus is typically a major feature of a syndrome referred to as Kinsbourne's infantile myoclonic encephalopathy, acute cerebellar encephalopathy, or infantile polymyoclonus. This syndrome, characterized by opsoclonus, cerebellar ataxia, hypotonia, and myoclonic jerks of the face and body, is frequently associated with neuroblastoma.

Spasmus nutans is a rapid, pendular, asymmetric horizontal nystagmus that varies in different directions of gaze. There is associated nodding of the head, and even an anomalous head tilt may occur. The nystagmus may disappear when the head is supine. Affected infants are normal. Generally the onset is between the ages of 6 weeks and 3 years. Spontaneous resolution in 2 to 3 months is the rule, although cases have persisted up to the age of 8 years. Spasmus nutans is distinguished from congenital nystagmus by its asymmetric nature, by its characteristic head nodding, and by its inevitable recovery, usually before the end of the third year.

Opticokinetic nystagmus (OKN) is produced by fixating a line on a rotating drum (railroad nystagmus). The slow phase is a following movement (in the direction of the turning drum), and the fast phase is a corrective movement. OKN is valuable in evaluating the presence of vision in infants and malingerers. It is also useful in localizing neurologic lesions. In parietal or occipital lobe lesions, for example, OKN is either poor or absent on rotating the drum toward the side of the lesion. In brainstem lesions there is usually a bilateral disturbance associated with a gaze palsy.

Ocular Myopathies

Myasthenia gravis may occur in a transient form in an infant whose mother has the disease. The infant exhibits flaccidity, droopy lids, and a poor suck for 2 to 3 weeks after birth. It is possible that a cholinesterase substance was transferred across the placenta, creating the state of muscle weakness in the infant. The usual onset of myasthenia gravis is in the second or third decade, but it can occur at any age.

Chronic progressive external ophthalmoplegia is a bilateral, usually symmetric, gradual external ophthalmoplegia (pupil and accommodation are not affected) and ptosis. In 50 percent of cases there is a family history, and transmission is usually dominant. Occasionally the disorder may be congenital, but usually the onset is in childhood or adolescence. Associated findings include retinitis pigmentosa (frequently involving only the posterior pole with a normal ERG), spinocerebellar atrophy, cardiac arrhythmias, weak face and pharyngeal muscles, pancreatic insufficiency, and testicular atrophy. Ptosis surgery must be avoided because of the inability to close the lids.

Myotonia congenita or Thomsen's disease is the congenital form of myotonic dystrophy. Symptoms of skeletal muscle myotonia and atrophy develop in childhood and may become worse at puberty; however, severe disability is rare. Eye signs are infrequent; they include ptosis and sluggish extraocular movements. Mental retardation is usual. Myotonic dystrophy, occurs in young adulthood, and eye involvement is a more prominent feature. Bilateral, anterior, and posterior cortical polychromatic opacities in the lens are almost pathognomonic. Other ocular findings include retinitis pigmentosa, ptosis, weak orbicularis, poorly reactive pupils, and low intraocular pressure.

Migraine

Migraine with associated visual symptoms and ophthalmoplegia is frequent in older children. Although it may occur in infancy, many cases begin at puberty. Familial cases are inherited as a dominant trait. Visual symptoms occurring with or without headaches include scintillating scotomas, homonomous scotomas, and even total hemianopsia. Characteristically the visual scotomas last 15 to 20 minutes and may be followed by a severe unilateral headache, which lasts from hours to days. Ophthalmoplegia may involve any of the ocular motor nerves, although recurring third nerve paralysis on the same side as the headache is most common. After several years of recurrent attacks, third nerve function may be permanently impaired.

References

Apt L: Headaches in infants and children. Int Ophthalmol Clin 2:859, 1962

Bienfama DC: Opsoclonus in infancy. Arch Ophthalmol 91:203, 1974

Caughey JE: Relationship of dystrophia myotonica (myotonic dystrophy) and myotonia congenita (Thomsen's disease). Neurology 8:469, 1958

Cogan DG: Neurology of the Visual System, 3rd ed. Springfield, Ill, Charles C Thomas, 1968

Ford FR: Diseases of the Nervous System in Infancy, Childhood and Adolescence, 5th ed. Springfield, Ill, Charles C Thomas, 1966

François J: Diagnosis of blindness in the infant. Ann Ophthalmol 2:533, 1970

Gass JDM: Serous detachment of the macula secondary to congenital pit of the optic nerve head. Am J Ophthalmol 67:821, 1969

Hoyt WF, Pont ME: Pseudopapilledema; anomalous elevation of optic disc; pitfalls in diagnosis and management. JAMA 181:191, 1962

Iverson HA: Hereditary optic atrophy. Arch Ophthalmol 59:850, 1958

Jayalakshmi D, McNair ST, Tucker S, Schaffer D: Infantile nystagmus: a prospective study of spasmus nutans, congenital nystagmus, and unclassified nystagmus of infancy. J Pediatr 77:177, 1970

Knox DL, Clark DB, Schuster FF: Benign VI nerve palsies in children. Pediatrics 40:560, 1967

Lloyd LA: Optic neuritis in children. Trans Can Ophthalmol Soc 21-22:108, 1959

McKeever GE: Myasthenia gravis in a mother and her unborn son. JAMA 147:320, 1951

McKinna A: Quinine induced hypoplasia of the optic nerve. Can J Ophthalmol 1:261, 1966

Merz M, Wojtowicz S: The Moebius syndrome. Am J Ophthalmol 63:837, 1967

Millichap JG: Benign intracranial hypertension and otitic hydrocephalus. Pediatrics 23:257, 1959

Pollack IP, Becker B: Hyaline bodies (drusen) of optic nerve. Am J Ophthalmol 54:651, 1962

Spaulding WL: Glioma of the optic nerve and its management. Am J Ophthalmol 46:654, 1958

Stanworth A: Ocular myopathies. Trans Ophthalmol Soc UK 83:515, 1963

Van Pelt W, Andermann F: On the early onset of ophthalmologic migraine. Am J Dis Child 107:628, 1964

Walsh FB, Hoyt WF: Clinical Neurophthalmology, Vols 1–3. Baltimore, Williams & Wilkins, 1969

STRABISMUS

Strabismus (squint, crossed eyes, walleye) affects about 3 percent of children. Early recognition of strabismus is essential for the restoration of vision and the establishment of binocular visual patterns. The earlier the strabismus therapy is begun, the better is the prognosis for both a functional and a cosmetic cure. No infant or child is too young to have an eye examination and to have treatment initiated. Children do not outgrow a constant monocular deviation. A child with crossed eyes or *esotropia* may look better upon becoming older because of the normal tendency for convergence tone to decrease with time, but amblyopia as an abnormal sensory visual function remains. Most children who apparently have outgrown their crossed eyes never had a true deviation. For example, eyes may appear esotropic because of epicanthal folds, which may create an illusion of crossed eyes.

Transient strabismus may be normal in the first 4 months of life, during the period of macular development. Any transient deviation after the age of 4 months, or a constant strabismus at *any* age, requires prompt referral to an ophthalmologist for diagnosis and therapy. It is significant that certain intraocular diseases (eg, retinoblastoma, toxocariasis, retrolental fibroplasia, and congenital cataract) may present early as transient or constant ocular deviation.

The fundamental disturbance in most cases of strabismus is an abnormal innervation from supranuclear sources. The nerves and the extraocular muscles usually are normal. Paralytic (noncomitant) types of strabismus are far less common in children than nonparalytic (comitant) types. Occasionally strabismus may be due to anisometropia, a difference in refractive error between the two eyes. In these cases the eye with the greatest refractive error becomes the deviating, and often amblyopic, eye.

DIAGNOSIS. Strabismus can be diagnosed in infants by observing the corneal light reflex when the patient fixes on a small light source. The light reflections should be in the center or just nasal of center in each pupil. In older children the more accurate *cover–uncover test* may be used. If when one eye is covered the other eye moves to fix on a light, the patient has strabismus. This test and the corneal light reflex test will reveal cases of strabismus not evident at first inspection. A visual acuity determination is an important part of the testing for strabismus. Amblyopia is not related to the size of the deviation; thus a small, inapparent deviation may lead to a profound loss of vision.

Neither physicians nor laymen are sufficiently aware that strabismus is one of the leading causes of monocular blindness and that in nearly every instance this blindness is preventable. Loss of vision in the deviating eye (lazy eye) of the strabismic child is termed *amblyopia ex anopsia*, or suppression amblyopia. Strabismic amblyopia originates from confusion and stimulus deprivation; the fovea of the nonpreferred eye perceives a confusing image that is overruled by the stronger foveal image of the preferred eye. Image incongruity and stimulus deprivation lead to neurophysiologic anomalies in the striate and prestriate cortex and morphologic changes in the lateral geniculate body. These changes have been confirmed in the primate (rhesus monkey)

and are assumed to occur in humans. The extent of visual loss in strabismic (suppression) amblyopia may range from a minimal decrease in acuity to legal blindness (20/200 or less).

Strabismic amblyopia treated early enough may be reversed. The most effective treatment of amblyopia is total occlusion of the preferred eye with a patch. The earlier this treatment is begun, the easier and more effective it is, and the least troublesome to the patient. In general, the age of 6 years is critical for arresting or reversing amblyopia of this type; beyond that age patching of the normal eye usually does not effect significant improvement in the vision of an eye that has been constantly deviated. Thus routine vision and strabismus screening at 4 years of age is urged. Amblyopic patients need to be followed into adolescence to detect and treat any recurrence of amblyopia in the successfully treated eye.

CLASSIFICATION. Strabismus may be internal (convergent, also called *esotropia*), external (divergent, *exotropia*), vertical (*hypertropia* when one eye is above the visual axis, hypotropia when one eye is lower), and occasionally torsional (*cyclotropia*). Frequently horizontal strabismus is complicated by a vertical component; this reduces the likelihood of a functional cure. In most cases of strabismus one eye is consistently deviated; this is known as monocular strabismus. A smaller number of patients, termed alternators, fix equally well with either eye. In general the monocular type is associated with amblyopia. The use of both eyes in the alternating variety permits vision development of both eyes.

Convergent strabismus (esotropia) in children may be congenital or acquired. Congenital esotropia is secondary to failure of proper development of binocular fusion associated with abnormal tonic innervation. This type of esotropia is usually well developed by the age of 4 to 6 months and is little influenced by any form of medical treatment. Surgery usually is performed before the age of 18 months.

Convergent strabismus of the acquired type is frequently accommodative in origin, thus indicating a disturbance in the intimate association of accommodation with convergence mediated by the brain. In an attempt to see clearly, the child must accommodate, and in so doing he exerts an abnormal degree of convergence. If the accommodative need can be satisfied in some fashion that does not require active accommodation, the associated overconvergence may be prevented. Glasses that remove the need for accommodation may be prescribed. The child then can see clearly and at the same time avoid the necessity for undue convergence. The fact that most children are hyperopic (farsighted), which requires extra accommodation, underlies the frequency of this form of strabismus. The onset of accommodative esotropia is from about 18 months to 4 years of age, corresponding to the maturation of the accommodation–convergence mechanism and to the developing interest of the child in his environment. Usually the child who is carried through the early years with suitable glasses will retain a natural binocular mechanism. Frequently the power of the glass prescribed may be somewhat excessive for correction of vision, but it prevents crossing of the visual axes. In time the overcorrection may be reduced or glasses may be eliminated completely. Additional means of treatment include bifocal glasses, which reduce the need for increased accommodation with near targets, and anticholinesterase drugs (miotics), which by their action on the ciliary body induce peripheral rather than central accommodation and thus lessen convergence. Surgery is not indicated in purely accommodative cases. In mixed types, surgery is restricted to the nonaccommodative portion of the deviation.

Divergent strabismus (exotropia) may be intermittent or constant. Intermittent exotropia has an early onset, often near birth, and is associated with little or no significant refractive error. The deviation occurs when the child looks at distant objects, and it is exaggerated when he is tired or daydreaming. The child may rub his eyes or close one eye when outdoors (a reaction to diplopia). Soon suppression of the deviating eye develops, and the deviation becomes more constant. Treatment consists of orthoptics (to combat suppression and build fusional amplitudes) and surgery. Many functional and cosmetic cures may result from surgery. A constant exotropia is almost invariably a surgical problem, whether it evolves from a previously intermittent divergent strabismus or occurs as a congenital anomaly or follows the loss of vision in the other eye. It is characteristic of a blind eye to become divergent in time.

Vertical strabismus (hypertropia or hypotropia) usually results from overaction or underaction of the vertical rectus and oblique muscles. The diagnosis of vertical muscle imbalance requires a sound knowledge of the anatomy and physiology of the extraocular muscles. Surgery is usually necessary to restore physiologic function of the vertical muscles. Surgery in strabismus may be unilateral or bilateral. As a rule, only a few days of hospitalization are necessary, and the operative risk is due primarily to general anesthesia. Convalescence of a week is sufficient before returning to full activity. The observation and care of the strabismic child do not end with surgery, but continue through the formative years until a stable binocular relationship has been firmly established.

Paralytic strabismus (noncomitant strabismus) is characterized by a deviation that varies in degree according to the direction of gaze and also according to whether the patient fixates with the good eye or with the affected eye. Total paralysis or partial paralysis (paresis) may affect a single muscle or group of muscles and usually is indicative of a neurogenic or myogenic lesion. Congenital anomalies and birth trauma may be causative. Paresis of a muscle may be evidenced by underaction as the eye rotates into its field of action (primary deviation), but more often an overaction of the yoke muscle in the good eye (secondary deviation) is noted. Surgery may be directed toward strengthening the weak muscle or weakening the overacting yoke muscle.

Ocular torticollis: In an effort to achieve binocular single vision or to assume a more favorable position of the eyes, the patient with a paretic lesion will often turn or tilt the head. Such head postures are often quite diagnostic. Head tilts are usually due to weakness of a vertical muscle or a superior oblique muscle, whereas head turns are due to paresis of the horizontal muscles. An important distinction should be made between ocular and congenital torticollis. Head tilts and head turns based on an ocular cause may be corrected by surgery of the extraocular muscles; occasionally medical measures alone suffice (prisms, corrective lenses).

References

Burian HM, von Noorden, GL: Binocular Vision and Ocular Motility: Theory and Management of Strabismus. St Louis, Mosby, 1974

Cogan DG: Neurology of the Ocular Muscles, 2nd ed. Springfield, Ill, Charles C Thomas, 1956

Duke-Elder S: Ocular motility and strabismus. In Duke-Elder S System of Ophthalmology, Vol VI. St Louis, Mosby, 1973

Gay AJ, Newman NM, Kettner JL, et al: Eye Movement Disorders. St Louis, Mosby, 1974

Manley DR: Strabismus. In Harley RD (ed): Pediatric Ophthalmology. Philadelphia, WB Saunders, 1974

Windsor CE, Hurtt J: Eye Muscle Problems in Childhood. St Louis, Mosby, 1974

REFRACTIVE ERRORS

Emmetropia is the term for the ideal condition in which, without accommodation, parallel rays of light (from infinity) are brought to a point focus on the retina. Very few eyes correspond to this ideal. At birth the eye is hyperopic (farsighted); that is, the increased curvature of the cornea cannot compensate for the smallness of the infant eye, and entering parallel rays of light are focused behind the eye. This *hyperopia* is 1 to 3 diopters in amount and remains stable or increases slightly until the age of 5 years. By the age of 6 years this physiologic hyperopia begins to decrease toward emmetropia, which is established at age 9 to 11 years. Moderate amounts of pathologic hyperopia may be overcome by the child's well-developed accommodative apparatus, and vision may be good. However, when the degree of hyperopia is unequal in the two eyes, the less hyperopic eye may become the preferred eye, since it requires less accommodative effort to see clearly, and the more hyperopic eye may become lazy or amblyopic (anisometropic amblyopia). Esotropia is frequently associated with hyperopia in childhood.

Myopia (nearsightedness) may begin to appear at age 9 to 11 years. It is often hereditary and is frequently associated with prematurity. The myopic eye has too much plus power, or is too long for its refractive power, and incident rays of light are brought to focus in front of the retina. Distance vision is blurred, but near vision may be normal. In most cases myopia tends to increase slowly until the individual stops growing in height and then remains unchanged. Two special forms of myopia may occur in children. Progressive or malignant myopia shows rapid progression each year until 20 years of age or beyond and is associated with vitreous and chorioretinal degeneration. High myopia of childhood results in 10 or more diopters of refractive error early in life. These children bump into things as soon as they learn to walk, and when examining objects they hold them close to their eyes. This type of myopia does not change significantly over the years.

Astigmatism is a condition in which rays of light are not refracted equally in all meridians, so that a point focus cannot be achieved. Astigmatism may be hyperopic or myopic. High degrees of oblique astigmatism may cause a tilting of the head. A child with astigmatism may hold reading matter close to the eyes to obtain a large, although blurred, retinal image.

Visual acuity should be checked routinely at about the age of 4 years, before starting school. Often a young child does not realize his vision is decreased, and he may not complain even if he has tired eyes (asthenopia). Behavior that may give clues to an uncorrected refractive error includes excessive blinking, frowning, squinting, tilting of the head when looking at objects, and frequent rubbing of the eyes. The child may hold books close to his face or avoid close work; he may skip words or lines, lose his place while reading, or read slowly; he may shut or cover one eye or exhibit general fatigue, drowsiness, or irritability after prolonged use of the eyes. Complaints of double vision, headaches, itching, burning, or watering of the eyes should alert the pediatrician to the possibility of decreased visual acuity.

TREATMENT.   Glasses are necessary to correct refractive errors (myopia, astigmatism, and higher amounts of hyperopia) in children or to reduce or correct the deviation in accommodative strabismus. The use of glasses does not increase a refractive error or prevent its progression; such changes occur irrespective of the wearing of glasses. Glasses serve to equalize and normalize vision, and where they are indicated they should be prescribed. Parental objections based on vanity or misconceptions should not be permitted to prevent a child from wearing glasses. The ability of contact lenses or atropine to inhibit the progression of the common type of myopia (school myopia) is doubted by most ophthalmologists.

Learning Disabilities

Learning disability has become a subject of considerable public concern. The inability of a child to read printed words with understanding is termed *dyslexia*. The term is used loosely to describe the condition of a child whose reading ability is two or more school grades below his age level. Approximately one-fifth of all children in the United States have some form of learning disability. Commonly the child with developmental dyslexia is a boy with normal intelligence and no physical (hearing, neurologic) defect who is brought to the physician because of his emotional reaction to his scholastic performance. Dyslexic children see and understand in ways different from those regarded as normal. They may reverse letters or the order of letters or words or demonstrate unusual spellings.

Most clues in word recognition are transmitted through our eyes to the brain. It seems natural, then, to attribute reading difficulties to defects in the eyes and vision. However, studies have shown that no eye defect produces dyslexia. In other words, eye defects do not cause reversals of letters or words. Children with developmental dyslexia have the same incidences of refractive errors, strabismus, and other eye abnormalities as normal children. Glasses should be prescribed if they are needed, but they are not a direct treatment for dyslexia. Methods to change hand or eye dominance and special eye exercises are claimed to be therapeutic by many nonmedical practitioners. There is no scientific evidence, however, that exercises of the eyes can improve perception or learning ability. The proper treatment of a dyslexic child should be left to educational scientists. The physician can contribute by correcting any physical disabilities that may interfere with function and by promptly referring such children to the appropriate educational facility. When dealing with a troublesome dyslexia problem optimally, the ophthalmologist should be a member of a team. The team may include the pediatrician, neurologist, otologist, psychologist, psychiatrist, social worker, and educator.

References

Flax N: Visual function in learning disabilities. J Learning Disabilities 1:551, Sept 1968

Goldberg HK, Drash PW: The disabled reader. J Pediatr Ophthalmol 5:11, 1968

Keeney AH, Keeney VT: Dyslexia: Diagnosis and Treatment of Reading Disorders. St Louis, Mosby, 1968

Sloane AE: Manual of Refraction. Boston, Little, Brown, 1970

THE ORBIT

Proptosis

The most frequent sign of disease of the orbit is proptosis. This term refers to a forward protrusion of the eye caused by a retrobulbar mass. *Exophthalmos* may be used synonymously, but is probably best used with reference to the condition seen in hyperthyroidism. A mass behind the eye may press on the optic nerve, producing papilledema and eventually optic atrophy. Extraocular movements may be impaired by involvement of nerves or direct interference with muscle action. Edema of the lids and chemosis are accompanied by variable degrees of orbital congestion. The cornea can suffer exposure damage if lid closure is inadequate.

The type of proptosis may give clues to the etiology. Intermittent proptosis is often due to a varix or vascular tumor in the orbit. Pulsating exophthalmos may result from an orbital aneurysm, meningocele, or carotid-cavernous fistula. The reducibility of the proptosis can be helpful. In general, inflammatory or malignant tumor masses are not compressible and do not allow the eye to be pushed back into the orbit.

The degree of proptosis should be measured with an exophthalmometer, because visual estimates may be misleading. A pseudoexophthalmos may be produced by a number of conditions, including lid retraction, shallow orbits, buphthalmos, and high myopia. Black persons commonly have shallow orbital formation and apparent proptosis. The average distance from the lateral orbital margin to the cornea is about 16 mm. A difference of more than 2 mm between the two eyes is considered significant. The evaluation of proptosis frequently includes x-rays of the orbits and optic foramina, orbital venography or angiography, and ultrasonography. A biopsy of an orbital mass may be necessary for diagnosis. The common causes of proptosis in children are listed in Table 4. This table can be used as a guide for discussing orbital diseases in children.

TABLE 4. Causes of Proptosis in Children

Developmental	Craniosynostosis, craniofacial dysostosis, mandibulofacial dysostosis, meningocele and encephalocele
Neoplastic	
Primary	Cavernous hemangioma, rhabdomyosarcoma, dermoid cyst, glioma of optic nerve, inflammatory pseudotumor
Secondary and metastatic	Lymphoma, leukemic infiltration, neurofibroma, retinoblastoma, neuroblastoma, chloroma
Traumatic	Orbital hemorrhage
Inflammatory	Orbital cellulitis (acute ethmoiditis), mucocele
Metabolic	Hyperthyroidism, reticuloendotheliosis (Hand-Schüller-Christian disease)

A number of *developmental anomalies of the skull and face* involve the orbit. Some have their origin in premature fusion of the cranial bones (craniosynostosis). Oxycephaly (tower skull), caused by fusion of both coronal and sagittal sutures, is associated with proptosis due to shallowness of the orbits. Divergent strabismus is common. Increased intracranial pressure leads in some cases to papilledema, followed by optic atrophy and severe visual loss. In plagiocephaly the ocular disturbance is usually asymmetric. Scaphocephaly less frequently involves the orbits, and visual impairment is rare. Crouzon's disease (craniofacial dysostosis) includes acrocephaly, marked proptosis or even prolapse of the globes, divergent strabismus, antimongoloid palpebral fissure obliquity, nystagmus, and optic atrophy. Apert's syndrome is similar to Crouzon's disease. Hypertelorism is an excessively wide separation of the eyes (greater than 33 mm between the two caruncles). Ocular findings include ptosis, inverse epicanthus, laterally displaced puncta, divergent strabismus, and optic atrophy. The finding of hypertelorism should also alert the pediatrician to Waardenburg's syndrome and Cornelia DeLange syndrome. Franceschetti's syndrome (Treacher-Collins syndrome) shows a variety of defects of the lids, facial bones, and ears. The complete form

includes antimongoloid palpebral fissure slant, symmetric colobomas of the lids, and abnormalities of the lashes. Three other related mandibulofacial dysostoses are oculoauriculovertebral dysplasia (Goldenhar's syndrome), Pierre Robin syndrome, and Hallerman-Streiff syndrome. The four syndromes represent abnormalities of the eyes and of the structures arising from the first and second brachial arches.

Of the *neoplasms* that may involve the orbit, hemangiomas are the most common. These are developmental tumors appearing at birth or during the first months of life. They occur in two forms: capillary hemangioma or strawberry mark, usually found on the lids, and cavernous hemangioma, commonly located in the orbit. These tumors may demonstrate a period of rapid growth early in life, during which time they may invade the orbit with proptosis. As a rule, spontaneous regression then ensues, and the tumor may completely disappear. Treatment usually is not indicated until natural improvement has reached its maximum, because conventional forms of therapy (surgery, irradiation, cryotherapy, sclerosing solutions) may lead to increased deformity. Systemic corticosteroid therapy has arrested some rapidly growing lesions.

Dermoid cysts are choristomas of misplaced ectoderm usually located at the outer end of the eyebrow in the upper lid. They are attached to periosteum and may extend back into the orbit and erode bone. Histologically they consist of a cyst lined by surface epidermis with skin appendages. The central cavity contains keratin debris, hair, and sebum. Rupture of these cysts into the subcutaneous tissue creates a severe granulomatous inflammation. For this reason, and for cosmetic purposes, dermoid cysts are usually removed surgically.

Rhabdomyosarcoma is the most common malignant tumor of the orbit in children. The average age of onset is 7 to 8 years, and white males are most often affected. The tumor arises from embryonic mesenchyme, usually in the upper and inner portion of the orbit, causing rapidly progressive downward and outward proptosis. Rhabdomyosarcoma is a highly malignant cancer that infiltrates the orbit deeply, often beyond the margins of attempted excision. Metastases appear in the lungs and bones. The prognosis is extremely poor, with most patients surviving less than 2 years. The best chance for a cure is early diagnosis and treatment. Improved therapeutic results have been reported with treatment that includes radiation therapy, systemic chemotherapy, and exenteration.

Approximately 7 percent of all pediatric orbital tumors are metastatic cancers. The primary site is often asymptomatic, so that proptosis may be the initial presentation of the tumor. In over 20 percent of patients with neuroblastoma of the adrenal cortex, for example, eye symptoms are the presenting complaint. The ocular findings include proptosis, hemorrhagic edema of the lids and conjunctiva, signs of necrosis and infection of the eyelids, ptosis, extraocular muscle palsies, papilledema, and optic atrophy. The proptosis may be unilateral or bilateral and is frequently rapid in onset. Lymphomas may be present in the orbit, particularly the African lymphoma of Burkitt. This tumor usually produces proptosis, as well as edema and ecchymoses of the lids.

One of the most common causes of proptosis in children is *bacterial infection of the ethmoid sinuses.* The infection readily extends into the cellular tissue of the orbit, producing cellulitis and proptosis. Chemosis, discharge, diplopia, and fixation of the eyeball may be present. As a rule, the condition responds satisfactorily to systemic antibiotics. Mucoceles are cystic herniations into the orbit arising from chronic inflammation of the ethmoid or, rarely in children, the frontal sinuses. They contain a gelatinous secretion that may become purulent. Mucoceles enlarge slowly without pain unless secondary infection is present. Treatment consists of surgical excision.

Hyperthyroidism is encountered less frequently in children than in adults, but it is still a common cause of exophthalmos. The exophthalmos is accompanied by upper lid retraction, tearing, foreign body sensation in the eyes, chemosis, lid edema, injection of the globes, and diplopia. The exophthalmos usually subsides slowly when the hyperthyroidism is treated. Malignant exophthalmos of the type seen in adults with hyperthyroidism is not observed in children.

Reticuloendotheliosis of the Hand-Schüller-Christian type may involve the orbits of children and young adults. Proptosis of one or both eyes may occur when the xanthomatous deposits characteristic of this disease accumulate in the orbital soft tissues. Eosinophilic granuloma rarely may localize in the ortibal bones, particularly in the upper temporal portion of the orbit. *Juvenile xanthogranuloma* is a cutaneous lesion of infants that may involve the orbit as well as the conjunctiva, iris, ciliary body, and lids. In the orbit, lesions are localized around the extraocular muscles, and histologically they consist of proliferating histiocytic cells with Touton giant cells and eosinophils. Spontaneous resolution of these lesions is the rule, but in some cases corticosteroids or irradiation have been required.

References

Blodi FC: Developmental anomalies of the skull affecting the eye. Arch Ophthalmol 57:593, 1957

Coleman DJ, Jack RL, Franzen LA: Ultrasonography in pediatric opthalmology. J Pediatr Ophtalmol 9:111, 1972

Crawford JS: The orbit. In The Eye of Childhood. Toronto Hospital for Sick Children: Chicago, Year Book, 1967

Feman SS, Apt L: Eye findings associated with pediatric malignancy. J Pediatr Ophtalmol 9:224, 1972

Frayer WC, Enterline HT: Embryonal rhabdomyosarcoma of the orbit in children and young adults. Arch Ophthalmol 62:203, 1959

Gaynes PM, Cohen GS: Juvenile xanthogranuloma of the orbit. Am J Ophthalmol 63:755, 1967

Iliff CE, Ossofsky H: Tumors of the Eye and Adnexa in Infancy and Childhood. Springfield, Ill, Charles C Thomas, 1962.

Porterfield JR: Orbital tumors in children. Int Ophthalmol Clin 2:319, 1962

Rees AB: Tumors of the Eye, 2nd ed. New York, Harper & Row, 1963

Richards RD: Congenital hemangioma of the orbit and lid. South Med J 67:498, 1974

Sagerman RH, Tretter P, Elsworth RM: The treatment of orbital rhabdomyosarcoma of children with primary radiation therapy. Am J Roetgenol Radium Ther Nucl Med 114:31, 1972

Sutow WW, Sullivan MP, Ried RH, Taylor HG, Griffith KM: Prognosis in childhood rhabdomyosarcoma. Cancer 25:1384, 1970

OCULAR TRAUMA

Ocular injuries require prompt and correct care if useful vision is to be saved. Examination of eye injuries in young children is usually difficult. If an adequate examination cannot be performed by the nonophthalmologic physician, the patient should be referred to an eye physician for further care. Local anesthesia and sedation may permit the pediatrician to attend to minor ocular trauma, such as a superficial conjunctival foreign body, but use of instruments in the eye should be avoided. In cases where the nature and extent of the injury are unknown, light general anesthesia will allow the opthhalmologist to perform a controlled and accurate examination. Testing the patient's visual acuity before treatment, if possible, is important for diagnostic, prognostic, and medicolegal reasons.

Foreign Bodies

Conjunctival foreign bodies can usually be removed easily by flushing with a stream of isotonic saline solution or by using a moistened cotton-tip applicator. The upper eyelid should be everted and inspected if the foreign body is not readily located. A local anesthetic will facilitate the examination.

Corneal foreign bodies generally cause more pain and congestion of the eye and are potentially more serious than conjunctival foreign bodies. Fluorescein stain may help to demonstrate the foreign body. If the foreign body cannot be removed with irrigation or a moist cotton applicator, the patient should be referred to an ophthalmologist. Broad-spectrum topical antibiotics should be used after the foreign body is removed. Patching is usually not necessary. In all cases the cornea should be reexamined in 24 hours to rule out an infection of the abraded area. Metallic foreign bodies frequently leave a localized rust stain (rust ring). This is best removed by the ophthalmologist under slit-lamp magnification.

Suspected or known intraocular foreign bodies should be referred immediately to an eye physician. It is possible for small high-speed foreign bodies to penetrate the eye, causing transient pain or no pain at all. X-rays may be helpful in confirming the suspicion of an intraocular foreign body.

Corneal Abrasions

Abrasions of the cornea result from traumatic removal of a portion of the surface epithelium. Fluorescein may be added to the eye and the extent of the corneal abrasion determined under cobalt blue light. In general, abrasions are very painful and are accompanied by marked blepharospasm, tearing, and photophobia. An initial instillation of a topical anesthetic will facilitate the examination. Treatment consists of the instillation of a broad-spectrum antibiotic preparation such as Neosporin or Chloromycetin and the application of a firm pressure patch for 24 hours. Most abrasions heal completely in this time. Young children may resist patching, and it can be omitted if necessary. All cases should be reexamined in 24 hours to rule out the possibility of infection. Topical anesthetics should never be dispensed for home use; they will delay epithelial healing, and they can cause serious toxic keratoconjunctivitis.

Contusions

Contusion injuries result from blunt trauma to the globe and adnexa. They may vary in severity from ecchymosis of the eyelid (black eye) to anterior chamber hemorrhage (hyphema), dislocated lens, vitreous hemorrhage, retinal detachment, or rupture of the globe. All cases of contusion injury should have a thorough ophthalmologic evaluation. What may appear to be a minor blunt injury to the eye or adnexa may in fact be a serious intraocular injury.

Lacerations

Lacerations involving the eyelid margin or lacrimal passages should be treated by an ophthalmologist. Failure to accurately approximate the cut edges of the lid margin will result in a permanent notching of the lid. Lacerations or perforating injuries of the globe are an ocular emergency. In such cases the lids and conjunctiva may be markedly swollen, the anterior chamber shallow or flat, and the pupil nonreactive; the intraocular contents may be seen presenting at the wound site. Since lid squeezing may cause expulsion of intraocular tissues, examination should be cautious and limited. The eye should be covered with a patch or shield, and immediate referral should be made to an eye physician.

Burns

Chemical burns of the conjunctiva and cornea should be treated at once by copious irrigation with water or isotonic saline solution. Acid burns are less serious than alkali burns, because the acid precipitates proteins and forms its own barrier to penetration. Alkaline agents, in contrast, have a lytic action and readily penetrate the cornea, causing rapid and severe damage. In cases of alkali burns irrigation must be carried out until the ophthalmologist arrives. Further treatment consists of local antibiotics, cycloplegics, and corticosteriods.

Thermal burns of the cornea with cigarette ashes, match heads, etc, are not usually serious and can be treated in the same manner as an abrasion.

Radiation burns in the form of ultraviolet light from the sun, sunlamps, or welding arcs can produce a diffuse superficial punctate keratitis that is very painful. The keratitis follows the radiation exposure by 8 to 10 hours. Treatment consists of firm bilateral patching for 24 to 48 hours.

Birth Injuries

Mechanical trauma to the eye and lids may occur during any delivery, but it is more common in prolonged and difficult deliveries or ones in which instrumentation is used. Some injury to the eye or adnexa occurs in 20 to 25 percent of births, but fortunately its extent is usually mild.

Corneal injury may result in a steamy opacity of the cornea secondary to edema. Ruptures in Descemet's membrane are seen as parallel lines in the posterior cornea. The condition is usually uniocular, and ecchymoses of the lids and subconjunctival hemorrhage may be associated. The corneal edema usually clears within a few days or weeks, but later in life high myopia, marked astigmatism, or conical cornea may result in severe visual impairment with amblyopia and strabismus.

The most common ocular birth injury is *retinal hemorrhage,* which has a reported incidence of 18 to 19 percent of all births. The etiology and significance of these hemorrhages are not known. Proposed causes include venous congestion of the head and neck secondary to prolonged and difficult labor, sudden release of intracranial pressure with birth, asphyxia, capillary fragility, impaired blood coagulability, constriction of the neck by the umbilical cord, or difficult instrument delivery, particularly vacuum extraction (50 percent of such cases have retinal hemorrhages). The firstborn (increased labor time) and the premature child (increased vessel fragility) develop retinal hemorrhages most often. The hemorrhages are bilateral in half the cases and occur in three forms: superficial flame-shaped hemorrhages close to the optic disc, large round hemorrhages near the optic disc, and small round or elongated hemorrhages adjacent to the macula or optic disc. Usually the hemorrhages are absorbed in 2 to 3 weeks without sequelae. Occasionally granular macular changes that could affect visual acuity are seen; actually this suggestion has never been confirmed. Large hemorrhages may organize into elevated scars that resemble tumors (massive retinal fibrosis). There is no apparent relationship between retinal hemorrhages and brain damage, but minor changes in the central nervous system may not be detectable.

Other intraocular injuries that have been rarely ascribed to birth trauma include hyphema, vitreous hemorrhage, cataract, iridodialysis, choroidal tears, and subluxation of the lens.

Minor injuries to the lids and conjunctiva are frequent. Edema, chemosis, ecchymoses, hematoma, and lacerations heal without sequelae. Lagophthalmos, the inability to close the eye, occurs occasionally in newborn infants. Usually it is unilateral and may be due to injury to the facial nerve from forceps pressure. The condition usually disappears within a week. Traumatic ptosis also occurs in newborn infants and usually disappears in a few days.

Orbital hemorrhage may produce proptosis and extraocular muscle palsies. A fracture of the orbit or the base of the skull may be associated. Optic atrophy and blindness can result. Compression of the orbit by mechanical forces can cause tearing or hemorrhage into the extraocular muscles. Transient or permanent muscle palsy may ensue. Rarely subluxation or luxation of the globe outside the palpebral aperture may occur from the use of forceps.

Damage to the cervical sympathetics by compression of the neck with forceps may produce congenital Horner's syndrome. This consists of ptosis, pseudoenophthalmos, miosis, heterochromia, and anhidrosis of the affected side of the face. It is often accompanied by manifestations of injury to the brachial plexus, which aids in differentiating it from intracranial hemorrhage as a cause of inequality in the size of the pupils.

The *ocular signs of intracranial hemorrhage* in newborn infants are pupillary dilation, ocular motor palsies, and retinal hemorrhage, which may be present at birth or shortly therafter. In infants, in contrast with adults, the pupillary reactions in intracranial hemorrhage are inconsistent, and the dilated pupil is not necessarily found on the side of the lesion.

Battered Child Syndrome

Ocular trauma may be the first sign or a prominent part of the symptomatology of the battered child syndrome. Approximately 40 percent of children who have been physically abused show evidence in the eyes. The most common ocular findings include retinal or subhyaloid hemorrhages (frequently with multiple skull fractures and subdural hematomas), periorbital swelling and ecchymoses, subconjunctival hemorrhage, hyphema, anisocoria, extraocular muscle palsies, retinal detachment, and papilledema. The possibility of child abuse must be considered in the differential diagnosis of ocular conditions in young children.

References

Chace RR, Merritt KK, Bellows M: Ocular findings in the newborn infant. Arch Ophthalmol 44:236, 1950

Duke-Elder S, MacFaul PA: Injuries. In Duke-Elder S (ed): System of Ophthalmology, Vol XIV. London, Henry Kimpton, 1972

Friendly DS: Ocular manifestations of physical child abuse. Trans Am Acad Ophthalmol Otolaryngol 75:318, 1971

Jensen AD, Smith RE, Olson MI: Ocular clues to child abuse. J Pediatr Ophthalmol 8:270, 1971

Leone CR Jr, Russell DA: Congenital Horner's syndrome. J Pediatr Ophthalmol 7:152, 1970

Mushin A, Morgan G: Ocular injury in the battered baby syndrome. Br J Ophthalmol 55:341, 1971

Schenker JG, Gombos GM: Retinal hemorrhage in the newborn. Obstet Gynecol 27:521, 1966

CHAPTER 32

Bones and Joints

FREDERIC N. SILVERMAN, *Associate Editor*

The skeletal system is more than a structural framework designed to support and protect soft tissues and to implement their activities, as in locomotion; it is an active reservoir of elements important in homeostasis, and it often accurately reflects responses to conditions that threaten the functional integrity of the body as a whole. In addition, it is subject to disorders that are restricted to, or chiefly manifested in, bone.

BONE DEVELOPMENT AND GROWTH

All bones begin as condensations of primitive connective tissue cells and their matrix, arising from meso-

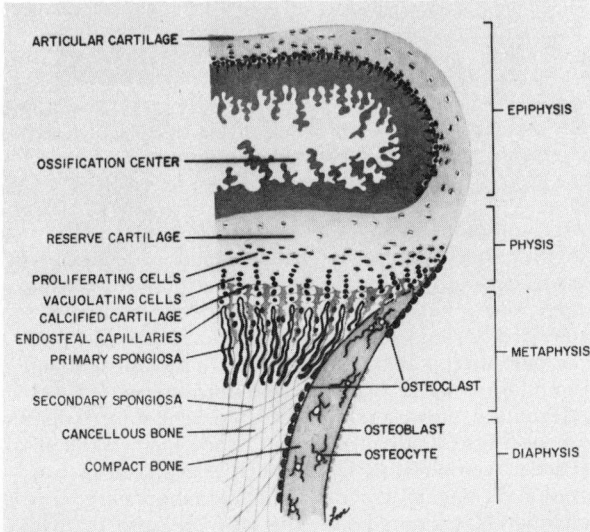

FIG. 1. Diagram of a representative cartilage–shaft junction. Growth occurs by proliferation of cartilage cells in the juxtametaphyseal portion of the physis. Vacuoles form around the older cells, which are aligned in columns in the axis of growth, and around the oldest cell the matrix calcifies. Endosteal capillaries and osteoclasts erode the horizontal walls of the vacuoles, and both osteolasts and osteoblasts accumulate along the residues of the vertical walls. Bone is laid down on these cores of calcified cartilage even as they are being eroded, and primary spongiosa is formed. The constant remodeling of bone trabeculae ultimately leads to disappearance of the last remnants of calcified cartilage, and this site marks the junction of metaphysis and diaphysis. Meanwhile the bone formed by the lateral growth and transformation of epiphyseal cartilage in the metaphysis is constricted by a ring of osteoclasts as well as by osteocyte-mediated resorption. The diaphysis grows in width by internal resorption of the cortex by osteoclasts and external apposition of bone by subperiosteal osteoblasts, and external apposition of bone by subperiosteal osteoblasts, some of which become incorporated in the bone to become osteocytes. (Adapted from Rubin: Dynamic Classification of Bone Dysplasias, 1964. Courtesy of Year Book Medical Publishers.)

derm. Fibrous cells and/or fibers increase predominantly in bones destined to become membranous, such as those of the cranial vault. Where cell proliferation predominates, matrix is formed and cartilage bones ultimately develop; these comprise the bulk of the skeleton. By condensation precartilage assumes the form of the ultimate bone structure within an envelope of oriented marginal mesenchymal cells, which becomes perichondrium. The oldest cartilage cells in the center of the long bones hypertrophy, the matrix calcifies, and a ring of osteoid is formed around the midshaft area. This ring quickly calcifies to form periosteal bone, and the perichondrium becomes osteoblast-lined periosteum. Cell masses then invade the central calcified cartilaginous matrix and change into bone-forming osteoblasts, vessels, and osteoclasts; these invade, break down, and remove calcified matrix and finally reconstruct bony trabeculae on residual cores of calcified cartilaginous matrix. The transformation of the cartilaginous model of the long-bone tissue proceeds toward both ends from the center, with simultaneous elongation of the subperiosteal bone, forming the diaphysis or shaft. Meanwhile, cartilage proliferation at the growing ends widens them as they elongate. A constriction of the widened ends of the shaft is accomplished by a ring of subperiosteal osteoclasts in that area, but also apparently by internal osteocytic resorption. The gentle terminal expansion of the long bones is the result of constrictive remodeling of the transverse dimensions of the growing bone even as longitudinal dimensions increase.

The longitudinal growth is accomplished by proliferation of cartilage cells of the physis (Fig. 1) in an orderly fashion and transformation of the surrounding matrix from calcified cartilage to bone by the same mechanisms that form the primary ossification center of the shaft. Secondary ossification centers make their appearance in the epiphyses of long bones* within a broad range of age beginning late in fetal life and extending to puberty. Their presence or absence is used in the estimation of bone age. At maturity the bone of the secondary ossification center has replaced all the cartilage of the epiphysis except that of the articular surface and has united with the bone of the shaft so that effective longitudinal growth ceases.

DISEASES OF BONES AND JOINTS

Disturbances in all stages of bone formation and growth, from defective mesenchymal condensation through cartilage–bone transformation to fusion of

---

By convention, a long bone has epiphyses at both ends, whereas a short bone has an epiphysis at only one end.

epiphysis and shaft, are often reflected in size, form, continuity, and radiodensity of individual bones or several bones as seen on radiography. Many of these deviations are described in this chapter. Certain systemic conditions with skeletal manifestations, such as scurvy, rickets, renal or metabolic disorders, tuberculous and syphilitic bone infections, and skeletal aspects of growth and development are described in other chapters. This section deals largely with disorders that affect primarily the skeletal system, and it is organized on a regional basis.

SKULL
FREDERIC N. SILVERMAN

CONGENITAL AND DEVELOPMENTAL ANOMALIES

Congenital and developmental defects of the skull may occur as isolated abnormalities or as part of a syndrome. Whenever a cranial abnormality is observed it is wise to search elsewhere for associated defects.

VARIATION IN SIZE.   An abnormally large head is properly designated *macrocrania* or *macrocephaly*. *Hydrocephalus* is a major cause of macrocrania. In infancy an enlarging head is often a presenting sign of subdural hematoma. Primary enlargement of the brain, in which an absolute increase in brain weight occurs, is called *megalencephaly;* it is associated with enlargement of the cranial cavity. In the brain the amount of tissue and the function are poorly correlated; as in hydrocephalus, children with megalencephalic macrocrania frequently are mentally retarded. Many children with neurofibromatosis have relative macrocrania. Megalencephalic macrocrania is also common in tuberous sclerosis, Hurler's syndrome, Tay-Sachs disease, and other storage diseases affecting the brain. Brain tumors cause cranial enlargement by obstructing cerebrospinal fluid pathways, producing hydrocephalus. *Pseudohydrocephalus* is disproportionate enlargement of the cranium with respect to the facial structures; it is most commonly seen in lateral projections of the skull in premature infants. A similar disproportion is observed in hypopituitary and Russell-Silver dwarfs and in some instances of the diencephalic syndrome. In the recovery phase of privational dwarfism, when cranial growth is rapid, widened sutures may simulate those of actively increased intracranial pressure. Macrocrania is a component of some generalized hyperostotic skeletal disorders; in achondroplasia it usually indicates hydrocephalus, but true megalencephaly may be present. In cerebral gigantism the head reaches adult size in early life.

Microcrania or *microcephaly* is an abnormally small head, frequently associated with or resulting from a primary developmental defect of the brain: microencephaly. Microcrania may be due to many causes, including premature synostosis of all the cranial sutures, prenatal infection (toxoplasmosis, cytomegalic inclusion disease, rubella), high levels of intrauterine radia-

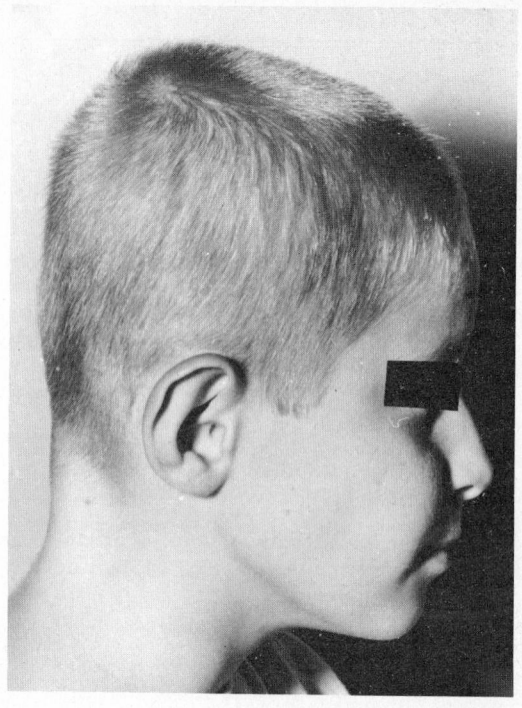

FIG. 2.   Postural flattening of skull in a child following prolonged recumbency resulting from congenital cardiac disease.

tion, and other causes of brain injury during fetal life or infancy. It is a common manifestation of syndromes associated with mental retardation; the majority of children whose head circumferences are more than two standard deviations below the mean are mentally subnormal. Microcrania is usual in Down's syndrome and is common in association with intrauterine growth retardation. However, underdevelopment at birth does not necessarily impair intellectual potential in the absence of complicating factors such as asphyxia or congenital disease. Macrocrania and microcrania are more adequately evaluated with the tape measure than by visual inspection or radiographic examination.

VARIATION IN SHAPE.   Abnormalities in shape may alter measurable circumference, but normal cranial volume may be retained as a result of compensatory changes in other dimensions. Thus, *postural flattening* due to prolonged recumbency in infancy may increase the vertical height of the skull at the expense of dimensions in the horizontal plane (Fig. 2). Mentally retarded children and those with neuromuscular defects are frequently unable to sit without support and may manifest marked postural flattening. Infants with normal mentality, but who have been maintained in dorsal recumbency by virtue of debilitating or prolonged illness, affective deprivation, or orthopedic appliances, may also develop postural flattening. Once the infant can sit and maintain the erect position, the deformity usually disappears spontaneously, provided brain growth is normal.

Craniosynostoses (p. 1977) are responsible for most clinically obvious variations in cranial shape that are persistent. Often they are associated with facial abnormalities. *Cranial bossing* (caput quadratum) of rickets and syphilitic hyperostoses are now rarely seen. Various hemolytic anemias, and occasionally simple iron-deficiency anemia, may demonstrate thickening of the vault that may alter its shape. Cephalhematoma (p. 1827) is the most common cause of circumscribed cranial swelling in the newborn period. Defects associated with meningocele or encephalocele are easily recognized (p. 1758). *Cranial asymmetry* is associated with congenital torticollis; in this condition asymmetry is seen as occipital flattening on the side opposite the affected sternocleidomastoid muscle and downward displacement of the eye, ear, and corner of the mouth on the same side. Mild cranial asymmetry occurs in association with some instances of anomalous parietal sutures. Polyostotic fibrous dysplasia may also provoke asymmetry of the skull. A wide cranial vault is commonly seen in osteogenesis imperfecta (p. 1930) and in cleidocranial dysostosi (p. 1996). Facial asymmetry occurs in the cri-du-chat syndrome and is progressive in Romberg's facial hemiatrophy. Wilderwanck's syndrome (cervicooculoacoustic syndrome) simulates facial asymmetry because of segmentation abnormalities of the cervical spine (Klippel-Feil anomaly), with torticollis and abducens paralysis with retraction of the bulb. Perceptive deafness is a feature of the condition. Neurofibromatosis (p. 2022) may be associated with cranial and facial asymmetry. Hemifacial microsomia is another cause of facial asymmetry and is considered by some to be a variant of Goldenhar's syndrome (oculoauriculovertebral dysplasia (p. 1971). Cherubism (p. 922) (familial fibrous dysplasia of the jaws), a special form of fibrous dysplasia almost exclusively affecting the jaws, is a cause of facial swelling in childhood. Mandibular swelling in Caffey's syndrome (infantile cortical hyperostosis) produces facial asymmetry at a much earlier age and is usually associated with bone lesions in the extremities (p. 2022).

Jaw cysts occur in the basal cell nevus syndrome, where they are associated with multiple cutaneous basal cell carcinomas, small pits in the palms, rib and vertebral deformities, and calcification in the falx cerebri. Siblings of patients with the syndrome have presented with brain tumors that have all been medulloblastomas.

CRANIOSYNOSTOSIS. Premature union of the cranial bones may take place before birth, which is considered to be the case if manifestations are observed prior to the second month of life. When intrauterine synostosis of the coronal and lambdoidal sutures is associated with congenital hydrocephalus, the newborn infant has a grotesque *trilobate cranium* that has been given the name cloverleaf skull. The association of cloverleaf skull with skeletal dysplasia resembling thanatophoric dwarfism has been described, but the exact nature of the generalized skeletal dysplasia is not yet certain. The range of normal variation in the time of postnatal closure of sutures has not been established, but there has been increasing opinion that closure may

begin normally in the second month of life. Premature closure of sutures has been attributed to developmental defects of the deformed base, to which dural fibers related to suture location are firmly attached.

Findings on direct inspection of the vault are not infrequently at variance with radiographic interpretations. Nevertheless, when premature union of cranial bones takes place during an age when growth of the brain is active, distortion occurs in patterns that frequently lead one to suspect which sutures are affected. If growth of the bony cranium is arrested at any one site and the cranial contents continue to enlarge, compensatory growth must occur at other sites.

It is now generally accepted that the sutures permit cranial growth rather than cause growth. The sutures do not function as growth sites as do the epiphyses of cartilaginous bones. Three basic assumptions, for which there is ample support, are helpful in understanding the cranial distortions produced by craniosynostoses: (1) specific growth of the cranial vault is dependent upon growth of the entire cranium; (2) growth occurs at the sutures in a direction perpendicular to the longitudinal axis of the suture; (3) premature closure of one small segment of a suture restricts growth as effectively as if the entire suture were involved. The implication is that bony continuity across a suture may not be demonstrated radiographically even though premature union has taken place. Premature synostosis of the cranial sutures has been observed in hypophosphatasia, in idiopathic hypercalcemia, in vitamin-D-resistant rickets, in privational rickets, and in children with hypothyroidism. It may occur as a complication following relief of increased intracranial pressure in hydrocephalus by a ventriculojugular shunt mechanism. In addition to the premature closure of the sutures, abnormal thickening of the skull vault and lamination of the diploë have been reported to be very frequent after operation for hydrocephalus. The clinical importance of craniosynostosis is related to (1) distortion, compression, and subsequent dysfunction of the brain and its nerves, (2) associated malformations of the brain, and (3) psychologic effects of cranial and facial deformities.

Clinical Forms. (Scaphocephaly). *Craniosynostosis of the sagittal suture* is the most common form; it constitutes about 50 percent of recorded cases. Lateral growth of the cranium is restricted, compensatory growth in length takes place and the skull becomes long and narrow (scaphocephaly) and may increase in height as well (Fig. 3).

ACROCEPHALY, OXYCEPHALY, PLAGIOCEPHALY. *Craniosynostosis of the coronal suture* is second in frequency; it results in a skull that is short in its anteroposterior diameter, but wide and high (acrocephaly or oxycephaly) (Fig. 4). Segmentation errors of the hands and feet functional or anatomic defects of the brain, facial deformity, and ocular hypertelorism are frequently associated anomalies. The shallow orbits lead to proptosis. Pressure on the optic nerves by the distorted bony structures may result in progressive blindness. Unilateral closure produces flattening of the forehead

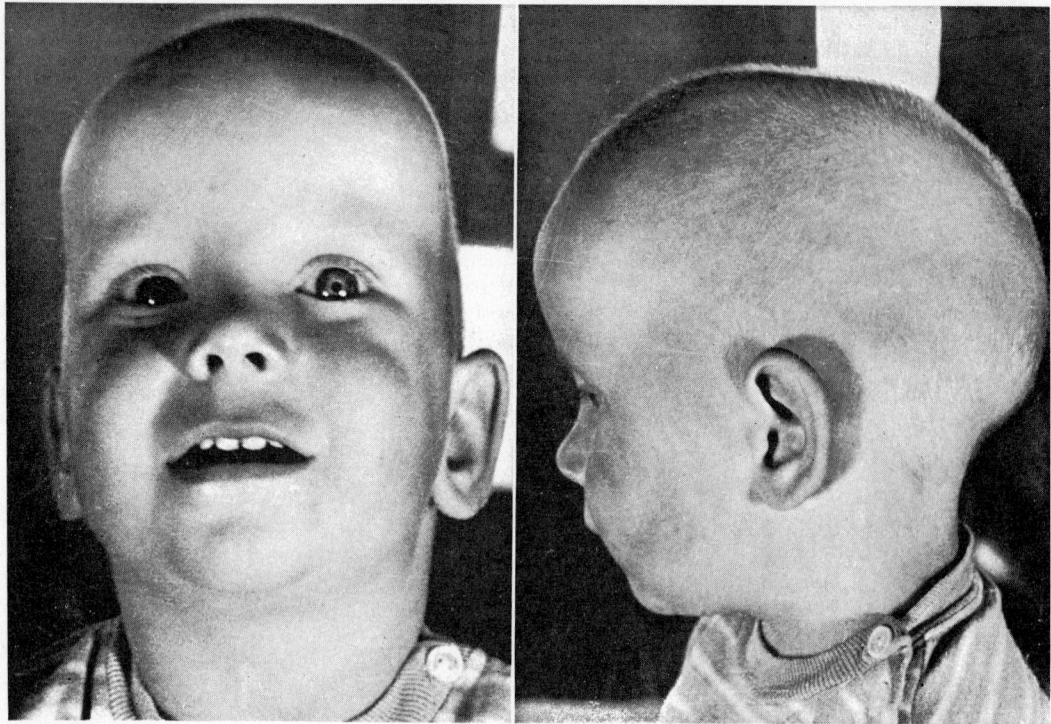

FIG. 3.   Premature synostosis of sagittal suture. The cranium is narrow, but it is high and elongated ventrodorsally. (From Silverman: Ohio Med J 50:131, 1954.)

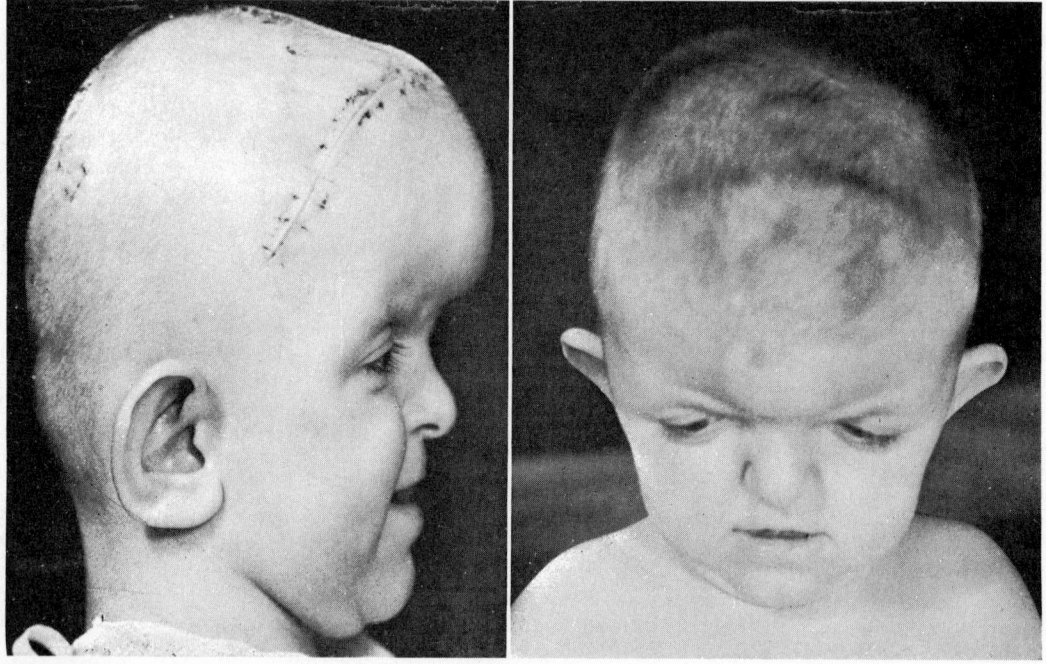

FIG. 4.   Premature synostosis of coronal suture. (Courtesy of Dr. Frank Mayfield.)

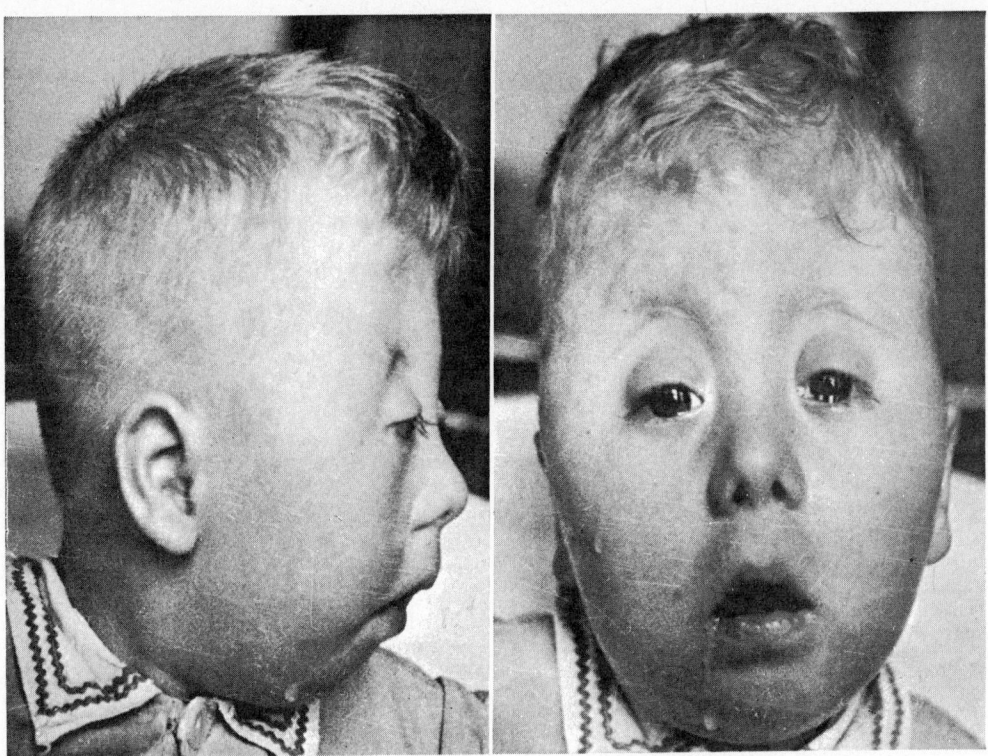

FIG. 5. Premature synostosis of coronal and sagittal sutures. (From Silverman: Ohio Med J 50:131, 1954.)

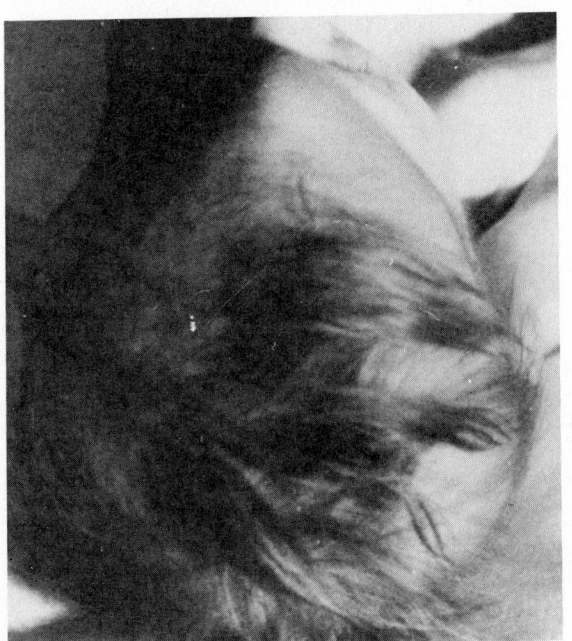
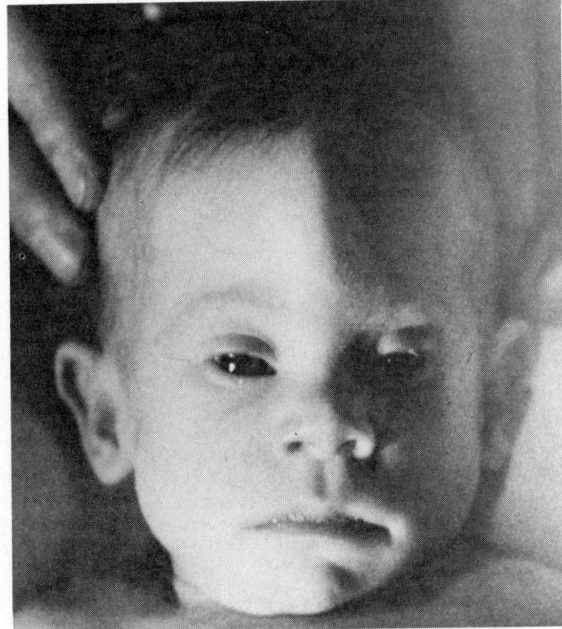

FIG. 6. Trigonocephaly: The triangular cranium is obvious when viewed from above, but the keellike forehead is made prominent when viewed frontally with side lighting. The mongoloid slope of the palpebral fissures may give an erroneous impression of Down's syndrome. This child was not mentally retarded.

on the affected side, with elevation of the ipsilateral orbit. Cranial asymmetry of this type is called plagiocephaly, but it can result from abnormal static forces, as in congenital torticollis, as well as from premature closure of one limb of a cranial suture that has bilateral components.

Combined sagittal and coronal suture involvement restricts cranial growth almost exclusively to the vertical axis of the skull. Consequently the cranium is high and narrow and almost comes to a point (Fig. 5). When all the cranial sutures are obliterated prematurely, growth of the skull is prevented in all directions, and microcrania and microcephaly result. Pedal and manual deformities, especially syndactyly, are common when both coronal and sagittal suture closures are involved, giving rise to acrocephalosyndactylies, such as Apert's syndrome (p. 1987), or acrocephalopolysyndactylies, of which Carpenter's syndrome (p. 1987) is the best example.

TRIGONOCEPHALY.   Trigonocephaly, a triangular-shaped head with a keellike protrusion of the forehead (Fig. 6), is associated with premature obliteration of the metopic suture and with hypoplasia of the ethmoid bone, which results in an abnormally narrowed distance between the medial walls of the orbits (orbital hypotelorism). A mongoloid slope of the palpebral fissures is commonly present, but trigonocephaly is rare in Down's syndrome. Surgical intervention is rarely employed in this particular craniosynostosis, except for cosmetic purposes.

CROUZON'S DISEASE.   In Crouzon's disease (crani-

ofacial dysostosis) the cranial deformity is associated with hypoplasia of the facial bones producing a characteristic facies (Fig. 7) with a high, wide skull flattened anteroposteriorly, exophthalmos and external strabismus, a beaked nose, a short upper lip combined with hypoplasia of the maxilla, and a protruding lower lip due to relative mandibular prognathism. Obstruction of the upper airway secondary to the hypoplastic maxilla may give rise to hypoxia and hypocapnia, with secondary pulmonary hypertension, cardiomegaly, and drowsiness.

Diagnosis.   In the majority of cases the diagnosis may be made or at least suspected at birth because of obvious skull deformity or common associated deformities. Palpation of the fontanelles and sutures may reveal obliteration of the normally softer areas or overlapping of bone that produces a ridge along the path of a suture. Radiography of the skull provides conclusive diagnosis only when bony continuity across a suture is demonstrated; demonstration of deformities secondary to the invisible suture abnormality is merely supportive evidence. When all sutures are obliterated and compensatory deformity cannot occur, a hammered-silver appearance is usually present that is generally considered to be indicative of increased intracranial pressure. However, measurements of cerebrospinal fluid pressure have been infrequently reported in craniosynostosis, and the results do not always agree. Evidence provided by flattened gyri, diminished amounts of cerebrospinal fluid, and forceful abrupt separation of bone when the last connecting fragment of bone is removed

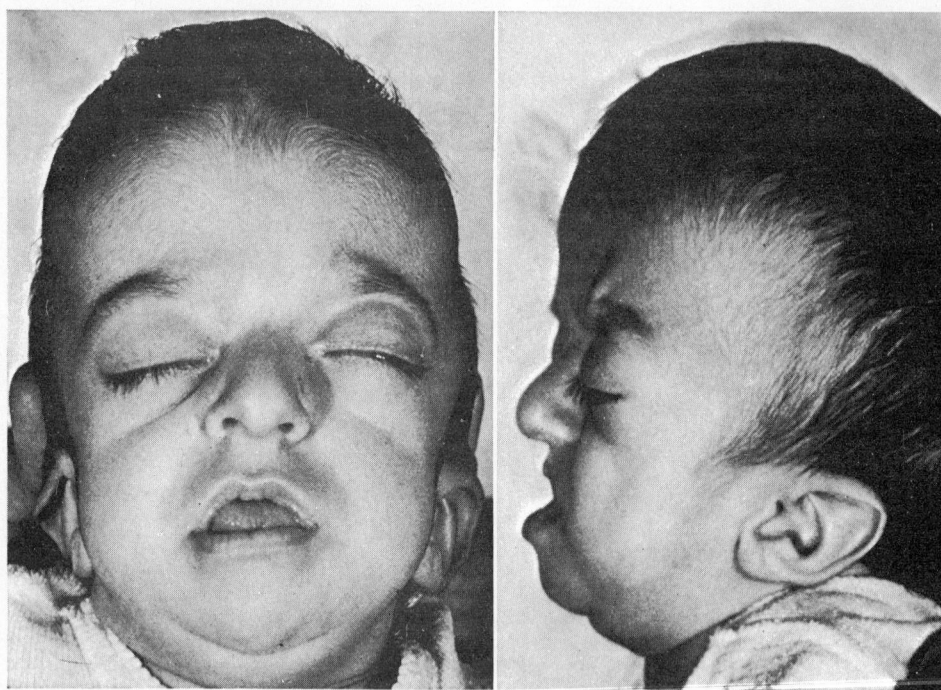

FIG. 7.   Crouzon's disease: craniosynostosis in association with hypoplasia of the maxilla and other deformities. Exophthalmos is seen even with the lids closed; also seen are prognathism and beaked nose.

during creation of an artificial suture indicates that increased intracranial pressure does exist in some instances.

Postural flattening of the skull and microcrania due to primary developmental or acquired defect of the brain must be differentiated from craniosynostosis. In the former there is often marked flattening in the occipital region, but little or no deformity in the region of the orbits; the coronal sutures are clearly shown to be open on roentgenographic examination. In microcrania due to defects of the brain, the skull is small because the stimulus of a growing brain is lacking. The sutures may close prematurely, but there is little or no cranial deformity, and signs of increased intracranial pressure are absent. In addition, the cranial bones may be unusually thick, and pneumatization of the paranasal sinuses and the temporal bone is often exaggerated.

Treatment.   The logical treatment for craniosynostosis is the surgical production of artificial sutures to permit normal, symmetric growth of the brain. At present, surgical treatment is recommended in instances of severe deformity or papilledema and in Crouzon's disease.

Tessier has pioneered in corrective surgical procedures for Crouzon's disease and other craniofacial dysostoses; the procedures require special craniofacial surgical expertise and involve a one-stage total osteotomy of the middle third of the face with forward displacement and fixation of the entire facial mass.

Since the rate of growth of the brain is very rapid during the first few years of life, lesser indications may be more important when a condition is recognized early. Considerable disagreement exists concerning the treatment of isolated sagittal suture synostosis, with claims that mental development and cosmetic results are not significantly affected by surgical treatment. In the other variants of craniosynostosis differences of opinion on management are not as sharp. Neurosurgeons reporting the largest series of cases tend to be more enthusiastic about the surgical results. In general the pediatrician must be guided by the experience of his neurosurgical colleagues and must recognize that the procedures are technically easier during the first 6 months of life than at later ages.

CRANIAL DEFECTS.   At birth as many as six fontanelles may be palpated or demonstrated radiographically in the normal infant skull (Fig. 8). Additional fontanelles may occur as normal variations in the metopic suture, and in the sagittal suture midway between the anterior and posterior fontanelles. However, these interparietal fontanelles tend to be seen more frequently in newborn infants with Down's syndrome and in various forms of intrauterine insults. Their slightly more frequent occurrence in premature infants has been cited as an indication of developmental retardation. Occasionally, continuity of unossified membrane is noted between midline fontanelles in otherwise normal children; in such instances closure of the fontanelles may be somewhat retarded without any adverse clinical findings. The speed and sequence of fontanelle closure are variable. The anterior fontanelle usually closes clinically during the first half of the second year of life, but it may close earlier. The posterior fontanelle is generally closed by the end of the second month and may even be closed at birth. The anterolateral fontanelles disappear during the first 3 months, and the posterolateral fontanelles during the second year. Localized defects of calvarial bone in the latter regions in neurofibromatosis may simulate persistence of posterolateral fontanelles. In as many as 35 percent of newborn infants, local areas of softening can be palpated, particularly in the parietal bone along the lambdoidal suture. These areas, when gently pressed, can be indented in the same fashion as a ping-pong ball—a normal condition in the first 3 months of life that is known as *craniotabes*. However, craniotabes occurs pathologi-

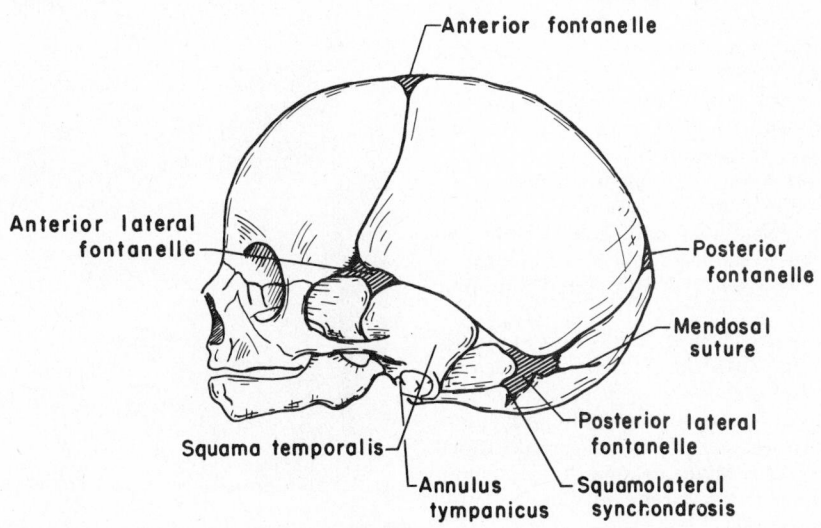

FIG. 8.   Normal fontanelles in newborn infant that may be palpated or visualized roentgenographically.

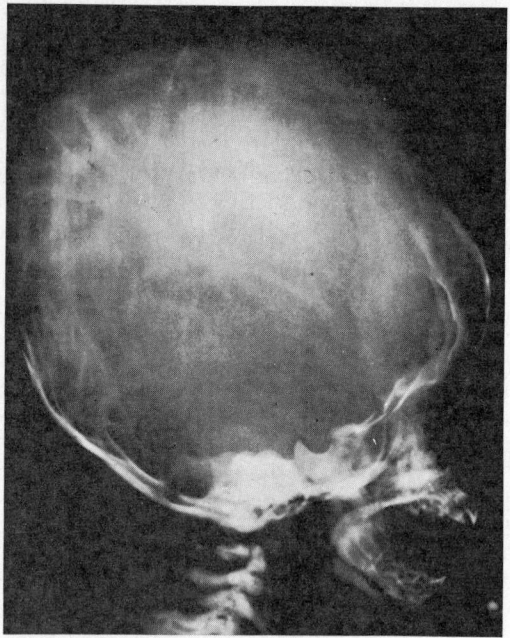

FIG. 9. Craniolacuna (Lückenschädel).

may lead to cerebral herniation into the orbit (orbital encephalocele) and produce pulsating exophthalmos. In the majority of cases neurofibromatosis is also present. Defects associated with meningocele and encephalocele are easily recognized; those associated with dermal sinuses extending intracranially may be shown only on radiography and occur most frequently in the occipital area near the torcular Herophili, where normally large channels for emissary vessels communicate with the dural sinuses. In occasional instances of idiopathic familial osteoarthropathy wide cranial sutures may be present; in one instance the cranial manifestations of the syndrome were observed to develop postnatally. The widened sutures may persist from birth, but in either case mineralization generally occurs by the end of the first decade of life.

In Hand-Schüller-Christian disease focal punched-out areas are commonly observed radiographically in the flat bones of the cranium (see Fig. 2, p. 1227). Epidermoidomas, which are intraosseous inclusions with epidermal elements, present radiographically as radiolucent defects with sharply demarcated sclerotic borders. Vascular malformations of the epicranium are occasionally associated with clinical and radiologic defects in the calvarium underneath the vascular soft tissue swellings. Cranial defects are also found in congenital generalized fibromatosis.

cally in rickets, hydrocephalus, and certain skeletal dystrophies, but even then it is rare after the first year.

Occasionally a defect is palpated that extends across the midline just anterior to the posterior fontanelle. Development of bone centrally divides the single defect into symmetric, bilateral parietal defects known as enlarged *parietal foramina;* they are without clinical significance, often persisting throughout life, and require no treatment. Their occurrence is strongly familial and suggests a dominant genetic trait. They must be differentiated from meningocele, histiocytosis X, epidermoidoma, localized infection, primary or metastatic neoplasm, and surgical defects.

Lacunar skull (Lückenschädel) describes the radiographic appearance of multiple large and small radiolucent areas (Fig. 9) in the skull of the infant with spina bifida, meningocele, or meningomyelocele. The Arnold-Chiari malformation is a common associated anomaly. The irregular mineralization of the skull, which causes the typical soap-bubble appearance of lacunar skull, usually disappears at 6 to 12 months of age, even when it is associated with spinal dysraphic syndromes.

In osteogenesis imperfecta (p. 2011) and in cleidocranial dysostosis (p. 2013) large cranial defects are present, and they may give the impression that there is no bone present. A large anterior fontanelle with extensions into adjacent sutures may persist in cleidocranial dysostosis even in adults. Mineralization of the cranium is also lacking in the severe and frequently fatal infantile form of hypophosphatasia.

Congenital defects in the roofs and walls of the orbits

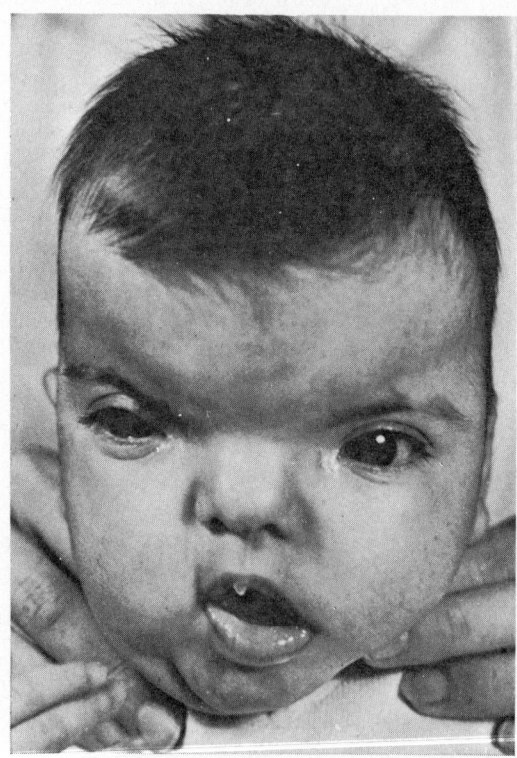

FIG. 10. Ocular hypertelorism; the child also has sagittal craniosynostosis. (Courtesy of Dr. Frank Mayfield.)

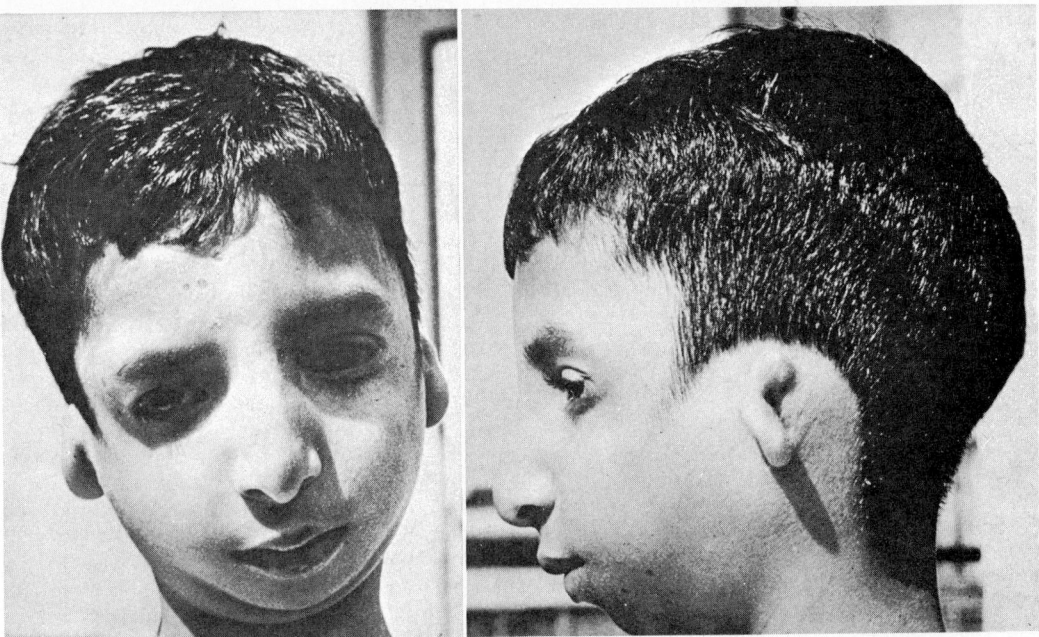

FIG. 11. Treacher-Collins syndrome (Franceschetti syndrome, mandibulofacial dysostosis): The deformities of the external ears and the hypoplastic mandible are clearly shown. The antimongoloid slant of the eyes can be recognized, but the defect of the lower lids (cloboma) is obscured by the heavy shadows.

MISCELLANEOUS ABNORMALITIES. *Ocular hypertelorism* is a rare, occasionally inherited, deformity of the anterior basilar portion of the cranium and the adjacent facial bones characterized by a conspicuous increase in the distance between the eyes (Fig. 10). The facial deformity is said to arise from overgrowth of the lesser wings of the sphenoid bone and underdevelopment of the greater wings, resulting in a simulation of the fetal cranial proportions. It frequently exists to a mild degree without any associated functional or anatomic abnormalities, but it is a common feature in many syndromes involving the face. Ocular hypertelorism is a prominent feature of the syndrome of hypogonadism and short stature called the fetal face syndrome. Occasionally ocular hyperterlorism is simulated by lateral displacement of the inner canthus (dystopia canthorum) without underlying bony abnormality, as in the Waardenburg syndrome. In severe forms there may be cleft lip, cleft palate, and even cleft nose; occasionally frontal lipomas or teratomas are present. The medial cleft face syndrome, as this group of malformations is known, is less frequently associated with intellectual deficit than is the group of medial cleft lip deformities associated with hypotelorism.

Orbital hypotelorism is characterized by an abnormal approximation of the medial walls of the orbits diagnosed radiographically. Clinically a relative excess of soft tissue between the palpebral fissures may give the impression of widely spaced eyes; epicanthal folds are frequently present. Relative hypotelorism is observed in Down's syndrome, regardless of the chromosomal abnormality. Orbital hypotelorism is present in trigono-

cephaly (Fig. 10) and in the cyclopia-arhinencephalia or holoprosencephaly group of cerebral malformations that are frequent in the trisomy 13–15 syndrome and are often associated with profound amentia and fatality in infancy.

In the Treacher-Collins or Franceschetti syndrome (mandibulofacial dysostosis) (Fig. 11) the lateral portions of the facial structure, particularly the zygomatic arches, are hypoplastic or absent, and the palpebral fissures have an antimongoloid slant. A defect is commonly present along the lower lid, the ears are deformed, and the mandible is hypoplastic. It has been suggested that these manifestations constitute a distinct entity: the first and second branchial arch syndrome. An antimongoloid slant of the palpebral fissures is also a significant feature of the Rubinstein-Taybi syndrome (p. 916). Hypoplasia of the mandible may produce serious respiratory distress and even retarded physical development when the associated glossoptosis is severe and occludes the pharyngeal airway. When a cleft palate is also present the condition is known as the Pierre Robin syndrome. the respiratory and feeding difficulties associated with a congenital small lower jaw and their treatment are described elsewhere (p. 1517).

ACQUIRED CRANIAL ABNORMALITIES

EFFECTS OF LABOR AND DELIVERY. In its passage through the birth canal, the fetal head undergoes characteristic distortion or *molding,* which increases the vertical dimensions of the head at the expense of the horizontal dimensions; the effects of the molding disappear within a few days. The following bone movements take place: The occipital bone bends as on a hinge at the cartilaginous junction immediately behind the foramen magnum, so that the parietal bones are squeezed superiorly. The parietal bones override one another centrally, the occipital posteriorly, and the frontal anteriorly and are widely separated from the squamosa of the temporal bones. Overlap is much more pronounced when the child is in the supine position than when in the lateral position. Resulting compression of the superior sagittal sinus has been observed angiographically in newborn infants. The possibility of serious consequences from a slowing of cerebral circulation and an increase in cerebral venous pressure as a result of sagittal sinus compression has been raised. In infants delivered by cesarean section, molding may be present only if the procedure was undertaken after the onset of labor.

CEPHALHEMATOMA. Prominent molding is frequently associated with neonatal cephalhematoma, which is a subperiosteal hemorrhage on the external surface of one or more calvarial bones. Because of the firm attachment of the periosteum to the sutures, the swelling caused by subperiosteal blood does not cross the sutures as it does in subgaleal hemorrhage or other subgaleal collections. Associated fractures may occur in as many as 25 percent of affected infants, but they are rarely of clinical significance. Calcification beneath the overlying periosteum will appear radiographically shortly after birth as irregular mottled densities or prominent external thickenings. Well-calcified cephalhematomas may be present at birth. They probably result from intrauterine mechanical pressure exerted by the calvarium impinging on the promontory of the sacrum. External thickenings of the calvarium from neonatal cephalhematoma may persist into the second decade; occasionally radiolucent areas indicate the site of fibrous rather than bony resolution of the neonatal cephalhematoma.

SKULL FRACTURES. Fractures of the skull are common in infancy and childhood. Radiographic examination is essential in identification of skull fractures, but failure to demonstrate a fracture does not exclude its. Gurdjian and associates have prepared charts for the prediction of fracture sites according to site of impact that permit selective positioning during radiographic examination. However, the curved surface of the calvarium and the superimposition of basal bones limit the usefulness of these techniques. Except in cases where there is a depressed fracture, radiographic documentation of fracture may provide information of great value concerning (1) degrees of injury to soft parts, particularly the brain; (2) location of the fracture with respect to vascular structures such as the dural sinuses and the middle meningeal vessels that are likely to produce subdural or epidural hemorrhage; (3) location of the fracture with respect to the intracranial air cavities (nasopharynx, paranasal sinuses, temporal bones, etc)

that provide direct communication with the outside and permit the introduction of infection into the cranial cavity; and (4) linear or diastatic (gaping) nature of the fracture. Diastatic fractures occur only if there are associated tears of the dura; under these circumstances cerebrospinal fluid may escape into the subdural space or into the subgaleal space and may produce leptomeningeal cysts under the area of the fracture. In addition, loss of integrity of the dura leaves the endocranial bone surface unprotected from the pulsating activities of the underlying brain and cerebrospinal fluid, and erosions may develop in association with subdural fluid collections that behave as space-occupying lesions. Rarely a fracture of this type enlarges progressively and forms a permanent cranial defect, usually associated with underlying cerebral focal atrophy and clinical sequelae such as paralyses, convulsions, and mental retardation.

In a hospital population of 4,465 children with head injuries, Harwood-Nash and associates found skull fracture in 26.6 percent, with 92 percent of the fractures evident radiographically. The parietal bone was most frequently involved. Although a third of the depressed fractures were associated with a dural tear, extradural hematomas and subdural hematomas were relatively uncommon. Extradural hematomas occurred with the same frequency in children with and without skull fracture, whereas subdural hematoma was twice as frequent without fracture as with fracture. Clinical and electroencephalographic evidences of injury to the central nervous system were found by Williams and associates in mentally retarded head-bangers. In addition, thickening of the calvarium, diastasis of the cranial sutures, soft tissue hematomas, intraocular calcification, and deformities of the external ears were noted.

Severe circulatory shock and unconsciousness are bad prognostic signs after head injury and should be treated immediately, even before undertaking any diagnostic radiography. The duration of unconsciousness is a rough index of the severity of the intracranial damage. The classic signs of epidural hemorrhage (unconsciousness, clear period, recurrence of unconsciousness) call for immediate neurosurgical intervention.

The wisdom of routine skull radiography in known or suspected cranial injuries may be questioned. The actual presence of a radiographically demonstrable fracture plays little role in the clinical management of the patient unless there is depression, injury to important vascular channels, or communication with the outside. In general the clinical information indicates whether these complications are to be expected. Clinical evidence of depression or of impact with a penetrating object, bleeding from the ear, ecchymoses in the mastoid region or orbits, and otorrhea or rhinorrhea constitute reasonable indications for radiologic examination of the cranium. Unconsciousness, which may be a reflection of the severity of the injury, could also be considered an indication. However, little may be gained by subjecting an unconscious and hypotensive child to the definite risk of multiple manipulations for radiography.

In the absence of localizing signs, such examination is best deferred until the clinical condition has stabilized. Without unconsciousness or any other localizing sign, and provided adequate clinical examination and repeated observation are available, radiography is probably not required. As a rule, radiographic studies of the cranium are often inconclusive, and they should not be a substitute for careful clinical examination of any child with head trauma.

Sequelae of skull fractures may include headaches, dizziness, disturbances of hearing, and neurologic defects, including epilepsy and mental retardation. Most of these are the consequence of complications of the fractures and are not due directly to the fractures.

The sudden increase of intraorbital pressure following a blow to the globe by a relatively blunt object such as a fist or a baseball can produce a fracture of the walls of the orbit, particularly the floor (roof of the maxillary sinus) termed a blowout fracture. The most common form consists of a fracture of the roof of the maxillary sinus with herniation of some of the orbital contents into the sinus. If the condition is not promptly recognized and treated, enophthalmos and persistent diplopia may occur when the initial edema and hemorrhage are resolved. Clinically the condition must be suspected following a direct blow to the eye or when diplopia, downward displacement of the eyeball, and anomalies of extraocular movements are found. Sensory disturbance of the skin supplied by the infraorbital nerve may be present. Radiographically the sinus on the affected side may be clouded, but a distinct depression of bone of the roof associated with a soft tissue shadow bulging downward into the sinus is diagnostic. In many instances laminograms are necessary to demonstrate the fracture and protrusion of orbital contents. Prompt reduction of the soft tissue herniation and elevation of the depressed bone are required in order to avoid the sequelae noted above.

CRANIAL NEOPLASMS. Primary neoplasms of the skull are rare. Osteochondromas occasionally arise from the cartilaginous bones of the face; even more rarely, Ewing's tumors may occur in the flat bones of the vault. Epidermal inclusion cysts (epidermoidoma) present as radiolucent defects that are usually rounded, with a sclerotic, sharp border; they are most frequent in the lateral aspects of the calvarium. In most instances they disappear with age; occasionally they may extend intracranially, producing signs of meningitis. Cranial reactions to adjacent tumors, such as meningiomas, include focal calcification, hyperostoses, increased vascularity, bone destruction, and pressure atrophy of bone adjacent to the meningioma. Destructive changes occur when rhabdomyosarcoma from the nasopharynx, ear, or orbit extends directly into the base; metastatic lesions of neuroblastoma may affect the calvarium as well as the base. Any or all of these lesions may be associated with widening of the sutures secondary to increased intracranial pressure. In neuroblastoma, however, focal proliferation of metastatic tumor in bone adjacent to the sutures may simulate sutural widening.

CRANIAL MANIFESTATIONS OF SYSTEMIC DISORDERS. The postural flattening and cranial bossing of rickets and syphilis have been described elsewhere (p. 2003). Thickening of the calvarium has also been documented as a consequence of long-term phenyroin (Dilantin) medication, probably related to the metabolic derangements that result in rachitic changes in the long bones. Cranial aberrations as a result of chronic hemolytic anemias are seen largely as radiographic observations, unless there is an intracranial vascular accident. Similar changes have been observed in chronic iron-deficiency anemia. The characteristic facies in Mediterranean anemia (thalassemia major) is produced by hyperplasia of the facial bones, particularly the maxilla and the zygoma, resulting in high cheekbones and a mongoloid appearance. Infections of the cranium are discussed in relation to the specific diseases in which they occur, such as syphilis, tuberculosis, and osteomyelitis.

New syndromes involving cranial features have recently appeared. The interested reader is referred to the monograph by Gorlin and Pindborg. Cranial features of skeletal dysplasias are covered in the section devoted to this group of conditions.

References

GENERAL

Bourne GH (ed): Biochemistry and Physiology of Bone, Vol III, 2nd ed. New York, Academic, 1971

Caffey J: Pediatric X-Ray Diagnosis, 6th ed. Chicago, Year Book, 1972

Chasler CN: Atlas of Roentgen Anatomy of the Newborn and Infant Skull. St Louis, Green, 1972

Köhler A: Borderlands of the Normal and Early Pathologic in Skeletal Roentgenology, 11th ed. (English translation by Wilk SP.) New York, Grune & Stratton, 1968

Murray RO, Jacobson HG: The Radiology of Skeletal Disorders. Baltimore, Williams & Wilkins, 1971

Newton TH, Potts DG: Radiology of the Skull and Brain. St Louis, Mosby, 1971

Rubin P: Dynamic Classification of Bone Dysplasias. Chicago, Year Book, 1964

Swischuk LE: The normal newborn skull. Semin Roentgenol 9:101, 1974
———— The growing skull. Semin Roentgenol 9:115, 1974

Warkany J: Congenital Malformations: Notes and Comments. Chicago, Year Book, 1971

CONGENITAL AND DEVELOPMENTAL ANOMALIES

Babson SG, Henderson NB: Fetal undergrowth: relation of head growth to later intellectual performance. Pediacrics 53:890, 1974

Capitanio M, Kirkpatrick JA: Widening of the cranial sutures. A roentgen observation during periods of accelerated growth in patients treated for deprivation dwarfism. Radiology 92:53, 1969

Dennis J, Rosenberg H, Alvord E Jr: Megalencephaly, internal hydrocephalus and other neurological aspects of achondroplasia. Brain 84:427, 1961

Dorst JP: Functional craniology: an aid in interpreting roentgenograms of the skull. Radiol Clin North Am 2:347, 1964

Holden JD: Russell-Silver dwarf. Dev Med Child Neurol 9:457, 1967

Jones PG: Torticollis in infancy and childhood. Springfield, Ill, Charles C Thomas, 1968

Nelson KB, Deutschberger J: Head size at 1 year as a predictor of 4 year I.Q. Dev Med Child Neurol 12:487, 1970

O'Connell EJ, Feldt RH, Stickler GB: Head circumference, mental retardation and growth failure. Pediatrics 36:62, 1965

Shapiro R: Anomalous parietal sutures and the bipartite parietal bone. Am J Roentgenol Radium Ther Nucl Med 115:569, 1972

Spitzer R, Rabinowitz JY, Wybach KC: A study of the abnormalities of the skull, teeth, and lenses in mongolism. Can Med Assoc J 84:567, 1961

Warkany J, Monroe BB, Sutherland BS: Intra-uterine growth retardation. Am J Dis Child 102:249, 1961

Weichert KA, et al: Macrocranium and neurofibromatosis. Radiology 107:163, 1973

CRANIOSYNOSTOSIS

Currarino G, Silverman FN: Orbital hypotelorism, arhinencephaly, and trigonocephaly. Radiology 74:206, 1960

Freeman JM, Borkowf S: Craniostenosis. Review on the literature and report of thirty-four cases. Pediatrics 30:57, 1962

Loop JW, Foltz EL: Craniostenosis and diploic lamination following operation for hydrocephalus. Acta Radiol 13:8, 1972

McLaurin RL, Matson DD: Importance of early surgical treatment of craniosynostosis: review of 36 cases treated during the first six months of life. Pediatrics 10:637, 1952

Moss ML: The pathogenesis of premature cranial synostosis in man. Acta Anat (Basel) 37:351, 1959

Riggs W Jr, Wilroy RS Jr, Etteldorf JN: Neonatal hyperthyroidism with accelerated skeletal maturation, craniosynostosis, and brachydactyly. Radiology 105:621, 1972

Shillito J Jr, Matson D: Craniosynostosis: a review of 519 surgical patients. Pediatrics 41:829, 1968

Tessier P: The definitive plastic surgical treatment of the severe facial deformities of craniofacial dysostosis. Crouzon's and Apert's diseases. Plast Reconstr Surg 48:419, 1971

Young RS, Pochaczevsky R, Leonidas JC, Wexler IB, Ratner H: Thanatophoric dwarfism and cloverleaf skull (Kleeblattschädel). Radiology 106:401, 1973

CRANIAL DEFECTS

Chamberlain DS, Whitaker J, Silverman FN: Idiopathic osteoarthropathy and cranial defects in children (familial idiopathic osteoarthropathy). Am J Roentgenol Radium Ther Nucl Med 93:408, 1965

Currarino G, Tierney RC, Giesel RG, Weihl C: Familial idiopathic osteoarthropathy. Am J Roentgenol Radium Ther Nucl Med 85:633, 1961

Matson DD, Ingraham FD: Intracranial complications of congenital dermal sinuses. Pediatrics 8:463, 1951

Morettin LB, Mueller E, Schreiber M: Generalized hamartomatosis (congenital generalized fibromatosis). Am J Roengenol Radium Ther Nucl Med 114:722, 1972

O'Rahilly R, Twohig MJ: Foramina parietalia permagna. Am J Roentgenol Radium Ther Nucl Med 67:551, 1952

Shopfner CE, Jabbour JT, Vallion RM: Craniolacunia. Am J Roentgenol Radium Ther Nucl Med 93:343, 1965

Taybi H, Silverman FN: Congenital defect of the bony orbit and pulsating exophthalmos. Am J Dis Child 92:138, 1956

MISCELLANEOUS ABNORMALITIES

DeMyer W, Zernan W, Palmer CG: The face predicts the brain: diagnostic significance of median facial anomalies for holoprosencephaly (arhinencephaly). Pediatrics 34:256, 1964

Gerald BE, Silverman FN: Normal and abnormal interorbital distances, with special reference to mongolism. Am J Roentgenol Radium Ther Nucl Med 95:154, 1965

Gorlin RJ, Pindborg JJ: Syndromes of the Head and Neck. New York, McGraw-Hill, 1964

Grabb WC: The first and second branchial arch syndrome. Plast Reconstr Surg 36:485, 1965

Kurlander GJ, DeMyer W, Campbell JA: Roentgenology of the median cleft face syndrome. Radiology 88:473, 1967

Robinow M, Silverman FN, Smith HD: A newly recognized dwarfing syndrome. Am J Dis Child 117:645, 1969

Schinzel A, Zellweger H, Grella A, Prader A: Fetal face syndrome with acral dysostosis. Helv paediatr Acta 29:55, 1974

ACQUIRED CRANIAL ABNORMALITIES

Gurdjian ES, Webster JE, Lissner HR: Observations on prediction of fracture site in head injury. Radiology 60:226, 1953

Harwood-Nash DC, Hendrick EB, Hudson AR: Significance of skull fractures in children: A study of 1,187 patients. Radiology 101:151, 1971

Hayes WG, Shopfner CE: Plain skull roentgenographic findings in infants and children with convulsions. Am J Dis Child 126:785, 1973

Kattan K: Calvarial thickening after Dilantin medication. Am J Roentgenol Radium Ther Nucl Med 110:102, 1970

Merten DF, Gooding CA, Newton TH: The radiographic features of meningiomas in childhood and adolescence. Pediatr Radiol 2:89, 1974

Moloy HC: Studies on head molding during labor. Am J Obstet Gynecol 44:762, 1942

Newton TH, Gooding CA: Superior sagittal sinus compression by neonatal calvarial molding. Radiology 115:635, 1975

Roberts F, Shopfner CE: Plain skull roentgenograms in children with head trauma. Am J Roentgenol Radium Ther Nucl Med 114:230, 1972

Williams JP, et al: Roentgenographic changes in head bangers. Acta Radiol (Stockh) 13:37, 1972

Young LW, et al: Rickets and anti-epileptic therapy. In Frame B, Parfitt AM, Duncan H (eds): Proceedings, International Symposium on Clinical Aspects of Metabolic Bone Disease. Amsterdam, Excerpta Medica, 1973

Zizmor J, Smith B. Fasano C, Converse JM: Roentgen diagnosis of blow-out fractures of the orbit. Am J Roentgenol Radium Ther Nucl Med 87:1009, 1962

EXTREMITIES

FREDERIC N. SILVERMAN

DEVELOPMENTAL ANOMALIES

In the growing skeleton of the infant or child any deviation from the expected normal should first be looked at as a possible anatomic variation. Comparison with the opposite extremity in the same radiographic projection is a wise precaution; reference texts on anatomic variants should be consulted in instances where asymmetry exists. A difference in size between the two sides of the body may represent *hemihypertrophy* or *hemiatrophy*. In some instances it is difficult or impossible to decide whether the large or the small side is the normal one. Generalized asymmetry may be an isolated malformation or it may be associated with other developmental anomalies on the affected side. Vascular or neurologic abnormalities are not uncommon; when unilateral lymphangiectasia is associated with unilateral or localized gigantism, clinically silent involvement of the lungs and bowel may be demonstrated by appropriate radiographic studies. Abnormalities of the lymphatic channels on the affected side may be shown by lymphangiography. Contrast material may collect in apparently unaffected bone as well as grossly affected bony structures, especially in films obtained 24 hours after the procedure.

Hemihypertrophy is associated with short stature and increased excretion or urinary gonadotropins in the Silver syndrome. Clinical manifestations overlap with those of a syndrome described by Russell. Therefore the combination of dwarfism, asymmetry, craniofacial disproportion (pseudohydrocephalus), and occasional anomalies of sexual development and/or abnormal urinary excretion of gonadotropins is best categorized in *Russell-Siver dwarfism*. The incidence of hemihypertrophy is increased in children with Wilms' tumor. Aniridia and hemihypertrophy also carry a high risk of associated Wilms' tumor, with no apparent relationship between the site of the tumor and the side of the somatic enlargement or ocular defect. Adrenal neoplasm and hepatoblastoma have also been reported in association with hemihypertrophy. *Localized hypertrophy* occurs in association with hemangiomas, neurofibromas, and lipomatosis.

Hypoplasias or malsegmentations are readily recognizable and may constitute problems in management. Hypoplasia of the femur has been reported in newborns of diabetic or prediabetic mothers. When this association also includes sacral hypoplasia or aplasia it is termed caudal regression syndrome. The occurrence of skeletal defects (*phocomelia*) following exposure of the pregnant mother to thalidomide has alerted physicians to the role of chemical as well as infectious agents in the production of defects.

Total absence of one, several, or all extremities is called *amelia*; *ectromelia* is an alternative term for the absence of a single extremity. In *hemimelia* the distal half (from elbow or knee) of an extremity is lacking, and a tapering stump is present. *Paraxial hemimelia* refers to the absence of a medial or lateral efficiency of the distal portions of any extremity and depending on its location, is designated ulnar, radial, tibial, or fibular. *Acheiria* is the congenital absence of a hand, *apodia* indicates the congenital absence of a foot, and *adactylia* is the congenital absence of the digits in any extremity. *Phocomelia* refers to the congenital absence of the portions of the limb between its root and its extremity, so that the hand or foot seems to arise directly from the trunk. Intrauterine amputations occur rarely; incomplete forms, in which circular grooves almost separate a digit or limb, are known as Streeter bands. The etiology of these is unknown. Local failure of growth is more likely than extrinsic pressure by amniotic bands. Hereditary factors have also been implicated.

Individual bones are occasionally absent; more frequently the defective bone is identified radiographically as a small oval or round osseous mass without functional structure. The fibula, radius, and femur are most frequently affected, in that sequence. When the fibula is absent, its vestiges contribute to lateral bowing of the tibia. Division of the dense band of undeveloped fibula is important for management of the deformity. Absence or hypoplasia of the radius is associated with radial deviation of the hand and frequently with absence or hypoplasia of the thumb.

Varying degrees of deformity have been observed by Fanconi and others in association with aplastic anemia, skin pigmentation, and other anomalies. Radial absence with preservation of the thumb is a feature of the syndrome of absent radius and thrombocytopenia. Deformity of the thumb in association with congenital heart disease, especially atrial septal defect, is known as the *Holt-Oram syndrome*, an autosomal dominant trait in which the thumb may be absent or may be a triphalangeal nonopposable fingerlike digit. Absence, hypoplasia, or habitual displacement of the patella is associated with the *iliac horn syndrome*, which in its fully developed form also includes arthrodysplasia of the elbows, ectodermal dysplasia of the nails (especially of the thumb and index finger), hornlike posterior growths of the ilium, and occasionally a familial form of nephritis.

Segmentation abnormalities of the fingers and toes are not uncommon components of recognizable syndromes. *Polydactyly*, the presence of more than the normal number of digits, usually occurs as a hereditary trait. The most common occurrence is that of a single accessory digit, often hypoplastic, attached to the ulnar side of the little finger; occasionally the thumb is duplicated. In some forms an entire extradigit may be present, with variable involvement of the phalanges and the associated metacarpal or metatarsal bones. The dichotomy is usually more prominent distally. The location of extradigits in relation to the radial (preaxial) or ulnar (postaxial) sides of the hand is of significance in syndrome identification. Thus postaxial polydactyly is a feature of the Laurence-Moon-Biedl syndrome, in association with obesity, hypogonadism, retinitis pigmentosa, and mental retardation. It also exists in the Ellis–van Creveld–syndrome (p. 2007) in association with chondrodystrophic changes, ectodermal dysplasia, and congenital heart disease.

Syndactyly is the partial or complete fusion of digits involving the soft tissues or bony structures, or both. In its mildest form it appears as a prominent web between adjacent digits. The observation of syndactyly in a newborn infant should warrant investigation for craniosynostoses, which are frequently associated, or for other associated dysmorphic syndromes. In Apert's syndrome (p. 916) the syndactyly usually involves the index, ring, and middle fingers and is complete, with bony as well as soft tissue fusion; there usually is but one nail for the conjoined mass of digits. In Carpenter's syndrome (p. 916) syndactyly is combined with polydactyly and craniosynostosis; the extra digit is on the radial side of the hand (preaxial), and the syndactyly is less severe than in Apert's syndrome. Individual nails are usually present for the almost completely fused digital mass. When syndactyly exists in the Laurence-Moon-Biedl syndrome the polydactylous digit is on the ulnar side of the hand or the fibular side of the foot. The combination of syndactyly associated with hypoplasia of the affected hand and absence of the sternal head of the pectoralis major and nipple on the same side is known as Poland syndactyly.

Abnormally elongated spidery fingers and toes (*arachnodactyly*) are components of Marfan's syndrome, congenital contractural arachnodactyly (with which it may be confused), and also homocystinuria. *Brachydactyly* (abnormally short digits) may result from shortness or absence of phalanges or metacarpal and metatarsal bones. Several hereditary forms have been described. Shortening of the third and fourth metacarpal bones is prominent in pseudohypoparathyroidism and in gonadal dysgenesis; it is also frequently an anatomic variant or a manifestation of primary skeletal dysplasia. Brachydactyly and brachymetacarpia may occur as isolated abnormalities; they are frequently classified among the peripheral dysostoses and are common manifestations of many forms of short-limbed dwarfism. Hypoplasia of the proximal phalanges of the great toes occurs in myositis ossificans progressiva and may appear before the soft tissue changes of the disease. Comparable deformitites occur in the hands.

Camptodactyly is a fixed flexion contracture of one or more fingers; it may be congenital or acquired, sporadic or familial. The proximal interphalangeal joint, most frequently that of the fifth digit, is most commonly affected. In 60 to 70 percent of the individuals the deformity is bilateral. *Clinodactyly* refers to incurving of the digit, usually associated with hypoplasia of the middle phalanx (brachymesophalangia). Curving of the terminal phalanx of the fifth digit is a manifestation of Kirner's anomaly, which appears to result from abnormal growth of the epiphyseal cartilage of the distal phalanx. In diastrophic dwarfism (p.2007) hypoplasia of the first metacarpal bone causes the thumb to arise at a more acute angle from the hand than is usual. In somatic trisomy syndromes there are various flexion contractures of fingers with overlapping. Radial-ulnar fusions are seen in some instances of Klinefelter's syndrome.

In children with the Duchenne type of muscular dystrophy the ratio of the maximal sagittal diameter of the fibula to the minimal sagittal diameter of the tibia is greater than in either normal children or children with other neuromuscular disturbances. The disparity apparently occurs as part of the disease and is not acquired as a consequence of abnormal neuromuscular stress. This so-called fibular sign has proved to be a helpful diagnostic and differential point. Changes are less marked in muscular dystrophies other than the Duchenne type.

PRENATAL BOWING OF TUBULAR BONES. Prenatal bowing of tubular bones in the extremities may be a consequence of faulty position of the fetus in utero. However, the condition may occur in successive pregnancies, and other than mechanical factors may at times be the cause. Bowing of the long bones is a feature of *congenital hypophosphatasia*. In most instances simple and multiple bowing deformities of the extremities are noted at birth, with skin pits or dimples at the summit of the bowing. In some of the children with hypophos-

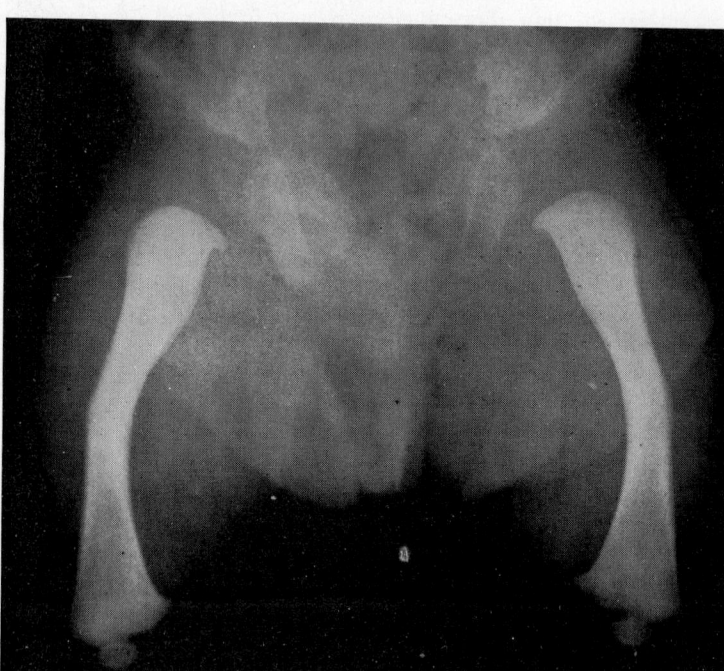

FIG. 12.   Congenital bowing of tubular bones. A dimple is present over the apex of the curve on the left thigh.

phatasia who are born with bowing deformities and dimples, other manifestations of hypophosphatasia are not present at birth, but develop some months later. Radiographic examination, which shows the bowing of the long bones, discloses cortical thickening on the inside of the curves (Fig. 12). The milder lesions gradually disappear after birth, and the affected bones are restored to normal. Moderately severe prenatal bowing of the femurs and tibias may persist as late as the seventh year. In severe cases plastic surgery may be required. Bowing is also common with congenital hypoplasia of the femur in offspring of diabetic mothers. It is also a constant feature in the so-called *campomelic syndrome*. This condition is usually discovered at birth because of small size for gestational age with extreme shortness and bowing of the extremities. Its outstanding radiographic features consist in the association of hypoplasia of the pelvis with bowing of the long tubular bones of the lower extremities, which differentiates it from achondroplasia. In addition, the face is flattened in this syndrome, and cleft palate occurs in about a third of the cases. Although the condition is generally lethal, deformities tend to regress in the rare patient who survives.

NONRACHITIC BOWLEGS. Nonrachitic bowlegs can be a cause of considerable parental concern if the usual history of retrogression in similarly affected siblings or other family members is not appreciated.

When the ankles are held together the medial surfaces of the knees are widely separated, and the calves even more so. Correction is usually spontaneous and its course can be followed radiographically. Rarely, and primarily in cases developing after the age of 6 years, the bowing tends to progress to a true tibia vara (a condition known as Blount's disease) and may require osteotomy for correction.

KNOCK-KNEE. Knock-knee is the opposite of bowleg and is seldom congenital; it usually makes its appearance after the child begins to walk, and it may be progressive. When it is not due to rickets or other metabolic disorders, generalized relaxation of ligamentous structures, including flatfoot deformity, is often present. During the period of growth, muscle training and minor orthopedic devices are preferable to surgical procedures in all but extreme cases. Progression of bowlegs and knock-knees to normal as a feature of normal growth and development has been described. However, when these deformities are due to dystrophies and dysplasias they are extremely difficult to correct.

CONGENITAL CLUBFOOT. The components of congenital clubfoot deformity include adduction of the forefoot, inversion of the calcaneus under the talus, and plantar flexion with equinus position at the ankle joint, all associated with relative rigidity in these abnormal positions (Fig. 13). Fixed clubfoot deformity requires orthopedic treatment; the marked clubfoot deformity

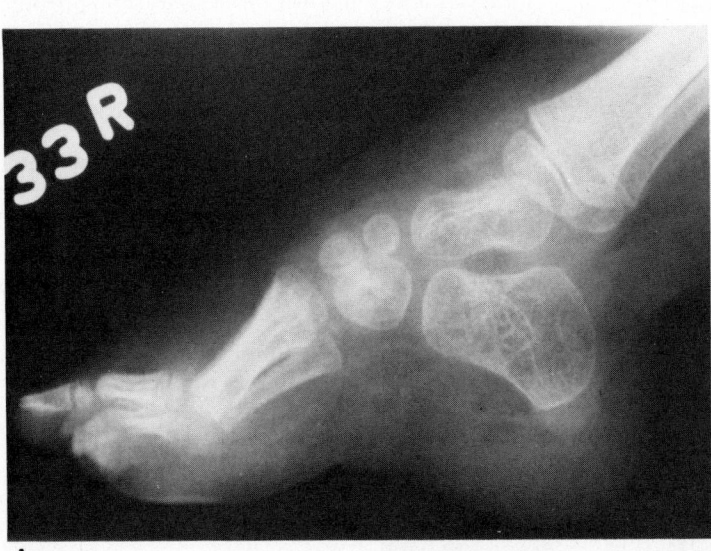

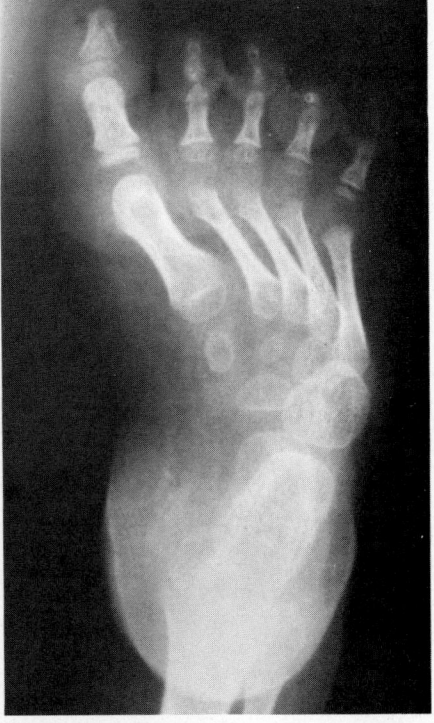

FIG. 13. Congenital clubfoot deformity in a girl 3 years 8 months of age. A. Lateral projection. The equinus position of the talus is indicated by its articulation with the tibia via its posterior surface rather than its dorsal surface. The planter flexion is reflected by the high arch and diminished angle between the axes of the calcaneus and the first metatarsal bone (normally 150 to 175 degrees; here about 121 degrees). B. Anteroposterior projection. The calcaneus is rotated under the talus (normal angle 25 to 50 degrees; here 15 degrees); the metatarsal bones are adducted (metatarsus varus).

occurring in association with diastrophic dwarfism (p. 2007) is extremely resistant to treatment and is probably an exception to this rule. Some infants who are born with one or both feet held in the clubbed position (or in the reverse position of abduction, eversion, and dorsiflexion) have passive motion of the foot through the normal full range. When it is released the foot resumes its clubbed attitude. In such infants manipulation through the full range of motion several times a day is the recommended treatment. Clubfoot deformity developing after birth may result from trauma, local disease, or neuromuscular disease such as poliomyelitis, myelodysplasia, or peroneal muscular atrophy.

FLATFOOT (PES PLANUS, PRONATED FEET, PES PLANOVALGUS). When the child first begins to walk, the marked thickness of the plantar fat pads causes the entire sole to touch the ground when bearing weight. In many instances the muscles supporting the inner side of the foot are actually weaker than their opponents, which causes some valgus deformity. The term valgus in this context refers to lateral displacement of the calcaneus (heel eversion) under the talus. Support for the head of the talus is consequently lost, and the anterior portion of the talus moves downward and medially, flattening the longitudinal arch. This condition is common and is referred to as physiologic flatfoot. It requires no treatment, for it soon corrects itself as the muscles increase in strength. After the age of 3 years the contour of the child's foot in weight bearing should resemble that of an adult.

True flatfoot deformity does not develop until some time after weight bearing begins, except in instances of pathologic ligamentous relaxation or in teratologic defects. In some instances ligamentous laxity exists elsewhere in the body and/or a familial history is elicited. Fatigue or pain in the feet is a frequent complaint. With the heel eversion, the forefoot twists outward and the line of weight bearing is directed to the first metatarsal bone, or even medial to it, rather than toward the second metatarsal bone, as it normally should. The valgus

position is obvious when the patient stands; on walking the child often automatically compensates and toes-in. The heel and sole of the shoe become unduly worn on the medial side. A double internal malleolus may be found on physical examination, the lowermost bony prominence being the head of the talus. Relatively simple lifts in the shoe or on the sole and mechanical devices to support the heel generally suffice to correct this condition.

Teratologic flatfoot deformity may occur in association with tarsal coalition (commonly a calcaneotalar bar) or in the so-called vertical talus, where there is a teratologic dislocation of the talonavicular joints such that the navicular bone articulates with the dorsal aspect of the talus and locks it into a plantar flexed vertical position (Figs. 14 and 15). The condition is now described under the term of congenital convex pes valgus and is referred to as *rocker-bottom feet.* It is not uncommon in meningomyelocele or as a complication of systemic disorders of the neuromuscular system and is a frequent component of autosomal trisomy syndromes. Its management is surgical.

TORSION OF LOWER EXTREMITIES. Twisting of the lower extremities on their longitudinal axes may be partial or total, lateral or medial, and congenital or acquired. Most cases appear to be acquired, and they are readily correctable. All acquired forms are believed to result from persistent positional stress. Sleeping prone in the frogleg position can produce lateral torsion of the femurs; sleeping in the fetal position can produce medial torsion of the tibias. Sitting on the floor with knees flexed and feet turned out (sitting between the feet) could be responsible for lateral torsion of the tibias and femurs; sitting on the feet could cause medial torsion of the tibias. The latter two positions will be recognized as common attitudes during television viewing.

The usual complaints are that children are either bowlegged or pigeon-toed in the medial torsions, or they have everted or even flat feet in the lateral variety.

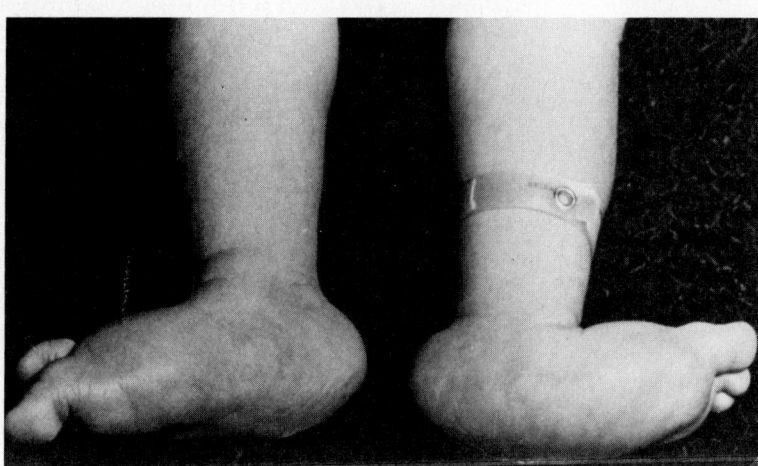

FIG. 14. Rocker-bottom feet due to vertical talus in 9-month-old infant (probably trisomy 18).

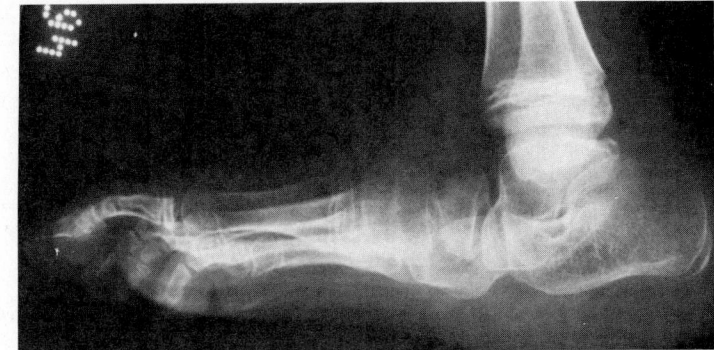

FIG. 15. Vertical talus in male with sacral agenesis (age 13.5 years). The navicular bone articulates with the dorsum of the talus, locking it in the vertical position.

The diagnosis is made by determining the extent of passive internal and external rotation. Normally the entire lower extremity can be rotated equally in both directions when the child lies in the supine position; when torsion exists rotation is restricted in the direction opposite to that of the torsion, and there is a dissociation between the position of the anterior aspect of the knees and the axis of the foot. In tibial torsion the feet turn in or out when the child sits with feet dangling. Children who habitually sit on their feet may in addition develop bony prominences and even callosities over the head of the talus and the anterior external corner of the calcaneus.

Radiography is usually not helpful, as the changes are greatest in the soft tissues. In severe medial tibial torsion there is a discrepancy between the positions of the upper and lower ends of the tibia and fibula, with the bones at knee level externally rotated while ankles are internally rotated. In very mild cases elimination of the posture habit may be all that is necessary for treatment. More severe cases require corrective manipulations under orthopedic guidance and minor appliances such as bars on shoes for sleeping, or even special shoes. Braces are rarely used, and surgical procedures are not indicated. As a general rule, conservative management will permit spontaneous regression in all common mild developmental deformities of the extremities in infancy and childhood. However, it is important that parents not be merely assured that the child will "outgrow" the condition; careful serial follow-up must be provided in all cases.

Acquired Conditions

Trauma

FRACTURE. Trauma is probably the most common cause of skeletal disease in childhood, with fracture as its most obvious manifestation. Fractures are often recognized clinically by the familiar triad of pain, swelling, and deformity; sometimes even careful radiographic examination immediately after injury may fail to disclose the fracture. Whenever a fracture is suspected clinically, competent radiographic examination should be obtained, including comparative examination of the injured and corresponding uninjured bones, both taken in identical position in two planes at right angles. The proximal and distal joints of a fractured bone should be included on the film. If two separate films are needed to show the proximal and distal joints there must be no change in position of the limb between the two exposures, and at least one film should be centered on the fracture site. Reduction of a fracture should be verified radiographically, and a final film is advisable when healing is believed to be completed.

Healing of fractures in children is generally prompt, and reconstitution of bone takes place rapidly enough that even major angulations readily correct. The longer the period between the time of fracture and cessation of bone growth (characterized by epiphyseal-diaphyseal union), the greater the chance of reconstitution. Rotational deformities and marked overriding or distortion require more careful correction then angulation, while injury to an epiphysis and its radiologically invisible cartilage tends to result in local disturbance of growth.

Spiral fracture of the tibia, which is frequent in childhood, may follow a fall; or the trauma may have gone unnoticed, and the child merely refuses to bear weight on one extremity. For optimal projection of the spiral fracture line on radiography, oblique as well as anteroposterior and lateral views may be necessary. The fracture is most commonly in the middle or distal third of the tibia and often lacks the sign of point tenderness; deformity or displacement seldom occurs because of the splinting action of the fibula. In cases with displacement, fracture of the opposite end of the adjacent fibula should be sought.

DISLOCATION. Dislocations may occur with or without fractures. As a general rule, one form of injury usually seems to protect against the other. Subluxation of the radial head is frequent, usually occurring when young children are dragged or lifted by the hand. The head of the radius partly escapes from the annular ligament. The forearm is usually held in moderate flexion at the elbow midway between pronation and supination and distinct tenderness is elicited over the region of the radial head. Reduction is readily accomplished by gentle pressure with the thumb over the radial head while and simultaneously extending the elbow very gently and supinating the forearm. Relief of symptoms is almost immediate. Sometimes the reduction is spontaneous, or it may occur during the manipulations involved in obtaining a radiograph (which is rarely helpful). Major dislocations generally occur following trauma of considerable force, such as a fall from a tree or a traffic accident. Acquired dislocations also occur as a result of neuromuscular malformations or injury, as in cerebral palsy and myelomeningoceles, where hip dislocation is quite common. Poliomyelitis was at one time a cause of acquired dislocation. Suppurative arthritis must always be considered when a dislocation occurs, particularly in an infant, because evidence of pain, limitation of motion, and even fever may be lacking.

EPIPHYSEAL SEPARATION.   Epiphyseal separations are common injuries in children. A fall on an outstretched arm that would produce a Colles' fracture in older children and adults usually results in a posterior displacement of the distal epiphysis of the radius together with a small fragment of the adjacent metaphysis. Mechanical reduction and cast immobilization are necessary. Although the possibility of epiphyseal injury and growth disturbance is greater than in a fracture of a shaft, adverse sequelae are infrequent.

Epiphyseal separation of the femoral head occurs in obese preadolescent or adolescent children; the condition may develop spontaneously and be manifested by pain, or it may occur with pain following unusual activity or injury. Hip pain at the time of injury warrants careful examination of both hips to detect demineralization of the femoral neck adjacent to the conjugating cartilage that precedes the slipping. Repositioning of the femoral head is often difficult, and the position is generally maintained by surgical introduction of a metallic nail along the course of the femoral neck into the femoral head.

Epiphyseal separations also occur with some frequency in adolescent and preadolescent children in shoulders, wrists, and other areas, as well as the hips. Displacement of the upper epiphysis of the humerus has been observed in a 14-year-old boy as a consequence of throwing a football. There is some experimental evidence suggesting that the vulnerability of the union between epiphysis and shaft is related to endocrine activity of puberty. The adolescent child who participates in athletics has an increased risk of injury to the growing epiphyses. This appears to be particularly true of obese children and tall, uncoordinated children. Fracture of the femoral epiphysis has been described in adolescent football players, thus emphasizing the point that epiphyseal separation may proceed to epiphyseal fracture. A practical classification of epiphyseal fractures has been provided by Salter and Harris. Sprains around weight-bearing joints in children must be carefully checked for possible epiphyseal injury. Reasonable supervision of children's athletic endeavors is important to help prevent injury.

BONE CONTUSION.   Contusions occur as a consequence of direct injury to bony structures. Usually there are no initial radiographic abnormalities. Subsequently subperiosteal hemorrhage that commonly accompanies the injury results in new bone formation under the elevated periosteum, which becomes visible radiographically about 2 to 3 weeks after the injury.

UNRECOGNIZED TRAUMA.   Sometimes trauma that is severe enough to produce fracture and reparative changes may not be recognized by those responsible for the child. Trauma at birth may not be appreciated in the absence of apparent difficulty at delivery; or the trauma incurred during play in which wrenching of extremities occurs may go unnoticed. Lack of recognition of the initial injury and ensuring lack of immobilization may lead to repetitive injury as a result of minor trauma. Repetition of injury is also promoted by the infant's inability to communicate information about the initial injury.

Repetitive injuries produce bizarre radiographic changes, usually within 12 to 14 days after the initial injury (Fig. 16). In tubular bones there are metaphyseal irregularities and frequently massive calcifying parosteal hematomas along the shafts and extending to the epiphyseal end of the shaft that resemble the calcifying hematomas of healing scurvy or even neoplasms. Even the histology of the new bone mass may simulate neoplasia and may lead to serious diagnostic error. The lesions differ from those of scurvy or other nutritional or metabolic disease in that in trauma the lesions are extensive at one end of a bone, while the other more rapidly growing end is normal, even when multiple bones are involved. In infants less than 6 months of age, scurvy is most unusual. Moreover, the vitamin C content of the blood can been measured. Hematologic disorders should also be ruled out.

Stress fractures occasionally seen in the upper third of the tibia or fibula are a form of unrecognized trauma sometimes described as fatigue fractures. They may cause limping or disinclination to bear weight on an extremity. Spiral fractures of the tibia (p. 1991) can also occur from unrecognized trauma. Delayed responses to partial avulsion of muscles from their attachment to tubular bones may subsequently give rise to myositis ossificans traumatica, which at times may simulate bone neoplasia. However, normal anatomic variations and developmental irregularities of mineralization in growing children should not be confused with traumatic lesions.

BATTERED CHILD.   (Chap. 15, p. 827). Children who are roughly handled by adults in play or in anger represent a large group of victims of trauma. In such circumstances the history of the initial trauma may be difficult or impossible to obtain because of unawareness, reluctance to incriminate oneself, or deliberate lying.

Generally the skeletal lesions of the battered child syndrome are identical to those previously described for unrecognized trauma. They are characterized not only by predilection for metaphyses and abundant subperiosteal new bone formation but by the different stages of injury and/or repair and by multiplicity of lesions. Spiral and transverse fractures of long bones

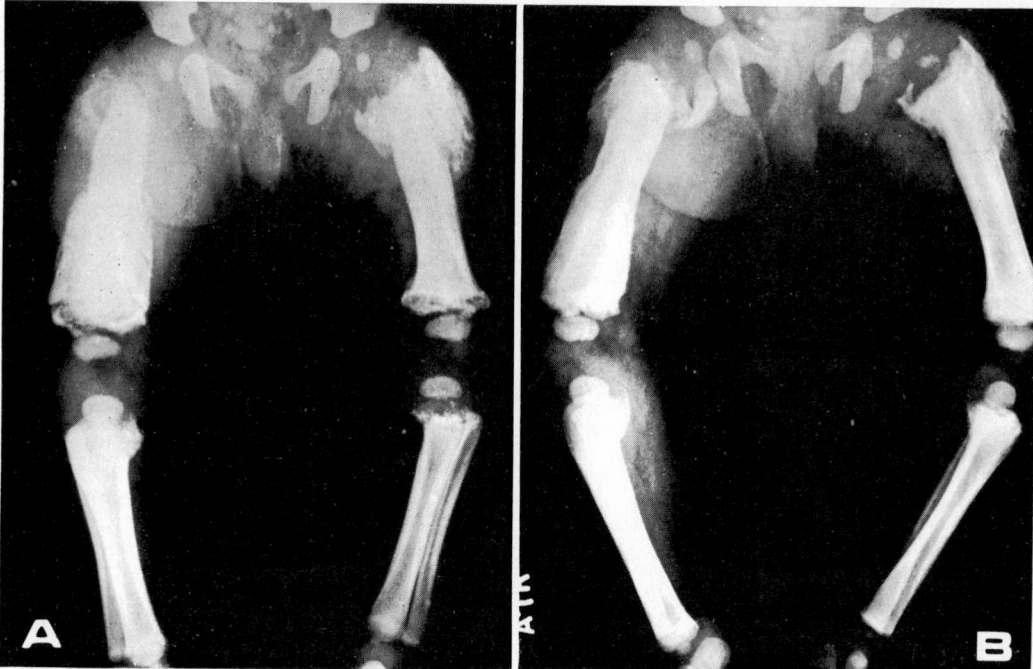

FIG. 16.   Reparative changes in unrecognized trauma in 7-month-old infant.

occurring as solitary injuries are more frequent than the classic epiphyseal-metaphyseal long bone fractures. Fractures of the lateral end of the clavicle, fractures of the ribs and scapula, and spinal fractures have been described.

Recognition of skeletal lesions due to child abuse is essential for three reasons: (1) Serious infection or neoplastic bone disease need not be considered, thereby eliminating potentially harmful, expensive, and time-consuming diagnostic procedures. (2) The victims can be removed from their dangerous environments. (3) The existence of such bone lesions should call attention to the possibility of subdural hematoma, a condition frequently associated with the skeletal lesions that is far more threatening than they are.

BONE ATROPHY.   Acquired bone atrophy may result from neuromuscular disease, from metabolic disorder, or, especially in children, from immobilization. Immobilization of the involved area results in prompt mobilization of calcium from the now inactive bones and secondary hypercalcemia, which can produce renal damage, hypertension, and convulsions. Physiotherapy to minimize inactivity is important in prevention as well as treatment of the immobilization syndrome. Children with vitamin-D-resistant hypophosphatemic rickets who are receiving large doses of vitamin D are especially susceptible to this condition when they are immobilized for osteotomies. Cortical bone increases in thickness through childhood; "atrophy" is related largely to inhibition or even reversal of this process. Cortical thick-

ness may be a more accurate indicator of nutritional status than size and number of the secondary ossification centers. Thus the nutritional status of a child with phenylketonuria managed by dietary restriction is best assessed by measurements of cortical thickness.

References

DEVELOPMENTAL ANOMALIES

Archibald RM, Finby N, DeVito F: Endocrine significance of short metacarpals. J Clin Endocrinol 19:1312, 1959

Blank E, Girdany BR: Symmetric bowing of the terminal phalanges of the fifth fingers in a family (Kirner's deformity). Am J Roentgenol Radium Ther Nucl Med 93:367, 1965

Caffey J: Prenatal bowing and thickening of tubular bones, with multiple cutaneous dimples in arms and legs; a congenital syndrome of mechanical origin. Am J Dis Child 74:543, 1947

Conway TJ: Prenatal bowing and angulation of long bones. Am J Dis Child 95:305, 1958

Hall JG, Levin J, Kuhn JP, Ottenheimer EJ, Van Berkum KAP, McKusick VA: Thrombocytopenia with absent radius (TAR). Medicine 48:411, 1969

Kaufman HJ (ed): Progress in Pediatric Radiology, Vol 4, Intrinsic Diseases of Bone. Basel, Karger, 1973

——— A new roentgen sign in pseudohypertrophic muscular dystrophy. Am J Roentgenol Radium Ther Nucl Med 89:970, 1963

Kellsey DC: Hypophosphatasia and congenital bowing of the long bones. JAMA 179:187, 1962

Kite JH: Torsion of the legs in young children. Clin Orthop 16:152, 1960

Langenskiöld A, Riska EB: Tibia vara (osteochondrosis deformans tibiae). J Bone Joint Surg [Am] 46:1405, 1964

Maroteaux P: The campomelic syndrome. In Kaufman HJ (ed): Progr Pediatr Radiol 4:578, 1973

Miller RW, Fraumeni JF Jr, Manning MD: Association of Wilm's tumor with aniridia, hemihypertrophy and other congenital malformations. N Engl J Med 270:922, 1964

Moseley JE, Moloshok RE, Freiberger RH: The Silver syndrome: congenital asymmetry, short stature and variations in sexual development, roentgen features. Am J Roentgenol Radium Ther Nucl Med 97:74, 1966

Poznanski AK: The Hand in Radiologic Diagnosis. Philadelphia, WB Saunders, 1974

Shopfner CE, Coin CG: Genu varus and valgus in children. Radiology 92:723, 1969

Silver HK, Kiyasu W, George J, Deamer W: Syndrome of congenital hemihypertrophy, shortness of stature, and elevated urinary gonadotropins. Pediatrics 12:368, 1953

ACQUIRED CONDITIONS

Caffey J: Multiple fractures in long bones of infants suffering from chronic subdural hematoma. Am J Roentgenol Radium Ther Nucl Med 56:163, 1946

Calhoun JD, Pierret G: Infantile coxa vara. Am J Roentgenol Radium Ther Nucl Med 115:561, 1972

Dodd K, Graubarth H, Rapoport S: Hypercalcemia nephropathy and encephalopathy following immobilization; case report. Pediatrics 6:124, 1950

Griffiths AL: Fatigue fracture of the fibula in childhood. Arch Dis Child 27:552, 1952

Helfer RE, Kempe CH (eds): The Battered Child, 2nd ed. Chicago, University of Chicago Press, 1974

Kelsey JL, Acheson RM, Keggi KJ: Body build of patients with slipped capital femoral epiphysis. Am J Dis Child 124:276, 1972

Kogutt MS, Swischuk LE, Fagan CJ: Patterns of injury and significance of uncommon fractures in the battered child syndrome. Am J Roentgenol Radium Ther Nucl Med 121:143, 1974

Larson RL, McMahan RO: The epiphyses and the childhood athlete. JAMA 196:607, 1968

Rogers LF, Jones S, Davis AR, Dietz G: "Clipping injury" fracture of the epiphysis in the adolescent football player: an occult lesion of the knee. Am J Roentgenol Radium Ther Nucl Med 121:69, 1974

Salter RB, Harris WR: Injuries involving the epiphyseal plate. J Bone Joint Surg [Am] 45:587, 1963

Silverman FN: Unrecognized trauma in infants, the battered child syndrome, and the syndrome of Ambroise Tardieu. Rigler lecture. Radiology 104:337, 1972

Tachdjian MO: Pediatric Orthopedics. Philadelphia, W B Saunders, 1972

AXIAL SKELETON

FREDERIC N. SILVERMAN

THORACIC CAGE

FUNNEL CHEST (PECTUS EXCAVATUM). The term funnel chest is applied to a congenital depression of variable depth in the lower portion of the sternum (Fig. 17). It is probably a consequence of a primary growth abnormality of the costal cartilages. The depressed sternum may compress the heart and displace the mediastinal structures posteriorly and to the left. The functional results of this deformity and its treatment are discussed elsewhere (p. 1592).

Functional cardiac murmurs commonly occur in association with congenital funnel chest. Similar murmurs are heard when the thoracic spatial relationships are disturbed in the straight-back syndrome, where an unusual straight alignment of the thoracic vertebrae and concomitant absence of physiologic posterior curvature of the dorsal spine limit the anteroposterior thoracic diameter from behind, much as a depressed sternum does.

PIGEON BREAST. Pigeon breast is, in effect, the reverse of funnel chest; the anteroposterior diameter of the thorax is increased by a ventral protrusion of the sternum and attached cartilages in the form of a sharp, often keellike projection. This deformity, which cosmetically may be more disturbing than funnel chest, occasionally occurs in association with other abnormalities, particularly of the vertebrae and ribs. It is seen more commonly as a localized, lower sternal protrusion in the presence of cardiac enlargement, particularly right ventricle hypertrophy. A special form of pigeon breast deformity results from premature union of the sternal segments, an anomaly also frequently associated with cardiac malformations and pulmonary hypertension.

Flaring of the lower rib cage is a deformity common in rickets; the horizontal grooves where the flare begins are known as *Harrison grooves*. In present-day practice this flaring is seen more frequently as a result of longstanding abdominal distension, as for example in chronic megacolon or in the celiac syndrome and in hypotonia of any etiology.

SPRENGEL'S DEFORMITY. Sprengel's deformity is a congenital failure of descent of the scapula, usually unilateral, that produces shoulder asymmetry. The involved scapula is higher and more medial than the normal scapula. The vertebral border of the scapula, which normally parallels the spine, inclines sharply caudally toward the spine. In some cases there is an anomalous bone connecting the medial border of the scapula to the spinous process of one or more cervical vertebrae; in other cases fibrous connections limit the lateral excursion of the scapula. Cervicodorsal scoliosis is almost always present, and anomalies of vertebrae (hemivertebrae, vertical fusions, and spina bifida) are frequently associated. Functionally there is inability to abduct the arm and raise it above the head. Surgical removal of restricting osseous or fibrous structures may produce both cosmetic and functional improvement. Confusion with various forms of short-neck deformities, such as those associated with the Klippel-Feil malformation (p. 1977) and the Wildervanck syndrome, (p. 1977) may be clarified by radiographic examination, although features common to the various conditions may make such differentiation difficult.

DEFECTS AND PROTRUSION. Congenital defects that are clinically visible and palpable as depressions in the thoracic wall occur as a result of maldevelopment of ribs; vertebral anomalies are usually present as well. Deformity of the thoracic wall occasionally occurs in association with hypoplasia of the pectoralis major, mammary hypoplasia, and costal cartilage defect. Rarely, failure of fusion of the lateral portions of the early fetal sternum leads to a midline defect, with retraction on inspiration. Congenital malformation of the heart may be present.

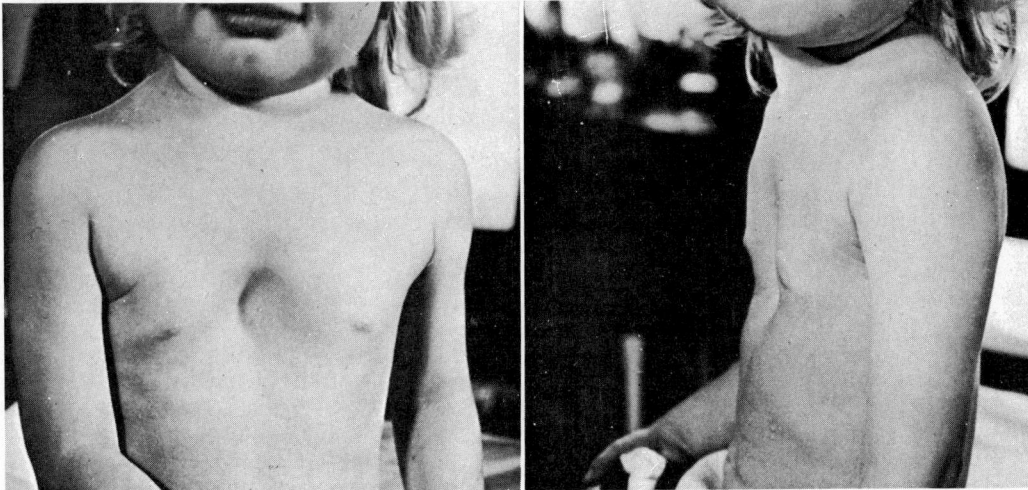

FIG. 17. Funnel chest deformity. (Courtesy of Dr. J. Holmsworth.)

A syndrome has been described that is characterized by a high omphalocele (between umbilicus and sternum) or gastroschisis, by defect of the anterior portion of the diaphragm, and by defect of the pericardium. A ventricular diverticulum may extend through the pericardial and diaphragmatic defects toward or through the umbilicus and present as a pulsating mass. Other thoracic wall protrusions commonly result from dyschondroplasias involving the costochondral junctions. They are invisible radiographically, although they are obvious clinically when composed of cartilage; evidence of dyschondroplasia elsewhere should suggest the diagnosis. The thorax is extremely narrow and is frequently associated with respiratory difficulties in Jeune's disease (*asphyxiating thoracic dystrophy*) and the Ellis–van Creveld syndrome; these are part of a group of skeletal dysplasias designated short-rib polydactyly syndromes. Deformities of the sternal ends of the ribs are frequent abnormalities of no clinical significance. However, forked rib deformities occur in association with the basal cell nevus syndrome in which, in addition, cysts of the jaw commonly occur and calcification of the falx occasionally occurs; medulloblastoma has also been reported in family members. Rib defects may be present in infants with the Pierre Robin syndrome (p. 917) and may contribute to their problems.

A rare affection of unknown cause that presents as painful or tender swelling of the costal cartilages is known as Tietze's syndrome. It may stimulate low-grade infections, trauma, or even tumor, but it has a self-limited course that lasts many months. Management includes reassurance and avoidance of unnecessary diagnostic or therapeutic measures.

VERTEBRAL COLUMN

The vertebral column forms a smooth curve in infancy when viewed laterally; several normal curves appear later as development proceeds from the stage of holding the head erect, to sitting, to ambulation. Posteriorly the spine is normally straight at all ages. Variations from the normal may include decrease or increase of normal curves and pathologic curves and protrusions. Subtle as well as obvious segmentation errors can be overlooked unless careful inspection of pedicles, spinous processes, and vertebral bodies is carried out.

SCOLIOSIS. Abnormal curvature that is usually lateral and is most obvious when viewed from behind is a very common orthopedic problem in childhood. It may result from congenital malformation of the vertebral column or from associated malformations such as Sprengel's deformity or hypoplasia of the femur. It was formerly a common result of poliomyelitis affecting spinal or extremity muscles. It may be a complication of other neuromuscular diseases such as spastic paralysis and muscular dystrophies. Many occur without obvious cause and are designated as idiopathic; some of these are possibly the result of clinically inapparent nervous system infections. Arteriovenous malformations have been demonstrated in some by aortography. Scoliosis is very common in neurofibromatosis, and it may be a manifestation of osteoid osteoma of the spine. Scoliosis is a component of several skeletal dysplasias, particularly diastrophic dwarfism, spondyloepiphyseal dysplasia, dysplasia epiphysealis punctata, and others. Kyphosis occurs occasionally in achondroplasia and is an important feature of metatropic dwarfism. Organicity of the scoliosis can be tested by observing the patient's spine after suspending him first by the arms, then by the legs. An abnormal curvature that persists during these maneuvers is not likely to improve spontaneously, but is almost certain to deteriorate progressively. Scoliosis may occur as a consequence of radiation therapy in infancy or childhood; occasionally the deformity is aggravated during the adolescent growth spurt.

All cases of scoliosis require competent orthopedic management. Surgical procedures such as excision of hemivertebrae or spine fusion have fairly clear indications and contraindications. Radiographic control of the progress of scoliosis is indispensable for management. Criteria for measuring angles have been described in detail in many publications on the subject; in any given patient identical criteria should be applied at each examination.

SCHEUERMANN'S DISEASE. Scheuermann's disease (juvenile kyphosis, juvenile roundback deformity), a progressive kyphosis, usually affects the dorsal spine and develops during adolescence. Originally considered an epiphysitis, it is now generally believed to be a consequence of rupture of thinned cartilaginous plates, with prolapse of intervertebral disk tissue into the cancellous bone of the vertebral bodies. Its primary cause has not been established, but there does appear to be some relationship to stress. Radiographically several adjacent vertebrae are involved, in contradistinction to the usual localization of infectious processes to one or two vertebrae. Early treatment by bracing and recumbency to minimize deformity is recommended.

CONGENITAL MALFORMATIONS. Malformations that are important in number and severity result from vertical and horizontal errors in segmentation. Vertical fusion of cervical vertebrae produces the *Klippel-Feil malformation,* which is characterized by a short neck, the head resting on the shoulders, limitation of head motion, low posterior hairline, and spina bifida at the affected level. Neurologic abnormalities, such as mirror movements of the upper extremities, are also occasionally present. Clinical confusion with Sprengel's deformity is not uncommon.

Spina bifida refers to a failure of fusion of the two lateral halves of the arch of the vertebra. In its mildest and clinically asymptomatic form (spina bifida occulta) the diagnosis is exclusively radiologic. The prevalence of radiographic defects in the sacral area diminishes with increasing age. For example, defects have been found in 22 percent of boys and 9 percent of girls between the ages of 7 and 8 years, contrasting with 4 percent of adult men and 1 percent of women. Undue importance has been attributed to the presence of lumbar spina bifida occulta in relation to disease of the urinary tract; the condition is as frequent in normal children as in those with urinary disease. In more severe forms (spina bifida vera) meningeal and neural elements may protrude posteriorly; neurologic deficit is usually present when neural elements occupy the protrusion (in meningomyelocele, but not in simple meningocele). In radiographs the incomplete neural arch is recognized by the increased distances between the pedicles. In some cases of spina bifida there is a bony, cartilaginous, or fibrous protrusion into the spinal canal from a vertebral body. The protrusion may transfix the spinal cord and aggravate any existing neurologic deficit, since longitudinal body growth alters the relationship of the transfixing spur to the spinal cord. Improvement in neurologic symptoms may follow surgical removal of the cord-splitting protrusion, whose action is indicated by the term diastematomyelia.

The *Arnold-Chiari malformation* and its intracranial complications should be suspected whenever meningomyelocele is present. Defects of union between the vertebral body and lateral masses, which are less readily demonstrated, may lead to anterolateral herniation of meninges at any level above the filum terminale and constitute the so-called anterior meningocele. Neuroenteric communications, a form of duplication of the intestine, have probably been mistaken for anterior meningoceles.

Hemivertebral deformities result from failure of development of one of the paired chondrification centers for vertebral bodies. They usually occur in the cervical and thoracic regions and often produce scoliosis. One sees partially mature development occurring haphazardly at successive levels on either side, and the final result is a jumble of malformed vertebrae, often out of line, with the vertebral bodies traversed here and there by vertical or diagonal fissures. The ribs share in the defect of segmentation; there may be 10 or 11 (or 13 or 14) ribs on one side, and fusion of some ribs is almost always found. Although there may be serious postural deformity, neurologic complications are rare. The condition is sometimes familial. Hemivertebral deformities are commonly associated with congenital malformations of the lungs, the heart, and the urinary tract, but they do not necessarily occur at the same level at which these malformed organs or systems are located.

Vertebral anomalies such as segmentation errors and hemivertebrae also occur in association with several fairly well defined syndromes. In Larsen's syndrome vertebral malformations are associated with congenital dislocation of the knees and other joints, a distinctive facies characterized by widely spaced eyes and frontal bossing and frequently by cleft palate. In Wildervanck's syndrome, a condition almost completely limited to females, a cervical Klippel-Feil anomaly is associated with congenital perceptive deafness and paralysis of the sixth nerve. Spina bifida may be a component of cleidocranial dysostosis. Anomalies of the spine and the ribs are seen in Waardenburg's syndrome (p. 895) and in the basal cell nevus syndrome. Goldenhar's syndrome (oculoauriculovertebral dysplasia) (p. 1952) is characterized by epibulbar dermoids, auricular appendages, and vertebral anomalies, including atloido-occipital fusion, wedge and block vertebra, hemivertebra, spina bifida, and/or scoliosis. Aplasia or hypoplasia of the odontoid process is common in Morquio's syndrome (mucopolysaccharidosis IV) (p. 1903), with atlantoaxial subluxation a serious complication that may lead to acute or chronic neurologic deficit, lower extremity weakness, or even paraplegia or death. A form of dwarfism in which virtually all vertebrae are hemivertebrae has been described under the name polydysspondyly. Sacral deformities are common with rectal atresia and imperforate anus. The existence of obvious vertebral abnormalities in a newborn warrants careful evaluation for a possible "high" form of rectal malformation.

Spondylolisthesis, a horizontal slipping of one vertebra, is most frequent at the level of the lumbosacral junction, with the fifth lumbar vertebral body moving anteriorly in relation to S-1. At one time it was thought always to result from a congenital weakness; now it is thought to result from stress factors on the pars interarticularis of the neural arch of L-5, with ensuing loss of osseous continuity. Reported instances in which osseous continuity has been reestablished provide strong support for an acquired rather than congenital origin. The back pain commonly seen in these defects (spondylolysis) may be related to the stress factor itself or to the adaptive changes on the opposite side, where hypertrophy and sclerosis of the pars interarticularis have been documented.

SPINAL FRACTURE AND DISLOCATION. Fracture of the cervical spine during delivery may in the newborn infant give rise to a clinical picture similar to amyotonia congenita. However, in the latter condition sensation and sphincter tone are preserved. In fracture of the cervical spine, contusion, laceration, and even total discontinuity of the spinal cord are responsible for the neurologic signs; contusion and avulsion of nerve roots secondary to marked head flexion during delivery probably play as significant a role. The marked displacements of skeletal structures, that during parturition caused these spinal cord and nerve injuries, may no longer be visualized at subsequent radiography.

Compression fractures of vertebral bodies and transverse or spinous process fractures occasionally occur in tetanus or following convulsive seizures of any other origin. In cervical injuries associated with marked forward flexion, the odontoid process may slowly "disappear," with an ultimate radiographic configuration simulating that of congenital absence of the odontoid process. Occasionally the odontoid process may persist as a separate ossicle without attachment to the body of the second cervical vertebra. Local disease such as osteomyelitis, leukemic infiltration, and histiocytosis may lead to compression fractures. It is now generally agreed that *Calvé vertebra plana* represents a compression fracture of a vertebral body affected with histiocytosis. A steplike depression of the central portion of the end plate of the vertebral body in sickle cell anemia, and occasionally in other hemolytic anemias, has been considered a form of depression fracture. Alternatively, it has been attributed to a focal growth disturbance secondary to chronic ischemia in the central area of the body. The spinal lesions in the hemolytic anemias are seldom of clinical significance, but are diagnostically helpful. Vertical fractures of cervical vertebral bodies may occur as a result of compression injuries, as in diving, and they may carry a bad prognosis because of associated cord damage and paraplegia. The Jefferson fracture, a bursting fracture of the ring that comprises the first cervical vertebra, is a special example of this type of injury.

Gross dislocations are easily recognized radiographically, *subluxations* are more difficult to recognize, if not impossible. A common problem following head and neck injury is the so-called subluxation of the cervical spine associated with acute torticollis. It has been shown that the radiographic appearance of subluxation may be induced at will by voluntary neck flexion mimicking torticollis. Since acute torticollis may result from various causes, including cervical adenitis, the diagnosis of subluxation is seldom if ever justified on radiographic grounds, and vigorous treatment (ie, casts, prolonged traction, immobilization) is wisely withheld until conservative measures have been tried. Acute torticollis may also be associated with calcification of the intervertebral disks, but a cause-and-effect relationship has not been proved in children. The latter condition is best considered an incidental observation without significance with respect to systemic disease. Rarely, calcified disk material may herniate and impinge on nerve roots or even on the spinal cord, in which case surgical intervention may be necessary.

Congenital torticollis is associated with fibrosis of a portion of a sternomastoid muscle that is present at birth or develops shortly thereafter; a tumor can frequently be palpated within the fibrotic muscle. The infant's head is generally inclined to the side of the affected muscle and rotated toward the opposite side. Cranial and facial asymmetry are common; both improve following relief of the torticollis. In a great majority of cases the deformity improves with conservative management, which may include gentle stretching of the affected muscle. In children in whom recovery does not take place by 6 months of age, surgical intervention can be considered, especially if facial deformity supervenes.

INFECTIONS. Tuberculosis of the spine (p. 469) has become uncommon in recent years. Tuberculin testing is of paramount importance in diagnosis, since the radiologic features of tuberculous osteitis are sometimes indistinguishable from those of nontuberculous osteitis. Therefore reliance on radiographic evidence alone for etiologic diagnosis of spinal lesions may be misleading. Benign osteitis of the spine exists in children; they may present with abdominal pain simulating intussusception or other acute intraabdominal disease. Furthermore, in two cases observed by the author, aspiration from the area of the lesion revealed hemolytic staphylococci that were sensitive to available antibiotics. The existence of freely communicating venous plexuses between the pelvic organs and the spine also explains the relationship between pelvic infection or surgery and subsequent osteitis. Although some nontuberculous lesions heal spontaneously, they are favorably influenced by restriction of activity. Antibiotics may be indicated.

PELVIS

Secondary ossification centers occur in considerable profusion in the pelvis and should not be confused with the manifestations of disease or injury. In girls crestal iliac centers usually appear within 6 months of the menarche. A corresponding developmental status may be inferred for males when this center is first noted. Radiographically, bridging of opposing pubic bones and "swelling" of the ischiopubic synchondroses are observed as part of normal growth and development.

Radiolucent defects separating the superior pubic ramus into medial and lateral portions are occasionally seen in newborn infants; they have no known clinical significance. Aseptic necroses of epiphyses in the hip are discussed under juvenile osteochrondroses (p. 2018).

Congenital malformations of consequence usually occur in association with systemic dysplasias or other malformations, and they may be helpful in establishing such diagnoses. Kaufmann's monograph is an extremely useful reference in this regard. Nonmineralization of the pubis is a manifestation of cleidocranial dysostosis in childhood; with increasing age, progressive mineralization takes place. Nonmineralization of the pubis should not be confused with actual pubic separation, which is found characteristically with exstrophy of the bladder, but also without bladder abnormality in instances of diastasis recti with ventral hernia. Congenital absence or hypoplasia of the sacrum is not uncommon; it is invariably associated with musculoskeletal abnormalities of the lower extremities and frequently with bladder or bowel dysfunction. A relationship with diabetes in the mother has been suggested, and relationships with congenital bowing of the femurs have also been postulated.

Sacrococcygeal teratomas are attached to the tip of the coccyx and present as mass lesions of the buttocks and presacral area. Frequently the greater portion of the mass is internal, and the tumor presents as a relatively small lesion externally. Characteristically the major portions of these structures lie anterior to the sacrum but may also protrude caudally. They may contain calcifications or actual dental structures and bone and may have variable density due to fat. The rectum is usually displaced anteriorly. Meningomyeloceles over the sacral area, with which they may be confused, generally lie posterior to the sacrum; often meningomyeloceles are not covered with skin. Lipomas and lipomeningoceles (lipoma penetrating the dura) also lie posterior to the sacrum and may demonstrate a fatty density. Rectal examination is of great importance in identifying the presacral location of sacrococcygeal teratomas. At surgery, because of their firm attachment to the coccyx, the portion to which the tumor is attached must be excised. Teratomas are potentially malignant, and some are actually malignant at the time of diagnosis.

Acetabular angles and their relationship to congenital dislocation of the hip are discussed on p. 2028. Flat acetabular roofs and wide ilia present in the first 6 months of life are radiographically diagnostic of Down's syndrome; steep acetabular roofs and narrow ilia occur in the newborn with trisomy 17–18.

Coxa vara, once a manifestation of rickets, is now recognized more frequently as a manifestation of metaphyseal dysostosis (p. 2008) as well as other skeletal dysplasias. It may also result from slipped capital femoral epiphysis, Legg-Perthes disease, and Legg-Perthes-like changes associated with systemic disorders such as Gaucher's disease and sickle cell anemia, as well as the head and neck changes that occasionally follow treatment of congenital dislocation of the hip.

Slipping of the femoral epiphysis (p. 2031) may occur about the time of adolescence, particularly in overweight males, and may cause considerable disability unless it is immediately and appropriately treated. The frequency of bilateral involvement warrants careful attention to the unaffected side.

Injuries to the pelvic bones usually result from trauma of considerable force. Those involving the hip joints may leave sequelae that affect locomotion. In addition, all injuries to the bony pelvis may damage important adjacent structures, particularly the urethra and rectum, as suggested by the presence of blood in the urine or feces. If the bladder contains gross blood after pelvic injury, it is best to allow the urine catheter to remain in the bladder for at least 24 to 48 hours. Cystourethrography is also indicated to demonstrate urethral laceration. After the latter procedure recatheterization may be difficult or impossible, and surgical drainage of the bladder may then become necessary.

Epiphyseal separations may occur in various portions of the pelvis as a consequence of self-inflicted trauma; one of the most common is avulsion of the nonunited ossification center of the ischial tuberosity following violent contraction of the hamstring muscles during strenuous activity in athletic teenagers. Initial local signs of pain are quickly forgotten, but recurrent pain and tenderness may lead to radiographic examination. The presence of irregular, and at times excessive, new bone formation may then lead to the erroneous diagnosis of neoplasm. The condition responds to conservative management; surgical intervention is unnecessary.

References

THORACIC CAGE

Cantrell JR, Haller JA, Ravitch MM: A syndrome of congenital defects involving the abdominal wall, sternum, diaphragm, pericardium and heart. Surg Gynecol Obstet 107:602, 1958

Currarino G, Silverman FN: Premature obliteration of the sternal sutures and pigeon breast deformity. Radiology 70:532, 1958

Miller KE, Allen RP, Davis WS: Rib gap defects with micrognathia: cerebro-costo-mandibular syndrome: Pierre Robin–like syndrome with rib dysplasia. Am J Roentgenol Radium Ther Nucl Med 114:253, 1972

Polgar G, Koop CE: Pulmonary function in pectus excavatum. Pediatrics 32:209, 1963

Spranger J, Grimm B, Weller M, Weissen Bacher G, Gibert E, Kepler R: Short rib-polydactyly (SRP) syndromes, types Majewski and Saldino-Noonan. Z Kinderheilkd 116:73, 1974

Wiedemann H-R: Tietze Syndrome (chondroosteopathia costalis tuberosa) im frühen Kindesalter. Helv Paediatr Acta 27:25, 1972

VERTEBRAL COLUMN

Bailey DK: Normal cervical spine in infants and children. Radiology 59:712, 1952

Ferguson AB: Roentgen Diagnosis of Extremities and Spine. New York, Hoeber, 1949

Freiberger RH: Osteoid osteoma of the spine. A cause of backache and scoliosis in children and young adults. Radiology 75:232, 1960

Jamison RC, Heimlich EM, Miethke JC, O'Loughlin BJ: Nonspecific spondylitis of infants and children. Radiology 77:355, 1961

Jones PG: Torticollis in Infancy and Childhood. Springfield, Ill, Charles C Thomas, 1968

Keim HA: The Milwaukee brace for treatment of scoliosis. J Pediatr 78:864, 1971

Lemire RJ, Graham CB, Beckwith JB: Skin covered sacrococcygeal masses in infants and children. J Pediatr 79:948, 1971

Mainzer F: Herniation of nucleus pulposus: rare complication of intervertebral disk calcification in children. Radiology 107:167, 1973

Melnick JC, Silverman FN: Intervertebral disk calcification in childhood. Radiology 80:399, 1963

Moes CAF, Hendrick EB: Diastematomyelia. J Pediatr 63:238, 1963

Passarge E, Lenz W: Syndrome of caudal regression in infants of diabetic mothers: observations of further cases. Pediatrics 37:672, 1966

Spiegel PG, Kengla KW, Isaacson AS, Wilson JC: Intervertebral disc space inflammation in children. J Bone Joint Surg [Am] 54:284, 1972

Townsend EH Jr, Rowe ML: Mobility of the upper cervical spine in health and disease. Pediatrics 10:567, 1952

Wilkinson RH, Hall JE: The sclerotic pedicle: tumor or pseudotumor? Radiology 111:683, 1974

Williams HJ, Pugh DG: Vertebral epiphysitis: a comparison of the clinical and roentgenologic findings. Am J Roentgenol Radium Ther Nucl Med 90:1236, 1963

Wiltse LL: The etiology of spondylolisthesis. J Bone Joint Surg [Am] 44:539, 1962

PELVIS

Blumel J, Evans EB, Eggers GWN: Partial and complete agenesis or malformation of the sacrum with associated anomalies; etiologic and clinical study with special reference to heredity; a preliminary report. J Bone Joint Surg [Am] 41:497, 1959

Caffey J: Achondroplasia of pelvis and lumbosacral spine. Am J Roentgenol Radium Ther Nucl Med 80:449, 1958

———— Ross SE: The ischiopubic syndhondrosis in healthy children. Am J Roentgenol Radium Ther Nucl Med 76:488, 1956

Kaufmann HJ: Röntgenbefunde am kindlichen Becken bei angeborenen Skelettaffektionen und chromosomalen Aberrationen. Stuttgart, Thieme, 1964

OSTEOMYELITIS

FREDERIC N. SILVERMAN AND MARTIN B. KLEIMAN

ETIOLOGY AND PATHOGENESIS. Osteomyelitis in children may be divided into two broad categories: (1) acute hematogenous osteomyelitis in which the pathogen reaches the bone marrow via the bloodstream; (2) osteomyelitis secondary to infection of contiguous structures, either from infected adjacent nonosseous tissue or through penetrating trauma or surgery.

Staphylococcus aureus is still the most common causative agent for acute hematogenous osteomyelitis in otherwise normal children beyond early infancy, although a distinct decrease in its relative frequency has been noted since the mid-1960s. However, *Staphylococcus aureus* still accounts for 70 to 90 percent of cases in most series, with group A β-hemolytic streptococci the next most frequent pathogen, especially in children under 2 years of age. *Staphylococcus epidermidias, Diplococcus Pneumoniac,* and *Haemophilus influenzae* are much less frequently involved. Enteric and other gram-negative organisms are encountered only rarely without

underlying disease beyond the neonatal period. Newborn infants and children with impaired host defenses due to malignancy, immunosuppression, congenital defects, or chronic acquired debilitating diseases, while susceptible to the same organisms as normal children, are more likely to develop infections with gram-negative organisms and also with organisms of low virulence that are not ordinarily pathogenic. Additional host factors may predispose to specific infections. Thus the predilection for *Salmonella* osteomyelitis of patients with sickle cell disease has been well documented. Finally, lack of sterile precautions and technique by the juvenile drug abuser quite commonly leads to septic foci caused by unusual organisms.

The organisms spreading from a contiguous focus vary with the site of the primary focus and the circumstances and method of contamination. Surgical manipulations in general tend to become complicated by staphylococcal infections, but urologic and bowel procedures often result in gram-negative infections. Such infections may occur at the local sites or they may be seeded at a distant focus by bacteremia. Procedures involving therapeutic foreign bodies predispose to infections with organisms that generally are of low virulence. Direct bacterial implantation by puncture wounds or bites may cause infections with common and/or unusual organisms in any child. Well-known examples are indolent *Pseudomonas* infections resulting from puncture wounds of the foot and gram-negative infections complicating femoral vein puncture in neonates and small infants. Mixed infections are exceptional in hematogenous osteomyelitis, but they are not unusual in osteomyelitis secondary to infection of contiguous structures. Mixed infections may also result from bites or other wounds contaminated by oral or upper respiratory flora. The agents of tuberculosis and syphilis cause special types of osteomyelitis, as do the mycotic organisms of histoplasmosis, coccidioidomycosis, blastomycosis, and actinomycosis. There have been reports of vaccinia and variola viruses and the agent of cat scratch disease causing osteomyelitis.

The anatomic factors affecting localization in acute hematogenous osteomyelitis are illustrated in Figure 18 (see also Fig. 1). Organisms enter the bloodstream from any site anywhere in the body and are introduced into the bone via its nutrient artery. Those organisms that reach the metaphyseal areas lodge in the region of the vascular loops that participate in the erosion of calcified epiphyseal cartilage. The end arteries that feed the loops continue directly into the capillaries which in turn empty into relatively dilated venous channels. Here the blood flow is slow and turbulent. It has been postulated that these conditions favor minute vascular occlusions and are quite favorable for bacterial growth, focal abscess formation, and frequent localization of the processes in children in the metaphyses of long bones. Stress factors and microtrauma may also play a role in the increased frequency of the disease in the larger bones of the lower extremities in children beyond 1 year of age. Although a history of injury is elicited with equal frequency in bone neoplasm, trauma is thought to

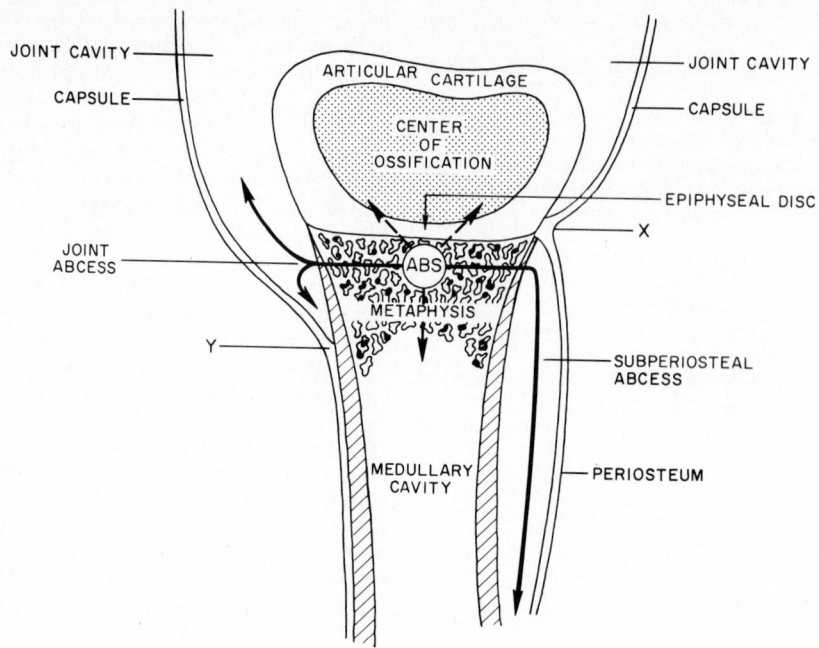

FIG. 18. Schematic representation of potential directions of spread of infection from a metaphyseal focus of osteomyelitis. X and Y mark sites of periosteal and capsular attachments when the metaphysis is extracapsular and intracapsular, respectively. See text for discussion. (Adapted from Kahn and Pritzger: Clin Orthop 96:12, 1973.)

be more contributory in osteomyelitis. The highest attack rate occurs between the ages of 5 years and 15 years. Most series have reported a preponderance of males.

In children under 1 year of age, lesions are often multiple; they may occur within epiphyses and metaphyses and frequently involve the adjacent joint. Trueta attributed the differences in localization within bone to the existence of vascular communications across the epiphyseal line in infants less than 18 months of age. Thus epiphyseal involvement in infancy may occur by direct extension from the metaphysis or by invasion from an adjacent septic joint. At about 18 months of age, however, these vascular connections have disappeared, and the blood supply to the epiphysis comes almost exclusively from peripheral vessels that also supply the periosteum and joint capsule.

The acute local inflammatory reaction is characterized by local accumulation of polymorphonuclear leukocytes and fibrin. Breakdown products of bacteria and cells damaged by ischemia liberate enzymes that cause necrosis of the marrow and probably of the surrounding bony trabeculae. The swelling of the inflammation is contained in a small space by the rigid bony envelope. Pressure increases with increasing amounts of exudate, thereby facilitating the extension of the infection to the medullary canal, to the canal system of the cortical bone, and directly through the extremely thin cortical bone at the junction of metaphysis and epiphysis. Finally, the infection reaches the periosteum,

which it elevates. While spreading along the shaft it may break through into the overlying soft tissues. Periosteal attachment at epiphyseal lines tends to prevent extension beyond this attachment. If the breakthrough to the periosteum involves a bone where metaphysis is partly intraarticular, such as the femoral neck, a septic joint infection occurs; otherwise the bone abscess tends to decompress and forms a soft tissue abscess. The elevated periosteum deprives the cortical bone of a significant portion of its blood supply. The devitalized bone becomes a *sequestrum* separated from the remainder of the bone and surrounded by pus. The sequestrum acts as a foreign body; it harbors bacteria, which cannot be reached by the antimicrobial agents and perpetuates the infection.

The periosteum is only loosely attached to the cortical bone in young children, particularly in infants. The cortical bone is also relatively thin in infants, and the purulent exudate frequently decompresses into the soft tissues in this age group. In older children intramedullary spread is more common because the bone and periosteum tend to restrain the infection.

Infections with organisms of low virulence, altered host defense mechanisms, and/or suboptimal antibiotic therapy sometimes lead to the development of subacute forms of osteomyelitis. Localization of an indolent abscess within bone gives rise to the *Brodie abscess* (p. 2001), whereas multiple small foci of disease and bone reaction are probably responsible for the Garré *sclerosing osteomyelitis* (p. 2001).

CLINICAL MANIFESTATIONS. The classic signs and symptoms of acute hematogenous osteomyelitis are fever of sudden onset, systemic toxicity, pain, and exquisite local tenderness. However, more frequently, especially early in the illness and in the very young child, the presentation is less typical, with vague nonspecific symptoms of fever and malaise and possibly a limp or favoring of an extremity. Meticulous, systematic, and repeated examinations may often be necessary to locate the focus or foci of infection. Occasionally, pain and tenderness are diffuse, making localization very difficult. The presentation of osteomyelitis in the neonatal period is even more variable. The newborn may present either with overwhelming sepsis without any local signs or, more commonly, with minimal systemic signs but obvious focal manifestations of swelling, tenderness, and decreased motion of the affected extremity. Potentially infective procedures such as femoral venipuncture may precede the disease in the neonatal period and in young infants, and joint involvement as well as multiple foci of osteomyelitis are common.

In the Brodie abscess or Garré sclerosing osteomyelitis, systemic symptoms are usually completely absent. Pain is almost always present and is occasionally worse at night, and limb motion may be limited. Tenderness and swelling are variable, and the brawny edema characteristic of acute osteomyelitis is absent. There are no diagnostic laboratory findings, and the diagnosis is generally made by biopsy and direct culture.

LABORATORY FINDINGS. Laboratory data vary with age, site, and severity and duration of symptoms. The leukocyte count is frequently elevated, with a shift to the left, and the erythrocyte sedimentation rate is also frequently accelerated. However, both of these tests can be within normal limits, especially in subacute infections, in localized infections of small bones and even in overwhelming sepsis. Blood cultures are positive and diagnostic in 50 percent of cases of acute hematogenous osteomyelitis.

Radiographic findings provide the most specific information; bone changes are seldom radiographically demonstrable until the second week of the disease. Alterations in the adjacent soft tissues can provide presumptive support for the diagnosis. Thickening of the deep soft tissues with obliteration of the intermuscular fascial planes is usually visible during the first week of the disease. The swelling of the deep tissues is revealed by the relative absence of thickened (edematous) septa in the subcutaneous fat external to the muscle masses. Comparison with the healthy extremity in identical position permits recognition of the early soft tissue changes. The earliest bone changes consist of focal areas of radiolucency that may include disappearance of both trabecular architecture and the thin metaphyseal cortex immediately adjacent to the epiphyseal line. Comparison of the same region from a previous film showing only soft tissue changes may be necessary to detect this early destructive phase. In the early phase of

osteomyelitis when no bone changes are present on radiography, bone scintigraphy (radio-nuclide imaging) using technetium Tc 99 m methylene diphosphonate can help in early detection and localization of the bone infection. It is a safe method which is recommended in the initial evaluation of children in whom osteomyelitis is suspected.

Toward the twelfth day after clinical onset, however, progressive destruction of bony architecture can be observed on radiography. At that time new bone formation under the elevated periosteum may make its appearance, and both production and destruction of bone then proceed to a degree that reflects the extent of the initial injury (Fig. 19). There is distinct lag between clinical recovery and x-ray evidence of improvement. Progressive destruction of bony tissue with extensive sequestrum and involucrum formation may continue and may go on to pathologic fracture, even in the face of clinical cure. This lag is related to the effects of antibiotics and to the nature of bone repair, which includes necrosis and removal as well as reorganization and repair. In infants the ease of decompression of the relatively thin cortex and its overlying periosteum frequently results in very little destructive change in the shaft of a bone, and productive changes seem to predominate. In the Brodie abscess or Garré sclerosing

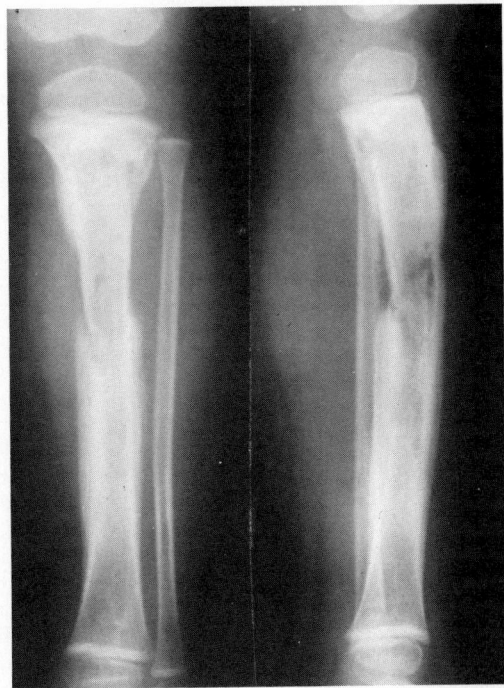

FIG. 19. Film 8-9 weeks after onset of osteomyelitis. The true extent of the spread of infection in and around the bone is shown by the sequestrum and involucrum formation. Note clarity of soft tissue shadows despite extensive postinfectious destructive and productive changes in bone.

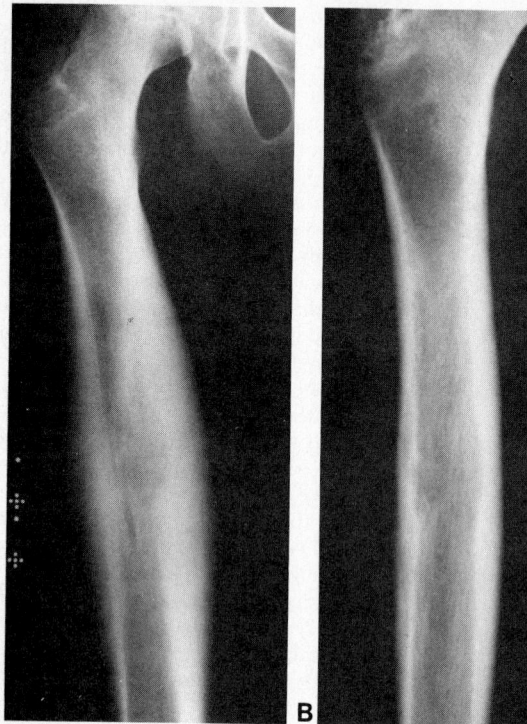

FIG. 20. Garré sclerosing osteomyelitis. A. Male 9 years old who had knee pain for 2 years and weight loss over preceding 9 months. Biopsy revealed chronic osteomyelitis. B. Same patient 3 years later; no symptoms. An osteoid osteoma could present in exactly the same fashion.

osteomyelitis (Fig. 20), the radiologic changes are much more indolent.

DIAGNOSIS. The differential diagnosis of osteomyelitis is quite broad and can be confusing, especially early in the course. Generalized sepsis is always a primary consideration, with the bone lesion representing only one of several metastatic foci. A diligent search must always be made for other sites of infections and for additional areas of bone involvement. Ewing's tumor may also present with systemic symptoms, malaise, fever, and leukocytosis, along with focal pain, swelling, and tenderness. The radiologic findings may be indistinguishable from those of osteomyelitis, and a biopsy may be necessary to make the diagnosis. Cellulitis, uncomplicated pyarthrosis, rheumatic fever, rheumatoid arthritis, accidental or intentional trauma, and even poliomyelitis are frequently difficult to differentiate early in the illness and are usually excluded with observation of the clinical and radiologic course. Bone infarct in sickle cell disease may present with clinical, laboratory, and radiologic findings similar to those of osteomyelitis. Repeated blood cultures may establish the diagnosis, but all too frequently direct culture may be the only way to differentiate the two. The hand-foot syndrome of sickle cell disease is usually separable on clinical grounds, despite radiologic changes suggesting osteomyelitis.

COMPLICATIONS. The complications of os-

teomyelitis include multiple metastatic foci. In young children, direct extension into an epiphysis and then into a joint may result in pyarthrosis; at any age direct extension into a joint and subsequently into the epiphysis can take place when the primary site of bone infection is located within the capsular attachments (Fig. 30). Pathologic fractures can occur and may result in deformity and even pseudarthrosis. Infection of the vertebrae may spread into the spinal canal, with secondary cord compression or meningitis. In osteomyelitis of cervical vertebra, prevertebral abscess may develop. Shortening of the affected bone may occur as a consequence of septic arthritis and damage to the epiphyseal cartilage; occasionally hyperemia may increase local growth. Chronic osteomyelitis is uncommon today because of the availability of antibiotic agents.

TREATMENT. As in the treatment of any closed-space infection, the principles of management include (1) prompt accurate diagnosis, (2) identification of the offending organism, (3) evacuation of pus and/or necrotic bone or tissue, and (4) appropriate high-dose intravenous antibiotic therapy. Whenever possible, bactericidal rather than bacteriostatic agents should be used. Delay in initiating treatment greatly increases the risks of immediate complications and of long-term sequelae. Therefore therapy should promptly be instituted after the appropriate cultures are obtained. Multiple blood cultures should always be taken before treatment. Where there is sufficient localization of disease, a direct culture should be obtained, either at the time of surgical drainage or by needle aspiration from an area of periosteal elevation or from areas of local drainage. Culture techniques should be applied that permit the isolation of aerobic and anaerobic bacteria, acid-fast organisms, and fungal agents. Examination of appropriately stained smears should always be made. If a surgical biopsy is obtained, appropriate histologic examination may also be helpful in establishing the diagnosis.

Initial therapy. The initial selection of antibiotics is determined by consideration of host factors, clinical presentation, and bacteriologic data from stained smears, if available. In any child without underlying pathology, *Staphylococcus* is still the most likely etiologic agent, and a penicillinase-resistant penicillin, such as methicillin or oxacillin, should be started at maximal dosage (200 to 300 mg/kg/24 hours) by the intravenous route, which will also provide coverage against other pyogenic cocci. In neonates or children with malignancy or impaired host defenses, it is recommended that in addition to methicillin or oxacillin, an aminoglycoside such as gentamicin be used against enteric gram-negative pathogens. In sickle cell disease, where bone infections due to *Salmonella* species occur with greater frequency, the antimicrobial regimen should also include either ampicillin, or chloramphenicol in areas where ampicillin-resistant organisms are known to be prevalent.

Further antibiotic therapy. Once the organism has been identified and specific sensitivities become available, the coverage should be adjusted accordingly (p. 408). Similarly, specific antituberculous therapy should be started if smears, skin tests, or associated findings suggest a diagnosis of tuberculosis (p. 478).

Duration of antibiotic therapy. Antibiotic treatment continued at maximal intravenous dosage for a minimum of 4 to 6 weeks has been shown to result in the fewest recurrences. During this period of treatment, progress should be monitored on repeated blood cultures and, if possible, wound cultures, together with the other important clinical and laboratory data: fever, systemic toxicity, local tenderness, leukocytosis, and sedimentation rate. Whenever possible, serum levels of antibiotics and serum bactericidal activity should be determined, especially if the clinical response is not satisfactory. At the present time short-term or oral antibiotic regimens are considered inadequate. In tuberculous osteitis antituberculous chemotherapy should be continued for at least 18 to 24 months. (p. 479).

Surgical therapy. Surgical drainage occupies an important place in therapy. If pus under pressure is allowed to spread it will cause increased tissue destruction. Furthermore, limited penetration of antibiotics into abscessed or devitalized bone may make purely medical management suboptimal. Indeed, viable organisms may be recovered for days after institution of seemingly adequate antibiotic treatment.

Surgical drainage is indicated at the outset of therapy if symptoms have been present for 48 to 72 hours or more and/or if there are obvious signs of abscess formation. Ferguson recommends incision over the affected metaphysis with opening of the periosteum to relieve any accumulated pus; stripping of the periosteum is to be avoided. If pus is not found the metaphysis is drilled, generally in three relatively adjacent areas. If pus is recovered a rectangular window of bone is removed from the cortex, the pus and/or granulomatous material is removed or curetted, and the wound is closed, after taking appropriate specimens for culture and biopsy. An arthrotomy should be performed in lesions that have extended into adjacent joints.

Where symptoms are of short duration and there are no signs of pus under pressure, medical management alone may be initiated as outlined. However, should systemic and local symptoms fail to subside after 48 to 72 hours of appropriate treatment, surgical drainage should be performed without further delay. Persistently positive blood cultures are also indications for surgical drainage and should also prompt a diligent search for additional foci of infection.

In osteomyelitis secondary to spread from contiguous foci, drainage and exploration are usually necessary, since symptoms are usually of long duration and these wounds not infrequently harbor foreign bodies. The subacute forms of osteomyelitis are usually diagnosed by biopsy, which when followed by curettage and combined with immobilization and antibiotic therapy is usually curative.

References

Capitanio MA, Kirkpatrick JA: Early roentgen observations in acute osteomyelitis. Am J Roentgenol Radium Ther Nucl Med 108:488, 1970

Ferguson AB Jr: Osteomyelitis in children. Clin Orthop 96:51, 1973

Gledhill RB: Subacute osteomyelitis in children. Clin Orthop 96:57, 1973

Hall JE, Silverstein EA: Acute hematogenous osteomyelitis. Pediatrics 31:1033, 1963

Kahn DS, PritzKer KPH: The pathophysiology of bone infection. Clin Orthop 96:12, 1973

McCracken GH Jr, Eichenwald HF: Antimicrobial therapy: therapeutic recommendations and a review of newer drugs. I. Therapy of infectious conditions. J Pediatr 85:297, 1974

Nelson JD: Antibiotic concentrations in septic joint effusions. N Engl J Med 284:349, 1971

Shandling B: Acute haematogenous osteomyelitis: a review of 300 cases treated during 1952–1959. S Afr Med J 34:520, 1960

Treves S, Khettry J, Broker FH, Wilkinson RH, Watts H: Osteomyelitis: early scintigraphic detection in children. Pediatrics 57:173, 1976.

Trueta J: The three types of acute haematogenous osteomyelitis: a clinical and vascular study. J Bone Joint Surg [Br] 41:671, 1959

Waldvogel FA, Medoff G, Swartz MN: Medical progress: osteomyelitis: a review of clinical features, therapeutic considerations, and unusual aspects. N Engl J Med 282:198, 260, 316, 1970

Weissberg ED, Smith AL, Smith DH: Clinical features of neonatal osteomyelitis. Pediatrics 53:505, 1974

SYSTEMIC AFFECTIONS OF THE SKELETON

FREDERIC N. SILVERMAN

HEREDITARY AND DEVELOPMENTAL CONDITIONS

Skeletal Dysplasias

Certain systemic dysplasias of the skeleton are clearly defined and obvious; others are more difficult to classify. Morphologic similarities do not necessarily reflect relationships in etiology or pathogenesis. However, until fundamental biochemical or other reproducible identifying data are available, morphologic criteria coupled with inheritance patterns appear to offer the best basis for the recognition of individual syndromes. Various classifications of skeletal dysplasias have been offered and are constantly being revised. Rubin, in his excellent monograph on bone dysplasias, postulates that they result from a specific alteration of the factors that cause bone to achieve its ultimate size, shape, and structure. By analysis of the alterations, defective factors can be identified, and relationships among various dysplasias can become the basis for a "dynamic" classification. Rubin's classification is shown in Table 1. Although this classification overlooks the probability of multifactorial genesis of some of these disorders, it is nevertheless a useful starting point for identification.

Rubin defines *dysplasia* as "a disturbance in bone form or modeling which assumes a disturbance in growth, intrinsic to bone." Depending upon the degree of growth disturbance, the dysplasia may be an aplasia, a hypoplasia, or a hyperplasia. *Dystrophy* is defined as "a disturbance in bone form or modeling which assumes a disturbance in nutrition or metabolism, extrinsic to bone." *Dysostosis* is defined as "a disturbance in bone

TABLE 1. Broad Classification and Terminology[a]

| | Dysplasia | | Dysostosis | Dystrophy |
	Hypoplasia (congenita and tarda)	Hyperplasia		
Epiphysis	Spondyloepiphyseal dysplasia Multiple epiphyseal dysplasia	Dysplasia epiphysalis hemimelica	Diastrophic dwarfism	Hypothyroidism
Physis	Achondroplasia Metaphyseal dysostosis	Hyperchondroplasia Enchondromatosis	Chondroectodermal dysplasia Dyschondrosteose	Hypopituitarism and hyperpituitarism Hurler's syndrome
Metaphysis	Hypophosphatasia Osteopetrosis Craniometaphyseal dysplasia	Multiple exostoses		Rachitiform disease Gaucher's disease Heavy-metal intoxication Hyperparathyroidism
Diaphysis	Osteogenesis imperfecta Idiopathic osteoporosis	Progressive diaphyseal dysplasia Hyperphosphatasemia	Cleidocranial dysostosis	Hormonal osteoporosis Vitamin A and D Intoxication

[a] From Rubin: Dynamic Classification of Bone Dysplasias, 1964. Courtesy of Year Book Medical Publishers.

form or modeling which assumes a disturbance or a defect in developmental ectodermal or mesenchymal tissues." These definitions are employed in the following discussion.

ACHONDROPLASIA. Achondroplasia is the most common and best known of the generalized skeletal dysplasias. Typical examples are seen in ancient Egyptian, Greek, and Roman art, as well as in the work of the sixteenth- and seventeenth-century painters. The reported incidence has varied from 1 in over 9,000 deliveries to 1 in slightly over 3,000 deliveries, but the diagnostic criteria used have been dissimilar. An autosomal-dominant type of inheritance is accepted for genetic counseling of affected individuals. Poor reproductivity, diminished longevity, and a fairly high spontaneous mutation rate may lead to difficulties in tracing the genetic features. It has been stated that advanced paternal age is a factor in the origin of new mutations for achondroplasia.

The basic morbid mechanism of achondroplasia is a failure of normal growth of the cells and the proliferative cartilage in the zones of growth, with defective endochondral bone formation everywhere in the skeleton. As a result, the long bones are shortened, and the round flat bones are reduced in size. In contrast, subperiosteal bone formation appears to proceed relatively normally, so that the cortical bone in all parts of the skeleton seems unaffected. However, measurements of cortical thickness indicates that the total osseous structure is actually deficient. The restriction in length of tubular bones is the most obvious feature. This selective disturbance in growth of the skeleton produces an individual in whom the extremities are disproportionately short in relation to the head and trunk. The roots or proximal bones of the extremities (humeri and femora), which normally grow most, are disproportionately short in relation to the distal bones; hence the characterization *rhizomelic dwarfism*.

The histologic features of the cartilage–shaft junction are presently under reinvestigation. The basic defect may be a quantitative rather than a qualitative decrease in the rate of endochondral ossification, but qualitative and quantitative differences may exist in different portions of the skeleton at the same time and at different times. The marked flaring of the metaphyses and the knobbed appearance of joints in some cases are considered by Rubin to be the consequences of disparity between appositional cartilage growth (width) and interstitial growth (length) of the epiphysis. The separation of all cases into either hypotrophic and hypertrophic forms histologically and radiographically has been challenged by the identification of *metatropic dwarfism* (see below) as a separate condition that probably includes almost all instances of hypertrophic chondrodystrophy.

Cranial deformities are a constant feature of classic achondroplasia. Individuals with normal skulls who have been incorrectly included in well-known monographs on chondrodystrophy almost certainly represent examples of other conditions, including various forms of spondyloepiphyseal dysplasia (p. 2008), metaphyseal dysostosis (p. 2008), and even vitamin-D-resistant rickets. The base of the cranium, preformed in cartilage, suffers from the same defective endochondral bone formation as do the long bones. The foramen magnum is small, a feature that may contribute to hydrocephalus and exaggerate the overgrowth of the calvarium that is necessary to accommodate the expanding brain. The forehead bulges over the base, and the nasal bone is anchored deep under the overlying forehead.

The disturbed growth of the vertebrae reduces the dimensions of the vertebral canal. Caffey has pointed out that in the frontal plane the interpediculate distance reflects this reduction, particularly in the areas (lower lumbar spine) where normally increased width is noted. The vertical height of vertebral bodies is less affected than are the sagittal and coronal diameters, both in the newborn period and throughout life. The restriction of space for the spinal cord makes this structure exceedingly vulnerable to trauma and to minor displacements.

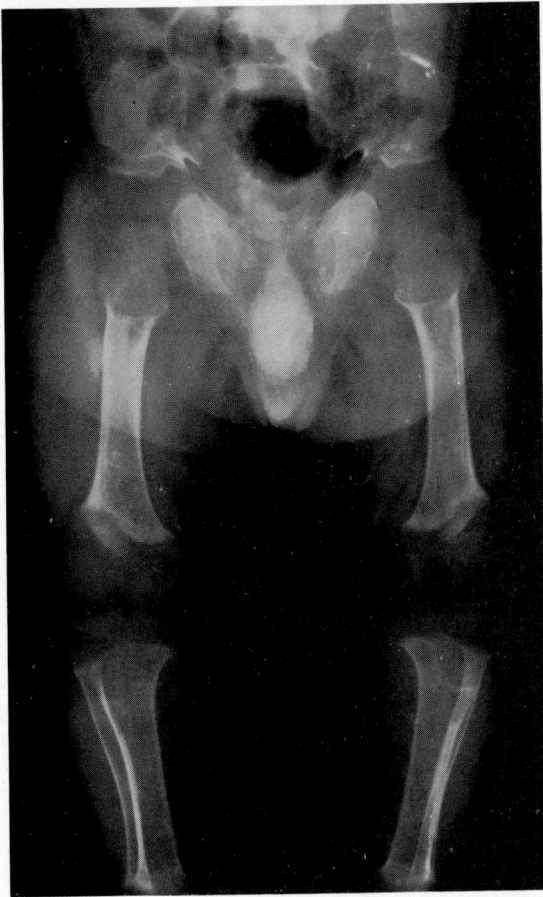

FIG. 21. Pelvis and lower extremities in achondroplasia. Note the small sacroliac notch.

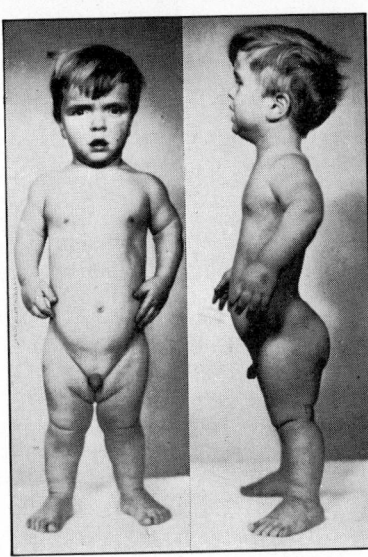

FIG. 22. Classic achondroplasia in a boy age 3 years 11 months.

In the pelvis the diminution in vertical height of the ilia due to decreased growth of the body of the ilium reduces the greater sciatic notch from a long smooth curve to a minute indentation in the medial border of the ilium (Fig. 21).

As in many other clearly defined syndromes, affected individuals from different families resemble each other much more than they resemble their unaffected siblings. The most striking clinical feature in children with achondroplasia is the extreme shortness of the extremities as compared with the length of the body (Fig. 22). The short upper extremities may scarcely extend below the iliac crests, instead of reaching halfway to the knees. In early infancy there appears to be too much soft tissue for the amount of bone, and the skin of the extremities is frequently thrown up into prominent folds. The fingers are short and stubby and of almost equal length; when placed on a flat surface they tend to diverge at the proximal interphalangeal joints (Fig. 23). The cranial involvement regularly results in prominence of the forehead and depression of the base of the nose. There is often marked prognathism, especially

with increasing age. A marked lumbar lordosis is present. The maximum height attained by achondroplastic dwarfs is often less than 3.5 feet. Some instances of hypochondroplasia, which simulates a very mild form of achondroplasia but may constitute a separate disease, probably account for the great variation in the severity of the disease reported in the literature. In achondroplasia puberty develops normally, and there is no impairment of reproductive function. In pregnant females cesarean section is required because of the deformity of the pelvis.

The mentality of the achondroplastic dwarf is more apt to be normal than not. Most affected individuals lead a normal life hampered only by the restrictions of stature and their distinctive appearance. Other forms of micromelic dwarfism may simulate achondroplasia in the newborn; these include *osteogenesis imperfecta* as a result of multiple fractures, *thanatophoric dwarfism, metatropic dwarfism, chondrodysplasia punctata, chondroectodermal dysplasia,* and others. The differential diagnosis is usu-

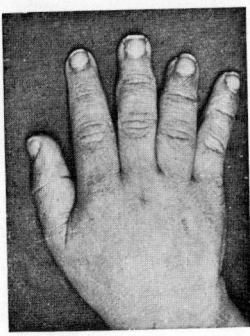

FIG. 23. Characteristic hand in achondroplasia.

ally simple if appropriate radiographs are available. Consistent involvement of the cranium and characteristic involvement of the pelvis and vertebral column serve to differentiate achondroplasia from other forms of micromelic dwarfism. Treatment of achondroplastic dwarfs with human growth hormone has not produced significant results.

ACHONDROGENESIS. Achondrogenesis is a rare lethal form of short-limbed dwarfism transmitted by autosomal recessive inheritance and characterized by absence of ossification of all vertebral structures in the lumbar area and absence of ossification centers for the vertebral bodies at the thoracic and cervical levels. There is failure of mineralization of the sacral, pubic, and ischial bones and the short, thick tubular bones of the extremities, which are expanded at their metaphyseal ends to form spurs. The term is no longer used for a nonlethal form of severe mesomelic dwarfism.

THANATOPHORIC DWARFISM. The separation of this condition from classic achondroplasia is generally recognized as valid. In contradistinction to achondroplasia, there is no attempt at column formation and no orderly progression of chondrocyte evolution. Clinically the patients are exaggerated achondroplastic dwarfs (Fig. 15, ch. 6); they either are born dead or survive only a few hours to days at the most. The early demise (*thanatophoros,* affinity for death) and the extreme micromelic dwarfism are associated with characteristic flat vertebral bodies and with short, thick, curved tubular bones; the usual increase in length of the fibula with respect to the tibia that is seen in achondroplasia is lacking. The severity of the clinical as well as the radiologic features separates thanatophoric dwarfism from achondroplasia. The genetic transmission of thanatophoric dwarfism is not known, but thus far all parents have been apparently normal; consequently a recessive mode of inheritance is possible. In one instance (Keats and associates) a thanatophoric dwarf was born with a normal fraternal twin. Other forms of lethal short-limbed dwarfism occur, some of which are described below in the section on chondroectodermal dysplasia.

METATROPIC DWARFISM. Metatropic dwarfism, which was identified by Maroteaux and his associates, probably represents the hyperplastic chondrodystrophy described by Kaufmann. At birth the affected infants resemble children with achondroplasia, because of their short extremities and prominent joints, but cranial involvement is questionable or entirely lacking. A small taillike appendage at the base of the spine is usually present. Radiographs show short tubular bones with markedly expanded metaphyses. The pelvis, although abnormal, differs from the achondroplastic pelvis in the size and shape of the body of the ilium (Fig. 24a). The strongest argument for the separation of metatropic dwarfism from achondroplasia is their later

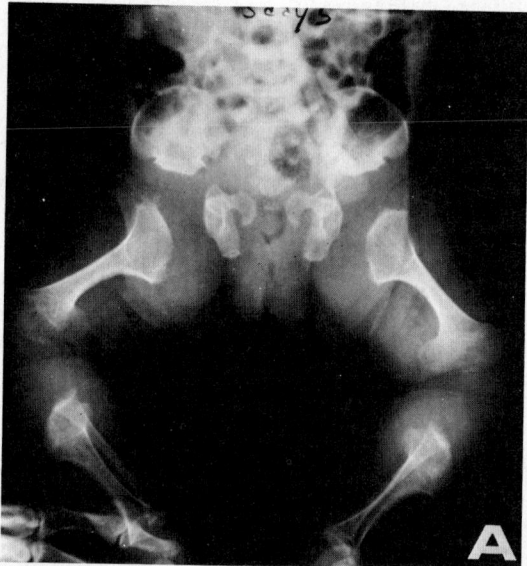

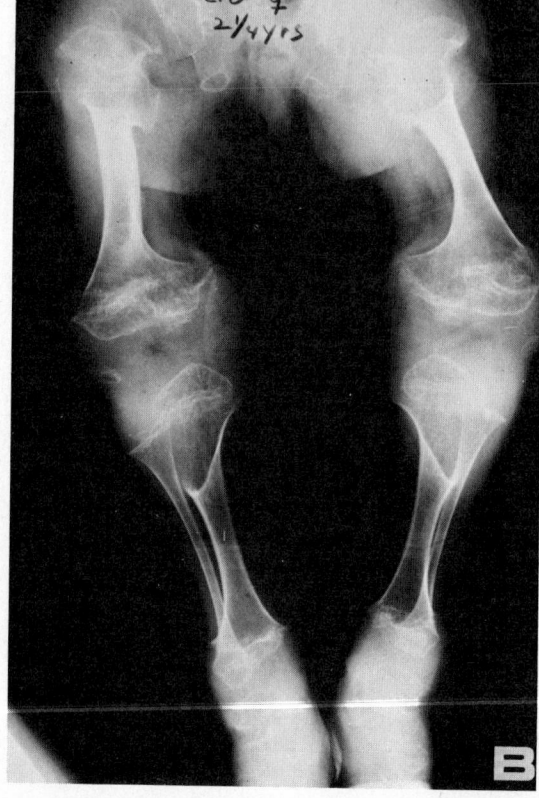

FIG. 24. A. Classic features of metatropic dwarfism in 3-day-old infant. At that time the child had a relatively long trunk and relatively short extremities and was thought to have achondroplasia in spite of a normal cranium. Radiographs demonstrated typical pelvic features and expanded ends of long bones characteristic of metatropic dwarfism. B. Same patient at age 2 years 3 months. The clinical deformities in the spine were becoming apparent and were reflected in the changes in the radiographic features of the lower extremities. (Courtesy of Dr. Chestley Yelton.)

development: achondroplastic infants become achondroplastic children and adults; children with the achondroplasialike proportions of metatropic dwarfism at birth become kyphotic, scoliotic, misshapen individuals with relatively short trunks and relatively long extremities (*metatropos*, affected by change).

DIASTROPHIC DWARFISM.   Diastrophic dwarfism is distinguished from achondroplasia in the newborn by the presence of congenital clubfoot deformity and proximal insertion of the thumbs (due to short first metacarpal bones). The ears may be deformed at birth or may develop blebs that subsequently lead to deformities resembling the cauliflower ear of the pugilist of earlier times. The characteristic cranial, vertebral, and pelvic changes of achondroplasia are absent. With increasing age the spine tends to become progressively scoliotic, a feature that together with the clubfoot deformity gives rise to the appellation diastrophic (*diastrophos*, twisted, contorted). Surgical procedures designed to prevent scoliosis or to correct the foot deformity are rarely successful, if ever. The condition is thought to be transmitted as an autosomal recessive trait. Adults with the condition are severely dwarfed.

CHONDROECTODERMAL DYSPLASIA.   Chondroectodermal dysplasia is also known as the *Ellis–van Creveld syndrome* and is characterized by (1) shortening of the long bones of the extremities due to failure of cartilaginous growth that simulates achondroplasia, (2) postaxial polydactylia, and (3) hypoplasia of the nails, teeth, and hair. In about a third of the cases congenital heart disease is present. The diagnosis is suggested when polydactyly and ectodermal dysplasia are noted in a child who appears to be achondroplastic. However, confusion with short-rib–polydactyly syndromes and asphyxiating thoracic dystrophy can occur. Pelvic features in chondroectodermal dysplasia include a longer sacroiliac spur than in achondroplasia, a prominent spur at the lateral margin of the acetabular roof, and a third spur between the two (Fig. 25). Identical features in the acetabular roof are present in Jeune's disease (see below). The tendency of the body of the ilium to mineralize as the child grows older works to normalize the pelvic configuration of the patient with chondroectodermal dysplasia, in contradistinction to the persistently and severely abnormal pelvis of the child with achondroplasia. This tendency probably accounts for reports of variable degrees of abnormality in the pelvis of patients with chondroectodermal dysplasia: the older the patient the less abnormal the pelvis. Premature appearance of ossification centers for the femoral heads is noted in about a third of the cases. In contradistinction to achondroplasia, the shortening of the extremities is more prominent in the distal portions than in the proximal (*acromelic* rather than *rhizomelic*). In the carpus, fusion of the capitate and hamate bones is common, and in the knee the proximal tibial epiphysis often has an eccentric, medially located ossification center. Ultimately a normal tibial plateau is formed. The skull and vertebral column show none of the growth disturbances

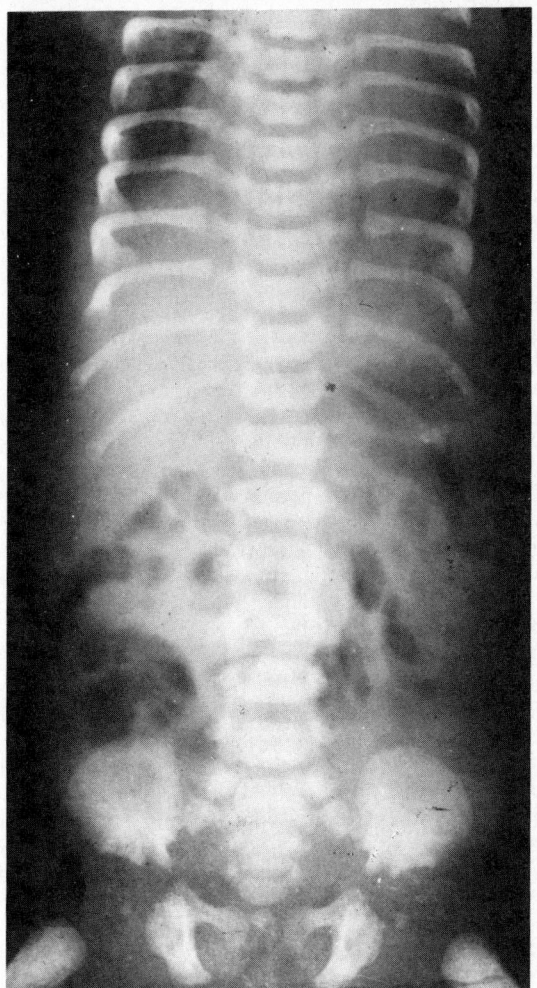

FIG. 25.   Chondroectodermal dysplasia in a newborn. The spine is relatively normal, but the ribs are very short and the trident appearance of the acetabular roofs is well developed. Ossification centers for the femoral heads are precociously developed. The identical appearance (ribs, spine, pelvis) can be seen in some instances of Jeune's syndrome (asphyxiating thoracic dystrophy).

of achondroplasia. The heredity follows an autosomal recessive pattern.

JEUNE'S DISEASE.   Jeune's disease (*asphyxiating thoracic dystrophy*) has many radiographic features in common with chondroectodermal dysplasia. The pelvic and rib changes are practically identical, including the medial, lateral, and central spurs of the acetabular roof, or "trident." Premature appearance of ossification centers for the femoral capital epiphyses also occurs. The extremities, when involved, have varying patterns of deformity; but none resembles those characteristic of chondroectodermal dysplasia, other than occasional instances of postaxial polydactylia (approximately 20 percent). Clinical manifestations are primarily related to respiratory difficulties, which may occasionally be improved by placing the child in the prone position. A sternal splitting procedure has been described that employs both grafts and external traction to increase the thoracic capacity, but in severe cases the thoracic cage appears to be too small to permit heart and lungs to sustain life.

At least two short-rib–polydactyly syndromes have been described that bear certain similarities to Jeune's disease as well as chondroectodermal dysplasia but that can be differentiated from them by both clinical and radiologic features. In the *Majewski syndrome* the polydactyly may be preaxial as well as postaxial. Cleft lip and cleft palate are present in the Majewski syndrome, but they have not been noted in chondroectodermal dysplasia or Jeune's disease; the same applies to gross abnormalities of form in the tibia and significant genital anomalies. The trident pelvis is not observed in the Majewski syndrome, but it exists in the *Saldino-Noonan syndrome* together with genital anomalies and imperforate anus. Both the Majewski syndrome and Saldino-Noonan syndrome are almost invariably lethal, while Jeune's syndrome and chondroectodermal dysplasia have a better life expectancy. All appear to be transmitted by autosomal recessive genes. There may be a high incidence of progressive renal failure in the few children who survive the infantile form of Jeune's disease.

METAPHYSEAL CHONDRODYSPLASIA. The term metaphyseal chondrodysplasia is preferred to the original term (metaphyseal dysostosis) because in this group of diseases the skeletal disorders are generally symmetric and generalized and are characterized by disturbances of endochondral bone formation manifested at the metaphyses. The outstanding radiographic feature of this group of disorders is irregular and inadequate mineralization of the primary zones of calcification and the metaphyses of tubular bones, with the changes resembling those of rickets. Confusion with vitamin-D-resistant rickets has occurred. The normal mineralization of the ossification centers in the shafts of the bone serves to identify metaphyseal chondrodysplasia, and the normal calcium, phosphorus, and alkaline phosphatase levels of the blood exclude rickets. Several forms of the condition can be recognized. One of the most distinct forms is the *Jansen type,* which features serious dwarfism, contracture deformities of hips and knees that result in a stance resembling that of the higher apes, and grossly expanded, cupped, irregularly mineralized metaphyses with normal or even somewhat enlarged epiphyseal ossification centers. The marked failure of mineralization of metaphyses is reminiscent of that seen in hypophosphatasia. However, in several reported cases the alkaline phosphatase level has been found elevated, and in others the calcium content of the serum has been elevated; but in general, diagnostic changes in chemical constituents of the blood have been lacking. The somewhat milder form of metaphyseal chondrodysplasia, the *Schmid type,* presents with dwarfism and metaphyseal irregularities resembling vitamin-D-resistant rickets, but with normal blood concentrations of calcium, phosphorus, and alkaline

phosphatase. A bilateral coxa vara is frequent. Some improvement in endochondral bone formation does take place with bed rest and with large doses of vitamin D. However, these large doses of vitamin D have resulted in toxic symptoms. The characteristic feature of this form of metaphyseal chondrodysplasia is marked bowing of the lower extremities.

McKusick has described a condition that is now known as metaphyseal chondrodysplasia, type McKusick (formerly *cartilage-hair hypoplasia*), among the Amish in Pennsylvania and Ohio. In addition to the metaphyseal changes, the head hair is sparse and fine and generally underpigmented. Metaphyseal chondrodysplasia has also been found in association with congenital pancreatic insufficiency and cyclic neutropenia. Some of these patients with exocrine pancreatic insufficiency have had siblings with diabetes mellitus. A form of metaphyseal chondrodysplasia with hereditary lymphopenic agammaglobulinemia has also been described. It is obvious that the radiographic observation of irregularities of mineralization in the metaphyses of major bones warrants careful evaluation of the patient for associated abnormalities in other body systems.

EPIPHYSEAL DYSPLASIA. In the group of epiphyseal dysplasias are included several conditions that are related largely through disproportionate involvement of epiphyseal ossification centers in the course of their development. Variable involvement of the vertebral column is prominent in many forms that are included in the term *spondyloepiphyseal dysplasias.* The various forms of stippled epiphyses are now included among the spondyloepiphyseal dysplasias. The prototype of this group, *chondrodysplasia punctata, Conradi-Hunermann type,* formerly called *dysplasia epiphysealis punctata* (Fig. 26), is usually recognized at birth because of asymmetric shortening of the limbs, joint contractures, and icthyosiform skin changes. Cataracts occur in somewhat under 20 percent of patients. If the patient survives the first month of life, asymmetric shortening of the limbs may become more prominent and scoliosis usually develops. Radiographically, punctate calcifications are present in the growth areas of cartilaginous bones, particularly the ends of the long bones. The stippling probably represents dystrophic calcification and may involve cartilage of the respiratory tree; it generally disappears by the end of the first year, but growth disturbance persists in those areas where the stippling has been most prominent. This particular form of chondrodysplasia punctata is considered to be transmitted by autosomal dominant inheritance. Some very mild variants exist in which calcification of cartilage may be followed by only minor deformity of affected carpal and tarsal areas and no restriction of growth of the major long bones.

Chondrodysplasia punctata, rhizomelic type, is a generally lethal form of the disease transmitted by autosomal recessive inheritance. These children all appear to be very similar, with flat faces and occasionally mongoloid features, but the stippling and shortening are rhizomelic in distribution and are symmetric. Cataracts are

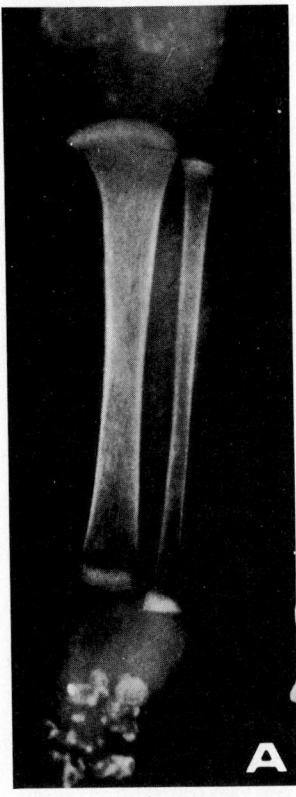
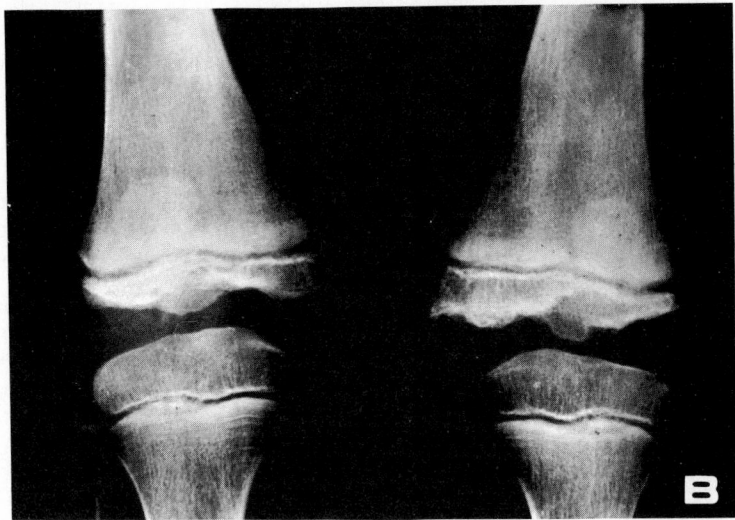

FIG. 26. An example of the Conradi-Huhnermann form of chondrodysplasia punctata. A. Patient at 2 months of age. B. Same patient at age 6 years. The flattened epiphyses resembled those in multiple epiphyseal dysplasia. Comparable transformations were present in other areas, especially in the wrists. Three members of two generations in this family were known to be affected.

present in almost two-thirds of cases. A characteristic radiolucent bar of cartilage can be seen in lateral projections of the spine separating the vertebral bodies into anterior and posterior centers; these ultimately unite if the patient survives.

Morquio's disease (mucopolysaccharidosis IV) is, from a morphologic standpoint, a spondyloepiphyseal dysplasia; biochemically it is one of the mucopolysaccharidoses (Chap. 30, p. 1898). The uniform platyspondyly and the severe dwarfism are also outstanding features of Morquio's disease. Corneal opacities become more prominent with increasing age, while mucopolysacchariduria tends to decrease. Of considerable clinical importance is the hypoplastic or absent odontoid process, which predisposes affected individuals to neurologic complications and even death.

A congenital form of spondyloepiphyseal dysplasia, *spondyloepiphyseal dysplasia congenita,* is characterized by short-trunk-type dwarfism, with short neck, pectus carinatum, and genu valgus. Approximately 50 percent of these patients have severe myopia, and they may develop retinal detachment. In the newborn infant radiographic examination shows retardation of ossification, with absence of ossification centers in the pubis and in the knee. The vertebral bodies are flat, and the lower dorsal and upper lumbar bodies are often wedged in the posterior portions; in later childhood anterior wedging is more common.

In *spondyloepiphyseal dysplasia tarda* short-trunk dwarfism manifests itself somewhat later in life. Transmission is generally considered to be X-linked recessive, but almost indistinguishable features have also been found in families with dominant autosomal inheritance. Flat and elongated vertebral bodies bulging toward each other on lateral projections and encroaching upon the intervertebral spaces are considered characteristic.

Multiple epiphyseal dysplasia (*dysplasia epiphysealis multiplex*) is a disease of older children in whom irregularities of epiphyseal ossification centers and round bones produce diagnostic changes. Long-term observation of children with stippled epiphyses (chondrodysplasia punctata) has shown them to develop features indistinguishable from those of dysplasia epiphysealis multiplex. Thus it has been postulated that the two conditions represent extremes of one syndrome in which the manifestations depend on the severity of the prenatal cartilaginous injury, but it is more likely that these two forms of epiphyseal dysplasia are separate entities.

The overlap of features in this group of diseases suggests both common causal factors (genes) and a common substrate on which they act (skeletal structures, particularly growing portions of the spine and long bones). In all instances evaluations of antecedents and

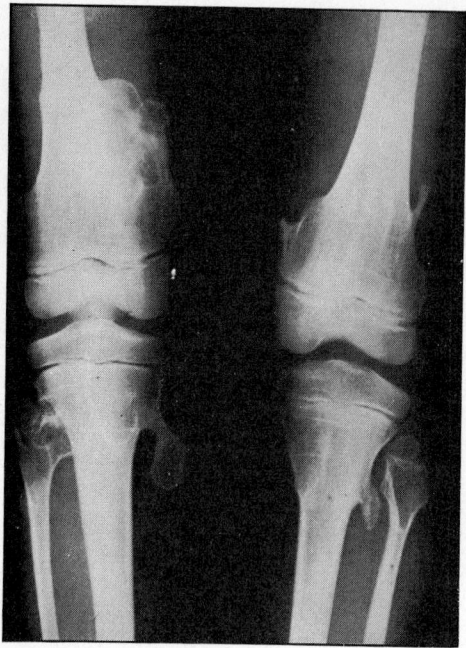

FIG. 27.   Multiple cartilaginous exostoses in the femora, tibias, and fibulas of a boy 5 years of age.

collaterals are important in establishing a probable diagnosis.

MULTIPLE CARTILAGINOUS EXOSTOSES.
Multiple cartilaginous exostoses (multiple hereditary exostoses, diaphyseal aclasis) may be considered a disorder of cartilaginous bone formation with epiosteal manifestations and a strong familial tendency. Characteristically, at the growing end of a bone, fragments of the cartilaginous epiphyseal line separate from the main body of cartilage and become incorporated in the bone of the shaft. The ectopic cartilage proliferates and changes into bone, forming a bony excrescence capped with cartilage that continues to grow, invariably away from the adjacent joint (Fig. 27), until cartilaginous growth ceases throughout the body. Knees and shoulders are most severely involved, but any bone may be affected, including vertebrae. The tumors are usually not present at birth, but make their appearance by 2 or 3 years of age and progress subsequently until cartilage growth ceases. Prior to the appearance of the tumors, radiographic examination of the skeleton may demonstrate no abnormalities whatsoever. Signs and symptoms arise from pressure of the bony masses on adjacent structures or from interference with joint action by sheer size or position. Treatment by excision is dictated by the severity of symptoms. Sarcomatous degeneration of the exostoses has been estimated to occur in 5 to 11 percent of cases. A sudden increase in growth of an osseous mass in the adult warrants careful evaluation for the possibility of this type of transformation.

ENCHONDROMATOSIS.   The effects of abnormal cartilage-bone growth may be more clearly understood if enchondromatosis (*Ollier's disease*) is considered analogous to multiple hereditary exostoses, with the exception that the masses of cartilage are proliferating within rather than upon the bone (enostosis rather than exostosis). The enosteal masses of cartilage are predominantly unilateral, but some bilateral involvement is usually present. The affected bones are short and bowed (Fig. 28). Disturbances of constriction occur, and they result from internal expansion of bone rather than from external excrescence. Bowing deformities may require surgical correction.

Maffucci's syndrome is the combination of muliple enchondromas with cavernous hemangiomas in which calcified phleboliths are commonly found on radiography. The condition manifests itself at or about puberty by the appearance of painless bluish nodules, usually on the hands and feet. Progressive enlargement takes place to form monstrous deformed limbs that are scarcely recognizable except for the presence of nails. The associated vascular and bony abnormalities are separate malformations. Gigantic deformities may require amputation.

In *metachondromatosis* features of both multiple exostoses and enchondromatosis are combined, and the cartilaginous tumors preferentially affect the hands and feet. Chondromas develop both inside and outside of the bone. The exostoses tend to grow toward the epiphysis, and both exostoses and enostoses may enlarge and subsequently resolve or disappear, or they may grow rapidly and produce marked limb deformities.

DYSCHONDROSTEOSIS.   The hereditary bone dysplasia dyschondrosteosis is transmitted as an autosomal dominant and is characterized by mesomelic dwarfism and a distal radio-ulnar wrist deformity that has been termed *Madelung's deformity*. Madelung's de-

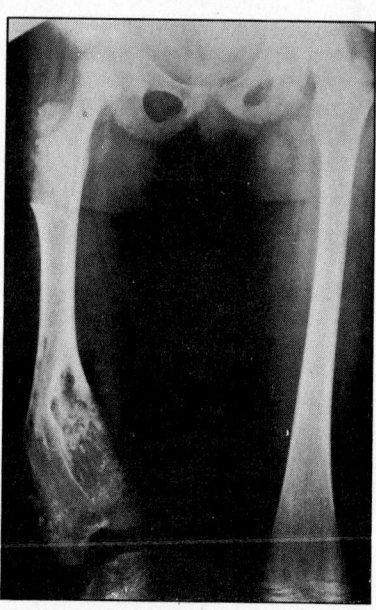

FIG. 28.   Ollier's enchondromatosis in a girl 5 years of age.

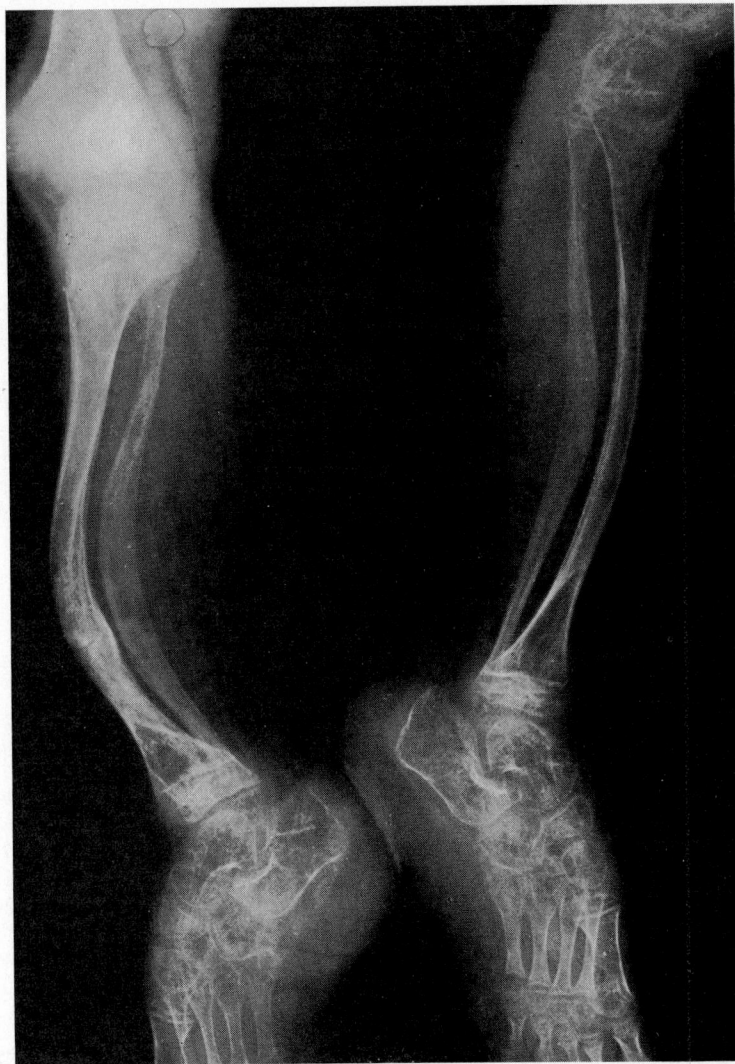

FIG. 29. Osteogenesis imperfecta in a boy 8 years of age. The bowing of the tibias and fibulas is secondary to fractures and callus formation. These changes are superimposed on a background of thin, brittle cortical walls, which is the primary change in osteogenesis imperfecta.

formity is characterized by bowing and disproportionate shortening of the radius, with dislocation or subluxation of the distal radio-ulnar articulation and dorsal prominence at the distal end of the ulna. It has been suggested that all instances of nontraumatic Madelung's deformity, without other obvious skeletal dysplasia such as hereditary exostoses and enchondromatosis, are nonetheless the result of generalized dysplasia with mild features. In addition, severe forms of mesomelic dwarfism, allegedly different from dyschondrosteosis, have been described. A possible relationship of all these entities has been suggested by the finding of typical Madelung's deformity in some members of a family in association with mesomelic dwarfism and the finding of severe mesomelic dwarfism in children born of parents with Madelung's deformity and/or short stature.

OSTEOGENESIS IMPERFECTA. Two forms of osteogenesis imperfecta that were previously thought to be separate entities are now thought to be different manifestations of a single basic disease. The *congenital* form is severe and usually occurs sporadically; it is characterized radiographically by ribbonlike bone shadows with almost countless fractures (Vrolik's disease). In *osteogenesis imperfecta tarda* (fragilitas ossium, osteopsathyrosis, Lobstein's disease), in which fractures appear later in life, there is marked bone atrophy with thinning of cortices associated with solitary fractures of individual bones in various stages of repair (Fig. 29) and secondary deformities. Also in the tarda form there may be one or more fractures present at birth, but the gracile appearance of the bones is very different from the total lack of modeling that characterizes the severe congenital form. In both forms inadequate mineralization

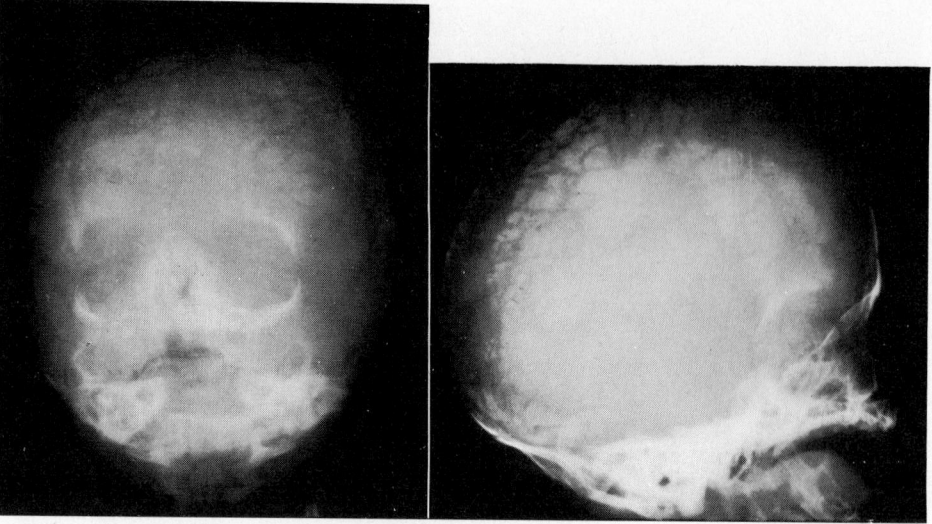

FIG. 30. Roentgenogram of skull in osteogenesis imperfecta showing the mosaic pattern of rarefaction at 1 week of age.

of the calvarium is seen, but it is most severe in the congenital form (Fig. 30). The entire calvarium at times appears to be formed by a network of sutures, and differentiation of any particular irregular suture from a fracture is virtually impossible. Possibly because the congenital form is rarely compatible with longevity, associated abnormalities are more commonly found in the tarda form; these include osteosclerosis with deafness, dental deficiencies of enamel and dentin (dentinogenesis imperfecta), and a characteristic blue color of the sclerae. Thinness or unusual translucency of the sclerae, which is said to be an expression of defective connective tissue, is responsible for the blue sclerae, which

may occur in individuals unaffected with skeletal abnormalities.

The clinical manifestations are almost exclusively related to the bone fractures. These can result not only from minor trauma but also from ordinary stresses of ambulation or even position changes, and they appear to be less painful than comparable fractures in normal individuals. As a general rule, the fractures tend to become less common after puberty. Endocrine therapy to induce early puberty has produced questionable results with regard to frequency of fractures. Healing of fractures takes place with exuberant calcifying callus formation, but refracture is common. As a result of the

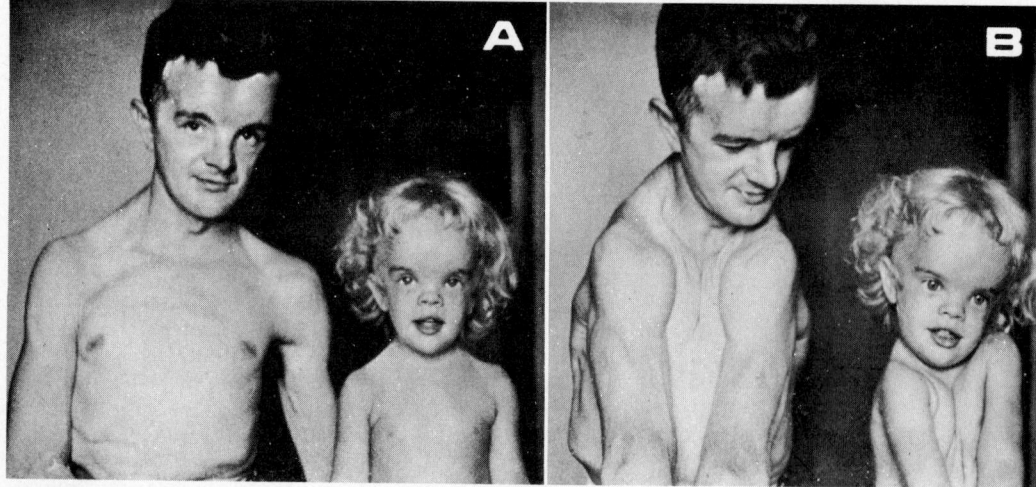

FIG. 31. A. Father and child with cleidocranial dysostosis. Note ocular hypertelorism, depression in center of father's forehead, and sloping shoulders. B. Approximation of shoulders made possible by defective formation of rudimentary clavicles.

recurring deforming fractures, dwarfism is usual and activity is often restricted. Compression fractures of the vertebral bodies are common, with the resulting vertebra plana contributing to diminished stature. Histologic examination of the bones reveals imperfectly formed and imperfectly calcified bone trabeculae and cortical deficiency and discontinuity. In older patients the cortex may become strikingly thickened, resulting in gracile, bent bones with thick cortices and narrow medullary cavities. Because of low serum pyrophosphatase levels and excessive urinary pyrophosphate excretion, therapy with magnesium salts has been recommended, since magnesium is the metallic ion in the pyrophosphatase enzyme. Studies are still progressing, but the initial enthusiasm for this form of therapy appears to be waning. Collagen synthesis by fibroblasts from patients with osteogenesis imperfecta is impaired, with measurements of bone turnover indicating excessive activity and suggesting a hypermetabolic state. At present no effective therapy other than good orthopedic management seems to be available.

CLEIDOCRANIAL DYSPLASIA. In cleidocranial dysplasia various structures other than clavicles and skull are also affected. In the classic form the teeth are defective, small, and poorly formed; deciduous teeth are retained well into adulthood. Mineralization of the pubis also takes place in adult life. However, nonmineralization of the pubis during childhood and adolescence, which is a frequent observation, produces no clinical signs and symptoms.

In the skull a large fontanelle tends to persist into late adolescence or early adult life. The skull may be so soft as to give the impression that there is no bone. The eyes are generally widely spaced, and the cranial vault seems to bulge forward and to each side of the facial area. Radiographically the inadequacy of mineralization is demonstrated by multiple small islands of bone density within the general membrane of the skull. After some time the islands enlarge and coalesce until mineralization of the skull is complete. The relative softness of the calvarium causes it to sag around the base, producing what has appropriately been described as a tam o'-shanter skull. Notwithstanding the softness of the calvarium, it rarely results in brain damage. Convulsive disorders and developmental neurologic abnormalities occasionally occur.

Ossification of the clavicles may be completely absent, or diminutive ossification centers may be found. Failure of development of the clavicles accounts for the characteristic ability of affected individuals to bring their shoulders together in front of the upper chest (Fig. 31). Ligamental laxity in other areas is not unusual, and both knock-knee deformity and genu recurvatum may occur. Spina bifida is common, and in many instances there are irregularities in the growing ends of the tubular bones not unlike those seen in metaphyseal chondrodysplasia. Certain individuals may demonstrate only some of the components; in fact, normal clavicles may be present. In questionable cases examination of other members of the family may assist in diagnosis, since the hereditary pattern is that of an autosomal dominant trait; however, about 25 percent of reported instances are sporadic.

Miscellaneous Dysplasias

DIAPHYSEAL DYSPLASIA. Diaphyseal dysplasia, a hyperostotic disease, affects primarily tubular bones, but it may involve the cranium and the vertebral column in well-developed cases. It usually begins between 2 and 6 years of age with gait disturbance, fatigability, and failure to gain weight. The involved long bones are symmetrically expanded as well as thickened. The external cortical thickening involves only the shafts; metaphyses and epiphyses are generally normal. Extensive involvement of the cranium and facial bones may produce a form of leontiasis ossea. Caffey has pointed out the enlargement of channels for nutrient vessels in the femur and tibia. Girdany has described a family with typical and severe cases as well as cases with only minimal external cortical thickening. He observed clinical improvement with increasing age in this family, and he has suggested that primary muscular involvement may be a part of the clinical picture.

Some confusion may occur with instances of hyperphosphatasemia, in which overproduction and overdestruction of bone and bone collagen takes place with resultant expansion of bones and cortical hyperostoses. The possibility that the latter progressively disabling condition may respond to treatment with thyrocalcitonin is worth noting.

METAPHYSEAL DYSPLASIA. Metaphyseal dysplasia (*Pyle's disease*) is characterized by failure of bone absorption in the metaphyses, so that the ends of the long bones are splayed (Fig. 32); the tibial curving commonly presents clinically as knock-knee. The tubular bones are longer than normal, and affected individuals are usually tall but have normal sitting height. Fractures may occur. Cranial involvement may be limited to slight thickening of the base of the skull without abnormality of the facial bones. However, cranial features of leontiasis ossea with massive swelling of cranial and facial bones have been reported in some patients who have been classified under *craniometaphyseal dysplasia*. The identity of these two conditions have not yet been established, notwithstanding the marked similarities in manifestations of splaying and elongation of tubular bones of the extremities.

MARFAN'S SYNDROME. In the past Marfan's syndrome was known as *arachnodactyly* because of the spiderlike elongated digits. However, McKusick has demonstrated that the typical gracile digits may be clinically inapparent. Furthermore, elongated digits may occur without the connective tissue disorder that constitutes Marfan's syndrome.

Marfan's syndrome is a generalized disorder of connective tissue with involvement of the eyes (ectopia lentis), the cardiovascular system (aortic aneurysm), and the osseous system (excessive length of tubular bones). The chief clinical features are the general elongation of the extremities. Even in individuals of stocky body build the condition may be present, characterized by an in-

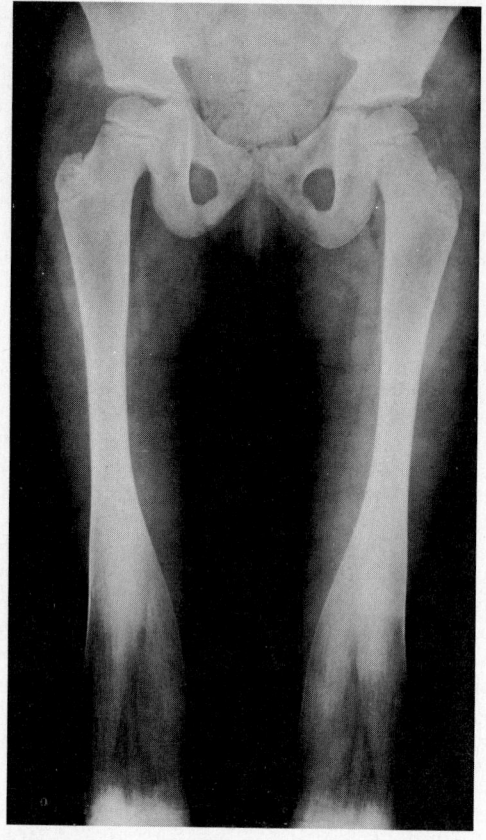 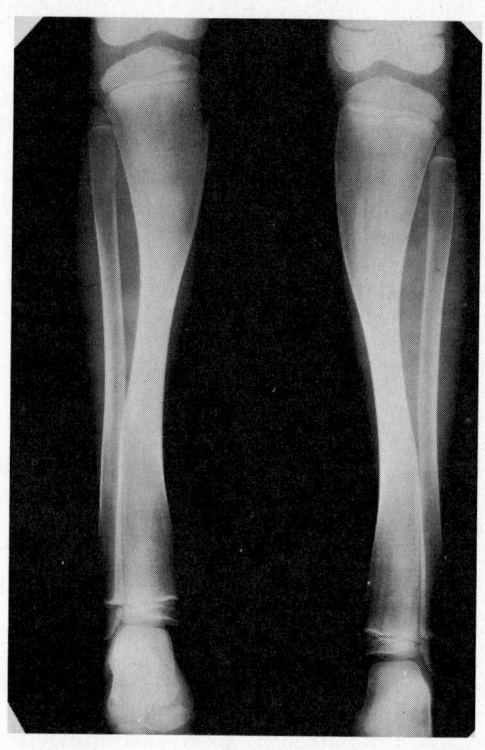

FIG. 32. Pyle's disease; photographs from original films of cases reported by Bakwin and Krida. (Courtesy of Dr. Harry Bakwin.)

crease in span (the distance between the tips of the middle fingers when the arms are fully extended at shoulder height) over vertical height. The ligaments are relaxed, so that joints are loose, and flat feet and scoliosis are common. Thoracic deformities (pectus excavatum and pectus carinatum) have been observed. The ectopia lentis is bilateral and is associated with tremor of the iris. Aortic aneurysm, which may lead to death in early adult life, results from degeneration of the media of the great vessels. Radiographically the narrow, elongated tubular bones are suggestive, but the diagnostic features include not only an absolute increase in length but also a disproportionate increase of the more distal bones: elongation of the forearms, for example, is disproportionately greater than that of the upper arms. Camptodactyly of the fifth finger occurs with some frequency. The condition is apparently transmitted as an autosomal dominant trait. Almost identical changes are seen in *homocystinuria;* the chief differential points are the almost universal mental retardation and the urinary excretion of homocystine in patients with homocystinuria. Homocystinuria is transmitted as an autosomal recessive trait.

Hecht and Beals have suggested that the original patient described by Marfan had a condition known as *congenital contractural arachnodactyly* rather than the syndrome currently known as Marfan's syndrome. Congenital contractural arachnodactyly is also transmitted as an autosomal dominant disorder. This condition in-

cludes arachnodactyly, contractures, and an ear deformity characterized by flattening of the helix and crumpling, but no known eye or cardiovascular involvement.

POLYOSTOTIC FIBROUS DYSPLASIA. Fibrous dysplasia with skin pigmentation and precocious puberty (*McCune-Albright disease*) may not ideally belong among the skeletal dysplasias, but it is included here because of the presence of interesting skeletal features. There are localized areas of fibrous dysplasia in bones, thus producing a washed-out uniform appearance with loss of trabecular architecture. These predominantly unilateral features are observed in several bones. Polyostotic fibrous dysplasia is generally associated with irregular pigmentation of the skin that is also predominantly unilateral, commonly on the same side as the bone lesions. In the cranium the bone tends to become thickened and increased in density with resulting cranial asymmetry. Precocious puberty has been described in females affected with the disease (Fig. 33) and in some males. Pathologic fractures through the areas of fibrous dysplasia may first call attention to the disease.

OSTEO-ONYCHODYSOSTOSIS. Also known as *nail-patella syndrome* and *iliac horn syndrome*, this condition is recognized clinically by inability to extend the elbows in an individual who has an ectodermal dysplasia involving the nails of at least the thumb and index finger. Other nails may be involved, but they become less

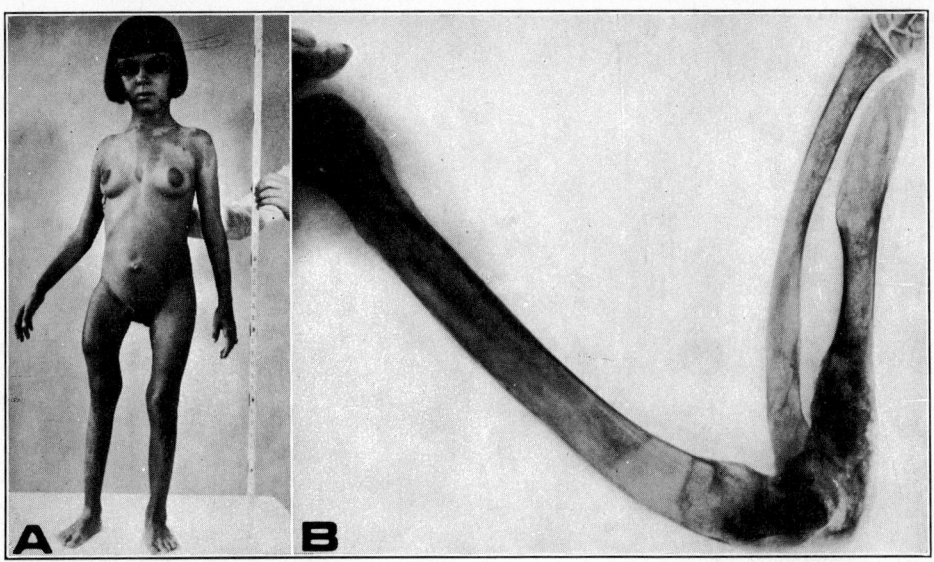

FIG. 33. Polyostotic fibrous dysplasia. A. Precocious puberty at age 5 years. B. Roentgenogram of bones of arm in osteodystrophia fibrosa. (From McCane and Brach: Am J Dis Child 54:806, 1937.)

severely affected toward the ulnar side of the hand. The knees have a broad, flat appearance resulting from congenital absence or hypoplasia of the patellas. Radiographically the radial heads are hypoplastic and dislocated, ossification centers for the patellas are either extremely small or absent, and bony excrescences (for which there does not appear to be any mammalian homologue) extend backward from the alae of the iliac bones. Occasionally they can be palpated clinically. The condition appears to be transmitted by an autosomal dominant gene that is closely linked to the locus determining the ABO blood group. Individuals with incomplete forms have been described in families in which an atypical form of nephritis is also prevalent.

HYPOPHOSPHATASIA. It is not clear whether hypophosphatasia itself is a true skeletal dysplasia or whether the characteristic hypophosphatasia results from other, more basic defects. In either event, low alkaline phosphatase levels in blood and tissues are associated with defective transformation of cartilage to bone, premature shedding of the deciduous teeth (often the feature that brings the child to the physician), and an abnormal metabolite (ethanolamine phosphate) in the urine. The condition is most severe in the newborn infant, who obviously has suffered in utero. These children are usually nonviable; they have practically no mineralized bone anywhere in the body and show failure to form primary spongiosa of an extremely severe degree. In infants over 6 months of age the mineralization of the skeleton is appreciably better, but the children fail to thrive. Separation of cranial sutures, bulging fontanelles, and bowing of the long bones are common manifestations. If the infant survives the clinical picture changes, the childhood forms of the condition are then

recognized. These resemble and have been confused with rickets because of defective gait, short stature, bowleg, enlargement of joints, and even rachitic rosary. As in rickets, radiographs demonstrate irregularities of mineralization in all areas where cartilage is changing into bone, especially in areas of most rapid growth. However, irregular islands of radiolucency characteristically extend into the shaft of the bone from the irregular epiphyseal line. There may be a history of fractures and of "rickets" during childhood. Premature closure of cranial sutures occurs in a large percentage of children. Teeth show aplasia, hypoplasia, or dysplasia of the cementum. Premature exfoliation is believed to be

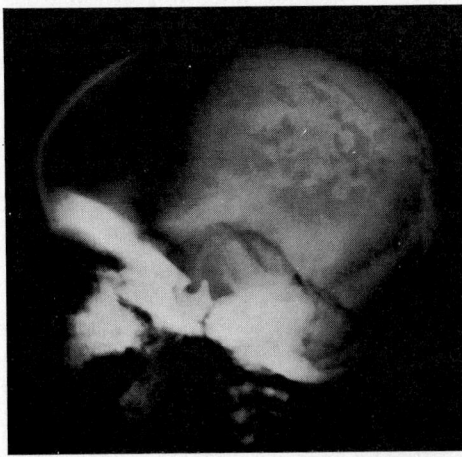

FIG. 34. Roentgenogram of skull of a boy with osteopetrosis (age 3 years 9 months).

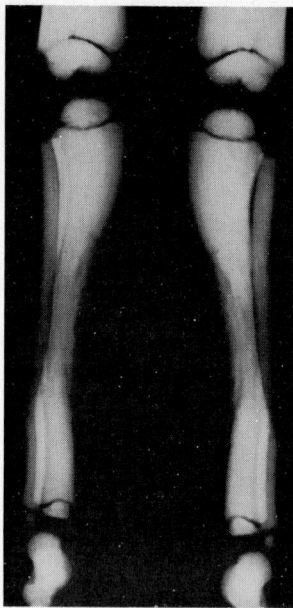

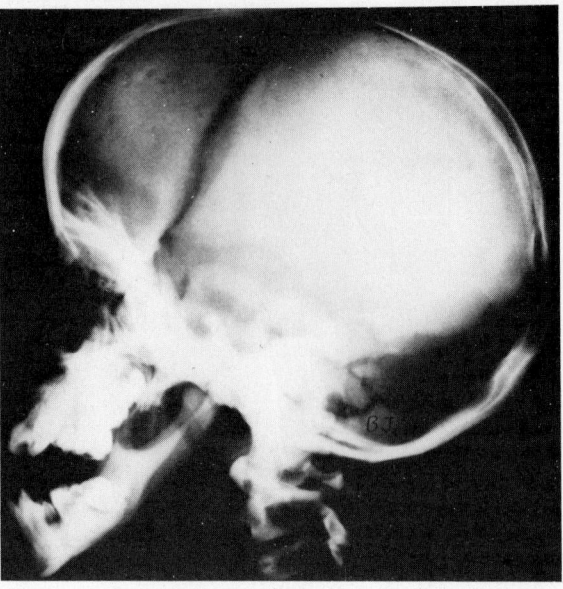

FIG. 35.   Roentgenogram of lower extremities of a boy with osteopetrosis (age 3 years 9 months).

FIG. 36.   Skull in pycnodysostosis (female, 12 years old). An open fontanelle, osteosclerosis, and an almost absent mandibular angle are characteristic. (Courtesy of Dr. Javier Lucaya.)

related to aplasia of cementum and may affect permanent as well as deciduous teeth. In adults the disease may be an incidental finding when a chemical analysis of the blood reveals a low alkaline phosphatase level; ethanolamine phosphate may also be present in the urine.

HYPERPHOSPHATASIA.   Frequently referred to as juvenile Paget's disease, hyperphosphatasia has clinical features in children quite comparable to those in adults. Bowing deformities of the legs and muscle weakness develop in childhood. Although thickening of the bones of the skull and of the face may take place, the cranial features are not as prominent clinically as in adults. In addition to the bowing, the long bones characteristically demonstrate extensive cortical hyperostoses, often with the appearance of active intraosseous reorganization. The alkaline phosphatase level of the serum is markedly and consistently elevated and serves to differentiate this condition from other hyperostotic conditions affecting the appendicular skeleton and the skull.

OSTEOPETROSIS.   Osteopetrosis (*Albers-Schönberg disease,* marble bones) is an osteosclerotic disorder that is commonly associated with anemia and deafness and is usually identified radiographically by marked increases in radiodensity of almost all the bones of the body, with disproportionate involvement of the long tubular bones and the base of the skull (Fig. 34). In spite of the radiodensity, the bones are relatively brittle, and fractures are common, particularly in the hip. In addition, constriction of the tubular bones is also disturbed, so that flaring of the distal ends of the growing shafts is a prominent feature in childhood (Fig. 35). Variations

in bone density extending in bands across the poorly constricted metaphysis suggest that there are periods of exacerbation and remission in the disease. Dental sepsis has been frequent, and osteomyelitis of the mandible was a common complication before antibiotics became available. Individuals surviving into adult life, although dwarfed, frequently recover from the myelosclerotic anemia that characterizes their course in infancy and childhood. Even the hepatosplenomegaly that is present in childhood tends to recede. The skeletal changes result from a persistence of primary spongiosa that is not properly eroded and remodeled. It would appear that some of the cases that have been reported in infancy represent instances of idiopathic hypercalcemia (p. 252) rather than osteopetrosis.

PYCNODYSOSTOSIS.   Maroteaux and Lamy have described a form of osteosclerotic dwarfism associated with fractures that has been confused with both osteogenesis imperfecta and osteopetrosis. Because of the dense bone, the term pycnodysostosis (*pyknos,* thick) was coined to describe it. Differential features include absence of severe anemia, loss of the angle of the mandible such that on radiography the ascending ramus is a direct continuation of the body of the mandible (Fig. 36), and hypoplasia of the terminal phalanges. The authors have postulated that Henri de Toulouse-Lautrec owed his short stature and his several bone fractures to pycnodysostosis rather than to osteogenesis imperfecta.

MEDULLARY STENOSIS.   Congenital medullary stenosis is a form of proportional dwarfism characterized by self-limited bouts of clinical tetany with hypocalcemia and hyperphosphatemia. On radiography of the skeleton there is an absolute decrease in size of tubular bones with disproportionately decreased shaft width due to extreme narrowness of the medullary cavities. The calvarial bones of the skull are thin, and the anterior fontanelle closes late. There are no signs of disease of associated organs. Medullary stenosis in metacarpal bones occurs to some degree in the normal population; it is more common in some Central American populations. The relationship of this developmental variation to the generalized disorder with systemic manifestations is not clear.

References

HEREDITARY AND DEVELOPMENTAL CONDITIONS

Bailey JA II: Disproportionate Short Stature: Diagnosis and Management. Philadelphia, WB Saunders, 1973

Bergsma D (ed): Skeletal Dysplasias. Miami, Symposia Specialists, 1974

Kaufmann HJ (ed): Progress in Pediatric Radiology, Vol IV, Intrinsic Diseases of Bones. Basel, Karger, 1973

McKusick VA: Mendelian Inheritance in Man, 3rd ed. Baltimore, Johns Hopkins University Press, 1971

Rubin P: Dynamic Classification of Bone Dysplasias. Chicago, Year Book, 1964

Spranger JW, Langer LO Jr, Wiedemann H-R: Bone Dysplasias. An Atlas of Constitutional Disorders of Skeletal Development. Philadelphia, WB Saunders, 1974

Warkany J: Congenital Malformations. Notes and Comments. Chicago, Year Book, 1971

ACHONDROPLASIA

Caffey J: Achondroplasia of the pelvis and lumbosacral spine. Am J Roentgenol Radium Ther Nucl Med 80:449, 1958

Cohen ME, Rosenthal AD, Matson DD: Neurological abnormalities in achondroplastic children. J Pediatr 71:367, 1967

Silverman FN: A differential diagnosis of achondroplasia. Radiol Clin North Am 2:223, 1968

——— Achondroplasia. In Kaufmann HJ (ed): Progress in Pediatric Radiology, Vol IV. Basel, Karger, 1973, p 94

ACHONDROGENESIS

Houston CS, Awen CF, Kent HD: Fatal neonatal dwarfism. J Can Assoc Radiol 23:45, 1972

Saldino RM: Lethal short limbed dwarfism: achondrogenesis and thanatophoric dwarfism. Am J Roentgenol Radium Ther Nucl Med 112:185, 1971

THANATOPHORIC DWARFISM

Keats TE, Rittervold HO, Michaelis LL: Thanatophoric dwarfism. Am J Roentgenol Radium Ther Nucl Med 108:473, 1970

Langer LO, Spranger J, Greinacher I, Herdman RC: Thanatophoric dwarfism. Radiology 92:285, 1969

Partington MW, Gonzales-Crussi F, Khakee SG, Wollin DG: Cloverleaf skull and thanatophoric dwarfism. Arch Dis Child 46:656, 1971

METATROPIC DWARFISM

Kaufmann E: Untersuchungen über die sogenannte foetale Rachitis (Chondrodystrophia foetalis). Berlin, Georg Reiner, 1892

Maroteaux P, Spranger J, Wiedemann H-R: Der metatropische Zwergwuchs. Arch Kinderheilkd 173:211, 1966

DIASTROPHIC DWARFISM

Langer LO: Diastrophic dwarfism in early infancy. Am J Roentgenol Radium Ther Nucl Med 93:399, 1965

Taber P, Freedman S, Lackey DA: Diastrophic dwarfism. In Kaufmann HJ (ed): Progress in Pediatric Radiology, Vol IV. Basel, Karger, 1973, p 152

CHONDROECTODERMAL DYSPLASIA

Caffey J: Chondroectodermal dysplasia (Ellis–van Creveld disease); report of 3 cases. Am J Roentgenol Radium Ther Nucl Med 68:875, 1952

Ellis RWB, Andrew JD: Chondroectodermal dysplasia. J Bone Joint Surg [Br] 44:626, 1962

——— van Creveld S: A syndrome characterized by ectodermal dysplasia, polydactyly, chondrodysplasia and congenital morbus cordis. Arch Dis Child 15:65, 1940

McKusick VA, Egeland JA, Eldridge R, Krusen DE: Dwarfism in the Amish. I. The Ellis–van Creveld syndrome. Bull Johns Hopkins Hospital 115:306, 1964

JEUNE'S DISEASE

Jequier J-C, Favreau-Ethier M, Gregoire H: Asphyxiating thoracic dysplasia. In Kaufmann HJ (ed): Progress in Pediatric Radiology, Vol IV. Basel, Karger, 1973, p 184

Jeune M, Carron R, Beraud C, Loaec Y: Polychondrodystrophie avec blocage thoracique d'evolution fatale. Pediatrie 9:390, 1954

Kaufmann HJ, Kirkpatrick JA: Jeune thoracic dysplasia. A spectrum of disorders? in Bergsma D (ed): Skeletal Dysplasias. Miami, Symposia Specialists, 1974

Spranger J, et al: Short rib-polydactyly (SRP) syndromes, types Majewski and Saldino-Noonan. Z Kinderheilkd 116:73, 1974

METAPHYSEAL CHONDRODYSPLASIA

Burke V, Colebatch JH, Anderson CM, Simons MJ: Association of pancreatic insufficiency and chronic neutropenia in childhood. Arch Dis Child 42:147, 1967

Evans R, Caffey J: Metaphyseal dysostosis resembling vitamin D refractory rickets. Am J Dis Child 95:640, 1958

Jansen M: Über atypische Chondrodystrophie (Achondroplasie) und über eine noch nicht beschriebene angeborene Wachstrumsstörung des Knochensystems: Metaphysäre Dysostosis. Z Orthop Chir 61:253, 1934

Kozlowski K: Metaphyseal dysostosis. Am J Roentgenol Radium Ther Nucl Med 91:602, 1964

McKusick VA, Eldridge R, Hostetler JA, Egeland JA, Ruangwit U: Dwarfism in the Amish. II. Cartilage-hair hypoplasia. Bull Johns Hopkins Hospital 116:285, 1965

Schmid F: Beitrag zur Dysostosis Enchondralis Metaphysaria. Monatsschr Kinderheilkd 97:393, 1949

Stephens FE: An achondroplastic mutation and the nature of its inheritance. J Hered 34:229, 1943

Sutcliffe J, Stanley P: Metaphyseal chondrodysplasias. In Kaufmann HJ (ed): Progress in Pediatric Radiology, Vol IV. Basel, Karger, 1973, p 250

EPIPHYSEAL DYSPLASIA

Ford N, Silverman FN, Kozlowski K: Spondyloepiphyseal dysplasia (pseudoachondroplastic type). Am J Roentgenol Radium Ther Nucl Med 86:462, 1961

Maroteaux P, Lamy M: La maladie de Morquio. Presse Med 71:2091, 1963

——— Wiedemann R, Spranger J, Kozlowski K, Lenzi L: Essai de Classification des Dysplasies Spondylo-épiphysaires. Lyon, France, SIMEP editions, 1968

Schenk EA, Haggerty J: Morquio's disease. A radiologic and morphologic study. Pediatrics 34:839, 1964

Silverman FN: Dysplasies épiphysaires: Entité protéiforme. Ann Radiol 4:833, 1961

Spranger J, Langer LO: Spondyloepiphyseal dysplasias. In Bergsma D (ed): Skeletal Dysplasias. Miami, Symposia Specialists, 1974, p 19
—————— Opitz JM, Bidder U: Heterogeneity of chondrodysplasia punctata. Humangenetik 11:190, 1971

MULTIPLE CARTILAGINOUS EXOSTOSES

Jaffe HL: Hereditary multiple exostosis. Arch Pathol 36:335, 1943
Solomon L: Hereditary multiple exostoses. J Bone Joint Surg [Br] 45:292, 1963

ENCHONDROMATOSIS

Carleton A, Elkington JSC, Greenfield JG, Robb-Smith AHT: Maffucci's syndrome (dyschondroplasia with haemangiomata). Q J Med 11:203, 1942
Margolis J: Ollier's disease. Arch Intern Med 103:297, 1959
Maroteaux P: La metachondromatose. Z Kinderheilkd 109:246, 1971

DYSCHONDROSTEOSIS

Herdman RC, Langer LO, Good RA: Dyschondrosteosis. J Pediatr 68:432, 1966
Silverman FN: Mesomelic dwarfism. In Kaufmann HJ (ed): Progress in Pediatric Radiology, Vol IV. Basel, Karger, 1973, p 546

OSTEOGENESIS IMPERFECTA

Cropp DJA, Myers DN: Physiological evidence of hypermetabolism in osteogenesis imperfecta. Pediatrics 49:375, 1972
Reilly FC, Brown DM: Morphological and biochemical studies in osteogenesis imperfecta. J Lab Clin Med 78:1000, 1971
Wright PB, Gernstetter SL, Greenblatt RB: Therapeutic acceleration of bone age in osteogenesis imperfecta; case report. J Bone Joint Surg [Am] 33:939, 1951

CLEIDOCRANIAL DYSPLASIA

Anspach WE, Huepel RC: Familial cleidocranial dysostosis (cleidal dysostosis); preosseous and dentinal dystrophy. Am J Dis Child 58:786, 1939
Bach C, Fauré C, Schaefer P, Jolly J: La dysostose cléidocranienne. Etude de six observations. Association à des manifestations neurologiques. An Pediatr 13:67, 1966
Forland M: Cleidocranial dysostosis. A review of the syndrome and report of a sporadic case with hereditary transmission. Am J Med 33:792, 1962

DIAPHYSEAL DYSPLASIA

Girdany BR: Engelmann's disease (progressive diaphyseal dysplasia). A nonprogressive familial form of muscular dystrophy with characteristic bone changes. Clin Orthop 14:102, 1959
Joseph J, LeFebvre J, Guy E, Job JC: Dysplasie cranio-diaphysaire progressive. Ann Radiol (Paris) 1:477, 1958
Neuhauser EBD, Schwachman H, Wittenberg MH, Cohen J: Progressive diaphyseal dysplasia. Radiology 51:11, 1948
Singleton EB, Thomas JR, Worthington WW, Hild JR: Progressive diaphyseal dysplasia (Engelmann's disease). Radiology 67:233, 1956

METAPHYSEAL DYSPLASIA

Bakwin H, Krida A: Familial metaphyseal dysplasia. Am J Dis Child 53:1521, 1937
Mori PA, Holt JF: Cranial manifestations of familial metaphyseal dysplasia. Radiology 66:335, 1956
Pyle E: A case of unusual bone development. J Bone Joint Surg 13:874, 1931

MARFAN'S SYNDROME

Hecht F, Beals RK: "New" syndrome of congenital contractural arachnodactyly originally described by Marfan in 1896. Pediatrics 49:574, 1972

MacLeod PM, Fraser FC: Congenital contractural arachnodactyly. Am J Dis Child 126:810, 1973
Schimke RN, McKusick VA, Huang T, Pollack AD: Homocystinuria. Studies of 20 families with 38 affected members. JAMA 193:711, 1965

POLYOSTOTIC FIBROUS DYSPLASIA

Albright F, Butler AM, Hampton AO, Smith P: Syndrome characterized by osteitis fibrosa disseminata, areas of pigmentation and endocrine dysfunction, with precocious puberty in females; report of five cases. N Engl J Med 216:727, 1937
McCune DJ, Bruch H: Osteodystrophia fibrosa; report of a case in which the condition was combined with precocious puberty, pathologic pigmentation of the skin and hyperthyroidism, with a review of the literature. Am J Dis Child 54:806, 1937

OSTEO-ONYCHODYSOSTOSIS

Carbonara P, Alpert M: Hereditary osteo-onychodysplasia (HOOD). Am J Med Sci 248:139, 1964
Doub H: Clinical observations and research (iliac horn syndrome). Radiology 59:578, 1952
Lawler SD, Renwick JH, Mosbech J, Wildervank LS, Hauge M: Linkage tests involving the P blood group locus and further data on the ABO:nail-patella linkage. Ann Hum Genet 22:342, 1958

HYPOPHOSPHATASIA

Currarino G, Neuhauser EBD, Reyersbach GC, Sobel E: Hypophosphatasia. Am J Roentgenol Radium Ther Nucl Med 78:392, 1957
Currarino G: Hypophosphatasia. In Kaufmann HJ (ed): Progress in Pediatric Radiology, Vol IV, Basel, Karger, 1973, p 469
McCance RA, Fairweather DVI, Barrett AM, Morrison AB: Genetic, clinical, biochemical and pathological features of hypophosphatasia. Q J Med 25:523, 1956
Ritchie GM: Hypophosphatasia: a metabolic disease with important dental manifestations. Arch Dis Child 39:584, 1964

HYPERPHOSPHATASIA

Caffey J: Familial hyperphosphatasemia with ateliosis and hypermetabolism of growing membranous bone; review of the clinical, radiographic and chemical features. Progr Pediat Radiol 4:438, 1973.
Fanconi G, Moreira G, Uehlinger E, Giedion A: Osteochalasia desmalis familiaris: hyperostosis corticalis deformans juvenilis, chronic idiopathic hyperphosphatasia, osteoectasia and macrocranium. Helv Paediatr Acta 19:279, 1964

OSTEOPETROSIS

Graham CB, Rudhe U, Eklof O: Osteopetrosis. Progr Pediat Radiol 4:375, 1973
Piatt AD, Erhard GA, Araj JS: Benign osteopetrosis; report of nine cases. Am J Roentgenol Radium Ther Nucl Med 76:1119, 1956

PYCNODYSOSTOSIS

Maroteaux P, Lamy M: The malady of Toulouse-Lautrec. JAMA 191:715, 1965

MEDULLARY STENOSIS

Caffey J: Congenital stenosis of medullary spaces in tubular bones and calvaria in two proportionate dwarfs, mother and son; coupled with transitory hypocalcemic tetany. Am J Roentgenol Radium Ther Nucl Med 100:1, 1967

POSTNATAL AND ACQUIRED CONDITIONS

Juvenile Osteochondroses

Irregularity of mineralization in an adult bone usually indicates replacement of normally mineralized structures by pathologic material. In the child, however, irregularity of mineralization is usually a stage in the transformation of cartilage to bone. At several sites in the growing skeleton delay in the appearance of ossification centers or damage to centers already present may result in structural alteration of the cartilage. Reossification then takes place over a period of many months, with variable residual deformities that are called the juvenile osteochondroses and that depend largely on local factors. Causes and pathogeneses are unknown, but a traumatic basis for at least some of them appears very likely. The subject has been confused because some of the reported series have included children whose irregular mineralization, although radiographically indistinguishable from that of an osteochondrosis, actually represents a stage of normal development. The absence of deformity in the final mineralized stage in such individuals has at times been attributed to various forms of treatment. It is obvious that critical reevaluation of both diagnosis and management of these conditions is necessary.

The usual clinical signs of osteochondroses are mild local tenderness, pain, swelling, and motor disability; constitutional signs are mild or absent. The frequency of these same complaints in active growing children warrants circumspection in making the diagnosis, even when the complaints are present in association with irregular mineralization. Examination of the opposite side, which frequently reveals bilateral symmetry of irregularities of mineralization, may be helpful in the recognition of anatomic variants. Most of the osteochondroses have been named after the authors who first described them. Only major and clearly defined entities will be discussed here; the References should be consulted for more extensive coverage.

COXA PLANA. Coxa plana *(Legg-Calvé-Perthes disease)* is by far the most important and the most serious of the juvenile osteochondroses. A limp that is usually intermittent and mild local pain that is often referred to the medial side of the ipsilateral knee are the principal and sometimes the only clinical manifestations. Limitation of abduction and of external rotation of the hip can often be demonstrated early during the active phase of the disease; these are usually lacking later. Constitutional signs are slight or absent. Significant percentages of cases are discovered incidental to radiologic examination such as intravenous pyelograms or bowel studies. In some children the symptoms are present for months prior to radiographic signs; in others the existence of well-advanced radiographic features at the time of the first complaints or shortly thereafter indicates a relatively long asymptomatic period.

Coxa plana rarely develops before 3 years of age; it is more frequent in boys than in girls in a ratio of about 6 to 1. The speed of its development and its regression appears to be unaffected by any form of treatment (Fig. 37). An active phase lasting approximately 18 months is characterized by initial faint sclerosis of the affected femoral head with some relative or even absolute radiolucency of the subjacent neck. Not uncommonly a curvilinear radiolucent shadow appears approximately 1 mm inside the convex projection of the subchondral aspect of the ossification center. In many cases this radiolucent shadow is seen only in a film taken with the femur in abduction and external rotation, and it appears to be related to the anterior portion of the ossification center. Caffey believes that this line is the consequence of direct traumatic compression of the femoral head by its acetabular roof and that ischemic necrosis is not the primary basis for Legg-Calvé-Perthes disease. He has also pointed out that generalized retardation of skeletal maturation is usually present and predisposes to the initial injury.

Following the subchondral epiphyseal fracture and the associated slight but regular lateral displacement of the femoral head in the acetabulum, the ossification center gradually flattens, develops irregular sclerosis and rarefaction, and increases in width. The subjacent neck often also increases in width, and adaptive changes in the acetabular fossa follow. Occasionally a destructive area in the femoral neck appears prior to diagnostic changes in the head. A period relatively quiescent radiographically, lasting about 12 months, follows the initial period of destruction, and then remineralization begins and progresses for approximately another 18 months. The ultimate shape of the femoral head is subject to wide variation. No convincing proof exists that prolonged periods of immobilization and abstinence from weight bearing significantly affect the end result. Nevertheless, avoidance of weight bearing would seem reasonable, at least while the child is symptomatic, and vigorous contact sports are probably best avoided. After a latent period of 10 to 20 years, osteoarthritic changes may develop in the hips if there is any degree of residual coxa plana or coxa magna deformity.

A form of epiphyseal dysplasia that simulates, and may actually progress to, Legg-Calvé-Perthes disease has been described by Meyer; it probably accounts for most of the cases found incidental to intravenous pyelograms or bowel studies. Thirty-two percent of the cases described by Meyer were bilateral, in contrast to the approximate 10 percent in Legg-Calvé-Perthes disease. Clinical signs are absent or extremely mild; the children tend to be younger than those with Legg-Calvé-Perthes disease, and radiologic diagnosis is usually made between 2 and 6 years of age. It differs primarily in that the irregularities of mineralization in the femoral capital epiphysis are a consequence of the *appearance* of an irregularly mineralized ossification center rather than the progressive dissolution and reconstitution of a well-developed ossification center. In Meyer's dysplasia the femoral heads frequently ossify from multiple separate centers of variable density that simulate the sclerotic, destructive phase of Legg-Calvé-Perthes disease as they coalesce. These patients require no treatment, although in general the orthopedist tends to be conservative and does limit weight bearing. Some of the instances of coxa plana–coxa magna that do follow this usually benign condition may be related to the delay in ossification that subjects the cartilage of the femoral head to stresses

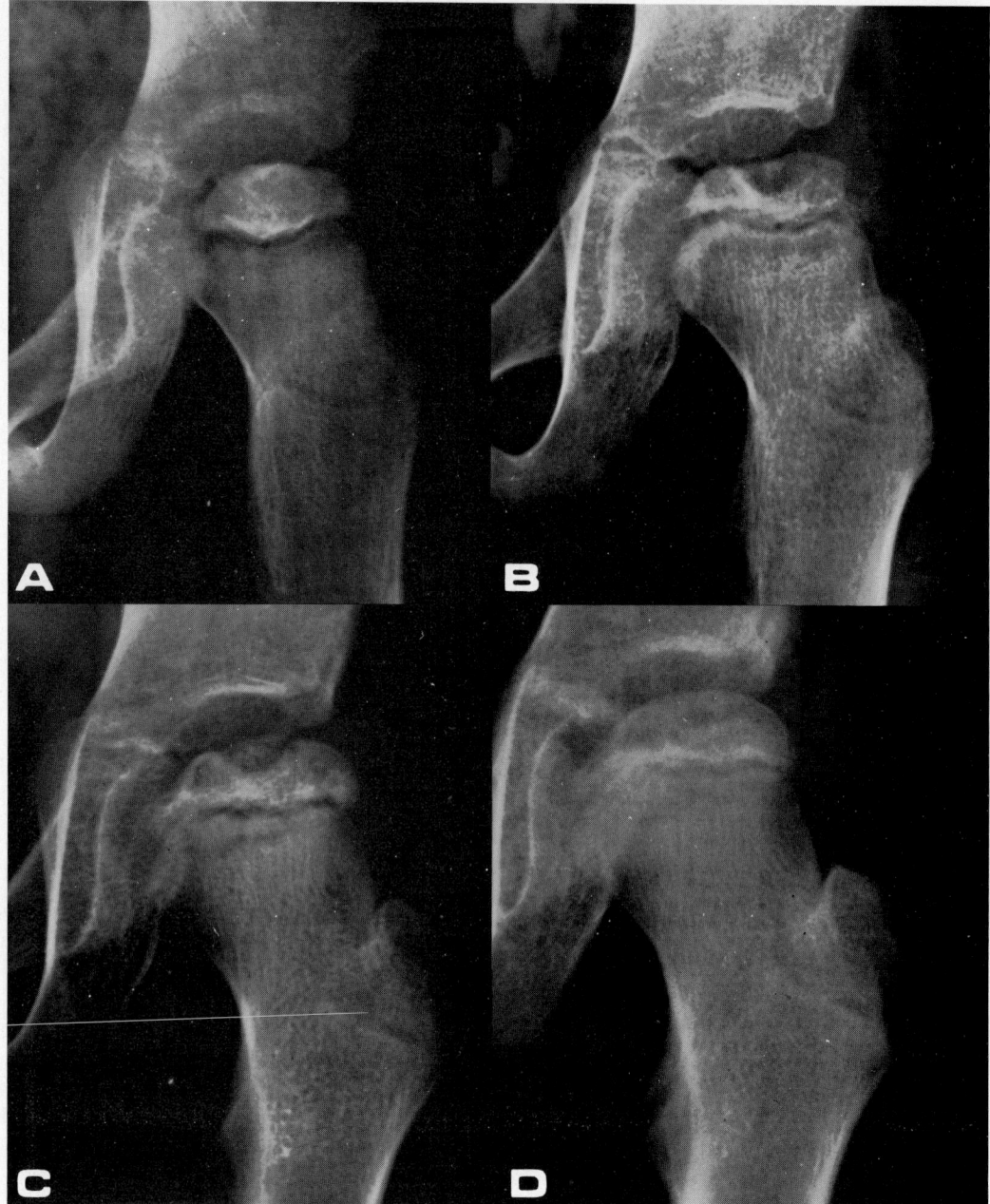

FIG. 37.   Serial films at approximately yearly intervals in 7-year-old boy with coxa plana who had a limp for 4.5 months prior to the first film. He was treated with bed rest for 7 months, followed by cast and crutches for about 1 year. Unrestricted activity was resumed 2 years 9 months after the first film.

different from those that obtain when an ossification center is present at the usual time. Meyer has indicated that whenever there is a distortion in the normal spherical shape of the femoral head following Legg-Calvé-Perthes disease or similar elements, the incidence of osteoarthritic changes in later life tends to increase. His investigations suggest that a good spherical head with no complications occurs more frequently in patients who have had no weight bearing and restricted activity during the early phases of the disease than in those who have had little or no treatment.

OSTEOCHONDROSIS OF TARSAL NAVICULAR. Osteochondrosis of the tarsal navicular (*Köhler's disease*) causes pain, tenderness, and swelling on the dorsum of the foot, usually between the ages of 3 and 8 years. Constitutional signs or symptoms are infrequent. The characteristic radiologic findings include irregular rarefaction and sclerosis with flattening and marginal expansion. Unfortunately the ossification center for the tarsal navicular normally makes its appearance during these same years, and it may from the very beginning have irregular sclerosis and apparent fragmentation. Measurement of the cartilage space between the anterior aspect of the talus and the cuneiform should indicate a diminution on the affected side if a pathologic process is present. Identical radiographic signs are not uncommonly observed on simultaneous examination of the healthy foot. The frequency of this disease is appreciably overestimated, and normal variations in development are often confused with it. Progressive demineralization of a tarsal navicular bone that has been normally mineralized is perhaps the only unequivocal radiographic feature.

OSTEOCHONDROSIS OF TUBEROSITY OF TIBIA. This osteochondrosis (*Osgood-Schlatter disease*) is generally believed to be a consequence of partial avulsion of the infrapatellar tendon from its insertion in the cartilaginous tuberosity. It develops most frequently between the ages of 10 and 15 years and is characterized by local swelling and tenderness, with pain on movement of the shank. On lateral radiography there should be soft tissue swelling over the region of the anterior tibial tubercle, thickening of the affected infrapatellar tendon when compared to the opposite side, and subsequently irregular deposition of calcium in the tendon and the adjacent tibial tubercle. Irregularity of mineralization without soft tissue swelling or thickening of the infrapatellar tendon is insufficient for a diagnosis.

OSTEOCHONDROSIS OF PATELLA. This osteochondrosis (*Syndig-Larson disease*) should be diagnosed only if there are *progressive* destructive radiographic changes in the patella in addition to distinct clinical signs. Irregular mineralization of the normal patella is the rule during the first 12 to 18 months of its ossification, and ossification from two or more centers is common even in older children. Pain and tenderness at the patella are the usual clinical signs.

PSEUDO-OSTEOCHONDROSES. The important pseudo-osteochondroses include *Blount's disease* (medial tibial condyle), *Calvé's disease* (single vertebral body), and *Scheuermann's disease* (several vertebrae and adjoining intervertebral disks).

In *Blount's disease* a failure of transformation of cartilage to bone at the medial aspect of the epiphyseal line produces a tilting of the medial half of the tibial plateau. The demineralized metaphysis beneath the epiphyseal ossification center develops a beak facing medially when viewed in the frontal plane and results in marked bowleg deformity. In early childhood nonrachitic deformities may develop even with a mild beak of the metaphysis; nevertheless, considerable and even complete spontaneous recovery can take place in children under 6 years of age, and osteotomy is recommended only in older children with prominent beaks and widely mineralized tibial epiphyses at the knee for whom spontaneous correction appears unlikely. The radiographic appearance of destruction in the medial spur of the tibia actually represents persistence of poorly developing epiphyseal cartilage.

Calvé described collapse of a single vertebral body in children between 2 and 11 years of age who had regional rigidity, tenderness, and kyphosis or scoliosis, usually in the lower dorsal or lumbar segments. The flattened vertebral body is visualized best in lateral projection and is unassociated with destructive changes in the intervertebral disks. In fact, adjacent to the anterior portion of the affected vertebra, which is compressed more than the posterior portion, the cartilage space of the intervertebral disk actually appears increased. Biopsies of collapsed vertebrae in young adults have clearly demonstrated that such lesions have been associated exclusively with eosinophilic granuloma. When identical lesions are observed in children, there are frequently other granulomatous lesions in the skeleton that on biopsy have the histologic features of Hand-Schüller-Christian disease or eosinophilic granuloma. Prognosis is uniformly good; complete clinical recovery is the rule, although anatomic recovery of the height of the vertebral body may not be achieved.

Scheuermann's adolescent kyphosis was once considered to result from ischemic necrosis of the epiphyseal ring ossification centers of the vertebral bodies, whereas Calvé's disease was originally considered an osteochondrosis of the primary center for the body. However, Schmorl was able to demonstrate that the primary lesion in Scheuermann's disease was fracture of the cartilaginous plates of the body, followed by protrusion of nucleus pulposus into the marrow cavity of the contiguous body and associated narrowing of the affected intervertebral disk. Because the posterior vertebral joints are secure, the disk herniation causes affected bodies to approximate each other anteriorly more than posteriorly. The resulting characteristic round-back deformity can be exaggerated as persistent unequal pressures on the vertebral bodies produce anterior wedging. The lesions of Scheuermann's disease usually develop between the ages of 10 and 20 years, more commonly in boys than in girls. Usually there is no pain or tenderness, and often the condition is first noted when parents or friends comment on "poor posture." In contradistinction to tuberculosis and Calvé's disease, several adjacent vertebrae are usually affected. Laminograms may be necessary to demonstrate the Schmorl nodes (intervertebral herniations of the nucleus pulposus). Prognosis is unpredictable. In some children the round-back deformity progresses to cause severe crippling; in others the deformity stabilizes, and mild deformity may actually disappear. Treatment is directed at prevention of further deformity, sometimes with the use of braces and generally avoiding unusual physical stress on the spine.

Miscellaneous Conditions

INFANTILE CORTICAL HYPEROSTOSIS. Infantile cortical hyperostosis is characterized by external cortical thickening of both long and flat bones in the fetus and younger infant. Its cause and pathogenesis are unknown. Fever and a high erythrocyte sedimentation rate are always present; however, bacterial, viral, and serologic studies have failed to identify a causal agent. Hypersensitivity to milk has been suggested as a cause, but this lacks scientific support. Increased platelet counts in several instances have suggested venous thrombotic phenomena as a causal mechanism. The presence of the disease in utero has been reported, as has its familial occurrence. It is generally accepted that the onset of the disease is limited to the fetus and infants younger than 6 months, but a chronic form of the condition may persist for years.

The disease develops in a previously healthy infant with sudden swelling of the lower part of the face, clavicles, scapulae, ribs, or extremities. Fever, hyperirritability, salivation, refusal of food, and pallor are common. The swelling is deep and firm and is fixed to the underlying bones, with neither discoloration of the easily movable overlying skin nor increased local heat. There is no local lymphadenopathy in any phase of the disease. Positive laboratory findings in the acute phase of the disease include acceleration of the erythrocyte sedimentation rate and increased alkaline phosphatase activity in serum. The course of the disease is highly variable in different patients as well as in individual lesions in a single patient. Unilateral proptosis has been reported in several instances. Erb's palsy may occur with involvement of the scapula alone or in combination with other bones, which may affect the brachial plexus by virtue of the early soft tissue inflammatory changes in the region of the shoulder girdle. Transient skull defects in association with otherwise typical manifestations of infantile cortical hyperostosis have also been noted. In some patients the disease may be limited to the lower jaw, with mild local and constitutional signs and with complete clinical recovery after a few weeks; in other patients most of the long bones of the body and their contiguous soft tissues are affected, with persistent high fever and extreme hyperirritability. Each individual lesion may have its own course; some may be involuting while others are evolving. A lesion may partially subside and then suddenly enlarge, with a severe local exacerbation. Complete clinical recovery is the rule after several weeks or months; however, the disease has lasted 2 or 3 years in several patients and as long as 7 years in one. Crippling residua have developed in the arms of one patient, and several patients have died of causes that are not clear.

The basic radiographic finding is an external thickening of the bony cortex. In some cases the mandible alone has been affected; in others the mandible and practically all of the tubular bones have been involved. In severe cases one or both scapulae have been thickened and sclerotic, and in one patient one ilium was similarly affected. Instances have been recorded where misdiagnoses of malignancy have led to mutilating surgery; these have occurred when lesions have been limited to the scapula and biopsy material has been misinterpreted. In long-standing cases the bones may become dilated and have large medullary cavities with thin cortical walls. The disease is generally self-limited, but severely ill patients may benefit from administration of cortisone or hydrocortisone, to which a prompt response usually can be anticipated. Recurrence of clinical signs and symptoms may be noted when steroid therapy is discontinued. Aspirin has been useful for symptomatic treatment. Caffey has recommended that steroid treatment be continued until 3 days after fever has subsided. Since response usually takes place within 72 hours, a period of 7 days is usually adequate for the initial treatment.

Identical clinical and radiologic sequences have been reported in an infant following smallpox vaccination; material reacting like vaccinia virus was obtained from a scapular biopsy. However, it is quite possible that this infant had both infantile cortical hyperostosis and generalized vaccinia and that a cause-and-effect relationship did not exist. Subperiosteal new bone formation has been reported in normal newborn infants as a developmental feature; the frequency of unrecognized traumatic periostitis must also be considered when cortical new bone formation is observed in young infants.

HYPERVITAMINOSIS A. In chronic poisoning by vitamin A, the onset of clinical signs is gradual and is characterized by such common complaints as pruritus, anorexia, and irritability. During the early phase the concentration of vitamin A in the blood is elevated, without associated bone lesions. The clinical picture first becomes suggestive when deep, tender, hard lumps appear in the extremities and in the occipital region of the skull; at this stage, usually 6 months or more after beginning ingestion of excessive amounts of vitamin A, hyperostoses can be demonstrated radiographically. Additional findings in some patients include fissures of the lips, loss of hair, jaundice, and enlargement of the liver. The diagnosis should be confirmed by measurement of the concentration of vitamin A in the blood, which is always increased, although to varying degrees. A careful history usually reveals the daily ingestion of vitamin A in excess of 50,000 units, often for the treatment of skin disorders. Recovery from the hypervitaminosis is rapid, and the patient's subjective symptoms usually disappear within 4 to 6 days after administration of vitamin A is discontinued. Preventive measures include instruction of mothers and physicians that vitamin A concentrates are potentially harmful. Except in rare circumstances the diet of the normally fed child contains adequate vitamin A and requires no supplementation.

Acute poisoning by vitamin A in infants is characterized by transitory bulging of the anterior fontanelle. This follows a massive single dose of vitamin A, usually of several hundred thousand units. Bulging of the fontanelle becomes evident after 12 hours and usually disappears after 36 hours. Vomiting is common. Ocular fundi and electroencephalography are normal. Instances of premature closure of cranial sutures have been observed subsequent to episodes of acute hypervitaminosis A.

PULMONARY OSTEOARTHROPATHY. Pulmonary osteoarthropathy may occur with conditions associated with hypoxia, with chronic pulmonary, liver, and enteric diseases, and occasionally without any associated or predisposing illness. Clubbing of the fingers and toes is most common in cyanotic heart disease. With empyema, clubbing may develop as early as 3 weeks after the onset of the primary disease; it usually subsides when the causative factor has been removed. Familial instances have been reported in association with either delayed closure of sutures or widening and subsequent slow remineralization of normal sutures, as well as with cutaneous eczematoid lesions and vague arthralgias.

PERIOSTEAL HYPEROSTOSIS WITH DYSPROTEINEMIA. Periosteal hyperostosis with dysproteinemia is manifested by febrile illness associated with severe pain in the extremities, bone tenderness, and radiographic evidence of widespread subperiosteal new bone formation in various bones, particularly the long bones. In many instances the plasma proteins are elevated. Elevated serum phosphate levels have been described without significant increase in alkaline phosphatase activity. The illness may last for months or years, but usually there is complete recovery.

DISEASES OF THE BLOOD. The skeletal system frequently reflects pathologic changes in the marrow. The skeletal symptoms may even at first distract attention from the primary disease in conditions such as leukemia and sickle cell anemia that may present with a rheumatic picture. The skeletal lesions may constitute incidental observations that are helpful in diagnosis; occasionally they are the first clues to the hematologic disorder. Leukemia, chronic hemolytic anemias, and hemophilia are disorders in which bone lesions are commonly encountered.

The frequency with which painful symmetric swellings of the hands and feet occur in sickle cell disease in infants has given rise to the term hand-foot syndrome. Swelling appears rapidly, persists for days or weeks, and is unassociated with hemolytic crises or obvious infection; in about 75 percent of cases reversible destructive and productive changes occur in the underlying bones. Similar radiographic changes have been observed in *Salmonella* infections associated with sickle cell disease, and they have even been described with gram-positive infections in individuals with normal hemoglobins. In severe instances of iron-deficiency anemias, changes comparable to those of the hemolytic anemias may be observed in the skull.

Angular depressions of the vertebral plates into the bodies, once thought to be specific for sickle cell disease, have been identified in other hematologic disorders and probably represent fractures of plates into vertebral bodies weakened by trabecular erosion subsequent to abnormal marrow activity. Bohrer has reported frequent epiphyseal-metaphyseal growth disturbances at the knees in patients with homozygous sickle cell anemia.

Clinical manifestations of "bone pain" and rheumatic symptoms occur in 50 percent of children with *leukemia,* and they may precede the development of diagnostic features in the blood. Local accumulations of leukemic cells are responsible for the destructive and productive bone lesions (Fig. 38) and probably for the pain. Leukemic lesions have been divided arbitrarily into four types: (1) transverse bands of diminished density at the growing ends of long bones; (2) focal areas of destruction, ranging from motheaten rarefaction to gross destruction with collapse of structure; (3) osteosclerosis; (4) subperiosteal new bone formation. Generally there is polyostotic involvement, and any bone may be affected. Vertebral body collapse has been observed as an initial manifestation of skeletal involvement. Pleural reactions may accompany rib lesions.

NEOPLASMS. Neoplasms may occur as a primary disease of skeletal structures, as neoplasia of nonosseous tissue in bone, or as metastatic lesions. Tumorlike irregularities are commonly seen in the growing bones of children in the course of normal development. These are common on the posterior aspect of the distal metaphysis of the femur, where they have been mistaken for periosteal sarcoma. Tumorlike bone production in the scapula in infantile cortical hyperostosis has been noted (p. 2022). Organic material such as thorns or other organic foreign bodies may produce reactions disturbingly similar to those of bone tumors.

The incidence of primary tumors increases with age. Specific tumors tend to occur with greater frequency at certain ages, although any tumor may occur over a fairly wide age range. Thus a bone tumor in a 9-year-old boy is more likely to be a sarcoma of the Ewing type and in a 16-year-old boy an osteogenic sarcoma. However, in all instances the definitive diagnosis rests on histologic examination in conjunction with radiographic features and the biologic behavior of the tumor.

Bone cysts are benign expanding lesions that occur most frequently in children between 6 and 12 years of age. They are most frequently recognized as a result of pathologic fracture or as a result of radiographic examination in a child without symptoms or with unrelated symptoms. A bone cyst usually appears to originate from a cartilaginous epiphyseal line, but it does not affect the epiphysis. Growth of the cyst continues as long as this attachment is maintained and skeletal growth continues. Recurrence may take place after surgical treatment if it is undertaken too early. Occasionally a pathologic fracture is curative.

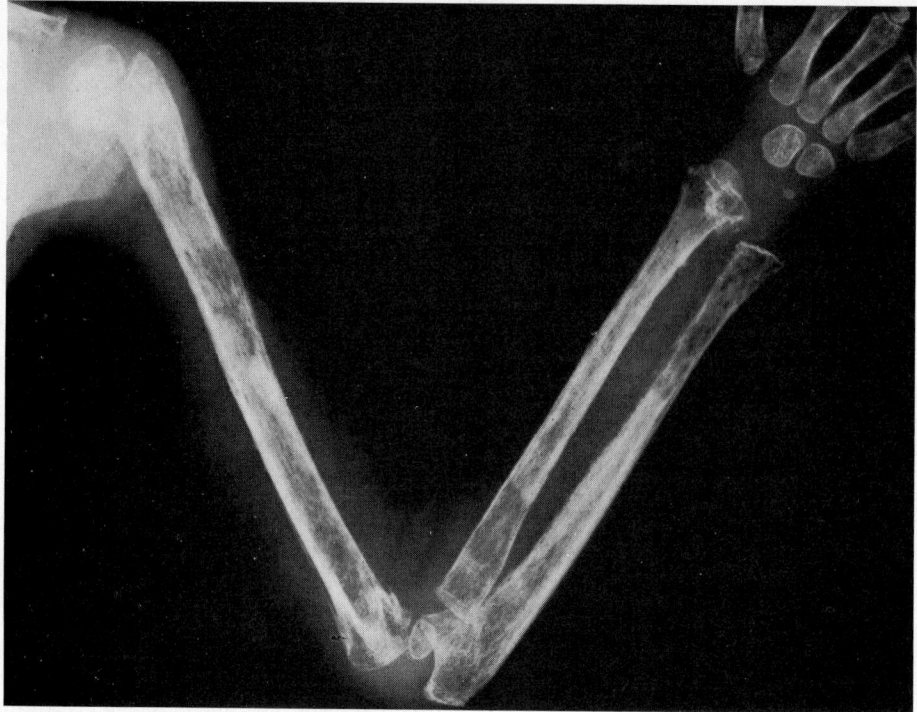

FIG. 38. Roentgenogram showing leukemic infiltration of the bones in a girl 3.5 years old.

Giant cell tumor occurs at a later age than bone cyst, usually in the late teenage years. It also differs from bone cyst in that the epiphysis is involved. Because giant cells are commonly found in areas of bone destruction, no matter what its cause, the diagnosis of giant cell tumor must be made with circumspection. It produces destruction of bone with little or no productive reaction. Aneurysmal bone cyst, which also produces destruction with little or no productive reaction, may be confused with giant cell tumor when the epiphyseal involvement and the age of the patient are not considered.

Other benign destructive lesions include *nonosteogenic fibroma* and *chondromyxoid fibroma*. These occur more frequently in the lower extremities than in the upper extremities; radiographic characteristics are similar and diagnosis is made by biopsy, which at times consists of the totally excised lesion. *Fibrous cortical defects* commonly occur in growing bone, particularly about the knee. They are generally asymptomatic incidental lesions, entirely benign, that are found on routine examination of the affected area. Multiple bone fibromas have been observed in infants who also had cutaneous fibromatosis and were thought to have neurofibromatosis with bone lesions. Several such patients have experienced spontaneous recovery with disappearance of both the cutaneous and osseous lesions.

Osteoid osteoma is regarded by many as a tumor. Others think it is infectious, notwithstanding the failure to identify any infectious agent. It is a small dense nidus of bone and osteoid tissue surrounded by vascular osteogenic tissue and is capable of producing an intense productive bone reaction. Clinically there is severe, boring local pain that is worse at night; the pain is said to respond to aspirin, and the administration of aspirin is reputed to be a diagnostic test. Symptoms are commonly relieved by excision of the nidus. Many cases that have been described as Garré's sclerosing osteomyelitis are now thought to have been examples of osteoid osteoma.

Among the malignant tumors of bone, osteogenic sarcoma and Ewing's tumor are encountered most frequently. *Ewing's tumor* may be productive or destructive of bone. The lamellated periosteal reaction, once considered pathognomonic, has no specific diagnostic value. The tumor usually occurs in children between 5 and 10 years of age; it is associated with pain and usually with regional soft tissue swelling. Any bone may be involved. The lesion metastasizes to lungs and to other bones. Microscopically, Ewing's sarcoma has been confused with neuroblastoma, and pathologists disagree about its exact nature. Clinically and radiologically it is most frequently confused with osteomyelitis. The condition is almost unknown in black children.

Osteogenic sarcoma is more common in children 10 to 15 years old. It also may arise in any bone, but the ends

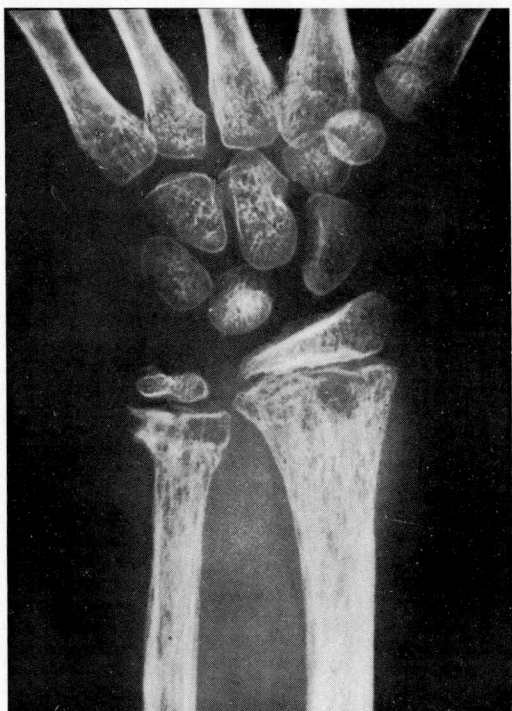

FIG. 39. Metastatic neuroblastoma in ulna and radius of a boy 9 years old.

of the shafts of the major long bones have a predilection. As the name indicates, it is generally a bone-producing tumor. New bone formation protrudes from the affected bone into the surrounding soft tissue. Some islands of bone are commonly found in the soft tissue, but they have no functional structure. In addition, destruction of preexisting bone almost always occurs, and in some instances this may predominate in the radiographic picture. Extension of tumor in the bone and its medullary cavity is invariably greater than can be demonstrated radiographically. Radical surgery and radiation are occasionally followed by "cure," but the rates of local recurrence or metastatic lesions (chiefly pulmonary) are disappointingly high, and the tumor is almost invariably associated with a fatal outcome.

Neuroblastoma frequently metastasizes to bone and produces destructive and reactive lesions in the appendicular skeleton (Fig. 39) indistinguishable from those of leukemia. In the skull, signs of actively increased pressure are often seen as the bony vault is thickened inward by the metastases. *Wilms' embryoma* of the kidney may also produce irregular destructive lesions when metastases to bone occur. *Neurofibromas* and *ganglioneuromas* cause bone changes by pressure erosion. However, pseudarthrosis in association with neurofibromatosis generally occurs without local tumor tissue. Scoliosis is common with neurofibromatosis, even in the absence of obvious bone lesions. Dumbbell tumors, in which relatively large intraspinal and extraspinal

masses of tumor communicate by a narrow isthmus through an intervertebral foramen, produce diagnostic enlargement of the foramen. *Metastatic embryonal rhabdomyosarcoma* may produce defective mineralization in the ends of the shafts of the major long bones that can resemble the lesions of neuroblastoma or leukemia. Vertebra plana secondary to metastatic rhabdomyosarcoma may simulate the vertebra plana of histiocytosis.

References

POSTNATAL AND ACQUIRED CONDITIONS

Bick EM, Copel JW: Longitudinal growth of the human vertebra; a contribution to human osteogeny. J Bone Joint Surg [Am] 32:803, 1950

Caffey J: The early roentgenographic changes in essential coxa plana; their significance in pathogenesis. Am J Roentgenol Radium Ther Nucl Med 103:620, 1968

Compere EL, Johnson WE, Coventry MB: Vertebra plana (Calvé's disease) due eosinophilic granuloma. J Bone Joint Surg [Am] 36:969, 1954

Harris VJ, Harris WS: Increased thickness of the fibula in Duchenne muscular dystrophy. Am J Roentgenol Radium Ther Nucl Med 98:744, 1966

Kaufmann HJ: New roentgen finding in pseudohypertrophic muscular dystrophy. Am J Roentgenol Radium Ther Nucl Med 89:970, 1963

Longeskiöld A: Tibia vara (osteochondrosis deformans tibiae); survey of 23 cases. Acta Chir Scand 103:1, 1952

Meyer J: Dysplasia epiphysealis capitis femoris. Acta Orthop Scand 34:183, 1964

——— Treatment of Legg-Calvé-Perthes' disease. Acta Orthop Scand [Suppl 86] 1966

Schmorl G, Junghanns H: The Human Spine in Health and Disease. New York, Grune & Stratton, 1959

Shopfner CE, Coin CG: Genu varus and valgus in children. Radiology 92:723, 1969

INFANTILE CORTICAL HYPEROSTOSIS

Caffey J: On some late skeletal changes in chronic infantile cortical hyperostosis. Radiology 59:651, 1952

——— Infantile cortical hyperostosis: a review of the clinical and radiographic features. Proc R Soc Med 50:347, 1957

Cochran W, Connolly JH, Thompson ID: Bone involvement after vaccination against smallpox. Br Med J 2:285, 1963

Goldbloom RB, Stein PB, Eisen A, McSheffrey JB, Brown BS, Wiglesworth FW: Idiopathic periosteal hyperostosis with dysproteinemia. A new clinical entity. N Engl J Med 274:873, 1966

Holtzman D: Infantile cortical hyperostosis of the scapula presenting as an ipsilateral Erb's palsy. J Pediatr 81:785, 1972

Iliff CE, Ossofsky HJ: Infantile cortical hyperostosis. An unusual cause of proptosis. Am J Ophthalmal 53:976, 1962

Keipert JA, Campbell PE: Recurrent hyperostosis of the clavicles: an undiagnosed syndrome. Aust Paediatr J 6:97, 1970

Melhem RE, Najjar SS, Khachadurian AK: Cortical hyperostosis with hyperphosphatemia: new syndrome? J Pediatr 77:986, 1970

Neuhauser EBD: Infantile cortical hyperostosis and skull defects. Postgrad Med 48:57, 1970

Pickering D, Cuddigan B: Infantile cortical hyperostosis associated with thrombocythemia. Lancet 2:464, 1969

Shopfner CE: Periosteal bone growth in normal infants. A preliminary report. Am J Roentgenol Radium Ther Nucl Med 97:154, 1966

Van Buskirk FW, Tampas JP, Peterson OS Jr: Infantile cortical hyperostosis: an inquiry into its familial aspects. Am J Roentgenol Radium Ther Nucl Med 85:613, 1961

HYPERVITAMINOSIS A

Knudson AG Jr, Rothman PE: Hypervitaminosis A; a review with a discussion of vitamin A. Am J Dis Child 85:316, 1959

Marie J, See G: Acute hypervitaminosis A of the infant, its clinical manifestations with benign acute hydrocephalus and pronounced bulge of fontanel; clinical and biologic study. Am J Dis Child 87:731, 1954

PULMONARY OSTEOARTHROPATHY

Chamberlain DS, Whitaker J, Silverman FN: Idiopathic osteoarthropathy and cranial defects in children (familial idiopathic osteoarthropathy). Am J Roentgenol Radium Ther Nucl Med 93:408, 1965

Currarino G, Tierney RC, Giesel RG, Weihl C: Familial idiopathic osteoarthropathy. Am J Roentgenol Radium Ther Nucl Med 85:633, 1961

DISEASES OF THE BLOOD

Bohrer SP: Growth disturbances of the distal femur following sickle-cell bone infarcts and/or osteomyelitis. Clin Radiol 25:221, 1974

Cassady JP, Berdon WE, Baker DH: The "typical" spine changes of sickle-cell anemia in a patient with thalassemia major (Cooley's anemia). Radiology 89:1065, 1967

Moseley JE: Bone Changes in Hematologic Disorders. New York, Grune & Stratton, 1963

Shahidi, NT, Diamond LK: Skull changes in infants with chronic iron deficiency anemia. N Engl J Med 202:137, 1960

Watson RJ, Burko H, Megas H, Robinson M: The hand-foot syndrome in sickle-cell disease in young children. Pediatrics 31:975, 1963

NEOPLASMS

Caffey J: Fibrous defects in cortical walls of growing tubular bones; their radiologic appearance, structure, prevalence, natural course and diagnostic significance. Adv Pediatr 7:13, 1955

———— Anderson D: Metastatic embryonal rhabdomyosarcoma in the growing skeleton. Am J Dis Child 95:581, 1958

Jaffey HL: Osteoid osteoma of bone. Radiology 45:319, 1945

Silverman FN: The skeletal lesions in leukemia. Am J Roentgenol Radium Ther Nucl Med 59:819, 1948

Silverstein MN, Kelly PJ: Leukemia with osteoarticular symptoms and signs. Ann Intern Med 59:637, 1963

Weston WJ: Thorn and twig-induced pseudotumors of bone and soft tissues. Br J Radiol 36:323, 1963

JOINTS

FREDERICK N. SILVERMAN AND MARTIN B. KLEIMAN

Discussions of acute pyarthrosis and the primary noninflammatory disorders of joints are included in this section. Discussed elsewhere are inflammatory joint conditions associated with specific infectious illnesses (Chap. 12) and involvement of the joints in connective tissue disorders (Chap. 11) and in gout (Chap. 14). The association of septic arthritis with acute osteomyelitis has already been discussed (p. 2002).

ACUTE PYARTHROSIS

FREDERIC N. SILVERMAN AND MARTIN B. KLEIMAN

The occurrence of bacterial joint infections (pyarthrosis, septic arthritis) in the absence of other associated infected primary foci warrants their consideration as a distinct clinical entity. Although they are now rarely life-threatening, their predilection for the large joints makes their sequelae a significant cause of persistent disability.

PATHOGENESIS AND ETIOLOGY. The pathogenesis of bacterial joint infections is not completely known, but it is thought that most pyarthroses are hematogenous in origin. The initial inflammatory focus is presumed to be in the synovium, from which the infection quickly spreads to involve the entire joint. Less frequently, infection results from direct penetrating wounds or spreads from involvement of adjacent soft tissue structures. Secondary pyarthrosis that extends from adjacent areas of osteomyelitis (p. 1999), accounts for a significant percentage of cases, especially in cases of hip involvement and in younger age groups.

When adequate cultures of joint fluid, blood, and other significant sites of infection are performed, a firm bacteriologic diagnosis is established in approximately 75 percent of cases. In the past, *Staphylococcus aureus* has been the most frequently encountered causative agent in the otherwise normal host in all age groups. The last decade, however, has seen a rising incidence of *Haemophilus influenzae* joint infections in infants and young children. The latter organism is now the most frequent etiologic agent in children under 2 years of age, while *Staphylococcus* remains the most frequent agent beyond this age. Since the population from which this has been reported has shown neither an increase in the attack rate of septic arthritis nor a rise in other type of *Haemophilus influenzae* infection, this change in disease pattern remains unexplained. Infections due to α- or β-hemolytic streptococci and the pneumococci do occur, but much less frequently, and the meningococci are rare. The rising incidence of venereal disease in all age groups has been accompanied by an increase in gonococcal joint infections, not only in adolescents but also in neonates and prepubescent children. Cases due to the gram-negative enteric organisms are seen in the first weeks of life, but they are quite rare in otherwise normal older infants and children.

Disease resulting from penetrating trauma, especially when associated with persistent foreign bodies, may result in infection with unusual organisms, both aerobic and anaerobic, including agents ordinarily of low virulence. Femoral venipuncture in the neonate and the small infant is well known for the frequency with which it is complicated by hip pyarthrosis. Additionally, both the neonate and the child whose antibacterial host defenses are altered by congenital or acquired defects, immunosuppressive therapy, or disseminated malignancy are subject to infection with unusual organisms. Other specific conditions, such as the presence of urinary tract infection or inflammatory bowel disease, may also predispose to infection of joints with the gram-negative enteric group of organisms.

CLINICAL MANIFESTATIONS. The majority of children with pyarthrosis present with fever and toxicity, as well as pain, swelling, and limitation of motion of the affected joint. This clinical picture may be altered in cases where antibiotics have been given inappropriately. The large joints are most frequently involved in isolated pyarthrosis, especially the knee and hip. Although the majority of cases are monoarticular, multiple joint involvement is seen occasionally and is especially frequent in gonococcal disease. A history of predisposing trauma, usually minor, is commonly elicited, but its role in pathogenesis is unclear.

COMPLICATIONS. The complications of untreated pyarthrosis arise directly from the accumulation of purulent material within the joint cavity that leads to rapid destruction of articular cartilage. If the joint is left untreated and/or undrained, it may even result in dislocation due to capsular distension. Portions of the bone entering into the joint may be destroyed, with resultant joint instability or ankylosis. The hip joint is most frequently involved in both the disease and the development of complications, since the vascular supply to the femoral head is easily compromised by the increased joint tension. Damage to epiphyses may result in growth disturbances and deformities caused by partial or complete premature epiphyseal fusion, especially when the septic arthritis originates from a contiguous site of osteomyelitis.

The diagnosis of septic arthritis is usually quite straightforward, provided that it is entertained and a joint aspirate is performed. As in acute osteomyelitis, the infected site may represent a metastatic focus of a systemic infection; therefore the possibility of other foci should be investigated. Contiguous osteomyelitis may be present, especially in infants under 18 months of age, in whom vascular communication exists between metaphysis and epiphysis, or in children of any age where the joint involved includes intracapsular metaphyses, as in the hip. The incidence of osteomyelitis in hip pyarthrosis is quite high.

DIAGNOSIS. Laboratory data that may be helpful are an elevated leukocyte count, usually with a shift, to the left and an accelerated erythrocyte sedimentation rate. The radiographic picture of a widened cartilage space, if present, offers strong support for the presence of an intra-articular effusion. However, the diagnosis is firmly established only by joint aspiration. The examination of joint fluid most commonly reveals numerous white blood cells (more than 20,000 cells/mm^3), with a predominance of polymorphonuclear leukocytes. Intra-articular glucose is frequently significantly depressed, well below half that of the simultaneous serum glucose. There is poor mucin clotting. A carefully stained smear of the fluid may show organisms. The fluid should be quickly inoculated (preferably at the bedside) onto culture media that support growth of both aerobic and anaerobic bacteria as well as fungal and mycobacterial agents. Simultaneous blood cultures should be obtained in addition to cultures of the joint fluid, since the purulent joint exudate can be inhibitory to bacterial growth. Cultures and examination of specimens taken from other infected sites (eg, cerebrospinal fluid, pleural fluid, vaginal or cervical smears) may also aid in early identification of a causative agent. The full differential diagnosis of acute arthritis is discussed elsewhere (Chap. 12). With hip involvement there may be diagnostic difficulties in differentiating idiopathic coxalgia (transient or toxic synovitis) (p. 2028) from pyarthrosis. The patient with idiopathic coxalgia is usually afebrile and nontoxic, with minimal signs of joint inflammation and normal leukocyte count and ery-

throcyte sedimentation rate. Yet examination of a joint aspirate may be necessary to exclude with certainty the diagnosis of septic joint. Disseminated gonococcal disease may affect a septic picture associated with mild to severe tenosynovitis; here blood cultures will yield organisms, while joint remains sterile. More commonly, however, gonococcal arthritis in children presents as a polyarthritis, sometimes migratory, where organisms are recovered from the joint fluid. Vaginal, cervical, or urethral cultures, and also cultures of suspicious skin lesions, may help to establish the gonococcal etiology of a septic joint, especially when joint cultures are sterile.

TREATMENT. Pyarthrosis is a medical emergency. Diagnostic joint aspiration should be performed without delay whenever intra-articular fluid is strongly suspected. Antibiotic therapy should be instituted immediately following examination of stained smears and collection of blood and other appropriate specimens for cultures and bacterial sensitivities.

The initial selection of antibiotics should be based primarily on the age of the patient, information from stained smears of joint fluid or material from other sites of infection, and any underlying host factors. As long as smears of the purulent material show no organisms, bactericidal therapy should be aimed at both the pyogenic cocci and *Haemophilus influenzae* in infants beyond the neonatal period and under 3 years of age. Initial therapy, pending reports of bacterial cultures and sensitivities, should include: 1) intravenous ampicillin (300 to 400 mg/kg/24 hours, in six divided doses) *or* chloramphenicol (150 mg/kg/24 hours) in those geographic locations where ampicillin resistance of *Haemophilus influenzae* has been documented, *and,* a β-lactamase resistant penicillin such as methicillin or oxacillin (200 to 300 mg/kg/24 hours, in six divided doses) also administered intravenously and directed against *Staphylococcus aureus* and other pyogenic cocci. In the newborn infant and in the child with impaired host defenses the antibiotic selection should also include an antibacterial agent, preferably an aminoglycoside such as gentamicin, against gram-negative enteric organisms. The initial selection of antibiotics will be more specific if smears provide early and unequivocal identification of the agent. When culture results and antibiotic sensitivities of the isolate become available, antibiotics should be adjusted accordingly.

The place of surgical drainage in therapy is less clear. Immediate incision and evacuation of pus is generally recommended in hip pyarthrosis, which also permits exploration of the femoral metaphysis and its drainage if osteomyelitis is discovered. In other joints, provided that therapy is instituted early, medical management alone or in combination with repeated needle aspiration is usually sufficient. Incision and drainage are indicated in case of contiguous areas of osteomyelitis, inadequate response to therapy, or thick loculated intra-articular exudate. With penetrating injury exploration of the joint space may be needed to remove the foreign body. Intra-articular instillation of antibiotics is not recommended, since adequate antibiotic levels have been demonstrated in inflamed joints.

The duration of intravenous antibiotic therapy for

isolated pyarthrosis should be at least 4 to 6 weeks in cases due to *Staphylococcus* or the gram-negative enteric organisms and 4 weeks for those due to the streptococci, *Haemophilus influenzae,* and pneumococci, provided there is a good clinical response. Therapy should be extended in the event that the response is inadequate. Joint infections due to gonococci or meningococci should be treated for 10 to 15 days. Radiographic examination should be repeated toward the projected end of the course of therapy. If there is evidence of osteomyelitis the minimum duration of therapy should be 6 weeks in all cases.

NONINFLAMMATORY DISORDERS

IDIOPATHIC COXALGIA.   (Toxic arthritis). It is not uncommon for children to develop acute hip pain and limitation of motion, particularly abduction and external rotation, with all symptoms abating spontaneously within 48 hours. At the onset the clinical features may suggest the diagnosis of coxa plana if the child is afebrile, or infectious arthritis if there is fever. There is no leukocytosis, and radiography is normal except for the displacement of the various intermuscular fat planes around the hip joint, which probably indicates muscular spasm and thickening rather than intra-articular effusion. The course is self-limited, and no therapy is necessary.

HEMARTHROSIS.   Hemarthrosis is uncommon in childhood except in association with blood dyscrasias, particularly hemophilia (Chap. 24). Pain, swelling, limitation of motion, and even fever may simulate infectious arthritis. Repeated episodes result in thickening of soft tissues, organization of unabsorbed blood, and deforming ankylosis. Subchondral hemorrhages directly into the bones may produce rounded defects of variable sizes. The chronic inflammation produces an acceleration of maturation and increase in size of the epiphyses of the affected joints.

DISLOCATION.   Dislocations occur as a result of congenital malformations, anomalies of fetal position, diseases of muscles and nerves, trauma, and infection.

Multiple dislocations occur in *Larsen's syndrome,* which includes anterior dislocation of the knee in addition to other dislocations, a peculiar facies, and frequently a cleft palate. Patterns of bony development in hands and feet demonstrable radiographically may be very helpful in the diagnosis.

Among the dislocations caused by trauma the most common is subluxation of the radial head ("pulled elbow"). This is seen in children between 1 year and 3 years of age following a sudden pull on the arm such as occurs in lifting. Pain is immediate, and the child usually refuses to move the arm, thus giving the erroneous impression of a neurologic injury. The forearm is held midway between pronation and supination. There is no swelling or discoloration and surprisingly little tenderness about the elbow. Radiographic examination is not particularly helpful, as gross dislocation is rarely present.

CONGENITAL   DISLOCATION   OF   HIP. Teratologic dislocation, in which there is gross congeni-

tal malformation involving the structures of the hip joint, is discussed on p. 00. The term congenital dislocation of the hip should be restricted to those cases occurring after the fourth month, when the hips are subjected to the stresses of weight bearing and locomotion. Prior to that time particularly in the newborn period, the condition is more accurately described as *dislocatability* of the hip.

PATHOGENESIS, EPIDERMIOLOGY.   For many years the most popular pathogenetic hypothesis has been that congenital dysplasia of the acetabulum and/or congenital (often familial) ligamentous laxity predispose to dislocation. Other investigators, particularly in Sweden, have postulated a delay in development of enzyme systems necessary for the degradation of transplacentally transmitted maternal hormones that causes ligamentous relaxation. Comparisons of urine hormone assays from newborn infants with hip dislocatability and those without the condition have been offered in support of the hypothesis. According to this theory, affected infants are unable to properly degrade maternal hormones until near the end of the first week of life. Because of ensuing ligamentous laxity, the femoral heads can be dislocated from the acetabular cavities when the femurs are extended and adducted (swaddling position). On flexion and abduction of the hips, the femoral heads can be induced to reenter the acetabular cavities. The entrance and exit of the femoral heads are responsible for the *clicks* in the Ortolani maneuver or the subluxation-provocation maneuver of Palmén and Coleman. If the position of the lower extremities favors dislocation of the femoral head from its acetabular cavity, and ligamentous resistance becomes normal when the delayed activity of enzymes begins in the second week, the dislocation becomes relatively fixed. Secondary atrophy of the acetabular fossa develops, and the classic appearance of acetabular dysplasia with congenital dislocation of the femur can be observed. The variability in development of an enzyme system necessary for degradation of the maternal enzymes has a counterpart in the variability in the development of other enzyme systems. Confirmation of this theory has not been forthcoming, but management based partly on this concept has reportedly been extremely successful and is said to have eliminated the disease in Sweden.

The lesion is six to seven times more frequent in girls than in boys, and the left hip is affected more frequently than the right. Black infants are rarely affected, and the incidence in other population groups is 1.5 in 1,000 live births. Local variations have been reported, and in some geographic areas there is a high familial incidence. Local areas of high incidence of congenital dislocation of the hip may be accounted for in part by local practices such as binding or swaddling, as well as by genetic factors in relation to maternal relaxing hormone production and timing of enzymatic degradation activity on the part of the newborn infant. Other cases may represent genetic factors related to congenital relaxation of ligaments, and described by Carter and Wilkinson.

CLINICAL MANIFESTATIONS.   Clinically, the older child usually walks with a marked limp, or even a wad-

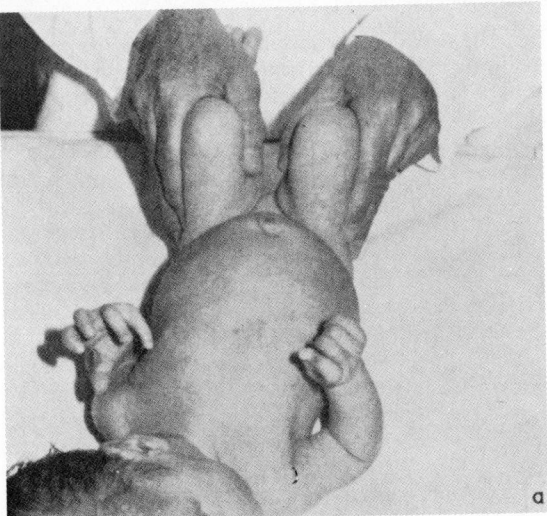

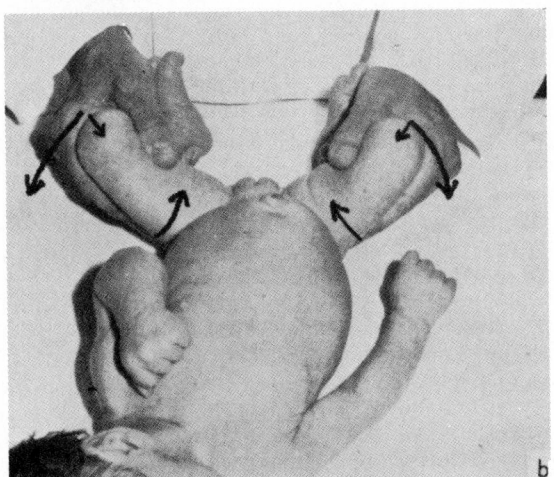

dling gait if both hips are involved. Shortening of the affected thigh and limitation of abduction and external rotation are important clinical findings. A positive Trendelenburg sign (lowering of the opposite gluteal fold when the patient bears his full weight on the affected limb) is easily demonstrated in older children. Asymmetry of skin folds in the thigh is so common in normal infants that this sign alone has little diagnostic value, although it does warrant further examination for dislocation or dislocatability of the hips.

For prevention of disability, the earlier the diagnosis is made and treatment is begun the greater the likelihood of cure. In the newborn period the *Ortolani maneuver* can identify the condition as the dislocated femoral head slips back into the acetabular fossa. In this procedure (Fig. 40) the examiner places the infant on his back on a firm surface. The legs are adducted with the hips and knees extended. The femurs are held between the thumb medially and the index and middle fingers laterally; the tips of the latter two should press against the greater trochanter. The knee joint usually then fits in the thenar portion of the examiner's palm. The legs are then flexed to 90 degrees at the hips and the knees. With one hand holding one lower extremity in this position, the other then abducts the other lower extremity into a frog-leg position, meanwhile pressing upward and forward with the tips of the fingers over the greater trochanter. With a normal infant, suitably relaxed, the abduction can be continued to 90 degrees without incident. In the child with a dislocated hip, a resistance may be encountered at about 60 degrees of flexion while the other leg is held fixed to stabilize the pelvis. Palmén and Coleman independently described a reverse procedure that would produce a dislocation not identified by the Ortolani maneuver. The initial stages of what Palmén

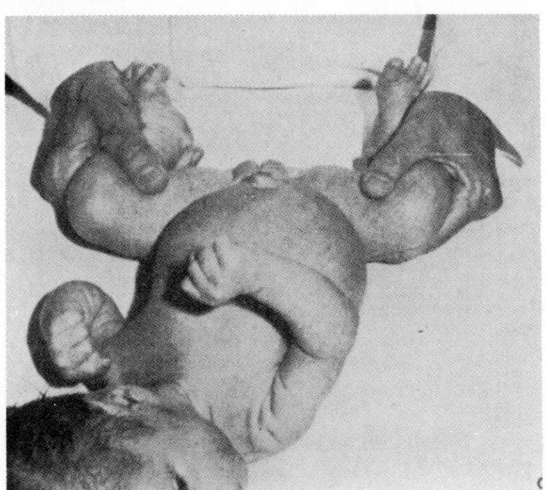

FIG. 40. Sequence of flexion and abduction of hips in the Ortolani maneuver. (From Palmén: Acta Paediatr Scand [Suppl 129] 50:1, 1961.)

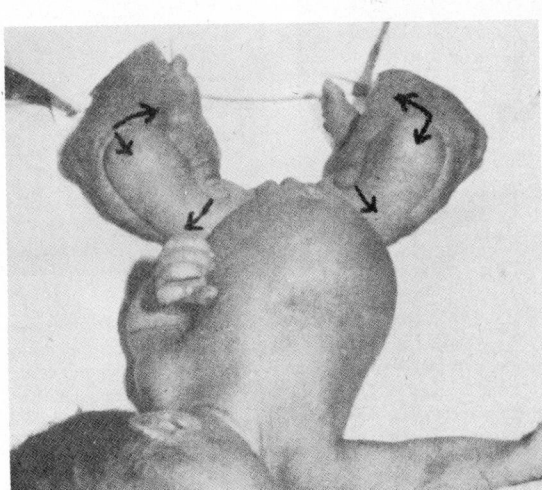

FIG. 41. Directions of forces exerted in the subluxation provocation maneuver (compare with Figure 40b). (From Palmén: Acta Paediatr Scand [Suppl 129] 50:1, 1961.)

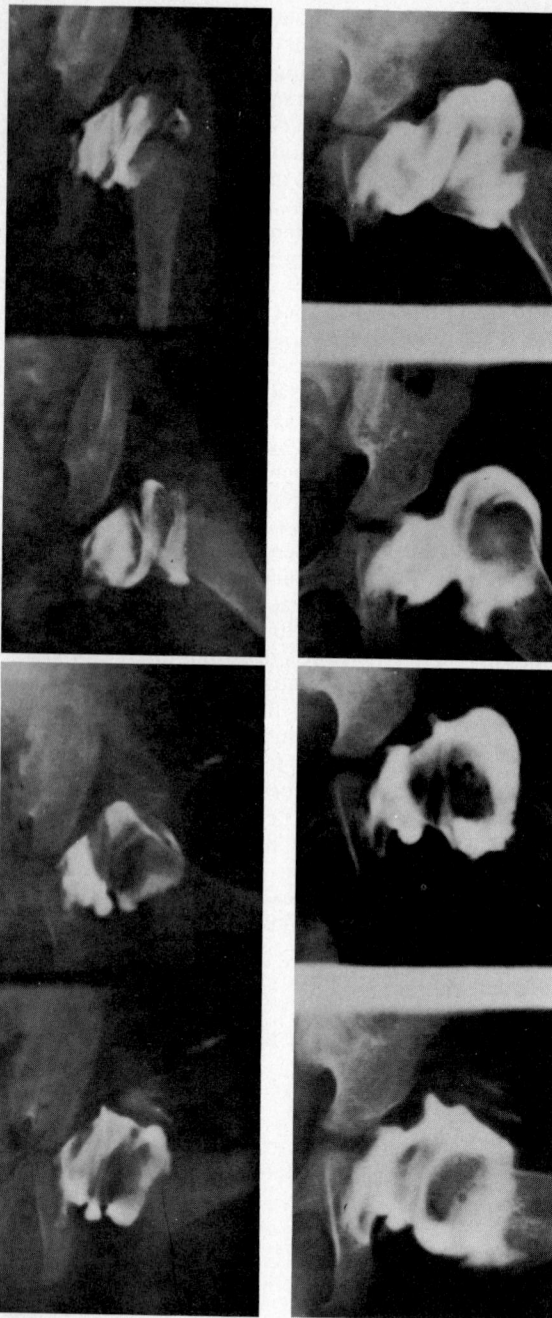

FIG. 42. Arthrograms in congenital dislocation of the hip. Left: female, age 7.5 weeks; spot films taken during manipulation. From top: neutral position; abduction; abduction and internal rotation; marked abduction and external rotation. Only in the bottom frame is cartilaginous head seated in acetabulum. Right: male, age 2 years. Hourglass contracture of capsule prevents entrance of head into acetabular cavity.

calls the *subluxation-provocation maneuver* are comparable to those of the Ortolani maneuver up to the point where abduction of the femurs is initiated. The femurs are abducted and flexed to only about 45 degrees and rotated slightly internally; the palms of the examiner are then pushed against the knees while the thumb presses outward on the internal aspects of the thighs (Fig. 41). A positive reaction is noted when the sensation of a jerk indicates that the femoral head has been displaced outward, upward, and backward from the acetabular fossa. The Ortolani maneuver then suffices for reduction.

RADIOGRAPHY. Unless there is gross dislocation, radiographic examination has little to offer in the newborn period. Acetabular angles, which were once considered of great diagnostic significance, are too variable to be relied on until at least the second half of the first year.

In cases first diagnosed as late as the end of the first year, and in which simple manipulative procedures do not replace the head firmly into the acetabular fossa, arthrograms (Fig. 42) may demonstrate the anatomic abnormalities of the capsule and labrum that preclude a satisfactory closed reduction. In cases diagnosed even later the acetabular cavity is shallow, and the ossification center for the femoral head on the affected side is small and lies at a higher level than the normal head on the opposite side. The femoral neck is usually anteverted; the proximal end of the femur is displaced laterally with respect to the acetabulum, as compared with the opposite side. A false acetabulum may be present in the ilium, which is usually hyperplastic (Fig. 43).

TREATMENTS. If a jerk of exit or entrance or both can be elicited in a newborn infant, the position of reduction is maintained by placing the child in a simple padded splint that holds the femurs in abduction and external rotation 24 hours a day for periods of 2 weeks to 3 months. Various splints, including the Frejka pillow splint, have been devised and are quite satisfactory. A large padded diaper may be utilized, but it is somewhat less secure in its effect. The splints or pads may be removed for bathing the baby, but they should be reapplied immediately. Usually within 2 to 3 weeks the entrance and exit clicks can no longer be elicited. After a period of 6 weeks, on the average, the splints are no longer needed and the joint is stable. Only if clinical signs persist at this time is radiographic examination necessary. In premature infants the clinical signs are extremely difficult to elicit, and it is probably wise to assess the range of motion of the hips at the time the infants is being discharged. Any limitation of abduction and external rotation or any abnormal clicks warrant radiographic examination.

Some infants who have been clinically and radiologically normal at birth have been shown conclusively to have develop dislocatability and even true dislocation around the fifth or sixth month of life. This is still early enough for the abduction splint management, which appears to be the most effective and least complicated form of therapy prior to the onset of ambulation.

In the treatment of older children with congenital dislocation of the hip, the soft tissues may be stretched

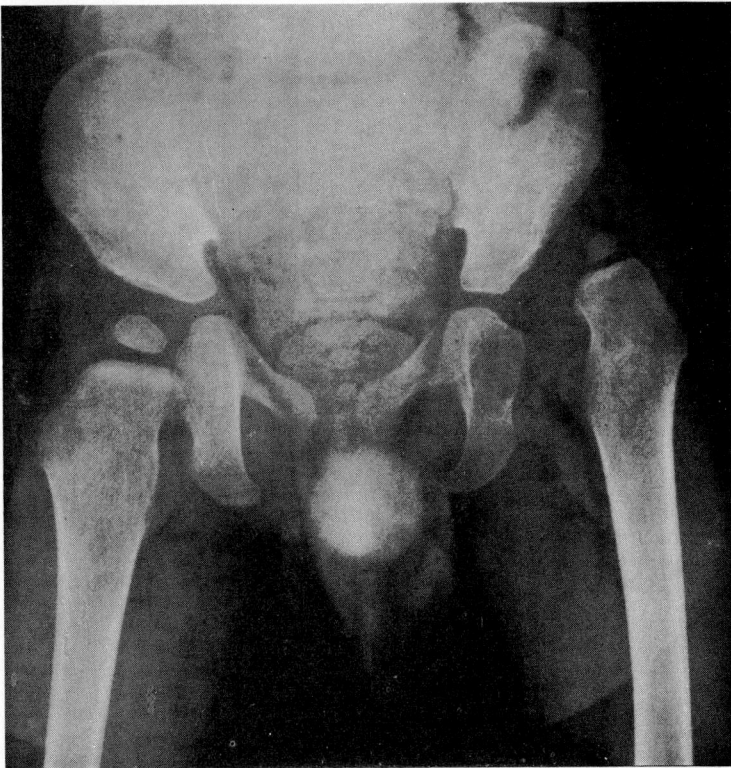

FIG. 43. Full dislocation of left hip in a girl 17 months old. All the components of Putti's triad are present. The acetabular roof is short and is tilted upward, with enlargement of the acetabular angle to 46 degrees. The femoral epiphyseal ossification center is small. The femur is displaced cephalad and laterad onto the iliac wing, where a shallow false acetabular cavity is already evident.

by traction, and by subsequent manipulation under anesthesia the femoral head can be replaced in the acetabular fossa. Plaster casts are usually required to maintain this position, because by that time the acetabulum has become quite shallow. In children who do not respond to relatively gently manipulative procedures, or whose arthrograms demonstrate complications to closed reduction, such as an hourglass capsule, interposition of the labrum, or accumulation of fat in the acetabulum, an open reduction is usually necessary.

With extensive abduction and external rotation the capsule of the hip is pulled tight and the vascular supply to the head may be compromised; aseptic necrosis of the femoral head has been reported in as many as 20 to 30 percent of older patients treated with rigid casts in marked abduction and external rotation. The ultimate fate of children with congenital dislocation of the hip is not known. Many who were treated by manipulative methods relatively late in childhood have developed coxa plana–coxa magna deformities and arthritic changes in middle adult life. Initial short-term follow-up of individuals treated in the newborn period by the more simple methods thus far suggests almost complete absence of complications or sequelae. Examination of the hips of the newborn infant for dislocatability by the maneuvers described should be an integral part of every newborn examination.

SLIPPED FEMORAL EPIPHYSIS. (p. 1998)

Slipped femoral epiphysis rarely occurs before 10 years or after 17 years of age. Boys are more frequently affected than girls, but only slightly so. Clinical manifestations are limited to pain in the affected hip and limb. In most cases, usually without any prior conspicuous injury, symptoms occur during ordinary activities such as walking and running; sometimes the pain has appeared in the morning after several hours of sleep. Diagnostic radiography shows the femoral head to be shifted medially and dorsally in relation to the end of the shaft. Often the radiolucent strip between the epiphyseal ossification center and the shaft is deepened. Some studies indicate that the primary change is fibrous degeneration of the cartilaginous plate that weakens the bone at that site and permits slipping of the epiphysis.

Treatment of slipped femoral epiphysis is surgical and is urgent. Bed rest must be instituted immediately to prevent the stresses of further weight bearing; most orthopedists insert metallic nails through the center of the femoral neck into the femoral head if it has been maintained in good position. If the femoral head has slipped appreciably, normalization of its position with respect to the femoral neck is attempted by manipulation prior to nailing. In every case careful attention must also be paid to the apparently healthy hip, because bilateral disease occurs in as many as 20 percent of patients.

References

ACUTE PYARTHROSIS

Almquist EE: The changing epidemiology of septic arthritis in children. Clin Orthop 68:96, 1970

Borella L, Goobar JE, Summit RL, Clark GM: Septic arthritis in childhood. J Pediatr 62:742, 1963

Butt WP: Radiology of the infected joint. Clin Orthop 96:136, 1973

Chacha PB: Suppurative arthritis of the hip joint in infancy. J Bone Joint Surg[Am] 53:538, 1971

Curtiss PH Jr: Joint infections: the pathophysiology of joint infections. Clin Orthop 96:129, 1973

Gillespie R: Septic arthritis of childhood. Clin Orthop 96:152, 1973

March AW, et al: Retroperitoneal abscess and septic arthritis of the hip in children: problem in differential diagnosis. J Bone Joint Surg [Am] 54:67, 1972

Nelson JD: Antibiotic concentrations in septic joint effusions. N Engl J Med 284:349, 1971

———— The bacterial etiology and antibiotic management of septic arthritis in infants and children. Pediatrics 50:437, 1972

Samilson RL, Bersani FA, Watkins MB: Acute suppurative arthritis in infants and children: the importance of early diagnosis and surgical drainage. Pediatrics 21:798, 1958

IDIOPATHIC COXALGIA

Monty CP: Prognosis of "observation hip" in children. Arch Dis Child 37:539, 1962

Reichman S: Roentgenologic soft tissue appearances in hip joint disease. Acta Radiol (Stockh) 6:167, 1967

Spock A: Transient synovitis of the hip joint in children. Pediatrics 24:1042, 1959

DISLOCATION

Poznanski AK: The Hand in Radiologic Diagnosis. Philadelphia, WB Saunders, 1974, p 319

Silverman FN: Larsen's syndrome: congenital dislocation of the knees and other joints, distinctive facies, and, frequently, cleft palate. Ann Radiol (Paris) 15:297, 1971

CONGENITAL DISLOCATION OF HIP

Andrén L: Instability of the pubic symphysis and congenital dislocation of the hip in newborns. Acta Radiol 54:123, 1960

Brecelj B: Congenital dysplasia of the hip. Final Report, Project 02.477.2 USDHEW, USPHS, MCHS, Ljubljana, Yugoslavia, May 1973

Caffey J, Ames R, Silverman WA, Ryder CT, Hough G: Contradiction of the congenital dysplasia–predislocation hypothesis of congenital dislocation of the hip through a study of the normal variation in acetabular angles at successive periods in infancy. Pediatrics 17:632, 1956

Carter CO, Wilkinson J: Persistent joint laxity and congenital dislocation of the hip. J Bone Joint Surg [Br] 46:40, 1964

Coleman S: Diagnosis of congenital dysplasia of the hip in the newborn infant. JAMA 162:548, 1956

Palmén K: Preluxation of the hip joint. Diagnosis and treatment in the newborn and the diagnosis of congenital dislocation of the hip joint in Sweden during the years 1948–1960. Acta Paediatr Scand Suppl 129, 1961

Silverman FN: Current concepts in diagnosis and management of congenital dislocation of the hip. Pediatrics 34:554, 1964

SLIPPED FEMORAL EPIPHYSIS

Johnston JA, Manson C, Mitchell CL: Epiphysiolysis. Am J Dis Child 92:337, 1956

Klein A, Joplin RJ, Reidy JA, Hanelin J: Roentgenographic features of slipped capital femoral epiphysis. Am J Roentgenol Radium Ther Nucl Med 66:361, 1951

Lacroix P, Verbrugge J: Slipping of the upper femoral epiphysis; a pathological study. J Bone Joint Surg [Am] 33:371, 1951

Index

Page numbers in **boldface type** refer to major headings.
Page numbers in *italic type* refer to illustrations and tables.

Infection
adrenal crisis of acute 1635-36
in children, bacteria causing *396-97*
disseminated, of gonococcal infections 439
ear **968-70**
with immunosuppressive therapy **412-14**
causative agents of 412, *413*
insulin requirement with 710
intercurrent 1654
in leukemia 1185-86
maternal-to-infant 503
nosocomial 414
of the premature and sick newborn 167
prenatal **124**
preventing 414
severe malnutrition and 216
in sickle cell disease **1151**, 1152-53
slow virus **594-96**, **1879-80**
steroids worsening 1654
superinfection 395
susceptibility to 379
treatment of, in marasmus 214
viral. *See* Viral infections
Infectious mononucleosis (IM) **539-42**, 957, 1093
neurologic complications of 1875-76
pharynx and 955
treatment of **958**
virus in primary encephalitis 1872
Inferiority versus industry 65
Inflammation
anti-inflammatory agents 1553
local 444
reduction in parenchyme because of **1577-80**
Inflammatory diseases of the gastrointestinal tract. *See* Gastrointestinal tract, inflammatory diseases
Influenza. *See also Haemophilus influenzae*
immunizations 512
vaccines 335, 549
viruses **547-49**
Infundibular hypertrophy 1415
INH. *See* Isoniazid
Initiative
examples of 70
guilt versus 65
Inguinal hernia **1035**
hydroceles and 32
Inhalant abuse **821-22**
Inhalation
of cleaning fluid 821-22
of humid air in pneumonia 454
injury in burns 777
provocation tests in asthma **339-40**
of tubercle bacilli 462
Inheritance
autosomal 272
sex influence on 273
multifactorial 293
sex-influenced 273, 292
X-linked 272-73
Inhibitory concentration, minimal 401
Injury
intentional, of children 73
nonaccidental **827-30**
Inositol 196
Inotropic effect 1407

INS (idiopathic nephrotic syndrome of childhood). *See* Nephrotic syndrome of childhood, idiopathic
Insect
bites **668**, 887-90
stings **361-62**
of bees and ants 666-67
Insecticide
in acquired aplastic anemia 1130
poisoning **793-95**
organophosphate **793-95**
Insomnia
in heroin withdrawal 812
as steroid complication 353
Inspiration, process of 1546-47, 1590
Inspiratory
capacity 1572, 1575
obstructions **1554-56**
pressure *1546*
reserve volume 1572
Inspissation of small bowel contents 1567
Insulin
caloric intake and 710
cell size and 100
deficiency 112
in diabetes 696-97, 702-5
in the endocrine system 718
in familial periodic paralysis 1888
fetal secretion of 106
obesity and 257
requirements
activity and 710
in adolescence 711
changing 708
infection and 710
response 353
sensitivity in short stature 1610
-specific staining techniques 723
tolerance tests 1624
growth hormone assay and 1637
types of 705
Intal. *See* Cromolyn sodium
Integration of physical and emotional changes 75
Integrity versus despair 66-67
Intellectual
assessment *1787*, 1791-92
development in the newborn 30
function, speech and 1741
Intelligence
quotient (IQ) 1767
Down's syndrome and 1768, 1778
intelligence tests and 1791-92
mental retardation and 1767-68
scores, increased 1791
tests 1767, *1787*, 1791-92
Interactional model of psychosocial development 61-62
Interalveolar inflammation, sites of *1581*
Intercostal muscles 1590
Interference
bacterial 495
physiologic 1390-91
Interferon
in antiviral therapy 515
in herpes simplex keratitis 1952
in influenza 549
in type IV hypersensitivity reactions 330

Microcephaly 1750-51, 1976
  alcohol and 1773
  causes of 1773
  in Cockayne's syndrome 1917
  diseases diagnosed by *1898*
  heroin and 1773
Microcornea 1951
Microcrania **916,** 1976
  craniosynostosis and 1981
Microcytosis in α-thalassemia 1160
Microencephaly 1976
Microfilariae 633, 634
Microglossia **922**
Micrognathia 146, **917**
Microlithiasis, pulmonary alveolar 1587
Micropenis 1726
Microphakia 1956
Microphthalmia 585
  congenital 146
Microphthalmos 1943, 1945
Microscopy
  bright-field 285
  fluorescence 431
Microsomia, hemifacial 1977
Microsporum infections 883-84
Microtubules in the liver **1065-66**
Micturation
  pattern of 1329
  syncope 1857
Middle adulthood as a stage of development 66
Middlebrook oleic acid agar 475
MIF. *See* Migration-inhibition factor
Migraine 1858-59, **1967.** *See also* Headache
  abdominal 369, 985, 1860
  depression and 1859
  epilepsy and 1859
  headaches 369-70
    serotonin and 370
  ophthalmologic 1858
  treatment of 1859
  vertigo and 1858
Migrainous neuralgia 1858
Migration
  cell, measurement of 308-9
  -inhibition factor (MIF) 302, 359
    macrophage migration and 308
    in type IV hypersensitivity reactions 330
Mikulicz syndrome 1184
Milia 144, **907**
Miliaria **901-2**
  crystallina 902
  rubra 144, 902
Miliary
  tubercles in histoplasmosis 615
  tuberculosis, acute 467-68
Milk(s)
  as allergen 367, 371
  allergy, adenoidal enlargement and 1555
  -associated gastroenteropathy 1006-7
  autoclaving 205
  boiled 205
  -borne disease 204
  breast 138
    alcohol and 204
    caloric value of 202

Milk(s) *(cont.)*
  breast *(cont.)*
    composition of 203, *205*
      conditions affecting 204
    drugs and 204
    emotional stresses and the secretion of 204
    fat in 204
    mineral constituents of *203*, 204
    nitrogen and 192
    protein in 203-4
    secretory IgA found in 300
    superiority of 202
    vitamin content of 204, *206*
  carbohydrates in various *1005*
  composition of natural *221*
  cow's
    allergies to 207
    composition of *205*
    constipation and 1012
    in gastrointestinal disorders 1007
    modification of 206
    vitamin content of *206*
  dried 207
  evaporated 207-8
  homogenized 207
  humanized 207
  intake of, in galactosemia 714
  microorganisms in 204
  minerals from, retention of *198*
  skim 207
  sterilization 205
  in tuberculosis 462
Miller-Abbott intestinal tube 1053
Milliequivalence 260
Milliosmolality 260
Millon reagent 233
Milontin (phensuximide) in epilepsy 1849, *1850*
Milroy's disease 906, 1001
Miltown. *See* Meprobamate
Milwaukee brace 943
Mineral(s)
  constituents of breast milk *203*, 204
  for milk, retention of *198*
  oil
    in constipation 1013
    in fissure in ano 990
  nutrition and **198-201**
Mineralization
  bone, irregular 2019-20
  of the cranium 1982
Mineralocorticoids. *See also* Aldosterone
  excess, in hypertension 1487
  renin levels and 1485
  replacement of 1640
Minimal brain dysfunction (MBD) **1764-66,** 1799-1800
  educating children with 1799-1801
  syndrome defined 1800
Minocycline 407
  in meningitis 426
  in meningococcal infections 449, 452
Minoxidil in hypertension 1491
Minute volume 1546
Miracidium 635
Miracil D (lucanthone) in schistosomiasis 637
Mirror writing 1765